DRUG FACTS AND COMPARISONS®

2012

DRUG FACTS AND COMPARISONS®

2012

Wolters Kluwer
Health

Facts & Comparisons®

Drug Facts and Comparisons,® 2012 Edition

Adapted from *Facts and Comparisons® eAnswers* online drug reference.

Manuscript indexed by Columbia Indexing Group, Las Vegas, Nevada.

ISBN-10: 1-57439-328-6
ISBN-13: 978-1-57439-328-6

Printed in the United States of America.

The information contained in *Drug Facts and Comparisons®* is available for licensing as source data. For more information on data licensing, please call 1-800-223-0554.

Wolters Kluwer Health
77 Westport Plaza, Suite 450
St. Louis, Missouri 63146-3125
Phone 314-216-2100 • 800-223-0554
Fax 314-878-5563
factsandcomparisons.com

DRUG FACTS AND COMPARISONS®

2012

Wolters Kluwer Health | Facts & Comparisons®

Facts & Comparisons™ Editorial Advisory Panel

Contributing Review Panel

Jonathan Abrams, MD
Professor of Medicine
Cardiology Division
University of New Mexico
Albuquerque, New Mexico

Danial E. Baker, PharmD, FASHP, FASCP
Associate Dean for Clinical Programs
Professor of Pharmacotherapy
Director, Drug Information Center
Washington State University
Spokane, Washington

Jimmy D. Bartlett, OD, DOS, ScD
Professor of Optometry, School of Optometry
Professor of Pharmacology, School of Medicine
University of Alabama at Birmingham
Birmingham, Alabama

Jeanelle Beltran, PharmD
Drug Information Consultant
Christchurch, New Zealand

Edward S. Bennett, OD, MSEd
Associate Professor
Co-Chief, Contact Lens Service
Director of Student Services
College of Optometry
University of Missouri – St. Louis
St. Louis, Missouri

Daniel L. Brown, PharmD
Director of Early Practice Education
Wingate University
School of Pharmacy
Wingate, North Carolina

Renay Bryant, RPh, BS Pharmacy
Drug Information Consultant
St. Louis, Missouri

R. Keith Campbell, RPh, FAPhA, FASHP, MBA, CDE
Associate Dean/Professor of Pharmacotherapy
Washington State University
College of Pharmacy
Pullman, Washington

Ielvin D. Cheitlin, MD
Imeritus Professor of Medicine
Iniversity of California, San Francisco, Cardiology Division
ormer Chief, Cardiology Division
an Francisco General Hospital
an Francisco, California

Santi Divvela, PharmD
linical Editor
hiladelphia, Pennsylvania

lchard J. Duma, MD, PhD
lrector, Department of nfectious Diseases
fectious Disease Division
llifax Medical Center
lytona Beach, Florida

lthryn M. Edwards, MD
e Chair for Clinical esearch
partment of Pediatrics
ofessor of Pediatrics
nderbilt University
hool of Medicine
shville, Tennessee

chael S. Edwards, harmD, MBA
istant Director, Pharmacy perations
Sidney Kimmel
omprehensive Cancer
enter at Johns Hopkins
hesda, Maryland

Mary J. Ferrill, PharmD, FASHP
Associate Dean for Academics and Professor
Wingate University
Lloyd L. Gregory School of Pharmacy
Palm Beach Atlantic University
West Palm Beach, Florida

Thomas A. Golper, MD
Professor of Medicine
Medical Director – Nephrology, Hypertension, and Diabetes Patient Care Center
Vanderbilt University Medical Center
Nashville, Tennessee

COL. John D. Grabenstein, RPh, PhD, FAPhA, FASHP, FRSH
Medical Service Corp.
Deputy Director for Clinical Operations
Military Vaccine Agency
U.S. Army Medical Command

Teena M. Halterman, RPh
Retail Staff Pharmacist
Chatham, Illinois

Edward A. Hartshorn, PhD
Professor
School of Allied Health Sciences
University of Texas Medical Branch
Galveston, Texas
Instructor
University of Texas Health Science Center
Houston, Texas

Siret D. Jaanus, PhD
Professor of Pharmacology
Southern California College of Optometry
Fullerton, California

Kimberly Johnson, BS, Pharm, RPh
Drug Information Consultant
Columbia, Illinois

Robert E. Kates, PharmD, PhD
President
Analytical Solutions, Inc.
Sunnyvale, California

Julio R. Lopez, PharmD
Chief, Pharmacy Service
VA Northern California Health Care System
Martinez, California

Richard M. Oksas, PharmD, MPh
Family Practice Pharmacist
Natividad Medical Center
Salinas, California

J. James Rowsey, MD
St. Luke's Cataract and Laser Institute
Tarpon Springs, Florida

Mary Beth Shirk, PharmD
Specialty Practice Pharmacist, Critical Care Medicine
Clinical Assistant Professor
The Ohio State University Medical Center
Columbus, Ohio

Udho Thadani, MD, MRCP, FRCP(C), FACC, FAHA
Professor Emeritus of Medicine
Cardiovascular Section
University of Oklahoma Health Sciences Center
Consultant Cardiologist, Oklahoma University Medical Center and VA Medical Center
Oklahoma City, Oklahoma

Phiyen Tra, PharmD
Drug Information Consultant
Dallas, Texas

Thom J. Zimmerman, MD, PhD
Emeritus Professor and Chairman
Department of Ophthalmology and Visual Sciences
Emeritus Professor of Pharmacology & Toxicology
University of Louisville School of Medicine
Global Ophthalmic Medical Director
Global Medical Affairs
Pharmacia Corporation
Louisville, Kentucky

Table of Contents

Foreword

Facts & Comparisons™, a part of Wolters Kluwer Health, has served the drug information needs of pharmacists and other health care professionals since its inception in 1946 by providing timely, accurate, comprehensive, unbiased, comparative information on prescription and nonprescription medications. *Drug Facts and Comparisons® (DFC),* our flagship product, is the primary source of drug information and the reference of choice for our many loyal subscribers because of its uncompromising editorial quality, reliability, and ease of use. *DFC* has remained unique among other drug information resources because of its organization by therapeutic use, providing single drug monographs with complete prescribing information as well as in-depth comparisons of closely related agents. Over the years, *DFC* has changed in size and scope, but the concept has never changed. That is why health care professionals continue to look to Facts & Comparisons™ to keep them abreast of important information in their practice.

In addition to the annual bound edition, *DFC* is also available as the popular monthly updated loose-leaf publication and as an annual pocket-size softbound abridged version. These versions allow customers to choose the format that is best suited to their practice site and workflow.

Customers who prefer the comprehensivenss, speed and efficiency of electronic products can access *DFC* through *Facts & Comparisons® eAnswers,* our electronic library of reference information, which is available on-line or CD ROM. In addition to *DFC,* other content sets available on *Facts and Comparisons® eAnswers* include *Drug Interaction Facts, A to Z Drug Facts, Brigg's Drugs in Pregnancy and Lactation, Off-Label Drug Facts, Med Facts* (patient drug information handouts), *Review of Natural Products, Cancer Chemotherapy,* and *Drug Identifier.* Recently, *Facts and Comparisons® eAnswers* has added more detailed product tables for certain drugs, which is based on Medi-Span data, and has added comparative efficacy information to some monographs regarding certain disease states. Information about *Facts & Comparisons® eAnswers,* can be accessed through www.factsandcomparisons.com. Facts & Comparisons™ also offers drug information for handheld personal data assistants, available for downloading at www.factsandcomparisons.com.

Drug Facts and Comparisons™ monographs are also integrated into Medi-Span's Drug Information Bridge, a pre-programmed application programming interface (API) that includes Medi-Span's drug files and clinical databases. The integration of the *DFC* referential content with Medi-Span's premier databases provides superior point-of-care solutions for our professional customers.

Facts & Comparisons™ takes our mission of providing drug information to health care professionals very seriously, which is why we continue to invest in technology, improve our current publications, and stay in contact with our customers to make sure we maintain the high standards we set many years ago when Erwin Kastrup, RPh, first developed this concept. We have many people to thank for helping us achieve these goals, including our Editorial Advisory Panel, reviewers, contributors, and our excellent, dedicated employees, but more than anything we want to thank our loyal subscribers who have helped us develop and improve our drug information publications that are so widely used today.

We are dedicated to maintaining the traditions that are important to both Facts & Comparisons™ and our customers, but we are also dedicated to evolving our products to meet the changing technologies and the changing needs of health care professionals. These goals only can be accomplished by responding to the comments and suggestions from our subscribers, which we encourage and appreciate. As always, let us know how we can better serve you and your drug information needs.

Cathy H. Reilly
Vice President and Publisher

Preface

As the premier publisher of drug information, Facts & Comparisons™ provides a broad range of print and electronic resources to fulfill the day-to-day needs of practicing health care professionals. *Drug Facts and Comparisons® (DFC)*, our flagship publication developed in 1946 by pharmacist Erwin K. Kastrup, was initially designed to provide objective information in a format that facilitated unbiased comparisons of drug products in a timely manner. After more than 60 years, the basic concepts remain the same. However, the content and presentation of material in *DFC* continues to evolve to reflect the changing needs of the health care environment.

The annual bound edition is one of several formats in which *DFC* is available. The original loose-leaf version is kept up to date through monthly print updates. An electronic version, updated continously, is available as part of *Facts & Comparisons® eAnswers* and can be accessed via www.factsandcomparisons.com.

Facts & Comparisons® eAnswers also provides full monographs with complete prescribing information for nearly every single agent drug product, while the print versions continue to present abbreviated drug monographs in instances where a class monograph exists.

The new 66th edition of *DFC* incorporates 23 new drugs: alcaftadine (*Lastacaft* by Vistakon Pharmaceuticals), azilsartan (*Edarbi* by Takeda), belimumab (*Benlysta* by Human Genome Sciences), cabazitaxel (*Jevtana* by Sanofi-Aventis), carglumic acid (*Carbaglu* by Accredo), ceftaroline fosamil monoacetate (*Teflaro* by Forest Pharmaceuticals), dabigatran etexilate mesylate (*Pradaxa* by Boehringer Ingelheim Pharmaceuticals), denosumab (*Prolia* by Amgen), eribulin mesylate (*Halaven* by Eisai), factor XIII concentrate (human) (*Corifact* by CSL Behring), fingolimod hydrochloride (*Gilenya* by Novartis), hexaminolevulinate hydrochloride (*Cysview* by GE Healthcare), hydroxyprogesterone caproate (*Makena* by Ther-Rx), iofluplane I 123 (*DaTscan* by GE Healthcare), ipilumamab (*Yervoy* by Bristol-Myers Squibb), lurasidone hydrochloride (*Latuda* by Sunovion), pegloticase (*Krystexxa* by Savient Pharmaceuticals), roflumilast (*Daliresp* by Forest Pharmaceuticals), sipuleucel-T (*Provenge* by Dendreon Corporation), spinosad (*Natroba* by ParaPRO/Pernix Therapeutics), tesamorelin acetate (*Egrifta* by EMD Serono), ulipristal acetate (*ella* by Watson Pharma), and vilazodone hydrochloride (*Viibryd* by Trovis Pharmaceuticals).

As this edition goes to press, we continue to update our database daily for use in future editions and formats of *DFC*. We also continue to expand our extensive library of drug information resources to remain the full service drug information provider that our customers have come to expect. However, this can only be accomplished with feedback from the loyal health care professionals who use our information on a daily basis. Comments, criticisms, and suggestions are always welcome and encouraged. Please call or visit us at www.factsandcomparisons.com.

Renee M. Wickersham
Senior Managing Editor,
Content Development

Kirsten K. Novak
Managing Editor

Introduction

Drug Facts and Comparisons® is a comprehensive drug information compendium. Organized by therapeutic drug class, the format is designed to provide a wide scope of drug information in a manner that facilitates evaluations and comparisons. A comprehensive index, a detailed table of contents for each chapter, and numerous cross references within monographs enable the reader to quickly locate needed information.

Editorial Policy

The principal editorial policy remains unchanged from the inception of *Drug Facts and Comparisons®* in 1945: Accurate, unbiased information; concise, standardized presentation; comparative, objective format; timely delivery. Review of FDA-approved product labeling, thousands of biomedical journal articles and textbooks, and policies and recommendations from many authoritative and official groups (eg, Centers for Disease Control; National Academy of Sciences; Joint National Committee on Detection, Evaluation, and Treatment of High Blood Pressure; National Heart, Lung and Blood Institute; American Thoracic Society; National Cancer Institute; FDA Office of Orphan Products Development; Food and Drug Administration) form the base of evaluation of information for *Drug Facts and Comparisons®*. (See the end of the Introduction for a list of references.)

Editorial policy is guided by the distinguished Facts & Comparisons™ Editorial Advisory Panel. This is an authoritative group of nationally and internationally recognized clinicians, scholars, scientists, physicians, pharmacists, and pharmacologists. In addition, many other prominent health care professionals serve on various expert panels and provide review in their specific areas of expertise for *Drug Facts and Comparisons®*. Indications and dosage recommendations are FDA-approved unless otherwise specified. Legitimate "Off-label" uses and dosages are included when appropriate and given special emphasis. They are intended to aid the health care professional in quickly identifying information regarding a specific off-label use. Inclusion of off-label drug information is intended for research purposes and not to be interpreted as a recommendation. The reader should always refer to primary literature for more comprehensive information prior to patient care decisions. In some instances, where noted, there is poor documentation to support the use. (See How to Use Drug Facts and Comparisons.) Input from an expert panel on drug interactions is also a feature.

This collection of wisdom and the world drug information literature is then molded and refined into the *Drug Facts and Comparisons®* database, monographs, and product listings. Many sources of drug information are constantly monitored so that *Drug Facts and Comparisons®* contains the most comprehensive, current drug information database available. There is not a more complete drug information compendium available presenting such clinical prescribing and drug product information.

Most of the products listed in *Drug Facts and Comparisons®* are protected by letters of patent, and their names are trademarked and registered by the firm whose name appears with the product. Identification of the product distributor is given in parentheses next to the brand name. The distributor may or may not be the actual manufacturer or fabricator of the final dosage form. When more than one company distributes a generic product, the generic product name is listed, followed by "Various, eg," in parentheses with a selected list of distributors. Listing of specific products is an indication only of market availability and is not an endorsement or recommendation. Most products listed have national or significant regional distribution.

Products that contain the same active ingredients are listed together for comparison and as an aid in product selection. However, drug product interchange is regulated by state laws; listing of products together does not imply that products are therapeutically equivalent or legally interchangeable. Cau-

tion is particularly advised when attempting to compare extended-release or delayed-release dosage forms.

How To Use *Drug Facts And Comparisons®*

Efficient use of *Drug Facts and Comparisons® (DFC)* requires an understanding of its organization and format.

Organization:

Information in *DFC* is organized by therapeutic use. Each of the 14 chapters is divided into groups and subgroups to facilitate comparisons of drugs and drug products with similar uses. The first page of each chapter provides a detailed outline, including page references of the information presented in that chapter.

Products most similar in content or use are listed together. This format of presenting the FACTS makes it easy to make COMPARISONS of identical, similar, or related products.

Drug Monographs:

Prescribing information is presented in comprehensive drug monographs. General information on a group of closely related drugs (eg, ACE inhibitors) may be presented in a group monograph. Specific information for each drug follows the product listing; often there are separate monographs for each route of administration. All monographs are divided into sections identified with bold titles for ease in locating the desired information.

Indications: All indications or uses listed are FDA-approved unless specifically designated as "off-label uses." Inclusion of off-label drug information is intended for research purposes and should not be interpreted as a recommendation.

Off-label uses – Some off-label uses include numbered documentation ratings. Definitions associated with each rating appear below.

Documentation Levels Used for Off-label Uses

Number	Documentation	Definition
1	Good	Efficacy, safety risks, and optimal dosing are clearly identified in appropriate population as evidenced by consistent favorable data from at least 1 well-designed, controlled trial and/or dramatic results from uncontrolled experiments supported by guidelines published by expert panels.
2	Fair	Therapy represents rational use as evidenced by *consistent favorable* clinical reports/trials but further study is needed due to at least 1 of the following factors: • Appropriate candidates for therapy have not been clearly identified. • Optimal dosage and duration of therapy have not been consistently studied or determined. • Some safety issues require further investigation (eg, bacterial resistance).
3	Significant safety concerns exist	Efficacy is evidenced by some clinical reports, but significant safety concerns (eg, adverse events or drug interactions) must be considered prior to use. Significant safety data have been identified by controlled or noncontrolled reports and/or FDA or manufacturer safety notifications (eg, black box warnings).

Documentation Levels Used for Off-label Uses		
Number	Documentation	Definition
4	Insufficient	Rational use cannot be established as evidenced by data in limited patient population (fewer than 30 patients) or inconsistent results. Assessment of appropriate patient population, dose, or efficacy cannot be adequately determined. In addition, significant safety data have been identified by FDA or manufacturer safety notifications (eg, black box warnings).
5	Poor	Use is not recommended based on data that indicate use is considered unsafe or noneffective.

Administration and Dosage: Dosage ranges and methods of administration are presented.

Off-label uses – When "off-label uses" with documentation ratings are listed in the Indications section, a summary of the corresponding dosing information will appear in the Administration and Dosage section. The documentation rating will be repeated (see Documentation Levels Used for Off-label Uses). Inclusion of dosing information for off-label uses is intended for research purposes and should not be interpreted as a recommendation.

Additional off-label information specific to dosing may also appear in the Administration and Dosage sections.

Actions: This section gives a brief summary of the known pharmacologic and pharmacokinetic properties.

Contraindications: This section specifies those conditions in which the drug should NOT be used.

Warnings and Precautions: These sections list conditions in which use of the drug may be hazardous, precautions to observe, and parameters to monitor during therapy.

Drug Interactions: A brief summary of documented, clinically significant drug-drug, drug-lab test and drug-food interactions is provided.

Adverse Reactions: Reported adverse reactions are presented. Incidence data on adverse effects are included when available.

Overdosage: The clinical manifestations of toxicity and treatment of overdosage are given for most agents.

Patient Information: Essential information required by the patient for safe and effective self-administration of the medication is included.

Index:

The alphabetical index includes page references for all drugs by their generic name, brand name, synonyms, common abbreviations and therapeutic group names. Generic names are listed in bold type face for easy identification.

Product Listings:

Individual products are listed at the beginning of each monograph. The format and components of the product listings are discussed below and illustrated on the opposite page.

NOTE: Products that contain the same active ingredients are listed together for comparison and as an aid in product selection. However, drug product interchange is regulated by state laws; listing of products together does not imply that products are therapeutically equivalent or legally interchangeable. Caution is particularly advised when attempting to compare extended-release or delayed-release dosage forms.

1. Products are grouped by dosage form and strength.
2. Brand name products with the same amount of active ingredient and in the same doseform are listed in alphabetical order.
3. The name of the distributor is given in parentheses next to the product name.
4. Products available by their generic name from multiple sources are indicated as available from (Various) distributors and in selected cases, examples of generic manufacturers are listed.
5. Package sizes are given for all dosage forms and strengths of each product.
6. Product identification imprint codes are listed in parentheses.
7. Cross references to the appropriate drug monograph(s) for complete prescribing information appear at the beginning of the monograph.
8. Controlled substances are designated by their schedule (*c-II, c-III, c-IV,* or *c-V*).
9. Distribution status of products is indicated as *Rx* or *otc* (products listed as *otc* may include nutritional or dietary supplements).
10. Sugar-free liquid preparations are designated by *sf.*
11. Combination products are listed in tables to facilitate comparisons. Products most similar in formulation are listed next to each other.
12. Products with identical active ingredients are listed together.

Aminopenicillins

AMOXICILLIN

		Product & Distributor	Dosage form	Description / Package
	Rx	**Amoxil** (SK-Beecham)	**Tablets**: 500 mg (as trihydrate)	(Amoxil 500). Film-coated. Capsule shape. Pink. In 20s, 100s, 500s
			875 mg (as trihydrate)	(Amoxil 875). Film coated, scored. Capsule shape. Pink. In 20s, 100s, 500s.
2	Rx	**Amoxicillin** (Various, eg, Biocraft, Major, Rugby, Teva, URL)	**Capsules**: 250 mg (as trihydrate) (1)	In 21s, 30s, 100s, 250s, 500s, 1000s and UD 45s and 100s.
2	Rx	**Amoxil** (SK-Beecham)		(Amoxil 250). Blue and pink. In 100s, 500s and UD 100s.
2	Rx	**Trimox** (Apothecon)		In 30s, 100s, 500s and UD 100s.
2, 3	Rx	**Wymox** (Wyeth-Ayerst)		(Wyeth 559). Gray and green. In 100s and 500s.
4	Rx	**Amoxicillin** (Various, eg, Biocraft, Major, Rugby, Teva, URL)	**Capsules**: 500 mg (as trihydrate)	(5) In 21s, 30s, 50s, 100s, 250s, 500s and UD 45s and 100s.
	Rx	**Amoxil** (SK-Beecham)		(6) (Amoxil 500). Blue and pink. In 100s, 500s and UD 100s.
	Rx	**Trimox** (Apothecon)		In 30s, 100s, 500s and UD 100s.
	Rx	**Wymox** (Wyeth-Ayerst)		(Wyeth 560). Gray and green. In 50s and 500s.
	Rx	**Amoxil Pediatric Drops** (SK-Beecham)	**Powder for Oral Suspension**: 50 mg/ml (as trihydrate) when reconstituted	Sucrose. Bubble gum flavor. In 15 and 30 ml.
	Rx	**Trimox Pediatric Drops** (Apothecon)		Sucrose. In 15 ml.
	Rx	**Amoxicillin** (Various, eg, Biocraft, Major, Teva, URL)	**Powder for Oral Suspension**: 125 mg/5 ml (as trihydrate) when reconstituted	In 80, 100, 150 and 200 ml.
	Rx	**Amoxil** (SK-Beecham)		Sucrose. Strawberry flavor. In 80, 100 and 150 ml and UD 5 ml.
	Rx	**Trimox** (Apothecon)		Sucrose. In 80, 100 and 150 ml.
	Rx	**Wymox** (Wyeth-Ayerst)		Sucrose. In 100 and 150 ml.
	Rx	**Amoxicillin** (Various, eg, Biocraft, Major, Teva, URL)	**Powder for Oral Suspension**: 250 mg/5 ml (as trihydrate) when reconstituted	In 80, 100, 150 and 200 ml.
	Rx	**Amoxil** (SK-Beecham)		Sucrose. Bubble gum flavor. In 80, 100 and 150 ml and UD 5 ml.
	Rx	**Trimox** (Apothecon)		Sucrose. In 80, 100 and 150 ml.
	Rx	**Wymox** (Wyeth-Ayerst)		Sucrose. In 100 and 150 ml.

7 — For complete prescribing information, refer to the Penicillins group monograph.

the advantage of more complete absorption than ampicillin, a 3-times a day regimen for most infections and less diarrhea than ampicillin.

COUGH PREPARATIONS

ANTITUSSIVE AND EXPECTORANT COMBINATIONS

Content given per tablet, 5 mL, or packet.

		Product & Distributor	Antitussive	Expectorant	Decongestant
11	*Rx*	**Levall Liquid**[1] (Athlon Pharmaceuticals[2])	20 mg carbetapentane citrate	100 mg guaifenesin	15 mg phenylephrine HCl
11, 12	*c-v*	**Dihistine Expectorant Liquid** (Alpharma)	10 mg codeine phosphate	100 mg guaifenesin	30 mg pseudoephedrine HCl
11, 12	*c-v*	**Guiatuss DAC Liquid**[1] (Various, eg, Alpharma, Ivax)			
11, 12	*c-v sf*	**Halotussin DAC Syrup**[1] (Watson Laboratories)			
11, 12	*c-v sf*	**Mytussin DAC Liquid**[1] (Morton Grove Pharmaceuticals)			
11, 12	*c-v*	**Novagest Expectorant with Codeine Liquid**[1] (Major)			
11	*c-iii*	**Nucofed Expectorant Syrup**[1] (Monarch)			
11, 8	*c-iii*	**Nucotuss Expectorant Syrup**[1] (Alpharma)	12.5% alcohol. In 473 mL.		
11	*c-v*	**Tussirex Syrup** (Scot-Tussin)	10 mg codeine phosphate	83.3 mg sodium citrate	4.17 mg phenylephrine HCl
11, 10	*c-v sf*	**Tussirex Sugar Free Liquid** (Scot-Tussin)			
11	*Rx*	**Donatussin Syrup**[1] (Laser)	7.5 mg dextromethorphan HBr	100 mg guaifenesin	10 mg phenylephrine HCl
11, 9	*otc sf*	**Tussex Cough Syrup**[1] (Alpharma)	10 mg dextromethorphan HBr	100 mg guaifenesin	5 mg phenylephrine HCl
11, 9	*Rx*	**Tussafed Ex Syrup**[1] (Everett Laboratories)	30 mg dextromethorphan HBr	200 mg guaifenesin	10 mg phenylephrine HCl
11	*otc*	**Guiatuss CF Syrup**[1] (Alpharma)	10 mg dextromethorphan HBr	100 mg guafenesin	30 mg pseudoephedrine HCl
11	*otc*	**Robafen CF Syrup**[1] (Major)			
11	*otc*	**Robitussin CF Syrup**[1] (Whitehall-Robins)			

References:

Product labeling; thousands of biomedical articles; policies, guidelines and recommendations from many authoritative groups; and textbooks are used to form the base of evaluation of information for *Drug Facts and Comparisons,* including the following:

Andrew S, Cranswick N, Hill S, et al, eds. *WHO Model Formulary for Children 2010.* Geneva, Switzerland: World Health Organization; 2010.

Aronoff GR, Bennett WM, Berns JS, et al. *Drug Prescribing information in Renal Failure: Dosing Guidelines for Adults and Children.* 5th ed. Philadelphia, PA: American College of Physicians; 2007.

Aronson, JK, ed. *Side Effects of Drugs Annual 31.* New York, NY: Elsevier; 2004.

Ash M, Ash I, comps. *Handbook of Pharmaceutical Additives.* 1st ed. Endicott, NY: Synapse Information Resources Inc; 1995.

Beers MH, ed. *The Merck Manual of Diagnosis and Therapy.* 17th ed. Whitehouse Station, NJ: Merck Research Laboratories; 1999.

Bernardi RR, DeSimone EM, Newton GD, et al, eds. *Handbook of Nonprescription Drugs.* 14th ed. Washington, DC: American Pharmaceutical Association; 2004.

Brand KA, Tierno H. *Renal Dosing. Hospital Pharmacy* [wall chart]. [published online]. St. Louis, MO: Wolters Kluwer Health Inc; 2009.

Briggs GG, Freeman RK, Yaffe SJ. *Drugs in Pregnancy and Lactation: A Reference Guide to Fetal and Neonatal Risk.* 8th ed. Philadelphia, PA: Wolters Kluwer Health/Lippincott Williams & Wilkins; 2008.

Briggs GG, Nageotte M, eds. *Diseases, Complications, and Drug Therapy in Obstetrics: A Guide for Clinicians.* Bethesda, MD: American Society of Health-System Pharmacists; 2009.

Brunton LL, Lazo JS, Parker KL, eds. *Goodman & Gilman's The Pharmacological Basis of Therapeutics.* 11th ed. New York, NY: McGraw-Hill; 2006.

Clinical Laboratory Tests: Values and Implications. 3rd ed. Springhouse, PA: Springhouse; 2001.

Cooper DH, Krainik AJ, Lubner SJ, Reno HE, eds. *The Washington Manual of Medical Therapeutics.* 32nd ed. Philadelphia, PA: Wolters Kluwer Health/Lippincott Williams & Wilkins; 2007.

Custer JW, Rau RE, eds. *The Harriet Lane Handbook: A Manual for Pediatric House Officers. The Harriet Lane Service, Children's Medical and Surgical Center of the Johns Hopkins Hospital.* 18th ed. Philadelphia, PA: Mosby/Elsevier; 2009.

Dickey RP. *Managing Contraceptive Pill Patients.* 13th ed. Dallas, TX: EMIS Inc; 2007.

DiPiro JT, Talbert RL, Yee GC, Matzke GR, Wells BG, Posey LM, eds. *Pharmacotherapy: A Pathophysiologic Approach.* 7th ed. New York, NY: McGraw-Hill Medical; 2008.

Drugs and Lactation Database [database online]. Bethesda, MD: National Library of Medicine.

Dusenbery SM, White A, eds. *The Washington Manual of Pediatrics.* Philadelphia, PA: Wolters Kluwer Health/Lipincott Williams & Wilkins; 2009.

Ellenhorn MJ. *Ellenhorn's Medical Toxicology.* 2nd ed. Baltimore, MD: Williams & Wilkins; 1997.

Fauci AS, Braunwald E, Kasper DL, et al, eds. *Harrison's Principles of Internal Medicine.* 14th ed. New York, NY: McGraw-Hill Medical; 1998.

Fick DM, Cooper JW, Wade WE, Walter JL, Maclean JR, Beers MH. Updating the Beers criteria for potentially inappropriate medication use in older adults: results of a US consensus panel of experts. *Arch Intern Med.* 2003;163(22):2716-2724.

Gaedeke MK. *Laboratory and Diagnostic Test Handbook.* Menlo Park, CA: Addison-Wesley Nursing; 1996.

Gilbert DN, Moellering RC, Eliopoulos GM, Chambers HF, Saag MS. *The Sanford Guide to Antimicrobial Therapy, 2009.* 39th ed. Sperryville, VA: Antimicrobial Therapy; 2009.

Hale TW. *Medications and Mothers' Milk: A Manual of Lactational Pharmacology.* 14th ed. Amarillo, TX. Hale Publishing; 2010.

Helms RA, Quan DJ, Herfindal ET, Gourley DR, eds. *Textbook of Therapeutics: Drug and Disease Management.* 8th ed. Philadelphia, PA: Lippincott Williams & Wilkins; 2006.

Humes HD, ed-in-chief; DuPont HL, Gardner LB, Griffin JW, et al, eds. *Kellley's Textbook of Internal Medicine.* 4th ed. Philadelphia, PA: Lippincott Williams & Wilkins; 2000.

Koda-Kimble MA, Young LY, Alldredge BK, et al, eds. *Applied Therapeutics: The Clinical Use of Drugs.* 8th ed. Philadelphia, PA: Wolters Kluwer Health/Lippincott Williams & Wilkins; 2005.

Kronenberg HM, Melmed S, Polonsky KS, Larsen PR, eds. *Williams Textbook of Endocrinology.* 9th ed. Philadelphia, PA: Saunders/Elsevier; 1998.

McEvoy GK, Snow EK, Miller J, Kester L, Welsh OH, eds. *AHFS Drug Information 2009.* Bethesda, MD: American Society of Health-System Pharmacists, Inc; 2009.

McMillan JA, Lee CK, Siberry GK, Dick JD, eds. *The Harriet Lane Handbook of Pediatric Antimicrobial Therapy.* Philadelphia, PA: Mosby/Elsevier; 2008.

McPherson RA, Pincus MR, eds. *Henry's Clinical Diagnosis and Management by Laboratory Methods.* 20th ed. Philadelphia, PA: Saunders; 2001.

Miaskowski C, Bair M. Chou R, et al. *Principles of Analgesic Use in the Treatment of Acute Pain and Cancer Pain.* 6th ed. Glenview, IL: American Pain Society; 2008.

National Heart, Lung, and Blood Institute. National Asthma Education and Prevention Program. *Expert Panel on the Management of Asthma. Expert Panel Report 3: Guidelines for the Diagnosis and Management of Asthma. Full Report 2007.* Bethesda, MD: US Department of Health and Human Services, National Institutes of Health, National Heart, Lung, and Blood Institute; 2007.

Patient Safety Analysis: High Risk Medication Measures – PDP/MA-PD Contracts Report User Guide: Burlingame, CA: Acumen, LLC; 2008.

Perry PJ, Alexander B, Liskow P, DeVane CL. *Psychotropic Drug Handbook.* 8th ed. Philadelphia, PA: Lippincott Williams & Wilkins; 2007.

Phelps SJ, Hak EB, Crill CM. *Pediatric Injectable Drugs (The Teddy Bear Book).* 9th ed. Bethesda, MD: American Society of Health-System Pharmacists; 2010.

Pickering LK, Baker CJ, Kimberlin DW, Long SS, eds. *Red Book: 2009 Report of the Committee on Infectious Diseases.* 27th ed. Elk Grove Village, IL: American Academy of Pediatrics; 2009.

Rakel RE, Bope ET, eds. *Conn's Current Therapy 2005.* Philadelphia, PA: Saunders; 2005.

Remington: The Science and Practice of Pharmacy. 21st ed. Philadelphia, PA: Lippincott Williams & Wilkins; 2006.

Repchinsky CE, ed. *CPS 2008: Compendium of Pharmaceuticals and Specialities.* Toronto, Canada: Canadian Pharmaceutical Association: 2008.

Shannon MW, Borron SW, Burns M. *Haddad and Winchester's Clinical Management of Poisoning and Drug Overdose.* 3rd ed. Philadelphia, PA: Saunders/Elsevier; 1998.

Sweetman SC, ed. *Martindale: The Complete Drug Reference.* 36th ed. London, England: Pharmaceutical Press; 2009.

Trissel LA. *Handbook on Injectable Drugs.* 15th ed. Bethesda, MD: American Society of Health-System Pharmacists; 2008.

USP DI Volume I: Drug Information for the Health Care Professional. Greenwood Village, CO: Thomson Micromedex; 2006.

USP DI Volume II: Advice for the Patient. Greenwood Village, CO: Thomson Micromedex; 2006.

USP Dictionary of USAN and International Drug Names. Rockville, MD: United States Pharmacopeial Convention Inc; 2009.

Wallach J. *Interpretation of Diagnostic Tests.* 7th ed. Philadelphia, PA: Wolters Kluwer Health/Lippincott Williams & Wilkins, 2000.

Wiffen P, Mitchell M, Snelling M, Stoner N. *Oxford Handbook of Clinical Pharmacy.* New York, NY: Oxford University Press; 2007.

Working Group on Antiretroviral Therapy and Medical Management of HIV-Infected Children. *Guidelines for the Use of Antiretroviral Agents inPediatric HIV infection.* February 23, 2009.

Young TE, Mangum B. *NeoFax 2009: A Manual of Drugs Used in Neonatal Care.* 22nd ed. Montvale, NJ: Thomson Reuters; 2009.

National Heart, Lung, and Blood Institute, National Asthma Education and Prevention Program. Expert Panel on the Management of Asthma. Expert Panel Report 3: Guidelines for the Diagnosis and Management of Asthma. Full Report 2007. Bethesda, MD: US Department of Health and Human Services, National Institutes of Health, National Heart, Lung, and Blood Institute; 2007.

Patient Safety Analysis: High Risk Medication Measures – PDP/MA-PD Contracts Report User Guide. Burlingame, CA: Acumen, LLC; 2008.

Perry PJ, Alexander B, Liskow BI, DeVane CL. Psychotropic Drug Handbook. 8th ed. Philadelphia, PA: Lippincott Williams & Wilkins; 2007.

Phelps SJ, Hak EB, Crill CM. Pediatric Injectable Drugs (The Teddy Bear Book). 9th ed. Bethesda, MD: American Society of Health-System Pharmacists; 2010.

Pickering LK, Baker CJ, Kimberlin DW, Long SS, eds. Red Book: 2009 Report of the Committee on Infectious Diseases. 27th ed. Elk Grove Village, IL: American Academy of Pediatrics; 2009.

Rakel RE, Bope ET, eds. Conn's Current Therapy 2005. Philadelphia, PA: Saunders; 2005.

Remington: The Science and Practice of Pharmacy. 21st ed. Philadelphia, PA: Lippincott Williams & Wilkins; 2006.

Repchinsky CE, ed. CPS 2008: Compendium of Pharmaceuticals and Specialties. Toronto, Canada: Canadian Pharmaceutical Association; 2008.

Shannon MW, Borron SW, Burns M. Haddad and Winchester's Clinical Management of Poisoning and Drug Overdose. 3rd ed. Philadelphia, PA: Saunders/Elsevier; 1998.

Sweetman SC, ed. Martindale: The Complete Drug Reference. 36th ed. London, England: Pharmaceutical Press; 2009.

Trissel LA. Handbook on Injectable Drugs. 15th ed. Bethesda, MD: American Society of Health-System Pharmacists; 2008.

USP DI Volume I: Drug Information for the Health Care Professional. Greenwood Village, CO: Thomson Micromedex; 2006.

USP DI Volume II: Advice for the Patient. Greenwood Village, CO: Thomson Micromedex; 2006.

USP Dictionary of USAN and International Drug Names. Rockville, MD: United States Pharmacopeial Convention Inc; 2008.

Wallach J. Interpretation of Diagnostic Tests. 8th ed. Philadelphia, PA: Wolters Kluwer Health/Lippincott Williams & Wilkins; 2006.

Walker R, Mitchell M, Snelling M, Stoner N. Oxford Handbook of Clinical Pharmacy. New York, NY: Oxford University Press; 2007.

Working Group on Antiretroviral Therapy and Medical Management of HIV-Infected Children. Guidelines for the Use of Antiretroviral Agents in Pediatric HIV Infection. February 23, 2009.

Young TE, Mangum B. NeoFax 2009: A Manual of Drugs Used in Neonatal Care. 22nd ed. Montvale, NJ: Thomson Reuters; 2009.

DIETARY REFERENCE INTAKES OF VITAMINS AND MINERALS

In 1941, the Food and Nutrition Board (FNB) of the Institute of Medicine, National Academy of Sciences, published the first edition of the Recommended Dietary Allowances (RDAs) to be used to evaluate the nutritional intakes of large populations. The primary purpose for the RDAs was to prevent diseases caused by nutritional deficiencies. Over the years, these guidelines were periodically updated and revised based on cumulative scientific evidence, and the tenth edition was published in 1989. In response to the growth of scientific knowledge regarding the roles of nutrients in human health, the FNB in partnership with Health Canada revised the RDAs and developed the Dietary Reference Intakes (DRIs).

The DRIs were published as a series of 8 reports from 1997 to 2005 and include the following nutrient reference values: Estimated Average Requirement (EAR), RDAs, Adequate Intake (AI), and Tolerable Upper Intake Level (UL). EAR refers to the intake value of a nutrient that is estimated to meet the nutritional needs by a specified indicator of adequacy in 50% of an age- and gender-specific group. RDAs are based on EARs and are estimated to meet the needs of most individuals (97% to 98%). AIs are used when an RDA cannot be determined. UL is the maximum amount of daily nutrient intake (from food, water, and supplements) that is likely to pose no risk of adverse reactions.

In the following DRI tables, the RDAs are in bold type and the AIs are in ordinary type followed by an asterisk (*). These values may be used as goals for individual intake. For healthy breast-fed infants, the AI represents mean intake. For all other life-stage groups, the AI is believed to cover the needs of all individuals, but a lack of data or uncertainty in the data prevent specifying with confidence the percentage of individuals covered by this intake.

DRIs: Recommended Intakes for Individuals (Vitamins)

Life-stage group	Vitamin A (mcg/d)[a]	Vitamin C (mg/d)	Vitamin D (mcg/d)[b,c]	Vitamin E (mg/d)[d]	Vitamin K (mcg/d)	Thiamine (mg/d)	Riboflavin (mg/d)	Niacin (mg/d)[e]	Vitamin B_6 (mg/d)	Folate (mcg/d)[f]	Vitamin B_{12} (mcg/d)	Pantothenic acid (mg/d)	Biotin (mcg/d)	Choline (mg/d)[g]
Infants														
0 to 6 mo	400*	40*	5*	4*	2*	0.2*	0.3*	2*	0.1*	65*	0.4*	1.7*	5*	125*
7 to 12 mo	500*	50*	5*	5*	2.5*	0.3*	0.4*	4*	0.3*	80*	0.5*	1.8*	6*	150*
Children														
1 to 3 y	300	15	5*	6	30*	0.5	0.5	6	0.5	150	0.9	2*	8*	200*
4 to 8 y	400	25	5*	7	55*	0.6	0.6	8	0.6	200	1.2	3*	12*	250*
Men														
9 to 13 y	600	45	5*	11	60*	0.9	0.9	12	1	300	1.8	4*	20*	375*
14 to 18 y	900	75	5*	15	75*	1.2	1.3	16	1.3	400	2.4	5*	25*	550*
19 to 30 y	900	90	5*	15	120*	1.2	1.3	16	1.3	400	2.4	5*	30*	550*
31 to 50 y	900	90	5*	15	120*	1.2	1.3	16	1.3	400	2.4	5*	30*	550*
51 to 70 y	900	90	10*	15	120*	1.2	1.3	16	1.7	400	2.4[h]	5*	30*	550*
70 y	900	90	15*	15	120*	1.2	1.3	16	1.7	400	2.4[h]	5*	30*	550*
Women														
9 to 13 y	600	45	5*	11	60*	0.9	0.9	12	1	300	1.8	4*	20*	375*
14 to 18 y	700	65	5*	15	75*	1	1	14	1.2	400[i]	2.4	5*	25*	400*
19 to 30 y	700	75	5*	15	90*	1.1	1.1	14	1.3	400[i]	2.4	5*	30*	425*
31 to 50 y	700	75	5*	15	90*	1.1	1.1	14	1.3	400[i]	2.4	5*	30*	425*
51 to 70 y	700	75	10*	15	90*	1.1	1.1	14	1.5	400	2.4[h]	5*	30*	425*
70 y	700	75	15*	15	90*	1.1	1.1	14	1.5	400	2.4[h]	5*	30*	425*
Pregnancy														
14 to 18 y	750	80	5*	15	75*	1.4	1.4	18	1.9	600[j]	2.6	6*	30*	450*
19 to 30 y	770	85	5*	15	90*	1.4	1.4	18	1.9	600[j]	2.6	6*	30*	450*
31 to 50 y	770	85	5*	15	90*	1.4	1.4	18	1.9	600[j]	2.6	6*	30*	450*
Lactation														
14 to 18 y	1,200	115	5*	19	75*	1.4	1.6	17	2	500	2.8	7*	35*	550*
19 to 30 y	1,300	120	5*	19	90*	1.4	1.6	17	2	500	2.8	7*	35*	550*
31 to 50 y	1,300	120	5*	19	90*	1.4	1.6	17	2	500	2.8	7*	35*	550*

NOTE: AIs are in ordinary type followed by an asterisk (*), and RDAs are in bold type.

[a] As retinol activity equivalents (RAEs). 1 RAE = retinol 1 mcg, β-carotene 12 mcg, α-carotene 24 mcg, or β-cryptoxanthin 24 mcg. The RAE for dietary provitamin A carotenoids is 2-fold greater than retinol equivalents (RE), whereas the RAE for preformed vitamin A is the same as RE.

[b] As cholecalciferol. Cholecalciferol 1 mcg = vitamin D 40 units.

[c] Values based on the absence of adequate exposure to sunlight.

[d] As α-tocopherol. α-Tocopherol includes *RRR*-α-tocopherol, the only form of α-tocopherol that occurs naturally in foods, and the *2R*-stereoisomeric forms of α-tocopherol (*RRR-*, *RSR-*, *RRS-*, and *RSS*-α-tocopherol) that occur in fortified foods and supplements. It does not include the *2S*-stereoisomeric forms of α-tocopherol (*SRR-*, *SSR-*, *SRS-*, and *SSS*-α-tocopherol), also found in fortified foods and supplements.

[e] Includes nicotinic acid amide, nicotinic acid (pyridine-3-carboxylic acid), and derivatives that exhibit the biological activity of nicotinamide. As niacin equivalents (NE). Niacin 1 mg = tryptophan 60 mg; 0 to 6 months = preformed niacin (not NE).

[f] As dietary folate equivalents (DFE). One DFE = food folate 1 mcg = folic acid 0.6 mcg from fortified food or as a supplement consumed with food = 0.5 mcg of a supplement taken on an empty stomach.

[g] Although AIs have been set for choline, there are few data to assess whether a dietary supply of choline is needed at all stages of the life-cycle, and it may be that the choline requirement can be met by endogenous synthesis at some of these stages.

[h] Because 10% to 30% of older people may malabsorb food-bound B_{12}, it is advisable for individuals older than 50 years of age to meet their RDA mainly by consuming foods fortified with B_{12} or a supplement containing B_{12}.

[i] In view of evidence linking folate intake with neural tube defects in the fetus, it is recommended that all women capable of becoming pregnant consume 400 mcg from supplements or fortified foods in addition to intake of food folate from a varied diet.

[j] It is assumed that women will continue consuming 400 mcg from supplements or fortified food until their pregnancy is confirmed and they enter prenatal care, which ordinarily occurs after the end of the periconceptional period—the critical time for formation of the neural tube.

DIETARY REFERENCE INTAKES OF VITAMINS AND MINERALS

	DRIs: Recommended Intakes for Individuals (Elements)														
Life-stage group	Calcium (mg/d)	Chromium (mcg/d)	Copper (mcg/d)	Fluoride (mg/d)	Iodine (mcg/d)	Iron (mg/d)[a]	Magnesium (mg/d)	Manganese (mg/d)	Molybdenum (mcg/d)	Phosphorus (mg/d)	Selenium (mcg/d)	Zinc (mg/d)[b]	Potassium (g/d)	Sodium (g/d)	Chloride (g/d)
Infants															
0 to 6 mo	210*	0.2*	200*	0.01*	110*	0.27*	30*	0.003*	2*	100*	15*	2*	0.4*	0.12*	0.18*
7 to 12 mo	270*	5.5*	220*	0.5*	130*	11	75*	0.6*	3*	275*	20*	3	0.7*	0.37*	0.57*
Children															
1 to 3 y	500*	11*	340	0.7*	90	7	80	1.2*	17	460	20	3	3*	1*	1.5*
4 to 8 y	800*	15*	440	1*	90	10	130	1.5*	22	500	30	5	3.8*	1.2*	1.9*
Men															
9 to 13 y	1,300*	25*	700	2*	120	8	240	1.9*	34	1,250	40	8	4.5*	1.5*	2.3*
14 to 18 y	1,300*	35*	890	3*	150	11	410	2.2*	43	1,250	55	11	4.7*	1.5*	2.3*
19 to 30 y	1,000*	35*	900	4*	150	8	400	2.3*	45	700	55	11	4.7*	1.5*	2.3*
31 to 50 y	1,000*	35*	900	4*	150	8	420	2.3*	45	700	55	11	4.7*	1.5*	2.3*
51 to 70 y	1,200*	30*	900	4*	150	8	420	2.3*	45	700	55	11	4.7*	1.3*	2*
70 y	1,200*	30*	900	4*	150	8	420	2.3*	45	700	55	11	4.7*	1.2*	1.8*
Women															
9 to 13 y	1,300*	21*	700	2*	120	8	240	1.6*	34	1,250	40	8	4.5*	1.5*	2.3*
14 to 18 y	1,300*	24*	890	3*	150	15	360	1.6*	43	1,250	55	9	4.7*	1.5*	2.3*
19 to 30 y	1,000*	25*	900	3*	150	18	310	1.8*	45	700	55	8	4.7*	1.5*	2.3*
31 to 50 y	1,000*	25*	900	3*	150	18	320	1.8*	45	700	55	8	4.7*	1.5*	2.3*
51 to 70 y	1,200*	20*	900	3*	150	8	320	1.8*	45	700	55	8	4.7*	1.3*	2*
70 y	1,200*	20*	900	3*	150	8	320	1.8*	45	700	55	8	4.7*	1.2*	1.8*
Pregnancy															
14 to 18 y	1,300*	29*	1,000	3*	220	27	400	2*	50	1,250	60	12	4.7*	1.5*	2.3*
19 to 30 y	1,000*	30*	1,000	3*	220	27	350	2*	50	700	60	11	4.7*	1.5*	2.3*
31 to 50 y	1,000*	30*	1,000	3*	220	27	360	2*	50	700	60	11	4.7*	1.5*	2.3*
Lactation															
14 to 18 y	1,300*	44*	1,300	3*	290	10	360	2.6*	50	1,250	70	13	5.1*	1.5*	2.3*
19 to 30 y	1,000*	45*	1,300	3*	290	9	310	2.6*	50	700	70	12	5.1*	1.5*	2.3*
31 to 50 y	1,000*	45*	1,300	3*	290	9	320	2.6*	50	700	70	12	5.1*	1.5*	2.3*

NOTE: AIs are in ordinary type followed by an asterisk (*) and RDAs are in bold type.

[a] Non-heme iron absorption is lower for those consuming vegetarian diets than for those eating nonvegetarian diets. Therefore, it has been suggested that the iron requirement for individuals consuming a vegetarian diet is approximately 2-fold greater than for individuals consuming a nonvegetarian diet.

[b] Zinc absorption is lower for those consuming vegetarian diets than for those eating nonvegetarian diets. Therefore, it has been suggested that the zinc requirement for individuals consuming a vegetarian diet is approximately 2-fold greater than for individuals consuming a nonvegetarian diet.

Fat-Soluble Vitamins

VITAMIN A

otc	Vitamin A (Various, eg, Freeda,[b] Naturally Vitamins[c])	Capsules; oral: 10,000 IU	In 100s, 250s, and 500s.
otc	Vitamin A (Various, eg, Freeda)	Capsules; oral: 15,000 IU[a]	In 100s and 250s.
Rx[d]	Vitamin A (Various, eg, Naturally Vitamins[c])	Capsules; oral: 25,000 IU	In 100s.
Rx	Aquasol A (Hospira)	Injection: 50,000 IU/mL[a]	In 2 mL vials.[e]

[a] As vitamin A palmitate.
[b] As vitamin A palmitate or beta carotene.
[c] As retinol.
[d] Some products may be available *otc* according to distributor discretion.
[e] With 0.5% chlorobutanol, polysorbate 80, butylated hydroxyanisole, and butylated hydroxytoluene.

VITAMIN A — ORAL

For additional information, refer to the Dietary Reference Intakes of Vitamins and Minerals table.

Indications

➤*Dietary supplement:* As a dietary supplement when vitamin A intake may be inadequate.

➤*Vitamin A deficiency:* Vitamin A may be used to treat Kwashiorkor and xerophthalmia, both conditions caused by vitamin A deficiency.

➤*Off-label uses:* Reduction in falciparum malaria episodes in children older than 12 months.

Administration and Dosage

➤*General dosing considerations:* In the past, the recommended daily allowance (RDA) for vitamin A has been expressed in units. This term units has been replaced by retinol activity equivalents (RAE) where 1 RAE = retinol 1 mcg, beta-carotene (from supplements) 0.2 mcg, beta-carotene (from food) 12 mcg, alpha-carotene 24 mcg, or beta-cryptoxanthin 24 mcg.

➤*Adults:*

Dietary supplement – 1 tablet or capsule daily.

➤*Administration:* Vitamin A absorption is enhanced if taken with food.

➤*Storage/Stability:* Store away from heat and direct light.

Actions

➤*Pharmacology:* Vitamin A comes in 2 different forms: Retinols and provitamins. Retinols are found in foods that come from animals (eg, meat, milk, eggs) and include retinol, retinal, and retinoic acid. Provitamins come from plants (which are then converted to vitamin A in the body) and include alpha-, beta- and gamma-carotene. Food processing may destroy some vitamins (eg, freezing may reduce the amount of vitamin A in foods). Remind patients the total amount of vitamin A includes what is received from foods that are eaten and from what is taken as a supplement.

Sources of vitamin A include 3 natural compounds from animal sources (retinol, retinal, and retinoic acid) and 3 provitamins from plants (alpha-, beta- and gamma-carotene). Sources rich in vitamin A include liver, butter, cheese, whole milk, egg yolk, meat, and fish. Plants that are good sources of beta-carotene include dark green leafy vegetables, carrots, sweet potatoes, squash, and cantaloupes.

Vitamin A activity is expressed in multiple ways (eg, units, retinol equivalents, retinol activity equivalents). Traditionally, food composition tables used "units" to express vitamin A, and used the following conversion factors: 1 mcg of retinol = 3.33 units of vitamin A activity from retinol. However, the use of "units" is no longer preferred when calculating and reporting the amount of dietary and supplemental vitamin A consumed.

Vitamin A derivatives are essential for vision, dental development, growth, hydrocortisone synthesis, epithelial tissue differentiation, embryonic development, and reproduction. Vitamin A is also required for maintenance of the mucous membranes of the eyes, skin, mouth, gastrointestinal tract, and genitourinary tract.

Physiological Roles of Vitamin A Derivatives

Vitamin A derivatives	Physiological role
Retinol	Supports the reproductive cycle
Retinal	Functions in the visual cycle
Retinoic acid	Promotes growth, differentiation, and maintenance of epithelial tissue
Beta-carotene	Visual adaptation to darkness

Deficiency – Vitamin A deficiency leads to suppressed mucus production resulting in irritation and infection. Common symptoms of vitamin A deficiency include nyctalopia (night blindness), keratomalacia (corneal necrosis), keratinization of the skin including secondary xerophthalmia, impaired resistance to infection, retardation of growth, thickening of bone, decreased production of cortical steroids, and fetal malformations. Vitamin A deficiency may also be associated with an increased susceptibility to bacterial, parasitic, and viral infections.

Conditions which may cause vitamin A deficiency: Biliary tract or pancreatic disease, sprue, hepatic cirrhosis, extreme dietary inadequacy, partial gastrectomy, and cystic fibrosis.

➤*Pharmacokinetics:*

Absorption/Distribution – Vitamin A is fat soluble; absorption from the proximal small intestine requires bile salts, pancreatic lipase and dietary fat. Retinol reaches a peak plasma concentration 4 hours after ingestion. Absorption for retinol preparations is greatest for aqueous preparations, intermediate for emulsions, and slowest for oil solutions. Water-miscible preparations should be used in patients where retinol absorption is reduced, such as in pancreatic/hepatic disease, intestinal disease/infections, and cystic fibrosis. Half of absorbed vitamin A is oxidized (or conjugated) and excreted in the feces and urine, while the other half is stored in the Kupffer cells of the liver, mainly as retinyl esters (eg, retinyl palmitate). Retinol is absorbed by intestinal cells through the presence of cellular retinol-binding protein (CRBPs), incorporated into chylomicrons, and transported to the liver.

In contrast to retinol, only 33% of beta-carotene is absorbed due to a high dependence on the presence of bile and absorbable fat in the intestinal tract. Only 50% of ingested beta-carotene is converted to retinol.

Normal serum vitamin A concentrations are 360 to 1200 mcg/L (retinol plasma range is 30 to 70 mcg/dL) and 270 to 753 Units/100 mL for carotenoids. The normal adult liver contains approximately 100 to 300 mcg/g (mostly as retinol palmitate), providing vitamin A requirements for 2 years. A plasma concentration less than 10 to 20 mcg/g or a retinoid hepatic concentration less than 5 to 20 mcg/g is associated with vitamin A deficiency. Plasma retinol concentrations are reduced in cystic fibrosis, alcohol-related cirrhosis, hepatic diseases, proteinuria, and febrile infections. Plasma retinol concentrations are elevated in patients with chronic renal disease.

Vitamin A absorption is enhanced if taken with food.

Metabolism/Excretion – Vitamin A is mobilized from liver stores and transported in the plasma as retinol bound to retinol-binding protein (RBP). RBP protects retinol from oxidation during transport. 11-cis-retinol is converted to 11-cis-retinal and combines with opsin (the rod pigment in the retina) to form rhodopsin, which is necessary for visual adaptation to darkness. Approximately 10% of vitamin A is not absorbed in the intestine and excreted in the feces.

Contraindications

Hypervitaminosis A; oral use in malabsorption syndrome; hypersensitivity; IV use.

Warnings/Precautions

➤*Prolonged administration:* Closely supervise prolonged administration over 25,000 IU/day. Evaluate vitamin A intake from fortified foods, dietary supplements, self-administered drugs, and prescription drug sources.

➤*Blood level assays:* Blood level assays are not a direct measure of liver storage. Liver storage should be adequate before discontinuing therapy.

➤*Multiple vitamin deficiency:* Single vitamin A deficiency is rare. Multiple vitamin deficiency is expected in any dietary deficiency.

➤*Acne:* Efficacy of large systemic doses of vitamin A (100,000 to 300,000 IU/day) in the treatment of acne has not been established. However, see topical retinoic acid (tretinoin) and isotretinoin monographs.

➤*Renal function impairment:* Vitamin A toxicity has been reported in chronic renal failure patients.

➤*Special risk:* Use vitamin A cautiously in patients who abuse alcohol or have kidney and liver disease or in patients being treated with etretinate or isotretinoin.

➤*Pregnancy: Category A.* (*Category C* in doses exceeding the RDA). The US RDA of vitamin A is 800 mcg retinol equivalents. Safety of amounts exceeding 5000 IU oral or 6000 IU parenteral daily during pregnancy has not been established. Avoid use of vitamin A in excess of the RDA during normal pregnancy. In pregnant women, vitamin A is necessary for the growth of a healthy fetus.

Animal reproduction studies have shown fetal abnormalities associated with overdosage in several species. One case of an infant with congenital renal anomalies has been reported. High doses and deficiency of vitamin A are considered to be *Category X.* Prolonged high doses of vitamin A (greater than 25,000 IU/day) have been associated with microtia, craniofacial and CNS anomalies, facial palsy, micro/anophthalmia, facial clefts, cardiac defects, limb reductions, GI atresia, and urinary tract defects.

➤*Lactation:* The US RDA of vitamin A is 1300 mcg retinol equivalents for nursing mothers in the first 6 months and 1200 mg retinol equivalents for the second 6 months. Human milk supplies sufficient vitamin A for infants unless maternal diet is grossly inadequate.

Drug Interactions

➤*Mineral oil:* Mineral oil may decrease the GI absorption of vitamin A.

Adverse Reactions

➤*Dermatologic:* Side effects involve the skin and mucous membranes and include cheilitis, facial dermatitis, dry mucous membranes, stratum corneum fragility, sticky skin, conjunctivitis, palmoplantar peeling, alopecia, pyogenic granuloma-like lesions in acne, paronychia, and corneal opacities.

VITAMIN A — ORAL

Overdosage

➤*Symptoms:* Toxicity manifestations depend on patient's age, dosage, and duration of administration.

Acute toxicity – Nausea, vomiting, drowsiness, headache, vertigo, and blurred vision in adults, or bulging fontanelles in infants.

Infants (less than 1 year old) – 100,000 IU/dose.

Children (1 to 6 years old) – 100,000 IU/dose.

Adults – Greater than 1,000,000 IU/dose.

Chronic toxicity – Hypercalcemia; dry scaly skin; bone pain; changes in texture of hair and nails, increased cerebrospinal pressure; pruritus; headache; nausea; irreversible bone changes (eg, demineralization); thinning of long bones; cortical hyperostosis, periostosis; premature closing of epiphyses.

Infants (3 to 6 months old) – 18,500 IU (water dispersed) daily for 1 to 3 months.

Adults – 1 million IU daily for 3 days, 50,000 IU daily for longer than 18 months, or 500,000 IU daily for 2 months.

Hypervitaminosis A syndrome (plasma retinol concentration greater than 100 mcg/dL) – Hypervitaminosis A syndrome generally manifests as a cirrhotic-like liver syndrome. The following have been reported as manifestations of chronic overuse:

CNS: Irritability; headache; vertigo; increased intracranial pressure as manifested by bulging fontanelles, papilledema and exophthalmos.

Dermatologic: Lip fissures; drying and cracking skin; alopecia; scaling; massive desquamation; increased pigmentation; generalized pruritus; erythema.

Musculoskeletal: Slow growth; hard tender cortical thickening over radius and tibia; migratory arthralgia; premature closure of epiphyses; bone pain.

Miscellaneous: Hypomenorrhea; hepatosplenomegaly; edema; leukopenia; vitamin A plasma levels greater than 1200 IU/dL; hypercalcemia; fatigue; malaise; lethargy; abdominal discomfort; jaundice; anorexia; vomiting.

➤*Treatment:* Treatment includes discontinuation of the retinoid. Desquamation and hyperostoses are evident for months. Bone malformations and liver damage may be irreversible.

Patient Information

Avoid prolonged use of mineral oil while taking this drug. Do not exceed recommended dosage, especially during pregnancy. Notify physician if signs of overdosage (eg, nausea, vomiting, drowsiness, headache, dizziness/feeling of whirling motion, blurred vision) or bulging fontanelles in infants occur.

VITAMIN A PALMITATE — INJECTION

For additional information, refer to the Dietary Reference Intakes of Vitamins and Minerals table.

Indications

➤*Vitamin A deficiency:* For the treatment of vitamin A deficiency.

The parenteral administration is indicated when the oral administration is not feasible as in anorexia, nausea, vomiting, pre- and postoperative conditions, or it is not available as in the "malabsorption syndrome" with accompanying steatorrhea.

➤*Off-label uses:* Reduction in falciparum malaria episodes in children older than 12 months of age.

Promyelocytic leukemia (retinoic acid); acne; diminishing malignant cell growth; enhancing the immune system; lower incidence of lung cancer and cardiovascular disease; reduction in mortality of HIV-infected children.

Administration and Dosage

➤*General dosing considerations:* In the past, the recommended daily allowance (RDA) for vitamin A was expressed in units. This term units has been replaced by retinol activity equivalents (RAE) where 1 RAE = retinol 1 mcg, beta-carotene (from supplements) 0.2 mcg, beta-carotene (from food) 12 mcg, alpha-carotene 24 mcg, or beta-cryptoxanthin 24 mcg.

➤*Adults:*

Vitamin A deficiency –

Usual dosage: 100,000 units/day intramuscularly (IM) for 3 days followed by 50,000 daily for 2 weeks.

Oral maintenance therapy: Follow-up therapy with an oral therapeutic multi-vitamin preparation, containing 10,000 to 20,000 units is recommended daily for 2 months. In malabsorption, the parenteral route must be used for an equivalent preparation.

➤*Children:*

Vitamin A deficiency –

1 to 8 years of age: 17,500 to 35,000 units/day IM for 10 days.

Infants: 7,500 to 15,000 units/day IM daily for 10 days.

Oral maintenance therapy: Use an oral therapeutic multi-vitamin preparation daily for 2 months. In malabsorption, the parenteral route must be used for an equivalent preparation.

- *Older than 8 years* – 10,000 to 20,000 units/day orally.
- *Younger than 8 years* – 5,000 to 10,000 units/day orally.

➤*Prolonged administration:* Avoid overdosage. Prolonged daily dose administration over 25,000 units vitamin A should be under close supervision.

➤*Administration:* For IM use.

➤*Storage/Stability:* Store at 2° to 8°C (36° to 46°F). Do not freeze. Protect from light.

Actions

➤*Pharmacology:* Beta-carotene, retinol, and retinal have effective and reliable vitamin A activity. Retinal and retinol are in chemical equilibrium in the body and have equivalent antixerophthalmic activity. Retinal combines with the rod pigment, opsin, in the retina to form rhodopsin, necessary for visual dark adaptation. Vitamin A prevents retardation of growth and preserves the epithelial cells' integrity. Normal adult liver storage is sufficient to satisfy 2 years' requirements of vitamin A.

Vitamin A is readily absorbed from the gastrointestinal tract, where the biosynthesis of vitamin A from beta-carotene takes place. Vitamin A absorption requires bile salts, pancreatic lipase, and dietary fat. It is transported in the blood to the liver by the chylomicron fraction of the lymph. Vitamin A is stored in Kupffer cells of the liver mainly as the palmitate. Normal serum vitamin A is 80 to 300 IU/per 100 mL (plasma range is 30 to 70 mcgdL) and for carotenoids 270 to 753 IU/per 100 mL. The normal adult liver contains approximately 100 to 300 mcg/g, mostly as retinol palmitate.

Contraindications

Intravenous administration; hypervitaminosis A; sensitivity to any of the ingredients in this preparation.

Warnings/Precautions

➤*Prolonged administration:* Avoid overdosage. Prolonged daily dose administration over 25,000 IU vitamin A should be under close supervision.

➤*Blood level assays:* Blood level assays are not a direct measure of liver storage. Liver storage should be adequate before discontinuing therapy.

➤*Multiple vitamin deficiency:* Single vitamin A deficiency is rare. Multiple vitamin deficiency is expected in any dietary deficiency.

➤*Pregnancy: Category X.* Safety of amounts exceeding 6,000 IU of vitamin A daily during pregnancy has not been established at this time. The use of vitamin A in excess of the recommended dietary allowance may cause fetal harm when administered to a pregnant woman. Animal reproduction studies have shown fetal abnormalities associated with overdosage in several species. Malformations of the central nervous system, the eye, the palate, and the urogenital tract are recorded. Vitamin A in excess of the recommended dietary allowance is contraindicated in women who are or may become pregnant. If vitamin A is used during pregnancy, or if the patient becomes pregnant while taking vitamin A, the patient should be apprised of the potential hazard to the fetus.

➤*Lactation:* The US Recommended Daily Allowance (RDA) of vitamin A (5,000 IU) is recommended for nursing mothers.

Drug Interactions

➤*Oral contraceptives:* Women on oral contraceptives have shown a significant increase in plasma vitamin A levels.

Adverse Reactions

See Overdosage. Anaphylactic shock and death have been reported using the intravenous route. Allergic reactions have been reported rarely with administration of vitamin A palmitate including 1 case of an anaphylactoid type reaction.

Overdosage

The following amounts have been found to be toxic orally. Toxicity manifestations depend on the age, dosage, size, and duration of administration.

➤*Acute toxicity:* Single dose (25,000 IU/kg body weight).

Infant – 350,000 IU.

Adult – Over 2 million IU.

➤*Chronic toxicity (4,000 units/kg body weight for 6 to 15 months):*

Infants 3 to 6 months old – 18,500 IU (water dispersed)/day for 1 to 3 months.

Adult – 1 million IU daily for 3 days; 50,000 Units daily for longer than 18 months; 500,000 IU daily for 2 months.

➤*Hypervitaminosis a syndrome:*

General manifestations – Fatigue, malaise, lethargy, abdominal discomfort, anorexia, and vomiting.

Specific manifestations –

Skeletal: Slow growth, hard tender cortical thickening over the radius and tibia, migratory arthralgia and premature closure of the epiphysis.

Central nervous system: Irritability, headache, and increased intracranial pressure as manifested by bulging fontanels, papilledema, and exophthalmos.

Dermatologic: Fissures of the lips, drying and cracking of the skin, alopecia, scaling, massive desquamation, and increased pigmentation.

Systemic: Hypomenorrhea, hepatosplenomegaly, jaundice, leukopenia, vitamin A plasma level over 1,200 IU/100 mL.

➤*Treatment:* The treatment of hypervitaminosis A consists of immediate withdrawal of the vitamin along with symptomatic and supportive treatment.

BETA-CAROTENE

otc sf	**Beta-Carotene** (Various, eg, Pharmavite, Tyson Nutraceuticals)	**Softgel capsule:** 15 mg (25,000 IU vitamin A)	In 60s and 100s.
otc	**Lumitene** (Tishcon Corp.)	**Capsule; oral:** 30 mg	Glucose. In 100s.

BETA-CAROTENE — ORAL

For additional information, refer to the Dietary Reference Intakes of Vitamins and Minerals table.

Indications

➤*Dietary supplement:* As a dietary supplement when vitamin A intake may be inadequate.

➤*Off-label uses:* Beta-carotene may also be used to treat or prevent a reaction to sun in patients with erythropoietic protoporphyria or polymorphous light eruption. Beta-carotene has a controversial role in lowering the incidence of cardiovascular disease and cancer, particularly lung cancer.

Administration and Dosage

➤*General dosing considerations:* In terms of vitamin A activity in supplements, 1 unit = beta-carotene 0.6 mcg or retinol 0.3 mcg.

In the past, the recommended daily allowance (RDA) for vitamin A was expressed in units. This term "units" has been replaced by retinol activity equivalents (RAE), where 1 RAE = retinol 1 mcg, beta-carotene (from supplements) 0.2 mcg, beta-carotene (from food) 12 mcg, alpha-carotene 24 mcg, or beta-cryptoxanthin 24 mcg.

➤*Adults:*

Dietary supplement – 1 capsule daily, preferably with a meal.

➤*Administration:* Take with a meal. Do not take with dairy products.

➤*Storage / Stability:* Store away from heat and direct light. Store in a cool, dry place. Do not freeze or refrigerate.

Actions

➤*Pharmacology:* Beta-carotene is a provitamin A carotenoid converted in the body to vitamin A (retinol), and is required for normal vision, gene expression, reproduction, embryonic development, immune function, and skin. A lack of vitamin A may cause a rare condition called night blindness, dry eyes, eye infections, skin problems, and slowed growth. Beta-carotene is also an immune system enhancer and antioxidant.

Beta-carotene is converted to retinol primarily in the intestinal mucosa.

Beta-carotene's antioxidant properties protect cell membranes from lipid preoxidation, alter the metabolism of carcinogens, and enhance immune function. By stimulating the release of natural killer cells, lymphocytes, and monocytes, beta-carotene helps the body resist precancerous changes. In contrast to vitamin A, beta-carotene exerts the greatest activity in the early, initiation phase of cancer.

➤*Pharmacokinetics:*

Absorption / Distribution – Bioavailability of beta-carotene depends on fat in the diet to act as a carrier and on bile in the intestinal tract for its absorption. Bioavailability is greatly decreased by steatorrhea, chronic diarrhea, and very low-fat diets. Approximately 50% of beta-carotene is converted to 2 molecules of retinol in the wall of the small intestine. Some retinal is further oxidized to retinoic acid. Once absorbed, carotenoids such as beta-carotene are transported via lymphatics to the liver where further conversion to vitamin A may occur.

Beta-carotene absorption is enhanced if taken with food.

Contraindications

Hypersensitivity to beta-carotene.

Warnings/Precautions

➤*Special risk:* Use beta-carotene cautiously in patients with eating disorders, kidney, or liver disease. These conditions may cause high blood levels of beta-carotene, which may increase the chance of side effects.

➤*Pregnancy: Category C.* Beta-carotene has not been studied in pregnant women.

Use only when clearly needed and when potential benefits outweigh potential hazards to the fetus. Beta-carotene use during pregnancy should not exceed 5000 IU of vitamin A.

➤*Lactation:* Avoid taking large amounts of a dietary supplement while breastfeeding. Beta-carotene has not been reported to cause problems in nursing babies.

It is not known whether this drug is excreted in breast milk. Exercise caution when administering to a nursing mother.

Adverse Reactions

➤*More common:* Yellowing of palms, hands, or soles of feet, and to a lesser extent the face (this may be a sign that the dose of beta-carotene as a nutritional supplement is too high).

➤*Rare:* Diarrhea; dizziness; joint pain; unusual bleeding or bruising.

Overdosage

➤*Symptoms:* Beta-carotene has been used at dosages of 180 mg/day or more without any adverse effects other than hypercarotenemia. Hypercarotenemia occurs when there is excessive unconverted carotene in the blood causing a yellow discoloration of the skin. Unrelated to jaundice because of the absence of scleral pigmentation, hypercarotenemia usually reverses upon discontinuation of the vitamin A source.

Patient Information

The presence of other medical problems may affect the use of beta-carotene. Tell your healthcare provider if you have any other medical problems, especially eating disorders, kidney disease, or liver disease. These conditions may cause high blood levels of beta-carotene, which may increase the chance for side effects.

Do not take with dairy products.

Skin may appear slightly yellow-orange while receiving beta-carotene therapy.

VITAMIN D

For additional information, refer to the Dietary Reference Intakes of Vitamins and Minerals table.

Indications

➤*Dietary supplement:*

Cholecalciferol – As a dietary supplement when vitamin D intake may be inadequate.

➤*Familial hypophosphatemia:*

Ergocalciferol – For the treatment of familial hypophosphatemia.

➤*Hypoparathyroidism:*

Calcitriol, ergocalciferol – For the treatment of hypoparathyroidism.

➤*Rickets:*

Ergocalciferol – For the treatment of refractory rickets, also known as vitamin D-resistant rickets.

➤*Secondary hyperparathyroidism (dialysis patients):*

Calcitriol, doxercalciferol – For the treatment of secondary hyperparathyroidism in patients with chronic kidney disease (CKD) on dialysis.

➤*Secondary hyperparathyroidism (predialysis patients):*

Calcitriol, doxercalciferol, paricalcitol – For the prevention and/or treatment of secondary hyperparathyroidism associated with CKD stage 3 and 4.

Administration and Dosage

Individualize dosage. The effectiveness of therapy is predicated on adequate daily intake of calcium either by calcium supplementation or proper dietary measures. Refer to the Recommended Dietary Allowances table for a complete listing.

Actions

➤*Pharmacology:* Vitamin D is a fat-soluble vitamin derived from natural sources (fish liver oils) or from conversion of provitamins (7-dehydrocholesterol and ergosterol). In humans, natural supplies of vitamin D depend on ultraviolet light for conversion of 7-dehydrocholesterol to vitamin D_3 or ergosterol to vitamin D_2. Following exposure to UV light, vitamin D_3 must then be converted to the active form of vitamin D (calcitriol) by the liver and kidneys. Vitamin D is hydroxylated by the hepatic microsomal enzymes to 25-hydroxyvitamin D_3 (25-]-D_3 or calcifediol). Calcifediol is hydroxylated primarily in the kidney to 1, 25-dihydroxy-vitamin D (1, 25-]$_2$-D_3 or calcitriol) and 24,25-dihydroxycholecalciferol (24,25-$(OH)_2D_3$). Doxercalciferol does not require activation by the kidneys. Calcitriol is believed to be the most active form of vitamin D_3 in stimulating intestinal calcium and phosphate transport.

One USP unit or one IU vitamin D activity is equal to 0.025 mcg vitamin D (1 mg = 40,000 units). "Vitamin D" refers to both ergocalciferol (D_2) and cholecalciferol (D_3). Vitamin D_2, essentially a plant vitamin, is used to fortify milk and cereals.

Dihydrotachysterol is a synthetic reduction product of tachysterol, a close isomer of vitamin D. Dihydrotachysterol is hydroxylated in liver to 25-hydroxydihydrotachy-sterol, the major circulating active form of the drug. It does not undergo further hydroxylation by kidney, and is the analog of 1,25-dihydroxy-vitamin D.

Paricalcitol is a synthetic vitamin D analog that reduces parathyroid hormone (PTH) levels. Paricalcitol suppresses PTH levels in patients with chronic renal failure (CRF) with no significant changes in the incidence of hypercalcemia or hyperphosphatemia when compared with placebo. However, the serum phosphorus, calcium, and calcium times phosphorus product (Ca x P) may increase when paricalcitol is administered.

Doxercalciferol is a synthetic vitamin D analog that undergoes metabolic activation in vivo to form 1α,25-dihydroxyvitamin D_2 (1α,25-$(OH)_2D_2$), a naturally occurring, biologically active form of vitamin D_2. Activation of doxercalciferol does not require involvement of the kidneys.

VITAMIN D

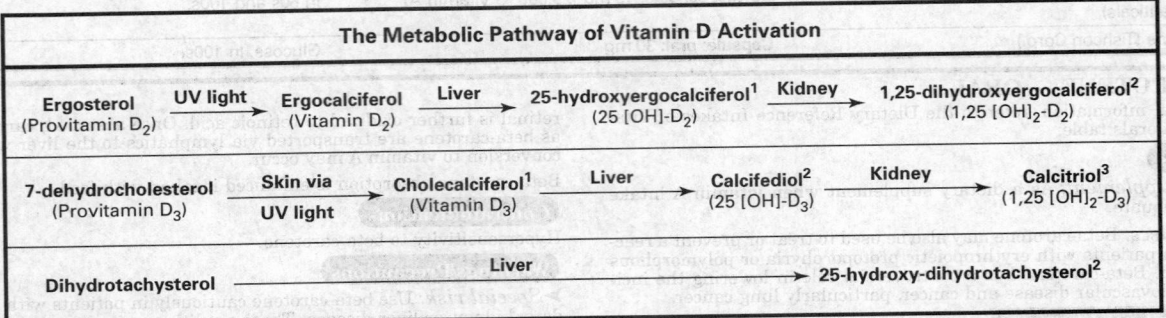

The Metabolic Pathway of Vitamin D Activation

Ergosterol (Provitamin D_2)	UV light →	Ergocalciferol (Vitamin D_2)	Liver →	25-hydroxyergocalciferol[1] (25 [OH]-D_2)	Kidney →	1,25-dihydroxyergocalciferol[2] (1,25 [OH]$_2$-D_2)
7-dehydrocholesterol (Provitamin D_3)	Skin via UV light →	Cholecalciferol[1] (Vitamin D_3)	Liver →	Calcifediol[2] (25 [OH]-D_3)	Kidney →	Calcitriol[3] (1,25 [OH]$_2$-D_3)
Dihydrotachysterol			Liver →			25-hydroxy-dihydrotachysterol[2]

[1] The kidney, in the absence of PTH, converts vitamin D_3 to 24,25$(OH)_2$-D_3, which is much less active than 1,25$(OH)_2$-D_3.
[2] Major transport form of vitamin D; minor intrinsic activity.
[3] Physiologically active forms.

Physiological function – Vitamin D is considered a hormone. Although not a natural human hormone, vitamin D_2 can substitute for D_3 in every metabolic step. Biologically active vitamin D metabolites control the intestinal absorption of dietary calcium, the tubular reabsorption of calcium by the kidney, and, in conjunction with parathyroid hormone (PTH), the mobilization of calcium from the skeleton. They act directly on bone cells (osteoblasts) to stimulate skeletal growth and on the parathyroid glands to suppress PTH synthesis and secretion. Vitamin D is also involved in magnesium metabolism.

Deficiency – Vitamin D deficiency leads to rickets in children and osteomalacia in adults. Vitamin D reverses symptoms of nutritional rickets.

➤*Pharmacokinetics:*

Absorption – Vitamin D is readily absorbed from the small intestine. Vitamin D_3 may be absorbed more rapidly and more completely than vitamin D_2. Bile is essential for adequate absorption. Absorption is reduced in liver or biliary disease. **Calcifediol**'s maximum concentration (C_{max}) is 4 hours following oral administration.

Distribution – Stored chiefly in the liver, vitamin D is also found in fat, muscle, skin, and bones. In plasma, it is bound to α globulins and albumin.

Metabolism – There is a 10- to 24-hour lag between administration of **ergocalciferol** and its onset of action. Maximal hypercalcemic effects occur ≈ 4 weeks after using a daily fixed dose; duration of action can be ≥ 2 months. Serum half-life of **calcifediol** is ≈ 16 days. Elimination half-life of **calcitriol**is 5 to 8 hours; pharmacologic activity persists for 3 to 5 days. **Dihydrotachysterol** has a rapid onset of effect and is less persistent after treatment cessation. **Paracalcitol** has a mean half-life of ≈ 15 hours. In healthy volunteers, peak blood levels of the major metabolite of **doxercalciferol**, 1α,25-$(OH)_2D_2$, has a mean half-life of ≈ 32 to 37 hours, with a range of up to 96 hours. Half-life in patients with end-stage renal disease on dialysis appear to be similar. The elimination half-life of **calcitriol** increased by at least twofold in chronic renal failure and hemodialysis patients compared with healthy subjects. Peak serum levels in patients with nephrotic syndrome were reached in 4 hours. For patients requiring hemodialysis, peak serum levels were reached in 8 to 12 hours; half-lives were estimated to be 16.2 and 21.9 hours, respectively.

Excretion – The primary route of vitamin D excretion is in the bile; only a small percentage is found in the urine.

Contraindications

Hypercalcemia; evidence of vitamin D toxicity; malabsorption syndrome; hypervitaminosis D; abnormal sensitivity to the effects of vitamin D; decreased renal function.

Warnings/Precautions

➤*Concomitant calcium administration:* Adequate dietary calcium is necessary for a clinical response to vitamin D therapy.

➤*Hypercalcemia:* Calcium phosphate may precipitate if the product of serum calcium multiplied by phosphate (Ca x P) exceeds 70. Progressive hypercalcemia due to overdosage of vitamin D and its metabolites may require emergency attention. Chronic hypercalcemia can lead to generalized vascular calcification, nephrocalcinosis and other soft tissue calcification. Radiographic or slit lamp evaluation of suspect anatomical regions may be useful for early detection.

In patients with normal renal function, chronic hypercalcemia may be associated with an increase in serum creatinine. While this is usually reversible, it is important to pay careful attention to factors that may lead to hypercalcemia.

A fall in serum alkaline phosphatase levels usually precedes hypercalcemia. Should hypercalcemia develop, discontinue the drug immediately. After achieving normocalcemia, readminister at a lower dosage.

➤*Bone lesions:* Adynamic bone lesions may develop if PTH levels are suppressed to abnormal levels (**calcitriol, paricalcitol**).

➤*Concomitant vitamin D intake:* Evaluate vitamin D ingested in fortified foods, dietary supplements, and other concomitantly administered drugs. It may be necessary to limit dietary vitamin D and its derivatives during treatment.

➤*Hypoparathyroidism:* May need calcium, parathyroid hormone, dihydrotachysterol.

➤*Hypersensitivity reactions:* Hypersensitivity to vitamin D may be one etiological factor in infants with idiopathic hypercalcemia. In these cases, severely restrict vitamin D intake.

➤*Tartrazine sensitivity:* Some of these products contain tartrazine, which may cause allergic-type reactions (including bronchial asthma) in susceptible individuals. Although the incidence of sensitivity is low, it is frequently seen in patients with aspirin hypersensitivity. Products containing tartrazine are identified in product listings.

➤*Renal function impairment:* The kidneys of uremic patients cannot adequately synthesize calcitriol, the active hormone formed from precursor vitamin D. Resultant hypocalcemia and secondary hyperparathyroidism are a major cause of the metabolic bone disease of renal failure.

The beneficial effect of calcitriol in renal osteodystrophy appears to result from correction of hypocalcemia and secondary hyperparathyroidism. It is uncertain whether calcitriol produces other independent beneficial effects. In patients with renal osteodystrophy accompanied by hyperphosphatemia, maintain a normal serum phosphorus level by dietary phosphate restriction or administration of aluminum gels to prevent metastatic calcification.

Because of the effect on serum calcium, administer to patients with renal stones only when potential benefits outweigh possible hazards.

➤*Special risk:* Use caution in patients, especially in the elderly with coronary disease, renal function impairment, and arteriosclerosis.

➤*Pregnancy: Category A* (*Category D* when used in doses that exceed the RDA) per Briggs' in *Pregnancy and Lactation*. Safety of vitamin D in amounts more than 400 IU/day is not established. Avoid doses greater than the RDA during a normal pregnancy. Animal studies have shown fetal abnormalities associated with hypervitaminosis D. Calcifediol and calcitriol are teratogenic in animals when given in doses several times the human dose. The offspring of a woman administered 17 to 36 mcg/day of calcitriol (17 to 36 times the recommended dose) during pregnancy manifested mild hypercalcemia in the first 2 days of life, which returned to normal at day 3. There are no adequate and well controlled studies in pregnant women; use during pregnancy only if the potential benefits outweigh the potential hazards to the fetus.

➤*Lactation:* Vitamin D is excreted in breast milk in limited amounts. In a mother given large doses of vitamin D, 25-hydroxycholecalciferol appeared in the milk and caused hypercalcemia in the child. Monitoring of the infant's serum calcium concentration was required. Do not nurse while taking **calcitriol**; otherwise, exercise caution when administering to a nursing mother.

➤*Children:* Safety and efficacy of vitamin D and its metabolites in children in doses exceeding the RDA and in children undergoing dialysis have not been established. Long-term *Rocaltrol* therapy is well-tolerated by pediatric patients not undergoing dialysis. Individualize pediatric doses and monitor under close medical supervision.

➤*Monitoring:* Dosage adjustment is required as soon as there is clinical improvement. Start therapy at the lowest possible dose, and do not increase without careful monitoring of the serum calcium. Estimate daily dietary calcium intake and adjust the intake when indicated. Patients with normal renal function taking calcitriol should avoid dehydration. Maintain adequate fluid intake. In vitamin D-resistant rickets, the range between therapeutic and toxic doses is narrow. When high therapeutic doses are used, follow progress with frequent serum and urinary calcium, phosphate, and blood urea nitrogen determinations.

Periodically monitor serum calcium, phosphate, magnesium, and alkaline phosphatase; monitor 24-hour urinary calcium and phosphate, especially in hypoparathyroid and dialysis patients. During the initial phase, determine serum calcium once or twice weekly. Maintain serum calcium levels between 9 and 10 mg/dL.

Paricalcitol – During the initial phase of therapy, frequently determine serum calcium and phosphate (eg, twice weekly). Once dosage has been established, measure serum calcium and phosphate at least monthly. Measurements of serum or plasma PTH are recommended every 3 months. An intact PTH (iPTH) assay is recommended for reliable detection of biologi-

VITAMIN D

cally active PTH. During dose adjustment of paricalcitol, laboratory tests may be required more frequently.

Drug Interactions

Vitamin D Drug Interactions

Precipitant drug	Object drug[a]		Description
Vitamin D	Antacids, magnesium-containing	↑	Hypermagnesemia may develop in patients on chronic renal dialysis.
Vitamin D	Digitalis glycosides	↑	Hypercalcemia in patients on digitalis may precipitate cardiac arrhythmias.
Vitamin D	Verapamil	↑	Atrial fibrillation has occurred when supplemental calcium and calciferol have induced hypercalcemia.
Cholestyramine	Vitamin D	↓	Intestinal absorption of vitamin D may be reduced.
Ketoconazole	Vitamin D	↓	Ketoconazole may inhibit both synthetic and catabolic enzymes of calcitriol. Reductions in serum endogenous calcitriol concentrations have been observed following the administration of 300 to 1200 mg/day ketoconazole for a week to healthy men.
Mineral oil	Vitamin D	↓	Absorption of vitamin D is reduced with prolonged use of mineral oil.
Phenytoin Phenobarbital	Vitamin D	↓	Endogenous synthesis of calcitriol will be inhibited. Higher doses of calcitriol may be necessary if these drugs are administered simultaneously.
Thiazide diuretics	Vitamin D	↑	Hypoparathyroid patients on vitamin D may develop hypercalcemia due to thiazide diuretics.

[a] ↑ = Object drug increased. ↓ = Object drug decreased.

Adverse Reactions

Early – Weakness; headache; somnolence; nausea; vomiting; dry mouth; constipation; muscle pain; bone pain; metallic taste.

Late – Polyuria; polydipsia; anorexia; irritability; weight loss; nocturia; mild acidosis; hypercalciuria; anemia; reversible azotemia, generalized vascular calcification, nephrocalcinosis; conjunctivitis (calcific); pancreatitis; photophobia; rhinorrhea; pruritus; hyperthermia; decreased libido; elevated BUN; albuminuria; hypercholesterolemia; elevated AST and ALT; ectopic calcification; hypertension; cardiac arrhythmias; overt psychosis (rare).

In clinical studies on hypoparathyroidism and pseudohypoparathyroidism, hypercalcemia was noted on at least one occasion in ≈ 1 in 3 patients and hypercalciuria in ≈ 1 in 7. Elevated serum creatinine levels were observed in ≈ 1 in 6 patients (approximately one half of whom had normal levels at baseline).

Occasional mild pain on injection has been observed (*Calcijex*).

Ergocalciferol – Hypercalciuria and mental retardation have been associated with ergocalciferol.

➤*Paricalcitol:*

Lab test abnormalities – **Paricalcitol** may reduce serum total alkaline phosphatase levels.

Miscellaneous – Discontinuation of therapy caused by any adverse event occurred in 6.5% of 62 patients treated with paricalcitol and 2% of 51 patients treated with placebo for 1 to 3 months.

Nausea (13%); vomiting (13%); edema (7%); chills, fever, flu, GI bleeding, lightheadedness, pneumonia, sepsis (5%); dry mouth, feeling unwell, palpitation (3%).

Overdosage

➤*Symptoms:* Administration of vitamin D to patients in excess of their daily requirements may cause hypercalcemia, hypercalciuria, and hyperphosphatemia. Concomitant high intake of calcium and phosphate may lead to similar abnormalities. **Dihydrotachysterol** may be toxic in doses as low as 25 mg/day, and is manifested by symptoms of hypercalcemia.

Hypercalcemia leads to anorexia, nausea, weakness, headache, somnolence, vomiting, dry mouth, metallic taste, weight loss, vague aches and stiffness, constipation, diarrhea, mental retardation, tinnitus, ataxia, hypotonia, depression, amnesia, disorientation, hallucinations, syncope, coma, anemia, and mild acidosis. Impairment of renal function may cause polyuria, nocturia, hypercalciuria, polydipsia, reversible azotemia, hypertension, nephrocalcinosis, generalized vascular calcification, irreversible renal insufficiency, or proteinuria. Widespread calcification of soft tissues, including heart, blood vessels, renal tubules, skin, and lungs may occur. Bone demineralization (osteoporosis) may occur in adults; decline in average linear growth rate and increased bone mineralization may occur in infants and children (dwarfism). Effects can persist ≥ 2 months after ergocalciferol treatment, 1 month after cessation of dihydrotachysterol therapy, 2 to 4 weeks for calcifediol and 2 to 7 days for calcitriol. Death may result from cardiovascular or renal failure. Obtain serum calcium levels at least weekly after all dosage changes and subsequent dosage titration. In patients receiving digitalis, obtain serial serum calcium determination, rate of urinary calcium excretion, and an assessment of ECG abnormalities due to hypercalcemia.

➤*Treatment:* Treatment of accidental overdose consists of general supportive measures. Refer to General Management of Acute Overdosage. If ingestion is discovered within a short time, emesis or gastric lavage may be beneficial. Mineral oil may promote fecal elimination.

Treatment of hypervitaminosis D with hypercalcemia consists of immediate withdrawal of vitamin D and calcium supplements, administration of a low-calcium diet, bed rest, administration of a laxative (mineral oil), attention to electrolyte imbalances, assessment of ECG abnormalities (critical in patients receiving digitalis), hemodialysis or peritoneal dialysis against a calcium-free dialysate, generous fluid intake, and urine acidification along with symptomatic and supportive treatment.

Hypercalcemic crisis with dehydration, stupor, coma, and azotemia requires more vigorous treatment. The first step is hydration; saline IV may quickly and significantly increase urinary calcium excretion. A loop diuretic (eg, furosemide) may be given with the saline infusion to further increase calcium excretion. Other measures include administration of citrates, sulfates, phosphates (do not administer with **paricalcitol**), corticosteroids, EDTA, possibly mithramycin and plicamycin. Persistent or markedly elevated serum calcium levels may be corrected by dialysis against a calcium-free dialysate. With appropriate therapy and when no permanent damage has occurred, recovery is probable.

Patient Information

Compliance with dosage instructions, diet, phosphate-binder use, and calcium supplementation is essential. Avoid use of nonprescription drugs, including magnesium-containing antacids, and natural products, unless such use has been discussed with a physician.

➤*Paricalcitol:* Instruct the patient that, to ensure effectiveness of paricalcitol therapy, it is important to adhere to a dietary regimen of calcium supplementation and phosphorus restriction. Appropriate types of phosphate-binding compounds may be needed; avoid excessive use of aluminum-containing compounds. Inform patients about the symptoms of elevated calcium.

Swallow whole; do not crush or chew.

Eating a balanced diet and periodic exposure to sunlight usually satisfies normal vitamin D requirements. Do not use vitamin supplements as a substitute for a balanced diet.

Notify physician if any of the following occurs: Weakness, lethargy, headache, anorexia, weight loss, nausea, vomiting, abdominal cramps, diarrhea, constipation, vertigo, excessive thirst, excessive urine output, dry mouth, or muscle or bone pain.

Avoid concurrent, prolonged use of mineral oil. If on chronic renal dialysis, avoid magnesium-containing antacids while taking these drugs. See Drug Interactions.

CALCITRIOL (1α,25 dihydroxycholecalciferol; 1,25 $[OH]_2D_3$)

Rx	**Calcitriol** (Teva)	**Capsules; oral:** 0.25 mcg	Mannitol, sorbitol. (93 and 657). Opaque red-brown and yellow-brown, oval. In 100s.
Rx	**Rocaltrol** (Validus)		Sorbitol, parabens. (Rocaltrol 0.25). Light orange. In 30s and 100s.
Rx	**Calcitriol** (Teva)	**Capsules; oral:** 0.5 mcg	Mannitol, sorbitol. (93 and 658). Opaque brown/pink. In 100s.
Rx	**Rocaltrol** (Validus)		Sorbitol, parabens. (Rocaltrol 0.5). Dark orange. In 100s.
Rx	**Calcitriol** (Roxane)	**Solution; oral:** 1 mcg/mL	In 15 mL with single-use graduated oral dispensers.
Rx	**Rocaltrol** (Validus)		In 15 mL bottle w/dispensers.
Rx	**Calcitriol** (aaiPharma)	**Injection:** 1 mcg/mL	Sodium chloride, EDTA. In 1 mL vials.
Rx	**Calcijex** (Abbott)		In 1 mL amps.[a]
Rx	**Calcitriol Injection** (aaiPharma)	**Injection:** 2 mcg/mL	Sodium chloride, EDTA. In 1 mL vials.

[a] With 4 mg polysorbate 20, 1.5 mg sodium chloride, 10 mg sodium ascorbate, 7.6 mg dibasic sodium phosphate, anhydrous, and EDTA.

CALCITRIOL — ORAL

For complete and comparative prescribing information, see the Vitamin D group monograph. For additional information, refer to the Dietary Reference Intakes of Vitamins and Minerals table.

Indications

➤*Predialysis patients:* Management of secondary hyperparathyroidism and resultant metabolic bone disease in patients with moderate to severe chronic renal failure (Ccr 15 to 55 mL/min) not yet on dialysis.

➤*Dialysis patients:* Management of hypocalcemia and the resultant metabolic bone disease in patients undergoing chronic renal dialysis.

➤*Hypoparathyroidism patients:* Management of hypocalcemia and its clinical manifestations in patients with postsurgical hypoparathyroidism, idiopathic hypoparathyroidism, and pseudohypoparathyroidism.

Administration and Dosage

➤*General dosing considerations:* The optimal daily dose of calcitriol must be carefully determined for each patient. Calcitriol therapy should always be started at the lowest possible dose and should not be increased without careful monitoring of serum calcium.

Oral calcitriol may normalize plasma ionized calcium in some uremic patients, yet fail to suppress parathyroid hyperfunction. In these individuals with autonomous parathyroid hyperfunction, oral calcitriol may be useful to maintain normocalcemia, but has not been shown to be adequate treatment for hyperparathyroidism.

Adjunct calcium therapy – The effectiveness of calcitriol therapy is predicated on the assumption that each patient is receiving an adequate but not excessive daily intake of calcium. Patients are advised to have a dietary intake of calcium at a minimum of 600 mg daily. The US RDA for calcium in adults is 800 to 1,200 mg. To ensure that each patient receives an adequate daily intake of calcium, a calcium supplement should either be prescribed or the patient should be instructed in proper dietary measures.

Because of improved calcium absorption from the GI tract, some patients on calcitriol may be maintained on a lower calcium intake. Patients who tend to develop hypercalcemia may require only low doses of calcium or no supplementation at all.

➤*Adults:*

Dialysis patients –

Initial dosage: 0.25 mcg/day.

Dosage titration: The dosage may be increased by 0.25 mcg/day at 4- to 8-week intervals if a satisfactory response in the biochemical parameters and clinical manifestations of the disease state are not observed. See Monitoring for additional recommendations.

Maintenance dosage: Patients with normal or only slightly reduced serum calcium levels may respond to calcitriol doses of 0.25 mcg every other day. Most patients undergoing hemodialysis respond to doses between 0.5 and 1 mcg/day.

Hypoparathyroidism – Malabsorption is occasionally noted in patients with hypoparathyroidism; hence, larger doses of calcitriol may be needed.

Initial dosage: 0.25 mcg/day given in the morning.

Dosage titration: The dose may be increased at 2- to 4-week intervals if a satisfactory response in the biochemical parameters and clinical manifestations of the disease are not observed. See Monitoring for additional recommendations.

Maintenance dosage: Most patients have responded to dosages of 0.5 to 2 mcg/day.

Predialysis patients –

Initial dosage: 0.25 mcg/day.

Dosage titration: The dosage may be increased if necessary to 0.5 mcg/day. See Monitoring for additional recommendations.

➤*Children:*

Hypoparathyroidism –

6 years of age and older: See Adults for dosing for children 6 years of age and older.

Predialysis patients –

3 years of age and older: See Adults for dosing for children 3 years of age and older.

Younger than 3 years of age: The initial dosage is 10 to 15 ng/kg/day. See Monitoring for additional recommendations.

➤*Elderly:* Dosing should be started cautiously, usually starting at the low end of the dosing range.

➤*Monitoring:* During the titration period of treatment with calcitriol, serum calcium levels should be checked at least twice weekly and, if hypercalcemia is noted, calcitriol should be immediately discontinued until normocalcemia ensues. When the optimal dosage of calcitriol has been determined, serum calcium levels should be checked every month (or as given below for individual indications). Samples for serum calcium estimation should be taken without a tourniquet.

Dialysis patients – Phosphorus, magnesium, and alkaline phosphatase should be determined periodically.

Hypoparathyroidism – Serum calcium, phosphorus, and 24-hour urinary calcium should be determined periodically.

Predialysis patients – Serum calcium, phosphorus, alkaline phosphatase, creatinine, and intact PTH (iPTH) should be determined initially. Thereafter, serum calcium, phosphorus, alkaline phosphatase, and creatine should be determined monthly for a 6-month period and then determined periodically. Intact PTH (iPTH) should be determined periodically every 3 to 4 months at the time of visits.

➤*Discontinuation of therapy:* Should hypercalcemia develop, the drug should be stopped immediately. During periods of hypercalcemia, serum calcium, and phosphate levels must be determined daily. When normal levels have been attained, treatment with calcitriol can be continued, at a daily dose 0.25 mcg lower than that previously used. An estimate of daily dietary calcium intake should be made and the intake adjusted when indicated.

➤*Storage/Stability:* Protect from light. Store at 25°C (77°F); excursions are permitted to 15° to 30°C (59° to 86°F).

CALCITRIOL — INJECTION

For complete and comparative prescribing information, see the Vitamin D group monograph. For additional information, refer to the Dietary Reference Intakes of Vitamins and Minerals table.

Indications

➤*Hypocalcemia:* Management of hypocalcemia in patients undergoing chronic renal dialysis. It has been shown to significantly reduce elevated parathyroid hormone (PTH) levels. Reduction of PTH has been shown to result in an improvement in renal osteodystrophy.

Administration and Dosage

➤*General dosing considerations:* The optimal dose of calcitriol injection must be carefully determined for each patient.

Adjunct calcium therapy – The effectiveness of calcitriol therapy is predicated on the assumption that each patient is receiving an adequate and appropriate daily intake of calcium. The recommended daily allowance (RDA) for calcium in adults is 800 mg. To ensure that each patient receives an adequate daily intake of calcium, the health care provider should either prescribe a calcium supplement or instruct the patient in proper dietary measures.

➤*Adults:*

Hypocalcemia –

Initial dosage: 1 mcg (0.02 mcg/kg) to 2 mcg administered 3 times weekly, approximately every other day. Doses as small as 0.5 mcg and as large as 4 mcg 3 times weekly have been used as an initial dose.

Dosage titration: If a satisfactory response is not observed, the initial dose may be increased by 0.5 to 1 mcg at 2- to 4-week intervals. During this titration period, serum calcium and phosphorus levels should be obtained at least twice weekly. If hypercalcemia or a serum calcium times phosphate product greater than 70 is noted, the drug should be immediately discontinued until these parameters are appropriate. Then, the calcitriol dose should be reinitiated at a lower dose. Doses may need to be reduced as the PTH levels decrease in response to the therapy. Thus, incremental dosing must be individualized and commensurate with PTH, serum calcium, and phosphorus levels. The following is a suggested approach in dose titration:

Calcitriol Injection Dose Titration

PTH levels	Calcitriol dose
The same or increasing	Increase
Decreasing by < 30%	Increase
Decreasing by > 30%, less than 60%	Maintain
Decreasing by > 60%	Decrease
1.5 to 3 times the upper limit of normal	Maintain

➤*Children:* The safety and effectiveness of calcitriol injection were examined in a 12-week randomized, double-blind, placebo-controlled study of 35 pediatric patients, 13 to 18 years of age, with end-stage renal disease on hemodialysis.

See Adults for dosing.

➤*Elderly:* Dose selection for an elderly patient should be made with caution, usually starting at the low end of the dosage range, reflecting the greater frequency of decreased hepatic, renal, or cardiac function, and of concomitant disease or other drug therapy.

➤*Monitoring:* Serum calcium, phosphorus, magnesium and alkaline phosphatase and 24-hour urinary calcium and phosphorus should be determined periodically. During the initial phase of the medication, serum calcium and phosphorus should be determined more frequently (twice weekly).

➤*Administration:* Intravenous.

➤*Storage/Stability:* Store at 15° to 30°C (59° to 86°F). Discard unused portion.

ERGOCALCIFEROL (D_2)

Ergocalciferol 1 mg provides 40,000 units of vitamin D activity.

otc	**Ergocalciferol Drops** (County Line Pharmaceuticals)	**Liquid; oral:** 8,000 units/mL	In 60 mL with dropper.[a]
otc	**Calciferol Drops** (Schwarz Pharma)		In 60 mL.[a]
otc	**Drisdol Drops** (Sanofi Pharm.)		In 60 mL.[a]
Rx	**Ergocalciferol** (Winthrop)	**Capsules; oral:** 50,000 units	Parabens, soybean oil. (E 50). Green, oval. In 50s.
Rx	**Vitamin D** (Pliva)		Soybean oil. (PA140). Green, oval. In 100s or 1,000s.
Rx	**Drisdol** (Sanofi Pharm.)		Tartrazine. (D92 W). In 50s.

[a] In propylene glycol.

ERGOCALCIFEROL — ORAL

For complete and comparative prescribing information, see the Vitamin D group monograph. For additional information, refer to the Dietary Reference Intakes of Vitamins and Minerals table.

Indications

➤*Hypoparathyroidism:* For the treatment of hypoparathyroidism.

➤*Rickets:* For the treatment of refractory rickets, also known as vitamin D-resistant rickets.

➤*Familial hypophosphatemia:* For the treatment of familial hypophosphatemia.

Administration and Dosage

➤*General dosing considerations:* The range between therapeutic and toxic doses is narrow. Dosage must be individualized under close medical supervision.

Ergocalciferol 1 mg provides 40,000 units of vitamin D activity.

Calcium intake should be adequate.

X-rays of the bones should be taken every month until condition is corrected and stabilized. Blood calcium and phosphorus determinations must be made every 2 weeks or more frequently if necessary.

➤*Adults:*

Hypoparathyroidism –

Usual dosage: 50,000 to 200,000 units daily.

Concomitant therapy: Calcium lactate 4 g 6 times per day.

Vitamin D-resistant rickets – 12,000 to 500,000 units daily.

➤*Storage/Stability:* Store at controlled room temperature between 15° and 30°C (59° to 86°F). Protect from light.

CHOLECALCIFEROL (D_3)

Cholecalciferol 1 mg provides 40,000 IU vitamin D activity.

otc sf	**Delta-D** (Freeda)	**Tablets; oral:** 400 units	In 250s and 500s.
otc sf	**Vitamin D_3** (Freeda)	**Tablets; oral:** 1,000 units	In 100s and 500s.
otc	**Maximum Strength D-2000** (21st Century)	**Tablets; oral:** 2,000 units	Gluten free. Calcium 180 mg. In 110s.
otc	**D-5000 Super Strength** (21st Century)	**Tablets; oral:** 5,000 units	Gluten free. Calcium 180 mg. In 110s.
otc	**D400** (Mason)	**Tablets, chewable; oral:** 400 units	Fructose, sucrose, sunflower oil, xylitol. Vanilla flavor. In 100s.
otc	**D3 Healthy Kids** (Mason)		Fructose, sucrose, sunflower oil. In 60s.
otc	**D1000** (Mason)	**Tablets, chewable; oral:** 1,000 units	Preservative free. Fructose, sucrose, sunflower oil, xylitol. Peach vanilla flavor. In 50s.
otc	**Ultra Strength D2000** (Mason Natural)	**Capsules; oral:** 2,000 units	In 60s.
otc	**D400** (Mason)	**Capsules, softgel; oral:** 400 units	Glycerin, soybean oil. In 100s.
otc	**High Potency D-1000** (Nature's Bounty)	**Capsules, softgel; oral:** 1,000 units	Glycerin, soybean oil. In 200s.
otc	**Advanced D5000** (Mason)	**Capsules, softgel; oral:** 5,000 units	Soybean oil. In 50s.
otc	**Maximum D3** (Pro-Pharma)	**Capsules; oral:** 10,000 units	In 5s.
otc sf	**D3–50** (Bio-Tech)	**Capsules; oral:** 50,000 units	Dye free, preservative free, sugar free, yeast free. In 100s.
otc sf	**Baby Ddrops** (J. R. Carlson Labs)	**Drops; oral:** 400 units per drop	Gluten free, preservative free, sugar free. In 11 mL.
otc sf	**Ddrops** (J. R. Carlson Labs)	**Drops; oral:** 1,000 units per drop	Gluten free, preservative free, sugar free. In 11 mL.
otc sf	**Ddrops** (J. R. Carlson Labs)	**Drops; oral:** 2,000 units per drop	Gluten free, preservative free, sugar free. In 11 mL.
otc	**Ultra Strength Vitamin D3** (Nature's Blend)	**Drops; oral:** 5,000 units per mL	Gluten free. Soybean oil, vitamin E. In 52.5 mL.
otc	**D^3 Spray** (Mason)	**Spray; oral:** 2,000 units	Vitamin E. Peppermint flavor. In 30 mL.

CHOLECALCIFEROL(D_3) — ORAL

For complete and comparative prescribing information, see the Vitamin D class monograph. For additional information, refer to the Dietary Reference Intakes of Vitamins and Minerals table.

Indications

➤*Dietary supplement:* As a dietary supplement when vitamin D intake may be inadequate.

Administration and Dosage

➤*General dosing considerations:* The US dietary reference intake is based on 1 mcg calciferol equaling 40 units vitamin D; cholecalciferol 1 mg provides 40,000 units of vitamin D activity.

➤*Adults:*

Dietary supplement –

Capsule/Tablet: 1 daily.

Drops: 1 drop (mL) daily.

Spray: 2 sprays under tongue.

Maximum D3: One capsule weekly.

➤*Children:* Safety and efficacy of vitamin D and its metabolites in children in doses exceeding the RDA and in children undergoing dialysis have not been established. Individualize pediatric doses and monitor under close medical supervision.

D3 Healthy Kids: Chew 1 tablet daily.

➤*Administration:* Swallow whole; do not crush or chew.

Shake spray well before use.

D3 Healthy Kids – Chew tablet before swallowing.

➤*Storage/Stability:* Store away from heat and direct light in a cool, dry place. Heat or moisture may cause the dietary supplement to break down.

PARICALCITOL

Rx	**Zemplar** (Abbott)	**Capsules:** 1 mcg	Alcohol, medium-chain triglycerides. (ZA). Gray, oval. In 30s.
		2 mcg	Alcohol, medium-chain triglycerides. (ZF). Orange-brown, oval. In 30s.
		4 mcg	Alcohol, medium-chain triglycerides. (ZK). Gold, oval. In 30s.
		Injection: 2 mcg/mL	In 1 mL single-dose *Fliptop* vials.
		5 mcg/mL	In 1 and 2 mL single-dose *Fliptop* vials.

PARICALCITOL — ORAL

For complete and comparative prescribing information, see the Vitamin D group monograph. For additional information, refer to the Dietary Reference Intakes of Vitamins and Minerals table.

Indications

➤*Hyperparathyroidism:* For the prevention and treatment of secondary hyperparathyroidism associated with chronic kidney disease (CKD) stage 3 and 4.

Administration and Dosage

➤*Adults:*

Hyperparathyroidism –

Initial dosage: The initial dose of paricalcitol is based on baseline intact parathyroid hormone (iPTH) levels.

Paricalcitol Oral Initial Dosage Recommendations

Baseline iPTH level	Daily dose	3 times weekly dosage[a]
≤ 500 pg/mL	1 mcg	2 mcg
more than 500 pg/mL	2 mcg	4 mcg

[a] To be administered not more often than every other day.

Dosage titration: Dosing must be individualized and based on serum or plasma iPTH levels, with monitoring of serum calcium and serum phosphorus. The following is a suggested titration approach.

Paricalcitol Oral Dosage Titration Recommendations

iPTH level relative to baseline	Paricalcitol dose	Dosage adjustment at 2- to 4-week intervals	
		Daily dosage	3 times weekly dosage[a]
The same or increased	Increase	1 mcg	2 mcg
Decreased less than 30%			
Decreased 30% to 60%	Maintain		
Decreased more than 60%	Decrease	1 mcg	2 mcg
iPTH less than 60 pg/mL			

[a] To be administered not more often than every other day.

If a patient is taking the lowest dose on the daily regimen and a dosage reduction is needed, the dosage can be decreased to 1 mcg 3 times a week. If a further dosage reduction is required, the drug should be withheld as needed and can be restarted at a lower dose.

If hypercalcemia or an elevated calcium-phosphorus product (Ca × P) is observed, the dose of paricalcitol should be reduced or interrupted until these parameters are normalized.

Concomitant therapy: If a patient is on a calcium-based phosphate binder, the binder dose may be decreased or withheld, or the patient may be switched to a non–calcium-based phosphate binder.

➤*Administration:* Paricalcitol may be administered daily or 3 times a week. When dosing 3 times weekly, the dose should be administered no more frequently than every other day. The average weekly doses for daily and 3 times weekly dosage regimens are similar.

Paricalcitol may be taken without regard to food.

➤*Storage/Stability:* Store at 25°C (77°F). Excursions permitted between 15° and 30°C (59° and 86°F).

PARICALCITOL — INJECTION

For complete and comparative prescribing information, see the Vitamin D group monograph. For additional information, refer to the Dietary Reference Intakes of Vitamins and Minerals table.

Indications

➤*Hyperparathyroidism:* For the prevention and treatment of secondary hyperparathyroidism associated with stage 5 chronic kidney disease.

Administration and Dosage

➤*General dosing considerations:* The currently accepted target range for intact parathyroid hormone (iPTH) levels in stage 5 chronic kidney disease patients is no more than 1.5 to 3 times the nonuremic upper limit of normal (ULN).

➤*Adults:*

Hyperparathyroidism –

Initial dosage: 0.04 to 0.1 mcg/kg (2.8 to 7 mcg) administered as an IV bolus dose no more frequently than every other day at any time during dialysis.

Dosage titration: If a satisfactory response is not observed, the dose may be increased by 2 to 4 mcg at 2- to 4-week intervals. During any dose-adjustment period, serum calcium and phosphorus levels should be monitored more frequently, and if an elevated calcium level or a calcium-phosphorous (Ca × P) product greater than 75 is noted, the drug dosage should be immediately reduced or interrupted until these parameters are normalized. Then, paricalcitol should be reinitiated at a lower dose. If a patient is on a calcium-based phosphate binder, the dose may be decreased or withheld, or the patient may be switched to a noncalcium-based phosphate binder. Doses may need to be decreased as the parathyroid hormone (PTH) levels decrease in response to therapy. Thus, incremental dosing must be individualized. The following is a suggested approach in dose titration:

Paricalcitol Injection Dosage Titration Recommendations

PTH level	Paricalcitol injection dose
The same or increasing	Increase
Decreasing by < 30%	Increase
Decreasing by > 30%, < 60%	Maintain
Decreasing by > 60%	Decrease
1.5 to 3 × the ULN	Maintain

➤*Administration:* Administer as an IV bolus.

➤*Storage/Stability:* Store at 25°C (77°F). Excursions are permitted to 15° to 30°C (59° to 86°F). After initial vial use, the contents of the multi-dose vial remain stable up to 7 days when stored at controlled room temperature. Discard unused portion.

DOXERCALCIFEROL

Rx	**Hectorol** (Genzyme)	**Capsules, softgel; oral:** 0.5 mcg	(g). Orange, oval. In 50s.
		1 mcg	Ethanol. (g). Peach, oval. In 50s.
		2.5 mcg	Ethanol. (g). Yellow, oval. In 50s.
		Injection, solution: 2 mcg/mL	100% ethanol 0.05 mL, disodium edetate 1.1. mg, sodium chloride 1.5 mg, sodium phosphate dibasic, sodium phosphate monobasic. In 2 mL amps.

DOXERCALCIFEROL — ORAL

For complete and comparative prescribing information, see the Vitamin D group monograph. For additional information, refer to the Dietary Reference Intakes of Vitamins and Minerals table.

Indications

➤*Secondary hyperparathyroidism (dialysis patients):* For the treatment of secondary hyperparathyroidism in patients with chronic kidney disease on dialysis.

➤*Secondary hyperparathyroidism (predialysis patients):* For the treatment of secondary hyperparathyroidism in patients with stage 3 or 4 chronic kidney disease.

Administration and Dosage

➤*General dosing considerations:* The optimal dose of doxercalciferol must be carefully determined for each patient. (See also Monitoring).

➤*Adults:*

Secondary hyperparathyroidism (dialysis patients) –

Maximum dose: 60 mcg/week (20 mcg administered 3 times a week at dialysis).

Initial dosage: 10 mcg administered 3 times weekly at dialysis (approximately every other day).

Dosage titration: The initial dose should be adjusted, as needed, in order to lower blood iPTH into the range of 150 to 300 pg/mL (see the following table). The dose may be increased at 8-week intervals by 2.5 mcg if iPTH is not lowered by 50% and fails to reach the target range. During titration, iPTH, serum calcium, and serum phosphorus levels should be obtained weekly. (Also see Monitoring).

Drug administration should be suspended if iPTH falls below 100 pg/mL and restarted 1 week later at a dose that is at least 2.5 mcg lower than the last administered dose. If hypercalcemia, hyperphosphatemia, or a serum calcium times serum phosphorus product greater than 55 mg^2/dL^2 is noted, the dose of doxercalciferol should be decreased or suspended and/or the dose of phosphate binders should be adjusted appropriately. If suspended, the drug should be restarted at a dose that is at least 2.5 mcg lower.

Dosing must be individualized and based on iPTH levels with monitoring of serum calcium and serum phosphorus levels. The following is a suggested approach in dose titration:

Initial Doxercalciferol Oral Dosing in Dialysis Patients

iPTH level	Doxercalciferol dosage
> 400 pg/mL	10 mcg 3 times per week at dialysis
	Dose titration
Above 300 pg/mL	Increase by 2.5 mcg at 8-week intervals as necessary
150 to 300 pg/mL	Maintain
< 100 pg/mL	Suspend for 1 week, then resume at a dose that is at least 2.5 mcg lower

Secondary hyperparathyroidism (predialysis patients) –

Maximum dose: 3.5 mcg once daily.

Initial dosage: 1 mcg once daily.

Dosage titration: The initial dose should be adjusted, as needed, in order to lower blood iPTH to within target ranges (see the following table). The dose may be increased at 2-week intervals by 0.5 mcg to achieve the target range of iPTH. (Also see Monitoring).

If hypercalcemia, hyperphosphatemia, or a serum calcium times phosphorus product greater than 55 mg^2/dL^2 is noted, the dose of doxercalciferol should be decreased or suspended and/or the dose of phosphate binders should be appropriately adjusted. If suspended, the drug should be restarted at a dose that is at least 0.5 mcg lower.

Dosing must be individualized and based on iPTH levels with monitoring of serum calcium and serum phosphorous levels. The following table provides a suggested approach to dose titration.

Initial Doxercalciferol Oral Dosing in Predialysis Patients

iPTH level	Doxercalciferol dose
> 70 pg/mL (stage 3) > 110 pg/mL (stage 4)	1 mcg once per day
Dose titration	
Above 70 pg/mL (stage 3) Above 110 pg/mL (stage 4)	Increase by 0.5 mcg at 2-week intervals as necessary
35 to 70 pg/mL (stage 3) 70 to 110 pg/mL (stage 4)	Maintain
< 35 pg/mL (stage 3) < 70 pg/mL (stage 4)	Suspend for 1 week, then resume at a dose that is at least 0.5 mcg lower

➤*Hepatic function impairment:* Use with caution.

➤*Therapeutic drug monitoring:* During titration, iPTH, serum calcium, and serum phosphorus levels should be obtained weekly. The following table provides the current recommended therapeutic target levels for iPTH in patients with chronic kidney disease.

Target Range of iPTH by Stage of Chronic Kidney Disease

Chronic kidney disease stage	Glomerular filtration rate (mL/min/1.73 m^2)	Target iPTH (pg/mL)
3	30 to 59	35 to 70
4	15 to 29	70 to 110
5	< 15 (or dialysis)	150 to 300

➤*Storage/Stability:* Store at 20° to 25°C (68° to 77°F).

DOXERCALCIFEROL — INJECTION

For complete and comparative prescribing information, see the Vitamin D group monograph. For additional information, refer to the Dietary Reference Intakes of Vitamins and Minerals table.

Indications

➤*Secondary hyperparathyroidism:* For the treatment of secondary hyperparathyroidism in adult patients with chronic kidney disease on dialysis.

Administration and Dosage

➤*General dosing considerations:* The optimal dose must be carefully determined for each patient.

➤*Adults:*

Secondary Hyperparathyroidism –

Initial dosage: 4 mcg administered as an IV bolus dose 3 times weekly at the end of dialysis (approximately every other day).

Dosage titration: The initial dose should be adjusted, as needed, in order to lower blood intact parathyroid hormone (iPTH) into the range of 150 to 300 pg/mL. The dose may be increased at 8-week intervals by 1 to 2 mcg if iPTH is not lowered by 50% and fails to reach the target range. Dosages higher than 18 mcg weekly have not been studied. During titration, iPTH, serum calcium, and serum phosphorus levels should be obtained weekly.

Drug administration should be suspended if iPTH falls below 100 pg/mL and restarted 1 week later at a dose that is at least 1 mcg lower than the last administered dose. If hypercalcemia, hyperphosphatemia, or a serum calcium times phosphorus product of greater than 55 mg^2/dL^2 is noted, doxercalciferol should be decreased or suspended and/or the dose of phosphate binders should be appropriately adjusted. If suspended, the drug should be restarted at a dose that is 1 mcg lower.

Dosing must be individualized and based on iPTH levels with monitoring of serum calcium and serum phosphorus levels. The following is a suggested approach for dose titration:

Initial Doxercalciferol Injection Dosing

iPTH level	Doxercalciferol dosage
> 400 pg/mL	4 mcg 3 times/week at the end of dialysis, or approximately every other day
	Dose titration
iPTH level	**Doxercalciferol dose**
Decreased by < 50% and above 300 pg/mL	Increase by 1 to 2 mcg at 8-week intervals as necessary
Decreased by > 50% and above 300 pg/mL	Maintain
150 to 300 pg/mL	Maintain
< 100 pg/mL	Suspend for 1 week, then resume at a dose that is at least 1 mcg lower

➤*Hepatic function impairment:* Use with caution.

➤*Therapeutic drug monitoring:* During titration, iPTH, serum calcium, and serum phosphorus levels should be obtained weekly.

➤*Administration:* Administer as an IV bolus.

➤*Storage/Stability:* Store at 15° to 25°C (59° to 77°F). Protect from light. Discard unused portion.

VITAMIN E

otc	**Vitamin E** (Various, eg, Freeda)	**Tablets; oral:** 100 units[a]	In 100s and 250s.
		200 units[a]	In 100s, 250s, and 500s.
		400 units[a]	In 100s, 250s, and 500s.
		500 units[a]	In 100s and 250s.
		800 units[a]	In 100s.
otc	**Vitamin E with Mixed Tocopherols** (Freeda)	**Tablets; oral:** 100 units[b]	In 100s and 250s.
		200 units[b]	In 100s and 250s.
		400 units[b]	In 100s, 250s, and 500s.
otc	**Vitamin E** (Various, eg, Apothecary, Goldline, Nature's Bounty)	**Capsules; oral:** 100 units[b]	In 100s.
		200 units[b]	In 100s.
		400 units[b]	In 100s and 250s.
		1000 units[b]	In 50s and 100s.
otc	**Mixed E 400 Softgels** (Naturally)	**Capsules; oral:** 400 units[b]	In 60s, 90s, and 180s.
otc sf	**Vita-Plus E** (Scot-Tussin)	**Capsules; oral:** 400 units[c]	In 50s.
otc	**d' ALPHA E 1000 Softgels** (Naturally)	**Capsules; oral:** 1000 units[a]	In 30s and 60s.
otc	**Mixed E 1000 Softgels** (Naturally)	**Capsules; oral:** 1000 units[b]	In 30s and 60s.
otc sf	**Natural E 200** (Mason)	**Capsules, softgels; oral:** 200 units	Preservative free, sugar free. In 100s.
otc	**Aquasol E** (Hospira)	**Drops; oral:** 15 units[d] per 0.3 mL	In 12 and 30 mL.
otc	**Aquavit-E** (Cypress)	**Drops; oral:** 15 units[d] per 0.3 mL	In 30 mL.
otc	**Vitamin E** (Freeda)	**Liquid; oral:** 15 units[b] per 30 mL	In 30, 60, and 120 mL.
otc sf	**Aqua-E** (Yasoo[e])	**Liquid; oral:** 30 units[f] per 1 mL	Gluten free, sugar free. PEG 1000. In 120 and 237 mL.
otc sf	**Nutr-E-Sol** (Advanced Nutritional Technology)	**Liquid; oral:** 798 units[b] per 30 mL	Dye free. In 473 mL.
otc sf	**Natural Vitamin E** (Freeda Vitamins)	**Liquid; oral:** 1,150 units[a] per 1.25 mL	Gluten free, lactose free, sugar free. In 114 mL.
otc	**E-Oil** (Nature's Bounty)	**Solution, concentrate; oral:** 100 units[c] per 0.25 mL	Corn oil, lemon oil, sesame oil, soybean oil, wheat germ oil. In 74 mL.

[a] As d-alpha tocopherol.
[b] Form of vitamin E unknown; content given in IU.
[c] As d-alpha tocopheryl acetate.
[d] As dl-alpha tocopheryl acetate.
[e] Yasoo Health, P.O. Box 3608, Johnson City, TN 37602; 1-888-469-2766; http://www.yasoo.com
[f] As d-alpha tocopherol, other tocopherols, and tocotrienols.

VITAMIN E — ORAL

For additional information, refer to the Dietary Reference Intakes of Vitamins and Minerals table.

Indications

➤*Dietary supplement:* As a dietary supplement when vitamin E intake may be inadequate.

➤*Off-label uses:*

Postherpetic neuralgia – [5] = Poor documentation. Use of vitamin E for treatment of postherpetic neuralgia (PHN) has only been studied in case series that showed inconsistent results. American Academy of Neurology clinical practice guidelines state that vitamin E is of no benefit in patients with PHN (level B, class II).

Other possible off-label uses – Vitamin E has been used in certain premature infants to reduce the toxic effects of oxygen therapy on the lung parenchyma (bronchopulmonary dysplasia) and the retina (retrolental fibroplasia). It has been investigated for the prevention of periventricular hemorrhage in premature infants.

It has also been used in cancer, skin conditions, sexual dysfunction, to reduce the incidence of non-fatal MI, to lower the incidence of coronary artery disease, aging, fibrocystic breast disease (cystic mastitis), to treat dapsone-associated hemolysis, arthritis, and tardive dyskinesia. Use of vitamin E in combination with vitamin A has been reported in the treatment of keratosis follicularis (Darier's disease), pityriasis rubra pilaris, ichthyosis, and acne. Use of vitamin E (400 IU) in combination with vitamin C (1 g/day) has resulted in significant risk reduction for preeclampsia during the second half of pregnancy.

Administration and Dosage

➤*General dosing considerations:* Vitamin E, also known as alpha-tocopherol, comes in different forms: RRR-alpha-tocopherol, the only form of alpha-tocopherol that occurs naturally in foods and the 2R-stereoisomeric forms of alpha-tocopherol (RRR-, RSR- RRS-, and RSS-alpha-tocopherol) that occur in fortified foods and supplements. Other commercially available forms include d- or dl-alpha tocopheryl acetate, d- or dl-alpha tocopherol, and d- or dl-alpha tocopheryl acid succinate.

In the past, the recommended daily allowance (RDA) for vitamin E had been expressed in units. The term units had been replaced by alpha tocopherol equivalents (alpha-TE) or milligrams (mg) of d-alpha tocopherol. One unit is equivalent to 1 mg of dl-alpha tocopherol acetate or 0.6 mg d-alpha tocopherol. Most products available in stores continue to be labeled in units. 1 mg alpha-tocopherol equivalents equals 1.5 units.

The RDA for vitamin E is based on the alpha-tocopherol form because it is the most active, or usable, form. Unlike other vitamins, the form of alpha-tocopherol made in the laboratory and found in supplements is not identical to the natural form, and is not quite as active as the natural form.

➤*Adults:*

Dietary supplement –

Tablets/capsules: Varies by product. Dosages range from 100 to 1,000 mg/day.

Drops (15 units/0.3 mL): 30 units (0.6 mL) daily.

Drops (100 units/0.25 mL): 100 units (5 drops or 0.25 mL) daily.

Off-label dosing –

➤*Children:*

Dietary supplement –

Drops (15 units/0.3 mL):

- *4 years and older* – 30 units (0.6 mL) daily.
- *1 to 3 years of age* – 10 units (0.2 mL) daily.
- *Younger than 1 year* – 5 units (0.1 mL) daily.

➤*Administration:* Swallow capsules whole; do not crush or chew. May take with a meal.

Drops may be mixed with any liquid of semi-liquid food (eg, milk, formulas, fruit juices, cereal, soups, desserts).

➤*Storage/Stability:* Store away from heat and direct light. Keep the oral liquid from freezing.

Actions

➤*Pharmacology:* Vitamin E is a fat-soluble vitamin with actions related to its antioxidant properties. Vitamin E protects cellular constituents from oxidation and prevents the formation of toxic oxidation products; it preserves red blood cell (RBC) wall integrity and protects RBCs against hemolysis; it stimulates a cofactor in steroid metabolism; inhibits prostaglandin production; and suppresses platelet aggregation. In combination with selenium, vitamin E protects cell membranes from oxidative damage.

There are 8 naturally occurring compounds with vitamin E activity; 4 are tocopherols and 4 are tocotrienols. Free d-alpha tocopherol is the most biologically active form of vitamin E. One IU of vitamin E activity is equivalent to 1 mg all- rac-alpha-tocopheryl acetate. Normal plasma levels of vitamin E are between 1 and 3 mg/dL in low-birth-weight infants. Infants receiving either oral or parenteral vitamin E should maintain serum vitamin levels less than 3.5 mg/dL. Sources of vitamin E include vegetables, oils, seeds, corn, soy, whole wheat flour, margarine, nuts, leafy vegetables, milk, eggs, and meats.

VITAMIN E — ORAL

Deficiency – Clinical deficiency of vitamin E is rare because adequate amounts are supplied in the normal diet. Symptoms of deficiency include ataxia, muscle weakness, nystagmus, and losses in touch and pain sensations. Low tocopherol levels have been noted in the following: Premature infants; malnourished infants with macrocyticanemia; prolonged fat malabsorption (ie, cystic fibrosis, hepatic cirrhosis, sprue); malabsorption syndromes (ie, celiac disease, GI resections); patients with abetalipoproteinemia. Vitamin E deficiency in premature infants may result in hemolytic anemia, thrombocytosis, and increased platelet aggregation. Vitamin E levels less than 0.5 mg/dL are suggestive of a deficiency.

Vitamin E requirements – The daily vitamin E requirement is related to the dietary intake of polyunsaturated fatty acids (PUFA), primarily linoleic acid. Vitamin E requirements may be increased in patients taking large doses of iron. Commercial infant formulas currently available provide an adequate ratio of vitamin E to PUFA; formulas for premature infants have a lower level of iron to preclude interference with vitamin E use. Thus, there is no longer a need to routinely administer vitamin E supplementation to prevent anemia.

➤*Pharmacokinetics:*

Absorption/Distribution – Vitamin E is 20% to 50% absorbed by intestinal epithelial cells in the small intestine. Bile and pancreatic juice are needed for tocopherol absorption. Absorption is increased when administered with medium-chain triglycerides. Distribution to tissues via the lymphatic system occurs as a lipoprotein complex. High concentrations of vitamin E are found in the adrenals, pituitary, testes, and thrombocytes.

Metabolism/Excretion – Vitamin E is stored unmodified in tissues (principally the liver and adipose tissue) and excreted via the feces. Excess vitamin E is converted to a lactone, esterified to glucuronic acid, and subsequently excreted in the urine.

Warnings/Precautions

➤*Pregnancy: Category A; Category C* if used in doses above the RDA(per Briggs' *Drugs in Pregnancy and Lactation.*) See Administration and Dosage for more information.

Refer to the Dietary Reference intakes of vitamins and minerals table.

➤*Lactation:* See Administration and Dosage for more information.

Refer to the Dietary Reference intakes of vitamins and minerals table.

➤*Children:* Vitamin E supplements may be recommended for premature infants with low levels of vitamin E.

See Overdosage for more information.

Drug Interactions

Vitamin E Drug Interactions

Precipitant drug	Object drug[a]		Description
Vitamin E	Anticoagulants, oral warfarin	↑	Vitamin E in high doses (greater than 4000 IU) may increase the hypoprothrombinemic effects of oral anticoagulants.
Vitamin E	Iron	↓	Vitamin E may impair the hematologic response to iron therapy in children with iron-deficiency anemia.

[a] ↑ = Object drug increased; ↓ = Object drug decreased.

Adverse Reactions

➤*Hypervitaminosis:* See Overdosage for more information.

Overdosage

➤*Symptoms:* Doses less than 2,000 IU are not likely to cause side effects. However, large doses (greater than 3,000 IU) have been noted to produce symptoms of hypervitaminosis E, which include nausea, weakness, intestinal cramps, headache, flatulence, diarrhea, thrombophlebitis, pulmonary embolism, severe fatigue syndrome, gynecomastia, breast tumors, increased cholesterol and triglycerides, decrease in serum thyroid hormone, and altered immunity.

Infants – Sepsis and necrotizing enterocolitis have been reported when vitamin E levels are maintained at 5 mg/dL in low-birth-weight infants.

Patient Information

Swallow capsules whole; do not crush or chew.

PHYTONADIONE (VITAMIN K)

otc	**Vitamin K** (Nature's Blend)	**Tablets; oral:** 0.1 mg	Gluten free, preservative free. In 100s.
Rx	**Mephyton** (Aton)	**Tablets; oral:** 5 mg	Lactose. (MSD 43 Mephyton). Yellow, scored. In 100s.
Rx	**Phytonadione** (Hospira)	**Injection, emulsion:** 2 mg per mL	Dextrose, 9 mg benzyl alcohol. In 0.5 mL ampul.
		10 mg/mL	Dextrose, 9 mg benzyl alcohol. In 1 mL ampul.

PHYTONADIONE (VITAMIN K) — ORAL

For additional information, refer to the Dietary Reference Intakes of Vitamins and Minerals table.

Indications

➤*Anticoagulant-induced prothrombin deficiency:* Anticoagulant-induced prothrombin deficiency caused by coumarin or indandione derivatives.

➤*Coagulation disorders:* Phytonadione is indicated in the following coagulation disorders which are due to faulty formation of factors II, VII, IX and X when caused by vitamin K deficiency or interference with vitamin K activity.

➤*Dietary Supplement:* As a dietary supplement.

➤*Hypoprothrombinemia:* Hypoprothrombinemia secondary to antibacterial therapy; hypoprothrombinemia secondary to administration of salicylates; hypoprothrombinemia secondary to obstructive jaundice or biliary fistulas but only if bile salts are administered concurrently, since otherwise the oral vitamin K will not be absorbed.

Administration and Dosage

➤*Adults:*

Anticoagulant-induced prothrombin deficiency – 2.5 to 10 mg or up to 25 mg (rarely 50 mg). May repeat in 12 to 48 hours.

Dietary Supplement – 0.1 mg daily.

Hypoprothrombinemia – 2.5 to 25 mg or more (rarely up to 50 mg).

➤*Children:*

Off-label dosing –

Anticoagulant (oral) overdosage: For major bleeding, the dosage is 5 mg, which may be repeated in 12 to 48 hours. If the INR is more than 8 but there is no bleeding or minor bleeding, then the dosage is 0.5 to 2.5 mg, which may be repeated in 12 to 48 hours.

Vitamin K deficiency: 2.5 to 5 mg/day.

➤*Administration:* The oral route should be avoided when the clinical disorder would prevent proper absorption. Bile salts must be given with the tablets when the endogenous supply of bile to the gastrointestinal tract is deficient.

➤*Storage/Stability:* Store at 25°C (77°F); excursions permitted to 15° to 30°C (59° to 86°F). Protect from light. Store container in carton until contents have been used.

Actions

➤*Pharmacology:* Phytonadione tablets possess the same type and degree of activity as does naturally-occurring vitamin K, which is necessary for the production via the liver of active prothrombin (factor II), proconvertin (factor VII), plasma thromboplastin component (factor IX), and Stuart factor (factor X). The prothrombin test is sensitive to the levels of three of these four factors (factors II, VII, and X). Vitamin K is an essential cofactor for a microsomal enzyme that catalyzes the post-translational carboxylation of multiple, specific, peptide-bound glutamic acid residues in inactive hepatic precursors of factors II, VII, IX, and X. The resulting gamma-carboxyglutamic acid residues convert the precursors into active coagulation factors that are subsequently secreted by liver cells into the blood.

In healthy animals and humans, phytonadione is virtually devoid of pharmacodynamic activity. However, in animals and humans deficient in vitamin K, the pharmacological action of vitamin K is related to its normal physiological function; that is, to promote the hepatic biosynthesis of vitamin K-dependent clotting factors.

➤*Pharmacokinetics:* Phytonadione is only absorbed from the GI tract via intestinal lymphatics in the presence of bile salts. Although initially concentrated in the liver, vitamin K is rapidly metabolized and very little tissue accumulation occurs. Little is known about the metabolic fate of vitamin K. Almost no free unmetabolized vitamin K appears in bile or urine.

Phytonadione tablets generally exert their effect within 6 to 10 hours.

Contraindications

Hypersensitivity to any component of this medication.

Warnings/Precautions

➤*Oral anticoagulant — induced hypoprothrombinemia:* An immediate coagulant effect should not be expected after administration of phytonadione. Phytonadione will not counteract the anticoagulant action of heparin.

When vitamin K_1 is used to correct excessive anticoagulant-induced hypoprothrombinemia, anticoagulant therapy still being indicated, the patient is again faced with the clotting hazards existing prior to starting the anticoagulant therapy. Phytonadione is not a clotting agent, but overzealous therapy with vitamin K_1 may restore conditions which originally permitted thromboembolic phenomena. Dosage should be kept as low as possible, and prothrombin time should be checked regularly as clinical conditions indicate.

➤*Hepatic function impairment:* Repeated large doses of vitamin K are not warranted in liver disease if the response to initial use of the vitamin is

PHYTONADIONE (VITAMIN K) — ORAL

unsatisfactory. Failure to respond to vitamin K may indicate a congenital coagulation defect or that the condition being treated is unresponsive to vitamin K.

➤*Pregnancy: Category C.* Animal reproduction studies have not been conducted with phytonadione. It is also not known whether phytonadione can cause fetal harm when administered to a pregnant woman or can affect reproduction capacity. Phytonadione should be given to a pregnant woman only if clearly needed.

➤*Lactation:* It is not known whether this drug is excreted in human milk. Because many drugs are excreted in human milk, caution should be exercised when phytonadione is administered to a nursing woman.

➤*Children:* Safety and effectiveness in pediatric patients have not been established with phytonadione. Hemolysis, jaundice, and hyperbilirubinemia in newborns, particularly in premature infants, have been reported with vitamin K.

➤*Monitoring:* Prothrombin time should be checked regularly as clinical conditions indicate.

Drug Interactions

Vitamin K Drug Interactions

Precipitant drug	Object drug[a]		Description
Vitamin K	Anticoagulants	⬇	Anticoagulant effects are antagonized by vitamin K. Temporary resistance to oral anticoagulants may result. It may be necessary to increase the anticoagulant dose.
Mineral oil	Vitamin K	⬇	Mineral oil may decrease GI absorption of vitamin K with concurrent oral administration.

[a] ⬇ = object drug decreased.

Adverse Reactions

➤*Hyperbilirubinemia:* Hyperbilirubinemia has been observed in the newborn following administration of parenteral phytonadione. This has occurred rarely and primarily with doses above those recommended.

Overdosage

The intravenous and oral LD_{50}s in the mouse are approximately 1.17 g/kg and greater than 24.18 g/kg, respectively.

PHYTONADIONE — INJECTION

For additional information, refer to the Dietary Reference Intakes of Vitamins and Minerals table.

WARNING

IV or IM use – Severe reactions, including fatalities, have occurred during and immediately after intravenous (IV) injection of phytonadione, even when precautions have been taken to dilute the phytonadione and to avoid rapid infusion. Severe reactions, including fatalities, also have been reported following intramuscular (IM) administration. Typically, these severe reactions have resembled hypersensitivity or anaphylaxis, including shock and cardiac or respiratory arrest. Some patients have exhibited these severe reactions on receiving phytonadione for the first time. Therefore, restrict the IV and IM routes to those situations where the subcutaneous route is not feasible and the serious risk involved is considered justified.

Indications

➤*Coagulation disorders:* Phytonadione is indicated in the following coagulation disorders which are due to faulty formation of factors II, VII, IX and X when caused by vitamin K deficiency or interference with vitamin K activity.

➤*Anticoagulant-induced prothrombin deficiency:* Phytonadione injection is indicated in anticoagulant-induced prothrombin deficiency caused by coumarin or indandione derivatives.

➤*Hemorrhagic disease of the newborn:* Prophylaxis and therapy of hemorrhagic disease of the newborn.

➤*Hypoprothrombinemia:* Hypoprothrombinemia secondary to factors limiting absorption or synthesis of vitamin K (eg, obstructive jaundice, biliary fistula, sprue, ulcerative colitis, celiac disease, intestinal resection, cystic fibrosis of the pancreas, regional enteritis), and other drug-induced hypoprothrombinemia where it is definitely shown that the result is due to interference with vitamin K metabolism (eg, salicylates, antibacterial therapy).

Administration and Dosage

➤*Adults:*

Anticoagulant-induced prothrombin deficiency – 2.5 to 10 mg or up to 25 mg (rarely 50 mg). May repeat in 6 to 8 hours.

Hypoprothrombinemia – 2.5 to 25 mg or more (rarely up to 50 mg).

➤*Children:*

Newborns –

Treatment of hemorrhagic disease: 1 mg subcutaneously or IM. Higher doses may be necessary if the mother has been receiving oral anticoagulants.

Prophylaxis of hemorrhagic disease: 0.5 to 1 mg IM dose within 1 hour of birth.

Off-label dosing –

Anticoagulant (oral) overdose:

• *Usual dose* – For major bleeding, the dosage is 5 mg, which may be repeated in 12 to 48 hours. If the INR is more than 8 but there is no bleeding or minor bleeding, then the dosage is 0.5 to 2.5 mg, which may be repeated in 12 to 48 hours. Phytonadione may be administered subcutaneously, IM or IV, but the subcutaneous route is the preferred route of administration.

• *Maximum dose* – 2 mg (infants); 5 to 10 mg (children).

Vitamin K deficiency: 1 to 2 mg as a single dose. May be administered subcutaneously (preferred), IM or IV.

➤*Preparation for administration:* Phytonadione may be diluted with sodium chloride 0.9% injection, dextrose 5% injection, or dextrose 5% and sodium chloride injection. Benzyl alcohol as a preservative has been associated with toxicity in newborns. Therefore, all of the above diluents should be preservative-free. Do not use other diluents. When dilutions are indicated, start administration immediately after mixture with the diluent, and discard unused portions of the dilution, as well as unused contents of the ampule.

➤*Administration:* Whenever possible, give phytonadione by the subcutaneous route. When IV administration is considered unavoidable, inject the drug very slowly, not exceeding 1 mg per minute.

➤*Storage / Stability:* Store at 15° to 30°C (59° to 86°F). Protect from light. Store ampules in tray until time of use.

Actions

➤*Pharmacology:* Phytonadione aqueous colloidal solution of vitamin K_1 for parenteral injection, possesses the same type and degree of activity as does naturally occurring vitamin K, which is necessary for the production via the liver of active prothrombin (factor II), proconvertin (factor VII), plasma thromboplastin component (factor IX), and Stuart factor (factor X). The prothrombin test is sensitive to the levels of 3 of these 4 factors: II, VII, and X. Vitamin K is an essential cofactor for a microsomal enzyme that catalyzes the post-translational carboxylation of multiple, specific, peptide-bound glutamic acid residues in inactive hepatic precursors of factors II, VII, IX, and X. The resulting gamma-carboxy-glutamic acid residues convert the precursors into active coagulation factors that are subsequently secreted by liver cells into the blood.

In healthy animals and humans, phytonadione is virtually devoid of pharmacodynamic activity. However, in animals and humans deficient in vitamin K, the pharmacological action of vitamin K is related to its normal physiological function, that is, to promote the hepatic biosynthesis of vitamin K-dependent clotting factors.

Contraindications

Hypersensitivity to any component of this medication.

Warnings/Precautions

➤*Benzyl alcohol:* Benzyl alcohol as a preservative in bacteriostatic sodium chloride injection has been associated with toxicity in newborns. Data are unavailable on the toxicity of other preservatives in this age group. There is no evidence to suggest that the small amount of benzyl alcohol contained in phytonadione, when used as recommended, is associated with toxicity.

➤*Aluminum:* This product may contain aluminum that may be toxic. Aluminum may reach toxic levels with prolonged parenteral administration if kidney function is impaired. Premature neonates are particularly at risk because their kidneys are immature, and they require large amounts of calcium and phosphate solutions, which contain aluminum.

➤*Oral anticoagulant — induced hypoprothrombinemia:* Do not expect an immediate coagulant effect after administration of phytonadione. It takes a minimum of 1 to 2 hours for measurable improvement in the prothrombin time. Whole blood or component therapy may also be necessary if bleeding is severe.

Phytonadione will not counteract the anticoagulant action of heparin.

When vitamin K_1 is used to correct excessive anticoagulant-induced hypoprothrombinemia, anticoagulant therapy still being indicated, the patient is again faced with the clotting hazards existing prior to starting the anticoagulant therapy. Phytonadione is not a clotting agent, but overzealous therapy with vitamin K_1 may restore conditions which originally permitted thromboembolic phenomena. Keep the dosage as low as possible, and check prothrombin time regularly as clinical conditions indicate.

➤*Renal function impairment:* Research indicates that patients with impaired kidney function, including premature neonates, who receive parenteral levels of aluminum at greater than 4 to 5 mcg/kg/day accumulate aluminum at levels associated with CNS and bone toxicity. Tissue loading may occur at even lower rates of administration.

PHYTONADIONE — INJECTION

➤*Hepatic function impairment:* Repeated large doses of vitamin K are not warranted in liver disease if the response to initial use of the vitamin is unsatisfactory. Failure to respond to vitamin K may indicate that the condition being treated is inherently unresponsive to vitamin K.

➤*Pregnancy: Category C.* Animal reproduction studies have not been conducted with phytonadione. It is also not known whether phytonadione can cause fetal harm when administered to a pregnant woman or can affect reproduction capacity. Give phytonadione to a pregnant woman only if clearly needed.

➤*Lactation:* It is not known whether this drug is excreted in human milk. Because many drugs are excreted in human milk, exercise caution when phytonadione is administered to a nursing woman.

➤*Children:* Benzyl alcohol has been reported to be associated with a fatal "gasping syndrome" in premature infants.

Hemolysis, jaundice, and hyperbilirubinemia in newborns, particularly in premature infants, may be related to the dose of phytonadione. Therefore, do not exceed the recommended dose.

➤*Monitoring:* Check prothrombin time regularly as clinical conditions indicate.

Drug Interactions

Vitamin K Injection Drug Interactions

Precipitant drug	Object drug[a]		Description
Vitamin K	Anticoagulants	⬇	Anticoagulant effects are antagonized by vitamin K. Temporary resistance to oral anticoagulants may result. It may be necessary to increase the anticoagulant dose.
Mineral oil	Vitamin K	⬇	Mineral oil may decrease GI absorption of vitamin K with concurrent oral administration.

[a] ⬇ = object drug decreased.

Adverse Reactions

➤*Parenteral administration:* Severe reactions, including fatalities, have occurred during and immediately after IV injection of phytonadione, even when precautions have been taken to dilute the phytonadione and to avoid rapid infusion. Severe reactions, including fatalities, also have been reported following IM administration. Typically, these severe reactions have resembled hypersensitivity or anaphylaxis, including shock and cardiac or respiratory arrest. Some patients have exhibited these severe reactions on receiving phytonadione for the first time. Therefore, restrict the IV and IM routes to those situations where the subcutaneous route is not feasible and the serious risk involved is considered justified.

➤*Allergic:* Keep in mind the possibility of allergic sensitivity, including an anaphylactoid reaction.

➤*Miscellaneous:* Transient "flushing sensations" and "peculiar" sensations of taste have been observed, as well as rare instances of dizziness, rapid and weak pulse, profuse sweating, brief hypotension, dyspnea, and cyanosis.

Pain, swelling, and tenderness at the injection site may occur. Infrequently, usually after repeated injection, erythematous, indurated, pruritic plaques have occurred; rarely, these have progressed to scleroderma-like lesions that have persisted for long periods. In other cases, these lesions have resembled erythema perstans.

Hyperbilirubinemia – Hyperbilirubinemia has been observed in the newborn following administration of phytonadione. This has occurred rarely and primarily with doses above those recommended.

Overdosage

The intravenous LD_{50} of phytonadione injection in the mouse is 41.5 and 52 mL/kg for the 0.2% and 1% concentrations, respectively.

THIAMIN (Vitamin B_1)

otc	**Thiamine Hydrochloride** (Various, eg, Goldline)	**Tablets:** 50 mg	In 100s and 250s.
		100 mg	In 100s, 250s, 1000s, and UD 100s.
		250 mg	In 100s, 250s.
otc	**Thiamilate** (Tyson)	**Tablets, enteric-coated:** 20 mg	In 100s.
Rx	**Thiamine Hydrochloride** (Various, eg, American Pharmaceutical Partners)	**Injection:** 100 mg/mL	≤ 9 mg benzyl alcohol. In 1 mL in 2 mL *Tubex* and 2 mL multiple-dose vials.

THIAMIN (Vitamin B_1) — ORAL

For additional information, refer to the Dietary Reference Intakes of Vitamins and Minerals table.

Indications

➤*Thiamin deficiency:* Treatment of thiamin deficiency.

➤*Off-label uses:* Oral thiamin has been studied as a mosquito repellant; further verification is needed.

Administration and Dosage

➤*General dosing considerations:* The need for thiamin is greater when the carbohydrate content of the diet is high.

➤*Adults:*

Thiamin deficiency – 1 tablet or capsule daily. A dosage of 0.5 mg/1,000 Kcal intake has also been suggested.

➤*Storage/Stability:* Store at room temperature in a dry place.

Actions

➤*Pharmacology:* Thiamin is a water-soluble vitamin. Sources include brewer's yeast, legumes, beef, pork, milk, liver, nuts, whole grains, enriched flour, and cereals. The primary functions of thiamin include metabolism of carbohydrates, maintenance of normal growth, transmission of nerve impulses, and acetylcholine synthesis.

Thiamin is essential for normal aerobic metabolism. Thiamin combines with adenosine triphosphate (ATP) and the enzyme thiamin diphosphokinase to form thiamin pyrophosphate, a coenzyme also known as cocarboxylase. Thiamin pyrophosphate is the active form of thiamin. It serves as a coenzyme in the carbohydrate metabolism for the decarboxylation of α keto acids (such as pyruvate) and α-ketoglutarate, as well as serving for the activity of transketolase in the pentose phosphate pathway.

➤*Pharmacokinetics:*

Absorption/Distribution – Thiamin is absorbed by a Na+ dependent active, carrier-mediated process at low concentrations in the jejunum and by passive diffusion in the jejunum and ileum at high concentrations. Maximum oral absorption is 8 to 15 mg/day. Oral absorption may be increased by administering in divided doses with food. Thiamin is mainly stored in the liver but is also found in the brain, kidney, heart, intestine, lung, spleen, and muscle. Tissue stores are saturated when intake exceeds the minimal requirement. For a complete listing of RDAs by age, sex, and condition, refer to the RDA table.

Metabolism/Excretion – Excess thiamin is excreted in the urine both as thiamin acetic acid and metabolites. Approximately 100 mcg/day of thiamin are excreted in the urine with a daily intake of 0.5 mg/1000 kcal. With normal renal function, 80% to 96% of an IV dose is excreted in the urine.

Contraindications

Hypersensitivity to thiamin.

Warnings/Precautions

➤*Multiple vitamin deficiency:* Simple vitamin B_1 deficiency is rare. Suspect multiple vitamin deficiencies.

➤*Hypersensitivity reactions:* Serious hypersensitivity/anaphylactic reactions can occur.

➤*Pregnancy: Category A* (parenteral). (*Category C* if used in doses greater than the RDA). Studies have not shown an increased risk of fetal abnormalities if administered during pregnancy. The possibility of fetal harm appears remote; however, use during pregnancy only if clearly needed.

➤*Lactation:* It is not known whether this drug is excreted in breast milk. Use with caution in nursing women.

Adverse Reactions

Feeling of warmth; pruritus; urticaria; weakness; sweating; nausea; restlessness; tightness of the throat; angioneurotic edema; cyanosis; pulmonary edema; hemorrhage into the GI tract; cardiovascular collapse; hypersensitivity; anaphylactic shock; death.

Overdosage

Hypersensitivity; anaphylactic shock. Doses of 500 mg/day for a month were administered without toxic effects.

THIAMINE — INJECTION

For additional information, refer to the Dietary Reference Intakes of Vitamins and Minerals table.

Indications

➤*Thiamine deficiency:* For the treatment of thiamin deficiency.

➤*Beriberi:* For the treatment of beriberi whether of the dry (major symptoms related to the nervous system) or wet (major symptoms related to the cardiovascular system) variety.

➤*General information:* Thiamine injection should be used where rapid restoration of thiamin is necessary, as in Wernicke's encephalopathy, infantile beriberi with acute collapse, cardiovascular disease due to thiamin deficiency, or neuritis of pregnancy if vomiting is severe. It is also indicated when giving IV dextrose to individuals with marginal thiamin status to avoid precipitation of heart failure. Thiamine HCl injection is also indicated in patients with established thiamin deficiency who cannot take thiamine orally due to coexisting severe anorexia, nausea, vomiting, or malabsorption. Thiamine HCl injection is not usually indicated for conditions of decreased oral intake or decreased GI absorption, because multiple vitamins should usually be given.

Administration and Dosage

➤*General dosing considerations:* Poor dietary habits should be corrected, and an abundant and well-balanced dietary intake should be prescribed.

➤*Adults:*

Beriberi – 10 to 20 mg IM 3 times daily for as long as 2 weeks. An oral therapeutic multivitamin preparation containing 5 to 10 mg thiamin administered daily for 1 month is recommended to achieve body tissue saturation.

"Wet" beriberi with myocardial failure: Must be treated as an emergency cardiac condition, and thiamine must be administered slowly IV in this situation.

Dextrose administration to patients with marginal thiamin status – 100 mg in each of the first few liters of IV fluid to avoid precipitating heart failure in patients with marginal thiamin status to whom dextrose is being administered.

Neuritis of pregnancy – 5 to 10 mg/day IM for patients in whom vomiting is severe enough to preclude adequate oral therapy.

Thiamin deficiency – IV doses as large as 100 mg/L to correct the deficiency as rapidly as possible. Continue parenteral doses at daily requirements only when GI disturbances prevent adequate oral absorption.

Wernicke-Korsakoff syndrome –

Initial dosage: 100 mg IV.

Maintenance dosage: 50 to 100 mg/day IM until the patient is consuming a regular, balanced diet.

➤*Children:*

Infantile beriberi – Infantile beriberi that is mild may respond to oral therapy, but if collapse occurs, doses of 25 mg may be given IV cautiously.

➤*Administration:* To be given IV or IM.

➤*Admixture compatibility:* Thiamin is unstable in neutral or alkaline solutions; do not use in combination with alkaline solutions (eg, carbonates, citrates, barbiturates, acetates, copper ions). Solutions containing sulfites are incompatible with thiamin as are other oxidizing and reducing agents. In vitro testing of thiamin 0.1% reduced activity of erythromycin estolate, kanamycin sulfate, and streptomycin sulfate.

➤*Storage/Stability:* Store between 15° and 30°C (59° and 86°F). Protect from light.

Actions

➤*Pharmacokinetics:* The requirement for thiamin is greater when the carbohydrate content of the diet is raised. Body depletion of vitamin B_1 can occur after ≈ 3 weeks of total absence of thiamin in the diet.

Absorption/Distribution – The water-soluble vitamins are widely distributed in both plants and animals. They are absorbed in man by both diffusion and active transport mechanisms. These vitamins are structurally diverse (derivatives of sugar, pyridine, purines, pyrimidine, organic acid complexes and nucleotide complex) and act as coenzymes, as oxidation-reduction agents, possibly as mitochondrial agents. Thiamin is distributed in all tissues. The highest concentrations occur in the liver, brain, kidney and heart. When thiamin intake is greatly in excess of need, tissue stores increase 2 to 3 times. If intake is insufficient, tissues become depleted of their vitamin content. Absorption of thiamin following IM administration is rapid and complete.

Metabolism/Excretion – Metabolism is rapid, and the excess is excreted in the urine. Thiamin combines with adenosine triphosphate (ATP) to form thiamin pyrophosphate, also known as cocarboxylase, a coenzyme. Its role in carbohydrate metabolism is the decarboxylation of pyruvic acid in the blood and α-ketoacids to acetaldehyde and carbon dioxide. Increased levels of pyruvic acid in the blood indicate vitamin B_1 deficiency.

Contraindications

A history of sensitivity to thiamin or to any of the ingredients in this drug is a contraindication (see Warnings).

Warnings/Precautions

➤*Wernicke's-Korsakoff syndrome:* Thiamin-deficient patients may experience a sudden onset or worsening of Wernicke's encephalopathy following glucose administration; in suspected thiamin deficiency, administer thiamin before or along with dextrose-containing fluids.

➤*Multiple vitamin deficiency:* Simple vitamin B_1 deficiency is rare. Multiple vitamin deficiencies should be suspected in any case of dietary inadequacy.

➤*Hypersensitivity reactions:* Serious hypersensitivity/anaphylactic reactions can occur, especially after repeated administration. Deaths have resulted from IV or IM administration of thiamin (see Adverse Reactions). Routine testing for hypersensitivity, in many cases, may not detect hypersensitivity. Nevertheless, a skin test should be performed on patients who are suspected of drug allergies or previous reactions to thiamin, and any positive responders should not receive thiamin by injection.

If hypersensitivity to thiamin is suspected (based on history of drug allergy or occurrence of adverse reactions after thiamin administration), administer one-hundredth of the dose intradermally and observe for 30 minutes. If no reaction occurs, full dose can be given; the patient should be observed for at least 30 minutes after injection. Be prepared to treat anaphylactic reactions regardless of the precautions taken.

Treatment of anaphylactic reactions includes maintaining a patent airway and the use of epinephrine, oxygen, vasopressors, steroids and antihistamines.

➤*Pregnancy: Category A.* Studies in pregnant women have not shown that thiamine hydrochloride increases the risk of fetal abnormalities if administered during pregnancy. If the drug is used during pregnancy, the possibility of fetal harm appears remote. Because studies cannot rule out the possibility of harm however, thiamine hydrochloride should be used during pregnancy only if clearly needed.

➤*Lactation:* It is not known whether this drug is excreted in human milk. Because many drugs are excreted in human milk, caution should be exercised when thiamine hydrochloride is administered to a nursing mother.

Adverse Reactions

➤*Hypersensitivity:* An occasional individual may develop a hypersensitivity or life-threatening anaphylactic reaction to thiamin, especially after repeated injection. Collapse and death have been reported.

➤*Local:* Some tenderness and induration may follow IM use (see Warnings).

➤*Miscellaneous:* A feeling of warmth, pruritus, urticaria, weakness, sweating, nausea, restlessness, tightness of the throat, angioneurotic edema, cyanosis, pulmonary edema, and hemorrhage into the GI tract have also been reported.

Overdosage

Parenteral doses of 100 to 500 mg singly have been administered without toxic effects. However, dosages exceeding 30 mg 3 times a day are not utilized effectively. When the body tissues are saturated with thiamin, it is excreted in the urine as pyrimidine. As the intake of thiamin is further increased, it appears unchanged in the urine.

Patient Information

The patient should be advised as to proper dietary habits during treatment so that relapses will be less likely to occur with reduction in dosage or cessation of injection therapy.

RIBOFLAVIN (B_2)

otc	**Vitamin B_2** (Nature's Blend)	**Tablets; oral:** 25 mg	Gluten free, preservative free. Polydextrose, sorbitol. In 100s.
otc	**Riboflavin** (Various, eg, Freeda)	**Tablets; oral:** 50 mg	In 100s and 250s.
		100 mg	In 100s and 250s.
otc	**B_2-400** (Bio-Tech)	**Capsules; oral:** 400 mg	Dye free, preservative free. In 100s.
otc	**Cyto B2** (Solace Nutrition)	**Powder; oral:** 343 mg per 1 g of powder	In 100 g.

RIBOFLAVIN — ORAL

For additional information, refer to the Dietary Reference Intakes of Vitamins and Minerals table.

Indications

➤*Riboflavin deficiency:* Riboflavin is used as a dietary supplement to treat and prevent riboflavin deficiency.

➤*Medical food (Cyto B2)*: For the dietary management of mitochondrial cytopathies or glutaric acidemia

➤*Off-label uses:* Lactic acidosis (with hepatic steatosis) in AIDS patients taking nucleoside reverse-transcriptase inhibitors (NRTI) has been successfully treated with riboflavin 50 mg.

Riboflavin is used for the treatment of infants with hyperbilirubinemia.

Riboflavin (400 mg) has been found to be an effective migraine prophylaxis in some patients.

Administration and Dosage

➤*Adults:*

Dietary supplemental – Varies by product. Dosages range from 25 to 400 mg/day.

Mitochondrial cytopathies or glutaric acidemia (Cyto B2) – The daily amount is based on age, body weight, and metabolic condition of the patient; consume in equal portions throughout the day. One level, unpacked, small scoop contains riboflavin 25 mg; 1 level, unpacked, large scoop contains riboflavin 100 mg.

➤*Children:*

Mitochondrial cytopathies or glutaric acidemia (Cyto B2) –

Older than 1 year: The daily amount is based on age, body weight, and metabolic condition of the patient; consume in equal portions throughout the day. One level, unpacked, small scoop contains riboflavin 25 mg; 1 level, unpacked, large scoop contains riboflavin 100 mg.

➤*Administration:*

Tablets/capsules – Some manufacturers recommend taking riboflavin with meals.

Cyto B2 – Consume directly by mouth or add to juices, beverages, or sprinkle on top of or mix into food.

➤*Storage/Stability:* Store away from heat and direct light. Do not store the powder in the refrigerator; use within 6 months of opening.

Actions

➤*Pharmacology:* Riboflavin is a water-soluble vitamin that functions as 2 coenzymes. Flavin adenine dinucleotide (FAD) and flavin mononucleotide (FMN) catalyze many oxidation-reduction reactions including glucose oxidation, amino acid deamination, and fatty acid breakdown. Sources of riboflavin include meats, poultry, fish, dairy products, broccoli, turnips, asparagus, spinach, and enriched and fortified grains, cereals, and bakery products.

➤*Pharmacokinetics:* Riboflavin is absorbed from the duodenum and is excreted with its metabolites in the urine. Small amounts of riboflavin are also excreted in the bile, feces, and sweat.

Warnings/Precautions

➤*Multiple vitamin deficiency:* Riboflavin deficiency seldom occurs alone and is often associated with deficiency of other vitamin deficiencies.

➤*Pregnancy:* Category A. (Category C in doses that exceed the RDA.)

See Administration and Dosage for more information.

➤*Lactation:* Riboflavin is excreted in breast milk.

See Administration and Dosage for more information.

Adverse Reactions

➤*GU:* Riboflavin may cause urine to have a more yellow color than normal, especially if large doses are taken. This is to be expected and is no cause for alarm. Usually, however, riboflavin does not cause any side effects.

Overdosage

Riboflavin is not toxic in humans because of the limited absorption from the GI tract.

Patient Information

Riboflavin may cause a yellow discoloration of the urine when taken in large doses.

PANTOTHENIC ACID (B_5)

otc sf	**Pantothenic Acid** (Various, eg, Freeda, Mason)	**Tablets; oral:** 100 mg	As d-calcium pantothenate. May contain calcium. In 100s.
otc sf	**Pantothenic Acid** (Various, eg, Freeda, Major)	200 mg	As d-calcium pantothenate. May contain calcium. In 100s and 250s.
otc sf	**Pantothenic Acid** (Various, eg, Freeda, Integrative Therapeutics, Rugby)	500 mg	As d-calcium pantothenate. May contain calcium. In 90s, 100s, and 250s.

PANTOTHENIC ACID (B_5) — ORAL

For complete prescribing information, refer to the Dietary Reference Intakes of Vitamins and Minerals table.

Indications

➤*Pantothenic acid deficiency:* As a dietary supplement to treat pantothenic acid deficiency.

Administration and Dosage

➤*Adults:*

Pantothenic acid deficiency – 1 or 2 tablets daily.

➤*Administration:* For oral use. Take with a meal.

➤*Storage/Stability:* Store at 15° to 30°C (59° to 86°F) in a cool, dry place, away from direct heat, light, and moisture.

Actions

➤*Pharmacology:* Pantothenic acid, a water-soluble vitamin, is a precursor of coenzyme A, which is a cofactor for a variety of enzyme-catalyzed reactions involving transfer of acetyl groups. Functions of pantothenic acid include oxidative metabolism of carbohydrates, gluconeogenesis, synthesis and degradation of fatty acids, and synthesis of steroids (cholesterol), steroid hormones, sphingosine, citrate, acetoacetate, and porphyrins. Sources of pantothenic acid include meat, poultry, fish, cereals, fruits, vegetables, milk, and egg yolks.

➤*Pharmacokinetics:*

Absorption/Distribution – Pantothenic acid is absorbed from the GI tract and is distributed to all tissues in concentrations ranging from 2 to 45 mcg/g.

Metabolism – Pantothenic acid is not degraded in the human body because the intake and the excretion are approximately equal.

Excretion – Approximately 70% of absorbed pantothenic acid is excreted in the urine.

Contraindications

Hypersensitivity to pantothenic acid.

Warnings/Precautions

➤*Pregnancy:* Category A. (Category C in doses that exceed the recommended dietary allowance).

➤*Lactation:* Pantothenic acid is excreted in breast milk. Milk concentrations are between 2 and 2.5 mg/L, with a weak correlation between maternal intake and milk levels. This corresponds to a daily dose of approximately 0.33 to 0.375 mg/kg/day for breast-feeding infants.

Per *Briggs' Drugs in Pregnancy and Lactation*, pantothenic acid is considered compatible with breast-feeding.

➤*Children:* Not indicated for use in children.

➤*Monitoring:* None well documented.

Drug Interactions

➤*Biotin:* Life-threatening eosinophilia pleuropericarditis has been reported with concurrent use.

Adverse Reactions

➤*Dermatologic:* Rash.

➤*GI:* Diarrhea at large doses.

Overdosage

No data available.

Patient Information

Advise patients to take with meals.

Advise patients not to take large doses of vitamins (megadoses or megavitamin therapy) while taking pantothenic acid tablets unless otherwise directed by their health care provider.

Advise patients to report any of the following severe adverse reactions to their health care provider immediately: severe allergic reactions (eg, rash, hives, difficultly breathing, tightness in the chest, swelling of the mouth face, lips, or tongue).

NIACIN (B_3; Nicotinic Acid)

otc[a]	**Nicotinic Acid (Niacin)** (Various, eg, Freeda, Goldline)	**Tablets; oral:** 50 mg	In 100s and 250s.
otc[a]	**Nicotinic Acid (Niacin)** (Various, eg, Freeda, Goldline)	**Tablets; oral:** 100 mg	In 100s and 250s.
otc sf	**Niacin No Flush** (Windmill)		Preservative free, sugar free. In 60s.
otc[a]	**Nicotinic Acid (Niacin)** (Various, eg, Goldline)	**Tablets; oral:** 250 mg	In 100s.
otc sf	**Niacin No Flush** (Windmill)		Preservative free, sugar free. In 60s.
otc[a]	**Nicotinic Acid (Niacin)** (Various, eg, Freeda, Goldline)	**Tablets; oral:** 500 mg	In 100s and 1,000s.
Rx	**Niacor** (Upsher-Smith)		Lactose. (W 901). White, scored. In 100s.
otc[a]	**Nicotinic Acid (Niacin)** (Various, eg, Naturally)	**Tablets, sustained-release; oral:** 500 mg	In 100s.
otc[a]	**Nicotinic Acid (Niacin)** (Various, eg, Freeda)	**Tablets, controlled-release; oral:** 250 mg	In 100s and 250s.
otc[a]	**Nicotinic Acid (Niacin)** (Various, eg, Goldline)	**Tablets, controlled-release; oral:** 500 mg	In 100s and 1,000s.
otc sf	**Nicotinic Acid (Niacin)** (Rugby)	**Tablets, controlled-release; oral:** 1,000 mg	Gluten free, preservative free, sugar free. In 100s.
otc[a] sf	**Slo-Niacin** (Upsher-Smith)	**Tablets, controlled-release; oral:** 250 mg	(250). Pink. In 100s.
		Tablets, controlled-release; oral: 500 mg	(500). Pink. In 100s.
		Tablets, controlled-release; oral: 750 mg	Pink. In 100s.
Rx	**Niaspan** (Abbott)	**Tablets, extended-release; oral:** 500 mg	(KOS/500). Off-white, capsule shape. In 100s.
		750 mg	(KOS/750). Off-white, capsule shape. In 100s.
		1000 mg	(KOS/1000). Off-white, capsule shape. In 100s.
otc sf	**Niacin Flush-Free** (Mason)	**Capsules; oral:** 750 mg	Preservative free, sugar free. Inositol 211.5 mg. In 50s.
otc[a]	**Nicotinic Acid (Niacin)** (Various)	**Capsules, extended-release; oral:** 250 mg	In 100s and 1,000s.
otc[a]	**Nicotinic Acid (Niacin)** (Various)	**Capsules, extended-release; oral:** 400 mg	In 100s.
otc[a]	**Nicotinic Acid (Niacin)** (Various)	**Capsules, sustained-release; oral:** 125 mg	In 100s.
otc[a]	**Nicotinic Acid (Niacin)** (Various)	**Capsules, sustained-release; oral:** 500 mg	In 100s.
otc	**Nicotinic Acid (Niacin)** (Various, eg, Goldline)	**Capsules, controlled-release; oral:** 250 mg	In 100s.
otc[a]	**Nicotinic Acid (Niacin)** (Various, eg, Goldline)	**Capsules, controlled-release; oral:** 500 mg	In 100s and 1,000s.

[a] Some products may be available *Rx*, according to distributor discretion. Most of these products are marketed as nutritional supplements.

NIACIN — ORAL

Also refer to the general discussion of these products in the Antihyperlipidemic Agents Introduction. For additional information, refer to the Dietary Reference Intakes of Vitamins and Minerals table.

Indications

➤*Niacin deficiency:* Treatment of niacin deficiency.

➤*Pellagra:* Prevention and treatment of pellagra.

➤*Hypercholesterolemia:* Adjunct to diet for the reduction of elevated total and LDL levels in patients with primary hypercholesterolemia when the response to diet and other nonpharmacologic measures alone has been inadequate.

➤*Hypertriglyceridemia (Types IV and V):* Adjunctive therapy for treatment in adult patients with very high serum triglyceride levels (Type IV and V hyperlipidemia) who present a risk of pancreatitis and who do not respond adequately to dietary control.

➤*Niacor*:

Hypercholesterolemia – Niacin, alone or in combination with a bile-acid binding resin, is indicated as an adjunct to diet for the reduction of elevated total and LDL cholesterolprimary levels in patients with hypercholesterolemia (Types IIa and IIb), (see classification of hyperlipoproteinemias) when the response to a diet restricted in saturated fat and cholesterol and other nonpharmacologic measures alone has been inadequate (see NCEP treatment guidelines).

Hypertriglyceridemia – Niacin is also indicated as adjunctive therapy for treatment of adult patients with very high serum triglyceride levels (Type IV and V hyperlipidemia; see table below) who present a risk of pancreatitis and who do not respond adequately to a determined dietary effort to control them.

➤*Niaspan*:

Hypercholesterolemia – Niacin extended-release tablets are indicated as an adjunct to diet for reduction of elevated TC, LDL-C, Apo B and TG levels, and to increase HDL-C in patients with primary hypercholesterolemia (heterozygous familial and nonfamilial) and mixed dyslipidemia (Frederickson Types IIa and IIb; see table), when the response to an appropriate diet has been inadequate.

Niacin extended-release tablets in combination with a bile acid binding resin is indicated as an adjunct to diet for reduction of elevated TC and LDL-C levels in adult patients with primary hypercholesterolemia (Type IIa, see table), when the response to an appropriate diet, or diet plus monotherapy, has been inadequate.

Combination therapy is not indicated as initial therapy.

Prevention of recurring MI – In patients with a history of MI and hypercholesterolemia, niacin is indicated to reduce the risk of recurrent nonfatal MI.

Atherosclerotic disease – In patients with a history of coronary artery disease (CAD) and hypercholesterolemia, niacin, in combination with a bile acid binding resin, is indicated to slow progression or promote regression of atherosclerotic disease.

Administration and Dosage

➤*General dosing considerations:* The flush response can be attenuated by slowly increasing the dose (eg, 100 mg 3 times a day each week), administering with food or milk, or by administering either a prostaglandin inhibitor, such as aspirin 325 mg 30 minutes prior to niacin administration, or sustained-release preparations.

Interchangeability – Do not substitute extended-release (modified-release, timed-release) nicotinic acid preparations for equivalent doses of immediate-release (crystalline) nicotinic acid. (See Warnings/Precautions.)

➤*Adults:*

Dietary supplement –

Slo-Niacin controlled-release tablets: Usual dosage is 250 to 500 mg daily, taken morning or evening, or as directed by health care provider. For the 750 mg tablets, divide the tablet in half. Before using more than 500 mg daily, consult your health care provider.

Niacin tablets, extended/sustained/timed-release capsules or tablets: 1 capsule or tablet daily, or as directed by health care provider.

Hyperlipidemia – 1 to 2 g 2 or 3 times daily. Do not exceed 6 g/day.

Pellagra – Up to 500 mg/day.

Niaspan –

Initial dosage: 500 mg at bedtime in order to reduce the incidence and severity of adverse reactions that may occur during early therapy.

Dosage titration: Doses should be individualized according to patient response. For weeks 1 to 4, the dosage is 500 mg at bedtime. For weeks 5 to 8, the dosage is 1,000 mg (2 tablets) at bedtime. After week 8, titrate to patient response and tolerance. If response to 1,000 mg daily is inadequate, increase dose to 1,500 mg daily; may subsequently increase dose to 2,000 mg daily. Daily dose should not be increased more than 500 mg in a 4-week period, and doses above 2,000 mg daily are not recommended. Women may respond at lower doses than men.

Maintenance dosage: 1,000 mg (two 500 mg tablets) to 2,000 mg (two 1,000 mg tablets or four 500 mg tablets) once daily at bedtime. Doses of more than 2,000 mg daily are not recommended.

Concomitant therapy: If lipid response to *Niaspan* extended-release tablets alone is insufficient or if higher doses of *Niaspan* extended-release tablets

NIACIN — ORAL

are not well tolerated, some patients may benefit from combination therapy with a bile-acid binding resin or an HMG-CoA reductase inhibitor.

• *Concomitant therapy with lovastatin* – Patients already receiving a stable dose of lovastatin who require further TG-lowering or HDL-raising (eg, to achieve NCEP non-HDL-C goals), may receive concomitant dosage titration with *Niaspan* per *Niaspan* recommended initial titration schedule (see Dosage Titration). For patients already receiving a stable dose of *Niaspan* who require further LDL-lowering (eg, to achieve NCEP LDL-C goals, see Dosage Titration section), the usual recommended starting dose of lovastatin is 20 mg once a day. Dose adjustments should be made at intervals of 4 weeks or more. Combination therapy with *Niaspan* and lovastatin should not exceed doses of 2,000 mg and 40 mg daily, respectively.

Discontinuation of therapy: If therapy is discontinued for an extended period, reinstitution of therapy should include a titration phase.

To reduce flushing: Flushing of the skin may be reduced in frequency or severity by pretreatment with aspirin (taken 30 minutes prior to dose) or another nonsteroidal anti-inflammatory drug. Tolerance to this flushing develops rapidly over the course of several weeks. Flushing, pruritus, and gastrointestinal distress are also greatly reduced by slowly increasing the dose of niacin and avoiding administration on an empty stomach.

Tablet interchangeability: Equivalent doses of *Niaspan* extended-release tablets should not be substituted for sustained-release (modified-release, timed-release) niacin preparations or immediate-release (crystalline) niacin. Patients previously receiving other niacin products should be started with the recommended *Niaspan* extended-release tablet titration schedule, and the dose should subsequently be individualized based on patient response. Single-dose bioavailability studies have demonstrated that *Niaspan* extended-release tablet strengths are not interchangeable.

Niacor –

Usual dosage: 1 to 2 g 2 or 3 times a day. Doses should be individualized according to the patient's response.

Initial dosage: Start with one-half tablet (250 mg) as a single daily dose following the evening meal.

Dosage titration: The frequency of dosing and total daily dose can be increased every 4 to 7 days until the desired LDL cholesterol or triglyceride level is achieved or the first-level therapeutic dose of 1.5 to 2 g/day is reached. If the patient's hyperlipidemia is not adequately controlled after 2 months at this level, the dosage can then be increased at 2- to 4-week intervals to 3 g/day (1 g 3 times per day). In patients with marked lipid abnormalities, a higher dose is occasionally required but generally should not exceed 6 g/day.

To reduce flushing: Flushing of the skin appears frequently and can be minimized by pretreatment with aspirin or another nonsteroidal anti-inflammatory drug. Tolerance to flushing develops rapidly over the course of several weeks. Flushing, pruritus, and gastrointestinal distress are also greatly reduced by slowly increasing the dose of nicotinic acid and avoiding administration on an empty stomach.

➤*Administration:*

OTC – Take with meals.

Extended-release products – Swallow whole; do not break, crush, or chew.

Niacor – Take following the evening meal.

Niaspan – Tablets should be taken at bedtime after a low-fat snack. Tablets should be taken whole and should not be broken, crushed, or chewed before swallowing.

Slo-Niacin – Niacin tablets may be broken on the score line, but should not be crushed or chewed. The inactive matrix of the tablet is not absorbed and may be excreted intact in the stool.

➤*Storage/Stability:* Store at room temperature, 20° to 25°C (68° to 77°F).

Slo-Niacin and *Niacor* – Store at room temperature, 15° to 30°C (59° to 86°F).

Actions

➤*Pharmacology:* Niacin, vitamin B_3, is the common name for nicotinic acid and niacinamide (nicotinamide). Nicotinic acid is present in the body as its active form, nicotinamide (niacinamide). Nicotinamide functions in the body as a component of 2 coenzymes: NAD (nicotinamide adenine dinucleotide, coenzyme I) and NADP (nicotinamide adenine dinucleotide phosphate, coenzyme II), which serve a role in oxidation-reduction reactions. Sources of niacin include niacinamide and tryptophan as well as liver, meat, fish, poultry, whole-grain and enriched breads and cereals, nuts, legumes, green vegetables, yeast, and potatoes. Approximately 60 mg of tryptophan is equivalent to 1 mg of niacin.

The mechanism by which niacin alters lipid profiles has not been well defined. It may involve several actions including partial inhibition of release of free fatty acids from adipose tissue, and increased lipoprotein lipase activity, which may increase the rate of chylomicron triglyceride removal from plasma. Niacin decreases the rate of hepatic synthesis of VLDL and LDL, and does not appear to affect fecal excretion of fats, sterols, or bile acids.

Nicotinic acid (but not nicotinamide) in gram doses produces an average 10% to 20% reduction in total and LDL cholesterol, a 30% to 70% reduction in triglycerides, and an average 20% to 35% increase in HDL cholesterol. The magnitude of individual lipid and lipoprotein responses may be influenced by the severity and type of underlying lipid abnormality. The increase in total HDL is associated with a shift in the distribution of HDL subfractions (as defined by ultra-centrifugation) with an increase in the HDL_2:HDL_3 ratio and an increase in apolipoprotein A-I content.

➤*Pharmacokinetics:*

Absorption –

Niaspan extended-release tablets: Niacin is rapidly and extensively absorbed (at least 60% to 76% of dose) when administered orally. To maximize bioavailability and reduce the risk of gastrointestinal (GI) upset, administration of *Niaspan* extended-release tablets with a low-fat meal or snack is recommended.

Single-dose bioavailability studies have demonstrated that *Niaspan* extended-release tablet strengths are not interchangeable.

Niacor tablets: Following an oral dose, the pharmacokinetic profile of nicotinic acid is characterized by rapid absorption from the gastrointestinal tract and a short plasma elimination half-life. At a 1 g dose, peak plasma concentrations of 15 to 30 mcg/mL are reached within 30 to 60 minutes.

Distribution –

Niaspan extended-release tablets: Studies using radiolabeled niacin in mice show that niacin and its metabolites concentrate in the liver, kidney and adipose tissue.

Metabolism –

Niaspan extended-release tablets: The pharmacokinetic profile of niacin is complicated due to rapid and extensive first-pass metabolism, which is species and dose-rate specific. In humans, 1 pathway is through a simple conjugation step with glycine to form nicotinuric acid (NUA). NUA is then excreted in the urine, although there may be a small amount of reversible metabolism back to niacin. The other pathway results in the formation of nicotinamide adenine dinucleotide (NAD). It is unclear whether nicotinamide is formed as a precursor to, or following the synthesis of, NAD. Nicotinamide is further metabolized to at least N-methylnicotinamide (MNA) and nicotinamide-N-oxide (NNO). MNA is further metabolized to 2 other compounds, N-methyl-2-pyridone-5-carboxamide (2PY) and N-methyl-4-pyridone-5-carboxamide (4PY). The formation of 2PY appears to predominate over 4PY in humans. At the doses used to treat hyperlipidemia, these metabolic pathways are saturable, which explains the nonlinear relationship between niacin dose and plasma concentrations following multiple-dose *Niaspan* extended-release tablet administration.

Nicotinamide does not have hypolipidemic activity; the activity of the other metabolites is unknown.

Excretion – Niacin and its metabolites are rapidly eliminated in the urine. Following single and multiple doses, approximately 60% to 76% of the niacin dose administered as *Niaspan* extended-release tablets were recovered in urine as niacin and metabolites; up to 12% was recovered as unchanged niacin after multiple dosing. The ratio of metabolites recovered in the urine was dependent on the dose administered.

Niacor tablets: Approximately 88% of an oral pharmacologic dose is eliminated by the kidneys as unchanged drug and nicotinuric acid, its primary metabolite.

The plasma elimination half-life of nicotinic acid ranges from 20 to 45 minutes.

Special populations –

Renal function impairment: There are no data in this population. *Niaspan* extended-release tablets should be used with caution in patients with renal disease.

Hepatic function impairment: No studies have been performed. *Niaspan* extended-release tablets should be used with caution in patients with a history of liver disease, who consume substantial quantities of alcohol, or have unexplained transaminase elevations. *Niaspan* extended-release tablets are contraindicated in patients with active liver disease.

Gender: Steady-state plasma concentrations of niacin and metabolites after administration of *Niaspan* are generally higher in women than in men, with the magnitude of the difference varying with dose and metabolite. Recovery of niacin and metabolites in urine, however, is generally similar for men and women, indicating that absorption is similar for both genders. The gender differences observed in plasma levels of niacin and its metabolites may be due to gender-specific differences in metabolic rate or volume of distribution. Data from the clinical trials suggest that women have a greater hypolipidemic response than men at equivalent doses of *Niaspan* extended-release tablets.

Contraindications

Niacin should not be administered unless recommended by and taken under the supervision of a physician if any of the following conditions exist: Gallbladder disease, gout, arterial bleeding, glaucoma, diabetes, impaired liver function, peptic ulcer, pregnancy, or lactation.

Known hypersensitivity to niacin or any component of this medication; significant or unexplained hepatic dysfunction; active peptic ulcer disease; arterial bleeding.

Warnings/Precautions

➤*Schizophrenia:* There is no evidence to support the use of nicotinic acid in the treatment of schizophrenia as part of what is referred to as "orthomolecular psychiatry".

➤*Heart disease:* Persons with heart disease, particularly those who have recurrent chest pain (angina) or who recently suffered a heart attack, should take niacin only under the supervision of a physician. Persons taking high blood pressure or cholesterol-lowering drugs should contact a physician before taking niacin because of possible interactions. Increased uric acid and glucose levels and abnormal liver function tests have been reported in persons taking daily doses of 500 mg or more of niacin.

Discontinue use if adverse reactions occur.

➤*Skeletal muscle effects:* Rare cases of rhabdomyolysis have been associated with concomitant administration of lipid-altering doses (greater than or equal to 1 g/day) of niacin and HMG-CoA reductase inhibitors. In clinical

NIACIN — ORAL

studies with a combination tablet of *Niaspan* and lovastatin, no cases of rhabdomyolysis and 1 suspected case of myopathy have been reported in 1079 patients who were treated with doses of up to 2000 mg of *Niaspan* and 40 mg of lovastatin daily for periods of up to 2 years. Physicians contemplating combined therapy with HMG-CoA reductase inhibitors and nicotinic acid should carefully weigh the potential benefits and risks and should carefully monitor patients for any signs and symptoms of muscle pain, tenderness, or weakness, particularly during the initial months of therapy and during any periods of upward dosage titration of either drug. Periodic serum creatine phosphokinase (CPK) and potassium determinations should be considered in such situations, but there is no assurance that such monitoring will prevent the occurrence of severe myopathy.

➤*Extended-release preparations:* Niacin extended-release tablet preparations should not be substituted for equivalent doses of immediate-release (crystalline) niacin. For patients switching from immediate-release niacin to niacin extended-release tablets, therapy with niacin extended-release tablets should be initiated with low doses (ie, 500 mg every night) and the niacin extended-release tablet dose should then be titrated to the desired therapeutic response.

➤*Hepatic effects:* Cases of severe hepatic toxicity, including fulminant hepatic necrosis, have occurred in patients who have substituted sustained-release (modified-release, timed-release) niacin products for immediate-release (crystalline) niacin at equivalent doses.

Niacin preparations, like some other lipid-lowering therapies, have been associated with abnormal liver tests. In 3 placebo-controlled clinical trials involving titration to final daily nicotinic acid doses ranging from 500 to 3000 mg, 245 patients received nicotinic acid for a mean duration of 17 weeks. No patient with normal serum transaminase levels (AST, ALT) at baseline experienced elevations to more than 3 times the upper limit of normal (ULN) during treatment with nicotinic acid. In these studies, fewer than 1% (2/245) of nicotinic acid patients discontinued due to transaminase elevations greater than 2 times the ULN.

In 3 safety and efficacy studies with a combination tablet of *Niaspan* and lovastatin involving titration to final daily doses (expressed as mg of *Niaspan*/mg of lovastatin) 500 mg/10 mg to 2500 mg/40 mg, 10 of 1028 patients (1%) experienced reversible elevations in AST/ALT to more than 3 times the ULN. Three of 10 elevations occurred at doses outside the recommended dosing limit of 2000 mg/40 mg; no patients receiving 1000 mg/20 mg had 3-fold elevations in AST/ALT.

In the placebo-controlled clinical trials and the long-term extension study, elevations in transaminases did not appear to be related to treatment duration; elevations in AST levels did appear to be dose related. Transaminase elevations were reversible upon discontinuation of nicotinic acid.

➤*Diabetes:* Diabetic patients may experience a dose-related rise in glucose intolerance, the clinical significance of which is unclear. Diabetic or potentially diabetic patients should be observed closely. Adjustment of diet or hypoglycemic therapy may be necessary.

➤*Flushing:* Flushing appears frequently with oral therapy and generally begins 20 minutes after ingestion and lasts 30 to 60 minutes. Flushing is transient and will usually subside after 3 to 6 weeks of continued therapy. The flush response can be attenuated by slowly increasing the niacin dose (100 mg 3 times daily each week), administering with food or milk, or by administering either a prostaglandin inhibitor, such as aspirin 325 mg 60 minutes prior to niacin administration, or sustained-release niacin preparations.

➤*Hyperlipidemia:* Before instituting therapy with niacin, an attempt should be made to control hyperlipidemia with appropriate diet, exercise, and weight reduction in obese patients, and to treat other underlying medical problems.

➤*Alcohol:* Use with caution in patients who consume substantial quantities of alcohol or have a history of liver disease.

➤*Heart disease:* Caution should also be used when niacin is used in patients with unstable angina or in the acute phase of MI, particularly when such patients are also receiving vasoactive drugs such as nitrates, calcium channel blockers, or adrenergic blocking agents.

➤*Gout:* Elevated uric acid levels have occurred with niacin therapy; therefore, use with caution in patients predisposed to gout.

➤*Renal/Hepatic function impairment:* Nicotinic acid should be used with caution in patients who have a history of liver disease. Active liver diseases or unexplained transaminase elevations are contraindications to the use of nicotinic acid.

Niaspan – Niacin is rapidly metabolized by the liver, and excreted through the kidneys. *Niaspan* extended-release tablets are contraindicated in patients with significant or unexplained hepatic dysfunction and should be used with caution in patients with renal dysfunction.

➤*Pregnancy: Category A* (*Category C* if used in doses above the RDA). Animal reproduction studies have not been conducted with niacin. It is not known whether nicotinic acid at doses typically used for lipid disorders can cause fetal harm when administered to pregnant women. If a woman receiving niacin or nicotinic acid for primary hypercholesterolemia (Types IIa or IIb) becomes pregnant, discontinue the drug. If a woman being treated with niacin or nicotinic acid for hypertriglyceridemia (Types IV or V) conceives, assess the benefits and risks of continued drug therapy on an individual basis.

➤*Lactation:* Niacin has been reported to be excreted in human milk. Because of the potential for serious adverse reactions in nursing infants from lipid-altering doses of nicotinic acid, a decision should be made whether to discontinue nursing or to discontinue the drug, taking into account the importance of the drug to the mother.

➤*Children:* Safety and effectiveness of niacin therapy in pediatric patients (less than or equal to 16 years for niacin extended-release tablets) have not been established. No studies in patients under 21 years of age have been conducted with niacin extended-release tablets.

➤*Lab test abnormalities:* In placebo-controlled trials, *Niaspan* extended-release tablets have been associated with small but statistically significant, dose-related reductions in phosphorus levels (mean of −13% with 2000 mg). Although these reductions were transient, phosphorus levels should be monitored periodically in patients at risk for hypophosphatemia.

➤*Monitoring:* Patients with a history of jaundice, hepatobiliary disease, or peptic ulcer should be observed closely during niacin therapy. Frequent monitoring of liver function tests and blood glucose should be performed to ascertain that the drug is producing no adverse effects on these organ systems.

Liver tests should be performed on all patients during therapy with niacin. Serum transaminase levels, including AST and ALT, should be monitored before treatment begins, every 6 to 12 weeks for the first year, and periodically thereafter (eg, at approximately 6-month intervals). Special attention should be paid to patients who develop elevated serum transaminase levels, and in these patients, measurements should be repeated promptly and then performed more frequently. If the transaminase levels show evidence of progression, particularly if they rise to 3 times the upper limit of normal and are persistent, or if they are associated with symptoms of nausea, fever, or malaise, the drug should be discontinued.

Drug Interactions

➤*HMG-CoA reductase inhibitors:* Rare cases of rhabdomyolysis have been associated with concomitant administration of lipid-altering doses (greater than or equal to 1 g/day) of niacin and HMG-CoA reductase inhibitors. In clinical studies with a combination tablet of *Niaspan* and lovastatin, no cases of rhabdomyolysis and 1 suspected case of myopathy have been reported in 1079 patients who were treated with doses of up to 2000 mg of *Niaspan* and 40 mg of lovastatin daily for periods of up to 2 years. Physicians contemplating combined therapy with HMG-CoA reductase inhibitors and nicotinic acid should carefully weigh the potential benefits and risks and should carefully monitor patients for any signs and symptoms of muscle pain, tenderness, or weakness, particularly during the initial months of therapy and during any periods of upward dosage titration of either drug. Periodic serum creatine phosphokinase (CPK) and potassium determinations should be considered in such situations, but there is no assurance that such monitoring will prevent the occurrence of severe myopathy.

➤*Anticoagulants: Niaspan* extended-release tablets have been associated with small but statistically significant dose-related reductions in platelet count (mean of −11% with 2000 mg). In addition, *Niaspan* extended-release tablets have been associated with small but statistically significant increases in prothrombin time (mean of approximately +4%); accordingly, patients undergoing surgery should be carefully evaluated. Caution should be observed when *Niaspan* extended-release tablets are administered concomitantly with anticoagulants; prothrombin time and platelet counts should be monitored closely in such patients.

➤*Antihypertensive therapy:* Niacin may potentiate the effects of ganglionic blocking agents and vasoactive drugs resulting in postural hypotension.

➤*Aspirin:* Concomitant aspirin may decrease the metabolic clearance of nicotinic acid. The clinical relevance of this finding is unclear.

➤*Alcohol or hot drinks:* Concomitant alcohol or hot drinks may increase the side effects of flushing and pruritus and should be avoided around the time of nicotinic acid ingestion.

➤*Bile-acid sequestrants:* An in vitro study was carried out investigating the niacin-binding capacity of colestipol and cholestyramine. About 98% of available niacin was bound to colestipol, with 10% to 30% binding to cholestyramine. These results suggest that 4 to 6 hours, or as great an interval as possible, should elapse between the ingestion of bile acid-binding resins and the administration of niacin extended-release tablets or other niacin products.

➤*Other sources of niacin:* Vitamins or other nutritional supplements containing large doses of niacin or related compounds such as nicotinamide may potentiate the adverse effects of niacin extended-release tablets or other niacin products.

➤*Drug/Lab test interactions:* Niacin may produce false elevations in some fluorometric determinations of plasma or urinary catecholamines. Niacin may also give false-positive reactions with cupric sulfate solution (Benedict's reagent) in urine glucose tests.

Adverse Reactions

➤*Miscellaneous:* Niacin may cause temporary flushing, itching and tingling, feelings of warmth and headache, particularly when beginning, increasing amount or changing brands of niacin. These effects seldom require discontinuing niacin use. Skin rash, upset stomach, and low blood pressure when standing are less common symptoms; if they persist, contact a physician.

➤*Niaspan* extended-release tablets: *Niaspan* extended-release tablets are generally well tolerated; adverse reactions have been mild and transient. In the placebo-controlled clinical trials, flushing episodes (ie, warmth, redness, itching or tingling) were the most common treatment-emergent adverse events (reported by as many as 88% of patients) for *Niaspan* extended-release tablets. Spontaneous reports suggest that flushing may also be accompanied by symptoms of dizziness, tachycardia, palpitations, shortness of breath, sweating, chills, or edema, which in rare cases may lead to syncope. In pivotal studies, fewer than 6% (14/245) of *Niaspan* extended-

NIACIN — ORAL

release tablet patients discontinued due to flushing. In comparisons of immediate-release niacin and *Niaspan* extended-release tablets, although the proportion of patients who flushed was similar, fewer flushing episodes were reported by patients who received *Niaspan* extended-release tablets. Following 4 weeks of maintenance therapy at daily doses of 1500 mg, the incidence of flushing over the 4-week period averaged 8.56 events per patient for IR niacin versus 1.88 following *Niaspan* extended-release tablets.

Other adverse reactions occurring in 5% or greater of patients treated with *Niaspan* extended-release tablets, at least remotely related to *Niaspan* extended-release tablets, are shown in the table below.

Niacin Treatment-Emergent Adverse Reactions by Dose Level in ≥ 5% of Patients; Reactions Considered at Least Remotely Related to Study Medication

	Placebo-controlled studies *Niaspan* extended-release tablets treatment[a]						
		Recommended daily maintenance doses				Greater than recommended daily doses	
Adverse reaction	Placebo (n = 157) %	500 mg[b] (n = 87) %	1,000 mg (n = 110) %	1,500 mg (n = 136) %	2,000 mg (n = 95) %	2,500 mg[b] (n = 49) %	3,000 mg[b] (n = 46) %
Headache	15%	5%[c]	9%	11%	8%	4%[c]	4%
Pain	3%	1%	2%	5%	3%	0%	2%
Pain, abdominal	3%	3%	2%	3%	5%	0%	0%
Diarrhea	8%	6%	7%	6%	8%	10%	11%
Dyspepsia	8%	2%	4%	5%	5%	6%	0%
Nausea	4%	2%	5%	3%	8%	10%	4%
Vomiting	2%	0%	2%	3%	8%[c]	8%	2%
Rhinitis	7%	2%	5%	4%	3%	0%	0%
Pruritus	1%	6%	less than 1%	3%	1%	0%	0%
Rash	less than 1%	5%	5%	4%	0%	0%	0%

[a] Pooled results from placebo-controlled studies; for *Niaspan* extended-release tablets, (n = 245) and mean treatment duration = 17 weeks. Number of *Niaspan* extended-release tablet patients (n) are not additive across doses.
[b] The 500 mg, 2500 mg and 3000 mg/day doses are outside the recommended daily maintenance dosing range.
[c] Significantly different from placebo at P ≤ 0.05; Chi-square test (cell sizes greater than 5), Fisher's Exact test (cell sizes less than or equal to 5). In general, the incidence of adverse events was higher in women compared to men.

➤*Niaspan* extended-release tablets: The following adverse reactions have also been reported with niacin products, either during clinical trials or in routine patient management.

Cardiovascular – Atrial fibrillation, and other cardiac arrhythmias; tachycardia; palpitations; orthostasis; syncope; hypotension.

CNS – Dizziness, insomnia.

Dermatologic – Hyperpigmentation; acanthosis nigricans; maculopapular rash; urticaria; dry skin; sweating.

Hematologic – Slight reductions in platelet counts and prolongation in prothrombin time.

GI – Activation of peptic ulcers and peptic ulceration; jaundice.

Lab test abnormalities – Elevations in serum transaminases, LDH, fasting glucose, uric acid, total bilirubin, and amylase; reductions in phosphorus.

Metabolic – Decreased glucose tolerance; gout.

Musculoskeletal – Myalgia.

Ophthalmic – Toxic amblyopia, cystoid macular edema.

Miscellaneous – Edema, asthenia, chills, migraine.

➤*Niacor* tablets:

Cardiovascular – Atrial fibrillation and other cardiac arrhythmias; orthostasis; hypotension.

CNS – Headache.

Dermatologic – Mild to severe cutaneous flushing; pruritus; hyperpigmentation; acanthosis nigricans; dry skin.

GI – Dyspepsia; vomiting; diarrhea; peptic ulceration; jaundice; abnormal liver function tests.

Metabolic – Decreased glucose-tolerance; hyperuricemia; gout.

Ophthalmic – Toxic amblyopia; cystoid macular edema.

Overdosage

➤*Treatment:* Supportive measures should be undertaken in the event of an overdosage.

Patient Information

➤*OTC:* Use of niacin may cause skin flushing, burning, itching, or rash.

May cause GI upset; take with meals.

Do not take more than 500 mg of niacin per day or switch to more than 250 mg of timed-release niacin per day, except under the supervision of a doctor.

Discontinue use and consult a physician immediately if any of the following symptoms occur: Persistent flu-like symptoms (nausea, vomiting, a general "not well" feeling); loss of appetite; a decrease in urine output associated with dark-colored urine; muscle discomfort such as tender, swollen muscles or muscle weakness; irregular heartbeat; or cloudy or blurry vision.

If you are pregnant or breastfeeding, consult with your doctor prior to use.

If dizziness (postural hypotension) occurs, avoid sudden changes in posture.

Extended-release products – Swallow whole; do not break, crush, or chew.

➤*Rx:* Cutaneous flushing and a sensation of warmth, especially of the face and upper body, may occur. Itching or tingling and headache also may occur. These effects are transient and usually subside with continued therapy.

Niaspan extended-release tablets – Take *Niaspan* extended-release tablets at bedtime after a low-fat snack. Administration on an empty stomach is not recommended.

Carefully follow the prescribed dosing regimen, including the recommended titration schedule, in order to minimize side effects.

Flushing is a common side effect of niacin therapy. Flushing may vary in severity, may last for several hours after dosing, and will, by taking *Niaspan* extended-release tablets at bedtime, most likely occur during sleep; however, if awakened by flushing at night, get up slowly, especially if feeling dizzy, feeling faint, or taking blood pressure medications.

Taking aspirin (approximately 30 minutes before taking *Niaspan* extended-release tablets) or a nonsteroidal anti-inflammatory drug (eg, ibuprofen) may minimize flushing.

Avoid ingestion of alcohol or hot drinks around the time of *Niaspan* extended-release tablets administration, to minimize flushing.

If *Niaspan* extended-release tablet therapy is discontinued for an extended length of time, the physician should be contacted prior to re-starting therapy; retitration is recommended.

Notify physician if they are taking vitamins or other nutritional supplements containing niacin or related compounds such as nicotinamide.

Notify physician if symptoms of dizziness occur. Avoid sudden changes in posture.

If diabetic, notify physician of changes in blood glucose.

Niaspan extended-release tablets should not be broken, crushed or chewed, but should be swallowed whole.

NIACINAMIDE (NICOTINAMIDE)

otc[a]	**Niacinamide (Nicotinamide)** (Various, eg, Freeda)	**Tablets:** 100 mg	In 100s and 250s.
		500 mg	In 100s and 250s.

[a] Some products may be available *Rx*, according to distributor discretion.

NIACINAMIDE — ORAL

For complete and comparative prescribing information, refer to the Niacin monograph. For additional information, refer to the Dietary Reference Intakes of Vitamins and Minerals table.

Indications

➤*Dietary supplement:* Niacinamide, 1 of 2 principle forms of niacin, is used as a dietary supplement when niacin intake may be inadequate.

➤*Pellagra:* Niacinamide is used in the prophylaxis and treatment of pellagra, a niacin deficiency condition. Symptoms of pellagra include stomach problems, sores in the mouth, anemia, and a triad of symptoms including dermatitis, diarrhea, and dementia.

➤*Off-label uses:* Treatment of several dermatologic conditions, including necrobiosis lipoidica, erythema multiforme, dermatitis herpetiformis, erythema elevatum diutinum, polymorphic light eruption, erythema induration, granuloma annulare, and psoriasis (500 mg 3 times daily).

Administration and Dosage

➤*General dosing considerations:* To treat deficiency, the dose is determined by the health care provider for each individual based on the severity of deficiency.

➤*Adults:*

Dietary supplement – 1 tablet daily.

➤*Administration:* Administer with food and liquid.

➤*Storage/Stability:* Store away from heat and direct light.

Actions

➤*Pharmacology:* Niacinamide is synonymous with nicotinamide, 3-pyridine carboxamide, and nicotinic acid amide. Nicotinic acid is present in the body as its active form, nicotinamide (niacinamide). Nicotinamide and nicotinic acid have identical vitamin activities, but they have very different pharmacological activities. Nicotinamide functions in the body as a component of 2 coenzymes: NAD (nicotinamide adenine dinucleotide, coenzyme I) and NADP (nicotinamide adenine dinucleotide phosphate, coenzyme II). These coenzymes participate in glycogenolysis, fatty metabolism, and tissue respiration. Although nicotinic acid and nicotinamide function identically as vitamins, their pharmacologic effects differ. Nicotinamide does not have the hypolipidemic or vasodilating effects characteristic of niacin (nicotinic acid). Nicotinamide has been shown to inhibit activated macrophage killing of beta cells in vitro and reduce induction of class II MHC protein on mouse beta cells.

Contraindications

Hepatic dysfunction; active peptic ulcer; hypersensitivity to nicotinamide or any ingredient.

Warnings/Precautions

➤*Special risk:* Use niacinamide cautiously in patients with diabetes mellitus, gout, liver disease, or stomach ulcers.

➤*Pregnancy:* *Category A*; *Category C* if used in doses above the RDA (per Briggs' *Drugs in Pregnancy and Lactation*). Avoid niacinamide use in excess of the RDA during normal pregnancy.

➤*Lactation:* Avoid niacinamide use in excess of the RDA during normal breastfeeding. Niacin, the precursor toniacinamide, is actively excreted into breast milk.

Adverse Reactions

➤*GI:* Nausea, vomiting, diarrhea, abdominal pain, dyspepsia.

➤*Hepatic:* Liver dysfunction at high doses.

Patient Information

Cutaneous flushing and a sensation of warmth, especially in the face, may occur. Itching or tingling and headache may also occur. These effects are transient and will usually subside with continued therapy.

May cause GI upset; take with meals.

Discontinue use and consult a physician immediately if any of the following symptoms occur: Persistent flu-like symptoms (nausea, vomiting, a general "not well" feeling; loss of appetite; a decrease in urine output associated with dark-colored urine; muscle discomfort such as tender, swollen muscles or muscle weakness; irregular heartbeat; or cloudy or blurry vision.

If dizziness (postural hypotension) occurs, avoid sudden changes in posture.

PYRIDOXINE HYDROCHLORIDE (B_6)

otc	**Vitamin B_6** (Various, eg, Freeda, Goldline, Nutro Labs)	**Tablets:** 50 mg	In 100s, 250s, and 1000s.
otc	**Vitamin B_6** (Various, eg, Freeda, Goldline, Naturally)	**Tablets:** 100 mg	In 100s and 250s.
otc	**Vitamin B_6** (Various, eg, Freeda)	**Tablets:** 250 mg	In 100s.
otc	**Vitamin B_6** (Various, eg, Naturally)	**Tablets:** 500 mg	In 100s.
otc	**Aminoxin** (Tyson & Assoc.)	**Tablets, enteric-coated:** 20 mg[a]	In 100s.
Rx	**Pyridoxine HCl** (Various)	**Injection:** 100 mg/mL[b]	In 1 mL vials.[c]

[a] As pyridoxal-5'-phosphate.
[b] As pyridoxine HCl.
[c] Also contains 5 mg chorobutanol anhydrous.

PYRIDOXINE HYDROCHLORIDE — ORAL

For additional information, refer to the Dietary Reference Intakes of Vitamins and Minerals table.

Indications

➤*Pyridoxine deficiency:* Pyridoxine is used as a dietary supplement to treat pyridoxine deficiency, including drug-induced deficiency (eg, isoniazid, hydralazine, oral contraceptives).

➤*Off-label uses:*

Palmar-plantar erythrodysesthesia syndrome – [2] = Fair documentation. Despite the lack of controlled data, this treatment appears to show promise with minimal side effects and would be recommended as there are few options available for patients with palmar-plantar erythrodysesthesia. (See Administration and Dosage.)

Tardive dyskinesia – [4] = Insufficient documentation. There is limited published information regarding the use of pyridoxine for the treatment of antipsychotic-induced tardive dyskinesia. Although initial data are promising, optimal dosing, dosing frequency, and best candidates have not been established. Larger trials are needed before this drug can be recommended for universal use. (See Administration and Dosage.)

Other possible off-label uses –

Hydrazine poisoning: Although experience is limited, reversal of neurologic symptoms and CNS depression have been reported.

Premenstrual syndrome (PMS): PMS has been treated with pyridoxine 40 to 500 mg/day, but with conflicting results.

Hyperoxaluria type I: Hyperoxaluria type I (and oxalate kidney stones) has been treated with pyridoxine in low doses (25 to 300 mg/day).

Nausea and vomiting in pregnancy: Pyridoxine may treat nausea and vomiting during pregnancy.

Carpal tunnel syndrome: 100 to 200 mg/day for greater than or equal to 12 weeks.

Administration and Dosage

➤*Adults:*

Pyridoxine deficiency – 100 to 200 mg daily.

Off-label dosing –

Palmar-plantar erythrodysesthesia syndrome: [2] = Fair documentation. 50 to 150 mg daily.

Tardive dyskinesia: [4] = Insufficient documentation. 100 to 400 mg per day for 4 to 8 weeks.

➤*Children:*

Off-label dosing –

Neuritis (drug-induced):

- *Usual dose* – 10 to 50 mg/day.
- *Prophylactic dosage* – 1 to 2 mg/kg/day.

Pyridoxine deficiency:

- *Initial dosage* – 5 to 25 mg/day for 3 weeks.
- *Maintenance dosage* – Following the initial dosage, the maintenance dosage is 1.5 to 2.5 mg/day.

Pyridoxine-dependent seizures:

- *Neonates and infants* –
  Initial dosage: 50 to 100 mg IM or IV push as a single dose.
  Maintenance dosage: 50 to 100 mg/day orally.

➤*Storage/Stability:* Store away from heat and direct light.

Actions

➤*Pharmacology:* Pyridoxine, pyridoxal, or pyridoxamine (in animals) are converted to the physiologically active forms of vitamin B6, pyridoxal phosphate and pyridoxamine phosphate.

Pyridoxine is a coenzyme in the metabolism of amino acids, glycogen, and sphingoid bases and necessary for normal breakdown of proteins, carbohydrates, and fats. Vitamin B_6 is essential to make hemoglobin and helps increase the amount of oxygen carried by hemoglobin. Vitamin B_6 is also involved in maintaining the health of the immune system including maintaining the health of lymphoid organs (thymus, spleen, and lymph nodes) that make white blood cells. Vitamin B_6 maintains normal levels of blood glucose by helping convert stored carbohydrates or other nutrients to glucose. Vitamin B_6 also is needed for the conversion of tryptophan to niacin.

Vitamin B_6 deficiency is extremely rare in humans; symptoms include ataxia, muscle weakness, nystagmus, and losses in touch and pain sensations.

➤*Pharmacokinetics:*

Absorption/Distribution – Vitamin B_6 is absorbed by passive diffusion in the jejunum and to a lesser extent in the ileum.

PYRIDOXINE HYDROCHLORIDE — ORAL

Metabolism/Excretion – Vitamin B_6 is converted to pyridoxal-5-phosphate in the liver and excreted mostly as 4-pyridoxic acid in the urine.

Contraindications

Sensitivity to pyridoxine.

Warnings/Precautions

➤*Pyridoxine deficiency:* Pyridoxine deficiency alone is rare; multiple vitamin deficiencies can be expected in any inadequate diet. Some drugs may result in increased pyridoxine requirements, including the following: Cycloserine, hydralazine, isoniazid, oral contraceptives, and penicillamine.

➤*Special risk:* Use pyridoxine cautiously in patients being treated with levodopa and phenytoin.

➤*Drug abuse and dependence:* Noted in adults withdrawn from 200 mg/day.

➤*Pregnancy: Category A* (*Category C* in doses that exceed the RDA). Avoid pyridoxine use in excess of the RDA during normal pregnancy. The RDA of pyridoxine is 1.9 mg/day during pregnancy.

➤*Lactation:* Vitamin B_6 is excreted in breast milk and is directly proportional to maternal intake. Convulsions have been reported in infants fed a pyridoxine-deficient diet. Neonatal seizures have been noted following birth in a mother consuming pyridoxine 80 mg/day or in infants whose mothers' breast milk contained 67 mcg/day (less than 20 ng/mL in a separate report). These seizures responded to pyridoxine therapy. Pyridoxine has been reported to inhibit lactation at oral doses of 600 mg/day.

Avoid pyridoxine use in excess of the RDA during normal breastfeeding. The RDA of pyridoxine is 2 mg/day for nursing mothers.

➤*Children:* Safety and efficacy have not been established for use in children in doses that exceed the RDA.

Drug Interactions

Pyridoxine Drug Interactions

Precipitant drug	Object drug[a]		Description
Pyridoxine	Levodopa	⬇	Pyridoxine reduces levodopa's effectiveness by increasing its peripheral metabolism; therefore, lower levels are available for CNS penetration.
Pyridoxine	Phenytoin	⬇	Phenytoin serum levels may be decreased.

[a] ⬇ = object drug decreased.

Adverse Reactions

Sensory neuropathic syndromes; unstable gait; numb feet; awkwardness of hands; perioral numbness; decreased sensation to touch, temperature, and vibration; paresthesia; photoallergic reaction; ataxia.

Overdosage

➤*Symptoms:* Patients receiving 2 to 7 g/day (or greater than 0.2 g/day for longer than 2 months) have developed sensory neuropathy with associated ataxia and numbness of the hands and feet. When pyridoxine is discontinued, symptoms will lessen. It may take 6 months for sensation to normalize.

PYRIDOXINE HYDROCHLORIDE — INJECTION

For additional information, refer to the Dietary Reference Intakes of Vitamins and Minerals table.

Indications

➤*Pyridoxine deficiency:* For the treatment of pyridoxine deficiency as seen in the following: Inadequate dietary intake, drug-induced deficiency, as from isoniazid (INH) or oral contraceptives, and inborn errors of metabolism, eg, vitamin B_6-dependent convulsions or vitamin B_6-responsive anemia.

The parenteral route is indicated when oral administration is not feasible as in anorexia, nausea and vomiting, and preoperative and postoperative conditions. It is also indicated when GI absorption is impaired.

➤*Off-label uses:*

Hydrazine poisoning – Although experience is limited, reversal of neurologic symptoms and CNS depression have been reported.

Premenstrual syndrome (PMS) – PMS has been treated with pyridoxine 40 to 500 mg/day, but with conflicting results.

Hyperoxaluria type I – Hyperoxaluria type I (and oxalate kidney stones) has been treated with pyridoxine in low doses (25 to 300 mg/day).

Administration and Dosage

➤*General dosing considerations:* The parenteral route is indicated when oral administration is not feasible as in anorexia, nausea and vomiting, and preoperative and postoperative conditions. It is also indicated when GI absorption is impaired.

➤*Adults:*

INH poisoning – An equal amount of pyridoxine to ingested INH should be given 4 g IV followed by 1 g IM every 30 minutes.

Pyridoxine deficiency –

Dietary deficiency:

- *Initial dosage* – 10 to 20 mg IM or IV daily for 3 weeks.
- *Maintenance dosage* – 2 to 5 mg orally daily for several weeks.

INH-induced deficiencies:

- *Usual dosage* – 100 mg IM or IV daily for 3 weeks.
- *Maintenance dosage* – 30 mg daily.
- *Vitamin B_6-dependency syndrome* – May require as much as 600 mg/day and a daily intake of 30 mg for life.

➤*Children:*

Off-label dosing –

Pyridoxine deficiency:

- *Initial dosage* – 5 to 25 mg/day IM or IV for 3 weeks.
- *Maintenance dosage* – 1.5 to 2.5 mg/day IM or IV.

Pyridoxine dependent seizures:

- *Younger than 1 year* –
  Initial dosage: 50 to 100 mg/dose IM or IV once.
  Maintenance dosage: 50 to 100 mg/day orally.

➤*Administration:* May be administered IM or IV. Use only if solution is clear and seal is intact.

➤*Storage/Stability:* Store between 15° and 30°C (59° and 86°F). Protect from light.

Actions

➤*Pharmacology:* Natural substances that have vitamin B_6 activity are pyridoxine in plants and pyridoxal or pyridoxamine in animals. All 3 are converted to pyridoxal phosphate by the enzyme pyridoxal kinase. The physiologically active forms of vitamin B_6 are pyridoxal phosphate (codecarboxylase) and pyridoxamine phosphate. Riboflavin is required for the conversion of pyridoxine phosphate to pyridoxal phosphate.

Vitamin B_6 acts as a coenzyme in the metabolism of protein, carbohydrate, and fat. In protein metabolism, it participates in the decarboxylation of amino acids, conversion of tryptophan to niacin or to serotonin (5-hydroxtryptamine), deamination, and transamination and transulfuration of amino acids. In carbohydrate metabolism, it is responsible for the breakdown of glycogen to glucose-1-phosphate.

➤*Pharmacokinetics:* The need for pyridoxine increases with the amount of protein in the diet. The tryptophan load test appears to uncover early vitamin B_6 deficiency by detecting xanthinurea. The average adult minimum daily requirement is about 1.25 mg. The dietary reference intake (DRI) is as much as 1.7 mg for adult males, 1.5 mg for adult females, 1.9 mg for pregnant women, and 2 mg for lactating women. The requirements are more in persons having certain genetic defects or those being treated with isonicotinic acid hydrazide (INHJ) or oral contraceptives.

Metabolism/Excretion – The total adult body pool consists of 16 to 25 mg of pyridoxine. Its half-life appears to be 15 to 20 days. Vitamin B_6 is degraded to 4-pyridoxic acid in the liver. This metabolite is excreted in the urine.

Contraindications

Sensitivity to pyridoxine or to any ingredient in this preparation.

Warnings/Precautions

➤*Multiple vitamin deficiency:* Single deficiency, as of pyridoxine alone, is rare. Multiple vitamin deficiency is to be expected in any inadequate diet.

➤*Oral contraceptives:* Women taking oral contraceptives may exhibit increased pyridoxine requirements.

➤*Drug abuse and dependence:* Symptoms of dependence have been noted in adults given only 200 mg daily, followed by withdrawal.

➤*Pregnancy: Category A.* The requirement for pyridoxine appears to be increased during pregnancy. Pyridoxine is sometimes of value in the treatment of nausea and vomiting of pregnancy.

➤*Lactation:* The need for pyridoxine is increased during lactation. It is not known whether this drug is excreted in human milk. Because many drugs are excreted in human milk, caution should be exercised when pyridoxine HCl is administered to a nursing woman.

➤*Children:* Safety and efficacy in children have not been established.

Drug Interactions

Pyridoxine Drug Interactions

Precipitant drug	Object drug[a]		Description
Pyridoxine	Levodopa	⬇	Pyridoxine reduces levodopa's effectiveness by increasing its peripheral metabolism; therefore, lower levels are available for CNS penetration.
Pyridoxine	Phenytoin	⬇	Phenytoin serum levels may be decreased.

[a] ⬇ = object drug decreased.

➤*Levodopa:* Pyridoxine supplements (greater than 5 mg/day) should not be given to patients receiving levodopa, because the action of the latter drug

PYRIDOXINE HYDROCHLORIDE — INJECTION

is antagonized by pyridoxine. However, this vitamin may be used concurrently in patients receiving a preparation containing both carbidopa and levodopa.

Adverse Reactions

Paresthesia, somnolence, and low serum folic acid levels have been reported.

Overdosage

➤*Symptoms:* Pyridoxine given to animals in amounts of 3 to 4 g/kg of body weight produces convulsions and death. In man, a dose of 25 mg/kg of body weight is well tolerated.

COBALAMIN (B_{12})
CYANOCOBALAMIN (B_{12})

otc	**Vitamin B_{12}** (Various, eg, Apothecary)	**Tablets; oral:** 100 mcg	In 100s.
otc	**Vitamin B_{12}** (Various, eg, Goldline)	**Tablets; oral:** 500 mcg	In 100s.
		1,000 mcg	In 100s.
otc	**Vitamin B_{12}** (Goldline)	**Tablets; oral:** 500 mcg	As crystalline cyanocobalamin. Pink. In 100s.
		1,000 mcg	As crystalline cyanocobalamin. Pink. In 100s.
otc	**Twelve Resin-K** (Key Company)	**Tablets; oral:** 1,000 mcg on resin.	In 60s, 250s, and 1000s.
otc sf	**B-12** (Mason Natural)	**Tablets, extended release; oral:** 1,500 mcg	Gluten free, preservative free, sugar free. In 60s.
otc	**Vitamin B_{12}** (Mason)	**Tablets; sublingual:** 1,000 mcg	Dextrose. In 100s.
otc	**Vitamin B_{12}** (Nature's Blend)	**Tablets; sublingual:** 2,500 mcg	Gluten free, preservative free. Sorbitol. In 100s.
otc	**Vitamin B_{12}** (Mason)	**Tablet; sublingual:** 5,000 mcg	As cyanocobalamin and 100 mcg dibencozide/coenzyme B-12. Mannitol. In 30s.
otc	**Vitamin B_{12}** (Freeda)	**Lozenges; oral:** 50 mcg	Sorbitol, mannitol. In 100s.
		100 mcg	In 100s.
		250 mcg	In 100s and 250s.
		500 mcg	In 100s and 250s.
Rx	**Nascobal** (Par)	**Spray, solution; intranasal:** 500 mcg per 0.1 mL (500 mcg/actuation)	Benzalkonium chloride. In 2.3 mL (8 doses/bottle).
otc	**Rapid B-12 Energy** (Mason)	**Spray, solution; sublingual:** 200 mcg per spray	Glycerin, potassium sorbate. Peppermint flavor. In 30 mL.
Rx	**Vitamin B_{12}** (Various, eg, Goldline)	**Injection, solution:** 100 mcg per mL	As crystalline cyanocobalamin. In 30 mL vials.
Rx	**Vitamin B_{12}** (Various, eg, American Regent, Geneva, Goldline, Major, Pasadena, Schein, Warner Chilcott)	**Injection, solution:** 1,000 mcg per mL	As crystalline cyanocobalamin. In 10 and 30 mL multi-dose vials.

CYANOCOBALAMIN — ORAL

For additional information, refer to the Dietary Reference Intakes of Vitamins and Minerals table.

Indications

➤*B_{12} deficiency:* Nutritional vitamin B $_{12}$ deficiency.

These products are NOT indicated for treatment of pernicious anemia.

Administration and Dosage

➤*Recommended Dietary Allowances (RDAs):* Adults, 2 mcg/day. For a complete listing of RDAs by age, sex, or condition, refer to the RDA table.

➤*Sublingual:*

Adults – 3 sprays under the tongue. Shake well before use.

➤*Nutritional supplement:* Dosage varies. See individual product literature.

Actions

➤*Pharmacology:* Vitamin B_{12} is essential to growth, cell reproduction, hematopoiesis, nucleic acid, and myelin synthesis. Sources of vitamin B_{12} include liver, meat, fish, and dairy products (eg, milk and cheese). Vitamin B_{12} is not present in foods of plant origin. Deficiency may result in megaloblastic anemia or pernicious anemia. Ten percent to 30% of Americans older than 60 years of age experience atrophic gastritis, resulting in an inability to absorb vitamin B_{12} bound to food protein. Because of enterohepatic recycling, patients who do not absorb, or have a diet deficient in, vitamin B_{12} may not see signs of deficiency for 3 to 5 years.

➤*Pharmacokinetics:* The parietal cells of the stomach secrete intrinsic factor, which regulates the amount of vitamin B_{12} absorbed in the terminal ileum. Simple diffusion is responsible for absorption when more than 30 mcg of vitamin B_{12} is ingested. Bioavailability of oral preparations is ≈ 25%. Vitamin B_{12} is primarily stored in the liver. Enterohepatic circulation plays a key role in recycling vitamin B_{12} from bile and other intestinal secretions. If plasma-binding proteins are saturated, excess free vitamin B_{12} will be excreted in the kidney.

Contraindications

Hypersensitivity to cyanocobalamin.

Warnings/Precautions

➤*Pregnancy: Category A.* (*Category C* in doses that exceed the RDA).

➤*Lactation:* Vitamin B_{12} is excreted into breast milk.

Overdosage

➤*Symptoms:* Vitamin B_{12} is essentially nontoxic in humans. Allergic reactions and hypersensitivity have been reported.

CYANOCOBALAMIN — INTRANASAL

For additional information, refer to the Dietary Reference Intakes of Vitamins and Minerals table.

Indications

➤*Vitamin B_{12} deficiency:*

CaloMist – For maintenance of vitamin B_{12} concentrations after normalization with intramuscular (IM) vitamin B_{12} therapy in patients with vitamin B_{12} deficiency who have no nervous system involvement.

Nascobal – For maintenance of normal hematologic status in pernicious anemia patients who are in remission following IM vitamin B_{12} therapy and who have no nervous system involvement.

Nascobal is also indicated as a supplement for other vitamin B_{12} deficiencies, including the following:

- Dietary deficiency of vitamin B_{12} occurring in strict vegetarians (isolated vitamin B_{12} deficiency is very rare);
- Malabsorption of vitamin B_{12} resulting from structural or functional damage to the stomach where intrinsic factor is secreted, or to the ileum where intrinsic factor facilitates B_{12} absorption. These conditions include HIV infection, AIDS, Crohn disease, tropical sprue, and nontropical sprue (idiopathic steatorrhea, gluten-induced enteropathy). Folate deficiency in these patients is usually more severe than vitamin B_{12} deficiency.
- Inadequate secretion of intrinsic factor resulting from lesions that destroy the gastric mucosa (ingestion of corrosives, extensive neoplasia) and conditions associated with a variable degree of gastric atrophy (eg, multiple sclerosis, HIV infection, AIDS, certain endocrine disorders, iron deficiency, subtotal gastrectomy). Total gastrectomy always produces vitamin B_{12} deficiency. Structural lesions leading to vitamin B_{12} deficiency include regional ileitis, ileal resections, and malignancies.
- Competition for vitamin B_{12} by intestinal parasites or bacteria. The fish tapeworm (*Diphyllobothrium latum*) absorbs huge quantities of vitamin B_{12} and infested patients often have associated gastric atrophy. The blind loop syndrome may produce deficiency of vitamin B_{12} or folate.
- Inadequate utilization of vitamin B_{12}. This may occur if antimetabolites for the vitamin are employed in the treatment of neoplasia.

CYANOCOBALAMIN — INTRANASAL

Administration and Dosage

➤*Adults:*

CaloMist – Initial dose is 1 spray in each nostril once daily (25 mcg per nostril, total daily dose 50 mcg). The dose should be increased to 1 spray in each nostril twice daily (total daily dose 100 mcg) for patients with an inadequate response to once-daily dosing.

Nascobal – Initial dose is 1 spray (500 mcg) administered in 1 nostril once weekly.

➤*Preparation for administration:*

CaloMist – The pump must be primed before the bottle is used for the first time. To prime the pump, place the nozzle between the first and second finger with the thumb on the bottom of the bottle. Pump the unit firmly and quickly then repeat this priming an additional 6 times for a total of 7 priming sprays. Now the nasal spray is ready for first-time use. If 5 or more days elapse since the last use, the pump must be re-primed with two re-priming sprays.

Nascobal – Before the first dose and administration, the pump must be primed. Remove the clear plastic cover and the plastic safety clip from the pump. To prime the pump, place the nozzle between the first and second finger with the thumb on the bottom of the bottle. Pump the unit firmly and quickly until the first appearance of spray, then prime the pump an additional 2 times. Now the nasal spray is ready for use. The unit must be re-primed before each dose. Prime the pump once immediately before each administration of doses 2 through 8.

➤*Administration:*

CaloMist – The dosing of *CaloMist* and other intranasal medications should be separated by several hours, and these patients should have more frequent monitoring of vitamin B_{12} concentrations because of the potential for erratic absorption.

Nascobal – *Nascobal* nasal spray should be administered at least 1 hour before or 1 hour after ingestion of hot foods or liquids. Periodic monitoring of serum B_{12} levels should be obtained to establish adequacy of therapy.

➤*Storage / Stability:* Protect from light. Keep *Nascobal* covered in carton until ready to use. Store upright at controlled room temperature (15° to 30°C; 59° to 86°F). Protect from freezing.

Actions

➤*Pharmacology:* Vitamin B_{12} is essential to growth, cell reproduction, hematopoiesis, and nucleoprotein and myelin synthesis. Cells characterized by rapid division (eg, epithelial cells, bone marrow, myeloid cells) appear to have the greatest requirements for vitamin B_{12}. Vitamin B_{12}can be converted to coenzyme B_{12} in tissues, and as such is essential for conversion of methylmalonate to succinate and synthesis of methionine from homocysteine, a reaction that also requires folate. In the absence of coenzyme B_{12}, tetrahydrofolate cannot be regenerated from its inactive storage form, 5-methyl tetrahydrofolate, and a functional folate deficiency occurs. Vitamin B_{12} also may be involved in maintaining sulfhydryl (SH) groups in the reduced form required by many SH-activated enzyme systems. Through these reactions, vitamin B_{12} is associated with fat and carbohydrate metabolism and protein synthesis. Vitamin B_{12} deficiency results in megaloblastic anemia, GI lesions, and neurologic damage that begins with an inability to produce myelin and is followed by gradual degeneration of the axon and nerve head.

Cyanocobalamin is the most stable and widely used form of vitamin B_{12}, and has hematopoietic activity apparently identical to that of the antianemia factor in purified liver extract. The following information, describing the clinical pharmacology of cyanocobalamin, has been derived from studies with injectable vitamin B_{12}.

Vitamin B_{12} is quantitatively and rapidly absorbed from IM and subcutaneous sites of injection. It is bound to plasma proteins and stored in the liver. Vitamin B_{12} is excreted in the bile and undergoes some enterohepatic recycling. Absorbed vitamin B_{12} is transported via specific B_{12} binding proteins, transcobalamin I and II, to the various tissues. The liver is the main organ for vitamin B_{12} storage.

Parenteral (IM) administration of vitamin B_{12} completely reverses the megaloblastic anemia and GI symptoms of vitamin B_{12} deficiency. The degree of improvement in neurologic symptoms depends on the duration and severity of the lesions, although progression of the lesions is immediately arrested.

GI absorption of vitamin B_{12} depends on the presence of sufficient intrinsic factor and calcium ions. Intrinsic factor deficiency causes pernicious anemia, which may be associated with subacute combined degeneration of the spinal cord. Prompt parenteral administration of vitamin B_{12} prevents progression of neurologic damage.

The average diet supplies about 4 to 15 mcg/day of vitamin B_{12} in a protein-bound form that is available for absorption after normal digestion. Vitamin B_{12} is not present in foods of plant origin, but is abundant in foods of animal origin. In people with normal absorption, deficiencies have been reported only in strict vegetarians who do not consume products of animal origin (including milk products or eggs).

Vitamin B_{12} is bound to intrinsic factor during transit through the stomach. Separation occurs in the terminal ileum in the presence of calcium, and vitamin B_{12} enters the mucosal cell for absorption. It is then transported by the transcobalamin binding proteins. A small amount (approximately 1% of the total amount ingested) is absorbed by simple diffusion, but this mechanism is adequate only with very large doses. Oral absorption is considered too unreliable for patients with pernicious anemia or other conditions resulting in malabsorption of vitamin B_{12}.

Colchicine, para-aminosalicylic acid, and heavy alcohol intake for longer than 2 weeks may produce malabsorption of vitamin B_{12}.

➤*Pharmacokinetics:*

Absorption – A 3-way crossover study in 25 fasting healthy subjects was conducted to compare the bioavailability of the B_{12} nasal spray to the B_{12} nasal gel and to evaluate the relative bioavailability of the nasal formulations as compared with the IM injection. The peak concentrations after administration of intranasal spray were reached in 1.25 ± 1.9 hours. The average peak concentration of B_{12} obtained after baseline correction following administration of intranasal spray was 757.96 ± 532.17 pg/mL. The bioavailability of the nasal spray relative to the IM injection was found to be 6.1%. The bioavailability of the B_{12} nasal spray was found to be 10% less than the B_{12} nasal gel. The 90% confidence intervals for the loge-transformed area under the curve from 0 to time t and maximum drug concentration was 71.71% to 114.19% and 71.6% to 118.66%, respectively.

In pernicious anemia patients, once weekly intranasal dosing with 500 mcg B_{12} gel resulted in a consistent increase in predose serum B_{12} levels during 1 month of treatment ($P < 0.003$) above that seen 1 month after 100 mcg IM dose.

Distribution – In the blood, B_{12} is bound to transcobalamin II, a specific B-globulin carrier protein, and is distributed and stored primarily in the liver and bone marrow.

Excretion – About 3 to 8 mcg of B_{12} is secreted into the GI tract daily via the bile. In healthy subjects with sufficient intrinsic factor, all but about 1 mcg is reabsorbed. When B_{12} is administered in doses that saturate the binding capacity of plasma proteins and the liver, the unbound B_{12} is rapidly eliminated in the urine. Retention of B_{12} in the body is dose-dependent. About 80% to 90% of an IM dose of up to 50 mcg is retained in the body; this percentage drops to 55% for a 100 mcg dose, and decreases to 15% when a 1,000 mcg dose is given.

Contraindications

Sensitivity to cobalt and/or vitamin B_{12} or to any component of this preparation.

Warnings/Precautions

➤*Leber disease:* Patients with early Leber disease (hereditary optic nerve atrophy) treated with vitamin B_{12} suffered severe and swift optic atrophy. Cyanocobalamin should not be used in these patients.

➤*Megaloblastic anemia:*

Nascobal – Hypokalemia and sudden death may occur in severe megaloblastic anemia that is treated intensely with vitamin B_{12}. Folic acid is not a substitute for vitamin B_{12}, although it may improve vitamin B_{12}–deficient megaloblastic anemia. Exclusive use of folic acid in treating vitamin B_{12}–deficient megaloblastic anemia could result in progressive and irreversible neurologic damage.

CaloMist – Megaloblastic anemia has many causes, including vitamin B_{12} deficiency and folate deficiency. Folic acid may result in a hematological response in patients with vitamin B_{12} deficiency, but will not prevent irreversible neurological manifestations. Vitamin B_{12} is not an appropriate treatment for folate deficiency.

Hypokalemia, thrombocytosis, and sudden death may occur when severe megaloblastic anemia is treated intensely with vitamin B_{12}. Carefully monitor serum potassium and platelet count in this setting.

➤*Blunted response to vitamin B_{12} therapy:* Blunted or impeded therapeutic response to vitamin B_{12} may be caused by such conditions as infection, uremia, drugs having bone marrow suppressant properties (eg, chloramphenicol), and concurrent iron or folic acid deficiency.

➤*Vitamin B_{12} deficiency:* Vitamin B_{12} deficiency that is allowed to progress for longer than 3 months may produce permanent degenerative lesions of the spinal cord. Dosages of folic acid of more than 0.1 mg/day may result in hematologic remission in patients with vitamin B_{12} deficiency. Neurologic manifestations will not be prevented with folic acid, and if not treated with vitamin B_{12}, irreversible damage will result.

If a patient is not properly maintained with intranasal vitamin B_{12}, IM vitamin B_{12} is necessary for adequate treatment of the patient. No single regimen fits all cases, and the status of the patient observed in follow-up is the final criterion for adequacy of therapy.

It may be possible to treat the underlying disease by surgical correction of anatomic lesions leading to small bowel bacterial overgrowth, expulsion of fish tapeworm, discontinuation of drugs leading to vitamin malabsorption, use of a gluten-free diet in nontropical sprue, or administration of antibiotics in tropical sprue. Such measures remove the need for long-term administration of vitamin B_{12}.

Requirements of vitamin B_{12} in excess of normal (because of pregnancy, thyrotoxicosis, hemolytic anemia, hemorrhage, malignancy, and hepatic and renal disease) can usually be met with intranasal or oral supplementation.

➤*Folate deficiency:* Dosages of vitamin B_{12} exceeding 10 mcg/day may produce a hematologic response in patients with folate deficiency. Indiscriminate administration may mask the true diagnosis.

Vitamin B_{12} is not a substitute for folic acid, and because it might improve folic acid deficient megaloblastic anemia, indiscriminate use of vitamin B_{12} could mask the true diagnosis.

➤*Hypokalemia and thrombocytosis:* Hypokalemia and thrombocytosis could occur upon conversion of severe megaloblastic to normal erythropoi-

CYANOCOBALAMIN — INTRANASAL

esis with vitamin B_{12} therapy. Therefore, carefully monitor serum potassium levels and platelet count during therapy.

➤*Polycythemia vera:* Vitamin B_{12} deficiency may suppress the signs of polycythemia vera. Treatment with vitamin B_{12} may unmask this condition.

➤*Nasal symptoms:* The effectiveness of intranasal cyanocobalamin in patients with nasal congestion, allergic rhinitis, and upper respiratory tract infections has not been determined. Defer treatment until symptoms have subsided. Patients with chronic nasal symptoms or significant nasal pathology are not ideal candidates for intranasal vitamin B_{12} therapy. If therapy is attempted in these patients, monitor vitamin B_{12} concentrations more frequently than in patients without nasal pathology because of the potential for erratic or blunted absorption.

➤*Hypersensitivity reactions:* Anaphylactic shock, death, and angioedema have been reported after parenteral vitamin B_{12} administration. No such reactions have been reported in clinical trials with *Nascobal* nasal spray, *Nascobal* nasal gel, or *CaloMist* nasal spray.

Test dose – An intradermal test dose of parenteral vitamin B_{12} is recommended before intranasal administration to patients suspected of cyanocobalamin sensitivity.

➤*Renal/Hepatic function impairment:* Patients with vitamin B_{12} deficiency and concurrent renal or hepatic disease may require increased doses or more frequent administration of vitamin B_{12} therapy.

➤*Pregnancy: Category C* (per manufacturer's prescribing information). *Category A* (when used in doses less than the recommended daily allowance per Brigg's *Drugs in Pregnancy and Lactation*). Animal reproduction studies have not been conducted with vitamin B_{12}. It is also not known whether vitamin B_{12} can cause fetal harm when administered to a pregnant woman or can affect reproduction capacity. Adequate and well-controlled studies have not been done in pregnant women; however, vitamin B_{12} is an essential vitamin and requirements are increased during pregnancy. The Food and Nutrition Board, National Academy of Sciences-National Research Council (NAS-NRC) recommends certain amounts of vitamin B_{12} to be consumed by women during pregnancy.

➤*Lactation:* Although vitamin B_{12} is an essential vitamin and requirements are increased during lactation, it is not known whether cyanocobalamin nasal spray can cause harm to an infant when administered to a breast-feeding woman. Vitamin B_{12} appears in the milk of breast-feeding mothers in concentrations that approximate the mother's vitamin B_{12} blood level. Vitamin B_{12} is considered to be compatible with breast-feeding according to the American Academy of Pediatrics. Exercise caution when cyanocobalamin nasal spray is administered to a breast-feeding woman. The Food and Nutrition Board, NAS-NRC, recommends certain amounts of vitamin B_{12} to be consumed by women during lactation.

➤*Children:*

Nascobal – Intake in pediatric patients should be in the amount recommended by the Food and Nutrition Board, NAS-NRC.

CaloMist – Because *CaloMist* nasal spray has not been studied in children, safety and effectiveness have not been established.

➤*Elderly:* In general, dose selection for an elderly patient should be cautious, usually starting at the low end of the dosing range, reflecting the greater frequency of decreased hepatic, renal, or cardiac function, and of concomitant disease or other drug therapy.

➤*Monitoring:* Obtain hematocrit, reticulocyte count, vitamin B_{12}, folate, and iron levels prior to treatment.

Nascobal – If folate levels are low, also administer folic acid. All hematologic parameters should be normal when beginning treatment.

Monitor vitamin B_{12} blood levels and peripheral blood counts 1 month after the start of treatment and then at 3- to 6-month intervals.

A decline in the serum levels of B_{12} after 1 month of treatment with B_{12} nasal spray may indicate that the dose needs to be adjusted upward. Patients should be seen 1 month after each dose adjustment. Continued low levels of serum B_{12} may indicate that the patient is not a candidate for this mode of administration.

Carefully monitor serum potassium levels and platelet count during therapy. Patients with pernicious anemia have about 3 times the incidence of stomach carcinoma when compared with the general population. Perform appropriate tests.

CaloMist – All hematologic parameters, including vitamin B_{12} concentrations, should be normal before initiating treatment with *CaloMist* nasal spray. Periodic monitoring of serum vitamin B_{12} concentrations must be obtained to confirm adequacy of therapy. Monitor vitamin B_{12} concentrations and complete blood counts 1 month after starting *CaloMist* nasal spray and then at 3- to 6-month intervals thereafter. Patients with boderline-low vitamin B_{12} concentrations (less than 300 ng/L) should also undergo measurement of methylmalonic acid and homocysteine concentrations, which are more sensitive measures of vitamin B_{12} deficiency in this setting. Patients with declining or abnormally low vitamin B_{12} concentrations, despite maximal doses of *CaloMist* nasal spray, should be switched back to IM vitamin B_{12} injections. Vitamin B_{12} deficiency that is inadequately treated for longer than 3 months may produce irreversible neurological damage.

Drug Interactions

➤*Bone marrow suppressants:* Bone marrow suppressants (eg, chloramphenicol) may blunt the therapeutic response to vitamin B_{12}.

➤*Drug/Lab test interactions:* Most antibiotics, methotrexate, or pyrimethamine invalidate folic acid and vitamin B_{12} diagnostic blood assays. The validity of diagnostic vitamin B_{12} or folic acid blood assays could be compromised by medications; consider this before relying on such tests for therapy.

Adverse Reactions

➤*Nascobal:* The incidence of adverse reactions described in the table below are based on data from a short-term clinical trial in vitamin B_{12}–deficient patients in hematologic remission receiving *Nascobal* gel for intranasal administration (n = 24) and IM vitamin B_{12} (n = 25). In the pharmacokinetic study comparing *Nascobal* nasal spray and *Nascobal* nasal gel, the incidence of adverse reactions was similar.

Nascobal Adverse Reactions

Adverse reactions	Vitamin B_{12} nasal gel 500 mcg (n = 24)	IM vitamin B_{12} 100 mcg (n = 25)
Cardiovascular		
Peripheral vascular disorder	0%	1%
CNS		
Abnormal gait	0%	1%
Anxiety	0%	1%[a]
Asthenia	1%	4%
Dizziness	0%	3%
Headache	2%[a]	11%
Hypesthesia	0%	1%
Incoordination	0%	2%[a]
Nervousness	0%	3%[a]
Paresthesia	1%	1%
GI		
Dyspepsia	0%	2%
Glossitis	1%	0%
Nausea	1%[a]	1%
Nausea and vomiting	0%	1%
Vomiting	0%	1%
Musculoskeletal		
Arthritis	0%	2%
Back pain	0%	1%
Myalgia	0%	1%
Respiratory		
Dyspnea	0%	1%
Rhinitis	1%[a]	2%
Miscellaneous		
Generalized pain	0%	3%
Infection[b]	4%	3%

[a] There may be a possible relationship between these adverse reactions and the study drugs. These adverse reactions could have also been produced by the patient's clinical state or other concomitant therapy.

[b] Sore throat, common cold.

The intensity of the reported adverse reactions following the administration of cyanocobalamin gel for intranasal administration were generally mild. A few adverse reactions of moderate intensity were reported following dosing with cyanocobalamin gel for intranasal administration (1 headache, 1 infection, and 1 paresthesia).

The majority of the reported adverse reactions following dosing with cyanocobalamin gel for intranasal administration were judged to be intercurrent events. For the other reported adverse reactions, the relationship to the study drug was judged as possible or remote. Of the adverse reactions judged to be of possible relationship to the study drug, headache, nausea, and rhinitis were reported following dosing with cyanocobalamin gel for intranasal administration.

➤*CaloMist:* The following data reflect exposure in 25 subjects (range, 27 to 82 years of age; 17 women; 21 white) with vitamin B_{12} deficiency (12 with pernicious anemia, 4 secondary to GI surgery, and 9 with unknown cause) who received *CaloMist* nasal spray 50 mcg daily for 8 weeks in an uncontrolled clinical trial. Prior to enrollment, all subjects were required to have normal vitamin B_{12} levels with IM vitamin B_{12} injections. One patient who completed the study developed epistaxis on day 12 of dosing and was noted to have irritation of the right nasal septum at study end. This patient had preexisting allergic rhinitis and required a doubling of the *CaloMist* nasal spray dose during the last week of the study because of declining vitamin B_{12} concentrations.

CYANOCOBALAMIN — INTRANASAL

CaloMist Adverse Reactions	
Adverse reactions	*CaloMist* nasal spray (N = 25)
CNS	
Dizziness	12%
Headache	12%
Hypersomnia	4%
Malaise	4%
Dermatologic	
Rash	8%
Musculoskeletal	
Arthralgia	12%
Back pain	4%
Respiratory	
Asthma	4%
Bronchitis	8%
Cough	4%
Epistaxis	4%
Nasal discomfort	8%
Nasopharyngitis	12%
Pharyngolaryngeal pain	4%
Postnasal drip	4%
Rhinorrhea	12%
Sinus headache	4%
Sinusitis	4%
Miscellaneous	
Influenza-like illness	4%
Pain	8%
Procedural pain	4%
Pyrexia	4%
Scab	4%
Tooth abscess	4%

➤*Postmarketing:* The following adverse reactions have been identified during postapproval use of cyanocobalamin. Because these reactions are reported voluntarily from a population of uncertain size, it is not always possible to reliably estimate their frequency or establish a causal relationship to drug exposure: angioedema and angioedema-like reactions.

Overdosage

No overdose has been reported.

Patient Information

➤*Nascobal*: Instruct patients with pernicious anemia that they will require weekly intranasal administration of *Nascobal* nasal spray for the remainder of their lives. Failure to do so will result in return of the anemia and in development of incapacitating and irreversible damage to the nerves of the spinal cord. Also, warn patients about the danger of taking folic acid in place of vitamin B_{12}, because the former may prevent anemia but allow progression of subacute combined degeneration of the spinal cord.

Hot foods may cause nasal secretions and a resulting loss of medication; therefore, tell patients to administer *Nascobal* nasal spray at least 1 hour before or 1 hour after ingestion of hot foods or liquids. A vegetarian diet that contains no animal products (including mild products or eggs) does not supply any vitamin B_{12}. Therefore, advise patients following such a diet to take *Nascobal* nasal spray weekly. The need for vitamin B_{12} is increased by pregnancy and lactation. Deficiency has been recognized in infants who were breastfed by vegetarian mothers, even though the mothers had no symptoms of deficiency at the time.

Because the nasal dosage forms of vitamin B_{12} have a lower absorption than IM dosage, nasal dosage forms are administered weekly, rather than the monthly IM dosage. At the end of a month, weekly nasal administration results in significantly higher serum vitamin B_{12} levels than after IM administration. The patient should also understand the importance of returning for follow-up blood tests every 3 to 6 months to confirm adequacy of the therapy.

Give careful instructions on the actuator assembly, priming of the actuator, and nasal administration of *Nascobal* nasal spray to the patient. Although instructions for patients are supplied with individual bottles, demonstrate procedures for use to each patient.

➤*CaloMist*: Patients with a chronic underlying cause of vitamin B_{12} deficiency will require indefinite administration of a vitamin B_{12} product, such as *CaloMist* nasal spray. Noncompliance or inadequate treatment with vitamin B_{12} therapy may result in recurrence of anemia and the development or worsening of irreversible neurological damage.

The dosing of *CaloMist* nasal spray and other intranasal medications should be separated by several hours.

Vitamin B_{12} concentrations should be monitored 1 month after *CaloMist* nasal spray initiation or dose change and every 3 to 6 months thereafter.

Give careful instructions on the priming of the actuator and nasal administration of *CaloMist* nasal spray to the patient, and demonstrate the procedures for use.

CYANOCOBALAMIN CRYSTALLINE — PARENTERAL

For additional information, refer to the Dietary Reference Intakes of Vitamins and Minerals table.

Administration and Dosage

➤*Pernicious anemia:* Parenteral therapy is required for life; oral therapy is not dependable. Administer 100 mcg daily for 6 or 7 days by IM or deep SC injection. If there is clinical improvement and a reticulocyte response, give the same amount on alternate days for 7 doses, then every 3 to 4 days for another 2 to 3 weeks. By this time, hematologic values should have become normal. Follow this regimen with 100 mcg monthly for life. Administer folic acid concomitantly if needed.

➤*Schilling test:* The flushing dose is 1,000 mcg IM.

➤*Off-label dosing:*

Other patients with vitamin B_{12} deficiency – In seriously ill patients, administer both vitamin B_{12} and folic acid. It is not necessary to withhold therapy until the precise cause of B_{12} deficiency is established. For hematologic signs, children may be given 10 to 50 mcg/day for 5 to 10 days followed by 100 to 250 mcg/dose every 2 to 4 weeks; for neurologic signs, 100 mcg/day for 10 to 15 days, then once or twice weekly for several months, possibly tapering to 250 to 1000 mcg monthly by 1 year.

IM or SC – 30 mcg daily for 5 to 10 days followed by 100 to 200 mcg monthly. Larger doses (eg, 1000 mcg) have been recommended, even though a larger amount is lost through excretion. However, it is possible that a greater amount is retained, allowing for fewer injections.

➤*Storage/Stability:* Protect from light. Avoid freezing.

COBALAMIN (B_{12})
HYDROXOCOBALAMIN

Rx	**Cyanokit** (Dey Labs)	**Injection, lyophilized powder for solution:** 2.5 g	In kits containing two 250 mL vials (2.5 g per vial), 2 sterile transfer spikes, and 1 sterile IV infusion set.
Rx	**Hydroxycobalamin** (Watson)	**Injection, solution:** 1,000 mcg/mL	As hydroxocobalamin acetate. May contain parabens. In 30 mL multidose vials.

HYDROXOCOBALAMIN — INJECTION

Indications

➤*Cyanide poisoning (Cyanokit only)*: For the treatment of known or suspected cyanide poisoning.

➤*Vitamin B_{12} deficiency (excludes Cyanokit)*: For the treatment of pernicious anemia, both uncomplicated and accompanied by nervous system involvement; dietary deficiency of vitamin B_{12} occurring in strict vegetarians and their breast-fed infants (isolated vitamin B_{12} deficiency is very rare); malabsorption of vitamin B_{12} resulting from structural or functional damage to the stomach (where intrinsic factor is secreted), or to the ileum, where intrinsic factor facilitates vitamin B_{12} absorption (these conditions include tropical and nontropical sprue [idiopathic steatorrhea, gluten-induced enteropathy]); inadequate secretion of intrinsic factor resulting from lesions that destroy the gastric mucosa (ingestion of corrosives, extensive neoplasia), and a number of conditions associated with a variable degree of gastric atrophy (eg, multiple sclerosis, certain endocrine disorders, iron deficiency, subtotal gastrectomy); competition for vitamin B_{12} by intestinal parasites or bacteria; inadequate utilization of vitamin B_{12}, which may occur if antimetabolites for the vitamin are employed in the treatment of neoplasia.

Total gastrectomy always produces vitamin B_{12} deficiency.

➤*Schilling test (excludes Cyanokit)*: For the Schilling test.

➤*Off-label uses:* Hydroxocobalamin has been used to prevent and to treat cyanide toxicity associated with sodium nitroprusside.

Administration and Dosage

➤*General dosing considerations:* Comprehensive treatment of acute cyanide intoxication requires support of vital functions. Hydroxocobalamin should be administered in conjunction with appropriate airway, ventilatory, and circulatory support.

In patients with Addisonian pernicious anemia, parenteral therapy with vitamin B_{12} is the recommended method of treatment and will be required for the remainder of the patient's life. Oral therapy is not dependable. In other

HYDROXOCOBALAMIN — INJECTION

patients with vitamin B_{12} deficiency, the duration of therapy and route of administration will depend on the cause and whether or not it is reversible.

➤*Adults:*

Cyanide poisoning – 5 g (ie, both 2.5 g vials) administered as an intravenous (IV) infusion over 15 minutes (approximately 15 mL/min [ie, 7.5 min/vial]).

Depending on the severity of the poisoning and the clinical response, a second dose of 5 g may be administered by IV infusion for a total dose of 10 g. The rate of infusion for the second dose may range from 15 minutes (for patients in extremis) to 2 hours as clinically indicated.

Schilling test – The flushing dose is 1,000 mcg intramuscularly (IM).

Vitamin B_{12} deficiency –

Initial dosage: 30 mcg IM daily for 5 to 10 days.

Maintenance dosage: 100 to 200 mcg IM monthly.

Dosage adjustment: If the patient is critically ill, or has neurologic disease, an infectious disease, or hypothyroidism, considerably higher doses may be indicated. However, current data indicate that the optimum obtainable neurologic response may be expected with a dosage of vitamin B_{12} sufficient to produce good hematologic response.

Conversion: Patients with normal intestinal absorption may be treated with an oral therapeutic multivitamin preparation containing vitamin B_{12} 15 mcg daily.

➤*Children:*

Vitamin B_{12} deficiency –

Initial dosage: A total of 1 to 5 mg over a period of 2 or more weeks in doses of 100 mcg IM.

Maintenance dosage: 30 to 50 mcg IM every 4 weeks.

Off-label dosing –

Cyanide poisoning:

- *Usual dose* – 70 mg/kg IV over 30 minutes as a single infusion.
- *Maximum dose* – 5 g.

➤*Preparation for administration:*

Cyanokit – Each 2.5 g vial of hydroxocobalamin for injection is to be reconstituted with 100 mL of diluent (not provided with hydroxocobalamin) using the supplied sterile transfer spike. The recommended diluent is sodium chloride 0.9% injection. Ringer's lactate injection and dextrose 5% injection have also been found to be compatible with hydroxocobalamin and may be used if sodium chloride 0.9% is not readily available. The line on each vial label represents 100 mL volume of diluent. Following the addition of diluent to the lyophilized powder, each vial should be repeatedly inverted or rocked, not shaken, for at least 30 seconds prior to infusion.

➤*Administration:*

Cyanide poisoning – Administer as an IV infusion over 15 minutes (approximately 15 mL/min). If a second dose is required, the rate of infusion may range from 15 minutes (for patients in extremis) to 2 hours as clinically indicated.

Vitamin B_{12} deficiency – Administer by IM injection only.

➤*Admixture compatibility:*

IV – Physical incompatibility (particle formation) and chemical incompatibility were observed with the mixture of hydroxocobalamin in solution with selected drugs that are frequently used in resuscitation efforts. Hydroxocobalamin is also chemically incompatible with sodium nitrite and sodium thiosulfate and has been reported to be incompatible with ascorbic acid. Consequently, these drugs should not be administered simultaneously through the same IV line as hydroxocobalamin.

Simultaneous administration of hydroxocobalamin and blood products (whole blood, packed red cells, platelet concentrate, and/or fresh frozen plasma) through the same IV line is not recommended. However, blood products and hydroxocobalamin can be administered simultaneously using separate IV lines (preferably on contralateral extremities, if peripheral lines are being used).

Exercise caution when administering other cyanide antidotes simultaneously with hydroxocobalamin because the safety of coadministration has not been established. If a decision is made to administer another cyanide antidote with hydroxocobalamin, do not administer these drugs concurrently in the same IV line.

➤*Storage/Stability:*

Cyanokit – Store at 25°C (77°F); excursions are permitted between 15° and 30°C (59° and 86°F).

Hydroxocobalamin may be exposed during short periods to the temperature variations of usual transport (15 days submitted to temperatures ranging from 5° to 40°C [41° to 104°F]), transport in the desert (4 days submitted to temperatures ranging from 5° to 60°C [41° to 140°F]), and freezing/defrosting cycles (15 days submitted to temperatures ranging from −20° to 40°C [−4° to 104°F]).

Once reconstituted, hydroxocobalamin is stable for up to 6 hours at temperatures not exceeding 40°C (104°F). Do not freeze. Any reconstituted product not used within 6 hours should be discarded.

IM – Store at 20° to 25°C (68° to 77°F). Protect from light.

Actions

➤*Pharmacology:* Vitamin B_{12} is essential to growth, cell reproduction, hematopoiesis, and nucleoprotein and myelin synthesis.

Cyanide poisoning – Cyanide is an extremely toxic poison. In the absence of rapid and adequate treatment, exposure to a high dose of cyanide can result in death within minutes due to the inhibition of cytochrome oxidase, resulting in arrest of cellular respiration. Specifically, cyanide binds rapidly with cytochrome a3, a component of the cytochrome c oxidase complex in mitochondria. Inhibition of cytochrome a3 prevents the cell from using oxygen and forces anaerobic metabolism, resulting in lactate production, cellular hypoxia, and metabolic acidosis. In massive acute cyanide poisoning, the mechanism of toxicity may involve other enzyme systems as well. Signs and symptoms of acute systemic cyanide poisoning may develop rapidly within minutes, depending on the route and extent of cyanide exposure.

The action of hydroxocobalamin in the treatment of cyanide poisoning is based on its ability to bind cyanide ions. Each hydroxocobalamin molecule can bind 1 cyanide ion by substituting it for the hydroxo ligand linked to the trivalent cobalt ion to form cyanocobalamin, which is then excreted in urine.

Pharmacodynamics: Administration of hydroxocobalamin to cyanide-poisoned patients with the attendant formation of cyanocobalamin resulted in increases in blood pressure and variable changes in heart rate upon initiation of hydroxocobalamin infusions.

➤*Pharmacokinetics:*

Absorption –

IM: Fifty percent of the administered dose of hydroxocobalamin disappears from the injection site in 2.5 hours.

Cyanokit: Dose-proportional pharmacokinetics were observed following single-dose IV administration of hydroxocobalamin 2.5 to 10 g in healthy volunteers. Mean free and total cobalamins-(III) maximal drug concentration (C_{max}) values of 113 and 579 mcg Eq/mL, respectively, were determined following a dose of hydroxocobalamin 5 g. Similarly, mean free and total cobalamins-(III) C_{max} values of 197 and 995 mcg Eq/mL, respectively, were determined following the dose of hydroxocobalamin 10 g.

Distribution – Hydroxocobalamin is bound to plasma proteins and stored in the liver.

Cyanokit: Following IV administration of hydroxocobalamin, significant binding to plasma proteins and low molecular weight physiological compounds occurs, forming various cobalamin-(III) complexes by replacing the hydroxo ligand. The low molecular weight cobalamins-(III) formed, including hydroxocobalamin, are termed "free cobalamins-(III)"; the sum of free and protein-bound cobalamins is termed "total cobalamins-(III)."

Excretion – Hydroxocobalamin is excreted in the bile and undergoes some enterohepatic recycling.

IM: Within 72 hours after injection of hydroxocobalamin 500 to 1,000 mcg, 16% to 66% of the injected dose may appear in the urine. The major portion is excreted within the first 24 hours.

Cyanokit: The predominant mean half-life of free and total cobalamins-(III) is approximately 26 to 31 hours at the 5 and 10 g dose levels.

The mean total amount of cobalamins-(III) excreted in urine during the collection period of 72 hours was approximately 60% of a 5 g dose and approximately 50% of a 10 g dose of hydroxocobalamin. Overall, the total urinary excretion was calculated to be at least 60% to 70% of the administered dose. The majority of the urinary excretion occurred during the first 24 hours, but red colored urine was observed for up to 35 days following IV infusion.

Contraindications

Hypersensitivity to any component of this medication.

Warnings/Precautions

➤*Diagnosis:* The validity of diagnostic vitamin B_{12} or folic acid blood assays could be compromised by medications, and this should be considered before relying on these tests for therapy.

➤*Polycythemia vera:* Vitamin B_{12} deficiency may suppress the signs of polycythemia vera. Treatment with vitamin B_{12} may unmask this condition.

➤*Folic acid therapy:* Folic acid is not a substitute for vitamin B_{12}, although it may improve vitamin B_{12}–deficient megaloblastic anemia. Exclusive use of folic acid in treating vitamin B_{12}–deficient megaloblastic anemia could result in progressive and irreversible neurological damage.

Vitamin B_{12} is not a substitute for folic acid and because it might improve folic acid–deficient megaloblastic anemia, indiscriminate use of vitamin B_{12} could mask the true diagnosis.

➤*Inadequate response:* Blunted or impeded therapeutic response to vitamin B_{12} may be due to such conditions as infection, uremia, drugs having bone marrow suppressant properties (eg, chloramphenicol), and concurrent iron or folic acid deficiency.

➤*Emergency patient management:* In addition to hydroxocobalamin, treatment of cyanide poisoning must include immediate attention to airway patency, adequacy of oxygenation and hydration, cardiovascular support, and management of any seizure activity. Consider decontamination measures based on the route of exposure.

➤*Blood pressure changes:* Many patients with cyanide poisoning will be hypotensive; however, elevations in blood pressure have also been observed in known or suspected cyanide poisoning victims.

Elevations in blood pressure (at least 180 mm Hg systolic or at least 110 mm Hg diastolic) were observed in approximately 18% of healthy subjects (not exposed to cyanide) receiving hydroxocobalamin 5 g and 28% of subjects receiving 10 g. Increases in blood pressure were noted shortly after the infusions were started; the maximal increase in blood pressure was observed toward the end of the infusion. These elevations were generally transient and returned to baseline levels within 4 hours of dosing.

HYDROXOCOBALAMIN — INJECTION

➤*Hypersensitivity reactions:* Use caution in the management of patients with known anaphylactic reactions to hydroxocobalamin or cyanocobalamin. Consider the use of alternative therapies if available.

Allergic reactions may include anaphylaxis, chest tightness, dyspnea, edema, pruritus, rash, and urticaria.

Allergic reactions, including angioneurotic edema, also have been reported in postmarketing experience.

➤*Photosensitivity:* Hydroxocobalamin absorbs visible light in the ultraviolet spectrum. It has potential to cause photosensitivity. Though it is not known if the skin redness caused by hydroxocobalamin predisposes to photosensitivity, advise patients to avoid direct sun while their skin remains discolored.

➤*Pregnancy: Category C.* Animal studies are insufficient with respect to effects on pregnancy and embryofetal development. There are no adequate and well-controlled studies in pregnant women. It is not known whether hydroxocobalamin can cause fetal harm when administered to a pregnant woman or can affect reproduction capacity. Use hydroxocobalamin during pregnancy only if the potential benefit justifies the potential risk to the fetus.

In a clinical study of the safety of hydroxocobalamin in healthy volunteers, a pregnant subject was inadvertently enrolled and administered hydroxocobalamin 5 g IV during her fourth week of gestation. Her pregnancy was uneventful, and she reported the birth of a healthy baby at term.

In a retrospective study of cyanide ingestion/inhalation, a female subject, 4 months pregnant, ingested an undetermined amount of potassium cyanide. She received hydroxocobalamin 10 g in addition to sodium thiosulfate in the first 24 hours postingestion. The fetus suffered intrauterine death, but it was suspected that this occurred prior to the ingestion of cyanide and administration of hydroxocobalamin. The mother survived without sequelae.

➤*Lactation:* It is not known whether hydroxocobalamin is excreted in human milk. However, because hydroxocobalamin may be administered in life-threatening situations, breast-feeding is not a contraindication to its use. Because many drugs are excreted in human milk, exercise caution following hydroxocobalamin administration to a breast-feeding woman. There are no data to determine when breast-feeding may be safely restarted following administration of hydroxocobalamin.

The World Health Organization classifies hydroxocobalamin for the treatment of vitamin B_{12} deficiency as compatible with breast-feeding.

➤*Children:*

Cyanokit – Safety and efficacy of hydroxocobalamin have not been established in this population. In non-US marketing experience, a dose of 70 mg/kg has been used to treat children.

➤*Monitoring:*

Vitamin B_{12} deficiency – Hypokalemia and thrombocytosis could occur on conversion of severe megaloblastic to normal erythropoiesis with vitamin B_{12} therapy. Therefore, carefully monitor serum potassium levels and platelet count during therapy. Closely observe serum potassium for the first 48 hours and administer potassium as necessary.

Cyanide poisoning – Though determination of blood cyanide concentration is not required for management of cyanide poisoning and should not delay treatment with hydroxocobalamin, collecting a pretreatment blood sample may be useful for documenting cyanide poisoning because sampling posthydroxocobalamin use may be inaccurate.

Drug Interactions

No formal drug interaction studies have been conducted with hydroxocobalamin.

➤*Drug/Lab test interactions:*

Cyanokit – Because of its deep red color, hydroxocobalamin has been found to interfere with colorimetric determinations of certain laboratory parameters (eg, clinical chemistry, coagulation, hematology, urine parameters). In vitro tests indicated that the extent and duration of the interference are dependent on numerous factors, such as the dose of hydroxocobalamin, analyte, methodology, analyzer, hydroxocobalamin concentration, and partially on the time between sampling and measurement.

Based on in vitro studies and pharmacokinetic data obtained in healthy volunteers, the following table describes laboratory interference that may be observed following a dose of hydroxocobalamin 5 g. Interference following a 10 g dose can be expected to last up to an additional 24 hours. The extent and duration of interference in cyanide-poisoned patients may differ. Results may vary substantially from 1 analyzer to another; therefore, use caution when reporting and interpreting laboratory results.

Laboratory Interference Observed With In Vitro Samples of Hydroxocobalamin Injection[a]

Laboratory parameters	No interference observed	Artificially increased[a]	Artificially decreased[a]	Unpredictable	Duration of interference
Clinical chemistry	Calcium Sodium Potassium Chloride Urea GGT[b]	Creatinine Bilirubin Triglycerides Cholesterol Total protein Glucose Albumin Alkaline phosphatase	ALT Amylase	Phosphate Uric acid AST Creatine kinase CK-MB[b] LDH[b]	24 hours with the exception of bilirubin (up to 4 days)
Hematology	Erythrocytes Hematocrit MVC[b] Leukocytes Lymphocytes Monocytes Eosinophils Neutrophils Platelets	Hemoglobin MCH[b] MCHC[b] Basophils			12 to 16 hours
Coagulation				aPTT[b] PT[b] (Quick or INR[b])	24 to 48 hours
Urinalysis		pH (with all doses) Glucose Protein Erythrocytes Leukocytes Ketones Bilirubin Urobilinogen Nitrite	pH (with equivalent doses of < 5 g)		48 hours up to 8 days; color changes may persist up to 28 days.

[a] ≥ 10% interference observed on at least 1 analyzer. Analyzers used the following: *ACL Futura* (Instrumentation Laboratory); *AxSYM/Architect* (Abbott); *BM Coasys[110]* (Boehringer Mannheim); *CellDyn 3,700* (Abbott); *Clinitek 500* (Bayer); *Cobas Integra 700, 400* (Roche); *Gen-S Coultronics, Hitachi 917, STA Compact, Vitros 950* (Ortho Diagnostics).

[b] GGT = gamma glutamyltransferase; CK-MB = creatine kinase muscle-band isoenyzme ; LDH = lactate dehydrogenase; MCV = mean cell volume; MCH = mean corpuscular hemoglobin; MCHC = mean corpuscular hemoglobin concentration; aPTT = activated partial thromboplastin time; PT = prothrombin time; INR = international normalized ratio.

Adverse Reactions

➤*Vitamin B_{12} deficiency:* Mild transient diarrhea, itching, transitory exanthema, feeling of swelling of entire body, anaphylaxis.

A few patients may experience pain after injection of hydroxocobalamin.

➤*Cyanide toxicity:*

Serious adverse reactions – Serious adverse reactions with hydroxocobalamin include allergic reactions and increases in blood pressure.

Healthy subjects –

Most frequent adverse reactions: Because of the dark red color of hydroxocobalamin, the 2 most frequently occurring adverse reactions were chromaturia (red colored urine), which was reported in all subjects receiving a 5 g dose or more, and erythema (skin redness), which occurred in most subjects receiving a 5 g dose or more.

Adverse reactions (5% or more):

Hydroxocobalamin Injection Adverse Reactions (> 5%)

Adverse reactions	Hydroxocobalamin 5 g (n = 66)	Placebo (n = 22)	Hydroxocobalamin 10 g (n = 18)	Placebo (n = 6)
Dermatologic				
Erythema	94%	0%	100%	0%
Rash[a]	20%	0%	44%	0%
Miscellaneous				
Blood pressure increased	18%	0%	28%	0%
Chromaturia (red colored urine)	100%	0%	100%	0%
Headache	6%	5%	33%	0%
Infusion-site reaction	6%	0%	39%	0%
Lymphocyte percent decreased	8%	0%	17%	0%
Nausea	6%	5%	11%	0%

[a] Rashes were predominately acneiform.

Other adverse reactions: In this study, the following adverse reactions were reported to have occurred in a dose-dependent fashion and with greater frequency than observed in placebo-treated cohorts: headache, increased blood pressure (particularly diastolic blood pressure), infusion-site reactions, nausea, and rash. All were mild to moderate in severity and resolved spontaneously when the infusion was terminated or with standard supportive therapies.

Other adverse reactions reported in this study and considered clinically relevant include the following:

- *CNS* – Dizziness, memory impairment, restlessness.
- *Dermatologic* – Pruritus, urticaria.
- *GI* – Abdominal discomfort, diarrhea, dyspepsia, dysphagia, hematochezia, vomiting.
- *Ophthalmic* – Eye irritation, eye redness, eye swelling.
- *Respiratory* – Dry throat, dyspnea, throat tightness.

HYDROXOCOBALAMIN — INJECTION

• *Miscellaneous* – Allergic reactions, chest discomfort, hot flush, peripheral edema.

Cyanide-poisoning victims –

Cardiovascular: Electrocardiogram repolarization abnormality, heart rate increased, ventricular extrasystoles.

Miscellaneous: Pleural effusion.

Overdosage

➤*Treatment:* No data are available about overdose with hydroxocobalamin in adults. If overdose occurs, direct treatment to the management of symptoms. Hemodialysis may be effective in such a circumstance but is only indicated in the event of significant hydroxocobalamin-related toxicity.

Patient Information

Cyanokit is indicated for cyanide poisoning, and patients will likely be unresponsive or may have difficulty in comprehending counseling information.

Advise patients that skin redness may last up to 2 weeks and urine coloration may last for up to 5 weeks after administration of *Cyanokit*. While it is not known if the skin redness predisposes to photosensitivity, advise patients to avoid direct sun while their skin remains discolored.

In some patients, an acneiform rash may appear anywhere from 7 to 28 days following *Cyanokit* treatment. This rash will usually resolve without treatment within a few weeks.

AMINOBENZOATE POTASSIUM

Rx	Potaba (Glenwood)	Tablets: 500 mg	In 100s and 1000s.
Rx	Aminobenzoate Potassium (Hope Pharm)	Capsules: 500 mg	In 250s.
Rx	Potaba (Glenwood)		In 250s and 1000s.
Rx	Potaba (Glenwood)	Envules (Powder): 2 g	In 50s.

AMINOBENZOATE POTASSIUM — ORAL

Indications

➤*Skin conditions:* "Possibly effective" in the treatment of scleroderma, dermatomyositis, morphea, linear scleroderma, pemphigus, and Peyronie's disease.

Administration and Dosage

➤*Adults:*

Scleroderma, morphea, linear scleroderma and Peyronie disease – 12 g/day, given in 4 to 6 divided doses. Tablets and capsules 500 mg are given at the rate of 4 tablets or capsules 6 times daily, or 6 tablets or capsules given 4 times daily usually with meals and at bedtime with a snack.

Dermatomyositis – 15 to 20 g/day, given in 4 to 6 divided doses.

➤*Children:*

Scleroderma, morphea, linear scleroderma, Peyronie disease, and dermatomyositis – 220 mg/kg/day, given in divided doses.

➤*Duration of therapy:* Therapy usually requires the maintenance of adequate dosage for 2 to 3 months.

➤*Administration:* Give with meals or a snack. Tablets must be dissolved in an adequate amount of liquid to prevent GI upset.

Actions

➤*Pharmacology:* Small amounts of para-aminobenzoate are present in cereal, eggs, milk, and meats. Detectable amounts are found in human blood, spinal fluid, urine, and sweat. It is suggested that aminobenzoate potassium has an antifibrosis action caused by mediation of increased oxygen uptake at the tissue level. Fibrosis is believed to occur from either too much serotonin or too little monoamine oxidase (MAO) activity over a period of time. MAO requires an adequate supply of oxygen to function properly. By increasing oxygen supply at the tissue level, aminobenzoate potassium may enhance MAO activity and prevent or cause regression of fibrosis.

Contraindications

Concurrent sulfonamide use.

Warnings/Precautions

➤*Anorexia or nausea:* If anorexia or nausea occurs, interrupt therapy until the patient is eating normally again to avoid hypoglycemia.

➤*Hypersensitivity reactions:* If a hypersensitivity reaction occurs, discontinue the drug. Refer to Management of Acute Hypersensitivity Reactions.

➤*Renal function impairment:* Use cautiously.

➤*Pregnancy: Category: Undetermined.* Aminobenzoate is considered a member of the vitamin B complex (thiamine [B_1], riboflavin [B_2], niacin [B_3], pantothenic acid [B_5], pyridoxine [B_6], B_{12} [cyanocobalamin], and folic acid). Members of the vitamin B complex are considered FDA *Category A* when used in the recommended daily allowance (RDA) doses (*Category C* used in doses exceeding RDA). Safety has not been established.

➤*Lactation:* Safety for use during lactation has not been established. Vitamins are naturally present in breast milk.

Adverse Reactions

Anorexia, nausea, fever, and rash have occurred infrequently and subside with omission of the drug. Desensitization can be accomplished and treatment resumed. Hepatotoxicity also has occurred.

Overdosage

➤*Symptoms:* Nausea and vomiting are the most common events associated with overdose. Drug fever, dermatitis, depression of the leukocyte count, and an alleged fatal case of toxic hepatitis have been reported.

VITAMIN C

Indications

➤*Ascorbic acid deficiency:* For ascorbic acid deficiency. Parenteral ascorbic acid supplementation may be necessary in the treatment of scurvy for patients with gastric disorders, patients with extensive injuries, surgical patients, and others who cannot take oral vitamins. Acute ascorbic acid deficiency may be associated with extensive injuries and other states of extreme stress. Vitamin C requirements are also significantly increased in certain diseases and conditions such as tuberculosis, hyperthyroidism, peptic ulcer, neoplastic disease, pregnancy, and lactation. Parenteral administration is desirable for patients with an acute deficiency or for those whose absorption of orally ingested ascorbic acid is uncertain.

➤*Off-label uses:* Vitamin C in high doses has been advocated for prevention of the common cold, for treatment of asthma, atherosclerosis, wounds, schizophrenia, and cancer; however, clinical data do not justify these uses.

Vitamin C (≥ 2 g/day) may be used as a urinary acidifier either alone or in combination with methenamine therapy. Data regarding the efficacy of ascorbic acid for this purpose are conflicting. Failure to significantly lower urine pH may be attributed to inadequate dosage (less than 2 g/day).

Vitamin C in doses of 150 mg or more have been used to control idiopathic methemoglobinemia (less effective than methylene blue).

Doses greater than the recommended RDA for vitamin C have been associated with a low incidence of senile cataract, cancer, coronary artery disease, and increase in HDL.

Risk reduction for pre-eclampsia in combination with vitamin E during the second half of pregnancy (1 g/day).

Topical – Topical vitamin C may photoprotect against UVR because of its antioxidant and anti-inflammatory properties.

Administration and Dosage

➤*General dosing considerations:* Ascorbic acid is usually administered orally. When oral administration is not feasible or when malabsorption is suspected, administer IM, IV, or subcutaneously. When given parenterally, utilization of the vitamin reportedly is best after IM administration, which is the preferred parenteral route.

Ascorbic acid injection is usually injected IM or subcutaneously. The solution has a pH of 5.5 to 7 and is not usually irritating to the tissues. The solution also may be injected intravenously, but a higher percentage of the drug will be excreted in the urine than when the subcutaneous or IM route is employed. When administered IV, slowly infuse ascorbic acid with large volume solutions. Add ascorbic acid to such solutions shortly before venoclysis; discard any of the mixture remaining after administration.

The blood level of ascorbic acid in normal persons ranges from 0.4 to 1.5 mg/100 mL.

➤*Adults:* Oral ascorbic acid is an over the counter product and therefore is not an approved product.

Recommended daily allowances –

Maximum dose: The Food and Nutrition Board has established upper limits for vitamin C that apply to both food and supplement intakes. Long-term intakes of vitamin C above the upper limit may increase the risk of adverse health effects. The upper limits do not apply to individuals receiving vitamin C for medical treatment, but such individuals should be under the care of a health care provider.

VITAMIN C

Tolerable Upper Intake Levels (ULs) for Vitamin C				
Age	Male	Female	Pregnancy	Lactation
0 to 12 months	Not possible to establish[a]	Not possible to establish[a]		
1 to 3 years	400 mg	400 mg		
4 to 8 years	650 mg	650 mg		
9 to 13 years	1,200 mg	1,200 mg		
14 to 18 years	1,800 mg	1,800 mg	1,800 mg	1,800 mg
19+ years	2,000 mg	2,000 mg	2,000 mg	2,000 mg

[a] Formula and food should be the only sources of vitamin C for infants.

Burns – In the treatment of burns, doses are governed by the extent of tissue injury.

Usual dosage: Deep and extensive burns may require 200 to 500 mg (0.4 to 1 mL) daily intravenously (IV) to maintain measurable blood concentrations. For severe burns, daily doses of 1 to 2 g IV are recommended.

Deficiency – It is difficult to establish an exact dosage of ascorbic acid suitable for the treatment of deficiencies. In general, therapeutic doses should substantially exceed the recommended daily dietary allowances for healthy persons.

Usual dosage: 100 to 250 mg IV (0.2 to 0.5 mL ascorbic acid), once or twice daily. If the deficiency is extreme, give 1 to 2 g IV (2 to 4 mL).

Maximum dose: There is no appreciable danger from excessive dosage because superfluous amounts of the vitamin are rapidly excreted in the urine.

Dosage adjustment: In other conditions in which the need for ascorbic acid is increased, 3 to 5 times the daily optimum allowances appear to be adequate.

Surgery –

Usual dosage: 300 to 500 mg daily IV for a week to 10 days, both preoperatively and postoperatively, are generally considered adequate, although considerably larger amounts have been recommended.

Doses of 1 to 2 g daily IV for 4 to 7 days may be given before operation in gastrectomy patients. Similar doses also have been used postoperatively to aid wound healing following extensive surgical procedures.

Off-label dosing –

Cancer: 10 g/day IV for 10 days followed by 10 g/day orally.

Cardiovascular disease:

- *Coronary heart disease prevention* – 400 mg/day.
- *Vasodilation* – 500 mg/day.
- *Hypertension* – 500 mg/day.

Gout prevention: 500 mg/day.

Lead toxicity: 1,000 mg/day.

➤*Children:*

Burns – See Adults for dosing.

Deficiency – See Adults for dosing.

Surgery – See Adults for dosing.

➤*Elderly:* Because maximizing blood levels of vitamin C may be important in protection against oxidative damage to cells and biological molecules, a vitamin C intake of at least 400 mg daily is particularly important for older adults who are at higher risk for chronic diseases caused, in part, by oxidative damage, such as heart disease, stroke, certain cancers, and cataract.

➤*Smokers:* The RDA for smokers is 100 mg/day because of an increased utilization of vitamin C. Although the IOM was unable to establish a specific vitamin C requirement for nonsmokers who are regularly exposed to secondhand smoke, these individuals should ensure that they meet the RDA for vitamin C.

➤*Preparation for administration:* The pharmacy bulk package is for use in a pharmacy admixture service only. A single entry through the vial closure should be made with a sterile dispensing set or transfer device. Multiple entries will increase the potential for microbial and particulate contamination. The pharmacy bulk container contains no preservative. Any unused portion must be discarded within 6 hours.

When using dispensing vials use aseptic technique. Dispense entire contents in aliquots under a laminar flow hood without delay or within 4 hours after entry or discard remaining contents after first withdrawal. Prepare stoppers with a suitable antiseptic solution. Do not use unless solution is clear and seal is intact.

Pressure may develop within the vial upon storage. Exercise care when withdrawing or relieve pressure by first inserting a sterile empty syringe into the vial, thus allowing pressure to equilibrate.

➤*Administration:* IM route is preferred; may administer IV or subcutaneously. Avoid rapid IV injection. IM injections may cause pain, local swelling, tenderness, and tissue necrosis.

➤*Admixture compatibility:* For IV injection, dilution into a large volume parenteral such as isotonic sodium chloride solution or glucose is recommended to minimize the adverse reactions associated with IV injection.

➤*Storage/Stability:*

Pharmacy bulk package and Cenolate – Store in refrigerator at 2° to 8°C (36° to 46°F). Do not allow to stand at room temperature before use. Failure to follow this caution may lead to excessive pressure inside the vial.

Vial – Store in carton until time of use. Store at controlled room temperature, not to exceed 23°C (73°F). Protect from light.

Actions

➤*Pharmacology:* Vitamin C is a water-soluble vitamin with antioxidant properties. Sources of vitamin C include citrus fruits (eg, lemons, limes), strawberries, tomatoes, cabbage greens, leafy vegetables, and melons.

Physiological Roles of Vitamin C	
Catecholamine biosynthesis	Stimulates peptide synthesis and hydroxylation of proline and lysine in collagen formation
Carnitine synthesis	Epinephrine synthesis
Conversion of folic acid to folinic acid	Facilitates GI iron absorption
Tyrosine metabolism	Dopamine hydroxylation to form norepinephrine

Ascorbic acid (vitamin C) has few strictly pharmacological actions. Administration in amounts greatly in excess of physiological requirements causes no demonstrable effects. The vitamin is an essential coenzyme for collagen formation, tissue repair, and synthesis of lipids and proteins. It acts both as a reducing agent and as an antioxidant and is necessary for many physiological functions (eg, metabolism of iron and folic acid, resistance to infection, preservation of blood vessel integrity).

Deficiency – Signs and symptoms of early deficiency include malaise, irritability, arthralgia, hyperkeratosis of hair follicles, nosebleed, and petechial hemorrhages. Prolonged deficiency leads to clinical scurvy.

Scurvy – Scurvy is characterized by degenerative changes in capillaries, bone, and connective tissues manifested as perifollicular hyperkeratotic papules, dry skin, ecchymosis, muscle weakness, loose teeth caused by gum inflammation, joint pain, easy bruising, and fatigue.

➤*Pharmacokinetics:*

Absorption/Distribution – Ascorbic acid is normally present in both plasma and cells. The absorbed vitamin is ubiquitous in all body tissues. The highest concentrations are found in glandular tissue, the lowest in muscle and stored fat.

Metabolism/Excretion – A major route of metabolism of ascorbic acid involves its conversion to urinary oxalate, presumably through intermediate formation of its oxidized product, dehydroascorbic acid.

Ascorbic acid is partially destroyed and partially excreted by the body. There is a renal threshold for vitamin C; the vitamin is excreted by the kidney in large amounts only when the plasma concentration exceeds this threshold, which is approximately 1.4 mg/100 mL. When the body is saturated with ascorbic acid, the plasma concentration will be about the same as that of the renal threshold: if further amounts are then administered, most of it escapes into the urine.

Warnings/Precautions

➤*Excessive vitamin C doses:* Diabetic patients, patients prone to recurrent renal calculi, those undergoing stool occult blood tests, and those on sodium-restricted diets or anticoagulant therapy should not take excessive doses of vitamin C over an extended period of time.

➤*Aluminum toxicity:* Some products contain aluminum that may be toxic. Aluminum may reach toxic levels with prolonged parenteral administration if kidney function is impaired. Premature neonates are particularly at risk because their kidneys are immature, and they require large amounts of calcium and phosphate solutions, which contain aluminum.

Research indicates that patients with impaired kidney function, including premature neonates, who receive parenteral levels of aluminum greater than 4 to 5 mcg/kg/day accumulate aluminum at levels associated with CNS and bone toxicity. Tissue loading may occur at even lower rates of administration.

➤*IV administration:* Avoid excessively rapid IV administration. Temporary faintness or dizziness may result.

➤*Tartrazine sensitivity:* Some of these products contain tartrazine, which may cause allergic-type reactions (including bronchial asthma) in susceptible individuals. Although the incidence of sensitivity is low, it is frequently seen in patients who also have aspirin hypersensitivity. Specific products containing tartrazine are identified in the product listings.

➤*Sulfite sensitivity:* Some of these products contain sulfites, which may cause allergic-type reactions in certain susceptible people. The overall prevalence of sulfite sensitivity in the general population is unknown and probably low. Sulfite sensitivity is seen more frequently in asthmatic than in nonasthmatic people.

➤*Pregnancy:* *Category C* (in doses greater than the RDA, per the manufacturer); *Category A* up to RDA, *Category C* (in doses greater than RDA, per Briggs'). High doses vitamin C taken during pregnancy have been reported to cause scurvy in infants removed from this environment at birth.

It is not known whether ascorbic acid can cause fetal harm or can affect reproduction capacity. Give to pregnant women only if clearly needed.

Mild to moderate vitamin C deficiency or excessive doses do not seem to pose a major risk to the mother or fetus. Because vitamin C is required for good maternal and fetal health and an increased demand for the vitamin occurs during pregnancy, intake up to the RDA is recommended.

Animal reproduction studies have not been conducted with ascorbic acid injection.

VITAMIN C

➤*Lactation:* Administer with caution to a breast-feeding mother.Ascorbic acid is excreted in breast milk.

Studies in well-nourished women consuming the RDA or more of vitamin C in their diets indicate that ingestion of greater amounts does not significantly increase levels of the vitamin in their milk. Even consumption of total vitamin C greater than 1,000 mg/day, 10 times the RDA, did not significantly increase milk concentrations or vitamin C intake of the infants.

Drug Interactions

➤*Urine acidification:* Acidification of the urine by ascorbic acid may cause precipitation of cysteine, urate, or oxalate stones and will alter the excretion of certain other drugs administered concurrently.

➤*Warfarin:* Large doses interfere with the anticoagulant effect of warfarin.

➤*Disulfiram:* Ascorbic acid has on occasion been used as a specific antidote for symptoms resulting from interaction between ethanol and disulfiram; it may be expected that the concurrent administration of ascorbic acid will interfere with the effectiveness of disulfiram given to patients to encourage abstention from alcohol.

➤*Bishydroxycoumarin:* Limited evidence suggests that ascorbic acid may influence the intensity and duration of action of bishydroxycoumarin.

➤*Drug/Lab test interactions:* Because ascorbic acid is a strong reducing agent, it interferes with numerous laboratory tests based on oxidation-reduction reactions. Diabetic patients taking more than 500 mg/day ascorbic acid may obtain false readings of their urinary glucose test. No exogenous ascorbic acid should be ingested for 48 to 72 hours before amine-dependent stool occult blood tests are conducted because false negative results may occur.

Adverse Reactions

Transient mild soreness may occur at the site of IM or SC injection. Rapid IV administration may cause temporary faintness or dizziness.

Overdosage

Nausea, vomiting, gout precipitation, rebound scurvy, increased iron absorption, impaired bacterial activity, and diarrhea (≥ 1 g). Monitor risk for developing renal calcium oxalate stones (1 to 3 g) due to excessive oxalate excretion produced by ascorbic acid metabolism.

ASCORBIC ACID

otc	**Ascorbic Acid** (Various, eg, Freeda, GNP)	**Tablets; oral:** 250 mg	In 100s and UD 100s.
otc	**C-250** (Nature's Bounty)		Gluten free, lactose free, sugar free. Preservative free. In 100s.
otc	**Ascorbic Acid** (Various, eg, Freeda, GNP[a])	**Tablets; oral:** 500 mg	In 100s, 250s, 500s, 1,000s, and UD 100s.
otc	**C-500** (Nature's Bounty)		Gluten free, lactose free, sugar free. Preservative free. In 100s, 250s, and 500s.
otc	**Ascorbic Acid** (Various, eg, Freeda, GNP[a])	**Tablets; oral:** 1,000 mg	In 100s and 250s.
otc	**Ascorbic Acid** (Various, eg, Major, Mason)	**Tablets, chewable; oral:** 500 mg	In 100s.
otc	**Ascorbic Acid** (Various, eg, Freeda, GNP, Major)	**Tablets, timed-release; oral:** 500 mg	In 100s, 250s, and 500s.
otc	**Complex C** (National Vitamin Company)		Gluten free, sugar free. Preservative free. Polydextrose. In 100s.
otc	**Ascorbic Acid** (Various, eg, Freeda, GNP, Major)	**Tablets, timed-release; oral:** 1,000 mg	In 100s, 250s, and 500s.
otc	**Complex C** (National Vitamin Co)		Gluten free, sugar free. Preservative free. Polydextrose. In 60s.
otc	**C-Gel** (JR Carlson)	**Capsules, softgels; oral:** 1,000 mg	In 60s, 100s, and 250s.
otc	**C-500** (Nature's Bounty)	**Capsules, timed-release; oral:** 500 mg	Gluten free, lactose free. Preservative free. Sucrose. In 100s.
otc	**N'ice** (Insight)	**Lozenges; oral:** 60 mg	Sugar free. Acesulfame potassium, menthol. Tangerine flavor. In 24s.
otc	**Ascorbic Acid** (Humco)	**Powder; oral:** 60 mg per ¼ tsp	In 113 and 454 g.
otc	**Vita-C** (Freeda)	**Powder; oral:** 1,000 mg per ¼ tsp	Gluten free, lactose free, sugar free. In 120 g and 1 lb.
otc	**Dull-C** (Freeda)	**Powder; oral:** 1,060 mg per ¼ tsp	Gluten free, lactose free, sugar free. In 120 g and 1 lb.
otc	**Ascocid** (Key Co)	**Powder; oral:** 5,000 mg per tsp	In 227 g.
otc	**Ascorbic Acid** (Various, eg, Hi-Tech, Rugby)	**Liquid; oral:** 500 mg per 5 mL	In 120, 473, and 480 mL.
Rx	**Ascorbic Acid** (Various, eg, American Regent, Bionich Pharma)	**Injection, solution:** 500 mg/mL	May contain edetate disodium. In 50 mL vials.
Rx	**Ascor L 500** (McGuff)		Edetate disodium 0.025%. Preservative free. In 50 mL.

[a] With or without rose hips.

For complete and comparative prescribing information, see the Vitamin C class monograph. For additional information, refer to the Dietary Reference Intakes of Vitamins and Minerals table.

ASCORBIC ACID — ORAL

Indications

➤*Ascorbic acid deficiency:* For ascorbic acid deficiency. Parenteral ascorbic acid supplementation may be necessary in the treatment of scurvy for patients with gastric disorders or extensive injuries, surgical patients, and others who cannot take oral vitamins. Acute ascorbic acid deficiency may be associated with extensive injuries and other states of extreme stress. Vitamin C requirements are also significantly increased in certain diseases and conditions, such as tuberculosis, hyperthyroidism, peptic ulcer, neoplastic disease, pregnancy, and lactation.

➤*Off-label uses:*

Urinary acidifier – [5] = Poor documentation. Clinical trials have produced inconsistent results, most of which do not recommend ascorbic acid as a urinary acidifier.

Other possible off-label uses – Vitamin C in high doses has been advocated for prevention of the common cold and treatment of asthma, atherosclerosis, wounds, schizophrenia, and cancer; however, clinical data do not justify these uses.

Vitamin C in doses of 150 mg or higher have been used to control idiopathic methemoglobinemia (less effective than methylene blue).

Doses greater than the recommended dietary allowances (RDAs) for vitamin C have been associated with a low incidence of senile cataract, cancer, coronary artery disease, and increase in high-density lipoprotein.

Risk reduction for preeclampsia in combination with vitamin E during the second half of pregnancy (1 g/day).

Administration and Dosage

➤*General dosing considerations:* Ascorbic acid is usually administered orally. When oral administration is not feasible or when malabsorption is suspected, administer intramuscularly, intravenously (IV), or subcutaneously.

The blood level of ascorbic acid in healthy persons ranges from 0.4 to 1.5 mg per 100 mL.

➤*Adults:*

Dietary reference intake for ascorbic acid –

19 years of age and older: 90 mg/day (males), 75 mg/day (females).
Pregnant females (19 to 50 years of age): 85 mg/day.
Lactating females (19 to 50 years of age): 120 mg/day.

Ascorbic acid supplement –

Scurvy: At least 10 mg/day.

Off-label dosing –

Cancer: 10 g/day IV for 10 days followed by 10 g/day orally.
Cardiovascular disease:
- *Coronary heart disease prevention* – 400 mg/day.
- *Vasodilation* – 500 mg/day.
- *Hypertension* – 500 mg/day.

Gout prevention: 500 mg/day.
Lead toxicity: 1,000 mg/day.

➤*Children:*

Dietary reference intake for ascorbic acid –

14 to 18 years of age: 75 mg/day (males), 65 mg/day (females).

ASCORBIC ACID — ORAL

- *Pregnant females* – 80 mg/day.
- *Lactating females* – 115 mg/day.

9 to 13 years of age: 45 mg/day.
4 to 8 years of age: 25 mg/day.
1 to 3 years of age: 15 mg/day.
30 days to 1 year of age: 6 mg/kg/day.

Scurvy – At least 10 mg/day.

➤*Elderly:* Because maximizing blood levels of vitamin C may be important in protection against oxidative damage to cells and biological molecules, a vitamin C intake of at least 400 mg daily is particularly important for older adults who are at higher risk for long-term diseases caused, in part, by oxidative damage, such as heart disease, stroke, certain cancers, and cataract.

➤*Smokers:* The RDA for smokers is 100 mg/day because of an increased utilization of vitamin C. Although the Institute of Medicine was unable to establish a specific vitamin C requirement for nonsmokers who are regularly exposed to second-hand smoke, these individuals should ensure they meet the RDA for vitamin C.

➤*Administration:* Administer with food.

➤*Storage/Stability:* Store at room temperature.

ASCORBIC ACID — INJECTION

Indications

➤*Ascorbic acid deficiency:* For ascorbic acid deficiency. Parenteral ascorbic acid supplementation may be necessary in the treatment of scurvy for patients with gastric disorders or extensive injuries, surgical patients, and others who cannot take oral vitamins. Acute ascorbic acid deficiency may be associated with extensive injuries and other states of extreme stress. Vitamin C requirements are also significantly increased in certain diseases and conditions, such as tuberculosis, hyperthyroidism, peptic ulcer, neoplastic disease, pregnancy, and lactation.

Parenteral administration is desirable for patients with an acute deficiency or for those whose absorption of orally ingested ascorbic acid is uncertain.

➤*Off-label uses:*

Urinary acidifier – [5] = Poor documentation. Clinical trials have produced inconsistent results, most of which do not recommend ascorbic acid as a urinary acidifier.

Other possible off-label uses – Vitamin C in high doses has been advocated for prevention of the common cold and treatment of asthma, atherosclerosis, wounds, schizophrenia, and cancer; however, clinical data do not justify these uses.

Vitamin C in doses of 150 mg or higher have been used to control idiopathic methemoglobinemia (less effective than methylene blue).

Doses greater than the recommended dietary allowances (RDAs) for vitamin C have been associated with a low incidence of senile cataract, cancer, and coronary artery disease and increase in high-density lipoprotein.

Risk reduction for preeclampsia in combination with vitamin E during the second half of pregnancy (1 g/day).

Administration and Dosage

➤*General dosing considerations:* Ascorbic acid is usually administered orally. When oral administration is not feasible or when malabsorption is suspected, administer intramuscularly (IM), intravenously (IV), or subcutaneously. When given parenterally, utilization of the vitamin reportedly is best after IM administration, which is the preferred parenteral route.

Ascorbic acid injection is usually administered IM or subcutaneously. The solution has a pH of 5.5 to 7 and is not usually irritating to the tissues. The solution also may be injected IV, but a higher percentage of the drug will be excreted in the urine than when the subcutaneous or IM route is employed.

There is no appreciable danger from excessive dosage because superfluous amounts of ascorbic acid are rapidly excreted in the urine.

The blood level of ascorbic acid in healthy persons ranges from 0.4 to 1.5 mg per 100 mL.

➤*Adults:*

Burns –

Usual dosage: Deep and extensive burns may require 200 to 500 mg (0.4 to 1 mL) daily to maintain measurable blood concentrations. For severe burns, daily doses of 1 to 2 g are recommended.

Deficiency –

Usual dosage: 100 to 250 mg (0.2 to 0.5 mL) once or twice daily. If the deficiency is extreme, give 1 to 2 g (2 to 4 mL).

Alternative dosage: In other conditions in which the need for ascorbic acid is increased, 3 to 5 times the daily optimum allowances appear to be adequate.

Surgery – 300 to 500 mg daily for a week to 10 days, both preoperatively and postoperatively, are generally considered adequate to enhance wound healing, although considerably larger amounts have been recommended.

Dosages of 1 to 2 g daily for 4 to 7 days may be given before operation in gastrectomy patients. Similar dosages also have been used postoperatively to aid wound healing following extensive surgical procedures.

Off-label dosing –

➤*Children:*

Burns – See Adults for dosing.

Deficiency – See Adults for dosing.

Surgery – See Adults for dosing.

➤*Elderly:* Because maximizing blood levels of vitamin C may be important in protection against oxidative damage to cells and biological molecules, a vitamin C intake of at least 400 mg daily is particularly important for older adults who are at higher risk for long-term diseases caused, in part, by oxidative damage, such as heart disease, stroke, certain cancers, and cataract.

➤*Smokers:* The RDA for smokers is 100 mg/day because of an increased utilization of vitamin C. Although the Institute of Medicine was unable to establish a specific vitamin C requirement for nonsmokers who are regularly exposed to secondhand smoke, these individuals should ensure that they meet the RDA for vitamin C.

➤*Preparation for administration:* The pharmacy bulk packages are for use in a pharmacy admixture service only. Use aseptic technique. Prepare stoppers with a suitable antiseptic solution. A single entry through the vial closure should be made with a sterile dispensing set or transfer device. Multiple entries will increase the potential for microbial and particulate contamination. Any unused portion must be discarded within 4 (dispensing vial) to 6 hours (*Ascor L 500*).

Pressure may develop within the vial upon storage. Exercise care when withdrawing from the vial or relieve pressure by first inserting a sterile empty syringe into the vial, thus allowing pressure to equilibrate.

For IV injection, dilution into a large volume parenteral, such as normal saline or glucose, is recommended to minimize the adverse reactions associated with IV injection. Ascorbic acid should be added to such solutions shortly before venoclysis.

➤*Administration:* IM route is preferred; may also administer IV or subcutaneously. When administered IV, infuse slowly; avoid rapid IV injection. IM injections may cause pain, local swelling, tenderness, and tissue necrosis.

➤*Storage/Stability:*

Ascor L 500 – Store in refrigerator at 2° to 8°C (36° to 46°F). Do not allow to stand at room temperature before use. Failure to follow this caution may lead to excessive pressure inside the vial.

Dispensing vial – Store in carton until time of use. Store below 23°C (73°F). Protect from light.

SODIUM ASCORBATE

Rx	**Cenolate** (Hospira)	**Injection, solution:** 500 mg/mL ascorbic acid	Preservative free. Equiv. to sodium ascorbate 562.5 mg/mL. Sodium hydrosulfite 5 mg. In 1 and 2 mL amps.

For complete prescribing information, refer to the Vitamin C class monograph. For additional information, refer to the Dietary Reference Intakes of Vitamin and Minerals table.

SODIUM ASCORBATE — INJECTION

Indications

➤*Ascorbic acid deficiency:* For ascorbic acid deficiency. Parenteral ascorbic acid may be necessary in the treatment of scurvy for patients with gastric disorders or extensive injuries, surgical patients, and others who cannot take vitamins. Acute ascorbic acid deficiency may be associated with extensive injuries and other states of extreme stress. Vitamin C requirements are also significantly increased in certain diseases and conditions, such as tuberculosis, hyperthyroidism, peptic ulcer, neoplastic disease, pregnancy, and lactation.

➤*Off-label uses:*

Urinary acidifier – [5] = Poor documentation. Clinical trials have produced inconsistent results, most of which do not recommend ascorbic acid as a urinary acidifier.

Other possible off-label uses – Vitamin C in high doses has been advocated for prevention of the common cold and treatment of asthma, atherosclerosis, wounds, schizophrenia, and cancer; however, clinical data do not justify these uses.

Vitamin C in doses of 150 mg or more has been used to control idiopathic methemoglobinemia (less effective than methylene blue).

Doses greater than the recommended dietary allowances (RDAs) for vitamin C have been associated with a low incidence of senile cataract, cancer, coronary artery disease, and increase in high-density lipoprotein.

SODIUM ASCORBATE — INJECTION

Risk reduction for preeclampsia in combination with vitamin E during the second half of pregnancy (1 g/day).

Administration and Dosage

➤*General dosing considerations:* The blood level of ascorbic acid in healthy persons ranges from 0.4 to 1.5 mg/100 mL.

There is no appreciable danger from excessive dosage because superfluous amounts of the vitamin are rapidly excreted in the urine.

➤*Adults:*

Ascorbic acid deficiency –

Usual dosage: 100 to 250 mg intravenously (IV) (0.2 to 0.5 mL), once or twice daily.

Alternative dosage: If the deficiency is extreme, give 1 to 2 g IV (2 to 4 mL).

Burns – Deep and extensive burns may require 200 to 500 mg (0.4 to 1 mL) daily IV to maintain measurable blood concentrations.

Surgery – Dosages of 1 to 2 g daily IV for 4 to 7 days may be given before operation in gastrectomy patients. Similar dosages also have been used postoperatively to aid wound healing following extensive surgical procedures.

Off-label dosing –

➤*Children:*

Ascorbic acid deficiency – See Adults for dosing.

Burns – See Adults for dosing.

Surgery – See Adults for dosing.

➤*Elderly:* Because maximizing blood levels of vitamin C may be important in protection against oxidative damage to cells and biological molecules, a vitamin C intake of at least 400 mg daily is particularly important for older adults who are at higher risk for long-term disease caused, in part, by oxidative damage, such as heart disease, stroke, certain cancers, and cataract.

➤*Smokers:* The RDA for smokers is 100 mg/day because of an increased utilization of vitamin C. Although the Institute of Medicine was unable to establish a specific vitamin C requirement for nonsmokers who are regularly exposed to secondhand smoke, these individuals should ensure that they meet the RDA for vitamin C.

➤*Preparation for administration:* For IV administration, add sodium ascorbate to large volume solutions shortly before venoclysis.

Because pressure may develop on long storage, take precautions to wrap the ampule in a protective covering while it is being opened.

➤*Administration:* Administer intramuscularly (IM) or subcutaneously. The solution also may be injected IV, but a higher percentage of the drug will be excreted in the urine than when the subcutaneous or IM route is employed. When administering IV, infuse slowly with large volume solutions.

➤*Storage/Stability:* Store in a refrigerator. Protect from light. Do not allow to stand at room temperature before use. Failure to follow this caution may lead to excessive pressure inside the ampule. Discard any mixture that remains after administration.

CALCIUM ASCORBATE

otc sf	**Calcium Ascorbate** (Freeda)	**Tablets:** 500 mg	75 mg calcium. Buffered. In 100s, 250s, and 500s.
otc sf	**Calcium Ascorbate** (Freeda)	**Powder:** 814 mg/¼ tsp	100 mg calcium/¼ tsp. Buffered. In 120 g and 1 lb.
otc	**Ascocid** (Key Company)	**Granules:** 4,000 mg/tsp (as vitamin C)	In 8 oz.

For complete and comparative prescribing information, see the Vitamin C group monograph. For additional information, refer to the Dietary Reference Intakes of Vitamins and Minerals table.

ASCORBIC ACID COMBINATIONS

otc	**SunKist Vitamin C** (Novartis)	**Tablets, chewable:** 60 mg vitamin C as sodium ascorbate and ascorbic acid	Sorbitol, sucrose, lactose. Orange flavor. In 11s.
otc sf	**Fruit C 100** (Freeda)	**Tablets, chewable:** 100 mg vitamin C as calcium ascorbate and ascorbic acid	In 250s.
otc sf	**Fruit C 200** (Freeda)	**Tablets, chewable:** 200 mg vitamin C as calcium ascorbate and ascorbic acid	Rose hips. In 100s and 250s.
otc	**Chewable Vitamin C** (Various, eg, Goldline)	**Tablets, chewable:** 250 mg vitamin C as sodium ascorbate and ascorbic acid	In 100s.
otc	**SunKist Vitamin C** (Novartis)		Fructose, sorbitol, sucrose, lactose. Orange flavor. In 60s.
otc	**Chewable Vitamin C** (Various, eg, Goldline)	**Tablets, chewable:** 500 mg vitamin C as sodium ascorbate and ascorbic acid	In 100s.
otc	**SunKist Vitamin C** (Novartis)		Fructose, sorbitol, sucrose, lactose. Orange flavor. In 75s.
otc	**Chew-C** (Key Company)		Sugar. Orange flavor. In 100s.
otc sf	**Fruit C 500** (Freeda)	**Tablets, chewable:** 500 mg vitamin C as calcium ascorbate and ascorbic acid	Rose hips. In 100s and 250s.
otc	**Vicks Vitamin C Drops** (Proctor and Gamble)	**Lozenges:** 25 mg vitamin C as sodium ascorbate and ascorbic acid	Sucrose, corn syrup. Orange flavor. In 20s.

For complete and comparative prescribing information, refer to the Vitamin C group monograph. For additional information, refer to the Dietary Reference Intakes of Vitamins and Minerals table.

BIOFLAVONOIDS (Vitamin P)

otc sf	**Pan C-500** (Freeda)	**Tablets:** 100 mg hesperidin, 100 mg citrus bioflavonoids, and 500 mg vitamin C	Sodium free. In 100s, 250s, and 500s.
otc sf	**C Factors "1000" Plus** (Solgar)	**Tablets:** 1000 mg vitamin C, 25 mg rose hips, 250 mg citrus bioflavonoids complex, 50 mg rutin, 25 mg hesperidin	Sodium free. In 50s.
otc sf	**Flavons** (Freeda)	**Tablets:** 500 mg bioflavonoids[a]	In 100s and 250s.
otc	**Tri-Super Flavons 1000** (Freeda)	**Tablets:** 1000 mg bioflavonoids	In 100s, 250s, and 500s.
otc	**Peridin-C** (Beutlich)	**Tablets:** 150 mg hesperidin complex, 50 mg hesperidin methyl cholcone (bioflavonoids), 200 mg ascorbic acid	In 100s and 500s.
otc sf	**Span C** (Freeda)	**Tablets:** 300 mg citrus bioflavonoids, 200 mg vitamin C (ascorbic acid and rose hips)[a]	In 100s, 250s, and 500s.
otc sf	**Flavons-500** (Freeda)	**Tablets:** 500 mg citrus bioflavonoids	In 100s and 250s.
otc sf	**Ester-C Plus 1000 mg Vitamin C** (Solgar)	**Tablets:** 1000 mg vitamin C, 200 mg citrus bioflavonoid complex, 25 mg acerola, 25 mg rutin, 25 mg rose hips, 125 mg calcium	Sodium free. In 90s.

Water-Soluble Vitamins

BIOFLAVONOIDS (Vitamin P)

otc	**Bioflex** (Advanced Generic)	**Tablet; oral**: 500 mg vitamin C, 50 mg citrus bioflavonoids, 25 mg hawthorn berry extract, 25 mg horsechestnut extract, 25 mg hesperidin complex, 40 mg rutin, 25 mg witch hazel extract	In 60s.
otc sf	**Quercetin** (Freeda)	**Tablets**: 50 mg quercetin (from eucalyptus)	Sodium free. In 100s and 250s.
		Tablets: 250 mg quercetin (from eucalyptus)	Sodium free. In 100s and 250s.
otc	**Amino-Opti-C** (Tyson)	**Tablets, sustained-release**: 1000 mg vitamin C, 250 mg lemon bioflavonoids. Rose hips powder, rutin, hesperidin[b]	In 100s.
otc sf	**Ester-C Plus Multi-Mineral** (Solgar)	**Capsules**: 425 mg vitamin C, 50 mg citrus bioflavonoid complex, 12.5 mg acerola, 12.5 mg rose hips, 5 mg rutin, 25 mg calcium, 13 mg magnesium, 12.5 mg potassium, 2.5 mg zinc	Sodium free. In 60s and 90s.
otc sf	**Ester-C Plus 500 mg Vitamin C** (Solgar)	**Capsules**: 500 mg vitamin C, 62 mg calcium, 25 mg citrus bioflavonoids, 10 mg acerola, 10 mg rose hips, 5 mg rutin	Sodium free. In 250s.

[a] Also contains calcium carbonate, calcium stearate.

[b] Also contains dicalcium phosphate, hydrogenated soybean oil.

BIOFLAVONOIDS (Vitamin P) — ORAL

Indications

➤*Dietary supplement:* Bioflavonoids may be used as a dietary supplement. Bioflavonoids help strengthen the capillaries, as well as increase the absorption of vitamin C.

➤*Off-label uses:* Bioflavonoids possess widespread activity. Some biological activities include the following: Anthelmintic, antimicrobial, antimalarial, antineoplastic, cytotoxic, mutagenic, carcinogenic, anticarcinogenic, antioxidant (free radical scavengers), inhibition of prostaglandin synthesis (anti-inflammatory), antiallergic, antiviral, antithrombotic, spasmolitic, and estrogenic. Certain flavonoids have been noted to increase lymphatic drainage and improve venous tone. Bioflavonoids are considered investigational in the treatment of HIV via HIV-1 reverse transcriptase, protease, and integrase inhibition. Unfortunately, many of these uses have not been tested in controlled clinical trials; therefore, there is little evidence that they are effective for any indication.

Administration and Dosage

➤*Adults:*

Dietary supplement –

Usual dosage: Dosage varies by product. To increase the absorption of vitamin C, the typical ratio is 500 mg vitamin C to 200 mg bioflavonoids taken once or twice daily with food.

• *Bioflex* – During the initial 60 day period take 3 tablets daily, 2 in the morning with food and 1 in the evening with food. After 60 days, take 1 in the morning and 1 in the evening with food, or as directed.

➤*Storage/Stability:* Store in a cool, dry place. Do not refrigerate.

Actions

➤*Pharmacology:* Flavonoids are naturally occurring, low-molecular-weight polyphenols of plant origin, historically named "vitamin P." More than 4000 naturally occurring flavonoids have been described. Groups of flavonoids include flavones, flavonols, flavanones, and flavanols, which differ by the number and positions of hydroxyl substituents in 2 aromatic rings. Flavonoids generally occur as aglycones, glycosides, and methylated derivatives. Flavonoids are present in fruits, vegetables, nuts, seeds, grains, tea, wine, stems, and flowers. Bioflavonoid refers to extracts of citrus including lemon, orange, mandarin, or grapefruit varieties. Bioflavonoids extracted from citrus contain a variety of flavonoids. The majority of citrus flavonoids are flavanones bound as glycosides.

Flavonoid Sources	
Flavonoid	Source
Naringin[a]	Grapefruit, pummelo
Narirutin[a]	Grapefruit
Hesperidin	Oranges, tangerines, lemons, limes
Ericotirin	Lemon, limes
Tangeretin	Tangerines, lemons, limes
Nobiletin	Tangerines, lemons, limes
Genistein	Soybeans
Quercetin	Onions, tomatoes, french beans, apples, berries, red wine

[a] Naringenin glycosides.

➤*Pharmacokinetics:*

Absorption/Distribution –

Quercetin: Quercetin peak levels are attained in less than 0.7 and 2.5 hours following onion and apple ingestion, respectively. Quercetin crosses the intestinal mucosa and is transported to the liver primarily bound to albumin.

Metabolism/Excretion –

Quercetin: Frequent intake of quercetin-rich food resulted in elimination half-lives of 23 hours for apples and 28 hours for onion sources. Quercetin undergoes methylation, sulphation, and glucuronidation to form various conjugates of quercetin. Multiple dosing of grapefruit and orange juice (containing 323 mg naringenin and 44 mg hesperidin) resulted in less than 25% urinary recovery.

Contraindications

None known.

Warnings/Precautions

➤*Pregnancy: Category: Undetermined.* Consult a health care provider.

➤*Lactation:* Vitamins are naturally present in breast milk. Consult a health care provider.

Drug Interactions

➤*Warfarin:* Use bioflavonoids cautiously in patients being treated with warfarin.

Patient Information

Notify your doctor if you go in for surgery because the presence of bioflavonoids can interfere with some medical tests.

FOLIC ACID AND DERIVATIVES (Folacin; Pteroylglutamic Acid; Folate)

otc[a]	**Folic Acid** (Various, eg, Fibertone, Major)	**Tablets; oral**: 0.4 mg	In 100s.
otc[a]	**Folic Acid** (Various, eg, Fibertone)	**Tablets; oral**: 0.8 mg	In 100s.
Rx	**Folic Acid** (Various, eg, Genetco, Goldline, Moore, Parmed, Qualitest)	**Tablets; oral**: 1 mg	In 30s, 100s, 1000s and UD 100s.
Rx sf	**Deplin** (Pamlab)	**Tablets; oral**: 7.5 mg	As L-methylfolate. Gluten free, lactose free, sugar free. (PAL 7.5). Lt. blue, round. In 30s, 90s.
Rx	**DuLeek-Dp 7.5** (Seton Pharmaceuticals)		As folate. (T545). White, round. In 30s and 90s.
Rx	**ViloFane-Dp** (Seton Pharmaceuticals)		Similar to L-methylfolate. (T545). White, round. In 30s and 90s.
Rx sf	**Deplin** (Pamlab)	**Tablets; oral**: 15 mg	As L-methylfolate. Gluten free, lactose free, sugar free. (deplin 15). Orange, round. In 90s.
Rx	**DuLeek-Dp 15** (Seton Pharmaceuticals)		As folate. (T505). Blue, oval. In 90s.

FOLIC ACID AND DERIVATIVES (Folacin; Pteroylglutamic Acid; Folate)

Rx	**Folic Acid** (American Pharmaceutical Partners)	**Injection:** 5 mg/mL	In 10 mL vials.[b]
Rx	**Folvite** (Lederle)		In 10 mL vials.[c]

[a] Although most folic acid products carry the *Rx* legend, products which provide 0.4 mg or less (or 0.8 mg for pregnant or lactating women) may be *otc* items.

[b] With 1.5% benzyl alcohol and EDTA.

[c] With 1.5% benzyl alcohol.

FOLIC ACID — ORAL

For additional information, refer to the.Dietary Reference Intakes of Vitamins and Minerals table

Indications

➤*Megaloblastic anemia:* For the treatment of megaloblastic anemias due to deficiency of folic acid (as may be seen in tropical or nontropical sprue) and in anemias of nutritional origin, pregnancy, infancy, or childhood.

Administration and Dosage

➤*General dosing considerations:* Doses greater than 0.1 mg should not be used unless anemia due to vitamin B12 deficiency has been ruled out or is being adequately treated with cobalamin.

Daily doses greater than 1 mg do not enhance the hematologic effect, and most of the excess is excreted unchanged in the urine.

When clinical symptoms have subsided and the blood picture has become normal, a daily maintenance dosage should be used.

In the presence of alcoholism, hemolytic anemia, anticonvulsant therapy, or chronic infection, the maintenance level may need to be increased.

➤*Adults:*

Megaloblastic anemia –

Usual dosage: Up to 1 mg daily. Resistant cases may require larger doses.

Maintenance dosage: Dose should never be less than 0.1 mg/day. Patients should be kept under close supervision and adjustment of maintenance level made if relapse appears imminent.

- *Adults* – 0.4 mg daily.
- *Pregnant and lactating women* – 0.8 mg daily.
- *Medical food* – 7.5 to 15 mg daily.

➤*Children:*

Megaloblastic anemia –

Usual dosage: Up to 1 mg daily. Resistant cases may require larger doses.

Maintenance dosage: Dose should never be less than 0.1 mg/day. Patients should be kept under close supervision and adjustment of maintenance level made if relapse appears imminent.

- *4 years of age and older* – 0.4 mg daily.
- *Less than 4 years of age* – 0.3 mg daily.
- *Infants* – 0.1 mg daily.

Off-label dosing –

11 years of age and older:

- *Initial dosage* – 1 mg/day.
- *Maintenance dosage* – 0.25 to 1 mg/day.

1 to 10 years of age:

- *Initial dosage* – 1 mg/day.
- *Maintenance dosage* – 0.1 to 0.4 mg/day.

Infants:

- *Maximum dose* – 50 mcg/day as an initial dose.
- *Initial dosage* – 15 mcg/kg/day.
- *Maintenance dosage* – 30 to 45 mcg/day.

➤*Storage/Stability:* Store at 15° to 30°C (59° to 86°F). Protect from light and moisture.

Actions

➤*Pharmacology:* Folic acid acts on megaloblastic bone marrow to produce a normoblastic marrow. In man, an exogenous source of folate is required for nucleoprotein synthesis and the maintenance of normal erythropoiesis. Folic acid is the precursor of tetrahydrofolic acid, which is involved as a cofactor for transformylation reactions in the biosynthesis of purines and thymidylates of nucleic acids. Impairment of thymidylate synthesis in patients with folic acid deficiency is thought to account for the defective deoxyribonucleic acid (DNA) synthesis that leads to megaloblast formation and megaloblastic and macrocytic anemias.

➤*Pharmacokinetics:*

Absorption/Distribution – Folic acid is absorbed rapidly from the small intestine, primarily from the proximal portion. Naturally occurring conjugated folates are reduced enzymatically to folic acid in the gastrointestinal tract prior to absorption. Folic acid appears in the plasma approximately 5 to 30 minutes after an oral dose; peak levels are generally reached within 1 hour. After intravenous administration, the drug is rapidly cleared from the plasma. Cerebrospinal fluid levels are several times greater than serum levels of the drug. Folic acid is metabolized in the liver to 7,8-dihydrofolic acid and eventually to 5,6,7,8-tetrahydrofolic acid with the aid of reduced diphosphopyridine nucleotide (DPNH) and folate reductases. Tetrahydrofolic acid is linked in the N^5 or N^{10} positions with formyl, hydroxymethyl, methyl, or formimino groups. N^5 formyltetrahydrofolic acid is leucovorin. Tetrahydrofolic acid derivatives are distributed to all body tissues but are stored primarily in the liver. Normal serum levels of total folate have been reported to be 5 to 15 ng/mL; normal cerebrospinal fluid levels are approximately 16 to 21 ng/mL. Normal erythrocyte folate levels have been reported to range from 175 to 316 ng/mL. In general, folate serum levels below 5 ng/mL indicate folate deficiency, and levels below 2 ng/mL usually result in megaloblastic anemia.

Metabolism/Excretion – After a single oral dose of 100 mcg of folic acid in a limited number of healthy adults, only a trace amount of the drug appeared in the urine. An oral dose of 5 mg in 1 study and a dose of 40 mcg/kg of body weight in another study resulted in approximately 50% of the dose appearing in the urine. After a single oral dose of 15 mg, up to 90% of the dose was recovered in the urine. A majority of the metabolic products appeared in the urine after 6 hours; excretion was generally complete within 24 hours. Small amounts of orally administered folic acid have also been recovered in the feces. Folic acid is also excreted in the milk of lactating mothers.

Contraindications

Previous intolerance to the drug.

Warnings/Precautions

➤*Pernicious anemia:* Folic acid in doses greater than 0.1 mg daily may obscure pernicious anemia in that hematologic remission can occur while neurologic manifestations remain progressive.

Administration of folic acid alone is improper therapy for pernicious anemia and other megaloblastic anemias in which vitamin B_{12} is deficient.

Except during pregnancy and lactation, folic acid should not be given in therapeutic doses greater than 0.4 mg daily until pernicious anemia has been ruled out. Patients with pernicious anemia receiving greater than 0.4 mg of folic acid daily who are inadequately treated with vitamin B_{12} may show reversion of the hematologic parameters to normal, but neurologic manifestations due to vitamin B_{12} deficiency will progress. Doses of folic acid exceeding the Recommended Dietary Allowance (RDA) should not be included in multivitamin preparations; if therapeutic amounts are necessary, folic acid should be given separately.

There is a potential danger in administering folic acid to patients with undiagnosed anemia, since folic acid may obscure the diagnosis of pernicious anemia by alleviating the hematologic manifestations of the disease while allowing the neurologic complications to progress. This may result in severe nervous system damage before the correct diagnosis is made. Adequate doses of vitamin B_{12} may prevent, halt, or improve the neurologic changes caused by pernicious anemia.

➤*Pregnancy: Category A.* Folic acid is usually indicated in the treatment of megaloblastic anemias of pregnancy. Folic acid requirements are markedly increased during pregnancy, and deficiency will result in fetal damage.

Studies in pregnant women have not shown that folic acid increases the risk of abnormalities if administered during pregnancy. If the drug is used during pregnancy, the possibility of fetal harm appears remote. Because studies cannot rule out the possibility of harm, however, folic acid should be used during pregnancy only if clearly needed.

➤*Lactation:* Folic acid is excreted in the milk of lactating mothers. During lactation, folic acid requirements are markedly increased; however, amounts present in human milk are adequate to fulfill infant requirements, although supplementation may be needed in low-birth-weight infants, in those who are breastfed by mothers with folic acid deficiency (50 mcg daily), or in those with infections or prolonged diarrhea.

Drug Interactions

Folic Acid Drug Interactions

Precipitant drug	Object drug[a]		Description
Aminosalicylic acid	Folic acid	⬇	Decreased serum folate levels may occur during concurrent use.
Contraceptives, oral	Folic acid	⬇	Oral contraceptives may impair folate metabolism and produce folate depletion, but the effect is mild and unlikely to cause anemia or megaloblastic changes.
Dihydrofolate reductase inhibitors (eg, methotrexate, trimethoprim)	Folic acid	⬇	A dihydrofolate reductase deficiency caused by administration of folic acid antagonists may interfere with folic acid utilization.
Sulfasalazine	Folic acid	⬇	Signs of folate deficiency have occurred.

FOLIC ACID — ORAL

Folic Acid Drug Interactions			
Precipitant drug	Object drug[a]		Description
Folic acid	Hydantoins	⬇	An increase in seizure frequency and a decrease in serum concentration to subtherapeutic levels have been reported in patients receiving folic acid (particularly 5 to 30 mg/day) with phenytoin. **Phenytoin** may cause a decrease in serum folate levels, and may produce symptoms of folic acid deficiency in 27% to 91% (but clinically important megaloblastic anemia in < 1%) of patients on long-term therapy. If folic acid is required, a higher dose of phenytoin may be needed.

[a] ⬇ = object drug decreased.

➤*Phenytoin and other anticonvulsant drugs:* There is evidence that the anticonvulsant action of phenytoin is antagonized by folic acid. A patient whose epilepsy is completely controlled by phenytoin may require increased doses to prevent convulsions if folic acid is given.

In an uncontrolled study, orally administered folic acid was reported to increase the incidence of seizures in some epileptic patients receiving phenobarbital, primidone, or phenytoin. Another investigator reported decreased phenytoin serum levels in folate-deficient patients receiving phenytoin who were treated with 5 mg or 15 mg of folic acid daily.

➤*Drugs causing folate deficiency:* Folate deficiency may result from increased loss of folate, as in renal dialysis or interference with metabolism (eg, folic acid antagonists such as methotrexate); the administration of anticonvulsants, such as phenytoin, primidone, and barbiturates, alcohol consumption and, especially, alcoholic cirrhosis; and the administration of pyrimethamine and nitrofurantoin.

➤*Drug/Lab test interactions:* False low serum and red cell folate levels may occur if the patient has been taking antibiotics, such as tetracycline, which suppress the growth of *Lactobacillus casei.*

Adverse Reactions

➤*CNS:* Other side effects reported in patients receiving 15 mg daily include altered sleep patterns, difficulty in concentrating, irritability, overactivity, excitement, mental depression, confusion, and impaired judgement.

➤*GI:* One patient experienced symptoms suggesting anaphylaxis following injection of the drug. GI side effects, including anorexia, nausea, abdominal distention, flatulence, and a bitter or bad taste, have been reported in patients receiving 15 mg of folic acid daily for 1 month.

➤*Hypersensitivity:* Allergic sensitization has been reported following oral administration of folic acid.

Folic acid is relatively nontoxic in man. Rare instances of allergic responses to folic acid preparations have been reported and have included erythema, skin rash, itching, general malaise, and respiratory difficulty due to bronchospasm.

➤*Miscellaneous:* Decreased vitamin B_{12} serum levels may occur in patients receiving prolonged folic acid therapy.

FOLIC ACID — INJECTION

For additional information, refer to the Dietary Reference Intakes of Vitamins and Minerals table.

Indications

➤*Megaloblastic anemia:* For the treatment of megaloblastic anemias due to a deficiency of folic acid as may be seen in tropical or nontropical sprue, in anemias of nutritional origin, pregnancy, infancy or childhood.

Administration and Dosage

➤*General dosing considerations:* Parenteral administration is not advocated but may be necessary in some individuals (eg, patients receiving parenteral or enteral alimentation). IM, IV and SC routes may be used if the disease is exceptionally severe or if GI absorption may be, or is known to be, impaired.

In the presence of alcoholism, hemolytic anemia, anticonvulsant therapy, or chronic infection, the maintenance level may need to be increased.

➤*Adults:*

Megaloblastic anemia –

Usual dosage: Up to 1 mg daily. Resistant cases may require larger doses.

Maintenance dosage: Dose should never be less than 0.1 mg/day. Patients should be kept under close supervision and adjustment of maintenance level made if relapse appears imminent.

- *Adults* – 0.4 mg daily.
- *Pregnant and lactating women* – 0.8 mg daily.

➤*Children:* The injection may contain benzyl alcohol. Benzyl alcohol has been reported to be associated with a fatal "gasping syndrome" in premature infants.

Megaloblastic anemia –

Usual dosage: Up to 1 mg daily. Resistant cases may require larger doses.

Maintenance dosage: Dose should never be less than 0.1 mg/day. Patients should be kept under close supervision and adjustment of maintenance level made if relapse appears imminent.

- *4 years of age and older* – 0.4 mg daily.
- *Younger than 4 years of age* – 0.3 mg daily.
- *Infants* – 0.1 mg daily.

Off-label dosing –

11 years of age and older:

- *Initial dosage* – 1 mg/day.
- *Maintenance dosage* – 0.25 to 1 mg/day.

1 to 10 years of age:

- *Initial dosage* – 1 mg/day.
- *Maintenance dosage* – 0.1 to 0.4 mg/day.

Infants:

- *Maximum dose* – 50 mcg/day as an initial dose.
- *Initial dosage* – 15 mcg/kg/day.
- *Maintenance dosage* – 30 to 45 mcg/day.

➤*Storage/Stability:* Store at 15° to 30°C (59° to 86°F).

Protect from light. Retain vial in carton until contents are used.

Actions

➤*Pharmacology:* In man, an exogenous source of folate is required for nucleoprotein synthesis and maintenance of normal erythropoiesis. Folic acid, whether given by mouth or parenterally, stimulates specifically the production of red blood cells, white blood cells and platelets in persons suffering from certain megaloblastic anemias.

Warnings/Precautions

➤*Pernicious anemia:* Folic acid in doses above 0.1 mg daily may obscure pernicious anemia in that hematologic remission can occur while neurological manifestations remain progressive.

Folic acid alone is improper therapy in the treatment of pernicious anemia and other megaloblastic anemias where vitamin B_{12} is deficient.

➤*Pregnancy:* *Category A; Category C* if used in doses above the RDA. Rapid transfer of folic acid to the fetus occurs in pregnancy. Folic acid is used in pregnant women. The RDA of folic acid in pregnant women is 0.6 mg/day (refer to the Dietary Reference Intakes of Vitamins and Minerals table).

➤*Lactation:* Folic acid is excreted in the milk of lactating mothers. The American Academy of Pediatrics classifies folic acid as compatible with breast-feeding. The RDA of folic acid in breast-feeding women is 0.5 mg/day (refer to the Dietary Reference Intakes of Vitamins and Minerals table).

Adverse Reactions

➤*Hypersensitivity:* Allergic sensitization has been reported following parenteral administration of folic acid.

For information on parenteral calcium products, refer to Intravenous Nutritional Therapy, Minerals section.

Indications

➤*Calcium deficiency:* As a dietary supplement when calcium intake may be inadequate. Conditions that may be associated with calcium deficiency include the following: Vitamin D deficiency, sprue, pregnancy and lactation, achlorhydria, chronic diarrhea, hypoparathyroidism, steatorrhea, menopause, renal failure, pancreatitis, hyperphosphatemia, and alkalosis. Some diuretics and anticonvulsants may precipitate hypocalcemia, which may validate calcium replacement therapy. Calcium salt therapy should not preclude the use of other corrective measures intended to treat the underlying cause of calcium depletion.

➤*Bone disorders:* For the treatment of osteoporosis, osteomalacia, and rickets.

➤*Tetany:* For the treatment of latent tetany.

➤*Premenstrual syndrome symptoms:* Calcium taken daily may help reduce typical premenstrual syndrome (PMS) symptoms such as bloating, cramps, fatigue, and moodiness.

➤*Calcium acetate (PhosLo):* Control of hyperphosphatemia in end-stage renal failure; does not promote aluminum absorption.

Administration and Dosage

➤*Recommended dietary allowances (RDAs):*

Men and women (19 to 24 years of age) – 1200 mg/day

Men and women (25 to 50 years of age) – 800 mg/day

Men and women (≥ 51 years of age) – 800 mg/day

➤*Dietary reference intakes (DRIs):*

Men and women (19 to 50 years of age) – 1000 mg/day

Men and women (older than 51 years of age) – 1200 mg/day

Pregnant and breastfeeding women – 1000 mg/day

➤*Dietary supplement:* The usual daily dose is 500 mg to 2 g, 2 to 4 times/day.

Calcium is recommended in doses of 1500 mg/day for men older than 65 years of age and for postmenopausal women not taking estrogen replacement therapy.

➤*PhosLo:* For adult dialysis patients, the initial dose is 2 tablets/capsules/gelcaps with each meal. The dosage may be increased gradually to bring the serum phosphate value less than 6 mg/dL, as long as hypercalcemia does not develop. Most patients require 3 to 4 tablets with each meal.

The recommended initial dose of the half-size (333.5 mg) *PhosLo* for the adult dialysis patient is 4 capsules with each meal. The dosage may be increased gradually to bring the serum phosphate value below 6 mg/dL, as long as hypercalcemia does not develop. Most patients require 6 to 8 capsules with each meal.

➤*Florical:* 1 capsule or tablet daily.

Actions

➤*Pharmacology:* Calcium is the fifth most abundant element in the body; the major fraction is in bone. It is essential for the functional integrity of the nervous and muscular systems, for normal cardiac function, for cell permeability, and for blood coagulation. It also functions as an enzyme cofactor and affects the secretory activity of endocrine and exocrine glands.

Adequate calcium intake is particularly important during periods of bone growth in childhood and adolescence and during pregnancy and lactation. An adequate supply of calcium is necessary in adults, especially those older than 40 years of age, to prevent a negative calcium balance, which may contribute to the development of osteoporosis.

Patients with advanced renal insufficiency (Ccr less than 30 mL/min) exhibit phosphate retention and some degree of hyperphosphatemia. The retention of phosphate plays a pivotal role in causing secondary hyperparathyroidism associated with osteodystrophy and soft-tissue calcification. Calcium acetate, when taken with meals, combines with dietary phosphate to form insoluble calcium phosphate, which is excreted in the feces.

Elemental Calcium Content of Calcium Salts[a]

Calcium salt	% Calcium	mEq Ca^{++}/g
Calcium glubionate	6.5	3.3
Calcium gluconate	9	4.5
Calcium lactate	13	6.5
Calcium citrate	21	10.6
Calcium acetate	25	12.6
Tricalcium phosphate	39	19.3
Calcium carbonate	40	20

[a] 1 mEq of elemental calcium = 20 mg

➤*Pharmacokinetics:*

Absorption – Calcium is absorbed from the GI tract by passive diffusion and active transport. Calcium must be in a soluble, ionized form for absorption to occur. Vitamin D is required for calcium absorption and increases the capability of the absorptive mechanisms. Calcium absorption is increased in the presence of food. Oral bioavailability in adults ranges from 25% to 35% when a 250 mg dose is given with a standardized breakfast. Absorption from milk was ≈ 29% under the same conditions. Calcium absorption varies with age, being highest during infancy (≈ 60%), decreasing to ≈ 28% in prepubertal children, and increasing again during puberty (≈ 34%). Fractional absorption remains at ≈ 25% in young adults, and increases during the last 2 trimesters of pregnancy. Calcium absorption decreases ≈ 0.21% annually in postmenopausal women and similarly in aging men.

Distribution – Calcium enters the extracellular fluid and is rapidly incorporated into skeletal tissue. Normal total serum calcium concentrations range from 9 to 10.4 mg/dL (4.5 to 5.2 mEq/L), but only ionized calcium is active. Calcium crosses the placenta and reaches higher concentrations in fetal blood than maternal blood. Calcium also is distributed in milk.

Excretion – Calcium is mainly excreted in the feces. Only small amounts are excreted in the urine. Urinary excretion of calcium may be as high as 250 to 300 mg/day in healthy adults who eat a regular diet. However, urinary excretion does not exceed 150 mg/day in patients on low calcium diets. Urinary excretion decreases with age, in the early stages of renal failure, and during pregnancy. Calcium also is excreted by the sweat glands.

Contraindications

Hypercalcemia, ventricular fibrillation.

Warnings/Precautions

➤*PhosLo:* End-stage renal failure patients may develop hypercalcemia when given calcium with meals. Do not give other calcium supplements concurrently with *PhosLo*. Chronic hypercalcemia may lead to vascular and other soft tissue calcification. Monitor serum calcium levels twice weekly during the early dose adjustment period. Do not allow serum calcium times phosphate product to exceed 66.

➤*GI effects:* Calcium salts may be irritating to the GI tract when administered orally and also may cause constipation.

➤*Hypercalcemia:* Hypercalcemia may occur when large doses of calcium are administered to patients with chronic renal failure. Mild hypercalcemia may exhibit as nausea, vomiting, anorexia, or constipation, with mental changes such as stupor, delirium, coma, or confusion. By reducing calcium intake, mild hypercalcemia is usually readily controlled.

➤*Renal calculi:* Recent evidence from studies in men 40 to 75 years of age with no history of kidney stones and women 34 to 59 years of age show that high dietary intake of calcium decreases the risk of symptomatic renal calculi, while intake of supplemental calcium may increase the risk of symptomatic stones. This conflicts with the previous theory that high calcium intake contributes to the risk of renal calculi.

➤*Calcium citrate:*

Renal function impairment – Avoid concurrent aluminum-containing antacids.

➤*Phenylketonurics:* Inform phenylketonuric patients that some of these products contain phenylalanine.

➤*Tartrazine sensitivity:* Some of these products contain tartrazine (FD&C Yellow No. 5), which may cause allergic-type reactions (including bronchial asthma) in susceptible individuals. Although the incidence of sensitivity is low, it is frequently seen in patients who also have aspirin hypersensitivity. Specific products containing tartrazine are identified in the product listings.

➤*Special risk:* Use calcium salts cautiously in patients with sarcoidosis, cardiac or renal disease, and in patients receiving cardiac glycosides.

➤*Pregnancy: Category C* (*PhosLo*). It is not known whether *PhosLo* can cause fetal harm when administered to a pregnant woman or can affect reproduction capacity. Give to a pregnant woman only if clearly needed. Adequate intake of calcium in pregnant women is 1,000 to 1,300 mg/day (refer to the Dietary Reference Intakes of Vitamins and Minerals).

➤*Lactation:* Adequate intake of calcium in breast-feeding women is 1,000 to 1,300 mg/day (refer to Dietary Reference Intakes of Vitamins and Minerals).

➤*Children:* Safety and efficacy in children have not been established (*PhosLo*).

➤*Monitoring:* Perform frequent determinations of serum calcium concentrations. Maintain serum calcium concentrations at 9 to 10.4 mg/dL (4.5 to 5.2 mEq/L). Do not allow levels to exceed 12 mg/dL.

Drug Interactions

Calcium Drug Interactions

Precipitant	Object drug[a]		Description
Calcium salts	Iron salts	⬇	GI absorption of iron may be reduced. In order to avoid a possible interaction, separate administration times whenever possible.
Calcium carbonate	Quinolones	⬇	GI absorption of quinolones may be decreased. The bioavailability of norfloxacin may be reduced; lomefloxacin and ofloxacin do not appear to be affected. Give antacids ≥ 6 hours before or 2 hours after the quinolone.
Calcium salts	Sodium polystyrene sulfonate	⬇	Coadministration in patients with renal impairment may result in an unanticipated metabolic alkalosis and a reduction of the resin's binding of potassium. Separate drugs by several hours.
Calcium salts	Tetracyclines	⬇	The absorption and serum levels of tetracyclines are decreased; a decreased anti-infective response may occur. Avoid simultaneous administration. Separate administration by 3 to 4 hours.
Calcium salts	Verapamil	⬇	Clinical effects and toxicities of verapamil may be reversed.

[a] ⬆ = Object drug increased. ⬇ = Object drug decreased.

Adverse Reactions

May cause constipation and headache. Mild hypercalcemia (Ca^{++} greater than 10.5 mg/dL) may be asymptomatic or manifest itself as anorexia, nausea, and vomiting. More severe hypercalcemia (Ca^{++} greater than 12 mg/dL) is associated with confusion, delirium, stupor, and coma.

Overdosage

Administration of *PhosLo* in excess of the appropriate daily dosage can cause severe hypercalcemia (see Adverse Reactions). Severe hypercalcemia can be treated by acute hemodialysis and discontinuing therapy.

Patient Information

Notify physician if any of the following occur: Anorexia, nausea, vomiting, constipation, abdominal pain, dry mouth, thirst, polyuria.

Inform phenylketonuric patients that some of these products contain phenylalanine.

Take with or following meals to enhance absorption.

Take with a large glass of water.

CALCIUM GLUCONATE

otc	**Calcium Gluconate** (Bio-Tech)	**Capsules; oral:** 500 mg	In 100s.
otc sf	**Calcium Gluconate** (Various, eg Mason, Southwood Pharmaceuticals)	**Tablets, chewable; oral:** 650 mg	Sugar free. In 30s, 60s, 90s, 100s, and 120s.
otc	**Calcium Gluconate** (Roxane)	**Tablets; oral:** 500 mg	Equivalent to elemental calcium 45 mg. In 100s, 1,000s, and UD 100s.
otc sf	**Calcium Gluconate** (Freeda)	**Tablets; oral:** ≈ 555.6 mg	Equivalent to elemental calcium 50 mg. Gluten free, sugar free. In 100s and 500s.
otc	**Calcium Gluconate** (Various, eg, Rugby)	**Tablets; oral:** 648 to 650 mg	Equivalent to elemental calcium 58.5 to 60 mg. In 100s and 1,000s.
otc	**Calcium Gluconate** (Various, eg, Rugby)	**Tablets; oral:** 972 to 975 mg	Equivalent to elemental calcium 87.75 to 90 mg. In UD 100s and 1,000s.
otc	**Cal-G** (Key)	**Capsules; oral:** 700 mg	Equivalent to elemental calcium 50 mg. Gluten free. In 100s and 250s.
otc sf	**Calcium Gluconate** (Freeda)	**Powder; oral:** 1,040 mg per 15 mL	Equivalent to elemental calcium 346.7 mg per 15 mL. Gluten free, sugar free. In 448 g.
Rx	**Calcium Gluconate** (Various, eg, American Regent, APP)	**Injection, solution:** 10%	Equivalent to elemental calcium 0.465 mEq/mL (9.3 mg). Preservative free. 10 and 50 mL single-dose vials and 100 and 200 mL pharmacy bulk vials.[a]

[a] Not for direct infusion; dilute prior to use.

CALCIUM GLUCONATE — ORAL

For complete and comparative prescribing information, refer to the Calcium class monograph. For additional information, refer to the Dietary Reference Intakes of Vitamins and Minerals table.

Indications

➤*Dietary supplement:* For use as a dietary calcium supplement.

Administration and Dosage

➤*Adults:*

Dietary supplement –

Capsules and tablets: 500 to 8,000 mg/day (as calcium gluconate) in divided doses, preferably 1 to 2 hours after meals.

➤*Administration:* Take capsules or tablets with food and liquid, preferable 1 to 2 hours after meals.

➤*Storage/Stability:* Store at room temperature. Do not expose to excessive heat or moisture.

CALCIUM GLUCONATE — INJECTION

For complete prescribing information, refer to the Calcium Gluconate individual and Calcium class monographs. For additional information, refer to the Dietary Reference Intakes of Vitamins and Minerals table.

Indications

➤*Adjunctive therapy:* Adjunctive treatment of rickets, osteomalacia, lead colic, and magnesium sulfate overdosage.

➤*Black widow spider bites:* For the treatment of black widow spider bites to relieve muscle cramping.

➤*Capillary permeability reduction:* To decrease capillary permeability in allergic conditions, nonthrombocytopenic purpura and exudative dermatoses such as dermatitis herpetiformis and for pruritus of eruptions caused by certain drugs.

➤*Cardiac toxicity associated with hyperkalemia:* In hyperkalemia, calcium gluconate may aid in antagonizing the cardiac toxicity provided the patient is not receiving digitalis therapy.

➤*Hypocalcemia:* To treat conditions arising from calcium deficiencies such as hypocalcemic tetany, hypocalcemia related to hypoparathyroidism and hypocalcemia due to rapid growth or pregnancy.

Administration and Dosage

➤*General dosing considerations:* The dose is dependent upon the individual requirements of the patient.

➤*Adults:*

Usual dosage – 500 mg to 2 g intravenously (IV) (5 to 20 mL of 10% solution).

➤*Children:*

Maximum dose – 200 mg (2 mL of 10% solution) for infants.

Usual dosage –

Children: 200 to 500 mg IV (2 to 5 mL of 10% solution).

Infants: Not more than 200 mg IV (not more than 2 mL of 10% solution).

➤*Preparation for administration:* If crystallization has occurred, warming in a 60° to 80°C (140° to 176°F) water bath for 15 to 30 minutes with occasional shaking may dissolve the precipitate. Cool to room temperature before use. The injection must be clear at the time of use.

Pharmacy bulk package – Pharmacy bulk package is not for direct infusion. The 100 mL pharmacy bulk package should be suspended (inverted) by its IV hang label in a laminar flow hood or biological safety cabinet. Prior to entering a pharmacy bulk package remove the flip-off seal and cleanse the rubber closure with a suitable antiseptic agent. Entry into the pharmacy bulk package must be made with a sterile transfer set or other sterile dispensing device and the contents dispensed in aliquots using aseptic technique. Use of a syringe needle is not recommended because it may cause leakage. Any unused portion must be discarded within 4 hours of the initial entry. The date and the time initially opened should be recorded in the space provided on the pharmacy bulk package label.

➤*Administration:* For use either by direct (slow) IV injection or by IV infusion. Not recommended for IM or subcutaneous use. Calcium gluconate injection must be administered slowly. When injected IV, inject through a small needle into a large vein in order to avoid too rapid an increase in serum calcium and extravasation of calcium solution into the surrounding tissue with resultant necrosis.

Calcium gluconate may be administered by intermittent infusion at a rate not exceeding 200 mg/min, or by continuous infusion.

➤*Extravasation:* Extravasation may occur during administration of calcium gluconate. If signs or symptoms of extravasation occur, stop the infusion immediately. If possible, withdraw 3 to 5 mL of blood to remove some of the drug. Remove the infusion needle. Delineate the infiltrated area on the patient's skin with a felt-tip marker. Hyaluronidase is an effective antidote for hyperosmolar drug infiltrations; administer promptly within the first few minutes to 1 hour after extravasation. Higher doses (150 units) have primarily been used in adults while lower doses (15 units) have been used in children. Administer hyaluronidase according to the following steps. Dilute hyaluronidase to desired concentration, depending on the dose and product used. (Note: Some products do not require dilution.) For example, if the total dose is 15 units, make 15 units/mL dilution. If the total dose is 150 units, make 150 units/mL dilution. Cleanse area with povidone-iodine. Inject hyaluronidase locally, subcutaneously or intradermally, using a 25-gauge needle or smaller. The dose is given as five 0.2 mL injections at the leading edge of the extravasation site. Change needle after each injection. Elevate for 48 hours above heart level using a sling or stockinette dressing with an observation window cut in the dressing. Avoid pressure or friction. Do not rub area. Observe for signs of increased erythema, pain, or skin necrosis. If increased symptoms occur, consult a plastic surgeon. Ensure that no medication is given distally to extravasation site. After 48 hours, encourage the patient to use the extremity normally to promote full range of motion.

➤*Admixture compatibility:* Calcium complexes tetracycline antibiotics, rendering them inactive. The 2 drugs should not be mixed for parenteral administration.

Do not reconstitute or mix ceftriaxone with a calcium-containing product, such as Ringer's or Hartmann's solution or parenteral nutrition containing calcium, because particulate formation can result.

Do not administer ceftriaxone and IV calcium-containing products including parenteral nutrition to any patient by the same or different infusion lines or sites within 48 hours of each other. Cases of fatal reactions with ceftriaxone-calcium precipitates in lungs and kidneys in neonates have been reported. Although most cases occurred with simultaneous administration of the 2

CALCIUM GLUCONATE — INJECTION

products, the interaction has also been reported when ceftriaxone and calcium-containing products were administered at different times and through different infusion lines. Based on 5 half-lives of ceftriaxone, there is a theoretical possibility that the interaction could occur up to 48 hours after ceftriaxone administration.

➤*Storage / Stability:* Store at 15° to 30°C (59° to 86°F). Do not freeze.

CALCIUM GLUBIONATE

otc	**Calcionate** (Various)	**Syrup:** 1.8 g/5 mL	In 473 mL.
otc	**Calciquid** (Breckenridge)		In 473 mL.

Complete and comparative prescribing information for these products begins in the Calcium group monograph. For additional information, refer to the Dietary Reference Intakes of Vitamins and Minerals table.

CALCIUM GLUBIONATE — ORAL

Indications

➤*Dietary supplement:* As a dietary supplement when calcium intake may be inadequate. Conditions that may be associated with calcium deficiency include the following: Vitamin D deficiency, sprue, pregnancy and lactation, achlorhydria, chronic diarrhea, hypoparathyroidism, steatorrhea, menopause, renal failure, pancreatitis, hyperphosphatemia, and alkalosis. Some diuretics and anticonvulsants may precipitate hypocalcemia, which may validate calcium replacement therapy. Calcium salt therapy should not preclude the use of other corrective measures intended to treat the underlying cause of calcium depletion.

➤*Other uses:* Oral calcium may also be used in the treatment of osteoporosis, osteomalacia, rickets, and latent tetany.

➤*PMS symptoms:* Calcium taken daily may help reduce typical premenstrual syndrome (PMS) symptoms such as bloating, cramps, fatigue, and moodiness.

Administration and Dosage

➤*Adults:*

Dietary supplement –

Usual dosage: 15 mL 3 times daily.

• *Pregnant or breast-feeding women* – 15 mL 4 times daily.

➤*Children:*

Dietary supplement –

4 years of age and older: 15 mL 3 times daily.

1 to younger than 4 years of age: 10 mL 3 times daily.

Younger than 12 months of age: 5 mL 5 times daily (may be given alone or mixed with juice or formula).

➤*Administration:* May be given alone or mixed with juice or formula.

➤*Storage / Stability:* Store between 15° and 30°C (59° and 86°F). Keep tightly closed.

CALCIUM LACTATE

otc	**Calcium Lactate** (Various, eg, Dixon-Shane)	**Tablets:** 648 to 650 mg (84.5 mg elemental calcium)	In 100s and 1000s.
otc	**Calcium Lactate** (Various, eg, Freeda)	**Tablets:** 100 mg elemental calcium	In 100s and 250s.
otc sf	**Cal-Lac** (Bio-Tech)	**Capsules:** 500 mg (96 mg elemental calcium)	In 100s.

Complete and comparative prescribing information for these products begins in the Calcium group monograph. For additional information, refer to the Dietary Reference Intakes of Vitamins and Minerals table.

CALCIUM LACTATE — ORAL

Indications

➤*Dietary supplement:* Calcium lactate is indicated as a dietary supplement when calcium intake may be inadequate. Conditions that may be associated with calcium deficiency include the following: Vitamin D deficiency, sprue, pregnancy and lactation, achlorhydria, chronic diarrhea, hypoparathyroidism, steatorrhea, menopause, renal failure, pancreatitis, hyperphosphatemia, and alkalosis. Some diuretics and anticonvulsants may precipitate hypocalcemia, which may validate calcium replacement therapy. Calcium salt therapy should not preclude the use of other corrective measures intended to treat the underlying cause of calcium depletion.

➤*Other uses:* Oral calcium may also be used in the treatment of osteoporosis, osteomalacia, rickets, and latent tetany.

➤*PMS symptoms:* Calcium taken daily may help reduce typical premenstrual syndrome (PMS) symptoms such as bloating, cramps, fatigue, and moodiness.

Administration and Dosage

➤*Adults:*

Dietary supplement – 250 to 600 mg of elemental calcium daily. Varies by product.

➤*Administration:* Take with or following meals to enhance absorption. Take with a large glass of water.

➤*Storage / Stability:* Store at room temperature. Do not expose to excessive heat or moisture.

CALCIUM CITRATE

otc	**Citracal** (Mission)	**Tablets:** 200 mg elemental calcium	(CITRACAL MPC). In 100s.
otc	**Citrus Calcium** (Rugby)	**Tablets:** 200 mg as calcium citrate	Lactose free. Coated. In 100s.
otc	**Calcium Citrate** (Various, eg, Freeda, Vitaline)	**Tablets:** 250 mg elemental calcium	In 100s, 120s, 250s, 500s, and 1,000s.
otc	**Cal-Citrate** (Bio-Tech)		In 250s.
otc	**Calcium Citrate** (Various, eg, Major)	**Tablets:** 950 mg	In 100s.
otc sf	**Cal-Cee** (Key Company)	**Tablets:** 1,150 mg (250 mg elemental calcium)	In 100s.
otc	**Cal-C-Caps** (Key Company)	**Capsules:** 180 mg elemental calcium	In 100s.
otc	**Cal-Citrate** (Bio-Tech)	**Capsules:** 225 mg elemental calcium	In 100s and 250s.
otc	**Calcium Citrate** (Various, eg, Freeda)	**Powder for oral suspension:** 760 mg elemental calcium/5 mL	In 454 g.

Complete prescribing information for these products begins in the Calcium group monograph. For additional information, refer to the Dietary Reference Intakes of Vitamins and Minerals table.

CALCIUM ACETATE

Rx	**Calphron** (Nephro-Tech)	**Tablets; oral:** 667 mg	169 mg elemental calcium. In 200s.
Rx	**Eliphos** (Hawthorn)		169 mg elemental calcium. PEG-8000. (CYP 910). White, round. In 200s.
Rx	**PhosLo** (Fresenius)	**Capsules; oral:** 667 mg	169 mg elemental calcium. Polyethylene glycol 8000. (PhosLo 667 mg). Blue/white. In 200s.
		Gelcaps; oral: 667 mg	169 mg elemental calcium. Polyethylene glycol 8000. (PhosLo 667 mg). Blue/white. In 200s.

Complete and comparative prescribing information for these products begins in the Calcium group monograph. For additional information, refer to the Dietary Reference Intakes of Vitamins and Minerals table.

CALCIUM ACETATE — ORAL

Indications

➤*Hyperphosphatemia:* Control of hyperphosphatemia in end-stage renal failure. Calcium acetate does not promote aluminum absorption.

Administration and Dosage

➤*General dosing considerations:* Calcium acetate therapy should always be started at a low dose and should not be increased without careful monitoring of serum calcium. An initial estimate of daily dietary calcium intake should be made and the intake adjusted as needed.

Patients with end stage renal failure may develop hypercalcemia when given calcium with meals. No other calcium supplements should be given concurrently with calcium acetate.

➤*Adults:*

Hyperphosphatemia –

Initial dosage: 2 capsules/tablets with each meal.

Dosage titration: The dosage may be increased gradually to bring the serum phosphate value below 6 mg/dL, as long as hypercalcemia does not develop.

Maintenance dosage: 3 to 4 capsules/tablets with each meal.

➤*Monitoring:* The serum calcium level should be monitored twice weekly during the early dose adjustment period. Serum phosphorus should also be determined periodically.

➤*Storage/Stability:* Store at 25°C (77°F); excursions permitted between 15° and 30°C (59° and 86°F).

TRICALCIUM PHOSPHATE (Calcium Phosphate, Tribasic)

otc sf	**Posture** (Inverness Medical Innovations)	**Tablets**: 600 mg elemental calcium	Preservative-free. In 90s.

Complete and comparative prescribing information for these products begins in the Calcium group monograph. For additional information, refer to the Dietary Reference Intakes of Vitamins and Minerals table.

CALCIUM CARBONATE

otc	**Calcium Carbonate** (Various, eg, Medirex, Vangard)	**Tablets; oral**: 500 mg (200 mg elemental calcium)	In 100s, 120s, and UD 100s.
otc	**Calcium Carbonate** (Various, eg, Major, Moore)	**Tablets; oral**: 600 mg (240 mg elemental calcium)	In 60s, 72s, 150s and UD 100s.
otc	**Calcium Carbonate** (Various, eg, Freeda, Lilly, Major, Roxane)	**Tablets; oral**: 648 to 650 mg (260 mg elemental calcium)	In 100s, 250s, 500s, and 1,000s.
otc	**Calcium Carbonate** (Various, eg, Roxane)	**Tablets; oral**: 1,250 mg (500 mg elemental calcium)	In 100s.
otc	**Cal-Carb Forte** (Vitaline)		Capsule shape, scored. In 100s.
otc	**Oyster Shell Calcium** (Various, eg, Major)		In 60s, 150s, 300s, 1,000s, and UD 100s.
otc	**Oysco 500** (Rugby)		As oyster shell calcium. In 60s and 250s.
otc sf	**Oyst-Cal 500** (Goldline)		As oyster shell calcium. Preservative free. Tartrazine. In 60s and 120s.
otc sf	**Os-Cal 500** (GlaxoSmithKline Consumer)		Oyster shell powder, corn syrup, parabens. In 75s.
otc	**Calcium Carbonate** (Various, eg, Major)	**Tablets; oral**: 1,500 mg (600 mg elemental calcium)	In 60s and 150s.
otc	**Calcium 600** (Various)		In 60s and 100s.
otc sf	**Caltrate 600** (Whitehall Robins)		Preservative free. (CALTRATE). In 60s.
otc	**Nephro-Calci** (Watson)		(RD26). White, oval, scored. In 100s.
otc	**Calci-Mix** (Watson)	**Capsules; oral**: 1,250 mg (500 mg elemental calcium)	In 100s.
otc	**Pepto Children's** (Procter & Gamble)	**Tablets, chewable; oral**: 400 mg (160 mg elemental calcium)	Sodium free. Mannitol, sorbitol, sugar. Bubble gum and watermelon flavors. In 24s.
otc	**Maalox Children's** (Novartis Consumer Health)		Aspartame, dextrose, maltodextrin, mannitol, 0.3 mg phenylalanine. Wild berry flavor. In 32s.
otc	**Mylanta Children's** (J&J/Merck)		Sorbitol. Bubble gum flavor. In 24s.
otc	**Trial Antacid** (Zee Medical)	**Tablets, chewable; oral**: 420 mg (168 mg elemental calcium)	Sorbitol. Spearmint flavor. In 24s.
otc	**Antacid Tablets** (Goldline)	**Tablets, chewable; oral**: 500 mg (200 mg elemental calcium)	Sucrose, ≤ 2 mg sodium.[a] Assorted flavors. In 150s.
otc	**Cal•Gest** (Rugby)		Dextrose. Assorted flavors. In 150s.
otc	**Dicarbosil** (BIRA)		Less than 2 mg sodium, 10 mEq ANC.[a] Peppermint flavor. White. In rolls of 12.
otc	**Equilet** (Mission)		≤ 0.35 mg sodium.[a] In 150s.
otc	**Maalox Antacid Barrier Maximum Strength** (Novartis)		Aspartame, sugar, mannitol, sucrose, 1.45 mg phenylalanine (mint flavor), 1.1 mg phenylalanine (cherry flavor), 23 mg sodium. In 65s.
otc	**Calcium Antacid Extra Strength** (Various, eg, Major)	**Tablets, chewable; oral**: 750 mg (300 mg elemental calcium)	In 96s.
otc	**Tums E-X** (GlaxoSmithKline Consumer)		Sucrose, talc. Mixed berry, assorted fruit, and sugar free orange (aspartame, less than 1 mg phenylalanine, sorbitol) flavors. In 96s.
otc	**Tums Calcium for Life PMS** (GlaxoSmithKline Consumer)		Sucrose. Strawberry flavor. In 120s.
otc	**Tums Kids** (GlaxoSmithKline Consumer)		Dextrose, gluten, maltodextrin, sorbitol, sucrose. Cherry flavor. In 36s.
otc	**Tums Smooth Dissolve** (GlaxoSmithKline)		Sorbitol, dextrose, sucrose (2 g sugar). In peppermint and assorted fruit flavors. In 45s.
otc	**Alka-Mints** (Bayer)	**Tablets, chewable; oral**: 850 mg (340 mg elemental calcium)	Sorbitol, sugar, less than 5 mg sodium.[a] (Alka-Mints). Assorted flavors and spearmint. In 75s.
otc	**Tums Ultra** (GlaxoSmithKline Consumer)	**Tablets, chewable; oral**: 1,000 mg (400 mg elemental calcium)	Sucrose, talc. Mint flavor. In 86s.
otc	**Rolaids Extra Strength Softchews** (Pfizer Consumer Health)	**Tablets, chewable; oral**: 1177 mg (470.8 mg elemental calcium)	Sucrose, corn syrup, corn syrup solids, nonfat dry milk. Vanilla creme and wild cherry flavors. In 18s.

CALCIUM CARBONATE

otc	**Calcium Carbonate** (Various, eg, Major, Roxane)	**Tablets, chewable; oral:** 1,250 mg (500 mg elemental calcium)	In 60s.
otc	**Cal-Carb Forte** (Vitaline)		Mint flavor. In 100s.
otc	**Calci-Chew** (Watson)		(RD05). Sugar. White. Cherry and assorted flavors. In 100s.
otc	**Os-Cal 500** (GlaxoSmithKline Consumer)		Dextrose. In 60s.
otc	**Tums Calcium for Life Bone Health** (GlaxoSmithKline Consumer)		In 90s.
otc	**Chooz** (Schering-Plough)	**Gum; oral:** 500 mg (200 mg elemental calcium)	Sucrose, glucose. Mint flavor. In 16s.
otc	**Surpass** (Wrigley)	**Gum; oral:** 300 mg (120 mg elemental calcium)	Aspartame, sorbitol. 3.9 mg phenylalanine. Wintergreen flavor. In 10s.
otc	**Surpass Extra Strength** (Wrigley)	**Gum; oral:** 450 mg (180 mg elemental calcium)	Aspartame, sorbitol, 3.9 mg phenylalanine. Fruit flavor. In 10s.
otc	**Calcium Carbonate** (Various, eg, Roxane)	**Suspension; oral:** 1,250 mg (500 mg elemental calcium)/5 mL	In 500 mL and UD 5 mL.
otc	**Calcium Carbonate** (Various, eg, Freeda, Humco)	**Powder; oral**	In 454 g.
otc	**TUMS Quik Pak** (Glaxo Consumer Health)	**Powder; oral:** 1,000 mg	Dextrose, maltodextrin, sorbitol, sucrose. Berry flavor. In 24s.

[a] Acid-neutralizing capacity and sodium content per tablet or 5 mL.

Complete and comparative prescribing information for these products begins in the Calcium group monograph. Also see the Antacids monograph in the Gastrointestinal Agents chapter. For additional information, refer to the Dietary Reference Intakes of Vitamins and Minerals table.

CALCIUM CARBONATE — ORAL

Indications

➤*Antacid:* For the relief of acid indigestion, heartburn, sour stomach, and upset stomach associated with these symptoms.

➤*Calcium supplementation:* May be used as a daily source of calcium for prevention of calcium deficiency; treatment of osteoporosis, osteomalacia, rickets, and latent tetany.

Calcium may be used as a dietary supplement when calcium intake may be inadequate. Conditions that may be associated with calcium deficiency include the following: Vitamin D deficiency, sprue, pregnancy and lactation, achlorhydria, chronic diarrhea, hypoparathyroidism, steatorrhea, menopause, renal failure, pancreatitis, hyperphosphatemia, and alkalosis. Some diuretics and anticonvulsants may precipitate hypocalcemia, which may validate calcium replacement therapy. Calcium salt therapy should not preclude the use of other corrective measures intended to treat the underlying cause of calcium depletion.

➤*Off-label uses:* Calcium taken daily may help reduce typical PMS symptoms such as bloating, cramps, fatigue, and moodiness. 1,000 to 1,200 mg daily for three menstrual cycles.

Administration and Dosage

➤*General dosing considerations:* Do not use the maximum dosage of this product for more than 2 weeks except under the advice and supervision of a health care provider.

➤*Adults:*

Antacid –

Tablets: Swallow or chew 2 to 4 tablets as symptoms occur. Repeat hourly if symptoms return or as directed by a health care provider.

Gum: Chew 1 to 2 tablets (calcium carbonate 500 to 1,000 mg) every 2 to 4 hours.

Calcium supplementation – 500 mg to 2 g 2 to 4 times/day. 1,500 mg/day for men older than 65 years of age and for postmenopausal women not taking estrogen-replacement therapy.

Gum: Chew 1 to 2 tablets after each meal.

Florical: One capsule or tablet daily.

Calci-Mix: One capsule daily as directed. Capsules may be swallowed whole or pulled apart and mixed with food and drink.

Oral suspension: 5 mL (1,250 mg, equivalent to elemental calcium 500 mg) 2 to 3 times daily with meals or as directed by a health care provider (except in unit dose quantities).

➤*Children:* For use as an antacid, see Adults for dosing for children 12 years of age and older.

Off-label dosing –

Antacid:

- *12 years of age and older –*
  Usual dosage: 1,000 mg to 3,000 mg as needed
  Maximum dose: 7,500 mg/day.
- *6 to 11 years of age –*
  Usual dosage: 800 mg as needed.
  Maximum dose: 2,400 mg/day.
- *2 to 5 years of age –*
  Usual dosage: 400 mg as needed.
  Maximum dose: 1,200 mg/day.

Hypocalcemia:

- *Children* – 45 to 65 mg/kg/day (dose expressed as elemental calcium) given in 4 divided doses.
- *Neonate –*
  Usual dosage: 20 to 150 mg/kg/day (dose expressed as elemental calcium). Doses should be divided and given every 4 to 6 hours.
  Maximum dose: 1 g/day (dose expressed as elemental calcium).

➤*Therapeutic drug monitoring:* Perform frequent determinations of serum calcium concentrations. Maintain serum calcium concentrations at 9 to 10.4 mg/dL (4.5 to 5.2 mEq/L). Do not allow levels to exceed 12 mg/dL.

➤*Administration:* Take with or following meals to enhance absorption. Take with a large glass of water.

➤*Storage/Stability:* Store at controlled room temperature between 15° and 30°C (59° and 86°F).

Oral suspension – Protect from freezing.

CALCIUM GLYCEROPHOSPHATE

otc	**Prelief** (AkPharma)	**Tablets; oral:** 340 mg (elemental calcium 65 mg, phosphorous 50 mg)	Magnesium stearate. White, capsule shape. In 120s.

CALCIUM GLYCEROPHOSPHATE — ORAL

Indications

➤*Heartburn:* For the relief of food-caused heartburn.

Administration and Dosage

Two tablets with each meal, snack, or beverage. Two tablets usually remove enough acid from most foods, but more can be taken if needed. For best results, tablets should be used on a daily basis.

CALCIUM MICROCRYSTALLINE HYDROXYAPATITE

otc	**Calcium Microcrystalline Hydroxyapatite** (Pure Encapsulations)	**Capsules; oral:** 150 mg	Bovine. Vitamin C. In 90s and 180s.
		300 mg	Bovine. Vitamin C. In 90s and 180s.

CALCIUM MICROCRYSTALLINE HYDROXYAPATITE — ORAL

Indications

➤*Supports bone health:* Supports bone mineral composition and reduces the risk of osteoporosis.

Administration and Dosage

➤*Adults:*

Supplement –

300 mg: 2 to 4 capsules/day, in divided doses.

150 mg: 2 to 6 capsules/day, in divided doses.

➤*Administration:* Take with or between meals.

➤*Storage/Stability:* Store at room temperature.

PHOSPHORUS

Contents given per tablet or 75 mL reconstituted liquid.

	Product and distributor	Phosphorus		Potassium		Sodium		Recommended adult dose	How supplied
		mg	mEq	mg	mEq	mg	mEq		
Rx	**Uro-KP-Neutral Tablets** (Star)	250	14.25	49.4	1.27	250.5	10.9	1 or 2 tablets 4 times/day with full glass of water	Lt. peach, capsule shape. Film-coated. In 100s.
Rx	**K-Phos Neutral Tablets** (Beach)	250	14.25	45	1.1	298	13		(Beach 1125). White, capsule shape. Film-coated. In 100s and 500s.
otc sf	**PHOS-NaK** (Cypress)	250	unknown	280	unknown	160	unknown	Mix 1 packet with 75 mL water or juice. Take 1 packet qid.	Fruit flavor. In 1.5 g packets (100s)

PHOSPHORUS REPLACEMENT PRODUCTS — ORAL

For information on parenteral phosphate, refer to the monograph in the IV Nutritional Therapy section. For additional information, refer to the Dietary Reference Intakes of Vitamins and Minerals table.

Indications

➤*Dietary supplement:* Dietary supplements of phosphorus, particularly if the diet is restricted or needs are increased.

➤*Phosphate deficiency: Neutra-Phos* and *Neutra-Phos-K* are useful in the treatment of children and adults with conditions associated with excessive renal phosphate loss or inadequate GI absorption of phosphate.

➤*Phosphate diabetes: Neutra-Phos* and *Neutra-Phos-K* are also useful as adjunct supplementation in the management of phosphate diabetes.

Administration and Dosage

➤*Adults:*

Phosphorous supplement –

K-Phos Neutral: 1 or 2 tablets 4 times/day. Take with a full glass of water with meals and at bedtime.

PHOS-NaK: Mix 1 packet with 75 mL water or juice. Take 1 packet 4 times/day.

➤*Children:*

Phosphorous supplement –

K-Phos Neutral:

• *Older than 4 years of age* – 1 tablet 4 times/day. Take with a full glass of water with meals and at bedtime.

PHOS-NaK:

• *4 years of age and older* – Mix 1 packet with 75 mL water or juice. Take 1 packet 4 times/day.

➤*Preparation for administration:*

PHOS-NaK – Mix 1 packet with 75 mL water or juice. Stir well and take promptly.

➤*Administration:*

K-Phos Neutral – Take with a full glass of water with meals and at bedtime.

➤*Storage/Stability:*

Powder – Store in a dry place. When reconstituted to solution, chill if desired.

Tablets – Keep tightly closed. Store at 20° to 25°C (68° to 77°F).

Actions

➤*Pharmacology:* Phosphorus has a number of important functions in the biochemistry of the body. The bulk of the body's phosphorus is located in the bones, where it plays a key role in osteoblastic and osteoclastic activities. Enzymatically catalyzed phosphate-transfer reactions are numerous and vital in the metabolism of carbohydrate, lipid, and protein, and a proper concentration of the anion is of primary importance in assuring an orderly biochemical sequence. In addition, phosphorus plays an important role in modifying steady-state tissue concentrations of calcium. Phosphate ions are important buffers of the intracellular fluid, and also play a primary role in the renal excretion of hydrogen ion.

➤*Pharmacokinetics:*

Absorption – Approximately ⅔ of phosphate consumed by adults is absorbed from the bowel, primarily through sodium-dependent active transport, although passive diffusion does play a role mainly within the jejunum and ileum. When reconstituted to an oral solution, phosphorus shows rapid absorption and utilization from the alimentary tract. Oral phosphate may allow serum levels to rise by as much as 1.5 mg/dL within 60 to 120 minutes after ingestion of 1000 mg phosphorus. The liquid products have an advantage over coated or uncoated tablets, as slow-dissolving tablets may cause local GI irritation or inflammation in sensitive individuals.

Metabolism – Phosphate metabolism is closely associated with calcium metabolism through vitamin D_1 parathyroid hormone, calcitonin, and the mineralization of osteoid. Reduction of plasma phosphate concentrations cause higher serum calcium levels and inhibit deposition of bone salt. An elevated plasma concentration of the phosphate anion promotes the effect of calcitonin on calcium deposition in bone.

Excretion – Over 90% of phosphate absorbed from the GI tract is excreted in the urine through filtration. The majority is then actively reabsorbed by the initial segment of the proximal tubule. A lesser amount is absorbed in the pars recta and/or loop of Henle, distal convulated tubule, and collecting duct. Phosphate excreted into the urine represents a difference between the amount filtered and amount reabsorbed. Tubule secretion is not known to occur in the mammalian kidney. Phosphate reduces levels of urinary calcium and elevates levels of urinary pyrophosphate inhibitor. Orthophosphates have been shown to decrease the crystallization of oxalate in the urine of calculous patients.

Contraindications

Addison's disease; hyperkalemia; acidification of urine in urinary stone disease; patients with infected urolithiasis or struvite stone formation; severely impaired renal function (less than 30% of normal); presence of hyperphosphatemia; hypersensitivity to active or inactive ingredients.

Warnings/Precautions

➤*Potential GI problems:* There have been reports in the literature of small bowel lesions with some long-acting and coated potassium tablets. Orthophosphates may cause dyspepsia in patients with a history of peptic ulcer; other modes of therapy may be necessary in such patients.

➤*Sodium/Potassium restriction:* Use with caution if patient is on a sodium- or potassium-restricted diet. These products provide significant amounts of sodium or potassium.

➤*Kidney stones:* Warn patients with kidney stones of the possibility of passing stones when phosphate therapy is started.

➤*Special risk:* Use with caution when the following medical problems exist: Cardiac disease (particularly in digitalized patients); acute dehydration; renal function impairment or chronic renal disease; extensive tissue breakdown; myotonia congenita; cardiac failure; cirrhosis of the liver or severe hepatic disease; peripheral and pulmonary edema; hypernatremia; hypertension; pre-eclampsia; hypoparathyroidism; osteomalacia; acute pancreatitis; rickets (rickets may benefit from phosphate therapy; however, use caution); severe adrenal insufficiency.

➤*Pregnancy: Category C.* It is not known whether this product can cause fetal harm or affect reproduction capacity when administered to a pregnant woman. Use only when clearly needed.

➤*Lactation:* It is not known whether this drug is excreted in breast milk. Exercise caution when administering to a nursing woman.

➤*Children:* For pediatric patients younger than 4 years of age, use only as directed by a physician.

➤*Monitoring:* The following determinations are important in patient monitoring (other tests may be warranted in some patients): Renal function; serum calcium; serum phosphorus; serum potassium; serum sodium. Monitor at periodic intervals during therapy.

PHOSPHORUS REPLACEMENT PRODUCTS — ORAL

Drug Interactions

Phosphate Drug Interactions			
Precipitant drug	Object drug[a]		Description
Androgens	Potassium and phosphate	↑	Androgens may cause retention of potassium and phosphate. Therefore, concurrent use with potassium phosphate may cause hyperkalemia or hyperphosphatemia.
Antacids	Phosphates	↓	Antacids containing magnesium, aluminum, or calcium may bind to phosphate and prevent its absorption.
Calcium Vitamin D	Phosphates	↓	The effects of phosphates may be antagonized in the treatment of hypercalcemia.
Iron supplements	Phosphate	↓	Iron-containing medications have the ability to bind phosphate and form an insoluble complex, thus preventing absorption.
Phosphate	Anorexiants	↓	Acidification of urine may increase elimination and decrease therapeutic effect of anorexiants.
Phosphate	Chlorpropamide (sulfonylurea)	↑	Acidification of urine may increase bioavailability of chlorpropamide and enhance the hypoglycemic actions.
Phosphate	Methadone	↓	Acidification of the urine increases renal clearance of methadone because of increased ionization.
Phosphate	Sympathomimetics	↓	Acidification of urine may increase elimination and decrease therapeutic effect of sympathomimetics.

[a] ↑ = Object drug increased. ↓ = Object drug decreased.

Adverse Reactions

Individuals may experience a mild laxative effect for the first few days. If this persists, reduce the daily intake until this effect subsides, or, if necessary, discontinue use.

GI upset (eg, diarrhea, nausea, stomach pain, vomiting) may occur with phosphate therapy. The following side effects have been reported less frequently: Headaches; dizziness; mental confusion; seizures; weakness or heaviness of legs; unusual tiredness or weakness; muscle cramps; numbness, tingling, pain, or weakness of hands or feet; numbness or tingling around lips; fast or irregular heartbeat; shortness of breath or troubled breathing; swelling of feet or lower legs; unusual weight gain; low urine output; unusual thirst; bone and joint pain. High serum phosphate levels may increase the incidence of extraskeletal calcification.

Magnesium

For more information on parenteral magnesium, refer to the IV Nutritional Therapy monograph in this chapter and the Anticonvulsant monograph in the CNS chapter.

Indications

➤*Magnesium dietary supplement:* As a dietary supplement.

Administration and Dosage

1 g Mg = 83.3 mEq (41.7 mmol).

➤*Dietary supplement:* 40 to 400 mg/day in divided doses. Refer to product labeling.

➤*Recommended dietary allowances (RDAs):*

Adult – Males, 270 to 400 mg; females, 280 to 300 mg. For a complete listing of RDAs by age, sex, and condition, refer to the RDA table.

Magnesium-containing antacids also may be used; refer to the Antacids monograph in the GI Agents chapter.

Actions

➤*Pharmacology:* Magnesium is the fourth most abundant mineral in the body and the second most abundant in muscles and other organs. Only potassium levels are higher than magnesium in soft tissues (non-bone tissues). Potassium cannot be retained in soft tissues and leaks out if magnesium is deficient. An adequate amount of magnesium also is required for the absorption and utilization of calcium, favoring the deposition of calcium in bone where it belongs and preventing deposition of calcium in the soft tissues and kidneys where it does not belong. Magnesium is required in adequate amount for the normal activity of 300 enzymes, including those involved in the transfer of energy from foods to physical and mental activities. It is a very important stabilizer of polynucleic acids, substances where genetic information is stored. Unstable nucleic acids predispose to cancer.

Warnings/Precautions

➤*Renal disease:* Do not use without health care provider supervision because of potential accumulation.

➤*Excessive dosage:* Excessive dosage may cause diarrhea and GI irritation.

➤*Heart disease:* Magnesium supplements may make this condition worse.

➤*Pregnancy: Category A.* It is unknown whether magnesium supplementation will harm a fetus or a breast-feeding child. Do not take this mineral without speaking with a health care provider if pregnant, planning a pregnancy, or breast-feeding. RDA of magnesium in pregnant women is 350 to 400 mg/day. (Refer to the Dietary Reference Intakes of Vitamins and Minerals table.)

➤*Lactation:* RDA of magnesium in a breast-feeding woman is 310 to 360 mg/day. (Refer to the Dietary Reference Intakes of Vitamins and Minerals table.)

Drug Interactions

Magnesium Drug Interactions			
Precipitant drug	Object drug[a]		Description
Magnesium salts	Aminoquinolines (eg, chloroquine)	↓	The absorption and therapeutic effect of the aminoquinolines may be decreased.
Magnesium salts	Nitrofurantoin	↓	Adsorption of nitrofurantoin onto magnesium salts may occur, decreasing the bioavailability and possibly the anti-infective effect of nitrofurantoin.
Magnesium salts	Penicillamine	↓	The GI absorption of penicillamine may be decreased, possibly decreasing its pharmacologic effects; however, this only has been reported for magnesium-containing antacids.
Magnesium salts	Tetracyclines	↓	The GI absorption and serum levels of tetracyclines may be decreased; a decreased antimicrobial response may occur.

[a] ↓ = Object drug decreased.

Overdosage

➤*Symptoms:* It is possible to overdose on any electrolyte if large quantities are given; magnesium is no exception. Administer magnesium cautiously, especially to patients with decreased renal function. The most common symptom of overdose is diarrhea. At serum levels between 3 to 5 mEq/L, there is a propensity for hypotension because of peripheral dilation. Severe hypotension may be seen at higher levels. Facial flushing may be seen, associated with a feeling of warmth or thirst. Nausea and vomiting may occur but are not always present. Lethargy, dysarthria, and drowsiness can appear when levels reach 5 to 7 mEq/L. Deep tendon reflexes are lost when levels reach 7 mEq/L. Shallow respirations, irregular brief periods of apnea, and, finally, prolonged apnea are expected when levels exceed 10 mEq/L. Coma occurs when serum levels are between 12 and 15 mEq/L. Finally, when levels exceed 15 to 20 mEq/L, cardiac arrest may be expected.

➤*Treatment:* Terminate exposure. Calcium administration improves many toxic symptoms. Forced diuresis intensifies the elimination of magnesium; hemodialysis is extremely effective at magnesium removal but is infrequently necessary in the absence of renal failure.

MAGNESIUM

otc	**Magnesium Gluconate** (Various, eg, Freeda)	**Tablets; oral:** elemental magnesium ≈ 27 mg	In 100s and 500s.
otc	**Magnesium** (Various, eg, Ivax)	**Tablets; oral:** elemental magnesium 30 mg	In 100s.
otc	**Magnesium** (Key Co)	**Tablets; oral:** elemental magnesium 80 mg	In 100s.
otc	**Magnesium Citrate** (Various, eg, Freeda)	**Tablets; oral:** elemental magnesium 100 mg	In 100s and 250s
otc	**Mag-200** (Optimox)	**Tablets; oral:** elemental magnesium 200 mg (as oxide)	300 mg PABA. In 120s.
otc	**Magnesium** (21st Century)	**Tablets; oral:** elemental magnesium 250 mg (as oxide)	Gluten free, preservative free. Calcium 47 mg. In 110s.
otc sf	**Mag-Ox 400** (Blaine)	**Tablets; oral:** magnesium oxide 400 mg (elemental magnesium 241.3 mg)	Sugar free. (BLAINE). In 120s, 1,000s, and UD 100s.
otc	**Magnesium Oxide** (Various, eg, Breckenridge, Cypress, Plus Pharma)		In 120s and 400s.
otc	**Maox 420** (Manne Co.)	**Tablets; oral:** magnesium oxide 420 mg (elemental magnesium 253 mg)	Tartrazine. 21 mEq acid neutralizing capacity per tablet. In 250s and 1,000s.
otc	**Mag-G** (Cypress)	**Tablets; oral:** magnesium gluconate dihydrate 500 mg (elemental magnesium 27 mg)	In 100s.
otc	**Magonate** (Fleming)		Ca 87.5 mg, P 66 mg (dibasic calcium phosphate dihydrate 376 mg). In 1,000s.
otc	**Magtrate** (Mission)	**Tablets; oral:** magnesium gluconate 500 mg (elemental magnesium 29 mg)	In 100s.
otc	**Magnesium Oxide** (Various, eg, Major)	**Tablets; oral:** magnesium oxide 500 mg (elemental magnesium 302 mg)	In 100s.
otc sf	**Maginex** (Logan Pharm)	**Tablets, enteric-coated; oral:** magnesium L-aspartate hydrochloride 615 mg (elemental magnesium 61 mg)	Sugar free. In blister pack 100s, UD 100s, and robot-ready 100s.
otc	**Slow-Mag** (Purdue)	**Tablets, enteric-coated; oral:** elemental magnesium 64 mg (as chloride hexahydrate)	Calcium carbonate. In 60s.
otc	**Mag-Tab SR** (Niche)	**Tablets, sustained-release; oral:** elemental magnesium 84 mg (as L-lactate dihydrate)	Lt. yellow, capsule shape, scored. In 60s, 100s, and 1,000s.
otc sf	**Uro-Mag** (Blaine)	**Capsules; oral:** magnesium oxide 140 mg (elemental magnesium 84.5 mg)	Sugar free. In 100s, 1,000s, and UD 100s.
otc	**Mag-Caps** (Genesis)	**Capsules; oral:** magnesium oxide ≈ 140 mg (elemental magnesium 85 mg)	In 100s.
otc sf	**Magonate Natal** (Fleming)	**Liquid; oral:** elemental magnesium 3.52 mg (as gluconate)/mL	Sugar free. In 480 mL.
otc	**Magonate** (Fleming)	**Liquid; oral:** magnesium gluconate dihydrate 1,000 mg per 5 mL (elemental magnesium 54 mg per 5 mL)	Sorbitol, magnesium carbonate. Melon flavor. In 473 mL.
otc	**Maginex DS** (Logan Pharm)	**Powder; oral:** magnesium L-aspartate hydrochloride 1,230 mg (elemental magnesium 122 mg)/packet	Preservative free. Sucrose. Lemon flavor. In 30s and robot-ready 30s.

For prescribing information for oral magnesium, refer to the Magnesium introduction. For more information on parenteral magnesium, refer to the IV Nutritional Therapy monograph in this chapter and the Anticonvulsant monograph in the CNS chapter.

MAGNESIUM GLUCONATE — ORAL

For additional information, refer to the Dietary Reference Intakes of Vitamins and Minerals table.

Indications

➤*Magnesium supplement:* Magnesium gluconate is a magnesium supplement for the maintenance of proper magnesium levels in the body. Magnesium gluconate is available as the magnesium gluconate chelate in both tablet and liquid forms.

Administration and Dosage

➤*General dosing considerations:* Two tablets or magnesium gluconate 5 mL (dihydrate) liquid contain elemental magnesium 54 mg. Magnesium 54 mg is 4.4 mEq.

➤*Adults:*

Magnesium supplement –

Initial dosage:

- *Liquid* – 5 to 10 mL of liquid the first day.
- *Tablets* – 2 to 4 tablets the first day.

Dosage titration: Increase daily dose until the stool becomes soft and remains so. With loose stool, reduce magnesium intake slightly. This titration regimen is done to prevent diarrhea and ensure proper magnesium homeostasis.

➤*Children:*

Magnesium supplement – Initiate at about half the adult dose and then titrate. (See Adults for more information.)

➤*Administration:* Administer with water on an empty stomach or at least 30 minutes before meals.

➤*Storage/Stability:* Store at 25°C (77°F); excursions are permitted to 15° to 30°C (59° to 86°F). Keep container tightly closed and protected from heat and moisture.

MAGNESIUM L-LACTATE DIHYDRATE — ORAL

For additional information, refer to the Dietary Reference Intakes of Vitamins and Minerals table.

Indications

➤*Heart diseases:* Studies have shown that people with low levels of magnesium are more prone to cardiovascular disease and sudden death than those who consume higher amounts of magnesium. Magnesium deficiencies may lead to hardening of the arteries, an increase in blood pressure, and irregular heart beats (ie, palpitations, arrhythmia) which can be life-threatening.

Many patients on diuretics are given potassium supplements. Its important to note that when people are losing potassium they are also losing magnesium. In most instances, patients who need potassium supplements also need magnesium supplements. Magnesium supplements replace the lost magnesium and help the body better utilize the potassium supplements.

➤*Diabetics:* Patients with diabetes are especially susceptible to magnesium deficiencies, which can lead to a host of complications. Diabetes causes increased excretion and decreased absorption of this mineral. Insulin deficiencies lead to more "wasting" of magnesium, and these deficiencies affect glucose tolerance and insulin resistance. Magnesium helps support insulin function and glucose metabolism.

The American Diabetes Association advises that an adequate supply of magnesium is essential to protect diabetics from developing cardiovascular diseases, and recommends that diabetics using diuretics on a long-term basis, or those having calcium or potassium deficiencies, congestive heart failure or a history of heart attack be tested/treated for magnesium deficiency.

Recent studies report other possible benefits of magnesium to include reducing platelet aggregation and helping maintain HDL ("good" cholesterol) levels.

MAGNESIUM L-LACTATE DIHYDRATE — ORAL

➤*Other conditions:* Clinicians have found that magnesium supplements are important for the following groups of patients with low magnesium levels: pregnancy (preeclampsia); patients receiving chemotherapy; transplant patients taking immunosuppressant drugs; patients with GI disorders such as inflammatory bowel disease; Crohn disease; malabsorption syndromes; people with migraine headaches; people who consume large quantities of alcohol.

➤*Off-label uses:* A pyridoxine/magnesium oxide combination has been used to prevent recurrence of calcium oxalate kidney stones.

Oral magnesium gluconate may be a cost-effective and clinically effective alternative to oral ritodrine as a tocolytic for continued inhibition of contractions following parenteral magnesium sulfate. Further study is needed.

Administration and Dosage

➤*General dosing considerations:* Two tablets provide magnesium 168 mg.

➤*Adults:*

Magnesium supplement – 1 or 2 tablets every 12 hours or as directed by a health care provider.

➤*Storage / Stability:* Store at 15° to 30°C (59° to 86°F).

MAGNESIUM OXIDE — ORAL

For additional information, refer to the Dietary Reference Intakes of Vitamins and Minerals table.

Indications

➤*Tablets:* Dietary supplement to increase daily intake of magnesium and for the relief of acid indigestion and upset stomach.

➤*Capsules:* Adult dietary supplement to increase daily intake of magnesium.

➤*Off-label uses:* A pyridoxine/magnesium oxide combination has been used to prevent recurrence of calcium oxalate kidney stones.

Administration and Dosage

➤*Adults:*

Antacid –

Tablets:

- *Usual dose* – 1 tablet 2 times a day.
- *Maximum dose* – 2 tablets/day.

Dietary supplement –

Capsules: 1 to 5 capsules daily.

Tablets: 1 to 2 tablets daily.

➤*Duration of therapy:* Do not use the maximum dosage for more than 2 weeks.

➤*Storage / Stability:* Store at 15° to 30°C (59° to 86°F).

MAGNESIUM CITRATE — ORAL

For additional information, refer to the Dietary Reference Intakes of Vitamins and Minerals table.

Indications

➤*Magnesium deficiency:* Magnesium is used as a magnesium supplement for the maintenance of proper magnesium levels in the body.

➤*Laxative:* For use as a hyperosmotic saline laxative.

Administration and Dosage

➤*Adults:*

Antacid – 1 tablet twice daily or as directed by a health care provider.

Dietary supplement – 2 tablets daily.

Laxative – 2 to 4 tablets daily, all at bedtime or individually throughout the day.

➤*Administration:* Magnesium supplements should be taken with meals and a full glass of water. Taking magnesium supplements on an empty stomach may cause diarrhea.

➤*Storage / Stability:* Store at room temperature, away from heat and direct light. Do not freeze or refrigerate.

MAGNESIUM ELEMENTAL — ORAL

Indications

➤*Magnesium supplement:* For the maintenance of proper magnesium levels in the body.

Administration and Dosage

➤*Adults:*

Dietary reference intake for elemental magnesium –

31 years of age and older: 420 mg/day (men); 320 mg/day (women).

19 to 30 years of age: 400 mg/day (men); 310 mg/day (women).

Pregnant women: 350 mg/day (19 to 30 years of age); 360 mg/day (31 to 50 years of age).

Breast-feeding women: 310 mg/day (19 to 30 years of age); 320 mg/day (31 to 50 years of age).

Hypomagnesemia –

Mild hypomagnesemia: Up to 240 mg/day in divided doses.

Severe hypomagnesemia: Up to 720 mg/day in divided doses.

➤*Children:*

Dietary reference intakes for elemental magnesium –

14 to 18 years of age: 410 mg/day (men); 360 mg/day (women).

9 to 13 years of age: 240 mg/day.

4 to 8 years of age: 130 mg/day.

1 to 3 years of age: 80 mg/day.

7 to 12 months of age: 75 mg/day (Adequate Intake value).

0 to 6 months of age: 30 mg/day (Adequate Intake value).

Hypomagnesemia – See Adults for dosing.

➤*Renal function impairment:* Do not use in patients with kidney disease or renal dysfunction without the supervision of a health care provider.

➤*Administration:* Should be taken with food.

➤*Storage / Stability:* Store at 15° to 30°C (59° to 86°F).

MAGNESIUM L-ASPARTATE HYDROCHLORIDE ORAL

Indications

➤*Magnesium supplement:* For the maintenance of proper magnesium levels in the body.

Administration and Dosage

➤*Adults:*

Magnesium supplement –

Maginex: Two tablets of magnesium L-aspartate 615 mg (magnesium 61 mg) up to 3 times daily.

Maginex DS: 1 packet of magnesium L-aspartate 1,230 mg (magnesium 122 mg) up to 3 times daily.

➤*Children:*

Magnesium supplement – See Adults for dosing.

➤*Renal function impairment:* Do not use in patients with kidney disease or renal dysfunction without the supervision of a health care provider.

➤*Administration:*

Maginex DS – Mix 1 packet in 120 mL of water or juice.

➤*Storage / Stability:* Store at 15° to 30°C (59° to 86°F).

SELENIUM

otc	**Selenium** (Various, eg, Major, Nature's Bounty, Windmill)	**Tablets; oral:** 50 mcg	In 100s.
otc sf	**Selenimin-50** (Key Co)		Film-coated. Sugar free and wheat free. In 100s.
otc sf	**Selenium** (Mason)	**Tablets; oral:** 100 mcg	In 100s.
otc sf	**Selenimin** (Key Co)	**Tablets; oral:** 125 mcg	Film-coated. Sugar free and wheat free. In 100s.
otc sf	**Selenium** (Various, eg, J.R. Carlson, Nature's Bounty, Windmill)	**Tablets; oral:** 200 mcg	In 50s, 60s, and 100s.
otc sf	**Selenimin-200** (Key Co)		Film-coated. Sugar free and wheat free. In 100s.
otc sf	**Selenium** (Major)	**Tablets, extended-release; oral:** 200 mcg	Contains wheat ingredients. Lactose free, preservative free, and sugar free. In 60s.
otc sf	**Selenium** (McGuff)	**Capsules; oral:** 100 mcg	Gluten free, preservative free, and sugar free. In 100s.
otc sf	**Se-100** (Bio-Tech Pharmacal)		Dye free, preservative free, and sugar free. In 100s.
otc	**Selenium** (Various, eg, J.R. Carlson)	**Capsules; oral:** 200 mcg	In 60s and 100s.
otc sf	**Selenicaps-200** (Key Co)		Sugar free and wheat free. In 100s.

SELENIUM — ORAL

Indications

➤*Selenium supplement:* As a nutritional supplement to prevent or treat selenium deficiency.

Administration and Dosage

➤*Adults:*

Selenium supplementation – 100 to 200 mcg/day, preferably with meals. The 50 mcg tablets may be taken as 1 tablet 4 times daily.

➤*Administration:* Take tablets with meals.

➤*Storage / Stability:* Store tightly closed in a cool, dry place. Avoid excessive heat.

Actions

➤*Pharmacology:* Selenium is an essential trace mineral that supports the immune system. As a component of the antioxidant enzyme glutathione peroxidase, selenium helps to protect cells from the harmful effects of free radicals. Selenium also spares vitamin E, which in turn boosts the cell's antioxidant defense system. Selenium plays a role in the structure of teeth.

➤*Pharmacokinetics:*

Absorption / Distribution – Selenium is readily absorbed from the GI tract and is then stored in the red blood cells, liver, spleen, heart, and nails.

Metabolism / Excretion – Once selenium reaches the tissues, it is converted to its active form. It is primarily excreted in the urine and, to a lesser extent, in the feces.

Contraindications

None well documented.

Warnings/Precautions

➤*Hypersensitivity reactions:* Some products contain yeast. Avoid administering these products in patients who are allergic to yeast.

➤*Pregnancy:* The recommended dietary allowance of selenium in pregnant women is 60 mcg/day. According to the manufacturers, selenium supplements are not intended for pregnant women. (Refer to the Dietary Reference Intakes of Vitamins and Minerals table.)

➤*Lactation:* The recommended dietary allowance of selenium in breast-feeding women is 70 mcg/day. According to the manufacturers, selenium supplements are not intended for breast-feeding women. (Refer to the Dietary Reference Intakes of Vitamins and Minerals table.)

Drug Interactions

None well documented.

Overdosage

➤*Symptoms:* Long-term exposure of selenium in high amounts may have toxic effects on the endocrine system, liver, GI tract, and skin (eg, nail and hair loss, dermatitis), and may also possibly cause neurotoxicity.

Symptoms of acute selenium overdose include GI effects (eg, vomiting), garlic breath odor or sour breath, restlessness, hypersalivation, muscle spasms, hemolysis, liver necrosis, cerebral edema, pulmonary edema, coma, and death.

Patient Information

Advise patients to take selenium with food.

Advise patients to consult with their health care provider before use if they are taking any medications.

Instruct patients to discontinue use and consult their health care provider if any adverse reactions occur.

Iron

IRON-CONTAINING PRODUCTS

For additional information, refer to the Dietary Reference Intakes of Vitamins and Minerals table.

> **WARNING**
>
> Accidental overdose of iron-containing products is a leading cause of fatal poisoning in children younger than 6 years of age. Keep products out of the reach of children. In case of accidental overdose, call a doctor or a poison control center immediately.

Indications

➤*Iron deficiency:* For the prevention and treatment of iron deficiency and iron deficiency anemias.

➤*Iron supplement:* As a dietary supplement for iron.

➤*Off-label uses:* Iron supplementation may be required by most patients receiving epoetin therapy. Failure to administer iron supplements (oral or intravenous [IV]) during epoetin therapy can impair the hematologic response to epoetin.

Administration and Dosage

Due to the availability of multiple salt forms, close attention is warranted when administering iron. Substitution of 1 salt for another without proper adjustment may result in serious over or under dosing.

Carbonyl iron and polysaccharide-iron complex are reported to be associated with fewer GI effects and are less toxic than other forms of iron.

The length of iron therapy depends upon the cause and severity of the iron deficiency. In general, approximately 4 to 6 months of oral iron therapy is required to reverse uncomplicated iron deficiency anemias. Iron therapy should increase hemoglobin levels by 1 g/week.

➤*Iron replacement therapy in deficiency states:* Iron doses are given as elemental iron.

Premature infants – 2 to 4 mg/kg/day given in 1 to 2 divided doses. Maximum dosage is 15 mg/day.

Children – 3 to 6 mg/kg/day given in 1 to 3 divided doses.

Adults – 150 to 300 mg/day given in 3 divided doses. Alternatively, 60 mg given 2 to 4 times/day may help lessen GI effects.

➤*Prevention of iron deficiency:*

Premature infants – 2 mg/kg/day given in 1 to 3 divided doses. Maximum dosage is 15 mg/day.

Children – 1 to 2 mg/kg/day given in 1 to 3 divided doses. Maximum dosage is 15 mg/day.

Adults – 60 mg/day given in 1 to 2 divided doses.

➤*Recommended dietary allowances (RDAs):* For a complete listing of RDAs, refer to the RDAs section of the Nutrients and Nutritionals chapter.

IRON-CONTAINING PRODUCTS

RDAs for Iron	
Patients	RDA for iron (mg/day)
Children	
7 to 12 months of age	11
1 to 3 years of age	7
4 to 8 years of age	10
Males	
9 to 13 years of age	8
14 to 18 years of age	11
≥ 19 years of age	8
Females	
9 to 13 years of age	8
14 to 18 years of age	15
19 to 50 years of age	18
older than 50 years of age	8
Pregnancy	27
Lactation	
≤ 18 years of age	10
≥ 19 years of age	9

➤*Iron supplementation:*

Pregnancy – Elemental iron 15 to 30 mg/day should be adequate to meet the daily requirement of the last 2 trimesters.

Actions

➤*Pharmacology:* Iron, an essential mineral, is a component of hemoglobin, myoglobin, and a number of enzymes (eg, cytochromes, catalase, peroxidase). The total body content of iron is approximately 50 mg/kg in men (3.5 g in the average 70 kg man), and 37 mg/kg in women. Iron is primarily stored as hemosiderin or aggregated ferritin, found in the reticuloendothelial system and hepatocytes. Approximately two thirds of total body iron is in the circulating red blood cell mass in hemoglobin, the major factor in oxygen transport.

Iron deficiency can affect muscle metabolism, heat production, and catecholamine metabolism and has been associated with behavioral or learning problems in children.

➤*Pharmacokinetics:*

Absorption/Distribution – The average dietary intake of iron is 12 to 20 mg/day for males and 8 to 15 mg/day for females; however, only approximately 10% of this iron is absorbed (1 to 2 mg/day) in individuals with adequate iron stores. Absorption is enhanced when storage iron is depleted or when erythropoiesis occurs at an increased rate.

Iron is primarily absorbed from the duodenum and jejunum. The ferrous salt form is absorbed 3 times more readily than the ferric form. The common ferrous salts (ie, sulfate, gluconate, fumarate) are absorbed almost on a milligram-for-milligram basis but differ in the content of elemental iron. Polysaccharide-complex is a product of ferric iron complexed to a low molecular weight polysaccharide. A radioisotope tracer study in humans demonstrated that absorption of polysaccharide-iron complex is comparable with that of ferrous sulfate. Sustained-release or enteric-coated preparations reduce the amount of available iron; absorption from these doseforms is reduced because iron is transported beyond the duodenum. Dose also influences the amount of iron absorbed. The amount of iron absorbed increases progressively with larger doses; however, the percentage absorbed decreases. Food can decrease the absorption of iron at least 50%; however, gastric intolerance may often necessitate administering the drug with food.

Excretion – Iron is transported via the blood and bound to transferrin. The daily loss of iron from urine, sweat, and sloughing of intestinal mucosal cells amounts to approximately 0.5 to 1 mg in healthy men. In menstruating women, approximately 1 to 2 mg is the normal daily loss.

Elemental Iron Content of Iron Salts	
Iron salt	% Iron
Ferrous fumarate	≈ 33
Ferrous gluconate	≈ 12
Ferrous sulfate	≈ 20
Ferrous sulfate, exsiccated (dried)	≈ 32

Contraindications

Hemochromatosis; hemosiderosis; hemolytic anemias; known hypersensitivity to any ingredient.

Warnings/Precautions

➤*Chronic iron intake:* Individuals with normal iron balance should not take iron chronically.

➤*Accidental overdose:* Accidental overdose of iron-containing products is a leading cause of fatal poisoning in children younger than 6 years of age. Keep this product out of reach of children.

➤*Intolerance:* Discontinue use if symptoms of intolerance appear.

➤*GI effects:* Occasional GI discomfort, such as nausea, may be minimized by taking with meals and by slowly increasing to the recommended dosage.

➤*Tartrazine sensitivity:* Some of these products contain tartrazine, which may cause allergic-type reactions (including bronchial asthma) in susceptible individuals. Although the incidence of tartrazine sensitivity in the general population is low, it is frequently seen in patients who also have aspirin hypersensitivity. Specific products containing tartrazine are identified in the product listings.

➤*Sulfite sensitivity:* Some of the products contain sulfites, which may cause allergic-type reactions (eg, hives, itching, wheezing, anaphylaxis) in certain susceptible people. Although the overall prevalence of sulfite sensitivity in the general population is probably low, it is seen more frequently in asthmatic or in atopic nonasthmatic people. Specific products containing sulfites are identified in the product listings.

➤*Pregnancy: Category A.* RDA of iron in pregnant women is 27 mg/day (refer to the Dietary Reference Intakes of Vitamins and Minerals table).

➤*Lactation:* RDA of iron in breast-feeding women is 9 to 10 mg/day (refer to the Dietary Reference Intakes of Vitamins and Minerals table).

Drug Interactions

Iron Salts Drug Interactions			
Precipitant drug	Object drug[a]		Description
Acetohydroxamic acid (AHA)	Iron salts	⬇	AHA chelates heavy metals, notably iron. The absorption of iron may be decreased. When iron is indicated, administer intramuscularly (IM).
Antacids	Iron salts	⬇	GI absorption of iron may be reduced.
Ascorbic acid	Iron salts	⬆	Ascorbic acid at doses ≥ 200 mg have been shown to enhance the absorption of iron ≥ 30%.
Calcium salts	Iron salts	⬇	GI absorption of iron may be reduced. When possible, separate administration times.
Chloramphenicol	Iron salts	⬆	Serum iron levels may be increased.
Digestive enzymes	Iron salts	⬇	The serum iron response to oral iron may be decreased by concomitant pancreatic extracts.
H_2 antagonists	Iron salts	⬇	GI absorption of iron may be reduced.
Proton pump inhibitors	Iron salts	⬇	GI absorption of iron may be reduced.
Trientine	Iron salts	⬇	The 2 agents inhibit the absorption of each other. If iron is needed, administer the agents at least 2 hours apart.
Iron salts	Trientine		
Iron salts	Captopril	⬇	Concomitant use within 2 hours may promote formation of inactive captopril disulfide dimer.
Iron salts	Cephalosporins (eg, cefdinir)	⬇	Iron supplements and foods fortified with iron may reduce the absorption of cefdinir 80% and 30%, respectively. If iron supplements are needed during cefdinir therapy, cefdinir should be taken 2 hours before or after the supplement. Iron-fortified infant formula (elemental iron 2.2 mg per 6 oz) has no effect on cefdinir absorption.
Iron salts	Fluoroquinolones (eg, ciprofloxacin)	⬇	GI absorption of fluoroquinolones may be decreased because of formation of iron-quinolone complex. Avoid coadministration of these drugs. (See individual fluoroquinolone monographs for administration recommendations.)
Iron salts	Levodopa	⬇	Levodopa appears to form chelates with iron salts, decreasing levodopa absorption and serum levels.
Iron salts	Levothyroxine	⬇	The efficacy of levothyroxine may be decreased, resulting in hypothyroidism. Avoid coadministration.
Iron salts	Methyldopa	⬇	Extent of methyldopa absorption may be decreased, possibly resulting in decreased efficacy.
Iron salts	Mycophenolate mofetil	⬇	Absorption of mycophenolate mofetil may be decreased. Avoid simultaneous administration.

IRON-CONTAINING PRODUCTS

Iron Salts Drug Interactions			
Precipitant drug	Object drug[a]		Description
Iron salts	Penicillamine	⬇	Marked reduction in GI absorption of penicillamine may occur, possibly because of chelation.
Iron salts	Tetracyclines	⬇	Concomitant use within 2 hours may decrease absorption and serum levels of tetracyclines.
Tetracyclines	Iron salts		Absorption of iron salts also may be decreased.
Iron salts	Thyroid hormones	⬇	Absorption of thyroid hormones may be decreased. Avoid coadministration.

[a] ⬆ = Object drug increased. ⬇ = Object drug decreased.

➤*Drug/Food interactions:* Administration of iron with food decreases the iron absorption by at least 50%.

Adverse Reactions

Iron-containing liquids may temporarily stain the teeth (enamel is not affected). Dilute the liquid and/or drink through a straw to reduce this possibility. When iron-containing drops are given to infants, the membrane covering the teeth may darken.

➤*GI:* Abdominal pain, constipation, diarrhea, GI irritation, nausea, vomiting. Stools may appear darker in color.

Overdosage

➤*Symptoms:* Symptoms may present when at least 20 mg/kg is ingested. Acute poisoning will produce symptoms in the following 4 stages:

1.) Within 6 hours: abdominal pain, coma, diminished tissue perfusion, dyspnea, fever, hyperglycemia, hypotension, lethargy, leukocytosis, metabolic acidosis, nausea, tarry stools, vomiting, weak-rapid pulse.
2.) If not immediately fatal, symptoms may subside within 12 to 24 hours.
3.) Symptoms return 12 to 48 hours after ingestion and may include the following: anuria, convulsions, death, diffuse vascular congestion, hyperthermia, metabolic acidosis, pulmonary edema, shock.
4.) If patient survives, in 2 to 6 weeks after ingestion pyloric or antral stenosis, hepatic cirrhosis, and CNS damage may be seen.

➤*Treatment:* Maintain proper airway, respiration, and circulation. Perform gastric lavage in patients who are candidates for GI decontamination. Systemic chelation therapy with deferoxamine is generally recommended for patients with serum iron levels greater than 350 to 500 mcg/dL or in patients with symptoms of iron toxicity. IM therapy may suffice, but severe poisoning (eg, shock, coma) may require IV administration (see deferoxamine mesylate in the Detoxification Agents section). Specific treatment for shock, convulsions, acidosis, and renal failure may be necessary. Treatment includes usual supportive measures. Refer to General Management of Acute Overdosage.

Patient Information

Inform patients to take on an empty stomach; if GI upset occurs, advise to take after meals or with food.

Advise patients not to take within 2 hours of antacids, tetracyclines, or fluoroquinolones.

Inform patients to drink liquid iron preparations in water or juice and through a straw to prevent tooth staining.

Inform patients that medication may cause black stools, constipation, or diarrhea.

Advise patients not to crush or chew sustained-release preparations.

FERROUS SULFATE

Ferrous sulfate – 20% elemental iron; ferrous sulfate exsiccated (dried) – approximately 30% elemental iron.

otc	**Ferrous Sulfate** (Magnus-Humphries Labs)	**Tablets; oral:** 27 mg	PEG. In 100s.
otc	**Feosol** (GlaxoSmithKline)	**Tablets; oral:** 200 mg (65 mg iron)	Exsiccated. Glucose. (Fe). In 100s.
otc	**Feratab** (Upsher-Smith)	**Tablets; oral:** 300 mg (60 mg iron)	Exsiccated. Red. In UD 100s.
otc	**Ferrous Sulfate** (Various, eg, Goldline, Upsher-Smith)	**Tablets; oral:** 325 mg (65 mg iron)	In 100s, 1,000s, and UD 100s.
otc	**Feosol** (GlaxoSmithKline)		Capsule shape. In 100s.
otc	**FeroSul** (Major)		Green or red. In 100s and 1,000s.
otc	**Ferrous Sulfate** (Various)	**Tablets, slow release; oral:** 160 mg (50 mg iron)	Exsiccated. In blister pack 60s.
otc	**Slow Release Iron** (Cardinal Health)		Exsiccated. Maltodextrin, mineral oil. In 30s.
otc	**Slow FE** (Novartis Consumer)	**Tablets, extended-release; oral:** 142 mg (45 mg iron)	Ascorbic acid, PEG. (SFE). In 30s, 60s, and 90s.
otc	**Ferrous Sulfate** (Various, eg, Goldline, Major, URL)	**Elixir; oral:** 220 mg per 5 mL (44 mg iron per 5 mL)	May contain alcohol. In 473 mL.
otc	**Ferrous Sulfate** (Hi-Tech)	**Drops; oral:** 15 mg iron per mL	Gluten free, lactose free. 0.2% alcohol, sodium bisulfite, sorbitol, sucrose. In 50 mL with dropper.
otc	**Enfamil Fer-In-Sol** (Mead Johnson Nutritionals)		Alcohol, sorbitol, sugar. In 50 mL.
otc	**Fer-Iron** (Rugby)		Alcohol 0.2%, lemon flavoring, sorbitol, sucrose. In 50 mL.
otc	**Ferrous Sulfate** (Pharmaceutical Associates)	**Liquid; oral:** 300 mg per 5 mL (60 mg iron per 5 mL)	Sucrose. Cinnamon flavor. In UD 100s of 5 mL each.

For complete and comparative prescribing information, refer to the Iron-Containing Products class monograph. For additional information, refer to the Dietary Reference Intakes of Vitamins and Minerals table.

FERROUS ASPARTATE

otc	**FE Aspartate** (Miller)	**Tablets:** 112 mg (18 mg elemental iron)/85 mg aspartic acid	In 90s.

FERROUS ASPARTATE — ORAL

For complete and comparative prescribing information, refer to the Iron-Containing Products group monograph. For additional information, refer to the Dietary Reference Intakes of Vitamins and Minerals table.

WARNING

Accidental overdose of iron-containing products is a leading cause of fatal poisoning in children younger than 6 years of age. Tell patients to keep this product out of the reach of children. Advise patients that in case of accidental overdose, they should call a health care provider or poison control center immediately.

Indications

➤*Dietary supplement:* For use as an iron dietary supplement.

Administration and Dosage

➤*General dosing considerations:* Ferrous aspartate 112 mg provides 18 mg of elemental iron.

➤*Adults:*

Dietary supplement – 1 tablet daily.

➤*Storage/Stability:* Store at 15° to 30°C (59° to 86°F).

FERROUS GLUCONATE

Approximately 12% elemental iron.

otc	**Ferrous Gluconate** (Various, eg, Goldline)	**Tablets**: 225 mg (27 mg iron)	In 100s.
otc	**Fergon** (Bayer)		In 100s.
otc	**Ferrous Gluconate** (Various, eg, Paddock Laboratories)	**Tablets**: 324 mg (38 mg iron)	In 100s.
otc	**Ferrous Gluconate** (Various, eg, Akyma Pharmaceuticals)	**Tablets**: 325 mg (36 mg iron)	In 1,000s.

For complete and comparative prescribing information, refer to the Iron-Containing Products group monograph. For additional information, refer to the Dietary Reference Intakes of Vitamins and Minerals table.

FERROUS FUMARATE

33% elemental iron.

otc	**Ferrous Fumarate** (Mission)	**Tablets**: 90 mg (29.5 mg iron)	Sugar. In 100s.
otc	**Ferrous Fumarate** (Various, eg, Cypress)	**Tablets**: 324 mg (106 mg iron)	In 100s.
otc	**Hemocyte** (U.S. Pharmaceutical Corp.)		In 30s and 100s.
otc	**Ferretts** (Pharmics)	**Tablets**: 325 mg (106 mg iron)	Polydextrose. (P-Fe). Red, oblong, scored. Film-coated. In 60s.
otc	**Ferro-Sequels** (Inverness Medical Innovations)	**Tablets, timed release**: 150 mg (50 mg iron)	Lactose, sodium docusate 100 mg. In 30s and 90s.

For complete and comparative prescribing information, refer to the Iron-Containing Products group monograph. For additional information, refer to the Dietary Reference Intakes of Vitamins and Minerals table.

CARBONYL IRON

Pure iron micro particles.

otc	**Feosol** (GlaxoSmithKline)	**Tablets; oral**: 45 mg iron	In 30s and 60s.
otc	**Ircon** (Kenwood)	**Tablets; oral**: 66 mg iron	In blister pack 100s.
otc	**Icar** (Hawthorn)	**Tablets, chewable; oral**: 15 mg carbonyl iron	Sorbitol. Grape flavor. In 60s.
otc	**Iron Chews** (Midlothian)	**Tablets, chewable; oral**: 15 mg carbonyl iron	Sorbitol. Grape flavor. In 60s.
otc	**Icar** (Hawthorn)	**Suspension; oral**: 15 mg carbonyl iron per 1.25 mL	Fructose, parabens. Grape and lemon flavors. In 118 mL.
otc	**Wee Care** (Centurion Labs)		Acesulfame K, glycerin, parabens, potassium sorbate, propylene glycol, sucralose. Wild cherry flavor. In 118 mL.

For complete and comparative prescribing information, refer to the Iron-Containing Products group monograph. For additional information, refer to the Dietary Reference Intakes of Vitamins and Minerals table.

POLYSACCHARIDE IRON COMPLEX

otc	**Niferex** (Ther-Rx)	**Capsules; oral**: 60 mg iron	Lactose. (THX 0134). Brown/Clear. In UD 100s.
otc	**Polysaccharide Iron Complex** (Various, eg, Contract Pharmacol Corp.)	**Capsules; oral**: 150 mg iron	In 100s.
otc	**Ferrex 150** (Various, eg, Breckenridge, Major)		In UD 100s.
otc	**iFerex 150** (Nnodum Pharmaceuticals)		(ziks 0203). Brown/orange. In 100s.
otc	**Myferon 150** (M.E. Pharmaceuticals)		In UD 100s.
otc	**Nu-Iron 150** (Merz)		Parabens, EDTA, castor oil, sucrose. In 100s.
otc	**Poly-Iron 150** (Cypress)		PEG, tartrazine. In 100s.
otc	**EZFE 200** (McNeil)	**Capsules; oral**: 200 mg iron	In 100s.

For complete and comparative prescribing information, refer to the Iron-Containing Products group monograph. For additional information, refer to the Dietary Reference Intakes of Vitamins and Minerals table.

MISCELLANEOUS IRON COMBINATIONS

otc	**Tandem** (US Pharmaceutical)	**Capsules**: 106 mg elemental Fe (as 162 mg ferrous fumarate, 115.2 mg polysaccharide iron complex)	(Tandem US). Lt. brown. In blister pack 90s.

MISCELLANEOUS IRON COMBINATIONS — ORAL

For complete prescribing information, refer to the Iron-Containing Products group monograph. For additional information, refer to the Dietary Reference Intakes of Vitamins and Minerals table.

IRON WITH VITAMIN C

Content given per capsule or tablet.

	Product and Distributor	Dose form	Fe (mg)	Vitamin C: Ascorbic Acid	Vitamin C: Sodium Ascorbate (mg)	Vitamin C: Calcium Ascorbate and Calcium Threonate (mg)	Other Content & How Supplied (mg)
otc	**Ferrex 150 Plus** (Breckenridge)	**Capsules**	150[a]	50			(B 303). Clear/yellow. In UD 100s.
otc	**Fero-Grad-500** (Abbott)	**Tablets, controlled release**	105[b]		500		Castor oil. In blister pack 30s.
otc	**Niferex-150** (Ther-Rx)	**Capsules**	150[c]			50	50 mg succinic acid. In 90s.
otc	**Vitelle Irospan** (Fielding)		65[d]	150			Sugar. In 60s.

IRON WITH VITAMIN C

	Product and Distributor	Dose form	Fe (mg)	Vitamin C: Ascorbic Acid	Vitamin C: Sodium Ascorbate (mg)	Vitamin C: Calcium Ascorbate and Calcium Threonate (mg)	Other Content & How Supplied (mg)
otc	**Vitron-C** (Heritage Consumer Products)	**Tablets**	66[e]	125			In 60s.

[a] From polysaccharide iron and ferrous bisglycinate.
[b] From ferrous sulfate.
[c] From ferrous asparto glycinate and polysaccharide iron complex.
[d] From ferrous sulfate exsiccated.
[e] From ferrous fumarate.

For complete prescribing information, refer to the Iron-Containing Products group monograph. For additional information, refer to the Dietary Reference Intakes of Vitamins and Minerals table.

IRON — PARENTERAL
FERUMOXYTOL

Rx	**Feraheme** (AMAG Pharmaceuticals)	**Injection, solution:** elemental iron 30 mg/mL	Mannitol 44 mg. Preservative free. In single-use vials.

FERUMOXYTOL — INJECTION

Indications

➤*Iron deficiency anemia:* For the treatment of iron deficiency anemia in adults with chronic kidney disease (CKD).

Administration and Dosage

➤*Adults:*

Iron deficiency anemia –

Usual dosage: 510 mg intravenously (IV) followed by a second 510 mg IV injection 3 to 8 days later.

Maintenance dosage: The recommended dose may be readministered to patients with persistent or recurrent iron deficiency anemia.

➤*Elderly:* Dose administration to an elderly patient should be cautious, reflecting the greater frequency of decreased hepatic, renal, or cardiac function, and of concomitant disease or other drug therapy.

➤*Renal function impairment:*

Hemodialysis – For patients receiving hemodialysis, administer ferumoxytol once the blood pressure is stable and the patient has completed at least 1 hour of hemodialysis.

➤*Therapeutic drug monitoring:* Monitor for signs and symptoms of hypotension following each ferumoxytol injection. Evaluate the hematologic response (hemoglobin, ferritin, iron, and transferrin saturation) at least 1 month following the second ferumoxytol injection.

➤*Administration:* Administer as an undiluted IV injection delivered at a rate of up to 1 mL/sec (30 mg/sec).

➤*Storage/Stability:* Store at 20° to 25°C (68° to 77°F). Excursions are permitted to 15° to 30°C (59° to 86°F).

Actions

➤*Pharmacology:* Ferumoxytol consists of a superparamagnetic iron oxide that is coated with a carbohydrate shell, which helps to isolate the bioactive iron from plasma components until the iron-carbohydrate complex enters the reticuloendothelial system macrophages of the liver, spleen, and bone marrow. The iron is released from the iron-carbohydrate complex within vesicles in the macrophages. Iron then enters the intracellular storage iron pool (eg, ferritin) or is transferred to plasma transferrin for transport to erythroid precursor cells for incorporation into hemoglobin.

➤*Pharmacokinetics:*

Absorption – The mean maximum observed plasma concentration (C_{max}) and time of maximum concentration (T_{max}) were 206 mcg/mL and 0.32 h, respectively. The C_{max} values increased with dose.

Distribution – The estimated value of volume of distribution following 2 doses of ferumoxytol 510 mg administered IV within 24 hours was 3.16 L. The volume of distribution was consistent with plasma volume.

Excretion – The half-life of feromyxytol is approximately 15 hours in humans. The estimated value of clearance following 2 doses of ferumoxytol 510 mg administered IV within 24 hours was 69.1 mL/h. The clearance was decreased by increasing the dose of ferumoxytol and the terminal half-life ($t_{½}$) values increased with dose.

Contraindications

Evidence of iron overload; hypersensitivity to ferumoxytol or any of its components; anemia not caused by iron deficiency.

Warnings/Precautions

➤*Hypotension:* Hypotension may follow ferumoxytol administration. In clinical studies, hypotension was reported in 1.9% of subjects, including 3 patients with serious hypotensive reactions. Monitor patients for signs and symptoms of hypotension following ferumoxytol administration.

➤*Iron overload:* Excessive therapy with parenteral iron can lead to excess storage of iron with the possibility of iatrogenic hemosiderosis. Regularly monitor the hematologic response during parenteral iron therapy. Do not administer ferumoxytol to patients with iron overload.

In the 24 hours following administration of ferumoxytol, laboratory assays may overestimate serum iron and transferrin-bound iron by also measuring the iron in the ferumoxytol complex.

➤*Magnetic resonance imaging:* Administration of ferumoxytol may transiently affect the diagnostic ability of magnetic resonance imaging (MRI). Conduct anticipated MRI studies prior to the administration of ferumoxytol. Alteration of MRI studies may persist for up to 3 months following the last ferumoxytol dose. If MRI is required within 3 months after ferumoxytol administration, use T1- or proton density-weighted magnetic resonance pulse sequences to minimize the ferumoxytol effects; do not perform MRI using T2-weighted pulse sequences earlier than 4 weeks after the administration of ferumoxytol. Maximum alteration of vascular MRI is anticipated to be evident for 1 to 2 days following ferumoxytol administration. Ferumoxytol will not interfere with X-ray, computed tomography (CT), positron emission tomography (PET), single photon emission computed tomography (SPECT), ultrasound, or nuclear medicine imaging.

➤*Hypersensitivity reactions:* Ferumoxytol may cause serious hypersensitivity reactions, including anaphylaxis and/or anaphylactoid reactions. In clinical studies, serious hypersensitivity reactions were reported in 0.2% of subjects receiving ferumoxytol. Other adverse reactions potentially associated with hypersensitivity (eg, pruritus, rash, urticaria, wheezing) were reported in 3.7% of these subjects. Observe patients for signs and symptoms of hypersensitivity for at least 30 minutes following ferumoxytol injection and only administer the drug when personnel and therapies are readily available for the treatment of hypersensitivity reactions.

➤*Pregnancy: Category C.* There are no studies of ferumoxytol in pregnant women. In animal studies, ferumoxytol caused decreased fetal weights and fetal malformations at maternally toxic doses of 13 to 15 times the human dose. Use ferumoxytol during pregnancy only if the potential benefit justifies the potential risk to the fetus.

In rats, administration of ferumoxytol at maternally toxic doses during organogenesis (ie, daily doses approximately 2 times the recommended 510 mg human dose on a mg/m^2 basis for 12 days) caused a decrease in fetal weights. The cumulative animal exposure was approximately 13 times the human therapeutic course of 1.02 g (on a mg/m^2 basis). In rabbits, administration of ferumoxytol at maternally toxic doses during organogenesis (ie, daily doses approximately 2 times the recommended 510 mg human dose on a mg/m^2 basis for 14 days) was associated with decreased fetal weights and external and/or soft tissue fetal malformations. The cumulative animal exposure was approximately 15 times the human therapeutic course of 1.02 g on a mg/m^2 basis.

In rabbits, no maternal or fetal effects of ferumoxytol were observed at daily doses of Fe 16.5 mg/kg during organogenesis for 14 days, approximately 1 time the recommended human dose of 510 mg on mg/m^2 basis. The cumulative animal exposure was approximately 7 times the human therapeutic course of 1.02 g on a mg/m^2 basis. Administration of ferumoxytol during organogenesis at maternally toxic doses of Fe 45 mg/kg/day (daily exposure approximately 2 times the recommended 510 mg human dose on a mg/m^2 basis) for 14 days (cumulative exposure approximately 15 times the human therapeutic course of 1.02 g on a mg/m^2 basis) caused decreased fetal weights and external and/or soft tissue fetal malformations.

➤*Lactation:* It is not known whether ferumoxytol is present in human milk. Because many drugs are excreted in human milk and because of the potential for adverse reactions in breast-feeding infants, decide whether to discontinue breast-feeding or to avoid ferumoxytol, taking into account the importance of ferumoxytol to the mother and the known benefits of breast-feeding.

➤*Children:* The safety and effectiveness of ferumoxytol in children have not been established.

➤*Elderly:* In general, be cautious in dose administration to elderly patients, reflecting the greater frequency of decreased hepatic, renal, or cardiac function, and of concomitant disease or other drug therapy.

➤*Monitoring:* Observe patients for signs and symptoms of hypersensitivity for at least 30 minutes following ferumoxytol injection and only administer the drug when personnel and therapies are readily available for the

FERUMOXYTOL — INJECTION

treatment of hypersensitivity reactions. Monitor patients for signs and symptoms of hypotension following ferumoxytol administration. Regularly monitor the hematologic response during parenteral iron therapy.

Drug Interactions

➤*Oral iron:* Ferumoxytol may reduce the absorption of concomitantly administered oral iron.

Adverse Reactions

Ferumoxytol Adverse Reactions (≥ 1%)		
Adverse reactions	Ferumoxytol 2 × 510 mg (n = 605)	Oral iron (n = 280)
Cardiovascular		
Chest pain	1.3%	0.7%
Edema	1.5%	1.4%
Hypotension	2.5%	0.4%
Peripheral edema	2%	3.2%
CNS		
Dizziness	2.6%	1.8%
Headache	1.8%	2.1%
Dermatologic		
Pruritus	1.2%	0.4%
Rash	1%	0.4%
GI		
Abdominal pain	1.3%	1.4%
Nausea	3.1%	7.5%
Vomiting	1.5%	5%
Musculoskeletal		
Back pain	1%	0%
Muscle spasms	1%	1.4%
Miscellaneous		
Cough	1.3%	1.4%
Dyspnea	1%	1.1%
Pyrexia	1%	0.7%

➤*Other adverse reactions:* Diarrhea (4%), constipation (2.1%), and hypertension (1%) have also been reported in ferumoxytol-treated patients.

➤*Discontinuation:* In clinical trials, adverse reactions leading to treatment discontinuation and occurring in 2 or more ferumoxytol-treated patients included chest pain, chronic renal failure, diarrhea, dizziness, ecchymosis, hypotension, increased serum ferritin level, infusion-site swelling, pruritus, and urticaria.

Overdosage

➤*Symptoms:* No data are available regarding overdosage of ferumoxytol in humans. Excessive dosages of ferumoxytol may lead to accumulation of iron in storage sites potentially leading to hemosiderosis. Do not administer ferumoxytol to patients with iron overload.

Patient Information

Question patients regarding any prior history of reactions to parenteral iron products.

Advise patients of the risks associated with ferumoxytol.

Advise patients to report any signs and symptoms of hypersensitivity that may develop during and following ferumoxytol administration, such as rash, itching, dizziness, light-headedness, swelling, and breathing problems.

IRON — PARENTERAL
IRON DEXTRAN

Rx	**INFeD** (Watson)	**Injection, solution:** 50 mg/mL[a]	In 2 mL single-dose vials.
Rx	**Dexferrum** (American Regent)		In 1 and 2 mL single-dose vials.

[a] Strength expressed as elemental iron.

IRON DEXTRAN — INJECTION

For additional information, refer to the Dietary Reference Intakes of Vitamins and Minerals table.

WARNING

Anaphylactic-type reactions – Anaphylactic-type reactions, including fatalities, have followed the parenteral administration of iron dextran injection. Have resuscitation equipment and personnel trained in the detection and treatment of anaphylactic-type reactions readily available during iron dextran administration.

Administer a test dose of iron dextran prior to the first therapeutic dose. If no signs or symptoms of anaphylactic-type reactions follow the test dose, administer the full therapeutic iron dextran dose. During all iron dextran administrations, observe for signs or symptoms of anaphylactic-type reactions. Fatal reactions have followed the test dose of iron dextran injection. Fatal reactions have also occurred in situations in which the test dose was tolerated.

Use iron dextran only in patients in whom clinical and laboratory investigations have established an iron-deficient state not amenable to oral iron therapy. Patients with a history of drug allergy or multiple drug allergies may be at increased risk of anaphylactic-type reactions to iron dextran.

Indications

➤*Iron deficiency:* For treatment of patients with documented iron deficiency in whom oral administration is unsatisfactory or impossible.

➤*Off-label uses:* Iron supplementation may be required by most patients receiving epoetin therapy. Failure to administer iron supplements (oral or intravenous [IV]) during epoetin therapy can impair the hematologic response to epoetin.

Administration and Dosage

➤*Maximum dose:*

Adults and children weighing 10 kg (22 lb) or more – 2 mL (100 mg of iron) daily according to the prescribing information.

Children weighing less than 10 kg (22 lb) – 1 mL (50 mg of iron) daily according to the prescribing information.

Infants weighing less than 5 kg (11 lb) – 0.5 mL (25 mg of iron) daily according to the prescribing information.

➤*General dosing considerations:* Discontinue oral iron prior to administration of iron dextran.

A test dose is required prior to the first administration. See Administration for more information.

Although there are significant variations in body build and weight distribution among men and women, the accompanying table and formula represent a convenient means for estimating the total iron required. This total iron requirement reflects the amount of iron needed to restore hemoglobin concentration to normal or near-normal levels plus an additional allowance to provide adequate replenishment of iron stores in most individuals with moderately or severely reduced levels of hemoglobin. It should be remembered that iron deficiency anemia will not appear until essentially all iron stores have been depleted. Therefore, therapy should aim at not only replenishment of hemoglobin iron but iron stores as well.

➤*Adults:*

Iron deficiency anemia

Total Iron Dextran Requirement for Hemoglobin Restoration and Iron Stores Replacement[a]									
Patient lean body weight		mL requirement of iron dextran injection based on observed hemoglobin of:							
kg	lb	3 (g/dL)	4 (g/dL)	5 (g/dL)	6 (g/dL)	7 (g/dL)	8 (g/dL)	9 (g/dL)	10 (g/dL)
5	11	3	3	3	3	2	2	2	2
10	22	7	6	6	5	5	4	4	3
15	33	10	9	9	8	7	7	6	5
20	44	16	15	14	13	12	11	10	9
25	55	20	18	17	16	15	14	13	12
30	66	23	22	21	19	18	17	15	14
35	77	27	26	24	23	21	20	18	17
40	88	31	29	28	26	24	22	21	19
45	99	35	33	31	29	27	25	23	21
50	110	39	37	35	32	30	28	26	24
55	121	43	41	38	36	33	31	28	26
60	132	47	44	42	39	36	34	31	28
65	143	51	48	45	42	39	36	34	31
70	154	55	52	49	45	42	39	36	33
75	165	59	55	52	49	45	42	39	35

IRON DEXTRAN — INJECTION

Total Iron Dextran Requirement for Hemoglobin Restoration and Iron Stores Replacement[a]									
Patient lean body weight		mL requirement of iron dextran injection based on observed hemoglobin of:							
kg	lb	3 (g/dL)	4 (g/dL)	5 (g/dL)	6 (g/dL)	7 (g/dL)	8 (g/dL)	9 (g/dL)	10 (g/dL)
80	176	63	59	55	52	48	45	41	38
85	187	66	63	59	55	51	48	44	40
90	198	70	66	62	58	54	50	46	42
95	209	74	70	66	62	57	53	49	45
100	220	78	74	69	65	60	56	52	47
105	231	82	77	73	68	63	59	54	50
110	242	86	81	76	71	67	62	57	52
115	253	90	85	80	75	70	64	59	54
120	264	94	88	83	78	73	67	62	57

[a] Table values were calculated based on a normal adult hemoglobin of 14.8 g/dL for weights of more than 15 kg (33 lb) and a hemoglobin of 12 g/dL for weights less than or equal to 15 kg (33 lb).

Alternatively, the total amount of iron dextran in mL required to treat anemia and replenish iron stores may be approximated as follows:

$$\text{Dose (mL)} = 0.0442\ (\text{desired Hb} - \text{observed Hb}) \times \text{LBW} + (0.26 \times \text{LBW})$$

Based on: desired Hb = the target Hb in g/dL.
Observed Hb = the patient's current hemoglobin in g/dL.
LBW = lean body weight in kg. Use a patient's lean body weight (or actual body weight if less than lean body weight) when determining dosage.

Iron replacement for blood loss: Some individuals sustain blood losses on an intermittent or repetitive basis. Such blood losses may occur periodically in patients with hemorrhagic diatheses (familial telangiectasia, hemophilia, GI bleeding) and on a repetitive basis from procedures such as renal hemodialysis. Direct iron therapy in these patients toward replacement of the equivalent amount of iron represented in the blood loss.

Quantitative estimates of the individual's periodic blood loss and hematocrit during the bleeding episode provide a convenient method for the calculation of the required iron dose.

The following formula is based on the approximation that 1 mL of normocytic, normochromic red cells contains 1 mg of elemental iron:

$$\text{Replacement iron (in mg)} = \text{blood loss (in mL)} \times \text{hematocrit}$$

➤*Children:*

Iron deficiency anemia –

Older than 4 months of age:

• *Children weighing more than 15 kg (33 lb)* – See Adults for dosing table.

• *Children weighing 5 to 15 kg (11 to 33 lb)* – See Adults for dosing table.

Alternatively, the total dose may be calculated:

$$\text{Dose (mL)} = 0.0442\ (\text{desired Hb} - \text{observed Hb}) \times W + (0.26 \times W)$$

Based on: desired Hb = the target Hb in g/dL. (Normal Hb for children 15 kg or less is 12 g/dL.)
W = weight in kg.

To calculate a patient's weight in kg when lb are known:

$$\text{Patient's weight in pounds}/2.2 = \text{weight in kg.}$$

Iron replacement for blood loss –

Older than 4 months of age: See Adults for dosing.

$$\text{Replacement iron (in mg)} = \text{blood loss (in mL)} \times \text{hematocrit}$$

Example: Blood loss of 500 mL with 20% hematocrit.

$$\text{Replacement iron} = 500 \times 0.2 = 100\ \text{mg.}$$

$$\text{Iron dextran dose} = 100\ \text{mg}/50 = 2\ \text{mL.}$$

Off-label dosing –

Iron deficiency in hemodialysis patients (chronic renal failure):

Iron Dextran for Iron Deficiency in Children on Hemodialysis	
Patient weight	IV dose[a]
> 20 kg	2 mL (100 mg)
10 to 20 kg	1 mL (50 mg)
< 10 kg	0.5 mL (25 mg)

[a] Each dose or dialysis × 10 doses. Iron dextran can also be administered at a dosage of 2 to 4 mg/kg (100 mg maximum) 3 times per week for 10 doses during erythropoietin therapy.

Iron deficiency in peritoneal dialysis patients (chronic renal failure):

Iron Dextran for Iron Deficiency in Children on Peritoneal Dialysis		
Patient weight	IV dose[a]	Volume of saline for infusion
> 20 kg	500 mg	250 mL
10 to 20 kg	250 mg	125 mL
< 10 kg	125 mg	75 mL

[a] To maintain adequate iron stores, this dose may be repeated.

➤*Administration:* The total amount of iron dextran required for the treatment of iron deficiency anemia or iron replacement for blood loss is determined from the Total Iron Dextran Requirement for Hemoglobin Restoration and Iron Stores Replacement table or appropriate formula.

Dexferrum should be administered IV only; *INFeD* may be administered by IV or intramuscular (IM) injection.

IV injection – Individual doses of 2 mL or less may be given on a daily basis until the calculated total amount required has been reached. Iron dextran is given undiluted at a slow gradual rate not to exceed 50 mg (1 mL) per minute.

Test dose: Prior to the first IV iron dextran therapeutic dose, administer an IV test dose of 0.5 mL. Administer the test dose at a gradual rate over at least 30 seconds (*INFeD*) or over at least 5 minutes (*Dexferrum*). Although anaphylactic reactions known to occur following iron dextran administration are usually evident within a few minutes, or sooner, it is recommended that a period of 1 hour or longer elapse before the remainder of the initial therapeutic dose is given.

IM injection (INFed only) – Iron dextran injection should be injected only into the muscle mass of the upper outer quadrant of the buttock (never into the arm or other exposed areas) and should be injected deeply, with a 2- or 3-inch 19- or 20-gauge needle. If the patient is standing, he/she should be bearing his/her weight on the leg opposite the injection site, or if in bed, the patient should be in the lateral position with the injection site uppermost. To avoid injection or leakage into the subcutaneous tissue, a Z-track technique (displacement of the skin laterally prior to injection) is recommended.

Test dose: Prior to the first IM iron dextran injection therapeutic dose, administer an IM test dose of 0.5 mL. Administer the test dose in the buttock using the same technique described in the following paragraph. If no adverse reactions are observed, iron dextran can be given according to the following schedule until the calculated total amount required has been reached. Although anaphylactic reactions known to occur following iron dextran injection administration are usually evident within a few minutes or sooner, it is recommended that at least 1 hour or longer elapse before the remainder of the initial therapeutic dose is given.

➤*Admixture compatibility:* Do not mix iron dextran with other medications or add to parenteral nutrition solutions for IV infusion.

➤*Storage / Stability:* Store at 20° to 25°C (68° to 77°F). Excursions are permitted for *Dexferrum* to between 15° and 30°C (59° and 86°F).

Actions

➤*Pharmacology:* Circulating iron dextran is removed from the plasma by cells of the reticuloendothelial system, which split the complex into its components of iron and dextran. The iron is immediately bound to the available protein moieties to form hemosiderin or ferritin, the physiological forms of iron, or, to a lesser extent, to transferrin. This iron, which is subject to physiological control, replenishes hemoglobin and depleted iron stores.

➤*Pharmacokinetics:*

Absorption / Distribution – After IM injection, iron dextran is absorbed from the injection site into the capillaries and the lymphatic system.

The major portion of IM injections of iron dextran is absorbed within 72 hours; most of the remaining iron is absorbed over the ensuing 3 to 4 weeks.

Metabolism / Excretion – Dextran, a polyglucose, is either metabolized or excreted. Negligible amounts of iron are lost via the urinary or alimentary pathways after administration of iron dextran.

Various studies involving IV administered ^{59}Fe iron dextran to iron-deficient subjects, some of whom had coexisting diseases, have yielded half-life values ranging from 5 hours to more than 20 hours. The 5-hour value was determined for ^{59}Fe iron dextran from a study that used laboratory methods to separate the circulating ^{59}Fe iron dextran from the transferrin-bound ^{59}Fe. The 20-hour value reflects a half-life determined by measuring total ^{59}Fe, both circulating and bound. It should be understood that these half-life values do not represent clearance of iron from the body. Iron is not easily eliminated from the body, and the accumulation of iron can be toxic.

Special populations –

Renal function impairment: Studies involving IV administered iron dextran to iron-deficient subjects who had coexisting end-stage renal disease and other clinical problems have yielded individual half-life values ranging from 9.4 to 87.4 hours. The average half-life value equaled 58.9 hours. These studies measured the total serum iron directly as well as the transferrin-bound iron, non-radio-isotopically. It should be understood that these half-life values do not represent clearance of iron from the body. Iron is not easily eliminated from the body, and accumulation of iron can be toxic.

• *Hemodialysis* – In vitro studies have shown that removal of iron dextran by dialysis is negligible. Six different dialyzer membranes were investigated (polysulphone, cuprophane, cellulose acetate, cellulose triacetate, polymethylmethacrilate, and polyacrylonitrile), including those considered high efficiency and high flux.

IRON DEXTRAN — INJECTION

Contraindications

Hypersensitivity to the product; all anemias not associated with iron deficiency.

Warnings/Precautions

➤*Anaphylactic-type reactions:* See the Warning box for more information.

The factors that affect the risk for anaphylactic-type reactions to iron dextran products are not fully known, but limited clinical data suggest the risk may be increased among patients with a history of drug allergy or multiple drug allergies. Additionally, concomitant use of angiotensin-converting enzyme (ACE) inhibitor drugs may increase the risk for reactions to an iron dextran product. The extent of risk for anaphylactic-type reactions following exposure to any specific iron dextran product is unknown and may vary among the products. Iron dextran products differ in chemical characteristics and may differ in clinical effects. Iron dextran products are not clinically interchangeable.

➤*Delayed reactions:* Large IV doses, such as those used with total dose infusions, have been associated with an increased incidence of adverse effects. The adverse effects frequently are delayed (1 to 2 days) reactions typified by one or more of the following symptoms: arthralgia, backache, chills, dizziness, moderate-to-high fever, headache, malaise, myalgia, nausea, and vomiting. The onset is usually 24 to 48 hours after administration, and symptoms generally subside within 3 to 4 days. The etiology of these reactions is not known. The potential for a delayed reaction must be considered when estimating the risk/benefit of treatment.

➤*Cardiovascular disease:* Adverse reactions experienced following administration of iron dextran may exacerbate cardiovascular complications in patients with preexisting cardiovascular disease.

➤*Infectious kidney disease:* Do not use this medication during the acute phase of infectious kidney disease.

➤*Hemosiderosis:* Unwarranted therapy with parenteral iron will cause excess storage of iron with the consequent possibility of exogenous hemosiderosis. Such iron overload is particularly apt to occur in patients with hemoglobinopathies and other refractory anemias that might be erroneously diagnosed as iron deficiency anemias.

➤*Rheumatoid arthritis:* Patients with rheumatoid arthritis may have an acute exacerbation of joint pain and swelling following the administration of iron dextran.

➤*Allergies/Asthma:* Use with caution in individuals with a history of significant allergies or asthma.

➤*Hypersensitivity reactions:* Anaphylaxis and other hypersensitivity reactions have been reported after uneventful test doses as well as therapeutic doses of iron dextran injection. Therefore, administer a test dose prior to the first administration of iron dextran.

Epinephrine should be immediately available in the event of acute hypersensitivity reactions (usual adult dose: 0.5 mL of a 1:1,000 solution, by subcutaneous or IM injection).

Patients using beta-blocking agents may not respond adequately to epinephrine. Isoproterenol or similar beta agonist agents may be required in these patients.

➤*Hepatic function impairment:* Use this preparation with extreme care in patients with serious impairment of liver function.

➤*Pregnancy: Category C.* Various animal studies and studies in pregnant humans have demonstrated inconclusive results with respect to the placental transfer of iron dextran as iron dextran. It appears that some iron does reach the fetus, but the form in which it crosses the placenta is not clear.

Teratogenic – Iron dextran has been shown to be teratogenic and embryocidal in mice, rats, rabbits, dogs, and monkeys when given in doses of about 3 times the maximum human dose.

No consistent adverse fetal effects were observed in mice, rats, rabbits, dogs, and monkeys at doses of 50 mg/kg or less of iron. Fetal and maternal toxicity has been reported in monkeys at a total IV dose of 90 mg/kg of iron over a 14-day period. Similar effects were observed in mice and rats upon administration of a single dose of 125 mg/kg of iron. Fetal abnormalities in rats and dogs were observed at doses of 250 mg/kg or more of iron. The animals used in these tests were not iron deficient. There are no adequate and well-controlled studies in pregnant women. Use during pregnancy only if the potential benefit justifies the potential risk to the fetus.

➤*Lactation:* Exercise caution when iron dextran is administered to a breast-feeding woman. Traces of unmetabolized iron dextran are excreted in human milk.

➤*Children:* Not recommended for use in infants younger than 4 months of age.

Reports in the literature from countries outside the United States (in particular, New Zealand) have suggested that the use of IM iron dextran in neonates has been associated with an increased incidence of gram-negative sepsis, primarily due to *Escherichia coli.*

➤*Monitoring:* Periodic hematologic determinations (hemoglobin and hematocrit) is a simple and accurate technique for monitoring hematological response and should be used as a guide in therapy. It should be recognized that iron storage may lag behind the appearance of normal blood morphology. Serum iron, total iron binding capacity, and percent saturation of transferrin are other important tests for detecting and monitoring the iron-deficient state.

After administration of iron dextran complex, evidence of a therapeutic response can be seen in a few days as an increase in the reticulocyte count.

Serum iron determinations (especially by colorimetric assays) may not be meaningful for 3 weeks following the administration of iron dextran. Serum ferritin peaks approximately 7 to 9 days after an IV dose of iron dextran and slowly returns to baseline after about 3 weeks.

Although serum ferritin is usually a good guide to body iron stores, the correlation of body iron stores and serum ferritin may not be valid in patients on chronic renal dialysis who are also receiving iron dextran complex.

Examination of the bone marrow for iron stores may not be meaningful for prolonged periods following iron dextran therapy because residual iron dextran may remain in the reticuloendothelial cells.

Drug Interactions

Iron Dextran Drug Interactions

Precipitant drug	Object drug[a]		Description
ACE inhibitors (eg, enalapril)	Iron dextran	↑	The risk of adverse systemic reactions to iron dextran may be increased. If an interaction is suspected, discontinue one of the agents.
Chloramphenicol	Iron dextran	↑	Serum iron levels may be increased because of decreased iron clearance and erythropoiesis due to direct bone marrow toxicity from chloramphenicol. If bone marrow suppression occurs, choose an alternative antimicrobial agent. If chloramphenicol must be continued, monitor iron stores and adjust the iron regimen as needed to avoid iron overload.

[a] ↑ = object drug increased.

➤*Drug/Lab test interactions:* Large doses of iron dextran (5 mL or more) have been reported to give a brown color to serum from a blood sample drawn 4 hours after administration.

The drug may cause falsely elevated values of serum bilirubin and falsely decreased values of serum calcium.

Bone scans involving 99m Tc-diphosphonate have been reported to show a dense, crescentic area of activity in the buttocks following the contour of the iliac crest, 1 to 6 days after IM injections of iron dextran.

Bone scans with 99m Tc-labeled bone-seeking agents, in the presence of high serum ferritin levels or following iron dextran infusions, have been reported to show reduction of bony uptake, marked renal activity, and excessive blood pool and soft tissue accumulation.

Adverse Reactions

➤*Cardiovascular:* Arrhythmias, bradycardia, cardiac arrest, chest pain, chest tightness, flushing, hypertension, hypotension, shock, tachycardia. Flushing and hypotension may occur from too rapid injections by the IV route.

➤*CNS:* Chills, convulsions, disorientation, dizziness, febrile episodes, headache, malaise, numbness, paresthesia, seizures, syncope, unconsciousness, unresponsiveness, weakness.

➤*Dermatologic:* Cyanosis, pruritus, purpura, rash, urticaria.

➤*GI:* Abdominal pain, diarrhea, nausea, vomiting.

➤*GU:* Hematuria.

➤*Hematologic/Lymphatic:* Leucocytosis, lymphadenopathy.

➤*Hypersensitivity:* Anaphylactic reactions have been reported with the use of iron dextran injection; on occasion, these reactions have been fatal. Such reactions, which occur most often within the first several minutes of administration, have been generally characterized by sudden onset of respiratory difficulty or cardiovascular collapse. Because fatal anaphylactic reactions have been reported after administration of iron dextran injection, give the drug only when resuscitation techniques and treatment of anaphylactic and anaphylactoid shock are readily available.

➤*Local:* Brown skin or underlying tissue discoloration (staining); local phlebitis at or near IV injection site; soreness or pain at or near IM injection site; atrophy/fibrosis, sterile abscess (IM injection site);

➤*Musculoskeletal:* Arthralgia, arthritis (may represent reactivation in patients with quiescent rheumatoid arthritis); backache; cellulitis; inflammation; myalgia; swelling.

➤*Respiratory:* Bronchospasm, dyspnea, respiratory arrest, wheezing.

➤*Miscellaneous:* Altered taste, shivering, sweating.

Delayed reactions – Arthralgia, backache, chills, dizziness, fever, headache, malaise, myalgia, nausea, vomiting.

Overdosage

➤*Symptoms:* Overdosage with iron dextran is unlikely to be associated with any acute manifestations. Dosages of iron dextran in excess of the

IRON DEXTRAN — INJECTION

requirements for restoration of hemoglobin and replenishment of iron stores may lead to hemosiderosis.

➤*Treatment:* Periodic monitoring of serum ferritin levels may be helpful in recognizing a deleterious progressive accumulation of iron resulting from impaired uptake of iron from the reticuloendothelial system in concurrent medical conditions such as chronic renal failure, Hodgkin disease, and rheumatoid arthritis. The median lethal dose of iron dextran in mice is not less than 500 mg/kg.

Patient Information

Advise patients of the potential adverse reactions associated with the use of iron dextran.

IRON — PARENTERAL

SODIUM FERRIC GLUCONATE COMPLEX

Rx	**Ferrlecit** (Sanofi Pharmaceuticals)	**Injection:** 62.5 mg per 5 mL (12.5 mg/mL) elemental iron	9 mg/mL of benzyl alcohol, 20% sucrose. In 5 mL amps.

SODIUM FERRIC GLUCONATE COMPLEX — INJECTION

For additional information, refer to the Dietary Reference Intakes of Vitamins and Minerals table.

Indications

➤*Iron deficiency:* For the treatment of iron deficiency anemia in patients 6 years of age and older undergoing chronic hemodialysis who are receiving supplemental epoetin therapy.

Administration and Dosage

➤*General dosing considerations:* The dosage of sodium ferric gluconate complex is expressed in milligrams of elemental iron. Each 5 mL ampule contains elemental iron 62.5 mg (12.5 mg/mL).

➤*Adults:*

Iron deficiency anemia – 125 mg (10 mL) per dose. The dose may be diluted in 100 mL of 0.9% sodium chloride and then administered by intravenous (IV) infusion over 1 hour, or it may be administered undiluted as a slow IV injection (at a rate of up to 12.5 mg/min). Most patients will require a minimum cumulative dose of 1 g elemental iron administered over 8 sessions at sequential dialysis treatments to achieve a favorable hemoglobin or hematocrit response. Patients may continue to require therapy with IV iron at the lowest dose necessary to maintain the target levels of hemoglobin, hematocrit, and laboratory parameters of iron storage within acceptable limits.

➤*Children:*

Iron deficiency –

6 years of age and older:

• *Usual dosage* – 1.5 mg/kg (0.12 mL/kg) diluted in 25 mL 0.9% sodium chloride and administered by IV infusion over 1 hour at 8 sequential dialysis sessions.

• *Maximum dose* – 125 mg/dose.

➤*Elderly:* Cautiously select dose for an elderly patient, usually starting at the low end of the dosing range, reflecting the greater frequency of decreased hepatic, renal, or cardiac function and of concomitant disease or other drug therapy.

➤*Administration:* Sodium ferric gluconate complex has been administered at sequential dialysis sessions by infusion or by slow IV injection during the dialysis session itself.

For adults, the dose may be diluted in 100 mL of 0.9% sodium chloride and then administered by intravenous (IV) infusion over 1 hour, or it may be administered undiluted as a slow IV injection (at a rate of up to 12.5 mg/min).

For children, the dose should be diluted in 25 mL 0.9% sodium chloride and administered by IV infusion over 1 hour.

➤*Admixture compatibility:* Do not mix with other medications or add to parenteral nutrition solutions for IV infusion. The compatibility of sodium ferric gluconate complex with IV infusion vehicles other than 0.9% sodium chloride has not been evaluated.

➤*Storage/Stability:* Store at 20° to 25°C (68° to 77°F); excursions permitted to 15° to 30°C (59° to 86°F). Do not freeze. Use immediately after dilution in saline.

Actions

➤*Pharmacology:* Sodium ferric gluconate complex in sucrose injection is a stable macromolecular complex used to replete the total body content of iron. Iron is critical for normal hemoglobin synthesis to maintain oxygen transport. Additionally, iron is necessary for metabolism and various enzymatic processes.

The total body iron content of an adult ranges from 2 to 4 g (approximately two thirds in hemoglobin and one third in reticuloendothelial storage [bone marrow, spleen, liver] bound to intracellular ferritin). The body highly conserves iron (daily loss of 0.03%), requiring supplementation of approximately 1 mg/day to replenish losses in healthy, nonmenstruating adults. The etiology of iron deficiency in hemodialysis patients is varied and can include increased iron use (eg, from epoetin therapy) and blood loss. The administration of exogenous epoetin increases red blood cell production and iron use. The increased iron use and blood losses in the hemodialysis patient may lead to absolute or functional iron deficiency. Iron deficiency is absolute when hematologic indicators of iron stores are low. Patients with functional iron deficiency do not meet laboratory criteria for absolute iron deficiency but demonstrate an increase in hemoglobin/hematocrit or a decrease in epoetin dosage with stable hemoglobin/hematocrit when parenteral iron is administered.

➤*Pharmacokinetics:*

Absorption/Distribution – In multiple, sequential, adult, single-dose IV studies, peak drug levels (C_{max}) varied significantly by dosage and by rate of administration with the highest C_{max} observed in the regimen in which 125 mg was administered in 7 minutes (19 mg/L). In single dose IV studies, pediatric patients receiving a dose of 1.5 mg/kg had a C_{max} and area under the curve (AUC) of 12.9 mg/L and 95 mg•h/L, respectively. Pediatric patients who received a dose of 3 mg/kg (maximum dose, 125 mg) had a C_{max} and AUC of 22.8 mg/L and 170.9 mg•h/L, respectively. The initial volume of distribution of 6 L corresponds well to calculated blood volume. The AUC for bound iron varied by dose from 17.5 mg•h/L (62.5 mg) to 35.6 mg•h/L (125 mg). Approximately 80% of drug bound iron was delivered to transferrin as a mononuclear ionic iron species within 24 hours of administration in each dosage regimen. Mean peak transferrin saturation did not exceed 100% and returned to near baseline by 40 hours after administration of each dosage regimen.

Metabolism/Excretion – The terminal elimination half-life for drug bound iron was approximately 1 hour for adults and 2 to 2.5 hours for pediatrics, varying by dose but not by rate of administration. Total clearance was 3.02 to 5.35 L/h. In vitro, less than 1% of the iron species within sodium ferric gluconate complex can be dialyzed through membranes with pore sizes corresponding to 12,000 to 14,000 daltons over a period of up to 270 minutes.

Contraindications

All anemias not associated with iron deficiency; hypersensitivity to sodium ferric gluconate complex or any of its inactive components; evidence of iron overload.

Warnings/Precautions

➤*Hypotension:* Hypotension associated with light-headedness, malaise, fatigue, weakness, or severe pain in the chest, back, flanks, or groin has been associated with administration of IV iron. These hypotensive reactions are not associated with signs of hypersensitivity and have usually resolved within 1 or 2 hours. Successful treatment may consist of observation or, if the hypotension causes symptoms, volume expansion.

➤*Benzyl alcohol:* This product contains benzyl alcohol, which has been associated with a fatal "gasping syndrome" in premature infants.

➤*Iron overload:* Iron is not easily eliminated from the body and accumulation can be toxic. Unnecessary therapy with parenteral iron will cause excess storage of iron with consequent possibility of iatrogenic hemosiderosis. Iron overload is particularly apt to occur in patients with hemoglobinopathies and other refractory anemias. Do not administer to patients with iron overload.

➤*Hypersensitivity reactions:* Serious hypersensitivity reactions have been rarely reported. One case of a life-threatening hypersensitivity reaction has been observed in a patient who received a single dose of sodium ferric gluconate complex in a postmarketing study. Three serious hypersensitivity reactions have been reported from the spontaneous reporting system (see Adverse Reactions).

➤*Pregnancy: Category B.* There are no adequate and well-controlled studies in pregnant women. Use during pregnancy only if the potential benefit justifies the potential risk to the fetus.

➤*Lactation:* It is not known whether this drug is excreted in breast milk. Because many drugs are excreted in human milk, exercise caution when administering to a breastfeeding woman.

➤*Children:* Safety and efficacy have not been established in pediatric patients younger than 6 years of age. Sodium ferric gluconate complex contains benzyl alcohol; therefore, do not use in neonates.

➤*Elderly:* Cautiously select dose for an elderly patient, usually starting at the low end of the dosing range, reflecting the greater frequency of decreased hepatic, renal, or cardiac function and of concomitant disease or other drug therapy.

Drug Interactions

➤*Oral iron preparations:* Coadministration of parenteral iron preparations may reduce absorption of oral iron preparations.

Adverse Reactions

➤*Hypotension:* (See Warnings). Of 226 renal dialysis patients exposed to sodium ferric gluconate complex, 3 (1.3%) patients experienced hypotensive events, which were accompanied by flushing in 2 patients. All completely reversed after 1 hour without sequelae.

SODIUM FERRIC GLUCONATE COMPLEX — INJECTION

Sodium ferric gluconate complex administered to patients during dialysis may cause transient hypotension. Administration may augment hypotension caused by dialysis.

Among the 126 patients evaluated in clinical studies, 1 patient experienced a transient decreased level of consciousness without hypotension. Another patient discontinued treatment prematurely because of dizziness, lightheadedness, diplopia, malaise, and weakness without hypotension that resulted in a 3- to 4-hour hospitalization for observation following drug administration. The syndrome resolved spontaneously.

➤*Hypersensitivity:* (See Warnings). In the single-dose, postmarketing safety study, 1 patient experienced a life-threatening hypersensitivity reaction (diaphoresis, nausea, vomiting, severe lower back pain, dyspnea, and wheezing for 20 minutes) following administration. There were 9 patients (0.8%) who had an adverse reaction that precluded further sodium ferric gluconate complex administration (drug intolerance). These included 1 life-threatening reaction, 6 allergic reactions (2 pruritus reactions and facial flushing, chills, dyspnea/chest pain, and rash), and 2 other reactions (hypotension and nausea). Another 2 patients (0.2%) experienced allergic reactions not deemed to represent drug intolerance (nausea/malaise and nausea/dizziness) following administration.

In multiple-dose studies, hypersensitivity events associated with sodium ferric gluconate complex resulting in premature study discontinuation occurred in 3 out of a total 88 (3.4%) treated patients. The first patient withdrew after the development of pruritus and chest pain following the test dose. The second patient, in the high-dose group, experienced nausea, abdominal and flank pain, fatigue, and rash following the first dose. The third patient, in the low-dose group, experienced a "red, blotchy rash" following the first dose. Of the 38 patients exposed, none reported hypersensitivity reactions.

Many chronic renal failure patients experience cramps, pain, nausea, rash, flushing, and pruritus.

➤*Other adverse reactions (adults):*

Cardiovascular – Hypotension (29%); hypertension (13%); syncope (6%); tachycardia (5%); angina pectoris; bradycardia; myocardial infarction; pulmonary edema; vasodilation.

CNS – Cramps (25%); dizziness (13%); fatigue, paresthesias (6%); agitation; somnolence.

Dermatologic – Pruritus (6%); increased sweating; rash.

GI – Diarrhea, nausea, vomiting (35%); abdominal pain (6%); anorexia; dyspepsia; eructation; flatulence; GI disorder; melena; rectal disorder.

Hematologic – Abnormal erythrocytes (11%); anemia; leukocytosis; lymphadenopathy.

Metabolic – Hyperkalemia (6%); generalized edema (5%); edema; hypervolemia; hypoglycemia; hypokalemia; leg edema; peripheral edema.

Musculoskeletal – Leg cramps (10%); arthralgia; myalgia.

Respiratory – Dyspnea (11%); coughing, upper respiratory tract infections (6%); pneumonia; rhinitis.

Special senses – Abnormal vision; conjunctivitis; ear disorder.

Miscellaneous – Injection-site reaction (33%); chest pain, pain (10%); asthenia, headache (7%); fever (5%); abscess; arm pain; back pain; carcinoma; chills; flu-like syndrome; infection; malaise; rigors; sepsis; urinary tract infection.

➤*Other adverse reactions (children):*

Cardiovascular – Hypertension (23%); hypotension (28% to 41%); tachycardia (13% to 21%); thrombosis (6%).

GI – Abdominal pain (3% to 15%); diarrhea (8%); nausea (6% to 12%); vomiting (9% to 12%).

Respiratory – Pharyngitis (6% to 12%); rhinitis (3% to 9%).

Miscellaneous – Fever (3% to 15%); headache (19% to 29%); infection (8%).

➤*Postmarketing:* Dry mouth, hemorrhage, hypertonia, nervousness.

Overdosage

➤*Symptoms:* Serum iron levels greater than 300 mcg/dL may indicate iron poisoning, which is characterized by abdominal pain, diarrhea, or vomiting that progresses to pallor or cyanosis, lassitude, drowsiness, hyperventilation due to acidosis, and cardiovascular collapse.

➤*Treatment:* Dosages in excess of iron needs may lead to accumulation of iron in iron storage sites and hemosiderosis. Periodic monitoring of laboratory parameters of iron storage may assist in recognition of iron accumulation. Do not administer sodium ferric gluconate complex in patients with iron overload. Sodium ferric gluconate complex is not dialyzable.

IRON — PARENTERAL
IRON SUCROSE

Rx	**Venofer** (Fresenius)	**Injection:** Elemental iron 20 mg/mL	Preservative free. 300 mg/mL sucrose 300 mg/mL (w/v). In 5 mL single-dose vials.

IRON SUCROSE — INJECTION

For additional information, refer to the Dietary Reference Intakes of Vitamins and Minerals table.

Indications

➤*Iron-deficiency anemia:* For the treatment of iron-deficiency anemia in the following patients:

- non-dialysis-dependent chronic kidney disease (NDD-CKD) patients receiving an erythropoietin
- NDD-CKD patients not receiving an erythropoietin
- hemodialysis-dependent chronic kidney disease (HDD-CKD) patients receiving an erythropoietin
- peritoneal dialysis-dependent chronic kidney disease (PDD-CKD) patients receiving an erythropoietin.

Administration and Dosage

➤*General dosing considerations:* The dosage of iron sucrose is expressed in terms of mg of elemental iron. Each mL contains elemental iron 20 mg.

Most CKD patients will require a minimum cumulative repletion dose of elemental iron 1,000 mg administered over sequential sessions to achieve a favorable hemoglobin response and to replenish iron stores (ferritin, transferrin saturation [TSAT]). Hemodialysis patients may continue to require therapy with iron sucrose or other intravenous (IV) iron preparations at the lowest dose necessary to maintain target levels of hemoglobin and laboratory parameters of iron storage within acceptable limits.

➤*Adults:*

Iron-deficiency anemia –

Hemodialysis dependent-chronic kidney disease patients: 100 mg per consecutive hemodialysis session for a total cumulative dose of 1,000 mg. Dose may be administered undiluted by slow IV injection over 2 to 5 minutes, or it may be diluted in a maximum of 100 mL of sodium chloride 0.9% and administered by IV infusion over a period of at least 15 minutes.

Nondialysis dependent-chronic kidney disease patients: Administer as a total cumulative dose of 1,000 mg over a 14-day period as a 200 mg slow IV injection undiluted over 2 to 5 minutes on 5 different occasions within the 14-day period.

Peritoneal dialysis dependent-chronic kidney disease patients: Administer as a total cumulative dose of 1,000 mg in 3 divided doses, given by slow IV infusion, within a 28-day period: 2 infusions of 300 mg over 1.5 hours 14 days apart, followed by one 400 mg infusion over 2.5 hours 14 days later. The iron sucrose dose should be diluted in a maximum of 250 mL of sodium chloride 0.9%.

➤*Preparation for administration:*

Hemodialysis dependent-chronic kidney disease patients – Dose may be given undiluted or diluted in a maximum of 100 mL of sodium chloride 0.9%.

Peritoneal dialysis dependent-chronic kidney disease patients – Dose should be diluted in a maximum of 250 mL of sodium chloride 0.9%.

➤*Administration:* Iron sucrose must only be administered IV either by slow injection or by infusion.

Hemodialysis dependent-chronic kidney disease patients – Dose may be administered undiluted by slow IV injection over 2 to 5 minutes, or it may diluted in a maximum of 100 mL of sodium chloride 0.9% and administered by IV infusion over a period of at least 15 minutes.

Nondialysis dependent-chronic kidney disease patients – Slowly administer IV injection undiluted over 2 to 5 minutes. There is limited experience with administration of an infusion of iron sucrose 500 mg, diluted in a maximum of 250 mL of sodium chloride 0.9% over a period of 3.5 to 4 hours on day 1 and 14; hypotension occurred in 2 of 30 patients treated.

Peritoneal dialysis dependent-chronic kidney disease patients – Infuse over 2.5 hours 14 days later. The iron sucrose dose should be diluted in a maximum of 250 mL of sodium chloride 0.9%.

➤*Storage/Stability:* Store in original carton at 25°C (77°F). Excursions are permitted to 15° to 30°C (59° to 86°F). Do not freeze. Contains no preservatives.

Actions

➤*Pharmacology:* Iron sucrose is used to replenish body iron stores in NDD-CKD patients receiving erythropoietin and in NDD-CKD patients not receiving erythropoietin, and in HDD-CKD and PDD-CKD patients receiving erythropoietin. Iron deficiency may be caused by blood loss during dialysis, increased erythropoiesis secondary to erythropoietin use, and insufficient absorption of iron from the GI tract. Iron is essential to the synthesis of hemoglobin to maintain oxygen transport and to the function and formation of other physiologically important heme and nonheme compounds. Most dialysis patients require IV iron to maintain sufficient iron stores.

➤*Pharmacokinetics:*

Absorption/Distribution – In healthy adults treated with IV doses of iron sucrose, its iron component exhibits first order kinetics. In healthy adults receiving IV doses of iron sucrose, its iron component appears to distribute mainly in blood and, to some extent, in extravascular fluid. Iron sucrose has a nonsteady state apparent volume of distribution of 10 L, and steady state apparent volume of distribution of 7.9 L. A study evaluating iron sucrose containing iron 100 mg labeled with $^{52}Fe/^{59}Fe$ in patients with iron deficiency shows that a significant amount of the administered iron distributes in the liver, spleen, and bone marrow and that the bone marrow is an iron-trapping compartment and not a reversible volume of distribution.

Metabolism/Excretion – Because iron disappearance from serum depends on the need for iron in the iron stores and iron-utilizing tissues of the body, serum clearance of iron is expected to be more rapid in iron-deficient patients treated with iron sucrose as compared with healthy individuals.

Following IV administration, iron sucrose is dissociated into iron and sucrose by the reticuloendothelial system. The sucrose component is eliminated mainly by urinary excretion with an elimination half-life of 6 hours and total clearance of 1.2 L/h. In a study evaluating a single IV dose of iron sucrose containing sucrose 1,510 mg and iron 100 mg in 12 healthy adults (9 women, 3 men; age range, 32 to 52 years), 68.3% of the sucrose was eliminated in urine in 4 hours and 75.4% in 24 hours. Some iron is also eliminated in the urine. Neither transferrin nor transferrin receptor levels changed immediately after the dose administration. In this study and another study evaluating a single IV dose of iron sucrose containing iron 500 to 700 mg in 26 anemic patients on erythropoietin therapy (23 women, 3 men; age range, 16 to 60 years), approximately 5% of the iron was eliminated in urine in 24 hours at each dose level.

Contraindications

Evidence of iron overload; known hypersensitivity to iron sucrose or any of its inactive components; anemia not caused by iron deficiency.

Warnings/Precautions

➤*Iron overload:* Because body iron excretion is limited and excess tissue iron can be hazardous, exercise caution to withhold iron administration in the presence of evidence of tissue iron overload. Dosages of iron sucrose in excess of iron needs may lead to accumulation of iron in storage sites, leading to hemosiderosis. Exercise particular caution to avoid overload where anemia unresponsive to treatment has been incorrectly diagnosed as iron deficiency anemia. Do not administer iron sucrose to patients with iron overload.

➤*Hypotension:* Hypotension has been reported frequently in HDD-CKD patients receiving IV iron. Hypotension also has been reported in NND- and PDD-CKD patients receiving IV iron. Hypotension following administration of iron sucrose may be related to rate of administration and total dose administered. Cautiously administer iron sucrose according to recommended guidelines.

➤*Hypersensitivity reactions:* See Adverse Reactions for more information.

➤*Pregnancy: Category B.* There are no adequate and well controlled studies in pregnant women. Because animal reproduction studies are not always predictive of human response, administer this drug during pregnancy only if clearly needed.

➤*Lactation:* Iron sucrose is excreted in milk of rats. It is not known whether this drug is excreted in human milk. Because many drugs are excreted in human milk, exercise caution when iron sucrose is administered to a breast-feeding woman.

➤*Children:* Safety and efficacy of iron sucrose in children have not been established.

➤*Elderly:* No overall differences in safety were observed between these subjects and younger subjects, and other reported clinical experience has not identified differences in responses between the elderly and younger patients, but greater sensitivity of some older individuals cannot be ruled out.

➤*Monitoring:* Patients receiving iron sucrose require periodic monitoring of hematologic and hematinic parameters (hemoglobin, hematocrit, serum ferritin, and transferrin saturation). Withhold iron therapy in patients with evidence of iron overload and discontinue use when serum ferritin levels equal or exceed established guidelines. Transferrin saturation values increase rapidly after IV administration of iron sucrose; thus, serum iron values may be reliably obtained 48 hours after IV dosing.

Drug Interactions

➤*Oral iron preparations:* Drug-drug interactions involving iron sucrose have not been studied. However, like other parenteral iron preparations, iron sucrose may be expected to reduce the absorption of concomitantly administered oral iron preparations.

Adverse Reactions

Iron Sucrose Adverse Reactions (≥ 2%) by Indication

	HDD-CKD	NDD-CKD		PDD-CKD	
Adverse reaction	Iron sucrose (n = 231)	Iron sucrose (n = 139)	Oral iron (n = 139)	Iron sucrose (n = 75)	Erythropoietin only (n = 46)
Any adverse reaction	78.8%	76.3%	73.4%	72%	65.2%
CNS					
Asthenia	2.2%	0.7%	2.2%	2.7%	0
Dizziness	6.5%	6.5%	1.4%	1.3%	4.3%
Fatigue	1.7%	3.6%	5.8%	0	4.3%
Headache	12.6%	2.9%	0.7%	4%	0
Hypoesthesia	0	0.7%	0.7%	0	4.3%
Cardiovascular					
Cardiac murmur	0.4%	2.2%	2.2%	0	0
Chest pain	6.1%	1.4%	0	2.7%	0
Hypertension	6.5%	6.5%	4.3%	8%	6.5%
Hypotension	39.4%	2.2%	0.7%	2.7%	2.2%
Dermatologic					
Pruritus	3.9%	2.2%	4.3%	2.7%	0
Rash	0.4%	1.4%	2.2%	0	2.2%
GI					
Abdominal pain	3.5%	1.4%	2.9%	4%	6.5%
Constipation	1.3%	4.3%	12.9%	4%	6.5%
Diarrhea	5.2%	7.2%	10.1%	8%	4.3%
Nausea	14.7%	8.6%	12.2%	5.3%	4.3%
Vomiting	9.1%	5%	8.6%	8%	2.2%
Local					
Catheter site infection	0	0	0	4%	8.7%
Infusion site burning	0	3.6%	0	0	0
Injection site extravasation	0	2.2%	0	0	0
Injection site pain	0	2.2%	0	0	0
Metabolic/Nutritional					
Fluid overload	3%	1.4%	0.7%	1.3%	0
Gout	0	2.9%	1.4%	0	0
Hyperglycemia	0	2.9%	0	0	2.2%
Hypoglycemia	0.4%	0.7%	0.7%	4%	0
Musculoskeletal					
Arthralgia	3.5%	1.4%	2.2%	4%	4.3%
Arthritis	0	0	0	0	4.3%
Back pain	2.2%	2.2%	3.6%	1.3%	4.3%
Muscle cramp	29.4%	0.7%	0.7%	2.7%	0
Myalgia	0	3.6%	0	1.3%	0
Pain in extremity	5.6%	4.3%	0	2.7%	6.5%
Respiratory					
Cough	3%	2.2%	0.7%	1.3%	0
Dyspnea	3.5%	3.6%	0.7%	1.3%	2.2%
Dyspnea exacerbated	0	2.2%	0.7%	0	0
Nasal congestion	0	1.4%	2.2%	1.3%	0
Nasopharyngitis	0.9%	0.7%	2.2%	2.7%	2.2%
Pharyngitis	0.4%	0	0	6.7%	0
Rhinitis allergic	0	0.7%	2.2%	0	0
Sinusitis	0	0.7%	0.7%	4%	0
Upper respiratory tract infection	1.3%	0.7%	1.4%	2.7%	2.2%
Special senses					
Conjunctivitis	0.4%	0	0	2.7%	0
Dysgeusia	0.9%	7.9%	0	0	0
Ear pain	0	2.2%	0.7%	0	0
Miscellaneous					
Edema	0.4%	6.5%	6.5%	0	2.2%
Fecal occult blood positive	0	1.4%	3.6%	2.7%	4.3%
Feeling abnormal	3%	0	0	0	0
Graft complications	9.5%	1.4%	0	0	0
Peripheral edema	2.6%	7.2%	5%	5.3%	10.9%
Peritoneal infection	0	0	0	8%	10.9%
Pyrexia	3%	0.7%	0.7%	1.3%	0

IRON SUCROSE — INJECTION

Iron Sucrose Adverse Reactions (≥ 2%) by Indication					
	HDD-CKD	NDD-CKD		PDD-CKD	
Adverse reaction	Iron sucrose (n = 231)	Iron sucrose (n = 139)	Oral iron (n = 139)	Iron sucrose (n = 75)	Erythropoietin only (n = 46)
Urinary tract infection NOS	0.4%	0.7%	5%	1.3%	2.2%

Drug-related adverse reactions reported by at least 2% of iron sucrose-treated patients are shown by dose group in the following table.

Iron Sucrose Adverse Reactions (≥ 2%) by Dose				
	HDD-CKD	NDD-CKD		PDD-CKD
Adverse reaction	100 mg (n = 231)	200 mg (n = 109)	500 mg (n = 30)	300 mg for 2 doses followed by 400 mg for 1 dose (n = 75)
Any adverse reaction	14.7%	23.9%	20%	10.7%
CNS				
Dizziness	0	2.8%	6.7%	0
Headache	0	2.8%	0	0
GI				
Diarrhea	0.9%	0	0	2.7%
Nausea	1.7%	2.8%	0	1.3%
Local				
Infusion site burning	0	3.7%	0	0
Injection site pain	0	2.8%	0	0
Miscellaneous				
Dysgeusia	0.9%	7.3%	3.3%	0
Hypotension	5.2%	0	6.7%	0
Peripheral edema	0	1.8%	6.7%	0

➤*HDD-CKD patients:* Adverse reactions, whether or not related to iron sucrose administration, reported more than 5% of treated patients from a total of 231 patients in HDD-CKD studies A, B, and C were as follows: hypotension (39.4%); muscle cramps (29.4%); nausea (14.7%); headache (12.6%); graft complications (9.5%); vomiting (9.1%); dizziness, hypertension (6.5%); chest pain (6.1%); diarrhea (5.2%).

Postmarketing –

Adverse reactions reported by more than 1% of 1,051 treated patients were congestive cardiac failure, sepsis, and dysgeusia.

➤*NDD-CKD patients:* In study D of 182 treated NDD-CKD patients, 91 were exposed to iron sucrose. Adverse reactions, whether or not related to iron sucrose, reported by at least 5% of the iron sucrose exposed patients were as follows: dysgeusia, peripheral edema (7.7%); constipation, diarrhea, dizziness, hypertension, nausea (5.5%).

One serious related adverse reaction was reported (hypotension and shortness of breath not requiring hospitalization in an iron sucrose patient). Two patients experienced possible hypersensitivity/allergic reactions (local edema/hypotension) during the study. Of the 5 patients who prematurely discontinued the treatment phase of the study because of adverse reactions (2 oral iron group and 3 iron sucrose group), 3 iron sucrose patients had reactions that were considered drug-related (hypotension, dyspnea, and nausea).

In an additional study of iron sucrose with varying erythropoietin doses in 96 treated NDD-CKD patients, adverse reactions, whether or not related to iron sucrose, reported by at least 5% of iron sucrose exposed patients are as follows: diarrhea, edema (16.5%); nausea (13.2%); vomiting (12.1%); arthralgia, back pain, dysgeusia, headache, hypertension (7.7%); dizziness (6.6%); extremity pain, injection site burning (5.5%).

No patient experienced a hypersensitivity/allergic reaction during the study. Of the patients who prematurely discontinued the treatment phase of the study because of adverse reactions (2.1% oral iron group and 12.5% iron sucrose group), only 1 patient (iron sucrose group) had reactions that were considered drug-related (anxiety, headache, and nausea). Ninety-one patients in this study were exposed to iron sucrose during the treatment or extending follow-up phase.

➤*PDD-CKD patients:* In study E of 121 treated PDD-CKD patients, 75 patients were exposed to iron sucrose. Adverse reactions, whether or not related to iron sucrose, reported by at least 5% of these patients are as follows: diarrhea, hypertension, nausea, peripheral edema, peritoneal infection, pharyngitis, and vomiting.

Of these 75 patients exposed to iron sucrose, 9 patients experienced serious adverse reactions as follows: peritoneal infection (2 patients) and 1 patient each with cardiopulmonary arrest, myocardial infarction, upper respiratory tract infection not otherwise specified (NOS), anemia, gangrene, hypovolemia, tuberculosis. None of these reactions were considered drug related. Two iron sucrose patients experienced a moderate hypersensitivity/allergic reaction (rash or swelling/itching) during the study.

The only drug-related adverse reaction to iron sucrose administration reported by at least 2% of patients was diarrhea.

Three patients in the iron sucrose study group discontinued study treatment because of adverse reactions (cardiopulmonary arrest, peritonitis and myocardial infarction, hypertension), which were considered to be not drug-related.

➤*Hypersensitivity:* In clinical studies, several patients experienced hypersensitivity reactions presenting with wheezing, dyspnea, hypotension, rashes, or pruritus. Serious episodes of hypotension occurred in 2 patients treated with iron sucrose 500 mg.

From the postmarketing spontaneous reporting system, there were 104 reports of anaphylactoid reactions, including patients who experienced serious or life-threatening reactions (anaphylactic shock, loss of consciousness or collapse, bronchospasm with dyspnea, or convulsion) associated with iron sucrose administration.

One hundred thirty (11%) of the 1,151 patients evaluated in the 4 US trials in HDD-CKD patients (studies A, B, and the 2 postmarketing studies) had prior other IV iron therapy and were reported to be intolerant (defined as precluding further use of the iron product). When these patients were treated with iron sucrose, there were no occurrences of adverse reactions that precluded further use of iron sucrose.

Overdosage

➤*Symptoms:* Symptoms associated with overdosage or infusing iron sucrose too rapidly included hypotension, dyspnea, headache, vomiting, nausea, dizziness, joint aches, paresthesia, abdominal and muscle pain, edema, and cardiovascular collapse.

➤*Treatment:* Most symptoms have been successfully treated with IV fluids, hydrocortisone, and/or antihistamines. Infusing the solution as recommended or at a slower rate may also alleviate symptoms.

MULTIVITAMINS WITH IRON

Content given per capsule, tablet, 5 mL liquid, or 1 mL drops.

	Product & Distributor	Fe mg	A units	D units	E units	B_1 mg	B_2 mg	B_3 mg	B_5 mg	B_6 mg	B_{12} mcg	C mg	Folate mg	Other Content	Excipients & How Supplied
Rx	**Nephron FA Tablets** (Nephro-Tech)	200[c]				1.5	1.7	20	10	10	6	40	1[d]	Biotin 300 mcg, docusate sodium 75 mg	In 100s.
Rx	**Ferrogel Forte Softgels** (Cypress)	151[c]									10	60	1[d]		Soybean oil. (CYP 189). In UD 100s.
Rx	**Chromagen Forte Tablets** (Ther-Rx)	151[e,f]									10	60	1[d]	Calcium threonate 0.8 mg, succinic acid 50 mg	Lactose. (Ther-Rx 197). Maroon, capsule shape. Film-coated. In 90s.
Rx	**Niferex-150 Forte Capsules** (Ther-Rx)	150[f,g]									25	60	1[d]	Calcium threonate 0.8 mg, succinic acid 50 mg	(THX 164). Red. In 90s.
Rx	**Fe-Tinic 150 Forte Capsules** (KV Pharm)	150[f,cc]									25	60	1[d]	Succinic acid 50 mg.	(THX 164). Red/Clear. In 90s.
Rx	**Maxaron Forte Capsules** (Centrix)	150[f,h]									25	60	1[d]	Calcium threonate	PEG. (Centrix 135). Orange. In 100s.
Rx	**Ferrex 150 Forte Capsules** (Breckenridge)	150[f,i]									25		1[d]		PEG. (B-198). Maroon. In UD 100s.
Rx	**Renatabs with Iron Tablets** (Hawthorn)	100[f,j]			5	1.5	1.7	20	10[k]	10	6	60	1[d]	D-biotin 300 mcg	*Multivitamin tablet*: Mineral oil. (HAW 160). Yellow, capsule shape. Film-coated. *Iron tablet*: Mineral oil, PEG. (HAW 161). Red, capsule shape. Film-coated. In UD 60s.
Rx	**Vitafol Syrup** (Hi-Tech)	100[l,m]						13.3		2	8.34		0.25[d]		Raspberry mint flavor. In 473 mL.
Rx	**Ferralet 90 Tablets** (Mission Pharmacal)	90[j]									12	120	1[d]	Docusate sodium 50 mg	(F5). Green, rectangular. Film-coated. In 90s.
Rx	**Chromagen FA Tablets** (Ther-Rx)	70[l,o]									10	150	1[d]	Calcium threonate 2 mg, succinic acid 75 mg,	Lactose, PEG. (Ther-Rx 199). Green, capsule shape. Film-coated. In 90s.
otc	**Gentle Iron Capsules** (Nature's Bounty)	28[p]									8	60	0.4[d]		In 90s.
Rx	**BiferaRx Tablets** (Alaven)	28[dd]									25		1[d]		PEG. (AP 85). Maroon, oval. Film-coated. In 90s.
otc	**Daily Multiple Vitamins with Iron Tablets** (Sundown Nutrition)[q]	18[c]	5,000[r]	400[s]	30[t]	1.5	1.7	20	10[u]	2	6	60	0.4[d]		Mannitol. In 100s.
otc	**Multi-Day Multivitamin Plus Iron Tablets** (Nature's Bounty)														Mannitol. In 100s and 365s.
otc	**One-Tablet-Daily with Iron Tablets** (Goldline)														Sodium free. Mannitol. In 100s.
otc	**Tab-A-Vite + Iron Tablets** (Major)														In 100s and 1,000s.
otc	**Once Daily Multi-Vitamin with Iron Tablets** (Prime)[v]	18[n]	5,000	400		2	2.5	20	1[k]	1	1	50			Sugar. In 100s and 1,000s.
otc	**Stress with Iron Tablets** (Major)	18[c]			30[t]	10	10	100	20[u]	5	12	500	0.4[d]	Biotin 45 mg	Coconut oil, mannitol. In 60s.
otc	**Animal Shapes + Iron Tablets** (Major)	15[c]	2,500[w]	400	15[t]	1.05	1.2	13.5		1.05	4.5	60	0.3[d]		Sodium 5 mg, sucrose, sugar
otc	**Flintstones Plus Iron Chewable Tablets** (Bayer)	15[c]	2,500[w]	400	15[x]	1.05	1.2	13.5		1.05	4.5	60	0.3[d]	Milk	Sodium 10 mg, sucrose, sugar < 1 g. In 60s.
otc	**Fruity Chews with Iron Chewable Tablets** (Goldline)	15[c]	2,500[r]	400[s]	15[t]	1	1	13.5		1.05	4.5	60	0.3[d]	Fish, soy	Mannitol, sodium 5 mg, sucrose, sugar < 1 g. In 100s.
otc	**Children's Chewable Vitamins + Iron Tablets** (Prime)	15[c]	2,500[y]	400[z]	15[t]	1.05	1.2	13.5		1.05	4.5	60	0.3[d]		Dextrose, sugar 0.6 g. In 100s and 1,000s.
otc	**S.S.S. Tonic Liquid** (S.S.S. Company[a])	11.1[b]				0.56	0.27	2.22						Ethyl alcohol 12%	Saccharin, sorbitol. In 300 mL.
otc	**Vita Drops with Iron Drops** (Major)	10[n]	1,500	400	5	0.5	0.6	8		0.4		35			Methylparaben, orange oil. Cherry flavor. In 50 mL.
otc	**Baby Vitamin with Iron Drops** (Goldline)	10[n]	1,500[aa]	400[z]	5[bb]	0.5	0.6	8		0.4		35			Methylparaben, orange oil. In 50 mL.
otc	**Tri-Vi-Sol with Iron Drops** (Mead Johnson)	10[f,n]	1,500[aa]	400[z]								35			Gluten free and lactose free. Fruit flavor. In 50 mL.

MULTIVITAMINS WITH IRON

	Product & Distributor	Fe mg	A units	D units	E units	B_1 mg	B_2 mg	B_3 mg	B_5 mg	B_6 mg	B_{12} mcg	C mg	Folate mg	Other Content	Excipients & How Supplied
otc	**Geritol with Ferrex 18 Tonic Liquid** (GlaxoSmithKline Consumer)	6				0.83	0.83	16.67	0.67	0.17				Choline bitartrate 16.7 mg, methionine 8.33 mg, soy	Alcohol 12%, sugar 2.3 g/5 mL. In 118 mL.
otc	**Senilezol Liquid** (Edwards)	1				0.42	0.42	1.67	0.83	0.17	0.83				Alcohol 15%, parabens, sucrose. In 473 mL.

[a] S.S.S. Company, 71 University Ave., Atlanta, GA 30315, 800-237-3843, http://www.ssspharmaceuticals.com.
[b] As ferric ammonium citrate.
[c] As ferrous fumarate.
[d] As folic acid.
[e] As ferrous fumarate and ferrous asparto glycinate.
[f] As elemental iron.
[g] As elemental polysaccharide iron and ferrous asparto glycinate.
[h] As elemental ferrous bisglycinate and polysaccharide iron.
[i] As polysaccharide iron.
[j] As carbonyl iron.
[k] As calcium pantothenate.
[l] As ferric pyrophosphate.
[m] Elemental iron 10.4 mg.
[n] As ferrous sulfate.
[o] As ferrous asparto glycinate.
[p] As ferrous bisglycinate.
[q] Sundown Nutrition, 90 Orville Dr., Bohemia, NY 11716, 888-848-2435, http://www.sundownnutrition.com.
[r] As retinyl acetate and beta-carotene.
[s] As ergocalciferol.
[t] As dl-alpha tocopheryl acetate.
[u] As d-calcium pantothenate.
[v] Prime Marketing, 1775 John R Rd., Troy, MI 48083-2512, 248-526-3700, http://www.primemarketinggroup.com.
[w] As vitamin A acetate and beta-carotene.
[x] As vitamin E acetate.
[y] As vitamin A acetate.
[z] As cholecalciferol.
[aa] As vitamin A palmitate.
[bb] As d-alpha tocopheryl succinate.
[cc] As polysaccharide iron complex.
[dd] As 22 mg polysaccharide iron complex and 6 mg heme iron polypeptide (bovine source).

For additional information, refer to the Dietary Reference Intakes of Vitamins and Minerals table.

IRON WITH VITAMIN B_{12} AND INTRINSIC FACTOR

Content given per capsule or tablet.

	Product & Distributor	Fe mg	B_{12}[a] mcg	IFC[b]	B_1 mg	B_2 mg	B_3 mg	C mg	FA mg	Other Content	How Supplied
Rx	**Hemax Caplet** (Pronova)	150[f]	60	amount unspecified				500	1	Cu, biotin 150 mg, docusate sodium 50 mg, vitamin E 30 units	French vanilla flavoring, maltodextrin, mineral oil, PEG, sodium benzoate. (HEMAX). Brown/Beige, oval, scored. In 90s.
otc	**Albafort Capsules** (Baroli)	110[c]	15	240 mg				100	0.8		In 100s.
Rx	**Foltrin Capsules** (Vitarine)	110[c]	15	240 mg				75	0.5		(E 5380). Maroon/red. In 100s and 1000s.
Rx	**TL Icon Capsules** (Trigen Labs)										(TL051). Red. In 60s.
Rx	**Multigen Caplets** (Breckenridge Pharmaceutical)	70[d]	10	50 mg desiccated stomach substance				152[e]		Succinic acid 75 mg	(B 543). Peach, capsule shape. Film-coated. In 90s.
Rx	**Vitagen Advance Caplets** (Midlothian)									Medium chain triglycerides, succinic acid 75 mg	Lactose, maltodextrin, polydextrose. (ML 550). Tan, capsule shape. Film-coated. In 90s.
Rx	**FeoGen Capsules** (Rising)	66	10	100 mg desiccated stomach substance				250			(115). Maroon. In UD 100s.

[a] B_{12} activity derived from cobalamin or liver.
[b] Intrinsic factor as concentrate or from stomach preparations.
[c] From ferrous fumarate.
[d] From ferrous asparto glycinate.
[e] As calcium ascorbate and calcium threonate.
[f] From carbonyl iron.

IRON WITH VITAMIN B_{12} AND INTRINSIC FACTOR — ORAL

Indications

➤*Absorption of vitamin B_{12}:* These products contain Intrinsic Factor derived from stomach extract to promote the absorption of vitamin B_{12}.

➤*Anemias:* For treatment of anemias that respond to hematinics, including pernicious anemia and other megaloblastic anemias and also iron deficiency anemia.

Warnings/Precautions

➤*Pregnancy: Category C* (*Foltrin*). Give to a pregnant woman only if clearly needed.

➤*Lactation:* Because many drugs are excreted in human milk, exercise caution when this drug is administered to a breast-feeding woman.

MANGANESE

otc sf	**Chelated Manganese** (Freeda)	**Tablets; oral:** 20 mg	In 100s, 250s and 500s.
		50 mg	In 100s, 250s and 500s.
otc	**Mangimin** (The Key Company)	**Capsules; oral:** 10 mg	In 100s.

MANGANESE — ORAL

For information on parenteral manganese, refer to the monograph in the IV Nutritional Therapy section. For additional information, refer to the Dietary Reference Intakes of Vitamins and Minerals table.

Indications

➤*Manganese deficiency:* As a dietary supplement to prevent or treat manganese deficiency.

Administration and Dosage

➤*General dosing considerations:* The need for manganese in human nutrition has been established, but because a lack of manganese is rare, there is no recommended daily allowance for it. For adults and adolescents, 2 to 5 mg/day via the diet is recommended.

➤*Adults:*

Manganese deficiency – 1 tablet daily.

➤*Storage/Stability:* Store at room temperature, away from heat and direct light. Do not freeze or refrigerate.

Actions

➤*Pharmacology:* Manganese is a cofactor in many enzyme systems; it stimulates synthesis of cholesterol and fatty acids in the liver and influences mucopolysaccharide synthesis. It is concentrated in mitochondria, primarily of the pituitary gland, pancreas, liver, kidney and bone.

Warnings/Precautions

➤*Special risk:* Use manganese cautiously in patients with biliary disease and liver disease.

➤*Pregnancy: Category: Undetermined*. Pregnant women should avoid manganese use in excess of the adequate intake. Adequate intake of manganese in pregnant women is 2 mg/d (refer to the Dietary Reference Intakes of Vitamins and Minerals table).

➤*Lactation:* Breast-feeding women should avoid manganese use in excess of the adequate intake. Adequate intake of manganese in breast-feeding women is 2.6 mg/d (refer to the Dietary Reference Intakes of Vitamins and Minerals table).

Patient Information

The presence of other medical problems may affect the use of manganese. Make sure to tell your healthcare provider if you have any other medical problems, especially biliary disease or liver disease.

Do not keep outdated dietary supplements or those no longer needed. Be sure that any discarded dietary supplement is out of the reach of children.

COPPER

otc	**Copper** (Freeda)	**Tablets; oral:** 2 mg	As copper gluconate. In 100s.
otc	**Coppermin** (Key Co)	**Tablets; oral:** 5 mg	In 100s.
otc sf	**Cu-5** (BioTech)	**Capsules; oral:** 5 mg	As copper sebicate. Dye free, preservative free, sugar free. In 100s.

COPPER — ORAL

For additional information, refer to the Dietary Reference Intakes of Vitamins and Minerals table.

Indications

➤*Copper supplementation:* As a nutritional supplement for the maintenance of proper copper levels in the body.

Administration and Dosage

➤*Children:*

Recommended dietary allowance –

14 to 18 years of age: 890 mcg/day.
9 to 13 years of age: 700 mcg/day.
4 to 8 years of age: 440 mcg/day.
1 to 3 years of age: 340 mcg/day.
7 to 12 months of age: 220 mcg/day (adequate intake).
0 to 6 months of age: 200 mcg/day (adequate intake).

➤*Storage/Stability:* Store in a cool dry place.

Contraindications

None well documented.

Warnings/Precautions

➤*Pregnancy: Category A*. It is unknown whether copper supplementation will harm a fetus. Women who are pregnant or planning to become pregnant should speak with a health care provider before taking this mineral. The RDA of copper in pregnant women is 1,000 mcg/day. (Refer to the Dietary Reference Intakes of Vitamins and Minerals table).

➤*Lactation:* It is unknown whether copper supplementation will harm a breast-feeding child. Breast-feeding women should speak with a health care provider before taking this mineral. The RDA of copper in breast-feeding women is 1,300 mcg/day. (Refer to the Dietary Reference Intakes of Vitamins and Minerals table.)

Zinc Supplements

For information on parenteral zinc, refer to the monograph in the IV Nutritional Therapy section. For additional information, refer to the Dietary Reference Intakes of Vitamins and Minerals table.

Indications

➤*Zinc deficiency:* As a dietary supplement; use to treat or prevent zinc deficiencies.

➤*Off-label uses:* For acrodermatitis enteropathica and delayed wound healing associated with zinc deficiency, doses of 220 mg zinc sulfate 3 times daily are used. Zinc sulfate has also been used to treat acne, rheumatoid arthritis and Wilson's disease. However, data conflict and are insufficient to recommend these uses.

In one study, zinc gluconate appeared to significantly shorten the duration of the common cold. Patients (n = 65) dissolved one tablet containing 23 mg zinc (one-half tablet for children) in the mouth every 2 hours until all symptoms were absent for 6 hours; 11% were asymptomatic within 12 hours, 22% within 24 hours. Zinc sulfate should not be used. Further study is needed.

Administration and Dosage

➤*Recommended dietary allowances (RDAs):* Adults, 12 to 15 mg. For a complete listing of RDAs by age, sex and condition, refer to the RDA table.

➤*Dietary supplement:* Average adult dose is 25 to 50 mg zinc daily. Take zinc with food to avoid gastric distress; however, some studies indicate that ingestion with some foods (eg, those that contain bran, phytates, protein, some minerals) may inhibit zinc absorption.

Actions

➤*Pharmacology:* Normal growth and tissue repair depend upon adequate zinc. Zinc acts as an integral part of several enzymes important to protein and carbohydrate metabolism.

Zinc deficiency – Zinc deficiency manifestations include: Anorexia; growth retardation; impaired taste and olfactory sensation; hypogonadism; alopecia; hepatosplenomegaly; dwarfism; rashes; cutaneous lesions; glossitis; stomatitis; blepharitis; paronychia; impaired healing.

➤*Pharmacokinetics:* Zinc salts are poorly absorbed from the GI tract; 20% to 30% of dietary zinc is absorbed. The major stores of zinc are in skeletal muscle and bone; zinc is also found in hair, nails, prostate, spermatazoa and choroid of the eye. The main excretion route is through the intestine. Only minor amounts are lost in urine (≈ 2%).

Contraindications

Pregnancy (see Warnings/Precautions); lactation.

Warnings/Precautions

➤*Excessive intake:* Excessive intake in healthy persons may be deleterious. Eleven healthy men who ingested 150 mg zinc twice daily for 6 weeks showed significant impairment of lymphocyte and polymorphonuclear leukocyte functions and a significant decrease in high-density lipoproteins (HDL). No clinical side effects were seen during the study.

➤*Do not exceed:* Do not exceed prescribed dosage; will cause emesis if administered in single 2 g doses.

➤*Pregnancy: Category C.* Although zinc deficiency during pregnancy has been associated with adverse perinatal outcomes, other studies report no such occurrences. Therefore, since zinc deficiency is very rare, the routine use of zinc supplementation during pregnancy is not recommended. The RDA of zinc in pregnant women is 11 to 12 mg/day (refer to the Dietary Reference Intakes of Vitamins and Minerals table).

➤*Lactation:* Breast milk concentrations of zinc decrease over time following delivery. The RDA of zinc in breast-feeding women is 12 to 13 mg/day (refer to the Dietary Reference Intakes of Vitamins and Minerals table).

Drug Interactions

Zinc Drug Interactions

Precipitant drug	Object drug [a]		Description
Zinc salts	Fluoroquinolones	⬇	The GI absorption and serum levels of some fluoroquinolones may be decreased, possibly resulting in a decreased anti-infective response.
Zinc salts	Tetracyclines	⬇	The GI absorption and serum levels of tetracyclines may be decreased, possibly resulting in a decreased anti-infective response. Doxycycline does not appear to be affected.

[a] ⬇ = object drug decreased.

➤*Drug/Food interactions:* Bran products (including brown bread) and some foods (eg, protein, phytates, some minerals) may decrease zinc absorption.

Adverse Reactions

Nausea; vomiting.

Overdosage

➤*Symptoms:* Nausea; severe vomiting; dehydration; restlessness; sideroblastic anemia (secondary to zinc-induced copper deficiency).

➤*Treatment:* Reduce dosage or discontinue to control symptoms.

Patient Information

If GI upset occurs, take with food, but avoid foods high in calcium, phosphorus or phytate.

ZINC SULFATE — ORAL

otc	**Zinc 15** (Mericon)	**Tablets:** 66 mg (15 mg zinc)	In 100s.
otc	**Orazinc** (Mericon)	**Tablets:** 110 mg (25 mg zinc)	In 100s.
otc	**Zinc Sulfate** (Various)	**Tablets:** 200 mg (45 mg zinc)	In 1000s.
Rx	**Zinc Sulfate** (Various)	**Capsules:** 220 mg (50 mg zinc)	In 100s, 1000s and UD 100s.
otc	**Orazinc** (Mericon)		In 100s and 1000s.
otc	**Verazinc** (Forest)		In 100s.
otc	**Zinc-220** (Alto)		(401).Pink and blue. In 100s, 1000s and UD 100s.
Rx	**Zincate** (Paddock)		In 100s and 1000s.

Complete and comparative prescribing information for these products begins in the Zinc Supplements group monograph. For additional information, refer to the Dietary Reference Intakes of Vitamins and Minerals table.

ZINC GLUCONATE (14.3% zinc)

otc	**Zinc Gluconate** (Various)	**Tablets; oral:** 10 mg	Equiv to 1.4 mg zinc. In 250s.
otc	**Zinc Gluconate** (Various, eg, Freeda)	**Tablets; oral:** 15 mg	Equiv to 2 mg zinc. In 250s.
otc	**Zinc Gluconate** (Various, eg, Major, Mission)	**Tablets; oral:** 50 mg	Equiv to 7 mg zinc. In 100s and 250s.
otc	**Zinc Gluconate** (Mericon)	**Lozenges; oral:** 10 mg	Cocoa powder, fructose, glycyrrhizic acid, powdered milk, sorbitol. In 50s.

Complete and comparative prescribing information for these products begins in the Zinc Supplements group monograph. For additional information, refer to the Dietary Reference Intakes of Vitamins and Minerals table.

ZINC ACETATE

Rx	**Galzin** (Gate Pharmaceuticals)	**Capsules; oral:** 25 mg	(93–215). Aqua blue. In 250s.
		50 mg	(93–208). Orange. In 250s.
otc	**Halls Zinc Defense** (Warner Lambert)	**Lozenges; oral:** 5 mg	Sugar. Cherry or peppermint flavor. In 24s.

Complete and comparative prescribing information for these products begins in the Zinc Supplements group monograph. For additional information, refer to the Dietary Reference Intakes of Vitamins and Minerals table.

ZINC COMBINATIONS

otc	**Zinc** (Zenith-Goldline)	**Lozenges:** 23 mg (zinc citrate/zinc gluconate)	Fructose. In 30s.

Complete and comparative prescribing information for these products begins in the Zinc Supplements group monograph. For additional information, refer to the Dietary Reference Intakes of Vitamins and Minerals table.

Indications

➤*Prevention of dental caries:* Both neutral and acidulated phosphate fluoride effectively control dental decay. Use where water supplies are low in fluoride (less than 0.7 ppm). Fluoride also controls rampant dental decay which frequently follows xerostomia-producing radiotherapy of head and neck tumors.

In communities without fluoridated water, the American Dental Association's Council on Dental Therapeutics recommends continuing fluoride supplements until the age of 13; the American Academy of Pediatrics recommends supplementation until 16 years of age.

➤*Off-label uses:* Sodium fluoride may be effective in treating osteoporosis. Doses (as fluoride) up to 60 mg daily or more are used in conjunction with calcium supplements, vitamin D or estrogen. However, large doses may result in a higher frequency of side effects. Some data suggest that doses less than 50 mg/day are efficacious with fewer adverse reactions. No commercially available products contain high sodium fluoride doses for this use; therefore a large number of tablets would be required to obtain this dosage. Fluoride supplementation is not recommended for the prophylaxis of osteoporosis due to the potential for increased incidence of fractures (see Precautions).

Administration and Dosage

Use according to directions accompanying the product.

Fluoride Dosage

Route/Age	Daily dose
Oral:	
Fluoride ion level in drinking water[a] *(less than 0.3 ppm):*	
Birth to 6 months	None
6 months to 3 years	0.25 mg/day[b]
3 to 6 years	0.5 mg/day
6 to 16 years	1 mg/day
Fluoride content of drinking water (0.3 - 0.6 ppm):	
Birth to 6 months	None
6 months to 3 years	None
3 to 6 years	0.25 mg/day
6 to 16 years	0.5 mg/day
Fluoride content of drinking water (greater than 0.6 ppm):	
Birth to 6 months	None
6 months to 3 years	None
3 to 6 years	None
6 to 16 years	None
Topical (rinse):	
Children (6 to 12 years)	5 to 10 mL[c]
Adults and children (older than 12 years of age)	10 mL[c]

[a] 1 ppm = 1 mg/L.
[b] 2.2 mg sodium fluoride contains 1 mg fluoride ion.
[c] Use once daily (*Point-Two*, once weekly) after thoroughly brushing teeth and rinsing mouth. Rinse around and between teeth for 1 minute, then spit out.

Actions

➤*Pharmacology:* Sodium fluoride acts systemically before tooth eruption, and topically posteruption, by increasing tooth resistance to acid dissolution, by promoting remineralization and by inhibiting the cariogenic microbial process. Acidulation provides greater topical fluoride uptake by dental enamel than neutral solutions. Phosphate protects enamel from demineralization by the acidulated formulation. Topical application of fluoride works superficially on enamel and plaque, and can reduce dental caries by 30% to 40%. Fluoride supplements may reduce the incidence of caries by up to 60%.

➤*Pharmacokinetics:* Fluoride is absorbed in the GI tract, lungs and skin. About 90% of oral fluoride is absorbed in the stomach. Absorption is related to solubility; sodium fluoride is almost completely absorbed. Calcium, iron or magnesium ions may delay absorption. Following ingestion, 50% of fluoride is deposited in bone and teeth. The major route of excretion is the kidneys; it is also excreted by sweat glands, the GI tract and in breast milk.

Contraindications

When the fluoride content of drinking water exceeds 0.7 ppm; low sodium or sodium free diets; hypersensitivity to fluoride. Do not use 1 mg tablets in children younger than 3 years old or when the drinking water fluoride content is ≥ 0.3 ppm. Do not use 1 mg/5 mL rinse (as a supplement) in children younger than 6 years old.

Warnings/Precautions

➤*Fractures:* Some epidemiological studies suggest that the incidence of certain types of bone fractures (crippling skeletal fluorosis) may be higher in some communities with naturally high or adjusted fluoride levels. However, other studies have not detected increased incidence of bone fractures. Crippling skeletal fluorosis is more common in parts of the world with high natural fluoride (greater than 10 ppm), but is extremely rare in the US.

➤*Mucositis:* Gingival tissues may be hypersensitive to some flavors or alcohol.

➤*Tartrazine sensitivity:* Some of these products contain tartrazine, which may cause allergic-type reactions (including bronchial asthma) in susceptible individuals. Although the incidence of tartrazine sensitivity in the general population is low, it is frequently seen in patients who also have aspirin hypersensitivity. Specific products containing tartrazine are identified in the product listings.

➤*Pregnancy:* Consult physician before using.

➤*Lactation:* Consult physician before using.

➤*Children:* See Contraindications.

Drug Interactions

➤*Drug/Food interactions:* Incompatibility of dairy foods with systemic fluoride has occurred due to formation of calcium fluoride, which is poorly absorbed.

Adverse Reactions

➤*Dermatologic:* Eczema; atopic dermatitis; urticaria; allergic rash and other idiosyncrasies (rare).

➤*Miscellaneous:* Gastric distress; headache; weakness. Rinses and gels containing stannous fluoride may produce surface staining of the teeth; this does not occur with nonstannous fluoride topical preparations. Acidulated fluoride may dull porcelain and composite restorations.

Overdosage

➤*Chronic overdosage:* Chronic overdosage of fluorides may result in dental fluorosis (a mottling of tooth enamel) and osseous changes.

➤*Acute overdosage:*

Symptoms – In children, acute ingestion of 10 to 20 mg sodium fluoride may cause excessive salivation and GI disturbances; 500 mg may be fatal. The oral lethal dose is 70 to 140 mg/kg (5 to 10 g in adults).

GI – Salivation, nausea, abdominal pain, vomiting and diarrhea are frequent due to conversion of sodium fluoride to corrosive hydrofluoric acid in the stomach.

CNS – Because of the calcium-binding effect of fluoride, CNS irritability, paresthesias, tetany, convulsions and respiratory and cardiac failure may occur. Fluoride has a direct toxic action on muscle and nerve tissue, and it interferes with many enzyme systems. Hypocalcemia, hypoglycemia and delayed hyperkalemia are frequent laboratory findings.

➤*Treatment:* Usual supportive measures. Refer to General Management of Acute Overdosage. Precipitate the fluoride by using gastric lavage with 0.15% calcium hydroxide. Administer IV glucose in saline for a forced diuresis; IV calcium may be indicated for tetany. Administer calcium IM (10 mL of 10% calcium gluconate, 5 mL in children) every 4 to 6 hours until recovery is complete. Maintain electrolytes, normal blood pH and adequate urine output. Removing fluoride with dialysis and hemoperfusion may also be beneficial.

Patient Information

➤*Tablets and drops:* Milk and other dairy products may decrease absorption of sodium fluoride; avoid simultaneous ingestion.

➤*Tablets:* Dissolve in the mouth, chew, swallow whole, add to drinking water or fruit juice or add to water for use in infant formulas or other food.

➤*Drops:* Take orally, undiluted, or mix with fluids or food.

➤*Rinses and gels:* Rinses and gels are most effective immediately after brushing or flossing and just prior to sleep. Expectorate any excess. Do not swallow. Do not eat, drink or rinse mouth for 30 minutes after application. Notify dentist if tooth enamel becomes discolored.

FLUORIDE — ORAL

Rx	**Sodium Flouride** (Breckenridge)	**Tablets, chewable; oral:** 0.25 mg (from 0.55 mg sodium fluoride)	Sucralose, xylitol. (SCI 1006). White to off-white, round. Orange flavor. In 120s.
Rx *sf*	**Fluor-A-Day** (Arbor Pharmaceuticals)		Sugar free. Maltodextrin, sorbitol, xylitol. Raspberry flavor. In 120s.
Rx *sf*	**Ludent** (Sancilio)		Dye free, sugar free. Sucralose, xylitol. (SCI 1015). White to off-white, round. Orange flavor. In 30s, 90s, and blister pack 30s.
Rx *sf*	**Luride Lozi-Tabs** (Colgate Oral Pharmaceuticals)		Sugar free. (COP 186). Vanilla flavor. In 120s.
Rx *sf*	**ReNaf** (River's Edge)		Sugar free. Cream, round. Vanilla flavor. In 120s and 1,000s.
Rx	**Sodium Fluoride**[a] (Various)	**Tablets, chewable; oral:** 0.5 mg (from 1.1 mg sodium fluoride)	In 1000s.S
Rx *sf*	**Fluor-A-Day** (Arbor Pharmaceuticals)		Sugar free. Maltodextrin, sorbitol, xylitol. Raspberry flavor. In 120s.
Rx	**Fluoritab** (Fluoritab)		Dye free. Pineapple flavor. In 1000s and 5000s.
Rx *sf*	**Ludent** (Sancilio)		Dye free, sugar free. Sucralose, xylitol. (SCI 1016). White to off-white, round. Orange flavor. In 30s, 90s, and blister pack 30s.
Rx *sf*	**Luride Lozi-Tabs** (Colgate Oral Pharmaceuticals)		Sugar free. (COP 014). Grape and assorted fruit flavors. In 120s. Grape also in 1200s.
Rx *sf*	**Pharmaflur 1.1** (Pharmics)		Sugar free. Grape flavor. In 120s.
Rx *sf*	**ReNaf** (River's Edge)		Sugar free. White, round. Grape flavor. In 120s and 1,000s.
Rx	**Sodium Fluoride**[a] (Various, eg, Major)	**Tablets, chewable; oral:** 1 mg (from 2.2 mg sodium fluoride)	In 100s, 1000s and UD 1000s.
Rx *sf*	**Fluor-A-Day** (Arbor Pharmaceuticals)		Sugar free. Maltodextrin, sorbitol, xylitol. Raspberry flavor. In 120s.
Rx	**Karidium** (Lorvic)		White. In 180s and 1000s.
Rx *sf*	**Ludent** (Sancilio)		Dye free, sugar free. Sucralose, xylitol. (SCI 1017). White to off-white, round. Orange flavor. In 30s, 90s, and blister pack 30s.
Rx *sf*	**Luride Lozi-Tabs** (Colgate Oral Pharmaceuticals)		Sugar free. (COP 006). Cherry and assorted fruit flavors. In 120s and 1000s. Cherry also in 5000s.
Rx *sf*	**Luride-SF Lozi-Tabs** (Colgate Oral Pharmaceuticals)		Sugar free. In 120s.
Rx *sf*	**Pharmaflur** (Pharmics)		Sugar free. Cherry flavor. In 1000s.
Rx *sf*	**Pharmaflur df** (Pharmics)		Dye free, sugar free. Cherry flavor. In 120s.
Rx *sf*	**ReNaf** (River's Edge)		Sugar free. Pink, round. Cherry flavor. In 120s and 1,000s.
Rx	**Fluoride** (Kirkman)	**Tablets; oral:** 1 mg (from 2.2 mg sodium fluoride)	In 1000s.
Rx *sf*	**Flura** (Kirkman)		Sugar free. In 100s and 1000s.
Rx	**Sodium Fluoride** (Various)	**Drops; oral:** 0.125 mg per drop (from ≈ 0.275 mg sodium fluoride)	In 30 mL.
Rx *sf*	**Fluor-A-Day** (Arbor Pharmaceuticals)		Sugar free. Methylparaben, xylitol. In 30 mL.
Rx *sf*	**Fluoritab** (Fluoritab)		Sugar free. In 30 mL.
Rx *sf*	**Sodium Fluoride** (Hi-Tech)	**Drops; oral:** 0.5 mg per mL (from 1.1 mg sodium fluoride)	Sugar free. In 50 mL.
Rx *sf*	**Luride** (Colgate)		Sugar free. Peach flavor. In 50 mL.
Rx *sf*	**SodiPhluor** (Kylemore)		Sugar free. Methylparaben, sucralose. Peach flavor. In 50 mL.
Rx *sf*	**Fluoride Loz** (Kirkman)	**Lozenges; oral:** 1 mg (from 2.2 mg sodium fluoride)	Sugar free. In 1000s.
Rx	**Flura-Loz** (Kirkman)		Raspberry flavor. In 100s and 1000s.
Rx *sf*	**Phos-Flur** (Novartis Consumer Health)	**Solution; oral:**[b] 0.2 mg per mL (from 0.44 mg sodium fluoride)	Sugar free. Cherry flavor. In 250, 500 mL & gal. Cinnamon (w/saccharin), grape, wintergreen flavors. In 500 mL.

[a] May be regular or chewable.

[b] May be used as a rinse or supplement.

Complete and comparative prescribing information begins in the Fluoride class monograph. For additional information, refer to the Dietary Reference Intakes of Vitamins and Minerals table.

FLUORIDE — TOPICAL

otc	ACT (Johnson & Johnson)	Liquid, rinse; dental: 0.02% (from 0.05% sodium fluoride)	7% alcohol. In 90, 360 and 480 mL.
otc	Fluorigard (Colgate-Palmolive)		6% alcohol. Tartrazine. In 180, 300 & 480 mL.
otc	Listerine Tooth Defense (Pfizer Cons Health)	Liquid, rinse; dental: 0.0221% sodium fluoride (0.01% fluoride)	21.6% alcohol, sorbitol, sucralose. Mint flavor. In 500 mL.
otc	Gel-Kam (Colgate-Palmolive)	Liquid, rinse; dental: 0.04% sodium fluoride	Mint, fruit and berry, bubblegum, and cinnamon flavors. In 4.3 and 7 oz.
otc sf	MouthKote F/R (Parnell)		Benzyl alcohol, sorbitol, menthol, EDTA. In 237 mL.
Rx	Fluorinse (Oral-B)	Liquid, rinse; dental: 0.09% (from 0.2% sodium fluoride)	Alcohol free. Mint and cinnamon flavors. In 480 mL.
Rx	Point-Two (Colgate Oral Pharmaceuticals)		6% alcohol. Mint flavor. In 240 mL and gal.
Rx	PreviDent Rinse (Colgate Oral Pharmaceuticals)	Liquid, rinse; dental: 0.2% neutral sodium fluoride	6% alcohol. Mint flavor. In 250 mL and gal (with pump dispenser).
Rx	Stannous Fluoride (Cypress)	Liquid, rinse concentrate; dental: 0.63% stannous fluoride	Mint flavor. In 122 g.
Rx	Gel-Kam (Colgate Oral)		Glycerin. Cinnamon and mint flavors. In 283 g.
Rx	PerioMed (Omnii)		Alcohol free. Tropical fruit, mint, and cinnamon flavors. In 4.3 and 7 oz.
otc	Gel-Kam (Colgate Oral)	Gel; dental: 0.1% (from 0.4% stannous fluoride)	Bubble gum, cinnamon, fruit and berry, and mint flavor. In 122 g and 105 g Dental Therapy-Pak.
otc	Gel-Tin (Young Dental)		Lime, grape, cinnamon, raspberry, mint and orange flavors. In 60 g.
otc	Stop (Oral-B)		Grape, cinnamon, bubblegum, piña colada and mint flavors. In 120 g.
otc	Stannous Fluoride (Cypress)	Gel; dental: 0.4% stannous fluoride	Parabens. Mint flavor. In 122 g.
otc	Just For Kids (3M ESPE)		Bubble gum flavor. In 121.9 g.
Rx	Karigel (Lorvic)	Gel; dental: 0.5% (from 1.1% sodium fluoride)	pH 5.6. Orange flavor. In 30, 130 and 250 g.
Rx	Karigel-N (Lorvic)		Neutral pH. In 24 and 120 g.
Rx	Prevident (Colgate Oral Pharmaceuticals)		Mint, berry, cherry and fruit sherbet flavors. In 24 and 60 g. Lime flavor in 60 g.
Rx	SF 1.1% (Cypress)		Parabens, saccharin, sorbitol. Mint flavor. In 56 g.
Rx	Thera-Flur (Colgate Oral Pharmaceuticals)	Gel; dental: 0.5% (from 1.1% sodium fluoride)	pH 4.5. Lime flavor. In 24 mL.
Rx	Thera-Flur-N (Colgate Oral Pharmaceuticals)		Neutral pH. In 24 mL.
Rx	DentaGel 1.1% (Rising Pharmaceuticals)	Gel; dental: 1.1% sodium fluoride	Saccharin, parabens, sorbitol. Fresh mint flavor. In 56 g.
Rx	NeutraGard Advanced (Pascal)		Wintermint flavor. In 60 g.
Rx	Luride (Colgate Oral)	Gel; dental: 1.2% (from sodium fluoride and hydrogen fluoride)	Mint flavor. In 7 g.
Rx	Prevident Plus (Novartis Consumer Health)		Mint, berry, cherry and fruit sherbet flavors. In 24 and 60 g. Lime flavor in 60 g.
Rx	Denta 5000 Plus (Rising Pharmaceuticals)	Cream; dental: 1.1%	Spearmint flavor. In 51 g (2s).
Rx	EtheDent (Ethex)		Sorbitol, saccharin. In 51 g.
Rx	PreviDent 5000 Plus (Novartis Consumer Health)		Sorbitol, saccharin. In spearmint and fruit flavors. In 51 g (1s and 2s).
Rx	SF 5000 Plus (Cypress Pharmaceutical)		Glycerin, saccharin, sorbitol. In 51 g.

Complete and comparative prescribing information for these products begins in the Fluoride group monograph. For additional information, refer to the Dietary Reference Intakes of Vitamins and Minerals table.

SODIUM CHLORIDE

otc	**Sustain** (Zee Medical)	**Tablets:** 220 mg sodium chloride, 18 mg calcium carbonate, 15 mg potassium chloride	In 24s.
otc	**Sodium Chloride** (Purepac)	**Tablets:** 650 mg	In 100s.
otc	**Sodium Chloride** (Various)	**Tablets:** 1 g	In 100s and 1000s.
otc	**Slo-Salt** (Mission)	**Tablets, slow release:** 600 mg	In 100s.
otc	**Slo-Salt-K** (Mission)	**Tablets, slow release:** 410 mg sodium chloride and 150 mg potassium chloride in wax matrix	In 1000s.

SODIUM CHLORIDE — ORAL

For additional information, refer to the Dietary Reference Intakes of Vitamins and Minerals table.

Indications

➤*Volume depletion:* Prevention or treatment of extracellular volume depletion, dehydration or sodium depletion.

➤*Heat prostration:* Aid in the prevention of heat prostration.

Administration and Dosage

➤*Adults:*

Heat prostration – Refer to specific product labeling for dosage guidelines.

Volume depletion – Refer to specific product labeling for dosage guidelines.

Warnings/Precautions

➤*Acclimatization:* Inappropriate salt administration in an effort to acclimatize to a hot environment can be dangerous. Balanced electrolytes and adequate hydration are essential.

➤*Salt tablets:* Salt tablets may pass through the GI tract undigested. Avoid their use in treating heat cramps since they may cause vomiting, pooling of oral fluids and potassium depletion. Use oral salt solutions instead.

➤*Supplementation:* Individuals with adequate dietary sodium intake and normal renal function should not require sodium chloride supplementation. Balanced electrolyte supplements may be preferred to prevent hypokalemia.

➤*Special risk:* Caution should be used in the presence of CHF, kidney dysfunction, peripheral or pulmonary edema or preeclampsia.

➤*Pregnancy:* *Category: Undetermined*. Seek professional advice before using these products while pregnant.

➤*Lactation:* Seek professional advice before using these products while breastfeeding.

Overdosage

➤*Symptoms:* Overdosage may cause serious electrolyte disturbances. Ingestion of large amounts of sodium chloride irritates the GI mucosa and may result in nausea, vomiting, diarrhea and abdominal cramps. Edema is a sign of excess total body sodium.

Manifestations of hypernatremia may include:

Neurologic – Irritability; restlessness; weakness; obtundation progressing to convulsions and coma.

Cardiovascular – Hypertension, tachycardia, fluid accumulation.

Respiratory – Pulmonary edema; respiratory arrest.

➤*Treatment:* Treatment includes usual supportive measures. Refer to General Management of Acute Overdosage. Use appropriate measures to empty the stomach. Magnesium sulfate may be given as a cathartic. Provide an adequate airway and ventilation. Maintain vascular volume and tissue perfusion.

POTASSIUM

Rx	**Potassium Chloride** (Various, eg, Abbott, Goldline, Warner Chilcott)	**Tablets, controlled release; oral:** 8 mEq (600 mg) potassium chloride in a wax matrix	In 100s and 1,000s.
Rx	**Klor-Con 8** (Upsher-Smith)		(KLOR–CON 8). Blue. Film coated. In 100s, 500s and UD 100s.
Rx	**Kaon Cl-10** (Savage)	**Tablets, controlled release; oral:** 10 mEq (750 mg) potassium chloride in a wax matrix	Sucrose. (10). Green. Sugar coated. Capsule shape. In 1000s and Stat-Pak 100s.
Rx	**Klor-Con 10** (Upsher-Smith)		(KLOR–CON 10).Yellow. Film coated. In 100s, 500s and UD 100s.
Rx	**Klotrix** (Bristol)		(KLOTRIX BL 10 meq 770). Orange. Film coated. In 100s, 1000s and UD 100s.
Rx	**K-Tab** (Abbott)		(NM A 101).Yellow. Film coated. Oval. In 100s, 1000s, 5000s and Abbo-Pac 100s.
Rx	**Potassium Chloride** (Watson Labs)	**Tablets, extended-release; oral:** 10 mEq potassium	(Andrx 710). Off-white, capsule shape. In 100s and 1,000s.
Rx	**Klor-Con M10** (Upsher-Smith)		From 750 mg potassium chloride. (KC M10). Oblong. In 90s, 100s, 1000s, and UD 100s.
Rx	**Klor-Con M15** (Upsher-Smith)	**Tablets, extended-release; oral:** 15 mEq potassium	From 1125 mg potassium chloride. (M 15). Oblong, scored. In 100s, 1000s, and UD 100s.
Rx	**Klor-Con M20** (Upsher-Smith)	**Tablets, extended-release; oral:** 20 mEq potassium	From 1500 mg potassium chloride. (KC M20). Oblong, scored. In 90s, 100s, 500s, 1000s, and UD 100s.
Rx	**Potassium Chloride** (Various, eg, Major)	**Tablets, extended release; oral:** 750 mg potassium chloride	Equivalent to 10 mEq potassium in a wax matrix. In 100s and 1000s.
Rx	**K-Dur 10** (Schering-Plough)	**Tablets, controlled release; oral:** 750 mg microencapsulated potassium chloride	Equivalent to 10 mEq potassium. (K-Dur 10). White. Oblong. In 100s and UD 100s.
Rx	**Potassium Chloride** (Ethex)	**Tablets, controlled release; oral:** 1,500 mg microencapsulated potassium chloride	Equivalent to 20 mEq potassium. (ETH 2 0). White to off-white, capsule shape. In 100s, 500s, 1,000s, and UD 100s.
Rx	**K-Dur 20** (Schering-Plough)		Equivalent to 20 mEq potassium. (20). White, scored. Oblong. In 100s, 500s, 1,000s and UD 100s.
otc	**Potassium** (Cardinal Health)	**Tablets; oral:** 99 mg potassium	As potassium gluconate. Film coated. In 100s.
otc	**Potassium Gluconate** (Various)	**Tablets; oral:** 500 mg potassium gluconate	83.45 mg potassium. In 100s and 1000s.
otc	**Potassium Gluconate** (Mission)	**Tablets; oral:** 595 mg potassium gluconate	99 mg potassium. In 100s.
Rx	**Effer-K** (Nomax)	**Tablets for solution, effervescent; oral:** 10 mEq potassium	As bicarbonate and citric acid. Sucralose (flavored only), dextrose, maltodextrin. (EK 10). Unflavored and cherry vanilla flavor. In 30s.
		20 mEq potassium	As bicarbonate and citric acid. Sucralose (flavored only), dextrose, maltodextrin. (EK 20). Unflavored and orange cream flavor. In 30s.
Rx *sf*	**Klorvess** (Sandoz)	**Tablets, effervescent; oral:** 20 mEq potassium	From potassium chloride and bicarbonate and lysine hydrochloride. Sodium free. Saccharin. White. In 60s and 1000s.
Rx	**K•Lyte/Cl 50** (Bristol)	**Tablets, effervescent; oral:** 50 mEq potassium	From potassium Cl and bicarbonate, l-lysine monohydrochloride, and citric acid. Saccharin, docusate sodium. Fruit punch or citrus flavors. In 30s & 100s.

POTASSIUM

Rx	**Effervescent Potassium** (Various)	**Tablets, effervescent; oral:** 25 mEq potassium	As bicarbonate and citrate. In 30s.
Rx	**Effer-K** (Nomax)		As bicarbonate and citrate. Saccharin. Orange or lime flavors. In 30s, 100s & 250s.
Rx sf	**Klor-Con/EF** (Upsher-Smith)		As bicarbonate and citrate. Saccharin. Orange flavor. In 30s and 100s.
Rx	**K•Lyte** (Bristol)		As bicarbonate and citrate. Saccharin, docusate sodium, dextrose. Orange or lime flavor. In 100s and 250s.
Rx	**Effervescent Potassium/Chloride** (Qualitest)	**Tablets, effervescent; oral:** 25 mEq potassium and chloride	From 1.5 g potassium chloride, 0.5 g potassium bicarbonate, 0.91 g l-lysine monohydrochloride, 0.55 g citric acid. Saccharin. Fruit-punch flavor. In 30s, 100s, and 250s.
Rx	**K•Lyte DS** (Bristol)	**Tablets, effervescent; oral:** 50 mEq potassium	From potassium bicarbonate and citrate and citric acid. Saccharin, docusate sodium, lactose. Orange or lime flavor. In 30s and 100s.
Rx	**Potassium Chloride** (Ethex)	**Capsules, extended-release; oral:** 8 mEq (600 mg) potassium chloride.	Microencapsulated particles. (ETHEX). Pale orange. In 100s and 500s.
Rx	**Micro-K Extencaps** (Ther-Rx)	**Capsules, controlled release; oral:** 600 mg potassium chloride	Equivalent to 8 mEq potassium. Microencapsulated particles. (Micro-K THER-RX 010). Orange. In 100s, 500s and UD 100s.
Rx	**Potassium Chloride** (Various, eg, EtheX, Goldline, Moore, Parmed, Warner-Chilcott)	**Capsules, controlled release; oral:** 10 mEq (750 mg) potassium chloride	Microencapsulated particles. In 100s and 500s.
Rx	**Micro-K 10 Extencaps** (Thera-Rx)		(Micro-K 10 AHR/ 5730). Orange/white. In 100s, 500s and UD 100s.
Rx	**Potassium Chloride** (Various, eg, Barre-National, Geneva, Major, Parmed, PBI, Schein)	**Liquid; oral:** 20 mEq/15 mL potassium and chloride (10% KCl)	In 473 and 3,785 mL.
Rx sf	**Cena-K** (Century)		In 473 and 3,785 mL.
Rx sf	**Potasalan** (Lannett)Potasalan		4% alcohol. Orange flavor. In 473 and 3,785 mL.
Rx	**Potassium Chloride** (Various, eg, Barre-National, Major, PBI)	**Liquid; oral:** 40 mEq/15 mL potassium and chloride (20% KCl)	In 473 and 3,785 mL.
Rx sf	**Kaon-Cl 20%** (Adria)		5% alcohol, saccharin. Cherry flavor. In 480 mL.
Rx	**Potassium Gluconate** (Various, eg, PBI)	**Liquid; oral:** 20 mEq/15 mL potassium	As potassium gluconate. In 118, 473, and 3,785 mL, and UD 5 and 15 mL (100s).
Rx sf	**Kaon** (Adria)		As potassium gluconate. 5% alcohol. Saccharin. Grape flavor. In 480 mL.
Rx	**Kaylixir** (Lannett)		As potassium gluconate. 5% alcohol. Saccharin. In 473 and 3,785 mL.
Rx	**Twin-K** (Boots)	**Liquid; oral:** 20 mEq/15 mL potassium	As potassium gluconate and potassium citrate. Sorbitol, saccharin. In 480 mL.
Rx sf	**Potassium Chloride** (Major)	**Solution; oral:** 20 mEq/15 mL	Sugar free. Glycerin, saccharin, sodium benzoate, sorbitol. Cherry flavor. In 473 mL.
Rx	**Potassium Chloride** (Various, eg, Schein)	**Powder; oral:** 20 mEq potassium chloride per packet	In 30s and 100s.
Rx sf	**Gen-K** (Goldline)		Orange/fruit flavor. In 30s.
Rx	**K-Lor** (Abbott)		Saccharin. Fruit flavor. In 30s and 100s.
Rx sf	**Klor-Con** (Upsher-Smith)		Saccharin. Fruit flavor. In 30s and 100s.
Rx sf	**Klor-Con/25** (Upsher-Smith)	**Powder; oral:** 25 mEq potassium chloride per packet	Saccharin. Fruit flavor. In 30s, 100s and 250s.
Rx	**K•Lyte/Cl** (Mead Johnson Nutritionals)	**Powder; oral:** 25 mEq potassium chloride per dose	Fruit punch flavor. In 225 g (30 doses).
Rx	**K-vescent Potassium Chloride** (Major)	**Powder; oral:** 20 mEq potassium and chloride	1.5 g potassium chloride. Saccharin. In 30 and 100 packets.

POTASSIUM — ORAL

For information on parenteral potassium, refer to the IV Nutritional Therapy section. For additional information, refer to the Dietary Reference Intakes of Vitamins and Minerals table.

Indications

➤*Hypokalemia:*

Treatment – Treatment of hypokalemia in the following conditions: With or without metabolic alkalosis; digitalis intoxication; familial periodic paralysis; diabetic acidosis; diarrhea and vomiting; surgical conditions accompanied by nitrogen loss, vomiting, suction drainage, diarrhea and increased urinary excretion of potassium; certain cases of uremia; hyperadrenalism; starvation and debilitation; corticosteroid or diuretic therapy.

Prevention – Prevention of potassium depletion when dietary intake is inadequate in the following conditions: Patients receiving digitalis and diuretics for congestive heart failure; significant cardiac arrhythmias; hepatic cirrhosis with ascites; states of aldosterone excess with normal renal function; potassium-losing nephropathy; certain diarrheal states.

➤*General information:* When hypokalemia is associated with alkalosis, use potassium chloride. When acidosis is present, use the bicarbonate, citrate, acetate or gluconate potassium salts.

➤*Off-label uses:* In patients with mild hypertension, the use of potassium supplements (24 to 60 mmol/day) appears to result in a long-term reduction of blood pressure.

Administration and Dosage

➤*Adults:*

Hypokalemia –

Prevention: 16 to 24 mEq/day.

Treatment: 40 to 100 mEq/day.

Potassium depletion – 40 to 100 mEq/day or more.

POTASSIUM — ORAL

➤*Children:*

Off-label dosing –

Hypokalemia: 1 to 4 mEq/kg/day divided 2 to 4 times daily.

➤*Administration:*

Liquid – Dilute in water or juice prior to administration.

Sustained release – Swallow whole; do not dissolve in the mouth or chew.

Actions

➤*Pharmacology:* Potassium, the principal intracellular cation of most body tissues, participates in a number of essential physiological processes, such as maintenance of intracellular tonicity and a proper relationship with sodium across cell membranes, cellular metabolism, transmission of nerve impulses, contraction of cardiac, skeletal and smooth muscle, acid-base balance and maintenance of normal renal function. Normal potassium serum levels range from 3.5 to 5 mEq/L. The active ion transport system maintains this gradient across the plasma membrane.

mEq/g of Various Potassium Salts

Potassium salt	mEq/g
Potassium gluconate	4.3
Potassium citrate	9.8
Potassium bicarbonate	10
Potassium acetate	10.2
Potassium chloride	13.4

Potassium homeostasis – The potassium concentration in extracellular fluid is normally 4 to 5 mEq/L; the concentration in intracellular fluid is approximately 150 to 160 mEq/L. Plasma concentration provides a useful clinical guide to disturbances in potassium balance. By producing large differences in the ratio of intracellular to extracellular potassium, relatively small absolute changes in extracellular concentration may have important effects on neuromuscular activity.

Despite wide variations in dietary intake of potassium (eg, 40 to 120 mEq/day), plasma potassium concentration is normally stabilized within the narrow range of 4 to 5 mEq/L by virtue of close renal regulation of potassium balance. Renal potassium excretion is accomplished largely by potassium secretion in the distal portion of the nephron; essentially all filtered potassium is reabsorbed in the proximal tubule. The potassium that appears in the urine is added to the filtrate by a distal process of sodium-cation exchange. Fecal excretion of potassium is normally only a few mEq per day and does not play a significant role in potassium homeostasis.

Natural potassium sources – Foods rich in potassium include: Beef; veal; ham; chicken; turkey; fish; milk; bananas; dates; prunes; raisins; avocado; watermelon; cantaloupes; apricots; molasses; beans; yams; broccoli; brussels sprouts; lentils; potatoes; spinach.

Hypokalemia – Gradual potassium depletion may occur whenever the rate of potassium loss through renal excretion or GI loss exceeds the rate of potassium intake. Potassium depletion is usually a consequence of prolonged therapy with oral diuretics, primary or secondary hyperaldosteronism, diabetic ketoacidosis, severe diarrhea (especially if associated with vomiting) or inadequate replacement during prolonged parenteral nutrition. Potassium depletion due to these causes is usually accompanied by a concomitant deficiency of chloride and is manifested by hypokalemia and metabolic alkalosis.

The use of potassium salts in patients receiving diuretics for uncomplicated essential hypertension is often unnecessary when such patients have a normal diet. However, if hypokalemia occurs, dietary supplementation with potassium-containing foods may be adequate. In more severe cases, potassium salt supplementation may be indicated.

Potassium depletion sufficient to cause 1 mEq/L drop in serum potassium requires a loss of about 100 to 200 mEq potassium from the total body store.

Symptoms: Weakness; fatigue; ileus; tetany; polydipsia; flaccid paralysis or impaired ability to concentrate urine (in advanced cases). ECG may reveal atrial and ventricular ectopy, prolongation of QT interval, ST segment depression, conduction defects, broad or flat T waves or appearance of U waves.

Contraindications

Severe renal impairment with oliguria or azotemia; untreated Addison's disease; hyperkalemia from any cause (eg, systemic acidosis, acute dehydration, extensive tissue breakdown); adynamia episodica hereditaria; acute dehydration; heat cramps; patients receiving potassium-sparing diuretics (spironolactone, triamterene or amiloride) or aldosterone-inhibiting agents. Wax matrix potassium chloride preparations have produced esophageal ulceration in cardiac patients with esophageal compression due to an enlarged left atrium; give potassium supplementation as a liquid preparation to these patients.

All solid oral dosage forms of potassium chloride are contraindicated in any patient in whom there is structural, pathological (eg, diabetic gastroparesis), or pharmacologic (use of anticholinergic agents or other agents with anticholinergic properties at sufficient doses to exert anticholinergic effects) cause for arrest or delay in tablet passage through the GI tract.

Warnings/Precautions

➤*Hyperkalemia:* In patients with impaired potassium excretion, potassium salts can produce hyperkalemia or cardiac arrest. This occurs most commonly in patients given IV potassium, but may also occur in patients given oral potassium. Potentially fatal hyperkalemia can develop rapidly and may be asymptomatic.

Hyperkalemia may be manifested only by an increased serum potassium concentration and characteristic ECG changes (eg, peaking of T waves, loss of P wave, depression of ST segment, prolongation of the QT interval, lengthened P-R interval, widened QRS complex). However, the following may also occur: Parasthesias; heaviness; muscle weakness and flaccid paralysis of the extremities; listlessness; mental confusion; decreased blood pressure; shock; cardiac arrhythmias; heart block.

In response to a rise in the concentration of body potassium, renal excretion of the ion is increased. With normal kidney function, it is difficult to produce potassium intoxication by oral administration. However, administer potassium supplements with caution, since the amount of deficiency and corresponding daily dose is unknown. Frequently monitor the clinical status, periodic ECG and serum potassium levels. This is particularly important in patients receiving digitalis and in patients with cardiac disease. There is a hazard in prescribing potassium in digitalis intoxication manifested by atrioventricular (AV) conduction disturbance.

➤*GI lesions:* Potassium chloride tablets have produced stenotic or ulcerative lesions of the small bowel and death. These lesions are caused by a concentration of potassium ion in the region of a rapidly dissolving tablet, which injures the bowel wall and produces obstruction, hemorrhage or perforation. The reported frequency of small bowel lesions is much less with wax matrix tablets (less than 1 per 100,000 patient-years) and microencapsulated tablets than with enteric coated tablets (40 to 50 per 100,000 patient-years). Upper GI bleeding, esophageal ulceration and stricture, gastric ulceration and lower GI ulceration have occurred with wax matrix preparations. The total number of GI lesions is less than 1 per 47,000 patient-years. Discontinue either type of tablet immediately and consider the possibility of bowel obstruction or perforation if severe vomiting, abdominal pain or distention or GI bleeding occurs.

Patients at greatest risk for developing potassium chloride-induced GI lesions include: The elderly, the immobile and those with scleroderma, diabetes mellitus, mitral valve replacement, cardiomegaly or esophageal stricture/compression.

Reserve slow release potassium chloride preparations for patients who cannot tolerate liquids or effervescent potassium preparations, or for patients in whom there is a problem of compliance with these preparations.

Some studies suggest the "microencapsulated" preparations are less likely to cause GI damage; however, evidence conflicts and a specific recommendation of one solid oral product over another (wax matrix or microencapsulated) cannot be made. Avoid enteric coated products.

➤*Metabolic acidosis and hyperchloremia:* In some patients (eg, those with renal tubular acidosis), potassium depletion is rarely associated with metabolic acidosis and hyperchloremia. Replace with potassium bicarbonate, citrate, acetate or gluconate.

➤*Hypokalemia:* Hypokalemia is ordinarily diagnosed by demonstrating potassium depletion in a patient and by a careful clinical history. In interpreting the serum potassium level, consider that acute alkalosis can produce hypokalemia in the absence of a deficit in total body potassium, while acute acidosis can increase the serum potassium concentration to the normal range, even in the presence of a reduced total body potassium. Treatment, particularly in the presence of cardiac disease, renal disease or acidosis, requires careful attention to acid-base balance and monitoring of serum electrolytes, ECG and clinical status of the patient.

The administration of concentrated dextrose or sodium bicarbonate may cause an intracellular potassium shift. This may cause hypokalemia which, in turn, may lead to serious cardiac arrhythmias.

Giving potassium to hypokalemic hypertensives may lower blood pressure.

➤*Renal function impairment:* Renal function impairment requires careful monitoring of the serum potassium concentration and appropriate dosage adjustment.

➤*Pregnancy: Category C.* It is not known whether potassium salts can cause fetal harm when administered to a pregnant woman or can affect reproduction capacity. Give to a pregnant woman only if clearly needed.

➤*Lactation:* It is not known whether this drug is excreted in breast milk. Exercise caution when administering to a nursing woman. The normal potassium content of breast milk is approximately 13 mEq/L. As long as body potassium is not excessive, the contribution of potassium salts should have little or no effect on the level of breast milk.

➤*Children:* Safety and efficacy for use in children have not been established.

➤*Monitoring:* When blood is drawn for analysis of plasma potassium, it is important to recognize that artificial elevations can occur after improper venipuncture technique or as a result of in vitro hemolysis of the sample.

Drug Interactions

Potassium Preparation Drug Interactions

Precipitant drug	Object drug[a]		Description
ACE inhibitors	Potassium preparations	↑	Concurrent use may result in elevated serum potassium concentrations in certain patients.
Anticholinergic agents (eg, atropine, scopolamine, hyoscyamine, clidinium)	Potassium preparations	↑	Anticholinergic agents may stop or delay passage of potassium tablets through the GI tract. Coadministration is contraindicated.

POTASSIUM — ORAL

Potassium Preparation Drug Interactions			
Precipitant drug	Object drug[a]		Description
Potassium-sparing diuretics	Potassium preparations	↑	Potassium-sparing diuretics will increase potassium retention and can produce severe hyperkalemia.
Potassium preparations	Digitalis	↑	In patients receiving digoxin, hypokalemia may result in digoxin toxicity. Therefore, use caution if discontinuing a potassium preparation in patients maintained on digoxin.

[a] ↑ = object drug increased

In addition, potassium citrate, a urinary alkalinizer, may affect the renal excretion and pharmacologic effects of various agents (refer to the Citrate and Citric Acid Solutions monograph).

Adverse Reactions

➤*Most common:* Nausea, vomiting, diarrhea, flatulence and abdominal discomfort due to GI irritation are best managed by diluting the preparation further, by taking with meals or by dose reduction.

➤*Rare:* Skin rash.

➤*Most severe:* Hyperkalemia; GI obstruction, bleeding, ulceration or perforation.

Overdosage

For symptoms and treatment of potassium overdosage and hyperkalemia, refer to the monograph in the IV Nutritional Therapy section.

Patient Information

May cause GI upset; take after meals or with food and with a full glass of water.

Do not chew or crush tablets; swallow whole.

Following release of potassium chloride, the expended wax matrix, which is not absorbable, can be found in the stool. This is no cause for concern.

Do not use salt substitutes concurrently, except on the advice of a physician.

Notify physician if tingling of the hands and feet, unusual tiredness or weakness, a feeling of heaviness in the legs, severe nausea, vomiting, abdominal pain or black stools (GI bleeding) occurs.

➤*Oral liquids, soluble powders and effervescent tablets:* Mix or dissolve completely in 3 to 8 ounces of cold water, juice or other suitable beverage and drink slowly.

ORAL ELECTROLYTE MIXTURES

		Electrolyte content									
	Product	Na+	K+	Cl−	Citrate	Ca++	Mg++	Phosphate	Other Content	Calories per fl. oz	How Supplied
otc	**Rehydralyte Solution** (Ross)	75[a]	20[a]	65[a]	30[a]				25 g/L dex-trose	3	In 240 mL ready-to-use.
otc	**Infalyte Oral Solution** (Mead Johnson)	50[a]	25[a]	45[a]	34[a]				30 g/L rice syrup solids	4.2	Fruit flavor. In ≈ 1 L ready-to-use.
otc	**Resol Solution** (Wyeth-Ayerst)	50[a]	20[a]	50[a]	34[a]	4[a]	4[a]	5[a]	20 g/L glu-cose	2.5	In 240 mL ready-to-use.
otc	**Naturalyte Solution** (UBI)	45[a]	20[a]	35[a]	48[a]				25 g/L dextrose		Unflavored, fruit or bubble gum flavors. In 240 mL and 1 L.
otc	**Pedialyte Solution** (Ross)	45[a]	20[a]	35[a]	30[a]				25 g/L dex-trose	3	Regular or fruit flavor. In 240 & 960 mL ready-to-use.
otc	**Pedialyte Freezer Pops** (Ross)	45[a]	20[a]	35[a]	30[a]				25 g/L dextrose, phenylalanine, aspartame	3	Grape, cherry, orange and blue raspberry flavors. In 2.1 fl oz ready-to-freeze pops (16s).
otc	**Temp Tab** (National Vitamin)	180[b]	15[b]	287[b]							Preservative- and sugar-free. In 100s.

[a] mEq/L

[b] Mg/tablet.

ORAL ELECTROLYTE MIXTURES — ORAL

For additional information, refer to the Dietary Reference Intakes of Vitamins and Minerals table.

Indications

➤*Fluid/Electrolyte depletion:* For maintenance of water and electrolytes following corrective parenteral therapy for severe diarrhea; for maintenance to replace mild to moderate fluid losses when food and liquid intake are discontinued; to restore fluid and minerals lost in diarrhea and vomiting in infants and children.

➤*Temp Tab:* For minimizing chronic fatigue, muscle cramps, or heat prostration because of excessive perspiration.

For use by people that are exposed to high temperatures which can cause heat fatigue.

Administration and Dosage

➤*Adults:*

Heat fatigue/prostration –

Temp Tab: 1 tablet up to 5 to 7 times/day, depending on working conditions.

➤*Children:*

Fluid/Electrolyte depletion –

Pedialyte/Rehydralyte: Offer frequently in amounts tolerated. Adjust total daily intake to meet individual needs, based on thirst and response to therapy. In the following table, suggested intakes for replacement are based on fluid losses of 5% or 10% of body weight, including maintenance requirement.

***Pedialyte/Rehydralyte* Dosage for Infants/Young Children**					
				Rehydralyte	
Age	Weight (approx.)		*Pedialyte* oz/day	Replacement for 5% dehydration (oz/day)	Replacement for 10% dehydration (oz/day)
2 wk	3.2 kg	7 lb	13 to 16	18 to 21	23 to 26
3 mo	6 kg	13 lb	28 to 32	38 to 42	48 to 52
6 mo	7.8 kg	17 lb	34 to 40	47 to 53	60 to 66
9 mo	9.2 kg	20 lb	38 to 44	53 to 59	68 to 74
1 yr	10.2 kg	23 lb	41 to 46	58 to 63	75 to 80
1.5 yr	11.4 kg	25 lb	45 to 50	64 to 69	83 to 88
2 yr	12.6 kg	28 lb	48 to 53	69 to 74	90 to 95
2.5 yr	13.6 kg	30 lb	51 to 56	74 to 79	97 to 102
3 yr	14.6 kg	32 lb	54 to 58	78 to 82	102 to 106
3.5 yr	16 kg	35 lb	56 to 60	83 to 87	110 to 114
4 yr	17 kg	38 lb	57 to 62	85 to 90	113 to 118

➤*Extemporaneous solution:*

Extemporaneous oral rehydration solution[a] (Developed by the World Health Organization)				
	Na+/Cl−	K+	Citrate	Glucose
Source	NaCl or table salt	KCl or potassium salt[b]	sodium bicarbonate (baking soda)	Glucose or sucrose (cane sugar)
Weight (g)	3.5	1.5	2.5	20[c]
Household measure	0.5 tsp	0.25 tsp	0.5 tsp	2 tbsp[d]
mmol/L	90/80	20	30	111

[a] To be added to 1 L water. Follow the health care provider's administration instructions.
[b] See potassium salt substitutes.
[c] If sucrose is used, 40 g.
[d] If sucrose is used, 4 tbsp.

➤*Administration:*

Temp Tab – Administer with 8 oz of water.

Actions

➤*Pharmacology:* Used properly, mixtures with electrolytes, water and glucose prevent dehydration or achieve rehydration, and maintain strength and feeling of well being. They contain sodium, chloride, potassium and bicarbonate to replace depleted electrolytes and restore acid-base balance. Glucose facilitates sodium transport, which aids in sodium and water absorption.

Contraindications

Severe, continuing diarrhea or other critical fluid losses; intractable vomiting; prolonged shock, renal dysfunction (anuria, oliguria). These require parenteral therapy.

Warnings/Precautions

➤*Pregnancy: Category: Undetermined*. Consult a health care provider before using in pregnant women.

➤*Lactation:* Consult a health care provider before using in breast-feeding women.

PERITONEAL DIALYSIS SOLUTIONS

	Product and Distributor	Icodextrin (g/liter)	Dextrose (g/liter)	Na+	Ca++	Mg++	Cl–	Lactate	Osmolarity (mOsm/liter)	How Supplied
Rx	**Dianeal Low Calcium w/1.5% Dextrose** (Baxter)	0	1.5	132	2.5	0.5	95	40	344	Preservative free. In 2,000, 2,500, 3,000, 5,000, and 6,000 mL *AMBU-FLEX II* containers.
Rx	**Dianeal Low Calcium w/2.5% Dextrose** (Baxter)	0	2.5	132	2.5	0.5	95	40	395	Preservative free. In 2,000, 2,500, 3,000, 5,000, and 6,000 mL *AMBU-FLEX II* and *AMBU-FLEX III* containers.
Rx	**Dianeal Low Calcium w/4.25 % Dextrose** (Baxter)	0	4.25	132	2.5	0.5	95	40	483	Preservative free. In 2,000, 2,500, 3,000, 5,000, and 6,000 mL *AMBU-FLEX II* and *AMBU-FLEX III* containers.
Rx	**UltraBag Dianeal PD-2 w/1.5% Dextrose** (Baxter)	0	1.5	132	3.5	0.5	96	40	346	Preservative free. In 1,500, 2,000, 2,500, and 3,000 mL *UltraBag* containers.
Rx	**Dianeal PD-2 w/1.5% Dextrose** (Baxter)									Preservative free. In 1,000, 2,000, 2,500, 3,000, 5,000, and 6,000 mL *AMBU-FLEX II* and *AMBU-FLEX III* containers and 250 and 500 mL *AMBU-FLEX III* containers.
Rx	**Dianeal PD-2 w/2.5% Dextrose** (Baxter)	0	2.5	132	3.5	0.5	96	40	396	Preservative free. In 1,000, 2,000, 2,500, 3,000, 5,000 and 6,000 mL *AMBU-FLEX II* and *AMBU-FLEX III* containers and 250 and 500 mL *AMBU-FLEX III* containers.
Rx	**UltraBag Dianeal PD-2 w/2.5% Dextrose** (Baxter)									Preservative free. In 1,500, 2,000, 2,500, and 3,000 mL *UltraBag* containers.
Rx	**UltraBag Dianeal PD-2 w/4.25% Dextrose** (Baxter)	0	4.25	132	3.5	0.5	96	40	485	Preservative free. In 1,500, 2,000, 2,500, and 3,000 mL *UltraBag* containers.
Rx	**Dianeal PD-2 w/4.25% Dextrose** (Baxter)									Preservative free. In 1,000, 2,000, 2,500, 3,000, 5,000 and 6,000 mL *AMBU-FLEX II* and *AMBU-FLEX III* containers and 500 mL *AMBU-FLEX III* containers.
Rx	**Dianeal PD-2 w/3.5% Dextrose** (Baxter)	0	3.5	132	3.5	0.5	96	40	447	Preservative free. In 2,500 mL *AMBU-FLEX III* containers.
Rx	**Dialyte Pattern LM w/1.5% Dextrose** (Gambro)	0	15	131	3.5	0.5	94	40	345	In 1000, 2000 and 4000 mL.
Rx	**Dialyte Pattern LM w/2.5% Dextrose** (Gambro)	0	25	131.5	3.5	0.5	94	40	395	In 1000, 2000 and 4000 mL.
Rx	**Dialyte Pattern LM w/4.25% Dextrose** (Gambro)	0	42.5	131.5	3.5	0.5	94	40	485	In 1000, 2000 and 4000 mL.
Rx	**Extraneal** (Baxter)	75	0	132	3.5	0.5	96	40	282-286	In 1.5, 2, and 2.5 L *Ultrabag* and 1.5, 2, and 2.5 L *Ambu-Flex*.

PERITONEAL DIALYSIS — INJECTION SOLUTIONS

Indications

➤*Renal failure:* For acute or chronic renal failure.

➤*Poisoning:* For acute poisoning by dialyzable toxins.

➤*Edema:* For intractable edema.

➤*Electrolyte deficiency:* For hyperkalemia and hypercalcemia.

➤*Elevated urea levels:* For azotemia and uremia.

➤*Hepatic coma:* For hepatic coma.

➤*General information:* Refer to manufacturer's package literature for specific prescribing information. Electrolyte content given in mEq/liter.

CITRATE AND CITRIC ACID SOLUTIONS

Rx	**Cytra-3** (Cypress)	**Syrup; oral**: 550 mg potassium citrate monohydrate, 500 mg sodium citrate dihydrate, 334 mg citric acid monohydrate per 5 mL (1 mEq potassium and 1 mEq sodium per mL and is equivalent to 2 mEq bicarbonate)	Sugar free. In 16 oz. bottles.
Rx	**Cytra-LC** (Cypress)	**Solution; oral**: 550 mg potassium citrate monohydrate, 500 mg sodium citrate dihydrate, 334 mg citric acid monohydrate per 5 mL (1 mEq potassium and 1 mEq sodium per mL and is equivalent to 2 mEq bicarbonate)	In 16 oz. bottles.
Rx	**Cytra-K** (Cypress)	**Solution; oral**: 1100 mg potassium citrate monohydrate and 334 mg citric acid monohydrate per 5 mL (2 mEq potassium per mL and is equivalent to 2 mEq bicarbonate)	Alcohol free. In 473 mL.
Rx	**Oracit** (Carolina Medical Products)	**Solution; oral**: 490 mg sodium citrate and 640 mg citric acid per 5 mL (1 mEq sodium per mL and is equivalent to 1 mEq bicarbonate)	Parabens. In 500 mL and UD 15 and 30 mL.
Rx sf	**Sodium Citrate/Citric Acid** (Pharmaceutical Associates)	**Solution; oral**: 500 mg sodium citrate dihydrate and 334 mg citric acid monohydrate per 5 mL (1 mEq sodium per mL and is equivalent to 1 mEq bicarbonate)	In 473 mL.
Rx	**Cytra-2** (Cypress)		Grape flavored. In 16 oz. bottles.
otc	**Naturalyte Oral Electrolyte Solution** (Unico)	**Solution; oral**: 20 mEq potassium, 30 mEq citrate (20 g dextrose, 5 g fructose, 35 mEq chloride, 45 mEq sodium)/L	In unflavored, artificial fruit, bubble gum, and grape flavors. In 1 liter.
Rx	**Taron-Crystals** (Trigen)	**Powder for solution; oral**: 3300 mg potassium citrate monohydrate and 1002 mg citric acid monohydrate per packet (30 mEq potassium and 30 mEq bicarbonate per reconstituted packet)	Sucralose. Blueberry flavor. In UD 4.32 g packets.

CITRATE AND CITRIC ACID SOLUTIONS — ORAL

Indications

➤*Chronic metabolic acidosis:* Treatment of chronic metabolic acidosis, particularly when caused by renal tubular acidosis.

➤*Urinary alkalinizer:* Conditions where long-term maintenance of an alkaline urine is desirable, in treatment of patients with uric acid and cystine calculi of the urinary tract and in conjunction with uricosurics in gout therapy to prevent uric acid nephropathy.

➤*Neutralizing buffer:* Nonparticulate neutralizing buffers.

Administration and Dosage

➤*Adults:*

Chronic metabolic acidosis – 15 to 30 mL of a liquid product diluted with a glass of water, administered after meals and before bedtime. For crystals, reconstitute 1 packet of crystals with cool water or juice and administer after meals and before bedtime. See also Off-label dosing.

Neutralizing buffer – A single dose of 15 mL diluted with 15 mL water.

Urinary alkalinizer – 15 to 30 mL of a liquid product diluted with a glass of water, administered after meals and before bedtime. For crystals, reconstitute 1 packet of crystals with cool water or juice and administer after meals and before bedtime. See also Off-label dosing.

Off-label dosing –

Alkalinizing agent/electrolyte supplement: 100 to 200 mEq of citrate daily administered in divided doses every 6 to 8 hours.

➤*Children:*

Chronic metabolic acidosis – 5 to 10 mL diluted with half a glass of water, after meals and before bedtime. See also Off-label dosing.

Neutralizing buffer – A single dose of 15 mL diluted with 15 mL water.

Urinary alkalinizer – 5 to 10 mL diluted with water, after meals and before bedtime. See also Off-label dosing.

Off-label dosing –

Alkalinizing agent/electrolyte supplement: 2 to 3 mEq of citrate per kg daily administered in divided doses every 6 to 8 hours.

➤*Monitoring:* Monitor urinary pH with Hydrion paper (pH 6 to 8) or Nitrazine paper (pH 4.5 to 7.5).

➤*Preparation for administration:* Dilute the liquid products prior to administration. For crystals, reconstitute 1 packet of crystals with 6 oz of cool water of juice and administer after meals and before bedtime.

➤*Administration:* Dilute in water before taking; follow with additional water, if desired. Palatability is enhanced if chilled before administration.

Children – The solution, not the crystals, is recommended for pediatric administration because dosage can be more easily regulated.

➤*Storage/Stability:* Keep tightly closed. Store at 20° to 25°C (68° to 77°F). Protect from excessive heat and freezing.

Actions

➤*Pharmacology:* Citrate and citric acid solutions are systemic and urinary alkalinizers. Preparations containing potassium citrate are preferred in patients requiring potassium or those who require sodium restriction. Conversely, sodium citrate may be administered when potassium is undesirable or contraindicated. Potassium citrate and sodium citrate are capable of buffering gastric acidity (pH greater than 2.5). The effects are essentially those of chlorides before absorption, and subsequently, those of bicarbonates.

➤*Pharmacokinetics:* Potassium citrate and sodium citrate are absorbed and metabolized to potassium bicarbonate and sodium bicarbonate, thus acting as systemic alkalinizers. The citric acid is metabolized to carbon dioxide and water; therefore, it has only a transient effect on systemic acid-base status. It functions as a temporary buffer component.

Oxidation is virtually complete; less than 5% of the citrates are excreted in the urine unchanged.

Contraindications

Severe renal impairment with oliguria, azotemia or anuria; untreated Addison disease; adynamia episodica hereditaria; acute dehydration; heat cramps; severe myocardial damage; hyperkalemia; sodium restricted patients.

Warnings/Precautions

➤*Urolithiasis:* Citrate mobilizes calcium from bones and increases its renal excretion; this, along with the elevated urine pH, may predispose to urolithiasis.

➤*Hyperkalemia/Alkalosis:* Patients with low urinary output and abnormal renal mechanisms may develop hyperkalemia or alkalosis, especially in the presence of hypocalcemia.

➤*Sodium salts:* Use cautiously in patients with cardiac failure, hypertension, impaired renal function, peripheral and pulmonary edema and preeclampsia. Monitor serum electrolytes, particularly the serum bicarbonate level, in patients with renal disease.

➤*GI effects:* Dilute with water to minimize GI injury associated with the oral ingestion of concentrated potassium salts. Take after meals to avoid saline laxative effect.

➤*Pregnancy: Category C.* In 4 animal species, no teratogenicity was observed with very high doses of citric acid. Citric acid is widely distributed in nature and is a key ingredient in intermediary metabolism.

➤*Lactation:* Exercise caution when administered to a breast-feeding woman.

Drug Interactions

Urinary Alkalinizer Drug Interactions

Precipitant drug	Object drug[a]		Description
Urinary alkalinizers (eg, potassium citrate, sodium citrate)	Chlorpropamide Lithium Methenamine Methotrexate Salicylates Tetracyclines	⬇	Urinary alkalinizers may increase the excretion and decrease the serum levels of these agents, possibly decreasing their pharmacologic effects.
Urinary alkalinizers (eg, potassium citrate, sodium citrate)	Anorexiants Flecainide Mecamylamine Quinidine Sympathomimetics	⬆	Urinary alkalinizers may decrease the excretion and increase the serum levels of these agents, possibly increasing their pharmacologic effects.

[a] ⬆ = object drug increased; ⬇ = object drug decreased.

Adverse Reactions

➤*Hyperkalemia:* Listlessness, weakness, mental confusion, tingling of extremities and other symptoms associated with high serum potassium. Hyperkalemia may exhibit the following ECG abnormalities: Disappearance of the P wave; widening or slurring of the QRS complex; changes of the ST segment; tall peaked T waves.

Overdosage

➤*Symptoms:* Overdosage with sodium salts may cause diarrhea, nausea, vomiting, hypernoia (excessive mental activity) and convulsions. Overdosage with potassium salts may cause hyperkalemia and alkalosis, especially in the presence of renal disease. Treat hyperkalemia immediately, because lethal levels can be reached in a few hours.

➤*Treatment:* For treatment of hyperkalemia, refer to the Potassium monograph in the IV Nutritional Therapy section; for treatment of sodium overdosage, refer to the Sodium Chloride monograph in the Salt Replacement Products section.

Patient Information

Dilute with water; follow with additional water, if desired.

Take after meals.

Notify physician if diarrhea, nausea, stomach pain, vomiting or convulsions occur.

SODIUM BICARBONATE

One g of sodium bicarbonate provides 11.9 mmol sodium and 11.9 mmol bicarbonate.

otc	**Sodium Bicarbonate** (Various)	**Tablets:** 325 mg	In 1,000s.
		650 mg	In 1,000s.
		Powder	In 120 and 300 g and 1 lb.

SODIUM BICARBONATE — ORAL

For information on parenteral sodium bicarbonate products, refer to the monograph in the IV Nutritional Therapy section. See also the Antacids group monograph.

Indications

➤*Antacid:* Sodium bicarbonate relieves acid indigestion, heartburn, sour stomach, and upset stomach associated with these symptoms.

➤*Alkalinizer:* Sodium bicarbonate may also be used for systemic or for urinary alkalinization.

➤*General information:* Sodium bicarbonate oral powder is not for injections.

Administration and Dosage

➤*General dosing considerations:* Each ½ teaspoonful of powder contains sodium 30 mg (0.7 g).

➤*Adults:*

Antacid –

Tablets:

- *Usual dose* – 1 to 4 tablets every 4 hours.
- *Maximum dose* – 24 tablets per day.

Oral powder:

- *Usual dose* – Take a level ½ teaspoonful in 120 mL of water every 2 hours up to maximum dosage.
- *Maximum dose* – 3 teaspoonfuls per day.

Systemic alkalinizer – In patients with severe metabolic acidosis, the initial dose should be 12 to 24 sodium bicarbonate 650 mg tablets (7,800 mg to 15,600 mg). Dissolve in 1 to 2 L of water and consume in 1 hour.

Urinary alkalinizer – The initial dose should be 6 sodium bicarbonate 650 mg tablets (3,900 mg), and then 2 to 4 tablets (1,300 mg to 2,600 mg) every 4 hours.

➤*Children:*

Antacid –

Oral powder:

- *6 years and older* –

  Usual dosage: Take a level ½ teaspoonful in 120 mL of water every 2 hours up to maximum dosage.

  Maximum dose: 3 teaspoonfuls per day.

➤*Elderly:*

Antacid –

Tablets:

- *Usual dose* – 1 to 2 tablets every 4 hours.
- *Maximum dose* – 12 tablets per day.

Oral powder:

- *Usual dose* – Take a level ½ teaspoonful in 120 mL of water every 2 hours up to maximum dosage.
- *Maximum dose* – 1.5 teaspoonfuls per day.

➤*Duration of therapy:* Do not use the maximum dose for more than 2 weeks.

➤*Preparation for administration:* Dissolve the powder in 120 mL of water. Tablets may be swallowed whole or dissolved in water prior to use.

➤*Storage / Stability:* Store between 15° and 30°C (59° and 86°F).

Warnings/Precautions

➤*Duration of treatment:* Do not use the maximum dose for more than 2 weeks.

➤*Sodium-restricted diet:* Do not use this product if you are on a sodium-restricted diet.

➤*Pregnancy: Category: Undetermined.* Pregnant women should ask a health professional before use.

➤*Lactation:* Nursing women should ask a health professional before use.

Overdosage

➤*Treatment:* In case of accidental ingestion, patients should seek professional assistance or should contact a poison control center immediately.

Patient Information

Ask a doctor or pharmacist before use if you are on a sodium-restricted diet or taking a prescription drug. Sodium bicarbonate may interact with certain prescription drugs.

Stop use and ask a doctor if your symptoms last more than 2 weeks.

If pregnant, ask a health professional before use.

If breast-feeding, ask a health professional before use.

AMINO ACIDS

GLUTAMIC ACID

otc	**Glutamic Acid** (Various, eg, Freeda)	**Tablets:** 500 mg	In 100s and 500s.
otc	**Glutamic Acid** (J.R. Carlson)	**Powder**	In 100 g bottles.

GLUTAMIC ACID — ORAL

Indications

➤*Dietary supplement:* For use as a dietary supplement.

Administration and Dosage

➤*Adults:*

Dietary supplement – 500 to 1,000 mg daily or as directed.

➤*Administration:* Take with liquids.

L-LYSINE

otc	**L-Lysine** (Various)	**Tablets:** 312 mg	In 100s.
otc	**Enisyl** (Person & Covey)	**Tablets:** 334 mg	In 100s.
otc	**L-Lysine** (Various, eg, Goldline, Moore, Mission, Pasadena, URL)	**Tablets:** 500 mg	In 100s.
otc	**Enisyl** (Person & Covey)		In 100s and 250s.
otc	**L-Lysine** (Approved Pharm.)	**Tablets:** 1000 mg	In 60s.
otc	**L-Lysine** (Various, eg, Miller, Tyson & Assoc.)	**Capsules:** 500 mg	In 100s and 250s.

L-LYSINE — ORAL

Indications

➤*Dietary supplement:* For use as a dietary supplement.

➤*Off-label uses:* Oral L-lysine has been promoted as treatment and as a prophylactic agent in herpes simplex infections; however, controlled studies do not support these claims.

Administration and Dosage

➤*Adults:*

Dietary supplement – 312 to 1,500 mg daily.

➤*Storage / Stability:* Store in a cool, dry place.

Actions

➤*Pharmacology:* An essential amino acid which improves utilization of vegetable proteins.

Warnings/Precautions

➤*Pregnancy: Category C* (per Briggs' *Drugs in Pregnancy and Lactation*). L-lysine is actively transported across the human placenta to the fetus.

➤*Lactation:* Supplementation of breast-feeding women with L-lysine will probably not result in significantly elevated levels of free lysine in milk.

METHIONINE

Refer to the Dermatologicals chapter for prescribing information.

THREONINE

otc	**Threonine** (Freeda)	**Tablets:** 500 mg	In 100s and 250s.

THREONINE — ORAL

Indications

➤*Dietary supplement:* For use as a dietary supplement.

Administration and Dosage

➤*Adults:*

Dietary supplement – 500 mg daily, preferably on an empty stomach.

➤*Storage/Stability:* Store away from heat and direct light.

Actions

➤*Pharmacology:* Threonine is an essential amino acid important for the formation of many proteins and tooth enamel, collagen, and elastin. It aids liver and lipotropic function when combined with aspartic acid and methionine. It metabolizes fat and prevents the build-up of fat in the liver, and is useful with intestinal disorders and indigestion.

Threonine is a precursor of glycine and serine. Threonine is an alcohol-containing amino acid that cannot be produced by metabolism and must be consumed in the diet. There are good levels of threonine in most meats, dairy foods, and eggs, and moderate levels in wheat germ, many nuts, beans, and seeds, as well as some vegetables.

Warnings/Precautions

➤*Pregnancy:* See Administration and Dosage for more information.

➤*Lactation:* See Administration and Dosage for more information.

AMINO ACIDS WITH VITAMINS AND MINERALS

otc	**Dequasine** (Miller)	**Tablets:** 20 mg L-lysine, 50 mg L-cysteine, 150 mg dL-methionine, 50 mg N-acetyl cysteine, 200 mg vitamin C, 40 mg Ca, 1 mg Cu, 5 mg Fe, 0.015 mg I, 20 mg K, 40 mg Mg, 5 mg Mn, 150 mcg Mo, 5 mg Zn. *Dose:* 1 tablet/day, or as recommended.	In 100s.
otc sf	**NeuroSlim** (NeuroGenesis)	**Capsules:** 500 mg dL-phenylalanine, 15 mg L-glutamine, 25 mg L-tyrosine, 10 mg L-carnitine, 10 mg L-arginine pyroglutamate, 10 mg ornithine aspartate, 0.033 mg Cr, 0.012 mg Se, 0.33 mg vitamin B_1, 0.5 mg B_2, 3.3 mg B_3, 0.012 mg B_5, 0.333 mg B_6, 1 mcg B_{12}, 5 IU E, 0.05 mg biotin, 0.066 mg FA, 1 mg Fe, 2.5 mg Zn, 35 mg Ca, 0.025 mg I, 0.33 mg Cu, 25 mg Mg. *Dose:* 2 capsules 3 times/day, 1 hour before or 2 hours after meals.	In 180s.
otc sf	**NeuRecovery-DA** (NeuroGenesis)	**Capsules:** 460 mg dL-phenylalanine, 25 mg L-glutamine, 333.3 IU vitamin A, 1.65 mg B_1, 0.85 mg B_2, 33 mg B_3, 15 mg B_5, 3 mg B_6, 5 mcg B_{12}, 0.065 mg FA, 100 mg C, 5 IU E, 0.05 mg biotin, 25 mg Ca, 0.01 mg Cr, 1.5 mg Fe, 25 mg Mg, 2.5 mg Zn. *Dose:* 2 capsules 3 times/day.	In 180s.
otc sf	**NeuRecovery-SA** (NeuroGenesis)	**Capsules:** 250 mg dL-phenylalanine, 150 mg L-tyrosine, 50 mg L-glutamine, 1.65 mg vitamin B_1, 2.5 mg B_2, 16.6 mg B_3, 15 mg B_5, 3.36 mg B_6, 5 mcg B_{12}, 0.067 mg FA, 100 mg C, 25 mg Ca, 1.5 mg Fe, 25 mg Mg, 5 mg Zn. *Dose:* ≤ 6 capsules/day.	In 180s.
otc	**A/G-Pro** (Miller)	**Tablets:** 542 mg protein hydrolysate, 50 mg L-lysine, 12.5 mg L-methionine, 0.33 mg vitamin B_6, 16.7 mg C, 1.66 mg iron. Cu, I, K, Mg, Mn, Zn. *Dose:* 2 tablets 3 times/day.	In 180s.
otc sf	**Jets** (Freeda)	**Tablets, chewable:** 300 mg L-lysine, 10 mg vitamin B_1, 5 mg B_6, 25 mcg B_{12}, 25 mg C.	In 100s.
otc sf	**Body Fortress Natural Amino** (Nature's Bounty)	**Tablets:** 1.67 g protein, 1500 mg lactalbumin hydrolysate *Dose:* 2 to 3 tablets with each meal and directly after each workout, or as directed.	Yeast and preservative free. In 150s.
otc sf	**Amina-21** (Miller)	**Capsules:** 556 mg free-form amino acids *Dose:* 1 or 2 capsules 3 times/day or as recommended.	In 100s and 300s.
otc	**PowerSleep** (Green Turtle Bay Vitamin Co.)	**Tablets:** 250 mg L-glutamine, 25 mg 5-HTP, 0.25 mg melatonin, 25 mg vitamin B_3, 5 mg B_6, 100 mg inositol, 25 mg Ca, 100 mg passion flower extract, 75 mg valerian powder *Dose:* 2 tablets 1 hour before bedtime.	In 60s.
otc sf	**PowerMate** (Green Turtle Bay Vitamin Co.)	**Tablets:** 25 mg N-acetyl-L-cysteine, 5 mg glutathione, 5000 IU vitamin A, 12.5 mg B_3, 250 mg C, 100 IU E, 2.5 mg Zn, 7.5 mcg Se, 5 mg ginkgo biloba, 100 mg green tea extract, 5 mg pine bark extract, 50 mg echinacea, 20 mg golden seal root, 2 mg coenzyme Q10 *Dose:* 2 tablets daily for 2 weeks/month.	Yeast free. In 50s.
otc	**EMF** (Wesley Pharmacal)	**Liquid:** Alanine, arginine, aspartic acid, cysteine, glutamic acid, glycine, histidine, hydroxylysine, hydroxyproline, isoleucineline, leucine, lysine, methionine, phenylalanine, proline, serine, threonine, tyrosine, valine, 15 g protein. *Dose:* 30 mL/day.	Sorbitol, saccharin. Cherry flavor. In qt.

Amino Acid Derivatives

LEVOCARNITINE (L-Carnitine)

Rx	**Levocarnitine** (Rising)	**Tablets:** 330 mg	(cor 160). White. In blisters of 90.
Rx	**Carnitor** (Sigma-Tau)		(CARNITOR ST). In 90s.
otc	**L-Carnitine** (Freeda Vitamins)	**Tablets:** 500 mg	In 50s and 100s.
otc	**L-Carnitine** (Various, eg, Miller Pharmacal Group, Nature's Bounty, Tyson, Watson)	**Capsules:** 250 mg	In 30s, 60s, and 100s.
Rx	**Levocarnitine** (Rising)	**Solution:** 100 mg/mL	Sucrose, parabens. Cherry flavor. In 118 mL.
Rx	**Carnitor** (Sigma-Tau)		Sucrose, parabens. Cherry flavor. In 118 mL.
Rx	**Levocarnitine** (Various, eg, American Regent, Bedford)	**Injection:** 200 mg/mL	In single-dose vials.
Rx	**Carnitor** (Sigma-Tau)		Preservative-free. In single-dose vials and amps.

LEVOCARNITINE — ORAL

Indications

➤*Primary systemic carnitine deficiency:* Treatment of primary systemic carnitine deficiency.

➤*Secondary carnitine deficiency:* For acute and chronic treatment of patients with an inborn error of metabolism which results in a secondary carnitine deficiency.

➤*Off-label uses:* Carnitine has been used to improve athletic performance and may be of use in valproate toxicity.

Administration and Dosage

➤*Adults:*

Primary systemic carnitine deficiency –

Oral solution:

• *Initial dosage* – 1 g/day (10 mL/day of levocarnitine 1 g per 10 mL oral solution).

• *Dosage titration* – Dosage should be increased slowly while assessing tolerance and therapeutic response.

• *Maintenance dosage* – 1 to 3 g/day for a 50 kg subject (10 to 30 mL/day of levocarnitine 1 g per 10 mL oral solution). Higher doses should be administered only with caution and only where clinical and biochemical considerations make it seem likely that higher doses will be of benefit.

Tablets (prescription only): 990 mg 2 or 3 times a day using the 330 mg tablets, depending on clinical response.

Secondary carnitine deficiency due to inborn error of metabolism – See Primary Systemic Carnitine Deficiency for dosing.

Dietary supplement –

Capsules (OTC): 1 capsule daily on an empty stomach.

Tablets: 1 tablet twice daily, preferable after meals.

➤*Children:*

Primary systemic carnitine deficiency –

Oral solution:

• *Maximum dose* – 3 g/day (30 mL/day of levocarnitine 1 g per 10 mL oral solution).

• *Initial dosage* – 50 mg/kg/day (0.5 mL/kg/day of levocarnitine 1 g per 10 mL oral solution).

• *Dosage titration* – Increase slowly to a maximum of 3 g/day (30 mL/day) while assessing tolerance and therapeutic response.

• *Maintenance dosage* – 50 to 100 mg/kg/day (0.5 to 1 mL/kg/day of 1 g per 10 mL solution levocarnitine oral solution). Higher doses should be administered only with caution and only where clinical and biochemical considerations make it seem likely that higher doses will be of benefit.

Tablets (prescription only):

• *Maximum dose* – 3 g/day.

• *Initial dosage* – 50 mg/kg/day.

• *Maintenance dosage* – 50 to 100 mg/kg/day in divided doses. The exact dosage will depend on clinical response.

Secondary carnitine deficiency due to inborn error of metabolism – See Primary Systemic Carnitine Deficiency for dosing.

Tablets (prescription only):

• *Maximum dose* – 3 g/day.

• *Initial dosage* – 50 mg/kg/day.

• *Maintenance dosage* – 50 to 100 mg/kg/day in divided doses. The exact dosage will depend on clinical response.

➤*Monitoring:* Monitoring should include periodic blood chemistries, vital signs, plasma carnitine concentrations and overall clinical condition.

➤*Administration:* GI reactions may result from a too-rapid consumption of carnitine. Levocarnitine oral solution may be consumed alone or dissolved in drink or other liquid food. Doses should be spaced evenly throughout the day (every 3 or 4 hours) preferably during or following meals and should be consumed slowly in order to maximize tolerance.

➤*Storage/Stability:* Store at (25°C [77°F]).

Actions

➤*Pharmacology:* Levocarnitine is a naturally occurring substance required in mammalian energy metabolism. It has been shown to facilitate long-chain, fatty-acid entry into cellular mitochondria, thereby delivering substrate for oxidation and subsequent energy production. Fatty acids are utilized as an energy substrate in all tissues except the brain. In skeletal and cardiac muscle, fatty acids are the main substrate for energy production.

Primary systemic carnitine deficiency – Primary systemic carnitine deficiency is characterized by low concentrations of levocarnitine in plasma, red blood cells, or tissues. It has not been possible to determine which symptoms are due to carnitine deficiency and which are due to an underlying organic acidemia, as symptoms of both abnormalities may be expected to improve with levocarnitine. The literature reports that carnitine can promote the excretion of excess organic or fatty acids in patients with defects in fatty acid metabolism or specific organic acidopathies that bioaccumulate acylCoA esters.

Secondary carnitine deficiency – Secondary carnitine deficiency can be a consequence of inborn errors of metabolism. Levocarnitine may alleviate the metabolic abnormalities of patients with inborn errors that result in accumulation of toxic organic acids. Conditions for which this effect has been demonstrated are the following: Glutaric aciduria II, methyl malonic aciduria, propionic acidemia, and medium chain fatty acylCoA dehydrogenase deficiency. Autointoxication occurs in these patients due to the accumulation of acylCoA compounds that disrupt intermediary metabolism. The subsequent hydrolysis of the acylCoA compound to its free acid results in acidosis which can be life-threatening. Levocarnitine clears the acylCoA compound by formation of acylcarnitine, which is quickly excreted. Carnitine deficiency is defined biochemically as abnormally low plasma concentrations of free carnitine, less than 20 mcmol/L at 1 week postterm and may be associated with low tissue or urine concentrations. Further, this condition may be associated with a plasma concentration ratio of acylcarnitine/levocarnitine greater than 0.4 or abnormally elevated concentrations of acylcarnitine in the urine. In premature infants and newborns, secondary deficiency is defined as plasma levocarnitine concentrations below age-related normal concentrations.

➤*Pharmacokinetics:*

Absorption/Distribution – The absolute bioavailability of levocarnitine from the 2 oral formulations of levocarnitine, calculated after correction for circulating endogenous plasma concentrations of levocarnitine, was 15.1 ± 5.3% for levocarnitine tablets and 15.9 ± 4.9% for levocarnitine oral solution.

In a relative bioavailability study in 15 healthy, adult, male volunteers, levocarnitine tablets were found to be bioequivalent to levocarnitine oral solution. Following 4 days of dosing with 6 tablets of levocarnitine 330 mg twice daily or 2 g of levocarnitine oral solution twice daily, the maximum plasma concentration (C_{max}) was about 80 mcmol/L, and the time to maximum plasma concentration (t_{max}) occurred at 3.3 hours.

Levocarnitine was not bound to plasma protein or albumin when tested at any concentration or with any species, including the human.

Metabolism/Excretion – In a pharmacokinetic study where 5 healthy, adult, male volunteers received an oral dose of [^{3}H-methyl]-L-carnitine following 15 days of a high-carnitine diet, and additional carnitine supplement, 58% to 65% of the administered radioactive dose was recovered in the urine and feces in 5 to 11 days. Maximum concentration of [^{3}H-methyl]-L-carnitine in serum occurred from 2 to 4.5 hours after drug administration. Major metabolites found were trimethylamine N-oxide, primarily in urine (8% to 49% of the administered dose) and [^{3}H]-γ-butyrobetaine, primarily in feces (0.44% to 45% of the administered dose). Urinary excretion of levocarnitine was about 4% to 8% of the dose. Fecal excretion of total carnitine was less than 1% of the administered dose.

After attainment of steady state following 4 days of oral administration of levocarnitine tablets (1980 mg every 12 hours) or oral solution (2000 mg every 12 hours) to 15 healthy male volunteers, the mean urinary excretion of levocarnitine during a single dosing interval (12 hours) was about 9% of the orally administered dose (uncorrected for endogenous urinary excretion).

Total body clearance of levocarnitine (Dose/AUC including endogenous baseline concentrations) was a mean of 4 L/hr.

Contraindications

None known.

Warnings/Precautions

➤*Oral solution:* Not for parenteral use. GI reactions may result from a too-rapid consumption of carnitine.

See Administration and Dosage for more information.

➤*Renal function impairment:* The safety and efficacy of oral levocarnitine has not been evaluated in patients with renal insufficiency. Chronic administration of high doses of oral levocarnitine in patients with severely compromised renal function or in ESRD patients on dialysis may result in accumulation of the potentially toxic metabolites, trimethylamine (TMA) and trimethylamine-N-oxide (TMAO), since these metabolites are normally excreted in the urine.

➤*Pregnancy: Category B.* There are no adequate and well-controlled studies in pregnant women. Because animal reproduction studies are not always predictive of human response, this drug should be used during pregnancy only if clearly needed.

➤*Lactation:* Levocarnitine supplementation in breast-feeding mothers has not been specifically studied.

Studies in dairy cows indicate that the concentration of levocarnitine in milk is increased following exogenous administration of levocarnitine. In breast-feeding mothers receiving levocarnitine, any risks to the child of excess carnitine intake need to be weighed against the benefits of levocarnitine supplementation to the mother. Consideration may be given to discontinuation of breast-feeding or of levocarnitine treatment.

➤*Children:* Levocarnitine may be used in infants and children.

➤*Monitoring:* Monitoring should include periodic blood chemistries, vital signs, plasma carnitine concentrations and overall clinical condition.

Adverse Reactions

➤*CNS:* Seizures have been reported to occur in patients with or without preexisting seizure activity receiving either oral or IV levocarnitine. In patients with preexisting seizure activity, an increase in seizure frequency or severity has been reported.

➤*GI:* Various mild GI complaints have been reported during the long-term administration of oral L- or D,L-carnitine; these include transient nausea and vomiting, abdominal cramps, and diarrhea. Mild myasthenia has been described only in uremic patients receiving D,L-carnitine. GI adverse reactions with levocarnitine oral solution dissolved in liquids might be avoided by a slow consumption of the solution or by a greater dilution. Decreasing the dosage often diminishes or eliminates drug-related patient body odor or GI symptoms when present. Tolerance should be monitored very closely dur-

LEVOCARNITINE — ORAL

ing the first week of administration, and after any dosage increases.

Overdosage

➤*Symptoms:* There have been no reports of toxicity from levocarnitine overdosage. Large doses of levocarnitine may cause diarrhea.

➤*Treatment:* Levocarnitine is easily removed from plasma by dialysis.

LEVOCARNITINE — INJECTION

Indications

➤*Secondary carnitine deficiency:* For the acute and chronic treatment of patients with an inborn error of metabolism which results in secondary carnitine deficiency.

➤*End-stage renal disease (ESRD):* For the prevention and treatment of carnitine deficiency in patients with end-stage renal disease who are undergoing dialysis.

➤*Primary systemic carnitine deficiency:* For treatment of primary systemic carnitine deficiency.

➤*Off-label uses:* Carnitine has been used to improve athletic performance and may be of use in valproate toxicity.

Administration and Dosage

➤*Adults:*

Carnitine deficiency in patients with end-stage renal disease requiring hemodialysis –

Initial dosage: 10 to 20 mg/kg dry body weight as a slow 2- to 3-minute IV bolus injection into the venous return line after each dialysis session. Initiation of therapy may be prompted by trough (predialysis) plasma levocarnitine concentrations that are below normal (40 to 50 mcmol/L).

Dosage adjustment: Dose adjustments should be guided by trough (predialysis) levocarnitine concentrations, and downward dose adjustments (eg, to 5 mg/kg after dialysis) may be made as early as the third or fourth week of therapy.

Secondary carnitine deficiency due to inborn error of metabolism – 50 mg/kg given as a slow, 2- to 3-minute IV bolus injection or by infusion. Often a loading dose is given in patients with severe metabolic crisis followed by an equivalent dose over the following 24 hours. It should be administered every 3 hours or every 4 hours, and never less than every 6 hours, either by infusion or by IV injection. All subsequent daily doses are recommended to be in the range of 50 mg/kg or as therapy may require. The highest dose administered has been 300 mg/kg.

Off-label dosing –

Valproic acid–induced hyperammonemia:

- *Loading dose* – 50 mg/kg IV.
- *Maintenance dosage* – Following the loading dose, administer 50 to 100 mg/kg/day IV divided every 8 hours. Repeat dosing is based on the patient's clinical status and blood ammonia levels.
- *Alternative dosage* – 50 mg/kg repeated every 6 hours for the first 24 hours, up to a total of 300 mg/kg/day.

➤*Children:* See Adults for dosing.

➤*Monitoring:* It is recommended that a plasma carnitine level be obtained prior to beginning this parenteral therapy. Weekly and monthly monitoring is recommended as well. This monitoring should include blood chemistries, vital signs, plasma carnitine concentrations (the plasma-free carnitine concentration should be between 35 and 60 mcmol/L) and overall clinical condition.

➤*Administration:* Administer as a slow, 2- to 3-minute bolus injection or by infusion.

➤*Admixture compatibility:* Levocarnitine injection is compatible and stable when mixed in parenteral solutions of sodium chloride 0.9% or lactated Ringer's in concentrations ranging from 250 mg/500 mL (0.5 mg/mL) to 4,200 mg/500 mL (8 mg/mL) and stored at room temperature (25°C [77°F]) for up to 24 hours in PVC plastic bags.

➤*Storage/Stability:* Store vials at 25°C (77°F). Retain vial in carton until time of use. Protect from light. Discard unused portion of an opened vial, as they contain no preservative

Actions

➤*Pharmacology:* Levocarnitine is a naturally occurring substance required in mammalian energy metabolism. It has been shown to facilitate long-chain, fatty-acid entry into cellular mitochondria, thereby delivering substrate for oxidation and subsequent energy production. Fatty acids are utilized as an energy substrate in all tissues except the brain. In skeletal and cardiac muscle, fatty acids are the main substrate for energy production.

Primary systemic carnitine deficiency – Primary systemic carnitine deficiency is characterized by low concentrations of levocarnitine in plasma, red blood cells (RBC), or tissues. It has not been possible to determine which symptoms are due to carnitine deficiency and which are due to the underlying organic acidemia, as symptoms of both abnormalities may be expected to improve with carnitine. The literature reports that levocarnitine can promote the excretion of excess organic or fatty acids in patients with defects in fatty acid metabolism or specific organic acidopathies that bioaccumulate acylCoA esters.

Secondary carnitine deficiency – Secondary carnitine deficiency can be a consequence of inborn errors of metabolism or iatrogenic factors such as hemodialysis. Levocarnitine may alleviate the metabolic abnormalities of patients with inborn errors that result in accumulation of toxic organic acids. Conditions for which this effect was demonstrated are as follows: Glutaric aciduria 2, methyl malonic aciduria, propionic acidemia, and medium chain fatty acylCoA dehydrogenase deficiency. Autointoxication occurs in these patients due to the accumulations of acylCoA compounds that disrupt intermediary metabolism. The subsequent hydrolysis of the acylCoA compound to its free acid results in acidosis that can be life-threatening. Levocarnitine clears the acylCoA compound by formation of acyl carnitine which is quickly excreted. Levocarnitine deficiency is defined biochemically as abnormally low plasma levels of free carnitine, less than 20 mcmol/L at 1 week postterm and may be associated with low tissue or urine concentrations. Further, this condition may be associated with a plasma-concentration ratio of acylcarnitine/levocarnitine greater than 0.4 or abnormally elevated concentrations of acylcarnitine in the urine. In premature infants and newborns, secondary deficiency is defined as plasma-free levocarnitine levels below age-related normal concentrations.

ESRD – ESRD patients on maintenance hemodialysis may have low plasma carnitine concentrations and an increased ratio of acylcarnitine/levocarnitine because of reduced intake of meat and dairy products, reduced renal synthesis and dialytic losses. Certain clinical conditions common in hemodialysis patients such as malaise, muscle weakness, cardiomyopathy and cardiac arrhythmias may be related to abnormal carnitine metabolism.

Pharmacokinetic and clinical studies with levocarnitine have shown that administration of levocarnitine to ESRD patients on hemodialysis results in increased plasma levocarnitine concentrations.

➤*Pharmacokinetics:*

Absorption – The plasma-concentration profiles of levocarnitine after a slow, 3-minute IV bolus dose of 20 mg/kg of levocarnitine were described by a 2-compartment model.

Distribution – Levocarnitine was not bound to plasma protein or albumin when tested at any concentration or with any species, including human.

Metabolism/Excretion – Following a single IV administration, approximately 76% of the levocarnitine dose was excreted in urine during the 0- to 24-hour interval. Using plasma concentrations uncorrected for endogenous levocarnitine, the mean distribution half-life was 0.585 hours and the mean apparent terminal elimination half-life was 17.4 hours.

Total body clearance of levocarnitine (dose/AUC including endogenous baseline concentrations) was a mean of 4 L/hr.

Special populations –

Renal function impairment: In a 9-week study, 12 ESRD patients undergoing hemodialysis for at least 6 months received levocarnitine 20 mg/kg, 3 times/wk after dialysis. Prior to initiation of levocarnitine therapy, mean plasma levocarnitine concentrations were approximately 20 mcmol/L predialysis and 6 mcmol/L postdialysis. The following table summarizes the pharmacokinetic data (mean ± SD mcmol/L) after the first dose of levocarnitine and after 8 weeks of levocarnitine therapy.

Levocarnitine Injection Therapy Pharmacokinetic Data (Mean ± SD mcmol/L)			
n = 12	Baseline	Single dose	8 weeks
C_{max}	-	1139 ± 240	1190 ± 270
Trough (predialysis, predose)	21.3 ± 7.7	68.4 ± 26.1	190 ± 55

After 1 week of levocarnitine therapy (3 doses), all patients had trough concentrations between 54 and 180 mcmol/L (normal 40 to 50 mcmol/L) and concentrations remained relatively stable or increased over the course of the study.

In a similar study in ESRD patients also receiving 20 mg/kg levocarnitine injection 3 times/week after hemodialysis, 12- and 24-week mean predialysis (trough) levocarnitine concentrations were 189 (n = 25) and 243 (n = 23) mcmol/L, respectively.

In a dose-ranging study in ESRD patients undergoing hemodialysis, patients received 10, 20, or 40 mg/kg levocarnitine 3 times/week following dialysis (n = 30 for each dose group). Mean ± SD trough levocarnitine concentrations (mcmol/L) by dose after 12 and 24 weeks of therapy in 12 patients are summarized in the following table:

Mean ± SD Trough Levocarnitine Injection Concentrations (mcmol/L) By Dose After 12 and 24 Weeks of Therapy		
	12 weeks	24 weeks
10 mg/kg	116 ± 69	148 ± 50
20 mg/kg	210 ± 58	240 ± 60
40 mg/kg	371 ± 111	456 ± 162

While the efficacy of levocarnitine to increase carnitine concentrations in patients with ESRD undergoing dialysis has been demonstrated, the effects of supplemental carnitine on the signs and symptoms of carnitine deficiency and on clinical outcomes in this population have not been determined.

Contraindications

None known.

LEVOCARNITINE — INJECTION

Warnings/Precautions

➤*Renal function impairment:* The safety and efficacy of oral levocarnitine have not been evaluated in patients with renal insufficiency. Chronic administration of high doses of oral levocarnitine in patients with severely compromised renal function or in ESRD patients on dialysis may result in accumulation of the potentially toxic metabolites, trimethylamine (TMA) and trimethylamine-N-oxide (TMAO), since these metabolites are normally excreted in the urine.

➤*Pregnancy: Category B.* There are no adequate and well-controlled studies in pregnant women. Because animal reproduction studies are not always predictive of human response, this drug should be used during pregnancy only if clearly needed.

➤*Lactation:* Levocarnitine supplementation in nursing mothers has not been specifically studied.

Studies in dairy cows indicate that the concentration of levocarnitine in milk is increased following exogenous administration of levocarnitine. In nursing mothers receiving levocarnitine, any risks to the child of excess carnitine intake need to be weighed against the benefits of levocarnitine supplementation to the mother. Consideration may be given to discontinuation of nursing or of levocarnitine treatment.

➤*Monitoring:* See Administration and Dosage for more information.

Adverse Reactions

Transient nausea and vomiting have been observed. Less frequent adverse reactions are body odor, nausea, and gastritis. An incidence for these reactions is difficult to estimate due to the confounding effects of the underlying pathology.

➤*Seizures:* Seizures have been reported to occur in patients with or without preexisting seizure activity receiving either oral or IV levocarnitine. In patients with preexisting seizure activity, an increase in seizure frequency or severity has been reported.

➤*Adverse reactions (≥ 5%):*

Levocarnitine Adverse Reactions with a Frequency ≥ 5% Regardless of Causality by Body System

Adverse reaction	Placebo (n = 63)	Levo-carnitine 10 mg (n = 34)	Levo-carnitine 20 mg (n = 62)	Levo-carnitine 40 mg (n = 34)	Levo-carnitine 10, 20 and 40 mg (n = 130)
Cardiovascular					
Arrhythmia	5	3	—	3	2
Atrial fibrillation	—	—	2	6	2
Cardiovascular disorder	6	3	5	6	5
Electro-cardiogram abnormal	—	3	—	6	2
Hemorrhage	6	9	2	3	4
Hypertension	14	18	21	21	20
Hypotension	19	15	19	3	14
Palpitations	—	3	8	—	5
Tachycardia	5	6	5	9	6
Vascular disorder	2	—	2	6	2
CNS					
Anxiety	5	—	2	—	1
Depression	3	6	5	6	5
Dizziness	11	18	10	15	13
Drug dependence	2	6	—	—	2
Hypertonia	5	3	—	—	1
Insomnia	6	3	6	—	4
Paresthesia	3	3	3	12	5
Vertigo	—	6	—	—	2
Dermatologic					
Pruritus	13	—	8	3	5
Rash	3	—	5	3	3
Endocrine					
Parathyroid disorder	2	6	2	6	4
GI					
Anorexia	3	3	5	6	5
Constipation	6	3	3	3	3
Diarrhea	19	9	10	35	16
Dyspepsia	10	9	6	—	5
GI disorder	2	3	—	6	2
Melena	3	6	—	—	2
Nausea	10	9	5	12	8
Stomach atony	5	—	—	—	—
Vomiting	16	9	16	21	15
GU					
Urinary tract infection	6	3	3	—	2
Kidney failure	5	6	6	6	6
Hematologic/lymphatic					
Anemia	3	3	5	12	6
Metabolic/nutritional					
Hypercalcemia	3	15	8	6	9
Hyperkalemia	6	6	6	6	6
Hypervolemia	17	3	3	12	5
Peripheral edema	3	6	5	3	5
Weight decrease	3	3	8	3	5
Weight increase	2	3	—	6	2
Musculoskeletal					
Leg cramps	13	—	8	—	4
Myalgia	6	—	—	—	—
Respiratory					
Bronchitis	—	—	5	3	3
Cough increase	16	—	10	18	9
Dyspnea	19	3	11	3	7
Pharyngitis	33	24	27	15	23
Respiratory disorder	5	—	—	—	—
Rhinitis	10	6	11	6	9
Sinusitis	5	—	2	3	2
Special senses					
Amblyopia	2	—	6	—	3
Eye disorder	3	6	3	—	3
Taste perversion	—	—	2	9	3
Miscellaneous					
Abdominal pain	17	21	5	6	9
Accidental injury	10	12	8	12	10
Allergic reaction	5	6	—	—	2
Asthenia	8	9	8	12	9
Back pain	10	9	8	6	8
Chest pain	14	6	15	12	12
Fever	5	6	5	12	7
Flu syndrome	40	15	27	29	25
Headache	16	12	37	3	22
Injection	17	15	10	24	15
Injection site reaction	59	38	27	38	33
Pain	49	21	32	35	30

Amino Acid Derivatives

LEVOCARNITINE — INJECTION

Overdosage

➤*Symptoms:* Large doses of levocarnitine may cause diarrhea.

There have been no reports of toxicity from levocarnitine overdosage.

➤*Treatment:* Levocarnitine is easily removed from plasma by dialysis.

LIPOTROPIC PRODUCTS

For additional information, refer to the Dietary Reference Intakes of Vitamins and Minerals table.

Actions

➤*Pharmacology:* The need for lipotropics in human nutrition is not established. The lipotropic factors choline, inositol and betaine, not proven therapeutically valuable, have been used for treatment of liver disorders and disturbed fat metabolism.

Choline (trimethylethanolamine), a component of the major phospholipid, lecithin, demonstrates lipotropic action, functions as a methyl group donor and is a precursor of the neurochemical transmitter acetylcholine. Choline and lecithin (because of its choline content) have been advocated for tardive dyskinesia, Huntington's chorea, Tourette's syndrome, Friedreich's ataxia, presenile dementia, fatty liver and cirrhosis. Intestinal bacteria metabolize choline to trimethylamine, which imparts an unpleasant odor to the breath and body. Lecithin does not produce this odor. Choline also causes clinical depression in some patients.

Inositol, an isomer of glucose, is present in cell membrane phospholipids and plasma lipoproteins. No specific role in human nutrition has been established.

Linoleic and linolenic acid are polyunsaturated fatty acids that serve as precursors of important biochemical compounds, such as arachidonic acid, which gives rise to a wide variety of prostaglandins. Linoleic acid is regarded as an essential fatty acid because it cannot be synthesized in vivo and because it has a defined metabolic significance; it helps support normal growth and development and prevent essential fatty acid deficiency (EFAD). The metabolic significance of linolenic acid is unclear. Use of these precursors to alter disease states requires more research.

CHOLINE

otc	**Choline** (Various, eg Nature's Bounty)	**Tablets; oral:** 650 mg	In 100s.
otc	**Choline** (Freeda)	**Powder:** ¼ tsp equals 375 mg choline	In 16 oz.
otc	**Choline Bitartrate** (Various, eg, Fibertone)	**Tablets; oral:** 250 mg	In 100s, 250s, 500s, 1000s.
		Powder	In 120 g and 1 lb.
Rx	**Choline Chloride** (Various)	**Powder**	In 120 and 500 g and 1 and 5 lb.
otc	**Choline Dihydrogen** Citrate (Freeda)	**Tablets; oral:** 650 mg	In 100s.
		Powder	In 120 g and 1 lb.
otc	**Choline Bitartrate** (Bio-Tech)	**Capsules; oral:** 648 mg	In 100s.
otc	**Choline-10** (Key Company)	**Tablets; oral:** 648 mg	In 100s and 250s.
otc	**Phosphatidyl Choline** (Miller)	**Capsules; oral:** 420 mg	In 100s.
		Tablets; oral: 65 mg	

CHOLINE — ORAL

Refer to additional information in the Lipotropic Products monograph. For additional information, refer to the Dietary Reference Intakes of Vitamins and Minerals table.

Indications

➤*Dietary supplement:* For use as a choline dietary supplement.

Administration and Dosage

➤*Adults:*

Dietary supplement – 1 or 2 tablets or capsules daily. Varies by product.

➤*Storage/Stability:* Store in a cool, dry place.

INOSITOL

otc	**Inositol** (Various, eg, Freeda, Nature's Bounty)	**Tablets:** 250 mg	In 100s.
		500 mg	In 100s.
		650 mg	In 90s and 100s.
		Powder: ¼ tsp equals 375 mg	In 25, 60, 100, 120, 500 g & lb.
otc *sf*	**Inositech** (Bio-tech)	**Capsules:** 324 mg	In 100s.

INOSITOL — ORAL

Refer to additional information in the Lipotropic Products monograph. For additional information, refer to the Dietary Reference Intakes of Vitamins and Minerals table.

LIPOTROPIC COMBINATIONS

otc	**Lecithin** (Various, eg, Nature's Bounty, West-Ward)	A source of choline, inositol, phosphorus, linoleic & linolenic acids	
		Capsules: 420 mg	In 60s.
		1.2 g	In 100s, 250s, 1000s.
		Tablets: 1.2 g	In 50s.
		Granules	In 210, 240, 420 g & lb.
		Liquid	In 480 mL.
otc	**PhosChol** (American Lecithin)	Phosphatidylcholine (highly purified lecithin)	
		Softgels: 565 mg	In 100s and 300s
		Softgels: 900 mg	In 100s and 300s.
		Liquid concentrate: 3000 mg/5 mL	In 240 and 480 mL.

LIPOTROPIC COMBINATIONS — ORAL

Refer to additional information in the Lipotropic Products monograph. For additional information, refer to the Dietary Reference Intakes of Vitamins and Minerals table.

Administration and Dosage

➤*Adults:*

Dietary supplement –

Lecithin: One to 2 capsules 1 to 3 times daily.

PhosChol: Two or 3 capsules per day.

➤*Storage/Stability:* Store at room temperature.

MULTIVITAMINS AND MINERALS WITH OMEGA-3 POLYUNSATURATED FATTY ACIDS

Content given per tablet or capsule.

	Product & Distributor	Omega -3 mg	N-3 Fat Content EPA mg	DHA mg	Ca[a] mg	Fe[b] mg	A units	D units	E units	B_1 mg	B_2 mg	B_3 mg	B_5 mg	B_6 mg	B_{12} mcg	C mg	Folate mg	Minerals	Other Content	Excipients & How Supplied
otc	**SuperEPA 2000 Softgels** (Advanced Nutritional Technology)	1,000	500	310					20[c]										Fish oil 1,250 mg, other omega-3 fatty acids 190 mg	In 90s.
Rx	**Lovaza Capsules** (GlaxoSmithKline)	900	465	375					4 mg[d]											Soybean oil. (Lovaza). Light yellow. In 60s and 120s.
otc	**Eskimo Kids Liquid** (Integrative Therapeutics)	800	270	180				100[e]	[f]											Gluten free. Canola,[g] fish, and soybean oils. Tutti-frutti flavor. In 105 mL bottles.
otc	**Sea-Omega 70 Capsules** (Rugby)	700	400	200					15[h]										Fish oil concentrate 1,100 mg, other omega-3 fatty acids 100 mg	Lemon oil. In 60s.
otc *sf*	**Coromega Packets** (Coromega)	650	350	230					3[i]							12				Gluten free. Fish oil, stevia leaf extract, vegetable oil. Orange flavor. In 90s.
otc *sf*	**Sea-Omega 50 Capsules** (Rugby)	500	300	200					1[i]										Fish oil 1,000 mg	Gluten free and preservative free. In 50s.
Rx	**Animi-3 Capsules** (PBM Pharmaceuticals)	500	35	350										12.5	500		1[j]		Phytosterols 200 mg	(Animi-3). Red, oblong. In 60s.
Rx	**Mi-Omega Capsules** (Nexgen Pharma)																			Fish oil, sunflower oil. (ML 500). Red, oblong. In 60s.
otc *sf*	**Sea-Omega 30 Capsules** (Rugby)	360	216	144					2[i]										Fish oil 1,200 mg	Gluten free and preservative free. In 100s.
otc	**Omega-3 Fish Oil Softgels** (Nature's Bounty)	340	180	120					1[i]										Fish oil 1,000 mg, other fatty acids 40 mg	In 50s.
otc	**Coromega Child Brain & Body Squeezer Packets** (Coromega)	284	36	200												11.6				Fish oil, safflower oil, stevia leaf extract, vegetable oil. Lemon-lime flavor. In 60s.
otc	**Protegra Cardio Softgels** (Inverness Medical)	250	45	30			5,000[k]		60[l]					6	12	250	0.8[j]	Cu, Mg, Mn, Se, Zn		Fish oil, soybean oil, hydrogenated soybean oil. In 60s.
otc	**Ocuvite Adult 50 + Softgel Capsules** (Bausch & Lomb)	150							30[c]							150		Cu, Zn	Lutein 6 mg	In 50s.
otc	**Ocuvite Adult Softgel Capsules** (Bausch & Lomb)	100							15[c]							100		Cu, Zn	Lutein 2 mg	In 50s.
otc	**Omega-3 Norwegian Cod Liver Oil Softgels** (Nature's Bounty)		110	100			2,664[m]	200[n]											Cod liver oil 1,000 mg	In 60s.
otc	**Omega-3 Norwegian Cod Liver Oil Softgels** (Nature's Bounty)		34	32			1,250[o]	135[o]											Cod liver oil 415 mg	In 100s.
otc	**Bayer Nutritional Science Vital & Sharp Mind Softgels** (Bayer HealthCare)			170						1.5	1.7	10	10	2	6		0.2[j]		Ginkgo biloba extract 180 mg	Fish oil. In 90s.

MULTIVITAMINS AND MINERALS WITH OMEGA-3 POLYUNSATURATED FATTY ACIDS

	Product & Distributor	Omega -3 mg	N-3 Fat Content EPA mg	DHA mg	Ca[a] mg	Fe[b] mg	A units	D units	E units	B_1 mg	B_2 mg	B_3 mg	B_5 mg	B_6 mg	B_{12} mcg	C mg	Folate mg	Minerals	Other Content	Excipients & How Supplied
otc sf	**Disney Princess Complete Children's MultiVitamin Chewable Tablets** (NatureSmart)			0.1	100	18[p]	5,000[q]	400[e]	30[r]	1.5	1.7	20	10	2	6	60	0.4[j]	Cu, I, Mg, Zn	Biotin 40 mcg	Dextrose, sucralose, xylitol. Grape, orange, and cherry flavors. In 60s.

[a] Calcium content expressed in mg elemental calcium.
[b] Iron content expressed in mg elemental iron.
[c] Form of vitamin E unknown; content given in units.
[d] Vitamin E content expressed in mg alpha-tocopherol.
[e] As cholecalciferol.
[f] Mixed tocopherols; amount not specified.
[g] Containing oleic acid, linoleic acid, and alpha-linolenic acid.
[h] As d-alpha-tocopherol and other mixed tocopherols.
[i] As d-alpha-tocopheryl.
[j] As folic acid.
[k] As beta-carotene.
[l] As d-alpha-tocopheryl acetate.
[m] As cod liver oil and retinyl palmitate.
[n] As cod liver oil and cholecalciferol.
[o] From cod liver oil.
[p] As ferrous sulfate.
[q] 70% (3,500 units) as beta-carotene and retinyl acetate.
[r] As dl-alpha-tocopheryl acetate.

For additional information, refer to the Dietary Reference Intakes of Vitamins and Minerals table.

OMEGA-3 (N-3) POLYUNSATURATED FATTY ACIDS — ORAL

Indications

➤*Dietary supplement:* As dietary supplements for patients at early risk of coronary artery disease primarily because of effects on platelets and lipids.

The American Heart Association recommends consumption of fish; however, it does not find justification for fish oil capsule supplementation.

Hypertriglyceridemia (Lovaza only*)* – As adjunct to diet to reduce triglyceride levels in adults with severe (500 mg/dL or more) hypertriglyceridemia.

Considerations: Place patients on appropriate lipid-lowering diet before instituting *Lovaza* and instruct patients to continue this diet during treatment.

Conduct laboratory studies to ascertain that the lipid levels are consistently abnormal before instituting *Lovaza* therapy. Make every attempt to control serum lipids with appropriate diet, exercise, weight loss in obese patients, and control of any medical problems such as diabetes mellitus and hypothyroidism that are contributing to the lipid abnormalities. If possible, discontinue medications known to exacerbate hypertriglyceridemia (eg, beta-blockers, thiazides, estrogens) if possible prior to consideration of triglyceride-lowering drug therapy.

Limitations: The effect of *Lovaza* on cardiovascular mortality and morbidity in patients with elevated triglycerides has not been determined.

➤*Off-label uses:* Omega-3 fatty acids have been studied as adjunctive treatment of rheumatoid arthritis (20 g/day has been used). These agents may also be of benefit in the treatment of psoriasis (10 to 15 g/day); however, data are conflicting. Omega-3 fatty acids (18 g/day) may be beneficial in preventing early restenosis after coronary angioplasty in combination with dipyridamole and aspirin in high-risk men.

Administration and Dosage

➤*General dosing considerations:* Assess triglyceride levels carefully before initiating therapy. Identify other causes (eg, diabetes mellitus, hypothyroidism, medications) of high triglyceride levels and manage as appropriate.

➤*Adults:*

Dietary supplement – 1 to 2 capsules 3 times daily with meals.

Hypertriglyceridemia (Lovaza only): 4 g/day as a single 4 g dose or as two 2 g doses. In clinical studies, *Lovaza* was administered with meals.

Patients should be placed on an appropriate lipid-lowering diet before receiving *Lovaza* and should continue this diet during treatment.

➤*Children:* Until further information is available, do not use omega-3 fatty acids in these patients.

➤*Administration:* Patients should be advised to swallow *Lovaza* capsules whole. Patients should not break open, crush, dissolve, or chew *Lovaza*.

➤*Storage/Stability:* Store *Lovaza* at 25°C (77°F); excursions are permitted between 15° and 30°C (59° and 86°F). Do not freeze.

Actions

➤*Pharmacology:* Cold water fish oils contain large amounts of omega-3 (N-3) polyunsaturated fatty acids, eicosapentaenoic acid (EPA) and docosahexaenoic acid (DHA). Diets high in omega-3 fatty acids may lower very low-density lipoproteins (VLDL), triglyceride and total cholesterol concentrations; increase concentrations of high-density lipoproteins (HDL); prolong bleeding times; decrease platelet aggregation; reduce plasma fibrinogen (data conflict); inhibit leukocyte function.

Studies on the effects of omega-3 fatty acids on the lipoproteins closely associated with atherosclerosis (LDL and HDL) show variable results and require further investigation.

Some studies have actually shown an increase in LDL-cholesterol levels in patients and healthy subjects receiving omega-3 fatty acids at doses currently recommended by the manufacturers (4.6 to 13.3 g/day). Although the optimal dose has not been established, significant effects of the omega-3 fatty acids may only be observed with 20 g or more per day. Some of the available products contain cholesterol and saturated fat, which may play a role in the increased LDL-cholesterol levels.

Patients on diets with high levels of fish oils have increased EPA levels and decreased arachidonic acid levels in plasma lipids and platelet membranes. Also, increased synthesis of prostaglandin I_3 and decreased platelet synthesis of thromboxane A_2 have been noted. Prostaglandin I_3, an antiaggregation substance, and thromboxane A_2, a potent stimulator of platelet aggregation and secretion, are usually in balance. It is believed EPA is utilized by vessel walls to synthesize prostaglandin I_3, and arachidonic acid is utilized by platelets to synthesize thromboxane A_2. Therefore, the higher EPA levels and lower arachidonic acid levels produced by a diet high in fish oils could cause decreased platelet aggregation. Vitamin E in the product could also contribute to decreased platelet aggregation.

Warnings/Precautions

➤*Diarrhea:* Diarrhea has occurred in patients taking 4 to 6 capsules per day.

➤*Bleeding:* Increased bleeding time and inhibition of platelet aggregation have occurred. Use caution in patients receiving **anticoagulants** or **aspirin**.

➤*Diabetes mellitus:* In one study the fasting and mean glucose levels increased and insulin secretion was impaired in six patients with type 2 diabetes mellitus following 1 month of omega-3 fatty acid administration (5.4 g/day). However, increased insulin sensitivity in type 2 diabetes mellitus patients has occurred. Use with caution in type 2 diabetes mellitus patients.

➤*Pregnancy: Category C.* There are no adequate and well-controlled studies in pregnant women. It is unknown whether omega-3 fatty acids can cause fetal harm when administered to a pregnant woman or can affect reproductive capacity. Omega-3 fatty acids should be used during pregnancy only if the potential benefit justifies the potential risk to the fetus.

Omega-3 acid ethyl esters have been shown to have an embryocidal effect in pregnant rats when given in doses resulting in exposures 7 times the recommended human dose of 4 g/day based on a body surface area comparison.

➤*Lactation:* It is not known whether omega-3 acid ethyl esters are excreted in human milk. Because many drugs are excreted in human milk, exercise caution when omega-3 fatty acids are administered to a woman who is breast-feeding.

ENZYMES

LACTASE ENZYME

otc	**Lactase Fast Acting** (Major)	**Tablets; oral:** 9,000 FCC lactase units	Fructose, dextrose, sugar. Capsule shape. In 32s.
otc	**Lactrase** (Schwarz Pharma)	**Capsules; oral:** 250 mg standardized enzyme lactase	(Kremers Urban 505). Orange/white. In 100s and blisterpack 10s and 30s.
otc	**DairyCare** (Plainview LLC)	**Capsules, delayed release; oral:** 190 mg *Lactobacillus acidophillus*, 15 mg lactase	In 60s.
otc	**Dairy Ease** (Blistex)	**Tablets, chewable; oral:** 3,000 FCC lactase units	Mannitol, sucrose. In 60s and 100s.
otc	**Lac-Dose** (Rugby		Dextrose, mannitol, sodium 12 mg. Capsule shape. In 50s.
otc	**Lactaid Fast Act** (McNeil Nutritionals)	**Tablets, chewable; oral:** 9,000 FCC lactase units	Mannitol, sucralose. In 32s.

LACTASE ENZYME — ORAL

Indications

➤*Lactose intolerance:* For persons who are lactose intolerant and experience gas, cramps, bloating or diarrhea from eating dairy foods, such as milk, ice cream, or cheese. Lactase enzyme dietary supplements aid in dairy food digestion in lactose-intolerant persons without gas, cramping, bloating, or diarrhea.

Lactase helps to prevent symptoms by breaking down milk sugar (lactose) and making dairy foods easier to digest.

Lactase is not a drug but a dietary supplement containing the natural lactase enzyme.

Lactase works naturally and may be used by patients 4 years of age and older.

Administration and Dosage

➤*General dosing considerations:* If the patient continues to eat dairy foods after 30 to 45 minutes, taking an additional tablet is recommended.

➤*Adults:*

Lactose intolerance –

9,000 units: Swallow or chew 1 or 2 tablets with the first bite of dairy foods. May be used with every meal or snack.

4,500 units: Swallow or chew 2 tablets with the first bite of dairy foods. May be used with every meal or snack.

3,000 units: Swallow or chew 3 tablets with the first bite of dairy foods. May be used with every meal or snack.

➤*Children:*

Lactose intolerance – See Adults for dosing in children 4 years and older.

➤*Storage/Stability:* Store below 25°C (77°F); do not refrigerate. Keep away from heat.

SACROSIDASE

Rx	**Sucraid** (Orphan Medical)	**Solution:** 8500 IU/mL	In 118 mL bottles (2) with 1 mL measuring scoop.

SACROSIDASE — ORAL

Indications

➤*Sucrase deficiency:* As oral replacement therapy of the genetically determined sucrase deficiency, which is part of congenital sucrase-isomaltase deficiency (CSID).

Administration and Dosage

➤*Adults:*

Sucrase deficiency – 2 mL (17,000 units) taken with each meal or snack. Dilute dose with 2 to 4 ounces of water or milk. (See Administration).

➤*Children:* Sarcosidase has been used in patients as young as 5 months of age.

Sucrase deficiency –

Patients weighing more than 15 kg: 2 mL (17,000 units) taken with each meal or snack. Dilute dose with 2 to 4 ounces of water, milk, or infant formula. (See Administration).

Patients weighing 15 kg or less: 1 mL (8,500 units) taken with each meal or snack. Dilute dose with 2 to 4 ounces of water, milk, or infant formula. (See Administration).

➤*Preparation for administration:* Dosage may be measured with the 1 mL measuring scoop (provided with product) or by drop count method (1 mL equals 22 drops from the sacrosidase container tip).

Dilute dose with 2 to 4 ounces of water, milk, or infant formula.

➤*Administration:* It is recommended that approximately half of the dosage be taken at the beginning of each meal or snack, and the remainder be taken at the end of each meal or snack.

The beverage or infant formula should be served cold or at room temperature. The beverage or infant formula should not be warmed or heated before or after addition of sacrosidase because heating is likely to decrease potency. Sacrosidase should not be reconstituted or consumed with fruit juice because its acidity may reduce the enzyme activity.

➤*Storage/Stability:* Store in a refrigerator at 2° to 8°C (36° to 46°F). Discard 4 weeks after first opening due to the potential for bacterial growth. Protect from heat and light.

Actions

➤*Pharmacology:* Congenital sucrase-isomaltase deficiency (CSID) is a chronic, autosomal recessive, inherited, phenotypically heterogenous disease with very variable enzyme activity. CSID is usually characterized by a complete or almost complete lack of endogenous sucrase activity, a very marked reduction in isomaltase activity, a moderate decrease in maltase activity and normal lactase levels.

Sucrase is naturally produced in the brush border of the small intestine, primarily the distal duodenum and jejunum. Sucrase hydrolyzes the disaccharide sucrose into its component monosaccharides, glucose and fructose. Isomaltase breaks down disaccharides from starch into simple sugars. Sacrosidase does not contain isomaltase.

In the absence of endogenous human sucrase, as in CSID, sucrose is not metabolized. Unhydrolyzed sucrose and starch are not absorbed from the intestine and their presence in the intestinal lumen may lead to osmotic retention of water. This may result in loose stools. Unabsorbed sucrose in the colon is fermented by bacterial flora to produce increased amounts of hydrogen, methane and water. As a consequence, excessive gas, bloating, abdominal cramps, nausea and vomiting may occur.

Chronic malabsorption of disaccharides may result in malnutrition. Undiagnosed/untreated CSID patients often fail to thrive and fall behind in their expected growth and development curves. Previously, the treatment of CSID has required the continual use of a strict sucrose-free diet.

CSID is often difficult to diagnose. Approximately 4 to 10% of pediatric patients with chronic diarrhea of unknown origin have CSID. Measurement of expired breath hydrogen under controlled conditions following a sucrose challenge (a measurement of excess hydrogen excreted in exhalation) in CSID patients has shown levels as great as 6 times that in healthy subjects.

A generally accepted clinical definition of CSID is that of a condition characterized by the following: Stool pH of less than 6, an increase in breath hydrogen of greater than 10 ppm when challenged with sucrose after fasting and a negative lactose breath test. However, because of the difficulties in diagnosing CSID, it may be warranted to conduct a short therapeutic trial (eg, one week) to assess response in patients suspected of having CSID.

Contraindications

Hypersensitivity to yeast, yeast products, or glycerin (glycerol).

Warnings/Precautions

➤*Severe wheezing:* Severe wheezing, 90 minutes after a second dose of sacrosidase, necessitated admission into the ICU for a 4-year old boy. The wheezing was probably caused by sacrosidase. He had asthma and was being treated with steroids. A skin test for sacrosidase was positive.

➤*Starch restriction:* Although sacrosidase provides replacement therapy for the deficient sucrase, it does not provide specific replacement therapy for the deficient isomaltase. Therefore, restricting starch in the diet may still be necessary to reduce symptoms as much as possible. The need for dietary starch restriction for patients using sacrosidase should be evaluated in each patient.

➤*CSID diagnosis:* The definitive test for diagnosis of CSID is the measurement of intestinal disaccharidases following small bowel biopsy.

Other tests used alone may be inaccurate: For example, the breath hydrogen test (high incidence of false-negatives) or oral sucrose tolerance test (high incidence of false positives). Differential urinary disaccharide testing has been reported to show good agreement with small intestinal biopsy for diagnosis of CSID.

It may sometimes be clinically inappropriate, difficult, or inconvenient to perform a small bowel biopsy or breath hydrogen test to make a definitive diagnosis of CSID. If the diagnosis of CSID is in doubt, it may be warranted to conduct a short therapeutic trial (eg, one week) with sacrosidase to assess response in a patient suspected of sucrase deficiency.

The effects of sacrosidase have not been evaluated in patients with secondary (acquired) disaccharidase deficiencies.

➤*Diabetics:* The use of sacrosidase will enable the products of sucrose hydrolysis (eg, glucose and fructose) to be absorbed. This fact must be carefully considered in planning the diet of diabetic CSID patients using sacrosidase.

➤*Hypersensitivity reactions:* Care should be taken to administer initial doses of sacrosidase near (within a few minutes' travel) a facility where acute hypersensitivity reactions can be adequately treated. Alternatively, the patient may be tested for hypersensitivity to sacrosidase through skin abrasion testing. Should symptoms of hypersensitivity appear, discontinue medication and initiate symptomatic and supportive therapy.

Skin testing as a rechallenge has been used to verify hypersensitivity in one asthmatic child who displayed wheezing after oral sacrosidase.

➤*Pregnancy: Category C.* Animal reproduction studies have not been conducted with sacrosidase. Sacrosidase is not expected to cause fetal harm when administered to a pregnant woman or to affect reproductive capacity. Sacrosidase should be given to a pregnant woman only if clearly needed.

➤*Lactation:* The sacrosidase enzyme is broken down in the stomach and intestines and the component amino acids and peptides are then absorbed as nutrients.

➤*Children:* Sacrosidase has been used in patients as young as 5 months of age. Evidence from one controlled trial in primarily pediatric patients shows that sacrosidase is safe and effective for the treatment of the genetically acquired sucrase deficiency, which is part of CSID.

Drug Interactions

➤*Drug/Food interactions:* Sacrosidase should not be reconstituted or consumed with fruit juice, since its acidity may reduce the enzyme activity.

Adverse Reactions

In clinical studies of up to 54 months duration, physicians treated a total of 52 patients with sacrosidase. The adverse experiences and respective number of patients reporting each event (in parenthesis) were as follows: abdominal pain (4), vomiting (3), nausea (2), diarrhea (2), constipation (2), insomnia (1), headache (1), nervousness (1), and dehydration (1).

Diarrhea and abdominal pain can be a part of the clinical presentation of the genetically determined sucrase deficiency, which is part of congenital sucrase-isomaltase deficiency (CSID).

➤*Hypersensitivity:* One asthmatic child experienced a serious hypersensitivity reaction (wheezing) probably related to sacrosidase (see Warnings). The event resulted in withdrawal of the patient from the trial but resolved with no sequelae.

➤*Most frequent adverse reactions:* The most frequent adverse reactions reported while taking sacrosidase were abdominal pain (8%) and vomiting (6%). One patient experienced a serious reaction; hypersensitivity (wheezing). This event resolved with no sequelae.

Overdosage

Overdosage with sacrosidase has not been reported.

Patient Information

Patients should be instructed to discard bottles of sacrosidase 4 weeks after first opening due to the potential for bacterial growth.

Sacrosidase is fully soluble with water, milk, and infant formula, but it is important to note that this product is sensitive to heat. Sacrosidase should not be reconstituted or consumed with fruit juice, since its acidity may reduce the enzyme activity.

PROBIOTIC PRODUCTS

otc	**Lactobacillin Acidophilus** (Nature's Blend)	**Capsules; oral:** 25 million units *Lactobacillus acidophilus*	Lactose. In 100s.
otc	**Intestinex** (A.G. Marin)	**Capsules; oral:** 100 million units *Lactobacillus acidophilus*	In 24s.
otc	**Acidophilus** (Nature's Bounty)	**Capsules; oral:** greater than 100 million units *Lactobacillus acidophilus*	Soybean oil, beeswax/ soybean oil mixture. In 100s.
otc	**Bacid** (Insight Pharmaceuticals)	**Capsules; oral:** Cultured strain ≥ 500 million viable *Lactobacillus acidophilus*	Mineral oil. In 50s and 100s.
otc	**Lacto-Key-100** (Key Company)	**Capsules; oral:** ≥ 1 billion CFU *Lactobacillus acidophilus*	In 60s, 120s, and 500s.
otc	**Probiotic Formula** (Rugby)	**Capsules; oral:** 2 billion CFU *Lactobacillus acidophilus*, 2 billion CFU *Lactobacillus salivarius*, 2 billion CFU *Lactobacillus plantarum*, 2 billion CFU *Lactobacillus casei*, 2 billion CFU *Bifidobacterium lactis*	In 30s.
otc	**SynBiotics-3** (NutraCea)	**Capsules; oral:** 4.5 billion CFU *Bifidobacterium longum, Lactobacillus rhamnosus* A, *Lactobacillus plantarum, Saccharomyces boulardii*	Maltodextrin. In 60s and UD 200s.
otc	**Florastor** (Biocodex)	**Capsules; oral:** 250 mg *Saccharomyces boulardii lyo*	Lactose. In 10s and 50s.
Rx	**VSL#3 The Living Shield** (Sigma-Tau)	**Capsules; oral:** Lyophilized lactic acid ≥ 225 billion units. *Streptococcus thermophilus, Bifidobacterium breve, Bifidobacterium longum, Bifidobacterium infantis, Lactobacillus acidophilus, Lactobacillus plantarum, Lactobacillus paracasei, Lactobacillus delbrueckii*	Gluten free. In 60s.
otc	**Culturelle** (Amerifit)	**Capsules; oral:** Lactobacillus GG 10 billion live cells	In 10s.
otc	**Ganeden Sustenex** (Ganeden)	**Capsules; oral:** Ganeden BC30 2 billion cells	Lactose free. In 30s.
otc	**Align Daily Probiotic Supplement** (Proctor & Gamble)	**Capsules; oral:** *Bifidobacterium infantis* 35624 4 mg	Lactose free. Sugar. In 28s.
otc	**Florastor Kids** (Biocodex)	**Powder; oral:** 250 mg *Saccharomyces boulardii lyo*	Lactose. Tutti-fruitti flavor. In 10s.
otc	**Lacto-Key-600** (Key Company)	**Capsules; oral:** ≥ 6 billion CFU *Lactobacillus acidophilus*	In 60s and 120s.
otc sf	**Kala** (Freeda)	**Tablets; oral:** 200 million units soy-based *Lactobacillus acidophilus*	In 100s, 250s, and 500s.
otc	**Floranex** (Rising)	**Tablets, chewable; oral:** 1 million CFU *Lactobacillus acidophilus* and *Lactobacillus bulgaricus*	Sucrose, lactose. In 50s.
otc	**Lactinex** (Becton Dickinson)	**Tablets, chewable; oral:** Mixed culture of *Lactobacillus acidophilus* and *Lactobacillus bulgaricus*	Lactose, sucrose, and mineral oil. In 50s.
otc	**ReZyst IM** (Zyber)	**Tablets, chewable; oral:** *Lactobacillus* and *Bifidobacterium* 150 mg	Sorbitol, sucralose, xytlitol. Berry flavor. In 60s.
otc	**Lactinex** (Becton Dickinson)	**Granules; oral:** Mixed culture of *Lactobacillus acidophilus* and *Lactobacillus bulgaricus*	In 1 g packets (12s).
otc	**Acidophilus** (Mason)	**Wafers; oral:** 20 million units *Lactobacillus acidophilus*	Preservative free. 1 g sugar. Vanilla-banana flavor. In 100s.
otc	**Acidophilus with Bifidus** (Various, eg, Mason, Nature's Bounty)	**Wafers; oral:** 1 billion units *Lactobacillus acidophilus* and *Lactobacillus bifidus*	1 g sugar. Strawberry flavor. In 100s.
otc	**Culturelle for Kids** (Amerifit)	**Powder; oral:** Lactobacillus GG 1 billion live cells	Lactose free, gluten free, preservative free. Mannitol, inulin. In 30s.
otc sf	**MoreDophilus** (Freeda)	**Powder; oral:** 4 billion units of acidophilus-carrot derivative per g	In 120 g.
otc	**Superdophilus** (Natren)	**Powder; oral:** 2 billion *Lactobacillus acidophilus* strain DDS-1 per g	In 37.5, 75, and 135 g.
otc	**VSL#3 DS Double Strength** (Sigma-Tau)	**Powder; oral:** Lyophilized lactic acid ≥ 900 billion units. *Streptococcus thermophilus, Bifidobacterium breve, Bifidobacterium longum, Bifidobacterium infantis, Lactobacillus acidophilus, Lactobacillus plantarum, Lactobacillus paracasei, Lactobacillus delbrueckii*	Gluten free. Maltose. In 20s.
otc	**VSL#3 The Living Shield** (Sigma-Tau)	**Powder; oral:** Lyophilized lactic acid ≥ 450 billion units. *Streptococcus thermophilus, Bifidobacterium breve, Bifidobacterium longum, Bifidobacterium infantis, Lactobacillus acidophilus, Lactobacillus plantarum, Lactobacillus paracasei, Lactobacillus delbrueckii*	Gluten free. Maltose. Lemon flavor. In 10s and 30s.
otc sf	**BioGaia** (Nutraceutics)	**Solution, concentrate; oral:** 100 million *Lactobacillus reuteri* Protectis per 5 drops	Preservative free, sugar free. Medium chain triglyceride oil, sunflower oil. In 5 mL.

LACTOBACILLUS ACIDOPHILUS — ORAL

Indications

➤*Restoration of intestinal flora: Lactobacillus acidophilus* has been found to be useful in the restoration and stabilization of normal intestinal flora.

➤*Off-label uses:*

Prevention of postantibiotic vulvovaginal candidiasis – [5] = Poor documentation. Initial data regarding the use of oral or vaginal lactobacillus to prevent postantibiotic vulvovaginitis indicate that this is not an effective means of therapy and it cannot be recommended.

Other possible off-label uses – The Food and Drug Administration has determined that *Lactobacillus acidophilus* ingredients are not generally recognized to be as safe and effective as antidiarrheal drug products.

Treatment of acute fever blisters (cold sores).

Administration and Dosage

The suggested use is 1 or 2 capsules daily or as directed by a physician.

➤*Storage / Stability: Lactobacillus acidophilus* products contain a specially prepared cultured strain on viable *Lactobacillus acidophilus* microorganisms which has been grown on rice and not milk. These microorganisms are encapsulated for stability and are viable for a year from the shipping date.

Actions

➤*Pharmacology:* This supplement is a viable culture of the naturally occurring metabolic products produced by *Lactobacillus acidophilus* and *Lactobacillus bulgaricus*.

LACTOBACILLUS ACIDOPHILUS — ORAL

Warnings/Precautions

➤*Duration:* Do not use for longer than 2 days unless directed by your health care provider.

➤*Fever:* Unless directed by a health care provider, do not use in the presence of high fever.

➤*Pregnancy: Category: Undetermined.* Consult a health care provider before using in pregnant women.

➤*Lactation:* Consult a health care provider before using in breast-feeding women.

➤*Children:* Unless directed by a health care provider, do not use in children younger than 3 years of age.

Patient Information

This supplement is recommended for diarrhea, fever, constipation, flatulence (excess gas pressure), anorexia (loss of appetite), emesis (vomiting), obesity. Many of these symptoms occur after antibiotic use, and many physicians recommend the use of yogurt or other sources of acidophilus subsequent to antibiotic treatment.

These *Lactobacillus acidophilus* microorganisms are encapsulated for stability and are viable for a year from the shipping date.

Lactobacillus acidophilus products contain no milk, soy, yeast or other allergens.

FLAVOCOXID

Rx	**Limbrel** (Primus)	**Capsules:** 250 mg	Maltodextrin. (LIMBREL 52001). Turquoise green. In 60s.
		500 mg	Maltodextrin. (LIMBREL 52002). Turquoise green with 2 white stripes. In 60s.

FLAVOCOXID — ORAL

Indications

➤*Osteoarthritis (OA):* For the clinical dietary management of the metabolic processes of OA, including associated inflammation.

➤*General information:* Flavocoxid has not been investigated for use in the clinical dietary management of rheumatoid arthritis, acute pain, or primary dysmenorrhea.

Administration and Dosage

➤*Adults:*

Osteoarthritis –

Usual dosage: 250 or 500 mg every 12 hours for a total of 500 to 1,000 mg daily.

Dosage adjustment: Dosage may be increased to 2 or more capsules every 12 hours.

➤*Administration:* May be taken with or without food. If the patient forgets to take the prescribed amount, they should take it as soon as they remember and then resume the normal schedule.

➤*Storage/Stability:* Store at 15° to 30°C (59° to 86°F). Protect from light and moisture. Dispense in a light-resistant container with a child-resistant closure.

Actions

➤*Pharmacology:* Flavocoxid acts by restoring and maintaining the balance of fatty acids in OA. Flavocoxid dampens arachidonic acid (AA) metabolism at relatively equal levels in the cyclooxygenase (COX) pathway (mediated by conversion of AA via the COX-1 and COX-2 enzymes), as well as inhibits the metabolism of AA by the 5-lipooxygenase (LOX) enzyme. This balanced inhibition of metabolism in the COX pathway yields relatively equal levels of thromboxanes, prostaglandins, and prostacyclins, which are key mediators of systemic organ function. Inhibition of these mediators in the COX pathway in conjunction with inhibition of leukotrienes in the LOX pathway results in a "dual inhibition" mechanism that manages inflammation with minimal effects on organ function. This balanced down-regulation of these enzymatic pathways is relatively weak when compared with the effects of traditional nonsteroidal antiinflammatory drugs (NSAIDs) and selective COX-2 inhibitors, thus allowing the body to produce AA metabolites at relatively equal levels to maintain physiologic function. Flavocoxid is not selective for either COX-1 or COX-2 enzymes. Inhibition of 5-LOX has been shown in cell-based assays to reduce the production of leukotriene B4 (LTB_4), an agent that fosters white blood cell chemotaxis and the subsequent release of histamines, reactive oxygen species (ROS), and proinflammatory cytokines. In addition, direct inhibition of the 5-LOX enzyme has been observed as well in enzymatic assays.

Flavocoxid also acts as a strong antioxidant to limit the oxidative conversion of AA by ROS to other damaging fatty acid products. Flavocoxid acts as an antioxidant to neutralize such ROS species as hydroxyl radical, superoxide anion radical, and hydrogen peroxide. Flavocoxid has demonstrated an oxygen radical absorbance capacity of 5,517 mcmolTE/g, as compared with vitamin E (1,100 mcmolTE/g) and vitamin C (5,000 mcmolTE/g).

➤*Pharmacokinetics:*

Absorption –

Food effects: Flavocoxid is safe taken with or without other foods. Taking flavocoxid 1 hour before or after meals may help to increase the absorption of the key ingredients. This observation is based upon a pharmacokinetic study in humans as well as in-market clinical experience in analyzing health care provider and patient product reports. Food does not affect the metabolism of flavocoxid and may buffer effects of slight indigestion.

Metabolism – Flavocoxid is primarily absorbed by albumin in the blood, and only a minor amount (less than 10%) is metabolized via glucuronidation and sulfation by hepatic metabolism involving CYP-450 isoenzymes. A primary ingredient constituent, baicalin, undergoes hydrolysis of the glucuronide moiety in the upper intestine via the action of intestinal flora and is absorbed as the aglycone, baicalein. Glucuronidation and sulfation of baicalein occur intrahepatically. In vitro CYP assays using a microsomal enzyme system demonstrated CYP inhibition to be nominal, ranging from 11% to 23% inhibition of selected isozymes when studied at a 10 mcM concentration.

Contraindications

Hypersensitivity to any component of flavocoxid or to flavonoids. Foods rich in flavonoid contents include colored fruits and vegetables, dark chocolate, tea (especially green tea), red wine, and Brazil nuts.

Warnings/Precautions

➤*GI effects:* Flavocoxid is expected to be safe on the stomach because of its mechanism of action, particularly its inhibition of 5-LOX and modest inhibition of COX-1. COX-1 inhibition causes the up-regulation of 5-LOX in the stomach, which converts AA to leukotrienes (particularly LTB_4). LTB_4 attracts white blood cells to the stomach mucosa, which cause and expand ulcerations. There are no specific controlled clinical trials examining flavocoxid's effect on the stomach in nonulcer or ulcer patients. In an open-label study of 24 patients taking an average of approximately 500 mg/day for a mean of 6.5 months, there was 1 observation of positive fecal occult blood in a patient with a history of hemorrhoids. Clinical experience by health care providers has shown flavocoxid to be well-tolerated in patients with a history of mild ulceration. Postmarketing surveillance has also shown that there has not been a single reported case of ulceration.

➤*Pregnancy: Category: Undetermined.* There are no formal studies among pregnant patients; as a precaution, flavocoxid is not recommended for pregnant patients.

➤*Lactation:* There are no formal studies among breast-feeding patients; as a precaution, flavocoxid is not recommended for breast-feeding patients.

➤*Children:* Because there are no formal studies among patients younger than 18 years of age, as a precaution, flavocoxid is not recommended for patients younger than 18 years of age.

Drug Interactions

➤*Drug/Food interactions:* See Actions for more information.

Adverse Reactions

Flavocoxid Adverse Reactions (≥ 2%)		
Flavocoxid 125 mg twice daily	Flavocoxid 250 mg twice daily	Placebo
Varicose veins (increase)	Psoriasis	Reduced flexibility
Hypertension (elevation)		
Fluid accumulation in the knee		
Psoriasis		

➤*Postmarketing:*

Flavocoxid Postmarketing Adverse Reactions		
	n	%
Cardiovascular		
Recurring heart palpitation	2	0.006%
CNS		
Light-headedness	1	0.003%
Dermatologic		
Hives	1	0.003%
Rash, itching	4	0.011%
GI		
Dyspepsia, heartburn	0	0%
Flatulence, bloating	2	0.006%
Nausea, vomiting	4	0.011%
GU		
Spontaneous abortion	1	0.003%
Musculoskeletal		
Joint pain	3	0.009%
Synovitis	3	0.009%

FLAVOCOXID — ORAL

Flavocoxid Postmarketing Adverse Reactions		
	n	%
Miscellaneous		
Edema	1	0.003%
Fever	2	0.006%
Flu-like symptoms, non-flu season	2	0.006%
Hot flashes	1	0.003%
Total	29	0.08%

Overdosage

➤*Treatment:* If an overdosage occurs, manage patients by systematic and supportive care as soon as possible following product consumption.

CAPRYLIDENE (CAPRYLIC TRIGLYCERIDE)

Rx	Axona[a] (Accera)	**Powder for solution; oral:** 40 g (20 g MCTs[b])	Acesulfame potassium, sucralose. Vanilla flavor. In 40 g packets. In 30s.[c]

[a] Caprylidene is a medical food that is generally recognized as safe (GRAS) (self-affirmed). For a substance to be GRAS, the Food and Drug Administration (FDA) requires that the substance be generally recognized, among experts qualified by scientific training and experience to evaluate its safety, as having been adequately shown through scientific procedures to be safe under the conditions of its intended use.

[b] MCTs = medium-chain triglycerides.

[c] Also contains potassium caseinate (milk-derived protein), maltodextrin, whey protein (milk-derived), sugar, sunflower oil, dimagnesium phosphate, tricalcium phosphate, dipotassium phosphate, soy lecithin, distilled monoglyceride, sodium ascorbate (vitamin C), silicon dioxide, natural vanilla bean extract, vitamin E acetate, vitamin A palmitate, zinc sulfate, pyridoxine hydrochloride (vitamin B_6), folic acid, and chromium chloride.

CAPRYLIDENE — ORAL

Indications

➤*Alzheimer disease:* For the clinical dietary management of the metabolic processes associated with mild to moderate Alzheimer disease (AD). Caprylidene is a medical food containing a proprietary formulation of MCTs, specifically caprylic triglyceride.

Administration and Dosage

➤*Adults:*

Alzheimer disease – 40 g/day (1 packet of caprylidene powder, containing 20 g of MCTs) during breakfast.

➤*Administration:* The contents of each packet of caprylidene should be added to 4 to 8 oz (118 to 236 mL) of water, as preferred, shaken until fully blended, and consumed immediately.

➤*Storage/Stability:* Store at 15° to 30°C (59° to 86°F), sealed and protected from light and moisture.

Actions

➤*Pharmacology:* Caprylidene provides a simple and safe method to induce hyperketonemia, thus providing an alternative energy substrate to glucose in the brains of patients with AD. After oral administration, caprylidene is processed by lipases in the gut, and the resulting medium-chain fatty acids (MCFAs) are absorbed into the portal vein. The MCFAs rapidly pass directly to the liver, where they undergo obligate oxidation. MCFAs enter the liver mitochondria as acyl-CoA, where they undergo beta-oxidation to form acetyl-CoA and acetoacetyl-CoA, which, when produced in excess, are combined to form 3-hydroxy-3-methyl-glutaryl-CoA (HMG-CoA). HMG-CoA is then acted on by HMG-CoA lyase to form acetoacetate and beta-hydroxybutyrate (BHB) (ie, ketone bodies). Since the liver does not use ketone bodies, they are released into the circulation to be used by extrahepatic tissues.

The ketone body BHB crosses the blood-brain barrier and is then taken up by neurons. Ketones are used in a concentration-dependent manner in the adult human brain, including the elderly brain, until circulating concentrations reach approximately 12 mM, at which point they saturate the oxidative machinery. In neurons, ketone bodies enter the mitochondria to produce a cascade effect on mitochondrial activity that increases mitochondrial efficiency and thereby reduces the generation of reactive oxygen species. Ketone bodies feed directly into the tricarboxylic acid (TCA) cycle in neurons and generate adenosine triphosphate (ATP), as well as increase pools of acetyl-CoA and acetylcholine. Ketone bodies are used by neurons even in the presence of abundant glucose.

MCTs are considered saturated fats, as are many long-chain triglycerides (LCTs). However, MCTs are metabolized differently from LCTs in that they do not significantly increase cholesterol levels and are not stored as fat. In a 14-day, open-label bridging study with caprylidene, no clinically significant changes in cholesterol, low-density lipoproteins (LDL), or high-density lipoproteins (HDL) were observed. In a 16-week, randomized, controlled study in 31 patients receiving a reduced-calorie diet containing olive oil or MCT oil (18 to 24 g daily), significant and comparable reductions in total cholesterol and LDL were observed in both study groups.

Contraindications

Allergy to milk or soy.

Warnings/Precautions

➤*Ketoacidosis:* Use caprylidene with caution in patients at risk for ketoacidosis (eg, alcoholism, poorly controlled diabetes).

➤*GI effects:* Caprylidene has demonstrated a favorable safety profile and was well tolerated in multiple clinical trials; however, more caprylidene subjects have experienced GI adverse reactions than have placebo subjects. The most prominent GI adverse reactions observed during clinical studies have been diarrhea, flatulence, and dyspepsia. Among the 172 subjects receiving caprylidene, 2 subjects with preexisting GI conditions developed serious adverse reactions, and for this reason, use caprylidene with caution in patients with a history of GI inflammatory conditions, such as irritable bowel syndrome (IBS), diverticular disease, chronic gastritis, and severe gastroesophageal reflux disease.

➤*Renal effects:* Mild increases in serum urea nitrogen (BUN), uric acid, or creatinine were occasionally observed among patients receiving caprylidene in 1 clinical trial; however, none of these increases exceeded 2.5 × upper limit of normal (ULN). Although none of the clinical investigators assessed these laboratory abnormalities as being clinically significant or as being associated with the development of adverse reactions, a possible relationship to caprylidene cannot be ruled out. Discuss using caprylidene with patients if they have a history of renal dysfunction.

➤*Elevated triglycerides:* Elevated triglyceride values were observed in some patients who presented with probable metabolic syndrome. Periodically monitor triglyceride levels in patients who meet at least 3 of the following 5 criteria indicative of metabolic syndrome: elevated waist circumference (at least 40 inches in men, at least 35 inches in women), BP at least 130/85 mm Hg, triglyceride at least 150 mg/dL, reduced fasting HDL (less than 40 mg/dL in men, less than 50 mg/dL in women), and fasting glucose at least 100 mg/dL.

➤*Hypersensitivity reactions:* Use caprylidene with caution in patients with known hypersensitivity to palm or coconut oil.

Caprylidene contains caseinate (milk-derived protein), whey (milk), and lecithin (soy). Do not use in patients allergic to these component ingredients or sources, that is, to milk or soy.

➤*Monitoring:* Periodically monitor triglyceride levels in patients receiving caprylidene who meet criteria indicative of metabolic syndrome.

Drug Interactions

No clinically important interactions have been observed. Use with caution in alcoholic patients because of possible risk of ketoacidosis.

➤*Drug/Lab test interactions:* No laboratory test abnormalities related to the use of caprylidene have been identified.

Adverse Reactions

➤*Single-administration study:* The first clinical study was a randomized, placebo-controlled, crossover-design study to measure the potential therapeutic events on memory of a single administration of caprylidene (40 to 80 g of MCTs) in 20 patients between 55 and 85 years of age and diagnosed with probable AD (n = 15) or mild cognitive impairment (MCI) (n = 5). Two subjects experienced adverse reactions primarily associated with the GI system, including nausea, abdominal discomfort, and diarrhea.

➤*Alzheimer disease study:* The second clinical study was a double-blind, randomized, 90-day, placebo-controlled study performed at multiple US clinical centers in a population of 152 patients with mild to moderate AD. Patients received 10 g of MCTs per day on days 1 to 7 and 20 g of MCTs per day on days 8 to 90. Seventy-six percent of caprylidene AD subjects experienced at least 1 adverse event during the course of the study, the majority of which were mild to moderate in severity. The most frequently reported adverse reactions involved the GI system, in which 48.8% of caprylidene and 27.3% of placebo subjects experienced 1 or more adverse reactions. The primary GI adverse reactions occurring more frequently in the caprylidene than in the placebo group consisted of diarrhea (24.4% vs 13.6%), flatulence (17.4% vs 7.6%), and dyspepsia (9.3% vs 4.5%).

Caprylidene Adverse Reactions (≥ 3%)[a]		
Adverse reactions	Caprylidene (n = 86)	Placebo (n = 66)
Any event	75.6%	62.1%
CNS		
Dizziness	7%	6.1%
Fatigue	3.5%	1.5%
Headache	5.8%	1.5%
GI		
Abdominal pain	4.7%	4.5%
Diarrhea	24.4%	13.6%
Dyspepsia	9.3%	4.5%

CAPRYLIDENE — ORAL

Caprylidene Adverse Reactions (≥ 3%)[a]		
Adverse reactions	Caprylidene (n = 86)	Placebo (n = 66)
Flatulence	17.4%	7.6%
Respiratory		
Coughing	3.5%	0%
Rhinitis	3.5%	3%
Miscellaneous		
Hypertension	4.7%	3%
Pain	3.5%	3%
Urinary tract infection	4.7%	4.5%

[a] Reported more frequently in caprylidene than in placebo patients.

➤*Bridging study:* The third clinical study was a 14-day, open-label, randomized trial performed at 4 US clinical centers in 66 healthy elderly volunteers. Three formulations of caprylidene were administered for 14 days either with a 7-day titration (7 days at 10 g of MCTs followed by 7 days at 20 g of MCTs) or without titration (14 days at 20 g of MCTs). The original formulation utilized in the double-blind AD study was compared with 2 formulations that contained different ratios of proteins to carbohydrates. Subjects within each cohort experienced comparable frequencies of adverse reactions, including those within the GI system. The most common adverse reactions, consisting of nausea (19.7%), abdominal distension (16.7%), flatulence (15.2%), and diarrhea (13.6%), were generally transient in nature and resolved without treatment. In addition, 7 subjects developed clinically significant increases in triglyceride values after caprylidene administration. Six of these 7 subjects were identified as having probable metabolic syndrome. Of note, dietary restrictions were not imposed during this study, and neither the quantity nor the quality of food consumption was monitored. Therefore, although a causal relationship to caprylidene was not determined, periodically monitor triglyceride levels in patients receiving caprylidene who meet criteria indicative of metabolic syndrome.

➤*GI:* In each of the 3 clinical studies, adverse reactions occurring within the GI system were the most commonly experienced events, and in general, the most frequently reported adverse reactions consisted of diarrhea, flatulence, and dyspepsia. Mild queasiness or nausea that was transient in nature was also occasionally reported, as were bloating and abdominal discomfort. In the double-blind AD study, the overall rate of severe GI events in caprylidene patients included diarrhea (5.8%), dyspepsia (2.3%), and flatulence (1.2%). In all but 2 cases, the diarrhea spontaneously resolved without treatment. The majority of GI events were mild to moderate in severity, and it was found that the severity of adverse reactions could be reduced if caprylidene was taken with food. In the double-blind AD study, the incidence of severe diarrhea declined from 9.7% to 3.1% following a change in mixing instructions (blending the original formulation of caprylidene with a meal replacement drink such as *Ensure* instead of water). The marketed formulation of caprylidene does not require mixing with *Ensure*.

In the double-blind AD study, a patient with AD 93 years of age with a history of IBS and intermittent diarrhea, along with multiple cardiac abnormalities, including left ventricular hypertrophy, died because of a GI bleed following 28 days of caprylidene administration. Also in the double-blind AD study, a patient 87 years of age with a history of diverticulitis and stomach ulcer was found to have a guaiac-positive stool when hospitalized for pneumonia. This patient was discharged from the hospital without sequelae. All of these events were likely to be related to the subject's underlying comorbidities; however, consider the possibility that caprylidene may exacerbate preexisting GI inflammatory processes.

➤*Renal:* In the double-blind AD clinical study, mean values in BUN, uric acid, or creatinine increased from screening values in the caprylidene group; however, none of the increased values in individual subjects exceeded 2.5 times the ULN. Five of 7 caprylidene AD subjects with notable elevations in BUN (more than 1.3 times ULN), uric acid (more than 1.2 times ULN), or creatinine (more than 1.33 times screening and more than the ULN) had abnormally high values at screening that were further increased at day 104. Among these subjects, 3 were noted to have had apparent urinary tract infections at study enrollment, and 1 had a history of renal failure requiring dialysis. These subjects with significant renal function test abnormalities were also noted to have BUN/creatinine ratios more than 15, a likely indication of dehydration. While the increases in these renal function tests appear to be related to either preexisting conditions or to dehydration, a relation to caprylidene cannot be entirely ruled out.

Overdosage

➤*Symptoms:* The dose-limiting toxicity with MCTs is known to be diarrhea.

➤*Treatment:* In the unlikely event of overusage of caprylidene, manage patients with systematic and supportive care as soon as possible after the overusage has occurred. Overusage symptoms could vary by patient. Severe episodic diarrhea may occur.

Patient Information

Caprylidene is a medical food product distributed by prescription, and must be used under the supervision of a health care provider. Instruct both the patients and their caregivers in the correct administration amount and schedule for caprylidene based on medical evaluation of the patient by the supervising health care provider.

Advise patients to take 1 packet of caprylidene once a day with breakfast. Contents of each packet of caprylidene should be added to 4 to 8 oz (118 to 236 mL) of water, as preferred, shaken until fully blended, and consumed immediately.

Counsel patients and their caregivers that mild GI symptoms (diarrhea, flatulence, dyspepsia, and feeling of unsettled stomach) may be experienced by some patients who take caprylidene. Remind patients who experience unacceptable GI adverse reactions to take caprylidene with food. Nonprescription medications such as simethicone, antacids, and antidiarrheals can be useful. Patients with persistent unacceptable GI adverse reactions may take one-half packet of caprylidene until adverse reactions have resolved and then resume taking a full packet of caprylidene.

MULTIVITAMINS

Content given per capsule, tablet, wafer, 5 mL liquid, or 1 mL drops.

	Product & Distributor	A units	D units	E units	B_1 mg	B_2 mg	B_3 mg	B_5 mg	B_6 mg	B_{12} mcg	C mg	Folate mg	Other Content	Excipients & How Supplied
otc	**A & D Softgel Capsules** (Nature's Bounty)	10,000[a]	400[b]											Soybean oil. In 100s.
otc sf	**Quintabs Tablets** (Freeda Vitamins)	5,000[c]	400[d]	50[e]	30	30	100	30	30	30	300	0.4[f]	Biotin 30 mcg	Gluten free, lactose free, and sugar free. In 100s and 250s.
otc	**Thera Caplets** (Auburn Pharmaceutical[v])	5,000	400[b]	30[g]	3	3.4	20	10	3	9	90	0.4	Biotin 30 mcg	Mineral oil, PEG, sucrose. In 100s.
otc	**Tab-A-Vite with Beta-Carotene Tablets** (Major)	5,000[h]	400[d]	30[g]	1.5	1.7	20	10	2	6	60	0.4[f]		In 100s.
otc sf	**One-Tablet-Daily Tablets** (Goldline)	5,000[i]	400[d]	30[g]	1.5	1.7	20	10	2	6	60	0.4[f]		Preservative free and sugar free. Mannitol, fish. In 1,000s.
otc	**Tab A Vite Essential with Beta Carotene Tablets** (Major)	5,000[j]	400[d]	30[g]	1.5	1.7	20	10	2	6	60	0.4[f]		Mannitol, fish ingredients. In 1,000s.
otc	**Sigtab Tablets** (Lee Pharmaceuticals)	5,000[h]	400	15	10.3	10	100	20	8	18	333	0.4[f]		PEG. In 90s.
otc	**Multi-Day with Beta-Carotene Tablets** (Nature's Bounty)	5,000[i]	400[b]	10[g]	1.5	1.7	20	10	2	6	60	0.4[f]		Mannitol, fish ingredients. In 365s.
otc	**Theravite Liquid** (Goldline)	5,000[l]	400[b]		10	10	100	21.4	4.1	5	200			Methylparaben, sugar. Cherry flavor. In 118 mL.
otc	**Thera Liquid** (Major)													Parabens, PEG, sucrose, sugar 2 g. Fruit flavor. In 118 mL.
otc	**Thera-Plus Liquid** (Hi-Tech)	5,000	400		10	10	100	21.4	4.1	5	200			Cherry flavoring, glycerin, methylparaben, sodium benzoate, sugar. In 118 mL.
otc	**Once-Daily Regular Formula Tablets** (Auburn Pharmaceutical[v])	5,000[m]	400[b]		2	2.5	20	1	1	1	50			Mineral oil, PEG. In 1,000s.
otc	**A & D Softgel Capsules** (Nature's Bounty)	5,000[n]	400[n]											Fish ingredients. In 100s.
otc	**One a Day Essential Tablets** (Bayer Health Care)	3,000[o]	400[d]	30[g]	1.5	1.7	20	10	2	6	60	0.4[f]		Dextrose, PEG, soy. In 130s.
otc	**Flintstones with Extra C Tablets** (Bayer Consumer)	2,500[h]	400	15[p]	1.05	1.2	13.5		1.05	4.5	250	0.3[f]		Fructose, milk, sodium 25 mg, sucrose, sugar (< 1 g). In 60s.
otc	**Fruity Chews Children's Chewable Tablets** (Goldline)	2,500[i]	400[d]	15[g]	1.05	1.2	13.5		1.05	4	60	0.3		Fish ingredients, mannitol, sucrose. In 100s.
otc	**Animal Shapes Children's Chewable Vitamins Tablets** (Major)	2,500[h]	400[d]	15[g]	1.05	1.2	13.5		1.05	4.5	60	0.3[f]		Hydrogenated cottonseed oil, sucrose. In 100s and 250s.
otc	**Children's Chewable Vitamins Tablets** (Auburn Pharmaceutical[v])	2,500[m]	400[b]	15[g]	1.05	1.2	13.5		1.05	4.5	60	0.3[f]		Dextrose, sugar, tartrazine. In 100s and 1,000s.
otc	**Daily Vitamins Syrup** (Rugby)	2,500[l]	400[b]	15[g]	1.05	1.2	13.5		1.05	4.5	60			High-fructose corn syrup, parabens, sugars 2.5 g. In 237 and 473 mL.
otc	**Cod Liver Oil Softgel Capsules** (Goldline)	2,500[q]	260[q]											Fish ingredients. In 100s.
otc	**Daily Vitamin Liquid** (Major)	2,250[l]	360[b]	13.5[g]	0.842	1.08	12.2		0.945	4.05	54			High-fructose corn syrup, parabens. Fruit flavor. In 473 mL.
otc sf	**Vitamin Liquid** (Goldline)													Alcohol free and sugar free. Methylparaben, saccharin. Lemon flavor. In 473 mL.
otc	**My First Flintstones Chewable Tablets** (Bayer Consumer Care)	1,998[h]	400	15[p]	1.05	1.2	10		1.05	4.5	60	0.3[f]		Invert sugar, sodium 10 mg, soybean oil, sucrose. In 100s.
otc	**Vitaball Vitamin Gumballs** (Amerifit Nutrition)	1,670[a]	400[b]	30[r]	1.5	1.7	20	10	2	6	60	0.4[f]	Biotin 45 mcg	Corn syrup, sucralose, sucrose. In 36s.
otc	**Vita Drops** (Major)	1,500	400	5	0.5	0.6	8		0.4	2	35			Ferrous sulfate[z], methylparaben, oil of orange. Cherry flavor. In 50 mL.
otc sf	**Baby Vitamin Drops** (Goldline)	1,500[l]	400[b]	5[e]	0.5	0.6	8		0.4	2	35			Alcohol free and sugar free. Ferrous sulfate[z], methylparaben, oil of orange. Cherry flavor. In 50 mL.
otc sf	**Polyvitamin Drops** (Rugby)	1,500[l]	400[b]	5[s]	0.5	0.6	8		0.4	2	35			Alcohol free and sugar free. Ferrous sulfate[z], methylparaben, oil of orange. Cherry flavor. In 50 mL.
Rx	**Tri-Vi-Sol Drops** (Mead Johnson)	1,500[l]	400[b]								35			Lactose free and gluten free. Fruit flavored. In 50 mL.
otc	**Tri-Vitamin Drops** (Rugby)	1,500[l]	400[b]								35			Methylparaben. Cherry flavor. In 50 mL.
otc	**Cod Liver Oil Softgel Capsules** (Rugby)	1,250[q]	130[q]											Fish ingredients. In 100s.
otc	**C & E Softgel Capsules** (Nature's Bounty)			400[t]							500			Soybean oil. Caramel color. In 50s and 100s.

MULTIVITAMINS

	Product & Distributor	A units	D units	E units	B_1 mg	B_2 mg	B_3 mg	B_5 mg	B_6 mg	B_{12} mcg	C mg	Folate mg	Other Content	Excipients & How Supplied
otc	**Cardiotek Tablets** (Stewart-Jackson Pharmacal[w])			200[g]					50	500	100	0.8[f]	L-arginine 75 mg	In 100s.
otc	**AllBee C-800 Caplets** (Inverness Medical)			45[g]	15	17	100	25	25	12	800	0.4[f]	Biotin 300 mcg	Dextrose, PEG. In 60s.
otc	**Stress Formula Tablets** (Various, eg, Goldline, Nature's Bounty)			30[g]	10	10	100	20	5	12	500	0.4[f]	Biotin 45 mcg	Fish ingredients, mannitol. In 60s.
otc	**Varisan Vitality Tablets** (Kramer-Novis)			25[p]	10		30		30	8	25		Citrus bioflavonoids 100 mg, Hammamelis virginian 100 mg, Hawthorne berries 100 mg, hesperidin 25 mg, horse chestnut 100 mg, rutin 40 mg	In 50s.
Rx	**Renatabs Tablets** (Hawthorn)			5	1.5	1.7	20	10	10	6	60	1[f]	d-Biotin 300 mcg	(HAW 160). Yellow, capsule shape. In 100s.
otc	**Neurodep Caps Capsules** (Medical Products Panamericana[x])				125				125	1,000				In 50s.
otc	**High-Potency Balanced B-100 Timed-Release Tablets** (Nature's Bounty)				100	100	100	100	100	100		0.4[f]	Biotin 100 mcg, choline bitartrate 100 mg, inositol 100 mg, PABA[y] 100 mg, proprietary blend (alfalfa, parsley, rice bran, soy lecithin, watercress) 1 mg	Mannitol. Extended release. In 50s, 60s, and 100s.
otc *sf*	**Balanced B-50 Tablets** (Major)				50	50	50	50	50	50		0.4[f]	Biotin 50 mcg, choline bitartrate 50 mg, inositol 50 mg, PABA 50 mg, natural food base (alfalfa, lecithin, parsley, rice bran, watercress) 2.5 mg	Gluten free, preservative free, and sugar free. Mannitol, sodium
otc *sf*	**Super Quints B-50 Tablets** (Freeda Vitamins)				50	50	50	50	50	50		0.4[f]	Biotin 50 mcg. Base 50 mg (containing choline, inositol, L-lysine, l-glutamic acid, l-glutamine, l-glycine, PABA)	Gluten free, lactose free, and sugar free. In 100s, 250s, and 500s.
otc	**High-Potency Balanced B-50 Tablets** (Nature's Bounty)				50	50	50	50	50	50		0.4[f]	Biotin 50 mcg, choline bitartrate 50 mg, inositol 50 mg, PABA 50 mg, proprietary blend (alfalfa, parsley, rice bran, soy lecithin, watercress) 2.5 mg	Hydrogenated vegetable oil, mannitol. In 50s and 100s.
otc *sf*	**Balanced B-100 Tablets** (Major)				100	100	100	100	100	100		0.1[f]	Biotin 100 mcg, choline bitartrate 12.5 mg, inositol 12.5 mg, PABA 12.5 mg, proprietary blend (alfalfa leaf powder, parsley leaf powder, rice bran defatted powder, soy lecithin granules, watercress leaf powder) 62.5 mg	Lactose free, preservative free, and sugar free. Mannitol, sodium
otc	**B-100 Ultra B-Complex Tablets** (Nature's Bounty)				100	100	100	100	100	100		0.1[f]	Biotin 100 mcg, choline bitartrate 12.5 mg, inositol 12.5 mg, PABA 12.5 mg, proprietary blend (alfalfa leaf powder, parsley leaf powder, rice bran defatted powder, soy lecithin granules, watercress leaf powder) 62.5 mg	Mannitol. In 50s.

MULTIVITAMINS

	Product & Distributor	A units	D units	E units	B_1 mg	B_2 mg	B_3 mg	B_5 mg	B_6 mg	B_{12} mcg	C mg	Folate mg	Other Content	Excipients & How Supplied
otc	**ThexForte Caplets** (Lee Pharmaceuticals)				25	15	100	10	5		500			In 75s.
Rx	**Strovite Tablets** (Everett Laboratories)				15	15	100	18	4	5	500	0.5[f]		Lactose, PEG, tartrazine. Lt. green, capsule shape. In 100s.
Rx	**Formula B Tablets** (Major)				15	15	100	18	4	5	500	0.5[f]		In 100s.
otc	**AllBee With C Caplets** (Inverness Medical)				15	10.2	50	10	5		300	0.4[f]	Biotin 300 mcg	PEG, tartrazine. In 130s.
otc	**Total B with C Caplets** (Major)				15	10.2	50	10	5		300			In 130s.
otc	**Superplex-T Tablets** (Major)				15	10	100	18.3	5	10	500			Sodium 65 mg. In 100s.
Rx	**Therobec Tablets** (Qualitest)				15	15	100	18	4	5	500	0.5		Mineral oil, PEG. In 100s.
otc	**Vitaline Biotin Forte Tablets** (Integrative Therapeutics)				10	10	40	10	25	10	100	0.8[f]	Biotin 5 mg	Soy lecithin. In 60s.
otc	**B Complex Plus B-12 Tablets** (Nature's Bounty)				7	14	4.5			25			Protease (as papain powder) 10 mg	Mannitol. In 90s.
otc	**Surbex-C Tablets** (Abbott)				4.96	5.4	27.2	8.28	1.85	4.5	225			Milk products, sodium 35 mg.
otc sf	**Apetigen Liquid** (Kramer-Novis)				3.33	3.33	66.67	6.67	0.67	8.33			Lysine (as L-lysine monohydrochloride) 206.33 mg	Alcohol free and sugar free. Castor oil, parabens, sorbitol. In 237 mL.
otc	**B-Complex with B-12 Tablets** (Major)				3	2	20	0.1	1	5				In 100s.
otc sf	**Full Spectrum B with Vitamin C Tablets** (Nature's Blend)				1.5	1.7	20	10	10	6	60	0.8[f]	Biotin 300 mcg	Preservative free and sugar free. In 100s.
Rx	**Nephro-Vite Rx Tablets** (Watson)				1.5	1.7	20	10	10	6	60	1[f]	d-Biotin 300 mcg	(RD 12). Yellow. Film-coated. In 100s.
Rx	**Rena-Vite Tablets** (Cypress)				1.5	1.7	20	10	10	6	60	0.8[f]	Biotin 300 mcg	Mineral oil. In 100s.
Rx sf	**DexFol Tablets** (Rising Pharmaceuticals)				1.5	1.5	20	10	50	1,000	60	5[f]	Biotin 300 mcg	Lactose free and sugar free. PEG. In 90s.
otc sf	**Nephronex Liquid** (Llorens)				1.5	1.7	20	10	10	10	60	0.9[f]	Biotin 300 mcg	Alcohol free, dye free, sugar free. Aspartame, parabens, phenylalanine. In 236.5 mL.
otc	**Nephro-Vite Tablets** (Rugby)				1.5	1.7	20	10	10	6	60	0.8[f]	d-Biotin 300 mcg	Lactose. In 100s.
Rx	**Renal Caps Softgel Capsules** (Cypress)				1.5	1.7	20	5	10	6	100	1[f]	Biotin 150 mcg	Soybean oil. (CYP 162). Opaque/black. In 100s.
Rx	**Rena-Vite Rx Tablets** (Cypress)				1.5	1.7	20	10	10	6	60	1[f]	Biotin 300 mcg	Mineral oil. Yellow. In 100s.
Rx sf	**Folbee Plus Tablets** (Breckenridge)				1.5	1.5	20	10	50	1,000	60	5[f]	Biotin 300 mcg	Lactose free and sugar free. Mineral oil. Yellow. Film-coated. In 90s.
otc	**Almebex Plus B_{12} Liquid** (Propharma)				1	2	5		1	8.33			Choline 33 mg	Alcohol free. Parabens, sucrose. Malt flavor. In 473 mL.
otc sf	**Cholinoid Capsules** (Goldline)				1	1	10	5	1	6	300		Choline (as choline bitartrate) 334 mg, inositol 334 mg, lemon bioflavonoids (fruit) 300 mg	Sugar free. Mannitol. In 100s.
Rx sf	**Cerefolin Tablets** (Pamlab)					5			50	1,000		5.635[k]		Gluten free, lactose free, and sugar free. (PAL M5) Blue. Film-coated. In 90s or 500s.
Rx sf	**Cardiotek Rx Tablets** (Stewart-Jackson Pharmacal[w])								50	500		2[f]	L-arginine 500 mg	Lactose free and sugar free. Orange, football-shape. Film-coated. In 30s.
Rx	**Metanx Tablets** (Pamlab)								35[cc]	2,000[aa]		3[bb]		In 90s and 500s.
otc	**TriCardio B Capsules** (Miller)								25	250		0.4[f]		In 60s.
Rx sf	**Foltx Tablets** (Pamlab)								25	2,000		2.5[f]		Lactose free and sugar free. PEG 400 and 8000. (PAL). Beige. Film-coated. In 90s.
Rx sf	**Folast** (Brookstone Pharmaceuticals)								25[cc]	2,000[aa]		2.8[k]		Gluten free, sugar free. (311). Purple, round, coated. In 90s.
Rx sf	**Folbic Tablets** (Breckenridge)								25	2,000		2.5[u]		Lactose free and sugar free. Mineral oil. (B 384). Rose color, oval. In 90s.
Rx sf	**Vita-Respa Tablets** (Respa)								25	1,300		2.2[u]		Dye free, lactose free, and sugar free. PEG. (Respa 913). Oval, scored. In 90s.
Rx	**Folgard Rx Tablets** (Upsher-Smith)								25	1,000		2.2[f]		PEG. (US 191). Yellow, oval. Film -coated. In 100s.

MULTIVITAMINS

	Product & Distributor	A units	D units	E units	B_1 mg	B_2 mg	B_3 mg	B_5 mg	B_6 mg	B_{12} mcg	C mg	Folate mg	Other Content	Excipients & How Supplied
otc	**Folgard Tablets** (Upsher-Smith)								10	115		0.8[f]		PEG. In 60s.
Rx sf	**Cerefolin NAC Caplets** (Pamlab)									2,000[aa]		5.6[k]	600 mg N-acetylcysteine	Gluten free, lactose free, sugar free. PEG, saccharin. (PAL 600). Blue, oval. In 90s and 500s.

[a] As retinyl palmitate.
[b] As cholecalciferol.
[c] As vitamin A palmitate and beta-carotene.
[d] As ergocalciferol.
[e] As d-alpha tocopheryl acid succinate.
[f] As folic acid.
[g] As dl-alpha tocopheryl acetate.
[h] As vitamin A acetate and beta-carotene.
[i] As retinyl acetate and beta-carotene.
[j] As retinyl-palmitate and beta-carotene.
[k] As L-methylfolate.
[l] As vitamin A palmitate.
[m] As vitamin A acetate.
[n] From fish liver oil.
[o] 17% as beta-carotene.
[p] As vitamin E acetate.
[q] As cod liver oil.
[r] As dl-tocopherol acetate.
[s] As d-alpha tocopheryl succinate.
[t] As d-alpha tocopherol plus d-beta, d-gamma, and d-delta tocopherols.
[u] As folacin.
[v] Auburn Pharmaceutical, 1775 John R, Troy, MI 48083; 800-222-5609, fax 248-526-3750; http://www.auburnpharm.com.
[w] Stewart-Jackson Pharmacal, 4587 Damascus Road, Memphis, TN 38118; 800-367-1395, http://www.sjpharma.com.
[x] Medical Products Panamericana, 647 West Flagler Street, Miami, FL 33130; 305-670-4416, fax 305-545-9592.
[y] PABA = para-aminobenzoic acid.
[z] Ferrous sulfate added as a stabilizer for cyanocobalamin.
[aa] As methylcobalamin.
[bb] As L-methylfolate calcium.
[cc] As pyridoxal-5′ phosphate.

For additional information, refer to the Dietary Reference Intakes of Vitamins and Minerals table.

MULTIVITAMINS WITH FLUORIDE

Content given per tablet or 1 mL.

	Product & Distributor	F[a] mg	A units	D units	E units	B_1 mg	B_2 mg	B_3 mg	B_6 mg	B_{12} mcg	C mg	Folate mg	Excipients & How Supplied
Rx	**Multi-Vitamin with Fluoride Chewable Tablets** (Vintage)	1	2,500[b]	400	15[c]	1.05	1.2	13.5	1.05	4.5	60	0.3[d]	PEG, sugar. In 100s.
	RE MultiVit with Fluoride Chewable Tablets 1 mg (River's Edge)	1	2,500	400	15	1.05	1.2	13.5	1.05	4.5	60	0.3[d]	(RE 366). Orange/red/purple. In 100s.
otc	**Multi-Vitamin with Fluoride Chewable Tablets** (Amide)	1	2,500[b]	400	15[e]	1.05	1.2	13.5	1.05	4.5	60	0.3[d]	Sucrose. In 100s.
Rx sf	**MVC Chewable Multivitamin with Fluoride** (Sancillo)	1	2,500[f]	400[g]	15[e]	1.05	1.2	13.5	1.05	4.5	60	0.3[d]	Sugar free, dye free. Sucralose. (SCI 1003) . White-speckled, hexagon shape. Orange flavor. In 100s and 1,000s.
Rx	**Tri-a-vite w/FL Chewable Tablets** (Major)	1	2,500	400							60		In 100s.
Rx	**Multi-Vitamin with Fluoride Chewable Tablets** (Vintage)	0.5	2,500[b]	400	15[c]	1.05	1.2	13.5	1.05	4.5	60	0.3[d]	PEG, sugar. In 100s.
Rx	**Multivite w/FL Chewable Tablets** (Major)	0.5	2,500	400	15	1.05	1.2	13.5	1.05	4.5	60	0.3[d]	In 100s.
otc	**Multi-Vitamin with Fluoride Chewable Tablets** (Amide)	0.5	2,500[b]	400	15[e]	1.05	1.2	13.5	1.05	4.5	60	0.3[d]	Sucrose. In 100s.
	RE MultiVit with Fluoride Chewable Tablets 0.50 mg (River's Edge)	0.5	2,500	400	15	1.05	1.2	13.5	1.05	4.5	60	0.3[d]	(RE 365). Orange/red/purple. In 100s.
Rx sf	**MVC Chewable Multivitamin with Fluoride** (Sancilio)	0.5	2,500[f]	400[g]	15[e]	1.05	1.2	13.5	1.05	4.5	60	0.3[d]	Sugar free, dye free. Sucralose. (SCI 1005). White-speckled, triangle shape. Orange flavor. In 100s and 1,000s.
Rx	**Multivitamin and Fluoride Drops** (Hi-Tech)	0.5	1,500[f]	400[g]	5[h]	0.5	0.6	8	0.4	2	35		Ferrous sulfate,[i] methylparaben, oil of orange. In 50 mL.
Rx	**PolyVitamin with Fluoride Drops** (Hi-Tech)												Ferrous sulfate.[i] In 50 mL.
Rx	**Multi-Vitamin with Fluoride Chewable Tablets** (Vintage)	0.25	2,500[b]	400	15[c]	1.05	1.2	13.5	1.05	4.5	60	0.3[d]	PEG, sugar. In 100s.
Rx	**Multi Vita-Bets with Fluoride Chewable Tablets** (Major)	0.25	2,500	400	15	1.05	1.2	13.5	1.05	4.5	60	0.3[d]	(A 150). Orange, cherry, grape flavors. In 100s.
otc	**Multi-Vitamin with Fluoride Chewable Tablets** (Amide)	0.25	2,500[b]	400	15[e]	1.05	1.2	13.5	1.05	4.5	60	0.3[d]	Sucrose. In 100s.
	RE MultiVit With Fluoride Chewable Tablets 0.25 mg (River's Edge)	0.25	2,500	400	15	1.05	1.2	13.5	1.05	4.5	60	0.3[d]	PEG, sugar. (RE 364). Orange/red/purple. Cherry/orange/grape flavor. In 100s.
Rx sf	**MVC Chewable Multivitamin with Fluoride** (Sancilio)	0.25	2,500[f]	400[g]	15[e]	1.05	1.2	13.5	1.05	4.5	60	0.3[d]	Sugar free, dye free. Sucralose. (SCI 1001). White-speckled, round. Orange flavor. In 100s and 1,000s.

MULTIVITAMINS WITH FLUORIDE

	Product & Distributor	F[a] mg	A units	D units	E units	B_1 mg	B_2 mg	B_3 mg	B_6 mg	B_{12} mcg	C mg	Folate mg	Excipients & How Supplied
Rx	**Multivitamin and Fluoride Drops** (Hi-Tech)	0.25	1,500[f]	400[g]	5[h]	0.5	0.6	8	0.4	2	35		Ferrous sulfate,[i] methylparaben, oil of orange. In 50 mL.
Rx	**Multi-Vit with Fluoride Drops** (Qualitest)												Glycerin. In 50 mL.
Rx	**PolyVitamin with Fluoride Drops** (Hi-Tech)												Ferrous sulfate.[i] In 50 mL.
Rx	**Tri-Vit with Fluoride Drops** (Qualitest)	0.25	1,500[f]	400[g]							35		In 50 mL.

[a] Fluoride content expressed in mg elemental fluoride.
[b] As vitamin A acetate.
[c] As vitamin E acetate.
[d] As folic acid.
[e] As dl-alpha-tocopheryl acetate.
[f] As vitamin A palmitate.
[g] As cholecalciferol.
[h] As d-alpha-tocopheryl acid succinate.
[i] Ferrous sulfate added as a stabilizer for cyanocobalamin.

For additional information, refer to theDietary Reference Intakes of Vitamins and Minerals table.

MULTIVITAMINS WITH MINERALS (INCLUDING IRON)

Content given per capsule, tablet, 5 mL liquid, or 1 mL drops.

	Product & Distributor	Fe[a] mg	Ca[b] mg	A units	D units	E units	B_1 mg	B_2 mg	B_3 mg	B_5 mg	B_6 mg	B_{12} mcg	C mg	Folate[c] mg	Other Minerals	Other Content	Excipients & How Supplied
Rx	**Folitab 500 Caplets** (Rising Pharmaceuticals)	525											500				
Rx	**Integra Plus Capsules** (US Pharmaceutical Corp)	327[d,i]					5	5	20	7	25	10	210[nnn]	1		Biotin	Gluten free. (US Integra Plus). Bright yellow/maroon. In 90s.
Rx	**Ferrocite Plus Capsules** (Breckenridge Pharmaceutical)	324[d]					10	6	30	10	5	15	200	1	Cu, Mg, Mn, Zn		Soy. (B 682). Pink. In 30s and 100s.
Rx	**Niferex Gold Tablets** (Ther-Rx)	200[h,i]										25	110	1	Zn		Lactose, PEG[iii], polydextrose. (Ther-Rx 162). Orange, oval, scored. Film-coated. In 90s.
Rx	**Vitagen Forte Caplets** (Midlothian Labs)	151[d,mmm]										10	60.8[ppp]	1		Succinic acid	Lactose, PEG. (ML 555). Dark brown. Film-coated. In 90s.
Rx	**Multigen Plus Capsules** (Breckenridge)															Succinic acid	Mineral oil, soy. (B 544). Brown, capsule shape. Film-coated. In 90s.
Rx	**Trimagen Forte Tablets** (Trigen)															Succinic acid	(MVC003). Lt. brown. Film-coated. In 90s.
Rx	**Pruvate 21/7 Tablets** (PruGen)	151[d,mmm]										10	200[ppp]	1		Succinic acid	Lactose, PEG, polydextrose. (101). Red, oval. Film-coated. In 21s. Lactose, PEG. (102). Purple, oval. Film-coated. In 7s.
Rx	**Rexavite 150 Capsules** (Midlothian Labs)	150[i,mmm]											50[ppp]			Succinic acid	(ML 397). Red/White. In 90s.
Rx	**Ferrex 150 Plus Capsules** (Breckenridge)															Succinic acid	PEG, tartrazine. (B703). White/ Orange. In 90s.
Rx	**Fe-Tinic 150 Forte Capsules** (Ethex)	150[i,qqq]										25	60	1		Succinic acid	(THX 164). Red/Clear. In 90s.
Rx	**Rexavite 150 Forte Capsules** (Midlothian Labs)	150[i,mmm]										25	60.8[ppp]	1		Succinic acid	(ML 395). Red/white. In 90s.
Rx	**Integra Capsules** (US Pharmaceutical Corp)																Gluten free. (US Integra). Red. In 90s.
Rx	**Integra F Capsules** (US Pharmaceutical Corp)																Gluten free. (US Integra-F). Maroon. In 90s.
Rx	**Ferrex 150 Forte Plus Capsules** (Breckenridge)															Succinic acid	PEG. (B 798). White/Orange. In 90s.
Rx	**Triferex 150 Forte Capsules** (Trigen)															Succinic acid	(MVC010). Red. In 90s.
Rx	**Tandem Plus Capsules** (US Pharmaceuticals)	106[d,i]					10	6	30	10	5	15	200	1	Cu, Mn, Zn		(Tandem Plus/US US US US US US US). Pink. In 90s.

MULTIVITAMINS WITH MINERALS (INCLUDING IRON)

	Product & Distributor	Fe[a] mg	Ca[b] mg	A units	D units	E units	B_1 mg	B_2 mg	B_3 mg	B_5 mg	B_6 mg	B_{12} mcg	C mg	Folate[c] mg	Other Minerals	Other Content	Excipients & How Supplied
Rx	**CenogenUltra Capsules** (US Pharm)	106[d]					10	6	30	10	5	15	200	1	Cu, Mn		(CENOGEN ULTRA/140). Blue/Pink. In UD 100s.
Rx	**Hematinic Plus Vitamins and Minerals Tablets** (Cypress)														Cu, Mg, Mn, Zn		In 100s.
Rx	**Ferrocite Plus Tablets** (Breckenridge)														Cu, Mg, Mn, Zn		PEG, mineral oil. (CPC 1325). Blue, capsule shape. Film-coated. In blister 100s.
Rx	**I-Fol Plus** (Breckenridge)	105					6	6	30	10	5	25	0.8				Mineral oil, PEG. In 60s.
Rx	**Ferralet 90 Tablets** (Mission Pharmacal)	90[r]										12	120	1		Docusate sodium	PEG. (F5). Green, rectangle shape. Film-coated. In 90s.
Rx	**FerraPlus 90 Tablets** (Trigen)																PEG. (TL012). Green, rectangle shape. Film-coated. In 90s.
Rx	**Trimagen FA** (Trigen)	70[mmm]										10	152	1		Succinic acid	(MCV004). Lt. brown. Film-coated. In 90s.
Rx	**Multifol Tablets** (Breckenridge)	65[d]	125[k]	6,000[zz]	400	30[e]	1.1	1.8	15		2.5	5	60	1			(B126). Purple, capsule shape. In UD 100s.
Rx	**Vitafol Caplets** (Everett)	65[d]	125[k]	6,000[zz]	400	30[f]	1.1	1.8	15		2.5	5	60	1			PEG. (EV0072). Pink. Film-coated. In UD 100s.
Rx	**Vitafol-PN Caplets** (Everett)	65[d]	125[k]	1,700[dd]	400[j]	30[e]	1.6	1.8	15		2.5	5	60	1	Mg, Zn		PEG. (EV0078). Lt. blue. In UD 100s.
Rx	**Vitafol-OB Caplets** (Everett)	65[d]	100[k]	2,700[g]	400[j]	30[e]	1.6	1.8	18		2.5	12	70	1	Cu, Mg, Zn		Polydextrose, PEG, sucrose, glucose. (EV 0079). Lt. blue. In UD 100s.
Rx	**Strong Start Tablets** (Ther-Rx)	35[d]	250[k]		6[j]	3.5[e]					50		50	1	Cu, Mg, Zn		(Ther-Rx 137). Orange. In UD 30s.
otc	**Iromin-G Tablets** (Mission)	29.5[n]	57[yy]	4,000[zz]	400[j]		4.8	2	10	1	20	2	100	0.8			PEG. Film-coated. In 100s.
otc sf	**Parvlex Tablets** (Freeda)	29[d]					20	20	20	10	10	50	60	0.4	Cu, Mn		Gluten free, lactose free, sugar free. In 100s.
otc	**Iron-Folic 500 Tablets** (Major)	28[d]	105				6	6	30	10	5	25	500	0.8			Sodium 65 mg. In 100s.
otc sf	**S.S.S. Tonic Tablets** (S.S.S. Company)	27[d]	100[ddd]			50[e]	7.5	7.5	50	10	12.5	12.5	300	0.2	Cu, Mg, Zn	Biotin	Preservative free, sugar free. In 20s.
otc	**Theravim-M Tablets** (Nature's Bounty)	27[d]	40[eee]	5,000[m]	400[j]	30[e]	3	3.4	20	10	3	9	90	0.4	Cr, Cu, I, K, Mg, Mn, Mo, P, Se, Zn	Biotin	Mannitol. Film-coated. In 130s.
otc	**Thera-M with Minerals Caplets** (Prime Marketing)	27[d]	40[qq]	5,000	400[j]	30[e]	3	3.4	20	10	3	9	90	0.4	Cl, Cr, Cu, I, K, Mg, Mn, Mo, P, Se, Zn	Biotin	Mineral oil, PEG, sucrose. In 130s and 500s.
Rx sf	**O-Cal F.A. Tablets** (Pharmics)	27[d]	200[k]	2,500[zz]	400[j]	30[l]	3	3	20		4	12	90	1	Cu, I, Mg, Zn		Dye free, gluten free, sugar free. Mineral oil, PEG. (Pharmics 00813). Oblong. Film-coated. In 100s.
Rx	**Formula B Plus Tablets** (Major)	27[d]		5,000		30[e]	20	20	100	25	25	50	500	0.8	Cr, Cu, Mg, Mn, Zn	Biotin	In 100s.
Rx	**Bacmin Tablets** (Marnel)	27[d]		5,000[zz]		30[e]	20	20	100	25	25	50	500	1	Cr, Cu, Mg, Mn, Se, Zn	Biotin, lemon bioflavonoids	PEG. (MMD). Dark red. In 30s and 100s.
otc	**Compete Tablets** (Mission)	27[n]		5,000[zz]	400[j]	43[q]	2	2.6	30		20	9	90	0.4	Zn		PEG. Film-coated. In 100s.
Rx	**Strovite Plus Caplets** (Everett)	27[d]		5,000[zz]		30[e]	20	20	100	25	25	50	500	0.8	Cr, Cu, Mg, Mn, Zn	Biotin	Mineral oil, PEG. (EV201). Dark red. In 100s.
otc sf	**Total Formula 2 Tablets** (Vitaline)	20[r]	100[o]	10,000[p]	400[j]	30[q]	15	15	25	25	25	25	100	0.4	B, Cr, Cu, I, K, Mg, Mn, Mo, Se, Si, V, Zn. Hesperidin complex, inositol, PABA[iii], rutin.	Biotin, citrus bioflavonoids, vitamin K	Gluten free, lactose free, preservative free, sugar free. In 60s.

MULTIVITAMINS WITH MINERALS (INCLUDING IRON)

	Product & Distributor	Fe[a] mg	Ca[b] mg	A units	D units	E units	B_1 mg	B_2 mg	B_3 mg	B_5 mg	B_6 mg	B_{12} mcg	C mg	Folate[c] mg	Other Minerals	Other Content	Excipients & How Supplied
otc sf	**Total Formula Tablets** (Vitaline)	20[r]	100[o]	7,500[s]	400[j]	30[q]	15	15	25	25	25	25	100	0.4	Cr, Cu, I, K, Mg, Mn, Mo, P, Se, V, Zn. Hesperidin complex, inositol, PABA, rutin.	Biotin, choline, citrus bioflavonoids, vitamin K	Gluten free, lactose free, preservative free, sugar free. Hydrogenated vegetable oil. soybean oil. In 90s.
otc	**One-Daily Tablets** (Geri-Care)	18		5,000	400		2	2.5	20	1	1	1	50				PEG. In 100s and 1,000s.
otc	**One a Day Women's Tablets** (Bayer Healthcare)	18[d]	450[k]	2,500[w]	800	30[e]	1.5	1.7	10	5	2	6	60	0.4	Cr, Cu, Mg, Mn, Se, Zn	Biotin, vitamin K	Maltodextrin, PEG, dextrose, glucose, soy, tartrazine. In 60s.
otc sf	**TabAVite Women's Tablets** (Major)	18[d]	450[k]	2,500[m]	400[j]	30[d]	1.5	1.7	10	5	2	6	60	0.4	Mg, Zn		Lactose free, preservative free, sugar free. Mannitol. In 60s.
otc	**One Daily Dieter's Support** (Bayer)	18[d]	300[k]	2,500[jj]	400[j]	30[e]	1.9	2.1	25	12.5	2.5	7.5	60	0.4	Cr, Cu, Mg, Mn, Se, Zn	Vitamin K	Dextrose, glucose, maltodextrin, PEG. In 100s.
otc	**TotalDay Tablets** (Nature's Blend)	18[n,t]	250[k,rrr,t]	25,000[g]	1,000[j]	100[e]	100	100	100	100	100	100	500	0.1	Cl, Cr, Cu, I, K, Mg, Mn, Mo, P, Se, Zn	Biotin, choline, citrus bioflavonoids complex, inositol, PABA, rutin	Maltodextrin, polydextrose. Timed release. In 120s.
otc	**Viactiv Caplets** (McNeil)	18[d]	200[k]	2,500[zz]	400[j]	33[e]	1.5	1.7	15	10	2	6	60	0.4	Cr, Cu, I, K, Mg, Mn, Mo, Se, Zn	Biotin, lutein, vitamin K	Polydextrose, glucose, PEG, sucralose. Film-coated. In 10s, 60s, 90s, and 120s.
otc	**Centrum Tablets** (Wyeth)	18[d]	200[k,pp]	3,500[g]	400[j]	30[e]	1.5	1.7	20	10	2	6	90	0.5	B, Cl, Cr, Cu, I, K, Mg, Mn, Mo, Ni, P, Se, Si, Sn, V, Zn	Biotin, lutein, lycopene, vitamin K	Hydrogenated palm oil, PEG, polyvinyl alcohol, sucrose. In 50s.
otc	**Viactiv Multi-Vitamin Flavor Glides Caplets** (McNeil Nutrition)	18	200	2,500	400	33	1.5	1.7	15	10	2	6	60	0.4	Cr, Cu, I, K, Mg, Mn, Mo, Se, Zn	Biotin, lutein, vitamin K	Glucose, maltodextrin, polydextrose, sucralose. Berry flavor. In 50s.
otc	**Myadec Tablets** (Pfizer Consumer)	18[d]	162[eee]	5,000[z]	400[oo]	30[e]	1.7	2	20	10	3	6	60	0.4	B, Cl, Cr, Cu, I, K, Mg, Mn, Mo, Ni, P, Se, Si, Sn, V, Zn	Biotin, soy, vitamin K	Glucose, PEG. In 130s.
otc	**Complete Daily with Lutein Tablets** (Rexall Sundown)	18[r]	162[bb]	5,000[aa]	400[j]	45[e]	1.9	2.1	25	12.5	2.5	7.5	120	0.4	B, Cl, Cr, Cu, I, K, Mg, Mn, Mo, Ni, P, Se, Si, Sn, V, Zn	Biotin, citrus bioflavonoids, lutein, vitamin K	Sugar, tartrizine. In 90s.
otc sf	**Certagen Tablets** (Ivax)	18[d]	162[bb]	5,000[m]	400[j]	30[e]	1.5	1.7	20	10	2	6	60	0.4	B, Cl, Cr, Cu, I, K, Mg, Mn, Mo, Ni, P, Se, Si, Sn, V, Zn	Biotin, lutein, vitamin K	Preservative free, sugar free. Mannitol, PEG. In 100s and 1,000s.
otc	**Complete Tablets** (Prime Marketing)	18	162	5,000[w]	400	30	1.5	1.7	20	10	2	6	60	0.4	B, Cl, Cr, Cu, I, K, Mg, Mn, Mo, Ni, P, Se, Si, Sn, V, Zn	Biotin, lutein, vitamin K	Mannitol, mineral oil, sucrose. In 130s.
otc	**SunVite Tablets** (Rexall Sundown)	18[d]	162[bb]	3,500[fff]	400[j]	30[e]	1.5	1.7	20	10	2	6	60	0.4	B, Cl, Cr, Cu, I, K, Mg, Mn, Mo, Ni, P, Se, Si, Sn, V, Zn	Biotin, lutein, lycopene, vitamin K	Mannitol, PEG. In 130s.
otc	**Advanced Formula Cerovite Tablets** (Rugby)	18[d]	162[cc]	3,500[m]	400	30[e]	1.5	1.7	20	10	2	6	60	0.4	B, Cl, Cr, Cu, I, K, Mg, Mn, Mo, Ni, P, Se, Si, Sn, V, Zn	Biotin, lutein, lycopene, soy, vitamin K	PEG. In 130s.
otc	**One a Day Maximum Tablets** (Bayer Healthcare)	18[d]	162[bb]	2,500[w]	400[oo]	30[e]	1.5	1.7	20	10	2	6	60	0.4	B, Cl, Cr, Cu, I, K, Mg, Mn, Mo, Ni, P, Se, Si, Sn, V, Zn	Biotin, vitamin K	Dextrose, PEG. In 100s.
otc	**Multi-Day plus Minerals Tablets** (Nature's Bounty)	18[d]	162[bb]	2,500[dd]	400[j]	30[e]	1.5	1.7	20	10	2	6	60	0.4	B, Cl, Cr, Cu, I, K, Mg, Mn, Mo, Ni, P, Se, Si, Sn, V, Zn	Biotin, vitamin K	In 100s.

MULTIVITAMINS WITH MINERALS (INCLUDING IRON)

	Product & Distributor	Fe[a] mg	Ca[b] mg	A units	D units	E units	B_1 mg	B_2 mg	B_3 mg	B_5 mg	B_6 mg	B_{12} mcg	C mg	Folate[c] mg	Other Minerals	Other Content	Excipients & How Supplied
otc	**Daily Multi Caplets** (Rexall Sundown)	18[d]	162[bb]	2,500[dd]	400[j]	30[e]	1.5	1.7	20	10	2	6	60	0.4	B, Cl, Cr, Cu, I, K, Mg, Mn, Mo, Ni, P, Se, Si, Sn, V, Zn	Biotin, vitamin K	In 100s.
otc sf	**One-Tablet-Daily with Minerals Tablets** (Ivax)	18[d]	162[bb]	2,500[m]	400[j]	30[e]	1.5	1.7	20	10	2	6	60	0.4	B, Cl, Cr, Cu, I, K, Mg, Mn, Mo, Ni, P, Se, Si, Sn, V, Zn	Biotin, vitamin K	Sugar free. In 100s.
otc sf	**TabAVite Maximum Tablets** (Major)	18[d]	162[k,eee]	2,500[fff]	400[j]	30[e]	1.5	1.7	20	10	2	6	60	0.4	B, Cl, Cr, Cu, I, K, Mg, Mn, Mo, Ni, P, Se, Si, Sn, V, Zn	Biotin, vitamin K	Lactose free, sugar free. In 60s.
otc	**Calcet Plus Tablets** (Mission)	18[d]	160[k]	5,000[zz]	400[j]	30[f]	2.25	2.55	30	15	3	9	500	0.8	Zn		PEG. Film-coated. In 60s.
otc	**CertaVite with Lutein Tablets** (Major)	18[d]	160[k]	5,000[g]	400	30[e]	1.5	1.7	20	10	2	6	60	0.4	B, Cl, Cr, Cu, I, K, Mg, Mn, Mo, Ni, P, Se, Si, Sn, V, Zn	Biotin, lutein, vitamin K	Mannitol. Sucrose. In 30s.
otc	**Cerovite Jr. Chewable Tablets** (Rugby)	18[d]	108[bb]	5,000[y]	400[j]	30[l]	1.5	1.7	20	10	2	6	60	0.4	Cr, Cu, I, Mg, Mn, Mo, P, Zn	Biotin, soy, vitamin K	Aspartame, phenylalanine 8 mg, sucrose, sugar. In 60s. Animal shapes.
otc	**Centrum Kids Dora the Explorer Chewable Tablets** (Wyeth)	18[r]	108[k]	3,500[dd]	400[oo]	30[e]	1.5	1.7	20	10	2	6	60	0.4	Cr, Cu, I, Mg, Mn, Mo, P, Zn	Biotin, vitamin K	Aspartame, dextrose, glucose, lactose, mannitol, phenylalanine, sucrose. Cherry, fruit punch, and orange flavors. In 60s.
otc	**Centrum Kids SpongeBob Squarepants Chewable Tablets** (Wyeth)	18[r]	108[k]	3,500[dd]	400[oo]	30[e]	1.5	1.7	20	10	2	6	60	0.4	Cr, Cu, I, Mg, Mn, Mo, P, Zn	Biotin, vitamin K	Aspartame, dextrose, glucose, lactose, mannitol, phenylalanine, sucrose. Cherry, fruit punch, and orange flavors. In 60s.
otc	**Centrum Chewable Tablets** (Wyeth)	18[r]	108[k]	3,500[dd]	400[oo]	30[e]	1.5	1.7	20	10	2	6	60	0.4	Cr, Cu, I, Mg, Mn, Mo, P, Zn	Biotin, vitamin K	Aspartame, glucose, lactose, dextrose, mannitol, phenylalanine, sucrose. Orange flavor. In 50s.
otc	**Centrum Kids Complete Tablets** (Wyeth)	18[r]	108[k]	3,500[dd]	400[ccc]	30[e]	1.5	1.7	20	10	2	6	60	0.4	Cr, Cu, I, Mg, Mn, Mo, P, Zn	Biotin, vitamin K	Aspartame, dextrose, lactose, mannitol, phenylalanine, sucrose, sugar. In 100s. Rugrat shapes.
otc	**Flintstones Complete Chewable Tablets** (Bayer Healthcare)	18[d]	100	3,000[ee]	400	30[l]	1.5	1.7	15	10	2	6	60	0.4	Cu, I, Mg, Na, P, Zn	Biotin, choline	Aspartame, hydrogenated vegetable oil, phenylalanine, sorbitol, soybean oil, sucrose, xylitol. In 60s, 150s, and 200s.
otc	**Centrum Performance Tablets** (Wyeth)	18[d]	100[k]	3,500[dd]	400[j]	60[e]	4.5	5.1	40	12	6	18	120	0.4	B, Cl, Cr, Cu, I, K, Mg, Mn, Mo, Ni, P, Se, V, Zn	Biotin, Ginkgo biloba leaf, ginseng root, vitamin K	Glucose, hydrogenated palm oil, PEG, polyvinyl alcohol, sucrose. In 45s.
otc	**Complete Energy Caplets** (Rexall Sundown)	18[r]	100[bb]	5,000[aa]	400[j]	60[e]	4.5	5.1	35	10	6	21	120	0.4	B, Cl, Cr, Cu, I, K, Mg, Mn, Mo, Ni, P, Se, Si, Sn, V, Zn	American ginseng extract, biotin, citrus bioflavonoids, Ginkgo biloba extract, guarana extract, lutein, vitamin K	In 60s.
otc	**Complete Winnie the Pooh Chewable Tablets** (NatureSmart)	18[ff]	100[bb]	5,000[gg]	400[j]	30[e]	1.5	1.7	20	10	2	6	60	0.4	Cu, I, Mg, Zn	Biotin	Dextrose, fructose, xylitol. Cherry, grape, and orange flavors. In 60s and 120s.
otc	**One-a-Day Kids Complete (Bugs Bunny and Friends) Chewable Tablets** (Bayer Healthcare)	18[d]	100	3,000[dd]	400	30[l]	1.5	1.7	15	10	2	6	60	0.4	Cu, I, Mg, P, Zn	Biotin	Aspartame, hydrogenated vegetable oil, phenylalanine, sorbitol, xylitol. In 60s.
otc	**One-a-Day Kids Complete (Scooby Doo) Chewable Tablets** (Bayer Healthcare)																

MULTIVITAMINS WITH MINERALS (INCLUDING IRON)

	Product & Distributor	Fe[a] mg	Ca[b] mg	A units	D units	E units	B_1 mg	B_2 mg	B_3 mg	B_5 mg	B_6 mg	B_{12} mcg	C mg	Folate[c] mg	Other Minerals	Other Content	Excipients & How Supplied
otc	**Vitamins To Go Maximum Tablets** (Rexall Sundown)	18[r]	777[bb]	5,000[m]	525[j]	445[e]	1.9	2.1	25	12.5	2.5	7.5	1,120	0.4	B, Cl, Cr, Cu, I, K, Mg, Mn, Mo, Na, Ni, P, Se, Sn, V, Zn	Biotin, citrus bioflavonoids, Eleuthro-Siberian root, lutein, rose hips, vitamin K	Soybean oil. In 30s.
otc sf	**Yelets Teenage Formula Tablets** (Freeda)	18[d]	60[ss]	5,000[hh]	400[oo]	30[q]	10	10	25	10	10	10	100	0.4	I, Mg, Mn, Se, Zn	Biotin, L-lysine	Gluten free, lactose free, sugar free. Kosher. In 100s.
otc sf	**High Potency Vitamins and Minerals Tablets** (Major)	18[d]	60[eee]	5,000[zz]	400[j]	30[e]	1.5	1.7	20	10	2	6	60	0.4	Cu, I, K, Mn, P, Zn	Soy	Gluten free, lactose free, preservative free, sugar free. In 100s.
otc	**Daily-Vite With Iron and Beta-Carotene Tablets** (Rugby)	18[d]		5,000[dd]	400[j]	30[e]	1.5	1.7	20	10	2	6	60	0.4			Dextrose, PEG, soy, sucrose. In 100s and 1,000s.
otc	**Geritol Complete Tablets** (GlaxoSmithKline Consumer Healthcare)	16	148	6,100[jj]	400	30	1.5	1.7	20	13	2	6.7	57	0.38	Cl, Cr, Cu, I, K, Mg, Mn, Mo, P, Se, Zn	Biotin, soy, vitamin K	In 100s.
otc	**Multilex T & M** (Rugby)	15[d]		10,000[kk]	400	5.5[e]	15	10	100	10	2	7.5	150		Cu, I, Mg, Mn, Zn		Lactose, PEG. In 100s.
otc sf	**Generix-T** (Ivax)	15[ff]	58[eee]	10,000[kk]	400[j]	5.5[e]	15	10	100	10	2	7	150		Cu, I, Mg, Mn, Zn		Sugar free. Mannitol. In 100s.
otc	**Fosfree** (Mission)	14.5[n]	175.5[yy]	1,500[zz]	150[j]		4.5	2	10.5	1	2.5	2	50				PEG. In 60s and 120s.
otc sf	**Monocaps** (Freeda)	14[d]	50[ss]	5,000[hh]	400	15[q]	15	15	40	15	15	15	120	0.4	Cu, I, Mg, Mn, Se, Zn	Biotin, L-lysine, lecithin, PABA	Gluten free, lactose free, sugar free. Kosher. In 100s, 250s, and 500s.
otc sf	**Superior 35 Tablets** (Mason)	12[n]	70	10,000[g]	400	100[e]	50	50	100	100	50	50	250	0.4	Cu, Cr, I, K, Mg, Mn, Mo, P, Se, Zn	Acerola, betaine, bioflavonoids, biotin, choline, desiccated liver, L-glutamic acid, hesperidin, inositol, L-lysine, PABA, rutin	Extended release. Gluten free, sugar free. In 60s.
otc	**Vigomar Forte Tablets** (Marlop)	12[d]		10,000	400[oo]	15	10	10	100	20	5	5	200		Cu, I, Mg, Mn, Zn		In 100s.
otc	**NanoVM 4-8 Years Powder** (Solace)	10[d]	800[qq]	1,332[dd]	200[j]	10[f]	0.6	0.6	8	3	0.6	1.2	25	0.2	Cr, Cu, I, K, Mg, Mn, Mo, P, Se, Zn	Biotin, vitamin K	In 100 g.
otc sf	**Vitalets Chewable Tablets** (Freeda)	10[d]	80[eee]	2,500[hh]	200[oo]	15[q]	0.75	0.85	10	5	1	3	40	0.2	Mg, Mn, P, Zn	Biotin	Gluten free, lactose free, sugar free. Mannitol, sorbitol. Orange, raspberry, and carob flavors. In 100s and 250s.
Rx	**Strovite Forte Caplets** (Everett)	10[d]		4,000[dd]	400[j]	60[e]	20	20	100	25	25	50	500	1	Cr, Cu, Mg, Mo, Se, Zn	Biotin	Mineral oil, PEG, sucrose. (EV0204). Dark green. Scored. In 100s.
otc sf	**Quintabs-M Tablets** (Freeda)	10[d]	30[cc]	5,000[hh]	400[oo]	50[q]	30	30	100	30	30	30	300	0.4	Cu, I, Mg, Mn, Se, Zn	Biotin, PABA	Gluten free, lactose free, sugar free. In 100s, 250s, and 500s.
otc	**Tri-Vi-Sol Drops** (Enfamil)	10[ff]		1,500[s]	400[j]								35				Gluten free, lactose free. Fruit flavor. In 50 mL bottles.
Rx	**Multivitamin Iron and Fluoride Drops** (Hi-Tech)	10[ff]		1,500	400[oo]	5[q]	0.5	0.6	8		0.4		35		Fluoride		Fruit flavor. In 50 mL with dropper.
Rx	**PolyVitamin with Fluoride 0.5 mg Drops** (Hi-Tech)	10[ff]		1,500	400[oo]	5[q]	0.5	0.6	8		0.4		35		Fluoride		In 50 mL.
Rx	**PolyVitamin with Fluoride 0.25 mg Drops** (Hi-Tech)	10[ff]		1,500	400[oo]	5[q]	0.5	0.6	8		0.4		35		Fluoride		In 50 mL.
otc	**Apetigen-Plus Tablets** (Kramer-Novis)	10[n]				30	15	8.5	80	20	8	6	225		Zn	Lysine	Sucrose. In 60s.
otc	**One a Day All-Day Energy Tablets** (Bayer Consumer)	9[d]	250[k]	3,500[uu]	400[j]	30[e]	3	3.4	40	10	4	12	60	0.4	B, Cl, Cr, Cu, I, K, Mg, Mn, Mo, Ni, Se, Si, Sn, V, Zn	Biotin, guarana blend, soy, vitamin K	Castor oil, glucose, PEG, polyvinyl alcohol, tartrazine. In 50s.

MULTIVITAMINS WITH MINERALS (INCLUDING IRON)

	Product & Distributor	Fe[a] mg	Ca[b] mg	A units	D units	E units	B_1 mg	B_2 mg	B_3 mg	B_5 mg	B_6 mg	B_{12} mcg	C mg	Folate[c] mg	Other Minerals	Other Content	Excipients & How Supplied
otc	**One a Day Active Tablets** (Bayer Consumer)	9[d]	110[k]	5,000[uu]	400[oo]	60[e]	4.5	5.1	40	10	6	18	120	0.4	B, Cl, Cr, Cu, I, K, Mg, Mn, Mo, Ni, Se, Si, Sn, V, Zn	American ginseng extract, biotin, soy, vitamin K	PEG, glucose. In 50s.
otc	**ProRenal Vital** (Nephroceuticals)	8[d]			800[j]		1.5	2	20	5	10	2.5	60	0.8	Cu, Se, Zn	Biotin	In 30s and 90s.
otc	**NanoVM 1-3 Years Powder** (Solace)	7[d]	500[qq]	1,000[dd]	200[j]	9[f]	0.5	0.5	6	2	0.5	0.9	15	0.15	Cr, Cu, K, I, Mg, Mn, Mo, P, Se, Zn	Biotin, vitamin K	In 100 g.
otc	**Ragus Tablets** (Miller)	6.67[n]	193.33[eee]	1,666.67	133.33	3.33	6.67	1	26.67	1.67	1.67	3	33.33		Cu, I, Mg, Mn, P, Zn	DL-methionine, L-lysine	In 100s.
otc sf	**Ultra Freeda with Iron Tablets** (Freeda)	6[d]	83.33[x]	1,666.67[s,w]	133.33[ccc]	66.67[q]	16.67	16.67	33.33	33.33	16.67	33.33	333.33	0.27	Cr, I, K, Mg, Mn, Mo, Se, Zn	Bioflavonoids, biotin, choline, inositol, PABA	Gluten free, lactose free, sugar free. In 90s and 180s.
otc	**Complere Tablets** (Miller)	5[ggg]	150[eee]	3,333.33	133.33	20[l]	5	5	16.67	5	5	5	66.67	0.03	Cr, Cu, I, K, Mg, Mn, P, Se, Zn	Biotin, DL-methionine, L-lysine	In 100s.
otc sf	**Hairvite Tablets** (Major)	4.5[t]	75[eee]	5,000[zz]		30[aaa]	2	4	35	50	2	6		0.4	I, Mn, Zn	Biotin, choline, inositol, PABA	Gluten free, sugar free, lactose free, preservative free. Hydrogenated cottonseed oil. In 50s.
otc	**Alka-Seltzer Plus Immunity Complex Effervescent Tablets** (Bayer)	4.5[ooo]		2,140[g]	350[j]	45[e]					6.5	9.6	1,000	0.4	Cu, Se, Zn	Sodium	Acesulfame K, aspartame, maltodextrin, phenylalanine, soy, sucrose, sulfites. In 10s and 20s.
otc sf	**Apetigen Plus Liquid** (Kramer-Novis)	4.17[n]					3.33	3.33	66.67	6.67	0.67	8.33			Zn	L-lysine	Alcohol free, sugar free. Castor oil, parabens, sorbitol. Orange flavor. In 240 mL.
otc sf	**Maximum Red Tablets** (Vitaline)	3.33[xx]	83[ww]	2,500[vv]	66.5[j]	66.5[q]	16.5	8	31.5	66.5	16.5	16.5	200	0.13	B, Cr, Cu, I, K, Mg, Mn, Mo, Na, Se, Si, V, Zn	Biotin, choline, citrus bioflavonoids, inositol, lysine, PABA	Gluten free, preservative free, sugar free. In 180s.
otc	**Sclerex Tablets** (Miller)	3.33[n]	8.33	833.33[s]	66.67	33.33	1.67	1.67	3.33	2.5	1.67	1.67	33.33	0.033	Cu, I, Mg, Mn, Zn	Inositol, succinate	In 60s.
otc sf	**Lysiplex Plus Liquid** (Kramer-Novis)	3.33[tt]		1666.67[s]			16.67[k]	5	16.67	16.67	16.67	16.67		0.27	Cu, Mo, Zn	Biotin, lysine	Sugar free. Parabens, sucralose. Orange flavor. In 178 and 474 mL.
otc sf	**Biotect Plus Liquid** (Advanced Generic)	3.33[sss]		1,666.67[s]	133.33	33.33[e]	16.67	16.67	16.67	16.67	16.67	16.67	166.67	0.33	Cr, Cu, Mg, Mn, Mo, Se, Zn	Biotin, choline, inositol, lysine	Alcohol free, dye free, sugar free. Acesulfame K, glycerin, methylparaben, polysorbate 80, xylitol. Strawberry flavor. In 473 mL.
Rx	**Strovite Forte Syrup** (Everett)	3.33[n]		1,333.33[hh]	133.33[j]	10[l]	5	5.67	33.33	8.33	6.67	6.67	100	0.33	Cr, Cu, Mg, Mn, Se, Zn	Biotin	In 473 mL.
otc	**Fortavit Liquid** (Portal)	3.33[ff]		166.67			16.67	16.67	16.67	16.67	16.67	15	83.33	0.3	Cu, Zn	Biotin, L-lysine	Gluten free. Parabens, saccharin. Cherry flavor. In 236 mL.
otc	**Gynovite Plus Tablets** (Optimox)	3[t]	83.33[u]	833.33[v]	66.67	66.67[q]	1.67	1.67	3.33	1.67	3.33	20.83	30	0.07	B, Cr, Cu, I, Mg, Mn, Se, Zn	Biotin, PABA, betaine, pancreatin 4x, inositol, hesperidin, rutin	In 180s.
otc	**Centrum Cardio Tablets** (Wyeth)	3[d]	54[pp]	1,750[y]	200[j]	15[e]	0.75	0.85	10	5	2.5	100	30	0.2	B, Cl, Cr, Cu, I, K, Mg, Mn, Mo, Ni, P, Se, Si, Sn, V, Zn	Biotin, phytosterols, soy, vitamin K	PEG, polyvinyl alcohol, sucrose. In 60s.
otc	**Androvite for Men Tablets** (Optimox)	3[t]		4,166.67[ii]	66.67[j]	66.67[q]	8.33	8.33	8.33	16.67	16.67	20.83	166.67	0.07	B, Cr, Cu, I, Mg, Mn, Se, Zn	Betaine, biotin, hesperidin, inositol, PABA, pancreatin 4x, rutin	In 80s.
otc	**Certagen Liquid** (Ivax)	3[n]		833.33[s]	133.33[j]	10[e]	0.5	0.57	6.67	3.33	0.67	2	20		Cr, I, Mn, Mo, Zn	Biotin	Edetate disodium, ethyl alcohol, parabens, sucrose, sugar. Fruit flavor. In 237 mL.
otc	**CertaVite Liquid** (Major)	3[n]		433.33[s]	133.33[j]	10[e]	0.5	0.57	6.67	3.33	0.67	2	20		Cr, I, Mn, Mo, Zn	Biotin	Alcohol, sucrose. Orange and lemon flavors. In 237 mL.

MULTIVITAMINS WITH MINERALS (INCLUDING IRON)

	Product & Distributor	Fe[a] mg	Ca[b] mg	A units	D units	E units	B_1 mg	B_2 mg	B_3 mg	B_5 mg	B_6 mg	B_{12} mcg	C mg	Folate[c] mg	Other Minerals	Other Content	Excipients & How Supplied
otc	**Centrum High Potency Liquid** (Wyeth)	3[n]		433.33[s]	133.33[j]	10[e]	0.5	0.57	6.67	3.33	0.67	2	20		Cr, I, Mn, Mo, Zn	Biotin	Ethyl alcohol, sucrose, sugar, PEG, castor oil. In 237 mL.
otc sf	**VITa-PMS Plus Tablets** (Cyclin)	2.5[t]	166.67[k]	666.67[s]	16.67[j]	16.67[hhh]	4.17	4.17	4.17	4.17	16.67	10.41	250	0.03	Cr, Cu, I, K, Mg, Mn, Se, Zn	Betaine, biotin, choline, citrus bioflavonoids, inositol, PABA, rutin, lipase, amylase and protease activity	Sugar free, lactose free. In 100s.
otc	**Theramill Plus Capsules** (Miller)	2.5[ll]	66.67[mm]	3,500[nn]	33.33	66.67[f]	12.5	6.33	33.33	16.67	16.67	16.67	166.67	0.07	B, Cr, Cu, I, K, Mg, Mn, Mo, Se, V, Zn	Bioflavonoids, biotin, choline, inositol, PABA, pantethine, pyridoxal 5 phosphate	In 180s.
otc sf	**VITa-PMS Tablets** (Rugby)	2.5[t]	20.84[t]	2083.83[s]	16.67[j]	16.67[hhh]	4.17	4.17	4.17	4.17	50	10.42	250	0.03	Cr, Cu, I, K, Mg, Mn, Se, Zn	Biotin, betaine, choline, citrus bioflavonoids, inositol, lipase, amylase and protease activity, PABA	Lactose free, sugar free. In 100s.
otc	**Geri-Vite Liquid** (Ivax)	2.5[n]					0.83	0.42	8.33	1.67	0.17	0.17			I, Mg, Mn, Zn	Choline	Alcohol 18%, sorbitol, saccharin, sugar. Sherry wine flavor. In 473 mL.
otc	**Geravim Liquid** (Major)	2.5[n]					0.83	0.42	8.33	1.67	0.17	0.17			I, Mg, Mn, Zn	Choline	Alcohol 18%, sucrose. Sherry wine flavor. In 473 mL.
otc	**Optivite PMT for Women Tablets** (Optimox)	2.5[t]	20.83	2083.33[rr]	16.7[j]	16.7[q]	4.17	4.17	4.17	4.17	50	10	250	0.03	Cr, I, K, Mg, Mn, Se, Zn	Biotin, choline, citrus bioflavonoids, betaine, pancreatin 4X, inositol, PABA, rutin	In 180s.
otc	**Mega VM-80 Tablets** (Nature's Bounty)	2[n]	19[bbb]	8,000[v]	400[j]	125[f]	80	80	80	80	80	80	250	0.4	B, Cr, Cu, I, K, Mg, Mn, Mo, Se, Zn	Alfalfa leaf powder, betaine, citrus bioflavonoids, biotin, coenzyme Q10, choline, garlic, hesperidin complex, inositol, Korean ginseng, PABA, parsley powder, pycnogenol, rice bran powder, rutin, watercress powder	In 60s.
otc sf	**Freedavite Tablets** (Freeda)	1.8[d]	20[cc]	5,000[hh]	400[oo]	30[q]	1.5	1.7	20	10	2	6	60	0.4	Cu, I, Mg, Mn, Se, Zn	Biotin	Sugar free, gluten free, lactose free. In 100s and 250s.

MULTIVITAMINS WITH MINERALS (INCLUDING IRON)

	Product & Distributor	Fe[a] mg	Ca[b] mg	A units	D units	E units	B_1 mg	B_2 mg	B_3 mg	B_5 mg	B_6 mg	B_{12} mcg	C mg	Folate[c] mg	Other Minerals	Other Content	Excipients & How Supplied
otc	**K-PAX Immune Support Capsules** (K-PAX)	1.125[jjj]	50[kkk]	1,250[jj]	25[j]	25[lll]	3.75	3.75	3.75	3.75	12.5	0.16	125	0.05	B, Cr, Cu, I, K, Mg, Mn, Mo, Se, Zn	N-acetyl-L-cysteine, acetyl-L-carnitine HCl, alpha lipoic acid, betaine HCl, biotin, choline, citrus bioflavo-noid complex, inositol (from soy), L-glutamic acid, mixed tocopherol blend	In 240s (60 packets of 8 capsules).

[a] Iron content expressed in mg elemental iron.
[b] Calcium content expressed in mg elemental calcium.
[c] As folic acid.
[d] As ferrous fumarate.
[e] As dl-alpha-tocopheryl acetate.
[f] As d-alpha-tocopherol acetate.
[g] As beta-carotene.
[h] As ferrous bis-glycinate chelate.
[i] As polysaccharide iron complex.
[j] As cholecalciferol.
[k] As calcium carbonate.
[l] As vitamin E acetate.
[m] As retinyl acetate and beta-carotene.
[n] As ferrous gluconate.
[o] As calcium carbonate, citrate, phosphate.
[p] As 50% from natural mixed carotenoids, 50% as palmitate.
[q] As d-alpha-tocopheryl succinate.
[r] As carbonyl iron.
[s] As palmitate.
[t] As amino acid chelate.
[u] As calcium citrate.
[v] As retinyl palmitate.
[w] 20% as beta-carotene.
[x] As calcium carbonate, ascorbate, and citrate.
[y] 29% as beta-carotene.
[z] 25% as beta-carotene.
[aa] As retinyl acetate and 40% as beta-carotene.
[bb] As dicalcium phosphate and calcium carbonate.
[cc] As calcium ascorbate and calcium carbonate.
[dd] As vitamin A acetate and beta-carotene.
[ee] 33% as beta-carotene.
[ff] As ferrous sulfate.
[gg] 78% as beta-carotene and retinyl acetate.
[hh] As vitamin A palmitate and beta-carotene.
[ii] As retinyl palmitate and 80% as beta-carotene.
[jj] 100% as beta-carotene.
[kk] As retinyl acetate.
[ll] As glycine chelate.
[mm] As citrate malate, glycinate, and oyster shell.
[nn] 71% as beta-carotene.
[oo] As ergocalciferol.
[pp] As dibasic calcium phosphate.
[qq] As tricalcium phosphate.
[rr] As retinyl palmitate and 60% as beta-carotene.
[ss] As calcium carbonate and calcium ascorbate.
[tt] As ferric ammonium citrate.
[uu] 40% as beta-carotene.
[vv] 66% as beta-carotene and as retinyl acetate.
[ww] As calcium carbonate and calcium citrate.
[xx] As ferrous succinate and iron chelate.
[yy] As calcium gluconate, lactate, carbonate.
[zz] As vitamin A acetate.
[aaa] As dl-alpha-tocopheryl acetate and d-mixed tocopheryls.
[bbb] As calcium carbonate, d-calcium pantothenate, and calcium phosphate.
[ccc] As ergocalciferol.
[ddd] As di and tricalcium phosphate.
[eee] As dicalcium phosphate.
[fff] As retinyl acetate and beta-carotene.
[ggg] As amino acid rice chelate.
[hhh] As d-alpha-tocopherol.
[iii] PEG = polyethylene glycol; PABA = paraaminobenzoic acid.
[jjj] As picolinate.
[kkk] As citrate, ascorbate, d-calcium pantothenate.
[lll] As d-alpha tocopherol succinate from soy.
[mmm] Ferrous asparto glycinate.
[nnn] As ProAscorb C.
[ooo] As ferrous lactate dihydrate.
[ppp] As calcium ascorbate and calcium threonate.
[qqq] As *Sumalate.*
[rrr] As calcium phosphate.
[sss] As ferric pyrophosphate.

For additional information, refer to the Dietary Reference Intakes of Vitamins and Minerals table.

MULTIVITAMINS WITH MINERALS (EXCEPT IRON)

Content given per capsule, tablet, packet, 5 mL liquid, and 1 mL drops.

	Product & Distributor	A units	D units	E units	B_1 mg	B_2 mg	B_3 mg	B_5 mg	B_6 mg	B_{12} mcg	C mg	Folate mcg	Minerals	Other Content	How Supplied
otc	**SAVision Eye Vitamin and Mineral Supplement Caplets** (Mason Vitamins)	25,000[f]		400[k]							500		Ca, Cu, Zn	Lutein 5 mg, zeaxanthin 1 mg.	Extended-release. Gluten free, preservative free, soy free. Sucrose. In 60s.
otc	**AquADEKS Softgels** (Yasoo Health)	18,167[a]	800[b]	150[c] and 80 mg[d]	1.5	1.7	10	12	1.9	12	75	200[e]	Se, Zn	Biotin 100 mcg, coenzyme Q_{10} 10 mg, vitamin K_1 700 mcg	PEG-1000. Dark brown, oblong. In 60s.
otc	**SourceCF Softgel Capsules** (SourceCF)	16,000[t]	1,000[b]	200[c]	1.5	1.7	20	12	1.9	6	100	200[e]	Zn	Biotin 100 mcg, vitamin K 800 mcg	Beeswax, soybean oil, sucralose, sucrose, vegetable oil. In 60s.
otc	**SourceCF Chewables** (SourceCF)	16,000[t]	1,000[b]	200[u]	1.5	1.7	10	12	1.9	6	100	200[e]	Zn	Biotin 100 mcg, vitamin K 800 mcg	Sucralose, sucrose. Bubble gum flavor. In 90s.
otc	**Ocuvite PreserVision Softgel Capsules** (Bausch & Lomb)	14,320[f]		200[g]							226		Cu, Zn		In 120s.
otc	**Macutek Tablets** (Zyber Pharmaceuticals)												Cu, Zn	Lutein 20 mg, zeaxanthin 4 mg	Dextrose, maltodextrin, sucralose, sucrose. Speckled beige. Orange flavor. In 90s.
otc	**Vitaline Total Formula 3 Tablets** (Integrative Therapeutics)	10,000[h]	400[b]	30[i]	15	15	25	25	25	25	100	400[e]	B, Ca, Cr, Cu, I, K, Mg, Mn, Mo, Se, Si, V, Zn	Biotin 300 mcg, choline 10 mg, citrus bioflavonoids complex 10 mg, hesperidin complex 10 mg, inositol 10 mg, rutin 10 mg, PABA[ccc] 8 mg	Soybean oil. In 60s.
otc	**Lipotriad Caplets** (Numark)	10,000[f]		60[k]	1.5	1.7	20	10	2	6	120	400[e]	Ca, Cu, Mn, Se, Zn	Lutein 250 mcg	Extended-release. Corn oil, cotton seed oil, mannitol, sucrose. In 60s.
otc	**ADEKs Caplets** (Axcan Scandipharm)	9,000[m]	400[b]	150[n]	1.2	1.3	10	10	1.5	12	60	200[e]	Zn	Biotin 50 mcg, vitamin K 150 mcg	Fructose. (ADEKs). Tan, scored. In 60s.
otc	**Oncovite Tablets** (Mission Pharmacal)	9,000[u]	400[b]	100[i]	0.34	0.5	5	2.3	25	1.6	500	400	Zn		PEG. Film-coated. In 100s.
Rx	**Vicap Forte Capsules** (Major)	8,000		50[g]	10	5	25	10	2	10	150	1,000[e]	Mg, Mn, Zn		Lactose. In 100s.
otc	**Ocuvite PreserVision Tablets** (Bausch & Lomb)	7,160[f]		100[k]							113		Cu, Zn		Lactose. In 240s.
otc	**Daily Multi 50+ Caplets** (Sundown[w])	6,000[o]	400[b]	60[k]	1.5	1.7	20	15	3	30	120	400[e]	B, Ca, Cl, Cr, Cu, I, K, Mg, Mn, Mo, Na, Ni, P, Se, Si, V, Zn	Billberry extract 10 mg, biotin 30 mcg, blueberry 10 mg, citrus bioflavonoids 25 mg, European elder 10 mg, lycopene 350 mcg, lutein 300 mcg, tin 15 mcg	Wheat ingredients. In 90s.
otc	**ICaps Tablets** (Alcon)	6,000[f]		60[k]		20					200		Cu, Mn, Se, Zn		Lactose free. PEG, sucrose. Film-coated. In 60s.
otc	**AquADEKs Pediatric Liquid** (Yasoo)	5,751[q]	400[b]	50[c] and 15[d]	0.6	0.6	6	3	0.6		45		Se, Zn	Biotin 15 mcg, coenzyme Q_{10} 2 mg, vitamin K 400 mcg	EDTA, sucralose. In 60 mL bottle with 1 mL graduated dropper.
Rx	**Glutofac-ZX Caplets** (Kenwood)	5,000[r]	400[b]	100[n]	20	20	100	10	25	2,500	200	2,800[e]	Cu, Cr, Mg, Mn, Se, Zn	Biotin 200 mcg, lutein 500 mcg, lycopene 500 mcg	Corn oil, mineral oil, sucrose. (GLUTOFAC-ZX). Lt. lime green. Film-coated. In 60s.
otc sf	**Therapeutic Tablets** (Goldline)	5,000	400[v]	30[k]	3	3.4	20	10	3	9	90	400	Ca	Biotin 30 mcg	Preservative free, sugar free. Mannitol. In 130s.
otc	**Thera Tablets** (Major)	5,000[u]	400[v]	30[k]	3	3.4	20	10	3	9	90	400[e]	Ca	Biotin 30 mcg	Mannitol. In 130s and 1,000s.
otc	**Once Daily Tablets** (HealthSenset)	5,000[dd]	400[b]		2	2.5	20	1	1	1	50		Ca		Mineral oil, PEG. In 100s.
otc	**Restore-X Powder for Solution** (Baxter)	5,000[x]		200[k]	6	6.8	80	40	8	35	500	400[e]	Cu, Mg, Se, Zn	L-arginine (as L-arginine and zinc arginate) 140 mg, L-glutamine 10 g, N-acetyl-L-cysteine 600 mg	In 20 g packets (60s).[y]
otc sf	**Antioxidant Formula Tablets** (Major)	5,000[f]		200[k]							250		Ca, Cu, Mn, Se, Zn		Lactose free, preservative free, sugar free. In 60s.

MULTIVITAMINS WITH MINERALS (EXCEPT IRON)

	Product & Distributor	A units	D units	E units	B_1 mg	B_2 mg	B_3 mg	B_5 mg	B_6 mg	B_{12} mcg	C mg	Folate mcg	Minerals	Other Content	How Supplied
otc sf	**Oxi-Freeda Tablets** (Freeda)	5,000[f]		150[z]	20	20	40	20	20	20	100		Ca, Se, Zn	L-glutathione 40 mg, L-cysteine 75 mg	Lactose free, sugar free. In 100s and 250s.
otc	**Protegra Softgel Capsules** (Inverness Medical)	5,000[f]		60[bb]							250		Cu, Mn, Se, Zn	Grape seed extract 50 mg	Sorbitol, soybean oil, vegetable oil. In 60s.
otc	**Eyetamins Caplets** (Sundown[w])	5,000[cc]		30[k]							60		Cu, Se, Si, Zn	Lutein 2 mg, zeaxanthin 95 mcg	In 60s.
otc	**OcuSoft VMS Tablets** (OcuSoft)	5,000[f]		30[bb]							60		Cu, Se, Si, Zn		Film-coated. In 60s.
otc	**Opti-gen Tablets** (Goldline)	5,000[f]		30[k]							60		Ca, Cu, P, Se, Zn		Milk and fish ingredients. In 60s.
otc	**SourceCF Drops** (SourceCF)	4,627	500	50	0.5	0.6			0.8	4	45		Zn	Biotin 15 mcg	In 60 mL.
otc	**Centrum Silver Chewable Tablets** (Wyeth)	4,000[ee]	400[b]	70[k]	2.2	2.7	12	10	7	25	75	500[e]	Ca, Cu, Cr, I, Mg, Mn, Mo, Ni, P, Se, Si, Sn, V, Zn	Biotin 45 mcg, lutein 250 mcg	Aspartame, lactose, mannitol, partially hydrogenated soybean oil, phenylalanine, sorbitol, sucrose. Citrus berry flavor. In 60s.
otc	**Oxiplen Capsules** (Medical Prod Panamericana)	3,750[f] and 1,250[ff]		100[gg]							250		Mn, Se, Zn	Catalase 25 mg, L-cysteine 0.25 mg, L-glutathione 6.25 mg, L-taurine 50 mg, super oxide dismutase 50 mg	In 60s.
otc	**Complete Senior Tablets** (HealthSense)	3,500[hh]	400[s]	45[g]	1.5	1.7	20	10	3	25	60	400[e]	B, Ca, Cl, Cr, Cu, I, K, Mg, Mn, Mo, Ni, P, Se, Si, V, Zn	Biotin 30 mcg, lutein 250 mcg, lycopene 300 mcg, vitamin K 10 mcg	Corn oil, mannitol, mineral oil, sucrose. In 60s.
otc	**One A Day Men's Health Formula Tablets** (Bayer)	3,500[ii]	400[v]	45[k]	1.2	1.7	16	5	3	18	90	400[e]	Ca, Cr, Cu, K, Mg, Mn, Se, Zn	Biotin 30 mcg, lycopene 600 mg, vitamin K 20 mcg	Dextrose, fish products, glucose, soy, sucrose. In 100s.
otc	**Daily Multivitamin Vital Body and Cells Formula Tablets** (Bayer)	3,500[kk]	400[b]	30[k]	1.5	1.7	20	10	3	6	60	400[e]	B, Ca, Cr, Cu, I, K, Mg, Mn, Mo, Ni, Se, Si, V, Zn	Alpha-lipoic acid 10 mg, biotin 45 mcg, pomegranate powder (whole fruit) 50 mg, vitamin K 80 mcg	Glucose, PEG, soy, tartrazine. In 60s and 100s.
otc	**Theramill Forte Capsules** (Miller)	3,500[ll]	33.33[s]	66.67[mm]	16.67	12.5	6.67[nn] and 26.67[oo]	16.67	16.67	12.5[pp] and 4.17[qq]	166.67	66.67[e]	B, Ca, Cr, I, K, Mg, Mn, Mo, Se, Si, V, Zn	Bioflavonoids (undiluted) 16.67 mg, biotin 50 mcg, choline bitartrate 12.5 mg, inositol 12.5 mg, PABA 8.33 mg, pantethine 4.17 mg, pyridoxyl 5 phosphate 4.17 mg	In 90s and 180s.
otc	**Dermavite Tablets** (GlaxoSmithKline)	3,500[hh]		60[k]		8.5			10		120	400	Ca, Cr, Cu, Mn, Se, Si, Zn	Biotin 600 mcg, lycopene 5 mg	Light mineral oil, mineral oil, sucrose. Film-coated. In 60s.
otc sf	**Kenwood Therapeutic Liquid** (Kenwood/Bradley)	3,333	133[s]	1.5[k]	2	1	20	2	0.33		50		Ca, K, Mg, Mn, P		Alcohol free, sugar free. In 240 mL.
otc	**ICaps Tablets** (Alcon Vision)	3,300[f]		75[k]		5					200		Ca, Cu, Mn, Se, Si, Zn	Lutein/Zeaxanthin 2 mg	Delayed-release. Lactose free. PEG, sucrose. Film-coated. In 120s.
Rx	**Strovite One Caplets** (Everett Labs)	3,000[ss]	1,000[b]	100[i]	20	5	25	12	25	50	300	1[e]	Cr, Cu, Mg, Mn, Se, Zn	Alpha-lipoic acid 15 mg, biotin 100 mcg, lutein 5 mg	Maltodextrin, soybean oil, sucrose. (EV 0207). White, capsule shape. In 90s.
Rx	**Strovite Advance Caplets** (Everett)	3,000[ss]	400[b]	100[n]	20	5	25	15	25	50	300	1,000[e]	Cr, Cu, Mg, Mn, Se, Zn	Alpha-lipoic acid 15 mg, biotin 100 mcg, lutein 5 mg	Mineral oil, sucrose. (EV 0208). In 100s.
Rx	**Nutravance Tablets** (Breckenridge)	3,000[ss]	400	100[n]	20	5	25	15	25	50	300	1,000[e]	Cr, Cu, Mg, Mn, Se, Zn	Alpha-lipoic acid 15 mg, biotin 100 mcg, lutein 5 mg	PEG. (B 128). White, oval. Film-coated. In 100s.
Rx	**Strovite Advance + D Caplets and Tablets** (Everett Laboratories)	3,000[ss]	400[d]; 600[b]	100[n]	20	5	25	15	25	50	300	1,000[e]	Cr, Cu, Mg, Mn, Se, Zn	Alpha lipoic acid 15 mg, biotin 100 mcg, lutein 5 mg	Glucose, sucrose. In UD 30s. *Caplet*: (EV 0208). White, oblong. *Tablet*: White, round.

MULTIVITAMINS WITH MINERALS (EXCEPT IRON)

	Product & Distributor	A units	D units	E units	B_1 mg	B_2 mg	B_3 mg	B_5 mg	B_6 mg	B_{12} mcg	C mg	Folate mcg	Minerals	Other Content	How Supplied
otc	**One A Day Women's 50+ Advantage Tablets** (Bayer)	2,500[tt]	800[b]	33[k]	4.5	3.4	20	15	6	25	60	400[e]	Ca,[jj] Cu, Cr, I, Mg, Mn, Mo, Se, Si, Zn	Biotin 30 mcg, Ginkgo biloba extract (leaf) 120 mg, vitamin K 20 mcg	Dextrose, glucose, PEG, soy, tartrazine. In 50s and 100s.
otc	**Centrum Silver Tablets** (Wyeth)	2,500[uu]	500[b]	50[k]	1.5	1.7	20	10	3	25	90	500[e]	B, Ca, Cl, Cr, Cu, I, K, Mg, Mn, Mo, Ni, P, Se, Si, V, Zn	Biotin 30 mcg, lutein 250 mcg, lycopene 300 mcg, vitamin K 30 mcg	Hydrogenated palm oil, PEG, sucrose. In 60s.
otc	**CertaVite Senior Tablets** (Major)	2,500[u]	400[b]	45[k]	1.5	1.7	20	10	3	25	60	400[e]	B, Ca, Cl, Cr, Cu, I, K, Mg, Mn, Mo, Ni, P, Se, Si, V, Zn	Biotin 30 mcg, lutein 250 mcg, vitamin K 10 mcg	In 60s, 90s, and 1,000s.
otc	**One A Day Men's 50+ Advantage Tablets** (Bayer)	2,500[tt]	400[b]	33[k]	4.5	3.4	20	15	6	25	120	400[e]	Ca,[jj] Cr, Cu, I, K, Mg, Mn, Mo, Se, Si, Zn	Biotin 30 mcg, Ginkgo biloba extract (leaf) 120 mg, lycopene 600 mcg, vitamin K 20 mcg	Glucose, PEG, sucrose. In 50s.
otc	**One A Day Cholesterol Plus Tablets** (Bayer)	2,500[kk]	400[v]	*30[k]	1.5	1.7	20	10	2	6	60	400[e]	B, Ca,[jj] Cr, Cu, I, K, Mg, Mn, Mo, Se, Si, Zn	Biotin 50 mcg, policosanol (*Saccharum officinarum* L.) 10 mg	PEG. In 50s.
otc	**Flintstones Plus Calcium Chewable Tablets** (Bayer)	2,500[tt]	400[s]	15[g]	1.05	1.2	13.5		1.05	4.5	60	300[e]	Ca,[jj] Na		Aspartame, phenylalanine, sorbitol. In 60s.
otc *sf*	**One A Day Kids Scooby-Doo Plus Calcium Chewable Tablets** (Bayer)												Ca,[jj] Na		Sugar free. Aspartame, phenylalanine, sorbitol. In 50s.
otc	**Daily Betic Tablets** (Optimum)	2,500	200[b]	30[i]	1.5	1.7	20	10	2.5	5	60	200[e]	Ca, Cr, I, K, Mg, Mn, Se, V, Zn	Alpha-lipoic acid 50 mg, biotin 75 mcg, lutein 250 mcg	PEG. In 60s.
otc *sf*	**PowerVites Tablets** (Green Turtle Bay)	2,500[f]	150[s]	12.5[g]	6.25	6.25	25	25	12.5	6.25	125	150[e]	B, Ca, Cr, Cu, K, Mg, Mn, Se, Zn	Bee pollen 125 mg, betaine hydrochloride 5 mg, biotin 25 mcg, choline bitartrate 12.5 mg, citrus bioflavonoids 12.5 mg, rutin 2.5 mg, hesperidin (citrus) 2.5 mg, inositol 6.25 mg, and PABA 6.25 mg	Lactose free, sugar free. In 100s and 200s.
otc *sf*	**Vitaline Maximum Blue Tablets** (Integrative Therapeutics)	2,500[vv]	16.5[b]	66.5[z]	16.5	8	31.5	66.5	16.5	16.5	200	133[e]	B, Ca, Cr, Cu, I, K, Mg, Mn, Mo, Na, Se, Si, V, Zn	Biotin 50 mcg, lysine (as L-lysine hydrochloride) 100 mg, choline 33 mg, inositol 16.5 mg, mixed bioflavonoids 50% (from citrus fruits) 16.5 mg, PABA 8 mg	Gluten free, lactose free, sugar free. Fractionated coconut oil, soybean oil. In 180s.
otc *sf*	**Vitaline Maximum Green Tablets** (Integrative Therapeutics)												B, Ca, Cr, I, K, Mg, Mn, Mo, Na, Se, Si, V, Zn	Biotin 50 mcg, lysine (as L-lysine hydrochloride) 100 mg, choline 33 mg, inositol 16.5 mg, mixed bioflavonoids 50% (from citrus fruits) 16.5 mg, PABA 8 mg	Gluten free, lactose free, sugar free. Fractionated coconut oil, soybean oil. In 180s.
otc	**Eye Health & Vitality Tablets** (Bayer Nutritional Science)	2,500[f]		200[k]							175		Ca, Cu, Na, Se, Si, Zn	Lutein/Zeaxanthin blend 3 mg, fruit/vegetable blend 50 mg	Soy, tartrazine. In 90s.
otc	**Cardenz Tablets** (Miller)	2,000	100[s]	5[g]			20		1.5	1	25		I, K, Mg, Si	Inositol 30 mg, PABA 9 mg	In 100s.
otc *sf*	**Ultra Freeda Tablets** (Freeda)	1,666.67[xx]	133.33[v]	66.67[z]	16.67	16.67	33.33	33.33	16.67	33.33	333.33	266 and 67[e]	Ca, Cr, I, K, Mg, Mn, Mo, Se, Si, Zn	Bioflavonoids 33.33 mg, biotin 100 mcg, base (containing choline, inositol, PABA) 100 mg	Gluten free, lactose free, sugar free. In 90s, 180s, and 270s.

MULTIVITAMINS WITH MINERALS (EXCEPT IRON)

	Product & Distributor	A units	D units	E units	B_1 mg	B_2 mg	B_3 mg	B_5 mg	B_6 mg	B_{12} mcg	C mg	Folate mcg	Minerals	Other Content	How Supplied
otc	**Hyalex Tablets** (Miller)	1,500	100[zz]	3[aaa]				5		2	30		Mg (oxide), Mg (p-aminobenzoate), Mg (salicylate), Zn		In 100s.
otc	**Biosupp Liquid** (Advanced Generic Corporation)	1,500[ff]	100[b]		6	2	30		2	10		800[e]	Mg, Zn	L-lysine 275 mg	Alcohol, parabens, sucrose. In 473 mL.
otc	**ProCycle Gold Tablets** (Women's Health America[t])	1,250[bbb]	100[b]	100[i]	2.5	2.5	5	2.5	5	31.25	62.5	200[e]	B, Ca, Cr, Cu, I, K, Mg, Mn, Se, Si, Zn	Biotin 100 mcg, proprietary blend 82 mg	Soy. In 120s.
otc sf	**Fiber Choice Chewable Tablets** (GlaxoSmithKline)	1,250	50[s]	15[k]	0.75	0.85	5	2.5	1	3	30	200[e]	Ca, Zn		Sugar free. Fish products, sorbitol. Cherry flavor. In 90s.
otc	**Hep-Forte Softgel Capsules** (Marlyn)	1,200[ff]		10[c]	1	1	10	2	0.5	1	10	60[e]	Zn	Biotin 3.3 mcg, choline 10 mg, inositol 10 mg, liver concentrate 65 mg, liver defatted 194 mg, liver fraction number two 65 mg, methionine 10 mg, yeast dried 65 mg	Soy, soybean oil. In 100s, 200s, and 500s.
otc	**Flintstones Gummies** (Bayer)	1,000[dd]	100[b]	10[g]				2.5	0.5	2.5	15	100[e]	I, Zn	Biotin 37.5 mcg, choline 19 mg, inositol 10 mcg	Glucose, sucrose, vegetable oil. In 60s and 150s.
otc	**Flintstones Sour Gummies** (Bayer)												I, Zn	Biotin 37.5 mcg, choline 19 mg, inositol 10 mcg	Glucose, sucrose, tartrazine. In 60s and 150s.
otc	**One A Day Kids Scooby-Doo Gummies** (Bayer)												I, Zn	Biotin 37.5 mcg, choline 15 mg, inositol 10 mcg	Glucose, sucrose, vegetable oil. In 50s.
otc	**Ocuvite Extra Tablets** (Bausch & Lomb)	1,000[f]		100[k]		3	40				300		Cu, Mn, Se, Zn	L-glutathione 5 mg, lutein 2 mg	In 50s.
otc	**Ocuvite Tablets** (Bausch & Lomb)	1,000[f]		60[k]							200		Cu, Se, Si, Zn	Lutein 2 mg	In 120s.
otc	**Disney Pixar Cars Gummies** (NatureSmart[l])	750[yy]	100[b]	7.5[k]				1.25	0.25	1.5	7.5	100[e]	Ca, I, Mg, Zn	Biotin 22.5 mcg, inositol 5 mcg	Lactose free, preservative free. Coconut oil, corn syrup, sugar. In 60s.
otc	**Disney Pixar Finding Nemo Gummies** (NatureSmart)												I, Mg, Na, Zn	Biotin 22.5 mcg, inositol 5 mcg	Corn syrup, sugar. In 60s.
otc	**Disney Winnie the Pooh Gummies** (NatureSmart)												Ca, I, Mg, Zn	Biotin 22.5 mcg, inositol 5 mcg	Coconut oil, corn syrup, sugar. In 60s.
otc	**The Amazing Spiderman Gummies** (Sundown[w])												I, Mg, Na, Zn	Biotin 22.5 mcg, inositol 5 mcg	Corn syrup, sugar. In 60s.
otc	**Dime Capsules** (Medical Products Panamericana)	625[f]		50[ww]	20				50	10	125	400[e]	Cr, Mg, Se, Zn	Alpha-lipoic acid 20 mg, biotin 25 mcg, L-carnitine 10 mg, L-taurine 50 mg	In 30s.
otc sf	**Zinc Lozenges with A & C Tablets** (National Vitamin)	500[dd]									100		Zn	Bee propolis 50 mg	Sugar free. Sorbitol. Cherry flavor. In 100s.
otc	**Diabetiks Tablets** (Green Turtle Bay)	250[f]		25[g]	10	1.25	7.5		6.25	22.5	75	75[e]	Cr, Cu, Mg, Mn, Mo, Se, Zn	Biotin 62.5 mcg, bilberry extract 25 mg, citrus bioflavonoids 6.25 mg, coenzyme Q_{10} 0.5 mg, Gingko biloba 5 mg, green tea extract 10 mg, huckleberry leaf 50 mg, L-carnitine-L-tartrate 3.75 mg, lipoic acid 2.5 mg, N-acetyl-L-cysteine 25 mg, pine bark extract 0.5 mg, taurine 187.5 mg	In 120s.
Rx	**Vital-D Tablets** (Nephro-Tech)		1,750[b]		1.5	1.7	20	10	10	6	60	1,000[e]	Si, Zn	Biotin 300 mcg	In 100s.

MULTIVITAMINS WITH MINERALS (EXCEPT IRON)

	Product & Distributor	A units	D units	E units	B_1 mg	B_2 mg	B_3 mg	B_5 mg	B_6 mg	B_{12} mcg	C mg	Folate mcg	Minerals	Other Content	How Supplied
otc	**D1000 Plus Tablets** (Mason)		1,000[b]						10	200		400[e]	Ca		PEG. In 60s.
otc	**Rx Support Heartburn & Acid Reflux Tablets** (Mason Vitamins)												Ca		PEG. In 60s.
otc	**Rx Support Heartburn & Acid Reflux Plus Aloe Tablets** (Mason Vitamins)												Ca	Aloe vera powder 100 mg	PEG. In 60s.
otc	**Prosteon Tablets** (Theralogix)		500										B, Ca, Mg, Sr	Vitamin K 25 mcg	In 240s.
Rx sf	**Corvite Free** (Vertical Pharmaceuticals)		400[b]	125	25	3.4	35	5	35	70	500	1.25[e]	Cr, Cu, Mg, Se, Zn	Alpha lipoic acid 10 mg, biotin 75 mcg, coenzyme Q_{10} 35 mg, lutein 400 mcg, lycopene 125 mcg	Dye free, gluten free, lactose free, sugar free. (VP030). White, oval. In 100s.
otc sf	**T-Vites Tablets** (Freeda)		400[v]		25	25	150	25	25	30	100	400[e]	K, Mg, Mn, Zn	Biotin 30 mcg	Gluten free, lactose free, sugar free. In 100s.
Rx sf	**Calafol Tablets** (Alaven)		400[b]						25	425		1,600[e]	Ca	Policosanol 5 mg	Dye free, lactose free, sugar free. (AP 99). Scored. In 90s.
otc	**Caltrate 600 + D Plus Minerals Chewable Tablets** (Wyeth)		400[b]										B, Ca, Cu, Mg, Mn, Zn		Dextrose, mineral oil, partially hydrogenated soybean oil, soy, sucrose. In 60s.
otc	**Caltrate 600 + D Plus Minerals Tablets** (Wyeth)												B, Ca, Cu, Mg, Mn, Zn		Sucrose. In 60s.
otc	**Pro-Cal Tablets** (Pro-Biotiks)		400								30		Ca, Mg, P		Levulose. In 120s and 240s.
otc	**Coral Calcium Plus Vitamin D & Magnesium Capsules** (Mason Vitamins)		400										Ca, Mg		Gluten free, preservative free, soy free. In 60s.
Rx	**Calcium-Folic Acid Plus D Chewable Wafers** (Brookstone)		300[b]						10	125		100[e]	B, Ca, Mg		Fructose. (BP 706). Brown, round. Chocolate flavor. Scored. In 60s.
Rx	**Calcifolic-D Wafers** (Everett)		300[b]						10	125		1,000[e]	B, Ca, Mg, Si		Fructose. Chocolate flavor. In 60s.
otc	**Os Cal Ultra Caplets** (GlaxoSmithKline)		200[b]	15[g]							60		B, Ca, Cu, Mg, Mn, Zn		Lactose, sucrose. In 120s.
otc	**Calcium Magnesium Zinc Caplets** (Nature's Bounty)		200[b]										Ca, Mg, Zn	Sodium 3.33 mg	Film-coated. In 100s.
otc	**Viactiv for Teens Chewable Tablets** (McNeil)												Ca	Sodium 15 mg, vitamin K 40 mcg	Corn syrup, hydrogenated palm kernel oil, nonfat milk, sugars 3 g. Fudge brownie flavor. In 60s.
otc sf	**OstiGen Melts** (U.S. Foods and Pharm)		150										Ca, Cu, K, Mg, P	Vitamin K, sodium 10 mg	Lactose free, sugar free. Maltitol. In chocolate, chocolate mint, and caramel flavors. In 30s and 90s.
otc sf	**Fem-Cal Plus Tablets** (Freeda)		133.33[v]										B, Ca, Mg, Mn, Si		Gluten free, lactose free, sugar free. In 100s and 250s.
otc	**Citracal Plus Tablets** (Mission)		125[b]						5				B, Ca, Cu, Mg, Mn, Zn		PEG. Film-coated. In 150s.
otc	**UpCal D Chewable Tablets** (Global Health)		125[b]										Ca, Mg		Sucralose. Fruit punch and cinnamon flavors. In 120s.
otc	**Calvite P & D Tablets** (Cypress)		120[b]										Ca, P		In 100s.
otc	**Dical-D Tablets** (Abbott)		120[s]										Ca, P.		Hydrogenated vegetable oil. In 100s.
otc	**ICaps MV Tablets** (Alcon)		100[b]	107.5[k]	0.375	2.5	2.5	2.5	0.5	1.5	128	100[e]	Ca, Cr, Cu, I, Mg, Mn, Mo, P, Se, Zn	Biotin 7.5 mcg, lutein 1.67 mg, lycopene 0.075 mg, vitamin K 6.25 mcg, zeaxanthin 0.83 mg	PEG, sucrose. Film-coated. In 50s and 100s.
otc sf	**Fem-Cal Tablets** (Freeda)		100[v]										B, Ca, Mg, Mn, Si		Gluten free, lactose free, sugar free. In 100s and 250s.

MULTIVITAMINS WITH MINERALS (EXCEPT IRON)

	Product & Distributor	A units	D units	E units	B_1 mg	B_2 mg	B_3 mg	B_5 mg	B_6 mg	B_{12} mcg	C mg	Folate mcg	Minerals	Other Content	How Supplied
otc sf	**Fem-Cal Citrate Tablets** (Freeda)		80[v]										B, Ca, Mg, Mn, Si		Gluten free, lactose free, sugar free. In 100s and 250s.
otc	**Joint and Bone Vitality Tablets** (Bayer Nutritional Science)		66.67[b]								20		Ca, Cu, Mn, Na	Chondroitin sulfate 400 mg, glucosamine hydrochloride 500 mg, vitamin K 26.67 mcg	In 30s and 60s.
otc	**Calcibon Suspension** (Kramer-Novis)		66.67[b]										B, Ca, Cu, Mg, Mn, Si, Zn		Aspartame, parabens, phenylalanine. Orange flavor. In 237 mL.
otc	**Preservision Lutein Softgel Capsules** (Bausch & Lomb)			200[g]							226		Cu, Zn	Lutein 5 mgs	In 50s.
otc	**Ecee Plus Tablets** (Edwards)			200[z]							100		Mg, Zn		In 100s.
Rx	**Udamin Caplets** (Kowa Pharm)			150[z], 34 mg[rr]					25	500		2,000[e]	Se, Zn	Lycopene complex 5 mg	Coconut oil, maltodextrin, PEG, polydextrose, soy protein. (PE220). Lt yellow, capsule shape. Film-coated. In 100s.
otc	**Ocuvite DF Tablets** (Bausch & Lomb)			100[g]	0.75		10		1		100			Alpha-lipoic acid 140 mg, genistein 25 mg	In 60s.
Rx sf	**Folpace Tablets** (Alaven)			100[i]					25	425		2,050[e]	Mg		Dye free, lactose free, sugar free. (AP 18). Scored. In 90s.
Rx	**BP Manuvite SP Caplets** (Brookstone)			75[z], 17 mg[rr]					12.5	250		1,000[e]	Se, Si, Zn	Lycopene complex 2.5 mcg, saw palmetto extract 320 mg	Sustained-release. PEG, polydextrose, soy protein. (BP SP). White. Film-coated. In 100s.
Rx	**Udamin SP Caplets** (Kowa Pharm)												Se, Zn	Lycopene complex 2.5 mcg, saw palmetto extract 320 mg	Maltodextrin, polydextrose, PEG, soy protein. (PE820). White, capsule shape. Film-coated. In 100s.
otc	**Z-Bec Caplets** (Inverness)			45[k]	15	10.2	100	25	10	6	600	400[e]	Zn	Biotin 300 mcg	PEG. In 60s.
otc	**Bee Zee Tablets** (Rugby)			45[dd]	15	10.2	100	25	10	6	600	400[e]	Zn	Biotin 300 mcg	Lactose, PEG. In 60s.
otc sf	**Z-Gen Tablets** (Goldline)			45[k]	15	10.2	100	25	10	6	600		Zn		Sugar free. Fish products, mannitol. In 60s.
otc	**Vita-Zinc Tablets** (Major)												Zn		In 60s.
Rx	**Renax 5.5 Caplets** (Everett)			35[g]	3	2	20	10	30	1	100	5,500[e]	Se, Zn	Biotin 300 mcg	Hydrogenated vegetable oil, PEG. (EV2755). Film-coated. In 90s.
Rx	**Renax Caplets** (Everett)			35[i]	3	2	20	10	15	12	50	2,500[e]	Se, Zn	Biotin 300 mcg	Hydrogenated vegetable oil, PEG. (EV 0300). Film-coated. In 90s.
otc sf	**Stress Formula With Zinc Tablets** (Goldline)			30[k]	10	10	100	20	5	12	500	400[e]	Ca, Cu, Si, Zn	Biotin 45 mcg	Preservative free, sugar free. Fish products. In 60s.
otc	**Stress Formula Tablets** (Major)												Ca, P, Si	Biotin 45 mcg	Fish products, mannitol, nuts. In 60s.
otc	**Stress Formula With Zinc Tablets** (Nature's Bounty)												Cu, Si, Zn	Biotin 45 mcg	Fish products, mannitol. In 60s.
Rx	**Dialyvite 3000 Tablets** (Hillestad)			30[z]	1.5	1.7	20	10	25	1	100	3,000[e]	Se, Zn	Biotin 300 mcg	(H). Lt. brown. In 90s.
otc	**Ocuvite Lutein Capsules** (Bausch & Lomb)			30[bb]							60		Cu, Si, Zn	Lutein 6 mg	Lactose. In 36s.
otc	**ProSight Lutein Capsules** (Major)			30[k]							60		Ca, Cu, Si, Zn	Lutein 6 mg.	In 36s.
otc	**Rutiplen C Capsules** (Medical Prod Panamericana)			25[g]							600		Zn	Citrus bioflavonoid complex 100 mg, rutin 50 mg	In 30s.
otc	**Varidin Forte Capsules** (Medical Prod Panamericana)			25[g]							125		Zn	Citrus bioflavonoids 25 mg, diosmin 150 mg, *Hammamelis virginiana* 25 mg, horse chestnut 100 mg, rutin 25 mg	In 60s.

MULTIVITAMINS WITH MINERALS (EXCEPT IRON)

	Product & Distributor	A units	D units	E units	B_1 mg	B_2 mg	B_3 mg	B_5 mg	B_6 mg	B_{12} mcg	C mg	Folate mcg	Minerals	Other Content	How Supplied
otc	**Aminobrain Forte Capsules** (Medical Prod Panamericana)			15^k	5		10		20	20		400^e	Cr, Mg, Se, Zn	Choline 25 mg, Ginkgo biloba 24/6 60 mg, glutamic acid 50 mg, phosphatidyl choline 25 mg, sodium glycerophosphate 32 mg	In 60s.
otc	**Dexatrim Max Slim Packs Fruit Fusion Powder Mix** (Chattem)			5.5^k	0.263	0.3	3.5	1.8	0.35	3	30	70^e	Ca, Cr, K, Mg, Mn	Caffeine 25 mg, ginsenosides 1 mg, green tea 45 mg, sodium 72 mg	Acesulfame K, dextrose, sucralose. In single-use packs (22s).
otc sf	**Time Release Balanced B-50 Tablets** (Major)				50	50	50	50	50	50		400^e	Ca, Si	Biotin 50 mcg, nutritional base (alfalfa, choline bitartrate, inositol, lecithin, PABA, parsley, rice bran, watercress) 50 mg	Lactose free, preservative free, sugar free. In 60s.
otc sf	**Complex B-50 Tablets** (21st Century HealthCare)				50	50	50	10	50	50		400^e	Ca	Biotin 50 mcg	Extended-release. Sugar free, preservative free. In 60s.
otc sf	**Viogen-C Capsules** (Goldline)				20	10	100	18.3	5		300		Mg, Si, Zn		Sugar free. Tartrazine. In 100s.
otc	**Dexatrim Max Caplets** (Chattem)				15	17	20	25	10	60			Ca, Cr	Asian ginseng root standardized extract 250 mg, green tea and oolong tea standardized leaf extracts 600 mg (90 mg epigallocatechin gallate, 200 mg caffeine)	Extended-release. Capsule shape. Film-coated. In 60s.
otc	**Therapeutic B with C Caplets** (Upsher-Smith)				15	10.2	50	10	5		300		Ca		In UD 100s.
otc sf	**High Potency B with C 300 mg Caplet** (Goldline)												Ca		Sugar free. In 130s.
otc	**Total B with C Tablets** (Major)												Ca		In 1,000s.
otc	**Vitaline Biotin Forte Tablets** (Integrative Therapeutics)				10	10		10	25	10	200	800^e	Si, Zn	Biotin 3 mg	Soy lecithin. In 60s.
otc sf	**Sunnie Tablets** (Green Turtle Bay)				2.5	2.5	6.25	12.5	2.5	25	125	100^e	Cu, Mg, Mn, Zn	Betain TMG 125 mg, biotin 12.5 mcg, choline bitartrate 6.25 mg, Gingko biloba (24% flavoglycosides 2.5 mg), inositol 6.25, L-glutamine 37.5 mg, PABA 2.5 mg, St. John's wort 225 mg	Lactose free, sugar free. In 120s.
Rx	**Dialyvite with Zinc Tablets** (Hillestad)				1.5	1.7	20	10	10	6	100	$1,000^e$	Zn	Biotin 300 mcg	In 100s.
Rx	**NephPlex Tablets** (Nephro-Tech)				1.5	1.7	20	10	10	6	60	$1,000^e$	Si, Zn	Biotin 300 mcg	In 100s.
otc	**Dialyvite 800 with Zinc 15 Tablets** (Hillestad)				1.5	1.7	20	10	10	6	60	800^e	Zn	Biotin 300 mcg	In 100s.
otc	**Dialyvite 800 with Zinc Tablets** (Hillstad)												Zn	Biotin 300 mcg	In 100s.
otc	**RenaPlex Tablets** (Nephro-Tech)												Si, Zn	Biotin 300 mg	In 100s.
otc sf	**B Complex With Vitamin B-12 Tablets** (Goldline)				1.5	1.7	20	10	2	6		400^e	Ca	Brewer's yeast 90 mg	Preservative free, sugar free. Mannitol. In 100s.
Rx sf	**Diatx Zn Tablets** (Centrix Pharmaceutical)				1.5	1.5	20	10	50	2,000	60	$5,000^e$	Cu, Si, Zn	d-biotin 300 mcg	Gluten free, lactose free, sugar free. PEG, tartrazine. (CEN 905). Round, yellow. Film-coated. In 90s.
Rx sf	**Folbee Plus CZ Tablets** (Breckenridge)				1.5	1.5	20	10	50	2,000	60	$5,000^{aa}$	Cu, Si, Zn	d-biotin 300 mcg	Lactose free, sugar free. Soy polysaccharide, tartrazine. (B528). Yellow-beige. Film-coated. In 90s.

MULTIVITAMINS WITH MINERALS (EXCEPT IRON)

	Product & Distributor	A units	D units	E units	B_1 mg	B_2 mg	B_3 mg	B_5 mg	B_6 mg	B_{12} mcg	C mg	Folate mcg	Minerals	Other Content	How Supplied
otc	**Dexatrim Max Slim Packs Powder Mix** (Chattem)				0.263	0.3	3.5	1.8	0.35	3	30	70	Cr, K, Mg, Mn	Caffeine 25 mg, green tea 45 mg, ginsenosides 1 mg, sodium 72 mg	Acesulfame K, dextrose, sucralose. In single-use packets (22s).
otc sf	**Advanced Ear Health Formula Caplets** (Mason)				0.33	1	3.33	1.66	1.66	300			Ca	Bioflavonoids 300 mg, choline 111.33 mg, inositol 111.33 mg	Sugar free. Capsule shape. In 100s.
otc	**Lipo-Flavonoid Caplets** (DSE Health)				0.3	1	3.3	1.67	0.3	1.67	100		Ca, Si	Bioflavonoids 100 mg, choline 111.33 mg, inositol 111.33 mg	PEG. In 100s.
otc	**Eldertonic Liquid** (Merz)				0.17	0.2	2.33	1	0.23	0.67			Mg, Mn, Zn		Alcohol, sorbitol, sucrose. In 465 mL.
Rx	**Invites Rx Tablets** (Breckenridge Pharmaceuticals)				1.5	1.7	20		10	6	60	1[e]	Zn	Biotin 300 mcg	(B 593). Beige. Film-coated. In 100s.
Rx	**Biomide 750 Tablets** (Brookstone[p])						750					500[e]	Cu, Zn		(AV 802). White. In 60s.
otc	**Mil Adregen Tablets** (Miller)							60	50		250		Si, Zn	Citrus bioflavonoids 25 mg, raw adrenal concentrate 250 mg, raw spleen concentrate 50 mg, raw thymus concentrate 50 mg	In 60s, 120s, 180s, and 500s.
otc	**Beelith Tablets** (Beach)								20				Mg		(Beach 1132). Golden yellow. Film-coated. In 100s.
otc	**Heart Vitality Tablets** (Bayer Nutritional Science)								1	3		200[e]	Ca,[jj] Si	Coenzyme Q_{10} 6 mg, phytosterols 1,000 mcg	In 60s.
Rx	**Magnebind 400 Rx Tablets** (Nephro-Tech)											1,000[e]	Ca, Mg		In 150s.
otc sf	**Ester-C 500 MG Tablets** (Mason Vitamins)											500	Ca	Citrus bioflavonoids 200 mg	Gluten free, preservative free, soy free, sugar free. In 60s.

[a] As 92% beta-carotene and 8% palmitate; beta-carotene 10 mg.
[b] As cholecalciferol.
[c] As d-alpha-tocopherol.
[d] As other mixed tocopherols.
[e] As folic acid.
[f] As beta-carotene.
[g] Form of vitamin E unknown; content given in units.
[h] As 50% from natural mixed carotenoids, 50% as palmitate.
[i] d-alpha tocopheryl succinate.
[j] Yasoo Health Inc, 2501 Aerial Center Parkway, Suite 205, Morrisville, North Carolina 27560, 919-439-2960, Fax: 919-388-4305, http://www.yasoo.com.
[k] As dl-alpha tocopheryl acetate.
[l] NatureSmart, Inc, 1500 East 128th Avenue, Thornton, Colorado 80241.
[m] As palmitate and 60% as beta-carotene.
[n] As succinate.
[o] As 50% beta-carotene and retinyl acetate.
[p] Brookstone Pharmaceuticals, LLC, 9005 Westside Parkway, Alpharetta, GA 30004, 678-325-5188, Fax: 678-746-0717, http://www.brookstonepharma.com.
[q] As 87% beta-carotene and 13% palmitate; beta-carotene 3 mg.
[r] As 50% beta-carotene and 50% acetate.
[s] Form of vitamin D unknown; content given in units.
[t] Women's Health America, Inc, 1289 Deming Way, Madison, WI 53717, 800-558-7046, Fax: 888-898-7412, http://womenshealth.com/home.
[u] As vitamin A acetate and beta-carotene.
[v] As ergocalciferol.
[w] Sundown Nutrition, 90 Orville Dr, Bohemia, NY 11716, 561-241-9400, http://www.sundownnutrition.com.
[x] As beta-carotene and with natural mixed carotenoids.
[y] Packet to be mixed into 6 to 8 ounces of juice, other liquid, or semisolid food, and stirred briskly.
[z] As d-alpha tocopheryl acid succinate.
[aa] As folacin.
[bb] As d-alpha tocopheryl acetate.
[cc] As retinyl acetate and 40% beta-carotene.
[dd] As acetate.
[ee] As 75% beta-carotene.
[ff] As palmitate.
[gg] As d-succinate.
[hh] 29% as beta-carotene.
[ii] As 14% beta-carotene.
[jj] As elemental calcium.
[kk] As 30% beta-carotene.
[ll] As 72% beta-carotene.
[mm] As d-alpha tocopherol acetate.
[nn] As niacin.
[oo] As niacinamide.
[pp] On ion exchange resin.
[qq] As dibencozide.
[rr] As other tocopheryls (d-gamma, d-delta, and d-beta).
[ss] As alpha-carotene, beta-carotene, cryptoxanthin, lutein, and zeaxanthin.
[tt] 20% as beta-carotene.
[uu] As 40% beta-carotene.
[vv] As 67% beta-carotene and as retinyl acetate.
[ww] As dl-acetate.
[xx] As A palmitate and 20% beta-carotene.
[yy] As retinyl palmitate.
[zz] As irradiated ergosterol.
[aaa] As dl-alpha tocopheryl.
[bbb] As 60% palmitate and 40% beta-carotene.
[ccc] PABA = para aminobenzoic acid.

For additional information, refer to the Dietary Reference Intakes of Vitamins and Minerals table.

MULTIMINERALS

Content given per tablet.

	Product & Distributor	Ca[a] mg	F[b] mg	Mg[c] mg	Other Content	Excipients & How Supplied
otc *sf*	**Mineral Zinc Tablets** (Mason)	122			Zinc 10 mg	Gluten free, preservative free, sugar free. In 100s.
otc	**Monocal Tablets** (Mericon)	250	3			In 100s.
otc	**MEGA MAG-CAL Tablets** (Freeda)	133.3		266.7		In 100s.
otc	**MAG-SR Plus Calcium Tablets** (Cypress)	106		64	Chloride 186.5 mg	Polyethylene glycol. In 60s.
otc	**MagneBind 300 Tablets** (Nephro-Tech)	101		86		In 150s.
otc	**Calcium & Magnesium Tablets** (Miller)	100		50		In 100s.
otc *sf*	**Calcium/Magnesium Tablets** (Windmill)	1,000		500		Preservative free, sugar free. In 60s.
otc	**Florical Capsules** (Mericon)	145	3.75			In 100s.
otc *sf*	**Magnesium Aspartate/Potassium Aspartate Capsules** (The Key Co.)			90	Potassium 90 mg	Sugar free. Clear. In 100s.
otc *sf*	**Blood Sugar Balance Tablets** (Mason)			200	Biotin 600 mcg, bitter melon 200 mg, chromium 48 mcg, ginkgo 120 mg, gymnema 300 mg, iron oxide, lipoic acid 150 mg, mineral oil, quercetin 50 mg, vanadium 40 mcg, zinc 30 mg	Gluten free, lactose free, preservative free, sugar free. PEG. In 60s.

[a] Calcium content expressed in mg elemental calcium.
[b] Fluoride content expressed in mg elemental fluoride.
[c] Magnesium content expressed in mg elemental magnesium.

For additional information, refer to the Dietary Reference Intakes of Vitamins and Minerals table.

PRENATAL VITAMINS WITH MINERALS

Content given per capsule or tablet.

	Product & Distributor	Folate mg	Ca mg	Fe mg	A units	D units	E units	B_1 mg	B_2 mg	B_3 mg	B_5 mg	B_6 mg	B_{12} mcg	C mg	Other Minerals	Omega-3 Acids & Other Content	Excipients & How Supplied
otc	**Neevo Caplets** (PAM LAB)	1.4[oo]	200	29[k]		400[d]	30[e]	3	3.4	20	7	2.6	500	80	Cu, Mg, Zn	Biotin 30 mcg	Gluten free. Polydextrose, PEG. (N). Pink, oval. In 90s and 500s.
otc	**Neevo DHA Capsules** (PAM LAB)	1.4[oo]	75	27[g]			30[e]					25	1	40		DHA 250 mg	Soybean oil. (NeevoDHA). Blue. In 30s.
Rx *sf*	**OB Complete Tablets** (Vertical)	1.25[a]		50[v]	2,100[f]	315[d]	20[w]	2	3.4	10		10	15	120	Cu, Mg, Zn		Gluten free, lactose free, sugar free. (VP010). Pink, capsule shape. In UD 100s.
Rx	**Elite OB** (Trigen)																(TL001). Pink, capsule shape. In 100s.
Rx	**Elite OB with DHA Tablets** (Trigen)	1.25[a]		28[g]		400[d]	30[ff]	2	3.4			10	15	120	Cu, Zn	Each softgel capsule contains omega-3 fatty acids (DHA and EPA) 200 mg.	(TL029). Annatto, capsule shape. In 60s.
Rx	**OB Complete with DHA Softgels** (Vertical)															DHA 200 mg	Annatto. In 60s.
Rx	**Se-Plete DHA Softgels** (Seton)															Omega-3 fatty acids (DHA and EPA)	Soybean oil. (VP022). Annatto. In 60s.
Rx	**PreNexa Capsules** (Upsher-Smith)	1.25[a]	160	27[g]		400[d]	30[o]					25		28		DHA 300 mg, docusate sodium 55 mg	Glycerin, palm kernel oil, sodium benzoate, soybean oil, sunflower oil. (Prenexa). Brown, opaque. In 30s.
Rx	**Taron Prenatal with DHA Capsules** (Trigen)	1.2[a]	160	30[g]		170[d]	30[e]					25		25		Docusate sodium < 55 mg, DHA 265 mg	(T543). Maroon, oval. In 30s.
Rx	**Se-Natal 90 Tablets** (Seton)	1[a]	250	90[g]	4,000[j]	400[h]	30[e]	3	3.4	20		20	12	120	Cu, I, Zn	Docusate sodium 50 mg	(MVC-008). Lt. brown, capsule shape. Film-coated. In 100s.
Rx	**Marnatal-F Plus Duo Pack Tablets and Licaps** (Marnel)	1[a]	250	60[k]	2,000[j]	400[d]	30[e]	3	3.4	20		5	12	100	Cu, I, Mg, Zn	Each *Licap* contains fish oil concentrate ultra refined TG 500 mg and omega-3 fatty acids 250 mg (EPA 150 mg, DHA 100 mg).	*Tablets:* Mineral oil, PEG. In unit-of-use 90s with 18 blister cards of 5 tablets and 5 *Licap* capsules.

PRENATAL VITAMINS WITH MINERALS

	Product & Distributor	Folate mg	Ca mg	Fe mg	A units	D units	E units	B_1 mg	B_2 mg	B_3 mg	B_5 mg	B_6 mg	B_{12} mcg	C mg	Other Minerals	Omega-3 Acids & Other Content	Excipients & How Supplied
Rx	**BP MultiNatal Plus Chewable Tablets** (Brookstone)	1[a]	250	40		6 mcg	3.5					2		50	Cu, Mg, Zn		Mannitol, sugar. (TL 014). Orange, oval. Orange flavor. In 30s.
Rx	**Vit C, Vit D, Vit E, Vit B, Folic Acid, Ca, Iron, Mg, Zn, and Cu 50-6-3.5-2-1-250-40-50-15-2 Chewable Tablets** (Brookstone)																Mannitol, sucralose, sugar. Orange, round. Orange flavor. In 30s.
Rx	**Vinate PN Care Tablets** (Breckenridge)	1[a]	250	30[p]		240[d]	3.5[e]	3	3.4	20		50	12	50	Cu, Mg, Zn	Docusate sodium 50 mg, succinic acid 35 mg	Maltodextrin, soy. (B584). Peach, oval. Film-coated. In 30s.
Rx	**Duet DHA with Ferrazone** (Xanodyne)	1	230	30[pp]	3,000[f]	410[d]	30[e]	1.8	4	20		28	12	130	Cu, Mg, Zn	Omega-3 fatty acids 440 mg (DHA 295 mg, EPA and DPA[oo] 145 mg) in 629 fish oil	*Tablets:* PEG, sucrose. (878). Yellow, oval. *Capsules:* (X1). Gold, oval. Enteric-coated. In 5 blister cards of 6 tablets and 6 capsules.
Rx	**Inatal Ultra Tablets** (Nnodum Pharmaceuticals)	1[a]	200	90[b]	2,700[f,i]	400[d]	30[e]	3	3.4	20		20	12	120	Cu, I, Zn	Docusate sodium 50 mg	Dye free. White, oval. In UD 10s.
Rx	**Inatal Advance Tablet** (Nnodum Pharmaceuticals)	1[a]	200	90[b]	2,700[f]	400[d]	30[e]	3	3.4	20		20	12	120	Cu, Mg, Zn	Docusate sodium 50 mg	Dye free. PEG. Oval. In UD 90s.
Rx	**TriAdvance Tablets** (Trigen)																(TL020). Green. In 90s.
Rx	**Prenatal AD Tablets** (Cypress)	1[a]	200	90[b]	2,700[f]	400[d]	30[e]	3	3.4	20		20	12	120	Cu, Mg, Zn	Docusate sodium 50 mg	(CYP194). Oval. Film-coated. In UD 90s.
Rx	**Ultra NatalCare Tablets** (ETHEX)	1[a]	200	90[b]	2,700[f,i]	400[d]	30[e]	3	3.4	20		20	12	120	Cu, I, Zn	Docusate sodium 50 mg	Dye free. Hydrogenated vegetable oil, lactose, sucrose. (ETHEX 292). Beige, oval, scored. In 100s.
Rx	**Vinate GT Tablets** (Breckenridge)	1[a]	200	90[b]	2,700[f]	400[d]	10[e]	3	3.4	20	6	20	12	120	Cu, Mg, Zn	Biotin 30 mcg, docusate sodium 50 mg	Mineral oil, sucrose. Purple, oval. In UD 90s.
Rx	**CitraNatal 90 DHA Tablet and Capsule Combination** (Mission Pharmacal)	1[a]	200	90[b]		400[d]	30[e]	3	3.4	20		20		120	Cu, I, Zn	Docusate sodium 50 mg. Each capsule contains DHA 250 mg.	In blister pack 6s with 5 tablets and 5 capsules. *Tablets:* (CN 90). Oval, scored.
Rx	**RE OB 90 + DHA** (River's Edge)														Cu, Zn	Docusate sodium 50 mg. Each softgel capsule contains DHA 250 mg.	Gluten free. In 30s. *Tablets:* (RE 338). Dark purple. *Capsules:* Pale yellow.
Rx	**Complete-RF Prenatal Tablets** (Trigen Laboratories)	1[a]	200	90[b]		400[d]	30[e]	3	3.4	20		20	12	120	Cu, Mg, Zn	Docusate sodium 50 mg	Dye free. PEG, polydextrose, vegetable oil. (44-338). White, oval. Film-coated. In 90s.
Rx	**Lactocal-F Tablets** (Laser)	1[a]	200	65[g]	4,000[j]	400	30[e]	3	3.4	20		5	12	100	Cu, I, Mg, Zn		Dye free. (LASER 179). Oval. Film-coated. In 100s.
Rx	**Trinatal Rx 1 Tablets** (Trigen)	1[a]	200	60[g]	4,000[r]	400[d]	15[e]	1.5	1.6	17	7	4	2.5	80	Cu, Mg, Zn	Biotin 30 mcg	PEG, polydextrose. (44175). White, oval. Film-coated. In 100s.
Rx	**Vinate One Tablets** (Breckenridge)	1[a]	200	60[g]	4,000[r]	400[d]	15[e]	1.5	1.6	17	7	4	2.5	80	Cu, Mg, Zn	Biotin 30 mcg	Maltodextrin, soy, sucrose. (B 566). Beige, oval. Film-coated. In 100s.
Rx	**Vit C, Vit E, Vit B1, B2, B3, B6, Folic Acid, B12, Ca, Fe, Zn, Cu 60-3-3-3.4-20-50-1-12-200-30-100-15-2 Tablets** (Brookstone)	1[a]	200	30[g]			30[e]	3	3.4	20		50	12	60	Cu, Mg, Zn		Lactose. Oblong, diamond shape. Yellow. Film-coated. In 30s.
Rx	**MultiNatal Plus Tablets** (Brookstone)																(MVC-001). Yellow, diamond shape. Film-coated. In 30s.
Rx	**Prenatabs RX Tablets** (Cypress)	1[a]	200	29[b]	4,000[f]	400[d]	30[e]	3	3	20	7	3	8	120	Cu, I, Mg, Zn	Biotin 30 mcg	(CYP 193). Oval. Film-coated. In 90s.
Rx	**RE-Nata 29 OB Prenatal Vitamin Tablets** (River's Edge)																PEG. (RE 394). White, oval. In 90s.
Rx	**Prenatabs FA Tablets** (Cypress)	1[a]	200	29[g]	4,000[f]	400[d]	30[e]	3	3	20		3	8	120	I, Zn		In 100s.

PRENATAL VITAMINS WITH MINERALS

	Product & Distributor	Folate mg	Ca mg	Fe mg	A units	D units	E units	B_1 mg	B_2 mg	B_3 mg	B_5 mg	B_6 mg	B_{12} mcg	C mg	Other Minerals	Omega-3 Acids & Other Content	Excipients & How Supplied
Rx	**Duet by Stuartnatal** (Xanodyne)	1[a]	200	29[aa]	3,000[f]	400[d]	30[e]	1.8	4	20		25	12	120	Cu, Mg, Zn	Each DHA softgel capsule contains 430 mg purified omega-3 fatty acids (295 mg DHA, EPA, and other omega-3 fatty acids).	*Tablets:* PEG, sucrose. (848). Yellow, oval. In 30s. *Capsules:* (XI). Golden, oval. In 30s.
Rx	**Duet DHA by StuartNatal** (Xanodyne)														Cu, Mg, Zn	Each DHA softgel capsule contains purified omega-3 fatty acids 430 mg (290 mg of DHA, EPA,[bb] and other omega-3 fatty acids).	*Tablets:* PEG, sucrose. (848). Yellow, oval. *Capsules:* Gold, oval. In unit-of-use 30s with 5 UD cards of 6 tablets and 6 capsules.
Rx	**Complete Natal DHA** (Trigen)	1[a]	200	29[cc]	3,000[f]	400[d]	30[e]	1.8	4	20		25	12	120	Cu, Mg, Zn	Each softgel capsule contains omega-3 fatty acids 250 mg, including DHA ≥ 200 mg.	*Tablets:* (01 030). Pale purple, oval. Film-coated. *Capsules:* Soybean oil. (01 030). Pale yellow. In unit-of-use 30s with 5 UD cards of 6 tablets and 6 capsules.
Rx	**Vinate II Tablets** (Breckenridge)	1[a]	200	29[t]	3,000[f]	400[d]	30[e]	1.8	4	20		25	12	120	Cu, Mg, Zn		Mineral oil, soy, sucrose. (B 178). Yellow, oval. Film-coated. In 100s.
Rx	**Vinate III Tablets** (Breckenridge)	1[a]	200	29[cc]	3,000[f]	400[d]	30[e]	1.8	4	20		25	12	120	Cu, Mg, Zn		Soy, sucrose. (B 378). Yellow, capsule shape. Film-coated. In 100s.
Rx	**Renate DHA** (River's Edge)	1[a]	200	29[cc]	3,000[f]	400[d]	30[e]	1.8	4	20		25	12	120	Cu, Mg, Zn	Each DHA softgel capsule contains omega-3 fatty acids 400 mg (275 mg of DHA , EPA,[bb] other omega-3 fatty acids).	*Tablets*: Preservative free. PEG, polydextrose, maltodextrin, sucrose. (RE 316). Dark pink. In UD 30s. *Capsules*: Soy. Dark brown. In 30s.
Rx	**PruEt DHA** (PruGen)	1[a]	200	29[aa]	3,000[f]	400[d]	30[e]	1.8	4	20		25	12	120	Cu, Mg, Zn	Each DHA softgel capsule contains purified omega-3 fatty acids 400 mg (275 mg DHA, EPA,[bb] other omega-3 fatty acids).	*Tablets*: (B 056). Off-white, oval. *Capsules*: Golden, oval. In UD 30s with blister card 6s of 5 tablets and 5 capsules.
Rx	**PruEt DHAec** (PruGen)	1[a]	200	29[aa]	3,000[f]	400[d]	3[e]	1.8	4	20		25	12	120	Cu, Mg, Zn	Each DHA softgel capsule contains purified omega-3 fatty acids 400 mg (275 mg DHA, EPA,[bb] other omega-3 fatty acids).	*Tablets:* (PE 669). Beige, oval. *Capsules*: Gold, oval. Enteric-coated. In unit-of-use 30s with 5 UD cards of 6 tablets and 6 capsules.
Rx	**Renate DHA Extra** (River's Edge)	1[a]	200	29[cc]	3,000[f]	400[d]	3[e]	1.8	4	20		25	12	120	Cu, Mg, Zn	Each softgel capsule contains purified omega-3 fatty acids 400 mg (275 mg DHA, EPA,[bb] and other omega-3 fatty acids).	*Tablets:* Gluten free, preservative free. PEG, maltodextrin, sucrose. (RE 340). Dark red, capsule shape. In UD 30s. *Capsules*: Soy. Dark brown. In 30s.
Rx	**Prenatal 19 Chewable Tablets** (Cypress)	1[a]	200	29[g]	1,000[f]	400[d]	30[e]	3	3	15	7	20	12	100	Zn		(CYP 197). Orange. Orange flavor. In 100s.
Rx	**Se-Natal 19 Tablets** (Seton)															Docusate sodium 25 mg	(TL019). Oblong. In 100s.
Rx	**Se-Natal 19 Chewable Tablets** (Seton)																(TL015). Multicolored, round. Orange flavor. In 100s.
Rx	**Prenatal 19 Tablets** (Cypress)															Docusate sodium 25 mg	(CYP196). Oval, scored. In 100s.
Rx	**Prenatabs OBN Tablets** (Cypress)	1[a]	200	29[b]		400[d]	30[e]	3	3	20		3	8	120	I, Zn		(CYP 176). Oval. Film-coated. In 90s.
Rx	**VitaSpire Tablets**(Trigen)																PEG, polydextrose, sucrose. (TL011). Blue, capsule shape. Film-coated. In 90s.
Rx	**Trinate Tablets** (Cypress)	1[a]	200	28[g]	3,000[f]	400[d]	22[e]	1.8	4	20		25	12	120	Cu, Mg, Zn		(CYP 192). Oval. Film-coated. In 100s.

PRENATAL VITAMINS WITH MINERALS

	Product & Distributor	Folate mg	Ca mg	Fe mg	A units	D units	E units	B_1 mg	B_2 mg	B_3 mg	B_5 mg	B_6 mg	B_{12} mcg	C mg	Other Minerals	Omega-3 Acids & Other Content	Excipients & How Supplied
Rx	**Gesticare Tablets** (Azur Pharma)	1[a]	200	28[g]		420	30	3	3	20		50	8	120	I, Zn	Choline	Maltodextrin, polydextrose. (P-114). Lt. pink, oblong. In 90s.
Rx	**Se-Care Gesture Tablets** (Seton)																(TL011). White, capsule shape. In 90s.
Rx	**Gesticare DHA** (Azur Pharma)	1[a]	200	28[g]		420	30	3	3	20		50	8	120	I, Zn	Choline, DHA 250 mg	*Tablets*: Maltodextrin, polydextrose. (P-114). Lt. pink, oblong. *Capsules*: Fish oils. In UD 30s with blister card 6s of 5 tablets and 5 capsules.
Rx	**Taron EC Calcium DHA Pack** (Trigen)														I, Zn	Choline, DHA 250 mg	Dextrose, maltodextrin, polydextrose. (T541). White, oblong. In 6 blister cards of 5 capsules and 5 tablets.
Rx	**Vinate-M Tablets** (Breckenridge)	1[a]	200	27[g]	5,000[j]	400[d]	30[e]	3	3.4	20	10	10	12	120	Cr, Cu, I, Mg, Mn, Mo, Se, Zn,	Biotin 30 mcg	Mineral oil, soy. In 100s.
Rx	**Prenatal Plus Iron Tablets** (Major)	1[a]	200	27[g]	4,000[f,j]	400[d]	22[e]	1.84	3	20		10	12	120	Cu, Zn		(G13). Yellow, oval. In 100s.
Rx	**PreNate Plus Tablets** (Boca)	1[a]	200	27[g]	4,000[f]	400[d]	22[e]	1.84	3	20		10	12	120	Cu, Zn		Maltodextrin, mineral oil, sucrose. In 100s.
Rx	**PrenaFirst Tablets** (Cypress)	1[a]	200	17[g]	4,000[f]	400[d]	30[e]	3	3	20		3	8	120	I, Zn		(CYP 178). Pink, oval. Film-coated. In 90s.
Rx	**BP FoliNatal Plus B Tablets** (Brookstone)	1[a]	200									75	12				Blue, oval. Film-coated. In 30s.
Rx	**Vit B6, Folic Acid, Vit B12 Tablets** (Brookstone)																Blue, oval. Film-coated. In 30s.
Rx	**Trimesis Rx Tablets** (Trigen)																(MVC005). Off white. Film-coated. In 30s.
Rx	**ComBi Rx** (Ethex)																PEG, polydextrose. (Ther-Rx 019). Blue, oval. Film-coated. In 30s.
Rx	**Folbecal Tablets** (Breckenridge)																Maltodextrin, mineral oil, soy. (B 077). White, oval. Film-coated. In 30s.
Rx	**VitaPhil One Caplets** (River's Edge)	1[a]	150	27[m]	3,000[f]	400[d]	30[e]	3	3.5	20	8	30	12	120	Cu, Mg, Zn	Biotin 30 mcg	Gluten free. PEG, soybean oil, sucrose. (RE288). Green, capsule shape. In 90s.
Rx	**Multivitamin with Minerals Capsules** (Lannett)	1[a]	150	27[mm]		170[d]	30[e]					25		25		Omega-3 fatty acids 300 mg, linoleic acid 30 mg, linolenic acid 30 mg	Parabens, sorbitol. (LCI 1637). Purple, oblong. In 30s.
Rx	**Cavan One Omega Capsules** (Seton)																(TL049). Maroon, oblong. In 30s.
Rx	**UltimateCare ONE Capsules** (Trigen)	1[a]	150	27[b,p]		170[d]	30[e]					25		25		Each softgel capsule contains omega-3 fatty acids 330 mg (DHA 260 mg, EPA 40 mg, ALA[ee] 30 mg) and linoleic acid 30 mg.	(TL049). Maroon. In 30s.
Rx	**Prenate DHA Softgel** (Sciele)	1[y]	140	27[g]		200[d]	10[e]					25	12	85	Mg	Omega-3 fatty acids 330 mg, DHA 300 mg	(Prenate DHA). Blue-green. In 30s.
Rx	**CitraNatal Assure** (Mission Pharmacal)	1[a]	125	35[b,c]		400[d]	30[e]	3	3.4	20		25		120	Cu, I, Zn	Docusate sodium 50 mg. Each capsule contains DHA 300 mg, EPA ≤ 0.75 mg.	*Tablet:* (0893). White, oval. Coated. *Capsule:* Clear. In blister pack 6s with 5 tablets and 5 capsules.
Rx	**Taron A Prenatal Pack with DHA** (Trigen)																*Tablet:* (T542). White, oblong. Coated. *Capsule:* Clear. In blister pack 6s with 5 tablets and 5 capsules.
Rx	**Vinate Calcium Tablets** (Breckenridge)	1[a]	125	27[b,c]	2,700[i]	400[d]	30[e]	3	3.4	20		20		120	Cu, I, Zn	Docusate sodium 50 mg	(B 469). Pink, oval, scored. Film-coated. In 100s.

PRENATAL VITAMINS WITH MINERALS

	Product & Distributor	Folate mg	Ca mg	Fe mg	A units	D units	E units	B_1 mg	B_2 mg	B_3 mg	B_5 mg	B_6 mg	B_{12} mcg	C mg	Other Minerals	Omega-3 Acids & Other Content	Excipients & How Supplied
Rx	**RE OB + DHA** (River's Edge)	1[a]	125	27[b,c]		400[d]	30[e]	3	3.4	20		20		120	Cu, I, Zn	Docusate sodium 50 mg. Each capsule contains DHA 250 mg.	*Tablets:* Gluten free, preservative free. (RE 337). Lt. purple. In 30s. *Capsules:* Pale yellow. In 30s.
Rx	**Foltabs Prenatal Plus DHA** (Midlothian Labs)														Cu, I, Zn	Docusate sodium 50 mg. Each capsule contains DHA 250 mg.	*Tablets:* (ML 160). White, oval, scored. In blister pack 6s with 5 tablets and 5 capsules.
Rx	**CitraNatal DHA Tablet and Capsule Combination** (Mission Pharmacal)														Cu, I, Zn	Docusate sodium 50 mg. Each capsule contains DHA 250 mg.	*Tablets:* (CN RX). Oval, scored. In blister pack 6s with 5 tablets and 5 capsules.
Rx	**CitraNatal Rx Tablets** (Mission)															Docusate sodium 50 mg	(CN RX). Oval, scored. In 90s.
Rx	**Complete-RF Prenatal Tablets** (Trigen)														Cu, Mg, Zn	Docusate sodium 50 mg	Dye free. PEG, polydextrose. (44-338). White, oval. Film-coated. In 90s.
Rx	**Tri Rx Tablets** (Trigen)														Cu, I, Zn		(TL021). Grey. Film-coated. In 90s.
Rx	**Foltabs Prenatal** (Midlothian Labs)														Cu, I, Zn		PEG. (ML 160). White, oval, scored. In 90s.
Rx	**Vinacal Prenatal Tablets** (Breckenridge)														Cu, I, Zn	Docusate sodium 50 mg, triglycerides	Sucrose. In 90s.
Rx	**Prenate Elite** (Sciele Pharma)	1[a]	120	27[g]	2,500[f]	400[d]	10[e]	3	3.4	20		20	12	80	Cu, I, Mg, Zn	Biotin 300 mcg, pantothenic acid 6 mg	Hydrogenated soybean oil, hydrogenated vegetable oil, polyvinyl alcohol, povidone, and sucrose. In 90s.
Rx *sf*	**Vitafol-OB+DHA Tablet and Gelcap Capsule Combination** (Everett Labs)	1[a]	100	65[g]	2,700[f]	400[d]	30[e]	1.6	1.8	18		2.5	12	70	Cu, Mg, Zn	Each capsule contains DHA 250 mg.	Gluten free, lactose free, sugar free. In UD 30s with blister card 6s of 5 tablets and 5 capsules. *Tablets:* PEG, polydextrose. (EV 0079). Lt. blue, capsule shape. *Capsules:* Orange flavor.
Rx	**BP Prenate Tablet and Capsule Combination** (Brookstone)	1[a]	100	30[b,c]	2,500[i]	425[d]	35[e]	5	4	25		25		100	Cu, I, Zn	Docusate sodium 75 mg. Each capsule contains DHA 275 mg.	*Tablet:* (BP PR PN RX). Oval, scored. In blister pack 6s of 5 tablets and 5 capsules.
Rx	**CRNatal Tablet and Capsule Combination** (Canopy Roads Pharmaceuticals)														Cu, I, Zn	Docusate sodium 75 mg. Each capsule contains DHA 275 mg.	*Tablet:* (CRNATAL PN RX). Oval, scored. In blister pack 6s with 5 tablets and 5 capsules.
Rx *sf*	**Atabex[EC] Caplets** (Advanced Medical Enterprises)	1[a]	100	29[b]	2,500[f]	400[d]	30[e]	1.5	3	20			12	120	Cu, Mg, Zn	Biotin 30 mcg, docusate sodium 40 mg	Gluten free, lactose free, sugar free. (ATABEX). Lt. blue, capsule shape. Enteric-coated. In 100s.
Rx	**OB-Natal One Capsules** (Lannett)	1[a]	100	27[b,p]	2,100[f]	800[d]	15[e]		1.5	10		50	15	25	I, Mg, Zn	Biotin 300 mcg, docusate sodium 50 mg, omega-3 fatty acids 500 mg (DHA 350 mg, EPA 100 mg, ALA[ee] 50 mg)	Parabens. (1766). Purple, oblong. In 30s.
Rx	**Natelle One Capsules** (Azure Pharma)	1[a]	100	27[g]			30[ff]					25		25		DHA 250 mg, EPA ≤ 0.625 mg	Soybean oil. (Natelle 1). Red. In 30s.
Rx	**UltimateCare ONE NF** (Trigen)	1[a]	100	27[b,p]		800[d]	15[e]		1.5	10		50		25	I, Mg, Zn	Biotin 300 mcg, docusate sodium 50 mg, omega-3 fatty acids 500 mg (DHA 350 mg, EPA[bb] 100 mg, ALA 50 mg)	Soy. Maroon. In 30s.

PRENATAL VITAMINS WITH MINERALS

	Product & Distributor	Folate mg	Ca mg	Fe mg	A units	D units	E units	B_1 mg	B_2 mg	B_3 mg	B_5 mg	B_6 mg	B_{12} mcg	C mg	Other Minerals	Omega-3 Acids & Other Content	Excipients & How Supplied
Rx	**VitaPhil + DHA** (River's Edge)	1[a]	100	26[t]	2,600[f]	420[d]	20[e]	3	3.5	20	8	30	12	120	Cu, Mg, Se, Zn	Choline, biotin 30 mcg. Each softgel capsule contains DHA 200 mg, EPA,[bb] and other omega-3 fatty acids.	*Tablets*: Gluten free. Maltodextrin, PEG, soy, sucrose. Green, capsule shape. In 30s and 90s. *Capsule*: (RE 341). Pale yellow. In 30s and 90s.
Rx	**VitaPhil + DHA 90** (River's Edge)															Choline, biotin 30 mcg. Each softgel capsule contains DHA 200 mg, EPA,[bb] and other omega-3 fatty acids.	*Tablets*: Gluten free. Maltodextrin, PEG, soy, sucrose. Green, capsule shape. In 30s and 90s. *Capsule*: (RE 341). Pale yellow. In 30s and 90s.
Rx	**Natelle-ez Tablets** (Azur Pharm)	1[a]	100	25[m]	2,700[f]	400[d]	20[n]	3	3.5	20	8	30	12	120	Cu, Mg, Se, Zn	Biotin 30 mcg, choline bitartrate 55 mg	(P-004). Lt. pink, capsule shape. Sugar-coated. In 90s.
Rx	**VitaPhil Tablets** (River's Edge)														Cu, Mg, Se, Zn	Biotin 30 mcg, choline bitartrate 55 mg	Sucrose, hydrogenated soybean oil. (RE259). Lt. green, capsule shape. In 90s.
Rx	**Tandem OB Capsule** (US Pharmaceutical)	1[a]		277.2[x]				10	6	30	10	5	15	200	Cu, Mg, Mn, Zn		(Tandem-OB US, US, US, US/US, US, US, US). Blue/pink. In 90s.
Rx	**Vinate IC Capsules** (Breckenridge)	1[a]		277.29[g,k]				10	6	30	10	5	15	200	Cu, Mg, Mn, Zn		Soy. (B 530). Blue/pink. In 90s.
Rx	**Se-Tan Plus Capsules** (Seton)														Cu, Mn, Zn		(T503). White. In 90s.
Rx	**Concept OB Capsules** (US Pharmaceutical)	1[a]		222.4[g,k]				5	5	20	7	25	10	210	Cu, Mg, Mn, Zn	Biotin 300 mcg	(US Concept OB). Pearl red. In 30s.
Rx	**Prenatal-U Capsules** (Cypress)	1[a]		106.5[g]				10	6	30	10	5	15	200	Cu, Mn		(CYP 179). Blue violet. In UD 100s.
Rx	**Concept DHA Capsules** (US Pharmaceutical)	1[a]		91.5[g,k]				2	3	1.8	5	25	12.5	25	Cu, Mg, Zn	Biotin 300 mcg, omega-3 fatty acids 200 mg (DHA 158 mg, EPA 39 mg).	(US Concept DHA). Persimmon. In 30s.
Rx	**NataFort Tablets** (Warner-Chilcott)	1[a]		60[u]	1,000[f,j]	400[d]	11[e]	2	3	20		10	12	120			Lactose. (NataFort). Film-coated. In 90s.
Rx	**Se-Tan DHA Capsules** (Seton)	1[a]		30[dd]								25		20		Omega-3 fatty acids 310.1 mg (DHA 215.12 mg, and EPA 53.46 mg) derived from at least 450 mg fish oil	(T513). Purple, oblong. In 90s.
Rx	**Tandem DHA Capsules** (US Pharmaceutical)																(Tandem DHA). Pink. In 90s.
Rx	**Docosavit Softgels** (River's Edge)	1[a]		30[g,k]								25		20		Omega-3 fatty acids 310.1 mg (DHA 215.12 mg, EPA[bb] 53.46 mg)	Gluten free, preservative free. Soy. Dark brown. In 90s.
Rx	**Obtrex Caplets** (Pronova)	1[a]		29[b]	2,700[f]	400[d]	18[e]	3	3.4	20		40	12	120	Mg, Se, Zn	Docusate sodium 50 mg	Mineral oil, parabens, sucrose. (OBX). Lt. orange. Enteric-coated. In 30s and 60s.
Rx	**Obtrex DHA** (Pronova)															Docusate sodium 50 mg. Each softgel capsule contains omega-3 fatty acids 387 mg (EPA[bb] 100 mg, DHA 250 mg).	*Tablets*: Maltodextrin, parabens, PEG, sucrose. (OBX). Orange. Enteric-coated. In 30s. *Capsules*: PEG. Amber, oval. In 30s.
Rx	**Select-OB Tablets** (Everett Laboratories)	1[a]		29[k]	1,700[f,j]	400[d]	30[e]	1.6	1.8	15		2.5	5	60	Mg, Zn		Fructose, hydrogenated vegetable oil, PEG, polydextrose. (EV 0077). Lt. blue, capsule shape. Berry flavor. In 90s.
Rx	**Select-OB + DHA Capsules** (Everett)															Each softgel capsule contains DHA 250 mg.	*Capsules*: Fructose, maltodextrin, PEG, polydextrose. Berry flavor. *Softgel*: Orange flavor. In blister pack 6s with 5 tablets and 5 capsules.

PRENATAL VITAMINS WITH MINERALS

	Product & Distributor	Folate mg	Ca mg	Fe mg	A units	D units	E units	B_1 mg	B_2 mg	B_3 mg	B_5 mg	B_6 mg	B_{12} mcg	C mg	Other Minerals	Omega-3 Acids & Other Content	Excipients & How Supplied
Rx	**NataChew Chewable Tablets** (Warner Chilcott)	1[a]		29[g]	1,000[f]	400[d]	11[e]	2	3	20		10	12	120			(WC 227). Speckled tan, scored. Wildberry flavor. In 90s.
Rx	**CompleteNate Chewable** (Trigen)																(TL014). Tan, round. In 90s.
Rx	**Gentex ADE Tablets** (Gentex Pharma)	1[a]		28[m]	2,000[j]	400[d]	25[e]	3	3	18	6	50	12	150	Cu, Mg, Zn	Choline, biotin 30 mcg	Sorbitol, mannitol. In 100s.
Rx	**VitaPhil Aide Caplets** (River's Edge)	1[a]		28[m]	2,000[f]	400[d]	25[e]	3	3	18	6	50	12	150	Cu, Mg, Zn	Choline, biotin 30 mcg	Gluten free, preservative free. PEG, sucrose. (RE302). Green, capsule shape. In 90s.
Rx	**Trifera OB Tablets** (Trigen)	1[a]		28[k,ll]		400[d]	10[e]	1.5	1.6	17	10	50	12		Cu, I, Se, Zn	Biotin 30 mcg	(MVC001). Off-white. Film-coated. In 90s.
Rx	**PreferaOB + DHA** (Alaven)	1[a]		22[k,nn]		400[d]	10[o]	1.5	1.6	17	10	50	12		Cu, I, Se, Zn	Biotin 30 mcg, DHA 200 mg	*Tablets:* Sucrose. (AP/88). Purple, oval. Film-coated. *Capsules:* Clear. In blister packs of 30 tablets and 30 softgels.
otc	**Prenavite Tablets** (Rugby)	0.8[a]	200	28[g]	4,000[f]	400[d]	30[e]	1.8	1.7	20		2.6	8	120	Zn		PEG, soy. In 100s.
Rx	**Stuart Prenatal Tablets** (Integrity)														Zn		PEG, sucrose. In 100s.
otc sf	**Prenatal S Tablets** (Ivax)	0.8[a]	200	27[g]	4,000[f,s]	400[d]	11[e]	1.84	1.7	18		2.6	4	100	Zn		Preservative free, sodium free, sugar free. Mannitol. Contains fish ingredients. In 100s.
otc	**Prenatal Tablets** (Prime Marketing)	0.8[a]	200	27[g]	4,000[f,j]	400[d]	11[e]	1.5	1.7	18		2.6	4	100	Zn		Mineral oil, sucrose. In 100s.
otc	**Mission Prenatal F.A. Tablets** (Mission)	0.8[a]	50	29.5[c]	4,000[j]	400[d]		4.7	2	10	1	10	2	100	Zn		PEG. Film-coated. In 100s.
otc	**Mission Prenatal H.P. Tablets** (Mission)	0.8[a]	50	29.5[c]	4,000[j]	400[d]		4	2	10	1	20	2	100			PEG. Film-coated. In 100s.
Rx sf	**PNV-DHA Plus Softgels** (Acella)	1.4[oo]	75	27[g]			30[o]					25	1	40		DHA 250 mg	Gluten free, lactose free, sugar free. Glycerin, lecithin oil, vegetable oil. (315). Blue opaque. In 30s.
otc	**Mission Prenatal Tablets** (Mission)	0.4[a]	50	29.5[c]	4,000[j]	400[d]		4.7	2	10	1	2.8	2	100			PEG. Film-coated. In 100s.
Rx	**PNV-Iron Tablets** (Acella Pharmaceuticals)	0.4[a]	200	29[k]		400[d]	30[e]	3	3.4	20	7	2.6	500	80	Cu, Mg, Zn	Biotin 30 mcg, L-methylfolate calcium 1 mg	Gluten free, lactose free. (314). Pink, oval. In 90s.
otc sf	**K.P.N. Prenatal with Extra Calcium Tablets** (Freeda)	0.267[a]	333.33	9[g]	666.67[i]	133.33[h]	10[jj]	2	2	6.67	5	1	2	33.33	Cu, Mg, Mn, Zn	Biotin 10 mcg. In a natural base containing 22 mg bioflavonoids and hesperidin.	Dye free, gluten free, lactose free, sugar free. In 100s and 250s.

PRENATAL VITAMINS WITH MINERALS

	Product & Distributor	Folate mg	Ca mg	Fe mg	A units	D units	E units	B_1 mg	B_2 mg	B_3 mg	B_5 mg	B_6 mg	B_{12} mcg	C mg	Other Minerals	Omega-3 Acids & Other Content	Excipients & How Supplied
otc sf	**A-Free Prenatal Tablets** (Freeda)	0.267[a]	333.33	9[g]		133.33[h]	10[ii]	2	2	10	5	1	2	33.33	Cu, Mg, Mn, Zn	Biotin 10 mcg. In a natural base containing 22 mg bioflavonoids and hesperidin.	Gluten free, lactose free, sugar free. In 100s.

[a] As folic acid.
[b] As carbonyl iron.
[c] As ferrous gluconate.
[d] As cholecalciferol.
[e] As dl-alpha-tocopheryl acetate.
[f] As beta-carotene.
[g] As ferrous fumarate.
[h] As ergocalciferol.
[i] As vitamin A palmitate.
[j] As vitamin A acetate.
[k] As polysaccharide iron complex.
[l] As 33% beta carotene.
[m] As ferrous (II)-bis-glycinate chelate.
[n] As dl-alpha-tocopherol succinate.
[o] As d-alpha tocopheryl acetate.
[p] As ferrous asparto glycinate.
[q] As 50% vitamin A acetate and 50% beta carotene.
[r] As acetate 3,600 units and beta carotene 400 units.
[s] As retinyl acetate.
[t] As ferrous bisglycinate.
[u] As ferrous sulfate 25 mg and carbonyl iron 35 mg.
[v] As ferronyl, micronized.
[w] As d-alpha succinate.
[x] As ferrous fumarate 162 mg and polysaccharide iron complex 115.2 mg.
[y] As L-methylfolate 600 mcg and folic acid 400 mcg.
[z] DHA = docosahexaenoic acid.
[aa] As ferrous bisglycinate hydrochloride and *Iron Aid.*
[bb] EPA = eicosapentaenoic acid.
[cc] As ferrous bisglycinate and iron protein succinylate.
[dd] As ferrous fumarate 15 mg and polysaccharide iron complex 15 mg.
[ee] ALA = alpha-linolenic acid.
[ff] As d-alpha tocopherol.
[gg] Calcium 150 mg in the capsule and 250 mg in the tablet.
[hh] Vitamin D_3 170 units in the capsule and 230 units in the tablet.
[ii] As d-alpha tocopherol acid succinate.
[jj] As d-alpha tocopherol succinate.
[kk] As carbonyl iron and *Sumalate* iron.
[ll] Heme iron complex.
[mm] As carbonyl iron and *Ferrochel* amino acid chelate.
[nn] Heme iron polypeptide as *Proferrin*-bovine source.
[oo] As L-methylfolate 1 mg and folic acid 400 mcg.
[pp] As sodium iron EDTA, *Ferrazone.*

For additional information, refer to the Dietary Reference Intakes of Vitamins and Minerals table.

CALCIUM WITH VITAMIN D

Content given per capsule, tablet, or packet.

	Product & Distributor	D units	Calcium (mg)	Other content	How Supplied
otc sf	**D-2000 Super Strength Softgel Capsules** (Nature's Bounty)	2,000[a]	115[g]		Gluten free, preservative free, sugar free. In 100s.
otc	**Calcium 500+D Tablets** (21st Century)	800[a]	1,000[f]		Preservative free. In 200s.
otc	**OsCal Extra D Caplets** (GlaxoSmithKline)	500[a]	500[c]		Gluten free. Alcohol, corn syrup, parabens, PEG, sucrose. Capsule shape. In 60s and 120s.
otc	**Calcium with Vitamin D_3 Tablets** (Rexall Sundown)	400[a]	1,000[f]	sodium 10 mg	Gluten free, preservative free. In 250s.
otc sf	**Calcium Citrate + D Caplets** (21st Century HealthCare)	400[a]	630[b]		Sugar free, preservative free. Capsule shape. In 120s.
otc	**Calcium 600 mg with Vitamin D Tablets** (Major)	400[a]	600[c]		In 60s and 150s.
otc	**Calcium 600 With Vitamin D Tablets** (Nature's Bounty)				In 60s and 250s.
otc	**Calcium 600-D Tablets** (Rugby)			sodium 5 mg	Maltodextrin, propylene glycol. In 60s.
otc	**Caltrate 600 + D Tablets** (Wyeth)			dl-alpha tocopherol, medium-chain triglycerides	Polyethylene glycol, polyvinyl alcohol, sucrose. In 60s.
otc	**Calcium 600 with Vitamin D Chewable Tablets** (Mason Vitamins)			Medium chain triglycerides, sodium 7 mg	Gluten free, preservative free, soy free. Coconut oil, corn syrup, sugar. Coffee mocha flavor. In 100s.
otc	**Calcium with D3 Tablets** (Nature Made)	200[a]	600[c]		Gluten free, preservative free. Glycerin, maltodextrin, mineral oil, PEG, soy. In 220s.
otc	**Calcium with D3 Liquid Softgels** (Nature Made)				Gluten free, preservative free. Glycerin, soy lecithin, soybean oil. In 100s.
otc	**Calcium with Vitamin D^3 Tablets** (Mason)	400[a]	500[f]		Maltodextrin, mineral oil, PEG, soy polysaccharide. In 100s.
otc	**Os Cal Caplets** (GlaxoSmithKline)	400[a]	500[c]	dl-alfa-tocopherol	Corn syrup, parabens, polyethylene glycol 3350, polyvinyl alcohol, sucrose. Film-coated. In 120s.
otc sf	**Os Cal Chewable Tablets** (GlaxoSmithKline)				Gluten free, sugar free. Aspartame, phenylalanine. Light lemon chiffon flavor. In 120s.

CALCIUM WITH VITAMIN D

	Product & Distributor	D units	Calcium (mg)	Other content	How Supplied
otc	**Calcium-500 Chewable Tablets** (Rugby)	200[a]	1,000[c]		Malted milk powder, nonfat dried milk, sugar, vanilla flavoring. In 60s.
otc	**UpCal D Powder** (Global Health)	250[a]	500[b]		Dextrose. In 2.5 g single-use packets.
otc *sf*	**Super Calcium 600 + Soy Caplets** (Mason Vitamins)	200[d]	600[c]	*NovaSoy* isoflavones 25 mg	Gluten free, preservative free, sugar free. Mineral oil, PEG, soy. Capsule shape. In 60s.
otc *sf*	**Calcarb 600 with Vitamin D Tablets** (Goldline)	200[a]	600[c]		Preservative free, sugar free. In 60s
otc	**Calcium 600 mg + D Tablets** (Major)				In 60s and 150s.
otc *sf*	**Calcium 600–D Tablets** (Rugby)				Sugar free. PEG, soy. In 60s.
otc	**Caltrate Colon Health Tablets** (Wyeth)			dl-alpha-tocopherol	Partially hydrogenated soybean oil, PEG, polydextrose, polyvinyl alcohol, sucrose. In 60s.
otc	**Calcium 600 mg with Vitamin D Tablets** (Cypress)	200[d]	600[c]		Mineral oil, PEG, soy polysaccharide. In 60s.
otc	**Citracal Tablets** (Bayer)	400[a]	500[b]		PEG. polyvinyl alcohol. Film-coated. In 150s.
otc	**Os Cal Caplets** (GlaxoSmithKline)	200[a]	500[c]		Gluten free. Corn syrup, parabens, PEG, polydextrose, tartrazine. Capsule shape. Film-coated. In 160s.
otc	**Oysco 500 + D Tablets** (Rugby)	200[a]	500[f]		In 60s and 1,000s.
otc	**Oyster Shell Calcium 500 mg + D Tablets** (Major)				Tartrazine. In 60s, 150s, 300s, and 1,000s.
otc	**Citrus Calcium + D Captabs** (Rugby)	200[a]	315[b]		Lactose free. PEG. Capsule shape. In 60s.
otc	**Citrus Calcium + D Tablets** (Rugby)	200[a]	200[b]		Lactose free. PEG. In 100s.
otc *sf*	**Oyst-Cal-D Tablets** (Goldline)	125[a]	250[f]		Preservative free, sugar free. Tartrazine. In 100s and 1,000s.
otc	**Oysco D Tablets** (Rugby)				PEG. In 100s, 250s, and 1,000s.
otc	**Oyster Shell Calcium with Vitamin D Tablets** (Major)				In 100s, 300s, and 1,000s.
otc	**Oyster Shell Calcium (Elemental) with Vitamin D Tablets** (Major)	125[d]	250[f]		In 100s.
otc	**Calcet Tablets** (Mission)	100[a]	150[e]		PEG, tartrazine. In 100s.

[a] As cholecalciferol.
[b] As calcium citrate.
[c] As calcium carbonate.
[d] Form of vitamin D unknown; content given in units.
[e] As calcium carbonate, calcium gluconate, and calcium lactate.
[f] As oyster shell.
[g] Form of calcium unknown.

For additional information, refer to the Dietary Reference Intakes of Vitamins and Minerals table.

AMINO ACID INJECTION (General formulations)

For a complete discussion of the use of protein substrates as a compound of intravenous nutritional therapy, refer to the IV Nutritional Therapy general monograph. For additional information, refer to the Dietary Reference Intakes of Vitamins and Minerals table.

Indications

➤*Nutritional supplement:* Six percent and 10% sulfite-free amino acid injections are indicated for the nutritional support of infants (including those of low birth weight) and young children requiring total parenteral nutrition (TPN) via either central or peripheral infusion routes. Parenteral nutrition with sulfite-free amino acid injections is indicated to prevent nitrogen and weight loss or treat negative nitrogen balance in infants and young children where the alimentary tract, by the oral, gastrostomy, or jejunostomy route, cannot or should not be used, or adequate protein intake is not feasible by these routes; gastrointestinal absorption of protein is impaired; or protein requirements are substantially increased, as with extensive burns. Dosage, route of administration, and concomitant infusion of nonprotein calories are dependent on various factors, such as nutritional and metabolic status of the patient, anticipated duration of parenteral nutritional support, and vein tolerance.

➤*Central venous nutrition:* Central venous infusion should be considered when amino acid solutions are to be admixed with hypertonic dextrose to promote protein synthesis in hypercatabolic or severely depleted infants, or those requiring long-term parenteral nutrition.

➤*Peripheral parenteral nutrition:* For moderately catabolic or depleted patients in whom the central venous route is not indicated, diluted amino acid solutions mixed with 5% to 10% dextrose solutions may be infused by peripheral vein, supplemented, if desired, with fat emulsion.

Administration and Dosage

➤*Nutritional support for children:* The objective of nutritional management of infants and young children is the provision of sufficient amino acid and caloric support for protein synthesis and growth.

The total daily dose of 6% and 10% sulfite-free amino acid injections depends on daily protein requirements and on the patient's metabolic and clinical response. The determination of nitrogen balance and accurate daily body weights, corrected for fluid balance, are probably the best means of assessing individual protein requirements. Dosage should also be guided by the patient's fluid intake limits and glucose and nitrogen tolerances, as well as by metabolic and clinical response.

➤*Protein allowances:* Recommendations for allowances of protein in infant nutrition have ranged from 2 to 4 g of protein per kilogram of body weight per day (2 to 4 g/kg/day). The recommended dosage of sulfite-free amino acid injections is 2 to 2.5 g of amino acids per kilogram of body weight per day (2 to 2.5 g/kg/day) for infants up to 10 kg. For infants and young children larger than 10 kg, the total dosage of amino acids should include the 20 to 25 g/day for the first 10 kg of body weight plus 1 to 1.25 g/day for each kg of body weight over 10 kg.

Typically, sulfite-free amino acid injections are admixed with 50% or 70% Dextrose Injection, supplemented with electrolytes and vitamins and administered continuously over a 24-hour period.

Total daily fluid intake should be appropriate for the patient's age and size. A fluid dose of 125 mL per kg body weight per day is appropriate for most infants on TPN. Although nitrogen requirements may be higher in severely hypercatabolic or depleted patients, provision of additional nitrogen may not be possible due to fluid intake limits, nitrogen, or glucose intolerance.

➤*Cysteine supplement:* Cysteine is considered to be an essential amino acid in infants and young children. An admixture of cysteine HCl to the TPN solution is therefore recommended. Based on clinical studies, the recommended dosage is 1 mmol of L-cysteine hydrochloride monohydrate per kilogram of body weight per day.

In many patients, provision of adequate calories in the form of hypertonic dextrose may require the administration of exogenous insulin to prevent hyperglycemia and glycosuria. To prevent rebound hypoglycemia, a solution containing 5% dextrose should be administered when hypertonic dextrose solutions are abruptly discontinued.

➤*Fat emulsion therapy:* Fat emulsion coadministration should be considered when prolonged (more than 5 days) parenteral nutrition is required in order to prevent essential fatty acid deficiency (EFAD). Serum lipids should be monitored for evidence of EFAD in patients maintained on fat-free TPN.

➤*Other electrolytes:* The provision of sufficient intracellular electrolytes, principally potassium, magnesium, and phosphate, is required for optimum utilization of amino acids. In addition, sufficient quantities of the major extracellular electrolytes sodium, calcium, and chloride, must be given. In patients with hyperchloremic or other metabolic acidoses, sodium and potassium may be added as the acetate salts to provide bicarbonate precursor. The electrolyte content of 6% and 10% sulfite-free amino acid injections must be considered when calculating daily electrolyte intake. Serum electrolytes, including magnesium and phosphorus, should be monitored frequently.

Appropriate vitamins, minerals and trace elements should also be provided.

➤*Central venous nutrition:* Hypertonic mixtures of amino acids and dextrose may be safely administered by continuous infusion through a central venous catheter with the tip located in the superior vena cava. Initial infusion rates should be slow, and gradually increased to the recommended 60 to 125 mL per kilogram of body weight per day. If administration rate should fall behind schedule, no attempt to "catch up" to planned intake should be made. In addition to meeting protein needs, the rate of administration, particularly during the first few days of therapy, is governed by the patient's glucose tolerance. Daily intake of amino acids and dextrose should be increased gradually to the maximum required dose as indicated by frequent determinations of glucose levels in blood and urine.

➤*Peripheral parenteral nutrition:* For patients in whom the central venous route is not indicated and who can consume adequate calories enterally, sulfite-free amino acid injections may be administered by peripheral vein with or without parenteral carbohydrate calories. Such infusates can be prepared by dilution with Sterile Water for Injection or 5% to 10% Dextrose Injection to prepare isotonic or slightly hypertonic solutions for peripheral infusion. It is essential that peripheral infusion be accompanied by adequate caloric intake.

Admixture incompatibility / compatibility – Sulfite-free amino acid injections may be admixed with solutions which contain phosphate or which have been supplemented with phosphate. The presence of calcium and magnesium ions in an additive solution should be considered when phosphate is also present, in order to avoid precipitation.

Care must be taken to avoid incompatible admixtures. Consult with pharmacist.

➤*Storage / Stability:* Protect from light until immediately prior to use. Do not remove container from overpouch until ready to use. Do not use if overpouch has been previously opened or damaged.

Exposure of pharmaceutical products to heat should be minimized. Avoid excessive heat. Protect from freezing. It is recommended that the product be stored at room temperature (25°C/77°F). Brief exposure up to 40°C (104°F) does not adversely affect the product.

Parenteral nutrition solutions should be used promptly after mixing. Any storage should be under refrigeration and limited to a brief period of time, preferably less than 24 hours.

Do not use unless solution is clear and seal is intact.

Actions

➤*Pharmacology:* Six percent and 10% sulfite-free amino acid injections provide a mixture of essential and nonessential amino acids as well as taurine and a soluble form of tyrosine, N-acetyl-L-tyrosine (NAT). This amino acid composition has been specifically formulated to provide a well-tolerated nitrogen source for nutritional support and therapy for infants and young children. When administered in conjunction with cysteine HCl, 6% and 10% amino acid injections result in the normalization of the plasma amino acid concentrations to a profile consistent with that of a breastfed infant.

The rationale for 6% and 10% amino acid injections is based on the observation of inadequate levels of essential amino acids in the plasma of infants receiving TPN using conventional amino acid solutions. These formulas were developed through the application of specific pharmacokinetic multiple regression analysis relating amino acid intake to the resulting plasma amino acid concentrations.

Clinical studies in infants and young children who required TPN therapy showed that infusion of 6% and 10% amino acid injections with a cysteine hydrochloride admixture resulted in a normalization of the plasma amino acid concentrations. In addition, weight gains, nitrogen balance, and serum protein concentrations were consistent with an improving nutritional status.

When infused with hypertonic dextrose as a calorie source, supplemented with cysteine hydrochloride, electrolytes, vitamins, and minerals, sulfite-free amino acid injections provide total parenteral nutrition in infants and young children, with the exception of essential fatty acids.

It is thought that the acetate from lysine acetate and acetic acid, under the conditions of parenteral nutrition, does not impact net acid-base balance when renal and respiratory functions are normal. Clinical evidence seems to support this thinking; however, confirmatory experimental evidence is not available.

The amount of chloride present in sulfite-free amino acid injections is not of clinical significance. The addition of cysteine hydrochloride will contribute to the chloride load.

The electrolyte content of any additives that are introduced should be carefully considered and included in total input computations.

Contraindications

Sulfite-free amino acid injections are contraindicated in patients with untreated anuria, hepatic coma, inborn errors of amino acid metabolism, including those involving branched chain amino acid metabolism such as maple syrup urine disease and isovaleric acidemia, or hypersensitivity to 1 or more amino acids present in the solution.

Warnings/Precautions

➤*Administration:* This injection is for compounding only, not for direct infusion.

➤*Azotemia:* Administration of amino acids in the presence of gastrointestinal bleeding may augment an already elevated blood urea nitrogen. Patients with azotemia from any cause should not be infused with amino acids without regard to total nitrogen intake.

➤*Fluid / solute overload:* Administration of IV fluids can cause fluid or solute overload, resulting in dilution of serum electrolyte concentrations, overhydration, congested states, or pulmonary edema. The risk of dilutional states is inversely proportional to the electrolyte concentrations of the solutions. The risk of solute overload causing congested states with peripheral and pulmonary edema is directly proportional to the electrolyte concentrations of the solution.

AMINO ACID INJECTION (General formulations)

➤*Hyperammonemia:* Hyperammonemia is of special significance in infants, as its occurrence in the syndrome caused by genetic metabolic defects is sometimes associated, although not necessarily in a causal relationship, with mental retardation. This reaction appears to be dose related and is more likely to develop during prolonged therapy. It is essential that blood ammonia be measured frequently in infants. The mechanisms of this reaction are not clearly defined but may involve genetic defects and immature or subclinically impaired liver function.

Conservative doses of amino acids should be given, dictated by the nutritional status of the patient. Should symptoms of hyperammonemia develop, amino acid administration should be discontinued and patient's clinical status reevaluated.

➤*Hypertonic solutions:* Strongly hypertonic nutrient solutions should be administered via an IV catheter placed in a central vein, preferably the superior vena cava.

➤*Ketone bodies:* Administration of amino acids without carbohydrates may result in the accumulation of ketone bodies in the blood. Correction of this ketonemia may be achieved by the administration of carbohydrates.

➤*Peripheral administration:* Peripheral administration of 6% and 10% sulfite-free amino acid injections requires appropriate dilution and provision of adequate calories. Care should be taken to ensure proper placement of the needle within the lumen of the vein. The venipuncture site should be inspected frequently for signs of infiltration. If venous thrombosis or phlebitis occurs, discontinue infusions or change infusion site and initiate appropriate treatment.

➤*Electrolyte supplementation:* Extraordinary electrolyte losses such as may occur during protracted nasogastric suction, vomiting, diarrhea, or gastrointestinal fistula drainage may necessitate additional electrolyte supplementation.

Metabolic acidosis can be prevented or readily controlled by adding a portion of the cations in the electrolyte mixture as acetate salts and, in the case of hyperchloremic acidosis, by keeping the total chloride content of the infusate to a minimum. Sulfite-free amino acid injections contain less than 3 mEq chloride per liter.

Sulfite-free amino acid injections contain no added phosphorus. Patients, especially those with hypophosphatemia, may require the addition of phosphate. To prevent hypocalcemia, calcium supplementation should always accompany phosphate administration. To ensure adequate intake, serum levels should be monitored frequently.

➤*Admixture incompatibilities:* To minimize the risk of possible incompatibilities arising from mixing this solution with other additives that may be prescribed, the final infusate should be inspected for cloudiness or precipitation immediately after mixing, prior to administration, and periodically during administration.

➤*Central venous nutrition:* Administration by central venous catheter should be used only by those familiar with this technique and its complications.

Central venous nutrition may be associated with complications which can be prevented or minimized by careful attention to all aspects of the procedure, including solution preparation, administration, and patient monitoring. It is essential that a carefully prepared protocol, based on current medical practices, be followed, preferably by an experienced team.

➤*Diabetes patients:* Special care must be taken when giving hypertonic dextrose to a diabetic or prediabetic patient. To prevent severe hyperglycemia in such patients, insulin may be required.

Administration of glucose at a rate exceeding the patient's utilization rate may lead to hyperglycemia, coma, and death.

➤*Renal function impairment:* Administration of amino acids in the presence of impaired renal function may augment an already elevated blood urea nitrogen.

➤*Hepatic function impairment:* Administration of amino acid solutions to a patient with hepatic insufficiency may result in plasma amino acid imbalances, hyperammonemia, prerenal azotemia, stupor and coma.

➤*Special risk:* Care should be taken to avoid circulatory overload, particularly in patients with cardiac insufficiency.

➤*Pregnancy: Category C.* Animal reproduction studies have not been conducted with 6% and 10% sulfite-free amino acid injections. It is also not known whether sulfite-free amino acid injections can cause fetal harm when administered to a pregnant woman or can affect reproduction capacity.

➤*Monitoring:* Clinical evaluation and periodic laboratory determinations are necessary to monitor changes in fluid balance, electrolyte concentrations, and acid-base balance during prolonged parenteral therapy or whenever the condition of the patient warrants such evaluation. Significant deviations from normal concentrations may require the use of additional electrolyte supplements.

Safe, effective use of parenteral nutrition requires a knowledge of nutrition as well as clinical expertise in recognition and treatment of the complications which can occur. Frequent evaluation and laboratory determinations are necessary for proper monitoring of parenteral nutrition. Studies should include blood sugar, serum proteins, kidney and liver function tests, electrolytes, hemogram, carbon dioxide content, serum osmolalities, blood cultures, and blood ammonia levels.

Adverse Reactions

If an adverse reaction does occur, discontinue the infusion, evaluate the patient, institute appropriate therapeutic countermeasures and save the remainder of the fluid for examination if deemed necessary.

➤*Infusion-related reactions:* Reactions reported in clinical studies as a result of infusion of the parenteral fluid were water weight gain, edema, increase in blood urea nitrogen (BUN), and mild acidosis.

➤*Reactions due to solution or administration technique:* Reactions which may occur because of the solution or the technique of administration include febrile response, infection at the site of injection, venous thrombosis or phlebitis extending from the site of injection, extravasation and hypervolemia.

➤*Local:* Local reaction at the infusion site, consisting of a warm sensation, erythema, phlebitis and thrombosis, have been reported with peripheral amino acid infusions, especially if other substances are also administered through the same site.

If electrolyte supplementation is required during peripheral infusion, it is recommended that additives be administered throughout the day in order to avoid possible venous irritation. Irritating additive medications may require injection at another site and should not be added directly to the amino acid infusate.

Symptoms may result from an excess or deficit of 1 or more of the ions present in the solution; therefore, frequent monitoring of electrolyte levels is essential.

➤*Phosphorus deficiency:* Phosphorus deficiency may lead to impaired tissue oxygenation and acute hemolytic anemia. Relative to calcium, excessive phosphorus intake can precipitate hypocalcemia with cramps, tetany and muscular hyperexcitability.

Overdosage

➤*Treatment:* In the event of a fluid or solute overload during parenteral therapy, reevaluate the patient's condition, and institute appropriate corrective treatment.

CRYSTALLINE AMINO ACID INFUSIONS

	Aminosyn 3.5% (Abbott)	Aminosyn II 3.5% (Abbott)	Aminosyn 5% (Abbott)	Aminosyn II 5% (Abbott)	Travasol 5.5% (Baxter)	TrophAmine 6% (McGaw)
Amino Acid Concentration	3.5%	3.5%	5%	5%	5.5%	6%
Nitrogen(g/100 ml)	0.55	0.54	0.79	0.77	0.925	0.93
Amino Acids (Essential) (mg/100 ml)						
Isoleucine	252	231	360	330	263	490
Leucine	329	350	470	500	340	840
Lysine	252	368	360	525	318	490
Methionine	140	60	200	86	318	200
Phenylalanine	154	104	220	149	340	290
Threonine	182	140	260	200	230	250
Tryptophan	56	70	80	100	99	120
Valine	280	175	400	250	252	470
Amino Acids (Nonessential) (mg/100 ml)						
Alanine	448	348	640	497	1140	320
Arginine	343	356	490	509	570	730
Histidine[1]	105	105	150	150	241	290
Proline	300	253	430	361	230	410
Serine	147	186	210	265		230
Taurine						15
Tyrosine	31	95	44	135	22	140
Aminoacetic Acid (Glycine)	448	175	640	250	1140	220
Glutamic Acid		258		369		300
Aspartic Acid		245		350		190
Cysteine						< 14
Electrolytes (mEq/L)						
Sodium	7	16.3		19.3		5
Potassium			5.4			
Chloride					22	< 3
Acetate	46	25.2	86	35.9	48	56
Phosphate (mM/L)						
Osmolarity (mOsm/L)	357	308	500	438	575	525
Supplied in (ml)	1000[2]	1000[3]	500[4] 1000[4]	500[3] 1000[3]	500[5] 1000[5] 2000[5]	500[6]
Labeled Indications						
Peripheral Parenteral Nutrition	Yes	Yes	Yes	Yes	Yes	Yes
Central TPN	No	No	Yes	Yes	Yes	Yes
Protein Sparing	Yes	Yes	Yes	Yes	Yes	No

	Aminosyn 7% (Abbott)	Aminosyn-PF 7% (Abbott)	Aminosyn II 7% (Abbott)	Aminosyn 8.5% (Abbott)
Amino Acid Concentration	7%	7%	7%	8.5%
Nitrogen (g/100 ml)	1.1	1.07	1.07	1.34
Amino Acids (Essential) (mg/100 ml)				
Isoleucine	510	534	462	620
Leucine	660	831	700	810
Lysine	510	475	735	624
Methionine	280	125	120	340
Phenylalanine	310	300	209	380
Threonine	370	360	280	460
Tryptophan	120	125	140	150
Valine	560	452	350	680
Amino Acids (Nonessential) (mg/100 ml)				
Alanine	900	490	695	1100
Arginine	690	861	713	850
Histidine[1]	210	220	210	260
Proline	610	570	505	750
Serine	300	347	371	370
Taurine		50		
Tyrosine	44	44	189	44
Aminoacetic Acid (Glycine)	900	270	350	1100
Glutamic Acid		576	517	
Aspartic Acid		370	490	
Cysteine				
Electrolytes (mEq/L)				
Sodium		3.4	31.3	
Potassium	5.4			5.4
Chloride				35
Acetate	105	32.5	50.3	90
Phosphate (mM/L)				
Osmolarity (mOsm/L)	700	586	612	850
Supplied in (ml)	500[4]	250[7] 500[7]	500[3]	500[4] 1000[4]
Labeled Indications				
Peripheral Parenteral Nutrition	Yes	Yes	Yes	Yes
Central TPN	Yes	Yes	Yes	Yes
Protein Sparing	Yes	No	Yes	Yes

	Aminosyn II 8.5% (Abbott)	Travasol 8.5 without electrolytes (Baxter)	FreAmine III 8.5% (B. Braun)
Amino Acid Concentration	8.5%	8.5%	8.5%
Nitrogen (g/100 ml)	1.3	1.43	
Amino Acids (Essential) (mg/100 ml)			
Isoleucine	561	406	590
Leucine	850	526	770
Lysine	893	492	620
Methionine	146	492	450
Phenylalanine	253	526	480
Threonine	340	356	340
Tryptophan	170	152	130
Valine	425	390	560
Amino Acids (Nonessential) (mg/100 ml)			
Alanine	844	1760	600
Arginine	865	880	810
Histidine[1]	255	372	240
Proline	614	356	950
Serine	450		500
Taurine			
Tyrosine	230	34	
Aminoacetic Acid (Glycine)	425	1760	1190
Glutamic Acid	627		
Aspartic Acid	595		
Cysteine			< 20
Electrolytes (mEq/L)			
Sodium	33.3		10
Potassium			
Chloride		34	< 3
Acetate	61.1	73	72
Phosphate (mM/L)			10
Osmolarity (mOsm/L)	742	890	810
Supplied in (ml)	500[3] 1000[3]	500[8] 1000[8] 2000[8]	500[9] 1000[9]
Labeled Indications			
Peripheral Parenteral Nutrition	Yes	Yes	Yes
Central TPN	Yes	Yes	Yes
Protein Sparing	Yes	Yes	Yes

Protein Substrates

CRYSTALLINE AMINO ACID INFUSIONS

	TrophAmine 10% (McGaw)	Aminosyn 10% (Abbott)	Aminosyn-PF 10% (Hospira)	Aminosyn II 10% (Hospira)	Aminosyn (pH6) 10% (Abbott)
Amino Acid Concentration	10%	10%	10%	10%	10%
Nitrogen (g/100 ml)	1.55	1.57	1.52	1.53	1.57
Amino Acids (Essential) (mg/100 ml)					
Isoleucine	820	720	760	660	720
Leucine	1400	940	1200	1000	940
Lysine	820	720	677	1050	720
Methionine	340	400	180	172	400
Phenylalanine	480	440	427	298	440
Threonine	420	520	512	400	520
Tryptophan	200	160	180	200	160
Valine	780	800	673	500	800
Amino Acids (Nonessential) (mg/100 ml)					
Alanine	540	1280	698	993	1280
Arginine	1200	980	1227	1018	980
Histidine[1]	480	300	312	300	300
Proline	680	860	812	722	860
Serine	380	420	495	530	420
Taurine	25		70		
Tyrosine	240	44	40	270	44
Aminoacetic Acid (Glycine)	360	1280	385	500	1280
Glutamic Acid	500		620	738	
Aspartic Acid	320		527	700	
Cysteine	< 16				
Electrolytes (mEq/L)					
Sodium	5		3.4	45.3	
Potassium		5.4			2.7
Chloride	< 3				
Acetate	97	148	46.3	71.8	111
Phosphate (mM/L)10					
Osmolarity (mOsm/L)	875	1000	829	873	993
Supplied in (ml)	500[6]	500[4] 1000[4]	1000[10]	500[3] 1000[3]	500[11] 1000[11]
Labeled Indications					
Peripheral Parenteral Nutrition	Yes	Yes	Yes	Yes	Yes
Central TPN	Yes	Yes	Yes	Yes	Yes
Protein Sparing	No	Yes	No	Yes	Yes

	Travasol 10% (Baxter)	FreAmine III 10% (McGaw)	Novamine (Clintec)	Novamine 15% (Clintec)	Aminosyn II 15% (Hospira)
Amino Acid Concentration	10%	10%	11.4%	15%	15%
Nitrogen (g/100 ml)	1.65	1.53	1.8	2.37	2.3
Amino Acids (Essential) (mg/100 ml)					
Isoleucine	600	690	570	749	990
Leucine	730	910	790	1040	1500
Lysine	580	730	900	1180	1575
Methionine	400	530	570	749	258
Phenylalanine	560	560	790	1040	447
Threonine	420	400	570	749	600
Tryptophan	180	150	190	250	300
Valine	580	660	730	960	750
Amino Acids (Nonessential) (mg/100 ml)					
Alanine	2070	710	1650	2170	1490
Arginine	1150	950	1120	1470	1527
Histidine[1]	480	280	680	894	450
Proline	680	1120	680	894	1083
Serine	500	590	450	592	795
Taurine					
Tyrosine	40		30	39	405
Aminoacetic Acid (Glycine)	1030	1400	790	1040	750
Glutamic Acid			570	749	1107
Aspartic Acid			330	434	1050
Cysteine		< 24			
Electrolytes (mEq/L)					
Sodium		10			62.7
Potassium					
Chloride	40	< 3			
Acetate	87	≈89	114	151	107.6
Phosphate (mM/L)		10			
Osmolarity (mOsm/L)	1000	≈ 950	1057	1388	1300
Supplied in (ml)	250[12,13] 500[12,13] 1000[12,13] 2000[12]	500[9] 1000[9]	500[14] 1000[14]	500[14] 1000[14]	2000[15]
Labeled Indications					
Peripheral Parenteral Nutrition	Yes	Yes	Yes	Yes	Yes
Central TPN	Yes	Yes	Yes	Yes	Yes
Protein Sparing	Yes	Yes	Yes	No	No

1 Histidine is considered an essential amino acid in infants and in renal failure.
2 With 7 mEq/L sodium from the antioxidant sodium hydrosulfite.
3 Includes 20 mg/dl sodium hydrosulfite.
4 Includes 5.4 mEq/L potassium from the antioxidant potassium metabisulfite.
5 With ≈ 3 mEq/L sodium bisulfite.
6 With < 50 mg sodium metabisulfite per 100 ml.
7 From the antioxidant sodium hydrosulfite.
8 With 3 mEq/L sodium bisulfite.
9 With < 0.1 g sodium bisulfite per 100 ml.
10 With 230 mg sodium hydrosulfite per 100 ml.
11 Potassium derived from the antioxidant potassium metabisulfite.
12 Acetate in Viaflex container = 60 mEq/L; osmolarity is 970 mOsm/L.
13 Sizes also come in Viaflex containers.
14 With 30 mg sodium metabisulfite.
15 With 60 mg sodium hydrosulfite per 100 ml.

CRYSTALLINE AMINO ACID INFUSIONS WITH ELECTROLYTES

	ProcalAmine (McGaw)	FreAmine III 3% w/Electrolytes (McGaw)	Aminosyn 3.5% M (Abbott)	Aminosyn II 3.5% M (Abbott)	3.5% Travasol w/Electrolytes (Clintec)	5.5% Travasol w/Electrolytes (Clintec)
Amino Acid Concentration	3%	3%	3.5%	3.5%	3.5%	5.5%
Nitrogen (g/100 ml)	0.46	0.46	0.55	0.54	0.591	0.925
Amino Acids (Essential) (mg/100 ml)						
Isoleucine	210	210	252	231	168	263
Leucine	270	270	329	350	217	340
Lysine	220	220	252	368	203	318
Methionine	160	160	140	60	203	318
Phenylalanine	170	170	154	104	217	340
Threonine	120	120	182	140	147	230
Tryptophan	46	46	56	70	63	99
Valine	200	200	280	175	161	252
Amino Acids (Nonessential) (mg/100 ml)						
Alanine	210	210	448	348	728	1140
Arginine	290	290	343	356	364	570
Histidine[1]	85	85	105	105	154	241
Proline	340	340	300	253	147	230
Serine	180	180	147	186		
Tyrosine			31	95	14	22
Glycine	420	420	448	175	728	1140
Glutamic Acid				258		
Aspartic Acid				245		
Cysteine	< 20	< 20				
Electrolytes (mEq/L)						
Sodium	35	35	47	36	25	70
Potassium	24	24.5	13	13	15	60
Magnesium	5	5	3	3	5	10
Chloride	41	41	40	37	25	70
Acetate	47	44	58	25	52	102
Phosphate (mM/L)	3.5	3.5	3.5	3.5	7.5	30
Osmolarity (mOsm/L)	735	≈ 405	477	425	450	850
Nonprotein Calories (g/100 ml) (glycerin)	3					
Supplied in (ml)	1000[2]	1000[3]	1000[4]	1000[5]	500[6] 1000[6]	500[6] 1000[6] 2000[6]
Labeled Indications						
Peripheral Parenteral Nutrition	Yes	Yes	Yes	Yes	Yes	Yes
Central TPN	No	No	No	No	No	Yes
Protein Sparing	Yes	Yes	Yes	Yes	Yes	Yes

	Aminosyn 7% w/Electrolytes (Abbott)	Aminosyn II 7% with Electrolytes (Abbott)	Aminosyn 8.5% w/Electrolytes (Abbott)	Aminosyn II 8.5% with Electrolytes (Abbott)	FreAmine III 8.5% w/Electrolytes (McGaw)	Travasol 8.5% w/Electrolytes (Hospira)	Aminosyn II 10% with Electrolytes (Abbott)
Amino Acid Concentration	7%	7%	8.5%	8.5%	8.5%	8.5%	10%
Nitrogen g/100 ml	1.1	1.07	1.34	1.3	1.3	1.43	1.53
Amino Acids (Essential) (mg/100 ml)							
Isoleucine	510	462	620	561	590	406	660
Leucine	660	700	810	850	770	526	1000
Lysine	510	735	624	893	620	492	1050
Methionine	280	120	340	146	450	492	172
Phenylalanine	310	209	380	253	480	526	298
Threonine	370	280	460	340	340	356	400
Tryptophan	120	140	150	170	130	152	200
Valine	560	350	680	425	560	390	500
Amino Acids (Nonessential) (mg/100 ml)							
Alanine	900	695	1100	844	600	1760	993
Arginine	690	713	850	865	810	880	1018
Histidine[1]	210	210	260	255	240	372	300
Proline	610	505	750	614	950	356	722

CRYSTALLINE AMINO ACID INFUSIONS WITH ELECTROLYTES

	Aminosyn 7% w/Electrolytes (Abbott)	Aminosyn II 7% with Electrolytes (Abbott)	Aminosyn 8.5% w/Electrolytes (Abbott)	Aminosyn II 8.5% with Electrolytes (Abbott)	FreAmine III 8.5% w/Electrolytes (McGaw)	Travasol 8.5% w/Electrolytes (Hospira)	Aminosyn II 10% with Electrolytes (Abbott)
Serine	300	371	370	450	500		530
Tyrosine	44	189	44	230		34	270
Glycine	900	350	1100	425	1190	1760	500
Glutamic Acid		517		627			738
Aspartic Acid		490		595			700
Cysteine					< 20		
Electrolytes (mEq/L)							
Sodium	70	76	70	80	60	70	87
Potassium	66	66	66	66	60	60	66
Magnesium	10	10	10	10	10	10	10
Chloride	96	86	98	86	60	70	86
Acetate	124	50	142	61	125	141	72
Phosphate (mM/L)	30	30	30	30	20	30	30
Osmolarity (mOsm/L)	1013	869	1160	999	1045	1160	1130
Supplied in (ml)	500[7]	500[8]	500[7]	500[8]	500[9] 1000[9]	500[6] 1000[6] 2000[6]	1000[8]
Labeled Indications							
Peripheral Parenteral Nutrition	Yes	Yes	Yes	Yes	Yes	Yes	Yes
Central TPN	Yes	Yes	Yes	Yes	Yes	Yes	Yes
Protein Sparing	Yes	Yes	Yes	Yes	Yes	Yes	Yes

[1] Histidine is considered an essential amino acid in infants and in renal failure.
[2] With < 50 mg K+ metabisulfite and 3 mEq Ca/L.
[3] With < 0.05 g of the antioxidant potassium metabisulfite.
[4] Includes 7 mEq/L sodium from the antioxidant sodium hydrosulfite.
[5] With 20 mg sodium hydrosulfite per 100 ml.
[6] With 3 mEq/L sodium bisulfite.
[7] Includes 5.4 mEq/L potassium from the antioxidant potassium metabisulfite.
[8] Includes sodium from the antioxidant sodium hydrosulfite.
[9] With < 0.1 g sodium bisulfite per 100 ml.

CRYSTALLINE AMINO ACID INFUSIONS WITH DEXTROSE

	Travasol 2.75% in 5% Dextrose[1] (Clintec)	Travasol 2.75% in 10% Dextrose[1] (Clintec)	Travasol 2.75% in 25% Dextrose[1] (Clintec)	Aminosyn II 3.5% in 5% Dextrose[1] (Hospira)	Aminosyn II 3.5% in 25% Dextrose[1] (Abbott)
Amino Acid Concentration	2.75%	2.75%	2.75%	3.5%	3.5%
Dextrose Concentration	5%	10%	25%	5%	25%
Nitrogen (g/100 ml)	0.46	0.46	0.46	0.54	0.54
Amino Acids (Essential) (mg/100 ml)					
Isoleucine	132	132	132	231	231
Leucine	170	170	170	350	350
Lysine	159	159	159	368	368
Methionine	159	159	159	60	60
Phenylalanine	170	170	170	104	104
Threonine	115	115	115	140	140
Tryptophan	50	50	50	70	70
Valine	126	126	126	175	175
Amino Acids (Nonessential) (mg/100 ml)					
Alanine	570	570	570	348	348
Arginine	285	285	285	356	356
Histidine[2]	120	120	120	105	105
Proline	115	115	115	252	252
Serine				186	186
Tyrosine	11	11	11	94	94
Aminoacetic Acid (Glycine)	570	570	570	175	175
Glutamic Acid				258	258
Aspartic Acid				245	245
Cysteine					
Electrolytes (mEq/L)					
Sodium				18	18
Potassium					

CRYSTALLINE AMINO ACID INFUSIONS WITH DEXTROSE

	Travasol 2.75% in 5% Dextrose[1] (Clintec)	Travasol 2.75% in 10% Dextrose[1] (Clintec)	Travasol 2.75% in 25% Dextrose[1] (Clintec)	Aminosyn II 3.5% in 5% Dextrose[1] (Hospira)	Aminosyn II 3.5% in 25% Dextrose[1] (Abbott)
Magnesium					
Chloride	11	11	11		
Acetate	16	16	16	25.2	25.2
Phosphate (mM/L)					
Osmolarity (mOsm/L)	530	785	1540	585	1515
Supplied in (ml)	500 ml with 500 ml dextrose	500 ml with 500 ml dextrose	500 ml with 500 ml dextrose	1000 ml with 1000 ml dextrose[3]	500 ml with 500 ml dextrose[3]
Labeled Indications					
Peripheral Parenteral Nutrition	Yes	Yes	Yes	Yes	No
Central TPN	Yes	Yes	Yes	No	Yes

	Travasol 4.25% in 5% Dextrose[1] (Clintec)	Aminosyn II 4.25% in 10% Dextrose[1] (Abbott)	Travasol 4.25% in 10% Dextrose[1] (Clintec)	Aminosyn II 4.25% in 20% Dextrose (Abbott)
Amino Acid Concentration	4.25%	4.25%	4.25%	4.25%
Dextrose Concentration	5%	10%	10%	20%
Nitrogen (g/100 ml)	0.7	0.65	0.7	0.65
Amino Acids (Essential) (mg/100 ml)				
Isoleucine	203	280	203	280
Leucine	263	425	263	425
Lysine	246	446	246	446
Methionine	246	73	246	73
Phenylalanine	263	126	263	126
Threonine	178	170	178	170
Tryptophan	76	85	76	85
Valine	195	212	195	212
Amino Acids (Nonessential) (mg/100 ml)				
Alanine	880	422	880	422
Arginine	440	432	440	432
Histidine[2]	186	128	186	128
Proline	178	307	178	307
Serine		225		225
Tyrosine	17	115	17	115
Aminoacetic Acid (Glycine)	880	212	880	212
Glutamic Acid		314		314
Aspartic Acid		298		298
Cysteine				
Electrolytes (mEq/L)				
Sodium		19		19
Potassium				
Magnesium				
Chloride	17		17	
Acetate	22	30.6	22	30.6
Phosphate (mM/L)				
Osmolarity (mOsm/L)	680	894	935	1295
Supplied in (ml)	500 ml with 500 ml dextrose	1000 ml w/1000 ml dextrose[3]	500 ml with 500 ml dextrose	1000 ml with 1000 ml dextrose[3]
Labeled Indications				
Peripheral Parenteral Nutrition	Yes	Yes	Yes	No
Central TPN	Yes	No	Yes	Yes

CRYSTALLINE AMINO ACID INFUSIONS WITH DEXTROSE

	Aminosyn II 4.25% in 25% Dextrose[1] (Abbott)	Travasol 4.25% in 25% Dextrose[1] (Clintec)	Aminosyn II 5% in 25% Dextrose[1] (Abbott)
Amino Acid Concentration	4.25%	4.25%	5%
Dextrose Concentration	25%	25%	25%
Nitrogen (g/100 ml)	0.65	0.65	0.77
Amino Acids (Essential) (mg/100 ml)			
Isoleucine	280	203	330
Leucine	425	263	500
Lysine	446	246	525
Methionine	73	246	86
Phenylalanine	126	263	149
Threonine	170	178	200
Tryptophan	85	76	100
Valine	212	195	250
Amino Acids (Nonessential) (mg/100 ml)			
Alanine	422	880	496
Arginine	432	440	509
Histidine[2]	128	186	150
Proline	307	178	361
Serine	225		265
Tyrosine	115	17	135
Aminoacetic Acid (Glycine)	212	880	250
Glutamic Acid	314		369
Aspartic Acid	298		350
Cysteine			
Electrolytes (mEq/L)			
Sodium	19		22.2
Potassium			
Magnesium			
Chloride		17	
Acetate	30.6	22	35.9
Phosphate (mM/L)			
Osmolarity (mOsm/L)	1536	1690	1539
Supplied in (ml)	750 and 1000 ml and 750 and 1000 ml dextrose[3]	500 ml with 500 ml dextrose[3]	500, 750 and 1000 ml and 500, 750 and 1000 ml dextrose[3]
Labeled Indications			
Peripheral Parenteral Nutrition	No	Yes	No
Central TPN	Yes	Yes	Yes

[1] Solution composition represents admixture of dual-chamber *Quick Mix* or *Nutrimix* container.

[2] Histidine is considered an essential amino acid in infants and in renal failure.

[3] With 30 mg sodium hydrosulfite per 100 ml.

CRYSTALLINE AMINO ACID INFUSIONS WITH ELECTROLYTES IN DEXTROSE

	Aminosyn II 3.5% M[1] in 5% Dextrose[2] (Abbott)	Aminosyn II 4.25% M[1] in 10% Dextrose[2] (Abbott)
Amino Acid Concentration	3.5%	4.25%
Dextrose Concentration	5%	10%
Nitrogen (g/100 ml)	0.535	0.65
Amino Acids (Essential) (mg/100 ml)		
Isoleucine	231	280
Leucine	350	425
Lysine	368	446
Methionine	60	73
Phenylalanine	104	126
Threonine	140	170
Tryptophan	70	85
Valine	175	212
Amino Acids (Nonessential) (mg/100 ml)		
Alanine	348	422
Arginine	356	432
Histidine[3]	105	128
Proline	252	307
Serine	186	225
Tyrosine	94	115
Aminoacetic Acid (Glycine)	175	212
Glutamic Acid	258	314
Aspartic Acid	245	298
Cysteine		
Electrolytes (mEq/L)		
Sodium	41	43.7
Potassium	13	13
Magnesium	3	3
Chloride	36.5	36.5
Acetate	25.1	30.5
Phosphorus (mM/L)	3.5	3.5
Osmolarity (mOsm/L)	616	919
Supplied in (ml)	500 and 1000 ml and 500 and 1000 ml dextrose[4]	500 ml and 500 ml dextrose[4]
Labeled Indications		
Peripheral Parenteral Nutrition	Yes	Yes
Central TPN	No	Yes
Protein Sparing	No	No

[1] With maintenance electrolytes.
[2] Solution composition represents admixture of *Nutrimix* dual-chamber container.
[3] Histidine is considered an essential amino acid in infants and in renal failure.
[4] With 30 mg sodium hydrosulfite per 100 ml.

AMINO ACID FORMULATIONS FOR RENAL FAILURE

	Aminosyn-RF 5.2% (Hospira)	Aminess 5.2% (Baxter)	5.4% NephrAmine (McGaw)	RenAmin (Baxter)
Amino Acid Concentration	5.2%	5.2%	5.4%	6.5%
Nitrogen (g/100 mL)	0.79	0.66	0.65	1
Amino Acids (Essential) (mg/100 mL)				
Isoleucine	462	525	560	500
Leucine	726	825	880	600
Lysine	535	600	640	450
Methionine	726	825	880	500
Phenylalanine	726	825	880	490
Threonine	330	375	400	380
Tryptophan	165	188	200	160
Valine	528	600	640	820
Histidine	429	412	250	420
Amino Acids (Nonessential) (mg/100 mL)				
Cysteine			< 20	
Arginine	600			630
Alanine				560
Proline				350
Glycine				300
Serine				300
Tyrosine				40
Electrolytes (mEq/L)				
Sodium			5	
Acetate	≈ 105	50	≈ 44	60
Potassium	5.4			
Chloride			< 3	31
Osmolarity (mOsm/L)	475	416	435	600
Supplied in (mL)	300[a]	400[b]	250[c]	250[d] 500[d]

[a] With 60 mg potassium metabisulfite per 100 mL.
[b] In 500 mL bottle.
[c] With less than 0.05 g sodium bisulfite per 100 mL.
[d] With ≈ 3 mEq sodium bisulfite.

AMINO ACID FORMULATIONS FOR RENAL FAILURE — INTRAVENOUS

For a complete discussion of the use of protein substrates for intravenous nutritional therapy, refer to the IV Nutritionals monograph. For additional information, refer to the .Dietary Reference Intakes of Vitamins and Minerals table

Indications

➤*Nutritional support:* For nutritional support of uremic patients, particularly when oral nutrition is impractical, not feasible or insufficient.

Essential amino acid injection does not replace dialysis and conventional supportive therapy in patients with renal failure. To promote urea reutilization, provide adequate calories with minimal amounts of essential amino acids and restrict the intake of nonessential nitrogen.

➤*Children:* Use with caution in pediatric patients, especially low birth weight infants, due to limited clinical experience. Laboratory and clinical monitoring must be extensive and frequent. Use a low initial dose and increase slowly.

The absence of arginine in *NephrAmine* and *Aminess* may accentuate the risk of hyperammonemia in infants. *Aminosyn-RF* and *RenAmin* contain arginine.

AMINO ACID FORMULATIONS FOR RENAL FAILURE — INTRAVENOUS

Administration and Dosage

Provide adequate calories simultaneously. Administer essential amino acid/dextrose mixtures by continuous infusion through a central venous catheter. Use slow initial infusion rates, generally 20 to 30 mL/hour for the first 6 to 8 hours. Increase by 10 mL/hour each 24 hours, up to a maximum of 60 to 100 mL/hour.

Administration rate is governed by the patient's nitrogen, fluid and glucose tolerance. Uremic patients are frequently glucose intolerant, especially in association with peritoneal dialysis, and may require exogenous insulin to prevent hyperglycemia. To prevent rebound hypoglycemia when hypertonic dextrose infusions are abruptly discontinued, administer a 5% dextrose solution.

➤*Adults:*

Aminosyn-RF – 300 to 600 mL. Mix 300 mL with 500 mL of 70% dextrose to provide a solution of 1.96% essential amino acids in 44% dextrose (calorie:nitrogen ratio = 504:1).

Aminess – 400 mL. Mix 400 mL with 500 mL of 70% dextrose to yield a solution of 2.3% essential amino acids in 39% dextrose (calorie:nitrogen ratio = 450:1).

NephrAmine – 250 to 500 mL. Mix 250 mL w/500 mL of 70% dextrose to yield solution of 1.8% essential amino acids in 47% dextrose (calorie: nitrogen ratio = 744:1).

RenAmin – 250 to 500 mL.

➤*Children:* Individualize dosage. A dosage of 0.5 to 1 g/kg/day will meet the requirements of the majority of pediatric patients. Use a low initial daily dosage and increase slowly; more than 1 g/kg/day is not recommended.

Actions

➤*Pharmacology:* Patients with renal decompensation have different amino acid requirements than those with normal renal function. Use in uremic patients is based on the minimal requirements for each of the 8 essential amino acids. These products contain histidine, an amino acid considered essential for infant growth and for uremic patients.

In renal failure, nonspecific nitrogen-containing compounds are broken down in the intestine. The ammonia formed is absorbed and incorporated by the liver into nonessential amino acids, provided essential amino acid requirements are being met. Exogenously supplying only essential amino acids allows urea nitrogen to be recycled which can serve as a precursor for nonessential amino acid synthesis. Therefore, administration to uremic patients, particularly those who are protein deficient, results in the utilization of retained urea, and may be followed by a drop in BUN and resolution of many azotemic symptoms.

Infusion of essential amino acids and hypertonic dextrose promotes protein synthesis, improves cellular metabolic balance, decreases the rate of rise of BUN and minimizes deterioration of serum potassium, magnesium and phosphorus balance in patients with impaired renal function. This therapy may decrease morbidity associated with acute renal failure and promote earlier return of renal function. Although controversial, these formulations may have no clinically significant advantage over the general formulations containing both essential and nonessential amino acids in most uremic patients.

AMINO ACID FORMULATIONS FOR HIGH METABOLIC STRESS — INTRAVENOUS

	STRESS FORMULATION		
	4% BranchAmin (Baxter)	FreAmine HBC 6.9% (McGaw)	Aminosyn-HBC 7% (Hospira)
Amino Acid Concentration	4%	6.9%	7%
Nitrogen (g/100 mL)	0.443	0.97	1.12
Amino Acids (Essential) (mg/100 mL)			
Isoleucine	1380	760	789
Leucine	1380	1370	1576
Lysine		410	265
Methionine		250	206
Phenylalanine		320	228
Threonine		200	272
Tryptophan		90	88
Valine	1240	880	789
Amino Acids (Nonessential) (mg/100 mL)			
Alanine		400	660
Arginine		580	507
Histidine[a]		160	154
Proline		630	448
Serine		330	221
Tyrosine			33
Glycine		330	660
Cysteine		< 20	
Electrolytes (mEq/L)			
Sodium		10	7[b]
Chloride		< 3	
Acetate		≈ 57	72
Phosphate (mM/L)			
Osmolarity (mOsm/L)	316	620	665
Supplied in (mL)	500	750[c,d]	500[b] 1000[b]
Labeled Indications			
Peripheral Parenteral Nutrition	Yes[e]	Yes	Yes
Central TPN	Yes[e]	Yes	Yes

[a] Histidine is considered an essential amino acid in infants and in renal failure.
[b] With 60 mg sodium hydrosulfite.
[c] With less than 100 mg sodium bisulfite/100 mL.
[d] In 1000 mL bottles.
[e] Must be admixed with a complete amino acid injection.

AMINO ACID FORMULATIONS FOR HIGH METABOLIC STRESS — INTRAVENOUS

For a complete discussion of the use of protein substrates as a compound of intravenous nutritional therapy, refer to the IV Nutritionals monograph. For additional information, refer to the Dietary Reference Intakes of Vitamins and Minerals table.

Indications

➤*Nitrogen imbalance:* To prevent nitrogen loss or treat negative nitrogen balance in adults if: (1) The alimentary tract, by oral, gastrostomy or jejunostomy route, cannot or should not be used, or adequate protein intake is not feasible by these routes; (2) GI protein absorption is impaired; or (3) nitrogen homeostasis is substantially impaired as with severe trauma or sepsis.

Administration and Dosage

➤*Adults:* Daily amino acid doses of ≈ 1.5 g/kg for adults with adequate calories generally satisfy protein needs and promote positive nitrogen balance. May need higher doses in severely catabolic states. Fat emulsion may help meet energy requirements.

➤*Severely catabolic patients:* For severely catabolic, depleted patients or those requiring long-term TPN, consider central venous nutrition. Start with infusates containing lower dextrose concentrations; gradually increase dextrose to estimated caloric needs as glucose tolerance increases. *FreAmine HBC* 750 mL and 250 mL 70% dextrose or 500 mL *Aminosyn-HBC* 7% and 500 mL concentrated dextrose, with added electrolytes, trace metals and vitamins, may be given over 8 hours. *BranchAmin* 4% must be admixed with a complete amino acid injection, with or without a concentrated caloric source.

➤*Moderately catabolic patients:* For moderately catabolic, depleted patients in whom central venous route is not indicated, may infuse diluted *FreAmine HBC* or *Aminosyn-HBC* 7% with minimal caloric supplementation by peripheral vein; supplement, if desired, with fat emulsion.

Usual administration of 4% BCAA Injection is used as a supplement to parenteral nutrition solutions to achieve an amino acid solution that is ≈ 50% w/w BCAA. One method for achieving this ratio is the admixture of two volumes of 4% BCAA Injection at 4 g/dL concentration with one volume of an amino acid solution of 8 to 10 g/dL concentration. The supplemental amino acid mixture is given with energy substrates to provide at least 35 kcal/kg ideal body weight as nonprotein calories.

AMINO ACID FORMULATIONS FOR HIGH METABOLIC STRESS — INTRAVENOUS

Actions

➤*Pharmacology:* These are mixtures of essential and nonessential amino acids with high concentrations of branched chain amino acids (BCAA): Isoleucine, leucine, valine.

Acute metabolic stress – Acute metabolic stress is characterized by increased urinary nitrogen excretion and hyperglycemia; glucose utilization and fat store mobilization are impaired. The primary substrates used to meet energy requirements of muscle are BCAAs.

AMINO ACID FORMULATION IN HEPATIC FAILURE/HEPATIC ENCEPHALOPATHY

	HEPATIC FORMULATION: HepatAmine (McGaw)
Amino Acid Concentration	8%
Nitrogen (g/100 mL)	1.2
Amino Acids (Essential) (mg/100 mL)	
Isoleucine	900
Leucine	1100
Lysine	610
Methionine	100
Phenylalanine	100
Threonine	450
Tryptophan	66
Valine	840
Amino Acids (Nonessential) (mg/100 mL)	
Alanine	770
Arginine	600
Histidine[a]	240
Proline	800
Serine	500
Tyrosine	
Glycine	900
Cysteine	< 20
Electrolytes (mEq/L)	
Sodium	10
Chloride	< 3
Acetate	≈ 62
Phosphate (mM/L)	10
Osmolarity (mOsm/L)	785
Supplied in (mL)	500[b]
Labeled Indications	
Peripheral Parenteral Nutrition	Yes
Central TPN	Yes

[a] Histidine is considered an essential amino acid in infants and in renal failure.
[b] With less than 100 mg sodium bisulfite/100 mL.

AMINO ACID FORMULATION IN HEPATIC FAILURE/HEPATIC ENCEPHALOPATHY — INTRAVENOUS

For additional information, refer to the Dietary Reference Intakes of Vitamins and Minerals table.

Indications

➤*Hepatic encephalopathy:* For the treatment of hepatic encephalopathy in patients with cirrhosis or hepatitis. Provides nutritional support for patients with these diseases of the liver who require parenteral nutrition and are intolerant of general purpose amino acid injections, which are contraindicated in patients with hepatic coma.

Administration and Dosage

Give 80 to 120 g amino acids (12 to 18 g nitrogen)/day. Typically, 500 mL *HepatAmine* with ≈ 500 mL 50% dextrose and electrolytes and vitamins is given over 8 to 12 hours. This results in total daily fluid intake of ≈ 2 to 3 L. Patients with fluid restrictions may only tolerate 1 to 2 L. Although nitrogen requirements may be higher in severely hypercatabolic or depleted patients, provision of additional nitrogen may not be possible due to fluid intake limits, nitrogen or glucose intolerance.

Use slow initial infusion rates; gradually increase to 60 to 125 mL/hr.

➤*Peripheral vein:* Peripheral vein administration is indicated with or without parenteral carbohydrate calories for patients in whom the central venous route is not indicated and who can consume adequate calories enterally. Prepare infusates by dilution of *HepatAmine* with Sterile Water for Injection or 5% to 10% Dextrose to prepare isotonic or slightly hypertonic solutions; accompany with adequate caloric supplementation.

Actions

➤*Pharmacology:* This formulation is a mixture of essential and nonessential amino acids with high concentrations of the BCAAs, isoleucine, leucine and valine.

Hepatic failure/Hepatic encephalopathy – Etiopathology of hepatic encephalopathy is unknown and multifactorial. Rationale for BCAA therapy is based on studies in which BCAA infusions reversed abnormal plasma amino acid pattern characterized by lower BCAA levels and elevated aromatic amino acids and methionine. Normalization of these amino acids improved mental status and EEG patterns. Nitrogen balance was significantly improved and mortality reduced in these typically protein-intolerant patients who received substantial amounts of protein equivalents.

CYSTEINE HYDROCHLORIDE

Rx	**Cysteine HCl** (Various, eg, Abbott, Gensia)	**Injection:** 50 mg per mL	In 10 mL additive syringe and single dose vials.

CYSTEINE HYDROCHLORIDE — INJECTION

For a complete discussion of the use of protein substrates as a component of intravenous nutritional therapy, refer to the IV Nutritionals monograph. For additional information, refer to the Dietary Reference Intakes of Vitamins and Minerals table.

Indications

➤*Cysteine supplement:* For use only after dilution as an additive to *Aminosyn* (a crystalline amino acid solution) to meet the IV amino acid nutritional requirements of infants receiving total parenteral nutrition.

Administration and Dosage

Use only after dilution in *Aminosyn*. Each 10 mL of cysteine HCl injection should be combined aseptically with 12.5 g of amino acids, such as that present in 250 mL of *Aminosyn* 5%. The admixture is then diluted with 250 mL of dextrose 50% or such lesser volume as indicated. Equal volumes of *Aminosyn* 5% and dextrose 50% produce a final solution which contains *Aminosyn* 2.5% in dextrose 25%, which is suitable for administration by central venous infusion. Administration of the final admixture should begin within 1 hour of mixing. Otherwise, the admixture should be refrigerated immediately and used within 24 hours of the time of mixing.

➤*Storage/Stability:* Store at controlled room temperature 15° to 30°C (59° to 86°F).

Actions

➤*Pharmacology:* Cysteine is synthesized from methionine via the transsulfuration pathway in the adult, but newborn infants lack the enzyme, cystathionase, necessary to effect this conversion. Therefore, cysteine HCl injection is generally considered to be an essential amino acid in infants.

Metabolism of cysteine produces pyruvate and inorganic sulfate as end products. Cysteine is introduced directly into the pathway of carbohydrate metabolism at the pyruvate stage with all 3 carbons convertible to glucose. The sulfur is primarily transformed to inorganic sulfate, which is introduced into complex polysaccharides among other structural components.

Contraindications

The contraindications, warnings, precautions, and adverse reactions associated with cysteine HCl injection additive are the same as those cited for *Aminosyn* 5%, given as part of a total parenteral nutrition program. This preparation should not be used in patients with hepatic coma or metabolic disorders involving impaired nitrogen utilization.

Warnings/Precautions

➤*Hyperammonemia:* Hyperammonemia is of special significance in infants, as it can result in mental retardation. Therefore, it is essential that blood ammonia levels be measured frequently in infants.

CYSTEINE HYDROCHLORIDE — INJECTION

Instances of asymptomatic hyperammonemia have been reported in patients without overt liver dysfunction. The mechanisms of this reaction are not clearly defined but may involve genetic defects and immature or subclinically impaired liver function.

➤*Aluminum toxicity:* This product contains aluminum that may be toxic. Aluminum may reach toxic levels with prolonged parenteral administration if kidney function is impaired. Premature neonates are particularly at risk because their kidneys are immature, and they require large amounts of calcium and phosphate solutions, which contain aluminum.

Research indicates that patients with impaired kidney function, including premature neonates, who receive parenteral levels of aluminum at greater than 4 to 5 mcg/kg/day accumulate aluminum at levels associated with central nervous system and bone toxicity. Tissue loading may occur at even lower rates of administration.

➤*Solutions with sodium:* Solutions containing sodium ion should be used with great care, if at all, in patients with congestive heart failure, severe renal insufficiency, and in clinical states in which there exists edema with sodium retention.

➤*Solutions with potassium:* Solutions which contain potassium ion should be used with great care, if at all, in patients with hyperkalemia, severe renal failure, and in conditions in which potassium retention is present.

➤*Solutions with acetate:* Solutions containing acetate ion should be used with great care in patients with metabolic or respiratory alkalosis. Acetate should be administered with great care in those conditions in which there is an increased level or an impaired utilization of this ion such as severe hepatic insufficiency.

➤*Renal/Hepatic function impairment:* Peripheral IV infusion of amino acids may induce a rise in blood urea nitrogen (BUN) especially in patients with impaired hepatic or renal function. Appropriate laboratory tests should be performed periodically and infusion discontinued if BUN levels exceed normal postprandial limits and continue to rise. It should be noted that a modest rise in BUN normally occurs as a result of increased protein intake.

Administration of amino acid solutions in the presence of impaired renal function may augment an increasing BUN, as does any protein dietary component.

Administration of amino acid solutions to a patient with hepatic insufficiency may result in serum amino acid imbalances, metabolic alkalosis, prerenal azotemia, hyperammonemia, stupor, and coma.

➤*Special risk:* Special care must be taken when administering hypertonic glucose to provide calories in diabetic or prediabetic patients.

IV feeding regimens which include amino acids should be used with caution in patients with a history of renal disease, pulmonary disease, or with cardiac insufficiency so as to avoid excessive fluid accumulation.

➤*Pregnancy: Category C.* Animal reproduction studies have not been conducted with cysteine HCl injection. It is also not known whether this additive can cause fetal harm when administered to pregnant women or can affect reproductive capacity.

Safe use during pregnancy has not been established, therefore, infusion of amino acids should be undertaken during pregnancy only when this is deemed essential to the patient's welfare, as judged by the physician. This medicine is not indicated for use in pregnant women.

➤*Lactation:* This medication is not indicated for use in breast-feeding women.

➤*Children:* The effect of infusion of amino acids, without dextrose, upon carbohydrate metabolism of children is not known at this time. Hyperammonemia is of special significance in infants, as it can result in mental retardation.

➤*Monitoring:* Frequent clinical evaluations and laboratory determinations are necessary for proper monitoring during administration. Blood studies should include glucose, urea nitrogen, serum electrolytes, ammonia, cholesterol, acid-base balance, serum proteins, kidney and liver function tests, osmolarity and hemogram. White blood count and blood cultures are to be determined if indicated. Urinary osmolarity and glucose should be determined frequently.

Nitrogen intake should be carefully monitored in patients with impaired renal function. For long-term total nutrition, or if a patient has inadequate fat stores, it is essential to provide adequate exogenous calories concurrently with the amino acids. Concentrated dextrose solutions are an effective source of such calories. Such strong hypertonic nutrient solutions should be administered through an indwelling IV catheter with the tip located in the superior vena cava.

Drug Interactions

➤*Tetracycline:* Because of its antianabolic activity, coadministration of tetracycline may reduce the nitrogen sparing effects of infused amino acids.

➤*Drug/Lab test interactions:* Do not withdraw venous blood for blood chemistries through the peripheral infusion site, as interference with estimations of nitrogen containing substances may occur.

Adverse Reactions

Local reactions consisting of a warm sensation, erythema, phlebitis, and thrombosis at the infusion site have occurred with peripheral intravenous infusion of amino acids, particularly if other substances, such as antibiotics, are also administered through the same site. In such cases, the infusion site should be changed promptly to another vein. Use of large peripheral veins, in-line filters, and slowing the rate of infusion may reduce the incidence of local venous irritation.

Electrolyte additives should be spread throughout the day. Irritating additive medications may need to be injected at another venous site.

Generalized flushing, fever, and nausea also have been reported during peripheral infusions of amino acid solutions.

Overdosage

Feeding regimens which include amino acids should be used with caution in patients with a history of renal disease, pulmonary disease, or with cardiac insufficiency to avoid excess fluid accumulation. In the event of overhydration or solute overload, reevaluate the patient and institute appropriate corrective measures.

TROMETHAMINE

Rx	**Tham** (Abbott)	**Injection:** 18 g (150 mEq) per 500 mL (0.3 M)	In 500 mL single dose container.[a]

[a] With acetic acid.

TROMETHAMINE — INJECTION

For additional information, refer to the Dietary Reference Intakes of Vitamins and Minerals table.

Indications

➤*Metabolic acidosis:* For the prevention and correction of metabolic acidosis.

Administration and Dosage

Tromethamine solution is administered by slow intravenous infusion, by addition to pump-oxygenator ACD blood or other priming fluid or by injection into the ventricular cavity during cardiac arrest. For infusion by peripheral vein, a large needle should be used in the largest antecubital vein or an indwelling catheter placed in a large vein of an elevated limb to minimize chemical irritation of the alkaline solution during infusion. Catheters are recommended.

Dosage and rate of administration should be carefully supervised to avoid overtreatment (alkalosis). Pretreatment and subsequent determinations of blood values (eg, pH, PCO_2, PO_2, glucose and electrolytes) and urinary output should be made as necessary to monitor dosage and progress of treatment. In general, dosage should be limited to an amount sufficient to increase blood pH to normal limits (7.35 to 7.45) and to correct acid-base derangements. The total quantity to be administered during the period of illness will depend upon the severity and progression of the acidosis. The possibility of some retention of tromethamine, especially in patients with impaired renal function, should be kept in mind.

The intravenous dosage of tromethamine solution (tromethamine injection) may be estimated from the buffer base deficit of the extracellular fluid in mEq/L determined by means of the Siggaard-Andersen nomogram. The following formula is intended as a general guide:

Tromethamine solution (mL of 0.3 M) Required = Body Weight (kg) × Base Deficit (mEq/L) × 1.1.

Factor of 1.1 accounts for an approximate reduction of 10% in buffering capacity due to the presence of sufficient acetic acid to lower pH of the 0.3 M solution to approximately 8.6).

The need for administration of additional tromethamine solution is determined by serial determinations of the existing base deficit.

➤*Acidosis associated with cardiac bypass surgery:* An adverse dose of approximately 9 mL/kg (324 mg/kg) has been used in clinical studies with tromethamine solution (tromethamine injection). This is equivalent to a total dose of 630 mL (189 mEq) for 70 kg patient. A total single dose of 500 mL (150 mEq) is considered adequate for most adults. Larger single doses (up to 1000 mL) may be required in unusually severe cases.

It is recommended that individual doses should not exceed 500 mg/kg (227 mg/lb) over a period of not less than 1 hour. Thus, for a 70 kg (154 pound) patient the dose should not exceed a maximum of 35 g per hour (1078 mL of a 0.3 M solution). Repeated determinations of pH and other clinical observations should be used as a guide to the need for repeat doses.

➤*Acidity of ACD blood in cardiac bypass surgery:* The pH of stored blood ranges from 6.80 to 6.22 depending upon the duration of storage. The amount of tromethamine solution used to correct this acidity ranges from 0.5 to 2.5 g (15 to 77 mL of a 0.3 M solution) added to each 500 mL of ACD

TROMETHAMINE — INJECTION

blood used for priming the pump-oxygenator. Clinical experience indicates that 2 g (62 mL of a 0.3 M solution) added to 500 mL of ACD blood is usually adequate.

➤*Acidosis associated with cardiac arrest:* In the treatment of cardiac arrest, tromethamine solution should be given at the same time that other standard resuscitative measures, including manual systole, are being applied. If the chest is open, tromethamine solution is injected directly into the ventricular cavity. From 2 to 6 g (62 to 185 mL of a 0.3 M solution) should be injected immediately. **Do not inject into the cardiac muscle.**

If the chest is not open, from 3.6 to 10.8 g (111 to 333 mL of a 0.3 M solution) should be injected immediately into a larger peripheral vein. Additional amounts may be required to control acidosis persisting after cardiac arrest is reversed.

➤*Admixture incompatibility:* Additives may be incompatible. Consult with pharmacist, if available. When introducing additives, use aseptic technique, mix thoroughly and do not store.

➤*Storage / Stability:* Protect from freezing and extreme heat.

Do not administer unless solution is clear and seal is intact. Discard unused portion.

Actions

➤*Pharmacology:* When administered intravenously as a 0.3 M solution, tromethamine act as a proton acceptor and prevents or corrects acidosis by actively binding hydrogen ions (H^+). It binds not only cations of fixed or metabolic acids, but also hydrogen ions of carbonic acid, thus increasing bicarbonate anion (HCO_3^-). Tromethamine also acts as an osmotic diuretic, increasing urine flow, urinary pH, and excretion of fixed acids, carbon dioxide and electrolytes. A significant fraction of tromethamine (30% at pH 7.4) is not ionized and therefore is capable of reaching equilibrium in total body water. This portion may penetrate cells and may neutralize acidic ions of the intracellular fluid.

➤*Pharmacokinetics:* The drug is rapidly eliminated by the kidney; 75% or more appears in the urine after 8 hours. Urinary excretion continues over a period of 3 days.

Contraindications

Anuria; uremia.

Warnings/Precautions

➤*Respiratory depression:* Large doses of tromethamine solution may depress ventilation, as a result of increased blood pH and reduced CO_2 concentration. Thus, dosage should be adjusted so that blood pH is not allowed to increase above normal. In situations in which respiratory acidosis may be present concomitantly with metabolic acidosis, the drug may be used with mechanical assistance to ventilation.

➤*Perivascular infiltration:* Care must be exercised to prevent perivascular infiltration since this can cause inflammation, necrosis and sloughing of tissue. Venospasm and intravenous thrombosis, which may occur during infusion, can be minimized by insuring that the injection needle is well within the largest available vein and that solutions are slowly infused. Intravenous catheters are recommended. If perivascular infiltration occurs, institute appropriate countermeasures. See Adverse Reactions.

➤*Administration:* Tromethamine solution for injection should be administered slowly and in amounts sufficient only to correct the existing acidosis, and to avoid overdosage and alkalosis.

➤*Hypoglycemia:* Overdosage in terms of total drug or too rapid administration, may cause hypoglycemia of a prolonged duration (several hours). Therefore, frequent blood glucose determinations should be made during and after therapy.

➤*Duration of therapy:* Because clinical experience has been limited generally to short-term use, the drug should not be administered for more than a period of 1 day except in a life-threatening situation.

➤*Fluid / solute overload:* The intravenous administration of tromethamine solution can cause fluid or solute overloading resulting in dilution of serum electrolyte concentrations, overhydration, congested states or pulmonary edema.

➤*Coagulation abnormalities:* While it has not been shown that the drug increases coagulation time in humans, this possibility should be kept in mind since this has been noted experimentally in dogs.

➤*Renal function impairment:* Extreme care should be exercised in patients with renal disease or reduced urinary output because of potential hyperkalemia and the possibility of a decreased excretion of tromethamine. In such patients, the drug should be used cautiously with electrocardiographic monitoring and frequent serum potassium determinations.

➤*Pregnancy: Category C.* Animal reproduction studies have not been conducted with tromethamine. It is also not known whether tromethamine can cause fetal harm when administered to a pregnant woman or can affect reproduction capacity. Tromethamine should be given to a pregnant woman only if clearly needed.

➤*Lactation:* Exercise caution when administering to a breast-feeding woman.

➤*Children:* Hypoglycemia may occur when this product is used in premature and even full-term neonates. See Adverse Reactions.

➤*Elderly:* Clinical studies of tromethamine solution did not include sufficient numbers of subjects aged 65 and over to determine whether they respond differently from younger subjects. Other reported clinical experience has not identified differences in response between the elderly and younger patients. In general, dose selection for an elderly patient should be cautious, usually starting at the low end of the dosing range, reflecting the greater frequency of decreased hepatic, renal, or cardiac function, and of concomitant disease or other drug therapy.

This drug is known to be substantially excreted by the kidney, and the risk of toxic reactions to this drug may be greater in patients with impaired renal function. Because elderly patients are more likely to have decreased renal function, care should be taken in dose selection, and it may be useful to monitor renal function.

➤*Monitoring:* Blood pH, PCO_2 bicarbonate, glucose and electrolyte determinations should be performed before, during and after administration of tromethamine solution.

Adverse Reactions

Generally, side effects have been infrequent.

➤*Hematologic:* Transient depression of blood glucose may occur.

➤*Local:* Extreme care should be taken to avoid perivascular infiltration. Local tissue damage and subsequent sloughing may occur if extravasation occurs. Chemical phlebitis and venospasm also have been reported.

➤*Respiratory:* Although the incidence of ventilatory depression is low, it is important to keep in mind that such depression may occur. Respiratory depression may be more likely to occur in patients who have chronic hypoventilation or those who have been treated with drugs which depress respiration. In patients with associated respiratory acidosis, tromethamine should be administered with mechanical assistance to ventilation.

➤*Miscellaneous:* Reactions which may occur because of the solution or the technique of administration include febrile response, infection at the site of injection, venous thrombosis or phlebitis extending from the site of injection, extravasation and hypervolemia.

If an adverse reaction does occur, discontinue the infusion, evaluate the patient, institute appropriate therapeutic countermeasures and save the remainder of the fluid for examination if deemed necessary.

Overdosage

➤*Symptoms:* Too rapid administration or excessive amounts of tromethamine may cause alkalosis, hypoglycemia, overhydration or solute overload.

➤*Treatment:* In the event of overdosage, discontinue the infusion, evaluate the patient and institute appropriate countermeasures.

DEXTROSE (d-GLUCOSE)

Rx	**D-2.5-W** (Various, eg, Abbott)	2.5%	In 1000 mL.
Rx	**D-5-W** (Various, eg, Abbott, IMS, McGaw)	5%	In 25, 50, 100, 150, 250, 500 and 1000 mL vials and 10 mL syringes, 25 mL fill in 150 mL, 50 mL fill in 250 mL and 100 mL fill in 250 mL vials.
Rx	**D-10-W** (Various, eg, Hospira, Solopak, Winthrop)	10%	In 3 mL amps, 250, 500 and 1000 mL vials, 17 mL fill in 20 mL, 500 mL fill in 1000 mL, and 1000 mL fill in 2000 mL vials.
Rx	**D-20-W** (Various, eg, Abbott)	20%	In 500 mL vials, 500 mL fill in 1000 mL and 1000 mL fill in 2000 mL.
Rx	**D-25-W** (Various, eg, Abbott, IMS)	25%	In 10 mL syringes.
Rx	**D-30-W** (Various, eg, Abbott, McGaw)	30%	In 500 and 1000 mL, 500 mL fill in 1000 mL and 1000 mL fill in 2000 mL.
Rx	**D-40-W** (Various, eg, Abbott, McGaw)	40%	In 500 and 1000 mL, 500 mL fill in 1000 mL and 1000 mL fill in 2000 mL.

Caloric Intake

DEXTROSE (d-GLUCOSE)

Rx	D-50-W (Various, eg, Abbott, IMS, McGaw, Pasadena)	50%	In 500, 1000 and 2000 mL and 50 mL amps, vials and syringes and 500 mL fill in 1000 mL and 1000 mL fill in 2000 mL.
Rx	D-60-W (Various, eg, Abbott, McGaw)	60%	In 500 and 1000 mL, 500 mL fill in 1000 mL and 1000 mL fill in 2000 mL.
Rx	D-70-W (Various, eg, Abbott, McGaw)	70%	In 70, 1000 and 2000 mL, 500 mL fill in 1000 mL and 1000 mL fill in 2000 mL.

DEXTROSE — INJECTION

Indications

➤*2.5%, 5%, and 10% solutions:* Used for peripheral infusion to provide calories whenever fluid and caloric replacement are required.

➤*25% (hypertonic) solutions):* Acute symptomatic episodes of hypoglycemia in the neonate or older infant to restore depressed blood glucose levels and control symptoms.

➤*50% solution:* Used in the treatment of insulin hypoglycemia (hyperinsulinemia or insulin shock) to restore blood glucose levels.

➤*10%, 20%, 30%, 40%, 50%, 60%, and 70% (hypertonic) solutions:* For infusion after admixture with amino acids or dilution with other compatible IV fluids to provide variable final dextrose concentrations for intravenous infusion in patients whose condition requires parenteral nutrition.

➤*Off-label uses:* Hypertonic solutions of 25% to 50% have been used as a sclerosing agent for the treatment of varicose veins, as an irritant to produce adhesive pleuritis and to reduce cerebrospinal pressure and cerebral edema caused by delirium tremens or acute alcohol intoxication.

Administration and Dosage

➤*General dosing considerations:* Dosage is dependent upon age, weight, clinical condition of the patient and laboratory determinations. Frequent laboratory determinations and clinical evaluation are essential to monitor changes in blood glucose and electrolyte concentrations, and fluid and electrolyte balance during prolonged parenteral therapy.

Fluid administration should be based on calculated maintenance or replacement fluid requirements for each patient.

➤*Adults:*

Fluid and caloric replacement (2.5%, 5%, and 10% solutions) – Individualize dosage.

Insulin-induced hypoglycemia (50% solution) – 10 to 25 g intravenously (IV). Repeated doses may be required in severe cases. Determine blood glucose before injecting dextrose. In emergencies, promptly administer without waiting for pretreatment test results.

Parenteral nutrition (10%, 20%, 30%, 40%, 50%, 60%, and 70% [hypertonic] solutions) – Concentrated dextrose in water is administered by slow IV infusion a) after admixture with amino acid solutions or b) after dilution with other compatible IV fluids. Dosage should be adjusted to meet the requirements of each individual patient.

➤*Children:* As reported in the literature, the dosage and constant infusion rate of IV dextrose must be selected with caution in children, particularly neonates and low birth weight infants, because of the increased risk of hyperglycemia/hypoglycemia.

Fluid and caloric replacement (2.5%, 5%, and 10% solutions) – Individualize dosage

Insulin-induced hypoglycemia (25% solution) – Determine blood glucose before injecting dextrose. In emergencies, promptly administer without waiting for pretreatment test results.

Children: There is no specific pediatric dose. The dose is dependent on weight, clinical condition, and laboratory results. Follow recommendations of appropriate pediatric reference text.

Neonates: 250 to 500 mg/kg/dose (5 to 10 mL of 25% dextrose in a 5 kg infant) to control acute symptomatic hypoglycemia.

Severe cases or older infants:: Larger or repeated single doses up to 10 or 12 mL of 25% dextrose may be required. Subsequent continuous IV infusion of 10% dextrose may be needed to stabilize blood glucose levels.

➤*Elderly:* Because elderly patients are more likely to have decreased renal function, care should be taken in dose selection, and it may be useful to monitor renal function.

➤*Renal function impairment:* Use with caution in patients with renal insufficiency.

➤*Extravasation:* Extravasation may occur during administration of dextrose (10% or higher). If signs or symptoms of extravasation occur, stop the infusion immediately. If possible, withdraw 3 to 5 mL of blood to remove some of the drug. Remove the infusion needle. Delineate the infiltrated area on the patient's skin with a felt-tip marker. Hyaluronidase is an effective antidote for hyperosmolar drug infiltrations; administer promptly within the first few minutes to 1 hour after extravasation. Higher doses (150 units) have primarily been used in adults, while lower doses (15 units) have been used in children. Administer hyaluronidase according to the following steps. Dilute hyaluronidase to desired concentration, depending on the dose and product used. (Note: Some products do not require dilution.) For example, if the total dose is 15 units, make 15 units/mL dilution. If the total dose is 150 units, make 150 units/mL dilution. Cleanse area with povidone-iodine. Inject hyaluronidase locally, subcutaneously, or intradermally, using a 25-gauge needle or smaller. The dose is given as five 0.2 mL injections at the leading edge of the extravasation site. Change needle after each injection. Elevate for 48 hours above heart level using a sling or stockinette dressing with an observation window cut in the dressing. Avoid pressure or friction. Do not rub area. Observe for signs of increased erythema, pain, or skin necrosis. If increased symptoms occur, consult a plastic surgeon. Ensure that no medication is given distally to extravasation site. After 48 hours, encourage the patient to use the extremity normally to promote full range of motion.

➤*Administration:* Do not administer concentrated solutions subcutaneously or intramuscularly (IM).

When a hypertonic solution is to be administered peripherally, it should be slowly infused through a small bore needle, placed well within the lumen of a large vein to minimize venous irritation. Carefully avoid infiltration.

The maximum rate at which dextrose can be infused without producing glycosuria is 0.5 g/kg of body weight per hour. About 95% of the dextrose is retained when infused at a rate of 0.8 g/kg per hour.

Significant hyperglycemia and possible hyperosmolar syndrome may result from too rapid administration.

In very low birth weight infants, excessive or rapid administration of dextrose injection may result in increased serum osmolality and possible intracerebral hemorrhage.

➤*Admixture compatibility:* Some additives may be incompatible. When introducing additives, use aseptic techniques. Mix thoroughly. Do not store.

Do not administer dextrose simultaneously with blood through the same infusion set because pseudoagglutination of red cells may occur.

➤*Storage/Stability:* Do not use unless solution is clear. Discard unused portion. Protect from freezing and extreme heat.

Actions

➤*Pharmacology:* Dextrose injection provides calories and is a source of water for hydration. It is capable of inducing diuresis depending on the clinical condition of the patient.

When administered intravenously, solutions containing carbohydrate in the form of dextrose restore blood glucose levels and provide calories. Carbohydrate in the form of dextrose may aid in minimizing liver glycogen depletion and exerts a protein sparing action. Dextrose injection undergoes oxidation to carbon dioxide and water.

Dextrose is readily metabolized, may decrease losses of body protein and nitrogen, promotes glycogen deposition, and decreases or prevents ketosis if sufficient doses are provided.

Caloric Content and Osmolarity of the Various Concentrations of Dextrose Injection

Dextrose concentration			
%	g/L	Caloric content (Cal/L)	Osmolarity (mOsm/L)
2.5	25	85	126
5	50	170	253
10	100	340	505
20	200	680	1,010
25	250	850	1,330
30	300	1,020	1,515
40	400	1,360	2,020
50	500	1,700	2,525
60	600	2,040	3,030
70	700	2,380	3,535

Contraindications

In diabetic coma while blood sugar is excessively high and in patients with hypersensitivity to corn products. When intracranial or intraspinal hemorrhage is present; in the presence of delirium tremens in dehydrated patients; in patients with severe hydration, anuria, hepatic coma, or glucose-galactose malabsorption syndrome.

Warnings/Precautions

➤*Fluid/solute overload:* The administration of intravenous solutions can cause fluid and/or solute overload resulting in dilution of serum electrolyte concentrations, overhydration, congested states or pulmonary edema. The risk of dilutional states is inversely proportional to the electrolyte concentration.

➤*Prolonged infusion:* Prolonged infusion of isotonic or hypotonic dextrose in water may increase the volume of extracellular fluid and cause water intoxication.

DEXTROSE — INJECTION

➤*Admixture incompatibility:* See Administration and Dosage for more information.

➤*Hypokalemia:* Excessive administration of potassium-free dextrose solutions may result in significant hypokalemia. Serum potassium levels should be maintained and potassium supplemented as required.

Hypokalemia may develop during parenteral administration of hypertonic dextrose solutions. Sufficient amounts of potassium should be added to dextrose solutions administered to fasting patients with good renal function, especially those on digitalis therapy.

➤*Hypertonic dextrose solutions:* Hypertonic dextrose solutions (above 5% concentration) should be given slowly, preferably through a small bore needle into a large vein, to minimize venous irritation. If infused via peripheral veins, thrombosis may result; therefore, administration via a central venous catheter is recommended.

➤*Rapid administration:* Concentrated dextrose in water should be administered only after suitable dilution. Hypertonic dextrose solutions should be given slowly. Significant hyperglycemia and possible hyperosmolar syndrome may result from too rapid administration. The physician should be aware of the symptoms of hyperosmolar syndrome, such as mental confusion and loss of consciousness, especially in patients with chronic uremia and those with known carbohydrate intolerance.

➤*Aluminum toxicity:* Dextrose injection contains aluminum that may be toxic. Aluminum may reach toxic levels with prolonged parenteral administration if kidney function is impaired. Premature neonates are particularly at risk because their kidneys are immature, and they require large amounts of calcium and phosphate solutions, which contain aluminum.

Dextrose injection contains no more than 25 mcg/L of aluminum.

Research indicates that patients with impaired kidney function, including premature neonates, who receive parenteral levels of aluminum at greater than 4 to 5 mcg/kg/day accumulate aluminum at levels associated with central nervous system and bone toxicity. Tissue loading may occur at even lower rates of administration.

➤*Concentrated solutions:* Some opacity of the plastic due to moisture absorption during sterilization process may be observed. This is normal and does not affect the solution quality or safety. The opacity will diminish gradually.

➤*Pumping device:* If administration is controlled by a pumping device, care must be taken to discontinue pumping action before the container runs dry or air embolism may result.

➤*Precipitation:* To minimize the risk of possible incompatibilities arising from mixing this solution with other additives that may be prescribed, the final infusate should be inspected for cloudiness or precipitation immediately after mixing, prior to administration, and periodically during administration.

➤*Diabetes mellitus:* Solutions containing dextrose should be used with caution in patients with overt or known subclinical diabetes mellitus or carbohydrate intolerance for any reason.

➤*Extravasation:* See Administration and Dosage for more information.

➤*Special risk:* These solutions should be used with care in patients with hypervolemia, renal insufficiency, urinary tract obstruction, or impending or frank cardiac decompensation.

➤*Pregnancy: Category C.* Animal reproduction studies have not been conducted with dextrose. It is also not known whether dextrose can cause fetal harm when administered to a pregnant woman or can affect reproduction capacity. Dextrose should be given to a pregnant woman only if clearly needed.

Dextrose crosses the placenta; however, insulin does not cross the placenta and the fetus is responsible for its own insulin production in response to the dextrose. Therefore, administer dextrose to a pregnant woman with caution. One report recommends an infusion rate of 3.5 to 7 g/hr since doses greater than 10 g/hr cause increases in fetal insulin.

Labor and delivery – As reported in the literature, dextrose solutions have been administered during labor and delivery. Caution should be exercised, and the fluid balance, glucose and electrolyte concentrations and acid-base balance, of both mother and fetus should be evaluated periodically or whenever warranted by the condition of the patient or fetus.

➤*Lactation:* Because many drugs are excreted in human milk, caution should be exercised when dextrose injections are administered to a nursing woman.

➤*Children:* The safety and effectiveness in the pediatric population are based on the similarity of the clinical conditions of the pediatric and adult populations. In neonates or very small infants the volume of fluid may affect fluid and electrolyte balance.

Serum glucose concentrations should be frequently monitored when dextrose is prescribed to pediatric patients, particularly infants, neonates, and low birth weight infants.

In very low birth weight infants, excessive or rapid administration of dextrose injection may result in increased serum osmolality and possible intracerebral hemorrhage.

➤*Elderly:* An evaluation of current literature revealed no clinical experience identifying differences in responses between the elderly and younger patients. In general, dose selection for an elderly patient should be cautious, usually starting at the low end of the dosing range, reflecting the greater frequency of decreased hepatic, renal, or cardiac function, and of concomitant disease or other drug therapy.

These drugs are known to be substantially excreted by the kidney, and the risk of toxic reactions to these drugs may be greater in patients with impaired renal function. Because elderly patients are more likely to have decreased renal function, care should be taken in dose selection, and it may be useful to monitor renal function.

➤*Monitoring:* Clinical evaluation and periodic laboratory determinations are necessary to monitor changes in fluid balance, electrolyte concentrations, and acid-base balance during prolonged parenteral therapy or whenever the condition of the patient warrants such evaluation. Significant deviations from normal concentrations may require tailoring of the electrolyte pattern, in these or alternative solutions.

Blood electrolyte monitoring is essential, and fluid and electrolyte imbalances should be corrected. Essential vitamins and minerals also should be provided as needed.

Hyperglycemia and glycosuria – To minimize hyperglycemia and consequent glycosuria, it is desirable to monitor blood and urine glucose and if necessary, add insulin. When concentrated dextrose infusion is abruptly withdrawn, it is advisable to follow with the administration of 5% or 10% dextrose to avoid rebound hypoglycemia.

Drug Interactions

➤*Corticosteroids:* Cautiously administer parenteral fluids, especially those containing sodium ions, to patients receiving corticosteroids or corticotropin.

Adverse Reactions

Reactions which may occur because of the solution or the technique of administration include febrile response, infection at the site of injection, venous thrombosis or phlebitis extending from the site of injection, extravasation and hypervolemia.

Too rapid infusion of hypertonic solutions may cause local pain and venous irritation. Rate of administration should be adjusted according to tolerance. Use of the largest peripheral vein and a small bore needle is recommended.

➤*Concentrated solutions:* Hyperosmolar syndrome, resulting from excessively rapid administration of concentrated dextrose may cause hypovolemia, dehydration, mental confusion, or loss of consciousness.

Reactions which may occur because of the solution or the technique of administration include febrile response, infection at the site of injection, venous thrombosis or phlebitis extending from the site of injection, extravasation and hypervolemia.

Overdosage

➤*Treatment:* In the event of a fluid or solute overload during parenteral therapy, reevaluate the patient's condition and institute appropriate corrective treatment.

ALCOHOL (ETHANOL) IN DEXTROSE INFUSIONS

	Product/Distributor	Cal/L	mOsm/L	How Supplied
Rx	**5% Alcohol and 5% Dextrose in Water** (Various, eg, Abbott)	450	1114	In 1000 mL.
Rx	**5% Alcohol and 5% Dextrose in Water** (McGaw)		1125	In 1000 mL.
Rx	**10% Alcohol and 5% Dextrose in Water** (McGaw)	720	1995	In 1000 mL.

ALCOHOL (ETHANOL) IN DEXTROSE INFUSIONS — INTRAVENOUS

For specific information on dextrose, refer to the individual monograph.

Indications

➤*Caloric/fluid supplement:* Increasing caloric intake and replenishing fluids.

➤*Off-label uses:*

Premature labor – Infusion of a 10% solution of ethyl alcohol IV causes a decrease in uterine activity during labor, presumably by inhibiting the release of oxytocin from the posterior pituitary, and has been used to prevent premature delivery. However, this use has largely been replaced by other therapies (eg, β-adrenergic therapy).

Administration and Dosage

➤*General dosing considerations:* Individualize dosage. The average adult can metabolize approximately 10 mL/h (200 mL of 5% solution or 100 mL of 10% solution).

➤*Adults:*

Caloric/fluid supplement – The usual dosage is 1 to 2 L and rarely exceeds 3 L of a 5% solution in a 24-hour period.

ALCOHOL (ETHANOL) IN DEXTROSE INFUSIONS — INTRAVENOUS

➤*Children:* Safety and efficacy are not established. However, children may be given 40 mL/kg/24 hours or from 350 to 1,000 mL, depending on size and clinical response.

➤*Administration:* Administer by slow IV infusion only and observe patient for restlessness or narcosis. Do not give subcutaneously.

➤*Storage / Stability:* Store at 25°C; however, brief exposure up to 40°C does not adversely affect the product. Exposure to heat should be minimized. Avoid excessive heat. Protect from freezing. Do not use unless solution is clear and seal is intact. Discard unused portion.

Actions

➤*Pharmacology:* Alcohol in dextrose solutions are an intravenous source of carbohydrate calories that restore blood glucose levels. Each mL of alcohol provides 5.6 calories; each gram of d–glucose monohydrate provides 3.4 calories. Dextrose may aid in minimizing liver glycogen depletion and exerts a protein-sparing action.

➤*Pharmacokinetics:* Ethyl alcohol is metabolized at a rate of ≈ 10 to 20 mL/hour. Sedative effects of alcohol occur if infusion rate exceeds metabolism rate. Dextrose (d-glucose) can be infused at a maximum of ≈ 0.5 to 0.85 g/kg/hour without producing significant glycosuria. Thus, the maximum rate that alcohol can be infused without producing sedative effects is well below maximum rate of dextrose utilization. Alcohol is metabolized (mostly in liver) to acetaldehyde or acetate; oxidation rate is linear with time. Starvation lowers metabolism rate and insulin increases it.

Contraindications

Epilepsy; urinary tract infection; alcoholism; diabetic coma.

Warnings/Precautions

➤*Diabetic patients:* Alcohol decreases blood sugar in these patients. In the untreated diabetic, the rate of alcohol metabolism is slowed.

➤*Vitamin deficiencies:* As a nutrient, alcohol supplies only calories; given alone it may cause or potentiate vitamin deficiencies and liver function disturbances.

➤*IV administration:* IV administration can cause fluid or solute overload resulting in dilution of serum electrolyte concentrations, overhydration, congested states or pulmonary edema.

➤*Pseudoagglutination / Hemolysis:* Do not administer simultaneously with blood because of possibility of pseudoagglutination or hemolysis.

➤*Administer slowly:* Administer slowly and observe patient for restlessness or narcosis.

➤*Gout:* Alcohol increases serum uric acid and can precipitate acute gout.

➤*Extravasation:* Avoid extravasation during IV administration; do not give SC.

➤*Renal / Hepatic function impairment:* Use alcohol cautiously.

➤*Special risk:* Use alcohol cautiously in shock, following cranial surgery and in actual or anticipated postpartum hemorrhage.

➤*Pregnancy:* *Category C.* It is not known whether alcohol can cause fetal harm when administered to a pregnant woman or can affect reproduction capacity. Use only when clearly needed. It crosses the placenta rapidly and enters fetal circulation.

Fetal Alcohol Syndrome (FAS) – Fetal alcohol syndrome (FAS), a pattern of fetal anomalies, is associated with chronic maternal alcohol consumption of 60 to 75 mL absolute alcohol (4 to 5 drinks) per day; mild FAS is associated with ingestion of as little as 30 mL per day. Features of FAS involve craniofacial, limb, growth, and CNS anomalies. Other reported problems involve cardiac and urogenital defects, liver abnormalities and hemangiomas. Behavioral problems may be long-term. Moderate drinking (more than 1 ounce absolute alcohol twice/week) is associated with second trimester spontaneous abortions.

Administration of alcohol prior to delivery may cause intoxication and depression of the newborn.

➤*Lactation:* Alcohol passes freely into breast milk approximately equivalent to maternal serum levels; however, effects on the infant are generally insignificant until maternal blood levels reach 300 mg/dL. The American Academy of Pediatrics considers alcohol use in the mother compatible with breastfeeding, although adverse effects may occur.

Alcohol may cause potentiation of severe hypoprothrombic bleeding, a pseudo-Cushing syndrome and a reduction in the milk-ejecting response.

➤*Children:* Safety and efficacy are not established. See Administration and Dosage.

➤*Monitoring:* Clinical evaluation and periodic laboratory determinations are necessary to monitor changes in electrolyte concentrations and fluid and acid-base balance.

Drug Interactions

The following interactions may occur with alcohol administration. Those interactions that may only occur with long-term oral alcohol ingestion have not been included.

Alcohol Drug Interactions

Precipitant drug	Object drug[a]		Description
Barbiturates Benzodiazepines Chloral hydrate Glutethimide Meprobamate Metoclopramide Phenothiazines	Alcohol	↑	Increased CNS depressant effects may occur.
Cephalosporins[b] Chlorpropamide Disulfiram Furazolidone Metronidazole Procarbazine	Alcohol	↑	A disulfiram-like reaction consisting of facial flushing, lightheadedness, weakness, sweating, tachycardia, nausea or vomiting may occur.
Alcohol	Antidiabetic agents (insulin, phenformin, sulfonylureas)	↑	Because of altered glucose metabolism, the pharmacologic effects of these agents may be increased by alcohol resulting in hypoglycemia. In addition, alcohol may contribute to the lactic acidosis that is sometimes observed following phenformin administration. Both hypo- and hyperglycemia have occurred with sulfonylureas and alcohol.
Alcohol	Bromocriptine	↑	Intolerance of bromocriptine due to the severity of side effects has occurred with concurrent alcohol.
Alcohol	Salicylates	↑	Alcohol may potentiate aspirin-induced GI blood loss and bleeding time prolongation.

[a] ↑ = object drug increased.
[b] Those agents with a methyltetrazolethiol moiety.

Adverse Reactions

Fever; injection site infection; venous thrombosis or phlebitis; extravasation; hypervolemia. These may occur because of the solution or administration technique.

Alcoholic intoxication may occur with too rapid infusion. Vertigo, flushing, disorientation (especially in elderly patients), or sedation may also occur. An alcoholic odor may be noted on the breath. Generally, these effects can be avoided by slowing the rate of infusion. Too rapid infusion of hypertonic solutions may cause local pain and, rarely, excessive vein irritation. Use the largest available peripheral vein and a well placed small bore needle.

Overdosage

In the event of alcoholic intoxication or sedation, slow the infusion or discontinue temporarily. If overhydration or solute overload occurs, reevaluate the patient and institute appropriate corrective measures.

FAT EMULSION

		Oil (%)		Fatty acid content (%)									
	Product & Distributor	Safflower	Soybean	Linoleic	Oleic	Palmitic	Linolenic	Stearic	Egg yolk phospholipids (%)	Glycerin (%)	Calories/mL	Osmolarity (mOsm/L)	How Supplied
Rx	**Intralipid[a] 20%** (Baxter)		20	50	26	10	9	3.5	1.2	2.25	2	260	In 50, 100, 250 and 500 mL.
Rx	**Intralipid[c] 30%** (Baxter)		30	44–62	19–30	7–14	4–11	1.4–5.5	1.2	1.7	3	200	In 500 mL.
Rx	**Liposyn II[b] 10%** (Hospira)	5	5	65.8	17.7	8.8	4.2	3.4	1.2	2.5	1.1	276	In 100, 200 and 500 mL.
Rx	**Liposyn II[b] 20%** (Hospira)	10	10	65.8	17.7	8.8	4.2	3.4	1.2	2.5	2	258	In 200 and 500 mL.
Rx	**Liposyn III[b] 10%** (Hospira)		10	54.5	22.4	10.5	8.3	4.2	1.2	2.5	1.1	284	In 100, 200 and 500 mL.
Rx	**Liposyn III[b] 20%** (Hospira)		20	54.5	22.4	10.5	8.3	4.2	1.2	2.5	2	292	In 200 and 500 mL.
Rx	**Liposyn III[a] 30%** (Hospira)		30	54.5	22.4	10.5	8.3	4.2	1.8	2.5	2.9	293	In 500 mL.

[a] Store at 20° to 25°C (68° to 77°F); do not freeze.
[b] Store at 30°C (86°F) or below; do not freeze.
[c] Should not be stored above 25°C (77°F); do not freeze.

FAT EMULSION — INTRAVENOUS

Refer to the general discussion beginning in the IV Nutritional Therapy monograph.

WARNING

Deaths in preterm infants – Death in preterm infants after infusion of IV fat emulsions have occurred. Autopsy findings included intravascular fat accumulation in the lungs. Treatment of premature and low birth weight infants with IV fat emulsion must be based on careful benefit-risk assessment. Strict adherence to the recommended total daily dose is mandatory; hourly infusion rate should be as slow as possible and should not exceed 1 g/kg in 4 hours. Premature and small for gestational age infants have poor clearance of IV fat emulsion and increased free fatty acid plasma levels following fat emulsion infusion; therefore, administer less than the maximum recommended doses in these patients to decrease the likelihood of IV fat overload. Monitor the infant's ability to eliminate the infused fat from the circulation (such as triglycerides or plasma free fatty acid levels). The lipemia must clear between daily infusions.

Indications

➤*Caloric/fatty acid source:* Source of calories and essential fatty acids for patients requiring parenteral nutrition for extended periods of time (usually for longer than 5 days).

Source of essential fatty acids when a deficiency occurs.

Administration and Dosage

➤*General dosing considerations:*

Total parenteral nutrition – Fat emulsion should comprise no more than 60% of the patient's total caloric intake, with carbohydrates and amino acids comprising the remaining 40% or more of caloric intake.

Essential fatty acid deficiency – To correct EFAD, supply 8% to 10% of the caloric intake by IV fat emulsion to provide an adequate amount of linoleic acid (4% of caloric intake as linoleate).

➤*Adults:*

Caloric/fatty acid source –

10%:

• *Maximum dose* – 2.5 g/kg/day.

• *Initial dosage* – 1 mL/min for the first 15 to 30 minutes.

• *Dosage titration* – If no adverse reactions occur, the infusion rate can be increased to 2 mL/min. Infuse only 500 mL the first day. If the patient has no untoward reactions, the dose can be increased on the following day.

20%:

• *Maximum dose* – 3 g/kg/day.

• *Initial dosage* – 0.5 mL/min for the first 15 to 30 minutes.

• *Dosage titration* – If no adverse reactions occur, the infusion rate can be increased to 1 mL/min. Infuse only 250 mL (*Liposyn II*) or 500 mL (*Intralipid*) the first day. If the patient has no untoward reactions, the dose can be increased on the following day.

30%:

• *Maximum dose* – 2.5 g/kg/day.

• *Initial dosage* – 0.1 g/min for the first 15 to 30 minutes.

• *Dosage titration* – If no untoward reactions occur, increase the infusion rate to 0.2 g fat/min. The admixture should not contain more than 330 mL of *Liposyn III 30%* or *Intralipid 30%* on the first day of therapy. If the patient has no untoward reactions, the dose can be increased on the following day.

➤*Children:*

Caloric/fatty acid source –

Older children:

• *10%* –

Maximum dose: 3 g/kg/day.

Initial dosage: 0.1 mL/min for the first 10 to 15 minutes.

Dosage adjustment: If no untoward reactions occur, increase rate to 1 mL/kg/h.

• *20% and 30%* –

Maximum dose: 3 g/kg/day.

Initial dosage: Up to 0.01 g/min for the first 10 to 15 minutes.

Dosage adjustment: If no untoward reactions occur, the rate can be changed to permit infusion of 0.1 g/kg/h.

Premature infants:

• *Maximum dose* – 3 g/kg/day according to the American Academy of Pediatrics. Hourly infusion rate should be as slow as possible and should not exceed 1 g/kg in 4 hours. (See Black Box Warning.)

• *Initial dosage* – 0.5 g/kg/day (5 mL *Intralipid 10%*, 2.5 mL *Intralipid 20%*, 1.7 mL *Liposyn III 30%* or *Intralipid 30%*).

• *Dosage adjustment* – May be increased in relation to the infant's ability to eliminate fat.

➤*Hepatic function impairment:* Use caution with patients with severe liver damage.

➤*Preparation for administration:* IV fat emulsions are compatible with dextrose and amino acids, when properly mixed, for use in TPN therapy. This is also referred to as all-in-one, 3-in-1, and triple-mix. The following proper mixing sequence must be followed to minimize pH-related problems by ensuring that typically acidic dextrose injections are not mixed with lipid emulsions alone: (1) transfer dextrose injection to the TPN admixture container; (2) transfer amino acid injection; (3) transfer the IV fat emulsion.

Amino acid injection, dextrose injection, and the IV fat emulsion may be simultaneously transferred to the admixture container. Use gentle agitation to avoid localized concentration effects. Additives must not be added directly to the fat emulsion and in no case should the fat emulsion be added to the TPN container first. Shake bags gently after each addition to minimize localized concentration. If evacuated glass containers are used, add the dextrose and amino acid injections first, followed by the fat emulsion and then additives. Shake bottles gently after each addition.

The prime destabilizers of emulsions are excessive acidity (low pH) and inappropriate electrolyte content. Carefully consider additions of divalent cations (calcium and magnesium), which cause emulsion instability. Amino acid solutions exert a buffering effect protecting the emulsion.

Inspect the admixture carefully for "breaking or oiling out" of the emulsion, which is described as the separation of the emulsion and can be visibly identified by a yellowish streaking or the accumulation of yellowish droplets in the admixed emulsion. Also examine the admixture for particulates. The admixture must be discarded if any of the above is observed.

Heparin may be added to activate lipoprotein lipase at a concentration of 1 or 2 units/mL of fat emulsion prior to administration.

Lipid-containing fluids have a propensity to extract phthalates from phthalate-plasticized polyvinyl chloride (PVC). Although the amount is very small and no adverse clinical effects have been reported from administration of such amounts of phthalate, consider administration through a nonphthalate infusion set. Commercially available products may be accompanied by nonphthalate infusion sets.

➤*Administration:* As part of TPN, administer IV via a peripheral vein or by central venous catheter.

In preterm infants, the hourly infusion rate should be as slow as possible and should not exceed 1 g/kg in 4 hours. (See Black Box Warning.)

Fat emulsion is supplied in single-dose containers; do not store partially used bottles or resterilize for later use. Do not use filters less than 1.2 microns. Do not use any bottle in which there appears to be separation of the emulsion.

Fat emulsions may be simultaneously infused with amino acid/dextrose mixtures by means of a Y-connector located near the infusion site using separate flow rate controls for each solution. Keep the lipid infusion line higher than the amino acid/dextrose line. Because the lipid emulsion has a lower specific gravity, it may be taken up into the amino acid/dextrose line.

Fat emulsions may also be infused through a separate peripheral site.

Lipids

FAT EMULSION — INTRAVENOUS

➤*Storage/Stability:* Use these admixtures promptly; refrigerate at 2° to 8°C (36° to 46°F) for 24 hours or less and use completely within 24 hours after removal from refrigeration. Do not freeze. If accidentally frozen, discard the bag.

Actions

➤*Pharmacology:* Intravenous fat emulsions are prepared from either soybean or safflower oil and provide a mixture of neutral triglycerides, predominantly unsaturated fatty acids. The major component of fatty acids are linoleic, oleic, palmitic, stearic and linolenic acids; see product listings for content. In addition, these products contain 1.2% egg yolk phospholipids as an emulsifier and glycerol to adjust tonicity. The emulsified fat particles are approximately 0.4 to 0.5 microns in diameter, similar to naturally occurring chylomicrons. IV fat emulsions are isotonic and may be given by central or peripheral venous routes.

These products are metabolized and utilized as a source of energy, causing an increase in heat production, decrease in respiratory quotient and an increase in oxygen consumption following use. The infused fat particles are cleared from the blood stream in a manner thought to be comparable to the clearing of chylomicrons.

Essential Fatty Acid Deficiency (EFAD) – Linoleic, linolenic and arachidonic acids are essential in humans. Linoleic acid, the metabolic precursor to both linolenic and arachidonic acid, cannot be synthesized in vivo. When there is a deficiency of linoleic acid, the enzyme system that converts linoleic acid to arachidonic acid (a tetraene) acts on oleic acid to synthesize eicosatrienoic acid (a triene) which lacks the physiologic functions of arachidonic acid. Biochemically, EFAD is defined as a triene to tetraene ratio greater than 0.4. Clinical manifestations of EFAD include scaly dermatitis, alopecia, growth retardation, poor wound healing, thrombocytopenia and fatty liver. IV fat emulsion prevents or reverses biochemical and clinical manifestations of EFAD.

Contraindications

Disturbance of normal fat metabolism such as pathologic hyperlipemia, lipoid nephrosis or acute pancreatitis, if accompanied by hyperlipemia. Egg yolk phospholipids are present; do not give to patients with severe egg allergies.

Warnings/Precautions

➤*Special risk patients:* Exercise caution in severe liver damage, pulmonary disease, anemia, blood coagulation disorders, or when there is danger of fat embolism.

➤*Jaundiced or premature infants:* Use with caution because free fatty acids displace bilirubin bound to albumin.

➤*Too rapid administration:* Too rapid administration can cause fluid or fat overloading. This can result in dilution of serum electrolyte concentrations, overhydration, pulmonary edema, impaired pulmonary diffusion capacity or metabolic acidosis.

➤*Pregnancy: Category C.* It is not known whether IV fat emulsions can cause fetal harm when administered to a pregnant woman or can affect reproduction capacity. Use only when clearly needed.

➤*Lactation:* No data regarding the use of IV fat emulsion in breast-feeding women are available.

➤*Monitoring:* When IV fat emulsion is administered, monitor the patient's capacity to eliminate the infused fat from the circulation. The lipemia must clear between daily infusions. Closely monitor the hemogram, blood coagulation, liver function tests, plasma lipid profile and platelet count (especially in neonates). Discontinue use if a significant abnormality in any of these parameters is attributed to therapy.

Adverse Reactions

Most frequent – Sepsis due to administration equipment and thrombophlebitis due to vein irritation from concurrently administered hypertonic solutions. These adverse reactions are inseparable from the TPN procedure with or without IV fat emulsion.

Less frequent (more directly related to IV fat emulsion) –

Immediate (acute): (Less than 1%) – Dyspnea; cyanosis; hyperlipemia; hypercoagulability; nausea; vomiting; headache; flushing; increase in temperature; sweating; sleepiness; chest and back pain; slight pressure over the eyes; dizziness; irritation at the infusion site; thrombocytopenia in neonates (rare).

Long-term (chronic): Hepatomegaly; jaundice due to central lobular cholestasis; splenomegaly; thrombocytopenia; leukopenia; transient increases in liver function tests; overloading syndrome (focal seizures, fever, leukocytosis, splenomegaly and shock).

The deposition of brown pigmentation in the reticuloendothelial system (the so-called "IV fat pigment") has occurred. Cause and significance of this phenomenon are unknown.

Overdosage

➤*Treatment:* Stop the infusion until visual inspection of the plasma, determination of triglyceride concentrations or measurement of plasma light-scattering activity by nephelometry indicates the lipid has cleared. Reevaluate the patient and institute appropriate corrective measures.

Vitamins, Parenteral

B VITAMINS — PARENTERAL

Content given per mL.

	Product & Distributor	B_1 mg	B_2 mg	B_3 mg	B_5 mg	B_6 mg	How Supplied
Rx	**Vitamin B Complex 100 Injection** (McGuff)	100	2	100	2	2	In 10 and 30 mL vials.[a]

[a] May contain benzyl alcohol.

B VITAMINS — PARENTERAL

For additional information, refer to the Dietary Reference Intakes of Vitamins and Minerals table.

B VITAMINS WITH VITAMIN C — PARENTERAL

Content given per mL.

	Product & Distributor	B_1 mg	B_2 mg	B_3 mg	B_5 mg	B_6 mg	B_{12} mcg	C mg	Other Content	How Supplied
Rx	**Lypholized Vitamin B Complex & Vitamin C with B_{12} Injection** (McGuff)									In 10 mL vials.

B VITAMINS WITH VITAMIN C — PARENTERAL

For additional information, refer to the Dietary Reference Intakes of Vitamins and Minerals table.

MULTIVITAMINS — PARENTERAL

	Product & Distributor	Content[a] given per	A IU	D IU	E IU	B_1 mg	B_2 mg	B_3 mg	B_5 mg	B_6 mg	B_{12} mcg	C mg	biotin mcg	FA mg	Other Content and How Supplied
Rx	**Berocca Parenteral Nutrition** (Roche)	1 mL	3300	200	10[b]	3	3.6	40	15	4	5	100	60	0.4	In 2 vial or ampule sets: Soln 1[c] (1 or 2 mL) and soln 2[c] (1 or 2 mL).
Rx	**M.V.I.-12 Injection** (Mayne)	5 mL													In 2 vial sets: Vial 1[d] (5 mL single dose or 50 mL multiple dose) and vial 2[e] (5 mL single dose or 50 mL multiple dose).
Rx	**M.V.I.-12 Unit Vial** (Mayne)	10 mL													In 10 mL two chambered vials.[d]

MULTIVITAMINS — PARENTERAL

	Product & Distributor	Content[a] given per	A IU	D IU	E IU	B_1 mg	B_2 mg	B_3 mg	B_5 mg	B_6 mg	B_{12} mcg	C mg	biotin mcg	FA mg	Other Content and How Supplied
Rx	**M.V.I. Pediatric** (Hospira)	5 mL	2300	400	7[b]	1.2	1.4	17	5	1	1	80	20	0.14	200 mcg vitamin K_1 and 375 mg mannitol. In single and multiple dose vials.[f]
Rx	**Cernevit-12** (Baxter Healthcare)	5 mL	3500	200	11.2[2]	3.51	4.14	46	17.25	4.53	5.5	125	60	414	In 5 mL single-dose vials.
Rx	**Infuvite Adult** (Baxter)	10 mL (after combining vials)	3300	200 IU D_3	10	6	3.6	40	15	6	5	200	60	600	150 mcg vitamin K. Polysorbate 80. In two 5 mL vials to be combined together.
Rx	**Infuvite Pediatric** (Baxter)	5 mL (after combining vials)	2300	400 IU D_3	7	1.2	1.4	17	5	1	1	80	20	140	0.2 mg vitamin K. Polysorbate 80. In two vials (4 mL and 1 mL to be combined together).
Rx	**B Complex with C and B-12 Injection** (Goldline)	1 mL				50	5	125	6	5	1,000	50			1% benzyl alcohol. In 10 mL multiple dose vials.

[a] After combining vials, if necessary.
[b] As dL-alpha tocopheryl acetate.
[c] With propylene glycol, EDTA and 1% benzyl alcohol.
[d] With propylene glycol, polysorbate 80 and polysorbate 20.
[e] With propylene glycol.
[f] With polysorbate 20 and polysorbate 80.

MULTIVITAMINS — PARENTERAL

For additional information, refer to the Dietary Reference Intakes of Vitamins and Minerals table.

CALCIUM

For information on oral calcium, refer to the Minerals, Oral section. For additional information, refer to the Dietary Reference Intakes of Vitamins and Minerals table.

Indications

➤*Hypocalcemia:* For a prompt increase in plasma calcium levels (eg, neonatal tetany and tetany due to parathyroid deficiency, vitamin D deficiency, alkalosis); prevention of hypocalcemia during exchange transfusions; conditions associated with intestinal malabsorption.

➤*Calcium chloride and gluconate:* Adjunctive therapy in the treatment of insect bites or stings, such as Black Widow spider bites to relieve muscle cramping; sensitivity reactions, particularly when characterized by urticaria; depression due to overdosage of magnesium sulfate; acute symptoms of lead colic; rickets; osteomalacia.

➤*Calcium chloride:* To combat the deleterious effects of severe hyperkalemia as measured by ECG, pending correction of increased potassium in the extracellular fluid.

Cardiac resuscitation – Particularly after open heart surgery, when epinephrine fails to improve weak or ineffective myocardial contractions.

➤*Calcium gluconate:* To decrease capillary permeability in allergic conditions, nonthrombocytopenic purpura and exudative dermatoses such as dermatitis herpetiformis; for pruritus of eruptions caused by certain drugs; in hyperkalemia, calcium gluconate may aid in antagonizing the cardiac toxicity, provided the patient is not receiving digitalis therapy.

➤*Off-label uses:* Calcium salts have been used to treat verapamil overdose, treat acute hypotension from verapamil and prevent initial hypotension in patients requiring verapamil for whom decreases in blood pressure could be detrimental.

Administration and Dosage

Elemental Calcium Content of Calcium Salts		
Salt	**% Calcium**	**mEq/g**
Calcium chloride	27.3	13.6
Calcium gluconate	9.3	4.65

Calcium gluconate is generally preferred over calcium chloride as it is less irritating.

➤*IV:* Warm solutions to body temperature and give slowly (0.5 to 2 mL/min); stop if patient complains of discomfort. Resume when symptoms disappear. Following injection, patient should remain recumbent for a short time. Repeated injections may be needed because of the rapid calcium excretion. Inject **calcium chloride** and **gluconate** through a small needle into a large vein to minimize venous irritation.

➤*IM administration:* IM administration of **calcium gluconate** may be tolerated; however, reserve this route for emergencies when technical difficulty makes IV injection impossible. Administer **calcium gluconate** only by the IV route and **calcium chloride** by the IV or intraventricular route.

➤*Admixture incompatibilities:* Calcium salts should not generally be mixed with carbonates, phosphates, sulfates or tartrates in parenteral admixtures; they are conditionally compatible with potassium phosphates, depending on concentration. Calcium ions will chelate tetracycline.

Actions

➤*Pharmacology:* Calcium is the fifth most abundant element in the body with greater than 99.5% of total body stores in skeletal bone. It is essential for the functional integrity of the nervous and muscular systems, for normal cardiac contractility and the coagulation of blood. It also functions as an enzyme cofactor and affects the secretory activity of endocrine and exocrine glands. Normal levels are 8.5 to 10.5 mg/dL.

Hypocalcemia –

Symptoms: Tetany; paresthesias; laryngospasm; muscle spasms; seizures (usually grand mal); irritability; depression; psychosis; prolonged QT interval; intestinal cramps and malabsorption; respiratory arrest. Prolonged hypocalcemia may be associated with ectodermal defects including the nails, skin and teeth.

➤*Pharmacokinetics:* Approximately 80% of body calcium is excreted in the feces as insoluble salts; urinary excretion accounts for the remaining 20%.

Contraindications

Hypercalcemia; ventricular fibrillation; digitalized patients.

Warnings/Precautions

➤*Extravasation:* **Calcium chloride** and **gluconate** can cause severe necrosis, sloughing and abscess formation with IM or SC administration. Take great care to avoid extravasation or accidental injection into perivascular tissues.

➤*Hypocalcemia of renal insufficiency:* **Calcium chloride** is an acidifying salt and is therefore usually undesirable for treating this condition.

➤*Cardiovascular effects:* It is particularly important to prevent a high concentration of calcium from reaching the heart because of the danger of cardiac syncope.

➤*Pregnancy:* *Category C.* It is not known whether this drug can cause fetal harm when given to a pregnant woman or can affect reproduction capacity. Use only when clearly needed.

➤*Lactation:* It is not known whether **calcium gluconate** is excreted in breast milk. Exercise caution when administering to a pregnant woman.

Drug Interactions

Calcium Drug Interactions			
Precipitant	**Object drug[a]**		**Description**
Thiazide diuretics	Calcium salts	⬆	Hypercalcemia resulting from renal tubular reabsorption, or bone release of calcium by thiazides may be amplified by exogenous calcium.

CALCIUM

Calcium Drug Interactions

Precipitant	Object drug[a]		Description
Calcium salts	Atenolol	↓	Mean peak plasma levels and bioavailability of atenolol may be decreased, possibly resulting in decreased beta blockade.
Calcium salts	Digitalis glycosides	↑	Inotropic and toxic effects are synergistic; arrhythmias may occur, especially if calcium is given IV. Avoid IV calcium in patients on digitalis glycosides; if necessary, give slowly in small amounts.
Calcium salts	Sodium polystyrene sulfonate	↓	Coadministration in patients with renal impairment may result in an unanticipated metabolic alkalosis and a reduction of the resin's binding of potassium.
Calcium salts	Verapamil	↓	Clinical effects and toxicities of verapamil may be reversed.

[a] ↑ = Object drug increased. ↓ = Object drug decreased.

➤*Drug/Lab test interactions:* Transient elevations of plasma 11-hydroxy-corticosteroid levels (Glenn-Nelson technique) may occur when IV calcium is administered, but levels return to control values after 1 hour. In addition, IV calcium gluconate can produce false-negative values for serum and urinary magnesium.

Adverse Reactions

IM administration – Local necrosis and abscess formation may occur with **calcium gluconate**, and severe necrosis and sloughing may occur with IM or SC administration of **calcium chloride**.

IV administration – Rapid IV administration may cause bradycardia, sense of oppression, tingling, metallic, calcium or chalky taste or "heat waves". Rapid IV **calcium gluconate** may cause vasodilation, decreased blood pressure, cardiac arrhythmias, syncope and cardiac arrest. **Calcium chloride** injections cause peripheral vasodilation and a local burning sensation; blood pressure may fall moderately.

Overdosage

➤*Symptoms:* Inadvertent systemic overloading with calcium ions can produce an acute hypercalcemic syndrome characterized by a markedly elevated plasma calcium level, weakness, lethargy, intractable nausea and vomiting, coma and sudden death.

➤*Treatment:* It may be life-saving to rapidly lower blood calcium to safe levels. It is now agreed the most effective therapy is IV sodium chloride infusion plus potent natriuretic agents, (eg, furosemide). Sodium competes with calcium for reabsorption in the distal renal tubule and furosemide potentiates this effect. Together they markedly increase renal calcium clearance and reduce hypercalcemia.

CALCIUM GLUCONATE

For complete prescribing information, refer to the Calcium Gluconate monograph in the Minerals section.

CALCIUM CHLORIDE

1 g (10 mL) contains 273 mg (13.6 mEq) calcium.

Rx	**Calcium Chloride** (Various, eg, Abbott, American Regent, IMS, Moore, VHA)	**Injection:** 10%	In 10 mL amps, vials and syringes.

For complete and comparative prescribing information, refer to the Calcium group monograph. For additional information, refer to the Dietary Reference Intakes of Vitamins and Minerals table.

CALCIUM PRODUCTS COMBINED — PARENTERAL

Rx	**Calphosan** (Glenwood)	**Injection:** 50 mg calcium glycerophosphate and 50 mg calcium lactate per 10 mL in sodium chloride solution (0.08 mEq Ca/mL)	In 60 mL vials.[a]

[a] With 0.25% phenol.

For complete and comparative prescribing information, refer to the Calcium group monograph. For additional information, refer to the Dietary Reference Intakes of Vitamins and Minerals table.

MAGNESIUM

Rx	**Magnesium Chloride** (Various, eg, American Regent, Bioniche Pharma, Merit)	**Injection, solution, concentrate:** 20% (200 mg/mL)	Equiv. to elemental magnesium 1.97 mEq/mL. May contain benzyl alcohol, sodium chloride, aluminum. In 50 mL multiple-dose vials.
Rx	**Chloromag** (Merit)		Equiv. to elemental magnesium 1.97 mEq/mL. Aluminum, benzyl alcohol 1%, sodium chloride 9 mg. In 50 mL multiple-dose vials.
Rx	**Magnesium Sulfate in Dextrose 5%** (Hospira)	**Injection, solution:** 1% (10 mg/mL)	Equiv. to elemental magnesium 0.081 mEq/mL. Dextrose 5 g. In 100 mL single-dose containers.
Rx	**Magnesium Sulfate in Dextrose 5%** (Hospira)	**Injection, solution:** 2% (20 mg/mL)	Equiv. to elemental magnesium 0.162 mEq/mL. Dextrose 5 g. In 500 and 1,000 mL single-dose containers.
Rx	**Magnesium Sulfate** (Various, eg, Hospira)	**Injection, solution:** 4% (40 mg/mL)	Equiv. to elemental magnesium 0.325 mEq/mL. In 50, 100, 500, and 1,000 mL single-dose containers.
Rx	**Magnesium Sulfate** (Various, eg, Hospira)	**Injection, solution:** 8% (80 mg/mL)	Equiv. to elemental magnesium 0.65 mEq/mL. In 50 mL single-dose containers.
Rx	**Magnesium Sulfate** (Various, eg, American Regent, APP Pharmaceuticals, Hospira)	**Injection, solution:** 50% (500 mg/mL)	Equiv. to elemental magnesium 4 mEq/mL. Preservative free. May contain aluminum. In 10 and 20 mL single-dose vials.

MAGNESIUM CHLORIDE — INJECTION

For information on oral magnesium, refer to the Minerals and Electrolytes, Oral section. For additional information, refer to the Dietary Reference Intakes of Vitamins and Minerals table.

Indications

➤*Magnesium deficiency:* As an electrolyte replenisher in patients with magnesium deficiencies.

Administration and Dosage

➤*General dosing considerations:* Magnesium chloride 1 g provides approximately elemental magnesium 120 mg (9.85 mEq).

During the period of parenteral therapy with magnesium salts, watch the patient carefully. Have a preparation of calcium readily available for intravenous (IV) administration as an antidote (see Overdosage). Caution must be observed to prevent exceeding the renal excretory capacity.

➤*Adults:*

Magnesium deficiency –

Usual dosage: 1 to 40 g daily as an IV infusion.

Duration of therapy: Serum magnesium levels should serve as a guide to continued dosage.

➤*Renal function impairment:* Contraindicated in patients with renal impairment.

➤*Therapeutic drug monitoring:* The normal magnesium serum level is 1.5 to 2.5 or 3 mEq/L. Monitor serum magnesium concentrations hourly for patients with severe hypomagnesemia. Once the serum concentration reaches 1.5 mEq/L and the symptoms resolve, monitor the serum concentrations every 6 to 12 hours for the next 24 hours. After the serum concentration remains stable in the normal range, obtain the serum concentration daily. (See also Monitoring.)

➤*Administration:* For IV infusion, use 4 g in 250 mL of dextrose 5% injection. Administer at a rate not exceeding 3 mL/min.

MAGNESIUM CHLORIDE — INJECTION

➤*Admixture compatibility:* It has been reported that magnesium may reduce the antibiotic activity of streptomycin, tetracycline, and tobramycin when given together.

The potential of incompatibility will often be in influenced by the changes in the concentration of reactants and the pH of the solutions.

➤*Storage/Stability:* Store at 15° to 30°C (59° to 86°F).

Actions

➤*Pharmacology:* Magnesium is the second most plentiful cation within cellular fluids. It is an important cofactor for enzymatic reactions and plays an important role in neurochemical transmission and muscular excitability. Deficits are accompanied by a variety of structural and functional disturbances. Normal plasma magnesium levels range from 1.5 to 2.5 or 3 mEq/L. As plasma magnesium rises above 4 mEq/L, the deep tendon reflexes are first decreased and then disappear as the plasma level approaches 10 mEq/L. At this level, respiratory paralysis may occur. Heart block may also occur at this or lower plasma levels of magnesium.

Magnesium deficiency – Predominant deficiency effects are neurological (eg, muscle irritability, clonic twitching, tremors). Hypocalcemia and hypokalemia often follow low serum levels of magnesium. While there are large stores of magnesium present intracellularly and in the bones of adults, these stores often are not mobilized sufficiently to maintain plasma levels. Parenteral magnesium therapy repairs the plasma deficit and causes deficiency symptoms and signs to cease.

➤*Pharmacokinetics:*

Absorption – IV administered magnesium is immediately absorbed.

Distribution – Approximately 1% to 2% of total body magnesium is located in the extracellular fluid space. Magnesium is about 30% protein bound to albumin.

Metabolism – Magnesium is not metabolized.

Excretion – Magnesium is excreted solely by the kidney at a rate proportioned to the serum concentration and glomerular filtration.

Contraindications

Renal impairment; marked myocardial disease; comatose patients.

Warnings/Precautions

➤*Aluminum toxicity:* Some products may contain aluminum that may be toxic. Aluminum may reach toxic levels with prolonged parenteral administration if kidney function is impaired. Premature neonates are particularly at risk because their kidneys are immature, and they require large amounts of calcium and phosphate solutions, which contain aluminum.

Research indicates that patients with impaired kidney function, including premature neonates, who receive parenteral levels of aluminum at more than 4 to 5 mcg/kg/day accumulate aluminum at levels associated with CNS and bone toxicity. Tissue loading may occur at even lower rates of administration.

➤*Flushing/Sweating:* Administer with caution if flushing and sweating occurs.

➤*Administration:* Observe the usual precautions for parenteral administration. Have a preparation of a calcium salt readily available for IV injection to counteract potential serious signs of magnesium intoxication. As long as deep tendon reflexes are active, it is probable that the patient will not develop respiratory paralysis.

➤*Renal function impairment:* Contraindicated in renal impairment.

➤*Pregnancy: Category C.* Animal reproduction studies have not been conducted. It is also not known whether magnesium can cause fetal harm when administered to a pregnant woman or can affect reproduction capacity. Give magnesium to a pregnant woman only if clearly needed. Long-term infusions of magnesium may be associated with sustained hypocalcemia in the fetus, resulting in congenital rickets. Neonatal neurologic depression may occur with respiratory depression, muscle weakness, and loss of reflexes. The toxicity is not usually correlated with cord serum magnesium levels. Carefully observe offspring of mothers treated with this drug close to delivery for signs of toxicity during the first 24 to 48 hours after birth. Caution is also advocated with the use of aminoglycoside antibiotics during this period.

➤*Lactation:* Magnesium is distributed into milk during parenteral magnesium sulfate administration. Therefore, use with caution when administering magnesium to breast-feeding women. Oral absorption of magnesium by the infant is poor, so maternal magnesium therapy is not expected to affect the breast-fed infant's serum magnesium. The American Academy of Pediatrics classifies magnesium sulfate as compatible with breast-feeding.

➤*Children:* Some products may contain benzyl alcohol. Benzyl alcohol has been associated with a fatal "gasping syndrome" in premature infants.

➤*Monitoring:* Monitor the serum magnesium concentration and the patient's clinical status. The normal serum level is 1.5 to 2.5 or 3 mEq/L. Carefully observe respiration and blood pressure during and after administration. Clinical indications of a safe dosage regimen include the presence of the patellar reflex (knee jerk) and absence of respiratory depression (approximately 16 or more breaths per minute). When repeated doses of the drug are given parenterally, knee jerk reflexes should be tested before each dose; if they are absent, do not give additional magnesium until they return. The strength of the deep tendon reflexes begins to diminish when magnesium levels exceed 4 mEq/L. Reflexes may be absent at magnesium 10 mEq/L, when respiratory paralysis is a potential hazard. Have an injectable calcium salt immediately available to counteract the potential hazards of magnesium intoxication.

Drug Interactions

Magnesium Drug Interactions

Precipitant drug	Object drug[a]		Description
Alcohol, aminoglycosides, amphotericin B, cisplatin, cyclosporine, digitalis, diuretics	Magnesium	⬇	Drug-induced renal losses of magnesium may occur. Use with caution and closely monitor magnesium concentrations.
Neuromuscular blocking agents (eg, pancuronium)	Magnesium	⬆	Additive or synergistic effects may result in excessive neuromuscular blockade. Coadminister with caution. Monitor for respiratory depression. Adjust the neuromuscular blocking agent dose as needed. Be prepared to provide life support.
Magnesium	Neuromuscular blocking agents (eg, pancuronium)		
Nifedipine	Magnesium	⬆	The risk of neuromuscular blockade and hypotension may be increased. Closely monitor the clinical response. Be prepared to provide supportive treatment or to discontinue one or both drugs if needed.
Magnesium	Nifedipine		

[a] ⬆ = object drug increased; ⬇ = object drug decreased.

Adverse Reactions

➤*Cardiovascular:* Flushing, sharply lowered blood pressure.

➤*Miscellaneous:* Hypothermia, respiratory depression, stupor, sweating.

Overdosage

➤*Symptoms:* Magnesium intoxication is manifested by a sharp drop in blood pressure and respiratory paralysis. Electrocardiograph changes may include prolonged PR interval, prolonged QRS complex, and prolonged QT interval. Disappearance of the patellar reflex is a useful clinical sign to detect the onset of magnesium intoxication.

As plasma magnesium rises above 4 mEq/L, the deep tendon reflexes are first decreased and then disappear as the plasma level approaches 10 mEq/L. At this level, respiratory paralysis may occur. Heart block also may occur at this or lower plasma levels of magnesium. Serum magnesium concentrations in excess of 12 mEq/L may be fatal.

➤*Treatment:* Provide artificial ventilation until a calcium salt (10 to 20 mL of a 5% solution, diluted with isotonic sodium chloride for injection if desired) can be injected IV to antagonize the effects of magnesium. For adults, a dose of 5 to 10 mEq of calcium gluconate 10% will usually reverse the respiratory depression and heart block. Physostigmine 0.5 to 1 mg administered subcutaneously may be helpful. Peritoneal dialysis and hemodialysis are also effective.

Hypermagnesemia in the newborn may require resuscitation and assisted ventilation via endotracheal intubation or intermittent positive pressure ventilation, as well as IV calcium.

Patient Information

Advise patients that this medication will be prepared and administered by a health care provider in a hospital setting.

Instruct patients to notify their health care provider if drowsiness, muscle weakness, sweating, flushing, or dizziness occurs.

MAGNESIUM SULFATE — INJECTION

For information on oral magnesium, refer to the Minerals and Electrolytes, Oral section. For additional information, refer to the Dietary Reference Intakes of Vitamins and Minerals table.

Indications

➤*Acute nephritis:* To control hypertension, encephalopathy, and convulsions in children with acute nephritis. However, try other drugs, such as barbiturates, reserpine, or hydralazine, first.

➤*Hyperalimentation:* In total parenteral nutrition (TPN), magnesium may be added to the nutrient admixture to correct or prevent hypomagnesemia that can arise during the course of therapy.

➤*Hypomagnesemia:* For replacement therapy in magnesium deficiency, especially in acute hypomagnesemia accompanied by signs of tetany similar to those observed in hypocalcemia. In such cases, the serum magnesium level is usually below the lower limit of normal (1.5 to 2.5 or 3 mEq/L), and the serum calcium level is normal (4.3 to 5.3 mEq/L) or elevated.

MAGNESIUM SULFATE — INJECTION

➤*Seizures in eclampsia/preeclampsia:* For the prevention and control of seizures (convulsions) in severe toxemia of pregnancy. When used judiciously, it effectively prevents and controls the convulsions of eclampsia without producing deleterious depression of the CNS of the mother or infant. However, other effective drugs are available for this purpose.

➤*Off-label uses:*

Premature labor – [5] = Poor documentation. Because of a lack of substantive evidence, long-term maintenance therapy with tocolytics is not recommended. Tocolytic therapy is recommended only as a method to prevent delivery long enough for a course of corticosteroids to be administered and for the patient to be transferred to an appropriate facility with the ability to care for a premature infant. The administration of magnesium for the treatment of premature labor appears to be of no benefit and may place the infant at risk for death and the mother at risk of adverse effects. (See Off-Label Dosing.)

Other possible off-label uses –

Severe asthma: In patients with asthma who respond poorly to beta-agonists, intravenous (IV) magnesium sulfate may be a beneficial adjunct for treatment of acute exacerbations of severe asthma (see also Off-label Dosing in Adults and Children).

Torsades de pointes: Magnesium may be considered for the treatment of torsades de pointes (see also Off-label Dosing in Adults and Children).

Barium poisoning: To counteract the muscle stimulating effects of barium poisoning. (See also Off-Label Dosing.)

Cerebral edema: For reduction of cerebral edema. (See also Off-Label Dosing.)

Paroxysmal atrial tachycardia: For the treatment of paroxysmal atrial tachycardia. (See also Off-Label Dosing.)

Administration and Dosage

➤*General dosing considerations:* Dosage of magnesium must be carefully adjusted according to individual requirements and response, and administration of the drug should be discontinued as soon as the desired effect is obtained.

During the period of parenteral therapy with magnesium salts, watch the patient carefully. Have a preparation of calcium, such as the gluconate or gluceptate, readily available for IV administration as an antidote (see Overdose).

In the treatment of deficiency states, caution must be observed to prevent exceeding the renal excretory capacity.

Magnesium sulfate 1 g provides approximately elemental magnesium 99 mg (8.12 mEq).

When repeated doses of the drug are given parenterally, knee jerk reflexes should be tested before each dose and, if they are absent, no additional magnesium should be given until they return.

➤*Adults:*

Seizures in eclampsia/preeclampsia – See also Off-Label Dosing for recommendations from the American College of Obstetricians and Gynecologists (ACOG).

Maximum dose: 30 to 40 g per 24 hours and less in anuric patients.

Initial dosage: 10 to 14 g. To accomplish this, an IV dose of 4 to 5 g in 250 mL of dextrose 5% injection or sodium chloride 0.9% injection or 4 g of magnesium/dextrose 5% injection may be infused, and, simultaneously, intramuscular (IM) doses of 8 to 10 g (4 or 5 g of the undiluted 50% solution in each buttock) are given. Alternatively, the initial IV dose of 4 g may be given by diluting the 50% solution to a 10% or 20% concentration; the diluted fluid (40 mL of a 10% solution or 20 mL of a 20% solution) may then be injected IV over a period of 3 to 4 minutes.

Maintenance dosage: 4 to 5 g (8 to 10 mL of the 50% undiluted solution) IM into alternate buttocks every 4 hours as needed, depending on the continuing presence of the patellar reflex and adequate respiratory function, and absence of signs of magnesium toxicity. Alternatively, after the initial IV dose, some health care providers administer 1 to 2 g/h by constant IV infusion.

Duration of therapy: Therapy should continue until paroxysms cease.

Hyperalimentation – 5 to 8 mEq of magnesium per L of TPN solution. Typical daily intakes range from 10 to 24 mEq/day. In TPN, maintenance requirements for magnesium are not precisely known.

Hypomagnesemia –

Usual dosage:

• *Mild hypomagnesemia* – 1 g (2 mL) IM of the undiluted 50% solution every 6 hours for 4 doses.

• *Severe hypomagnesemia* – See also Off-Label Dosing for recommendations from the American Heart Association (AHA).

Up to 246 mg/kg (0.5 mL/kg) IM of the undiluted 50% solution within a period of 4 hours if necessary, or 5 g (10 mL) can be added to 1 L of dextrose 5% injection or sodium chloride 0.9% injection for slow IV infusion over a 3-hour period.

Off-label dosing –

Asthma (life-threatening exacerbations or those that stay in the severe category after 1 hour of intensive conventional therapy): 1.2 to 2 g IV over 20 minutes, according to guidelines.

Barium poisoning: 1 to 2 g IV to counteract the muscle-stimulating effects of barium poisoning.

Cerebral edema: 2.5 g (25 mL of a 10% solution) IV for reduction of cerebral edema.

Paroxysmal atrial tachycardia: 3 to 4 g (30 to 40 mL of a 10% solution) IV over 30 seconds with extreme caution. Magnesium should be used only if simpler measures have failed and there is no evidence of myocardial damage.

Severe or symptomatic hypomagnesemia: According to AHA/American College of Cardiology (ACC) guidelines, give 1 to 2 g IV over 5 to 60 minutes. If seizures are present, give 2 g IV over 10 minutes.

Seizures in eclampsia: The following dosage regimen is according to ACOG guidelines.

• *Initial dosage* – 4 to 6 g diluted in 100 mL of compatible fluid and administered IV over 15 to 20 minutes.

• *Maintenance dosage* – 2 g/h continuous IV infusion.

Torsades de pointes: The following dosages are according to AHA/ACC guidelines. If associated with cardiac arrest, 1 to 2 g diluted in 10 mL of dextrose 5% injection administered IV/intraosseous over 5 to 20 minutes. If torsades de pointes is intermittent and not associated with cardiac arrest, dilute 1 to 2 g in 50 to 100 mL of dextrose 5% injection and administer over 5 to 60 minutes.

➤*Children:*

Hyperalimentation – 0.25 to 0.6 mEq/kg/day. In TPN, maintenance requirements for magnesium are not precisely known.

Nephritic seizures – 20 to 40 mg/kg (0.1 to 0.2 mL/kg) of a 20% solution IM as needed to control seizures.

Off-label dosing –

Asthma (life-threatening exacerbations or those that stay in the severe category after 1 hour of intensive conventional therapy):

• *Usual dose* – According to guidelines, the dosage is 25 to 75 mg/kg IV over 20 minutes every 4 to 6 hours for 3 or 4 doses; repeat as needed.

• *Maximum dose* – 2 g/dose.

Hypomagnesemia:

• *Usual dose* – 25 to 50 mg/kg IV/intraosseous over 10 to 20 minutes every 4 to 6 hours for 3 or 4 doses; repeat as needed.

• *Maximum dose* – 2 g.

Torsades de pointes:

• *Usual dose* – According to AHA/ACC guidelines, the dosage is 25 to 50 mg/kg IV/intraosseous over several minutes.

• *Maximum dose* – 2 g.

➤*Renal function impairment:*

Severe renal impairment –

Usual dosage: The dose should be lower and frequent serum magnesium concentrations must be obtained. Consider reducing the dosage by 50%.

Maximum dose: 20 g per 48 hours.

➤*Therapeutic drug monitoring:* Normal plasma magnesium levels range from 1.5 to 2.5 or 3 mEq/L. Effective anticonvulsant serum levels range from 2.5 or 3 to 7.5 mEq/L (6 mg/100 mL). Monitor serum magnesium concentrations hourly for patients with severe hypomagnesemia. Once the serum concentration reaches 1.5 mEq/L and the symptoms resolve, monitor the serum concentrations every 6 to 12 hours for the next 24 hours. After the serum concentration remains stable in the normal range, obtain the serum concentration daily. (See also Monitoring in Warnings/Precautions.)

➤*Preparation for administration:* Solutions for IV infusion must be diluted to a concentration of 20% or less prior to administration. The diluents commonly used are dextrose 5% injection and sodium chloride 0.9% injection. Deep IM injection of the undiluted 50% solution is appropriate for adults, but the solution should be diluted to a 20% or less concentration prior to such injection in children (See Seizures in Eclampsia/Preeclampsia for additional preparation techniques).

➤*Administration:* Magnesium 4%, 8%, and magnesium/dextrose 5% solutions are for IV administration only. Both IV and IM administration are appropriate for magnesium 50% solution; must be diluted prior to IV administration. IM administration is painful and should be reserved for those patients with limited IV access and severe hypomagnesemia. IV bolus administration may cause flushing, sweating, and warm sensation, and should be avoided, if possible. Do not use flexible container in series connections.

The rate of IV injection should generally not exceed 150 mg/min (1.5 mL of a 10% concentration, 7.5 mL of a 2% concentration, or its equivalent), except in severe eclampsia with seizures.

➤*Admixture compatibility:* Magnesium in solution may result in a precipitate formation when mixed with solutions containing alcohol (in high concentrations), alkali carbonates and bicarbonates, alkali hydroxides, arsenates, barium, clindamycin phosphate, calcium, heavy metals, hydrocortisone sodium succinate, phosphates, polymyxin B sulfate, procaine hydrochloride, salicylates, strontium, or tartrates.

The potential incompatibility will often be influenced by the changes in the concentration of reactants and the pH of the solutions.

It has been reported that magnesium may reduce the antibiotic activity of streptomycin, tetracycline, and tobramycin when given together.

➤*Storage/Stability:* Store at 20° to 25°C (68° to 77°F). Protect from freezing. Discard unused portion. Any unused portion of the 50% solution remaining in the container should be discarded within 24 hours of initial use.

Actions

➤*Pharmacology:* Magnesium is the second most plentiful cation of the intracellular fluids. It is an important cofactor for enzymatic reactions and plays an important role in neurochemical transmission and muscular excitability. Deficits are accompanied by a variety of structural and functional disturbances. Normal plasma magnesium levels range from 1.5 to 2.5 or 3 mEq/L. As plasma magnesium rises above 4 mEq/L, the deep tendon reflexes are first decreased and then disappear as the plasma level approaches 10 mEq/L. At this level, respiratory paralysis may occur. Heart block also may occur at this or lower plasma levels of magnesium.

MAGNESIUM SULFATE — INJECTION

Hyperalimentation – As a nutritional adjunct in hyperalimentation, the precise mechanism of action for magnesium is uncertain. Early symptoms of hypomagnesemia (less than 1.5 mEq/L) may develop as early as 3 to 4 days, or within weeks.

Magnesium deficiency – Predominant deficiency effects are neurological (eg, muscle irritability, clonic twitching, tremors). Hypocalcemia and hypokalemia often follow low serum levels of magnesium. While there are large stores of magnesium present intracellularly and in the bones of adults, these stores often are not mobilized sufficiently to maintain plasma levels. Parenteral magnesium therapy repairs the plasma deficit and causes deficiency symptoms and signs to cease.

Anticonvulsant – Magnesium prevents or controls convulsions by blocking neuromuscular transmission and decreasing the amount of acetylcholine liberated at the end-plate by the motor nerve impulse. Magnesium is said to have a depressant effect on the CNS, but it does not adversely affect the mother, fetus, or neonate when used as directed in eclampsia or preeclampsia.

➤*Pharmacokinetics:*

Absorption – With IV administration, the onset of anticonvulsant action is immediate and lasts about 30 minutes. Following IM administration, the onset of action occurs in about 1 hour and persists for 3 to 4 hours.

Distribution – Approximately 1% to 2% of total body magnesium is located in the extracellular fluid space. Magnesium is 30% bound to albumin.

Metabolism – Magnesium is not metabolized.

Excretion – Magnesium is excreted solely by the kidney at a rate proportional to the serum concentration and glomerular filtration.

Special populations –

Renal function impairment: Magnesium is excreted solely by the kidney. In patients with severe renal insufficiency, lower the dose and obtain frequent serum magnesium levels.

Contraindications

Toxemia of pregnancy during the 2 hours preceding delivery.

Warnings/Precautions

➤*Aluminum toxicity:* Some of these products may contain aluminum that may be toxic. Aluminum may reach toxic levels with prolonged parenteral administration if kidney function is impaired. Premature neonates are particularly at risk because their kidneys are immature and they require large amounts of calcium and phosphate solutions, which contain aluminum.

Research indicates that patients with impaired kidney function, including premature neonates, who receive parenteral levels of aluminum at more than 4 to 5 mcg/kg/day accumulate aluminum at levels associated with CNS and bone toxicity. Tissue loading may occur at even lower rates of administration.

➤*Flushing / Sweating:* Administer with caution if flushing and sweating occurs.

➤*Hypermagnesemia:* The principle hazard in parenteral magnesium therapy is the production of abnormally high levels of magnesium in the plasma. Such high levels may cause flushing, sweating, hypotension, circulatory collapse, and depression of cardiac and CNS function. The most immediate danger to life is respiratory depression.

As plasma magnesium rises above 4 mEq/L, the deep tendon reflexes are first decreased and then disappear as the plasma level approaches 10 mEq/L. At this level, respiratory paralysis may occur. Heart block also may occur at this or lower plasma levels of magnesium. Serum magnesium concentrations in excess of 12 mEq/L may be fatal.

During the period of parenteral therapy with magnesium salts, watch the patient carefully. Have a preparation of calcium, such as the gluconate or gluceptate, readily available for IV administration as an antidote.

➤*Administration:* IV use in eclampsia should be reserved for immediate control of life-threatening convulsions. Magnesium 50% solution must be diluted to a concentration of 20% or less prior to IV infusion. Rate of administration should be slow and cautious to avoid producing hypermagnesemia. The 50% solution also should be diluted to 20% or less for IM injection in infants and children. (see Administration and Dosage.)

➤*Renal function impairment:* Because magnesium is removed from the body solely by the kidneys, parenteral use in the presence of renal insufficiency may lead to magnesium intoxication. Some of these products may contain aluminum. Patients with impaired kidney function who receive parenteral levels of aluminum at more than 4 to 5 mcg/kg/day accumulate aluminum at levels associated with CNS and bone toxicity. Use caution in patients with renal impairment. (See Administration and Dosage.)

➤*Pregnancy: Category A* per manufacturer's prescribing information. *Category B* per Briggs' *Drugs in Pregnancy and Lactation*. Studies in pregnant women have not shown that magnesium increases the risk of fetal abnormalities if administered during all trimesters of pregnancy. Long-term infusions of magnesium may be associated with sustained hypocalcemia in the fetus, resulting in congenital rickets. Neonatal neurologic depression may occur with respiratory depression, muscle weakness, and loss of reflexes. The toxicity is not usually correlated with cord serum magnesium levels. Carefully observe offspring of mothers treated with this drug close to delivery for signs of toxicity during the first 24 to 48 hours after birth. Caution is also advocated with the use of aminoglycoside antibiotics during this period. If this drug is used during pregnancy, the possibility of fetal harm appears remote. However, because studies cannot rule out the possibility of harm, use magnesium during pregnancy only if clearly needed.

When administered by continuous IV infusion (especially for more than 24 hours preceding delivery) to control convulsions in toxemic mothers, the newborn may show signs of magnesium toxicity, including neuromuscular or respiratory depression. Hypermagnesemia in the newborn may require resuscitation and assisted ventilation via endotracheal intubation or intermittent positive pressure ventilation as well as IV calcium. Carefully observe offspring of mothers treated with this drug close to delivery for signs of toxicity during the first 24 to 48 hours after birth.

➤*Lactation:* Because magnesium is distributed into milk during parenteral magnesium administration, use the drug with caution in breast-feeding women. Oral absorption of magnesium by the infant is poor, so maternal magnesium therapy is not expected to affect the breast-fed infant's serum magnesium. The American Academy of Pediatrics classifies magnesium as compatible with breast-feeding.

➤*Children:* See Administration and Dosage for more information.

➤*Elderly:* Elderly patients may require reduced dosage because of impaired renal function.

➤*Monitoring:* Monitor the serum concentration of magnesium and the patient's clinical status. The normal serum level is 1.5 to 2.5 or 3 mEq/L.

Maintain urine output at a level of 100 mL every 4 hours. Carefully observe respiration and blood pressure during and after administration Clinical indications of a safe dosage regimen include the presence of the patellar reflex (knee jerk) and absence of respiratory depression (approximately 16 or more breaths per minute). Serum magnesium levels usually sufficient to control convulsions range from 2.5 to 5 mEq/L (3 to 6 mg per 100 mL). The strength of the deep tendon reflexes begins to diminish when magnesium levels exceed 4 mEq/L. Reflexes may be absent at magnesium 10 mEq/L, where respiratory paralysis is a potential hazard. An injectable calcium salt should be immediately available to counteract the potential hazards of magnesium intoxication in eclampsia. (See also Therapeutic Drug Monitoring.)

Drug Interactions

Magnesium Drug Interactions

Precipitant drug	Object drug[a]		Description
Alcohol, aminoglycosides, amphotericin B, cisplatin, cyclosporine, digitalis, diuretics	Magnesium	⬇	Drug-induced renal losses of magnesium may occur. Use with caution and closely monitor magnesium concentrations.
Neuromuscular blocking agents (eg, pancuronium)	Magnesium	⬆	Additive or synergistic effects may result in excessive neuromuscular blockade. Coadminister with caution. Monitor for respiratory depression. Adjust the neuromuscular blocking agent dose as needed. Be prepared to provide life support.
Magnesium	Neuromuscular blocking agents (eg, pancuronium)		
Nifedipine	Magnesium	⬆	The risk of neuromuscular blockade and hypotension may be increased. Closely monitor the clinical response. Be prepared to provide supportive treatment or to discontinue one or both drugs if needed.
Magnesium	Nifedipine		

[a] ⬆ = object drug increased; ⬇ = object drug decreased.

Adverse Reactions

➤*Cardiovascular:* Circulatory collapse, cardiac depression, hypotension.

➤*Dermatologic:* Flushing, sweating.

➤*Musculoskeletal:* Depressed reflexes, flaccid paralysis.

➤*Miscellaneous:* CNS depression, hypothermia, hypocalcemia with signs of tetany, respiratory paralysis.

Overdosage

➤*Symptoms:* Magnesium intoxication is manifested by a sharp drop in blood pressure and respiratory paralysis. Disappearance of the patellar reflex is a useful clinical sign to detect the onset of magnesium intoxication. Electrocardiograph changes may include prolonged PR interval, prolonged QRS complex, and prolonged QT interval.

As plasma magnesium rises above 4 mEq/L, the deep tendon reflexes are first decreased and then disappear as the plasma level approaches 10 mEq/L. At this level, respiratory paralysis may occur. Heart block also may occur at this or lower plasma levels of magnesium. Serum magnesium concentrations in excess of 12 mEq/L may be fatal.

➤*Treatment:* In the event of overdosage, artificial ventilation must be provided until a calcium salt can be injected IV to antagonize the effects of magnesium.

In adults, IV administration of 5 to 10 mEq of calcium gluconate 10% will usually reverse respiratory depression or heart block due to magnesium intoxication. In extreme cases, peritoneal or hemodialysis may be required.

MAGNESIUM SULFATE — INJECTION

Hypermagnesemia in the newborn may require resuscitation and assisted ventilation via endotracheal intubation or intermittent positive pressure ventilation, as well as IV calcium.

Patient Information

Advise patients that this medication will be prepared and administered by a health care provider in a hospital setting.

Instruct patients to notify their health care provider if drowsiness, muscle weakness, sweating, flushing, or dizziness occurs.

PHOSPHATE

Rx	**Potassium Phosphate** (Various, eg, Abbott, American Regent)	**Injection:** Provides phosphate 3 mM and potassium 4.4 mEq per mL	In 5, 10, 15, 30, and 50 mL vials.
Rx	**Sodium Phosphate** (Various, eg, American Regent, Hospira)	**Injection, solution, concentrate:** Provides phosphate 3 mM and sodium 4 mEq per mL	In 5, 15, and 50 mL vials.

SODIUM PHOSPHATES — INJECTION

For additional information, refer to the Dietary Reference Intakes of Vitamins and Minerals table.

Indications

➤*Hypophosphatemia:* As a source of phosphate, for addition to large volume intravenous (IV) fluids, to prevent or correct hypophosphatemia in patients with restricted or no oral intake. It is also useful as an additive for preparing specific parenteral fluid formulas when the needs of the patient cannot be met by standard electrolyte or nutrient solutions.

Administration and Dosage

➤*General dosing considerations:* The concomitant amount of sodium (4 mEq/mL) must be calculated into total electrolyte dose of prepared solutions.

Phosphate 1 mmol = phosphorous 31 mg.

➤*Adults:*

Hypophosphatemia –

Usual dosage: The dose and rate of administration are dependent upon the individual needs of the patient.

Total parenteral nutrition: In patients on total parenteral nutrition (TPN), approximately 10 to 15 mmol of phosphorus (equivalent to 310 to 465 mg elemental phosphorus) per liter bottle of TPN solution containing dextrose 250 g is usually adequate to maintain normal serum phosphorus, although larger amounts may be required in hypermetabolic states. The amount of sodium and phosphorus that accompanies the addition of sodium phosphate also should be kept in mind and, if necessary, serum sodium levels should be monitored.

Off-label dosing –

Hypophosphatemia:

- *Mild hypophosphatemia (serum phosphorus 2.3 to 3 mg/dL)* – 0.16 mmol/kg. Administer at a rate no faster than 7.5 mmol/h.
- *Moderate hypophosphatemia (serum phosphorus 1.6 to 2.2 mg/dL)* – 0.32 mmol/kg. Administer at a rate no faster than 7.5 mmol/h.
- *Severe hypophosphatemia (serum phosphorous less than 1.6 mg/dL)* – 0.64 mmol/kg. Administer at a rate no faster than 7.5 mmol/h.
- *TPN* – 20 to 40 mmol/day.

➤*Children:*

Hypophosphatemia –

Usual dosage: The dose and rate of administration are dependent upon the individual needs of the patient.

Total parenteral nutrition: The suggested dose of phosphorus for infants receiving TPN is 1.5 to 2 mmol/kg/day.

Off-label dosing –

Hypophosphatemia:

- *Acute* – 0.16 to 0.32 mmol/kg per dose IV over 6 hours.
- *Maintenance dosage* – 0.5 to 1.5 mmol/kg per dose IV over 24 hours.
- *Total parenteral nutrition –*
  - *Preterm neonates:* 1 to 2 mmol/kg/day.
  - *Infants/Children:* 0.5 to 2 mmol/kg/day.
  - *Adolescents and children weighing more than 50 kg:* 10 to 40 mmol per day.

➤*Elderly:* Because elderly patients are more likely to have decreased renal function, care should be taken in dose selection, and it may be useful to monitor renal function.

➤*Renal function impairment:* Sodium ions and phosphorus are known to be substantially excreted by the kidney, and the risk of toxic reactions to this drug may be greater in patients with impaired renal function.

➤*Preparation for administration:* All or part of the contents of 1 or more vials may be added to other IV fluids to provide any desired number of millimoles of phosphate and milliequivalents of sodium.

➤*Administration:* Sodium phosphates injection is administered IV only after dilution and thorough mixing in a larger volume of fluid. The dose and rate of administration are dependent upon the individual needs of the patient.

➤*Storage/Stability:* Store at controlled room temperature 15° to 30°C (59° to 86°F).

Do not administer unless the solution is clear and the seal is intact. Discard any unused portion.

Actions

➤*Pharmacology:* Phosphorus in the form of organic and inorganic phosphate has a variety of important biochemical functions in the body, and is involved in many significant metabolic and enzyme reactions in almost all organs and tissues. It exerts a modifying influence on the steady state of calcium levels, a buffering effect on acid-base equilibrium, and a primary role in the renal excretion of hydrogen ion.

Phosphorus, present in large amounts in erythrocytes and other tissue cells, plays a significant intracellular role in the synthesis of high-energy organic phosphates. It has been shown to be essential to maintain red cell glucose utilization, lactate production, and the concentration of both erythrocyte adenosine triphosphate (ATP) and 2, 3 diphosphoglycerate (DPG), and must be deemed as important to other tissue cells. Hypophosphatemia should be avoided during periods of TPN or other lengthy periods of IV infusions. It has been suggested that patients receiving TPN receive 20 mEq phosphate (13 mmol phosphate)/1,000 kcal from dextrose. Serum phosphorus levels should be regularly monitored and appropriate amounts of phosphorus should be added to the infusions to maintain healthy serum phosphorus levels. IV infusion of inorganic phosphorus may be accompanied by a decrease in the serum level and urinary excretion of calcium. The healthy level of serum phosphorus is 3 to 4.5 mg per 100 mL in adults; 4 to 7 mg per 100 mL in children.

➤*Pharmacokinetics:* IV infused phosphorus not taken up by the tissues is excreted almost entirely in the urine. Plasma phosphorus is believed to be filterable by the renal glomeruli, and the major portion of filtered phosphorus (more than 80%) is actively reabsorbed by the tubules. Many modifying influences tend to alter the amount excreted in the urine.

Contraindications

High phosphorus or low calcium levels; hypernatremia.

Warnings/Precautions

➤*Parenteral administration:* Sodium phosphates injection must be diluted and thoroughly mixed before use.

To avoid phosphorus intoxication, infuse solutions containing sodium phosphate slowly. Infusing high concentrations of phosphorus may result in a reduction of serum calcium and symptoms of hypocalcemic tetany. Calcium levels should be monitored.

➤*Sodium retention:* Solutions containing sodium ion should be used with great care, if at all, in patients with congestive heart failure, those with severe renal insufficiency, and those in clinical states in which edema with sodium retention exists.

➤*Aluminum toxicity:* This product may contain aluminum that may be toxic. Aluminum may reach toxic levels with prolonged parenteral administration if kidney function is impaired. Premature neonates are particularly at risk because their kidneys are immature and they require large amounts of calcium and phosphate solutions, which contain aluminum.

➤*Renal function impairment:* In patients with diminished renal function, administration of solutions containing sodium ions may result in sodium retention.

➤*Special risk:* Use with caution in patients with renal impairment, cirrhosis, or cardiac failure, or in conjunction with other edematous medications. It should not be used with sodium-retaining medications.

➤*Pregnancy:* Category C. Animal reproduction studies have not been conducted with sodium phosphate. It is also not known whether sodium phosphate can cause fetal harm when administered to a pregnant woman or can affect reproduction capacity. Sodium phosphate should be given to a pregnant woman only if clearly needed.

➤*Lactation:* It is not known whether this drug is excreted in human milk. Because many drugs are excreted in human milk, caution should be exercised when sodium phosphate is administered to a breast-feeding woman.

➤*Children:* The safety and efficacy of sodium phosphate have been established in children (neonates, infants, children, and adolescents).

➤*Elderly:* An evaluation of current literature revealed no clinical experience identifying differences in response between elderly and younger patients. In general, dose selection for an elderly patient should be cautious, usually starting at the low end of the dosing range, reflecting the greater frequency of decreased hepatic, renal, or cardiac function, and of concomitant disease or other drug therapy.

Minerals

SODIUM PHOSPHATES — INJECTION

Sodium ions and phosphorus ions are known to be substantially excreted by the kidney, and the risk of toxic reactions may be greater in patients with impaired renal function. Because elderly patients are more likely to have decreased renal function, care should be taken in dose selection, and it may be useful to monitor renal function.

➤*Monitoring:* Phosphate replacement therapy with sodium phosphate should be guided primarily by serum inorganic phosphate levels and the limits imposed by the accompanying sodium (Na+) ion. Frequent monitoring of serum sodium, phosphorus, and calcium levels, as well as renal function, is recommended.

Drug Interactions

➤*Thiazides:* Concurrent use with thiazides may cause renal damage.

➤*Corticosteroids and corticotropin:* Caution must be exercised in the administration of parenteral fluids, especially those containing sodium ion, to patients receiving corticosteroids or corticotropin.

Adverse Reactions

Adverse reactions involve the possibility of combined sodium and phosphorus intoxication from overdosage.

Phosphorus intoxication results in hypocalcemic tetany.

Overdosage

➤*Symptoms:* Phosphorus intoxication results in a reduction of serum calcium, and the symptoms are those of hypocalcemic tetany.

➤*Treatment:* In the event of overdosage, discontinue infusions containing sodium phosphate immediately and institute corrective therapy to restore depressed serum calcium and to reduce elevated serum sodium levels.

Electrolytes

SODIUM CHLORIDE

otc	**Sodium Chloride 0.45%** (Dey)	**Injection, solution:** 0.45% sodium chloride	Preservative free. Sodium 77 mEq/L, chloride 77 mEq/L, ≈ 155 mOsm/L. In single-use 3 and 5 mL vials.
Rx	**Sodium Chloride 0.45% (½ Normal Saline)** (Various, eg, Abbott)		Sodium 77 mEq/L, chloride 77 mEq/L, ≈ 155 mOsm/L. In 25, 50, 150, 250, 500 and 1000 mL.
otc	**Sodium Chloride 0.9%** (Dey)	**Injection, solution:** 0.9% sodium chloride	Preservative free. Sodium 154 mEq/L, chloride 154 mEq/L, and ≈ 310 mOsm/L. In 3, 5, and 15 mL.
Rx	**Sodium Chloride 0.9% (Normal Saline)** (Various, eg, American Regent, Gensia, Hospira, Smith & Nephew SoloPak)		Sodium 154 mEq/L, chloride 154 mEq/L, and ≈ 310 mOsm/L. In 1, 2, 2.5, 3, 5, 10, 20, 25, 30, 50, 100, 150, 250, 500, 1000 mL and 2 mL fill in 3 mL.[a]
Rx	**Sodium Chloride 3%** (Various)	**Injection, solution:** 3% sodium chloride	Sodium 513 mEq/L, chloride 513 mEq/L, and 1030 mOsm/L. In 500 mL.
Rx	**Sodium Chloride 5%** (Various, eg, Abbott)	**Injection, solution:** 5% sodium chloride	Sodium 855 mEq/L, chloride 855 mEq/L, and 1710 mOsm/L. In 500 mL.
Rx	**Sodium Chloride** (Various, eg, Hospira)	**Injection, solution, concentrate:** 14.6%	In 250 mL.
Rx	**Sodium Chloride** (Various, eg, Hospira)	**Injection, solution, concentrate:** 23.4%	In 100 mL.

[a] May contain benzyl alcohol 9 mg.

SODIUM CHLORIDE — INJECTION

For information on oral sodium chloride, refer to Minerals and Electrolytes, Oral section. For additional information, refer to the Dietary Reference Intakes of Vitamins and Minerals table.

Indications

➤*0.45% and 0.9% flexible plastic containers:* IV solutions containing sodium chloride are indicated for parenteral replenishment of fluid and sodium chloride as required by the clinical condition of the patient.

➤*0.9% syringe:* Sodium chloride injection, 0.9% is intended for use in flushing the indwelling venipuncture device where the medication to be administered is incompatible with heparin.

➤*0.45% and 0.9% vial:* Sodium chloride injection, 0.45% and 0.9% preparations are indicated for diluting or dissolving drugs for intramuscular (IM), intravenous (IV) or subcutaneous injection or for inhalation according to instructions of the manufacturer of the drug to be administered.

Also indicated for use in flushing of IV catheters and for tracheal lavage.

➤*3% and 5% concentrates:* These IV solutions are indicated for use in adults and children as sources of electrolytes and water for hydration.

Sodium chloride injections, 3% and 5% are of particular value in severe salt depletion when rapid electrolyte restoration is of paramount importance. The low salt syndrome may occur in the presence of heart failure, renal impairment, during surgery, and postoperatively. In these conditions, chloride loss frequently exceeds sodium loss.

These hypertonic sodium chloride solutions are also indicated for the following clinical conditions: hyponatremia and hypochloremia due to electrolyte and fluid loss replaced with sodium-free fluids; drastic dilution of extracellular body fluid following excessive water intake sometimes resulting from multiple enemas or perfusion of irrigating fluids into open venous sinuses during transurethral prostatic resections; emergency treatment of severe salt depletion due to excess sweating, vomiting, diarrhea, and other conditions.

➤*14.6% concentrate:* For use as an electrolyte replenisher in parenteral fluid therapy. It serves as an IV sodium supplement in hyponatremia or low salt syndrome, as an additive for total parenteral nutrition (TPN), and as an additive for carbohydrate-containing IV fluids.

Toxicity secondary to intestinal obstruction is usually accompanied by a marked reduction in serum chloride, and sodium chloride supplements can have a lifesaving effect. Symptoms of sodium chloride deficiency are very similar to those of Addison's disease, and large doses of sodium chloride will produce temporary alleviation of symptoms. Other disorders where sodium chloride is of clinical benefit include extensive burns, failure of gastric secretion, and postoperative intestinal paralysis.

➤*23.4% concentrate:* As an additive in parenteral fluid therapy for use in patients who have special problems of sodium electrolyte intake or excretion. It is intended to meet the specific requirement of the patient with unusual fluid and electrolyte needs. After available clinical and laboratory information is considered and correlated, determine the appropriate number of milliequivalents of concentrated sodium chloride injection and dilute for use.

Administration and Dosage

➤*General dosing considerations:* Dosage is to be directed by a physician and is dependent on age, weight, clinical condition of the patient, and laboratory determinations. Frequent laboratory determinations and clinical evaluation are essential to monitor changes in blood glucose and electrolyte concentrations, and fluid and electrolyte balance during prolonged parenteral therapy.

Fluid administration should be based on calculated maintenance or replacement fluid requirements for each patient.

➤*Adults:*

Additive in parenteral fluid therapy –

23.4% concentrate: The dosage is predicted on the specific requirement of the patient after necessary clinical and laboratory information is considered and correlated.

Diluting or dissolving drugs for IM, IV, or subcutaneous injection or for inhalation –

0.45% and 0.9% vial: Consult the manufacturer's instructions for choice of vehicle, appropriate dilution or volume for dissolving the drugs to be injected, including the route and rate of injection.

Electrolyte replenisher in parenteral fluid therapy –

14.6% concentrate: The actual dose administered depends upon specific patient requirements, which are usually determined by review of serial blood samples and clinical evaluation.

- *Maintenance dosage* – 33 to 40 mEq/L on the assumption the patient will receive 2 to 3 L of fluid/day.

Total parenteral nutrition: Patients should usually receive 120 mEq of sodium/day (range, 75 to 180 mEq/day).

Flushing of IV catheters and for tracheal lavage –

0.9% vial / syringe: Prior to and after administration of the medication, the IV catheter should be flushed in its entirety. Use in accordance with any warnings or precautions appropriate to the medication being administered.

Flushing the indwelling venipuncture device –

0.9% vial / syringe: Prior to and after administration of the medication, the IV injection device must be flushed in its entirety with 2 mL (one cartridge). Use in accordance with any warnings or precautions appropriate to the medication being administered.

SODIUM CHLORIDE — INJECTION

Parenteral replenishment of fluid and sodium chloride –

0.45% and 0.9% flexible plastic containers: The dose is dependent upon the age, weight, and clinical condition of the patient.

Sources of electrolytes and water for hydration –

3% and 5% concentrates:

• *Maximum dose* – 100 mL/hour or 400 mL/24 hours.

• *Dosage adjustment* – Before additional amounts are given, the serum electrolyte concentrations, including chloride and bicarbonate, should be determined to evaluate the need for more sodium chloride.

➤*Children:* For use in newborns, only preservative-free sodium chloride 0.9% injection should be used. (See Warnings/Precautions.)

Additive in parenteral fluid therapy –

14.6% concentrate: Preterm infants typically receive 3 to 4 mEq/kg/day.

Off-label dosing –

Maximum concentration: 154 mEq/L via peripheral line; 5% sodium chloride via a central line.

Sodium Chloride Injection Off-Label Dosing in Children

Indication	Concentration	Dosage
Hypotension/shock	0.9%	20 mL/kg infused rapidly. Up to 80 mL/kg may be required in the first hour. Continuously assess for fluid overload.
Moderate to severe dehydration	0.9%	20 mL/kg infused over 20 to 60 min. May be repeated in severe dehydration. Follow with fluid deficit replacement (% dehydration × weight [kg] over 24 hours).
Severe traumatic brain injury	1.5%	Infuse to obtain serum sodium concentration of 145 to 150 mEq/L.
	3%	0.1 to 1 mL/kg/h titrated to an intracranial pressure of less than 20 mm Hg.
Symptomatic hyponatremia	3%	*Initial dosage:* Infusion rate should increase sodium concentration by 1 mEq/L/h until symptoms resolve. Approximately 1 mL/kg of sodium chloride 3% will raise the serum sodium by 1 mEq/L. Severe symptoms (eg, seizures) may require more aggressive therapy. *Maintenance dosage:* Adjust infusion to increase serum sodium concentration by up to 10 to 12 mEq/L/day. Frequent monitoring of serum sodium concentrations is essential. Sodium deficit (mEq) = 0.6 × weight (kg) × (desired serum sodium [usually 135 mEq/L] − measured serum sodium).

➤*Preparation for administration:*

0.45% and 0.9% flexible plastic containers – Tear outer wrap at notch and remove solution container. If supplemental medication is desired, follow directions to add medication before preparing for administration. Some opacity of the plastic due to moisture absorption during the sterilization process may be observed. This is normal and does not affect the solution quality or safety. The opacity will diminish gradually.

1.) Close flow control clamp of administration set.
2.) Remove cover from outlet port at bottom of container.
3.) Insert piercing pin of administration set into port with a twisting motion until the set is firmly seated. See full directions on administration set carton.
4.) Suspend container from hanger.
5.) Squeeze and release drip chamber to establish proper fluid level in chamber.
6.) Open flow control clamp and clear air from set. Close clamp.
7.) Attach set to venipuncture device. If device is not indwelling, prime and make venipuncture.
8.) Regulate rate of administration with flow control clamp.

To add medication:

1.) Prepare additive port.
2.) Using aseptic technique and an additive delivery needle of appropriate length, puncture resealable additive port at target area, inner diaphragm and inject. Withdraw needle after injecting medication.
3.) The additive port may be protected by covering with an additive cap.
4.) Mix container contents thoroughly.

3% and 5% concentrates –

Directions for use of Excel container: Tear overwrap down at notch and remove solution container. Check for minute leaks by squeezing solution container firmly. If leaks are found, discard solution as sterility may be impaired. If supplemental medication is desired, follow directions to add medication before preparing for administration.

Remove plastic protector from sterile set port at bottom of container. Attach administration set. Refer to complete directions accompanying set.

• *To add medication before solution administration –*

1.) Prepare medication site.
2.) Using syringe with 18- to 22-gauge needle, puncture medication port and inner diaphragm and inject.
3.) Squeeze and tap ports while ports are upright and mix solution and medication thoroughly.

• *To add medication during solution administration –*

1.) Close clamp on the set.
2.) Prepare medication site.
3.) Using syringe with 18- to 22-gauge needle of appropriate length (at least ⅝ inch), puncture resealable medication port and inner diaphragm and inject.
4.) Remove container from IV pole or turn to an upright position.
5.) Evacuate both ports by tapping and squeezing them while container is in the upright position.
6.) Mix solution and medication thoroughly.
7.) Return container to in use position and continue administration.

14.6% concentrate –

Recommended directions for use of the pharmacy bulk package: Use aseptic technique:

1.) Perform all manipulations in an appropriate laminar flow hood.
2.) Aseptically remove aluminum overseal.
3.) Insert piercing pin of sterile transfer set and suspend unit in a laminar flow hood. Insertion of a piercing pin into the outlet port only once in a pharmacy bulk package solution. Once the outlet site has been entered, the withdrawal of container contents should be completed promptly in one continuous operation. Should this not be possible, a maximum time of 4 hours from transfer set pin or implement insertion is permitted to complete fluid transfer operations (ie, discard container no later than 4 hours after initial closure puncture).
4.) Sequentially dispense aliquots of 14.6% sodium chloride injection into IV containers using appropriate transfer set.

23.4% concentrate – The concentrate is strongly hypertonic and must be diluted prior to administration.

The appropriate volume is withdrawn for proper dilution. Having determined the milliequivalents of sodium chloride to be added, divide by 4 to calculate the number of mL of concentrated solution to be used. Withdraw this volume aseptically and transfer this additive solution into appropriate IV solutions such as dextrose 5% injection.

Directions for dispensing from 100 mL pharmacy bulk package — not for direct infusion: The 100 mL pharmacy bulk package is for use in a pharmacy admixture service only. Suspend the 100 mL pharmacy bulk package (inverted) by its IV hang label in a laminar flow hood or biological safety cabinet. Prior to entering a pharmacy bulk package, remove the flip-off seal and cleanse the rubber closure with a suitable antiseptic agent. Entry into the pharmacy bulk package must be made with a sterile transfer set or other sterile dispensing device and the contents dispensed in aliquots using aseptic technique. Use of a syringe needle is not recommended as it may cause leakage. Any unused portion must be discarded within 4 hours after initial entry. The date and the time initially opened should be recorded in the space provided on the pharmacy bulk package label.

➤*Administration:*

0.45% and 0.9% flexible plastic containers – Do not use flexible container in series connections.

3% and 5% concentrates – For IV administration using sterile equipment. It is recommended that IV administration apparatus be replaced at least once every 24 hours.

Do not use plastic containers in series connection.

If administration is controlled by a pumping device, care must be taken to discontinue pumping action before the container runs dry or air embolism may result.

When a hypertonic solution is to be administered peripherally, it should be slowly infused through a small bore needle, placed well within the lumen of a large vein to minimize venous irritation. Carefully avoid infiltration.

14.6% concentrate – Administer IV, but only after dilution in a larger volume of fluid.

23.4% concentrate – The properly diluted solutions may be given IV or subcutaneously.

➤*Admixture compatibility:* Before sodium chloride injection is used as a vehicle for the administration of a drug, specific references should be checked for any possible incompatibility.

➤*Storage/Stability:* Avoid excessive heat. Protect from freezing. Store at 15° to 30°C (59° to 86°F).

3% and 5% concentrates – Store at room temperature, 25°C (77°F); brief exposure up to 40°C (104°F) does not adversely affect the product.

Actions

➤*Pharmacology:* Solutions which provide combinations of hypotonic or isotonic concentrations of sodium chloride are suitable for parenteral maintenance or replacement of water and electrolyte requirements.

Sodium, the major cation of the extracellular fluid, functions primarily in the control of water distribution, fluid balance, and osmotic pressure of body fluids. Sodium is also associated with chloride and bicarbonate in the regulation of the acid-base equilibrium of body fluid.

SODIUM CHLORIDE — INJECTION

Chloride, the major extracellular anion, closely follows the metabolism of sodium, and changes in the acid-base balance of the body are reflected by changes in the chloride concentration.

Water balance is maintained by various regulatory mechanisms. Water distribution depends primarily on the concentration of electrolytes in the body compartments and sodium (Na^+) plays a major role in maintaining physiologic equilibrium. Sodium chloride is an electrolyte replenisher. Sodium is the principal cation of extracellular fluid. With a normal plasma concentration of 142 mEq/L, sodium comprises more than 90% of the total plasma cations. While sodium can diffuse across membranes, the intracellular sodium concentration is maintained at a much lower level than extracellular concentrations, the so-called "sodium pump." Compensation for loss of intracellular potassium occurs through an increase in intracellular sodium. Sodium is the principal ion that determines osmotic pressure of interstitial fluids and the degree of tissue hydration.

Adult serum chloride values typically range from 100 to 106 mEq/L. Serum chloride levels decrease in metabolic alkalosis, as serum bicarbonate levels generally increase. In parenteral nutrition when acidosis occurs, it is common practice to reduce chloride intake by substituting acetate salts in place of chloride salts.

Contraindications

Hypernatremic and fluid retention syndromes. Elevated, normal, or only slightly decreased plasma electrolyte concentrations, or when additives of sodium and chloride could be clinically detrimental.

Warnings/Precautions

➤*Fluid/solute overload:* The risk of dilutional states is inversely proportional to the electrolyte concentrations of administered parenteral solutions. The risk of solute overload causing congested states with peripheral and pulmonary edema is directly proportional to the electrolyte concentrations of such solutions.

Excessive amounts of sodium chloride by any route may cause hypokalemia and acidosis. Excessive amounts by the parenteral route may precipitate congestive heart failure and acute pulmonary edema, especially in patients with cardiovascular disease and in patients receiving corticosteroids or corticotropin or drugs that may give rise to sodium retention.

Excessive infusion of hypertonic sodium chloride solutions may supply more sodium and chloride than normally found in serum and can exceed normal tolerance, resulting in hypernatremia. Infusion of excess chloride ions may cause a loss of bicarbonate, resulting in an acidifying effect.

➤*Sodium retention:* Solutions containing sodium ions should be used with great care, if at all, in patients with congestive heart failure, severe renal insufficiency, and in clinical states in which there exists edema with sodium retention.

➤*Hypokalemia:* Excessive administration of potassium-free solutions may result in significant hypokalemia.

➤*Surgical patients:* Surgical patients should seldom receive salt-containing solutions immediately following surgery unless factors producing salt depletion are present. Because renal retention of salt occurs during surgery, additional electrolytes given intravenously may result in fluid retention, edema and circulatory overload.

➤*3% and 5% concentrates:* These are very concentrated hypertonic sodium chloride solutions. Infuse very slowly with constant observation of the patient to avoid pulmonary edema.

➤*14.6% and 23.4% concentrates:* Sodium chloride injection is hypertonic and must be diluted prior to administration. Inadvertent direct injection or absorption of concentrated sodium chloride solution may give rise to sudden hypernatremia and such complications as cardiovascular shock, central nervous system disorders, extensive hemolysis and cortical necrosis of the kidneys and severe local tissue necrosis (if administered extravascularly).

➤*Aluminum toxicity (23.4% concentrate):* This product contains aluminum that may be toxic. Aluminum may reach toxic levels with prolonged parenteral administration if kidney function is impaired. Premature neonates are particularly at risk because their kidneys are immature, and they require large amounts of calcium and phosphate solutions, which contain aluminum.

Research indicates that patients with impaired kidney function, including premature neonates, who receive parenteral levels of aluminum at greater than 4 to 5 mcg/kg/day accumulate aluminum at levels associated with central nervous system and bone toxicity. Tissue loading may occur at even lower rates of administration.

➤*Electrolyte losses:* Extraordinary electrolyte losses may occur during protracted nasogastric suction, vomiting, diarrhea, or gastrointestinal fistula drainage and may necessitate additional electrolyte supplementation.

Additional essential electrolytes, minerals, and vitamins should be supplied as needed.

➤*0.9%:*

Children – For use in newborns, when a sodium chloride solution is required for preparation or diluting medications or in flushing intravenous catheters, only preservative free sodium chloride injection, 0.9% should be used.

➤*Renal function impairment:* In patients with diminished renal function, administration of solutions containing sodium may result in sodium retention. The intravenous administration of this solution (after appropriate dilution) can cause fluid or solute overloading resulting in dilution of other serum electrolyte concentrations, overhydration, congested states or pulmonary edema.

➤*Special risk:*

3% and 5% concentrates – These solutions should be used with care in patients with hypervolemia, renal insufficiency, urinary tract obstruction, or impending or frank cardiac decompensation.

Care should be exercised in administering solutions containing sodium to patients with renal or cardiovascular insufficiency, with or without congestive heart failure, particularly if they are postoperative or elderly. Special caution should be used in administering sodium-containing solutions to patients with severe renal impairment, cirrhosis of the liver or other edematous or sodium-retaining states.

➤*Pregnancy:* Category C. Animal reproduction studies have not been conducted with sodium chloride injection. It is also not known whether sodium chloride can cause fetal harm when administered to a pregnant woman or can affect reproduction capacity. Sodium chloride should be given to a pregnant woman only if clearly needed.

➤*Lactation:* It is not known whether sodium chloride injection is excreted in human milk. Because many drugs are excreted in human milk, caution should be exercised when sodium chloride is administered to a nursing woman.

➤*Children:* Safety and efficacy of sodium chloride injection have not been established in pediatric patients. Its limited use in pediatric patients has been inadequate to fully define proper dosage and limitations for use.

0.45% and 0.9% flexible plastic containers – The safety and efficacy in the pediatric population are based on the similarity of the clinical conditions of the pediatric and adult populations. In neonates or very small infants, the volume of fluid may affect fluid and electrolyte balance.

➤*Monitoring:* Clinical evaluation and periodic laboratory determinations are necessary to monitor changes in fluid balance, electrolyte concentrations and acid-base balance during prolonged parenteral therapy or whenever the condition of the patient warrants such evaluation.

Drug Interactions

➤*Corticosteroids and corticotropin:* Caution must be exercised in the administration of parenteral fluids, especially those containing sodium ions to patients receiving corticosteroids or corticotropin.

Adverse Reactions

➤*Reactions due to solution or technique of administration:* Reactions which may occur because of the solution or the technique of administration include febrile response, infection at the site of injection, venous thrombosis or phlebitis extending from the site of injection, extravasation and hypervolemia.

➤*Too rapid infusion:* Too rapid infusion of hypertonic solutions may cause local pain and venous irritation. Rate of administration should be adjusted according to tolerance. Use the largest peripheral vein and a well-placed small bore needle is recommended.

Ion excess/deficit – Symptoms may result from an excess or deficit of 1 or more of the ions present in the solution; therefore, frequent monitoring of electrolyte levels is essential.

If infused in large amounts, chloride ions may cause a loss of bicarbonate ions, resulting in an acidifying effect.

Hypernatremia – Hypernatremia may be associated with edema and exacerbation of congestive heart failure due to the retention of water, resulting in an expanded extracellular fluid volume.

➤*14.6% concentrate:* Sodium overload can occur with intravenous infusion of excessive amounts of sodium-containing solutions.

Under rapid infusion – Overzealous administration can result in edema and symptoms resembling congestive heart failure.

Postoperative salt intolerance – Signs of postoperative salt intolerance include cellular dehydration, weakness, disorientation, anorexia, nausea, distention, deep respiration, oliguria, and increased BUN. If an adverse reaction does occur, discontinue the infusion, evaluate the patient, institute appropriate therapeutic countermeasures, and save the remainder of the fluid for examination if deemed necessary.

Overdosage

➤*Symptoms:* Excessive administration of sodium chloride injection may result in electrolyte imbalance with water retention, edema, loss of potassium, and aggravation of an existing acidosis.

Excessive sodium chloride intake is accompanied by excretion of crystalloids, in an attempt to maintain normal osmotic pressure. Increased excretion of potassium and bicarbonate can result in acidosis. There is also a rapid elimination of any foreign salt, such as iodide and bromide, being used therapeutically.

When used as a diluent, solvent or intravascular flushing solution, this parenteral preparation is unlikely to pose a threat of sodium chloride or fluid overload except possibly in very small infants.

➤*Treatment:* In the event of a fluid or solute overload during parenteral therapy, reevaluate the patient's condition and institute appropriate corrective treatment.

POTASSIUM SALTS

For information on oral potassium, refer to Mineral and Electrolytes, Oral section. For information on potassium phosphate, refer to specific monograph in this section. For additional information, refer to the Dietary Reference Intakes of Vitamins and Minerals table.

Indications

➤*Hypokalemia:* Prevention and treatment of moderate or severe potassium deficit when oral replacement therapy is not feasible.

➤*Potassium acetate:* Potassium acetate is useful as an additive for preparing specific IV fluid formulas when patient needs cannot be met by standard electrolyte or nutrient solutions.

Also indicated for marked loss of GI secretions by vomiting, diarrhea, GI intubation or fistulas; prolonged diuresis; prolonged parenteral use of potassium-free fluids (eg, normal saline, dextrose solutions); diabetic acidosis, especially during vigorous insulin and dextrose treatment; metabolic alkalosis; attacks of hereditary or familial periodic paralysis; hyperadrenocorticism; primary aldosteronism; overmedication with adrenocortical steroids, testosterone or corticotropin; healing phase of scalds or burns; cardiac arrhythmias, especially due to digitalis glycosides.

Administration and Dosage

mEq/g of Various Potassium Salts

Potassium salt	mEq/g
Potassium acetate	10.2
Potassium chloride	13.4
Dibasic potassium phosphate[a]	11.5
Monobasic potassium phosphate[a]	7.3

[a] Commercial preparations of potassium phosphate injection contain a mixture of both mono- and dibasic salts (see Potassium Phosphate monograph).

➤*Do not administer undiluted potassium:* Potassium preparations must be diluted with suitable large volume parenteral solutions, mixed well and given by slow IV infusion.

Too rapid infusion of hypertonic solutions may cause local pain and, rarely, vein irritation. Adjust rate of administration according to tolerance. Use of the largest peripheral vein and a small bore needle is recommended.

The usual additive dilution of potassium chloride is 40 mEq/L of IV fluid. The maximum desirable concentration is 80 mEq/L, although extreme emergencies may dictate greater concentrations.

In critical states, potassium chloride may be administered in saline (unless saline is contraindicated) since dextrose may lower serum potassium levels by producing an intracellular shift.

Avoid "layering" of potassium by proper agitation of the prepared IV solution. Do not add potassium to an IV bottle in the hanging position.

Individualize dosage. Guide dosage and rate of infusion by ECG and serum electrolyte determinations. The following may be used as a guide:

Potassium Dosage/Rate of Infusion Guidelines

Serum K+	Maximum infusion rate	Maximum concentration	Maximum 24 hour dose
> 2.5 mEq/L	10 mEq/hr	40 mEq/L	200 mEq
< 2 mEq/L	40 mEq/hr	80 mEq/L	400 mEq

Add electrolytes to the mixed solutions only after considering electrolytes already present and potential incompatibilities such as calcium and phosphate or sulfate.

➤*Children:* IV infusion up to 3 mEq/kg or 40 mEq/m^2/day. Adjust volume of administered fluids to body size.

Actions

➤*Pharmacology:* The principal intracellular cation, potassium is essential for maintenance of intracellular tonicity; transmission of nerve impulses; contraction of cardiac, skeletal and smooth muscle; and maintenance of normal renal function. Potassium participates in carbohydrate utilization and protein synthesis and is critical in regulating nerve conduction and muscle contraction, particularly in the heart.

Hypokalemia – Gradual potassium depletion occurs via renal excretion, through GI loss or because of inadequate intake (excretion greater than intake). Depletion usually results from diuretic therapy, primary or secondary hyperaldosteronism, diabetic ketoacidosis, severe diarrhea (especially if associated with vomiting) or inadequate replacement during prolonged parenteral nutrition.

Potassium depletion sufficient to cause 1 mEq/L drop in serum potassium requires a loss of about 100 to 200 mEq of potassium from the total body store.

Symptoms: Weakness; fatigue; ileus; polydipsia; flaccid paralysis or impaired ability to concentrate urine (in advanced cases).

ECG may reveal premature atrial and ventricular contractions, prolongation of QT interval, ST segment depression, broad and flat T waves or appearance of U waves. Severe cases may lead to muscular weakness, paralysis, respiratory failure.

➤*Pharmacokinetics:* Normally about 80% to 90% of potassium intake is excreted in urine with the remainder voided in stool and, to a small extent, in perspiration. Kidneys do not conserve potassium well; during fasting or in patients on a potassium-free diet, potassium loss from the body continues, resulting in potassium depletion. A deficiency of either potassium or chloride will lead to a deficit of the other.

Contraindications

Diseases where high potassium levels may be encountered; hyperkalemia; renal failure and conditions in which potassium retention is present; oliguria or azotemia; anuria; crush syndrome; severe hemolytic reactions; adrenocortical insufficiency (untreated Addison's disease); adynamica episodica hereditaria; acute dehydration; heat cramps; hyperkalemia from any cause; early postoperative oliguria except during GI drainage.

Warnings/Precautions

➤*Potassium intoxication:* Do not infuse rapidly. High plasma concentrations of potassium may cause death through cardiac depression, arrhythmias or arrest. Monitor potassium replacement therapy whenever possible by continuous or serial ECG. In addition to ECG effects, local pain and phlebitis may result when a greater than 40 mEq/L concentration is infused.

Renal impairment or adrenal insufficiency – Renal impairments or adrenal insufficiency may cause potassium intoxication. Potassium salts can produce hyperkalemia and cardiac arrest. Potentially fatal hyperkalemia can develop rapidly and be asymptomatic. Use with great caution, if at all.

➤*Concentrated potassium:* Concentrated potassium solutions are for IV admixtures only; do not use undiluted. Direct injection may be instantaneously fatal.

➤*Metabolic alkalosis:* Potassium depletion is usually accompanied by an obligatory loss of chloride resulting in hypochloremic metabolic alkalosis. Treat the underlying cause of potassium depletion and administer IV potassium chloride.

Use solutions containing acetate ion carefully in metabolic or respiratory alkalosis, and when there is an increased level or impairment of utilization of this ion.

➤*Metabolic acidosis:* Treat associated hypokalemia with an alkalinizing potassium salt (eg, bicarbonate, citrate, gluconate, acetate).

➤*Musculoskeletal / Cardiac effects:* When serum sodium or calcium concentration is reduced, moderate elevation of serum potassium may cause toxic effects on the heart and skeletal muscle. Weakness and later paralysis of voluntary muscles, with consequent respiratory distress and dysphagia, are generally late signs, sometimes significantly preceding dangerous or fatal cardiac toxicity.

➤*Fluid / Solute overload:* IV administration can cause fluid or solute overloading resulting in dilution of serum electrolyte concentrations, overhydration, congested states or pulmonary edema.

The risk of dilutional states is inversely proportional to the electrolyte concentration of administered parenteral solutions. The risk of solute overload causing congested states with peripheral and pulmonary edema is directly proportional to the electrolyte concentrations of such solutions.

➤*Renal function impairment:* Normal kidney function permits safe potassium therapy. Although temporary elevation of serum potassium level due to renal insufficiency secondary to dehydration or shock may mask an intracellular potassium deficit, do not replenish potassium until renal function is reestablished by overcoming dehydration and shock. Discontinue potassium-containing solutions if signs of renal insufficiency develop during infusions.

➤*Special risk:* Use with caution in the presence of cardiac disease, particularly in digitalized patients or in the presence of renal disease, metabolic acidosis, Addison's disease, acute dehydration, prolonged or severe diarrhea, familial periodic paralysis, hypoadrenalism, hyperkalemia, hyponatremia and myotonia congenita.

➤*Pregnancy: Category C.* It is not known whether potassium salts can cause fetal harm when administered to a pregnant woman or can affect reproduction capacity. Give to a pregnant woman only if clearly needed.

➤*Lactation:* Exercise caution when administering to a nursing woman.

➤*Monitoring:* Close medical supervision with frequent ECGs and serum potassium determinations. Plasma levels are not necessarily indicative of tissue levels.

Drug Interactions

Potassium Preparation Drug Interactions

Precipitant drug	Object drug[a]		Description
ACE inhibitors	Potassium preparations	⬆	Concurrent use may result in elevated serum potassium concentrations in certain patients.
Potassium-sparing diuretics/ potassium-containing salt substitutes	Potassium preparations	⬆	Potassium-sparing diuretics and potassium-containing salt substitutes will increase potassium retention and can produce severe hyperkalemia.
Potassium preparations	Digitalis	⬆	In patients on digoxin, hypokalemia may result in digoxin toxicity. Use caution if discontinuing a potassium preparation in patients maintained on digoxin.

[a] ⬆ = Object drug increased.

POTASSIUM SALTS

Adverse Reactions

Hyperkalemia – Adverse reactions involve the possibility of potassium intoxication. Signs and symptoms include: Paresthesias of extremities; flaccid paralysis; muscle or respiratory paralysis; areflexia; weakness; listlessness; mental confusion; weakness and heaviness of legs; hypotension; cardiac arrhythmias; heart block; ECG abnormalities such as disappearance of P waves, spreading and slurring of the QRS complex with development of a biphasic curve and cardiac arrest. See Overdosage.

➤*GI:* Nausea; vomiting; abdominal pain; diarrhea.

Reactions due to solution or technique of administration – Febrile response; infection at injection site; venous thrombosis; phlebitis extending from injection site; extravasation; hypervolemia; hyperkalemia; venospasm.

Overdosage

If excretory mechanisms are impaired or if potassium is administered too rapidly IV, potentially fatal hyperkalemia can result (see Contraindications and Warnings). It is important to consider the entire clinical picture and not rely solely on potassium levels since only extracellular potassium can be measured, yet intracellular potassium accounts for 98% of the total body amount.

➤*Symptoms:* Mild (greater than 5.5 to 6.5 mEq/L) to moderate (greater than 6.5 to 8 mEq/L) hyperkalemia may be asymptomatic and manifested only by increased serum potassium concentration and characteristic ECG changes. Other symptoms include muscular weakness, progressing to flaccid quadriplegia and respiratory paralysis; however, these generally do not develop unless potassium concentrations exceed 8 mEq/L. Dangerous cardiac arrhythmias often occur before onset of complete paralysis. Note that hyperkalemia produces symptoms paradoxically similar to those of hypokalemia.

ECG – Progressive increase in height and peaking of T waves; lowering of the R wave; decreased amplitude and ultimate disappearance of P waves; prolongation of PR interval and QRS complex; shortening of the QT interval; and finally, ventricular fibrillation and death.

➤*Treatment:* Terminate potassium administration. Monitor ECG. Infusion of combined dextrose and insulin in a ratio of 3 g dextrose to 1 unit regular insulin may be administered to shift potassium into cells. Administer sodium bicarbonate 50 to 100 mEq IV to reverse acidosis and also produce an intracellular shift. Give 10 to 100 mL calcium gluconate or calcium chloride 10% to reverse ECG changes. To remove potassium from the body use sodium polystyrene sulfonate resin or hemodialysis or peritoneal dialysis.

In digitalized patients, too rapid lowering of serum potassium can cause digitalis toxicity (see Drug Interactions).

POTASSIUM CHLORIDE

Rx	**Potassium Chloride** (Various, eg, APP, Hospira)	**Injection, solution, concentrate:** 2 mEq/mL	Equiv. to 149 mg/mL of potassium chloride. In 250 and 500 mL pharmacy bulk packages.
Rx	**Potassium Chloride** (Various, eg, APP, B. Braun, Hospira)	**Injection, solution, concentrate:** 10 mEq	Equiv. to 149 mg/mL of potassium chloride. In 5 and 10 mL single-dose vials and 50 and 100 mL flexible plastic containers.
Rx	**Potassium Chloride** (Various, eg, APP, Hospira)	**Injection, solution, concentrate:** 20 mEq	Equiv. to 149 mg/mL of potassium chloride. In 10 mL single-dose vials and 50 and 100 mL flexible plastic containers.
Rx	**Potassium Chloride** (Various, eg, APP, Hospira)	**Injection, solution, concentrate:** 30 mEq	Equiv. to 149 mg/mL of potassium chloride. In 15 mL single-dose vials and 100 mL flexible plastic containers.
Rx	**Potassium Chloride** (Various, eg, APP, Hospira, McGuff)	**Injection, solution, concentrate:** 40 mEq	Equiv. to 149 mg/mL of potassium chloride. In 20 and 30 mL single-dose vials and 100 mL flexible plastic containers.
Rx	**Potassium Chloride** (Various, eg, APP, McGuff)	**Injection, solution, concentrate:** 60 mEq	Equiv. to 149 mg/mL of potassium chloride. Parabens. In 30 mL multiple-use vials.

POTASSIUM CHLORIDE — INJECTION

For additional information, refer to the Dietary Reference Intakes of Vitamins and Minerals table.

Indications

➤*Hypokalemia:* Treatment of potassium deficiency states when oral replacement is not feasible.

Administration and Dosage

➤*General dosing considerations:* Continuous cardiac monitoring and frequent serum potassium determinations are essential to avoid hyperkalemia and cardiac arrest.

➤*Adults:*

Hypokalemia –

Serum potassium level greater than 2.5 mEq/L: Give at a rate not to exceed 10 mEq/h and in a concentration of up to 40 mEq/L. The 24-hour total dose should not exceed 200 mEq.

Serum potassium level less than 2 mEq/L and electrocardiographic changes or muscle paralysis: Infuse very cautiously at a rate of up to 40 mEq/h. As much as 400 mEq may be administered in a 24-hour period.

➤*Children:*

Off-label dosing –

Hypokalemia: 0.5 to 1 mEq/kg/h for 1 to 2 hours.

➤*Renal function impairment:* Contraindicated in patients with renal failure. Administration of potassium may cause potassium intoxication and life-threatening hyperkalemia.

➤*Preparation for administration:* In critical conditions, potassium may be administered in saline (unless contraindicated) rather than in dextrose-containing fluids because dextrose may lower serum potassium levels.

Potassium chloride concentrate must be diluted before administration. Care must be taken to ensure there is complete mixing of the potassium with the large volume fluid, particularly if soft or bag-type containers are used.

➤*Administration:* Administer intravenously (IV) only with a calibrated infusion device at a slow, controlled rate. Because pain associated with peripheral infusion of potassium chloride has been reported, whenever possible, administration via a central route is recommended for dilution by the blood stream and avoidance of extravasation. Highest concentrations (300 and 400 mEq/L) should be exclusively administered via a central route. Use of a final filter is recommended during administration when possible. Do not use flexible containers in series connection.

➤*Extravasation:* Extravasation may occur during administration of potassium chloride. If signs or symptoms of extravasation occur, stop the infusion immediately. If possible, withdraw 3 to 5 mL of blood to remove some of the drug. Remove the infusion needle. Delineate the infiltrated area on the patient's skin with a felt-tip marker. Hyaluronidase is an effective antidote for hyperosmolar drug infiltrations; administer promptly within the first few minutes to 1 hour after extravasation. Higher doses (150 units) have primarily been used in adults while lower doses (15 units) have been used in children. Administer hyaluronidase according to the following steps. Dilute hyaluronidase to desired concentration, depending on the dose and product used. (Note: Some products do not require dilution.) For example, if the total dose is 15 units, make 15 units/mL dilution. If the total dose is 150 units, make 150 units/mL dilution. Cleanse area with povidone-iodine. Inject hyaluronidase locally, subcutaneously or intradermally, using a 25-gauge needle or smaller. The dose is given as five 0.2 mL injections at the leading edge of the extravasation site. Change needle after each injection. Elevate for 48 hours above heart level using a sling or stockinette dressing with an observation window cut in the dressing. Avoid pressure or friction. Do not rub area. Observe for signs of increased erythema, pain, or skin necrosis. If increased symptoms occur, consult a plastic surgeon. Ensure that no medication is given distally to extravasation site. After 48 hours, encourage the patient to use the extremity normally to promote full range of motion.

➤*Admixture compatibility:* Do not add supplementary medication. Such use could result in air embolism due to residual air being drawn from the primary container before administration of the fluid from the secondary container is completed.

➤*Storage/Stability:* Store at 20° to 25°C (68° to 77°F). Protect from freezing. Avoid excessive heat. Discard unused portion of pharmacy bulk containers after 4 hours.

POTASSIUM ACETATE

Rx	**Potassium Acetate** (Various, eg, Abbott, American Regent, IMS)	**Injection:** 2 mEq/mL	In 20, 50 and 100 mL vials.
Rx	**Potassium Acetate** (Various)	**Injection:** 4 mEq/mL	In 50 mL vials.

POTASSIUM ACETATE — INJECTION

For additional information, refer to the Dietary Reference Intakes of Vitamins and Minerals table.

Indications

➤*Hypokalemia:* Treatment of potassium deficiency states when oral replacement therapy is not feasible.

➤*General information:* The solution is intended as an alternative to potassium chloride to provide potassium (K^+) for addition to large volume infusion fluids for intravenous (IV) use.

Administration and Dosage

➤*General dosing considerations:* Potassium acetate injections are concentrated solutions and must be diluted prior to administration. (See Preparation for Administration.)

The dose and rate of administration are dependent upon the individual condition of each patient. Electrocardiograph (ECG) and serum potassium should be monitored as a guide to dosage.

➤*Adults:*

Hypokalemia – The dose and rate of administration are dependent upon the individual condition of each patient. The normal daily potassium requirement for adults is 40 to 80 mEq per 24 hr.

➤*Children:*

Hypokalemia – The dose and rate of administration are dependent upon the individual condition of each patient. The normal daily potassium requirement for children is 2 to 3 mEq/kg/hr. The normal daily potassium requirement for newborns is 2 to 6 mEq/kg/hr.

➤*Preparation for administration:* Potassium acetate injection must be diluted before administration.

Withdraw the calculated volume aseptically and transfer to appropriate IV fluids to provide the desired number of milliequivalents of potassium (K^+) with an equal number of milliequivalents of acetate (CH_3COO^-).

➤*Administration:* Administer slowly IV. The infusion rate should not exceed 1 mEq/kg/hr to avoid potassium intoxication.

➤*Storage/Stability:* Store between 15° to 30°C (59° to 86°F).

SODIUM BICARBONATE

Rx	**Sodium Bicarbonate** (Hospira)	**Injection:** 4.2% (0.5 mEq/mL)	In 10 mL (5 mEq) syringes.
Rx	**Sodium Bicarbonate** (American Pharmaceutical Partners)		In 10 mL (5 mEq) *Bristoject* syringes.
Rx	**Sodium Bicarbonate** (Hospira)	**Injection:** 5% (0.6 mEq/mL)	In 500 mL[a] (297.5 mEq).
Rx	**Sodium Bicarbonate** (Baxter)		In 500 mL (297.5 mEq).
Rx	**Sodium Bicarbonate** (McGaw)		In 500 mL[a] (297.5 mEq).
Rx	**Sodium Bicarbonate** (Hospira)	**Injection:** 7.5% (0.9 mEq/mL)	In 50 mL (44.6 mEq) amps and 50 mL (44.6 mEq) syringes.
Rx	**Sodium Bicarbonate** (American Regent)		In 50 mL (44.6 mEq) vials.
Rx	**Sodium Bicarbonate** (American Pharmaceutical Partners)		In 50 mL (44.6 mEq) single-dose vials, 50 mL (44.6 mEq) *Bristoject* syringes and 200 mL (179 mEq) *MaxiVials.*
Rx	**Sodium Bicarbonate** (Hospira)	**Injection:** 8.4% (1 mEq/mL)	In 50 mL (50 mEq) fliptop vials and 10 mL (10 mEq) and 50 mL (50 mEq) syringes.
Rx	**Sodium Bicarbonate** (American Regent)		In 50 mL (50 mEq) vials.
Rx	**Sodium Bicarbonate** (American Pharmaceutical Partners)		In 50 mL (50 mEq) vials and 10 and 50 mEq *Bristoject* syringes.
Rx	**Neut** (Abbott)	**Neutralizing Additive Solution**[2]: 4% (0.48 mEq/mL)	In 5 mL (2.4 mEq) fliptop and pintop vials.[a]
Rx	**Sodium Bicarbonate** (American Pharmaceutical Partners)	**Neutralizing Additive Solution**[b]: 4.2% (0.5 mEq/mL)	In 5 mL fill in 6 mL vials (2.5 mEq).

[a] With EDTA.

[b] For use as a neutralizing additive solution to acidic large volume parenterals.

SODIUM BICARBONATE — INJECTION

For information on oral sodium bicarbonate, refer to Systemic Alkalinizers. For additional information, refer to the Dietary Reference Intakes of Vitamins and Minerals table.

Indications

➤*Metabolic acidosis:* In severe renal disease, uncontrolled diabetes, circulatory insufficiency due to shock, anoxia or severe dehydration, extracorporeal circulation of blood, cardiac arrest and severe primary lactic acidosis where a rapid increase in plasma total CO_2 content is crucial. Treat metabolic acidosis in addition to measures designed to control the cause of the acidosis (eg, insulin in uncomplicated diabetes, blood volume restoration in shock). Since an appreciable time interval may elapse before all ancillary effects occur, bicarbonate therapy is indicated to minimize risks inherent to acidosis itself.

At one time it was suggested to administer bicarbonate during cardiopulmonary resuscitation following cardiac arrest; however, recent evidence suggests that little benefit is provided and its use may be detrimental. For treatment of acidosis in this clinical situation, concentrate efforts on restoring ventilation and blood flow. According to the American Heart Association guidelines, use as a last resort after other standard measures have been utilized.

➤*Urinary alkalinization:* In the treatment of certain drug intoxications (eg, salicylates, lithium) and in hemolytic reactions requiring alkalinization of urine to diminish nephrotoxicity of blood pigments.

➤*Severe diarrhea:* Severe diarrhea, which is often accompanied by a significant loss of bicarbonate.

➤*Neutralizing additive solution:* To reduce the incidence of chemical phlebitis and patient discomfort due to vein irritation at or near the infusion siteby raising the pH of intravenous (IV) acid solutions.

➤*Off-label uses:*

Prevention of contrast media nephrotoxicity – [2] = Fair documentation. The use of sodium bicarbonate hydration appears to be beneficial as a preventive agent for radiocontrast-induced nephrotoxicity. Initial data suggest that this agent may be particularly useful for populations known to be at increased risk for contrast nephrotoxicity (eg, those with diabetes mellitus, reduced renal function). This limited study was single center and terminated early. However, it should be recognized that the adverse reaction profile of this drug is minimal when used short term. (See Administration and Dosage.)

Administration and Dosage

➤*General dosing considerations:* Exercise particular care when administering sodium-containing solutions to elderly or postoperative patients with renal or cardiovascular insufficiency, with or without CHF.

➤*Adults:*

Cardiac arrest – Bicarbonate administration in this situation may be detrimental. (See Indications.) Administer according to results of arterial blood pH and $PaCO_2$ and calculation of base deficit. Flush IV lines before and after use.

Usual dosage: A rapid IV dose of 200 to 300 mEq of bicarbonate, given as a 7.5% or 8.4% solution. Observe caution where rapid infusion of large quantities of bicarbonate is indicated. Bicarbonate solutions are hypertonic and may produce an undesirable rise in plasma sodium concentration. In cardiac arrest, however, the risks from acidosis exceed those of hypernatremia.

In emergencies, administer 300 to 500 mL of 5% sodium bicarbonate injection as rapidly as possible without overalkalinizing the patient. To avoid overalkalinizing a patient whose own body mechanisms for correcting metabolic acidosis may be maximally stimulated, only one-third to one-half of the calculated dose is administered as rapidly as indicated by the patient's cardiovascular and fluid balance status. Then, redetermine serum pH and bicarbonate concentration.

Metabolic acidosis (less urgent forms) – It is unwise to attempt full correction of a low total CO_2 content during the first 24 hours, since this may accompany an unrecognized alkalosis due to delayed readjustment of ventilation to normal. Thus, achieving total CO_2 content of about 20 mEq/L

SODIUM BICARBONATE — INJECTION

at the end of the first day will usually be associated with a normal blood pH. Further modification of the acidosis to completely normal values usually occurs in the presence of normal kidney function when and if the cause of the acidosis can be controlled. Total CO_2 brought to normal or above normal within the first day may be associated with grossly alkaline blood pH.

Usual dosage: Sodium bicarbonate injection may be added to other IV fluids. The amount of bicarbonate to be given over a 4- to 8-hour period is approximately 2 to 5 mEq/kg, depending on the severity of the acidosis as judged by the lowering of total CO_2 content, blood pH, and clinical condition. Initially, an infusion of 2 to 5 mEq/kg over 4 to 8 hours will produce improvement in the acid-base status of the blood.

Alternative dosage: Alternatively, estimates of the initial dose of sodium bicarbonate may be based on the following equation:

0.5 (L/kg) × body weight (kg) × desired increase in serum HCO_3(mEq/L) = bicarbonate dose (mEq) or 0.5 (L/kg) × body weight (kg) × base deficit (mEq/L) = bicarbonate dose (mEq).

The next step of therapy is dependent on the clinical response of the patient. If severe symptoms have abated, reduce frequency of administration and dose.

If the CO_2 plasma content is unknown, a safe average dose of sodium bicarbonate is 5 mEq (420 mg)/kg.

Metabolic acidosis (severe forms) – Administer 90 to 180 mEq/L (≈ 7.5 to 15 g) at a rate of 1 to 1.5 L during the first hour. Adjust to patient's needs for further management.

Neutralizing additive solution – One vial of neutralizing additive solution added to 1 L of any of the commonly used parenteral solutions, including dextrose, sodium chloride, Ringer's, etc, will increase the pH to a more physiologic range (specific pH may vary slightly).

Note: Some products such as amino acid solutions and multiple electrolyte solutions containing dextrose will not be brought to near physiologic pH by the addition of sodium bicarbonate neutralizing additive solution. This is due to the relatively high buffer capacity of these fluids.

Off-label dosing –

Prevention of contrast media nephrotoxicity: [2] = Fair documentation. Sodium bicarbonate (154 mEq/L) was administered at 3 mL/kg/h for 1 hour before contrast administration, followed by an infusion of 1 mL/kg/h for 6 hours after the procedure.

➤*Children:*

Cardiac arrest –

Younger than 2 years of age: 4.2% solution for IV administration at a rate not to exceed 8 mEq/kg/day to guard against the possibility of producing hypernatremia, decreasing CSF pressure and inducing intracranial hemorrhage.

- *Maximum dose* – 8 mEq/kg/day.
- *Initial dosage* – 1 to 2 mEq/kg/min given over 1 to 2 minutes followed by 1 mEq/kg every 10 minutes of arrest. If base deficit is known, give calculated dose of 0.3 × kg × base deficit. If only 7.5% or 8.4% sodium bicarbonate is available, dilute 1:1 with 5% dextrose in water before administration.

Metabolic acidosis (less urgent forms) –

Older children: See Adults for dosing.

➤*Preparation for administration:*

IV administration – For IV administration, suitable concentrations range from 1.5% (isotonic) to 8.4% (undiluted), depending on the clinical condition and requirements of the patient. Suitable dilution can be calculated from the following formula:

$$conc_1 \times volume_1 = conc_2 \times volume_2$$

Thus, 8.4% × 50 mL = 1.5% × 280 mL; or 7.5% × 50 mL = 1.5% × 250 mL; or 4.2% × 10 mL = 1.5% × 28 mL.

The diluent may be sterile water for injection, sodium chloride injection, 5% dextrose or other standard electrolyte solutions.

Subcutaneous administration – For subcutaneous administration, an isotonic solution (1.5%) of sodium bicarbonate can be prepared by diluting 1 mL (84 mg) of 8.4% solution with 4.6 mL sterile water for injection. For 7.5% solution, dilute 1 mL (75 mg) with 4 mL sterile water for injection. For 4.2% solution, dilute 1 mL (42 mg) with 1.8 mL sterile water for injection.

Neutralizing additive solution – Administer this solution promptly. When introducing additives, mix thoroughly and do not store.

➤*Administration:* Administer IV or subcutaneous following dilution to isotonicity (1.5%).

If administration is controlled by a pumping device, discontinue pumping action before the container runs dry or air embolism may result.

Replace administration apparatus at least once every 24 hours.

➤*Extravasation:* Extravasation may occur during administration of sodium bicarbonate 8.4%. If signs or symptoms of extravasation occur, stop the infusion immediately. If possible, withdraw 3 to 5 mL of blood to remove some of the drug. Remove the infusion needle. Delineate the infiltrated area on the patient's skin with a felt-tip marker. Hyaluronidase is an effective antidote for hyperosmolar drug infiltrations; administer promptly within the first few minutes to 1 hour after extravasation. Higher doses (150 units) have primarily been used in adults while lower doses (15 units) have been used in children. Administer hyaluronidase according to the following steps. Dilute hyaluronidase to desired concentration, depending on the dose and product used. (Note: Some products do not require dilution.) For example, if the total dose is 15 units, make 15 units/mL dilution. If the total dose is 150 units, make 150 units/mL dilution. Cleanse area with povidone-iodine. Inject hyaluronidase locally, subcutaneously or intradermally, using a 25-gauge needle or smaller. The dose is given as five 0.2 mL injections at the leading edge of the extravasation site. Change needle after each injection. Elevate for 48 hours above heart level using a sling or stockinette dressing with an observation window cut in the dressing. Avoid pressure or friction. Do not rub area. Observe for signs of increased erythema, pain, or skin necrosis. If increased symptoms occur, consult a plastic surgeon. Ensure that no medication is given distally to extravasation site. After 48 hours, encourage the patient to use the extremity normally to promote full range of motion.

➤*Admixture compatibility:*

Compatibilities – The diluent may be sterile water for injection, sodium chloride injection, 5% dextrose or other standard electrolyte solutions.

Incompatibilities – Avoid adding sodium bicarbonate to parenteral solutions containing calcium, except where compatibility is established; precipitation or haze may result. Norepinephrine and dobutamine are incompatible.

➤*Storage/Stability:* Store at 15° to 30°C (59° to 86°F). Avoid excessive heat. Protect from freezing. Brief exposure up to 40°C does not adversely affect the product.

Actions

➤*Pharmacology:* Increases plasma bicarbonate; buffers excess hydrogen ion concentration; raises blood pH; reverses the clinical manifestations of acidosis.

One g sodium bicarbonate provides 11.9 mEq each of sodium and bicarbonate.

➤*Pharmacokinetics:* Sodium bicarbonate in water dissociates to provide sodium (Na^+) and bicarbonate (HCO_3^-) ions. Sodium is the principal cation of extracellular fluid. Bicarbonate is a normal constituent of body fluids and normal plasma level ranges from 24 to 31 mEq/L. Plasma concentration is regulated by the kidney. Bicarbonate anion is considered "labile" since, at a proper concentration of hydrogen ion (H^+), it may be converted to carbonic acid (H_2CO_3), then to its volatile form, carbon dioxide (CO_2), excreted by lungs. Normally, a ratio of 1:20 (carbonic acid: bicarbonate) is present in extracellular fluid. In a healthy adult with normal kidney function, almost all the glomerular filtered bicarbonate ion is reabsorbed; less than 1% is excreted in urine.

Contraindications

Losing chloride by vomiting or from continuous GI suction; receiving diuretics known to produce a hypochloremic alkalosis; metabolic and respiratory alkalosis; hypocalcemia in which alkalosis may produce tetany, hypertension, convulsions or congestive heart failure (CHF); when sodium use could be clinically detrimental.

➤*Neutralizing additive solution:* Do not use as a systemic alkalinizer.

Warnings/Precautions

➤*Cardiac effects:*

Cardiac arrest – The risk of rapid infusion must be weighed against the potential for fatality due to acidosis.

CHF – Since sodium accompanies bicarbonate, use cautiously in patients with CHF or other edematous or sodium-retaining states.

➤*Fluid/Solute overload:* IV administration can cause fluid or solute overloading resulting in dilution of serum electrolyte concentrations, overhydration, congested states or pulmonary edema. The risk of dilutional states is inversely proportional to the electrolyte concentrations of administered parenteral solutions. The risk of solute overload causing congested states with peripheral and acute pulmonary edema is directly proportional to the electrolyte concentrations of such solutions. Rapid or excessive administration of Sodium Bicarbonate Injection may produce tetany due to a decrease in ionized calcium and hypokalemia as potassium reenters the cells. Hypertonic solutions may cause vein damage. Avoid extravasation.

➤*Neonates and children (younger than 2 years old):* Rapid injection (10 mL/min) of hypertonic sodium bicarbonate solutions may produce hypernatremia, a decrease in cerebrospinal fluid pressure and possible intracranial hemorrhage. Do not administer more than 8 mEq/kg/day. A 4.2% solution is preferred for such slow administration.

➤*Avoid overdosage and alkalosis:* Avoid overdosage and alkalosis by giving repeated small doses and periodic monitoring by appropriate laboratory tests.

➤*Potassium depletion:* Potassium depletion may predispose to metabolic alkalosis, and coexistent hypocalcemia may be associated with carpopedal spasm as the plasma pH rises. Minimize by treating electrolyte imbalances prior to or concomitantly with bicarbonate.

➤*Chloride loss:* Patients losing chloride by vomiting or GI intubation are more susceptible to developing severe alkalosis if given alkalinizing agents.

➤*Neutralizing additive solution:* Administer this solution promptly. When introducing additives, mix thoroughly and do not store. Raising pH of IV fluids with neutralizing additive solution will only reduce incidence of chemical irritation caused by infusate; it will not diminish any foreign body effects caused by needle or catheter.

Extraordinary electrolyte losses such as may occur during protracted nasogastric suction, vomiting, diarrhea or GI fistula drainage may necessitate additional electrolyte supplementation.

➤*Extravasation:* See Administration and Dosage for more information.

SODIUM BICARBONATE — INJECTION

➤*Renal function impairment:* Administration of solutions containing sodium ions may result in sodium retention. Use with caution. Also use cautiously in oliguria or anuria.

➤*Pregnancy: Category C.* It is not known whether sodium bicarbonate can cause fetal harm when administered to a pregnant woman. Use only if clearly needed.

➤*Lactation:* It is not known whether this drug is excreted in breast milk. Exercise caution when administering to a nursing woman.

➤*Elderly:* Exercise particular care when administering sodium-containing solutions to elderly or postoperative patients with renal or cardiovascular insufficiency, with or without CHF.

➤*Monitoring:* Adverse reactions may result from an excess or deficit of one or more of the ions in the solution; frequent monitoring of electrolyte levels is essential.

Drug Interactions

Sodium Bicarbonate Drug Interactions

Precipitant drug	Object drug[a]		Description
Sodium bicarbonate	Chlorpropamide Lithium Methotrexate Salicylates Tetracyclines	⬇	The renal clearance of these agents may be increased due to alkalinization of the urine, possibly resulting in a decreased pharmacologic effect.
Sodium bicarbonate	Anorexiants Flecainide Mecamylamine Quinidine Sympathomimetics	⬆	The renal clearance of these agents may be decreased due to alkalinization of the urine, possibly resulting in increased pharmacologic or toxic effects.

[a] ⬆ = Object drug increased. ⬇ = Object drug decreased.

Adverse Reactions

If an adverse reaction does occur, discontinue the infusion, evaluate the patient, institute appropriate therapeutic countermeasures and save the remainder of the fluid for examination if deemed necessary.

➤*Clinical cellulitis:* Extravasation of IV hypertonic solutions of sodium bicarbonate may cause chemical cellulitis (because of their alkalinity), with tissue necrosis, ulceration or sloughing at the site of infiltration. Prompt elevation of the part, warmth and local injection of lidocaine or hyaluronidase are recommended to prevent sloughing.

Rapid infusion – Too rapid infusion of hypertonic solutions may cause local pain and venous irritation. Adjust the rate of administration according to tolerance. Use of the largest peripheral vein and a well placed small bore needle is recommended.

Too rapid or excessive administration may result in hypernatremia and alkalosis accompanied by hyperirritability or tetany. Hypernatremia may be associated with edema and exacerbation of CHF due to the retention of water, resulting in an expanded extracellular fluid volume.

Reactions due to solution or administration technique – Reactions that may occur because of the solution or the technique of administration include febrile response, infection at the site of injection, venous thrombosis or phlebitis extending from the injection site, extravasation and hypervolemia.

Overdosage

➤*Symptoms:* Excessive or too rapid administration may produce alkalosis. Severe alkalosis may be accompanied by hyperirritability or tetany.

➤*Treatment:* Discontinue sodium bicarbonate. Control symptoms of alkalosis by rebreathing expired air from a paper bag or rebreathing mask or, if more severe, by parenteral injections of calcium gluconate (to control tetany and hyperexcitability). Correct severe alkalosis by IV infusion of 2.14% ammonium chloride solution, except in patients with hepatic disease, in whom ammonia use is contraindicated. Sodium chloride (0.9%) IV or potassium chloride may be indicated if there is hypokalemia.

SODIUM LACTATE

Rx	**1/6 Molar Sodium Lactate** (Various, eg, Hospira, Baxter)	**Injection:** 167 mEq/L each of sodium and lactate ions	In 500 and 1000 mL.

SODIUM LACTATE — INJECTION

Complete and comparative prescribing information for these products begins in the Sodium Bicarbonate monograph. For additional information, refer to the Dietary Reference Intakes of Vitamins and Minerals table.

Indications

➤*Metabolic acidosis:* As a source of bicarbonate for prevention or control of mild to moderate metabolic acidosis in patients with restricted oral intake whose oxidative processes are not seriously impaired.

Administration and Dosage

➤*General dosing considerations:* All or part of the contents of 1 or more vials (50 mEq in 10 mL) may be added to other intravenous (IV) solutions to provide any desired number of milliequivalents of lactate anion (with the same number of milliequivalents of sodium). The contents of 1 vial (50 mEq in 10 mL) added to 290 mL of a nonelectrolyte solution or of sterile water for injection will provide 300 mL of an approximately isotonic (1/6 molar) concentration of sodium lactate (1.9%), containing 167 mEq/L each of sodium and lactate anion.

Must be diluted before administration.

➤*Adults:*

Metabolic acidosis – 50 mEq is administered IV only after addition to a larger volume of fluid. The amount of sodium ion and lactate ion to be added to larger volume IV fluids should be determined in accordance with the electrolyte requirements of each individual patient.

➤*Administration:* Sodium lactate injection is administered IV and must be suitably diluted before infusion to avoid a sudden increase in the level of sodium or lactate. Too rapid administration and overdosage should be avoided.

➤*Storage/Stability:* Store at 15° to 30°C (59° to 86°F). Discard unused portion.

Actions

➤*Pharmacology:* Lactate anion ($CH_3CH(OH)COO^-$) serves the important purpose of providing "raw material" for subsequent regeneration of bicarbonate (HCO_3^- and thus acts as a source (alternate) of bicarbonate when normal production and utilization of lactic acid is not impaired as a result of disordered lactate metabolism. Lactate anion is usually present in extracellular fluid at a level of less than 1 mEq/L, but may attain a level of 10 mEq/L during exercise. It is seldom measured as such and thus is one of the "unmeasured anions" ("anion gap") in determinations of the ionic composition of plasma.

Since metabolic conversion of lactate to bicarbonate is dependent on the integrity of cellular oxidative processes, lactate may be inadequate or ineffective as a source of bicarbonate in patients suffering from acidosis associated with shock or other disorders involving reduced perfusion of body tissues. When oxidative activity is intact, 1 to 2 hours time is required for conversion of lactate to bicarbonate.

The sodium (Na^+) ion combines with bicarbonate ion produced from carbon dioxide of the body and thus retains bicarbonate to combat metabolic acidosis (bicarbonate deficiency). The normal plasma level of lactate ranges from 0.9 to 1.9 mEq/L.

Contraindications

Hypernatremia or fluid retention. It should not be used in conditions in which lactate levels are increased (eg, shock, congestive heart failure, respiratory alkalosis) or in which utilization of lactate is diminished (eg, anoxia, beriberi). Not for use in the treatment of lactic acidosis.

Warnings/Precautions

➤*Sodium solutions:* Solutions containing sodium ions should be used with great care, if at all, in patients with congestive heart failure, severe renal insufficiency, and in clinical states in which there exists edema with sodium retention.

➤*Fluid/solute overload:* The IV administration of this solution (after appropriate dilution) can cause fluid or solute overloading resulting in dilution of other serum electrolyte concentrations, overhydration, congested states, or pulmonary edema.

➤*Hypokalemia:* Excessive administration of potassium-free solutions may result in significant hypokalemia.

➤*Severe acidosis:* It is not intended nor effective for correcting severe acidotic states which require immediate restoration of plasma bicarbonate levels. Sodium lactate has no advantage over sodium bicarbonate and may be detrimental in the management of lactic acidosis.

➤*Administration:* Sodium lactate injection must be suitably diluted before infusion to avoid a sudden increase in the level of sodium or lactate. Too rapid administration and overdosage should be avoided.

➤*Sodium-retaining states:* The potentially large loads of sodium given with lactate require that caution be exercised in patients with congestive heart failure or other edematous or sodium-retaining states, as well as in patients with oliguria or anuria.

➤*Lactase solution:* Solutions containing lactate ions should be used with caution as excess administration may result in metabolic alkalosis.

➤*Renal function impairment:* In patients with diminished renal function, administration of solutions containing sodium ions may result in sodium retention.

➤*Pregnancy: Category C.* Animal reproduction studies have not been conducted with sodium lactate. It is also not known whether sodium lactate can cause fetal harm when administered to a pregnant woman or can affect reproduction capacity. Sodium lactate should be given to a pregnant woman only if clearly needed.

➤*Lactation:* There is no information regarding sodium lactate in breast-feeding women.

SODIUM LACTATE — INJECTION

Drug Interactions

➤*Corticosteroids or corticotropin:* Caution must be exercised in the administration of parenteral fluids especially those containing sodium ions, to patients receiving corticosteroids or corticotropin.

Adverse Reactions

Adverse reactions to sodium lactate are essentially limited to overdosage of either sodium or lactate ions.

Overdosage

➤*Treatment:* In the event of overdosage, discontinue infusion containing sodium lactate immediately and institute corrective therapy as indicated to reduce elevated serum sodium levels and restore acid-base balance if necessary.

SODIUM ACETATE

Rx	**Sodium Acetate** (Various, eg, Abbott, American Regent)	**Injection:** 2 mEq each of sodium and acetate per mL (16.4%)	In 20, 50 and 100 mL vials.
Rx	**Sodium Acetate** (Various, eg, American Regent)	**Injection:** 4 mEq each of sodium and acetate per mL (32.8%)	In 50 and 100 mL vials.

SODIUM ACETATE — INJECTION

Complete and comparative prescribing information for these products begins in the Sodium Bicarbonate monograph. For additional information, refer to the Dietary Reference Intakes of Vitamins and Minerals table.

Indications

➤*Hyponatremia:* As a source of sodium for addition to large volume IV fluids to prevent or correct hyponatremia in patients with restricted or no oral intake. It is also useful as an additive for preparing specific IV fluid formulas when the needs of the patient cannot be met by standard electrolyte or nutrient solutions.

Administration and Dosage

➤*General dosing considerations:* Sodium acetate injections are concentrated solutions and must be diluted prior to administration. (See Preparation for Administration.)

Sodium replacement therapy should be guided primarily by the serum sodium level.

➤*Adults:*

Hyponatremia – The dose and rate of administration are dependent upon the individual needs of the patient. Serum sodium should be monitored as a guide to dosage.

➤*Preparation for administration:* Using aseptic technique, all or part of the contents of 1 or more vials may be added to other intravenous (IV) fluids to provide any desired number of milliequivalents (mEq) of sodium with an equal number of acetate.

➤*Administration:* Sodium acetate is administered IV only after dilution in a larger volume of fluid.

To avoid sodium overload and water retention, infuse sodium-containing solutions slowly.

➤*Storage/Stability:* Store at 15° to 30°C (59° to 86°F).

Actions

➤*Pharmacology:* Sodium (NA^+) is the principal cation of extracellular fluid. It comprises more than 90% of total cations at its normal plasma concentration of approximately 140 mEq/L. The sodium ion exerts a primary role in controlling total body water and its distribution.

Acetate (CH_3COO^-), a source of hydrogen ion acceptors, is an alternate source of bicarbonate (HCO_3^-) by metabolic conversion in the liver. This has been shown to proceed readily, even in the presence of severe liver disease.

Contraindications

Hypernatremia or fluid retention.

Warnings/Precautions

➤*Administration:* Sodium acetate must be diluted before use.

To avoid sodium overload and water retention, infuse sodium-containing solutions slowly.

➤*Sodium solutions:* Solutions containing sodium ions should be used with great care, if at all, in patients with congestive heart failure, severe renal insufficiency and in clinical states in which there exists edema with sodium retention.

➤*Acetate solutions:* Solutions containing acetate ions should be used with great care in patients with metabolic or respiratory alkalosis. Acetate should be administered with great care in those conditions in which there is an increased level or an impaired utilization of this ion, such as severe hepatic insufficiency.

Solutions containing acetate ions should be used with caution as excess administration may result in metabolic alkalosis.

➤*Fluid/solute overload:* The IV administration of this solution (after appropriate dilution) can cause fluid or solute overloading resulting in dilution of other serum electrolyte concentrations, overhydration, congested states, or pulmonary edema. Excessive administration of potassium free solutions may result in significant hypokalemia.

➤*Sodium retaining states:* Caution should be exercised in administering sodium-containing solutions to patients with severe renal function impairment, cirrhosis, cardiac failure or other edematous or sodium-retaining states, as well as in patients with oliguria or anuria.

➤*Renal function impairment:* In patients with diminished renal function, administration of solutions containing sodium ions may result in sodium retention.

➤*Pregnancy: Category C.* Animal reproduction studies have not been conducted with sodium acetate. It is also not known whether sodium acetate can cause fetal harm when administered to a pregnant woman or can affect reproduction capacity. Sodium acetate should be given to a pregnant woman only if clearly needed.

➤*Lactation:* It is not known whether this drug is excreted in breast milk. Exercise caution when administering to a breast-feeding woman.

➤*Children:* Sodium acetate is not intended for pediatric use.

➤*Monitoring:* Sodium replacement therapy should be guided primarily by the serum sodium level.

Drug Interactions

➤*Corticosteroids or corticotropin:* Caution must be exercised in the administration of parenteral fluids, especially those containing sodium ions, to patients receiving corticosteroids or corticotropin.

Overdosage

➤*Treatment:* In the event of overdosage, discontinue infusion-containing sodium acetate immediately and institute corrective therapy as indicated to reduce elevated serum sodium levels and restore acid-base balance, if necessary.

AMMONIUM CHLORIDE

Rx	**Ammonium Chloride** (Hospira)	**Injection:** 26.75% (5 mEq/mL) To be diluted before infusion	In 20 mL (100 mEq) vials.[a]

[a] With 2 mg EDTA.

AMMONIUM CHLORIDE — INJECTION

Indications

➤*Hypochloremia/metabolic alkalosis:* Treatment of patients with hypochloremic states and metabolic alkalosis.

Administration and Dosage

➤*Adults:*

Hypochloremia/metabolic alkalosis – Dosage is dependent upon the condition and tolerance of the patient. Solutions for IV infusion should not exceed a concentration of 1% to 2% of ammonium chloride.

➤*Monitoring:* Dosage should be monitored by repeated serum bicarbonate determinations.

➤*Preparation for administration:* Ammonium chloride injection must be diluted before use. It is recommended that the contents of 1 to 2 vials (100 to 200 mEq) be added to 500 or 1,000 mL of isotonic (0.9%) sodium chloride injection.

➤*Administration:* The rate of IV infusion should not exceed 5 mL/min in adults (approximately 3 hours for infusion of 1,000 mL). IV administration should be slow to avoid local irritation and toxic effects.

➤*Storage/Stability:* Store at 15° to 30°C (59° to 86°F). When exposed to low temperatures, concentrated solutions of ammonium chloride may crystallize. If crystals are observed, the vial should be warmed to room temperature in a water bath prior to use. Do not administer unless the solution is clear and seal is intact. Discard unused portion.

AMMONIUM CHLORIDE — INJECTION

Actions

➤*Pharmacology:* The ammonium ion (NH_4^+) in the body plays an important role in the maintenance of acid-base balance. The kidney uses ammonium (NH_4^+) in place of sodium (Na^+) to combine with fixed anions in maintaining acid-base balance, especially as a homeostatic compensatory mechanism in metabolic acidosis.

When a loss of hydrogen ions (H^+) occurs and serum chloride (Cl^-) decreases, sodium is made available for combination with bicarbonate (HCO_3^-). This creates an excess of sodium bicarbonate ($NaHCO_3$) which leads to a rise in blood pH and a state of metabolic alkalosis.

The therapeutic effects of ammonium chloride depend upon the ability of the kidney to utilize ammonia in the excretion of an excess of fixed anions and the conversion of ammonia to urea by the liver, thereby liberating hydrogen (H^+) and chloride (Cl^-) ions into the extracellular fluid.

One g of ammonium chloride provides 18.7 mEq of chloride.

Contraindications

Severe impairment of renal or hepatic function; metabolic alkalosis due to vomiting of hydrochloric acid is accompanied by loss of sodium (excretion of sodium bicarbonate in the urine).

Warnings/Precautions

➤*Ammonium toxicity:* Patients receiving ammonium chloride should be constantly observed for symptoms of ammonia toxicity (pallor, sweating, retching, irregular breathing, bradycardia, cardiac arrhythmias, local and general twitching, tonic convulsions and coma).

➤*Respiratory acidosis:* It should be used with caution in patients with high total CO_2 and buffer base secondary to primary respiratory acidosis.

➤*Administration:* IV administration should be slow to avoid local irritation and toxic effects.

➤*Pregnancy: Category C* per manufacturer's prescribing information. *Category B* per Briggs' *Drugs in Pregnancy and Lactation*. Animal reproduction studies have not been conducted with ammonium chloride. It is also not known whether ammonium chloride can cause fetal harm when administered to a pregnant woman or can affect reproduction capacity. Ammonium chloride should be given to a pregnant woman only if clearly needed. When consumed in large quantities at term, ammonium chloride may cause acidosis in the mother and the fetus. In some cases, the decreased pH and CO_2, increased lactic acid, and reduced oxygen saturation were as severe as those seen with fatal apnea neonatorum. However, the newborns did not appear to be in distress.

➤*Lactation:* Per Briggs' *Drugs in Pregnancy and Lactation*, ammonium chloride is probably compatible with breast-feeding.

Adverse Reactions

Rapid intravenous administration of ammonium chloride may be accompanied by pain or irritation at the site of injection or along the venous route.

If an adverse reaction does occur, discontinue the infusion, evaluate the patient, institute appropriate therapeutic countermeasures and save the remainder of the fluid for examination if deemed necessary.

➤*Reactions due to solution or administration technique:* Reactions which may occur because of the solution or the technique of administration include febrile response, infection at the site of injection, venous thrombosis or phlebitis extending from the site of injection, extravasation and hypervolemia (from large volume diluent).

Overdosage

➤*Symptoms:* Overdosage of ammonium chloride has resulted in a serious degree of metabolic acidosis, disorientation, confusion and coma.

➤*Treatment:* Should metabolic acidosis occur following overdosage, the administration of an alkalinizing solution such as sodium bicarbonate or sodium lactate will serve to correct the acidosis.

Trace Metals

Refer to the Trace Elements section for information on oral iodine, manganese, and zinc. Iodine is used as a thyroid agent and as an expectorant (see monographs in Thyroid Drugs section). For additional information, refer to the Dietary Reference Intakes of Vitamins and Minerals table.

Indications

➤*Total parenteral nutrition:* Supplement to intravenous (IV) solutions given for total parenteral nutrition (TPN).

Administration helps to maintain serum levels of essential trace metals (zinc, copper, chromium, and manganese) and to prevent depletion of endogenous stores and symptoms of subsequent deficiency.

Administration and Dosage

Administer IV after dilution. Frequently monitor plasma levels and clinical status.

➤*Admixture compatibility:* Trace metals are usually physically compatible together, and with the electrolytes usually present in the amino acid/dextrose solution used for TPN.

Actions

➤*Pharmacology:*

Chromium – Trivalent chromium is part of glucose tolerance factor, an essential activator of insulin-mediated reactions. Chromium helps maintain normal glucose metabolism and peripheral nerve function.

Serum chromium is bound to transferrin (siderophilin). Administration of chromium supplements to chromium deficient patients can result in normalization of the glucose tolerance curve from the diabetic-like curve typical of chromium deficiency. This response is viewed as a more meaningful indicator than serum chromium levels.

Copper – Copper serves as a cofactor for serum ceruloplasmin, an oxidase necessary for proper formation of the iron carrier protein, transferrin. Copper also helps maintain normal rates of red and white blood cell formation. The daily turnover of copper through ceruloplasmin is approximately 0.5 mg.

Scorbutic type bone changes seen in infants fed exclusively with copper-poor cow's milk are believed to be due to decreased activity of ascorbate oxidase, a cupro enzyme.

Iodine – Absorption from the GI tract is rapid and complete. Skin and lungs can also absorb iodine. On administration, iodide equilibrates in extracellular fluids and although all body cells contain iodide, it is specifically concentrated by the thyroid gland, which is estimated to contain 7 to 8 mg total iodine.

Other important organs to take up iodide are salivary glands, gastric mucosa, choroid plexus, skin, hair, mammary glands and placenta. Iodine in saliva and gastric mucosal secretions is reabsorbed and recycled. The circulating iodine is hormonal thyroxine of which 30 to 70 mcg is protein bound and 0.5 mcg is free thyroxine.

Manganese – Manganese serves as an activator for several enzymes. During minimal intake, 20 mcg/day is retained. Manganese is bound to a specific transport protein, transmanganin, and is widely distributed, but it concentrates in mitochondria-rich tissues such as brain, kidney, pancreas and liver.

Ancillary routes for manganese excretion include pancreatic juice, or reabsorption into the lumen of the duodenum, jejunum, or ileum.

Molybdenum – Molybdenum is a constituent of the enzymes xanthine oxidase, sulfite oxidase and aldehyde oxidase. Tissue storage of molybdenum varies with the intake levels and is affected by the amount of copper and sulfate in the diet. Consistent levels are observed in liver, kidney and adrenal cortex.

Selenium – Selenium is part of glutathione peroxidase which protects cell components from oxidative damage due to peroxides produced in cellular metabolism.

Pediatric conditions, Keshan disease and Kwashiorkor have been associated with low dietary intake of selenium. The conditions are endemic to geographic areas with low selenium soil content. Dietary supplementation with selenium salts reduces the incidence of the conditions among affected children.

Zinc – Zinc serves as a cofactor for more than 70 different enzymes. Zinc facilitates wound healing, helps maintain normal growth rates, normal skin hydration and the senses of taste and smell. Zinc resides in muscle, bone, skin, kidney, liver, pancreas, retina, prostate and particularly in the red and white blood cells. Zinc binds to plasma albumin, α_2–macroglobulin and some plasma amino acids including histidine, cysteine, threonine, glycine and asparagine.

Zinc is eliminated via the intestine and kidneys. Consider the possibility of retention in patients with malfunctioning excretory routes.

At plasma levels less than 20 mcg/dL, dermatitis followed by alopecia has been reported for TPN patients. The following table summarizes deficiency symptoms excretion routes and normal plasma levels for various trace metals. The serum level at which deficiency symptoms appear for many of these elements is not well defined.

Trace Metals: Deficiency/Excretion/Plasma Levels

Trace metal	Symptoms of deficiency	Excretion	Normal plasma levels
Copper	Leukopenia, neutropenia, anemia, decreased ceruloplasmin levels, impaired transferrin formation, secondary iron deficiency, skeletal abnormalities, defective tissue formation.	Bile (80%), intestinal wall (16%), urine (4%)	80-163 mcg/dL
Chromium	Impaired glucose tolerance, peripheral neuropathy, ataxia, confusion.	Kidneys (3-50 mcg/day), bile	1-5 mcg/L[a]
Iodine	Impaired thyroid function, goiter, cretinism.	Kidneys, bile	0.5-1.5 mcg/dL
Manganese	Nausea, vomiting, weight loss, dermatitis, changes in growth and hair color.	Bile; if obstruction present, then pancreatic juice or return to intestinal lumen. Urine (negligible)	6-12 mcg/L (whole blood)
Molybdenum	Tachycardia, tachypnea, headache, night blindness, nausea, vomiting, central scotomas, edema, lethargy, disorientation, coma, hypermethioninemia, hypouricemia, hypouricuria, low urinary excretion of inorganic sulfate and elevated urinary excretion of thiosulfate.	Primarily renal, some biliary	nd
Selenium	Muscle pain & tenderness, cardiomyopathy, Kwashiorkor, Keshan disease.	Urine, feces, lungs, skin	nd[b]
Zinc	Diarrhea, apathy, depression, parakeratosis, hypogeusia, anorexia, dysosmia, geophagia, hypogonadism, growth retardation, anemia, hepatosplenomegaly, impaired wound healing.	90% in stools; urine, perspiration	100 ± 12 mcg/dL

[a] Not considered a meaningful index of tissue stores.
[b] nd = No data

Contraindications

Do not give undiluted by direct injection into a peripheral vein because of the potential for infusion phlebitis and tissue irritation, and potential to increase renal loss of minerals from a bolus injection.

Warnings/Precautions

➤*Aluminum:* Products may contain aluminum that may be toxic. Aluminum may reach toxic levels with prolonged parenteral administration if renal function is impaired. Premature neonates are particularly at risk because their kidneys are immature and they require large amounts of calcium and phosphate solutions, which contain aluminum.

Research indicates that patients with impaired kidney function, including premature neonates, who receive parenteral levels of aluminum at more than 4 to 5 mcg/kg/day accumulate aluminum at levels associated with CNS and bone toxicity. Tissue loading may occur at even lower rates of administration.

➤*Biliary tract obstruction:* Copper and manganese are eliminated via the bile. In patients with severe hepatic dysfunction and/or biliary tract obstruction, decreasing or omitting copper and manganese supplements entirely may be necessary.

➤*Wilson's disease:* Avoid administering **copper** supplements to patients with this genetic disorder of copper metabolism.

➤*Decreased serum levels:* Administration of **copper** in the absence of **zinc** and of zinc in the absence of copper may cause decreases in plasma levels. Perform periodic determinations of plasma zinc and copper for subsequent administrations.

➤*Copper deficiency:* **Molybdenum** promotes tissue **copper** mobilization and increases urinary copper excretion; excessive amounts produce a copper deficiency. Frequently check the metabolism of copper in patients receiving molybdenum.

➤*Multiple trace element solutions:* Multiple trace element solutions present a risk of overdosage when the need for one trace element is appreciably higher than that for the other trace elements in the formulation. Administration of trace metals as separate entities may be required.

➤*Replacement trace metal therapy:* Replacement trace metal therapy beyond maintenance requirements may be necessary in protracted vomiting or diarrhea, in patients with fistula drainage or nasogastric suction or in acute catabolic states.

➤*Diabetes mellitus:* In assessing the contribution of chromium supplements to maintenance of glucose homeostasis, consider that the patient may be diabetic.

➤*Iodine:* Iodine is readily absorbed through skin, lungs and mucous membranes. Give consideration to the environment, topical skin disinfection and wound treatment practices with surgical swabs and solutions containing iodine and povidone iodine. Air in the coastal areas is known to contain more iodine than inland areas.

➤*Benzyl alcohol:* Some of these products contain benzyl alcohol, which has been associated with a fatal gasping syndrome in premature infants.

➤*Hypersensitivity reactions:* Sensitization to **iodides** and deaths due to anaphylactic shock after use have occurred (see Adverse Reactions). Evaluate patient for hypersensitivity before initiating TPN. If patient develops a reaction, withdraw TPN immediately and institute appropriate measures. Refer to Management of Acute Hypersensitivity.

➤*Renal function impairment:* In renal failure, give consideration to accumulation of trace metals where the excretion route is compromised.

➤*Hepatic function impairment:* Copper and manganese are eliminated via the bile. In patients with severe hepatic dysfunction and/or biliary tract obstruction, decreasing or omitting copper and manganese supplements entirely may be necessary.

➤*Pregnancy: Category C.* It is not known whether trace metals can cause fetal harm or can affect reproductive capacity. Give to a pregnant woman only if clearly needed.

Molybdenum crosses the placenta. Presence of **selenium** in placenta and umbilical cord blood has been reported.

➤*Lactation:* It is unknown whether these trace elements will harm a breast-feeding child. Instruct breast-feeding women to speak to a health care provider before taking any trace elements (refer to the Dietary Reference Intake of Vitamins and Minerals table).

➤*Monitoring:* Frequent determinations of serum levels of the various trace elements are suggested as a guideline for adjusting the dosage or completely omitting the solution.

Adverse Reactions

Symptoms of toxicity are unlikely to occur at recommended doses.

Hypersensitivity to **iodides** may result in angioneurotic edema, cutaneous and mucosal hemorrhages, fever, arthralgia, lymph node enlargement and eosinophilia. (See Warnings.)

Overdosage

➤*Chromium:* Nausea, vomiting, GI ulcers, renal/hepatic damage, convulsions, coma.

➤*Copper:* Prostration, behavior change, diarrhea, progressive marasmus, hypotonia, photophobia, hepatic damage and peripheral edema have occurred with a serum copper level of 286 mcg/dL. Penicillamine is an effective antidote.

➤*Iodine:* Symptoms of chronic poisoning include metallic taste, sore mouth, increased salivation, coryza, sneezing, swelling of the eyelids, severe headache, pulmonary edema, tenderness of salivary glands, acneiform skin lesions and skin eruptions. Abundant fluid and salt intake helps in elimination of iodides.

➤*Manganese:* Manganese toxicity in TPN patients has not been reported.

➤*Molybdenum:* Gout-like syndrome with increased blood levels of molybdenum, uric acid and xanthine oxidase.

No data on treatment of molybdenosis in humans is available. Among animals, treatment with copper, sulfate ions and tungsten enhances excretion of molybdenum. The sulfur-containing amino acids, methionine and cysteine, may afford limited protection.

➤*Selenium:* Toxicity symptoms include hair loss, weak nails, dermatitis, dental defects, GI disorders, nervousness, mental depression, metallic taste, vomiting and garlic odor of breath and sweat. Acute poisoning due to ingestion has resulted in death with histopathological changes including fulminating peripheral vascular collapse, internal vascular congestion, diffusely hemorrhagic, congested and edematous lungs and brick-red color gastric mucosa. Death was preceded by coma. No effective antidote is known.

➤*Zinc:* Single IV doses of 1 to 2 mg/kg have been given to adult leukemic patients without toxic manifestations. However, acute toxicity was reported in an adult when 10 mg zinc was infused over 1 hour on each of 4 consecutive days. Profuse sweating, decreased consciousness, blurred vision, tachycardia (140/min) and marked hypothermia (94.2°F) on the fourth day were accompanied by a serum zinc concentration of 207 mcg/dL. Symptoms abated within 3 hours.

Patients receiving an inadvertent overdose (50 to 70 mg zinc/day) developed hyperamylasemia (557 to 1850 Klein units; normal, 130 to 310).

Death resulted from 1683 mg zinc IV over 60 hours to a 72-year-old patient. Symptoms included hypotension (80/40 mm Hg), pulmonary edema, diarrhea, vomiting, jaundice and oliguria with a serum zinc level of 4184 mcg/dL.

Calcium supplements may confer a protective effect against zinc toxicity.

ZINC

Rx	**Zinc Sulfate** (American Regent)	**Injection, solution:** 1 mg/mL	As zinc sulfate 2.46 mg/mL. Preservative free. In 10 mL single-use vials.
Rx	**Concentrated Zinc Sulfate** (American Regent)	**Injection, solution, concentrate:** 5 mg/mL	As zinc sulfate 12.32 mg/mL. Preservative free. In 5 mL vials.

ZINC SULFATE — INJECTION

For complete and comparative prescribing information, refer to the Zinc Supplements class monograph. For additional information, refer to the Trace Metals class monograph and the Dietary Reference Intakes of Vitamins and Minerals table.

Indications

➤*Zinc supplement:* As a supplement to intravenous (IV) solutions given for total parenteral nutrition (TPN). Administration helps to maintain plasma zinc levels and to prevent depletion of endogenous stores.

Administration and Dosage

➤*General dosing considerations:* Zinc sulfate 2.46 mg/mL provides zinc 1 mg/mL.

Zinc sulfate 12.32 mg/mL provides zinc 5 mg/mL.

Zinc sulfate injection should not be given undiluted by direct injection. (See Administration.)

➤*Adults:*

Zinc supplementation in metabolically stable patients receiving TPN – Zinc 2.5 to 4 mg/day added to the TPN. An additional 2 mg/day is suggested for acute catabolic states. For the stable adult with fluid loss from the small bowel, an additional zinc 12.2 mg/liter of TPN solution, or an additional zinc 17.1 mg/kg of stool or ileostomy is recommended.

➤*Children:*

Zinc supplementation in patients receiving TPN –

Full-term infants and children up to 5 years of age: Zinc 100 mcg/kg/day added to TPN.

Premature infants (birth weight less than 1,500 g) up to 3 kg in body weight: Zinc 300 mcg/kg/day added to TPN.

➤*Monitoring:* Frequent monitoring of zinc blood levels is suggested for patients receiving more than the usual maintenance dosage of zinc. Normal plasma levels for zinc vary from approximately 88 to 112 mcg per 100 mL.

➤*Preparation for administration:* Aseptically add zinc sulfate injection to TPN solution under a laminar flow hood.

➤*Administration:* Zinc sulfate injection should not be given undiluted by direct injection into a peripheral vein because of the potential for infusion phlebitis and the potential to increase renal loss of zinc from a bolus injection.

➤*Admixture compatibility:* Zinc is physically compatible with the electrolytes and vitamins usually present in amino acid/dextrose solutions used for TPN.

➤*Storage/Stability:* Store at 15° to 30°C (59° to 86°F).

Actions

➤*Pharmacology:* Zinc has been identified as a cofactor for more than 70 different enzymes, including alkaline phosphatase, lactic dehydrogenase, and both RNA and DNA polymerase. Zinc facilitates wound healing and helps maintain normal growth rates, normal skin hydration, and the senses of taste and smell.

Providing zinc during TPN prevents development of the following deficiency symptoms: anorexia, dysosmia, geophagia, growth retardation, hepatosplenomegaly, hypogeusia, hypogonadism, and parakeratosis. At plasma levels less than 20 mcg per 100 mL, dermatitis followed by alopecia has been reported for TPN patients.

Contraindications

Do not give undiluted by direct injection into a peripheral vein because of the likelihood of infusion phlebitis and the potential to increase renal loss of zinc from a bolus injection.

Warnings/Precautions

➤*Aluminum toxicity:* This product contains aluminum, which may be toxic. Aluminum may reach toxic levels with prolonged parenteral administration if kidney function is impaired. Premature neonates are particularly at risk because their kidneys are immature, and they require large amounts of calcium and phosphate solutions, which contain aluminum.

Research indicates that patients with impaired kidney function, including premature neonates, who receive parenteral levels of aluminum at greater than 4 to 5 mcg/kg/day accumulate aluminum at levels associated with CNS and bone toxicity. Tissue loading may occur at even lower rates of administration.

➤*Concomitant copper therapy:* Administration of zinc in the absence of copper may cause a decrease in serum copper levels. Periodic determination of serum copper as well as zinc are suggested as a guideline for subsequent zinc administration.

➤*Renal function impairment:* This product contains aluminum that may be toxic. Aluminum may reach toxic levels with prolonged parenteral administration if kidney function is impaired. (See Aluminum Toxicity.)

Zinc is eliminated via the intestine and kidneys. Consider the possibility of retention in patients with malfunctioning excretory routes.

➤*Pregnancy: Category C.* Safety for use in pregnancy has not been established. Use of zinc in women of childbearing potential requires that anticipated benefits be weighed against possible hazards. The recommended dietary allowance of zinc in pregnancy is 11 mg/day (19 to 50 years of age) or 12 mg/day (14 to 18 years of age) (refer to the Dietary Reference Intakes of Vitamins and Minerals table).

➤*Lactation:* Safety for use in lactation has not been established. The recommended dietary allowance of zinc in breast-feeding women is 12 mg/day (19 to 50 years of age) or 13 mg/day (14 to 18 years of age) (refer to the Dietary Reference Intakes of Vitamins and Minerals table).

➤*Children:* This product contains aluminum, which may be toxic. Premature neonates are particularly at risk because their kidneys are immature, and they require large amounts of calcium and phosphate solutions, which contain aluminum. (See Aluminum Toxicity.)

➤*Monitoring:* Periodic determination of serum copper as well as zinc are suggested as a guideline for subsequent zinc administration.

Adverse Reactions

The amount of zinc present in zinc sulfate injection is very small; symptoms of toxicity from zinc are considered unlikely to occur.

Overdosage

➤*Symptoms:* Symptoms of zinc overdosage resulting from oral ingestion of zinc sulfate in large amounts (30 and 44 g, respectively) have resulted in death. Symptoms include nausea, vomiting, dehydration, electrolyte imbalances, dizziness, abdominal pain, lethargy, and incoordination. Single IV doses of zinc 1 to 2 mg/kg body weight have been given to adults with leukemia without toxic manifestations. Normal plasma levels for zinc vary from approximately 88 to 112 mcg per 100 mL. Plasma levels sufficient to produce symptoms of toxic manifestations in humans are not known.

➤*Treatment:* Calcium supplements may confer a protective effect against zinc toxicity.

COPPER

Rx	**Copper** (Hospira)	**Injection:** 0.4 mg/mL (as 1.07 mg cupric Cl)	In 10 mL vials.
Rx	**Cupric Sulfate** (American Regent)	**Injection:** 0.4 mg/mL (as 1.57 mg sulfate)	In 10 mL vials.

COPPER — INJECTION

Complete and comparative prescribing information begins in the Trace Metals group monograph. For additional information, refer to the Dietary Reference Intakes of Vitamins and Minerals table.

Indications

➤*Copper supplement:* Copper is indicated for use as a supplement to IV solutions given for total parenteral nutrition (TPN).

Administration and Dosage

Copper contains 0.4 mg copper/mL and is administered IV only after dilution. The additive should be diluted in a volume of fluid not less than 100 mL.

➤*Adults:* The suggested additive dosage is 0.5 to 1.5 mg copper/day (1.25 to 3.75 mL/day).

➤*Children:* The suggested additive dosage is 20 mcg copper/kg/day (0.05 mL/kg/day).

➤*Storage/Stability:* Store at controlled room temperature 15° to 30°C (59° to 86°F).

Do not use unless the solution is clear and the seal is intact. Solution contains no preservatives; discard unused portion immediately after admixture procedure is completed.

MANGANESE

Rx	**Manganese Chloride** (Hospira)	**Injection, solution:** 0.1 mg/mL	As manganese chloride 0.36 mg/mL. Preservative free. In 10 mL vials.
Rx	**Manganese Sulfate** (American Regent)	**Injection, solution:** 0.1 mg/mL	As manganese sulfate 0.308 mg/mL. Preservative free. In 10 mL single-dose vials.

MANGANESE — INJECTION

For complete and comparative prescribing information, refer to the Trace Metals class monograph. For additional information, refer to the Dietary Reference Intakes of Vitamins and Minerals table.

Indications

➤*Manganese supplement:* As a supplement to intravenous (IV) solutions given for total parenteral nutrition (TPN). Administration helps to maintain manganese plasma levels and to prevent depletion of endogenous stores and subsequent deficiency symptoms.

Administration and Dosage

➤*General dosing considerations:* Manganese chloride 0.36 mg/mL provides manganese 0.1 mg/mL.

Manganese sulfate 0.308 mg/mL provides manganese 0.1 mg/mL.

Manganese injection should not be given undiluted by direct injection. (See Administration.)

➤*Adults:*

Manganese supplementation in adults receiving TPN – 0.15 to 0.8 mg/day of manganese added to the TPN.

➤*Children:*

Manganese supplementation in adults receiving TPN – 2 to 10 mcg/kg/day of manganese added to TPN.

➤*Hepatic function impairment:* Liver dysfunction and/or biliary dysfunction (eg, biliary tract obstruction) may require omission or reduction of manganese doses because it is primarily eliminated in the bile.

➤*Monitoring:* Periodic monitoring of manganese plasma levels is suggested as a guideline for subsequent administration.

➤*Preparation for administration:* Aseptically add manganese injection to the TPN solution under a laminar flow hood; it should be used promptly and in a single operation without any repeated penetrations. Solution contains no preservatives; discard unused portion immediately after procedure is completed.

➤*Administration:* Manganese injection should not be given undiluted by direct injection into a peripheral vein because of the potential for infusion phlebitis.

Direct intramuscular (IM) or IV injection of manganese chloride is contraindicated because the acidic pH of the solution may cause considerable tissue irritation.

➤*Admixture compatibility:* Manganese is physically compatible with the electrolytes and vitamins usually present in amino acid/dextrose solutions used for TPN.

➤*Storage/Stability:* Store at 15° to 30°C (59° to 86°F).

MOLYBDENUM

Rx	**Ammonium Molybdate** (American Regent)	**Injection, solution:** 25 mcg/mL	As ammonium molybdate 46 mcg/mL. In 10 mL single-dose vials.

MOLYBDENUM AMMONIUM MOLYBDATE — INJECTION

For complete and comparative prescribing information, refer to the Trace Metals class monograph. For additional information, refer to the Dietary Reference Intakes of Vitamins and Minerals table.

Indications

➤*Molybdenum supplement:* For use as a supplement to total parenteral nutrition (TPN) solutions to help prevent depletion of endogenous molybdenum stores and subsequent deficiency syndromes.

Administration and Dosage

➤*General dosing considerations:* Ammonium molybdate 46 mcg/mL injection provides molybdenum 25 mcg/mL.

Ammonium molybdate injection should not be given undiluted by direct injection. (See Administration.)

➤*Adults:*

Molybdenum supplementation in metabolically stable patients receiving TPN – 20 to 120 mcg/day of molybdenum added to the TPN.

Molybdenum deficiency state resulting from prolonged TPN support – 163 mcg/day of molybdenum for 21 days has reversed deficiency symptoms in an adult without toxicity.

➤*Children:*

Molybdenum supplementation in metabolically stable children receiving TPN – Calculate the additive dosage level by extrapolation from the adult dosage recommendation.

➤*Renal function impairment:* Molybdenum is excreted in urine and bile. Molybdenum supplements may need to be adjusted, reduced, or omitted in patients with renal dysfunction.

➤*Hepatic function impairment:* Molybdenum is excreted in urine and bile. Molybdenum supplements may need to be adjusted, reduced, or omitted in patients with bile duct obstruction.

➤*Monitoring:* Monitoring of sulfur and purine metabolism is suggested. Frequently monitor blood copper levels during molybdenum administration because copper and molybdenum are antagonistic to each other.

➤*Preparation for administration:* Aseptically add ammonium molybdate injection to the TPN solution under a laminar flow hood.

➤*Administration:* Ammonium molybdate injection should not be given undiluted by direct injection into a peripheral vein because of the potential for infusion phlebitis. Ammonium molybdate injection is a hypotonic solution and should be administered in admixtures only.

➤*Admixture compatibility:* Molybdate is physically compatible with the electrolytes and other trace elements usually present in amino acid/dextrose solutions used for TPN.

➤*Storage/Stability:* Store at 20° to 25°C (68° to 77°F); excursions are permitted between 15° and 30°C (59° and 86°F).

CHROMIUM

Rx	**Chromic Chloride** (Hospira)	**Injection, solution:** 4 mcg/mL	As chromic chloride 20.5 mcg/mL. Preservative free. In 10 mL vials.
Rx	**Chromic Chloride** (American Regent)		As chromic chloride 20.5 mcg/mL. Preservative free. In 10 mL single-use vials.

CHROMIC CHLORIDE — INJECTION

For complete and comparative prescribing information, refer to the Trace Metals class monograph. For additional information, refer to the Dietary Reference Intakes of Vitamins and Minerals table.

Indications

➤*Chromium supplement:* As a supplement to intravenous (IV) solutions given for total parenteral nutrition (TPN). Administration helps to maintain chromium serum levels and to prevent depletion of endogenous stores and subsequent deficiency symptoms.

Administration and Dosage

➤*General dosing considerations:* Chromic chloride 20.5 mcg/mL injection provides chromium 4 mcg/mL.

Chromic chloride injection should not be given undiluted by direct injection. (See Administration.)

➤*Adults:*

Chromium supplementation in patients receiving TPN – 10 to 15 mcg/day of chromium added to TPN. The metabolically stable adult with intestinal fluid loss may require chromium 20 mcg/day, with frequent monitoring of blood levels as a guideline for subsequent administration.

➤*Children:*

Chromium supplementation in patients receiving TPN – 0.14 to 0.2 mcg/kg/day of chromium added to TPN.

➤*Renal function impairment:* Chromium is excreted by the kidneys. Chromium supplements may need to be adjusted, reduced, or omitted in patients with renal impairment.

➤*Preparation for administration:* Aseptically add chromic chloride injection to the TPN solution under a laminar flow hood; it should be used promptly and in a single operation without any repeated penetrations. The

CHROMIC CHLORIDE — INJECTION

solution contains no preservatives; discard unused portion immediately after procedure is completed.

➤*Administration:* Chromium chloride injection should not be given undiluted by direct injection into a peripheral vein because of the potential for infusion phlebitis.

Direct intramuscular (IM) or intravenous (IV) injection of chromic chloride is contraindicated because the acidic pH of the solution may cause considerable tissue irritation.

➤*Admixture compatibility:* Chromium is physically compatible with the electrolytes and vitamins usually present in amino acid/dextrose solutions used for TPN.

➤*Storage/Stability:* Store at 15° to 30°C (59° to 86°F).

SELENIUM

Rx	**Selenium** (American Regent)	**Injection, solution:** 40 mcg/mL (as selenious acid 65.4 mcg/mL)	In 10 mL single-dose vials.

SELENIOUS ACID — INJECTION

For complete and comparative prescribing information, refer to the Trace Metals class monograph. For additional information, refer to the Dietary Reference Intakes of Vitamins and Minerals table.

Indications

➤*Selenium supplement:* As a supplement to intravenous (IV) solutions given for total parenteral nutrition (TPN).

Administration and Dosage

➤*General dosing considerations:* Selenious acid 65.4 mcg/mL provides selenium 40 mcg/mL.

➤*Adults:*

Metabolically stable patients receiving total parenteral nutrition – Selenium 20 to 40 mcg/day added to TPN.

In adults with selenium deficiency states resulting from long-term TPN support, IV selenium as selenomethionine or selenious acid 100 mcg/day for a period of 24 and 31 days, respectively, has been reported to reverse deficiency symptoms without toxicity.

➤*Children:*

Metabolically stable patients receiving total parenteral nutrition – Selenium 3 mcg/kg/day added to TPN.

➤*Renal function impairment:* Renal dysfunction may require adjusted, reduced, or omitted selenium supplementation.

➤*Therapeutic drug monitoring:* Periodic monitoring of selenium plasma levels is suggested as a guideline for subsequent administration. The normal whole blood range for selenium is approximately 10 to 37 mcg per 100 mL.

➤*Preparation for administration:* Aseptically add selenium injection to the TPN solution under a laminar flow hood.

➤*Administration:* Selenium injection should not be given undiluted by direct injection into a peripheral vein because of the potential for infusion phlebitis.

➤*Admixture compatibility:* Selenium is physically compatible with the electrolytes and other trace elements usually present in amino acid/dextrose solutions used for TPN.

➤*Storage/Stability:* Store between 20° and 25°C (68° and 77°F); excursions are permitted between 15° and 30°C (59° and 86°F).

SODIUM IODIDE

Rx	**Iodopen** (American Pharmaceutical Partners)	**Injection, solution:** 100 mcg/mL	As sodium iodide 118 mcg. In 10 mL single-dose vials.

SODIUM IODIDE — INJECTION

For complete and comparative prescribing information, refer to the Trace Metals class monograph. For additional information, refer to the Dietary Reference Intakes of Vitamins and Minerals table.

Indications

➤*Iodine supplement:* For use as a supplement to intravenous solutions given for total parenteral nutrition (TPN). Administration of sodium iodide injection in TPN solutions helps to prevent depletion of endogenous iodine stores and subsequent deficiency symptoms.

Administration and Dosage

➤*General dosing considerations:* Sodium iodide 118 mcg/mL provides iodine 100 mcg/mL.

Sodium iodide injection should not be given undiluted by direct injection. (See Administration.)

➤*Adults:*

Iodine supplementation in metabolically stable patients receiving TPN – 1 to 2 mcg/kg/day of iodine (healthy adults, 75 to 150 mcg/day) added to TPN.

For pregnant and breast-feeding women, the suggested dosage is 2 to 3 mcg/kg/day of iodine.

➤*Children:*

Iodine supplementation in metabolically stable patients receiving TPN – For growing children, the dosage is 2 to 3 mcg/kg/day of iodine added to TPN.

➤*Renal function impairment:* Iodine is eliminated in the urine. Iodine supplements may need to be adjusted, reduced, or omitted in patients with renal dysfunction.

➤*Monitoring:* Periodic monitoring of thyroid function is suggested as a guideline for adjusting dosage level.

➤*Preparation for administration:* Aseptically add chromic chloride injection to the TPN solution under a laminar flow hood.

➤*Administration:* Sodium iodide injections should not be given undiluted by direct injection into a peripheral vein because of the potential for infusion phlebitis. Sodium iodide is a hypotonic solution and should be administered in admixtures only.

➤*Admixture compatibility:* Iodine is physically compatible with the electrolytes and other trace elements usually present in amino acid/dextrose solutions used for TPN.

➤*Storage/Stability:* Store at 20° to 25°C (68° to 77°F).

TRACE METAL COMBINATIONS

Content given per mL solution.

	Product & Distributor	Chromium (as chloride) mcg	Copper (as sulfate) mg	Manganese (as sulfate) mg	Selenium (as selenious acid) mcg	Zinc (as sulfate) mg	How Supplied
Rx	**Multitrace-4 Neonatal** (American Regent)	0.85	0.1	0.025		1.5	In 2 mL single-dose vials.
Rx	**Multitrace-4 Pediatric** (American Regent)	1	0.1	0.025		1	Preservative free. In 3 mL single-dose vials.
Rx	**Trace Elements 4 Pediatric** (American Regent)	1	0.1	0.03		0.5	In 10 mL multidose vials.[b]
Rx	**Multitrace-4** (American Regent)	4	0.4	0.1		1	In 10 mL multidose vials.[b]
Rx	**Multitrace-5** (American Regent)	4	0.4	0.1	20	1	In 10 mL multidose vials.[b]
Rx	**4 Trace Elements** (Hospira)	6	0.42[a]	0.37[a]		1.67[a]	Preservative free. In 5 mL vial.[c]
Rx	**Multitrace-4 Concentrate** (American Regent)	10	1	0.5		5	In 1 mL single-dose vials and 10 mL multidose vials.[b]
Rx	**Multitrace-5 Concentrate** (American Regent)	10	1	0.5	60	5	In 1 mL single-dose and 10 mL multidose vials.[b]

[a] As chloride.
[b] With 0.9% benzyl alcohol.
[c] With sodium chloride 9 mg/mL.

Trace Metals

TRACE METAL COMBINATIONS — INJECTION

Complete and comparative prescribing information begins in the Trace Metals group monograph. For additional information, refer to the Dietary Reference Intakes of Vitamins and Minerals table.

Administration and Dosage

See manufacturers' product labeling for individual dosing information.

Therapeutic supplements to provide replacement for extraordinary losses of individual trace metals may be added.

➤*General dosing considerations:* Periodic monitoring of plasma levels of chromium, copper, manganese, and zinc is suggested as a guideline for administration.

Normal plasma range for copper is approximately 80 to 160 mcg per 100 mL; the normal plasma levels for zinc vary from approximately 88 to 112 mcg per 100 mL.

➤*Adults:*

Total parenteral nutrition supplement –

4 Trace Elements: 5 mL/day in metabolically stable adult TPN patients.

Trace Elements 4 Pediatric:

- *Chromium –*
  - *Metabolically stable adults:* 10 to 15 mcg/day.
  - *Intestinal fluid loss:* 20 mcg/day with frequent monitoring of blood levels as a guideline for subsequent administration.
- *Copper* – 0.5 to 1.5 mg/day in metabolically stable adults.
- *Manganese* – 0.15 to 0.8 mg/day in metabolically stable adults.
- *Zinc –*
  - *Metabolically stable adults:* 2.5 to 4 mg/day.
  - *Acute catabolic states:* 4.5 to 6 mg/day.
  - *Fluid loss from the small bowel:* An additional 12.2 mg/L of small bowel fluid lost or an additional zinc 17.1 mg/kg of stool or ileostomy output.

➤*Children:*

Total parenteral nutrition supplement –

Trace Elements 4 Pediatric:

- *Chromium* – 0.14 to 0.2 mcg/kg/day.
- *Copper* – 20 mcg/kg/day.
- *Manganese* – 2 to 10 mcg/kg/day.
- *Zinc –*
  - *Full-term infants and children:* 100 mcg/kg/day.
  - *Preterm infants (birth weight less than 1,500 g) up to 3 kg in body weight:* 300 mcg/kg/day.

➤*Preparation for administration:* Aseptic addition of the solution to the TPN solution under a laminar flow hood is recommended.

➤*Administration: Trace Elements 4 Pediatric* should only be administered after dilution to a minimum of 1:200.

4 Trace Elements solution is administered IV only after dilution.

➤*Admixture compatibility:* The trace elements present in the solution are physically compatible with the electrolytes and vitamins usually present in the amino acid/dextrose solution used for TPN.

Do not use syringes, needles, or IV sets containing aluminum parts that may come in contact with trace elements solution, for preparation or administration. Aluminum reacts and dissolves in acid media.

Intravenous Replenishment Solutions

COMBINED ELECTROLYTE SOLUTIONS

Electrolyte content given in mEq/L.

	Product and distributor	Na^+	K^+	Ca^{++}	Mg^{++}	Cl^-	Lactate	Acetate	Gluconate	Phosphate	Osmolarity (mOsm/L)	How supplied
Rx	**Normosol-M**[a] (Abbott)	40	13		3	40		16			109	In 1000 mL single-dose container.
Rx	**Ringer's Injection** (Various, eg, Abbott, Baxter, B. Braun)	≈ 147	4	≈ 4		≈ 156					≈ 310	In 500 and 1000 mL.
Rx	**Lactated Ringer's Injection** (Various, eg, Abbott, Baxter, B. Braun)	130	4	≈ 3		≈ 109	28				≈ 274	In 250, 500, and 1000 mL.
Rx	**Plasma-Lyte R**[b] (Baxter)	140	10	5	3	103	8	47			312	In 1000 mL.
Rx	**Isolyte S pH 7.4** (B. Braun)	141	5		3	98		27	23	1	295	Preservative free. In 500 and 1000 mL.
Rx	**Normosol-R**[c] (Hospira)	140	5		3	98		27	23		294	Preservative free. In 500 and 1000 mL single-dose containers.
Rx	**Normosol-R pH 7.4** (Abbott)										295	Preservative free. In 500 and 1000 mL single-dose containers.
Rx	**Plasma-Lyte 148**[b] (Baxter)										294	In 500 and 1000 mL.
Rx	**Plasma-Lyte A pH 7.4** (Baxter)										294	In 500 and 1000 mL.
Rx	**Potassium Chloride in 0.9% Sodium Chloride Injection** (Various, eg, Baxter, B. Braun)	154	20			174					≈ 350	In 1000 mL.
		154	40			194					≈ 390	In 1000 mL.

[a] pH ≈ 6.
[b] pH ≈ 5.5.
[c] pH ≈ 6.6.

COMBINED ELECTROLYTE SOLUTIONS — INTRAVENOUS

For additional information, refer to the Dietary Reference Intakes of Vitamins and Minerals table.

Indications

➤*Hydration:* For use in adults and children as a source of electrolytes and water for hydration. Additives to the solutions may help prevent certain electrolyte deficiencies in patients receiving prolonged parenteral fluid therapy (eg, magnesium) or act as alkalinizing agents.

➤*Extracellular fluid volume loss: Normosol-R* and *Normosol R pH 7.4* are indicated for replacement of acute extracellular fluid volume losses in surgery, trauma, burns, or shock. Both can be used as adjunctive therapy to restore decreased circulatory volume in patients with moderate blood loss.

➤*Transfusions: Normosol-R pH 7.4* also is indicated for use in starting blood (eg, as a priming solution for infusion sets) or as a diluent in packed red blood cell transfusions.

COMBINED ELECTROLYTE CONCENTRATES

Electrolyte content given in mEq/20 mL or mEq/25 mL after dilution.

	Product and distributor	Na^+	K^+	Ca^{++}	Mg^{++}	Cl^-	Acetate	Gluconate	Osmolarity (mOsm/L)	How supplied
Rx	**Lypholyte**[a] (American Pharmaceutical Partners)	25	≈ 40	5	8	≈ 33	≈ 41	5	≈ 7562	In 20 and 40 mL single-dose vials, and 100 and 200 mL *Maxivials*.[b]
Rx	**Multilyte-40**[c] (American Pharmaceutical Partners)								≈ 6015	In 25 mL single-dose vials.
Rx	**Nutrilyte**[a] (American Regent)								≈ 7562	In 20 mL single-dose vials and 100 mL.[b]
Rx	**Lypholyte-II**[a] (American Pharmaceutical Partners)	35	20	4.5	5	35	29.5		≈ 6200	In 20 and 40 mL single-dose vials and 100 and 200 mL *Maxivials*[b].
Rx	**TPN Electrolytes**[a] (Hospira)	35	20	4.5	5	35	29.5		6220	In 100 mL vials.[b]
Rx	**Nutrilyte II**[a] (American Regent)	35	20	4.5	5	35	29.5		≈ 6212	In 20 mL single-dose vials and 100 mL vials.[b]

Intravenous Replenishment Solutions

COMBINED ELECTROLYTE CONCENTRATES

	Product and distributor	Na^+	K^+	Ca^{++}	Mg^{++}	Cl^-	Acetate	Gluconate	Osmolarity (mOsm/L)	How supplied
Rx	**TPN Electrolytes II**[a] (Hospira)	18	18	4.5	5	35	10.5		4320	In 20 mL single-dose and additive syringes.
Rx	**TPN Electrolytes III**[a] (Hospira)	25	40.6	5	8	33.5	40.6	5	7520	In 100 mL vials.[b]
Rx	**Hyperlyte CR**[a] (B. Braun)	25	20	5	5	30	30		5500	In 250 mL *Super-Vials*.[b]
Rx	**Multilyte-20**[c] (American Pharmaceutical Partners)	25	20	5	5	30	25		≈ 4205	In 25 mL single-dose vials.

[a] In mEq/20 mL.
[b] Pharmacy bulk packaging.
[c] In mEq/25 mL.

For additional information, refer to the Dietary Reference Intakes of Vitamins and Minerals table.

COMBINED ELECTROLYTE CONCENTRATES — INTRAVENOUS

Indications

➤*Parenteral nutrition:* To facilitate amino acid utilization and maintain electrolyte balance in adults receiving parenteral nutritional solutions containing amino acids, dextrose, and other sources of calories administered by central or peripheral venous infusion. Also indicated for electrolyte replacement in adult parenteral therapy patients.

Administration and Dosage

➤*General dosing considerations:* These concentrated solutions are not for direct infusion. They are for prescription compounding of IV admixtures only. Dilute to appropriate strength with suitable IV fluid prior to administration.

Osmolarity is based on the concentrate.

➤*Adults:*

Parenteral nutrition – 20 to 25 mL added to 1 L of amino acid/dextrose solution (TPN).

➤*Children:* Not intended for use in children.

➤*Preparation for administration:* These concentrated solutions are not for direct infusion. Add to 1 L of amino acid/dextrose solution (TPN).

➤*Administration:* Not for direct infusion. For prescription compounding of IV admixtures only. Administer by central or peripheral venous infusion after diluting to appropriate strength.

➤*Storage/Stability:* Store at 15° to 30°C (59° to 86°F).

DEXTROSE-ELECTROLYTE SOLUTIONS

Electrolyte content given in mEq/L.

	Product and distributor	Dextrose (g/L)	Calories (Cal/L)	Na^+	K^+	Ca^{++}	Mg^{++}	Cl^-	Phosphate	Lactate	Acetate	Gluconate	Osmolarity (mOsm/L)	How supplied
Rx	**Ionosol-T and 5% Dextrose Injection** (Hospira)	50		40	35			40	15[a]	20			432	In 500 and 1,000 mL.
Rx	**Ionosol B and 5% Dextrose Injection** (Hospira)	50		57	25		5	49	7[a]	25			426	In 500 and 1,000 mL single-dose containers.
Rx	**Dextrose 2.5% with 0.45% Sodium Chloride** (Various, eg, Abbott, Baxter, B. Braun)	25	85	77				77					280	In 500 and 1000 mL.
Rx	**Dextrose 3.3% and 0.3% Sodium Chloride** (B. Braun)	33	110	51				51					270	In 250, 500, and 1000 mL.
Rx	**Dextrose 5% with 0.2% Sodium Chloride** (Various, eg, Baxter, B. Braun)	50	170	34				34					≈ 320	In 250, 500, and 1000 mL.
Rx	**Dextrose 5% and 0.225% Sodium Chloride** (Hospira)	50	170	38.5				38.5					329	In 250, 500, and 1000 mL.
Rx	**Dextrose 5% with 0.3% Sodium Chloride** (Hospira)	50	170	51				51					355	In 250, 500, and 1000 mL.
Rx	**Dextrose 5% with 0.33% Sodium Chloride** (Various, eg, Baxter, B. Braun)	50	170	56				56					365	In 250, 500, and 1000 mL.
Rx	**Dextrose 5% with 0.45% Sodium Chloride** (Various, eg, Hospira, Baxter, B. Braun)	50	170	77				77					≈ 405	In 250, 500, and 1000 mL.
Rx	**Dextrose 5% with 0.9% Sodium Chloride** (Various, eg, Hospira, Baxter, B. Braun)	50	170	154				154					≈ 560	In 250, 500, and 1000 mL.
Rx	**Dextrose 10% with 0.2% Sodium Chloride** (Various, eg, B. Braun)	100	340	34				34					575	In 250 mL.
Rx	**Dextrose 10% with 0.225% Sodium Chloride** (Abbott)	100	340	38.5				38.5					582	In 250 and 500 mL.
Rx	**Dextrose 10% with 0.45% Sodium Chloride** (B. Braun)	100	340	77				77					660	In 1000 mL.
Rx	**Dextrose 10% and 0.9% Sodium Chloride** (Various, eg, Baxter, B. Braun)	100	340	154				154					813-815	In 500 and 1000 mL.
Rx	**Potassium Chloride in 5% Dextrose and Lactated Ringer's** (Baxter)	50	170	130	24	3		129		28			565	In 1000 mL.
		50	170	130	44	3		149		28			605	In 1000 mL.
Rx	**Potassium Chloride in 5% Dextrose and Lactated Ringer's** (Hospira)	50	179	130	24	2.7		129		28			563	In 1000 mL.
		50	179	130	44	2.7		149		28			604	In 1000 mL.
Rx	**Potassium Chloride in 5% Dextrose** (Various, eg, Baxter, B. Braun, Hospira)	50	170		10			10					≈ 272	In 1000 mL.
		50	170		20			20					292-295	In 1000 mL.
		50	170		30			30					310-312	In 1000 mL.
		50	170		40			40					330-333	In 500 and 1000 mL.
Rx	**Potassium Chloride in 3.3% Dextrose and 0.3% Sodium Chloride** (B. Braun)	33	110	51	20			71					310	In 1000 mL.

DEXTROSE-ELECTROLYTE SOLUTIONS

	Product and distributor	Dextrose (g/L)	Calories (Cal/L)	Na^+	K^+	Ca^{++}	Mg^{++}	Cl^-	Phosphate	Lactate	Acetate	Gluconate	Osmolarity (mOsm/L)	How supplied
Rx	**Potassium Chloride in 5% Dextrose and 0.2% Sodium Chloride** (Various, eg, Baxter, B. Braun)	50	170	34	10			44					≈ 340	In 1000 mL.
		50	170	34	20			54					≈ 360	In 250, 500, and 1000 mL.
		50	170	34	30			64					≈ 380	In 1000 mL.
		50	170	34	40			74					≈ 400	In 1000 mL.
Rx	**Potassium Chloride in 5% Dextrose and 0.33% Sodium Chloride** (Various, eg, Baxter, B. Braun)	50	170	56	20			76					405	In 500 and 1000 mL.
		50	170	56	30			86					425	In 1000 mL.
		50	170	56	40			96					446	In 1000 mL.
Rx	**Potassium Chloride in 5% Dextrose and 0.45% Sodium Chloride** (Various, eg, Baxter, B. Braun)	50	170	77	10			87					≈ 425	In 1000 mL.
		50	170	77	20			97					445-447	In 500 and 1000 mL.
		50	170	77	30			107					≈ 465	In 1000 mL.
		50	170	77	40			117					487-490	In 1000 mL.
Rx	**Potassium Chloride in 5% Dextrose and 0.9% Sodium Chloride** (Various, eg, Baxter, B. Braun)	50	170	154	20			174					≈ 600	In 1000 mL.
		50	170	154	40			194					≈ 640	In 1000 mL.
Rx	**Potassium Chloride in 10% Dextrose and 0.2% Sodium Chloride** (B. Braun)	100	340	34	20			54					615	In 250 mL.
Rx	**Dextrose 5% and Electrolyte No. 75** (Baxter)	50	180	40	35			48	15	20			402	In 250, 500, and 1000 mL.
Rx	**Isolyte M in 5% Dextrose** (B. Braun)	50	170	36	35			49	15		20		390	In 500 and 1000 mL
Rx	**Ringer's in 5% Dextrose** (Various, eg, Abbott, Baxter, B. Braun)	50	170	≈147	4	≈4.5		≈156					≈560	In 500 and 1000 mL.
Rx	**Half-Strength Lactated Ringer's in 2.5% Dextrose** (Various, eg, Abbott, Baxter, B. Braun)	25	85-89	≈65.5	2	≈1.5		≈55		14			≈264	In 250, 500, and 1000 mL.
Rx	**Lactated Ringer's in 5% Dextrose** (Various, eg, Abbott, Baxter, B. Braun)	50	170	130	4	≈ 3		109-112		28			525-530	In 250, 500, and 1000 mL.
Rx	**Dextrose 5% and Electrolyte No. 48** (Baxter)	50	180	25	20		3	24	3	23			348	In 250 mL.
Rx	**Isolyte H in 5% Dextrose** (B. Braun)	50	170	39	13		3	44			16		360	In 1000 mL.
Rx	**Normosol-M and 5% Dextrose** (Hospira)	50	170	40	13		3	40			16		363	In 500 and 1000 mL.
Rx	**Plasma-Lyte 56 and 5% Dextrose** (Baxter)													In 500 and 1000 mL.
Rx	**Isolyte P in 5% Dextrose** (B. Braun)	50	170	23	20		3	29	3		23		340	In 250, 500, and 1000 mL.
Rx	**Isolyte S with 5% Dextrose** (B. Braun)	50	170	140	5		3	106			27	23	550	In 1000 mL.
Rx	**Normosol-R and 5% Dextrose** (Abbott)	50	185	140	5		3	98			27	23	547	In 500 and 1000 mL.
Rx	**Plasma-Lyte 148 and 5% Dextrose** (Baxter)	50	190	140	5		3	98			27	23	547	In 500 and 1000 mL.
Rx	**Dextrose 10% and Electrolyte No. 48** (Baxter)	100	350	25	20		3	24	3	23			600	In 250 mL.[b]
Rx	**Isolyte R in 5% Dextrose** (B. Braun)	50	170	39	16	5	3	46			24		375	In 1000 mL.
Rx	**Plasma-Lyte M and 5% Dextrose** (Baxter)	50	180	40	16	5	3	40		12	12		377	In 500 and 1000 mL.
Rx	**Plasma-Lyte R and 5% Dextrose** (Baxter)	50	180	140	10	5	3	103		8	47		564	In 1000 mL.[b]

[a] Millimoles per liter.

[b] With sodium bisulfite.

DEXTROSE-ELECTROLYTE SOLUTIONS — INJECTION

For additional information, refer to the Dietary Reference Intakes of Vitamins and Minerals table.

Indications

➤*Parenteral nutrition:* For use as a parenteral source of electrolytes, calories, or water for hydration.

➤*Alkalinizing agent:* For use as an alkalinizing agent.

INVERT SUGAR-ELECTROLYTE SOLUTIONS

Electrolyte content given in mEq/L.

	Product and distributor	Invert Sugar (g/L)	Calories (Cal/L)	Na+	K+	Mg++	Cl-	Phosphate	Lactate	Osmolarity (mOsm/L)	How supplied
Rx	**Multiple Electrolytes and 5% Travert** (Baxter)	50	196	56	25	6	56	12.5	25	449	In 1000 mL.[a]
Rx	**Multiple Electrolytes and 10% Travert** (Baxter)	100	384	56	25	6	56	12.5	25	726	In 1000 mL.[a]

[a] With sodium 5 mEq/L sodium bisulfite.

INVERT SUGAR-ELECTROLYTE SOLUTIONS — INTRAVENOUS

Refer to dextrose monograph for further information. For additional information, refer to the Dietary Reference Intakes of Vitamins and Minerals table.

Indications

➤*Parenteral nutrition:* Used as a source of calories and hydration. Invert sugar is composed of equal parts of dextrose and fructose and shares the same actions and caloric value. Any supposed advantage of using invert sugar solutions would be from the fructose component.

Erythropoiesis-Stimulating Agents

EPOETIN ALFA, RECOMBINANT (Erythropoietin; EPO)

Rx	**Epogen** (Amgen)	**Injection, solution**: 2,000 units/mL	In 1 mL single-dose vials.[a]
Rx	**Procrit** (Ortho Biotech)		In 1 mL single-dose vials.[a]
Rx	**Epogen** (Amgen)	**Injection, solution**: 3,000 units/mL	In 1 mL single-dose vials.[a]
Rx	**Procrit** (Ortho Biotech)		In 1 mL single-dose vials.[a]
Rx	**Epogen** (Amgen)	**Injection, solution**: 4,000 units/mL	In 1 mL single-dose vials.[a]
Rx	**Procrit** (Ortho Biotech)		In 1 mL single-dose vials.[a]
Rx	**Epogen** (Amgen)	**Injection, solution**: 10,000 units/mL	In 1 mL single-dose vials[a] and 2 mL multidose vials.[b]
Rx	**Procrit** (Ortho Biotech)		In 1 mL single-dose vials[a] and 2 mL multidose vials.[b]
Rx	**Epogen** (Amgen)	**Injection, solution**: 20,000 units/mL	In 1 mL multidose vials.[b]
Rx	**Procrit** (Ortho Biotech)		In 1 mL multidose vials.[b]
Rx	**Procrit** (Ortho Biotech)	**Injection, solution**: 40,000 units/mL	In 1 mL single-dose vials.[a]

[a] Preservative free. Also contains albumin (human) 2.5 mg/mL.

[b] Preserved with benzyl alcohol 1%. Also contains albumin (human) 2.5 mg/mL.

EPOETIN ALFA RECOMBINANT — INJECTION

WARNING

Increased mortality, serious cardiovascular and thromboembolic events, and increased risk of tumor progression or recurrence –

Renal failure: Patients experienced greater risks for death and serious cardiovascular (CV) events when administered erythropoiesis-stimulating agents (ESAs) to target higher versus lower hemoglobin levels (13.5 vs 11.3 g/dL; 14 vs 10 g/dL) in 2 clinical studies. Individualize dosing to achieve and maintain hemoglobin levels within the range of 10 to 12 g/dL.

Cancer:
- ESAs shortened overall survival and/or increased the risk of tumor progression or recurrence in some clinical studies in patients with breast, non–small cell lung, head and neck, lymphoid, and cervical cancers.
- To decrease these risks, as well as the risk of serious CV and thrombovascular events, use the lowest dose needed to avoid red blood cell (RBC) transfusions.
- Use ESAs only for treatment of anemia caused by concomitant myelosuppressive chemotherapy.
- ESAs are not indicated for patients receiving myelosuppressive therapy when the anticipated outcome is cure.
- Discontinue following the completion of a chemotherapy course.

Perisurgery: Epoetin alfa increased the rate of deep venous thromboses in patients not receiving prophylactic anticoagulation. Consider deep venous thrombosis prophylaxis.

See also Warnings/Precautions, Indications, and Administration and Dosage for more information.

Indications

➤*Anemia in cancer patients on chemotherapy:* For the treatment of anemia caused by the effect of coadministered chemotherapy based on studies that have shown a reduction in the need for RBC transfusions in patients with metastatic, nonmyeloid malignancies receiving chemotherapy for a minimum of 2 months. Studies to determine whether epoetin alfa increases mortality or decreases progression-free/recurrence-free survival are ongoing.

Epoetin alfa is not indicated for patients receiving myelosuppressive therapy when the anticipated outcome is cure because of the absence of studies that adequately characterize the impact of epoetin alfa on progression-free and overall survival.

➤*Anemia in chronic renal failure patients:* For the treatment of anemia associated with chronic renal failure (CRF), including patients on dialysis (end-stage renal disease) and patients not on dialysis. To elevate or maintain the RBC level (as manifested by hematocrit or hemoglobin determinations) and to decrease the need for transfusions in these patients.

Nondialysis patients with symptomatic anemia considered for therapy should have a hemoglobin of less than 10 g/dL.

➤*Anemia in zidovudine-treated, HIV-infected patients:* For the treatment of anemia related to therapy with zidovudine in HIV-infected patients. To elevate or maintain the RBC level (as manifested by hematocrit or hemoglobin determinations) and to decrease the need for transfusions in these patients.

➤*Reduction of allogeneic blood transfusion in surgery patients:* For the treatment of anemic patients (hemoglobin of more than 10 to less than or equal to 13 g/dL) who are at high risk for perioperative blood loss from elective, noncardiac, nonvascular surgery to reduce the need for allogeneic blood transfusions.

➤*Off-label uses:*

Uremic pruritus – [4] = Insufficient documentation. Data regarding epoetin in the treatment of uremic pruritus are limited. In addition, pruritus improvement in one study may have been related to increases in mean hemoglobin rather than decreases in plasma histamine levels. Thus, further larger, controlled trials are needed before this drug can be recommended for the treatment of uremic pruritus.

Other possible off-label uses – Anemia associated with critically ill patients, congestive heart failure (CHF), chronic disease (eg, rheumatoid arthritis), postpartum anemia, sickle cell disease, thalassemia, multiple myeloma, Jehovah's witnesses, radiation treatment, epidermolysis bullosa, porphyria; for athletic enhancement, sexual dysfunction, and transfusional iron overload.

Administration and Dosage

➤*General dosing considerations:* Epoetin alfa dosing regimens are different for each of the indications described in this section.

Individually titrate to achieve and maintain hemoglobin levels between 10 and 12 g/dL. (See also Monitoring in Warnings/Precautions.)

Iron evaluation and supplementation – Prior to and during epoetin alfa therapy, evaluate the patient's iron status, including transferrin saturation (serum iron divided by iron-binding capacity) and serum ferritin. Virtually all patients will eventually require supplemental iron to increase or maintain transferrin saturation to levels that will adequately support erythropoiesis stimulated by epoetin alfa. Provide all surgery patients with adequate iron supplementation throughout the course of therapy.

➤*Adults:*

Anemia in cancer patients on chemotherapy – Although no specific serum erythropoietin level has been established that predicts which patients would be unlikely to respond to epoetin alfa therapy, treatment of patients with grossly elevated serum erythropoietin levels (eg, more than 200 milliunits/mL) is not recommended.

Hemoglobin should be monitored on a weekly basis in patients receiving epoetin alfa therapy until hemoglobin becomes stable. The dose of epoetin alfa should be titrated for each patient to achieve and maintain the lowest hemoglobin level sufficient to avoid the need for blood transfusion. Do not initiate therapy at hemoglobin levels of 10 g/dL or higher.

Initial dosage: 150 units/kg subcutaneously 3 times per week or 40,000 units subcutaneously weekly.

Dosage adjustment:

Epoetin Alfa Dosage Guidelines for Adult Cancer Patients on Chemotherapy	
Starting dose:	150 units/kg subcutaneously 3 times per week or 40,000 units subcutaneously once weekly
Reduce dose by 25% when:	Hemoglobin reaches a level needed to avoid transfusion or increases > 1 g/dL in any 2-week period.
Withhold dose if:	Hemoglobin exceeds a level needed to avoid transfusion. Restart at 25% below the previous dose when hemoglobin approaches a level for which transfusions may be required.
Increase dose if:	
3-times-per-week dosing: Increase dosage to 300 units/kg 3 times per week if:	Response is not satisfactory (no reduction in transfusion requirements or rise in hemoglobin) after 4 weeks to achieve and maintain the lowest hemoglobin level sufficient to avoid the need for RBC transfusion.
Weekly dosing: Increase to 60,000 units subcutaneously weekly:	Response is not satisfactory (no increase in hemoglobin by ≥ 1 g/dL after 4 weeks of therapy, in the absence of an RBC transfusion) to achieve and maintain the lowest hemoglobin level sufficient to avoid the need for RBC transfusion.
Discontinue:	If after 8 weeks of therapy, there is no response as measured by hemoglobin levels or if transfusions are still required.

Discontinuation of therapy: Discontinue epoetin alfa if after 8 weeks of therapy there is no response as measured by hemoglobin levels or if transfusions are still required. Discontinue epoetin alfa following completion of a chemotherapy course.

EPOETIN ALFA RECOMBINANT — INJECTION

Anemia in chronic renal failure patients – Individualize dosage to achieve and maintain hemoglobin levels between 10 and 12 g/dL. The dose of epoetin alfa should be reduced as the hemoglobin approaches 12 g/dL or increases by more than 1 g/dL in any 2-week period. If hemoglobin excursions outside the recommended range occur, the epoetin alfa dose should be adjusted as described in the following table.

During therapy, hematologic parameters should be monitored regularly.

Epoetin Alfa Dosage Guidelines for Adults With CRF	
Starting dose:	50 to 100 units/kg 3 times per week given IV[a] or subcutaneously. IV route is recommended in patients on hemodialysis.
Increase dose by 25% if:	Hemoglobin is < 10 g/dL and has not increased by 1 g/dL after 4 weeks of therapy or hemoglobin decreases below 10 g/dL.
Reduce dose by 25% when:	Hemoglobin approaches 12 g/dL or hemoglobin increases by > 1 g/dL in any 2-week period.

[a] IV = intravenous.

Maintenance dosage: The maintenance dose must be individualized for each patient on dialysis.

• *Adults not on dialysis* – In adult patients with CRF not on dialysis, the dose should be individualized to maintain hemoglobin levels between 10 and 12 g/dL. Epoetin alfa dosages of 75 to 150 units/kg/week have been shown to maintain hematocrits of 36% to 38% for up to 6 months.

• *Adults on hemodialysis* – In the US, phase 3, multicenter trial in patients on hemodialysis, the median dosage was 75 units/kg 3 times per week, with a range of 12.5 to 525 units/kg 3 times/week. Almost 10% of patients required a dose of 25 units/kg or less, and approximately 10% of patients required more than 200 units/kg 3 times per week to maintain their hematocrit in the suggested target range.

Dosage adjustment: Increases in dose should not be made more frequently than once a month. If the hemoglobin is increasing and approaching 12 g/dL, the dose should be reduced by approximately 25%. If the hemoglobin continues to increase, the dose should be temporarily withheld until the hemoglobin begins to decrease, at which point therapy should be reinitiated at a dose approximately 25% below the previous dose. If the hemoglobin increases by more than 1 g/dL in a 2-week period, the dose should be decreased by approximately 25%.

If the increase in the hemoglobin is less than 1 g/dL over 4 weeks and iron stores are adequate, the dose of epoetin alfa may be increased by approximately 25% of the previous dose. Further increases may be made at 4-week intervals until the specified hemoglobin is obtained.

If the transferrin saturation is more than 20%, the dose of epoetin alfa may be increased. Such dose increases should not be made more frequently than once a month, unless clinically indicated, because the response time of the hemoglobin to a dose increase can be 2 to 6 weeks. Hemoglobin should be measured twice weekly for 2 to 6 weeks following dose increases.

For patients whose hemoglobin does not attain a level within the range of 10 to 12 g/dL despite the use of appropriate epoetin alfa dose titrations over a 12-week period:

- do not administer higher epoetin alfa doses and use the lowest dose that will maintain a hemoglobin level sufficient to avoid the need for recurrent RBC transfusions,
- evaluate and treat for other causes of anemia, and
- thereafter, hemoglobin should continue to be monitored and, if responsiveness improves, epoetin alfa dose adjustments should be made as described in the previous table; discontinue epoetin alfa if responsiveness does not improve and the patient needs recurrent RBC transfusions.

Concomitant therapy: If the transferrin saturation is less than 20%, supplemental iron should be administered.

Anemia in zidovudine-treated, HIV-infected patients – Prior to beginning epoetin alfa, it is recommended that the endogenous serum erythropoietin level be determined (prior to transfusion). Available evidence suggests that patients receiving zidovudine with endogenous serum erythropoietin levels of more than 500 milliunits/mL are unlikely to respond to therapy with epoetin alfa. The dose of epoetin alfa should be titrated for each patient to achieve and maintain the lowest hemoglobin level sufficient to avoid the need for blood transfusion, not to exceed 12 g/dL.

Initial dosage: For adult patients with serum erythropoietin levels of 500 milliunits/mL or less who are receiving a dose of zidovudine 4,200 mg/week or less, the recommended starting dose of epoetin alfa is 100 units/kg as an IV or subcutaneous injection 3 times per week for 8 weeks.

Dosage titration: During the dose adjustment phase of therapy, the hemoglobin should be monitored weekly. If the response is not satisfactory in terms of reducing transfusion requirements or increasing hemoglobin after 8 weeks of therapy, the dosage of epoetin alfa can be increased by 50 to 100 units/kg 3 times per week. Response should be evaluated every 4 to 8 weeks thereafter and the dose adjusted accordingly by 50 to 100 units/kg increments 3 times per week. If patients have not responded satisfactorily to an epoetin alfa dosage of 300 units/kg 3 times per week, it is unlikely that they will respond to higher doses of epoetin alfa.

Maintenance dosage: After attainment of the desired response (ie, reduced transfusion requirements, increased hemoglobin), the dose of epoetin alfa should be titrated to maintain the response based on factors such as variations in the zidovudine dose and the presence of intercurrent infectious or inflammatory episodes. If the hemoglobin exceeds 12 g/dL, the dose should be discontinued until the hemoglobin drops below 11 g/dL. The dose should be reduced by 25% when treatment is resumed and then titrated to maintain the desired hemoglobin.

Reduction of allogeneic blood transfusion in surgery patients – Prior to initiating treatment with epoetin alfa, a hemoglobin should be obtained to establish that it is more than 10 to less than or equal to 13 g/dL.

Usual dosage: 300 units/kg/day subcutaneously for 10 days before surgery, on the day of surgery, and for 4 days after surgery.

Alternative dosage: 600 units/kg subcutaneously in once-weekly doses (21, 14, and 7 days before surgery), plus a fourth dose on the day of surgery.

Concomitant therapy: All patients should receive adequate iron supplementation. Iron supplementation should be initiated no later than the beginning of treatment with epoetin alfa and should continue throughout the course of therapy. Strongly consider deep venous thrombosis prophylaxis.

Off-label dosing –

Uremic pruritus: [4] = Insufficient documentation. Initial dosage of 36 units/kg 3 times per week at the end of the dialysis session. The dosage is reduced to 18 units/kg 3 times per week once hematocrit reaches or exceeds 30%.

➤*Children:*

Anemia in cancer patients on chemotherapy – See Adults for more information.

In a randomized, double-blind, placebo-controlled, multicenter study in anemic children 5 to 18 years of age receiving chemotherapy for the treatment of various childhood malignancies, there was no evidence of an improvement in health-related quality of life, including no evidence of an effect on fatigue, energy, or strength in patients receiving epoetin alfa compared with those receiving placebo.

5 years of age and older:

• *Maximum dose* – 60,000 units weekly.

• *Initial dosage* – 600 units/kg IV weekly.

• *Dosage adjustment* –

Epoetin Alfa Dosage Guidelines for Children With Cancer on Chemotherapy	
Starting dose:	600 units/kg IV weekly (maximum, 40,000 units)
Reduce dose by 25% when:	Hemoglobin reaches a level needed to avoid transfusion or increases > 1 g/dL in any 2 weeks.
Withhold dose if:	Hemoglobin exceeds a level needed to avoid transfusion and restart at 25% below the previous dose when the hemoglobin approaches a level for which transfusions may be required.
Increase dose to 900 units/kg IV (maximum, 60,000 units) if:	Response is not satisfactory (no increase in hemoglobin by ≥ 1 g/dL after 4 weeks of therapy, in the absence of a RBC transfusion) to achieve and maintain the lowest hemoglobin level sufficient to avoid the need for RBC transfusion.
Discontinue:	If after 8 weeks of therapy, there is no response as measured by hemoglobin levels or if transfusions are still required.

• *Discontinuation of therapy* – Discontinue epoetin alfa if after 8 weeks of therapy there is no response, as measured by hemoglobin levels, or if transfusions are still required. Discontinue epoetin alfa following completion of a chemotherapy course.

Anemia in chronic renal failure patients – See Adults for more information.

1 month and older (on dialysis) or 3 months and older (not on dialysis):

Epoetin Alfa Dosage Guidelines for Children With CRF	
Starting dose:	50 units/kg 3 times a week given IV or subcutaneously. (IV route is recommended in patients on hemodialysis.)
Increase dose by 25% if:	Hemoglobin is < 10 g/dL and has not increased by 1 g/dL after 4 weeks of therapy or hemoglobin decreases below 10 g/dL.
Reduce dose by 25% when:	Hemoglobin approaches 12 g/dL or hemoglobin increases by >1 g/dL in any 2-week period.

• *Maintenance dosage* – The maintenance dose must be individualized for each patient on dialysis. In pediatric hemodialysis and peritoneal dialysis patients, the median maintenance dosage was 167 units/kg/week (49 to 447 units/kg/week) and 76 units/kg per week (24 to 323 units/kg/week) administered in divided doses (3 times per week or twice per week), respectively, to achieve the target range of 30% to 36%.

• *Dosage adjustment* – See Adults for more information.

• *Concomitant therapy* – See Adults for more information.

If the transferrin saturation is less than 20%, supplemental iron should be administered.

Anemia in zidovudine-treated, HIV-infected patients – See Adults for more information.

EPOETIN ALFA RECOMBINANT — INJECTION

8 months of age and older: Published literature has reported the use of epoetin alfa in 20 zidovudine-treated, anemic, HIV-infected children 8 months to 17 years of age treated with 50 to 400 units/kg subcutaneously or IV, 2 to 3 times per week. Increases in hemoglobin levels and reticulocyte counts and decreases in or elimination of blood transfusions were observed.

➤*Elderly:* Individualize dose selection and adjustment for an elderly patient to achieve and maintain the target hematocrit.

See Adults for dosing.

➤*Preparation for administration:*

1.) Do not shake. It is not necessary to shake epoetin alfa. Prolonged vigorous shaking may denature any glycoprotein, rendering it biologically inactive.
2.) Protect the solution from light.
3.) Using aseptic techniques, attach a sterile needle to a sterile syringe. Remove the flip top from the vial containing epoetin alfa and wipe the septum with a disinfectant. Insert the needle into the vial and withdraw into the syringe an appropriate volume of solution.
4.) Do not dilute or administer in conjunction with other drug solutions. However, at the time of subcutaneous administration, preservative-free epoetin alfa from single-use vials may be admixed in a syringe with bacteriostatic sodium chloride 0.9% injection with benzyl alcohol 0.9% (bacteriostatic saline) at a 1:1 ratio using aseptic technique. The benzyl alcohol in the bacteriostatic saline acts as a local anesthetic, which may ameliorate the subcutaneous injection-site discomfort. Admixing is not necessary when using the multidose vials of epoetin alfa containing benzyl alcohol.

➤*Administration:* Epoetin alfa may be given as an IV or subcutaneous injection. In patients on hemodialysis, the IV route is recommended. While the administration of epoetin alfa is independent of the dialysis procedure, epoetin alfa may be administered into the venous line at the end of the dialysis procedure to obviate the need for additional venous access.

Patients who have been judged competent by their health care provider to self-administer epoetin alfa without medical or other supervision may give themselves an IV or subcutaneous injection.

➤*Admixture compatibility:* Do not dilute or administer in conjunction with other drug solutions. However, at the time of subcutaneous administration, preservative-free epoetin alfa from single-use vials may be admixed in a syringe with bacteriostatic sodium chloride 0.9% injection with benzyl alcohol 0.9% (bacteriostatic saline) at a 1:1 ratio.

➤*Storage/Stability:* Store at 2° to 8°C (36° to 46°F). Do not freeze or shake. Protect from light. Store multidose vials at 2° to 8°C (36° to 46°F) after initial entry and between doses. Discard 21 days after initial entry.

Actions

➤*Pharmacology:* Erythropoietin is a glycoprotein that stimulates RBC production. It is produced in the kidney and stimulates the division and differentiation of committed erythroid progenitors in the bone marrow. Epoetin alfa, a 165 amino acid glycoprotein manufactured by recombinant DNA technology, has the same biological effects as endogenous erythropoietin. It has a molecular weight of 30,400 daltons and is produced by mammalian cells into which the human erythropoietin gene has been introduced. The product contains the identical amino acid sequence of isolated natural erythropoietin.

Endogenous production of erythropoietin is normally regulated by the level of tissue oxygenation. Hypoxia and anemia generally increase the production of erythropoietin, which in turn stimulates erythropoiesis. In healthy subjects, plasma erythropoietin levels range from 0.01 to 0.03 units/mL and increase up to 100- to 1,000-fold during hypoxia or anemia. In contrast, in patients with CRF, production of erythropoietin is impaired, and this erythropoietin deficiency is the primary cause of their anemia.

➤*Pharmacokinetics:*

Absorption/Distribution – After subcutaneous administration, peak plasma levels are achieved within 5 to 24 hours.

A pharmacokinetic study comparing 150 units/kg subcutaneously 3 times/week with a dosing regimen of 40,000 units/week subcutaneously weekly was conducted for 4 weeks in healthy subjects (n = 12) and for 6 weeks in anemic cancer patients (n = 32) receiving cyclic chemotherapy. There was no accumulation of serum erythropoietin after the 2 dosing regimens during the study period. The 40,000 units weekly regimen had a higher maximum drug concentration (C_{max}) (3- to 7-fold), longer time to maximum concentration (T_{max}) (2- to 3-fold), higher area under the curve (AUC_{0-168h}) (2- to 3-fold) of erythropoietin, and lower clearance (50%) than the 150 units/kg 3 times/week regimen.

After the dosing of 150 units/kg 3 times/week, the values of T_{max} and clearance were similar (13.3 ± 12.4 vs 14.2 ± 6.7 hours; 20.2 ± 15.9 vs 23.6 ± 9.5 mL/h/kg) between week 1 when patients were receiving chemotherapy (n = 14) and week 3 when patients were not receiving chemotherapy (n = 4). Differences were observed after the dosing of 40,000 units weekly, with longer T_{max} (38 ± 18 hours) and lower clearance (9.2 ± 4.7 mL/h/kg) during week 1 when patients were receiving chemotherapy (n = 18), compared with those (22 ± 4.5 hours; 13.9 ± 7.6 mL/h/kg) during week 3 when patients were not receiving chemotherapy (n = 7).

Metabolism/Excretion – In adults and children with CRF, the elimination half-life of plasma erythropoietin after IV-administered epoetin alfa ranges from 4 to 13 hours. The half-life is approximately 20% longer in patients with CRF than in healthy subjects. The half-life is similar between adults with serum creatinine level greater than 3 and not on dialysis and those maintained on dialysis.

In anemic cancer patients, the average elimination half-life ($t_{1/2}$) was similar (40 hours; range, 16 to 67 hours) after both dosing regimens (150 units/kg subcutaneously 3 times/week or 40,000 units subcutaneously weekly).

Special populations –

Children: Limited data are available in neonates. A study of 7 preterm, very low birth weight neonates and 10 healthy adults given IV erythropoietin suggested that distribution volume was approximately 1.5 to 2 times higher in preterm neonates than in healthy adults, and clearance was approximately 3 times higher in preterm neonates than in healthy adults.

Contraindications

Uncontrolled hypertension; known hypersensitivity to mammalian cell-derived products; known hypersensitivity to albumin (human).

Warnings/Precautions

➤*Benzyl alcohol:* The multidose preserved formulation contains benzyl alcohol. Benzyl alcohol has been reported to be associated with an increased incidence of neurological and other complications in premature infants, which are sometimes fatal.

➤*Increased mortality, serious cardiovascular and thromboembolic reactions:*

Cancer patients – An increased incidence of thrombotic events has also been observed in patients with cancer treated with erythropoietic agents.

In a randomized, controlled study (referred to as the BEST study) with another ESA in 939 women with metastatic breast cancer receiving chemotherapy, patients received weekly epoetin alfa or placebo for up to a year. This study was designed to show that survival was superior when an ESA was administered to prevent anemia (maintain hemoglobin levels between 12 and 14 g/dL or hematocrit between 36% and 42%). The study was terminated prematurely when interim results demonstrated that a higher mortality at 4 months (8.7% vs 3.4%) and a higher rate of fatal thrombotic events (1.1% vs 0.2%) in the first 4 months of the study were observed among patients treated with epoetin alfa. Based on Kaplan-Meier estimates, at the time of study termination, the 12-month survival was lower in the epoetin alfa group than in the placebo group (70% vs 76%; hazard ratio [HR], 1.37; 95% confidence interval [CI], 1.07 to 1.75; $P = 0.012$).

Chronic renal failure patients – Patients with CRF experienced greater risk for death and serious CV reactions when administered ESAs to target higher versus lower hemoglobin levels (13.5 vs 11.3 g/dL; 14 vs 10 g/dL) in 2 clinical studies. Patients with CRF and an insufficient hemoglobin response to ESA therapy may be at even greater risk for CV events and mortality than other patients. Epoetin alfa and other ESAs increased the risks for death and serious CV events in controlled clinical trials of patients with cancer. These events included myocardial infarction (MI), stroke, CHF, and hemodialysis vascular access thrombosis. A rate of hemoglobin rise of more than 1 g/dL over 2 weeks may contribute to these risks.

During hemodialysis, patients treated with epoetin alfa may require increased anticoagulation with heparin to prevent clotting of the artificial kidney.

Other thrombotic events (eg, cerebrovascular accident, MI, transient ischemic attack) have occurred in clinical trials at an annualized rate of less than 0.04 events per patient-year of epoetin alfa therapy. These trials were conducted in patients with CRF (whether on dialysis or not) in whom the target hematocrit was 32% to 40%. However, the risk of thrombotic events, including vascular access thrombosis, was significantly increased in patients with ischemic heart disease or CHF receiving epoetin alfa therapy with the goal of reaching a healthy hematocrit (42%), compared with a target hematocrit of 30%. Closely monitor patients with preexisting CV disease.

Zidovudine-treated, HIV-infected patients – Epoetin alfa therapy has not been linked to exacerbation of thrombotic events in HIV-infected patients. However, the clinical data do not rule out an increased risk for serious CV events.

Surgery patients – An increased incidence of deep vein thrombosis in patients receiving epoetin alfa undergoing surgical orthopedic procedures has been observed. In a randomized, controlled study (referred to as the SPINE study), 681 adult patients not receiving prophylactic anticoagulation and undergoing spinal surgery received either 4 doses of epoetin alfa 600 units/kg (7, 14, and 21 days before surgery and the day of surgery) and standard of care treatment or standard of care treatment alone. Preliminary analysis showed a higher incidence of deep vein thrombosis, determined by color flow duplex imaging or clinical symptoms, in the epoetin alfa group (16 [4.7%] patients) compared with the standard of care group (7 [2.1%] patients). In addition, 12 patients in the epoetin alfa group and 7 patients in the standard of care group had other thrombotic vascular events. Strongly consider deep venous thrombosis prophylaxis when ESAs are used for the reduction of allogeneic RBC transfusions in surgical patients.

Increased mortality also was observed in a randomized, placebo-controlled study of epoetin alfa in adult patients who were undergoing coronary artery bypass surgery (7 deaths in 126 patients randomized to epoetin alfa vs no deaths among 56 patients receiving placebo). Four of these deaths occurred during the period of study drug administration, and all 4 deaths were associated with thrombotic events. ESAs are not approved for reduction of allogeneic RBC transfusions in patients scheduled for cardiac surgery.

➤*Increased mortality and/or increased risk of tumor progression or recurrence:* Erythropoiesis-stimulating agents resulted in decreased locoregional control/progression-free survival and/or overall survival. These findings were observed in studies of patients with advanced head and neck cancer receiving radiation therapy (cancer studies 5 and 6), in patients receiving chemotherapy for metastatic breast cancer (cancer study 1) or lymphoid malignancy (cancer study 2), and in patients with non–small cell lung

EPOETIN ALFA RECOMBINANT — INJECTION

cancer or various malignancies who were not receiving chemotherapy or radiotherapy (cancer studies 7 and 8).

Decreased overall survival – Mortality at 4 months (8.7% vs 3.4%) was significantly higher in the epoetin alfa arm in the cancer study 1 (the BEST study). The most common investigator-attributed cause of death within the first 4 months was disease progression; 28 of 41 deaths in the epoetin alfa arm and 13 of 16 deaths in the placebo arm were attributed to disease progression. Investigator-assessed time to tumor progression was not different between the 2 groups. Survival at 12 months was significantly lower in the epoetin alfa arm (70% vs 76%; HR, 1.37; 95% CI, 1.07 to 1.75; $P = 0.012$).

Cancer study 2 was a phase 3, double-blind, randomized (darbepoetin alfa vs placebo) study conducted in 344 anemic patients with lymphoid malignancy receiving chemotherapy. With a median follow-up of 29 months, overall mortality rates were significantly higher among patients randomized to darbepoetin alfa compared with placebo (HR, 1.36; 95% CI, 1.02 to 1.82).

Cancer study 7 was a phase 3, multicenter, randomized (epoetin alfa vs placebo), double-blind study in which patients with advanced non–small cell lung cancer receiving only palliative radiotherapy or no active therapy were treated with epoetin alfa to achieve and maintain hemoglobin levels between 12 and 14 g/dL. Following an interim analysis of 70 of 300 patients planned, a significant difference in survival in favor of the patients on the placebo arm of the trial was observed (median survival, 63 vs 129 days; HR, 1.84; $P = 0.04$).

Cancer study 8 was a phase 3, double-blind, randomized (darbepoetin alfa vs placebo), 16-week study in 989 anemic patients with active malignant disease, neither receiving nor planning to receive chemotherapy or radiation therapy. There was no evidence of a statistically significant reduction in proportion of patients receiving RBC transfusions. The median survival was shorter in the darbepoetin alfa treatment group (8 months) compared with the placebo group (10.8 months) (HR, 1.3; 95% CI, 1.07 to 1.57).

Decreased progression-free survival and overall survival – Cancer study 3 (the PREPARE study) was a randomized, controlled study in which darbepoetin alfa was administered to prevent anemia in 733 women receiving neoadjuvant breast cancer treatment. An interim analysis was performed after a median follow-up of approximately 3 years, at which time the survival rate was lower (86% vs 90%; HR, 1.42; 95% CI, 0.93 to 2.18) and relapse-free survival rate was lower (72% vs 78%; HR, 1.33; 95% CI, 0.99 to 1.79) in the darbepoetin alfa–treated arm compared with the control arm.

Cancer study 4 (protocol GOG 191) was a randomized, controlled study that enrolled 114 of a planned 460 cervical cancer patients receiving chemotherapy and radiotherapy. Patients were randomized to receive epoetin alfa to maintain hemoglobin between 12 and 14 g/dL or to transfusion support as needed. The study was terminated prematurely because of an increase in thromboembolic events in epoetin alfa–treated patients compared with control (19% vs 9%). Both local recurrence (21% vs 20%) and distant recurrence (12% vs 7%) were more frequent in the epoetin alfa–treated group compared with control. Progression-free survival at 3 years was lower in the epoetin alfa–treated group compared with control (59% vs 62%; HR, 1.06; 95% CI, 0.58 to 1.91). Overall survival at 3 years was lower in the epoetin alfa–treated group compared with control (61% vs 71%; HR, 1.28; 95% CI, 0.68 to 2.42).

Cancer study 5 was a randomized, controlled study in 351 patients with head and neck cancer in which epoetin beta or placebo was administered to achieve target hemoglobin of 14 and 15 g/dL for women and men, respectively. Locoregional progression-free survival was significantly shorter in patients receiving epoetin beta (HR, 1.62; 95% CI, 1.22 to 2.14; $P = 0.0008$), with a median of 406 days for epoetin beta versus 745 days for placebo. Overall survival was significantly shorter in patients receiving epoetin beta (HR, 1.39; 95% CI, 1.05 to 1.84; $P = 0.02$).

Decreased locoregional control – Cancer study 6 (DAHANCA 10) was conducted in 522 patients with primary squamous cell carcinoma of the head and neck receiving radiation therapy randomized to darbepoetin alfa with radiotherapy or radiotherapy alone. An interim analysis in 484 patients demonstrated that locoregional control at 5 years was significantly shorter in patients receiving darbepoetin alfa (RR, 1.44; 95% CI, 1.06 to 1.96; $P = 0.02$). Overall survival was shorter in patients receiving darbepoetin alfa (RR, 1.28; 95% CI, 0.98 to 1.68; $P = 0.08$).

➤*Pure red cell aplasia:* Cases of pure red cell aplasia and severe anemia, with or without other cytopenias, associated with neutralizing antibodies to erythropoietin, have been reported in patients treated with epoetin alfa. This has been reported predominantly in patients with CRF receiving epoetin alfa by subcutaneous administration. Evaluate any patient who develops a sudden loss of response to epoetin alfa accompanied by severe anemia and low reticulocyte count for the etiology of loss of effect, including the presence of neutralizing antibodies to erythropoietin. If antierythropoietin antibody–associated anemia is suspected, withhold epoetin alfa and other erythropoietic proteins. Contact the manufacturer to perform assays for binding and neutralizing antibodies. Permanently discontinue epoetin alfa in patients with antibody-mediated anemia. Do not switch patients to other erythropoietic proteins because antibodies may cross-react.

➤*Transmission of infectious agents:* Epoetin alfa contains albumin, a derivative of human blood. Based on effective donor screening and product manufacturing processes, it carries an extremely remote risk for transmission of viral diseases. A theoretical risk for transmission of Creutzfeldt-Jakob disease (CJD) also is considered extremely remote. No cases of transmission of viral diseases or CJD have ever been identified for albumin.

➤*Hypertension:* Do not treat patients with uncontrolled hypertension with epoetin alfa; control blood pressure adequately before initiation of therapy. Although there do not appear to be any direct pressor effects of epoetin alfa, blood pressure may rise during epoetin alfa therapy.

➤*Seizures:*

Cancer patients – In double-blind, placebo-controlled trials, 3.2% (2/63) of patients treated with epoetin alfa 3 times a week and 2.9% (2/68) of placebo-treated patients had seizures. Seizures in 1.6% (1/63) of patients treated with epoetin alfa 3 times per week occurred in the context of a significant increase in blood pressure and hematocrit from baseline values. However, both patients treated with epoetin alfa also had underlying CNS pathology, which may have been related to seizure activity.

In a placebo-controlled, double-blind trial utilizing weekly dosing with epoetin alfa, 1.2% (2/168) of safety-evaluable patients treated with epoetin alfa and 1% (1/165) of placebo-treated patients had seizures. Seizures in patients treated with weekly epoetin alfa occurred in the context of a significant increase in hemoglobin from baseline values; however, significant increases in blood pressure were not seen. These patients may have had other CNS pathology.

Chronic renal failure patients – Seizures have occurred in patients with CRF participating in epoetin alfa clinical trials.

In adult patients on dialysis, there was a higher incidence of seizures during the first 90 days of therapy (occurring in approximately 2.5% of patients) compared with later time points.

Given the potential for an increased risk of seizures during the first 90 days of therapy, closely monitor blood pressure and the presence of premonitory neurologic symptoms. Caution patients to avoid potentially hazardous activities, such as driving or operating heavy machinery, during this period.

While the relationship between seizures and the rate of rise of hemoglobin is uncertain, it is recommended that the dose of epoetin alfa be decreased if the hemoglobin increase exceeds 1 g/dL in any 2-week period.

Zidovudine-treated, HIV-infected patients – In double-blind studies, a single seizure has been experienced by a patient treated with epoetin alfa.

➤*Hematologic effects:* Exacerbation of porphyria has been observed rarely in patients with CRF treated with epoetin alfa. However, epoetin alfa has not caused increased urinary excretion of porphyrin metabolites in healthy volunteers, even in the presence of a rapid erythropoietic response. Nevertheless, use epoetin alfa with caution in patients with known porphyria.

Measure hemoglobin in patients with CRF twice a week; measure hemoglobin in zidovudine-treated, HIV-infected and cancer patients once a week until hemoglobin has been stabilized, and measure periodically thereafter.

Allow sufficient time to determine a patient's responsiveness to a dosage of epoetin alfa before adjusting the dose. Because of the time required for erythropoiesis and red cell half-life, an interval of 2 to 6 weeks may occur between the time of a dose adjustment (initiation, increase, decrease, or discontinuation) and a significant change in hemoglobin.

In order to avoid reaching the suggested target hemoglobin too rapidly or exceeding the suggested target range (hemoglobin of 10 to 12 g/dL), follow the guidelines for dose and frequency of dose adjustments.

For patients who respond to epoetin alfa with a rapid increase in hemoglobin (eg, more than 1 g/dL in any 2-week period), reduce the dose of epoetin alfa because of the possible association of the excessive rate of rise of hemoglobin with an exacerbation of hypertension.

The elevated bleeding time characteristic of CRF decreases toward normal after correction of anemia in adult patients treated with epoetin alfa. Reduction of bleeding time also occurs after correction of anemia by transfusion.

➤*Bone marrow fibrosis:* Bone marrow fibrosis is a known complication of CRF in humans and may be related to secondary hyperparathyroidism or unknown factors. The incidence of bone marrow fibrosis was not increased in a study of adult patients on dialysis who were treated with epoetin alfa for 12 to 19 months compared with the incidence of bone marrow fibrosis in a matched group of patients who had not been treated with epoetin alfa.

➤*Iron evaluation:* During epoetin alfa therapy, absolute or functional iron deficiency may develop. Functional iron deficiency with normal ferritin levels but low transferrin saturation is presumably because of the inability to mobilize iron stores rapidly enough to support increased erythropoiesis. Transferrin saturation should be at least 20%, and ferritin should be at least 100 ng/mL.

Prior to and during epoetin alfa therapy, evaluate the patient's iron status, including transferrin saturation (serum iron divided by iron-binding capacity) and serum ferritin. Virtually all patients will eventually require supplemental iron to increase or maintain transferrin saturation to levels that will adequately support erythropoiesis stimulated by epoetin alfa. Provide all surgery patients being treated with epoetin alfa with adequate iron supplementation throughout the course of therapy in order to support erythropoiesis and avoid depletion of iron stores.

➤*Chronic renal failure patients:*

Diet – Reinforce the importance of compliance with dietary and dialysis prescriptions.

Hyperkalemia – In patients with CRF, hyperkalemia is not uncommon. In US studies in patients on dialysis, hyperkalemia has occurred at an annualized rate of approximately 0.11 episodes per patient-year of epoetin alfa therapy, often in association with poor compliance to medication, diet, and/or dialysis.

Dialysis management – Therapy with epoetin alfa results in an increase in hematocrit and a decrease in plasma volume, which could affect dialysis efficiency. In studies to date, the resulting increase in hematocrit did not appear to adversely affect dialyzer function or the efficiency of high-flux

EPOETIN ALFA RECOMBINANT — INJECTION

hemodialysis. During hemodialysis, patients treated with epoetin alfa may require increased anticoagulation with heparin to prevent clotting of the artificial kidney.

Patients who are marginally dialyzed may require adjustments in their dialysis prescription. As with all patients on dialysis, regularly monitor serum chemistry values (including serum urea nitrogen [BUN], creatinine, phosphorus, and potassium) in patients treated with epoetin alfa to ensure the adequacy of the dialysis prescription.

➤*Immunogenicity:* As with all therapeutic proteins, there is the potential for immunogenicity. Neutralizing antibodies to erythropoietin, in association with pure red cell aplasia or severe anemia (with or without other cytopenias), have been reported in patients receiving epoetin alfa during postmarketing experience.

➤*Hypersensitivity reactions:* Attend the parenteral administration of any biologic product with appropriate precautions in case allergic or other untoward reactions occur. In clinical trials, while transient rashes were occasionally observed concurrently with epoetin alfa therapy, no serious allergic or anaphylactic reactions were reported.

There have been rare reports of potentially serious allergic reactions, including urticaria with associated respiratory symptoms or circumoral edema, or urticaria alone. Most reactions occurred in situations in which a causal relationship could not be established. Symptoms recurred with rechallenge in a few instances, suggesting that allergic reactivity may occasionally be associated with epoetin alfa therapy. If an anaphylactoid reaction occurs, immediately discontinue epoetin alfa and initiate appropriate therapy.

➤*Renal function impairment:* In adult patients with CRF not on dialysis, closely monitor renal function and fluid and electrolyte balance. In patients with CRF not on dialysis, placebo-controlled studies of progression of renal function impairment over periods of more than 1 year have not been completed. In shorter-term trials in patients with CRF not on dialysis, changes in creatinine and creatinine clearance were not significantly different in patients treated with epoetin alfa compared with placebo-treated patients. Analysis of the slope of 1/serum creatinine versus time plots in these patients indicates no significant change in the slope after the initiation of epoetin alfa therapy.

➤*Pregnancy: Category C.* Epoetin alfa has been shown to have adverse reactions in rats when given in doses 5 times the human dose. There are no adequate and well-controlled studies in pregnant women. However, it appears that the benefits of epoetin alfa outweigh the risks. Epoetin alfa does not cross the placenta and does not seem to present a major risk to the fetus. Only use epoetin alfa during pregnancy if the potential benefit justifies the potential risk to the fetus.

In studies in female rats, there were decreases in body weight gain, delays in appearance of abdominal hair, delayed eyelid opening, delayed ossification, and decreases in the number of caudal vertebrae in the F1 fetuses of the 500 units/kg group. In female rats treated IV, there was a trend for slightly increased fetal wastage at doses of 100 and 500 units/kg.

In some female patients, menses have resumed following epoetin alfa therapy; discuss the possibility of pregnancy and the need for contraception evaluation.

➤*Lactation:* Postnatal observations of the live offspring (F1 generation) of female rats treated with epoetin alfa during gestation and lactation revealed no effect of epoetin alfa at doses of up to 500 units/kg. There were, however, decreases in body weight gain, delays in appearance of abdominal hair, delayed eyelid opening, and decreases in the number of caudal vertebrae in the F1 fetuses of the 500 units/kg group. There were no epoetin alfa–related effects on the F2 generation fetuses.

It is not known whether epoetin alfa is excreted in human milk. However, epoetin alfa is not expected to pass into human milk. If epoetin alfa did pass through to an infant, the infant would digest the epoetin alfa. Epoetin alfa is considered to be compatible with breast-feeding.

Because many drugs are excreted in human milk, exercise caution when epoetin alfa is administered to a breast-feeding woman.

➤*Children:*

Children on dialysis – Epoetin alfa is indicated in infants (1 month to 2 years of age), children (2 to 12 years of age), and adolescents (12 to 16 years of age) for the treatment of anemia associated with CRF requiring dialysis. Safety and efficacy in children younger than 1 month of age have not been established. The safety data from these studies show that there is no increased risk to children with CRF on dialysis when compared with the safety profile of epoetin alfa in adult patients with CRF. Published literature provides supportive evidence of the safety and efficacy of epoetin alfa in children with CRF on dialysis.

Children not requiring dialysis – Published literature has reported the use of epoetin alfa in 133 children 3 months to 20 years of age with anemia associated with CRF not requiring dialysis, treated with 50 to 250 units/kg subcutaneously or IV once weekly to 3 times per week. Dose-dependent increases in hemoglobin and hematocrit were observed with reductions in transfusion requirements.

HIV-infected children – Published literature has reported the use of epoetin alfa in 20 zidovudine-treated, anemic, HIV-infected children 8 months to 17 years of age treated with 50 to 400 units/kg subcutaneously or IV 2 to 3 times per week. Increases in hemoglobin levels and reticulocyte counts and decreases in or elimination of blood transfusions were observed.

Children with cancer on chemotherapy – The safety and efficacy of epoetin alfa were evaluated in a randomized, double-blind, placebo-controlled, multicenter study in anemic children 5 to 18 years of age receiving chemotherapy for the treatment of various childhood malignancies. There was no evidence of an improvement in health-related quality of life, including no evidence of an effect on fatigue, energy, or strength in patients receiving epoetin alfa compared with those receiving placebo.

Benzyl alcohol – The multidose preserved formulation contains benzyl alcohol. Benzyl alcohol has been reported to be associated with an increased incidence of neurological and other complications that are sometimes fatal in premature infants.

➤*Elderly:* Individualize dose selection and adjustment for an elderly patient to achieve and maintain the target hematocrit.

➤*Lab test abnormalities:*

Chronic renal failure patients – During clinical trials, modest increases were seen in platelets and white blood cell counts. While these changes were statistically significant, they were not clinically significant, and the values remained within normal ranges.

During clinical trials in adult patients on dialysis, modest increases were seen in BUN, creatinine, phosphorus, and potassium. In some adult patients with CRF not on dialysis treated with epoetin alfa, modest increases in serum uric acid and phosphorus were observed. While changes were statistically significant, the values remained within the ranges normally seen in patients with CRF.

➤*Monitoring:* Take special care to closely monitor and aggressively control blood pressure in patients treated with epoetin alfa, particularly in patients with an underlying history of hypertension or CV disease, or who are in the perioperative period.

Closely monitor patients with preexisting CV disease.

Prior to and during epoetin therapy, evaluate the patient's iron stores, including transferrin saturation (serum iron divided by iron-binding capacity) and serum ferritin. Transferrin saturation should be at least 20%, and ferritin should be at least 100 ng/mL.

Given the potential for an increased risk of seizures during the first 90 days of therapy, closely monitor blood pressure and the presence of premonitory neurologic symptoms.

Cancer patients on chemotherapy – Monitor hemoglobin on a weekly basis until hemoglobin becomes stable.

Chronic renal failure patients – Determine the hemoglobin twice a week until it has stabilized in the suggested target range and the maintenance dose has been established. After any dose adjustment, also determine the hemoglobin twice weekly for at least 2 to 6 weeks until it has been determined that the hemoglobin has stabilized in response to the dose change. Then monitor the hemoglobin at regular intervals.

Regularly perform a complete blood cell count (CBC) with differential and platelet count.

Regularly monitor serum chemistry values (including BUN, creatinine, phosphorus, potassium, and uric acid).

Monitor blood pressure and hemoglobin in patients with CRF not requiring dialysis no less frequently than for patients maintained on dialysis. Closely monitor renal function and fluid and electrolyte balance.

Zidovudine-treated, HIV-infected patients – During the dose-adjustment phase of therapy, monitor the hemoglobin weekly.

Surgery patients – Prior to initiating treatment with epoetin alfa, obtain a hemoglobin to establish that it is more than 10 and less than or equal to 13 g/dL.

Drug Interactions

None known.

Adverse Reactions

For more information on bone marrow fibrosis, hematologic effects (eg, porphyria), hypersensitivity/allergic reactions, hypertension, increased mortality, pure red cell aplasia, seizures, serious CV events (eg, death, hospitalization from CHF, MI, stroke), and thromboembolic reactions, refer to the Warnings/Precautions section.

➤*Cancer patients on chemotherapy:*

Epoetin Alfa Adverse Reactions in Cancer Patients on Chemotherapy (> 10%)

Adverse reaction	Epoetin alfa (n = 63)	Placebo (n = 68)
CNS		
Asthenia	13%	16%
Dizziness	5%	12%
Paresthesia	11%	6%
GI		
Diarrhea	21%[a]	7%
Nausea	17%[a]	32%
Vomiting	17%	15%

EPOETIN ALFA RECOMBINANT — INJECTION

Epoetin Alfa Adverse Reactions in Cancer Patients on Chemotherapy (> 10%)		
Adverse reaction	Epoetin alfa (n = 63)	Placebo (n = 68)
Respiratory		
Shortness of breath	13%	9%
Upper respiratory tract infection	11%	4%
Miscellaneous		
Edema	17%[a]	1%
Fatigue	13%	15%
Pyrexia	29%	19%
Trunk pain	3%[a]	16%

[a] Statistically significant.

➤*Chronic renal failure patients:*

Epoetin Alfa Adverse Reactions in CRF Patients (> 5% or significant)		
Adverse reaction	Epoetin alfa (n = 200)	Placebo (n = 135)
Cardiovascular		
CVA/TIA[a]	0.4%	0.6%
Hypertension	24%	19%
MI	0.4%	1.1%
CNS		
Asthenia	7%	12%
Dizziness	7%	13%
Headache	16%	12%
Seizure	1.1%	1.1%
GI		
Diarrhea	9%	6%
Nausea	11%	9%
Vomiting	8%	5%
Miscellaneous		
Arthralgias	11%	6%
Chest pain	7%	9%
Clotted access	7%	2%
Death	0%	1.7%
Edema	9%	10%
Fatigue	9%	14%
Skin reaction (administration site)	7%	12%

[a] CVA = cerebrovascular accident; TIA = transient ischemic attack.

Adults on dialysis – In the US epoetin alfa studies in patients on dialysis (more than 567 patients), the incidence (number of reactions per patient-year) of the most frequently reported adverse reactions were the following: hypertension (0.75%), tachycardia (0.31%), nausea/vomiting (0.26%), clotted vascular access (0.25%), shortness of breath (0.14%), diarrhea (0.11%), hyperkalemia (0.11%), and headache (0.4%). Other reported reactions occurred at a rate of less than 0.1 reactions per patient per year.

Children with chronic renal failure – In children with CRF on dialysis, the pattern of most adverse reactions was similar to that found in adults. Additional adverse reactions reported during the double-blind phase in more than 10% of children in either treatment group were the following: abdominal pain; constipation; cough; dialysis access complications, including access infections and peritonitis in those receiving peritoneal dialysis; fever; pharyngitis; and upper respiratory tract infection. The rates are similar between the treatment groups for each reaction.

Other adverse reactions – Reactions reported to have occurred within several hours of administration of epoetin alfa were rare, mild, and transient, and included injection-site stinging in dialysis patients and flu-like symptoms, such as arthralgias and myalgias.

Hypertension – Increases in blood pressure have been reported in clinical trials, often during the first 90 days of therapy. On occasion, hypertensive encephalopathy and seizures have been observed in patients with CRF treated with epoetin alfa. When data from all patients in the US, phase 3, multicenter trial were analyzed, there was an apparent trend of more reports of hypertensive adverse reactions in patients on dialysis with a faster rate of rise of hematocrit (more than 4 hematocrit points in any 2-week period).

Seizures – There have been 47 seizures in 1,010 patients on dialysis treated with epoetin alfa in clinical trials, with an exposure of 986 patient-years for a rate of approximately 0.048 reactions per patient-year. However, there appeared to be a higher rate of seizures during the first 90 days of therapy (occurring in approximately 2.5% of patients) compared with subsequent 90-day periods. The baseline incidence of seizures in the untreated dialysis population is difficult to determine; it appears to be in the range of 5% to 10% per patient-year.

Thrombotic reactions – In clinical trials in which the maintenance hematocrit was 35% ± 3% on epoetin alfa, clotting of the vascular access (arteriovenous [AV] shunt) has occurred at an annualized rate of approximately 0.25 events per patient-year, and other thrombotic reactions (eg, CVA, MI, pulmonary embolism, TIA) occurred at a rate of 0.04 reactions per patient-year. In a separate study of 1,111 untreated dialysis patients, clotting of the AV shunt occurred at a rate of 0.5 events per patient-year. However, in patients with CRF on hemodialysis who also had clinically evident ischemic heart disease or CHF, the risk of AV shunt thrombosis was higher (39% vs 29%; $P < 0.001$), and MI, vascular ischemic reactions, and venous thrombosis were increased in patients targeted to a hematocrit of 42% ± 3% compared with those maintained at 30% ± 3%.

In patients treated with commercial epoetin alfa, there have been rare reports of serious or unusual thromboembolic reactions, including microvascular thrombosis, migratory thrombophlebitis, pulmonary embolus, and thrombosis of the retinal artery and temporal and renal veins. A causal relationship has not been established.

Hypersensitivity – There have been no reports of serious allergic reactions or anaphylaxis associated with epoetin alfa administration during clinical trials. Skin rashes and urticaria have been observed rarely and, when reported, have generally been mild and transient in nature.

See Warnings/Precautions for more information.

➤*Zidovudine-treated, HIV-infected patients:*

Epoetin Alfa Adverse Reactions in Zidovudine-Treated, HIV-Infected Patients (≥10%)		
Adverse reaction	Epoetin alfa (n = 144)	Placebo (n = 153)
CNS		
Asthenia	11%	14%
Dizziness	9%	10%
Headache	19%	14%
Dermatologic		
Rash	16%	8%
Skin reaction, medication site	10%	7%
GI		
Diarrhea	16%	18%
Nausea	15%	12%
Respiratory		
Cough	18%	14%
Respiratory congestion	15%	10%
Shortness of breath	14%	13%
Miscellaneous		
Fatigue	25%	31%
Pyrexia	38%	29%

Hypersensitivity – Two zidovudine-treated, HIV-infected patients had urticarial reactions within 48 hours of their first exposure to study medication. One patient was treated with epoetin alfa, and one was treated with placebo (epoetin alfa vehicle alone). Both patients had positive immediate skin tests against their study medication with a negative saline control. The basis for this apparent preexisting hypersensitivity to components of the epoetin alfa formulation is unknown but may be related to HIV-induced immunosuppression or prior exposure to blood products.

Seizures – In double-blind and open-label trials of epoetin alfa in zidovudine-treated, HIV-infected patients, 10 patients experienced seizures. In general, these seizures appear to be related to underlying pathology, such as meningitis or cerebral neoplasms, not epoetin alfa therapy.

➤*Surgery patients:*

Epoetin Alfa Adverse Reactions in Surgery Patients (≥ 10%)					
Adverse reaction	Epoetin alfa 300 units/kg (n = 112)[a]	Epoetin alfa 100 units/kg (n = 101)[a]	Placebo (n = 103)[a]	Epoetin alfa 600 units/kg (n = 73)[b]	Epoetin alfa 300 units/kg (n = 72)[b]
CNS					
Anxiety	7%	2%	11%	11%	4%
Dizziness	12%	9%	12%	11%	21%
Headache	13%	11%	9%	10%	19%
Insomnia	13%	16%	13%	21%	18%
Cardiovascular					
Deep venous thrombosis	10%	3%	5%	0%[c]	0%[c]
Hypertension	10%	11%	10%	5%	10%
Dermatologic					
Pruritus	16%	16%	14%	14%	22%
Skin pain	18%	18%	17%	5%	4%
Skin reaction, medication site	25%	19%	22%	26%	29%

EPOETIN ALFA RECOMBINANT — INJECTION

Epoetin Alfa Adverse Reactions in Surgery Patients (≥ 10%)					
Adverse reaction	Epoetin alfa 300 units/kg (n = 112)[a]	Epoetin alfa 100 units/kg (n = 101)[a]	Placebo (n = 103)[a]	Epoetin alfa 600 units/kg (n = 73)[b]	Epoetin alfa 300 units/kg (n = 72)[b]
GI					
Constipation	43%	42%	43%	51%	53%
Diarrhea	10%	7%	12%	10%	6%
Dyspepsia	9%	11%	6%	7%	8%
Nausea	48%	43%	45%	45%	58%
Vomiting	22%	12%	14%	21%	29%
Miscellaneous					
Edema	6%	11%	8%	11%	7%
Pyrexia	51%	50%	60%	47%	42%
Urinary tract infection	12%	3%	11%	11%	8%

[a] Study including patients undergoing orthopedic surgery treated with epoetin alfa or placebo for 15 days.
[b] Study including patients undergoing orthopedic surgery treated with epoetin alfa 600 units/kg/week × 4 or 300 units/kg daily × 15.
[c] Determined by clinical symptoms.

Thrombotic/Vascular reactions – In 3 double-blind, placebo-controlled orthopedic surgery studies, the rate of deep venous thrombosis was similar among epoetin alfa–treated and placebo-treated patients in the recommended population of patients with a pretreatment hemoglobin of more than 10 to less than or equal to 13 g/dL. However, in 2 of 3 orthopedic surgery studies, the overall rate (all pretreatment hemoglobin groups combined) of deep vein thrombosis detected by postoperative ultrasonography and/or surveillance venography was higher in the group treated with epoetin alfa than in the placebo-treated group (11% vs 6%). This finding was attributable to the difference in deep vein thrombosis rates observed in the subgroup of patients with pretreatment hemoglobin of more than 13 g/dL.

In the orthopedic surgery study of patients with pretreatment hemoglobin of more than 10 to less than or equal to 13 g/dL that compared 2 dosing regimens (600 units/kg/week × 4 and 300 units/kg daily × 15), 4 (5%) subjects in the epoetin alfa 600 units/kg/week group and no subjects in the 300 units/kg daily group had a thrombotic vascular reaction during the study period.

In a study examining the use of epoetin alfa in 182 patients scheduled for coronary artery bypass graft surgery, 23% of patients treated with epoetin alfa and 29% treated with placebo experienced thrombotic/vascular reactions. There were 4 deaths among the epoetin alfa–treated patients that were associated with a thrombotic/vascular reaction.

Overdosage

➤*Symptoms:* The expected manifestations of epoetin alfa overdosage include signs and symptoms associated with an excessive and/or rapid increase in hemoglobin concentration, including any of the CV reactions described in the previous sections.

➤*Treatment:* Closely monitor patients receiving an overdose of epoetin alfa for CV reactions and hematologic abnormalities. Manage polycythemia acutely with phlebotomy, as clinically indicated. Following resolution of the effects caused by epoetin alfa overdose, accompany reintroduction of epoetin therapy with close monitoring for evidence of rapid increases in hemoglobin concentration (more than 1 g/dL per 14 days). In patients with an excessive hematopoietic response, reduce the epoetin alfa dose in accordance with the recommendations described in the Administration and Dosage section.

Patient Information

Inform patients of the increased risks of mortality, serious CV reactions, thromboembolic reactions, and increased risk of tumor progression or recurrence. In those situations in which the health care provider determines that a patient or their caregiver can safely and effectively administer epoetin alfa at home, instruct the patient as to the proper dosage and administration.

Inform patients of the possible adverse reactions of epoetin alfa and of the signs and symptoms of an allergic drug reaction, and advise them of appropriate actions. If home use is prescribed for a home dialysis patient, thoroughly instruct the patient in the importance of proper disposal and caution against the reuse of needles, syringes, or drug product.

A puncture-resistant container for the disposal of used syringes and needles should be available to the patient; provide guidance on disposal of the full container.

In some women, menses have resumed following epoetin alfa therapy; discuss the possibility of pregnancy and the need for contraception evaluation.

Caution patients to avoid potentially hazardous activities, such as driving or operating heavy machinery, during this period.

DARBEPOETIN ALFA

Rx	**Aranesp** (Amgen)	**Injection, solution**[a]: 25 mcg per 0.42 mL	Preservative free. In single-dose prefilled *SureClick* autoinjector and *SingleJect* syringes.[b]
		25 mcg/mL	Preservative free. In single-dose vials.
		40 mcg per 0.4 mL	Preservative free. In single-dose prefilled *SureClick* autoinjector and *SingleJect* syringes.[b]
		40 mcg/mL	Preservative free. In single-dose vials.
		60 mcg per 0.3 mL	Preservative free. In single-dose prefilled *SureClick* autoinjector and *SingleJect* syringes.[b]
		60 mcg/mL	Preservative free. In single-dose vials.
		100 mcg per 0.5 mL	Preservative free. In single-dose prefilled *SureClick* autoinjector and *SingleJect* syringes.[b]
		100 mcg/mL	Preservative free. In single-dose vials.
		150 mcg per 0.3 mL	Preservative free. In single-dose prefilled *SureClick* autoinjector and *SingleJect* syringes.[b]
		150 mcg per 0.75 mL	Preservative free. In single-dose vials.
		200 mcg per 0.4 mL	Preservative free. In single-dose prefilled *SureClick* autoinjector and *SingleJect* syringes.[b]
		200 mcg/mL	Preservative free. In single-dose vials.
		300 mcg per 0.6 mL	Preservative free. In single-dose prefilled *SureClick* autoinjector and *SingleJect* syringes.[b]
		300 mcg/mL	Preservative free. In single-dose vials.
		500 mcg/mL	Preservative free. In single-dose vials and single-dose prefilled *SureClick* autoinjector and *SingleJect* syringes.[b]

[a] Each mL contains 0.05 mg of polysorbate 80 and is formulated at pH 6.2 ± 0.2 with sodium phosphate monobasic monohydrate 2.12 mg, sodium phosphate dibasic anhydrous 0.66 mg, sodium chloride 8.18 mg, and water for injection.

[b] The needle cover of the prefilled syringe contains natural rubber (a derivative of latex).

DARBEPOETIN ALFA — INJECTION

WARNING

Increased mortality, serious cardiovascular and thromboembolic events, and increased risk of tumor progression or recurrence –

Renal failure: Patients experienced greater risks for death and serious cardiovascular events when administered erythropoiesis-stimulating agents (ESAs) to target higher versus lower hemoglobin levels (13.5 vs 11.3 g/dL; 14 vs 10 g/dL) in 2 clinical studies. Individualize dosing to achieve and maintain hemoglobin levels within the range of 10 to 12 g/dL.

WARNING (cont.)

Cancer:

- ESAs shortened overall survival and/or increased the risk of tumor progression or recurrence in some clinical studies in patients with breast, non–small cell lung, head and neck, lymphoid, and cervical cancers.
- To decrease these risks, as well as the risk of serious cardiovascular and thrombovascular events, use the lowest dose needed to avoid red blood cell (RBC) transfusion.
- Use ESAs only for treatment of anemia caused by concomitant myelosuppressive chemotherapy.
- ESAs are not indicated for patients receiving myelosuppressive therapy when the anticipated outcome is cure.
- Discontinue following the completion of a chemotherapy course.

DARBEPOETIN ALFA — INJECTION

Indications

➤*Anemia associated with chronic renal failure:* For the treatment of anemia associated with chronic renal failure, including patients on dialysis and patients not on dialysis.

➤*Anemia associated with nonmyeloid malignancies caused by chemotherapy:* For the treatment of anemia caused by the effect of coadministered chemotherapy based on studies that have shown a reduction in the need for RBC transfusions in patients with metastatic, nonmyeloid malignancies.

➤*Off-label uses:* Anemia associated with malignancy.

Administration and Dosage

➤*General dosing considerations:* Individualize dosing to achieve and maintain hemoglobin levels within the range of 10 to 12 g/dL.

For patients converting from epoetin alfa, see Conversion from epoetin alfa to darbepoetin alfa.

➤*Adults:*

Anemia associated with chronic renal failure –

Initial dosage: 0.45 mcg/kg body weight as a single intravenous (IV) or subcutaneous injection once weekly. In patients on hemodialysis, the IV route is recommended. Alternatively, in patients not receiving dialysis, an initial dose of 0.75 mcg/kg may be administered subcutaneously as a single injection once every 2 weeks.

Maintenance dosage: The dose should be individualized to maintain hemoglobin levels within the range of 10 to 12 g/dL.

In the maintenance phase, darbepoetin alfa may continue to be administered as a single injection once weekly or once every 2 weeks. For many patients, the appropriate maintenance dose will be lower than the starting dose. Chronic renal failure patients not on dialysis, in particular, may require lower maintenance doses.

Dosage adjustment: The dose should be adjusted for each patient to achieve and maintain hemoglobin levels within the range of 10 to 12 g/dL. If hemoglobin excursions outside the recommended range occur, the dose should be adjusted as described. Increases in dose should not be made more frequently than once a month.

If the hemoglobin is increasing and approaching 12 g/dL, the dose should be reduced by approximately 25%. If the hemoglobin continues to increase, doses should be temporarily withheld until the hemoglobin begins to decrease, at which point therapy should be reinitiated at a dose approximately 25% below the previous dose. If the hemoglobin increases by more than 1 g/dL in a 2-week period, the dose should be decreased by approximately 25%.

If the increase in hemoglobin is less than 1 g/dL over 4 weeks and iron stores are adequate, the dose of darbepoetin alfa may be increased by approximately 25% of the previous dose. Further increases may be made at 4-week intervals until the specified hemoglobin is obtained.

For patients whose hemoglobin does not attain a level within the range of 10 to 12 g/dL, despite the use of appropriate darbepoetin alfa dose titrations over a 12-week period:

- do not administer higher darbepoetin alfa doses and use the lowest dose that will maintain a hemoglobin level sufficient to avoid the need for recurrent red blood cell transfusions,
- evaluate and treat for other causes of anemia, and
- thereafter, hemoglobin should continue to be monitored and, if responsiveness improves, darbepoetin alfa dose adjustments should be made as previously described. Discontinue darbepoetin alfa if responsiveness does not improve and the patient needs recurrent RBC transfusions.

Conversion: For patients converting from epoetin alfa, see Conversion from epoetin alfa to darbepoetin alfa.

Anemia associated with nonmyeloid malignancies caused by chemotherapy –

Initial dosage: 2.25 mcg/kg subcutaneously weekly or 500 mcg subcutaneously once every 3 weeks.

Therapy should not be initiated at hemoglobin levels of 10 g/dL or more.

Dosage adjustment: For both dosing schedules, the dose should be adjusted for each patient to maintain the lowest hemoglobin level sufficient to avoid the need for RBC transfusion. If the rate of hemoglobin increase is more than 1 g/dL per 2-week period or when the hemoglobin reaches a level needed to avoid transfusion, the dose should be reduced by 40% of the previous dose. If the hemoglobin exceeds a level needed to avoid transfusion, darbepoetin alfa should be temporarily withheld until the hemoglobin approaches a level for which transfusions may be required. At this point, therapy should be reinitiated at a dose 40% below the previous dose.

For patients receiving weekly administration, if there is less than a 1 g/dL increase in hemoglobin after 6 weeks of therapy, the dose of darbepoetin alfa should be increased up to 4.5 mcg/kg.

Conversion: For patients converting from epoetin alfa, see Conversion from epoetin alfa to darbepoetin alfa.

Discontinuation of therapy: Discontinue darbepoetin alfa if, after 8 weeks of therapy, there is no response as measured by hemoglobin levels or if transfusions are still required.

Discontinue darbepoetin alfa following the completion of a chemotherapy course.

➤*Children:*

Anemia associated with chronic renal failure –

1 year of age and older:

• *Initial dosage* – The starting weekly dosage should be estimated on the basis of the weekly epoetin alfa dosage at the time of substitution (see Conversion from epoetin alfa to darbepoetin alfa). For children receiving a weekly epoetin alfa dosage of less than 1,500 units/week, the available data are insufficient to determine a darbepoetin alfa conversion dosage. Because of variability, doses should be titrated to achieve and maintain hemoglobin levels within the range of 10 to 12 g/dL. Because of the longer serum half-life, darbepoetin alfa should be administered less frequently than epoetin alfa. Darbepoetin alfa should be administered once per week if a patient was receiving epoetin alfa 2 to 3 times weekly. Darbepoetin alfa should be administered once every 2 weeks if a patient was receiving epoetin alfa once per week. The route of administration (IV or subcutaneous) should be maintained.

• *Maintenance dosage* – See Adults for more information.

The dose should be individualized to maintain hemoglobin levels within the range of 10 to 12 g/dL.

In the maintenance phase, darbepoetin alfa may continue to be administered as a single injection once weekly or once every 2 weeks. For many patients, the appropriate maintenance dose will be lower than the starting dose. Chronic renal failure patients not on dialysis, in particular, may require lower maintenance doses.

• *Dosage adjustment* – See Adults for more information.

• *Conversion* – For patients converting from epoetin alfa, see Conversion from epoetin alfa to darbepoetin alfa.

➤*Conversion from epoetin alfa to darbepoetin alfa:* The starting weekly dosage of darbepoetin alfa for adults and children should be estimated on the basis of the weekly epoetin alfa dosage at the time of substitution. For children receiving a weekly epoetin alfa dosage of less than 1,500 units/week, the available data are insufficient to determine a darbepoetin alfa conversion dosage. Because of variability, doses should be titrated to achieve and maintain hemoglobin levels within the range of 10 to 12 g/dL. Because of the longer serum half-life, darbepoetin alfa should be administered less frequently than epoetin alfa. Darbepoetin alfa should be administered once per week if a patient was receiving epoetin alfa 2 to 3 times weekly. Darbepoetin alfa should be administered once every 2 weeks if a patient was receiving epoetin alfa once per week. The route of administration (IV or subcutaneous) should be maintained.

Estimated Darbepoetin Alfa Starting Dosages Based on Previous Epoetin Alfa Dosage

Previous weekly epoetin alfa dosage (units/week)	Weekly starting darbepoetin alfa dosage (mcg/week)	
	Adults	Children
< 1,500	6.25	[a]
1,500 to 2,499	6.25	6.25
2,500 to 4,999	12.5	10
5,000 to 10,999	25	20
11,000 to 17,999	40	40
18,000 to 33,999	60	60
34,000 to 89,999	100	100
≥ 90,000	200	200

[a] For children receiving a weekly epoetin alfa dosage of < 1,500 units/week, the available data are insufficient to determine a darbepoetin alfa conversion dosage.

➤*Monitoring:* When darbepoetin alfa therapy is initiated or adjusted, the hemoglobin should be followed weekly until stabilized and monitored at least monthly thereafter. During therapy, hematological parameters should be monitored regularly.

➤*Preparation for administration:* Do not dilute darbepoetin alfa. Vigorous shaking or exposure to light may denature darbepoetin alfa, causing it to become biologically inactive. Darbepoetin alfa contains no preservative. Discard any unused portion. Do not pool unused portions from the vials or prefilled syringes. Do not use the vial, prefilled syringe, or autoinjector more than 1 time.

Do not use any vials, prefilled syringes, or auto-injectors exhibiting particulate matter or discoloration.

Autoinjector – The prefilled *SureClick* autoinjector is designed to deliver the full dose. The completion of the injection is signaled by an audible click. Removal of the autoinjector from the injection site automatically extends a needle cover.

➤*Administration:* Administer IV or subcutaneously. In hemodialysis patients, the IV route is recommended.

Autoinjectors are for subcutaneous administration only. Because the autoinjectors are designed to deliver the full content, autoinjectors should only be used for patients who need the full dose.

➤*Admixture compatibility:* Do not administer in conjunction with other drug solutions.

➤*Storage / Stability:* Store at 2° to 8°C (36° to 46°F). Do not freeze or shake. Protect from light.

After removing from the refrigerator, protect from room light until administration. Vigorous shaking or exposure to light may denature darbepoetin alfa, causing it to become biologically inactive. Always store vials and prefilled syringes or autoinjectors in their cartons until use.

Actions

➤*Pharmacology:* Darbepoetin alfa stimulates erythropoiesis by the same mechanism as endogenous erythropoietin. A primary growth factor for erythroid development, erythropoietin is produced in the kidney and released

DARBEPOETIN ALFA — INJECTION

into the bloodstream in response to hypoxia. In responding to hypoxia, erythropoietin interacts with progenitor stem cells to increase RBC production. Production of endogenous erythropoietin is impaired in patients with chronic renal failure, and erythropoietin deficiency is the primary cause of their anemia. Increased hemoglobin levels are not generally observed until 2 to 6 weeks after initiating treatment with darbepoetin alfa. In patients with cancer receiving concomitant chemotherapy, the etiology of anemia is multifactorial.

➤*Pharmacokinetics:*

Absorption/Distribution – Following IV administration in chronic renal failure patients receiving dialysis, darbepoetin alfa serum concentration-time profiles were biphasic, with a distribution half-life of approximately 1.4 hours.

Following subcutaneous administration of darbepoetin alfa to chronic renal failure patients (receiving or not receiving dialysis), absorption was slow and peak concentrations occurred at 48 hours (range, 12 to 72 hours). The bioavailability of darbepoetin alfa in chronic renal failure patients receiving dialysis after subcutaneous administration was 37% (range, 30% to 50%).

Peak concentrations were observed at 90 hours (range, 71 to 123 hours) after a dose of 2.25 mcg/kg and at 71 hours (range, 28 to 120 hours) after a dose of 6.75 mcg/kg. When administered on a once-every-3-weeks schedule, 48-hour postdose darbepoetin alfa levels after the fourth dose were similar to those after the first dose.

Excretion – In chronic renal failure patients receiving dialysis, the average half-life was 46 hours (range, 12 to 89 hours), and, in chronic renal failure patients not receiving dialysis, the average half-life was 70 hours (range, 35 to 139 hours). Darbepoetin alfa apparent clearance was approximately 1.4 times faster on average in patients receiving dialysis compared with patients not receiving dialysis.

Following IV administration in chronic renal failure patients receiving dialysis, the mean terminal half-life was 21 hours. When administered IV, the terminal half-life of darbepoetin alfa was approximately 3-fold longer than epoetin alfa. Following the first subcutaneous dose of 6.75 mcg/kg (equivalent to 500 mcg for a 74 kg patient) in patients with cancer, the mean terminal half-life was 74 hours (range, 24 to 144 hours).

Special populations –
Children: Following a single subcutaneous dose, the average bioavailability was 54% (range, 32% to 70%), which was higher than that obtained in adult chronic renal failure patients on dialysis.

Contraindications

Uncontrolled hypertension; hypersensitivity to the active substance or any of the excipients.

Warnings/Precautions

➤*Increased mortality, serious cardiovascular and thromboembolic events:* Patients with chronic renal failure experienced greater risks for death and serious cardiovascular events when administered ESAs to target higher versus lower hemoglobin levels (13.5 vs 11.3 g/dL; 14 vs 10 g/dL) in 2 clinical studies. Patients with chronic renal failure and an insufficient hemoglobin response to ESA therapy may be at an even greater risk for cardiovascular events and mortality than other patients. Darbepoetin alfa and other ESAs increased the risks for death and serious cardiovascular events in controlled clinical trials of patients with cancer. These events included MI, stroke, CHF, and hemodialysis vascular access thrombosis. A rate of hemoglobin rise of more than 1 g/dL over 2 weeks may contribute to these risks.

See the Warning box for more information.

➤*Increased mortality and/or increased risk of tumor progression or recurrence:* ESAs resulted in decreased locoregional control/progression-free survival and/or overall survival. These findings were observed in studies of patients with advanced head and neck cancer receiving radiation therapy, in patients receiving chemotherapy for metastatic breast cancer or lymphoid malignancy, and in patients with non–small cell lung cancer or various malignancies who were not receiving chemotherapy or radiotherapy.

➤*Hypertension:* Darbepoetin alfa should not be used to treat patients with uncontrolled hypertension; adequately control blood pressure before initiation of therapy. Blood pressure may rise during treatment of anemia with darbepoetin alfa or epoetin alfa. In darbepoetin alfa clinical trials, approximately 40% of patients with chronic renal failure required initiation or intensification of antihypertensive therapy during the early phase of treatment when the hemoglobin was increasing. Hypertensive encephalopathy and seizures have been observed in patients with chronic renal failure who were treated with darbepoetin alfa or epoetin alfa.

Take special care to closely monitor and control blood pressure in patients treated with darbepoetin alfa. During darbepoetin alfa therapy, advise patients of the importance of compliance with antihypertensive therapy and dietary restrictions. If blood pressure is difficult to control by pharmacologic or dietary measures, reduce or withhold the dose of darbepoetin alfa. A clinically significant decrease in hemoglobin may not be observed for several weeks.

➤*Seizures:* Seizures have occurred in patients with chronic renal failure participating in clinical trials of darbepoetin alfa and epoetin alfa. During the first several months of therapy, closely monitor for the presence of premonitory neurologic symptoms. While the relationship between seizures and the rate of rise of hemoglobin is uncertain, it is recommended that the dose of darbepoetin alfa be decreased if the hemoglobin increase exceeds 1 g/dL in any 2-week period.

➤*Pure red cell aplasia (PRCA):* Cases of PRCA and severe anemia, with or without other cytopenias, associated with neutralizing antibodies to erythropoietin have been reported in patients treated with darbepoetin alfa. This has been reported predominantly in patients with chronic renal failure receiving darbepoetin alfa by subcutaneous administration. Evaluate any patient who develops a sudden loss of response to darbepoetin alfa accompanied by severe anemia and low reticulocyte count for the etiology of loss of effect, including the presence of neutralizing antibodies to erythropoietin. If antierythropoietin antibody–associated anemia is suspected, withhold darbepoetin alfa and other erythropoietic proteins. Contact the manufacturer (1-800-772-6436) to perform assays for binding and neutralizing antibodies. Permanently discontinue darbepoetin alfa in patients with antibody-mediated anemia. Do not switch patients to other erythropoietic proteins because antibodies may crossreact.

➤*Compromised erythropoietic response:* A lack of response or failure to maintain a hemoglobin response with darbepoetin alfa doses within the recommended dosing range should prompt a search for causative factors. Exclude or correct deficiencies of folic acid, iron, or vitamin B_{12}. Depending on the clinical setting, intercurrent infections, inflammatory or malignant processes, osteofibrosis cystica, occult blood loss, hemolysis, severe aluminum toxicity, and bone marrow fibrosis may compromise an erythropoietic response. In the absence of another etiology, evaluate the patient for evidence of PRCA and test sera for the presence of antibodies to erythropoietin.

➤*Hematology:* Allow sufficient time to determine a patient's responsiveness to a dose of darbepoetin alfa before adjusting the dose. Because of the time required for erythropoiesis and the RBC half-life, an interval of 2 to 6 weeks may occur between the time of a dose adjustment (ie, initiation, increase, decrease, discontinuation) and a significant change in hemoglobin.

In order to prevent the hemoglobin from exceeding the recommended target (12 g/dL) or rising too rapidly (more than 1 g/dL in 2 weeks), follow the guidelines for dose and frequency of dose adjustments (see Administration and Dosage).

➤*Chronic renal failure patients not requiring dialysis:* Patients with chronic renal failure not yet requiring dialysis may require lower maintenance doses of darbepoetin alfa than patients receiving dialysis. Though predialysis patients generally receive less frequent monitoring of blood pressure and laboratory parameters than dialysis patients, predialysis patients may be more responsive to the effects of darbepoetin alfa and require judicious monitoring of blood pressure and hemoglobin. Closely monitor renal function and fluid and electrolyte balance.

➤*Patients transitioning to dialysis:* During the transition period onto dialysis, carefully monitor hemoglobin and blood pressure; patients may need to have their maintenance doses adjusted to maintain hemoglobin levels within the range of 10 to 12 g/dL.

➤*Dialysis management:* Therapy with darbepoetin alfa results in an increase in RBCs and a decrease in plasma volume, which could reduce dialysis efficiency; patients who are marginally dialyzed may require adjustments in their dialysis prescription.

➤*Immunogenicity:* As with all therapeutic proteins, there is a potential for immunogenicity. Neutralizing antibodies to erythropoietin, in association with PRCA or severe anemia (with or without other cytopenias), have been reported in patients receiving darbepoetin alfa during postmarketing experience.

➤*Latex allergy:* The needle cover of the prefilled syringe contains dry natural rubber (a derivative of latex), which may cause allergic reactions in individuals sensitive to latex.

➤*Hypersensitivity reactions:* There have been rare reports of potentially serious allergic reactions, including skin rash and urticaria, associated with darbepoetin alfa. Symptoms have recurred with rechallenge, suggesting a causal relationship exists in some instances. If a serious allergic or anaphylactic reaction occurs, immediately and permanently discontinue darbepoetin alfa and administer appropriate therapy.

➤*Special risk:* The safety and efficacy of darbepoetin alfa therapy have not been established in patients with underlying hematologic diseases (eg, hemolytic anemia, sickle cell anemia, thalassemia, porphyria).

➤*Pregnancy: Category C.* When darbepoetin alfa was administered IV to rats and rabbits during gestation, no evidence of a direct embryotoxic, fetotoxic, or teratogenic outcome was observed at dosages of up to 20 mcg/kg/day. The only adverse reaction observed was a slight reduction in fetal weight, which occurred at dosages causing exaggerated pharmacological effects in the dams (1 mcg/kg/day and higher). An increase in postimplantation fetal loss was observed in studies assessing fertility.

IV injection of darbepoetin alfa to female rats every other day from day 6 of gestation through day 23 of lactation at doses of 2.5 mcg/kg/dose and higher resulted in offspring (F1 generation) with decreased body weights, which correlated with a low incidence of deaths, as well as delayed eye opening and delayed preputial separation.

There are no adequate and well-controlled studies in pregnant women. Use darbepoetin alfa during pregnancy only if the potential benefit justifies the potential risk to the fetus.

➤*Lactation:* It is not known whether darbepoetin alfa is excreted in human milk. Because many drugs are excreted in human milk, exercise caution when administering darbepoetin alfa to a breast-feeding woman.

➤*Children:*

Children with chronic renal failure – A study of the conversion from epoetin alfa to darbepoetin alfa among children with chronic renal failure older than 1 year of age showed similar safety and efficacy to the findings

DARBEPOETIN ALFA — INJECTION

from adult conversion studies. Safety and efficacy in the initial treatment of anemic children with chronic renal failure or in the conversion from another erythropoietin to darbepoetin alfa in children with chronic renal failure younger than 1 year of age have not been established.

Children with cancer – The safety and efficacy of darbepoetin alfa in children with cancer have not been established.

➤*Monitoring:* After initiation of darbepoetin alfa therapy, determine the hemoglobin weekly until it has stabilized and the maintenance dose has been established. After a dose adjustment, determine the hemoglobin weekly for at least 4 weeks until it has been determined that the hemoglobin has stabilized in response to the dose change. Then monitor the hemoglobin at regular intervals.

In order to ensure effective erythropoiesis, evaluate iron status for all patients before and during treatment because the majority of patients will eventually require supplemental iron therapy. Supplemental iron therapy is recommended for all patients whose serum ferritin is less than 100 mcg/L or whose serum transferrin saturation is less than 20%.

Closely monitor blood pressure and the presence of premonitory neurologic symptoms during the first several months of therapy. Closely monitor renal function and electrolyte balance in patients with chronic renal failure not requiring dialysis.

Drug Interactions

None known.

Adverse Reactions

➤*Chronic renal failure:*

Adults –

Serious adverse reactions: In all studies, the most frequently reported serious adverse reactions with darbepoetin alfa were infection, CHF, angina pectoris/cardiac chest pain, thrombosis vascular access, and cardiac arrhythmia/cardiac arrest.

• *Most frequent adverse reactions* – The most frequently reported adverse reactions resulting in clinical intervention (eg, discontinuation of darbepoetin alfa, adjustment in dosage, or the need for concomitant medication to treat an adverse reaction symptom) were infection, hypertension, hypotension, and muscle spasm.

Darbepoetin Alfa Adverse Reactions in Chronic Renal Failure Patients (≥ 5%)

Adverse reaction	Darbepoetin alfa (N = 1,801)
Cardiovascular	
Acute MI	2%
Angina pectoris/cardiac chest pain	8%
Cardiac arrhythmias/cardiac arrest	8%
CHF	5%
Hypertension	20%
Hypotension	20%
Stroke	2%
Thrombosis vascular access	6%
Transient ischemic attack	≤ 1%
CNS	
Asthenia	5%
Dizziness	7%
Fatigue	9%
Headache	15%
Seizure	1%
GI	
Abdominal pain	10%
Constipation	5%
Diarrhea	14%
Nausea	11%
Vomiting	14%
Musculoskeletal	
Arthralgia	9%
Back pain	7%
Limb pain	8%
Muscle spasm	17%
Respiratory	
Bronchitis	5%
Cough	9%
Dyspnea	10%
Upper respiratory tract infection	15%
Miscellaneous	
Access hemorrhage	7%
Access infection	6%
Chest pain	7%
Death	6%
Fever	7%
Fluid overload	6%
Infection[a]	24%
Influenza-like symptoms	6%
Injection-site pain	6%
Peripheral edema	10%
Pruritus	6%

[a] Infection includes abscess, bacteremia, peritonitis, pneumonia, and sepsis.

Thrombotic events – See Warnings/Precautions for more information.

Children –

Most serious adverse reactions: In an open-label, randomized study, darbepoetin alfa was administered to 81 children with chronic renal failure who had stable hemoglobin concentrations while previously receiving epoetin alfa. In this study, the most frequently reported serious adverse reactions with darbepoetin alfa were fever and dialysis-access infection.

• *Most common adverse reactions* – The most commonly reported adverse reactions were cough, fever, headache, hypertension, hypotension, injection-site pain, and upper respiratory tract infection.

• *Discontinuation of therapy* – Darbepoetin alfa administration was discontinued because of injection-site pain in 2 patients and moderate hypertension in a third patient.

➤*Cancer patients receiving chemotherapy:*

Serious adverse reactions – The most frequently reported serious adverse reactions included death (10%), fever (4%), dehydration (3%), pneumonia (3%), dyspnea (2%), and vomiting (2%).

Most common adverse reactions – The most commonly reported adverse reactions were diarrhea, dyspnea, edema, fatigue, fever, nausea, and vomiting.

Discontinuation of therapy – The most frequently reported reasons for discontinuation of darbepoetin alfa were asthenia, death, discontinuation of the chemotherapy, dyspnea, GI hemorrhage, pneumonia, and progressive disease.

Darbepoetin Alfa Adverse Reactions in Patients on Chemotherapy (≥ 5%)

Adverse reaction	Darbepoetin alfa (n = 873)	Placebo (n = 221)
Cardiovascular		
Hypertension	3.7%	3.2%
Pulmonary embolism	1.3%	0%
Thrombosis[a]	5.6%	4.1%
Thrombotic events	6.2%	4.1%
CNS		
Dizziness	14%	8%
Fatigue	33%	30%
Headache	12%	9%
Seizures[b]	0.6%	0.5%
GI		
Constipation	18%	17%
Diarrhea	22%	12%
Metabolic/Nutritional		
Dehydration	5%	3%
Edema	21%	10%
Musculoskeletal		
Arthralgia	13%	6%
Myalgia	8%	5%
Miscellaneous		
Fever	19%	16%
Rash	7%	3%

[a] Thrombosis includes the following: deep thrombophlebitis, deep venous thrombosis, thromboembolism, thrombophlebitis, thrombosis, and venous thrombosis.

[b] Seizures include the following preferred terms: seizures, seizures local, and tonic-clonic seizures.

➤*Thrombotic and cardiovascular events:* Overall, the incidence of thrombotic events was 6.2% for darbepoetin alfa and 4.1% for placebo. However, the following events were reported more frequently in darbepoetin

DARBEPOETIN ALFA — INJECTION

alfa–treated patients than in placebo controls: pulmonary embolism, thromboembolism, thrombophlebitis (deep and/or superficial), and thrombosis. In addition, edema of any type was more frequently reported in darbepoetin alfa–treated patients (21%) than in patients who received placebo (10%).

Overdosage

➤*Symptoms:* The expected manifestations of darbepoetin alfa overdosage include signs and symptoms associated with an excessive and/or rapid increase in hemoglobin concentration, including any of the cardiovascular reactions previously described.

➤*Treatment:* Closely monitor patients receiving an overdosage of darbepoetin alfa for cardiovascular reactions and hematologic abnormalities. Acutely manage polycythemia with phlebotomy, as clinically indicated. Following resolution of the effects caused by darbepoetin alfa overdosage, accompany reintroduction of darbepoetin alfa therapy by close monitoring for evidence of rapid increases in hemoglobin concentration (more than 1 g/dL per 14 days). In patients with an excessive hematopoietic response, reduce the darbepoetin alfa dose.

Patient Information

Inform patients of the increased risks of mortality, serious cardiovascular reactions, thromboembolic reactions, and increased risk of tumor progression or recurrence. Inform patients of the possible side effects of darbepoetin alfa and be instructed to report them to the prescribing physician.

Inform patients of the signs and symptoms of allergic drug reactions and be advised of appropriate actions.

Counsel patients on the importance of compliance with their darbepoetin alfa treatment, dietary and dialysis prescriptions, and the importance of judicious monitoring of blood pressure and hemoglobin concentration should be stressed.

In those rare cases where it is determined that a patient can safely and effectively administer darbepoetin alfa at home, provide appropriate instruction on the proper use of darbepoetin alfa for patients and their caregivers.

Caution patients and caregivers against the reuse of needles, syringes, or drug product, and be thoroughly instructed in their proper disposal. A puncture-resistant container for the disposal of used syringes and needles should be made available to the patient.

Inform patients that the needle cover on the prefilled syringe contains dry natural rubber (a derivative of latex), which should not be handled by persons sensitive to latex.

METHOXY POLYETHYLENE GLYCOL-EPOETIN BETA

Rx	**Mircera** (Hoffmann-La Roche[a])	**Injection, solution:** 50 mcg per 0.3 mL	Preservative free. In single-use prefilled syringes. In packs of 1.
		50 mcg/mL	Preservative free. In single-use vials. In packs of 1 or 12.
		75 mcg per 0.3 mL	Preservative free. In single-use prefilled syringes. In packs of 1.
		100 mcg per 0.3 mL	Preservative free. In single-use prefilled syringes. In packs of 1.
		100 mcg/mL	Preservative free. In single-use vials. In packs of 1 or 12.
		150 mcg per 0.3 mL	Preservative free. In single-use prefilled syringes. In packs of 1.
		200 mcg per 0.3 mL	Preservative free. In single-use prefilled syringes. In packs of 1.
		200 mcg/mL	Preservative free. In single-use vials. In packs of 1 or 12.
		250 mcg per 0.3 mL	Preservative free. In single-use prefilled syringes. In packs of 1.
		300 mcg/mL	Preservative free. In single-use vials. In packs of 1 or 12.
		400 mcg per 0.6 mL	Preservative free. In single-use prefilled syringes. In packs of 1.
		400 mcg/mL	Preservative free. In single-use vials. In packs of 1 or 12.
		600 mcg per 0.6 mL	Preservative free. In single-use prefilled syringes. In packs of 1.
		600 mcg/mL	Preservative free. In single-use vials. In packs of 1 or 12.
		800 mcg per 0.6 mL	Preservative free. In single-use prefilled syringes. In packs of 1.
		1,000 mcg/mL	Preservative free. In single-use vials. In packs of 1 or 12.

[a] Hoffmann La-Roche Inc., 340 Kingsland Street, Nutley, New Jersey 07110-1199.

METHOXY POLYETHYLENE GLYCOL-EPOETIN BETA — INJECTION

WARNING

Increased mortality, serious cardiovascular and thromboembolic events, and tumor progression –

Renal failure: Patients experienced greater risks for death and serious cardiovascular events when administered erythropoiesis-stimulating agents (ESAs) to target higher versus lower hemoglobin levels (13.5 vs 11.3 g/dL; 14 vs 10 g/dL) in 2 clinical studies. Individualize dosing to achieve and maintain hemoglobin levels within the range of 10 to 12 g/dL.

Cancer: Methoxy polyethylene glycol-epoetin beta is not indicated for the treatment of anemia caused by cancer chemotherapy. A dose-ranging study of methoxy polyethylene glycol-epoetin beta was terminated early because of significantly more deaths among patients receiving methoxy polyethylene glycol-epoetin beta than another ESA. Other studies of ESAs in patients with cancer displayed the following findings: ESAs shortened overall survival and/or time to tumor progression in clinical studies in patients with advanced breast, head and neck, lymphoid, and non–small cell lung malignancies when dosed to a target hemoglobin of 12 g/dL or more; the risks of shortened survival and tumor promotion have not been excluded when ESAs are dosed to target a hemoglobin of less than 12 g/dL.

Indications

➤*Anemia associated with chronic renal failure (CRF):* For the treatment of anemia associated with CRF in adults, including patients on dialysis and patients not on dialysis.

Administration and Dosage

➤*General dosing considerations:* The dose of methoxy polyethylene glycol-epoetin beta should be reduced as the hemoglobin approaches 12 g/dL or if it increases by more than 1 g/dL in any 2-week period. (See Dosage adjustment).

During therapy, hematological parameters should be monitored regularly. (See Monitoring).

Individualize dosing to achieve and maintain hemoglobin levels within the range of 10 to 12 g/dL.

➤*Adults:*

Anemia associated with chronic renal failure (CRF) –

Patients not currently treated with an ESA: 0.6 mcg/kg body weight administered as a single intravenous (IV) or subcutaneous injection once every 2 weeks.

Methoxy polyethylene glycol-epoetin beta should be dosed to achieve and maintain hemoglobin between 10 and 12 g/dL. Once the hemoglobin has been maintained within this range, methoxy polyethylene glycol-epoetin beta may be administered once monthly using a dose that is twice that of the every-2-week dose and subsequently titrated as necessary.

Patients currently treated with an ESA: Methoxy polyethylene glycol-epoetin beta can be administered once every 2 weeks or once monthly to patients whose hemoglobin has been stabilized by treatment with an ESA. The dose may be given as a single IV or subcutaneous injection and should be based on the total weekly ESA dose at the time of conversion.

Methoxy Polyethylene Glycol-Epoetin Beta Starting Doses for Patients Currently Receiving an ESA

Previous weekly epoetin alfa dose (units/week)	Previous weekly darbepoetin alfa dose (mcg/week)	Methoxy polyethylene glycol-epoetin beta dose: Once monthly (mcg/month)	Methoxy polyethylene glycol-epoetin beta dose: Once every 2 weeks (mcg/every 2 weeks)
< 8,000	< 40	120	60
8,000 to 16,000	40 to 80	200	100
> 16,000	> 80	360	180

• *Dosage adjustment –* Dose adjustments should be made more often than once a month. A significant change in hemoglobin may not be observed for several weeks after the dose is adjusted. If a dose adjustment is necessary to maintain the recommended hemoglobin level, the dose may be increased or decreased by approximately 25%, as needed.

During methoxy polyethylene glycol-epoetin beta therapy, if the increase in hemoglobin is greater than 1 g/dL in 2 weeks or if the hemoglobin is increasing and approaching 12 g/dL, the dose should be reduced by approximately 25%. If the hemoglobin continues to increase, methoxy polyethylene glycol-epoetin beta should be discontinued until the hemoglobin begins to

METHOXY POLYETHYLENE GLYCOL-EPOETIN BETA — INJECTION

decrease. Methoxy polyethylene glycol-epoetin beta may then be restarted at a dose approximately 25% below the previously administered dose.

For patients not converted from another ESA, if the increase in hemoglobin is less than 1 g/dL over the initial 4 weeks of treatment and iron stores are adequate, the dose of methoxy polyethylene glycol-epoetin beta may be increased by approximately 25%.

If a dose of methoxy polyethylene glycol-epoetin beta is missed, administer the missed dose as soon as possible and restart methoxy polyethylene glycol-epoetin beta at the prescribed dosing frequency.

• *Monitoring* – When therapy is initiated or adjusted, the hemoglobin should be monitored every 2 weeks until stabilized, and every 2 to 4 weeks thereafter. For patients whose hemoglobin does not attain a level within the range 10 to 12 g/dL despite the use of appropriate methoxy polyethylene glycol-epoetin beta dose titrations over a 12-week period, consider the following: do not administer higher methoxy polyethylene glycol-epoetin beta doses and use the lowest dose that will maintain a hemoglobin level sufficient to avoid the need for recurrent red blood cell transfusions; evaluate and treat for other causes of anemia; thereafter, continue to monitor the hemoglobin level, and if responsiveness improves, make methoxy polyethylene glycol-epoetin beta dose adjustments as described previously; discontinue methoxy polyethylene glycol-epoetin beta if responsiveness does not improve and the patient needs recurrent red blood cell transfusions.

➤*Preparation for administration:* Methoxy polyethylene glycol-epoetin beta is packaged as single-use vials and prefilled syringes and contains no preservatives. Discard any unused portion. Do not pool unused portions from the vials or prefilled syringes. Do not use the vial or prefilled syringe more than 1 time.

Always store the vials or prefilled syringes in their original cartons. Vigorous shaking or prolonged exposure to light should be avoided.

➤*Administration:* Administer either IV or subcutaneously. The IV route is recommended for patients receiving hemodialysis because the IV route may be less immunogenic. When administering subcutaneously, inject in the abdomen, arm, or thigh.

For administration using the prefilled syringe, the plunger must be fully depressed during injection in order for the needle guard to activate. Following administration, remove the needle from the injection site and then release the plunger to allow the needle guard to move up until the entire needle is covered.

➤*Admixture compatibility:* Do not mix methoxy polyethylene glycol-epoetin beta with any parenteral solution.

➤*Storage/Stability:* The recommended storage temperature is at 2° to 8°C (36° to 46°F). Do not freeze or shake. Protect from light.

Storage of vials over the recommended temperature (2° to 8°C [36° to 46°F]), when necessary, is permissible only for temperatures up to 25°C (77°F) and for no more than 7 days.

Storage of prefilled syringes over the recommended temperature (2° to 8°C [36° to 46°F]), when necessary, is permissible only for temperatures up to 25°C (77°F) and for no more than 30 days.

Actions

➤*Pharmacology:* Methoxy polyethylene glycol-epoetin beta is an erythropoietin receptor activator with greater activity in vivo as well as increased half-life, in contrast to erythropoietin. A primary growth factor for erythroid development, erythropoietin is produced in the kidney and released into the bloodstream in response to hypoxia. In responding to hypoxia, erythropoietin interacts with erythroid progenitor cells to increase red cell production. Production of endogenous erythropoietin is impaired in patients with CRF, and erythropoietin deficiency is the primary cause of their anemia.

Pharmacodynamics – Following a single dose of methoxy polyethylene glycol-epoetin beta in CRF patients, the onset of hemoglobin increase (defined as an increase greater than 0.4 g/dL from baseline) was observed 7 to 15 days following initial dose administration.

➤*Pharmacokinetics:*

Absorption – The pharmacokinetics of methoxy polyethylene glycol-epoetin beta were studied in anemic patients with CRF including patients on dialysis and not on dialysis. The maximum serum concentrations of methoxy polyethylene glycol-epoetin beta were observed 72 hours (median value) following the subcutaneous administration. The absolute bioavailability of methoxy polyethylene glycol-epoetin beta after the subcutaneous administration was 62%.

In CRF patients receiving multiple methoxy polyethylene glycol-epoetin beta doses, pharmacokinetics were studied after the first dose and on week 9 and week 19 or 21. Multiple dosing was found to have no effect on clearance, volume of distribution, or bioavailability of methoxy polyethylene glycol-epoetin beta. Based on population analyses of the clinical studies, methoxy polyethylene glycol-epoetin beta did not accumulate following administration every 4 weeks. However, when methoxy polyethylene glycol-epoetin beta was administered every 2 weeks, blood concentrations at steady state increased by 12%.

The site of subcutaneous injection (abdomen, arm, or thigh) had no clinically important effects on the pharmacokinetics or pharmacodynamics of methoxy polyethylene glycol-epoetin beta in healthy volunteers.

Excretion – Following an IV administration of methoxy polyethylene glycol-epoetin beta 0.4 mcg/kg body weight to CRF patients receiving peritoneal dialysis, the observed terminal half-life was 134 ± 65 hours (mean ± standard deviation), and the total systemic clearance was 0.49 ± 0.18 mL/h/kg. Following a subcutaneous administration of methoxy polyethylene glycol-epoetin beta 0.8 mcg/kg to CRF patients receiving peritoneal dialysis, the terminal half-life was 139 ± 67 hours.

Contraindications

Uncontrolled hypertension; history of hypersensitivity or allergy to the drug.

Warnings/Precautions

➤*Increased mortality and serious cardiovascular and thromboembolic events:*

Anemia associated with CRF – Patients experienced greater risks for death and serious cardiovascular events when administered ESAs to target higher versus lower hemoglobin levels (13.5 vs 11.3 g/dL; 14 vs 10 g/dL) in 2 clinical studies. Patients with CRF and an insufficient hemoglobin response to ESA therapy may be at even greater risk for cardiovascular events and mortality than other patients. These events included myocardial infarction, stroke, congestive heart failure, and hemodialysis vascular access thrombosis. A rate of hemoglobin rise of more than 1 g/dL over 2 weeks may contribute to these risks.

In a randomized prospective trial, 1,432 anemic CRF patients who were not undergoing dialysis were assigned to epoetin alfa treatment targeting a maintenance hemoglobin concentration of 13.5 or 11.3 g/dL. A major cardiovascular event (death, myocardial infarction, stroke, or hospitalization for congestive heart failure) occurred among 125 (18%) of the 715 patients in the higher hemoglobin group compared with 97 (14%) among the 717 patients in the lower hemoglobin group (hazard ratio [HR], 1.3; 95% confidence interval [CI], 1 to 1.7; $P = 0.03$).

Increased risk for serious cardiovascular events was also reported from a randomized, prospective trial of 1,265 hemodialysis patients with clinically evident cardiac disease (ischemic heart disease or congestive heart failure). In this trial, patients were assigned to epoetin alfa treatment targeted to a maintenance hemoglobin of either 14 ± 1 g/dL or 10 ± 1 g/dL. Higher mortality (35% vs 29%) was observed in the 634 patients randomized to a target hemoglobin of 14 g/dL than in the 631 patients randomized to a target hemoglobin of 10 g/dL. The reason for the increased mortality observed in this study is unknown; however, the incidence of nonfatal myocardial infarction, vascular access thrombosis, and other thrombotic events was also higher in the group randomized to a target hemoglobin of 14 g/dL.

Anemia caused by other conditions – The safety and efficacy of methoxy polyethylene glycol-epoetin beta have not been established for use among patients with anemia caused by cancer chemotherapy or for reduction in the need for allogeneic red blood cell transfusion in the perisurgical setting. In these conditions, clinical trials of ESAs have shown risks for thrombotic events and/or mortality.

In a randomized, controlled study (referred to as Cancer Study 1, the Bone Estrogen Strength Training [BEST] study) with another ESA in 939 women with metastatic breast cancer receiving chemotherapy, patients received either weekly epoetin alfa or placebo for up to a year. This study was designed to show that survival was superior when an ESA was administered to prevent anemia (maintain hemoglobin levels between 12 and 14 g/dL or hematocrit between 36% and 42%). The study was terminated prematurely when interim results demonstrated that a higher mortality at 4 months (8.7% vs 3.4%) and a higher rate of fatal thrombotic events (1.1% vs 0.2%) in the first 4 months of the study were observed among patients treated with epoetin alfa. Based on Kaplan-Meier estimates, at the time of study termination, the 12-month survival was lower in the epoetin alfa group than in the placebo group (70% vs 76%; HR, 1.37; 95% CI, 1.07 to 1.75; $P = 0.012$).

A systematic review of 57 randomized controlled trials (including Cancer Studies 1 and 3, the BEST and "ENHANCE" studies) evaluating 9,353 patients with cancer compared ESAs plus red blood cell transfusion with red blood cell transfusion alone for prophylaxis or treatment of anemia in cancer patients with or without concurrent antineoplastic therapy. An increased relative risk (RR) of thromboembolic events (RR, 1.67; 95% CI, 1.35 to 2.06; 35 trials and 6,769 patients) was observed in ESA-treated patients. An overall survival HR of 1.08 (95% CI, 0.99 to 1.18; 42 trials and 8,167 patients) was observed in ESA-treated patients.

An increased incidence of deep vein thrombosis (DVT) in patients receiving epoetin alfa undergoing surgical orthopedic procedures has been observed. In a randomized, controlled study (referred to as the SPINE study), 681 adult patients not receiving prophylactic anticoagulation and undergoing spinal surgery received epoetin alfa and standard of care (SOC) treatment, or SOC treatment alone. Preliminary analysis showed a higher incidence of DVT, determined by either Color Flow Duplex Imaging or by clinical symptoms, in the epoetin alfa group (16 [4.7%] patients) compared with the SOC group (7 [2.1%] patients). In addition, 12 patients in the epoetin alfa group and 7 patients in the SOC group had other thrombotic vascular events.

Increased mortality was observed in a randomized, placebo-controlled study of epoetin alfa in adult patients who were undergoing coronary artery bypass surgery (7 deaths in 126 patients randomized to epoetin alfa vs no deaths among 56 patients receiving placebo). Four of these deaths occurred during the period of study drug administration, and all 4 deaths were associated with thrombotic events.

➤*Increased mortality and/or tumor progression:* A dose-ranging trial of methoxy polyethylene glycol-epoetin beta in 153 patients who were undergoing chemotherapy for non-small cell lung cancer was terminated prematurely because significantly more deaths occurred among patients receiving methoxy polyethylene glycol-epoetin beta than another ESA.

ESAs, when administered to target a hemoglobin of greater than 12 g/dL, shortened the time to tumor progression in patients with advanced head and neck cancer receiving radiation therapy (Cancer Studies 3 and 4 [DAHANCA 10]). ESAs also shortened survival in patients with metastatic breast cancer (Cancer Study 1) and in patients with lymphoid malignancy (Cancer Study 2)

METHOXY POLYETHYLENE GLYCOL-EPOETIN BETA — INJECTION

receiving chemotherapy when administered to target a hemoglobin of approximately 12 g/dL or more. In addition, ESAs shortened survival in patients with non–small cell lung cancer and in a study enrolling patients with various malignancies who were not receiving chemotherapy or radiotherapy; in these 2 studies, ESAs were administered to target a hemoglobin of approximately 12 g/dL or more (Cancer Studies 5 and 6). Although studies evaluated hemoglobin targets of approximately 12 g/dL or more in these tumor types, the risks of shortened survival and tumor progression have not been excluded when ESAs are dosed to target a hemoglobin of less than 12 g/dL.

Decreased overall survival – Cancer Study 1 (the BEST study), which was previously described, showed that mortality at 4 months (8.7% vs 3.4%) was significantly higher in the epoetin alfa arm. The most common investigator-attributed cause of death within the first 4 months was disease progression; 28 of 41 deaths in the epoetin alfa arm and 13 of 16 deaths in the placebo arm were attributed to disease progression. Investigator assessed time to tumor progression was not different between the 2 groups. Survival at 12 months was significantly lower in the epoetin alfa arm (70% vs 76%; HR, 1.37; 95% CI, 1.07 to 1.75; $P = 0.012$).

Cancer Study 2 was a phase 3, double-blind, randomized (darbepoetin alfa vs placebo) study conducted in 344 anemic patients with lymphoid malignancy receiving chemotherapy. With a median follow-up of 29 months, overall mortality rates were significantly higher among patients randomized to darbepoetin alfa compared with placebo (HR, 1.36; 95% CI, 1.02 to 1.82).

Cancer Study 5 was a phase 3, multicenter, randomized (epoetin alfa vs placebo), double-blind study in which patients with advanced non–small cell lung cancer receiving only palliative radiotherapy or no active therapy were treated with epoetin alfa to achieve and maintain hemoglobin levels between 12 and 14 g/dL. Following an interim analysis of 70 of 300 patients planned, a significant difference in survival in favor of the patients on the placebo arm of the trial was observed (median survival, 63 vs 129 days; HR, 1.84; $P = 0.04$).

Cancer Study 6 was a phase 3, double-blind, randomized (darbepoetin alfa vs placebo), 16-week study in 989 anemic patients with active malignant disease, neither receiving nor planning to receive chemotherapy or radiation therapy. There was no evidence of a statistically significant reduction in proportion of patients receiving red blood cell transfusions. The median survival was shorter in the darbepoetin alfa treatment group (8 months) compared with the placebo group (10.8 months; HR, 1.30; 95% CI, 1.07 to 1.57).

Decreased LRPFS and overall survival – Cancer Study 3 (the "ENHANCE" study) was a randomized, controlled study in 351 head and neck cancer patients in which epoetin beta or placebo was administered to achieve target hemoglobins of 14 and 15 g/dL for women and men, respectively. LRPFS was significantly shorter in patients receiving epoetin beta (HR, 1.62; 95% CI, 1.22 to 2.14; $P = 0.0008$) with a median of 406 days epoetin beta versus 745 days placebo. Overall survival was significantly shorter in patients receiving epoetin beta (HR, 1.39; 95% CI, 1.05 to 1.84; $P = 0.02$).

Decreased locoregional control – Cancer Study 4 (DAHANCA 10) was conducted in 522 patients with primary squamous cell carcinoma of the head and neck receiving radiation therapy randomized to darbepoetin alfa with radiotherapy or radiotherapy alone. An interim analysis on 484 patients demonstrated that locoregional control at 5 years was significantly shorter in patients receiving darbepoetin alfa (RR, 1.44; 95% CI, 1.06 to 1.96; $P = 0.02$). Overall survival was shorter in patients receiving darbepoetin alfa (RR, 1.28; 95% CI, 0.98 to 1.68; $P = 0.08$).

➤*Hypertension:* Adequately control blood pressure before initiation of methoxy polyethylene glycol-epoetin beta therapy. Take special care to closely monitor and control blood pressure during methoxy polyethylene glycol-epoetin beta therapy, especially in patients with a history of cardiovascular disease or hypertension. If blood pressure is difficult to control by pharmacologic or dietary measures, reduce or withhold the dose of methoxy polyethylene glycol-epoetin beta.

In methoxy polyethylene glycol-epoetin beta clinical studies, approximately 27% of patients with CRF, including patients on dialysis and not on dialysis, required intensification of antihypertensive therapy. Hypertensive encephalopathy and/or seizures have been observed in patients with CRF treated with methoxy polyethylene glycol-epoetin beta.

➤*Seizures:* Seizures have occurred in patients participating in methoxy polyethylene glycol-epoetin beta clinical studies. During the first several months of therapy, closely monitor blood pressure and the presence of premonitory neurologic symptoms. While the relationship between seizures and the rate of rise of hemoglobin is uncertain, decrease or withhold the dose of methoxy polyethylene glycol-epoetin beta if the hemoglobin increases more than 1 g/dL in any 2-week period.

➤*Pure red cell aplasia (PRCA):* PRCA and severe anemia, with or without other cytopenias, have been associated with the development of neutralizing antibodies to erythropoietin in patients treated with ESAs. PRCA occurred predominantly in patients with CRF receiving an ESA by subcutaneous administration. PRCA was not observed in clinical studies of methoxy polyethylene glycol-epoetin beta.

Any patient who develops a sudden loss of response to methoxy polyethylene glycol-epoetin beta accompanied by severe anemia and low reticulocyte count should be evaluated for the etiology of the altered hemoglobin response, including evaluation for the development of neutralizing antibodies to erythropoietin. Obtain serum samples at least a month after the last methoxy polyethylene glycol-epoetin beta administration to prevent interference of methoxy polyethylene glycol-epoetin beta with the assay. If anti-erythropoietin antibody–associated anemia is suspected, withhold methoxy polyethylene glycol-epoetin beta and other erythropoietic proteins. Contact the manufacturer at 1-800-526-6367 to perform assays for antibodies.

Permanently discontinue methoxy polyethylene glycol-epoetin beta in patients with antibody-mediated anemia. Do not switch patients to other erythropoietic proteins because antibodies may cross-react.

➤*Lack or loss of response:* The lack of a hemoglobin response or failure to maintain a hemoglobin response with methoxy polyethylene glycol-epoetin beta doses within the recommended dosing range should prompt a search for causative factors. Exclude or correct deficiencies of iron, folic acid, and vitamin B_{12}.

Intercurrent infections, malignancy, inflammation, occult blood loss, hemolysis, severe aluminum toxicity, osteitis fibrosis cystica, underlying hematological disease (eg, thalassemia, refractory anemia, myelodysplastic disorders), or bone marrow fibrosis may also compromise the hemoglobin response. In the absence of another etiology, evaluate the patient for evidence of PRCA, including tests for the presence of antibodies to erythropoietin.

➤*Hematologic effects:* Allow sufficient time to determine a patient's response to a methoxy polyethylene glycol-epoetin beta dose before adjusting the subsequent doses. Because of the time required for erythropoiesis and the red blood cell life span, an interval of 2 to 6 weeks may occur between the time of a dose adjustment (initiation, increase, decrease, or discontinuation) and a significant change in hemoglobin. To prevent the hemoglobin from exceeding 12 g/dL or rising too rapidly (greater than 1 g/dL in 2 weeks), follow the guidelines for dose and frequency of dose adjustments.

Average platelet counts decreased approximately 7% among patients receiving methoxy polyethylene glycol-epoetin beta in clinical studies, with most patients maintaining platelet counts within normal levels. The decrease in platelet counts occurred immediately following methoxy polyethylene glycol-epoetin beta initiation, and the levels remained stable thereafter. At least 1 postbaseline platelet count below 100×10^9/L was observed in 7.5% of patients treated with methoxy polyethylene glycol-epoetin beta and 4.4% of patients treated with another ESA.

➤*Allergic reactions:* Serious allergic reactions, consisting of tachycardia, pruritus, and rash, have been reported in patients treated with methoxy polyethylene glycol-epoetin beta. If a serious allergic or anaphylactic reaction occurs because of methoxy polyethylene glycol-epoetin beta, immediately and permanently discontinue treatment and administer appropriate therapy.

➤*Patients with CRF not requiring dialysis:* Patients with CRF not requiring dialysis may require lower maintenance doses of methoxy polyethylene glycol-epoetin beta than patients receiving dialysis. Patients who are not receiving dialysis may be more responsive to the effects of methoxy polyethylene glycol-epoetin beta and require judicious monitoring of blood pressure and hemoglobin. Also, closely monitor renal function and fluid electrolyte balance.

➤*Dialysis management:* Therapy with methoxy polyethylene glycol-epoetin beta results in an increase in red blood cells and a decrease in plasma volume, which could reduce dialysis efficiency; patients who are marginally dialyzed may require adjustments in their dialysis prescription.

➤*Pregnancy: Category C.* When methoxy polyethylene glycol-epoetin beta was administered subcutaneously to rats and rabbits during gestation, bone malformation was observed in both species at 50 mcg/kg once every 3 days. This effect was observed as missing caudal vertebrae resulting in a thread-like tail in one rat fetus, absent first digit metacarpal and phalanx on each forelimb resulting in absent polex in one rabbit fetus, and fused fourth and fifth cervical vertebrae centra in another rabbit fetus. Dose-related reduction in fetal weights was observed in both rats and rabbits. At doses of 5 mcg/kg and higher once every 3 days, methoxy polyethylene glycol-epoetin beta caused exaggerated pharmacodynamic effects in dams. Once-weekly doses of methoxy polyethylene glycol-epoetin beta of up to 50 mcg/kg/dose given to pregnant female rats did not adversely affect pregnancy parameters, natural delivery, or litter observations. Increased deaths and significant reduction in growth rate of F1 generation were observed during lactation and early postweaning period. However, no remarkable effect on reflex, physical and cognitive development, or reproductive performance was observed in F1 generation of any dose groups.

There are no adequate and well-controlled studies in pregnant women. Methoxy polyethylene glycol-epoetin beta should be used during pregnancy only if the potential benefit justifies the potential risk to the fetus.

➤*Lactation:* It is not known whether methoxy polyethylene glycol-epoetin beta is excreted into human breast milk. In one study in rats, methoxy polyethylene glycol-epoetin beta was excreted into maternal milk. Because many drugs are excreted in human milk, exercise caution when administering methoxy polyethylene glycol-epoetin beta to a breast-feeding woman.

➤*Children:* The safety and efficacy of methoxy polyethylene glycol-epoetin beta in children have not been established.

➤*Elderly:* In general, dose selection for an elderly patient should be cautious, usually starting at the low end of the dosing range, reflecting the greater frequency of decreased hepatic, renal, or cardiac function, and of concomitant disease or other drug therapy.

➤*Monitoring:* To ensure effective erythropoiesis, evaluate iron status for all patients before and during treatment. Provide supplemental iron therapy for patients whose serum ferritin is below 100 mcg/L or whose serum transferrin saturation is below 20%.

During methoxy polyethylene glycol-epoetin beta therapy, monitor hemoglobin every 2 weeks until the hemoglobin level has stabilized between 10 and 12 g/dL and the maintenance methoxy polyethylene glycol-epoetin beta dose

METHOXY POLYETHYLENE GLYCOL-EPOETIN BETA — INJECTION

has been established. The hemoglobin should then be monitored at least monthly. If a patient requires a dose adjustment or is switched to methoxy polyethylene glycol-epoetin beta from another ESA, monitor hemoglobin every 2 weeks until the hemoglobin level has stabilized.

Monitor and control blood pressure during methoxy polyethylene glycol-epoetin beta therapy, especially in patients with a history of cardiovascular disease or hypertension.

Drug Interactions

None known.

Adverse Reactions

The following serious adverse reactions are discussed in greater detail in the Warnings and Precautions section: hypertension; increased mortality and/or tumor progression; pure red cell aplasia; increased mortality; seizures; serious cardiovascular and thromboembolic events.

The most commonly reported adverse reactions were hypertension, diarrhea, nasopharyngitis, headache, and upper respiratory tract infection. The most common adverse reactions that led to treatment discontinuation in the methoxy polyethylene glycol-epoetin beta clinical studies included the following: anemia, concomitant termination of other CRF therapy, coronary artery disease, hypertension, and septic shock.

➤*Clinical trials experience:* Some of the adverse reactions reported are typically associated with CRF or recognized complications of dialysis and may not necessarily be attributable to methoxy polyethylene glycol-epoetin beta therapy. Adverse reaction rates did not importantly differ between patients receiving methoxy polyethylene glycol-epoetin beta and those receiving another ESA.

The following table summarizes the most frequent adverse reactions (5% or more) in patients treated with methoxy polyethylene glycol-epoetin beta.

Methoxy Polyethylene Glycol-Epoetin Beta Adverse Reactions (≥ 5%)	
Adverse reaction	Patients treated with methoxy polyethylene glycol-epoetin beta (n = 1,789)
Cardiovascular	
Arteriovenous fistula site complication	5%
Arteriovenous fistula thrombosis	5%
Hypertension	13%
Hypotension	5%
Procedural hypotension	8%
CNS	
Headache	9%
GI	
Constipation	5%
Diarrhea	11%
Vomiting	6%
GU	
Urinary tract infection	5%
Metabolic/Nutritional	
Fluid overload	7%
Musculoskeletal	
Back pain	6%
Muscle spasms	8%
Respiratory	
Cough	6%
Nasopharyngitis	11%
Upper respiratory tract infection	9%
Miscellaneous	
Pain in extremity	5%

In the controlled trials, the rates of serious adverse reactions did not importantly differ between patients receiving methoxy polyethylene glycol-epoetin beta and another ESA (38% vs 42%) except for the occurrence of serious GI hemorrhage (1.2% vs 0.2%). Serious hemorrhagic adverse reactions of all types occurred among 5% and 4% of patients receiving methoxy polyethylene glycol-epoetin beta or another ESA, respectively.

➤*Immunogenicity:* As with all therapeutic proteins, there is a potential for immunogenicity. Neutralizing antibodies to erythropoietin, in association with PRCA or severe anemia (with or without other cytopenias), have been reported in patients receiving other ESAs during postmarketing experience. Compared with subcutaneous administration, the IV route of administration may lessen the risk for development of antibodies to methoxy polyethylene glycol-epoetin beta.

Overdosage

➤*Symptoms:* The expected manifestations of methoxy polyethylene glycol-epoetin beta overdosage include signs and symptoms associated with an excessive and/or rapid increase in hemoglobin concentration, including any of the cardiovascular events described in Warnings and Precautions.

➤*Treatment:* Closely monitor patients receiving an overdosage of methoxy polyethylene glycol-epoetin beta for cardiovascular events and hematologic abnormalities. Manage polycythemia acutely with phlebotomy, as clinically indicated. Following resolution of the effects caused by methoxy polyethylene glycol-epoetin beta overdosage, accompany reintroduction of methoxy polyethylene glycol-epoetin beta therapy with close monitoring for evidence of rapid increases in hemoglobin concentration (greater than 1 g/dL per 14 days). In patients with an excessive hematopoietic response, reduce the methoxy polyethylene glycol-epoetin beta dose in accordance with the recommendations described in Administration and Dosage.

Patient Information

Inform patients of the need for regular blood pressure monitoring and laboratory tests for hemoglobin to lessen the risks for mortality and serious cardiovascular events.

Inform patients of the possible adverse reactions of methoxy polyethylene glycol-epoetin beta, including injection-site reactions, allergic reactions, and potential problems due to excessive increases in blood hemoglobin levels.

Inform patients of the signs and symptoms of injection-site and allergic reactions.

Inform patients of the importance of compliance with any prescribed dietary restrictions, dialysis regimens, or medications, including antihypertensive medications.

Thrombopoietin Mimetic Agents

ROMIPLOSTIM

Rx	Nplate (Amgen)	**Injection, lyophilized powder for solution:** 250 mcg	Mannitol, sucrose, L-histidine, polysorbate 20. In 250 mcg single-use vials. Preservative free.
		500 mcg	Mannitol, sucrose, L-histidine, polysorbate 20. In 500 mcg single-use vials. Preservative free.

ROMIPLOSTIM — INJECTION

Indications

➤*Thrombocytopenia:* For the treatment of thrombocytopenia in patients with chronic immune (idiopathic) thrombocytopenic purpura (ITP) who have had an insufficient response to corticosteroids, immunoglobulins, or splenectomy. Romiplostim should be used only in patients with ITP whose degree of thrombocytopenia and clinical condition increases the risk for bleeding. Romiplostim should not be used in an attempt to normalize platelet counts.

Administration and Dosage

➤*General dosing considerations:* Use the lowest dose of romiplostim to achieve and maintain a platelet count of at least 50×10^9/L as necessary to reduce the risk for bleeding. Romiplostim should not be used in an attempt to normalize platelet counts.

Only health care providers enrolled in the romiplostim NEXUS (Network of Experts Understanding and Supporting *Nplate* and Patients) program may prescribe romiplostim. Romiplostim must be administered by the enrolled health care provider or under their direction.

➤*Adults:*

Thrombocytopenia –

Maximum dose: 10 mcg/kg weekly.

Initial dosage: 1 mcg/kg based on actual body weight.

Dosage adjustment: Use the actual body weight at initiation of therapy, then adjust the weekly dose of romiplostim by increments of 1 mcg/kg until the patient achieves a platelet count of at least 50×10^9/L as necessary to reduce the risk for bleeding; do not exceed a maximum weekly dose of 10 mcg/kg. In clinical studies, most patients who responded to romiplostim achieved and maintained platelet counts of at least 50×10^9/L with a median dose of 2 mcg/kg.

During romiplostim therapy, assess complete blood cell counts (CBCs), including platelet count and peripheral blood smears, weekly until a stable platelet count (at least 50×10^9/L for at least 4 weeks without dose adjustment) has been achieved. Obtain CBCs, including platelet counts and peripheral blood smears, monthly thereafter.

Adjust the dose as follows:

- If the platelet count is less than 50×10^9/L, increase the dose by 1 mcg/kg.

ROMIPLOSTIM — INJECTION

- If platelet count is more than 200 × 10^9/L for 2 consecutive weeks, reduce the dose by 1 mcg/kg.
- If platelet count is more than 400 × 10^9/L, do not dose. Continue to assess the platelet count weekly. After the platelet count has fallen to less than 200 × 10^9/L, resume romiplostim at a dose reduced by 1 mcg/kg.

Concomitant therapy: Romiplostim may be used with other medical ITP therapies, such as corticosteroids, danazol, azathioprine, immunoglobulin intravenous (IV), and anti-D immunoglobulin. If the patient's platelet count is at least 50 × 10^9/L, medical ITP therapies may be reduced or discontinued.

Discontinuation of therapy: Discontinue romiplostim if the platelet count does not increase to a level sufficient to avoid clinically important bleeding after 4 weeks of romiplostim therapy at the maximum weekly dose of 10 mcg/kg. Obtain CBCs, including platelet counts, weekly for at least 2 weeks following discontinuation of romiplostim.

➤*Preparation for administration:* Romiplostim is supplied in single-use vials that must be reconstituted as outlined in the following table and administered using a syringe with 0.01 mL graduations. Using aseptic technique, reconstitute romiplostim with preservative-free sterile water for injection, as described in the following table. Do not use bacteriostatic water for injection.

Reconstitution of Romiplostim Single-Use Vials

Romiplostim single-use vial	Total vial content of romiplostim		Sterile water for injection[a]		Deliverable product and volume	Final concentration
250 mcg	375 mcg	add	0.72 mL	=	250 mcg in 0.5 mL	500 mcg/mL
500 mcg	625 mcg	add	1.2 mL	=	500 mcg in 1 mL	500 mcg/mL

[a] Use preservative-free sterile water for injection.

Gently swirl and invert the vial to reconstitute. Avoid excess or vigorous agitation; do not shake. Generally, dissolution of romiplostim takes less than 2 minutes. The reconstituted romiplostim solution should be clear and colorless.

➤*Administration:* Administer as a weekly subcutaneous injection. Because the injection volume may be very small, use a syringe with graduations to 0.01 mL.

To determine the injection volume to be administered, first identify the patient's total dose in micrograms (mcg) using the dosing information previously mentioned. For example, a 75 kg patient initiating therapy at 1 mcg/kg will begin with a dose of 75 mcg. Next, calculate the volume of romiplostim solution that is given to the patient by dividing the microgram dose by the concentration of the reconstituted romiplostim solution (500 mcg/mL). For this patient example, the 75 mcg dose is divided by 500 mcg/mL, resulting in an injection volume of 0.15 mL.

➤*Storage / Stability:* Store romiplostim vials in their carton to protect from light until time of use. Keep romiplostim vials refrigerated at 2° to 8°C (36° to 46°F). Do not freeze.

Reconstituted romiplostim can be kept at room temperature (25°C [77°F]) or refrigerated at 2° to 8°C (36° to 46°F) for up to 24 hours prior to administration. Protect the reconstituted product from light. Discard any unused portion. Do not pool unused portions from the vials. Do not administer more than 1 dose from a vial.

Actions

➤*Pharmacology:* Romiplostim increases platelet production through binding and activation of the thrombopoietin (TPO) receptor, a mechanism analogous to endogenous TPO.

Pharmacodynamics – In clinical studies, treatment with romiplostim resulted in dose-dependent increases in platelet counts. After a single subcutaneous dose of romiplostim 1 to 10 mcg/kg in patients with chronic ITP, the peak platelet count was 1.3 to 14.9 times greater than the baseline platelet count over a 2- to 3-week period. The platelet counts were more than 50 × 10^9/L for 7 out of 8 patients with chronic ITP who received 6 weekly doses of romiplostim 1 mcg/kg.

➤*Pharmacokinetics:* In the long-term extension study in patients with ITP receiving weekly treatment of romiplostim subcutaneously, the pharmacokinetics of romiplostim over the dose range of 3 to 15 mcg/kg indicated that peak serum concentrations of romiplostim were observed about 7 to 50 hours postdose (median, 14 hours). The serum concentrations varied among patients and did not correlate with the dose administered.

Excretion – Half-life values ranged from 1 to 34 days (median, 3.5 days). The elimination of serum romiplostim is in part dependent on the TPO receptor on platelets. As a result, for a given dose, patients with high platelet counts are associated with low serum concentrations and vice versa.

Contraindications

None known.

Warnings/Precautions

➤*Bone marrow effects:* Romiplostim administration increases the risk for development or progression of reticulin fiber deposition within the bone marrow. In clinical studies, romiplostim was discontinued in 4 of the 271 patients because of bone marrow reticulin deposition. Six additional patients had reticulin observed upon bone marrow biopsy. All 10 patients with bone marrow reticulin deposition had received romiplostim doses of at least 5 mcg/kg, and 6 received doses of at least 10 mcg/kg. Progression to marrow fibrosis with cytopenias was not reported in the controlled clinical studies. In the extension study, 1 patient with ITP and hemolytic anemia developed marrow fibrosis with collagen during romiplostim therapy. Clinical studies have not excluded a risk of bone marrow fibrosis with cytopenias.

Prior to initiation of romiplostim, examine the peripheral blood smear closely to establish a baseline level of cellular morphologic abnormalities. Following identification of a stable romiplostim dose, examine peripheral blood smears and CBCs monthly for new or worsening morphological abnormalities (eg, teardrop and nucleated red blood cells, immature white blood cells) or cytopenia(s). If the patient develops new or worsening morphological abnormalities or cytopenia(s), discontinue treatment with romiplostim and consider a bone marrow biopsy, including staining for fibrosis.

➤*Discontinuation:* Discontinuation of romiplostim may result in thrombocytopenia of greater severity than was present prior to romiplostim therapy. This worsened thrombocytopenia may increase the patient's risk of bleeding, particularly if romiplostim is discontinued while the patient is on anticoagulants or antiplatelet agents. In clinical studies of patients with chronic ITP who had romiplostim discontinued, 4 of 57 patients developed thrombocytopenia of greater severity than was present prior to romiplostim therapy. This worsened thrombocytopenia resolved within 14 days. Following discontinuation of romiplostim, obtain weekly CBCs, including platelet counts, for at least 2 weeks and consider alternative treatments for worsening thrombocytopenia, according to current treatment guidelines.

➤*Thrombotic / Thromboembolic effects:* Thrombotic/thromboembolic complications may result from excessive increases in platelet counts. Excessive doses of romiplostim or medication errors that result in excessive romiplostim doses may increase platelet counts to a level that produces thrombotic/thromboembolic complications. In controlled clinical studies, the incidence of thrombotic/thromboembolic complications was similar between romiplostim and placebo. To minimize the risk for thrombotic/ thromboembolic complications, do not use romiplostim in an attempt to normalize platelet counts. Follow the dose adjustment guidelines to achieve and maintain a platelet count of at least 50 × 10^9/L.

➤*Lack or loss of response:* Hyporesponsiveness or failure to maintain a platelet response with romiplostim should prompt a search for causative factors, including neutralizing antibodies to romiplostim or bone marrow fibrosis. To detect antibody formation, submit blood samples to Amgen (1-800-772-6436). Amgen will assay these samples for antibodies to romiplostim and TPO. Discontinue romiplostim if the platelet count does not increase to a level sufficient to avoid clinically important bleeding after 4 weeks at the highest weekly dose of 10 mcg/kg.

➤*Malignancies:* Romiplostim stimulation of the TPO receptor on the surface of hematopoietic cells may increase the risk for hematologic malignancies. In controlled clinical studies among patients with chronic ITP, the incidence of hematologic malignancy was low and similar between romiplostim and placebo. In a separate single-arm clinical study of 44 patients with myelodysplastic syndrome (MDS), 11 patients were reported as having possible disease progression, among whom 4 patients had confirmation of acute myelogenous leukemia (AML) during follow-up. Romiplostim is not indicated for the treatment of thrombocytopenia due to MDS or any cause of thrombocytopenia other than chronic ITP.

➤*Distribution program:* Romiplostim is available only through a restricted distribution program called the romiplostim NEXUS program. Under the romiplostim NEXUS program, only health care providers and patients registered with the program are able to prescribe, administer, and receive romiplostim. This program provides educational materials and a mechanism for the proper use of romiplostim. To enroll in the romiplostim NEXUS program, call 1-877-675-2831. Prescribers and patients are required to understand the risks of romiplostim therapy. Prescribers are required to understand the information in the prescribing information and be able to:

- Educate patients on the benefits and risks of treatment with romiplostim, ensure that the patient receives the *Medication Guide*, instruct them to read it, and encourage them to ask questions when considering romiplostim. Patients may be educated by the enrolled prescriber or a health care provider under that prescriber's direction.
- Review the romiplostim NEXUS program health care provider enrollment form, sign the form, and return the form according to romiplostim NEXUS program instructions.
- Review the romiplostim NEXUS program patient enrollment form, answer all questions, obtain the patients signature on the romiplostim NEXUS program patient enrollment form, place the original signed form in the patients medical record, send a copy according to romiplostim NEXUS program instructions, and give a copy to the patient.
- Report any serious adverse reactions associated with the use of romiplostim to the romiplostim NEXUS program call center at 1-877-675-2831 or to the Food and Drug Administration MedWatch program at 1-800-332-1088.
- Report serious adverse reactions observed in patients receiving romiplostim, including reactions actively solicited at 6-month intervals.

➤*Immunogenicity:* As with all therapeutic proteins, patients may develop antibodies to the therapeutic protein. Patients were screened for immunogenicity to romiplostim using a BIAcore-based biosensor immunoassay. This assay is capable of detecting both high- and low-affinity binding antibodies that bind to romiplostim and cross-react with TPO. The samples from patients that tested positive for binding antibodies were further evaluated for neutralizing capacity using a cell-based bioassay.

In clinical studies, the incidence of preexisting antibodies to romiplostim was 8% (17/225), and the incidence of binding antibody development during romiplostim treatment was 10% (23/225). The incidence of preexisting antibodies to endogenous TPO was 5% (12/225), and the incidence of binding antibody development to endogenous TPO during romiplostim treatment

ROMIPLOSTIM — INJECTION

was 5% (12/225). Of the patients with positive antibodies to romiplostim or to TPO, 1 (0.4%) patient had neutralizing activity to romiplostim and none had neutralizing activity to TPO. No correlation was observed between antibody activity and clinical effectiveness or safety.

Immunogenicity assay results are highly dependent on the sensitivity and specificity of the assay used in detection and may be influenced by several factors, including sample handling, concomitant medications, and underlying disease. For these reasons, comparison of incidence of antibodies to romiplostim with the incidence of antibodies to other products may be misleading.

➤*Renal function impairment:* Use romiplostim with caution in this population.

➤*Hepatic function impairment:* Use romiplostim with caution in this population.

➤*Pregnancy: Category C.* There are no adequate and well-controlled studies of romiplostim use in pregnant women. In animal reproduction and developmental toxicity studies, romiplostim crossed the placenta, and adverse fetal reactions included thrombocytosis, postimplantation loss, and an increase in pup mortality. Use romiplostim during pregnancy only if the potential benefit to the mother justifies the potential risk to the fetus.

In rat and rabbit developmental toxicity studies, no evidence of fetal harm was observed at romiplostim doses up to 11 times (rats) and 82 times (rabbit) the maximum human dose (MHD) based on systemic exposure. In mice at doses 5 times the MHD, reductions in maternal body weight and increased postimplantation loss occurred.

In a prenatal and postnatal development study in rats at doses 11 times the MHD, there was an increase in perinatal pup mortality. Romiplostim crossed the placental barrier in rats and increased fetal platelet counts at clinically equivalent and higher doses.

Pregnancy registry – A pregnancy registry has been established to collect information about the effects of romiplostim use during pregnancy. Health care providers are encouraged to register pregnant patients, or pregnant women may enroll themselves by calling 1-877-675-2831.

➤*Lactation:* It is not known whether romiplostim is excreted in human milk; however, human immunoglobulin G is excreted in human milk. Published data suggest that breast milk antibodies do not enter the neonatal and infant circulation in substantial amounts. Because many drugs are excreted in human milk and because of the potential for serious adverse reactions in breast-feeding infants from romiplostim, a decision should be made whether to discontinue breast-feeding or romiplostim, taking into account the importance of romiplostim to the mother and the known benefits of breast-feeding.

➤*Children:* Safety and effectiveness in children (younger than 18 years of age) have not been established.

➤*Elderly:* In general, dose adjustment for an elderly patient should be cautious, reflecting the greater frequency of decreased hepatic, renal, or cardiac function, and of concomitant disease or other drug therapy.

➤*Monitoring:* Monitor CBCs, including platelet counts and peripheral blood smears, prior to initiation, throughout, and following discontinuation of romiplostim therapy. Prior to the initiation of romiplostim, examine the peripheral blood differential to establish the baseline extent of red and white blood cell abnormalities. Obtain CBCs, including platelet counts and peripheral blood smears, weekly during the dose adjustment phase of romiplostim therapy and then monthly following establishment of a stable romiplostim dose. Obtain CBCs, including platelet counts, weekly for at least 2 weeks following discontinuation of romiplostim.

Drug Interactions

None known.

Adverse Reactions

➤*Serious adverse reactions:* Serious adverse reactions associated with romiplostim in clinical studies were bone marrow reticulin deposition and worsening thrombocytopenia after romiplostim discontinuation. See Warnings and Precautions for more information.

➤*Common adverse reactions:* In the placebo-controlled studies, headache was the most commonly reported adverse drug reaction, occurring in 35% of patients receiving romiplostim and 32% of patients receiving placebo. Headaches were usually of mild or moderate severity.

Romiplostim Adverse Drug Reactions (≥ 5%)

Adverse reactions	Romiplostim (n = 84)	Placebo (n = 41)
CNS		
Dizziness	17%	0%
Insomnia	16%	7%
Paresthesia	6%	0%
GI		
Abdominal pain	11%	0%
Dyspepsia	7%	0%
Musculoskeletal		
Arthralgia	26%	20%
Myalgia	14%	2%
Pain in extremity	13%	5%
Shoulder pain	8%	0%

Overdosage

➤*Symptoms:* In the event of overdose, platelet counts may increase excessively and result in thrombotic/thromboembolic complications.

➤*Treatment:* Discontinue romiplostim and monitor platelet counts. Reinitiate treatment with romiplostim in accordance with dosing and administration recommendations.

Patient Information

Prior to treatment, patients should fully understand the risks and benefits of romiplostim. Inform patients that the risks associated with long-term administration of romiplostim are unknown and that they must enroll in the romiplostim NEXUS Program, which provides for the proper use of romiplostim in ITP patients.

Inform patients of the following risks and considerations for romiplostim:

- Romiplostim can only be administered by a health care provider who is enrolled in the romiplostim NEXUS program or a health care provider under their direction.
- Romiplostim therapy is administered to achieve and maintain a platelet count of at least 50×10^9/L as necessary to reduce the risk for bleeding; romiplostim is not used to normalize platelet counts.
- Following discontinuation of romiplostim, thrombocytopenia and risk of bleeding that is worse than that experienced prior to the romiplostim therapy may develop.
- Romiplostim therapy increases the risk of reticulin fiber formation within the bone marrow, and further fiber formation may progress to marrow fibrosis. Detection of peripheral blood cell abnormalities may necessitate a bone marrow examination.
- Too much romiplostim may result in excessive platelet counts and a risk for thrombotic/thromboembolic complications.
- Romiplostim stimulates certain bone marrow cells to make platelets and may increase the risk for progression of underlying MDS or hematologic malignancies.
- Platelet counts and CBCs, including peripheral blood smears, must be performed weekly until a stable romiplostim dose has been achieved; thereafter, platelet counts and CBCs, including peripheral blood smears, must be performed monthly while taking romiplostim.
- Patients must be closely monitored with weekly platelet counts and CBCs for at least 2 weeks following romiplostim discontinuation.
- Even with romiplostim therapy, patients should continue to avoid situations or medications that may increase the risk for bleeding.

FILGRASTIM (Granulocyte Colony Stimulating Factor; G-CSF)

Rx	**Neupogen** (Amgen)	**Injection:** 300 mcg/mL[a]	Preservative free. In 1 and 1.6 mL single-dose vials.
		Injection: 300 mcg per 0.5 mL[b]	Preservative free. In 0.5 mL and 0.8 mL prefilled syringes.

[a] With 0.59 mg acetate, 50 mg sorbitol, 0.004% *Tween* 80 and 0.035 mg Na/mL in water for injection.

[b] With 0.295 mg acetate, 25 mg sorbitol, 0.004% *Tween* 80, and 0.0175 mg Na/mL in water for injection.

FILGRASTIM — INJECTION

Indications

➤*Cancer patients:*

Myelosuppressive chemotherapy – To decrease the incidence of infection, as manifested by febrile neutropenia, in patients with nonmyeloid malignancies receiving myelosuppressive anticancer drugs associated with a significant incidence of severe neutropenia with fever. A complete blood count (CBC) and platelet count should be obtained prior to chemotherapy, and twice a week (see Precautions, Monitoring) during filgrastim therapy to avoid leukocytosis and to monitor the neutrophil count. In phase 3 clinical studies, filgrastim therapy was discontinued when the ANC was greater than or equal to 10,000/mm^3 after the expected chemotherapy-induced nadir.

Acute myeloid leukemia (AML) receiving induction or consolidation chemotherapy – For reducing the time to neutrophil recovery and the duration of fever, following induction or consolidation chemotherapy treatment of adults with AML.

Bone marrow transplant – To reduce the duration of neutropenia and neutropenia-related clinical sequelae (eg, febrile neutropenia) in patients with nonmyeloid malignancies undergoing myeloablative chemotherapy followed by marrow transplantation. It is recommended that CBCs and plate-

FILGRASTIM — INJECTION

let counts be obtained at a minimum of 3 times a week (see Precautions, Monitoring) following marrow infusion to monitor the recovery of marrow reconstitution.

Peripheral blood progenitor cell (PBPC) collection and therapy – For the mobilization of hematopoietic progenitor cells into the peripheral blood for collection by leukapheresis. Mobilization allows for the collection of increased numbers of progenitor cells capable of engraftment compared with collection by leukapheresis without mobilization or bone marrow harvest. After myeloablative chemotherapy, the transplantation of an increased number of progenitor cells can lead to more rapid engraftment, which may result in a decreased need for supportive care.

➤*Severe chronic neutropenia (SCN):* For chronic administration to reduce the incidence and duration of sequelae of neutropenia (eg, fever, infections, oropharyngeal ulcers) in symptomatic patients with congenital neutropenia, cyclic neutropenia, or idiopathic neutropenia. It is essential that serial CBCs with differential and platelet counts and an evaluation of bone marrow morphology and karyotype be performed prior to initiation of filgrastim therapy (see Warnings/Precautions). The use of filgrastim prior to confirmation of SCN may impair diagnostic efforts and may thus impair or delay evaluation and treatment of an underlying condition, other than SCN, causing the neutropenia.

➤*Off-label uses:*

Neutropenic fever – [2] = Fair documentation. The American Society of Clinical Oncology and the Infectious Diseases Society of America support the limited use of filgrastim in adult cancer patients with febrile neutropenia who are at high risk for infection-associated complications or who have prognostic factors indicative of a poor clinical outcome. Evidence regarding the use of this granulocyte colony-stimulating factor (G-CSF) in cancer patients is conflicting, and benefit may be related to patient-specific characteristics (eg, chemotherapy regimen, age, comorbid disease states, performance status). More research is needed to determine the effect of filgrastim on patient morbidity and mortality.

Other possible off-label uses – Treatment of graft failure after bone marrow transplantation; neutropenia associated with myelodysplastic syndrome; hairy cell leukemia; aplastic anemia; AIDS; zidovudine- and other drug-induced neutropenias.

Administration and Dosage

➤*Adults:*

Bone marrow transplant –

Initial dosage: 10 mcg/kg/day given as an intravenous (IV) infusion of 4 or 24 hours or as a continuous 24-hour subcutaneous infusion. Administer the first dose at least 24 hours after cytotoxic chemotherapy and at least 24 hours after bone marrow infusion.

Dosage titration: If the absolute neutrophil count (ANC) is greater than 1,000/mm^3 for 3 consecutive days, reduce the dose to 5 mcg/kg/day. If, at any time during dosing with 5 mcg/kg/day, the ANC decreases to less than 1,000/mm^3, the filgrastim dose should be increased to 10 mcg/kg/day, and the above steps repeated. If the ANC remains greater than 1,000 mm^3 for 3 more consecutive days, filgrastim should be discontinued. If the ANC decreases to less than 1,000/mm^3, filgrastim should be resumed at 5 mcg/kg/day.

Myelosuppressive chemotherapy –

Usual dosage: 4 to 8 mcg/kg/day.

Initial dosage: 5 mcg/kg/day as a single daily subcutaneous bolus injection by short IV infusion (15 to 30 minutes) or by continuous subcutaneous or continuous IV infusion. Administer no earlier than 24 hours after the administration of cytotoxic chemotherapy. Do not administer in the period 24 hours before the administration of chemotherapy.

Dosage titration: Increase in increments of 5 mcg/kg for each chemotherapy cycle, according to the duration and severity of the ANC nadir.

Duration of therapy: Administer daily for up to 2 weeks, until the ANC has reached 10,000/mm^3 following the expected chemotherapy-induced neutrophil nadir. The duration of filgrastim therapy needed to attenuate chemotherapy-induced neutropenia may be dependent on the myelosuppressive potential of the chemotherapy regimen employed. Discontinue if the ANC surpasses 10,000/mm^3 after the expected chemotherapy-induced neutrophil nadir.

Monitoring: A CBC and platelet count should be obtained before instituting filgrastim therapy and monitored twice weekly during therapy.

Peripheral blood progenitor cell (PBPC) collection and therapy –

Usual dosage: 10 mcg/kg/day subcutaneously as a bolus or a continuous infusion.

Dosage adjustment: Dose modification should be considered for those patients who develop a white blood cell (WBC) count greater than 100,000/mm^3.

Duration of therapy: Give for at least 4 days before the first leukapheresis procedure and continue until the last leukapheresis. Although the optimal duration of filgrastim administration and leukapheresis schedule have not been established, administration of filgrastim for 6 to 7 days with leukaphereses on days 5, 6, and 7 was found to be safe and effective.

Monitoring: Neutrophil counts should be monitored after 4 days of filgrastim.

Severe chronic neutropenia (SCN) – Administer filgrastim to those patients in whom a diagnosis of congenital, cyclic, or idiopathic neutropenia has been definitively confirmed. Other diseases associated with neutropenia should be ruled out.

Usual dosage:

- *Congenital neutropenia* – 6 mcg/kg/day.
- *Cyclic neutropenia* – 2.1 mcg/kg/day.
- *Idiopathic neutropenia* – 1.2 mcg/kg/day.

Initial dosage:

- *Congenital neutropenia* – 6 mcg/kg twice daily subcutaneously every day.
- *Idiopathic or cyclic neutropenia* – 5 mcg/kg as a single injection subcutaneously every day.

Dosage adjustment: ANC should not be used as the sole indication of efficacy. Adjust the dose based on the patient's clinical course and ANC. In rare instances, patients with congenital neutropenia have required filgrastim doses of 100 mcg/kg/day and more.

Duration of therapy: Chronic daily administration is required to maintain clinical benefit.

Off-label dosing –

Neutropenic fever: [2] = Fair documentation. Filgrastim should be given subcutaneously 24 to 72 hours after administration of myelotoxic chemotherapeutic agents. Recommended dosing in adults is 5 mcg/kg daily until an ANC of at least 2 to 3 × 10^9/L is reached.

➤*Children:*

Off-label dosing

Off-label dosing in children:

Filgrastim Off-Label Dosing in Children

Indication	Dosage
Aplastic anemia	400 to 1,200 mcg/m^2/day for 2 weeks
Bone marrow transplantation	5 to 10 mcg/kg/day. Administer ≥ 24 hours after chemotherapy and ≥ 24 hours after bone marrow infusion. If the ANC is > 1,000/mm^3 for 3 consecutive days, reduce the dose to 5 mcg/kg/day. If the ANC remains > 1,000/mm^3 for 3 more consecutive days, filgrastim should be discontinued. If the ANC decreases to < 1,000/mm^3, filgrastim should be resumed at 5 mcg/kg/day.
Cancers (acute lymphocytic leukemia, non-Hodgkin lymphoma, Wilms tumor neuroblastoma [advanced-stage], rhabdomyosarcoma, CNS tumors, acute myelogenous leukemia)	5 to 17 mcg/kg/day
Congenital neutropenia or agranulocytosis	3 to 15 mcg/kg/day subcutaneously as a single dose or divided twice daily, or 10 to 30 mcg/kg/day as an intermittent infusion ≤ 60 mcg/kg/day as a continuous infusion
Mobilization of PBPCs	10 to 24 mcg/kg/day subcutaneously for 3 to 5 days before PBPC apheresis
Neutropenia and sepsis in neonates	5 to 10 mcg/kg once or twice daily for 3 to 6 days
Neutropenia/neutrophil dysfunction caused by glycogen storage disease type 1b	3 to 8 mcg/kg/day for ≤ 290 days or 3 to 7.5 mcg/kg/day subcutaneously for 6 to 12 months
Postchemotherapy neutropenia	5 to 17 mcg/kg/day

➤*Preparation for administration:* If required, filgrastim may be diluted in dextrose 5%. Filgrastim diluted to concentrations between 5 and 15 mcg/mL should be protected from adsorption to plastic materials by the addition of albumin (human) to a final concentration of 2 mg/mL. When diluted in dextrose 5% or dextrose 5% plus albumin (human), filgrastim is compatible with glass bottles, polyvinyl chloride and polyolefin IV bags, and polypropylene syringes. Dilution of filgrastim to a final concentration of less than 5 mcg/mL is not recommended at any time.

➤*Admixture compatibility:* Do not dilute with saline at any time; product may precipitate.

➤*Storage/Stability:* Store at 2° to 8°C (36° to 46°F). Avoid shaking. Prior to injection, filgrastim may be allowed to reach room temperature for a maximum of 24 hours. Any vial or prefilled syringe left at room temperature for more than 24 hours should be discarded.

Actions

➤*Pharmacology:* Colony-stimulating factors are glycoproteins which act on hematopoietic cells by binding to specific cell-surface receptors and stimulating proliferation, differentiation commitment, and some end-cell functional activation.

Endogenous G-CSF is a lineage-specific, colony-stimulating factor which is produced by monocytes, fibroblasts, and endothelial cells. G-CSF regulates

FILGRASTIM — INJECTION

the production of neutrophils within the bone marrow and affects neutrophil-progenitor proliferation, differentiation, and selected end-cell functional activation (including enhanced phagocytic ability, priming of the cellular metabolism associated with respiratory burst, antibody-dependent killing, and the increased expression of some functions associated with cell surface antigens). G-CSF is not species-specific and has been shown to have minimal direct in vivo or in vitro effects on the production of hematopoietic cell types other than the neutrophil lineage.

➤*Pharmacokinetics:*

Absorption/Distribution – Absorption and clearance of filgrastim follows first-order pharmacokinetic modeling without apparent concentration dependence. A positive linear correlation occurred between the parenteral dose and both the serum concentration and area under the concentration-time curves (AUCs). Continuous IV infusion of 20 mcg/kg of filgrastim over 24 hours resulted in mean and median serum concentrations of approximately 48 and 56 ng/mL, respectively. SC administration of 3.45 mcg/kg and 11.5 mcg/kg resulted in maximum serum concentrations of 4 and 49 ng/mL, respectively, within 2 to 8 hours. The volume of distribution averaged 150 mL/kg in both healthy subjects and cancer patients.

Excretion – The elimination half-life, in both healthy subjects and cancer patients, was approximately 3.5 hours. Clearance rates of filgrastim were approximately 0.5 to 0.7 mL/minute/kg. Single parenteral doses or daily IV doses, over a 14-day period, resulted in comparable half-lives. The half-lives were similar for IV administration (231 minutes, following doses of 34.5 mcg/kg) and for SC administration (210 minutes, following filgrastim doses of 3.45 mcg/kg). Continuous 24-hour IV infusions of 20 mcg/kg over an 11- to 20-day period produced steady-state serum concentrations of filgrastim with no evidence of drug accumulation over the time period investigated.

Contraindications

Hypersensitivity to *E. coli*-derived proteins, filgrastim, or any component of the product.

Warnings/Precautions

➤*Patients with SCN:* The safety and efficacy of filgrastim in the treatment of neutropenia due to other hematopoietic disorders (eg, myelodysplastic syndrome [MDS]) have not been established. Care should be taken to confirm the diagnosis of SCN before initiating filgrastim therapy.

MDS and AML have been reported to occur in the natural history of congenital neutropenia without cytokine therapy. Cytogenetic abnormalities, transformation to MDS, and AML have also been observed in patients treated with filgrastim for SCN. Based on available data, including a postmarketing surveillance study, the risk of developing MDS and AML appears to be confined to the subset of patients with congenital neutropenia (see Adverse Reactions). Abnormal cytogenetics and MDS have been associated with the eventual development of myeloid leukemia. The effect of filgrastim on the development of abnormal cytogenetics, and the effect of continued filgrastim administration in patients with abnormal cytogenetics or MDS are unknown. If a patient with SCN develops abnormal cytogenetics or myelodysplasia, the risks and benefits of continuing filgrastim should be carefully considered.

➤*Simultaneous use with chemotherapy and radiation therapy:* The safety and efficacy of filgrastim given simultaneously with cytotoxic chemotherapy have not been established. Because of the potential sensitivity of rapidly dividing myeloid cells to cytotoxic chemotherapy, do not use filgrastim in the period 24 hours before through 24 hours after the administration of cytotoxic chemotherapy (see Administration and Dosage).

The efficacy of filgrastim has not been evaluated in patients receiving chemotherapy associated with delayed myelosuppression (eg, nitrosoureas) or with mitomycin C or with myelosuppressive doses of antimetabolites such as 5-fluorouracil.

The safety and efficacy of filgrastim have not been evaluated in patients receiving concurrent radiation therapy. Simultaneous use of filgrastim with chemotherapy and radiation therapy should be avoided.

➤*Potential effect on malignant cells:* Filgrastim is a growth factor that primarily stimulates neutrophils. However, the possibility that filgrastim can act as a growth factor for any tumor type cannot be excluded. In a randomized study evaluating the effects of filgrastim vs placebo in patients undergoing remission induction for AML, there was no significant difference in remission rate, disease-free or overall survival.

The safety of filgrastim in chronic myeloid leukemia (CML) and myelodysplasia has not been established.

When filgrastim is used to mobilize PBPC, tumor cells may be released from the marrow and subsequently collected in the leukapheresis product. The effect of reinfusion of tumor cells has not been well studied, and the limited data available are inconclusive.

➤*Leukocytosis:*

Cancer patients receiving myelosuppressive chemotherapy – White blood cell counts of greater than or equal to 100,000/mm^3 were observed in approximately 2% of patients receiving filgrastim at doses above 5 mcg/kg/day. There were no reports of adverse events associated with this degree of leukocytosis. In order to avoid the potential complications of excessive leukocytosis, a CBC is recommended twice a week during filgrastim therapy (see Monitoring).

➤*Premature discontinuation of filgrastim therapy:*

Cancer patients receiving myelosuppressive chemotherapy – A transient increase in neutrophil counts is typically seen 1 to 2 days after initiation of filgrastim therapy. However, for a sustained therapeutic response, filgrastim therapy should be continued following chemotherapy until the post nadir ANC reaches 10,000/mm^3. Therefore, the premature discontinuation of filgrastim therapy, prior to the time of recovery from the expected neutrophil nadir, is generally not recommended (see Administration and Dosage).

➤*Hypersensitivity reactions:* Allergic-type reactions occurring on initial or subsequent treatment have been reported in less than 1 in 4000 patients treated with filgrastim. These have generally been characterized by systemic symptoms involving at least 2 body systems, most often skin (rash, urticaria, facial edema), respiratory (wheezing, dyspnea), and cardiovascular (hypotension, tachycardia). Some reactions occurred on initial exposure. Reactions tended to occur within the first 30 minutes after administration and appeared to occur more frequently in patients receiving filgrastim IV. Rapid resolution of symptoms occurred in most cases after administration of antihistamines, steroids, bronchodilators, or epinephrine. Symptoms recurred in more than half the patients who were rechallenged.

➤*Pregnancy: Category C.* Filgrastim has been shown to have adverse effects in pregnant rabbits when given in doses 2 to 10 times the human dose. Since there are no adequate and well-controlled studies in pregnant women, the effect, if any, of filgrastim on the developing fetus or the reproductive capacity of the mother is unknown. However, the scientific literature describes transplacental passage of filgrastim when administered to pregnant rats during the latter part of gestation and apparent transplacental passage of filgrastim when administered to pregnant humans by less than or equal to 30 hours prior to preterm delivery (less than or equal to 30 weeks gestation). Filgrastim should be used during pregnancy only if the potential benefit justifies the potential risk to the fetus.

In rabbits, increased abortion and embryolethality were observed in animals treated with filgrastim at 80 mcg/kg/day. Filgrastim administered to pregnant rabbits at doses of 80 mcg/kg/day during the period of organogenesis was associated with increased fetal resorption, genitourinary bleeding, developmental abnormalities, decreased body weight, live births, and food consumption. External abnormalities were not observed in the fetuses of dams treated at 80 mcg/kg/day. Reproductive studies in pregnant rats have shown that filgrastim was not associated with lethal, teratogenic, or behavioral effects on fetuses when administered by daily IV injection during the period of organogenesis at dose levels up to 575 mcg/kg/day.

In segment III studies in rats, offspring of dams treated at greater than 20 mcg/kg/day exhibited a delay in external differentiation (detachment of auricles and descent of testes) and slight growth retardation, possibly due to lower body weight of females during rearing and nursing. Offspring of dams treated at 100 mcg/kg/day exhibited decreased body weights at birth, and a slightly reduced 4-day survival rate.

➤*Lactation:* It is not known whether filgrastim is excreted in human milk. Because many drugs are excreted in human milk, caution should be exercised if filgrastim is administered to a nursing woman.

➤*Children:* In a phase 3 study to assess the safety and efficacy of filgrastim in the treatment of SCN, 120 patients with a median age of 12 years were studied. Of the 120 patients, 12 were infants (1 month to 2 years of age), 47 were children (2 to 12 years of age), and 9 were adolescents (12 to 16 years of age). Additional information is available from a SCN postmarketing surveillance study, which includes long-term follow-up of patients in the clinical studies and information from additional patients who entered directly into the postmarketing surveillance study. Of the 531 patients in the surveillance study as of December 31, 1997, 32 were infants, 200 were children, and 68 were adolescents (see Indications, Precautions, Administration and Dosage).

Pediatric patients with congenital types of neutropenia (Kostmann's syndrome, congenital agranulocytosis, or Schwachman-Diamond syndrome) have developed cytogenetic abnormalities and have undergone transformation to MDS and AML while receiving chronic filgrastim treatment. The relationship of these events to filgrastim administration is unknown (see Warnings and Adverse Reactions).

Long-term follow-up data from the postmarketing surveillance study suggest that height and weight are not adversely affected in patients who received up to 5 years of filgrastim treatment. Limited data from patients who were followed in the phase 3 study for 1.5 years did not suggest alterations in sexual maturation or endocrine function.

The safety and efficacy in neonates and patients with autoimmune neutropenia of infancy have not been established.

In the cancer setting, 12 pediatric patients with neuroblastoma have received up to 6 cycles of cyclophosphamide, cisplatin, doxorubicin, and etoposide chemotherapy concurrently with filgrastim; in this population, filgrastim was well-tolerated. There was 1 report of palpable splenomegaly associated with filgrastim therapy; however, the only consistently reported adverse event was musculoskeletal pain, which is no different from the experience in the adult population.

➤*Lab test abnormalities:* In clinical trials, the following laboratory results were observed:

- Cyclic fluctuations in the neutrophil counts were frequently observed in patients with congenital or idiopathic neutropenia after initiation of filgrastim therapy.
- Platelet counts were generally at the upper limits of normal prior to filgrastim therapy. With filgrastim therapy, platelet counts decreased but usually remained within normal limits (see Adverse Reactions).
- Early myeloid forms were noted in peripheral blood in most patients, including the appearance of metamyelocytes and myelocytes. Promyelocytes and myeloblasts were noted in some patients.

FILGRASTIM — INJECTION

- Relative increases were occasionally noted in the number of circulating eosinophils and basophils. No consistent increases were observed with filgrastim therapy.
- As in other trials, increases were observed in serum uric acid, lactic dehydrogenase, and serum alkaline phosphatase.

➤*Monitoring:* Left upper abdominal pain or shoulder tip pain accompanied by rapid increase in spleen size should be carefully monitored due to the rare but serious risk of splenic rupture.

Cancer patients receiving myelosuppressive chemotherapy – A CBC and platelet count should be obtained prior to chemotherapy, and at regular intervals (twice a week) during filgrastim therapy. Following cytotoxic chemotherapy, the neutrophil nadir occurred earlier during cycles when filgrastim was administered, and WBC differentials demonstrated a left shift, including the appearance of promyelocytes and myeloblasts. In addition, the duration of severe neutropenia was reduced, and was followed by an accelerated recovery in the neutrophil counts. Therefore, regular monitoring of WBC counts, particularly at the time of the recovery from the postchemotherapy nadir, is recommended in order to avoid excessive leukocytosis.

Cancer patients receiving bone marrow transplant – Frequent CBCs and platelet counts are recommended (at least 3 times a week) following marrow transplantation.

Patients with SCN – During the initial 4 weeks of filgrastim therapy and during the 2 weeks following any dose adjustment, a CBC with differential and platelet count should be performed twice weekly. Once a patient is clinically stable, a CBC with differential and platelet count should be performed monthly during the first year of treatment. Thereafter, if clinically stable, routine monitoring with regular CBCs (ie, as clinically indicated but at least quarterly) is recommended. Additionally, for those patients with congenital neutropenia, annual bone marrow and cytogenetic evaluations should be performed throughout the duration of treatment (see Warnings and Adverse Reactions).

Hematologic effects – In studies of filgrastim administration following chemotherapy, most reported side effects were consistent with those usually seen as a result of cytotoxic chemotherapy (see Adverse Reactions). Because of the potential of receiving higher doses of chemotherapy (ie, full doses on the prescribed schedule), the patient may be at greater risk of thrombocytopenia, anemia, and nonhematologic consequences of increased chemotherapy doses (please refer to the monograph information for the specific chemotherapy agents used). Regular monitoring of the hematocrit and platelet count is recommended. Furthermore, care should be exercised in the administration of filgrastim in conjunction with other drugs known to lower the platelet count. In septic patients receiving filgrastim, the physician should be alert to the possibility of adult respiratory distress syndrome, due to the possible influx of neutrophils at the site of inflammation.

There have been rare reports (less than 1 in 7000 patients) of cutaneous vasculitis in patients treated with filgrastim. In most cases, the severity of cutaneous vasculitis was moderate or severe. Most of the reports involved patients with SCN receiving long-term filgrastim therapy. Symptoms of vasculitis generally developed simultaneously with an increase in the ANC and abated when the ANC decreased. Many patients were able to continue filgrastim at a reduced dose.

Drug Interactions

Drug interactions between filgrastim and other drugs have not been fully evaluated. Drugs which may potentiate the release of neutrophils, such as lithium, should be used with caution.

Adverse Reactions

➤*Cancer patients receiving myelosuppressive chemotherapy:* In clinical trials involving greater than 350 patients receiving filgrastim following nonmyeloablative cytotoxic chemotherapy, most adverse reactions were the sequelae of the underlying malignancy or cytotoxic chemotherapy. In all phase 2 and 3 trials, medullary bone pain, reported in 24% of patients, was the only consistently observed adverse reaction attributed to filgrastim therapy. This bone pain was generally reported to be of mild-to-moderate severity, and could be controlled in most patients with nonnarcotic analgesics; infrequently, bone pain was severe enough to require narcotic analgesics. Bone pain was reported more frequently in patients treated with higher doses (20 to 100 mcg/kg/day) administered IV, and less frequently in patients treated with lower SC doses of filgrastim (3 to 10 mcg/kg/day).

In the randomized double-blind, placebo-controlled trial of filgrastim therapy following combination chemotherapy in patients (n = 207) with small cell lung cancer, the following adverse events were reported during blinded cycles of study medication (placebo or filgrastim at 4 to 8 mcg/kg/day). Events are reported as exposure-adjusted since patients remained on double-blind filgrastim a median of 3 cycles vs 1 cycle for placebo.

Filgrastim Adverse Reactions in Patients Receiving Myelosuppressive Chemotherapy

Adverse reaction	Filgrastim (n = 384) Patient cycles	Placebo (n = 257) Patient cycles
Nausea/vomiting	57%	64%
Skeletal pain	22%	11%
Alopecia	18%	27%
Diarrhea	14%	23%
Neutropenic fever	13%	35%
Mucositis	12%	20%
Fever	12%	11%
Fatigue	11%	16%
Anorexia	9%	11%
Dyspnea	9%	11%
Headache	7%	9%
Cough	6%	8%
Skin rash	6%	9%
Chest pain	5%	6%
Generalized weakness	4%	7%
Sore throat	4%	9%
Stomatitis	5%	10%
Constipation	5%	10%
Pain (unspecified)	2%	7%

In this study, there were no serious, life-threatening, or fatal adverse reactions attributed to filgrastim therapy. Specifically, there were no reports of flu-like symptoms, pleuritis, pericarditis, or other major systemic reactions to filgrastim.

Spontaneously reversible elevations in uric acid, lactate dehydrogenase, and alkaline phosphatase occurred in 27% to 58% of 98 patients receiving blinded filgrastim therapy following cytotoxic chemotherapy; increases were generally mild to moderate. Transient decreases in blood pressure (less than $^{90}/_{60}$ mmHg), which did not require clinical treatment, were reported in 7 of 176 patients in phase 3 clinical studies following administration of filgrastim. Cardiac events (myocardial infarctions [MIs], arrhythmias) have been reported in 11 of 375 cancer patients receiving filgrastim in clinical trials; the relationship to filgrastim therapy is unknown. No evidence of interaction of filgrastim with other drugs was observed in the course of clinical trials (see Drug Interactions).

There has been no evidence for the development of antibodies or of a blunted or diminished response to filgrastim in treated patients, including those receiving filgrastim daily for almost 2 years.

➤*Patients with acute myeloid leukemia:* In a randomized phase 3 clinical trial, 259 patients received filgrastim, and 262 patients received placebo postchemotherapy. Overall, the frequency of all reported adverse events was similar in both the filgrastim and placebo groups (83% vs 82% in induction 1; 61% vs 64% in consolidation 1). Adverse events reported more frequently in the filgrastim-treated group included the following: Petechiae (17% vs 14%); epistaxis (9% vs 5%); transfusion reactions (10% vs 5%). There were no significant differences in the frequency of these reactions.

There were a similar number of deaths in each treatment group during induction (25 filgrastim vs 27 placebo). The primary causes of death included infection (9 vs 18), persistent leukemia (7 vs 5), and hemorrhage (6 vs 3). Of the hemorrhagic deaths, 5 cerebral hemorrhages were reported in the filgrastim group and 1 in the placebo group. Other serious nonfatal hemorrhagic events were reported in the respiratory tract (4 vs 1), skin (4 vs 4), GI tract (2 vs 2), urinary tract (1 vs 1), ocular (1 vs 0), and other nonspecific sites (2 vs 1). While nineteen (7%) patients in the filgrastim group and five (2%) patients in the placebo group experienced severe or fatal hemorrhagic events, overall, hemorrhagic adverse events were reported at a similar frequency in both groups (40% vs 38%). The time to transfusion-independent platelet recovery and the number of days of platelet transfusions were similar in both groups.

➤*Cancer patients receiving bone marrow transplant (BMT):* In clinical trials, the reported adverse effects were those typically seen in patients receiving intensive chemotherapy followed by BMT. The most common events reported in both control and treatment groups included stomatitis, nausea, and vomiting, generally of mild-to-moderate severity and were considered unrelated to filgrastim. In the randomized studies of BMT involving 167 patients who received study drug, the following events occurred more frequently in patients treated with filgrastim than in controls: Nausea (10% vs 4%); vomiting (7% vs 3%); hypertension (4% vs 0%); rash (12% vs 10%); peritonitis (2% vs 0%). None of these events were reported by the investigator to be related to filgrastim. One event of erythema nodosum was reported moderate in severity and possibly related to filgrastim.

Generally, adverse reactions observed in nonrandomized studies were similar to those seen in randomized studies, occurred in a minority of patients, and were of mild-to-moderate severity. In 1 study (n = 45), 3 serious adverse events reported by the investigator were considered possibly related to filgrastim. These included 2 events of renal insufficiency and 1 event of capillary leak syndrome. The relationship of these events to filgrastim remains unclear since they occurred in patients with culture-proven infection with clinical sepsis who were receiving potentially nephrotoxic antibacterial and antifungal therapy.

➤*Cancer patients undergoing PBPC collection and therapy:* In clinical trials, 126 patients received filgrastim for PBPC mobilization. In this setting, filgrastim was generally well tolerated. Adverse events related to filgrastim consisted primarily of mild-to-moderate musculoskeletal symp-

FILGRASTIM — INJECTION

toms, reported in 44% of patients. These symptoms were predominantly events of medullary bone pain (33%). Headache was reported related to filgrastim in 7% of patients. Transient increases in alkaline phosphatase related to filgrastim were reported in 21% of the patients who had serum chemistries measured; most were mild to moderate.

All patients had increases in neutrophil counts during mobilization, consistent with the biological effects of filgrastim. Two patients had a WBC count greater than 100,000/mm^3. No sequelae were associated with any grade of leukocytosis.

Sixty-five percent (65%) of patients had mild-to-moderate anemia, and 97% of patients had decreases in platelet counts; 5 patients (out of 126) had decreased platelet counts to less than 50,000/mm^3. Anemia and thrombocytopenia have been reported to be related to leukapheresis; however, the possibility that filgrastim mobilization may contribute to anemia or thrombocytopenia has not been ruled out.

➤*Patients with SCN:* Mild-to-moderate bone pain was reported in approximately 33% of patients in clinical trials. This symptom was readily controlled with nonnarcotic analgesics. Generalized musculoskeletal pain was also noted in higher frequency in patients treated with filgrastim. Palpable splenomegaly was observed in approximately 30% of patients. Abdominal or flank pain was seen infrequently, and thrombocytopenia (less than 50,000/mm^3) was noted in 12% of patients with palpable spleens. Fewer than 3% of all patients underwent splenectomy, and most of these had a history of splenomegaly. Fewer than 6% of patients had thrombocytopenia (less than 50,000/mm^3) during filgrastim therapy, most of whom had a history of thrombocytopenia. In most cases, thrombocytopenia was managed by filgrastim dose reduction or interruption. An additional 5% of patients had platelet counts between 50,000 to 100,000/mm^3. There were no associated serious hemorrhagic sequelae in these patients. Epistaxis was noted in 15% of patients treated with filgrastim, but was associated with thrombocytopenia in 2% of patients. Anemia was reported in approximately 10% of patients, but in most cases appeared to be related to frequent diagnostic phlebotomy, chronic illness, or concomitant medications. Other adverse reactions infrequently observed and possibly related to filgrastim therapy were the following: Injection site reaction, rash, hepatomegaly, arthralgia, osteoporosis, cutaneous vasculitis, hematuria/proteinuria, alopecia, and the exacerbation of some preexisting skin disorders (eg, psoriasis).

Cytogenetic abnormalities, transformation to MDS, and AML have been observed in patients treated with filgrastim for SCN (see Warnings). As of December 31, 1997, data were available from a postmarketing surveillance study of 531 SCN patients with an average follow-up of 4 years. Based on analysis of these data, the risk of developing MDS and AML appears to be confined to the subset of patients with congenital neutropenia. A life-table analysis of these data revealed that the cumulative risk of developing leukemia or MDS by the end of the eighth year of filgrastim treatment in a patient with congenital neutropenia was 16.5% (95% confidence interval [CI] = 9.8%, 23.3%); this represents an annual rate of approximately 2%. Cytogenetic abnormalities, most commonly involving chromosome 7, have been reported in patients treated with filgrastim who had previously documented normal cytogenetics. It is unknown whether the development of cytogenetic abnormalities, MDS, or AML is related to chronic daily filgrastim administration, or to the natural history of congenital neutropenia. It is also unknown if the rate of conversion in patients who have not received filgrastim is different from that of patients who have received filgrastim. Routine monitoring through regular CBCs is recommended for all SCN patients. Additionally, annual bone marrow and cytogenetic evaluations are recommended in all patients with congenital neutropenia (see Precautions).

Overdosage

➤*Symptoms:* In cancer patients receiving filgrastim as an adjunct to myelosuppressive chemotherapy, it is recommended, to avoid the potential risks of excessive leukocytosis, that filgrastim therapy be discontinued if the ANC surpasses 10,000/mm^3 after the chemotherapy-induced ANC nadir has occurred. Doses of filgrastim that increase the ANC beyond 10,000/mm^3 may not result in any additional clinical benefit.

The maximum tolerated dose of filgrastim has not been determined. Efficacy was demonstrated at doses of 4 to 8 mcg/kg/day in the phase 3 study of nonmyeloablative chemotherapy. Patients in the BMT studies received up to 138 mcg/kg/day without toxic effects, although there was a flattening of the dose-response curve above daily doses of greater than 10 mcg/kg/day.

In filgrastim clinical trials of cancer patients receiving myelosuppressive chemotherapy, WBC counts greater than 100,000/mm^3 have been reported in less than 5% of patients, but were not associated with any reported adverse clinical effects.

➤*Treatment:* In cancer patients receiving myelosuppressive chemotherapy, discontinuation of filgrastim therapy usually results in a 50% decrease in circulating neutrophils within 1 to 2 days, with a return to pretreatment levels in 1 to 7 days.

Patient Information

In those situations in which the physician determines that the patient can safely and effectively self-administer filgrastim, the patient should be instructed as to the proper dosage and administration. Patients should be referred to the "Information for Patients" labeling included with each dispensing carton of filgrastim. This patient information, however, is not intended to be a disclosure of all known or possible effects. If home use is prescribed, patients should be thoroughly instructed in the importance of proper disposal and cautioned against the reuse of needles, syringes, or drug product. A puncture-resistant container for the disposal of used syringes and needles should be available to the patient. The full container should be disposed of according to the directions provided by the physician.

PEGFILGRASTIM

Rx	**Neulasta** (Amgen)	**Injection, solution:** 10 mg/mL	Preservative free. In dispensing pack containing single-dose syringe with needle.

PEGFILGRASTIM — INJECTION

Indications

➤*Myelosuppressive chemotherapy:* To decrease the incidence of infection, as manifested by febrile neutropenia, in patients with nonmyeloid malignancies receiving myelosuppressive anticancer drugs associated with a clinically significant incidence of febrile neutropenia.

Administration and Dosage

➤*Adults:* 6 mg subcutaneously once per chemotherapy cycle.

➤*Children:* The 6 mg fixed-dose formulation should not be used in infants, children, or smaller adolescents weighing less than 45 kg. For children weighing more than 45 kg, administer 6 mg subcutaneously once per chemotherapy cycle.

➤*Administration:* Pegfilgrastim should not be administered in the period between 14 days before and 24 hours after administration of cytotoxic chemotherapy.

Avoid shaking the syringe.

➤*Storage/Stability:* Store refrigerated between 2° and 8°C (36° and 46°F); syringes should be kept in their carton to protect from light until time of use. Before injection, pegfilgrastim may be allowed to reach room temperature for a maximum of 48 hours, but should be protected from light. Pegfilgrastim left at room temperature for more than 48 hours should be discarded. Freezing should be avoided; however, if accidentally frozen, pegfilgrastim should be allowed to thaw in the refrigerator before administration. If frozen a second time, pegfilgrastim should be discarded.

Actions

➤*Pharmacology:* Both filgrastim and pegfilgrastim are colony-stimulating factors that act on hematopoietic cells by binding to specific cell surface receptors, thereby stimulating proliferation, differentiation, commitment, and end-cell functional activation. Studies on cellular proliferation, receptor binding, and neutrophil function demonstrate that filgrastim and pegfilgrastim have the same mechanism of action. Pegfilgrastim has reduced renal clearance and prolonged persistence in vivo as compared with filgrastim.

➤*Pharmacokinetics:* The pharmacokinetics and pharmacodynamics of pegfilgrastim were studied in 379 patients with cancer. The pharmacokinetics of pegfilgrastim were nonlinear in cancer patients and clearance decreased with increases in dose. Neutrophil receptor binding is an important component of the clearance of pegfilgrastim, and serum clearance is directly related to the number of neutrophils. For example, the concentration of pegfilgrastim declined rapidly at the onset of neutrophil recovery that followed myelosuppressive chemotherapy. In addition to numbers of neutrophils, body weight appeared to be a factor. Patients with higher body weights experienced higher systemic exposure to pegfilgrastim after receiving a dose normalized for body weight. A large variability in the pharmacokinetics of pegfilgrastim was observed in cancer patients.

Excretion – The half-life of pegfilgrastim ranged from 15 to 80 hours after subcutaneous injection.

Contraindications

Hypersensitivity to pegfilgrastim or filgrastim.

Warnings/Precautions

➤*Peripheral blood progenitor cell mobilization:* The safety and efficacy of pegfilgrastim for peripheral blood progenitor cell (PBPC) mobilization have not been evaluated in adequate and well-controlled studies. Do not use pegfilgrastim for PBPC mobilization.

➤*Splenic rupture:* Splenic rupture, including fatal cases, has been reported following the administration of pegfilgrastim and its parent compound, filgrastim. In patients receiving pegfilgrastim who report left upper abdominal and/or shoulder tip pain, evaluate for an enlarged spleen or splenic rupture.

➤*Acute respiratory distress syndrome:* Acute respiratory distress syndrome (ARDS) has been reported in patients receiving pegfilgrastim, and is postulated to be secondary to an influx of neutrophils to sites of inflammation in the lungs. In patients receiving pegfilgrastim who develop fever, lung infiltrates, or respiratory distress, evaluate for the possibility of ARDS. In the event that ARDS occurs, discontinue pegfilgrastim and/or withhold until resolution of ARDS, and give patients appropriate medical management for this condition.

➤*Sickle cell disorders:* Severe sickle cell crises have been associated with the use of pegfilgrastim in patients with sickle cell disorders. Severe sickle cell crises, in some cases resulting in death, have also been associated with filgrastim, the parent compound of pegfilgrastim. Only health care providers qualified by specialized training or experience in the treatment of patients with sickle cell disorders should prescribe pegfilgrastim for such patients, and only after careful consideration of the potential risks and benefits.

PEGFILGRASTIM — INJECTION

➤*Use with chemotherapy and/or radiation therapy:* Do not administer pegfilgrastim in the period between 14 days before and 24 hours after administration of cytotoxic chemotherapy because of the potential for an increase in sensitivity of rapidly dividing myeloid cells to cytotoxic chemotherapy.

➤*Potential effect on malignant cells:* Pegfilgrastim is a growth factor that primarily stimulates neutrophils and neutrophil precursors; however, the granulocyte colony-stimulating factor (G-CSF) receptor through which pegfilgrastim and filgrastim act has been found on tumor cell lines, including some myeloid, T-lymphoid, lung, head and neck, and bladder tumor cell lines. The possibility that pegfilgrastim can act as a growth factor for any tumor type cannot be excluded. Use of pegfilgrastim in myeloid malignancies and myelodysplasia has not been studied. In a randomized study comparing the effects of the parent compound of pegfilgrastim, filgrastim, with placebo in patients undergoing remission induction and consolidation chemotherapy for acute myeloid leukemia, important differences in remission rate between the 2 arms were excluded. Disease-free survival and overall survival were comparable; however, the study was not designed to detect important differences in these end points.

➤*Bone imaging:* Increased hematopoietic activity of the bone marrow in response to growth factor therapy has been associated with transient positive bone-imaging changes. Consider this when interpreting bone-imaging results.

➤*Immunogenicity:* As with all therapeutic proteins, there is a potential for immunogenicity. Binding antibodies to pegfilgrastim were detected using a BIAcore assay. The approximate limit of detection for this assay is 500 ng/mL. Preexisting binding antibodies were detected in approximately 6% (51/849) of patients with metastatic breast cancer. Four of 521 pegfilgrastim-treated subjects who were negative at baseline developed binding antibodies to pegfilgrastim following treatment. None of these 4 patients had evidence of neutralizing antibodies detected using a cell-based bioassay.

The detection of antibody formation is highly dependent on the sensitivity and specificity of the assay, and the observed incidence of antibody positivity in an assay may be influenced by several factors, including sample handling, concomitant medications, and underlying disease. Therefore, comparison of the incidence of antibodies to pegfilgrastim with the incidence of antibodies to other products may be misleading.

Cytopenias resulting from a neutralizing antibody response to exogenous growth factors have been reported on rare occasions in patients treated with other recombinant growth factors. There is a theoretical possibility that an antibody directed against pegfilgrastim may crossreact with endogenous G-CSF, resulting in immune-mediated neutropenia, but this has not been observed in clinical studies.

➤*Hypersensitivity reactions:* Allergic reactions to pegfilgrastim, manifesting as anaphylaxis, angioedema, or urticaria, have been reported in postmarketing experience. The majority of reported reactions occurred upon initial exposure. In some cases, symptoms recurred with rechallenge. In rare cases, allergic reactions, including anaphylaxis, recurred within days after initial antiallergic treatment was discontinued. If a serious allergic reaction occurs, administer appropriate therapy, with close patient follow-up over several days. Permanently discontinue pegfilgrastim in patients with serious allergic reactions.

➤*Pregnancy: Category C.* Pegfilgrastim has been shown to have adverse effects in pregnant rabbits when administered subcutaneously every other day during gestation at doses as low as 50 mcg/kg/dose (approximately 4-fold higher than the recommended human dose). Decreased maternal food consumption accompanied by a decreased maternal body weight gain and decreased fetal body weights were observed at 50 to 1,000 mcg/kg/dose. Pegfilgrastim doses of 200 and 250 mcg/kg/dose resulted in an increased incidence of abortions. Increased postimplantation loss because of early resorptions was observed at doses of 200 to 1,000 mcg/kg/dose, and decreased numbers of live rabbit fetuses were observed at pegfilgrastim doses of 200 to 1,000 mcg/kg/dose, given every other day.

Subcutaneous injections of pegfilgrastim of up to 1,000 mcg/kg/dose every other day during the period of organogenesis in rats were not associated with an embryotoxic or fetotoxic outcome. However, an increased incidence (compared with historical controls) of wavy ribs was observed in rat fetuses at 1,000 mcg/kg/dose every other day. Very low levels (less than 0.5%) of pegfilgrastim crossed the placenta when administered subcutaneously to pregnant rats every other day during gestation.

There are no adequate and well-controlled studies in pregnant women. Use pegfilgrastim during pregnancy only if the potential benefit to the mother justifies the potential risk to the fetus.

➤*Lactation:* It is not known whether pegfilgrastim is excreted in human milk. Because many drugs are excreted in human milk, exercise caution when pegfilgrastim is administered to a breast-feeding woman.

➤*Children:* The safety and effectiveness of pegfilgrastim in children have not been established. Do not use the 6 mg fixed-dose single-use syringe formulation in infants, children, or smaller adolescents weighing less than 45 kg.

➤*Monitoring:* To assess a patient's hematologic status and ability to tolerate myelosuppressive chemotherapy, obtain a complete blood cell count and platelet count before chemotherapy is administered. Perform regular monitoring of hematocrit value and platelet count.

Drug Interactions

➤*Lithium:* Drugs such as lithium may potentiate the release of neutrophils; ensure that patients receiving lithium and pegfilgrastim have more frequent monitoring of neutrophil counts.

Adverse Reactions

➤*Clinical trial experience:*

Placebo-controlled trials –

Pegfilgrastim Adverse Reactions (≥ 10%[a])		
Adverse reaction	Pegfilgrastim (n = 467)	Placebo (n = 461)
CNS		
Asthenia	13%	11%
Headache	16%	14%
GI		
Constipation	10%	6%
Diarrhea	29%	28%
Vomiting	13%	11%
Musculoskeletal		
Arthralgia	16%	13%
Bone pain[b]	31%	26%
Myalgia	21%	18%
Miscellaneous		
Alopecia	48%	47%
Peripheral edema	12%	10%
Pyrexia (not including febrile neutropenia)	23%	22%

[a] Events occurring in ≥ 10% of pegfilgrastim-treated patients and at a higher incidence compared with placebo-treated patients.
[b] Bone pain is limited to the specified adverse reaction term "bone pain."

➤*Active-controlled trials:*

CNS – Dizziness, headache, insomnia (15% to 72%).

Dermatologic – Alopecia (15% to 72%).

GI – Abdominal pain, anorexia, constipation, diarrhea, dyspepsia, fatigue, mucositis, nausea, stomatitis, taste perversion, vomiting (15% to 72%).

Musculoskeletal – Myalgia, skeletal pain (15% to 72%).

Miscellaneous – Arthralgia, fever, generalized weakness, granulocytopenia, neutropenic fever, peripheral edema (15% to 72%).

Bone pain – In the placebo-controlled study, the incidence of bone pain was 57% in pegfilgrastim-treated patients compared with 50% in placebo-treated patients. Bone pain was generally reported to be of mild to moderate severity.

Among patients experiencing bone pain, approximately 37% of pegfilgrastim-treated and 31% of placebo-treated patients utilized nonnarcotic analgesics, and 10% of pegfilgrastim-treated and 9% of placebo-treated patients utilized narcotic analgesics.

Lab abnormalities: In clinical studies, leukocytosis (white blood cell [WBC] counts of more than 100×10^9/L) was observed in less than 1% of 932 patients with nonmyeloid malignancies receiving pegfilgrastim. Leukocytosis was not associated with any adverse effects.

➤*Postmarketing:*

Dermatologic – Generalized erythema and flushing; Sweet syndrome (acute febrile neutrophilic dermatosis).

Miscellaneous – Allergic reactions; ARDS; injection-site reactions (pain, induration, and local erythema); sickle cell crisis; splenic rupture.

Overdosage

➤*Symptoms:* The maximum amount of pegfilgrastim that can be safely administered in single or multiple doses has not been determined. Single doses of 300 mcg/kg have been administered subcutaneously to 8 healthy volunteers and 3 patients with non–small cell lung cancer without serious adverse reactions. These subjects experienced a mean maximum absolute neutrophil count (ANC) of 55×10^9/L, with a corresponding mean maximum WBC of 67×10^9/L. The absolute maximum ANC observed was 96×10^9/L, with a corresponding absolute maximum WBC of 120×10^9/L. The duration of leukocytosis ranged from 6 to 13 days.

➤*Treatment:* Consider leukapheresis in the management of symptomatic patients.

SARGRAMOSTIM (Granulocyte Macrophage Colony Stimulating Factor; GM-CSF)

Rx	Leukine (Genzyme)	**Powder for injection, lyophilized:** 250 mcg	Preservative-free. In vials.[a]
		Injection solution: 500 mcg/mL	1.1% benzyl alcohol. In multiple use vials.[a]

[a] With 40 mg mannitol, 10 mg sucrose, 1.2 mg tromethamine per mL.

SARGRAMOSTIM — INJECTION

Indications

➤*Following induction chemotherapy in acute myelogenous leukemia:* For use following induction chemotherapy in older adult patients with acute myelogenous leukemia (AML) to shorten time to neutrophil recovery and to reduce the incidence of severe and life-threatening infections and infections resulting in death. The safety and efficacy of sargramostim have not been assessed in patients with AML under 55 years of age.

➤*Mobilization and following transplantation of autologous peripheral blood progenitor cells:* For the mobilization of hematopoietic progenitor cells into peripheral blood for collection by leukapheresis. Mobilization allows for the collection of increased numbers of progenitor cells capable of engraftment as compared with collection without mobilization. After myeloablative chemotherapy, the transplantation of an increased number of progenitor cells lead to more rapid engraftment, which result in a decreased need for supportive care. Myeloid reconstitution is further accelerated by administration of sargramostim following peripheral blood progenitor cell transplantation.

➤*Myeloid reconstitution after autologous bone marrow transplantation (BMT):* For acceleration of myeloid recovery in patients with non-Hodgkin lymphoma (NHL), acute lymphoblastic leukemia (ALL), and Hodgkin disease undergoing autologous BMT. After autologous BMT in patients with NHL, ALL, or Hodgkin disease, sargramostim has been found to be safe and effective in accelerating myeloid engraftment, decreasing median duration of antibiotic administration, reducing the median duration of infectious episodes, and shortening the median duration of hospitalization. Hematologic response to sargramostim can be detected by complete blood count (CBC) with differential performed twice per week.

➤*Myeloid reconstitution after allogeneic bone marrow transplantation:* For acceleration of myeloid recovery in patients undergoing allogeneic BMT from HLA-matched related donors. Sargramostim has been found to be safe and effective in accelerating myeloid engraftment, reducing the incidence of bacteremia and other culture positive infections, and shortening the median duration of hospitalization.

➤*Bone marrow transplantation failure or engraftment delay:* In patients who have undergone allogeneic or autologous BMT in whom engraftment is delayed or has failed. Sargramostim has been found to be safe and effective in prolonging survival of patients who are experiencing graft failure or engraftment delay, in the presence or absence of infection, following autologous or allogeneic BMT. Survival benefit may be relatively greater in those patients who demonstrate one or more of the following characteristics: autologous BMT failure or engraftment delay, no previous total body irradiation, malignancy other than leukemia or a multiple organ failure (MOF) score of 2 or less. Hematologic response to sargramostim can be detected by CBC with differential performed twice weekly.

➤*Off-label uses:*

Crohn disease – [2] = Fair documentation. Initial data from a limited number of trials suggest sargramostim may be of benefit in the treatment of Crohn disease; however, it is associated with a high incidence of mild yet transient adverse events. Larger, controlled trials are needed to determine its role in the treatment of Crohn disease.

Drug-induced neutropenia – [2] = Fair documentation. A large number of case reports have consistently demonstrated a decreased time to neutrophil count recovery with the possibility of decreased mortality when growth factors are administered to patients with drug-induced neutropenia or agranulocytosis. Because of the infrequency of drug-induced neutropenia or agranulocytosis, it is doubtful that a well-designed clinical trial will be performed. Consideration of individual patient characteristics is important because of the medication cost, potential adverse effects, and uncertainty of effect.

Neutropenia associated with myelodysplastic syndromes – [2] = Fair documentation. Although neutrophil counts can be increased in patients with myelodysplastic syndromes, outcome data are lacking. American Society of Clinical Oncology and National Comprehensive Cancer Network recommend the use of white blood cell growth factors, such as sargramostim, in patients with myelodysplastic syndromes and severe neutropenia who experience recurrent or resistant infections. Without good quality-controlled studies in neutropenic patients with myelodysplastic syndromes, frequency and duration of therapy are unclear. More information is needed to further define sargramostim's place in therapy.

Oral mucositis – [4] = Insufficient documentation. Sargramostim is a novel approach to the prevention and treatment of oral mucositis in patients being treated for cancer. A variety of trials have been performed using growth factors (eg, sargramostim) with inconsistent results, which has prevented the recommendation of its use on a large scale. Higher-quality studies are needed to further define sargramostim's role in the prevention and management of oral mucositis.

Other possible off-label uses – Melanoma, wound healing, stomatitis, vaccine adjuvancy; adjunct to high-dose chemotherapy;aplastic anemia; zidovudine and other drug-induced neutropenia.

Administration and Dosage

➤*General dosing considerations:* In order to avoid potential complications of excessive leukocytosis (white blood cell [WBC] count more than 50,000 cells/mm^3 or absolute neutrophil count [ANC] more than 20,000 cells/mm^3) a complete blood count (CBC) with differential is recommended twice a week during sargramostim therapy. Sargramostim treatment should be interrupted or the dose reduced 50% if the ANC exceeds 20,000 cells/mm^3.

➤*Adults:*

Neutrophil recovery following chemotherapy in acute myelogenous leukemia –

Usual dosage: 250 mcg/m^2/day administered intravenously (IV) over a 4-hour period starting approximately on day 11 or 4 days following the completion of induction chemotherapy, if the day 10 bone marrow is hypoplastic with less than 5% blasts. If a second cycle of induction chemotherapy is necessary, sargramostim should be administered approximately 4 days after the completion of chemotherapy if the bone marrow is hypoplastic with less than 5% blasts.

Duration of therapy: Continue until an ANC of more than 1,500/mm^3 for 3 consecutive days or a maximum of 42 days.

Discontinuation of therapy: Discontinue immediately if leukemic regrowth occurs. If a severe adverse reaction occurs, the dose can be reduced 50% or temporarily discontinued until the reaction abates.

Mobilization of peripheral blood progenitor cells –

Usual dosage: 250 mcg/m^2/day administered IV over 24 hours or subcutaneously once daily. Dosing should continue at the same dose through the period of peripheral blood progenitor cells (PBPC) collection. The optimal schedule for PBPC collection has not been established. In clinical studies, collection of PBPC was usually begun by day 5 and performed daily until protocol specified targets were achieved.

Dosage adjustment: If the WBC is more than 50,000 cells/mm^3, the sargramostim dose should be reduced 50%. If adequate numbers of progenitor cells are not collected, other mobilization therapy should be considered.

Postperipheral blood progenitor cells transplantation – 250 mcg/m^2/day administered IV over 24 hours or subcutaneously once daily beginning immediately following infusion of progenitor cells and continuing until an ANC greater than 1,500/mm^3 for 3 consecutive days is attained.

Myeloid reconstitution after autologous or allogeneic bone marrow transplantation –

Usual dosage: 250 mcg/m^2/day administered IV over a 2-hour period beginning 2 to 4 hours after bone marrow infusion, and not less than 24 hours after the last dose of chemotherapy or radiotherapy. Patients should not receive sargramostim until the postmarrow infusion ANC is less than 500 cells/mm^3.

Duration of therapy: Sargramostim should be continued until an ANC greater than 1,500/mm^3 for 3 consecutive days is attained.

Discontinuation of therapy: If a severe adverse reaction occurs, the dose can be reduced 50% or temporarily discontinued until the reaction abates. Sargramostim should be discontinued immediately if blast cells appear or disease progression occurs.

Bone marrow transplantation failure or engraftment delay –

Usual dosage: 250 mcg/m^2/day for 14 days as a 2-hour IV infusion. The dose can be repeated after 7 days off therapy if engraftment has not occurred. If engraftment still has not occurred, a third course of 500 mcg/m^2/day for 14 days may be tried after another 7 days off therapy. If there is still no improvement, it is unlikely that further dose escalation will be beneficial.

Discontinuation of therapy: If a severe adverse reaction occurs, the dose can be reduced 50% or temporarily discontinued until the reaction abates. Sargramostim should be discontinued immediately if blast cells appear or disease progression occurs.

Off-label dosing –

Crohn disease: [2] = Fair documentation. Used as monotherapy or as combination therapy at doses ranging from 4 to 6 mcg/kg daily as a subcutaneous injection.

Drug-induced neutropenia: [2] = Fair documentation. Used as monotherapy at doses of approximately 300 mcg daily administered by subcutaneous injection until levels reach 0.5×10^9 cells/L or higher.

Neutropenia associated with myelodysplastic syndromes: [2] = Fair documentation. 250 mcg/m^2 daily as a subcutaneous injection used intermittently as monotherapy.

Oral mucositis: [4] = Insufficient documentation. 4 mcg/kg daily as a subcutaneous injection used as monotherapy.

➤*Preparation for administration:*

1.) Sargramostim liquid is formulated as a sterile, preserved (1.1% benzyl alcohol), injectable solution (500 mcg/mL) in a vial. Lyophilized sargramostim is a sterile, white, preservative-free powder (250 mcg) that requires reconstitution with 1 mL sterile water for injection, or 1 mL bacteriostatic water for injection.
2.) Lyophilized sargramostim (250 mcg) should be reconstituted aseptically with 1 mL of diluent. The contents of vials reconstituted with different diluents should not be mixed together. Previously reconstituted solutions mixed with freshly reconstituted solutions must be administered within 6 hours following mixing. Preparations containing benzyl alcohol (including sargramostim liquid and lyophilized sargramostim reconstituted with bacteriostatic water for injection) should not be used in neonates (see Storage and Warnings/Precautions).
3.) During reconstitution the diluent should be directed at the side of the vial and the contents gently swirled to avoid foaming during dissolution. Avoid excessive or vigorous agitation; do not shake.
4.) Sargramostim should be used for subcutaneous injection without further dilution. Dilution for IV infusion should be performed in sodium chloride 0.9% injection. If the final concentration of sargramostim is below 10 mcg/mL, albumin (human) at a final concentration of 0.1% should be added to the saline prior to addition of sargramostim to prevent adsorption to the components of the drug delivery system. To obtain a final concentration of albumin 0.1% (human), add albumin 1 mg (human) per 1 mL sodium chloride 0.9% injection (eg, use 1 mL albumin 5% [human] in 50 mL sodium chloride 0.9% injection).

SARGRAMOSTIM — INJECTION

5.) An in-line membrane filter should not be used for IV infusion of sargramostim.
6.) In the absence of compatibility and stability information, no other medication should be added to infusion solutions containing sargramostim. Use only sodium chloride 0.9% injection to prepare IV infusion solutions.
7.) Aseptic technique should be employed in the preparation of all sargramostim solutions. To ensure correct concentration following reconstitution, care should be exercised to eliminate any air bubbles from the needle hub of the syringe used to prepare the diluent. Parenteral drug products should be inspected visually for particulate matter and discoloration prior to administration whenever solution and container permit.

➤*Administration:* Administer IV or subcutaneously per indication.

➤*Storage/Stability:* The sterile, preserved, injectable solution; the sterile powder; the reconstituted solution; and the diluted solution for injection should be refrigerated at 2° to 8°C (36° to 46°F). Do not freeze or shake. Do not use beyond the expiration date printed on the vial.

Sterile water for injection (without preservative) – Sargramostim vials contain no antibacterial preservative, and therefore solutions prepared with sterile water for injection should be administered as soon as possible, and within 6 hours following reconstitution or dilution for IV infusion. The vial should not be re-entered or reused. Do not save any unused portion for administration more than 6 hours following reconstitution.

Bacteriostatic water for injection (benzyl alcohol 0.9%) – Reconstituted solutions prepared with bacteriostatic water for injection (benzyl alcohol 0.9%) may be stored for up to 20 days at 2° to 8°C (36° to 46°F) prior to use. Discard reconstituted solution after 20 days.

Actions

➤*Pharmacology:* Granulocyte-macrophage colony stimulating factor (GM-CSF) belongs to a group of growth factors termed colony stimulating factors that support survival, clonal expansion, and differentiation of hematopoietic progenitor cells. GM-CSF induces partially committed progenitor cells to divide and differentiate in the granulocyte-macrophage pathways.

GM-CSF is also capable of activating mature granulocytes and macrophages. GM-CSF is a multilineage factor and, in addition to dose-dependent effects on the myelomonocytic lineage, can promote the proliferation of megakaryocytic and erythroid progenitors. However, other factors are required to induce complete maturation in these 2 lineages. The various cellular responses (division, maturation, activation) are induced through GM-CSF binding to specific receptors expressed on the cell surface of target cells.

In vitro studies of sargramostim in human cells – The biological activity of GM-CSF is species-specific. Consequently, in vitro studies have been performed on human cells to characterize the pharmacological activity of sargramostim. In vitro exposure of human bone marrow cells to sargramostim at concentrations ranging from 1 to 100 ng/mL results in the proliferation of hematopoietic progenitors and in the formation of pure granulocyte, pure macrophage, and mixed granulocyte-macrophage colonies. Chemotactic, anti-fungal and anti-parasitic activities of granulocytes and monocytes are increased by exposure to sargramostim in vitro. Sargramostim increases the cytotoxicity of monocytes toward certain neoplastic cell lines and activates polymorphonuclear neutrophils to inhibit the growth of tumor cells.

Antibody formation – Serum samples collected before and after sargramostim treatment from 214 patients with a variety of underlying diseases have been examined for the presence of antibodies. Neutralizing antibodies were detected in 5 of 214 patients (2.3%) after receiving sargramostim by continuous IV infusion (3 patients) or subcutaneous injection (2 patients) for 28 to 84 days in multiple courses. All 5 patients had impaired hematopoiesis before the administration of sargramostim and consequently the effect of the development of anti-GM-CSF antibodies on normal hematopoiesis could not be assessed. Drug-induced neutropenia, neutralization of endogenous GM-CSF activity and diminution of the therapeutic effect of sargramostim secondary to formation of neutralizing antibody remain a theoretical possibility.

➤*Pharmacokinetics:* Pharmacokinetic profiles have been analyzed in controlled studies of 24 healthy men. Liquid and lyophilized sargramostim, at the recommended dose of 250 mcg/m^2, have been determined to be bioequivalent based on the statistical evaluation of AUC. When sargramostim (either liquid or lyophilized) was administered IV over 2 hours to healthy volunteers, the mean beta half-life was approximately 60 minutes. Peak concentrations of GM-CSF were observed in blood samples obtained during or immediately after completion of sargramostim infusion. For sargramostim liquid, the mean maximum concentration (C_{max}) was 5 ng/mL, the mean clearance rate was approximately 420 mL/min/m^2 and the mean $AUC_{0-\infty}$ was 640 ng/mL min. Corresponding results for lyophilized sargramostim in the same subjects were mean C_{max} of 5.4 ng/mL, mean clearance rate of 431 mL/min/m^2, and mean $AUC_{0-\infty}$ of 677 ng/mL•min. GM-CSF was last detected in blood samples obtained at 3 or 6 hours. When sargramostim (either liquid or lyophilized) was administered subcutaneously to healthy volunteers, GM-CSF was detected in the serum at 15 minutes, the first sample point. The mean beta half-life was approximately 162 minutes. Peak levels occurred at 1 to 3 hours postinjection, and sargramostim remained detectable for up to 6 hours after injection. The mean C_{max} was 1.5 ng/mL. For sargramostim liquid, the mean clearance was 549 mL/min/m^2 and the mean $AUC_{0-\infty}$ was 549 ng/mL•min. For lyophilized sargramostim, the mean clearance was 529 mL/min/m^2 and the mean $AUC_{0-\infty}$ was 501 ng/mL•min.

Contraindications

In patients with excessive leukemic myeloid blasts in the bone marrow or peripheral blood (≥ 10%); hypersensitivity to GM-CSF, yeast-derived products or any component of the product; concomitant use with chemotherapy and radiotherapy.

Because of the potential sensitivity of rapidly dividing hematopoietic progenitor cells, sargramostim should not be administered simultaneously with cytotoxic chemotherapy or radiotherapy or within 24 hours preceding or following chemotherapy or radiotherapy. In 1 controlled study, patients with small cell lung cancer received sargramostim and concurrent thoracic radiotherapy and chemotherapy or the identical radiotherapy and chemotherapy without sargramostim. The patients randomized to sargramostim had significantly higher incidence of adverse events, including higher mortality and a higher incidence of grade 3 and 4 infections and grade 3 and 4 thrombocytopenia.

Warnings/Precautions

➤*Benzyl alcohol:* Benzyl alcohol is a constituent of sargramostim liquid and bacteriostatic water for injection diluent. Benzyl alcohol has been reported to be associated with a fatal gasping syndrome in premature infants. Liquid solutions containing benzyl alcohol (including sargramostim liquid) or lyophilized sargramostim reconstituted with bacteriostatic water for injection (0.9% benzyl alcohol) should not be administered to neonates (see Children and Administration and Dosage).

➤*Fluid retention:* Edema, capillary leak syndrome, pleural or pericardial effusion have been reported in patients after sargramostim administration. In 156 patients enrolled in placebo-controlled studies using sargramostim at a dose of 250 mcg/m^2/day by 2-hour IV infusion, the reported incidences of fluid retention (sargramostim versus placebo) were as follows: Peripheral edema, 11% versus 7%; pleural effusion, 1% versus 0%; and pericardial effusion, 4% versus 1%. Capillary leak syndrome was not observed in this limited number of studies; based on other uncontrolled studies and reports from users of marketed sargramostim, the incidence is estimated to be less than 1%. In patients with preexisting pleural and pericardial effusions, administration of sargramostim may aggravate fluid retention; however, fluid retention associated with or worsened by sargramostim has been reversible after interruption or dose reduction of sargramostim with or without diuretic therapy. Sargramostim should be used with caution in patients with preexisting fluid retention, pulmonary infiltrates, or congestive heart failure.

➤*Respiratory symptoms:* Sequestration of granulocytes in the pulmonary circulation has been documented following sargramostim infusion, and dyspnea has been reported occasionally in patients treated with sargramostim. Special attention should be given to respiratory symptoms during or immediately following sargramostim infusion, especially in patients with preexisting lung disease. In patients displaying dyspnea during sargramostim administration, the rate of infusion should be reduced by half. If respiratory symptoms worsen despite infusion rate reduction, the infusion should be discontinued. Subsequent IV infusions may be administered following the standard dose schedule with careful monitoring. Use caution when administering sargramostim to patients with hypoxia.

➤*Cardiovascular symptoms:* Occasional transient supraventricular arrhythmia has been reported in uncontrolled studies during sargramostim administration, particularly in patients with a previous history of cardiac arrhythmia. However, these arrhythmias have been reversible after discontinuation of sargramostim. Use caution when administering sargramostim to patients with preexisting cardiac disease.

➤*Hypersensitivity reactions:* Parenteral administration of recombinant proteins should be attended by appropriate precautions in case an allergic or untoward reaction occurs. Serious allergic or anaphylactic reactions have been reported. If any serious allergic or anaphylactic reaction occurs, immediately discontinue sargramostim therapy and initiate appropriate therapy.

➤*First dose effect:* A syndrome characterized by respiratory distress, hypoxia, flushing, hypotension, syncope, or tachycardia has been reported following the first administration of sargramostim in a particular cycle. These signs have resolved with symptomatic treatment and usually do not recur with subsequent doses in the same cycle of treatment.

➤*Hematologic effects:* Stimulation of marrow precursors with sargramostim may result in a rapid rise in white blood cell (WBC) count. If the ANC exceeds 20,000 cells/mm^3 or if the platelet count exceeds 500,000/mm^3, interrupt sargramostim administration or reduce the dose by half. Base the decision to reduce the dose or interrupt treatment on the clinical condition of the patient. Excessive blood counts have returned to normal or baseline levels within 3 to 7 days following cessation of sargramostim therapy. Perform twice weekly monitoring of CBC with differential (including examination for the presence of blast cells) to preclude development of excessive counts.

➤*Growth factor potential:* Sargramostim is a growth factor that primarily stimulates normal myeloid precursors. However, the possibility that sargramostim can act as a growth factor for any tumor type, particularly myeloid malignancies, cannot be excluded. Because of the possibility of tumor growth potentiation, exercise precaution when using this drug in any malignancy with myeloid characteristics.

Should disease progression be detected during sargramostim treatment, discontinue sargramostim therapy.

Sargramostim has been administered to patients with myelodysplastic syndromes (MDS) in uncontrolled studies without evidence of increased relapse rates. Controlled studies have not been performed in patients with MDS.

➤*Use in patients receiving purged bone marrow:* Sargramostim is effective in accelerating myeloid recovery in patients receiving bone marrow

SARGRAMOSTIM — INJECTION

purged by anti-B lymphocyte monoclonal antibodies. Data obtained from uncontrolled studies suggest that if in vitro marrow purging with chemical agents causes a significant decrease in the number of responsive hematopoietic progenitors, the patient may not respond to sargramostim. When the bone marrow purging process preserves a sufficient number of progenitors (more than 1.2×10^4/kg), a beneficial effect of sargramostim on myeloid engraftment has been reported.

➤*Use in patients previously exposed to intensive chemotherapy/radiotherapy:* In patients who before autologous BMT, have received extensive radiotherapy to hematopoietic sites for the treatment of primary disease in the abdomen or chest, or have been exposed to multiple myelotoxic agents (alkylating agents, anthracycline antibiotics, antimetabolites), the effect of sargramostim on myeloid reconstitution may be limited.

➤*Use in patients with malignancy undergoing sargramostim-mobilized PBPC collection:* When using sargramostim to mobilize PBPC, the limited in vitro data suggest that tumor cells may be released and reinfused into the patient in the leukapheresis product. The effect of reinfusion of tumor cells has not been well studied and the data are inconclusive.

➤*Renal/Hepatic function impairment:* In some patients with preexisting renal or hepatic dysfunction enrolled in uncontrolled clinical trials, administration of sargramostim has induced elevation of serum creatinine or bilirubin and hepatic enzymes. Dose reduction or interruption of sargramostim administration has resulted in a decrease to pretreatment values. However, in controlled clinical trials the incidences of renal and hepatic dysfunction were comparable between sargramostim (250 mcg/m²/day by 2-hour IV infusion) and placebo-treated patients. Monitoring of renal and hepatic function in patients displaying renal or hepatic dysfunction prior to initiation of treatment is recommended at least every other week during sargramostim administration.

➤*Pregnancy: Category C.* Animal reproduction studies have not been conducted with sargramostim. It is not known whether sargramostim can cause fetal harm when administered to a pregnant woman or can affect reproductive capability. Give sargramostim to a pregnant woman only if clearly needed.

➤*Lactation:* It is not known whether sargramostim is excreted in human milk. Because many drugs are excreted in human milk, administer sargramostim to a nursing woman only if clearly needed.

➤*Children:* Safety and effectiveness in children have not been established; however, available safety data indicate that sargramostim does not exhibit any greater toxicity in children than adults. A total of 124 pediatric subjects between the ages of 4 months and 18 years of age have been treated with sargramostim in clinical trials at doses ranging from 60 to 1,000 mcg/m²/day intravenously and 4 to 1,500 mcg/m²/day subcutaneously. In 53 pediatric patients enrolled in controlled studies at a dose of 250 mcg/m²/day by 2-hour IV infusion, the type and frequency of adverse events were comparable with those reported for the adult population. Do not administer liquid solutions containing benzyl alcohol (including sargramostim liquid) or lyophilized sargramostim reconstituted with bacteriostatic water for injection (0.9% benzyl alcohol) to neonates.

➤*Lab test abnormalities:* Sargramostim can induce variable increases in WBC or platelet counts. In order to avoid potential complications of excessive leukocytosis (WBC greater than 50,000 cells/mm³; ANC greater than 20,000 cells/mm³), a CBC is recommended twice weekly during sargramostim therapy.

➤*Monitoring:* Monitoring of renal and hepatic function in patients displaying renal or hepatic dysfunction prior to initiation of treatment is recommended at least biweekly during sargramostim administration. Body weight and hydration status should be carefully monitored during sargramostim administration.

Drug Interactions

Interactions between sargramostim and other drugs have not been fully evaluated. Use caution when administering drugs that may potentiate the myeloproliferative effects of sargramostim (eg, lithium, corticosteroids).

Adverse Reactions

➤*Autologous and allogeneic BMT:* Sargramostim is generally well tolerated. In 3 placebo-controlled studies enrolling a total of 156 patients after autologous BMT or PBPC transplantation, reactions reported in at least 10% of patients who received IV sargramostim or placebo were as follows:

Sargramostim AuBMT Adverse Reactions		
Adverse reactions	Sargramostim (n = 79)	Placebo (n = 77)
Cardiovascular		
Hemorrhage	23%	30%
CNS		
CNS disorder	11%	16%
Dermatologic		
Alopecia	73%	74%
Rash	44%	38%
GI		
Nausea	90%	96%
Diarrhea	89%	82%
Vomiting	85%	90%
Anorexia	54%	58%
GI disorder	37%	47%
GI hemorrhage	27%	33%
Stomatitis	24%	29%
Liver damage	13%	14%
GU		
Urinary tract disorder	14%	13%
Kidney function abnormal	8%	10%
Hematologic/lymphatic		
Blood dyscrasia	25%	27%
Metabolic/nutritional		
Edema	34%	35%
Peripheral edema	11%	7%
Respiratory		
Dyspnea	28%	31%
Lung disorder	20%	23%
Miscellaneous		
Fever	95%	96%
Mucous membrane disorder	75%	78%
Asthenia	66%	51%
Malaise	57%	51%
Sepsis	11%	14%

No significant differences were observed between sargramostim and placebo-treated patients in the type or frequency of laboratory abnormalities, including renal and hepatic parameters. In some patients with preexisting renal or hepatic dysfunction enrolled in uncontrolled clinical trials, administration of sargramostim has induced elevation of serum creatinine or bilirubin and hepatic enzymes (see Warnings). In addition, there was no significant difference in relapse rate and 24 month survival between the sargramostim and placebo-treated patients. In the placebo-controlled trial of 109 patients after allogeneic BMT, reactions reported in at least 10% of patients who received IV sargramostim or placebo were the following:

Sargramostim Allogeneic BMT Adverse Reactions		
Adverse reaction	Sargramostim (n = 53)	Placebo (n = 56)
CNS		
Paresthesia	11%	13%
Insomnia	11%	9%
Anxiety	11%	2%
Dermatologic		
Rash	70%	73%
Alopecia	45%	45%
Pruritus	23%	13%
GI		
Diarrhea	81%	66%
Nausea	70%	66%
Vomiting	70%	57%
Stomatitis	62%	63%
Anorexia	51%	57%
Dyspepsia	17%	20%
Hematemesis	13%	7%
Dysphagia	11%	7%
GI hemorrhage	11%	5%
Constipation	8%	11%
GU		
Hematuria	9%	21%
Hematologic/Lymphatic		
Thrombocytopenia	19%	34%
Leukopenia	17%	29%
Petechia	6%	11%
Agranulocytosis	6%	11%

SARGRAMOSTIM — INJECTION

Sargramostim Allogeneic BMT Adverse Reactions		
Adverse reaction	Sargramostim (n = 53)	Placebo (n = 56)
Laboratory abnormalities[a]		
High glucose	41%	49%
Low albumin	27%	36%
High BUN	23%	17%
Low calcium	2%	7%
High cholesterol	17%	8%
Metabolic/Nutritional		
Bilirubinemia	30%	27%
Hyperglycemia	25%	23%
Peripheral edema	15%	21%
Increased creatinine	15%	14%
Hypomagnesemia	15%	9%
Increased ALT	13%	16%
Edema	13%	11%
Increased alkaline phosphatase	8%	14%
Musculoskeletal		
Bone pain	21%	5%
Arthralgia	11%	4%
Ophthalmic		
Eye hemorrhage	11%	0%
Cardiovascular		
Hypertension	34%	32%
Tachycardia	11%	9%
Respiratory		
Pharyngitis	23%	13%
Epistaxis	17%	16%
Dyspnea	15%	14%
Rhinitis	11%	14%
Miscellaneous		
Fever	77%	80%
Abdominal pain	38%	23%
Headache	36%	36%
Chills	25%	20%
Pain	17%	36%
Asthenia	17%	20%
Chest pain	15%	9%
Back pain	9%	18%

[a] Grade 3 and 4 laboratory abnormalities only. Denominators may vary due to missing laboratory measurements.

There were no significant differences in the incidence or severity of GVHD, relapse rates and survival between the sargramostim and placebo-treated patients.

Adverse reactions observed for the patients treated with sargramostim in the historically controlled BMT failure study were similar to those reported in the placebo-controlled studies. In addition, headache (26%), pericardial effusion (25%), arthralgia (21%) and myalgia (18%) were also reported in patients treated with sargramostim in the graft failure study.

In uncontrolled Phase I/II studies with sargramostim in 215 patients, the most frequent adverse events were fever, asthenia, headache, bone pain, chills and myalgia. These systemic events were generally mild or moderate and were usually prevented or reversed by the administration of analgesics and antipyretics such as acetaminophen. In these uncontrolled trials, other infrequent events reported were dyspnea, peripheral edema, and rash.

Reports of reactions occurring with marketed sargramostim include arrhythmia, fainting, eosinophilia, dizziness, hypotension, injection site reactions, pain (including abdominal, back, chest, and joint pain), tachycardia, thrombosis, and transient liver function abnormalities.

In patients with preexisting edema, capillary leak syndrome, pleural or pericardial effusion, administration of sargramostim may aggravate fluid retention (see Warnings). Body weight and hydration status should be carefully monitored during sargramostim administration.

Adverse reactions observed in pediatric patients in controlled studies were comparable to those observed in adult patients.

➤*Acute myelogenous leukemia:* Adverse reactions reported in at least 10% of patients who received sargramostim or placebo were the following:

Sargramostim AML Adverse Reactions		
Adverse reactions	Sargramostim (n = 52)	Placebo (n = 47)
Cardiovascular		
Hemorrhage	29%	43%
Hypertension	25%	32%
Cardiac	23%	32%
Hypotension	13%	26%
CNS		
Neuro-clinical	42%	53%
Neuromotor	25%	26%
Neuropsychiatric	15%	26%
Neurosensory	6%	11%
Dermatologic		
Skin	77%	45%
Alopecia	37%	51%
GI		
Nausea	58%	55%
Liver	77%	83%
Diarrhea	52%	53%
Vomiting	46%	34%
Stomatitis	42%	43%
Anorexia	13%	11%
Abdominal distention	4%	13%
GU		
Genitourinary	50%	57%
Hematologic/Lymphatic		
Coagulation	19%	21%
Respiratory		
Pulmonary	48%	64%
Metabolic/Nutritional		
Metabolic	58%	49%
Edema	25%	23%
Miscellaneous		
Fever (no infection)	81%	74%
Infection	65%	68%
Weight loss	37%	28%
Weight gain	8%	21%
Chills	19%	26%
Allergy	12%	15%
Sweats	6%	13%

Nearly all patients reported leukopenia, thrombocytopenia and anemia. The frequency and type of adverse reactions observed following induction were similar between sargramostim and placebo groups. The only significant difference in the rates of these adverse reactions was an increase in skin associated reactions in the sargramostim group (P = 0.002). No significant differences were observed in laboratory results, renal or hepatic toxicity. No significant differences were observed between the sargramostim and placebo-treated patients for adverse reactions following consolidation. There was no significant difference in response rate or relapse rate.

In a historically controlled study of 86 patients with acute myelogenous leukemia (AML), the sargramostim treated group exhibited an increased incidence of weight gain (P = 0.007), low serum proteins and prolonged prothrombin time (P = 0.02) when compared to the control group. Two sargramostim treated patients had progressive increase in circulating monocytes and promonocytes and blasts in the marrow which reversed when sargramostim was discontinued. The historical control group exhibited an increased incidence of cardiac events (P = 0.018), liver function abnormalities (P = 0.008), and neurocortical hemorrhagic events (P = 0.025).

Overdosage

➤*Symptoms:* The maximum amount of sargramostim that can be safely administered in single or multiple doses has not been determined. Doses up to 100 mcg/kg/day (4000 mcg/m^2/day or 16 times the recommended dose) were administered to 4 patients in a Phase I uncontrolled clinical study by continuous IV infusion for 7 to 18 days. Increases in WBC up to 200,000 cells/mm^3 were observed. Adverse reactions reported were dyspnea, malaise, nausea, fever, rash, sinus tachycardia, headache and chills. All these reactions were reversible after discontinuation of sargramostim.

➤*Treatment:* In case of overdosage, sargramostim therapy should be discontinued and the patient carefully monitored for WBC increase and respiratory symptoms.

PLERIXAFOR

Rx	**Mozobil** Genzyme	**Injection, solution:** 20 mg/mL	Sodium chloride 5.9 mg. Preservative free. Single-use vial.

PLERIXAFOR — INJECTION

Indications

➤*Peripheral stem cell collection and transplantation:* In combination with granulocyte colony-stimulating factor (G-CSF) to mobilize hematopoietic stem cells (HSCs) to the peripheral blood for collection and subsequent autologous transplantation in patients with non-Hodgkin lymphoma (NHL) and multiple myeloma.

Administration and Dosage

➤*General dosing considerations:* Dosage adjustment in patients with a creatinine clearance (CrCl) of 50 mL/min or less is recommended (see Renal Function Impairment).

➤*Adults:*

Peripheral stem cell collection and transplantation –

Usual dosage: 0.24 mg/kg body weight by subcutaneous injection. Begin treatment with plerixafor after the patient has received G-CSF once daily for 4 days. Administer plerixafor approximately 11 hours prior to initiation of apheresis for up to 4 consecutive days.

Maximum dose: 40 mg/day.

Concomitant therapy: Administer daily morning doses of G-CSF 10 mcg/kg for 4 days prior to the first evening dose of plerixafor and on each day prior to apheresis.

➤*Elderly:* In general, take care in dose selection for elderly patients because of the greater frequency of decreased renal function with advanced age. Dosage adjustment in elderly patients with a CrCl of 50 mL/min or less is recommended (see Renal Function Impairment).

➤*Renal function impairment:*

Recommended Dosage of Plerixafor in Patients With Renal Function Impairment

Estimated CrCl (mL/min)	Plerixafor dosage
> 50	0.24 mg/kg once daily (not to exceed 40 mg/day)
≤ 50	0.16 mg/kg once daily (not to exceed 27 mg/day)
Hemodialysis	Insufficient information to make dosage recommendation.

➤*Preparation for administration:* Use the patient's actual body weight to calculate the volume of plerixafor to be administered. Each vial delivers 1.2 mL of 20 mg/mL solution, and the volume to be administered to patients should be calculated from the following equation:

0.012 × patient's actual body weight (kg) = volume to be administered (mL).

In clinical studies, plerixafor dose has been calculated based on actual body weight in patients up to 175% of ideal body weight. Plerixafor dose and treatment of patients weighing more than 175% of ideal body weight have not been investigated.

➤*Administration:* Administer by subcutaneous injection.

➤*Storage/Stability:* Store at 25°C (77°F); excursions are permitted between 16° and 30°C (59° and 86°F). Any unused drug remaining after injection must be discarded.

Actions

➤*Pharmacology:* Plerixafor, a hematopoietic stem cell mobilizer, is an inhibitor of the CXCR4 chemokine receptor and blocks binding of its cognate ligand, stromal cell-derived factor-1α (SDF-1α). SDF-1α and CXCR4 are recognized to play a role in the trafficking and homing of human HSCs to the marrow compartment. Once in the marrow, stem cell CXCR4 can act to help anchor these cells to the marrow matrix, either directly via SDF-1α or through the induction of other adhesion molecules. Treatment with plerixafor resulted in leukocytosis and elevations in circulating hematopoietic progenitor cells in mice, dogs, and humans. CD34+ cells mobilized by plerixafor were capable of engraftment with long-term repopulating capacity for up to 1 year in canine transplantation models.

➤*Pharmacokinetics:* A population pharmacokinetic analysis incorporated plerixafor data from 63 subjects (patients with NHL, patients with multiple myeloma, subjects with varying degrees of renal impairment, and healthy subjects) who received a single subcutaneous dose (0.04 to 0.24 mg/kg) of plerixafor. A 2-compartment disposition model with first order absorption and elimination was found to adequately describe the plerixafor concentration-time profile. Significant relationships between clearance and CrCl, as well as between central volume of distribution and body weight, were observed.

The population pharmacokinetic analysis showed that the mg/kg-based dosage results in an increased plerixafor exposure ($AUC_{0\text{-}24h}$) with increasing body weight. There is limited experience with the 0.24 mg/kg dose of plerixafor in patients weighing more than 160 kg. Therefore the dose should not exceed that of a 160 kg patient (ie, 40 mg/day if CrCl is more than 50 mL/min and 27 mg/day if CrCl is 50 mL/min or less).

Absorption – Peak plasma concentrations occurred at approximately 30 to 60 minutes after a subcutaneous dose.

Distribution – Plerixafor is bound to human plasma proteins up to 58%. The apparent volume of distribution of plerixafor in humans is 0.3 L/kg demonstrating that plerixafor is largely confined to, but not limited to, the extravascular fluid space.

Metabolism – The metabolism of plerixafor was evaluated with in vitro assays. Plerixafor is not metabolized as shown in assays using human liver microsomes or human primary hepatocytes and does not exhibit inhibitory activity in vitro towards the major drug metabolizing cytochrome P450 enzymes (1A2, 2C9, 2C19, 2D6, and 3A4/5). In in vitro studies with human hepatocytes, plerixafor does not induce CYP1A2, CYP2B6, or CYP3A4 enzymes. These findings suggest that plerixafor has a low potential for involvement in CYP-450–dependent drug-drug interactions.

Excretion – The major route of elimination of plerixafor is urinary. Following a 0.24 mg/kg dose in healthy volunteers with normal renal function, approximately 70% of the dose was excreted in the urine as the parent drug during the first 24 hours following administration. In studies with healthy subjects and patients, the terminal half-life in plasma ranged between 3 and 5 hours. The ability of plerixafor to act as a substrate or as an inhibitor of P-glycoprotein has not been investigated. The distribution half-life was estimated to be 0.3 hours and the terminal population half-life was 5.3 hours in patients with normal renal function.

Special populations –

Renal function impairment: Following a single 0.24 mg/kg subcutaneous dose, plerixafor clearance was reduced in subjects with varying degrees of renal impairment and was positively correlated with CrCl. The mean $AUC_{0\text{-}24h}$ of plerixafor in subjects with mild (CrCl 51 to 80 mL/min), moderate (CrCl 31 to 50 mL/min), and severe (CrCl of less than 31 mL/min) renal impairment was 7%, 32%, and 39%, respectively, higher than healthy subjects with normal renal function. Renal impairment had no effect on C_{max}. A population pharmacokinetic analysis indicated an increased exposure ($AUC_{0\text{-}24h}$) in patients with moderate and severe renal impairment compared with patients with CrCl of greater than 50 mL/min. These results support a dose reduction of one-third in patients with moderate to severe renal impairment (CrCl 50 mL/min or less) in order to match the exposure in patients with normal renal function. The population pharmacokinetic analysis showed that the mg/kg-based dosage results in an increased plerixafor exposure ($AUC_{0\text{-}24h}$) with increasing body weight; therefore, if CrCl is 50 mL/min or less, the dosage should not exceed 27 mg/day.

Contraindications

None known.

Warnings/Precautions

➤*Leukemia:* For the purpose of HSC mobilization, plerixafor may cause mobilization of leukemic cells and subsequent contamination of the apheresis product. Therefore, plerixafor is not intended for HSC mobilization and harvest in patients with leukemia.

➤*Hematologic effects:*

Leukocytosis – Administration of plerixafor in conjunction with G-CSF increases circulating leukocytes as well as HSC populations. Monitor white blood cell counts during plerixafor use. Exercise clinical judgment when administering plerixafor to patients with peripheral blood neutrophil counts above 50,000/mcL.

Thrombocytopenia – Thrombocytopenia has been observed in patients receiving plerixafor. Monitor platelet counts in all patients who receive plerixafor and then undergo apheresis.

➤*Tumor cell mobilization:* When plerixafor is used in combination with G-CSF for HSC mobilization, tumor cells may be released from the marrow and subsequently collected in the leukapheresis product. The effect of potential reinfusion of tumor cells has not been well studied.

➤*Splenic enlargement:* Higher absolute and relative spleen weights associated with extramedullary hematopoiesis were observed following prolonged (2 to 4 weeks) daily plerixafor subcutaneous administration in rats at doses approximately 4-fold higher than the recommended human dose based on body surface area. The effect of plerixafor on spleen size in patients was not specifically evaluated in clinical studies. Evaluate individuals receiving plerixafor in combination with G-CSF who report left upper abdominal pain and/or scapular or shoulder pain for splenic integrity.

➤*Renal function impairment:* In patients with moderate and severe renal impairment (CrCl of 50 mL/min or less), reduce the dose of plerixafor by one-third to 0.16 mg/kg. (See also Actions and Administration/Dosage.)

➤*Pregnancy: Category D.* Plerixafor may cause fetal harm when administered to a pregnant woman. There are no adequate and well-controlled studies in pregnant women using plerixafor. Advise women of childbearing potential to avoid becoming pregnant while receiving treatment with plerixafor. If this drug is used during pregnancy, or if the patient becomes pregnant while taking this drug, apprise the patient of the potential hazard to the fetus.

Plerixafor was teratogenic in animals. Plerixafor administered to pregnant rats induced embryo-fetal toxicities, including fetal death, increased resorption and postimplantation loss, decreased fetal weights, anophthalmia, shortened digits, cardiac interventricular septal defect, ringed aorta, globular heart, hydrocephaly, dilatation of olfactory ventricles, and retarded skeletal development. Embryo-fetal toxicities occurred mainly at a dose of

PLERIXAFOR — INJECTION

90 mg/m^2 (approximately 10 times the recommended human dose of 0.24 mg/kg when compared on a mg/m^2 basis or 10 times the AUC in subjects with normal renal function who received a single dose of 0.24 mg/kg).

➤*Lactation:* It is not known whether plerixafor is excreted in human milk. Because many drugs are excreted in human milk and because of the potential for serious adverse reactions in breast-feeding infants from plerixafor, a decision should be made whether to discontinue breast-feeding or the drug, taking into account the importance of the drug to the mother.

➤*Children:* The safety and effectiveness of plerixafor in children have not been established in controlled clinical studies.

➤*Elderly:* Because plerixafor is mainly excreted by the kidney, no dose modifications are necessary in elderly individuals with normal renal function. In general, take care in dose selection for elderly patients because of the greater frequency of decreased renal function with advanced age. Dosage adjustment in elderly patients with a CrCl of 50 mL/min or less is recommended.

➤*Monitoring:* Monitor white blood cell counts during plerixafor use. Exercise clinical judgment when administering plerixafor to patients with peripheral blood neutrophil counts higher than 50,000/mcL. Monitor platelet counts in all patients who receive plerixafor and then undergo apheresis. Evaluate individuals receiving plerixafor in combination with G-CSF who report left upper abdominal pain and/or scapular or shoulder pain for splenic integrity. Monitor patients for vasovagal reactions following administration.

Drug Interactions

➤*Nephrotoxic drugs:* Because plerixafor is primarily eliminated by the kidneys, coadministration of plerixafor with drugs that reduce renal function or compete for active tubular secretion may increase serum concentrations of plerixafor or the coadministered drug. The effects of coadministration of plerixafor with other drugs that are renally eliminated or are known to affect renal function have not been evaluated.

Adverse Reactions

For more information on the potential for tumor cell mobilization in leukemia patients, increased circulating leukocytes and decreased platelet counts, and potential for splenic enlargement, refer to Warnings/Precautions.

➤*Common adverse reactions:* The most common adverse reactions (at least 10%) reported in patients who received plerixafor in conjunction with G-CSF regardless of causality and more frequent with plerixafor than placebo during HSC mobilization and apheresis were diarrhea, nausea, fatigue, injection-site reactions, headache, arthralgia, dizziness, and vomiting.

➤*Clinical trial data:*

Plerixafor Adverse Reactions (≥5%)						
	Plerixafor and G-CSF (n = 301)			Placebo and G-CSF (n = 292)		
Adverse reaction	All grades[a]	Grade 3	Grade 4	All grades	Grade 3	Grade 4
CNS						
Dizziness	11%	0%	0%	6%	0%	0%
Fatigue	27%	0%	0%	25%	0%	0%
Headache	22%	< 1%	0%	21%	1%	0%
Insomnia	7%	0%	0%	5%	0%	0%
GI						
Diarrhea	37%	< 1%	0%	17%	0%	0%
Flatulence	7%	0%	0%	3%	0%	0%
Nausea	34%	1%	0%	22%	0%	0%
Vomiting	10%	< 1%	0%	6%	0%	0%
Miscellaneous						
Arthralgia	13%	0%	0%	12%	0%	0%
Injection-site reactions	34%	0%	0%	10%	0%	0%

[a] Grades based on criteria from the World Health Organization.

➤*Injection-site reactions:* In the randomized studies, 34% of patients with NHL or multiple myeloma had mild to moderate injection-site reactions at the site of subcutaneous administration of plerixafor. These included erythema, hematoma, hemorrhage, induration, inflammation, irritation, pain, paresthesia, pruritus, rash, swelling, and urticaria.

➤*Other adverse reactions (less than 5%):* Other adverse reactions that occurred in less than 5% of patients but were reported as related to plerixafor during HSC mobilization and apheresis included abdominal pain, hyperhidrosis, abdominal distention, dry mouth, erythema, stomach discomfort, malaise, hypoesthesia oral, constipation, dyspepsia, and musculoskeletal pain.

➤*Other adverse reactions (less than 1%):* Mild to moderate systemic reactions were observed in less than 1% of patients approximately 30 minutes after plerixafor administration. Reactions included 1 or more of the following: urticaria (n = 2), periorbital swelling (n = 2), dyspnea (n = 1), or hypoxia (n = 1). Symptoms generally responded to treatments (eg, antihistamines, corticosteroids, hydration or supplemental oxygen), or resolved spontaneously.

Vasovagal reactions, orthostatic hypotension, and/or syncope can occur following subcutaneous injections. In plerixafor oncology and healthy volunteer clinical studies, less than 1% of subjects experienced vasovagal reactions following subcutaneous administration of plerixafor doses of 0.24 mg/kg or less. The majority of these reactions occurred within 1 hour of plerixafor administration. Because of the potential for these reactions, take appropriate precautions.

Overdosage

➤*Symptoms:* Based on limited data at doses above the recommended dose of 0.24 mg/kg subcutaneously, the frequency of GI disorders, vasovagal reactions, orthostatic hypotension, and/or syncope may be higher.

Patient Information

Advise patients of the signs and symptoms of potential systemic reactions such as urticaria, periorbital swelling, dyspnea, or hypoxia during and following plerixafor injection.

Instruct patients to inform a health care provider immediately if symptoms of vasovagal reactions such as orthostatic hypotension or syncope occur during or shortly after their plerixafor injection.

If patients experience itching, rash, or reaction at the site of injection, instruct them to notify a health care provider because these symptoms have been treated with nonprescription medications during clinical trials.

Inform patients that plerixafor may cause GI disorders, including diarrhea, nausea, vomiting, flatulence, and abdominal pain. Tell patients how to manage specific GI disorders and to inform their health care provider if severe events occur following plerixafor injection.

Advise women with reproductive potential to use effective contraceptive methods during plerixafor use.

OPRELVEKIN (Interleukin 11; IL-11)

Rx	**Neumega** (Wyeth)	**Injection, lyophilized, powder for solution:** 5 mg	1.6 mg dibasic sodium phosphate heptahydrate, 0.55 mg monobasic sodium phosphate monohydrate. Preservative free. In single-dose vials with diluent.

OPRELVEKIN — INJECTION

WARNING

Allergic reactions, including anaphylaxis – Oprelvekin has caused allergic or hypersensitivity reactions, including anaphylaxis. Permanently discontinue administration of oprelvekin in any patient who develops an allergic or hypersensitivity reaction.

Indications

➤*Thrombocytopenia prevention:* For the prevention of severe thrombocytopenia and the reduction of the need for platelet transfusions following myelosuppressive chemotherapy in adult patients with nonmyeloid malignancies who are at high risk of severe thrombocytopenia. Efficacy was demonstrated in patients who had experienced severe thrombocytopenia following the previous chemotherapy cycle. Oprelvekin is not indicated following myeloablative chemotherapy. The safety and efficacy of oprelvekin have not been established in children.

Administration and Dosage

➤*Adults:*

Thrombocytopenia, prevention –

Usual dosage: 50 mcg/kg given once daily. Initiate dosing 6 to 24 hours after the completion of chemotherapy.

Duration of therapy: Monitor platelet counts periodically to assess the optimal duration of therapy. Continue dosing until the post nadir platelet count is at least 50,000/mcL. In controlled clinical studies, doses were administered in courses of 10 to 21 days. Dosing beyond 21 days per treatment course is not recommended.

Discontinuation of therapy: Discontinue treatment with oprelvekin at least 2 days before starting the next planned cycle of chemotherapy.

➤*Renal function impairment:* The recommended dose of oprelvekin in adults with severe renal function impairment (creatinine clearance [CrCl] less than 30 mL/min) is 25 mcg/kg. An estimate of the patient's CrCl in mL/min is required.

OPRELVEKIN — INJECTION

➤*Preparation for administration:* Oprelvekin is a sterile, white, preservative-free, lyophilized powder for subcutaneous injection upon reconstitution. Reconstitute oprelvekin (5 mg vials) aseptically with 1 mL of sterile water for injection (without preservative). The reconstituted oprelvekin solution is clear, colorless, and isotonic, with a pH of 7, and contains oprelvekin 5 mg/mL. Do not reenter or reuse the single-use vial. Discard any unused portion of either reconstituted oprelvekin solution or sterile water for injection.

Because neither oprelvekin powder for injection nor its accompanying diluent, sterile water for injection, contains a preservative, use oprelvekin within 3 hours of reconstitution.

➤*Administration:* Administer subcutaneously as a single injection in either the abdomen, thigh, or hip (or upper arm if not self-injecting).

➤*Storage / Stability:* Store lyophilized oprelvekin and diluent in a refrigerator at 2° to 8°C (36° to 46°F). Protect from light. Do not freeze. Reconstituted oprelvekin must be used within 3 hours of reconstitution and can be stored in the vial either at 2° to 8°C (36° to 46°F) or at room temperature up to 25°C (77°F). Do not freeze or shake the reconstituted solution.

Actions

➤*Pharmacology:* The primary hematopoietic activity of oprelvekin is stimulation of megakaryocytopoiesis and thrombopoiesis. Oprelvekin has shown potent thrombopoietic activity in animal models of compromised hematopoiesis, including moderately to severely myelosuppressed mice and nonhuman primates. In these models, oprelvekin improved platelet nadirs and accelerated platelet recoveries compared with controls.

Preclinical trials have shown that mature megakaryocytes that develop during in vivo treatment with oprelvekin are ultrastructurally normal. Platelets produced in response to oprelvekin were morphologically and functionally normal and possessed a normal lifespan.

IL-11 also has been shown to have nonhematopoietic activities in animals, including the following: the regulation of intestinal epithelium growth (enhanced healing of GI lesions), inhibition of adipogenesis, induction of acute phase protein synthesis, inhibition of proinflammatory cytokine production by macrophages, and stimulation of osteoclastogenesis and neurogenesis. Nonhematopoietic pathologic changes observed in animals include fibrosis of tendons and joint capsules, periosteal thickening, papilledema, and embryotoxicity.

IL-11 is produced by bone marrow stromal cells and is part of the cytokine family that shares the gp130 signal transducer. Primary osteoblasts and mature osteoclasts express mRNAs for both IL-11 receptor (IL-11R alpha) and gp130. Both bone-forming and bone-resorbing cells are potential targets of IL-11.

Pharmacodynamics – In a study in which oprelvekin was administered to nonmyelosuppressed cancer patients, daily subcutaneous dosing for 14 days with oprelvekin increased the platelet count in a dose-dependent manner. Platelet counts began to increase relative to baseline between 5 and 9 days after the start of dosing with oprelvekin. After cessation of treatment, platelet counts continued to increase for up to 7 days and then returned toward baseline within 14 days. No change in platelet reactivity as measured by platelet activation in response to adenosine diphosphate and platelet aggregation in response to adenosine diphosphate, epinephrine, collagen, ristocetin, and arachidonic acid has been observed in association with oprelvekin treatment.

In a randomized, double-blind, placebo-controlled study in healthy volunteers, subjects receiving oprelvekin had a mean increase in plasma volume of more than 20%, and all subjects receiving oprelvekin had at least a 10% increase in plasma volume. Red blood cell volume decreased similarly (because of repeated phlebotomy) in the oprelvekin and placebo groups. As a result, whole blood volume increased approximately 10%, and hemoglobin concentration decreased approximately 10% in subjects receiving oprelvekin compared with subjects receiving placebo. Mean 24-hour sodium excretion decreased, and potassium excretion did not increase, in subjects receiving oprelvekin compared with subjects receiving placebo.

➤*Pharmacokinetics:*

Absorption / Distribution – The absolute bioavailability of oprelvekin was more than 80%. In a study in which multiple subcutaneous doses of 25 and 50 mcg/kg were administered to cancer patients receiving chemotherapy, oprelvekin did not accumulate, and clearance of oprelvekin was not impaired following multiple doses.

In preclinical studies in rats, radiolabeled oprelvekin was rapidly cleared from the serum and distributed to highly perfused organs.

The pharmacokinetics of oprelvekin have been evaluated in healthy adults and cancer patients receiving chemotherapy. In a study in which a single 50 mcg/kg subcutaneous dose was administered to 18 healthy men, the peak serum concentration (C_{max}) of 17.4 ± 5.4 ng/mL (mean ± standard deviation [SD]) was reached at 3.2 ± 2.4 hours (time to maximum concentration [T_{max}]) following dosing.

Excretion – The terminal half life was 6.9 ± 1.7 hours. The kidney was the primary route of elimination. The amount of intact oprelvekin in urine was low, indicating that the molecule was metabolized before excretion.

Special populations –

Renal function impairment: In a clinical study, a single dose of oprelvekin was administered to subjects with severe renal function impairment (CrCl less than 30 mL/min). The mean ± SD values for C_{max} and area under the curve (AUC) were 30.8 ± 8.6 ng/mL and 373 ± 106 ng•h/mL, respectively. When compared with control subjects in this study with healthy renal function, the mean C_{max} was 2.2-fold higher, and the mean AUC was 2.6-fold (95% confidence interval [CI], 1.7% to 3.8%) higher in the subjects with severe renal function impairment. In the subjects with severe renal function impairment, clearance was approximately 40% of the value seen in subjects with healthy renal function. The average terminal half-life was similar in subjects with severe renal function impairment and those with healthy renal function.

A second clinical study of 24 subjects with varying degrees of renal function also was performed and confirmed the results observed in the first study. Single 50 mcg/kg subcutaneous and intravenous (IV) doses were administered in a randomized fashion. As the degree of renal function impairment increased, the oprelvekin AUC increased, although half-life remained unchanged. In the 6 patients with severe impairment, the mean ± SD C_{max} and AUC were 23.6 ± 6.7 ng/mL and 373 ± 55.2 ng•h/mL, respectively, compared with 13.1 ± 3.8 ng/mL and 195 ± 49.3 ng•h/mL, respectively, in the 6 subjects with healthy renal function. A comparable increase in exposure was observed after IV administration of oprelvekin.

The pharmacokinetic studies suggest that overall exposure to oprelvekin increases as renal function decreases, indicating that a 50% dose reduction of oprelvekin is warranted for patients with severe renal function impairment. No dosage reduction is required for smaller changes in renal function.

Children: In a dose-escalation phase 1 study, oprelvekin also was administered to 43 children (age, 8 months to 18 years) and 1 adult patient receiving ifosfamide, carboplatin, etoposide (ICE) chemotherapy. Administered doses ranged from 25 to 125 mcg/kg. Analysis of data from 40 children showed that C_{max}, T_{max}, and terminal half-life were comparable with that in adults. The mean AUC for children (8 months to 18 years of age) receiving 50 mcg/kg was approximately half that achieved in healthy adults receiving 50 mcg/kg. Available data suggest that clearance of oprelvekin decreases with increasing age.

Contraindications

Hypersensitivity to oprelvekin or any component of the product.

Warnings/Precautions

➤*Myeloablative chemotherapy:* Oprelvekin is not indicated following myeloablative chemotherapy. In a randomized, placebo-controlled, phase 2 study, the efficacy of oprelvekin was not demonstrated. In this study, a statistically significant increased incidence in edema, conjunctival bleeding, hypotension, and tachycardia was observed in patients receiving oprelvekin as compared with placebo.

➤*Fluid retention:* Oprelvekin is known to cause serious fluid retention that can result in peripheral edema, dyspnea on exertion, pulmonary edema, capillary leak syndrome, atrial arrhythmias, and exacerbation of preexisting pleural effusions. Severe fluid retention, some cases resulting in death, was reported following recent bone marrow transplantation in patients who have received oprelvekin. Use with caution in patients with clinically evident congestive heart failure, patients receiving aggressive hydration, patients who may be susceptible to developing congestive heart failure, patients with a history of heart failure who are well compensated and receiving appropriate medical therapy, and patients who may develop fluid retention as a result of associated medical conditions or whose medical condition may be exacerbated by fluid retention.

➤*Dilutional anemia:* Moderate decreases in hemoglobin concentration, hematocrit, and red blood cell count (approximately 10% to 15%) without a decrease in red blood cell mass have been observed. These changes are predominantly because of an increase in plasma volume (dilutional anemia) that is primarily related to renal sodium and water retention. The decrease in hemoglobin concentration typically begins within 3 to 5 days of the initiation of oprelvekin and is reversible over approximately a week following discontinuation of oprelvekin.

➤*Cardiovascular effects:* Oprelvekin use is associated with cardiovascular reactions, including arrhythmias and pulmonary edema. Cardiac arrest has been reported, but the causal relationship to oprelvekin is uncertain. Use with caution in patients with a history of atrial arrhythmias, and only after consideration of the potential risks in relation to anticipated benefit. In clinical trials, cardiac reactions, including atrial arrhythmias (atrial fibrillation or atrial flutter), occurred in 23 of 157 (15%) patients treated with oprelvekin at doses of 50 mcg/kg. Arrhythmias were usually brief in duration; conversion to sinus rhythm typically occurred spontaneously or after rate-control drug therapy. Approximately 11 of 24 (50%) patients who were rechallenged had recurrent atrial arrhythmias. Clinical sequelae, including stroke, have been reported in patients who experienced atrial arrhythmias while receiving oprelvekin.

The mechanism for induction of arrhythmias is not known. Oprelvekin was not directly arrhythmogenic in animal models. In some patients, development of atrial arrhythmias may be because of increased plasma volume associated with fluid retention.

In the postmarketing setting, ventricular arrhythmias have been reported, generally occurring within 2 to 7 days of initiation of treatment.

➤*CNS effects:* Stroke has been reported in the setting of patients who develop atrial fibrillation/flutter while receiving oprelvekin. Patients with a history of stroke or transient ischemic attack also may be at increased risk for these reactions.

➤*Papilledema:* Papilledema has been reported in 10 of 405 (2%) patients receiving oprelvekin in clinical trials following repeated cycles of exposure. The incidence was higher (16% [7/43]) in children than in adults (1% [3/362]). Nonhuman primates treated with oprelvekin at a dose of 1,000 mcg/kg subcutaneously once daily for 4 to 13 weeks developed papilledema that was not associated with inflammation or any other histologic abnormality and was reversible after dosing was discontinued. Use oprelvekin with caution in patients with preexisting papilledema, or with

OPRELVEKIN — INJECTION

tumors involving the CNS because it is possible that papilledema could worsen or develop during treatment. Changes in visual acuity and/or visual field defects ranging from blurred vision to blindness can occur in patients with papilledema taking oprelvekin.

➤*Chronic administration:* Oprelvekin has been administered safely using the recommended dosing schedule for up to 6 cycles following chemotherapy. The safety and efficacy of chronic administration of oprelvekin have not been established. Continuous dosage (2 to 13 weeks) in nonhuman primates produced joint capsule and tendon fibrosis and periosteal hyperostosis. The relevance of these findings to humans is unclear.

➤*Timing of therapy:* Begin dosing with oprelvekin 6 to 24 hours following the completion of chemotherapy dosing. The safety and efficacy of oprelvekin given immediately prior to or concurrently with cytotoxic chemotherapy or initiated at the time of expected nadir have not been established.

➤*Duration:* The efficacy of oprelvekin has not been evaluated in patients receiving chemotherapy regimens of more than 5 days duration or regimens associated with delayed myelosuppression (eg, nitrosoureas, mitomycin-C).

➤*Hypersensitivity reactions:* In the postmarketing setting, oprelvekin has caused allergic or hypersensitivity reactions, including anaphylaxis. The administration of oprelvekin should be attended by appropriate precautions in case allergic reactions occur. In addition, counsel patients about the symptoms for which they should seek medical attention. Signs and symptoms reported included edema of the face, tongue, or larynx; shortness of breath; wheezing; chest pain; hypotension (including shock); dysarthria; loss of consciousness; mental status changes; rash; urticaria; flushing; and fever. Reactions occurred after the first dose or subsequent doses of oprelvekin. Permanently discontinue oprelvekin in any patient who develops an allergic or hypersensitivity reaction.

➤*Renal function impairment:* Oprelvekin is eliminated primarily by the kidneys. The pharmacokinetics of oprelvekin were studied in subjects with varying degrees of renal function impairment. $AUC_{0-\infty}$, C_{max}, and absolute bioavailability were significantly increased in subjects with severe renal function impairment (CrCl less than 30 mL/min). There were no significant changes in the pharmacokinetic parameters in subjects with mild or moderate impairment. A significant decrease in the hemoglobin concentration was noted on day 2 after a single dose of oprelvekin in subjects with all degrees of renal function impairment. By day 14, the hemoglobin was decreased only in patients with severe renal function impairment. Fluid retention associated with oprelvekin treatment has not been studied in patients with renal function impairment, but carefully monitor fluid balance in these patients.

➤*Pregnancy: Category C.* Oprelvekin has been shown to have embryocidal effects in pregnant rats and rabbits when given in doses of 0.2 to 20 times the human dose. There are no adequate and well-controlled studies of oprelvekin in pregnant women. Use oprelvekin during pregnancy only if the potential benefit justifies the potential risk to the fetus.

Oprelvekin has been tested in studies of fertility, early embryonic development, and prenatal and postnatal development in rats, and in studies of organogenesis (teratogenicity) in rats and rabbits. Parental toxicity has been observed when oprelvekin is given at doses of 2 to 20 times the human dose (at least 100 mcg/kg/day) in the rat and 0.02 to 2 times the human dose (at least 1 mcg/kg/day) in the rabbit. Findings in pregnant rats consisted of transient hypoactivity and dyspnea after administration (maternal toxicity), as well as prolonged estrus cycle, increased early embryonic deaths, and decreased numbers of live fetuses. In addition, low fetal body weights and a reduced number of ossified sacral and caudal vertebrae (ie, retarded fetal development) occurred in rats at 20 times the human dose. Findings in pregnant rabbits consisted of decreased (fecal/urine) eliminations (the only toxicity noted at 1 mcg/kg/day in dams) as well as decreased food consumption, body weight loss, abortion, increased embryonic and fetal deaths, and decreased numbers of live fetuses. No teratogenic effects of oprelvekin were observed in rabbits at doses of up to 0.6 times the human dose (30 mcg/kg/day).

Adverse reactions in the first-generation offspring of rats given oprelvekin at maternally toxic doses at least 2 times the human dose (at least 100 mcg/kg/day) during gestation and lactation included increased newborn mortality, decreased viability index on day 4 of lactation, and decreased body weights during lactation. In rats given 20 times the human dose (1,000 mcg/kg/day) during both gestation and lactation, maternal toxicity and growth retardation of the first-generation offspring resulted in an increased rate of fetal death of the second-generation offspring.

➤*Lactation:* It is not known if oprelvekin is excreted in human milk. Because many drugs are excreted in human milk and because of the potential for serious adverse reactions in breast-feeding infants from oprelvekin, decide whether to discontinue breast-feeding or oprelvekin, taking into account the importance of the drug to the mother.

➤*Children:* A safe and effective dose of oprelvekin has not been established in children.

Studies in animals were predictive of the effect of oprelvekin on developing bone in children. In growing rodents treated with 100, 300, or 1,000 mcg/kg/day for a minimum of 28 days, thickening of femoral and tibial growth plates that did not completely resolve after a 28-day nontreatment period was noted. A nonhuman primate toxicology study of oprelvekin animals treated for 2 to 13 weeks at doses of 10 to 1,000 mcg/kg showed partially reversible joint capsule and tendon fibrosis and periosteal hyperostosis. An asymptomatic, laminated periosteal reaction in the diaphyses of the femur, tibia, and fibula has been observed in one patient during pediatric studies involving multiple courses of oprelvekin treatment. The relationship of these findings to treatment with oprelvekin is unclear. No studies have been performed to assess the long-term effects of oprelvekin on growth and development.

➤*Monitoring:* Obtain a complete blood cell count prior to chemotherapy and at regular intervals during oprelvekin therapy. Monitor platelet counts during the time of the expected nadir and until adequate recovery has occurred (postnadir counts at least 50,000/mcL).

During dosing with oprelvekin, monitoring of fluid balance and appropriate medical management is advised.

Perform close monitoring of fluid and electrolyte status in patients receiving chronic diuretic therapy. Sudden deaths have occurred in oprelvekin-treated patients receiving chronic diuretic therapy and ifosfamide who developed severe hypokalemia.

Monitor preexisting fluid collections, including pericardial effusions or ascites. Consider drainage if medically indicated.

Drug Interactions

None known.

Adverse Reactions

Because clinical trials are conducted under widely varying conditions, adverse reaction rates observed in the clinical studies of a drug cannot be directly compared with rates in the clinical studies of another drug and may not reflect the rates observed in practice. The adverse reaction information from clinical trials does, however, provide a basis for identifying the adverse reactions that appear to be related to drug use and for approximating rates.

In general, the incidence and type of adverse reactions were similar between oprelvekin 50 mcg/kg and the placebo groups. The most frequently reported serious adverse reactions were neutropenic fever, syncope, atrial fibrillation, fever, and pneumonia. The most commonly reported adverse reactions were edema, dyspnea, tachycardia, conjunctival injection, palpitations, atrial arrhythmias, and pleural effusions. The most frequently reported adverse reactions resulting in clinical intervention (eg, discontinuation of oprelvekin, adjustment in dosage, need for concomitant medication to treat an adverse reaction symptom) were atrial arrhythmias, syncope, dyspnea, congestive heart failure, and pulmonary edema. Selected adverse reactions that occurred in at least 10% of oprelvekin-treated patients are listed in the following table.

Oprelvekin Adverse Reactions (%)

Adverse reaction	Placebo (n = 67)	50 mcg/kg (n = 69)
Cardiovascular		
Atrial fibrillation/flutter[a]	1%	12%
Palpitations[a]	3%	14%
Syncope	6%	13%
Tachycardia[a]	3%	20%
Vasodilatation	9%	19%
CNS		
Dizziness	28%	38%
Headache	36%	41%
Insomnia	27%	33%
Dermatologic		
Rash	16%	25%
GI		
Diarrhea	33%	43%
Mucositis	37%	43%
Nausea/Vomiting	70%	77%
Oral moniliasis[a]	1%	14%
Respiratory		
Cough increased	22%	29%
Dyspnea[a]	22%	48%
Pharyngitis	16%	25%
Pleural effusion[a]	0%	10%
Rhinitis	31%	42%
Special senses		
Conjunctival injection[a]	3%	19%
Miscellaneous		
Edema[a]	15%	59%
Fever	28%	36%
Neutropenic fever	42%	48%

[a] Occurred in significantly more oprelvekin-treated than placebo-treated patients.

➤*Children:* In a phase 1, single-arm, dose-escalation study, 43 children were treated with oprelvekin at doses ranging from 25 to 125 mcg/kg/day following ICE chemotherapy. All patients required platelet transfusions, and the lack of a comparator arm made the study design inadequate to assess efficacy. The projected effective dose (based on comparable AUC observed for the effective dose in healthy adults) in children appears to exceed the maximum tolerated pediatric dose of 50 mcg/kg/day. Papilledema was dose limiting and occurred in 16% of children.

The most common adverse reactions seen in pediatric studies included tachycardia (84%), conjunctival injection (57%), radiographic and echocardiographic evidence of cardiomegaly (21%), and periosteal changes (11%). These reactions occurred at a higher frequency in children than in adults. The incidence of other adverse reactions was generally similar to those observed using oprelvekin 50 mcg/kg in the randomized studies in adults receiving chemotherapy.

➤*Other adverse reactions:* The following adverse reactions also occurred more frequently in cancer patients receiving oprelvekin than in those receiving placebo: blurred vision, dehydration, exfoliative dermatitis, eye hemor-

OPRELVEKIN — INJECTION

rhage, paresthesia, and skin discoloration. Other than a higher incidence of severe asthenia in oprelvekin-treated patients (10 [14%] in oprelvekin patients vs 2 [3%] in placebo patients), the incidence of severe or life-threatening adverse reactions was comparable in the oprelvekin and placebo treatment groups.

Two patients with cancer treated with oprelvekin experienced sudden death, which the investigator considered possibly or probably related to oprelvekin. Both deaths occurred in patients with severe hypokalemia (less than 3 mEq/L) who had received high doses of ifosfamide and were receiving daily doses of a diuretic.

Other serious reactions associated with oprelvekin were papilledema and cardiovascular reactions, including atrial arrhythmias and stroke. In addition, cardiomegaly was reported in children.

The following adverse reactions, occurring in at least 10% of patients, were observed at equal or greater frequency in placebo-treated patients: abdominal pain, anorexia, alopecia, asthenia, bone pain, chills, constipation, dyspepsia, ecchymosis, infection, myalgia, nervousness, and pain. The incidence of fever, neutropenic fever, flu-like symptoms, thrombocytosis, and thrombotic events; the average number of units of red blood cells transfused per patient; and the duration of neutropenia less than 500/mcL were similar in the oprelvekin 50 mcg/kg and placebo groups.

➤*Immunogenicity:* In clinical studies that evaluated the immunogenicity of oprelvekin, 2 of 181 (1%) patients developed antibodies to oprelvekin. In one of these 2 patients, neutralizing antibodies to oprelvekin were detected in an unvalidated assay. The clinical relevance of the presence of these antibodies is unknown. In the postmarketing setting, cases of allergic reactions, including anaphylaxis, have been reported. The presence of antibodies to oprelvekin was not assessed in these patients.

➤*Lab test abnormalities:* The most common laboratory abnormality reported in patients in clinical trials was a decrease in hemoglobin concentration predominantly as a result of expansion of the plasma volume. The increase in plasma volume also is associated with a decrease in the serum concentration of albumin and several other proteins (eg, transferrin and gamma globulins). A parallel decrease in calcium without clinical effects has been documented.

After daily subcutaneous injections, treatment with oprelvekin resulted in a 2-fold increase in plasma fibrinogen. Other acute-phase proteins also increased. These protein levels returned to normal after dosing with oprelvekin was discontinued. Von Willebrand factor concentrations increased with a normal multimer pattern in healthy subjects receiving oprelvekin.

➤*Postmarketing:* The following adverse reactions have been reported during the postmarketing use of oprelvekin: allergic reactions; anaphylaxis/anaphylactoid reactions; capillary leak syndrome; injection-site reactions described as dermatitis, pain, and discoloration; optic neuropathy; papilledema; renal failure; ventricular arrhythmias; visual disturbances ranging from blurred vision to blindness.

Overdosage

➤*Symptoms:* Doses of oprelvekin of more than 125 mcg/kg have not been administered to humans. While clinical experience is limited, doses of oprelvekin more than 50 mcg/kg may be associated with an increased incidence of cardiovascular reactions in adult patients.

➤*Treatment:* If an overdose of oprelvekin is administered, discontinue oprelvekin and closely observe the patient for signs of toxicity. Base reinstitution of oprelvekin therapy upon individual patient factors (eg, evidence of toxicity, continued need for therapy).

Patient Information

Use oprelvekin under the guidance and supervision of a health care provider. However, when the health care provider determines that oprelvekin may be used outside of the hospital or office setting, instruct persons who will be administering oprelvekin as to the proper dose and the method for reconstituting and administering oprelvekin. Give each dose at about the same time each day. If a dose is missed, instruct patients to continue with the next scheduled dose. If home use is prescribed, instruct patients in the importance of proper disposal and caution against the reuse of needles, syringes, drug product, and diluent. Instruct patients to use a puncture-resistant container for the disposal of used needles.

Inform patients of the most serious and common adverse reactions associated with oprelvekin administration, including those symptoms related to allergic or hypersensitivity reactions. Advise patients to immediately seek medical attention if any of the following signs or symptoms develop: chest pain; confusion; difficulty breathing, swallowing, or talking; drowsiness; fever; flushing; hives; itching; light-headedness; loss of consciousness; rash; shortness of breath; swelling of the face, tongue, or throat; throat tightness; and/or wheezing. Mild to moderate peripheral edema and shortness of breath on exertion can occur within the first week of treatment and may continue for the duration of administration of oprelvekin.

Advise patients who have preexisting pleural or other effusions or a history of congestive heart failure to contact their health care provider for worsening of dyspnea. Most patients who receive oprelvekin develop anemia. Advise patients to contact their health care provider if symptoms attributable to atrial arrhythmia develop.

Advise women of childbearing potential of the possible risks to the fetus on oprelvekin.

Thrombopoietin Receptor Agonist

ELTROMBOPAG

Rx	**Promacta** (GlaxoSmithKline)	**Tablets; oral:** 25 mg	As eltrombopag olamine. Mannitol. (GS NX3 25). Orange, round. Film-coated. In 30s.
		50 mg	As eltrombopag olamine. Mannitol. (GS UFU 50). Blue, round. Film-coated. In 30s.
		75 mg	As eltrombopag olamine. Mannitol. (GS FFS 75). Pink, round. Film-coated. In 30s.

ELTROMBOPAG OLAMINE — ORAL

WARNING

Hepatotoxicity – Eltrombopag may cause hepatotoxicity.

Measure serum ALT, AST, and bilirubin prior to initiation of eltrombopag, every 2 weeks during the dose adjustment phase, and monthly following establishment of a stable dose. If bilirubin is elevated, perform fractionation. Evaluate abnormal serum liver tests with repeat testing within 3 to 5 days. If the abnormalities are confirmed, monitor serum liver tests weekly until the abnormality(ies) resolve, stabilize, or return to baseline levels. Discontinue eltrombopag if ALT levels increase to 3 times the upper limit of normal (ULN) and are progressive, persistent for 4 weeks or more, accompanied by increased direct bilirubin, or accompanied by clinical symptoms of liver injury or evidence for hepatic decompensation.

Because of the risk for hepatotoxicity and other risks, eltrombopag is available only through a restricted distribution program called PROMACTA CARES. Under PROMACTA CARES, only prescribers, pharmacies, and patients registered with the program are able to prescribe, dispense, and receive eltrombopag. To enroll in PROMACTA CARES, call 1-877-9-PROMACTA (1-877-977-6622).

Indications

➤*Thrombocytopenia:* For the treatment of thrombocytopenia in patients with chronic immune (idiopathic) thrombocytopenic purpura (ITP) who have had an insufficient response to corticosteroids, immunoglobulins, or splenectomy. Eltrombopag should be used only in patients with ITP whose degree of thrombocytopenia and clinical condition increases the risk for bleeding. Eltrombopag should not be used in an attempt to normalize platelet counts.

Administration and Dosage

➤*Maximum dose:*

Adults – 75 mg daily according to the prescribing information.

➤*General dosing considerations:* Only prescribers enrolled in PROMACTA CARES may prescribe eltrombopag.

Do not use eltrombopag in an attempt to normalize platelet counts.

Modify the dosage regimen of concomitant ITP medications, as medically appropriate, to avoid excessive increases in platelet counts during therapy with eltrombopag.

Do not administer more than 1 dose of eltrombopag within any 24-hour period.

➤*Adults:*

Thrombocytopenia – Use the lowest dose of eltrombopag to achieve and maintain a platelet count of at least 50×10^9/L as necessary to reduce the risk for bleeding.

Maximum dose: 75 mg daily according to the prescribing information.

Initial dosage: 50 mg once daily.

Dosage adjustment: Dose adjustments are based upon the platelet count response.

Dose Adjustments of Eltrombopag

Platelet count result	Dose adjustment or response
$< 50 \times 10^9$/L following ≥ 2 weeks of eltrombopag	Increase daily dose by 25 mg to a max of 75 mg/day.
$\geq 200 \times 10^9$/L to $\leq 400 \times 10^9$/L at any time	Decrease the daily dose by 25 mg. Wait 2 weeks to assess the effects of this and any subsequent dose adjustments.

ELTROMBOPAG OLAMINE — ORAL

Dose Adjustments of Eltrombopag	
Platelet count result	Dose adjustment or response
> 400 × 10^9/L	Stop eltrombopag; increase the frequency of platelet monitoring to twice weekly. Once the platelet count is ^{9}/L, reinitiate therapy at a daily dose reduced by 25 mg.
> 400 × 10^9/L after 2 weeks of therapy at lowest dose of eltrom-bopag	Permanently discontinue eltrombopag.

➤*Children:* The safety and efficacy of eltrombopag in children have not been established.

➤*Hepatic function impairment:* For patients with moderate or severe hepatic impairment, initiate eltrombopag at a reduced dosage of 25 mg once daily.

➤*East Asian ancestry (eg, Chinese, Japanese, Taiwanese, Korean):* Initiate eltrombopag at a reduced dosage of 25 mg once daily.

➤*Monitoring:* Monitor liver tests (ALT, AST, and bilirubin) prior to initiation of eltrombopag and throughout therapy with eltrombopag. If bilirubin is elevated, perform fractionation. During therapy with eltrombopag, assess complete blood cell counts (CBCs), including platelet count and peripheral blood smears, weekly until a stable platelet count has been achieved. Obtain CBCs, including platelet counts and peripheral blood smears, monthly thereafter. Monitor CBCs, including platelet counts, for at least 4 weeks following discontinuation of eltrombopag. In clinical studies, platelet counts generally increased within 1 to 2 weeks after starting eltrombopag and decreased within 1 to 2 weeks after discontinuing eltrombopag.

➤*Discontinuation of therapy:* Discontinue eltrombopag if the platelet count does not increase to a level sufficient to avoid clinically important bleeding after 4 weeks of therapy with eltrombopag at the maximum daily dose of 75 mg. Excessive platelet count responses or important liver test abnormalities also necessitate discontinuation of eltrombopag.

➤*Administration:* Take eltrombopag on an empty stomach (1 hour before or 2 hours after a meal). Allow at least a 4-hour interval between eltrombopag and other medications (eg, antacids), calcium-rich foods (eg, dairy products and calcium fortified juices), or supplements containing polyvalent cations such as iron, calcium, aluminum, magnesium, selenium, and zinc.

➤*Storage/Stability:* Store at 25°C (77°F); excursions are permitted between 15° and 30°C (59° and 86°F).

Actions

➤*Pharmacology:* Eltrombopag is an orally bioavailable, small-molecule thrombopoietin (TPO)-receptor agonist that interacts with the transmembrane domain of the human TPO-receptor and initiates signaling cascades that induce proliferation and differentiation of megakaryocytes from bone marrow progenitor cells.

➤*Pharmacokinetics:*

Absorption –

Eltrombopag Geometric Mean Steady-State Pharmacokinetic Parameters (95% CI)[a]	
Regimen of eltrombopag	$AUC_{(0-\tau)}$ (mcg•h/mL)
50 mg once daily (n = 34)	91.9 (73.6 to 115)
75 mg once daily (n = 26)	146 (122 to 176)

[a] CI = confidence interval; AUC = area under the curve.

Eltrombopag is absorbed with a peak concentration occurring 2 to 6 hours after oral administration. Based on urinary excretion and biotransformation products eliminated in feces, the oral absorption of drug-related material following administration of a single 75 mg solution dose was estimated to be at least 52%.

In a clinical study, administration of a single 75 mg dose of eltrombopag with a polyvalent cation-containing antacid (1,524 mg aluminum hydroxide, 1,425 mg magnesium carbonate, and sodium alginate) decreased plasma eltrombopag $AUC_{0-\infty}$ and maximal concentration (C_{max}) by 70%. The contribution of sodium alginate to this interaction is not known.

Effect of food: An open-label, randomized, crossover study was conducted to assess the effect of food on the bioavailability of eltrombopag. A standard high-fat breakfast significantly decreased plasma eltrombopag $AUC_{0-\infty}$ by approximately 59% and C_{max} by 65% and delayed time to C_{max} (T_{max}) by 1 hour. The calcium content of this meal may have also contributed to this decrease in exposure.

Distribution – The concentration of eltrombopag in blood cells is approximately 50% to 79% of plasma concentrations based on a radiolabel study. In vitro studies suggest that eltrombopag is highly bound to human plasma proteins (more than 99%). Eltrombopag is not a substrate for P-glycoprotein or OATP1B1.

Metabolism – Absorbed eltrombopag is extensively metabolized, predominantly through pathways including cleavage, oxidation, and conjugation with glucuronic acid, glutathione, or cysteine. In a human radiolabel study, eltrombopag accounted for approximately 64% of plasma radiocarbon $AUC_{0-\infty}$. Metabolites due to glucuronidation and oxidation were also detected. In vitro studies suggest that CYP1A2 and 2C8 are responsible for the oxidative metabolism of eltrombopag. UGT1A1 and UGT1A3 are responsible for the glucuronidation of eltrombopag.

Excretion – The predominant route of eltrombopag excretion is via feces (59%), and 31% of the dose is found in the urine. Unchanged eltrombopag in feces accounts for approximately 20% of the dose; unchanged eltrombopag is not detectable in urine. The plasma elimination half-life of eltrombopag is approximately 21 to 32 hours in healthy subjects and 26 to 35 hours in ITP patients.

Special populations –

Hepatic function impairment: Plasma eltrombopag $AUC_{0-\infty}$ was 41% higher in subjects with mild hepatic impairment, and 80% to 93% higher in subjects with moderate to severe hepatic impairment compared with healthy subjects. A corresponding reduction in apparent clearance was also reported. The impact of hepatic impairment was highly variable between subjects. Unbound eltrombopag (active) concentrations for this highly protein bound drug was not measured.

Gender: Results from a population pharmacokinetic model suggest that men have a 27% greater apparent eltrombopag clearance than women, after adjustment for the body weight difference.

Race: Based on noncompartment analysis and population pharmacokinetic analysis, plasma eltrombopag exposure was approximately 70% higher in some Asian subjects of Japanese, Chinese, Taiwanese, and Korean ancestry (ie, East Asian) with ITP as compared with non-Asian subjects who were predominantly white. In addition, the pharmacodynamic response to eltrombopag was qualitatively similar in the Asian subjects, but the absolute pharmacodynamic response was somewhat greater.

An approximately 40% higher systemic eltrombopag exposure in healthy black subjects was noted in at least 1 clinical pharmacology study. The effect of black ethnicity on exposure and related safety and efficacy of eltrombopag has not been established.

Contraindications

None known.

Warnings/Precautions

➤*Hepatotoxicity:* Eltrombopag administration may cause hepatotoxicity. In the controlled clinical studies, 1 patient experienced grade 4 (National Cancer Institute Common Terminology Criteria for Adverse Events [NCI-CTCAE] toxicity scale) elevations in serum liver test values during therapy with eltrombopag, worsening of underlying cardiopulmonary disease, and death. No patients in the placebo group experienced grade 4 liver test abnormalities. Overall, serum liver test abnormalities (predominantly grade 2 or less in severity) were reported in 10% and 8% of the eltrombopag and placebo groups, respectively. In the controlled studies, 2 (1%) patients treated with eltrombopag and 2 (3%) patients in the placebo group discontinued treatment due to hepatobiliary laboratory abnormalities. Seven of the patients treated with eltrombopag in the controlled studies with hepatobiliary laboratory abnormalities were reexposed to eltrombopag in the extension study. Six of these patients again experienced liver test abnormalities (predominantly grade 1) resulting in discontinuation of eltrombopag in 1 patient. In the extension study, 1 additional patient had eltrombopag discontinued because of liver test abnormalities (grade 3 or less).

See the Warning box for more information.

Reinitiating treatment with eltrombopag is not recommended. If the potential benefit for reinitiating eltrombopag treatment is considered to outweigh the risk for hepatotoxicity, then cautiously reintroduce eltrombopag and measure serum liver tests weekly during the dose adjustment phase. If liver tests abnormalities persist, worsen or recur, then permanently discontinue eltrombopag.

➤*Bone marrow reticulin formation/bone marrow fibrosis:* Eltrombopag is a TPO receptor agonist; TPO-receptor agonists increase the risk for development or progression of reticulin fiber deposition within the bone marrow.

In the extension study, 7 patients had reticulin fiber deposition reported in bone marrow biopsies, including 2 patients who also had collagen fiber deposition. The fiber deposition was not associated with cytopenias and did not necessitate discontinuation of eltrombopag. However, clinical studies have not excluded a risk of bone marrow fibrosis with cytopenias.

Prior to initiation of eltrombopag, examine the peripheral blood smear closely to establish a baseline level of cellular morphologic abnormalities. Following identification of a stable dose of eltrombopag, examine peripheral blood smears and CBCs monthly for new or worsening morphological abnormalities (eg, teardrop and nucleated red blood cells, immature white blood cells) or cytopenia(s). If the patient develops new or worsening morphological abnormalities or cytopenia(s), discontinue treatment with eltrombopag and consider a bone marrow biopsy, including staining for fibrosis.

➤*Discontinuation:* Discontinuation of eltrombopag may result in thrombocytopenia of greater severity than was present prior to therapy with eltrombopag. This worsened thrombocytopenia may increase the patient's risk of bleeding, particularly if eltrombopag is discontinued while the patient is on anticoagulants or antiplatelet agents. In the controlled clinical studies, transient decreases in platelet counts to levels lower than baseline

ELTROMBOPAG OLAMINE — ORAL

were observed following discontinuation of treatment in 10% and 6% of the eltrombopag and placebo groups, respectively. Serious hemorrhagic events requiring the use of supportive ITP medications occurred in 3 severely thrombocytopenic patients within 1 month following the discontinuation of eltrombopag; none were reported among the placebo group.

Following discontinuation of eltrombopag, obtain weekly CBCs, including platelet counts for at least 4 weeks and consider alternative treatments for worsening thrombocytopenia, according to current treatment guidelines.

➤*Thrombotic/thromboembolic complications:* Thrombotic/thromboembolic complications may result from excessive increases in platelet counts. Excessive doses of eltrombopag or medication errors that result in excessive doses of eltrombopag may increase platelet counts to a level that produces thrombotic/thromboembolic complications. In the controlled clinical studies, 1 thrombotic/thromboembolic complication was reported within the groups that received eltrombopag and none within the placebo groups. Seven patients experienced thrombotic/thromboembolic complications in the extension study. Use caution when administering eltrombopag to patients with known risk factors for thromboembolism (eg, factor V Leiden, ATIII deficiency, antiphospholipid syndrome). To minimize the risk for thrombotic/thromboembolic complications, do not use eltrombopag in an attempt to normalize platelet counts. Follow the dose adjustment guidelines to achieve and maintain a platelet count of 50×10^9/L or more.

➤*Malignancies:* Eltrombopag stimulation of the TPO receptor on the surface of hematopoietic cells may increase the risk for hematologic malignancies. In the controlled clinical studies, patients were treated with eltrombopag for a maximum of 6 weeks and during this period no hematologic malignancies were reported. One hematologic malignancy (non-Hodgkin lymphoma) was reported in the extension study. Eltrombopag is not indicated for the treatment of thrombocytopenia due to causes of thrombocytopenia (eg, myelodysplasia, chemotherapy) other than chronic ITP.

➤*Cataracts:* In the controlled clinical studies, cataracts developed or worsened in 5 (5%) patients who received 50 mg eltrombopag daily and 2 (3%) placebo-group patients. In the extension study, cataracts developed or worsened in 4% of patients who underwent ocular examination prior to therapy with eltrombopag. Cataracts were observed in toxicology studies of eltrombopag in rodents. Perform a baseline ocular examination prior to administration of eltrombopag and, during therapy with eltrombopag, regularly monitor patients for signs and symptoms of cataracts.

➤*Distribution program:* Eltrombopag is available only through a restricted distribution program called PROMACTA CARES. Under PROMACTA CARES, only prescribers, pharmacies, and patients registered with the program are able to prescribe, dispense, and receive eltrombopag. This program provides educational materials and a mechanism for the proper use of eltrombopag. To enroll in PROMACTA CARES, call 1-877-977-6622. Prescribers and patients are required to understand the risks of therapy with eltrombopag. Prescribers are required to understand the information in the prescribing information and be able to:

- Educate patients on the benefits and risks of treatment with eltrombopag, ensure that patients receive the Medication Guide, instruct them to read it, and encourage them to ask questions when considering eltrombopag. Patients may be educated by the enrolled prescriber or a health care provider under that prescriber's direction.
- Review the PROMACTA CARES Prescriber Enrollment Forms, sign the form, and return the form according to PROMACTA CARES Program instructions.
- As part of the initial prescription process for eltrombopag, obtain the patient's signature on the Patient Enrollment and Consent form, sign it, place the original signed form in the patient's medical record, send a copy to PROMACTA CARES, and give a copy to the patient.
- Report any serious adverse reactions associated with the use of eltrombopag to PROMACTA CARES Call Center at 1-877-977-6622 or to the FDA's MedWatch Program at 1-800-FDA-1088 (1-800-332-1088).
- Report serious adverse reactions observed in patients receiving eltrombopag, including reactions actively solicited at 6-month intervals.

➤*Renal function impairment:* The safety and efficacy of eltrombopag in patients with varying degrees of renal function have not been established. Closely monitor patients with impaired renal function when administering eltrombopag.

➤*Hepatic function impairment:* The disposition of eltrombopag was compared in patients with hepatic impairment with subjects with normal hepatic function. Apparent clearance of eltrombopag was reduced by approximately 50% in patients with moderate and severe (as indicated by the Child-Pugh method) hepatic impairment. In this clinical study that did not evaluate protein binding effects, the half-life of eltrombopag was prolonged 2-fold in patients with moderate and severe hepatic impairment.

Exercise caution when administering eltrombopag to patients with hepatic disease. For patients with moderate and severe hepatic impairment, initiate eltrombopag at a reduced dosage of 25 mg once daily.

➤*Pregnancy:* Category C. There are no adequate and well-controlled studies of eltrombopag use in pregnancy. In animal reproduction and developmental toxicity studies, there was evidence of embryolethality and reduced fetal weights at maternally toxic doses. Use eltrombopag during pregnancy only if the potential benefit to the mother justifies the potential risk to the fetus.

If eltrombopag is indicated, the maternal benefit appears to outweigh the unknown embryo-fetal risk, and the drug should not be withheld because of pregnancy.

Eltrombopag was administered orally to pregnant rats in an embryofetal development study at 10, 20, or 60 mg/kg/day (0.8, 2, and 7 times the human clinical exposure, respectively, based on AUC). Decreases in maternal body weight gain and food consumption occurred in the 60 mg/kg/day dosage group. At this maternally toxic dose, male and female fetal weights were significantly reduced (6% to 7%) and there was a slight increase in the presence of cervical ribs, a fetal variation.

In an early embryonic development study, female rats received eltrombopag at doses of 0.8, 2, and 7 times the human clinical exposure (based on AUC). Increased pre- and postimplantation loss and reduced fetal weight were observed at the highest dose that also caused maternal toxicity.

In an embryofetal development study, pregnant rats received eltrombopag at doses of 0.8, 2, and 7 times the human clinical exposure (based on AUC). Decreased fetal weights and a slight increase in the presence of cervical ribs were observed at the highest dose that also caused maternal toxicity. However, no evidence of major structural malformations was observed.

In an embryofetal development study in pregnant rabbits treated with oral eltrombopag doses of 0.1, 0.3, and 0.6 times the human clinical exposure (based on AUC) no evidence of fetotoxicity, embryolethality, or teratogenicity was observed.

In a pre- and postnatal developmental toxicity study in pregnant rats (F0), no adverse reactions on maternal reproductive function or on the development of the offspring (F1) were observed at doses up to 2 times the human clinical exposure (based on AUC). Eltrombopag was detected in the plasma of offspring (F1). The plasma concentrations in pups increased with dose (0.8 and 2 times the human clinical exposure based on AUC) following administration of drug to the F0 dams.

Pregnancy registry – A pregnancy registry has been established to collect information about the effects of eltrombopag during pregnancy. Health care providers are encouraged to register pregnant patients, or pregnant women may enroll themselves in the eltrombopag pregnancy registry by calling 1-888-825-5249.

➤*Lactation:* It is not known whether eltrombopag is excreted in human milk. The molecular weight (about 443 for the free acid) and the long elimination half-life suggest that the drug will be excreted into breast milk, but the high protein binding should limit the amount excreted. Because many drugs are excreted in human milk and because of the potential for serious adverse reactions in breast-feeding infants from eltrombopag, decide whether to discontinue breast-feeding or eltrombopag, taking into account the importance of eltrombopag to the mother and the known benefits of breast-feeding.

➤*Children:* The safety and efficacy of eltrombopag in children have not been established.

➤*Elderly:* In general, be cautious in dose adjustment for an elderly patient, reflecting the greater frequency of decreased hepatic, renal, or cardiac function, and of concomitant disease or other drug therapy.

➤*Monitoring:* Monitor CBCs, including platelet counts and peripheral blood smears, prior to initiation, throughout, and following discontinuation of therapy with eltrombopag. Prior to the initiation of eltrombopag, examine the peripheral blood differential to establish the extent of red and white blood cell abnormalities. Obtain CBCs, including platelet counts and peripheral blood smears, weekly during the dose adjustment phase of therapy with eltrombopag, and then monthly following establishment of a stable dose of eltrombopag. Obtain CBCs, including platelet counts, weekly for at least 4 weeks following discontinuation of eltrombopag.

Monitor serum liver tests (ALT, AST, and bilirubin) prior to initiation of eltrombopag, every 2 weeks during the dose adjustment phase and monthly following establishment of a stable dose. If bilirubin is elevated, perform fractionation. If abnormal levels are detected, repeat the tests within 3 to 5 days. If the abnormalities are confirmed, monitor serum liver tests weekly until the abnormality(ies) resolve, stabilize, or return to baseline levels. Discontinue eltrombopag for the development of important liver test abnormalities.

Perform a baseline ocular examination prior to administration of eltrombopag and, during therapy with eltrombopag, regularly monitor patients for signs and symptoms of cataracts.

Drug Interactions

Eltrombopag Drug Interactions

Precipitant drug	Object drug[a]		Description
CYP1A2 inhibitors (eg, ciprofloxacin, fluvoxamine)	Eltrombopag	⬆	In vitro studies demonstrate that CYP1A2 and CYP2C8 are involved in the oxidative metabolism of eltrombopag. Monitor patients for signs and symptoms of excessive eltrombopag exposure when eltrombopag is coadministered with these moderate or strong inhibitors of CYP1A2 or CYP2C8.
CYP2C8 inhibitors (eg, gemfibrozil, trimethoprim)	Eltrombopag	⬆	

ELTROMBOPAG OLAMINE — ORAL

Eltrombopag Drug Interactions			
Precipitant drug	Object drug[a]		Description
Polyvalent cations (eg, aluminum, calcium, iron, selenium, zinc)	Eltrombopag	↓	Eltrombopag chelates polyvalent cations in foods, mineral supplements, and antacids. Coadministration of eltrombopag with an antacid (eg, aluminum hydroxide, magnesium carbonate, sodium alginate) decreased plasma eltrombopag systemic exposure by 70%. Eltrombopag must not be taken within 4 hours of any medications containing polyvalent cations.
Eltrombopag	Acetaminophen, narcotics, nonsteroidal anti-inflammatory drugs	↑	Monitor patients closely for signs or symptoms of excessive exposure to these drugs when coadministered with eltrombopag.
Eltrombopag	OATP1B1 substrates (eg, atorvastatin, benzylpenicillin, fluvastatin, methotrexate, nateglinide, pravastatin, repaglinide, rifampin, rosuvastatin)	↑	Eltrombopag is an inhibitor of the organic anion transporting polypeptide OATP1B1 and can increase the systemic exposure of other drugs that are substrates of this transporter. In a clinical study of healthy adult subjects, administration of a single dose of rosuvastatin following repeated daily eltrombopag dosing increased plasma rosuvastatin $AUC_{0-\infty}$ by 55% and C_{max} by 103%. Use caution with coadministration. Monitor patients closely for signs and symptoms of excessive exposure to the drugs that are substrates of OATP1B1 and consider reduction of the dose of these drugs. In clinical trials with eltrombopag, a dose reduction of rosuvastatin by 50% was recommended for coadministration with eltrombopag.

[a] ↑ = object drug increased; ↓ = object drug decreased.

➤*Drug/Food interactions:* A standard high-fat breakfast significantly decreased plasma eltrombopag $AUC_{0-\infty}$ by approximately 59% and C_{max} by 65% and delayed T_{max} by 1 hour. The calcium content of this meal may have also contributed to this decrease in exposure.

Eltrombopag must not be taken within 4 hours of any medications or products containing polyvalent cations, such as dairy products, to avoid significant reduction in eltrombopag absorption due to chelation.

Adverse Reactions

In clinical studies, hemorrhage was the most common serious adverse reaction and most hemorrhagic reactions followed discontinuation of eltrombopag. Other serious adverse reactions included liver test abnormalities and thrombotic/thromboembolic complications.

Eltrombopag Adverse Reactions		
Adverse reactions	Eltrombopag 50 mg (n = 106)	Placebo (n = 67)
GI		
Dyspepsia	2%	0%
Nausea	6%	4%
Vomiting	4%	3%
Hematological/Lymphatic		
Ecchymosis	2%	1%
Thrombocytopenia	2%	0%
Hepatic		
Increased ALT	2%	0%
Increased AST	2%	0%
Special senses		
Cataract	3%	1%
Conjunctival hemorrhage	2%	1%
Miscellaneous		
Menorrhagia	4%	1%
Myalgia	3%	1%
Paresthesia	3%	1%

Overdosage

➤*Animal toxicology:* Eltrombopag is phototoxic and photoclastogenic in vitro. In vitro photoclastogenic effects were observed only at cytotoxic drug concentrations (15 mcg/mL or more) and at ultraviolet (UV) light exposure intensity (30 minimal erythematous dose [MED]). No evidence of in vitro photoclastogenicity was observed at higher drug concentrations (up to 58.4 mcg/mL) and UV light exposure of 15 MED. There was no evidence of in vivo cutaneous phototoxicity in mice, photo-ocular toxicity in rats, or photo-ocular toxicity in mice at exposures up to 11, 6, and 7 times the human clinical exposure based on the AUC, respectively.

Treatment-related cataracts were detected in rodents in a dose- and time-dependent manner. At 7 times or more the human clinical exposure based on AUC, cataracts were observed in mice after 6 weeks and in rats after 28 weeks of dosing. At 5 times or greater the human clinical exposure based on AUC, cataracts were observed in mice after 13 weeks and in rats after 39 weeks of dosing. Cataracts were not observed in dogs after 52 weeks of dosing (3 times the human clinical exposure based on AUC). The clinical relevance of these findings is unknown.

Renal tubular toxicity was observed in studies up to 14 days in duration in mice and rats at exposures that were generally associated with morbidity and mortality. Tubular toxicity was also observed in a 2-year oral carcinogenicity study in mice at dosages of 25, 75, and 150 mg/kg/day. The exposure at the lowest dose was 1.4 times the human clinical exposure based on AUC. No similar effects were observed after 13 weeks at exposures greater than those associated with renal changes in the 2-year study, suggesting that this effect is both dose- and time-dependent. Renal tubular toxicity was not observed in rats in a 2-year carcinogenicity study or in dogs after 52 weeks at exposures 5 and 3 times the human clinical exposure based on AUC, respectively.

Eltrombopag produced hepatocellular hypertrophy in mice (7 times the human clinical exposure based on AUC), rats (5 times the human clinical exposure based on AUC), rabbits (1.4 times the human clinical exposure based on AUC), and dogs (4 times the human clinical exposure based on AUC) and hepatocellular vacuolation in rats (2 times the human clinical exposure based on AUC).

➤*Symptoms:* In the event of overdose, platelet counts may increase excessively and result in thrombotic/thromboembolic complications. In 1 report, a subject ingested eltrombopag 5,000 mg and experienced rash, bradycardia, ALT/AST elevations, and fatigue.

➤*Treatment:* In case of an overdose, consider oral administration of a metal cation-containing preparation, such as calcium, aluminum, or magnesium preparations, to chelate eltrombopag and thus limit absorption. Closely monitor platelet counts. Reinitiate treatment with eltrombopag in accordance with dosing and administration recommendations.

In 1 report, a subject ingested 5,000 mg of eltrombopag and was treated with gastric lavage, oral lactulose, intravenous fluids, omeprazole, atropine, furosemide, calcium, dexamethasone, and plasmapheresis. The patient's platelet count increased to a maximum of 929×10^9/L at 13 days following the ingestion. The abnormal platelet count and liver test abnormalities persisted for 3 weeks. After 2 months follow-up, all events had resolved without sequelae.

Hemodialysis is not expected to enhance the elimination of eltrombopag because eltrombopag is not significantly renally excreted and is highly bound to plasma proteins.

Patient Information

Instruct patients to read the FDA-approved Medication Guide.

Prior to treatment, ensure that patients fully understand the risks and benefits of eltrombopag. Inform patients that the risks associated with long-term administration of eltrombopag are unknown and that they must enroll in PROMACTA CARES, which provides for the proper use of eltrombopag in ITP patients.

Inform patients of the following risks and considerations for eltrombopag:

- Therapy with eltrombopag is administered to achieve and maintain a platelet count of at least 50×10^9/L as necessary to reduce the risk for bleeding; eltrombopag is not used to normalize platelet counts.
- Therapy with eltrombopag may be associated with hepatobiliary laboratory abnormalities. Monitor serum liver tests (ALT, AST, and bilirubin) prior to initiation of eltrombopag, every 2 weeks during the dose adjustment phase, and monthly following establishment of a stable dose. If bilirubin is elevated, perform fractionation.
- Advise patients to report any of the following signs and symptoms of liver problems to their health care provider right away: yellowing of the skin or the whites of the eyes (jaundice), unusual darkening of the urine, unusual tiredness, right upper stomach area pain.
- Following discontinuation of eltrombopag, thrombocytopenia and risk of bleeding may develop that is worse than that experienced prior to therapy with eltrombopag, particularly if eltrombopag is discontinued while the patient is on anticoagulants or antiplatelet agents.
- Therapy with eltrombopag increases the risk of reticulin fiber formation within the bone marrow, and further fiber formation may progress to marrow fibrosis. Detection of peripheral blood cell abnormalities may necessitate a bone marrow examination.
- Too much eltrombopag may result in excessive platelet counts and a risk for thrombotic/thromboembolic complications.
- Eltrombopag stimulates certain bone marrow cells to make platelets and may increase the risk for progression of underlying myelodysplastic syndromes or hematological malignancies.

Thrombopoietin Receptor Agonist

ELTROMBOPAG OLAMINE — ORAL

- Platelet counts and CBCs, including peripheral blood smears, must be performed weekly until a stable dose of eltrombopag has been achieved; thereafter, platelet counts and CBCs, including peripheral blood smears, must be performed monthly while taking eltrombopag.
- Patients must be closely monitored with weekly platelet counts and CBCs for at least 4 weeks following discontinuation of eltrombopag.
- Even during therapy with eltrombopag, advise patients to continue to avoid situations or medications that may increase the risk for bleeding.
- Patients must be advised to keep at least a 4 hour interval between eltrombopag and foods, mineral supplements, and antacids which contain polyvalent cations, such as iron, calcium, aluminum, magnesium, selenium, and zinc.

ANTIPLATELET AGENTS

Aggregation Inhibitors

CILOSTAZOL

Rx	**Cilostazol** (Various, eg, Andrx, Teva)	**Tablets**: 50 mg	In 60s.
Rx	**Pletal** (Otsuka America Pharmaceuticals)		(PLETAL 50). White, triangular. In 60s
Rx	**Cilostazol** (Various, eg, Andrx, Eon, Teva)	**Tablets**: 100 mg	In 60s and 500s.

CILOSTAZOL — ORAL

WARNING

Cilostazol and several of its metabolites are inhibitors of phosphodiesterase (PDE) 3. Several drugs with this pharmacologic effect have caused decreased survival compared with placebo in patients with class III to IV congestive heart failure. Cilostazol is contraindicated in patients with congestive heart failure of any severity.

Indications

➤*Intermittent claudication:* For the reduction of symptoms of intermittent claudication, as indicated by an increased walking distance.

Administration and Dosage

➤*Adults:*

Intermittent claudication –

Usual dosage: 100 mg twice daily taken at least 30 minutes before or 2 hours after breakfast and dinner.

Duration of therapy: Patients may respond as early as 2 to 4 weeks after the initiation of therapy, but treatment for up to 12 weeks may be needed before a beneficial effect is experienced.

Concomitant therapy: A dosage of 50 mg twice daily should be considered during coadministration of CYP3A4 inhibitors (eg, diltiazem, erythromycin, itraconazole, ketoconazole) and during coadministration of CYP2C19 inhibitors (eg, omeprazole).

Discontinuation of therapy: The available data suggest that the dosage of cilostazol can be reduced or discontinued without rebound (ie, platelet hyperaggregability).

➤*Storage/Stability:* Store cilostazol tablets at 25°C (77°F); excursions are permitted to between 15° and 30°C (59° and 86°F).

Actions

➤*Pharmacology:* The mechanism of the effects of cilostazol on the symptoms of intermittent claudication is not fully understood. Cilostazol and several of its metabolites are cyclic adenosine monophosphate (cAMP) PDE 3 inhibitors, inhibiting PDE activity and suppressing cAMP degradation with a resultant increase in cAMP in platelets and blood vessels, leading to inhibition of platelet aggregation and vasodilation, respectively.

Cilostazol reversibly inhibits platelet aggregation induced by a variety of stimuli, including thrombin, adenosine diphosphate (ADP), collagen, arachidonic acid, epinephrine, and shear stress. Effects on circulating plasma lipids have been examined in patients taking cilostazol. After 12 weeks, as compared with placebo, cilostazol 100 mg twice daily produced a reduction in triglycerides of 29.3 mg/dL (15%) and an increase in high-density lipoprotein cholesterol of 4 mg/dL (approximately 10%).

Cilostazol affects both vascular beds and cardiovascular function. It produces nonhomogeneous dilation of vascular beds, with greater dilation in femoral beds than in vertebral, carotid, or superior mesenteric arteries. Renal arteries were not responsive to the effects of cilostazol.

In dogs or cynomolgous monkeys, cilostazol increased heart rate, myocardial contractile force, and coronary blood flow as well as ventricular automaticity, as would be expected for a PDE 3 inhibitor. Left ventricular contractility was increased at doses required to inhibit platelet aggregation. Atrio ventricular conduction was accelerated. In humans, heart rate increased in a dose-proportional manner by a mean of 5.1 and 7.4 beats per minute in patients treated with 50 and 100 mg twice daily, respectively. In 264 patients evaluated with Holter monitors, numerically more cilostazol-treated patients had increases in ventricular premature beats and nonsustained ventricular tachycardia events than did placebo-treated patients; the increases were not dose-related.

➤*Pharmacokinetics:*

Absorption – Cilostazol is absorbed after oral administration. A high-fat meal increases absorption, with an approximately 90% increase in a maximum plasma concentration (C_{max}) and a 25% increase in the area under the plasma concentration-time curve (AUC). Absolute bioavailability is not known.

Distribution – Cilostazol is 95% to 98% protein bound, predominantly to albumin. The mean percent binding for 3,4-dehydro–cilostazol is 97.4% and for 4'-trans-hydroxy–cilostazol is 66%.

Metabolism/Excretion – Cilostazol is extensively metabolized by hepatic cytochrome P-450 enzymes, mainly 3A4, and, to a lesser extent, 2C19, with metabolites largely excreted in urine. Two metabolites are active, with 1 metabolite (3,4-dehydro–cilostazol) appearing to account for at least 50% of the pharmacologic (PDE 3 inhibition) activity after administration of cilostazol. Pharmacokinetics are approximately dose proportional. Cilostazol and its active metabolites have apparent elimination half-lives of about 11 to 13 hours. Cilostazol and its active metabolites accumulate about 2-fold with chronic administration and reach steady-state blood levels within a few days.

Following oral administration of radio-labeled cilostazol 100 mg, 56% of the total analytes in plasma was cilostazol, 15% was 3,4-dehydro–cilostazol (4 to 7 times as active as cilostazol), and 4% was 4'-trans-hydroxy-cilostazol (one fifth as active as cilostazol). The primary route of elimination was via the urine (74%), with the remainder excreted in the feces (20%). No measurable amount of unchanged cilostazol was excreted in the urine, and less than 2% of the dose was excreted as 3,4-dehydro–cilostazol. About 30% of the dose was excreted in the urine as 4'-trans-hydroxy–cilostazol. The remainder was excreted as other metabolites, none of which exceeded 5%. There was no evidence of induction of hepatic microenzymes.

Special populations –

Renal function impairment: The free fraction of cilostazol was 27% higher in subjects with renal function impairment than in healthy volunteers. The total pharmacologic activity of cilostazol and its metabolites was similar in subjects with mild to moderate renal impairment and in healthy subjects. Severe renal function impairment increases metabolite levels and alters protein binding of the parent and metabolites. The expected pharmacologic activity, based on plasma concentrations and relative to PDE 3 inhibiting potency of parent drug and metabolites, appeared little changed.

Patients on dialysis have not been studied, but it is unlikely that cilostazol can be removed efficiently by dialysis because of its high protein binding (95% to 98%).

Special caution is advised when cilostazol is used in patients with severe renal function impairment: (estimated creatine clearance less than 25 mL/min).

Smokers: Population pharmacokinetic analysis suggests that smoking decreased cilostazol exposure by about 20%.

Patients with intermittent claudication due to peripheral arterial disease (PAD): The pharmacokinetics of cilostazol and its 2 major active metabolites were similar in healthy subjects and patients with intermittent claudication due to PAD.

Contraindications

➤*Congestive heart failure:* Cilostazol and several of its metabolites are inhibitors of PDE 3. Several drugs with this pharmacologic effect have caused decreased survival compared with placebo in patients with class III to IV congestive heart failure. Cilostazol is contraindicated with patients with congestive heart failure of any severity.

➤*Other contraindications:* In patients with hemostatic disorders or active pathologic bleeding, such as bleeding peptic ulcer and intracranial bleeding. Cilostazol inhibits platelet aggregation in a reversible manner, and in patients with known or suspected hypersensitivity to any of its components.

Warnings/Precautions

➤*Congestive heart failure:* Cilostazol is contraindicated in patients with congestive heart failure. In patients without congestive heart failure, the long-term effects of PDE 3 inhibitors (including cilostazol) are unknown. Patients in the 3- to 6-month placebo-controlled trials of cilostazol were relatively stable (no recent myocardial infarction or strokes, no rest pain or other signs of rapidly progressing disease), and only 19 patients died (0.7% in the placebo group and 0.8% in the cilostazol group). The calculated relative risk of death of 1.2 has a wide 95% confidence limit (0.5 to 3.1). There are no data as to longer-term risk or risk in patients with more severe underlying heart disease.

➤*Hematologic effects:* Rare cases of thrombocytopenia or leukopenia progressing to agranulocytosis have been reported when cilostazol was not immediately discontinued. The agranulocytosis, however, was reversible on discontinuation of cilostazol.

➤*Pregnancy: Category C.* In a rat developmental toxicity study, oral administration of cilostazol 1,000 mg/kg/day was associated with decreased fetal weights and increased incidences of cardiovascular, renal, and skeletal anomalies (eg, ventricular septal, aortic arch, and subclavian artery abnor-

CILOSTAZOL — ORAL

malities; renal pelvic dilation; 14th rib; retarded ossification). At this dose, systemic exposure to unbound cilostazol in nonpregnant rats was about 5 times the exposure in humans given the MRHD. Increased incidences of ventricular septal defect and retarded ossification were also noted at 150 mg/kg/day (5 times the MRHD on a systemic exposure basis). In a rabbit developmental toxicity study, an increased incidence of retardation of ossification of the sternum was seen at dosages as low as 150 mg/kg/day. In nonpregnant rabbits given 150 mg/kg/day, exposure to unbound cilostazol was considerably lower than that seen in humans given the MRHD, and exposure to 3,4-dehydro–cilostazol was barely detectable.

When cilostazol was administered to rats during late pregnancy and lactation, an increased incidence of stillbirth and decreased birth weights of offspring was seen at dosages of 150 mg/kg/day (5 times the MRHD on a systemic exposure basis).

There are no adequate and well-controlled studies in pregnant women.

➤*Lactation:* Transfer of cilostazol into milk has been reported in experimental animals (rats). Because of the potential risk to breast-feeding infants, decide whether to discontinue breast-feeding or cilostazol.

➤*Children:* The safety and efficacy of cilostazol in children have not been established.

➤*Elderly:* Of the total number of subjects (N = 2,274) in clinical studies of cilostazol, 56% were 65 years of age and older, while 16% were 75 years of age and older.

Drug Interactions

Cilostazol Drug Interactions

Precipitant drug	Object drug[a]		Description
Clopidogrel	Cilostazol	↑	Additive effects on bleeding times not determined. Monitor bleeding times during coadministration.
CYP3A4 inhibitors (eg, erythromycin, ketoconazole)	Cilostazol	↑	Concurrent use may increase the systemic exposure of cilostazol and/or its major metabolites. Consider a reduced dose of cilostazol.
CYP2C19 (eg, omeprazole)	Cilostazol	↑	Concurrent use may increase the systemic exposure of cilostazol and/or its major metabolites. Consider a reduced dose of cilostazol.
Diltiazem	Cilostazol	↑	Diltiazem 180 mg decreased the clearance of cilostazol by approximately 30% and increased the C_{max} and AUC approximately 30% and 40%, respectively.
Aspirin	Cilostazol	↑	Coadministration of aspirin with cilostazol increased the inhibition of platelet aggregation compared to either product alone. Coadministration had no clinically significant impact on PT, aPTT, or bleeding time.
Cilostazol	Aspirin		
Lovastatin	Cilostazol	↓	The coadministration of lovastatin with cilostazol decreased cilostazol $C_{ss, max}$ and AUC by 15%. There is also a decrease, although nonsignificant, in cilostazol metabolite concentrations. Coadministration increases lovastatin AUC by approximately 70%.
Cilostazol	Lovastatin	↑	

[a] ↑ = Object drug increased; ↓ = Object drug decreased.

➤*Drug/Food interactions:* Grapefruit juice increased the C_{max} of cilostazol by approximately 50%, but had no effect on AUC. A high-fat meal increases absorption with an approximately 90% increase in C_{max} and a 25% increase in the AUC.

Adverse Reactions

Adverse reactions were assessed in 8 placebo-controlled clinical trials involving 2,274 patients exposed to either 50 or 100 mg of cilostazol twice daily (n = 1,301) or placebo (n = 973), with a median treatment duration of 127 days for patients on cilostazol and 134 days for patients on placebo.

The only adverse reaction resulting in discontinuation of therapy in greater than or equal to 3% of patients treated with cilostazol 50 or 100 mg twice daily was headache, which occurred with an incidence of 1.3%, 3.5%, and 0.3% in patients treated with cilostazol 50 mg twice daily, 100 mg twice daily, or placebo, respectively. Other frequent causes of discontinuation included palpitation and diarrhea, both 1.1% for cilostazol (all doses) versus 0.1% for placebo.

Cilostazol Adverse Reactions (≥2%)

Adverse reaction	Cilostazol 50 mg twice daily (n = 303)	Cilostazol 100 mg twice daily (n = 998)	Placebo (n = 973)
Cardiovascular			
Palpitation	5%	10%	1%
Tachycardia	4%	4%	1%
CNS			
Dizziness	9%	10%	6%
Headache	27%	34%	14%
Vertigo	3%	1%	1%
GI			
Abdominal pain	4%	5%	3%
Abnormal stools	12%	15%	4%
Diarrhea	12%	19%	7%
Dyspepsia	6%	6%	4%
Flatulence	2%	3%	2%
Nausea	6%	7%	6%
Metabolic/Nutritional			
Peripheral edema	9%	7%	4%
Musculoskeletal			
Back pain	6%	7%	6%
Myalgia	2%	3%	2%
Respiratory			
Cough increased	3%	4%	3%
Pharyngitis	7%	10%	7%
Rhinitis	12%	7%	5%
Miscellaneous			
Infection	14%	10%	8%

➤*Other Adverse Reactions:* Other adverse reactions seen with an incidence of greater than or equal to 2%, but occurring in the placebo group at least as frequently as in the 100 mg twice-daily group, were as follows:

Cardiovascular – Angina pectoris, hypertension.

CNS – Hypesthesia, paresthesia.

Dermatologic – Rash.

GI – Vomiting.

GU – Hematuria, urinary tract infection.

Respiratory – Bronchitis, dyspnea.

Miscellaneous – Arthritis, asthenia, flu syndrome, leg cramps. Less frequent adverse reactions (less than 2%) that were experienced by patients exposed to cilostazol 50 or 100 mg twice daily in the 8 controlled clinical trials, and that occurred at a greater frequency in the 100 mg twice-daily group than in the placebo group, regardless of suspected drug relationship, were as follows:

➤*Cardiovascular:* Atrial fibrillation, atrial flutter, cerebral infarct, cerebral ischemia, congestive heart failure, heart arrest, hemorrhage, hypotension, myocardial infarction, myocardial ischemia, nodal arrhythmia, postural hypotension, supraventricular tachycardia, syncope, varicose vein, vasodilation, ventricular extrasystoles, ventricular tachycardia.

➤*CNS:* Anxiety, insomnia, malaise, neuralgia.

➤*Dermatologic:* Dry skin, furunculosis, skin hypertrophy, urticaria.

➤*Endocrine:* Diabetes mellitus.

➤*GI:* Anorexia, cholelithiasis, colitis, duodenal ulcer, duodenitis, esophageal hemorrhage, esophagitis, gastritis, gastroenteritis, gum hemorrhage, hematemesis, increased gamma-glutamyltransferase, melena, peptic ulcer, periodontal abscess, rectal hemorrhage, stomach ulcer, tongue edema.

➤*GU:* Albuminuria, cystitis, urinary frequency, vaginal hemorrhage, vaginitis.

➤*Hematologic/Lymphatic:* Anemia, ecchymosis, iron deficiency anemia, polycythemia, purpura.

➤*Metabolic/Nutritional:* Gout, hyperlipemia, hyperuricemia, increased creatinine.

➤*Musculoskeletal:* Arthralgia, bone pain, bursitis, neck rigidity.

➤*Respiratory:* Asthma, epistaxis, hemoptysis, pneumonia, sinusitis.

➤*Special senses:* Amblyopia, blindness, conjunctivitis, diplopia, ear pain, eye hemorrhage, retinal hemorrhage, tinnitus.

➤*Miscellaneous:* Chills, face edema, fever, generalized edema, pelvic pain, retroperitoneal hemorrhage.

➤*Postmarketing:* The following events have been reported spontaneously from worldwide postmarketing experience since the launch of cilostazol in the United States.

CILOSTAZOL — ORAL

Cardiovascular – Subacute thrombosis. (These cases of subacute thrombosis occurred in patients treated with aspirin and "off-label" use of cilostazol for prevention of thrombotic complication after coronary stenting.)

Torsades de pointes, QTc prolongation. (Torsades de pointes and QTc prolongation occurred in patients with cardiac disorders [eg, complete atrioventricular block, cardiac failure, bradycardia] when treated with cilostazol. Cilostazol was used "off label" because of its positive chronotropic action.)

CNS – Cerebral hemorrhage, cerebrovascular accident, intracranial hemorrhage.

Dermatologic – Hemorrhage subcutaneous; pruritus; skin eruptions including, skin drug eruption (dermatitis medicamentosa), Stevens-Johnson syndrome.

GI – GI hemorrhage.

Hematologic/Lymphatic – Agranulocytosis, bleeding tendency, granulocytopenia, leukopenia, platelet count decreased, thrombocytopenia, white blood cell count decreased.

Hepatic – Hepatic dysfunction/abnormal liver function tests, jaundice.

Lab test abnormalities – Blood glucose increased, blood uric acid increased, increase in serum urea nitrogen (BUN) abnormalities (serum urea increased).

Respiratory – Interstitial pneumonia, pulmonary hemorrhage.

Miscellaneous – Chest pain, extradural hematoma, hot flashes, subdural hematoma pain.

Overdosage

➤*Symptoms:* Information on acute overdosage with cilostazol in humans is limited. The signs and symptoms of an acute overdose can be anticipated to be those of excessive pharmacologic effect, including the following: severe headache, diarrhea, hypotension, tachycardia, and possibly cardiac arrhythmias.

The oral median lethal dose of cilostazol is greater than 5 g/kg in mice and rats and greater than 2 g/kg in dogs.

Animal toxicity – Repeated oral administration of cilostazol to dogs (greater than or equal to 30 mg/kg/day for 52 weeks, greater than or equal to 150 mg/kg/day for 13 weeks, and 450 mg/kg/day for 2 weeks) produced cardiovascular lesions that included endocardial hemorrhage, hemosiderin deposition and fibrosis in the left ventricle, hemorrhage in the right atrial wall, hemorrhage and necrosis of the smooth muscle in the wall of the coronary artery, intimal thickening of the coronary artery, and coronary arteritis and periarteritis. At the lowest dose associated with cardiovascular lesions in the 52-week study, systemic exposure (AUC) to unbound cilostazol was less than that seen in humans at the MRHD of 100 mg twice daily. Similar lesions have been reported in dogs following the administration of other positive inotropic agents (including PDE 3 inhibitors) or vasodilation agents. No cardiovascular lesions were seen in rats following 5 or 13 weeks of administration of cilostazol at dosages up to 1,500 mg/kg/day. At this dose, systemic exposures (AUCs) to unbound cilostazol were only about 1.5 and 5 times (male and female rats, respectively) the exposure seen in humans at the MRHD. Cardiovascular lesions were also not seen in rats following 52 weeks of administration of cilostazol at dosages up to 150 mg/kg/day. At this dose, systemic exposures (AUCs) to unbound cilostazol were about 0.5 and 5 times (male and female rats, respectively) the exposure in humans at the MRHD. In female rats, cilostazol AUCs were similar at 150 and 1,500 mg/kg/day. Cardiovascular lesions were also not observed in monkeys after oral administration of cilostazol for 13 weeks at dosages up to 1,800 mg/kg/day. While this dose of cilostazol produced pharmacologic effects in monkeys, plasma cilostazol levels were less than those seen in humans given the MRHD and those seen in dogs given doses associated with cardiovascular lesions.

➤*Treatment:* Carefully observe the patient and provide supportive treatment. Since cilostazol is highly protein bound, it is unlikely that it can be efficiently removed by hemodialysis or peritoneal dialysis.

Patient Information

Advise patients to read the package information for cilostazol carefully before starting therapy and to reread it each time therapy is renewed in case the information has changed.

Advise patients to take cilostazol at least 30 minutes before or 2 hours after food.

Inform patients that the beneficial effects of cilostazol on the symptoms of intermittent claudication may not be immediate. Although the patient may experience benefits in 2 to 4 weeks after initiation of therapy; however, treatment for up to 12 weeks may be required before a beneficial effect is experienced.

Inform patients about the uncertainty concerning cardiovascular risk in long-term use or in patients with severe underlying heart disease.

CLOPIDOGREL

Rx	**Plavix** (Bristol-Myers Squibb)	**Tablets; oral:** 75 mg	Equivalent to clopidogrel bisulfate 97.875 mg. Castor oil, mannitol, PEG-6000. (75 1171). Pink, round. Film-coated. In 30s, 90s, 500s, and UD 100s.
		300 mg	Equivalent to clopidogrel bisulfate 391.5 mg. Castor oil, mannitol, PEG-6000. (300 1332). Pink, oblong. Film-coated. In UD 30s.

CLOPIDOGREL BISULFATE — ORAL

WARNING

Diminished effectiveness in poor metabolizers – The effectiveness of clopidogrel is dependent on its activation to an active metabolite by the cytochrome P450 (CYP-450) system, principally CYP2C19. Poor metabolizers treated with clopidogrel at recommended doses exhibit higher cardiovascular event rates following acute coronary syndrome or percutaneous coronary intervention (PCI) than patients with normal CYP2C19 function. Tests are available to identify a patient's CYP2C19 genotype and can be used as an aid in determining therapeutic strategy. Consider alternative treatment or treatment strategies in patients identified as CYP2C19 poor metabolizers.

Indications

➤*Acute coronary syndrome:*

Unstable angina/non–ST-segment elevation myocardial infarction – For patients with non–ST-segment elevation acute coronary syndrome (unstable angina/non–ST-elevation myocardial infarction [MI]), including patients who are to be managed medically and those who are to be managed with coronary revascularization, clopidogrel has been shown to decrease the rate of a combined end point of cardiovascular death, MI, or stroke, as well as the rate of a combined end point of cardiovascular death, MI, stroke, or refractory ischemia.

ST-segment elevation acute myocardial infarction – For patients with ST-elevation MI, clopidogrel has been shown to reduce the rate of death from any cause and the rate of a combined end point of death, reinfarction, or stroke. The benefit for patients who undergo primary percutaneous coronary intervention is unknown.

➤*Recent myocardial infarction, recent stroke, or established peripheral arterial disease:* For patients with a history of recent MI, recent stroke, or established peripheral arterial disease, clopidogrel has been shown to reduce the rate of a combined end point of new ischemic stroke (fatal or not), new MI (fatal or not), and other vascular death.

➤*Off-label uses:*

Loading dose regimen in patients undergoing coronary stent placement – [1] = Good documentation. Although there appears to be a clear benefit of using a loading dose regimen of clopidogrel with aspirin to prevent cardiac adverse events in patients who have received coronary stent implantation, the optimal loading dose and administration timing have yet to be defined. (See Administration and Dosage.)

Other possible off-label uses – In a small study, clopidogrel was effective for the treatment of arterial ischemic stroke in children. Clopidogrel was also an effective antiplatelet therapy in children with a cardiac condition and at risk for arterial thrombosis (ie, a systemic to pulmonary artery shunt or another cardiac condition with a risk for arterial thrombosis, including a stent placement).

Administration and Dosage

➤*Adults:*

Acute coronary syndrome –

Non–ST-elevation myocardial infarction:

- *Initial dosage* – A single 300 mg loading dose.
- *Maintenance dosage* – 75 mg once daily.
- *Concomitant therapy* – Aspirin 75 to 325 mg once daily.

ST-elevation myocardial infarction:

- *Usual dosage* – 75 mg once daily. Clopidogrel may be initiated with or without a loading dose.
- *Concomitant therapy* – Administer in combination with aspirin 75 to 325 mg once daily, with or without thrombolytics.

Recent myocardial infarction, recent stroke, or established peripheral arterial disease – 75 mg once daily.

Off-label dosing –

Loading dose regimen in patients undergoing coronary stent placement: Loading doses range from 150 to 600 mg, followed by daily dosing of 75 or 150 mg. In all studies evaluating clinical outcomes of post-stent implementation, loading doses have been either 150 or 300 mg, followed by 75 mg daily. Loading doses have been administered from 3 to 24 hours preprocedure or within 24 hours postprocedure.

➤*Children:*

Off-label dosing –

Arterial ischemic stroke:

- *1 month of age and older* – 1 mg/kg/day (up to 75 mg) was the dose studied in a small prospective clinical trial in children (mean, 8.8 years of age). The risk of intracranial bleeding is increased when given concomitantly with aspirin.

CLOPIDOGREL BISULFATE — ORAL

Cardiac condition at risk for arterial thrombosis:

• *24 months of age and younger* – 0.2 mg/kg/day was found to be an effective dose to achieve platelet inhibition in children with a cardiac condition and at risk for arterial thrombosis (ie, a systemic to pulmonary artery shunt or another cardiac condition with a risk for arterial thrombosis, including a stent placement).

➤*Elderly:* See Adults for dosing.

➤*CYP2C19 poor metabolizers:* CYP2C19 poor metabolizer status is associated with diminished antiplatelet response to clopidogrel. Although a higher dose regimen (600 mg loading dose followed by 150 mg once daily) in poor metabolizers increases antiplatelet response, an appropriate dose regimen for this patient population has not been established in clinical outcome trials.

➤*Discontinuation of therapy:* If a patient is to undergo surgery and an antiplatelet effect is not desired, discontinue clopidogrel 5 days prior to surgery.

Avoid lapses in therapy, and if clopidogrel must be temporarily discontinued, restart as soon as possible. Premature discontinuation of clopidogrel may increase the risk of cardiovascular events.

➤*Administration:* Administer with or without food.

➤*Storage/Stability:* Store at 25°C (77°F); excursions are permitted between 15° and 30°C (59° and 86°F).

Actions

➤*Pharmacology:* Clopidogrel is an inhibitor of platelet activation and aggregation through the irreversible binding of its active metabolite to the $P2Y_{12}$ class of adenosine diphosphate (ADP) receptors on platelets.

Clopidogrel must be metabolized by CYP-450 enzymes to produce the active metabolite that inhibits platelet aggregation. The active metabolite of clopidogrel selectively inhibits the binding of ADP to its platelet $P2Y_{12}$ receptor and the subsequent ADP-mediated activation of the glycoprotein IIb/IIIa complex, thereby inhibiting platelet aggregation. This action is irreversible. Consequently, platelets exposed to clopidogrel's active metabolite are affected for the remainder of their lifespan (approximately 7 to 10 days). Platelet aggregation induced by agonists other than ADP is also inhibited by blocking the amplification of platelet activation by released ADP.

Pharmacodynamics – Dose-dependent inhibition of platelet aggregation can be seen 2 hours after single oral doses of clopidogrel. Repeated dosages of clopidogrel 75 mg/day inhibit ADP-induced platelet aggregation on the first day, and inhibition reaches steady state between day 3 and day 7. At steady state, the average inhibition level observed with a dosage of clopidogrel 75 mg/day was between 40% and 60%. Platelet aggregation and bleeding time gradually return to baseline values after treatment is discontinued, generally in about 5 days.

➤*Pharmacokinetics:*

Absorption/Distribution – After single and repeated oral dosages of 75 mg/day, clopidogrel is rapidly absorbed. Absorption is at least 50%, based on urinary excretion of clopidogrel metabolites.

Effect of food: Clopidogrel can be administered with or without food. In a study in healthy male subjects when clopidogrel 75 mg/day was given with a standard breakfast, mean inhibition of ADP-induced platelet aggregation was reduced by less than 9%. The active metabolite area under the curve (AUC_{0-24}) was unchanged in the presence of food, while there was a 57% decrease in active metabolite maximum concentration (C_{max}). Similar results were observed when a clopidogrel 300 mg loading dose was administered with a high-fat breakfast.

Metabolism/Excretion – Clopidogrel is a prodrug and is metabolized to a pharmacologically active metabolite and inactive metabolites.

Clopidogrel is extensively metabolized by 2 main metabolic pathways: one mediated by esterases and leading to hydrolysis into an inactive carboxylic acid derivative (85% of circulating metabolites) and one mediated by multiple CYP-450 enzymes. Cytochromes first oxidize clopidogrel to a 2-oxo-clopidogrel intermediate metabolite. Subsequent metabolism of the 2-oxo-clopidogrel intermediate metabolite results in formation of the active metabolite, a thiol derivative of clopidogrel. This metabolic pathway is mediated by CYP2C19, CYP3A, CYP2B6, and CYP1A2. The active thiol metabolite binds rapidly and irreversibly to platelet receptors, thus inhibiting platelet aggregation for the lifespan of the platelet.

The C_{max} of the active metabolite is twice as high following a single clopidogrel 300 mg loading dose as it is after 4 days of a 75 mg maintenance dose. C_{max} occurs approximately 30 to 60 minutes after dosing. In the 75 to 300 mg dose range, the pharmacokinetics of the active metabolite deviates from dose proportionality, increasing the dose by a factor of 4 results in 2- and 2.7-fold increases in C_{max} and AUC, respectively.

Following an oral dose of ^{14}C-labeled clopidogrel in humans, approximately 50% of total radioactivity was excreted in urine and approximately 46% in feces over 5 days postdosing. After a single oral dose of 75 mg, clopidogrel has a half-life of approximately 6 hours. The half-life of the active metabolite is approximately 30 minutes.

Special populations –

Renal function impairment: After repeated dosages of clopidogrel 75 mg/day, patients with severe (creatinine clearance [CrCl] from 5 to 15 mL/min) and moderate (CrCl from 30 to 60 mL/min) renal impairment showed low (25%) inhibition of ADP-induced platelet aggregation.

Hepatic function impairment: After repeated dosages of clopidogrel 75 mg/day for 10 days in patients with severe hepatic impairment, inhibition of ADP-induced platelet aggregation was similar to that observed in healthy subjects.

Elderly: Patients 75 years of age and older and younger healthy patients had similar effects on platelet aggregation.

Gender: In a small study comparing men and women, less inhibition of ADP-induced platelet aggregation was observed in women.

CYP2C19 poor metabolizers: CYP2C19 is involved in the formation of the active metabolite and the 2-oxo-clopidogrel intermediate metabolite. Clopidogrel active metabolite pharmacokinetics and antiplatelet effects, as measured by ex vivo platelet aggregation assays, differ according to CYP2C19 genotype. Genetic variants of other CYP-450 enzymes may also affect the formation of clopidogrel's active metabolite.

Contraindications

Hypersensitivity (eg, anaphylaxis) to the drug or any component of the product; active pathological bleeding, such as peptic ulcer or intracranial hemorrhage.

Warnings/Precautions

➤*CYP2C19 poor metabolizers:* Clopidogrel is a prodrug. Inhibition of platelet aggregation by clopidogrel is entirely caused by an active metabolite. The metabolism of clopidogrel to its active metabolite can be impaired by genetic variations in CYP2C19 and by concomitant medications that interfere with CYP2C19. Avoid concomitant use of clopidogrel and drugs that inhibit CYP2C19 activity.

➤*Risk of bleeding:* Thienopyridines, including clopidogrel, increase the risk of bleeding. If a patient is to undergo surgery and an antiplatelet effect is not desired, discontinue clopidogrel 5 days prior to surgery. In patients who stopped therapy more than 5 days prior to coronary artery bypass graft (CABG), the rates of major bleeding were similar (event rate, 4.4% clopidogrel plus aspirin; 5.3% placebo plus aspirin). In patients who remained on therapy within 5 days of CABG, the major bleeding rate was 9.6% for clopidogrel plus aspirin and 6.3% for placebo plus aspirin.

Thienopyridines inhibit platelet aggregation for the lifetime of the platelet (7 to 10 days); therefore, withholding a dose will not be useful in managing a bleeding event or the risk of bleeding associated with an invasive procedure. Because the half-life of clopidogrel's active metabolite is short, it may be possible to restore hemostasis by administering exogenous platelets; however, platelet transfusions within 4 hours of the loading dose or 2 hours of the maintenance dose may be less effective.

➤*Ischemic events:* In patients with recent transient ischemic attack (TIA) or stroke who are at high risk for recurrent ischemic reactions, the combination of aspirin and clopidogrel has not been shown to be more effective than clopidogrel alone, but the combination has been shown to increase major bleeding.

➤*Thrombotic thrombocytopenic purpura:* Thrombotic thrombocytopenic purpura, sometimes fatal, has been reported following use of clopidogrel, sometimes after a short exposure (less than 2 weeks). Thrombotic thrombocytopenic purpura is a serious condition that can be fatal and requires urgent treatment, including plasmapheresis (plasma exchange). It is characterized by thrombocytopenia, microangiopathic hemolytic anemia (schistocytes [fragmented red blood cells] seen on peripheral smear), neurological findings, renal impairment, and fever.

➤*Renal function impairment:* Experience is limited in patients with moderate and severe renal impairment.

➤*Hepatic function impairment:* No dosage adjustment is necessary in patients with hepatic impairment.

➤*Pregnancy:* *Category B.* It is not known if the inactive parent drug or its active or inactive metabolites cross the placenta, though the relatively low molecular weight suggests that some passage should be expected. This lack of human information prevents an accurate assessment, but the known benefits to a woman appear to outweigh the unknown fetal risks. Therefore, if a patient's condition requires clopidogrel, the treatment should not be withheld because of pregnancy.

There are, however, no adequate and well-controlled studies in pregnant women. Because animal reproduction studies are not always predictive of a human response, use clopidogrel during pregnancy only if clearly needed.

Reproduction studies performed in rats and rabbits at dosages of up to 500 and 300 mg/kg/day (65 and 78 times, respectively, the recommended daily human dose on an mg/m^2 basis) revealed no evidence of impaired fertility or fetotoxicity as a result of clopidogrel.

➤*Lactation:* Studies in rats have shown that clopidogrel and/or its metabolites are excreted in milk. The molecular weight of the inactive parent drug (approximately 420 for the bisulfate) suggests that some drug is excreted into breast milk. The effect of this possible exposure on a breast-feeding infant is unknown. Because many drugs are excreted in human milk and because of the potential for serious adverse reactions in breast-feeding infants, decide whether to discontinue breast-feeding or the drug, taking into account the importance of the drug to the mother.

➤*Children:* Safety and efficacy in children have not been established.

➤*Monitoring:* Because of the risk of bleeding and undesirable hematological effects, promptly consider blood cell count determination and/or other appropriate testing whenever such suspected clinical symptoms arise during the course of treatment.

Drug Interactions

➤*CYP-450 system:* Clopidogrel is metabolized to its active metabolite in part by CYP2C19. Concurrent use of drugs that inhibit the activity of this enzyme reduce plasma concentrations of the active metabolite of clopidogrel and reduce platelet inhibition. Avoid drugs that inhibit CYP2C19 (eg, omeprazole).

CLOPIDOGREL BISULFATE — ORAL

➤*Proton pump inhibitors (eg, omeprazole):* The American College of Cardiology, the American College of Gastroenterology, and the American Heart Association recommend the use of proton pump inhibitors (PPIs) to reduce the risk of GI bleeding in patients who are at high risk for GI bleeding and are receiving antiplatelet therapy. Patients at high risk for GI bleeding are defined as those with a history of GI bleeding; advanced age; concurrent use of anticoagulants, steroids, or NSAIDs, including aspirin; and those with *Helicobacter pylori* infection. However, patients who are not at high risk for bleeding achieve little benefit from concurrent use of a PPI with clopidogrel. If a PPI is needed in a patient at lower risk for GI bleeding, a drug that is not a strong or moderate CYP2C19 inhibitor, such as pantoprazole, should be considered, because omeprazole may interfere with the metabolic (CYP2D19) conversion of clopidogrel to its active metabolite. There are conflicting data on the clinical impact of concurrent use of clopidogrel and PPIs. However, the prescribing information recommends against concurrent use of omeprazole and clopidogrel.

Clopidogrel Drug Interactions

Precipitant drug	Object drug[a]		Description
Aspirin	Clopidogrel	↑	Clopidogrel and aspirin are coadministered in the treatment of acute coronary syndrome. Risk of life-threatening bleeding (eg, intracranial and GI hemorrhage) may be increased in high-risk patients with TIA or ischemic stroke. Avoid use of aspirin in high-risk patients with recent ischemic stroke or TIA who are receiving clopidogrel.
CYP2C19 inhibitors (eg, cimetidine, esomeprazole, etravirine, felbamate, fluconazole, fluoxetine, fluvoxamine, ketoconazole, omeprazole, ticlopidine, voriconazole)	Clopidogrel	↓	CYP2C19 inhibitors may decrease the pharmacologic effects of clopidogrel by decreasing metabolism to the active metabolite. Avoid coadministration of CYP2C19 inhibitors with clopidogrel.
Macrolide and related antibiotics (eg, erythromycin, telithromycin)	Clopidogrel	↓	The antiplatelet effect of clopidogrel may be inhibited by certain macrolide and related antibiotics. Monitor platelet function when starting or stopping macrolide and related antibiotics. Adjust the clopidogrel dose as needed. Because azithromycin does not inhibit CYP3A4 , it may be a useful alternative.
NSAIDs	Clopidogrel	↑	Coadministration of clopidogrel with naproxen was associated with increased occult GI blood loss. Administer NSAIDs and clopidogrel with caution.
PPIs (eg, esomeprazole, omeprazole)	Clopidogrel	↓	Controlled studies are needed to determine the magnitude of this interaction with each PPI and clopidogrel. The antiplatelet activity of clopidogrel may be decreased by PPIs. Certain PPIs (eg, omeprazole) may interfere with the metabolic (CYP2C19) conversion of clopidogrel to its active metabolite. If a PPI is clearly indicated in a patient receiving clopidogrel, use with caution. An antacidor H_2 receptor antagonist (eg, ranitidine) may be a safer alternative. Cimetidine inhibits CYP2C19 and is not recommended.
Rifamycins (eg, rifampin)	Clopidogrel	↑	The antiplatelet effect of clopidogrel may be enhanced by rifamycins. Carefully monitor platelet function when starting, stopping, or changing the rifamycin dose. Adjust the clopidogrel dose as needed.

Clopidogrel Drug Interactions

Precipitant drug	Object drug[a]		Description
Warfarin	Clopidogrel	↔	Because of the increased risk of bleeding, coadminister warfarin and clopidogrel with caution.
Clopidogrel	Warfarin		
Clopidogrel	Bupropion	↑	Bupropion plasma concentrations may be elevated, increasing the pharmacologic effects and adverse reactions. Closely monitor patients. Adjust the bupropion dose as needed when clopidogrel is started or stopped.

[a] ↑ = object drug increased; ↓ = object drug decreased; ↔ = undetermined clinical effect.

➤*Drug/Food interactions:* In a study in healthy men when clopidogrel 75 mg/day was given with a standard breakfast, mean inhibition of ADP-induced platelet aggregation was reduced less than 9%. The active metabolite AUC was unchanged by food, while the active metabolite C_{max} was reduced 57%. However, clopidogrel can be administered without regard to food.

Adverse Reactions

For more information on thrombotic thrombocytopenic purpura and bleeding, see Warnings/Precautions.

➤*Hemorrhagic:*

CURE study – In CURE, clopidogrel use with aspirin was associated with an increase in major bleeding (primarily GI and at puncture sites) compared with placebo plus aspirin. The incidence of intracranial hemorrhage (0.1%) and fatal bleeding (0.2%) was the same in both groups. Other bleeding events that were reported more frequently in the clopidogrel group were epistaxis, hematuria, and bruise.

The overall incidence of bleeding in patients receiving clopidogrel and aspirin in CURE is described in the following table.

Clopidogrel Bleeding Adverse Reactions in CURE

Adverse reactions	Clopidogrel (+ aspirin)[a] (n = 6,259)	Placebo (+ aspirin)[a] (n = 6,303)	P value
Major bleeding[b]	3.7%[c]	2.7%[d]	0.001
Life-threatening bleeding	2.2%	1.8%	0.13
Fatal	0.2%	0.2%	
5 g/dL hemoglobin drop	0.9%	0.9%	
Requiring surgical intervention	0.7%	0.7%	
Hemorrhagic strokes	0.1%	0.1%	
Requiring inotropes	0.5%	0.5%	
Requiring transfusion (≥ 4 units)	1.2%	1%	
Other major bleeding	1.6%	1%	0.005
Significantly disabling	0.4%	0.3%	
Intraocular bleeding with significant loss of vision	0.05%	0.03%	
Requiring 2 to 3 units of blood	1.3%	0.9%	
Minor bleeding[e]	5.1%	2.4%	< 0.001

[a] Other standard therapies were used as appropriate.
[b] Life-threatening and other major bleeding.
[c] Major bleeding event rates for clopidogrel + aspirin were dose-dependent on aspirin:
[d] Major bleeding event rate for placebo + aspirin was dose-dependent on aspirin: < 100 mg = 2%; 100 to 200 mg = 2.3%; > 200 mg = 4%. Major bleeding event rates for placebo + aspirin by age were
[e] Led to interruption of study medication.

Ninety-two percent of the patients in the CURE study received heparin or low molecular weight heparin, and the rate of bleeding in these patients was similar to the overall results.

COMMIT study – In COMMIT, similar rates of major bleeding were observed in the clopidogrel and placebo groups, both of which also received aspirin.

Clopidogrel Bleeding Adverse Reactions in COMMIT

Adverse reactions	Clopidogrel (+ aspirin) (n = 22,961)	Placebo (+ aspirin) (n = 22,891)	P value
Major[a] noncerebral or cerebral bleeding[b]	0.6%	0.5%	0.59
Major noncerebral	0.4%	0.3%	0.48
Fatal	0.2%	0.2%	0.9
Hemorrhagic stroke	0.2%	0.2%	0.91
Fatal	0.2%	0.2%	0.81

CLOPIDOGREL BISULFATE — ORAL

Clopidogrel Bleeding Adverse Reactions in COMMIT			
Adverse reactions	Clopidogrel (+ aspirin) (n = 22,961)	Placebo (+ aspirin) (n = 22,891)	*P* value
Other noncerebral bleeding (nonmajor)	3.6%	3.1%	0.005
Any noncerebral bleeding	3.9%	3.4%	0.004

[a] Major bleeds are cerebral bleeds or noncerebral bleeds thought to have caused death or that required transfusion.
[b] The relative rate of major noncerebral or cerebral bleeding was independent of age. Event rates for clopidogrel + aspirin by age were < 60 years of age = 0.3%, ≥ 60 to < 70 years of age = 0.7%, ≥ 70 years of age = 0.8%. Reaction rates for placebo + aspirin by age were < 60 years of age = 0.4%, ≥ 60 to < 70 years of age = 0.6%, ≥ 70 years of age = 0.7%.

CAPRIE (clopidogrel vs aspirin) – In CAPRIE, GI hemorrhage occurred at a rate of 2% in those taking clopidogrel versus 2.7% in those taking aspirin; bleeding requiring hospitalization occurred in 0.7% and 1.1%, respectively. The incidence of intracranial hemorrhage was 0.4% for clopidogrel compared with 0.5% for aspirin.

Other bleeding events that were reported more frequently in the clopidogrel group were epistaxis and hematoma.

➤*Other adverse reactions:* In CURE and CHARISMA, which compared clopidogrel plus aspirin with aspirin alone, there was no difference in the rate of adverse reactions (other than bleeding) between clopidogrel and placebo.

In CAPRIE, which compared clopidogrel with aspirin, pruritis was more frequently reported in those taking clopidogrel. No other difference in the rate of adverse events (other than bleeding) was reported.

➤*Postmarketing:*

Cardiovascular – Hypotension.

CNS – Confusion, fatal intracranial bleeding, hallucinations, taste disorders.

Dermatologic – Angioedema, bullous dermatitis, eczema, erythema multiforme, lichen planus, maculopapular or erythematous rash, Stevens-Johnson syndrome, skin bleeding, toxic epidermal necrolysis, urticaria.

GI – Colitis (including lymphocytic or ulcerative colitis), GI and retroperitoneal hemorrhage with fatal outcome, pancreatitis, stomatitis.

GU – Increased creatinine levels, glomerulopathy.

Hematologic – Agranulocytosis, aplastic anemia/pancytopenia, thrombotic thrombocytopenic purpura.

Hepatic – Abnormal liver function tests, acute liver failure, hepatitis (noninfectious).

Hypersensitivity – Anaphylactoid reactions, hypersensitivity reactions, serum sickness.

Musculoskeletal – Arthralgia, arthritis, musculoskeletal bleeding, myalgia.

Respiratory – Bronchospasm, interstitial pneumonitis, respiratory tract bleeding.

Special senses – Conjunctival, ocular, and retinal bleeding.

Miscellaneous – Cardiovasculitis, fever, hemorrhage of operative wound.

Overdosage

➤*Symptoms:* Platelet inhibition by clopidogrel is irreversible and will last for the life of the platelet. Overdose following clopidogrel administration may result in bleeding complications. A single oral dose of clopidogrel at 1,500 or 2,000 mg/kg was lethal to mice and rats and at 3,000 mg/kg to baboons. Symptoms of acute toxicity were vomiting, difficulty breathing, GI hemorrhage, and prostration in animals.

➤*Treatment:* Based on biological plausibility, platelet transfusion may restore clotting ability.

Patient Information

Advise patients that it may take longer than usual to stop bleeding and that they may bruise and/or bleed more easily when they take clopidogrel or clopidogrel combined with aspirin. Patients should report any unusual excessive or prolonged bleeding or blood in their stool or urine to their health care provider.

Instruct patients to inform their health care provider and dentist that they are taking clopidogrel and/or any other product known to affect bleeding before any surgery or any invasive procedure is scheduled and before any new drug is taken.

Inform patients to take clopidogrel exactly as prescribed and not to discontinue clopidogrel without first discussing it with the health care provider who prescribed clopidogrel.

Inform patients that thrombotic thrombocytopenic purpura is a rare but serious condition that has been reported with clopidogrel and other drugs in this class of drugs.

Instruct patients to get prompt medical attention if they experience any of the following symptoms that cannot otherwise be explained: fever, weakness, extreme skin paleness, purple skin patches, yellowing of the skin or eyes, or neurologic changes.

Ask patients to list all prescription medications, nonprescription medications, or dietary supplements they are taking or planning to take, including prescription or nonprescription omeprazole, so the health care provider knows about other treatments that may affect how clopidogrel works (eg, warfarin, NSAIDs).

PRASUGREL

Rx	**Effient** (Eli Lilly and Company)	**Tablets; oral:** 5 mg	Equiv. to prasugrel hydrochloride 5.49 mg. Mannitol. (5 MG 4760). Yellow, elongated hexagonal. Film-coated. In 7s and 30s.
		10 mg	Equiv. to prasugrel hydrochloride 10.98 mg. Mannitol. (10 MG 4759). Beige, elongated hexagonal. Film-coated. In 30s and UD 90s.

PRASUGREL HYDROCHLORIDE — ORAL

WARNING

Bleeding risk – Prasugrel can cause significant, sometimes fatal, bleeding.

Do not use prasugrel in patients with active pathological bleeding or a history of transient ischemic attack (TIA) or stroke.

In patients 75 years of age and older, prasugrel is generally not recommended because of the increased risk of fatal and intracranial bleeding and uncertain benefit, except in high-risk situations (patients with diabetes or a history of prior myocardial infarction [MI]) in which its effect appears to be greater and its use may be considered.

Do not start prasugrel in patients likely to undergo urgent coronary artery bypass graft (CABG) surgery. When possible, discontinue prasugrel at least 7 days prior to any surgery.

Additional risk factors for bleeding include body weight less than 60 kg, propensity to bleed, and concomitant use of medications that increase the risk of bleeding (eg, warfarin, heparin, fibrinolytic therapy, long-term use of nonsteroidal anti-inflammatory drugs [NSAIDs]).

Suspect bleeding in any patient who is hypotensive and has recently undergone coronary angiography, percutaneous coronary intervention (PCI), CABG, or other surgical procedures in the setting of prasugrel.

If possible, manage bleeding without discontinuing prasugrel. Discontinuing prasugrel, particularly in the first few weeks after acute coronary syndrome (ACS), increases the risk of subsequent cardiovascular events.

Indications

➤*Acute coronary syndrome:* To reduce the rate of thrombotic cardiovascular events (including stent thrombosis) in patients with ACS who are to be managed with PCI as follows: patients with unstable angina or non–ST segment elevation MI (NSTEMI); patients with ST elevation MI (STEMI) when managed with primary or delayed PCI.

Administration and Dosage

➤*Adults:*

Acute coronary syndrome –

Usual dosage:
- *Weight 60 kg or more* – 10 mg once daily.
- *Weight less than 60 kg* – 5 mg once daily should be considered.

Loading dose: 60 mg single dose.

Concomitant therapy: Prasugrel should also be taken with aspirin 75 to 325 mg daily.

➤*Elderly:* Use of prasugrel is generally not recommended in patients 75 years of age and older except in high-risk situations (diabetes and history of MI) in which its effect appears to be greater and its use may be considered.

➤*Discontinuation of therapy:* Discontinue prasugrel for active bleeding, elective surgery, stroke, or TIA.

In patients who are managed with PCI and stent placement, premature discontinuation of any antiplatelet medication, including thienopyridines, conveys an increased risk of stent thrombosis, MI, and death. Patients who require premature discontinuation of a thienopyridine will be at an increased risk for cardiac events. Avoid lapses in therapy, and if thienopyridines must be temporarily discontinued because of an adverse event(s), restart therapy as soon as possible.

➤*Administration:* May be administered with or without food. Do not break the tablet.

PRASUGREL HYDROCHLORIDE — ORAL

➤*Storage/Stability:* Store at 25°C (77°F); excursions are permitted between 15° and 30°C (59° and 86°F). Dispense and keep the product in its original container.

Actions

➤*Pharmacology:* Prasugrel is a thienopyridine class inhibitor of platelet activation and aggregation through the irreversible binding of its active metabolite to the $P2Y_{12}$ class of adenosine diphosphate receptors on platelets.

➤*Pharmacokinetics:*

Absorption/Distribution – Following oral administration, at least 79% of the dose is absorbed. The absorption is rapid, with peak plasma concentrations (C_{max}) of the active metabolite occurring approximately 30 minutes after dosing. The active metabolite's exposure (area under the curve [AUC]) increases slightly more than proportionally over the dose range of 5 to 60 mg. Repeated daily doses of 10 mg do not lead to accumulation of the active metabolite. The active metabolite is bound about 98% to human serum albumin. The major inactive metabolites are highly bound to human plasma proteins. The estimates of apparent volume of distribution of prasugrel's active metabolite ranged from 44 to 68 L.

Effect of food: In a study of healthy subjects given a single 15 mg dose, the AUC of the active metabolite was unaffected by a high-fat, high-calorie meal, but C_{max} was decreased by 49% and time to C_{max} (T_{max}) was increased from 0.5 to 1.5 hours. Prasugrel can be administered without regard to food.

Metabolism/Excretion – Prasugrel is a prodrug and is not detected in plasma following oral administration. It is rapidly hydrolyzed in the intestine to a thiolactone, which is then converted to the active metabolite by a single step, primarily by cytochrome P450 (CYP-450) 3A4 and CYP2B6, and to a lesser extent by CYP2C9 and CYP2C19. Estimates of apparent clearance ranged from 112 to 166 L/h in healthy subjects and patients with stable atherosclerosis. The active metabolite has an elimination half-life of about 7 hours (range, 2 to 15 hours). The active metabolite is metabolized to 2 inactive compounds by S-methylation or conjugation with cysteine. Approximately 68% of the prasugrel dose is excreted in the urine and 27% in the feces as inactive metabolites.

Special populations –

Renal function impairment: In patients with end-stage renal disease, exposure to the active metabolite, both C_{max} and AUC ($0\text{-}t_{last}$), was approximately half that in healthy controls and patients with moderate renal impairment.

Elderly: In Trial to Assess Improvement in Therapeutic Outcomes by Optimizing Platelet Inhibition With Prasugrel (TRITON-TIMI 38), the mean exposure (AUC) of the active metabolite was 19% higher in patients 75 years of age and older than in patients younger than 75 years of age.

Race: In clinical pharmacology studies, after adjusting for body weight, the AUC of the active metabolite was approximately 19% higher in Chinese, Japanese, and Korean subjects than in white subjects.

Body weight: The mean exposure (AUC) to the active metabolite is approximately 30% to 40% higher in subjects with a body weight of less than 60 kg than in those weighing 60 kg or more.

Contraindications

Active pathological bleeding, such as peptic ulcer or intracranial hemorrhage; prior TIA or stroke; hypersensitivity (eg, anaphylaxis) to prasugrel or any component of the product.

Warnings/Precautions

➤*Risk of bleeding:* Thienopyridines, including prasugrel, increase the risk of bleeding. With the dosing regimens used in TRITON-TIMI 38, thrombosis in MI (TIMI) major (clinically overt bleeding associated with a fall in hemoglobin of at least 5 g/dL, or intracranial hemorrhage) and TIMI minor (overt bleeding associated with a fall in hemoglobin of at least 3 g/dL but less than 5 g/dL) bleeding events were more common on prasugrel than on clopidogrel.

See the Warning box for more information.

Other risk factors for bleeding are the following: 75 years of age and older (because of the risk of bleeding, including fatal bleeding, and uncertain effectiveness in patients 75 years of age and older, use of prasugrel is generally not recommended in these patients, except in high-risk situations [patients with diabetes or history of MI] in which its effect appears to be greater and its use may be considered); CABG or other surgical procedure; body weight less than 60 kg (consider a lower [5 mg] maintenance dose); propensity to bleed (eg, recent trauma, recent surgery, recent or recurrent GI bleeding, active peptic ulcer disease, severe hepatic impairment); medications that increase the risk of bleeding (eg, oral anticoagulants, long-term use of NSAIDs, fibrinolytic agents). Aspirin and heparin were commonly used in TRITON-TIMI 38.

Thienopyridines inhibit platelet aggregation for the lifetime of the platelet (7 to 10 days), so withholding a dose will not be useful in managing a bleeding event or the risk of bleeding associated with an invasive procedure. Because the half-life of prasugrel's active metabolite is short relative to the lifetime of the platelet, it may be possible to restore hemostasis by administering exogenous platelets; however, platelet transfusions within 6 hours of the loading dose or 4 hours of the maintenance dose may be less effective.

➤*CABG surgery–related bleeding:* See the Warning box for more information.

Of the 437 patients who underwent CABG during TRITON-TIMI 38, the rates of CABG-related TIMI major or minor bleeding were 14.1% in the prasugrel group and 4.5% in the clopidogrel group. The higher risk of bleeding events in patients treated with prasugrel persisted for up to 7 days from the most recent dose of study drug. For patients receiving a thienopyridine within 3 days prior to CABG, the frequencies of TIMI major or minor bleeding were 26.7% in the prasugrel group compared with 5% in the clopidogrel group. For patients who received their last dose of thienopyridine within 4 to 7 days prior to CABG, the frequencies decreased to 11.3% in the prasugrel group and 3.4% in the clopidogrel group.

CABG-related bleeding may be treated with transfusion of blood products, including packed red blood cells and platelets. However, platelet transfusions within 6 hours of the loading dose or 4 hours of the maintenance dose may be less effective.

➤*Prior transient ischemic attack or stroke:* Prasugrel is contraindicated in patients with a history of prior TIA or stroke. In TRITON-TIMI 38, patients with a history of TIA or ischemic stroke (more than 3 months prior to enrollment) had a higher rate of stroke on prasugrel (6.5%; of which, 4.2% were thrombotic stroke and 2.3% were intracranial hemorrhage) than on clopidogrel (1.2%, all thrombotic). In patients without such a history, the incidence of stroke was 0.9% (0.2%, intracranial hemorrhage) and 1% (0.3%, intracranial hemorrhage) with prasugrel and clopidogrel, respectively. Patients with a history of ischemic stroke within 3 months of screening and patients with a history of hemorrhagic stroke at any time were excluded from TRITON-TIMI 38. Patients who experience a stroke or TIA while on prasugrel generally should have therapy discontinued.

➤*Discontinuation of therapy:* See Administration and Dosage for more information.

➤*Thrombotic thrombocytopenic purpura:* Thrombotic thrombocytopenic purpura (TTP) has been reported with the use of prasugrel. TTP can occur after a brief exposure (less than 2 weeks). TTP is a serious condition that can be fatal and requires urgent treatment, including plasmapheresis (plasma exchange). TTP is characterized by thrombocytopenia, microangiopathic hemolytic anemia (schistocytes [fragment red blood cells] seen on peripheral smear), neurological findings, renal dysfunction, and fever.

➤*Low body weight:* In TRITON-TIMI 38, 4.6% of patients treated with prasugrel had body weight less than 60 kg. Individuals with body weight less than 60 kg had an increased risk of bleeding and an increased exposure to the active metabolite of prasugrel.

See Administration and Dosage for more information.

➤*Hepatic function impairment:* The pharmacokinetics and pharmacodynamics of prasugrel in patients with severe hepatic disease have not been studied, but such patients are generally at a higher risk of bleeding.

➤*Pregnancy: Category B.* There are no adequate and well-controlled studies of prasugrel use in pregnant women. Reproductive and developmental toxicology studies in rats and rabbits at doses of up to 30 times the recommended therapeutic exposures in humans (based on plasma exposures to the major circulating human metabolite) revealed no evidence of fetal harm; however, animal studies are not always predictive of a human response. Use prasugrel during pregnancy only if the potential benefit to the mother justifies the potential risk to the fetus.

➤*Lactation:* It is not known whether prasugrel is excreted in human milk; however, metabolites of prasugrel were found in rat milk. Because many drugs are excreted in human milk, use prasugrel during breast-feeding only if the potential benefit to the mother justifies the potential risk to the breast-feeding infant.

➤*Children:* Safety and effectiveness in children have not been established.

➤*Elderly:* Patients 75 years of age and older who received prasugrel had an increased risk of fatal bleeding events (1%) compared with patients who received clopidogrel (0.1%). In patients 75 years of age and older, symptomatic intracranial hemorrhage occurred in 0.8% of patients who received prasugrel and in 0.3% who received clopidogrel. Because of the risk of bleeding and because effectiveness is uncertain in patients 75 years of age and older, use of prasugrel is generally not recommended in these patients, except in high-risk situations (diabetes and history of MI) in which its effect appears to be greater and its use may be considered.

➤*Monitoring:* Monitor patient for bleeding or unusual bruising.

Drug Interactions

Prasugrel Drug Interactions

Precipitant drug	Object drug[a]		Description
Aspirin	Prasugrel	⬆	Aspirin 150 mg daily did not alter inhibition of platelet aggregation by the active metabolite of prasugrel; however, bleeding time was increased. Aspirin 75 to 325 mg daily can be administered with prasugrel.
CYP3A inhibitors (eg, ciprofloxacin, clarithromycin, diltiazem, grapefruit juice, indinavir, ketoconazole, verapamil)	Prasugrel	⬇	Ketoconazole 400 mg daily did not affect prasugrel-mediated inhibition of platelet aggregation or the AUC or T_{max} of the active metabolite. However, the C_{max} of prasugrel and its metabolite decreased 34% and 46%, respectively. This was not expected to have a clinically important effect on the pharmacokinetics of the active metabolite of prasugrel.

PRASUGREL HYDROCHLORIDE — ORAL

Prasugrel Drug Interactions			
Precipitant drug	Object drug[a]		Description
Drugs that elevate gastric pH (eg, ranitidine, lansoprazole)	Prasugrel	↓	Coadministration of ranitidine or lansoprazole with prasugrel decreased the C_{max} of the prasugrel active metabolite 14% and 29%, respectively, but did not change the AUC or T_{max}. Prasugrel can be administered with drugs that elevate gastric pH.
Fibrinolytic therapy (eg, tenecteplase)	Prasugrel	↑	The risk of bleeding is increased. Use with caution and closely monitor clinical response.
Prasugrel	Fibrinolytic therapy (eg, tenecteplase)		
Heparin	Prasugrel	↑	The risk of bleeding is increased. A single intravenous dose of unfractionated heparin 100 units/kg did not alter coagulation or prasugrel-mediated inhibition of platelet aggregation; however, bleeding time was increased. Heparin can be administered with prasugrel.
Prasugrel	Heparin		
NSAIDs (eg, ibuprofen)	Prasugrel	↑	Coadministration of prasugrel and long-term use of NSAIDs may increase the risk of bleeding. Use with caution.
Prasugrel	NSAIDs (eg, ibuprofen)		
Warfarin	Prasugrel	↑	Coadministration of prasugrel with warfarin 15 mg prolonged bleeding time. The risk of bleeding is increased. Use with caution. Closely monitor clinical and laboratory parameters and adjust therapy as needed.
Prasugrel	Warfarin		
Prasugrel	CYP2B6 substrates (eg, bupropion, cyclophosphamide, nevirapine, propofol)	↓	In healthy subjects, prasugrel decreased exposure to the active metabolite of bupropion (hydroxybupropion) by 23%, an amount not considered to be clinically important. Therefore, it is not anticipated that prasugrel will affect the pharmacokinetics of drugs that are primarily metabolized by CYP2B6.

[a] ↑ = object drug increased; ↓ = object drug decreased.

➤*Drug/Food interactions:* See Actions for more information.

Adverse Reactions

➤*Discontinuation of treatment:* The rate of study drug discontinuation because of adverse reactions was 7.2% for prasugrel and 6.3% for clopidogrel. Bleeding was the most common adverse reaction leading to study drug discontinuation for both drugs (2.5% for prasugrel and 1.4% for clopidogrel).

➤*Bleeding:*

Bleeding unrelated to CABG surgery –

Prasugrel Non-CABG–Related Bleeding[a] Adverse Reactions	Prasugrel (n = 6,741)	Clopidogrel (n = 6,716)	*P* value
TIMI major or minor bleeding	4.5%	3.4%	*P* = 0.002
TIMI major bleeding[b]	2.2%	1.7%	*P* = 0.029
Life-threatening	1.3%	0.8%	*P* = 0.015
Fatal	0.3%	0.1%	–
Symptomatic intracranial hemorrhage	0.3%	0.3%	–
Requiring inotropes	0.3%	0.1%	–
Requiring surgical intervention	0.3%	0.3%	–
Requiring transfusion (≥ 4 units)	0.7%	0.5%	–
TIMI minor bleeding[b]	2.4%	1.9%	*P* = 0.022

[a] Patients may be counted in more than 1 row.
[b] See Warnings/Precautions for more information.

Prasugrel Bleeding Rates for Non-CABG–Related Bleeding by Weight and Age	Major/Minor		Fatal	
	Prasugrel	Clopidogrel	Prasugrel	Clopidogrel
Weight < 60 kg (n = 308 prasugrel, n = 356 clopidogrel)	10.1%	6.5%	0%	0.3%
Weight ≥ 60 kg (n = 6,373 prasugrel, n = 6,299 clopidogrel)	4.2%	3.3%	0.3%	0.1%
Age < 75 years (n = 5,850 prasugrel, n = 5,822 clopidogrel)	3.8%	2.9%	0.2 %	0.1%
Age ≥ 75 years (n = 891 prasugrel, n = 894 clopidogrel)	9%	6.9%	1%	0.1%

Bleeding related to CABG –

Prasugrel CABG-Related Bleeding[a] Adverse Reactions	Prasugrel (n = 213)	Clopidogrel (n = 224)
TIMI major or minor bleeding	14.1%	4.5%
TIMI major bleeding	11.3%	3.6%
Fatal	0.9%	0%
Reoperation	3.8%	0.5%
Transfusion of 5 units or more	6.6%	2.2%
Intracranial hemorrhage	0%	0%
TIMI minor bleeding	2.8%	0.9%

[a] Patients may be counted in more than 1 row.

Other bleeding adverse reactions – Hemorrhagic reactions reported as adverse reactions in TRITON-TIMI 38 were, for prasugrel and clopidogrel, respectively: epistaxis (6.2%, 3.3%), GI hemorrhage (1.5%, 1%), hemoptysis (0.6%, 0.5%), subcutaneous hematoma (0.5%, 0.2%), postprocedural hemorrhage (0.5%, 0.2%), retroperitoneal hemorrhage (0.3%, 0.2%), pericardial effusion/hemorrhage/tamponade (0.3%, 0.2%), and retinal hemorrhage (0%, 0.1%).

➤*Malignancies:* During TRITON-TIMI 38, newly diagnosed malignancies were reported in 1.6% and 1.2% of patients treated with prasugrel and clopidogrel, respectively. The sites contributing to the differences were primarily colon and lung. It is unclear if these observations are causally related or are random occurrences.

➤*Nonhemorrhagic adverse reactions:* In TRITON-TIMI 38, common and other important nonhemorrhagic adverse reactions were, for prasugrel and clopidogrel, respectively: severe thrombocytopenia (0.06%, 0.04%), anemia (2.2%, 2%), abnormal hepatic function (0.22%, 0.27%), allergic reactions (0.36%, 0.36%), and angioedema (0.06%, 0.04%).

Prasugrel Non-Hemorrhagic Adverse Reactions (≥ 2.5%) Adverse reactions	Prasugrel (n = 6,741)	Clopidogrel (n = 6,716)
Cardiovascular		
Atrial fibrillation	2.9%	3.1%
Bradycardia	2.9%	2.4%
Hypertension	7.5%	7.1%
Hypotension	3.9%	3.8%
CNS		
Dizziness	4.1%	4.6%
Fatigue	3.7%	4.8%
Headache	5.5%	5.3%
GI		
Diarrhea	2.3%	2.6%
Nausea	4.6%	4.3%
Respiratory		
Cough	3.9%	4.1%
Dyspnea	4.9%	4.5%
Miscellaneous		
Back pain	5%	4.5%
Hypercholesterolemia/Hyperlipidemia	7%	7.4%
Leukopenia (< 4 × 10^9 WBC/L)[a]	2.8%	3.5%
Noncardiac chest pain	3.1%	3.5%
Pain in extremity	2.6%	2.6%
Peripheral edema	2.7%	3%

PRASUGREL HYDROCHLORIDE — ORAL

Prasugrel Non-Hemorrhagic Adverse Reactions (≥ 2.5%)		
Adverse reactions	Prasugrel (n = 6,741)	Clopidogrel (n = 6,716)
Pyrexia	2.7%	2.2%
Rash	2.8%	2.4%

[a] WBC = white blood cell.

➤*Postmarketing:* Hypersensitivity reactions (including anaphylaxis), thrombocytopenia, TTP.

Overdosage

➤*Symptoms:* Platelet inhibition by prasugrel is rapid and irreversible, lasting for the life of the platelet, and is unlikely to be increased in the event of an overdose.

➤*Treatment:* Platelet transfusion may restore clotting ability. The prasugrel active metabolite is not likely to be removed by dialysis.

Patient Information

Advise patients to take prasugrel exactly as prescribed and remind patients not to discontinue prasugrel without first discussing it with the health care provider who prescribed prasugrel.

Inform patients that they will bruise and bleed more easily; it will take longer than usual to stop bleeding; and to report any unanticipated, prolonged, or excessive bleeding or blood in their stool or urine.

Inform patients that TTP is a rare but serious condition that has been reported with prasugrel.

Instruct patients to get prompt medical attention if they experience any of the following symptoms that cannot otherwise be explained: extreme skin paleness, fever, neurological changes, purple skin patches, weakness, or yellowing of the skin or eyes.

Instruct patients to inform health care providers and dentists that they are taking prasugrel before any invasive procedure is scheduled. Tell the health care provider performing the invasive procedure to talk to the health care prescriber before stopping prasugrel.

Ask patients to list all prescription medications, nonprescription medications, or dietary supplements they are taking or plan to take so the health care provider knows about other treatments that may affect bleeding risk (eg, warfarin, NSAIDs).

TICLOPIDINE HYDROCHLORIDE

Rx	**Ticlopidine HCl** (Various, eg, Apotex Corp., Teva)	**Tablets:** 250 mg	In 30s, 60s, 100s, 500s, and 1000s.
Rx	**Ticlid** (Syntex)		(Ticlid 250). White. Oval. Film coated. In 30s, 60s, and 500s.

TICLOPIDINE HYDROCHLORIDE — ORAL

WARNING

Ticlopidine HCl can cause life-threatening hematological adverse reactions, including neutropenia/agranulocytosis and thrombotic thrombocytopenic purpura (TTP) and aplastic anemia.

Neutropenia/agranulocytosis – Among 2048 patients in clinical trials, there were 50 cases (2.4%) of neutropenia (less than 1200 neutrophils/mm^3), and the neutrophil count was below 450/mm^3 in 17 of these patients (0.8% of the total population).

TTP – One case of TTP was reported during clinical trials. Based on postmarketing data, US physicians reported about 100 cases between 1992 and 1997. Based on an estimated patient exposure of 2 million to 4 million, and assuming an event reporting rate of 10% (the true rate is not known), the incidence of ticlopidine-associated TTP may be as high as 1 case in every 2000 to 4000 patients exposed.

Aplastic anemia – Aplastic anemia was not seen during clinical trials in stroke patients, but US physicians reported about 50 cases between 1992 and 1998. Based on an estimated patient exposure of 2 million to 4 million, and assuming an event reporting rate of 10% (the true rate is not known), the incidence of ticlopidine-associated aplastic anemia may be as high as 1 case in every 4000 to 8000 patients exposed.

Monitoring of clinical and hematologic status – Severe hematologic adverse reactions may occur within a few days of the start of therapy. The incidence of TTP peaks after about 3 to 4 weeks of therapy and neutropenia peaks at approximately 4 to 6 weeks. The incidence of aplastic anemia peaks after about 4 to 8 weeks of therapy. The incidence of the hematologic adverse reactions declines thereafter. Only a few cases of neutropenia, TTP, or aplastic anemia have arisen after more than 3 months of treatment.

Hematological adverse reactions cannot be reliably predicted by any identified demographic or clinical characteristics. During the first 3 months of treatment, patients receiving ticlopidine HCl must, therefore, be hematologically and clinically monitored for evidence of neutropenia or TTP. If any such evidence is seen, ticlopidine HCl should be immediately discontinued.

Indications

➤*Stroke:* To reduce the risk of thrombotic stroke (fatal or nonfatal) in patients who have experienced stroke precursors, and in patients who have had a completed thrombotic stroke. Because ticlopidine is associated with a risk of life-threatening blood dyscrasias, including thrombotic thrombocytopenic purpura (TTP), neutropenia/agranulocytosis and aplastic anemia, ticlopidine should be reserved for patients who are intolerant or allergic to aspirin therapy or who have failed aspirin therapy.

➤*Stent thrombosis, adjunctive therapy:* As adjunctive therapy with aspirin to reduce the incidence of subacute stent thrombosis in patients undergoing successful coronary stent implantation.

Administration and Dosage

➤*Adults:*

Stroke – 250 mg twice daily taken with food.

Coronary artery stenting – 250 mg twice daily taken with food and with antiplatelet doses of aspirin for up to 30 days of therapy following successful stent implantation.

➤*Renal function impairment:* For patients with renal impairment, it may be necessary to reduce the dosage of ticlopidine or discontinue it altogether if hemorrhagic or hematopoietic problems are encountered.

➤*Hepatic function impairment:* Since ticlopidine is metabolized by the liver, dosing of ticlopidine or other drugs metabolized in the liver may require adjustment upon starting or stopping concomitant therapy. Because of limited experience in patients with severe hepatic disease and who may have bleeding diatheses, the use of ticlopidine is not recommended in this population.

➤*Administration:* Administration of ticlopidine with food is recommended to maximize GI tolerance. In controlled trials, ticlopidine was taken with meals.

Administer twice a day.

➤*Storage/Stability:* Store at 15° to 30°C (59° to 86°F).

Actions

➤*Pharmacology:* When taken orally, ticlopidine HCl causes a time- and dose-dependent inhibition of both platelet aggregation and release of platelet granule constituents, as well as a prolongation of bleeding time. The intact drug has no significant in vitro activity at the concentrations attained in vivo; and, although analysis of urine and plasma indicates at least 20 metabolites, no metabolite which accounts for the activity of ticlopidine has been isolated.

Ticlopidine HCl, after oral ingestion, interferes with platelet membrane function by inhibiting ADP-induced platelet-fibrinogen binding and subsequent platelet-platelet interactions. The effect on platelet function is irreversible for the life of the platelet, as shown both by persistent inhibition of fibrinogen binding after washing platelets ex vivo and by inhibition of platelet aggregation after resuspension of platelets in buffered medium.

Pharmacodynamics – In healthy volunteers over the age of 50, substantial inhibition (greater than 50%) of ADP-induced platelet aggregation is detected within 4 days after administration of ticlopidine HCl 250 mg twice daily, and maximum platelet aggregation inhibition (60% to 70%) is achieved after 8 to 11 days. Lower doses cause less, and more delayed, platelet aggregation inhibition, while doses above 250 mg twice daily give little additional effect on platelet aggregation but an increased rate of adverse effects. The dose of 250 mg twice daily is the only dose that has been evaluated in controlled clinical trials.

After discontinuation of ticlopidine HCl, bleeding time and other platelet function tests return to normal within 2 weeks, in the majority of patients.

At the recommended therapeutic dose (250 mg twice daily), ticlopidine HCl has no known significant pharmacological actions in man other than inhibition of platelet function and prolongation of the bleeding time.

➤*Pharmacokinetics:*

Absorption – After oral administration of a single 250 mg dose, ticlopidine HCl is rapidly absorbed, with peak plasma levels occurring at approximately 2 hours after dosing and is extensively metabolized. Absorption is greater than 80%.

The oral bioavailability of ticlopidine is increased by 20% when taken after a meal. Administration of ticlopidine HCl with food is recommended to maximize GI tolerance. In controlled trials, ticlopidine HCl was taken with meals.

Distribution – Ticlopidine HCl binds reversibly (98%) to plasma proteins, mainly to serum albumin and lipoproteins. The binding to albumin and lipoproteins is nonsaturable over a wide concentration range. Ticlopidine also binds to alpha-1 acid glycoprotein. At concentrations attained with the recommended dose, only 15% or less ticlopidine in plasma is bound to this protein.

Excretion – Ticlopidine HCl is metabolized extensively by the liver; only trace amounts of intact drug are detected in the urine. Following an oral

TICLOPIDINE HYDROCHLORIDE — ORAL

dose of radioactive ticlopidine HCl administered in solution, 60% of the radioactivity is recovered in the urine and 23% in the feces. Approximately ⅓ of the dose excreted in the feces is intact ticlopidine HCl, possibly excreted in the bile. Ticlopidine HCl is a minor component in plasma (5%) after a single dose, but at steady-state is the major component (15%). Approximately 40% to 50% of the radioactive metabolites circulating in plasma are covalently bound to plasma proteins, probably by acylation.

Clearance of ticlopidine decreases with age. Steady-state trough values in elderly patients (mean age 70 years) are about twice those in younger volunteer populations.

Ticlopidine HCl displays nonlinear pharmacokinetics and clearance decreases markedly on repeated dosing. In older volunteers the apparent half-life of ticlopidine after a single 250 mg dose is about 12.6 hours; with repeat dosing at 250 mg twice daily, the terminal elimination half-life rises to 4 to 5 days and steady-state levels of ticlopidine HCl in plasma are obtained after approximately 14 to 21 days.

Special populations –

Renal function impairment: Patients with mildly (Ccr 50 to 80 mL/min) or moderately (Ccr 20 to 50 mL/min) impaired renal function were compared to healthy subjects (Ccr 80 to 150 mL/min) in a study of the pharmacokinetic and platelet pharmacodynamic effects of ticlopidine HCl (250 mg twice daily) for 11 days. Concentrations of unchanged ticlopidine HCl were measured after a single 250 mg dose and after the final 250 mg dose on Day 11.

AUC values of ticlopidine increased by 28% and 60% in mild and moderately impaired patients, respectively, and plasma clearance decreased by 37% and 52%, respectively, but there were no statistically significant differences in ADP-induced platelet aggregation. In this small study (26 patients), bleeding times showed significant prolongation only in the moderately impaired patients.

Hepatic function impairment: The effect of decreased hepatic function on the pharmacokinetics of ticlopidine HCl was studied in 17 patients with advanced cirrhosis. The average plasma concentration of ticlopidine in these subjects was slightly higher than that seen in older subjects in a separate trial. In patients with severe liver impairment, ticlopidine HCl is contraindicated.

Contraindications

Hypersensitivity to the drug; presence of hematopoietic disorders such as neutropenia and thrombocytopenia or a history of TTP or aplastic anemia; presence of a hemostatic disorder or active pathological bleeding (such as bleeding peptic ulcer or intracranial bleeding); patients with severe liver impairment.

Warnings/Precautions

➤*Hematological effects:*

Neutropenia – Neutropenia may occur suddenly. Bone marrow examination typically shows a reduction in myeloid precursors. After withdrawal of ticlopidine, the neutrophil count usually rises to greater than 1200/mm^3 within 1 to 3 weeks.

Thrombocytopenia – Rarely, thrombocytopenia may occur in isolation or together with neutropenia.

Thrombotic thrombocytopenic purpura (TTP) – TTP is characterized by thrombocytopenia, microangiopathic hemolytic anemia (schistocytes [fragmented RBCs] seen on peripheral smear), neurological findings, renal dysfunction, and fever. The signs and symptoms can occur in any order, in particular, clinical symptoms may precede laboratory findings by hours or days. With prompt treatment (often including plasmapheresis), 70% to 80% of patients will survive with minimal or no sequelae. Because platelet transfusions may accelerate thrombosis in patients with TTP on ticlopidine, they should, if possible, be avoided.

Aplastic anemia – Aplastic anemia is characterized by anemia, thrombocytopenia and neutropenia together with a bone marrow examination that shows decreases in the precursor cells for red blood cells, white blood cells, and platelets. Patients may present with signs or symptoms suggestive of infection, in association with low white blood cell and platelet counts. Prompt treatment, which may include the use of drugs to stimulate the bone marrow, can minimize the mortality associated with aplastic anemia.

Monitoring for hematologic adverse reactions – See Warnings/Precautions for more information.

➤*Other hematological effects:* Rare cases of agranulocytosis, pancytopenia or aplastic anemia have been reported in postmarketing experience, some of which have been fatal. All forms of hematological adverse reactions are potentially fatal.

➤*Cholesterol elevation:* Ticlopidine HCl therapy causes increased serum cholesterol and triglycerides. Serum total cholesterol levels are increased 8% to 10% within 1 month of therapy and persist at that level. The ratios of the lipoprotein subfractions are unchanged.

➤*GI bleeding:* Ticlopidine HCl prolongs template bleeding time. The drug should be used with caution in patients who have lesions with a propensity to bleed (such as ulcers). Drugs that might induce such lesions should be used with caution in patients on ticlopidine HCl.

➤*Renal function impairment:* There is limited experience in patients with renal impairment. Decreased plasma clearance, increased AUC values and prolonged bleeding times can occur in renally impaired patients. In controlled clinical trials, no unexpected problems have been encountered in patients having mild renal impairment, and there is no experience with dosage adjustment in patients with greater degrees of renal impairment. Nevertheless, for renally impaired patients, it may be necessary to reduce the dosage of ticlopidine or discontinue it altogether if hemorrhagic or hematopoietic problems are encountered.

See Actions for more information.

➤*Hepatic function impairment:* Since ticlopidine is metabolized by the liver, dosing of ticlopidine HCl or other drugs metabolized in the liver may require adjustment upon starting or stopping concomitant therapy. Because of limited experience in patients with severe hepatic disease, who may have bleeding diatheses, the use of ticlopidine HCl is not recommended in this population.

See Actions for more information.

➤*Special risk:* Ticlopidine HCl should be used with caution in patients who may be at risk of increased bleeding from trauma, surgery or pathological conditions. If it is desired to eliminate the antiplatelet effects of ticlopidine HCl prior to elective surgery, the drug should be discontinued 10 to 14 days prior to surgery. Several controlled clinical studies have found increased surgical blood loss in patients undergoing surgery during treatment with ticlopidine. In TASS and CATS it was recommended that patients have ticlopidine discontinued prior to elective surgery. Several hundred patients underwent surgery during the trials, and no excessive surgical bleeding was reported.

Prolonged bleeding time is normalized within 2 hours after administration of 20 mg IV methylprednisolone. Platelet transfusions may also be used to reverse the effect of ticlopidine HCl on bleeding. Because platelet transfusions may accelerate thrombosis in patients with TTP on ticlopidine, they should, if possible, be avoided.

➤*Pregnancy: Category B.* There are no adequate and well-controlled studies in pregnant women. Because animal reproduction studies are not always predictive of a human response, this drug should be used during pregnancy only if clearly needed.

➤*Lactation:* Studies in rats have shown ticlopidine is excreted in the milk. It is not known whether this drug is excreted in human milk. Because many drugs are excreted in human milk and because of the potential for serious adverse reactions in nursing infants from ticlopidine, a decision should be made whether to discontinue nursing or to discontinue the drug, taking into account the importance of the drug to the mother.

➤*Children:* Safety and efficacy in pediatric patients have not been established.

➤*Elderly:* Clearance of ticlopidine is somewhat lower in elderly patients and trough levels are increased. The major clinical trials with ticlopidine HCl were conducted in an elderly population with an average age of 64 years. Of the total number of patients in the therapeutic trials, 45% of patients were over 65 years old and 12% were over 75 years old. No overall differences in efficacy or safety were observed between these patients and younger patients, and other reported clinical experience has not identified differences in responses between the elderly and younger patients, but greater sensitivity of some older individuals cannot be ruled out.

Per the Beers list, ticlopidine has been shown to be no better than aspirin in preventing clotting and may be considerably more toxic. Safer, more effective alternatives exist.

➤*Lab test abnormalities:*

Liver function – Ticlopidine HCl therapy has been associated with elevations of alkaline phosphatase, bilirubin, and transaminases, which generally occurred within 1 to 4 months of therapy initiation. In controlled clinical trials in stroke patients, the incidence of elevated alkaline phosphatase (greater than 2 times upper limit of normal [ULN]) was 7.6% in ticlopidine patients, 6% in placebo patients and 2.5% in aspirin patients. The incidence of elevated AST (greater than 2 times ULN) was 3.1% in ticlopidine patients, 4% in placebo patients and 2.1% in aspirin patients. No progressive increases were observed in closely monitored clinical trials (eg, no transaminase greater than 10 times the ULN was seen), but most patients with these abnormalities had therapy discontinued. Occasionally, patients had developed minor elevations in bilirubin.

Postmarketing experience includes rare individuals with elevations in their transaminases and bilirubin to greater than 10 × above upper limits of normal. Based on postmarketing and clinical trial experience, liver function testing, including ALT, AST, and GGT, should be considered whenever liver dysfunction is suspected, particularly during the first 4 months of treatment.

➤*Monitoring:* Starting just before initiating treatment and continuing through the third month of therapy, patients receiving ticlopidine HCl must be monitored every 2 weeks. Because of ticlopidine's long plasma half-life, patients who discontinue ticlopidine during this 3-month period should continue to be monitored for 2 weeks after discontinuation. More frequent monitoring, and monitoring after the first 3 months of therapy, is necessary only in patients with clinical signs (eg, signs or symptoms suggestive of infection) or laboratory signs (eg, neutrophil count less than 70% of the baseline count, decrease in hematocrit or platelet count) that suggest incipient hematological adverse reactions.

Clinically, fever might suggest either neutropenia, TTP or aplastic anemia; TTP might also be suggested by weakness, pallor, petechiae or purpura, dark urine (due to blood, bile pigments, or hemoglobin) or jaundice, or neurological changes. Patients should be told to discontinue ticlopidine HCl and to contact the physician immediately upon the occurrence of any of these findings.

Laboratory monitoring should include a complete blood count, with special attention to the absolute neutrophil count (WBC × percent neutrophils), platelet count, and the appearance of the peripheral smear. Ticlopidine is occasionally associated with thrombocytopenia unrelated to TTP or aplastic anemia. Any acute, unexplained reduction in hemoglobin or platelet count

TICLOPIDINE HYDROCHLORIDE — ORAL

should prompt further investigation for a diagnosis of TTP, and the appearance of schistocytes (fragmented RBCs) on the smear should be treated as presumptive evidence of TTP. A simultaneous decrease in platelet count and WBC count should prompt further investigation for a diagnosis of aplastic anemia. If there are laboratory signs of TTP, or aplastic anemia, or if the neutrophil count is confirmed to be less than 1200/mm^3, then the drug should be discontinued.

Drug Interactions

The dose of drugs with low therapeutic ratios metabolized by hepatic microsomal enzymes may require adjustment to maintain optimal therapeutic blood levels when starting or stopping concomitant therapy with ticlopidine.

Ticlopidine Drug Interactions

Precipitant drug	Object drug[a]		Description
Antacids	Ticlopidine	↓	Giving ticlopidine after antacids has resulted in an 18% decrease in ticlopidine plasma levels.
Cimetidine	Ticlopidine	↑	Chronic cimetidine administration has reduced the clearance of a single ticlopidine dose by 50%.
Ticlopidine	Aspirin	↑	Ticlopidine potentiated the effect of aspirin on collagen-induced platelet aggregation. Ticlopidine-mediated inhibition of ADP-induced platelet aggregation is not affected. Coadministration is not recommended.
Ticlopidine	Digoxin	↓	Digoxin plasma levels may decrease slightly (≈ 15%).
Ticlopidine	Phenytoin	↑	Elevated phenytoin plasma levels with associated somnolence and lethargy have been reported. Exercise caution when administering with ticlopidine. Remeasuring phenytoin levels may be useful.
Ticlopidine	Theophylline	↑	Theophylline elimination half-life was significantly increased (from 8.6 to 12.2 hr) with a comparable reduction in total plasma clearance.

[a] ↑ = Object drug increased. ↓ = Object drug decreased.

Therapeutic doses of ticlopidine HCl caused a 30% increase in the plasma half-life of antipyrine and may cause analogous effects on similarly metabolized drugs. Therefore, the dose of drugs metabolized by hepatic microsomal enzymes with low therapeutic ratios or being given to patients with hepatic impairment may require adjustment to maintain optimal therapeutic blood levels when starting or stopping concomitant therapy with ticlopidine. Studies of specific drug interactions yielded the following results:

➤*Anticoagulant drugs:* The tolerance and safety of coadministration of ticlopidine HCl with heparin, oral anticoagulants or fibrinolytic agents have not been established. In trials for cardiac stenting, patients received heparin and ticlopidine tablets concomitantly for approximately 12 hours. If a patient is switched from an anticoagulant or fibrinolytic drug to ticlopidine HCl, the former drug should be discontinued prior to ticlopidine HCl administration.

➤*Aspirin and other NSAIDs:* Ticlopidine potentiates the effect of aspirin or other NSAIDs on platelet aggregation. The safety of concomitant use of ticlopidine with aspirin or other NSAIDs has not been established. The safety of concomitant use of ticlopidine and aspirin beyond 30 days has not been established. Aspirin did not modify the ticlopidine-mediated inhibition of ADP-induced platelet aggregation, but ticlopidine potentiated the effect of aspirin on collagen-induced platelet aggregation. Caution should be exercised in patients who have lesions with a propensity to bleed, such as ulcers. Long-term concomitant use of aspirin and ticlopidine is not recommended.

➤*Propranolol:* In vitro studies demonstrated that ticlopidine does not alter the plasma protein binding of propranolol. However, the protein binding interactions of ticlopidine and its metabolites have not been studied in vivo. Caution should be exercised in coadministering this drug with ticlopidine HCl.

➤*Drug/Food interactions:* See Administration and Dosage for more information.

Adverse Reactions

Adverse reactions were relatively frequent, with greater than 50% of patients reporting at least one. Most (30% to 40%) involved the GI tract. Most adverse effects are mild, but 21% of patients discontinued therapy because of an adverse reaction, principally diarrhea, rash, nausea, vomiting, GI pain and neutropenia. Most adverse effects occur early in the course of treatment, but a new onset of adverse effects can occur after several months.

The incidence rates of adverse reactions listed in the following table were derived from multicenter, controlled clinical trials described above comparing ticlopidine HCl, placebo and aspirin over study periods of up to 5.8 years. Adverse events considered by the investigator to be probably drug related that occurred in at least 1% of patients treated with ticlopidine HCl are shown in the following table:

Percent of Patients With Adverse Reactions in Ticlopidine Controlled Studies[a]

Adverse reaction	Ticlopidine HCl (n = 2048)	Aspirin (acetylsalicylic acid) (n = 1527)	Placebo (n = 536)
Any reactions	60% (20.9%)	53.2% (14.5%)	34.3% (6.1%)
Diarrhea	12.5% (6.3%)	5.2% (1.8%)	4.5% (1.7%)
Nausea	7% (2.6%)	6.2% (1.9%)	1.7% (0.9%)
Dyspepsia	7% (1.1%)	9% (2%)	0.9% (0.2%)
Rash	5.1% (3.4%)	1.5% (0.8%)	0.6% (0.9%)
GI pain	3.7% (1.9%)	5.6% (2.7%)	1.3% (0.4%)
Neutropenia	2.4% (1.3%)	0.8 (0.1%)	1.1% (0.4%)
Purpura	2.2% (0.2%)	1.6% (0.1%)	0% (0%)
Vomiting	1.9% (1.4%)	1.4% (0.9%)	0.9% (0.4%)
Flatulence	1.5% (0.1%)	1.4% (0.3%)	0% (0%)
Pruritus	1.3% (0.8%)	0.3% (0.1%)	0% (0%)
Dizziness	1.1% (0.4%)	0.5% (0.4%)	0% (0%)
Anorexia	1% (0.4%)	0.5% (0.3%)	0% (0%)
Abnormal liver function test	1% (0.7%)	0.3% (0.3%)	0% (0%)

[a] Incidence of discontinuation, regardless of relationship to therapy, is shown in parentheses.

➤*Dermatologic:* Ticlopidine has been associated with a maculopapular or urticarial rash (often with pruritus). Rash usually occurs within 3 months of initiation of therapy with a mean onset time of 11 days. If drug is discontinued, recovery occurs within several days. Many rashes do not recur on drug rechallenge. There have been rare reports of severe rashes, including Stevens-Johnson syndrome, erythema multiforme and exfoliative dermatitis.

➤*GI:* Ticlopidine HCl therapy has been associated with a variety of GI complaints including diarrhea and nausea. The majority of cases are mild, but about 13% of patients discontinued therapy because of these. They usually occur within 3 months of initiation of therapy and typically are resolved within 1 to 2 weeks without discontinuation of therapy. If the effect is severe or persistent, therapy should be discontinued. In some cases of severe or bloody diarrhea, colitis was later diagnosed.

➤*Hematologic:* Neutropenia/thrombocytopenia, TTP, aplastic anemia, leukemia, agranulocytosis, eosinophilia, pancytopenia, thrombocytosis and bone marrow depression have been reported.

Hemorrhagic – Ticlopidine HCl has been associated with increased bleeding, spontaneous posttraumatic bleeding and perioperative bleeding including, but not limited to, GI bleeding. It has also been associated with a number of bleeding complications such as ecchymosis, epistaxis, hematuria and conjunctival hemorrhage.

Intracerebral bleeding was rare in clinical trials with ticlopidine HCl, with an incidence no greater than that seen with comparator agents (ticlopidine 0.5%, aspirin 0.6%, placebo 0.75%). It has also been reported postmarketing.

➤*Less frequent adverse reactions (probably related):* Clinical adverse experiences occurring in 0.5% to 1% of patients in the controlled trials include the following:

CNS – Headache.

Dermatologic – Urticaria.

GI – GI fullness.

Hematologic – Epistaxis.

Special senses – Tinnitus.

Miscellaneous – Asthenia, pain.

➤*Postmarketing experience:*

Miscellaneous – In addition, the following rarer, relatively serious events have also been reported from postmarketing experience: Hemolytic anemia with reticulocytosis, immune thrombocytopenia, hepatitis, hepatocellular jaundice, cholestatic jaundice, hepatic necrosis, hepatic failure, peptic ulcer, renal failure, nephrotic syndrome, hyponatremia, vasculitis, sepsis, angioedema, allergic pneumonitis and anaphylaxis, systemic lupus (positive ANA), peripheral neuropathy, serum sickness, arthropathy and myositis.

Overdosage

➤*Symptoms:* One case of deliberate overdosage with ticlopidine HCl has been reported by a foreign postmarketing surveillance program. A 38-year-old male took a single 6000 mg dose of ticlopidine HCl (equivalent to 24 standard 250 mg tablets). The only abnormalities reported were increased bleeding time and increased ALT. No special therapy was instituted and the patient recovered without sequelae.

Patient Information

Patients should be told that a decrease in the number of white blood cells (neutropenia) or platelets (thrombocytopenia) can occur with ticlopidine HCl, especially during the first 3 months of treatment and that neutropenia, if it is severe, can result in an increased risk of infection. They should be told it is critically important to obtain the scheduled blood tests to detect neutropenia or thrombocytopenia. Patients should also be reminded to contact their physicians if they experience any indication of infection such as fever, chills, or sore throat, any of which might be a consequence of neutropenia.

TICLOPIDINE HYDROCHLORIDE — ORAL

Thrombocytopenia may be part of a syndrome called TTP. Symptoms and signs of TTP, such as fever, weakness, difficulty speaking, seizures, yellowing of skin or eyes, dark or bloody urine, pallor or petechiae (pinpoint hemorrhagic spots on the skin), should be reported immediately.

All patients should be told that it may take them longer than usual to stop bleeding when they take ticlopidine HCl and that they should report any unusual bleeding to their physician. Patients should tell physicians and dentists that they are taking ticlopidine HCl before any surgery is scheduled and before any new drug is prescribed.

Patients should be told to promptly report side effects of ticlopidine HCl such as severe or persistent diarrhea, skin rashes or subcutaneous bleeding or any signs of cholestasis, such as yellow skin or sclera, dark urine, or light-colored stools.

Patients should be told to take ticlopidine HCl with food or just after eating in order to minimize GI discomfort.

Glycoprotein IIb/IIIa Inhibitors

Indications

➤*Acute coronary syndrome:* For the treatment of acute coronary syndrome, including patients who are to be managed medically and those undergoing percutaneous coronary intervention (PCI). See individual monographs for specific indications.

Actions

➤*Pharmacology:* Tirofiban and eptifibatide are antagonists of the platelet glycoprotein (GP) IIb/IIIa receptor, the major platelet surface receptor involved in platelet aggregation. GP IIb/IIIa is found only on platelets and their progenitors. Activation of its receptor function leads to the binding of fibrinogen and von Willebrand's factor to platelets and thus, platelet aggregation. These agents reversibly prevent fibrinogen, von Willebrand's factor, and other adhesion ligands from binding to the GP IIb/IIIa receptor, thereby inhibiting platelet aggregation. They inhibit ex vivo platelet aggregation in a dose- and concentration-dependent manner. Inhibition persists over the duration of the maintenance infusion and is reversible following infusion cessation.

➤*Pharmacokinetics:*

Absorption / Distribution – The recommended regimen of a loading infusion followed by a maintenance infusion produces an early peak plasma concentration that is similar to the steady-state concentration during the infusion. Steady state is reportedly achieved within 4 to 6 hours with eptifibatide. In patients with coronary artery disease, the plasma clearance of tirofiban ranges from 152 to 267 mL/min; renal clearance accounts for 39% of plasma clearance. The steady-state volume of distribution ranges from 22 to 42 L. Unbound fraction of tirofiban in human plasma is 35%, whereas eptifibatide is 75% unbound (25% bound).

Metabolism / Excretion – The half-life is approximately 2 hours for tirofiban and approximately 2.5 hours for eptifibatide. Metabolism appears to be limited. Clearance of eptifibatide in patients with coronary artery disease is 55 to 58 mL/kg/hr. These agents are cleared from the plasma largely by renal excretion, approximately 65% for tirofiban and approximately 50% for eptifibatide.

Special populations –

Renal function impairment: Plasma clearance of **tirofiban** is significantly decreased (more than 50%) in patients with creatinine clearance less than 30 mL/min, including patients requiring hemodialysis (see Administration and Dosage). Tirofiban is removed by hemodialysis.

Elderly: Plasma clearance of **tirofiban** is approximately 19% to 26% lower in elderly (older than 65 years of age) patients with coronary artery disease than in younger (65 years of age and under) patients.

Contraindications

Hypersensitivity to any component of the product; active internal bleeding or a history of bleeding diathesis within the previous 30 days; a history of thrombocytopenia following prior exposure to tirofiban; history of stroke within 30 days or any history of hemorrhagic stroke; major surgical procedure or severe physical trauma within the previous month; severe hypertension (systolic blood pressure over 180 mmHg [tirofiban], over 200 mmHg [eptifibatide] or diastolic blood pressure over 110 mmHg); concomitant use of another parenteral GP IIb/IIIa inhibitor, a history of intracranial hemorrhage, intracranial neoplasm, arteriovenous malformation or aneurysm, history, symptoms, or findings suggestive of aortic dissection, acute pericarditis (tirofiban). A platelet count less than 100,000/mm^3, serum creatinine 2 or more mg/dL (for the 180 mcg/kg bolus and the 2 mcg/kg/min infusion) or 4 or more mg/dL (for the 135 mcg/kg bolus and the 0.5 mcg/kg/min infusion), dependency on renal dialysis (eptifibatide).

Warnings/Precautions

➤*Bleeding:* Major and minor bleeding events are the most common complications encountered during therapy with tirofiban and eptifibatide. Most major bleeding occurs at the arterial access site for cardiac catheterization.

Use with caution in patients with a platelet count less than 150,000/mm^3 and in patients with hemorrhagic retinopathy.

Because these agents inhibit platelet aggregation, use caution when employed with other drugs that affect hemostasis (eg, warfarin, thrombolytics, NSAIDs, dipyridamole, ticlopidine, clopidogrel). The safety of tirofiban when used in combination with thrombolytic agents has not been established. Study regimens (n = 180) of eptifibatide administered concomitantly with the approved "accelerated" regimen of alteplase did not increase the incidence of major bleeding or transfusion compared with the incidence seen when alteplase was given alone. At high study infusion rates (1.3 mcg/kg/min and 2 mcg/kg/min), eptifibatide was associated with an increase in the incidence of bleeding and transfusions compared with the incidence seen when streptokinase was given alone.

During therapy, monitor patients for potential bleeding. When bleeding cannot be controlled with pressure, discontinue infusion of the GP IIb/IIIa inhibitor and heparin.

➤*Percutaneous coronary intervention:*

Care of the femoral artery access site – Therapy with tirofiban and eptifibatide is associated with increases in bleeding rates particularly at the site of arterial access for femoral sheath placement. Take care when attempting vascular access that only the anterior wall of the femoral artery is punctured. Prior to pulling the sheath, discontinue heparin for 3 to 4 hours and document activated clotting time (ACT) less than 180 seconds or APTT less than 45 seconds. Obtain proper hemostasis after removal of the sheaths using standard compressive techniques followed by close observation. While the vascular sheath is in place, maintain patients on complete bed rest with the head of the bed elevated 30° and the affected limb restrained in a straight position. Achieve sheath hemostasis at least 4 hours before hospital discharge.

Minimize vascular and other trauma – Minimize other arterial and venous punctures, IM injections, and the use of urinary catheters, nasotracheal intubation, and nasogastric tubes. When obtaining IV access, avoid noncompressible sites (eg, subclavian or jugular veins).

➤*Renal function impairment:* Patients with severe renal insufficiency (creatinine clearance less than 30 mL/min) showed decreased plasma clearance of **tirofiban**. Reduce the dosage of tirofiban in these patients (see Administration and Dosage).

Dose adjustment is unnecessary for **eptifibatide** in mild to moderate renal impairment; no data are available for severe impairment or dialysis.

➤*Pregnancy: Category B.* Tirofiban crosses the placenta in pregnant rats and rabbits. There are no adequate and well-controlled studies in pregnant women. Use during pregnancy only if clearly needed.

➤*Lactation:* It is not known whether GP IIb/IIIa inhibitors are excreted in breast milk. However, significant levels of tirofiban were shown to be present in rat milk. Because of the potential for adverse effects on the nursing infant, decide whether to discontinue nursing or discontinue the drug, taking into account the importance of the drug to the mother.

➤*Children:* Safety and efficacy in pediatric patients have not been established.

➤*Elderly:* Elderly patients receiving **tirofiban** with heparin or heparin alone had a higher incidence of bleeding complications than younger patients. The incremental risk of bleeding in patients treated with tirofiban in combination with heparin compared with heparin alone was similar regardless of age; however, the incremental risk of **eptifibatide**-associated bleeding was greater in the older patients. The overall incidence of nonbleeding adverse events was higher in older patients both for tirofiban with heparin and heparin alone. No dose adjustment is recommended.

➤*Monitoring:* Monitor platelet counts, hemoglobin, hematocrit, serum creatinine, and PT/APTT prior to treatment, within 6 hours following the loading infusion, and at least daily thereafter during therapy with tirofiban (or more frequently if there is evidence of significant decline). In eptifibatide patients undergoing PCI, also measure the ACT. Maintain the APTT between 50 and 70 seconds unless PCI is to be performed; during PCI, maintain the ACT between 300 and 350 seconds. If the patient experiences a platelet decrease to less than 100,000/mm^3, perform additional platelet counts to exclude pseudothrombocytopenia. If thrombocytopenia is confirmed, discontinue GP IIb/IIIa inhibitors and heparin, and appropriately monitor and treat the condition.

To monitor unfractionated heparin, monitor APTT 6 hours after the start of the heparin infusion; adjust heparin to maintain APTT at approximately 2 times control.

Drug Interactions

Glycoprotein IIb/IIIa Inhibitor Drug Interactions

Precipitant drug	Object drug[a]		Description
Aspirin Heparin	GP IIb/IIIa inhibitors	⬆	Concurrent use with heparin and aspirin has been associated with an increase in bleeding compared with heparin and aspirin alone. Use caution when using with other drugs that affect hemostasis (eg, warfarin) (see Warnings).
Levothyroxine Omeprazole	Tirofiban	⟷	Concomitant administration increased tirofiban clearance. Clinical significance is unknown.

[a] ⬆ = Object drug increased. ⟷ = Undetermined clinical effect.

Adverse Reactions

➤*Bleeding:* The most common drug-related adverse event reported during therapy was bleeding (see Warnings).

In clinical trials, incidence of major bleeding ranged from 1.4% to 2.2% (vs 0.8% to 1.6% with heparin alone) for **tirofiban** and 4.4% to 10.8% for **eptifibatide**. Incidence of minor bleeding was 10.5% to 12% (vs 6.3% to 8% with heparin alone) for tirofiban and 10.5% to 14.2% for eptifibatide.

Intracranial bleeding in 1 study was 0.1% for **tirofiban** with heparin and 0.3% for heparin alone. The overall incidence of stroke was 0.5% to 0.7% in patients receiving **eptifibatide** and 0.7% to 0.8% in placebo patients. The incidences of retroperitoneal bleeding for tirofiban with heparin and heparin alone were 0% to 0.6% and 0.1% to 0.3%, respectively. The incidences of major GI and GU bleeding for tirofiban with heparin were 0.1% to 0.2% and 0% to 0.1%, respectively.

Female and elderly patients receiving **tirofiban** with heparin or heparin alone had a higher incidence of bleeding complications than male patients or younger patients. The incremental risk of bleeding in patients treated with tirofiban in combination with heparin over the risk in patients treated with heparin alone was comparable regardless of age or gender. No dose adjustment is recommended.

Tirofiban Hydrochloride Injection Nonbleeding Adverse Reactions (> 1%)

Adverse reaction	Tirofiban + Heparin (n = 1953)	Heparin (n = 1887)
Bradycardia	4	3
Dissection, coronary artery	5	4
Dizziness	3	2
Edema/Swelling	2	1
Pain, leg	3	2
Pain, pelvic	6	5
Reaction, vasovagal	2	1
Sweating	2	1

Other nonbleeding side effects reported at more than a 1% rate with **tirofiban** administered concomitantly with heparin were nausea, fever, and headache; these side effects were reported at a similar rate in the heparin group.

The only serious nonbleeding adverse event that occurred at a rate of at least 1% and was more common with **eptifibatide** than placebo (7% vs 6%) was hypotension.

➤*Lab test abnormalities:* Decreases in hemoglobin (2.1%) and hematocrit (2.2%) were observed in the group receiving **tirofiban** compared with 3.1% and 2.6%, respectively, in the heparin group. Increases in the presence of urine and fecal occult blood also were observed (10.7% and 18.3%, respectively) in the group receiving tirofiban compared with 7.8% and 12.2%, respectively, in the heparin group.

Patients treated with **tirofiban** with heparin were more likely to experience decreases in platelet counts than the control group. These decreases were reversible upon discontinuation of tirofiban. The incidence of thrombocytopenia and platelet transfusions were similar between patients treated with **eptifibatide** and placebo.

Overdosage

➤*Symptoms:* In clinical trials, inadvertent overdosage with tirofiban occurred at doses 5 times or less and 2 times the recommended dose for bolus administration and loading infusion, respectively. Inadvertent overdosage occurred in doses 9.8 times or less than the 0.15 mcg/kg/min maintenance infusion rate.

The most frequently reported manifestation of overdosage was bleeding, primarily minor mucocutaneous bleeding events and minor bleeding at the sites of cardiac catheterization (see Warnings).

➤*Treatment:* Treat tirofiban overdosage by assessment of the patient's clinical condition and cessation or adjustment of the drug infusion as appropriate. Tirofiban can be removed by hemodialysis.

TIROFIBAN HYDROCHLORIDE

Rx	Aggrastat (Merck)	Injection: 50 mcg/mL	Preservative-free. In 250[a] and 500 mL[b] single-dose *IntraVia* containers.
		Injection, concentrate: 250 mcg/mL	Preservative-free. In 25 and 50 mL vials.[c]

[a] With 2.25 g sodium chloride and 135 mg sodium citrate dihydrate.
[b] With 4.5 g sodium chloride and 270 mg sodium citrate dihydrate.
[c] With 8 mg sodium chloride and 2.7 mg sodium citrate dihydrate.

TIROFIBAN HYDROCHLORIDE — INJECTION

For complete and comparative prescribing information, refer to the Glycoprotein IIb/IIIa Inhibitors group monograph.

Indications

➤*Acute coronary syndrome:* Tirofiban, in combination with heparin, is indicated for the treatment of acute coronary syndrome, including patients who are to be managed medically and those undergoing percutaneous transluminal coronary angioplasty (PTCA) or atherectomy. In this setting, tirofiban has been shown to decrease the rate of a combined endpoint of death, new myocardial infarction (MI) or refractory ischemia/repeat cardiac procedure.

Administration and Dosage

➤*Adults:*

Acute coronary syndrome –

Usual dosage: Initial rate of 0.4 mcg/kg/min IV for 30 minutes and then continued at 0.1 mcg/kg/min.

The information below is provided as a guide to dosage adjustment by weight.

Tirofiban Hydrochloride Injection Dosage Adjustment by Weight

Patient weight (kg)	Most patients: 30-minute loading infusion rate (mL/hr)	Most patients: Maintenance infusion rate (mL/hr)
30 to 37	16	4
38 to 45	20	5
46 to 54	24	6
55 to 62	28	7
63 to 70	32	8
71 to 79	36	9
80 to 87	40	10
88 to 95	44	11
96 to 104	48	12
105 to 112	52	13
113 to 120	56	14
121 to 128	60	15
129 to 137	64	16
138 to 145	68	17
146 to 153	72	18

Duration of therapy: In PRISM-PLUS, tirofiban was administered in combination with heparin for 48 to 108 hours. The infusion should be continued through angiography and for 12 to 24 hours after angioplasty or atherectomy.

Concomitant therapy: In the clinical studies, patients received aspirin, unless it was contraindicated, and heparin.

➤*Renal function impairment:* Patients with severe renal insufficiency (creatinine clearance less than 30 mL/min) should receive half the usual rate of infusion.

Tirofiban Hydrochloride Injection Recommended Dosage for Renal Impairment

Patient weight (kg)	Severe renal impairment: 30-minute loading infusion rate (mL/hr)	Severe renal impairment: Maintenance infusion rate (mL/hr)
30 to 37	8	2
38 to 45	10	3
46 to 54	12	3
55 to 62	14	4
63 to 70	16	4
71 to 79	18	5
80 to 87	20	5
88 to 95	22	6
96 to 104	24	6
105 to 112	26	7
113 to 120	28	7
121 to 128	30	8
129 to 137	32	8
138 to 145	34	9
146 to 153	36	9

➤*Preparation for administration:*

Concentrate – Tirofiban concentrated injection is first diluted to the same strength as tirofiban injection premixed as follows: Withdraw and discard 100 mL from a 500 mL bag of sterile 0.9% sodium chloride or 5% dextrose in water and replace this volume with 100 mL of tirofiban injection (from two 50 mL vials), or withdraw and discard 50 mL from a 250 mL bag of sterile 0.9% sodium chloride or 5% dextrose in water and replace this volume with

TIROFIBAN HYDROCHLORIDE — INJECTION

50 mL of tirofiban injection (from one 50 mL vial), to achieve a final concentration of 50 mcg/mL. Mix well prior to administration.

Premixed – Tirofiban injection premixed is supplied as 500 mL of sodium chloride 0.9% containing tirofiban 50 mcg/mL. It is supplied in plastic containers (PL 2408 plastic). To open the container, first tear off its dust cover. The plastic may be somewhat opaque because of moisture absorption during sterilization; the opacity will diminish gradually. Check for leaks by squeezing the inner bag firmly; if any leaks are found, the sterility is suspect and the solution should be discarded. Do not use unless the solution is clear and the seal is intact. Suspend the container from its eyelet support, remove the plastic protector from the outlet port, and attach a conventional administration set.

➤*Administration:* Administer IV. Tirofiban and heparin can be administered through the same IV catheter.

Tirofiban is intended for IV delivery using sterile equipment and technique. Do not add other drugs or remove solution directly from the bag with a syringe. Do not use plastic containers in series connections; such use can result in air embolism by drawing air from the first container if it is empty of solution. Any unused solution should be discarded.

➤*Admixture compatibility:*

Compatibility – Tirofiban may be administered in the same IV line as dopamine, lidocaine, potassium chloride, and famotidine injection. Tirofiban and heparin can be administered through the same IV catheter.

Incompatibility – Tirofiban should not be administered in the same IV line as diazepam.

➤*Storage / Stability:*

Concentrate – Store at 25°C (77°F), with excursions permitted between 15° to 30°C (59° to 86°F). Do not freeze. Protect from light during storage.

Premixed – Store at 25°C (77°F), with excursions permitted between 15° to 30°C (59° to 86°F). Do not freeze. Protect from light during storage.

EPTIFIBATIDE

Rx **Integrilin** (Schering)	**Injection for solution:** 0.75 mg/mL	In 100 mL vials.
	2 mg/mL	In 10 and 100 mL vials.

EPTIFIBATIDE — INJECTION

For complete and comparative prescribing information, refer to the Glycoprotein IIb/IIIa Inhibitors group monograph.

Indications

➤*Acute coronary syndrome:* For the treatment of patients with acute coronary syndrome (unstable angina [UA]/non-ST-segment elevation myocardial infarction [NSTEMI]), including patients who are to be managed medically and those undergoing percutaneous coronary intervention (PCI). In this setting, eptifibatide has been shown to decrease the rate of a combined endpoint of death or new myocardial infarction.

➤*Patients undergoing PCI:* For the treatment of patients undergoing PCI, including those undergoing intracoronary stenting. In this setting, eptifibatide has been shown to decrease the rate of a combined endpoint of death, new myocardial infarction, or need for urgent intervention.

Administration and Dosage

➤*General dosing considerations:* Patients requiring thrombolytic therapy should have eptifibatide infusions stopped.

➤*Adults:*

Acute coronary syndrome –

Usual dosage: 180 mcg/kg as an IV bolus as soon as possible following diagnosis, followed by a continuous infusion of 2 mcg/kg/min until hospital discharge or initiation of coronary artery bypass graft (CABG) surgery, up to 72 hours. If a patient is to undergo a PCI while receiving eptifibatide, the infusion should be continued up to hospital discharge, or for up to 18 to 24 hours after the procedure, whichever comes first, allowing for up to 96 hours of therapy.

Concomitant therapy:

• *Aspirin* – 160 to 325 mg orally (by mouth) initially and daily thereafter.

• *Heparin* – Target activated partial thromboplastin time (aPTT) 50 to 70 seconds during medical management for the following:

• If weight is greater than or equal to 70 kg, 5,000 units bolus followed by infusion of 1,000 units/h.

• If weight is less than 70 kg, 60 units/kg bolus followed by infusion of 12 units/kg/h.

Target activated clotting time (ACT) 200 to 300 seconds during PCI for the following:

• If heparin is initiated prior to PCI, additional boluses during PCI to maintain an ACT target of 200 to 300 seconds.

• Heparin infusion after the PCI is discouraged.

Percutaneous coronary intervention:

• *Usual dosage* – 180 mcg/kg as an IV bolus administered immediately before the initiation of PCI followed by a continuous infusion of 2 mcg/kg/min and a second 180 mcg/kg bolus 10 minutes after the first bolus. Infusion should be continued until hospital discharge, or for up to 18 to 24 hours, whichever comes first. A minimum of 12 hours of infusion is recommended.

• *Concomitant therapy* –

Aspirin: 160 to 325 mg orally (by mouth) 1 to 24 hours prior to PCI and daily thereafter.

Heparin: Target ACT 200 to 300 seconds for the following:

• 60 units/kg bolus initially in patients not treated with heparin within 6 hours prior to PCI.

• Additional boluses during PCI to maintain ACT within target.

• Heparin infusion after the PCI is strongly discouraged.

• *Discontinuation of therapy* – In patients who undergo coronary artery bypass graft surgery, eptifibatide infusion should be discontinued prior to surgery.

➤*Renal function impairment:* Total drug clearance is decreased by approximately 50% and steady-state plasma eptifibatide concentrations are doubled in patients with an estimated creatinine clearance (CrCl) less than 50 mL/min (using the Cockroft-Gault equation). Therefore, the infusion dose should be reduced to 1 mcg/kg/min in such patients. If an estimated CrCl is not available, the infusion dose should be reduced in patients with a serum creatinine greater than 2 mg/dL. There has been no clinical experience in patients dependent on dialysis.

Acute coronary syndrome – 180 mcg/kg IV bolus as soon as possible following diagnosis, immediately followed by a continuous infusion of 1 mcg/kg/min in patients with CrCl less than 50 mL/min or serum creatinine greater than 2 mg/dL.

Percutaneous coronary intervention – 180 mcg/kg IV bolus administered immediately before the initiation of the procedure, immediately followed by a continuous infusion of 1 mcg/kg/min and a second 180 mcg/kg bolus administered 10 minutes after the first. Administer in patients with a CrCl less than 50 mL/min or serum creatinine greater than 2 mg/dL.

➤*Administration:* Eptifibatide is to be administered by volume according to patient weight. Patients should receive eptifibatide according to the following table:

Eptifibatide Dosing Charts by Weight

Patient weight		180 mcg/kg bolus volume	2 mcg/kg/min infusion volume		1 mcg/kg/min infusion volume	
kg	lb	(from 2 mg/mL vial)	(from 2 mg/mL 100 mL vial)	(from 0.75 mg/mL 100 mL vial)	(from 2 mg/mL 100 mL vial)	from 0.75 mg/mL 100 mL vial)
37 to 41 kg	81 to 91 lb	3.4 mL	2 mL/h	6 mL/h	1 mL/h	3 mL/h
42 to 46 kg	92 to 102 lb	4 mL	2.5 mL/h	7 mL/h	1.3 mL/h	3.5 mL/h
47 to 53 kg	103 to 117 lb	4.5 mL	3 mL/h	8 mL/h	1.5 mL/h	4 mL/h
54 to 59 kg	118 to 130 lb	5 mL	3.5 mL/h	9 mL/h	1.8 mL/h	4.5 mL/h
60 to 65 kg	131 to 143 lb	5.6 mL	3.8 mL/h	10 mL/h	1.9 mL/h	5 mL/h
66 to 71 kg	144 to 157 lb	6.2 mL	4 mL/h	11 mL/h	2 mL/h	5.5 mL/h
72 to 78 kg	158 to 172 lb	6.8 mL	4.5 mL/h	12 mL/h	2.3 mL/h	6 mL/h
79 to 84 kg	173 to 185 lb	7.3 mL	5 mL/h	13 mL/h	2.5 mL/h	6.5 mL/h
85 to 90 kg	186 to 198 lb	7.9 mL	5.3 mL/h	14 mL/h	2.7 mL/h	7 mL/h
91 to 96 kg	199 to 212 lb	8.5 mL	5.6 mL/h	15 mL/h	2.8 mL/h	7.5 mL/h
97 to 103 kg	213 to 227 lb	9 mL	6 mL/h	16 mL/h	3 mL/h	8 mL/h
104 to 109 kg	228 to 240 lb	9.5 mL	6.4 mL/h	17 mL/h	3.2 mL/h	8.5 mL/h
110 to 115 kg	241 to 253 lb	10.2 mL	6.8 mL/h	18 mL/h	3.4 mL/h	9 mL/h
116 to 121 kg	254 to 267 lb	10.7 mL	7 mL/h	19 mL/h	3.5 mL/h	9.5 mL/h
> 121 kg	> 267 lb	11.3 mL	7.5 mL/h	20 mL/h	3.7 mL/h	10 mL/h

Bolus – The bolus dose(s) of eptifibatide should be withdrawn from the 10 mL vial into a syringe. The bolus dose(s) should be administered by IV push.

Continuous infusion – Immediately following the bolus dose administration, a continuous infusion of eptifibatide should be initiated. When using an IV infusion pump, eptifibatide should be administered undiluted directly from the 100 mL vial. The 100 mL vial should be spiked with a vented infusion set. Care should be taken to center the spike within the circle on the stopper top.

➤*Admixture compatibility:*

Compatibility – Eptifibatide may be administered in the same IV line as alteplase, atropine, dobutamine, heparin, lidocaine, meperidine, metoprolol, midazolam, morphine, nitroglycerin, or verapamil.

Eptifibatide may be administered in the same IV line with 0.9% NaCl or 0.9% NaCl/5% dextrose. With either vehicle, the infusion may also contain up to 60 mEq/L of potassium chloride. No incompatibilities have been observed with IV administration sets. No compatibility studies have been performed with PVC bags.

Incompatibility – Eptifibatide should not be administered through the same IV line as furosemide.

➤*Storage / Stability:* Vials should be stored refrigerated at 2° to 8°C (36° to 46°F). Vials may be transferred to room temperature storage for a period not to exceed 2 months. Upon transfer, vial cartons must be marked

EPTIFIBATIDE — INJECTION

by the dispensing pharmacist with a "discard by" date (2 months from the transfer date or the labeled expiration date, whichever comes first).

Protect from light until administration. Discard any unused portion left in the vial.

Store at controlled room temperature 25°C (77°F); excursions are permitted between 15° and 30°C (59° and 86°F).

ABCIXIMAB

Rx	**ReoPro** (Lilly)	**Injection:** 2 mg/mL	In buffered solution of 0.01 molar (M) sodium phosphate and 0.15 M sodium chloride. Preservative free. In 5 mL single-use vials.

ABCIXIMAB — INJECTION

Indications

➤*Adjunct to percutaneous coronary intervention (PCI):* Adjunct to PCI for the prevention of cardiac ischemic complications in patients undergoing PCI and in patients with unstable angina not responding to conventional medical therapy when PCI is planned within 24 hours.

➤*General information:* Abciximab is intended for use with aspirin and heparin and has been studied only in that setting.

➤*Off-label uses:*

Acute ischemic stroke – [4] = Insufficient documentation. Guidelines state that intravenous (IV) administration of glycoprotein IIb/IIIa inhibitors such as abciximab is not recommended outside of clinical trials (class III, level of evidence B). Some patients respond to an IV glycoprotein IIb/IIIa inhibitor, but compared with placebo, the results generally show no difference for most outcome measures.

Early treatment of acute myocardial infarction – [1] = Good documentation. Early abciximab administration before PCI in patients with ST-segment elevation myocardial infarction (STEMI) is recommended in American College of Cardiology/American Heart Association practice guidelines.

Other possible off-label uses – For the early treatment of acute myocardial infarction (MI). Abciximab has been shown to facilitate the rate and extent of thrombolysis when combined with low-dose alteplase or low-dose reteplase.

Administration and Dosage

➤*Adults:*

Adjunct to percutaneous coronary intervention –

Usual dosage: 0.25 mg/kg intravenous (IV) bolus administered 10 to 60 minutes before the start of percutaneous coronary intervention (PCI), followed by a continuous IV infusion of 0.125 mcg/kg/min (to a maximum of 10 mcg/min) for 12 hours.

Maximum dose: 10 mcg/min.

Alternative dosage: Patients with unstable angina not responding to conventional medical therapy and who are planned to undergo PCI within 24 hours may be treated with an abciximab 0.25 mg/kg IV bolus followed by an 18- to 24-hour IV infusion of 10 mcg/min, concluding 1 hour after the PCI.

Concomitant therapy: The safety and efficacy of abciximab have only been investigated with coadministration of heparin and aspirin.

Discontinuation of therapy: In the event of serious bleeding that cannot be controlled by compression, abciximab and heparin should be discontinued immediately.

In patients with failed PCIs, the continuous infusion of abciximab should be stopped because there is no evidence for abciximab efficacy in this setting.

Off-label dosing –

Acute ischemic stroke: [4] = Insufficient documentation. An initial bolus of abciximab 0.25 mg/kg given IV, followed by a 12-hour infusion of 0.125 mcg/kg/min (maximum, 10 mcg/min).

Early treatment of acute myocardial infarction: [1] = Good documentation. 0.25 mg/kg by IV bolus, given 10 to 60 minutes before the start of PCI, followed by a continuous infusion of 0.125 mcg/kg/min (maximum, 10 mcg/min) for 12 hours.

➤*Elderly:* See Adults for dosing.

➤*Administration:*

Bolus – Withdraw the necessary amount of abciximab for bolus injection into a syringe. Filter the bolus injection using a sterile, nonpyrogenic, low-protein-binding 0.2 or 5 mcm syringe filter (millipore SLGVO25LS or SLSVO25LS, or equivalent).

Continuous infusion – Withdraw the necessary amount of abciximab for the continuous infusion into a syringe. Inject into an appropriate container of sterile saline 0.9% or dextrose 5% and infuse at the calculated rate via a continuous infusion pump. The continuous infusion should be filtered upon admixture using a sterile, nonpyrogenic, low-protein-binding 0.2- or 5-mcm syringe filter (millipore SLGVO25LS or SLSVO25LS, or equivalent) or upon administration using an inline, sterile, nonpyrogenic, low-protein-binding 0.2- or 0.22-mcm filter (Abbott #4524 or equivalent). Discard the unused portion at the end of the infusion.

Hypersensitivity reactions – Hypersensitivity reactions should be anticipated whenever protein solutions such as abciximab are administered. Epinephrine, dopamine, theophylline, antihistamines, and corticosteroids should be available for immediate use. If symptoms of an allergic reaction or anaphylaxis appear, the infusion should be stopped and appropriate treatment given.

➤*Admixture compatibility:* Abciximab should be administered in a separate IV line whenever possible and not mixed with other medications.

➤*Storage / Stability:* Vials should be stored at 2° to 8°C (36° to 46°F). Do not freeze. Do not shake. Do not use beyond the expiration date. Discard any unused portion left in the vial.

Actions

➤*Pharmacology:* Abciximab binds to the intact platelet GPIIb/IIIa receptor, which is a member of the integrin family of adhesion receptors and the major platelet surface receptor involved in platelet aggregation. Abciximab inhibits platelet aggregation by preventing the binding of fibrinogen, von Willebrand factor, and other adhesive molecules to GPIIb/IIIa receptor sites on activated platelets. The mechanism of action is thought to involve steric hindrance or conformational effects to block access of large molecules to the receptor rather than direct interaction with the RGD (arginine-glycine-aspartic acid) binding site of GPIIb/IIIa.

Abciximab binds with similar affinity to the vitronectin receptor, also known as the $\alpha_v\beta_3$ integrin. The vitronectin receptor mediates the procoagulant properties of platelets and the proliferative properties of vascular endothelial and smooth muscle cells. In in vitro studies using a model cell line derived from melanoma cells, abciximab blocked $\alpha_v\beta_3$-mediated effects, including cell adhesion (50% inhibitory concentration $[IC_{50}] = 0.34$ mcg/mL). At concentrations that provide greater than 80% GPIIb/IIIa receptor blockade in vivo, but above the in vivo therapeutic range, abciximab more effectively blocked the burst of thrombin generation that followed platelet activation than select comparator antibodies that inhibit GPIIb/IIIa alone. The relationship of these in vitro data to clinical efficacy is unknown.

Abciximab also binds to the activated Mac-1 receptor on monocytes and neutrophils. In in vitro studies, abciximab and 7E3 immunoglobulin G blocked Mac-1 receptor function, as evidenced by inhibition of monocyte adhesion. In addition, the degree of activated Mac-1 expression on circulating leukocytes and the numbers of circulating leukocyte-platelet complexes has been shown to be reduced in patients treated with abciximab compared with control patients. The relationship of these in vitro data to clinical efficacy is uncertain.

Pharmacodynamics – In humans, IV administration of single bolus doses of abciximab from 0.15 to 0.3 mg/kg produced rapid dose-dependent inhibition of platelet function, as measured by ex vivo platelet aggregation in response to adenosine diphosphate or by prolongation of bleeding time. At the 2 highest doses (0.25 and 0.3 mg/kg) at 2 hours post injection (the first time point evaluated), more than 80% of the GPIIb/IIIa receptors were blocked and platelet aggregation in response to adenosine diphosphate 20 mcM was almost abolished. The median bleeding time increased to over 30 minutes at both doses compared with a baseline value of approximately 5 minutes.

In humans, IV administration of a single bolus dose of 0.25 mg/kg followed by a continuous infusion of 10 mcg/min for periods of 12 to 96 hours produced sustained high-grade GPIIb/IIIa receptor blockade (80% or more) and inhibition of platelet function (ex vivo platelet aggregation in response to adenosine diphosphate 5 or 20 mcM less than 20% of baseline and bleeding time more than 30 minutes) for the duration of the infusion in most patients. Similar results were obtained when a weight-adjusted infusion dose (0.125 mcg/kg/min to a maximum of 10 mcg/min) was used in patients weighing up to 80 kg. Results in patients who received the 0.25 mg/kg bolus followed by a 5 mcg/min infusion for 24 hours showed a similar initial receptor blockade and inhibition of platelet aggregation, but the response was not maintained throughout the infusion period. The onset of abciximab-mediated platelet inhibition following a 0.25 mg/kg bolus and 0.125 mcg/kg/min infusion was rapid, and platelet aggregation was reduced to less than 20% of baseline in 8 of 10 patients at 10 minutes after treatment initiation.

Low levels of GPIIb/IIIa receptor blockade are present for more than 10 days following cessation of the infusion. After discontinuation of abciximab infusion, platelet function gradually returns to normal. Bleeding time returned to 12 minutes or less within 12 hours following the end of infusion in 15 of 20 patients (75%) and within 24 hours in 18 of 20 patients (90%). Ex vivo platelet aggregation in response to adenosine diphosphate 5 mcM returned to 50% or more of baseline within 24 hours following the end of infusion in 11 of 32 patients (34%) and within 48 hours in 23 of 32 patients (72%). In response to adenosine diphosphate 20 mcM, ex vivo platelet aggregation returned to 50% or more of baseline within 24 hours in 20 of 32 patients (62%) and within 48 hours in 28 of 32 patients (88%).

➤*Pharmacokinetics:*

Absorption – IV administration of a 0.25 mg/kg bolus dose of abciximab followed by continuous infusion of 10 mcg/min (or a weight-adjusted infusion of 0.125 mcg/kg/min to a maximum of 10 mcg/min) produces approximately constant free-plasma concentrations throughout the infusion.

Excretion – Following IV bolus administration, free-plasma concentrations of abciximab decrease rapidly with an initial half-life of less than 10 minutes and a second phase half-life of about 30 minutes, probably related to rapid binding to the platelet GPIIb/IIIa receptors. Platelet function generally recovers over the course of 48 hours, although abciximab remains in the circulation for 15 days or more in a platelet-bound state. At

ABCIXIMAB — INJECTION

the termination of the infusion period, free-plasma concentrations fall rapidly for approximately 6 hours then decline at a slower rate.

Contraindications

Active internal bleeding; administration of oral anticoagulants within 7 days unless prothrombin time is 1.2 or less times control; bleeding diathesis; history of cerebrovascular accident (CVA) within 2 years, or CVA with a significant residual neurological deficit; intracranial neoplasm, arteriovenous malformation, or aneurysm; recent (within 6 weeks) GI or GU bleeding of clinical significance; known hypersensitivities to any component of this product or to murine proteins; presumed or documented history of vasculitis; recent (within 6 weeks) major surgery or trauma; severe uncontrolled hypertension; thrombocytopenia (less than 100,000 cells/mcL); use of IV dextran before PCI or intent to use it during an intervention.

Warnings/Precautions

➤*Bleeding:* Abciximab has the potential to increase the risk of bleeding, particularly in the presence of anticoagulation (eg, from heparin, other anticoagulants, or thrombolytics).

The risk of major bleeds due to abciximab therapy is increased in patients receiving thrombolytics; weigh this risk against the anticipated benefits.

Should serious bleeding occur that is not controllable with pressure, stop the infusion of abciximab and any concomitant heparin.

To minimize the risk of bleeding with abciximab, it is important to use a low-dose, weight-adjusted heparin regimen, a weight-adjusted abciximab bolus and infusion, strict anticoagulation guidelines, careful vascular access-site management, discontinuation of heparin after the procedure, and early femoral arterial sheath removal.

Therapy with abciximab requires careful attention to all potential bleeding sites (including catheter insertion sites, arterial and venous puncture sites, cutdown sites, needle puncture sites, and GI, GU, pulmonary [alveolar], and retroperitoneal sites).

Minimize arterial and venous punctures, intramuscular injections, and use of urinary catheters, nasotracheal intubation, nasogastric tubes, and automatic blood pressure cuffs. When obtaining IV access, avoid noncompressible sites (eg, subclavian or jugular veins). Consider saline or heparin locks for blood drawing. Document and monitor vascular puncture sites. Provide gentle care when removing dressings.

Femoral artery access site – Arterial access-site care is important to prevent bleeding. Take care when attempting vascular access so that only the anterior wall of the femoral artery is punctured, avoiding a Seldinger (through and through) technique for obtaining sheath access. Avoid femoral vein sheath placement unless needed. While the vascular sheath is in place, maintain patients on complete bed rest with the head of the bed 30° or less and the affected limb restrained in a straight position. Patients may be medicated for back/groin pain as necessary.

Discontinuation of heparin immediately upon completion of the procedure and removal of the arterial sheath within 6 hours is strongly recommended if activated partial thromboplastin time (APTT) is 50 seconds or less or ACT is 175 seconds or less. In all circumstances, discontinue heparin at least 2 hours prior to arterial sheath removal.

Following sheath removal, apply pressure to the femoral artery for at least 30 minutes using either manual compression or a mechanical device for hemostasis. Apply a pressure dressing following hemostasis. Maintain the patient on bed rest for 6 to 8 hours following sheath removal or discontinuation of abciximab, or 4 hours following discontinuation of heparin, whichever is later. Remove the pressure dressing prior to ambulation. Frequently check the sheath insertion site and distal pulses of affected leg(s) while the femoral artery sheath is in place and for 6 hours after femoral artery sheath removal. Measure any hematoma and monitor for enlargement.

The following conditions have been associated with an increased risk of bleeding and may be additive with the effect of abciximab in the angioplasty setting: PCI within 12 hours of the onset of symptoms for acute MI, prolonged PCI (lasting more than 70 minutes), and failed PCI.

➤*Thrombocytopenia:* Thrombocytopenia, including severe thrombocytopenia, has been observed with abciximab administration. Monitor platelet counts prior to, during, and after treatment with abciximab. Differentiate between decreases in platelet count and true thrombocytopenia and pseudothrombocytopenia. If true thrombocytopenia is verified, discontinue abciximab immediately and monitor and treat the condition appropriately.

In clinical trials, patients who developed thrombocytopenia were followed with daily platelet counts until their platelet count returned to normal. Heparin and aspirin were discontinued for platelet counts below 60,000 cells/mcL and platelets were transfused for a platelet count below 50,000 cells/mcL. Most cases of severe thrombocytopenia (less than 50,000 cells/mcL) occurred within the first 24 hours of abciximab administration.

In a registry study of abciximab readministration, a history of thrombocytopenia associated with prior use of abciximab was predictive of an increased risk of recurrent thrombocytopenia. Readministration within 30 days was associated with an increased incidence and severity of thrombocytopenia, as was a positive human antichimeric antibody (HACA) test at baseline, compared with the rates seen in studies with first administration.

➤*Restoration of platelet function:* In the event of serious uncontrolled bleeding or the need for emergency surgery, discontinue abciximab. If platelet function does not return to normal, it may be restored, at least in part, with platelet transfusions.

➤*Readministration:* Administration of abciximab may result in HACA formation, which could potentially cause allergic or hypersensitivity reactions (including anaphylaxis), thrombocytopenia, or diminished benefit upon readministration of abciximab.

Readministration of abciximab to patients undergoing PCI was assessed in a registry that included 1,342 treatments in 1,286 patients. Most patients were receiving their second abciximab exposure; 15% were receiving the third or subsequent exposure. The overall rate of HACA positivity prior to the readministration was 6% and increased to 27% post-readministration. There were no reports of serious allergic reactions or anaphylaxis. Thrombocytopenia was observed at higher rates in the readministration study than in the phase 3 studies of first-time administration, suggesting that readministration may be associated with an increased incidence and severity of thrombocytopenia.

➤*Concomitant therapy:* In the EPIC, EPILOG, CAPTURE, and EPISTENT trials, abciximab was used concomitantly with heparin and aspirin. Because abciximab inhibits platelet aggregation, employ caution when it is used with other drugs that affect hemostasis, including thrombolytics, oral anticoagulants, nonsteroidal anti-inflammatory drugs, dipyridamole, and ticlopidine.

In the EPIC trial, there was limited experience with the administration of abciximab with low molecular weight dextran. Low molecular weight dextran was usually given for the deployment of a coronary stent, for which oral anticoagulants were also given. In the 11 patients who received low molecular weight dextran with abciximab, 5 had major bleeding events and 4 had minor bleeding events. None of the 5 placebo patients treated with low molecular weight dextran had a major or minor bleeding event.

Because of observed synergistic effects on bleeding, use abciximab therapy judiciously in patients who have received systemic thrombolytic therapy. The GUSTO V trial randomized patients with acute MI to treatment with combined abciximab and half-dose reteplase, or full-dose reteplase alone. In this trial, the incidence of moderate or severe nonintracranial bleeding was increased in patients receiving abciximab and half-dose reteplase versus those receiving reteplase alone (4.6% vs 2.3%, respectively).

➤*Hypersensitivity reactions:* Allergic reactions, including anaphylaxis (sometimes fatal), have been reported rarely in patients treated with abciximab. Patients with allergic reactions should receive appropriate treatment. Treatment of anaphylaxis should include immediate discontinuation of abciximab administration and initiation of resuscitative measures.

Patients with HACA titers may have allergic or hypersensitivity reactions when treated with other diagnostic or therapeutic monoclonal antibodies.

➤*Pregnancy: Category C.* Animal reproduction studies have not been conducted with abciximab. It is also not known whether abciximab can cause fetal harm when administered to a pregnant woman or can affect reproduction capacity. Only give abciximab to a pregnant woman if clearly needed.

➤*Lactation:* It is not known whether this drug is excreted in human milk or absorbed systemically after ingestion. Because many drugs are excreted in human milk, exercise caution when abciximab is administered to a breast-feeding woman.

➤*Children:* Safety and effectiveness in children have not been studied.

➤*Monitoring:* Monitor platelet counts prior to treatment, 2 to 4 hours following the bolus dose of abciximab, and at 24 hours or prior to discharge, whichever is first. If a patient experiences an acute platelet decrease (eg, a platelet decrease to less than 100,000 cells/mcL and a decrease of at least 25% from pretreatment value), determine additional platelet counts. Continue platelet monitoring until platelet counts return to normal.

To exclude pseudothrombocytopenia, a laboratory artifact due to in vitro anticoagulant interaction, draw blood samples in 3 separate tubes containing ethylenediaminetetraacetic acid (EDTA), citrate, and heparin, respectively. A low platelet count in EDTA but not in heparin and/or citrate is supportive of a diagnosis of pseudothrombocytopenia.

Before infusion of abciximab, measure platelet count, prothrombin time, ACT, and APTT to identify preexisting hemostatic abnormalities.

Based on an integrated analysis of data from all studies, utilize the following guidelines to minimize the risk for bleeding:

- When abciximab is initiated 18 to 24 hours before PCI, maintain the APTT between 60 and 85 seconds during the abciximab and heparin infusion period.
- During PCI, maintain the ACT between 200 and 300 seconds.
- If anticoagulation is continued in these patients following PCI, maintain the APTT between 55 and 75 seconds.
- Check the APTT or ACT prior to arterial sheath removal. Do not remove the sheath unless APTT is 50 seconds or less or ACT is 175 seconds or less.

Drug Interactions

➤*Thrombolytics, anticoagulants, and other antiplatelet agents:* Because abciximab inhibits platelet aggregation, employ caution when it is used with other drugs that affect hemostasis, including thrombolytics, oral anticoagulants, nonsteroidal anti-inflammatory drugs, dipyridamole, and ticlopidine.

Adverse Reactions

➤*Bleeding:* Abciximab has the potential to increase the risk of bleeding, particularly in the presence of anticoagulation (eg, from heparin, other anticoagulants, or thrombolytics).

In the EPIC trial, in which a non–weight-adjusted, longer-duration heparin dose regimen was used, the most common complication during abciximab therapy was bleeding during the first 36 hours. The incidences of major

ABCIXIMAB — INJECTION

bleeding, minor bleeding, and transfusion of blood products were significantly increased. Major bleeding occurred in 10.6% of patients in the abciximab bolus-plus-infusion arm compared with 3.3% of patients in the placebo arm. Minor bleeding was seen in 16.8% of abciximab bolus-plus-infusion patients and 9.2% of placebo patients. Approximately 70% of abciximab-treated patients with major bleeding had bleeding at the arterial access site in the groin. Abciximab-treated patients also had higher incidences of major bleeding reactions from GI, GU, retroperitoneal, and other sites.

Subgroup analyses in the EPIC and CAPTURE trials showed that non-CABG major bleeding was more common in abciximab patients weighing 75 kg or less. In the EPILOG and EPISTENT trials, which used weight-adjusted heparin dosing, the non-CABG major bleeding rates for abciximab-treated patients did not differ substantially by weight subgroup.

Pulmonary alveolar hemorrhage has been rarely reported during use of abciximab. This can present with any or all of the following symptoms in close association with abciximab administration: hypoxemia, alveolar infiltrates on chest x-ray, hemoptysis, or an unexplained drop in hemoglobin.

Abciximab Non-CABG Bleeding in Trials of PCI (EPILOG, EPISTENT, and CAPTURE)

	Placebo[a] (n = 1,748)	Abciximab + low-dose heparin[b] (n = 2,525)	Abciximab + standard-dose heparin[c] (n = 918)
EPILOG and EPISTENT			
Major[d]	18 (1%)	21 (0.8%)	17 (1.9%)
Minor	46 (2.6%)	82 (3.2%)	70 (7.6%)
Requiring transfusion[e]	15 (0.9%)	13 (0.5%)	7 (0.8%)
CAPTURE			
	Placebo[f] (n = 635)		Abciximab[f] (n = 630)
Major[d]	12 (1.9%)		24 (3.8%)
Minor	13 (2%)		30 (4.8%)
Requiring transfusion[e]	9 (1.4%)		15 (2.4%)

[a] Standard-dose heparin with or without stent (EPILOG and EPISTENT).
[b] Low-dose heparin with or without stent (EPILOG and EPISTENT).
[c] Standard-dose heparin (EPILOG).
[d] Patients who had bleeding in more than 1 classification are counted only once according to the most severe classification. Patients with multiple bleeding reactions of the same classification are also counted once within that classification.
[e] Patients with major non-CABG bleeding who received packed red blood cells or whole blood transfusion.
[f] Standard-dose heparin (CAPTURE).

➤*Thrombocytopenia:* In the clinical trials, patients treated with abciximab were more likely than patients treated with placebo to experience decreases in platelet counts.

Among patients in the EPILOG and EPISTENT trials who were treated with abciximab plus low-dose heparin, the proportion of patients with any thrombocytopenia (platelets less than 100,000 cells/mcL) ranged from 2.5% to 3%. The incidence of severe thrombocytopenia (platelets less than 50,000 cells/mcL) ranged from 0.4% to 1%, and platelet transfusions were required in 0.9% to 1.1%, respectively. Modestly lower rates were observed among patients treated with placebo plus standard-dose heparin. Overall higher rates were observed among patients in the EPIC and CAPTURE trials treated with abciximab plus longer duration heparin: 2.6% to 5.2% were found to have any thrombocytopenia, 0.9% to 1.7% had severe thrombocytopenia, and 2.1% to 5.5% required platelet transfusion, respectively.

In a readministration registry study of patients receiving a second or subsequent exposure to abciximab, the incidence of any degree of thrombocytopenia was 5%, with an incidence of profound thrombocytopenia of 2% (less than 20,000 cells/mcL). Factors associated with an increased risk of thrombocytopenia were a history of thrombocytopenia on previous abciximab exposure, readministration within 30 days, and a positive HACA assay prior to the readministration.

Among 14 patients who had thrombocytopenia associated with a prior exposure to abciximab, 7 (50%) had recurrent thrombocytopenia. In 130 patients with a readministration interval of 30 days or less, 25 (19%) developed thrombocytopenia. Severe thrombocytopenia occurred in 19 of these patients. Among the 71 patients who had a positive HACA assay at baseline, 11 (15%) developed thrombocytopenia, 7 of which were severe.

➤*Allergic reactions:* There have been rare reports of allergic reactions, some of which were anaphylaxis.

➤*Immunogenicity:* As with all therapeutic proteins, there is a potential for immunogenicity. In the EPIC, EPILOG, and CAPTURE trials, positive HACA responses occurred in approximately 5.8% of patients receiving a first exposure to abciximab. No increase in hypersensitivity or allergic reactions was observed with abciximab treatments.

In a study of readministration of abciximab for patients, the overall rate of HACA positivity prior to the readministration was 6% and increased post-readministration to 27%. Among the 36 subjects receiving a fourth or greater abciximab exposure, HACA positive assays were observed post-readministration in 16 subjects (44%). There were no reports of serious allergic reactions or anaphylaxis. HACA-positive status was associated with an increased risk of thrombocytopenia.

➤*Other adverse reactions:* The following table shows adverse reactions other than bleeding and thrombocytopenia from the combined EPIC, EPILOG, and CAPTURE trials that occurred in patients in the bolus-plus-infusion arm at an incidence of more than 0.5% higher than in those treated with placebo.

Abciximab Adverse Reactions

Adverse reaction	Placebo (n = 2,226)	Bolus + infusion (n = 3,111)
Cardiovascular		
Bradycardia	79 (3.5%)	140 (4.5%)
Hypotension	230 (10.3%)	447 (14.4%)
CNS		
Headache	122 (5.5%)	200 (6.4%)
GI		
Abdominal pain	49 (2.2%)	97 (3.1%)
Nausea	255 (11.5%)	423 (13.6%)
Vomiting	152 (6.8%)	226 (7.3%)
Miscellaneous		
Back pain	304 (13.7%)	546 (17.6%)
Chest pain	208 (9.3%)	356 (11.4%)
Peripheral edema	25 (1.1%)	49 (1.6%)
Puncture-site pain	58 (2.6%)	113 (3.6%)

➤*Additional adverse reactions:* The following additional adverse reactions from the EPIC, EPILOG, and CAPTURE trials were reported by investigators for patients treated with a bolus plus infusion of abciximab at incidences that were less than 0.5% higher than those for patients in the placebo arm.

Cardiovascular – Ventricular tachycardia (1.4%); pseudoaneurysm (0.8%); palpitation (0.5%); arteriovenous fistula (0.4%); incomplete atrioventricular (AV) block (0.3%); nodal arrhythmia (0.2%); complete AV block, embolism (limb), thrombophlebitis (0.1%).

CNS – Dizziness (2.9%); anxiety (1.7%); abnormal thinking (1.3%); agitation, asthenia (0.7%); hypesthesia (0.6%); confusion (0.5%); muscle contractions (0.4%); coma, hypertonia (0.2%); diplopia (0.1%).

GI – Dyspepsia (2.1%); diarrhea (1.1%); dry mouth, enlarged abdomen, ileus (0.1%); gastroesophageal reflux (0.1%).

GU – Urinary retention (0.7%); abnormal renal function, dysuria (0.4%); cystalgia, frequent micturition, prostatitis, urinary incontinence (0.1%).

Hematologic/Lymphatic – Anemia (1.3%); leukocytosis (0.5%); petechiae (0.2%).

Musculoskeletal – Myalgia (0.2%).

Respiratory – Pneumonia, rales (0.4%); bronchitis, bronchospasm, pleural effusion (0.3%); pleurisy, pulmonary embolism (0.2%); rhonchi (0.1%).

Miscellaneous – Pain (5.4%); sweating increased (1%); incisional pain (0.6%); pruritus (0.5%); abnormal vision, edema (0.3%); abscess, cellulitis, peripheral coldness, wound (0.2%); bullous eruption, diabetes mellitus, drug toxicity, hyperkalemia, inflammation, injection-site pain, pallor (0.1%).

Overdosage

There has been no experience of overdosage in human clinical trials.

Patient Information

Advise patients that abciximab may reduce the number of blood cells that are needed for clotting. Patients should report any unusual bleeding, bruising, or blood in stools.

ANAGRELIDE HYDROCHLORIDE

Rx	**Anagrelide Hydrochloride** (Various, eg, IVAX, Roxane)	**Capsules:** 0.5 mg	In 100s and 500s.
Rx	**Agrylin** (Shire)		Lactose. (S 063). White, opaque. In 100s.
Rx	**Anagrelide Hydrochloride** (Various, eg, IVAX, Roxane)	**Capsules:** 1 mg	In 100s and 500s.

ANAGRELIDE HYDROCHLORIDE — ORAL

Indications

➤*Thrombocythemia:* For the treatment of patients with thrombocythemia, secondary to myeloproliferative disorders, to reduce the elevated platelet count and the risk of thrombosis and to ameliorate associated symptoms including thrombohemorrhagic events.

Administration and Dosage

➤*General dosing considerations:* Treatment with anagrelide should be initiated under close medical supervision.

Patients with known or suspected heart disease, renal insufficiency, or hepatic dysfunction should be monitored closely.

Maintenance dosing is not expected to be different between adult and pediatric patients.

➤*Adults:*

Thrombocythemia –

Maximum dose: Dose should not exceed 10 mg/day or 2.5 mg in a single dose.

Initial dosage: 0.5 mg 4 times daily or 1 mg 2 times daily, which should be maintained for at least 1 week.

Maintenance dosage: Typically, platelet count begins to respond within 7 to 14 days at the proper dosage. The time to complete response, defined as platelet count less than or equal to 600,000/mcL, ranged from 4 to 12 weeks. Most patients will experience an adequate response at a dosage of 1.5 to 3 mg/day.

Dosage adjustment: Dosage should be adjusted to the lowest effective dosage required to reduce and maintain platelet count below 600,000/mcL, and ideally to the normal range. The dosage should be increased by not more than 0.5 mg/day in any 1 week.

➤*Children:*

Thrombocythemia –

Maximum dose: See Adults.

Initial dosage: Starting dosages in children have ranged from 0.5 mg/day to 0.5 mg 4 times daily. Because there are limited data on the appropriate starting dosage for children, an initial dosage of 0.5 mg/day is recommended.

Maintenance dosage: See Adults.

Dosage adjustment: See Adults.

➤*Hepatic function impairment:* It is recommended that patients with moderate hepatic impairment start anagrelide therapy at a dosage of 0.5 mg/day and be maintained for a minimum of 1 week with careful monitoring of cardiovascular effects. The dosage increment must not exceed more than 0.5 mg/day in any 1 week. The potential risks and benefits of anagrelide therapy in a patient with mild and moderate impairment of hepatic function should be assessed before treatment is commenced. Use of anagrelide in patients with severe hepatic impairment has not been studied. Use of anagrelide in patients with severe hepatic impairment is contraindicated.

➤*Storage/Stability:* Store at 25°C (77°F) in a light-resistant container. Excursions permitted to 15° to 30°C (59° to 86°F).

Actions

➤*Pharmacology:* The mechanism by which anagrelide reduces blood platelet count is still under investigation. Studies in patients support a hypothesis of dose-related reduction in platelet production resulting from a decrease in megakaryocyte hypermaturation. In blood withdrawn from healthy volunteers treated with anagrelide, a disruption was found in the postmitotic phase of megakaryocyte development and a reduction in megakaryocyte size and ploidy. At therapeutic doses, anagrelide does not produce significant changes in white cell counts or coagulation parameters, and may have a small, but clinically insignificant effect on red cell parameters. Anagrelide inhibits cyclic AMP phosphodiesterase III (PDE III). PDE III inhibitors can also inhibit platelet aggregation. However, significant inhibition of platelet aggregation is observed only at doses of anagrelide higher than those required to reduce platelet count.

➤*Pharmacokinetics:*

Absorption/Distribution – The available plasma concentration time data at steady state in patients showed that anagrelide does not accumulate in plasma after repeated administration.

There were no apparent differences between patient groups (pediatric vs adult patients) for T_{max} and $t_{½}$ for anagrelide, 3-hydroxy anagrelide, or RL603.

Pharmacokinetic data obtained from healthy volunteers comparing the pharmacokinetics of anagrelide in the fed and fasted states showed that administration of an anagrelide 1 mg dose with food decreased the C_{max} 14% and increased the area under the curve (AUC) 20%.

Metabolism/Excretion – Following oral administration of ^{14}C-anagrelide in people, more than 70% of radioactivity was recovered in urine. Based on limited data, there appears to be a trend toward dose linearity between doses of 0.5 and 2 mg. At fasting and at a dose of anagrelide 0.5 mg, the plasma half-life is 1.3 hours. Two major metabolites have been identified (RL603 and 3-hydroxy anagrelide).

Special populations –

Hepatic function impairment: A pharmacokinetic study at a single dose of anagrelide 1 mg in subjects with moderate hepatic impairment showed an 8-fold increase in total exposure (AUC) to anagrelide.

Children: Pharmacokinetic data from pediatric (range, 7 to 14 years of age) and adult (range, 16 to 86 years of age) patients with thrombocythemia secondary to a myeloproliferative disorder indicate that dose and body weight-normalized exposure, C_{max}, and AUC of anagrelide were lower in the pediatric patients compared with the adult patients (C_{max} 48%, AUC_t 55%).

Contraindications

Severe hepatic impairment. Exposure to anagrelide is increased 8-fold in patients with moderate hepatic impairment. Use of anagrelide in patients with severe hepatic impairment has not been studied.

Warnings/Precautions

➤*Cardiovascular:* Use anagrelide with caution in patients with known or suspected heart disease, and only if the potential benefits of therapy outweigh the potential risks. Because of the positive inotropic effects and side effects of anagrelide, a pretreatment cardiovascular examination is recommended along with careful monitoring during treatment. In humans, therapeutic doses of anagrelide may cause cardiovascular effects, including vasodilation, tachycardia, palpitations, and congestive heart failure.

➤*Cessation of treatment:* In general, interruption of anagrelide treatment is followed by an increase in platelet count. After sudden stoppage of anagrelide therapy, the increase in platelet count can be observed within 4 days.

➤*Blood pressure:* In 9 subjects receiving a single 5 mg dose of anagrelide, standing blood pressure fell an average of 22/15 mm Hg, usually accompanied by dizziness. Only minimal changes in blood pressure were observed following a dose of 2 mg.

➤*Hepatic function impairment:* Exposure to anagrelide is increased 8-fold in patients with moderate hepatic impairment. Use of anagrelide in patients with severe hepatic impairment has not been studied. Assess the potential risks and benefits of anagrelide therapy in a patient with mild and moderate hepatic impairment before treatment begins. In patients with moderate hepatic impairment, dose reduction is required; carefully monitor patients for cardiovascular effects.

➤*Pregnancy: Category C.*

Nonteratogenic – A fertility and reproductive performance study performed in female rats revealed that anagrelide at oral dosages of 60 mg/kg/day (360 mg/m²/day, 49 times the MRHD based on body surface area) or higher disrupted implantation and exerted adverse effect on embryo/fetal survival.

A perinatal and postnatal study performed in female rats revealed that anagrelide at oral dosages of 60 mg/kg/day (360 mg/m²/day, 49 times the MRHD based on body surface area) or higher produced delay or blockage of parturition, deaths of nondelivering pregnant dams and their fully developed fetuses, and increased mortality in the pups born.

Five women became pregnant while on anagrelide treatment at dosages of 1 to 4 mg/day. Treatment was stopped as soon as they realized that they were pregnant. All delivered healthy babies. There are no adequate and well-controlled studies in pregnant women. Use anagrelide during pregnancy only if the potential benefit justifies the potential risk to the fetus.

Anagrelide is not recommended in women who are or may become pregnant. If this drug is used during pregnancy, or if the patient becomes pregnant while taking this drug, apprise the patient of the potential harm to the fetus. Instruct women of childbearing potential that they must not be pregnant and that they should use contraception while taking anagrelide. Anagrelide may cause fetal harm when administered to a pregnant woman.

➤*Lactation:* It is not known whether this drug is excreted in human milk. Because many drugs are excreted in human milk and because of the potential for serious adverse reactions in breast-feeding infants from anagrelide, decide whether to discontinue breast-feeding or discontinue the drug, taking into account the importance of the drug to the mother.

➤*Children:* The frequency of adverse reactions observed in pediatric patients was similar to adult patients. The most common adverse reactions observed in pediatric patients were fever, epistaxis, headache, and fatigue during 3 months of anagrelide treatment in the study. Adverse reactions that had been reported in these pediatric patients prior to the study and were considered to be related to anagrelide treatment based on retrospective review were palpitation, headache, nausea, vomiting, abdominal pain, back pain, anorexia, fatigue, and muscle cramps. Episodes of increased pulse rate and decreased systolic or diastolic blood pressure beyond the normal ranges in the absence of clinical symptoms were observed in some patients. Reported adverse reactions were consistent with the known pharmacological profile of anagrelide and the underlying disease. There were no apparent trends or differences in the types of adverse reactions observed between the pediatric patients compared with those of the adult patients. No overall difference in dosing and safety were observed between pediatric and adult patients.

In another open-label study, anagrelide had been used successfully in 12 pediatric patients (range, 6.8 to 17.4 years of age; 6 men and 6 women), including 8 patients with ET, 2 patients with CML, 1 patient with PV, and 1

ANAGRELIDE HYDROCHLORIDE — ORAL

patient with OMPD. Patients were started on therapy with 0.5 mg 4 times daily up to a maximum daily dose of 10 mg. The median duration of treatment was 18.1 months with a range of 3.1 to 92 months. Three patients received treatment for more than 3 years. Other adverse reactions reported in spontaneous reports and literature reviews include anemia, cutaneous photosensitivity, and elevated leukocyte count.

➤*Monitoring:* Anagrelide therapy requires close clinical supervision of the patient. While the platelet count is being lowered (usually during the first 2 weeks of treatment), monitor blood counts (hemoglobin, white blood cells), liver function (AST, ALT), and renal function (serum creatinine, serum urea nitrogen [BUN]).

Closely monitor patients with known or suspected heart disease, renal insufficiency, or hepatic dysfunction.

To monitor the effect of anagrelide and prevent the occurrence of thrombocytopenia, platelet counts should be performed every 2 days during the first week of treatment and at least weekly thereafter until the maintenance dosage is reached.

Drug Interactions

Anagrelide Drug Interactions

Precipitant drug	Object drug[a]		Description
CYP1A2 inhibitors (eg, theophylline)	Anagrelide	↑	Anagrelide demonstrates some limited inhibitory activity towards CYP1A2, which may present a theoretical potential for interaction with other coadministered medicinal products sharing that clearance mechanism.
Sucralfate	Anagrelide	↓	There is a single case report that suggests that sucralfate may interfere with anagrelide absorption.
Anagrelide	Aspirin	↑	Anagrelide slightly enhanced the inhibition of platelet aggregation by aspirin.
Anagrelide	Cyclic AMP PDE III (eg, milrinone, enoximone, amrinone, olprinone, cilostazol)	↑	Anagrelide is an inhibitor of cyclic AMP PDE III. The effects of medicinal products with similar properties may be exacerbated by anagrelide.

[a] ↑ = Object drug increased. ↓ = Object drug decreased.

Adverse Reactions

Analysis of the adverse reactions in a population consisting of 942 patients in 3 clinical trials diagnosed with myeloproliferative diseases of varying etiology (ET: 551; PV: 117; OMPD: 274) has shown that all disease groups have the same adverse reaction profile. While most reported adverse reactions during anagrelide therapy have been mild in intensity and have decreased in frequency with continued therapy, serious adverse reactions were reported in these patients. These included the following: atrial fibrillation, cardiomegaly, cardiomyopathy, cerebrovascular accident, complete heart block, congestive heart failure, gastric/duodenal ulceration, myocardial infarction, pancreatitis, pericardial effusion, pericarditis, pleural effusion, pulmonary fibrosis, pulmonary hypertension, pulmonary infiltrates, and seizure.

Of the 942 patients treated with anagrelide for a mean duration of approximately 65 weeks, 161 (17%) were discontinued from the study because of adverse reactions or abnormal laboratory test results. The most common adverse reactions for treatment discontinuation were abdominal pain, diarrhea, edema, headache, and palpitation. Overall, the occurrence rate of all adverse reactions was 17.9 per 1,000 treatment days. The occurrence rate of adverse reactions increased at higher dosages of anagrelide.

➤*Adverse reactions with an incidence of 5% or more:*

Cardiovascular – Palpitations (26.1%); tachycardia (7.5%).

CNS – Headache (43.5%); asthenia (23.1%); dizziness (15.4%); paresthesia (5.9%).

Dermatologic – Rash, including urticaria (8.3%); pruritus (5.5%).

GI – Diarrhea (25.7%); nausea (17.1%); abdominal pain (16.4%); flatulence (10.2%); vomiting (9.7%); anorexia (7.7%); dyspepsia (5.2%).

Respiratory – Dyspnea (11.9%).

Miscellaneous – Edema (20.6%); pain, other (15%); fever (8.9%); peripheral edema (8.5%); chest pain (7.8%); pharyngitis (6.8%); malaise (6.4%); cough (6.3%); back pain (5.9%).

➤*Events with an incidence of 1% to less than 5%:*

Cardiovascular – Angina pectoris, arrhythmia, cardiovascular disease, heart failure, hypertension, postural hypotension, syncope, thrombosis, vasodilation.

CNS – Amnesia, confusion, depression, insomnia, migraine, nervousness, somnolence.

Dermatologic – Alopecia, skin disease.

GI – Aphthous stomatitis, constipation, eructation, gastritis, GI distress, GI hemorrhage, melena.

GU – Dysuria, hematuria.

Hematologic/Lymphatic – Anemia, ecchymosis, lymphadenopathy, thrombocytopenia.

Platelet counts below 100,000/mcL occurred in 84 patients (ET: 35; PV: 9; OMPD: 40), reduction below 50,000/mcL occurred in 44 patients (ET: 7; PV: 6; OMPD: 31) while on anagrelide therapy. Thrombocytopenia promptly recovered upon discontinuation of anagrelide.

Hepatic – Elevated liver enzymes were observed in 3 patients (ET: 2; OMPD: 1) during anagrelide therapy.

Musculoskeletal – Arthralgia, leg cramps, myalgia.

Renal – Renal abnormalities occurred in 15 patients (ET: 10; PV: 4; OMPD: 1). Six ET patients, 4 PV patients, and 1 with OMPD experienced renal failure (approximately 1%) while on anagrelide treatment; in 4 cases, the renal failure was considered to be possibly related to anagrelide treatment. The remaining 11 were found to have preexisting renal impairment. Doses ranged from 1.5 to 6 mg/day, with exposure periods of 2 to 12 months. No dose adjustment was required because of renal insufficiency.

Respiratory – Asthma, bronchitis, epistaxis, pneumonia, respiratory disease, rhinitis, sinusitis.

Special senses – Abnormal vision, amblyopia, diplopia, tinnitus, visual field abnormality.

Miscellaneous – Chills, dehydration, flu symptoms, hemorrhage, photosensitivity.

Overdosage

➤*Symptoms:* There are no reports of overdosage with anagrelide. Platelet reduction from anagrelide therapy is dose-related; therefore, thrombocytopenia, which can potentially cause bleeding, is expected from overdosage. If overdosage occurs, cardiac and CNS toxicity also can be expected.

➤*Treatment:* In case of overdosage, close clinical supervision of the patient is required; this especially includes monitoring of the platelet count for thrombocytopenia. Decrease or stop dosage, as appropriate, until the platelet count returns to within the normal range.

DIPYRIDAMOLE

Rx	**Dipyridamole** (Various, eg, Barr, Genetco, Moore)	Tablets: 25 mg	In 90s, 100s, 500s, 1000s, 5000s and UD 100s,
Rx	**Persantine** (Boehringer Ingelheim)		(Bl/17). Orange, sugar coated. In 100s, 1000s and UD 100s.
Rx	**Dipyridamole** (Various, eg, Barr, Genetco, Moore)	Tablets: 50 mg	In 100s, 500s, 1000s and UD 100s,
Rx	**Persantine** (Boehringer Ingelheim)		(Bl/18). Orange, sugar coated. In 100s, 1000s and UD 100s.
Rx	**Dipyridamole** (Various, eg, Barr, Genetco, Moore)	Tablets: 75 mg	In 100s, 500s, 1000s and UD 100s.
Rx	**Persantine** (Boehringer Ingelheim)		(Bl/19). Orange, sugar coated. In 100s, 500s and UD 100s.

DIPYRIDAMOLE — ORAL

Indications

➤*Thromboembolic complications:* As an adjunct to coumarin anticoagulants in the prevention of postoperative thromboembolic complications of cardiac valve replacement.

➤*Off-label uses:* At one time, dipyridamole was indicated as a "possibly effective" long-term therapy for chronic angina pectoris. The FDA, however, has withdrawn approval for this indication.

Dipyridamole in combination with aspirin has been commonly used in the prevention of myocardial reinfarction and reduction of mortality post MI. However, combination therapy appears to be no more beneficial than the use of aspirin alone.

Dipyridamole has been used in children with Kawasaki disease as an alternative to aspirin when Reye syndrome is of concern (eg, influenza or varicella infection occurs) (See Administration and Dosage).

Administration and Dosage

➤*Adults:*

Adjunctive use in prophylaxis of thromboembolism after cardiac valve replacement – 75 to 100 mg 4 times daily as an adjunct to the usual warfarin therapy.

➤*Children:*

12 years of age and older – See Adults for dosing.

Off-label dosing –

Alternative to aspirin in treatment of patients with Kawasaki disease: 4 mg/kg orally divided in 3 doses.

➤*Storage/Stability:* Store at 25°C (77°F); excursions are permitted to 15° to 30°C (59° to 86°F). Keep out of the reach of children.

DIPYRIDAMOLE — ORAL

Actions

➤*Pharmacology:* It is believed that platelet reactivity and interaction with prosthetic cardiac valve surfaces, resulting in abnormally shortened platelet survival time, is a significant factor in thromboembolic complications occurring in connection with prosthetic heart valve replacement.

Dipyridamole tablets have been found to lengthen abnormally shortened platelet survival time in a dose-dependent manner.

Dipyridamole inhibits the uptake of adenosine into platelets, endothelial cells, and erythrocytes in vitro and in vivo; the inhibition occurs in a dose-dependent manner at therapeutic concentrations (0.5 to 1.9 mcg/mL). This inhibition results in an increase in local concentrations of adenosine which acts on the platelet A_2-receptor, thereby stimulating platelet adenylate cyclase and increasing platelet cyclic-3',5'-adenosine monophosphate (cAMP) levels. Via this mechanism, platelet aggregation is inhibited in response to various stimuli such as platelet activating factor (PAF), collagen, and adenosine diphosphate (ADP).

Dipyridamole inhibits phosphodiesterase (PDE) in various tissues. While the inhibition of cAMP-PDE is weak, therapeutic levels of dipyridamole inhibit cyclic-3',5'-guanosine monophosphate-PDE (cGMP-PDE), thereby augmenting the increase in cGMP produced by endothelium-derived relaxing factor (EDRF), now identified as nitric oxide.

Hemodynamics – In dogs, intraduodenal doses of dipyridamole of 0.5 to 4 mg/kg produced dose-related decreases in systemic and coronary vascular resistance leading to decreases in systemic blood pressure and increases in coronary blood flow. Onset of action was in about 24 minutes and effects persisted for about 3 hours.

Similar effects were observed following IV dipyridamole in doses ranging from 0.025 to 2 mg/kg.

In man, the same qualitative hemodynamic effects have been observed. However, acute intravenous administration of dipyridamole may worsen regional myocardial perfusion distal to partial occlusion of coronary arteries.

➤*Pharmacokinetics:*

Absorption/Distribution – Following an oral dose of dipyridamole tablets, the average time to peak concentration is about 75 minutes. The decline in plasma concentration following a dose of dipyridamole tablets fits a 2-compartment model. The alpha half-life (the initial decline following peak concentration) is approximately 40 minutes. The beta half-life (the terminal decline in plasma concentration) is approximately 10 hours. Dipyridamole is highly bound to plasma proteins.

Metabolism/Excretion – It is metabolized in the liver where it is conjugated as a glucuronide and excreted with the bile.

Contraindications

Hypersensitivity to dipyridamole or any of the other components.

Warnings/Precautions

➤*Hepatic effects:* Elevations of hepatic enzymes and hepatic failure have been reported in association with dipyridamole administration.

➤*Special risk:*

Coronary artery disease – Dipyridamole has a vasodilatory effect and should be used with caution in patients with severe coronary artery disease (eg, unstable angina, recently sustained MI). Chest pain may be aggravated in patients with underlying coronary artery disease who are receiving dipyridamole.

Hypotension – Dipyridamole tablets should be used with caution in patients with hypotension since it can produce peripheral vasodilation.

➤*Pregnancy:* Category B.

Teratogenic – There are no adequate and well-controlled studies in pregnant women. Because animal reproduction studies are not always predictive of human response, this drug should be used during pregnancy only if clearly needed.

➤*Lactation:* As dipyridamole is excreted in human milk, caution should be exercised when dipyridamole tablets are administered to a nursing woman.

➤*Children:* Safety and effectiveness in the pediatric population below the age of 12 years have not been established.

➤*Elderly:* Per the Beers list, dipyridamole may cause orthostatic hypotension. Dipyridamole is considered a high risk medication for the elderly according to the Centers of Medicare and Medicaid Services.

➤*Lab test abnormalities:* Dipyridamole has been associated with elevated hepatic enzymes.

Drug Interactions

➤*Adenosine:* Dipyridamole has been reported to increase the plasma levels and cardiovascular effects of adenosine. Adjustment of adenosine dosage may be necessary.

➤*Cholinesterase inhibitors:* Dipyridamole may counteract the anticholinesterase effect of cholinesterase inhibitors, thereby potentially aggravating myasthenia gravis.

Adverse Reactions

Adverse reactions at therapeutic doses are usually minimal and transient. On long-term use of dipyridamole tablets initial side effects usually disappear.

Dipyridamole Adverse Reactions in 2 Heart Valve Replacement Trials

Adverse reaction	Dipyridamole tablets/warfarin (n = 147)	Placebo/warfarin (n = 170)
Dizziness	13.6%	8.2%
Abdominal distress	6.1%	3.5%
Headache	2.3%	0%
Rash	2.3%	1.1%

When dipyridamole tablets were administered concomitantly with warfarin, bleeding was no greater in frequency or severity than that observed when warfarin was administered alone.

➤*Other reactions from uncontrolled studies:*

Miscellaneous – Other reactions from uncontrolled studies include diarrhea, vomiting, flushing and pruritus. In addition, angina pectoris has been reported rarely, and there have been rare reports of liver dysfunction. On those uncommon occasions when adverse reactions have been persistent or intolerable, they have ceased on withdrawal of the medication.

➤*Postmarketing experience:*

Miscellaneous – In postmarketing reporting experience, there have been rare reports of hypersensitivity reactions (eg, rash, urticaria, severe bronchospasm, angioedema), laryngeal edema, fatigue, malaise, myalgia, arthritis, nausea, dyspepsia, paresthesia, hepatitis, thrombocytopenia, alopecia, cholelithiasis, hypotension, palpitation, and tachycardia.

Overdosage

➤*Symptoms:* Hypotension, if it occurs, is likely to be of short duration, but a vasopressor drug may be used if necessary. Symptoms of acute toxicity included ataxia, decreased locomotion and diarrhea in rodents and emesis, ataxia and depression in dogs.

In case of real or suspected overdose, seek medical attention or contact a poison control center immediately. Careful medical management is essential. Based upon the known hemodynamic effects of dipyridamole, symptoms such as warm feeling, flushes, sweating, restlessness, feeling of weakness, and dizziness may occur. A drop in blood pressure and tachycardia might also be observed.

➤*Treatment:* Symptomatic treatment is recommended, possibly including vasopressor drug. Gastric lavage should be considered. Administration of xanthine derivatives (eg, aminophylline) may reverse the hemodynamic effects of dipyridamole overdose. Since dipyridamole tablets are highly protein bound, dialysis is not likely to be of benefit.

Antiplatelet Combination Agents

DIPYRIDAMOLE AND ASPIRIN

Rx	**Aggrenox** (Boehringer Ingelheim)	**Capsules:** 200 mg extended-release dipyridamole/25 mg aspirin	Lactose, sucrose. (01A). Red/Ivory. In 60s.

DIPYRIDAMOLE AND ASPIRIN — ORAL

For more information, refer to the individual monographs for dipyridamole and aspirin.

Indications

➤*Stroke:* To reduce the risk of stroke in patients who have had transient ischemia of the brain or complete ischemic stroke due to thrombosis.

Administration and Dosage

➤*General dosing considerations:* Do not interchange with individual components of aspirin and dipyridamole tablets.

➤*Adults:*

Stroke – 1 capsule given orally twice daily.

➤*Children:* Safety and efficacy of dipyridamole and aspirin combination capsules in pediatric patients have not been studied. Because of the aspirin component, use of this product in the pediatric population is not recommended.

➤*Renal function impairment:* Avoid aspirin in patients with severe renal failure (glomerular filtration rate less than 10 mL/min).

➤*Hepatic function impairment:* Avoid aspirin in patients with severe hepatic function impairment.

➤*Administration:* Administer 1 capsule in the morning and 1 capsule in the evening. Swallow whole; do not crush or chew.

➤*Storage/Stability:* Store at 25°C (77°F). Protect from excessive moisture.

Actions

➤*Pharmacology:* Antithrombotic action is the result of the additive antiplatelet effects of dipyridamole and aspirin.

Dipyridamole inhibits the uptake of adenosine into platelets, endothelial cells, and erythrocytes in vitro and in vivo; the inhibition occurs in a dose-dependent manner at therapeutic concentrations (0.5 to 1.9 mcg/mL). This inhibition results in an increase in local concentrations of adenosine that

DIPYRIDAMOLE AND ASPIRIN — ORAL

acts on the platelet A_2-receptor thereby stimulating platelet adenylate cyclase and increasing platelet cyclic-3′,5′-adenosine monophosphate (cAMP) levels. Platelet aggregation is inhibited in response to various stimuli such as platelet activation factor, collagen, and adenosine diphosphate (ADP). Dipyridamole inhibits phosphodiesterase (PDE) in various tissues. While the inhibition of cAMP-PDE is weak, therapeutic levels of dipyridamole inhibit cyclic-3′,5′-guanosine monophosphate-PDE (cGMP-PDE), thereby augmenting the increase in cGMP produced by endothelium-derived relaxing factor (now identified as nitric oxide).

Aspirin inhibits platelet aggregation by irreversible inhibition of platelet cyclooxygenase and thus inhibits the generation of thromboxane A_2, a powerful inducer of platelet aggregation and vasoconstriction.

➤*Pharmacokinetics:*

Absorption –

Dipyridamole: Peak plasma levels of dipyridamole are achieved approximately 2 hours after administration of a daily dose of 400 mg dipyridamole and aspirin combination (given as 200 mg twice daily). The peak plasma concentration at steady-state is approximately 1.98 mcg/mL and the steady state trough concentration is approximately 0.53 mcg/mL.

Aspirin: Peak plasma levels of aspirin are achieved approximately 0.63 hours after administration of a 50 mg aspirin daily dose from dipyridamole and aspirin combination (given as 25 mg twice daily). The peak plasma concentration at steady-state is approximately 319 ng/mL. Aspirin undergoes moderate hydrolysis to salicylic acid in the liver and the GI wall, with 50% to 75% of an administered dose reaching the systemic circulation as intact aspirin.

Distribution –

Dipyridamole: Dipyridamole is highly lipophilic; however, it has been shown that the drug does not cross the blood-brain barrier to any significant extent in animals. The steady-state volume of distribution of dipyridamole is approximately 92 L. Approximately 99% of dipyridamole is bound to plasma proteins, predominantly to α1-acid glycoprotein and albumin.

Aspirin: Aspirin is poorly bound to plasma proteins and its apparent volume of distribution is low (10 L). Its metabolite, salicylic acid, is highly bound to plasma proteins, but its binding is concentration-dependent (nonlinear). At low concentrations (less than 100 mcg/mL), approximately 90% of salicylic acid is bound to albumin. Salicylic acid is widely distributed to all tissues and fluids in the body, including the CNS, breast milk, and fetal tissues.

Metabolism/Excretion –

Dipyridamole: Dipyridamole is metabolized in the liver, primarily by conjugation with glucuronic acid, of which monoglucuronide, which has low pharmacodynamic activity, is the primary metabolite. In plasma, approximately 80% of the total amount is present as parent compound and 20% as monoglucuronide. Most of the glucuronide metabolite (approximately 95%) is excreted via bile into the feces, with some evidence of enterohepatic circulation. Renal excretion of parent compound is negligible and urinary excretion of the glucuronide metabolite is low (approximately 5%). With IV treatment of dipyridamole, a triphasic profile is obtained: A rapid alpha phase with a half-life of approximately 3.4 minutes, a beta phase with a half-life of approximately 39 minutes, (which, together with the alpha phase accounts for approximately 70% of the total area under the curve, AUC), and a prolonged elimination phase λ_Z with a half-life of approximately 15.5 hours.

Aspirin: Aspirin is rapidly hydrolized in plasma to salicylic acid with a half-life of 20 minutes. Plasma levels of aspirin are essentially undetectable 2 to 2.5 hours after dosing, and peak salicylic acid concentration occurs 1 hour (range, 0.5 to 2 hours) after aspirin administration. Salicylic acid is primarily conjugated in the liver to form salicyluric acid, a phenolic glucuronide, an acyl glucuronide, and a number of minor metabolites. Salicylate metabolism is saturable and the total body clearance decreases at higher serum concentrations because of the limited ability of the liver to form both salicyluric acid and phenolic glucuronide. Following toxic doses (10 to 20 g), the plasma half-life may increase to more than 20 hours.

The elimination of acetylsalicylic acid follows first-order kinetics with the dipyridamole and aspirin combination and has a half-life of 0.33 hours. The half-life of salicylic acid is 1.71 hours. Both values correspond well with data from the literature at a lower dose which state a resultant half-life of approximately 2 to 3 hours. At higher doses, the elimination of salicylic acid follows zero-order kinetics (ie, the rate of elimination is constant in relation to plasma concentration) with an apparent half-life of 6 or more hours. Renal excretion of unchanged drug depends upon urinary pH. As urinary pH rises above 6.5, the renal clearance of free salicylate increases from less than 5% to more than 80%. Following therapeutic doses, approximately 10% is excreted as salicylic acid and 75% as salicyluric acid, as the phenolic and acyl glucuronides, in urine.

Special populations –

Renal function impairment: No changes were observed in the pharmacokinetics of **dipyridamole** or its glucuronide metabolite with creatinine clearances ranging from approximately 15 mL/min to greater than 100 mL/min if data were corrected for differences in age. Avoid **aspirin** in patients with severe renal failure (glomerular filtration rate less than 10 mL/min).

Hepatic function impairment: In a study conducted with an IV formulation of **dipyridamole**, patients with mild-to-severe hepatic insufficiency showed no change in plasma concentrations of dipyridamole but showed an increase in the pharmacologically inactive monoglucuronide metabolite. Dipyridamole can be dosed without restriction as long as there is no evidence of hepatic failure. Avoid **aspirin** in patients with severe hepatic function impairment.

Elderly: Plasma concentrations (determined as AUC) of dipyridamole in healthy elderly subjects more than 65 years of age were approximately 40% higher than in subjects less than 55 years of age receiving treatment with the dipyridamole and aspirin combination.

Contraindications

Hypersensitivity to dipyridamole, aspirin, or any of the other product components.

➤*Allergy:* Aspirin is contraindicated in patients with a known allergy to NSAIDs and in patients with asthma, rhinitis, and nasal polyps. Aspirin may cause severe urticaria, angioedema, or bronchospasms (asthma).

➤*Reye's syndrome:* Do not use in children or teenagers with viral infections with or without fever. There is a risk of Reye's syndrome with concomitant use of aspirin in certain viral illnesses.

Warnings/Precautions

➤*Alcohol:* Counsel patients who consume approximately 3 alcoholic drinks every day about the bleeding risks involved with chronic, heavy alcohol use while taking **aspirin**.

➤*Coagulation abnormalities:* Even low doses of **aspirin** can inhibit platelet function leading to an increase in bleeding time. This can adversely affect patients with inherited or acquired bleeding disorders (eg, liver disease, vitamin K deficiency).

➤*GI side effects:* GI side effects include stomach pain, heartburn, nausea, vomiting, and gross GI bleeding. Minor upper GI symptoms, such as dyspepsia, are common and can occur anytime during therapy. Watch for signs of ulceration and bleeding, even in the absence of previous GI symptoms. Inform patients about the signs and symptoms of GI side effects and what steps to take if they occur.

➤*Peptic ulcer disease:* Avoid using **aspirin**, which can cause gastric mucosal irritation and bleeding in patients with a history of active peptic ulcer disease.

➤*Hepatic effects:* Elevations of hepatic enzymes and hepatic failure have been reported in association with **dipyridamole** administration.

➤*Individual component interchangeability:* Dipyridamole and aspirin combination is not interchangeable with the individual components of aspirin and dipyridamole tablets.

➤*Coronary artery disease:* Due to the vasodilatory effect of **dipyridamole**, use with caution in patients with severe coronary artery disease (eg, unstable angina, recently sustained MI). Chest pain may be aggravated in patients with underlying coronary artery disease who are receiving dipyridamole. For stroke or transient ischemic attack patients for whom **aspirin** is indicated to prevent recurrent MI or angina pectoris, the aspirin in this product may not provide adequate treatment for the cardiac indications.

➤*Hypotension:* **Dipyridamole** can produce peripheral vasodilation; use with caution in patients with hypotension.

➤*Risk of bleeding:* In 1 study, the incidence of GI bleeding was 68 patients (4.1%) in the dipyridamole and aspirin combination group, 36 patients (2.2%) in the dipyridamole group, 52 patients (3.2%) in the aspirin group, and 34 patients (2.1%) in the placebo groups. The incidence of intracranial hemorrhage was 9 patients (0.6%) in the dipyridamole and aspirin combination group, 6 patients (0.5%) in the dipyridamole group, 6 patients (0.4%) in the aspirin group, and 7 patients (0.4%) in the placebo groups.

➤*Renal function impairment:* Avoid aspirin in patients with severe renal failure (glomerular filtration rate less than 10 mL/min).

➤*Pregnancy: Category B* (dipyridamole); *Category D* (aspirin). Reproduction studies have been performed with the dipyridamole and aspirin combination in a ratio of 1:4.4 in rats and rabbits and have revealed no teratogenic evidence at doses of up to 405 mg/kg/day in rats and 135 mg/kg/day in rabbits. However, treatment with the dipyridamole and aspirin combination at 405 mg/kg/day induced abortion in rats. The doses of dipyridamole at 75 mg/kg/day represent 1.5 times the recommended human dose on a body surface area (BSA) basis. In these studies, aspirin itself was teratogenic at doses of 330 mg/kg/day (1980 mg/m²/day) in rats (eg, spina bifida, exencephaly, microphthalmia, coelosomia) and 110 mg/kg/day (1320 mg/m²/day) in rabbits (eg, congested fetuses, agenesis of skull and upper jaw, generalized edema with malformation of the head, diaphanous skin). The doses of aspirin at 330 mg/kg/day in rats and at 110 mg/kg/day in rabbits were approximately 54 and 36 times the recommended human dose, respectively, on a BSA basis.

There are no adequate and well-controlled studies in pregnant women. Use this combination during pregnancy only if the potential benefit justifies the risk to the fetus. Because of the aspirin component, avoid the combination in the third trimester of pregnancy.

➤*Lactation:* Dipyridamole and aspirin are excreted in human breast milk in low concentrations. Exercise caution when dipyridamole and aspirin combination capsules are administered to a nursing woman.

➤*Children:* Safety and efficacy of dipyridamole and aspirin combination capsules in pediatric patients have not been studied. Because of the aspirin component, use of this product in the pediatric population is not recommended.

➤*Elderly:* Per the Beers list, extended release dipyridamole may cause hypotension in elderly patients with artificial heart valves.

➤*Lab test abnormalities:* **Aspirin** has been associated with elevated hepatic enzymes, blood urea nitrogen and serum creatinine, hyperkalemia, proteinuria, and prolonged bleeding time. **Dipyridamole** has been associated with elevated hepatic enzymes.

DIPYRIDAMOLE AND ASPIRIN — ORAL

Over the course of 24 months, patients treated with dipyridamole and aspirin combination therapy showed a decline (mean change from baseline) in hemoglobin of 0.25 g/dL, hematocrit of 0.75%, and erythrocyte count of $0.13 \times 10^6/mm^3$.

Drug Interactions

No drug-drug interaction studies were conducted with the combination of dipyridamole and aspirin. The following drug interactions are representative of the literature for each agent (dipyridamole or aspirin).

Dipyridamole and Aspirin Oral Combination Drug Interactions

Precipitant drug	Object drug[a]		Description
Dipyridamole	Adenosine	↑	Dipyridamole increases the plasma levels and cardiovascular effects of adenosine. Adjust adenosine dose as necessary.
Aspirin	ACE inhibitors	↓	Due to the indirect effect of aspirin on the renin-angiotensin conversion pathway, the hyponatremic and hypotensive effects of ACE inhibitors may be diminished by concomitant administration of aspirin.
Aspirin	Acetazolamide	↑	Concurrent use can lead to high serum concentrations of acetazolamide (and toxicity) due to competition at the renal tubule for secretion.
Aspirin	Anticoagulants	↑	Patients on anticoagulation therapy are at increased risk for bleeding because of effects on platelets. Aspirin can displace warfarin from protein binding sites, leading to prolongation of the prothrombin time and the bleeding time. Aspirin can also increase the anticoagulant activity of heparin, increasing bleeding risk.
Aspirin	Anticonvulsants (hydantoins, valproic acid)	↑	Increased free fraction of valproic acid, possibly leading to toxic effects of valproic acid, has occurred. The pharmacologic and toxic effects of hydantoins may be increased by coadministration of high doses of salicylates.
Aspirin	Beta blockers	↓	The hypotensive effects of beta blockers may be diminished by concomitant aspirin because of inhibition of renal prostaglandins, leading to decreased renal blood flow and salt and fluid retention.
Dipyridamole	Cholinesterase inhibitors	↓	Dipyridamole may counteract the anticholinesterase effect of cholinesterase inhibitors, thereby potentially aggravating myasthenia gravis.
Aspirin	Diuretics	↓	The effectiveness of diuretics in patients with underlying renal or cardiovascular disease may be diminished by concomitant aspirin because of inhibition of renal prostaglandins, leading to decreased renal blood flow and salt and fluid retention.
Aspirin	Methotrexate	↑	Salicylates can inhibit renal clearance of methotrexate, leading to bone marrow toxicity, especially in the elderly or renally impaired.
Aspirin	NSAIDs	↑	The concurrent use of aspirin with other NSAIDs may increase bleeding or lead to decreased renal function.
Aspirin	Oral hypoglycemics	↑	Moderate doses of aspirin may increase the effectiveness of oral hypoglycemic drugs, leading to hypoglycemia.
Aspirin	Uricosuric agents (eg, probenecid, sulfinpyrazone)	↓	Salicylates antagonize the uricosuric action of uricosuric agents.

[a] ↑ = Object drug increased. ↓ = Object drug decreased.

Adverse Reactions

Dipyridamole and Aspirin Oral Combination Therapy Adverse Events (%)

	Individual treatment group (n = 6602)			
Adverse reaction	Dipyridamole/ Aspirin combination (n = 1650)	ER[a]-DP alone (n = 1654)	ASA alone (n = 1649)	Placebo (n = 1649)
% of patients with ≥ 1 on-treatment adverse event	79.9	78.9	80.2	70.1
CNS				
Headache	39.2	38.3	33.8	32.9
Amnesia	2.4	2.4	3.5	2.1
Convulsions	1.7	0.9	1.7	1.6
Anorexia	1.2	1	0.6	0.9
Somnolence	1.2	0.8	1.1	0.5
Confusion	1.1	0.5	1.3	0.9
GI				
Abdominal pain	17.5	15.4	15.9	14.5
Dyspepsia	18.4	17.4	18.1	16.7
Nausea	16	15.4	12.7	14.1
Vomiting	8.4	7.8	6.1	7.2
Diarrhea	12.7	15.5	6.8	9.8
Melena	1.9	0.6	1.2	0.8
Rectal hemorrhage	1.6	1.3	1	0.8
GI hemorrhage	1.2	0.3	0.9	0.4
Hemorrhoids	1	0.8	0.6	0.6
Hematologic				
Hemorrhage NOS[b]	3.2	1.5	2.8	1.5
Epistaxis	2.4	1	2.7	1.5
Anemia	1.6	1	1.2	0.5
Purpura	1.4	0.5	0.5	0.4
Musculoskeletal				
Arthralgia	5.5	4.5	5.5	4.6
Arthritis	2.1	1.5	1	1.2
Myalgia	1.2	1	0.7	0.7
Arthrosis	1.1	1.3	0.8	0.8
Respiratory				
Coughing	1.5	1.1	1.9	1.3
Upper respiratory tract infection	1	0.5	1	0.8
Miscellaneous				
Pain	6.4	5.3	6.2	6
Fatigue	5.8	5.6	5.9	5.5
Back pain	4.6	4.7	4.5	3.9
Accidental injury	2.5	1.5	3.1	2.2
Asthenia	1.8	1.1	1	1.1
Neoplasm NOS[b]	1.7	1	1.4	1.2
Cardiac failure	1.6	1	1.8	1.5
Malaise	1.6	1.4	1.6	1.3
Syncope	1	0.8	1	0.5

[a] Extended release.
[b] NOS = Not otherwise specified.

Adverse reactions that occurred in less than 1% of patients treated with dipyridamole and aspirin combination therapy and that were medically judged to be possibly related to either dipyridamole or aspirin are listed below.

➤*Cardiovascular:* Hypotension; tachycardia; palpitation; arrhythmia; supraventricular tachycardia.

➤*CNS:* Coma; dizziness; paresthesia; cerebral hemorrhage; intracranial hemorrhage; subarachnoid hemorrhage; agitation.

➤*Dermatologic:* Pruritus; urticaria.

➤*GI:* Gastritis; ulceration; perforation.

➤*Hematologic:* Hematoma; gingival bleeding.

➤*Hepatic:* Cholelithiasis; jaundice; abnormal hepatic function.

➤*Metabolic/Nutritional:* Hyperglycemia; thirst.

DIPYRIDAMOLE AND ASPIRIN — ORAL

➤*Respiratory:* Hyperpnea; asthma; bronchospasm; hemoptysis; pulmonary edema.

➤*Special senses:* Tinnitus; deafness; taste loss. Patients with high frequency hearing loss may have difficulty perceiving tinnitus. In these patients, tinnitus cannot be used as a clinical indication of salicylism.

➤*Miscellaneous:* Allergic reaction; fever; flushing; uterine hemorrhage; renal insufficiency and failure; hematuria.

➤*Postmarketing reports:* The following is a list of additional adverse reactions that have been reported either in the literature or are from postmarketing spontaneous reports for either dipyridamole or aspirin.

Dermatologic – Rash; alopecia; angioedema; Stevens-Johnson syndrome.

GI – Pancreatitis; Reye's syndrome; hematemesis.

GU – Prolonged pregnancy and labor; stillbirths; lower birth weight infants; antepartum and postpartum bleeding; interstitial nephritis; papillary necrosis; proteinuria.

Hematologic – Prolongation of the prothrombin time; disseminated intravascular coagulation; coagulopathy; thrombocytopenia.

Hepatic – Hepatitis; hepatic failure.

Hypersensitivity – Acute anaphylaxis; laryngeal edema.

Lab test abnormalities – Hyperkalemia; metabolic acidosis; respiratory alkalosis; hypokalemia.

Metabolic/Nutritional – Hypoglycemia; dehydration.

Respiratory – Tachypnea; dyspnea.

Miscellaneous – Hypothermia; chest pain; angina pectoris; cerebral edema; hearing loss; rhabdomyolysis; allergic vasculitis.

Overdosage

Because of the dose ratio of dipyridamole to aspirin, overdosage of the dipyridamole and aspirin combination is likely to be dominated by signs and symptoms of dipyridamole overdose. In case of real or suspected overdose, seek medical attention or contact a Poison Control Center immediately.

➤*Symptoms:*

Dipyridamole – Based upon the known hemodynamic effects of dipyridamole, symptoms such as warm feeling, flushes, sweating, restlessness, feeling of weakness, and dizziness may occur. A drop in blood pressure and tachycardia might also be observed.

Aspirin – Salicylate toxicity may result from acute ingestion (overdose) or chronic intoxication. The early signs of salicylic overdose (salicylism), including tinnitus (ringing in the ears), occur at plasma concentrations approaching 200 mcg/mL. Plasma concentrations of aspirin greater than 300 mcg/mL are clearly toxic. Severe toxic effects are associated with levels greater than 400 mcg/mL. A single lethal dose of aspirin in adults is not known with certainty but death may be expected at 30 g.

➤*Treatment:*

Dipyridamole – Symptomatic treatment is recommended, possibly including a vasopressor drug. Consider gastric lavage. Because dipyridamole is highly protein bound, dialysis is not likely to be of benefit.

Aspirin – Treatment consists primarily of supporting vital functions, increasing salicylate elimination, and correcting the acid-base disturbance. Gastric emptying or lavage are recommended as soon as possible after ingestion, even if the patient has vomited spontaneously. After lavage or emesis, administration of activated charcoal (as a slurry) is beneficial, if less than 3 hours have passed since ingestion. Do not employ charcoal absorption prior to emesis and lavage.

Severity of aspirin intoxication is determined by measuring the blood salicylate level. Closely follow acid-base status with serial blood gas and serum pH measurements. Maintain fluid and electrolyte balance.

In severe cases, hyperthermia and hypervolemia are the major immediate threats to life. Sponge children with tepid water. Administer replacement fluid IV and augment with correction of acidosis. Monitor plasma electrolytes and pH to promote alkaline diuresis of salicylate if renal function is normal. Infusion of glucose may be required to control hypoglycemia.

Hemodialysis and peritoneal dialysis can be performed to reduce the body drug content. In patients with renal insufficiency or in cases of life-threatening intoxication, dialysis is usually required. Exchange transfusion may be indicated in infants and young children.

Patient Information

Counsel patients who consume 3 or more alcoholic drinks every day about the bleeding risks involved with chronic, heavy alcohol use while taking **aspirin**.

Inform patients about the signs and symptoms of GI side effects and what steps to take if they occur.

Avoid using **aspirin**, which can cause gastric mucosal irritation and bleeding in patients with a history of active peptic ulcer disease.

Aspirin is contraindicated in patients with known allergy to NSAIDs and in patients with asthma, rhinitis, and nasal polyps. Aspirin may cause severe urticaria, angioedema, or bronchospasm (asthma).

Do not use in children or teenagers with viral infections with or without fever. There is a risk of Reye's syndrome with concomitant use of **aspirin** in certain viral illnesses.

ANTICOAGULANTS

Blood coagulation resulting in the formation of a stable fibrin clot involves a cascade of proteolytic reactions involving the interaction of clotting factors, platelets, and tissue materials. Clotting factors (see table) exist in the blood in inactive form and must be converted to an enzymatic or activated (a) form before the next step in the clotting mechanism can be stimulated. Each factor is stimulated in turn until an insoluble fibrin clot is formed.

Two separate pathways, intrinsic and extrinsic, lead to the formation of a fibrin clot. Both pathways must function for hemostasis.

➤*Intrinsic pathway:* All the protein factors necessary for coagulation are present in circulating blood. Clot formation may take several minutes and is initiated by activation of factor XII.

➤*Extrinsic pathway:* Coagulation is activated by release of tissue thromboplastin, a factor not found in circulating blood. Clotting occurs in seconds because factor III bypasses the early reactions.

Refer to the complete coagulation pathway.

Anticoagulants used therapeutically include fractionated and unfractionated heparin, warfarin (a coumarin derivative), and anisindione (an indandione derivative).

Blood Clotting Factors		
Factor	Synonym	Vitamin K-dependent
I	Fibrinogen	no
II	Prothrombin	yes
III	Tissue thromboplastin, tissue factor	no
IV	Calcium	no
V	Labile factor, proaccelerin	no
VII	Proconvertin	yes
VIII	Antihemophilic factor, AHF	no
IX	Christmas factor, plasma thromboplastin component, PTC	yes
X	Stuart factor, Stuart-Prower factor	yes
XI	Plasma thromboplastin antecedent, PTA	no
XII	Hageman factor	no
XIII	Fibrin stabilizing factor, FSF	no
HMW-K	High molecular weight kininogen, Fitzgerald factor	no
PL	Platelets or phospholipids	no
PK	Prekallikrein, Fletcher factor	no
Protein C[a]		yes
Protein S[b]		yes

[a] Partially responsible for inhibition of the extrinsic pathway. Inactivates factors V and VIII and promotes fibrinolysis. Activity declines following warfarin administration.
[b] A cofactor to accelerate the anticoagulant activity of protein C. Decreased levels occur following warfarin administration.

COAGULATION PATHWAY

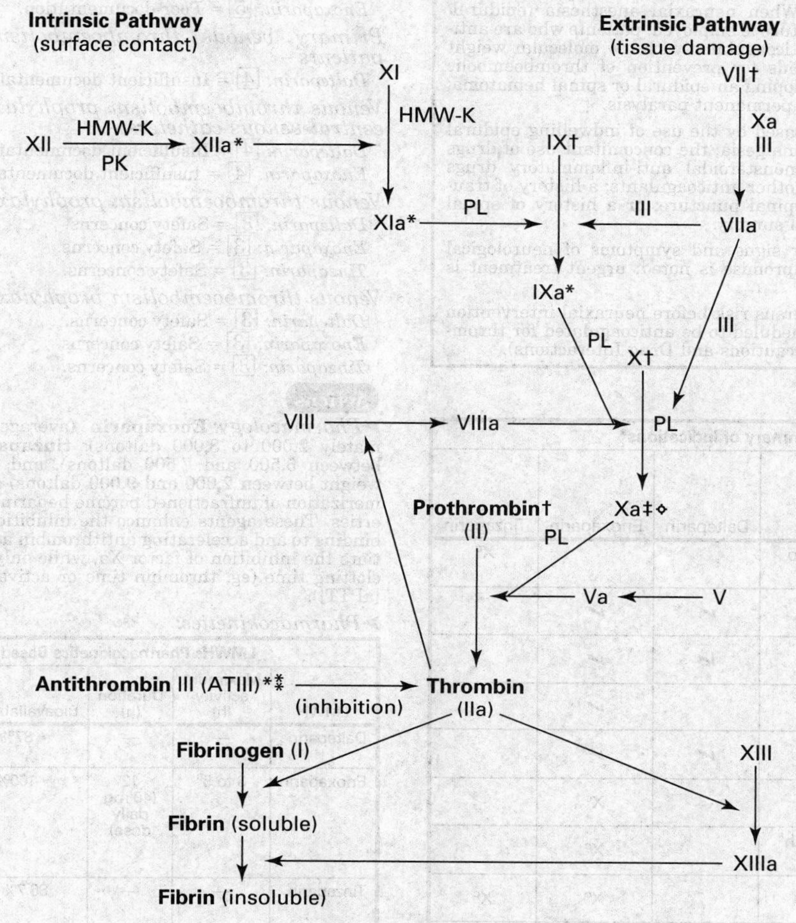

* Major site of activity for unfractionated heparin
† Site of activity for warfarin and anisindione
‡ Major site of activity for fractionated heparin
⁑ Minor site of activity for fractionated heparin
◇ Minor site of activity for unfractionated heparin

WARNING

Spinal/Epidural hematomas – When neuraxial anesthesia (epidural/spinal anesthesia) or spinal puncture is employed, patients who are anticoagulated or scheduled to be anticoagulated with low molecular weight heparins (LMWHs) or heparinoids for prevention of thromboembolic complications are at risk of developing an epidural or spinal hematoma, which can result in long-term or permanent paralysis.

The risk of these events is increased by the use of indwelling epidural catheters for administration of analgesia; the concomitant use of drugs affecting hemostasis, such as nonsteroidal anti-inflammatory drugs (NSAIDs), platelet inhibitors, or other anticoagulants; a history of traumatic or repeated epidural or spinal puncture; or a history of spinal deformity, spinal injury, or spinal surgery.

Frequently monitor patients for signs and symptoms of neurological impairment. If neurological compromise is noted, urgent treatment is necessary.

Consider the potential benefit versus risk before neuraxial intervention in patients anticoagulated or scheduled to be anticoagulated for thromboprophylaxis (see Warnings/Precautions and Drug Interactions).

Indications

LMWHs—Summary of Indications[a]

Indications ✓ = FDA approved X = off-label use	Dalteparin	Enoxaparin	Tinzaparin
Prophylaxis of DVT that may lead to PE[b]			X[c]
In patients undergoing abdominal surgery	✓	✓	
In patients undergoing hip replacement surgery	✓	✓	
In patients undergoing knee replacement surgery		✓	
In patients with severely restricted mobility during acute illness	✓	✓	
In patients undergoing surgery, moderate risk		X[c]	
In patients undergoing surgery, high risk		X[c]	
In patients undergoing orthopedic surgery		X[c]	X[c]
In patients undergoing hip fracture surgery			X[c]
In patients undergoing neurosurgery			X[c]
Treatment of DVT with or without PE[d]		✓[d]	✓
Prophylaxis of ischemic complications in unstable angina and non–Q-wave MI[e]	✓	✓[e]	
Primary venous thromboembolism prophylaxisin cancer patients	X[c]		
Venous thromboembolism prophylaxis in cancer patients with central venous catheters	X[c]	X[c]	
Venous thromboembolism prophylaxis in general surgery	X[f]	X[f]	X[f]
Venous thromboembolism prophylaxis in gynecologic surgery	X[f]	X[f]	X[f]
Prevention of exercise-induced bronchoconstriction		X[f]	
Acute STEMI		✓[e]	
Extended treatment of symptomatic venous thromboembolism in cancer patients to reduce recurrence	✓		

[a] FDA = Food and Drug Administration; PE = pulmonary embolism; DVT = deep vein thrombosis; MI = myocardial infarction; STEMI = ST-segment elevation myocardial infarction.
[b] In patients at risk for thromboembolic complications.
[c] Insufficient documentation.
[d] In conjunction with warfarin therapy.
[e] In conjunction with aspirin therapy.
[f] Safety concerns.

➤*Off-label uses:* Refer to individual monographs for further information.

Prevention of exercise-induced bronchoconstriction –
Enoxaparin: [5] = Poor documentation.

Primary venous thromboembolism prophylaxis in cancer patients –
Dalteparin: [4] = Insufficient documentation.

Venous thromboembolism prophylaxis in cancer patients with central venous catheters –
Dalteparin: [4] = Insufficient documentation.
Enoxaparin: [4] = Insufficient documentation.

Venous thromboembolism prophylaxis in general surgery –
Dalteparin: [3] = Safety concerns.
Enoxaparin: [3] = Safety concerns.
Tinzaparin: [3] = Safety concerns.

Venous thromboembolism prophylaxis in gynecologic surgery –
Dalteparin: [3] = Safety concerns.
Enoxaparin: [3] = Safety concerns.
Tinzaparin: [3] = Safety concerns.

Actions

➤*Pharmacology:* **Enoxaparin** (average molecular weight is approximately 2,000 to 8,000 daltons), **tinzaparin** (average molecular weight between 5,500 and 7,500 daltons), and **dalteparin** (average molecular weight between 2,000 and 9,000 daltons) are LMWHs obtained by depolymerization of unfractioned porcine heparin. They have antithrombotic properties. These agents enhance the inhibition of factor Xa and thrombin by binding to and accelerating antithrombin activity. They preferentially potentiate the inhibition of factor Xa, while only slightly affecting thrombin and clotting time (eg, thrombin time or activated partial thromboplastin time [aPTT]).

➤*Pharmacokinetics:*

LMWHs Pharmacokinetics Based on Anti-Xa Activity[a,b]

LMWH	Maximum activity (h)	Duration (h)	Bioavailability	T_{max} (h)	Vd	Terminal t½ (h)
Dalteparin	—	—	≈ 87%	4	40 to 60 mL/kg	3 to 5
Enoxaparin	3 to 5[c]	12 (40 mg daily dose)	≈ 100%	3 to 4.5	4.3 L	4.5 (single dose) 7 (repeated doses)
Tinzaparin	—	—	86.7%	3.7 (single dose)	3.1 to 5 L	3 to 4

[a] T_{max} = time to maximal concentration; Vd = apparent volume of distribution; t½ = half-life.
[b] Information listed without regard to dosage or indication.
[c] Maximum anti–factor Xa and antithrombin activities.

Metabolism/Excretion – LMWHs are primarily metabolized in the liver by desulfation and/or depolymerization to lower molecular weight species with much reduced biological potency. Total renal clearance of active and nonactive **enoxaparin** fragments represents 40% of the dose, with 10% being active fragments.

Special populations –

Renal function impairment:

• *Dalteparin* – In patients with chronic renal insufficiency requiring hemodialysis, the mean terminal half-life of anti–factor Xa activity may be considerably longer; therefore, greater accumulation can be expected in these patients.

• *Enoxaparin* – Anti–factor Xa exposure represented by area under the curve (AUC) at steady state is marginally increased in mild (creatinine clearance [CrCl] 50 to 80 mL/min) and moderate (CrCl 30 to 50 mL/min) renal impairment. In patients with severe renal impairment (CrCl less than 30 mL/min), the AUC is significantly increased, on average, by 65%.

• *Tinzaparin* – Clearance is reduced in patients with moderate (CrCl 30 to 50 mL/min) and severe (CrCl less than 30 mL/min) renal impairment. Patients with severe renal impairment exhibited a 24% reduction in tinzaparin clearance.

Elderly:

• *Enoxaparin* – The day 10 mean AUC was approximately 15% greater than the mean day 1 AUC value.

Weight:

• *Enoxaparin* – When non–weight-adjusted enoxaparin dosing was administered, it was found that after a single subcutaneous 40 mg dose, anti–factor Xa exposure was 52% higher in low-weight women (less than 45 kg) and 27% higher in low-weight men (less than 57 kg).

• *Tinzaparin* – Weight-based dosing is appropriate for heavy/obese patients.

Contraindications

Hypersensitivity to LMWHs, heparin, or pork products; hypersensitivity to sulfites or benzyl alcohol (multidose vials); history of heparin-induced thrombocytopenia (**dalteparin** and **tinzaparin**); active major bleeding; thrombocytopenia associated with positive in vitro tests for antiplatelet antibody in the presence of a LMWH.

Do not give **dalteparin** to patients undergoing regional anesthesia for unstable angina, non–Q-wave MI, or prolonged VTE prophylaxis.

Warnings/Precautions

➤*Route of administration:* For subcutaneous administration only; do not administer intramuscularly.

➤*Interchangeability:* LMWHs cannot be used interchangeably (unit for unit) with other LMWHs or unfractionated heparin.

➤*Spinal/Epidural hematomas:* As with other anticoagulants, rare cases of neuraxial, spinal, or epidural hematomas have been reported with the concurrent use of LMWHs and spinal/epidural anesthesia or spinal puncture, resulting in long-term or permanent paralysis. The risk of these events may be higher with the use of postoperative indwelling epidural catheters or by the concomitant use of additional drugs, such as NSAIDs, that affect hemostasis (see Warning Box).

➤*Hemorrhage:* Use LMWHs, like other anticoagulants, with extreme caution in patients who have an increased risk of hemorrhage, such as those with severe uncontrolled hypertension; bleeding diathesis; diabetic retinopathy; bacterial endocarditis; congenital or acquired bleeding disorders (including hepatic failure and amyloidosis); active ulceration and angiodysplastic GI disease; hemorrhagic stroke or shortly after brain, spinal, or ophthalmological surgery; or in patients treated concomitantly with platelet inhibitors. As with other anticoagulants, bleeding can occur at any site during therapy with a LMWH. Search for a bleeding site if an unexpected drop in hematocrit, hemoglobin, or blood pressure occurs.

Hemorrhage in some cases has been reported to result in death or permanent disability. If severe hemorrhage occurs, discontinue the LMWH.

Major hemorrhages, including retroperitoneal and intracranial bleeding, have been reported. Some of these cases have been fatal.

Discontinue agents that might affect hemostasis (eg, oral anticoagulants, platelet inhibitors) prior to therapy with LMWHs. Concomitant use may increase the risk of hemorrhage. Monitor the patient closely if coadministration cannot be avoided (see Drug Interactions).

➤*Thrombocytopenia:* The incidence of thrombocytopenia with platelet counts between 50,000/mm^3 and 100,000/mm^3 was 1.3% in patients treated with **enoxaparin**, 1% with **tinzaparin**, and less than 1% with **dalteparin**. Severe thrombocytopenia (platelet count less than 50,000/mm^3) occurred in 0.13% of tinzaparin-treated patients and 0.1% of enoxaparin-treated patients.

Use extreme caution in patients with a history of heparin-induced thrombocytopenia. Do not use dalteparin or tinzaparin in these patients. Closely monitor thrombocytopenia of any degree. If the platelet count falls to less than 100,000/mm^3, discontinue the LMWH.

Cases of thrombocytopenia with disseminated thrombosis also have been observed in clinical practice with LMWHs, including dalteparin and tinzaparin. Some of these cases were complicated by organ infarction with secondary organ dysfunction or limb ischemia and have resulted in death.

➤*Priapism:* Priapism has been reported from postmarketing surveillance of **tinzaparin** as a rare occurrence. In some cases, surgical intervention was required.

➤*Special risk patients:* Use with care in patients with bleeding diathesis, uncontrolled arterial hypertension, or a history of recent GI ulceration or bleeding, hypertensive or diabetic retinopathy, hemorrhage, and severe liver or kidney insufficiency.

➤*Thromboembolic event:* If a thromboembolic event occurs despite LMWH prophylaxis, discontinue the drug and initiate appropriate therapy.

➤*Mechanical prosthetic heart valves:* The use of **enoxaparin** has not been adequately studied for thromboprophylaxis or long-term use in patients with mechanical prosthetic heart valves. Isolated cases of prosthetic heart valve thrombosis have been reported in patients with mechanical prosthetic heart valves who have received enoxaparin for thromboprophylaxis. Some of these cases were pregnant women in whom thrombosis led to maternal and fetal deaths. Insufficient data, the underlying disease, and the possibility of inadequate anticoagulation complicate the evaluation of these cases. Women with mechanical prosthetic heart valves may be at higher risk for thromboembolism during pregnancy and, when pregnant, have a higher rate of fetal loss from stillbirth, spontaneous abortion, and premature delivery. Therefore, frequent monitoring of peak and trough anti–factor Xa levels and dose adjustment may be needed.

➤*Low-weight patients:* An increase in exposure of **enoxaparin** with prophylactic dosages (less than 45 kg) and low-weight men (less than 57 kg) has been observed. Observe all such patients carefully for signs and symptoms of bleeding.

➤*Benzyl alcohol:* The multidose vials of **dalteparin**, **enoxaparin**, and **tinzaparin** contain benzyl alcohol as a preservative. Benzyl alcohol has been associated with a fatal "gasping syndrome" in premature infants (when large amounts have been administered [99 to 405 mg/kg/day]). Because benzyl alcohol may cross the placenta, do not use LMWHs preserved with benzyl alcohol in pregnant women.

➤*Sulfite sensitivity:* **Tinzaparin** contains metabisulfite, a sulfite that may cause allergic-type reactions, including anaphylactic symptoms and life-threatening asthmatic episodes, in certain susceptible people. The overall prevalence of sulfite sensitivity in the general population is unknown and probably low. Sulfite sensitivity is seen more frequently in asthmatic than in nonasthmatic people.

➤*Renal/Hepatic function impairment:* Delayed elimination of LMWHs may occur with severe liver or kidney insufficiency. Use with caution.

In patients with renal impairment, there is an increase in exposure of **enoxaparin**. Use with care and observe all such patients carefully for signs and symptoms of bleeding. Because exposure of enoxaparin is significantly increased in patients with severe renal impairment (CrCl less than 30 mL/min), a dosage adjustment is recommended for therapeutic and prophylactic dose ranges.

➤*Pregnancy: Category B.* There are no adequate and well-controlled studies in pregnant women. There were 72 hemorrhagic events (11 serious) in 63 women. There were 14 cases of neonatal hemorrhage. A few spontaneous postmarketing fetal deaths have been reported in **enoxaparin**-treated patients. Use during pregnancy only if clearly needed. See Warnings/Precautions for pregnant women with mechanical prosthetic heart valves.

There have been cases reported of cleft palate, optic nerve hypoplasia, trisomy 21 (Down) syndrome, and cutis aplasia of the scalp in infants of women who received **tinzaparin** during pregnancy. A cause-and-effect relationship has not been established.

There have been reports of fetal death/miscarriage in pregnant women receiving tinzaparin who had high-risk pregnancies or a history of spontaneous abortion. Approximately 6% of pregnancies were complicated by fetal distress. There have been spontaneous reports of 1 case each of pulmonary hypoplasia or muscular hypotonia in infants of women receiving tinzaparin during pregnancy. A cause-and-effect relationship to the previously described observations has not been established.

Approximately 10% of pregnant women receiving tinzaparin experienced significant vaginal bleeding. A cause-and-effect relationship has not been established.

If tinzaparin is used during pregnancy, or if the patient becomes pregnant while taking this drug, apprise the patient of the potential hazards to the fetus.

➤*Lactation:* Limited published data indicate that dalteparin is minimally excreted in human milk. It is not known whether enoxaparin and tinzaparin are excreted in breast milk. In studies in which **tinzaparin** was administered subcutaneously to lactating rats, very low levels of tinzaparin were found in breast milk. Exercise caution when administering to a breast-feeding woman.

➤*Children:* Safety and efficacy in children have not been established.

➤*Elderly:* Delayed elimination of **enoxaparin** and **tinzaparin** may occur. Use with caution.

The incidence of bleeding complications was higher in elderly patients compared with younger patients when enoxaparin injection was administered at dosages of 1.5 mg/kg once a day or 1 mg/kg every 12 hours. The risk of enoxaparin-associated bleeding increased with age. Serious adverse events increased with age for patients receiving enoxaparin injection. Careful attention to dosing intervals and concomitant medications (especially antiplatelet medications) is advised. Consider monitoring of elderly patients with low body weight (less than 45 kg) and those predisposed to decreased renal function.

➤*Lab test abnormalities:* Asymptomatic reversible increases in AST and ALT levels have occurred in patients treated with LMWHs and heparin (see Adverse Reactions). Because ALT determinations are important in the differential diagnosis of MI, liver disease, and pulmonary emboli, interpret elevations that might be caused by LMWHs with caution.

➤*Monitoring:* Perform periodic complete blood cell counts, including platelet counts and hematocrit or hemoglobin and stool occult blood tests, during the course of treatment. Closely monitor thrombocytopenia of any degree. If the platelet count falls below 100,000/mm^3, discontinue the LMWH (see Warnings/Precautions). No special monitoring of blood clotting times (eg, aPTT) is needed. At recommended prophylaxis doses, routine coagulation tests such as PT and aPTT are relatively insensitive measures of activity and are, therefore, unsuitable for monitoring. Anti–factor Xa may be used to monitor the anticoagulant effect in patients with significant renal impairment or if abnormal coagulation parameters or bleeding should occur. Monitor patients with low body weight (less than 45 kg in women or less than 57 kg in men), those predisposed to decreased renal function, and pregnant women for signs and symptoms of bleeding.

Monitor patients frequently for signs and symptoms of neurologic impairment.

Drug Interactions

➤*Antithrombin:* The risk of severe bleeding may be increased when coadministered with dalteparin, enoxaparin, or tinzaparin.

➤*Anticoagulants/Platelet inhibitors:* Use LMWHs with care in patients receiving oral anticoagulants or platelet inhibitors (eg, aspirin; salicylates; NSAIDs, including ketorolac tromethamine, dipyridamole, sulfinpyrazone, dextran, ticlopidine, and clopidogrel) and thrombolytics because of increased risk of bleeding. Unless needed, discontinue agents that may enhance the risk of hemorrhage prior to initiation of **enoxaparin** therapy. If coadministration is essential, use close clinical and laboratory monitoring of these patients. Aspirin, unless contraindicated, is recommended in patients treated for unstable angina or non–Q-wave MI.

➤*Selective serotonin reuptake inhibitors (fluoxetine):* The risk of severe bleeding may be increased when coadministered with dalteparin, enoxaparin, or tinzaparin.

Adverse Reactions

LMWH Adverse Reactions (%)[a]			
Adverse reaction	Dalteparin	Enoxaparin	Tinzaparin
Hemorrhagic events			
Clinically significant bleeding[b]	0% to 3.6%	0% to 4%	0.8%
Hemorrhage	—	0% to 13%	1.5%
Injection-site hematoma	0.2% to 7.1%	✓[c]	16%
Wound hematoma	0% to 3.4%	—	✓
Nonhemorrhagic events			
Cardiovascular			
Angina pectoris	—	—	≥ 1%
Hypertension	—	—	≥ 1%
Hypotension	—	—	≥ 1%
Pulmonary embolism	—	—	2.3%
Tachycardia	—	—	≥ 1
CNS			
Confusion	—	2.2%	≥ 1%
Dizziness	—	—	≥ 1%
Insomnia	—	—	≥ 1%
Headache	—	—	1.7%
Dermatologic			
Bullous eruption	—	—	≥ 1%
Erythematous rash	—	—	≥ 1%
Pruritus/Rash	✓	✓	≥ 1%
Skin disorder	—	—	≥ 1%
GI			
Abdominal pain	—	—	0.8%
Constipation	—	—	1.3%
Diarrhea	—	2.2%	0.6%
Dyspepsia	—	—	≥ 1%
Flatulence	—	—	≥ 1%
GI disorder (NOS[d])	—	—	≥ 1%
Nausea	—	< 1% to 3%	1.7%
Vomiting	—	—	1%
GU			
Dysuria	—	—	≥ 1%
Hematuria	2.9%	< 1 to 2%	1%
Urinary retention	—	—	≥ 1%
Urinary tract infection	—	—	3.7%
Hematologic			
Anemia	—	< 2% to 16%	≥ 1%
Hematoma	—	✓	≥ 1%
Thrombocythemia	—	✓	—
Thrombocytopenia	< 1%	2.8%	≥ 1%
Respiratory			
Dyspnea	—	3.3%	1.2%
Epistaxis	—	—	1.9%
Pneumonia	—	—	≥ 1%
Respiratory disorder	—	—	≥ 1%
Miscellaneous			
Allergic reactions[e]	✓	✓	✓
Back pain, pain	—	—	1.5%
Cerebrovascular accident	—	—	—
Chest pain	—	—	2.3%
Edema	—	1% to 2%	—
Fever	✓	0% to 8%	1.5%
Healing impaired	—	—	≥ 1%
Infection	—	—	≥ 1%
Injection-site reactions	✓	✓	✓
Peripheral edema	—	0% to 6%	—
Thrombophlebitis, deep	—	—	≥ 1%
Thrombophlebitis, leg deep	—	—	≥ 1%

[a] Data pooled from several studies and are not necessarily comparable. Percentages listed without regard to specific dosage or indication.
[b] Defined as overt bleeding resulting in a decrease in hemoglobin of 2 g/dL or more, transfusion of 2 or more units of blood, intracranial, intraocular, retroperitoneal, or intra-articular bleeding or moderate to severe bleeding that required discontinuation from the study or required an invasive diagnostic or therapeutic procedure.
[c] ✓ = occurs; incidence unknown.
[d] NOS = not otherwise specified.
[e] Includes maculopapular rash, vesiculobullous rash, urticaria, and bullous eruption.

➤*Hemorrhagic complications:* Fatal or nonfatal hemorrhage from any tissue or organ can occur. The signs, symptoms, and severity will vary according to the location and degree or extent of the bleeding. Hemorrhagic complications may present as, but are not limited to, paralysis; paresthesia; headache, chest, abdomen, joint, muscle, or other pain; dizziness; shortness of breath or difficulty breathing or swallowing; swelling; weakness; hypotension; shock; or coma. Therefore, consider the possibility of hemorrhage when evaluating the condition of any anticoagulated patient with complaints that do not indicate an obvious diagnosis.

➤*Lab test abnormalities:* Asymptomatic increases in transaminase levels (AST and ALT) greater than 3 times the upper limit of normal of the laboratory reference range have been reported in 1.7% to 8.8% and 4.3% to 13% of patients, respectively, during treatment with LMWHs. Similar significant increases in transaminase levels have been observed in patients treated with heparin. Such elevations are fully reversible and are rarely associated with increases in bilirubin. Because transaminase determinations are important in the differential diagnosis of MI, liver disease, and pulmonary emboli, interpret elevations that might be caused by LMWHs with caution.

➤*Dalteparin:*

Hematologic – Since 1985, there have been more than 15 reports of epidural or spinal hematoma formation with concurrent use of dalteparin and spinal/epidural anesthesia or spinal puncture (see Warnings/Precautions). The majority of patients had postoperative indwelling epidural catheters placed for analgesia or received additional drugs affecting hemostasis. In some cases, the hematomas caused long-term or permanent paralysis (partial or complete).

Miscellaneous – Pain at the injection site (4.5% to 12%); few cases of anaphylactoid reactions.

Postmarketing – Alopecia, skin necrosis.

➤*Enoxaparin:*

Cardiovascular – Heart failure (0.95%); atrial fibrillation (0.7%).

Local – Injection-site hemorrhage (3% to 5%); injection-site pain (2%); injection-site reactions (eg, mild local irritation, pain, hematoma, ecchymosis, erythema).

Respiratory – Pneumonia (0.82%); lung edema (0.7%).

Postmarketing – Anaphylactoid reactions; cutaneous vasculitis; epidural or spinal hematoma; hyperkalemia; hyperlipidemia; hypersensitivity; hypertriglyceridemia; local reaction at injection site (eg, nodules, inflammation, oozing); purpura; skin necrosis; systemic allergic reactions; thrombocytosis, thrombocytopenia with thrombosis; vesiculobullous rash.

➤*Tinzaparin:*

Cardiovascular – Cardiac arrhythmia, dependent edema, MI/coronary thrombosis, thromboembolism.

Dermatologic – Bullous eruption, erythematous rash, maculopapular rash, purpura, skin disorder, skin necrosis.

Hematologic – Anorectal bleeding, cerebral/intracranial bleeding, ecchymosis, GI hemorrhage, granulocytopenia, hemarthrosis, hematemesis, hemopericardium, injection-site bleeding, melena, retroperitoneal/intra-abdominal bleeding, vaginal hemorrhage.

Approximately 10% of pregnant women receiving tinzaparin experienced significant vaginal bleeding. A cause-and-effect relationship has not been established.

Local – Cellulitis, ecchymosis, hematoma, mild local irritation, pain.

Miscellaneous – Allergic reaction, anaphylactic/anaphylactoid reactions, cellulitis (local), congenital anomaly, fetal death, fetal distress, neoplasm.

Postmarketing – Abscess, acute febrile reaction, agranulocytosis, allergic purpura, angioedema, cholestatic hepatitis, cutis aplasia of the scalp (fetal/neonatal), epidermal necrolysis, hemoptysis, increase in hepatic enzymes, ischemic necrosis, necrosis, neonatal hypotonia, ocular hemorrhage, pancytopenia, peripheral ischemia, priapism, rectal bleeding, Stevens-Johnson syndrome, thrombocythemia, urticaria.

There has been at least 1 case of spinal epidural hematoma with tinzaparin at a therapeutic dose in a patient who had not received neuraxial anesthesia or spinal puncture.

Overdosage

➤*Symptoms:* An excessive amount of a LMWH may lead to dose-related hemorrhagic complications.

➤*Treatment:* Effects of LMWHs may generally be stopped by the slow IV injection of protamine sulfate (1% solution) at a dose of 1 mg for every 100 anti-Xa units of **dalteparin** and **tinzaparin** or 1 mg for every 1 mg of **enoxaparin** if enoxaparin was administered in the previous 8 hours. An infusion of 0.5 mg of protamine/mg of enoxaparin may be administered if enoxaparin was administered more than 8 hours prior to the protamine administration. A second infusion of protamine 0.5 mg per 100 anti-Xa units of dalteparin and tinzaparin or per 1 mg of enoxaparin may be administered if the aPTT measured 2 to 4 hours after the first infusion remains prolonged. After 12 hours of the enoxaparin injection, protamine administration may not be required. Even with these additional doses of protamine, the aPTT may remain more prolonged than would usually be found following administration of conventional heparin. In all cases, the anti–factor Xa activity is never completely neutralized (maximum, approximately 60% to 75%). Take particular care to avoid overdosage with protamine.

Administration of protamine sulfate can cause severe hypotensive and anaphylactoid reactions. Because fatal reactions, often resembling anaphylaxis, have been reported, give protamine only when resuscitation techniques and treatment of anaphylactic shock are readily available.

Patient Information

Advise patients who have had neuraxial anesthesia or spinal puncture, especially if they are taking concomitant NSAIDs, platelet inhibitors, or other anticoagulants, to watch for signs and symptoms of spinal or epidural hematoma (eg, tingling, numbness, muscular weakness) and to notify their health care provider immediately if any of these symptoms occur.

Instruct patients to contact their health care provider if they experience bleeding, bruising, dizziness, light-headedness, itching, rash, fever, swelling, or difficulty breathing.

Instruct patients to notify their health care provider if they are pregnant, planning to become pregnant, or are breast-feeding.

Instruct patients to change the injection site daily.

Instruct patients to use proper injection technique; instruct them to inject under the skin, not into muscle.

To minimize bruising, advise patients not to rub the injection site after completion of injection.

DALTEPARIN SODIUM

Rx	**Fragmin** (Eisai)	**Injection, solution:** 2,500 units per 0.2 mL[a]	As dalteparin sodium 16 mg per 0.2 mL. Preservative free. In 0.2 mL single-dose prefilled syringes with 27-gauge × ½ in needle.
		5,000 units per 0.2 mL[a]	As dalteparin sodium 32 mg per 0.2 mL. Preservative free. In 0.2 mL single-dose prefilled syringes with 27-gauge × ½ in needle.
		7,500 units per 0.3 mL[a]	As dalteparin sodium 48 mg per 0.3 mL. Preservative free. In 0.3 mL single-dose prefilled syringes with 27-gauge × ½ in needle.
		10,000 units per 0.4 mL[a]	As dalteparin sodium 64 mg per 0.4 mL. Preservative free. In 0.4 mL single-dose prefilled syringes with 27-gauge × ½ in needle.
		10,000 units/mL[a]	As dalteparin sodium 64 mg/mL. Preservative free. In 1 mL single-dose, graduated syringes with 27-gauge × ½ in needle.
		12,500 units per 0.5 mL[a]	As dalteparin sodium 80 mg per 0.5 mL. Preservative free. In 0.5 mL single-dose prefilled syringes with 27-gauge × ½ in needle.
		15,000 units per 0.6 mL[a]	As dalteparin sodium 96 mg per 0.6 mL. Preservative free. In 0.6 mL single-dose prefilled syringes with 27-gauge × ½ in needle.
		18,000 units per 0.72 mL[a]	As dalteparin sodium 115.2 mg per 0.72 mL. Preservative free. In 0.72 mL single-dose prefilled syringes with 27-gauge × ½ in needle.
		95,000 units per 3.8 mL[a]	As dalteparin sodium 160 mg/mL. Benzyl alcohol 14 mg/mL. In 3.8 mL multidose vials.
		95,000 units per 9.5 mL[a]	As dalteparin sodium 64 mg/mL. Benzyl alcohol 14 mg/mL. In 9.5 mL multidose vials.

[a] Anti–factor Xa international units.

DALTEPARIN SODIUM — INJECTION

For complete and comparative prescribing information, refer to the Low Molecular Weight Heparins class monograph.

WARNING

Spinal/Epidural hematomas – Epidural or spinal hematomas may occur in patients who are anticoagulated with low molecular weight heparins or heparinoids and are receiving neuraxial anesthesia or undergoing spinal puncture. These hematomas may result in long-term or permanent paralysis. Consider these risks when scheduling patients for spinal procedures. Factors that can increase the risk of developing epidural or spinal hematomas in these patients include use of indwelling epidural catheters; concomitant use of other drugs that affect hemostasis, such as nonsteroidal anti-inflammatory drugs (NSAIDs), platelet inhibitors, or other anticoagulants; a history of traumatic or repeated epidural or spinal punctures; or a history of spinal deformity or spinal injury.

Monitor patients frequently for signs and symptoms of neurological impairment. If neurological compromise is noted, urgent treatment is necessary. Consider the benefits and risks before neuraxial intervention in patients anticoagulated or to be anticoagulated for thromboprophylaxis.

Indications

➤*Deep vein thrombosis prophylaxis:* For the prophylaxis of deep vein thrombosis (DVT), which may lead to pulmonary embolism in patients undergoing hip replacement surgery, in patients undergoing abdominal surgery who are at risk for thromboembolic complications, and in medical patients who are at risk for thromboembolic complications caused by severely restricted mobility during acute illness.

➤*Symptomatic venous thromboembolism:* For the extended treatment of symptomatic venous thromboembolism (VTE) (proximal DVT and/or pulmonary embolism) to reduce the recurrence of VTE in patients with cancer. Dalteparin is not indicated for the acute treatment of VTE.

➤*Unstable angina/non–Q-wave myocardial infarction:* For the prophylaxis of ischemic complications in unstable angina and non–Q-wave myocardial infarction (MI), when coadministered with aspirin therapy.

➤*Off-label uses:*

Primary venous thromboembolism prophylaxis in cancer patients – [4] = Insufficient documentation. Although primary prophylaxis with dalteparin or other anticoagulants is not recommended for all ambulatory cancer patients, cancer patients with other indications for anticoagulation should receive therapy.

Venous thromboembolism prophylaxis in cancer patients with central venous catheters – [4] = Insufficient documentation. Studies to date suggest that the rate of symptomatic central venous catheter (CVC)–associated VTE in patients with cancer is only 2% to 4%, which may be too low to warrant routine thromboprophylaxis even if it were efficacious. Conflicting results have been observed in trials evaluating prevention of CVC-induced VTE. Although prophylaxis of CVC-induced VTE with dalteparin or other anticoagulants is not recommended for all cancer patients, cancer patients with other indications for anticoagulation should receive therapy.

Venous thromboembolism prophylaxis in general surgery – [3] = Safety concerns. American College of Chest Physicians (ACCP) prevention of VTE guidelines noted that most general surgeries present a moderate risk of VTE. Low molecular weight heparins/heparinoids, such as dalteparin, were clearly shown to reduce DVT and pulmonary embolism after general surgery.

Venous thromboembolism prophylaxis in gynecologic surgery – [3] = Safety concerns. ACCP guidelines noted that most gynecologic surgeries present a moderate risk of VTE. Patients at moderate and high risk for VTE from gynecologic surgery should receive routine thromboprophylaxis with a low molecular weight heparin/heparinoid such as dalteparin, low-dose unfractionated heparin, fondaparinux, mechanical methods, or a combination of pharmacologic and mechanical thromboprophylaxis strategies.

Administration and Dosage

➤*Adults:*

Deep vein thrombosis prophylaxis –

Abdominal surgery:

• *Usual dosage* – 2,500 units administered by subcutaneous injection once daily, starting 1 to 2 hours prior to surgery and repeated once daily postoperatively.

High-risk patients (eg, malignant disorder): 5,000 units subcutaneously the evening before surgery, then once daily postoperatively. Alternatively, in patients with malignancy, 2,500 units of dalteparin can be administered subcutaneously 1 to 2 hours before surgery followed by 2,500 units subcutaneously 12 hours later, and then 5,000 units once daily postoperatively.

• *Duration of therapy* – 5 to 10 days postoperatively.

Hip-replacement surgery:

• *Usual dosage* –

Dalteparin Dosing Options for Patients Undergoing Hip Replacement Surgery

	Dose of dalteparin to be given subcutaneously			
Timing of first dose of dalteparin	10 to 14 h before surgery	Within 2 h before surgery	4 to 8 h after surgery[a]	Postoperative period[b]
Postoperative start	—	—	2,500 units[c]	5,000 units once daily
Preoperative start, day of surgery	—	2,500 units	2,500 units[c]	5,000 units once daily
Preoperative start, evening before surgery[d]	5,000 units	—	5,000 units	5,000 units once daily

[a] Or later, if hemostasis has not been achieved.
[b] Up to 14 days of treatment was well tolerated in controlled clinical trials, where the usual duration of treatment was 5 to 10 days postoperatively.
[c] Allow a minimum of 6 h between this dose and the dose to be given on postoperative day 1. Adjust the timing of the dose on postoperative day 1 accordingly.
[d] Allow approximately 24 h between doses.

• *Duration of therapy* – The usual duration of administration is 5 to 10 days after surgery; up to 14 days of treatment with dalteparin have been well tolerated in clinical trials.

DALTEPARIN SODIUM — INJECTION

Patients with severely restricted mobility during acute illness:

• *Usual dosage* – 5,000 units administered by subcutaneous injection once daily.

• *Duration of therapy* – In clinical trials, the usual duration of administration was 12 to 14 days.

Symptomatic venous thromboembolism –

Patients with cancer and symptomatic venous thromboembolism:

• *Month 1 –*

Usual dosage: For the first 30 days of treatment, administer dalteparin 200 units/kg total body weight subcutaneously once daily.

Dalteparin Dose to Be Administered Subcutaneously by Patient Weight During the First Month		
Body weight (lb)	Body weight (kg)	Dalteparin dose (units) (prefilled syringe) once daily
≤ 124	≤ 56	10,000
125 to 150	57 to 68	12,500
151 to 181	69 to 82	15,000
182 to 216	83 to 98	18,000
≥ 217	≥ 99	18,000

Maximum dose: The total daily dose should not exceed 18,000 units.

• *Months 2 to 6 –*

Usual dosage: Administer approximately 150 units/kg subcutaneously once daily during months 2 through 6.

Dalteparin Dose to Be Administered Subcutaneously by Patient Weight During Months 2 to 6		
Body weight (lb)	Body weight (kg)	Dalteparin dose (units) (prefilled syringe) once daily
≤ 124	≤ 56	7,500
125 to 150	57 to 68	10,000
151 to 181	69 to 82	12,500
182 to 216	83 to 98	15,000
≥ 217	≥ 99	18,000

Maximum dose: The total daily dose should not exceed 18,000 units.

• *Dosage adjustment –*

Thrombocytopenia: In patients receiving dalteparin who experience platelet counts between 50,000 and 100,000/mm^3, reduce the daily dose of dalteparin by 2,500 units until the platelet count recovers to at least 100,000/mm^3. In patients receiving dalteparin who experience platelet counts less than 50,000/mm^3, dalteparin should be discontinued until the platelet count recovers above 50,000/mm^3.

Unstable angina/non–Q-wave myocardial infarction –

Usual dosage: 120 units/kg of body weight, but not more than 10,000 units, subcutaneously every 12 hours with concurrent oral aspirin (75 to 165 mg/day) therapy.

Volume of Dalteparin to Be Administered by Patient Weight		
Body weight (lb)	Body weight (kg)	Volume of dalteparin (mL)[a]
< 110	< 50	0.55
110 to 131	50 to 59	0.65
132 to 153	60 to 69	0.75
154 to 175	70 to 79	0.9
176 to 197	80 to 89	1
≥ 198	≥ 90	1

[a] Calculated volume based on the 9.5 mL (10,000 units/mL) multidose vial.

Maximum dose: Not more than 10,000 units, subcutaneously every 12 hours.

Duration of therapy: Treatment should be continued until the patient is clinically stabilized. The usual duration of administration is 5 to 8 days.

Concomitant therapy: Concurrent aspirin therapy is recommended except when contraindicated.

Off-label dosing –

Primary venous thromboembolism prophylaxis in cancer patients: [4] = Insufficient documentation. 2,500 to 5,000 units once daily by subcutaneous injection.

Venous thromboembolism prophylaxis in cancer patients with CVC: [4] = Insufficient documentation. 2,500 or 5,000 units once daily by subcutaneous injection.

Venous thromboembolism prophylaxis in general surgery: [3] = Safety concerns. 2,500 units once daily by subcutaneous injection, starting 1 to 2 hours prior to surgery and repeated once daily postoperatively until hospital discharge.

In patients with other risk factors, such as cancer, that place them at high risk of VTE, the recommended dose is 5,000 units subcutaneously the evening before surgery, then once daily postoperatively at least until hospital discharge. Alternatively, in patients with malignancy, dalteparin 2,500 units can be administered 1 to 2 hours before surgery followed by 2,500 units 12 hours later, and then 5,000 units once daily postoperatively at least until hospital discharge.

For selected high-risk general surgery patients, including some who have undergone major cancer surgery or have previously experienced VTE, consider continuing dalteparin for up to 28 days after hospital discharge.

Venous thromboembolism prophylaxis in gynecologic surgery: [3] = Safety concerns. 2,500 units once daily by subcutaneous injection, starting 1 to 2 hours prior to surgery and repeated once daily postoperatively.

In patients with other risk factors, such as cancer, that place them at high risk of VTE, the recommended dose is 5,000 units subcutaneously the evening before surgery, then once daily postoperatively. Alternatively, in patients with malignancy, 2,500 units of dalteparin can be administered subcutaneously 1 to 2 hours before surgery followed by 2,500 units by subcutaneous injection 12 hours later, and then 5,000 units once daily postoperatively.

All patients who have major gynecologic surgery should receive thromboprophylaxis at least until hospital discharge. For patients undergoing major gynecologic surgery who are at high risk for VTE, including patients with a history of VTE or patients who had surgery for cancer, consider continuing dalteparin therapy for up to 28 days after hospital discharge.

➤*Renal function impairment:* Use with caution in patients with severe renal impairment.

Renal function impairment in extended treatment of acute symptomatic venous thromboembolism in patients with cancer – In patients with severe renal impairment (creatinine clearance less than 30 mL/min), monitoring for anti–factor Xa levels is recommended to determine the appropriate dalteparin dose. Target anti–factor Xa range is 0.5 to 1.5 units/mL. When monitoring anti–factor Xa in these patients, sampling should be performed 4 to 6 hours after dalteparin dosing and only after the patient has received 3 to 4 doses.

➤*Hepatic function impairment:* Use with caution in patients with severe hepatic impairment.

➤*Administration:* Dalteparin is administered by subcutaneous injection. It must not be administered by intramuscular (IM) injection.

Subcutaneous injection technique – Patients should be sitting or lying down and dalteparin administered by deep subcutaneous injection. Dalteparin may be injected in a U-shape area around the navel, the upper outer side of the thigh, or the upper outer quadrangle of the buttock. The injection site should be varied daily. When the area around the navel or the thigh is used, using the thumb and forefinger, you must lift up a fold of skin while giving the injection. The entire length of the needle should be inserted at a 45° to 90° angle.

Instructions for using the prefilled single-dose syringes preassembled with needle-guard devices –

Fixed-dose syringes: To ensure delivery of the full dose, do not expel the air bubble from the prefilled syringe before injection. Hold the syringe assembly by the open sides of the device. Remove the needle shield. Insert the needle into the injection area as instructed. Depress the plunger of the syringe while holding the finger flange until the entire dose has been given. The needle guard will not be activated unless the entire dose has been given. Remove needle from the patient. Let go of the plunger and allow the syringe to move up inside the device until the entire needle is guarded. Discard the syringe assembly in approved containers.

Graduated syringes: Hold the syringe assembly by the open sides of the device. Remove the needle shield. With the needle pointing up, prepare the syringe by expelling the air bubble and then continuing to push the plunger to the desired dose or volume, discarding the extra solution in an appropriate manner. Insert the needle into the injection area as previously instructed. Depress the plunger of the syringe while holding the finger flange until the entire dose remaining in the syringe has been given. The needle guard will not be activated unless the entire dose has been given. Remove the needle from the patient. Let go of the plunger and allow syringe to move up inside the device until the entire needle is guarded. Discard the syringe assembly in approved containers.

➤*Admixture compatibility:* Dalteparin injection should not be mixed with other injections or infusions unless specific compatibility data are available that support such mixing.

➤*Storage/Stability:* Store at 20° to 25°C (68° to 77°F). After first penetration of the rubber stopper, store the multidose vials at room temperature for up to 2 weeks. Discard any unused solution after 2 weeks.

Low Molecular Weight Heparins (LMWHs)

ENOXAPARIN SODIUM

Rx	**Enoxaparin Sodium** (Sandoz)	**Injection, solution:** 30 mg per 0.3 mL[a]	Preservative free. In single-dose prefilled syringes with a 27-gauge × ½-inch needle.
	Lovenox (Sanofi-Aventis)		Preservative free. In single-dose prefilled syringes with a 27-gauge × ½-inch needle.
Rx	**Enoxaparin Sodium** (Sandoz)	**Injection, solution:** 40 mg per 0.4 mL[a]	Preservative free. In single-dose prefilled syringes with a 27-gauge × ½-inch needle.
	Lovenox (Sanofi-Aventis)		Preservative free. In single-dose prefilled syringes with a 27-gauge × ½-inch needle.
Rx	**Enoxaparin Sodium** (Sandoz)	**Injection, solution:** 60 mg per 0.6 mL[a]	Preservative free. In graduated, single-dose prefilled syringes with a 27-gauge × ½-inch needle.
	Lovenox (Sanofi-Aventis)		Preservative free. In graduated, single-dose prefilled syringes with a 27-gauge × ½-inch needle.
Rx	**Enoxaparin Sodium** (Sandoz)	**Injection, solution:** 80 mg per 0.8 mL[a]	Preservative free. In graduated, single-dose prefilled syringes with a 27-gauge × ½-inch needle.
	Lovenox (Sanofi-Aventis)		Preservative free. In graduated, single-dose prefilled syringes with a 27-gauge × ½-inch needle.
Rx	**Enoxaparin Sodium** (Sandoz)	**Injection, solution:** 100 mg per 1 mL[a]	Preservative free. In graduated, single-dose prefilled syringes with a 27-gauge × ½-inch needle.
	Lovenox (Sanofi-Aventis)		Preservative free. In graduated, single-dose prefilled syringes with a 27-gauge × ½-inch needle.
Rx	**Enoxaparin Sodium** (Sandoz)	**Injection, solution:** 120 mg per 0.8 mL[b]	Preservative free. In graduated, single-dose prefilled syringes with a 27-gauge × ½-inch needle.
	Lovenox (Sanofi-Aventis)		Preservative free. In graduated, single-dose prefilled syringes with a 27-gauge × ½-inch needle.
Rx	**Enoxaparin Sodium** (Sandoz)	**Injection, solution:** 150 mg per 1 mL[b]	Preservative free. In graduated, single-dose prefilled syringes with a 27-gauge × ½-inch needle.
	Lovenox (Sanofi-Aventis)		Preservative free. In graduated, single-dose prefilled syringes with a 27-gauge × ½-inch needle.
Rx	**Lovenox** (Sanofi-Aventis)	**Injection, solution:** 300 mg per 3 mL[a]	Benzyl alcohol 15 mg/mL. In 3 mL multidose vials.

[a] Approximate anti–factor Xa activity of 1,000 units per 0.1 mL (with reference to the World Health Organization [WHO] First International Low Molecular Weight Heparin [LMWH] Reference Standard).

[b] Approximate anti–factor Xa activity of 1,500 units per 0.1 mL (with reference to the WHO First International LMWH Reference Standard).

ENOXAPARIN SODIUM — INJECTION

For complete and comparative prescribing information, refer to the Low Molecular Weight Heparins (LMWHs) class monograph.

WARNING

Spinal/Epidural hematomas – Epidural or spinal hematomas may occur in patients who are anticoagulated with LMWHs or heparinoids and are receiving neuraxial anesthesia or undergoing spinal puncture. These hematomas may result in long-term or permanent paralysis. Consider these risks when scheduling patients for spinal procedures.

Factors that can increase the risk of developing epidural or spinal hematomas in these patients include use of indwelling epidural catheters; concomitant use of other drugs that affect hemostasis, such as nonsteroidal anti-inflammatory drugs (NSAIDs), platelet inhibitors, and other anticoagulants; a history of traumatic or repeated epidural or spinal punctures; and a history of spinal deformity or spinal surgery.

Monitor patients frequently for signs and symptoms of neurological impairment. If neurological compromise is noted, urgent treatment is necessary.

Consider the benefits and risks before neuraxial intervention in patients anticoagulated or to be anticoagulated for thromboprophylaxis.

Indications

➤*Acute ST-segment elevation myocardial infarction:* For the treatment of acute ST-segment elevation myocardial infarction (STEMI) in patients receiving thrombolysis and being managed medically or with percutaneous coronary intervention (PCI).

➤*Prophylaxis of deep vein thrombosis:* For the prophylaxis of deep vein thrombosis (DVT), which may lead to pulmonary embolism in patients undergoing abdominal surgery who are at risk for thromboembolic complications; patients undergoing hip replacement surgery, during and following hospitalization; patients undergoing knee replacement surgery; and medical patients who are at risk for thromboembolic complications because ofseverely restricted mobility during acute illness.

➤*Prophylaxis of ischemic complications of unstable angina/non–Q-wave myocardial infarction:* For the prophylaxis of ischemic complications of unstable angina/non–Q-wave MI, when coadministered with aspirin.

➤*Treatment of acute deep vein thrombosis:* For the inpatient treatment of acute DVT with or without pulmonary embolism, when administered in conjunction with warfarin; for the outpatient treatment of acute DVT without pulmonary embolism, when administered in conjunction with warfarin.

➤*Off-label uses:*

Prevention of exercise-induced bronchoconstriction – [5] = Poor documentation. Enoxaparin and heparin produce similar inhibitory effects on exercise-induced bronchoconstriction (EIB). The inability of enoxaparin to protect against methacholine-induced bronchoconstriction suggests that its action is not based on direct effect of the airway smooth muscle. Despite these effects, the use of this agent cannot be recommended for routine EIB control because there are several alternatives readily available.

Venous thromboembolism prophylaxis in cancer patients with central venous catheters – [4] = Insufficient documentation. Studies to date suggest that the rate of symptomatic central venous catheter (CVC)–associated venous thromboembolism (VTE) in patients with cancer is only 2% to 4%, which may be too low to warrant routine thromboprophylaxis even if prophylaxis was efficacious. Conflicting results have been observed in the studies evaluating prophylaxis of catheter-related VTE. Although prophylaxis of CVC-induced VTE with enoxaparin or other anticoagulants is not recommended for all cancer patients, cancer patients with other indications for anticoagulation should receive therapy. For example, patients with cancer who undergo surgical procedures should receive routine thromboprophylaxis as indicated by the type of surgery. In addition, patients with cancer who are bedridden because of acute illness should receive routine prophylaxis, as would be indicated in the absence of a cancer diagnosis.

Venous thromboembolism prophylaxis in general surgery – [3] = Safety concerns. American College of Chest Physicians (ACCP) guidelines for prevention of VTE noted that most general surgeries present a moderate risk of VTE. In the absence of special factors that pose a high risk of bleeding, routine thromboprophylaxis is recommended for most patients. LMWHs such as enoxaparin were clearly shown to reduce DVT and pulmonary embolism after general surgery. Potential advantages of enoxaparin over low-dose unfractionated heparin include once-daily administration and a lower risk of heparin-induced thrombocytopenia. In patients at a high risk of bleeding, mechanical thromboprophylaxis methods are preferred. In patients at a very high risk of VTE, such as cancer surgery patients, enoxaparin administration for up to 28 days after hospital discharge may reduce the incidence of VTE.

Venous thromboembolism prophylaxis in gynecologic surgery – [3] = Safety concerns. ACCP guidelines noted that most gynecologic surgeries present a moderated risk of VTE. Patients at moderate and high risk for VTE from gynecologic surgery should receive routine thromboprophylaxis with a LMWH/heparinoid such as enoxaparin, low-dose unfractionated heparin, fondaparinux, mechanical methods, or a combination of pharmacologic and mechanical thromboprophylaxis strategies. Potential advantages of enoxaparin over low-dose unfractionated heparin include once-daily administration and a lower risk of heparin-induced thrombocytopenia. In patients at a very high risk of VTE, such as cancer surgery patients, enoxaparin administration for up to 28 days after hospital discharge may be considered on a case-by-case basis; however, additional studies are needed to identify the precise population of gynecologic surgery patients who will benefit from extended thromboprophylaxis.

ENOXAPARIN SODIUM — INJECTION

Administration and Dosage

➤*General dosing considerations:* All patients should be evaluated for a bleeding disorder before administration, unless the medication is needed urgently.

Dosing adjustment is required for patients with severe renal impairment (creatinine clearance [CrCl] less than 30 mL/min). (See Renal Function Impairment.)

➤*Adults:*

Acute ST-segment elevation myocardial infarction –

Usual dosage: Single intravenous (IV) bolus of 30 mg plus a 1 mg/kg subcutaneous dose, followed by 1 mg/kg subcutaneously every 12 hours (maximum, 100 mg for the first 2 doses only, followed by 1 mg/kg dosing for the remaining doses).

When administered in conjunction with a thrombolytic (fibrin-specific or nonfibrin-specific), enoxaparin should be given between 15 minutes before and 30 minutes after the start of fibrinolytic therapy.

Maximum dose: 100 mg for the first 2 doses.

Duration of therapy: In a pivotal clinical study, the enoxaparin treatment duration was 8 days or until hospital discharge, whichever came first. An optimal duration of treatment is not known, but it is likely to be longer than 8 days.

Concomitant therapy: All patients should receive aspirin as soon as they are identified as having STEMI and should be maintained with 75 to 325 mg once daily unless contraindicated.

Percutaneous coronary intervention: If the last subcutaneous administration was given less than 8 hours before balloon inflation, no additional dosing is needed. If the last subcutaneous administration was given more than 8 hours before balloon inflation, an IV bolus of enoxaparin 0.3 mg/kg should be administered.

Prophylaxis of deep vein thrombosis –

Abdominal surgery:

- *Usual dosage* – 40 mg subcutaneously once daily, with the initial dose given 2 hours prior to surgery.
- *Duration of therapy* – 7 to 10 days; up to 12 days has been administered in clinical trials.

Hip or knee replacement surgery:

- *Usual dosage* – 30 mg subcutaneously every 12 hours. Provided that hemostasis has been established, the initial dose should be given 12 to 24 hours after surgery.
- *Alternative dosage* – For hip replacement surgery, 40 mg subcutaneously once daily given initially 12 (±3) hours prior to surgery may be considered. Following the initial phase of thromboprophylaxis in hip replacement surgery, continued prophylaxis with enoxaparin 40 mg subcutaneously once daily for 3 weeks is recommended.
- *Duration of therapy* – 7 to 10 days; up to 14 days has been administered in clinical trials.

Medical patients during acute illness:

- *Usual dosage* – 40 mg subcutaneously once a day.
- *Duration of therapy* – 6 to 11 days; up to 14 days has been administered in a controlled clinical trial.

Prophylaxis of ischemic complications of unstable angina/non–Q-wave myocardial infarction –

Usual dosage: 1 mg/kg subcutaneously every 12 hours.

Duration of therapy: Minimum of 2 days and continued until clinical stabilization. The usual duration of treatment is 2 to 8 days; up to 12.5 days has been administered in clinical trials.

Concomitant therapy: Aspirin 100 to 325 mg orally once daily.

Treatment of acute deep vein thrombosis –

Usual dosage: In outpatient treatment of patients with acute DVT without pulmonary embolism, 1 mg/kg subcutaneously every 12 hours.

In inpatient treatment of patients with acute DVT with or without pulmonary embolism, 1 mg/kg subcutaneously every 12 hours or 1.5 mg/kg subcutaneously once daily at the same time every day.

Duration of therapy: Therapy should be continued for a minimum of 5 days and until a therapeutic oral anticoagulant effect has been achieved (international normalization ratio [INR], 2 to 3). The average duration of therapy is 7 days; up to 17 days has been administered in controlled clinical trials.

Concomitant therapy: Warfarin should be initiated when appropriate (usually within 72 hours of enoxaparin).

Off-label dosing –

Venous thromboembolism prophylaxis in cancer patients with central venous catheters: [4] = Insufficient documentation. 40 mg by subcutaneous injection once daily. Enoxaparin was initiated 2 hours before CVC insertion and continued for 6 weeks.

Venous thromboembolism prophylaxis in general surgery: [3] = Safety concerns. 40 mg once daily administered by subcutaneous injection, with the initial dose given 2 hours prior to surgery. The usual duration of administration is until hospital discharge or for 7 to 10 days.

For selected high-risk general surgery patients, including some who have undergone major cancer surgery or have previously experienced VTE, consider continuing enoxaparin for up to 28 days after hospital discharge.

Venous thromboembolism prophylaxis in gynecologic surgery: [3] = Safety concerns. 40 mg once per day administered by subcutaneous injection, with the initial dose given 2 hours prior to surgery. All patients who have major gynecologic surgery should receive thromboprophylaxis at least until hospital discharge.

For patients undergoing major gynecologic surgery who are at high risk for VTE, including patients with a history of VTE or who had surgery for cancer, consider continuing enoxaparin therapy for up to 28 days after hospital discharge.

➤*Children:*

Off-label dosing –

Thrombosis prophylaxis:

- *2 months of age and older* – 0.5 mg/kg subcutaneously every 12 hours.
- *Younger than 2 months of age* – 0.75 mg/kg subcutaneously every 12 hours.

Thrombosis treatment:

- *Usual dose –*

  2 months of age and older: 1 mg/kg subcutaneously every 12 hours.

  Younger than 2 months of age: 1.5 mg/kg subcutaneously every 12 hours.

  Preterm infants younger than 2 months of age: May require higher doses to achieve therapeutic anti–factor Xa concentrations; 2 mg/kg subcutaneously every 12 hours has been recommended.

- *Dosage adjustment –*

Enoxaparin Thrombosis Treatment Dosage Adjustments in Children Based on Anti–Factor Xa Concentrations

Anti–factor Xa concentration	Dosage adjustment	Timing of next dosage	Repeat anti–factor Xa level
< 0.35 units/mL	Increase dose 25%	On time	4 h after next dose
0.35 to 0.46 units/mL	Increase dose 10%	On time	4 h after next dose
0.5 to 1 unit/mL	No change	On time	Every other day[a]
1.1 to 1.5 units/mL	Decrease dose 20%	On time	4 h after next dose
1.6 to 2 units/mL	Decrease dose 30%	Delay dose 3 h	4 h after next dose
> 2 units/mL	Decrease dose 40%	Delay dose until anti–factor Xa	Every 12 h until anti–factor Xa [b]

[a] Some references recommend repeating the anti–factor Xa level the following day and then 1 week later 4 hours postdose.
[b] Some references recommend repeating anti–factor Xa level 4 hours after next dose.

Therapeutic monitoring: Draw anti–factor Xa concentrations 4 to 6 hours after a subcutaneous dose. Therapeutic anti–factor Xa levels are 0.1 to 0.4 units/mL for prophylactic dosages and 0.5 to 1 unit/mL for treatment dosages.

➤*Elderly:*

Acute ST-segment elevation myocardial infarction –

75 years of age and older: Do not use an initial IV bolus. Initiate dosing with 0.75 mg/kg subcutaneously every 12 hours (maximum, 75 mg for the first 2 doses only, followed by 0.75 mg/kg dosing for the remaining doses).

➤*Renal function impairment:*

Severe renal impairment –

Enoxaparin Dosage Regimens for Patients With Severe Renal Impairment (CrCl

Indication	Dosage regimen
Acute STEMI in patients < 75 years of age, when administered in conjunction with aspirin	30 mg single IV bolus plus a 1 mg/kg dose subcutaneously followed by 1 mg/kg subcutaneously once daily
Acute STEMI in patients ≥ 75 years of age, when administered in conjunction with aspirin	1 mg/kg subcutaneously once daily (no initial bolus)
Prophylaxis of DVT: abdominal surgery, hip or knee replacement surgery, medical patients during acute illness	30 mg subcutaneously once daily
Prophylaxis of ischemic complications of unstable angina/non–Q-wave MI, when coadministered with aspirin	1 mg/kg subcutaneously once daily
Treatment of acute DVT with or without pulmonary embolism, when administered in conjunction with warfarin (inpatient)	1 mg/kg subcutaneously once daily
Treatment of acute DVT without pulmonary embolism, when administered in conjunction with warfarin (outpatient)	1 mg/kg subcutaneously once daily

➤*Administration:* For subcutaneous use or IV bolus injection. Enoxaparin must not be administered by intramuscular (IM) injection.

For subcutaneous administration, patients may self-inject only if their health care provider determines that it is appropriate, and with medical follow-up as necessary. The use of a tuberculin syringe or equivalent is recommended when using multidose vials to ensure withdrawal of the appropriate volume of drug.

Subcutaneous injection – Patients should be lying down, and enoxaparin should be administered by deep subcutaneous injection. To avoid the loss of drug when using the 30 and 40 mg prefilled syringes, do not expel the air bubble from the syringe before the injection. Administration should be alternated between the left and right anterolateral and left and right pos-

ENOXAPARIN SODIUM — INJECTION

terolateral abdominal wall. The whole length of the needle should be introduced into a skin fold held between the thumb and forefinger; the skin fold should be held throughout the injection. To minimize bruising, do not rub the injection site after completion of the injection.

IV (bolus) injection – For IV injection, the multidose vial should be used. Enoxaparin should be administered through an IV line. To avoid the possible mixture with other drugs, the IV access chosen should be flushed with a sufficient amount of saline or dextrose solution prior to and following the IV bolus administration to clear the port of the drug.

➤*Admixture compatibility:* Enoxaparin should not be mixed or coadministered with other injections or infusions. For IV use, enoxaparin can be mixed with normal saline solution (0.9%) or dextrose 5% in water.

➤*Storage/Stability:* Store at 25°C (77°F); excursions are permitted to 15° to 30°C (59° to 86°F). Do not store the multidose vials for more than 28 days after the first use.

TINZAPARIN SODIUM

Rx	**Innohep** (Leo Pharma)	**Injection, solution**: 20,000 units/mL[a]	Sodium metabisulfite 3.1 mg/mL, benzyl alcohol 10 mg/mL. In 2 mL multidose vials.

[a] Anti-factor Xa international units.

TINZAPARIN SODIUM — INJECTION

For complete and comparative prescribing information, refer to the Low Molecular Weight Heparins class monograph.

WARNING

Spinal/Epidural hematomas – Epidural or spinal hematomas may occur in patients who are anticoagulated with low molecular weight heparins (LMWHs) or heparinoids and are receiving neuraxial anesthesia or undergoing spinal puncture. These hematomas may result in long-term or permanent paralysis. Consider these risks when scheduling patients for spinal procedures. Factors that can increase the risk of developing epidural or spinal hematomas in these patients include use of indwelling epidural catheters; concomitant use of other drugs that affect hemostasis, such as nonsteroidal anti-inflammatory drugs (NSAIDs), platelet inhibitors, or other anticoagulants; a history of traumatic or repeated epidural or spinal punctures; and a history of spinal deformity or spinal surgery.

Monitor patients frequently for signs and symptoms of neurological impairment. If neurological compromise is noted, urgent treatment is necessary. Consider the benefits and risks before neuraxial intervention in patients anticoagulated or to be anticoagulated for thromboprophylaxis.

Indications

➤*Deep vein thrombosis:* Treatment of acute symptomatic deep vein thrombosis (DVT), with or without pulmonary embolism (PE), when administered in conjunction with warfarin.

➤*Off-label uses:*

Venous thromboembolism prophylaxis in general surgery – [3] = Safety concerns. American College of Chest Physicians (ACCP) guidelines noted that most general surgeries present a moderate risk of venous thromboembolism (VTE). In the absence of special risk factors that pose a high risk of bleeding, routine thromboprophylaxis would be recommended for most patients. LMWHs/heparinoids such as tinzaparin were clearly shown to reduce DVT and PE after general surgery. Potential advantages of tinzaparin over low-dose unfractionated heparin include once-daily administration and a lower risk of heparin-induced thrombocytopenia. In patients at a high risk of bleeding, mechanical thromboprophylaxis methods are preferred. In patients at a very high risk of VTE, such as cancer surgery patients, tinzaparin administration for up to 28 days after hospital discharge may reduce the incidence of VTE.

Venous thromboembolism prophylaxis in gynecologic surgery – [3] = Safety concerns. ACCP guidelines noted that most gynecologic surgeries present a moderate risk of VTE. Patients at moderate and high risk of VTE from gynecologic surgery should receive routine thromboprophylaxis with a LMWH/heparinoid such as tinzaparin, low-dose unfractionated heparin, fondaparinux, mechanical methods, or a combination of pharmacologic and mechanical thromboprophylaxis strategies. Potential advantages of tinzaparin over low-dose unfractionated heparin include once-daily administration and a lower risk of heparin-induced thrombocytopenia. In patients at a very high risk of VTE, such as cancer surgery patients, tinzaparin administration for up to 28 days after hospital discharge may be considered on a case-by-case basis; however, additional studies are needed to identify the precise population of gynecologic surgery patients who will benefit from extended thromboprophylaxis.

Other possible off-label uses – Prophylaxis of DVT, which may lead to PE, in patients undergoing orthopedic surgery, hip fracture surgery, or neurosurgery at risk of thromboembolic complications.

Administration and Dosage

➤*General dosing considerations:* Evaluate all patients for bleeding disorders before administration of tinzaparin.

➤*Adults:*

Deep vein thrombosis –

Usual dosage: 175 anti-factor Xa (anti-Xa) units/kg of body weight, administered subcutaneously once daily for at least 6 days and until the patient is adequately anticoagulated with warfarin (international normalized ratio [INR] of at least 2 for 2 consecutive days).

Tinzaparin Dosing for Treatment of Deep Vein Thrombosis

Body weight (kg)	175 units/kg subcutaneously once daily 20,000 units/mL	
	Dose (units)	Amount (mL)
31 to 36	6,000	0.3
37 to 42	7,000	0.35
43 to 48	8,000	0.4
49 to 53	9,000	0.45
54 to 59	10,000	0.5
60 to 65	11,000	0.55
66 to 70	12,000	0.6
71 to 76	13,000	0.65
77 to 82	14,000	0.7
83 to 88	15,000	0.75
89 to 93	16,000	0.8
94 to 99	17,000	0.85
100 to 105	18,000	0.9
106 to 110	19,000	0.95
111 to 116	20,000	1
117 to 122	21,000	1.05
123 to 128	22,000	1.1
129 to 133	23,000	1.15
134 to 139	24,000	1.2
140 to 145	25,000	1.25
146 to 150	26,000	1.3
151 to 156	27,000	1.35
157 to 162	28,000	1.4

It is necessary to calculate the appropriate tinzaparin dose for patient weights not displayed in the table. Use the following equation to calculate the volume (mL) of tinzaparin 175 anti-factor Xa units/kg subcutaneous dose for treatment of DVT:

Patient weight (kg) × 0.00875 mL/kg = volume to be given (mL) subcutaneously.

Concomitant therapy: Initiate warfarin therapy when appropriate (usually within 1 to 3 days of tinzaparin initiation).

Because tinzaparin may theoretically affect the prothrombin time (PT)/INR, draw blood for PT/INR determination just prior to the next scheduled dose of tinzaparin for patients receiving tinzaparin and warfarin.

Off-label dosing –

Venous thromboembolism prophylaxis in general surgery: [3] = Safety concerns. 3,500 units administered by subcutaneous injection once per day started preoperatively. The usual duration of administration is until hospital discharge or for 7 days. For selected high-risk general surgery patients, including some who have undergone major cancer surgery or have previously experienced VTE, consider continuing tinzaparin for up to 28 days after hospital discharge.

Venous thromboembolism prophylaxis in gynecologic surgery: [3] = Safety concerns. 3,500 units by subcutaneous injection once daily, started just before surgery. All patients who have major gynecologic surgery should receive thromboprophylaxis at least until hospital discharge. For patients undergoing major gynecologic surgery who are at high risk of VTE, including patients with a history of VTE or patients who had surgery for cancer, consider continuing tinzaparin therapy for up to 28 days after hospital discharge.

➤*Elderly:* Use with extreme caution in elderly patients with renal impairment.

➤*Preparation for administration:* Use an appropriately calibrated syringe to ensure the correct volume of drug is withdrawn from the vials.

Low Molecular Weight Heparins (LMWHs)

TINZAPARIN SODIUM — INJECTION

➤*Administration:* Administer tinzaparin by subcutaneous injection. Do not administer by intramuscular or intravenous (IV) injection.

Position patients either lying down (supine) or sitting, and administer tinzaparin by deep subcutaneous injection. Alternate administration between left and right anterolateral and left and right posterolateral abdominal wall. Vary the injection site daily. Introduce the whole length of the needle into a skin fold held between the thumb and forefinger; hold the skin fold throughout the injection. To minimize bruising, do not rub the injection site after completion of the injection.

➤*Admixture compatibility:* Do not mix with other injections or infusions.

➤*Storage/Stability:* Store at 25°C (77°F); excursions are permitted between 15° and 30°C (59° and 86°F).

Heparin

Rx	**Heparin Sodium**[a] (Various, eg, APP, Hospira)	**Injection, solution:** 1,000 units/mL	In 1 mL vials.
Rx	**Heparin Sodium**[a] (Various, eg, APP)	**Injection, solution:** 2,000 units per 2 mL (1,000 units/mL)	In 2 mL vials.
Rx	**Heparin Sodium**[a] (Various, eg, APP, Hospira)	**Injection, solution:** 10,000 units per 10 mL (1,000 units/mL)	In 10 mL vials.
Rx	**Heparin Sodium**[a] (Various, eg, APP, Hospira)	**Injection, solution:** 30,000 units per 30 mL (1,000 units/mL)	In 30 mL vials.
Rx	**Heparin Sodium**[a] (Various, eg, Hospira)	**Injection, solution:** 10,000 units per 5 mL (2,000 units/mL)	In 5 mL vials.
Rx	**Heparin Sodium**[a] (Various, eg, Hospira)	**Injection, solution:** 25,000 units per 10 mL (2,500 units/mL)	In 10 mL vials.
Rx	**Heparin Sodium**[a] (Various, eg, APP, Baxter)	**Injection, solution:** 5,000 units/mL	In 1 mL vials.
Rx	**Heparin Sodium**[a] (Various, eg, Baxter, Hospira)	**Injection, solution:** 50,000 units per 10 mL (5,000 units/mL)	In 10 mL vials.
Rx	**Heparin Sodium**[a] (Various, eg, APP, Baxter, Hospira)	**Injection, solution:** 10,000 units/mL	In 1 mL vials.
Rx	**Heparin Sodium**[a] (Various, eg, Baxter)	**Injection, solution:** 40,000 units per 4 mL (10,000 units/mL)	In 4 mL vials.
Rx	**Heparin Sodium**[a] (Various, eg, APP)	**Injection, solution:** 50,000 units per 5 mL (10,000 units/mL)	In 5 mL vials.
Rx	**Heparin Sodium**[a] (Various, eg, APP)	**Injection, solution:** 20,000 units/mL	In 1 mL vials.
Rx	**Heparin Sodium**[a] **in Dextrose 5% Injection** (Various, eg, Baxter, B. Braun, Hospira)	**Injection, solution:** 20,000 units per 500 mL (40 units/mL)	In 500 mL containers.
		12,500 units per 250 mL (50 units/mL)	In 250 mL containers.
		25,000 units per 500 mL (50 units/mL)	In 500 mL containers.
		25,000 units per 250 mL (100 units/mL)	In 250 mL containers.
Rx	**Heparin Sodium**[a] **in Sodium Chloride 0.45% Injection** (Hospira)	**Injection, solution:** 12,500 units per 250 mL (50 units/mL)	In 250 mL.
		25,000 units per 500 mL (50 units/mL)	In 500 mL.
		25,000 units per 250 mL (100 units/mL)	In 250 mL.
Rx	**Heparin Sodium**[a] **in Sodium Chloride 0.9% Injection** (Baxter, Hospira)	**Injection, solution:** 1,000 units per 500 mL (2 units/mL)	In 500 mL.
		2,000 units per 1,000 mL (2 units/mL)	In 1,000 mL.
Rx	**Heparin I.V. Flush**[a] (Medefil)	**Injection, solution:** 1 unit/mL	In 1 mL prefilled syringes.
Rx	**Heparin I.V. Flush**[a] (Medefil)	**Injection, solution:** 2 units per 2 mL (1 unit/mL)	In 2 mL prefilled syringes.
Rx	**Heparin I.V. Flush**[a] (Medefil)	**Injection, solution:** 2.5 units per 2.5 mL (1 unit/mL)	In 2.5 mL prefilled syringes.
Rx	**Heparin I.V. Flush**[a] (Medefil)	**Injection, solution:** 3 units per 3 mL (1 unit/mL)	In 3 mL prefilled syringes.
Rx	**Heparin I.V. Flush**[a] (Medefil)	**Injection, solution:** 5 units per 5 mL (1 unit/mL)	In 5 mL prefilled syringes.
Rx	**Heparin I.V. Flush**[a] (Medefil)	**Injection, solution:** 10 units per 10 mL (1 unit/mL)	In 10 mL prefilled syringes.
Rx	**Heparin I.V. Flush**[a] (Medefil)	**Injection, solution:** 1 unit/mL	In 1 mL prefilled syringes.
Rx	**Heparin Lock Flush**[a] (Various, eg, APP, Hospira)	**Injection, solution:** 10 units/mL	In 1 mL.
Rx	**Heparin I.V. Flush**[a] (Medefil)		In 1 mL prefilled syringes.
Rx	**Heparin Lock Flush**[a] (Various, eg, Hospira)	**Injection, solution:** 20 units per 2 mL (10 units/mL)	May contain benzyl alcohol or parabens. In 2 mL.
Rx	**Heparin I.V. Flush**[a] (Medefil)		In 2 mL prefilled syringes.
Rx	**Heparin I.V. Flush**[a] (Medefil)	**Injection, solution:** 25 units per 2.5 mL (10 units/mL)	In 2.5 mL prefilled syringes.
Rx	**Heparin Lock Flush**[a] (Various, eg, Hospira)	**Injection, solution:** 30 units per 3 mL (10 units/mL)	May contain benzyl alcohol or parabens. In 3 mL.
Rx	**Heparin I.V. Flush**[a] (Medefil)		In 3 mL prefilled syringes.
Rx	**Monoject PreFill Advanced**[a] (Kendall)		Preservative free. In 3 mL prefilled syringes.
Rx	**Heparin Lock Flush**[a] (Various, eg, Hospira)	**Injection, solution:** 50 units per 5 mL (10 units/mL)	May contain benzyl alcohol or parabens. In 5 mL.
Rx	**Heparin I.V. Flush**[a] (Medefil)		In 5 mL prefilled syringes.
Rx	**Monoject PreFill Advanced**[a] (Kendall)		Preservative free. In 5 mL prefilled syringes.
Rx	**Heparin Lock Flush**[a] (Various, eg, APP)	**Injection, solution:** 100 units per 10 mL (10 units/mL)	May contain benzyl alcohol or parabens. In 10 mL.
Rx	**Heparin I.V. Flush**[a] (Medefil)		In 10 mL prefilled syringes.
Rx	**Hepflush-10**[a] (APP)		Preservative free. In 10 mL single-dose vial.
Rx	**Monoject PreFill Advanced**[a] (Kendall)		Preservative free. In 10 mL prefilled syringes.
Rx	**Heparin Lock Flush**[a] (Various, eg, APP, Hospira)	**Injection, solution:** 100 units/mL	May contain benzyl alcohol or parabens. In 1 mL.
Rx	**Heparin I.V. Flush**[a] (Medefil)		In 1 mL prefilled syringes.
Rx	**Heparin Lock Flush**[a] (Various, eg, Hospira)	**Injection, solution:** 200 units per 2 mL (100 units/mL)	May contain benzyl alcohol or parabens. In 2 mL.
Rx	**Heparin I.V. Flush**[a] (Medefil)		In 2 mL prefilled syringes.
Rx	**Heparin I.V. Flush**[a] (Medefil)	**Injection, solution:** 250 units per 2.5 mL (100 units/mL)	In 2.5 mL prefilled syringes.

Heparin			
Rx	Heparin Lock Flush[a] (Various, eg, Hospira)	Injection, solution: 300 units per 3 mL (100 units/mL)	May contain benzyl alcohol or parabens. In 3 mL.
Rx	Heparin I.V. Flush[a] (Medefil)		In 3 mL prefilled syringes.
Rx	Monoject PreFill Advanced[a] (Kendall)		Preservative free. In 3 mL prefilled syringes.
Rx	Heparin Lock Flush[a] (Various, eg, APP, Hospira)	Injection, solution: 500 units per 5 mL (100 units/mL)	May contain benzyl alcohol or parabens. In 5 mL.
Rx	Heparin I.V. Flush[a] (Medefil)		In 5 mL prefilled syringes.
Rx	Monoject PreFill Advanced[a] (Kendall)		Preservative free. In 5 mL prefilled syringes.
Rx	Heparin I.V. Flush[a] (Medefil)	Injection, solution: 1,000 units per 10 mL (100 units/mL)	In 10 mL prefilled syringes.

[a] From porcine intestinal mucosa.

HEPARIN SODIUM — INJECTION

Indications

➤*Anticoagulation:* For anticoagulant therapy in prophylaxis and treatment of venous thrombosis and its extension, in low-dose regimen for prevention of postoperative deep venous thrombosis (DVT) and pulmonary embolism (PE) in patients undergoing major abdominothoracic surgery who are at risk of developing thromboembolic disease, for prophylaxis and treatment of PE, in atrial fibrillation with embolization, for diagnosis and treatment of acute and chronic consumptive coagulopathies (disseminated intravascular coagulation), for prevention of clotting in arterial and cardiac surgery, and for prophylaxis and treatment of peripheral arterial embolism.

Heparin may also be employed as an anticoagulant in blood transfusions, extracorporeal circulation, dialysis procedures, and in blood samples for laboratory purposes.

➤*Off-label uses:* According to the antithrombotic guidelines from the American College of Chest Physicians (ACCP), heparin is recommended as an anticoagulant in several conditions, such as the following: acute DVT of the legs, acute DVT of the upper extremity, acute PE, superficial vein thrombosis, patients with atrial fibrillation undergoing cardioversion, nonbacterial thrombotic endocarditis and systemic or pulmonary emboli, cerebral venous sinus thrombosis, non–ST-segment elevation acute coronary syndrome (NSTE ACS), acute ST-segment elevation myocardial infarction (MI), including patients undergoing primary percutaneous coronary intervention, unstable angina, acute arterial emboli or thrombosis, and patients undergoing major vascular reconstruction. See the ACCP antithrombotic guidelines for more details. See also Administration and Dosage.

Administration and Dosage

➤*General dosing considerations:* All patients should be screened prior to heparin treatment to rule out bleeding disorders.

Potency changes – According to the Food and Drug Administration (FDA), heparin manufactured after October 1, 2009 will be approximately 10% less potent than heparin manufactured prior to that date. This is because of the *United States Pharmacopeia* (USP) revising the heparin monograph. The revised USP monograph will include a new USP reference standard and test method that is used to determine the potency of the drug. The monograph change will also harmonize the USP unit dose with the World Health Organization (WHO) International Standard (IS) unit dose. However, harmonization of the standard will result in an approximately 10% reduction in the potency of the heparin marketed in the United States.

The change in heparin potency may have clinical significance in some situations, such as when heparin is administered as a bolus intravenous (IV) dose and an immediate anticoagulant effect is clinically important. In such situations, health care providers should consider the change in potency of heparin when making decisions about what dose to administer. The change in heparin potency is expected to be less clinically significant when it is administered subcutaneously because of the low and highly variable bioavailability of heparin when administered by this route. Health care providers should also be aware of the decrease in heparin potency as they monitor the anticoagulant effect of the drug; more heparin may be required to achieve and maintain the desired level of anticoagulation in some patients.

The potency change may require more frequent or intensive activated partial thromboplastin time (aPTT) or activated clotting time (ACT) monitoring.

In April 2010, the FDA announced the following information. Laboratory studies performed at the request of the FDA have shown that heparin made under the new USP monograph ("new heparin") has approximately 10% less blood-thinning (anticoagulant) activity compared with heparin prepared using the previous ("old") USP monograph. The results of these studies reinforce the FDA's previous recommendation for health care providers to exercise clinical judgment in determining the dose of heparin for a patient and consider the clinical circumstances where the potency decrease may require dosage adjustments and more frequent monitoring. Health care providers may wish to consider not using the products interchangeably.

The ACCP did not revise their antithrombotic guidelines as a result of this potency change. Health care providers should be aware that larger doses of heparin will be required to achieve therapeutic levels of anticoagulation and to guide heparin infusions based on anticoagulation tests (eg, aPTT, ACT, or thrombin clotting time [TCT]). In situations in which fixed doses of heparin are administered with clinical monitoring (but not laboratory monitoring), heparin doses may or may not need to be increased to maintain circuit patency. Also, health care providers may or may not notice a decrease in efficacy when heparin is administered as fixed doses without laboratory or clinical monitoring. Those health care providers who use large, weight-adjusted, fixed doses of heparin for the treatment of acute venous thromboembolism may be particularly impacted.

For heparin products made according to the new standard, most manufacturers will include an "N" in the lot number or following the expiration date. Products manufactured by Hospira can be identified by the number "82" or higher (eg, 83, 84) at the start of their lot numbers.

Product verification – Always read the product label carefully to verify that the correct product name and strength have been selected. Fatal medication errors have occurred when higher dose heparin 10,000 units/mL injection was inadvertently administered instead of the lower dose of heparin 10 units/mL lock flush solution. Do not use heparin sodium injection as a catheter lock flush product.

Dosage adjustment – The dosage should be adjusted according to the patient's coagulation test results. See also Monitoring.

➤*Adults:*

General dosing guidelines – Although dosage must be adjusted for the individual patient according to the results of suitable laboratory tests, the following dosage schedules may be used as guidelines. See also Off-Label Uses for dosing recommendations from the ACCP antithrombotic guidelines.

Heparin Dosage Guidelines

Method of administration	Frequency	Recommended dose (based on 150 lb [68 kg] patient)
Deep, subcutaneous (intrafat) injection. A different site should be used for each injection to prevent the development of massive hematoma.	Initial dose	5,000 units by IV injection, followed by 10,000 to 20,000 units of a concentrated solution subcutaneously
	Every 8 hours or	8,000 to 10,000 units of a concentrated solution
	every 12 hours	15,000 to 20,000 units of a concentrated solution
Intermittent IV injection	Initial dose	10,000 units, either undiluted or in 50 to 100 mL of sodium chloride 0.9% injection or dextrose 5% injection
	Every 4 to 6 hours	5,000 to 10,000 units, either undiluted or in 50 to 100 mL of sodium chloride 0.9% injection or dextrose 5% injection
Continuous IV infusion	Initial dose	5,000 units by IV injection
	Continuous	20,000 to 40,000 units per 24 hours diluted in sodium chloride 0.9% injection or dextrose 5% injection (or in any compatible solution) for infusion

Clot prevention during cardiovascular surgery – An initial dose of not less than 150 units/kg for patients undergoing total body perfusion for open-heart surgery. Frequently, a dose of 300 units/kg is used for procedures estimated to last less than 60 minutes or 400 units/kg for those estimated to last more than 60 minutes.

Prophylaxis of postoperative thromboembolism (low-dose heparin) – A number of well-controlled clinical trials have demonstrated that low-dose heparin prophylaxis, given just prior to and after surgery, will reduce the incidence of postoperative DVT in the legs (as measured by the I-125 fibrinogen technique and venography) and of clinical PE.

Such prophylaxis should be reserved for patients older than 40 years of age who are undergoing major surgery. Patients with bleeding disorders and those having brain or spinal cord surgery, spinal anesthesia, eye surgery, or potentially sanguineous operations should be excluded, as should patients receiving oral anticoagulants or platelet-active drugs. The value of such prophylaxis in hip surgery has not been established.

Prior to initiating heparin treatment, the health care provider should rule out bleeding disorders by appropriate history and laboratory tests, and appropriate coagulation tests should be repeated just prior to surgery.

HEPARIN SODIUM — INJECTION

Coagulation test values should be normal or only slightly elevated at these times. There is usually no need for daily monitoring of the effect of low-dose heparin in patients with normal coagulation parameters.

A concentrated solution of heparin is recommended.

Usual dosage: 5,000 units administered 2 hours before surgery and 5,000 units administered every 8 to 12 hours thereafter for 7 days or until the patient is fully ambulatory, whichever is longer. Administer by deep subcutaneous injection in the arm or abdomen with a fine needle (25- to 26-gauge) to minimize tissue trauma.

If clinical evidence of thromboembolism develops despite low-dose prophylaxis, full therapeutic doses of anticoagulants should be given unless contraindicated.

Discontinuation of therapy: The possibility of increased bleeding during surgery or postoperatively should be kept in mind. If such bleeding occurs, discontinuance of heparin and neutralization with protamine are advisable.

Off-label dosing –

Acute deep vein thrombosis of the legs or upper extremity:

• *Continuous IV heparin* – The following recommendation is preferred over administration of IV boluses throughout treatment.

Initial dosage: IV bolus of 80 units/kg or 5,000 units.

Maintenance dosage: Follow initial dosage with continuous IV infusion. Start infusion with 18 units/kg/h or 1,300 units/h (or at least 32,000 units/day).

Dosage adjustment: Adjust dosage to maintain an aPTT that corresponds to plasma heparin levels of 0.3 to 0.7 units/mL anti-Xa activity (by amidolytic assay).

• *Subcutaneous heparin (monitored)* –

Initial dosage: 17,500 units (or 250 units/kg) administered subcutaneously twice daily.

Dosage adjustment: Adjust dosage to maintain an aPTT that corresponds to plasma heparin levels of 0.3 to 0.7 units/mL anti-Xa activity measured 6 hours postinjection.

• *Subcutaneous administration (fixed-dose, unmonitored)* –

Initial dosage: 333 units/kg administered subcutaneously.

Maintenance dosage: Follow initial dosage with 250 units/kg administered subcutaneously twice daily.

Acute pulmonary embolism:

• *Continuous IV heparin* – The following recommendation is preferred over administration of IV boluses throughout treatment.

Initial dosage: IV bolus of 80 units/kg or 5,000 units.

Maintenance dosage: Follow initial dosage with continuous IV infusion. Start infusion with 18 units/kg/h or 1,300 units/h (or at least 32,000 units/day).

Dosage adjustment: Adjust dosage to maintain an aPTT that corresponds to plasma heparin levels of 0.3 to 0.7 units/mL anti-Xa activity (by amidolytic assay).

• *Subcutaneous heparin (monitored)* –

Initial dosage: 17,500 units (or 250 units/kg) administered subcutaneously twice daily.

Dosage adjustment: Adjust dosage to maintain an aPTT that corresponds to plasma heparin levels of 0.3 to 0.7 units/mL anti-Xa activity measured 6 hours postinjection.

• *Subcutaneous administration (fixed-dose, unmonitored)* –

Initial dosage: 333 units/kg administered subcutaneously.

Maintenance dosage: Follow initial dosage with 250 units/kg administered subcutaneously twice daily.

Non–ST-segment elevation acute coronary syndrome:

• *Maximum dose* – 5,000 units (initial dose); 1,000 units/h (maintenance infusion).

• *Initial dosage* – 60 to 70 units/kg (up to 5,000 units) IV.

• *Maintenance dosage* – Follow the initial dose with 12 to 15 units/kg/h (up to 1,000 units/h). The aPTT should be maintained between 50 and 70 seconds. Heparin is also recommended in patients with NSTE ACS who will undergo an early invasive treatment.

Acute ST-segment elevation myocardial infarction:

• *Patients receiving streptokinase* – For patients weighing more than 80 kg, the heparin dosage is 5,000 units administered as an IV bolus followed by 1,000 units/h. For patients weighing less than 80 kg, the heparin dosage is 5,000 units administered as an IV bolus followed by 800 units/h. The target aPTT should be 50 to 75 seconds.

Alternatively, heparin may be administered subcutaneously at a dosage of 12,500 units every 12 hours.

• *Patients receiving alteplase, tenecteplase, or reteplase* – Administration of weight-adjusted heparin is recommended. A bolus dose of 60 units/kg (up to 4,000 units) followed by 12 units/kg/h (up to 1,000 units/h). Dosage should be adjusted to maintain an aPTT of 50 to 70 seconds for 48 hours.

• *Patients undergoing primary percutaneous coronary intervention* – For patients receiving a glycoprotein IIb/IIIa, the periprocedural heparin dosage is 50 to 70 units/kg with a target activated clotting time of over 200 seconds. For patients not receiving a glycoprotein IIb/IIIa, the periprocedural heparin dosage is 60 to 100 units/kg with a target activated clotting time of 250 to 350 seconds.

Unstable angina:

• *Maximum dose* – 5,000 units (initial dose); 1,000 units/h (maintenance infusion).

• *Initial dosage* – 60 to 70 units/kg (up to 5,000 units) IV.

• *Maintenance dosage* – Follow the initial dose with 12 to 15 units/kg/h (up to 1,000 units/h).

Patients with atrial fibrillation (for at least 48 hours or unknown duration) undergoing cardioversion: IV heparin with a target PTT of 60 seconds (range, 50 to 70 seconds) is recommended.

Patients with atrial fibrillation (duration of less than 48 hours) undergoing cardioversion: Cardioversion may be performed without prolonged anticoagulation. However, anticoagulation with IV heparin (with a target PTT of 60 seconds [range, 50 to 70 seconds]) should be started in patients with no contraindications to anticoagulation.

Emergency cardioversion in hemodynamically unstable patient: IV heparin with a target PTT of 60 seconds (range, 50 to 70 seconds) is recommended.

Nonbacterial thrombotic endocarditis and systemic or pulmonary emboli: Full-dose IV heparin treatment is recommended.

Superficial vein thrombosis: Intermediate doses of IV heparin for at least 4 weeks is recommended.

➤*Children:*

Thrombosis – Follow the recommendations of appropriate pediatric reference texts. In general, the following dosage schedule may be used as a guideline.

Initial dosage: 50 units/kg (IV infusion).

Maintenance dosage: 100 units/kg (IV infusion) every 4 hours or 20,000 units/m^2 per 24 hours continuously.

Off-label dosing –

Anticoagulation: The following are general dosing regimens. See the ACCP antithrombotic guidelines for more specific information.

• *Maximum dose* – 7,500 units (initial bolus); 1,600 units (initial infusion).

• *Initial dosage* – 75 units/kg administered as an IV bolus over 10 minutes.

• *Maintenance dosage* –

Neonates and infants: 28 units/kg/h.

Children: 20 units/kg/h.

Older children: 18 units/kg/h.

• *Alternative dosage* – Administration by IV infusion is preferred. If intermittent injection is elected, then the dosage is 75 to 100 units/kg administered IV every 4 hours.

➤*Elderly:* Patients older than 60 years of age may require lower doses of heparin.

➤*Pregnant women:*

Acute venous thromboembolism – Adjusted-dose heparin is recommended. Heparin may be administered as an IV bolus followed by a continuous infusion to maintain the aPTT within the therapeutic range or heparin may be administered subcutaneously and the dosage adjusted to maintain the aPTT (6 hours after injection) within the therapeutic range. Initial therapy should be administered for at least 5 days. Heparin maintenance therapy should be continued throughout pregnancy and then discontinued at least 24 hours prior to elective labor induction. See guidelines for additional information regarding prevention of recurrent venous thromboembolism in pregnant women.

Management of venous thromboembolism – It is recommended that heparin substitute the vitamin K antagonist.

Women with mechanical valves – It is recommended that adjusted-dose heparin be administered either throughout the pregnancy or until the thirteenth week with substitution by warfarin until heparin is resumed close to delivery. Heparin should be administered subcutaneously every 12 hours in doses adjusted to maintain the mid-interval aPTT at least twice the control or to attain an anti-Xa heparin level of 0.35 to 0.7 units/mL.

➤*Prevention in blood transfusion:* Addition of heparin 400 to 600 units per 100 mL of whole blood is usually employed to prevent coagulation. Usually, 7,500 units of heparin are added to 100 mL of sodium chloride 0.9% injection (or 75,000 units per 1,000 mL of sodium chloride 0.9% injection) and mixed, and from this sterile solution, 6 to 8 mL is added per 100 mL of whole blood.

➤*Prevention in laboratory samples:* Addition of heparin 70 to 150 units per 10 to 20 mL sample of whole blood is usually employed to prevent coagulation of the sample. Leukocyte counts should be performed on heparinized blood within 2 hours after addition of the heparin. Heparinized blood should not be used for isoagglutinin, complement, erythrocyte fragility tests, or platelet counts.

➤*Monitoring:* When heparin is given by continuous IV infusion, the coagulation time should be determined approximately every 4 hours in the early stages of treatment. When the drug is administered intermittently by IV injection, coagulation tests should be performed before each injection during the early stages of treatment and at appropriate intervals thereafter. Dosage is considered adequate when the aPTT is 1.5 to 2 times normal or when the whole blood clotting time is elevated approximately 2.5 to 3 times the control value. After deep subcutaneous (intrafat) injections, tests for adequacy of dosage are best performed on samples drawn 4 to 6 hours after the injections.

According to ACCP antithrombotic guidelines, an aPTT range that correlates with a heparin level of 0.3 to 0.7 units anti-Xa (or 0.2 to 0.4 units by protamine titration) should be used when treating venous thrombosis. Although the therapeutic range for coronary indications is currently unknown, the ACCP guidelines suggest that a heparin level that is 10% lower than that used for venous thromboembolism should be considered.

➤*Converting to oral anticoagulant:* When an oral anticoagulant of the coumarin or similar type is to begin in patients already receiving heparin, baseline and subsequent tests of prothrombin activity must be determined at a time when heparin activity is too low to affect the prothrombin time. This is about 5 hours after the last IV bolus and 24 hours after the last subcutaneous dose. If continuous IV heparin infusion is used, prothrombin time can usually be measured at any time.

HEPARIN SODIUM — INJECTION

In converting from heparin to an oral anticoagulant, the dose of the oral anticoagulant should be the usual initial amount; thereafter, prothrombin time should be determined at the usual intervals. To ensure continuous anticoagulation, it is advisable to continue full heparin therapy for several days after the prothrombin time has reached the therapeutic range. Heparin therapy may then be discontinued without tapering.

➤*Preparation for administration:* When heparin is added to an infusion solution for continuous IV administration, the container should be inverted at least 6 times to ensure adequate mixing and prevent pooling of the heparin in the solution.

Slight discoloration does not alter potency. Do not use if solution is discolored or contains a precipitate.

➤*Administration:* Heparin is not effective by oral administration and should be given by intermittent IV injection (after dilution), IV infusion or deep subcutaneous (intrafat) (ie, above the iliac crest or abdominal fat layer) injection. Use a fine needle (25 to 26 gauge) for subcutaneous administration to minimize tissue trauma. Avoid the intramuscular (IM) route of administration because of the frequent occurrence of hematoma at the injection site.

➤*Admixture compatibility:* Compatible with sodium chloride 0.9% injection and dextrose 5% injection.

➤*Storage / Stability:* Store at 20° to 25°C (68° to 77°F).

Actions

➤*Pharmacology:* Heparin inhibits reactions that lead to the clotting of blood and the formation of fibrin clots both in vitro and in vivo. Heparin acts at multiple sites in the normal coagulation system. Small amounts of heparin in combination with antithrombin III (heparin cofactor) can inhibit thrombosis by inactivating activated factor X and inhibiting the conversion of prothrombin to thrombin. Once active thrombosis has developed, larger amounts of heparin can inhibit further coagulation by inactivating thrombin and preventing the conversion of fibrinogen to fibrin. Heparin also prevents the formation of a stable fibrin clot in inhibiting the activation of the fibrin stabilizing factor.

Bleeding time is usually unaffected by heparin. Clotting time is prolonged by full therapeutic doses of heparin; in most cases, it is not measurably affected by low doses of heparin.

Heparin does not have fibrinolytic activity; therefore, it will not lyse existing clots.

➤*Pharmacokinetics:*

Absorption / Distribution – Peak plasma levels of heparin are achieved 2 to 4 hours following subcutaneous administration, although there are considerable individual variations. Loglinear plots of heparin plasma concentrations with time for a wide range of dose levels are linear, suggesting the absence of zero order processes.

Heparin is extensively protein bound. It does not cross the placental barrier and is not excreted into breast milk.

Metabolism / Excretion – Liver and the reticuloendothelial system are the sites of biotransformation. The biphasic elimination curve, a rapidly declining alpha phase (half-life, 10 minutes) and after 40 years of age, a slower beta phase, indicates uptake in organs. The absence of a relationship between anticoagulant half-life and concentration half-life may reflect factors such as protein binding of heparin. An average half-life of 1.5 hours (range, 1 to 6 hours) has been reported. Heparin is excreted in the urine, primarily as metabolites.

Special populations –

Renal function impairment: The half-life may be slightly prolonged.

Hepatic function impairment: Half-life may be either increased or decreased in patients with liver impairment.

Elderly: Patients older than 60 years of age, following similar doses of heparin, may have higher plasma levels of heparin and longer aPTTs compared with patients younger than 60 years of age.

Contraindications

Severe thrombocytopenia; patients in whom suitable blood coagulation tests (eg, the whole blood clotting time, PTT) cannot be performed at appropriate intervals [this contraindication refers to full-dose heparin; there is usually no need to monitor coagulation parameters in patients receiving low-dose heparin]); uncontrollable active bleeding state, except when due to disseminated intravascular coagulation;hypersensitivity to heparin.

Do not administer heparin sodium injection, USP (porcine), preserved with benzyl alcohol to neonates, infants, pregnant women, or breast-feeding mothers. Benzyl alcohol has been associated with serious adverse reactions and death, particularly in children. Use heparin sodium injection, USP (porcine), preservative free, in these populations when indicated.

Warnings/Precautions

➤*Potency changes:* See Administration and Dosage for more information.

➤*Benzyl alcohol:* Do not administer heparin sodium injection, USP (porcine), preserved with benzyl alcohol to neonates, infants, pregnant women, or breast-feeding mothers. Benzyl alcohol has been associated with serious adverse reactions and death, particularly in children. Use heparin sodium injection, USP (porcine), preservative free, when indicated, in these populations.

➤*Fatal medication errors:* Do not use heparin sodium injection as a "catheter lock flush" product. Heparin injection is supplied in vials containing various strengths of heparin, including vials that contain a highly concentrated solution of 10,000 units in 1 mL. Fatal hemorrhages have occurred in children because of medication errors in which heparin sodium 1 mL injection vials were confused with 1 mL "catheter lock flush" vials. Carefully examine all heparin vials to confirm the correct vial choice prior to administration of the drug.

➤*Hemorrhage:* Hemorrhage can occur at virtually any site in patients receiving heparin. An unexplained fall in hematocrit, fall in blood pressure, or any other unexplained symptom should lead to serious consideration of a hemorrhagic event.

Use heparin with extreme caution in disease states in which there is increased danger of hemorrhage. Some of the conditions in which increased danger of hemorrhage exists are as follows:

Cardiovascular – Subacute bacterial endocarditis, severe hypertension.

Surgical – During and immediately following spinal tap or spinal anesthesia, or major surgery, especially involving the brain, spinal cord, or eye.

Hematologic – Conditions associated with increased bleeding tendencies, such as hemophilia, thrombocytopenia, and some vascular purpuras.

GI – Ulcerative lesions and continuous tube drainage of the stomach or small intestine.

Other – Menstruation, liver disease with impaired hemostasis.

➤*Thrombocytopenia:* Thrombocytopenia has been reported to occur in patients receiving heparin with a reported incidence of 0% to 30%. Obtain platelet counts at baseline and periodically during heparin administration. Mild thrombocytopenia (count greater than 100,000/mm^3) may remain stable or reverse even if heparin is continued. However, closely monitor thrombocytopenia of any degree. If the count falls below 100,000/mm^3 or if recurrent thrombosis develops, discontinue the heparin product, and if necessary, administer an alternative anticoagulant.

➤*Heparin-induced thrombocytopenia and heparin-induced thrombocytopenia and thrombosis:* Heparin-induced thrombocytopenia is a serious antibody-mediated reaction resulting from irreversible aggregation of platelets. Heparin-induced thrombocytopenia may progress to the development of venous and arterial thromboses, a condition referred to as heparin-induced thrombocytopenia and thrombosis (white clot syndrome). Thrombotic events may also be the initial presentation for heparin-induced thrombocytopenia and thrombosis. These serious thromboembolic events include DVT, PE, cerebral vein thrombosis, limb ischemia, stroke, MI, mesenteric thrombosis, renal arterial thrombosis, skin necrosis, gangrene of the extremities that may lead to amputation, and possibly death. Closely monitor thrombocytopenia of any degree. If the count falls below 100,000/mm^3 or if recurrent thrombosis develops, promptly discontinue the heparin product and consider alternative anticoagulants if patients require continued anticoagulation.

➤*Delayed onset of heparin-induced thrombocytopenia and heparin-induced thrombocytopenia and thrombosis:* Heparin-induced thrombocytopenia as well as heparin-induced thrombocytopenia and thrombosis can occur up to several weeks after the discontinuation of heparin therapy. Evaluate patients presenting with thrombocytopenia or thrombosis after discontinuation of heparin for heparin-induced thrombocytopenia and heparin-induced thrombocytopenia and thrombosis.

➤*Heparin resistance:* Increased resistance to heparin is frequently encountered in fever, thrombosis, thrombophlebitis, infections with thrombosing tendencies, myocardial infarction, cancer, and in postsurgical patients.

➤*Hypersensitivity reactions:* Only give the drug to patients with documented hypersensitivity to heparin in clearly life-threatening situations.

➤*Pregnancy:* *Category C.* No reports linking the use of heparin during gestation with congenital defects have been located. Other problems, at times lethal to the fetus or neonate, may be related to heparin or to the severe maternal disease necessitating anticoagulant therapy. Animal reproduction studies have not been conducted with heparin. It is also not known whether heparin can cause fetal harm when administered to a pregnant woman or can affect reproduction capacity. Give heparin to a pregnant woman only if clearly needed.

Benzyl alcohol – Do not administer heparin sodium injection, USP (porcine), preserved with benzyl alcohol, to pregnant women. When indicated, administer heparin sodium injection, USP (porcine), preservative free, to pregnant women.

➤*Lactation:* Heparin is not excreted in human milk and is considered to be compatible with breast-feeding.

Benzyl alcohol – Do not administer heparin sodium injection, USP (porcine), preserved with benzyl alcohol, to breast-feeding mothers. When indicated, administer preservative-free heparin sodium injection, USP (porcine) to breast-feeding mothers.

➤*Children:* Some heparin injection formulations contain benzyl alcohol as a preservative. Benzyl alcohol has been reported to be associated with a fatal "gasping syndrome" in premature neonates and infants. The "gasping syndrome," (characterized by CNS depression, metabolic acidosis, gasping respirations, and high levels of benzyl alcohol and its metabolites found in the blood and urine) has been associated with benzyl alcohol dosages more than 99 mg/kg/day in neonates and low birth weight neonates. Additional symptoms may include gradual neurological deterioration, seizures, intracranial hemorrhage, hematologic abnormalities, skin breakdown, hepatic and renal failure, hypotension, bradycardia, and cardiovascular collapse. Premature and low birth weight infants, as well as patients receiving high dosages, may be more likely to develop toxicity.

HEPARIN SODIUM — INJECTION

➤*Elderly:* A higher incidence of bleeding has been reported in patients older than 60 years of age, especially women. Clinical studies indicate that lower doses of heparin may be indicated in these patients.

➤*Monitoring:* When heparin is administered in therapeutic amounts, regulate its dosage by frequent blood coagulation tests. If the coagulation test is unduly prolonged or if hemorrhage occurs, discontinue heparin promptly.

Periodic platelet counts, hematocrits, and tests for occult blood in stool are recommended during the entire course of heparin therapy, regardless of the route of administration.

Drug Interactions

Heparin Drug Interactions

Precipitant drug	Object drug[a]		Description
Activated protein C (eg, drotrecogin alfa, activated)	Heparin	↑	The risk of bleeding may be increased. Use with caution. Close clinical and laboratory monitoring are indicated.
Antihistamines, digitalis, nicotine, nitroglycerin (IV), tetracycline	Heparin	↓	May partially counteract the anticoagulant action of heparin sodium. Monitor the coagulation status of the patient and adjust the heparin dose as needed.
Antithrombin	Heparin	↑	Pharmacologic effects of heparin may be increased. Close clinical and laboratory monitoring (aPTT and/or anti-Xa) are indicated. Adjust the heparin as needed. Reduced doses of heparin are recommended when coadministered with antithrombin III.
Cephalosporins (eg, cefazolin, ceftriaxone)	Heparin	↑	Several parenteral cephalosporins have caused coagulopathies; this might be additive with heparin, possibly increasing the risk of bleeding. Monitor for bleeding and coagulopathies. If an interaction is suspected, reduce the dose or discontinue one or both drugs.
Direct thrombin inhibitors (eg, desirudin)	Heparin	↑	The risk of bleeding may be increased. Concurrent use is not recommended.
Penicillins, parenteral (eg, ampicillin, penicillin G)	Heparin	↑	Parenteral penicillins can produce alterations in platelet aggregation and coagulation tests. These effects might be additive with heparin, possibly increasing the risk of bleeding. Avoid excessive doses of parenteral penicillin during concurrent use of heparin. Closely monitor coagulation status and adjust the heparin dose as needed.
Platelet inhibitors (eg, aspirin, dextran, dipyridamole, hydroxychloroquine, NSAIDs[b] [eg, ibuprofen, indomethacin], ticlopidine)	Heparin	↑	An increased risk of bleeding is possible during coadministration due to interference with platelet aggregation. Use with caution. In addition, heparin may reduce indomethacin efficacy when used to induce closure of a patent ductus arteriosus.
Heparin	Platelet inhibitors (ie, indomethacin)	↓	
Streptokinase	Heparin	↓	Relative resistance to heparin anticoagulation following administration of streptokinase as a systemic thrombolytic agent may occur. Use more frequent aPTT to guide dosage adjustments.
Heparin	Alteplase	↑	The risk of serious bleeding may be increased. Use with caution in any condition for which serious bleeding constitutes an important hazard. Starting anticoagulant therapy within 24 hours of treatment with IV administered alteplase for the treatment of ischemic stroke is not recommended.
Heparin	Palifermin	↑	Plasma concentrations and pharmacologic effects of palifermin may be increased. Avoid coadministration. Rinse IV infusion lines maintained with heparin with normal saline before and after palifermin administration.
Heparin	Warfarin	↔	Heparin may prolong the 1-stage prothrombin time. In patients receiving warfarin, ≥ 5 hours after the last IV heparin dose should elapse before blood is drawn if a valid prothrombin time is to be obtained.

[a] ↑ = object drug increased; ↓ = object drug decreased; ↔ = undetermined clinical effect.
[b] NSAIDs = nonsteroidal anti-inflammatory drugs.

➤*Drug/Lab test interactions:* Significant elevations of aminotransferase (AST and ALT) levels have occurred in a high percentage of patients. Cautiously interpret aminotransferase increases that might be caused by heparin.

Adverse Reactions

➤*Hematologic:*

Hemorrhage – Hemorrhage is the chief complication that may result from heparin therapy. An overly prolonged clotting time or minor bleeding during therapy can usually be controlled by withdrawing the drug. GI or urinary tract bleeding during anticoagulant therapy may indicate the presence of an underlying occult lesion. Bleeding can occur at any site, but certain specific hemorrhagic complications may be difficult to detect:

1.) Adrenal hemorrhage, with resultant acute adrenal insufficiency, has occurred during anticoagulant therapy. Therefore, discontinue such treatment in patients who develop signs and symptoms of acute adrenal hemorrhage and insufficiency. Initiation of corrective therapy should not depend on laboratory confirmation of the diagnosis since any delay in an acute situation may result in the patient's death.
2.) Ovarian (corpus luteum) hemorrhage developed in a number of women of reproductive age receiving short- or long-term anticoagulant therapy. If unrecognized, this complication may be fatal.
3.) Retroperitoneal hemorrhage.

Thrombocytopenia – Thrombocytopenia has been reported to occur in patients receiving heparin with a reported incidence of 0% to 30%. While often mild and of no obvious clinical significance, thrombocytopenia can be accompanied by severe thromboembolic complications, such as skin necrosis, gangrene of the extremities that may lead to amputation, MI, PE, stroke, and possibly death.

➤*Hypersensitivity:* Generalized hypersensitivity reactions have been reported, with chills, fever, and urticaria as the most usual manifestations, and anaphylactoid reactions (including shock), asthma, headache, lacrimation, nausea, rhinitis, and vomiting occurring more rarely. Itching and burning, especially on the plantar side of the feet may occur.

Certain episodes of painful, ischemic, and cyanosed limbs have in the past been attributed to allergic vasospastic reactions. Whether these are identical to the thrombocytopenia-associated complications remains to be determined.

➤*Local:* Erythema, hematoma, local irritation, mild pain, or ulceration may follow deep subcutaneous (intrafat) injection of heparin. These complications are much more common after IM use, and such use is not recommended.

➤*Miscellaneous:* Osteoporosis following long-term administration of high doses of heparin, cutaneous necrosis after systemic administration, suppression of aldosterone synthesis, delayed transient alopecia, priapism, and rebound hyperlipemia on discontinuation of heparin have also been reported.

➤*Lab test abnormalities:* Significant elevations of aminotransferase (AST and ALT) levels have occurred in a high percentage of patients (and healthy subjects) who have received heparin.

Overdosage

➤*Symptoms:* Bleeding is the chief sign of heparin overdosage. Nosebleeds, blood in urine, or tarry stools may be noted as the first sign of bleeding. Easy bruising or petechial formations may precede frank bleeding.

➤*Treatment:* When clinical circumstances (bleeding) require reversal of heparinization, protamine sulfate (1% solution) by slow infusion will neutralize heparin. Administer no more than protamine 50 mg very slowly in any 10-minute period. Each milligram of protamine sulfate neutralizes approximately 100 heparin units. The amount of protamine required decreases over time as heparin is metabolized. Although the metabolism of heparin is complex, it may, for the purpose of choosing a protamine dose, be assumed to have a half-life of about 30 minutes after IV injection.

Administration of protamine can cause severe hypotensive and anaphylactoid reactions. Because fatal reactions often resembling anaphylaxis have been reported, give the drug only when resuscitation techniques and treatment of anaphylactoid shock are readily available.

HEPARIN SODIUM — INJECTION

Patient Information

Instruct patients to report signs/symptoms of thrombocytopenia or hemorrhage.

If self administered, teach patient the proper technique and placement of injections and the importance of rotating the injection sites.

HEPARIN SODIUM AND SODIUM CHLORIDE — INJECTION

Indications

➤*Anticoagulation:* Atrial fibrillation with embolization; diagnosis and treatment of acute and chronic consumption coagulopathies (disseminated intravascular coagulation [DIC]); prevention of clotting in arterial and heart surgery; prophylaxis and treatment of peripheral arterial embolism; very low-dose heparin is used as an anticoagulant in extracorporeal circulation and dialysis procedures; to maintain catheter patency.

➤*Off-label uses:* According to the antithrombotic guidelines from the American College of Chest Physicians (ACCP), heparin is recommended as an anticoagulant in several conditions, such as the following: acute deep vein thrombosis (DVT) of the legs, acute DVT of the upper extremity, acute pulmonary embolism, superficial vein thrombosis, patients with atrial fibrillation undergoing cardioversion, nonbacterial thrombotic endocarditis and systemic or pulmonary emboli, cerebral venous sinus thrombosis, non–ST-segment elevation acute coronary syndrome (NSTE ACS), acute ST-segment elevation myocardial infarction (MI) including patients undergoing primary percutaneous coronary intervention, unstable angina, acute arterial emboli or thrombosis, and patients undergoing major vascular reconstruction. See the ACCP antithrombotic guidelines for more details. See also Administration and Dosage.

Administration and Dosage

➤*General dosing considerations:*

Potency changes – According to the Food and Drug Administration (FDA), heparin manufactured after October 1, 2009 will be approximately 10% less potent than heparin manufactured prior to that date. This is because of the United States Pharmacopeia (USP) revising the heparin monograph. The revised USP monograph will include a new USP reference standard and test method that is used to determine the potency of the drug. The monograph change will also harmonize the USP unit dose with the World Health Organization (WHO) International Standard (IS) unit dose. However, harmonization of the standard will result in an approximately 10% reduction in the potency of the heparin marketed in the United States.

The change in heparin potency may have clinical significance in some situations, such as when heparin is administered as a bolus intravenous (IV) dose and an immediate anticoagulant effect is clinically important. In such situations health care providers should consider the change in potency of heparin when making decisions about what dose to administer. The change in heparin potency is expected to be less clinically significant when it is administered subcutaneously because of the low and highly variable bioavailability of heparin when administered by this route. Health care providers should also be aware of the decrease in heparin potency because they monitor the anticoagulant effect of the drug; more heparin may be required to achieve and maintain the desired level of anticoagulation in some patients.

The potency change may require more frequent or intensive activated partial thromboplastin time (aPTT) or activated clotting time (ACT) monitoring.

Product verification – Always read the product label carefully to verify that the correct product name and strength have been selected. Fatal medication errors have occurred when higher dosage heparin 10,000 units/mL injection was inadvertently administered instead of the lower dosage of heparin 10 units/mL lock flush solution.

Dosage adjustment – The dosage should be adjusted according to the patient's coagulation test results. See also Monitoring.

➤*Adults:*

Anticoagulation – Although dosage must be adjusted for the individual patient according to the results of suitable laboratory tests, the following dosage schedules may be used as guidelines. See also Off-Label Uses for dosing recommendations from the ACCP antithrombotic guidelines.

Heparin in Sodium Chloride Dosage Guidelines in Adults

Method of administration	Frequency	Recommended dose (based on 150 lb [68 kg] patient)
Intermittent IV injection	Initial dose	10,000 units, either undiluted or in 50 to 100 mL of sodium chloride 0.45% injection
	Every 4 to 6 hours	5,000 to 10,000 units, either undiluted or in 50 to 100 mL of sodium chloride 0.45% injection
Continuous IV infusion	Initial dose	5,000 units by IV injection
	Continuous	20,000 to 40,000 units per 24 hours in sodium chloride 0.45% injection

Clot prevention during cardiovascular surgery – An initial dose of not less than 150 units/kg given IV for patients undergoing total body perfusion for open-heart surgery. Frequently, a dose of 300 units/kg is used for procedures estimated to last less than 60 minutes or 400 units/kg for those estimated to last more than 60 minutes.

Catheter patency – 6 units/h (3 mL/h of the 2 units/mL formulation) has been found to be satisfactory, although the rate of infusion is dependent upon age, weight, clinical condition of the patient, and the procedure being employed.

Off-label dosing –

Acute deep vein thrombosis of the legs or upper extremity: The following continuous infusion recommendation is preferred over administration of IV boluses throughout treatment.

- *Initial dosage* – IV bolus of 80 units/kg or 5,000 units.
- *Maintenance dosage* – Follow initial dosage with continuous IV infusion. Start infusion with 18 units/kg/h or 1,300 units/h (or at least 32,000 units/day).
- *Dosage adjustment* – Adjust dosage to maintain an aPTT that corresponds to plasma heparin levels of 0.3 to 0.7 units/mL anti-Xa activity (by amidolytic assay).

Acute pulmonary embolism: The following continuous infusion recommendation is preferred over administration of IV boluses throughout treatment.

- *Initial dosage* – IV bolus of 80 units/kg or 5,000 units.
- *Maintenance dosage* – Follow initial dosage with continuous IV infusion. Start infusion with 18 units/kg/h or 1,300 units/h (or at least 32,000 units/day).
- *Dosage adjustment* – Adjust dosage to maintain an aPTT that corresponds to plasma heparin levels of 0.3 to 0.7 units/mL anti-Xa activity (by amidolytic assay).

Non–ST-segment elevation acute coronary syndrome:

- *Maximum dose* – 5,000 units (initial dose); 1,000 units/h (maintenance infusion).
- *Initial dosage* – 60 to 70 units/kg (up to 5,000 units) IV.
- *Maintenance dosage* – Follow the initial dose with 12 to 15 units/kg/h (up to 1,000 units/h). The aPTT should be maintained between 50 and 70 seconds. Heparin is also recommended in patients with NSTE ACS who will undergo an early invasive treatment.

Acute ST-segment elevation myocardial infarction:

- *Patients receiving streptokinase* – For patients weighing more than 80 kg, the heparin dosage is 5,000 units administered as an IV bolus followed by 1,000 units/h. For patients weighing less than 80 kg, the heparin dosage is 5,000 units administered as an IV bolus followed by 800 units/h. The target aPTT should be 50 to 75 seconds.
- *Patients receiving alteplase, tenecteplase, or reteplase* – Administration of weight-adjusted heparin is recommended. A bolus dose of 60 units/kg (up to 4,000 units) followed by 12 units/kg/h (up to 1,000 units/h). Adjust dosage to maintain an aPTT of 50 to 70 seconds for 48 hours.
- *Patients undergoing primary percutaneous coronary intervention* – For patients receiving a glycoprotein IIb/IIIa, the periprocedural heparin dosage is 50 to 70 units/kg with a target activated clotting time of over 200 seconds. For patients not receiving a glycoprotein IIb/IIIa, the periprocedural heparin dosage is 60 to 100 units/kg with a target activated clotting time of 250 to 350 seconds.

Unstable angina:

- *Maximum dose* – 5,000 units (initial dose); 1,000 units/h (maintenance infusion).
- *Initial dosage* – 60 to 70 units/kg (up to 5,000 units) IV.
- *Maintenance dosage* – Follow the initial dose with 12 to 15 units/kg/h (up to 1,000 units/h).

Patients with atrial fibrillation (for at least 48 hours or unknown duration) undergoing cardioversion: IV heparin with a target PTT of 60 seconds (range, 50 to 70 seconds) is recommended.

Patients with atrial fibrillation (duration of less than 48 hours) undergoing cardioversion: Cardioversion may be performed without prolonged anticoagulation. However, anticoagulation with IV heparin (with a target PTT of 60 seconds [range, 50 to 70 seconds]) should be started in patients with no contraindications to anticoagulation.

Emergency cardioversion in hemodynamically unstable patient: IV heparin with a target PTT of 60 seconds (range, 50 to 70 seconds) is recommended.

Nonbacterial thrombotic endocarditis and systemic or pulmonary emboli: Full-dose IV heparin treatment is recommended.

Superficial vein thrombosis: Intermediate doses of IV heparin for at least 4 weeks is recommended.

➤*Children:*

Thrombosis – Follow the recommendations of appropriate pediatric reference texts. In general, the following dosage schedule may be used as a guideline.

Initial dosage: 50 units/kg (IV infusion).

Maintenance dosage: 100 units/kg (IV infusion) every 4 hours or 20,000 units/m^2 per 24 hours continuously.

Off-label dosing –

Anticoagulation: The following are general dosing regimens. See the ACCP antithrombotic guidelines for more specific information.

- *Maximum dose* – 7,500 units (initial bolus); 1,600 units (initial infusion).
- *Initial dosage* – 75 units/kg administered as an IV bolus over 10 minutes.

HEPARIN SODIUM AND SODIUM CHLORIDE — INJECTION

• *Maintenance dosage* –

Neonates and infants: 28 units/kg/h.

Children: 20 units/kg/h.

Older children: 18 units/kg/h.

• *Alternative dosage* – Administration by IV infusion is preferred. If intermittent injection is elected, then the dosage is 75 to 100 units/kg administered IV every 4 hours.

➤*Elderly:* Patients older than 60 years of age may require lower doses of heparin.

➤*Pregnant women:*

Acute venous thromboembolism – Adjusted-dose heparin is recommended. Heparin may be administered as an IV bolus followed by a continuous infusion to maintain the aPTT within the therapeutic range. Initial therapy should be administered for at least 5 days. Heparin maintenance therapy should be continued throughout pregnancy and then discontinued at least 24 hours prior to elective labor induction. See guidelines for additional information regarding prevention of recurrent venous thromboembolism in pregnant women.

Management of venous thromboembolism – It is recommended that heparin substitute the vitamin K antagonist.

Women with mechanical valves – It is recommended that adjusted-dose heparin be administered either throughout the pregnancy or until week 13, with substitution by warfarin until heparin is resumed close to delivery.

➤*Monitoring:* When heparin is given by continuous IV infusion, determine the coagulation time approximately every 4 hours in the early stages of treatment. When the drug is administered intermittently by IV injection, perform coagulation tests before each injection during the early stages of treatment and at appropriate intervals thereafter. Dosage is considered adequate when the aPTT is 1.5 to 2 times normal or when the whole blood clotting time is elevated approximately 2.5 to 3 times the control value.

According to ACCP antithrombotic guidelines, use an aPTT range that correlates with a heparin level of 0.3 to 0.7 units anti-Xa (or 0.2 to 0.4 units by protamine titration) when treating venous thrombosis. Although the therapeutic range for coronary indications is currently unknown, the ACCP guidelines suggest that a heparin level that is 10% lower than that used for venous thromboembolism should be considered.

➤*Converting to oral anticoagulant:* When an oral anticoagulant of the coumarin or similar type is to begin in patients already receiving heparin, baseline and subsequent tests of prothrombin activity must be determined at a time when heparin activity is too low to affect the prothrombin time. If continuous IV heparin infusion is used, prothrombin time can usually be measured at any time.

In converting from heparin to an oral anticoagulant, the dose of the oral anticoagulant should be the usual initial amount; thereafter, determine prothrombin time at the usual intervals. To ensure continuous anticoagulation, it is advisable to continue full heparin therapy for several days after the prothrombin time has reached the therapeutic range. Heparin therapy may then be discontinued without tapering.

➤*Preparation for administration:* Slight discoloration does not alter potency. Do not use if solution is discolored or contains a precipitate.

➤*Administration:* Heparin in sodium chloride injection is not intended for IM use and is not effective by oral administration; administer by IV infusion or intermittent IV injection. Do not use as a "catheter lock flush" product.

As the dosage of solutions of heparin sodium must be titrated to individual patient response, additive medications should not be delivered via this solution.

➤*Admixture compatibility:* No additives should be made to heparin in sodium chloride.

➤*Storage/Stability:* Store at 20° to 25°C (68° to 77°F). Protect from freezing.

HEPARIN SODIUM IN 5% DEXTROSE — INJECTION

Indications

➤*Anticoagulation:* As a continuous intravenous (IV) infusion following an initial IV therapeutic dose of heparin. For anticoagulant therapy in prophylaxis and treatment of venous thrombosis and its extension; for prophylaxis and treatment of pulmonary embolism (PE); in atrial fibrillation with embolization; for diagnosis and treatment of acute and chronic consumptive coagulopathies (disseminated intravascular coagulation [DIC]); for prevention of clotting in arterial and heart surgery; and in prophylaxis and treatment of peripheral arterial embolism; in extracorporeal arterial circulation and dialysis procedures.

➤*Off-label uses:* According to the antithrombotic guidelines from the American College of Chest Physicians (ACCP), heparin is recommended as an anticoagulant in several conditions, such as the following: acute deep vein thrombosis (DVT) of the legs, acute DVT of the upper extremity, acute PE, superficial vein thrombosis, patients with atrial fibrillation undergoing cardioversion, nonbacterial thrombotic endocarditis and systemic or pulmonary emboli, cerebral venous sinus thrombosis, non–ST-segment elevation acute coronary syndrome (NSTE ACS), acute ST-segment elevation myocardial infarction (MI), including patients undergoing primary percutaneous coronary intervention, unstable angina, acute arterial emboli or thrombosis, and patients undergoing major vascular reconstruction. See the ACCP antithrombotic guidelines for more details. See also Administration and Dosage.

Administration and Dosage

➤*General dosing considerations:*

Potency changes – According to the Food and Drug Administration (FDA), heparin manufactured after October 1, 2009 will be approximately 10% less potent than heparin manufactured prior to that date. This is because of the United States Pharmacopeia (USP) revising the heparin monograph. The revised USP monograph will include a new USP reference standard and test method that is used to determine the potency of the drug. The monograph change will also harmonize the USP unit dose with the World Health Organization (WHO) International Standard (IS) unit dose. However, harmonization of the standard will result in an approximately 10% reduction in the potency of the heparin marketed in the United States.

The change in heparin potency may have clinical significance in some situations, such as when heparin is administered as a bolus IV dose and an immediate anticoagulant effect is clinically important. In such situations, health care providers should consider the change in potency of heparin when making decisions about what dose to administer. The change in heparin potency is expected to be less clinically significant when it is administered subcutaneously because of the low and highly variable bioavailability of heparin when administered by this route. Health care providers should also be aware of the decrease in heparin potency because they monitor the anticoagulant effect of the drug; more heparin may be required to achieve and maintain the desired level of anticoagulation in some patients.

The potency change may require more frequent or intensive activated partial thromboplastin time (aPTT) or activated clotting time (ACT) monitoring.

Product verification – Always read the product label carefully to verify that the correct product name and strength have been selected. Fatal medication errors have occurred when higher dosage heparin 10,000 units/mL injection was inadvertently administered instead of the lower dosage of heparin 10 units/mL lock flush solution.

Dosage adjustment – The dosage should be adjusted according to the patient's coagulation test results. See also Monitoring.

➤*Adults:*

Anticoagulation – Although dosage must be adjusted for the individual patient according to the results of suitable laboratory tests, the following dosage schedules may be used as guidelines. See also Off-Label Dosing for dosing recommendations from the ACCP antithrombotic guidelines.

Heparin in Dextrose 5% Dosage Guidelines

Method of administration	Frequency	Recommended dose (based on 150 lb [68 kg] patient)
Continuous IV infusion	Initial dose	5,000 units by IV injection
	Continuous	20,000 to 40,000 units per 24 hours

Off-label dosing –

Acute deep vein thrombosis of the legs or upper extremity: The following continuous infusion recommendation is preferred over administration of IV boluses throughout treatment.

• *Initial dosage* – IV bolus of 80 units/kg or 5,000 units.

• *Maintenance dosage* – Follow initial dosage with continuous IV infusion. Start infusion with 18 units/kg/h or 1,300 units/h (or 32,000 units/day).

• *Dosage adjustment* – Adjust dosage to maintain an aPTT that corresponds to plasma heparin levels of 0.3 to 0.7 units/mL anti-Xa activity (by amidolytic assay).

Acute pulmonary embolism: The following continuous infusion recommendation is preferred over administration of IV boluses throughout treatment.

• *Initial dosage* – IV bolus of 80 units/kg or 5,000 units.

• *Maintenance dosage* – Follow initial dosage with continuous IV infusion. Start infusion with 18 units/kg/h or 1,300 units/h (or at least 32,000 units/day).

• *Dosage adjustment* – Adjust dosage to maintain an aPTT that corresponds to plasma heparin levels of 0.3 to 0.7 units/mL anti-Xa activity (by amidolytic assay).

Non–ST-segment elevation acute coronary syndrome:

• *Maximum dose* – 5,000 units (initial dose); 1,000 units/h (maintenance infusion).

• *Initial dosage* – 60 to 70 units/kg (up to 5,000 units) IV.

• *Maintenance dosage* – Follow the initial dose with 12 to 15 units/kg/h (up to 1,000 units/h). The aPTT should be maintained between 50 and 70 seconds. Heparin is also recommended in patients with NSTE ACS who will undergo an early invasive treatment.

Acute ST-segment elevation myocardial infarction:

• *Patients receiving streptokinase* – For patients weighing more than 80 kg, the heparin dosage is 5,000 units administered as an IV bolus followed by 1,000 units/h. For patients weighing less than 80 kg, the heparin dosage is 5,000 units administered as an IV bolus followed by 800 units/h. The target aPTT should be 50 to 75 seconds.

• *Patients receiving alteplase, tenecteplase, or reteplase* – Administration of weight-adjusted heparin is recommended. A bolus dose of 60 units/kg (up to 4,000 units) followed by 12 units/kg/h (up to 1,000 units/h). Dosage should be adjusted to maintain an aPTT of 50 to 70 seconds for 48 hours.

• *Patients undergoing primary percutaneous coronary intervention* –

HEPARIN SODIUM IN 5% DEXTROSE — INJECTION

For patients receiving a glycoprotein IIb/IIIa, the periprocedural heparin dosage is 50 to 70 units/kg with a target activated clotting time of over 200 seconds. For patients not receiving a glycoprotein IIb/IIIa, the periprocedural heparin dosage is 60 to 100 units/kg with a target activated clotting time of 250 to 350 seconds.

Unstable angina:

• *Maximum dose* – 5,000 units (initial dose); 1,000 units/h (maintenance infusion).

• *Initial dosage* – 60 to 70 units/kg (up to 5,000 units) IV.

• *Maintenance dosage* – Follow the initial dose with 12 to 15 units/kg/h (up to 1,000 units/h).

Patients with atrial fibrillation (for at least 48 hours or unknown duration) undergoing cardioversion: IV heparin with a target PTT of 60 seconds (range, 50 to 70 seconds) is recommended.

Patients with atrial fibrillation (duration of less than 48 hours) undergoing cardioversion: Cardioversion may be performed without prolonged anticoagulation. However, anticoagulation with IV heparin (with a target PTT of 60 seconds [range, 50 to 70 seconds]) should be started in patients with no contraindications to anticoagulation.

Emergency cardioversion in hemodynamically unstable patient: IV heparin with a target PTT of 60 seconds (range, 50 to 70 seconds) is recommended.

Nonbacterial thrombotic endocarditis and systemic or pulmonary emboli: Full-dose IV heparin treatment is recommended.

Superficial vein thrombosis: Intermediate doses of IV heparin for at least 4 weeks is recommended.

➤*Children:*

Thrombosis – Follow the recommendations of appropriate pediatric reference texts. In general, the following dosage schedule may be used as a guideline.

Initial dosage: 50 units/kg (IV infusion).

Maintenance dosage: 100 units/kg (IV infusion) every 4 hours or 20,000 units/m^2 per 24 hours continuously.

Off-label dosing –

Anticoagulation: The following are general dosing regimens. See the ACCP antithrombotic guidelines for more specific information.

• *Maximum dose* – 7,500 units (initial bolus); 1,600 units (initial infusion).

• *Initial dosage* – 75 units/kg administered as an IV bolus over 10 minutes.

• *Maintenance dosage* –

Neonates and infants: 28 units/kg/h.

Children: 20 units/kg/h.

Older children: 18 units/kg/h.

• *Alternative dosage* – Administration by IV infusion is preferred. If intermittent injection is elected, then the dosage is 75 to 100 units/kg administered IV every 4 hours.

➤*Elderly:* Patients older than 60 years of age may require lower doses of heparin.

➤*Pregnant women:*

Acute venous thromboembolism – Adjusted-dose heparin is recommended. Heparin may be administered as an IV bolus followed by a continuous infusion to maintain the aPTT within the therapeutic range. Initial therapy should be administered for at least 5 days. Heparin maintenance therapy should be continued throughout pregnancy and then discontinued at least 24 hours prior to elective labor induction. See guidelines for additional information regarding prevention of recurrent venous thromboembolism in pregnant women.

Management of venous thromboembolism – It is recommended that heparin substitute the vitamin K antagonist.

Women with mechanical valves – It is recommended that adjusted-dose heparin be administered either throughout the pregnancy or until the thirteenth week with substitution by warfarin until heparin is resumed close to delivery.

➤*Monitoring:* When heparin is given by continuous IV infusion, the coagulation time should be determined approximately every 4 hours in the early stages of treatment. When the drug is administered intermittently by IV injection, coagulation tests should be performed before each injection during the early stages of treatment and at appropriate intervals thereafter. Dosage is considered adequate when the aPTT is 1.5 to 2 times normal or when the whole blood clotting time is elevated approximately 2.5 to 3 times the control value.

According to ACCP antithrombotic guidelines, an aPTT range that correlates with a heparin level of 0.3 to 0.7 units anti-Xa (or 0.2 to 0.4 units by protamine titration) should be used when treating venous thrombosis. Although the therapeutic range for coronary indications is currently unknown, the ACCP guidelines suggest that a heparin level that is 10% lower than that used for venous thromboembolism should be considered.

➤*Converting to oral anticoagulant:* When an oral anticoagulant of the coumarin or similar type is to begin in patients already receiving heparin, baseline and subsequent tests of prothrombin activity must be determined at a time when heparin activity is too low to affect the prothrombin time. This is approximately 5 hours after the last IV bolus and 24 hours after the last subcutaneous dose. If continuous IV heparin infusion is used, prothrombin time can usually be measured at any time.

In converting from heparin to an oral anticoagulant, the dose of the oral anticoagulant should be the usual initial amount; thereafter, prothrombin time should be determined at the usual intervals. To ensure continuous anticoagulation, it is advisable to continue full heparin therapy for several days after the prothrombin time has reached the therapeutic range. Heparin therapy may then be discontinued without tapering.

➤*Preparation for administration:* Slight discoloration does not alter potency. Do not use if solution is discolored or contains a precipitate.

➤*Administration:* Heparin in dextrose is not effective by oral administration and should be given by continuous IV infusion. Do not use as a "catheter lock flush" product. Products should not be infused under pressure.

Heparin is not intended for intramuscular (IM) use.

If administration is controlled by a pumping device, care must be taken to discontinue pumping action before the container runs dry or air embolism may result.

These solutions are intended for IV administration using sterile equipment. It is recommended that any unused heparin solution and IV administration apparatus be replaced at least once every 24 hours.

Dextrose solutions with low electrolyte concentrations should not be administered simultaneously with blood through the same administration set because of the possibility of pseudoagglutination or hemolysis. The bag container label for these solutions bears the statement: Do not administer simultaneously with blood.

➤*Admixture compatibility:* Do not admix with other drugs.

➤*Storage/Stability:* Store at 25°C (77°F); however, brief exposure up to 40°C (104°F) does not adversely affect the product. Avoid excessive heat. Protect from freezing.

ANTITHROMBIN

Rx	**Thrombate III** (Talecris)	**Injection, lyophilized powder for solution:** 500 units (human)	Preservative free. Sodium 110 to 210 mEq/L. In single-use vials with 10 mL of sterile water for injection.
Rx	**ATryn** (Ovation)	**Injection, lyophilized powder for solution:** 1,750 units (recombinant)	Preservative free. Sodium chloride 79 mg, sodium citrate 26 mg. In single-dose vials.

ANTITHROMBIN — INJECTION

Indications

➤*Antithrombin (human):*

Antithrombin III deficiency – Antithrombin III (human) (AT-III) is indicated for the treatment of patients with hereditary AT-III deficiency in connection with surgical or obstetrical procedures or when they suffer from thromboembolism.

➤*Antithrombin (recombinant):*

Prevention of thromboembolic events – For the prevention of perioperative and peripartum thromboembolic events in patients with hereditary antithrombin deficiency.

Administration and Dosage

➤*General dosing considerations:* The dosage of AT recombinant is to be individualized based on the patients pretreatment functional AT activity level (expressed in percent of normal) and body weight (expressed in kilograms) and using therapeutic drug monitoring.

As a general recommendation, the therapeutic program may be utilized as a starting program for treatment.

The goal of treatment is to restore and maintain functional AT activity levels between 80% to 120% of normal (0.8 to 1.2 units/mL).

➤*Adults:*

Antithrombin deficiency –

Antithrombin (human): Dosage should be determined using the following formula:

$$\text{units required} = \frac{[\text{desired} - \text{baseline AT-III level}]^{a}}{1.4} \times \text{weight (kg)}$$

[a] (expressed as % normal level based on functional AT-III assay)

• *Loading dose* – An initial loading dose of AT-III (human) calculated to elevate the plasma AT-III level to 120%, assuming an expected rise over the baseline plasma AT-III level of 1.4% (functional activity) per unit per kg of AT-III (human) administered. Thus, if an individual has a baseline AT-III of 57%, the initial AT-III (human) dose would be (120 − 57)/1.4 = 45 units/kg.

• *Maintenance dosage* – Plasma levels between 80% to 120% may be maintained by administration of maintenance doses of 60% of the initial

ANTITHROMBIN — INJECTION

loading dose administered every 24 hours. Make adjustments in the maintenance dose and/or interval between doses based on actual plasma AT-III levels achieved.

• *Dosage adjustment* – Measure preinfusion and 20 minutes postinfusion (peak) plasma AT-III levels following the initial loading dose, plasma AT-III level after 12 hours, then preceding the next infusion (trough level). Subsequently measure AT-III levels preceding and 20 minutes after each infusion until predictable peak and trough levels have been achieved, generally between 80% to 120%.

In some situations (eg, following surgery hemorrhage, acute thrombosis, during intravenous (IV) heparin administration), the half-life of AT-III (human) has been reported to be shortened. In such conditions, monitor plasma AT-III levels more frequently, and administer AT-III (human) as necessary.

• *Duration of therapy* – When an infusion of AT-III (human) is indicated for a patient with hereditary deficiency to control an acute thrombotic episode or to prevent thrombosis following surgical or obstetrical procedures, it is desirable to raise the AT-III level to normal and maintain this level for 2 to 8 days, depending on the indication for treatment, type and extent of surgery, patient's medical condition, past history, and health care provider's judgment.

• *Concomitant therapy* – Coadministration of heparin should be based on the medical judgement of the health care provider.

Antithrombin (recombinant):

• *Loading dose* – Treatment should be initiated prior to delivery or approximately 24 hours prior to surgery to ensure that the plasma AT level is in the target range at that time.

Pregnant women: Loading dose (units) = (100 − baseline AT activity level)/1.3 × body weight (kg).

Surgical patients: Loading dose (units) = (100 − baseline AT activity level)/2.3 × body weight (kg).

• *Maintenance dosage* –

Pregnant women: Maintenance dosage (units/h) = (100 − baseline AT activity level)/5.4 × body weight (kg).

Surgical patients: Maintenance dosage (units/h) = (100 − baseline AT activity level)/10.2 × body weight (kg).

• *Dosage adjustment* – AT activity monitoring is required for proper treatment. Check AT activity once or twice per day with dose adjustments accordingly.

Antithrombin Activity Monitoring and Dose Adjustment

Initial monitor time	AT level	Dose adjustment	Recheck AT level
2 h after initiation of treatment	< 80%	Increase 30%	2 h after each dose adjustment
	80% to 120%	None	6 h after initiation of treatment or dose adjustment
	> 120%	Decrease 30%	2 h after each dose adjustment

Because surgery or delivery may rapidly decrease the AT activity levels, check the AT level just after surgery or delivery. If AT activity level is below 80%, an additional bolus dose may be administered to rapidly restore decreased AT activity level. In such instances, the loading dose formula should be used, utilizing in the calculation the last available AT activity result. Thereafter, restart the maintenance dose at the same rate of infusion as before the bolus.

• *Duration of therapy* – Continue treatment until adequate follow-on anticoagulation is established.

➤*Elderly:* In general, dose selection for an elderly patient should be cautious, usually starting at the low end of the dosing range, reflecting the greater frequency of decreased hepatic, renal, or cardiac function, and of concomitant disease or other drug therapy.

➤*Therapeutic drug monitoring:* It is recommended that following an initial dose of AT-III (human), plasma levels of AT-III be initially monitored at least every 12 hours and before the next infusion of AT-III to maintain plasma AT-III levels more than 80%. In some situations (eg, following surgery, hemorrhage, acute thrombosis, during IV heparin administration), the half-life of AT-III (human) has been reported to be shortened. In such conditions, plasma AT-III levels should be monitored more frequently, and AT-III (human) administered as necessary.

➤*Preparation for administration:*

Antithrombin (human) – Reconstitute AT-III (human) with sterile water for injection and bring it to room temperature prior to administration. Filter AT-III (human) through a sterile filter needle as supplied in the package prior to use, and administer within 3 hours following reconstitution. Do not refrigerate after reconstitution.

Vacuum transfer: Carefully follow aseptic technique. All needles and vial tops that come into contact with the product to be administered via the IV route should not come into contact with any nonsterile surface. Discard any contaminated needles by placing them in a puncture-proof container, and use new equipment.

1.) After removing all items from the box, warm the sterile water (diluent) to room temperature (25°C; 77°F).
2.) Remove the plastic flip tops from each vial. Cleanse vial tops (gray stoppers) with alcohol swab and allow surface to dry. After cleaning, do not allow anything to touch the stopper.
3.) Carefully remove the plastic sheath from the short end of the transfer needle. Insert the exposed needle into the diluent vial to the hub.
4.) Carefully grip the sheath of the other end of the transfer needle and twist to remove it.
5.) Invert the diluent vial and insert the attached needle into the concentrate vial at a 45° angle. This will direct the stream of diluent against the wall of the concentrate vial and minimize foaming. the vacuum will draw the diluent into the concentrate vial (If vacuum is lost in the concentrate vial, use a sterile syringe to remove the sterile water from the diluent vial and inject it into the concentration vial, directing the stream of fluid against the wall of the vial).
6.) When diluent transfer is complete, remove the diluent vial and transfer needle.
7.) Immediately after adding the diluent, swirl continuously until completely dissolved. Some foaming may occur, but attempt to avoid excessive foaming. The vial should then be visually inspected for particulate matter and discoloration prior to administration.
8.) Clean the top of the vial of reconstituted AT-III (human) again with alcohol swab and let surface dry.
9.) Attach the filter needle (from the package) to sterile syringe. Withdraw the AT-III (human) solution into the syringe through the filter needle.
10.) Remove the filter needle from the syringe and place with an appropriate injection or butterfly need for administration. Discard filter needle into a puncture-proof container.
11.) If the same patient is using more than 1 vial of AT-III (human), the contents of multiple vials may be drawn into the same syringe through the filter needles provided.

Antithrombin (recombinant) –

1.) Bring vials to room temperature no more than 3 hours prior to reconstitution.
2.) Reconstitute with 10 mL sterile water for injection (not supplied with AT) immediately prior to use. Do not shake.
3.) Do not use solution containing visible particulates or if it is discolored or cloudy.
4.) Draw solution from one or more vials into a sterile disposable syringe for IV administration or add solution to an infusion bag containing 0.9% sterile sodium chloride for injection (eg, dilute solution to obtain a concentration of 100 units/mL).
5.) Administer using an infusion set with a 0.22 micron pore-size, in-line filter.
6.) Administer contents of infusion syringes or dilute solution within 8 to 12 hours of preparation when stored at 68° to 77°F (20° to 25°C).
7.) Discard unused product in accordance with local requirements.

➤*Administration:*

Antithrombin (human) – Administer only by the IV route. Adapt the rate of administration to the response of the individual patient; administration of the entire dose in 10 to 20 minutes is generally well tolerated.

Once reconstituted, give AT (human) alone, without mixing with other agents or diluting solutions.

Antithrombin (recombinant) – For IV use as a continuous infusion only after reconstitution.

Administer loading dose as a 15 minute IV infusion, immediately followed by a continuous infusion of the maintenance dose.

➤*Storage / Stability:*

Antithrombin (human) – Store under 25°C (77°F). Avoid freezing because breakage of the diluent bottle might occur.

Antithrombin (recombinant) – Store refrigerated at between 2° and 8°C (36° and 46°F). Discard unused portions. Infusion syringes or diluted solutions are stable within 8 to 12 hours of preparation when stored at 68° to 77°F) (20° to 25°C).

Actions

➤*Pharmacology:*

Antithrombin (human) – AT-III, an alpha$_2$-glycoprotein of molecular weight 58,000, is normally present in human plasma at a concentration of approximately 12.5 mg/dL, and is the major plasma inhibitor of thrombin. Inactivation of thrombin by AT-III occurs by formation of a covalent bond resulting in an inactive 1:1 stoichiometric complex between the 2, involving an interaction of the active serine of thrombin and an arginine reactive site on AT-III. AT-III is also capable of inactivating other components of the coagulation cascade, including factors IXa, Xa, XIa, and XIIa, as well as plasmin.

The neutralization rate of serine proteases by AT-III proceeds slowly in the absence of heparin, but is greatly accelerated in the presence of heparin. As the therapeutic antithrombotic effect in vivo of heparin is mediated by AT-III, heparin is ineffective in the absence or near absence of AT-III.

Antithrombin (recombinant) – AT plays a central role in the regulation of hemostasis. AT is the principal inhibitor of thrombin and factor Xa, the serine proteases that play pivotal roles in blood coagulation. AT neutralizes the activity of thrombin and factor Xa by forming a complex that is rapidly removed from the circulation. The ability of AT to inhibit thrombin and factor Xa can be enhanced by more than 300- to 1,000-fold when AT is bound to heparin.

Pharmacodynamics: Hereditary AT deficiency causes an increased risk of venous thromboembolism. During high-risk situations, such as surgery or trauma or for pregnant women during the peripartum period, the risk of development of venous thromboembolisms as compared with the healthy population in these situations is increased by a factor 10 to 50.

In patients with hereditary AT deficiency, AT restores (normalizes) plasma AT activity levels during perioperative and peripartum periods.

ANTITHROMBIN — INJECTION

➤*Pharmacokinetics:*

Antithrombin (human) – In clinical studies of AT-III (human) conducted in 10 asymptomatic subjects with hereditary deficiency of AT-III, the mean in vivo recovery of AT-III was 1.6% per unit per kg administered based on immunologic AT-III assays, and 1.4% per unit per kg administered based on functional AT-III assays. The mean 50% disappearance time (the time to fall to 50% of the peak plasma level following an initial administration) was approximately 22 hours, and the biologic half-life was 2.5 days based on immunologic assays and 3.8 days based on functional assays of AT-III. These values are similar to the half-life for radiolabeled AT-III (human) reported in the literature of 2.8 to 4.8 days.

Antithrombin (recombinant) – In an open-label, single-dose pharmacokinetic study, men and women (18 years of age and older) with hereditary AT deficiency, received AT (recombinant) 50 units/kg (n = 9; all women) or AT (recombinant) 100 units/kg (n = 6; 2 men and 4 women) IV. These patients were not in high-risk situations. The baseline corrected pharmacokinetic parameters for AT (recombinant) are summarized in the following table.

Antithrombin (Recombinant) Baseline Corrected Mean Pharmacokinetic Parameters (%CV)[a]

Parameter	50 units/kg	100 units/kg
Cl (mL/h/kg)	9.6 (34.4%)	7.2 (15.3%)
Half-life (h)	11.6 (84.7%)	17.7 (60.9%)
MRT (h)	16.2 (74.9%)	20.5 (40.2%)
V_{ss} (mL/kg)	126.2 (37.4%)	156.1 (43.4%)

[a] CV = coefficient of variation; Cl = clearance; MRT = mean residence time; V_{ss} = apparent volume of distribution steady state.

Incremental recovery [mean (%CV)] was 2.24 (20.2) and 1.94 (14.8) %/units/kg for 50 and 100 units/kg, respectively.

As compared with plasma-derived AT, AT (recombinant) has a shorter half-life and more rapid clearance (approximately 9 and 7 times, respectively).

Pharmacokinetics may be influenced by concomitant heparin administration, as well as surgical procedures, delivery, or bleeding. Perform AT activity monitoring to properly treat such patients.

Special populations –

Pregnancy: Population pharmacokinetic analysis of hereditary deficient patients in a high-risk situation revealed that the Cl and volume of distribution in pregnant patients were 1.38 L/h and 14.3 L, respectively, which are higher than nonpregnant patients (0.67 L/h and 7.7 L, respectively). Therefore, use the distinct dosing formula for surgical and pregnant patients (see Administration and Dosage).

Contraindications

➤*Antithrombin (human):* None known.

➤*Antithrombin (recombinant):* Known hypersensitivity to goat and goat milk proteins.

Warnings/Precautions

➤*Viral infections:* AT-III (human) is made from human plasma. Products made from human plasma may contain infectious agents, such as viruses and, theoretically, the Creutzfeldt-Jakob (CJD) agent, that can cause disease. The risk that such products will transmit an infectious agent has been reduced by screening plasma donors for prior exposure to certain viruses, testing for the presence of certain current virus infections, and inactivating or removing certain viruses. Despite these measures, such products can still potentially transmit disease. There is also the possibility that unknown infectious agents may be present in such products. Individuals who receive infusions of blood or plasma products may develop signs or symptoms of some viral infections, particularly hepatitis C. Discuss the risks and benefits of this product with the patient before prescribing or administering.

Report all infections possibly transmitted by this product to the manufacturer at 1-800-520-2807.

➤*Antithrombin III deficiency diagnosis:* Base the diagnosis of hereditary AT-III deficiency on a clear family history of venous thrombosis as well as decreased plasma AT-III levels, and the exclusion of acquired deficiency.

➤*Coagulation monitoring tests:* The anticoagulant effect of drugs that use AT to exert their anticoagulation may be altered when AT (recombinant) is added or withdrawn. To avoid excessive or insufficient anticoagulation, perform coagulation tests suitable for the anticoagulant used (eg, activated partial thromboplastin time [aPTT] and anti–factor Xa activity) regularly, at close intervals, in particular in the first hours following the start or withdrawal of AT (recombinant). Additionally, monitor the patients for the occurrence of bleeding or thrombosis in such situation.

➤*Immunogenicity:* For AT (recombinant), a potential safety issue is the development of an immunological reaction to the recombinant protein or any of the potential contaminating proteins. Assays were developed and used to detect antibodies directed against AT (recombinant), goat AT, or goat milk proteins. No confirmed specific immunological reaction was seen in any of the patients tested, nor were there any clinical adverse events that might indicate such a response.

➤*Hypersensitivity reactions:* Allergic-type hypersensitivity reactions are possible with AT (recombinant). Patients must be closely monitored and carefully observed for any symptoms throughout the infusion period. Inform patients of the early signs of hypersensitivity reactions, including hives, generalized urticaria, tightness of the chest, wheezing, hypotension, and anaphylaxis. If these symptoms occur during administration, treatment must be discontinued immediately and emergency treatment administered.

➤*Pregnancy:*

Antithrombin (human) – *Category B*. It is not known whether AT-III (human) can cause fetal harm when administered to a pregnant woman or can affect reproduction capacity. The molecular weight of the protein, about 58,000, should prevent passive diffusion of AT (human) to the embryo or fetus. Because animal reproduction studies are not always predictive of human response, use this drug during pregnancy only if clearly needed.

Antithrombin (recombinant) – *Category C*. There are no adequate and well-controlled studies in pregnant women. Because animal reproductive studies are not always predictive of human response, use this drug during pregnancy only if clearly needed.

In rats, a dose of AT (recombinant) 210 mg/kg/day (5 to 6 times the human dose for pregnant women) administered during most of the pregnancy and entire lactation showed a slight but statistically significant increase in pup mortality in day 1 through day 4 when compared with concurrent control (90% compared with 94% viability index for 210 mg/kg/day vs control). This slight statistical difference does not reflect a true treatment-related effect. This same dose was shown to be safe in a second rat study when administered around parturition and during lactation where the no-adverse-effect level for dam and pups was 210 mg/kg/day.

Labor and delivery – AT (recombinant) is indicated for the treatment of pregnant women during the peripartum period. Pregnant patients who need a surgical procedure other than cesarean section are to be treated according to the dosing formulae for pregnant patients.

➤*Lactation:* No reports describing the use of AT-III during lactation have been located. The high molecular weight of the protein (about 58,000) suggests that it will not be excreted into breast milk. However, even if small amounts did enter the milk, they likely would be digested in the infant's stomach. Therefore, the risk to a breast-feeding infant appears to be nil.

Antithrombin (human) – The high molecular weight of the protein (58,000) suggests that it will not be excreted into breast milk. Even if small amounts did enter the milk, they likely would be digested in the infant's stomach.

Antithrombin (recombinant) – AT (recombinant) will be present in breast milk at levels estimated to be 1/50 to 1/100 of its concentration in the blood. This level is the same as that estimated to be present in breast milk of healthy lactating women, which is not known to be harmful to breast-fed neonates. However, exercise caution when AT is administered to a breast-feeding woman. Use only if clearly needed.

➤*Children:*

Antithrombin (human) – Safety and effectiveness in children have not been established. Measure the AT-III level in neonates of parents with hereditary AT-III deficiency immediately after birth. (Fatal neonatal thromboembolism, such as aortic thrombi in children of women with hereditary AT-III deficiency, has been reported.)

Plasma levels of AT-III are lower in neonates than adults, averaging approximately 60% in healthy term infants. AT-III levels in premature infants may be much lower. Low plasma AT-III levels, especially in a premature infant, therefore, do not necessarily indicate hereditary deficiency. It is recommended that testing and treatment with AT-III of neonates be discussed with an expert on coagulation.

Antithrombin (recombinant) – Safety and effectiveness in children have not been established.

➤*Elderly:* In general, be cautious in dose selection for an elderly patient, usually starting at the low end of the dosing range, reflecting the greater frequency of decreased hepatic, renal, or cardiac function, and of concomitant disease or other drug therapy.

➤*Monitoring:*

Antithrombin (human) – It is recommended that AT-III plasma levels be monitored during the treatment period. Functional levels of AT-III in plasma may be measured by amidolytic assays using chromogenic substrates, or by clotting assays.

Antithrombin (recombinant) – Perform coagulation tests regularly, at close intervals, in particular in the first hours following the start or withdrawal of antithrombin (recombinant) if the patient is on an anticoagulant.

Additionally, monitor for bleeding or thrombosis in such situations. Closely monitor and observe patients for hypersensitivity reactions throughout the infusion period.

Drug Interactions

➤*Anticoagulants:* The anticoagulant effect of heparin and low–molecular weight heparin is enhanced by AT. The half-life of AT may be altered by concomitant treatment with these anticoagulants caused by an altered AT turnover. Thus, coadministration of AT with heparin, low–molecular weight heparin, or other anticoagulants that use AT to exert their anticoagulant effect must be monitored clinically and biologically.

Adverse Reactions

➤*Antithrombin (human):* In clinical studies involving AT-III (human), adverse reactions were reported in association with 17 of the 340 infusions during the clinical studies. Included were dizziness (7), chest tightness (3), nausea (3), foul taste in mouth (3), chills (2), cramps (2), shortness of breath (1), chest pain (1), film over eye (1), light-headedness (1), bowel fullness (1), hives (1), fever (1), and oozing and hematoma formation (1). If adverse reactions are experienced, decrease the infusion rate or, if indicated, interrupt the infusion until symptoms abate.

ANTITHROMBIN — INJECTION

➤*Antithrombin (recombinant):* The serious adverse reaction that has been reported in clinical studies is hemorrhage (intra-abdominal, hemarthrosis, and postprocedural). The most common adverse reactions reported in clinical trials at a frequency of at least 5% are hemorrhage and infusion-site reaction. Adverse reactions that occurred in 2% of the total population (N = 47) in clinical trials in patients with hereditary AT deficiency are application-site pruritus, feeling hot, hemarthrosis, hematoma, hematuria, hepatic enzymes abnormal, intra-abdominal hemorrhage, and noncardiac chest pain.

Overdosage

None reported.

Patient Information

Inform patients that allergic-type hypersensitivity reactions are possible and instruct them to inform their health care provider about any past or present known hypersensitivity to goats or goat milk proteins prior to treatment with AT (recombinant). Inform patients of the early signs of hypersensitivity reactions, including hives, generalized urticaria, tightness of the chest, wheezing, hypotension, and anaphylaxis and to notify their health care provider immediately if these events develop.

Inform patients about the risk of bleeding when AT is administered with other anticoagulants and instruct them to notify their health care provider of any bleeding events while on treatment with AT.

DABIGATRAN ETEXILATE

Rx	**Pradaxa** (Boehringer Ingelheim Pharmaceuticals)	**Capsules; oral:** 75 mg	Equiv. to dabigatran etexilate mesylate 86.48 mg. (R75). Lt. blue/cream opaque. In 60s and UD 60s.
		150 mg	Equiv. to dabigatran etexilate mesylate 172.95 mg. (R150). Lt. blue/cream opaque. In 60s and UD 60s.

DABIGATRAN ETEXILATE MESYLATE — ORAL

Indications

➤*Stroke/Systemic embolism prevention:* To reduce the risk of stroke and systemic embolism in patients with nonvalvular atrial fibrillation.

Administration and Dosage

➤*Adults:*

Stroke/Systemic embolism prevention –

Usual dosage: 150 mg twice daily.

Missed dose: If a dose of dabigatran is not taken at the scheduled time, the dose should be taken as soon as possible on the same day; the missed dose should be skipped if it cannot be taken at least 6 hours before the next scheduled dose. The dose should not be doubled to make up for a missed dose.

➤*Renal function impairment:*

Creatinine clearance 15 to 30 mL/min – 75 mg twice daily.

Creatinine clearance less than 15 mL/min or dialysis – Dosing recommendations cannot be provided.

➤*Conversion:*

Warfarin – When converting patients from warfarin to dabigatran, discontinue warfarin and start dabigatran when the international normalized ratio (INR) is below 2.

When converting from dabigatran to warfarin, adjust the starting time of warfarin based on creatinine clearance (CrCl) as follows: for CrCl greater than 50 mL/min, start warfarin 3 days before discontinuing dabigatran; for CrCl 31 to 50 mL/min, start warfarin 2 days before discontinuing dabigatran; for CrCl 15 to 30 mL/min, start warfarin 1 day before discontinuing dabigatran; and for CrCl less than 15 mL/min, no recommendations can be made.

Because dabigatran can contribute to an elevated INR, the INR will better reflect warfarin's effect after dabigatran has been stopped for at least 2 days.

Parenteral anticoagulants – For patients currently receiving a parenteral anticoagulant, start dabigatran 0 to 2 hours before the time that the next dose of the parenteral drug was to have been administered or at the time of discontinuation of a continuously administered parenteral drug (eg, intravenous [IV] unfractionated heparin).

For patients currently taking dabigatran, wait 12 hours (CrCl 30 mL/min or more) or 24 hours (CrCl less than 30 mL/min) after the last dose of dabigatran before initiating treatment with a parenteral anticoagulant.

➤*Invasive or surgical procedures:* If possible, discontinue dabigatran 1 to 2 days (CrCl 50 mL/min or more) or 3 to 5 days (CrCl less than 50 mL/min) before invasive or surgical procedures because of the increased risk of bleeding. Consider longer times for patients undergoing major surgery, spinal puncture, or placement of a spinal or epidural catheter or port, in whom complete hemostasis may be required.

➤*Administration:* Swallow the capsules whole. Breaking, chewing, or emptying the contents of the capsule can result in increased exposure. Take with or without food.

➤*Storage/Stability:* Store at 25°C (77°F); excursions are permitted between 15° and 30°C (59° and 86°F). Once the bottle is opened, the product must be used within 30 days. Store in the original package to protect from moisture.

Actions

➤*Pharmacology:* Dabigatran and its acyl glucuronides are competitive, direct thrombin inhibitors. Because thrombin (serine protease) enables the conversion of fibrinogen into fibrin during the coagulation cascade, its inhibition prevents the development of a thrombus. Free and clot-bound thrombin and thrombin-induced platelet aggregation are inhibited by the active moieties.

➤*Pharmacokinetics:*

Absorption – Dabigatran etexilate mesylate is absorbed as the dabigatran etexilate ester. The ester is then hydrolyzed, forming dabigatran, the active moiety. The absolute bioavailability of dabigatran is approximately 3% to 7%. Dabigatran is a substrate of the efflux transporter P-glycoprotein (P-gp). After oral administration of dabigatran in healthy volunteers, maximum plasma concentrations (C_{max}) occur at 1 hour postadministration in the fasted state.

The oral bioavailability of dabigatran increases by 75% when the pellets are taken without the capsule shell compared with the intact capsule formulation. Therefore, do not break, chew, or open dabigatran capsules before administration.

Effect of food: Coadministration of dabigatran with a high-fat meal delays the time to C_{max} by approximately 2 hours, but has no effect on the bioavailability of dabigatran. Dabigatran may be administered with or without food.

Distribution – Dabigatran is approximately 35% bound to human plasma proteins. The red blood cell to plasma partitioning of dabigatran measured as total radioactivity is less than 0.3. The volume of distribution of dabigatran is 50 to 70 L. Given twice daily, dabigatran's accumulation factor is approximately 2.

Metabolism – After oral administration, dabigatran etexilate is converted to dabigatran. The cleavage of the dabigatran etexilate by esterase-catalyzed hydrolysis to the active principal dabigatran is the predominant metabolic reaction. Dabigatran is not a substrate, inhibitor, or inducer of cytochrome P450 enzymes. Dabigatran is subject to conjugation-forming pharmacologically active acyl glucuronides. Four positional isomers, 1-O-, 2-O-, 3-O-, and 4-O-acylglucuronide, exist, and each accounts for less than 10% of total dabigatran in plasma. The glucoronides and dabigatran have similar pharmacological activity.

Excretion – Dabigatran is eliminated primarily in the urine. Renal clearance of dabigatran is 80% of total clearance after IV administration. After oral administration of radiolabeled dabigatran, 7% of radioactivity is recovered in urine and 86% in feces. The half-life of dabigatran in healthy subjects is 12 to 17 hours.

Special populations –

Renal function impairment: An open, parallel-group, single-center study compared dabigatran pharmacokinetics in healthy subjects and patients with mild to moderate renal impairment receiving a single dose of dabigatran 150 mg. Based on pharmacokinetic modeling, estimated exposure to dabigatran increases with the severity of renal impairment. Similar findings were observed in the Randomized Evaluation of Long-Term Anticoagulant Therapy (RE-LY) trial.

Dabigatran Pharmacokinetic Parameters by Renal Function

Renal function	CrCl	Increase in AUC[a]	Increase in C_{max}	Half-life
Normal	80 mL/min	1×	1×	13 h
Mild	50 mL/min	1.5×	1.1×	15 h
Moderate	30 mL/min	3.2×	1.7×	18 h

[a] AUC = area under the curve.

Contraindications

Active pathological bleeding; history of a serious hypersensitivity reaction to dabigatran (eg, anaphylactic reaction, anaphylactic shock).

Warnings/Precautions

➤*Bleeding:* Dabigatran increases the risk of bleeding and can cause significant and sometimes fatal bleeding. Risk factors for bleeding include the use of drugs that increase the risk of bleeding in general (eg, antiplatelet agents, heparin, fibrinolytic therapy, chronic use of nonsteroidal anti-inflammatory drugs [NSAIDs]) and labor and delivery. Promptly evaluate any signs or symptoms of blood loss (eg, a drop in hemoglobin and/or hematocrit, hypotension). Discontinue dabigatran in patients with active pathological bleeding.

In the RE-LY study, a life-threatening bleed (bleeding that met 1 or more of the following criteria: fatal, symptomatic intracranial bleed; reduction in

DABIGATRAN ETEXILATE MESYLATE — ORAL

hemoglobin of at least 5 g/dL; transfusion of at least 4 units of blood; associated with hypotension requiring the use of IV inotropic agents; or necessitating surgical intervention) occurred at an annualized rate of 1.5% and 1.8% for dabigatran 150 mg and warfarin, respectively.

➤*Discontinuation:* Discontinuing anticoagulants, including dabigatran, for active bleeding, elective surgery, or invasive procedures places patients at an increased risk of stroke. Avoid lapses in therapy. If anticoagulation with dabigatran must be temporarily discontinued for any reason, restart therapy as soon as possible.

➤*Renal function impairment:* See Administration and Dosage for more information.

➤*Pregnancy: Category C.* There are no adequate and well-controlled studies in pregnant women.

Dabigatran has been shown to decrease the number of implantations when male and female rats were treated at a dose of 70 mg/kg (about 2.6 to 3 times the human exposure at the maximum recommended human dose [MRHD] of 300 mg/day based on AUC comparisons) prior to mating and up to implantation (gestation day 6). Treatment of pregnant rats after implantation with dabigatran at the same dose increased the number of dead offspring and caused excess vaginal/uterine bleeding close to parturition. Although dabigatran increased the incidence of delayed or irregular ossification of fetal skull bones and vertebrae in the rat, it did not induce major malformations in rats or rabbits.

Labor and delivery – Consider the risks of bleeding and stroke in using dabigatran in this setting.

Death of offspring and mother rats during labor in association with uterine bleeding occurred during treatment of pregnant rats from implantation (gestation day 7) to weaning (lactation day 21) with dabigatran at a dose of 70 mg/kg (about 2.6 times the human exposure at the MRHD of 300 mg/day based on AUC comparisons).

➤*Lactation:* It is not known whether dabigatran is excreted in human milk. Because many drugs are excreted in human milk, exercise caution when dabigatran is administered to a breast-feeding woman.

➤*Children:* Safety and effectiveness of dabigatran in children have not been established.

➤*Elderly:* The risk of stroke and bleeding increase with age, but the risk-benefit profile is favorable in all age groups.

➤*Monitoring:* Monitor for signs of bleeding throughout therapy.

Drug Interactions

Dabigatran Drug Interactions

Precipitant drug	Object drug[a]		Description
Amiodarone	Dabigatran	⬆	Administration of a single dose of amiodarone 600 mg increased the dabigatran AUC and C_{max} 58% and 50%, respectively. The increased exposure was mitigated by a 65% increase in dabigatran renal clearance. The increase in renal clearance may persist after amiodarone discontinuation because of the long half-life of amiodarone. No change in dabigatran trough concentration was observed.
Clopidogrel	Dabigatran	⬆	Concurrent use of dabigatran with a loading dose of clopidogrel 300 or 600 mg increased the dabigatran AUC and C_{max} 30% and 40%, respectively. Coadministration resulted in no further prolongation of capillary bleeding times compared with clopidogrel monotherapy.
Drugs that increase the risk of bleeding (eg, antiplatelet agents [eg, clopidogrel], fibrinolytic therapy [alteplase], heparin, chronic use of NSAIDs [eg, ibuprofen])	Dabigatran	⬆	The risk of severe and sometimes fatal bleeding may be increased. Monitor for any signs or symptoms of blood loss (eg, drop in hemoglobin, hypotension). Discontinue dabigatran in patients with active pathologic bleeding.
Ketoconazole	Dabigatran	⬆	Single-dose administration of ketoconazole increased dabigatran AUC and C_{max} 138% and 135%, respectively. Multiple-dose administration increased the AUC and C_{max} 153% and 149%, respectively.
Quinidine	Dabigatran	⬆	When dabigatran was administered for 3 days with and without pretreatment with quinidine 200 mg every 2 hours up to 1,000 mg, coadministration of quinidine increased the dabigatran AUC and C_{max} 53% and 56%, respectively.
Rifamycins (eg, rifampin)	Dabigatran	⬇	Dabigatran exposure may be reduced, decreasing the efficacy. Pretreatment with rifampin 600 mg once daily for 7 days decreased the dabigatran AUC and C_{max} 66% and 67%, respectively. Seven days after discontinuing rifampin, dabigatran exposure was close to healthy. Avoid concurrent use of rifampin.
Verapamil	Dabigatran	⬆	Coadministration may increase dabigatran AUC and C_{max}. The extent of the increase depends on the verapamil formulation and time of administration. If verapamil is present in the gut when dabigatran is taken, dabigatran exposure will increase and the greatest increase (2.4-fold) is observed when a single dose of verapamil extended release is taken 1 hour prior to dabigatran. If verapamil is taken 2 hours after dabigatran, the increase is negligible. No important changes in dabigatran trough concentrations were observed.

[a] ⬆ = object drug increased; ⬇ = object drug decreased.

➤*Drug/Food interactions:* See Actions for more information.

Adverse Reactions

➤*Discontinuation:* The rates of adverse reactions leading to treatment discontinuation were 21% for dabigatran 150 mg and 16% for warfarin. The most frequent adverse reactions leading to discontinuation of dabigatran were bleeding and GI events (eg, dyspepsia, nausea, upper abdominal pain, GI hemorrhage, diarrhea).

➤*Bleeding:* Major bleeds fulfilled 1 or more of the following criteria: bleeding associated with a reduction in hemoglobin of at least 2 g per deciliter or leading to a transfusion of at least 2 units of blood, or symptomatic bleeding in a critical area or organ (intraocular, intracranial, intraspinal or intramuscular with compartment syndrome, retroperitoneal bleeding, intra-articular bleeding, or pericardial bleeding). A life-threatening bleed met 1 or more of the following criteria: fatal, symptomatic intracranial bleed, reduction in hemoglobin of at least 5 g per deciliter, transfusion of at least 4 units of blood, associated with hypotension requiring the use of IV inotropic agents, or necessitating surgical intervention. Intracranial hemorrhage included intracerebral (hemorrhagic stroke), subarachnoid, and subdural bleeds.

Dabigatran Serious Bleeding Events[a] (per 100 Patient-Years)

	Dabigatran 150 mg twice daily	Warfarin	Hazard ratio (95% CI[b])
Randomized patients	6,076	6,022	
Patient-years	12,033	11,794	
Intracranial hemorrhage	0.3%	0.8%	0.41 (0.28 to 0.6)
Life-threatening bleed	1.5%	1.9%	0.80 (0.66 to 0.98)
Major bleed	3.3%	3.6%	0.93 (0.81 to 1.07)
Any bleed	16.6%	18.4%	0.91 (0.85 to 0.96)

[a] Patients contributed multiple events and events were counted in multiple categories.
[b] CI = confidence interval.

The risk of major bleeds was similar with dabigatran 150 mg and warfarin across major subgroups defined by baseline characteristics, with the exception of age, where there was a trend towards a higher incidence of major bleeding on dabigatran (hazard ratio, 1.2; 95% CI, 1 to 1.4) for patients 75 years of age and older.

There was a higher rate of major GI bleeds in patients receiving dabigatran 150 mg than in patients receiving warfarin (1.6% vs 1.1%, respectively, with a hazard ratio vs warfarin of 1.5; 95% CI, 1.2 to 1.9) and a higher rate of any GI bleeds (6.1% vs 4%, respectively).

DABIGATRAN ETEXILATE MESYLATE — ORAL

➤*GI:* Patients on dabigatran 150 mg had an increased incidence of GI adverse reactions (35% vs 24% on warfarin). These were commonly dyspepsia (including abdominal pain upper, abdominal pain, abdominal discomfort, and epigastric discomfort) and gastritis-like symptoms (including gastroesophageal reflux disease [GERD], esophagitis, erosive gastritis, gastric hemorrhage, hemorrhagic gastritis, hemorrhagic erosive gastritis, and GI ulcer).

➤*Hypersensitivity:* In the RE-LY study, drug hypersensitivity (including urticaria, rash, and pruritus), allergic edema, anaphylactic reaction, and anaphylactic shock were reported in less than 0.1% of patients receiving dabigatran.

Overdosage

➤*Symptoms:* Accidental overdose may lead to hemorrhagic complications.

➤*Treatment:* There is no antidote to dabigatran etexilate or dabigatran. In the event of hemorrhagic complications, initiate appropriate clinical support, discontinue treatment with dabigatran, and investigate the source of bleeding. Dabigatran is primarily excreted in the urine; therefore, maintain adequate diuresis. Dabigatran can be dialyzed (protein binding is low), with the removal of about 60% of drug over 2 to 3 hours; however, data supporting this approach are limited. Consider surgical hemostasis or the transfusion of fresh frozen plasma or red blood cells. There is some experimental evidence to support the role of activated prothrombin complex concentrates (eg, factor VIII inhibitor bypassing activity), recombinant factor VIIa, or concentrates of coagulation factors II, IX, or X; however, their usefulness in clinical settings has not been established. Consider administration of platelet concentrates in cases where thrombocytopenia is present or long-acting antiplatelet drugs have been used. Measurement of activated partial thromboplastin time or ecarin clotting time may help guide therapy.

Patient Information

Remind patients not to discontinue dabigatran without talking to the health care provider who prescribed it.

Advise patients not to chew or break the capsules before swallowing them and not to open the capsules and take the pellets alone (eg, sprinkled over food or into beverages).

Advise patients that if they miss a dose to take it as soon as possible on the same day; instruct patients to skip the missed dose if it cannot be taken at least 6 hours before the next scheduled dose. Instruct patients to not double the dose to make up for a missed dose.

Inform patients that they may bleed more easily or longer and to call their health care provider for any signs or symptoms of bleeding.

Instruct patients to seek emergency care right away if they have any of the following, which may be a sign or symptom of serious bleeding: unusual bruising (bruises that appear without known cause or that get bigger); pink or brown urine; red or black, tarry stools; coughing up blood; or vomiting blood or vomit that looks like coffee grounds.

Instruct patients to call their health care provider or to get prompt medical attention if they experience any signs or symptoms of bleeding: pain, swelling, or discomfort in a joint; headaches, dizziness, or weakness; reoccurring nose bleeds; unusual bleeding from gums; bleeding from a cut that takes a long time to stop; or menstrual bleeding or vaginal bleeding that is heavier than normal.

Instruct patients to call their health care provider if they experience any signs or symptoms of dyspepsia or gastritis: dyspepsia (upset stomach), burning, or nausea; abdominal pain or discomfort; or epigastric discomfort or GERD (gastric indigestion).

Instruct patients to inform their health care provider that they are taking dabigatran before any invasive procedure (including dental procedures) is scheduled.

Ask patients to list all prescription medications, over-the-counter medications, or dietary supplements they are taking or plan to take so their health care provider knows about other treatments that may affect bleeding risk (eg, aspirin, NSAIDs) or dabigatran exposure.

DESIRUDIN

Rx	**Iprivask** (Canyon Pharmaceuticals)	**Powder for injection, lyophilized:** 15 mg	Preservative free. In single-use vials with diluent.[a]

[a] Diluent includes 0.6 mL mannitol (3%) in water for injection.

DESIRUDIN — INJECTION

WARNING

Spinal/Epidural hematomas – When neuraxial anesthesia (epidural/spinal anesthesia) or spinal puncture is employed, patients anticoagulated or scheduled to be anticoagulated with selective inhibitors of thrombin such as desirudin may be at risk of developing an epidural or spinal hematoma which can result in long-term or permanent paralysis.

The risk of these events may be increased by the use of indwelling spinal catheters for administration of analgesia or by the concomitant use of drugs affecting hemostasis such as nonsteroidal anti-inflammatory drugs (NSAIDs), platelet inhibitors, or other anticoagulants. Likewise with such agents, the risk appears to be increased by traumatic or repeated epidural or spinal puncture.

Patients should be frequently monitored for signs and symptoms of neurological impairment. If neurological compromise is noted, urgent treatment is necessary.

The physician should consider the potential benefit versus risk before neuraxial intervention, in patients anticoagulated or to be anticoagulated for thromboprophylaxis.

Indications

➤*Deep vein thrombosis, prophylaxis:* Desirudin is indicated for the prophylaxis of deep vein thrombosis, which may lead to pulmonary embolism, in patients undergoing elective hip-replacement surgery.

Administration and Dosage

➤*General dosing considerations:* All patients should be evaluated for bleeding disorder risk before prophylactic administration of desirudin. Any agent which may enhance the risk of hemorrhage should be discontinued prior to initiation of desirudin therapy. These agents include medications such as dextran 40, systemic glucocorticoids, thrombolytics, and anticoagulants.

➤*Adults:*

Deep vein thrombosis, prophylaxis –

Hip-replacement surgery:

• *Usual dosage* – 15 mg every 12 hours administered by subcutaneous injection, with the initial dose given up to 5 to 15 minutes prior to surgery, but after induction of regional block anesthesia, if used.

• *Duration of therapy* – Up to 12 days administration (average duration 9 to 12 days) of desirudin has been well tolerated in controlled clinical trials.

➤*Renal function impairment:*

Desirudin Use in Renal Function Impairment

Degree of renal insufficiency	Creatinine clearance (mL/min/1.73 m^2 body surface area)	aPTT monitoring and dosing instructions
Moderate	≥ 31 to 60	Initiate therapy at 5 mg every 12 hours by subcutaneous injection. Monitor aPTT and serum creatinine at least daily. If aPTT exceeds 2 times control: 1) Interrupt therapy until the value returns to less than 2 times control. 2) Resume therapy at a reduced dose guided by the initial degree of aPTT abnormality.
Severe	< 31	Initiate therapy at 1.7 mg every 12 hours. Monitor aPTT and serum creatinine at least daily. If aPTT exceeds 2 times control: 1) Interrupt therapy until the value returns to less than 2 times control. 2) Consider further dose reductions guided by the initial degree of aPTT abnormality.

DESIRUDIN — INJECTION

➤*Preparation for administration:*

1.) Reconstitution should be carried out under sterile conditions.
2.) Reconstitute each vial with 0.5 mL of provided diluent (mannitol USP [3%] in water for injection). Once reconstituted, each 0.5 mL contains 15.75 mg of desirudin
3.) Shake the vial gently until the drug is fully reconstituted.
4.) Reconstituted desirudin is a clear colorless solution. Inspect desirudin visually for particulate matter and discoloration prior to administration. Do not use solutions that are cloudy or contain particles.
5.) Use a syringe with a 26- or 27-gauge needle which is approximately ½ inch in length to withdraw all of the reconstituted solution (15.75 mg desirudin/0.5 mL) and inject the entire contents of the syringe subcutaneous, which will deliver 15 mg.
6.) The reconstituted solution should be used immediately; however, it is stable for up to 24 hours when stored at room temperature and protected from light. Discard any unused solution appropriately.

➤*Administration:* Desirudin is administered by subcutaneous injection. It must not be administered by IM injection.

Subcutaneous injection technique – Select a syringe with a 26- or 27-gauge needle which is approximately ½ inch in length for administration of desirudin. Withdraw the entire reconstituted solution (15.75 mg desirudin/0.5 mL) into the syringe and inject the total volume subcutaneous.

Patients should be sitting or lying down, and desirudin injection should be administered by deep subcutaneous injection. Administration should be alternated between the left and right anterolateral and left and right posterolateral thigh or abdominal wall. The whole length of the needle should be introduced into a skin fold held between the thumb and forefinger; the skin fold should be held throughout the injection. To minimize bruising, do not rub the injection site after completion of the injection.

➤*Admixture compatibility:* Desirudin should not be mixed with other injections, solvents, or infusions.

➤*Storage/Stability:* Store unopened vials or ampules at 25°C (77°F); excursions permitted between 15° and 30°C (59° and 86°F). Protect from light.

Actions

➤*Pharmacology:* Desirudin is a selective inhibitor of free circulating and clot-bound thrombin. The anticoagulant properties of desirudin are demonstrated by its ability to prolong the clotting time of human plasma. One molecule of desirudin binds to 1 molecule of thrombin and thereby blocks the thrombogenic activity of thrombin. As a result, all thrombin-dependent coagulation assays are affected. Activated partial thromboplastin time (aPTT) is a measure of the anticoagulant activity of desirudin and increases in a dose-dependent fashion. The pharmacodynamic effect of desirudin on proteolytic activity of thrombin was assessed as an increase in aPTT. A mean peak aPTT prolongation of about 1.38 times baseline value (range 0.58 to 3.41) was observed following SC twice-daily injections of 15 mg desirudin. Thrombin time (TT) frequently exceeds 200 seconds even at low plasma concentrations of desirudin, which renders this test unsuitable for routine monitoring of desirudin therapy. At therapeutic serum concentrations, desirudin has no effect on other enzymes of the hemostatic system such as factors IXa, Xa, kallikrein, plasmin, tissue plasminogen activator, or activated protein C. In addition, it does not display any effect on other serine proteases, such as the digestive enzymes trypsin, chymotrypsin, or on complement activation by the classical or alternative pathways.

➤*Pharmacokinetics:*

Absorption – Pharmacokinetic parameters were calculated based on plasma concentration data obtained by a nonspecific enzyme-linked immunosorbent assay (ELISA) method that does not discriminate between native desirudin and its metabolites. It is not known if the metabolites are pharmacologically active.

The absorption of desirudin is complete when administered SC at doses of 0.3 mg/kg or 0.5 mg/kg. Following SC administration of single doses of 0.1 to 0.75 mg/kg, plasma concentrations of desirudin increased to a maximum level (C_{max}) between 1 and 3 hours. Both C_{max} and area-under-the-curve (AUC) values are dose proportional.

Distribution – The pharmacokinetic properties of desirudin following IV administration are well described by a 2- or 3- compartment disposition model. Desirudin is distributed in the extracellular space with a volume of distribution at steady state of 0.25 L/kg, independent of the dose. Desirudin binds specifically and directly to thrombin, forming an extremely tight, noncovalent complex with an inhibition constant of approximately 2.6×10^{-13} M. Thus, free or protein bound desirudin immediately binds circulating thrombin. The pharmacological effect of desirudin is not modified when coadministered with highly protein-bound drugs (greater than 99%).

Metabolism – Human and animal data suggest that desirudin is primarily eliminated and metabolized by the kidney. The total urinary excretion of unchanged desirudin amounts to 40% to 50% of the administered dose. Metabolites lacking 1 or 2 C-terminal amino acids constitute a minor proportion of the material recovered from urine (less than 7%). There is no evidence for the presence of other metabolites. This indicates that desirudin is metabolized by stepwise degradation from the C-terminus probably catalyzed by carboxypeptidase(s) such as carboxypeptidase A, originating from the pancreas. Total clearance of desirudin is approximately 1.5 to 2.7 mL/min/kg following either SC or IV administration and is independent of dose. This clearance value is close to the glomerular filtration rate.

Excretion – The elimination of desirudin from plasma is rapid after IV administration, with approximately 90% of the dose disappearing from the plasma within 2 hours of the injection. Plasma concentrations of desirudin then decline with a mean terminal elimination half-life of 2 to 3 hours. After SC administration, the mean terminal elimination half-life is also approximately 2 hours.

Special populations –

Renal function impairment: In a pharmacokinetic study of renally impaired subjects, subjects with mild (creatinine clearance [Ccr] between 61 and 90 mL/min/1.73 m² body surface area), moderate (Ccr between 31 and 60 mL/min/1.73 m² body surface area), and severe (Ccr below 31 mL/min/1.73 m² body surface area) renal insufficiency, were administered a single IV dose of 0.5, 0.25, or 0.125 mg/kg desirudin, respectively. This resulted in mean dose-normalized AUC_{effect} ($AUC_{0\text{-}60th}$ for aPTT prolongation) increases of approximately 3-, and 9-fold for the moderate and severe renally impaired subjects, respectively, compared with healthy individuals. In subjects with mild renal impairment, there was no increase in AUC_{effect} compared with healthy individuals. In subjects with severe renal insufficiency, terminal elimination half-lives were prolonged up to 12 hours compared with 2 to 4 hours in healthy volunteers or subjects with mild-to-moderate renal insufficiency. Dose adjustments are recommended in certain circumstances in relation to the degree of impairment or degree of aPTT abnormality.

Age/Gender: The mean plasma clearance of desirudin in patients greater than or equal to 65 years of age (n = 12; 110 mL/min) is approximately 28% lower than in patients younger than 65 years of age (n = 8; 153 mL/min). Population pharmacokinetics conducted in 301 patients undergoing elective total hip replacement indicate that age or gender do not affect the systemic clearance of desirudin when renal creatinine clearance is considered. This drug is substantially excreted by the kidney, and the risk of adverse events due to it may be greater in patients with impaired renal function. Because elderly patients are more likely to have decreased renal function, care should be taken in dose selection, and it may be useful to monitor renal function. Dosage adjustment in the case of moderate and severe renal impairment is necessary.

Contraindications

Hypersensitivity to natural or recombinant hirudins; active bleeding or irreversible coagulation disorders.

Warnings/Precautions

➤*Hemorrhagic events:* Desirudin is not intended for IM injection, as local hematoma formation may result.

Desirudin, like other anticoagulants, should be used with caution in patients with increased risks of hemorrhage such as those with recent major surgery, organ biopsy or puncture of a noncompressible vessel within the last month; a history of hemorrhagic stroke, intracranial or intraocular bleeding including diabetic (hemorrhagic) retinopathy; recent ischemic stroke, severe uncontrolled hypertension, bacterial endocarditis, a known hemostatic disorder (congenital or acquired [eg, hemophilia, liver disease]) or a history of GI or pulmonary bleeding within the past 3 months.

Bleeding can occur at any site during therapy with desirudin. An unexplained fall in hematocrit or blood pressure should lead to a search for a bleeding site.

➤*Spinal/epidural anesthesia:* As with other anticoagulants, there is a risk of neuraxial hematoma formation with the concurrent use of desirudin and spinal/epidural anesthesia, which has the potential to result in long term or permanent paralysis. The risk may be greater with the use of postoperative indwelling catheters or the concomitant use of additional drugs affecting hemostasis such as nonsteroidal anti-inflammatory drugs (NSAIDs), platelet inhibitors or other anticoagulants. The risk may also be increased by traumatic or repeated neuraxial puncture.

To reduce the potential risk of bleeding associated with the concurrent use of desirudin and epidural or spinal anesthesia/analgesia, the pharmacokinetic profile of the drug should be considered when scheduling or using epidural or spinal anesthesia in proximity to desirudin administration. The physician should consider placement of the catheter prior to initiating desirudin and removal of the catheter when the anticoagulant effect of desirudin is low.

Should the physician decide to administer anticoagulation in the context of epidural/spinal anesthesia, extreme vigilance and frequent monitoring must be exercised to detect any signs and symptoms of neurological impairment such as midline back pain, sensory and motor deficits (numbness or weakness in lower limbs), bowel or bladder dysfunction. Patients should be instructed to inform their physicians immediately if they experience any of the above signs or symptoms. If signs or symptoms of spinal hematoma are suspected, urgent diagnosis and treatment including spinal cord decompression should be initiated.

The physician should consider the potential benefit versus risk before neuraxial intervention in patients anticoagulated or to be anticoagulated for thromboprophylaxis.

Interchangeability – Desirudin cannot be used interchangeably with other hirudins as they differ in manufacturing process and specific biological activity (ATUs). Each of these medicines has its own instructions for use.

➤*Hypersensitivity reactions:*

Antibodies/reexposure – Antibodies have been reported in patients treated with hirudins. Potential for cross-sensitivity to hirudin products cannot be excluded. Irritative skin reactions were observed in 9/322 volunteers exposed to desirudin by SC injection or IV bolus or infusion in single or multiple administrations of the drug. Allergic events were reported in less than 2% of patients who were administered desirudin in phase III clinical trials. Allergic events were reported in 1% of patients receiving unfractionated heparin and 1% of patients receiving enoxaparin. Hirudin-specific IgE evaluations may not be indicative of sensitivity to desirudin as this test was not always positive in the presence of symptoms. Very rarely, antihirudin

DESIRUDIN — INJECTION

antibodies have been detected upon reexposure to desirudin. Fatal anaphylactoid reactions have been reported during hirudin therapy.

➤*Renal function impairment:* Desirudin must be used with caution in patients with renal impairment, particularly in those with moderate and severe renal impairment (creatinine clearance less than or equal to 60 mL/min/1.73 m^2 body surface area). Dose reductions by factors of 3 and 9 are recommended for patients with moderate and severe renal impairment respectively. In addition, daily aPTT and serum creatinine monitoring are recommended for patients with moderate or severe renal impairment.

➤*Hepatic function impairment:* No information is available about the use of desirudin in patients with hepatic insufficiency/liver injury. Although desirudin is not significantly metabolized by the liver, hepatic impairment or serious liver injury (eg, liver cirrhosis) may alter the anticoagulant effect of desirudin due to coagulation defects secondary to reduced generation of vitamin K-dependent coagulation factors. Desirudin should be used with caution in these patients.

➤*Pregnancy: Category C.* Teratology studies have been performed in rats at SC doses in a range of 1 to 15 mg/kg/day (about 0.3 to 4 times the recommended human dose based on body surface area) and in rabbits at IV doses in a range of 0.6 to 6 mg/kg/day (about 0.3 to 3 times the recommended human dose based on body surface area) and have revealed desirudin to be teratogenic. Observed teratogenic findings were omphalocele, asymmetric and fused sternebrae, edema, shortened hind limbs in rats; and spina bifida, malrotated hind limb, hydrocephaly, gastroschisis in rabbits. There are no adequate and well-controlled studies in pregnant women. Desirudin should be used during pregnancy only if the potential benefit justifies the potential risk to the fetus.

➤*Lactation:* It is not known whether desirudin is excreted in human milk. Because many drugs are excreted in human milk, caution should be exercised when desirudin is administered to a nursing woman.

➤*Children:* Safety and efficacy in pediatric patients have not been established.

➤*Elderly:* In 3 clinical studies of desirudin, the percentage of patients greater than 65 years of age treated with 15 mg of desirudin SC every 12 hours was 58.5%, while 20.8% were 75 years of age or older. Elderly patients treated with desirudin had a reduction in the incidence of VTE similar to that observed in the younger patients, and a slightly lower incidence of VTE compared to those patients treated with heparin or enoxaparin.

Regarding safety, in the clinical studies the incidence of hemorrhage (major or otherwise) in patients 65 years of age or older was similar to that in patients less than 65 years of age. In addition, the elderly had a similar incidence of total, treatment-related, or serious adverse events compared to those patients less than 65 years of age. Serious adverse events occurred more frequently in patients 75 years of age or older as compared to those less than 65 years of age. In general, 15 mg desirudin every 12 hours can be used safely in the geriatric population as in the population of patients younger than 65 years of age so long as renal function is adequate.

➤*Monitoring:* Activated partial thromboplastin time (aPTT) should be monitored daily in patients with increased risk of bleeding or renal impairment. Serum creatinine should be monitored daily in patients with renal impairment. Peak aPTT should not exceed 2 times control. Should peak aPTT exceed this level, dose reduction is advised, based on the degree of aPTT abnormality. If necessary, therapy with desirudin should be interrupted until aPTT falls to less than 2 times control, at which time treatment with desirudin can be resumed at a reduced dose). Thrombin time (TT) is not a suitable test for routine monitoring of desirudin therapy. Dose adjustments based on serum creatinine may be necessary.

Drug Interactions

Desirudin Drug Interactions

Precipitant drug	Object drug[a]		Description
Thrombolytics (eg, alteplase, streptokinase), Glucocorticoids Dextran	Desirudin	↑	Concomitant treatment with thrombolytics may increase the risk of bleeding. Discontinue before initiations of desirudin therapy.
Anticoagulants (eg, heparin [unfractionated, and LMWH])	Desirudin	↑	During prophylaxis of venous thromboembolism, concomitant treatment is not recommended. The effects include prolongation of aPTT. As with other anticoagulants, desirudin should be used with caution.
Antiplatelets and glycoprotein IIb/IIIa antagonists (eg, salicylates, NSAIDs, ketorolac, acetylsalicylic acid, triclopidine, dipyridamole, sulfinpyrazone, clopidogrel, abciximab)	Desirudin	↑	Use with caution in conjunction with desirudin

[a] ↑ = Object drug increased.

Adverse Reactions

In the phase II and III clinical studies, desirudin was administered to 2159 patients undergoing elective hip-replacement surgery to determine the safety and efficacy of desirudin in preventing VTE in this population. Below is the safety profile of the desirudin 15 mg (every 12 hours) regimen from these 5 multicenter clinical trials.

Hemorrhagic events –

Hemorrhage in Patients Undergoing Hip-Replacement Surgery Receiving Desirudin

	Dosing regimen		
	Desirudin 15 mg every 12 hours SC (n = 1561) n (%)	Heparin 5000 IU every 8 hours SC (n = 501) n (%)	Enoxaparin 40 mg every day SC (n = 1036) n (%)
Patients with any hemorrhage [a]	464 (30%)	111 (22%)	341 (33%)
Patients with serious hemorrhage [b]	41 (3%)	15 (3%)	21 (2%)
Patients with major hemorrhage [c]	13 (< 1%)	0 (0%)	2 (< 1%)

[a] Includes hematomas which occurred at an incidence of 6% in the desirudin and enoxaparin treatment groups and 5% in the heparin treatment group.
[b] Bleeding complications were considered serious if perioperative transfusion requirements exceeded 5 units of whole blood or packed red cells, or if total transfusion requirements up to postoperative day 6 inclusive exceeded 7 units of whole blood or packed red cells, or total blood loss up to postoperative day 6 inclusive exceeded 3500 mL.
[c] Bleeding complications were considered major if the hemorrhage was overt and it produced a fall in hemoglobin of greater than or equal to 2 g/dL or if it lead to a transfusion of 2 or more units of whole or packed cells outside the perioperative period (the time from start of surgery until up to 12 hours after) and retroperitoneal, intracranial, intraocular, intraspinal, or occurred in a major prosthetic joint.

Nonhemorrhagic reactions –

Adverse Reactions Occurring at ≥ 2% in Desirudin-Treated Patients Undergoing Hip-replacement Surgery[a,b]

Body system (Preferred term)	Desirudin 15 mg every 12 hours SC (n = 1561) n (%)	Heparin 5000 IU every 8 hours SC (n = 501) n (%)	Enoxaparin 40 mg every day SC (n = 1036) n (%)
Injection site mass	56 (4%)	32 (6%)	7 (< 1%)
Wound secretion	59 (4%)	23 (5%)	34 (3%)
Anemia	51 (3%)	11 (2%)	37 (4%)
Deep thrombophlebitis	24 (2%)	41 (8%)	22 (2%)
Nausea	24 (2%)	5 (< 1%)	10 (< 1%)

[a] Represents reactions reported while on treatment, excluding unrelated adverse reactions.
[b] All hemorrhages that occurred are included in Adverse Reactions.

Related adverse reactions with a frequency of less than 2% and greater than 0.2% (in decreasing order of frequency) – Thrombosis, hypotension, leg edema, fever, decreased hemoglobin, hematuria, dizziness, epistaxis, vomiting, impaired healing, cerebrovascular disorder, leg pain, hematemesis.

➤*Hypersensitivity:* In clinical studies, allergic events were reported less than 2% overall and in 2% of patients who were administered 15 mg desirudin.

Postmarketing – In addition to adverse reactions reported from clinical trials the following adverse reactions have been identified during postapproval use of desirudin. These events were reported voluntarily from a population of unknown size and the frequency of occurrence cannot be determined precisely: Rare reports of major hemorrhages, some of which were fatal, and anaphylactic/anaphylactoid reactions.

DESIRUDIN — INJECTION

Overdosage

➤*Animal pharmacology and toxicology:*

General toxicity – Desirudin produced bleeding, local inflammation, and granulation at injection sites in rat and dog toxicity studies. In a 28-day study in rhesus monkeys, there was also evidence of SC bleeding and local inflammation at the injection sites. In addition, desirudin was immunogenic in dogs and formed antibody complexes resulting in prolonged half-life and accumulation. Desirudin showed sensitization potential in guinea pig immediate and delayed hypersensitivity models.

➤*Treatment:* In case of overdose, most likely reflected in hemorrhagic complications or suggested by excessively high aPTT values, desirudin therapy should be discontinued. Emergency procedures should be instituted as appropriate (for example, determination of aPTT and other coagulation levels, hemoglobin, the use of blood transfusion or plasma expanders).

No specific antidote for desirudin is available; however, the anticoagulant effect of desirudin is partially reversible using thrombin-rich plasma concentrates while aPTT levels can be reduced by the IV administration of 0.3 mcg/kg DDAVP (desmopressin). The clinical effectiveness of DDAVP in treating bleeding due to desirudin overdose has not been studied. In an open, pilot, dose-ascending study to assess safety, the highest dose of desirudin (40 mg every 12 hours) caused excessive hemorrhage.

LEPIRUDIN

Rx	**Refludan** (Hoechst-Marion Roussel)	**Powder for injection:** 50 mg	Mannitol. Freeze-dried. In boxes of 10.

LEPIRUDIN — INJECTION

Indications

➤*Thrombocytopenia, heparin-induced:* Lepirudin is indicated for anticoagulation in patients with heparin-induced thrombocytopenia (HIT) and associated thromboembolic disease in order to prevent further thromboembolic complications.

Administration and Dosage

➤*General dosing considerations:* A patient baseline aPTT should be determined prior to initiation of therapy with lepirudin because lepirudin should not be started in patients presenting with a baseline aPTT ratio of 2.5 or more, in order to avoid initial overdosing.

Normally, the initial dosage depends on the patient's body weight. This is valid up to a body weight of 110 kg.

➤*Adults:*

Heparin-induced thrombocytopenia –

Maximum dose:

• *Adults* – Initial bolus dose of 44 mg, initial infusion dose of 16.5 mg/h according to the prescribing information.

Initial dosage: 0.4 mg/kg body weight (up to 110 kg) slow IV (eg, over 15 to 20 seconds) as a bolus dose, followed by 0.15 mg/kg body weight (up to 110 kg)/h as a continuous IV infusion for 2 to 10 days or longer if clinically needed.

In patients with a body weight exceeding 110 kg, the initial dosage should not be increased beyond the 110 kg body weight dose.

Dosage adjustment: In general, the dosage (infusion rate) should be adjusted according to the aPTT ratio.

Any aPTT ratio out of the target range is to be confirmed at once before drawing conclusions with respect to dose modifications, unless there is a clinical need to react immediately.

If the confirmed aPTT ratio is above the target range, the infusion should be stopped for 2 hours. At restart, the infusion rate should be decreased by 50% (no additional IV bolus should be administered). The aPTT ratio should be determined again 4 hours later.

If the confirmed aPTT ratio is below the target range, the infusion rate should be increased in steps of 20%. The aPTT ratio should be determined again 4 hours later.

In general, an infusion rate of 0.21 mg/kg/h should not be exceeded without checking for coagulation abnormalities that might be preventive of an appropriate aPTT response.

Duration of therapy: 2 to 10 days or longer if clinically needed.

Concomitant thrombolytic therapy: Initial IV bolus, 0.2 mg/kg body weight; continuous IV infusion, 0.1 mg/kg body weight/hour.

Clinical trials in HIT patients have provided only limited information on the combined use of lepirudin and thrombolytic agents. The dosage regimen of lepirudin was used in a total of 9 HIT patients in the historically controlled clinical trials (HAT-1 and HAT-2) studies who presented with thromboembolic complications (TECs) at baseline and were started on both lepirudin and thrombolytic therapy (rt-PA, urokinase or streptokinase).

Special attention should be paid to the fact that thrombolytic agents per se may increase the aPTT ratio. Therefore, aPTT ratios with a given plasma level of lepirudin are usually higher in patients who receive concomitant thrombolysis than in those who do not.

Conversion to oral anticoagulation: If a patient is scheduled to receive coumarin derivatives (vitamin K antagonists) for oral anticoagulation after lepirudin therapy, the dose of lepirudin should first be gradually reduced in order to reach an aPTT ratio just above 1.5 before initiating oral anticoagulation. Coumarin derivatives should be initiated only when platelet counts are normalizing. The intended maintenance dose should be started with no loading dose. To avoid prothrombotic effects when initiating coumarin, continue parenteral anticoagulation for 4 to 5 days. The parenteral agent can be discontinued when the INR stabilizes within the desired target range.

➤*Renal function impairment:*

Dosage adjustment – Dose adjustments should be based on CrCl values, whenever available, as obtained from a reliable method (24-hour urine sampling). If CrCl is not available, the dose adjustments should be based on the serum creatinine.

Usual dosage – In all patients with renal insufficiency, the bolus dose is to be reduced to 0.2 mg/kg body weight. The standard initial infusion rate given in initial dosage and IV infusion must be reduced according to the recommendations given in the following data. Additional aPTT monitoring is highly recommended.

Reduction of Lepirudin Infusion Rate in Patients With Renal Impairment

CrCl (mL/min)	Serum creatinine (mg/dL)	Adjusted infusion rate	
		% of standard initial infusion rate	(mg/kg/h)
45 to 60 mL/min	1.6 to 2 mg/dL	50%	0.075 mg/kg/h
30 to 44 mL/min	2.1 to 3 mg/dL	30%	0.045 mg/kg/h
15 to 29 mL/min	3.1 to 6 mg/dL	15%	0.0225 mg/kg/h
Below 15 mL/min[a]	Above 6 mg/dL[a]	Avoid or stop infusion[a]	

[a] In hemodialysis patients or in case of acute renal failure (CrCl below 15 mL/min or serum creatinine above 6 mg/dL), infusion of lepirudin is to be avoided or stopped. Additional IV bolus doses of 0.1 mg/kg body weight should be considered every other day only if the aPTT ratio falls below the lower therapeutic limit of 1.5.

➤*Monitoring Therapy:* The target range for the aPTT ratio during treatment (therapeutic window) should be 1.5 to 2.5. Data from clinical trials in HIT patients suggest that with aPTT ratios higher than this target range, the risk of bleeding increases, while there is no incremental increase in clinical efficacy.

Lepirudin should not be started in patients presenting with a baseline aPTT ratio of 2.5 or more, in order to avoid initial overdosing.

The first aPTT determination for monitoring treatment should be done 4 hours after start of the lepirudin infusion.

Follow-up aPTT determinations are recommended at least once daily, as long as treatment with lepirudin is ongoing.

More frequent aPTT monitoring is highly recommended in patients with renal impairment or serious liver injury or with an increased risk of bleeding.

➤*Preparation for administration:* Reconstitution and further dilution are to be carried out under sterile conditions:

- For reconstitution, sterile water for injection or sodium chloride 0.9% injection are to be used.
- For further dilution, sodium chloride injection or dextrose 5% injection are suitable.
- For rapid, complete reconstitution, inject 1 mL of diluent into the vial and shake it gently. After reconstitution, a clear, colorless solution is usually obtained in a few seconds, but definitely in less than 3 minutes.
- Parenteral drug products should be inspected visually for particulate matter and discoloration prior to administration whenever solution and container permit. Do not use solutions that are cloudy or contain particles.
- The reconstituted solution is to be used immediately. It remains stable for up to 24 hours at room temperature (eg, during infusion).
- The preparation should be warmed to room temperature before administration.
- Discard any unused solution appropriately.

Initial IV bolus – For IV bolus injection, use a solution with a concentration of 5 mg/mL.

Preparation of a lepirudin solution with a concentration of 5 mg/mL: Reconstitute 1 vial (50 mg of lepirudin) with 1 mL of sterile water for injection or sodium chloride 0.9% injection.

The final concentration of 5 mg/mL is obtained by transferring the contents of the vial into a sterile, single-use syringe (of at least 10 mL capacity) and diluting the solution to a total volume of 10 mL, using sterile water for injection, sodium chloride 0.9% injection, or dextrose 5% injection.

The final solution is to be administered according to body weight (see the following table and Initial dose section.)

IV injection of the bolus is to be carried out slowly (eg, over 15 to 20 seconds).

Standard Bolus Injection Volumes According to Body Weight for a 5 mg/mL Lepirudin Concentration

Body weight (kg)	Injection volume	
	Dosage 0.4 mg/kg	Dosage 0.2 mg/kg[a]
50 kg	4 mL	2 mL
60 kg	4.8 mL	2.4 mL

LEPIRUDIN — INJECTION

Standard Bolus Injection Volumes According to Body Weight for a 5 mg/mL Lepirudin Concentration		
	Injection volume	
Body weight (kg)	Dosage 0.4 mg/kg	Dosage 0.2 mg/kg[a]
70 kg	5.6 mL	2.8 mL
80 kg	6.4 mL	3.2 mL
90 kg	7.2 mL	3.6 mL
100 kg	8 mL	4 mL
≥ 110 kg	8.8 mL	4.4 mL

[a] Dosage recommended for all patients with renal insufficiency.

IV infusion – For continuous IV infusion, solutions with concentration of 0.2 or 0.4 mg/mL may be used.

Preparation of a lepirudin solution with a concentration of 0.2 or 0.4 mg/mL: Reconstitute 2 vials (each containing 50 mg of lepirudin) with 1 mL each using either sterile water for injection or sodium chloride 0.9% injection.

The final concentrations of 0.2 or 0.4 mg/mL are obtained by transferring the contents of both vials into an infusion bag containing 500 or 250 mL of sodium chloride 0.9% injection or dextrose 5% injection.

The infusion rate (mL/h) is to be set according to body weight.

Standard Lepirudin Infusion Rates According to Body Weight		
	Infusion rate at 0.15 mg/kg/h	
Body weight (kg)	500 mL infusion bag 0.2 mg/mL	250 mL infusion bag 0.4 mg/mL
50 kg	38 mL/h	19 mL/h
60 kg	45 mL/h	23 mL/h
70 kg	53 mL/h	26 mL/h
80 kg	60 mL/h	30 mL/h
90 kg	68 mL/h	34 mL/h
100 kg	75 mL/h	38 mL/h
≥ 110 kg	83 mL/h	41 mL/h

➤*Administration:* Administer as a slow IV bolus dose (eg, over 15 to 20 seconds), followed by continuous IV infusion.

➤*Admixture compatibility:* Lepirudin should not be mixed with other drugs except for sterile water for injection, sodium chloride 0.9% injection, or dextrose 5% injection.

➤*Storage/Stability:* Store unopened vials between 2° and 25°C (36° and 77°F). Once reconstituted, use lepirudin immediately.

Actions

➤*Pharmacology:* The pharmacodynamic effect of lepirudin on the proteolytic activity of thrombin was routinely assessed as an increase in aPTT. This was observed with increasing plasma concentrations of lepirudin, with no saturable effect up to the highest tested dose (0.5 mg/kg body weight IV bolus). Thrombin time (TT) frequently exceeded 200 seconds even at low plasma concentrations of lepirudin, which renders this test unsuitable for routine monitoring of lepirudin therapy.

The pharmacodynamic response defined by the aPTT ratio (aPTT at a time after lepirudin administration over an aPTT reference value, usually median of the laboratory normal range for aPTT) depends on plasma drug levels which in turn depend on the individual patient's renal function. For patients undergoing additional thrombolysis, elevated aPTT ratios were already observed at low lepirudin plasma concentrations, and further response to increasing plasma concentrations was relatively flat. In other populations, the response was steeper. At plasma concentrations of 1500 ng/mL, aPTT ratios were nearly 3 for healthy volunteers, 2.3 for patients with heparin-induced thrombocytopenia, and 2.1 for patients with deep venous thrombosis.

➤*Pharmacokinetics:*

Absorption/Distribution – The pharmacokinetic properties of lepirudin following IV administration are well described by a 2-compartment model. Distribution is essentially confined to extracellular fluids and is characterized by an initial half-life of approximately 10 minutes. Elimination follows a first-order process and is characterized by a terminal half-life of about 1.3 hours in young healthy volunteers. As the IV dose is increased over the range of 0.1 to 0.4 mg/kg, the maximum plasma concentration and the area-under-the-curve increase proportionally.

Metabolism/Excretion – Lepirudin is thought to be metabolized by release of amino acids via catabolic hydrolysis of the parent drug. However, conclusive data are not available. About 48% of the administered dose is excreted in the urine, which consists of unchanged drug (35%) and other fragments of the parent drug.

The systemic clearance of lepirudin is proportional to the glomerular filtration rate or creatinine clearance. Dose adjustment based on creatinine clearance is recommended. In patients with marked renal insufficiency (creatinine clearance below 15 mL/min) and on hemodialysis, elimination half-lives are prolonged up to 2 days.

The systemic clearance of lepirudin in women is about 25% lower than in men. In elderly patients, the systemic clearance of lepirudin is 20% lower than in younger patients. This may be explained by the lower creatinine clearance in elderly patients compared to younger patients.

The table below summarizes systemic clearance (Cl) and volume of distribution at steady state (Vss) of lepirudin for various study populations.

Cl and Vss of Lepirudin		
	Cl (mL/min) mean (% CV[a])	Vss (L) mean (% CV[a])
Healthy young subjects (n = 18, age 18 to 60 years)	164 (19.3%)	12.2 (16.4%)
Healthy elderly subjects (n = 10, age 65 to 80 years)	139 (22.5%)	18.7 (20.6%)
Renally impaired patients (n = 16, creatinine clearance below 80 mL/min)	61 (89.4%)	18 (41.1%)
HIT[b] patients (n = 73)	114 (46.8%)	32.1 (98.9%)

[a] CV is coefficient of variation.
[b] HIT is heparin-induced thrombocytopenia.

Contraindications

Known hypersensitivity to hirudins or to any of the components in lepirudin (rDNA) for injection.

Warnings/Precautions

➤*Hemorrhagic events:* As with other anticoagulants, hemorrhage can occur at any site in patients receiving lepirudin. An unexpected fall in hemoglobin, fall in blood pressure or any unexplained symptom should lead to consideration of a hemorrhagic event. While patients are being anticoagulated with lepirudin, the anticoagulation status should be monitored closely using an appropriate measure such as the aPTT.

Intracranial bleeding following concomitant thrombolytic therapy with rt-PA or streptokinase may be life-threatening. There have been reports of intracranial bleeding with lepirudin in the absence of concomitant thrombolytic therapy.

For patients with increased risk of bleeding, a careful assessment weighing the risk of lepirudin administration vs its anticipated benefit has to be made by the treating physician.

In particular, this includes the following conditions: recent puncture of large vessels or organ biopsy; anomaly of vessels or organs; recent cerebrovascular accident, stroke, intracerebral surgery, or other neuraxial procedures; severe uncontrolled hypertension; bacterial endocarditis; advanced renal impairment (see Renal impairment); hemorrhagic diathesis; recent major surgery; recent major bleeding (eg, intracranial, gastrointestinal, intraocular, or pulmonary bleeding); recent active peptic ulcer.

➤*Antibodies:* Formation of antihirudin antibodies was observed in about 40% of HIT patients treated with lepirudin. This may increase the anticoagulant effect of lepirudin possibly due to delayed renal elimination of active lepirudin-antihirudin complexes. Therefore, strict monitoring of aPTT is necessary also during prolonged therapy. No evidence of neutralization of lepirudin or of allergic reactions associated with positive antibody test results was found.

➤*Reexposure:* During the HAT-1 and HAT-2 studies, a total of 13 patients were reexposed to lepirudin. One of these patients experienced a mild allergic skin reaction during the second treatment cycle. In postmarketing experience, anaphylaxis after reexposure has been reported.

➤*Hypersensitivity reactions:* There have been reports of allergic and hypersensitivity reactions, including anaphylactic reactions. Serious anaphylactic reactions that have resulted in shock or death have been reported. These reactions have been reported during initial administration or upon second or subsequent reexposure(s).

➤*Renal function impairment:* With renal impairment, relative overdose might occur even with standard dosage regimen. Therefore, the bolus dose and the rate of infusion must be reduced in patients with known or suspected renal insufficiency.

➤*Hepatic function impairment:* Serious liver injury (eg, liver cirrhosis) may enhance the anticoagulant effect of lepirudin due to coagulation defects secondary to reduced generation of vitamin K-dependent coagulation factors.

➤*Pregnancy: Category B.* There are no adequate and well-controlled studies in pregnant women. Because animal reproduction studies are not always predictive of human response, this drug should be used during pregnancy only if clearly needed.

Lepirudin (1 mg/kg) by IV administration crosses the placental barrier in pregnant rats. It is not known whether the drug crosses the placental barrier in humans.

Following IV administration of lepirudin at 30 mg/kg/day (180 mg/m^2/day, 1.2 times the recommended maximum human total daily dose based on body surface area) during organogenesis and perinatal-postnatal periods, pregnant rats showed an increased maternal mortality due to undetermined causes.

➤*Lactation:* It is not known whether lepirudin is excreted in human milk. Because many drugs are excreted in human milk and because of the potential for serious adverse reactions in nursing infants from lepirudin, a deci-

LEPIRUDIN — INJECTION

sion should be made whether to discontinue nursing or to discontinue the drug, taking into account the importance of the drug to the mother.

➤*Children:* Safety and effectiveness in pediatric patients have not been established. In the HAT-2 study, two children, an 11-year-old girl and a 12-year-old boy, were treated with lepirudin. Both children presented with TECs at baseline. Lepirudin doses given ranged from 0.15 mg/kg/hr to 0.22 mg/kg/hr for the girl, and from 0.1 mg/kg/hr (in conjunction with urokinase) to 0.7 mg/kg/hr for the boy. Treatment with lepirudin was completed after 8 and 58 days, respectively, without serious adverse events.

➤*Lab test abnormalities:* In general, the dosage (infusion rate) should be adjusted according to the aPTT ratio (patient aPTT at a given time over an aPTT reference value, usually median of the laboratory normal range for aPTT). Other thrombin-dependent coagulation assays are changed by lepirudin.

Drug Interactions

Lepirudin Drug Interactions

Precipitant drug	Object drug[a]		Description
Thrombolytics (eg, alteplase, streptokinase)	Lepirudin	⬆	Concomitant treatment with thrombolytics may increase the risk of bleeding complications and considerably enhance the effect of lepirudin on aPTT prolongation.
Coumarin derivatives (vitamin K antagonists)	Lepirudin	⬆	Concomitant treatment with coumarin derivatives and drugs that affect platelet function may increase the risk of bleeding.

[a] ⬆ = Object drug increased.

Adverse Reactions

➤*Adverse events reported in HIT patients:* The following safety information is based on all 198 patients treated with lepirudin in the HAT-1 and HAT-2 studies. The safety profile of 113 lepirudin patients from these studies who presented with TECs at baseline is compared to 91 such patients in the historical control.

Hematologic –

Hemorrhagic events: Bleeding was the most frequent adverse event observed in patients treated with lepirudin. The following table gives an overview of all hemorrhagic events which occurred in at least 2 patients. Patients may have suffered more than one event.

Overview of Hemorrhagic Events in Lepirudin Studies

Hemorrhagic events	HAT-1 HAT-2 (all patients) (n = 198)	Patients with TECs: Lepirudin (n = 113)	Patients with TECs: Historical control (n = 91)
Bleeding from puncture sites and wounds	14.1%	10.6%	4.4%
Anemia or isolated drop in hemoglobin	13.1%	12.4%	1.1%
Other hematoma and unclassified bleeding	11.1%	10.6%	4.4%
Hematuria	6.6%	4.4%	0%
GI and rectal bleeding	5.1%	5.3%	6.6%
Epistaxis	3%	4.4%	1.1%
Hemothorax	3%	0%	1.1%
Vaginal bleeding	1.5%	1.8%	0%
Intracranial bleeding	0%	0%	2.2%

Other hemorrhagic events (hemoperitoneum, hemoptysis, liver bleeding, lung bleeding, mouth bleeding, retroperitoneal bleeding) each occurred in one individual among all 198 patients treated with lepirudin.

Miscellaneous –

Nonhemorrhagic events: The following table gives an overview of the most frequently observed nonhemorrhagic events. Patients may have suffered more than 1 event.

Overview of the Most Frequently Observed Nonhemorrhagic Events in Lepirudin Studies

Adverse reaction	HAT-1 HAT-2 (all patients) (n = 198)	Patients with TECs: Lepirudin (n = 113)	Patients with TECs: Historical control (n = 91)
Fever	6.1%	4.4%	8.8%
Abnormal liver function	6.1%	5.3%	0%
Pneumonia	4%	4.4%	5.5%
Sepsis	4%	3.5%	5.5%
Allergic skin reactions	3%	3.5%	1.1%
Heart failure	3%	1.8%	2.2%
Abnormal kidney function	2.5%	1.8%	4.4%
Unspecified infections	2.5%	1.8%	1.1%
Multiorgan failure	2%	3.5%	0%
Pericardial effusion	1%	0%	1.1%
Ventricular fibrillation	1%	0%	0%

➤*Adverse events reported in other populations:* The following safety information is based on a total of 2302 individuals who were treated with lepirudin in clinical pharmacology studies (n = 323) or for clinical indications other than HIT (n = 1979).

Intracranial bleeding – Intracranial bleeding was the most serious adverse reaction found in populations other than HIT patients. It occurred in patients with acute myocardial infarction who were started on both lepirudin and thrombolytic therapy with rt-PA or streptokinase. The overall frequency of this potentially life-threatening complication among patients receiving both lepirudin and thrombolytic therapy was 0.6% (7 out of 1134 patients). Although no intracranial bleeding was observed in 1168 subjects or patients who did not receive concomitant thrombolysis, there have been postmarketing reports of intracranial bleeding with lepirudin (rDNA) for injection in the absence of concomitant thrombolytic therapy.

Allergic –

Allergic or Suspected Allergic Reactions in non-HIT Patients Treated with Lepirudin

Airway reactions (cough, bronchospasm, stridor, dyspnea)	common
Unspecified allergic reactions	uncommon
Skin reactions (pruritus, urticaria, rash, flushes, chills)	uncommon
General reactions (anaphylactoid or anaphylactic reactions)	uncommon
Edema (facial edema, tongue edema, larynx edema, angioedema)	rare

The Council for International Organization of Medical Sciences (CIOMS) III standard categories are used for classification frequencies:

CIOMS III Standard Categories

Very common	10% or more
Common (frequent)	1% to < 10%
Uncommon (infrequent)	0.1% to < 1%
Rare	0.01% to < 0.1%
Very rare	0.01% or less

About 53% (n = 46) of all allergic reactions or suspected allergic reactions occurred in patients who concomitantly received thrombolytic therapy (eg, streptokinase) for acute myocardial infarction and/or contrast media for coronary angiography.

➤*Adverse events from postmarketing reports:* Serious anaphylactic reactions that have resulted in shock or death have been reported.

Intracranial bleeding has been reported in patients treated with lepirudin, with or without concomitant thrombolytic therapy. Although no intracranial bleeding was observed in clinical trials in those patients who did not receive concomitant thrombolytic therapy, there have been postmarketing reports of intracranial bleeding in patients who received lepirudin without concomitant thrombolytic therapy.

Overdosage

➤*General toxicity:* Lepirudin caused bleeding in animal toxicity studies.

➤*Symptoms:* In case of overdose (eg, suggested by excessively high aPTT values) the risk of bleeding is increased.

➤*Treatment:* No specific antidote for lepirudin is available. If life-threatening bleeding occurs and excessive plasma levels of lepirudin are suspected, the following steps should be followed:

1.) Immediately STOP lepirudin administration.
2.) Determine aPTT and other coagulation levels as appropriate.
3.) Determine hemoglobin and prepare for blood transfusion.
4.) Follow the current guidelines for treating patients with shock.

Individual clinical case reports and in vitro data suggest that either hemofiltration or hemodialysis (using high-flux dialysis membranes with a cutoff point of 50,000 daltons, eg, AN/69) may be useful in this situation. In studies in pigs, the application of von Willebrand Factor (vWF, 66 IU/kg body weight) markedly reduced the bleeding time. The clinical significance of this data is unknown.

Thrombin Inhibitor

ARGATROBAN

Rx	Argatroban (GlaxoSmithKline)	**Injection, solution, concentrate:** 100 mg/mL	D-sorbitol 750 mg, dehydrated alcohol 1,000 mg. In 2.5 mL single-use vials.

ARGATROBAN — INJECTION

Indications

➤*Heparin-induced thrombocytopenia / heparin-induced thrombosis-thrombocytopenia syndrome:* As an anticoagulant for prophylaxis or treatment of thrombosis in patients with heparin-induced thrombocytopenia (HIT)/heparin-induced thrombosis-thrombocytopenia syndrome (HITTS).

➤*Percutaneous coronary intervention in heparin-induced thrombocytopenia / heparin-induced thrombosis-thrombocytopenia syndrome:* As an anticoagulant in patients with or at risk for HIT undergoing percutaneous coronary intervention (PCI).

Administration and Dosage

➤*Maximum dose:* 10 mcg/kg/min for the treatment of heparin-induced thrombocytopenia/heparin-induced thrombosis-thrombocytopenia syndrome according to the prescribing information. There is no well-established maximum dose for the other approved indication according to the prescribing information.

➤*Adults:*

Heparin-induced thrombocytopenia / heparin-induced thrombosis-thrombocytopenia syndrome – Before administering argatroban, discontinue heparin therapy and obtain a baseline activated partial thromboplastin time (aPTT).

In general, therapy with argatroban is monitored using the aPTT. Tests of anticoagulant effects (including the aPTT) typically attain steady-state levels within 1 to 3 hours following initiation of argatroban. Dose adjustment may be required to attain the target aPTT.

Maximum dose: Not to exceed 10 mcg/kg/min.

Initial dosage: See the following table.

2 mcg/kg/min, administered as a continuous infusion. Check the aPTT during HIT or HITTS therapy 2 hours after initiation of therapy to confirm that the aPTT is within the desired therapeutic range.

Dosage adjustment: After the initial dose of argatroban, the dose can be adjusted as clinically indicated (not to exceed 10 mcg/kg/min), until the steady-state aPTT is 1.5 to 3 times the initial baseline value (not to exceed 100 seconds).

Argatroban Doses and Infusion Rates for 2 mcg/kg/min for Patients With HIT/HITTS (1 mg/mL Final Concentration)[a]

Body weight (kg)	Dose (mcg/min)	Infusion rate (mL/h)
50	100	6
60	120	7
70	140	8
80	160	10
90	180	11
100	200	12
110	220	13
120	240	14
130	260	16
140	280	17

[a] HIT/HITTS = heparin-induced thrombocytopenia/heparin-induced thrombosis-thrombocytopenia syndrome.

Percutaneous coronary intervention in heparin-induced thrombocytopenia / heparin-induced thrombosis-thrombocytopenia syndrome – Therapy with argatroban is monitored using activated clotting time (ACT). ACTs should be obtained before dosing, 5 to 10 minutes after bolus dosing and after change in the infusion rate, and at the end of the PCI procedure. Additional ACTs should be drawn approximately every 20 to 30 minutes during a prolonged procedure.

Initial dosage: See the following table.

An infusion of argatroban should be started at 25 mcg/kg/min, and a bolus of 350 mcg/kg administered via a large bore intravenous (IV) line over 3 to 5 minutes. Check ACT 5 to 10 minutes after the bolus dose is completed. The procedure may proceed if the ACT is more than 300 seconds.

Dosage adjustment: See the following table.

If the ACT is less than 300 seconds, administer an additional IV bolus dose of 150 mcg/kg, increase the infusion dose to 30 mcg/kg/min, and check the ACT 5 to 10 minutes later.

If the ACT is more than 450 seconds, decrease the infusion rate to 15 mcg/kg/min, and check the ACT 5 to 10 minutes later. Once a therapeutic ACT (between 300 and 450 seconds) has been achieved, continue this infusion dose for the duration of the procedure.

Recommended Doses and Infusion Rates of Argatroban for Patients Undergoing Percutaneous Coronary Intervention (1 mg/mL Final Concentration)[a]

	For ACT 300 to 450 seconds initial dosage[b] 25 mcg/kg/min			If ACT < 300 seconds dosage adjustment[c] 30 mcg/kg/min			If ACT > 450 seconds dosage adjustment 15 mcg/kg/min	
Body weight (kg)	Bolus dose (mcg)	Infusion dose (mcg/min)	Infusion rate (mL/h)	Bolus dose (mcg)	Infusion dose (mcg/min)	Infusion rate (mL/h)	Infusion dose (mcg/min)	Infusion rate (mL/h)
50	17,500	1,250	75	7,500	1,500	90	750	45
60	21,000	1,500	90	9,000	1,800	108	900	54
70	24,500	1,750	105	10,500	2,100	126	1,050	63
80	28,000	2,000	120	12,000	2,400	144	1,200	72
90	31,500	2,250	135	13,500	2,700	162	1,350	81
100	35,000	2,500	150	15,000	3,000	180	1,500	90
110	38,500	2,750	165	16,500	3,300	198	1,650	99
120	42,000	3,000	180	18,000	3,600	216	1,800	108
130	45,500	3,250	195	19,500	3,900	234	1,950	117
140	49,000	3,500	210	21,000	4,200	252	2,100	126

[a] Note: 1 mg = 1,000 mcg; 1 kg = 2.2 lbs.
[b] Initial IV bolus dose of 350 mcg/kg should be administered.
[c] Additional IV bolus dose of 150 mcg/kg should be administered if ACT < 300 seconds.

In case of dissection, impending abrupt closure, thrombus formation during the procedure, or inability to achieve or maintain an ACT over 300 seconds, additional bolus doses of 150 mcg/kg may be administered and the infusion dose increased to 40 mcg/kg/min. Check the ACT after each additional bolus or change in the rate of infusion.

Continued anticoagulation after percutaneous coronary intervention: If a patient requires anticoagulation after the procedure, argatroban may be continued but at a lower infusion dose (see previous HIT/HITTS section).

➤*Children:* Initial argatroban infusion doses are lower for seriously ill children compared with adults with healthy hepatic function.

➤*Hepatic function impairment:*

Heparin-induced thrombocytopenia / heparin-induced thrombosis-thrombocytopenia syndrome – For adult patients with HIT and hepatic function impairment, reduce the initial dose of argatroban. For adult patients with moderate hepatic function impairment, an initial dose of 0.5 mcg/kg/min is recommended, based on the approximate 4-fold decrease in argatroban clearance relative to those with healthy hepatic function. Closely monitor the aPTT and adjust the dosage as clinically indicated.

Heparin-induced thrombocytopenia / heparin-induced thrombosis-thrombocytopenia syndrome patients undergoing percutaneous coronary intervention – Carefully titrate argatroban until the desired level of anticoagulation is achieved.

➤*Conversion to oral anticoagulant therapy:*

Initiating oral anticoagulant therapy – Once the decision is made to initiate oral anticoagulant therapy, recognize the potential for combined effects on international normalized ratio (INR) with coadministration of argatroban and warfarin. A loading dose of warfarin should not be used. Initiate therapy using the expected daily dose of warfarin. To avoid prothrombotic effects and ensure continuous anticoagulation when initiating warfarin, it is suggested that argatroban and warfarin therapy be overlapped. There are insufficient data available to recommend the duration of the overlap.

Coadministration of warfarin and argatroban at doses of up to 2 mcg / kg / min – Use of argatroban with warfarin results in prolongation of INR beyond that produced by warfarin alone. To avoid prothrombotic effects and ensure continuous anticoagulation when initiating warfarin, it is suggested that warfarin be coadministered before discontinuing argatroban. There are insufficient data available to recommend the duration of the coadministration. The previously established relationship between INR and bleeding risk is altered. The combination of argatroban and warfarin does not cause further reduction in the vitamin K–dependent factor Xa activity than that seen with warfarin alone. The relationship between INR obtained on combined therapy and INR obtained on warfarin alone is dependent on the dose of argatroban and the thromboplastin reagent used. The INR value on warfarin alone (INR_W) can be calculated from the INR value on combination argatroban and warfarin therapy.

The INR should be measured daily while argatroban and warfarin are coadministered. In general, with doses of argatroban of up to 2 mcg/kg/min, argatroban can be discontinued when the INR is greater than 4 on combined therapy. After argatroban is discontinued, repeat the INR measurement in 4 to 6 hours. If the repeat INR is below the desired therapeutic range, resume the infusion of argatroban and repeat the procedure daily until the desired therapeutic range on warfarin alone is reached.

ARGATROBAN — INJECTION

Coadministration of warfarin and argatroban at doses of greater than 2 mcg/kg/min – For doses of greater than 2 mcg/kg/min, the relationship of INR between warfarin alone to the INR on warfarin plus argatroban is less predictable. In this case, in order to predict the INR on warfarin alone, temporarily reduce the dose of argatroban to a dose of 2 mcg/kg/min. Repeat the INR on argatroban and warfarin 4 to 6 hours after reduction of the argatroban dose and follow the process previously outlined for administering argatroban at doses of up to 2 mcg/kg/min.

➤*Preparation for administration:* Each 2.5 mL vial contains argatroban 250 mg and, as supplied, is a concentrated drug (100 mg/mL) that must be diluted 100-fold prior to infusion. Argatroban should be diluted in sodium chloride 0.9% injection, dextrose 5% injection, or Ringer's lactate injection, to a final concentration of 1 mg/mL. The contents of each 2.5 mL vial should be diluted 100-fold by mixing with 250 mL of diluent. Use 250 mg (2.5 mL) per 250 mL of diluent or 500 mg (5 mL) per 500 mL of diluent. The reconstituted solution must be mixed by repeated inversion of the diluent bag for 1 minute. Upon preparation, the solution may show slight but brief haziness because of the formation of microprecipitates that rapidly dissolve upon mixing. The pH of the IV solution prepared as recommended is 3.2 to 7.5.

Argatroban is a clear, colorless to pale yellow, slightly viscous solution. If the solution is cloudy or if an insoluble precipitate is noted, the vial should be discarded.

➤*Administration:* Administer IV.

➤*Admixture compatibility:* Argatroban should not be mixed with other drugs prior to dilution in a suitable IV fluid.

No significant potency losses have been noted following simulated delivery of the solution through IV tubing.

➤*Storage/Stability:* Store the vials in original cartons at room temperature, 25°C (77°F); excursions are permitted to 15° to 30°C (59° to 86°F). Do not freeze. Retain in the original carton to protect from light.

Solutions prepared as recommended are stable at 25°C (77°F), with excursions permitted to 15° to 30°C (59° to 86°F) in ambient indoor light for 24 hours; therefore, light-resistant measures, such as foil protection for IV lines, are unnecessary. Solutions are physically and chemically stable for up to 96 hours when protected from light and stored at controlled room temperature, 20° to 25°C (68° to 77°F), or in refrigerated conditions, 5° ± 3°C (41° ± 5°F). Do not expose prepared solutions to direct sunlight.

Actions

➤*Pharmacology:* Argatroban is a direct thrombin inhibitor that reversibly binds to the thrombin active site. Argatroban does not require the cofactor antithrombin III for antithrombotic activity. Argatroban exerts its anticoagulant effects by inhibiting thrombin-catalyzed or thrombin-induced reactions, including fibrin formation; activation of coagulation factors V, VIII, and XIII; activation of protein C; and platelet aggregation.

Argatroban is highly selective for thrombin, with an inhibitory constant (K_1) of 0.04 mcM. At therapeutic concentrations, argatroban has little or no effect on related serine proteases (trypsin, factor Xa, plasmin, and kallikrein).

Argatroban is capable of inhibiting the action of both free and clot-associated thrombin.

Argatroban does not interact with heparin-induced antibodies. Evaluation of sera from 12 healthy subjects and 8 patients who received multiple doses of argatroban did not reveal antibody formation to argatroban.

Because argatroban is a direct thrombin inhibitor, coadministration of argatroban and warfarin produces a combined effect on the laboratory measurement of the INR. However, compared with warfarin monotherapy, concurrent therapy exerts no additional effect on vitamin K–dependent factor Xa activity.

The relationship between INR on co-therapy and warfarin alone is dependent on the dose of argatroban and the thromboplastin reagent used. This relationship is influenced by the international sensitivity index (ISI) of the thromboplastin. Thromboplastins with higher ISI values result in higher INRs on combined therapy of warfarin and argatroban. These data are based on results obtained in healthy individuals.

Pharmacodynamics – When argatroban is administered by continuous infusion, anticoagulant effects and plasma concentrations of argatroban follow similar predictable temporal response profiles, with low intersubject variability. Immediately upon initiation of argatroban infusion, anticoagulant effects are produced as plasma argatroban concentrations begin to rise. Steady-state levels of both drug and anticoagulant effect are typically attained within 1 to 3 hours and are maintained until the infusion is discontinued or the dosage adjusted. Steady-state plasma argatroban concentrations increase proportionally with dose (for infusion doses of up to 40 mcg/kg/min in healthy subjects) and are well correlated with steady-state anticoagulant effects. For infusion doses of up to 40 mcg/kg/min, argatroban increases (in a dose-dependent fashion) the aPTT, the ACT, the prothrombin time (PT), the INR, and the thrombin time (TT) in healthy volunteers and cardiac patients..

➤*Pharmacokinetics:*

Distribution – Argatroban distributes mainly in the extracellular fluid, as evidenced by an apparent steady-state volume of distribution of 174 mL/kg (12.18 L in an adult weighing 70 kg). Argatroban is 54% bound to human serum proteins, with binding to albumin and alpha-1 acid glycoprotein at 20% and 34%, respectively.

Metabolism – The main route of argatroban metabolism is hydroxylation and aromatization of the 3-methyltetrahydroquinoline ring in the liver. The formation of each of the 4 known metabolites is catalyzed in vitro by the human liver microsomal CYP-450 enzymes CYP3A4/5. The primary metabolite (M1) exerts 3- to 5-fold weaker anticoagulant effects than argatroban. Unchanged argatroban is the major component in plasma. The plasma concentrations of M1 range between 0% and 20% of that of the parent drug. The other metabolites (M2 to M4) are only in very low quantities in the urine and have not been detected in plasma or feces. These data, together with the lack of effect of erythromycin (a potent CYP3A4/5 inhibitor), on argatroban pharmacokinetics suggest that CYP3A4/5-mediated metabolism is not an important elimination pathway in vivo.

There is no interconversion of the 21-(R):21-(S) diastereoisomers. The plasma ratio of these diastereoisomers is unchanged by metabolism or hepatic function impairment, remaining constant at 65:35 (± 2%).

Excretion – Total body clearance is approximately 5.1 mL/kg/min (0.31 L/kg/h) for infusion doses of up to 40 mcg/kg/min. The terminal elimination half-life of argatroban ranges between 39 and 51 minutes.

Argatroban is excreted primarily in the feces, presumably through biliary secretion. In a study in which ^{14}C-argatroban (5 mcg/kg/min) was infused for 4 hours into healthy subjects, approximately 65% of the radioactivity was recovered in the feces within 6 days of the start of infusion, with little or no radioactivity subsequently detected. Approximately 22% of the radioactivity appeared in the urine within 12 hours of the start of infusion. Little or no additional urinary radioactivity was subsequently detected. Average percent recovery of unchanged drug, relative to total dose, was 16% in urine and at least 14% in feces.

Special populations –

Hepatic function impairment: Decrease the dosage of argatroban in patients with hepatic function impairment. Patients with hepatic function impairment were not studied in PCI trials. At a dose of 2.5 mcg/kg/min, hepatic function impairment is associated with decreased clearance and increased elimination half-life of argatroban (to 1.9 mL/kg/min and 181 minutes, respectively, for patients with a Child-Pugh score higher than 6).

Children: Argatroban clearance is decreased in seriously ill children. Pharmacokinetic parameters of argatroban were characterized in a population pharmacokinetic/pharmacodynamic analysis with sparse data from 15 seriously ill children. Clearance in children (0.16 L/h/kg) was 50% lower compared with healthy adults (0.31 L/h/kg). Four children with elevated bilirubin (secondary to cardiac complications or hepatic function impairment) had, on average, 80% lower clearance (0.03 L/h/kg) when compared with children with normal bilirubin levels.

Contraindications

Overt major bleeding; hypersensitivity to this product or any of its components.

Warnings/Precautions

➤*Route of administration:* Argatroban is intended for IV administration. Discontinue all parenteral anticoagulants before administration of argatroban.

➤*Hemorrhage:* Hemorrhage can occur at any site in the body in patients receiving argatroban. If the patient has an unexplained fall in hematocrit, fall in blood pressure, or any other unexplained symptom, consider occurrence of a hemorrhagic event. Use argatroban with extreme caution in disease states and other circumstances in which there is an increased danger of hemorrhage. These include the following: severe hypertension; immediately following lumbar puncture; spinal anesthesia; major surgery, especially involving the brain, spinal cord, or eye; hematologic conditions associated with increased bleeding tendencies (eg, congenital or acquired bleeding disorders) and GI lesions (eg, ulcerations).

➤*Hepatic function impairment:* Exercise caution when administering argatroban to patients with hepatic function impairment; start with a lower dose and carefully titrate until the desired level of anticoagulation is achieved. Achievement of steady-state aPTT levels may take longer and require more argatroban dose adjustments in patients with hepatic function impairment compared with patients with healthy hepatic function. Also, upon cessation of argatroban infusion in patients with hepatic function impairment, full reversal of anticoagulant effects may require longer than 4 hours because of decreased clearance and increased elimination half-life of argatroban. Avoid use of high doses of argatroban in PCI patients with clinically significant hepatic disease or AST/ALT levels of 3 or more times the upper limit of normal. Such patients were not studied in PCI trials.

➤*Pregnancy: Category B.* There are no adequate and well-controlled studies in pregnant women. Because animal reproduction studies are not always predictive of human response, use this drug during pregnancy only if clearly needed.

It is not known if argatroban crosses the human placenta. Expect exposure of the embryo/fetus because of the low molecular weight (about 527 for the hydrated form).

➤*Lactation:* Experiments in rats show that argatroban is detected in milk. It is not known whether this drug is excreted in human milk. The molecular weight (about 527 for the hydrated form), low metabolism, and moderate serum protein binding suggest that the drug will be excreted into breast milk, especially as it is given as a continuous infusion. Because many drugs are excreted in human milk and because of the potential for serious adverse reactions in breast-feeding infants from argatroban, decide whether to discontinue breast-feeding or the drug, taking into account the importance of the drug to the mother.

Argatroban is expected to be excreted into human breast milk. The effects of this exposure on a breast-feeding infant are unknown, but oral absorption is probably poor.

ARGATROBAN — INJECTION

➤*Children:* The safety and effectiveness of argatroban, including the appropriate anticoagulation goals and duration of therapy, have not been established among children.

Argatroban was studied among 18 seriously ill children who required an alternative to heparin anticoagulation. Most patients were diagnosed with HIT or suspected HIT. Age ranges of patients were younger than 6 months of age (n = 8), 6 months to younger than 8 years of age (n = 6), and 8 to 16 years of age (n = 4). All patients had serious underlying conditions and were receiving multiple concomitant medications. Thirteen patients received argatroban solely as a continuous infusion (no bolus dose). Dosing was initiated in the majority of these 13 patients at 1 mcg/kg/min. Dosing was titrated as needed to achieve and maintain an aPTT of 1.5 to 3 times the baseline value. Most patients required multiple dose adjustments to maintain anticoagulation parameters within the desired range. During the 30-day study period, thrombotic events occurred during argatroban administration to 2 patients and following argatroban discontinuation in 3 other patients. Major bleeding occurred among 2 patients; 1 patient experienced an intracranial hemorrhage after 4 days of argatroban therapy in the setting of sepsis and thrombocytopenia. Another patient completed 14 days of argatroban treatment in the study but experienced an intracranial hemorrhage while receiving argatroban following completion of the study treatment period.

When argatroban is used among seriously ill children with HIT/HITTS who require an alternative to heparin and who have healthy hepatic function, initiate a continuous infusion of argatroban at a dose of 0.75 mcg/kg/min. Initiate the infusion at a dose of 0.2 mcg/kg/min among seriously ill children with hepatic function impairment. Check the aPTT 2 hours after the initiation of the argatroban infusion and adjust the dose to achieve the target aPTT. These dose recommendations are based upon a goal of aPTT prolongation of 1.5 to 3 times the baseline value and avoidance of an aPTT longer than 100 seconds. Increments of 0.1 to 0.25 mcg/kg/min for children with healthy hepatic function and increments of 0.05 mcg/kg/min or lower for children with hepatic function impairment may be considered by dose selection must take into account multiple factors, including the current argatroban dose, the current aPTT, target aPTT, and the clinical status of the patient. These dose recommendations are based upon a goal of aPTT prolongation of 1.5 to 3 times the baseline value and avoidance of an aPTT longer than 100 seconds.

➤*Elderly:* In the clinical studies of adult patients with HIT or HITTS, the effectiveness of argatroban was not affected by age.

➤*Monitoring:* Anticoagulation effects associated with argatroban infusion at doses of up to 40 mcg/kg/min correlated with increases of the aPTT.

In clinical trials in PCI, the ACT was used for monitoring argatroban activity during the procedure. Obtain ACTs before dosing, 5 to 10 minutes after bolus dosing, after change in infusion rate, and at the end of the PCI procedure. Draw additional ACTs approximately every 20 to 30 minutes during a prolonged procedure.

In general, therapy with argatroban is monitored using the aPTT. Tests of anticoagulant effects (including the aPTT) typically attain steady-state levels within 1 to 3 hours following initiation of argatroban. Dose adjustment may be required to attain the target aPTT. Check the aPTT during HIT or HITTS therapy 2 hours after initiation of therapy to confirm that the aPTT is within the desired therapeutic range.

Alternative approaches for monitoring concurrent argatroban and warfarin therapy are described in the following information. Measure INR daily while argatroban and warfarin are coadministered. In general, with doses of argatroban of up to 2 mcg/kg/min, argatroban can be discontinued when the INR is more than 4 on combined therapy. After argatroban is discontinued, repeat the INR measurement in 4 to 6 hours. If the repeat INR is lesser than the desired therapeutic range, resume the infusion of argatroban and repeat the procedure daily until the desired therapeutic range on warfarin alone is reached. The relationship between INR obtained on combined therapy and INR obtained on warfarin alone is dependent on the dose of argatroban and the thromboplastin reagent used.

For doses of more than 2 mcg/kg/min, the relationship of INR on warfarin alone to the INR on warfarin plus argatroban is less predictable. In this case, in order to predict the INR on warfarin alone, temporarily reduce the dose of argatroban to a dose of 2 mcg/kg/min. Repeat the INR on argatroban and warfarin 4 to 6 hours after reduction of the argatroban dose and follow the process previously outlined for administering argatroban at doses of up to 2 mcg/kg/min.

Drug Interactions

Argatroban Drug Interactions

Precipitant drug	Object drug[a]		Description
Anticoagulants (eg, heparin, warfarin)	Argatroban	⬆	Concomitant use of argatroban and warfarin results in prolongation of the PT and INR. The use of heparin is contraindicated in patients with HIT.
Antiplatelet agents (eg, clopidogrel, NSAIDs, salicylates)	Argatroban	⬆	Concomitant treatment with antiplatelet agents may increase the risk of bleeding.
Glycoprotein IIb/IIIa antagonists (epifibatide, tirofiban)	Argatroban	⬌	The safety and effectiveness of argatroban with glycoprotein IIb/IIIa antagonists have not been established.
Argatroban	Glycoprotein IIb/IIIa antagonists (epifibatide, tirofiban)		
Thrombolytics (eg, alteplase, streptokinase)	Argatroban	⬆	Concomitant treatment with thrombolytics may increase the risk of bleeding.

[a] ⬆ = object drug increased; ⬌ = undetermined clinical effect.

Adverse Reactions

➤*Heparin-induced thrombocytopenia/heparin-induced thrombosis-thrombocytopenia syndrome:*

Hemorrhagic adverse reactions – Major bleeding was defined as bleeding that was overt and associated with a hemoglobin decrease of 2 g/dL or more, that led to a transfusion of 2 or more units, or that was intracranial, retroperitoneal, or into a major prosthetic joint. Minor bleeding was overt bleeding that did not meet the criteria for major bleeding.

The following table gives an overview of the most frequently observed hemorrhagic reactions, presented separately by major and minor bleeding, sorted by decreasing occurrence among argatroban-treated HIT/HITTS patients.

Argatroban Hemorrhagic Adverse Reactions in HIT/HITTS Patients[a]

Hemorrhagic adverse reaction	Argatroban-treated patients (n = 568)	Historical control (n = 193)
Major hemorrhagic reactions[b]		
Overall bleeding	5.3%	6.7%
GI	2.3%	1.6%
GU and hematuria	0.9%	0.5%
Decreased hemoglobin/hematocrit	0.7%	0%
Multisystem hemorrhage and disseminated intravascular coagulation	0.5%	1%
Limb and below-the-knee amputation stump	0.5%	0%
Intracranial hemorrhage	0%[c]	0.5%
Minor hemorrhagic reactions[b]		
GI	14.4%	18.1%
GU and hematuria	11.6%	0.8%
Decreased hemoglobin/hematocrit	10.4%	0%
Groin	5.4%	3.1%
Hemoptysis	2.9%	0.8%
Brachial	2.4%	0.8%

[a] HIT/HITTS = Heparin-induced thrombocytopenia/heparin-induced thrombosis-thrombocytopenia syndrome.
[b] Patients may have experienced more than 1 adverse reaction.
[c] One patient experienced intracranial hemorrhage 4 days after discontinuation of argatroban and following therapy with urokinase and oral anticoagulation.

Nonhemorrhagic adverse reactions (2% or more) – The following table gives an overview of the most frequently observed nonhemorrhagic reactions (2% or more) among argatroban-treated patients.

Argatroban Nonhemorrhagic Adverse Reactions in HIT/HITTS Patients (≥ 2%)[a,b]

Adverse reaction	Argatroban-treated patients (n = 568)	Historical control (n = 193)
Cardiovascular		
Atrial fibrillation	3%	11.4%
Cardiac arrest	5.8%	3.1%
Cerebrovascular disorder	2.3%	4.1%
Hypotension	7.2%	2.6%
Ventricular tachycardia	4.8%	3.1%
GI		
Abdominal pain	2.6%	1.6%
Diarrhea	6.2%	1.6%
Nausea	4.8%	0.5%
Vomiting	4.2%	0%

ARGATROBAN — INJECTION

Argatroban Nonhemorrhagic Adverse Reactions in HIT/HITTS Patients (≥ 2%)[a,b]		
Adverse reaction	Argatroban-treated patients (n = 568)	Historical control (n = 193)
GU		
Abnormal renal function	2.8%	4.7%
Urinary tract infection	4.6%	5.2%
Respiratory		
Coughing	2.8%	1.6%
Dyspnea	8.1%	8.8%
Pneumonia	3.3%	9.3%
Miscellaneous		
Fever	6.9%	2.1%
Infection	3.7%	3.6%
Pain	4.6%	3.1%
Sepsis	6%	12.4%

[a] HIT/HITTS = Heparin-induced thrombocytopenia/heparin-induced thrombosis-thrombocytopenia syndrome.
[b] Patients may have experienced more than 1 adverse reaction.

➤*Heparin-induced thrombocytopenia/heparin-induced thrombosis-thrombocytopenia syndrome patients undergoing percutaneous coronary intervention:*

Hemorrhagic adverse reactions – Major bleeding was defined as bleeding that was overt and associated with a hemoglobin decrease of 5 g/dL or more, that led to a transfusion of 2 or more units, or that was intracranial, retroperitoneal, or into a major prosthetic joint.

The rate of major bleeding reactions and intracranial hemorrhage in the PCI trials was 1.8% and in the placebo arm of the Evaluation in PTCA to Improve Long-Term Outcome with Abciximab GP IIb/IIIa Blockade Study (EPILOG) trial (placebo plus standard dose, weight-adjusted heparin) was 3.1%.

Argatroban Hemorrhagic Adverse Reactions in HIT/HITTS Patients Undergoing PCI[a]	
Hemorrhagic adverse reaction	Argatroban-treated patients (n = 112)[b]
Major hemorrhagic reactions[c]	
Retroperitoneal	0.9%
GI	0.9%
Intracranial	0%
Minor hemorrhagic reactions[c]	
Groin (bleeding or hematoma)	3.6%
GI (includes hematemesis)	2.6%
GU (includes hematuria)	1.8%
Decrease in hemoglobin and/or hematocrit	1.8%
CABG[d] (coronary arteries)	1.8%
Access site	0.9%
Hemoptysis	0.9%
Other	0.9%

[a] HIT/HITTS = heparin-induced thrombocytopenia/heparin-induced thrombosis-thrombocytopenia syndrome; PCI = percutaneous coronary intervention.
[b] 91 patients who underwent 112 interventions.
[c] Patients may have experienced more than 1 adverse reaction.
[d] CABG = coronary artery bypass graft.

Nonhemorrhagic adverse reactions (more than 2%) – The following table gives an overview of the most frequently observed nonhemorrhagic reactions (more than 2%), sorted by decreasing frequency of occurrence among argatroban-treated PCI patients.

Argatroban Nonhemorrhagic Adverse Reactions in HIT/HITTS Patients Undergoing PCI (≥ 2%)[a,b]		
Adverse reaction	Argatroban procedures[b] (n = 112)[c]	Controls (n = 2,226)[d]
Cardiovascular		
Bradycardia	4.5%	3.5%
Hypotension	10.7%	10.3%
Myocardial infarction	3.6%	NR[e]
GI		
Abdominal pain	3.6%	2.2%
Nausea	7.1%	11.5%
Vomiting	6.3%	6.8%
Miscellaneous		
Back pain	8%	13.7%
Chest pain	15.2%	9.3%
Fever	3.6%	< 0.5%
Headache	5.4%	5.5%

[a] HIT/HITTS = heparin-induced thrombocytopenia/heparin-induced thrombosis-thrombocytopenia syndrome; PCI = percutaneous coronary intervention.
[b] Patients may have experienced more than 1 adverse reaction.
[c] 91 patients who underwent 112 interventions.
[d] Controls from Evaluation of c7E3 fragment antigen binding in the Prevention of Ischemic Complications, EPILOG, and Chimeric 7E3 Antiplatelet Therapy in Unstable angina Refractory to standard treatment trials.
[e] NR = not reported.

Serious adverse reactions – There were 22 serious adverse reactions in 17 PCI patients (19.6% in 112 interventions). The types of reactions, which are listed regardless of relationship to treatment, are shown in the following table. The table lists the serious adverse reactions occurring in argatroban-treated HIT/HITTS patients undergoing PCI.

Argatroban Serious Adverse Reactions in HIT/HITTS Patients Undergoing PCI[a,b]	
Serious adverse reaction	Argatroban procedures[c] (n = 112)
Cardiovascular	
Angina pectoris	1.8%
Aortic stenosis	0.9%
Arterial thrombosis	0.9%
Cerebrovascular disorder	0.9%
Coronary occlusion	1.8%
Coronary thrombosis	1.8%
Myocardial infarction	3.5%
Myocardial ischemia	1.8%
Vascular disorder	0.9%
GI	
GI disorder (gastroesophageal reflux disease)	0.9%
GI hemorrhage	0.9%
Respiratory	
Lung edema	0.9%
Miscellaneous	
Chest pain	0.9%
Fever	0.9%
Retroperitoneal hemorrhage	0.9%

[a] HIT/HITTS = heparin-induced thrombocytopenia/heparin-induced thrombosis-thrombocytopenia syndrome; PCI = percutaneous coronary intervention.
[b] Individual reactions may also have been reported elsewhere (see previous tables).
[c] 91 patients underwent 112 procedures. Some patients may have experienced more than 1 reaction.

➤*Adverse reactions reported in other populations:*

Allergic – One hundred fifty-six allergic reactions or suspected allergic reactions were observed in 1,127 individuals treated with argatroban in clinical pharmacology studies or for various clinical indications. About 95% (148/156) of these reactions occurred in patients who concomitantly received thrombolytic therapy (eg, streptokinase) for acute myocardial infarction and/or contrast media for coronary angiography.

Allergic reactions or suspected allergic reactions in populations other than HIT/HITTS patients include (in descending order of frequency [The Council for International Organization of Medical Sciences III standard categories are used for classification of frequencies.]):

- airway reactions (coughing, dyspnea): 10% or more;
- skin reactions (rash, bullous eruption): 1% to less than 10%;
- general reactions (vasodilation): 1% to 10%.

Intracranial bleeding – The overall frequency of intracranial bleeding among patients with acute myocardial infarction receiving argatroban and thrombolytic therapy (streptokinase or tissue plasminogen activator) was 1% (8/810 patients). Intracranial bleeding was not observed in 317 subjects or patients who did not receive concomitant thrombolysis.

ARGATROBAN — INJECTION

Intracranial bleeding was also observed in a prospective, placebo-controlled study of argatroban in patients who had onset of acute stroke within 12 hours of study entry. Symptomatic intracranial hemorrhage was reported in 5 of 117 (4.3%) patients who received argatroban at 1 to 3 mcg/kg/min and in none of the 54 patients who received placebo. Asymptomatic intracranial hemorrhage occurred in 5 (4.3%) and 2 (3.7%) of the patients, respectively.

Overdosage

➤*Animal toxicology:* Single IV doses of argatroban at 200, 124, 150, and 200 mg/kg were lethal to mice, rats, rabbits, and dogs, respectively.

The symptoms of acute toxicity in mice were clonic convulsions, coma, loss of righting reflex, paralysis of hind limbs, and tremors.

➤*Symptoms:* Excessive anticoagulation, with or without bleeding, may be controlled by discontinuing argatroban or by decreasing the argatroban infusion dosage. In clinical studies at therapeutic levels, anticoagulation parameters generally return to baseline within 2 to 4 hours after discontinuation of the drug. Reversal of anticoagulant effect may take longer in patients with hepatic function impairment.

➤*Treatment:* No specific antidote to argatroban is available. If life-threatening bleeding occurs and excessive plasma levels of argatroban are suspected, discontinue argatroban immediately and determine aPTT and other coagulation tests. Provide symptomatic and supportive therapy to the patient. When argatroban was administered as a continuous infusion (2 mcg/kg/min) prior to and during a 4-hour hemodialysis session, approximately 20% of argatroban was cleared through dialysis.

Patient Information

Inform patients that this medicine may cause dizziness. They should not drive, operate machinery, or do anything else that could be dangerous until they know how they react to this medicine.

Advise patients that this medicine may reduce the number of clot-forming cells (platelets) in their blood. To prevent bleeding, advise patients to avoid situations in which bruising or injury may occur. Tell patients to report any unusual bleeding, bruising, blood in stools, or dark, tarry stools to their health care provider.

Tell patients to check with their health care provider if any of these most common adverse reactions persist or become bothersome: diarrhea, injection-site reactions (eg, minor bleeding, redness, discomfort), nausea, pain, or vomiting.

Tell patients to notify their health care provider right away if any of the following severe adverse reactions occur: severe allergic reactions (difficulty breathing; hives; rash; swelling of the mouth, face, lips, or tongue; tightness in the chest); chest pain; coffee-ground vomit; confusion; dizziness; fast, slow, or irregular heartbeat; fever; one-sided weakness; pain (especially in the pelvis or legs); pink- or red-colored urine; slurred speech; swelling; trouble breathing; vision problems; or vomiting of blood.

BIVALIRUDIN

Rx	**Angiomax** (Medicines Company)	**Powder for injection, lyophilized:** 250 mg	In single-use vials.

BIVALIRUDIN — INJECTION

Indications

➤*Concomitant aspirin therapy:* Bivalirudin is intended for use with aspirin and has been studied only in patients receiving concomitant aspirin.

The safety and efficacy of bivalirudin have not been established in patients with acute coronary syndromes who are not undergoing percutaneous transluminal coronary angioplasty (PTCA) or percutaneous coronary intervention (PCI).

➤*PCI:* Bivalirudin with provisional use of glycoprotein IIb/IIIa inhibitor (GPIIb/IIIa inhibitor) is indicated for use as an anticoagulant in patients undergoing PCI.

➤*PTCA:* Bivalirudin is indicated for use as an anticoagulant in patients with unstable angina undergoing PTCA.

➤*Heparin-induced thrombocytopenia / heparin-induced thrombocytopenia and thrombosis syndrome (HIT / HITTS):* Bivalirudin is indicated for patients with, or at risk of, HIT/HITTS undergoing PCI.

Administration and Dosage

➤*Dosage:* The recommended dosage of bivalirudin is an intravenous (IV) bolus dose of 0.75 mg/kg. This should be followed by an infusion of 1.75 mg/kg/h for the duration of the PCI procedure. Five minutes after the bolus dose has been administered, an activated clotting time (ACT) should be performed and an additional bolus of 0.3 mg/kg should be given if needed.

GPIIb/IIIa inhibitor administration should be considered in the event that any of the following conditions are present: decreased thrombosis in myocardial infarction (TIMI) flow (0 to 2) or slow reflow; dissection with decreased flow; new or suspected thrombus; persistent residual stenosis; distal embolization; unplanned stent; suboptimal stenting; side branch closure; abrupt closure; clinical instability; prolonged ischemia.

HIT / HITTS – The recommended dose of bivalirudin in patients with HIT/HITTS undergoing PCI is an IV bolus dose of 0.75 mg/kg. This should be followed by a continuous infusion at a rate of 1.75 mg/kg/h for the duration of the procedure.

Continuation of the infusion following PCI for up to 4 hours postprocedure is optional, at the discretion of the treating health care provider. After 4 hours, an additional IV infusion of bivalirudin may be initiated at a rate of 0.2 mg/kg/h for up to 20 hours, if needed. Bivalirudin is intended for use with aspirin (300 to 325 mg daily) and has been studied only in patients receiving concomitant aspirin.

The dose to be administered is adjusted according to the patient's weight (see the following table).

Bivalirudin Dosing

Weight (kg)	5 mg/mL concentration: Bolus 0.75 mg/kg (mL)	5 mg/mL concentration: Infusion 1.75 mg/kg/h (mL/h)	0.5 mg/mL concentration: Subsequent low-rate infusion 0.2 mg/kg/h (mL/h)
43 to 47	7	16	18
48 to 52	7.5	17.5	20
53 to 57	8	19	22
58 to 62	9	21	24
63 to 67	10	23	26
68 to 72	10.5	24.5	28
73 to 77	11	26	30
78 to 82	12	28	32
83 to 87	13	30	34
88 to 92	13.5	31.5	36
93 to 97	14	33	38
98 to 102	15	35	40
103 to 107	16	37	42
108 to 112	16.5	38.5	44
113 to 117	17	40	46
118 to 122	18	42	48
123 to 127	19	44	50
128 to 132	19.5	45.5	52
133 to 137	20	47	54
138 to 142	21	49	56
143 to 147	22	51	58
148 to 152	22.5	52.5	60

➤*Preparation for administration:* Bivalirudin is intended for IV injection and infusion after dilution. To each 250 mg vial, add 5 mL of sterile water for injection. Gently swirl until all material is dissolved. Each reconstituted vial should be further diluted in 50 mL of 5% dextrose in water or 0.9% sodium chloride for injection to yield a final concentration of 5 mg/mL (eg, 1 vial in 50 mL; 2 vials in 100 mL; 5 vials in 250 mL). The dose to be administered is adjusted according to the patient's weight, see the Bivalirudin Dosing table.

If the low-rate infusion is used after the initial infusion, a lower concentration bag should be prepared. In order to prepare this bag, reconstitute the 250 mg vial with 5 mL of sterile water for injection. Gently swirl until all material is dissolved. Each reconstituted vial should be further diluted in 500 mL of 5% dextrose in water or 0.9% sodium chloride for injection to yield a final concentration of 0.5 mg/mL. The infusion rate to be administered should be selected from the subsequent low-rate infusion column in the previous table.

➤*IV compatibilities / incompatibilities:* Bivalirudin should be administered via an IV line. No incompatibilities have been observed with glass bottles or polyvinyl chloride bags and administration sets. The following drugs should not be administered in the same IV line with bivalirudin because they resulted in haze formation, microparticulate formation, or gross precipitation when mixed with bivalirudin: alteplase, amiodarone, amphotericin B, chlorpromazine, diazepam, prochlorperazine edisylate, reteplase, streptokinase, and vancomycin. Dobutamine was compatible at concentrations up to 4 mg/mL but incompatible at a concentration of 12.5 mg/mL.

BIVALIRUDIN — INJECTION

Parenteral drug products should be inspected visually for particulate matter and discoloration prior to administration. Preparations of bivalirudin containing particulate matter should not be used. Reconstituted material will be a clear to slightly opalescent, colorless to slightly yellow solution.

➤*Renal function impairment:* The infusion dose of bivalirudin may need to be reduced and anticoagulant status monitored in patients with renal function impairment. Patients with moderate renal function impairment (creatinine clearance [Ccr], 30 to 59 mL/min) should receive 1.75 mg/kg/h. If the Ccr is less than 30 mL/min, reduction of the infusion rate to 1 mg/kg/h should be considered. If a patient is on hemodialysis, the infusion should be reduced to 0.25 mg/kg/h. No reduction in the bolus dose is needed.

➤*Storage/Stability:* Store bivalirudin dosage units at 20° to 25°C (68° to 77°F); excursions to 15° to 30°C (59° to 86°F) permitted.

Do not freeze reconstituted or diluted bivalirudin. Reconstituted material may be stored at 2° to 8°C (36° to 46°F) for up to 24 hours. Diluted bivalirudin with a concentration between 0.5 and 5 mg/mL is stable at room temperature for up to 24 hours. Discard any unused portion of reconstituted solution remaining in the vial.

Actions

➤*Pharmacology:* Bivalirudin directly inhibits thrombin by specifically binding both to the catalytic site and to the anion-binding exosite of circulating and clot-bound thrombin. Thrombin is a serine proteinase that plays a central role in the thrombotic process, acting to cleave fibrinogen into fibrin monomers and to activate factor XIII to factor XIIIa, allowing fibrin to develop a covalently cross-linked framework that stabilizes the thrombus; thrombin also activates factors V and VIII, promoting further thrombin generation, and activates platelets, stimulating aggregation and granule release. The binding of bivalirudin to thrombin is reversible as thrombin slowly cleaves the bivalirudin-Arg_3-Pro_4 bond, resulting in recovery of thrombin active site functions.

In in vitro studies, bivalirudin inhibited both soluble (free) and clot-bound thrombin, was not neutralized by products of the platelet-release reaction, and prolonged the activated partial thromboplastin time (aPTT), thrombin time (TT), and prothrombin time (PT) of normal human plasma in a concentration-dependent manner. The clinical relevance of these findings is unknown.

Pharmacodynamics – In healthy volunteers and patients (with 70% or more vessel occlusion undergoing routine angioplasty), bivalirudin exhibits linear dose- and concentration-dependent anticoagulant activity as evidenced by prolongation of the ACT, aPTT, PT, and TT. IV administration of bivalirudin produces an immediate anticoagulant effect. Coagulation times return to baseline approximately 1 hour following cessation of bivalirudin administration.

In 291 patients with 70% or more vessel occlusion undergoing routine angioplasty, a positive correlation was observed between the dose of bivalirudin and the proportion of patients achieving ACT values of 300 or 350 seconds. At a bivalirudin dose of 1 mg/kg IV bolus plus 2.5 mg/kg/h IV infusion for 4 hours, followed by 0.2 mg/kg/h, all patients reached maximal ACT values greater than 300 seconds.

➤*Pharmacokinetics:*

Distribution – Bivalirudin does not bind to plasma proteins (other than thrombin) or to red blood cells.

Metabolism/Excretion – Bivalirudin is cleared from plasma by a combination of renal mechanisms and proteolytic cleavage, with a half-life in patients with healthy renal function of 25 minutes.

Special populations –

Renal function impairment:

Bivalirudin Pharmacokinetic Parameters in Patients with Renal Function Impairment[a]

Renal function (GFR, mL/min)	Clearance (mL/min/kg)	Half-life (min)
Normal renal function (≥ 90 mL/min)	3.4	25
Mild renal impairment (60 to 89 mL/min)	3.4	22
Moderate renal impairment (30 to 59 mL/min)	2.7	34
Severe renal impairment (10 to 29 mL/min)	2.8	57
Dialysis-dependent patients (off dialysis)	1	3.5 h

[a] Monitor the ACT in renally impaired patients.

The disposition of bivalirudin was studied in PTCA patients with mild and moderate renal function impairment and in patients with severe renal function impairment. Drug elimination was related to glomerular filtration rate (GFR). Total body clearance was similar for patients with healthy renal function and with mild renal impairment (60 to 89 mL/min). Clearance was reduced approximately 20% in patients with moderate and severe renal impairment and was reduced approximately 80% in dialysis-dependent patients. See the following table for pharmacokinetic parameters. For patients with renal function impairment, monitor the ACT. Bivalirudin is hemodialyzable. Approximately 25% is cleared by hemodialysis.

Administration – Bivalirudin exhibits linear pharmacokinetics following IV administration to patients undergoing PTCA. In these patients, a mean steady-state bivalirudin concentration of 12.3 ± 1.7 mcg/mL is achieved following an IV bolus of 1 mg/kg and a 4-hour 2.5 mg/kg/h IV infusion.

Contraindications

Active major bleeding; hypersensitivity to bivalirudin or its components.

Warnings/Precautions

➤*Hematologic effects:* Bivalirudin is not intended for intramuscular administration. Although most bleeding associated with the use of bivalirudin in PCI occurs at the site of arterial puncture, hemorrhage can occur at any site. An unexplained fall in blood pressure or hematocrit, or any unexplained symptom, should lead to serious consideration of a hemorrhagic event and cessation of bivalirudin administration.

➤*Brachytherapy:* An increased risk of thrombus formation has been associated with the use of bivalirudin in gamma brachytherapy, including fatal outcomes.

Use caution when bivalirudin is used as the antithrombin during brachytherapy procedures. Operators are advised to maintain meticulous catheter technique, with frequent aspiration and flushing, paying special attention to minimizing conditions of stasis within the catheter or vessels.

➤*Antidote:* There is no known antidote to bivalirudin. Bivalirudin is hemodialyzable.

➤*Immunogenicity/Reexposure:* Among 494 subjects who received bivalirudin in clinical trials and were tested for antibodies, 2 subjects had treatment-emergent positive bivalirudin antibody tests. Neither subject demonstrated clinical evidence of allergic or anaphylactic reactions, and repeat testing was not performed. Nine additional patients who had initial positive tests were negative on repeat testing.

➤*Renal function impairment:* The disposition of bivalirudin was studied in PTCA patients with mild and moderate renal function impairment and in patients with severe renal function impairment. Drug elimination was related to GFR. Total body clearance was similar for patients with healthy renal function and with mild renal impairment (60 to 89 mL/min). Clearance was reduced approximately 20% in patients with moderate and severe renal impairment and was reduced approximately 80% in dialysis-dependent patients.

➤*Special risk:* Use bivalirudin with caution in patients with disease states associated with an increased risk of bleeding.

➤*Pregnancy: Category B.* Bivalirudin is intended for use with aspirin. Because of the possible adverse reactions on the neonate and the potential for increased maternal bleeding, particularly during the third trimester, use bivalirudin and aspirin together during pregnancy only if clearly needed.

There are no adequate and well-controlled studies in pregnant women. Because animal reproduction studies are not always predictive of human response, use this drug during pregnancy only if clearly needed.

➤*Lactation:* It is not known whether bivalirudin is excreted in human milk. Because many drugs are excreted in human milk, exercise caution when bivalirudin is administered to a breast-feeding woman.

➤*Children:* The safety and efficacy of bivalirudin in pediatric patients have not been established.

➤*Elderly:* In studies of patients undergoing PCI, 44% were 65 years of age and older, and 12% were older than 75 years of age. Elderly patients experienced more bleeding events than younger patients. Patients treated with bivalirudin experienced fewer bleeding events in each age stratum, compared with heparin.

Drug Interactions

Bivalirudin does not exhibit binding to plasma proteins (other than thrombin) or red blood cells.

➤*Hematological agents:* In clinical trials in patients undergoing PTCA/PCI, coadministration of bivalirudin with heparin, warfarin, thrombolytics, or GPIIb/IIIa inhibitors was associated with increased risks of major bleeding events compared with patients not receiving these concomitant medications. There is no experience with coadministration of bivalirudin and plasma expanders such as dextran.

Adverse Reactions

➤*Bleeding:*

Major Hematologic Outcomes in the Bivalirudin REPLACE-2 Study (Safety Population)

Hematologic events	Bivalirudin plus "provisional" GPIIb/IIIa inhibitor[a] (n = 2,914)	Heparin plus GPIIb/IIIa inhibitor (n = 2,987)	*P* value
Protocol-defined major hemorrhage[b]	2.3%	4%	< 0.001
Protocol-defined minor hemorrhage[c]	13.6%	25.8%	< 0.001
TIMI-defined bleeding[d]			
Major	0.6%	0.9%	0.259
Minor	1.3%	2.9%	< 0.001

BIVALIRUDIN — INJECTION

Major Hematologic Outcomes in the Bivalirudin REPLACE-2 Study (Safety Population)			
Hematologic events	Bivalirudin plus "provisional" GPIIb/IIIa inhibitor[a] (n = 2,914)	Heparin plus GPIIb/IIIa inhibitor (n = 2,987)	*P* value
Non-access site bleeding			
Retroperitoneal bleeding	0.2%	0.5%	0.069
Intracranial bleeding	< 0.1%	0.1%	1
Access site bleeding			
Sheath site bleeding	0.9%	2.4%	< 0.001
Thrombocytopenia[e]			
< 100,000/mm³	0.7%	1.7%	< 0.001
< 50,000/mm³	0.3%	0.6%	0.039
Transfusions			
Red blood cells (RBC)	1.3%	1.9%	0.08
Platelets	0.3%	0.6%	0.095

[a] GPIIb/IIIa inhibitors were administered to 7.2% of patients in the bivalirudin plus "provisional" GPIIb/IIIa inhibitor group.
[b] Defined as the occurrence of any of the following: intracranial bleeding, retroperitoneal bleeding, a transfusion of 2 units or more of blood/blood products, a fall in hemoglobin greater than 4 g/dL, whether or not bleeding site is identified, spontaneous or nonspontaneous blood loss with a decrease in hemoglobin greater than 3 g/dL.
[c] Defined as observed bleeding that does not meet the criteria for major hemorrhage.
[d] TIMI major bleeding is defined as: intracranial, or a fall in adjusted hemoglobin (Hgb) greater than 5 g/dL or hematocrit of greater than 15%; TIMI minor bleeding is defined as a fall in adjusted hemoglobin of 3 to less than 5 g/dL or a fall in adjusted hematocrit of 9% to less than 15%, with a bleeding site such as hematuria, hematemesis, hematomas, retroperitoneal bleeding, or a decrease in hemoglobin of greater than 4 g/dL with no bleeding site.
[e] If less than 100,000/mm³ and greater than 25% reduction from baseline, or less than 50,000/mm³.

Bivalirudin Major Bleeding and Transfusions: All Patients[a]		
Hematologic event	Bivalirudin (n = 2,161)	Heparin (n = 2,151)
Number (%) patients with major hemorrhage[b]	79 (3.7%)	199 (9.3%)
with ≥ 3 g/dL fall in hemoglobin	41 (1.9%)	124 (5.8%)
with ≥ 5 g/dL fall in hemoglobin	14 (0.6%	47 (2.2%)
Retroperitoneal bleeding	5 (0.2%)	15 (0.7%)
Intracranial bleeding	1 (< 0.1%)	2 (< 0.1%)
Required transfusion	43 (2%)	123 (5.7%)

[a] No monitoring of ACT (or PTT) was done after a target ACT was achieved.
[b] Major hemorrhage was defined as the occurrence of any of the following: intracranial bleeding, retroperitoneal bleeding, clinically overt bleeding with a decrease in hemoglobin greater than or equal to 3 g/dL or leading to a transfusion of greater than or equal to 2 units of blood. This table includes data from the entire hospitalization period.

➤*Other adverse reactions:* Adverse reactions observed in clinical trials are similar between the bivalirudin-treated patients and the control groups. Adverse reactions seen are those typical of PCI trials.

Bivalirudin Adverse Reactions (> 5%)		
Adverse reaction	Bivalirudin (n = 2,161)	Heparin (n = 2,151)
Cardiovascular		
Bradycardia	118 (5%)	164 (8%)
Hypertension	135 (6%)	115 (5%)
Hypotension	262 (12%)	371 (17%)
CNS		
Headache	264 (12%)	225 (10%)
Insomnia	142 (7%)	139 (6%)
Nervousness	102 (5%)	87 (4%)
GI		
Abdominal pain	103 (5%)	104 (5%)
Dyspepsia	100 (5%)	111 (5%)
Nausea	318 (15%)	347 (16%)
Vomiting	138 (6%)	169 (8%)
GU		
Urinary retention	89 (4%)	98 (5%)
Miscellaneous		
Anxiety	127 (6%)	140 (7%)
Back pain	916 (42%)	944 (44%)
Fever	103 (5%)	108 (5%)
Injection-site pain	174 (8%)	274 (13%)
Pain	330 (15%)	358 (17%)
Pelvic pain	130 (6%)	169 (8%)

➤*Other adverse reactions:* Serious, nonbleeding adverse reactions were experienced in 2% of 2,161 bivalirudin-treated patients and 2% of 2,151 heparin-treated patients. The following individual serious, nonbleeding adverse reactions were rare (greater than 0.1% to less than 1%) and similar in incidence between bivalirudin- and heparin-treated patients.

Cardiovascular – Hypotension, syncope, vascular anomaly, ventricular fibrillation.

CNS – Cerebral ischemia, confusion, facial paralysis.

GU – Kidney failure, oliguria.

Respiratory – Lung edema.

Miscellaneous – Fever, infection, sepsis. In the double-blind, randomized REPLACE-2 trial described above that compared bivalirudin plus "provisional" GPIIb/IIIa inhibitor with heparin plus GPIIb/IIIa inhibitor, similar adverse reactions were reported in both treatment groups:

Bivalirudin Adverse Reactions (≥ 2%)		
Adverse reaction	Bivalirudin plus "provisional" GPIIb/IIIa inhibitor (n = 2,914)	Heparin plus GPIIb/IIIa inhibitor (n = 2,987)
Cardiovascular		
Angina pectoris	155 (5.3%)	156 (5.2%)
Hypotension	91 (3.1%)	120 (4%)
CNS		
Headache	75 (2.6%)	83 (2.8%)
GI		
Nausea	86 (3%)	96 (3.2%)
Miscellaneous		
Back pain	268 (9.2%)	263 (8.8%)
Chest pain	68 (2.3%)	69 (2.3%)
Injection-site pain	80 (2.7%)	80 (2.7%)
Pain	98 (3.4%)	72 (2.4%)

Postmarketing – The following reactions have been reported: fatal bleeding; hypersensitivity and allergic reactions, including very rare reports of anaphylaxis; thrombus formation during PCI with and without intracoronary brachytherapy, including reports of fatal outcomes.

Overdosage

➤*Symptoms:* Single bolus doses of bivalirudin up to 7.5 mg/kg have been reported without associated bleeding or other adverse reactions. Discontinuation of bivalirudin leads to a gradual reduction in anticoagulant effects caused by metabolism of the drug.

➤*Treatment:* In case of overdosage, discontinue bivalirudin immediately and closely monitor the patient for signs of bleeding. Bivalirudin is hemodialyzable. There is no known antidote to bivalirudin.

FONDAPARINUX SODIUM

Rx	**Arixtra** (GlaxoSmithKline)	**Injection:** 2.5 mg per 0.5 mL	Preservative free. In single-dose, prefilled syringes with 27-gauge needle. In 10s.
		5 mg per 0.4 mL	Preservative free. In single-dose, prefilled syringes with 27-gauge needle. In 10s.
		7.5 mg per 0.6 mL	Preservative free. In single-dose, prefilled syringes with 27-gauge needle. In 10s.
		10 mg per 0.8 mL	Preservative free. In single-dose, prefilled syringes with 27-gauge needle. In 10s.

FONDAPARINUX SODIUM — INJECTION

WARNING

Spinal/Epidural hematomas – When neuraxial anesthesia (epidural/spinal anesthesia) or spinal puncture is employed, patients anticoagulated or scheduled to be anticoagulated with low molecular weight heparins (LMWHs), heparinoids, or fondaparinux for prevention of thromboembolic complications are at risk of developing an epidural or spinal hematoma that can result in long-term or permanent paralysis.

The risk of these events is increased by the use of indwelling epidural catheters for administration of analgesia or by the concomitant use of drugs affecting hemostasis, such as nonsteroidal anti-inflammatory drugs (NSAIDs), platelet inhibitors, or other anticoagulants. The risk also appears to be increased by traumatic or repeated epidural or spinal puncture.

Frequently monitor patients for signs and symptoms of neurological impairment. If neurologic compromise is noted, urgent treatment is necessary.

Consider the potential benefit versus risk before neuraxial intervention in patients anticoagulated or scheduled to be anticoagulated for thromboprophylaxis. Use fondaparinux injection, like other anticoagulants, with extreme caution in conditions with increased risk of hemorrhage, such as congenital or acquired bleeding disorders; active ulcerative and angiodysplastic GI disease; hemorrhagic stroke; or shortly after brain, spinal, or ophthalmological surgery; or in patients treated concomitantly with platelet inhibitors.

Indications

➤*Prophylaxis of deep vein thrombosis (DVT):* For the prophylaxis of DVT, which may lead to pulmonary embolism (PE):

- in patients undergoing hip fracture surgery, including extended prophylaxis;
- in patients undergoing hip replacement surgery;
- in patients undergoing knee replacement surgery;
- in patients undergoing abdominal surgery who are at risk for thromboembolic complications.

➤*Treatment of acute DVT:* For the treatment of acute DVT when administered in conjunction with warfarin.

➤*Treatment of acute PE:* For the treatment of acute PE when administered in conjunction with warfarin when initial therapy is administered in the hospital.

➤*Off-label uses:*

Venous thromboembolism prophylaxis in general surgery – [3] = Safety concerns. American College of Chest Physicians (ACCP) guidelines on prevention of VTE noted that most general surgeries present a moderate risk of VTE. In the absence of special factors that pose a high risk of bleeding, routine thromboprophylaxis would be recommended for most patients. The ACCP guideline authors concluded that fondaparinux was as effective and safe as low molecular weight heparins for pharmacologic thromboprophylaxis in patients undergoing general surgery. Advantages of fondaparinux include its excellent bioavailability after subcutaneous administration, long half-life, and lack of variability in response, which allow for once-daily fixed dosing without laboratory monitoring. In addition, fondaparinux does not cross-react with heparin-induced thrombocytopenia antibodies and may be used safely in patients with heparin-induced thrombocytopenia. Fondaparinux also does not appear to affect bone-like unfractionated heparin or low molecular weight heparins. A limitation to use is that fondaparinux is contraindicated in patients with renal insufficiency characterized by a creatinine clearance of less than 30 mL/min. In patients at high risk of bleeding, mechanical thromboprophylaxis methods are preferred over fondaparinux.

Administration and Dosage

➤*General dosing considerations:* Fondaparinux is intended for use under a health care provider's guidance. Patients may self-inject only if their health care providers determine that it is appropriate and with medical follow-up as necessary. Provide proper training in subcutaneous injection technique.

If thrombotic events occur despite fondaparinux prophylaxis, initiate appropriate therapy.

Fondaparinux prophylactic therapy is contraindicated in patients with body weight less than 50 kg undergoing hip fracture, hip replacement, knee replacement surgery, and abdominal surgery.

➤*Adults:*

Deep vein thrombosis prophylaxis following hip fracture or hip or knee replacement surgeries –

Usual dosage: 2.5 mg administered by subcutaneous injection once daily. After hemostasis has been established, give the initial dose 6 to 8 hours after surgery. Administration before 6 hours after surgery has been associated with an increased risk of major bleeding.

Duration of therapy: The usual duration of administration is 5 to 9 days; up to 11 days administration has been tolerated.

In patients undergoing hip fracture surgery, an extended prophylaxis course of up to 24 additional days is recommended. In patients undergoing hip fracture surgery, a total of 32 days (perioperative and extended prophylaxis) has been tolerated.

Deep vein thrombosis prophylaxis following abdominal surgery –

Weighing at least 50 kg:

- *Usual dosage* – 2.5 mg administered by subcutaneous injection once daily after hemostasis has been established. The initial dose should be given 6 to 8 hours after surgery. Administration before 6 hours after surgery has been associated with an increased risk of major bleeding.
- *Duration of therapy* – The usual duration of administration is 5 to 9 days; up to 10 days of fondaparinux injection has been administered.

Deep vein thrombosis –

Usual dosage: Continue fondaparinux injection treatment for at least 5 days and until a therapeutic oral anticoagulant effect is established (international normalized ratio [INR] 2 to 3).

- *Body weight less than 50 kg* – 5 mg subcutaneous once daily.
- *Body weight 50 to 100 kg* – 7.5 mg subcutaneous once daily.
- *Body weight greater than 100 kg* – 10 mg subcutaneous once daily.

Duration of therapy: The usual duration of administration of fondaparinux is 5 to 9 days; up to 26 days of fondaparinux injection has been administered.

Concomitant therapy: Initiate concomitant treatment with warfarin as soon as possible, usually within 72 hours.

Pulmonary embolism – See Deep vein thrombosis for dosing.

Off-label dosing –

Venous thromboembolism prophylaxis in general surgery: [3] = Safety concerns. 2.5 mg administered by subcutaneous injection once daily after hemostasis has been established. The initial dose should be given no earlier than 6 to 8 hours after surgery to reduce the risk of major bleeding. The usual duration of administration is 5 to 9 days.

➤*Renal function impairment:* Fondaparinux injection is contraindicated in patients with severe renal impairment (CrCl less than 30 mL/min). Use fondaparinux with caution in patients with moderate renal impairment (CrCl 30 to 50 mL/min).

➤*Administration:* Administer injection according to the recommended regimen, especially with respect to the timing of the first dose after surgery. In the hip fracture, hip replacement, knee replacement, or abdominal surgery clinical studies, the administration of fondaparinux less than 6 hours after surgery has been associated with an increased risk of major bleeding.

Fondaparinux is administered by subcutaneous injection. Administer in the fatty tissue, alternating injection sites (eg, between the left and right anterolateral or the left and right posterolateral abdominal wall). It must not be administered by intramuscular injections.

Fondaparinux injection is provided in a single-dose, prefilled syringe affixed with an automatic needle protection system. To avoid the loss of drug when using the prefilled syringe, do not expel the air bubble from the syringe before the injection.

➤*Admixture compatibility:* Do not mix with other injections or infusions.

➤*Storage/Stability:* Store at 25°C (77°F); excursions permitted between 15° and 30°C (59° and 86°F).

Actions

➤*Pharmacology:* The antithrombotic activity of fondaparinux is the result of antithrombin III (ATIII)-mediated selective inhibition of factor Xa. By selectively binding to ATIII, fondaparinux potentiates (about 300 times) the innate neutralization of factor Xa by ATIII. Neutralization of factor Xa interrupts the blood coagulation cascade and inhibits thrombin formation and thrombus development.

Fondaparinux does not inactivate thrombin (activated factor II) and has no known effect on platelet function. At the recommended dose, fondaparinux does not affect fibrinolytic activity or bleeding time.

Anti-Xa activity – The pharmacodynamics/pharmacokinetics of fondaparinux are derived from fondaparinux plasma concentrations quantified via anti-factor Xa activity. Only fondaparinux can be used to calibrate the

FONDAPARINUX SODIUM — INJECTION

anti-Xa assay. (The international standards of heparin or LMWH are not appropriate for this use.) As a result, the activity of fondaparinux is expressed as milligrams (mg) of the fondaparinux calibrator. The anti-Xa activity of the drug increases with increasing drug concentration, reaching maximum values in approximately 3 hours.

➤*Pharmacokinetics:*

Absorption – Fondaparinux administered by subcutaneous injection is rapidly and completely absorbed (absolute bioavailability is 100%). Following a single subcutaneous dose of fondaparinux 2.5 mg in young male subjects, C_{max} of 0.34 mg/L is reached in approximately 2 hours. In patients undergoing treatment with fondaparinux injection 2.5 mg once daily, the peak steady-state plasma concentration is, on average, 0.39 to 0.5 mg/L and is reached approximately 3 hours postdose. In these patients, the minimum steady-state plasma concentration is 0.14 to 0.19 mg/L. In patients with symptomatic DVT and PE undergoing treatment with fondaparinux injection 5 mg (body weight less than 50 kg), 7.5 mg (body weight 50 to 100 kg), and 10 mg (body weight greater than 100 kg) once daily, the body-weight-adjusted doses provide similar mean steady-state peaks and minimum plasma concentrations across all body weight categories. The mean peak steady-state plasma concentration is in the range of 1.2 to 1.26 mg/L. In these patients, the mean minimum steady-state plasma concentration is in the range of 0.46 to 0.62 mg/L.

Distribution – In healthy adults, intravenously (IV) or subcutaneously administered fondaparinux distributes mainly in blood and only to a minor extent in extravascular fluid as evidenced by steady state and nonsteady state apparent volume of distribution of 7 to 11 L. Similar fondaparinux distribution occurs in patients undergoing elective hip surgery or hip fracture surgery. In vitro, fondaparinux is highly (at least 94%) and specifically bound to ATIII and does not bind significantly to other plasma proteins (including platelet factor 4 [PF4]) or red blood cells.

Metabolism – In vivo metabolism of fondaparinux has not been investigated since the majority of the administered dose is eliminated unchanged in urine in individuals with normal kidney function.

Excretion – In individuals with normal kidney function, fondaparinux is eliminated in urine mainly as unchanged drug. In healthy individuals up to 75 years of age, up to 77% of a single subcutaneous or IV fondaparinux dose is eliminated in urine as unchanged drug in 72 hours. The elimination half-life is 17 to 21 hours.

Special populations –

Renal function impairment: Fondaparinux elimination is prolonged in patients with renal impairment because the major route of elimination is urinary excretion of unchanged drug. In patients undergoing prophylaxis following elective hip surgery or hip fracture surgery, the total clearance of fondaparinux is approximately 25% lower in patients with mild renal impairment (creatinine clearance [Ccr] 50 to 80 mL/min), approximately 40% lower in patients with moderate renal impairment (Ccr 30 to 50 mL/min) and approximately 55% lower in patients with severe renal impairment (less than 30 mL/min) compared with patients with normal renal function. A similar relationship between fondaparinux clearance and extent of renal impairment was observed in DVT treatment patients.

Elderly: Fondaparinux elimination is prolonged in patients older than 75 years of age. In studies evaluating 2.5 mg fondaparinux prophylaxis in hip fracture surgery or elective hip surgery, the total clearance of fondaparinux was approximately 25% lower in patients older than 75 years of age as compared with patients younger than 65 years of age. A similar relationship between fondaparinux clearance and age was observed in DVT treatment patients.

Patients weighing less than 50 kg: Total clearance of fondaparinux is decreased by approximately 30% in patients weighing less than 50 kg. Fondaparinux prophylactic therapy is contraindicated in patients with body weight less than 50 kg undergoing hip fracture, hip replacement, knee replacement surgery, and abdominal surgery. During the randomized clinical trials of prophylaxis in the perioperative period following hip fracture, hip replacement, or knee replacement surgery, occurrence of major bleeding was doubled in patients with body weight less than 50 kg compared with those with body weight greater than or equal to 50 kg (5.4% vs 2.1%). In the clinical trial in patients undergoing abdominal surgery, the major bleeding rate was also higher in patients with a body weight less than 50 kg as compared with those with a body weight of at least 50 kg (5.3% vs 3.3%), respectively.

Contraindications

Fondaparinux injection is contraindicated in patients with severe renal impairment (Ccr less than 30 mL/min). Fondaparinux is eliminated primarily by the kidneys, and such patients are at increased risk for major bleeding episodes.

Fondaparinux prophylactic therapy is contraindicated in patients with body weight less than 50 kg undergoing hip fracture, hip replacement, knee replacement surgery, or abdominal surgery. During the randomized clinical trials of prophylaxis in the perioperative period following hip fracture, hip replacement, or knee replacement surgery, occurrence of major bleeding was doubled in patients with a body weight less than 50 kg compared with those with a body weight greater than or equal to 50 kg (5.4% vs 2.1%). In the clinical trial in patients undergoing abdominal surgery, the major bleeding rate was also higher in patients with a body weight less than 50 kg as compared with those with a body weight of 50 kg or greater (5.3% vs 3.3%), respectively.

The use of fondaparinux is contraindicated in patients with active major bleeding, bacterial endocarditis, in patients with thrombocytopenia associated with a positive in vitro test for antiplatelet antibody in the presence of fondaparinux, or in patients with known hypersensitivity to fondaparinux.

Warnings/Precautions

➤*Interchangeability:* Fondaparinux injection cannot be used interchangeably (unit for unit) with heparin, LMWHs, or heparinoids, as they differ in manufacturing process, anti-Xa and anti-IIa activity, units, and dosage. Each of these medicines has its own instructions for use.

➤*Hemorrhage:* See the Warning box for more information.

➤*Neuraxial anesthesia and postoperative indwelling epidural catheter use:* See the Warning box for more information.

➤*Thrombocytopenia:* Thrombocytopenia can occur with the administration of fondaparinux. Moderate thrombocytopenia (platelet counts between 100,000/mm^3 and 50,000/mm^3) occurred at a rate of 3% in patients given fondaparinux 2.5 mg in the perioperative hip fracture, hip replacement, or knee replacement surgery, and abdominal surgery clinical trials. Severe thrombocytopenia (platelet counts less than 50,000/mm^3) occurred at a rate of 0.2% in patients given fondaparinux 2.5 mg in these clinical trials. During extended prophylaxis, no cases of moderate or severe thrombocytopenia were reported.

Moderate thrombocytopenia occurred at a rate of 0.5% in patients given the fondaparinux treatment regimen in the DVT and PE treatment clinical trials. Severe thrombocytopenia occurred at a rate of 0.04% in patients given the fondaparinux treatment regimen in the DVT and PE treatment clinical trials.

Closely monitor thrombocytopenia of any degree. If the platelet count falls below 100,000/mm^3, discontinue fondaparinux.

➤*Renal function impairment:*

Hip fracture, hip replacement, and knee replacement surgeries – Major bleeding in patients receiving prophylactic therapy in hip fracture, hip replacement, or knee replacement surgery occurred in 1.6% (25/1,565) of patients with normal renal function, in 2.4% (31/1,288) with mild renal impairment, in 3.8% (19/504) with moderate renal impairment, and in 4.8% (4/83) with severe renal impairment. When fondaparinux was used according to the recommended timing of the first injection (6 to 8 hours after surgery), major bleeding occurred in 1.8% (16/905) of patients with normal renal function, in 2.2% (15/675) with mild renal impairment, in 2.3% (6/265) with moderate renal impairment, and in 0% (0/40) with severe renal impairment.

Abdominal surgery – Major bleeding in patients receiving prophylactic therapy in abdominal surgery occurred in 2.1% (13/606) of patients with normal renal function, in 3.6% (22/613) with mild renal impairment, in 6.7% (12/179) with moderate renal impairment, and in 7.1% (1/14) with severe renal impairment. When fondaparinux was used according to the recommended timing of the first injection (6 to 8 hours after surgery), major bleeding occurred in 2.1% (10/467) of patients with normal renal function, in 3.3% (16/481) with mild renal impairment, in 5.8% (8/137) with moderate renal impairment, and in 7.7% (1/13) with severe renal impairment.

Treatment of DVT and PE – Major bleeding in patients receiving treatment for DVT and PE occurred in 0.4% (4/1,132) of patients with normal renal function, in 1.6% (12/733) with mild renal impairment, in 2.2% (7/318) with moderate renal impairment, and in 7.3% (4/55) with severe renal impairment.

Use fondaparinux with caution in patients with moderate renal impairment (Ccr 30 to 50 mL/min). Periodically assess renal function in patients receiving fondaparinux. Immediately discontinue the drug in patients who develop severe renal impairment while on therapy. After discontinuation of fondaparinux, its anticoagulant effects may persist for 2 to 4 days in patients with normal renal function (ie, at least 3 to 5 half-lives). The anticoagulant effects of fondaparinux may persist even longer in patients with renal impairment.

➤*Special risk:* Use fondaparinux injection with care in patients with a bleeding diathesis, uncontrolled arterial hypertension, or a history of recent GI ulceration, diabetic retinopathy, and hemorrhage.

➤*Pregnancy: Category B.* There are no adequate and well-controlled studies in pregnant women. Because animal reproduction studies are not always predictive of human response, use this drug during pregnancy only if clearly needed.

➤*Lactation:* Fondaparinux was found to be excreted in the milk of lactating rats. However, it is not known whether this drug is excreted in human milk. Because many drugs are excreted in human milk, exercise caution when fondaparinux is administered to a nursing mother.

➤*Children:* Safety and effectiveness of fondaparinux in pediatric patients have not been established.

➤*Elderly:* Use fondaparinux injection with caution in elderly patients. Over 3,000 patients, 65 years of age and older, have received 2.5 mg fondaparinux in randomized clinical trials. Over 1,200 patients, 65 years of age and older, have received the fondaparinux treatment regimen in the DVT and PE treatment clinical trials. The efficacy of fondaparinux in the elderly (65 years of age and older) was similar to that seen in younger patients (younger than 65 years). In the perioperative hip fracture, hip replacement, or knee replacement surgery clinical trials with patients receiving fondaparinux 2.5 mg the risk of fondaparinux-associated major bleeding increased with age: 1.8% (23/1,253) in patients younger than 65 years, 2.2% (24/1,111) in those 65 to 74 years, and 2.7% (33/1,227) in those 75 years or older. Serious adverse reactions increased with age for patients receiving fondaparinux. In patients undergoing 3 weeks of extended prophylaxis following 1 week of perioperative prophylaxis after hip fracture surgery, the incidence of major bleeding was 1.9% (1/52) in patients younger than 65 years of age, 1.4% (1/71) in those 65 to 74 years, and 2.9% (6/204) in those 75 years of age or older. In the abdominal surgery clinical

FONDAPARINUX SODIUM — INJECTION

trial, the risk of fondaparinux-associated major bleeding increased with age: 3% (19/644) in patients younger than 65 years of age, 3.2% (16/507) in those 65 to 74 years of age, and 5% (14/282) in those 75 years of age and older. In the DVT and PE treatment clinical trials with patients receiving the fondaparinux treatment regimen, the risk of fondaparinux-associated major bleeding increased with age: 0.6% (7/1151) in patients younger than 65 years of age, 1.6% (9/560) in those 65 to 74 years of age, and 2.1% (12/583) in those 75 years of age or older. Careful attention to dosing directions and concomitant medications (especially antiplatelet medication) is advised.

Fondaparinux is substantially excreted by the kidney, and the risk of toxic reactions to fondaparinux may be greater in patients with impaired renal function. Because elderly patients are more likely to have decreased renal function, it may be useful to monitor renal function.

➤*Monitoring:* Frequently monitor patients for signs and symptoms of neurological impairment.

Periodic routine complete blood counts (including platelet count), serum creatinine level, and stool occult blood tests are recommended during the course of treatment with fondaparinux injection.

When administered at the recommended doses, routine coagulation tests such as prothrombin time (PT) and activated partial thromboplastin time (aPTT) are relatively insensitive measures of fondaparinux activity, and are therefore, unsuitable for monitoring.

The anti-factor Xa activity of fondaparinux can be measured by anti-Xa assay using the appropriate calibrator (fondaparinux). Since the international standards of heparin or LMWH are not appropriate calibrators, the activity of fondaparinux is expressed in milligrams (mg) of the fondaparinux and cannot be compared with activities of heparin or LMWHs.

Because routine coagulation tests such as PT and aPTT are relatively insensitive measures of fondaparinux activity and international standards of heparin or LMWH are not calibrators to measure anti-factor Xa activity of fondaparinux, if during fondaparinux therapy unexpected changes in coagulation parameters or major bleeding occurs, discontinue fondaparinux.

Drug Interactions

Discontinue agents that may enhance the risk of hemorrhage prior to initiation of fondaparinux therapy. If coadministration is essential, close monitoring may be appropriate.

➤*Coumarin:* In an in vitro study in human liver microsomes, inhibition of CYP2A6 hydroxylation of coumarin by fondaparinux (200 mcM [ie, 350 mg/L]) was 17% to 28%. Inhibition of the other isozymes evaluated (CYPs 2A1, 2C9, 2C19, 2D6, 3A4, and 3E1) was 0% to 16%. Since fondaparinux does not markedly inhibit CYP450s (CYP1A2, CYP2A6, CYP2C9, CYP2C19, CYP2D6, CYP2E1, or CYP3A4) in vitro, fondaparinux is not expected to significantly interact with other drugs in vivo by inhibition of metabolism mediated by these isozymes.

Adverse Reactions

➤*Hemorrhage:* During fondaparinux administration, the most common adverse reactions were bleeding complications.

Hip fracture, hip replacement, and knee replacement surgery –

Fondaparinux Major Bleeding Episodes[a] in Randomized, Controlled, Hip Fracture, Hip Replacement, and Knee Replacement Surgery Studies

Indications	Perioperative prophylaxis (day 1 to day 7 ± 1 postsurgery): 2.5 mg Fondaparinux subcutaneously once daily	Perioperative prophylaxis: Enoxaparin[b,c]	Extended prophylaxis (day 8 to day 28 ± 2 postsurgery): 2.5 mg Fondaparinux subcutaneously once daily	Extended prophylaxis: Placebo subcutaneously once daily
Hip fracture	18/831 (2.2%)	19/842 (2.3%)	8/327 (2.4%)[d]	2/329 (0.6%)
Hip replacement	67/2,268 (3%)	55/2,597 (2.1%)		
Knee replacement	11/517 (2.1%)[e]	1/517 (0.2%)		

[a] Major bleeding was defined as clinically overt bleeding that was (1) fatal, (2) bleeding at critical site (eg, intracranial, retroperitoneal, intra-ocular, pericardial, spinal, into adrenal gland), (3) associated with reoperation at operative site, or (4) with a bleeding index (BI) greater than or equal to 2 calculated as [number of whole blood or packed red blood cell units transfused ± [(prebleeding) − (post-bleeding)] hemoglobin (g/dL) values].
[b] Enoxaparin dosing regimen: 30 mg every 12 hours or 40 mg once daily.
[c] Not approved for use in patients undergoing hip fracture surgery.
[d] During noncomparative, unblinded, perioperative prophylaxis, major bleeding was reported in 22/737 (3%) patients. Fifteen of these 22 patients continued to receive fondaparinux in extended prophylaxis. After randomization, 4/327 (1.2%) patients experienced major bleeding for the first time.
[e] *P*-value vs enoxaparin: less than 0.01, 95% CI, [1.1% to 3.3%] in fondaparinux group versus [0% to 1.1%] in enoxaparin group.

Fondaparinux Bleeding Across Randomized, Controlled Hip Fracture, Hip Replacement and Knee Replacement Surgery Studies

Bleeding incidents	Perioperative prophylaxis (day 1 to day 7 ± 1 postsurgery): 2.5 mg Fondaparinux subcutaneously once daily (n = 3,616)	Perioperative prophylaxis: Enoxaparin[a,b] (n = 3,956)	Extended prophylaxis (day 8 to day 28 ± 2 postsurgery): 2.5 mg Fondaparinux subcutaneously once daily (n = 327)	Extended prophylaxis: Placebo subcutaneously once daily (n = 329)
Major bleeding[c]	96 (2.7%)	75 (1.9%)	8 (2.4%)[d]	2 (0.6%)
Fatal bleeding	0 (0%)	1 (< 0.1%)	0 (0%)	0 (0%)
Non-fatal bleeding at critical site	0 (0%)	1 (< 0.1%)	0 (0%)	0 (0%)
Re-operation due to bleeding	12 (0.3%)	10 (0.3%)	2 (0.6%)	2 (0.6%)
BI ≥ 2[e]	84 (2.3%)	63 (1.6%)	6 (1.8%)	0 (0%)
Minor bleeding[f]	109 (3%)	116 (2.9%)	5 (1.5%)	2 (0.6%)

[a] Enoxaparin dosing regimen: 30 mg every 12 hours or 40 mg once daily.
[b] Not approved for use in patients undergoing hip fracture surgery.
[c] Major bleeding was defined as clinically overt bleeding that was (1) fatal, (2) bleeding at critical site (eg, intracranial, retroperitoneal, intra-ocular, pericardial, spinal, into adrenal gland), (3) associated with reoperation at operative site, or (4) with a BI greater than or equal to 2.
[d] During noncomparative, unblinded, perioperative prophylaxis, 2 fatal bleeds were reported (1 in a 50 kg patient, 1 in a severe renal failure patient).
[e] BI greater than or equal to 2: overt bleeding associated only with a BI greater than or equal to 2 calculated as [number of whole blood or packed red blood cell units transfused + [(prebleeding) − (postbleeding)] hemoglobin (g/dL) values].
[f] Minor bleeding was defined as clinically overt bleeding that was not major.

A separate analysis of major bleeding across all randomized, controlled, perioperative, prophylaxis, clinical studies of hip fracture, hip replacement, or knee replacement surgery according to the time of the first injection of fondaparinux after surgical closure was performed in patients who received fondaparinux only postoperatively. In this analysis the incidences of major bleeding were as follows: less than 4 hours was 4.8% (5/104), 4 to 6 hours was 2.3% (28/1,196), 6 to 8 hours was 1.9% (38/1,965). In all studies, the majority (greater than or equal to 75%) of the major bleeding events occurred during the first 4 days after surgery.

Abdominal surgery:

FondaparinuxMajor Bleeding Episodes[a] in Randomized, Controlled, Abdominal Surgery Study

Bleeding incidents	Fondaparinux 2.5 mg subcutaneously once daily (n = 1,433)	Dalteparin 5,000 units subcutaneously once daily (n = 1, 425)
Major bleeding	49 (3.4%)	34 (2.4%)
Fatal bleeding	2 (0.1%)	2 (0.1%)
Nonfatal bleeding at critical site	0 (0%)	0 (0%)
Other nonfatal major bleeding		
Surgical site	38 (2.7%)	26 (1.8%)
Nonsurgical site	9 (0.6%)	6 (0.4%)
Minor bleeding[b]	31 (2.2%)	23 (1.6%)

[a] Major bleeding was defined as bleeding that was (1) fatal, (2) bleeding at the surgical site leading to intervention, (3) nonsurgical bleeding at a critical site (eg, intracranial, retroperitoneal, intraocular, pericardial, spinal, into adrenal gland) or leading to an intervention, and/or with a bleeding index (BI) ≥ 2. (BI ≥ 2 calculated as [number of whole blood or packed red blood cell units transfused + [(prebleeding) − (postbleeding)] hemoglobin (g/dL) values].)
[b] Minor bleeding was defined as clinically overt bleeding that was not major.

A separate analysis of major bleeding according to the time of the first injection of fondaparinux after surgical closure was performed. In this analysis, the incidences of major bleeding were as follows: less than 6 hours was 3.4% (9/263) and 6 to 8 hours was 2.9% (32/1,112).

Treatment of DVT and PE –

Fondaparinux Bleeding[a] in DVT and PE Treatment Studies

Bleeding incidents	Fondaparinux treatment regimen (n = 2,294)	1 mg/kg enoxaparin subcutaneously every 12 hours (n = 1,101)	Heparin aPTT adjusted IV (n = 1,092)
Major bleeding[b]	28 (1.2%)	13 (1.2%)	12 (1.1%)
Fatal bleeding	3 (0.1%)	0 (0%)	1 (0.1%)
Nonfatal bleeding at a critical site	3 (0.1%)	0 (0%)	2 (0.2%)
Intracranial bleeding	3 (0.1%)	0 (0%)	1 (0.1%)
Retroperitoneal bleeding	0 (0%)	0 (0%)	1 (0.1%)

FONDAPARINUX SODIUM — INJECTION

Fondaparinux Bleeding[a] in DVT and PE Treatment Studies			
Bleeding incidents	Fondaparinux treatment regimen (n = 2,294)	1 mg/kg enoxaparin subcutaneously every 12 hours (n = 1,101)	Heparin aPTT adjusted IV (n = 1,092)
Clinically overt bleeding with a 2 g/dL fall in hemoglobin and/ or leading to transfusion of PRBC or whole blood ≥ 2 units	22 (1%)	13 (1.2%)	10 (0.9%)
Minor bleeding[c]	70 (3.1%)	33 (3%)	57 (5.2%)

[a] Bleeding rates are during the study drug treatment period (approximately 7 days). Patients were also treated with vitamin K antagonists initiated within 72 hours after the first study drug administration.
[b] Major bleeding was defined as clinically overt: and/or contributing to death - and/or in a critical organ including intracranial, retroperitoneal, intraocular, spinal, pericardial, or adrenal gland - and/or associated with a fall in hemoglobin level greater than or equal to 2 g/dL - and/or leading to a transfusion greater than or equal to 2 units of packed red blood cells or whole blood.
[c] Minor bleeding was defined as clinically overt bleeding that was not major.

Thrombocytopenia – Thrombocytopenia can occur with the administration of fondaparinux. Moderate thrombocytopenia (platelet counts between 100,000/mm^3 and 50,000/mm^3) occurred at a rate of 2.9% in patients given fondaparinux 2.5 mg in the perioperative hip fracture, hip replacement, or knee replacement surgery clinical trials. Severe thrombocytopenia (platelet counts less than 50,000/mm^3) occurred at a rate of 0.2% in patients given fondaparinux 2.5 mg in these clinical trials. During extended prophylaxis, no cases of moderate or severe thrombocytopenia were reported.

Moderate thrombocytopenia occurred at a rate of 0.5% in patients given the fondaparinux treatment regimen in the DVT and PE treatment clinical trials. Severe thrombocytopenia occurred at a rate of 0.04% in patients given the fondaparinux treatment regimen in the DVT and PE treatment clinical trials.

Closely monitor thrombocytopenia of any degree. If the platelet count falls below 100,000/mm^3, discontinue fondaparinux.

➤*Local:* Mild local irritation (injection site bleeding, rash and pruritus) may occur following subcutaneous injection of fondaparinux.

➤*Elevations of serum aminotransferases:* In the perioperative prophylaxis randomized clinical trials of 7 ± 2 days asymptomatic increases in AST and ALT aminotransferase levels greater than 3 times the upper limit of normal of the laboratory reference range have been reported in 1.7% and 2.6% of patients, respectively, during treatment with fondaparinux 2.5 mg injection versus 3.2% and 3.9%, of patients, respectively, during treatment with enoxaparin 30 mg every 12 hours or enoxaparin 40 mg once daily. Such elevations are fully reversible and are rarely associated with increases in bilirubin. In the extended prophylaxis clinical trial no significant differences in AST and ALT between fondaparinux 2.5 mg injection and placebo-treated patients were observed.

In the DVT and PE treatment clinical trials asymptomatic increases in AST and ALT aminotransferase levels greater than 3 times the upper limit of normal of the laboratory reference range have been reported in 0.7% and 1.3% of patients, respectively, during treatment with the fondaparinux injection treatment regimen. In comparison, these increases have been reported in 4.8% and 12.3%, of patients, respectively, in the DVT treatment trial during treatment with enoxaparin 1 mg/kg every 12 hours, and in 2.9% and 8.7% of patients, respectively, in the PE treatment trial during treatment with aPTT adjusted heparin.

Since aminotransferase determinations are important in the differential diagnosis of myocardial infarction, liver disease, and pulmonary emboli, interpret elevations that might be caused by drugs like fondaparinux with caution.

➤*Other adverse reactions:*

Adverse Reactions in Fondaparinux, Enoxaparin, or Placebo-Treated Patients in Randomized, Controlled, Surgery Studies (≥ 2%)				
	Perioperative prophylaxis (day 1 to day 7 ± 1 postsurgery)		Extended prophylaxis (day 8 to day 28 ± 2 postsurgery)	
Adverse reactions	2.5 mg fondaparinux subcutaneously once daily (n = 3,616)	Enoxaparin[a,b] (n = 3,956)	2.5 mg fondaparinux subcutaneously once daily (n = 327)	Placebo subcutaneously once daily (n = 329)
Cardiovascular				
Hypotension	126 (3.5%)	125 (3.2%)	1 (0.3%)	0 (0%)
CNS				
Confusion	113 (3.1%)	132 (3.3%)	4 (1.2%)	1 (0.3%)
Dizziness	131 (3.6%)	165 (4.2%)	2 (0.6%)	0 (0%)
Headache	72 (2%)	97 (2.5%)	0 (0%)	2 (0.6%)
Insomnia	179 (5%)	214 (5.4%)	3 (0.9%)	1 (0.3%)
Dermatologic				
Bullous eruption[c]	112 (3.1%)	102 (2.6%)	0 (0%)	1 (0.3%)
Purpura	128 (3.5%)	137 (3.5%)	0 (0%)	0 (0%)
Rash	273 (7.5%)	329 (8.3%)	2 (0.6%)	4 (1.2%)
Surgical site reaction	29 (0.8%)	41 (1%)	5 (1.5%)	8 (2.4%)
GI				
Constipation	309 (8.5%)	416 (10.5%)	6 (1.8%)	7 (2.1%)
Diarrhea	90 (2.5%)	102 (2.6%)	6 (1.8%)	8 (2.4%)
Dyspepsia	87 (2.4%)	102 (2.6%)	1 (0.3%)	2 (0.6%)
Nausea	409 (11.3%)	484 (12.2%)	1 (0.3%)	4 (1.2%)
Vomiting	212 (5.9%)	236 (6%)	2 (0.6%)	4 (1.2%)
GU				
Urinary retention	106 (2.9%)	117 (3%)	0 (0%)	1 (0.3%)
Urinary tract infection	136 (3.8%)	135 (3.4%)	13 (4%)	13 (4%)
Hematologic				
Anemia	707 (19.6%)	670 (16.9%)	5 (1.5%)	4 (1.2%)
Hematoma	103 (2.8%)	109 (2.8%)	7 (2.1%)	1 (0.3%)
Hypokalemia	152 (4.2%)	164 (4.1%)	0 (0%)	0 (0%)
Postoperative hemorrhage	85 (2.4%)	69 (1.7%)	2 (0.6%)	2 (0.6%)
Miscellaneous				
Edema	313 (8.7%)	348 (8.8%)	3 (0.9%)	2 (0.6%)
Fever	491 (13.6%)	610 (15.4%)	1 (0.3%)	4 (1.2%)
Pain	62 (1.7%)	101 (2.6%)	0 (0%)	0 (0%)
Wound drainage increased	161 (4.5%)	184 (4.7%)	2 (0.6%)	0 (0%)

[a] Enoxaparin dosing regimen: 30 mg every 12 hours or 40 mg once daily.
[b] Not approved for use in patients undergoing hip fracture surgery.
[c] Localized blister coded as bullous eruption.

Adverse Reactions in Fondaparinux- or Dalteparin-Treated Patients Undergoing Abdominal Surgery (≥ 2%)		
Adverse reaction	Fondaparinux 2.5 mg subcutaneously once daily (n = 1,433)	Dalteparin 5,000 units subcutaneously once daily (n = 1,425)
Cardiovascular		
Hypertension	35 (2.4%)	41 (2.9%)
Dermatologic		
Postoperative wound infection	70 (4.9%)	69 (4.8%)
Surgical site reaction	46 (3.2%)	40 (2.8%)
GI		
Vomiting	31 (2.2%)	26 (1.8%)
Hematologic		
Anemia	35 (2.4%)	26 (1.8%)
Postoperative hemorrhage	61 (4.3%)	42 (2.9%)
Respiratory		
Pneumonia	33 (2.3%)	23 (1.6%)
Miscellaneous		
Fever	53 (3.7%)	54 (3.8%)

Selective Factor Xa Inhibitor

FONDAPARINUX SODIUM — INJECTION

Adverse Reactions in Fondaparinux, Enoxaparin, or Heparin-treated Patients Across VTE Treatment Studies (≥ 2%)

Adverse reaction	Fondaparinux (n = 2,294)	Enoxaparin (n = 1,101)	Heparin (n = 1,092)
Cardiovascular			
Chest pain	33 (1.4%)	8 (0.7%)	26 (2.4%)
CNS			
Anxiety	18 (0.8%)	8 (0.7%)	22 (2%)
Headache	104 (4.5%)	37 (3.4%)	65 (6%)
Insomnia	86 (3.7%)	19 (1.7%)	75 (6.9%)
GI			
Abdominal pain	33 (1.4%)	14 (1.3%)	28 (2.6%)
Constipation	106 (4.6%)	32 (2.9%)	93 (8.5%)
Diarrhea	43 (1.9%)	22 (2%)	27 (2.5%)
Nausea	76 (3.3%)	29 (2.6%)	53 (4.9%)
Vomiting	26 (1.1%)	14 (1.3%)	27 (2.5%)
GU			
Urinary tract infection	53 (2.3%)	20 (1.8%)	24 (2.2%)
Hematologic			
Anemia	28 (1.2%)	3 (0.3%)	23 (2.1%)
Epistaxis	30 (1.3%)	12 (1.1%)	41 (3.8%)
Prothrombin decreased	30 (1.3%)	3 (0.3%)	34 (3.1%)
Hepatic			
ALT increased	4 (0.2%)	31 (2.8%)	3 (0.3%)
AST increased	7 (0.3%)	47 (4.3%)	8 (0.7%)
Hepatic enzymes increased	7 (0.3%)	52 (4.7%)	30 (2.7%)
Hepatic function abnormal	10 (0.4%)	14 (1.3%)	24 (2.2%)

Adverse Reactions in Fondaparinux, Enoxaparin, or Heparin-treated Patients Across VTE Treatment Studies (≥ 2%)

Adverse reaction	Fondaparinux (n = 2,294)	Enoxaparin (n = 1,101)	Heparin (n = 1,092)
Metabolic/Nutritional			
Hypokalemia	25 (1.1%)	2 (0.2%)	23 (2.1%)
Respiratory			
Coughing	48 (2.1%)	7 (0.6%)	26 (2.4%)
Miscellaneous			
Back pain	30 (1.3%)	11 (1%)	34 (3.1%)
Bruise	24 (1%)	24 (2.2%)	14 (1.3%)
Fever	81 (3.5%)	32 (2.9%)	47 (4.3%)
Leg pain	31 (1.4%)	10 (0.9%)	22 (2%)

Overdosage

➤*Symptoms:* There is no known antidote for fondaparinux injection. Overdose of fondaparinux may lead to hemorrhagic complications.

➤*Treatment:* Overdosage associated with bleeding complications should lead to treatment discontinuation and initiation of appropriate therapy. Data obtained in patients undergoing chronic intermittent hemodialysis suggest that fondaparinux clearance can increase by 20% during hemodialysis.

Patient Information

Advise patients not to take any aspirin or NSAIDs without consulting a doctor. The risk of bleeding is increased when taken with fondaparinux.

Administer as a subcutaneous injection. Instruct patient on proper injection technique.

Advise patients to notify a doctor immediately if any unusual bleeding or symptoms occur (eg, bruising, petechiae, hematuria, nosebleeds, black, tarry stools).

Inform patients that regular visits to a doctor or clinic are needed to monitor therapy.

Coumarin Anticoagulants

WARFARIN SODIUM

Rx	**Warfarin Sodium** (Various, eg, Barr, Taro)	**Tablets; oral:** 1 mg	In 100s, 1,000s, 5,000s, and UD 100s.
Rx	**Coumadin** (Bristol-Myers Squibb)		Lactose. (COUMADIN 1). Pink, scored. In 100s, 1,000s, and UD 100s.
Rx	**Jantoven** (Upsher-Smith)		Lactose. (WRF 1 832). Pink, scored. In 100s, 1,000s, and UD 100s.
Rx	**Warfarin Sodium** (Various, eg, Barr, Taro)	**Tablets; oral:** 2 mg	In 100s, 1,000s, 5,000s, and UD 100s.
Rx	**Coumadin** (Bristol-Myers Squibb)		Lactose. (COUMADIN 2). Lavender, scored. In 100s, 1,000s, and UD 100s.
Rx	**Jantoven** (Upsher-Smith)		Lactose. (WRF 2 832). Lavender, scored. In 100s, 1,000s, and UD 100s.
Rx	**Warfarin Sodium** (Various, eg, Barr, Taro)	**Tablets; oral:** 2.5 mg	In 100s, 1,000s, 5,000s, and UD 100s.
Rx	**Coumadin** (Bristol-Myers Squibb)		Lactose. (COUMADIN 2½). Green, scored. In 100s, 1,000s, and UD 100s.
Rx	**Jantoven** (Upsher-Smith)		Lactose. (WRF 2½ 832). Green, scored. In 100s, 1,000s, and UD 100s.
Rx	**Warfarin Sodium** (Various, eg, Barr, Taro)	**Tablets; oral:** 3 mg	In 100s, 1,000s, 5,000s, and UD 100s.
Rx	**Coumadin** (Bristol-Myers Squibb)		Lactose. (COUMADIN 3). Tan, scored. In 100s, 1,000s, and UD 100s.
Rx	**Jantoven** (Upsher-Smith)		Lactose. (WRF 3 832). Tan, scored. In 100s, 1,000s, and UD 100s.
Rx	**Warfarin Sodium** (Various, eg, Barr, Taro)	**Tablets; oral:** 4 mg	In 100s, 1,000s, 5,000s, and UD 100s.
Rx	**Coumadin** (Bristol-Myers Squibb)		Lactose. (COUMADIN 4). Blue, scored. In 100s, 1,000s, and UD 100s.
Rx	**Jantoven** (Upsher-Smith)		Lactose. (WRF 4 832). Blue, scored. In 100s, 1,000s, and UD 100s.
Rx	**Warfarin Sodium** (Various, eg, Barr, Taro)	**Tablets; oral:** 5 mg	In 100s, 1,000s, 5,000s, and UD 100s.
Rx	**Coumadin** (Bristol-Myers Squibb)		Lactose. (COUMADIN 5). Peach, scored. In 100s, 1,000s, and UD 100s.
Rx	**Jantoven** (Upsher-Smith)		Lactose. (WRF 5 832). Peach, scored. In 100s, 1,000s, and UD 100s.
Rx	**Warfarin Sodium** (Various, eg, Barr, Taro)	**Tablets; oral:** 6 mg	In 100s, 1,000s, 5,000s, and UD 100s.
Rx	**Coumadin** (Bristol-Myers Squibb)		Lactose. (COUMADIN 6). Teal, scored. In 100s, 1,000s, and UD 100s.
Rx	**Jantoven** (Upsher-Smith)		Lactose. (WRF 6 832). Teal, scored. In 100s, 1,000s, and UD 100s.
Rx	**Warfarin Sodium** (Various, eg, Barr, Taro)	**Tablets; oral:** 7.5 mg	In 100s, 1,000s, and UD 100s.
Rx	**Coumadin** (Bristol-Myers Squibb)		Lactose. (COUMADIN 7½). Yellow, scored. In 100s and UD 100s.
Rx	**Jantoven** (Upsher-Smith)		Lactose. (WRF 7½ 832). Yellow, scored. In 100s, 500s, and UD 100s.
Rx	**Warfarin Sodium** (Various, eg, Barr, Taro)	**Tablets; oral:** 10 mg	In 100s, 1,000s, and UD 100s.
Rx	**Coumadin** (Bristol-Myers Squibb)		Dye free. Lactose. (COUMADIN 10). Scored. In 100s and UD 100s.
Rx	**Jantoven** (Upsher-Smith)		Dye free. Lactose. (WRF 10 832). Scored. In 100s, 500s, and UD 100s.
Rx	**Coumadin** (Bristol-Myers Squibb)	**Injection, lyophilized, powder for solution:** 5.4 mg (2 mg/mL when reconstituted)	Mannitol. Preservative free. In single-use 5 mg vials.

WARFARIN SODIUM — ORAL

WARNING

Bleeding risk – Warfarin can cause major or fatal bleeding. Bleeding is more likely to occur during the starting period and with a higher dose (resulting in a higher international normalized ratio [INR]). Risk factors for bleeding include high intensity of anticoagulation (INR of more than 4), 65 years of age and older, highly variable INRs, history of GI bleeding, hypertension, cerebrovascular disease, serious heart disease, anemia, malignancy, trauma, renal function impairment, concomitant drugs, and long duration of warfarin therapy. Regular monitoring of INR should be performed on all treated patients. Those at high risk of bleeding may benefit from more frequent INR monitoring, careful dose adjustment to desired INR, and a shorter duration of therapy. Patients should be instructed about prevention measures to minimize risk of bleeding and to report immediately to health care provider signs and symptoms of bleeding.

Indications

➤*Recurrent myocardial infarction (MI)/thromboembolic event:* To reduce the risk of death, recurrent MI, and thromboembolic events such as stroke or systemic embolization after MI.

➤*Thromboembolic complications:* For the prophylaxis and/or treatment of the thromboembolic complications associated with atrial fibrillation and/or cardiac valve replacement.

➤*Venous thrombosis/pulmonary embolism:* For the prophylaxis and/or treatment of venous thrombosis and its extension, and pulmonary embolism.

➤*Off-label uses:*

Primary venous thromboembolism prophylaxis in cancer patients – [4] = Insufficient documentation. Although primary prophylaxis with warfarin or other anticoagulants was not recommended for all ambulatory cancer patients, cancer patients with other indications for anticoagulation should receive therapy. For example, patients with cancer who undergo surgical procedures should receive routine thromboprophylaxis as indicated by the type of surgery. In addition, patients with cancer who are bedridden because of acute illness should receive routine prophylaxis, as would be indicated in the absence of a cancer diagnosis. Additional clinical trials evaluating warfarin for primary venous thromboembolism (VTE) prophylaxis in cancer patients may be able to resolve the conflicting results observed to date and identify the patient population most likely to benefit from therapy.

Venous thromboembolism prophylaxis in cancer patients with central venous catheters – [4] = Insufficient documentation. Studies to date suggest that the rate of symptomatic central venous catheter (CVC)–associated VTE in patients with cancer is only 2% to 4%, which may be too low to warrant routine thromboprophylaxis even if thromboprophylaxis were efficacious. Conflicting results have been observed in the studies evaluating prophylaxis for catheter-related VTE. The American College of Chest Physicians guideline authors speculated that even if higher warfarin doses could produce more consistent beneficial results, the higher doses would pose an unacceptable risk of major bleeding. Although prophylaxis of CVC-induced VTE with warfarin or other anticoagulants was not recommended for all cancer patients, cancer patients with other indications for anticoagulation should receive therapy. For example, patients with cancer who undergo surgical procedures should receive routine thromboprophylaxis as indicated by the type of surgery. In addition, patients with cancer who are bedridden because of acute illness should receive routine prophylaxis, as would be indicated in the absence of a cancer diagnosis.

Administration and Dosage

➤*General dosing considerations:* The dosage and administration of warfarin must be individualized for each patient according to the particular patient's prothrombin time (PT)/INR response to the drug.

An INR of more than 4 appears to provide no additional therapeutic benefit in most patients and is associated with a higher risk of bleeding.

Use of a large loading dose may increase the incidence of hemorrhagic and other complications, does not offer more rapid protection against thrombi formation, and is not recommended.

Consider lower initiation and maintenance doses for patients with certain genetic variations in CYP2C9 and VKORC1 enzymes, as well as for elderly and/or debilitated patients and patients with a potential to exhibit greater than expected PT/INR response to warfarin.

➤*Adults:*

Anticoagulation –

Initial dosage: 2 to 5 mg daily.

Maintenance dosage: 2 to 10 mg daily. The individual dose and interval should be gauged by the patient's prothrombin response. Acquired or inherited warfarin resistance is rare, but should be suspected if large daily doses of warfarin are required to maintain a patient's PT/INR within a normal therapeutic range.

Dosage adjustment: Base dosage adjustment on PT/INR determinations.

Duration of therapy: In general, anticoagulant therapy should be continued until the danger of thrombosis and embolism has passed.

See Monitoring for more information.

Conversion from heparin therapy: Because the anticoagulant effect of warfarin is delayed, heparin is preferred initially for rapid anticoagulation. Conversion to warfarin may begin concomitantly with heparin therapy or may be delayed 3 to 6 days. To ensure continuous anticoagulation, it is advisable to continue full-dose heparin therapy and overlap warfarin therapy with heparin for 4 to 5 days, until warfarin has produced the desired therapeutic response as determined by PT/INR. When warfarin has produced the desired PT/INR or prothrombin activity, heparin may be discontinued. Warfarin may increase the activated partial thromboplastin time (aPTT) test, even in the absence of heparin. A severe elevation (more than 50 seconds) in aPTT with a PT/INR in the desired range has been identified as an indication of increased risk of postoperative hemorrhage. During initial therapy with warfarin, the interference with heparin anticoagulation is of minimal clinical significance.

• *Monitoring* – As heparin may affect the PT/INR, patients receiving both heparin and warfarin should have blood for PT/INR determination drawn at least 5 hours after the last intravenous (IV) bolus dose of heparin, 4 hours after cessation of a continuous IV infusion of heparin, or 24 hours after the last subcutaneous heparin injection.

Missed dose: The anticoagulant effect of warfarin persists beyond 24 hours. If the patient forgets to take the prescribed dose of warfarin at the scheduled time, the dose should be taken as soon as possible on the same day. The patient should not take the missed dose by doubling the daily dose to make up for missed doses, but should refer back to his or her health care provider.

Off-label dosing –

Primary venous thromboembolism prophylaxis in cancer patients: [4] = Insufficient documentation. 1 mg orally each day, adjusted to maintain an international normalized ratio (INR) of 1.3 to 1.9.

In the one published clinical trial to date, treatment was initiated either concurrently with chemotherapy or within 4 weeks of starting chemotherapy and was continued until 1 week after chemotherapy was completed. The mean daily dose was 2.6 mg, and the mean duration of warfarin therapy was 181 days. INR was checked every 2 weeks during the first 6 weeks of therapy, and then approximately every 2 to 3 weeks when patients received chemotherapy.

Venous thromboembolism prophylaxis in cancer patients with central venous catheter: [4] = Insufficient documentation. 1 mg per day orally as a fixed dose.

In clinical trials, therapy was continued either for 90 days or until the CVC was removed, the patient died, or the patient developed a symptomatic, radiographically confirmed CVC-associated thrombosis.

➤*Children:*

Off-label dosing –

30 days and older: The following recommendations are to achieve an INR between 2 and 3.

• *Usual dose* – Approximately 0.1 mg/kg once daily; range, 0.05 to 0.34 mg/kg/day.

Warfarin Sodium Oral Unlabeled Dosing in Children

	Loading dose (day 1)
Baseline INR 1 to 1.3	0.2 mg/kg/dose (maximum dose, 10 mg)
	Loading dose (days 2 to 4)
INR 1.1 to 1.3	Repeat day 1 loading dose
INR 1.4 to 1.9	50% of day 1 loading dose
INR 2 to 3	50% of day 1 loading dose
INR 3.1 to 3.5	25% of day 1 loading dose
INR greater than 3.5	Hold doses until INR is less than 3.5 and restart according to maintenance dose guidelines
	Maintenance dose
INR 1.1 to 1.4	Increase previous dose by 20%
INR 1.5 to 1.9	Increase previous dose by 10%
INR 2 to 3	No change
INR 3.1 to 3.5	Decrease previous dose by 10%
INR greater than 3.5	Hold doses until INR is less than 3.5 and restart at 20% less than the last dose

➤*Elderly:* Lower initiation and maintenance doses of warfarin are recommended. (See Warnings/Precautions.)

➤*Management of nontherapeutic INRs:*

Management of Nontherapeutic INRs

INR	Significant bleeding	Rapid reversal	Intervention
< 5	No	No	Lower or omit a dose; resume therapy at lower dose when INR is in therapeutic range. If the INR is only minimally greater than the therapeutic range, no dose reduction may be required.

WARFARIN SODIUM — ORAL

Management of Nontherapeutic INRs			
INR	Significant bleeding	Rapid reversal	Intervention
≥ 5 but < 9	No	No	Omit next few doses, monitor INR more frequently, resume therapy at a lower dose when INR is in the therapeutic range.
	Yes	No	Omit dose, give ≤ 5 mg of vitamin K_1 orally.
	Yes	Yes	Give 2 to 4 mg of vitamin K_1 orally, decrease in INR within 24 hours. If INR is still high, give additional dose of 1 to 2 mg of vitamin K_1 orally.
≥ 9	No	No	Hold warfarin therapy, administer 5 to 10 mg of vitamin K_1 orally; decrease in INR within 24 to 48 hours; monitor INR frequently, repeat dose if necessary. Resume therapy at lower dose when INR is in therapeutic range.
Serious bleeding at any elevation of INR	Yes	Yes	Hold warfarin therapy. Give 10 mg of vitamin K_1 slow IV infusion. May repeat dose every 12 hours, supplement with plasma or prothrombin complex concentrate.
Life-threatening bleeding	Yes	Yes	Hold warfarin therapy. Give prothrombin complex concentrate supplemented with 10 mg of vitamin K_1 slow IV. Repeat if necessary.

➤*Monitoring:*

Post-MI – In most health care settings, moderate- and low-risk patients with an MI should be treated with aspirin alone. In health care settings in which meticulous INR monitoring is standard and routinely accessible, for both high- and low-risk patients after MI, long-term (up to 4 years), high-intensity oral warfarin (target INR, 3.5; range, 3 to 4) without concomitant aspirin or moderate-intensity oral warfarin (target INR, 2.5; range, 2 to 3) with aspirin is recommended. For high-risk patients with MI, including those with a large anterior MI, those with significant heart failure, those with intracardiac thrombus visible on echocardiography, and those with a history of thromboembolic event, therapy with combined moderate-intensity (INR, 2 to 3) oral warfarin plus low-dose aspirin (100 mg/day or less) for 3 months after the MI is suggested. The 7th ACCP recommends an INR of 2.5 to 3.5 to prevent recurrent MI.

Acute MI – The 7th ACCP recommends an INR of 2 to 3.

Atrial fibrillation – Either moderately high INR (2 to 4.5) or low INR (1.4 to 3). The 7th ACCP recommends an INR of 2 to 3.

Mechanical and bioprosthetic heart valves – For patients with a St. Jude Medical (St. Paul, MN) bileaflet valve in the aortic position, a target INR of 2.5 (range, 2 to 3) is recommended. For patients with tilting disk valves and bileaflet mechanical valves in the mitral position, the 7th ACCP recommends a target INR of 3 (range, 2.5 to 3.5). For patients with caged ball or caged disk valves, a target INR of 2.5 (range, 2 to 3) in combination with aspirin 75 to 100 mg/day is recommended. For patients with bioprosthetic valves, warfarin therapy with a target INR of 2.5 (range, 2 to 3) is recommended for valves in the mitral position and is suggested for valves in the aortic position for the first 3 months after valve insertion.

Venous thromboembolism (including deep vein thrombosis and pulmonary embolism) – For patients with a first episode of deep vein thrombosis (DVT) or pulmonary embolism secondary to a transient (reversible) risk factor, treatment with warfarin for 3 months is recommended. For patients with a first episode of idiopathic DVT or pulmonary embolism, warfarin is recommended for at least 6 to 12 months. For patients with 2 or more episodes of documented DVT or pulmonary embolism, indefinite treatment with warfarin is suggested. For patients with a first episode of DVT or pulmonary embolism who have documented antiphospholipid antibodies or who have 2 or more thrombophilic conditions, treatment for 12 months is recommended and indefinite therapy is suggested. For patients with a first episode of DVT or pulmonary embolism who have documented deficiency of antithrombin, deficiency of protein C or S, or the factor V Leiden or prothrombin 20210 gene mutation, homocystinemia, or high factor VIII levels (more than 90th percentile of normal), treatment for 6 to 12 months is recommended and indefinite therapy is suggested for idiopathic thrombosis. The risk-benefit should be reassessed periodically in patients who receive indefinite anticoagulant treatment. The dose of warfarin should be adjusted to maintain a target INR of 2.5 (INR range, 2 to 3) for all treatment durations. These recommendations are supported by the 7th ACCP guidelines.

Recurrent systemic embolism and other indications – A moderate dose regimen (INR, 2 to 3) is recommended.

➤*Storage/Stability:* Store at 15° to 30°C (59° to 86°F). Protect from light.

Actions

➤*Pharmacology:* Warfarin and other coumarin anticoagulants act by inhibiting the synthesis of vitamin K–dependent clotting factors, which include factors II, VII, IX, and X, and the anticoagulant proteins C and S.

The resultant in vivo effect is a sequential depression of factor VII, protein C, factor IX, protein S, and factors X and II activities. Vitamin K is an essential cofactor for the postribosomal synthesis of the vitamin K–dependent clotting factors. The vitamin promotes the biosynthesis of γ-carboxyglutamic acid residues in the proteins, which are essential for biological activity.

Warfarin is thought to interfere with clotting factor synthesis by inhibition of the C1 subunit of the vitamin K epoxide reductase (VKORC1) enzyme complex, thereby reducing the regeneration of vitamin K_1 epoxide. The degree of depression is dependent upon the dosage administeredand in part by the patient's VKORC1 genotype. Therapeutic doses of warfarin decrease the total amount of the active form of each vitamin K–dependent clotting factor made by the liver by approximately 30% to 50%.

Anticoagulants have no direct effect on an established thrombus, nor do they reverse ischemic tissue damage. However, once a thrombus has occurred, the goal of anticoagulant treatment is to prevent further extension of the formed clot and prevent secondary thromboembolic complications that may result in serious and possibly fatal sequelae.

Warfarin is a racemic mixture of the R- and S-enantiomers. The S-enantiomer exhibits 2 to 5 times more anticoagulant activity than the R-enantiomer in humans, but generally has a more rapid clearance.

➤*Pharmacokinetics:*

Absorption – Warfarin is essentially completely absorbed after oral administration with peak concentration generally attained within the first 4 hours.

An anticoagulation effect generally occurs within 24 hours after drug administration. However, peak anticoagulant effect may be delayed 72 to 96 hours. The duration of action of a single dose of racemic warfarin is 2 to 5 days. The effects of warfarin may become more pronounced as effects of daily maintenance doses overlap.

Distribution – There are no differences in the apparent volumes of distribution after IV and oral administration of single doses of warfarin. Warfarin distributes into a relatively small apparent volume of distribution of about 0.14 L/kg. A distribution phase lasting 6 to 12 hours is distinguishable after rapid IV or oral administration of an aqueous solution. Using a one-compartment model and assuming complete bioavailability, estimates of the volumes of distribution of R- and S-warfarin are similar to each other and to that of the racemate. Concentrations in fetal plasma approach the maternal values, but warfarin has not been found in human milk. Approximately 99% of the drug is bound to plasma proteins.

Metabolism – The elimination of warfarin is almost entirely by metabolism. Warfarin is stereoselectively metabolized by hepatic microsomal enzymes (CYP-450) to inactive hydroxylated metabolites (predominant route) and by reductases to reduced metabolites (warfarin alcohols). The warfarin alcohols have minimal anticoagulant activity. The metabolites are principally excreted into the urine, and to a lesser extent into the bile. The metabolites of warfarin that have been identified include dehydrowarfarin, 2 diastereoisomer alcohols, and 4-, 6-, 7-, 8- and 10-hydroxywarfarin. The CYP-450 isozymes involved in the metabolism of warfarin include 2C9, 2C19, 2C8, 2C18, 1A2, and 3A4. 2C9 is likely to be the principal form of human liver P-450, which modulates the in vivo anticoagulant activity of warfarin.

Excretion – The terminal half-life of warfarin after a single dose is approximately 1 week; however, the effective half-life ranges from 20 to 60 hours, with a mean of about 40 hours. The clearance of R-warfarin is generally half that of S-warfarin; thus, as the volumes of distribution are similar, the half-life of R-warfarin is longer than that of S-warfarin. The half-life of R-warfarin ranges from 37 to 89 hours, while that of S-warfarin ranges from 21 to 43 hours. Studies with radiolabeled drug have demonstrated that up to 92% of the orally administered dose is recovered in urine. Very little warfarin is excreted unchanged in urine. Urinary excretion is in the form of metabolites.

Special populations –

Hepatic function impairment: Hepatic function impairment can potentiate the response to warfarin through impaired synthesis of clotting factors and decreased metabolism of warfarin.

Elderly: Patients 60 years of age and older appear to exhibit greater than expected PT/INR response to the anticoagulant effects of warfarin. The cause of the increased sensitivity to the anticoagulant effects of warfarin in this age group is unknown. This increased anticoagulant effect from warfarin may be due to a combination of pharmacokinetic and pharmacodynamic factors. Racemic warfarin clearance may be unchanged or reduced with increasing age. Limited information suggests there is no difference in the clearance of S-warfarin in elderly subjects versus younger subjects. However, there may be a slight decrease in the clearance of R-warfarin in elderly subjects as compared with younger subjects. Therefore, as patient age increases, a lower dose of warfarin is usually required to produce a therapeutic level of anticoagulation.

Race: Asian patients may require lower initiation and maintenance doses of warfarin. One noncontrolled study conducted in 151 Chinese outpatients reported a mean daily warfarin requirement of 3.3 ± 1.4 mg to achieve an INR of 2 to 2.5. These patients were stabilized on warfarin for various indications. Patient age was the most important determinant of warfarin requirement in Chinese patients with a progressively lower warfarin requirement with increasing age.

WARFARIN SODIUM — ORAL

Contraindications

Pregnancy (see Warnings/Precautions); hemorrhagic tendencies or blood dyscrasias; recent or contemplated surgery of the CNS, eye, or traumatic surgery resulting in large open surfaces; bleeding tendencies associated with active ulceration or overt bleeding of: the GI, GU, or respiratory tracts; cerebrovascular hemorrhage; aneurysms-cerebral, dissecting aorta; pericarditis and pericardial effusions, or bacterial endocarditis; threatened abortion, eclampsia and preeclampsia; inadequate laboratory facilities; unsupervised patients with senility, alcoholism, or psychosis or other lack of patient cooperation; spinal puncture and other diagnostic or therapeutic procedures with potential for uncontrollable bleeding; major regional, lumbar block anesthesia, malignant hypertension; known hypersensitivity to warfarin or to any other components of this product.

Warnings/Precautions

➤*Hemorrhage/Necrosis:* The most serious risks associated with anticoagulant therapy with warfarin are hemorrhage in any tissue or organ and, less frequently (less than 0.1%), necrosis and/or gangrene of skin and other tissues. Observe increased caution when warfarin is administered in the presence of any predisposing condition for which added risk of hemorrhage, necrosis, and/or gangrene is present.Hemorrhage and necrosis have in some cases been reported to result in death or permanent disability. Necrosis appears to be associated with local thrombosis and usually appears within a few days of the start of anticoagulant therapy. In severe cases of necrosis, treatment through debridement or amputation of the affected tissue, limb, breast, or penis has been reported. Careful diagnosis is required to determine whether necrosis is caused by an underlying disease. Discontinue warfarin therapy when warfarin is suspected to be the cause of developing necrosis and consider heparin therapy for anticoagulation. Although various treatments have been attempted, no treatment for necrosis has been considered uniformly effective. See the following sections for information on predisposing conditions. These and other risks associated with anticoagulant therapy must be weighed against the risk of thrombosis or embolization in untreated cases.

➤*Atheroemboli/Microemboli:* Anticoagulation therapy with warfarin may enhance the release of atheromatous plaque emboli, thereby increasing the risk of complications from systemic cholesterol microembolization, including "purple toes syndrome." Discontinuation of warfarin therapy is recommended when such phenomena are observed.

Systemic atheroemboli and cholesterol microemboli can present with a variety of signs and symptoms, including purple toes syndrome; livedo reticularis; rash; gangrene; abrupt and intense pain in the leg, foot, or toes; foot ulcers; myalgia; penile gangrene; abdominal pain; flank or back pain; hematuria; renal function impairment; hypertension; cerebral ischemia; spinal cord infarction; pancreatitis; symptoms simulating polyarteritis; or any other sequelae of vascular compromise due to embolic occlusion. The most commonly involved visceral organs are the kidneys, followed by the pancreas, spleen, and liver. Some cases have progressed to necrosis or death.

➤*Purple toes syndrome:* Purple toes syndrome is a complication of oral anticoagulation characterized by a dark, purplish or mottled color of the toes, usually occurring between 3 to 10 weeks, or later, after the initiation of therapy with warfarin or related compounds. Major features of this syndrome include purple color of plantar surfaces and sides of the toes that blanches on moderate pressure and fades with elevation of the legs, pain and tenderness of the toes, and waxing and waning of the color over time. While the purple toes syndrome is reported to be reversible, some cases progress to gangrene or necrosis, which may require debridement of the affected area or may lead to amputation.

➤*Heparin-induced thrombocytopenia:* Warfarin should be used with caution in patients with heparin-induced thrombocytopenia and deep vein thrombosis (DVT). Cases of venous limb ischemia, necrosis, and gangrene have occurred in patients with heparin-induced thrombocytopenia and DVT when heparin treatment was discontinued and warfarin therapy was started or continued. In some patients, sequelae have included amputation of the involved area and/or death.

➤*Laboratory control:* The PT reflects the depression of vitamin K–dependent factors VII, X, and II. A system of standardizing the PT in oral anticoagulant control was introduced by the World Health Organization in 1983. It is based upon the determination of an INR, which provides a common basis for communication of PT results and interpretations of therapeutic ranges. Determine PT daily after the administration of the initial dose until PT/INR results stabilize in the therapeutic range. Base intervals between subsequent PT/INR determinations upon the health care provider's judgment of the patient's reliability and response to warfarin in order to maintain the individual within the therapeutic range. Acceptable intervals for PT/INR determinations are normally within the range of 1 to 4 weeks after a stable dosage has been determined. To ensure adequate control, it is recommended that additional PT tests are done when other warfarin products are interchanged with warfarin tablets, as well as whenever other medications are initiated, discontinued, or taken irregularly.

Safety and efficacy of warfarin therapy can be improved by increasing the quality of laboratory control. Reports suggest that in usual care monitoring, patients are in therapeutic range only 33% to 64% of the time. Time in therapeutic range is significantly greater (56% to 93%) in patients managed by anticoagulation clinics, among self-testing and self-monitoring patients, and in patients managed with the help of computer programs. Self-testing patients had fewer bleeding events than patients in usual care.

➤*Enhanced anticoagulant effects:* Endogenous factors that may be responsible for increased PT/INR response include blood dyscrasias, cancer, collagen vascular disease, congestive heart failure (CHF), diarrhea, elevated temperature, hepatic disorders (eg, infectious hepatitis, jaundice), hyperthyroidism, poor nutritional state, steatorrhea, and vitamin K deficiency.

➤*Decreased anticoagulant effects:* Endogenous factors that may be responsible for decreasing the PT/INR response include edema, hereditary coumarin resistance, hyperlipidemia, hypothyroidism, and nephrotic syndrome.

➤*Hypersensitivity reactions:* Minor and severe allergic/hypersensitivity reactions and anaphylactic reactions have been reported.

➤*Special risk:*

Considerations for increased bleeding risk – Warfarin is a narrow therapeutic range (index) drug, and additional caution should be observed when warfarin is administered to certain patients. Reported risk factors for bleeding include high intensity of anticoagulation (INR more than 4), 65 years of age or older, highly variable INRs, history of GI bleeding, hypertension, cerebrovascular disease, serious heart disease, anemia, malignancy, trauma, renal function impairment, concomitant drugs, and long duration of warfarin therapy. Identification of risk factors for bleeding and certain genetic variations in CYP2CP and VKORC1 in a patient may increase the need for more frequent INR monitoring and the use of lower warfarin doses. Bleeding is more likely to occur during the starting period and with a higher dose of warfarin (resulting in a higher INR).

Intramuscular (IM) injections of concomitant medications should be confined to the upper extremities, which permits easy access for manual compression, inspections for bleeding, and use of pressure bandages.

The decision to administer anticoagulants in the following conditions must be based upon clinical judgment in which the risks of anticoagulant therapy are weighed against the benefits: lactation; severe to moderate hepatic or renal function impairment; infectious diseases or disturbances of intestinal flora: sprue, antibiotic therapy; trauma that may result in internal bleeding; surgery or trauma resulting in large exposed raw surfaces; indwelling catheters; severe to moderate hypertension; polycythemia vera; vasculitis; severe diabetes.

Protein C deficiency: Hereditary or acquired deficiencies of protein C or its cofactor, protein S, have been associated with tissue necrosis following warfarin administration. Not all patients with these conditions develop necrosis, and tissue necrosis occurs in patients without these deficiencies. Inherited resistance to activated protein C has been described in many patients with venous thromboembolic disorders but has not yet been evaluated as a risk factor for tissue necrosis. The risk associated with these conditions, both for recurrent thrombosis and for adverse reactions, is difficult to evaluate because it does not appear to be the same for everyone. Decisions about testing and therapy must be made on an individual basis. It has been reported that concomitant anticoagulation therapy with heparin for 5 to 7 days during initiation of therapy with warfarin may minimize the incidence of tissue necrosis. Discontinue warfarin therapy when warfarin is suspected to be the cause of developing necrosis; heparin therapy may be considered for anticoagulation. Patients with CHF may exhibit greater than expected PT/INR response to warfarin, thereby requiring more frequent laboratory monitoring and reduced doses of warfarin.

➤*Pregnancy: Category X* per manufacturer's prescribing information. *Category D* per Briggs' *Drugs in Pregnancy and Lactation*.

Warfarin is contraindicated in women who are or may become pregnant because the drug passes through the placental barrier and may cause fatal hemorrhage to the fetus in utero. Furthermore, there have been reports of birth malformations in children born to mothers who have been treated with warfarin during pregnancy.

Embryopathy characterized by nasal hypoplasia with or without stippled epiphyses (chondrodysplasia punctata) has been reported in pregnant women exposed to warfarin during the first trimester. CNS abnormalities, including dorsal midline dysplasia characterized by agenesis of the corpus callosum, Dandy-Walker malformation, and midline cerebellar atrophy, also have been reported. Ventral midline dysplasia, characterized by optic atrophy, and eye abnormalities have been observed. Mental retardation, blindness, and other CNS abnormalities have been reported in association with second- and third-trimester exposure. Although rare, teratogenic reports following in utero exposure to warfarin include urinary tract anomalies such as single kidney, asplenia, anencephaly, spina bifida, cranial nerve palsy, hydrocephalus, cardiac defects and congenital heart disease, polydactyly, deformities of toes, diaphragmatic hernia, corneal leukoma, cleft palate, cleft lip, schizencephaly, and microcephaly.

Spontaneous abortion and stillbirth are known to occur and a higher risk of fetal mortality is associated with the use of warfarin. Low birth weight and growth retardation have also been reported.

Carefully evaluate women of childbearing potential who are candidates for anticoagulant therapy and critically review the indications with the patient. If the patient becomes pregnant while taking this drug, apprise her of the potential risks to the fetus, and discuss the possibility of termination of the pregnancy in light of those risks.

➤*Lactation:* Based on very limited published data, warfarin has not been detected in the breast milk of mothers treated with warfarin. The same limited published data report that some breast-fed infants whose mothers were treated with warfarin had prolonged PTs, although not as prolonged as those of the mothers. Undertake the decision to breast-feed only after careful consideration of the available alternatives. Carefully monitor women who are breast-feeding and anticoagulated with warfarin so that recommended PT/INR values are not exceeded. It is prudent to perform coagulation tests and to evaluate vitamin K status before advising women taking warfarin to breast-feed. Effects in premature infants have not been evaluated.

➤*Children:* Safety and effectiveness in children younger than 18 years of age have not been established in randomized, controlled clinical trials. How-

WARFARIN SODIUM — ORAL

ever, the use of warfarin in children is well-documented for the prevention and treatment of thromboembolic events. Difficulty achieving and maintaining therapeutic PT/INR ranges in children has been reported. More frequent PT/INR determinations are recommended because of possible changing warfarin requirements.

➤*Elderly:* Patients 60 years of age or older appear to exhibit greater than expected PT/INR response to the anticoagulant effects of warfarin. Warfarin is contraindicated in any unsupervised patient with senility. Observe caution with administration of warfarin to elderly patients in any situation or physical condition where added risk of hemorrhage is present. Lower initiation and maintenance doses of warfarin are recommended for elderly patients.

➤*Monitoring:* It cannot be emphasized too strongly that treatment of each patient is a highly individualized matter. Warfarin, a narrow therapeutic range (index) drug, may be affected by factors such as other drugs and dietary vitamin K. Control dosage by periodic determinations of PT/INR or other suitable coagulation tests. Determinations of whole blood clotting and bleeding times are not effective measures for control of therapy. Heparin prolongs the one-stage PT.

Patients with CHF may exhibit greater than expected PT/INR response to warfarin, thereby requiring more frequent laboratory monitoring and reduced doses of warfarin.

Periodic determination of PT/INR is essential. Numerous factors, alone or in combination, including changes in diet, medications, botanicals (herbals), and genetic variations in the CYP2C9 and VKORC1 enzymes, may influence the response of the patient to warfarin.

It is generally good practice to monitor the patient's response with additional PT/INR determinations in the period immediately after discharge from the hospital and whenever other medications, including herbals, are initiated, discontinued, or taken irregularly.

Because a patient may be exposed to a combination of endogenous and exogenous factors, the net effect of warfarin on PT/INR response may be unpredictable. More frequent PT/INR monitoring is therefore advisable. Medications of unknown interaction with coumarins are best regarded with caution. When these medications are started or stopped, more frequent PT/INR monitoring is advisable.

Very carefully monitor women who are breast-feeding and anticoagulated with warfarin so that recommended PT/INR values are not exceeded. It is prudent to perform coagulation tests and to evaluate vitamin K status before advising women taking warfarin to breast-feed.

Drug Interactions

Careful monitoring and appropriate dosage adjustments will usually permit combination therapy. Critical times during therapy will usually permit combination therapy. Critical times during therapy occur when an interacting drug is added or discontinued from a patient stabilized on anticoagulants.

Oral Anticoagulant Drug Interactions

Precipitant drug	Object drug[a]		Description
Acetaminophen	Anticoagulants	⬆	These agents may increase the anticoagulant effect. The risk of bleeding may be increased. The mechanism of the interaction is unknown or complicated.
Androgens			
Anabolic steroids (eg, danazol, oxandrolone, oxymethalone, stanozol)			
Anticoagulants (eg, argatroban, bivalirudin, dicumarol, lepirudin)			
Antineoplastic agents (eg, capecitabine, cyclophosphamide, fluorouracil, gefitinib)			
Beta-blockers (eg, atenolol, propranolol)			
Cephalosporins, parenteral (eg, cefamandole, cefazolin, cefoperazone, cefotetan, cefoxitin, ceftriaxone)			
Chenodiol			
Chlorpropamide			
Cisapride			
Dextran			
Dextrothyroxine			
Diazoxide			

Oral Anticoagulant Drug Interactions

Precipitant drug	Object drug[a]		Description
Disulfiram	Anticoagulants	⬆	These agents may increase the anticoagulant effect. The risk of bleeding may be increased. The mechanism of the interaction is unknown or complicated.
Felbamate			
Fibric acids (eg, fenofibrate, gemfibrozil)			
Flutamide			
Glucagon			
Halothane			
Heparin			
Influenza virus vaccine			
Isonazid			
Levamisole			
Methyldopa			
Methylphenidate			
Mineral oil			
NSAIDs[b], COX-2 selective			
Orlistat			
Pentoxifylline			
Propoxyphene			
Quinolines (eg, ciprofloxacin, levofloxacin, norfloxacin, ofloxacin)			
Ropinirole			
Selective COX-2 inhibitors (eg, celecoxib, rofecoxib, valdecoxib)			
SSRIs[b,c] (ie, fluoxetine, fluvoxamine, paroxetine, sertraline)			
Tamoxifen			
Thrombolytics (eg, streptokinase, tissue plasminogen activator, urokinase)			
Thyroid hormones (eg, levothyroxine, liothyonine, thyroid)			
Tolbutamide			
Tolterodine			
Tramadol			
Trastuzumab			
Zafirlukast			
Zileuton			
Allopurinol	Anticoagulants	⬆	These agents may increase the anticoagulant effect of warfarin by inhibition of the anticoagulant's hepatic metabolism. The risk of bleeding may be increased.
Amiodarone			
Azole antifungals (eg, fluconazole, itraconazole, miconazole[d])			
Chloramphenicol			
Cimetidine			
HMG-CoA reductase inhibitors (ie, fluvastatin, lovastatin, simvastatin)			
Isofamide[e]			
Leflunomide			

WARFARIN SODIUM — ORAL

Oral Anticoagulant Drug Interactions

Precipitant drug	Object drug[a]		Description
Metronidazole	Anticoagulants	↑	These agents may increase the anticoagulant effect of warfarin by inhibition of the anticoagulant's hepatic metabolism. The risk of bleeding may be increased.
Omeprazole			
Phenylbutazone[e]			
Propafenone			
Proton pump inhibitors (eg, esomeprazole, lansoprazole, omeprazole, pentoprazole, rabeprazole)			
Quinidine			
Quinine			
Sulfonamides (eg, sulfamethazole, sulfisoxazole, trimethoprim, sulfamethoxazole)			
Sulfinpyrazone			
Macrolide antibiotics (eg, azithromycin, clarithromycin, erythromycin)	Anticoagulants	↑	These agents may increase the anticoagulant effect by reducing body clearance of warfarin. The risk of bleeding may be increased.
Loop diuretics (ie, ethacrynic acid, furosemide)	Anticoagulants	↑	These agents may increase the anticoagulant effect of warfarin caused by displacement from binding sites. The risk of bleeding may be increased.
Meflaquine			
Nalidixic acid			
Valproate			
Aminoglycosides, oral	Anticoagulants	↑	These agents may increase the anticoagulant effect of warfarin through an interference with vitamin K. The risk of bleeding may be increased.
Fish oil			
Neomycin			
Tetracyclines (eg, doxycycline, tetracycline)			
Vitamin E			
Aminosalicylic acid	Anticoagulants	↑	These agents may increase the anticoagulant effect of warfarin and increase the risk of bleeding because of effects on platelet function, and, in the case of NSAIDs, GI irritant effects.
Diflunisal			
Methylsalicylate ointment, topical			
NSAIDs (eg, diclofenac, fenoprofen, ibuprofen, indomethacin, ketoprofen, ketorolac, mefenamic acid, naproxen, oxaprozin, piroxicam, sulindac)			
Olsalazine			
Penicillins, high-dose IV (eg, penicillin G, piperacillin, ticarcillin)			
Salicylates			
Ticlopidine			

Oral Anticoagulant Drug Interactions

Precipitant drug	Object drug[a]		Description
Alcohol[f]	Anticoagulants	↑↓	Increased and decreased PT/INR responses have been reported. May increase or decrease the anticoagulant effect of warfarin; the mechanism is unknown.
Atorvastatin			
Chloral hydrate			
Cholestyramine[g]			
Corticosteroids			
Cyclophosphamide			
Methimazole			
Moricizine			
Hydantoins (eg, phenytoin)			
Pravastatin			
Prednisone			
Propylthiouracil			
Ranitidine			
Ascorbic acid, high doses	Anticoagulants	↓	These agents may decrease the anticoagulant effect of warfarin. The mechanism of the interaction is unknown.
Chlordiazepoxide			
Clozapine			
Contraceptives, oral[h]			
Cyclosporine[i]			
Estrogens			
Ethchlorvynol			
Griseofluvin			
Haloperidol			
Isotretinoin			
Menthol			
Meprobamate			
Mesalamine			
Paraldehyde			
Protease inhibitors (eg, indinavir, ritonavir)			
Raloxifene			
Ribavirin			
Trazodone			
Aminoglutethimide	Anticoagulants	↓	These agents may decrease the anticoagulant effect of warfarin (because of the induction of the anticoagulant's hepatic microsomal enzyme).
Aprepitant			
Barbituates (eg, aminobarbital, butabarbital, pentobarbital, phenobarbital, secobarbital)			
Bosentan			
Carbamazepine			
Dicloxacillin[j]			
Glutethimide			
Mitotane			
Nafcillin[j]			
Nevirapine			
Primidone			
Rifamycins			
Terbinafine			

WARFARIN SODIUM — ORAL

Oral Anticoagulant Drug Interactions			
Precipitant drug	Object drug[a]		Description
Spironolactone[k]	Anticoagulants	↓	These agents may decrease the anticoagulant effect of warfarin by various mechanisms (eg, possible decreased absorption or increased elimination)
Sucralfate			
Thiazide diuretics (eg, chlorthalidone)[k]			
Thiopurines (eg, azathioprine)[l]			
Ubiquinone			
Vitamin K[m]			

[a] ↑ = object drug increased; ↓ = object drug decreased.
[b] NSAIDs = nonsteroidal anti-inflammatory drugs; SSRIs = selective serotonin reuptake inhibitors.
[c] Bleeding has been reported with fluoxetine alone.
[d] Miconazole includes both intravaginal and systemic formulations.
[e] May also displace the anticoagulant from protein binding sites.
[f] Chronic consumption may increase the clearance of the anticoagulant; moderate to small doses do not alter the anticoagulant effect.
[g] Reduced anticoagulant absorption and possibly increased elimination.
[h] Rarely, increased risk of thromboembolism; this is in contrast to intended effect.
[i] Cyclosporine levels may also be decreased.
[j] Associated with warfarin resistance.
[k] Diuretic-induced hemoconcentration of clotting factors.
[l] Thiopurine-induced increase in synthesis or activation of prothrombin.
[m] Vitamin K overcomes interference of vitamin K–dependent clotting factors by anticoagulants.

➤*Herbal medicines:* Exercise caution when herbal medicines are taken concomitantly with warfarin.

Specific herbals reported to affect warfarin therapy include the following:

- Bromelains, danshen, dong quai (*Angelica sinensis*), garlic, *Ginkgo biloba*, ginseng, and cranberry products are associated most often with an increase in the effects of warfarin.
- Coenzyme Q_{10} (ubidecarenone) and St. John's wort are associated most often with a decrease in the effects of warfarin. Conversely, other herbals may have coagulant properties when taken alone or may decrease the effects of warfarin.

Some herbals may cause bleeding events when taken alone (eg, garlic, *Ginkgo biloba*) and may have anticoagulant, antiplatelet, and/or fibrinolytic properties. These effects would be expected to be additive to the anticoagulant effects of warfarin. Conversely, other herbals may have coagulant properties when taken alone or may decrease the effects of warfarin.

Some herbals that may affect coagulation are listed in the following table; however, this list should not be considered all-inclusive. Many herbals have several common names and scientific names. The most widely recognized common botanical names are listed.

Herbals That Contain Coumarins With Potential Anticoagulant Effects		
Agrimony[a]	Cassia[b]	Parsley
Alfalfa	Celery	Passion flower
Angelica (dong quai)	Chamomile (German and Roman)	Prickly ash (Northern)
Aniseed	Dandelion[b]	Quassia
Arnica	Fenugreek	Red clover
Asafoetida	Horse chestnut	Sweet clover
Bogbean[c]	Horseradish	Sweet woodruff
Boldo	Licorice[b]	Tonka beans
Buchu	Meadowsweet[c]	Wild carrot
Capsicum[d]	Nettle	Wild lettuce

[a] Contains coumarins, has antiplatelet properties, and may have coagulant properties because of possible vitamin K content.
[b] Contains coumarins and has antiplatelet properties.
[c] Contains coumarins and salicylates.
[d] Contains coumarins and has fibrinolytic properties.

Miscellaneous Herbals With Anticoagulant Properties	
Bladder wrack (*Fucus*)	Pau d'arco

Herbals That Contain Salicylate and/or Have Antiplatelet Properties		
Agrimony[a]	Dandelion[b]	Meadowsweet[c]
Aloe gel	Feverfew	Onion[d]
Aspen	Garlic[d]	Policosanol
Black cohosh	German sarsaparilla	Poplar
Black haw	Ginger	Senega
Bogbean[c]	*Ginkgo biloba*	Tamarind
Cassia[b]	Ginseng (*Panax*)[d]	Willow
Clove	Licorice[b]	Wintergreen

[a] Contains coumarins, has antiplatelet properties, and may have coagulant properties because of possible vitamin K content. Contains salicylate and has anticoagulant properties.
[b] Contains coumarins and has antiplatelet properties.
[c] Contains coumarins and salicylates.
[d] Has antiplatelet and fibrinolytic properties.

Herbals With Fibrinolytic Properties		
Bromelains	Garlic[b]	Inositol nicotinate
Capsicum[a]	Ginseng (*Panax*)[b]	Onion[b]

[a] Contains coumarins and has fibrinolytic properties.
[b] Has antiplatelet and fibrinolytic properties.

Herbals with Coagulant Properties	
Agrimony[a]	Mistletoe
Goldenseal	Yarrow

[a] Contains coumarins, has antiplatelet properties, and may have coagulant properties because of possible vitamin K content.

➤*Drug/Food interactions:* Vitamin K–rich vegetables may decrease the anticoagulant effects of warfarin by interfering with absorption. Patients should minimize consumption of vitamin K–rich foods (eg, broccoli, spinach, seaweed, turnip greens), nutritional supplements, or enteral nutrition. Mango has been shown to increase warfarin's effect.

Adverse Reactions

➤*Cardiovascular:* Angina syndrome, hypotension, purple toes syndrome, syncope, systemic cholesterol microembolization, vasculitis.

➤*CNS:* Asthenia; coma; dizziness; fatigue; headache; lethargy; loss of consciousness; paresthesia, including feeling cold and chills.

➤*Dermatologic:* Alopecia; necrosis of skin and other tissues; pruritus; rash and dermatitis, including bullous eruptions; urticaria.

➤*GI:* Abdominal pain, including cramping; diarrhea; flatulence/bloating; nausea; taste perversion; vomiting.

➤*GU:* Priapism has been associated with anticoagulant administration; however, a causal relationship has not been established.

➤*Hematologic:* Fatal or nonfatal hemorrhage from any tissue or organ. This is a consequence of the anticoagulant effect. The signs, symptoms, and severity will vary according to the location and degree or extent of the bleeding. Hemorrhagic complications may present as paralysis; paresthesia; headache; chest, abdomen, joint, muscle, or other pain; dizziness; shortness of breath; difficult breathing or swallowing; unexplained swelling; weakness; hypotension; or unexplained shock. Therefore, consider the possibility of hemorrhage in evaluating the condition of any anticoagulated patient with complaints that do not indicate an obvious diagnosis. Bleeding during anticoagulant therapy does not always correlate with PT/INR. Bleeding that occurs when the PT/INR is within the therapeutic range warrants diagnostic investigation because it may unmask a previously unsuspected lesion (eg, tumor, ulcer). Anemia.

➤*Hepatic:* Cholestatic hepatic injury, elevated liver enzymes, hepatitis, jaundice.

➤*Hypersensitivity:* Hypersensitivity/allergic reactions, including anaphylactic reactions.

➤*Respiratory:* Rare events of tracheal or tracheobronchial calcification have been reported in association with long-term warfarin therapy. The clinical significance of this event is unknown.

➤*Miscellaneous:* Chest pain, cold intolerance, edema, fever, malaise, pain, pallor.

Overdosage

➤*Symptoms:* Suspected or overt abnormal bleeding (eg, appearance of blood in stools or urine, excessive bruising or persistent oozing from superficial injuries, excessive menstrual bleeding, hematuria, melena, petechiae) are early manifestations of anticoagulation beyond a safe and satisfactory level.

➤*Treatment:* Excessive anticoagulation with or without bleeding may be controlled by discontinuing warfarin therapy and, if necessary, by administration of oral or parenteral vitamin K_1.

Such use of vitamin K_1 reduces response to subsequent warfarin therapy. Patients may return to a pretreatment thrombotic status following the rapid reversal of a prolonged PT/INR. Resumption of warfarin administration reverses the effect of vitamin K, and a therapeutic PT/INR can again be obtained by careful dosage adjustment. If rapid anticoagulation is indicated, heparin may be preferable for initial therapy.

If minor bleeding progresses to major bleeding, give 5 to 25 mg (rarely up to 50 mg) of parenteral vitamin K_1. In emergency situations of severe hemorrhage, clotting factors can be returned to normal by administering 200 to 500 mL of fresh whole blood or fresh frozen plasma, or by giving commercial factor IX complex.

A risk of hepatitis and other viral diseases is associated with the use of these blood products. Factor IX complex is also associated with an increased risk of thrombosis. Therefore, use these preparations in exceptional or life-threatening bleeding episodes secondary to warfarin overdosage.

Do not use purified factor IX preparations because they cannot increase the levels of prothrombin, factor VII, and factor X, which are also depressed along with the levels of factor IX as a result of warfarin treatment. Packed red blood cells may also be given if significant blood loss has occurred. Carefully monitor infusions of blood or plasma to avoid precipitating pulmonary edema in elderly patients or patients with heart disease.

Patient Information

The objective of anticoagulant therapy is to decrease the clotting ability of the blood so that thrombosis is prevented, while avoiding spontaneous bleed-

WARFARIN SODIUM — ORAL

ing. Effective therapeutic levels with minimal complications are in part dependent upon cooperative and well-instructed patients who communicate effectively with their health care provider.

Advise patients that strict adherence to prescribed dosage schedule is necessary.

Instruct patients not to take or discontinue any other medication, including salicylates (eg, aspirin, topical analgesics) and other nonprescription medications, and herbal products (eg, bromelains, coenzyme Q_{10}, danshen, dong quai, garlic, *Ginkgo biloba*, ginseng, St. John's wort), except on advice of the health care provider.

Instruct patients to avoid alcohol consumption.

Advise patients to not take warfarin during pregnancy and to not become pregnant while taking it.

Advise patients to avoid any activity or sport that may result in traumatic injury.

Advise patients that PT tests and regular visits to their health care provider or clinic are needed to monitor therapy.

Instruct patients to carry identification stating that warfarin is being taken.

If the prescribed dose of warfarin is forgotten, instruct patients to notify their health care provider immediately. Instruct patients to take the dose as soon as possible on the same day, but do not take a double dose of warfarin the next day to make up for missed doses.

The amount of vitamin K in food may affect therapy with warfarin. Advise patients to eat a healthy, balanced diet maintaining a consistent amount of vitamin K. Instruct patients to avoid drastic changes in dietary habits, such as eating large amounts of green leafy vegetables. Instruct patients to avoid intake of cranberry juice or any other cranberry products. Encourage patients to notify health care provider if any of these products are part of their normal diet.

Instruct patients to contact their health care provider to report any illness, such as diarrhea, infection, or fever.

Advise patients to notify their health care provider immediately if any unusual bleeding or symptoms occur. Signs and symptoms of bleeding include pain, swelling, or discomfort; prolonged bleeding from cuts; increased menstrual flow or vaginal bleeding; nosebleeds; bleeding of gums from brushing; unusual bleeding or bruising; red or dark brown urine; red or tar black stools; headache; dizziness; or weakness.

If therapy with warfarin is discontinued, caution patients that the anticoagulant effects of warfarin may persist for about 2 to 5 days.

Inform patients that all warfarin products represent the same medication and should not be taken concomitantly, as overdosage may result.

WARFARIN SODIUM — INJECTION

WARNING

Bleeding risk – Warfarin can cause major or fatal bleeding. Bleeding is more likely to occur during the starting period and with a higher dose (resulting in a higher international normalized ratio [INR]). Risk factors for bleeding include high intensity of anticoagulation (INR of more than 4), 65 years of age and older, highly variable INRs, history of GI bleeding, hypertension, cerebrovascular disease, serious heart disease, anemia, malignancy, trauma, renal function impairment, concomitant drugs, and long duration of warfarin therapy. Regular monitoring of INR should be performed on all treated patients. Those at high risk of bleeding may benefit from more frequent INR monitoring, careful dose adjustment to desired INR, and a shorter duration of therapy. Patients should be instructed about prevention measures to minimize risk of bleeding and to report immediately to health care provider signs and symptoms of bleeding.

Indications

➤*Recurrent myocardial infarction (MI)/thromboembolic event:* To reduce the risk of death, recurrent MI, and thromboembolic events such as stroke or systemic embolization after MI.

➤*Thromboembolic complications:* For the prophylaxis and/or treatment of the thromboembolic complications associated with atrial fibrillation and/or cardiac valve replacement.

➤*Venous thrombosis/pulmonary embolism:* For the prophylaxis and/or treatment of venous thrombosis and its extension, and pulmonary embolism.

Administration and Dosage

➤*General dosing considerations:* Warfarin injection provides an alternate administration route for patients who cannot receive oral drugs. The IV dosages would be the same as those that would be used orally.

The dosage and administration of warfarin must be individualized for each patient according to the particular patient's prothrombin time (PT)/INR response to the drug.

Use of a large loading dose may increase the incidence of hemorrhagic and other complications, does not offer more rapid protection against thrombi formation, and is not recommended.

An INR of more than 4 appears to provide no additional therapeutic benefit in most patients and is associated with a higher risk of bleeding.

Consider lower initiation and maintenance doses for patients with certain genetic variations in CYP2C9 and VKORC1 enzymes, as well as for elderly and/or debilitated patients and patients with a potential to exhibit greater than expected PT/INR response to warfarin.

➤*Adults:*

Anticoagulation –

Initial dosage: 2 to 5 mg daily.

Maintenance dosage: 2 to 10 mg daily. The individual dose and interval should be gauged by the patient's prothrombin response. Acquired or inherited warfarin resistance is rare, but should be suspected if large daily doses of warfarin are required to maintain a patient's PT/INR within a normal therapeutic range.

Duration of therapy: In general, anticoagulant therapy should be continued until the danger of thrombosis and embolism has passed.

See Monitoring for more information.

Conversion from heparin therapy: Since the anticoagulant effect of warfarin is delayed, heparin is preferred initially for rapid anticoagulation. Conversion to warfarin may begin concomitantly with heparin therapy or may be delayed 3 to 6 days. To ensure continuous anticoagulation, it is advisable to continue full-dose heparin therapy and overlap warfarin therapy with heparin for 4 to 5 days, until warfarin has produced the desired therapeutic response as determined by PT/INR. When warfarin has produced the desired PT/INR or prothrombin activity, heparin may be discontinued. Warfarin may increase the activated partial thromboplastin time (aPTT) test, even in the absence of heparin. A severe elevation (more than 50 seconds) in aPTT with a PT/INR in the desired range has been identified as an indication of increased risk of postoperative hemorrhage. During initial therapy with warfarin, the interference with heparin anticoagulation is of minimal clinical significance.

• *Monitoring* – As heparin may affect the PT/INR, patients receiving both heparin and warfarin should have blood for PT/INR determination drawn at least 5 hours after the last intravenous (IV) bolus dose of heparin, 4 hours after cessation of a continuous IV infusion of heparin, or 24 hours after the last subcutaneous heparin injection.

➤*Elderly:* Lower initiation and maintenance doses of warfarin are recommended for elderly patients. (See Warnings/Precautions.)

➤*Hepatic function impairment:* May require dosage adjustments. (See Actions.)

➤*Monitoring:*

Post-MI – In health care settings in which meticulous INR monitoring is standard and routinely accessible, for both high- and low-risk patients after MI, long-term (up to 4 years), high-intensity oral warfarin (target INR, 3.5; range, 3 to 4) without concomitant aspirin or moderate-intensity oral warfarin (target INR, 2.5; range, 2 to 3) with aspirin is recommended. For high-risk patients with MI, including those with a large anterior MI, those with significant heart failure, those with intracardiac thrombus visible on echocardiography, and those with a history of thromboembolic event, therapy with combined moderate-intensity (INR, 2 to 3) oral warfarin plus low-dose aspirin (100 mg/day or less) for 3 months after the MI is suggested.

Atrial fibrillation – Either moderately high INR (2 to 4.5) or low INR (1.4 to 3). The 7th ACCP recommends an INR of 2 to 3.

Mechanical and bioprosthetic heart valves – For patients with a St. Jude Medical (St. Paul, MN) bileaflet valve in the aortic position, a target INR of 2.5 (range, 2 to 3) is recommended. For patients with tilting disk valves and bileaflet mechanical valves in the mitral position, the 7th ACCP recommends a target INR of 3 (range, 2.5 to 3.5). For patients with caged ball or caged disk valves, a target INR of 2.5 (range, 2 to 3) in combination with aspirin 75 to 100 mg/day is recommended. For patients with bioprosthetic valves, warfarin therapy with a target INR of 2.5 (range, 2 to 3) is recommended for valves in the mitral position and is suggested for valves in the aortic position for the first 3 months after valve insertion.

Venous thromboembolism (including deep vein thrombosis and pulmonary embolism) – For patients with a first episode of deep vein thrombosis (DVT) or pulmonary embolism secondary to a transient (reversible) risk factor, treatment with warfarin for 3 months is recommended. For patients with a first episode of idiopathic DVT or pulmonary embolism, warfarin is recommended for at least 6 to 12 months. For patients with 2 or more episodes of documented DVT or pulmonary embolism, indefinite treatment with warfarin is suggested. For patients with a first episode of DVT or pulmonary embolism who have documented antiphospholipid antibodies or who have 2 or more thrombophilic conditions, treatment for 12 months is recommended and indefinite therapy is suggested. For patients with a first episode of DVT or pulmonary embolism who have documented deficiency of antithrombin, deficiency of protein C or S, or the factor V Leiden or prothrombin 20210 gene mutation, homocystinemia, or high factor VIII levels (more than 90th percentile of normal), treatment for 6 to 12 months is recommended and indefinite therapy is suggested for idiopathic thrombosis. The risk-benefit should be reassessed periodically in patients who receive indefinite anticoagulant treatment. The dose of warfarin should be adjusted to maintain a target INR of 2.5 (INR range, 2 to 3) for all treatment durations. These recommendations are supported by the 7th ACCP guidelines.

Recurrent systemic embolism and other indications – A moderate dose regimen (INR, 2 to 3) is recommended for these patients.

➤*Preparation for administration:* Reconstitute the vial with 2.7 mL of sterile water for injection.

➤*Administration:* Administer as a slow bolus injection over 1 to 2 minutes into a peripheral vein. It is not recommended for intramuscular administration.

WARFARIN SODIUM — INJECTION

➤*Storage/Stability:* Store at 15° to 30°C (59° to 86°F). Protect from light. Keep the vial in box until used. After reconstitution, store at 15° to 30°C (59° to 86°F) and use within 4 hours. Do not refrigerate. Discard any unused solution.

Actions

➤*Pharmacology:* Warfarin and other coumarin anticoagulants act by inhibiting the synthesis of vitamin K–dependent clotting factors, which include factors II, VII, IX, and X, and the anticoagulant proteins C and S.

The resultant in vivo effect is a sequential depression of factor VII, protein C, factor IX, protein S, and factors X and II activities. Vitamin K is an essential cofactor for the postribosomal synthesis of the vitamin K–dependent clotting factors. The vitamin promotes the biosynthesis of γ-carboxyglutamic acid residues in the proteins, which are essential for biological activity.

Warfarin is thought to interfere with clotting factor synthesis by inhibition of the C1 subunit of the vitamin K epoxide reductase (VKORC1) enzyme complex, thereby reducing the regeneration of vitamin K_1 epoxide. The degree of depression is dependent upon the dosage administeredand, in part, by the patient's VKORC1 genotype. Therapeutic doses of warfarin decrease the total amount of the active form of each vitamin K–dependent clotting factor made by the liver by approximately 30% to 50%.

Anticoagulants have no direct effect on an established thrombus, nor do they reverse ischemic tissue damage. However, once a thrombus has occurred, the goal of anticoagulant treatment is to prevent further extension of the formed clot and prevent secondary thromboembolic complications, which may result in serious and possibly fatal sequelae.

Warfarin is a racemic mixture of the R- and S-enantiomers. The S-enantiomer exhibits 2 to 5 times more anticoagulant activity than the R-enantiomer in humans, but generally has a more rapid clearance.

➤*Pharmacokinetics:*

Absorption – Warfarin is essentially completely absorbed after oral administration, with peak concentration generally attained within the first 4 hours.

An anticoagulation effect generally occurs within 24 hours after drug administration. However, peak anticoagulant effect may be delayed 72 to 96 hours. The duration of action of a single dose of racemic warfarin is 2 to 5 days. The effects of warfarin may become more pronounced as effects of daily maintenance doses overlap.

Distribution – There are no differences in the apparent volumes of distribution after IV and oral administration of single doses of warfarin solution. Warfarin distributes into a relatively small apparent volume of distribution of about 0.14 L/kg. A distribution phase lasting 6 to 12 hours is distinguishable after rapid IV or oral administration of an aqueous solution. Using a one-compartment model and assuming complete bioavailability, estimates of the volumes of distribution of R- and S-warfarin are similar to each other and to that of the racemate. Concentrations in fetal plasma approach the maternal values, but warfarin has not been found in human milk. Approximately 99% of the drug is bound to plasma proteins.

Metabolism – The elimination of warfarin is almost entirely by metabolism. Warfarin is stereoselectively metabolized by hepatic microsomal enzymes (CYP-450) to inactive hydroxylated metabolites (predominant route) and by reductases to reduced metabolites (warfarin alcohols). The warfarin alcohols have minimal anticoagulant activity. The metabolites are principally excreted into the urine, and to a lesser extent into the bile. The metabolites of warfarin that have been identified include dehydrowarfarin; 2 diastereoisomer alcohols; and 4-, 6-, 7-, 8- and 10-hydroxywarfarin. The CYP-450 isozymes involved in the metabolism of warfarin include 2C9, 2C19, 2C8, 2C18, 1A2, and 3A4. 2C9 is likely to be the principal form of human liver P-450, which modulates the in vivo anticoagulant activity of warfarin.

Excretion – The terminal half-life of warfarin after a single dose is approximately 1 week; however, the effective half-life ranges from 20 to 60 hours, with a mean of about 40 hours. The clearance of R-warfarin is generally half that of S-warfarin; thus, as the volumes of distribution are similar, the half-life of R-warfarin is longer than that of S-warfarin. The half-life of R-warfarin ranges from 37 to 89 hours, while that of S-warfarin ranges from 21 to 43 hours. Studies with radiolabeled drug have demonstrated that up to 92% of the orally administered dose is recovered in urine. Very little warfarin is excreted unchanged in urine. Urinary excretion is in the form of metabolites.

Special populations –

Hepatic function impairment: Hepatic function impairment can potentiate the response to warfarin through impaired synthesis of clotting factors and decreased metabolism of warfarin.

Elderly: Patients 60 years of age or older appear to exhibit greater than expected PT/INR response to the anticoagulant effects of warfarin. The cause of the increased sensitivity to the anticoagulant effects of warfarin in this age group is unknown. This increased anticoagulant effect from warfarin may be due to a combination of pharmacokinetic and pharmacodynamic factors. Racemic warfarin clearance may be unchanged or reduced with increasing age. Limited information suggests there is no difference in the clearance of S-warfarin in elderly subjects versus younger subjects. However, there may be a slight decrease in the clearance of R-warfarin in elderly subjects as compared with younger subjects. Therefore, as patient age increases, a lower dose of warfarin is usually required to produce a therapeutic level of anticoagulation.

Race: Asian patients may require lower initiation and maintenance doses of warfarin. One noncontrolled study conducted in 151 Chinese outpatients reported a mean daily warfarin requirement of 3.3 ± 1.4 mg to achieve an INR of 2 to 2.5. These patients were stabilized on warfarin for various indications. Patient age was the most important determinant of warfarin requirement in Chinese patients with a progressively lower warfarin requirement with increasing age.

Contraindications

Pregnancy (see Warnings/Precautions); hemorrhagic tendencies or blood dyscrasias; recent or contemplated surgery of the CNS, eye, or traumatic surgery resulting in large open surfaces; bleeding tendencies associated with active ulceration or overt bleeding of: the GI, GU, or respiratory tracts; cerebrovascular hemorrhage; aneurysms-cerebral, dissecting aorta; pericarditis and pericardial effusions; bacterial endocarditis; threatened abortion, eclampsia, and preeclampsia; inadequate laboratory facilities; unsupervised patients with senility, alcoholism, or psychosis, or other lack of patient cooperation; spinal puncture and other diagnostic or therapeutic procedures with potential for uncontrollable bleeding; major regional, lumbar block anesthesia; malignant hypertension; known hypersensitivity to warfarin or to any other components of this product.

Warnings/Precautions

➤*Hemorrhage/Necrosis:* The most serious risks associated with anticoagulant therapy with warfarin are hemorrhage in any tissue or organ and, less frequently (less than 0.1%), necrosis and/or gangrene of skin and other tissues.

Observe increased caution when warfarin is administered in the presence of any predisposing condition where added risk of hemorrhage, necrosis, and/or gangrene is present.

Hemorrhage and necrosis have in some cases been reported to result in death or permanent disability. Necrosis appears to be associated with local thrombosis and usually appears within a few days of the start of anticoagulant therapy. In severe cases of necrosis, treatment through debridement or amputation of the affected tissue, limb, breast, or penis has been reported. Careful diagnosis is required to determine whether necrosis is caused by an underlying disease. Discontinue warfarin therapy when warfarin is suspected to be the cause of developing necrosis and consider heparin therapy for anticoagulation. Although various treatments have been attempted, no treatment for necrosis has been considered uniformly effective. See the following sections for information on predisposing conditions. These and other risks associated with anticoagulant therapy must be weighed against the risk of thrombosis or embolization in untreated cases.

➤*Atheroemboli/Microemboli:* Anticoagulation therapy with warfarin may enhance the release of atheromatous plaque emboli, thereby increasing the risk of complications from systemic cholesterol microembolization, including "purple toes syndrome." Discontinuation of warfarin therapy is recommended when such phenomena are observed.

Systemic atheroemboli and cholesterol microemboli can present with a variety of signs and symptoms, including purple toes syndrome; livedo reticularis; rash; gangrene; abrupt and intense pain in the leg, foot, or toes; foot ulcers; myalgia; penile gangrene; abdominal pain; flank or back pain; hematuria; renal function impairment; hypertension; cerebral ischemia; spinal cord infarction; pancreatitis; symptoms simulating polyarteritis; or any other sequelae of vascular compromise due to embolic occlusion. The most commonly involved visceral organs are the kidneys, followed by the pancreas, spleen, and liver. Some cases have progressed to necrosis or death.

➤*Purple toes syndrome:* Purple toes syndrome is a complication of oral anticoagulation characterized by a dark, purplish or mottled color of the toes, usually occurring between 3 to 10 weeks, or later, after the initiation of therapy with warfarin or related compounds. Major features of this syndrome include purple color of plantar surfaces and sides of the toes that blanches on moderate pressure and fades with elevation of the legs; pain and tenderness of the toes; and waxing and waning of the color over time. While the purple toes syndrome is reported to be reversible, some cases progress to gangrene or necrosis, which may require debridement of the affected area or may lead to amputation.

➤*Heparin-induced thrombocytopenia:* Use warfarin with caution in patients with heparin-induced thrombocytopenia and deep vein thrombosis (DVT). Cases of venous limb ischemia, necrosis, and gangrene have occurred in patients with heparin-induced thrombocytopenia and DVT when heparin treatment was discontinued and warfarin therapy was started or continued. In some patients, sequelae have included amputation of the involved area or death.

➤*Enhanced anticoagulant effects:* Endogenous factors that may be responsible for increased PT/INR response include blood dyscrasias, cancer, collagen vascular disease, congestive heart failure (CHF), diarrhea, elevated temperature, hepatic disorders (eg, infectious hepatitis, jaundice), hyperthyroidism, poor nutritional state, steatorrhea, and vitamin K deficiency.

➤*Decreased anticoagulant effects:* Endogenous factors that may be responsible for decreasing the PT/INR response include edema, hereditary coumarin resistance, hyperlipidemia, hypothyroidism, and nephrotic syndrome.

➤*Hypersensitivity reactions:* Minor and severe allergic/hypersensitivity reactions and anaphylactic reactions have been reported.

➤*Special risk:* Warfarin is a narrow therapeutic range (index) drug; observe additional caution when warfarin is adminsitered to certain patients. Reported risk factors for bleeding include high intensity of anticoagulation (INR more than 4), 65 years of age or older, highly variable INRs, history of GI bleeding, hypertension, cerebrovascular disease, serious heart disease, anemia, malignancy, trauma, renal function impairment, concomitant drugs, and long duration of warfarin therapy. Identification of risk factors for bleeding and certain genetic variations in CYP2CP and VKORC1 in

WARFARIN SODIUM — INJECTION

a patient may increase the need for more frequent INR monitoring and the use of lower warfarin doses. Bleeding is more likely to occur during the starting period and with a higher dose of warfarin (resulting in a higher INR).

Confine IM injections of concomitant medications to the upper extremities, which permits easy access for manual compression, inspections for bleeding, and use of pressure bandages.

The decision to administer anticoagulants in the following conditions must be based upon clinical judgment in which the risks of anticoagulant therapy are weighed against the benefits: lactation; severe to moderate hepatic or renal function impairment; infectious diseases or disturbances of intestinal flora; sprue, antibiotic therapy; trauma that may result in internal bleeding; surgery or trauma resulting in large exposed raw surfaces; indwelling catheters; severe to moderate hypertension; polycythemia vera; vasculitis; severe diabetes.

Protein C deficiency – Hereditary or acquired deficiencies of protein C or its cofactor, protein S, have been associated with tissue necrosis following warfarin administration. Not all patients with these conditions develop necrosis, and tissue necrosis occurs in patients without these deficiencies. Inherited resistance to activated protein C has been described in many patients with venous thromboembolic disorders but has not yet been evaluated as a risk factor for tissue necrosis. The risk associated with these conditions, both for recurrent thrombosis and for adverse reactions, is difficult to evaluate since it does not appear to be the same for everyone. Decisions about testing and therapy must be made on an individual basis. It has been reported that concomitant anticoagulation therapy with heparin for 5 to 7 days during initiation of therapy with warfarin may minimize the incidence of tissue necrosis. Discontinue warfarin therapy when warfarin is suspected to be the cause of developing necrosis; consider heparin therapy for anticoagulation.

Patients with CHF may exhibit greater than expected PT/INR response to warfarin, thereby requiring more frequent laboratory monitoring and reduced doses of warfarin.

➤*Pregnancy: Category X* per manufacturer's prescribing information. *Category D* per Briggs' *Drugs in Pregnancy and Lactation*.

Warfarin is contraindicated in women who are or may become pregnant because the drug passes through the placental barrier and may cause fatal hemorrhage to the fetus in utero. Furthermore, there have been reports of birth malformations in children born to mothers who have been treated with warfarin during pregnancy.

Embryopathy characterized by nasal hypoplasia with or without stippled epiphyses (chondrodysplasia punctata) has been reported in pregnant women exposed to warfarin during the first trimester. CNS abnormalities, including dorsal midline dysplasia characterized by agenesis of the corpus callosum, Dandy-Walker malformation, and midline cerebellar atrophy, also have been reported. Ventral midline dysplasia, characterized by optic atrophy, and eye abnormalities have been observed. Mental retardation, blindness, and other CNS abnormalities have been reported in association with second- and third-trimester exposure. Although rare, teratogenic reports following in utero exposure to warfarin include urinary tract anomalies such as single kidney, asplenia, anencephaly, spina bifida, cranial nerve palsy, hydrocephalus, cardiac defects and congenital heart disease, polydactyly, deformities of toes, diaphragmatic hernia, corneal leukoma, cleft palate, cleft lip, schizencephaly, and microcephaly.

Spontaneous abortion and stillbirth are known to occur and a higher risk of fetal mortality is associated with the use of warfarin. Low birth weight and growth retardation have also been reported.

Carefully evaluate women of childbearing potential who are candidates for anticoagulant therapy and critically review the indications with the patient. If the patient becomes pregnant while taking this drug, apprise her of the potential risks to the fetus, and discuss the possibility of termination of the pregnancy in light of those risks.

➤*Lactation:* Based on very limited published data, warfarin has not been detected in the breast milk of mothers treated with warfarin. The same limited published data report that some breast-fed infants, whose mothers were treated with warfarin, had prolonged PTs, although not as prolonged as those of the mothers. Undertake the decision to breast-feed only after careful consideration of the available alternatives. Women who are breast-feeding and anticoagulated with warfarin should be very carefully monitored so that recommended PT/INR values are not exceeded. It is prudent to perform coagulation tests and to evaluate vitamin K status before advising women taking warfarin to breast-feed. Effects in premature infants have not been evaluated.

➤*Children:* Safety and effectiveness in children younger than 18 years of age have not been established in randomized, controlled clinical trials. However, the use of warfarin in children is well documented for the prevention and treatment of thromboembolic events. Difficulty achieving and maintaining therapeutic PT/INR ranges in children has been reported. More frequent PT/INR determinations are recommended because of possible changing warfarin requirements.

➤*Elderly:* Patients 60 years of age or older appear to exhibit greater than expected PT/INR response to the anticoagulant effects of warfarin. Warfarin is contraindicated in any unsupervised patient with senility. Observe caution with administration of warfarin to elderly patients in any situation or physical condition where added risk of hemorrhage is present. Lower initiation and maintenance doses of warfarin are recommended for elderly patients.

➤*Monitoring:* It cannot be emphasized too strongly that treatment of each patient is a highly individualized matter. Warfarin, a narrow therapeutic range (index) drug, may be affected by factors such as other drugs and dietary vitamin K. Dosage should be controlled by periodic determinations of PT/INR or other suitable coagulation tests. Determinations of whole blood clotting and bleeding times are not effective measures for control of therapy. Heparin prolongs the one-stage PT.

Patients with CHF may exhibit greater than expected PT/INR response to warfarin, thereby requiring more frequent laboratory monitoring and reduced doses of warfarin.

Periodic determination of PT/INR is essential. Numerous factors, alone or in combination, including changes in diet, medications, herbals, and genetic variations in the CYP2C9 and VKORC1 enzymes, may influence the response of the patient to warfarin.

It is generally good practice to monitor the patient's response with additional PT/INR determinations in the period immediately after discharge from the hospital and whenever other medications, including herbals, are initiated, discontinued, or taken irregularly.

Because a patient may be exposed to a combination of the previous factors, the net effect of warfarin on PT/INR response may be unpredictable. More frequent PT/INR monitoring is therefore advisable. Medications of unknown interaction with coumarins are best regarded with caution. When these medications are started or stopped, more frequent PT/INR monitoring is advisable.

Very carefully monitor women who are breast-feeding and anticoagulated with warfarin so that recommended PT/INR values are not exceeded. It is prudent to perform coagulation tests and to evaluate vitamin K status before advising women taking warfarin to breast-feed.

Drug Interactions

Careful monitoring and appropriate dosage adjustments usually will permit combination therapy. Critical times during therapy usually will permit combination therapy. Critical times during therapy occur when an interacting drug is added or discontinued from a patient stabilized on anticoagulants.

Injection Anticoagulant Drug Interactions

Precipitant drug	Object drug[a]		Description
Acetaminophen	Anticoagulants	↑	These agents may increase the anticoagulant effect. The risk of bleeding may be increased. The mechanism of the interaction is unknown or complicated.
Androgens			
Anabolic steroids (eg, danazol, oxandrolone, oxymethalone, stanozol)			
Anticoagulants (eg, argatroban, bivalirudin, dicumarol, lepirudin)			
Antineoplastic agents (eg, capecitabine, cyclophosphamide, fluorouracil, gefitinib)			
Beta-blockers (eg, atenolol, propranolol)			
Cephalosporins, parenteral (eg, cefamandole, cefazolin, cefoperazone, cefotetan, cefoxitin, ceftriaxone)			
Chenodiol			
Chlorpropamide			
Cisapride			
Dextran			
Dextrothyroxine			
Diazoxide			
Disulfiram			
Felbamate			
Fibric acids (eg, fenofibrate, gemfibrozil)			
Flutamide			
Glucagon			

WARFARIN SODIUM — INJECTION

Injection Anticoagulant Drug Interactions

Precipitant drug	Object drug[a]		Description
Halothane	Anticoagulants	↑	These agents may increase the anticoagulant effect. The risk of bleeding may be increased. The mechanism of the interaction is unknown or complicated.
Heparin			
Influenza virus vaccine			
Isonazid			
Levamisole			
Methyldopa			
Methylphenidate			
Mineral oil			
NSAIDs[b], COX-2 selective			
Orlistat			
Pentoxifylline			
Propoxyphene			
Quinlones (eg, ciprofloxacin, levofloxacin, norfloxacin, ofloxacin)			
Ropinirole			
Selective COX-2 inhibitors (eg, celecoxib, rofecoxib, valdecoxib)			
SSRIs[b,c] (eg, fluoxetine, fluvoxamine, paroxetine, sertraline)			
Tamoxifen			
Thrombolytics (ie, streptokinase, tissue plasminogen activator, urokinase)			
Thyroid hormones (eg, levothyroxine, liothyonine, thyroid)			
Tolbutamide			
Tolterodine			
Tramadol			
Trastuzumab			
Zafirlukast			
Zileuton			

Injection Anticoagulant Drug Interactions

Precipitant drug	Object drug[a]		Description
Allopurinol	Anticoagulants	↑	These agents may increase the anticoagulant effect of warfarin by inhibition of the anticoagulant's hepatic metabolism. The risk of bleeding may be increased.
Amiodarone			
Azole antifungals (eg, fluconazole, itraconazole, miconazole[d])			
Chloramphenicol			
Cimetidine			
HMG-CoA reductase inhibitors (ie, fluvastatin, lovastatin, simvastatin)			
Isofamide[e]			
Leflunomide			
Metronidazole			
Omeprazole			
Phenylbutazone[e]			
Propafenone			
Proton pump inhibitors (eg, esomeprazole, lansoprazole, omeprazole, pentoprazole, rabeprazole)			
Quinidine			
Quinine			
Sulfonamides (eg, sulfamethazole, sulfisoxazole, trimethoprim, sulfamethoxazole)			
Sulfinpyrazone			
Macrolide antibiotics (eg, azithromycin, clarithromycin, erythromycin)	Anticoagulants	↑	These agents may increase the anticoagulant effect by reducing body clearance of warfarin. The risk of bleeding may be increased.
Loop diuretics (ie, ethacrynic acid, furosemide)	Anticoagulants	↑	These agents may increase the anticoagulant effect of warfarin caused by displacement from binding sites. The risk of bleeding may be increased.
Meflaquine			
Nalidixic acid			
Valproate			
Aminoglycosides, oral	Anticoagulants	↑	These agents may increase the anticoagulant effect of warfarin through an interference with vitamin K. The risk of bleeding may be increased.
Fish oil			
Neomycin			
Tetracyclines (eg, doxycycline, tetracycline)			
Vitamin E			
Aminosalicylic acid	Anticoagulants	↑	These agents may increase the anticoagulant effect of warfarin and increase the risk of bleeding because of effects on platelet function, and, in the case of NSAIDs, GI irritant effects.
Diflunisal			
Methylsalicylate ointment, topical			
NSAIDs (eg, diclofenac, fenoprofen, ibuprofen, indomethacin, ketoprofen, ketorolac, mefenamic acid, naproxen, oxaprozin, piroxicam, sulindac)			

WARFARIN SODIUM — INJECTION

Injection Anticoagulant Drug Interactions			
Precipitant drug	Object drug[a]		Description
Olsalazine	Anticoagulants	↑	These agents may increase the anticoagulant effect of warfarin and increase the risk of bleeding because of effects on platelet function, and, in the case of NSAIDs, GI irritant effects.
Penicillins, high-dose IV (eg, penicillin G, piperacillin, ticarcillin)			
Salicylates			
Ticlopidine			
Alcohol[f]	Anticoagulants	↑↓	Increased and decreased PT/INR responses have been reported. May increase or decrease the anticoagulant effect of warfarin; the mechanism is unknown.
Atorvastatin			
Chloral hydrate			
Cholestyramine[g]			
Corticosteroids			
Cyclophosphamide			
Hydantoins (eg, phenytoin)			
Methimazole			
Moricizine			
Pravastatin			
Prednisone			
Propylthiouracil			
Ranitidine			
Ascorbic acid, high doses	Anticoagulants	↓	These agents may decrease the anticoagulant effect of warfarin. The mechanism of the interaction is unknown.
Chlordiazepoxide			
Clozapine			
Contraceptives, oral[h]			
Cyclosporine[i]			
Estrogens			
Ethchlorvynol			
Griseofluvin			
Haloperidol			
Isotretinoin			
Menthol			
Meprobamate			
Mesalamine			
Paraldehyde			
Protease inhibitors (eg, indinavir, ritonavir)			
Raloxifene			
Ribavirin			
Trazodone			
Aminoglutethimide	Anticoagulants	↓	These agents may decrease the anticoagulant effect of warfarin (because of the induction of the anticoagulant's hepatic microsomal enzyme).
Aprepitant			
Barbituates (eg, aminobarbital, butabarbital, pentobarbital, phenobarbital, secobarbital)			
Bosentan			
Carbamazepine			
Dicloxacillin[j]			
Glutethimide			
Mitotane			
Nafcillin[j]			
Nevirapine			
Primidone			
Rifamycins			
Terbinafine			

Injection Anticoagulant Drug Interactions			
Precipitant drug	Object drug[a]		Description
Spironolactone[k]	Anticoagulants	↓	These agents may decrease the anticoagulant effect of warfarin by various mechanisms (eg, possible decreased absorption or increased elimination)
Sucralfate			
Thiazide diuretics (eg, chlorthalidone)[k]			
Thiopurines (eg, azathioprine)[l]			
Vitamin K[m]			
Ubiquinone			

[a] ↑ = object drug increased; ↓ = object drug decreased.
[b] NSADs = nonsteroidal anti-inflammatory drugs; SSRIs = selective serotonin reuptake inhibitors.
[c] Bleeding has been reported with fluoxetine alone.
[d] Miconazole includes both intravaginal and systemic formulations.
[e] May also displace the anticoagulant from protein binding sites.
[f] Chronic consumption may increase the clearance of the anticoagulant; moderate to small doses do not alter the anticoagulant effect.
[g] Reduced anticoagulant absorption and possibly increased elimination.
[h] Rarely, increased risk of thromboembolism; this is in contrast to intended effect.
[i] Cyclosporine levels may also be decreased.
[j] Associated with warfarin resistance.
[k] Diuretic-induced hemoconcentration of clotting factors.
[l] Thiopurine-induced increase in synthesis or activation of prothrombin.
[m] Vitamin K overcomes interference of vitamin K–dependent clotting factors by anticoagulants.

➤*Herbal medicines:* Exercise caution when herbal medicines are taken concomitantly with warfarin.

Specific herbals reported to affect warfarin therapy include the following:

- Bromelains, danshen, dong quai (*Angelica sinensis*), garlic, *Ginkgo biloba*, ginseng, and cranberry products are associated most often with an increase in the effects of warfarin.
- Coenzyme Q_{10} (ubidecarenone) and St. John's wort are associated most often with a decrease in the effects of warfarin.

Some herbals may cause bleeding events when taken alone (eg, garlic, *Ginkgo biloba*) and may have anticoagulant, antiplatelet, and/or fibrinolytic properties. These effects would be expected to be additive to the anticoagulant effects of warfarin. Conversely, other herbals may have coagulant properties when taken alone or may decrease the effects of warfarin.

Some herbals that may affect coagulation are listed in the following table; however, this list should not be considered all-inclusive. Many herbals have several common names and scientific names. The most widely recognized common botanical names are listed.

Herbals That Contain Coumarins With Potential Anticoagulant Effects		
Agrimony[a]	Cassia[b]	Parsley
Alfalfa	Celery	Passion flower
Angelica (dong quai)	Chamomile (German and Roman)	Prickly ash (Northern)
Aniseed	Dandelion[b]	Quassia
Arnica	Fenugreek	Red clover
Asafoetida	Horse chestnut	Sweet clover
Bogbean[c]	Horseradish	Sweet woodruff
Boldo	Licorice[b]	Tonka beans
Buchu	Meadowsweet[c]	Wild carrot
Capsicum[d]	Nettle	Wild lettuce

[a] Contains coumarins, has antiplatelet properties, and may have coagulant properties because of possible vitamin K content.
[b] Contains coumarins and has antiplatelet properties.
[c] Contains coumarins and salicylates.
[d] Contains coumarins and has fibrinolytic properties.

Miscellaneous Herbals With Anticoagulant Properties	
Bladder wrack (*Fucus*)	Pau d'arco

Herbals That Contain Salicylate and/or Have Antiplatelet Properties		
Agrimony[a]	Dandelion[b]	Meadowsweet[c]
Aloe gel	Feverfew	Onion[d]
Aspen	Garlic[d]	Policosanol
Black cohosh	German sarsaparilla	Poplar
Black haw	Ginger	Senega
Bogbean[c]	*Ginkgo biloba*	Tamarind
Cassia[b]	Ginseng (*Panax*)[d]	Willow
Clove	Licorice[b]	Wintergreen

[a] Contains coumarins, has antiplatelet properties, and may have coagulant properties because of possible vitamin K content.
[b] Contains coumarins and has antiplatelet properties.
[c] Contains coumarins and salicylates.
[d] Has antiplatelet and fibrinolytic properties.

WARFARIN SODIUM — INJECTION

Herbals With Fibrinolytic Properties		
Bromelains	Garlic[b]	Inositol nicotinate
Capsicum[a]	Ginseng (*Panax*)[b]	Onion[b]

[a] Contains coumarins and has fibrinolytic properties.
[b] Has antiplatelet and fibrinolytic properties.

Herbals With Coagulant Properties	
Agrimony[a]	Mistletoe
Goldenseal	Yarrow

[a] Contains coumarins, has antiplatelet properties, and may have coagulant properties because of possible vitamin K content.

➤*Drug/Food interactions:* Vitamin K–rich vegetables may decrease the anticoagulant effects of warfarin by interfering with absorption. Patients should minimize consumption of vitamin K–rich foods (eg, spinach, seaweed, broccoli, turnip greens) or nutritional supplements, or enteral nutrition. Mango has been shown to increase warfarin's effect.

Adverse Reactions

➤*Cardiovascular:* Angina syndrome, hypotension, purple toes syndrome, syncope, systemic cholesterol microembolization, vasculitis.

➤*CNS:* Asthenia; coma; dizziness; fatigue; headache; lethargy; loss of consciousness; paresthesia, including feeling cold and chills.

➤*Dermatologic:* Alopecia; necrosis of skin and other tissues; pruritus; rash and dermatitis, including bullous eruptions; urticaria.

➤*GI:* Abdominal pain, including cramping; diarrhea; flatulence/bloating; nausea; taste perversion; vomiting.

➤*GU:* Priapism has been associated with anticoagulant administration; however, a causal relationship has not been established.

➤*Hematologic:* Fatal or nonfatal hemorrhage from any tissue or organ. This is a consequence of the anticoagulant effect. The signs, symptoms, and severity will vary according to the location and degree or extent of the bleeding. Hemorrhagic complications may present as paralysis; paresthesia; headache; chest, abdomen, joint, muscle, or other pain; dizziness; shortness of breath; difficult breathing or swallowing; unexplained swelling; weakness; hypotension; or unexplained shock. Therefore, consider the possibility of hemorrhage in evaluating the condition of any anticoagulated patient with complaints that do not indicate an obvious diagnosis. Bleeding during anticoagulant therapy does not always correlate with PT/INR. Bleeding that occurs when the PT/INR is within the therapeutic range warrants diagnostic investigation because it may unmask a previously unsuspected lesion (eg, tumor, ulcer). Anemia.

➤*Hepatic:* Cholestatic hepatic injury, elevated liver enzymes, hepatitis, jaundice.

➤*Hypersensitivity:* Hypersensitivity/allergic reactions, including anaphylactic reactions.

➤*Respiratory:* Rare events of tracheal or tracheobronchial calcification have been reported in association with long-term warfarin therapy. The clinical significance of this event is unknown.

➤*Miscellaneous:* Chest pain, cold intolerance, edema, fever, malaise, pain, pallor.

Overdosage

➤*Symptoms:* Suspected or overt abnormal bleeding (eg, appearance of blood in stools or urine, hematuria, excessive menstrual bleeding, melena, petechiae, excessive bruising or persistent oozing from superficial injuries) are early manifestations of anticoagulation beyond a safe and satisfactory level.

➤*Treatment:* Excessive anticoagulation with or without bleeding may be controlled by discontinuing warfarin therapy and, if necessary, by administration of oral or parenteral vitamin K_1.

Such use of vitamin K_1 reduces response to subsequent warfarin therapy. Patients may return to a pretreatment thrombotic status following the rapid reversal of a prolonged PT/INR. Resumption of warfarin administration reverses the effect of vitamin K, and a therapeutic PT/INR can again be obtained by careful dosage adjustment. If rapid anticoagulation is indicated, heparin may be preferable for initial therapy.

If minor bleeding progresses to major bleeding, give 5 to 25 mg (rarely up to 50 mg) of parenteral vitamin K_1. In emergency situations of severe hemorrhage, clotting factors can be returned to normal by administering 200 to 500 mL of fresh whole blood or fresh frozen plasma, or by giving commercial factor IX complex.

A risk of hepatitis and other viral diseases is associated with the use of these blood products. Factor IX complex is also associated with an increased risk of thrombosis. Therefore, use these preparations in exceptional or life-threatening bleeding episodes secondary to warfarin overdosage.

Do not use purified factor IX preparations because they cannot increase the levels of prothrombin, or factor VII and X, which are also depressed along with the levels of factor IX as a result of warfarin treatment. Packed red blood cells may also be given if significant blood loss has occurred. Carefully monitor infusions of blood or plasma to avoid precipitating pulmonary edema in elderly patients or patients with heart disease.

Patient Information

The objective of anticoagulant therapy is to decrease the clotting ability of the blood so that thrombosis is prevented, while avoiding spontaneous bleeding. Effective therapeutic levels with minimal complications are in part dependent upon cooperative and well-instructed patients who communicate effectively with their health care provider.

Advise patients that strict adherence to prescribed dosage schedule is necessary.

Instruct patients not to take or discontinue any other medication, including salicylates (eg, aspirin and topical analgesics) and other nonprescription medications, and herbal products (eg, bromelains, coenzyme Q_{10}, danshen, dong quai, garlic, *Ginkgo biloba*, ginseng, St. John's wort), except on advice of the health care provider.

Instruct the patient to avoid alcohol consumption.

Advise patients to not take warfarin during pregnancy and to not become pregnant while taking it.

Advise patients to avoid any activity or sport that may result in traumatic injury.

Advise patients that PT tests and regular visits to physician or clinic are needed to monitor therapy.

Instruct patients to carry identification stating that warfarin is being taken.

Inform patients that if the prescribed dose of warfarin is forgotten, to notify their health care provider immediately. Instruct patients to take the dose as soon as possible on the same day, but not to take a double dose of warfarin the next day to make up for missed doses.

The amount of vitamin K in food may affect therapy with warfarin. Instruct patients to eat a healthy, balanced diet maintaining a consistent amount of vitamin K. Advise patients to avoid drastic changes in dietary habits, such as eating large amounts of green leafy vegetables. Advise patients to also avoid intake of cranberry juice or any other cranberry products. Instruct patients to notify their health care provider if any of these products are part of their normal diet.

Instruct patients to contact their health care provider to report any illness, such as diarrhea, infection, or fever.

Advise patients to notify their health care provider immediately if any unusual bleeding or symptoms occur. Signs and symptoms of bleeding include pain, swelling, or discomfort; prolonged bleeding from cuts; increased menstrual flow or vaginal bleeding; nosebleeds; bleeding of gums from brushing; unusual bleeding or bruising; red or dark brown urine; red or tar black stools; headache; dizziness; or weakness.

Caution patients that if therapy with warfarin is discontinued, the anticoagulant effects of warfarin may persist for about 2 to 5 days.

Inform patients that all warfarin products represent the same medication and should not be taken concomitantly, as overdosage may result.

PROTAMINE SULFATE

Rx	Protamine Sulfate (Various, eg, American Pharmaceutical Partners)	Injection: 10 mg/mL	Preservative-free. In 5 and 25 mL vials.

PROTAMINE SULFATE — INJECTION

Indications

➤*Heparin overdose:* Treatment of heparin overdosage.

Administration and Dosage

➤*Adults:*

Heparin overdose –
Usual dosage: 50 mg.

Alternative dosage: Because heparin disappears rapidly from the circulation, the dose of protamine required also decreases rapidly with the time elapsed following IV injection of heparin. For example, if the protamine is administered 30 minutes after the heparin, one-half the usual dose may be sufficient.

➤*Children:*

Off-label dosing –
Heparin overdose:

Protamine Dosage in Children With Heparin Overdose

Time since last heparin dose received	Protamine dose
< 30 min	1 mg/100 units heparin received
30 to 60 min	0.5 to 0.75 mg/100 units heparin received
60 to 120 min	0.375 to 0.5 mg/100 units heparin received
> 120 min	0.25 to 0.375 mg/100 units heparin received

Enoxaparin overdose:

Protamine Dosage in Children With Enoxaparin Overdose

Time since last enoxaparin dose	Enoxaparin dose
< 8 h	1 mg/1 mg enoxaparin received
8 to 12 h	0.5 mg/1 mg enoxaparin received
> 12 h	Protamine not required

An infusion of protamine 0.5 mg per enoxaparin 1 mg may be administered if enoxaparin was administered more than 8 hours prior to the protamine administration, or if it has been determined that a second dose of protamine is required. The second infusion of protamine 0.5 mg per enoxaparin 1 mg may be administered if the aPTT measured 2 to 4 hours after the first infusion remains prolonged.

➤*Preparation for administration:* Protamine is intended for injection without further dilution; however, if further dilution is desired, D5-W or normal saline may be used.

➤*Administration:* Protamine should be given by very slow IV injection over a 10-minute period.

➤*Admixture compatibility:* Protamine should not be mixed with other drugs without knowledge of their compatibility because protamine has been shown to be incompatible with certain antibiotics, including several of the cephalosporins and penicillins.

➤*Storage/Stability:* Store at controlled room temperature, 15° to 30°C (59° to 86°F). Do not permit to freeze. Diluted solutions should not be stored because they contain no preservative.

Actions

➤*Pharmacology:* When administered alone, protamine has an anticoagulant effect. However, when it is given in the presence of heparin (which is strongly acidic), a stable salt is formed and the anticoagulant activity of both drugs is lost.

➤*Pharmacokinetics:*

Absorption/Distribution – Protamine sulfate has a rapid onset of action. Neutralization of heparin occurs within 5 minutes after IV administration of an appropriate dose of protamine sulfate.

Metabolism – Although the metabolic fate of the heparin-protamine complex has not been elucidated, it has been postulated that protamine sulfate in the heparin-protamine complex may be partially metabolized or may be attacked by fibrinolysin, thus freeing heparin.

Contraindications

Previous intolerance to the drug.

Warnings/Precautions

➤*Hyperheparinemia or bleeding:* Hyperheparinemia or bleeding has been reported in experimental animals and in some patients 30 minutes to 18 hours after cardiac surgery (under cardiopulmonary bypass) in spite of complete neutralization of heparin by adequate doses of protamine sulfate at the end of the operation. It is important to keep the patient under close observation after cardiac surgery. Additional doses of protamine sulfate should be administered if indicated by coagulation studies, such as the heparin titration test with protamine and the determination of plasma thrombin time.

➤*Anticoagulant effect:* Because of the anticoagulant effect of protamine, it is unwise to give more than 100 mg over a short period unless a larger dose is clearly needed.

➤*Previous exposure to protamine:* Previous exposure to protamine through use of protamine-containing insulins or during heparin neutralization may predispose susceptible individuals to the development of untoward reactions from the subsequent use of this drug. Reports of the presence of antiprotamine antibodies in the sera of infertile or vasectomized men suggest that some of these individuals may react to the use of protamine sulfate.

➤*Hypersensitivity reactions:* Too-rapid administration of protamine sulfate can cause severe hypotensive and anaphylactoid reactions (see Administration and Dosage and Warnings). Facilities to treat shock should be available.

Patients with a history of allergy to fish may develop hypersensitivity reactions to protamine, although to date no relationship has been established between allergic reactions to protamine and fish allergy.

Fatal anaphylaxis has been reported in one patient with no history of allergies.

➤*Pregnancy: Category C.* Animal reproduction studies have not been conducted with protamine sulfate. It is also not known whether protamine sulfate can cause fetal harm when administered to a pregnant woman or can affect reproduction capacity. Protamine sulfate should be given to a pregnant woman only if clearly needed.

➤*Lactation:* It is not known whether this drug is excreted in human milk. Because many drugs are excreted in human milk, caution should be exercised when protamine sulfate is administered to a nursing woman.

➤*Children:* Safety and effectiveness in children have not been established.

Drug Interactions

➤*Antibiotics:* Protamine sulfate has been shown to be incompatible with certain antibiotics, including several of the cephalosporins and penicillins (see Administration and Dosage).

Adverse Reactions

➤*Cardiovascular:* The IV administration of protamine sulfate may cause a sudden fall in blood pressure and bradycardia.

Back pain has been reported in conscious patients undergoing such procedures as cardiac catheterization.

Severe and potentially irreversible circulatory collapse associated with MI and reduced cardiac output can also occur. The mechanism(s) of this reaction and the role played by concurrent factors are unclear.

High-protein, noncardiogenic pulmonary edema associated with the use of protamine has been reported in patients on cardiopulmonary bypass who are undergoing cardiovascular surgery. The etiologic role of protamine in the pathogenesis of this condition is uncertain, and multiple factors have been present in most cases. The condition has been reported in association with administration of certain blood products, other drugs, cardiopulmonary bypass alone, and other etiologic factors. It is difficult to treat, and it can be life-threatening. Because fatal anaphylactic and anaphylactoid reactions have been reported after the administration of protamine sulfate, the drug should be given only when resuscitation techniques and treatment of anaphylactic and anaphylactoid shock are readily available.

➤*Hypersensitivity:* Severe adverse reactions have been reported including: Anaphylaxis that resulted in severe respiratory distress, circulation collapse and capillary leak (see Warnings). Fatal anaphylaxis has been reported in one patient with no prior history of allergies; anaphylactoid reactions with circulatory collapse, capillary leak, and noncardiogenic pulmonary edema; acute pulmonary hypertension.

Complement activation by the heparin-protamine complexes, release of lysosomal enzymes from neutrophils, and prostaglandin and thomboxane generation have been associated with the development of anaphylactoid reactions.

➤*Miscellaneous:* Other reactions include transitory flushing and feeling of warmth, dyspnea, nausea, vomiting and lassitude.

Overdosage

The median lethal dose of protamine sulfate is 100 mg/kg in mice. Serum concentrations of protamine sulfate are not clinically useful. Information is not available on the amount of drug in a single dose that is associated with overdosage or is likely to be life-threatening.

➤*Symptoms:* Overdose of protamine sulfate may cause bleeding. Protamine has a weak anticoagulant effect due to an interaction with platelets and with many proteins including fibrinogen. This effect should be distinguished from the rebound anticoagulation that may occur 30 minutes to 18 hours following the reversal of heparin with protamine.

Rapid administration of protamine is more likely to result in bradycardia, dyspnea, a sensation of warmth, flushing, and severe hypotension. Hypertension has also occurred.

PROTAMINE SULFATE — INJECTION

➤*Treatment:* To obtain up-to-date information about the treatment of overdose, a good resource is your certified regional poison control center. In managing overdosage, consider the possibility of multiple drug overdoses, interaction among drugs and unusual drug kinetics in your patient.

Replace blood loss with blood transfusions of fresh frozen plasma.

If the patient is hypotensive, consider fluids, epinephrine, dobutamine, or dopamine.

THROMBOLYTIC AGENTS

Tissue Plasminogen Activators

ALTEPLASE RECOMBINANT

Rx	**Activase** (Genentech)	**Lyophilized powder for injection**[a]: 50 mg (29 million units)	In vials with diluent (50 mL sterile water for injection) and vacuum.
		100 mg (58 million units)	In vials with diluent (100 mL sterile water for injection) and 1 transfer device.
Rx	**Cathflo Activase** (Genentech)	**Lyophilized powder for injection**[a]: 2 mg	In vials.

[a] With L-arginine, phosphoric acid, and polysorbate 80.

ALTEPLASE RECOMBINANT — INJECTION

Indications

➤*Acute myocardial infarction (AMI) (Activase only):* For the management of AMI in adults for the improvement of ventricular function following AMI, the reduction of the incidence of congestive heart failure, and the reduction of mortality associated with AMI. Initiate treatment as soon as possible after the onset of AMI symptoms.

➤*Acute ischemic stroke (AIS) (Activase only):* For the management of AIS in adults for improving neurological recovery and reducing the incidence of disability. Initiate treatment only within 3 hours after the onset of stroke symptoms and after exclusion of intracranial hemorrhage (ICH) by a cranial computerized tomography (CT) scan or other diagnostic imaging method sensitive for the presence of hemorrhage (see Contraindications).

➤*Pulmonary embolism (PE) (Activase only):* For the management of acute massive PE in adults for the lysis of acute PE, defined as obstruction of blood flow to a lobe or multiple segments of the lungs, and for the lysis of PE accompanied by unstable hemodynamics (eg, failure to maintain blood pressure without supportive measures).

Confirm the diagnosis by objective means such as pulmonary angiography or noninvasive procedures such as lung scanning.

➤*Restoration of function to central venous access device (Cathflo Activase only):* For the restoration of function to central venous access devices as assessed by the ability to withdraw blood.

➤*Off-label uses:*

Frostbite – [4] = Insufficient documentation. A small, open-label trial indicates that alteplase therapy may provide benefit as adjunctive therapy in the management of severe frostbite. However, the study used a variety of doses and administration routes (eg, intra-arterial, intravenous [IV]). (See Administration and Dosage.)

Hemolytic uremic syndrome (children) – [4] = Insufficient documentation. Although rationale exists for the use of alteplase in hemolytic uremic syndrome, no clinical trials were identified to support its use. Randomized, controlled trials are needed to determine efficacy, safety, dosing, and duration of therapy for specific patient populations before the use of alteplase can be recommended.

Kidney cortex necrosis – [5] = Poor documentation. No evidence was found that supports the use of alteplase in prevention or treatment of kidney cortex necrosis. Therefore, the use of alteplase for this indication is not recommended.

Pleural effusion (parapneumonic) – [4] = Insufficient documentation. Preliminary data suggest that alteplase administration into the pleural space may be effective in maintaining pleural tube patency and may allow for efficient drainage. However, these data are limited to 2 published case reports. (See Administration and Dosage.)

Retinal artery occlusion/retinal vein occlusion – [3] = Safety concerns. Initial data from clinical trials show that administration of tissue plasminogen activator (TPA) may be beneficial in the treatment of central retinal artery occlusion (CRAO) or central retinal vein occlusion (CRVO). IV administration has shown visual acuity improvement; however, adverse effects with systemic use may outweigh the benefits of therapy. Intravitreal and intraarterial administration have also demonstrated visual improvements with less systemic adverse effects. Because CRAO and CRVO are associated with a high risk of permanent visual impairment, further controlled studies are needed to determine the role of alteplase compared with standard therapy, and to establish appropriate patient populations (including CRAO vs CRVO), dosages, and routes of administration for this indication.

Administration and Dosage

➤*Adults:*

Acute ischemic stroke (Activase only) –

Usual dosage: 0.9 mg/kg (not to exceed 90 mg total dose) infused over 60 minutes with 10% of the total dose administered as an initial IV bolus over 1 minute.

Maximum dose: Doses greater than 0.9 mg/kg may be associated with an increased incidence of ICH. Do not use doses greater than 0.9 mg/kg (maximum, 90 mg) in the management of acute ischemic stroke.

Concomitant therapy: The safety and efficacy of this regimen with coadministration of heparin and aspirin during the first 24 hours after symptom onset have not been investigated.

Acute myocardial infarction (Activase only) – Do not use a dose of 150 mg because it has been associated with an increase in intracranial bleeding.

Usual dosage: Administer as soon as possible after the onset of symptoms.

• *Accelerated infusion* – The safety and efficacy of this accelerated infusion of alteplase regimen have only been investigated with coadministration of heparin and aspirin.

Patients weighing more than 67 kg: 100 mg as a 15 mg IV bolus, followed by 50 mg infused over the next 30 minutes, and then 35 mg infused over the next 60 minutes.

Patients weighing 67 kg or less: 15 mg IV bolus, followed by 0.75 mg/kg infused over the next 30 minutes not to exceed 50 mg, and then 0.5 mg/kg over the next 60 minutes not to exceed 35 mg.

• *3-hour infusion* – The recommended dose is 100 mg administered as 60 mg (34.8 million units) in the first hour (with 6 to 10 mg administered as a bolus), 20 mg (11.6 million units) over the second hour, and 20 mg (11.6 million units) over the third hour. For smaller patients (less than 65 kg), a dose of 1.25 mg/kg administered over 3 hours, as described above, may be used.

Maximum dose: The recommended total dose is based upon patient weight, not to exceed 100 mg.

Concomitant therapy: Although the use of anticoagulants during and following alteplase administration has not been fully studied, heparin has been administered concomitantly for 24 hours or longer in more than 90% of patients. Aspirin and/or dipyridamole has been given either during or following heparin treatment (see Drug Interactions).

Pulmonary embolism (Activase only) –

Usual dosage: 100 mg administered by IV infusion over 2 hours.

Concomitant therapy: Institute or reinstitute heparin therapy near the end of or immediately following the alteplase infusion when the partial thromboplastin time or thrombin time returns to twice normal or less.

Restoration of function to central venous access device (Cathflo Activase only) –

Usual dosage: Instill into dysfunctional catheter at a concentration of 1 mg/mL. If catheter function is not restored in 120 minutes after 1 dose, a second dose may be instilled.

• *Patients weighing 30 kg or more* – Use 2 mg in 2 mL.

• *Patients weighing 10 kg or more to less than 30 kg* – Use 110% of the internal lumen volume of the catheter, not to exceed 2 mg in 2 mL.

Off-label dosing –

Frostbite: [4] = Insufficient documentation. 0.15 mg/kg IV bolus, followed by a 0.15 mg/kg/h infusion over 6 hours, up to a maximum of 100 mg. All patients were rescanned after treatment and received a second course of therapy (6-hour infusion) if significant improvement was not noted. Following the completion of the alteplase infusion, all patients were started on IV heparin until the partial thromboplastin time was 2 times the control. Warfarin was started 3 to 5 days after alteplase and continued for an additional 4 weeks.

Pleural effusion (parapneumonic): [4] = Insufficient documentation.

• *Adults* – 16 mg per 100 mL normal saline injected into the chest tube and tube clamped for 2 hours. Dose repeated once daily for 6 days.

• *Retrospective reviews* – 4 mg per 30 to 50 mL saline infused via chest tube into pleural space, clamped for 1 hour and left to drain at a suction pressure of −20 cm H_2O. This dose was empirically selected and is twice the standard dose used to unblock central venous catheters. Patients received doses early at a median of 4 hours (range, 0 to 21 hours) after diagnosis or late at a median of 64 hours (range, 28 to 195 hours) after discharge. In a retrospective review of children, 0.1 mg/kg (maximum dose of 6 mg) was diluted in 25 to 100 mL normal saline. The volume was arbitrarily selected based on the age and size of the patient and an estimate of the volume of pleural space to be treated.

Retinal artery occlusion/retinal vein occlusion: [3] = Safety concerns. 100 mg IV over 6 hours (40 mg the first hour, 20 mg the second hour, 10 mg in hours 3 to 6); 75 to 100 mcg given via intravitreal administration; or 3 mg aliquots intraarterially, up to 20 mg, over 35 minutes.

➤*Children:*

Restoration of function to central venous access device (Cathflo Activase only) –

Older than 2 years of age or weighing more than 10 kg: See Adults.

ALTEPLASE RECOMBINANT — INJECTION

Off-label dosing –

Hemolytic uremic syndrome: [4] = Insufficient documentation. 0.2 mg/kg/h IV for 5 hours and 0.05 mg/kg/h for 14 days thereafter has been used.

Pleural effusion (parapneumonic): [4] = Insufficient documentation.

• *Case report: 16 months* – 2 mg infused via catheter into the pleural space and tube clamped for 4 hours. Dose repeated 4 times during 6 days.

• *Retrospective reviews* – See Adults.

➤*Renal function impairment:* The risks of alteplase therapy may be increased and should be weighed against the anticipated benefits in patients with hemostatic defects including those secondary to severe renal disease.

➤*Hepatic function impairment:* The risks of alteplase therapy may be increased and should be weighed against the anticipated benefits in patients with hemostatic defects including those secondary to severe hepatic disease or significant hepatic dysfunction.

➤*Preparation for administration:*

Reconstitution – Reconstitute only with sterile water for injection without preservatives. Do not use bacteriostatic water for injection.

The reconstituted preparation results in a colorless to pale yellow, transparent solution.

Slight foaming upon reconstitution is usual; standing undisturbed for several minutes is usually sufficient to allow dissipation of any large bubbles.

50 mg vial: Do not use if vacuum is not present. Reconstitute with a large-bore needle (eg, 18-gauge), directing the stream of sterile water for injection into the lyophilized cake.

100 mg vial: Use transfer device provided for reconstitution. 100 mg vials do not contain vacuum.

May be administered as reconstituted at 1 mg/mL.

As an alternative, the reconstituted solution may be further diluted immediately before administration with an equal volume of sodium chloride 0.9% injection or dextrose 5% injection to yield a concentration of 0.5 mg/mL.

➤*Administration:* For IV administration only.

➤*Admixture compatibility:* Do not add other medications to infusion solution.

➤*Storage/Stability:* Store lyophilized alteplase at controlled room temperature not to exceed 30°C (86°F) or under refrigeration (2° to 8°C; 36° to 46°F). During extended storage, protect from excessive exposure to light. Discard any unused solution.

The solution may be used for direct IV administration within 8 hours following reconstitution when stored between 2° and 30°C (36° and 86°F). Avoid excessive agitation during dilution; mix by gentle swirling or slow inversion. Do not use other infusion solutions.

Actions

➤*Pharmacology:* Alteplase, a tissue plasminogen activator (tPA) produced by recombinant DNA, is synthesized using the complementary DNA for natural human tissue-type plasminogen activator obtained from a human melanoma cell line. Biological potency, determined by an in vitro clot lysis assay, is expressed in international units. The specific activity is 580,000 units/mg.

Alteplase is an enzyme (serine protease) that has the property of fibrin-enhanced conversion of plasminogen to plasmin. It produces limited conversion of plasminogen in the absence of fibrin. When introduced into the systemic circulation at pharmacologic concentration, alteplase binds to fibrin in a thrombus and converts the entrapped plasminogen to plasmin. This initiates local fibrinolysis with limited systemic proteolysis. Following administration of 100 mg, there is a decrease (16% to 36%) in circulating fibrinogen. In a controlled trial, 8 of 73 patients (11%) receiving alteplase (1.25 mg/kg over 3 hours) experienced a decrease in fibrinogen to below 100 mg/dL.

➤*Pharmacokinetics:*

Absorption/Distribution – Because of its large molecular size, alteplase cannot easily diffuse across biological membranes and must be given parenterally, usually IV. Maximal plasma concentrations of 3 to 4 mg/L are achieved after standard administration of 90 to 100 mg doses. Steady-state concentrations for the initial infusion period were 45% higher when administered in an accelerated regimen.

Metabolism/Excretion – Alteplase is cleared rapidly from plasma at a rate of 380 to 570 mL/min, primarily by the liver. More than 50% of the drug present in plasma is cleared within 5 minutes after the infusion has been terminated, and approximately 80% is cleared within 10 minutes. Initial volume of distribution is 2.8 to 4.6 L, and it approximately doubles at steady state. Total body clearance is 34.3 to 38.4 L/h.

Contraindications

Hypersensitivity to alteplase or any of the components.

➤*AMI or PE (Activase only):* Active internal bleeding; history of cerebrovascular accident; recent intracranial or intraspinal surgery or trauma; intracranial neoplasm, arteriovenous malformation, or aneurysm; bleeding diathesis; severe uncontrolled hypertension.

➤*AIS (Activase only):* Evidence of ICH on pretreatment evaluation; suspicion of subarachnoid hemorrhage; recent (within 3 months) intracranial or intraspinal surgery, serious head trauma, or previous stroke; history of ICH; uncontrolled hypertension at time of treatment (eg, greater than 185 mm Hg systolic or greater than 110 mm Hg diastolic); seizure at the onset of stroke; active internal bleeding; intracranial neoplasm, arteriovenous malformation, or aneurysm; bleeding diathesis.

➤*Bleeding diathesis:* Bleeding diathesis includes, but is not limited to: Current use of oral anticoagulants (eg, warfarin sodium) with prothrombin time (PT) longer than 15 seconds; administration of heparin within 48 hours preceding stroke onset with an elevated activated partial thromboplastin time (aPTT) at presentation; platelet count below 100,000/mm^3.

Warnings/Precautions

➤*Bleeding:* Bleeding is the most common complication. The bleeding associated with thrombolytic therapy can be divided into 2 broad categories:

1.) Internal bleeding involving intracranial or retroperitoneal sites or the GI, GU, or respiratory tracts.
2.) Superficial or surface bleeding, observed mainly at invaded or disturbed sites (eg, venous cutdowns, arterial punctures, sites of recent surgical intervention).

The concomitant use of heparin anticoagulation may contribute to the bleeding. Some of the hemorrhagic episodes occurred 1 or more days after alteplase effects had dissipated but while heparin therapy was continuing.

As fibrin is lysed during alteplase therapy, bleeding from recent puncture sites may occur. Therefore, thrombolytic therapy requires careful attention to all potential bleeding sites (including catheter insertion sites, arterial and venous puncture sites, cutdown sites, and needle puncture sites). Avoid IM injections and nonessential handling of the patient during treatment with alteplase. Perform venipunctures carefully and only as required. Minimize arterial and venous punctures.

Should an arterial puncture be necessary during an infusion, it is preferable to use an upper extremity vessel accessible to manual compression. Apply pressure for at least 30 minutes, apply a pressure dressing, and check the puncture site frequently for bleeding evidence. Avoid noncompressible arterial puncture (ie, avoid internal jugular and subclavian venous punctures to minimize noncompressible site bleeding).

If serious bleeding (not controllable by local pressure) occurs, immediately terminate alteplase infusion and any concomitant heparin. Protamine can be given to reverse heparin effects.

In the following conditions, the risks of alteplase therapy may be increased and should be weighed against the anticipated benefits: recent major surgery (eg, coronary artery bypass graft, obstetrical delivery, organ biopsy, previous puncture of noncompressible vessels); cerebrovascular disease; recent GI or GU bleeding; recent trauma; hypertension: systolic BP 175 mm Hg or more or diastolic BP 110 mm Hg or more; likelihood of left heart thrombus (eg, mitral stenosis with atrial fibrillation); acute pericarditis; subacute bacterial endocarditis; hemostatic defects including those secondary to severe hepatic or renal disease; significant hepatic dysfunction; pregnancy; diabetic hemorrhagic retinopathy or other hemorrhagic ophthalmic conditions; septic thrombophlebitis or occluded AV cannula at seriously infected site; advanced age (eg, older than 75 years of age); patients currently receiving oral anticoagulants (eg, warfarin sodium); any other condition in which bleeding constitutes a significant hazard or would be particularly difficult to manage because of its location.

➤*Cholesterol embolism:* Cholesterol embolism has been reported rarely in patients treated with all thrombolytic agents; the incidence is unknown. This serious condition, which can be lethal, is associated with invasive vascular procedures (eg, cardiac catheterization, angiography, vascular surgery) or anticoagulant therapy. Clinical features of cholesterol embolism may include livedo reticularis, "purple toe" syndrome, acute renal failure, gangrenous digits, hypertension, pancreatitis, MI, cerebral infarction, spinal cord infarction, retinal artery occlusion, bowel infarction, and rhabdomyolysis.

➤*Arrhythmias:* Coronary thrombolysis may result in arrythmias associated with reperfusion. These arrhythmias (such as sinus bradycardia, accelerated idioventricular rhythm, ventricular premature depolarizations, ventricular tachycardia) are not different from those often seen in the ordinary course of AMI and may be managed with standard antiarrhythmic measures. Have antiarrhythmic therapy for bradycardia or ventricular irritability available when alteplase infusions are administered.

➤*PE:* The treatment of PE with alteplase has not been shown to constitute treatment of underlying deep vein thrombosis. Consider the possible risk of re-embolization caused by lysis of underlying deep venous thrombi.

➤*AMI:* In AMI patients who are at low risk of death from cardiac causes (ie, no previous myocardial infarction, Killip class I) and who have high blood pressure at the time of presentation, the risk for stroke may offset the survival benefit produced by thrombolytic therapy.

➤*AIS:* The risks of alteplase therapy to treat AIS may be increased in the following conditions and should be weighed against the anticipated benefits: Severe neurological deficit (eg, NIHSS greater than 22) at presentation (increases risk of ICH) and major early infarct signs on a CT scan (eg, substantial edema, mass effect, or midline shift).

In patients without recent use of oral anticoagulants or heparin, initiate alteplase treatment prior to the availability of coagulation study results. However, discontinue infusion if either a pretreatment PT longer than 15 seconds or an elevated aPTT is identified.

In AIS, neither the incidence of ICH nor the benefits of therapy are known in patients treated with alteplase more than 3 hours after the onset of symptoms. Therefore, do not treat patients with AIS more than 3 hours after symptom onset. Because of the increased risk for misdiagnosis of AIS, special diligence is required in making this diagnosis in patients whose blood glucose values are less than 50 mg/dL or greater than 400 mg/dL.

➤*Neurological deficit:* The safety and efficacy of treatment with alteplase in patients with minor neurological deficit or with rapidly improving symp-

ALTEPLASE RECOMBINANT — INJECTION

toms prior to the start of alteplase administration has not been evaluated; therefore, treatment with alteplase is not recommended.

➤*Infection (Cathflo Activase* only): Use with caution in the presence of suspected infection in a catheter. Use during infection may release a localized infection into the systemic circulation.

➤*Hypersensitivity reaction:* There is no experience with readministration of alteplase. If an anaphylactoid reaction occurs, discontinue the infusion immediately and initiate appropriate therapy. Refer to Management of Acute Hypersensitivity Reactions.

Readministration – Sustained antibody formation in patients receiving 1 dose of alteplase has not been documented, but readminister with caution. Detectable antibody levels (single point measurement) were reported in 1 patient but subsequent antibody test results were negative.

➤*Pregnancy: Category C.* Alteplase has been shown to have an embryocidal effect because of an increased postimplantation loss rate in rabbits when administered by IV at doses approximately 100 times (3 mg/kg) the human dose. There are no adequate and well-controlled studies in pregnant women. Use during pregnancy only if the potential benefit justifies the potential risk to the fetus.

➤*Lactation:* It is not known whether alteplase is excreted in human milk. Exercise caution when administering to nursing women.

➤*Children:* Safety and efficacy of alteplase in pediatric patients have not been established (*Activase*); safety and efficacy in patients younger than 2 years of age or who weigh less than 10 kg have not been established (*Cathflo Activase*).

➤*Lab test abnormalities:* During therapy, if coagulation tests or measures of fibrinolytic activity are performed, the results may be unreliable unless specific precautions are taken to prevent in vitro artifacts. Alteplase present in blood in pharmacologic concentrations remains active in vitro. This can lead to degradation of fibrinogen in blood samples removed for analysis. Collection of blood samples in the presence of aprotinin (150 to 200 units/mL) can, to some extent, mitigate this phenomenon.

➤*Monitoring:* With coadministration of heparin or aspirin, monitor for bleeding especially at arterial puncture sites. Control and monitor blood pressure frequently during and following alteplase administration to manage AIS.

Heparin has been given with and after alteplase infusions to reduce risk of rethrombosis. Either heparin or alteplase may cause bleeding complications; carefully monitor for bleeding, especially at arterial puncture sites.

Drug Interactions

➤*Anticoagulants:* A potential increased risk exists when alteplase is used concomitantly with heparin and vitamin K antagonists.

➤*Drugs affecting platelet function:* Drugs that alter platelet function (ie, aspirin, dipyridamole, and abciximab) may increase the risk of bleeding if administered prior to or after alteplase therapy.

➤*Nitroglycerin:* Concomitant use decreases alteplase concentrations, therefore decreasing thrombolytic effect. Avoid use of nitroglycerin with alteplase.

Adverse Reactions

Bleeding (most frequent) – Should serious bleeding in a critical location (intracranial, GI, retroperitoneal, pericardial) occur, immediately discontinue alteplase therapy along with any concomitant therapy with heparin.

Incidence of Significant Bleeding with Alteplase for 3-Hour Infusion Regimen

Site of bleeding	Total dose ≤ 100 mg/3 h
GI	5%
GU	4%
Ecchymosis	1%
Retroperitoneal	< 1%
Epistaxis	< 1%
Gingival	< 1%

The incidence of ICH in AMI patients treated with alteplase is as follows:

Incidence of Intracranial Bleeding in AMI Patients with Alteplase

Dose	Patients	%
100 mg, 3 hours	3,272	0.4
≤ 100 mg, accelerated	10,396	0.7
150 mg	1,779	1.3
1 to 1.4 mg/kg	237	0.4

Accelerated infusion – All strokes (1.6%); nonfatal stroke (0.9%); hemorrhagic stroke (0.7%). The incidence of all strokes, as well as that for hemorrhagic stroke, increased with increasing age.

Hypersensitivity – Allergic-type reactions (eg, anaphylactoid reaction, laryngeal edema, orolingual angioedema, rash, and urticaria) have been reported. Most reports were of patients treated for AIS and some from treatment for AMI. Many of these patients received concomitant angiotensin-converting enzyme inhibitors (ACEIs). Most cases resolved with prompt treatment.

Other adverse reactions (Activase only) –

AMI: Arrhythmia; AV block; cardiogenic shock; heart failure; cardiac arrest; recurrent ischemia; myocardial reinfarction; myocardial rupture; electromechanical dissociation; pericardial effusion; pericarditis; mitral regurgitation; cardiac tamponade; thromboembolism; pulmonary edema; nausea and/or vomiting; hypotension; fever.

PE: Pulmonary re-embolization; pulmonary edema; pleural effusion; thromboembolism; hypotension; fever.

AIS: Cerebral edema; cerebral herniation; seizure; new ischemic stroke.

Other adverse reactions (Cathflo Activase only) – GI bleeding; sepsis; venous thrombosis; death; major hemorrhage; ICH; pulmonary emboli; arterial emboli; injection-site hemorrhage; upper extremity deep venous thrombosis.

RETEPLASE RECOMBINANT

Rx	**Retavase** (Centocor)	**Powder for injection, lyophilized:** 10.4 units (18.1 mg)	Preservative-free. In kits[a] and half-kits.[b]

[a] Each kit includes a package insert, 2 single-use reteplase vials of 10.4 units (18.1 mg), 2 single-use diluent vials for reconstitution (10 mL sterile water for injection), 2 sterile 10 mL syringes, 2 sterile dispensing pins, 4 sterile needles, and 2 alcohol swabs.

[b] Each half-kit includes a package insert, 1 single-use reteplase vial 10.4 units (18.1 mg), 1 single-use diluent vial for reconstitution (10 mL sterile water for injection), and a sterile dispensing pin.

RETEPLASE RECOMBINANT — INJECTION

Indications

➤*Acute myocardial infarction (AMI):* For use in the management of AMI in adults for the improvement of ventricular function following AMI, the reduction of the incidence of congestive heart failure and the reduction of mortality associated with AMI. Initiate treatment as soon as possible after the onset of AMI symptoms.

➤*Off-label uses:*

Occluded catheters – [2] = Fair documentation. Based on limited data, reteplase appears to be a safe and effective local thrombolytic for occluded catheters. Because the commercial product is preservative free, perform aseptic dilutions to prevent microbial contamination. (See Administration and Dosage.)

Other possible off-label uses – Thrombolytic treatment of acute and chronic deep venous thrombosis (DVT); treatment of massive pulmonary embolism with a double bolus; use in conjunction with heparin and percutaneous transluminal angioplasty (PTA) in the treatment of thrombosed polytetrafluoroethylene hemodialysis arteriovenous grafts (AVGs).

Administration and Dosage

➤*Adults:*

Acute myocardial infarction –

Usual dosage: Administer as a 10 + 10 unit double-bolus injection. Two 10 unit bolus injections are required for a complete treatment. Administer each bolus as an IV injection over 2 minutes. Give the second bolus 30 minutes after initiation of the first bolus injection.

Concomitant therapy: Although the value of anticoagulants and antiplatelet drugs during and following administration of reteplase has not been studied, heparin has been administered concomitantly in greater than 99% of patients. Aspirin has been given either during and/or following heparin treatment. Studies assessing the safety and efficacy of reteplase without adjunctive therapy with heparin and aspirin have not been performed.

Off-label dosing –

Occluded catheters: [2] = Fair documentation. 0.4 units/lumen with a dwell time of 20 to 30 minutes. In abstract data, longer dwell times were allowed (60 minutes) if patency was not achieved after the first 30 minutes, and repeat doses were administered if occlusion was not cleared after 60 minutes. In one clinical trial, doses were reconstituted with sterile water for injection without preservative and frozen in 3 mL syringes for up to 30 days (at −8°C). Once thawed, doses were further diluted with isotonic sodium chloride solution to provide volumes that would fill the catheter lumen (1.3 to 1.6 mL).

➤*Preparation for administration:* Reconstitute using the diluent and dispensing pin provided with reteplase. It is important that reteplase be reconstituted only with the supplied sterile water for injection (without preservatives). The reconstituted preparation results in a colorless solution containing reteplase 1 unit/mL. Slight foaming upon reconstitution is not unusual; allowing the vial to stand undisturbed for several minutes is usually sufficient to allow dissipation of any large bubbles.

Reconstitution instructions –

Reteplase kit and reteplase half-kit: Use aseptic technique throughout.

1.) Withdraw 10 mL of sterile water for injection from the supplied vial into a sterile 10 mL syringe.
2.) Open the package containing the dispensing pin. Remove the protective cap from the luer lock port of the dispensing pin and connect the sterile 10 mL syringe to the dispensing pin. Remove the protective flip-cap from 1 vial of reteplase.

RETEPLASE RECOMBINANT — INJECTION

3.) Remove the protective cap from the spike end of the dispensing pin, and insert the spike into the vial of reteplase until the security clips lock onto the vial. Transfer the 10 mL of sterile water for injection through the dispensing pin into the vial of reteplase.
4.) With the dispensing pin and syringe still attached to the vial, swirl the vial gently to dissolve the reteplase. Do not shake.
5.) Withdraw 10 mL of reteplase reconstituted solution back into the syringe. A small amount of solution will remain in the vial due to overfill.
6.) Detach the syringe from the dispensing pin, and attach a sterile needle.
7.) The 10 mL bolus dose is now ready for administration.

Safely discard all used reconstitution components and the empty reteplase vial according to institutional procedures.

➤*Administration:* Reteplase is for IV administration only. Administer each bolus as an IV injection over 2 minutes.

Give each bolus injection via an IV line in which no other medication is being simultaneously injected or infused. No other medication should be added to the injection solution containing reteplase.

➤*Admixture compatibility:* Heparin and reteplase are incompatible when combined in solution. Do not administer heparin and reteplase simultaneously in the same IV line. If reteplase is to be injected through an IV line containing heparin, flush a normal saline or 5% dextrose solution through the line prior to and following the reteplase injection.

➤*Storage/Stability:* Store reteplase at 2° to 25°C (36° to 77°F). The box should remain sealed until use to protect the lyophilisate from exposure to light.

Because reteplase contains no antibacterial preservatives, reconstitute it immediately before use. When reconstituted as directed, the solution may be used within 4 hours when stored at 2° to 30°C (36° to 86°F).

Actions

➤*Pharmacology:* Reteplase is a recombinant plasminogen activator which catalyzes the cleavage of endogenous plasminogen to generate plasmin. Plasmin in turn degrades the fibrin matrix of the thrombus, thereby exerting its thrombolytic action. In a controlled trial, 36 of 56 patients treated for an acute myocardial infarction (AMI) had a decrease in fibrinogen levels to below 100 mg/dL by 2 hours following the administration of reteplase as a double-bolus IV injection (10 + 10 unit) in which 10 unit (17.4 mg) was followed 30 minutes later by a second bolus of 10 unit (17.4 mg). The mean fibrinogen level returned to the baseline value by 48 hours.

➤*Pharmacokinetics:*

Metabolism/Excretion – Based on the measurement of thrombolytic activity, reteplase is cleared from plasma at a rate of 250 to 450 mL/min, with an effective half-life of 13 to 16 minutes. Reteplase is cleared primarily by the liver and kidney.

Contraindications

Active internal bleeding; history of cerebrovascular accident; recent intracranial or intraspinal surgery or trauma; intracranial neoplasm, arteriovenous malformation, or aneurysm; known bleeding diathesis; severe uncontrolled hypertension

Warnings/Precautions

➤*Arterial puncture:* Should an arterial puncture be necessary during the administration of reteplase, it is preferable to use an upper extremity vessel that is accessible to manual compression. Apply pressure for at least 30 minutes, apply a pressure dressing, and frequently check the puncture site for evidence of bleeding.

➤*Bleeding:* The most common complication encountered during reteplase therapy is bleeding. The sites of bleeding include both internal bleeding sites (intracranial, retroperitoneal, GI, GU, or respiratory) and superficial bleeding sites (venous cutdowns, arterial punctures, sites of recent surgical intervention). The concomitant use of heparin anticoagulation may contribute to bleeding. In clinical trials, some of the hemorrhage episodes occurred 1 or more days after the effects of reteplase had dissipated, but while heparin therapy was continuing. Should serious bleeding (not controllable by local pressure) occur, immediately terminate concomitant anticoagulant therapy. In addition, do not give the second bolus of reteplase if serious bleeding occurs before it is administered.

Injection sites – As fibrin is lysed during reteplase therapy, bleeding from recent puncture sites may occur. Therefore, thrombolytic therapy requires careful attention to all potential bleeding sites (including catheter insertion sites, arterial and venous puncture sites, cutdown sites, and needle puncture sites). Noncompressible arterial puncture must be avoided and internal jugular and subclavian venous punctures should be avoided to minimize bleeding from noncompressible sites.

IM injections – Avoid IM injections and nonessential handling of the patient during treatment with reteplase. Perform venipunctures carefully and only as required.

High-risk conditions – Carefully evaluate each patient being considered for therapy with reteplase and weigh anticipated benefits against the potential risks associated with therapy. In the following conditions, the risks of reteplase therapy may be increased and should be weighed against the anticipated benefits: recent major surgery (eg, coronary artery bypass graft, obstetrical delivery, organ biopsy); previous puncture of noncompressible vessels; cerebrovascular disease; recent GI or GU bleeding; recent trauma; hypertension: systolic BP greater than or equal to 180 mm Hg and/or diastolic BP greater than or equal to 110 mm Hg; high likelihood of left heart thrombus (eg, mitral stenosis with atrial fibrillation); acute pericarditis; subacute bacterial endocarditis; hemostatic defects including those secondary to severe hepatic or renal disease; severe hepatic or renal dysfunction; pregnancy; diabetic hemorrhagic retinopathy or other hemorrhagic ophthalmic conditions; septic thrombophlebitis or occluded AV cannula at a seriously infected site; advanced age; patients currently receiving oral anticoagulants (eg, warfarin sodium); any other condition in which bleeding constitutes a significant hazard or would be particularly difficult to manage because of its location.

➤*Cholesterol embolization:* Cholesterol embolism has been reported rarely in patients treated with thrombolytic agents; the true incidence is unknown. This serious condition, which can be lethal, is also associated with invasive vascular procedures (eg, cardiac catheterization, angiography, vascular surgery) and/or anticoagulant therapy. Clinical features of cholesterol embolism may include livedo reticularis, "purple toe" syndrome, acute renal failure, gangrenous digits, hypertension, pancreatitis, myocardial infarction, cerebral infarction, spinal cord infarction, retinal artery occlusion, bowel infarction, and rhabdomyolysis.

➤*Arrhythmias:* Coronary thrombolysis may result in arrhythmias associated with reperfusion. These arrhythmias (such as sinus bradycardia, accelerated idioventricular rhythm, ventricular premature depolarizations, ventricular tachycardia) are not different from those often seen in the ordinary course of AMI and should be managed with standard antiarrhythmic measures. Antiarrhythmic therapy for bradycardia and/or ventricular irritability should be available when reteplase is administered.

➤*General:* Implement standard management of MI concomitantly with reteplase treatment. Minimized arterial and venous punctures. In addition, do not give the second bolus of reteplase if the serious bleeding occurs before it is administered. In the event of serious bleeding, terminate any concomitant heparin immediately. Heparin effects can be reversed by protamine.

➤*Readministration:* There is no experience with patients receiving repeat courses of therapy with reteplase. Reteplase did not induce the formation of reteplase specific antibodies in any of the approximately 2,400 patients who were tested for antibody formation in clinical trials. If an anaphylactoid reaction occurs, do not give the second bolus of reteplase, and initiate appropriate therapy.

➤*Pregnancy: Category C.* Reteplase has been shown to have an abortifacient effect in rabbits when given in doses 3 times the human dose (0.86 unit/kg). Reproduction studies performed in rats at doses less than or equal to 15 times the human dose (4.31 unit/kg) revealed no evidence of fetal anomalies; however, reteplase administered to pregnant rabbits resulted in hemorrhaging in the genital tract, leading to abortions in mid-gestation. There are no adequate and well-controlled studies in pregnant women. The most common complication of thrombolytic therapy is bleeding, and certain conditions, including pregnancy, can increase this risk. Use reteplase during pregnancy only if the potential benefit justifies the potential risk to the fetus.

➤*Lactation:* It is not known whether reteplase is excreted in human milk. Because many drugs are excreted in human milk, exercise caution when reteplase is administered to a nursing woman.

➤*Children:* Safety and efficacy of reteplase in children have not been established.

➤*Monitoring:* Because heparin, aspirin, or reteplase may cause bleeding complications, careful monitoring for bleeding is advised, especially at arterial puncture sites.

Drug Interactions

The interaction of reteplase with other cardioactive drugs has not been studied. In addition to bleeding associated with heparin and vitamin K antagonists, drugs that alter platelet function (such as aspirin, dipyridamole, and abciximab) may increase the risk of bleeding if administered prior to or after reteplase therapy.

➤*Use of antithrombotics:* Heparin and aspirin have been administered concomitantly with and following the administration of reteplase in the management of AMI. Because heparin, aspirin, or reteplase may cause bleeding complications, careful monitoring for bleeding is advised, especially at arterial puncture sites.

➤*Drug/Lab test interactions:* Administration of reteplase may cause decreases in plasminogen and fibrinogen. During reteplase therapy, if coagulation tests and/or measurements of fibrinolytic activity are performed, the results may be unreliable unless specific precautions are taken to prevent in vitro artifacts. Reteplase is an enzyme that when present in blood in pharmacologic concentrations remains active under in vitro conditions. This can lead to degradation of fibrinogen in blood samples removed for analysis. Collection of blood samples in the presence of PPACK (chloromethylketone) at 2 mm concentrations was used in clinical trials to prevent in vitro fibrinolytic artifacts.

Adverse Reactions

➤*Bleeding:* The most frequent adverse reaction associated with reteplase is bleeding. The types of bleeding events associated with thrombolytic therapy may be broadly categorized as either intracranial hemorrhage or other types of hemorrhage.

- Intracranial hemorrhage. In the INJECT clinical trial the rate of in-hospital, intracranial hemorrhage among all patients treated with reteplase was 0.8% (23 of 2,965 patients). As seen with reteplase and other thrombolytic agents, the risk for intracranial hemorrhage is increased in patients with advanced age or with elevated blood pressure.

RETEPLASE RECOMBINANT — INJECTION

- Other types of hemorrhage. The incidence of other types of bleeding events in clinical studies of reteplase varied depending upon the use of arterial catheterization or other invasive procedures and whether the study was performed in Europe or the USA. The overall incidence of any bleeding event in patients treated with reteplase in clinical studies (n = 3,805) was 21.1%. The rates for bleeding events, regardless of severity, for the 10 + 10 unit reteplase regimen from controlled clinical studies are summarized in the following table.

➤*Reteplase hemorrhage rates:*

Reteplase RecombinantHemorrhage Rates			
	INJECT	RAPID 1 and RAPID 2	
Bleeding site	Europe (n = 2,965)	US (n = 210)	Europe (n = 113)
Anemia, site unknown	2.6%	1.4%	0.9%
GI	2.5%	9%	1.8%
GU	1.6%	9.5%	0.9%
Injection site[a]	4.6%	48.6%	19.5%

[a] Includes the arterial catheterization site (all patients in the RAPID studies underwent arterial catheterization).

In these studies the severity and sites of bleeding events were comparable for reteplase and the comparison thrombolytic agents.

Should serious bleeding in a critical location (intracranial, GI, retroperitoneal, pericardial) occur, immediately terminate any concomitant heparin. In addition, do not give the second bolus of reteplase if the serious bleeding occurs before it is administered. Death and permanent disability are not uncommonly reported in patients who have experienced stroke (including intracranial bleeding) and other serious bleeding episodes.

Fibrin which is part of the hemostatic plug formed at needle puncture sites will be lysed during reteplase therapy. Therefore, reteplase therapy requires careful attention to potential bleeding sites (eg, catheter insertion sites, arterial puncture sites).

➤*Allergic:* Among the 2,965 patients receiving reteplase in the INJECT trial, serious allergic reactions were noted in 3 patients, with 1 patient experiencing dyspnea and hypotension. No anaphylactoid reactions were observed among the 3,856 patients treated with reteplase in initial clinical trials. In an ongoing clinical trial 2 anaphylactoid reactions have been reported among approximately 2,500 patients receiving reteplase.

➤*Miscellaneous:* Patients administered reteplase as treatment for MI have experienced many events which are frequent sequelae of myocardial infarction and may or may not be attributable to reteplase therapy. These events include cardiogenic shock, arrhythmias (eg, sinus bradycardia, accelerated idioventricular rhythm, ventricular premature depolarizations, supraventricular tachycardia, ventricular tachycardia, ventricular fibrillation), AV block, pulmonary edema, heart failure, cardiac arrest, recurrent ischemia, reinfarction, myocardial rupture, mitral regurgitation, pericardial effusion, pericarditis, cardiac tamponade, venous thrombosis and embolism, and electromechanical dissociation. These events can be life-threatening and may lead to death. Other adverse events have been reported, including nausea and/or vomiting, hypotension, and fever.

TENECTEPLASE RECOMBINANT

Rx	TNKase (Genentech)	Powder for Injection, lyophilized: 50 mg	In vials[a] with one 10 mL vial of sterile water for injection and syringe.

[a] With 0.55 g L-arginine, 0.17 g phosphoric acid, 4.3 mg polysorbate 20.

TENECTEPLASE RECOMBINANT — INJECTION

Indications

➤*Acute myocardial infarction (AMI):* For use in the reduction of mortality associated with AMI. Treatment should be initiated as soon as possible after the onset of AMI symptoms.

Administration and Dosage

➤*Adults:*

Acute myocardial infarction –

Usual dosage:

Tenecteplase Dose Information		
Patient weight (kg)	Tenecteplase (mg)	Volume tenecteplase[a] to be administered (mL)
< 60	30	6
≥ 60 to < 70	35	7
≥ 70 to < 80	40	8
≥ 80 to < 90	45	9
≥ 90	50	10

[a] From 1 vial of tenecteplase reconstituted with 10 mL of sterile water for injection.

A single bolus dose should be administered over 5 seconds based on patient weight. Treatment should be initiated as soon as possible after the onset of AMI symptoms.

Maximum dose: The recommended total dose should not exceed 50 mg and is based upon patient weight.

Concomitant therapy: The safety and efficacy of tenecteplase has only been investigated with concomitant administration of heparin and aspirin.

➤*Elderly:* In elderly patients, the benefits of tenecteplase on mortality should be carefully weighed against the risk of increased adverse events, including bleeding.

➤*Preparation for administration:* Because tenecteplase contains no antibacterial preservatives, it should be reconstituted immediately before use. If the reconstituted tenecteplase is not used immediately, refrigerate the tenecteplase vial at 2° to 8°C (36° to 46°F) and use within 8 hours.

Read all instructions completely before beginning reconstitution and administration.

1.) Remove the shield assembly from the supplied *B-D* 10 cc syringe with *TwinPak* Dual Cannula Device (see figure) and aseptically withdraw 10 mL of sterile water for injection from the supplied diluent vial using the red hub cannula syringe filling device. Do not use bacteriostatic water for injection. Do not discard the shield assembly.
2.) Inject the entire contents of the syringe (10 mL) into the tenecteplase vial directing the diluent stream into the powder. Slight foaming upon reconstitution is not unusual; any large bubbles will dissipate if the product is allowed to stand undisturbed for several minutes.
3.) Gently swirl until contents are completely dissolved. Do not shake. The reconstituted preparation results in a colorless to pale yellow transparent solution containing tenecteplase at 5 mg/mL at a pH of approximately 7.3. The osmolality of this solution is approximately 290 mOsm/kg.
4.) Determine the appropriate dose of tenecteplase and withdraw this volume (in milliliters) from the reconstituted vial with the syringe. Any unused solution should be discarded.
5.) Once the appropriate dose of tenecteplase is drawn into the syringe, stand the shield vertically on a flat surface (with green side down) and passively recap the red hub cannula.
6.) Remove the entire shield assembly, including the red hub cannula, by twisting counter clockwise. Note: The shield assembly also contains the clear-ended blunt plastic cannula; retain for split septum IV access.

➤*Administration:* Tenecteplase is for intravenous administration only. Reconstituted tenecteplase should be administered as a single IV bolus over 5 seconds. Tenecteplase may be administered as reconstituted at 5 mg/mL.

Although the supplied syringe is compatible with a conventional needle, this syringe is designed to be used with needleless IV systems. From the information below, follow the instructions applicable to the IV system in use.

- Split septum IV system: Remove the green cap. Attach the clear-ended blunt plastic cannula to the syringe. Remove the shield and use the blunt plastic cannula to access the split septum injection port. Because the blunt plastic cannula has 2 side ports, air or fluid expelled through the cannula will exit in two sideways directions; direct away from face or mucous membranes.
- *Luer-Lok system:* Connect syringe directly to IV port.
- Conventional needle (not supplied in this kit): Attach a large bore needle, eg, 18 gauge, to the syringe's universal *Luer-Lok*.

➤*Admixture compatibility:* Precipitation may occur when tenecteplase is administered in an IV line containing dextrose. Dextrose-containing lines should be flushed with a saline-containing solution prior to and following single bolus administration of tenecteplase.

➤*Storage/Stability:* Store lyophilized tenecteplase at controlled room temperature not to exceed 30°C (86°F) or under refrigeration 2° to 8°C (36° to 46°F).

Actions

➤*Pharmacology:* Tenecteplase is a modified form of human tissue plasminogen activator (tPA) that binds to fibrin and converts plasminogen to plasmin. In the presence of fibrin, in vitro studies demonstrate that tenecteplase conversion of plasminogen to plasmin is increased relative to its conversion in the absence of fibrin. This fibrin specificity decreases systemic activation of plasminogen and the resulting degradation of circulating fibrinogen as compared to a molecule lacking this property. Following administration of 30, 40, or 50 mg of tenecteplase, there are decreases in circulating fibrinogen (4% to 15%) and plasminogen (11% to 24%). The clinical significance of fibrin-specificity on safety (eg, bleeding) or efficacy has not been established. Biological potency is determined by an in vitro clot lysis assay and is expressed in tenecteplase-specific units. The specific activity of tenecteplase has been defined as 200 units/mg.

➤*Pharmacokinetics:* In patients with acute myocardial infarction (AMI), tenecteplase administered as a single bolus exhibits a biphasic disposition from the plasma. Tenecteplase was cleared from the plasma with an initial half-life of 20 to 24 minutes. The terminal phase half-life of tenecteplase was 90 to 130 minutes. In 99 of 104 patients treated with tenecteplase, mean plasma clearance ranged from 99 to 119 mL/min.

TENECTEPLASE RECOMBINANT — INJECTION

The initial volume of distribution is weight related and approximates plasma volume. Liver metabolism is the major clearance mechanism for tenecteplase.

Contraindications

Tenecteplase therapy in patients with acute myocardial infarction is contraindicated in the following situations because of an increased risk of bleeding (see Warnings): active internal bleeding; history of cerebrovascular accident; intracranial or intraspinal surgery or trauma within 2 months; intracranial neoplasm, arteriovenous malformation, or aneurysm; known bleeding diathesis; severe uncontrolled hypertension.

Warnings/Precautions

➤*Bleeding:* The most common complication encountered during tenecteplase therapy is bleeding. The type of bleeding associated with thrombolytic therapy can be divided into two broad categories:

- Internal bleeding, involving intracranial and retroperitoneal sites, or the gastrointestinal, genitourinary, or respiratory tracts.
- Superficial or surface bleeding, observed mainly at vascular puncture and access sites (eg, venous cutdowns, arterial punctures) or sites of recent surgical intervention.

Should serious bleeding (not controlled by local pressure) occur, any concomitant heparin or antiplatelet agents should be discontinued immediately.

In clinical studies of tenecteplase, patients were treated with both aspirin and heparin. Heparin may contribute to the bleeding risks associated with tenecteplase. The safety of the use of tenecteplase with other antiplatelet agents has not been adequately studied (see Drug Interactions). Intramuscular injections and nonessential handling of the patient should be avoided for the first few hours following treatment with tenecteplase. Venipunctures should be performed and monitored carefully.

Should an arterial puncture be necessary during the first few hours following tenecteplase therapy, it is preferable to use an upper extremity vessel that is accessible to manual compression. Pressure should be applied for at least 30 minutes, a pressure dressing applied, and the puncture site checked frequently for evidence of bleeding.

High-risk patients – Each patient being considered for therapy with tenecteplase should be carefully evaluated and anticipated benefits weighed against potential risks associated with therapy. In the following conditions, the risk of tenecteplase therapy may be increased and should be weighed against the anticipated benefits:

- Recent major surgery, eg, coronary artery bypass graft, obstetrical delivery, organ biopsy, previous puncture of noncompressible vessels
- Cerebrovascular disease
- Recent gastrointestinal or genitourinary bleeding
- Recent trauma
- Hypertension: Systolic BP at least 180 mmHg and/or diastolic BP at least 110 mmHg
- High likelihood of left heart thrombus (eg, mitral stenosis with atrial fibrillation)
- Acute pericarditis
- Subacute bacterial endocarditis
- Hemostatic defects, including those secondary to severe hepatic or renal disease
- Severe hepatic dysfunction
- Pregnancy
- Diabetic hemorrhagic retinopathy or other hemorrhagic ophthalmic conditions
- Septic thrombophlebitis or occluded AV cannula at seriously infected site
- Advanced age (see Warnings, Elderly)
- Patients currently receiving oral anticoagulants (eg, warfarin sodium)
- Recent administration of GP IIb/IIIa inhibitors
- Any other condition in which bleeding constitutes a significant hazard or would be particularly difficult to manage because of its location

➤*Cholesterol embolization:* Cholesterol embolism has been reported rarely in patients treated with all types of thrombolytic agents; the true incidence is unknown. This serious condition, which can be lethal, is also associated with invasive vascular procedures (eg, cardiac catheterization, angiography, vascular surgery) and/or anticoagulant therapy. Clinical features of cholesterol embolism may include livedo reticularis, "purple toe" syndrome, acute renal failure, gangrenous digits, hypertension, pancreatitis, myocardial infarction, cerebral infarction, spinal cord infarction, retinal artery occlusion, bowel infarction, and rhabdomyolysis.

➤*Arrhythmias:* Coronary thrombolysis may result in arrhythmias associated with reperfusion. These arrhythmias (such as sinus bradycardia, accelerated idioventricular rhythm, ventricular premature depolarizations, ventricular tachycardia) are not different from those often seen in the ordinary course of acute myocardial infarction and may be managed with standard antiarrhythmic measures. It is recommended that antiarrhythmic therapy for bradycardia and/or ventricular irritability be available when tenecteplase is administered.

➤*General information:* Standard management of myocardial infarction should be implemented concomitantly with tenecteplase treatment. Arterial and venous punctures should be minimized. Noncompressible arterial puncture must be avoided and internal jugular and subclavian venous punctures should be avoided to minimize bleeding from the noncompressible sites. In the event of serious bleeding, heparin and antiplatelet agents should be discontinued immediately. Heparin effects can be reversed by protamine.

➤*Readministration:* Readministration of plasminogen activators, including tenecteplase, to patients who have received prior plasminogen activator therapy has not been systematically studied. Three of 487 patients tested for antibody formation to tenecteplase had a positive antibody titer at 30 days. The data reflect the percentage of patients whose test results were considered positive for antibodies to tenecteplase in a radioimmunoprecipitation assay, and are highly dependent on the sensitivity and specificity of the assay. Additionally, the observed incidence of antibody positivity in an assay may be influenced by several factors including sample handling, concomitant medications, and underlying disease. For these reasons, comparison of the incidence of antibodies to tenecteplase with the incidence of antibodies to other products may be misleading. Although sustained antibody formation in patients receiving one dose of tenecteplase has not been documented, readministration should be undertaken with caution. If an anaphylactic reaction occurs, appropriate therapy should be administered.

➤*Pregnancy: Category C.* Tenecteplase has been shown to elicit maternal and embryo toxicity in rabbits given multiple IV administrations. In rabbits administered 0.5, 1.5, and 5 mg/kg/day, vaginal hemorrhage resulted in maternal deaths. Subsequent embryonic deaths were secondary to maternal hemorrhage and no fetal anomalies were observed. Tenecteplase does not elicit maternal and embryo toxicity in rabbits following a single IV administration. Thus, in developmental toxicity studies conducted in rabbits, the no observable effect level (NOEL) of a single IV administration of tenecteplase on maternal or developmental toxicity was 5 mg/kg (approximately 8 to 10 times the human dose). There are no adequate and well-controlled studies in pregnant women. Tenecteplase should be given to pregnant women only if the potential benefits justify the potential risk to the fetus.

➤*Lactation:* It is not known if tenecteplase is excreted in human milk. Because many drugs are excreted in human milk, caution should be exercised when tenecteplase is administered to a breast-feeding woman.

➤*Children:* The safety and efficacy of tenecteplase in pediatric patients have not been established.

➤*Elderly:* Of the patients in ASSENT-2 who received tenecteplase, 4,958 (59%) were under the age of 65; 2256 (27%) were between the ages of 65 and 74; and 1244 (15%) were 75 and over. The 30-day mortality rates by age were 2.5% in patients under the age of 65, 8.5% in patients between the ages of 65 and 74, and 16.2% in patients age 75 and over. The ICH rates were 0.4% in patients under the age of 65, 1.6% in patients between the ages of 65 and 74, and 1.7% in patients age 75 and over. The rates of any stroke were 1% in patients under the age of 65, 2.9% in patients between the ages of 65 and 74, and 3% in patients age 75 and over. Major bleeding rates, defined as bleeding requiring blood transfusion or leading to hemodynamic compromise, were 3.1% in patients under the age of 65, 6.4% in patients between the ages of 65 and 74, and 7.7% in patients age 75 and over. In elderly patients, the benefits of tenecteplase on mortality should be carefully weighed against the risk of increased adverse events, including bleeding.

Drug Interactions

Formal interaction studies of tenecteplase with other drugs have not been performed. Patients studied in clinical trials of tenecteplase were routinely treated with heparin and aspirin. Anticoagulants (such as heparin and vitamin K antagonists) and drugs that alter platelet function (such as acetylsalicylic acid, dipyridamole, and GP IIb/IIIa inhibitors) may increase the risk of bleeding if administered prior to, during, or after tenecteplase therapy.

➤*Drug/Lab test interactions:* During tenecteplase therapy, results of coagulation tests and/or measures of fibrinolytic activity may be unreliable unless specific precautions are taken to prevent in vitro artifacts. Tenecteplase is an enzyme that, when present in blood in pharmacologic concentrations, remains active under in vitro conditions. This can lead to degradation of fibrinogen in blood samples removed for analysis.

Adverse Reactions

➤*Allergic:* Allergic-type reactions (eg, anaphylaxis, angioedema, laryngeal edema, rash, urticaria) have rarely (less than 1%) been reported in patients treated with tenecteplase. Anaphylaxis was reported in less than 0.1% of patients treated with tenecteplase; however, causality was not established. When such reactions occur, they usually respond to conventional therapy.

➤*Hematologic:* The most frequent adverse reaction associated with tenecteplase is bleeding (see Warnings).

Should serious bleeding occur, concomitant heparin and antiplatelet therapy should be discontinued. Death or permanent disability can occur in patients who experience stroke or serious bleeding episodes.

For tenecteplase-treated patients in ASSENT-2, the incidence of intracranial hemorrhage was 0.9% and any stroke was 1.8%. The incidence of all strokes, including intracranial bleeding, increases with increasing age (see Warnings).

Tenecteplase vs Activase ASSENT-2 Non-ICH Bleeding Events

Bleeding events	Tenecteplase (n = 8,461)	Accelerated activase (n = 8,488)	Relative risk tenecteplase/activase (95% CI)
Major bleeding[a]	4.7%	5.9%	0.78 (0.69, 0.89)
Minor bleeding	21.8%	23%	0.94 (0.89, 1)

TENECTEPLASE RECOMBINANT — INJECTION

Tenecteplase vs Activase ASSENT-2 Non-ICH Bleeding Events			
Bleeding events	Tenecteplase (n = 8,461)	Accelerated activase (n = 8,488)	Relative risk tenecteplase/activase (95% CI)
Units of transfused blood			
Any	4.3%	5.5%	0.77 (0.67, 0.89)
1 to 2	2.6%	3.2%	
> 2	1.7%	2.2%	

[a] Major bleeding is defined as bleeding requiring blood transfusion or leading to hemodynamic compromise.

Nonintracranial major bleeding and the need for blood transfusions were lower in patients treated with tenecteplase.

Types of major bleeding reported in 1% or more of the patients were hematoma (1.7%) and gastrointestinal tract (1%). Types of major bleeding reported in less than 1% of the patients were urinary tract, puncture site (including cardiac catheterization site), retroperitoneal, respiratory tract, and unspecified. Types of minor bleeding reported in 1% or more of the patients were hematoma (12.3%), urinary tract (3.7%), puncture site (including cardiac catheterization site) (3.6%), pharyngeal (3.1%), GI tract (1.9%), epistaxis (1.5%), and unspecified (1.3%).

➤*Miscellaneous:* The following adverse reactions have been reported among patients receiving tenecteplase in clinical trials. These reactions are frequent sequelae of the underlying disease, and the effect of tenecteplase on the incidence of these events is unknown.

These events include cardiogenic shock, arrhythmias, atrioventricular block, pulmonary edema, heart failure, cardiac arrest, recurrent myocardial ischemia, myocardial reinfarction, myocardial rupture, cardiac tamponade, pericarditis, pericardial effusion, mitral regurgitation, thrombosis, embolism, and electromechanical dissociation. These events can be life-threatening and may lead to death. Nausea and/or vomiting, hypotension, and fever have also been reported.

Human Protein C

DROTRECOGIN ALFA (ACTIVATED)

Rx	Xigris (Eli Lilly)	Injection, lyophilized, powder for solution: 5 mg	Preservative free. 40.3 mg sodium chloride, 31.8 mg sucrose. In single-use vials.
		20 mg	Preservative free. 158.1 mg sodium chloride, 124.9 mg sucrose. In single-use vials.

DROTRECOGIN ALFA (ACTIVATED) — INJECTION

Indications

➤*Sepsis:* For the reduction of mortality in adult patients with severe sepsis (sepsis associated with acute organ dysfunction) who have a high risk of death (eg, as determined by the Acute Physiology and Chronic Health Evaluation [APACHE] II score).

Drotrecogin alfa is not indicated in adult patients with severe sepsis and a lower risk of death. Safety and efficacy have not been established in children with severe sepsis.

Administration and Dosage

➤*Adults:*

Sepsis –

Usual dosage: Administer intravenously (IV) at an infusion rate of 24 mcg/kg/h (based on actual body weight) for a total duration of infusion of 96 hours. If the infusion is interrupted, restart drotrecogin alfa at the 24 mcg/kg/h infusion rate.

Dosage adjustment: Dose adjustment based on clinical or laboratory parameters is not recommended.

Discontinuation of therapy: In the event of clinically important bleeding, immediately stop the infusion.

➤*Elderly:* See Adults for dosing.

➤*Preparation for administration:*

1.) Use appropriate aseptic technique during the preparation of drotrecogin alfa for IV administration.
2.) Calculate the approximate amount of drotrecogin alfa needed based upon the patient's actual body weight and duration of this infusion period. The maximum duration of infusion from one preparation step is 12 hours. Multiple infusion periods will be needed to cover the entire 96-hour duration of administration.

mg of drotrecogin alfa = (patient weight, kg) × 24 mcg/kg/h × (hours of infusion) ÷ 1,000

Note: Round the actual amount of drotrecogin alfa to be prepared to the nearest 5 mg increment to avoid discarding reconstituted drotrecogin alfa.

3.) Determine the number of vials of drotrecogin alfa needed to make up this amount.
4.) Reconstitute each vial of drotrecogin alfa with sterile water for injection. The 5 mg vials must be reconstituted with 2.5 mL and the 20 mg vials with 10 mL. Slowly add sterile water for injection to the vial and avoid inverting or shaking the vial. Gently swirl each vial until the powder is completely dissolved. The resulting drotrecogin alfa concentration of the solution is 2 mg/mL.
5.) Drotrecogin alfa contains no antibacterial preservatives; immediately prepare the IV solution after reconstitution of the drotrecogin alfa in the vial(s). If the reconstituted vial is not used immediately, it may be stored at controlled room temperature, 20° to 25°C (68° to 77°F), but must be used within 3 hours.
6.) Inspect the reconstituted drotrecogin alfa for particulate matter and discoloration before further dilution. Do not use vials if particulate matter is visible or if the solution is discolored.
7.) Administer drotrecogin alfa via a dedicated IV line or a dedicated lumen of a multilumen central venous catheter. The only other solutions that can be administered through the same line are sodium chloride 0.9%, Ringer's lactate, dextrose, or dextrose and sodium chloride injections.
8.) Avoid exposing drotrecogin alfa solutions to heat and/or direct sunlight. Studies conducted at the recommended concentrations indicate that the drotrecogin alfa IV solution is compatible with glass infusion bottles and infusion bags and syringes made of polyvinylchloride, polyethylene, polypropylene, or polyolefin.

Dilution and administration for an IV infusion pump –

1.) Complete preparation and administration steps 1 through 8, then complete the next 6 steps.
2.) The solution of reconstituted drotrecogin alfa must be further diluted into an infusion bag containing sodium chloride 0.9% injection to a final concentration between 0.1 and 0.2 mg/mL. Bag volumes between 50 and 250 mL are typical.
3.) Confirm that the intended bag volume will result in an acceptable final concentration.

Final concentration, mg/mL = (actual drotrecogin alfa amount, mg) ÷ (bag volume, mL)

Note: If the calculated final concentration is not between 0.1 and 0.2 mg/mL, select a different bag volume and recalculate the final concentration.

4.) Slowly withdraw the reconstituted drotrecogin alfa solution from the vial(s) and add the reconstituted drotrecogin alfa into the infusion bag of sodium chloride 0.9% injection. When injecting the drotrecogin alfa into the infusion bag, direct the stream to the side of the bag to minimize the agitation of the solution. Gently invert the infusion bag to obtain a homogeneous solution. Do not transport the infusion bag using mechanical transport systems, such as pneumatic-tube systems, which may cause vigorous agitation of the solution.
5.) Calculate the actual duration of the infusion period for the diluted drotrecogin alfa.

Infusion period, hours = (actual drotrecogin alfa amount, mg) × 1,000 ÷ (patient weight, kg) ÷ 24 mcg/kg/h

6.) Account for the added volume of reconstituted drotrecogin alfa (drotrecogin alfa 0.5 mL/mg used) and the volume of bag saline solution removed (if saline solution is removed prior to adding the reconstituted drotrecogin alfa).

Final bag volume, mL = starting bag volume, mL + reconstituted drotrecogin alfa volume, mL − saline volume removed (if any), mL

7.) Calculate the actual infusion rate of the diluted drotrecogin alfa.

Infusion rate, mL/h = final bag volume, mL ÷ infusion period, hours

8.) After preparation for an IV infusion pump, use the IV solution at controlled room temperature, 20° to 25°C (68° to 77°F) within 14 hours. If the IV solution is not administered immediately, the solution may be stored refrigerated at 2° to 8°C (36° to 46°F) for up to 12 hours. If the prepared solution is refrigerated prior to administration, the maximum time limit for use of the IV solution, including preparation, refrigeration, and administration, is 24 hours.

Dilution and administration for a syringe pump –

1.) Complete preparation and administration steps 1 through 8, then complete the next 7 steps.
2.) The solution of reconstituted drotrecogin alfa must be further diluted with sodium chloride 0.9% injection to a final concentration between 0.1 and 1 mg/mL.

DROTRECOGIN ALFA (ACTIVATED) — INJECTION

3.) Confirm that the intended volume will result in an acceptable final concentration.

Final concentration, mg/mL = (actual drotrecogin alfa amount, mg) ÷ (solution volume, mL)

Note: If the calculated final concentration is not between 0.1 and 1 mg/mL, select a different solution volume and recalculate the final concentration.

4.) Slowly withdraw the reconstituted drotrecogin alfa solution from the vial(s) into a syringe that will be used in the syringe pump. Into the same syringe, slowly withdraw sodium chloride 0.9% injection to obtain the desired final volume of diluted drotrecogin alfa. Gently invert and/or rotate the syringe to obtain a homogenous solution.

5.) Calculate the actual duration of the infusion period for the diluted drotrecogin alfa.

Infusion period, hours = (actual drotrecogin alfa amount, mg) × 1,000 ÷ (patient weight, kg) ÷ 24 mcg/kg/h

6.) Calculate the actual infusion rate of the diluted drotrecogin alfa.

Infusion rate, mL/h = (solution volume, mL) ÷ (infusion period, hours)

7.) When administering drotrecogin alfa using a syringe pump at low concentrations (less than approximately 0.2 mg/mL) at low flow rates (less than approximately 5 mL/h), the infusion set must be primed for approximately 15 minutes at a flow rate of approximately 5 mL/h.

8.) After preparation for a syringe pump, the IV solution should be used at controlled room temperature, 20° to 25°C (68° to 77°F), within 12 hours. The maximum time limit for use of the IV solution, including preparation and administration, is 12 hours.

➤*Administration:* Administer reconstituted and diluted solution via IV infusion pump or syringe pump.

Dose escalation or bolus doses of drotrecogin alfa are not recommended.

➤*Admixture compatibility:* The only other solutions that can be administered through the same line are sodium chloride 0.9%, Ringers lactate, dextrose, or dextrose and sodium chloride injections.

Drotrecogin alfa IV solution is compatible with glass infusion bottles and infusion bags and syringes made of polyvinylchloride, polyethylene, polypropylene, or polyolefin.

➤*Storage/Stability:* Store drotrecogin alfa in a refrigerator at 2° to 8°C (36° to 46°F). Do not freeze. Protect unreconstituted vials of drotrecogin alfa from light. Retain in the carton until time of use.

If the reconstituted vial is not used immediately, it may be stored at controlled room temperature, 20° to 25°C (68° to 77°F), but must be used within 3 hours.

IV infusion pump – After preparation for an IV infusion pump, use the IV solution at controlled room temperature, 20° to 25°C (68° to 77°F), within 14 hours. If the IV solution is not administered immediately, the solution may be stored refrigerated at 2° to 8°C (36° to 46°F) for up to 12 hours. If the prepared solution is refrigerated prior to administration, the maximum time limit for use of the IV solution, including preparation, refrigeration, and administration, is 24 hours.

Syringe pump – After preparation for a syringe pump, the IV solution should be used at controlled room temperature, 20° to 25°C (68° to 77°F) within 12 hours. The maximum time limit for use of the IV solution, including preparation and administration, is 12 hours.

Actions

➤*Pharmacology:* Activated protein C exerts an antithrombotic effect by inhibiting factors Va and VIIIa. In vitro data indicate that activated protein C may have indirect profibrinolytic activity through its ability to inhibit plasminogen activator inhibitor-1 and may exert an anti-inflammatory effect by limiting the chemotactic response of leukocytes to inflammatory cytokines, an inhibitory process mediated by leukocyte cell surface activated protein C receptor. In addition, in vivo data suggest activated protein C may reduce interactions between leukocytes and the microvascular endothelium. In vitro bacterial phagocytosis by neutrophils and monocytes is not affected.

Pharmacodynamics – The specific mechanisms by which drotrecogin alfa exerts its effect on survival in patients with severe sepsis are not completely understood. In patients with severe sepsis, drotrecogin alfa infusions of 48 or 96 hours produced dose-dependent declines in D-dimer and interleukin-6. Compared with placebo, drotrecogin alfa-treated patients experienced more rapid declines in D-dimer, plasminogen activator inhibitor-1 levels, thrombin-antithrombin levels, prothrombin F1.2, and interleukin-6; more rapid increases in protein C and antithrombin levels; and normalization of plasminogen. As assessed by infusion duration, the maximum observed pharmacodynamic effect of drotrecogin alfa on D-dimer levels occurred at the end of 96 hours of infusion for the 24 mcg/kg/h treatment group.

➤*Pharmacokinetics:*

Absorption/Distribution – Drotrecogin alfa and endogenous activated protein C are inactivated by endogenous plasma protease inhibitors. Plasma concentrations of endogenous activated protein C in healthy subjects and patients with severe sepsis are usually below detection limits. The median steady-state concentration (C_{ss}) of 45 ng/mL (interquartile range, 35 to 62 ng/mL) was attained within 2 hours after starting infusion. In the majority of patients, plasma concentrations of drotrecogin alfa fell below the assay's quantitation limit of 10 ng/mL within 2 hours after stopping infusion.

In patients with severe sepsis, drotrecogin alfa infusions of 12 to 30 mcg/kg/h rapidly produce C_{ss} proportional to infusion rates.

Metabolism/Excretion – In one study, median clearance of drotrecogin alfa was 40 L/h (interquartile range, 27 to 52 L/h). Plasma clearance of drotrecogin alfa in patients with severe sepsis is approximately 50% higher than in healthy subjects.

Contraindications

Hypersensitivity to drotrecogin alfa or any component of this product; active internal bleeding; recent (within 3 months) hemorrhagic stroke; recent (within 2 months) intracranial or intraspinal surgery, or severe head trauma; trauma with an increased risk of life-threatening bleeding; presence of an epidural catheter; intracranial neoplasm or mass lesion or evidence of cerebral herniation.

Warnings/Precautions

➤*Bleeding:* Bleeding is the most common serious adverse reaction associated with drotrecogin alfa therapy. Carefully evaluate each patient being considered for therapy with drotrecogin alfa and weigh the anticipated benefits against the potential risks associated with therapy.

Certain conditions, many of which led to exclusion from studies, are likely to increase the risk of bleeding with drotrecogin alfa therapy. For individuals with one or more of the following conditions, carefully consider the increased risk of bleeding when deciding whether to use drotrecogin alfa therapy:

- concurrent therapeutic dosing of heparin to treat an active thrombotic or embolic event
- platelet count less than 30,000 × 10^6/L, even if the platelet count is increased after transfusions
- prothrombin time (PT) - international normalized ratio (INR) of more than 3
- recent (within 6 weeks) GI bleeding
- recent administration (within 3 days) of thrombolytic therapy
- recent administration (within 7 days) of oral anticoagulants or glycoprotein IIb/IIIa inhibitors
- recent administration (within 7 days) of aspirin of more than 650 mg/day or other platelet inhibitors
- recent (within 3 months) ischemic stroke
- intracranial arteriovenous malformation or aneurysm
- known bleeding diathesis
- chronic severe hepatic disease
- any other condition in which bleeding constitutes a significant hazard or would be particularly difficult to manage because of its location.

Should clinically important bleeding occur, immediately stop the infusion of drotrecogin alfa. Carefully assess continued use of other agents affecting the coagulation system. Once adequate hemostasis has been achieved, continued use of drotrecogin alfa may be reconsidered.

Invasive procedures increase the risk for bleeding among patients receiving drotrecogin alfa (see Invasive Procedures).

➤*Immunogenicity:* As with all therapeutic proteins, there is a potential for immunogenicity. The incidence of antibody development in patients receiving drotrecogin alfa has not been adequately determined because the assay sensitivity is inadequate to reliably detect all potential antibody responses. One study patient developed antibodies to drotrecogin alfa without clinical sequelae. Another study patient who developed antibodies to drotrecogin alfa developed superficial and deep vein thrombi during the study and died of multiorgan failure on day 36 posttreatment, but the relationship of this reaction to antibody is not clear.

➤*Invasive procedures:* Minimize invasive procedures, including arterial and central venous punctures, in order to decrease the risk of serious bleeding. Avoid noncompressible puncture sites. Discontinue drotrecogin alfa 2 hours prior to the performance of invasive surgical procedures or other procedures associated with special risk of bleeding. Once adequate hemostasis has been achieved, initiation of drotrecogin alfa may be reconsidered 12 hours after major invasive procedures or surgery or restarted immediately after uncomplicated, less invasive procedures.

➤*Prophylactic heparin:* In a randomized study of prophylactic heparin versus placebo in 1,935 adult patients with severe sepsis treated with drotrecogin alfa, mortality and the rate of serious adverse reactions were increased in the subgroup of 434 patients whose low-dose heparin was stopped on study entry by randomization to placebo. This finding was based on prospectively defined exploratory subgroup analyses; however, the explanation for the finding is unclear.

➤*Readministration:* Drotrecogin alfa has not been readministered to patients with severe sepsis.

➤*Single organ dysfunction and recent surgery:* Among the small number of patients enrolled in the PROWESS study with single organ dysfunction and recent surgery (surgery within 30 days prior to study treatment), all-cause mortality was numerically higher in the drotrecogin alfa group (28-day: 10/49; in-hospital: 14/48) compared with the placebo group (28-day: 8/49; in-hospital: 8/47).

In an analysis of the subset of patients with single organ dysfunction and recent surgery from a separate, randomized, placebo-controlled study (ADDRESS) of septic patients not at a high risk of death, all-cause mortality was also higher in the drotrecogin alfa group (28-day: 67/323; in-hospital: 76/325) compared with the placebo group (28-day: 44/313; in-hospital: 62/314).

Patients with single organ dysfunction and recent surgery may not be at high risk of death irrespective of the APACHE II score and, therefore, not among the indicated population.

DROTRECOGIN ALFA (ACTIVATED) — INJECTION

➤*Pregnancy: Category C.* Animal reproductive studies have not been conducted with drotrecogin alfa. It is not known whether drotrecogin alfa can cause fetal harm when administered to a pregnant woman or affect reproduction capacity. Administer drotrecogin alfa to a pregnant woman only if clearly needed.

➤*Lactation:* It is not known whether drotrecogin alfa is excreted in human milk or absorbed systemically after ingestion. Because many drugs are excreted in human milk and because of the potential for adverse reactions in the breast-feeding infant, decide whether to discontinue breast-feeding or the drug, taking into account the importance of the drug to the mother.

➤*Children:* Data from a placebo-controlled trial in 477 patients did not establish the efficacy of drotrecogin alfa in children.

There was a higher rate of CNS bleeding in the drotrecogin alfa versus the placebo group. Over the infusion period (study days 0 to 6), the number of patients experiencing CNS bleeding was 5 versus 1 for the overall population (drotrecogin alfa vs placebo), with 4 of the 5 reactions in the drotrecogin alfa group occurring in patients 60 days of age or younger or 3 kg or less. Fatal CNS bleeding reactions, serious bleeding reactions (over the infusion period and over the 28-day study period), serious adverse reactions, and major amputations were similar in the drotrecogin alfa and placebo groups.

➤*Lab test abnormalities:* Most patients with severe sepsis have a coagulopathy that is commonly associated with prolongation of activated partial thromboplastin time (APTT) and PT. Drotrecogin alfa may variably prolong APTT. Therefore, APTT cannot be used reliably to assess the status of the coagulopathy during drotrecogin alfa infusion. Drotrecogin alfa has minimal effect on PT, and PT can be used to monitor the status of the coagulopathy in these patients.

Drug Interactions

➤*Drugs that affect hemostasis:* There is an increased risk of bleeding with drotrecogin alfa; employ caution when drotrecogin alfa is used with other drugs that affect hemostasis.

➤*Drug/Lab test interactions:* Because drotrecogin alfa may affect APTT assays, drotrecogin alfa present in plasma samples may interfere with one-stage coagulation assays based on APTT (eg, factor VIII, IX, and XI assays). This interference may result in an apparent factor concentration that is lower than the true concentration. Drotrecogin alfa present in plasma samples does not interfere with one-stage factor assays based on PT (eg, factor II, V, VII, and X assays).

Adverse Reactions

➤*Bleeding:* Bleeding is the most common adverse reaction associated with drotrecogin alfa.

In one study, serious bleeding reactions were observed during the 28-day study period in 3.5% of drotrecogin alfa-treated and 2% of placebo-treated patients, respectively. The difference in serious bleeding between drotrecogin alfa-treated patients and placebo-treated patients occurred primarily during the infusion period and is shown in the following table. Serious bleeding reactions were defined as any intracranial hemorrhage, any life-threatening or fatal bleed, any bleeding reaction requiring the administration of 3 units or more of packed red blood cells per day for 2 consecutive days, or any bleeding reaction assessed as a serious adverse reaction.

Drotrecogin Alfa Serious Bleeding Event by Site of Hemorrhage (%)[a]

Site of hemorrhage	Drotrecogin alfa (n = 850)	Placebo (n = 840)
GI	0.6%	0.5%
GU	0.2%	0%
Intraabdominal	0.2%	0.4%
Intracranial	0.2%	0%
Intrathoracic	0.5%	0%
Retroperitoneal	0.4%	0%
Skin/Soft tissue	0.1%	0%
Miscellaneous[b]	0.1%	0.1%
Total	2.4%	1%

[a] The study drug infusion period is defined as the date of initiation of the study drug to the date of study drug discontinuation plus the next calendar day.
[b] Patients requiring the administration of 3 units or more of packed red blood cells per day for 2 consecutive days without an identified site of bleeding.

In the PROWESS study, 2 cases of intracranial hemorrhage occurred during the infusion period for drotrecogin alfa-treated patients, and no cases were reported in the placebo patients. The incidence of intracranial hemorrhage during the 28-day study period was 0.2% for drotrecogin alfa-treated patients and 0.1% for placebo-treated patients. Intracranial hemorrhage has been reported in patients receiving drotrecogin alfa in non–placebo-controlled trials with an incidence of approximately 1% during the infusion period. The risk of intracranial hemorrhage may be increased in patients with risk factors for bleeding, such as severe coagulopathy and severe thrombocytopenia.

In the PROWESS study, 25% of drotrecogin alfa-treated patients and 18% of placebo-treated patients experienced at least 1 bleeding reaction during the 28-day study period. In both treatment groups, the majority of bleeding reactions were ecchymoses or GI tract bleeding.

Additional information on adverse reactions has been obtained in a controlled study of patients not at high risk of death (study 2) and an open label, uncontrolled study of 2,378 adult patients with severe sepsis that enrolled both patients at high risk of death and those not at high risk of death (study 3). The incidence rates and nature of treatment-associated adverse reactions in study 2 were generally similar to those seen in study 1. In study 3, serious bleeding occurred in 3.6% of patients during the infusion period and 6.5% during the 28-day study period. Intracranial hemorrhage occurred among 0.6% of patients during the infusion period and 1.5% within 28 days. Most of the postinfusion intracranial hemorrhage reactions occurred within 1 week of the drotrecogin alfa infusion; the relationship of these reactions to drotrecogin alfa is uncertain.

➤*Other adverse reactions:* Patients administered drotrecogin alfa as treatment for severe sepsis experienced many reactions that are potential sequelae of severe sepsis and may or may not be attributable to drotrecogin alfa therapy. In clinical trials, there were no types of nonbleeding adverse reactions, suggesting a causal association with drotrecogin alfa.

Overdosage

➤*Symptoms:* In postmarketing experience, a limited number of medication errors have been reported of excessive rate of drotrecogin alfa infusion for short periods of time (median, 2 hours). No unexpected adverse reactions were observed during the overdose period. However, this information is insufficient to assess whether drotrecogin alfa overdose is associated with an increased hemorrhage risk beyond that observed with drotrecogin alfa administered at the recommended dose.

➤*Treatment:* There is no known antidote for drotrecogin alfa. In case of overdose, stop the infusion immediately and monitor closely for hemorrhagic complications.

Patient Information

Advise patients that this medicine may cause serious bleeding and that each patient should weigh the benefits against the potential risks associated with therapy.

PROTEIN C CONCENTRATE (HUMAN)

Rx	**Ceprotin** (Baxter)	**Injection, lyophilized, powder for solution:** 500 units	In single-dose vials.[a]
		1,000 units	In single-dose vials.[a]

[a] Each single-dose vial contains the following excipients: 8 mg/mL human albumin, 4.4 mg/mL trisodium citrate dihydrate, and 8.8 mg/mL sodium chloride when reconstituted with the appropriate amount of diluent.

PROTEIN C CONCENTRATE (HUMAN) — INJECTION

Indications

➤*Severe congenital protein C deficiency:* For patients with severe congenital protein C deficiency for the prevention and treatment of venous thrombosis and purpura fulminans; as congenital protein C replacement therapy for children and adults.

Administration and Dosage

➤*General dosing considerations:* Treatment with protein C concentrate should be initiated under the supervision of a health care provider experienced in replacement therapy with coagulation factors/inhibitors where monitoring of protein C activity is feasible.

The dose, administration frequency, and duration of treatment with protein C concentrate depend on the severity of the protein C deficiency, the patient's age, the clinical condition of the patient, and the patient's plasma level of protein C. Therefore, the dose regimen should be adjusted according to the pharmacokinetic profile for each individual patient.

In patients receiving prophylactic administration of protein C concentrate, higher peak protein C activity levels may be warranted in situations of an increased risk of thrombosis (such as infection, trauma, or surgical intervention). Maintenance of trough protein C activity levels above 25% is recommended.

➤*Adults:*

Severe congenital protein C deficiency –

Initial dosage: 100 to 120 units/kg for determination of recovery and half-life is recommended for acute episodes and short-term prophylaxis. Subsequently, the dose should be adjusted to maintain a target peak protein C activity of 100%. See table below.

Intermediate dosage: See table below.

Maintenance dosage: See table below.

PROTEIN C CONCENTRATE (HUMAN) — INJECTION

After resolution of the acute episode, continue the patient on the same dose to maintain trough protein C activity level above 25% for the duration of treatment.

Protein C concentrate dosing schedule –

Protein C Concentrate Dosing Schedule[a]			
	Initial dose[b]	Subsequent 3 doses[b]	Maintenance dose[b]
Acute episode/ short-term prophylaxis[c]	100 to 120 units/kg	60 to 80 units/kg every 6 hours	45 to 60 units/kg every 6 or 12 hours
Long-term prophylaxis	NA[d]	NA	45 to 60 units/kg every 12 hours

[a] Dosing is based upon a pivotal clinical trial of 15 patients.
[b] The dose regimen should be adjusted according to the pharmacokinetic profile for each individual.
[c] Protein C concentrate should be continued until desired anticoagulation is achieved.
[d] NA = not applicable.

➤*Children:*

Severe congenital protein C deficiency – See Adults for dosing.

➤*Initiation of vitamin K antagonists:* In patients starting treatment with oral anticoagulants belonging to the class of vitamin K antagonists, a transient hypercoagulable state may arise before the desired anticoagulant effect becomes apparent. This transient effect may be explained by the fact that protein C, itself a vitamin K–dependent plasma protein, has a shorter half-life than most of the vitamin K–dependent proteins (ie, factor II, IX, and X).

In the initial phase of treatment, the activity of protein C is more rapidly suppressed than that of the procoagulant factors. For this reason, if the patient is switched to oral anticoagulants, protein C replacement must be continued until stable anticoagulation is obtained. Although warfarin-induced skin necrosis can occur in any patient during the initiation of treatment with oral anticoagulant therapy, individuals with severe congenital protein C deficiency are particularly at risk.

During the initiation of oral anticoagulant therapy, it is advisable to start with a low dose of the anticoagulant and adjust this incrementally, rather than use a standard loading dose of the anticoagulant.

➤*Therapeutic drug monitoring:* The measurement of protein C activity using a chromogenic assay is recommended for the determination of the patient's plasma level of protein C before and during treatment with protein C activity. The half-life of protein C activity may be shortened in certain clinical conditions such as acute thrombosis, purpura fulminans, and skin necrosis. In the case of an acute thrombotic event, it is recommended that protein C activity measurements be performed immediately before the next injection until the patient is stabilized. After the patient is stabilized, continue monitoring the protein C levels to maintain the trough protein C level above 25%.

Patients treated during the acute phase of their disease may display much lower increases in protein C activity. Coagulation parameters should also be checked; however, in clinical trials, data were insufficient to establish correlation between protein C activity levels and coagulation parameters.

➤*Preparation for administration:*
- Bring the protein C concentrate (powder) and sterile water for injection (diluent) to room temperature.
- Remove caps from the protein C concentrate and diluent vials.
- Cleanse stoppers with germicidal solution, and allow them to dry prior to use.
- Remove protective covering from one end of the double-ended transfer needle and insert exposed needle through the center of the diluent vial stopper.
- Remove protective covering from the other end of the double-ended transfer needle. Invert diluent vial over the upright protein C concentrate vial; then rapidly insert the free end of the needle through the protein C concentrate vial stopper at its center. The vacuum in the vial will draw in the diluent. If there is no vacuum in the vial, do not use the product, and contact 1-888-237-7684.
- Disconnect the 2 vials by removing the needle from the diluent vial stopper. Then, remove the transfer needle from the protein C concentrate vial. Gently swirl the vial until all powder is dissolved. Be sure that the protein C concentrate is completely dissolved; otherwise, active materials will be removed by the filter needle.

After reconstitution, the solution is colorless to slightly yellowish and clear to slightly opalescent and essentially free from visible particles. Do not use the product if the solution does not meet these criteria. Protein C concentrate should be administered at room temperature not more than 3 hours after reconstitution.
- Attach the filter needle to a sterile, disposable syringe and draw back the plunger to admit air into the syringe.
- Insert the filter needle into the vial of reconstituted protein C concentrate.
- Inject air into the vial and then withdraw the reconstituted protein C concentrate into the syringe.
- Remove and discard the filter needle in a hard-walled sharps container for proper disposal. Filter needles are intended to filter the contents of a single vial of protein C concentrate only.
- Attach a suitable needle or infusion set with winged adapter and inject intravenously (IV).

➤*Administration:* Protein C concentrate is administered by IV injection after reconstitution of the powder for solution for injection with sterile water for injection. Allergic-type hypersensitivity reactions are possible.

Protein C concentrate should be administered at a maximum injection rate of 2 mL/min except for children with a body weight of less than 10 kg, for whom the injection rate should not exceed a rate of 0.2 mL/kg/min.

➤*Storage/Stability:* Protein C concentrate is stable for 3 years when stored refrigerated at 2 to 8C (36 to 46F). Do not freeze, in order to prevent damage to the diluent vial. Store the vial in the original carton to protect it from light. The reconstituted solution should be used within 3 hours of reconstitution.

Actions

➤*Pharmacology:* Protein C is the precursor of a vitamin K–dependent anticoagulant glycoprotein (serine protease) that is synthesized in the liver. It is converted by the thrombin/thrombomodulin-complex on the endothelial cell surface to activated protein C (APC). APC is a serine protease with potent anticoagulant effects, especially in the presence of its cofactor protein S. APC exerts its effect by the inactivation of the activated forms of factors V and VIII, which leads to a decrease in thrombin formation. APC has also been shown to have profibrinolytic effects.

The protein C pathway provides a natural mechanism for control of the coagulation system and prevention of excessive procoagulant responses to activating stimuli. A complete absence of protein C is not compatible with life. A severe deficiency of this anticoagulant protein causes a defect in the control mechanism and leads to unchecked coagulation activation, resulting in thrombin generation and intravascular clot formation with thrombosis.

Pharmacodynamics – In clinical studies, the IV administration of protein C concentrate demonstrated a temporary increase, within approximately half an hour of administration, in plasma levels of protein C. Replacement of protein C in protein C–deficient patients is expected to control or, if given prophylactically, to prevent thrombotic complications.

➤*Pharmacokinetics:*

Pharmacokinetics of Protein C Concentrate in Subjects With Severe Congenital Protein C Deficiency[a]					
Pharmacokinetic parameter	N	Median	95% CI for median	Min	Max
C_{max} (units/dL)	21	110	106 to 127	40	141
T_{max} (h)	21	0.5	0.5 to 1.05	0.17	1.33
Incremental recovery[b] (units/dL)/(units/kg)	21	1.42	1.32 to 1.59	0.5	1.76
Initial half-life (h)	21	7.8	5.4 to 9.3	3	36.1
Terminal half-life (h)	21	9.9	7 to 12.4	4.4	15.8
Half-life by the noncompartmental approach (h)	21	9.8	7.1 to 11.6	4.9	14.7
$AUC_{0-\infty}$ units•h/dL	21	1,500	1,289 to 1,897	344	2,437
MRT (h)	21	14.1	10.3 to 16.7	7.1	21.3
Clearance (dL/kg/h)	21	0.0533	0.0428 to 0.0792	0.0328	0.2324
Volume of distribution at steady state (dL/kg)	21	0.74	0.7 to 0.89	0.44	1.65

[a] CI = confidence interval; C_{max} = maximum concentration after infusion; T_{max} = time at maximum concentration; $AUC_{0-\infty}$ = area under the curve from 0 to infinity; MRT = mean residence time.
[b] Incremental recovery = maximum increase in protein C concentration following infusion divided by dose.

Absorption – The protein C plasma activity was measured by chromogenic and/or clotting assay. C_{max} and AUC appeared to increase dose-linearly between 40 and 80 units/kg. The median incremental recovery was 1.42 (]/]) after IV administration of protein C concentrate.

Excretion – The median half-lives, based on noncompartmental method, ranged from 4.9 to 14.7 hours, with a median of 9.8 hours. In patients with acute thrombosis, both the increase in protein C plasma levels as well as half-life may be considerably reduced.

Special populations –

Children: The pharmacokinetic profile in children has not been formally assessed. Limited data suggest that the pharmacokinetics of protein C concentrate may be different between very young children and adults. The systemic exposure (maximal drug concentration [C_{max}] and [AUC]) may be considerably reduced because of a faster clearance, a larger volume of distribution, and/or a shorter half-life of protein C in very young children than in older subjects. This fact must be considered when a dosing regimen for children is determined. Individualize doses based upon protein C activity levels.

Contraindications

None known.

Warnings/Precautions

➤*Transmission of infectious agents:* Protein C concentrate is made from human plasma. Products made from human plasma may contain infectious agents, such as viruses, that can cause disease. The risk that such products will transmit an infectious agent has been reduced by screening plasma donors for prior exposure to certain viruses, by testing for the presence of

PROTEIN C CONCENTRATE (HUMAN) — INJECTION

certain current virus infections, and by inactivating and/or removing a broad range of viruses during manufacture.

Despite these measures, such products can still potentially transmit disease. Because this product is made from human blood, it may carry a risk of transmitting infectious agents (eg, viruses and, theoretically, the Creutzfeldt-Jakob disease agent). All infections thought by a health care provider to have possibly been transmitted by this product should be reported by the health care provider to 1-866-888-2472. The health care provider should discuss the risks and benefits of this product with the patient.

Some viruses, such as human parvovirus B19 (B19V) or hepatitis A, are particularly difficult to remove or inactivate. B19V most seriously affects pregnant women (fetal infection) or immune-compromised individuals. Symptoms of B19V infection include fever, drowsiness, chills, and runny nose followed about 2 weeks later by a rash and joint pain. Evidence of hepatitis A may include several days to weeks of poor appetite, tiredness, and low-grade fever followed by nausea, vomiting, and abdominal pain. Dark urine and a yellowed complexion are also common symptoms. Encourage patients to consult their health care provider if such symptoms appear.

Consider appropriate vaccination (hepatitis A and B) for patients in regular and/or repeated receipt of human plasma–derived protein C.

➤*Bleeding episodes:* Several bleeding episodes have been observed in clinical studies. Concurrent anticoagulant medication may have been responsible for these bleeding episodes. However, it cannot be completely ruled out that the administration of protein C concentrate further contributed to these bleeding events.

Simultaneous administration of protein C concentrate and tissue plasminogen activator (tPA) may further increase the risk of bleeding from tPA.

➤*Heparin-induced thrombocytopenia (HIT):* Protein C concentrate contains trace amounts of heparin that may lead to HIT. Determine the platelet count immediately and consider discontinuation of protein C concentrate.

➤*Low-sodium diet:* Inform patients on a low-sodium diet that the quantity of sodium in the maximum daily dose of protein C concentrate exceeds 200 mg. Closely monitor patients with renal function impairment for sodium overload.

➤*Hypersensitivity reactions:* Protein C concentrate may contain traces of mouse protein and/or heparin as a result of the manufacturing process. Allergic reactions to mouse protein and/or heparin cannot be ruled out. If symptoms of a hypersensitivity/allergic reaction occur, discontinue the injection/infusion. In case of anaphylactic shock, the current medical standards for treatment are to be observed.

➤*Pregnancy: Category C.* Animal reproduction studies have not been conducted with protein C concentrate. It is also not known whether protein C concentrate can cause fetal harm when administered to a pregnant woman or can affect reproduction capacity. Protein C concentrate has not been studied for use in pregnancy.

Labor and delivery – There has been one report of protein C concentrate exposure during labor and delivery with no adverse outcome. Protein C concentrate has not been studied for use during labor and delivery.

➤*Lactation:* It is not known whether protein C concentrate is excreted in human milk. Protein C concentrate has not been studied for use in breast-feeding mothers.

➤*Children:* Neonatal and pediatric subjects were included in several retrospective and prospective studies evaluating the safety and efficacy of protein C concentrate. Subjects were enrolled from as early as 2 days of age throughout adolescence.

➤*Monitoring:* Closely monitor patients with renal function impairment for sodium overload.

Drug Interactions

➤*tPA:* Simultaneous administration of protein C concentrate and tPA may further increase the risk of bleeding from tPA.

Adverse Reactions

The most serious and common adverse reactions related to protein C concentrate treatment observed were hypersensitivity or allergic reactions (itching and rash) and light-headedness.

The safety profile of protein C concentrate was based on 121 patients from clinical studies and compassionate use in severe congenital protein C deficiency. Duration of exposure ranged from 1 day to 8 years. One patient experienced hypersensitivity/allergic reactions (itching and rash) and light-headedness, which were determined by the investigator to be related to protein C concentrate.

No inhibiting antibodies to protein C concentrate have been observed in clinical studies. However, the potential for developing antibodies cannot be ruled out.

Overdosage

➤*Animal toxicity:*

Citrate toxicity – Protein C concentrate contains trisodium citrate dihydrate (TCD) 4.4 mg/mL of reconstituted product. Studies in mice evaluating 1,000-unit vials reconstituted with 10 mL vehicle followed by dosing at 30 mL/kg (TCD 132 mg/kg) and 60 mL/kg (TCD 264 mg/kg) resulted in signs of citrate toxicity (dyspnea, slowed movement, hemoperitoneum, lung and thymus hemorrhage, and renal pelvis dilation).

➤*Symptoms:* No symptoms of overdose with protein C concentrate have been reported.

The maximum infusion rate administered in clinical studies were doses of up to 600 units/kg body weight (BW)/day (150 units/kg BW every 6 hours) of protein C concentrate. There have been no overdosages of protein C concentrate reported during clinical studies. In long-term prophylactic treatment of doses of up to 291.7 units/kg BW/day, no adverse reactions were reported.

Patient Information

Inform patients of the early signs of hypersensitivity reactions, including hives, generalized urticaria, tightness of the chest, wheezing, hypotension, and anaphylaxis, because the risk of an allergic-type hypersensitivity reaction cannot be excluded. In addition, protein C concentrate may contain traces of mouse protein or heparin as a result of the manufacturing process. Allergic reactions to mouse protein or heparin cannot be ruled out. If symptoms of hypersensitivity/allergic reaction occur, patients should immediately discontinue the injection/infusion and inform their health care provider as soon as possible.

Prior to reconstitution, protect protein C concentrate from light.

Reconstitute the lyophilized protein C concentrate powder with the supplied diluent (sterile water for injection) using the sterile transfer needle. Gently swirl the vial until all of the powder is dissolved.

Visually inspect the solution for discoloration and particulate matter. The reconstituted solution should be colorless to slightly yellowish and clear to slightly opalescent and essentially free from visible particles. Protein C concentrate should not be administered if discoloration or particulate matter is observed. The solution is drawn through the sterile filter needle into a sterile disposable syringe.

The reconstituted solution contains no preservatives and is intended for single use only. Once reconstituted, it is recommended that the product be administered by IV injection within 3 hours. All unused solution, empty vials, and used needles must be discarded appropriately.

UROKINASE

Rx	**Abbokinase** (Abbott)	**Powder for injection, lyophilized**: 250,000 IU/vial	Preservative free. 25 mg mannitol, 25 mg albumin (human), 50 mg sodium chloride. In vials.

UROKINASE — INJECTION

Indications

➤*Catheter:* Urokinase for catheter clearance is indicated for the restoration of patency to IV catheters, including central venous catheters, obstructed by clotted blood or fibrin.

➤*Injection:*

Pulmonary embolism –

Urokinase is indicated in adults: For the lysis of acute massive pulmonary emboli, defined as obstruction of blood flow to a lobe or multiple segments.

For the lysis of pulmonary emboli accompanied by unstable hemodynamics (ie, failure to maintain blood pressure without supportive measures). The diagnosis should be confirmed by objective means, such as pulmonary angiography via an upper extremity vein, or noninvasive procedures such as lung scanning.

Angiographic and hemodynamic measurements demonstrate a more rapid improvement with lytic therapy than with heparin therapy.

Coronary artery thrombosis – Urokinase has been reported to lyse acute thrombi obstructing coronary arteries, associated with evolving transmural MI. The majority of patients who received urokinase by intracoronary infusion within 6 hours following onset of symptoms showed recanalization of the involved vessel.

It has not been established that intracoronary administration of urokinase during evolving transmural MI results in salvage of myocardial tissue, nor that it reduces mortality. The patients who might benefit from this therapy cannot be defined.

Administration and Dosage

➤*General dosing considerations:* At the end of urokinase therapy, treatment with heparin by continuous IV infusion is recommended to prevent recurrent thrombosis. Heparin treatment, without a loading dose, should not begin until the thrombin time has decreased to less than twice the normal control value (approximately 3 to 4 hours after completion of the infusion). See the heparin monograph for proper use of heparin. This should then be followed by oral anticoagulants in the conventional manner.

Urokinase treatment should be instituted soon after onset of pulmonary embolism. Delay in instituting therapy may decrease the potential for optimal efficacy.

UROKINASE — INJECTION

➤*Adults:*

Coronary artery thrombosis –

Usual dosage: Infuse into the occluded artery at a rate of 4 mL/min (6,000 units/min) for periods up to 2 hours. Average total dose is 500,000 units.

Duration of therapy: Continue therapy until the artery is maximally opened, usually 15 to 30 minutes after the initial opening.

Concomitant therapy: 2,500 to 10,000 units heparin IV bolus before administering urokinase. It is advisable to continue heparin after the artery has been opened.

Monitoring: To determine response to urokinase therapy, periodic angiography during the infusion is recommended. It is suggested that the angiography be repeated at approximately 15 minute intervals.

Pulmonary embolism –

Loading dose: 2,000 units/pound (4,400 units/kg) at a rate of 90 mL/h over a period of 10 minutes.

Maintenance dosage: Continuous infusion of 2,000 units/pound/h (4,400 units/kg/h) at a rate of 15 mL/h for 12 hours.

Concomitant therapy: Because some urokinase admixture will remain in the tubing at the end of an infusion pump delivery cycle, the following flush procedure should be performed to insure that the total dose of urokinase is administered. A solution of 0.9% sodium chloride injection or 5% dextrose injection approximately equal in amount to the volume of the tubing in the infusion set should be administered via the pump to flush the urokinase admixture from the entire length of the infusion set. The pump should be set to administer the flush solution at the continuous infusion rate of 15 mL/h.

➤*Therapeutic drug monitoring:* Following the infusion, coagulation parameters should be determined.

➤*Preparation for administration:*

Catheter – Preparation of solution (univial)

1.) Remove protective cap. Turn plunger-stopper a quarter turn and press to force diluent into lower chamber.
2.) Roll and tilt to effect solution. Use only a clear, essentially colorless solution.
3.) Sterilize top of stopper with a suitable germicide.
4.) Insert needle through the center of stopper until tip is barely visible. Withdraw dose.

Thin translucent filaments may occasionally occur in reconstituted urokinase vials, but do not indicate any decrease in potency of this product. It is recommended that vigorous shaking be avoided during reconstitution; roll and tilt to enhance reconstitution.

Injection – Reconstitute urokinase for injection by aseptically adding 5 mL of sterile water for injection to 1 vial for lysis of pulmonary emboli or 3 vials for lysis of coronary artery thrombi. It is important that urokinase be reconstituted only with sterile water for injection without preservatives. Bacteriostatic water for injection should not be used.

To minimize formation of filaments, avoid shaking the vial during reconstitution. Roll and tilt the vial to enhance reconstitution. The solution may be terminally filtered (eg, through a 0.45 micron or smaller cellulose membrane filter). No other medication should be added to this solution.

➤*Administration:*

Catheter – When the following procedure is used to clear a central venous catheter, the patient should be instructed to exhale and hold his breath any time the catheter is not connected to IV tubing or a syringe. This is to prevent air from entering the open catheter.

Aseptically disconnect the IV tubing connection at the catheter hub and attach an empty 10 mL syringe. Determine occlusion of the catheter by gently attempting to aspirate blood from the catheter with the 10 mL syringe. If aspiration is not possible, remove the 10 mL syringe and attach a syringe filled with an amount of prepared urokinase for catheter clearance solution equal to the internal volume of the catheter. Slowly and gently inject the urokinase solution into the catheter. Aseptically remove the syringe and connect a 5 mL syringe to the catheter. Wait at least 5 minutes before attempting to aspirate the drug and residual clot with the empty syringe. Repeat aspiration attempts every 5 minutes. If the catheter is not open within 30 minutes, the catheter may be capped allowing urokinase solution to remain in the catheter for an additional 30 to 60 minutes before again attempting to aspirate. A second injection of urokinase for catheter clearance may be necessary in resistant cases.

When patency is restored, aspirate 4 to 5 mL of blood to ensure removal of all drug and residual clot. Remove the blood-filled syringe and replace it with a 10 mL syringe filled with 0.9% sodium chloride injection. The catheter should then be gently irrigated with this solution to ensure patency of the catheter. After the catheter has been irrigated, remove the 10 mL syringe and aseptically reconnect sterile IV tubing to the catheter hub.

Injection –

Coronary artery thrombosis: Add the contents of the 3 reconstituted urokinase vials to 500 mL of 5% dextrose injection. The resulting solution admixture will have a concentration of approximately 1,500 units/mL. No other medication should be added to the solution.

Pulmonary embolism: Prior to infusing, dilute the reconstituted urokinase with 0.9% sodium chloride injection or 5% dextrose injection.

Urokinase Dose Preparation: Pulmonary Embolism

Patient weight (pounds)	Total dose[a] urokinase (units)	Number of vials of urokinase	Volume of urokinase after reconstitution (mL)[b]	+	Volume of diluent (mL)	=	Final volume (mL)
81 to 90	2,250,000	9	45		150		195
91 to 100	2,500,000	10	50		145		195
101 to 110	2,750,000	11	55		140		195
111 to 120	3,000,000	12	60		135		195
121 to 130	3,250,000	13	65		130		195
131 to 140	3,500,000	14	70		125		195
141 to 150	3,750,000	15	75		120		195
151 to 160	4,000,000	16	80		115		195
161 to 170	4,250,000	17	85		110		195
171 to 180	4,500,000	18	90		105		195
181 to 190	4,750,000	19	95		100		195
191 to 200	5,000,000	20	100		95		195
201 to 210	5,250,000	21	105		90		195
211 to 220	5,500,000	22	110		85		195
221 to 230	5,750,000	23	115		80		195
231 to 240	6,000,000	24	120		75		195
241 to 250	6,250,000	25	125		70		195
	Loading dose				Dose for 12-hour period		
Infusion rate:	15 mL/10 min[c]				15 mL/h for 12 hours		

[a] Loading dose + dose administered during 12-hour period.
[b] After addition of 5 mL of sterile water for injection, per vial (see Preparation).
[c] Pump rate = 90 mL/h.

Administered using a constant infusion pump that is capable of delivering a total volume of 195 mL.

➤*Storage/Stability:* Reconstituted solution should be used immediately after reconstitution. Discard any unused portion.

Catheter – Store powder below 25°C (77°F). Avoid freezing.

Injection – Store powder at 2° to 8°C (36° to 46°F).

Actions

➤*Pharmacology:* Urokinase is an enzyme (protein) produced by the kidney, and found in the urine. There are 2 forms of urokinase which differ in molecular weight but have similar clinical effects. Urokinase, intended for use as a thrombolytic agent, is the low molecular weight form. Urokinase acts on the endogenous fibrinolytic system. It converts plasminogen to the enzyme plasmin. Plasmin degrades fibrin clots as well as fibrinogen and some other plasma proteins.

Information about the pharmacokinetic properties in man is limited. Urokinase administered by intravenous infusion is rapidly cleared by the liver with an elimination half-life for biologic activity of 12.6 ± 6.2 minutes and a distribution volume of 11.5 L. Small fractions of the administered dose are excreted in bile and urine. Although the pharmacokinetics of exogenously administered urokinase have not been characterized in patients with hepatic impairment, endogenous urokinase-type plasminogen activator plasma levels are elevated 2- to 4-fold in patients with moderate to severe cirrhosis. Thus, reduced urokinase clearance in patients with hepatic impairment might be expected.

Intravenous infusion of urokinase in doses recommended for lysis of pulmonary embolism is followed by increased fibrinolytic activity in the circulation. This effect disappears within a few hours after discontinuation, but a decrease in plasma levels of fibrinogen and plasminogen and an increase in the amount of circulating fibrin and fibrinogen degradation products may persist for 12 to 24 hours. There is a lack of correlation between embolus resolution and changes in coagulation and fibrinolytic assay results.

Treatment with urokinase demonstrated more improvement on pulmonary angiography, lung perfusion scanning, and hemodynamic measurements within 24 hours than did treatment with heparin. Lung perfusion scanning showed no significant treatment-associated difference by day 7.

Information based on patients treated with fibrinolytics for pulmonary embolus suggests that improvement in angiographic and lung perfusion scans is lessened when treatment is instituted more than several days (eg, 4 to 6 days) after onset.

Catheter – When used as directed for IV catheter clearance, only small amounts of urokinase may reach the circulation; therefore, therapeutic serum levels are not expected to be achieved. Nevertheless, one should be aware of the clinical pharmacology of urokinase.

Contraindications

Contraindicated in patients with a history of hypersensitivity to the product.

Because thrombolytic therapy increases the risk of bleeding, urokinase is contraindicated in the following situations: Active internal bleeding; recent (within 2 months) cerebrovascular accident; recent (within 2 months) intracranial or intraspinal surgery; recent trauma, including cardiopulmonary resuscitation; intracranial neoplasm, arteriovenous malformation, or aneurysm; known bleeding diathesis; severe uncontrolled arterial hypertension.

UROKINASE — INJECTION

There have been no reports, however, that would suggest a contraindication for the use of urokinase for IV catheter clearance.

Warnings/Precautions

➤*Catheter:* Excessive pressure should be avoided when urokinase solution is injected into the catheter. Such force could cause rupture of the catheter or expulsion of the clot into the circulation. During attempts to determine catheter occlusion, vigorous suction should not be applied due to possible damage to the vascular wall or collapse of soft-wall catheters.

Catheters may be occluded by substances other than fibrin clots such as drug precipitates. Urokinase solution is not effective in such cases and there is the possibility that the substances may be forced into the vascular system.

➤*Injection:*

Bleeding – The aim of urokinase is the production of sufficient amounts of plasmin for lysis of intravascular deposits of fibrin; however, fibrin deposits that provide hemostasis, for example, at sites of needle puncture, will also lyse and bleeding from such sites may occur.

The risk of serious bleeding is increased with use of urokinase. Fatalities due to hemorrhage, including intracranial and retroperitoneal, have been reported in association with urokinase therapy.

Concurrent administration of urokinase with other thrombolytic agents, anticoagulants, or agents inhibiting platelet function may further increase the risk of serious bleeding.

Urokinase therapy requires careful attention to all potential bleeding sites (including catheter insertion sites, arterial and venous puncture sites, cutdown sites, and other needle puncture sites).

IM injections and nonessential handling of the patient must be avoided during treatment with urokinase. Venipunctures should be performed carefully and as infrequently as possible.

Should an arterial puncture be necessary (except for intracoronary administration), upper extremity vessels are preferable. Pressure should be applied for at least 30 minutes, a pressure dressing applied, and the puncture site checked frequently for evidence of bleeding.

In the following conditions, the risks of therapy may be increased and should be weighed against the anticipated benefits:

1.) Recent (within 10 days) major surgery, obstetrical delivery, organ biopsy, or previous puncture of noncompressible vessels.
2.) Recent (within 10 days) serious GI bleeding or high likelihood of a left heart thrombus (eg, mitral stenosis with atrial fibrillation).
3.) Subacute bacterial endocarditis.
4.) Hemostatic defects, including those secondary to severe hepatic or renal disease.
5.) Pregnancy.
6.) Cerebrovascular disease.
7.) Diabetic hemorrhagic retinopathy.
8.) Any other condition in which bleeding might constitute a significant hazard or be particularly difficult to manage because of its location.

When internal bleeding occurs, it may be more difficult to manage than that which occurs with conventional anticoagulant therapy. Should potentially serious spontaneous bleeding (not controllable by direct pressure) occur, the infusion of urokinase should be terminated immediately, and measures to manage the bleeding implemented. Serious blood loss may be managed with volume replacement, including packed red blood cells. Dextran should not be used. When appropriate, fresh frozen plasma or cryoprecipitate may be considered to reverse the bleeding tendency.

Cholesterol embolization: Cholesterol embolism has been reported rarely in patients treated with all types of thrombolytic agents; the true incidence is unknown. This serious condition, which can be lethal, is also associated with invasive vascular procedures (eg, cardiac catheterization, angiography, vascular surgery) or anticoagulant therapy. Clinical features of cholesterol embolism may include livedo reticularis, "purple toe" syndrome, acute renal failure, gangrenous digits, hypertension, pancreatitis, myocardial infarction, cerebral infarction, spinal cord infarction, retinal artery occlusion, bowel infarction, and rhabdomyolysis.

Product source and formulation with albumin: Urokinase is made from human neonatal kidney cells grown in tissue culture. Products made from human source material may contain infectious agents, such as viruses, that can cause disease. The risk that urokinase will transmit an infectious agent has been reduced by screening donors for prior exposure to certain viruses, by testing donors for the presence of certain current virus infections, by testing for certain viruses during manufacturing, and by inactivating or removing certain viruses during manufacturing. Despite these measures, urokinase may carry a risk of transmitting infectious agents, including those that cause the Creutzfeldt-Jakob disease (CJD) or other diseases not yet known or identified; thus, the risk of transmission of infectious agents cannot be totally eliminated. A theoretical risk for transmission of Creutzfeldt-Jakob disease (CJD) is considered extremely remote.

This product is formulated in 5% albumin, a derivative of human blood. Based on effective donor screening and product manufacturing processes, albumin carries an extremely remote risk for transmission of viral diseases. A theoretical risk for transmission of Creutzfeldt-Jakob disease (CJD) also is considered extremely remote. No cases of transmission of viral diseases or CJD have ever been identified for albumin.

All infections thought by a physician possibly to have been transmitted by this product should be reported by the physician or other healthcare provider to the manufacturer.

Anticoagulants – Concurrent use of anticoagulants with IV administration of urokinase is not recommended. However, concurrent use of heparin may be required during intracoronary administration of urokinase. A clinical study with concurrent use of heparin and urokinase during intracoronary administration has demonstrated no tendency toward increased bleeding that would not be attributable to the procedure or urokinase alone. Nevertheless, careful monitoring for excessive bleeding is advised.

Arrhythmias – Rapid lysis of coronary thrombi has been reported occasionally to cause atrial or ventricular dysrhythmias as a result of reperfusion requiring immediate treatment. Careful monitoring for arrhythmias should be maintained during and immediately following intracoronary administration of urokinase.

➤*Hypersensitivity reactions:* Postmarketing reports of hypersensitivity reactions have included anaphylaxis (with rare reports of fatal anaphylaxis), bronchospasm, orolingual edema and urticaria. There have also been reports of other infusion reactions which have included 1 or more of the following: Fever or chills/rigors, hypoxia, cyanosis, dyspnea, tachycardia, hypotension, hypertension, acidosis, back pain, vomiting, and nausea. Reactions generally occurred within 1 hour of beginning urokinase infusion. Patients who exhibit reactions should be closely monitored and appropriate therapy instituted.

Infusion reactions generally respond to discontinuation of the infusion or administration of intravenous antihistamines, corticosteroids, or adrenergic agents.

Antipyretics which inhibit platelet function (aspirin and other nonsteroidal antiinflammatory agents) may increase the risk of bleeding and should not be used for treatment of fever.

➤*Pregnancy: Category B.* Reproduction studies have been performed in mice and rats at doses up to 1,000 times the human therapeutic dose and have revealed no evidence of impaired fertility or harm to the fetus due to urokinase. There are, however, no adequate and well-controlled studies in pregnant women. Because animal reproduction studies are not always predictive of human response, this drug should be used during pregnancy only if clearly needed.

➤*Lactation:* It is not known whether this drug is excreted in human milk. Because many drugs are excreted in human milk, caution should be exercised when urokinase is administered to a nursing woman.

➤*Children:* Safety and efficacy in children have not been established.

➤*Elderly:* Clinical studies of urokinase did not include sufficient numbers of subjects 65 years of age and older to determine whether they respond differently from younger subjects. Urokinase should be used with caution in elderly patients.

➤*Lab test abnormalities:*

Injection – Before commencing thrombolytic therapy, obtain a hematocrit, platelet count, and a thrombin time (TT), activated partial thromboplastin time (aPTT), or prothrombin time (PT). If heparin has been given, it should be discontinued unless it is to be used in conjunction with urokinase for intracoronary administration. TT or aPTT should be less than twice the normal control value before thrombolytic therapy is started.

During the infusion, coagulation tests and/or measures of fibrinolytic activity may be performed if desired. Results do not, however, reliably predict either efficacy or a risk of bleeding. The clinical response should be observed frequently, and vital signs (ie, pulse, temperature, respiratory rate, and blood pressure) should be checked at least every 4 hours. The blood pressure should not be taken in the lower extremities to avoid dislodgment of possible deep vein thrombi.

Following the IV infusion, before (re)instituting heparin, the TT or aPTT should be less than twice the upper limits of normal. Following intracoronary infusion of urokinase, blood coagulation parameters should be determined and heparin therapy continued as appropriate.

➤*Monitoring:*

Injection – Careful monitoring for excessive bleeding is advised and careful monitoring for arrhythmias should be maintained during and immediately following intracoronary administration of urokinase.

Drug Interactions

Anticoagulants and agents that alter platelet function (such as aspirin, other nonsteroidal antiinflammatory agents, dipyridamole, and GP IIb/IIIa inhibitors) may increase the risk of serious bleeding.

Administration of urokinase prior to, during, and after other thrombolytic agents may increase the risk of serious bleeding.

Because of concomitant use of urokinase with agents that alter coagulation, inhibit platelet function, or are thrombolytic may further increase the potential for bleeding complications, careful monitoring for bleeding is recommended.

The interaction of urokinase with other drugs has not been studied and is not known.

Adverse Reactions

The most serious adverse reactions reported with urokinase administration include fatal hemorrhage and anaphylaxis.

➤*Hematologic:* Bleeding is the most frequent adverse reaction associated with urokinase and can be fatal. In controlled clinical studies using a 12-hour infusion of urokinase for the treatment of pulmonary embolism (UPET and USPET), bleeding resulting in at least a 5% decrease in hematocrit was reported in 52 of 141 urokinase-treated patients. Significant bleeding events requiring transfusion of greater than 2 units of blood were observed during the 14-day study period in 3 of 141 urokinase-treated patients in these studies. Multiple bleeding events may have occurred in an individual patient. Most bleeding occurred at sites of external incisions and

Thrombolytic Enzyme

UROKINASE — INJECTION

vascular puncture, with lesser frequency in gastrointestinal, genitourinary, intracranial, retroperitoneal, and intramuscular sites.

➤*Sources of information on adverse reactions:* There are limited well-controlled clinical studies performed using urokinase. The adverse reactions described in the following sections reflect both the clinical use of urokinase in the general population and limited controlled study data. Because post-marketing reports of adverse reactions are voluntary and the population is of uncertain size, it is not always possible to reliably estimate the frequency of the reaction or establish a causal relationship to drug exposure.

Allergic – Rare cases of fatal anaphylaxis have been reported. In controlled clinical trials, allergic reaction was reported in 1 of 141 patients (less than 1%).

The following allergic-type reactions have been observed in clinical trials or postmarketing experience: Bronchospasm, orolingual edema, urticaria, skin rash, and pruritus.

Infusion reaction symptoms include hypoxia, cyanosis, dyspnea, tachycardia, hypotension, hypertension, acidosis, fever or chills/rigors, back pain, vomiting, and nausea.

Hematologic – The following reactions have been associated with urokinase for injection in doses recommended for lysis of pulmonary embolism and may also occur with intracoronary artery infusion.

The type of bleeding associated with thrombolytic therapy can be placed into 2 broad categories: Superficial or surface bleeding, observed mainly at invaded or disturbed sites (eg, venous cutdowns, arterial punctures, sites of recent surgical intervention) or internal bleeding (eg, the GI tract, GU tract, vagina, or IM, retroperitoneal, or intracranial sites).

Several fatalities due to intracranial or retroperitoneal hemorrhage have occurred during thrombolytic therapy.

Should serious bleeding occur, urokinase infusion should be discontinued and, if necessary, blood loss and reversal of the bleeding tendency can be effectively managed with whole blood (fresh blood preferable), packed red blood cells and cryoprecipitate or plasma. Dextran and hetastarch should not be used. Although the use of aminocaproic acid in humans as an antidote for urokinase has not been documented, it may be considered in an emergency situation.

Immunogenicity – The immunogenicity of urokinase has not been studied.

➤*Miscellaneous:* Other adverse events occurring in patients receiving urokinase therapy in clinical studies, regardless of causality, include myocardial infarction, recurrent pulmonary embolism, hemiplegia, stroke, decreased hematocrit, substernal pain, thrombocytopenia, and diaphoresis.

Additional adverse reactions reported from postmarketing experience include cardiac arrest, vascular embolization (cerebral and distal) including cholesterol emboli, cerebral vascular accident, pulmonary edema, reperfusion ventricular arrhythmias, and chest pain. A cause and effect relationship has not been established.

ANTISICKLING AGENTS

HYDROXYUREA

For complete and comparative prescribing and other indications information, refer to the Hydroxyurea monograph in the Antineoplastics chapter.

PROTEIN C1 INHIBITORS

C1 INHIBITOR, HUMAN

Rx	**Berinert** (CSL Behring)	**Injection, lyophilized powder for solution:** 500 units	Preservative free. In single-use vials.[a]
Rx	**Cinryze** (Lev Pharmaceuticals)	**Injection, lyophilized powder for solution:** 500 units	Preservative free. In single-use vials.[b]

[a] Contains total protein 50 to 80 mg, glycine 85 to 115 mg, sodium chloride 70 to 100 mg, and sodium citrate 25 to 35 mg per vial.

[b] Contains sodium chloride 4.1 mg/mL, sucrose 21 mg/mL, trisodium citrate 2.6 mg/mL, L-valine 2 mg/mL, L-alanine 1.2 mg/mL, and L-threonine 4.5 mg/mL.

C1 INHIBITOR, HUMAN — INJECTION

Indications

➤*Hereditary angioedema:*

Berinert – For the treatment of acute abdominal or facial attacks of hereditary angioedema in adult and adolescent patients.

Cinryze – For routine prophylaxis against angioedema attacks in adolescent and adult patients with hereditary angioedema.

Administration and Dosage

➤*General dosing considerations:*

Berinert – Use either the *Mix2Vial* transfer set provided or a commercially available double-ended needle and vented filter spike.

➤*Adults:*

Hereditary angioedema –

Berinert: 20 units per kg body weight by intravenous (IV) injection.

Cinryze: 1,000 units (2 vials) IV every 3 or 4 days.

➤*Children:*

Hereditary angioedema –

13 years of age and older: See Adults for dosing.

➤*Preparation for administration:*

Berinert – Ensure that the vial and diluent vial are at room temperature. Place the C1 inhibitor vial, diluent vial, and *Mix2Vial* transfer set on a flat surface. Remove the flip caps from the vials. Treat the vial stoppers with the alcohol swab provided and allow to dry prior to opening the *Mix2Vial* transfer set package. Open the *Mix2Vial* transfer set package by peeling away the lid. Leave the *Mix2Vial* transfer set in the clear package. Place the diluent vial on a flat surface and hold the vial tight. Grip the *Mix2Vial* transfer set together with the clear package and snap the blue end of the *Mix2Vial* transfer set onto the diluent vial stopper at a 90° angle. Carefully remove the clear package from the *Mix2Vial* transfer set. Make sure to only pull up the clear package and not the *Mix2Vial* transfer set.

With the C1 inhibitor vial placed firmly on a flat surface, invert the diluent vial with the *Mix2Vial* transfer set attached and snap the transparent adapter onto the C1 inhibitor vial stopper at a 90° angle. The diluent will automatically transfer into the C1 inhibitor vial. With the diluent and C1 inhibitor vial still attached to the *Mix2Vial* transfer set, gently swirl the C1 inhibitor vial to ensure that the C1 inhibitor is fully dissolved. Do not shake the vial.

With one hand, grasp the C1 inhibitor side of the *Mix2Vial* transfer set and with the other hand grasp the blue diluent-side of the *Mix2Vial* transfer set and unscrew the set into 2 pieces. Draw air into an empty, sterile syringe. While the C1 inhibitor vial is upright, screw the syringe to the *Mix2Vial* transfer set. Inject air into the C1 inhibitor vial. While keeping the syringe plunger pressed, invert the system upside down and draw the concentrate into the syringe by pulling the plunger back slowly. Now that the concentrate has been transferred into the syringe, firmly grasp the barrel of the syringe (keeping the plunger facing down) and unscrew the syringe from the *Mix2Vial* transfer set. Attach the syringe to a suitable IV administration set. If the same patient is to receive more than 1 vial, the contents of multiple vials may be pooled in a single administration device (eg, syringe). A new unused *Mix2Vial* transfer set should be used for each C1 inhibitor vial.

Cinryze – Bring the C1 inhibitor and sterile water for injection to room temperature if refrigerated. Remove caps from the vials. Cleanse stoppers with germicidal solution and allow them to dry prior to use. Remove protective covering from one end of the double-ended transfer needle and insert exposed needle through the center of the diluent vial stopper. Remove protective covering from the other end of the double-ended transfer needle. Invert diluent vial containing 5 mL of sterile water for injection over the upright and slightly angled C1 inhibitor vial; then rapidly insert the free end of the needle through the C1 inhibitor vial stopper at its center. The vacuum in the vial will draw in the diluent. If there is no vacuum in the vial, do not use the product. Disconnect the 2 vials by removing the needle from the C1 inhibitor vial stopper and discard the diluent vial along with the transfer needle directly into the sharps container. Gently swirl the C1 inhibitor vial until all powder is dissolved. Be sure that C1 inhibitor is completely dissolved. One vial of reconstituted C1 inhibitor contains 5 mL of C1 inhibitor at a concentration of 100 units/mL. Reconstitute 2 vials of C1 inhibitor for 1 dose.

Attach the filter needle to a sterile, disposable syringe and draw back the plunger to admit air into the syringe. Insert the filter needle into the vial of reconstituted C1 inhibitor. Inject air into the vial and then withdraw the reconstituted solution into the syringe. This should be repeated with a second vial of C1 inhibitor to make the complete dose. Remove and discard the filter needle in a hard-walled sharps container for proper disposal. Filter needles are intended to filter the contents of a single dose (2 vials) of *Cinryze* only.

➤*Administration:*

Berinert – For IV use only by a separate infusion line. Administer by slow IV injection at a rate of approximately 4 mL/min.

Cinryze – Administer at room temperature within 3 hours after reconstitution. Attach a suitable needle or infusion set with winged adapter, and inject IV. Administer at an infusion rate of 1 mL/min over 10 minutes.

➤*Admixture compatibility:* Do not mix with other medicinal products or other materials.

➤*Storage/Stability:*

Berinert – Store at 2° to 25°C (36° to 77°F). Keep in its original carton until ready to use. Do not freeze. Protect from light. Any product that has

C1 INHIBITOR, HUMAN — INJECTION

been reconstituted should be used promptly. When reconstitution is carried out using aseptic technique, administration may begin within 8 hours provided the solution has been stored at up to 25°C (77°F). Do not refrigerate or freeze the reconstituted solution. Discard partially used vials.

Cinryze – Store at 2° to 25°C (36° to 77°F). Do not freeze. Do not use if frozen. Store the vial in the original carton to protect it from light. The reconstituted solution must be used within 3 hours of reconstitution. Any vial that has been entered should be used promptly.

Actions

➤*Pharmacology:* C1 esterase inhibitor is a normal constituent of human plasma and belongs to the group of serine protease inhibitors (serpins) that includes antithrombin III, alpha-protease inhibitor, alpha-antiplasmin, and heparin cofactor II. As with the other inhibitors in this group, C1 esterase inhibitor has an important inhibiting potential on several of the major cascade systems of the human body including the complement system, the intrinsic coagulation (contact) system, the fibrinolytic system, and the coagulation cascade. Regulation of these systems is performed through the formation of complexes between the proteinase and the inhibitor, resulting in inactivation of both and consumption of the C1 esterase inhibitor.

C1 esterase inhibitor, which is usually activated during the inflammatory process, inactivates its substrate by covalently binding to the reactive site. C1 esterase inhibitor is the only known inhibitor for the subcomponent of the complement component 1 (C1r), C1s, coagulation factor XIIa, and kallikrein. Additionally, C1 esterase inhibitor is the main inhibitor for coagulation factor XIa of the intrinsic coagulation cascade.

Hereditary angioedema patients have low levels of endogenous or functional C1 esterase inhibitor. Although the events that induce attacks of angioedema in hereditary angioedema patients are not well defined, it has been postulated that increased vascular permeability and the clinical manifestation of hereditary angioedema attacks may be primarily mediated through contact system activation. Suppression of contact system activation by C1 esterase inhibitor through the inactivation of plasma kallikrein and factor XIIa is thought to modulate this vascular permeability by preventing the generation of bradykinin.

Administration of C1 inhibitor to patients with C1 esterase inhibitor deficiency replaces the missing or malfunctioning protein in patients. The plasma concentration of C1 esterase inhibitor in healthy volunteers is approximately 270 mg/L.

➤*Pharmacokinetics:*

Berinert –

Adults:

Pharmacokinetic Parameters of C1 Inhibitor in Adults (N = 35)[a]

Pharmacokinetic parameters	Unadjusted for baseline	Adjusted for baseline
$AUC_{(0-t)}$ (h ×units/mL)[b]	27.5 ± 8.5 (15.7 to 44.7)	12.8 ± 6.7 (3.9 to 34.7)
CL (mL/h/kg)	0.6 ± 0.17 (0.34 to 0.96)	1.44 ± 0.67 (0.43 to 3.85)
V_{ss} (mL/kg)	18.6 ± 4.9 (11.1 to 27.6)	35.4 ± 10.5 (14.1 to 56.1)
Half-life (h)	21.9 ± 1.7 (16.5 to 24.4)	18.4 ± 3.5 (7.4 to 22.8)
MRT (h)	31.5 ± 2.4 (23.7 to 35.2)	26.4 ± 5 (10.7 to 33)

[a] AUC = area under the curve; CL = clearance; V_{ss} = volume steady state; MRT = mean residence time.
[b] Based on a 15 unit/kg dose; numbers in parentheses are range.

Children:

Pharmacokinetic Parameters of C1 Inhibitor in Children (N = 5)

Pharmacokinetic parameters	Unadjusted for baseline	Adjusted for baseline
$AUC_{(0-t)}$ (h × units/mL)[a]	25.45 ± 5.8 (16.8 to 31.7)	9.78 ± 4.37 (4.1 to 15.2)
CL (mL/hr/kg)	0.62 ± 0.17 (0.47 to 0.89)	1.9 ± 1.1 (0.98 to 3.69)
V_{ss} (mL/kg)	19.8 ± 4 (16.7 to 26.1)	38.8 ± 8.9 (31.9 to 54)
Half-life (h)	22.4 ± 1.6 (20.3 to 24.4)	16.7 ± 5.8 (7.4 to 22.5)
MRT (h)	32.3 ± 2.3 (29.3 to 35.2)	24 ± 8.3 (10.7 to 32.4)

[a] Based on a 15 unit/kg dose. Numbers in parentheses are range.

Cinryze –

C1 Inhibitor Mean Pharmacokinetic Parameters[a,b]

Pharmacokinetic parameters	Single dosage[c]	Double dosage[d]
$C_{baseline}$ (units/mL)	0.31 ± 0.2 (n = 12)	0.33 ± 0.2 (n = 12)
C_{max} (units/mL)	0.68 ± 0.08 (n = 12)	0.85 ± 0.12 (n = 13)
T_{max} (h)	3.9 ± 7.3 (n = 12)	2.7 ± 1.9 (n = 13)
$AUC_{(0-t)}$ (units•h/mL)	74.5 ± 30.3 (n = 12)	95.9 ± 19.6 (n = 13)
CL (mL/min)	0.85 ± 1.07 (n = 7)	1.17 ± 0.78 (n = 9)
Half-life (h)	56 ± 36 (n = 7)	62 ± 38 (n = 9)

[a] $C_{baseline}$ = baseline concentrations; C_{max} = maximal drug concentrations; T_{max} = time to C_{max}.
[b] One unit is equal to the mean C1 inhibitor concentration of 1 mL of normal human plasma.
[c] Single dose = 1,000 units.
[d] Double dose = 1,000 units followed by a second 1,000 units 60 minutes later.

Contraindications

Life-threatening immediate hypersensitivity reactions to C1 esterase inhibitor preparation, including anaphylaxis.

Warnings/Precautions

➤*Thrombotic events:* Thrombotic events have been reported in association with C1 inhibitor products when used off-label and at higher than labeled doses. Animal studies supported a concern about the risk of thrombosis from IV administration of C1 esterase inhibitor products.

➤*Human plasma:* Because C1 inhibitor is made from human blood, it may carry a risk of transmitting infectious agents (ie, viruses and, theoretically, the Creutzfeldt-Jakob disease [CJD] agent). All infections thought to have been possibly transmitted by C1 inhibitor should be reported by the health care provider to the manufacturer. Discuss the risks and benefits of this product with the patient before prescribing or administering.

The risk that such products will transmit an infectious agent has been reduced by screening plasma donors for prior exposure to certain viruses, by testing for the presence of certain current virus infections, and by processes demonstrated to inactivate and/or remove certain viruses during manufacturing.

Despite these measures, such products may still potentially transmit disease. There is also the possibility that unknown infectious agents may be present in such products.

Since 1979, a few suspected cases of viral transmission have been reported with the use of C1 inhibitor outside the United States, including cases of acute hepatitis C. From the incomplete information available from these cases, it was not possible to determine with certainty if the infections were or were not related to prior administration of C1 inhibitor.

➤*Hypersensitivity reactions:* Severe hypersensitivity reactions may occur. The signs and symptoms of hypersensitivity reactions may include the appearance of hives, urticaria, tightness of the chest, wheezing, hypotension, and/or anaphylaxis experienced during or after injection of C1 inhibitor.

Because hypersensitivity reactions may have symptoms similar to hereditary angioedema attacks, carefully consider treatment methods.

In case of hypersensitivity, discontinue C1 inhibitor infusion immediately and institute appropriate treatment. Ensure epinephrine is immediately available for treatment of acute severe hypersensitivity reaction.

➤*Pregnancy: Category C.* No animal data are available. No adequate and well-controlled studies were conducted in pregnant women. It is not known whether C1 inhibitor can cause fetal harm when administered to a pregnant woman or can affect reproduction capacity. Give C1 inhibitor to a pregnant woman only if clearly needed.

➤*Lactation:* It is not known whether C1 inhibitor is excreted in human breast milk. Because many drugs are excreted in human breast milk, exercise caution when C1 is administered to a breast-feeding woman.

➤*Children:*

Berinert – Safety and efficacy of C1 inhibitor in children (0 to 12 years of age) have not been established. There was an insufficient number of subjects in this age group to determine whether they respond differently from older subjects. The safety and efficacy of C1 inhibitor were evaluated in 5 children (3 to 12 years of age) and in 8 adolescent subjects (13 to 16 years of age).

Cinryze – The safety and effectiveness of C1 inhibitor have not been established in neonates, infants, or children. Three of the 24 subjects in the study were younger than 18 years of age (9, 14, and 16 years of age).

➤*Monitoring:* Monitor all patients for thrombotic and hypersensitivity reactions.

Drug Interactions

None well documented.

Adverse Reactions

➤*Berinert:*

Serious adverse reactions – The most serious adverse reaction reported in subjects in clinical studies who received C1 inhibitor was an increase in the severity of pain associated with hereditary angioedema.

Common adverse reactions – The most common adverse reactions that have been reported in more than 4% of subjects receiving C1 inhibitor in clinical studies were subsequent hereditary angioedema attack, headache, abdominal pain, nausea, muscle spasms, pain, diarrhea, and vomiting.

Placebo-controlled clinical study: The treatment-emergent serious adverse reactions that occurred in 5 subjects in the RCT were laryngeal edema, facial attack with laryngeal edema, swelling (shoulder and chest), exacerbation of hereditary angioedema, and laryngospasm.

C1 INHIBITOR, HUMAN — INJECTION

C1 Inhibitor Injection Adverse Reactions Occurring Up to 4 hours After Initial Infusion (> 4%)[a,b]		
Adverse reactions	C1 inhibitor 20 units/kg (n = 43)	Placebo (n = 42)
CNS		
Headache	0%	4.8%
GI		
Abdominal pain	4.7%	7.1%
Diarrhea	0%	9.5%
Dysgeusia	4.7%	0%
Nausea	7%	11.9%
Vomiting	2.3%	7.1%

[a] The study protocol specified that adverse events that began within 72 hours of blind study medication administration were to be classified as at least possibly related to study medication (ie, adverse reactions).

[b] The following abdominal symptoms were identified in the protocol as associated with hereditary angioedema abdominal attacks: abdominal pain, bloating, cramps, nausea, vomiting, and diarrhea.

C1 Inhibitor Injection Adverse Reactions Occurring Up to 72 hours After Infusion of Initial or Rescue Medication (> 4%)[a,b]		
Adverse reactions	C1 inhibitor[c] 20 units/kg (n = 43)	Placebo[c] (n = 42)
GI		
Abdominal pain	7%	11.9%
Diarrhea	0%	19%
Dysgeusia	4.7%	2.4%
Nausea	7%	26.2%
Vomiting	2.3%	16.7%
Musculoskeletal		
Back pain	0%	4.8%
Muscle spasms	2.3%	9.5%
Miscellaneous		
Facial pain	0%	4.8%
Headache	7%	11.9%
Pain	2.3%	9.5%

[a] The study protocol specified that adverse events that began within 72 hours of blind study medication administration were to be classified as at least possibly related to study medication (ie, adverse reactions).

[b] If a subject experienced no relief or insufficient relief of symptoms within 4 hours after infusion, investigators had the option to administer a blind second infusion (rescue treatment) of C1 inhibitor (20 units/kg for the placebo group, 10 units/kg for the 10 units/kg group), or placebo (for the 20 units/kg group).

[c] Adverse reactions following either initial treatment and/or blind rescue treatment. Because more subjects in the placebo randomization group than in the C1 inhibitor randomization group received rescue treatment, the median observation period in this analysis for subjects randomized to placebo was slightly longer than for subjects randomized to receive C1 inhibitor.

C1 Inhibitor Injection Adverse Reactions Occurring 7 to 9 Days After Infusion (> 4%)[a]	
Adverse reactions	Percent of subjects reporting adverse reactions (n = 108)
GI	
Abdominal pain[b]	6.5%
Diarrhea[b]	4.6%
Nausea[b]	6.5%
Vomiting[b]	4.6%
Miscellaneous	
Headache	11.1%
Hereditary angioedema	11.1%
Muscle spasms	5.6%
Pain	5.6%

[a] Includes subjects in the placebo group who received C1 inhibitor 20 units/kg as rescue study medication.

[b] These symptoms were identified in the protocol as related to the underlying disease. Any increase in intensity or new occurrence of these symptoms after study medication administration was considered to be an adverse reaction.

Extension study:

C1 Inhibitor Injection Adverse Reactions Occurring Up to 72 Hours or 9 Days After Infusion (> 4%)		
Adverse reactions	Subjects reporting adverse reactions ≤ 72 hours (n = 56)	Subjects reporting adverse reactions ≤ 9 days (n = 56)
Miscellaneous		
Abdominal pain	5.4%	5.4%
Headache	5.4%	7.1%
Hereditary angioedema	3.6%	7.1%
Nasopharyngitis	3.6%	5.4%

➤*Cinryze:*

Serious adverse reactions – The most serious adverse reactions observed in clinical studies have been death due to noncatheter-related foreign body embolus, preeclampsia resulting in emergency C-section, stroke, and exacerbation of hereditary angioedema attacks, none of which have been considered drug related.

Common adverse reactions – The most common drug-related adverse reactions observed at a rate of 5% or more were headache, rash, sinusitis, and upper respiratory tract infections.

Routine prophylaxis –

C1 Inhibitor Injection Adverse Reactions in Routine Prophylaxis		
Adverse reactions	Number of adverse reactions	Number of subjects (N = 24)
Dermatologic		
Pruritus	2	2
Rash	7	5
Musculoskeletal		
Back pain	2	2
Limb injury	2	2
Pain in extremity	2	2
Respiratory		
Bronchitis	2	2
Sinusitis	8	5
Upper respiratory tract infection	3	3
Viral upper respiratory tract infection	5	3
Miscellaneous		
Headache	4	4

➤*Postmarketing:*

Berinert – Adverse reactions reported in Europe since 1979 in patients receiving C1 inhibitor for treatment of hereditary angioedema include hypersensitivity/anaphylactic reactions, a few suspected cases of viral transmission including cases of acute hepatitis C, injection-site pain, injection-site redness, chills, and fever.

Hypersensitivity/Anaphylactic reactions, shock, pain upon injection, redness at injection site, chills, and fever have been attributed to C1 inhibitor during post-approval use outside the United States.

Overdosage

➤*Symptoms:*

Berinert – The development of thrombosis has been reported after doses exceeding 20 units/kg body weight of C1 inhibitor in newborns and young children with congenital heart anomalies during or after cardiac surgery under extracorporeal circulation when used off-label.

Patient Information

Inform patients to immediately report signs and symptoms of thrombosis to their health care provider, such as new onset swelling and pain in the limbs or abdomen, new onset chest pain, shortness of breath, loss of sensation or motor power, or altered consciousness or speech.

Inform patients of the early signs of hypersensitivity reactions, including hives (itchy white elevated patches), tightness of the chest, wheezing, hypotension, and anaphylaxis. Advise patients to discontinue use of C1 inhibitor and contact their health care provider if these symptoms occur.

Advise women to notify their health care provider if they become pregnant or intend to become pregnant during C1 inhibitor therapy.

Advise patients to notify their health care provider if they are breast-feeding or plan to breast-feed.

Based on their current regimen, advise patients to bring an adequate supply of C1 inhibitor for routine prevention when traveling. Advise patients to consult with their health care provider prior to travel.

Advise patient that, because C1 inhibitor is made from human blood, it may carry a risk of transmitting infectious agents (ie, viruses, and, theoretically,

C1 INHIBITOR, HUMAN — INJECTION

the CJD agent). The risk of transmitting disease has been reduced, but not eliminated, by carefully selecting blood donors, testing donors for infections, and inactivating or removing most viruses during the manufacturing process. Inform patients of the risks and benefits of C1 inhibitor before prescribing or administering to the patient.

KALLIKREIN INHIBITOR

ECALLANTIDE

Rx	**Kalbitor** (Dyax Corp)[a]	**Injection, solution:** 10 mg/mL	Preservative free. In single-use vials.[b,c]

[a] 300 Technology Square, Cambridge, MA 02139; 1-617-225-2500 (phone); 1-617-225-2501 (fax).

[b] Also contains disodium hydrogen orthophosphate (dihydrate) 0.76 mg, monopotassium phosphate 0.2 mg, potassium chloride 0.2 mg, and sodium chloride 8 mg.

[c] Produced in *Pichia pastoris* yeast cells by recombinant DNA technology.

ECALLANTIDE — INJECTION

WARNING

Anaphylaxis has been reported after administration of ecallantide. Because of the risk of anaphylaxis, ecallantide should only be administered by a health care provider with appropriate medical support to manage anaphylaxis and hereditary angioedema. Health care providers should be aware of the similarity of symptoms between hypersensitivity reactions and hereditary angioedema, and patients should be monitored closely. Do not administer ecallantide to patients with known clinical hypersensitivity to ecallantide.

Indications

➤*Hereditary angioedema:* For treatment of acute attacks of hereditary angioedema in patients 16 years of age and older.

Administration and Dosage

➤*Adults:*

Hereditary angioedema – 30 mg (3 mL) given subcutaneously in three 10 mg (1 mL) injections. If the attack persists, an additional dose of 30 mg may be administered within a 24-hour period.

➤*Children:*

Hereditary angioedema –

16 years of age and older: See Adults for dosing.

➤*Elderly:* In general, dose selection for an elderly patient should be cautious, usually starting at the low end of the dosing range, reflecting the greater frequency of decreased hepatic, renal, or cardiac function, and of concomitant disease or other drug therapy.

➤*Preparation for administration:* Using aseptic technique, withdraw 1 mL (10 mg) of ecallantide from the vial using a large bore needle. Change the needle on the syringe to a needle suitable for subcutaneous injection. The recommended needle size is 27 gauge.

➤*Administration:* Inject ecallantide into the skin of the abdomen, thigh, or upper arm.

The injection site for each of the injections may be in the same or in different anatomic locations (abdomen, thigh, or upper arm). There is no need for site rotation. Injection sites should be separated by at least 2 inches (5 cm) and away from the anatomical site of attack.

➤*Storage/Stability:* Refrigerate at 2° to 8°C (36° to 46°F). Store vials removed from refrigeration below 30°C (86°F) and use them within 14 days or return to refrigeration until use.

Protect vials from light until use.

Actions

➤*Pharmacology:* Hereditary angioedema is a rare genetic disorder caused by mutations to C1-esterase-inhibitor (C1-INH) located on chromosome 11q and inherited as an autosomal dominant trait. Hereditary angioedema is characterized by low levels of C1-INH activity and low levels of C4. C1-INH functions to regulate the activation of the complement and intrinsic coagulation (contact system pathway) and is a major endogenous inhibitor of plasma kallikrein. The kallikrein-kinin system is a complex proteolytic cascade involved in the initiation of both inflammatory and coagulation pathways. One critical aspect of this pathway is the conversion of high molecular weight (HMW) kininogen to bradykinin by the protease plasma kallikrein. In hereditary angioedema, normal regulation of plasma kallikrein activity and the classical complement cascade is therefore not present. During attacks, unregulated activity of plasma kallikrein results in excessive bradykinin generation. Bradykinin is a vasodilator that is thought by some to be responsible for the characteristic hereditary angioedema symptoms of localized swelling, inflammation, and pain.

Ecallantide is a potent (Ki = 25 pM), selective, reversible inhibitor of plasma kallikrein. Ecallantide binds to plasma kallikrein and blocks its binding site, inhibiting the conversion of HMW kininogen to bradykinin. By directly inhibiting plasma kallikrein, ecallantide reduces the conversion of HMW kininogen to bradykinin, and thereby treats symptoms of the disease during acute episodic attacks of hereditary angioedema.

Pharmacodynamics – The effect of ecallantide on activated partial thromboplastin time (aPTT) was measured because of potential effect on the intrinsic coagulation pathway. Prolongation of aPTT has been observed following intravenous (IV) dosing of ecallantide at doses of at least 20 mg/m^2. At 80 mg administered IV in healthy subjects, aPTT values were prolonged approximately 2-fold over baseline values and returned to normal by 4 hours postdose.

➤*Pharmacokinetics:*

Absorption – Following the administration of a single 30 mg subcutaneous dose of ecallantide to healthy subjects, a mean (± standard deviation) maximum plasma concentration of 586 ± 106 ng/mL was observed approximately 2 to 3 hours postdose. The mean area under the concentration-time curve (AUC) was 3,017 ± 402 ng•h/mL.

Distribution – The volume of distribution was 26.4 ± 7.8 L.

Excretion – Plasma clearance was 153 ± 20 mL/min. Following administration, plasma concentration declined with a mean elimination half-life of 2 ± 0.5 hours. Ecallantide is a small protein (7,054 daltons) and renal elimination in the urine of treated subjects has been demonstrated.

Contraindications

Known clinical hypersensitivity to ecallantide.

Warnings/Precautions

➤*Immunogenicity:* In the ecallantide hereditary angioedema program, patients developed antibodies to ecallantide. Rates of seroconversion increased with exposure to ecallantide over time. Overall, 7.4% of patients seroconverted to anti-ecallantide antibodies. Neutralizing antibodies to ecallantide were determined in vitro to be present in 4.7% of patients.

Anti-ecallantide and anti-*P. pastoris* immunoglobulin antibodies were also detected. Patients who seroconvert may be at a higher risk of a hypersensitivity reaction. The long-term effects of antibodies to ecallantide are not known.

The test results for the ecallantide program were determined using one of two assay formats: enzyme-linked immunosorbent assay and bridging electrochemiluminescence (ECL). As with all therapeutic proteins, there is a potential for immunogenicity with the use of ecallantide. The incidence of antibody formation is highly dependent on the sensitivity and specificity of the assay. Additionally, the observed incidence of antibody (including neutralizing antibody) positivity in an assay may be influenced by several factors, including assay methodology, sample handling, timing of sample collection, concomitant medications, and underlying disease. For these reasons, comparison of the incidence of antibodies to ecallantide with the incidence of antibodies to other products may be misleading.

➤*Hypersensitivity reactions:* Potentially serious hypersensitivity reactions, including anaphylaxis, have occurred in patients treated with ecallantide. In 255 hereditary angioedema patients treated with IV or subcutaneous ecallantide in clinical studies, 10 (3.9%) patients experienced anaphylaxis. For the subgroup of 187 patients treated with subcutaneous ecallantide, 5 (2.7%) patients experienced anaphylaxis. Symptoms associated with these reactions have included chest discomfort, flushing, pharyngeal edema, pruritus, rhinorrhea, sneezing, nasal congestion, throat irritation, urticaria, wheezing, and hypotension. These reactions occurred within the first hour after dosing.

Other adverse reactions indicative of hypersensitivity reactions included the following: pruritus (5.1%), rash (3.1%), and urticaria (2%).

Observe patients for an appropriate period of time after administration of ecallantide, taking into account the time to onset of anaphylaxis.

See the Warning box for more information.

➤*Pregnancy: Category C.* There are no adequate and well-controlled trials of ecallantide in pregnant women. Ecallantide has been shown to cause developmental toxicity in rats, but not rabbits. Because animal reproductive studies are not always predictive of human response, use ecallantide during pregnancy only if clearly needed.

In rats, IV ecallantide at an IV dose approximately 13 times the maximum recommended human dose (MRHD) on a mg/kg basis caused increased numbers of early resorptions and percentages of resorbed conceptuses per litter in the presence of mild maternal toxicity. No development toxicity was observed in rats that received an IV dose approximately 8 times the MRHD on a mg/kg basis. There were no adverse effects of ecallantide on embryofetal development in rats that received subcutaneous doses up to approximately 2.4 times the MRHD on an AUC basis, and in rabbits that received IV doses up to approximately 6 times the MRHD on an AUC basis.

➤*Lactation:* It is not known whether ecallantide is excreted in human milk. Exercise caution when ecallantide is administered to a breast-feeding woman.

➤*Children:* Safety and effectiveness of ecallantide in patients younger than 16 years of age have not been established.

➤*Monitoring:* Observe patients for an appropriate period of time after administration of ecallantide, taking into account the time to onset of anaphylaxis.

ECALLANTIDE — INJECTION

Drug Interactions

None well documented.

Adverse Reactions

➤*Clinical trials:* Overall, the most common adverse reactions in 255 patients with hereditary angioedema were headache (16.1%), nausea (12.9%), fatigue (11.8%), diarrhea (10.6%), upper respiratory tract infection (8.2%), injection-site reactions (7.4%), nasopharyngitis (5.9%), vomiting (5.5%), pruritus (5.1%), upper abdominal pain (5.1%), and pyrexia (4.7%). Anaphylaxis was reported in 3.9% of patients with hereditary angioedema. Injection-site reactions were characterized by local bruising, erythema, pain, irritation, pruritus, and/or urticaria.

Ecallantide Adverse Reactions (≥ 3%)[a]		
	Ecallantide (n = 100)	Placebo (n = 81)
GI		
Diarrhea	4%	4%
Nausea	5%	1%
Miscellaneous		
Headache	8%	7%
Injection-site reactions	3%	1%
Nasopharyngitis	3%	0%
Pyrexia	4%	0%

[a] Patients experiencing more than 1 event with the same preferred term are counted only once for that preferred term.

Overdosage

➤*Animal toxicology:* Ecallantide has been shown to cause developmental toxicity in rats, but not rabbits. Treatment of rats with an IV dosage of 15 mg/kg/day (approximately 13 times the MRHD on a mg/kg basis) caused increased numbers of early resorptions and percentages of resorbed conceptuses per litter in the presence of mild maternal toxicity. However, no development toxicity was observed in rats that received an IV dosage of 10 mg/kg/day (approximately 8 times the MRHD on a mg/kg basis). Ecallantide was not teratogenic in rats at subcutaneous dosages of up to 20 mg/kg/day (approximately 2.4 times the MRHD on an AUC basis) and rabbits that received IV dosages of up to 5 mg/kg/day (approximately 6 times the MRHD on an AUC basis).

No deaths occurred in monkeys that received IV or subcutaneous doses of up to 25 mg/kg (approximately 22 times the MRHD on an AUC basis).

There have been no reports of overdose with ecallantide. Hereditary angioedema patients have received single doses of up to 90 mg IV without evidence of dose-related toxicity.

Patient Information

Advise patients that ecallantide may cause anaphylaxis and other hypersensitivity reactions.

Advise patients that ecallantide should be administered by a health care provider with appropriate medical support to manage anaphylaxis and hereditary angioedema.

Instruct patients who have known clinical hypersensitivity to ecallantide not to receive additional doses of ecallantide.

Advise patients to consult the Medication Guide for additional information regarding the risk of anaphylaxis and other hypersensitivity reactions.

HEMORRHEOLOGIC AGENTS

PENTOXIFYLLINE

Rx	**Pentoxifylline** (Copley)	**Tablets, controlled-release:** 400 mg	Film-coated. In 100s, 500s, and bulk pack 5000s.
Rx	**Trental** (Hoechst Marion Roussel)		(Trental). Pink. Film coated. Oblong. In 100s and bulk pack 5000s.
Rx	**Pentoxifylline Extended-Release** (Purepac)	**Tablets, extended-release:** 400 mg	In 100s, 500s and 1000s.

PENTOXIFYLLINE — ORAL

Indications

➤*Intermittent claudication:* For the treatment of intermittent claudication on the basis of chronic occlusive arterial disease of the limbs. Pentoxifylline can improve function and symptoms but is not intended to replace more definitive therapy, such as surgical bypass, or removal of arterial obstructions when treating peripheral vascular disease.

➤*Off-label uses:*

Aphthous stomatitis – [4] = Insufficient documentation. Preliminary data from noncontrolled trials suggest that pentoxifylline may be effective in preventing recurrence or providing symptomatic relief in patients with minor to severe recurrent aphthous stomatitis. However, a small controlled trial revealed a significant benefit only in the reduction of median ulcer size after 2 months of therapy. Thus, the use of this agent as first-line therapy is not recommended until large controlled trials validate its place in therapy. (See Administration and Dosage.)

Mucositis (chemotherapy induced) – [5] = Poor documentation. Limited data suggest that pentoxifylline is not useful in the treatment or prevention of chemotherapy-induced mucositis. Because other more effective alternatives are available, this therapy is not recommended for this indication.

Prevention of altitude sickness – [4] = Insufficient documentation. The published experience with pentoxifylline use for prevention of high-altitude sickness is limited to small, controlled trials that assessed indirect measurements for high-altitude sickness instead of clinical parameters. Because of the absence of clear clinical benefit and the availability of other established agents for high-altitude sickness prophylaxis, the use of pentoxifylline cannot be recommended at this time. (See Administration and Dosage.)

Stomatitis (chemotherapy induced) – [5] = Poor documentation. Data from controlled trials indicate that pentoxifylline is not beneficial in the prevention of chemotherapy- or immunosuppressant-induced stomatitis.

Other possible off-label uses – Pentoxifylline was found superior to placebo in improving psychopathological symptoms in patients with cerebrovascular insufficiency. The drug has also been studied in diabetic angiopathies and neuropathies, transient ischemic attacks, leg ulcers, sickle cell thalassemias, strokes, asthenozoospermia, acute and chronic hearing disorders, severe idiopathic recurrent aphthous stomatitis (400 mg 3 times a day for 1 month), eye circulation disorders, and Raynaud phenomenon.

Administration and Dosage

➤*Adults:*

Intermittent claudication –

Usual dosage: 400 mg 3 times a day with meals.

Dosage adjustment: Digestive and central nervous system side effects are dose related. If patients develop these effects, it is recommended that the dosage be lowered to 1 tablet twice a day (800 mg/day). If side effects persist at this lower dosage, discontinue the administration of pentoxifylline.

Duration of therapy: While the effect of pentoxifylline may be seen within 2 to 4 weeks, it is recommended that treatment be continued for at least 8 weeks. Efficacy has been demonstrated in double-blind clinical studies of 6 month's duration.

Off-label dosing –

Aphthous stomatitis: [4] = Insufficient documentation. 400 mg 3 times daily for 1 to 6 months.

Prevention of altitude sickness: [4] = Insufficient documentation. 400 mg 3 times per day throughout the stay at high altitude.

➤*Renal function impairment:*

CrCl greater than 50 mL/min – Give the usual dose every 8 to 12 hours.

CrCl 10 to 50 mL/min – Give the usual dose every 12 to 24 hours.

CrCl less than 10 mL/min – Give the usual dose every 24 hours.

Peritoneal dialysis – Give the usual dose every 24 hours.

➤*Storage/Stability:* Store between 15° and 30°C (59° and 86°F). Dispense in well-closed, light-resistant containers. Protect blisters from light.

Actions

➤*Pharmacology:* Pentoxifylline and its metabolites improve the flow properties of blood by decreasing its viscosity. In patients with chronic peripheral arterial disease, this increases blood flow to the affected microcirculation and enhances tissue oxygenation. The precise mode of action of pentoxifylline and the sequence of events leading to clinical improvement are still to be defined. Pentoxifylline administration has been shown to produce dose-related hemorrheologic effects, lowering blood viscosity, and improving erythrocyte flexibility. Leukocyte properties of hemorrheologic importance have been modified in animal and in vitro human studies. Pentoxifylline has been shown to increase leukocyte deformability and to inhibit neutrophil adhesion and activation. Tissue oxygen levels have been shown to be significantly increased by therapeutic doses of pentoxifylline in patients with peripheral arterial disease.

➤*Pharmacokinetics:*

Absorption/Distribution – After oral administration in aqueous solution pentoxifylline is almost completely absorbed. It undergoes a first-pass effect and the various metabolites appear in plasma very soon after dosing. Peak plasma levels of the parent compound and its metabolites are reached within 1 hour. The major metabolites are Metabolite I (1-]-3,7-dimethylxanthine) and Metabolite V (1-]-3,7-dimethylxanthine), and plasma levels of these metabolites are 5 and 8 times greater, respectively, than pentoxifylline.

PENTOXIFYLLINE — ORAL

After administration of the 400 mg controlled-release pentoxifylline tablet, plasma levels of the parent compound and its metabolites reach their maximum within 2 to 4 hours and remain constant over an extended period of time. Coadministration of pentoxifylline tablets with meals resulted in an increase in mean C_{max} and AUC by about 28% and 13% for pentoxifylline, respectively. C_{max} for Metabolite I also increased by about 20%. The controlled release of pentoxifylline from the tablet eliminates peaks and troughs in plasma levels for improved gastrointestinal tolerance.

Metabolism/Excretion – Following oral administration of aqueous solutions containing 100 to 400 mg of pentoxifylline, the pharmacokinetics of the parent compound and Metabolite I are dose-related and not proportional (nonlinear), with half-life and area under the blood-level time curve (AUC) increasing with dose. The elimination kinetics of Metabolite V are not dose-dependent. The apparent plasma half-life of pentoxifylline varies from 0.4 to 0.8 hours and the apparent plasma half-lives of its metabolites vary from 1 to 1.6 hours. There is no evidence of accumulation or enzyme induction (cytochrome P450) following multiple oral doses.

Excretion is almost totally urinary; the main biotransformation product is Metabolite V. Essentially no parent drug is found in the urine. Despite large variations in plasma levels of parent compound and its metabolites, the urinary recovery of Metabolite V is consistent and shows dose proportionality. Less than 4% of the administered dose is recovered in feces. Food intake shortly before dosing delays absorption of an immediate-release dosage form but does not affect total absorption. The pharmacokinetics and metabolism of pentoxifylline have not been studied in patients with renal and/or hepatic dysfunction, but AUC was increased and elimination rate decreased in an older population (60 to 68 years) compared to younger individuals (22 to 30 years).

Contraindications

Recent cerebral and/or retinal hemorrhage; previous intolerance to this product or methylxanthines such as caffeine, theophylline, and theobromine.

Warnings/Precautions

➤*Arterial disease of the limbs:* Patients with chronic occlusive arterial disease of the limbs frequently show other manifestations of arteriosclerotic disease. Pentoxifylline has been used safely for treatment of peripheral arterial disease in patients with concurrent coronary artery and cerebrovascular diseases, but there have been occasional reports of angina, hypotension, and arrhythmia. Controlled trials do not show that pentoxifylline causes such adverse effects more often than placebo, but, as it is a methylxanthine derivative, it is possible some individuals will experience such responses.

➤*Pregnancy: Category C.* Teratogenicity studies have been performed in rats and rabbits using oral doses up to 576 and 264 mg/kg, respectively. On a weight basis, these doses are 24 and 11 times the MRHD; on a body-surface-area basis, they are 4.2 and 3.5 times the MRHD. No evidence of fetal malformation was observed. Increased resorption was seen in rats of the 576 mg/kg group. There are no adequate and well controlled studies in pregnant women. Use pentoxifylline during pregnancy only if the potential benefit justifies the potential risk to the fetus.

➤*Lactation:* Pentoxifylline and its metabolites are excreted in human milk. Because of the potential for tumorigenicity shown for pentoxifylline in rats, a decision should be made whether to discontinue nursing or discontinue the drug, taking into account the importance of the drug to the mother.

➤*Children:* Safety and effectiveness in pediatric patients have not been established.

➤*Monitoring:* Patients on warfarin should have more frequent monitoring of prothrombin times, while patients with other risk factors complicated by hemorrhage (eg, recent surgery, peptic ulceration, cerebral and/or retinal bleeding) should have periodic examinations for bleeding including, hematocrit and/or hemoglobin.

Drug Interactions

➤*Anticoagulants:* Although a causal relationship has not been established, there have been reports of bleeding and/or prolonged prothrombin time in patients treated with pentoxifylline with and without anticoagulants or platelet aggregation inhibitors. Patients on warfarin should have more frequent monitoring of prothrombin times, while patients with other risk factors complicated by hemorrhage (eg, recent surgery, peptic ulceration) should have periodic examinations for bleeding including, hematocrit and/or hemoglobin.

➤*Theophylline:* Concomitant administration of pentoxifylline and theophylline-containing drugs leads to increased theophylline levels and theophylline toxicity in some individuals. Closely monitor such patients for signs of toxicity and have their theophylline dosage adjusted as necessary.

➤*Antihypertensives:* Pentoxifylline has been used concurrently with antihypertensive drugs, beta blockers, digitalis, diuretics, antidiabetic agents, and antiarrhythmics, without observed problems. Small decreases in blood pressure have been observed in some patients treated with pentoxifylline; periodic systemic blood pressure monitoring is recommended for patients receiving concomitant antihypertensive therapy. If indicated, reduce the dosage of the antihypertensive agents.

Adverse Reactions

Clinical trials were conducted using either controlled-release pentoxifylline tablets for up to 60 weeks or immediate-release pentoxifylline capsules for up to 24 weeks. Dosage ranges in the tablet studies were 400 mg twice daily to 3 times daily and in the capsule studies, 200 to 400 mg 3 times daily. The data below summarize the incidence (in percent) of adverse reactions considered drug related, as well as the numbers of patients who received controlled-release pentoxifylline tablets, immediate-release pentoxifylline capsules, or the corresponding placebos. The incidence of adverse reactions was higher in the capsule studies (where dose related increases were seen in digestive and nervous system side effects) than in the tablet studies. Studies with the capsule include domestic experience, whereas studies with the controlled-release tablets were conducted outside the US.

Pentoxifylline Incidence of Adverse Reactions

Adverse reaction	Controlled-release tablets (commercially available)		Immediate-release capsules (used only for controlled clinical trials)	
	Pentoxifylline	Placebo	Pentoxifylline	Placebo
(Number of patients at risk)	(321)	(128)	(177)	(138)
Discontinued for side effect	3.1%	0	9.6%	7.2%
Cardiovascular				
Angina/ chest pain	0.3%	-	1.1%	2.2%
Arrhythmia/palpitation	-	-	1.7%	0.7%
Flushing	-	-	2.3%	0.7%
CNS				
Agitation/nervousness	-	-	1.7%	0.7%
Blurred vision	-	-	2.3%	1.4%
Dizziness	1.9%	3.1%	11.9%	4.3%
Drowsiness	-	-	1.1%	5.8%
Headache	1.2%	1.6%	6.2%	5.8%
Insomnia	-	-	2.3%	2.2%
Tremor	0.3%	0.8%	-	-
GI				
Abdominal discomfort	-	-	4%	1.4%
Belching/flatus/ bloating	0.6%	-	9%	3.6%
Diarrhea	-	-	3.4%	2.9%
Dyspepsia	2.8%	4.7%	9.6%	2.9%
Nausea	2.2%	0.8%	28.8%	8.7%
Vomiting	1.2%	-	4.5%	0.7%

➤*Other reactions less than 1%:* Pentoxifylline has been marketed in Europe and elsewhere since 1972. In addition to the above symptoms, the following have been reported spontaneously since marketing or occurred in other clinical trials with an incidence of less than 1%; the causal relationship was uncertain:

Cardiovascular – Dyspnea, edema, hypotension.

CNS – Anxiety, aseptic meningitis, confusion, depression, seizures.

Dermatologic – Angioedema, brittle fingernails, pruritus, rash, urticaria.

GI – Anorexia, cholecystitis, constipation, dry mouth/thirst.

Respiratory – Epistaxis, flu-like symptoms, laryngitis, nasal congestion.

Special senses – Blurred vision, conjunctivitis, earache, scotoma.

Miscellaneous – Bad taste, excessive salivation, leukopenia, malaise, sore throat/swollen neck glands, weight change.

➤*Rare events:* A few rare events have been reported spontaneously worldwide since marketing in 1972. Although they occurred under circumstances in which a causal relationship with pentoxifylline could not be established, they are listed to serve as information for physicians:

Cardiovascular – Anaphylactoid reactions, angina, arrhythmia, tachycardia.

GI – Hepatitis, jaundice, increased liver enzymes.

Hematologic/Lymphatic – Aplastic anemia, decreased serum fibrinogen, leukemia, pancytopenia, purpura, thrombocytopenia.

Overdosage

➤*Symptoms:* Overdosage with pentoxifylline has been reported in pediatric patients and adults. Symptoms appear to be dose related. A report from a poison control center on 44 patients taking overdoses of enteric-coated pentoxifylline tablets noted that symptoms usually occurred 4 to 5 hours after ingestion and lasted about 12 hours. The highest amount ingested was 80 mg/kg; flushing, hypotension, convulsions, somnolence, loss of consciousness, fever, and agitation occurred. All patients recovered.

➤*Treatment:* In addition to symptomatic treatment and gastric lavage, special attention must be given to supporting respiration, maintaining systemic blood pressure, and controlling convulsions. Activated charcoal has been used to absorb pentoxifylline in patients who have overdosed.

COAGULATION FACTOR VIIa, RECOMBINANT

Rx	**NovoSeven RT** (Novo Nordisk)	**Injection, lyophilized powder for solution:** 1 mg	Preservative free. In single-use vials with histidine diluent.[a]
		2 mg	Preservative free. In single-use vials with histidine diluent.[a]
		5 mg	Preservative free. In single-use vials with histidine diluent.[a]
		8 mg	Preservative free. In single-use vials with histidine diluent.[a]

[a] After reconstitution with the appropriate volume of histidine diluent, each vial contains approximately 1 mg/mL of coagulation factor VIIa (corresponding to 1,000 mcg/mL), 2.3 mg/mL of sodium chloride, 1.5 mg/mL of calcium chloride dihydrate, 1.3 mg/mL of glycylglycine, 0.1 mg/mL of polysorbate 80, 25 mg/mL of mannitol, 10 mg/mL of sucrose, 0.5 mg/mL of methionine, and 1.6 mg/mL of histidine.

COAGULATION FACTOR VIIa, RECOMBINANT — INJECTION

Indications

➤*Bleeding episodes:* For the treatment of bleeding episodes in hemophilia A or B patients with inhibitors to factor VIII or factor IX and in patients with acquired hemophilia.

For the prevention of bleeding in surgical interventions or invasive procedures in hemophilia A or B patients with inhibitors to factor VIII or factor IX and in patients with acquired hemophilia.

For the treatment of bleeding episodes in patients with congenital factor VII deficiency.

For the prevention of bleeding in surgical interventions or invasive procedures in patients with congenital factor VII deficiency.

Administration and Dosage

➤*General dosing considerations:* Evaluation of hemostasis should be used to determine the effectiveness of coagulation factor VIIa and to provide a basis for modification of the coagulation factor VIIa treatment schedule; coagulation parameters do not necessarily correlate with or predict the effectiveness of coagulation factor VIIa.

➤*Adults:*

Acquired hemophilia – 70 to 90 mcg/kg by slow bolus injection repeated every 2 to 3 hours until hemostasis is achieved. The minimum effective dose in acquired hemophilia has not been determined.

Hemophilia A or B patients with inhibitors to factor VIII or factor IX –

Bleeding episodes:

• *Usual dosage* – 90 mcg/kg every 2 hours by slow bolus infusion until hemostasis is achieved, or until the treatment has been judged to be inadequate.

Doses between 35 and 120 mcg/kg have been used successfully in clinical trials for hemophilia A or B patients with inhibitors to factor VIII or factor IX.

For patients treated for joint or muscle bleeds, a decision on outcome was reached for a majority of patients within 8 doses, although more doses were required for severe bleeds. A majority of patients who reported adverse reactions received more than 12 doses.

• *Dosage adjustment* – Both the dose and administration interval may be adjusted based on the severity of the bleeding and the degree of hemostasis achieved. The minimal effective dose has not been established.

• *Duration of therapy* – The appropriate duration of posthemostatic dosing has not been studied. For severe bleeds, dosing should continue at 3- to 6-hour intervals after hemostasis is achieved to maintain the hemostatic plug. The biological and clinical effects of prolonged elevated levels of factor VIIa have not been studied; therefore, the duration of posthemostatic dosing should be minimized, and patients should be appropriately monitored by a health care provider experienced in the treatment of hemophilia during this time period.

Surgical interventions:

• *Initial dosage* – 90 mcg/kg by slow bolus injection immediately before the intervention and repeated at 2-hour intervals for the duration of the surgery.

• *Duration of therapy* – For minor surgery, postsurgical dosing by bolus infusion should occur at 2-hour intervals for the first 48 hours, then at 2- to 6-hour intervals until healing has occurred. For major surgery, postsurgical dosing by bolus injection should occur at 2-hour intervals for 5 days, followed by 4-hour intervals until healing has occurred. Additional bolus doses should be administered if required.

Congenital factor VII deficiency –

Bleeding episodes: 15 to 30 mcg/kg by slow bolus injection every 4 to 6 hours until hemostasis is achieved. Effective treatment has been achieved with doses as low as 10 mcg/kg. Dose and frequency of injections should be adjusted to each individual. The minimal effective dose has not been determined.

The healthy factor VII plasma concentration is 0.5 mcg/mL. Factor VII levels of 15% to 25% (0.075 to 0.125 mcg/mL) are generally sufficient to achieve healthy hemostasis. For example, a 70 kg individual with factor VII deficiency (plasma volume of approximately 3,000 mL) would thus require recombinant factor VIIa 3.2 to 5.4 mcg/kg to secure hemostasis, assuming 100% recovery; however, because the mean plasma recovery for recombinant factor VIIa is 20% for factor VII-deficient patients, a recombinant factor VIIa dose range of 16 to 27 mcg/kg would be required to achieve sufficient factor VII plasma levels for hemostasis, which is consistent with the recommended dose range.

Surgical interventions: See Bleeding Episodes for dosing.

➤*Children:* See Adults for dosing.

➤*Concomitant use with other formulations:* Concomitant use of coagulation factor VIIa with other formulations (eg, *NovoSeven*) is not recommended because of the potential dosing errors based on different concentrations.

➤*Preparation for administration:* Calculate the coagulation factor VIIa dosage needed and select the appropriate vial package, which contains 1 vial of coagulation factor VIIa powder and 1 vial of the histidine diluent required to prepare reconstituted coagulation factor VIIa solution.

Reconstitute only with the histidine diluent provided; do not reconstitute with sterile water or other diluent. Perform reconstitution using the following procedures:

1.) Always use aseptic technique.
2.) Bring coagulation factor VIIa powder and the specified volume of histidine diluent to room temperature, but not above 37°C (98.6°F). The specified volume of diluent corresponding to the amount of coagulation factor VIIa is as follows: 1 mg vial + 1.1 mL of histidine diluent, 2 mg vial + 2.1 mL of histidine diluent, 5 mg vial + 5.2 mL of histidine diluent. After reconstitution with the specified volume of diluent, each vial contains approximately 1 mg/mL of coagulation factor VIIa.
3.) Remove caps from the vials to expose the central portion of the rubber stopper. Cleanse the rubber stoppers with an alcohol swab and allow them to dry prior to use.
4.) Draw back the plunger of a sterile syringe (attached to sterile needle) and admit air into the syringe. It is recommended to use syringe needles of gauge size 20 to 26.
5.) Insert the needle of the syringe into the histidine diluent vial. Inject air into the vial and withdraw the quantity required for reconstitution.
6.) Insert the syringe needle containing the diluent into the vial through the center of the rubber stopper, aiming the needle against the side so that the stream of liquid runs down the vial wall (the vial does not contain a vacuum). Do not inject the diluent directly onto the coagulation factor VIIa powder.
7.) Gently swirl the vial until all the material is dissolved. The reconstituted solution is a clear, colorless solution that may be stored at room temperature or refrigerated for up to 3 hours after reconstitution.

➤*Administration:* For intravenous (IV) bolus injection only. Administer as a slow bolus injection over 2 to 5 minutes, depending on the dose administered.

Administration should take place within 3 hours after reconstitution. Any unused solution should be discarded.

➤*Admixture compatibility:* Coagulation factor VIIa should not be mixed with infusion solutions.

➤*Storage/Stability:* Prior to reconstitution, keep refrigerated or store between 2° and 25°C (36° and 77°F). Do not freeze. Store protected from light. After reconstitution, store at room temperature or refrigerated for up to 3 hours. Do not freeze or store in syringes.

Actions

➤*Pharmacology:* Recombinant coagulation factor VIIa, when complexed with tissue factor, can activate coagulation factor X to factor Xa, as well as coagulation factor IX to factor IXa. Factor Xa, in complex with other factors, then converts prothrombin to thrombin, which leads to the formation of a hemostatic plug by converting fibrinogen to fibrin and thereby inducing local hemostasis. This process may also occur on the surface of active platelets.

➤*Pharmacokinetics:*

Hemophilia A or B – Single-dose pharmacokinetics of coagulation factor VIIa (17.5, 35, and 70 mcg/kg) exhibited dose-proportional behavior in 15 subjects with hemophilia A or B. Factor VII clotting activities were measured in plasma drawn prior to and during a 24-hour period after coagulation factor VIIa administration.

Congenital factor VII deficiency – Single-dose pharmacokinetics of coagulation factor VIIa in congenital factor VII deficiency at doses of 15 and 30 mcg/kg showed no significant difference with regard to dose-independent parameters.

Absorption/Distribution –

Hemophilia A or B: The median apparent volume of distribution at steady state was 103 mL/kg (range, 78 to 139 mL/kg).

Congenital factor VII deficiency: Volume of distribution at steady state was 280 to 290 mL/kg.

Metabolism/Excretion –

Hemophilia A or B: Median clearance was 33 mL/kg/h (range, 27 to 49 mL/kg/h). The median residence time was 3 hours (range, 2.4 to 3.3 hours), and the half-life was 2.3 hours (range, 1.7 to 2.7 hours). The median in vivo plasma recovery was 44% (30% to 71%).

Congenital factor VII deficiency: Total body clearance was 70.8 to 79.1 mL/h × kg, mean residence time was 3.75 to 3.8 hours, and half-life was 2.82 to 3.11 hours. The mean in vivo plasma recovery was approximately 20% (18.9% to 22.2%).

Contraindications

None known.

COAGULATION FACTOR VIIa, RECOMBINANT — INJECTION

Warnings/Precautions

➤*Thrombotic events:* The extent of the risk of thrombotic adverse reactions after treatment with coagulation factor VIIa in patients with hemophilia and inhibitors to factor VIII or factor IX is not known but is considered to be low. Patients with disseminated intravascular coagulation (DIC), advanced atherosclerotic disease, crush injury, septicemia, or concomitant treatment with activated or nonactivated prothrombin complex concentrates may have an increased risk of developing thrombotic events because of circulating tissue factor or predisposing coagulopathy. When there is laboratory confirmation of intravascular coagulation or presence of clinical thrombosis, reduce the dosage or stop the treatment, depending on the patient's symptoms.

The extent of the risk of arterial and venous thromboembolic adverse reactions after treatment with coagulation factor VIIa in patients without hemophilia is also not known. A clinical study in elderly nonhemophilia intracerebral hemorrhage patients indicated a potential increased risk of arterial thromboembolic adverse reactions with use of coagulation factor VIIa, including cerebral ischemia and/or infarction, myocardial infarction (MI), and myocardial ischemia. Safety and effectiveness have not been established in these settings.

➤*Prolonged administration:* Because of limited clinical studies that clearly address the effect of posthemostatic dosing, exercise caution when coagulation factor VIIa is used for prolonged dosing.

➤*Concomitant use with other formulations:* Concomitant use of coagulation factor VIIa with other formulations (eg, *NovoSeven*) is not recommended because of the potential dosing errors based on different concentrations.

➤*Hypersensitivity reactions:* Administer coagulation factor VIIa with caution in patients with known hypersensitivity to the drug or any of its components, or in patients with known hypersensitivity to mouse, hamster, or bovine proteins.

➤*Pregnancy: Category C.* Treatment of rats and rabbits with coagulation factor VIIa in reproduction studies has been associated with mortality at doses of up to 6 mg/kg and 5 mg/kg, respectively. At 6 mg/kg in rats, the abortion rate was 0 of 25 litters; in rabbits at 5 mg/kg, the abortion rate was 2 of 25 litters. Twenty-three of 25 female rats given coagulation factor VIIa 6 mg/kg gave birth successfully; however, 2 of the 23 litters died during the early period of lactation. No evidence of teratogenicity was observed after dosing with coagulation factor VIIa. There are no adequate and well-controlled studies in pregnant women. Use coagulation factor VIIa during pregnancy only if the potential benefit justifies the potential risk to the fetus.

➤*Lactation:* It is not known whether coagulation factor VIIa is excreted in breast milk. Because many drugs are excreted in breast milk, and because of the potential for serious adverse reactions in breast-feeding infants, decide whether to discontinue breast-feeding or the drug, taking into account the importance of the drug to the mother.

➤*Lab test abnormalities:* Laboratory coagulation parameters may be used as an adjunct to the clinical evaluation of hemostasis in monitoring the efficacy and treatment schedule of coagulation factor VIIa, although these parameters have shown no direct correlation to achieving hemostasis. Assays of prothrombin time (PT), activated partial thromboplastin time (aPTT), and plasma factor VII clotting activity may give different results with different reagents. Treatment with coagulation factor VIIa has been shown to produce the following characteristics:

PT – In patients with hemophilia A or B with inhibitors to factor VIII or factor IX, the PT shortened to an approximately 7-second plateau at a plasma factor VII clotting level of approximately 5 units/mL. For plasma factor VII clotting levels of more than 5 units/mL, there is no further change in PT.

aPTT – While administration of coagulation factor VIIa shortens the prolonged aPTT in hemophilia A or B patients with inhibitors to factor VIII or factor IX, normalization has usually not been observed in doses shown to induce clinical improvement. Data indicate that clinical improvement was associated with a shortening of aPTT of 15 to 20 seconds.

Plasma factor VII clotting – Plasma factor VII clotting levels were measured 2 hours after administration of coagulation factor VIIa 35 and 90 mcg/kg following 2 days of dosing at 2-hour intervals. Average steady-state levels were 11 and 28 units/mL for the 2 dose levels, respectively.

➤*Monitoring:* Monitor patients for signs or symptoms of activation of the coagulation system or thrombosis. When there is laboratory confirmation of intravascular coagulation or the presence of clinical thrombosis, reduce the dosage or stop the treatment, depending on the patient's symptoms.

Monitor factor VII–deficient patients for PT and factor VII coagulant activity before and after administration. If the factor VIIa activity fails to reach the expected level, PT is not corrected, or bleeding is not controlled after treatment with the recommended doses, suspect antibody formation and perform analysis for antibodies.

Drug Interactions

➤*Coagulation factor concentrates:* The risk of a potential interaction between coagulation factor VIIa and coagulation factor concentrates has not been adequately evaluated in preclinical or clinical studies. Avoid simultaneous use of activated prothrombin complex concentrates or prothrombin complex concentrates.

Adverse Reactions

➤*Serious adverse reactions:* The most serious adverse reactions observed in patients receiving coagulation factor VIIa were thrombotic reactions; however, the extent of the risk of thrombotic adverse reactions after treatment with coagulation factor VIIa in individuals with hemophilia and inhibitors to factor VIII or factor IX is considered to be low.

➤*Common adverse reactions:* The most common adverse reactions observed in clinical studies for all labeled indications of coagulation factor VIIa were arthralgia, edema, headache, hemorrhage, hypertension, hypotension, injection-site reaction, nausea, pain, pyrexia, rash, and vomiting.

➤*Hemophilia A or B patients with inhibitors to factor VIII or factor IX:*

Coagulation Factor VIIa Adverse Reactions in Hemophilia A or B Patients With Inhibitors to Factor VIII or Factor IX (≥ 2%)

Adverse reaction	Number of episodes reported (n = 1,939 treatments)	Number of unique patients (n = 298 patients)
Cardiovascular		
Hypertension	9	6
Hematologic		
Fibrinogen plasma decreased	10	5
Hemarthrosis	14	8
Hemorrhage NOS[a]	15	8
Miscellaneous		
Fever	16	13

[a] NOS = not otherwise specified.

Other adverse reactions (1%) – Reactions that were reported in 1% of patients and were considered to be at least possibly or of unknown relationship to coagulation factor VIIa administration were abnormal renal function, allergic reaction, arthrosis, bradycardia, coagulation disorder, decreased prothrombin, decreased therapeutic response, DIC, edema, headache, hypotension, increased fibrinolysis, injection-site reaction, pain, pneumonia, pruritus, purpura, rash, and vomiting.

Serious adverse reactions – Serious adverse reactions that were probably or possibly related, or where the relationship to coagulation factor VIIa was not specified, occurred in 14 of the 298 (4.7%) patients. Six of these 14 patients died of the following conditions: anesthesia complications during proctoscopy, renal failure complicating a retroperitoneal bleed, ruptured abscess leading to sepsis and DIC, pneumonia, splenic hematoma and GI bleeding, and worsening of chronic renal failure. In the 298 hemophilia patients, thrombosis was reported in 2 patients.

➤*Surgery studies:* In the randomized, double-blind, parallel-group study, 6 patients experienced serious adverse reactions; 2 of these patients had reactions that were considered probably or possibly related to study medication (ie, acute postoperative hemarthrosis, internal jugular thrombosis). No deaths occurred during the study.

➤*Congenital factor VII deficiency:* In the compassionate/emergency use programs, 28 adverse reactions in 13 patients and 10 serious adverse reactions in 9 patients were reported. Nonserious adverse reactions in the compassionate/emergency use programs were single reactions in 1 patient, except for fever (3 patients), intracranial hemorrhage (3 patients), and pain (2 patients). The most common serious adverse reaction in the compassionate/emergency programs was serious bleeding in critically ill patients. All 9 patients with serious adverse reactions died. One adverse reaction (localized phlebitis) was reported in the literature. No adverse reactions were reported in the pharmacokinetics study reports or the HTRS registry. No thromboembolic complications were reported for these 75 patients.

Isolated cases of factor VII–deficient patients developing antibodies against factor VII were reported after treatment with coagulation factor VIIa. These patients had previously been treated with human plasma and/or plasma–derived factor VII. In some cases, the antibodies showed an inhibitory effect in vitro.

➤*Acquired hemophilia:* Of 139 patients, 10 experienced 12 serious adverse reactions that were of possible, probable, or unknown relationship to treatment with coagulation factor VIIa. Thrombotic serious adverse reactions included angina pectoris, cerebral infarction, cerebral ischemia, deep vein thrombosis, MI, and pulmonary embolism. Additional serious adverse reactions included shock and subdural hematoma.

Data collected for mortality in the compassionate use programs, the HTRS registry, and the publications spanning a 10-year period were overall 32 of 139 (23%). Deaths were due to arrhythmias (2), cardiovascular failure (4), hemorrhage (10), neoplasia (4), respiratory failure (3), sepsis (2), thrombotic reactions (2), trauma (1), and unknown causes (4).

➤*Postmarketing:* The following additional adverse reactions were reported after the use of coagulation factor VIIa in both labeled and unlabeled indications that included individuals with situational coagulopathy and without known coagulopathy: high D-dimer levels and consumptive coagulopathy, isolated hypersensitivity reactions (eg, anaphylactic reactions), and thromboembolic reactions (eg, arterial thrombosis, cerebral infarction and/or ischemia, deep vein thrombosis, MI, myocardial ischemia, related pulmonary embolism, thrombophlebitis).

Additional data on the adverse reaction profile in general and regarding the frequency of thrombotic reactions in particular is being collected through a

COAGULATION FACTOR VIIa, RECOMBINANT — INJECTION

postmarketing surveillance program. The HTRS registry surveillance program is designed to collect data on all uses of coagulation factor VIIa to expand the base of experience regarding the use of coagulation factor VIIa. All prescribers can obtain information regarding contribution of patient data to this program by calling 1-877-362-7355.

Overdosage

➤*Symptoms:* Dose-limiting toxicities of coagulation factor VIIa have not been investigated in clinical trials. The following are examples of accidental overdose. One hemophilia B patient (16 years of age, 68 kg) received a single dose of 352 mcg/kg and 1 hemophilia A patient (2 years of age, 14.6 kg) received doses ranging from 246 to 986 mcg/kg on 5 consecutive days. There were no reported complications in either case. A newborn girl with congenital factor VII deficiency was administered an overdose of coagulation factor VIIa (single dose, 800 mcg/kg). Following additional administration of coagulation factor VIIa and various plasma products, antibodies against coagulation factor VIIa were detected but no thrombotic complications were reported. A factor VII–deficient man (83 years of age, 111.1 kg) received 2 doses of 324 mcg/kg (10 to 20 times the recommended dose) and experienced a thrombotic reaction (occipital stroke). Do not intentionally increase the recommended dose schedule, even in the case of lack of effect, because of the absence of information on the additional risk that may be incurred.

Patient Information

Inform patients receiving coagulation factor VIIa of the benefits and risks associated with treatment.

Warn patients about the early signs of hypersensitivity reactions, including anaphylaxis, hives, hypotension, tightness of the chest, urticaria, and wheezing. Although bleeding can cause similar symptoms, also warn patients about the signs of thrombosis, including altered consciousness or speech, loss of sensation or motor power, new onset chest pain, new onset swelling and pain in the limbs or abdomen, or shortness of breath.

ANTIHEMOPHILIC FACTOR, HUMAN (Factor VIII; AHF)

Rx	**Monoclate-P** (CSL Behring LLC)	**Injection, lyophilized powder for solution:** 250 units of AHF (human)	Heat-treated, monoclonal antibody purified. Albumin (human) ≈ 1% to 2%, mannitol 0.8%, sodium, histidine, ≤ 50 ng of murine monoclonal antibody per 100 AHF units. In kits with single-dose 10 mL vials and diluent.
Rx	**Koate-DVI** (Talecris)		Solvent/Detergent-treated, heat-treated. Albumin (human) ≤ 10 mg/mL, PEG, glycine, aluminum ≤ 1 mcg/mL, histidine. In kits with single-dose bottles and diluent (sterile water for injection).
Rx	**Monoclate-P** (CSL Behring LLC)	**Injection, lyophilized powder for solution:** 500 units of AHF (human)	Heat-treated, monoclonal antibody purified. Albumin (human) ≈ 1% to 2%, mannitol 0.8%, sodium, histidine, ≤ 50 ng of murine monoclonal antibody per 100 AHF units. In kits with single-dose 10 mL vials and diluent.
Rx	**Koate-DVI** (Talecris)		Solvent/Detergent-treated, heat-treated. Albumin (human) ≤ 10 mg/mL, PEG, glycine, aluminum ≤ 1 mcg/mL, histidine. In kits with single-dose bottles and diluent (sterile water for injection).
Rx	**Monoclate-P** (CSL Behring LLC)	**Injection, lyophilized powder for solution:** 1,000 units of AHF (human)	Heat-treated, monoclonal antibody purified. Albumin (human) ≈ 1% to 2%, mannitol 0.8%, sodium, histidine, ≤ 50 ng of murine monoclonal antibody per 100 AHF units. In kits with single-dose 20 mL vials and diluent.
Rx	**Koate-DVI** (Talecris)		Solvent/Detergent-treated, heat-treated. Albumin (human) ≤ 10 mg/mL, PEG, glycine, aluminum ≤ 1 mcg/mL, histidine. In kits with single-dose bottles and diluent (sterile water for injection).
Rx	**Monoclate-P** (CSL Behring LLC)	**Injection, lyophilized powder for solution:** 1,500 units of AHF (human)	Heat-treated, monoclonal antibody purified. Albumin (human)≈ 1% to 2%, mannitol 0.8%, sodium, histidine, ≤ 50 ng of murine monoclonal antibody per 100 AHF units. In kits with single-dose 20 mL vials and diluent.
Rx	**Alphanate** (Grifols)	**Injection, lyophilized powder for solution:** As labeled (≥ 5 units of AHF (human)/mg of total protein)	Solvent/Detergent-treated, heat-treated. Albumin (human) 0.3 to 0.9 g per 100 mL, glycine, heparin, histidine, arginine, PEG, sodium. In kits with single-dose vials and diluent (sterile water for injection).
Rx	**Hemofil M** (Baxter)	**Injection, powder for solution:** 2 to 20 units of AFH (human)/mg of total protein	Method M, monoclonal antibody purified, solvent/detergent treated. Albumin (human) ≤ 12.5 mg/mL, PEG 3350, histidine, glycine, and ≤ 0.1 ng of mouse protein per AHF unit. In kits with single-dose bottles and diluent (10 mL of sterile water for injection).

ANTIHEMOPHILIC FACTOR, HUMAN

Indications

➤*Classical hemophilia:* For the prevention and control of hemorrhagic episodes in patients with classical hemophilia (hemophilia A), in which there is a demonstrated deficiency of activity of the plasma clotting factor, factor VIII, or in patients with acquired factor VIII deficiency.

Antihemophilic factor (AHF) (human) provides a means of temporarily replacing the missing clotting factor in order to control or prevent bleeding episodes or in order to perform emergency and elective surgery on individuals with hemophilia. AHF (human) contains naturally occurring von Willebrand factor (vWF), which is copurified as part of the manufacturing process.

AHF (human) can be of significant therapeutic value in patients with acquired factor VIII inhibitors not exceeding 10 Bethesda units/mL. However, in such uses, control the dosage by frequent laboratory determinations of circulating AHF.

AHF (human) is not effective in controlling the bleeding of patients with von Willebrand disease, and therefore is not approved for such use.

Administration and Dosage

➤*General dosing considerations:* Incorrect diagnosis, inappropriate dosage, method of administration, and biological differences in individual patients could reduce the efficacy of this product or even result in an ill effect following its use. It is important that this product is stored properly, the directions for use are followed carefully during use, the risk of transmitting viruses is carefully weighed before the product is prescribed, and that plasma factor VIII levels are measured in initial treatment situations or if clinical response appears inadequate.

Potency – AHF potency (factor VIII coagulant activity [VIII:c]) is expressed in units on the product label. One unit approximates the activity in 1 mL of normal human plasma. Replacement therapy studies have shown a linear dose-response relationship with a 2% to 2.5% increase in factor VIII activity for each unit of VIII:c per kilogram of body weight transfused, from which an approximate factor of 0.5 units/kg can be calculated.

The high purity of AHF has been thought to influence the difficulty of producing an accurate potency measurement. Experiments have shown that to achieve accurate activity levels, such a potency assay should be conducted using plastic test tubes and pipets as well as substrate containing normal levels of vWF.

Calculation of dosage –

Alphanate: The following formula provides a guide for dosage calculation (the plasma factor VIII may vary depending upon the age, weight, severity of hemorrhage, or surgical procedure of the patient):

Body weight (in kg) × 0.5 units/kg × factor VIII increase desired (%) = number of VIII:c units required.

Example:

50 kg × 0.5 units/kg × 30 (% increase) = 750 units VIII:c

Hemofil M: The expected in vivo peak AHF (human) level (expressed as units/dL of plasma or percent of normal) can be calculated by multiplying the dose administered per kilogram body weight (units/kg) by 2. This calculation is based on the clinical finding that is supported by data from the collaborative study of in vivo recovery and survival with 15 different lots of AHF (human) on 56 hemophiliac patients that demonstrated a mean peak recovery point above the mean preinfusion baseline of about 2 units/dL per infused unit/kg body weight. Examples:

1.) A dose of 1,750 AHF (human) units administered to a 70 kg patient (ie, 25 units/kg [1,750/70], should be expected to cause a peak postinfusion AHF [human] increase of 25 × 2 = 50 units/dL [50% of normal]).
2.) A peak level of 70% is required in a 40 kg child. In this situation, the dose would be 70/2 × 40 = 1,400 units.

ANTIHEMOPHILIC FACTOR, HUMAN

Koate-DVI: The in vivo percent elevation in factor VIII level can be estimated by multiplying the dose of AHF (human) per kilogram of body weight (units/kg) by 2%. This method of calculation is based on clinical findings and is illustrated in the following examples.

$$\text{Expected \% factor VIII increase} = \frac{[\text{\# units administered} \times 2\% \text{ per units/kg}]}{\text{body weight (kg)}}$$

Example for a 70 kg adult:

$$\frac{[1{,}400 \text{ units} \times 2\% \text{ per units/kg}]}{70 \text{ kg}} = 40\%$$

Or

$$\text{Dosage required (units)} = \frac{[\text{body weight (kg)} \times \text{desired \% factor VIII increase}]}{2\% \text{ per units/kg}}$$

Example for a 15 kg child:

$$\frac{[15 \text{ kg} \times 100\%]}{2\% \text{ per units/kg}} = 750 \text{ units required}$$

Monoclate-P: As a general rule, 1 unit of AHF activity per kilogram will increase the circulating AHF level by 2%. The following formula provides a guide of dosage calculations for adults and children:

Number of AHF units required = body weight (in kg) × desired factor VIII increase (% normal) × 0.5

➤*Adults:*

Classical hemorrhage –

Mild hemorrhage:

• *Alphanate* – Can usually be treated with a single administration of AHF (human) sufficient to raise the plasma factor VIII level to 20% to 30%.

• *Hemofil M* – For early hemarthrosis, muscle bleeding, or oral bleeding, a dose of AHF sufficient to achieve a level of 20% to 40% of normal should be given. Begin infusion every 12 to 24 hours for 1 to 3 days until the bleeding episode as indicated by pain is resolved or healing is achieved.

• *Koate-DVI* – Mild superficial or early hemorrhages may respond to a single dose of 10 units/kg, leading to an in vivo rise of approximately 20% in the factor VIII level. Therapy need not be repeated unless there is evidence of further bleeding.

• *Monoclate-P* – Minor hemorrhagic episodes will generally subside with a single infusion if a level of 30% or more is attained.

Moderate hemorrhage:

• *Alphanate* – Can usually be treated with a single administration of AHF (human) sufficient to raise the plasma factor VIII level to 20% to 30%.

• *Hemofil M* – For more extensive hemarthrosis, muscle bleed, or hematoma, a dose of AHF sufficient to achieve a level of 30% to 60% of normal should be given. Repeat infusion every 12 to 24 hours for usually 3 days or more until pain and disability are resolved.

• *Koate-DVI* – For more serious bleeding episodes (eg, definite hemarthroses, known trauma), the factor VIII level should be raised to 30% to 50% by administering approximately 15 to 25 units/kg. If further therapy is required, repeated doses of 10 to 15 units/kg every 8 to 12 hours may be given.

• *Monoclate-P* –

Initial dosage: For more serious hemorrhages and minor surgical procedures, the patient's factor VIII level should be raised to 30% to 50% of normal, which usually requires an initial dose of 15 to 25 units/kg.

Maintenance dosage: If further therapy is required, a maintenance dose is 10 to 15 units/kg every 8 to 12 hours.

Severe hemorrhage:

• *Alphanate* – The patient's plasma factor VIII level should be raised to 30% to 50%. Infusions are generally required at twice-daily intervals over several days.

• *Hemofil M* – For life-threatening bleeds (eg, head injury, throat bleeding, severe abdominal pain), a dose of AHF sufficient to achieve a level of 60% to 100% of normal should be given. Repeat infusion every 8 to 24 hours until threat is resolved.

• *Koate-DVI* –

Initial dosage: In patients with life-threatening bleeding or possible hemorrhage involving vital structures (eg, CNS, retropharyngeal and retroperitoneal spaces, iliopsoas sheath), the factor VIII level should be raised to 80% to 100% of normal in order to achieve hemostasis. This may be achieved in most patients with an initial AHF (human) dose of 40 to 50 units/kg.

Maintenance dosage: 20 to 25 units/kg every 8 to 12 hours.

• *Monoclate-P* –

Initial dosage: In hemorrhages near vital organs (neck, throat, subperitoneal), it may be desirable to raise the factor VIII level to 80% to 100% of normal, which can be achieved with an initial dose of 40 to 50 units/kg.

Maintenance dosage: 20 to 25 units/kg every 8 to 12 hours.

Surgery:

• *Alphanate* – Requires that postoperatively the factor VIII level be raised to 50% to 80% and maintained at or above 30% for approximately 2 weeks.

• *Hemofil M* – For minor surgical procedures, a dose of AHF sufficient to achieve a level of 60% to 80% of normal should be given. A single infusion plus oral antifibrinolytic therapy within 1 hour is sufficient in approximately 70% of cases.

For major surgical procedures, a dose of AHF sufficient to achieve a level of 80% to 100% of normal should be given pre- and postoperatively. Repeat infusion every 8 to 24 hours depending on state of healing.

• *Koate-DVI* – For major surgical procedures, the factor VIII level should be raised to approximately 100% by giving a preoperative dose of 50 units/kg. The level should be checked to ensure that the expected level is achieved before the patient goes to surgery. In order to maintain hemostatic levels, repeat infusions may be necessary every 6 to 12 hours initially and for a total of 10 to 14 days until healing is complete. The intensity of factor VIII replacement therapy required depends on the type of surgery and postoperative regimen employed. For minor surgical procedures, less intensive treatment schedules may provide adequate hemostasis.

• *Monoclate-P* – For surgical procedures, a dose of AHF sufficient to achieve a level 80% to 100% of normal should be given an hour prior to surgery. A second dose, half the size of the priming dose, should be given 5 hours after the first dose. Factor VIII levels should be maintained at a daily minimum of at least 30% for a period of 10 to 14 days postoperatively.

Dental extractions:

• *Alphanate* – The factor VIII level should be raised to 50% immediately prior to the procedure; additional AHF (human) may be given if bleeding recurs.

• *Hemofil M* – A dose of AHF sufficient to achieve a level of 60% to 80% of normal should be given prior to procedure. A single infusion plus oral antifibrinolytic therapy within 1 hour is sufficient in approximately 70% of cases.

Prophylactic –

Alphanate: In patients with severe factor VIII deficiency who experience frequent hemorrhages, AHF (human) may be administered prophylactically on a daily or every other day schedule to raise the factor VIII level to approximately 15%.

Koate-DVI: Factor VIII concentrates may also be administered on a regular schedule for prophylaxis of bleeding.

➤*Children:*

Classical hemophilia –

Alphanate:

• *17 years of age and older* – See Adults for dosing.

➤*Elderly:* Dose selection should be cautious, reflecting the greater frequency of decreased hepatic, renal, or cardiac function, and of concomitant disease or other drug therapy. Dosing should be appropriate to the clinical situation.

➤*Therapeutic drug monitoring:* Factor VIII levels should be monitored periodically to evaluate individual patient response to the dosage regimen. Although dosage can be estimated by these calculations, it is strongly recommended that whenever possible, appropriate laboratory tests, including serial AHF assays, be performed on the patient's plasma at suitable intervals to ensure that adequate AHF levels have been reached and are maintained.

For major surgical procedures, factor III levels should be checked throughout the perioperative course to ensure adequate replacement therapy. The careful control of the substitution therapy is especially important in cases of major surgery or life-threatening hemorrhages. Other dosage regimens have been proposed that describe continuous maintenance therapy.

➤*Administration:* AHF (human) is for IV administration only. The product must be administered within 3 hours after reconstitution.

Alphanate – Perform venipuncture and administer slowly at a rate not exceeding 10 mL/min.

Monoclate-P – Administer solution IV at a rate (approximately 2 mL/min) comfortable to the patient. Administer at room temperature; do not refrigerate after reconstitution. Discard any unused contents into the appropriate safety container.

Following reconstitution with the supplied diluent, AHF (human) should be administered IV within 3 hours after reconstitution to avoid the potential ill effect of any inadvertent bacterial contamination occurring during reconstitution.

Rate of administration – The rate of administration should be adapted to the response of the individual patient, but administration of the entire dose in 5 to 10 minutes is generally well tolerated. Preparations of AHF can be administered at a rate of up to 10 mL per minute with no significant reactions. The pulse rate should be determined before and during administration of AHF (human). If a significant increase occurs, reducing the rate of administration or temporarily halting the injection usually allows the symptoms to disappear promptly.

Handling/Disposal – Nursing personnel and others who administer this material should exercise appropriate caution when handling AHF (human) because of the risk of exposure to viral infection. Discard any unused contents into the appropriate safety container. Discard administration equipment after single use into the appropriate safety container. Do not resterilize components. Place needles in sharps container after single use. Discard all equipment, including any reconstituted AHF (human) product, in accordance with biohazard procedures.

➤*Storage/Stability:*

Alphanate – Store between 2° and 8°C (36° and 46°F). Do not freeze to prevent damage to diluent vial. May be stored at, but not to exceed, 30°C (86°F) for up to 2 months. When removed from refrigeration, record the removal date on the space provided on the carton.

Hemofil M – AHF (human) can be stored under refrigeration, between 2° and 8°C (36° and 46°F), or at room temperature, not to exceed 30°C (86°F) until the expiration date noted on the package. Avoid freezing to prevent damage to the diluent bottle. Do not refrigerate after reconstitution. Administer not more than 3 hours after reconstitution.

ANTIHEMOPHILIC FACTOR, HUMAN

Koate-DVI – Store under refrigeration, between 2° and 8°C (36° and 46°F). Storage of lyophilized powder at room temperature up to 25°C (77°F) for 6 months, such as in home treatment situations, may be done without loss of activity. Freezing should be avoided because breakage of the diluent bottle might occur.

Monoclate-P – When stored at refrigerator temperature, between 2° and 8°C (36° and 46°F), AHF (human) is stable for the period indicated by the expiration date on its label. Within this period, AHF (human) may be stored at, but not to exceed, 25°C (77°F) for up to 6 months. Avoid freezing, which may damage the container for the diluent.

Actions

➤*Pharmacology:* Hemophilia A is a hereditary bleeding disorder characterized by deficient coagulant activity of the specific plasma protein clotting factor, factor VIII. In afflicted individuals, hemorrhages may occur spontaneously or after only minor trauma. Surgery on such individuals is not feasible without first correcting the clotting abnormality. The administration of AHF (human) provides an increase in plasma levels of factor VIII and can temporarily correct the coagulation defect in these patients.

After infusion of AHF (human), there is usually an instantaneous rise in the coagulant level, followed by an initial rapid decrease in activity, and then a subsequent much slower rate of decrease in activity. The early rapid phase may represent the time of equilibration with the extravascular compartment, and the second or slow phase of the survival curve presumably is the result of degradation and reflects the true biologic half-life of the infused AHF (human).

AHF is a protein found in normal plasma, which is necessary for clot formation. The administration of AHF provides an increase in plasma levels of AHF and can temporarily correct the coagulation defect of patients with hemophilia A (classical hemophilia). The administration of AHF will also correct deficiencies caused by circulating inhibitors when the inhibitor level does not exceed 10 Bethesda units/mL.

VIII:c is the coagulant portion of the factor VIII complex circulating in plasma. It is noncovalently associated with the von Willebrand protein responsible for vWF activity. These 2 proteins have distinct biochemical and immunological properties and are under separate genetic control. VIII:c acts as a cofactor for factor IX to activate factor X in the intrinsic pathway of blood coagulation. Hemophilia A, a hereditary disorder of blood coagulation caused by decreased levels of VIII:c, results in profuse bleeding into joints, muscles, or internal organs as a result of a trauma. AHF (human) provides an increase in plasma levels of antihemophilic factor, thereby enabling temporary correction of hemophilia A bleeding.

AHF (human) is a constituent of normal plasma and is required for clotting. The administration of AHF (human) temporarily increases the plasma level of this clotting factor, thus minimizing the hazard of hemorrhage. The solvent/detergent treatment process has been shown to provide a high level of virus kill without compromising protein structure and function. The susceptibility of human pathogenic viruses, such as the human immunodeficiency viruses and hepatitis viruses, as well as marker viruses, such as Sindbis virus and vesicular stomatitis virus (VSV), to inactivation by organic solvent/detergent treatment has been discussed in the literature.

In vitro inactivation studies to evaluate the solvent/detergent treatment step used in the manufacture of AHF (human) employed an assay with a sensitivity of 2 logs of virus for the marker viruses VSV and Sindbis virus. The studies demonstrated a log kill of at least 4.1 for VSV and at least 4.7 for Sindbis virus. At least 11.1 logs of HIV-1 and at least 6.1 logs of HIV-2 were inactivated by the solvent/detergent treatment step. The number of viral particles inactivated by the process represents the maximum amount of virus added initially to the sample, thus the results of the study indicate that all the added HIV virus was killed.

In another study, the dry heat cycle of 80°C (176°F) for 72 hours of the AHF (human) manufacturing process was shown to inactivate at least 5.8 logs of hepatitis A virus (HAV). In a different study, the following steps in the manufacturing process of AHF (human) were evaluated for virus reduction/removal capability: precipitation with PEG 3.5%, solvent/detergent treatment with tri-n-butyl phosphate 0.3% and polysorbate 80 1%, heparin-actigel-ALD chromatography, lyophilization of factor VIII, and heat treatment at 80°C (176°F) for 72 hours. The following viruses were used in these studies: bovine herpesvirus (BHV), bovine viral diarrhea (BVD), human poliovirus Sabin type 2 (POL), canine parvovirus (CPV), and HIV-1.

The following table summarizes the reduction factors for each virus evaluated for each viral inactivation/removal step validated in the manufacturing process of AHF (human). However, no treatment method has yet been shown capable of totally eliminating all potential infective virus in preparations of coagulation factor concentrates.

Virus Reduction Factor During the Manufacture of AHF (Human)

Virus reduction (log_{10})	Processing step					
	3.5% PEG precipitation	Solvent/ Detergent treatment	Column chromato-graphy	Lyophilization of factor VIII	Dry heat cycle[a]	Total log removal
BHV		≥ 8	7.6	1.3	2.1	≥ 19
BVD	< 1	≥ 4.5	< 1	< 1	≥ 4.9	≥ 9.4
POL	3.3	–	< 1	3.4	≥ 2.5	≥ 9.2
CPV	1.2	–	< 1	< 1	4.1	5.3
VSV	–	≥ 4.1	–	–	–	≥ 4.1
Sindbis	–	≥ 4.7	–	–	–	≥ 4.7

Virus Reduction Factor During the Manufacture of AHF (Human)

Virus reduction (log_{10})	Processing step					
	3.5% PEG precipitation	Solvent/ Detergent treatment	Column chromato-graphy	Lyophilization of factor VIII	Dry heat cycle[a]	Total log removal
HIV-1	< 1	≥ 11.1	≥ 2	–	–	≥ 13.1
HIV-2	–	≥ 6.1	–	–	–	≥ 6.1
HAV	–	–	–	2.1	≥ 5.8	≥ 7.9

[a] At 80°C (176°F) over 72 hours.

➤*Pharmacokinetics:* Following the administration of AHF (human) during clinical trials, the mean in vivo half-life of factor VIII observed in 12 adult subjects with severe hemophilia A was 17.9 ± 9.6 hours. In this same study, the in vivo recovery was 96.7 ± 14.5% at 10 minutes postinfusion. Recovery at 10 minutes postinfusion was also determined as 2.4 ± 0.4 units factor VIII rise/dL plasma per units factor VIII infused/kg body weight.

Clinical evaluation of AHF (human) concentrate for its half-life characteristics in hemophilic patients showed it to be comparable with other commercially available AHF (human) concentrates. The mean half-life obtained from 6 patients was 17.5 hours with a mean recovery of 1.9 units/dL rise/unit/kg. The half-life of AHF, method M, monoclonal purified, administered to factor VIII–deficient patients has been shown to be 14.8 ± 3 hours.

Contraindications

Known hypersensitivity to mouse protein (*Hemofil M* and *Monoclate-P*).

Warnings/Precautions

➤*Infectious disease transmission:* AHF (human) is made from human plasma. Products made from human plasma may contain infectious agents, such as viruses, that can cause disease. The risk that such products will transmit an infectious agent has been reduced by screening plasma donors for prior exposure to certain viruses, testing for the presence of certain current virus infections, and inactivating and/or removing certain viruses. The manufacturing procedure for AHF (human) includes processing steps designed to reduce further the risk of viral transmission. Stringent procedures utilized at plasma collection centers, plasma testing laboratories, and fractionation facilities are designed to reduce the risk of viral transmission. The primary viral reduction step of the AHF (human) manufacturing process is the heat treatment of the purified, stabilized aqueous solution at 60°C (140°F) for 10 hours. In addition, the purification procedure (several precipitation steps) used in the manufacture of AHF (human) also provides viral reduction capacity.

Because this product is made from human blood, it may carry a risk of transmitting infectious agents (eg, viruses, and, theoretically, the Creutzfeldt-Jakob disease agent) despite these measures. There is also the possibility that unknown infectious agents may be present in such products. All infections thought by a health care provider possibly to have been transmitted by this product should be reported by the health care provider to the manufacturer. Discuss the risks and benefits of this product with the patient before prescribing or administering it.

Individuals who receive infusions of blood or plasma products may develop signs and/or symptoms of some viral infections, particularly hepatitis C. Incubation in a solvent detergent mixture during the manufacturing process is designed to reduce the risk of transmitting viral infection. However, scientific opinion encourages hepatitis A and hepatitis B vaccinations for patients with hemophilia at birth or at the time of diagnosis. It is emphasized that hepatitis B vaccination is essential for patients with hemophilia, and it is recommended that this be done at birth or diagnosis. Hepatitis A vaccination is also recommended for hemophilic patients who are hepatitis A seronegative.

➤*Formation of inhibitors to factor VIII:* Some patients develop inhibitors to factor VIII. Factor VIII inhibitors are circulating antibodies (ie, globulins) that neutralize the procoagulant activity of factor VIII. No studies have been conducted with AHF (human) to evaluate inhibitor formation. Therefore, it is not known whether there are greater, lesser, or the same risks of developing inhibitors due to the use of this product than there are with other AHF preparations. Patients with these inhibitors may not respond to treatment with AHF (human), or the response may be much less than would otherwise be expected; therefore, larger doses of AHF (human) are often required. The management of bleeding in patients with inhibitors requires careful monitoring, especially if surgical procedures are indicated.

If the AHF content of the patient's plasma fails to reach expected levels or if bleeding is not controlled after apparently adequate dosage, suspect the presence of inhibitor. By appropriate laboratory procedures, the presence of inhibitor can be demonstrated and quantified in terms of AHF units neutralized by each milliliter of plasma or by the total estimated plasma volume. If the inhibitor is at low levels (ie, less than 10 Bethesda units/mL), after administration of sufficient AHF units to neutralize the inhibitor, additional AHF units will elicit the predicted response.

➤*Hemolysis:* AHF (human) contains blood group–specific isoagglutinins; however, processing significantly reduces the presence of blood group–specific antibodies in the final product. Nevertheless, when large or frequent doses are required in patients of blood groups A, B, or AB, monitor the patient by means of hematocrit and direct Coombs test for signs of intravascular hemolysis and falling hematocrit. If this condition occurs, thus leading to progressive hemolytic anemia, consider administration of serologically compatible type O red blood cells or administration of AHF (human) produced from group-specific plasma.

ANTIHEMOPHILIC FACTOR, HUMAN

➤*Hepatitis and AIDS:* Product administration and handling of the infusion set and needles must be done with caution. Percutaneous puncture with a needle contaminated with blood can transmit infectious viruses, including HIV (AIDS) and hepatitis. Obtain immediate medical attention if injury occurs.

➤*Vasomotor reactions:* Do not administer AHF (human) at a rate exceeding 10 mL/min. Rapid administration of a factor VIII concentrate may result in vasomotor reactions.

➤*Latex sensitivity:* Certain components used in the packaging of *Hemofil M* and *Koate-DVI* contain natural rubber latex.

➤*Surgery:* Patients affected with classical hemophilia frequently require therapy following minor accidents. Surgery, when required in such individuals, must be preceded by temporary corrections of the clotting abnormality. Surgical prophylaxis in severe AHF deficiency can be accomplished with an appropriately dosed presurgical IV bolus of AHF (human), followed by intermittent maintenance doses.

➤*Hypersensitivity reactions:*

Formation of antibodies to mouse protein (Hemofil M and Monoclate-P) – Although no hypersensitivity reactions have been observed, because AHF (human) contains trace amounts of mouse protein, the possibility exists that patients treated with AHF (human) may develop hypersensitivity to the mouse proteins.

➤*Pregnancy: Category C.* Animal reproduction studies have not been conducted with AHF (human). It is not known whether AHF (human) can cause fetal harm when administered to a pregnant woman or can affect reproduction capacity. Give AHF (human) to a pregnant woman only if clearly needed.

➤*Lactation:* Currently there are no data available on the excretion of AHF (human) into breast milk; however, because of the large molecular weight of the drug, it is highly unlikely.

➤*Children:* The safety and effectiveness of *Monoclate-P* for the treatment of hemophilia A have been demonstrated in 33 children. As in adults, dose children based upon weight. The safety and effectiveness of *Alphanate* in children 16 years of age and younger have not been studied. *Koate-DVI* has not been studied in children. *Koate-HP*, solvent/detergent–treated AHF (human), has been used extensively in children.

Across a well-controlled half-life and recovery clinical trial in patients previously treated with factor VIII concentrates for hemophilia A, the 1 child receiving solvent/detergent–treated *Alphanate* responded similarly when compared with 12 adult patients. Spontaneous adverse reaction reports with *Koate-HP* for pediatric use were within the experience of those reports for adult use.

➤*Elderly:* In general, use caution in dose selection for an elderly patient, reflecting the greater frequency of decreased hepatic, renal, or cardiac function, and of concomitant disease or other drug therapy. Dosing should be appropriate to the clinical situation.

➤*Monitoring:* Determine the pulse rate before and during administration of AHF. If a significant increase occurs, reducing the rate of administration or temporarily halting the injection usually allows the symptoms to disappear promptly.

Although dosage can be estimated by the calculations in the Administration and Dosage section, it is strongly recommended that whenever possible, appropriate laboratory tests be performed on the patient's plasma at suitable intervals to ensure that adequate AHF levels have been reached and are maintained.

AHF (human) is intended for treatment of bleeding disorders arising from a deficiency in factor VIII. Prove this deficiency prior to administering AHF (human).

Drug Interactions

None well documented.

Adverse Reactions

Occasionally, mild reactions may occur following the administration of AHF (human), such as allergic reactions, chills, nausea, or stinging at the infusion site. In some cases, inhibitors of factor VIII may occur. If a reaction is experienced and the patient requires additional AHF (human), administer product from a different lot.

➤*Alphanate*: Massive doses of AHF (human) have rarely resulted in acute hemolytic anemia, increased bleeding tendency, or hyperfibrinogenemia.

➤*Hemofil M*: The protein in greatest concentration in AHF (human) is albumin (human). Reactions associated with albumin are extremely rare, although chills, fever, nausea, or urticaria have been reported.

➤*Koate-DVI*: Ten adverse reactions related to 7 infusions were observed during a total of 1,053 infusions performed during a clinical study of AHF (human), for a frequency of 0.7% infusions associated with adverse reactions. All reactions were mild and included blurred vision, headache, jittery feeling, nausea, stomach ache, and tingling in the arm, ear, and face.

Overdosage

None reported.

Patient Information

Some viruses, such as parvovirus B19 or hepatitis A, are particularly difficult to remove or inactivate at this time. Parvovirus B19 most seriously affects pregnant women, or immune-compromised individuals.

Inform patients that although the overwhelming number of hepatitis A and parvovirus B19 cases are community-acquired, there have been reports of these infections associated with the use of some plasma-derived products. Therefore, be alert to the potential symptoms of parvovirus B19 and hepatitis A infections and inform patients receiving plasma-derived products to report potential symptoms promptly.

Advise patients that symptoms of parvovirus B19 infection include fever, drowsiness, chills, and runny nose followed about 2 weeks later by a rash and joint pain. Evidence of hepatitis A may include several days to weeks of poor appetite, tiredness, and low-grade fever, followed by nausea, vomiting, and pain in the belly. Dark urine and a yellowed complexion are also common symptoms. Encourage patients to consult their health care provider if such symptoms appear.

Inform patients of the early signs and symptoms of hypersensitivity reactions, including hives, generalized urticaria, tightness of the chest, dyspnea, wheezing, faintness, hypotension, and anaphylaxis, and advise them to discontinue use of the concentrate and contact their health care provider and/or seek immediate emergency care, depending on the severity of the reaction, if these symptoms occur.

ANTIHEMOPHILIC FACTOR, RECOMBINANT

Rx	**Helixate FS** (CSL Behring LLC)	**Injection, lyophilized powder for solution:** 250 units of AHF (recombinant)	Preservative and albumin free. Solvent/Detergent treated, monoclonal antibody purified. Sucrose 28 mg, glycine, histidine, sodium. In kits with single-dose bottles and diluent (2.5 mL of sterile water for injection).
Rx	**Kogenate FS** (Bayer)		Preservative and albumin free. Solvent/Detergent treated, monoclonal antibody purified. Sucrose 28 mg, glycine, histidine, polysorbate 80, sodium. In kits with single-use vials and diluent (2.5 mL of sterile water for injection).
Rx	**Recombinate** (Baxter)		Preservative free. Monoclonal antibody purified. Albumin (human) ≤ 12.5 mg/mL, von Willebrand factor ≤ 2 ng per AHF unit, histidine, PEG 3350, sodium. In kits with single-dose vials and diluent (10 mL of sterile water for injection).
Rx	**ReFacto** (Wyeth)		Preservative and albumin free. Sucrose, L-histidine. In kits with single-use vials and diluent (4 mL of sodium chloride 0.9%).
Rx	**Xyntha** (Wyeth)		Preservative free, plasma/albumin free. Solvent/Detergent treated, nanofiltrated. Sucrose, L-histidine. In kits with single-use vials and diluent (4 mL of sodium chloride 0.9%).
Rx	**Advate** (Baxter)	**Injection, powder for solution:** 250 units of AHF (recombinant)	Preservative and plasma/albumin free. Solvent/Detergent treated, monoclonal antibody purified. von Willebrand factor ≤ 2 ng per AHF unit, glutathione, histidine, sodium. In kits with single-dose vials and diluent (5 mL of sterile water for injection).

ANTIHEMOPHILIC FACTOR, RECOMBINANT

Rx	**Helixate FS** (CSL Behring LLC)	**Injection, lyophilized powder for solution:** 500 units of AHF (recombinant)	Preservative and albumin free. Solvent/Detergent treated, monoclonal antibody purified. Sucrose 28 mg, glycine, histidine, sodium. In kits with single-use bottles and diluent (2.5 mL of sterile water for injection).
Rx	**Kogenate FS** (Bayer)		Preservative and albumin free. Solvent/Detergent treated, monoclonal antibody purified. Sucrose 28 mg, glycine, histidine, polysorbate 80, sodium. In kits with single-dose vials and diluent (2.5 mL of sterile water for injection).
Rx	**Recombinate** (Baxter)		Preservative free. Monoclonal antibody purified. Albumin (human) ≤ 12.5 mg/mL, von Willebrand factor ≤ 2 ng per AHF unit, histidine, PEG 3350, sodium. In kits with single-dose vials and diluent (10 mL of sterile water for injection).
Rx	**ReFacto** (Wyeth)		Preservative and albumin free. Sucrose, L-histidine. In kits with single-use vials and diluent (4 mL of sodium chloride 0.9%).
Rx	**Xyntha** (Wyeth)		Preservative free, plasma/albumin free. Solvent/Detergent treated, nanofiltrated. Sucrose, L-histidine. In kits with single-use vials and diluent (4 mL of sodium chloride 0.9%).
Rx	**Advate** (Baxter)	**Injection, powder for solution:** 500 units of AHF (recombinant)	Preservative and plasma/albumin free. Solvent/Detergent treated, monoclonal antibody purified. Von Willebrand factor ≤ 2 ng per AHF unit, glutathione, histidine, sodium. In kits with single-dose vials and diluent (5 mL of sterile water for injection).
Rx	**Helixate FS** (CSL Behring LLC)	**Injection, lyophilized powder for solution:** 1,000 units of AHF (recombinant)	Preservative and albumin free. Solvent/Detergent treated, monoclonal antibody purified. Sucrose 28 mg, glycine, histidine, sodium. In kits with single-dose bottles and diluent (2.5 mL of sterile water for injection).
Rx	**Kogenate FS** (Bayer)		Preservative and albumin free. Solvent/Detergent treated, monoclonal antibody purified. Sucrose 28 mg, glycine, histidine, polysorbate 80, sodium. In kits with single-use vials and diluent (2.5 mL of sterile water for injection).
Rx	**Recombinate** (Baxter)		Preservative free. Monoclonal antibody purified. Albumin (human) ≤ 12.5 mg/mL, von Willebrand factor ≤ 2 ng per AHF unit, histidine, PEG 3350, sodium. In kits with single-dose vials and diluent (10 mL of sterile water for injection).
Rx	**ReFacto** (Wyeth)		Preservative and albumin free. Sucrose, L-histidine. In kits with single-use vials and diluent (4 mL of sodium chloride 0.9%).
Rx	**Xyntha** (Wyeth)		Preservative free, plasma/albumin free. Solvent/Detergent treated, nanofiltrated. Sucrose, L-histidine. In kits with single-use vials and diluent (4 mL of sodium chloride 0.9%).
Rx	**Advate** (Baxter)	**Injection, powder for solution:** 1,000 units of AHF (recombinant)	Preservative and plasma/albumin free. Solvent/Detergent treated, monoclonal antibody purified. von Willebrand factor ≤ 2 ng per AHF unit, glutathione, histidine, sodium. In kits with single-dose vials and diluent (5 mL of sterile water for injection).
Rx	**Advate** (Baxter)	**Injection, powder for solution:** 1,500 units of AHF (recombinant)	Preservative and plasma/albumin free. Solvent/Detergent treated, monoclonal antibody purified. von Willebrand factor ≤ 2 ng per AHF unit, glutathione, histidine, sodium. In kits with single-dose vials and diluent (5 mL of sterile water for injection).
Rx	**Helixate FS** (CSL Behring LLC)	**Injection, lyophilized powder for solution:** 2,000 units of AHF (recombinant)	Preservative and albumin free. Solvent/Detergent treated, monoclonal antibody purified. Sucrose 56 mg, glycine, histidine, sodium. In kits with single-dose bottles and diluent (5 mL of sterile water for injection).
Rx	**Kogenate FS** (Bayer)		Preservative and albumin free. Solvent/Detergent treated, monoclonal antibody purified. Sucrose 52 mg, glycine, histidine, polysorbate 80, sodium. In kits with single-use vials and diluent (5 mL of sterile water for injection).
Rx	**ReFacto** (Wyeth)		Preservative and albumin free. Sucrose, L-histidine. In kits with single-use vials and diluent (4 mL of sodium chloride 0.9%).
Rx	**Xyntha** (Wyeth)		Preservative free, plasma/albumin free. Solvent/Detergent treated, nanofiltrated. Sucrose, L-histidine. In kits with single-use vials and diluent (4 mL of sodium chloride 0.9%).
Rx	**Advate** (Baxter)	**Injection, powder for solution:** 2,000 units of AHF (recombinant)	Preservative and plasma/albumin free. Solvent/Detergent treated, monoclonal antibody purified. von Willebrand factor ≤ 2 ng per AHF unit, glutathione, histidine, sodium. In kits with single-dose vials and diluent (5 mL of sterile water for injection).
Rx	**Advate** (Baxter)	**Injection, powder for solution:** 3,000 units of AHF (recombinant)	Preservative and plasma/albumin free. Solvent/Detergent treated, monoclonal antibody purified. von Willebrand factor ≤ 2 ng per AHF unit, glutathione, histidine, sodium. In kits with single-dose vials and diluent (5 mL of sterile water for injection).
Rx	**Xyntha** (Wyeth)	**Injection, lyophilized powder for solution:** 3,000 units of AHF (recombinant)	Preservative free, plasma/albumin free. Solvent/Detergent treated, nanofiltrated. L-histidine, polysorbate 80, sucrose. In kits with single-use vials and diluent (4 mL of sodium chloride 0.9%).
Rx	**Kogenate FS** (Bayer)		Preservative and albumin free. Solvent/Detergent treated, monoclonal antibody purified. Sucrose 52 mg, glycine, histidine, polysorbate 80, sodium. In kits with single-use vials and diluent (5 mL of sterile water for injection).

ANTIHEMOPHILIC FACTOR, RECOMBINANT

Indications

➤*Classical hemophilia:* For the prevention and control of bleeding episodes in hemophilia A (classical hemophilia); for the perioperative management of patients with hemophilia A; surgical prophylaxis in patients with hemophilia A (congenital factor VIII deficiency or classic hemophilia); for short-term routine prophylaxis to reduce the frequency of spontaneous bleeding episodes.

Administration and Dosage

➤*General dosing considerations:* rAHF must be administered by the intravenous (IV) route. The reconstituted product must be administered within 3 hours after reconstitution.

Some patients with low-titer inhibitors (less than 10 Bethesda units) can be successfully treated with factor VIII preparations without a resultant anamnestic rise in inhibitor titer. Factor VIII levels and clinical response to treatment must be assessed to ensure adequate response. Use of alternative treatment products, such as factor IX complex concentrates, AHF (porcine),

ANTIHEMOPHILIC FACTOR, RECOMBINANT

recombinant factor VIIa, or anti-inhibitor coagulant complex, may be necessary for patients with anamnestic responses to factor VIII treatment and/or high-titer inhibitors.

Other dosage regimens have been proposed, including one that describes continuous maintenance therapy.

Calculation of dosage – The expected in vivo peak increase in factor VIII levels expressed as units/dL of plasma or percent of normal can be estimated by multiplying the dose administered per kilogram of body weight (units/kg) by 2. This calculation is based on the clinical findings of several pharmacokinetic studies of rAHF concentrates and is supported by the data generated by 223 pharmacokinetic studies with *Advate* (419 with *Recombinate*) in 107 study subjects (67 with *Recombinate*). These pharmacokinetic data demonstrated a peak postinfusion recovery of approximately 1.5 to 2.5 units/dL per units/kg above the preinfusion baseline.

Examples (assuming patient's baseline factor VIII level is less than 1% of normal):

1.) A dose of rAHF 1,750 units administered to a 70 kg patient should be expected to result in a peak postinfusion factor VIII increase of 50 units/dL (50% of normal).
2.) A peak level of 70% is required in a 40 kg child. In this situation, the appropriate dose would be

$$\frac{70 \text{ units/dL}}{[2 \text{ units/dL} \div \text{units/kg}] \times 40 \text{ kg}} = 1{,}400 \text{ units.}$$

The in vivo percent elevation in factor VIII levels can be estimated by multiplying the dose of rAHF per kilogram of body weight (units/kg) by 2. This method of calculation is based on clinical findings with the use of plasma-derived and rAHF products and is illustrated in the following examples.

$$\text{Expected \% factor VIII increase} = \frac{[\text{\# units administered} \times 2\% \text{ per units/kg}]}{\text{body weight (kg)}}$$

Example for a 70 kg adult:

$$\frac{[1{,}400 \text{ units} \times 2\% \text{ per units/kg}]}{70 \text{ kg}} = 40\%$$

Or

$$\text{Dosage required (units)} = \frac{[\text{body weight (kg)} \times \text{desired \% factor VIII increase}]}{2\% \text{ per units/kg}}$$

Example for a 15 kg child:

$$\frac{[15 \text{ kg} \times 100\%]}{2\% \text{ per units/kg}} = 750 \text{ units required}$$

The calculation of the required dosage of factor VIII is based upon the empirical finding that, on average, 1 international unit of factor VIII per kilogram of body weight raises the plasma factor VIII activity by approximately 2 units/dL per units/kg administered. The required dosage is determined using the following formula:

Required units = body weight (kg) × desired factor VIII rise (units/dL or % of normal) × 0.5 (units/kg per units/dL)

Although dosage can be estimated by the calculations above, it is strongly recommended that whenever possible, appropriate laboratory tests, including serial factor VIII assays, be performed on the patient's plasma at suitable intervals to ensure that adequate factor VIII levels have been reached and are maintained.

The dosage necessary to achieve hemostasis depends upon the type and severity of the bleeding episode, according to the following general guidelines.

It is recommended that individual factor VIII values for recovery and, if clinically indicated, other pharmacokinetic characteristics be used to guide dosing and administration. Although dosage can be estimated by the calculations above, it is strongly recommended that whenever possible, appropriate laboratory tests, including serial factor VIII assays, be performed on the patient's plasma at suitable intervals to ensure that adequate factor VIII levels have been reached and are maintained.

➤*Adults:*

Classical hemophilia –

Bleeding prophylaxis:

• *Helixate FS* – rAHF concentrates may be administered on a regular schedule for prophylaxis of bleeding as reported by Nilsson et al.

• *Kogenate FS* – rAHF concentrates may be administered on a regular schedule for prophylaxis of bleeding as reported by Nilsson et al.

• *ReFacto* – Administer twice a week for short-term routine prophylaxis to prevent or reduce the frequency of spontaneous musculoskeletal hemorrhage in patients with hemophilia A. In some cases, especially children, shorter dosage intervals or higher doses may be necessary.

Mild hemorrhage:

• *Advate* – A dose of rAHF sufficient to achieve a level of 20% to 40% of normal should be given for hemarthrosis, muscle bleeding episodes, or mild oral bleeding episodes. Begin infusions every 12 to 24 hours for 1 to 3 days until the bleeding episode is resolved (as indicated by relief of pain) or healing is achieved.

• *Helixate FS* – 10 to 20 units/kg of rAHF to achieve a level of 20% to 40% of normal for superficial, early hemorrhages and hemorrhages into joints. Repeat dose if there is evidence of further bleeding.

• *Kogenate FS* – See *Helixate FS* for dosing.

• *Recombinate* – See *Advate* for dosing.

• *ReFacto* – A dose of rAHF sufficient to achieve a level of 20% to 40% of normal should be given for early hemarthrosis, minor muscle bleeding, or oral bleeding. Begin infusions every 12 to 24 hours as necessary until resolved for at least 1 day, depending upon the severity of the hemorrhage.

• *Xyntha* – See *ReFacto* for dosing.

Moderate hemorrhage:

• *Advate* – A dose of rAHF sufficient to achieve a level of 30% to 60% of normal should be given for more extensive hemarthrosis, muscle bleeding, or hematoma. Repeat infusions every 12 to 24 hours for (usually) 3 days or more until pain and disability are resolved.

• *Helixate FS* – 15 to 30 units/kg of rAHF to achieve a level of 30% to 60% of normal for moderate to major hemorrhage (hemorrhages into muscles, hemorrhages into the oral cavity, definite hemarthrosis, known trauma). Repeat 1 dose at 12 to 24 hours if needed.

• *Kogenate FS* – See *Helixate FS* for dosing.

• *Recombinate* – See *Advate* for dosing.

• *ReFacto* – A dose of rAHF sufficient to achieve a level of 30% to 60% of normal should be given for hemorrhages into muscles, mild trauma capitis, minor operations (including tooth extraction), and hemorrhages into oral cavity. Repeat infusion every 12 to 24 hours for 3 to 4 days or until adequate local hemostasis is achieved.

• *Xyntha* – See *ReFacto* for dosing.

Major hemorrhage:

• *Advate* – A dose of rAHF sufficient to achieve a level of 60% to 100% of normal should be given for life-threatening bleeding episodes such as head injury, throat bleeding episodes, or severe abdominal pain. Repeat infusions every 8 to 24 hours until resolution of the bleeding episode has occurred.

• *Helixate FS* – 40 to 50 units/kg of rAHF to achieve a level of 80% to 100% of normal for major to life-threatening hemorrhages (intracranial, intra-abdominal, or intrathoracic hemorrhages; GI bleeding; CNS bleeding; bleeding in the retroperitoneal or retropharyngeal spaces or iliopsoas sheath), fractures, and head trauma. Repeat a dose of 20 to 25 units/kg every 8 to 12 hours.

• *Kogenate FS* – See *Helixate FS* for dosing.

• *Recombinate* – See *Advate* for dosing.

• *ReFacto* – A dose of rAHF sufficient to achieve a level of 60% to 100% of normal should be given for GI bleeding; intracranial, intra-abdominal, or intrathoracic hemorrhages; fractures; and major operations. Repeat infusions every 8 to 24 hours until threat is resolved or, in the case of surgery, until adequate local hemostasis is achieved.

• *Xyntha* – A dose of rAHF sufficient to achieve a level of 60% to 100% of normal should be given for GI bleeding; intracranial, intra-abdominal, or intrathoracic hemorrhages; and fractures. Repeat infusion every 8 to 24 hours until bleeding is resolved.

Surgery:

• *Advate* –

Minor: A dose of rAHF sufficient to achieve a level of 60% to 100% of normal should be given for minor surgery, including tooth extraction. Give a single bolus infusion beginning within 1 hour of the operation, with optional additional dosing every 12 to 24 hours as needed to control bleeding. For dental procedures, adjunctive therapy may be considered.

Major: A dose of rAHF sufficient to achieve a level of 80% to 120% pre- and postoperatively should be given. For bolus infusion replacement, repeat infusions every 8 to 24 hours, depending on the desired level of factor VIII and state of wound healing.

• *Helixate FS* –

Major: 50 units/kg preoperatively to raise the factor VIII level to approximately 100% activity before surgery begins. May repeat as necessary after 6 to 12 hours initially and for a total of 10 to 14 days until healing is complete.

• *Kogenate FS* –

Major: See *Helixate FS* for dosing.

• *Recombinate* –

Minor: Administer a single infusion to achieve a peak postinfusion factor VIII activity of 60% to 80% of normal in combination with oral antifibrinolytic therapy for minor surgery, including tooth extraction. Starting the infusion within 1 hour of the procedure is sufficient for approximately 70% of cases.

Major: Administer a single infusion to achieve a peak postinfusion factor VIII activity of 80% to 100% pre- and postoperatively. Repeat infusion every 8 to 24 hours, depending on state of healing.

• *ReFacto* –

Major: A dose of rAHF sufficient to achieve a level of 60% to 100% of normal should be given. Repeat infusion every 8 to 24 hours until adequate local hemostasis is achieved in the case of surgery.

• *Xyntha* –

Minor: Administer a single infusion to achieve a peak postinfusion factor VIII activity of 30% to 60% of normal for minor operations, including tooth extraction. Repeat infusion every 12 to 24 hours for 3 to 4 days or until adequate local hemostasis is achieved. For tooth extraction, a single infusion plus oral antifibrinolytic therapy within 1 hour may be sufficient.

Major: Administer a single infusion to achieve a peak postinfusion factor VIII activity of 60% to 100% of normal. Repeat infusion every 8 to 24 hours in the case of surgery, until adequate local hemostasis and wound healing are achieved.

➤*Children:*

Classical hemophilia –

Bleeding prophylaxis:

• *Helixate FS* – 25 units/kg of body weight every other day.

• *Kogenate FS* – See Adults for dosing.

ANTIHEMOPHILIC FACTOR, RECOMBINANT

- *ReFacto* – See Adults for dosing.

Mild hemorrhage:
- *Helixate FS* – See Adults for dosing.
- *Kogenate FS* – See Adults for dosing.
- *Recombinate* – See Adults for dosing.
- *ReFacto* – See Adults for dosing.

Moderate hemorrhage:
- *Helixate FS* – See Adults for dosing.
- *Kogenate FS* – See Adults for dosing.
- *Recombinate* – See Adults for dosing.
- *ReFacto* – See Adults for dosing.

Major hemorrhage:
- *Helixate FS* – See Adults for dosing.
- *Kogenate FS* – See Adults for dosing.
- *Recombinate* – See Adults for dosing.
- *ReFacto* – See Adults for dosing.

Surgery:
- *Helixate FS* – See Adults for dosing.
- *Kogenate FS* – See Adults for dosing.
- *Recombinate* – See Adults for dosing.
- *ReFacto* – See Adults for dosing.

➤*Elderly:* Dose selection should be individualized.

➤*Therapeutic drug monitoring:* Although dose can be estimated by the previous calculations, it is highly recommended that whenever possible appropriate laboratory tests, including serial factor VIII activity assays, be performed on the patient's plasma at suitable intervals to ensure that adequate factor VIII levels have been reached and are maintained.

➤*Preparation for administration:* Patients should follow the specific reconstitution and administration procedures provided by their health care provider. The procedures are provided as general guidelines for the reconstitution and administration of rAHF.

rAHF when reconstituted contains polysorbate 80, which is known to increase the rate of di-(2-ethylhexyl)(phthalate (DEHP) extraction from polyvinyl chloride (PVC). This should be considered during the preparation and administration of rAHF, including storage time elapsed in a PVC container following reconstitution. It is important that the administration and dosage instructions be followed closely.

➤*Administration:* It is recommended to use the administration set provided. Administer by IV infusion after reconstitution with the supplied diluent.

Rate of administration – The rate of administration should be adapted to the response of the individual patient, but administration of the entire dose in 5 to 10 minutes or less is well tolerated. After reconstitution, rAHF should be injected IV over several minutes. The rate of administration should be determined by the patient's comfort level.

Bolus infusion (Advate/Recombinate) – A dose of rAHF should be administered over a period of 5 minutes or less (maximum infusion rate, 10 mL/min). The pulse rate should be determined before and during administration of rAHF. Should a significant increase in pulse rate occur, reducing the rate of administration or temporarily halting the injection usually allows the symptoms to disappear promptly.

➤*Admixture compatibility:*

ReFacto/Xyntha – In the absence of incompatibility studies, reconstituted rAHF should not be administered in the same tubing or container with other medicinal products. In vitro studies suggest that factor VIII may adsorb to the internal surfaces of some infusion equipment.

➤*Storage/Stability:*

Advate – Refrigerate (2° to 8°C [36° to 46°F]) in powder form. May be stored at room temperature (up to 30°C [86°F]) for a period of up to 6 months, not to exceed the expiration date. After storage at room temperature, the product must not be returned to the refrigerator. Avoid freezing to prevent damage to the diluent vial.

Helixate FS/Kogenate FS – Store under refrigeration (2° to 8°C [36° to 46°F]). Product may also be stored at room temperature not exceeding 25°C (77°F) for up to 3 months, such as in home treatment situations. Do not freeze. Protect from extreme exposure to light; store the lyophilized powder in the carton prior to use.

Recombinate – Refrigerate (2° to 8°C [36° to 46°F]) or store at room temperature, not exceeding 30°C (86°F). Avoid freezing to prevent damage to the diluent vial.

ReFacto/Xyntha – Refrigerate at a temperature of 2° to 8°C (36° to 46°F). It may also be stored at room temperature, not exceeding 25°C (77°F) for up to 3 months until the expiration date. The patient should write in the space provided on the outer carton the date the product was placed at room temperature. At the end of the 3-month period, the product should not be put back into the refrigerator, but should be used immediately or discarded. The diluent syringe may be stored at 2° to 25°C (36° to 77°F). Freezing should be avoided to prevent damage to the prefilled diluent syringe. During storage, avoid prolonged exposure of rAHF vial to light. The product after reconstitution does not contain a preservative and should be used within 3 hours.

Actions

➤*Pharmacology:* Factor VIII is the specific clotting factor deficient in patients with hemophilia A (classical hemophilia). Hemophilia A is a genetic bleeding disorder characterized by hemorrhages that may occur spontaneously or after minor trauma. The administration of rAHF provides an increase in plasma levels of factor VIII and can temporarily correct the coagulation defect in these patients.

rAHF provides a means of temporarily replacing the missing clotting factor in order to correct or prevent bleeding episodes, or in order to perform emergency or elective surgery in hemophiliac patients.

Activated factor VIII acts as a cofactor for activated factor IX, accelerating the conversion of factor X to activated factor X. Activated factor X converts prothrombin into thrombin. Thrombin then converts fibrinogen into fibrin and a clot is formed. Factor VIII activity is greatly reduced in patients with hemophilia A and therefore replacement therapy is necessary.

The administration of rAHF increases plasma levels of factor VIII activity and can temporarily correct the coagulation defect in hemophilia A patients.

➤*Pharmacokinetics:*

Advate – The pharmacokinetics of rAHF were investigated in a phase 2/3 multicenter, pivotal study of previously treated subjects. In addition, an interim analysis comparing the pharmacokinetics of rAHF at the onset of treatment and after a period of at least 75 exposure days was performed in the context of an ongoing continuation study in subjects who completed treatment in the multicenter, pivotal phase 2/3 study. Postinfusion levels and clearance of factor VIII during the perioperative period were examined in an interim analysis of subjects from the pivotal and continuation studies who were enrolled in an ongoing phase 2/3 surgical study. Finally, the pharmacokinetics of rAHF were investigated in an interim analysis of an ongoing study of previously treated children younger than 6 years of age.

A randomized, crossover pharmacokinetic comparison of rAHF produced at a pilot-scale facility in Orth, Austria (the test article) and *Recombinate* (the control article) was conducted in the context of the pivotal phase 2/3 study. Study subjects were initially infused with 1 of the 2 preparations at a dose of 50 ± 5 units/kg body weight while in a nonbleeding state.

The second study preparation was infused in a nonbleeding state at 50 ± 5 units/kg after a washout period of 72 hours to 4 weeks following the first study infusion. The order in which each study preparation was administered was assigned by randomization. Pharmacokinetic parameters (area under the factor VIII plasma concentration versus time curve [AUC], maximal postinfusion factor VIII level [C_{max}], in vivo recovery, half-life, clearance, mean residence time, and volume of distribution in steady state [V_{ss}]) were calculated from factor VIII activity measurements in blood samples obtained immediately before and at standardized time intervals up to 48 hours following each infusion.

A total of 56 study subjects were enrolled and randomized. Of these, 50 (modified intent-to-treat population) received both infusions of study medication and had sufficient pharmacokinetic data for the comparison of *Advate* and *Recombinate*. Thirty subjects (per-protocol population) received both pharmacokinetic infusions of study medication and had data for all pharmacokinetic time points.

Pharmacokinetic Parameters of *Advate* and *Recombinate* (Per-Protocol Analysis) (Mean ± SD)[a]

Parameter	*Recombinate* (n = 30)	*Advate* (n = 30)
$AUC_{0-48\ h}$ (units•h/dL)	1,530 ± 380	1,534 ± 436
In vivo recovery (units/dL per units/kg)[b]	2.59 ± 0.52	2.41 ± 0.5
Half-life	11.24 ± 2.53	11.98 ± 4.28
C_{max} (units/dL)	129 ± 27	120 ± 26
Mean residence time (h)	14.52 ± 3.81	15.68 ± 6.21
V_{ss} (dL/kg)	0.46 ± 0.1	0.47 ± 0.1
Clearance (dL/kg/h)	0.03 ± 0.01	0.03 ± 0.01

[a] $AUC_{0-48\ h}$ = AUC from 0 to 48 hours postinfusion; SD = standard deviation.
[b] Calculated as C_{max} baseline factor VIII divided by the dose in units/kg, where C_{max} is the maximal postinfusion factor VIII measurement.

For the pharmacokinetic parameters $AUC_{0-48\ h}$ and in vivo recovery, the 90% confidence intervals (CI) for the ratios of the mean values for the test and control articles were within the preestablished limits of 0.8 and 1.25 for both the per-protocol (n = 30) study populations. This was also true in the intent-to-treat study (n = 50) population for the total AUC and in vivo recovery. In addition, in vivo recovery at the onset of treatment and after 75 exposure days was compared for 62 subjects. Results of this analysis indicated no significant change in vivo recovery at the onset of treatment and after at least 75 exposure days.

Additionally, the pharmacokinetics of rAHF produced at the Orth facility were compared with those of rAHF produced at a commercial-scale facility in Neuchatel, Switzerland. For the pharmacokinetic parameters $AUC_{0-48\ h}$ and in vivo recovery, the 90% CI for the ratios of the mean values for the test and control articles were within the preestablished limits of 0.8 and 1.25 for both the per-protocol and intent-to-treat study populations.

The phase 2/3 continuation study provided a means for examining potential changes in all pharmacokinetic parameters of rAHF at the onset of treatment and after a period of at least 75 exposure days. This comparison utilized data for rAHF produced in the Orth facility obtained at the onset of treatment on the pivotal phase 2/3 study with data for rAHF produced in the Neuchatel facility obtained in the continuation study. A total of 13 of 34 eligible subjects were included in an interim per-protocol analysis. Ninety-five percent CI calculated for the ratios of the mean values for $AUC_{0-48\ h}$ and in vivo recovery before and after at least 75 exposure days indicated no evidence of a difference in the pharmacokinetics of rAHF at the 2 time points.

ANTIHEMOPHILIC FACTOR, RECOMBINANT

Pharmacokinetic Parameters for *Advate* Before and After At Least 75 Exposure Days (N = 13)

Parameter	Parameters at the onset of treatment[a]				Parameters after ≥ 75 exposure days[b]			
	Mean	SD	Min	Max	Mean	SD	Min	Max
$AUC_{0-48\ h}$ (units•h/dL)	1,315	405	876	2,314	1,262	497	831	2,731
C_{max} (units/dL)	111	23	77	151	111	25	73	151
Adjusted recovery (units/dL per units/kg)	2.24	0.47	1.54	3.02	2.2	0.51	1.46	3.06
Total AUMC[c] (units•h^2/dL)	21,000	14,486	8,597	63,038	19,171	13,171	8,478	58,978
Half-life	11.1	2.72	8.38	17.96	10.89	1.37	9.24	13.92
Clearance (dL/[kg•h])	0.04	0.01	0.02	0.06	0.04	0.01	0.01	0.06
Mean residence time (h)	13.95	4.02	8.63	23.38	13.54	2.98	8.04	19.58
V_{ss} (dL/kg)	0.51	0.1	0.37	0.67	0.55	0.12	0.32	0.73

[a] Data from the phase 2/3 pivotal study for rAHF produced in Orth.
[b] Data from the phase 2/3 continuation study for rAHF produced in Neuchatel.
[c] AUMC = area under the first moment curve.

In an interim analysis of data from 10 of 25 planned subjects in the phase 2/3 surgery study, the target factor VIII level was met or exceeded in all cases following a single loading dose ranging from 48 to 69.8 units/kg.

Helixate FS/Kogenate FS – Pharmacokinetic studies were conducted in 20 patients with severe hemophilia A in North America. In this comparative pharmacokinetic study, rAHF was shown to be similar to its predecessor product rAHF (albumin). Mean factor VIII recovery measured 10 minutes following infusion was 2.1 ± 0.3% per units/kg for rAHF and 2.4 ± 0.7% per units/kg for rAHF (plasma-derived). The 2 recoveries were not statistically different (CI, 0.815 to 1.01). The mean biological half-life of recombinant factor VIII formulated with sucrose is similar to the predecessor product, with a mean of approximately 13 hours, which has previously been shown to be similar to plasma-derived AHF. The activated partial thromboplastin time shortened appropriately with both recombinant factor VIII and recombinant factor VIII formulated with sucrose. The recovery and half-life data for recombinant factor VIII formulated with sucrose were unchanged after 24 weeks of exclusive treatment, indicating continued efficacy and no evidence of factor VIII inhibition. The mean factor VIII recovery measured 10 minutes following a dose of recombinant factor VIII formulated with sucrose in 37 patients (after 24 weeks of treatment with recombinant factor VIII formulated with sucrose) was 2.1% per units/kg, which was unchanged from factor VIII recovery determined at baseline and at weeks 4 and 12.

Recombinate – Pharmacokinetic studies of 69 patients revealed the circulating mean half-life for rAHF to be 14.6 ± 4.9 hours (n = 67), which was not statistically significantly different from plasma-derived AHF (human). The mean half-life of plasma-derived AHF (human) was 14.7 ± 5.1 hours (n = 61). The actual baseline recovery observed with rAHF was 123.9 ± 47.7 units/dL (n = 23), which is significantly higher than the actual plasma-derived AHF (human) baseline recovery of 101.7 ± 31.6 units/dL (n = 61). However, the calculated ratio of actual to expected recovery with rAHF (121.2 ± 48.9%) is not different on average from plasma-derived AHF (human) (123.4 ± 16.4%).

ReFacto – In a crossover pharmacokinetic study of 18 previously treated patients using the chromogenic assay, the circulating mean half-life for rAHF was 14.8 ± 5.6 hours (range, 7.6 to 28.5 hours), which was not statistically significantly different from plasma-derived AHF (human), which had a mean half-life of 13.7 ± 3.7 hours (range, 8.8 to 25.1 hours). Mean incremental recovery (K-value) of rAHF in plasma was 2.4 ± 0.4 units/dL per units/kg (range, 1.9 to 3.3 units/dL per units/kg). This was comparable with the mean incremental recovery observed in plasma for plasma-derived AHF, which was 2.3 ± 0.3 units/dL per units/kg (range, 1.7 to 2.9 units/dL per units/kg). Results of a comparative study that evaluated the effect of phospholipids on the 1-stage clotting and chromogenic assays showed that the 1-stage clotting assay gave results that were approximately 50% of the values obtained with the chromogenic assay.

In 2 additional clinical studies, pharmacokinetic parameters were evaluated for previously treated patients and previously untreated patients. In previously treated patients (n = 101; median age, 26 ± 12 years), rAHF had a mean incremental recovery at week 0 of 2.4 ± 0.4 units/dL per units/kg (range, 1.1 to 3.8 units/dL per units/kg). In measurements over 4 years of use (month 3 [n = 90], month 6 [n = 87], month 12 [n = 88], month 24 [n = 70], month 36 [n = 64], and month 48 [n = 52]), mean incremental recovery was reproducible and ranged from 2.3 to 2.5 units/dL per units/kg. A subset of 37 study subjects had evaluable pharmacokinetic profiles at both baseline and month 12. The 90% CI for the ratios of the mean values of month 12 to baseline AUC_T, AUC_∞, and K-value were well within the bioequivalence window of 80% to 125%, demonstrating the stability of these pharmacokinetic parameters over 1 year. In previously untreated patients (n = 59; median age, 10 ± 8.3 months), rAHF had a lower mean incremental recovery at week 0 of 1.5 ± 0.6 units/dL per units/kg (range, 0.2 to 2.8 units/dL per units/kg) as compared with previously treated patients. The mean incremental recovery for previously untreated patients was stable over time (5 visits during a 2-year period) and ranged from 1.5 to 1.8 units/dL per units/kg of rAHF. Population pharmacokinetic modeling using data from 44 previously untreated patients led to a mean estimated half-life of rAHF in previously untreated patients of 8 ± 2.2 hours.

ReFacto Pharmacokinetic Parameters

Parameter	Baseline				Month 12			
	Mean	SD	Min	Max	Mean	SD	Min	Max
C_{max} (units/mL)	1.17	0.24	0.55	1.9	1.2	0.29	0.84	2.31
AUC_T (units•h/mL)	13.6	3.4	6	21.1	14	4.7	7.8	32.4
Half-life	10.6	2.5	6.8	17.2	11.4	3.5	6.6	20.1
AUC∞ (h•units/mL)	15.4	4.5	7.6	28.1	16.5	5.7	8.8	33.5
Clearance (mL/h/kg)	3.53	1.03	1.78	6.6	3.37	1.08	1.49	5.66
Mean residence time (h)	15	3.4	9.8	24.7	16.1	4.6	9.7	27.8
V_{ss} (mL/kg)	50.9	13	36.9	99	51.1	11.4	21.3	83.2
K-value (units/dL per units/kg)	2.34	0.49	1.1	3.8	2.4	0.58	1.67	4.61

Xyntha – In a pivotal crossover clinical study, 30 evaluable previously treated patients (12 years of age and older) received a single infusion of 50 units/kg of rAHF followed by a full-length recombinant factor VIII (*Advate*) or a single infusion of full-length recombinant factor VIII followed by rAHF in a randomized crossover design. The 1-stage clotting assay method was used to determine the concentrations of these 2 products in blood. rAHF was shown to be pharmacokinetically equivalent to full-length recombinant factor VIII as the 90% CI for rAHF to full-length recombinant factor VIII ratios of the mean values of C_{max} and AUC_∞ were within preestablished limits of 80% to 125%.

In addition, 25 previously treated patients received a single infusion of 50 units/kg of rAHF for a 6-month follow-up pharmacokinetic study. The pharmacokinetic parameters were comparable between baseline and month 6, indicating no time-dependent changes in the pharmacokinetic properties of rAHF; the 90% CI for rAHF 6-month to baseline ratios of the mean values of C_{max} and AUC_∞ were within preestablished limits of 80% to 125%.

Xyntha Pharmacokinetic Parameters

Parameter	Initial visit (crossover phase, n = 30)	Month 6 (follow-up phase, n = 25)
C_{max} (units/mL)	1.08 ± 0.22	1.24 ± 0.42
AUC∞ (h•units/mL)	13.5 ± 5.6	15 ± 7.5
Half-life	11.2 ± 5	11.8 ± 6.2[a]
Clearance (mL/h/kg)	4.51 ± 2.23	4.04 ± 1.87
K-value (units/dL per units/kg)	2.15 ± 0.44	2.47 ± 0.84
In vivo recovery (%)	103 ± 21	116 ± 40

[a] One subject was excluded from the calculation because of the lack of a well-defined terminal phase.

Special populations –

Children:

• *Advate* – A total of 54 subjects 16 years of age and younger have been treated across all studies of rAHF to date. Interim pharmacokinetic data for 34 subjects (per-protocol analysis population) 16 years of age and younger were obtained from a combined dataset comprising subjects 10 to 16 years of age treated in the phase 2/3 pivotal study and subjects enrolled and treated in the ongoing study of previously treated children younger than 6 years of age. Among these, 0 were neonates (birth to younger than 1 month of age), 2 were infants (1 month to younger than 2 years of age), 15 were children (2 to 12 years of age), and 17 were adolescents (12 to 16 years of age).

Pharmacokinetic parameters were not significantly different for the different age categories. The mean (± SD) plasma half-life was 11.21 ± 2.92 hours (range, 8.31 to 24.7 hours). The mean $AUC_{0-48\ h}$ was 1,363 ± 440 units•h/dL. The mean values for C_{max} and adjusted recovery were 109 ± 23 units/dL and 2.17 ± 0.44 units/dL per units/kg, respectively.

Advate Pharmacokinetic Parameters in Previously Treated Children (Per-Protocol Analysis) (N = 34)

Parameter	Mean	SD	Min	Max
$AUC_{0-48\ h}$ (units•h/dL)	1,363	440	792	2,398
C_{max} (units/dL)	109	23	62	181
Adjusted recovery (units/dL per units/kg)	2.17	0.44	1.23	3.39
Total AUMC (units•h^2/dL)	22,545	18,198	7,989	109,633
Half-life (h)	11.21	2.92	8.31	24.7
Clearance (dL [kg•h])	0.04	0.01	0.01	0.06
Mean residence time (h)	14.24	4.52	8.94	34.25
V_{ss} (dL/kg)	0.51	0.1	0.27	0.71

• *Xyntha* – The pharmacokinetics of *Xyntha* were studied in 7 previously treated patients 12 to 16 years of age. Pharmacokinetic parameters in these patients were similar to those obtained for adults after a dose of 50 units/kg. For these 7 patients, the mean (± SD) C_{max} and AUC_∞ were 1.09 ± 0.21 units/mL and 11.5 ± 5.2 units•h/mL, respectively. The mean clearance

ANTIHEMOPHILIC FACTOR, RECOMBINANT

and plasma half-life values were 5.23 ± 2.36 mL/h/kg and 8.03 ± 2.44 hours (range, 3.52 to 10.6 hours), respectively. The mean K-value and in vivo recoveries were 2.18 ± 0.41 units/dL per units/kg and 112 ± 23%, respectively.

Contraindications

Known intolerance or allergic reactions to constituents of the preparation; known hypersensitivity to mouse or hamster protein; known hypersensitivity to bovine protein (*Recombinate*); patients who have manifested life-threatening immediate hypersensitivity reactions, including anaphylaxis, to the product.

Warnings/Precautions

➤*Antibody formation to factor VIII:* The formation of neutralizing antibodies to factor VIII (factor VIII inhibitors) is a known complication in the management of individuals with hemophilia A. Inhibitor formation is especially common in young children with severe hemophilia during their first years of treatment or in patients of any age who have received little previous treatment with factor VIII. Nonetheless, inhibitor formation may occur at any time in the treatment of a patient with hemophilia A. The reported prevalence of these antibodies in previously untreated patients who were administered rAHF products over several years is 20.7% to 31.7%; the reported prevalence of these antibodies in patients receiving plasma-derived factor VIII is 10% to 20%. These inhibitors are invariably of the immunoglobulin G (IgG) isotype, and the factor VIII inhibitory activity is expressed as Bethesda units/mL of plasma. Carefully monitor patients treated with rAHF for the development of factor VIII inhibitors by appropriate clinical observations and laboratory tests. If expected factor VIII activity plasma levels are not attained or if bleeding is not controlled with an appropriate dose, perform an assay to determine if a factor VIII inhibitor is present. If detected, titer inhibitors in Bethesda units.

Factor VIII inhibitor testing was performed throughout all studies in the rAHF (plasma/albumin-free) method clinical program. Among 136 treated subjects 10 years of age and older, all of whom had at least 150 exposure days to factor VIII products at study entry, 102 had at least 75 exposure days to rAHF. None of these subjects developed an inhibitor. One subject who had less than 50 exposure days to rAHF while on study developed an inhibitor. This subject manifested a low-titer inhibitor (2 Bethesda units by the Bethesda assay) after 26 rAHF exposure days. Eight weeks later, the inhibitor was no longer detectable and in vivo recovery was normal at 1 and 3 hours after infusion of *Recombinate* rAHF. For the group comprising all subjects with at least 75 exposure days to rAHF and the single subject who developed an inhibitor, the 95% CI (Poisson distribution) for the risk of developing an inhibitor to factor VIII was 0.02% to 5.4%.

An interim analysis of inhibitor development in 15 of 50 planned children younger than 6 years of age who had at least 50 prior exposure days to factor VIII at study entry was conducted. No subject completed 50 exposure days to rAHF. Ten of the 15 enrolled subjects completed at least 10 exposure days to rAHF or 120 total days on study; among this subset, there were no inhibitors.

Over the investigational period, none of the 69 previously treated individuals, without an inhibitor at entry into the study, developed an inhibitor. In the previously untreated patient group, there were 73 eligible patients with factor VIII levels less than or equal to 2% who received at least 1 rAHF treatment (median days, 100; range, 3 to 821) and who were tested for inhibitor after treatment with rAHF. Of this group, 23 individuals developed detectable inhibitor (median days, 10; range, 3 to 69) and of these, 8 patients showed a titer more than 10 Bethesda units.

Activity-neutralizing antibodies (inhibitors) have been detected in patients receiving factor VIII–containing products. Low-titer inhibitors are common in previously untreated patients and in previously treated patients on factor VIII products, as are high-titer inhibitors in previously untreated patients. High-titer inhibitors, which are generally rare in previously treated patients, have been reported in previously treated patients on rAHF.

➤*Hepatitis and AIDS:* AHF is prepared from human plasma; the risk of transmitting hepatitis or AIDS is present. The individual units of plasma are nonreactive when tested for hepatitis B surface antigen. In addition, these products are heated during manufacturing to reduce the risk of hepatitis transmission (including some non-A, non-B hepatitis).

Patients who have not received multiple infusions of blood or plasma products are very likely to develop signs or symptoms of some viral infections, especially non-A, non-B hepatitis after introduction of clotting factor concentrates. For such patients, especially those with mild hemophilia, use single-donor products. For patients with moderate or severe hemophilia who have received numerous infusions of blood or blood products, the risk of hepatitis is small.

HIV is the virus believed to cause AIDS. Donor screening tests for antibodies to HIV are available and are used to screen donated blood. Positive tests are further screened. Antibodies develop in infected individuals within 2 to 3 months of infection.

➤*Lack of effect:* Reports of less than expected or lack of effect following infusion of rAHF, mainly in prophylaxis patients, have been received during the clinical trials and in the postmarketing setting. The reported less than expected or lack of effect has been described as unexpected bleeding into target joints, bleeding into new joints, or a subjective feeling by the patient of new-onset bleeding. Less than expected or lack of effect and/or low factor VIII recovery has been reported in patients with inhibitors but also in patients who had no evidence of inhibitors. When switching to rAHF, it is important to closely monitor each patient's clinical hemostatic response and plasma VIII:c following administration of the product and to titrate the dose accordingly to ensure an adequate therapeutic response. Monitoring plasma VIII:c is particularly important in the setting of surgical prophylaxis and major bleeds.

➤*Latex sensitivity:* Certain components used in the packaging of this product contain natural rubber latex.

➤*Hypersensitivity reactions:*

Formation of antibodies to mouse or hamster protein – rAHF contains trace amounts of mouse IgG (maximum of 0.1 ng/units of rAHF), hamster (CHO) proteins (maximum of 1.5 ng/units of rAHF), and bovine protein (*Recombinate* only: maximum of rAHF 1 ng body surface area/units). As such, there exists a remote possibility that patients treated with this product may develop hypersensitivity to these nonhuman mammalian proteins.

In the phase 2/3 pivotal study of rAHF, serum samples were tested by enzyme immunoassays at baseline and after every 15 ± 2 exposure days, for the presence of antibodies to CHO protein and mouse IgG. Regression analysis of assay results was conducted to evaluate trends in levels of antibodies to heterologous proteins as a function of time on study. Four study subjects showed a statistically significant increasing trend in the levels of anti-CHO (n = 1) or anti–mouse IgG (n = 3) antibody levels over the course of the study. A fifth study subject showed a marked increase in anti–mouse IgG antibodies coincident with the 60- and 75-exposure day interval study visits. None of these subjects exhibited adverse reactions or other study findings consistent with an allergic or hypersensitivity response.

Assays to detect seroconversion to mouse and hamster protein were conducted on all patients in clinical studies. No patient has developed specific antibodies to these proteins after commencing study, and no animal protein–associated serious allergic reactions have been observed with recombinant factor VIII formulated with sucrose infusions. Although no such reactions were observed, inform patients of the possibility of a hypersensitivity reaction to mouse and/or hamster protein and alert them to the early signs of such a reaction (eg, hives, hypotension, localized or generalized urticaria, wheezing). Advise patients to discontinue use of the product and contact their health care provider if such symptoms occur.

Allergic and anaphylactic reactions – Among patients treated with AHF concentrates, cases of hypotension, urticaria, and chest tightness in association with hypersensitivity reactions have been reported in the literature. Very rare cases of allergic and anaphylactic reactions have been reported with the predecessor product rAHF (plasma-derived), particularly in very young patients or patients who have previously reacted to other factor VIII concentrates. Serious anaphylactic reactions require immediate emergency treatment with resuscitative measures, such as the administration of epinephrine and oxygen.

As with any IV protein product, allergic-type hypersensitivity reactions are possible. Inform patients of the early signs of hypersensitivity reactions, including hives, generalized urticaria, tightness of the chest, wheezing, hypotension, and anaphylaxis. Advise patients to discontinue use of the product and contact their health care provider if these symptoms occur.

➤*Pregnancy: Category C.* Animal reproduction studies have not been conducted with rAHF. It is also not known whether rAHF can cause fetal harm when administered to a pregnant woman or affect reproduction capacity. Use rAHF during pregnancy only if clearly indicated.

➤*Lactation:* It is not known whether this drug is excreted into human milk; however, because of the large molecular weight, it is highly unlikely. Because many drugs are excreted into human milk, exercise caution if rAHF is administered to breast-feeding mothers. Use rAHF during lactation only if clearly indicated.

➤*Children:*

Helixate FS/Kogenate FS/Recombinate/ReFacto – rAHF is appropriate for use in children of all ages, including neonates, infants, and adolescents. Safety and efficacy studies have been performed in previously treated children and adolescents and in previously untreated neonates, infants, and children. rAHF is similar to rAHF (plasma-derived) in its biological activity and may be used in children in the same manner.

Advate/Xyntha – Use of *Advate* is being examined in the context of an ongoing study of previously treated subjects younger than 6 years of age and in a planned study of previously untreated subjects with severe or moderately severe hemophilia A. In addition, children between 10 and 16 years of age were treated on the phase 2/3 pivotal study, and those older than 5 years of age were eligible for treatment on the ongoing phase 2/3 surgery study.

A study of *Xyntha* in previously untreated patients younger than 6 years of age is currently ongoing.

➤*Elderly:* Clinical trials with rAHF did not include sufficient numbers of patients 65 years of age and older to be able to determine whether they respond differently from younger patients. However, clinical experience with rAHF (plasma-derived) and other AHF products has not identified differences between the elderly and younger patients. As with any patient receiving rAHF, individualize dose selection for an elderly patient.

➤*Monitoring:* Monitor patients using rAHF for the development of factor VIII inhibitors. If the patient's plasma factor VIII level fails to increase as expected or if bleeding is not controlled after adequate dosing, suspect the presence of an inhibitor. By performing the appropriate laboratory procedures, the presence of an inhibitor can be demonstrated and quantified in terms of the number of Bethesda units/mL (ie, the amount of factor VIII activity neutralized by 1 mL of patient plasma). If the inhibitor is present at levels less than 10 Bethesda units/mL, the administration of additional AHF concentrate may neutralize the inhibitor, and may permit an appropriate hemostatic response. The close monitoring of plasma factor VIII levels by laboratory assays is necessary in this situation.

ANTIHEMOPHILIC FACTOR, RECOMBINANT

Inhibitor titers above 10 Bethesda units/mL are likely to make the control of hemostasis with AHF concentrates either impossible or impractical because of the very large dose required. In addition, the inhibitor titer may rise following AHF infusion as a result of an anamnestic response to factor VIII. The treatment or prevention of bleeding in such patients requires the use of alternative therapeutic approaches and agents.

Precise monitoring of the replacement therapy by means of coagulation analysis (plasma factor VIII activity) is recommended, particularly for surgical intervention.

When monitoring a patient's factor VIII activity levels during treatment, the available clinical data suggest that either assay may be used. Most patients in clinical trials were monitored with the 1-stage clotting assay. It is necessary to adhere to the incubation/activation times and other test conditions as specified by the assay manufacturers.

Drug Interactions

None known.

Adverse Reactions

➤*Advate*: Across all clinical studies, a total of 1,304 adverse reactions were reported among 128 of the 150 subjects who received at least 1 infusion of rAHF. Of the 1,304 adverse reactions, 696 were reported among 85 subjects older than 16 years of age and 608 were reported among 43 subjects 16 years of age and younger.

***Advate* Adverse Reactions (≥ 10%)**		
Adverse reaction	Events (n)	Subjects (% evaluable[a])
CNS		
Headache NOS[b]	138	29.3%
GI		
Pharyngolaryngeal pain	22	11.3%
Musculoskeletal		
Arthralgia	74	23.3%
Respiratory		
Cough	37	15.3%
Nasopharyngitis	32	14.7%
Miscellaneous		
Accident NOS	62	17.3%
Fall	25	12.7%
Limb injury NOS	195	34.7%
Pyrexia	37	16.7%

[a] Percent relative to 150, the total number of subjects across all studies who received at least 1 infusion of rAHF.
[b] NOS = not otherwise specified.

Eighteen of the 1,304 adverse reactions were deemed serious; none were related to the study medication. There were no deaths. Among the 1,286 nonserious adverse reactions, only 28 in 12 subjects were judged by the investigator to be related to the study drug. Severity ratings among the 28 events were mild in 8 cases, moderate in 16 cases, and severe in 4 cases. Mild cases included the following: dysgeusia (3); pruritus, dizziness, catheter-related infection, rigors, and headache NOS (1). Moderate cases included the following: dizziness, hot flushes (2); dysgeusia, headache NOS, diarrhea NOS, edema lower limb, sweating increased, nausea, dyspnea, abdominal pain upper, chest pain, bleeding tendency (recorded as prolonged bleeding after postoperative drain removal on the case report form), hematocrit decreased, joint swelling (1). Severe cases included headache NOS, pyrexia, hematoma NOS, and coagulation factor VIII decreased (1).

The unexpected decreased coagulation factor VIII levels occurred in 1 subject during continuous infusion of rAHF following surgery (postoperative days 10 to 14). Hemostasis was maintained at all times during this period and both plasma factor VIII levels and clearance rates returned to appropriate levels by postoperative day 15. Factor VIII inhibitor assays performed after completion of continuous infusion and at study termination were negative.

Factor VIII inhibitor testing was performed throughout all studies in the rAHF (plasma/albumin-free) method clinical program. Among 136 treated subjects 10 years of age and older, all of whom had at least 150 exposure days to factor VIII products at study entry, 102 had at least 75 exposure days to rAHF. None of these subjects developed an inhibitor.

One subject who had less than 50 exposure days to rAHF while on study developed an inhibitor. This subject manifested a low-titer inhibitor (2 Bethesda units by the Bethesda assay) after 26 rAHF exposure days. Eight weeks later, the inhibitor was no longer detectable, and in vivo recovery was normal at 1 and 3 hours after infusion of *Recombinate*.

For the group comprising all subjects with at least 75 exposure days to rAHF and the single subject who developed an inhibitor, the 95% CI (Poisson distribution) for the risk of developing an inhibitor to factor VIII was 0.02% to 5.4%.

➤*Helixate FS/Kogenate FS*: During the clinical studies conducted in previously treated patients, 109 adverse reactions were reported in the course of 4,160 infusions (2.6%). Only 13 reactions were reported by the investigator as at least remotely related to study drug. Another 7 reactions were nonassessable. Thus, 20 reactions in 11 patients were considered to be either nonassessable, or at least remotely related to rAHF administration, for an incidence of 0.5% relative to the number of infusions administered.

Reactions that were at least remotely drug-related included the following: local injection-site reactions, dizziness, rash (2); unusual taste in the mouth, mild increase in blood pressure, pruritus, depersonalization, nausea, and rhinitis (1). No factor VIII inhibitors have developed in the 72 previously treated patients with severe hemophilia A who have received rAHF for a mean of 54 exposure days.

In clinical studies with previously untreated patients and minimally treated patients (children), 18 adverse reactions were reported by the clinical investigators as at least possibly related to the study drug, including the expected complication of inhibitor development in 8 patients, a forearm bleed following venipuncture, constipation, adenopathy, rash, anemia and pallor in 1 inhibitor patient with gastroenteritis, and serous otitis media.

➤*Recombinate*: During the clinical trials conducted in the previously treated patient group, there were 13 infusion-related minor adverse reactions reported out of 10,446 infusions (0.12%). One patient experienced flushing and nausea during his first infusion that abated on decreasing the infusion rate. A second patient experienced mild fatigue during and following 1 infusion, and a third patient had a series of 11 nosebleeds with a periodicity associated with the infusions.

The protein in greatest concentration in rAHF is albumin (human). Reactions associated with IV administration of albumin are extremely rare, although nausea, fever, chills, or urticaria have been reported. Other allergic reactions could be encountered in the use of the factor VIII preparation.

➤*ReFacto*: In phase 3 clinical studies of rAHF involving a total of 218 study subjects (113 previously treated patients, 101 previously untreated patients, and 4 previously treated patients who participated in the surgery study only), more than 138 million units were administered during a total of 75,757 exposure days. The 113 previously treated patients in the long-term previously treated patient study were given a medium of 327 injections (range, 4 to 1,769 injections) over a median of 313 exposure days (range, 4 to 1,312 days). The 101 previously untreated patients in the long-term previously untreated patient study were given a median of 218 injections (range, 1 to 1,476 injections) over a median of 197 exposure days (range, 1 to 1,466 days).

Administration – As with the IV administration of any protein product, the following reactions may be observed after administration: chills, fever, flushing, headache, lethargy, manifestations of allergic reactions, nausea, or vomiting. During phase 3 clinical studies with rAHF, 278 adverse reactions were probably or possibly related or of unknown relation to therapy with 80,370 infusions (0.35% of infusions) in 109 of 218 (50%) study subjects.

Adverse reactions (at least 1%) – Adverse reactions reported by at least 1% of study subjects are presented in the following 2 tables for previously treated patients and previously untreated patients, respectively. One of 218 subjects experienced hypotension that was mild in severity and considered probably related to the administration of rAHF.

***ReFacto* Adverse Reactions in Previously Treated Patients (≥ 1%)**		
Adverse reaction[a]	Event (n = 145)	Subjects (n = 113)
CNS		
Asthenia	1.4%	1.8%
Chills	1.4%	1.8%
Dizziness	2.8%	3.5%
Headache	3.4%	3.5%
GI		
Nausea	17.2%	4.4%
Taste perversion	2.1%	2.7%
Hematologic/Lymphatic		
CHO AB lab increase (ELISA[b])	13.1%	14.2%
Factor VIII AB lab increase (ELISA)	2.8%	3.5%
Hemorrhage	1.4%	1.8%
Mouse IgG AB increase (ELISA)	2.8%	3.5%
Miscellaneous		
Dyspnea	4.1%	1.8%
Injection-site pain	3.4%	1.8%
Pruritus	23.4%	1.8%

[a] Includes reactions for 113 previously treated patients during their participation in the long-term study and surgery study. The 4 previously treated patients who participated in the surgery study had no adverse reactions that were study drug related.
[b] ELISA = enzyme-linked immunosorbent assay.

***ReFacto* Adverse Reactions in Previously Untreated Patients (≥ 1%)**		
Adverse reaction[a]	Events (n = 133)	Subjects (n = 101)
CNS		
Asthenia	0.8%	1%
Somnolence	0.8%	1%

ANTIHEMOPHILIC FACTOR, RECOMBINANT

ReFacto Adverse Reactions in Previously Untreated Patients (≥ 1%)		
Adverse reaction[a]	Events (n = 133)	Subjects (n = 101)
CV		
Hypotension	0.8%	1%
Vasodilation	0.8%	1%
Dermatologic		
Rash	0.8%	1%
Urticaria	0.8%	1%
GI		
Abdominal pain	0.8%	1%
Anorexia	0.8%	1%
Diarrhea	0.8%	1%
GI hemorrhage	0.8%	1%
Nausea	0.8%	1%
Hematologic/Lymphatic		
CHO AB lab increase (ELISA)	15%	16.8%
Factor VIII inhibitor	24.1%	31.7%
Factor VIII AB lab increase (ELISA)	23.3%	25.7%
Hemorrhage	0.8%	1%
Mouse IgG AB increase (ELISA)	12.8%	11.9%
Metabolic/Nutritional		
AST increased	0.8%	1%
Edema	0.8%	1%
Miscellaneous		
Anaphylactic reaction	0.8%	1%
Arthralgia	0.8%	1%
Catheter infection	0.8%	1%
Catheter miscellaneous	0.8%	1%
Catheter thrombosis	1.5%	2%
Fever	4.5%	5.9%
Infection	0.8%	1%
Injection-site reaction	0.8%	1%
Pain	1.5%	2%
Rhinitis	0.8%	1%
Urinary tract infection	1.5%	1%

[a] Includes events for 101 previously untreated patients during their participation in the long-term study and surgery study.

If any adverse reaction takes place that is thought to be related to administration of rAHF, the rate of infusion should be decreased or stopped.

Rate of infusion –

Antibody formation: Inhibitor development is a known adverse reaction associated with the treatment of patients with hemophilia A. In addition to the 1 report of a high-titer inhibitor in the clinical study of previously treated patients, there have been reports of high-titer inhibitors in previously treated patients in the postmarketing setting. High- and low-titer inhibitors have been reported in previously untreated patients in clinical trials and the postmarketing setting.

Other adverse reactions: Other adverse reactions that were reported during the clinical trials that were assessed by the investigator and the sponsor as unlikely to be related to rAHF administration included dyspnea (3), rash (2), pruritus (1), neuropathy (1), arm weakness (1), and thrombophlebitis of upper arm (1).

➤*Xyntha:* In study 1 (safety and efficacy study), the most frequently reported treatment-emergent adverse reaction was headache (24%). Other adverse reactions reported in 5% or more of subjects were nausea (6%); and diarrhea, asthenia, and pyrexia (5%). No subject developed anti-CHO or anti-TN8.2 antibodies.

In study 2 (surgery study), the most frequently reported treatment-emergent adverse reaction was pyrexia (41%). Other adverse reactions reported in 5% or more of subjects were headache and nausea (9%); and diarrhea, vomiting, and asthenia (5%). The adverse reactions reported in either study were considered mild or moderate in severity.

Immunogenicity – In study 1, the incidence of factor VIII inhibitors to rAHF was the primary safety end point. Two subjects with inhibitors were observed in 89 (2.2%) subjects who completed at least 50 exposure days. These results were consistent with the prespecified end point that no more than 2 inhibitors may be observed in at least 81 subjects.

In a Bayesian statistical analysis, results from this study were used to update previously treated patient results from a prior supporting study using rAHF manufactured at the initial facility, where 1 de novo and 2 recurrent inhibitors were observed in 110 subjects, and the experience with predecessor product (1 inhibitor in 113 subjects). This Bayesian analysis indicates that the population (true) inhibitor rate for rAHF, the estimate of the 95% upper limit of the true inhibitor rate, was 4.17%.

Bayesian Posterior Distribution of Inhibitor Rate for rAHF							
				Posterior beta distribution characteristics			
Factor VIII inhibitor Nijmegan result (BU/mL)	Inhibitors (n)	Subjects analyzed (n)	Observed inhibitor rate	Alpha[a]	Beta[b]	Posterior probability[c]	95% upper limit of inhibitor rate (%)[d]
≥ 0.6	2	89	2.25%	4.5	197	0.9613	4.17

[a] Prior alpha of 2.5 plus the number of observed inhibitors.
[b] Prior beta of 110 plus the number of subjects analyzed minus the number of observed inhibitors.
[c] Posterior probability is the probability that the true inhibitor rate is less than the upper acceptable limit of 4.4%. A posterior probability greater than 0.95 is deemed acceptable.
[d] The 95% upper limit of the true inhibitor rate (the maximum rate calculated with at least 95% probability) based on the posterior distribution. An inhibitor rate of less than 4.4% is deemed acceptable.

➤*Postmarketing:*

Helixate FS/Kogenate FS – The following reactions are principally derived from postmarketing experience and publications, and accurate rate estimates are generally not possible. Among patients treated with the predecessor products, very rare cases of serious allergic reactions and anaphylactic reactions have been reported, particularly in very young patients or patients who had previously reacted to other factor VIII concentrates. Individual cases of hypotension have been very rarely reported. Rare cases of urticaria have also been reported. Although such serious reactions have not been reported with the use of rAHF, it is likely that these may also occur. Rare cases of dyspnea have been reported with rAHF.

Overdosage

No symptoms of overdosage have been reported.

Patient Information

Discuss the risks and benefits of this product with patients.

Allergic-type hypersensitivity reactions with rAHF are possible. Inform patients of the early signs of hypersensitivity reactions, including hives, generalized urticaria, tightness of the chest, wheezing, hypotension, and anaphylaxis. Advise patients to discontinue use of the product and contact their health care provider if these symptoms occur.

Advise patients to contact their health care provider or treatment facility for further treatment and/or assessment if they experience a lack of a clinical response to factor VIII replacement therapy because this may be a manifestation of an inhibitor.

Advise women to notify their health care provider if they become pregnant, intend to become pregnant during therapy, or are breast-feeding.

Based on their current regimen, advise individuals with hemophilia using rAHF to bring an adequate supply of rAHF for anticipated treatment when traveling. Advise patients to consult with their health care provider prior to travel.

ANTI-INHIBITOR COAGULANT COMPLEX

Rx	Feiba NF[a] (Baxter)	**Injection, lyophilized powder for solution**: 500 units/vial	Heparin free. Nanofiltered and vapor heated. Sodium chloride 8 mg/mL, trisodium citrate 4 mg/mL. In single-dose vials with *Baxject* needleless transfer device. With 20 or 50 mL of diluent.
		1,000 units/vial	Heparin free. Nanofiltered and vapor heated. Sodium chloride 8 mg/mL, trisodium citrate 4 mg/mL. In single-dose vials with *Baxject* needleless transfer device. With 20 or 50 mL of diluent.
		2,500 units/vial	Heparin free. Nanofiltered and vapor heated. Sodium chloride 8 mg/mL, trisodium citrate 4 mg/mL. In single-dose vials with *Baxject* needleless transfer device. With 20 or 50 mL of diluent.

[a] Certain components of the packaging material contain dry natural rubber latex.

ANTI-INHIBITOR COAGULANT COMPLEX — INJECTION

WARNING

Thrombotic/Thromboembolic events – Thrombotic and thromboembolic events have been reported during postmarketing surveillance following infusion of anti-inhibitor coagulant complex, particularly following the administration of high doses and/or in patients with thrombotic risk factors.

Indications

➤*Hemorrhage:* For the control of spontaneous bleeding episodes or to cover surgical interventions in hemophilia A and B patients with inhibitors.

Administration and Dosage

➤*General dosing considerations:* Give high doses only as long as necessary to stop the bleeding.

If clinical signs of intravascular coagulation occur (eg, changes in blood pressure or pulse rate, respiratory distress, chest pain, cough), stop the infusion and initiate appropriate diagnostic and therapeutic measures.

Certain components of the packaging material contain dry natural rubber latex.

➤*Adults:*

Hemorrhage –

Usual dosage: 50 to 100 units/kg intravenously (IV) at 12-hour intervals.

Maximum dose: 100 units/kg/single dose or 200 units/kg/daily dose.

Concomitant therapy: Do not use antifibrinolytics until 12 hours after administration of anti-inhibitor coagulant complex.

Joint hemorrhage:

- *Initial dosage* – 50 units/kg IV at 12-hour intervals.
- *Dosage titration* – May increase to 100 units/kg IV at 12-hour intervals.
- *Duration of therapy* – Continue until clear signs of clinical improvement appear, such as relief of pain, reduction of swelling, or mobilization of the joint.

Mucous membrane bleeding:

- *Initial dosage* – 50 units/kg IV at 6-hour intervals under careful monitoring (visible bleeding site, repeated measurements of the patient's hematocrit).
- *Dosage titration* – If hemorrhage does not stop, may increase to 100 units/kg IV at 6-hour intervals.

Other severe hemorrhages: 100 units/kg IV at 12-hour intervals. Sometimes anti-inhibitor coagulant complex may be indicated at 6-hour intervals until clear clinical improvement is achieved.

Serious soft tissue hemorrhage: 100 units/kg IV at 12-hour intervals.

➤*Children:*

31 days of age and older – See Adults for dosing.

➤*Preparation for administration:* Allow the unopened vials of anti-inhibitor coagulant complex (concentrate) and sterile water for injection (diluent) to reach room temperature (not above 37°C [98°F]). Remove caps from the concentrate and diluent vials to expose central portions of the rubber stoppers.

Open the *Baxject* device package by peeling away the lid without touching the inside. Do not remove the device from the package. Turn the package over and insert the plastic spike through the diluent stopper. Grip the package at its edge and pull the package off the device. Turn the system over, so that the vial is on top. Quickly insert the other plastic spike into the anti-inhibitor coagulant complex stopper. The vacuum will draw the diluent into the anti-inhibitor coagulant complex vial. The connection of the 2 vials should be done expeditiously to close the open fluid pathway created by the first insertion of the spike to the diluent vial. Swirl gently until anti-inhibitor coagulant complex is completely dissolved. Do not refrigerate after reconstitution.

After complete reconstitution of anti-inhibitor coagulant complex, its injection or infusion should be commenced as promptly as practicable, but it must be completed within 3 hours following reconstitution.

Plastic luer lock syringes are recommended for use with this product because protein, such as anti-inhibitor coagulant complex, tends to stick to the surface of all-glass syringes. Turn the *Baxject* device handle down towards the anti-inhibitor coagulant complex concentrate vial and remove the cap attached to the syringe connection of the *Baxject* device. Draw air into the syringe, connect the syringe to the *Baxject* device, and inject air into the concentrate vial. While keeping the syringe plunger in place, turn the system upside down (concentrate vial now on top). Draw the concentrate into the syringe by pulling the plunger back slowly. Turn the *Baxject* handle to its original position (facing sideways). Disconnect the syringe and attach a suitable needle to inject or infuse IV.

➤*Administration:* The solution must be given by IV injection or IV drip infusion, and the maximum injection or infusion rate must not exceed 2 units/kg/minute.

➤*Storage/Stability:* Store at 2° to 8°C (36° to 46°F). Within the indicated shelf life, the product may be stored at room temperature (not exceeding 25°C [77°F]) for up to 6 months. After storage at room temperature, the product must not be returned to the refrigerator. If the product is transferred from the refrigerator to room temperature, it expires at the end of the 6-month period or at the end of shelf life, whichever comes earliest. Record the date on the package prior to shifting the product at room temperature. Avoid freezing, which may damage the diluent vial.

After complete reconstitution, injection or infusion must be completed within 3 hours. Do not refrigerate after reconstitution.

Actions

➤*Pharmacology:* Anti-inhibitor coagulant complex is a sterile human plasma fraction with factor VIII inhibitor–bypassing activity. In vitro, anti-inhibitor coagulant complex shortens the activated partial thromboplastin time of plasma containing factor VIII inhibitor.

Contraindications

Known normal coagulation mechanism; the treatment of bleeding episodes resulting from coagulation factor deficiencies in the absence of inhibitors to coagulation factor VIII or coagulation factor IX; patients with significant signs of disseminated intravascular coagulation (DIC).

Warnings/Precautions

➤*Thrombotic/Thromboembolic events:* Thrombotic and thromboembolic events (including DIC, venous thrombosis, pulmonary embolism, myocardial infarction [MI], and stroke) have been reported, particularly following high doses and/or in patients with thrombotic risk factors. Always consider the possible presence of such risk factors in patients with congenital and acquired hemophilia. Thromboembolic events are well recognized potential complications of anti-inhibitor coagulant complex infusion. Many of these events occurred with doses above 200 units/kg/day or in patients with other risk factors of thromboembolic events. Do not exceed a single dose of 100 units/kg and a daily dose of 200 units/kg unless the severity of bleeding warrants and justifies the use of higher doses. Give high doses of anti-inhibitor coagulant complex only as long as absolutely necessary to stop bleeding. Patients with DIC, advanced atherosclerotic disease, crush injury, septicemia, or concomitant treatment with recombinant factor VIIa have an increased risk of developing thrombotic events due to circulating tissue factor or predisposing coagulopathy. Use anti-inhibitor coagulant complex with particular caution and only if there are no therapeutic alternatives in patients at risk of DIC, arterial or venous thrombosis, or with existing thrombotic conditions (eg, acute myocardial infarction, venous thrombosis). Anti-inhibitor coagulant complexes should not be given to patients with significant signs of DIC of fibrinolysis. Use caution when administering anti-inhibitor coagulant complex to patients with an increased risk of thromboembolic complications. These include, but are not limited to, patients with a history of coronary heart disease, DIC, and postoperative immobilization. In each of these situations, weigh the potential benefit of treatment with anti-inhibitor coagulant complex against the risk of these complications.

➤*Potential disease transmission:* Anti-inhibitor coagulant complex is made from human plasma. Products made from plasma may contain infectious agents, such as viruses, that can cause disease. The risk that such products will transmit an infectious agent has been reduced by effective donor screening, testing for the presence of certain current virus infections, and inactivating and/or removing certain viruses. Despite these measures, such products can still potentially transmit disease. Because this product is made from human blood, it may carry a risk of transmitting infectious agents (eg, viruses, theoretically the Creutzfeldt-Jacob disease agent). Individuals who receive infusions of blood or plasma products may develop signs and/or symptoms of some viral infections, particularly non-A, non-B hepatitis. Report all infections thought possibly to have been transmitted by this product to the manufacturer.

➤*Concomitant antifibrinolytics:* It has been reported that anti-inhibitor coagulant complex and antifibrinolytics have been given simultaneously without complications. No adequate and well-controlled studies of the combined or sequential use of anti-inhibitor coagulant complex and recombinate factor VIIa or antifibrinolytics have been conducted. Consider the possibility of thrombotic events when systemic antifibrinolytics, such as tranexamic acid and aminocaproic acid, are used during treatment with anti-inhibitor coagulant complex. It is, however, recommended not to use antifibrinolytics until 12 hours after the administration of anti-inhibitor coagulant complex.

➤*Anamnestic responses:* Anamnestic responses with rises in factor VIII inhibitor titer have been observed in 20% of the cases.

ANTI-INHIBITOR COAGULANT COMPLEX — INJECTION

➤*Nonhemophilic patients:* Nonhemophilic patients with acquired inhibitors against factors VIII, IX, or XII may have both a bleeding tendency and an increased risk of thrombosis at the same time.

➤*Hypersensitivity reactions:* Allergic reactions, including severe anaphylactoid reactions, have been reported. If signs and symptoms of severe allergic reactions occur, immediately discontinue administration and provide appropriate supportive care. Make epinephrine and other appropriate medications available to treat allergic reactions.

➤*Hepatic function impairment:* Use with caution when administering to patients with an increased risk of thromboembolic complications, including patients with liver disease. Weigh the potential benefit of treatment against the risk.

➤*Pregnancy: Category C.* Animal reproduction studies have not been conducted with anti-inhibitor coagulant complex. It is also not known whether anti-inhibitor coagulant complex can cause fetal harm when administered to a pregnant woman or can affect reproduction capacity. Give anti-inhibitor coagulant complex to a pregnant woman only if clearly needed.

➤*Lactation:* No information regarding the use of anti-inhibitor coagulant complex during breast-feeding is available.

➤*Children:* No data are available regarding the use of anti-inhibitor coagulant complex in newborns. Use with caution when administering to patients with an increased risk of thromboembolic complications, including neonates. Weigh the potential benefit of treatment against the risk of complications.

➤*Elderly:* Use with caution when administering to patients with an increased risk of thromboembolic complications, including elderly patients. Weigh the potential benefit of treatment against the risk of complications.

➤*Monitoring:* Monitor for development of signs or symptoms of DIC, acute coronary ischemia, and signs and symptoms of other thrombotic and thromboembolic events. If clinical signs of intravascular coagulation occur (eg, changes in blood pressure or pulse rate, respiratory distress, chest pain, cough), stop the infusion promptly and initiate appropriate diagnostic and therapeutic measures. Laboratory indications of DIC are decreased fibrinogen, decreased platelet count, or the presence of fibrin-fibrinogen degradation products. Other indications of DIC include significantly prolonged thrombin time, prothrombin time, or partial thromboplastin time.

Drug Interactions

None well documented.

Adverse Reactions

➤*Postmarketing:*

Cardiovascular – Blood pressure decreased, DIC, embolism, MI.

Thrombotic events have been identified through postmarketing surveillance following anti-inhibitor coagulant complex use for each of the approved indications. The incidence of thrombotic events cannot be determined from postmarketing data.

CNS – Hypoaesthesia, hypoaesthesia facial.

Hypersensitivity – Anaphylactic reaction, hypersensitivity.

Miscellaneous – Injection-site pain, urticaria.

Overdosage

➤*Symptoms:* Overdosage of anti-inhibitor coagulant complex may increase the risk of thromboembolism, DIC, or MI.

Patient Information

Discuss the risks and benefits of this product with the patient.

Some viruses, such as parvovirus B19 or hepatitis A, are particularly difficult to remove or inactivate at this time. Parvovirus B19 most seriously affects pregnant women or immune-compromised individuals. Symptoms of parvovirus B19 infection include fever, drowsiness, chills, and runny nose, followed by a rash and joint pain approximately 2 weeks later. Evidence of hepatitis A may include several days to weeks of poor appetite, tiredness, and low-grade fever, followed by nausea, vomiting, and pain in the belly. Dark urine and a yellowed complexion are also common symptoms. Encourage patients to consult their health care provider if such symptoms appear.

FACTOR IX

Rx	**AlphaNine SD** (Grifols)	**Injection, lyophilized powder for solution:** ≥ 150 units of factor IX (human)/mg protein[a]	Solvent/detergent-treated. Virus-filtered. With heparin, dextrose, polysorbate 80, and tri(n-butyl) phosphate. In kits with single-dose vials and diluent (10 mL sterile water for injection).
Rx	**BeneFIX** (Wyeth)	**Injection, lyophilized powder for solution:** 250 units of factor IX (recombinant)[a]	Preservative free. With glycine, L-histidine, polysorbate 80, and sucrose. In kits with single-dose vial and diluent.
		Injection, lyophilized powder for solution: 500 units of factor IX (recombinant)[a]	
		Injection, lyophilized powder for solution: 1,000 units of factor IX (recombinant)[a]	
		Injection, lyophilized powder for solution: 2,000 units of factor IX (recombinant)[a]	
Rx	**Mononine** (CSL Behring)	**Injection, lyophilized powder for solution:** ≈ 500 units of factor IX (human)	Monoclonal antibody purified. With histidine, mannitol, polysorbate 80, and ≤ 50 ng of mouse protein per 100 factor IX activity units. In kits with single-dose vials and diluent (sterile water for injection).
		Injection, lyophilized powder for solution: ≈ 1,000 units of factor IX (human)[a]	

[a] Actual factor IX activity in units is stated on the label of each vial.

FACTOR IX — INJECTION

Indications

➤*Factor IX deficiency (hemophilia B [Christmas disease]):* For the prevention and control of bleeding in patients with factor IX deficiency (hemophilia B [Christmas disease]). *BeneFIX* is also indicated to control and prevent bleeding in these patients in surgical settings.

Administration and Dosage

➤*General dosing considerations:* Dosage and duration of treatment for all factor IX products depend on the severity of the factor IX deficiency, the location and extent of bleeding, and the patient's clinical condition, age, and recovery of factor IX.

The factor IX level of each patient should be monitored frequently during replacement therapy.

➤*Adults:*

Factor IX deficiency (hemophilia B [Christmas disease]) –

AlphaNine SD: Each vial is labeled with the total units expressed as international units of factor IX, which is referenced to the World Health Organization International Standard. One unit approximates the activity of 1 mL of pooled normal human plasma.

• *Usual dosage* – The amount of *AlphaNine SD* required to establish hemostasis will vary with each patient and depend upon the circumstances. The following formula may be used as a guide in determining the number of units to be administered.

Body weight (kg) × desired increase in factor IX (%) × 1 unit/kg = number of factor IX units required.

AlphaNine SD Dosage Guidelines

Type of hemorrhage or surgical event	Examples	Treatment guidelines
Minor hemorrhages	Bruises, cuts or scrapes, uncomplicated joint hemorrhage	Factor IX levels should be brought to ≥ 20% to 30% (factor IX 20 to 30 units/kg twice daily) until hemorrhage stops and healing has been achieved (1 to 2 days).
Moderate hemorrhages	Nose bleeds, mouth and gum bleeds, dental extractions, hematuria	Factor IX levels should be brought to 25% to 50% (factor IX 25 to 50 units/kg twice daily) until healing has been achieved (average, 2 to 7 days).
Major hemorrhages	Joint and muscle hemorrhages (especially in the large muscles), major trauma, hematuria, intracranial and intraperitoneal bleeding	Factor IX levels should be brought to 50% for ≥ 3 to 5 days (factor IX 30 to 50 units/kg twice daily). Following this treatment period, factor IX levels should be maintained at 20% (factor IX 20 units/kg twice daily) until healing has been achieved. Major hemorrhages may require treatment for up to 10 days.

FACTOR IX — INJECTION

AlphaNine SD Dosage Guidelines		
Type of hemorrhage or surgical event	Examples	Treatment guidelines
Surgery		Prior to surgery, factor IX levels should be brought to 50% to 100% of normal (factor IX 50 to 100 units/kg twice daily). For the next 7 to 10 days, or until healing has been achieved, patients should be maintained at 50% to 100% factor IX levels (factor IX 50 to 100 units/kg twice daily).

• *Dosage adjustment* – Dosing requirements and frequency of dosing is calculated on the basis of an initial response of 1% factor IX increase achieved per unit of factor IX infused per kg body weight and an average half-life for factor IX of 18 hours. If dosing studies have revealed that a particular patient exhibits a lower response, the dose should be adjusted accordingly.

BeneFIX:

• *Usual dosage* – The method of calculating the factor IX dose is shown in the following equation.

Number of factor IX units required = body weight (kg) × desired factor IX increase (% or units/dL) × reciprocal of observed recovery (units/kg per units/dL).

In previously treated adults, on average, 1 unit of *BeneFIX* per kilogram of body weight increased the circulating activity of factor IX by 0.78 ± 0.19 (range, 0.39 to 1.2) units/dL. The method of dose estimation is illustrated in the following example. If 0.78 units/dL average increase of factor IX per unit/kg body weight administered is used, then:

Number of factor IX units required = body weight (kg) × desired factor IX increase (% or units/dL) × 1.3 (units/kg per units/dL).

In the presence of an inhibitor, higher doses may be required.

BeneFIX Dosing Guidelines			
Type of hemorrhage	Circulating factor IX activity required (% or [units/dL])	Dosing interval (hours)	Duration of therapy (days)
Minor			
Uncomplicated hemarthroses, superficial muscle, or soft tissue	20 to 30	12 to 24	1 to 2
Moderate			
Intramuscular or soft tissue with dissection, mucous membranes, dental extractions, or hematuria	25 to 50	12 to 24	Treat until bleeding stops and healing begins; about 2 to 7 days.
Major			
Pharynx, retropharynx, retroperitoneum, CNS, surgery	50 to 100	12 to 24	7 to 10

• *Dosage titration* – Doses should be titrated using the factor IX activity and pharmacokinetic parameters, such as half-life and recovery, as well as taking the clinical situation into consideration in order to adjust the dose as appropriate.

Titrate the initial dose upward if necessary to achieve the desired clinical response. As with some plasma-derived factor IX products, subjects at the low end of the observed factor IX recovery may require upward dosage adjustment to as much as 2 times the initial empirically calculated dose in order to achieve the intended rise in circulating factor IX activity.

Mononine:

• *Usual dosage* – As a general rule, 1 unit of factor IX activity per kg can be expected to increase the circulating level of factor IX by 1% (units/dL) of normal. The following formula provides a guide to dosage calculations:

Number of factor IX units required = body weight (kg) × desired factor IX increase (% or units/dL) × 1 unit/kg (units/kg per units/dL).

The amount of *Mononine* to be infused, as well as the frequency of infusions, will vary with each patient and with the clinical situation.

As a general rule, the level of factor IX required for treatment of different conditions is described in the following information. Recovery of the loading dose varies from patient to patient. *Mononine* administered in doses of at least 75 units/kg were well tolerated. In the presence of an inhibitor to factor IX, higher doses of *Mononine* might be necessary to overcome the inhibitor. No data on the treatment of patients with inhibitors to factor IX with *Mononine* are available.

Mononine Dosage Guidelines		
	Minor spontaneous hemorrhage, prophylaxis	Major trauma or surgery
Desired levels of factor IX for hemostasis	15% to 25% (or units/dL)	25% to 50% (or units/dL)
Initial loading dose to achieve desired level	Up to 20 to 30 units/kg	Up to 75 units/kg
Frequency of dosing	Once; repeated in 24 hours if necessary	Every 18 to 30 h, depending on half-life and measured factor IX levels
Duration of treatment	Once; repeated if necessary	Up to 10 days, depending on nature of insult

• *Dosage titration* – Doses administered should be titrated to the patient's response.

➤*Children:*

Factor IX deficiency (hemophilia B [Christmas disease]) –

BeneFIX:

• *15 years of age or older* – See Adults for dosing.

• *Younger than 15 years of age* –

Usual dosage: In children, on average, 1 unit of *BeneFIX* per kilogram of body weight increased the circulating activity of factor IX by 0.7 ± 0.3 (range, 0.2 to 2.1 units/dL; median, 0.6 units/dL per units/kg). The method of dose estimation is illustrated in the following example. If 0.7 units/dL average increase of factor IX per units/kg body weight administered is used, then:

number of factor IX units required (units) = body weight (kg) × desired factor IX increase (% or units/dL) × 1.4 (units/kg per units/dL).

Mononine: See Adults for dosing.

➤*Preparation for administration:*

AlphaNine SD – Use aseptic technique.

1.) Warm diluent (sterile water for injection) and concentrate (*AlphaNine SD*) to at least room temperature (but not above 37°C).
2.) Remove plastic caps from the diluent and concentrate vials.
3.) Swab the exposed stopper surface with a cleansing agent such as alcohol. Do not leave excess cleansing agent on the stoppers.
4.) Remove the cover from one end of the double-ended transfer needle. Insert the exposed end of the needle through the center of the stopper in the diluent vial.
5.) Remove the plastic cap from the other end of the double-ended transfer needle now seated in the stopper of the diluent vial. To reduce any foaming, invert the vial of diluent and insert the exposed end of the needle through the center of the stopper in the concentrate vial at an angle, making certain that the diluent vial is always above the concentrate vial. The angle of insertion directs the flow of diluent against the side of the concentrate vial. There should be enough vacuum in the vial to transfer all of the diluent.
6.) Disconnect the 2 vials by removing the transfer needle from the diluent vial stopper. Remove the double-ended transfer needle from the concentrate vial and discard the needle into the appropriate safety container.
7.) Let the vial stand until contents are in solution, then gently swirl until all concentrate is dissolved. Reconstitution requires less than 5 minutes.
8.) Do not shake the contents of the vial. Do not invert the concentrate vial until ready to withdraw contents.
9.) Use as soon as possible after reconstitution.
10.) After reconstitution, parenteral drug products should be inspected visually for particulate matter and discoloration prior to administration, whenever solution and container permit. When reconstitution procedure is strictly followed, a few small particles may occasionally remain. The microaggregate filter will remove particles and the labeled potency will not be reduced.

BeneFIX – Reconstitute lyophilized powder for injection with the supplied diluent (sodium chloride 0.234% solution) from the prefilled syringe provided. Once the diluent has been injected into the vial, gently rotate the vial until all powder is dissolved.

After reconstitution, the solution is drawn back into the syringe. The solution should be clear and colorless. The solution should be discarded if visible particulate matter or discoloration is observed.

Administer within 3 hours of reconstitution. The reconstituted solution may be stored at room temperature prior to administration.

BeneFIX, when reconstituted, contains polysorbate 80, which is known to increase the rate of di-(2-ethylhexyl)phthalate (DEHP) extraction from polyvinyl chloride (PVC). This should be considered during the preparation and administration of *BeneFIX*, including storage time elapsed in a PVC container following reconstitution.

Mononine –

1.) Warm both the diluent and *Mononine* in unopened vials to room temperature (not above 37°C [98°F]).
2.) Remove the caps from both vials to expose the central portions of the rubber stoppers.
3.) Treat the surface of the rubber stoppers with antiseptic solution and allow them to dry.

FACTOR IX — INJECTION

4.) Using aseptic technique, insert one end of the double-end needle into the rubber stopper of the diluent vial. Invert the diluent vial and insert the other end of the double-end needle into the rubber stopper of the *Mononine* vial. Direct the diluent, which will be drawn in by vacuum, over the entire surface of the *Mononine* cake. (In order to ensure transfer of all the diluent, adjust the position of the tip of the needle in the diluent vial to the inside edge of the diluent stopper.) Rotate the vial to ensure complete wetting of the cake during the transfer process.
5.) Remove the diluent vial to release the vacuum, then remove the double-ended needle from the *Mononine* vial.
6.) Gently swirl the vial until the powder is dissolved and the solution is ready for administration. The concentrate routinely and easily reconstitutes within 1 minute. To ensure sterility, *Mononine* should be administered within 3 hours of reconstitution.
7.) Filter the product prior to use as described in Administration.

➤*Administration:*

AlphaNine SD – Administer intravenously (IV) slowly at a rate not exceeding 10 mL/min.

Administer promptly following reconstitution. Administration of *AlphaNine SD* within 3 hours of reconstitution is recommended to avoid the potential ill effect of any inadvertent bacterial contamination occurring during reconstitution. Discard any unused contents into the appropriate safety container.

Administration by syringe: Use aseptic technique.
1.) Peel cover from micro-aggregate filter spike package and securely install the syringe into the exposed luer inlet of the filter, using a slight clockwise twisting motion.
2.) Remove filter spike from packaging. Remove protective cover from the spike end of the filter spike.
3.) Pull back the plunger, drawing sufficient air into the syringe to allow reconstituted product to be withdrawn as described in the next step.
4.) Insert the spike end of the filter into the reconstituted concentrate vial. Inject air and withdraw the reconstituted product from the vial into the syringe.
5.) Remove the filter spike from the syringe; discard the filter spike and the empty concentrate vial into the appropriate safety container. Attach the syringe to an infusion set, and expel air from the syringe and infusion set. Perform venipuncture and administer slowly at a rate not exceeding 10 mL/min.
6.) If the patients is to receive more than 1 vial of concentrate, the infusion set will allow administration of multiple vials to be performed with a single venipuncture.
7.) Discard all administration equipment after use into the appropriate safety container. Do not reuse.

BeneFIX – After reconstitution, *BeneFIX* should be injected IV over several minutes. The rate of administration should be determined by the patient's comfort level.

Administer using the infusion set provided in the kit, and the prefilled diluent syringe provided or a single sterile disposable plastic syringe. In addition, the solution should be withdrawn from the vial using the vial adapter.

Note: Agglutination of red blood cells in the tubing/syringe has been reported with the administration of *BeneFIX*. No adverse reactions have been reported in association with this observation. To minimize the possibility of agglutination, it is important to limit the amount of blood entering the tubing. Blood should not enter the syringe. If red blood cell agglutination is observed in the tubing or syringe, discard all material (tubing, syringe, and *BeneFIX* solution) and resume administration with a new package.

Mononine – The rate of administration should be determined by the response and comfort of the patient; IV dosage administration rates of up to 225 units/min have been regularly tolerated without incident. When reconstituted as directed (ie, to approximately 100 units/mL), *Mononine* should be administered at a rate of approximately 2 mL/min.

Plastic disposable syringes are recommended with *Mononine* solution. The ground glass surfaces of all glass syringes tend to stick with solutions of this type. Please note, this concentrate is supplied with a self-venting filter spike.
1.) Using aseptic technique, attach the vented filter spike to a sterile disposable syringe. Caution: the use of other, nonvented filter needles or spikes without the proper procedure may result in an air lock and prevent the complete transfer of the concentrate. Caution: do not inject air into the *Mononine* vial. The self-venting feature of the vented filter spike precludes the need to inject air in order to facilitate withdrawal of the reconstituted solution. The injection of air could cause partial product loss through the vent filter.
2.) Insert the vented filter spike into the stopper of the *Mononine* vial, invert the vial, and position the filter spike so that the orifice is at the inside edge of the stopper.
3.) Withdraw the reconstituted solution into the syringe.
4.) Discard the filter spike. Perform venipuncture using the enclosed winged needle with microbore tubing. Attach the syringe to the luer end of the tubing. Caution: use of other winged needles without microbore tubing, although compatible with the concentrate, will result in a larger retention of solution within the winged infusion set.

➤*Storage / Stability:* Store unreconstituted vials under refrigeration (2° to 8°C [35° to 46°F]). *AlphaNine SD* and *Mononine* may be stored at room temperature up to 25°C (77°F) (*Mononine*) or up to 30°C (86°F) (*AlphaNine SD*) for up to 1 month. *BeneFIX* may be stored at room temperature up to 25°C (77°F) for up to 6 months. Do not freeze diluent.

After reconstitution, use products within 3 hours.

Actions

➤*Pharmacology:* Factor IX is activated by factor VII/tissue factor complex in the extrinsic coagulation pathway, as well as by factor XIa in the intrinsic coagulation pathway. Activated factor IX, in combination with activated factor VIII, activates factor X. This ultimately results in the conversion of prothrombin to thrombin. Thrombin then converts fibrinogen to fibrin, and a clot can be formed.

Factor IX is the specific clotting factor deficient in patients with hemophilia B and in patients with acquired factor IX deficiencies. The administration of factor IX (human or recombinant) increases factor IX plasma levels and can temporarily correct the anticoagulation defect in these patients.

➤*Pharmacokinetics:*

AlphaNine SD – Eighteen patients with severe to moderate hemophilia B each received a single infusion of factor IX 40 to 50 units/kg body weight of *AlphaNine SD*. Following the administration of *AlphaNine SD*, the mean half-life of factor IX observed was approximately 21 hours. This half-life value was computed using the biphasic linear regression model recommended by the International Society of Thrombosis and Hemostasis. The half-life obtained for the solvent-detergent treated product is comparable with that of *AlphaNine* (approximately 19 hours) as well as the range of 18 to 36 hours reported for factor IX complex preparations. The mean recovery observed in clinical trials was approximately 48% and was comparable with that of *AlphaNine* (approximately 51%).

BeneFIX – The mean (± standard deviation [SD]) incremental recovery (K-value) value was 0.73 ± 0.2 units/dL per unit/kg. The mean (±SD) area under the curve (AUC) value was 940 ± 237 units•h/dL. The mean (±SD) half-life value was 22.4 ± 5.3 hours. The pharmacokinetic parameters were followed up in 23 previously treated patients (12 years of age and older) after reported administration for 6 months and found to be unchanged compared with those obtained at the initial evaluation. The K-values, determined by age, were on average 0.78 ± 0.19 units/dL per units/kg (range, 0.39 to 1.2 units/dL per units/kg) for those older than 15 years (n = 16), and 0.66 ± 0.16 units/dL per units/kg (range, 0.44 to 0.92 units/dL per units/kg) for those 15 years of age and younger (n = 7).

Children: Nineteen previously treated children (range, 4 to 15 years of age) underwent pharmacokinetic evaluations for up to 24 months. The mean increase in circulating factor IX activity was 0.7 ± 0.2 units/dL per units/kg infused (range, 0.3 to 1.1 units/dL per units/kg; median, 0.6 units/dL per units/kg). The mean biological half-life was 20.2 ± 4 hours (range, 14 to 28 hours).

Mononine – Infusion of *Mononine* into 10 subjects with severe or moderate hemophilia B has shown a mean recovery of 0.67 units/dL rise per units/kg body weight infused and a mean half-life of 22.6 hours. After 6 months of experience with repeated infusions performed on the 9 subjects who remained in the study, it was shown that the half-life and recovery was maintained at a level comparable with that found with the initial infusion. The 6-month data showed a mean recovery of 0.68 units/dL rise per units/kg body weight infused and a mean half-life of 25.3 hours. The data show no statistically significant differences between the initial and 6-month values.

Contraindications

Known hypersensitivity to mouse protein (*Mononine*) or hamster protein (*BeneFIX*).

None known (*AlphaNine SD*).

Warnings/Precautions

➤*Human plasma:* Because factor IX (human) products are made from pooled human plasma, they may carry a risk of transmitting infectious agents (eg, viruses) and, theoretically, the Creutzfeldt-Jakob disease agent. The risk that such products will transmit an infectious agent has been reduced by screening plasma donors for prior exposure to certain viruses, by testing for the presence of certain current viral infections, and by inactivating and/or removing certain viruses during manufacturer. Stringent procedures, utilized at plasma collection centers, plasma testing laboratories, and fractionation facilities are designed to reduce the risk of virus transmission. Despite these measures, such products may still potentially contain human pathogenic agents, including those not yet know or identified. Thus the risk of transmission of infectious agents cannot be totally eliminated. Any infections thought by a health care provider possibly to have been transmitted by one of these products should be reported to the manufacturer. Discuss the risks and benefits of these products with the patient.

Individuals who receive infusions of blood or plasma products may develop signs and/or symptoms of some viral infections, particularly non–A, non–B hepatitis. Scientific opinion encourages hepatitis B and hepatitis A vaccinations at birth or at diagnosis for patients with hemophilia.

➤*Thromboembolic complications:* Since the use of factor IX complex concentrates (which contain high amounts of factors II, VII, IX, and X) has historically been associated with the development of thromboembolic complications, the use of factor IX–containing products may be potentially hazardous in patients with signs of fibrinolysis and in patients with disseminated intravascular coagulation (DIC). Because of the potential risk of thromboembolic complications, exercise caution when administering these products to patients with liver disease, postoperative patients, neonates, or patients at risk for thromboembolic phenomena or DIC. In each of these situations, weigh the benefit of treatment against the risk of these complications.

Following administration of factor IX to surgery patients and individuals with known liver disease, closely observe the patient for signs or symptoms of potential DIC. Continued administration should be left to the discretion of the health care provider.

➤*Administration:* In order to minimize the possibility of thrombogenic complications, strictly follow dosing guidelines.

Do not administer *AlphaNine SD* at a rate exceeding 10 mL/min. Rapid administration may result in vasomotor reactions.

FACTOR IX — INJECTION

➤*Nephrotic syndrome:* Nephrotic syndrome has been reported following attempted immune tolerance induction with factor IX products in hemophilia B patients with factor IX inhibitors and a history of allergic reactions to factor IX. The safety and efficacy of using factor IX in attempted immune tolerance induction have not been established.

➤*Renal effects:* Twelve days after a dose of *BeneFIX* for a bleeding episode, one hepatitis C antibody positive patient developed a renal infarct. The relationship of the infarct to prior administration of *BeneFIX* is uncertain but was judged to be unlikely by the investigator. The patient continued to be treated with *BeneFIX*.

➤*Hypersensitivity reactions:* Hypersensitivity and allergic-type hypersensitivity reactions, including anaphylaxis, have been reported for all factor IX products. Frequently, these events have occurred in close temporal association with the development of factor IX inhibitors. Inform patients of the early symptoms and signs of hypersensitivity reactions, including hives, generalized urticaria, angioedema, chest tightness, dyspnea, wheezing, faintness, hypotension, tachycardia, and anaphylaxis. Advise patients to discontinue use of the product, contact their health care provider, and/or seek immediate emergency care, depending on the severity of the reactions, if any of these symptoms occur.

Activity-neutralizing antibodies (inhibitors) have been detected in patients receiving factor IX–containing products. Monitor patients for the development of factor IX inhibitors. Patients with these inhibitors may be at increased risk of anaphylaxis upon subsequent challenge with factor IX. Evaluate patients experiencing allergic reactions for the presence of inhibitor.

Preliminary information suggests a relationship may exist between the presence of major deletion mutations in a patients factor IX gene and an increased risk of inhibitor formation and of acute hypersensitivity reactions. Observe closely patients known to have major deletion mutations of the factor IX gene for signs and symptoms of acute hypersensitivity reactions, particularly during the early phases of initial exposure to product. In view of the potential for allergic reactions with factor IX concentrates, the initial (approximately 10 to 20) administrations of factor IX should be performed under medical supervision where proper medical care for allergic reactions could be provided.

In previously treated patients, it is possible that anaphylaxis may occur after a median exposure of 11 days. Monitor these patients closely between the 10th and 12th exposure day.

➤*Pregnancy: Category C.* Animal reproduction studies have not been conducted with factor IX. It is not known whether factor IX can cause fetal harm when administered to a pregnant woman or if it can affect reproduction capacity. Give to a pregnant woman only if clearly needed.

➤*Lactation:* Lactation studies have not been conducted.

➤*Children:*

AlphaNine SD – Clinical trials for safety and effectiveness in children 16 years of age and younger have not been conducted.

BeneFIX – Safety, effectiveness, and pharmacokinetic studies have been evaluated in previously treated and untreated children (see Actions).

Mononine – Evaluation of the safety and effectiveness of *Mononine* treatment in 51 children between 1 day and 20 years of age, as a part of virus safety trials and trials for surgery, trauma, or spontaneous bleeding, showed that excellent hemostasis was achieved with no thrombotic complications. Included in the experience with patients 0 to 20 years of age are 2 long-term virus safety studies demonstrating lack of virus transmission. Dosing in children is based on body weight and generally based on the same guidelines as for adults.

➤*Elderly:* Clinical studies of factor IX did not include sufficient numbers of subjects 65 years of age and older to determine whether they respond differently from younger subjects. As with any patient receiving factor IX, individualize dose selection for an elderly patient.

➤*Monitoring:* Monitoring the factor IX activity using the factor IX activity assay is advised. Following administration of factor IX to surgery patients and individuals with known liver disease, closely observe the patient for signs or symptoms of potential DIC. Monitor patients for the development of factor IX inhibitors. Patients with these inhibitors may be at increased risk of anaphylaxis upon subsequent challenge with factor IX.

Drug Interactions

None known.

Adverse Reactions

For more information on thromboembolic complications, nephrotic syndrome, renal effects, and hypersensitivity, refer to the Warnings/Precautions section.

➤*Cardiovascular:* Potential risk for thromboembolic episodes (see Warnings/Precautions).

➤*GI:* Nausea, vomiting.

➤*Hypersensitivity:* Allergic reactions (see Warnings/Precautions), hives.

If evidence of an acute hypersensitivity reaction is observed, promptly stop the infusion and administer appropriate counter measures and supportive therapy.

➤*Local:* Stinging or burning at the infusion site.

If any reaction takes place that is thought to be related to the administration of factor IX, decrease or stop the infusion. For most reactive individuals, slowing the infusion rate relieves the symptoms. For those highly reactive individuals, a different lot may be satisfactory.

➤*Miscellaneous:* Chills, fever, flushing, headache, lethargy, tingling.

Mononine – In a clinical study with *Mononine* in previously untreated hemophilia B patients, 5 patients experienced ALT elevations. Serologic tests for hepatitis A, hepatitis B, hepatitis C, cytomegalovirus, and Epstein-Barr virus were negative.

➤*Postmarketing:* Anaphylaxis, angioedema, cyanosis, dyspnea, hypotension, inadequate factor IX recovery, inadequate therapeutic response, inhibitor development, laryngeal edema, thrombosis.

➤*BeneFIX:*

Previously treated patients –

One subject discontinued *BeneFIX* because of pulmonary allergic-type symptoms.

BeneFIX Adverse Reactions Reported for Previously Treated Patients[a]

Adverse reactions	Total number of events[b] (n = 129)	Percent of patients from which the reports originated (n = 65)	Percent of infusions temporally associated with the reaction[c] (n = 7,573)
Total	131	41.5%	2.2%
CNS			
Dizziness	7	7.7%	0.11%
Drowsiness	1	1.5%	0.01%
Headache	10	10.8%	0.17%
Dermatologic			
Flushing	3	3.1%	0.05%
Hives	3	3.1%	0.04%
Rash	6	7.7%	0.09%
GI			
Diarrhea	1	1.5%	0.01%
Nausea	27	6.2%	0.36%
Taste perversion (altered taste)	14	4.6%	0.25%
Vomiting	1	1.5%	0.01%
Local			
Cellulitis at the IV site	1	1.5%	0.09%
Injection-site pain	10	6.2%	0.21%
Injection-site reaction	11	7.7%	0.16%
Phlebitis at the IV site	1	1.5%	0.09%
Respiratory			
Dry cough	1	1.5%	0%
Hypoxia (urge to cough with hypoxemia)	11	1.5%	0.15%
Lung disorder	1	1.5%	0.01%
Miscellaneous			
Allergic reaction	1	1.5%	0.01%
Allergic rhinitis	7	4.6%	0.12%
Chest tightness	1	1.5%	0.05%
Factor IX inhibitor[d]	1	1.5%	0.03%
Fever	2	3.1%	0.03%
Pain (burning sensation in the jaw and skull)	6	1.5%	0.09%
Renal infarct[e]	1	1.5%	0.01%
Shaking	2	3.1%	0.01%
Visual disturbance	1	1.5%	0.01%

[a] More than 1 event in the table could have been associated with an infusion; however, the total represents the actual number of infusions given.
[b] With a definite, probable, possible, or unknown relation to therapy.
[c] Reaction occurring within 72 hours of infusion.
[d] Low titer transient inhibitor information.
[e] The renal infarct developed in hepatitis C antibody–positive patient 12 days after a dose of *BeneFIX* for a bleeding episode. The relationship of the infarct to the prior administration of *BeneFIX* is uncertain.

FACTOR IX — INJECTION

Previously untreated patients –

BeneFIX Adverse Reactions Reported for Previously Untreated Patients[a]			
Adverse reactions	Total number of events[b] (n = 22)	Percent of patients from which the reports originated (n = 63)	Percent of infusions temporally associated with the reaction[c] (n = 5,538)
Total	22	17.5%	0.6%
Dermatologic			
Photosensitivity reaction	1	1.6%	0%
Rash (body rash)	1	1.6%	0.02%
Urticaria (hives)	3	4.8%	0.05%
Laboratory test abnormality			
Elevated ALT	1	1.6%	0%
Elevated AST	1	1.6%	0%
Increased alkaline phosphatase	1	1.6%	0.05%
Injection-site reaction	1	1.6%	0.04%
Respiratory			
Asthma	1	1.6%	0.02%
Dyspnea (respiratory distress)	2	3.2%	0.04%
Miscellaneous			
Chills (rigors)	1	1.6%	0.05%
Diarrhea	5	1.6%	0.2%
Factor IX inhibitor[d]	2	3.2%	0.07%
HAV seroconversion[e]	1	1.6%	0.04%
Parvovirus B19 seroconversion[f]	1	1.6%	0.02%

[a] More than 1 event in the table could have been associated with an infusion; however, the total represents the actual number of infusions given.
[b] With a definite, probable, possible, or unknown relation to therapy.
[c] Reaction occurring within 72 hours of infusion.
[d] Two subjects developed high titer inhibitor formation during treatment with *BeneFIX*.
[e] Relationship of HAV seroconversion to BeneFIX is unknown. HAV seroconversion was noted on 2 occasions in a single patient but was negative at final visit. The patients had no laboratory or clinical findings associated with active infection.
[f] Relationship of Parvovirus B seroconversion to BeneFIX is unknown. It was unlikely that seroconversion was related to *BeneFIX* because of the frequency of community acquired infection and viral safeguards built into the manufacturing process.

Patient Information

Inform patients of the early symptoms and signs of hypersensitivity reactions, including hives, generalized urticaria, tightness of the chest, dyspnea, wheezing, faintness, hypotension, and anaphylaxis. Advise patients to discontinue use of the product and contact their health care provider and/or seek immediate emergency care, depending on the severity of the reaction, if these symptoms occur.

Some viruses, such as the parvovirus B19 or hepatitis A, are particularly difficult to remove or inactivate at this time. Parvovirus B19 may most seriously affect sero-negative pregnant women or immunocompromised individuals. Although the overwhelming number of hepatitis A cases are community acquired, there have been reports of these infections associated with the use of such plasma derived products. Therefore, be alert to the potential symptoms of hepatitis A infections and inform patients under supervision receiving plasma-derived products to report potential symptoms promptly.

Evidence of hepatitis A may include several days to weeks of poor appetite, tiredness, and low-grade fever followed by nausea, vomiting, or pain in the belly. Dark urine and a yellowed complexion are also common symptoms. Encourage patients to consult a health care provider if such symptoms occur.

FACTOR IX COMPLEX

Rx	**Bebulin VH** (Baxter)	**Injection, lyophilized, powder for solution**: Factors IX, II, X, and low amounts of VII (human)[a]	Vapor heated. With heparin. In kits with single-dose vials and diluent (sterile water for injection).[b]
Rx	**Profilnine SD** (Grifols)	**Injection, lyophilized, powder for solution**: Factors IX, II, X, and low amounts of VII (human)[a]	Solvent/Detergent treated. Preservative free. In kits with single-dose vials and diluent (sterile water for injection).

[a] Actual factor IX activity in units is stated on the label of each vial.
[b] Also contains dry natural rubber latex.

FACTOR IX COMPLEX — INJECTION

Indications

➤*Factor IX deficiency (hemophilia B [Christmas disease]):* For the prevention and control of bleeding in patients with factor IX deficiency (hemophilia B [Christmas disease]).

Administration and Dosage

➤*General dosing considerations:*

Bebulin VH – As a general rule, 1 international unit of factor IX activity/kg will increase the plasma level of factor IX by 0.8%. Accordingly, the following formula is provided for dosage calculations:

body weight (kg) × desired factor IX increase (% of normal) ×1.2 = number of factor IX units required

It must be emphasized that the response to treatment will vary from patient to patient and that, occasionally, larger doses than those derived from the above formula will be required, particularly if treatment is delayed.

Exact dosage determination should be based on localization and extent of hemorrhage and the level of factor IX to be achieved.

It must be emphasized that, particularly with severe hemorrhage and major surgery, close laboratory monitoring of the factor IX level is required to determine proper dosage.

Profilnine SD – A 1% increase in factor IX (0.01 unit)/units administered/kg can be expected. The amount of *Profilnine SD* required to establish hemostasis will vary with each patient and depend on the circumstances. The following formula may be used as a guide in determining the number of units to be administered:

body weight (kg) × 1 unit/kg × desired increase in plasma factor IX (%) = number of factor IX units required

In normal clinical practice, there is variability among patients and their clinical condition. Therefore, the factor IX level of each patient should be monitored frequently during replacement therapy.

➤*Adults:*

Factor IX deficiency (hemophilia B [Christmas disease]) –

Bebulin VH:

• *Dental extraction* – For tooth extraction, the same initial dose as for minor surgery is recommended (see surgical procedures table below). Generally, 1 infusion will be sufficient. In case of extraction of several teeth, replacement therapy for up to 1 week may be necessary using the same dose as for minor surgery.

• *Minor/moderate/major hemorrhage* – Approximate factor IX levels, typical initial doses, and the average duration of treatment are suggested in the following table. For minor bleeding, a single dose will usually be sufficient; otherwise, a second dose may be given after 24 hours. More severe hemorrhage will require the administration of several doses at approximately 24-hour intervals. For maintenance therapy, usually two-thirds of the initial dose is infused.

Bebulin VH Dosing Guidelines According to Bleeding Type			
Type of bleeding	Approximate factor IX level (% normal)	Typical initial dose (units/kg)	Average duration of treatment (days)
Minor Early hemarthrosis, minor epistaxis, gingival bleeding, mild hematuria	20	25 to 35	1
Moderate Severe joint bleeding, early hematoma, major open bleeding, minor trauma, minor hemoptysis, hematemesis, melena, major hematuria	40	40 to 55	2 or until adequate wound healing

FACTOR IX COMPLEX — INJECTION

Bebulin VH Dosing Guidelines According to Bleeding Type			
Type of bleeding	Approximate factor IX level (% normal)	Typical initial dose (units/kg)	Average duration of treatment (days)
Major Severe hematoma, major trauma, severe hemoptysis, hematemesis, melena	≥ 60[a]	60 to 70	2 to 3 or until adequate wound healing

[a] For patient predisposing to thrombosis see the Warnings/Precautions section.

Bebulin VH Dosing According to Surgery Type						
	Day of operation		Initial postoperative period (week 1 to 2)		Late postoperative period (week 3 on)	
Type of surgery	Approximate factor IX level (% normal)	Dose (units/kg)	Approximate factor IX level (% normal)	Dose (units/kg)	Approximate factor IX level (% normal)	Dose (units/kg)
Major	≥ 60[a]	70 to 95	60 to 20	70 to 35	20	35 to 25
Minor	40 to 60	50 to 60	40 to 20	55 to 25	N/A[b]	N/A

[a] For patients predisposing to thrombosis see Warnings/Precautions section.

[b] N/A = not applicable.

Profilnine SD:

• *Dental extractions* – The factor IX level should be raised to 50% immediately prior to the procedure; additional factor IX complex may be given if bleeding recurs.

• *Mild/moderate/major hemorrhage* – Mild to moderate hemorrhages may usually be treated with a single administration sufficient to raise the plasma factor IX level to 20% to 30%. In the event of more serious hemorrhage, the patient's plasma factor IX level should be raised by 30% to 50%. Infusions are generally required daily.

• *Surgery* – Surgery in patients with factor IX deficiency requires that the factor IX level be raised to 30% to 50% for at least 1 week following operation.

➤Children:

Factor IX deficiency (hemophilia B [Christmas disease]) – *Profilnine SD*:

• *17 years of age and older* – See Adults for dosing.

➤Preparation for administration:

Bebulin VH – Bebulin VH should be reconstituted immediately before administration. The solution does not contain a preservative and must be used within 3 hours of reconstitution. Do not refrigerate after reconstitution.

For reconstitution, proceed as follows:

1.) Warm both diluent and concentrate in unopened vials to room temperature (not above 37°C [98°F]).
2.) Remove caps from both vials to expose central portions of the rubber stoppers.
3.) Clean exposed surface of the rubber stoppers with germicidal solution and allow to dry.
4.) Using aseptic technique, remove protective covering from 1 end of the double-ended needle and insert the exposed end through the diluent vial stopper.
5.) Remove protective covering from the other end of the double-ended needle, taking care not to touch the exposed end. Invert diluent vial over the concentrate vial, then insert free end of the needle through the concentrate vial stopper. Diluent will be drawn into the concentrate vial by vacuum.
6.) Disconnect the 2 vials by removing needle from the concentrate vial stopper. Gently agitate or rotate the concentrate vial until all material is dissolved.

After reconstituting the concentrate as previously described, attach the enclosed filter needle to a sterile disposable syringe using aseptic technique. Insert filter needle through the concentrate vial stopper. Inject air and withdraw solution into the syringe. Remove and discard filter needle. Attach a suitable intravenous (IV) needle or infusion set with winged adapter.

Profilnine SD –

1.) Warm diluent (sterile water for injection) and concentrate (*Profilnine SD*) to at least room temperature (but not above 37°C [98.6°F]).
2.) Remove plastic cap from both the diluent and concentrate vials.
3.) Swab the exposed stopper surfaces with a cleansing agent, such as alcohol. Do not leave excess cleansing agent on the stoppers.
4.) Remove plastic cover from 1 end of the double-ended needle. Insert the exposed end of the needle through the center of the stopper in the diluent vial.
5.) Remove plastic cap from the other end of the double-ended needle now seated in the stopper of the diluent vial. Hold concentrate vial in one hand, invert vial of diluent in the other hand, and push the second end of the needle through the center of the stopper in the concentrate vial, making certain that the diluent vial is always above the concentrate vial. There should be enough vacuum in the concentrate vial to transfer all of the diluent.
6.) Disconnect the 2 vials by removing the needle from the diluent vial stopper. Remove the double-ended needle from the concentrate vial and discard the needle. Gently swirl the concentrate vial until all concentrate is dissolved. Reconstitution requires less than 10 minutes. After reconstitution, parenteral drug products should be visually inspected for particulate matter and discoloration prior to administration, whenever solution and container permit. When the reconstitution procedure is strictly followed, a few small particles may occasionally remain. The microaggregate filter will remove particles and the labeled potency will not be reduced.
7.) Discard all infusion equipment after use. Do not reuse.

• *Prophylactic treatment* – Prophylactic doses of 20 to 30 units/kg administered once, or preferably up to twice a week, have been shown to significantly reduce the frequency of spontaneous hemorrhage. It is, however, recommended that prophylactic dosage regimens be tailored to individual needs.

• *Surgical procedures* – Dosage guidelines for surgical procedures are suggested in the following table. The preoperative loading dose should be administered 1 hour prior to surgery. Depending on the type of surgery, replacement therapy has to be continued over 1 to several weeks until adequate wound healing is achieved. The average treatment interval will initially be 12 hours; in the later postoperative period, 24 hours is generally adequate.

➤Administration:

Bebulin VH – Administer the solution IV at a rate comfortable to the patient (maximum rate, 2 mL/min).

Profilnine SD – Administer IV, promptly following reconstitution with the supplied diluent. Although *Profilnine SD* is stable for at least 3 hours at room temperature after reconstitution, prompt administration is recommended to avoid the ill effect of any inadvertent bacterial contamination occurring during reconstitution. *Profilnine SD* may be administered by injection (plastic disposable syringe only) or infusion. Administer at room temperature; do not refrigerate after reconstitution and discard any unused contents.

Always use aseptic technique.

1.) Peel cover from the microaggregate filter package and securely install the syringe into the exposed luer inlet of the filter, using a slight clockwise twisting motion.
2.) Remove the filter from the packaging. Remove the protective cover from the spike end of the filter.
3.) Pull back the plunger, drawing sufficient air into the syringe to allow reconstituted product to be withdrawn as described in the following step.
4.) Insert the spike end of the filter into the reconstituted concentrate vial. Inject air and draw the reconstituted product from the vial into the syringe.
5.) Remove and discard the filter from the syringe. Attach the syringe to an infusion set. Expel air from the syringe and infusion set. Perform venipuncture and administer slowly.
6.) If the patient is to receive more than 1 vial of concentrate, the infusion set will allow administration of multiple vials to be performed with a single venipuncture.
7.) Discard all administration equipment after use. Do not reuse.

Handling/Disposal – Exercise appropriate caution in handling because of the risk of exposure to viral infection.

Discard any unused contents. Discard administration equipment after single use. Do not resterilize components. Do not reuse components.

➤Storage/Stability: Store unreconstituted vials under refrigeration (2° to 8°C [35° to 46°F]). *Profilnine SD* may be stored at room temperature, up to 30°C (86°F) for up to 1 month. Do not freeze diluent.

After reconstitution, use products within 3 hours. Do not refrigerate after reconstitution.

Actions

➤Pharmacology: Factor IX complex products are a mixture of vitamin K–dependent clotting factors found in normal plasma. The administration of factor IX complex provides an increase in plasma levels of factor IX and can temporarily correct the coagulation defect of patients with factor IX deficiency. Plasma levels of factors II and X will also be increased by *Bebulin VH* and *Proplex T*.

➤Pharmacokinetics:

Bebulin VH – In vivo recovery of *Bebulin VH* was determined by investigators in Germany, Japan, and the United States using the former International Standard World Health Organization 72/32 and was found to be 53.3% ± 9.6%, 57.5% ± 21.8%, and 53.24% ± 16.95%, respectively. In the same studies, using different methodologies, half-lives were determined to be 19.4 ± 3.8 hours, 24.6 ± 3.2 hours, and 19.97 ± 8.24 hours, respectively.

FACTOR IX COMPLEX — INJECTION

Profilnine SD – A clinical study, which evaluated 12 subjects with hemophilia B, indicated that following administration of *Profilnine SD*, factor IX in vivo half-life is 24.68 ± 8.29 hours, and recovery is 1.15 ± 0.16 units/dL per units infused per kg of body weight.

Administration of factor IX complex can result in higher than normal levels of factor II because of its significantly longer half-life.

Contraindications

None known.

Warnings/Precautions

➤*Human plasma:* Because factor IX complex products are made from pooled human plasma, they may carry a risk of transmitting infectious agents (eg, viruses) and, theoretically, the Creutzfeldt-Jakob disease agent. The risk that such products will transmit an infectious agent has been reduced by screening plasma donors for prior exposure to certain viruses, by testing for the presence of certain current viral infections, and by inactivating and/or removing certain viruses during the manufacturing process. Stringent procedures, utilized at plasma collection centers, plasma testing laboratories, and fractionation facilities are designed to reduce the risk of virus transmission. Despite these measures, such products can still potentially transmit disease. There is also the possibility that unknown infectious agents may be present in such products. Report all infections possibly to have been transmitted by one of these products to the manufacturer. Discuss the risks and benefits of these products with the patient.

Individuals who receive infusions of blood or plasma products may develop signs and/or symptoms of some viral infections, particularly non-A, non-B hepatitis. Scientific opinion encourages hepatitis B and hepatitis A vaccinations at birth or diagnosis for patients with hemophilia.

➤*Thromboembolic complications:* The risk of thromboembolic complications, including disseminated intravascular coagulation (DIC) and hyperfibrinolysis, is present with the administration of factor IX complex, particularly in the postoperative period and in patients with risk factors predisposing them to thrombosis.

In patients undergoing surgery and in patients with known liver disease, thrombosis and DIC are serious and potentially fatal adverse reactions associated with the administration of factor IX complex concentrates. Infrequent but consistent reports have been described that indicate that patients are at greater risk of developing thrombosis and DIC in the periods following surgery. Cases have also been cited that indicate that patients with liver disease may be predisposed to thrombosis or DIC when treated with factor IX complex. Although the available data is limited, only administer *Profilnine SD* to patients when the beneficial effects of use outweigh the serious risk of potential hypercoagulation.

The use of high doses of prothrombin complex concentrates has been reported to be associated with instances of myocardial infarction, DIC, venous thrombosis, and pulmonary embolism.

If signs of intravascular coagulation, thrombosis, or emboli occur, which include changes in blood pressure and pulse rate, respiratory distress, chest pain, and cough, promptly stop the infusion. In general, the risk of enhancing DIC may be reduced by raising the patient's factor VII or IX level to not more than about 50% of normal. If the need exists to raise the patient's factor IX or VII level higher than 50% of normal, monitor infusion of material to detect signs and symptoms of DIC.

➤*Administration:* Do not administer *Profilnine SD* at a rate exceeding 10 mL/min. Rapid administration may result in vasomotor reactions.

➤*Parvovirus and hepatitis A:* Some viruses, such as parvovirus B19 or hepatitis A, are particularly difficult to remove or inactivate at this time. Parvovirus B19 most seriously affects pregnant women or immune-compromised individuals. Symptoms of parvovirus B19 infection include fever, drowsiness, chills, and runny nose followed approximately 2 weeks later by a rash and joint pain. Evidence of hepatitis A may include several days to weeks of poor appetite, tiredness, and low-grade fever followed by nausea, vomiting, and pain in the stomach. Dark urine and a yellowed complexion are also common symptoms. Encourage patients to consult their health care provider if such symptoms appear.

➤*Latex sensitivity:* Certain components used in the packaging of some of these products contain natural rubber latex, which may cause an allergic reaction in sensitive individuals.

➤*Hypersensitivity reactions:* If evidence of an acute hypersensitivity reaction is observed, promptly stop the infusion and administer appropriate counter measures and supportive therapy.

➤*Hepatic function impairment:* Take special caution in patients with preexisting liver disease.

➤*Pregnancy: Category C.* Animal reproduction studies have not been conducted with factor IX complex. It is not known whether factor IX complex can cause fetal harm when administered to a pregnant woman or can affect reproduction capacity. Give to a pregnant woman only if clearly needed.

➤*Children:*

Profilnine SD – Clinical trials for safety and efficacy in children 16 years of age and younger have not been conducted.

➤*Monitoring:* Monitor the factor IX level frequently during replacement therapy.

Drug Interactions

None known.

Adverse Reactions

For most reactive individuals, slowing the infusion rate relieves the symptoms. For those highly reactive individuals, a different lot may be satisfactory.

➤*Cardiovascular:* DIC, thrombosis.

➤*CNS:* Headache, somnolence.

➤*GI:* Nausea, vomiting.

➤*Hypersensitivity:* Rare occurrences of anaphylactoid or anaphylactic reactions (eg, anaphylactic shock, dyspnea, fever, nausea, retching, urticarial rashes).

➤*Miscellaneous:* Chills, fever, flushing, lethargy, tingling, urticaria.

Patient Information

Inform patients of the early symptoms and signs of hypersensitivity reaction, including hives, generalized urticaria, chest tightness, dyspnea, wheezing, faintness, hypotension, and anaphylaxis. Advise patients to discontinue use of the product and contact their health care provider and/or seek immediate emergency care, depending on the severity of the reaction, if these symptoms occur.

Some viruses, such as parvovirus B19 or hepatitis A, are particularly difficult to remove or inactivate at this time. Parvovirus B19 most seriously affects pregnant women or immune-compromised individuals. Symptoms of parvovirus B19 infection include fever, drowsiness, chills, and runny nose followed about 2 weeks later by a rash and joint pain. Evidence of hepatitis A may include several days to weeks of poor appetite, tiredness, and low-grade fever, followed by nausea, vomiting, and pain in the stomach. Dark urine and a yellowed complexion are also common symptoms. Encourage patients to consult their health care provider if such symptoms appear.

FACTOR XIII CONCENTRATE (HUMAN)

Rx	**Corifact** (CSL Behring)	**Injection, lyophilized powder for solution:** 1,000 to 1,600 units[a]	Preservative free. In kits with single-dose vials[b] and diluent.

[a] The actual units of potency of factor XIII are stated on each vial label and carton.

[b] Each single-dose vial contains human albumin 120 to 200 mg, total protein 120 to 320 mg, glucose 80 to 120 mg.

FACTOR XIII CONCENTRATE (HUMAN) — INJECTION

Indications

➤*Congenital factor XIII deficiency:* For routine prophylactic treatment of congenital factor XIII deficiency.

Administration and Dosage

➤*General dosing considerations:* Factor XIII dosing regimen should be individualized based on body weight, laboratory values, and the patient's clinical condition.

➤*Adults:*

Congenital factor XIII deficiency –

Initial dosage: 40 units/kg by slow intravenous (IV) injection at a rate not to exceed 4 mL/min.

Dosage adjustment: Recommended dosing adjustments of ± 5 units/kg should be based on trough factor XIII activity levels and the patient's clinical condition.

Factor XIII Dose Adjustment Using the Berichrom Activity Assay

Factor XIII activity trough level (%)	Dosage adjustment
One trough level of < 5%	Increase by 5 units/kg
Trough level of 5% to 20%	No change
Two trough levels of > 20%	Decrease by 5 units/kg
One trough level of > 25%	Decrease by 5 units/kg

Subsequent dosing: Dosing should be guided by the most recent trough factor XIII activity level, with dosing every 28 days (4 weeks) to maintain a trough factor XIII activity level of approximately 5% to 20%.

➤*Children:* See Adults for dosing.

➤*Preparation for administration:* Reconstitute with provided sterile water for injection and gently swirl; do not shake. Ensure that the factor XIII vial and diluent vial are at room temperature prior to reconstitution. Factor XIII is for single use only and contains no preservatives. The solution must be used within 4 hours after reconstitution. Discard partially used vials.

➤*Administration:* Administer by slow IV injection at a rate not exceeding 4 mL/min. The reconstituted solution should be brought to room temperature before infusion. Administer though a separate infusion line.

➤*Admixture compatibility:* Do not mix factor XIII with other medicinal products.

To screen for specific compatibilities, see *Trissel's IV-Check*.

FACTOR XIII CONCENTRATE (HUMAN) — INJECTION

➤*Storage/Stability:* Store in a refrigerator at 2° to 8°C (36° to 46°F). Factor XIII is stable for 24 months. Store in original carton to protect from light. Do not freeze. May be stored at room temperature not to exceed 25°C (77°F) for up to 6 months; do not return the product to the refrigerator after it is stored at room temperature.

This product does not contain a preservative. The product must be used within 4 hours after reconstitution. Do not refrigerate or freeze the reconstituted solution.

Actions

➤*Pharmacology:* Factor XIII is an endogenous plasma glycoprotein consisting of 2 A-subunits and 2 B-subunits. Factor XIII circulates in blood and is present in platelets, monocytes, and macrophages. Factor XIII appears in 2 forms, a heterotetrameric (A_2B_2) plasma protein with a molecular weight of about 320 kDa and a homodimeric (A_2) cellular form. Factor XIII is a proenzyme that is activated, in the presence of calcium ion, by thrombin cleavage of the A-subunit to become activated factor XIII (factor XIIIa). Intracellularly, the homodimeric form of only the A-subunits (A_2) is found. The B-subunits in plasma have no enzymatic activity and function as carrier molecules for the A-subunits. They stabilize the structure of the A-subunits and protect them from proteolysis.

Factor XIIIa promotes cross-linking of fibrin during coagulation and is essential to the physiological protection of the clot against fibrinolysis. Factor XIIIa is a transglutaminase enzyme that catalyzes the cross-linking of the fibrin alpha- and gamma-chains for fibrin stabilization and renders the fibrin clot more elastic and resistant to fibrinolysis. Factor XIIIa also cross-links alpha$_2$-plasmin inhibitor to the alpha-chain of fibrin, resulting in protection of the fibrin clot from degradation by plasmin. Cross-linked fibrin is the end result of the coagulation cascade, and provides tensile strength to a primary hemostatic platelet plug.

Pharmacodynamics – In clinical studies, the IV administration of factor XIII demonstrated an increase in plasma levels of factor XIII lasting approximately 28 days.

In the pharmacokinetic study, after the third 40 units/kg dose (steady state), the mean increase in factor XIII activity levels was 83% with a range of 48% to 114% over the baseline.

➤*Pharmacokinetics:* Each subject received factor XIII IV 40 units/kg every 28 days for a total of 3 doses administered at approximately 250 units/min. Blood samples for doses 1 and 2 were drawn from patients to determine the factor XIII activity level at baseline and 30 and 60 minutes after the infusion. Following the infusion of the third dose of factor XIII, blood samples were drawn at regular intervals up to 28 days to determine the pharmacokinetic parameters.

Factor XIII Pharmacokinetic Parameters (N = 13) by Berichrom Assay Method - Baseline Adjusted Values[a]	
Parameters	Mean ± SD
$AUC_{ss, (0-inf)}$ (units•h/mL)	184 ± 65.78
$C_{ss, max}$ (units/mL)[b]	0.9 ± 0.2
$C_{ss, min}$ (units/mL)[b]	0.05 ± 0.05
T_{max} (h)	1.7 ± 1.44
Half-life (days)	6.6 ± 2.29
CL (mL/h/kg)	0.25 ± 0.09
V_{ss} (mL/kg)	51.1 ± 12.61
MRT (days)	10 ± 3.45

[a] $AUC_{ss, (0-inf)}$ = area under the plasma concentration curve from time 0 to infinity at steady state; $C_{ss, max}$ = peak concentration at steady state; $C_{ss, min}$ = trough concentration at steady state; T_{max} = time to peak concentration; CL = clearance; V_{ss} = volume of distribution at steady state; MRT = mean residence time; SD = standard deviation.
[b] 100% activity corresponds to 1 unit/mL.

Contraindications

History of anaphylactic or severe systemic reactions to human plasma-derived products or to any components in factor XIII.

Warnings/Precautions

➤*Immunogenicity:* Development of inhibitory antibodies against factor XIII has been detected in patients receiving factor XIII. Monitor patients for possible development of inhibitory antibodies. Presence of inhibitory antibodies may manifest as an inadequate response to treatment. If expected plasma factor XIII activity levels are not attained, or if breakthrough bleeding occurs while receiving prophylaxis, an assay that measures factor XIII inhibitory antibody concentrations should be performed. One case of inhibitory antibodies against factor XIII has been reported in the clinical studies. Cases of inhibitory antibodies against factor XIII in patients with congenital factor XIII deficiency have also been reported in postmarketing surveillance.

➤*Thromboembolic events:* Thromboembolic complications have been reported in postmarketing surveillance. Carefully assess benefits and risks in pregnant women because of their hypercoagulable state and potential for increased risk of thromboembolic events.

➤*Transmission of infectious agents:* Factor XIII is made from human plasma. Because this product is made from human blood, it may carry a risk of transmitting infectious agents (eg, viruses) and, theoretically, the Creutzfeldt-Jakob disease (CJD) agent. There is also the possibility that unknown infectious agents may be present in such products. The risk that such products could transmit viruses has been reduced by screening plasma donors for prior exposure to certain viruses, by testing for the presence of certain current virus infections, and by inactivating and removing certain viruses during manufacture. Despite these measures, such products may still potentially transmit disease.

Consider appropriate vaccination (against hepatitis A and B virus) for patients in regular/repeated receipt of factor XIII. All infections thought by a health care provider to have been possibly transmitted by this product should be reported by a health care provider to the CSL Behring Pharmacovigilance Department at 1-866-915-6958 or FDA at 1-800-332-1088 or http://www.fda.gov/medwatch.

➤*Hypersensitivity reactions:* Hypersensitivity reactions (including allergy, rash, pruritus, and erythema) have been observed with factor XIII. If signs or symptoms of anaphylaxis or hypersensitivity reactions (including urticaria, rash, tightness of the chest, wheezing, and hypotension) occur, immediately discontinue administration and institute appropriate treatment.

➤*Pregnancy: Category C.* Animal reproduction studies have not been conducted with factor XIII. Safety and effectiveness in pregnancy have not been established. Administer to a pregnant woman only if clearly needed.

➤*Lactation:* It is not known whether factor XIII is excreted in human milk. Use factor XIII only if clearly needed when treating breast- feeding women.

➤*Children:* Of the 187 unique subjects in the factor XIII clinical studies, 90 were subjects younger than 16 years at the time of enrollment (younger than 1 month, n = 2; 1 month to younger than 2 years, n = 14; 2 to 11 years, n = 52; 12 to younger than 16 years, n = 22). In the pharmacokinetic study, 5 of the 14 subjects ranged in age from 2 to younger than 16 years. Subjects younger than 16 years had a shorter half-life (5.7 ± 1 day) and faster clearance (0.29 ± 0.12 mL/h/kg) compared to adults (half-life, 7.1 ± 2.74 days; clearance, 0.22 ± 0.07 mL/h/kg). The number of subjects younger than 16 years limits the statistical interpretation. There were no apparent differences in the safety profile in children as compared to adults. All children were treated for congenital factor XIII deficiency.

➤*Elderly:* The safety and efficacy of factor XIII in elderly patients have not been established due to an insufficient number of subjects.

➤*Monitoring:* Monitoring of patients' trough factor XIII activity level is recommended during treatment with factor XIII.

If breakthrough bleeding occurs, or if expected peak plasma factor XIII activity levels are not attained, perform an investigation to determine the presence of factor XIII inhibitory antibodies.

Drug Interactions

Do not mix factor XIII concentrate (human) with other drugs and administer through a separate infusion line.

Adverse Reactions

In the 12-week prospective, open-label, multicenter, pharmacokinetic and safety study conducted in 7 women and 7 men with congenital factor XIII deficiency, ranging in age from 5 to 42 years (3 children, 2 adolescents, and 9 adults), there were no reports of deaths, life-threatening events, or adverse reactions that led to discontinuation or withdrawal from the study. No breakthrough bleeding episodes were reported in this study.

➤*Most common adverse reactions:*

Adverse reactions (more than 2% following first study infusion) – Abdominal pain, arthralgia, contusion, diarrhea, epistaxis, fever, flu-like syndrome, head injury, headache, hematoma, joint injury, limb injury, rash, road traffic accident, upper respiratory tract infection, vomiting.

Adverse reactions (more than 1% following treatment) – Arthralgia, hypersensitivity reactions (including allergy, erythema, pruritus, and rash), chills/rise in temperature, elevated thrombin-antithrombin levels, headache, increase in hepatic enzymes.

Immunogenicity – A case of neutralizing antibodies against factor XIII was reported in the ongoing postmarketing clinical study. The patient received prophylactic treatment with factor XIII for 10 years. Concomitant medications included interferon for hepatitis C infection. This patient presented with bruising, and postinfusion factor XIII levels were found to be lower than expected. Over several weeks, factor XIII recovery values decreased, so the dose and frequency of treatments were increased. Neutralizing antibodies to factor XIII were detected, interferon treatment was discontinued, and the subject underwent plasmapheresis. Within a month, neutralizing antibodies were no longer detectable, factor XIII recovery levels improved, and the previous prophylactic regimen was resumed.

➤*Postmarketing:* The following adverse reactions were spontaneously reported after administration of factor XIII during postmarketing surveillance outside the United States since 1993.

Cardiovascular – Thrombosis, embolism.

Hypersensitivity – Allergic/anaphylactic reaction (including alteration in blood pressure, chills, cutaneous reactions, dyspnea, fever, and nausea).

Miscellaneous – Factor XIII inhibitor formation, pyrexia, transmission of an infectious agent via medicinal products (causality to factor XIII could not be established for any virus transmission case report) made from human plasma.

Overdosage

No overdose reported.

Patient Information

Inform patients of the signs and symptoms of allergic hypersensitivity reactions, such as urticaria, rash, tightness of the chest, wheezing, hypotension, and/or anaphylaxis experienced during or after injection of factor XIII.

Inform patients of the signs and symptoms of immunogenicity, such as breakthrough bleeding.

FACTOR XIII CONCENTRATE (HUMAN) — INJECTION

Inform patients of signs and symptoms of thrombosis, such as limb or abdomen swelling and/or pain, chest pain, shortness of breath, loss of sensation or motor power, altered consciousness, vision, or speech.

Advise patients that because factor XIII is made from human blood, it may carry a risk of transmitting infectious agents (eg, viruses, and theoretically, the CJD agent).

ANTIHEMOPHILIC FACTOR COMBINATIONS

ANTIHEMOPHILIC FACTOR/von WILLEBRAND FACTOR COMPLEX (Factor VIII/VWF; AHF/VWF)

Rx	**Humate-P** (CSL Behring)	**Injection, lyophilized powder for solution:** AHF 250 units and VWF:RCo 600 units per vial[a]	In single-dose vials with 5 mL diluent, filter transfer set for reconstitution, and a vented filter spike for withdrawal.
		AHF 500 units and VWF:RCo 1,200 units per vial[a]	In single-dose vials with 10 mL diluent, filter transfer set for reconstitution, and a vented filter spike for withdrawal.
		AHF 1,000 units and VWF:RCo 2,400 units per vial[a]	In single-dose vials with 15 mL diluent, filter transfer set for reconstitution, and a vented filter spike for withdrawal.
Rx	**Wilate** (Octapharma USA)	**Injection, lyophilized powder for solution:** VWF:RCo 450 units and AHF 450 units per vial[b]	Preservative free. In single-dose vials and a vial of diluent, transfer device, and an infusion set.
		VWF:RCo 900 units and AHF 900 units per vial[c]	Preservative free. In single-dose vials and a vial of diluent, transfer device, and an infusion set.

[a] Heat treated. Upon reconstitution with the volume of diluent provided, each milliliter contains factor VIII activity 40 to 80 units, von Willebrand factor:ristocetin cofactor (VWF:RCo) activity 72 to 224 units, glycine 15 to 33 mg, sodium citrate 3.5 to 9.3 mg, sodium chloride 2 to 5.3 mg, albumin (human) 8 to 16 mg, other proteins 2 to 14 mg, and total proteins 10 to 30 mg. Contains anti-A and anti-B blood group isoagglutinins.

[b] Heat treated. Upon reconstitution with the volume of diluent provided (water for injection with 0.1% polysorbate 80), each vial contains VWF:RCo 450 units, factor VIII 450 units, and total protein 7.5 mg or less. Each vial also contains glycine 50 mg, sucrose 50 mg, sodium chloride 117 mg, sodium citrate 14.7 mg, and calcium chloride 0.8 mg.

[c] Heat treated. Upon reconstitution with the volume of diluent provided (water for injection with 0.1% polysorbate 80), each vial contains VWF:RCo 900 units, factor VIII 900 units, and total protein (≤ 15 mg). Each vial also contains glycine 100 mg, sucrose 100 mg, sodium chloride 234 mg, sodium citrate 29.4 mg, and calcium chloride 1.5 mg.

ANTIHEMOPHILIC FACTOR/von WILLEBRAND FACTOR COMPLEX (Factor VIII/VWF; AHF/VWF) — INJECTION

Indications

➤*Hemophilia A (Humate-P only)*: In adult patients for treatment and prevention of bleeding in hemophilia A (classical hemophilia).

➤*von Willebrand disease:*

Humate-P – In adults and children with von Willebrand disease for treatment of spontaneous and trauma-induced bleeding episodes and prevention of excessive bleeding during and after surgery. This applies to patients with severe von Willebrand disease as well as patients with mild to moderate von Willebrand disease in which use of desmopressin is known or suspected to be inadequate.

Wilate – For the treatment of spontaneous and trauma-induced bleeding episodes in patients with severe von Willebrand disease as well as patients with mild or moderate von Willebrand disease in whom the use of desmopressin is known or suspected to be ineffective or contraindicated.

Administration and Dosage

➤*General dosing considerations:* Strongly consider administration of hepatitis A and hepatitis B vaccines to persons receiving plasma derivatives. Potential risks and benefits of vaccination should be carefully weighed by the health care provider and discussed with the patient.

Treatment should be initiated under the supervision of a health care provider experienced in the treatment of coagulation disorders.

Each vial contains the labeled amount in units of von Willebrand factor activity as measured with the ristocetin cofactor assay (VWF:RCo) and coagulation factor VIII (FVIII) activity measured with the chromogenic substrate assay.

The number of units of VWF:RCo and FVIII activities administered is expressed in units, which are related to the current World Health Organization (WHO) standards for VWF and FVIII products. VWF:RCo and FVIII activities in plasma are expressed either as a percentage (relative to normal human plasma) or in units (relative to the International Standards for VWF:RCo and FVIII activities in plasma).

The careful control of replacement therapy is especially important in life-threatening hemorrhages. When using a FVIII-containing von Willebrand disease product, the treating health care provider should be aware that continued treatment may cause an excessive rise in FVIII activity.

➤*Adults:*

Hemophilia A –

Humate-P:

• *Usual dosage* –

AHF/VWF Adult Dosage Recommendations for the Treatment of Hemophilia A

Hemorrhagic event	Dosage (AHF units/kg)
Minor hemorrhage: •Early joint or muscle bleed •Severe epistaxis	Loading dose, 15 units/kg to achieve factor VIII:C[a] plasma level of approximately 30% of normal; 1 infusion may be sufficient. If needed, half of the loading dose may be given once or twice daily for 1 to 2 days.
Moderate hemorrhage: •Advanced joint or muscle bleed •Neck, tongue, or pharyngeal hematoma (without airway compromise) •Tooth extraction •Severe abdominal pain	Loading dose, 25 units/kg to achieve factor VIII:C plasma level of approximately 50% of normal, followed by 15 units/kg every 8 to 12 hours for first 1 to 2 days to maintain factor VIII:C plasma level at 30% of normal, and then the same dose once or twice a day for a total of up to 7 days, or until adequate wound healing.
Life-threatening hemorrhage: •Major operations •GI bleeding •Neck, tongue, or pharyngeal hematoma with potential for airway compromise •Intracranial, intra-abdominal, or intrathoracic bleeding •Fractures	Initially 40 to 50 units/kg, followed by 20 to 25 units/kg every 8 hours to maintain factor VIII:C plasma level at 80% to 100% of normal for 7 days, then continue the same dose once or twice a day for another 7 days in order to maintain the factor VIII:C level at 30% to 50% of normal.

[a] Factor VIII:C = plasma factor VIII activity.

• *Dosage adjustment* – In all cases, the dose should be adjusted individually by clinical judgement of the potential for compromise of a vital structure and by frequent monitoring of factor VIII activity in the patient's plasma.

von Willebrand disease –

Humate-P:

• *Usual dosage* – The dosage should be adjusted according to the extent and location of bleeding. As a rule, 40 to 80 units of VWF:RCo (corresponding to 17 to 33 units of factor VIII in AHF/VWF) per kilogram body weight are given every 8 to 12 hours. Repeat doses are administered for as long as needed based on repeat monitoring of appropriate clinical and laboratory measures. Expected levels of VWF:RCo are based on an expected in vivo recovery of 2 units/dL rise per unit/kg of VWF:RCo administered. The administration of 1 unit of factor VIII per kilogram body weight can be expected to lead to a rise in circulating VWF:RCo of approximately 5 units/dL.

VWF:RCo Dosing Recommendations for Adults for the Treatment of von Willebrand disease

Classification of von Willebrand disease	Hemorrhage	Dosage (VWF:RCo units/kg)
Type 1		
Mild, if desmopressin is inappropriate (baseline VWF:RCo activity typically > 30%)	Major (eg, severe or refractory epistaxis, GI bleeding, CNS trauma, traumatic hemorrhage)	Loading dose, 40 to 60 units/kg, then 40 to 50 units/kg every 8 to 12 hours for 3 days to keep the trough level of VWF:RCo > 50%; then 40 to 50 units/kg daily for a total of up to 7 days of treatment.

ANTIHEMOPHILIC FACTOR/von WILLEBRAND FACTOR COMPLEX (Factor VIII/VWF; AHF/VWF) — INJECTION

VWF:RCo Dosing Recommendations for Adults for the Treatment of von Willebrand disease

Classification of von Willebrand disease	Hemorrhage	Dosage (VWF:RCo units/kg)
Moderate or severe (baseline VWF:RCo activity typically < 30%)	Minor (eg, epistaxis, oral bleeding, menorrhagia)	40 to 50 units/kg (1 or 2 doses).
	Major (eg, severe or refractory epistaxis, GI bleeding, CNS trauma, hemarthrosis, traumatic hemorrhage)	Loading dose, 50 to 75 units/kg, then 40 to 60 units/kg every 8 to 12 hours for 3 days to keep the trough level of VWF:RCo > 50%; then 40 to 60 units/kg/day for a total of up to 7 days of treatment. Factor VIII:C levels should be monitored and maintained according to the guidelines for hemophilia A therapy. See the previous table.
Types 2 (all variants) and 3		
	Minor (clinical indications above)	40 to 50 units/kg (1 or 2 doses).
	Major (clinical indications above)	Loading dose, 60 to 80 units/kg, then 40 to 60 units/kg every 8 to 12 hours for 3 days to keep the trough level of VWF:RCo > 50%; then 40 to 60 units/kg/day for a total of up to 7 days of treatment. Factor VIII:C levels should be monitored and maintained according to the guidelines for hemophilia A therapy.

Wilate: In von Willebrand disease type 3 patients, especially in those with GI bleedings, higher doses may be required.

AHF/VWF Dosing for Treatment of Minor and Major Hemorrhages

Type of hemorrhages	Loading dose (units VFW:RCo/kg body weight)	Maintenance dosage (units VWF:RCo/kg body weight)	Therapeutic goal
Minor hemorrhages	20 to 40 units/kg	20 to 30 units/kg every 12 to 24 hours[a]	VWF:RCo and FVIII activity trough levels of > 30%
Major hemorrhages	40 to 60 units/kg	20 to 40 units/kg every 12 to 24 hours[a]	VWF:RCo and FVIII activity trough levels of > 50%

[a] Treatment guidelines apply to all von Willebrand disease types. This may need to be continued for up to 3 days for minor hemorrhages and 5 to 7 days for major hemorrhages.

Repeat doses are administered for as long as needed based upon repeat monitoring of appropriate clinical and laboratory measures. Although dose can be estimated by the previously described guidelines, it is highly recommended that, whenever possible, appropriate laboratory tests be performed on the patient's plasma at suitable intervals to ensure that adequate VWF:RCo and FVIII activity levels have been reached and are maintained.

In the unlikely event that a patient who is actively bleeding should miss a dose, it may be appropriate to adopt a dosage depending on the level of coagulation factors measured, extent of the bleeding, and patient's clinical condition.

Prevention of excessive bleeding during and after surgery in von Willebrand disease –

Loading dose –

AHF/VWF Loading Dose for Adults for the Prevention of Excessive Bleeding During and After Surgery

Type of surgery	VWF:RCo target peak plasma level	Factor VIII:C target peak plasma level	Calculation of loading dose (to be administered 1 to 2 hours before surgery)
Major	100 units/dL	80 to 100 units/dL	Δ[a] VWF:RCo × body weight (kg)/ in vivo recovery[b] = units VWF:RCo required If the incremental in vivo recovery is not available, assume an in vivo recovery of 2 units/dL per unit/kg and calculate the loading dose as follows: (100 − baseline plasma VWF:RCo) × body weight (kg)/2 In the case of emergency surgery, administer a dose of 50 to 60 units/kg.
Minor/Oral[c]	50 to 60 units/dL	40 to 50 units/dL	Δ[a] VWF:RCo × body weight (kg)/ in vivo recovery[b] = units VWF:RCo required

[a] Δ = target peak plasma VWF:RCo − baseline plasma VWF:RCo.
[b] In vivo recovery = incremental recovery as measured in the patient.
[c] Oral surgery is defined as removal of < 3 teeth, if the teeth are nonmolars and have no bony involvement. Removal of > 1 impacted wisdom tooth is considered major surgery because of the expected difficulty of the surgery and the expected blood loss, particularly in subjects with type 2A or type 3 von Willebrand disease. Removal of > 2 teeth is considered major surgery in all patients.

Attaining a target peak factor VIII:C plasma level of 80 to 100 units of factor VIII:C/dL for major surgery and 40 to 50 units of factor VIII:C/dL for minor surgery or oral surgery might require additional dosing with AHF/VWF. Because the ratio of VWF:RCo to factor VIII:C activity in AHF/VWF is 2.4:1, any additional dosing will increase VWF:RCo proportionally more than factor VIII:C. Assuming an incremental in vivo recovery of 2 units of VWF:RCo/dL per unit/kg infused, additional dosing to increase factor VIII:C in plasma will also increase plasma VWF:RCo by approximately 5 units/dL for each unit/kg of factor VIII:C administered.

Maintenance dose – The initial maintenance dose for the prevention of excessive bleeding during and after surgery should be half the loading dose, irrespective of additional dosing required to meet factor VIII:C targets.

VWF:RCo and Factor VIII:C Maintenance Doses for Adults for the Prevention of Excessive Bleeding During and After Surgery

Type of surgery	VWF:RCo target trough plasma levels[a]		Factor VIII:C target trough plasma levels[a]		Minimum duration of treatment
	Up to 3 days following surgery	After day 3	Up to 3 days following surgery	After day 3	
Major	> 50 units/dL	> 30 units/dL	> 50 units/dL	> 30 units/dL	72 hours
Minor	≥ 30 units/dL			> 30 units/dL	48 hours
Oral[b]	≥ 30 units/dL	—	—	> 30 units/dL	8 to 12 hours[c]

[a] Trough levels for either coagulation factor should not exceed 100 units/dL.
[b] Oral surgery is defined as removal of < 3 teeth, if the teeth are nonmolars and have no bony involvement. Removal of > 1 impacted wisdom tooth is considered major surgery because of the expected difficulty of the surgery and the expected blood loss, particularly in subjects with type 2A or type 3 von Willebrand disease. Removal of > 2 teeth is considered major surgery in all patients.
[c] At least 1 maintenance dose following surgery based on individual pharmacokinetic values.

Based on individual pharmacokinetic-derived half-lives, the frequency of maintenance doses is generally every 8 or 12 hours; patients with shorter half-lives may require dosing every 6 hours. In the absence of pharmacokinetic data, it is recommended that AHF/VWF be administered initially every 8 hours, with further adjustments determined by monitoring trough coagulation factor levels.

Dosage adjustment: When hemostatic levels are judged insufficient or trough levels are outside the recommended range, consider modifying the administration interval and/or the dose. It is advisable to monitor trough VWF:RCo and factor VIII:C levels at least once daily in order to adjust AHF/VWF dosing as needed to avoid excessive accumulation of coagulation factors.

Duration of therapy: The duration of treatment generally depends on the type of surgery performed but must be assessed for individual patients based on their hemostatic response.

➤*Children:*

von Willebrand disease –

Humate-P: See Adults for dosing.

Wilate:

- *5 to 16 years of age* – See Adults for dosing.

ANTIHEMOPHILIC FACTOR/von WILLEBRAND FACTOR COMPLEX (Factor VIII/VWF; AHF/VWF) — INJECTION

Prevention of excessive bleeding during and after surgery in von Willebrand disease –

Humate-P: See Adults for dosing.

➤*Preparation for administration:*

Humate-P –

1.) Before infusion, ensure that AHF/VWF and diluent are at room temperature.
2.) Remove caps from both vials to expose central portions of the rubber stoppers.
3.) Treat surface of rubber stoppers with the alcohol swab provided and allow to dry prior to opening the *Mix2Vial* package.
4.) Open the *Mix2Vial* package by peeling away the lid. To maintain sterility, leave the *Mix2Vial* in the clear outer packaging. Place the diluent vial on an even surface and hold the vial tight. Grip the *Mix2Vial* together with the clear packaging and firmly snap the blue end onto the diluent stopper.
5.) While holding onto the diluent vial, carefully remove the clear outer packaging from the *Mix2Vial* set. Make sure to only pull up the clear outer packaging and not the *Mix2Vial* set.
6.) With the product vial firmly on a surface, invert the diluent vial with set attached and firmly snap the transparent adapter onto the product vial stopper. The diluent will automatically transfer into the product vial. To ensure product sterility, AHF/VWF should be administered within 3 hours after reconstitution.
7.) With the diluent and product vial still attached, gently swirl the product vial to ensure the product is fully dissolved. Do not shake vial.
8.) With one hand, grasp the product side of the *Mix2Vial* set and with the other hand, grasp the blue diluent side of the *Mix2Vial* set and unscrew the set into 2 pieces.
9.) Draw air into an empty sterile syringe. Plastic disposable syringes are recommended. While the product vial is upright, screw the syringe to the *Mix2Vial* set. Inject air into the product vial. While keeping the syringe plunger pressed, invert the system upside down and draw the concentrate into the syringe by pulling the plunger back slowly.
10.) Now that the concentrate has been transferred into the syringe, firmly grasp the barrel of the syringe (keeping the syringe plunger facing down) and unscrew the syringe from the *Mix2Vial*. Attach the syringe to a venipuncture set.
11.) If the same patient is to receive concentrate from more than 1 vial, the contents of 2 vials may be drawn into the same syringe through a separate unused *Mix2Vial* set before attaching the vein needle.
12.) Parenteral drug products should be inspected visually for particulate matter and discoloration prior to administration, whenever solution and container permit. When the reconstitution procedure is precisely followed, it is not uncommon for a few small flakes or particles to remain. The *Mix2Vial* set provided with AHF/VWF should remove those particles, and this should not influence dosage calculations.

Wilate – *Wilate* is provided with a *Mix2Vial* transfer device for reconstitution of the freeze-dried powder in diluent, a 10 mL syringe, an infusion set, and 2 alcohol swabs.

Instructions for reconstitution:

1.) Warm the powder and diluent in the closed vials up to room temperature. This temperature should be maintained during reconstitution. If a water bath is used for warming, care must be taken to avoid water coming into contact with the rubber stoppers (latex free) or the caps of the vials. The temperature of the water bath should not exceed 37°C (98°F).
2.) Remove the caps from the concentrate vial and the diluent vial and clean the rubber stoppers with an alcohol swab.
3.) Peel away the lid of the outer package of the *Mix2Vial* transfer set. To maintain sterility, leave the *Mix2Vial* device in the clear outer packaging. Place the diluent vial on a level surface and hold the vial firmly. Take the *Mix2Vial* in its outer package and invert it over the diluent vial. Push the blue plastic cannula of the *Mix2Vial* firmly through the rubber stopper of the diluent vial. While holding onto the diluent vial, carefully remove the outer package from the *Mix2Vial*, being careful to leave the *Mix2Vial* attached firmly to the diluent vial.
4.) With the concentrate vial held firmly on a level surface, quickly invert the diluent vial with the *Mix2Vial* attached and push the transparent plastic cannula end of the *Mix2Vial* firmly through the stopper of the concentrate vial. The diluent will be drawn into the concentrate vial by the vacuum.
5.) With both vials still attached, gently swirl the product vial to ensure the product is fully dissolved to a clear solution. Once the contents of the vial are completely dissolved, firmly hold both the transparent and blue parts of the *Mix2Vial*. Unscrew the *Mix2Vial* into 2 separate pieces and discard the empty diluent vial and the blue part of the *Mix2Vial*.

The powder should be reconstituted only directly before injection. As *Wilate* contains no preservatives, the solution should be used immediately after reconstitution.

The solution is clear to slightly opalescent. If the concentrate fails to dissolve completely or an aggregate is formed, the preparation must not be used.

Instructions for injection:

1.) With the vial still upright, attach a plastic disposable syringe to the *Mix2Vial* (transparent plastic part). Invert the system and draw the reconstituted solution into the syringe.
2.) Once solution has been transferred into the syringe, firmly hold the barrel of the syringe (keeping the syringe plunger facing down) and detach the *Mix2Vial* from the syringe. Discard the *Mix2Vial* (transparent plastic part) and empty the vial.
3.) Clean the intended injection site with an alcohol swab.
4.) Attach a suitable infusion needle to the syringe.

Any unused product or waste material should be disposed of in accordance with local requirements.

➤*Administration:* For intravenous (IV) administration only. Plastic disposable syringes are recommended for withdrawal and administration of AHF/VWF solution. Protein solutions of this type tend to adhere to the ground glass surface of all-glass syringes.

Inject the solution at a slow speed of 2 to 4 mL/min (maximally 4 mL/min) IV with a venipuncture set or another suitable injection set.

As a precautionary measure, the patient's pulse rate should be measured before and during the injection. If a marked increase in the pulse rate occurs, the injection speed must be reduced or the administration must be interrupted.

➤*Admixture compatibility: Wilate* must not be mixed with other medicinal products or administered simultaneously with other IV preparations in the same infusion set.

➤*Storage / Stability:*

Humate-P – When stored up to 25°C (77°F), AHF/VWF is stable for the period indicated by the expiration date on its label. Avoid freezing. Do not refrigerate after reconstitution. To ensure product sterility, AHF/VWF should be administered within 3 hours after reconstitution.

Wilate – Store vials in the original container for up to 36 months at 2° to 8°C (36° to 46°F) protected from light from the date of manufacture. Within this period, the vials may be stored for a period of up to 6 months at room temperature (maximum of 25°C [77°F]). The starting date of room temperature storage should be clearly recorded on the product carton. Once stored at room temperature, the product must not be returned to the refrigerator. The shelf-life then expires after storage at room temperature, or the expiration date on the product vial, whichever is earliest. Do not freeze.

Reconstitute the powder only directly before injection. Use the solution immediately after reconstitution. Use the reconstituted solution on one occasion only, and discard any remaining solution.

Actions

➤*Pharmacology:*

Wilate – VWF and FVIII are normal constituents of human plasma. The AHF/VWF complex consists of 2 different noncovalently bound proteins (factor VIII) and von Willebrand factor). Factor VIII is an essential cofactor in activation of factor X, leading ultimately to formation of thrombin and fibrin. VWF is a multimeric protein with 2 key functions. It is an adhesive molecule, which mediates the binding between platelets and damaged subendothelial tissues. It is also a carrier protein, involved in the transport and stabilization of FVIII. Patients suffering from von Willebrand disease have a deficiency or abnormality of VWF. This reduction in VWF concentration in the bloodstream results in a correspondingly low FVIII activity and an abnormal platelet function, thereby resulting in excessive bleeding. The VWF in AHF/VWF is derived from normal human plasma and is expected to behave in the same way as endogenous VWF. Thus, administration of VWF allows correction of the hemostatic abnormalities in von Willebrand disease patients at 2 levels: the VWF reestablishes platelet adhesion to the vascular subendothelium at the site of vascular damage (as it binds both to the vascular subendothelium and to the platelet membrane), providing primary hemostasis, as shown by the shortening of the bleeding time. This effect occurs immediately. The VWF induces correction of the associated FVIII deficiency in von Willebrand disease. Administered IV, VWF binds endogenous FVIII (which is produced normally by the patient) and, by stabilizing this factor, avoids its rapid degradation. This action is slightly delayed. However, administration of a FVIII-containing VWF preparation like AHF/VWF rapidly restores the FVIII activity level to normal. The activity of VWF is measured as VWF:RCo.

➤*Pharmacokinetics:*

Absorption / Distribution –

Humate-P:

• *Hemophilia A* – After IV injection of AHF/VWF in humans, there is a rapid increase of plasma factor VIII activity (factor VIII:C), followed by a rapid decrease in activity and a subsequent slower rate of decrease in activity.

• *von Willebrand disease* – Pharmacokinetic studies of AHF/VWF have been performed with cohorts of patients in the nonbleeding state. Wide intersubject variability was observed in pharmacokinetic values obtained from these studies.

The pharmacokinetics of AHF/VWF were evaluated in a prospective US study in 41 subjects in the nonbleeding state prior to a surgical procedure. Subjects received 60 units of VWF:RCo/kg body weight of AHF/VWF. Sixteen patients had type I von Willebrand disease, 2 had type 2A, 4 had type 2B, 6 had type 2M, and 13 had type 3. The median in vivo recovery for VWF:RCo activity was 2.4 units/dL per units/kg (range, 1.1 to 4.2). High molecular weight multimers were measured in 13 subjects with type 3 von Willebrand disease; 11 had absent or barely detectable multimers at baseline. Of those 11 subjects, all had some high molecular weight multimers present 24 hours after infusion of AHF/VWF.

Pharmacokinetics were also evaluated in a European study in 28 subjects in the nonbleeding state prior to a surgical procedure. Subjects received 80 units of VWF:RCo/kg body weight of AHF/VWF. Ten subjects had type I von Willebrand disease, 10 had type 2A, 1 had type 2M, and 7 had type 3. The volume of distribution at steady state was 59 mL/kg (range, 32 to 290 mL/kg). The median in vivo recovery for VWF:RCo activity was 1.9 units/dL per unit/kg (range, 0.6 to 4.5). Infusion of AHF/VWF corrected the defect of the multimer pattern in subjects with types IIA and III von Willebrand disease. High molecular weight multimers were detectable until at least 8 hours after infusion.

ANTIHEMOPHILIC FACTOR/von WILLEBRAND FACTOR COMPLEX (Factor VIII/VWF; AHF/VWF) — INJECTION

Wilate: An open-label, prospective, randomized, controlled, 2-arm, crossover phase 2 study with *Wilate* and a comparator product was conducted at 6 sites in the United States. In this study, pharmacokinetic profiles of *Wilate* were determined by FVIII activity, VWF:RCo, VWF:Ag, and VWF:CB.

Each of 22 subjects with inherited von Willebrand disease (type 1, n = 6; type 2, n = 9 [6 type 2A, 1 type 2B, and 2 type 2M]; and type 3, n = 7) received an IV bolus dose of *Wilate* containing approximately 40 units of VWF:RCo/kg body weight. Twenty subjects completed the study as per protocol.

Pharmacokinetic Parameters of VWF:RCo: Mean ± SD (Range)[a]

Parameters	VWD type 1 (n = 5)	VWD type 2 (n = 9)	VWD type 3 (n = 6)	Total (n = 20)
C_{max} (units/dL)	74 ± 13 (62 to 91)	77 ± 18 (40 to 100)	79 ± 13 (65 to 102)	76 ± 15 (40 to 102)
$AUC_{0\text{-}inf}$ (units•h/dL)	1,633 ± 979 (984 to 3,363)	1,172 ± 421 (571 to 1,897)	995 ± 292 (527 to 1,306)	1,235 ± 637 (527 to 3,363)
V_{ss} (mL/kg)	81.7 ± 38.5 (15.3 to 74.2)	76.6 ± 35.4 (45.3 to 158.8)	49.4 ± 16.7 (29.7 to 67.1)	69.7 ± 33.2 (29.7 to 158.8)
MRT (h)	32.7 ± 25.8 (15.3 to 74.2)	19.7 ± 5.6 (9.9 to 27.1)	11.9 ± 2.9 (9.2 to 15.9)	17.4 ± 4.5 (10.2 to 28.8)
Recovery (% units/kg)	1.8 ± 0.2 (1.5 to 2)	1.8 ± 0.5 (1 to 2.4)	2.1 ± 0.3 (1.8 to 2.6)	2 ± 0.5 (1 to 2.7)

[a] SD = standard deviation; C_{max} = peak concentration; AUC = area under curve; V_{ss} = volume of distribution at steady state; MRT = mean residence time.

The pharmacokinetics parameters reported in the previous table are based on VWF:RCo values obtained using a modified Behring Coagulation System (BCS) analytical method. The modified BCS was used because of its validated lower variability compared with the standard BCS. The measured concentrations (units VWF:RCo/mL) are higher by the modified BCS than by the standard BCS analytical method, which is used in some clinical laboratories. Dose adjusted C_{max} and AUC determined by this modified BCS method are approximately 1.5 times higher than those by the standard BCS method. No difference has been found in incremental recovery.

Pharmacokinetic Parameters of FVIII:C: Mean ± SD (Range) – Chromogenic

Parameters	VWD type 1 (n = 5)	VWD type 2 (n = 8)[a]	VWD type 3 (n = 6)	Total (n = 19)[a]
C_{max} (units/dL)	117.1± 12.1 (103 to 135)	147.2 ± 32.6 (102 to 206)	120 ± 23 (91 to 148)	112 ± 23 (59 to 148)
$AUC_{0\text{-}inf}$ (units•h/dL)	1,187 ± 382 (523 to 1,483)	1,778 ± 1,430 (544 to 4,821)	2,670 ± 854 (1,874 to 3,655)	2,290 ± 1,045 (464 to 4,424)
V_{ss} (mL/kg)	95 ± 53.8 (57.1 to 190)	79.5 ± 23.1 (52.8 to 116.2)	44.2 ± 10.4 (31.8 to 57.1)	72.4 ± 36.2 (31.8 to 190)
MRT (hrs)	24.1 ± 5.5 (17.2 to 31.5)	35.1 ± 14.2 (17.5 to 61.6)	23 ± 3.7 (18 to 27.7)	28.4 ± 11.1 (17.2 to 61.6)
Recovery (% units/kg)	1.9 ± 0.5 (1.1 to 2.5)	2.2 ± 0.4 (1.6 to 2.8)	2.5 ± 0.5 (2 to 3)	2.2 ± 0.5 (1.1 to 3)

[a] One subject with implausible long half-life is not included in the summary table, except for recovery result.

Excretion –

Humate-P:

• *Hemophilia A* – Studies with AHF/VWF in hemophilic patients have demonstrated a mean half-life of 12.2 hours (range, 8.4 to 17.4 hours).

• *von Willebrand disease* – One study evaluated 41 subjects in the nonbleeding state prior to a surgical procedure in a prospective US study. The median terminal half-life of VWF:RCo was 11 hours (range, 3.5 to 33.6 hours), excluding 5 subjects with a half-life exceeding the blood sampling time of 24 or 48 hours. The median clearance was 3.1 mL/h/kg (range, 1 to 16.6 mL/h/kg). A second European study evaluated 28 subjects in the nonbleeding state prior to a surgical procedure. The median terminal half-life of VWF:RCo was 10 hours (range, 2.8 to 28.3 hours), excluding 1 subject with a half-life exceeding the blood sampling time of 48 hours. The median clearance was 4.8 mL/h/kg (range, 2.1 to 53 mL/h/kg).

Wilate:

Pharmacokinetic Parameters of VWF:RCo: Mean ± SD (Range)

Parameters	VWD type 1 (n = 5)	VWD type 2 (n = 9)	VWD type 3 (n = 6)	Total (n = 20)
Half-life (h)	24.7 ± 17.9 (11.2 to 48.5)	15.3 ± 6.3 (6 to 26.4)	9.1 ± 2.6 (5.7 to 12.9)	15.8± 11 (5.7 to 48.5)
CL[a] (mL/h/kg)	3.1 ± 1.1 (1.2 to 4.1)	4.1 ± 1.7 (2 to 7.1)	4.2 ± 1.4 (3 to 6.6)	3.7± 1.5 (1.8 to 8.8)

[a] CL = clearance.

Pharmacokinetic Parameters of FVIII:C: Mean ± SD (Range) – Chromogenic

Parameters	VWD type 1 (n = 5)	VWD type 2 (n = 8)[a]	VWD type 3 (n = 6)	Total (n = 19)[a]
Half-life (h)	17.5 ± 4.9 (10.9 to 23.8)	23.6 ± 8.3 (12.6 to 34.7)	16.1 ± 3.1 (11.8 to 20.1)	19.6 ± 6.9 (10.9 to 34.7)
CL (mL/h/kg)	4.4 ± 3.7 (2.5 to 11)	2.5 ± 0.9 (1.2 to 3.5)	2 ± 0.6 (1.4 to 2.8)	2.9 ± 2.1 (1.2 to 11)

[a] One subject with implausible long half-life is not included in the summary table, except for recovery result.

Contraindications

History of anaphylactic or severe systemic response to AHF or VWF preparations; known hypersensitivity to any of its components.

Warnings/Precautions

➤*Thromboembolic events:* Thromboembolic events have been reported in patients with von Willebrand disease receiving coagulation AHF/VWF complex replacement therapy, especially in the setting of known risk factors for thrombosis. Early reports might indicate a higher incidence in women. In addition, endogenous high levels of factor VIII have also been associated with thrombosis but no causal relationship has been established. In all patients with von Willebrand disease in situations of high thrombotic risk receiving coagulation factor replacement therapy, exercise caution and consider antithrombotic measures.

When using a FVIII-containing VWF product, be aware that continued treatment may cause an excessive rise in FVIII activity. Monitor plasma levels of VWF:RCo and FVIII activities in patients receiving AHF/VWF to avoid sustained excessive VWF and FVIII activity levels, which may increase the risk of thrombotic events.

➤*Inhibitor formation:* Patients with von Willebrand disease, especially those with type 3, may potentially develop neutralizing antibodies (inhibitors) to VWF. If a patient develops inhibitor to VWF (or FVIII), the condition will manifest itself as an inadequate clinical response. Thus, if the expected VWF activity plasma levels are not attained, or if bleeding is not controlled with an adequate dose or repeated dosing, perform an appropriate assay to determine if a VWF inhibitor is present. In patients with antibodies against VWF, VWF is not effective and infusion of this protein may lead to severe adverse reactions. Consider other therapeutic options for such patients. Health care providers with experience in the care of patients with hemostatic disorders should direct their management. In all such cases, it is recommended that a center specialized in bleeding disorders be contacted.

Because inhibitor antibodies may occur concomitantly with anaphylactic reactions, also evaluate patients experiencing an anaphylactic reaction for the presence of inhibitors.

➤*Transmission of infectious agents:* AHF/VWF is made from human plasma. Products made from human plasma may contain infectious agents, such as viruses, that can cause disease. Because AHF/VWF is made from human blood, it may carry a risk of transmitting infectious agents (eg, viruses) and, theoretically, the Creutzfeldt-Jakob disease agent. There is also the possibility that unknown infectious agents may be present in such products. The risk that such products will transmit an infectious agent has been reduced by screening plasma donors for prior exposure to certain viruses, by testing for the presence of certain current viral infections, and by inactivating and/or removing certain viruses during manufacture. Stringent procedures, utilized at plasma collection centers, plasma testing laboratories, and fractionation facilities, are designed to reduce the risk of virus transmission. The primary virus reduction step of the AHF/VWF manufacturing process is the heat treatment of the purified, stabilized aqueous solution at 60°C for 10 hours (ie, pasteurization). In addition, the purification procedure, which includes several precipitation steps and an adsorption step used in the manufacture of AHF/VWF, also provides virus reduction capacity. Despite these measures, such products may still potentially contain human pathogenic agents, including those not yet known or identified. Thus, the risk of transmission of infectious agents cannot be totally eliminated. Report any infections thought possibly to have been transmitted by this product to the manufacturer.

Record the batch number of the product every time *Wilate* is administered to a patient, and consider appropriate vaccination (against hepatitis A and B virus) of patients in regular/repeated receipt of *Wilate*.

➤*Identification of clotting deficiency:* It is important to determine that the coagulation disorder is caused by factor VIII or VWF deficiency because no benefit in treating other deficiencies can be expected.

➤*Isoagglutinin:* This AHF/VWF preparation contains blood group isoagglutinins (anti-A and anti-B). When very large or frequently repeated doses are needed, as when inhibitors are present or when presurgical and postsurgical care is involved, monitor patients of blood groups A, B, and AB for signs of intravascular hemolysis and decreasing hematocrit values, and treat them appropriately as required.

➤*Hypersensitivity reactions:* Hypersensitivity or allergic reactions (which may include angioedema, burning and stinging at the infusion site, chills, flushing, generalized urticaria, headache, hives, hypotension, lethargy, nausea, restlessness, tachycardia, tightness of the chest, tingling, vomiting, and wheezing) have been observed upon use of AHF/VWF and may, in some cases, progress to severe anaphylaxis (including shock) with or without fever. Closely monitor patients receiving AHF/VWF and carefully observe for any symptoms throughout the infusion period.

Inform patients of the early signs of hypersensitivity reactions, including hives, generalized urticaria, tightness of the chest, wheezing, hypotension, and anaphylaxis. If allergic symptoms occur, instruct patients to discontinue the administration immediately and contact their health care provider.

ANTIHEMOPHILIC FACTOR/von WILLEBRAND FACTOR COMPLEX (Factor VIII/VWF; AHF/VWF) — INJECTION

Because inhibitor antibodies may occur concomitantly with anaphylactic reactions, also evaluate patients experiencing an anaphylactic reaction for the presence of inhibitors.

➤*Pregnancy: Category C.* Animal reproduction studies have not been conducted with AHF/VWF. It is also not known whether AHF/VWF can cause fetal harm when administered to a pregnant woman or can affect reproduction capacity. Administer AHF/VWF to a pregnant woman only if clearly needed.

Labor and delivery – AHF/VWF has not been studied in labor or delivery. It should be administered to VWF-deficient women at labor or delivery only if clearly indicated.

➤*Lactation:* AHF/VWF has not been studied in lactating women.

➤*Children:*

Hemophilia A –

Humate-P: Adequate and well-controlled studies with long-term evaluation of joint damage have not been done in children. Joint damage may result from suboptimal treatment of hemarthroses. For immediate control of bleeding for hemophilia A, the general recommendations for dosing and administration for adults may be referenced.

von Willebrand disease –

Humate-P: The safety and efficacy of AHF/VWF for the treatment of von Willebrand disease were demonstrated in 26 pediatric patients, including infants, children, and adolescents, but have not yet been evaluated in neonates. The safety of AHF/VWF for the prevention of excessive bleeding during and after surgery was demonstrated in 8 children (3 to 15 years of age) with von Willebrand disease. Of the 34 pediatric subjects studied for both treatment of von Willebrand disease and prevention of excessive bleeding during and after surgery, 4 were infants (1 month to younger than 2 years of age), 23 were children (2 to 12 years of age), and 7 were adolescents (13 to 15 years of age).

As in adults, children should be dosed based on weight (kg).

Wilate: Eleven pediatric patients with von Willebrand disease between 5 to 16 years of age (eight type 3, one type 2, two type 1) were treated with AHF/VWF for 234 bleeding episodes in clinical studies. These studies showed that 88% of the bleeding episodes were treated successfully in this population. No dose adjustment is needed for pediatric patients, as administered dosages were similar to those used in the adult population.

➤*Monitoring:* Monitor the factor VIII levels of patients with von Willebrand disease receiving AHF/VWF using standard coagulation tests, especially in cases of surgery. Also give strong consideration to monitoring VWF:RCo levels in patients with von Willebrand disease receiving AHF/VWF for the prevention of excessive bleeding during and after surgery. It is advisable to monitor trough VWF:RCo and factor VIII:C levels at least once daily in order to adjust the dosage of AHF/VWF as needed to avoid excessive accumulation of coagulation factors, which may increase the risk of thrombotic events.

Monitor for development of VWF and FVIII inhibitors. Perform assays to determine whether VWF and/or FVIII inhibitor(s) is present if bleeding is not controlled with the expected dose of AHF/VWF.

Drug Interactions

None well documented.

Adverse Reactions

➤*Humate-P*:

Serious adverse reactions – The most serious adverse reaction observed in patients receiving AHF/VWF is anaphylaxis. Thromboembolic events have also been observed in patients receiving AHF/VWF for the treatment of von Willebrand disease.

Common adverse reactions – Although few adverse reactions have been reported in clinical studies and in the postmarketing setting in patients receiving AHF/VWF for treatment of hemophilia A and von Willebrand disease, the most commonly reported are allergic-anaphylactic reactions (including chest tightness, edema, pruritus, rash, shock, and urticaria). For patients undergoing surgery, the most common adverse reactions are postoperative wound or injection-site bleeding.

Thromboembolic events – Thromboembolic events have also been observed in patients receiving AHF/VWF for the treatment of von Willebrand disease. Reports of thromboembolic events in patients with von Willebrand disease with other thrombotic risk factors receiving coagulation factor replacement therapy have been obtained from spontaneous reports, published literature, and a European clinical study. Early reports might indicate a higher incidence in women. In some cases, inhibitors to coagulation factors may occur. However, no inhibitor formation was observed in any of the clinical trials.

Treatment of von Willebrand disease – Allergic symptoms, including allergic reaction, urticaria, chest tightness, rash, pruritus, and edema, were reported in 6% of patients in a Canadian retrospective study. Four percent of patients experienced 7 adverse reactions that were considered to have a possible or probable relationship to the product. These included chills, paresthesia, phlebitis, pruritus, rash, urticaria, and vasodilation. All were mild in intensity, with the exception of a moderate case of pruritus.

In a prospective, open-label safety and efficacy study of AHF/VWF in patients with von Willebrand disease with serious life- or limb-threatening bleeding or undergoing emergency surgery, 10% of patients experienced 9 adverse reactions. These were mild vasodilation (1/9), allergic reactions (2/9), pruritus (1/9), and paresthesia (2/9); moderate peripheral edema (1/9) and extremity pain (1/9); and severe pseudothrombocytopenia (platelet clumping with a false low reading) (1/9). AHF/VWF was discontinued in the subject who experienced peripheral edema and extremity pain.

von Willebrand disease patients undergoing surgery –

Common adverse reactions: Among the 63 patients with von Willebrand disease who received AHF/VWF for prevention of excessive bleeding during and after surgery, including 1 patient who underwent colonoscopy without the planned polypectomy, the most common adverse reactions were postoperative hemorrhage (35 reactions in 19 patients, with 5 patients experiencing bleeding at up to 3 different sites), postoperative nausea (15 subjects), and postoperative pain (11 subjects).

• *Postoperative hemorrhagic adverse reactions* –

AHF/VWF Postoperative Hemorrhagic Adverse Reactions in von Willebrand Patients

Adverse reaction	Surgical procedure category	Number of patients/reactions	Onset[a] (number of reactions)		Severity (number of reactions)		
			On	Post	Mild	Moderate	Severe
Wound/Injection-site bleeding	Major	8/11	7	4	9	—	2
	Minor	2/2	2	—	1	1	—
	Oral	2/6	—	6	3	3	—
Epistaxis	Major	4/4	2	2	3	1	—
	Minor	1/1	1	—	1	—	—
Cerebral hemorrhage/ subdural hematoma	Major	1/2	2[b]	—	—	2	—
GI bleeding	Major	1/3	3[c]	—	—	2	1
Menorrhagia	Major	1/1	1[d]	—	—	1	—
Groin bleed	Oral	1/1	—	1	1	—	—
Ear bleed	Major	1/1	1	—	1	—	—
Hemoptysis	Major	1/1	1	—	1	—	—
Hematuria	Major	1/1	1	—	1	—	—
Shoulder bleed	Major	1/1	1	—	1	—	—

[a] On = on-therapy; onset while receiving AHF/VWF or within 1 day of completing AHF/VWF administration. Post = posttherapy; onset at least 1 day after completing AHF/VWF administration.
[b] Reported as serious adverse reactions after intracranial surgery.
[c] Two of these reactions reported as serious adverse reactions occurring after gastrojejunal bypass.
[d] Reported as serious adverse reaction requiring hysterectomy after hysteroscopy and dilation and curettage.

ANTIHEMOPHILIC FACTOR/von WILLEBRAND FACTOR COMPLEX (Factor VIII/VWF; AHF/VWF) — INJECTION

• *Nonhemorrhagic adverse reactions* – The following table lists the nonhemorrhagic adverse reactions reported in at least 2 subjects, regardless of causality, and the adverse reactions that were possibly related to AHF/VWF. Pulmonary embolus possibly related to AHF/VWF occurred in 1 elderly subject who underwent bilateral knee replacement.

AHF/VWF Nonhemorrhagic Adverse Reactions in Surgical von Willebrand disease

Adverse reaction	Number of patients with an adverse reaction possibly related to AHF/VWF	Number of patients with an adverse reaction regardless of causality[a]
Cardiovascular		
Chest pain	—	3
Pulmonary embolus[b]	1	1
Thrombophlebitis[b]	1	1
CNS		
Dizziness	1	5
Headache	1	4
Insomnia	—	2
Dermatologic		
Increased sweating	—	3
Pruritus	—	3
Rash	1	1
GI		
Abdominal pain	—	3
Constipation	—	7
Nausea	1	15
Vomiting	1	3
GU		
Urinary retention	—	4
Urinary tract infection	—	2
Miscellaneous		
Anemia/Decreased hemoglobin	—	2
Back pain	—	2
Facial edema	—	2
Fever	—	4
Increased ALT	1	1
Infection	—	3
Pain	—	11
Sore throat	—	2
Surgery	—	3

[a] Occurring in 2 or more patients.
[b] These events occurred in separate patients.

Eight patients experienced 10 postoperative serious adverse reactions: one with subdural hematoma and intracerebral bleeding following intracranial surgery related to an underlying cerebrovascular abnormality; one with 2 occurrences of GI bleeding following gastrojejunal bypass; and one each with facial edema, infection, menorrhagia requiring hysterectomy following hysteroscopy and dilation and curettage, pulmonary embolus, pyelonephritis, and sepsis.

➤*Wilate*: The most serious adverse reactions to treatment with AHF/von Willebrand disease in patients with von Willebrand disease have been hypersensitivity reactions.

There were 92 von Willebrand disease patients who received *Wilate* on 5,676 occasions, including clinical studies that involved prophylactic use, treatment on demand, surgery, and pharmacokinetics. Their safety data showed that the most common adverse reactions were urticaria and dizziness (each with 2 patients; 2.2%). There were also 4 (4.4%) patients who showed seroconversion for antibodies to parvovirus B19 not accompanied by clinical signs of disease. Seroconversion has not been reported since implementation of minipool testing of plasma used for the manufacture of *Wilate*.

➤*Postmarketing:* Adverse reactions reported in patients receiving AHF/VWF for treatment of von Willebrand disease or hemophilia A are allergic-anaphylactic reactions (including chest tightness, edema, pruritus, rash, shock, and urticaria), development of inhibitors to factor VIII, and hemolysis. Additional adverse reactions reported for von Willebrand disease are chills and fever, dyspnea, nausea, vomiting, cough, hypervolemia, and thromboembolic complications.

Patient Information

Advise patients that some viruses, such as parvovirus B19 or hepatitis A, are particularly difficult to remove or inactivate at this time. Parvovirus B19 may most seriously affect pregnant women or immune-compromised individuals.

Inform patients that although the overwhelming number of hepatitis A and parvovirus B19 cases are community acquired, there have been reports of these infections associated with the use of some plasma-derived products. Therefore, be alert to the potential symptoms of parvovirus B19 and hepatitis A infections, and inform patients receiving plasma-derived products to report potential symptoms promptly.

Advise patients that symptoms of parvovirus B19 may include low-grade fever, rash, arthralgias, and transient symmetric, nondestructive arthritis. Diagnosis is often established by measuring B19-specific immunoglobulin M (IgM) and IgG antibodies. Symptoms of hepatitis A include anorexia, fatigue, jaundice, low-grade fever, nausea, and vomiting. A diagnosis may be established by determination of specific IgM antibodies.

Inform patients of the early signs of hypersensitivity reactions, including hives, generalized urticaria, tightness of the chest, wheezing, hypotension, and anaphylaxis. If allergic symptoms occur, instruct patients to discontinue the administration immediately and contact their health care provider.

Inform patients that undergoing multiple treatments with AHF/VWF may increase the risk of thrombotic events, thereby requiring frequent monitoring of plasma VWF:RCo and FVIII activities.

Inform patients that there is a potential of developing inhibitors to VWF, leading to an inadequate clinical response. Thus, if the expected VWF activity plasma levels are not attained, or if bleeding is not controlled with an adequate dose or repeated dosing, advise patients to contact their treating health care provider.

Inform patients that despite procedures for screening donors and plasma as well as those for inactivation or removal of infectious agents, the possibility of transmitting infective agents with plasma-derived products cannot be totally excluded.

HEMOSTATICS

Systemic

AMINOCAPROIC ACID

Rx	**Aminocaproic Acid** (VersaPharm)	**Tablets; oral:** 500 mg	(VP 045). White, scored. In 100s.
Rx	**Amicar** (Xanodyne)		(XP A 10). White, round, scored. In 100s.
Rx	**Amicar** (Xanodyne)	**Tablets; oral:** 1,000 mg	(XP A 20). White, oblong, scored. In 100s.
Rx	**Aminocaproic Acid** (VersaPharm)	**Solution; oral:** 250 mg/mL	Saccharin, sorbitol, parabens. Raspberry flavor. In 237 and 473 mL.
Rx	**Amicar** (Xanodyne)		Parabens, edetate disodium 0.3%, saccharin, sorbitol. Raspberry flavor. In 473 mL.
Rx	**Aminocaproic Acid** (Various, eg, American Regent, Hospira)	**Injection:** 250 mg/mL	In 20 mL vials.

AMINOCAPROIC ACID — ORAL

Indications

➤*Excessive bleeding:* Aminocaproic acid is useful in enhancing hemostasis when fibrinolysis contributes to bleeding. In life-threatening situations, fresh whole blood transfusions, fibrinogen infusions, and other emergency measures may be required.

➤*Off-label uses:*

Amegakaryocytic thrombocytopenic hemorrhage – [4] = Insufficient documentation. Initial data from case reports suggest that aminocaproic acid may be beneficial in controlling acute bleeding episodes and reducing the need for platelet transfusions in patients with amegakaryocytic thrombocytopenia. However, larger, controlled trials are needed to verify results and determine optimal dosing. (See Administration and Dosage.)

Other possible off-label uses – Oral or intravenous (IV) aminocaproic acid, 36 g/day in 6 divided doses, has been used to prevent recurrence of subarachnoid hemorrhage (SAH).

To abort and prevent attacks of hereditary angioneurotic edema.

In patients with acute promyelocytic leukemia who develop coagulopathy associated with low levels of alpha-2 – plasmin inhibitor.

To reduce postsurgical bleeding complications in patients undergoing cardiopulmonary bypass procedures (eg, 5 g IV followed by 1 g/h infusions for 6 to 8 hours).

Administration and Dosage

➤*General dosing considerations:* If the patient is able to take medication by mouth, an identical dosage regimen (to the injection) may be followed by administering aminocaproic acid tablets or aminocaproic acid syrup, 25%.

AMINOCAPROIC ACID — ORAL

➤*Adults:*

Excessive bleeding –

Initial dosage: 5 g to be administered during the first hour of treatment.

Maintenance dosage: A continuing rate of 1 g (tablet) or 1.25 g (syrup) per hour. This method of treatment would ordinarily be continued for about 8 hours or until the bleeding situation has been controlled.

Off-label dosing –

Amegakaryocytic thrombocytopenic hemorrhage: [4] = Insufficient documentation. A variety of oral and IV doses were used. For long-term therapy, doses ranging from 2 to 24 g/day were studied for as long as 13 months.

➤*Renal function impairment:* Administer with caution.

➤*Hepatic function impairment:* Administer with caution.

➤*Storage/Stability:* Store between 15° to 30°C (59° to 86°F). Dispense in tight containers. Do not freeze.

Actions

➤*Pharmacology:* The fibrinolysis-inhibitory effects of aminocaproic acid appear to be exerted principally via inhibition of plasminogen activators and to a lesser degree through antiplasmin activity.

➤*Pharmacokinetics:*

Absorption – In adults, oral absorption appears to be a zero-order process with an absorption rate of 5.2 g/hr. The mean lag time in absorption is 10 minutes. After a single oral dose of 5 g, absorption was complete (F = 1). Mean ± SD peak plasma concentrations (164 ± 28 mcg/mL) were reached within 1.2 ± 0.45 hours. A single IV dose has a duration of action of less than 3 hours.

Distribution – After oral administration, the apparent volume of distribution was estimated to be 23.1 ± 6.6 L (mean ± SD). Correspondingly, the volume of distribution after intravenous administration has been reported to be 30 ± 8.2 L. After prolonged administration, aminocaproic acid has been found to distribute throughout extravascular and intravascular compartments of the body, penetrating human red blood cells as well as other tissue cells.

Excretion – Renal excretion is the primary route of elimination, whether aminocaproic acid is administered orally or intravenously. Sixty-five percent of the dose is recovered in the urine as unchanged drug and 11% of the dose appears as the metabolite adipic acid. Renal clearance (116 mL/min) approximates endogenous creatinine clearance. The total body clearance is 169 mL/min. The terminal elimination half-life for aminocaproic acid is approximately 2 hours.

Contraindications

Evidence of an active intravascular clotting process.

When there is uncertainty as to whether the cause of bleeding is primary fibrinolysis or disseminated intravascular coagulation (DIC), this distinction must be made before administering aminocaproic acid because aminocaproic acid administered to a patient with DIC may produce potentially fatal thrombus formation.

Aminocaproic acid must not be used in the presence of DIC without concomitant heparin.

Warnings/Precautions

➤*Upper urinary tract bleeding:* In patients with upper urinary tract bleeding, aminocaproic acid administration has been known to cause intrarenal obstruction in the form of glomerular capillary thrombosis or clots in the renal pelvis and ureters. For this reason, aminocaproic acid should not be used in hematuria of upper urinary tract origin, unless the possible benefits outweigh the risk.

➤*Skeletal muscle weakness:* Rarely, skeletal muscle weakness with necrosis of muscle fibers has been reported following prolonged administration. Clinical presentation may range from mild myalgias with weakness and fatigue to a severe proximal myopathy with rhabdomyolysis, myoglobinuria, and acute renal failure. Muscle enzymes, especially creatine phosphokinase (CPK) are elevated. CPK levels should be monitored in patients on long-term therapy. Aminocaproic acid administration should be stopped if a rise in CPK is noted. Resolution follows discontinuation of aminocaproic acid; however, the syndrome may recur if aminocaproic acid is restarted.

➤*Cardiac/Hepatic lesions:* The possibility of cardiac muscle damage should also be considered when skeletal myopathy occurs. One case of cardiac and hepatic lesions observed in man has been reported. The patient received 2 g of aminocaproic acid every 6 hours for a total dose of 26 g. Death was due to continued cerebrovascular hemorrhage. Necrotic changes in the heart and liver were noted at autopsy.

➤*Hyperfibrinolysis:* Aminocaproic acid inhibits both the action of plasminogen activators and to a lesser degree, plasmin activity. The drug should not be administered without a definite diagnosis and/or laboratory finding indicative of hyperfibrinolysis (hyperplasminemia).

Fibrinolysis is a normal process, presumably active at all times to ensure the fluidity of blood. Inhibition of fibrinolysis by aminocaproic acid may theoretically result in clotting or thrombosis. However, there is no definite evidence that administration of aminocaproic acid has been responsible for the few reported cases of intravascular clotting which followed this treatment. Rather, it appears that such intravascular clotting was most likely due to the patient's preexisting clinical condition, eg, the presence of DIC. It has been postulated that extravascular clots formed in vivo may not undergo spontaneous lysis as do normal clots.

➤*Neurological events:* Reports have appeared in the literature of an increased incidence of certain neurological deficits such as hydrocephalus, cerebral ischemia, or cerebral vasospasm associated with the use of antifibrinolytic agents in the treatment of subarachnoid hemorrhage (SAH). All of these events have also been described as part of the natural course of SAH, or as a consequence of diagnostic procedures such as angiography. Drug relatedness remains unclear.

➤*Thrombophlebitis:* Thrombophlebitis, a possibility with all intravenous therapy, should be guarded against by strict attention to the proper insertion of the needle and the fixing of its position.

➤*Thrombosis:* Epsilon-aminocaproic acid should not be administered with Factor IX Complex concentrates or Anti-Inhibitor Coagulant concentrates, as the risk of thrombosis may be increased.

➤*Special risk:*

Cardiac, hepatic or renal disease – Administer with caution to these patients. Animal pathology has shown endocardial hemorrhages, myocardial fat degeneration, and kidney concretions.

Subendocardial hemorrhages have been observed in dogs given intravenous infusions of 0.2 times the maximum human therapeutic dose of aminocaproic acid and in monkeys given 8 times the maximum human therapeutic dose of aminocaproic acid.

Fatty degeneration of the myocardium has been reported in dogs given intravenous doses of aminocaproic acid at 0.8 to 3.3 times the maximum human therapeutic dose and in monkeys given intravenous doses of aminocaproic acid at 6 times the maximum human therapeutic dose.

➤*Pregnancy: Category C.* Animal teratological studies have not been conducted with aminocaproic acid. It is also not known whether aminocaproic acid can cause fetal harm when administered to a pregnant woman or can affect reproduction capacity. Aminocaproic acid should be given to a pregnant woman only if clearly needed.

➤*Lactation:* It is not known whether this drug is excreted in human milk. Because many drugs are excreted in human milk, caution should be exercised when aminocaproic acid is administered to a nursing woman.

➤*Children:* Safety and effectiveness in pediatric patients have not been established.

➤*Lab test abnormalities:* The use of aminocaproic acid should be accompanied by tests designed to determine the amount of fibrinolysis present. There are presently available: general tests such as those for the determination of the lysis of a clot of blood or plasma; and more specific tests for the study of various phases of fibrinolytic mechanisms.

These latter tests include both semiquantitative and quantitative techniques for the determination of profibrinolysin, fibrinolysin, and antifibrinolysin.

Drug Interactions

➤*Oral contraceptives or estrogens:* An increase in clotting factors leading to a hypercoagulable state may be produced by coadministration.

➤*Drug/Lab test interactions:* Prolongation of the template bleeding time has been reported during continuous intravenous infusion of aminocaproic acid at dosages exceeding 24 g/day. Platelet function studies in these patients have not demonstrated any significant platelet dysfunction. However, in vitro studies have shown that at high concentrations (7.4 mmol/L or 0.97 mg/mL and greater) EACA inhibits ADP and collagen-induced platelet aggregation, the release of ATP and serotonin, and the binding of fibrinogen to the platelets in a concentration-response manner. Following a 10 g bolus of aminocaproic acid, transient peak plasma concentrations of 4.6 mmol/L or 0.6 mg/mL have been obtained. The concentration of aminocaproic acid necessary to maintain inhibition of fibrinolysis is 0.99 mmol/L or 0.13 mg/mL. Administration of a 5 g bolus followed by 1 to 1.25 g/hr should achieve and sustain plasma levels of 0.13 mg/mL. Thus, concentrations which have been obtained in vivo clinically in patients with normal renal function are considerably lower than the in vitro concentrations found to induce abnormalities in platelet function tests. However, higher plasma concentrations of aminocaproic acid may occur in patients with severe renal failure.

Serum potassium may be elevated by aminocaproic acid, especially in patients with impaired renal function.

Adverse Reactions

Aminocaproic acid is generally well tolerated. The following adverse experiences have been reported:

➤*Cardiovascular:* Bradycardia; hypotension; peripheral ischemia; thrombosis.

➤*CNS:* Confusion; convulsions; delirium; dizziness; hallucinations; intracranial hypertension; stroke; syncope. Two cases of convulsions following IV administration have been reported.

➤*Dermatologic:* Pruritus; rash.

➤*GI:* Abdominal pain; diarrhea; nausea; vomiting.

➤*GU:* BUN increased; renal failure.

➤*Hematologic:* Agranulocytosis; coagulation disorder; leukopenia; thrombocytopenia.

➤*Hypersensitivity:* Allergic and anaphylactoid reactions; anaphylaxis.

➤*Local:* Injection site reactions; pain and necrosis.

➤*Musculoskeletal:* CPK increased; muscle weakness; myalgia; myopathy (see Warnings); myositis; rhabdomyolysis.

AMINOCAPROIC ACID — ORAL

➤*Respiratory:* Dyspnea; nasal congestion; pulmonary embolism.

➤*Special senses:* Tinnitus; vision decreased; watery eyes.

➤*Miscellaneous:* Edema; headache; malaise.

There have been some reports of dry ejaculation during the period of aminocaproic acid treatment. These have been reported to date only in hemophilia patients who received the drug after undergoing dental surgical procedures. However, this symptom resolved in all patients within 24 to 48 hours of completion of therapy.

There have been reports of an increased incidence of certain neurological deficits (eg, hydrocephalus, cerebral ischemia, cerebral vasospasm) associated with use of fibrinolytic agents in the treatment of SAH. All of these events have also been described as part of the natural course of SAH, or as a consequence of diagnostic procedures such as angiography. Drug relatedness remains unclear.

Overdosage

A few cases of acute overdosage with aminocaproic acid have been reported with the injection formulation. See the aminocaproic acid injection monograph for specific details.

The intravenous and oral LD_{50} of aminocaproic acid were 3 and 12 g/kg, respectively, in the mouse and 3.2 and 16.4 g/kg, respectively, in the rat. An intravenous infusion dose of 2.3 g/kg was lethal in the dog. On intravenous administration, tonic-clonic convulsions were observed in dogs and mice. No treatment for overdosage is known, although evidence exists that aminocaproic acid is removed by hemodialysis and may be removed by peritoneal dialysis. Pharmacokinetic studies have shown that total body clearance of aminocaproic acid is markedly decreased in patients with severe renal failure.

AMINOCAPROIC ACID — INJECTION

Indications

➤*Excessive bleeding:* Aminocaproic acid is useful in enhancing hemostasis when fibrinolysis contributes to bleeding. In life-threatening situations, fresh whole blood transfusions, fibrinogen infusions, and other emergency measures may be required.

➤*Off-label uses:*

Amegakaryocytic thrombocytopenic hemorrhage – [4] = Insufficient documentation. Initial data from case reports suggest that aminocaproic acid may be beneficial in controlling acute bleeding episodes and reducing the need for platelet transfusions in patients with amegakaryocytic thrombocytopenia. However, larger, controlled trials are needed to verify results and determine optimal dosing. (See Administration and Dosage.)

Postsurgical bleeding complication – [2] = Fair documentation. Guidelines are available recommending the use of aminocaproic acid to decrease blood loss during cardiac surgeries. Although this drug has been shown to decrease total blood loss, it has not consistently reduced the need for blood transfusions in patients undergoing various surgeries. Administering aminocaproic acid throughout the perioperative period has been shown to be more beneficial than giving it solely postoperatively to decrease bleeding complications. (See Administration and Dosage.)

Other possible off-label uses – Oral or intravenous (IV) aminocaproic acid, 36 g/day in 6 divided doses, has been used to prevent recurrence of subarachnoid hemorrhage (SAH).

To abort and prevent attacks of hereditary angioneurotic edema.

In patients with acute promyelocytic leukemia who develop coagulopathy associated with low levels of alpha-2–plasmin inhibitor.

Administration and Dosage

➤*General dosing considerations:* Rapid injection of aminocaproic acid injection undiluted into a vein is not recommended (see Administration).

➤*Adults:*

Excessive bleeding –

Usual dosage: For the treatment of acute bleeding syndromes due to elevated fibrinolytic activity, it is suggested that 16 to 20 mL (4 to 5 g) of aminocaproic acid injection in 250 mL of diluent be administered by infusion during the first hour of treatment, followed by a continuing infusion at the rate of 4 mL (1 g) per hour in 50 mL of diluent. This method of treatment would ordinarily be continued for about 8 hours or until the bleeding situation has been controlled.

Maximum dose: Administration of more than 30 g per 24 hours is not recommended.

Initial dosage: 5 g, followed by 1 to 1.25 g hourly, should achieve and sustain drug plasma levels at 0.13 mg/mL. This is the concentration apparently necessary for inhibition of fibrinolysis.

Off-label dosing –

Amegakaryocytic thrombocytopenic hemorrhage: [4] = Insufficient documentation. A variety of oral and IV doses were used. For long-term therapy, doses ranging from 2 to 24 g/day were studied for as long as 13 months.

Postsurgical bleeding complication: [2] = Fair documentation. A variety of doses have been used, depending on the type of surgery. The following are common regimens.

- *Preoperatively for cardiac surgery* –
  Loading dose: 100 mg/kg given over 30 minutes.
  Maintenance dosage: 1 g/h started before the surgical procedure, with 10 g incorporated into the cardiopulmonary bypass solution.
- *Postoperatively for cardiac surgery* –
  Loading dose: 5 g.
  Maintenance dosage: 1.25 g/h for 4 hours.
- *Orthopedic surgery* –
  IV bolus: 5 to 10 g or 150 mg/kg before surgery.
  Maintenance dose: 5 g or 12.5 to 15 mg/kg/h prior to or during the procedure for 3 to 5 hours.

➤*Renal function impairment:* Administer with caution.

➤*Hepatic function impairment:* Administer with caution.

➤*Administration:* Aminocaproic acid injection is administered by infusion, utilizing the usual compatible intravenous vehicles. Rapid injection of aminocaproic acid injection undiluted into a vein is not recommended. Hypotension, bradycardia, or arrhythmia may result.

➤*Admixture compatibility:* Compatible with the following IV vehicles: sterile water for injection, sodium chloride for injection, dextrose 5% or Ringer's injection. Although sterile water for injection is compatible for IV injection, the resultant solution is hypo-osmolar.

➤*Storage/Stability:* Store between 15° and 30°C (59° and 86°F). Do not freeze.

Actions

➤*Pharmacology:* The fibrinolysis-inhibitory effects of aminocaproic acid appear to be exerted principally via inhibition of plasminogen activators and to a lesser degree through antiplasmin activity.

➤*Pharmacokinetics:*

Distribution – After oral administration, the apparent volume of distribution was estimated to be 23.1 ± 6.6 L (mean ± SD). Correspondingly, the volume of distribution after intravenous administration has been reported to be 30 ± 8.2 L. After prolonged administration, aminocaproic acid has been found to distribute throughout extravascular and intravascular compartments of the body, penetrating human red blood cells as well as other tissue cells.

Metabolism – A single IV dose has a duration of action less than 3 hours.

Excretion – Renal excretion is the primary route of elimination, whether aminocaproic acid is administered orally or intravenously. Sixty-five percent of the dose is recovered in the urine as unchanged drug and 11% of the dose appears as the metabolite adipic acid. Renal clearance (116 mL/min) approximates endogenous creatinine clearance. The total body clearance is 169 mL/min. The terminal elimination half-life for aminocaproic acid is approximately 2 hours.

Contraindications

Evidence of an active intravascular clotting process.

When there is uncertainty as to whether the cause of bleeding is primary fibrinolysis or disseminated intravascular coagulation (DIC), this distinction must be made before administering aminocaproic acid because aminocaproic acid administered to a patient with DIC may produce potentially fatal thrombus formation.

Aminocaproic acid must not be used in the presence of DIC without concomitant heparin.

Warnings/Precautions

➤*Upper urinary tract bleeding:* In patients with upper urinary tract bleeding, aminocaproic acid administration has been known to cause intrarenal obstruction in the form of glomerular capillary thrombosis or clots in the renal pelvis and ureters. For this reason, aminocaproic acid should not be used in hematuria of upper urinary tract origin, unless the possible benefits outweigh the risk.

Subendocardial hemorrhages have been observed in dogs given intravenous infusions of 0.2 times the maximum human therapeutic dose of aminocaproic acid and in monkeys given 8 times the maximum human therapeutic dose of aminocaproic acid.

Fatty degeneration of the myocardium has been reported in dogs given intravenous doses of aminocaproic acid at 0.8 to 3.3 times the maximum human therapeutic dose and in monkeys given intravenous doses of aminocaproic acid at 6 times the maximum human therapeutic dose.

➤*Skeletal muscle weakness:* Rarely, skeletal muscle weakness with necrosis of muscle fibers has been reported following prolonged administration. Clinical presentation may range from mild myalgias with weakness and fatigue to a severe proximal myopathy with rhabdomyolysis, myoglobinuria, and acute renal failure. Muscle enzymes, especially creatine phosphokinase (CPK) are elevated. CPK levels should be monitored in patients on long-term therapy. Aminocaproic acid administration should be stopped if a rise in CPK is noted. Resolution follows discontinuation of aminocaproic acid; however, the syndrome may recur if aminocaproic acid is restarted.

➤*Cardiac and hepatic lesions:* The possibility of cardiac muscle damage should also be considered when skeletal myopathy occurs. One case of cardiac and hepatic lesions observed in man has been reported. The patient received 2 g of aminocaproic acid every 6 hours for a total dose of 26 g. Death was due to continued cerebrovascular hemorrhage. Necrotic changes in the heart and liver were noted at autopsy.

AMINOCAPROIC ACID — INJECTION

➤*Benzyl alcohol:* Aminocaproic acid injection contains benzyl alcohol as a preservative and is not recommended for use in newborns.

➤*Hyperfibrinolysis:* Aminocaproic acid inhibits both the action of plasminogen activators and to a lesser degree, plasmin activity. The drug should not be administered without a definite diagnosis or laboratory finding indicative of hyperfibrinolysis (hyperplasminemia).

Fibrinolysis is a normal process, presumably active at all times to ensure the fluidity of blood. Inhibition of fibrinolysis by aminocaproic acid may theoretically result in clotting or thrombosis. However, there is no definite evidence that administration of aminocaproic acid has been responsible for the few reported cases of intravascular clotting which followed this treatment. Rather, it appears that such intravascular clotting was most likely due to the patient's preexisting clinical condition, eg, the presence of DIC. It has been postulated that extravascular clots formed in vivo may not undergo spontaneous lysis as do normal clots.

➤*Neurologic events:* Reports have appeared in the literature of an increased incidence of certain neurological deficits such as hydrocephalus, cerebral ischemia, or cerebral vasospasm associated with the use of antifibrinolytic agents in the treatment of subarachnoid hemorrhage (SAH). All of these events have also been described as part of the natural course of SAH, or as a consequence of diagnostic procedures such as angiography. Drug relatedness remains unclear.

➤*Thrombophlebitis:* Thrombophlebitis, a possibility with all intravenous therapy, should be guarded against by strict attention to the proper insertion of the needle and the fixing of its position.

➤*Thrombosis:* Thrombosis with severe sequelae (acute myocardial infarction, gangreno) has been rarely reported in patients with hemophilia receiving combined treatment with Factor IX concentrate and aminocaproic acid. Aminocaproic acid should not be administered concomitantly with prothrombin complex concentrates or with activated prothrombin concentrates unless the increased risk of thrombosis is outweighed by the anticipated clinical benefit.

Epsilon-aminocaproic acid should not be administered with Factor IX complex concentrates or anti-inhibitor coagulant concentrates, as the risk of thrombosis may be increased.

➤*Special risk:*

Cardiac, hepatic, or renal disease – Administer with caution to these patients. Animal pathology has shown endocardial hemorrhages, myocardial fat degeneration, and kidney concretions.

➤*Pregnancy: Category C.* Animal teratological studies have not been conducted with aminocaproic acid. It is also not known whether aminocaproic acid can cause fetal harm when administered to a pregnant woman or can affect reproduction capacity. Aminocaproic acid should be given to a pregnant woman only if clearly needed.

➤*Lactation:* It is not known whether this drug is excreted in human milk. Because many drugs are excreted in human milk, caution should be exercised when aminocaproic acid is administered to a nursing woman.

➤*Children:* Safety and effectiveness in pediatric patients have not been established.

➤*Lab test abnormalities:* The use of aminocaproic acid should be accompanied by tests designed to determine the amount of fibrinolysis present. There are presently available: General tests such as those for the determination of the lysis of a clot of blood or plasma; and more specific tests for the study of various phases of fibrinolytic mechanisms.

These latter tests include both semiquantitative and quantitative techniques for the determination of profibrinolysin, fibrinolysin, and antifibrinolysin.

Drug Interactions

➤*Drug/Lab test interactions:* Prolongation of the template bleeding time has been reported during continuous IV infusion of aminocaproic acid at dosages exceeding 24 g/day. Platelet function studies in these patients have not demonstrated any significant platelet dysfunction. However, in vitro studies have shown that at high concentrations (7.4 mMol/L or 0.97 mg/mL or greater) EACA inhibits ADP and collagen-induced platelet aggregation, the release of ATP and serotonin, and the binding of fibrinogen to the platelets in a concentration-response manner. Following a 10 g bolus of aminocaproic acid, transient peak plasma concentrations of 4.6 mMol/L or 0.6 mg/mL have been obtained. The concentration of aminocaproic acid necessary to maintain inhibition of fibrinolysis is 0.99 mMol/L or 0.13 mg/mL. Administration of a 5 g bolus followed by 1 to 1.25 g/hr should achieve and sustain plasma levels of 0.13 mg/mL. Thus, concentrations which have been obtained in vivo clinically in patients with normal renal function are considerably lower than the in vitro concentrations found to induce abnormalities in platelet function tests. However, higher plasma concentrations of aminocaproic acid may occur in patients with severe renal failure.

Adverse Reactions

Aminocaproic acid is generally well tolerated. The following adverse reactions have been reported:

➤*Cardiovascular:* Bradycardia; hypotension; peripheral ischemia; thrombosis.

➤*CNS:* Confusion; convulsions; delirium; dizziness; hallucinations; intracranial hypertension; stroke; syncope.

➤*Dermatologic:* Pruritus; rash.

➤*GI:* Abdominal pain; diarrhea; nausea; vomiting.

➤*GU:* BUN increased; renal failure.

➤*Hematologic:* Agranulocytosis; coagulation disorder; leukopenia; thrombocytopenia.

➤*Hypersensitivity:* Allergic and anaphylactoid reactions; anaphylaxis.

➤*Local:* Injection site reactions; pain and necrosis.

➤*Musculoskeletal:* CPK increased; muscle weakness; myalgia; myopathy; myositis; rhabdomyolysis.

➤*Respiratory:* Dyspnea; nasal congestion; pulmonary embolism.

➤*Special senses:* Tinnitus; vision decreased; watery eyes.

➤*Miscellaneous:* Edema; headache; malaise.

There have been some reports of dry ejaculation during the period of aminocaproic acid treatment. These have been reported to date only in hemophilia patients who received the drug after undergoing dental surgical procedures. However, this symptom resolved in all patients within 24 to 48 hours of completion of therapy.

There have been reports of an increased incidence of certain neurological deficits (eg, hydrocephalus, cerebral ischemia, cerebral vasospasm) associated with use of fibrinolytic agents in the treatment of SAH. All of these events have also been described as part of the natural course of SAH, or as a consequence of diagnostic procedures such as angiography. Drug relatedness remains unclear.

Overdosage

➤*Symptoms:* A few cases of acute overdosage with aminocaproic acid administered intravenously have been reported. The effects have ranged from no reaction to transient hypotension to severe acute renal failure leading to death. One patient with a history of brain tumor and seizures experienced seizures after receiving an 8 g bolus injection of aminocaproic acid. The single dose of aminocaproic acid causing symptoms of overdosage or considered to be life-threatening is unknown. Patients have tolerated doses as high as 100 grams while acute renal failure has been reported following a dose of 12 g.

➤*Treatment:* The intravenous and oral LD_{50} of aminocaproic acid were 3 and 12 g/kg, respectively, in the mouse and 3.2 and 16.4 g/kg, respectively, in the rat. An intravenous infusion dose of 2.3 g/kg was lethal in the dog. On intravenous administration, tonic-clonic convulsions were observed in dogs and mice. No treatment for overdosage is known, although evidence exists that aminocaproic acid is removed by hemodialysis and may be removed by peritoneal dialysis. Pharmacokinetic studies have shown that total body clearance of aminocaproic acid is markedly decreased in patients with severe renal failure.

FIBRINOGEN CONCENTRATE (HUMAN)

Rx	**RiaSTAP** (CSL Behring)	**Injection; lyophilized powder for solution:** ≈ 1 g (900 to 1,300 mg)	Preservative free. Albumin 400 to 700 mg. In single-use vials.

FIBRINOGEN CONCENTRATE (HUMAN) — INJECTION

Indications

➤*Fibrinogen deficiency:* For the treatment of acute bleeding episodes in patients with congenital fibrinogen deficiency, including afibrinogenemia and hypofibrinogenemia.

Administration and Dosage

➤*General dosing considerations:* Fibrinogen dosing, duration of dosing, and frequency of administration should be individualized based on the extent of bleeding, laboratory values, and the clinical condition of the patient.

Monitoring of patient's fibrinogen level is recommended during treatment.

➤*Adults:*

Fibrinogen deficiency –

Usual dosage:

• *Baseline fibrinogen level is known* – Dose should be individually calculated for each patient based on the target plasma fibrinogen level, based on the type of bleeding, actual measured plasma fibrinogen level, and body weight using the following formula:

$$\frac{\text{Target level (mg/dL)} - \text{measured level (mg/dL)}}{\text{1.7 (mg/dL per mg/kg body weight)}}$$

• *Fibrinogen dose when baseline fibrinogen level is not known* – 70 mg per kg of body weight administered intravenously (IV). A target fibrinogen level of 100 mg/dL should be maintained until hemostasis is obtained.

FIBRINOGEN CONCENTRATE (HUMAN) — INJECTION

➤*Children:*

Fibrinogen deficiency –

16 years of age and older: See Adults for dosing.

➤*Preparation for administration:* Do not use fibrinogen beyond the expiration date. Fibrinogen contains no preservative. Use aseptic technique when preparing and reconstituting fibrinogen.

Reconstitute fibrinogen at room temperature as follows:

1.) Remove the cap from the vial to expose the central portion of the rubber stopper.
2.) Clean the surface of the rubber stopper with an antiseptic solution and allow it to dry.
3.) Using an appropriate transfer device or syringe, transfer 50 mL of sterile water for injection into the vial.
4.) Gently swirl the vial to ensure the drug is fully dissolved. Do not shake the vial.

After reconstitution, the fibrinogen solution should be colorless and clear to slightly opalescent. Inspect visually for particulate matter and discoloration prior to administration. Do not use if the solution is cloudy or contains particulates. Do not freeze fibrinogen solution. Discard partially used vials.

Fibrinogen is stable for 24 hours after reconstitution when stored at 20° to 25°C (68° to 77°F) and should be administered within this time period.

➤*Administration:* Administer fibrinogen at room temperature by slow IV injection at a rate not exceeding 5 mL per minute.

➤*Admixture compatibility:* Do not mix fibrinogen with other medicinal products or IV solutions, and administer through a separate injection site.

➤*Storage / Stability:* When stored at temperatures of 2° to 25°C (36° to 77°F), fibrinogen is stable for the period indicated by the expiration date on the carton and vial label (up to 30 months). Keep fibrinogen in its original carton until ready to use. Do not freeze. Protect from light. After reconstitution, fibrinogen solution is stable for 24 hours when stored at 20° to 25°C and should be administered within this time period.

Actions

➤*Pharmacology:* Fibrinogen (factor I) is a soluble plasma glycoprotein with a molecular weight of approximately 340 kDa. The native molecule is a dimer and consists of 3 pairs of polypeptide chains (Aα, Bβ and γ). Fibrinogen is a physiological substrate of 3 enzymes: thrombin, factor XIIIa, and plasmin.

During the coagulation process, thrombin cleaves the Aα and Bβ chains, releasing fibrinopeptides A and B (FPA and FPB, respectively). FPA is separated rapidly and the remaining molecule is a soluble fibrin monomer (fibrin I). The slower removal of FPB results in formation of fibrin II, which is capable of polymerization that occurs by aggregation of fibrin monomers. The resulting fibrin is stabilized in the presence of calcium ions and by activated factor XIII, which acts as a transglutaminase. Factor XIIIa–induced cross-linking of fibrin polymers renders the fibrin clot more elastic and more resistant to fibrinolysis. Cross-linked fibrin is the end result of the coagulation cascade and provides tensile strength to a primary hemostatic platelet plug and structure to the vessel wall.

Pharmacodynamics – Administration of fibrinogen to patients with congenital fibrinogen deficiency replaces the missing, or low, coagulation factor. Normal levels are in the range of 200 to 450 mg/dL.

➤*Pharmacokinetics:* A prospective, open-label, uncontrolled, multicenter pharmacokinetic study was conducted in 5 females and 9 males with congenital fibrinogen deficiency (afibrinogenemia), ranging in age from 8 to 61 years (2 children, 3 adolescents, 9 adults). Each subject received a single IV dose of fibrinogen 70 mg/kg. Blood samples were drawn from the patients to determine the fibrinogen activity at baseline and up to 14 days after the infusion.

The incremental in vivo recovery was determined from levels obtained up to 4 hours after infusion. The median incremental in vivo recovery was 1.7 mg/dL (range, 1.3 to 2.73 mg/dL) increase per mg/kg. The median in vivo recovery indicates that a dose of 70 mg/kg will increase patients' fibrinogen plasma concentration by approximately 120 mg/dL.

The pharmacokinetic analysis using fibrinogen antigen data (ELISA) was concordant with the fibrinogen activity (Clauss assay).

Pharmacokinetic Parameters (n = 14) for Fibrinogen Activity[a]	
Parameters	Mean ± SD (range)
Half-life (hours)	78.7 ± 18.13 (55.73 to 117.26)
C_{max} (mg/dL)	140 ± 27 (100 to 210)
AUC for dose of 70 mg/kg (mg•h/mL)	124.3 ± 24.16 (81.73 to 156.4)
Clearance (mL/h/kg)	0.59 ± 0.13 (0.45 to 0.86)
Mean residence time (hours)	92.8 ± 20.11 (66.14 to 126.44)
Volume of distribution at steady state (mL/kg)	52.7 ± 7.48 (36.22 to 67.67)

[a] SD = standard deviation; C_{max} = maximum plasma concentration; AUC = area under the curve.

Special populations –

Children: Subjects younger than 16 years of age (n = 4) had shorter half-lives (69.9 ± 8.5 hours) and faster clearance (0.73 ± 0.14 mL/h/kg) compared with subjects older than 16 years of age. The number of subjects younger than 16 years of age in this study limits statistical interpretations.

Gender: No statistically relevant difference was observed between males and females for fibrinogen activity.

Contraindications

Severe, immediate hypersensitivity reactions, including anaphylaxis to fibrinogen or its components.

Warnings/Precautions

➤*Thrombosis:* Thrombosis may occur spontaneously in patients with congenital fibrinogen deficiency with or without the use of fibrinogen replacement therapy. Thromboembolic events have been reported in patients treated with fibrinogen. Weigh the benefits of fibrinogen administration versus the risk of thrombosis. Monitor patients receiving fibrinogen for signs and symptoms of thrombosis.

➤*Transmissible infectious agents:* Fibrinogen is made from human plasma. Products made from human plasma may contain infectious agents (eg, viruses and theoretically the Creutzfeldt-Jakob disease [CJD] agent) that can cause disease. The risk that such products will transmit an infectious agent has been reduced by screening plasma donors for prior exposure to certain viruses, by testing for the presence of certain current virus infections, and by a process demonstrated to inactivate and/or remove certain viruses during manufacturing. Despite these measures, such products may still potentially transmit disease. There is also the possibility that unknown infectious agents may be present in such products. Report all infections thought to possibly have been transmitted by this product to the manufacturer at 1-866-915-6958.

➤*Hypersensitivity reactions:* Allergic reactions may occur. If symptoms of allergic or early signs of hypersensitivity reactions (including hives, generalized urticaria, tightness of the chest, wheezing, hypotension, and anaphylaxis) occur, immediately discontinue fibrinogen administration. The treatment required depends on the nature and severity of the reaction.

➤*Pregnancy:* Category C. Animal reproduction studies have not been conducted with fibrinogen. It is not known whether fibrinogen can cause fetal harm when administered to a pregnant woman or can affect reproduction capacity. Use fibrinogen during pregnancy only if clearly needed.

➤*Lactation:* Fibrinogen has not been studied in breast-feeding mothers with congenital fibrinogen deficiency.

➤*Children:* Fibrinogen studies have included subjects younger than 16 years of age. In the pharmacokinetic study, 2 children (8 and 11 years of age) and 3 adolescents (12, 14, and 16 years of age) were studied. Subjects younger than 16 years of age (n = 4) had shorter half-lives (69.9 ± 8.5 hours) and faster clearance (0.7 ± 0.1 mg/L) compared with adults (half-life, 82.3 ± 20 hours; clearance, 0.53 ± 0.1 mg/L). The number of subjects younger than 16 years of age in this study limits statistical interpretation.

➤*Elderly:* The safety and efficacy of fibrinogen in elderly patients has not been studied. There were an insufficient number of subjects in this age group to determine whether they respond differently from younger subjects.

➤*Monitoring:* Monitor patients receiving fibrinogen for signs and symptoms of thrombosis.

Drug Interactions

None known.

Adverse Reactions

➤*Serious adverse reactions:* The most serious adverse reactions reported in clinical studies or through postmarketing surveillance following fibrinogen treatment were allergic-anaphylactic reactions and thromboembolic episodes, including arterial thrombosis, deep vein thrombosis, myocardial infarction, and pulmonary embolism.

➤*Common adverse reactions:* The most common adverse reactions observed in more than 1 subject in clinical studies (frequency greater than 1%) were fever and headache.

The most common adverse reactions reported in clinical studies or through postmarketing surveillance following fibrinogen treatment are allergic reactions and generalized reactions such as chills, nausea, and vomiting.

➤*Postmarketing:* Adverse reactions reported in patients receiving fibrinogen for treatment of fibrinogen deficiency include allergic-anaphylactic reactions (eg, dyspnea, rash); general reactions, such as chills, fever, nausea, vomiting; and thromboembolic complications, such as deep vein thrombosis, myocardial infarction, and pulmonary embolism.

The following adverse reactions, identified by system organ class, have shown a possible causal relationship with fibrinogen.

Allergic – Anaphylaxis, dyspnea, rash.

Cardiovascular – Pulmonary embolism, thromboembolism.

Miscellaneous – Chills, fever, nausea, vomiting.

Patient Information

Inform patients of the early signs of allergic or hypersensitivity reactions to fibrinogen, including hives, chest tightness, wheezing, hypotension, and anaphylaxis. Advise them to notify their health care provider immediately if they experience any of these symptoms.

Inform patients that thrombosis with or without embolization may be caused by underlying fibrinogen deficiency and has been reported with the use of fibrinogen. Advise them to report any symptoms of thrombotic events, such as unexplained pleuritic, chest, and/or leg pain or edema, hemoptysis, dyspnea, tachypnea, or unexplained neurologic symptoms, to their health care provider immediately.

Inform patients that fibrinogen is made from human plasma (part of the blood) and may contain infectious agents that can cause disease (eg, viruses

Systemic

FIBRINOGEN CONCENTRATE (HUMAN) — INJECTION

and, theoretically, the CJD agent). Explain that the risk that fibrinogen may transmit an infectious agent has been reduced by screening the plasma donors, by testing the donated plasma for certain virus infections, and by a process demonstrated to inactivate and/or remove certain viruses during manufacturing. Symptoms of a possible virus infection include headache, fever, nausea, vomiting, weakness, malaise, diarrhea, or, in the case of hepatitis, jaundice.

TRANEXAMIC ACID

Rx	**Lysteda** (Ferring)	**Tablets; oral:** 650 mg	(XP650). White, oval. In 30s, 100s, 500s, and UD 30s.
Rx	**Cyklokapron** (Pfizer)	**Injection:** 100 mg/mL	In 10 mL amps.

TRANEXAMIC ACID — ORAL

Indications

➤*Cyclic heavy menstrual bleeding:* For the treatment of cyclic heavy menstrual bleeding.

Administration and Dosage

➤*Adults:*

Cyclic heavy menstrual bleeding – Two 650 mg tablets taken 3 times daily (3,900 mg/day) for a maximum of 5 days during monthly menstruation.

➤*Renal function impairment:* In patients with renal impairment, the plasma concentration of tranexamic acid increased as serum creatinine concentration increased. Dosage adjustment is needed in patients with serum creatinine concentration higher than 1.4 mg/dL.

Dosage of Tranexamic Acid Oral in Patients With Renal Impairment

Serum creatinine (mg/dL)	Adjusted dose	Total daily dose
Creatinine > 1.4 and ≤ 2.8	1,300 mg 2 times a day for a maximum of 5 days during menstruation	2,600 mg
Creatinine > 2.8 and ≤ 5.7	1,300 mg once a day for a maximum of 5 days during menstruation	1,300 mg
Creatinine > 5.7	650 mg once a day for a maximum of 5 days during menstruation	650 mg

➤*Administration:* Tranexamic acid may be administered without regard to meals.

Tablets should be swallowed whole and not chewed or broken apart.

➤*Storage/Stability:* Store at 25°C (77°); excursions are permitted to 15° to 30°C (59° to 86°F).

Actions

➤*Pharmacology:* Tranexamic acid is a synthetic lysine amino acid derivative, which diminishes the dissolution of hemostatic fibrin by plasmin. In the presence of tranexamic acid, the lysine receptor binding sites of plasmin for fibrin are occupied, preventing binding to fibrin monomers, thus preserving and stabilizing fibrin's matrix structure.

The antifibrinolytic effects of tranexamic acid are mediated by reversible interactions at multiple binding sites within plasminogen. Native human plasminogen contains 4 to 5 lysine binding sites with low affinity for tranexamic acid (K_d = 750 mcmol/L) and 1 with high affinity (K_d = 1.1 mcmol/L). The high affinity lysine site of plasminogen is involved in its binding to fibrin. Saturation of the high affinity binding site with tranexamic acid displaces plasminogen from the surface of fibrin. Although plasmin may be formed by conformational changes in plasminogen, its binding to and dissolution of the fibrin matrix is inhibited.

➤*Pharmacokinetics:*

Absorption – After single oral dose of two 650 mg tablets of tranexamic acid, the peak plasma concentration (C_{max}) occurred at approximately 3 hours (T_{max}). The absolute bioavailability of tranexamic acid in women 18 to 49 years of age is approximately 45%. Following administration of multiple oral doses (two 650 mg tablets 3 times daily) of tranexamic acid for 5 days, the mean C_{max} increased by approximately 19% and the mean area under the curve (AUC) remained unchanged, compared with single oral dose administration (two 650 mg tablets). Plasma concentrations reached steady state at the 5th dose of tranexamic acid on day 2.

Tranexamic Acid Oral Pharmacokinetic Parameters[a]

Parameter	Arithmetic mean (CV%)	
	Single dose	Multiple dose
C_{max} (mcg/mL)	13.83 (32.14)	16.41 (26.19)
AUC_{tldc} (mcg•h/mL)	77.96 (31.14)	77.67 (29.39)
AUC_{inf} (mcg•h/mL)	80.19 (30.43)	—
T_{max} (h)[b]	2.5 (1 to 5)	2.5 (2 to 3.5)
t½ (h)	11.08 (16.94)	—

[a] AUC_{tldc} = area under the drug concentration curve from time 0 to time of last determinable concentration; $AUC_{0\text{-}tau}$ (mcg•h/mL) = area under the drug concentration curve from time 0 to 8 hours; AUC_{inf} = area under the drug concentration curve from time 0 to infinity; t½ = terminal elimination half-life.
[b] Data presented as median (range).

Effect of food: Tranexamic acid may be administered without regard to meals. Single dose administration (two 650 mg tablets) of tranexamic acid with food increased both C_{max} and AUC by 7% and 16%, respectively.

Distribution – Tranexamic acid is 3% bound to plasma proteins with no apparent binding to albumin. Initially, the volume of distribution of tranexamic acid is 0.18 L/kg and steady-state apparent volume of distribution is 0.39 L/kg.

Tranexamic acid crosses the placenta. The concentration in cord blood after an intravenous (IV) injection of 10 mg/kg to pregnant women is about 30 mg/L, as high as in the maternal blood.

Tranexamic acid concentration in cerebrospinal fluid is about one tenth of the plasma concentration.

The drug passes into the aqueous humor of the eye achieving a concentration of approximately one tenth of plasma concentrations.

Metabolism – A small fraction of the tranexamic acid is metabolized.

Excretion – Tranexamic acid is eliminated by urinary excretion primarily via glomerular filtration with more than 95% of the dose excreted unchanged. Excretion of tranexamic acid 10 mg/kg is about 90% at 24 hours after IV administration. Most of the elimination after IV administration occurred during the first 10 hours, giving an apparent elimination half-life of approximately 2 hours. The mean terminal half-life of tranexamic acid is approximately 11 hours. Plasma clearance of tranexamic acid is 110 to 116 mL/min.

Special populations –

Renal function impairment: The effect of renal impairment on the disposition of oral tranexamic acid has not been evaluated. Urinary excretion following a single IV injection of tranexamic acid declines as renal function decreases. Following a single IV injection of tranexamic acid 10 mg/kg in 28 patients, the 24-hour urinary fractions of tranexamic acid with serum creatinine concentrations 1.4 to 2.8, 2.8 to 5.7, and greater than 5.7 mg/dL were 51%, 39%, and 19%, respectively. The 24-hour tranexamic acid plasma concentrations for these patients demonstrated a direct relationship to the degree of renal impairment. Therefore, dose adjustment is needed in patients with renal impairment.

Contraindications

Active thromboembolic disease (eg, cerebral thrombosis, deep vein thrombosis, pulmonary embolism); a history of thrombosis or thromboembolism, including retinal vein or artery occlusion; an intrinsic risk of thrombosis or thromboembolism (eg, hypercoagulopathy, thrombogenic cardiac rhythm disease, thrombogenic valvular disease); known hypersensitivity to tranexamic acid.

Warnings/Precautions

➤*Thrombosis/Thromboembolism:* Venous and arterial thrombosis or thromboembolism, as well as cases of retinal artery and retinal vein occlusions, have been reported with tranexamic acid.

➤*Ocular effects:* Retinal venous and arterial occlusion has been reported in patients using tranexamic acid. Instruct patient to report visual and ocular symptoms promptly. In the event of such symptoms, instruct patient to discontinue tranexamic acid immediately and refer to an ophthalmologist for a complete ophthalmic evaluation, including dilated retinal examination, to exclude the possibility of retinal venous or arterial occlusion. Ligneous conjunctivitis also has been reported in patients taking tranexamic acid. The conjunctivitis resolved following cessation of the drug.

➤*Subarachnoid hemorrhage:* Cerebral edema and cerebral infarction may be caused by use of tranexamic acid in women with subarachnoid hemorrhage.

➤*Hypersensitivity reactions:* A case of severe allergic reaction to tranexamic acid was reported in the clinical trials, involving a subject who experienced dyspnea, tightening of her throat, and facial flushing that required emergency medical treatment. A case of anaphylactic shock has also been reported, involving a patient who received an IV bolus of tranexamic acid.

TRANEXAMIC ACID — ORAL

➤*Renal function impairment:* The effect of renal impairment on the pharmacokinetics of oral tranexamic acid has not been studied. Because tranexamic acid is primarily eliminated via the kidneys by glomerular filtration with more than 95% excreted as unchanged in the urine, dosage adjustment in patients with renal impairment is necessary.

➤*Hepatic function impairment:* The effect of hepatic impairment on the pharmacokinetics of tranexamic acid has not been studied. Because only a small fraction of the drug is metabolized, dosage adjustment in patients with hepatic impairment is not necessary.

➤*Pregnancy: Category B.* Tranexamic acid is not indicated for use in pregnant women. There are no adequate and well-controlled studies in pregnant women. Reproduction studies have been performed in mice, rats, and rabbits and have revealed no evidence of impaired fertility or harm to the fetus caused by tranexamic acid. However, tranexamic acid is known to cross the placenta and appears in cord blood at concentrations approximately equal to the maternal concentration.

➤*Lactation:* Tranexamic acid is present in breast milk at a concentration of about one hundredth of the corresponding serum concentration. Use tranexamic acid during lactation only if clearly needed.

➤*Children:* Tranexamic acid is indicated for women of reproductive age and is not intended for use in premenarcheal girls. Tranexamic acid has not been studied in adolescents younger than 18 years of age with heavy menstrual bleeding.

➤*Elderly:* Tranexamic acid is indicated for women of reproductive age and is not intended for use by postmenopausal women.

➤*Monitoring:* Monitor for symptoms of severe allergic reaction and changes in vision.

Drug Interactions

Tranexamic Acid Drug Interactions

Precipitant Drug	Object Drug[a]		Description
Tissue plasminogen activators	Tranexamic acid	↓	Coadministration may decrease the efficacy of both tranexamic acid and tissue plasminogen activators. Use with caution. Additional clinical monitoring is warranted.
Tranexamic acid	Tissue plasminogen activators		
Tranexamic acid	Factor IX complex concentrates or anti-inhibitor coagulant concentrates	↑	Coadministration of tranexamic acid and factor IX complex concentrates or anti-inhibitor coagulant concentrates may increase the risk of thrombosis. Avoid coadministration.
Tranexamic acid	Hormonal contraceptives	↑	Coadministration of tranexamic acid and hormonal contraceptives may exacerbate the increased thrombotic risk associated with combination hormonal contraceptives. Coadminister only if there is a strong medical need and if the benefit of treatment outweighs the potential for the increased risk of a thrombotic event. Additional clinical monitoring is warranted.
Tranexamic acid	Tretinoin	↑	Coadministration of tretinoin with tranexamic acid may increase the risk of severe thromboembolic reactions. Use with caution. Additional clinical monitoring is warranted.

[a] ↑ = object drug increased; ↓ = object drug decreased.

➤*Drug/Food interactions:* A single dose administration of tranexamic acid 1,300 mg with food increased the C_{max} and AUC 7% and 16%, respectively. However, tranexamic acid may be given without regard to meals.

Adverse Reactions

➤*Short-term studies:*

Adverse reactions (at least 5%) –

Tranexamic Acid Oral Adverse Reactions (≥ 5%)

Adverse reactions	Tranexamic acid 3,900 mg/day (n = 232)	Placebo (n = 139)
Total number of adverse reactions	1,500	923
Subjects with ≥ 1 adverse reaction	89.7%	87.8%
CNS		
Fatigue	5.2%	4.3%
Headache[a]	50.4%	46.8%
Migraine	6%	5.8%
Musculoskeletal		
Arthralgia[b]	6.9%	5%
Back pain	20.7%	15.1%
Muscle cramps and spasms	6.5%	5.8%
Musculoskeletal pain[c]	11.2%	2.9%
Miscellaneous		
Abdominal pain[d]	19.8%	18%
Anemia	5.6%	3.6%
Nasal and sinus symptoms[e]	25.4%	17.3%

[a] Includes headache and tension headache.
[b] Arthralgia includes joint stiffness and swelling.
[c] Musculoskeletal pain includes musculoskeletal discomfort and myalgia.
[d] Abdominal pain includes abdominal tenderness and discomfort.
[e] Nasal and sinus symptoms include nasal, respiratory tract and sinus congestion, sinusitis, acute sinusitis, sinus headache, allergic sinusitis and sinus pain, and multiple allergies and seasonal allergies.

➤*Long-term studies:*

Discontinuation of therapy – A total of 12.4% of the subjects withdrew because of adverse reactions in the 2 open-label studies. A total of 2.1% of the subjects in the long-term, open-label, extension study withdrew because of adverse reactions.

Adverse reactions – The types and severity of adverse reactions in these 2 long-term open-label trials were similar to those observed in the double-blind, placebo-controlled studies, although the percentage of subjects reporting them was greater in the 27-month study, most likely because of the longer study duration.

Hypersensitivity – A case of severe allergic reaction to tranexamic acid was reported in the extension trial, involving a subject on her fourth cycle of treatment who experienced dyspnea, tightening of her throat, and facial flushing that required emergency medical treatment.

➤*Postmarketing:*

Cardiovascular – Thromboembolic events (eg, acute renal cortical necrosis, central retinal artery and vein obstruction, cerebral thrombosis, deep vein thrombosis, pulmonary embolism).

CNS – Dizziness.

GI – Diarrhea, nausea, vomiting.

Hypersensitivity – Allergic skin reactions, anaphylactic shock, anaphylactoid reactions.

Special senses – Impaired color vision, other visual disturbances.

Overdosage

➤*Symptoms:* There are no known cases of intentional overdose with oral tranexamic acid and no subjects in the clinical program took more than 2 times the prescribed amount of oral tranexamic acid in a 24-hour period (more than 7,800 mg/day). However, cases of overdose of other forms of tranexamic acid have been reported. Based on these reports, symptoms of overdose may include GI (diarrhea, nausea, vomiting); hypotensive (eg, orthostatic symptoms); thromboembolic (arterial, embolic, venous); visual impairment; mental status changes; myoclonus; or rash.

➤*Treatment:* No specific information is available on the treatment of overdose with tranexamic acid. In the event of overdose, employ the usual supportive measures (eg, clinical monitoring, supportive therapy) as dictated by the patient's clinical status.

Patient Information

Instruct patients that the usual schedule is to take 2 tablets with liquids 3 times a day during menstruation. Instruct patients not to exceed 3 doses (6 tablets) in a 24-hour period or to take for longer than 5 days in any menstrual cycle.

Inform patients that they should immediately stop tranexamic acid if they notice any eye symptoms or change in their vision. Instruct them to report any such problems promptly to their health care provider and to follow-up with an ophthalmologist for a complete ophthalmic evaluation, including dilated retinal examination of the retina.

Inform patients that they should stop tranexamic acid and seek immediate medical attention if they notice symptoms of a severe allergic reaction (eg, shortness of breath, throat tightening).

Instruct patients that common adverse effects of tranexamic acid include abdominal pain, anemia, back pain, fatigue, headache, joint pain, migraine, muscle cramps, musculoskeletal pain, and sinus and nasal symptoms.

Advise patients to contact their health care provider if their heavy menstrual bleeding symptoms persist or worsen.

Remind patients to read the patient labeling carefully before starting therapy and with each refill.

TRANEXAMIC ACID — INJECTION

Indications

➤*Hemorrhage:* In patients with hemophilia for short-term use (2 to 8 days) to reduce or prevent hemorrhage and reduce the need for replacement therapy during and following tooth extraction.

➤*Off-label uses:*

Gastrointestinal hemorrhage – [3] = Safety concerns. Although trials have generally produced favorable outcomes, the lack of consistency with respect to the major outcomes of death, surgery, and transfusion requirements may have contributed to the low adoption of tranexamic acid for treatment of GI hemorrhage. A meta-analysis found that all-cause mortality with tranexamic acid was lower than with placebo; however, tranexamic acid does have the potential to cause fatal thromboembolism, which may further limit use. Additional studies are needed to determine the optimal dosing regimen.

Hereditary angioneurotic edema – Because hereditary angioneurotic edema is relatively rare, the use of tranexamic acid in treating this disorder has been established through expert consensus and review of case reports and small case series. Guidelines recommend tranexamic acid or epsilon-aminocaproic acid as first-line therapy. Although the evidence of risk is low, regular eye examinations are recommended during long-term therapy. Liver function should also be monitored every 6 months.

Hereditary angioneurotic edema (adults): [1] = Good documentation.

Hereditary angioneurotic edema (children): [1] = Good documentation.

Prevention of perioperative bleeding – [3] = Safety concerns. Results of tranexamic trials for reducing bleeding and transfusion after surgery have been consistently favorable, but doses varied widely. Additional study is required to determine the optimal dose.

Prevention of rebleeding after subarachnoid hemorrhage – [3] = Safety concerns. Use of tranexamic acid to prevent rebleeding is recommended in selected situations only, such as patients who are at low risk of vasospasm and patients who would benefit from delaying surgery. Routine use is not recommended because of a lack of overall improvement in outcomes; an increased incidence of cerebral ischemia offsets the benefits of decreased rebleeding.

Other possible off-label uses – Tranexamic acid has been used for many hemostatic purposes, including trauma. It has also been used to treat primary or intrauterine device–induced menorrhagia, gastric and intestinal hemorrhage, and recurrent epistaxis. Tranexamic acid has been used with systemic therapy topically as a mouthwash to reduce bleeding after oral surgery in patients on anticoagulant therapy. The drug also inhibits hyperfibrinolysis during thrombolytic treatment with plasminogen activators.

Administration and Dosage

➤*Adults:*

Dental extraction in patients with hemophilia –

Usual dosage: 10 mg/kg IV together with replacement therapy immediately before tooth extraction, then following tooth extraction 10 mg/kg 3 to 4 times daily.

Duration of therapy: May be used for 2 to 8 days.

Off-label dosing –

Gastrointestinal hemorrhage: [3] = Safety concerns. 3 to 6 g/day IV in divided doses every 6 to 8 hours for 2 to 3 days, followed by 3 to 6 g/day orally for an additional 3 to 5 days.

Hereditary angioneurotic edema (adults): [1] = Good documentation.

- *Long-term prophylaxis* – 1 to 1.5 g 2 to 3 times per day, reducing to 0.5 g once or twice per day and continued indefinitely.
- *Short-term prophylaxis* – 1 g 4 times per day for 48 hours before and after the procedure.
- *Emergency treatment of acute attacks* – 1 g 4 times daily for 48 hours.

Hereditary angioneurotic edema (children): [1] = Good documentation.

- *Long-term prophylaxis* – 1 to 2 g per day, depending on age and size; 50 mg/kg/day is a typical dose, and alternate-day or twice-weekly regimens are recommended.
- *Short-term prophylaxis* – 500 mg 4 times per day for 48 hours before and after the procedure.

Prevention of perioperative bleeding: [3] = Safety concerns. 2.5 to 100 mg/kg as an IV loading dose, followed by maintenance dosages of 0.25 to 4 mg/kg/h for 1 to 12 hours.

Prevention of rebleeding after subarachnoid hemorrhage: [3] = Safety concerns. The most commonly assessed dosage was 6 g IV each day in 6 divided doses of 1 g each for 3 weeks. Dosages ranged from 4 to 9 g per day and were continued from 10 days to 6 weeks. In some studies, patients were transitioned to daily oral doses of 6 g after 2 to 4 weeks.

➤*Children:*

Dental extraction in patients with hemophilia – See Adults for dosing.

➤*Renal function impairment:*

Moderate to Severe Renal Function Impairment Dosage of Tranexamic Acid Injection[a]	
Serum creatinine (mcmol/L)	IV dosage
120 to 250 (1.36 to 2.83 mg/dL)	10 mg/kg twice daily
250 to 500 (2.83 to 5.66 mg/dL)	10 mg/kg daily
> 500 (> 5.66 mg/dL)	10 mg/kg every 48 hours or 5 mg/kg every 24 hours

[a] IV = intravenous.

➤*Administration:* Administer IV.

➤*Admixture compatibility:*

Compatibility – For IV infusion, tranexamic acid injection may be mixed with most solutions for infusion such as electrolyte solutions, carbohydrate solutions, amino acid solutions and Dextran solutions. The mixture should be prepared the same day the solution is to be used. Heparin may be added to tranexamic acid injection.

Incompatibility – Tranexamic acid injection should not be mixed with blood. The drug is a synthetic amino acid, and should not be mixed with solutions containing penicillin.

➤*Storage/Stability:* Store tranexamic injection at 15° to 30°C (59° to 86°F).

Actions

➤*Pharmacology:*

Electrophysiology – Tranexamic acid is a competitive inhibitor of plasminogen activation, and at much higher concentrations, a noncompetitive inhibitor of plasmin, ie, actions similar to aminocaproic acid. Tranexamic acid is about 10 times more potent in vitro than aminocaproic acid.

Tranexamic acid binds more strongly than aminocaproic acid to both the strong and weak receptor sites of the plasminogen molecule in a ratio corresponding to the difference in potency between the compounds. Tranexamic acid in a concentration of 1 mg/mL does not aggregate platelets in vitro.

Tranexamic acid in concentrations up to 10 mg/mL blood has no influence on the platelet count, the coagulation time or various coagulation factors in whole blood or citrated blood from healthy subjects. On the other hand, tranexamic acid in concentrations of 10 mg and 1 mg/mL blood prolongs the thrombin time.

The plasma protein binding of tranexamic acid is about 3% at therapeutic plasma levels and seems to be fully accounted for by its binding to plasminogen. Tranexamic acid does not bind to serum albumin.

➤*Pharmacokinetics:*

Distribution – After an intravenous dose of 1 g, the plasma concentration time curve shows a triexponential decay with a half-life of about 2 hours for the terminal elimination phase. The initial volume of distribution is about 9 to 12 L.

Tranexamic acid passes through the placenta. The concentration in cord blood after an intravenous injection of 10 mg/kg to pregnant women is about 30 mg/L, as high as in the maternal blood. Tranexamic acid diffuses rapidly into joint fluid and the synovial membrane. In the joint fluid the same concentration is obtained as in the serum. The biological half-life of tranexamic acid in the joint fluid is about 3 hours.

The concentration of tranexamic acid in a number of other tissues is lower than in blood. In breast milk the concentration is about one-hundredth of the serum peak concentration. Tranexamic acid concentration in cerebrospinal fluid is about one-tenth of that of the plasma. The drug passes into the aqueous humor, the concentration being about one-tenth of the plasma concentration.

Tranexamic acid has been detected in semen where it inhibits fibrinolytic activity but does not influence sperm migration.

Metabolism – Only a small fraction of the drug is metabolized.

Excretion – Urinary excretion is the main route of elimination via glomerular filtration. Overall renal clearance is equal to overall plasma clearance (110 to 116 mL/min) and more than 95% of the dose is excreted in the urine as the unchanged drug. Excretion of tranexamic acid is about 90% at 24 hours after intravenous administration of 10 mg per kg body weight. After oral administration of 10 to 15 mg per kg body weight, the cumulative urinary excretion at 24 hours is 39% and at 48 hours, 41% of the ingested dose or 78% and 82% of the absorbed material.

An antifibrinolyic concentration of tranexamic acid remains in different tissues for about 17 hours, and in the serum up to 7 to 8 hours.

Contraindications

Acquired defective color vision, since this prohibits measuring one endpoint that should be followed as a measure of toxicity (see Warnings); subarachnoid hemorrhage (anecdotal experience indicates that cerebral edema and cerebral infarction may be caused by tranexamic acid in such patients); active intravascular clotting.

TRANEXAMIC ACID — INJECTION

Warnings/Precautions

➤*Visual abnormalities and retinal degeneration:* Focal areas of retinal degeneration have developed in cats, dogs and rats following intravenous tranexamic acid at doses between 250 to 1600 mg/kg/day (6 to 40 times the recommended usual human dose) from 6 days to 1 year. The incidence of such lesions has varied from 25% to 100% of animals treated and was dose-related. At lower doses some lesions have appeared to be reversible.

Limited data in cats and rabbits showed retinal changes in some animals with doses as low as 126 mg/kg/day (only about 3 times the recommended human dose) administered for several days to 2 weeks.

No retinal changes have been reported or noted in eye examinations in patients treated with tranexamic acid for weeks to months in clinical trials.

However, visual abnormalities, often poorly characterized, represent the most frequently reported postmarketing adverse reaction in Sweden. For patients who are to be treated continually for longer than several days, an ophthalmological examination, including visual acuity, color vision, eye-ground and visual fields, is advised, before commencing and at regular intervals during the course of treatment. Tranexamic acid should be discontinued if changes in examination results are found.

➤*Ureteral obstruction:* Ureteral obstruction due to clot formation in patients with upper urinary tract bleeding has been reported in patients treated with tranexamic acid.

➤*Thrombosis/Thromboembolism:* Venous and arterial thrombosis or thromboembolism has been reported in patients treated with tranexamic acid. In addition, cases of central retinal artery and central retinal vein obstruction have been reported.

Patients with a previous history of thromboembolic disease may be at increased risk for venous or arterial thrombosis.

Tranexamic acid should not be administered concomitantly with factor IX complex concentrates or anti-inhibitor coagulant concentrates, as the risk of thrombosis may be increased.

➤*Disseminated intravascular coagulation (DIC):* Patients with DIC who require treatment with tranexamic acid, must be under strict supervision of a physician experienced in treating this disorder.

➤*Renal function impairment:* The dose of tranexamic acid should be reduced in patients with renal insufficiency because of the risk of accumulation (see Administration and Dosage).

➤*Pregnancy: Category B.* There are no adequate and well-controlled studies in pregnant women. However, tranexamic acid is known to pass the placenta and appears in cord blood at concentrations approximately equal to maternal concentration. Because animal reproduction studies are not always predictive of human response, this drug should be used during pregnancy only if clearly needed.

➤*Lactation:* Tranexamic acid is present in the mother's milk at a concentration of about a hundredth of the corresponding serum levels. Caution should be exercised when tranexamic acid is administered to a nursing woman.

➤*Children:* The drug has had limited use in pediatric patients, principally in connection with tooth extraction. The limited data suggest that dosing instructions for adults can be used for pediatric patients needing tranexamic acid therapy.

Drug Interactions

Tranexamic Acid Drug Interactions			
Precipitant Drug	Object Drug[a]		Description
Tissue plasminogen activators	Tranexamic acid	⬇	Coadministration may decrease the efficacy of both tranexamic acid and tissue plasminogen activators. Use with caution. Additional clinical monitoring is warranted.
Tranexamic acid	Tissue plasminogen activators		
Tranexamic acid	Factor IX complex concentrates or anti-inhibitor coagulant concentrates	⬆	Coadministration of tranexamic acid and factor IX complex concentrates or anti-inhibitor coagulant concentrates may increase the risk of thrombosis. Avoid coadministration.
Tranexamic acid	Hormonal contraceptives	⬆	Coadministration of tranexamic acid and hormonal contraceptives may exacerbate the increased thrombotic risk associated with combination hormonal contraceptives. Coadminister only if there is a strong medical need and if the benefit of treatment outweighs the potential for the increased risk of a thrombotic event. Additional clinical monitoring is warranted.
Tranexamic acid	Tretinoin	⬆	Coadministration of tretinoin with tranexamic acid may increase the risk of severe thromboembolic reactions. Use with caution. Additional clinical monitoring is warranted.

[a] ⬆ = object drug increased; ⬇ = object drug decreased.

➤*Drug/Food interactions:* A single dose administration of tranexamic acid 1,300 mg with food increased the C_{max} and AUC 7% and 16%, respectively. However, tranexamic acid may be given without regard to meals.

Adverse Reactions

➤*Cardiovascular:* Hypotension has been reported occasionally. Hypotension has been observed when intravenous injection is too rapid. To avoid this response, the solution should not be injected more rapidly than 1 mL/min.

➤*GI:* GI disturbances (nausea, vomiting, diarrhea) may occur but disappear when the dosage is reduced.

➤*Miscellaneous:* Giddiness.

➤*Worldwide postmarketing reports:* Thromboembolic events (eg, deep vein thrombosis, pulmonary embolism, cerebral thrombosis, and central retinal artery and vein obstruction) have been rarely reported in patients receiving tranexamic acid for indications other than hemorrhage prevention in patients with hemophilia. However, due to the spontaneous nature of the reporting of medical events and the lack of controls, the actual incidence and causal relationship of drug and event cannot be determined.

Overdosage

There is no known case of overdosage of tranexamic acid injection.

➤*Symptoms:* Symptoms of overdosage may be nausea, vomiting, orthostatic symptoms or hypotension.

APROTININ

Rx	**Trasylol** (Bayer Pharmaceuticals)	**Injection:** 10,000 KIU[a]/mL	In 100 and 200 mL vials.[b]

[a] KIU = Kallikrein Inhibitor Units.

[b] With 9 mg sodium chloride/mL.

APROTININ — INJECTION

WARNING

Anaphylactic or anaphylactoid reactions are possible when aprotinin is administered. Hypersensitivity reactions are rare in patients with no prior exposure to aprotinin. The risk of anaphylaxis is increased in patients who are re-exposed to aprotinin-containing products. The benefit of aprotinin to patients undergoing primary coronary artery bypass graft (CABG) surgery should be weighed against the risk of anaphylaxis should a second exposure to aprotinin be required (see Warnings and Precautions).

Indications

➤*Hemorrhage, coronary artery bypass graft surgery:* Aprotinin is indicated for prophylactic use to reduce perioperative blood loss and the need for blood transfusion in patients undergoing cardiopulmonary bypass in the course of coronary artery bypass graft surgery.

Administration and Dosage

➤*General dosing considerations:* Aprotinin is supplied as a solution containing 10,000 kallikrein inhibitor units (KIU/mL), which is equal to 1.4 mg/mL.

Aprotinin given prophylactically in regimen A and regimen B (half regimen A) to patients undergoing coronary artery bypass graft (CABG) surgery significantly reduced the donor blood transfusion requirement relative to placebo treatment.

Both regimens include a 1 mL test dose, a loading dose, a dose to be added while recirculating the priming fluid of the cardiopulmonary bypass circuit (pump prime dose), and a constant infusion dose.

In low risk patients there is no difference in efficacy between regimens A and B. Therefore, the dosage used (A vs B) is at the discretion of the practitioner.

Total doses of more than 7 million KIU have not been studied in controlled trials.

APROTININ — INJECTION

➤*Adults:*

Hemorrhage, coronary artery bypass graft surgery –

Test dose:
- *Regimen A* – 1 mL (1.4 mg or 10,000 KIU)
- *Regimen B* – 1 mL (1.4 mg or 10,000 KIU)

Loading dose:
- *Regimen A* – 200 mL (280 mg or 2 million KIU)
- *Regimen B* – 100 mL (140 mg or 1 million KIU)

Pump prime dose:
- *Regimen A* – 200 mL (280 mg or 2 million KIU)
- *Regimen B* – 100 mL (140 mg or 1 million KIU)

Constant infusion dose:
- *Regimen A* – 50 mL/hr (70 mg/h or 500,000 KIU/h)
- *Regimen B* – 25 mL/hr (35 mg/h or 250,000 KIU/h)

➤*Administration:* All intravenous doses of aprotinin should be administered through a central line. Do not administer any other drug using the same line.

Test dose – The 1 mL test dose should be administered intravenously at least 10 minutes before the loading dose.

Loading dose – With the patient in a supine position, the loading dose is given slowly over 20 to 30 minutes, after induction of anesthesia but prior to sternotomy. In patients with known previous exposure to aprotinin, the loading dose should be given just prior to cannulation.

Constant infusion dose – When the loading dose is complete, it is followed by the constant infusion dose, which is continued until surgery is complete and the patient leaves the operating room.

Pump prime dose – The pump prime dose is added to the recirculating priming fluid of the cardiopulmonary bypass circuit, by replacement of an aliquot of the priming fluid, prior to the institution of cardiopulmonary bypass.

➤*Admixture compatibility:* To avoid physical incompatibility of aprotinin and heparin when adding to the pump prime solution, each agent must be added during recirculation of the pump prime to assure adequate dilution prior to admixture with the other component.

➤*Storage/Stability:* Aprotinin should be stored between 2° and 25°C (36° and 77°F). Protect from freezing.

Actions

➤*Pharmacology:* Aprotinin is a broad-spectrum protease inhibitor which modulates the systemic inflammatory response (SIR) associated with cardiopulmonary bypass (CPB) surgery. SIR results in the interrelated activation of the hemostatic, fibrinolytic, cellular and humoral inflammatory systems. Aprotinin, through its inhibition of multiple mediators (eg, kallikrein, plasmin) results in the attenuation of inflammatory responses, fibrinolysis, and thrombin generation.

Aprotinin inhibits pro-inflammatory cytokine release and maintains glycoprotein homeostasis. In platelets, aprotinin reduces glycoprotein loss (eg, GpIb, GpIIb/IIIa), while in granulocytes it prevents the expression of pro-inflammatory adhesive glycoproteins (eg, CD11b).

The effects of aprotinin use in CPB involves a reduction in inflammatory response which translates into a decreased need for allogeneic blood transfusions, reduced bleeding, and decreased mediastinal re-exploration for bleeding.

➤*Pharmacokinetics:* The studies comparing the pharmacokinetics of aprotinin in healthy volunteers, cardiac patients undergoing surgery with cardiopulmonary bypass, and women undergoing hysterectomy suggest linear pharmacokinetics over the dose range of 50,000 KIU to 2 million KIU. After IV injection, rapid distribution of aprotinin occurs into the total extracellular space, leading to a rapid initial decrease in plasma aprotinin concentration. Following this distribution phase, a plasma half-life of about 150 minutes is observed. At later time points, (ie, beyond 5 hours after dosing) there is a terminal elimination phase with a half-life of about 10 hours.

Average steady state intraoperative plasma concentrations were 137 KIU/mL (n = 10) after administration of the following dosage regimen: 1 million KIU IV loading dose, 1 million KIU into the pump prime volume, 250,000 KIU per hour of operation as continuous intravenous infusion (Regimen B). Average steady state intraoperative plasma concentrations were 250 KIU/mL in patients (n = 20) treated with aprotinin during cardiac surgery by administration of Regimen A (exactly double Regimen B): 2 million KIU IV loading dose, 2 million KIU into the pump prime volume, 500,000 KIU per hour of operation as continuous intravenous infusion.

Following a single IV dose of radiolabeled aprotinin, approximately 25% to 40% of the radioactivity is excreted in the urine over 48 hours. After a 30 minute infusion of 1 million KIU, about 2% is excreted as unchanged drug. After a larger dose of 2 million KIU infused over 30 minutes, urinary excretion of unchanged aprotinin accounts for approximately 9% of the dose.

Animal studies have shown that aprotinin is accumulated primarily in the kidney. Aprotinin, after being filtered by the glomeruli, is actively reabsorbed by the proximal tubules in which it is stored in phagolysosomes. Aprotinin is slowly degraded by lysosomal enzymes. The physiological renal handling of aprotinin is similar to that of other small proteins (eg, insulin).

Contraindications

Hypersensitivity to aprotinin.

Warnings/Precautions

➤*Reexposure to aprotinin:* In a retrospective review of 387 European patient records with documented reexposure to aprotinin, the incidence of hypersensitivity/anaphylactic reactions was 2.7%. Two patients who experienced hypersensitivity/anaphylactic reactions subsequently died, 24 hours and 5 days after surgery, respectively. The relationship of these 2 deaths to aprotinin is unclear. This retrospective review also showed that the incidence of a hypersensitivity or anaphylactic reaction following reexposure is increased when the reexposure occurs within 6 months of the initial administration (5% for reexposure within 6 months and 0.9% for reexposure of more than 6 months). Other smaller studies have shown that in case of reexposure, the incidence of hypersensitivity/anaphylactic reactions may reach the 5% level.

Before initiating treatment with aprotinin in a patient with a history of exposure to aprotinin or products containing aprotinin, the recommendations below should be followed to manage a potential hypersensitivity or anaphylactic reaction:

1.) Have standard emergency treatments for hypersensitivity or anaphylactic reactions readily available in the operating room (eg, epinephrine, corticosteroids).
2.) Administration of the test dose and loading dose should be done only when the conditions for rapid cannulation (if necessary) are present.
3.) Delay the addition of aprotinin into the pump prime solution until after the loading dose has been safely administered. Additionally, administration of H_1 and H_2 blockers 15 minutes before the test dose may be considered.

➤*Test dose:* All patients treated with aprotinin should first receive a test dose to assess the potential for allergic reactions. The test dose of 1 mL aprotinin should be administered intravenously at least 10 minutes prior to the loading dose. However, even after the uneventful administration of the initial 1 mL test-dose, the therapeutic dose may cause an anaphylactic reaction. If this happens the infusion of aprotinin should immediately be stopped, and standard emergency treatment for anaphylaxis be applied. It should be noted that hypersensitivity/anaphylactic reactions can also occur in connection with application of the test dose (see Warnings). In reexposure cases, IV administration of an antihistamine is recommended shortly before the loading dose of aprotinin.

➤*Loading dose:* The loading dose of aprotinin should be given intravenously to patients in the supine position over a 20 to 30 minute period. Rapid intravenous administration of aprotinin can cause a transient fall in blood pressure (see Administration and Dosage).

➤*Hypersensitivity reactions:* Anaphylactic or anaphylactoid reactions are possible when aprotinin is administered. Hypersensitivity reactions are rare in patients with no prior exposure to aprotinin. Hypersensitivity reactions can range from skin eruptions, itching, dyspnea, nausea, and tachycardia to fatal anaphylactic shock with circulatory failure. If a hypersensitivity reaction occurs during injection or infusion of aprotinin, administration should be stopped immediately and emergency treatment should be initiated. It should be noted that severe (fatal) hypersensitivity/anaphylactic reactions can also occur in connection with application of the 1 mL test dose. Even when a second exposure to aprotinin has been tolerated without symptoms, a subsequent administration may result in severe hypersensitivity/anaphylactic reactions.

➤*Special risk:*

Allergic reactions – Patients with a history of allergic reactions to drugs or other agents may be at greater risk of developing a hypersensitivity or anaphylactic reaction upon exposure to aprotinin (see Warnings).

Use in patients undergoing deep hypothermic circulatory arrest – Two US case control studies have reported contradictory results in patients receiving aprotinin while undergoing deep hypothermic circulatory arrest in connection with surgery of the aortic arch.

Renal failure/mortality: The first study showed an increase in both renal failure and mortality compared to age-matched historical controls. Similar results were not observed, however, in a second case control study. The strength of this association is uncertain because there are no data from randomized studies to confirm or refute these findings.

➤*Pregnancy: Category B.* There are no adequate and well-controlled studies in pregnant women. Because animal reproduction studies are not always predictive of human response, this drug should be used during pregnancy only if clearly needed.

➤*Lactation:* Not applicable.

➤*Children:* Safety and effectiveness in pediatric patient(s) have not been established.

➤*Elderly:* Of the total of 3083 subjects in clinical studies of aprotinin, 1100 (35.7%) were 65 and over, while 297 (9.6%) were 75 and over. Of patients 65 years and older, 479 (43.5%) received Regimen A and 237 (21.5%) received Regimen B. No overall differences in safety or effectiveness were observed between these subjects and younger subjects for either dose regimen, and other reported clinical experience has not identified differences in responses between the elderly and younger patients.

APROTININ — INJECTION

Drug Interactions

Aprotinin Drug Interactions			
Precipitant drug	Object drug[a]		Description
Aprotinin	Captopril	⬇	In a study of nine patients with untreated hypertension, aprotinin IV infused in a dose of 2 million KIU over 2 hours blocked the acute hypotensive effect of 100 mg captopril.
Aprotinin	Fibrinolytic agents	⬇	Aprotinin is known to have antifibrinolytic activity and, therefore, may inhibit the effects of fibrinolytic agents.
Aprotinin	Heparin	⬆	Aprotinin, in the presence of heparin, has been found to prolong the activated clotting time. However, aprotinin should not be viewed as a heparin-sparing agent.

[a] ⬆ = Object drug increased. ⬇ = Object drug decreased.

➤*Laboratory monitoring of anticoagulation during cardiopulmonary bypass:* Aprotinin prolongs whole blood clotting times by a different mechanism than heparin. In the presence of aprotinin, prolongation is dependent on the type of whole blood clotting test employed. If an ACT is used to determine the effectiveness of heparin anticoagulation, the prolongation of the ACT by aprotinin may lead to an overestimation of the degree of anticoagulation, thereby leading to inadequate anticoagulation. During extended extracorporeal circulation, patients may require additional heparin, even in the presence of ACT levels that appear adequate.

Methods to maintain adequate anticoagulation – In patients undergoing CPB with aprotinin therapy, 1 of the following methods may be employed to maintain adequate anticoagulation:

ACT: An activated clotting time (ACT) is not a standardized coagulation test, and different formulations of the assay are affected differently by the presence of aprotinin. The test is further influenced by variable dilution effects and the temperature experienced during cardiopulmonary bypass. It has been observed that kaolin-based ACTs are not increased to the same degree by aprotinin as are diatomaceous earth-based (celite) ACTs. Although protocols vary, a minimal celite ACT of 750 seconds or kaolin ACT of 480 seconds, independent of the effects of hemodilution and hypothermia, is recommended in the presence of aprotinin. Consult the manufacturer of the ACT test regarding the interpretation of the assay in the presence of aprotinin.

Fixed heparin dosing: A standard loading dose of heparin, administered prior to cannulation of the heart, plus the quantity of heparin added to the prime volume of the cardiopulmonary bypass (CPB) circuit, should total at least 350 IU/kg. Additional heparin should be administered in a fixed-dose regimen based on patient weight and duration of CPB.

Heparin titration: Protamine titration, a method that is not affected by aprotinin, can be used to measure heparin levels. A heparin dose response, assessed by protamine titration, should be performed prior to administration of aprotinin to determine the heparin loading dose. Additional heparin should be administered on the basis of heparin levels measured by protamine titration. Heparin levels during bypass should not be allowed to drop below 2.7 U/mL (2 mg/kg) or below the level indicated by heparin dose response testing performed prior to administration of aprotinin. In patients treated with aprotinin, the amount of protamine administered to reverse heparin activity should be based on the actual amount of heparin administered, and not on the ACT values.

Adverse Reactions

Studies of patients undergoing CABG surgery, either primary or repeat, indicate that aprotinin is generally well tolerated. The adverse events reported are frequent sequelae of cardiac surgery and are not necessarily attributable to aprotinin therapy. Adverse events reported, up to the time of hospital discharge, from patients in US placebo-controlled trials are listed in the following table. The table lists only those events that were reported in 2% or more of the aprotinin treated patients without regard to causal relationship.

Aprotinin Adverse Reactions (≥ 2%)		
Adverse reaction	Aprotinin (n = 2002)	Placebo (n = 1084)
Any event	76%	77%
Cardiovascular		
Arrhythmia	4%	3%
Atrial arrhythmia	3%	3%
Atrial fibrillation	21%	23%
Atrial flutter	6%	5%
Heart failure	5%	4%
Hypertension	4%	5%
Hypotension	8%	10%
Myocardial infarct	6%	6%
Pericarditis	5%	5%
Peripheral edema	5%	5%
Supraventricular tachycardia	4%	3%
Tachycardia	6%	7%
Ventricular extrasystoles	6%	4%
Ventricular tachycardia	5%	4%
CNS		
Confusion	4%	4%
Insomnia	3%	4%
Dermatologic		
Rash	2%	2%
GI		
Constipation	4%	5%
Diarrhea	3%	2%
Liver function tests abnormal	3%	2%
Nausea	11%	9%
Vomiting	3%	4%
GU		
Kidney function abnormal	3%	2%
Urinary retention	3%	3%
Urinary tract infection	2%	2%
Hematologic/Lymphatic		
Anemia	2%	8%
Metabolic/Nutritional		
Creatine phosphokinase increased	2%	1%
Musculoskeletal		
Any event	2%	3%
Respiratory		
Asthma	2%	3%
Atelectasis	5%	6%
Dyspnea	4%	4%
Hypoxia	2%	1%
Lung disorder	8%	8%
Pleural effusion	7%	9%
Pneumothorax	4%	4%
Miscellaneous		
Asthenia	2%	2%
Chest pain	2%	2%
Fever	15%	14%
Infection	6%	7%

In comparison to the placebo group, no increase in mortality in patients treated with aprotinin was observed. Additional events of particular interest from controlled US trials with an incidence of less than 2%, are listed below:

Aprotinin Adverse Reactions (< 2%)		
Adverse reaction	Aprotinin (n = 2002)	Placebo (n = 1084)
Thrombosis	1%	0.6%
Shock	0.7%	0.4%
Cerebrovascular accident	0.7%	2.1%
Thrombophlebitis	0.2%	0.5%
Deep thrombophlebitis	0.7%	1%
Lung edema	1.3%	1.5%
Pulmonary embolus	0.3%	0.6%
Kidney failure	1%	0.6%
Acute kidney failure	0.5%	0.6%
Kidney tubular necrosis	0.8%	0.4%

➤*Additional events, incidence between 1% and 2%:* Listed below are additional events, from controlled US trials with an incidence between 1% and 2%, and also from uncontrolled, compassionate use trials and spontaneous postmarketing reports. Estimates of frequency cannot be made for spontaneous postmarketing reports.

Cardiovascular – Ventricular fibrillation, heart arrest, bradycardia, congestive heart failure, hemorrhage, bundle branch block, myocardial isch-

APROTININ — INJECTION

emia, ventricular tachycardia, heart block, pericardial effusion, ventricular arrhythmia, shock, pulmonary hypertension (1% to 2%).

CNS – Agitation, dizziness, anxiety, convulsion (1% to 2%).

Dermatologic – Skin discoloration (spontaneous postmarketing reports).

GI – Dyspepsia, gastrointestinal hemorrhage, jaundice, hepatic failure (1% to 2%).

GU – Oliguria, kidney failure, acute kidney failure, kidney tubular necrosis (1% to 2%).

Hematologic/Lymphatic – Although thrombosis was not reported more frequently in aprotinin versus placebo-treated patients in controlled trials, it has been reported in uncontrolled trials, compassionate use trials, and spontaneous postmarketing reporting. These reports of thrombosis encompass the following terms: Thrombosis, occlusion, arterial thrombosis, coronary occlusion, embolus, pulmonary embolus, thrombophlebitis, deep thrombophlebitis, cerebrovascular accident, cerebral embolism (1% to 2%); pulmonary thrombosis (spontaneous postmarketing reports). Other hematologic events reported include leukocytosis, thrombocytopenia, coagulation disorder (which includes disseminated intravascular coagulation), decreased prothrombin (1% to 2%).

Metabolic/Nutritional – Hyperglycemia, hypokalemia, hypervolemia, acidosis (1% to 2%).

Musculoskeletal – Arthralgia (1% to 2%).

Respiratory – Pneumonia, apnea, increased cough, lung edema (1% to 2%).

Miscellaneous – Sepsis, death, multisystem organ failure, immune system disorder (1% to 2%); hemoperitoneum (spontaneous postmarketing reports).

➤*Myocardial infarction:* In the pooled analysis of all patients undergoing CABG surgery, there was no significant difference in the incidence of investigator-reported myocardial infarction (MI) in aprotinin-treated patients as compared to placebo-treated patients. However, because no uniform criteria for the diagnosis of myocardial infarction were utilized by investigators, this issue was addressed prospectively in 3 later studies (2 studies evaluated Regimen A, Regimen B, and Pump Prime Regimen; 1 study evaluated only Regimen A), in which data were analyzed by a blinded consultant employing an algorithm for possible, probable or definite MI. Utilizing this method, the incidence of definite myocardial infarction was 5.9% in the aprotinin-treated patients versus 4.7% in the placebo-treated patients. This difference in the incidence rates was not statistically significant. Data from these 3 studies are summarized below.

Incidence of Myocardial Infarctions with Aprotinin

Treatment	Definite MI %	Definite or probable MI %	Definite, probable, or possible MI
Pooled data from 3 studies that evaluated Regimen A			
Aprotinin regimen A (n = 646)	4.6	10.7	14.1
Placebo (n = 661)	4.7	11.3	13.4
Pooled data from 2 studies that evaluated Regimen B and Pump Prime Regimen			
Aprotinin Regimen B (n = 241)	8.7	15.9	18.7
Aprotinin Pump Prime Regimen (n = 239)	6.3	15.7	18.1
Placebo (n = 240)	6.3	15.1	15.8

➤*Graft patency:* In a recently completed multicenter, multinational study to determine the effects of aprotinin Regimen A vs placebo on saphenous vein graft patency in patients undergoing primary CABG surgery, patients were subjected to routine postoperative angiography. Of the 13 study sites, 10 were in the United States and 3 were non-US centers (Denmark 1, Israel 2). The results of this study are summarized below.

Incidence of Graft Closure, Myocardial Infarction and Death With Aprotinin

	Overall closure rates[a]		Incidence of MI[b]	Incidence of death[c]
	All centers (n = 703), %	US centers (n = 381), %	All centers (n = 831), %	All centers (n = 870), %
Aprotinin	15.4	9.4	2.9	1.4
Placebo	10.9	9.5	3.8	1.6
CI for the difference (%) (drug-placebo)	(1.3, 9.6)[d]	(−3.8, 5.9)[d]	(−3.3, 1.5)[e]	(−1.9, 1.4)[e]

[a] Population: All patients with assessable saphenous vein grafts.
[b] Population: All patients assessable by blinded consultant.
[c] All patients.
[d] 90%; per protocol.
[5] 95%; not specified in protocol.

Although there was a statistically significantly increased risk of graft closure for aprotinin-treated patients compared to patients who received placebo (p = 0.035), further analysis showed a significant treatment by site interaction for 1 of the non-US sites vs the US centers. When the analysis of graft closures was repeated for US centers only, there was no statistically significant difference in graft closure rates in patients who received aprotinin vs placebo. These results are the same whether analyzed as the proportion of patients who experienced at least 1 graft closure postoperatively or as the proportion of grafts closed. There were no differences between treatment groups in the incidence of myocardial infarction as evaluated by the blinded consultant (2.9% aprotinin vs 3.8% placebo) or of death (1.4% aprotinin vs 1.6% placebo) in this study.

➤*Hypersensitivity:* See Warnings. Hypersensitivity and anaphylactic reactions during surgery were rarely reported in US controlled clinical studies in patients with no prior exposure to aprotinin (1/1424 patients or less than 0.1% on aprotinin vs 1/861 patients or 0.1% on placebo). In case of reexposure the incidence of hypersensitivity/anaphylactic reactions has been reported to reach the 5% level. A review of 387 European patient records involving reexposure to aprotinin showed that the incidence of hypersensitivity or anaphylactic reactions was 5% for reexposure within 6 months and 0.9% for reexposure greater than 6 months.

➤*Lab test abnormalities:*

Serum creatinine – Data pooled from all patients undergoing CABG surgery in US placebo-controlled trials showed no statistically or clinically significant increase in the incidence of postoperative renal dysfunction in patients treated with aprotinin. The incidence of serum creatinine elevations greater than 0.5 mg/dL above pretreatment levels was 9% in the aprotinin group vs 8% in the placebo group (p = 0.248), while the incidence of elevations greater than 2 mg/dL above baseline was only 1% in each group (p = 0.883). In the majority of instances, postoperative renal dysfunction was not severe and was reversible. Patients with baseline elevations in serum creatinine were not at increased risk of developing postoperative renal dysfunction following aprotinin treatment.

Serum transaminases – Data pooled from all patients undergoing CABG surgery in US placebo-controlled trials showed no evidence of an increase in the incidence of postoperative hepatic dysfunction in patients treated with aprotinin. The incidence of treatment-emergent increases in ALT (formerly SGPT) greater than 1.8 times the upper limit of normal was 14% in both the aprotinin and placebo-treated patients (P = 0.687), while the incidence of increases greater than 3 times the upper limit of normal was 5% in both groups (P = 0.847).

Other laboratory findings – The incidence of treatment-emergent elevations in plasma glucose, AST (formerly SGOT), LDH, alkaline phosphatase, and CPK-MB was not notably different between aprotinin - and placebo- treated patients undergoing CABG surgery. Significant elevations in the partial thromboplastin time (PTT) and celite activated clotting time (celite ACT) are expected in aprotinin-treated patients in the hours after surgery due to circulating concentrations of aprotinin, which are known to inhibit activation of the intrinsic clotting system by contact with a foreign material (eg, celite), a method used in these tests (see Laboratory monitoring of anticoagulation during cardiopulmonary bypass.)

Overdosage

The maximum amount of aprotinin that can be safely administered in single or multiple doses has not been determined. Doses up to 17.5 million KIU have been administered within a 24 hour period without any apparent toxicity. There is 1 poorly documented case, however, of a patient who received a large, but not well determined, amount of aprotinin (in excess of 15 million KIU) in 24 hours. The patient, who had preexisting liver dysfunction, developed hepatic and renal failure postoperatively and died. Autopsy showed hepatic necrosis and extensive renal tubular and glomerular necrosis. The relationship of these findings to aprotinin therapy is unclear.

THROMBIN

Rx	**Evithrom**[a] (J&J Wound Management)	**Solution, frozen; topical**: 800 to 1,200 units/mL	In 2, 5, or 20 mL single-use vials.
Rx	**Recothrom**[b] (ZymoGenetics)	**Powder for solution, lyophilized; topical**: 1,000 units/mL	Preservative free. PEG. In 5,000 and 20,000 units single-use vials with diluent and 20,000 units Spray Applicator Kits.
Rx	**Thrombin-JMI**[c] (King Pharmaceuticals)		Preservative free. In 5,000 units vials and Epistaxis Kits with diluent; 20,000 units vials, Pump Spray Kits, and Syringe Spray Kits with diluent.
Rx	**Thrombi-Pad 3 × 3**[c] (King Pharmaceuticals)	**Pad, lyophilized; topical**: 200 units	Preservative free. In single-use 1s.
Rx	**Thrombi-Gel 10**[c] (King Pharmaceuticals)	**Pad, lyophilized; topical**: 1,000 units	Preservative free. 0.2 mg or less of residual formaldehyde. In single-use 10s.
Rx	**Thrombi-Gel 40**[c] (King Pharmaceuticals)		Preservative free. 0.2 mg or less of residual formaldehyde. In single-use 5s.
Rx	**Thrombi-Gel 100**[c] (King Pharmaceuticals)	**Pad, lyophilized; topical**: 20,000 units	Preservative free. 0.2 mg or less of residual formaldehyde. In single-use 5s.

[a] Human origin.
[b] Produced via recombinant DNA technology from genetically modified Chinese hamster ovary (CHO) cell line.
[c] Bovine origin.

THROMBIN — TOPICAL

WARNING

The use of topical bovine thrombin preparations has occasionally been associated with abnormalities in hemostasis ranging from asymptomatic alterations in laboratory determinations, such as prothrombin time (PT) and partial thromboplastin time (PTT), to severe bleeding or thrombosis, which rarely have been fatal. These hemostatic effects appear to be related to the formation of antibodies against bovine thrombin and/or factor V, which in some cases may cross-react with human factor V, potentially resulting in factor V deficiency. Repeated clinical applications of topical bovine thrombin increase the likelihood that antibodies against thrombin and/or factor V may be formed. Consultation with an expert in coagulation disorders is recommended if a patient exhibits abnormal coagulation laboratory values, abnormal bleeding, or abnormal thrombosis following the use of topical thrombin. Any interventions should consider the immunologic basis of this condition. Patients with antibodies to bovine thrombin preparations should not be reexposed to these products.

Indications

➤*Hemostasis:*

Evithrom, Recothrom, Thrombin-JMI – As an aid to hemostasis whenever oozing blood and minor bleeding from capillaries and small venules is accessible and control of bleeding by standard surgical techniques is ineffective or impractical. In various types of surgery, solutions of thrombin may be used in conjunction with an absorbable gelatin sponge for hemostasis.

➤*Thrombi-Gel, Thrombi-Pad*: As a trauma dressing for temporary control of moderate to severe bleeding wounds and for the control of surface bleeding from vascular access sites and percutaneous catheters and tubes.

Administration and Dosage

➤*General dosing considerations:* Do not use *Thrombi-Pad 3 × 3* as a replacement for absorbable hemostats. This product contains nonabsorbable materials and is not intended to be left in the body.

➤*Adults:*

Hemostasis – The amount of thrombin required will vary, depending on the size and number of bleeding sites and the method of application.

Evithrom: As an approximate guide, volumes of up to 10 mL were used in clinical studies when human thrombin was used in conjunction with an absorbable gelatin sponge.

Thrombin-JMI: Where bleeding is profuse, as from abraded surfaces of liver or spleen, concentrations of 1,000 units/mL may be required. For general use in plastic surgery, dental extractions, skin grafting, etc, solutions containing approximately 100 units/mL are frequently used.

➤*Children:*

Hemostasis –

Evithrom: See Adults for dosing.

➤*Preparation for administration:*

Frozen solution – Thaw the frozen solution before administration in 1 of the following ways: 1 day in the refrigerator or 1 hour at room temperature. The 2 and 5 mL vials can only thaw for 10 minutes at 37°C. Do not exceed 37°C and do not leave vial for longer than 10 minutes at this temperature.

Remove the flip-off plastic cap from the vial to expose the rubber stopper. Using a sterile needle and syringe, draw the solution from the vial. Alternatively, remove the rubber stopper (by removing the metal pull tab) to transfer the solution into a sterile container.

Powder for solution –

Bovine origin: Reconstitute with sterile isotonic saline at a recommended concentration of 1,000 to 2,000 units/mL. Intermediate strengths to suit the needs of the case may be prepared by diluting the thrombin with an appropriate volume of sterile isotonic saline. In many situations, it may be advantageous to use in a dry form on oozing surfaces.

In instances where a concentration of approximately 1,000 units/mL is desired, the contents of the vial of sterile isotonic saline diluent may be transferred into the thrombin container with a sterile syringe or sterile transfer device.

If the transfer device is used for reconstitution, transfer the diluent according to the following directions: remove the plastic cap off of the diluent vial. Remove the *Tyvek* cover from the transfer device container; do not remove the device from the package. Seat the blue end of the device on the diluent vial, pushing down until the spike penetrates the diaphragm and the device snaps in place. Flip the plastic cover up on the thrombin container; do not remove the cover and aluminum seal. Remove the plastic package from the transfer device, taking care not to touch the exposed end of the device. Invert the vial of diluent and insert the clear end of the transfer device into the diaphragm of the thrombin container.

• *Pump spray kit* – Remove the outer lid by pulling up at the indicated edge. The inner tray is sterile and suitable for introduction into any operating field. Remove the cover on inner tray to expose sterile contents. Reconstitute to desired potency by introducing sterile isotonic saline with a sterile syringe or a sterile transfer device. If the transfer device is used, follow the previously described procedure. When the powder is completely dissolved, open vial by flipping up metal and tearing counterclockwise. Remove the rubber diaphragm from vial. Remove pump with protective cap from tray and snap onto vial. Remove protective cap and attach actuator. Do not transfer spray pump to another vial.

• *Epistaxis kit* – Remove the outer lid by pulling up at the indicated edge. The inner tray is sterile and suitable for introduction into any operating field. Remove the cover on the inner tray to expose sterile contents. Using the sterile syringe equipped with a transfer device, draw the desired amount of saline diluent from the vial into the syringe. Inject the saline diluent into the thrombin vial. When the thrombin is completely dissolved, draw the solution into the syringe. Remove the syringe from the transfer device by turning the syringe counter clockwise. Affix the nasal drug delivery device onto the syringe by pushing the device down onto the thrombin solution–filled syringe and turn clockwise until the nasal drug delivery device locks into place.

• *Syringe spray kit* – Remove the outer lid by pulling up at the indicated edge. The inner tray is sterile and suitable for introduction into any operating field. Remove the cover on the inner tray to expose sterile contents. Using the sterile syringe equipped with a transfer device, draw the desired amount of saline diluent from the vial into the syringe. Inject the saline diluent into the thrombin vial. When the powder is completely dissolved, draw the solution into the syringe. Remove the syringe from the transfer device by turning syringe counterclockwise. Affix spray tip by pushing down and turning clockwise until the spray tip locks in place.

Recombinant:

• *5,000 unit vial* – Remove the flip-off cap from the top of the thrombin vial. Attach the needle-free transfer device and snap it into place on the vial by placing the vial flat on a surface and attaching the transfer device straight into the center of the vial stopper. Attach the prefilled diluent syringe to the needle-free transfer device. Inject the 5 mL of diluent from the syringe into the product vial. Keep the syringe plunger depressed. Do not reuse the diluent syringe for transfer of the reconstituted product. Remove and discard the diluent syringe. Gently swirl and invert the product vial until the powder is completely dissolved (avoid excessive agitation). Apply the preprinted "Do Not Inject" label to the sterile, empty transfer syringe provided, then draw up the solution.

• *20,000 unit vial* – Remove the flip-off cap from the top of the thrombin and the diluent vials. Attach a needle-free transfer device (1 each) to the thrombin and diluent vials and snap them into place by placing the vial flat on a surface and attaching the transfer device straight into the center of the vial stopper. Open the sterile, empty 20 mL syringe package and attach the preprinted "Do Not Inject" label. Attach the labeled 20 mL syringe to the needle-free transfer device on the diluent vial (injection of air into the diluent vial may facilitate withdrawal of the diluent). Draw up 20 mL of diluent from the vial into the syringe. Remove the diluent-filled syringe from the diluent vial and attach it to the transfer device on the thrombin vial. Transfer the 20 mL of the diluent from the syringe into the thrombin vial; the vacuum in the vial facilitates transfer. Leave the syringe attached and gen-

THROMBIN — TOPICAL

tly swirl the vial and invert the thrombin vial until the powder is completely absorbed (avoid excessive agitation). With the same syringe, draw up the thrombin solution.

- *Pad* – Pad is supplied sterile; do not resterilize.

  Thrombi-Gel: Open the foil pouch and transfer the tray into the sterile field. Peel back the lid of the tray completely. If desired, the pad can be cut or rolled to desired shape before wetting. For *Thrombi-Gel 10*, apply up to 3 mL of sterile isotonic sodium chloride 0.9% solution for injection or sterile water for injection. For *Thrombi-Gel 40*, apply up to 10 mL of sterile isotonic sodium chloride 0.9% solution for injection or sterile water for injection. For *Thrombi-Gel 100*, apply up to 20 mL of sterile isotonic sodium chloride 0.9% solution for injection or sterile water for injection. The wetted pad should be kneaded to thoroughly saturate and remove trapped air bubbles.

  Thrombi-Pad 3 × 3: Open the foil pouch and remove the pad. The pad may be used dry or wet. If wetting the pad, apply up to 10 mL of sterile isotonic sodium chloride 0.9% solution to the pad.

➤*Administration:* For topical use only. Do not inject solution. Topically apply on the surface of bleeding tissue only. The recipient surface should be sponged (not wiped) or suctioned free of blood before thrombin is applied. A spray may be used or the surface may be flooded using a sterile syringe and small gauge needle. The most effective hemostasis results occur when the thrombin topical mixes freely with the blood as soon as it reaches the surface. Sponging of the treated surfaces should be avoided to ensure that the clot remains securely in place.

Adjunct therapy with absorbable gelatin sponge – Prepare thrombin solution to desired strength. Transfer solution from syringe to a sterile bowl or basin. Immerse sponge of desired size and shape in solution. Knead the sponge vigorously with moistened, gloved fingers to remove trapped air, thereby facilitating saturation of the sponge. Remove the saturated sponge(s) and squeeze gently to remove excess solution. Apply saturated sponge to bleeding area in a single layer. Hold in place with pledget of cotton or a small gauze sponge until hemostasis occurs.

Epistaxis kit – Insert the nasal drug delivery device into the naris and spray the solution onto the nasal mucosa by depressing the syringe plunger using mild or moderate pressure. If feasible, the bleeding site on the patient's nasal mucosa may be placed in a dependent position during administration. After administration, the device may be removed immediately or briefly held in the nasal passage.

Pad – Place the wetted pad directly over the source of bleeding and apply adjunct manual compression until hemostasis is achieved.

The *Thrombi-Pad 3 × 3* may be left in place for up to 24 hours. Upon removal, do not disrupt the clot by physical manipulation. If the pad adheres to the placement site, gently irrigate the pad with nonheparinized saline and carefully remove.

Pump spray kit – To spray, hold vial upright or at a slight angle. Several strokes of the pump may be required to expel the solution.

Syringe spray kit – To spray, depress the syringe plunger in a normal fashion to dispense the solution through the tip in a fine spray.

➤*Storage/Stability:*

Evithrom – Store frozen vials at −18°C (−64°F) or colder for up to 2 years. Unopened thawed vials can be stored at 2° to 8°C (36° to 46°F) for up to 30 days or at room temperature for up to 24 hours. Do not refreeze. Do not refrigerate once at room temperature. Discard unused content.

Recothrom – Store vials at 2° to 25°C (36° to 77°F). Reconstituted solutions may be stored for up to 24 hours at 2° to 25°C (36° to 77°F). Discard reconstituted solution after 24 hours. Discard unused contents.

Thrombin-JMI – Store vials at 2° to 25°C (36° to 77°F). Solutions should be used promptly upon removal from the container. However, the solution may be refrigerated at 2° to 8°C (36° to 46°F) for up to 24 hours or may be stored at room temperature for up to 8 hours following reconstitution. Discard unused contents.

Thrombin-Gel, Thrombi-Pad – Store at 2° to 25°C (36° to 77°F) in a cool, dry place. Discard *Thrombi-Gel* 3 hours and *Thrombi-Pad* 1 hour after preparation.

Actions

➤*Pharmacology:* Thrombin is a highly specific serine protease that promotes clot formation and hemostasis and acts locally when applied topically to a site of bleeding. Thrombin efficiently activates platelets and catalyzes the conversion of fibrinogen to fibrin, which are steps that are essential for blood clot formation. The fibrin clot is stabilized by cross-linking, occurring as a result of activation of the patient's endogenous factor XIII, which requires the presence of calcium.

Contraindications

➤*Evithrom*: Known anaphylactic or severe systemic reaction to human blood products; injection directly into the circulatory system; for the treatment of severe or brisk arterial bleeding.

➤*Recothrom*: Known hypersensitivity to thrombin, hamster proteins, or any component of the product; injection directly into the circulatory system; for the treatment of massive or brisk arterial bleeding.

➤*Thrombi-Gel*: Known hypersensitivity to any component of the product (including material of bovine origin); use in the closure of skin incisions.

➤*Thrombi-Pad*: Known sensitivity to bovine-derived materials.

➤*Thrombin-JMI*: Know sensitivity to any component of the product and/or material of bovine origin.

Warnings/Precautions

➤*Thrombosis:* Potential risk of thrombosis if absorbed systemically.

➤*Human plasma:* Because *Evithrom* is made from human plasma, it may carry a risk of transmitting infectious agents, such as viruses, and theoretically, the Creutzfeidt-Jakob disease (CJD) agent. The risk of transmitting an infectious agent has been reduced by screening plasma donors for prior exposure to certain viruses, by testing for the presence of certain current virus infections and by inactivating and removing certain viruses. Despite these measures, such products can still potentially transmit disease. There is also the possibility that unknown infectious agents may be present in such products. The health care provider should discuss the risks and benefits of this product with the patient. To report suspected adverse reactions, contact ETHICON Customer Support Center at 877-384-4266 or FDA at 1-800-FDA-1088 or http://www.fda.gov/medwatch.

➤*Infection:* *Thrombi-Gel* and *Thrombi-Pad* should not be used in the presence of infection. It should be used with caution in contaminated areas of the body.

➤*Administration:* Because of its action in the clotting mechanism, thrombin must not be injected or otherwise allowed to enter large blood vessels. Extensive intravascular clotting and even death may result. *Thrombi-Gel* should not be used in the closure of skin incisions because it may interfere with the healing of skin edges. This is due to mechanical interposition of gelatin and is not secondary to intrinsic interference with wound healing. Do not use *Thrombi-Pad 3 × 3* as a replacement for absorbable hemostats. This product contains nonabsorbable materials and is not intended to be left in the body.

➤*Immunogenicity:*

Recothrom – Treatment with thrombin (recombinant) resulted in a statistically significantly lower incidence of specific antiproduct antibody development. 1.5% (95% confidence interval [CI], 0% to 4%) of the patients in the thrombin (recombinant) arm development specific antithrombin product antibodies (1 patient also developed anti-CHO host cell protein antibodies). No patients developed antibodies to pro-thrombin activator. Twenty-two percent of patients (95% CI, 16% to 28%) in the bovine thrombin arm developed specific antibodies to bovine thrombin product. None of the antibodies in the thrombin (recombinant) group neutralized native human thrombin. Antibodies against bovine thrombin product were not tested for neutralization of native human thrombin. Development of antibodies in either group did not lead to any adverse reactions such as excessive bleeding.

At baseline in the phase 3 study, 1.5% of patients in the thrombin (recombinant) group had positive anti-product antibody titers compared with 5% of patients in the bovine thrombin group. Of the patients who had detectable anti-product antibodies at baseline, 0 of 3 in the thrombin (recombinant) group and 8 of 10 in the bovine thrombin group exhibited 1 or more titer unit (10-fold or more) increases in antibody levels after study treatment.

In phase 2 studies incidence of antibody development following treatment with thrombin (recombinant) was 1.2% (95% CI, 0% to 6.5%) compared with 2.4% (95% CI, 0.1% to 12.9%) for placebo.

Evithrom – In the clinical study, serum samples were collected at baseline and at 5 weeks postsurgery for evaluation of antibodies to bovine. Thrombin, bovine factor V/Va, human thrombin, and human factor V/Va. Samples were collected at both time points for 81.3% of the patients. The enzyme-linked immunosorbent assay (ELISA) data were adjudicated by a panel of experts blinded to treatment assignment. After reviewing all data, the panel used an algorithm for assigning outcomes for each antigen: seroconversion negative or seroconversion positive.

The protocol did not specify any comparative analysis for immunogenicity data, only descriptive statistics. The adjudicated results show that 3.3% of the patients treated with human thrombin developed antibodies to any of the 4 antigens, compared with 12.7% of the patients developing antibodies in the control group (bovine thrombin). A total of 7.94% of the patients treated with bovine thrombin (control group) developed antibodies to bovine thrombin, and 9.52% of these patients developed antibodies to bovine factor V/Va. A few control patients had antibodies that cross-reacted with human thrombin, but none had antibodies that cross-reacted with human factor V/Va. None of the patients treated with human thrombin developed detectable antibodies to human thrombin or to human factor V/Va.

➤*Hypersensitivity reactions:* In patients with known hypersensitivity to snake proteins, there may be a potential for allergic reaction to thrombin (recombinant).

➤*Pregnancy:* *Category C.* Animal reproduction studies have not been conducted with thrombin. Adequate and well-controlled studies in pregnant women have not been performed. It is not known whether thrombin can cause fetal harm when administered to a pregnant woman or can affect reproduction capacity. Thrombin should be given to a pregnant woman only if clearly indicated.

Reproductive studies performed in rats with the combination of TnBP and *Triton-X 100* (components of human thrombin) at dosages of up to approximately 600-fold human dosage of TnBP (900 mcg/kg/day) and 3,000-fold human dosage of the *Triton-X 100* (4,500 mcg/kg/day) resulted in increased postimplantation loss and an increased number of late resorptions. Other studies performed with combinations of TnBP (300-fold human dosage, 450 mcg/kg/day) and *Triton-X 100* (1,500-fold human dosage, 2,250 mcg/kg/day) resulted in increased resorption rates, decreased fetal body weights, and an increased number of runts. No embryofetal adverse reactions were observed at dosages of up to of 300 mcg/kg/day TnBP and 1,500 mg/kg day *Triton-X 100*, 200-fold and 1,000-fold the human dose, respectively.

THROMBIN — TOPICAL

➤*Lactation:* The safety of human thrombin for use during breast-feeding has not been established. Use only if clearly needed.

➤*Children:* Safety and effectiveness in children have not been established for *Recothrom, Thrombin-JMI, Thrombi-Gel,* or *Thrombi-Pad.*

Evithrom – Of the 155 patients undergoing liver surgery who were treated in adequate and well-controlled studies of *Evicil fibrin sealant (human)* in which human thrombin is a component, 8 were children. Of these, 5 were less than 2 years of age and 3 were between 2 and 12 years of age. Use of human thrombin in children is supported by these data and by extrapolation of findings for safety and efficacy in adults.

Adverse Reactions

➤*Recothrom:*

Common adverse reactions – The most common adverse reactions were incision site complication (63% for both treatment groups), procedural pain (recombinant 29%; bovine 34%), and nausea (recombinant 28%; bovine 35%).

Serious adverse reactions – Serious adverse reactions were reported by 18% of patients treated with thrombin (recombinant) and 22% with thrombin (bovine).

Other adverse reactions –

Thrombin (Recombinant) Adverse Reactions		
Adverse reactions	Thrombin (recombinant) (n = 205)	Thrombin (bovine) (n = 206)
Any reaction	60%	56%
Cardiovascular		
Cardiac	20%	18%
Thromboembolic	6%	5%
Miscellaneous		
Bleeding	13%	12%
Hypersensitivity	15%	18%
Nausea and vomiting	33%	40%
Other infection	13%	15%
Postoperative wound infection	9%	11%

[a] Adverse reactions were included in categories based on a blinded review of the investigator verbatim and coded terms.

➤*Evithrom:*

Most common adverse reactions – The most common adverse reactions reported were procedural complications and pruritus.

Serious adverse reactions – At least 1 serious adverse reaction was reported for 17% of patients treated with human thrombin and 11% of patients treated with bovine thrombin. The adverse reactions reported were associated with postsurgical complications (eg, wound infection 2% for *Evithrom* and 1.3% for bovine thrombin) and the medical condition of the patient and were not considered related to study drug. 1.3% of patients in the human thrombin group experienced a treatment emergent severe adverse reaction: respiratory arrest and postprocedural hematoma (in 1 patient) and extradural hematoma. Three patients in the bovine thrombin group experienced a treatment emergent severe adverse reaction: hyperhidrosis, pyrexia, and postprocedural hematoma. None of the adverse reactions reported were considered causality related to human thrombin administration.

Hypersensitivity – Anaphylactic reactions may occur in rare cases. No adverse reactions of this type were reported during the conduct of the clinical trials. Mild reactions can be managed with antihistamines. Severe hypotensive reactions require immediate intervention using current principles of shock therapy.

Adverse reactions (2% or more) –

Human Thrombin Adverse Reactions (> 2%)			
Adverse reactions	Human thrombin (n = 153)	Bovine thrombin (n = 152)	Total (n = 305)
Lab test abnormalities	7.2%	9.2%	8.2%
Activated partial thromboplastin time increased	2.6%	5.3%	3.9%
International normalized ratio increased	2.6%	3.3%	3%
Lymphocyte count decreased	2.6%	1.3%	2%
Prothrombin time prolonged	2.6%	5.3%	3.9%
Neutrophil count increased	2%	1.3%	1.6%
Pruritus	0.7%	2%	1.3%
Site conditions	0	2%	1%

➤*Bovine thrombin:*

Hypersensitivity – Allergic reactions may be encountered in persons known to be sensitive to bovine materials. Inhibitory antibodies which interfere with hemostasis may develop in a small percentage of patients.

Patient Information

Inform patients that, if absorbed systemically, thrombin could potentially cause blood clotting disorders.

Encourage patients to consult their health care provider for any new or unusual symptoms.

Advise patients using human thrombin of the following: some viruses such as hepatitis A virus and parvovirus B19 are particularly difficult to remove or inactivate. Parvovirus B19 most seriously affects pregnant women or immunocompromised individuals. Symptoms of parvovirus B19 infection include fever, drowsiness, chills, and runny nose followed approximately 2 weeks by a rash and joint pain. Evidence of hepatitis A may include several days to weeks of poor appetite, fatigue, and low-grade fever followed by nausea, vomiting, and abdominal pain. Dark urine and yellowed complexion are also common symptoms. Encourage patients to consult their health care provider if such symptoms appear.

FIBRIN SEALANT, HUMAN (FIBRINOGEN/THROMBIN)

	Product/Distributor	Surface Area[a]	Total Fibrinogen (Human) Content	Total Thrombin (Human) Content	How Supplied
Rx	**TachoSil** (Baxter)	9.5 cm × 4.8 cm	337.4 mg	123.1 units	In 1s.
		4.8 cm × 4.8 cm	170.5 mg	62.2 units	In 2s.
		3 cm × 2.5 cm	55.5 mg	20.3 units	In 1s and 5s.

[a] Each fibrin sealant patch contains per cm^2: human fibrinogen range, 3.6 to 7.4 mg (5.5 mg); human thrombin range, 1.3 to 2.7 units (2 units); equine collagen and human albumin.

FIBRIN SEALANT, HUMAN (FIBRINOGEN/THROMBIN) — TOPICAL

Indications

➤*Adjunct to hemostasis:* As an adjunct to hemostasis for use in cardiovascular surgery when control of bleeding by standard surgical techniques (such as suture, ligature, or cautery) is ineffective or impractical.

Administration and Dosage

➤*General dosing considerations:* When applying fibrin sealant, use precaution because the white, inactive side of fibrin sealant may also adhere to surgical instruments (eg, forceps) or gloves covered with blood because of the affinity of collagen to blood. Premoisten surgical instruments and gloves with saline solution to reduce the adherence.

➤*Adults:*

Adjunct to hemostasis –

Usual dosage: The selection and number of patches to be applied should be determined by the size of the bleeding area to be treated. Select the appropriate patch so that it extends 1 to 2 cm beyond the margins of the wound. The patch can be cut to the correct size and shape if desired. If more than 1 patch is used, overlap patches by at least 1 cm.

Maximum dose: Do not exceed 7 patches sized 9.5 × 4.8 cm, 14 patches sized 4.8 × 4.8 cm, or 42 patches sized 3 × 2.5 cm.

➤*Preparation for administration:* Prior to application, cleanse the area to be treated to remove disinfectants and other fluids. The fibrinogen and thrombin proteins can be denatured by alcohol, iodine, or heavy metal ions. If any of these substances have been used to clean the wound area, thoroughly irrigate the area before the application of the patch.

Fibrin sealant comes ready to use in sterile packages and must be handled accordingly. Use only undamaged packages because resterilization is not possible. When in the operating room, the outer aluminum foil pouch may be opened in a nonsterile environment. The inner sterile blister must be opened in a sterile environment. Remove the fibrin sealant patch from the blister, which can be used as a container for premoistening of the patch, if needed.

➤*Administration:* Apply on the surface of tissue only. Do not use intravascularly. Apply the yellow, active side of the patch directly to the bleeding area wet or dry. Hold in place with gentle pressure applied through moistened gloves or a moist pad for at least 3 minutes. If applied wet, premoisten in saline 0.9% solution for no more than 1 minute and then apply immediately. In the case of a wet tissue surface (eg, oozing bleeding) fibrin sealant may be applied without premoistening.

After gently holding fibrin sealant to the bleeding area for at least 3 minutes, remove the gloved hand or moistened pad carefully from the patch. To avoid pulling the patch loose, first place a premoistened surgical instrument at one end of the patch before relieving the pressure. Gentle irrigation may also aid in removing the premoistened pad or gloved hand without removing the patch from the bleeding area.

FIBRIN SEALANT, HUMAN (FIBRINOGEN/THROMBIN) — TOPICAL

Leave fibrin sealant in place once it adheres to organ tissue. Remove unattached fibrin sealant patches (or part of) and replace with new patches.

➤*Storage/Stability:* Store between 2° and 25°C (36° and 77°F). Do not freeze. Discard unused, opened packages of fibrin sealant. Fibrin sealant cannot be resterilized once removed from the inner pouch.

Actions

➤*Pharmacology:* Fibrin sealant contains human fibrinogen and human thrombin as a dried coating on the surface of an equine collagen patch. When fibrin sealant is in contact with physiological fluids, the components of the coating dissolve and partly diffuse into the wound surface. Soluble fibrinogen is transformed into fibrin by the enzymatic action of thrombin, which polymerizes into a fibrin clot that adheres the collagen patch to the wound surface and achieves hemostasis. Fibrin sealant exhibits flexibility to accommodate for the physiological movements of tissues and organs and can withstand pressures of up to 61.4 hPa (46.1 mm Hg).

➤*Pharmacokinetics:*

Absorption/Distribution – Because fibrin sealant is applied only topically, systemic exposure or distribution to other organs or tissues is not expected.

Contraindications

Known anaphylactic or severe systemic reaction to human blood products or horse proteins; intravascular administration.

Warnings/Precautions

➤*Administration:* Do not apply fibrin sealant intravascularly. Intravascular application may result in life-threatening thromboembolic events. Do not leave fibrin sealant in an infected or contaminated space because it may potentiate an existing infection. When placing fibrin sealant into cavities or closed spaces, avoid overpacking because this may cause compression of underlying tissue. Use only the minimum amount necessary to achieve hemostasis. Carefully remove or reposition unattached pieces of fibrin sealant, if medically necessary.

➤*Arterial bleeding:* Do not use fibrin sealant for the treatment of severe or brisk arterial bleeding because fibrin sealant has not been evaluated in this treatment.

➤*Primary hemostasis:* Do not use fibrin sealant as the primary mode to control hemostasis. Fibrin sealant is not intended as a substitute for meticulous surgical technique and the proper application of suture, ligature, or other conventional procedures for hemostasis.

➤*Transmission of infectious agents:* The active substances of fibrin sealant are made from human plasma. Products made from human plasma may contain infectious agents, such as viruses, that can cause disease. The risk that such products will transmit an infectious agent has been reduced by screening plasma donors for prior exposure to certain viruses, by testing for the presence of certain virus infections, and by inactivating and removing certain viruses. Despite these measures, such products can still potentially transmit disease. Because this product is made from human blood, it may carry a risk of transmitting infectious agents (eg, viruses), and, theoretically, the Creutzfeldt-Jakob disease agent. Report all infections thought by a health care provider possibly to have been transmitted by this product to the manufacturer at 1-800-423-2862. Discuss the risks and benefits of this product with the patient.

Some viruses, such as parvovirus B19, are particularly difficult to remove or inactivate at this time. Parvovirus B19 most seriously affects pregnant women (fetal infection), immune-compromised individuals, or individuals with an increased erythropoiesis (eg, hemolytic anemia).

➤*Hypersensitivity reactions:* Hypersensitivity or allergic/anaphylactoid reactions may occur. Symptoms associated with allergic anaphylactic reactions include flush, urticaria, pruritus, nausea, drop in blood pressure, tachycardia or bradycardia, dyspnea, severe hypotension, and anaphylactic shock. These reactions may occur in patients receiving fibrin sealant for the first time or may increase with repetitive applications. In the event of hypersensitivity reactions, discontinue administration. Mild reactions can be managed with antihistamines. Severe hypotensive reactions require immediate intervention using current principles of shock therapy.

➤*Pregnancy:* *Category C.* Animal reproduction studies still have not been conducted with fibrin sealant. There are no adequate and well-controlled studies in pregnant women. It is also not known whether fibrin sealant can cause fetal harm when administered to a pregnant woman or can affect reproduction capacity. Some viruses, such as parvovirus B19, are particularly difficult to remove or inactivate at this time. Parvovirus B19 most seriously affects pregnant women (fetal infection). Administer fibrin sealant to pregnant women only if clearly needed.

➤*Lactation:* It is not known whether this drug is excreted in human breast milk. Because many drugs are excreted in human milk, exercise caution when administering fibrin sealant to breast-feeding women.

➤*Children:* The safety and effectiveness of fibrin sealant in children undergoing cardiovascular surgery have not been established.

➤*Elderly:* Greater susceptibility of some older patients to adverse reactions cannot be ruled out.

Drug Interactions

None well documented.

Adverse Reactions

➤*Most common adverse reactions:* The most common adverse reactions reported in greater than 5% of patients were atrial fibrillation and pyrexia. Atrial fibrillation was reported in 6.1% of fibrin sealant cases (5.9% of controls) and pyrexia in 5.8% of fibrin sealant cases (4.9% of controls).

In the cardiovascular study, the most frequently reported adverse reactions were atrial fibrillation (29% in the fibrin sealant group and 24.6% in the comparator group) and pleural effusion (22.6% in the fibrin sealant group and 19.3% in the comparator group).

➤*Adverse reactions (5% or more):*

Fibrin Sealant Adverse Reactions (≥ 5%)

Adverse reactions	Fibrin sealant (n = 62)[a]	Comparator (n = 57)[a]
At least 1 adverse reaction[b]	74.2%	75.4%
Cardiovascular		
Atrial fibrillation	29%	24.6%
Pericardial effusion	4.8%	7%
Pleural effusion	22.6%	19.3%
Tachyarrhythmia	6.5%	7%
Miscellaneous		
Hemorrhagic anemia	8.1%	10.5%
Postprocedural hemorrhage	4.8%	5.3%
Pyrexia	6.5%	5.3%

[a] As treated population (safety data set).
[b] The table presents the number of patients experiencing at least 1 adverse reaction (regardless of causality). At each level of patient summarization, please note that a patient is counted once regardless of whether the patient had 1 or more reactions reported.

➤*Postmarketing:*

Cardiovascular – Phlebitis, thrombosis.

GU – Renal artery thrombosis, renal failure.

Hematologic – Eosinophilia, hematoma, hemorrhage, postprocedural hemorrhage, splenic hemorrhage

Hepatic – Biloma, hepatitis C, portal vein thrombosis.

Respiratory – Hemothorax, laryngeal edema, postprocedural pulmonary embolism, respiratory distress.

Miscellaneous – Abscess, drug ineffective, catheter-related complication, foreign body trauma, granuloma, inflammation, multiorgan failure, mydriasis, nerve compression, parathyroid disorder, pyrexia.

Patient Information

Advise patients that because fibrin sealant is made from human blood, it may carry a risk of transmitting infectious agents (eg, viruses, and, theoretically, the Creutzfeldt-Jakob disease agent).

Instruct patients to consult their health care provider if symptoms of B19 virus infection appear (eg, fever, drowsiness, chills, and runny nose followed about 2 weeks later by a rash and joint pain).

MICROFIBRILLAR COLLAGEN HEMOSTAT

Rx	**Hemopad** (Astra)	**Fibrous absorbable collagen hemostat:** 2.5 cm x 5 cm, 5 cm x 8 cm and 8 cm x 10 cm	In 10s.

MICROFIBRILLAR COLLAGEN HEMOSTAT — TOPICAL

Indications

➤*Hemostasis:* Used in surgical procedures as an adjunct to hemostasis when control of bleeding by ligature or conventional procedures is ineffective or impractical.

Administration and Dosage

➤*General dosing considerations:* Moistening or wetting with saline or thrombin impairs its hemostatic efficacy. It should be used dry.

➤*Adults:*

Hemostasis –

Capillary bleeding: 1 g is usually sufficient for a 50 cm² area. Thicker coverage is required for more brisk bleeding.

Control of oozing from cancellous bone: Pack firmly into the spongy bone surface. After 5 to 10 minutes, tease excess away; this can usually be accomplished with blunt forceps and is facilitated by wetting with sterile 0.9% saline solution and irrigation. If breakthrough bleeding occurs in areas of thin application, apply additional hemostat. The amount required depends on the severity of bleeding.

MICROFIBRILLAR COLLAGEN HEMOSTAT — TOPICAL

➤*Administration:* This product should not be resterilized. It is not for injection or intraocular use. Discard any unused portion.

Fibrous form – Must be applied directly to the source of bleeding. Because of its adhesiveness, it may seal over the exit site of deeper hemorrhage and conceal an underlying hematoma, as in penetrating liver wounds.

Surface preparation: Compress with dry sponges immediately prior to application of the dry product, then apply pressure over the hemostat with a dry sponge; the length of time varies with the force and severity of bleeding. A minute may suffice for capillary bleeding (eg, skin graft donor sites, dermatologic curettage), but 3 to 5 minutes or more may be required for brisk bleeding (eg, splenic tears) or high pressure leaks in major artery suture holes.

Application: Adheres to wet gloves, instruments or tissue surfaces. To facilitate handling, use dry smooth forceps. Do not use gloved fingers to apply pressure.

Nonwoven web form – In neurosurgical and other procedures, apply small squares to bleeding areas; then cover the sites with moist cottonoid patties. To prevent wetting of the microfibullar collagen hemostat, and to apply needed pressure, hold a suction tip against the cottonoid for one to several minutes, depending on the briskness of bleeding. After 5 to 10 minutes, remove excess microfibullar collagen hemostat by teasing and irrigation.

Actions

➤*Pharmacology:* Microfibrillar collagen hemostat (MCH) is an absorbable topical hemostatic agent prepared as a dry, sterile, fibrous, water insoluble, partial hydrochloric acid salt of purified bovine corium collagen.

In contact with a bleeding surface, MCH attracts platelets that adhere to the fibrils and undergo the release phenomenon to trigger aggregation of platelets into thrombi in the interstices of the fibrous mass. The effect on platelet adhesion and aggregation is not inhibited by heparin in vitro. Platelets of patients with clinical thrombasthenia do not adhere to the hemostat in vitro. However, in clinical trials, it was effective in 50 of 68 patients receiving aspirin. It cannot control bleeding due to systemic coagulation disorders. Institute appropriate therapy to correct the underlying coagulopathy prior to use of the drug. It is tenaciously adherent to surfaces wet with blood, but excess material not involved in the hemostatic clot may be removed by teasing or irrigation, usually without restarting bleeding.

MCH stimulates a mild, chronic cellular inflammatory response. When implanted in animal tissues, it is absorbed in less than 84 days and does not predispose to stenosis at vascular anastomotic sites. These findings have not been confirmed in humans. In human studies of hemostasis in osteotomy cuts, it does not interfere with bone regeneration or healing.

Contraindications

Closure of skin incisions; it may interfere with the healing of the skin edges due to simple mechanical interposition of dry collagen.

Bone surfaces to which prosthetic materials are to be attached with methylmethacrylate adhesives. By filling porosities of cancellous bone, MCH may significantly reduce the bond strength of methylmethacrylate adhesives.

Warnings/Precautions

➤*Sterilization:* MCH is inactivated by autoclaving. Ethylene oxide reacts with bound hydrochloric acid to form ethylene chlorohydrin.

➤*Infection:* The presence of the hemostat does not enhance or initiate experimental staphylococcus wound infections to a greater or lesser extent than control agents. The effects on experimental wounds contaminated with a gram-negative aerobic rod and an anaerobic non-spore-forming bacteria are currently under investigation. Use in contaminated wounds may enhance infection.

➤*Excess material:* After several minutes, remove excess material; this is usually possible without the reinitiation of active bleeding. Failure to remove excess material may result in bowel adhesion or mechanical pressure sufficient to compromise the ureter. In otolaryngological surgery, precautions against aspiration should include removal of all excess dry material and thorough irrigation of the pharynx.

➤*Antibodies:* Contains a low level of intercalated bovine serum protein that reacts immunologically as does beef serum albumin (BSA). Increases in anti-BSA titer have been observed following treatment. About two-thirds of individuals exhibit antibody titers because of ingestion of food products of bovine origin. Intradermal skin tests have occasionally shown weak positive reactions to BSA or MCH, but these have not been correlated with IgG titers to BSA. Tests have failed to demonstrate clinically significant elicitation of antibodies of the IgE class against BSA following therapy.

➤*Blood from operative sites:* Fragments of MCH may pass through filters of blood scavenging systems. Therefore, avoid reintroduction of blood from operative sites treated with MCH.

➤*Autologous blood salvage circuits:* MCH should not be used in conjunction with autologous blood salvage circuits.

➤*Handling:* Avoid spillage on nonbleeding surfaces, particularly in abdominal or thoracic viscera.

➤*Pregnancy: Category undetermined*. There are no well controlled studies in pregnant women. Safety for use during pregnancy has not been established. Use only when clearly needed and when the potential benefits outweigh the potential hazards to the fetus.

➤*Lactation:* There is no information available regarding this medication in breast-feeding women.

Adverse Reactions

Most serious – Potentiation of infection (including abscess formation, hematoma, wound dehiscenceand mediastinitis). Adhesion formation; allergic reaction; foreign body reaction; subgaleal seroma (single case).

The use of MCH in dental extraction sockets increases the incidence of alveolalgia. Transient laryngospasm due to aspiration of dry materials has been reported following use in tonsillectomy.

ABSORBABLE GELATIN SPONGE

Rx	**Gelfoam** (Upjohn)	**Sponges**: Size 12: 2 x 6 cm x 3 or 7 mm	In 4s and 12s (7 mm only).
		Size 50: 8 x 6.25 cm	In 4s.
		Size 100: 8 x 12.5 cm	In regular and compressed. In 6s.
		Size 200: 8 x 25 cm	In 6s.
		Packs: Size 2: 40 x 2 cm	In single jars.
		Size 6: 40 x 6 cm	In 6s.
		Dental pk: Size 4: 2 x 2 cm	In 15s.
		Prostatectomy cones: Size 13: 5″ diameter	In 6s.
		Size 18: 7″ diameter	In 6s.

ABSORBABLE GELATIN — SPONGE

Indications

➤*Hemostasis:* For use in surgical procedures as an adjunct to hemostasis when control of bleeding by ligature or conventional procedures is ineffective or impractical.

Also used in oral and dental surgery as an aid in providing hemostasis.

In open prostatic surgery, insertion into the prostatic cavity provides hemostasis.

Administration and Dosage

➤*Adults:*

Hemostasis – See Administration.

➤*Administration:*

Dentistry – When used dry, roll between fingers and lightly compress to diameter of cavity or socket. After insertion, apply light finger pressure for 1 or 2 min. When used moist, immerse in NaCl solution, then remove, squeeze thoroughly to remove air bubbles and replace in solution where it will swell to original size. Take from solution, blot on sterile gauze to remove excess fluid and place in cavity or wound.

Hemostasis – Apply dry or saturated with NaCl injection. When bleeding is controlled, leave pieces in place. Because sponge causes little more cellular infiltration than the blood clot, the wound may be closed over it. When applied, the sponge will stay in place until it liquefies. When applied dry, compress pieces before application to bleeding surface, then hold in place with moderate pressure for 10 to 15 seconds. When used with saline solutions, immerse in solution, withdraw, squeeze to remove the air bubbles present and replace in solution where it will swell to original size. If it does not, remove and knead vigorously until all air is expelled. Leave piece wet, or blot to dampness on gauze, and apply to bleeding point. Hold in place with moderate pressure with a cotton pledget or small gauze sponge until hemostasis results.

Prostatectomy cones – These are designed for use with the Foley bag catheter.

➤*Storage/Stability:* Once package is opened, contents are subject to contamination.

Actions

➤*Pharmacology:* A sterile, pliable surgical sponge prepared from purified gelatin solution and capable of absorbing and holding many times its weight of whole blood.

ABSORBABLE GELATIN — SPONGE

When implanted into tissues, it is absorbed completely within 4 to 6 weeks without inducing excessive scar tissue formation. When applied to bleeding areas of nasal, rectal or vaginal mucosa, it completely liquefies within 2 to 5 days.

Contraindications

Closure of skin incisions (may interfere with the healing of skin edges); control of postpartum bleeding or menorrhagia.

Warnings/Precautions

➤*Sterilization:* Do not resterilize by heat, since heating may change absorption time. Ethylene oxide is not recommended for resterilization; it may be trapped in the interstices of the foam and trace amounts may cause burns or irritation to tissue.

➤*Infection:* Not recommended in the presence of infection. If signs of infection or abscess develop in the area where the sponge has been placed, reoperation may be necessary to remove the infected material and allow drainage.

➤*Compression:* Sponge may expand and impinge on nearby structures. When placing into cavities or closed tissue spaces, use minimal preliminary compression; avoid overpacking.

➤*Pregnancy:* Category: Undetermined.

➤*Lactation:* There is no information regarding breast-feeding women.

Adverse Reactions

Sponge may form infection and abscess (see Precautions). Giant cell granuloma in the brain has occurred at implantation site, as well as brain and spinal cord compression due to sterile fluid accumulation. Excessive fibrosis and prolonged fixation of the tendon were seen when the sponge was used at a tendon juncture.

ABSORBABLE GELATIN FILM

Rx	**Gelfilm** (Upjohn)	**Film:** 100 mm x 125 mm	In 1s.
Rx	**Gelfilm Ophthalmic** (Upjohn)	**Film:** 25 mm x 50 mm	In 6s.

ABSORBABLE GELATIN — FILM

Indications

➤*Neurosurgery:* As a dural substitute; absorbable gelatin film is nonconducive to undue inflammatory reaction and absorbable at a rate slow enough to permit dural regeneration and healing of the arachnoid layer. Its use in patients undergoing craniotomies reportedly prevented the development of meningocerebral adhesions, thereby reducing the risk of postoperative sequelae.

➤*Thoracic surgery:* In the repair of pleural defects in connection with thoracotomies, thoracoplasties and extrapleural procedures, implantation has been followed by minimal tissue reaction and subsequent closure of the defect by ingrowth of regenerating pleural and fibrous tissue across the gradually resorbed implant.

➤*Ocular surgery:* In glaucoma filtration operations (ie, iridencleisis and trephination), extraocular muscle surgery and diathermy or scleral "buckling" operations for retinal detachment. There is a remarkable lack of cellular reaction to the film implanted subconjunctivally or used as a seton into the anterior chamber. Evidence shows that implants help prevent formation of adhesions between contiguous ocular structures.

Administration and Dosage

➤*Adults:*

Neurosurgery –

Covering dural defects: Place over the surface of the brain. Tuck the edges of the implant beneath the dura and the wound; close the wound in the usual manner. If desired, the film can be sutured loosely to the dura. The moist film tears easily.

Ocular surgery –

As a seton in iridencleisis: Place a small piece (approximately 4 mm × 10 mm) over the prolapsed iris pillar parallel to the limbus; Tenon's capsule and the conjunctiva are then closed with continuous absorbable sutures closely spaced to ensure tight wound closure.

Diathermy or scleral "buckling" operations: Place film over the sclera, then suture the muscle and the conjunctiva over the underlying film.

Extraocular muscle surgery: Place film over and beneath the muscle before Tenon's capsule and the conjunctiva are closed in layers.

Thoracic surgery –

Covering pleural defects: Place over the defect and anchor in place by means of small interrupted sutures.

➤*Preparation for administration:* Immerse in sterile saline solution; soak until quite pliable; cut to the desired size and shape.

➤*Storage/Stability:* Once the envelopes have been opened, contents are subject to contamination. To ensure sterility, use immediately after withdrawal from the envelope. Store at 15° to 30°C (59° to 86°F).

Actions

➤*Pharmacology:* A sterile, absorbable gelatin film for use in neurosurgery, thoracic and ocular surgery.

In the dry state, absorbable gelatin film has the appearance and texture of cellophane of equivalent thickness; when moistened, it assumes a rubbery consistency and can then be cut to the desired size and fitted to rounded or irregular surfaces. The rate of absorption after implantation ranges from 1 to 6 months, depending on the size of the implant and the site of implantation. Pleural and muscle implants are completely absorbed in 8 to 14 days; dural and ocular implants usually require at least 2 to 5 months for complete absorption. The absence of undue tissue reactions, with the consequent decreased likelihood of developing adhesions, has been of particular value in the case of dural and ocular implants.

Contraindications

Because the rate of absorption is likely to be increased in the presence of purulent exudation, do not implant in grossly contaminated or infected surgical wounds.

Warnings/Precautions

➤*Pregnancy:* Category: Undetermined.

There is no information in pregnant patients.

➤*Lactation:* There is no information in breast-feeding patients.

OXIDIZED CELLULOSE

Rx	**Oxycel** (Becton-Dickinson)	**Pads:** 3" x 3", 8 ply **Pledgets:** 2" x 1" x 1" **Strips:** 18" x 2", 4 ply	In 10s.
Rx	**Surgicel** (Johnson & Johnson)	**Strips:** 2" x 14" 4" x 8" 2" x 3" ½" x 2"	In 1s.
		Surgical Nu-knit: 1" x 1" 3" x 4" 6" x 9"	In 1s.

OXIDIZED CELLULOSE — TOPICAL

Indications

➤*Hemorrhage:* Used adjunctively in surgical procedures to assist in the control of capillary, venous and small arterial hemorrhage when ligation or other conventional methods of control are impractical or ineffective. Also indicated for use in oral surgery and exodontia.

Administration and Dosage

➤*Adults:*

Hemorrhage – Withdraw hemostat from the container with dry, sterile forceps. Minimal amounts of an appropriate size are laid on the bleeding site or held firmly against the tissues until hemostasis is obtained.

➤*Children:* See Adults for dosing.

➤*Storage/Stability:* Discard opened, unused oxidized cellulose. It cannot be resterilized.

Actions

➤*Pharmacology:* An absorbable hemostatic agent prepared from cellulose by a special process that converts it into polyanhydroglucuronic acid (cellulosic acid). Oxidation of cellulose yields an absorbable product of known acidity, soluble in alkali.

Provides hemostatic action when applied to sites of bleeding. The mechanism of action is not completely understood, but it appears to be a physical effect rather than any alteration of the normal physiologic clotting mecha-

OXIDIZED CELLULOSE — TOPICAL

nism. Upon contact with blood, oxidized cellulose becomes a dark reddish-brown or almost black, tenacious, adhesive mass. It conforms and adheres readily to the bleeding surface. After 24 to 48 hours, it becomes gelatinous and can be removed, usually without causing additional bleeding. If left in situ, absorption depends on several factors, including the amount used, degree of saturation with blood and the tissue bed.

Oxidized cellulose swells upon contact with blood; the resultant pressure adds to its hemostatic action. It does not enter the normal clotting mechanism; however, within a few minutes of contact with blood, it forms an artificially produced clot in the bleeding area.

Bactericidal effects – The hemostat is bactericidal in vitro against many gram-positive and gram-negative organisms including aerobes and anaerobes: *Staphylococcus aureus, S. epidermidis, Micrococcus luteus, Streptococcus pyogenes* Groups A and B, *S. salivarius, Bacillus subtilis, Proteus vulgaris, Corynebacterium xerosis, Mycobacterium phlei, Clostridium tetani, Branhamella catarrhalis, Escherichia coli, Klebsiella aerogenes, Lactobacillus* sp, *Salmonella enteritidis, Shigella dysenteriae, Serratia marcescens, C. perfringens, Bacteroides fragilis, Enterococcus, Enterobacter cloacae, Pseudomonas aeruginosa, P. stutzeri* and *Proteus mirabilis*. In contrast to other hemostatic agents, it does not tend to enhance experimental infection.

Contraindications

Packing or wadding as a hemostatic agent; packing or implantation in fractures or laminectomies (it interferes with bone regeneration and can cause cyst formation); control of hemorrhage from large arteriesor on nonhemorrhagic serous oozing surfaces since body fluids other than whole blood (eg, serum) do not react with oxidized cellulose to produce satisfactory hemostatic effects; do not use around the optic nerve and chiasm; as a wrap in vascular surgery because it has a stenotic effect.

Warnings/Precautions

➤*Sterilization:* Do not autoclave; autoclaving causes physical breakdown.

➤*Surgery:* Not intended as a substitute for careful surgery and proper use of sutures and ligatures.

➤*Contaminated wound:* Closing oxidized cellulose in a contaminated wound without drainage may lead to complications and should be avoided.

➤*Application/Removal:* The hemostatic effect is greater when applied dry; therefore, do not moisten with water or saline. Do not impregnate with materials such as buffering or hemostatic substances. Its hemostatic effect is not enhanced by the addition of thrombin; the activity of thrombin is destroyed by the low pH of the product. If used temporarily to line the cavity of large open wounds, place so as not to overlap the skin edges.

May be left in situ when necessary, but remove it once hemostasis is achieved. It must always be removed if used in, around or in proximity to foramina in bone, areas of bony confine, the spinal cord or the optic nerve and chiasm; by swelling, it may cause nerve damage by pressure in a bony confine. Paralysis has been reported when used around the spinal cord, particularly in surgery for herniated intervertebral disc. Remove from open wounds by forceps or by irrigation with sterile water or saline solution after bleeding has stopped.

➤*Infections:* Although it is bactericidal against a wide range of pathogenic microorganisms, it is not a substitute for systemic antimicrobial agents to control or prevent postoperative infections. Do not impregnate with anti-infective agents.

➤*Packing:* Apply by loosely packing against the bleeding surface. Avoid wadding or packing tightly, especially within the bony enclosure of the CNS and within other relatively rigid cavities where swelling may interfere with normal function or possibly cause necrosis.

➤*Use sparingly:* To control bleeding in open reduction of fractures and in cancellous bone, use sparingly. To minimize the possibility of interference with callus formation and the theoretical chance of cyst formation, remove any excess after bleeding is controlled.

➤*Urological procedures:* Use minimal amounts and exercise care to prevent plugging of the urethra, ureter or catheter.

➤*Concomitant therapy:* Since absorption is prevented in chemically cauterized areas, its use should not be preceded by application of silver nitrate or any other escharotic chemicals.

➤*Otorhinolaryngologic surgery:* Exercise care so that none of the material is aspirated by the patient (eg, when controlling hemorrhage after tonsillectomy; controlling epistaxis).

➤*Pregnancy:* Category: *Undetermined*. There are no data regarding oxidized cellulose in pregnancy.

➤*Lactation:* There are no data regarding the use of oxidized cellulose in breast-feeding.

Adverse Reactions

Encapsulation of fluid and foreign body reactions, with or without infection, have been reported.

Possible prolongation of drainage in cholecystectomies and difficulty passing urine per urethra after prostatectomy have been reported. There has been one report of a blocked ureter after kidney resection.

Burning has been reported when applied after nasal polyp removal and after hemorrhoidectomy. Headache, burning, stinging and sneezing in epistaxis and other rhinological procedures and stinging when applied on surface wounds (varicose ulcerations, dermabrasions and donor sites) have also been reported. These are believed to be due to the low pH of the product.

Intestinal obstruction has occurred, due to transmigration of a bolus of oxidized cellulose from gallbladder bed to terminal ileum or to adhesions in a loop of denuded intestine to which oxidized cellulose had been applied.

➤*Miscellaneous:* Necrosis of nasal mucous membraneor perforation of nasal septum due to tight packing; urethral obstruction following retropubic prostatectomy and introduction of oxidized cellulose within enucleated prostatic capsule.

PLASMA EXPANDERS

Plasma Protein Fractions

Indications

➤*General information: Unless the condition responsible for the hypoproteinemia can be corrected, albumin in any form can provide only symptomatic relief or supportive treatment.*

➤*Shock:* For shock due to burns, trauma, surgery and infections; in the treatment of injuries of such severity that shock, although not immediately present, is likely to ensue; in other similar conditions where the restoration of blood volume is urgent.

In cases in which there has been a considerable loss of red blood cells, transfusion with whole blood or red blood cells is indicated.

For the earliest emergency treatment of shock, it may be more convenient to have 25% normal serum albumin available because it is so highly concentrated. However, the concentrated solution depends (for its maximum osmotic effect) on holding additional fluids in the circulation, which are drawn from the tissues or administered separately; if patient is dehydrated, maximum effect cannot be obtained without additional fluids. Therefore, for routine hospital use, normal serum albumin 5% may be preferred, as maximum osmotic effect is obtained with no additional fluids.

Albumin 25% with appropriate crystalloids may offer therapeutic advantages in oncotic deficits or in long-standing shock where treatment has been delayed. Removal of ascitic fluid from the patient with cirrhosis may cause changes in cardiovascular function and even result in hypovolemic shock.

➤*Burns:* Albumin 5% or plasma protein 5% may be used in conjunction with adequate infusions of crystalloid to prevent hemoconcentration and to combat the water, protein and electrolyte losses which usually follow serious burns. After 24 hours, albumin 25% can be used to maintain plasma colloid osmotic pressure.

➤*Hypoproteinemia:* In clinical situations usually associated with a low concentration of plasma protein and, consequently, a reduced volume of circulating blood.

Normal serum albumin 5% or plasma protein fraction 5% may be used in hypoproteinemic patients, providing sodium restriction is not a problem. If sodium restriction is imperative, use 25% normal serum albumin.

For acute complications of chronic hypoproteinemia, use albumin 25% possibly in conjunction with a diuretic.

➤*Adult respiratory distress syndrome (ARDS):* This syndrome is characterized by deficient oxygenation caused by pulmonary interstitial edema complicating shock and postsurgical conditions. When clinical signs are those of hypoproteinemia with a fluid volume overload, albumin 25%, together with a diuretic, may play a role in therapy.

➤*Cardiopulmonary bypass:* Preoperative dilution of the blood using albumin and crystalloid is safe and well tolerated. Although the limit to which the hematocrit and plasma protein concentration can be safely lowered has not been defined, it is common to achieve a hematocrit of 20% and a plasma albumin concentration of 2.5 g/100 mL.

➤*Acute liver failure with or without coma:* Administration of albumin may serve the double purpose of supporting the colloid osmotic pressure of the plasma as well as binding excess plasma bilirubin. Albumin 25% may be considered.

➤*Sequestration of protein rich fluids:* This occurs in such conditions as acute peritonitis, pancreatitis, mediastinitis and extensive cellulitis. The magnitude of loss into the third space may require treatment of reduced volume or oncotic activity with albumin.

➤*Erythrocyte resuspension:* Albumin may be required to avoid excessive hypoproteinemia during certain types of exchange transfusion or with the use of very large volumes of previously frozen or washed red cells.

➤*Acute nephrosis:* Certain patients may not respond to cyclophosphamide or steroid therapy. A loop diuretic and albumin 25% may help control the edema and the patient may then respond to steroid treatment.

➤*Renal dialysis:* Albumin 25% may be of value in treating shock or hypotension.

➤*Hyperbilirubinemia and erythroblastosis fetalis:* Albumin can be a useful adjunct in exchange transfusions; it reduces the necessity for re-exchange and increases the amount of bilirubin removed with each transfusion, lessening the risk of kernicterus.

Actions

➤*Pharmacology:* The plasma protein fractions include plasma protein fraction 5% (83% albumin with alpha and beta globulins), normal serum albumin 5% and normal serum albumin 25%.

The albumin fraction of human blood has two known functions: Maintenance of plasma colloid osmotic pressure and carrier of intermediate metabolites in the transport and exchange of tissue products. It comprises about 50% to 60% of the plasma proteins and provides approximately 70% to 80% of their colloid osmotic pressure. Thus, it is important in regulating the volume of circulating blood; its loss is critical, particularly in shock with hemorrhage or reduced plasma volume. When plasma volume is reduced, an adequate amount of albumin quickly restores the volume in most instances. Twenty-five grams of albumin is the osmotic equivalent of approximately 2 units (500 mL) of fresh frozen plasma; or 100 mL of normal serum albumin 25% provides about as much plasma protein as does 500 mL plasma or 2 pints whole blood. Normal serum albumin 5% is osmotically equivalent to an approximately equal volume of citrated plasma. The 25% albumin solution is osmotically equivalent to 5 times the volume of citrated plasma.

Plasma protein fraction is effective in the maintenance of a normal blood volume, but it has not been proven effective to maintain oncotic pressure. When the circulating blood volume has been depleted, the hemodilution following albumin administration persists for many hours. In individuals with normal blood volume, it usually lasts only a few hours. The half-life of albumin is 15 to 20 days with a turnover of approximately 15 g per day.

Albumin 5% increases the circulating plasma volume by approximately equal to the amount infused. Albumin 25% draws about 3.5 times its volume of additional fluid into the circulation within 15 minutes except when the patient is dehydrated. Both 5% and 25% decrease blood viscosity.

There is no evidence that normal serum albumin (human) interferes with normal coagulation mechanisms. Antibodies, especially isoagglutinins, have been removed, enabling the product to be used without regard to the patient's blood group or blood factors.

Unlike whole blood or plasma, plasma protein fractions are free of the danger of homologous serum hepatitis, because these solutions are heat treated at 60°C (140°F) for 10 hours; thus, the possibility of transmitting serum hepatitis is reduced to a minimum. No crossmatching is required and the absence of cellular elements removes the risk of sensitization with repeated infusions.

Contraindications

A history of allergic reactions to albumin; severe anemia; cardiac failure; the presence of normal or increased intravascular volume; patients on cardiopulmonary bypass.

In chronic nephrosis, infused albumin is promptly excreted by the kidneys with no relief of the chronic edema or effect on the underlying renal lesion. It is of occasional use in the rapid "priming" diuresis of nephrosis. Similarly, in hypoproteinemic states associated with chronic cirrhosis, malabsorption, protein losing enteropathies, pancreatic insufficiency and undernutrition, the infusion of albumin as a source of protein nutrition is not justified.

Warnings/Precautions

➤*Concomitant blood administration:* When large quantities of albumin are given, supplement with or replace by whole blood to combat relative anemia.

Not a substitute for whole blood in situations where the oxygen carrying capacity of whole blood is required in addition to plasma volume expansion. Contains no recognized blood coagulating factors and should not be used for control of hemorrhage due to deficiencies or defects in the clotting mechanism.

➤*Hypotension:* Rapid infusion (greater than 10 mL/min) may produce hypotension. Monitor blood pressure during use and slow or discontinue infusion if hypotension occurs. Vasopressors may also help correct the hypotension.

➤*Hemorrhage:* Supplement albumin with hemodilution. When circulating blood volume has been reduced, hemodilution following the administration of albumin persists for many hours. In patients with a normal blood volume, hemodilution lasts for a much shorter period.

➤*Shock:* Monitor blood pressure frequently. Widening of the pulse pressure is correlated with an increase in stroke volume or cardiac output.

➤*Dehydration:* Patients with marked dehydration require additional fluids.

➤*Special risk patients:* Use with caution in patients with hepatic or renal failure because of the added protein load.

Certain patients (eg, those with congestive cardiac failure, renal insufficiency or with stabilized chronic anemia) are at risk of developing circulatory overload. Rapid infusion may cause vascular overload with resultant pulmonary edema. Monitor for signs of increased venous pressure.

Use caution in patients with low cardiac reserve or with no albumin deficiency. A rapid increase in plasma volume may cause circulatory embarrassment or pulmonary edema.

➤*Pregnancy:* *Category C.* Safety for use has not been established. Use only when clearly needed and when the potential benefits outweigh the hazards to the fetus.

➤*Lactation:* Excretion into breast milk is unknown.

➤*Monitoring:* The quick rise in blood pressure that may follow administration of albumin after injuries or surgery necessitates observation to detect bleeding points that may have failed to bleed at the lower blood pressure; otherwise, new hemorrhage and shock may occur.

Adverse Reactions

Allergic or pyrogenic reactions – Such reactions are characterized primarily by fever and chills. Flushing, urticaria, back pain, headache, rash, nausea, vomiting, increased salivation and febrile reactions, tachycardia, hypotension, and changes in respiration, pulse and blood pressure have also been reported. If such reactions occur, discontinue the infusion and institute appropriate therapy.

➤*Cardiovascular:* Hypotension (see Warnings/Precautions). In addition, rapid administration may result in vascular overload, dyspnea and pulmonary edema.

PLASMA PROTEIN FRACTION

Rx	**Plasmanate** (Talecris)	**Injection:** 5%	In 50 and 250 mL vials.
Rx	**Plasma-Plex** (Centeon)		In 50, 250, and 500 mL vials with injection set.
Rx	**Protenate** (Baxter Healthcare)		In 250 and 500 mL vials.

PLASMA PROTEIN FRACTION (HUMAN) — INJECTION

For complete and comparative prescribing information, refer to the Plasma Protein Fractions group monograph.

Indications

➤*Treatment of shock:* Treatment of shock due to burns, crushing injuries, abdominal emergencies, and any other cause where there is a predominant loss of plasma fluids and not red blood cells. It is also effective in the emergency treatment of shock due to hemorrhage. Following the emergency phase of therapy, blood transfusions may be indicated depending on the severity of the blood loss.

Infants and small children – Found to be very useful in the initial therapy of shock due to dehydration and infection.

Administration and Dosage

➤*Adults:*

Treatment of shock – The usual minimum effective dose in adults is 250 to 500 mL.

➤*Preparation for administration:* First, swab the stopper with iodine tincture, followed by a sterile antiseptic swab.

Only 16-gauge needles or dispensing pins should be used with 20 mL vial sizes and larger. Needles or dispensing pins should only be inserted within the stopper area delineated by the raised ring. The stopper should be penetrated perpendicular to the plane of the stopper within the ring.

➤*Administration:* Administration should be by vein and preferably through an area of skin at some distance from any site of infection or trauma.

As with any plasma expander, the rate should be adjusted or slowed according to the clinical response and rising blood pressure.

➤*Admixture compatibility:* Plasma protein fraction (human) is compatible with the usual carbohydrate and electrolyte solutions.

➤*Storage/Stability:* Store at room temperature not exceeding 30°C (86°F). Solution that has been frozen should not be used.

ALBUMIN HUMAN (Normal Serum Albumin)

Rx	**Albuminar-5** (ZLB Behring)	**Injection:** 5%	In 50 and 1,000 mL vials.
Rx	**Albutein 5%** (Grifols)		In 250 and 500 mL vials.
Rx	**Normal Serum Albumin (Human) 5% Solution** (Immuno-US)		In 50, 250, and 500 mL vials with IV set.
Rx	**Plasbumin-5** (Talecris)		In 50, 250, and 500 mL vials.
Rx	**Plasbumin-20** (Talecris)	**Injection:** 20%	In 50 and 100 mL vials.

ALBUMIN HUMAN (Normal Serum Albumin)

Rx	**Albuminar-25** (ZLB Behring)	**Injection**: 25%	In 20 mL vials.
Rx	**Albutein 25%** (Grifols)		In 20, 50, and 100 mL vials.
Rx	**Human Albumin Grifols** (Grifols)		In 50 and 100 mL vials.
Rx	**Normal Serum Albumin (Human) 25% Solution** (Immuno-US)		In 20, 50, and 100 mL vials with IV set.
Rx	**Plasbumin-25** (Talecris)		In 20, 50, and 100 mL vials.

ALBUMIN HUMAN — INJECTION

For complete and comparative prescribing information, refer to the Plasma Protein Fractions group monograph.

Indications

➤*Hypovolemic shock:*

25% and 20% solutions – For emergency treatment of hypovolemic shock.

Albumin (human) 25% and 20% solutions are hyperoncotic and on intravenous (IV) infusion will expand the plasma volume by an additional amount, 3 to 4 times the volume actually administered, by withdrawing fluid from the interstitial spaces, provided the patient is normally hydrated interstitially or there is interstitial edema. If the patient is dehydrated, additional crystalloids must be given, or, alternatively, albumin (human) 5% solution, should be used. The patient's hemodynamic response should be monitored and the usual precautions against circulatory overload observed. The total dose should not exceed the level of albumin found in the healthy individual (ie, about 2 g/kg body weight) in the absence of active bleeding). Although albumin (human) 5% solution is to be preferred for the usual volume deficits, albumin (human) 25% or 20% solution with appropriate crystalloids may offer therapeutic advantages in oncotic deficits or in longstanding shock where treatment has been delayed.

Removal of ascitic fluid from a patient with cirrhosis may cause changes in cardiovascular function and even result in hypovolemic shock. In such circumstances, the use of an albumin infusion may be required to support the blood volume.

5% solution – For the treatment of hypovolemic shock.

➤*Hypoproteinemia (with or without edema):*

25% and 20% solutions – During major surgery, patients can lose over half of their circulating albumin, with the attendant complications of oncotic deficit. A similar situation can occur in sepsis or intensive-care patients. Treatment with albumin (human) 25% or 20% solutions may be of value in such cases.

5% solution – For treatment in conditions in which there is severe hypoalbuminemia. However, unless the pathologic condition responsible for the hypoalbuminemia can be corrected, administration of albumin can afford only symptomatic or supportive relief.

➤*Cardiopulmonary bypass:*

25% and 20% solutions – With the relatively small priming volume required with modern pumps, preoperative dilution of the blood using albumin and crystalloid has been shown to be safe and well tolerated. Although the limit to which the hematocrit and plasma protein concentration can be safely lowered has not been defined, it is common practice to adjust the albumin and crystalloid pump prime to achieve a hematocrit of 20% and a plasma albumin concentration of 2.5 g per 100 mL in the patient.

5% solution – May be used as an adjunct in cardiopulmonary bypass procedures.

➤*Renal dialysis:*

25% and 20% solutions – Although not part of the regular regimen of renal dialysis, albumin (human) 25% or 20% solutions may be of value in the treatment of shock or hypotension in these patients. The usual volume administered is about 100 mL, taking particular care to avoid fluid overload, as these patients are often fluid overloaded and cannot tolerate substantial volumes of salt solution.

5% solution – May be used as an adjunct in hemodialysis.

Note – In those conditions in which the colloid requirement is high, and there is less need for fluid, albumin should be administered as a 25% solution.

➤*Burn therapy:*

25% and 20% solutions – An optimal therapeutic regimen with respect to the administration of colloids, crystalloids, and water following extensive burns has not been established. During the first 24 hours after sustaining thermal injury, large volumes of crystalloids are infused to restore the depleted extracellular fluid volume. Beyond 24 hours, albumin (human) 25% or 20% solutions can be used to maintain plasma colloid osmotic pressure.

➤*Adult respiratory distress syndrome:*

25% and 20% solutions – Adult respiratory distress syndrome (ARDS) is characterized by deficient oxygenation caused by pulmonary interstitial edema complicating shock and postsurgical conditions. When clinical signs are those of hypoproteinemia with a fluid volume overload, albumin (human) 25% or 20% solution together with a diuretic may play a role in therapy.

➤*Acute liver failure:*

25% and 20% solutions – In the uncommon situation of rapid loss of liver function with or without coma, administration of albumin may serve the double purpose of supporting the colloid osmotic pressure of the plasma as well as binding excess plasma bilirubin.

➤*Sequestration of protein-rich fluids:*

25% and 20% solutions – Sequestration of protein-rich fluids occurs in such conditions as acute peritonitis, pancreatitis, mediastinitis, and extensive cellulitis. The magnitude of loss into the third space may require treatment of reduced volume or oncotic activity with an infusion of albumin.

➤*Erythrocyte resuspension:*

25% and 20% solutions – Albumin may be required to avoid excessive hypoproteinemia during certain types of exchange transfusion or with the use of very large volumes of previously frozen or washed red cells. About 25 g of albumin per liter of erythrocytes is commonly used, although the requirements in preexistent hypoproteinemia or hepatic impairment can be greater. Albumin human 25% or 20% solutions are added to the isotonic suspension of washed red cells immediately prior to transfusion.

➤*Acute nephrosis:*

25% and 20% solutions – Certain patients with acute nephrosis may not respond to cyclophosphamide or steroid therapy. The steroids may even aggravate the underlying edema. In this situation, a loop diuretic and 100 mL of albumin (human) 25% or 20% solutions repeated daily for 7 to 10 days may be helpful in controlling the edema, and the patient may then respond to steroid treatment.

➤*Pediatric use:*

25% and 20% solutions –

Neonatal hemolytic disease: The administration of albumin (human) 25% or 20% solutions may be indicated prior to exchange transfusion in order to bind free bilirubin, thus lessening the risk of kernicterus. A dosage of 1 g/kg body weight is given about 1 hour prior to exchange transfusion. Caution must be observed in hypervolemic infants.

5% solution – The pediatric use of albumin (human) 5% solution has not been clinically evaluated. Therefore, physicians should weigh the risks and benefits of the use of albumin (human) 5% solution in the pediatric population.

➤*Situations in which albumin administration is not warranted:* In chronic nephrosis, infused albumin is promptly excreted by the kidneys, with no relief of the chronic edema or effect on the underlying renal lesion. It is of occasional use in the rapid "priming" diuresis of nephrosis. Similarly, in hypoproteinemic states associated with chronic cirrhosis, malabsorption, protein losing enteropathies, pancreatic insufficiency, and undernutrition, the infusion of albumin as a source of protein nutrition is not justified.

Administration and Dosage

➤*General dosing considerations:* The pediatric use of albumin (human) 5% solution has not been clinically evaluated. Therefore, health care providers should weigh the risks and benefits of the use of albumin (human) 5% solution in children.

Unless the pathologic condition responsible for the hypoalbuminemia can be corrected, administration of albumin can afford only symptomatic or supportive relief in hypoproteinemia (with or without edema).

➤*Adults:*

Acute nephrosis –

25% and 20% solutions: Certain patients with acute nephrosis may not respond to cyclophosphamide or steroid therapy. The steroids may even aggravate the underlying edema. In this situation, a loop diuretic and 100 mL of albumin (human) 25% or 20% solutions repeated daily for 7 to 10 days may be helpful in controlling the edema, and the patient may then respond to steroid treatment.

Burns –

25% and 20% solutions:

• *Usual dosage* – After a burn injury (usually beyond 24 hours), there is a close correlation between the amount of albumin infused and the resultant increase in plasma colloid osmotic pressure. The aim should be to maintain the plasma albumin concentration in the region of 2.5 ± 0.5 g per 100 mL, with a plasma oncotic pressure of 20 mm Hg (equivalent to a total plasma protein concentration of 5.2 g per 100 mL). This is best achieved by the IV administration of albumin (human) 25% or 20% solutions.

• *Duration of therapy* – The duration of therapy is decided by the loss of protein from the burned areas and in the urine. In addition, oral or parenteral feeding with amino acids should be initiated because the long-term administration of albumin should not be considered as a source of nutrition.

Cardiopulmonary bypass –

5%, 25%, and 20% solutions: Although the limit to which the hematocrit and plasma protein concentration can be safely lowered has not been defined, it is common practice to adjust the albumin and crystalloid pump prime to achieve a hematocrit of 20% and a plasma albumin concentration of 2.5 g per 100 mL in the patient.

Erythrocyte resuspension –

25% and 20% solutions: About 25 g of albumin per liter of erythrocytes is commonly used, although the requirements in preexisting hypoproteinemia or hepatic impairment can be greater. Albumin (human) 25% or 20% solu-

ALBUMIN HUMAN — INJECTION

tions are added to the isotonic suspension of washed red blood cells immediately prior to transfusion.

Hypoproteinemia with or without edema –
25% and 20% solutions: The usual daily dose is 50 to 75 g. Patients with severe hypoproteinemia who continue to lose albumin may require larger quantities. Because hypoproteinemic patients usually have approximately normal blood volumes, the rate of administration of albumin (human) 25% or 20% solutions should not exceed 2 mL/min because more rapid injection may precipitate circulatory embarrassment and pulmonary edema.

Hypovolemic shock –
Usual dosage:
• *25% and 20% solutions* – For treatment of hypovolemic shock, the volume administered and the speed of infusion should be adapted to the response of the individual patient.
• *5% solution* – The total dosage will vary with the individual. In adults, an initial infusion of 500 mL is suggested. Additional amounts may be administered as clinically indicated.
In the treatment of the patient in shock with greatly reduced blood volume, albumin (human) 5% solution may be administered as rapidly as necessary to improve the clinical condition and restore normal blood volume. This may be repeated in 15 to 30 minutes if the initial dose fails to prove adequate. In the patient with a slightly low or normal blood volume, the rate of administration should be 1 to 2 mL/min.
Maximum dose: The total dose should not exceed the level of albumin found in healthy individuals (ie, about 2 g/kg body weight) in the absence of active bleeding.

Renal dialysis –
25% and 20% solutions: The usual volume administered is about 100 mL, taking particular care to avoid fluid overload because these patients are often fluid overloaded and cannot tolerate substantial volumes of salt solution.

➤*Children:*

Hypoproteinemia with or without edema –
25% and 20% solutions: The usual daily dose is 25 g. Patients with severe hypoproteinemia who continue to lose albumin may require larger quantities. Because hypoproteinemic patients usually have approximately normal blood volumes, the rate of administration of albumin (human) 25% or 20% solutions should not exceed 2 mL/min because more rapid injection may precipitate circulatory embarrassment and pulmonary edema.

Hypovolemic shock –
5% solution: The pediatric use of albumin (human) 5% solution has not been clinically evaluated. The dosage will vary with the clinical state and body weight of the individual. Typically, a dose one-quarter to one-half the adult dose may be administered, or dosage may be calculated on the basis of 0.6 to 1 g/kg of body weight (12 to 20 mL of human albumin 5% solution). The usual rate of administration in children should be one-quarter the adult rate.

Neonatal hemolytic disease –
25% and 20% solutions: A dosage of 1 g/kg body weight is given about 1 hour prior to exchange transfusion. Caution must be observed in hypervolemic infants.

➤*Preparation for administration:* Remove seal to expose stopper. Always swab stopper top immediately with a suitable antiseptic prior to entering vial.

Only 16-gauge needles or dispensing pins should be used with 20 mL vial sizes and larger. Needles or dispensing pins should only be inserted within the stopper area delineated by the raised ring. The stopper should be penetrated perpendicular to the plane of the stopper within the ring.

5% solution –
Directions for use (250 and 500 mL with administration set): Flip off plastic cap on the top of the vial and expose rubber stopper. Cleanse exposed rubber stopper with a suitable germicidal solution, being sure to remove any excess. Observe aseptic technique and prepare sterile IV equipment as follows. Close clamp on administration set (delivers approximately 15 drops/mL); with bottle upright, thrust piercing pin straight through stopper center. Do not twist or angle; immediately invert bottle to automatically establish proper fluid level in drip chamber (half full); attach infusion set to administration set, open clamp, and allow solution to expel air from tubing and needle, then close clamp; make venipuncture and adjust flow.

Discard all administration equipment after use. Discard any unused contents.

➤*Administration:* Albumin (human) 25%, 20%, and 5% solutions are administered IV.

The volume of the total dose and the rate of infusion depend on the patient's condition and response.

25% and 20% solutions – Albumin (human) 25% and 20% solutions may be administered either undiluted or diluted in sodium chloride 0.9% or dextrose 5% in water. If sodium restriction is required, albumin (human) 25% or 20% solutions should only be administered either undiluted or diluted in a sodium-free carbohydrate solution such as dextrose 5% in water.

➤*Admixture compatibility:* Albumin may be administered either in conjunction with or combined with other parenteral products such as whole blood, plasma, saline, glucose, or sodium lactate.

➤*Storage/Stability:* A number of factors beyond manufacturer control could reduce the efficacy of the product or even result in an adverse reaction following its use. These include improper storage and handling of the product after it leaves the manufacturer, diagnosis, dosage, method of administration, and biological differences in individual patients. Because of these factors, it is important that this product is stored properly and that the directions be followed carefully during use.

Solutions of albumin (human) should not be used if they appear turbid or if there is sediment in the bottle. Do not begin administration more than 4 hours after the container has been entered. Discard unused portion.

Solutions that have been frozen should not be used. Vials that are cracked or have been previously entered or damaged should not be used, as this may have allowed the entry of microorganisms. Albumin (human) 25%, 20%, and 5% solutions contain no preservative.

5% solution – Albumin (human) 5% solution is stable for 3 years, providing storage temperature does not exceed 30°C (89°F). Protect from freezing.

25% and 20% solutions – Store at room temperature not exceeding 30°C (86°F). Do not freeze. Do not use after expiration date.

PLASMA EXPANDERS

HETASTARCH (Hydroxyethyl Starch; HES)

Rx	**Hespan** (B. Braun Medical)	**Injection, solution:** 6 g per 100 mL in sodium chloride 0.9%	In 500 mL IV[a] infusion bottles.
Rx	**6% Hetastarch** (Hospira)		In 500 mL single-dose containers.
Rx	**Voluven** (Hospira)		In 500 mL polyolefin bags.

[a] IV = intravenous.

HETASTARCH (Hydroxyethyl Starch; HES) — INJECTION

Indications

➤*Hypovolemia:* For the treatment and prophylaxis of hypovolemia.

It is not a substitute for red blood cells or coagulation factors in plasma.

➤*Leukapheresis (Hespan only):* Adjunct to improve harvesting and increase yield of granulocytes.

Administration and Dosage

➤*Adults:*

Hypovolemia –
Hespan:
• *Usual dosage* – 500 to 1,000 mL.
• *Maximum dose* – Total dosage does not usually exceed 1,500 mL/day (20 mL/kg).
In acute hemorrhagic shock, rates approaching 20 mL/kg/h may be used.
Voluven: Up to *Voluven* 50 mL injection per kg of body weight per day (equivalent to hydroxyethyl starch 3 g and sodium 7.7 mEq per kg of body weight). This dose is equivalent to *Voluven* 3,500 mL injection for a 70 kg patient.

Leukapheresis –
Hespan (only): In continuous flow centrifugation (CFC) procedures, 250 to 700 mL is typically infused at a constant fixed ratio of 1:8 to 1:13 to venous whole blood.

➤*Children:*

Hypovolemia –
Voluven: Limited clinical data on the use of *Voluven* injection in children are available. In 41 children including newborn to infants (younger than 2 years), a mean dose of 16 ± 9 mL/kg was administered. The dosage in children should be adapted to the individual patient colloid needs, taking into account the disease state, as well as the hemodynamic and hydration status. The safety and efficacy of *Voluven* injection have not been established in the age group of 2 to 12 years of age. Use of *Voluven* injection in children older than 12 years of age is supported by evidence from adequate and well-controlled studies of *Voluven* injection in adults and by data from children younger than 2 years of age.

➤*Preparation for administration:*

Hespan – Use aseptic technique.
1.) Close flow-control clamp of administration set.
2.) Twist off plug from port designated "infusion set port."
3.) Insert spike of infusion set into port with a twisting motion until the set is firmly seated.
4.) Suspend container from hanger.
5.) Follow manufacturer's recommended procedures for the administration set.
6.) Discontinue administration and notify health care provider immediately if patient exhibits signs of adverse reactions.

General recommendations: Do not use plastic container in series connection. If administration is controlled by a pumping device, care must be taken to discontinue pumping action before the container runs dry or air embolism may result.

HETASTARCH (Hydroxyethyl Starch; HES) — INJECTION

This solution is intended for IV administration using sterile equipment. It is recommended that the IV administration apparatus be replaced at least once every 24 hours.

If administration is by pressure infusion, all air should be withdrawn or expelled from the bag through the medication port prior to infusion.

Directions for use of Excel container: As a precaution, review these directions before administering to the patient:

• *Visual checking* –

1.) Do not remove the plastic infusion container from its overwrap until immediately before use.
2.) While the overwrap is intact, identify the solution as *Hespan*, the lot number, and the expiration date.
3.) Check that the solution is clear.
4.) Inspect the intact unit for signs of obvious damage. If present, the unit should not be used.

Removal of overwrap: To open overwrap, tear at any notch located at either end of unit. After removing the overwrap, check for any leakage by squeezing the container firmly. If any leaks are found, discard the unit because sterility may be impaired.

Leukapheresis: 250 to 700 mL of *Hespan* to which citrate anticoagulant has been added is typically administered by aseptic addition to the input line of the centrifugation apparatus at a ratio of 1:8 to 1:13 to venous whole blood. The *Hespan* and citrate should be thoroughly mixed to ensure effective anticoagulation of blood as it flows through the leukapheresis machine.

Voluven –

Directions for the use of Voluven injection:

1.) Check the solution composition, lot number, and expiry date, and inspect the container for damage or leakage; if damaged, do not use.
2.) Use opening aid to remove overwrap.
3.) Identify the blue infusion (administration) port.
4.) Break off the blue tamper-evident cover from the *Freeflex* infusion port.
5.) Close the roller clamp. Insert the spike until the clear plastic collar of the port meets the shoulder of the spike.
6.) Use a nonvented standard infusion set and close air inlet.
7.) Hang the bag on the infusion stand. Press drip chamber to get fluid level. Prime the infusion set. Connect and adjust the flow rate. Do not remove the *Freeflex* IV container from its overwrap until immediately before use.

Voluven injection should be used immediately after insertion of the administration set. Do not vent. If administered by pressure infusion, air should be withdrawn or expelled from the bag through the medication/administration port prior to infusion. It is recommended that administration sets be changed at least once every 24 hours.

Discontinue the infusion if an adverse reaction occurs.

For single use only. Discard unused portion.

➤*Administration:* Administer by IV infusion only. Total dosage and rate of infusion depend upon the amount of blood lost and the resultant hemoconcentration.

Voluven – The daily dose and rate of infusion depend on the patient's blood loss, on the maintenance and restoration of hemodynamics, and on the hemodilution (dilution effect). *Voluven* injection can be administered repetitively over several days.

The initial 10 to 20 mL should be infused slowly, keeping the patient under close observation because of possible anaphylactoid reactions.

➤*Admixture compatibility:* When stored at room temperature, *Hespan* admixtures of 500 to 560 mL with citrate concentrations up to 2.5% were compatible for 24 hours.

The safety and compatibility of additives other than citrate have not been established.

➤*Storage/Stability:*

Hespan – Exposure of pharmaceutical products to heat should be minimized. Avoid excessive heat. Protect from freezing. It is recommended that the product be stored at room temperature (25°C [77°F]); however, brief exposure up to 40°C (104°F) does not adversely affect the product.

Voluven – Store at 15° to 25°C (59° to 77°F). Do not freeze.

Actions

➤*Pharmacology:* Hetastarch (HES) is a complex mixture of ethoxylated amylopectin molecules of various sizes; average molecular weight (MW) is 450,000 (range, 10,000 to more than 1 million). Colloidal properties of 6% HES approximate those of human albumin. After IV infusion, plasma volume expands slightly in excess of volume infused and decreases over 24 to 36 hours. Hemodynamic status will decrease after 24 hours. Adding HES to whole blood increases the erythrocyte sedimentation rate and improves the efficiency of granulocyte collection by centrifugal means.

➤*Pharmacokinetics:* Molecules less than 50,000 MW are rapidly eliminated renally; approximately 33% appear in urine in 24 hours. Larger molecules are broken down; approximately 90% of the dose is eliminated (average half-life, 17 days; the remainder has a half-life of 48 days). The hydroxyethyl group remains intact and attached to glucose units when excreted.

Contraindications

Severe bleeding disorders; severe cardiac failure; renal failure with oliguria or anuria.

Warnings/Precautions

➤*Blood/Plasma substitute:* Not a substitute for blood or plasma, as it does not have oxygen-carrying capacity or contain plasma proteins (eg, coagulation factors).

➤*Coagulation effects:* Large volumes may alter coagulation and result in transient prolongation of prothrombin time (PT), partial thromboplastin time (PTT), bleeding and clotting times, decreased hematocrit and excessive dilution of plasma proteins.

➤*Leukapheresis:* Slight declines in platelet count and hemoglobin levels have been observed in donors undergoing repeated leukapheresis procedures due to the volume expanding effects of hetastarch. Hemoglobin levels usually return to normal within 24 hours. Hemodilution by hetastarch and saline may also result in 24 hour declines of total protein, albumin, calcium, and fibrinogen values.

➤*Hypersensitivity reactions:* Anaphylactoid reactions (periorbital edema, urticaria, wheezing) have been reported. If these occur, discontinue the drug. If necessary, give antihistamines. See Management of Acute Hypersensitivity Reactions. Also, use caution when administering HES to a person allergic to corn.

➤*Special risk:* The possibility of circulatory overload exists. Take special care in patients with impaired renal clearance and when the risk of pulmonary edema or congestive heart failure is increased. Indirect bilirubin levels increased in two subjects receiving multiple infusions; levels returned to normal by 96 hours after infusion. Total bilirubin remained normal. Use caution in liver disease.

➤*Pregnancy: Category C.* Safety for use has not been established. Use only when clearly needed and when potential benefits outweigh potential hazards to the fetus.

➤*Lactation:* It is not known whether hetastarch is excreted in breast milk. Exercise caution when administering to a breast-feeding woman.

➤*Children:* Safety and efficacy have not been established.

➤*Monitoring:* During leukapheresis, monitor CBC, total leukocyte and platelet counts, leukocyte differential count, hemoglobin, hematocrit, PT and PTT.

Adverse Reactions

Vomiting; mild temperature elevation; chills; itching; submaxillary and parotid glandular enlargement; mild influenza-like symptoms; headache; muscle pain; peripheral edema of the lower extremities; allergic reactions (see Warnings).

DEXTRAN, LOW MOLECULAR WEIGHT (Dextran 40)

Rx	**Dextran 40** (McGaw)	**Injection:** 10% dextran 40 in 0.9% sodium chloride	In 500 mL.
Rx	**Gentran 40** (Baxter)		In 500 mL.
Rx	**10% LMD** (Hospira)		In 500 mL.
Rx	**Rheomacrodex** (Medisan)		In 500 mL.
Rx	**Dextran 40** (McGaw)	**Injection:** 10% dextran 40 in 5% dextrose	In 500 mL.
Rx	**Gentran 40** (Baxter)		In 500 mL.
Rx	**10% LMD** (Hospira)		In 500 mL.
Rx	**Rheomacrodex** (Medisan)		In 500 mL.

DEXTRAN, LOW MOLECULAR WEIGHT (Dextran 40) — INJECTION

Indications

➤*Shock:* Adjunctive treatment of shock or impending shock due to hemorrhage, burns, surgery or other trauma. The solution is for emergency treatment when whole blood products are not available; it is not a substitute for whole blood or plasma proteins.

➤*Priming fluid:* As a priming fluid, either as the sole primer or as an additive, in pump oxygenators during extracorporeal circulation.

➤*Deep venous thrombosis (DVT)/Pulmonary embolism (PE) prophylaxis:* Prophylaxis against DVT and PE in patients undergoing procedures associated with a high incidence of thromboembolic complications, such as hip surgery.

DEXTRAN, LOW MOLECULAR WEIGHT (Dextran 40) — INJECTION

Administration and Dosage

➤*Adults:*

Shock, adjunctive therapy –

Usual dosage: The first 10 mL/kg should be infused rapidly, with the remaining dose being administered more slowly. Monitor the central venous pressure frequently during the initial infusion.

Maximum dose: Total dosage during the first 24 hours should not exceed 20 mL/kg. Should therapy continue beyond 24 hours, total daily dosage should not exceed 10 mL/kg, and therapy should not continue beyond 5 days.

Duration of therapy: Therapy should not continue beyond 5 days.

Hemodiluent in extracorporeal circulation –

Usual dosage: Generally, 10 to 20 mL/kg are added to the perfusion circuit. The dosage employed in the priming fluid will vary with the volume of pump oxygenator employed. It may be added as sole primer or as an additive.

Maximum dose: Do not exceed total dosage of 20 mL/kg; this can be limited and controlled by adding other priming fluids.

Venous thrombosis/thromboembolism, prophylactic therapy –

Usual dosage: In general, initiate treatment during surgery. Administer 500 to 1,000 mL (approximately 10 mL/kg) on the day of the operation.

Maintenance dosage: Continue treatment at a dose of 500 mL/day for an additional 2 to 3 days. Thereafter, and according to the risk of complications, 500 mL may be administered every second or third day during the period of risk for up to 2 weeks.

Duration of therapy: Up to 2 weeks.

➤*Children:* The best guide is the body weight or surface area, and the total dosage should not exceed 20 mL/kg.

➤*Elderly:* Use solutions containing sodium ions with great care, if at all, in clinical states in which edema exists with sodium retention (particularly in elderly patients).

➤*Renal function impairment:* In patients with diminished renal function, use of solutions containing sodium ions may result in sodium retention. Excessive doses may precipitate renal failure.

➤*Administration:* For IV use only.

➤*Storage/Stability:* Store at a constant temperature between 15° to 30°C (59° to 86°F). Protect from freezing.

Actions

➤*Pharmacology:* Dextran 40 is a branched polysaccharide plasma-volume expander with an average molecular weight of 40,000 (range 10,000 to 90,000). A 2.5% solution of dextran 40 is equivalent in colloid osmotic pressure to normal plasma. Generally, plasma volume is increased onefold to twofold over the volume of dextran 40 infused. The extent and duration of volume expansion produced will depend on the preexisting blood volume, rate of infusion and rate of dextran clearance by the kidneys.

➤*Pharmacokinetics:* Dextran 40 is evenly distributed in the vascular system. Its distribution according to molecular weight shifts toward higher molecular weights as the smaller molecules are excreted by the kidney. Approximately 50% administered to a normovolemic subject is excreted in the urine within 3 hours, 60% within 6 hours and 75% within 24 hours. The remaining 25% is partially hydrolyzed and excreted in the urine, partially excreted in the feces and partially oxidized. Unexcreted dextran molecules diffuse into the extravascular compartment and are temporarily taken up by the reticuloendothelial system. Some of these molecules are returned to the intravascular compartment via the lymphatics. Dextran is slowly degraded to glucose by the enzyme dextranase.

Adjunctive therapy in shock – Enhances blood flow, particularly in the microcirculation, by a combination of the following mechanisms: Increases blood volume, venous return and cardiac output; decreases blood viscosity and peripheral vascular resistance; reduces aggregation of erythrocytes and other cellular elements of blood by coating them and maintaining their electronegative charges.

Administration to a patient in shock usually increases blood volume, central venous pressure, cardiac output, stroke volume, arterial blood pressure, pulse pressure, capillary perfusion, venous return and urinary output; it also decreases blood viscosity, heart rate, peripheral resistance and mean transit time and prevents or reverses cellular aggregation. Hematocrit is lowered in proportion to the infusion volume.

The intense but relatively short-lived plasma expansion volume produced by dextran 40 is advantageous in the treatment of early shock because it acts rapidly to correct hypovolemia while allowing control of the plasma volume. If overexpansion occurs, the discontinuation of the infusion will result in a decline in plasma volume due to loss of dextran from the intravascular space.

Priming solution for extracorporeal circulation – Dextran 40's advantages over homologous blood and other priming fluids include: Decreased destruction of erythrocytes and platelets; reduced intravascular hemagglutination; maintenance of electronegativity of erythrocytes and platelets.

Prophylaxis against venous thrombosis, thromboembolism – The infusion of dextran 40 during and after surgical trauma reduces the incidence of DVT and PE in surgical patients subject to procedures with a high incidence of thromboembolic complications. Dextran 40 simultaneously inhibits mechanisms essential to thrombus formation such as vascular stasis and platelet adhesiveness, and alters the structure and lysability of fibrin clots.

Dextran 40 increases cardiac output, arterial, venous and microcirculatory flow and reduces mean transit time, chiefly by expanding plasma volume, by reducing blood viscosity through hemodilution and by reducing red cell aggregation.

Contraindications

Hypersensitivity to dextran; marked hemostatic defects of all types (eg, thrombocytopenia, hypofibrinogenemia), including those caused by drugs (eg, heparin, warfarin); marked cardiac decompensation; renal disease with severe oliguria or anuria.

Decreased urinary output, secondary to shock, is not a contraindication unless there is no improvement in urine output after the initial dose.

If administration of sodium or chloride could be clinically detrimental, 10% Dextran in 0.9% Sodium Chloride Injection is contraindicated.

Warnings/Precautions

➤*Fluid imbalance:* These products are colloid hypertonic solutions and will attract water from the extravascular space. Poorly hydrated patients will need additional fluid therapy. If given in excess, vascular overload could occur. This can be avoided by monitoring central venous pressure.

Administration of dextran IV can cause fluid or solute overloading, resulting in dilution of serum electrolyte concentrations, overhydration, congested states or pulmonary edema. The risk of dilutional states is inversely proportional to electrolyte concentrations of administered parenteral solutions.

➤*Hemorrhage:* Use with caution in patients with active hemorrhage; the increase in perfusion pressure and improved microcirculatory flow may result in additional blood loss.

Avoid administering infusions that exceed the recommended dose, as a dose-related increase in the incidence of wound hematoma, wound seroma, wound bleeding, distant bleeding (hematuria and melena) and pulmonary edema has been observed.

➤*Hematologic effects:* Use with caution in patients with thrombocytopenia. Hematocrit should not be depressed below 30% by volume. When large volumes of dextran are administered, plasma protein levels will be decreased. Do not give dextran 40 to patients with marked thrombocytopenia or hypofibrinogenemia.

In individuals with normal hemostasis, dosages of up to 15 mL/kg or more than 1000 mL may prolong bleeding time and decrease coagulation due to depressed platelet function. Dosages in this range also markedly decrease factor VIII; they also decrease factors V and IX to a slightly greater degree than would be expected from hemodilution alone. Because these changes tend to be more pronounced following trauma or major surgery, observe all patients for early signs of bleeding complications.

➤*Bleeding complications:* Observe patients for early signs of bleeding complications, particularly following surgery, major trauma or if anticoagulant drugs are being administered.

➤*Hypersensitivity reactions:* Antigenicity of dextrans is directly related to their degree of branching. Because dextran 40 has a low degree of branching, it is relatively free of antigenic effect. Hypersensitivity reactions have, however, been reported (see Adverse Reactions). Infrequently, severe and fatal anaphylactoid reactions (eg, marked hypotension, cardiac and respiratory arrest) have been reported. Most of these reactions occurred early in the infusion period in patients not previously exposed to IV dextran and have appeared after administration of as little as 10 mL. Stop infusion immediately if an anaphylactoid reaction is imminent. Refer to Management of Acute Hypersensitivity Reactions. In circulatory collapse due to anaphylaxis, institute rapid volume substitution with an agent other than dextran. Dextran 1 is indicated for prophylaxis of serious anaphylactic reactions to dextran infusions.

➤*Renal function impairment:* Renal excretion causes elevation of the specific gravity of the urine. In the presence of adequate urine flow, only minor elevations occur, but in patients with diminished urine flow, urine viscosity and specific gravity can be increased markedly. As osmolarity is only slightly affected by the presence of dextran molecules, assess a patient's state of hydration by determination of urine or serum osmolarity. If signs of dehydration are noted, administer additional fluids. An osmotic diuretic such as mannitol is useful in maintaining adequate urine flow.

Renal failure, sometimes irreversible, has been reported. While the preexisting clinical condition of these patients could account for the oliguria or anuria, it is possible that dextran use may have contributed to its development. Evidence of tubular vacuolization (osmotic nephrosis) has been found following administration. The exact clinical significance is unknown.

In patients with diminished renal function, use of solutions containing sodium ions may result in sodium retention. Excessive doses may precipitate renal failure.

➤*Special risk:* Use solutions containing sodium ions with great care, if at all, in patients with congestive heart failure, severe renal insufficiency, in clinical states in which edema exists with sodium retention (particularly in postoperative or elderly patients) and in patients receiving corticosteroids.

Use dextrose-containing solutions with caution in overt or known subclinical diabetes mellitus.

➤*Pregnancy:* Category C. Safety for use during pregnancy has not been established. Use only when clearly needed and when the potential benefits outweigh the potential hazards to the fetus.

➤*Lactation:* It is not known whether this drug is excreted in breast milk. Exercise caution when dextran 40 is administered to a nursing woman.

DEXTRAN, LOW MOLECULAR WEIGHT (Dextran 40) — INJECTION

➤*Monitoring:* Urine output should be carefully monitored. Usually, an increase in urine output occurs in oliguric patients after administration. If no increase is observed after the infusion of 500 mL, discontinue the drug until adequate diuresis develops spontaneously or can be induced by other means.

Exercise care to prevent a depression of the hematocrit below 30%.

Infusion of dextran may lead to excessive dilution of red blood cells and plasma proteins, dilution of other blood constituents (platelets, fibrinogen) or dilutional acidosis caused by dilution of the bicarbonate ion.

Drug Interactions

➤*Drug/Lab test interactions:* Blood sugar determinations that employ high concentrations of acid (acetic or sulfuric) may cause hydrolysis of dextran; falsely elevated glucose assays may be reported in patients receiving dextran. In other laboratory tests, the presence of dextran may result in the development of turbidity, which can interfere with bilirubin assays in which alcohol has been employed, in total protein assays employing biuret reagent and in blood sugar determinations with the ortho-toluidine method. Consider withdrawal of blood for chemical laboratory tests prior to initiating therapy.

Blood typing and crossmatching procedures employing enzyme techniques may give unreliable readings if the samples are taken after infusion. Other blood typing and crossmatching procedures are not affected. Draw blood samples for the above determinations prior to initiating infusion or, alternatively, inform the laboratory that the patient has received dextran so that suitable assay methods can be applied.

Occasional abnormal renal and hepatic function values have been reported following IV use. The specific effect on renal and hepatic function could not be determined, as most of these patients had also undergone surgery or cardiac catheterization.

Adverse Reactions

➤*Hypersensitivity:* Mild cutaneous eruptions, generalized urticaria, hypotension, nausea, vomiting, headache, dyspnea, fever, tightness of the chest, bronchospasm, wheezing and, rarely, anaphylactoid (allergic) shock (see Warnings).

➤*Miscellaneous:* Reactions which may occur because of the solution or the technique of administration include febrile response, infection at the injection site, venous thrombosis or phlebitis extending from the injection site, extravasation and hypervolemia.

Hypernatremia may be associated with edema and exacerbation of congestive heart failure due to the retention of water, resulting in expanded extracellular fluid volume.

If solutions containing sodium chloride are infused in large volumes, chloride ions may cause a loss of bicarbonate ions, resulting in an acidifying effect.

DEXTRAN, HIGH MOLECULAR WEIGHT (Dextran 70)

Rx	**Dextran 70** (McGaw)	**Injection:** 6% dextran 70 in 0.9% sodium chloride	In 500 mL.
Rx	**Gentran 70** (Baxter)		In 500 mL.
Rx	**Macrodex** (Medisan)		In 500 mL.
Rx	**Macrodex** (Medisan)	**Injection:** 6% dextran 70 in 5% dextrose	In 500 mL.

DEXTRAN, HIGH MOLECULAR WEIGHT (Dextran 70) — INJECTION

Indications

➤*Shock:* Treatment of shock or impending shock due to surgery or other trauma, hemorrhage or burns. Intended for emergency treatment only when whole blood or blood products are not available; do not regard as a substitute for whole blood or plasma proteins. It should not replace other forms of therapy known to be of value in the treatment of shock.

Administration and Dosage

➤*General dosing considerations:* Total dose and rate of infusion depend on the magnitude of fluid loss and the resultant hemoconcentration.

➤*Adults:*

Shock –

Usual dosage: 500 to 1,000 mL, which may be given at a rate of 20 to 40 mL/min in an emergency.

Maximum dose: 20 mL/kg during the first 24 hours.

➤*Children:*

Shock – The best guide to dosage is the body weight or surface area of the patient; total dosage should not exceed 20 mL/kg.

➤*Renal function impairment:* Use solutions containing sodium ions with great care, if at all, in patients with severe renal insufficiency. Circulatory overload may occur. Exercise special care in patients with impaired renal clearance.

➤*Administration:* Administer by IV infusion only.

➤*Admixture compatibility:* No additives should be delivered via plasma volume expanders.

➤*Storage/Stability:* The solution has no bacteriostat; discard partially used containers. The solution must be clear. Store at a constant temperature not more than 25°C (77°F).

Actions

➤*Pharmacology:* Dextrans are synthetic polysaccharides used to approximate the colloidal properties of albumin. Dextran 70 has an average molecular weight (MW) of 70,000 (range 20,000 to 200,000). Dextran 70 improves blood pressure, pulse rate, respiratory exchange and renal function in patients with hypovolemia or hypotensive shock. IV infusion results in an expansion of plasma volume slightly in excess of volume infused and decreases from this maximum over the next 24 hours. This plasma volume expansion improves hemodynamic status for 24 hours or more.

➤*Pharmacokinetics:* Dextran molecules below 50,000 molecular weight are eliminated by renal excretion, with approximately 50% appearing in the urine in 24 hours in the normovolemic patient. The remaining dextran is enzymatically degraded to glucose at a rate of about 70 to 90 mg/kg/day. This is a variable process.

Contraindications

Hypersensitivity to dextran; marked hemostatic defects of all types (thrombocytopenia, hypofibrinogenemia, etc), including those induced by drugs; marked cardiac decompensation; renal disease with severe oliguria or anuria; severe congestive heart failure, pulmonary edema and severe bleeding disorders; where use of sodium or chloride could be clinically detrimental.

Warnings/Precautions

➤*Fluid imbalance:* Fluid or solute overloading may occur, resulting in dilution of serum electrolyte concentrations, overhydration, congested states (CHF) and peripheral or pulmonary edema. The risk of dilutional states is inversely proportional to the electrolyte concentration of administered parenteral solutions.

The risk of solute overload causing congested states with peripheral and pulmonary edema is directly proportional to electrolyte concentrations of such solutions.

➤*Hematologic effects:* In individuals with normal hemostasis, dosages approximating 15 mL/kg or more than 1000 mL prolong bleeding time and decrease coagulation due to depressed platelet function; use with caution in patients with thrombocytopenia. Such dosages also markedly decrease factor VIII and decrease factor V and factor IX more than would be expected from hemodilution alone. These changes tend to be more pronounced following trauma or major surgery; observe patients for early signs of bleeding complications. Transient prolongation of bleeding time may occur following doses greater than 1000 mL, particularly if the patient is on concomitant anticoagulation therapy. Take care to prevent depression of hematocrit below 30% by volume. When large volumes of dextran are given, plasma protein level will be decreased.

➤*Bleeding complications:* Observe patients for early signs of bleeding complications, particularly following surgery or major trauma, or if anticoagulant drugs are being administered.

➤*Hypersensitivity reactions:* Severe and fatal anaphylactoid reactions (eg, marked hypotension, cardiac and respiratory arrest) have occurred early in the infusion period in patients not previously exposed to IV dextran. Stop infusion immediately if an anaphylactoid reaction is imminent, provided that other means of sustaining the circulation are available. Refer to Management of Acute Hypersensitivity Reactions. In circulatory collapse due to anaphylaxis, institute rapid volume substitution with an agent other than dextran. Antihistamines may be effective in relieving some symptoms. Dextran 1 is indicated for prophylaxis of serious anaphylactic reactions associated with dextran infusions.

➤*Special risk:* Use solutions containing sodium ions with great care, if at all, in patients with congestive heart failure, pulmonary edema, severe renal insufficiency, patients receiving corticosteroids or corticotropin and in clinical states in which edema exists with sodium retention. Circulatory overload may occur. Exercise special care in patients with impaired renal clearance.

Exercise care in patients with pathological abdominal conditions and in those undergoing bowel surgery.

➤*Pregnancy:* *Category C.* Safety for use during pregnancy has not been established. There are no adequate and well controlled studies in pregnant women. Use only when clearly needed and when potential benefits outweigh potential hazards.

➤*Lactation:* It is not known whether this drug is excreted in breast milk. Exercise caution when administering to a nursing woman.

➤*Monitoring:* Urine output should be carefully observed. An increase in urine output usually occurs in oliguric patients after the administration of dextran. If no increase is observed after the infusion of 500 mL of dextran, discontinue the drug until adequate diuresis develops spontaneously or can be provoked by other means.

DEXTRAN, HIGH MOLECULAR WEIGHT (Dextran 70) — INJECTION

Monitoring central venous blood pressure is recommended to detect overexpansion of blood volume. When signs of overexpansion appear, discontinuing IV infusion allows blood volume to readjust and decline, primarily by loss of fluid to urine.

Drug Interactions

➤*Drug/Lab test interactions:* Blood sugar determinations that employ high concentrations of acid (acetic or sulfuric) may cause hydrolysis of dextran; falsely elevated glucose assays may be reported in patients receiving dextran. In other laboratory tests, the presence of dextran may result in the development of turbidity, which can interfere with bilirubin assays in which alcohol has been employed, in total protein assays employing biuret reagent and in blood sugar determinations with the ortho-toluidine method.

Blood typing and crossmatching procedures employing enzyme techniques may give unreliable readings if the samples are taken after infusion. If blood is drawn after the infusion, the saline-agglutination and indirect antiglobulin methods may be used for typing and crossmatching. Draw blood samples for the above determinations prior to initiating infusion or, alternatively, inform the laboratory that the patient has received dextran so that suitable assay methods can be applied.

Adverse Reactions

➤*Infusion technique:* Reactions which may occur because of the solution or the technique of administration include febrile response, infection at the injection site, venous thrombosis or phlebitis extending from the injection site, extravasation and hypervolemia. If a reaction develops, discontinue use and treat accordingly.

➤*Hypersensitivity:* Allergic reactions include urticaria, nasal congestion, wheezing, tightness of the chest, dyspnea, mild hypotension and, rarely, anaphylactoid (allergic) shock (see Warnings).

➤*Miscellaneous:* Sudden marked hypotension; nausea; vomiting; fever; joint pains.

Hypernatremia may be associated with edema and exacerbation of congestive heart failure due to water retention, resulting in expanded extracellular fluid volume.

If solutions containing sodium chloride are infused in large volumes, chloride ions may cause a loss of bicarbonate ions, resulting in an acidifying effect.

HEMIN

HEMIN

Rx	Panhematin (Ovation)	**Injection, lyophilized powder for solution:** 313 mg hemin[a]	Preserved free. With 300 mg sorbitol. In single-dose vials.

[a] When mixed with sterile water for injection, each 43 mL provides the equivalent of approximately 301 mg hematin (7 mg/mL).

HEMIN — INJECTION

WARNING

Hemin for injection should only be used by health care providers experienced in the management of porphyrias in hospitals in which the recommended clinical and laboratory diagnostic and monitoring techniques are available.

Consider hemin therapy after an appropriate period of alternate therapy (ie, glucose 400 g/day for 1 to 2 days).

Indications

➤*Porphyria:* For the amelioration of recurrent attacks of acute intermittent porphyria temporally related to the menstrual cycle in susceptible women. Manifestations such as abnormal mental status, hypertension, mild to progressive neurologic signs, pain, and tachycardia may be controlled in selected patients.

Similar findings have been reported in other patients with acute intermittent porphyria, porphyria variegata, and hereditary coproporphyria. Hemin is not indicated in porphyria cutanea tarda.

Administration and Dosage

➤*General dosing considerations:* Before administering hemin for injection, consider alternate therapy (ie, glucose 400 g/day for 1 to 2 days). If improvement is unsatisfactory for the treatment of acute attacks of porphyria, administer an IV infusion of hematin.

➤*Adults:*

Porphyria –

Usual dosage: 1 to 4 mg/kg/day of hematin as an IV infusion over a period of 10 to 15 minutes for 3 to 14 days, based on clinical signs. In more severe cases, this dose may be repeated no earlier than every 12 hours.

Maximum dose: 6 mg/kg in any 24-hour period.

Duration of therapy: 3 to 14 days.

➤*Children:*

16 years of age and older – See Adults for dosing.

➤*Renal function impairment:* Strictly follow recommended dosage guidelines. Reversible renal shutdown has been observed when an excessive hematin dose (12.2 mg/kg) was administered in a single infusion. No worsening of renal function has been seen with use of recommended dosages.

➤*Preparation for administration:* Reconstitute by adding 43 mL of sterile water for injection to the dispensing vial. Immediately after adding diluent, shake well for a period of 2 to 3 minutes to aid dissolution.

Because reconstituted hemin is not transparent, any undissolved particulate matter is difficult to see; therefore, terminal filtration through a sterile 0.45-micron or smaller filter is recommended.

After reconstitution, each mL contains the equivalent of approximately 7 mg of hematin. The drug may be administered directly from the vial.

After the first withdrawal from the vial, any solution remaining must be discarded.

➤*Administration:* Administer as an IV infusion over a period of 10 to 15 minutes. Use a large arm vein or a central venous catheter to avoid phlebitis.

Hemin Dosage Calculation Table
1 mg hematin equivalent = 0.14 mL
2 mg hematin equivalent = 0.28 mL
3 mg hematin equivalent = 0.42 mL
4 mg hematin equivalent = 0.56 mL

➤*Admixture compatibility:* Do not add any drug or chemical agent to a hemin fluid admixture unless its effect on the chemical and physical stability has first been determined.

➤*Storage/Stability:* Because this product contains no preservative and undergoes rapid chemical decomposition in solution, do not reconstitute until immediately before use. Refrigerate lyophilized powder at 2° to 8°C (36° to 46°F) until time of use. Discard any unused portion.

Actions

➤*Pharmacology:* Hemin for injection is an enzyme inhibitor derived from processed red blood cells. Hemin was known previously as hematin. The term hematin has been used to describe the chemical reaction product of hemin and sodium carbonate solution. Hemin is an iron-containing metalloporphyrin.

Heme acts to limit the hepatic and/or marrow synthesis of porphyrin, which is likely due to inhibition of δ-aminolevulinic acid synthetase, the enzyme that limits the rate of the porphyrin/heme biosynthetic pathway. However, the exact mechanism by which hematin produces symptomatic improvement in patients with acute episodes of the hepatic porphyrias is not known.

Hemin therapy for the acute porphyrias is not curative. After discontinuation of treatment, symptoms generally return, although remission may be prolonged. Some neurological symptoms have improved weeks to months after therapy, although little or no response was noted at the time of treatment.

➤*Pharmacokinetics:* Following IV administration of hematin in nonjaundiced patients, an increase in fecal urobilinogen can be observed, which is roughly proportional to the amount of hematin administered. This suggests an enterohepatic pathway as at least 1 route of elimination. Bilirubin metabolites also are excreted in the urine following hematin injections.

Contraindications

Hypersensitivity to hemin.

Warnings/Precautions

➤*Transmission of viral disease:* Hemin is made from human blood. Products made from human blood may contain infectious agents, such as viruses, that can cause disease. The risk that such products will transmit an infectious agent has been reduced by screening blood donors for prior exposure to certain viruses, testing for the presence of certain current virus infections, and inactivating certain viruses. Despite these measures, such products can still potentially transmit disease. There is also the possibility that unknown infectious agents may be present in such products. Report all infections thought to possibly have been transmitted by this product to the manufacturer (1-800-455-1141). Discuss the risks and benefits of this product with the patient.

HEMIN — INJECTION

Because this product is made from human blood, it may carry a risk of transmitting infectious agents (eg, viruses) and, theoretically, the Creutzfeldt-Jakob disease agent.

➤*Neuronal damage:* Clinical benefit depends on prompt administration. Attacks of porphyria may progress to irreversible neuronal damage. Hemin therapy is intended to prevent an attack from reaching the critical stage of neuronal degeneration. This agent is not effective in repairing neuronal damage.

➤*Renal effects:* Strictly follow recommended dosage guidelines. Reversible renal shutdown has been observed when an excessive hematin dose (12.2 mg/kg) was administered in a single infusion. Oliguria and increased nitrogen retention occurred, although the patient remained asymptomatic. No worsening of renal function has been seen with use of recommended dosages.

➤*Phlebitis:* Utilize a large arm vein or a central venous catheter for administration of hemin to avoid the possibility of phlebitis.

➤*Diagnostic tests:* Before beginning therapy, diagnose the presence of acute porphyria using the following criteria: presence of clinical symptoms and positive Watson-Schwartz or Hoesch test.

A negative Watson-Schwartz or Hoesch test indicates a porphyric attack is highly unlikely. When in doubt, quantitative measures of δ-aminolevulinic acid and porphobilinogen in serum or urine may aid in diagnosis.

➤*Pregnancy: Category C.* Animal reproduction studies have not been conducted with hematin. It is also not known whether hematin can cause fetal harm when administered to a pregnant woman or can affect reproduction capacity. For this reason, do not give hemin to a pregnant woman unless the expected benefits are sufficiently important to the health and welfare of the patient to outweigh the unknown hazard to the fetus.

➤*Lactation:* It is not known whether hemin for injection is excreted in breast milk. Because many drugs are excreted in human milk, exercise caution when hemin is administered to a breast-feeding woman.

➤*Children:* Safety and effectiveness for use in children younger than 16 years of age have not been established.

➤*Elderly:* In general, be cautious with dose selection for an elderly patient, usually starting at the low end of the dosing range, reflecting the greater frequency of decreased hepatic, renal, or cardiac function and of concomitant disease or other drug therapy.

➤*Monitoring:* Urinary concentrations of the following compounds may be monitored during hemin therapy. Drug effect will be demonstrated by a decrease of 1 or more of the following compounds: δ-aminolevulinic acid, uroporphyrinogen, porphobilinogen corproporphyrin.

Drug Interactions

Hemin Drug Interactions			
Precipitant drug	Object drug[a]		Description
Barbiturates Estrogens Steroid metabolites	Hemin	↔	These agents increase the activity of δ-amino-levulinic acid synthetase. Because hemin therapy limits the rate of porphyria/heme biosynthesis, possibly by inhibiting the enzyme δ-aminolevulinic acid synthetase, avoid concurrent use of these agents.
Hemin	Anticoagulants	↑	Hemin has exhibited transient, mild anticoagulant effects during clinical studies; therefore, avoid concurrent anticoagulant therapy. The extent and duration of the hypocoagulable state have not been established.

[a] ↑ = object drug increased; ↔ = undetermined clinical effect.

Adverse Reactions

Phlebitis – Phlebitis with or without leukocytosis and with or without mild pyrexia has occurred after administration of hematin through small arm veins.

➤*Renal:* Reversible renal shutdown has occurred with administration of excessive doses.

Postmarketing – There have been postmarketing and literature reports of thrombocytopenia and coagulopathy (including prolonged prothrombin time [PT] and prolonged partial thromboplastin time [PTT]) in patients receiving hemin. The initial literature report described coagulopathy occurring in a patient receiving hematin therapy. This patient exhibited prolonged PT, PTT, thrombocytopenia, mild hypofibrinogenemia, mild elevation of fibrin split products, and a 10% fall in hematocrit.

Overdosage

➤*Symptoms:* Reversible renal shutdown has been observed in a case in which an excessive hematin dose (12.2 mg/kg) was administered in a single infusion.

➤*Treatment:* Treatment of this case consisted of ethacrynic acid and mannitol.

WARNING

Estrogens have been reported to increase the risk of endometrial carcinoma in postmenopausal women – Studies have shown an increased risk of endometrial cancer in postmenopausal women exposed to exogenous estrogens for more than 1 year. The risk of endometrial cancer in estrogen users was 4.5 to 13.9 times higher than in nonusers and appears to depend on duration of treatment and dose. Therefore, when estrogens are used for the treatment of menopausal symptoms, use the lowest dose and discontinue medication as soon as possible. When prolonged treatment is indicated, reassess the patient at least semiannually by endometrial sampling to determine the need for continued therapy.

Close clinical surveillance of women taking estrogens is important. Adequate diagnostic measures, including endometrial sampling when indicated, should be undertaken to rule out malignancy in all cases of undiagnosed persistent or recurring abnormal vaginal bleeding.

There is no evidence that natural estrogens are more or less hazardous than synthetic estrogens at equiestrogenic doses.

Do not use estrogens during pregnancy – Estrogen therapy during pregnancy is associated with an increased risk of congenital defects in the reproductive organs of the fetus and possibly other birth defects. Studies of women who received diethylstilbestrol (DES) during pregnancy have shown that female offspring have an increased risk of vaginal adenosis, squamous cell dysplasia of the uterine cervix, and clear cell vaginal cancer later in life; male offspring have an increased risk of urogenital abnormalities and possibly testicular cancer later in life.

There is no indication for estrogen therapy during pregnancy or during the immediate postpartum period. Estrogens are ineffective for the prevention or treatment of threatened or habitual abortion. Estrogens are not indicated for the prevention of postpartum breast engorgement.

If estrogens are used during pregnancy, or if the patient becomes pregnant while taking estrogens, inform her of the potential risks to the fetus.

Cardiovascular and other risks – Do not use estrogens with or without progestins for the prevention of cardiovascular disease.

The Women's Health Initiative (WHI) reported increased risks of MI, stroke, invasive breast cancer, pulmonary emboli, and deep vein thrombosis in postmenopausal women during 5 years of treatment with conjugated equine estrogens 0.625 mg combined with medroxyprogesterone acetate 2.5 mg relative to placebo. Other doses of conjugated estrogens and medroxyprogesterone acetate and other combinations of estrogens and progestins were not studied in the WHI and, in the absence of comparable data, these risks should be assumed to be similar. Because of these risks, prescribe estrogens with or without progestins at the lowest effective doses and for the shortest duration consistent with treatment goals and risks for the individual woman.

Dementia – The Women's Health Initiative Memory Study (WHIMS), a substudy of WHI, reported increased risk of developing probable dementia in postmenopausal women 65 years of age or older during 4 years of treatment with conjugated estrogens plus medroxyprogesterone acetate relative to placebo. It is unknown whether this finding applies to younger postmenopausal women or to women taking estrogen alone therapy.

Indications

➤*Contraception/Hormone replacement therapy/Palliative therapy in cancer patients:* Estrogens are most commonly used as a component of combination contraceptives or as hormone replacement therapy in postmenopausal women. Benefits in postmenopausal women include relief of moderate to severe vasomotor symptoms and decreased risk of osteoporosis. Hormone replacement therapy also may be used in vaginal and vulvar atrophy and in hypoestrogenism caused by hypogonadism, castration, or primary ovarian failure. Less commonly, select breast or prostate cancer patients with advanced disease may receive estrogens as palliative therapy. Refer to individual agents for specific indications.

➤*Off-label uses:* Refer to individual monographs for further information.

Alzheimer disease – [5] = Poor documentation.

Traumatic brain injury – [4] = Insufficient documentation.

Other possible off-label uses – In the treatment of Turner syndrome (ovarian dysgenesis), estrogen therapy replicates the events of puberty.

Administration and Dosage

Refer to individual agents for specific administration and dosage recommendations.

➤*Moderate to severe vasomotor symptoms and/or moderate to severe symptoms of vulvar and vaginal atrophy associated with menopause:* Start at the lowest dose and discontinue as promptly as possible. Attempts to discontinue or taper medication should be made at 3- to 6-month intervals. Therapy may be given continuously with no interruption in therapy or in cyclical regimens (such as 25 days on followed by 5 days off drug) as is medically appropriate on an individualized basis.

➤*Hypoestrogenism caused by hypogonadism, castration, or primary ovarian failure:* Therapy usually is given cyclically (such as 3 weeks on and 1 week off). Adjust dose depending on severity of symptoms and patient responsiveness.

➤*Osteoporosis prevention:* Therapy may be given continuously with no interruption in therapy or in cyclical regimens (such as 25 days on followed by 5 days off drug) as is medically appropriate on an individualized basis. Discontinuation of therapy may re-establish the natural rate of bone loss.

➤*Prostate cancer (advanced androgen-dependent):* For palliation only. The effectiveness of therapy can be judged by phosphatase determinations as well as by symptomatic improvement of the patient.

➤*Breast cancer (metastatic):* For palliation only. Therapy usually is given for at least 3 months.

➤*Concomitant progestin therapy when a woman has not had a hysterectomy:* Addition of a progestin for 10 or more days of a cycle of estrogen has lowered the incidence of endometrial hyperplasia. Morphological and biochemical studies of endometrium suggest that 10 to 14 days of progestin are needed to provide maximal maturation of the endometrium and to reduce the likelihood of any hyperplastic changes. It is not established whether this will provide protection from endometrial carcinoma. There may be additional risks with the inclusion of progestin in estrogen replacement regimens, including possible increased risk of breast cancer; adverse effects on carbohydrate and lipid metabolism (lowering HDL and raising LDL); impairment of glucose tolerance; possible enhancement of mitotic activity in breast epithelial tissue, although few epidemiological data are available to address this point. Choice of progestin, regimen, and dosage may be important in minimizing risks.

Actions

➤*Pharmacology:* Estrogens occur naturally in several forms. The primary source of estrogen in normally cycling adult women is the ovarian follicle, which secretes 70 to 500 mcg of estradiol daily, depending on the phase of the menstrual cycle. This is converted primarily to estrone, which circulates in roughly equal proportion to estradiol, and to small amounts of estriol. After menopause, most endogenous estrogen is produced by conversion of androstenedione, secreted by the adrenal cortex, to estrone by peripheral tissues. Thus, estrone—especially in its sulfate ester form—is the most abundant circulating estrogen in postmenopausal women. Although circulating estrogens exist in a dynamic equilibrium of metabolic interconversions, estradiol is the principal intracellular human estrogen and is substantially more potent than estrone or estriol at the receptor.

Estrogens, important in developing and maintaining the female reproductive system and secondary sex characteristics, promote growth and development of the vagina, uterus, and fallopian tubes. With other hormones, such as pituitary hormones and progesterone, they cause enlargement of the breasts through promotion of ductal growth, stromal development, and the accretion of fat. Estrogens are intricately involved with other hormones, especially progesterone, in the processes of the ovulatory menstrual cycle and pregnancy and affect release of pituitary gonadotropins. Indirectly, they contribute to the following: Shaping of the skeleton; maintenance of tone and elasticity of urogenital structures; changes in epiphyses of long bones that allow for pubertal growth spurt and its termination; growth of axillary and pubic hair; pigmentation of nipples and genitals.

Menstruation – Decline of estrogenic activity at the end of the menstrual cycle can induce menstruation, although cessation of progesterone secretion is the most important factor in the mature ovulatory cycle. However, in the preovulatory or nonovulatory cycle, estrogen is the primary determinant of the onset of menstruation.

Menopause – After menopause, estradiol secretion from the ovaries ceases and the primary circulating estrogen is estrone. Estrone has approximately one-third the estrogenic potency of estradiol, but the estrone concentrations are about 4-fold that of estradiol after menopause.

Osteoporosis – Immobilization and prolonged bed rest produce rapid bone loss, while weight-bearing exercise has been shown to reduce bone loss and to increase bone mass. The optimal type and amount of physical activity that would prevent osteoporosis have not been established.

Estrogen reduces bone resorption and retards or halts postmenopausal bone loss. Studies have shown an approximately 60% reduction in hip and wrist fractures in women whose estrogen replacement began within a few years of menopause. Studies also suggest that estrogen reduces the rate of vertebral fractures. Even when started as late as 6 years after menopause, estrogen prevents further loss of bone mass but does not restore it to premenopausal levels.

➤*Pharmacokinetics:*

Absorption/Distribution – Estrogens used in therapy are well absorbed through the skin, mucous membranes, and GI tract. When applied for a local action, absorption is usually sufficient to cause systemic effects. When conjugated with aryl and alkyl groups for parenteral administration, the rate of absorption of oily preparations is slowed with a prolonged duration of action, such that a single IM injection of estradiol valerate or estradiol cypionate is absorbed over several weeks. Conjugated estrogens are well absorbed from the GI tract after release from the drug formulation. The tablet releases conjugated estrogens slowly over several hours. The distribution of exogenous estrogens is similar to that of endogenous estrogens. Estrogens are widely distributed in the body and are generally found in higher concentration in the sex hormone target organs. Estrogens circulate in the blood largely bound to sex hormone-binding globulin (SHBG) and albumin.

Transdermal system: In contrast to oral estradiol, the skin metabolizes estradiol via the transdermal system only to a small extent. Therefore, transdermal use produces therapeutic serum levels of estradiol with lower circulating levels of estrone and estrone conjugates and requires smaller total doses.

Metabolism/Excretion – When given orally, naturally occurring estrogens and their esters are extensively metabolized (first-pass effect) and circulate primarily as estrone sulfate, with smaller amounts of other conjugated and unconjugated estrogenic species. This results in limited oral potency. By contrast, synthetic estrogens, such as ethinyl estradiol and the nonsteroidal estrogens, are degraded very slowly in the liver and other tissues, which results in their high intrinsic potency. Estrogen drug products administered by non-oral routes are not subject to first-pass metabolism but also undergo significant hepatic uptake, metabolism, and enterohepatic recycling.

Metabolic conversion of estrogens occurs primarily in the liver (first-pass effect) but also at local target tissue sites. Complex metabolic processes result in a dynamic equilibrium of circulating conjugated and unconjugated estrogenic forms that are continually interconverted, especially between estrone and estradiol and between esterified and nonesterified forms. A certain proportion of the estrogen is excreted into the bile and then reabsorbed from the intestine. During this enterohepatic recirculation, estrogens are desulfated and resulfated and undergo degradation through conversion to less active estrogens (estriol and other estrogens), oxidation to nonestrogenic substances (catecholestrogens, which interact with catecholamine metabolism, especially in the CNS), and conjugation with glucuronic acids (which are then rapidly excreted in the urine).

Contraindications

Known or suspected breast cancer, except in appropriately selected patients being treated for metastatic disease; known or suspected estrogen-dependent neoplasia; undiagnosed abnormal genital bleeding; active deep vein thrombosis, PE, or a history of these conditions; active or recent (eg, within past year) arterial thromboembolic disease (eg, stroke, MI); active thrombophlebitis or thromboembolic disorders; history of thrombophlebitis, thrombosis or thromboembolic disorders associated with previous estrogen use (except when used in treatment of breast or prostatic malignancy); known or suspected pregnancy (see Warning Box); porphyria (estradiol vaginal tablets only); hypersensitivity to any product component.

Warnings/Precautions

➤*Induction of malignant neoplasms:*

Endometrial cancer – The use of unopposed estrogens in women with intact uteri has been associated with an increased risk of endometrial cancer. The reported endometrial cancer risk among unopposed estrogen users is about 2- to 12-fold greater than in nonusers and appears dependent on duration of treatment and on estrogen dose. Most studies show no significant increased risk associated with use of estrogens for less than 1 year. The greatest risk appears associated with prolonged use, with increased risks of 15- to 24-fold for 5 to 10 years or more and this risk has been shown to persist for at least 8 to 15 years after estrogen therapy is discontinued.

Clinical surveillance of all women taking estrogen/progestin combinations is important. Adequate diagnostic measures, including endometrial sampling when indicated, should be undertaken to rule out malignancy in all cases of undiagnosed persistent or recurring abnormal vaginal bleeding. There is no evidence that the use of natural estrogens results in a different endometrial risk profile than synthetic estrogens of equivalent estrogen dose. Adding a progestin to postmenopausal estrogen therapy has been shown to reduce the risk of endometrial hyperplasia, which may be a precursor to endometrial cancer.

Breast cancer – Estrogen and estrogen/progestin therapy in postmenopausal women have been associated with an increased risk of breast cancer. In the 0.625 mg conjugated equine estrogens plus 2.5 mg medroxyprogesterone acetate per day substudy of the WHI, 26% of the women reported prior use of estrogen alone and/or estrogen/progestin combination hormone therapy. After a mean follow-up of 5.6 years during the clinical trial, the overall relative risk of invasive breast cancer was 1.24 (95% confidence interval 1.01 to 1.54), and the overall absolute risk was 41 vs 33 cases per 10,000 women-years, for estrogen plus progestin compared with placebo. among women who reported prior use of hormone therapy, the relative risk of invasive breast cancer was 1.86, and absolute risk was 46 vs 25 cases per 10,000 women-years, for estrogen plus progestin compared with placebo. Among women who reported no prior use of hormone therapy, the relative risk of invasive breast cancer was 1.09, and the absolute risk was 40 vs 36 cases per 10,000 women-years for estrogen plus progestin compared with placebo. In the WHI trial invasive breast cancers were larger and diagnosed at a more advanced stage in the estrogen plus progestin group compared with the placebo group. Metastatic disease was rare with no apparent difference between the 2 groups. Other prognostic factors such as histologic subtype, grade, and hormone receptor status did not differ between the groups.

A postmenopausal woman without a uterus who requires estrogen should receive estrogen-alone therapy and should not be exposed unnecessarily to progestins. All postmenopausal women should receive yearly breast exams by a health care provider and perform monthly breast self-examinations. In addition, mammography examinations should be scheduled based on patient age and risk factors.

Ovarian cancer – Use of estrogen-only products, in particular for 10 years or more, has been associated with an increased risk of ovarian cancer in some epidemiological studies. Other studies did not show a significant association. Data are insufficient to determine whether there is an increased risk with combined estrogen/progestin therapy in postmenopausal women.

➤*Gallbladder disease:* There is a 2-fold to 4-fold increase in risk of gallbladder disease requiring surgery in women receiving postmenopausal estrogens.

➤*Cardiovascular disorders:* Estrogen and estrogen/progestin therapy have been associated with an increased risk of cardiovascular events (eg, MI and stroke, venous thrombosis, PE [venous thromboembolism (VTE)]). Should any of these occur or be suspected, discontinue estrogens immediately.

Risk factors for cardiovascular disease (eg, hypertension, diabetes mellitus, tobacco use, hypercholesterolemia, obesity) should be managed appropriately.

CHD – In the 0.625 mg conjugated equine estrogens per day substudy of the WHI, an increase in the number of MIs and strokes has been observed compared with placebo. These observations are preliminary and the study is continuing.

In the 0.625 mg conjugated equine estrogens plus 2.5 mg medroxyprogesterone acetate per day substudy of the WHI, an increased risk of CHD events (defined as nonfatal MI and CHD death) was observed compared with placebo (37 vs 30 per 10,000 person-years). The increase in risk was observed in year 1 and persisted.

In the same substudy of the WHI, an increased risk of stroke also was observed compared with placebo (29 vs 21 per 10,000 person-years). The increase in risk was observed after the first year and persisted.

In postmenopausal women with documented heart disease (n = 2763; average age, 66.7 years) a controlled clinical trial of secondary prevention of cardiovascular disease (Heart and Estrogen/progestin Replacement Study; HERS) treatment with 0.625 mg conjugated equine estrogens plus 2.5 mg medroxyprogesterone acetate per day demonstrated no cardiovascular benefit. During an average follow-up of 4.1 years, treatment with 0.625 mg conjugated equine estrogens plus 2.5 mg medroxyprogesterone acetate per day did not reduce the overall rate of CHD events in postmenopausal women with established CHD. There were more CHD events in the 0.625 mg conjugated equine estrogens plus 2.5 mg medroxyprogesterone acetate per day-treated group than in the placebo group in year 1, but not during subsequent years.

Large doses of estrogen (5 mg conjugated estrogens per day), comparable with those used to treat cancer of the prostate and breast, have been shown in a large prospective clinical trial in men to increase the risks of nonfatal MI, PE, and thrombophlebitis.

VTE – In the 0.625 mg conjugated equine estrogens per day substudy of the WHI, an increase in VTE has been observed compared with placebo. These observations are preliminary, and the study is continuing.

In the 0.625 mg conjugated equine estrogens plus 2.5 mg medroxyprogesterone acetate per day substudy of the WHI, a 2-fold greater rate of VTE, including deep venous thrombosis and PE, was observed compared with placebo. The rate of VTE was 34 per 10,000 woman-years in the 0.625 mg conjugated equine estrogens plus 2.5 mg medroxyprogesterone acetate per day group compared with 16 per 10,000 woman-years in the placebo group. The increase in VTE risk was observed during the first year and persisted.

If feasible, discontinue estrogens at least 4 to 6 weeks before surgery of the type associated with an increased risk of thromboembolism or during periods of prolonged immobilization.

➤*Dementia:* In the WHIMS, 4,532 generally healthy postmenopausal women 65 years of age and older were studied, of whom 35% were 70 to 74 years of age and 18% were 75 years of age or older. After an average follow-up of 4 years, 40 women being treated with 0.625 mg conjugated estrogens plus 2.5 mg medroxyprogesterone acetate (1.8%, n = 2,229) and 21 women in the placebo group (0.9%, n = 2,303) received diagnoses of probable dementia. The relative risk for estrogen/progestin vs placebo was 2.05 (95% confidence interval 1.21 to 3.48), and was similar for women with and without histories of menopausal hormone use before WHIMS. The absolute risk of probable dementia for estrogen/progestin vs placebo was 45 vs 22 cases per 10,000 women-years, and the absolute excess risk for estrogen/progestin was 23 cases per 10,000 women-years. It is unknown whether these findings apply to younger postmenopausal women.

The results of the estrogen alone substudy of the WHIMS have not been reported. It is unknown whether these findings apply to estrogen alone therapy.

➤*Hepatic adenoma:* Benign hepatic adenomas appear to be associated with the use of oral contraceptives (OCs). Although benign and rare, they may rupture and may cause death through intra-abdominal hemorrhage. Such lesions have not been reported in association with other estrogen or progestogen preparations but should be considered in estrogen users having abdominal pain and tenderness, abdominal mass, or hypovolemic shock. Hepatocellular carcinoma also has been reported in women taking estrogen-containing OCs. The relationship of this malignancy to these drugs is not known.

➤*Familial hyperlipoproteinemia:* Estrogen therapy may be associated with elevations of plasma triglycerides leading to pancreatitis and other complications in patients with familial defects of lipoprotein metabolism.

➤*Hypercalcemia:* Estrogens may lead to severe hypercalcemia in patients with breast cancer and bone metastases. If this occurs, discontinue the drug and take appropriate measures to reduce the serum calcium level.

➤*Glucose tolerance:* A worsening of glucose tolerance has been observed in a significant percentage of patients on estrogen-containing OCs. Carefully observe diabetic patients receiving estrogen.

➤*Visual abnormalities:* Retinal vascular thrombosis has been reported in patients receiving estrogens. Discontinue medication pending examination if there is sudden partial or complete loss of vision or a sudden onset of proptosis, diplopia, or migraine. If examination reveals papilledema or retinal vascular lesions, discontinue estrogens.

➤*Hypothyroidism:* Estrogen administration leads to increased thyroid-binding globulin (TBG) levels. Patients with normal thyroid function can compensate for the increased TBG by making more thyroid hormone, thus maintaining free T_4 and T_3 serum concentrations in the normal range. Patients dependent on thyroid hormone replacement therapy who are also receiving estrogens may require increased doses of their thyroid replacement therapy. Monitor thyroid function in these patients in order to maintain their free thyroid hormone levels in an acceptable range.

➤*Depression:* OCs appear to be associated with an increased incidence of mental depression. Although it is not clear whether this is caused by the estrogenic or progestogenic component of the contraceptive, carefully observe patients with a history of depression.

➤*Uterine leiomyomata:* Pre-existing uterine leiomyomata may increase in size during estrogen use.

➤*Elevated blood pressure:* In a small number of case reports, substantial increases in blood pressure have been attributed to idiosyncratic reactions to estrogens. In a large, randomized, placebo-controlled clinical trial, a generalized effect of estrogen therapy on blood pressure was not seen. Monitor blood pressure at regular intervals with estrogen use.

➤*Hypercoagulability:* Some studies have shown that women taking estrogen replacement therapy have hypercoagulability, primarily related to decreased antithrombin activity. This effect appears dose- and duration-dependent and is less pronounced than that associated with oral contraceptive use. Also, postmenopausal women tend to have increased coagulation parameters at baseline compared with premenopausal women. There is some suggestion that low-dose postmenopausal mestranol may increase the risk of thromboembolism, although the majority of studies (of primarily conjugated estrogens users) report no such increase. There is insufficient information on hypercoagulability in women who have had previous thromboembolic disease. Therefore, do not use in people with active thrombophlebitis or thromboembolic disorders or in people with a history of such disorders associated with estrogen use (except in treatment of malignancy).

➤*History/Physical exam:* Before initiating estrogens, take complete medical and family history. Pretreatment and periodic history and physical exams every 12 months should include blood pressure, breasts, abdomen, pelvic organs, and a Papanicolaou smear. Generally, do not prescribe for longer than 1 year between physical examinations.

➤*Vaginal products:* Estradiol vaginal ring may not be suitable for women with narrow, short, or stenosed vaginas. Narrow vagina, vaginal stenosis, prolapse, and vaginal infections are conditions that make the vagina more susceptible to estradiol vaginal ring-caused irritation or ulceration. Women with signs or symptoms of vaginal irritation should alert their physician.

Vaginal infection is generally more common in postmenopausal women because of the lack of the normal flora of fertile women, especially lactobacillus, and the subsequent higher pH. Treat vaginal infections with appropriate antimicrobial therapy before initiation of therapy. If a vaginal infection develops during use of the estradiol vaginal ring, remove the ring and reinsert only after the infection has been appropriately treated.

Conjugated estrogens vaginal cream exposure has been reported to weaken latex condoms. Consider its potential to weaken and contribute to the failure of condoms, diaphragms, or cervical caps made of latex or rubber.

➤*Excessive estrogenic stimulation:* Certain patients may develop undesirable manifestations of excessive estrogenic stimulation (eg, abnormal or excessive uterine bleeding, mastodynia). Advise the pathologist of estrogen therapy when relevant specimens are submitted.

➤*Fluid retention:* Estrogens may cause some degree of fluid retention; conditions that might be influenced by this factor (eg, asthma, epilepsy, migraine, cardiac or renal dysfunction) require careful observation.

➤*Calcium and phosphorus metabolism:* Calcium and phosphorus metabolism is influenced by estrogens; use caution in metabolic bone diseases associated with hypercalcemia or in renal insufficiency. Use estrogens with caution in individuals with severe hypocalcemia.

➤*Endometrial hyperplasia:* Prolonged unopposed estrogen therapy may increase risk of endometrial hyperplasia.

➤*Exacerbations of other conditions:* Endometriosis may be exacerbated with administration of estrogen therapy. Estrogen therapy also may cause an exacerbation of asthma, diabetes mellitus, epilepsy, migraine, or porphyria; use with caution in patients with these conditions.

➤*Benzyl alcohol:* Benzyl alcohol, contained in some of these products as a preservative, has been associated with a fatal "gasping syndrome" in premature infants.

➤*Tartrazine sensitivity:* Some of these products contain tartrazine (FD&C Yellow No. 5), which may cause allergic-type reactions (including bronchial asthma) in susceptible individuals. Although the incidence of sensitivity is low, it is frequently seen in patients who also have aspirin hypersensitivity. Specific products containing tartrazine are identified in the product listings.

➤*Hepatic function impairment:* Exercise caution in patients with a history of cholestatic jaundice associated with past estrogen use or with pregnancy and, in the case of recurrence, discontinue medication. Estrogens may be poorly metabolized in impaired liver function; use with caution.

➤*Pregnancy: Category X.* Do not use estrogens during pregnancy. See Warning Box.

➤*Lactation:* Estrogens have been shown to decrease the quantity and quality of breast milk and detectable amounts are excreted in breast milk. Administer only when clearly needed.

➤*Children:* Estrogen therapy has been used for the induction of puberty in adolescents with some forms of pubertal delay. Safety and efficacy in pediatric patients have not otherwise been established.

Large and repeated doses of estrogen over an extended period of time have been shown to accelerate epiphyseal closure, which could result in short adult stature if treatment is initiated before the completion of physiologic puberty in normally developing children. If estrogen is administered to patients whose bone growth is not complete, periodic monitoring of bone maturation and effects on epiphyseal centers is recommended during estrogen administration.

Estrogen treatment of prepubertal girls also induces premature breast development and vaginal cornification and may induce vaginal bleeding. In boys, estrogen treatment may modify the normal pubertal process and induce gynecomastia.

➤*Elderly:* Per the Beers list, evidence of the carcinogenic (breast and endometrial cancer) potential and lack of cardioprotective effect in older women is a concern with oral estrogens. Estrogens (**conjugated estrogen**, **estropipate**, **esterified estrogen**) are considered high risk medication for the elderly according to the Centers of Medicare and Medicaid Services.

➤*Lab test abnormalities:* Certain endocrine and liver function tests may be affected by estrogen-containing OCs. Expect the following similar changes with larger doses:

Increased sulfobromophthalein retention.

Increased prothrombin time, partial thromboplastin time, platelet aggregation time, platelet count, and factors II, VII, VIII, IX, X, XII, VII-X complex, II-VII-X complex, and β-thromboglobulin; decreased antithrombin III, antifactor Xa; increased fibrinogen, plasminogen, and norepinephrine-induced platelet aggregability.

Increased thyroid binding globulin (TBG) leading to increased circulating total thyroid hormone, as measured by protein bound iodine (PBI), T_4 by column or T_4 or T_3 by radioimmunoassay. Free T_3 resin uptake is decreased, reflecting the elevated TBG; free T_4 and free T_3 concentration is unaltered.

Impaired glucose tolerance; decreased pregnanediol excretion; reduced response to metyrapone test; reduced serum folate concentration; increased serum triglyceride and phospholipid concentration.

Other binding proteins may be elevated in serum (ie, corticosteroid binding globulin [CBG], SHBG), leading to increased circulating corticosteroids and sex steroids, respectively. Free or biologically active hormone concentrations are unchanged. Other plasma proteins may be increased (angiotensinogen/renin substrate, α-1-antitrypsin, ceruloplasmin).

Increased plasma HDL and HDL-2 subfraction concentrations, reduced LDL cholesterol concentration levels, increased triglyceride levels.

Drug Interactions

Refer to the drug interaction section in the Oral Contraceptives group monograph for more information.

Estrogen Drug Interactions

Precipitant drug	Object drug[a]		Description
Estrogens	Anticoagulants, oral	↓	Estrogens may theoretically reduce the effect of anticoagulants.
Estrogens	Antidepressants, tricyclic	↔	Pharmacologic effects of these agents may be altered by estrogens; the effects of this interaction may depend on the dose of the estrogen. An increased incidence of toxic reactions also may occur.
Estrogens	Corticosteroids	↑	An increase in the pharmacologic and toxicologic effects of corticosteroids may occur via inactivation of hepatic P-450 enzyme.
Estrogens	Thyroid hormones	↓	In hypothyroid women, estrogens may increase serum thyroxine-binding globulin concentrations, therefore changing serum thyroxine and thyrotropin concentrations. Thyroid hormone requirements may be increased.
CYP 3A4 inducers Barbiturates Carbamazepine Rifampin St. John's wort	Estrogens	↓	Coadministration may reduce plasma concentrations of estrogens, possibly resulting in a decrease in therapeutic effects and/or changes in the uterine bleeding profile.
CYP 3A4 inhibitors Itraconazole Ketoconazole Macrolide antibiotics Ritonavir	Estrogens	↑	Coadministration may increase plasma concentrations of estrogens and may result in side effects.

Estrogen Drug Interactions			
Precipitant drug	Object drug[a]		Description
Hydantoins	Estrogens	⬇	Breakthrough bleeding, spotting, and pregnancy have resulted when these medications were used concurrently. A loss of seizure control also has been suggested and may be caused by fluid retention.
Estrogens	Hydantoins		
Topiramate	Estrogens	⬇	Topiramate may increase the metabolism of estrogens, decreasing their efficacy.

[a] ⬆ = Object drug increased. ⬇ = Object drug decreased. ⬌ = Undetermined clinical effect.

➤*Drug/Food interactions:* Grapefruit juice may inhibit CYP3A4-mediated estrogen metabolism, increasing plasma concentrations of estrogens and possibly resulting in side effects.

Adverse Reactions

See Warnings regarding induction of neoplasia, adverse effects on the fetus, increased incidence of gallbladder disease, hypercalcemia, cardiovascular disease, elevated blood pressure, and adverse effects similar to those of OCs.

➤*Cardiovascular:* Venous thromboembolism; pulmonary embolism; syncope; deep and superficial venous thrombosis; thrombophlebitis; MI; stroke; increased blood pressure.

➤*CNS:* Headache; migraine; dizziness; mental depression; chorea; insomnia; anxiety; emotional lability; nervousness; mood disturbances; irritability; exacerbation of epilepsy; fatigue; sinus headache; tension headaches.

➤*Dermatologic:* Chloasma or melasma (may persist when drug is discontinued); erythema nodosum/multiforme; hemorrhagic eruption; dermatitis; skin hypertrophy; loss of scalp hair; hirsutism; pruritus; rash; pruritus ani; acne.

➤*GI:* Nausea; vomiting; abdominal cramps/pain; bloating; cholestatic jaundice; pancreatitis; diarrhea; dyspepsia; flatulence; gastritis; gastroenteritis; enlarged abdomen; hemorrhoids; increased incidence of gallbladder disease; constipation.

➤*GU:* Breakthrough bleeding; abnormal withdrawal bleeding; spotting; change in menstrual flow; dysmenorrhea; premenstrual-like syndrome; amenorrhea during and after treatment; vaginal candidiasis; change in cervical ectropion and degree of cervical secretion; cystitis-like syndrome; urinary tract infection; leukorrhea; vaginitis; vaginal discomfort/pain; vaginal hemorrhage; asymptomatic genital bacterial growth; genital moniliasis; cystitis; dysuria; genital pruritus; genital eruption; urinary incontinence; endometrial hyperplasia; increase in size of uterine leiomyomata/fibromyomata; ovarian cancer; endometrial cancer; micturition frequency; urethral disorder; vaginosis fungal; vaginal discharge.

➤*Local:* Redness/erythema and irritation at application site with the estradiol transdermal system; rash (rare).

➤*Ophthalmic:* Steepening of corneal curvature; intolerance to contact lenses; retinal vascular thrombosis.

➤*Respiratory:* Upper respiratory tract infection; sinusitis; rhinitis; bronchitis; pharyngitis; nasopharyngitis; cough; nasal congestion; pharyngolaryngeal pain.

➤*Miscellaneous:* Aggravation of porphyria; edema; changes in libido; breast pain, tenderness, enlargement, or secretion; galactorrhea; fibrocystic breast changes; breast cancer; reduced carbohydrate tolerance; pain; hypersensitivity reactions; increase or decrease in weight; back pain; arthritis; arthralgia; skeletal pain; flu-like symptoms; hot flushes; allergy; chest pain; leg edema; otitis media; toothache; tooth disorder; infection; accidental injury; asthenia; anemia; paresthesia; leg cramps; anaphylactoid/anaphylactic reactions (including urticaria and angioedema); hypocalcemia; exacerbation of asthma; increased triglycerides; neck pain; neck rigidity; candidal infection; fungal infection; herpes simplex; fluid retention.

Overdosage

Serious ill effects have not been reported following ingestion of large doses of estrogen-containing OCs by young children. Overdosage of estrogen may cause nausea and vomiting; withdrawal bleeding may occur in females.

Patient Information

Patient package insert is available with products.

Estrogens increase the chances of getting cancer of the uterus. Report any unusual vaginal bleeding right away. Vaginal bleeding after menopause may be a warning sign of cancer of the uterus.

Do not use estrogens with or without progestins to prevent heart disease, heart attacks, or strokes. Using estrogens with or without progestins may increase the chances of heart attacks, strokes, breast cancer, and blood clots.

Notify physician if any of the following occur: Pain in the calves; sharp chest pain or sudden shortness of breath; coughing blood; abnormal vaginal bleeding; missed menstrual period or suspected pregnancy; lumps in the breast; severe headache or vomiting; dizziness or fainting; vision or speech disturbance; weakness or numbness in an arm or leg; abdominal pain, swelling, or tenderness; yellowing of the skin or eyes; depression.

ESTRADIOL TRANSDERMAL

Rx	**Menostar** (Berlex)	**Patch; transdermal**: 0.014 mg/24 h	1 mg total estradiol. 3.25 cm^2. In 4s.
Rx	**Estradiol Transdermal System** (Mylan)	**Patch; transdermal**: 0.025 mg/24 h	0.97 mg total estradiol. 7.75 cm^2. In 4s.
Rx	**Alora** (Watson)		0.77 mg total estradiol. 9 cm^2. In calendar packs (8 systems).
Rx	**Climara** (Bayer)		2 mg total estradiol. 6.5 cm^2. In 4s.
Rx	**Vivelle-Dot** (Novartis)		0.39 mg total estradiol. 2.5 cm^2. In calendar packs (8s and 24s).
Rx	**Estradiol Transdermal System** (Mylan)	**Patch; transdermal**: 0.0375 mg/24 h	1.46 mg total estradiol. 11.625 cm^2. In 4s.
Rx	**Climara** (Bayer)		2.85 mg total estradiol. 9.375 cm^2. In 4s.
Rx	**Vivelle** (Novartis)		3.28 mg total estradiol. 11 cm^2. In calendar packs (8 and 24 systems).
Rx	**Vivelle-Dot** (Novartis)		0.585 mg total estradiol. 3.75 cm^2. In calendar packs (8 systems).
Rx	**Estradiol Transdermal System** (Mylan)	**Patch; transdermal**: 0.05 mg/24 h	1.94 mg total estradiol. 15.5 cm^2. In 4s.
Rx	**Alora** (Watson)		1.5 mg total estradiol. 18 cm^2. In calendar packs (8s).
Rx	**Climara** (Bayer)		3.8 mg total estradiol. 12.5 cm^2. In 4s.
Rx	**Estraderm** (Novartis)		4 mg total estradiol. 10 cm^2. In calendar packs (8 and 24 systems).
Rx	**Vivelle** (Novartis)		4.33 mg total estradiol. 14.5 cm^2. In calendar packs (8 and 24 systems).
Rx	**Vivelle-Dot** (Novartis)		0.78 mg total estradiol. 5 cm^2. In calendar packs (8 systems).
Rx	**Estradiol Transdermal System** (Mylan)	**Patch; transdermal**: 0.06 mg/24 h	2.33 mg total estradiol. 18.6 cm^2. In 4s.
Rx	**Climara** (Bayer)		4.55 mg total estradiol. 15 cm^2. In 4s.
Rx	**Estradiol Transdermal System** (Mylan)	**Patch; transdermal**: 0.075 mg/24 h	2.91 mg total estradiol. 23.25 cm^2. In 4s.
Rx	**Alora** (Watson)		2.3 mg total estradiol. 27 cm^2. In calendar packs (8 systems).
Rx	**Climara** (Bayer)		5.7 mg total estradiol. 18.75 cm^2. In 4s.
Rx	**Vivelle** (Novartis)		6.57 mg total estradiol. 22 cm^2. In calendar packs (8 and 24 systems).
Rx	**Vivelle–Dot** (Novartis)		1.17 mg total estradiol. 7.5 cm^2. In calendar packs (8 systems).

ESTRADIOL TRANSDERMAL

Rx	**Estradiol Transdermal System** (Mylan)	**Patch; transdermal:** 0.1 mg/24 h	3.88 mg total estradiol. 31 cm^2. In 4s.
Rx	**Alora** (Watson)		3.1 mg total estradiol. 36 cm^2. In calendar packs (8 systems).
Rx	**Climara** (Bayer)		7.6 mg total estradiol. 25 cm^2. In 4s.
Rx	**Estraderm** (Novartis)		8 mg total estradiol. 20 cm^2. In calendar packs (8 and 24 systems).
Rx	**Vivelle** (Novartis)		8.66 mg total estradiol. 29 cm^2. In calendar packs (8 and 24 systems).
Rx	**Vivelle-Dot** (Novartis)		1.56 mg total estradiol. 10 cm^2. In calendar packs (8 systems).
Rx	**Elestrin** (Azur Pharma)	**Gel; topical:** estradiol 0.06% (estradiol 0.52 mg per 0.87 g unit dose)	Edetate disodium, ethanol. In a 144 g metered-dose pump that delivers 100 metered doses of approximately 0.87 g/pump.
Rx	**EstroGel** (Ascend Therapeutics)	**Gel; topical:** estradiol 0.06% (estradiol 0.75 mg per 1.25 g unit dose)	Alcohol. In 50 g pump that delivers 32 metered 1.25 g doses.
Rx	**Divigel** (Upsher-Smith)	**Gel; topical:** estradiol 0.1%	Ethanol. In 0.25, 0.5, and 1 g per single-dose foil packet.[a] In carton of 30 packets.
Rx	**Estrasorb** (Graceway)	**Emulsion; topical:** estradiol 2.5 mg/g	Soybean oil, ethanol. In 1.74 g pouches.
Rx	**Evamist** (Ther-Rx)	**Spray, solution; topical:** estradiol 1.7% (estradiol 1.53 mg/spray)	Alcohol, octisalate. In 8.1 mL metered-dose pump that delivers 56 sprays of 90 mcL.

[a] Corresponding to estradiol 0.25, 0.5, and 1 mg, respectively.

ESTRADIOL — TRANSDERMAL PATCH

For complete and comparative prescribing information, refer to the Estrogens group monograph.

WARNING

Estrogens increase the risk of endometrial cancer – Close clinical surveillance of all women taking estrogens is important. Use adequate diagnostic measures, including endometrial sampling when indicated, to rule out malignancy in all cases of undiagnosed persistent or recurring abnormal vaginal bleeding. There is currently no evidence that "natural" estrogens results in a different endometrial risk profile than synthetic estrogens at equivalent estrogen dose(s).

Cardiovascular and other risks – Do not use estrogens with or without progestins for the prevention of cardiovascular disease or dementia.

The Women's Health Initiative (WHI) study reported increased risks of myocardial infarction (MI), stroke, invasive breast cancer, pulmonary emboli (PE), and deep vein thrombosis in postmenopausal women during 5 years of treatment with conjugated equine estrogens 0.625 mg combined with medroxyprogesterone acetate 2.5 mg relative to placebo.

The Women's Health Initiative Memory Study (WHIMS), a substudy of WHI, reported increased risk of developing probable dementia in postmenopausal women 65 years of age or older during 4 years of treatment with oral conjugated estrogens plus medroxyprogesterone acetate relative to placebo. It is unknown whether this finding applies to younger postmenopausal women or to women taking estrogen alone therapy.

Other doses of conjugated estrogens with medroxyprogesterone, and other combinations of estrogens and progestins were not studied in the WHI and, in the absence of comparable data, these risks should be assumed to be similar. Because of these risks, prescribe estrogens with or without progestins at the lowest effective doses and for the shortest duration consistent with treatment goals and risks for the individual woman.

Indications

➤*Vasomotor symptoms (except Menostar)*: Treatment of moderate to severe vasomotor symptoms associated with menopause.

➤*Vulvular/Vaginal atrophy (except Menostar)*: Treatment of moderate to severe symptoms of vulvar and vaginal atrophy associated with menopause. When prescribing solely for the treatment of symptoms of vulvar and vaginal atrophy, consider topical vaginal products.

➤*Hypoestrogenism (except Menostar)*: Treatment of hypoestrogenism because of hypogonadism, castration, or primary ovarian failure.

➤*Prevention of postmenopausal osteoporosis:* When prescribing solely for the prevention of postmenopausal osteoporosis, consider therapy only for women at significant risk of osteoporosis. Carefully consider nonestrogen medications. The mainstays for decreasing the risk of postmenopausal osteoporosis are weight-bearing exercise, adequate calcium and vitamin D intake, and when indicated, pharmacologic therapy. Postmenopausal women require an average of 1,500 mg/day of elemental calcium. Therefore, when not contraindicated, calcium supplementation may be helpful for women with suboptimal dietary intake. Vitamin D supplementation of 400 to 800 units/day may also be required to ensure adequate daily intake in postmenopausal women.

Administration and Dosage

➤*General dosing considerations:* For women who have a uterus, undertake adequate diagnostic measures, such as endometrial sampling, when indicated, to rule out malignancy in cases of undiagnosed persistent or recurring abnormal vaginal bleeding.

Initiate prophylactic therapy to prevent postmenopausal bone loss with the lowest available dosage as soon as possible after menopause.

➤*Adults: Alora, Estraderm, Vivelle,* and *Vivelle-Dot* are applied twice per week. *Climara* and *Menostar* last for 7 days and are applied once per week.

Estradiol transdermal therapy may be given continuously in patients who do not have an intact uterus. In those patients with an intact uterus, transdermal estradiol may be given on a cyclic schedule (eg, 3 weeks on drug, followed by 1 week off drug); *Vivelle* may be given continuously or on a cyclic schedule (eg, 3 weeks on drug, followed by 1 week off drug) with a progestin.

Hypoestrogenism –

Initial dosage: 0.025 to 0.05 mg/day. *Alora, Estraderm, Vivelle,* and *Vivelle-Dot* are applied twice per week; *Climara* and *Menostar* are applied once per week.

Dosage adjustment: Adjust the dosage as necessary to control symptoms. Choose the lowest dose and regimen that will control symptoms. In order to use the lowest dosage necessary for the control of symptoms, do not make decisions to increase dosage until after the first month of therapy.

Duration of therapy: Discontinue the medication as promptly as possible. Make attempts to taper or discontinue the medication at 3- to 6-month intervals.

Osteoporosis prevention –

Initial dosage: 0.025 mg/day is the minimum dosage that has been shown to be effective. *Alora, Estraderm, Vivelle,* and *Vivelle-Dot* are applied twice per week; *Climara* and *Menostar* are applied once per week.

Dosage adjustment: The dosage may be adjusted if necessary.

Discontinuation of therapy: Discontinuation may reestablish bone loss at a rate comparable with the immediate postmenopausal period.

Vasomotor symptoms associated with menopause –

Initial dosage: 0.025 to 0.05 mg/day. *Alora, Estraderm, Vivelle,* and *Vivelle-Dot* are applied twice per week; *Climara* and *Menostar* are applied once per week.

Dosage adjustment: Adjust the dosage as necessary to control symptoms. Choose the lowest dose and regimen that will control symptoms. In order to use the lowest dosage necessary for the control of symptoms, do not make decisions to increase dosage until after the first month of therapy.

Duration of therapy: Discontinue the medication as promptly as possible. Make attempts to taper or discontinue the medication at 3- to 6-month intervals.

Vulvar and vaginal atrophy associated with menopause –

Initial dosage: 0.025 to 0.05 mg/day. *Alora, Estraderm, Vivelle,* and *Vivelle-Dot* are applied twice per week; *Climara* and *Menostar* are applied once per week.

Dosage adjustment: Adjust the dosage as necessary to control symptoms. Choose the lowest dose and regimen that will control symptoms. In order to use the lowest dosage necessary for the control of symptoms, do not make decisions to increase dosage until after the first month of therapy.

Duration of therapy: Discontinue the medication as promptly as possible. Make attempts to taper or discontinue the medication at 3- to 6-month intervals.

➤*Concomitant progestin therapy:* When estrogen is prescribed for a postmenopausal woman with a uterus, initiate progestin also to reduce the risk of endometrial cancer. A woman without a uterus does not need progestin.

It is recommended that women who have a uterus and are being treated with *Menostar* receive a progestin for 14 days every 6 to 12 months and undergo an endometrial biopsy at yearly intervals or as clinically indicated.

➤*Conversion from oral estrogens:* In women not currently taking oral estrogens, treatment with transdermal estradiol may be initiated at once. In women who are currently taking oral estrogen, initiate treatment with transdermal estradiol 1 week after withdrawal of oral hormone therapy, or sooner if menopausal symptoms reappear in less than 1 week.

➤*Duration of therapy:* Limit use of estrogen alone or in combination with a progestin to the shortest duration consistent with treatment goals and risks for the individual woman. Reevaluate patients periodically as clinically appropriate (eg, 3- to 6-month intervals) to determine whether treatment is still necessary.

➤*Administration: Alora, Estraderm, Vivelle,* and *Vivelle-Dot* are applied twice per week. *Climara* and *Menostar* last for 7 days and are applied once per week.

ESTRADIOL — TRANSDERMAL PATCH

Application of system – Place the adhesive side of the transdermal system on a clean, dry area of the lower abdomen, femoral triangle (upper inner thigh), upper arm, upper quadrant of the buttock, or outer aspect of the hip. Place the adhesive side of *Menostar* on a clean, dry area of the lower abdomen only. The site selected should be one that is not exposed to sunlight. Do not apply to or near the breasts or other parts of the body. Replace the transdermal system once or twice weekly, depending on the product specification. The sites of application must be rotated, with an interval of at least 1 week allowed between applications to a particular site. The area selected should not be oily, damaged, or irritated. Avoid the waistline because tight clothing may rub the patch off. Also avoid application to areas where sitting would dislodge the patch. Apply the patch immediately after opening the pouch and removing the protective liner. Press the patch firmly in place with the palm of the hand for approximately 10 seconds, making sure there is good contact, especially around the edges. If the patch lifts, apply pressure to maintain adhesion.

In the unlikely event that a patch should fall off, the same patch may be reapplied (except *Climara* or *Menostar*). If necessary, a new patch may be applied. In the event that a *Climara* or a *Menostar* system falls off, apply a new system for the remainder of the 7-day dosing interval. Wear only 1 system at any one time during the 7-day dosing interval. In either case, continue the original treatment schedule.

If a patient has forgotten to apply a patch, she should apply a new patch as soon as possible. Apply the new patch on the original treatment schedule. The interruption of treatment in women might increase the likelihood of breakthrough bleeding, spotting, and recurrence of symptoms. Wear only 1 patch at any given time. Swimming, bathing, or using a sauna while using the transdermal system may decrease the adhesion of the patch and the delivery of estradiol.

Removal of the transdermal system – Carefully and slowly remove the system to avoid irritation of the skin. Should any adhesive remain on the skin after removal of the system, allow the area to dry for 15 minutes. Then gently rub the area with an oil-based cream or lotion to remove the adhesive residue. Used patches still contain some active hormones. Carefully fold each patch in half so that it sticks to itself before throwing it away.

➤*Storage/Stability:* Store at 25°C (77°F). Do not store above 30°C (86°F). Do not store unpouched. Apply immediately upon removal from the protective pouch. Discard used estradiol transdermal systems in household trash in a manner that prevents accidental application or ingestion by children, pets, or others.

ESTRADIOL — TRANSDERMAL MISCELLANEOUS

For complete and comparative prescribing information, refer to the Estrogens class monograph.

WARNING

Endometrial cancer – Close clinical surveillance of all women taking estrogen is important. Undertake adequate diagnostic measures, including endometrial sampling when indicated, to rule out malignancy in all cases of undiagnosed persistent or recurring abnormal vaginal bleeding. There is no evidence that the use of "natural" estrogens results in a different endometrial risk profile than synthetic estrogens at equivalent estrogenic doses.

Cardiovascular and other risks – Do not use estrogens with or without progestins for the prevention of cardiovascular disease or dementia.

The Women's Health Initiative (WHI) estrogen-alone substudy reported increased risks of stroke and deep vein thrombosis (DVT) in postmenopausal women (50 to 79 years of age) during 6.8 and 7.1 years, respectively, of treatment with daily oral conjugated estrogens 0.625 mg, relative to placebo.

The estrogen-plus-progestin WHI substudy reported increased risks of myocardial infarction (MI), stroke, invasive breast cancer, pulmonary emboli (PE), and DVT in postmenopausal women (50 to 79 years of age) during 5.6 years of treatment with daily oral conjugated estrogens 0.625 mg combined with medroxyprogesterone acetate 2.5 mg, relative to placebo.

The WHI Memory Study (WHIMS), a substudy of the WHI, reported increased risk of developing probable dementia in postmenopausal women 65 years of age and older during 5.2 years of treatment with daily conjugated estrogens 0.625 mg alone and during 4 years of treatment with daily conjugated estrogens 0.625 mg combined with medroxyprogesterone acetate 2.5 mg, relative to placebo. It is unknown whether this finding applies to younger postmenopausal women.

Other doses of conjugated estrogens with medroxyprogesterone acetate, and other combinations of estrogens and progestins, were not studied in the WHI and, in the absence of comparable data, assume these risks to be similar. Because of these risks, estrogens with or without progestins should be prescribed at the lowest effective doses and for the shortest duration consistent with treatment goals and risks for the individual woman.

Indications

➤*Vasomotor symptoms associated with menopause:* For the treatment of moderate to severe vasomotor symptoms associated with menopause.

➤*Vulvar/Vaginal atrophy associated with menopause (EstroGel only):* For the treatment of moderate to severe symptoms of vulvar and vaginal atrophy associated with menopause. When prescribing solely for the treatment of symptoms of vulvar and vaginal atrophy, consider topical vaginal products.

Administration and Dosage

➤*General dosing considerations:* For women with a uterus, adequate diagnostic measures, such as endometrial sampling, when indicated, should be undertaken to rule out malignancy in case of undiagnosed persistent or recurring abnormal vaginal bleeding.

➤*Adults:*

Vasomotor symptoms associated with menopause –

Gel:

• *Divigel* –

Initial dosage: 0.25 g applied once daily to the skin of either the right or left upper thigh.

Maintenance dosage: 0.25 to 1 g applied once daily to the skin of either the right or left upper thigh. Use the lowest effective dose.

Dosage adjustment: Subsequent dosage adjustments may be made based upon the individual patient response. This dose should be periodically reassessed by the health care provider.

• *Elestrin* –

Usual dosage: Apply 1 pump of gel per day (0.87 g/day) to the upper arm.

Dosage adjustment: Subsequent dose adjustment may be made based upon the patient's response. This dose should be periodically reassessed by the health care provider.

• *EstroGel* – 1.25 g applied at the same time each day over the entire area on the inside and outside of the arm from wrist to shoulder. The lowest effective dose has not been determined.

Spray:

• *Initial dosage* – 1 spray per day applied each morning to the inner surface of the forearm, starting near the elbow.

• *Maintenance dosage* – 1 to 3 sprays per day applied each morning to the inner surface of the forearm, starting near the elbow.

• *Dosage adjustment* – Dosage adjustment should be guided by the clinical response.

Emulsion: 3.48 g applied once daily to both legs each morning. The lowest effective dose has not been determined.

Vulvar and vaginal atrophy associated with menopause –

EstroGel: 1.25 g applied at the same time each day over the entire area on the inside and outside of the arm from wrist to shoulder. The lowest effective dose has not been determined.

➤*Concomitant progestin therapy:* When estrogen is prescribed for a postmenopausal woman with a uterus, also initiate a progestin to reduce the risk of endometrial cancer. A woman without a uterus does not need progestin.

➤*Duration of therapy:* Use of estrogen, alone or in combination with a progestin, should be with the lowest effective dose and for the shortest duration consistent with treatment goals and risks for the individual women. Reevaluate patients periodically as clinically appropriate (eg, at 3- to 6-month intervals) to determine if treatment is still necessary.

➤*Administration:*

Gel –

Divigel: Apply *Divigel* once daily to the skin of either the right or left upper thigh. The application surface area should be about 5 × 7 inches (approximately the size of 2 palm prints). Apply the entire contents of a unit dose packet each day. To avoid potential skin irritation, apply *Divigel* to the right or left upper thigh on alternating days. Do not apply *Divigel* to the face, breasts, or irritated skin, or in or around the vagina. After application, allow the gel to dry before dressing. Do not wash the application site within 1 hour after application. Avoid eye contact. Wash hands after application.

Elestrin: Prime the pump (10 depressions) before the first use. *Elestrin* is applied once daily to the upper arm. Never apply to the breast or in or around the vagina. Allow the gel to dry for 5 minutes or more before dressing. Try to keep the area dry for as long as possible. Do not apply sunscreen to the area where the gel was applied for at least 25 minutes or where the gel was applied for 7 or more consecutive days. Wash hands after application.

EstroGel: For the 50 g pump, prime 3 times before using the pump. Discard the unused gel after priming. Apply the gel at the same time each day. Apply the gel to clean, dry, unbroken skin. Never apply directly to the breast. Apply the gel to 1 arm and spread the gel as thinly as possible over the entire area on the inside and outside of the arm from wrist to shoulder. Allow the gel to dry for up to 5 minutes before dressing. Wash hands after applying the gel.

Spray – Before applying the first dose from a new applicator, prime the pump by spraying 3 sprays with the cover on. Hold the container upright and vertical for spraying. Apply 1, 2, or 3 sprays each morning to adjacent, non-overlapping areas on the inner surface of the forearm, starting near the elbow. Apply to clean, dry, unbroken skin. Never apply directly to the breast or in or around the vagina. Hold the applicator upright and rest the plastic cone flat against the skin so there are no gaps between the cone and the skin. Depress the pump fully once. If 2 or 3 sprays are needed, then move the cone to an area of the skin next to but not touching the area of the previous spray. Do not massage or rub into the skin. Allow sprays to dry for approximately 2 minutes, and do not wash the site for 30 minutes. Do not apply the spray to skin surfaces other than the forearm.

Emulsion – Open each foil-laminated pouch individually. Apply in a comfortable sitting position to clean, dry skin on both legs each morning. Do not

ESTRADIOL — TRANSDERMAL MISCELLANEOUS

apply to any skin that appears to be red or irritated. Apply the entire contents of the pouch to the top of the left thigh. Using 1 hand, rub the emulsion into the entire left thigh and left calf for 3 minutes or until thoroughly absorbed. Rub any excess emulsion remaining on both hands on the buttocks. Open the second pouch and repeat the previous steps on the right leg. Allow the application areas to dry completely before covering with clothing. Wash hands after application. Do not apply sunscreen and the emulsion at the same time.

➤*Storage/Stability:* Alcohol and alcohol-based liquids and gels are flammable. Avoid fire, flame, or smoking until the spray or gel has dried.

Gel/Emulsion – Store at 20° to 25°C (68° to 77°F); excursions are permitted to 15° to 30°C (59° to 86°F). Do not freeze.

Spray – Store at 25°C (77°F); excursions are permitted to 15° to 30°C (59° to 86°F). Do not freeze.

ESTRADIOL

Rx	**Femtrace** (Warner Chilcott)	**Tablets:** 0.45 mg estradiol acetate	Lactose. (WC 389). Cream. In 100s.
Rx	**Estradiol** (Various, eg, Geneva, Mylan)	**Tablets:** 0.5 mg micronized estradiol	May contain lactose. In 100s.
Rx	**Estrace** (Warner Chilcott)		Lactose. (021 MJ). White, scored. In 100s.
Rx	**Gynodiol** (Novavax Inc.)		Lactose. (0768). Lavender, scored. In 30s and 100s.
Rx	**Femtrace** (Warner Chilcott)	**Tablets:** 0.9 mg estradiol acetate	Lactose. (WC 390). White. In 100s.
Rx	**Estradiol** (Various, eg, Geneva, Mylan)	**Tablets:** 1 mg micronized estradiol	May contain lactose. In 100s and 500s.
Rx	**Estrace** (Warner Chilcott)		Lactose. (755 MJ). Lavender, scored. In 100s, 500s.
Rx	**Gynodiol** (Novavax Inc.)		Lactose. (1259). Rose, scored. In 30s and 100s.
Rx	**Gynodiol** (Novavax Inc.)	**Tablets:** 1.5 mg micronized estradiol	Lactose. (0158). Aqua, scored. In 30s and 100s.
Rx	**Femtrace** (Warner Chilcott)	**Tablets:** 1.8 mg estradiol acetate	Lactose. (WC 391). Yellow. In 100s.
Rx	**Estradiol** (Various, eg, Geneva, Mylan)	**Tablets:** 2 mg micronized estradiol	May contain lactose. In 100s and 500s.
Rx	**Estrace** (Warner Chilcott)		Lactose, tartrazine. (756 MJ). Turquoise, scored. In 100s and 500s.
Rx	**Gynodiol** (Novavax Inc.)		Lactose. (0748). Blue, scored. In 30s and 100s.

ESTRADIOL — ORAL

For complete and comparative prescribing information, refer to the Estrogens group monograph.

WARNING

Endometrial cancer – Estrogens increase the risk of endometrial cancer. Close clinical surveillance of all women taking estrogens is important. Undertake adequate diagnostic measures, including endometrial sampling when indicated, to rule out malignancy in all cases of undiagnosed persistent or recurring abnormal vaginal bleeding.

Cardiovascular and other risks – Do not use estrogens with or without progestins for the prevention of cardiovascular disease.

The Women's Health Initiative (WHI) study reported increased risks of myocardial infarction (MI), stroke, invasive breast cancer, pulmonary emboli, and deep vein thrombosis (DVT) in postmenopausal women (50 to 79 years of age) during 5 years of treatment with oral conjugated estrogens 0.625 mg combined with medroxyprogesterone acetate 2.5 mg relative to placebo.

The Women's Health Initiative Memory Study (WHIMS), a substudy of WHI, reported increased risk of developing probable dementia in postmenopausal women 65 years of age or older during 4 years of treatment with oral conjugated estrogens combined with medroxyprogesterone acetate relative to placebo.

Because of these risks, prescribe estrogens with or without progestins at the lowest effective doses and for the shortest duration consistent with treatment goals and risks for the individual woman.

Indications

➤*Breast cancer (except Femtrace)*: For palliation only in appropriately selected women and men with metastatic disease.

➤*Hypoestrogenism caused by hypogonadism, castration, or primary ovarian failure (except Femtrace)*: Treatment of hypoestrogenism caused by hypogonadism, castration, or primary ovarian failure.

➤*Moderate to severe vasomotor symptoms:* Treatment of moderate to severe vasomotor symptoms associated with menopause.

➤*Osteoporosis prevention (except Femtrace)*: For the prevention of osteoporosis.

➤*Prostate cancer (except Femtrace)*: For palliation only in advanced androgen-dependent prostate carcinoma.

➤*Vulval and vaginal atrophy (except Femtrace)*: Treatment of vulval and vaginal atrophy associated with menopause.

➤*Off-label uses:*

Alzheimer disease – [5] = Poor documentation. Prospective, controlled studies have failed to confirm a beneficial effect of estrogen therapy in the progression of Alzheimer disease, and there is some evidence of potential harm. Because of the serious risks associated with estrogen administration and lack of clear benefit, estrogen cannot be recommended for the treatment of the cognitive symptoms of Alzheimer disease.

Administration and Dosage

➤*Adults:*

Breast cancer – 10 mg 3 times daily for at least 3 months. For palliation only.

Hypoestrogenism caused by hypogonadism, castration, or primary ovarian failure –

Initial dosage: 1 to 2 mg daily. Determine the minimal effective dose by titration.

Dosage adjustment: Adjust dose as necessary to control presenting symptoms.

Osteoporosis prevention –

Usual dosage: Administer 0.5 mg/day cyclically (eg, 23 days on and 5 days off) as soon as possible after menopause. Adjust dosage if necessary to control concurrent menopausal symptoms. Discontinuation may re-establish natural rate of bone loss.

Concomitant therapy: Calcium, exercise, and nutrition are also important in preventing and managing osteoporosis.

Prostate cancer – 1 to 2 mg 3 times daily. For palliation only. Judge the efficacy of therapy by phosphatase determinations and symptomatic improvement of the patient.

Vasomotor symptoms associated with menopause –

Initial dosage: Initiate treatment at the lowest dose. Titrate to determine the minimal effective dose.

- *Estradiol acetate* – Administer once daily.
- *Micronized estradiol* – Administer cyclically (eg, 3 weeks on and 1 week off).

Duration of therapy: Use the lowest dose and for the shortest duration consistent with treatment goals and risks for the individual woman. Periodically reevaluate patients as clinically appropriate (eg, 3- to 6-month intervals) to determine if treatment is still necessary. Attempt to discontinue or taper medication at 3- to 6-month intervals.

Vulval and vaginal atrophy associated with menopause –

Initial dosage: Initiate treatment at the lowest dose. Titrate to determine the minimal effective dose.

- *Estradiol acetate* – Administer once daily.
- *Micronized estradiol* – Administer cyclically (eg, 3 weeks on and 1 week off).

Duration of therapy: Use the lowest dose and for the shortest duration consistent with treatment goals and risks for the individual woman. Periodically reevaluate patients as clinically appropriate (eg, 3- to 6-month intervals) to determine if treatment is still necessary. Attempt to discontinue or taper medication at 3- to 6-month intervals.

Off-label dosing –

➤*Concomitant progestin therapy:* When estrogen is prescribed for a postmenopausal woman with a uterus, also initiate progestin to reduce the risk of endometrial cancer. A woman without a uterus does not need progestin.

➤*Storage/Stability:* Store at controlled room temperature, 15° to 30°C (59° to 86°F). Dispense in a tight, light-resistant container.

ESTRADIOL VALERATE

Rx	**Estradiol Valerate** (Sandoz)	**Injection:** 10 mg per mL	In 5 mL multidose vials.[a]
Rx	**Delestrogen** (JHP)		In 5 mL multidose vials.[a]
Rx	**Estradiol Valerate** (Sandoz)	**Injection:** 20 mg per mL	In 5 mL multidose vials.[b]
Rx	**Delestrogen** (JHP)		In 5 mL multidose vials.[b]
Rx	**Estradiol Valerate** (Sandoz)	**Injection:** 40 mg per mL	In 5 mL multidose vials.[b]
Rx	**Delestrogen** (JHP)		In 5 mL multidose vials.[b]

[a] In sesame oil with chlorobutanol.

[b] In castor oil with benzyl benzoate and benzyl alcohol.

ESTRADIOL VALERATE — INJECTION

For complete and comparative prescribing information, refer to the Estrogens group monograph.

WARNING

Estrogens increase the risk of endometrial cancer – Close clinical surveillance of all women taking estrogens is important. Adequate diagnostic measures, including endometrial sampling when indicated, should be undertaken to rule out malignancy in all cases of undiagnosed persistent or recurrent abnormal vaginal bleeding. There is no evidence that "natural" estrogens results in a different endometrial risk profile than synthetic estrogens at equivalent estrogen doses.

Cardiovascular and other risks – Estrogens with and without progestins should not be used for the prevention of cardiovascular disease.

The Women's Health Initiative (WHI) study reported increased risks of myocardial infarction, stroke, invasive breast cancer, pulmonary emboli, and deep vein thrombosis in postmenopausal women during 5 years of treatment with conjugated equine estrogens (CE 0.625 mg) combined with medroxyprogesterone acetate (MPA 2.5 mg) relative to placebo. Other doses of conjugated estrogens with medroxyprogesterone, and other combinations of estrogens and progestins were not studied in the WHI and, in the absence of comparable data, these risks should be assumed to be similar. Because of these risks, estrogens with or without progestins should be prescribed at the lowest effective doses and for the shortest duration consistent with treatment goals and risks for the individual woman.

Indications

➤*Menopause/Hypoestrogenism/Prostate cancer:* Estradiol valerate injection is indicated for the treatment of the following: moderate to severe vasomotor symptoms associated with menopause; hypoestrogenism caused by hypogonadism, castration, or primary ovarian failure; advanced androgen-dependent carcinoma of the prostate (for palliation only); vulval and vaginal atrophy associated with the menopause. When prescribing solely for the treatment of vulvar and vaginal atrophy, topical vaginal products should be considered.

Administration and Dosage

➤*General dosing considerations:* Patients should be started at the lowest effective dose for the indication.

For women who have a uterus, adequate diagnostic measures, such as endometrial sampling, when indicated, should be undertaken to rule out malignancy in cases of undiagnosed persistent or recurring abnormal vaginal bleeding.

➤*Adults:*

Advanced androgen-dependent carcinoma of the prostate – 30 mg or more administered IM every 1 or 2 weeks. For palliation only.

Hypoestrogenism caused by hypogonadism, castration, or primary ovarian failure – 10 to 20 mg IM every 4 weeks.

Vasomotor symptoms associated with menopause – 10 to 20 mg IM every 4 weeks.

Vulval and vaginal atrophy associated with menopause – 10 to 20 mg IM every 4 weeks.

➤*Concomitant progestin therapy:* When estrogen is prescribed for a postmenopausal woman with a uterus, progestin should also be initiated to reduce the risk of endometrial cancer. A woman without a uterus does not need progestin.

➤*Duration of therapy:* Use of estrogen, alone or in combination with a progestin, should be limited to the shortest duration consistent with treatment goals and risks for the individual woman, and medication should be discontinued as promptly as possible. Patients should be reevaluated periodically as clinically appropriate (eg, 3- to 6-month intervals) to determine if treatment is still necessary, and attempts to discontinue or taper medication should be made.

➤*Preparation for administration:* Storage at low temperatures may result in the separation of some crystalline material that redissolves readily on warming. A dry needle and syringe should be used. Use of a wet needle or syringe may cause the solution to become cloudy; however, this does not affect the potency of the material. By virtue of the low viscosity of the vehicles, the various preparations of estradiol may be administered with a small gauge needle.

➤*Administration:* Care should be taken to inject deeply into the upper, outer quadrant of the gluteal muscle following the usual precautions for IM administration. Because the 40 mg potency provides a high concentration in a small volume, particular care should be taken to administer the full dose.

➤*Storage/Stability:* Store at room temperature.

CONJUGATED ESTROGENS

Tablets and injection contain a mixture of conjugated equine estrogens obtained exclusively from natural sources that include sodium estrone sulfate, sodium equilin sulfate, sodium sulfate conjugates, 17α-dihydroequilin, 17α-estradiol, and 17β-dihydroequilin.

Rx	**Premarin** (Wyeth)	**Tablets; oral:** 0.3 mg	Lactose, sucrose. Green, oval. In 100s and 1,000s.
		0.45 mg	Lactose, sucrose. Blue, oval. In 100s.
		0.625 mg	Lactose, sucrose. Maroon, oval. In 100s and 1,000s.
		0.9 mg	Lactose, sucrose. White, oval. In 100s.
		1.25 mg	Lactose, sucrose. Yellow, oval. In 100s and 1,000s.
Rx	**Premarin Intravenous** (Wyeth)	**Injection, lyophilized cake for solution:** 25 mg	In *Secules* vials,[a] each with 5 mL of sterile diluent.

[a] With lactose 200 mg, simethicone 0.2 mg, and sodium citrate 12.2 mg.

CONJUGATED ESTROGENS — ORAL

For complete and comparative prescribing information, refer to the Estrogens group monograph.

WARNING

Endometrial cancer – Adequate diagnostic measures, including endometrial sampling when indicated, should be undertaken to rule out malignancy in all cases of undiagnosed persistent or recurring abnormal vaginal bleeding.

Cardiovascular and other risks – Estrogens with or without progestins should not be used for the prevention of cardiovascular disease or dementia.

The estrogen-alone substudy of the Women's Health Initiative (WHI) reported increased risks of stroke and deep vein thrombosis (DVT) in postmenopausal women 50 to 79 years of age during 6.8 and 7.1 years, respectively, of treatment with daily oral conjugated estrogens 0.625 mg, relative to placebo.

The estrogen-plus-progestin substudy of WHI reported increased risks of myocardial infarction (MI), stroke, invasive breast cancer, pulmonary embolism (PE), and DVT in postmenopausal women 50 to 79 years of age during 5.6 years of treatment with daily conjugated estrogen 0.625 mg combined with medroxyprogesterone 2.5 mg, relative to placebo.

The WHI Memory Study (WHIMS), a substudy of WHI, reported an increased risk of developing probable dementia in postmenopausal women 65 years of age or older during 5.2 years of treatment with daily conjugated estrogens 0.625 mg alone and during 4 years of treatment with daily conjugated estrogens 0.625 mg combined with medroxyprogesterone 2.5 mg relative to placebo. It is unknown whether this finding applies to younger postmenopausal women.

In the absence of comparable data, these risks should be assumed to be similar for other doses of conjugated estrogens and medroxyprogesterone, and other combinations and dosage forms of estrogens and progestins. Because of these risks, estrogens with or without progestins should be prescribed at the lowest effective doses and for the shortest duration consistent with treatment goals and risks for the individual woman.

Indications

➤*Breast cancer:* For the treatment of breast cancer (for palliation only) in appropriately selected women and men with metastatic disease.

➤*Hypoestrogenism:* For the treatment of hypoestrogenism caused by hypogonadism, castration, or primary ovarian failure.

➤*Osteoporosis:* For the prevention of postmenopausal osteoporosis (loss of bone mass). When prescribing solely for the prevention of postmenopausal osteoporosis, therapy should only be considered for women at significant risk of osteoporosis and for whom non-estrogen medications are not considered to be appropriate.

➤*Prostate cancer:* For the treatment of advanced androgen-dependent prostatic carcinoma (for palliation only).

➤*Vasomotor symptoms:* For the treatment of moderate to severe vasomotor symptoms associated with menopause.

➤*Vulvular/Vaginal atrophy:* For the treatment of moderate to severe symptoms of vulvar and vaginal atrophy associated with menopause. When prescribing solely for the treatment of symptoms of vulvar and vaginal atrophy, topical vaginal products should be considered.

➤*Off-label uses:*

Alzheimer disease – [5] = Poor documentation. Prospective, controlled studies have failed to confirm a beneficial effect of estrogen therapy in the progression of Alzheimer disease, and there is some evidence of potential harm. Because of the serious risks associated with estrogen administration and lack of clear benefit, estrogen cannot be recommended for the treatment of the cognitive symptoms of Alzheimer disease.

Traumatic brain injury – [4] = Insufficient documentation. The Neurobehavioral Guidelines Working Group authors concluded that more supporting evidence was needed before estrogen could be recommended as a therapeutic option for aggression after traumatic brain injury.

Administration and Dosage

➤*General dosing considerations:* For women with a uterus, adequate diagnostic measures, such as endometrial sampling, when indicated, should be undertaken to rule out malignancy in cases of undiagnosed persistent or recurring abnormal vaginal bleeding.

When prescribing solely for the prevention of postmenopausal osteoporosis, therapy should be considered only for women at significant risk of osteoporosis and for whom non-estrogen medications are not considered to be appropriate.

➤*Adults:*

Breast cancer – 10 mg 3 times daily for at least 3 months. For palliation only.

Female hypoestrogenism –

Female hypogonadism: 0.3 to 0.625 mg daily, administered cyclically (eg, 3 weeks on and 1 week off). Doses are adjusted depending on the severity of symptoms and responsiveness of the endometrium.

In clinical studies of delayed puberty due to female hypogonadism, breast development was induced by doses as low as 0.15 mg. The dosage may be gradually titrated upward at 6- to 12-month intervals as needed to achieve appropriate bone age advancement and eventual epiphyseal closure. Clinical studies suggest that doses of 0.15, 0.3, and 0.6 mg are associated with mean ratios of bone age advancement to chronological age progression of 1.1, 1.5, and 2.1, respectively. Available data suggest that chronic dosing with 0.625 mg is sufficient to induce artificial cyclic menses with sequential progestin treatment and to maintain bone mineral density (BMD) after skeletal maturity is achieved.

Female castration or primary ovarian failure: 1.25 mg/day cyclically. Adjust dosage according to severity of symptoms and patient response. For maintenance, adjust to lowest effective level.

Osteoporosis prevention –

Initial dosage: Patients should be treated with the lowest effective dose. Generally, women should be started at 0.3 mg daily. Therapy may be given continuously with no interruption in therapy, or in cyclical regimens (eg, 25 days on drug followed by 5 days off drug), as is medically appropriate on an individualized basis.

Dosage adjustment: Subsequent dosage adjustment may be made based on the individual clinical and BMD responses. This dose should be periodically reassessed by the health care provider.

Prostate cancer – 1.25 to 2.5 mg 3 times daily. For palliation only. Effectiveness of therapy can be judged by phosphatase determinations as well as by symptomatic improvement.

Vasomotor symptoms and/or vulvar/vaginal atrophy associated with menopause –

Initial dosage: Patients should be treated with the lowest effective dose. Generally, women should be started on 0.3 mg/day. Therapy may be given continuously with no interruption, or in cyclical regimens (eg, 25 days on drug followed by 5 days off drug), as is medically appropriate on an individualized basis.

Dosage adjustment: Subsequent dosage adjustments may be made based on individual patient response. This dose should be periodically reassessed by the health care provider.

Off-label dosing –

Traumatic brain injury: [4] = Insufficient documentation. 0.625 mg/day of estrogen initially, increased to 1.25 mg/day. The form of estrogen was not provided in the case report. The duration of therapy has not been reported. Long-term administration may be required, however, to maintain symptom control.

➤*Concomitant progestin therapy:* When estrogen is prescribed for a postmenopausal woman with a uterus, also initiate progestin to reduce the risk of endometrial cancer. A woman without a uterus does not need progestin.

➤*Duration of therapy:* Limit the use of estrogen, alone or in combination with a progestin, to the lowest effective dose and shortest duration consistent with treatment goals and risks for the individual woman. Periodically re-evaluate patients as clinically appropriate (eg, at 3- to 6-month intervals) to determine if treatment is still necessary.

➤*Administration:* Conjugated estrogens can be taken without regard to meals.

➤*Storage/Stability:* Store at room temperature (20° to 25°C; 68° to 77°F); excursions are permitted between 15° and 30°C (59° and 86°F). Dispense in a well-closed container.

CONJUGATED ESTROGENS — INJECTION

For complete and comparative prescribing information, refer to the Estrogens group monograph.

WARNING

Endometrial cancer – Adequate diagnostic measures, including endometrial sampling when indicated, should be undertaken to rule out malignancy in all cases of undiagnosed persistent or recurring abnormal vaginal bleeding.

Cardiovascular and other risks – Estrogens with or without progestin should not be used for prevention of cardiovascular disease or dementia.

The estrogen-alone substudy of the Women's Health Initiative (WHI) reported increased risks of stroke and deep vein thrombosis (DVT) in postmenopausal women 50 to 79 years of age during 6.8 and 7.1 years, respectively, of treatment with daily oral conjugated estrogens 0.625 mg, relative to placebo.

The estrogen-plus-progestin substudy of WHI reported increased risks of myocardial infarction (MI), stroke, invasive breast cancer, pulmonary embolism (PE), and DVT in postmenopausal women 50 to 79 years of age during 5.6 years of treatment with daily conjugated estrogens 0.625 mg combined with medroxyprogesterone 2.5 mg, relative to placebo.

The WHI Memory Study (WHIMS), a substudy of WHI, reported an increased risk of developing probable dementia in postmenopausal women 65 years of age and older during 5.2 years of treatment with daily conjugated estrogens 0.625 mg alone, and during 4 years of treatment with conjugated estrogens 0.625 mg combined with medroxyprogesterone 2.5 mg, relative to placebo. It is unknown whether this finding applies to younger postmenopausal women.

In the absence of comparable data, these risks should be assumed to be similar for other doses of conjugated estrogens and medroxyprogesterone, and other combinations and dosage forms of estrogens and progestin. Because of these risks, estrogens with or without progestin should be prescribed at the lowest effective doses and for the shortest duration consistent with treatment goals and risks for the individual woman.

Indications

➤*Uterine bleeding:* For the treatment of abnormal uterine bleeding caused by hormonal imbalance in the absence of organic pathology. Conjugated estrogens intravenous (IV) is for short-term use only to provide a rapid and temporary increase in estrogen levels.

Administration and Dosage

➤*Adults:*

Uterine bleeding – One 25 mg injection, IV or intramuscularly (IM). IV use is preferred because more rapid response can be expected from this mode of administration. Repeat in 6 to 12 hours if necessary. The use of conjugated estrogens does not preclude the advisability of other appropriate measures.

➤*Preparation for administration:* Reconstitute with 5 mL of sterile water for injection. Introduce the diluent slowly against the side of the *Secule* vial and agitate gently. Do not shake violently. Use immediately after reconstitution.

➤*Administration:* For IV or IM injection. The usual precautionary measures governing IV administration should be adhered to. Injection should be made slowly to obviate the occurrence of flushes.

➤*Admixture compatibility:* Infusion of conjugated estrogens with other agents is not generally recommended. In emergencies, however, when an infusion has already been started, it may be expedient to make the injection into the tubing just distal to the infusion needle. If so used, compatibility of solutions must be considered.

Compatibility – Conjugated estrogens is compatible with isotonic sodium chloride solution, dextrose, and invert sugar solutions.

Incompatibility – It is not compatible with protein hydrolysate, ascorbic acid, or any solution with an acid pH.

➤*Storage/Stability:* Store in the refrigerator, between 2° and 8°C (36° and 46°F).

ESTERIFIED ESTROGENS

These products contain 75% to 85% sodium estrone sulfate and 6% to 15% sodium equilin sulfate, in such proportion that the total of these 2 components is not less than 90% of the total esterified estrogens content.

Rx	**Menest** (Monarch)	**Tablets:** 0.3 mg	Lactose. (M72). Yellow, oblong. Film-coated. In 100s.
		0.625 mg	Lactose. (M73). Orange, oblong. Film-coated. In 100s.
		1.25 mg	Lactose. (M74). Green, oblong. Film-coated. In 100s.
		2.5 mg	Lactose. (M75). Pink, oblong. Film-coated. In 50s.

ESTERIFIED ESTROGENS — ORAL

For complete prescribing information, refer to the Estrogens group monograph.

WARNING

Estrogens have been reported to increase the risk of endometrial carcinoma – Three independent case control studies have shown an increased risk of endometrial cancer in postmenopausal women exposed to exogenous estrogens for prolonged periods. This risk was independent of the other known risk factors for endometrial cancer. These studies are further supported by the finding that incidence rates of endometrial cancer have increased sharply since 1969 in 8 different areas of the United States with population-based cancer reporting systems, an increase which may be related to the rapidly expanding use of estrogens during the last decade.

The 3 case control studies reported that the risk of endometrial cancer in estrogen users was about 4.5 to 13.9 times higher than in nonusers. The risk appears to depend on both duration of treatment and on estrogen dose. In view of these findings, when estrogens are used for the treatment of menopausal symptoms, the lowest dose that will control symptoms should be utilized and medication should be discontinued as soon as possible. When prolonged treatment is medically indicated, the patient should be reassessed on at least a semiannual basis to determine the need for continued therapy. Although the evidence must be considered preliminary, 1 study suggests that cyclic administration of low doses of estrogen may carry less risk than continuous administration; it therefore appears prudent to utilize such a regimen.

Close clinical surveillance of all women taking estrogens is important. In all cases of undiagnosed persistent or recurring abnormal vaginal bleeding, adequate diagnostic measures should be undertaken to rule out malignancy.

There is no evidence at present that "natural" estrogens are more or less hazardous than "synthetic" estrogens at equiestrogenic doses.

WARNING (cont.)

Estrogens should not be used during pregnancy – The use of female sex hormones, both estrogens and progestagens, during early pregnancy may seriously damage the offspring. It has been shown that females exposed in utero to diethylstilbestrol, a nonsteroidal estrogen, have an increased risk of developing in later life a form of vaginal or cervical cancer that is ordinarily extremely rare. The risk has been estimated as not more than 4/1,000 exposures. Furthermore, a high percentage of such exposed women (from 30% to 90%) have been found to have vaginal adenosis, epithelial changes of the vagina and cervix. Although these changes are histologically benign, it is not known whether they are precursors of malignancy. Although similar data are not available with the use of other estrogens, it cannot be presumed they would not induce similar changes. Several reports suggest an association between intrauterine exposure to female sex hormones and congenital anomalies, including congenital heart defects and limb reduction defects. One case control study estimated a 4.7-fold increased risk of limb reduction defects in infants exposed in utero to sex hormones (oral contraceptives, hormone withdrawal tests for pregnancy, or attempted treatment for threatened abortion). Some of these exposures were very short and involved only a few days of treatment. The data suggest that the risk of limb reduction defects in exposed fetuses is somewhat less than 1/1,000. In the past, female sex hormones have been used during pregnancy in an attempt to treat threatened or habitual abortion. There is considerable evidence that estrogens are ineffective for these indications, and there is no evidence from well-controlled studies that progestagens are effective for these uses. If esterified estrogens tablets are used during pregnancy, or if the patient becomes pregnant while taking this drug, she should be apprised of the potential risks to the fetus, and the advisability of pregnancy continuation.

Indications

➤*Menopause:* For the treatment of moderate to severe vasomotor symptoms associated with menopause. (There is no evidence that estrogens are effective for nervous symptoms or depression which might occur during menopause, and they should not be used to treat these conditions.)

➤*Atrophic vaginitis:* For the treatment of atrophic vaginitis.

➤*Kraurosis vulvae:* For the treatment of kraurosis vulvae.

➤*Female hypogonadism:* For the treatment of female hypogonadism.

ESTERIFIED ESTROGENS — ORAL

➤*Female castration:* For the treatment of female castration.

➤*Primary ovarian failure:* For the treatment of primary ovarian failure.

➤*Breast cancer:* For palliation in appropriately selected women and men with metastatic breast cancer only.

➤*Prostatic carcinoma:* For palliative therapy of advanced prostatic carcinoma only.

➤*General information:* Esterified estrogens tablets have not been shown to be effective for any purpose during pregnancy and its use may cause severe harm to the fetus (see Warning Box).

➤*Off-label uses:*

Traumatic brain injury – [4] = Insufficient documentation. The Neurobehavioral Guidelines Working Group authors concluded that more supporting evidence was needed before estrogen could be recommended as a therapeutic option for aggression after traumatic brain injury.

Administration and Dosage

➤*General dosing considerations:* When estrogen is prescribed for a postmenopausal woman with a uterus, a progestin should also be initiated to reduce the risk of endometrial cancer. A woman without a uterus does not need progestin.

Use of estrogen, alone or in combination with a progestin, should be with the lowest effective dose and for the shortest duration consistent with treatment goals and risks. Patients should be started at the lowest dose.

Patients should be reevaluated periodically as clinically appropriate (eg, 3- to 6-month intervals) to determine if treatment is still necessary.

For women who have a uterus, adequate diagnostic measures, such as endometrial sampling, when indicated, should be undertaken to rule out malignancy in cases of undiagnosed persistent or recurring abnormal vaginal bleeding.

➤*Adults:*

Female castration –
Usual dosage: 1.25 mg daily, cyclically.
Dosage adjustment: Adjust dosage upward or downward according to severity of symptoms and response of the patient.

Female hypogonadism –
Usual dosage: 2.5 to 7.5 mg daily, in divided doses for 20 days, followed by a rest period of 10 days' duration. If bleeding does not occur by the end of this period, the same dosage schedule is repeated.

The number of courses of estrogen therapy necessary to produce bleeding may vary depending on responsiveness of the endometrium.

Dosage adjustment: If bleeding occurs before the end of the 10-day period, begin a 20-day estrogen-progestin cyclic regimen with esterified estrogens tablets, 2.5 to 7.5 mg daily in divided doses, for 20 days. During the last 5 days of estrogen therapy, give an oral progestin. If bleeding occurs before this regimen is concluded, therapy is discontinued and may be resumed on the fifth day of bleeding.

Inoperable progressing metastatic breast cancer – 10 mg 3 times daily for a period of at least 3 months.

Inoperable progressing prostatic cancer – 1.25 to 2.5 mg 3 times daily. The effectiveness of therapy can be judged by phosphatase determinations as well as by symptomatic improvement of the patient.

Moderate to severe menopausal vasomotor symptoms –
Usual dosage: 1.25 mg daily. Administration should be cyclic (eg, 3 weeks on and 1 week off).
Initial dosage: If the patient has not menstruated within the last 2 months or more, cyclic administration is started arbitrarily. If the patient is menstruating, cyclic administration is started on day 5 of bleeding.
Discontinuation of therapy: Attempts to discontinue or taper medication should be made at 3- to 6-month intervals.

Moderate to severe menopausal vulvar and vaginal atrophy –
Usual dosage: 0.3 to 1.25 mg or more daily, depending upon the tissue response of the individual patient. Administration should be cyclic (eg, 3 weeks on and 1 week off).
Discontinuation of therapy: Attempts to discontinue or taper medication should be made at 3- to 6-month intervals.

Primary ovarian failure – See Female castration.

Off-label dosing –
Traumatic brain injury: [4] = Insufficient documentation. 0.625 mg/day of estrogen initially, increased to 1.25 mg/day. The form of estrogen was not provided in the case report. The duration of therapy has not been reported. However, long-term administration may be required to maintain symptom control.

➤*Duration of therapy:*

Given cyclically for short term use only – Moderate to severe vasomotor symptoms; moderate to severe symptoms of vulvar and vaginal atrophy.

Given cyclically – Female hypogonadism; female castration; primary ovarian failure.

Given chronically (palliative care) – Inoperable progressing prostatic cancer; inoperable progressing breast cancer.

➤*Storage/Stability:* No storage info provided.

ESTROPIPATE (Piperazine Estrone Sulfate)

Estropipate is a natural substance prepared from crystalline estrone solubilized as the sulfate and stabilized with piperazine.

Rx	**Estropipate** (Various, eg, Mylan, Watson)	**Tablets:** 0.625 mg sodium estrone sulfate (equiv. to 0.75 mg estropipate)	In 30s, 100s, and 500s.
Rx	**Estropipate** (Various, eg, Mylan, Watson)	**Tablets:** 1.25 mg sodium estrone sulfate (equiv. to 1.5 mg estropipate)	In 30s, 100s, and 500s.
Rx	**Estropipate** (Various, eg, Watson)	**Tablets:** 2.5 mg sodium estrone sulfate (equiv. to 3 mg estropipate)	In 30s, 100s, and 500s.
Rx	**Ogen** (Pharmacia)		Lactose. (U 3774). Blue, scored. In 100s.
Rx	**Estropipate** (Various, eg, Watson)	**Tablets:** 5 mg sodium estrone sulfate (equiv. to 6 mg estropipate)	In 30s, 100s, and 500s.

ESTROPIPATE — ORAL

For complete prescribing information, refer to the Estrogens group monograph.

WARNING

Estrogens have been reported to increase the risk of endometrial carcinoma in postmenopausal women – Close clinical surveillance of all women taking estrogens is important. Adequate diagnostic measures, including endometrial sampling when indicated, should be undertaken to rule out malignancy in all cases of undiagnosed persistent or recurring abnormal vaginal bleeding. There is no evidence that "natural" estrogens are more or less hazardous than "synthetic" estrogens at equiestrogenic doses.

Estrogens should not be use during pregnancy – There is no indication for estrogen therapy during pregnancy or during the immediate postpartum period. Estrogens are ineffective for the prevention or treatment of threatened or habitual abortion. Estrogens are not indicated for the prevention of postpartum breast engorgement.

Estrogen therapy during pregnancy is associated with an increased risk of congenital defects in the reproductive organs of the fetus, and possibly other birth defects. Studies of women who received diethylstilbestrol (DES) during pregnancy have shown that female offspring have an increased risk of vaginal adenosis, squamous cell dysplasia of the uterine cervix, and clear cell vaginal cancer later in life; male offspring have an increased risk of urogenital abnormalities and possibly testicular cancer later in life. The 1985 DES Task Force concluded that use of DES during pregnancy is associated with a subsequent increased risk of breast cancer in the mothers, although a causal relationship remains unproven and the observed level of excess risk is similar to that for a number of other breast cancer risk factors.

Indications

➤*Menopause/Hypoestrogenism/Osteoporosis prevention:* Treatment of moderate to severe vasomotor symptoms associated with menopause; treatment of vulval and vaginal atrophy; treatment of hypoestrogenism due to hypogonadism, castration or primary ovarian failure; prevention of osteoporosis.

➤*General information:* Because estrogen administration is associated with risk, selection of patients should ideally be based on prospective identification of risk factors for developing osteoporosis. Unfortunately, there is no certain way to identify those women who will develop osteoporotic fractures. Most prospective studies of efficacy for this indication have been carried out in white menopausal women, without stratification by other risk factors, and tend to show a universally salutary effect on bone. Thus, patient selection must be individualized based on the balance of risks and benefits. A more favorable risk/benefit ratio exists in a hysterectomized woman because she has no risk of endometrial cancer (see Warning Box).

➤*Off-label uses:*

Traumatic brain injury – [4] = Insufficient documentation. The Neurobehavioral Guidelines Working Group authors concluded that more supporting evidence was needed before estrogen could be recommended as a therapeutic option for aggression after traumatic brain injury.

Administration and Dosage

➤*General dosing considerations:* For treatment of moderate to severe vasomotor symptoms and vulval and vaginal atrophy associated with menopause, the lowest dose and regimen that will control symptoms should be chosen and medication should be discontinued as promptly as possible.

ESTROPIPATE — ORAL

For female hypoestrogenism, the lowest dose that will control symptoms should be chosen.

➤*Adults:*

Female hypoestrogenism caused by castration –

Usual dosage: 1.5 to 9 mg/day may be given for the first 3 weeks of a theoretical cycle, followed by a rest period of 8 to 10 days.

Dosage adjustment: Adjust dosage upward or downward according to severity of symptoms and response of the patient.

Female hypoestrogenism caused by hypogonadism –

Usual dosage: 1.5 to 9 mg/day may be given for the first 3 weeks of a theoretical cycle, followed by a rest period of 8 to 10 days. If bleeding does not occur by the end of this period, the same dosage schedule is repeated.

Duration of therapy: The number of courses of estrogen therapy necessary to produce bleeding may vary depending on the responsiveness of the endometrium.

Concomitant therapy: If satisfactory withdrawal bleeding does not occur, an oral progestogen may be given in addition to estrogen during the third week of the cycle.

Female hypoestrogenism caused by primary ovarian failure – See Female Hypoestrogenism Caused by Castration for dosing.

Moderate to severe vasomotor symptoms –

Usual dosage: 0.75 mg to 6 mg/day.

Dosage adjustment: If the patient has not menstruated within the last 2 months or more, cyclic administration is started arbitrarily. If the patient is menstruating, cyclic administration is started on day 5 of bleeding.

Discontinuation of therapy: Medication should be discontinued as promptly as possible. Attempts to discontinue or taper medication should be made at 3- to 6-month intervals.

Prevention of osteoporosis – 0.75 mg/day for 25 days of a 31-day cycle per month.

Vulval and vaginal atrophy –

Usual dosage: 0.75 mg to 6 mg/day, depending upon the tissue response of the individual patient. Administer cyclically.

Discontinuation of therapy: Medication should be discontinued as promptly as possible. Attempts to discontinue or taper medication should be made at 3- to 6-month intervals.

Off-label dosing –

Traumatic brain injury: [4] = Insufficient documentation. 0.625 mg/day of estrogen initially, increased to 1.25 mg/day. The form of estrogen was not provided in the case report. The duration of therapy has not been reported. Long-term administration may be required, however, to maintain symptom control.

➤*Monitoring:* Treated patients with an intact uterus should be monitored closely for signs of endometrial cancer and appropriate diagnostic measures should be taken to rule out malignancy in the event of persistent or recurring abnormal vaginal bleeding.

➤*Storage/Stability:* Store at 15° to 30°C (59° to 86°F).

SYNTHETIC CONJUGATED ESTROGENS, A

Rx	**Cenestin** (Barr/Duramed)	**Tablets:** 0.3 mg	Lactose. (dp 41). Green. Film-coated. In 30s, 100s, and 1,000s.
		0.45 mg	Lactose. (dp 46). Orange. Film-coated. In 30s, 100s, and 1,000s.
		0.625 mg	Lactose. (dp 42). Red. Film-coated. In 30s, 100s, and 1,000s.
		0.9 mg	Lactose. (dp 43). White. Film-coated. In 30s, 100s, and 1,000s.
		1.25 mg	Lactose. (dp 44). Blue. Film-coated. In 30s, 100s, and 1,000s.

SYNTHETIC CONJUGATED ESTROGENS, A — ORAL

For complete prescribing information, refer to the Estrogens group monograph.

WARNING

Estrogens increase the risk of endometrial cancer – The use of unopposed estrogens in women with intact uteri has been associated with an increased risk of endometrial cancer. The reported endometrial cancer risk among unopposed estrogen users is about 2- to 12-fold higher than in nonusers, and appears dependent on duration of treatment and on estrogen dose. Most studies show no significant increased risk associated with use of estrogens for less than 1 year. The greatest risk appears associated with prolonged use, with increased risks of 15- to 24-fold for 5 to 10 years or more, and this risk has been shown to persist for at least 8 to 15 years after estrogen therapy is discontinued.

Clinical surveillance of all women taking estrogen/progestin combinations is important. Undertake adequate diagnostic measures, including endometrial sampling when indicated to rule out malignancy in all cases of undiagnosed persistent or recurring abnormal vaginal bleeding. There is no evidence that the use of natural estrogens results in a different endometrial risk profile than synthetic estrogens of equivalent estrogen dose. Adding a progestin to estrogen therapy has been shown to reduce the risk of endometrial hyperplasia, which may be a precursor to endometrial cancer.

Cardiovascular and other risks – Estrogens, with and without progestins, should not be used for the prevention of cardiovascular disease.

The Women's Health Initiative (WHI) study reported increased risks of myocardial infarction, stroke, invasive breast cancer, pulmonary emboli, and deep vein thrombosis in postmenopausal women (50 to 79 years of age) during 5 years of treatment with conjugated equine estrogens (CEE 0.625 mg) combined with medroxyprogesterone acetate (MPA 2.5 mg) relative to placebo. Other doses of conjugated estrogens with medroxyprogesterone, and other combinations of estrogens and progestins were not studied in the WHI and, in the absence of comparable data, these risks should be assumed to be similar. Because of these risks, prescribe estrogens, with or without progestins, in the lowest effective doses and for the shortest duration consistent with treatment goals and risks for the individual woman.

Indications

➤*Vasomotor symptoms:* This medication is indicated for the treatment of moderate to severe vasomotor symptoms associated with menopause (ie, 0.45 mg, 0.625 mg, 0.9 mg, 1.25 mg).

➤*Vulvar/Vaginal atrophy:* This medication is indicated for the treatment of moderate to severe symptoms of vulvar and vaginal atrophy associated with the menopause (ie, 0.3 mg). When prescribing solely for the treatment of symptoms of vulvar and vaginal atrophy, consider topical vaginal products.

➤*Off-label uses:*

Traumatic brain injury – [4] = Insufficient documentation. The Neurobehavioral Guidelines Working Group authors concluded that more supporting evidence was needed before estrogen could be recommended as a therapeutic option for aggression after traumatic brain injury.

Administration and Dosage

➤*General dosing considerations:* For women who have a uterus, undertake adequate diagnostic measures, such as endometrial sampling, when indicated, to rule out malignancy in cases of undiagnosed persistent or recurring abnormal vaginal bleeding.

When prescribing solely for the treatment of symptoms of vulvar and vaginal atrophy, consider topical vaginal products.

➤*Adults:*

Vasomotor symptoms – Start with 0.45 mg daily and titrate dose based on response.

Vulvar/Vaginal atrophy – 0.3 mg daily.

Off-label dosing –

Traumatic brain injury: [4] = Insufficient documentation. 0.625 mg/day of estrogen initially, increased to 1.25 mg/day. The form of estrogen was not provided in the case report. The duration of therapy has not been reported. Long-term administration may be required, however, to maintain symptom control.

➤*Concomitant progestin therapy:* When estrogen is prescribed for a postmenopausal woman with a uterus, also initiate progestin to reduce the risk of endometrial cancer. A woman without a uterus does not need progestin.

➤*Duration of therapy:* Limit use of estrogen, alone or in combination with a progestin, to the shortest duration consistent with treatment goals and risks for the individual woman. Periodically reevaluate patients as clinically appropriate (eg, 3- to 6-month intervals) to determine if treatment is still necessary.

➤*Administration:* Administer without regard to meals. Administer with food if GI upset occurs.

➤*Storage/Stability:* Store at 20° to 25°C (68° to 77°F); excursions are permitted to 15° to 30°C (59° to 86°F).

SYNTHETIC CONJUGATED ESTROGENS, B

Rx	Enjuvia (Barr/Duramed)	Tablets; oral[a]: 0.3 mg	EDTA, PEG, lactose. (E1). Oval. Film-coated. In 100s.
		0.45 mg	EDTA, PEG, lactose. (E2). Mauve, oval. Film-coated. In 100s.
		0.625 mg	EDTA, PEG, lactose. (E3). Pink, oval. Film-coated. In 100s.
		0.9 mg	EDTA, PEG, lactose. (E4). Light blue-green, oval. Film-coated. In 100s.
		1.25 mg	EDTA, PEG, lactose. (E4). Yellow, oval. Film-coated. In 100s.

[a] Tablets contain a blend of 10 synthetic estrogenic substances: sodium estrone sulfate, sodium equilin sulfate, sodium 17α-dihydroequilin sulfate, sodium 17α-estradiol sulfate, sodium 17β-dihydroequilin sulfate, sodium 17α-dihydroequilenin sulfate, sodium 17β-dihydroequilenin sulfate, sodium equilenin sulfate, sodium 17β-estradiol sulfate, and sodium $\Delta^{8,9}$-dehydroestrone sulfate.

SYNTHETIC CONJUGATED ESTROGENS, B — ORAL

For complete prescribing information, refer to the Estrogens group monograph.

WARNING

Estrogens increase the risk of endometrial cancer – Close clinical surveillance of all women taking estrogens is important. Adequate diagnostic measures, including endometrial sampling when indicated, should be undertaken to rule out malignancy in all cases of undiagnosed persistent or recurring abnormal vaginal bleeding. There is no evidence that the use of "natural" estrogens results in a different endometrial risk profile than synthetic estrogens at equivalent estrogen doses.

Cardiovascular and other risks – Estrogens with or without progestins should not be used for the prevention of cardiovascular disease or dementia.

The estrogen-alone substudy of the Women's Health Initiative (WHI) reported increased risks of stroke and deep vein thrombosis (DVT) in postmenopausal women (50 to 79 years of age) during 6.8 and 7.1 years, respectively, of treatment with oral conjugated estrogens (0.625 mg) alone per day, relative to placebo.

The estrogen-plus-progestin substudy of the WHI reported increased risks of myocardial infarction (MI), stroke, invasive breast cancer, pulmonary emboli, and DVT in postmenopausal women (50 to 79 years of age) during 5.6 years of treatment with oral conjugated estrogens (0.625 mg) combined with medroxyprogesterone acetate (2.5 mg) per day, relative to placebo.

The WHI Memory Study (WHIMS), a substudy of the WHI study, reported increased risk of developing probable dementia in postmenopausal women 65 years of age and older during 5.2 years of treatment with conjugated estrogen 0.625 mg alone and during 4 years of treatment with conjugated estrogen 0.625 mg combined with medroxyprogesterone acetate 2.5 mg, relative to placebo. It is unknown whether this finding applies to younger postmenopausal women.

Other doses of conjugated estrogens and medroxyprogesterone, and other combinations and dosage forms of estrogens and progestins, were not studied in the WHI clinical trials, and in the absence of comparable data, these risks should be assumed to be similar. Because of these risks, estrogens with or without progestins should be prescribed at the lowest effective doses and for the shortest duration consistent with treatment goals and risks for the individual woman.

Indications

➤*Vaginal dryness/vulvar and vaginal atrophy (0.3 mg only):* For the treatment of moderate to severe vaginal dryness and pain with intercourse and symptoms of vulvar and vaginal atrophy, associated with menopause.

➤*Vasomotor symptoms:* For the treatment of moderate to severe vasomotor symptoms associated with menopause.

➤*Off-label uses:*

Traumatic brain injury – [4] = Insufficient documentation. The Neurobehavioral Guidelines Working Group authors concluded that more supporting evidence was needed before estrogen could be recommended as a therapeutic option for aggression after traumatic brain injury.

Administration and Dosage

➤*General dosing considerations:* For women who have a uterus, undertake adequate diagnostic measures, such as endometrial sampling, when indicated, to rule out malignancy in cases of undiagnosed persistent or recurring abnormal vaginal bleeding.

When prescribing solely for the treatment of moderate to severe vaginal dryness and pain during intercourse, topical vaginal products should be considered.

➤*Adults:*

Vaginal dryness/vulvar and vaginal atrophy – 0.3 mg once daily.

Vasomotor symptoms – Start at 0.3 mg once daily. Subsequent dosage adjustment may be made based upon the individual patient response.

Off-label dosing –

Traumatic brain injury: [4] = Insufficient documentation. 0.625 mg/day of estrogen initially, increased to 1.25 mg/day. The form of estrogen was not provided in the case report. The duration of therapy has not been reported. Long-term administration may be required, however, to maintain symptom control.

➤*Concomitant progestin therapy:* When estrogen is prescribed for a postmenopausal woman with a uterus, initiate a progestin to reduce the risk of endometrial cancer. A woman without a uterus does not need a progestin.

➤*Duration of therapy:* Prescribe estrogen, alone or in combination with a progestin, at the lowest effective dose and for the shortest duration consistent with treatment goals and risks for the individual woman. Adjust dose by clinical response rather than by serum hormone levels (eg, estradiol, follicle-stimulating hormone [FSH]). Reevaluate patients periodically as clinically appropriate (eg, at 3- to 6-month intervals) to determine if treatment is still necessary.

➤*Administration:* Administer without regard to meals. Administer with food if GI upset occurs.

➤*Storage/Stability:* Store at 20° to 25°C (68° to 77°F).

ESTRADIOL CYPIONATE

Rx	Depo-Estradiol (Pfizer U.S.)	Injection: 5 mg /mL	In 5 mL vials.[a]

[a] In cottonseed oil with 5.4 mg chlorobutanol.

ESTRADIOL CYPIONATE — INJECTION

For complete prescribing information, refer to the Estrogens group monograph.

WARNING

Estrogens have been reported to increase the risk of endometrial carcinoma in postmenopausal women – Close clinical surveillance of all women taking estrogens is important. Adequate diagnostic measures including endometrial sampling when indicated, should be undertaken to rule out malignancy in all cases of undiagnosed persistent or recurring abnormal vaginal bleeding. There is currently no evidence that "natural" estrogens are more or less hazardous than "synthetic" estrogens at equi-estrogenic doses.

Estrogens should not be used during pregnancy – There is no indication for estrogen therapy during pregnancy or during the immediate postpartum period. Estrogens are ineffective for the prevention or treatment of threatened or habitual abortion. Estrogens are not indicated for the prevention of postpartum breast engorgement.

WARNING (cont.)

Estrogen therapy during pregnancy is associated with an increased risk of congenital defects in the reproductive organs of the fetus, and possibly other birth defects. Studies of women who received diethylstilbestrol (DES) during pregnancy have shown that female offspring have an increased risk of vaginal adenosis, squamous cell dysplasia of the uterine cervix, and clear cell vaginal cancer later in life; male offspring have an increased risk of urogenital abnormalities and possibly testicular cancer later in life. The 1985 DES Task force concluded that use of DES during pregnancy is associated with a subsequent increased risk of breast cancer in the mothers, although a causal relationship remains unproven and the observed level of excess risk is similar to that for a number of other breast cancer risk factors.

Indications

➤*Hypoestrogenism/Menopause:* Hypoestrogenism caused by hypogonadism; moderate to severe vasomotor symptoms associated with the menopause. (There is no evidence that estrogens are effective for nervous symptoms or depression that might occur during menopause, and they should not be used to treat these conditions.)

ESTRADIOL CYPIONATE — INJECTION

Administration and Dosage

➤*Adults:*

Hypoestrogenism caused by hypogonadism – 1.5 to 2 mg injected IM at monthly intervals.

Vasomotor symptoms associated with menopause –

Usual dosage: 1 to 5 mg injected IM every 3 to 4 weeks.

Duration of therapy: The lowest dose and regimen that will control symptoms should be chosen and medication should be discontinued as promptly as possible. Attempts to discontinue or taper medication should be made at 3- to 6-month intervals.

Vulval and vaginal atrophy associated with menopause –

Usual dosage: 1 to 5 mg injected IM every 3 to 4 weeks.

Duration of therapy: The lowest dose and regimen that will control symptoms should be chosen and medication should be discontinued as promptly as possible. Attempts to discontinue or taper medication should be made at 3- to 6-month intervals.

➤*Preparation for administration:* Warming and shaking the vial should redissolve any crystals that may have formed during storage at temperatures lower than recommended.

➤*Administration:* Administer IM only.

➤*Storage / Stability:* Store at 20° to 25°C (68° to 77°F).

ESTROGENS, VAGINAL

CONJUGATED ESTROGENS

Rx	**Premarin Vaginal** (Wyeth-Ayerst)	**Cream; vaginal:** conjugated estrogens 0.625 mg/g	Benzyl and cetyl alcohols, mineral oil. In 42.5 g with calibrated applicator.

CONJUGATED ESTROGENS — VAGINAL

WARNING

Estrogens increase the risk of endometrial cancer – There is an increased risk of endometrial cancer in a woman with a uterus who uses unopposed estrogens. Adding a progestin to estrogen therapy has been shown to reduce the risk of endometrial hyperplasia, which may be a precursor to endometrial cancer. Undertake adequate diagnostic measures, including directed or random endometrial sampling when indicated, to rule out malignancy in postmenopausal women with undiagnosed persistent or recurring abnormal genital bleeding.

Cardiovascular disorders and probable dementia – Do not use estrogen-alone therapy for the prevention of cardiovascular disease or dementia.

The Women's Health Initiative (WHI) estrogen-alone substudy reported increased risks of stroke and deep vein thrombosis (DVT) in postmenopausal women (50 to 79 years of age) during 7.1 years of treatment with daily oral conjugated estrogens 0.625 mg relative to placebo.

The Women's Health Initiative Memory Study (WHIMS) estrogen-alone ancillary study of WHI reported an increased risk of developing probable dementia in postmenopausal women 65 years of age and older during 5.2 years of treatment with daily conjugated estrogens 0.625 mg alone, relative to placebo. It is unknown whether this finding applies to younger postmenopausal women.

In the absence of comparable data, these risks should be assumed to be similar for other doses of conjugated estrogens and other dosage forms of estrogens.

Prescribe estrogens with or without progestins at the lowest effective doses and for the shortest duration consistent with treatment goals and risks for the individual woman.

Cardiovascular disorders, breast cancer, and probable dementia for estrogen plus progestin therapy – Do not use estrogen plus progestin therapy for the prevention of cardiovascular disease or dementia.

The WHI estrogen plus progestin substudy reported increased risks of DVT, pulmonary embolism, stroke, and myocardial infarction in postmenopausal women (50 to 79 years of age) during 5.6 years of treatment with daily oral conjugated estrogens 0.625 mg combined with medroxyprogesterone acetate 2.5 mg, relative to placebo.

The WHI estrogen plus progestin substudy also demonstrated an increased risk of invasive breast cancer.

The WHIMS estrogen plus progestin ancillary study of the WHI reported an increased risk of developing probable dementia in postmenopausal women 65 years of age and older during 4 years of treatment with daily conjugated estrogens 0.625 mg combined with medroxyprogesterone acetate 2.5 mg, relative to placebo. It is unknown whether this finding applies to younger postmenopausal women.

In the absence of comparable data, assume these risks to be similar for other doses of conjugated estrogens and medroxyprogesterone acetate, and other combinations and dosage forms of estrogens and progestins.

Prescribe estrogens with or without progestins at the lowest effective doses and for the shortest duration consistent with treatment goals and risks for the individual woman.

Indications

➤*Atrophic vaginitis:* For the treatment of atrophic vaginitis.

➤*Dyspareunia (Premarin only):* For the treatment of moderate to severedyspareunia, a symptom of vulvar and vaginal atrophy caused by menopause.

➤*Kraurosis vulvae:* For the treatment of kraurosis vulvae.

➤*Off-label uses:* For the treatment of nonspecific vulvovaginitis in prepubertal girls. (See Administration and Dosage.)

Administration and Dosage

➤*General dosing considerations:* Generally, when estrogen is prescribed for a postmenopausal woman with a uterus, also consider a progestin to reduce the risk of endometrial cancer.

A woman without a uterus does not need a progestin. In some cases, however, hysterectomized women with a history of endometriosis may need a progestin.

➤*Adults:*

Atrophic vaginitis and kraurosis vulvae – 0.5 to 2 g daily, intravaginally, depending on the severity of the condition. The lowest dose that will control symptoms should be chosen and medication should be discontinued as promptly as possible. Administration should be cyclic (eg, 3 weeks on and 1 week off).

Dyspareunia (Premarin only) – 0.5 g is administered intravaginally in a twice-weekly (eg, Monday and Thursday) continuous regimen or in a cyclic regimen of 21 days of therapy followed by 7 days off of therapy.

➤*Children:*

Off-label dosing –

Nonspecific vulvovaginitis (prepubertal girls): Improved hygienic measures should be recommended first. In persistent cases, application of conjugated estrogens cream to the vulva for 2 to 3 weeks may be beneficial. Application of a topical estrogen cream may also help to thicken the epithelium, thus making it more resistant to infections.

➤*Duration of therapy:* Use of conjugated estrogens vaginal cream, alone or in combination with a progestin, should be limited to the shortest duration consistent with treatment goals and risks for the individual woman. Patients should be reevaluated periodically as clinically appropriate (eg, at 3- to 6-month intervals) to determine if treatment is still necessary.

➤*Administration:* Administer intravaginally.

➤*Storage / Stability:* Store between 20° and 25°C (68° and 77°F); excursions permitted between 15° and 30°C (59° and 86°F).

ESTRADIOL ACETATE

Rx	**Femring** (Warner Chilcott)	**Ring; vaginal:** estradiol acetate 0.05 mg/day[a]	In single packs.
		estradiol acetate 0.1 mg/day[b]	In single packs.

[a] Central core contains estradiol acetate 12.4 mg that releases 0.05 mg/day for 3 months. Dimensions: outer diameter, 56 mm; cross-sectional diameter, 7.6 mm; core diameter, 2 mm.

[b] Central core contains estradiol acetate 24.8 mg that releases 0.1 mg/day for 3 months. Dimensions: outer diameter, 56 mm; cross-sectional diameter, 7.6 mm; core diameter, 2 mm.

ESTRADIOL ACETATE — VAGINAL

For complete prescribing information, refer to the Estrogens group monograph.

WARNING

Estrogens increase the risk of endometrial cancer – Close clinical surveillance of all women taking estrogens is important. Adequate diagnostic measures, including endometrial sampling when indicated, should be undertaken to rule out malignancy in all cases of undiagnosed persistent or recurring abnormal vaginal bleeding. There is no evidence that the use of "natural" estrogens results in a different endometrial risk profile than synthetic estrogens at equivalent estrogen doses.

Cardiovascular and other risks – Estrogens with and without progestins should not be used for the prevention of cardiovascular disease.

The Women's Health Initiative (WHI) study reported increased risks of myocardial infarction, stroke, invasive breast cancer, pulmonary emboli, and deep vein thrombosis in postmenopausal women during 5 years of treatment with conjugated equine estrogens 0.625 mg combined with medroxyprogesterone acetate 2.5 mg relative to placebo. Other doses of conjugated estrogens with medroxyprogesterone acetate, and other combinations of estrogens and progestins were not studied in the WHI and, in the absence of comparable data, these risks should be assumed to be similar. Because of these risks, estrogens with or without progestins should be prescribed at the lowest effective doses and for the shortest duration consistent with treatment goals and risks for the individual woman.

Indications

➤*Menopause:* Moderate to severe vasomotor symptoms associated with menopause; moderate to severe symptoms of vulvar and vaginal atrophy associated with the menopause. When prescribing solely for the treatment of symptoms of vulvar and vaginal atrophy, other vaginal products should be considered.

Administration and Dosage

➤*General dosing considerations:* Patients should be started at the lowest dose.

For women who have a uterus, adequate diagnostic measures, such as endometrial sampling, when indicated, should be undertaken to rule out malignancy in cases of undiagnosed persistent or recurring abnormal vaginal bleeding.

➤*Adults:*

Usual dosage – 0.05 to 0.1 mg daily. Vaginal ring should remain in place for 3 months and then be replaced.

➤*Concomitant progestin therapy:* When estrogen is prescribed for a postmenopausal woman with a uterus, progestin should also be initiated to reduce the risk of endometrial cancer. A woman without a uterus does not need progestin.

➤*Duration of therapy:* Use of estrogen, alone or in combination with a progestin, should be limited to the shortest duration consistent with treatment goals and risks for the individual woman. Patients should be reevaluated periodically as clinically appropriate (eg, 3- to 6-month intervals) to determine if treatment is still necessary. (See Boxed Warning).

➤*Administration:* Hands should be thoroughly washed before and after ring insertion.

Instructions for use –

Vaginal ring insertion: Insert upon removal from the protective pouch. The opposite sides of the vaginal ring should be pressed together and inserted into the vagina. The exact position is not critical to its function. When the vaginal ring is in place, the patient should not feel anything. If the patient feels discomfort, the vaginal ring is probably not far enough inside the vagina. Gently push estradiol acetate vaginal ring further into the vagina.

The patient should not feel the vaginal ring when it is in place and it should not interfere with sexual intercourse. Straining upon bowel movement may make the vaginal ring move down in the lower part of the vagina. If so, it may be repositioned with a finger.

If the vaginal ring is expelled totally from the vagina, it should be rinsed in lukewarm water and reinserted by the patient (or health care provider if necessary).

Vaginal ring removal: The vaginal ring may be removed by looping a finger through the ring and pulling it out.

➤*Storage/Stability:* Store at 25°C (77°F); excursions permitted to 15° to 30°C (59° to 86°F).

ESTRADIOL

Rx	**Vagifem** (Novo Nordisk)	**Tablets; vaginal**: estradiol 10 mcg	Equiv. to estradiol hemihydrate 10.3 mcg. Lactose. White, round. Film-coated. In single-use applicators of 8s and 18s.
		estradiol 25 mcg	Equiv. to estradiol hemihydrate 25.8 mcg. Lactose. White, round. Film-coated. In single-use applicators of 8s and 18s.
Rx	**Estrace Vaginal** (Warner Chilcott)	**Cream; vaginal**: estradiol 0.1 mg/g	Stearyl alcohol, EDTA, methylparaben. In 42.5 g with calibrated applicator.
Rx	**Estring** (Pharmacia)	**Ring; vaginal**: estradiol 2 mg[a]	In single packs.

[a] Releases estradiol, approximately 7.5 mcg per 24 hours, in a consistent, stable manner over 90 days. Dimensions: outer diameter, 55 mm; cross-sectional diameter, 9 mm; core diameter, 2 mm.

ESTRADIOL — VAGINAL

For complete prescribing information, refer to the Estrogens group monograph.

WARNING

Estrogens have been reported to increase the risk of endometrial carcinoma in postmenopausal women – Close clinical surveillance of all women taking estrogens is important. Adequate diagnostic measures, including endometrial sampling when indicated, should be undertaken to rule out malignancy in all cases of undiagnosed persistent or recurring abnormal vaginal bleeding. There is no evidence that "natural" estrogens are more or less hazardous than "synthetic" estrogens at equiestrogenic doses.

Three independent, case-controlled studies have reported an increased risk of endometrial cancer in postmenopausal women exposed to exogenous estrogens for more than 1 year. This risk was independent of the other known risk factors for endometrial cancer. These studies are further supported by the finding that incidence rates of endometrial cancer have increased sharply since 1969 in 8 different areas of the United States with population-based, cancer-reporting systems, an increase which may be related to the rapidly expanding use of estrogens during the last decade.

The 3 case-controlled studies reported that the risk of endometrial cancer in estrogen users was about 4.5 to 13.9 times higher than in nonusers. The risk appears to depend on both duration of treatment and on estrogen dose. In view of these findings, when estrogens are used for the treatment of menopausal symptoms, the lowest dose that will control symptoms should be utilized and medication should be discontinued as soon as possible. When prolonged treatment is medically indicated, the patient should be reassessed, on at least a semiannual basis, to determine the need for continued therapy.

WARNING (cont.)

Estrogens should not be used during pregnancy – There is no indication for estrogen therapy during pregnancy or during the immediate postpartum period. Estrogens are ineffective for the prevention or treatment of threatened or habitual abortion. Estrogens are not indicated for the prevention of postpartum breast engorgement.

Estrogen therapy during pregnancy is associated with an increased risk of congenital defects in the reproductive organs of the fetus, and possibly other birth defects. Studies of women who received diethylstilbestrol (DES) during pregnancy have shown that female offspring have an increased risk of vaginal adenosis, squamous cell dysplasia of the uterine cervix, and clear cell vaginal cancer later in life; male offspring have an increased risk of urogenital abnormalities and possibly testicular cancer later in life. The 1985 DES Task Force concluded that use of DES during pregnancy is associated with subsequent increased risk of breast cancer in the mothers; although, a causal relationship remains unproven, and the observed level of excess risk is similar to that for a number of other breast cancer risk factors.

Indications

➤*Vaginal cream:* Estradiol vaginal cream is indicated in the treatment of vulval and vaginal atrophy.

➤*Vaginal tablets:* Estradiol vaginal tablets are indicated for the treatment of atrophic vaginitis.

➤*Vaginal ring:* Estradiol vaginal ring is indicated for the treatment of urogenital symptoms associated with postmenopausal atrophy of the vagina (eg, dryness, burning, pruritus, dyspareunia) and/or the lower urinary tract (urinary urgency and dysuria).

ESTRADIOL — VAGINAL

Administration and Dosage

➤*General dosing considerations:* Patients with intact uteri should be monitored closely for signs of endometrial cancer, and appropriate diagnostic measures should be taken to rule out malignancy in the event of persistent or recurring abnormal vaginal bleeding.

For treatment of vulval and vaginal atrophy and atrophic vaginitis associated with the menopause, the lowest dose and regimen that will control symptoms should be chosen.

➤*Adults:*

Vaginal cream –

Vulval and vaginal atrophy:

• *Usual dosage* – 2 to 4 g (marked on the applicator or delivered via 1 g tubes) daily for 1 or 2 weeks, then gradually reduced to one-half initial dosage for a similar period.

• *Maintenance dosage* – 1 g, 1 to 3 times a week, may be used after restoration of the vaginal mucosa has been achieved.

Vaginal ring –

Urogenital symptoms associated with menopause: One vaginal ring inserted vaginally as deeply as possible into the upper one third of the vaginal vault. The ring is to remain in place continuously for 3 months, after which it is to be removed and, if appropriate, replaced by a new ring.

Vaginal tablets –

Atrophic vaginitis:

• *Initial dosage* – One vaginal tablet, inserted vaginally, once daily for 2 weeks. It is advisable to have the patient administer treatment at the same time each day.

• *Maintenance dosage* – One vaginal tablet, inserted vaginally, twice weekly.

➤*Duration of therapy:* The need to continue therapy should be assessed by the health care provider with the patient. Attempts to discontinue or taper medication should be made at 3- to 6-month intervals. For treatment of vulval and vaginal atrophy and atrophic vaginitis associated with the menopause, the medication should be discontinued as promptly as possible.

➤*Administration:*

Vaginal ring –

Ring insertion: The ring should be pressed into an oval and inserted into the upper third of the vaginal vault. The exact position is not critical. When the vaginal ring is in place, the patient should not feel anything. If the patient feels discomfort, the vaginal ring is probably not far enough inside. Gently push the vaginal ring further into the vagina.

The vaginal ring should be left in place continuously for 90 days and then, if continuation of therapy is deemed appropriate, replaced by a new vaginal ring. Retention of the ring for greater than 90 days does not represent overdosage but will result in progressively greater underdosage with the attendant risk of loss of efficacy and increasing risk of vaginal infections and/or erosions.

The patient should not feel the vaginal ring when it is in place and it should not interfere with sexual intercourse. Straining at defecation may make the vaginal ring move down in the lower part of the vagina. If so, it may be pushed up again with a finger.

If the vaginal ring is expelled totally from the vagina, it should be rinsed in lukewarm water and reinserted by the patient (or health care provider/nurse if necessary).

Ring removal: The vaginal ring may be removed by hooking a finger through the ring and pulling it out.

Vaginal tablet – The vaginal tablet is gently inserted into the vagina as far as it can comfortably go without force, using the supplied applicator.

➤*Storage/Stability:*

Vaginal cream – Store at room temperature. Protect from temperatures in excess of 40°C (104°F).

Vaginal ring and tablets – Store at controlled room temperature 15° to 30°C (59° to 86°F).

Selective Estrogen Receptor Modulator

RALOXIFENE HYDROCHLORIDE

Rx	**Evista** (Eli Lilly)	**Tablets; oral:** 60 mg	Equiv. to 55.71 mg free base. Lactose. (LILLY 4165). Elliptical. Film-coated. In 2,000s and unit-of-use 30s and 100s.

RALOXIFENE HYDROCHLORIDE — ORAL

WARNING

Increased risk of venous thromboembolism (VTE) and death from stroke – Increased risk of deep vein thrombosis and pulmonary embolism have been reported with raloxifene. Women with active VTE or a history of VTE should not take raloxifene.

Increased risk of death caused by stroke occurred in a trial in postmenopausal women with documented coronary heart disease or increased risk for major coronary reactions. Consider the risk-benefit balance in women at risk for stroke.

Indications

➤*Osteoporosis treatment and prevention:* For the treatment and prevention of osteoporosis in postmenopausal women.

➤*Reduction in the risk of invasive breast cancer in postmenopausal women with osteoporosis:* For the reduction in risk of invasive breast cancer in postmenopausal women with osteoporosis.

➤*Reduction in the risk of invasive breast cancer in postmenopausal women at high risk of invasive breast cancer:* For the reduction in risk of invasive breast cancer in postmenopausal women at high risk of invasive breast cancer.

➤*Off-label uses:* For the treatment of uterine leiomyomas (with gonadotropin-releasing hormone [GnRH] agonist therapy); treatment of pubertal gynecomastia; the prevention of bone loss in men with prostate cancer (with GnRH agonist therapy).

Administration and Dosage

➤*Adults:*

Osteoporosis –

Usual dosage: 60 mg daily.

Concomitant therapy: Supplemental calcium and/or vitamin D should be added to the diet if daily intake is inadequate. Postmenopausal women require an average elemental calcium intake of 1,500 mg/day. Total daily intake of calcium higher than 1,500 mg has not demonstrated additional bone benefits, while daily intake higher than 2,000 mg has been associated with increased risk of adverse reactions, including hypercalcemia and kidney stones.

The recommended intake of vitamin D is 400 to 800 units per day. Patients at increased risk for vitamin D insufficiency (eg, older than 70 years of age, nursing home–bound, chronically ill) may need additional vitamin D supplements. Patients with GI malabsorption syndromes may require higher doses of vitamin D supplementation, and measurement of 25-hydroxyvitamin D should be considered.

Reduction in the risk of invasive breast cancer –

Usual dosage: 60 mg daily.

Duration of therapy: Not known.

➤*Administration:* May be administered any time of day without regard to meals.

➤*Storage/Stability:* Store between 20° and 25°C (68° and 77°F); excursions permitted between 15° and 30°C (59° and 86°F).

Handling and disposal – Raloxifene is a hormonal agent and is considered a teratogen and potential mutagen. Follow safe handling procedures when preparing, administering, or dispensing raloxifene.

Actions

➤*Pharmacology:* Raloxifene is an estrogen agonist/antagonist, commonly referred to as a selective estrogen receptor modulator (SERM). The biological actions of raloxifene are largely mediated through binding to estrogen receptors (ER). This binding results in activation of estrogenic pathways in some tissues (agonism) and blockade of estrogenic pathways in others (antagonism). The agonistic or antagonistic action of raloxifene depends on the extent of recruitment of coactivators to ER target gene promoters.

Raloxifene appears to act as an estrogen agonist in bone. It decreases resorption of bone and bone turnover, increases bone mineral density (BMD), and decreases fracture incidence. Preclinical data demonstrate that raloxifene is an estrogen antagonist in uterine and breast tissues. These results are consistent with findings in clinical trials, which suggest that raloxifene lacks estrogen-like effects on the uterus and breast tissue.

➤*Pharmacokinetics:*

Raloxifene Pharmacokinetic Parameters in Healthy Postmenopausal Women[a]

	C_{max}[b] (ng/mL)/(mg/kg)	Half-life (h)	$AUC_{0-\infty}$[b] (ng•h/mL)/(mg/kg)	CL/F (L/kg•h)	V/F (L/kg)
Single dose					
Mean	0.5	27.7	27.2	44.1	2,348
CV (%)	52	10.7 to 273[c]	44	46	52
Multiple dose					
Mean	1.36	32.5	24.2	47.4	2,583
CV (%)	37	15.8 to 86.6[c]	36	41	56

[a] C_{max} = maximal plasma concentration; AUC = area under the curve; CL = clearance; CV = coefficient of variation; F = bioavailability; V = volume of distribution.
[b] Data normalized for dose in milligrams and body weight in kilograms.
[c] Range of observed half-life.

Absorption – Raloxifene is absorbed rapidly after oral administration. Approximately 60% of an oral dose is absorbed, but presystemic glucuronide conjugation is extensive. Absolute bioavailability of raloxifene is 2%. The time to reach average C_{max} and bioavailability are functions of systemic interconversion and enterohepatic cycling of raloxifene and its glucuronide metabolites.

RALOXIFENE HYDROCHLORIDE — ORAL

Food effects: Administration of raloxifene with a standardized, high-fat meal increases the absorption of raloxifene (C_{max} 28% and AUC 16%) but does not lead to clinically meaningful changes in systemic exposure. Raloxifene can be administered without regard to meals.

Distribution – Following oral administration of single raloxifene doses ranging from 30 to 150 mg, the apparent volume of distribution is 2,348 L/kg and is not dose dependent. Raloxifene and the monoglucuronide conjugates are highly (95%) bound to plasma proteins. Raloxifene binds to both albumin and alpha-1-acid glycoprotein but not to sex steroid–binding globulin.

Metabolism – Biotransformation and disposition of raloxifene in humans have been determined following oral administration of ^{14}C-labeled raloxifene. Raloxifene undergoes extensive first-pass metabolism to the following glucuronide conjugates: raloxifene-4′-glucuronide, raloxifene-6-glucuronide, and raloxifene-6, 4′-diglucuronide. No other metabolites have been detected, providing strong evidence that raloxifene is not metabolized by CYP-450 pathways. Unconjugated raloxifene comprises less than 1% of the total radiolabeled material in plasma. The terminal log-linear portions of the plasma concentration curves for raloxifene and the glucuronides are generally parallel. This is consistent with interconversion of raloxifene and the glucuronide metabolites.

Following intravenous (IV) administration, raloxifene is cleared at a rate approximating hepatic blood flow. Apparent oral clearance is 44.1 L/kg•h. Raloxifene and its glucuronide conjugates are interconverted by reversible systemic metabolism and enterohepatic cycling, thereby prolonging its plasma elimination half-life to 27.7 hours after oral dosing.

Results from single oral doses of raloxifene predict multiple-dose pharmacokinetics. Following chronic dosing, clearance ranges from 40 to 60 L/kg•h. Increasing doses of raloxifene (ranging from 30 to 150 mg) result in slightly less than a proportional increase in the AUC.

Excretion – Raloxifene is primarily excreted in the feces, and less than 0.2% is excreted unchanged in the urine. Less than 6% of the raloxifene dose is eliminated in the urine as glucuronide conjugates.

Special populations –

Renal function impairment: When a single dose of raloxifene 120 mg was administered to 10 men with renal function impairment (7 with moderate function impairment, creatinine clearance [CrCl] 31 to 50 mL/min; 3 with severe function impairment, CrCl 30 mL/min or less) and to 10 healthy men (CrCl more than 80 mL/min), plasma raloxifene concentrations were 122% ($AUC_{0-\infty}$) higher in patients with renal function impairment than those of healthy volunteers. Use raloxifene with caution in patients with moderate or severe renal function impairment.

Hepatic function impairment: Apparent clearance of raloxifene was reduced 56%, and the half-life of raloxifene was not altered in patients with mild hepatic function impairment. Plasma raloxifene concentrations were approximately 150% higher than those in healthy volunteers and correlated with total bilirubin concentrations. The pharmacokinetics of raloxifene have not been studied in patients with moderate or severe hepatic function impairment. Use raloxifene with caution in patients with hepatic function impairment.

Contraindications

Pregnant women or women who may become pregnant; breast-feeding women; women with active VTE or a history of VTE, including deep vein thrombosis, pulmonary embolism, and retinal vein thrombosis.

Warnings/Precautions

➤*VTE:* In clinical trials, raloxifene-treated women had an increased risk of VTE (deep vein thrombosis and pulmonary embolism). Other venous thromboembolic reactions could also occur. A less serious reaction, superficial thrombophlebitis, also has been reported more frequently with raloxifene than with placebo. The greatest risk for deep vein thrombosis and pulmonary embolism occurs during the first 4 months of treatment, and the magnitude of risk appears to be similar to the reported risk associated with use of hormone therapy. Because immobilization increases the risk for venous thromboembolic reactions independent of therapy, discontinue raloxifene at least 72 hours prior to and during prolonged immobilization (eg, postsurgical recovery, prolonged bed rest), and resume raloxifene therapy only after the patient is fully ambulatory. In addition, advise women taking raloxifene to move about periodically during prolonged travel. Consider the risk-benefit balance in women at risk of thromboembolic disease for other reasons (eg, active malignancy, congestive heart failure, superficial thrombophlebitis).

➤*Death caused by stroke:* In a clinical trial of postmenopausal women with documented coronary heart disease or at increased risk for coronary reactions, an increased risk of death caused by stroke was observed after treatment with raloxifene. During an average follow-up of 5.6 years, 59 (1.2%) raloxifene-treated women died because of a stroke compared with 39 (0.8%) placebo-treated women (22 vs 15 per 10,000 women-years; HR 1.49; 95% CI, 1 to 2.24; $P = 0.0499$). There was no statistically significant difference between treatment groups in the incidence of stroke (249 [4.9%] in raloxifene vs 224 [4.4%] placebo). Raloxifene had no significant effect on all-cause mortality. Consider the risk-benefit balance in women at risk for stroke, such as atrial fibrillation, cigarette smoking, hypertension, prior stroke or transient ischemic attack.

➤*Cardiovascular disease:* Do not use raloxifene for the primary or secondary prevention of cardiovascular disease. In a clinical trial of postmenopausal women with documented coronary heart disease or at increased risk for coronary reactions, no cardiovascular benefit was demonstrated after treatment with raloxifene for 5 years.

➤*Premenopausal use:* There is no indication for premenopausal use of raloxifene. Safety of raloxifene in premenopausal women has not been established, and its use is not recommended.

➤*Hypertriglyceridemia:* Limited clinical data suggest that some women with histories of marked hypertriglyceridemia (more than 5.6 mmol/L or more than 500 mg/dL) in response to treatment with oral estrogen or estrogen plus progestin may develop increased levels of triglycerides when treated with raloxifene. Monitor serum triglycerides in women with this medical history when they are taking raloxifene.

➤*History of breast cancer:* Raloxifene has not been adequately studied in women with a history of breast cancer.

➤*Use in men:* There is no indication for the use of raloxifene in men. Raloxifene has not been adequately studied in men, and its use is not recommended.

➤*Unexplained uterine bleeding:* Investigate any unexplained uterine bleeding as clinically indicated. Raloxifene- and placebo-treated groups had similar incidences of endometrial proliferation.

➤*Breast abnormalities:* Investigate any unexplained breast abnormality occurring during raloxifene therapy. Raloxifene does not eliminate the risk of breast cancer.

➤*Renal function impairment:* Use raloxifene with caution in patients with moderate or severe renal function impairment. Safety and efficacy have not been established in patients with moderate or severe renal function impairment.

➤*Hepatic function impairment:* Use raloxifene with caution in patients with hepatic function impairment. Safety and efficacy have not been established in patients with hepatic function impairment.

➤*Pregnancy: Category X.* Raloxifene is contraindicated in pregnancy and in women who may become pregnant. Raloxifene may cause fetal harm when administered to a pregnant woman. If this drug is used during pregnancy or if the patient becomes pregnant while taking this drug, apprise the patient of the potential hazard to the fetus.

In rabbit studies, abortion and a low rate of fetal heart anomalies (ventricular septal defects) occurred in rabbits at doses of 0.1 mg/kg or more (0.04 times or more than the human dose based on BSA, mg/m^2), and hydrocephaly was observed in fetuses at doses of 10 mg/kg or more (4 times or more than the human dose based on BSA, mg/m^2). In rat studies, retardation of fetal development and developmental abnormalities (eg, kidney cavitation wavy ribs) occurred at doses of 1 mg/kg or more (0.2 times or more than the human dose based on surface area, mg/m^2). Treatment of rats at doses of 0.1 to 10 mg/kg (0.02 to 1.6 times the human dose based on BSA, mg/m^2) during gestation and lactation produced effects that included delayed and disrupted parturition, decreased neonatal survival and altered physical development, sex- and age-specific reductions in growth and changes in pituitary hormone content, and decreased lymphoid compartment size in offspring. At 10 mg/kg, raloxifene disrupted parturition, which resulted in maternal and progeny death and morbidity. Effects in adult offspring (4 months of age) included uterine hypoplasia and reduced fertility; however, no ovarian or vaginal pathology was observed.

➤*Lactation:* Raloxifene is contraindicated in breast-feeding women. Treatment of rats at doses of 0.1 to 10 mg/kg (0.02 to 1.6 times the human dose based on surface area, mg/m^2) during gestation and lactation produced effects that included delayed and disrupted parturition; decreased neonatal survival and altered physical development; sex- and age-specific reductions in growth and changes in pituitary hormone content; and decreased lymphoid compartment size in offspring.

It is not known whether raloxifene is excreted in human milk. Because many drugs are excreted in human milk, exercise caution when raloxifene is administered to a breast-feeding woman.

➤*Children:* Safety and effectiveness in children have not been established.

➤*Monitoring:* Advise patients that they should have breast exams and mammograms before starting therapy and should continue regular breast exams and mammograms after beginning therapy. Monitor serum triglycerides in patients with hypertriglyceridemia.

Drug Interactions

Raloxifene Drug Interactions

Precipitant drug	Object drug[a]		Description
Ampicillin	Raloxifene	⬇	Peak raloxifene levels and the overall extent of absorption are reduced 28% and 14%, respectively, with coadministration of ampicillin. However, systemic exposure and elimination rate of raloxifene were not affected. Therefore, raloxifene can be coadministered with ampicillin.
Cholestyramine	Raloxifene	⬇	Raloxifene absorption and enterohepatic cycling was reduced 60%; avoid coadministration.

RALOXIFENE HYDROCHLORIDE — ORAL

Raloxifene Drug Interactions			
Precipitant drug	Object drug[a]		Description
Highly protein-bound drugs (eg, diazepam, diazoxide, lidocaine)	Raloxifene	↑	Raloxifene is more than 95% bound to plasma proteins. Use caution when raloxifene is coadministered with other highly protein-bound drugs.
Raloxifene	Systemic estrogens	↔	The safety of concomitant use of raloxifene with systemic estrogens has not been studied, and its use is not recommended.
Raloxifene	Warfarin	↓	In single-dose studies, 10% decreases in prothrombin time (PT) have been observed. Monitor PT closely.

[a] ↑ = object drug increased; ↓ = object drug decreased; ↔ = undetermined clinical effect.

➤*Drug/Food interactions:* See Actions for more information.

Adverse Reactions

➤*Osteoporosis treatment:* The most serious adverse reaction related to raloxifene was VTE (deep venous thrombosis, pulmonary embolism, and retinal vein thrombosis). During an average of study-drug exposure of 2.6 years, VTE occurred in about 1 of 100 raloxifene-treated patients. Twenty-six raloxifene-treated women had a VTE compared with 11 placebo-treated women; the HR was 2.4 (95% CI, 1.2 to 4.5), and the highest VTE risk was during the initial months of treatment.

Common adverse reactions considered to be related to raloxifene therapy were hot flashes and leg cramps. Hot flashes occurred in about 1 in 10 patients on raloxifene and were most commonly reported during the first 6 months of treatment and were not different from placebo thereafter. Leg cramps occurred in about 1 in 14 patients on raloxifene.

➤*Osteoporosis prevention:* Common adverse reactions considered to be drug related were hot flashes and leg cramps. Hot flashes occurred in about 1 in 4 patients on raloxifene versus about 1 in 6 on placebo. The first occurrence of hot flashes was most commonly reported during the first 6 months of treatment.

Raloxifene Adverse Reactions in Osteoporosis Clinical Trials (≥ 2%)

	Treatment		Prevention	
Adverse reaction	Raloxifene (n = 2,557)	Placebo (n = 2,576)	Raloxifene (n = 581)	Placebo (n = 584)
Cardiovascular				
Hot flashes	9.7%	6.4%	24.6%	18.3%
Migraine	[a]	[a]	2.4%	2.1%
Syncope	2.3%	2.1%	[b]	[b]
Varicose vein	2.2%	1.5%	[a]	[a]
CNS				
Depression	[a]	[a]	6.4%	6%
Headache	9.2%	8.5%	[a]	[a]
Hypesthesia	2.1%	2%	[a]	[a]
Insomnia	[a]	[a]	5.5%	4.3%
Neuralgia	2.4%	1.9%	[b]	[b]
Vertigo	4.1%	3.7%	[a]	[a]
Dermatologic				
Rash	[a]	[a]	5.5%	3.8%
Sweating	2.5%	2%	3.1%	1.7%
GI				
Diarrhea	7.2%	6.9%	[a]	[a]
Dyspepsia	[a]	[a]	5.9%	5.8%
Flatulence	[a]	[a]	3.1%	2.4%
Gastroenteritis	[b]	[b]	2.6%	2.1%
GI disorder	[a]	[a]	3.3%	2.1%
Nausea	8.3%	7.8%	8.8%	8.6%
Vomiting	4.8%	4.3%	3.4%	3.3%
GU				
Cystitis	4.6%	4.5%	3.3%	3.1%
Endometrial disorder[c]	[b]	[b]	3.1%	1.9%
Leukorrhea	[a]	[a]	3.3%	1.7%
Urinary tract disorder	2.5%	2.1%	[a]	[a]
Urinary tract infection	[a]	[a]	4%	3.9%
Uterine disorder[c,d]	3.3%	2.3%	[a]	[a]
Vaginal hemorrhage	2.5%	2.4%	[a]	[a]
Vaginitis	[a]	[a]	4.3%	3.6%
Metabolic/nutritional				
Peripheral edema	5.2%	4.4%	3.3%	1.9%
Weight gain	[a]	[a]	8.8%	6.8%
Musculoskeletal				
Arthralgia	15.5%	14%	10.7%	10.1%
Arthritis	[a]	[a]	4%	3.6%
Myalgia	[a]	[a]	7.7%	6.2%
Tendon disorder	3.6%	3.1%	[a]	[a]
Respiratory				
Bronchitis	9.5%	8.6%	[a]	[a]
Increased cough	9.3%	9.2%	6%	5.7%
Laryngitis	[b]	[b]	2.2%	1.4%
Pharyngitis	5.3%	5.1%	7.6%	7.2%
Pneumonia	[a]	[a]	2.6%	1.5%
Rhinitis	10.2%	10.1%	[a]	[a]
Sinusitis	7.9%	7.5%	10.3%	6.5%
Miscellaneous				
Chest pain	[a]	[a]	4%	3.6%
Conjunctivitis	2.2%	1.7%	[a]	[a]
Fever	3.9%	3.8%	3.1%	2.6%
Flu syndrome	13.5%	11.4%	14.6%	13.5%
Infection	[a]	[a]	15.1%	14.6%
Leg cramps	7%	3.7%	5.9%	1.9%

[a] Placebo incidence ≥ raloxifene incidence.
[b] Less than 2% incidence and more frequent with raloxifene.
[c] Includes only patients with an intact uterus. Prevention trials: raloxifene, n = 354; placebo, n = 364; treatment trial: raloxifene, n = 1,948; placebo, n = 1,999.
[d] Actual terms most frequently referred to endometrial fluid.

➤*Comparison of raloxifene and hormone therapy:*

Raloxifene Adverse Reactions in Osteoporosis Prevention Clinical Trials (≥ 2%)[a]

Adverse reaction	Raloxifene (n = 317)	Continuous combined hormone therapy[b] (n = 96)	Cyclic hormone therapy[c] (n = 219)
GI			
Abdominal pain	6.6%	10.4%	18.7%
Flatulence	1.6%	12.5%	6.4%
GU			
Breast pain	4.4%	37.5%	29.7%
Vaginal bleeding[d]	6.2%	64.2%	88.5%
Miscellaneous			
Chest pain	2.8%	0%	0.5%
Hot flashes	28.7%	3.1%	5.9%
Infection	11%	0%	6.8%

[a] These data are from blinded and open-label studies.
[b] Continuous combined hormone therapy = conjugated estrogens 0.625 mg plus medroxyprogesterone 2.5 mg.
[c] Cyclic hormone therapy = conjugated estrogens 0.625 mg for 28 days with concomitant medroxyprogesterone 5 mg or norgestrel 0.15 mg on days 1 through 14 or 17 through 28.
[d] Includes only patients with an intact uterus. Raloxifene, n = 290; continuous combined hormone therapy, n = 67; cyclic hormone therapy, n = 217.

➤*Postmenopausal women at increased risk for major coronary reactions:* Adverse reactions reported more frequently in the raloxifene-treated women than in placebo-treated women included peripheral edema (14.1% raloxifene vs 11.7% placebo), muscle spasms/leg cramps (12.1% raloxifene vs 8.3% placebo), hot flashes (7.8% raloxifene vs 4.7% placebo), venous thromboembolic reactions (2% raloxifene vs 1.4% placebo), and cholelithiasis (3.3% raloxifene vs 2.6% placebo).

➤*Postmarketing:* Adverse reactions reported since market introduction include retinal vein occlusion, stroke, and death associated with VTE (all very rare).

Overdosage

➤*Symptoms:* Adverse reactions were reported in approximately half of the adults who took raloxifene 180 mg or more and included leg cramps and dizziness. Two children 18 months of age each ingested raloxifene 180 mg. In

RALOXIFENE HYDROCHLORIDE — ORAL

these 2 children, symptoms reported included ataxia, diarrhea, dizziness, flushing, rash, tremor, and vomiting, as well as elevation in alkaline phosphatase.

Patient Information

Instruct patients to read the Medication Guide before starting therapy with raloxifene and reread it each time the prescription is refilled.

For osteoporosis treatment or prevention, instruct patients to take supplemental calcium and/or vitamin D, if daily dietary intake is inadequate. Instruct patients at increased risk for vitamin D insufficiency (eg, age older than 70 years, nursing home–bound, chronically ill, or with GI malabsorption syndromes) to take additional vitamin D if needed. Consider weight-bearing exercise along with the modification of certain behavioral factors, such as cigarette smoking and/or alcohol consumption, if these factors exist.

Discontinue raloxifene at least 72 hours prior to and during prolonged immobilization (eg, postsurgical recovery, prolonged bed rest). Advise patients to avoid prolonged restrictions of movement during travel because of the increased risk of venous thromboembolic reactions.

Raloxifene may increase the incidence of hot flashes and is not effective in reducing hot flashes or flushes associated with estrogen deficiency. In some asymptomatic patients, hot flashes may occur upon beginning raloxifene therapy.

Use of raloxifene is associated with the reduction of the risk of invasive breast cancer in postmenopausal women. Raloxifene has not been shown to reduce the risk of noninvasive breast cancer. When considering treatment, discuss the potential benefits and risks of raloxifene treatment with patients.

Raloxifene is not indicated for the treatment of invasive breast cancer or reduction of the risk of recurrence. Advise patients that they should have breast exams and mammograms before starting raloxifene and should continue regular breast exams and mammograms, in keeping with good medical practice, after beginning treatment with raloxifene.

Progestins

For progestins recommended only for antineoplastic action in endometrial carcinoma, see megestrol acetate and medroxyprogesterone acetate monographs in the Antineoplastics chapter.

WARNING

Progestins and estrogens should not be used for the prevention of cardiovascular disease.

The Women's Health Initiative (WHI) study reported increased risks of myocardial infarction, stroke, invasive breast cancer, pulmonary emboli, and deep vein thrombosis in postmenopausal women (50 to 79 years of age) during 5 years of treatment with oral conjugated estrogens (CE 0.625 mg) combined with medroxyprogesterone acetate (MPA 2.5 mg) relative to placebo.

The Women's Health Initiative Memory Study (WHIMS), a sub-study of WHI, reported increased risk of developing probable dementia in postmenopausal women 65 years of age or older during 4 years of treatment with oral conjugated estrogens plus medroxyprogesterone acetate relative to placebo. It is unknown whether this finding applies to younger postmenopausal women.

Other doses of oral conjugated estrogens with medroxyprogesterone and other combinations and dosage forms of estrogens and progestins were not studied in the WHI clinical trials. In the absence of comparable data and product-specific studies, the relevance of the WHI findings to other products has not been established. Therefore, the risks should be assumed to be similar for all estrogen and progestin products. Because of these risks, estrogens with or without progestins should be prescribed at the lowest effective doses and for the shortest duration consistent with treatment goals and risks for the individual woman.

Indications

➤*Amenorrhea:* Primary and secondary.

➤*Abnormal uterine bleeding:* Abnormal uterine bleeding caused by hormonal imbalance in the absence of organic pathology, such as fibroids or uterine cancer.

➤*Endometriosis:* Norethindrone only.

➤*AIDS wasting syndrome:* Megestrol acetate suspension only.

➤*Infertility (progesterone gel only):* Progesterone supplementation or replacement as part of an Assisted Reproductive Technology (ART) treatment for infertile women with progesterone deficiency.

➤*Off-label uses:* Refer to individual monographs for further information.

Hot flashes –

Megestrol: [3] = Safety concerns.

Other possible off-label uses – Adding progestin for at least 7 days of a cycle of estrogen replacement for menopause has lowered incidence of endometrial hyperplasia. Morphological and biochemical endometrium studies suggest 10 to 13 days of progestin provide maximal maturation of endometrium and eliminate any hyperplastic changes. It is not clear whether this provides protection from endometrial carcinoma. There may be additional risks with progestin in estrogen replacement regimens, including adverse effects on carbohydrate and lipid metabolism. Choice of progestin and dosage may be important in minimizing these adverse effects.

Megestrol: Appetite stimulant for cachexia in advanced cancer.

Progesterone: Progesterone suppositories (rectal or vaginal, 200 to 400 mg twice daily) have been used in premenstrual syndrome (PMS). Some studies report no improvements in PMS symptoms with progesterone suppositories vs placebo; however, these studies may have had methodologic flaws. One controlled trial suggested oral progesterone (100 mg in the morning, 200 mg at night for 10 days during the luteal phase) improved PMS symptoms. Further controlled studies are needed.

Progesterone has been used successfully in premature labor in late stages of pregnancy. Progesterone suppositories have been used during the luteal phase to the end of the first trimester to decrease spontaneous abortions in previous aborters and in anovulatory women receiving clomiphene citrate or human menopausal gonadotropins, and in luteal phase defects to improve fertility (see Warning Box).

Actions

➤*Pharmacology:* Progesterone, a principle of corpus luteum, is the primary endogenous progestational substance. Progestins (progesterone and derivatives) transform proliferative endometrium into secretory endometrium. Progesterone is necessary to increase endometrial receptivity for implantation of an embryo. Once an embryo is implanted, progesterone acts to maintain the pregnancy. They inhibit (at the usual dose range) or facilitate through positive feedback the secretion of pituitary gonadotropins, which in turn prevents follicular maturation and ovulation or alternatively promotes it for the "primed" follicle. They also inhibit spontaneous uterine contractions as well as other smooth muscles throughout the body. Progestins may demonstrate some anabolic or androgenic activity.

Several investigators have reported on the appetite-enhancing property of megestrol acetate and its possible use in cachexia. The precise mechanism by which megestrol produces effects in anorexia and cachexia is unknown.

➤*Pharmacokinetics:*

Gel –

Multiple Dose Pharmacokinetics of Progesterone Gel

Parameter	Twice daily dosing for 12 days	Once daily dosing for 12 days
C_{max} (ng/ml)	14.57	15.97
C_{avg} (ng/ml)	11.6	8.99
T_{max} (hr)	3.55	5.4
AUC (ng•hr/ml)	138.72	391.98
t½ (hr)	25.91	45

Mean Single Dose Relative Bioavailability of Progesterone: Gel vs IM

Parameter	8% gel	90 mg IM
C_{max} (ng/ml)	14.87	53.76
$C_{avg\ 0\text{-}24}$ (ng/ml)	6.98	28.98
$AUC_{0\text{-}96}$ (ng•hr/ml)	296.78	1378.91
T_{max} (hr)	6.8	9.2
T½ (hr)	34.8	19.6

Absorption/Distribution –

Oral: Progestins are rapidly absorbed from the GI tract and undergo prompt hepatic degradation. Maximum concentration is achieved in 1 to 2 hours. During the first 6 hours after ingestion, half-life is approximately 2 to 3 hours; half-life is approximately 8 to 9 hours thereafter. Metabolites, present for several days after an oral dose, are excreted in the urine.

IM: Following IM administration, progesterone in oil is rapidly absorbed and undergoes rapid metabolism. Half-life is a few minutes. Effective concentrations of long-acting forms can be maintained for 3 to 6 months. Maximum concentration occurs in approximately 24 hours with a half-life of approximately 10 weeks.

Gel: Because of the gel's sustained release properties, progesterone absorption is prolonged with an absorption half-life of approximately 25 to 50 hours, and an elimination half-life of 5 to 20 minutes. Progesterone is extensively bound to serum proteins (approximately 96% to 99%), primarily to serum albumin and corticosteroid binding globulin.

Metabolism/Excretion –

Oral/IM: The major urinary metabolite of oral progesterone is 5β-pregnan-3α, 20α-diol glucuronide. Progesterone undergoes biliary and renal elimination. Following an injection of labeled progesterone, 50% to 60% of the excretion of progesterone metabolites occurs via the kidney; approximately 10% occurs via the bile and feces, the second major excretory pathway. Overall recovery of labeled material accounts for 70% of an administered dose, with the remainder of the dose not characterized with respect to elimination. Only a small portion of unchanged progesterone is excreted in the bile.

Contraindications

Hypersensitivity to progestins; thrombophlebitis, thromboembolic disorders, cerebral hemorrhage, or patients with a history of these conditions; impaired liver function or disease; carcinoma of the breast or genital organs;

undiagnosed vaginal bleeding; missed abortion; as a diagnostic test for pregnancy; prophylactic use to avoid weight loss (megestrol acetate suspension).

Warnings/Precautions

➤*Ophthalmologic effects:* Discontinue medication pending examination if there is a sudden partial or complete loss of vision or if there is sudden onset of proptosis, diplopia, or migraine. If papilledema or retinal vascular lesions occur, discontinue use.

➤*Thrombotic disorders:* Thrombotic disorders (eg, thrombophlebitis, cerebrovascular disorders, retinal thrombosis, pulmonary embolism) occasionally occur in patients taking progestins; be alert to the earliest manifestations of the disease. If these occur or are suspected, discontinue the drug immediately. However, this has not been shown to occur more often than that seen in a control group.

➤*HIV-infected women:* Although **megestrol** has been used extensively in women for endometrial and breast cancers, its use in HIV-infected women has been limited.

➤*Pretreatment physical examination:* Pretreatment physical examination should include breasts and pelvic organs, as well as Papanicolaou smear. Advise the pathologist of progestin therapy when relevant specimens are submitted. In cases of irregular vaginal bleeding, consider nonfunctional causes. Adequately diagnose all cases of vaginal bleeding.

➤*Fluid retention:* Fluid retention may occur; therefore, conditions influenced by this factor (epilepsy, migraine, asthma, cardiac or renal dysfunction) require careful observation.

➤*Depression:* Observe patients who have a history of psychic depression and discontinue the drug if depression recurs to a serious degree.

➤*Glucose tolerance:* A decrease in glucose tolerance has been observed in a small percentage of patients on estrogen-progestin combination drugs. The mechanism of this decrease is not known. For this reason, carefully observe diabetic patients receiving progestin therapy.

➤*Menopause:* The age of the patient constitutes no absolute limiting factor although treatment with progestins may mask the onset of the climacteric.

➤*Causes of weight loss:* Institute therapy with **megestrol** for weight loss only after treatable causes of weight loss are sought and addressed. These treatable causes include possible malignancies, systemic infections, GI disorders affecting absorption and endocrine, renal or psychiatric diseases.

➤*Benzyl alcohol:* Benzyl alcohol, contained in some of these products as a preservative, has been associated with a fatal "gasping syndrome" in premature infants.

➤*Pregnancy:* *Category D* (**progesterone** injection); *Category X* (**norethindrone acetate**). Use is not recommended (see Warning Box). Progesterone gel is used to support embryo implantation and maintain pregnancies as part of ART treatments.

Fertility impairment – Medroxyprogesterone acetate at high doses is an antifertility drug. High doses would be expected to impair fertility until the cessation of treatment.

➤*Lactation:* Detectable amounts of progestins enter the milk of mothers receiving these agents. The effect on the nursing infant has not been determined.

Medroxyprogesterone does not adversely affect lactation and may increase milk production and duration of lactation if given in the puerperium.

➤*Children:* Safety and efficacy of **megestrol acetate suspension** in children have not been established.

➤*Lab test abnormalities:* Laboratory test results of hepatic function, coagulation tests (increase in prothrombin, Factors VII, VIII, IX and X), thyroid, metyrapone test and endocrine functions, may be affected by progestins.

Drug Interactions

Progestins Drug Interactions			
Precipitant drug	Object drug[a]		Description
Aminoglutethimide	Medroxyprogesterone	⬇	Aminoglutethimide may increase the hepatic metabolism of medroxyprogesterone, possibly decreasing its therapeutic effects.
Rifampin	Norethindrone	⬇	Rifampin may reduce the plasma levels of norethindrone via hepatic microsomal enzyme induction, possibly decreasing its pharmacologic effects.

[a] ⬇ = Object drug decreased.

➤*Pregnanediol:* Pregnanediol determination may be altered by the use of progestins.

Adverse Reactions

For information concerning adverse reactions associated with combined estrogen-progestin therapy, refer to the Oral Contraceptives group monograph.

➤*General:*

CNS – Insomnia; somnolence; mental depression.

Dermatologic – Rash (allergic) with and without pruritus; acne; melasma or chloasma. **Progesterone** is irritating at the injection site whether the oil or aqueous vehicle is used; however, the aqueous preparation is particularly painful.

GI – Changes in weight (increase or decrease); nausea.

GU – Breakthrough bleeding; spotting; change in menstrual flow; amenorrhea; changes in cervical eversion, cervical secretions; galactorrhea.

Miscellaneous – Breast changes (tenderness); masculinization of the female fetus; edema; cholestatic jaundice; pyrexia; hirsutism.

➤*Medroxyprogesterone acetate:*

Miscellaneous – Sensitivity reactions ranging from pruritus and urticaria to generalized rash; alopecia; hirsutism.

➤*Progesterone gel:*

Progesterone Gel Adverse Reactions (%)		
Adverse reaction	90 mg once daily	90 mg twice daily
CNS		
Somnolence	27	-
Headache	17	13
Nervousness	16	-
Depression	11	-
Libido decreased	10	-
Dizziness	-	5
GI		
Constipation	27	-
Nausea	22	7
Diarrhea	8	-
Vomiting	5	-
GU		
Breast enlargement	40	-
Breast pain	-	13
Moniliasis, genital	-	7
Vaginal discharge	-	7
Dyspareunia	6	-
Miscellaneous		
Nocturia	13	-
Arthralgia	8	-
Pruritus	-	5
Perineal pain	17	-
Cramps	-	15
Abdominal pain	12	-
Pain	-	8
Bloating	-	7

➤*Additional adverse events reported in women at a frequency less than 5% include the following:*

CNS – Emotional lability; insomnia.

Dermatologic – Acne; pruritus.

GI – Dyspepsia; eructation; flatulence.

GU – Dysuria; micturition frequency; UTI.

Miscellaneous – Allergy; fatigue; fever; influenza-like symptoms; water retention; asthma; back pain; leg pain; sinusitis; upper respiratory tract infection.

➤*Megestrol acetate suspension:*

Megestrol Adverse Reactions (%)[a]		
Adverse reaction	Megestrol	Placebo
Diarrhea	8 to 15	8 to 15
Impotence	4 to 14	≤ 3
Rash	2 to 12	3 to 9
Flatulence	≤ 10	3 to 9
Hypertension	≤ 8	0
Asthenia	2 to 6	3 to 8
Insomnia	≤ 6	0
Nausea	≤ 5	3 to 9
Anemia	≤ 5	≤ 6
Fever	2 to 6	3
Libido decreased	≤ 5	≤ 3
Dyspepsia	≤ 4	≤ 5
Hyperglycemia	≤ 6	≤ 3
Headache	≤ 10	3 to 6
Pain	≤ 6	5 to 6
Vomiting	≤ 6	3 to 9
Pneumonia	≤ 3	3 to 6
Urinary frequency	≤ 2	≤ 5

[a] Data pooled from several studies. Percentages listed for megestrol without regard to specified dosage.

➤*Other adverse reactions reported in 1% to 3% of patients on megestrol include the following:*

Cardiovascular – Cardiomyopathy; palpitation.

CNS – Paresthesia; confusion; convulsion; depression; neuropathy; hypesthesia; abnormal thinking.

Dermatologic – Alopecia; herpes; pruritus; vesiculobullous rash; sweating; skin disorder.

GI – Constipation; dry mouth; hepatomegaly; increased salivation; oral moniliasis.

GU – Albuminuria; urinary incontinence; urinary tract infection; gynecomastia.

Respiratory – Dyspnea; cough; pharyngitis; lung disorder.

Miscellaneous – Leukopenia; amblyopia; LDH increased; edema; peripheral edema; abdominal pain; chest pain; infection; moniliasis; sarcoma.

Patient Information

Patient package insert is available with product.

If GI upset occurs, take with food.

➤*Diabetic patients:* Glucose tolerance may be decreased; monitor urine sugar closely and report any abnormalities to physician.

Notify physician if pregnancy is suspected or if any of the following occurs: Sudden severe headache; visual disturbance; numbness in an arm or leg.

➤*Vaginal gel:* Do not use concurrently with other local intravaginal therapy. If other local intravaginal therapy is to be used concurrently, administer ≥ 6 hours before or after progesterone gel.

PROGESTERONE

Rx	**Prometrium** (Solvay)	**Capsules, micronized soft gel; oral:** 100 mg	Glycerin, peanut oil. (SV). Round, peach. In 100s.
		200 mg	Glycerin, peanut oil. (SV2). Oval, pale yellow. In 100s.
Rx	**Progesterone in Oil** (Various, eg, APP, Watson)	**Injection:** 50 mg/mL	May contain sesame oil, benzyl alcohol. In 10 mL multidose vials.
Rx	**Crinone** (Watson Labs)	**Gel; vaginal:** 4% (45 mg)	Glycerin, mineral oil, palm oil. In single-use, prefilled applicator. In 6s.
Rx	**Prochieve** (Columbia Labs)		Glycerin, mineral oil, palm oil. In single-use, prefilled applicator. In 6s.
Rx	**Crinone** (Watson Labs)	**Gel; vaginal:** 8% (90 mg)	Glycerin, mineral oil, palm oil. In single-use, prefilled applicator. In 15s.
Rx	**Endometrin** (Ferring Pharmaceuticals)	**Insert, micronized; vaginal:** 100 mg	(FPI 100). Oblong. UD with 21 vaginal applicators. In 21s.

PROGESTERONE — ORAL

For complete and comparative prescribing information, refer to the Progestins class monograph.

WARNING

Progestins plus estrogens should not be used for the prevention of cardiovascular disease or dementia.

The Women's Health Initiative (WHI) estrogen plus progestin substudy reported increased risks of myocardial infarction (MI), stroke, pulmonary embolism, and deep vein thrombosis in postmenopausal women (50 to 79 years of age) during 5.6 years of treatment with daily oral conjugated estrogens 0.625 mg combined with medroxyprogesterone acetate 2.5 mg relative to placebo.

The WHI estrogen plus progestin substudy also demonstrated an increased risk of invasive breast cancer.

The Women's Health Initiative Memory Study (WHIMS) estrogen plus progestin ancillary study of the WHI reported an increased risk of developing probable dementia in postmenopausal women 65 years of age and older.

Indications

➤*Endometrial hyperplasia:* For use in the prevention of endometrial hyperplasia in nonhysterectomized postmenopausal women who are receiving conjugated estrogens tablets.

➤*Secondary amenorrhea:* For use in secondary amenorrhea.

Administration and Dosage

➤*Adults:*

Prevention of endometrial hyperplasia – 200 mg/day as a single dose at bedtime for 12 days sequentially per 28-day cycle for postmenopausal women with a uterus who are receiving daily conjugated estrogens tablets.

Secondary amenorrhea – 400 mg/day as a single dose at bedtime for 10 days.

➤*Hepatic function impairment:* Contraindicated in patients with known liver dysfunction or disease.

➤*Administration:* Some women may experience difficulty swallowing progesterone capsules. For these women, progesterone capsules should be taken with a glass of water while in the standing position.

➤*Storage/Stability:* Store at 25°C (77°F); excursions are permitted from 15° to 30°C (59° to 86°F). Dispense in tight, light-resistant container. Protect from excessive moisture.

PROGESTERONE — VAGINAL

For complete and comparative prescribing information, refer to the Progestins group monograph.

Indications

➤*Assisted reproductive technology (ART):*

Progesterone gel (8% only) – For progesterone supplementation or replacement as part of an ART treatment for infertile women with progesterone deficiency.

Progesterone insert – To support embryo implantation and early pregnancy by supplementation of corpus luteal function as part of an ART treatment program for infertile women.

➤*Secondary amenorrhea:*

Progesterone gel – The 4% gel is for the treatment of secondary amenorrhea, and the 8% gel is for women who have failed to respond to treatment with the 4% gel.

Administration and Dosage

➤*Adults:*

Vaginal gel –

Assisted reproductive technology:

• *Duration of therapy* – If pregnancy occurs, continue treatment up to 10 to 12 weeks until placental autonomy is achieved.

• *Progesterone supplementation* – 90 mg (1 applicatorful of 8% gel) vaginally once daily in women who require progesterone supplementation.

• *Progesterone replacement* – 90 mg (1 applicatorful of 8% gel) vaginally twice daily in women with partial or complete ovarian failure, who require progesterone replacement.

Secondary amenorrhea:

• *Initial dosage* – 45 mg (1 applicatorful of 4% gel) vaginally every other day for up to a total of 6 doses.

• *Dosage adjustment* – For women who fail to respond, a trial of 90 mg (1 applicatorful of 8% gel) every other day up to a total of 6 doses may be instituted. It is important to note that a dosage increase from the 4% gel can only be accomplished by using the 8% gel. An increase in the volume of gel administered does not increase the amount of progesterone absorbed.

Vaginal insert –

Assisted reproductive technology: 100 mg administered vaginally 2 or 3 times daily starting at oocyte retrieval and continuing for up to 10 weeks total duration.

➤*Storage/Stability:* Store at 25°C (77°F); excursions are permitted to 15° to 30°C (59° to 86°F).

PROGESTERONE — INJECTION

For complete and comparative prescribing information, refer to the Progestins group monograph.

Indications

➤*Amenorrhea and abnormal uterine bleeding:* For the treatment of amenorrhea and abnormal uterine bleeding caused by hormonal imbalance in the absence of organic pathology, such as submucous fibroids or uterine cancer.

Administration and Dosage

➤*Adults:*

Amenorrhea – 5 to 10 mg/day intramuscular (IM) for 6 to 8 consecutive days. If there has been sufficient ovarian activity to produce a proliferative endometrium, one can expect withdrawal bleeding 48 to 72 hours after the last injection. This may be followed by spontaneous normal cycles.

PROGESTERONE — INJECTION

Functional uterine bleeding –

Usual dosage: 5 to 10 mg/day IM for 6 doses. Bleeding may be expected to cease within 6 days. If menstrual flow begins during the course of injections of progesterone, the injections are discontinued.

Concomitant therapy: When estrogen is given as well, the administration of progesterone is begun after 2 weeks of estrogen therapy.

➤*Hepatic function impairment:* Because progesterone is metabolized by the liver, use in patients with hepatic function impairment or liver disease is contraindicated.

➤*Administration:* Progesterone is administered by IM injection. It differs from other commonly used steroids in that it is irritating at the place of injection. This is true whether the preparation is an oil or an aqueous vehicle. The latter is particularly painful.

➤*Storage/Stability:* Store at 15° to 30°C (59° to 86°F).

HYDROXYPROGESTERONE CAPROATE

Rx	**Makena** (Ther-Rx)	**Injection, solution:** 250 mg/mL	Castor oil, benzyl alcohol, benzyl benzoate. In 5 mL multidose vials.

HYDROXYPROGESTERONE CAPROATE — INJECTION

Indications

➤*Preterm birth:* To reduce the risk of preterm birth in women with a singleton pregnancy who have a history of singleton spontaneous preterm birth.

Administration and Dosage

➤*Adults:*

Preterm birth –

Usual dosage: 250 mg administered intramuscularly (IM) once weekly (every 7 days). Begin treatment between 16 weeks, 0 days and 20 weeks, 6 days of gestation.

Duration of therapy: Continue administration once weekly until week 37 (through 36 weeks, 6 days) of gestation or delivery, whichever occurs first.

➤*Children:* See Adults for dosing in adolescents 16 years and older.

➤*Preparation for administration:* Draw up 1 mL of drug into a 3 mL syringe with an 18-gauge needle. Change the needle to a 21-gauge 1½ inch needle.

➤*Administration:* After preparing the skin, inject IM in the upper outer quadrant of the gluteus maximus. The solution is viscous and oily. Slow injection (over 1 minute or longer) is recommended.

Apply pressure to the injection site to minimize bruising and swelling.

Discard any unused product 5 weeks after first use.

➤*Storage/Stability:* Store at 15° to 30°C (59° to 86°F). Use within 5 weeks after first use. Protect vial from light and store upright in its box.

MEDROXYPROGESTERONE ACETATE

Rx	**Medroxyprogesterone Acetate** (Various, eg, Barr, Greenstone)	**Tablets:** 2.5 mg	In 30s, 90s, 100s, 500s and 1000s.
Rx	**Provera** (Pharmacia & Upjohn)		(PROVERA 2.5). Lactose, sucrose. Orange, scored. In 30s and 100s.
Rx	**Medroxyprogesterone Acetate** (Various, eg, Barr, Greenstone)	**Tablets:** 5 mg	In 30s, 100s, 500s and 1000s.
Rx	**Provera** (Pharmacia & Upjohn)		(PROVERA 5). Lactose, sucrose. White, scored. Hexagonal. In 30s and 100s.
Rx	**Medroxyprogesterone Acetate** (Various, eg, Barr, Geneva, Greenstone)	**Tablets:** 10 mg	In 30s, 40s, 50s, 100s, 250s and 500s.
Rx	**Provera** (Pharmacia & Upjohn)		(PROVERA 10). Lactose, sucrose. White, scored. In 30s, 100s, 500s and UD 10s.

MEDROXYPROGESTERONE ACETATE — ORAL

For complete and comparative prescribing information, refer to the Progestins group monograph. Parenteral medroxyprogesterone acetate is used as an antineoplastic agent; refer to the monograph in the Antineoplastics section.

Indications

➤*Secondary amenorrhea:* Secondary amenorrhea and abnormal uterine bleeding due to hormonal imbalance in the absence of organic pathology, such as fibroids or uterine cancer.

➤*Endometrial hyperplasia:* To reduce the incidence of endometrial hyperplasia in nonhysterectomized postmenopausal women receiving conjugated estrogen 0.625 mg.

➤*Off-label uses:* Treatment of advanced breast cancer.

Administration and Dosage

➤*Adults:*

Abnormal uterine bleeding caused by hormonal imbalance in the absence of organic pathology –

Usual dosage: 5 or 10 mg daily for 5 to 10 days, beginning day 16 or 21 of the menstrual cycle.

Alternative dosage: To produce an optimum secretory transformation of an endometrium that has been adequately primed with endogenous or exogenous estrogen, give 10 mg daily for 10 days, beginning day 16 of the cycle.

Discontinuation of therapy: Withdrawal bleeding usually occurs 3 to 7 days after discontinuing therapy. Patients with recurrent episodes of abnormal uterine bleeding may benefit from planned menstrual cycling with medroxyprogesterone acetate.

Endometrial hyperplasia – 5 or 10 mg daily for 12 to 14 consecutive days per month, beginning day 1 or 16 of the cycle.

Secondary amenorrhea –

Usual dosage: 5 or 10 mg daily for 5 to 10 days. Start therapy any time.

Alternative dosage: A dose for inducing an optimum secretory transformation of an endometrium that has been adequately primed with endogenous or exogenous estrogen is 10 mg daily for 10 days.

Discontinuation of therapy: Withdrawal bleeding usually occurs 3 to 7 days after therapy ends.

➤*Renal function impairment:* Because progestogens may cause some degree of fluid retention, conditions that might be influenced by this factor such as renal dysfunction require careful observation.

➤*Hepatic function impairment:* For patients with mild to moderate degree of hepatic impairment, a lower dose of medroxyprogesterone acetate or a less frequent administration should be considered.

Medroxyprogesterone acetate is contraindicated in patients with severe hepatic disease.

➤*Storage/Stability:* Store at 20° to 25°C (68° to 77°F).

NORETHINDRONE ACETATE

Rx	**Norethindrone** (Barr)	**Tablets; oral:** 5 mg	Scored. In 50s.
Rx	**Aygestin** (Duramed)		(5 AYGESTIN B/424). Lactose. Oval, scored. In 50s and blister pack 10s.

NORETHINDRONE ACETATE — ORAL

For complete and comparative prescribing information, refer to the Progestins group monograph.

Indications

➤*Amenorrhea:* For the treatment of secondary amenorrhea.

➤*Endometriosis:* For the treatment of endometriosis.

➤*Uterine bleeding:* For the treatment of abnormal uterine bleeding caused by hormonal imbalance in the absence of organic pathology such as submucous fibroids or uterine cancer.

Administration and Dosage

➤*Adults:*

Amenorrhea – 2.5 to 10 mg may be given daily for 5 to 10 days to produce secretory transformation of an endometrium that has been adequately primed with either endogenous or exogenous estrogen.

Progestins

NORETHINDRONE ACETATE — ORAL

Endometriosis –

Initial dosage: 5 mg daily for 2 weeks.

Dosage titration: Increase by 2.5 mg/day every 2 weeks until 15 mg/day of norethindrone is reached. Therapy may be held at this level for 6 to 9 months or until annoying breakthrough bleeding demands temporary termination.

Uterine bleeding – See Amenorrhea for dosing.

➤*Hepatic function impairment:* Contraindicated in patients with impaired liver function or liver disease.

➤*Administration:* Administer once daily, without regard to meals. Administer with food if GI upset occurs.

➤*Storage / Stability:* Store at 20° to 25°C (68° to 77°F).

MEGESTROL ACETATE

Rx	**Megestrol Acetate** (Various, eg, UDL)	**Tablets:** 20 mg	In 100s and UD 100s.
Rx	**Megestrol Acetate** (Various, eg, Major, UDL)	**Tablets:** 40 mg	In 100s, 500s, UD 100s, and blister package 25s.
Rx	**Megace** (Bristol-Myers Oncology)		Lactose. Lt. blue, scored. In 250s and 500s.
Rx	**Megestrol Acetate** (Various, eg, Roxane, Teva)	**Suspension:** 40 mg/mL	Alcohol, sorbitol, sucrose. In 240 mL.
Rx	**Megace** (Bristol-Myers Oncology)		≤ 0.06% alcohol, sucrose. Lemon-lime flavor. In 240 mL.
Rx	**Megace ES** (Par Pharmaceutical, Inc.)	**Suspension:** 125 mg/mL	≤ 0.06% alcohol, sucrose. Lemon-lime flavor. In 150 mL.

MEGESTROL ACETATE — ORAL

For complete and comparative prescribing information, refer to the Progestins group monograph.

Indications

➤*Tablets:* For the palliative treatment of advanced carcinoma of the breast or endometrium (recurrent, inoperable, or metastatic disease). It should not be used in lieu of currently accepted procedures such as surgery, radiation, or chemotherapy.

➤*Oral suspension:* For the treatment of anorexia, cachexia, or an unexplained, significant weight loss in patients with a diagnosis of acquired immunodeficiency syndrome (AIDS).

➤*Off-label uses:*

Hot flashes – [3] = Safety concerns. One investigative group has stated that megestrol acetate is the recommended treatment for hot flashes in patients with prostate cancer who have undergone androgen deprivation therapy. Another group has suggested that use for this indication is reasonable but encourages health care providers to review the potential risks with patients. (See Administration and Dosage.)

Other possible off-label uses – Appetite stimulant for cachexia in advanced cancer.

Administration and Dosage

➤*Adults:*

Anorexia, cachexia, or unexplained, significant weight loss in AIDS patients – The initial dosage is 800 mg/day (20 mL/day) of the oral suspension (40 mg/mL) or 625 mg/day (5 mL/day) of the extra strength oral suspension (125 mg/mL).

In clinical trials evaluating different dose schedules, daily doses of 400 and 800 mg/day of the 40 mg/mL oral suspension were found to be clinically effective.

Breast cancer –

Usual dosage: 160 mg/day (40 mg 4 times a day; tablets only). For palliation only.

Duration of therapy: At least 2 months of continuous treatment is considered an adequate period for determining the efficacy of megestrol.

Endometrial carcinoma –

Usual dosage: 40 to 320 mg/day in divided doses (tablets only). For palliation only.

Duration of therapy: At least 2 months of continuous treatment is considered an adequate period for determining the efficacy of megestrol acetate.

Off-label dosing –

Hot flashes: [3] = Safety concerns. 40 mg daily (20 mg twice daily). One follow-up study demonstrated that continued beneficial effects were maintained with chronic dosing of 20 mg/day or less. Once benefits are recognized, the dose may be tapered to the lowest effective dose.

➤*Preparation for administration:* Megestrol is a hormonal agent and is also considered a teratogen. Follow safe handling procedures when preparing, administering, or dispensing megestrol.

➤*Administration:* Shake oral suspension well before using.

➤*Storage / Stability:*

Tablets – Store at 25°C (77°F); excursions permitted to 15° to 30°C (59° to 86°F). Protect from temperatures above 40°C (104°F).

Oral suspension – Store megestrol acetate oral suspension between 15° to 25°C (59° to 77°F) and dispense in a tight container. Protect from heat.

Estrogen/Progestin Combinations

ESTROGEN/PROGESTIN COMBINATIONS

Rx	**Prempro** (Wyeth)	**Tablets; oral:** Conjugated estrogens 0.3 mg/medroxyprogesterone acetate 1.5 mg	Lactose, sucrose. (Prempro 0.3/1.5). Cream, oval. In blister card 28s.
		Conjugated estrogens 0.45 mg/ medroxyprogesterone acetate 1.5 mg	Lactose, sucrose. (Prempro 0.45/1.5). Gold, oval. In blister card 28s.
		Conjugated estrogens 0.625 mg/ medroxyprogesterone acetate 2.5 mg	Lactose, sucrose. (Prempro). Peach, oval. In blister card 28s.
		Conjugated estrogens 0.625 mg /medroxyprogesterone acetate 5 mg	Lactose, sucrose. (W 0.625/5). Lt. blue, oval. In blister card 28s.
Rx	**Premphase** (Wyeth)	**Tablets; oral:** Conjugated estrogens 0.625 mg; conjugated estrogens 0.625 mg/medroxyprogesterone acetate 5 mg	Lactose, sucrose. (PREMARIN 0.625). **Estrogen only:** Maroon, oval. **Estrogen/ Progestin:** (W 0.625/5). Lt. blue, oval. In blister card 28s (14 of each tablet).
Rx	**Angeliq** (Bayer)	**Tablets; oral:** Estradiol 1 mg/drospirenone 0.5 mg	Lactose. (CK). Pink, round. Film-coated. In blister pack 28s.
Rx	**Femhrt** (Warner Chilcott)	**Tablets; oral:** Ethinyl estradiol 2.5 mcg/ norethindrone acetate 0.5 mg	Lactose. (PD 145). White, oval. In 90s and blister card 28s.
Rx	**Femhrt** (Warner Chilcott)	**Tablets; oral:** Ethinyl estradiol 5 mcg/ norethindrone acetate 1 mg	Lactose. (PD 144). White, D-shaped. In 90s and blister card 28s.
Rx	**Jinteli** (Teva)		Lactose. (b 125). White, round. In 90s and blister card 28s.
Rx	**Activella** (Novo Nordisk)	**Tablets; oral:** Estradiol 0.5 mg/ norethindrone acetate 0.1 mg	Lactose. (NOVO 291). White, round. Film-coated. In dial pack 28s.
Rx	**Estradiol & Norethindrone Acetate** (Breckenridge)	**Tablets; oral:** Estradiol 1 mg/ norethindrone acetate 0.5 mg	May contain lactose. In blister pack 28s.
Rx	**Mimvey** (Teva)		Lactose. (b 34). White, round. Film-coated. In blister card 28s.
Rx	**Activella** (Novo Nordisk)		Lactose. (NOVO 288). White, round. Film-coated. In dial pack 28s.

ESTROGEN/PROGESTIN COMBINATIONS

Rx	**Prefest** (Duramed)	**Tablets; oral:** Estradiol 1 mg; estradiol 1 mg/norgestimate 0.09 mg	Lactose. **Estradiol only:** (P 93). Peach, round. **Estradiol/Norgestimate:** (P 92). White, round. In blister card 30s (15 of each tablet).
Rx	**Climara Pro** (Bayer)	**Patch; transdermal:** Estradiol 0.045 mg/levonorgestrel 0.015 mg per day	4.4 mg total estradiol and 1.39 mg total levonorgestrel per transdermal system. 22 cm^2. In 4s.
Rx	**CombiPatch** (Novartis)	**Patch; transdermal:** Estradiol 0.05 mg/norethindrone acetate 0.14 mg per day	0.62 mg total estradiol and 2.7 mg total norethindrone acetate per transdermal system. 9 cm^2. In 8s.
		Estradiol 0.05 mg/norethindrone acetate 0.25 mg per day	0.51 mg total estradiol and 4.8 mg total norethindrone acetate per transdermal system. 16 cm^2. In 8s.

ESTROGEN/PROGESTIN COMBINATIONS — ORAL

For additional information, refer to the Estrogens class monograph and the Progestins class monograph. Consider the information given for oral contraceptives (see class monograph) when using these products.

WARNING

Estrogens and progestins should not be used for the prevention of cardiovascular disease or dementia.

The estrogen-plus-progestin substudy of the Women's Health Initiative (WHI) reported increased risks of myocardial infarction (MI), stroke, invasive breast cancer, pulmonary emboli, and deep vein thrombosis (DVT) in postmenopausal women (50 to 79 years of age) during 5.6 years of treatment with oral conjugated estrogens 0.625 mg combined with medroxyprogesterone acetate 2.5 mg/day, relative to placebo.

The estrogen-alone substudy of the WHI reported increased risks of stroke and DVT in postmenopausal women (50 to 79 years of age) during 6.8 and 7.1 years, respectively, of treatment with oral conjugated estrogens 0.625 mg/day, relative to placebo.

There is an increased risk of endometrial cancer in a woman with a uterus who uses unopposed estrogens. Adding a progestin to estrogen therapy has been shown to reduce the risk of endometrial hyperplasia, which may be a precursor to endometrial cancer. Undertake adequate diagnostic measures, including directed or random endometrial sampling when indicated, to rule out malignancy in postmenopausal women with undiagnosed persistent or recurring abnormal genital bleeding.

The Women's Health Initiative Memory Study (WHIMS), a substudy of the WHI study, reported increased risk of developing probable dementia in postmenopausal women 65 years of age and older during 4 years of treatment with conjugated estrogens 0.625 mg combined with medroxyprogesterone 2.5 mg and during 5.2 years of treatment with conjugated estrogens 0.625 mg alone, relative to placebo. It is unknown whether this finding applies to younger postmenopausal women.

Other doses of oral conjugated estrogens with medroxyprogesterone acetate, and other combinations and dosage forms of estrogens and progestins were not studied in the WHI clinical trials; in the absence of comparable data, these risks should be assumed to be similar. Because of these risks, prescribe estrogens with or without progestins at the lowest effective doses and for the shortest duration consistent with treatment goals and risks for the individual woman.

Indications

➤*Moderate to severe vasomotor symptoms:* For treatment of moderate to severe vasomotor symptoms associated with menopause.

➤*Moderate to severe vulvar and vaginal atrophy (except Femhrt and Activella 0.5 mg/0.1 mg):* For treatment of moderate to severe symptoms of vulvar and vaginal atrophy associated with menopause.

When prescribing solely for the treatment of symptoms of vulvar and vaginal atrophy, consider topical vaginal products.

➤*Osteoporosis prevention (except Angeliq):* For prevention of postmenopausal osteoporosis.

When prescribing solely for the prevention of postmenopausal osteoporosis, consider therapy only for women at significant risk of osteoporosis; carefully consider nonestrogen medications.

Administration and Dosage

➤*General dosing considerations:* Patients should be started at the lowest dose.

For women who have a uterus, adequate diagnostic measures, such as endometrial sampling, when indicated, should be undertaken to rule out malignancy in cases of undiagnosed persistent or recurring abnormal vaginal bleeding. Patients should be evaluated for breast abnormalities in accordance with good clinical practice.

Use of estrogen, alone or in combination with a progestin, should be limited to the lowest effective dose available and to the shortest duration consistent with treatment goals and risks for the individual woman.

➤*Adults:*

Moderate to severe vasomotor symptoms –

Usual dosage:

• *Activella, Angeliq, Femhrt, Mimvey,* and *Prempro* – One tablet daily.

• *Prefest* – One estradiol 1 mg (peach) tablet daily for 3 days, followed by 1 estradiol 1 mg/norgestimate 0.09 mg (white) tablet daily for 3 days. This regimen is repeated continuously without interruption.

• *Premphase* – One conjugated estrogens 0.625 mg (maroon) tablet once daily on days 1 through 14 and 1 conjugated estrogens 0.625 mg/medroxyprogesterone 5 mg (light blue) tablet taken once daily on days 15 through 28.

Moderate to severe vulvar and vaginal atrophy (except Femhrt and Activella 0.5 mg/0.1 mg) – See Moderate to Severe Vasomotor Symptoms for dosing.

When used solely for the treatment of symptoms of vulval and vaginal atrophy, consider topical vaginal products.

Osteoporosis prevention (except Angeliq) – See Moderate to Severe Vasomotor Symptoms for dosing.

➤*Children:* Not indicated for use in children.

➤*Renal function impairment:* *Angeliq* is contraindicated in patients with renal insufficiency.

➤*Hepatic function impairment:* Contraindicated in patients with liver dysfunction or disease.

➤*Discontinuation of therapy:* Reevaluate patients at 3- to 6-month intervals to determine the need for continued treatment.

➤*Storage/Stability:* Store at 20° to 25°C (68° to 77°F). Store in a dry place protected from light.

ESTROGEN/PROGESTIN COMBINATIONS — TRANSDERMAL

For complete and comparative prescribing information, refer to the Estrogen/Progestin Combinations Oral monograph. For additional information, refer to the Estrogens class monograph and the Progestins class monograph.

WARNING

Estrogens and progestins should not be used for the prevention of cardiovascular disease or dementia.

The Women's Health Initiative (WHI) study reported increased risks of myocardial infarction (MI), stroke, invasive breast cancer, pulmonary emboli, and deep vein thrombosis (DVT) in postmenopausal women 50 to 79 years of age during 5 years of treatment with oral conjugated equine estrogens 0.625 mg combined with medroxyprogesterone acetate 2.5 mg relative to placebo.

The WHI study reported increased risks of stroke and DVT in postmenopausal women 50 to 79 years of age during 6.8 years of treatment with oral conjugated estrogens 0.625 mg relative to placebo.

The Women's Health Initiative Memory Study (WHIMS), a substudy of WHI, reported increased risk of developing probable dementia in postmenopausal women 65 years of age and older during 4 years of treatment with oral conjugated estrogens 0.625 mg plus medroxyprogesterone 2.5 mg and during 5.2 years of treatment with conjugated estrogens 0.625 mg alone, relative to placebo. It is unknown whether this finding applies to younger postmenopausal women.

WARNING (cont.)

Other doses of oral conjugated estrogens with medroxyprogesterone acetate, and other combinations and dosage forms of estrogens and progestins were not studied in the WHI clinical trials and, in the absence of comparable data, these risks should be assumed to be similar. Because of these risks, prescribe estrogens with or without progestins at the lowest effective doses and for the shortest duration consistent with treatment goals and risks for the individual woman.

Indications

➤*Moderate to severe vasomotor symptoms:* For treatment of moderate to severe vasomotor symptoms associated with the menopause.

➤*Moderate to severe vulvar and vaginal atrophy (CombiPatch only):* For treatment of moderate to severe symptoms of vulvar and vaginal atrophy associated with the menopause.

When prescribing solely for the treatment of symptoms of vulvar and vaginal atrophy, consider topical vaginal products.

➤*Hypoestrogenism (CombiPatch only):* For treatment of hypoestrogenism due to hypogonadism, castration, or primary ovarian failure.

➤*Osteoporosis prevention (Climara Pro only):* For prevention of postmenopausal osteoporosis.

ESTROGEN/PROGESTIN COMBINATIONS — TRANSDERMAL

When prescribing solely for the prevention of postmenopausal osteoporosis, consider therapy only for women at significant risk of osteoporosis; carefully consider nonestrogen medications.

Administration and Dosage

➤*General dosing considerations:* Use of estrogen alone or in combination with a progestin should be limited to the shortest duration and the lowest effective dose consistent with treatment goals and risks for the individual woman.

Patients should be started at the lowest dose.

For women who have a uterus, adequate diagnostic measures, such as endometrial sampling, when indicated, should be undertaken to rule out malignancy in cases of undiagnosed persistent or recurring abnormal vaginal bleeding.

➤*Adults:*

Moderate to severe vasomotor symptoms –

Usual dosage: Treatment of postmenopausal symptoms is usually initiated during the menopausal stage when vasomotor symptoms occur. Women currently using continuous estrogen or combination estrogen/progestin therapy should complete the current cycle of therapy before initiating *Climara Pro* or *CombiPatch* therapy. Women often experience withdrawal bleeding at the completion of the cycle. The first day of this bleeding would be an appropriate time to begin transdermal therapy.

• *Continuous combined regimen* – The transdermal system is worn continuously on the lower abdomen. A new system should be applied once weekly (*Climara Pro*) or twice weekly (*CombiPatch*) during a 28-day cycle. Irregular bleeding may occur particularly in the first 6 months, but generally decreases with time, and often to an amenorrheic state.

• *Continuous sequential regimen (CombiPatch* only) – *CombiPatch* can be applied as a sequential regimen in combination with an estradiol-only transdermal delivery system. In this treatment regimen, an estradiol 0.05 mg/day (nominal delivery rate) transdermal system (*Vivelle*) is worn for the first 14 days of a 28-day cycle, replacing the system twice weekly according to product directions. For the remaining 14 days of the 28-day cycle, *CombiPatch* estradiol 0.05 mg/norethindrone 0.14 mg/day (9 cm^2) transdermal system should be applied to the lower abdomen. Additionally, an estradiol 0.05 mg/norethindrone 0.25 mg/day (16 cm^2) system is available if a greater progestin dose is desired. The *CombiPatch* system should be replaced twice weekly during this period in the cycle. Women should be advised that monthly withdrawal bleeding often occurs.

Moderate to severe vulvar and vaginal atrophy (CombiPatch only) – See Moderate to Severe Vasomotor Symptoms for dosing.

Hypoestrogenism (CombiPatch only) – See Moderate to Severe Vasomotor Symptoms for dosing.

Osteoporosis prevention (Climara Pro only) – See Moderate to Severe Vasomotor Symptoms for dosing.

➤*Hepatic function impairment:* Contraindicated in patients with liver dysfunction of disease.

➤*Concomitant progestin therapy:* When estrogen therapy is prescribed for a postmenopausal woman with a uterus, a progestin should be initiated to reduce the risk of endometrial cancer. A woman without a uterus does not need progestin.

➤*Discontinuation of therapy:* Reevaluate patients periodically as clinically appropriate (eg, 3- to 6-month intervals) to determine whether treatment is still necessary.

➤*Administration:*

Application – Place on a smooth (fold-free), clean, dry area of the skin on the lower abdomen. Do not apply to or near the breasts. The area selected should not be oily (which can impair adherence of the system), damaged, or irritated. The waistline should be avoided because tight clothing may rub the system off or modify drug delivery. The sites of application must be rotated, with an interval of at least 1 week allowed between applications to the same site.

After opening the pouch, remove one side of the protective liner, taking care not to touch the adhesive part of the transdermal delivery system with the fingers. Immediately apply the transdermal delivery system to a smooth (fold-free) area of skin on the lower abdomen. Remove the second side of the protective liner and press the system firmly in place with the hand for at least 10 seconds, making sure there is good contact, especially around the edges.

Care should be taken that the system does not become dislodged during bathing and other activities. If a system should fall off, the same system may be reapplied to another area of the lower abdomen. If necessary, a new transdermal system may be applied, in which case, the original treatment schedule should be continued. Only one system should be worn at any one time during the 1-week (*Climara Pro*) or 3- to 4-day (*CombiPatch*) dosing interval.

Once in place, the transdermal system should not be exposed to the sun for prolonged periods of time.

Removal – Removal of the system should be done carefully and slowly to avoid irritation of the skin. If any adhesive remains on the skin after removal of the system, allow the area to dry for 15 minutes, then gently rubbing the area with an oil-based cream or lotion should remove the adhesive residue.

Used patches still contain some active hormones. Each patch should be carefully folded in half so that it sticks to itself before throwing it away.

➤*Storage/Stability:* Store *Climara Pro* at 20° to 25°C (68° to 77°F); excursions are permitted to 15° to 30°C (59° to 85°F).

Prior to dispensing to the patient, store *CombiPatch* refrigerated at 2° to 8°C (36° to 46°F). After dispensing to the patient, *CombiPatch* can be stored at room temperature below 25°C (77°F) for up to 6 months. When *CombiPatch* is dispensed to the patient, place an expiration date on the label. The date should not exceed 6 months from the date of sale or the expiration date, whichever comes first. Store the systems in the sealed foil pouch. Do not store the system in areas where extreme temperatures can occur.

ESTROGEN/ANDROGEN COMBINATIONS

Rx	**Esterified Estrogens and Methyltestosterone H.S.** (Various, eg, Breckenridge, Interpharm, Lannett)	**Tablets; oral:** 0.625 mg esterified estrogens and 1.25 mg methyltestosterone	May contain lactose. In 100s and 1,000s.
Rx	**Covaryx H.S.** (Centrix)		Lactose, tartrazine. (C020). Lt. pink, capsule shape. Film-coated. In 100s.
Rx	**Estratest H.S.** (Solvay)		Lactose, sucrose, parabens. (SOLVAY 1023). Lt. green, capsule shape. Sugar coated. In 100s.
Rx	Esterified Estrogens and Methyltestosterone (Various, eg, (Breckenridge, Interpharm, Lannett)	**Tablets; oral:** 1.25 mg esterified estrogens and 2.5 mg methyltestosterone	May contain lactose. In 100s and 1,000s.
Rx	**Covaryx** (Centrix)		Lactose, tartrazine. (C010) Lt. yellow, capsule shape. Film-coated. In 100s.
Rx	**Estratest** (Solvay)		Lactose, sucrose, parabens. (SOLVAY 1026). Dk. green, capsule shape. Sugar-coated. In 100s and 1000s.

ESTROGEN/ANDROGEN COMBINATIONS — ORAL

For complete and comparative prescribing information, refer to the Estrogens and Androgens class monographs.

WARNING

Estrogens have been reported to increase the risk of endometrial carcinoma.

Close clinical surveillance of all women taking estrogens is important. In all cases of undiagnosed, persistent, or recurring abnormal vaginal bleeding, adequate diagnostic measures should be undertaken to rule out malignancy.

Do not use estrogens during pregnancy.

The use of female sex hormones, estrogens and progestogens, during early pregnancy may seriously damage the offspring.

Refer to the Warning Box in the Estrogens group monograph for more information.

Indications

➤*Moderate to severe vasomotor symptoms:* Moderate to severe vasomotor symptoms associated with menopause in patients not improved with estrogens alone.

Administration and Dosage

➤*General dosing considerations:* Use the lowest dose that will control symptoms and discontinue medication as promptly as possible.

➤*Adults:*

Moderate to severe vasomotor symptoms –

Usual dosage: One of the esterified estrogens 1.25 mg/methyltestosterone 2.5 mg tablets or 1 or 2 of the esterified estrogens 0.625 mg/methyltestosterone 1.25 mg tablets daily, as recommended by the health care provider. Administer cyclically (3 weeks on and 1 week off) for short-term use only.

Discontinuation of therapy: Make attempts to discontinue or taper medication at 3- to 6-month intervals.

➤*Monitoring:* Closely monitor treated patients with an intact uterus for signs of endometrial cancer and take appropriate diagnostic measures to rule out malignancy in the event of persistent or recurring abnormal vaginal bleeding.

➤*Storage/Stability:* Store at 15° to 30°C (59° to 86°F).

Warnings/Precautions

➤*Pregnancy: Category X.* These medications are contraindicated for use in pregnant women because of the possibility of masculinization of the female fetus.

➤*Lab test abnormalities:* Methyltestosterone should not be used in breast-feeding mothers because of the possibility of masculinization of the female breast-fed infant.

CONTRACEPTIVES, ORAL

WARNING

Smoking – Cigarette smoking increases the risk of serious cardiovascular side effects from oral contraceptives (OCs). This risk increases with age and with heavy smoking (at least 15 cigarettes daily) and is quite marked in women older than 35 years of age. Women who use OCs should not smoke.

Indications

➤*Acne vulgaris (Ortho Tri-Cyclen and Estrostep only):* For the treatment of moderate acne vulgaris in females at least 15 years of age who have no known contraindications to oral contraceptive therapy and who desire contraception, have achieved menarche, and are unresponsive to topical antiacne medications.

➤*Contraception:* For the prevention of pregnancy.

Because of the positive association between the amount of estrogen and progestin in OCs and the risk of vascular disease and thromboembolism, minimizing exposure to these agents is in keeping with good principles of therapeutics. For any particular combination, prescribe the dosage regimen that contains the least amount of estrogen and progestin compatible with a low failure rate and needs of the individual patient. Start new patients on preparations containing estrogen 35 mcg or less.

➤*Emergency contraception (Plan B and Preven only):* For prevention of pregnancy following unprotected intercourse or a known or suspected contraceptive failure. To obtain efficacy, have the patient take the first dose as soon as possible within 72 hours of intercourse. The second dose must be taken 12 hours later.

➤*Premenstrual dysphoric disorder (PMDD) (YAZ only):* For treatment of symptoms of PMDD in women who choose to use an oral contraceptive as their method of contraception. The effectiveness of *YAZ* for PMDD when used for more than 3 menstrual cycles has not been evaluated.

Administration and Dosage

➤*Acne vulgaris:* The timing of dosing with *Ortho Tri-Cyclen* or *Estrostep* for acne should follow the guidelines for use of *Ortho Tri-Cyclen* or *Estrostep* as an OC. The dosage regimen for treatment of facial acne uses a 21-day active and a 7-day inert schedule. Have the patient take 1 active tablet daily for 21 days followed by 1 inert for 7 days. After 28 tablets have been taken, the patient should start a new course the next day.

➤*Contraception:*

Progestin-only – One tablet every day at the same time. Administration is continuous, with no interruption between pill packs. Every time a pill is taken late, especially if a pill is missed, pregnancy is more likely.

Missed dose: If the patient is more than 3 hours late or misses at least 1 tablet, she should take the missed pill as soon as remembered, then go back to taking progestin-only products (POPs) at the regular time, while being sure to use a backup method (eg, condom, spermicide) every time she has sexual intercourse for the next 48 hours.

Combined –

Sunday-start packaging: If the instructions recommend starting the regimen on Sunday, inform the patient to take the first tablet on the first Sunday after menstruation begins. If menstruation begins on Sunday, she should take the first tablet on that day.

21-day regimen: For day-1 start, the first day of menstrual bleeding should be counted as day 1. The cycle is to take 1 tablet per day for 21 days; no tablets are taken for 7 days. Whether bleeding has stopped or not, the patient should start a new course of the 21-day regimen. Withdrawal flow will normally occur approximately 3 days after the last tablet is taken. The patient must follow the schedule whether flow occurs as expected, or whether spotting or breakthrough bleeding (BTB) occurs during the cycle.

28-day regimen: To eliminate the need to count the days between cycles, some products contain 7 inert or iron-containing tablets to permit continuous daily dosage during the entire 28-day cycle. For patients who require estrogen during the latter part of the cycle or require a longer duration of estrogen/progestin therapy, please see the Monophasic Oral Contraceptives for more information.

84-day regimen: The dosage of *Seasonale* and *Seasonique* is 1 active tablet per day for 84 consecutive days, followed by 7 days of white (inert) tablets (*Seasonale*) or 7 yellow (ethinyl estradiol) tablets (*Seasonique*). Withdrawal bleeding should occur during the 7 days following discontinuation of active tablets. During the first cycle, the patient should not place contraceptive reliance on *Seasonale* or *Seasonique* until an active tablet has been taken daily for 7 consecutive days; the patient should use a nonhormonal backup method of birth control (such as condoms or spermicide) during those 7 days. The patient should consider the possibility of ovulation and conception prior to initiation of medication.

The patient begins her next and all subsequent 91-day courses of tablets without interruption on the same day of the week on which she began her first course, following the same schedule. If in any cycle the patient starts tablets later than the proper day, she should protect herself against pregnancy by using a nonhormonal backup method of birth control until she has taken an active tablet daily for 7 consecutive days.

Biphasic, triphasic, and 4-phasic OCs: Have the patient follow the instructions on the dispensers or packs; these are clearly marked, usually indicating where to start on the regimen and in what order to take the pills (usually marked with arrows), along with the appropriate week numbers. If there is any question, detailed instructions are provided in the specific package insert. As with the monophasic OCs, 1 tablet is taken each day; however, as the color of the tablet changes, the strength of the tablet also changes (the estrogen/progestin ratio varies).

Missed active dose: For information on missed doses of 4-phasic OCs, refer to the 4-Phasic Contraceptives, Oral monograph.

While there is little likelihood of ovulation occurring if only 1 tablet is missed, the possibility of spotting or bleeding is increased. The possibility of ovulation occurring increases with each successive day that scheduled tablets are missed. This is particularly likely to occur if at least 2 consecutive tablets are missed. Any time at least 1 active tablets have been missed, the patient should use another method of contraception for the balance of the cycle until tablets have been taken for 7 consecutive days. If a patient forgets to take at least 1 tablet, the following is suggested:

- *One active tablet –* Have the patient take this as soon as remembered or she should take 2 tablets the next day; alternatively, the patient can take 1 tablet, discard the other missed tablet, continue as scheduled, and use another form of contraception until menses.
- *Two consecutive active tablets –* The patient should take 2 tablets as soon as remembered with the next pill at the usual time or she should take 2 tablets daily for the next 2 days, then resume the regular schedule. The patient should use an additional form of contraception for the 7 days after pills are missed , preferably for the remainder of the cycle. If 2 active pills are missed in a row in the third week and the patient is a Sunday starter, 1 pill should be taken every day until Sunday. On Sunday, the rest of the pack should be discarded and a new pack of pills started that same day. If 2 active pills are missed in a row in the third week and the patient is a day-1 starter, the rest of the pill pack should be discarded and a new pack started that same day. Menses may not occur this month but this is expected. However, if menses do not occur 2 months in a row, the health care provider or clinic should be contacted because of the possibility of pregnancy.
- *Three consecutive active tablets –* If the patient is a Sunday starter, she should keep taking 1 pill every day until Sunday. On Sunday, the rest of the pack should be discarded and a new pack of pills started that same day. If she is a day-1 starter, the rest of the pill pack should be discarded and a new

CONTRACEPTIVES, ORAL

pack started that same day. Menses may not occur this month, but this is expected. However, if menses do not occur 2 months in a row, the health care provider or clinic should be contacted because of the possibility of pregnancy. Pregnancy may result from sexual intercourse during the 7 days after the pills are missed. The patient should use another birth control method (eg, condoms, foam) as a backup method for those 7 days.

Switching pills – If switching from the combined pills to POPs, the patient should take the first POP the day after the last active combined pill is finished. She should not take any of the 7 inactive pills from the combined pill pack. Many women have irregular periods after switching to POPs; this is normal and to be expected. If switching from POPs to the combined pills, the patient should take the first active combined pill on the first day of menses, even if the POP pack is not finished. If switching to another brand of POPs, she should start the new brand any time. If the patient is breastfeeding, she can switch to another method of birth control at any time, except she should not switch to the combined pills until breastfeeding is stopped or until at least 6 months after delivery.

Bleeding – Bleeding that resembles menstruation occurs rarely. Persistent bleeding not controlled by this method indicates the need for re-examination of the patient; consider nonhormonal causes. If pathology has been excluded, time or a change to another formulation may solve the problem.

Missed menstrual period – If the patient has not adhered to the prescribed dosage regimen, consider possible pregnancy after the first missed period; withhold OCs until ruling out pregnancy and use a nonhormonal method of contraception. If the patient has adhered to the prescribed regimen and misses 2 consecutive periods, rule out pregnancy before continuing the contraceptive regimen.

After several months of treatment, menstrual flow may reduce to a point of virtual absence. This reduced flow may occur as a result of medication and is not indicative of pregnancy.

Postpartum administration – Postpartum administration in non-breast-feeding mothers may begin at the first postpartum examination (4 to 6 weeks), regardless of whether spontaneous menstruation has occurred. Have the patient consider the possibility of ovulation and conception prior to initiation of medication. Also, the patient should start no earlier than 4 to 6 weeks after a midtrimester pregnancy termination. Immediate postpartum use is associated with increased risk of thromboembolism. If possible, breast-feeding mothers should defer taking OCs until the infant is weaned (see Warnings/Precautions).

If fully breastfeeding (not giving baby any food or formula), start the patient on POPs 6 weeks after delivery. If partially breastfeeding (giving baby some food or formula), the patient should start taking POPs by 3 weeks after delivery.

In the nonlactating mother, *Seasonale* may be initiated no earlier than day 28 postpartum for contraception because of the increased risk for thromboembolism. When the tablets are administered in the postpartum period, the increased risk of thromboembolic disease associated with the postpartum period must be considered. Advise the patient to use a nonhormonal backup method for the first 7 days of tablet-taking. However, if intercourse has already occurred, consider the possibility of ovulation and conception prior to initiation of medication. *Seasonale* may be initiated immediately after a first-trimester abortion; if the patient starts *Seasonale* immediately, additional contraceptive measures are not needed.

Dosage adjustments – Side effects noted during the initial cycles may be transient; if they continue, dosage adjustments may be indicated. Many side effects are related to the potency of the estrogen or progestin in the products. The following table summarizes these dose-related side effects.

Achieving Proper Hormonal Balance in an Oral Contraceptive

Estrogen		Progestin	
Excess	Deficiency	Excess	Deficiency
Nausea, bloating Cervical mucorrhea, polyposis Melasma Hypertension Migraine headache Breast fullness or tenderness Edema	Early or mid-cycle breakthrough bleeding Increased spotting Hypomenorrhea	Increased appetite Weight gain Tiredness, fatigue Hypomenorrhea Acne, oily scalp[a] Hair loss, hirsutism[a] Depression Monilial vaginitis Breast regression	Late breakthrough bleeding Amenorrhea Hypermenorrhea

[a] Result of androgenic activity of progestins.

Pharmacological Effects of Progestins Used in Oral Contraceptives[a]

	Progestin	Estrogen	Androgen
Desogestrel	++++	0	+++
Dienogest	No data	No data	No data
Levonorgestrel	++++	0	++++
Norgestrel	+++	0	+++
Ethynodiol diacetate	++	+++	+
Norgestimate	++	0	++
Norethindrone acetate	++	++	++
Norethindrone	++	++	++

[a] *Symbol Key: ++++ – pronounced effect; +++ – moderate effect; ++ – low effect; + – slight effect; 0 – no effect*

Minimize the effects listed in the table by adjusting the estrogen/progestin balance or dosage. The following table categorizes products by their estrogenic, progestational, and androgenic activity. Because overall activity is influenced by the interaction of components, including androgenic and antiestrogenic activity, it is difficult to precisely classify products; placement in the table is only approximate. Differences between products within a group are probably not clinically significant.

Estimated Relative Oral Contraceptive Progestin/Estrogen/Androgen Activity

	Ingredients	Brand-name examples	Progestin activity	Estrogen activity	Androgen activity
Monophasic	0.1 mg levonorgestrel/ 20 mcg EE[a]	*Alesse, Aviane, Lessina, Levlite*	Low	Low	Low
	0.25 mg norgestimate/35 mcg EE	*Ortho-Cyclen, Sprintec*		Intermediate	
	0.5 mg norethindrone/35 mcg EE	*Brevicon, Modicon, Necon 0.5/35, Nortrel 0.5/35*		High	
	0.4 mg norethindrone/35 mcg EE	*Ovcon-35*			
	0.15 mg levonorgestrel/30 mcg EE	*Levlen, Levora, Nordette, Portia*	Intermediate	Low	Intermediate
	0.3 mg norgestrel/30 mcg EE	*Cryselle, Lo-Ovral, Low-Ogestrel*			
	1 mg norethindrone/50 mcg mestranol	*Necon 1/50, Norinyl 1+50, Ortho-Novum 1/50*		Intermediate	
	1 mg norethindrone/35 mcg EE	*Necon 1/35, Norinyl 1+35, Nortrel 1/35, Ortho-Novum 1/35*		High	
	1 mg norethindrone/50 mcg EE	*Ovcon-50*			
	1 mg norethindrone acetate/20 mcg EE	*Loestrin 21 1/20, Loestrin Fe 1/20, Microgestin Fe 1/20*	High	Low	
	1.5 mg norethindrone acetate/30 mcg EE	*Loestrin 21 1.5/30, Loestrin Fe 1.5/30, Microgestin Fe 1.5/30*			High
	1 mg ethynodiol diacetate/35 mcg EE	*Demulen 1/35, Zovia 1/35E*			Low
	Desogestrel/EE 0.15 mg-20 mcg and EE 10 mcg	*Kariva, Mircette*			
	0.15 mg desogestrel/30 mcg EE	*Apri, Desogen, Ortho-Cept*	High	Intermediate	
	1 mg ethynodiol diacetate/50 mcg EE	*Demulen 1/50, Zovia 1/50E*			
	0.5 mg norgestrel/50 mcg EE	*Ovral, Ogestrel*		High	High
	3 mg drospirenone/30 mcg EE	*Yasmin*	No data	Intermediate[b]	None[b]

CONTRACEPTIVES, ORAL

Estimated Relative Oral Contraceptive Progestin/Estrogen/Androgen Activity

	Ingredients	Brand-name examples	Progestin activity	Estrogen activity	Androgen activity
Biphasic	Norethindrone/EE 0.5-35/1-35 mg-mcg	*Necon 10/11, Ortho-Novum 10/11*	Intermediate	High	Low
Triphasic	Norgestimate/EE 0.18-25/0.215-25/0.25-25 mg-mcg	*Ortho Tri-Cyclen Lo*	Low	Low	
	Levonorgestrel/EE 0.05-30/0.075-40/0.125-30 mg-mcg	*Enpresse, Tri-Levlen, Triphasil, Trivora*		Intermediate	
	Norgestimate/EE 0.18-35/0.215-35/0.25-35 mg-mcg	*Ortho Tri-Cyclen*			
	Norethindrone/EE 0.5-35/1-35/0.5-35 mg-mcg	*Tri-Norinyl*		High	
	Norethindrone/EE 0.5-35/0.75-35/1-35 mg-mcg	*Necon 7/7/7, Ortho-Novum 7/7/7*	Intermediate		
	Norethindrone/EE 1-20/1-30/1-35 mg-mcg	*Estrostep 21, Estrostep Fe*	High	Low	Intermediate
	Desogestrel/EE 0.1-25/0.125-25/0.15-25 mg-mcg	*Cyclessa*			Low
4-phasic	Dienogest/estradiol valerate 0-3/2-2/3-2/0-1 mg-mg	*Natazia*	No data	Low	No data

[a] EE = ethinyl estradiol.
[b] Preclinical studies have shown that drospirenone has no androgenic, estrogenic, glucocorticoid, antiglucocorticoid, or antiandrogenic activity.

➤*Emergency contraception (Plan B and Preven only):* The *Preven* emergency contraceptive kit contains a pregnancy test. This test can be used to verify an existing pregnancy resulting from intercourse that occurred earlier in the current menstrual cycle or the previous cycle. If a positive pregnancy result is obtained, advise the patient not to take the pills in the kit.

Take the initial 1 (*Plan B*) or 2 (*Preven*) pills as soon as possible but within 72 hours of unprotected intercourse. This is followed by the second dose of 1 (*Plan B*) or 2 (*Preven*) pills 12 hours later. Emergency contraception can be used at any time during the menstrual cycle. If the user vomits within 1 hour of taking either dose of the medication, she should contact her health care professional to discuss whether or not to repeat that dose or take an antinausea medication. Emergency contraceptive pills are not indicated for ongoing pregnancy protection and should not be used as a woman's routine form of contraception.

Actions

➤*Pharmacology:* OCs include estrogen-progestin combinations and POPs.

Progestin-only – Progestin-only oral contraceptives prevent conception by suppressing ovulation in approximately 50% of users, thickening the cervical mucus to inhibit sperm penetration, lowering the midcycle luteinizing hormone (LH) and follicle-stimulating hormone (FSH) peaks, slowing the movement of the ovum through the fallopian tubes, and altering the endometrium.

Combination OCs – Combination OCs inhibit ovulation by suppressing the gonadotropins, FSH, and LH. Additionally, alterations in the genital tract, including cervical mucus (which inhibits sperm penetration) and the endometrium (which reduces the likelihood of implantation), may contribute to contraceptive effectiveness.

These products differ in the type and relative potency of the components and in the relative predominance of estrogenic or progestational activity. Their ultimate effects are related to combined estrogenic, progestational, androgenic, and antiestrogenic effects.

Progestins may modify the effects of estrogens; these effects depend on the type or amount of progestin present and the ratio of progestin to estrogen. Dosage, potency, length of administration, and concomitant estrogen administration contribute to total progestational potency, making it difficult to establish equivalent doses of progestins. The total estrogenic potency of an OC is based on the combined effects of the estrogen and the estrogenic/antiestrogenic/androgenic effect of the progestin.

See the table in Administration and Dosage for a summary of the effects of the various progestins. Although not in the table, note that drospirenone is a spironolactone analog with antimineralocorticoid activity. Preclinical studies have shown that drospirenone has no androgenic, estrogenic, glucocorticoid, antiglucocorticoid, or antiandrogenic activity. Nonclinical studies in animals and in vitro have shown that dienogest is devoid of estrogenic, androgenic, glucocorticoid, and mineralocorticoid activities.

Contraceptive efficacy – In a study comparing the efficacy and safety of *Plan B* (1 tablet of levonorgestrel 0.75 mg taken within 72 hours of intercourse and 1 tablet taken 12 hours later) with the Yuzpe regimen (2 tablets of levonorgestrel 0.25 mg and ethinyl estradiol 0.05 mg taken within 72 hours of intercourse and 2 tablets taken 12 hours later), *Plan B* was at least as effective as the Yuzpe regimen in preventing pregnancy. After a single act of intercourse, the expected pregnancy rate of 8% (with no contraception) was reduced to approximately 1% with *Plan B*. Thus, *Plan B* reduced the expected number of pregnancies by 89%.

If 100 women used emergency contraceptive pills (ECPs) correctly in 1 month, approximately 2 women would become pregnant after a single act of intercourse. The use of ECPs results in a 75% reduction in the number of pregnancies expected if no ECPs were used after unprotected intercourse. Some clinical trials have shown that efficacy was greatest when ECPs were taken within 24 hours of unprotected intercourse; the efficacy decreases somewhat during each subsequent 24-hour period.

ECPs are not as effective as other forms of contraception. Efficacy in most cases depends greatly upon degree of compliance and user reliability. No other contraceptive drug or device, except levonorgestrel implant and medroxyprogesterone injection, approaches the efficacy of the combined OCs. For effectiveness rates of other contraceptive methods, refer to the following table.

Pregnancy Rates for Various Means of Contraception (%)[a]

Method of contraception	Lowest expected[b]	Typical[c]
Oral contraceptives		3
Combined	0.1	5
Progestin-only	0.5	5
Mechanical/Chemical		
Levonorgestrel implant	0.09	0.09
Medroxyprogesterone injection	0.3	0.3
IUD		
Progesterone	1.5	2
Copper T 380A	0.8	0.6
LNg 20	0.1	0.1
Cervical cap		
Parous	26	40
Nulliparous	9	20
Condom		
Without spermicide	3	14
With spermicide[d]	1.8	4 to 6
Spermicide alone	6	26
Diaphragm (with spermicidal cream or gel)	6	20
Female condom	5	21
Periodic abstinence (ie, rhythm; all methods)	1 to 9	25
Sterility		
Vasectomy	0.1	0.15
Tubal ligation	0.5	0.5
No contraception	85	85

[a] During first year of continuous use.
[b] Best guess of percentage expected to experience an accidental pregnancy among couples who initiate a method and use it consistently and correctly.
[c] A "typical" couple who initiate a method and experience an accidental pregnancy.
[d] Used as a separate product (not in condom package).

There are 4 types of combination OCs: monophasic, biphasic, triphasic, and 4-phasic. The biphasic and triphasic OCs are intended to deliver hormones in a fashion similar to physiologic processes.

Monophasic – There is a fixed dosage of estrogen to progestin throughout the cycle.

Biphasic – The amount of estrogen remains the same for the first 21 days of the cycle. A decreased progestin:estrogen ratio in the first half of the cycle allows endometrial proliferation. An increased ratio in the second half provides adequate secretory development.

Triphasic – The estrogen amount remains the same while the progestin changes, or the dose of both estrogen and progestin change during the cycle.

4-phasic – The dose of both estrogen and progestin changes during the cycle.

Noncontraceptive health benefits – The following health benefits related to the use of combination OCs are supported by epidemiological studies that largely utilized OC formulations containing estrogen doses of ethinyl estradiol 35 mcg or more or mestranol 50 mcg.

Effects on menses: Increased menstrual cycle regularity, decreased blood loss and decreased incidence of iron deficiency anemia, decreased incidence of dysmenorrhea.

Effects related to inhibition of ovulation: Decreased incidence of functional ovarian cysts and ectopic pregnancies.

CONTRACEPTIVES, ORAL

Other effects: Decreased incidence of fibroadenomas and fibrocystic disease of the breast, acute pelvic inflammatory disease, endometrial cancer, ovarian cancer, maintenance of bone density, and decreased symptomatic endometriosis.

➤*Pharmacokinetics:*

Estrogens – Ethinyl estradiol is rapidly absorbed with peak concentrations attained within 2 hours. It undergoes considerable first-pass elimination. Mestranol is demethylated to ethinyl estradiol. Ethinyl estradiol is 97% to 98% bound to plasma albumin. Half-life varies from 6 to 20 hours. It is excreted in bile and urine as conjugates and undergoes some enterohepatic recirculation. Estradiol valerate peak concentrations are attained within approximately 6 hours with 60% bound to plasma albumin. Estradiol undergoes extensive first-pass effect and metabolites are mainly excreted in the urine. The terminal half-life is approximately 14 hours.

Progestins – Peak concentrations of norethindrone occur 0.5 to 4 hours after oral administration; it undergoes first-pass metabolism with an overall bioavailability of approximately 65%. Levonorgestrel reaches peak concentrations between 0.5 to 2 hours, does not undergo a first-pass effect, and is completely bioavailable. Norethindrone and levonorgestrel are chiefly metabolized by reduction followed by conjugation. Desogestrel is rapidly and completely absorbed and converted into 3-keto-desogestrel, the biologically active metabolite. Relative bioavailability is approximately 84%. Maximum concentrations of the metabolite are reached at approximately 1.4 hours. Norgestimate is well absorbed; peak serum concentrations are observed within 2 hours followed by a rapid decline to levels generally below assay within 5 hours. However, a major metabolite, 17-deacetyl norgestimate, appears rapidly in serum with concentrations greatly exceeding that of the parent. Both norethynodrel and ethynodiol diacetate are converted to norethindrone. Peak serum concentrations of drospirenone are reached 1 to 3 hours after administration. Progestins are bound to albumin (79% to 95%) and to sex hormone binding globulin (except drospirenone). Terminal half-life of the progestins are as follows: Norethindrone, 5 to 14 hours; levonorgestrel, 11 to 45 hours; desogestrel (metabolite), 38 ± 20 hours; norgestimate (metabolite), 12 to 30 hours; drospirenone, 30 hours. Progestin-only administration results in lower steady-state serum progestin levels and a shorter elimination half-life than coadministration with estrogens. Bioavailability of dienogest is about 91%, maximum serum concentrations are reached at approximately 1 hour, and the terminal half-life is approximately 14 hours.

Contraindications

Thrombophlebitis; thromboembolic disorders (eg, valvular heart disease with thrombogenic complications or atrial fibrillation); history of deep vein thrombophlebitis or pulmonary embolism; cerebral vascular disease; MI; coronary artery disease; known or suspected breast carcinoma or estrogen-dependent neoplasia; carcinoma of endometrium; hepatic adenomas/carcinomas (see Warnings/Precautions); undiagnosed abnormal genital bleeding; known or suspected pregnancy (see Warnings/Precautions); cholestatic jaundice of pregnancy/jaundice with prior pill use; hypersensitivity to any component of the product; acute liver disease; uncontrolled hypertension; headaches with focal neurological symptoms; diabetes with vascular complications; major surgery with prolonged immobility.

➤*Natazia:* Smoking, if older than 35 years of age; inherited or acquired hypercoagulopathies.

➤*Yasmin:* Renal insufficiency, hepatic dysfunction, adrenal insufficiency, heavy smoking (at least 15 cigarettes daily) and older than 35 years of age.

Warnings/Precautions

➤*Smoking:* Cigarette smoking increases the risk of serious cardiovascular side effects from OCs. This risk increases with age and with heavy smoking (at least 15 cigarettes daily) and is quite marked in women older than 35 years of age. Women who use OCs should not smoke.

➤*Hyperkalemia: Yasmin* contains the progestin drospirenone that has antimineralocorticoid activity, including the potential for hyperkalemia in high-risk patients, comparable with spironolactone 25 mg. *Yasmin* should not be used in patients with conditions that predispose to hyperkalemia (eg, renal insufficiency, hepatic dysfunction, adrenal insufficiency). Women receiving daily, long-term treatment for chronic conditions or diseases with medications that may increase serum potassium should have their serum potassium level checked during the first treatment cycle. Drugs that may increase serum potassium include ACE inhibitors, angiotensin-II receptor antagonists, potassium-sparing diuretics, heparin, aldosterone antagonists, and NSAIDs.

➤*Risks of OC use:* The use of OCs is associated with increased risk of thromboembolism, stroke, MI, hypertension, hepatic neoplasia, and gallbladder disease, although risk of serious morbidity or mortality is very small in healthy women without underlying risk factors. Risk of morbidity/mortality increases significantly in the presence of other underlying risk factors such as hypertension, hyperlipidemias, obesity, and diabetes.

➤*Mortality:* Mortality associated with all methods of birth control is low and below that associated with childbirth, with the exception of OC use in women at least 35 years of age who smoke and at least 40 years of age who do not smoke. In 1989, the Fertility and Maternal Health Drugs Advisory Committee concluded that although cardiovascular disease risk may be increased with OC use in healthy nonsmoking women older than 40 years of age (even with the newer low-dose formulations), there also are greater potential health risks associated with pregnancy in older women and with the alternative surgical and medical procedures that may be necessary if such women do not have access to effective and acceptable means of contraception. Therefore, the committee recommended that the benefits of low-dose OC use by healthy nonsmoking women older than 40 years of age may outweigh the possible risks. Of course, like all women, older women who take oral contraceptives should take an oral contraceptive that contains the least amount of estrogen and progestin that is compatible with a low failure rate and individual patient needs.

➤*Thromboembolism:* Be alert to the earliest symptoms of thromboembolic and thrombotic disorders. Should any of these occur or be suspected, discontinue the drug immediately.

In 1998, the American College of Obstetrics and Gynecology Committee on Gynecologic Practice reconfirmed that the risks of nonfatal venous thromboembolism for healthy, nonpregnant nonusers of OCs is 4 cases per 100,000 woman-years versus 10 to 15 cases per 100,000 woman-years and 20 to 30 cases per 100,000 woman-years for users of second- and third-generation OCs, respectively. The risk for pregnant women is 60 cases per 100,000 woman-years. The committee confirms that the risk of nonfatal venous thrombosis with third-generation OCs (desogestrel, gestodene, and norgestimate) is 2 to 3 times the risk of second-generation OCs. The risk of development of deep vein thrombosis was found to be 2 to 5 times higher with low-estrogen, desogestrel-containing OCs than with second-generation monophasic and triphasic preparations. The committee stated that the decision regarding the use of third-generation OCs should be left to the clinician and patient because they might have benefit in some cases (eg, patients requiring suppression of ovarian androgens or those with conditions for which they might be advantageous).

MI – MI risk associated with OC use is increased. This risk is primarily in smokers or women with other underlying risk factors for coronary artery disease such as hypertension, hypercholesterolemia, morbid obesity, and diabetes. The risk is very low in women younger than 30 years of age. It is estimated that the relative risk of heart attack for current OC users is 2 to 6.

Long-term use – Data suggest that the increased risk of MI persists after discontinuation of long-term OC use; the highest risk group includes women 40 to 49 years of age who used OCs for at least 5 years.

Smoking – Smoking in combination with OC use has been shown to contribute substantially to the incidence of MIs in women in their mid-30s or older, with smoking accounting for the majority of excess cases. Mortality rates associated with circulatory disease have been shown to increase substantially in smokers, especially in those at least 35 years of age who use OCs.

Cerebrovascular diseases – OCs increase the risk of cerebrovascular events (thrombotic and hemorrhagic strokes), although, in general, the risk is greatest in hypertensive women older than 35 years of age who also smoke. Relative risk of thrombotic strokes ranges from 3 (normotensive users) to 14 (severe hypertensive users). Relative risk of hemorrhagic stroke for OC users is 1.2 for nonsmokers, 7.6 for smokers, 1.8 for normotensives, and 25.7 for severe hypertensives; for nonuser smokers, risk is 2.6. The attributable risk also is greater in older women.

Vascular disease – A positive association is observed between the amount of estrogen and progestin in OCs and the risk of vascular disease. A decline in serum high-density lipoproteins (HDL) has occurred with progestins and has been associated with an increased incidence of ischemic heart disease. Because estrogens increase HDL cholesterol, the net effect depends on a balance achieved between doses of estrogen and progestin and the activity of the progestin used in the contraceptives.

Age – The risk of cerebrovascular and circulatory disease in OC users is substantially increased in women at least 35 years of age with other risk factors (eg, smoking, uncontrolled hypertension, hypercholesterolemia [LDL 190], obesity, diabetes). Mortality rates associated with circulatory disease have been shown to increase substantially in smokers older than 35 years of age and nonsmokers older than 40 years of age among women who use OCs. Current clinical practice involves use of lower-estrogen dose formulations combined with careful restriction of OC use to women who do not have the various risk factors listed.

Postsurgical thromboembolism – Risk is increased 2- to 4-fold. If possible, discontinue OCs at least 4 weeks before and 2 weeks after surgery and during and following prolonged immobilization because OCs are associated with an increased risk of thromboembolism.

Subarachnoid hemorrhage – Subarachnoid hemorrhage has been increased by OC use. Smoking alone increases the incidence of these accidents; smoking and OC use appear to work together to produce a combined risk greater than either alone.

Persistence of risk – An increased risk may persist for at least 6 years after discontinuation of OC use for cerebrovascular disease and at least 9 years for MI in users 40 to 49 years of age who had used OCs at least 5 years; this risk was not demonstrated in other age groups. This information is based on studies that used OC formulations containing at least estrogen 50 mcg.

NOTE – The associations between OCs and cardiovascular disease are based on epidemiological studies whose conclusions have been criticized for the following reasons: National trends of cardiovascular mortality are incompatible with these risk estimates; excess deaths may not be attributable entirely to smoking; the clinical diagnosis of thromboembolism is often unreliable.

➤*Ocular lesions:* Ocular lesions such as retinal thrombosis have been associated with the use of OCs. Discontinue medication if there is unexplained loss of vision, onset of proptosis or diplopia, papilledema, or retinal vascular lesions. Immediately undertake appropriate diagnostic therapeutic measures.

➤*Carcinoma:* Numerous epidemiological studies have been performed on the incidence of breast, endometrial, ovarian, and cervical cancer in women using OCs. While there are conflicting reports, the overall evidence in the

CONTRACEPTIVES, ORAL

literature suggests that use of OCs is not associated with an increase in the risk of developing breast cancer, regardless of age and parity of first use. The Cancer and Steroid Hormone study also showed no latent effect on the risk of breast cancer for at least a decade following long-term use. Some studies have shown an increased relative risk of developing breast cancer, particularly at a younger age and apparently related to duration of use. These studies have predominantly involved combined oral contraceptives; there is insufficient data to determine whether the use of POPs similarly increases the risk. Women with breast cancer should not use OCs because the role of female hormones in breast cancer has not been fully determined. Most studies have not shown such a risk; methodologies of earlier studies have been questioned. According to the CDC, there is a small subset of premenopausal-associated breast cancers, but there is no proof of cause and effect; there is no association with the postmenopausal variety.

Some studies suggest that OC use has been associated with an increase in the risk of cervical intraepithelial neoplasia in some populations of women. There is insufficient data to determine whether the use of POPs increases the risk of developing cervical intraepithelial neoplasia. There continues to be controversy about the extent to which such findings may be because of differences in sexual behavior and other factors. Other epidemiologic studies have suggested an increased risk of cervical dysplasia and carcinoma.

In spite of many studies of the relationship between OC use and breast and cervical cancers, a cause and effect relationship has not been established.

Studies have reported an increased risk of endometrial carcinoma associated with the prolonged use of estrogen in postmenopausal women. However, the risk appears to be decreased in OC users because of the progestin component. In fact, there is a protective effect; users appear about half as likely to develop ovarian and endometrial cancer as women who have never used OCs. The protective effect from endometrial cancer lasts up to 15 years after the pills are stopped.

There appears to be no increased risk of breast cancer in OC users or any subgroup of users, although the CDC states that there may be an association with a subset of young, premenopausal users. There is no increased risk of breast cancer in OC users with prior benign breast disease. Another study suggests that use prior to the first full-term pregnancy was associated with a significant relative risk of breast cancer especially when OC use began before 25 years of age.

Close clinical surveillance of all women taking OCs is essential; they should be reexamined at least once a year. In all cases of undiagnosed persistent or recurrent abnormal vaginal bleeding, rule out malignancy. Monitor women with a strong family history of breast cancer or who have breast nodules, fibrocystic disease of the breast, cervical dysplasia, or abnormal mammograms.

➤*Hepatic lesions (eg, adenomas, focal nodular hyperplasia, hepatocellular carcinoma):* Benign and malignant hepatic adenomas have been associated with the use of OCs, but this is a relatively rare disease. Severe abdominal pain, shock, or death may be caused by rupture and hemorrhage of a liver tumor. Fortunately, this is quite rare; there may be some association with higher-dose mestranol preparations or duration (greater after at least 4 years) of OC use. While hepatic adenoma is uncommon, consider it in women presenting with abdominal pain and tenderness, abdominal mass, or shock. A few cases of hepatocellular carcinoma have been reported in women taking OCs long-term; however, an association has not been established.

➤*Gallbladder disease:* Earlier studies have reported an increased risk of gallbladder surgery in OC users. More recent studies, however, have shown that the relative risk of developing gallbladder disease among OC users may be minimal. These recent findings may be related to the use of OC formulations containing lower estrogen and progestin doses.

➤*Carbohydrate metabolism:* Glucose tolerance may decrease, which is directly related to estrogen dose. Progestins increase insulin secretion and create insulin resistance. These effects vary with different agents. However, OCs appear to have no effect on fasting blood glucose in nondiabetic women. Observe prediabetic and diabetic patients receiving OCs. In a recent study, OC users were less likely to develop diabetes than nonusers.

➤*Lipid profile:* A small proportion of women will have persistent hypertriglyceridemia while using OCs. Changes in serum triglycerides and lipoprotein levels have been reported in OC users.

➤*Elevated blood pressure:* Elevated blood pressure and hypertension may occur within a few months of beginning use. The prevalence increases with the duration of use and age. Incidence of hypertension may directly correlate with increasing dosages of progestin.

Encourage women with a history of hypertension, renal disease, or hypertension-related diseases during pregnancy to use another method of contraception. Monitor these patients if they choose to use OCs. Discontinue the OC if elevated blood pressure occurs. High blood pressure returns to normal in most women after OC discontinuation.

➤*Headaches:* Onset or exacerbation of migraine or development of headache with focal neurological symptoms of a new pattern that is recurrent, persistent, or severe, requires OC discontinuation and evaluation.

➤*Bleeding irregularities:* BTB and spotting are sometimes encountered in OC patients, especially during the first 3 months of use. BTB, spotting, and amenorrhea are frequent reasons for discontinuing OCs. The type and dose of progestin may be important. In BTB, consider nonhormonal causes. In undiagnosed persistent or recurrent abnormal vaginal bleeding, rule out pregnancy or malignancy. If amenorrhea occurs, rule out pregnancy. If pathology has been excluded, time or formulation change may resolve the problem. Changing to an OC with a higher estrogen content may minimize menstrual irregularity, but consider the increased risk of thromboembolic disease. Consider short-term estrogen supplements.

It was thought that women with a history of oligomenorrhea or secondary amenorrhea or young women without regular cycles may tend to remain anovulatory or become amenorrheic after discontinuation of OCs; however, this is not certain. Other factors may play a role in the development of amenorrhea after OC withdrawal, including stress, previous menstrual irregularity, psychiatric conditions, and marked weight loss. Also, the incidence may have been much higher when higher-dose products were used more regularly. Advise patients of this possibility.

Seasonale – When prescribing *Seasonale*, the convenience of fewer planned menses (4 annually instead of 13 annually) should be weighed against the inconvenience of increased intermenstrual bleeding and/or spotting. More *Seasonale* subjects, compared with subjects on the 28-day cycle regimen enrolled in a clinical trial, discontinued prematurely for unacceptable bleeding (7.7% with *Seasonale* versus 1.8% of 28-day cycle regimen).

Progestin-only products – Episodes of irregular, unpredictable spotting, and BTB within the first year are the most frequently encountered side effects and are the major reasons why women discontinue OC use.

➤*Risks of use immediately preceding pregnancy:* Some extensive epidemiological studies have revealed no increased risk of birth defects in OC users prior to pregnancy.

➤*Menopause:* Treatment with OCs may mask the onset of the climacteric.

➤*Angioedema:* In women with hereditary angioedema, exogenous estrogens may induce of exacerbate symptoms of angioedema.

➤*Lipid disorders:* Closely follow women taking OCs who are being treated for hyperlipidemias. Some progestins may elevate LDL levels and decrease HDL levels (see Warnings), making hyperlipidemia control more difficult. Consider withholding the OC if the dyslipidemia does not respond (ie, LDL of 190).

HDL and total cholesterol may be increased, LDL may be increased or decreased, while LDL/HDL ratio may be decreased and triglycerides unchanged.

➤*Uterine fibroids:* Pre-existing uterine leiomyomata (uterine fibroids) may increase in size. However, there is no evidence of this with low-dose OCs. In addition, data indicate that the risk of developing uterine fibroids is actually reduced with OC use.

➤*Depression:* The incidence of depression in OC users ranges from less than 5% to 30%. Pyridoxine deficiency may be a factor in the depression. Pyridoxine 25 to 50 mg per day has been recommended. In patients with a history of depression, discontinue if depression recurs to a serious degree. Patients becoming significantly depressed should discontinue medication to determine if the symptom is drug-related.

➤*Fluid retention:* OCs may cause fluid retention; prescribe with caution and monitor patients with conditions that might be aggravated by fluid retention (eg, convulsive disorders; migraine syndrome; asthma; cardiac, hepatic, or renal dysfunction).

➤*Hepatic disease:* Patients with a history of jaundice during pregnancy have an increased risk of recurrence of jaundice; if jaundice develops, discontinue use. Steroid hormones may be poorly metabolized in patients with liver dysfunction; administer with caution.

➤*Contact lenses:* Contact lens wearers who develop changes in vision or lens tolerance should be assessed by an ophthalmologist; consider temporary or permanent cessation of wear.

➤*Serum folate levels:* Serum folate levels may be depressed by therapy. Although OCs may impair folate metabolism, the effect is mild and unlikely to cause anemia or megaloblastic changes in women who have a good dietary folate intake. Because the pregnant woman is predisposed to folate deficiency, a woman who becomes pregnant shortly after stopping therapy may have a greater chance of developing folate deficiency and its attendant complications. Folic acid supplements are recommended.

➤*Chloasma:* Chloasma may occasionally occur, especially in women with a history of chloasma gravidarum. Women with a tendency to chloasma should avoid exposure to the sun or ultraviolet radiation while taking OCs.

➤*Acute intermittent porphyria:* Estrogens have been reported to precipitate attacks of acute intermittent porphyria; use with caution in susceptible patients.

➤*Vomiting/Diarrhea:* Several cases of OC failure have been reported in association with vomiting or diarrhea. If significant GI disturbance occurs, a backup method of contraception for the remainder of the cycle is recommended.

➤*Pancreatitis:* Women with hypertriglyceridemia, or a family history thereof, may be at an increased risk of pancreatitis when using OCs.

➤*Sexually transmitted diseases (STDs):* Advise patients that OCs do not protect against HIV infection and other STDs.

➤*Body mass index:* The efficacy of *Natazia* in women with a body mass index of more than 30 kg/m^2 has not been evaluated.

➤*Tartrazine sensitivity:* Some of these products contain tartrazine, which may cause allergic-type reactions (including bronchial asthma) in susceptible individuals. Although the incidence of tartrazine sensitivity in the general population is low, it is frequently seen in patients who also have aspirin hypersensitivity. Specific products containing tartrazine are identified in the product listings.

CONTRACEPTIVES, ORAL

➤*Pregnancy:* *Category X.* Rule out pregnancy before initiating or continuing OCs and always consider it if withdrawal bleeding does not occur. Rule out pregnancy before continuing OCs for any patient who has missed 2 consecutive periods. If the patient has not adhered to the prescribed schedule, consider the possibility of pregnancy at the time of the first missed period and withhold further use until pregnancy has been ruled out. If pregnancy is confirmed, apprise the patient of the potential risks to the fetus. The majority of recent studies do not indicate a teratogenic effect, particularly cardiac anomalies and limb reduction defects, when OCs are taken inadvertently during early pregnancy.

The use of female sex hormones (eg, estrogens) during early pregnancy may seriously damage the offspring (see the Warning Box in the Estrogens monograph). However, there is no conclusive evidence that OC use is associated with an increase in birth defects when taken inadvertently during early pregnancy. Previously, a few studies reported that OCs might be associated with birth defects, but these findings have not been seen in more recent studies. Nevertheless, do not use during pregnancy unless clearly necessary.

Do not administer OCs to induce withdrawal bleeding as a test for pregnancy.

Do not use OCs during pregnancy to treat threatened or habitual abortion.

Ectopic pregnancy – Ectopic pregnancy, as well as intrauterine pregnancy, may occur in contraceptive failures.

The incidence of ectopic pregnancies for progestin-only OC users is 5 per 1,000 women-years. Up to 10% of pregnancies reported in clinical studies of progestin-only OC users are extrauterine. Although symptoms of ectopic pregnancy should be watched for, a history of ectopic pregnancy need not be considered a contraindication for use of this contraceptive method. Health care providers should be alert to the possibility of an ectopic pregnancy in women who become pregnant or complain of lower abdominal pain while on progestin-only OCs.

Fertility impairment – Fertility impairment may occur in women discontinuing OCs; however, impairment diminishes with time. In nulliparous women 25 to 29 years of age, the effect is negligible after 48 months. Among nulliparous women 30 to 34 years of age, impairment persists up to 72 months and appears more severe. For parous women, the effect is negligible and short-lived after cessation of contraception.

The limited available data indicated a rapid return of normal ovulation and fertility following discontinuation of progestin-only OCs.

➤*Lactation:* Combination OCs given in the postpartum period may interfere with lactation, decreasing the quantity and quality of breast milk. Furthermore, a small amount of OC steroids is excreted in breast milk. A few adverse effects on the breast-feeding infant have been reported, including jaundice and breast enlargement. If possible, defer use until the infant has been weaned; however, in some situations, breast-feeding is the only real alternative (see Administration and Dosage).

Small amounts of progestin pass into the breast milk resulting in steroid levels in infant plasma of 1% to 6% of maternal plasma levels.

➤*Children:* Safety and efficacy has been established in women of reproductive age. Safety and efficacy are expected to be the same for postpubertal adolescents 16 years of age or younger. Use of these products before menarche is not indicated.

➤*Monitoring:* It is good medical practice for all women to have annual history and physical examinations, including women using OCs. Physical examination may be deferred until after initiation of OCs if requested by the patient and judged appropriate by the health care provider. The physical exam should evaluate blood pressure, breasts, abdomen, and pelvic organs, including Pap smear. Perform preventative measures (ie, ensure up to date vaccinations) and screening, which should include total and HDL cholesterol within 5-year intervals. Advise the pathologist of OC therapy when relevant specimens are submitted. Do not prescribe for more than 1 year without another physical exam.

Drug Interactions

Oral Contraceptive Drug Interactions

Precipitant drug	Object drug[a]		Description
Antibiotics	Contraceptives, hormonal	↓	Coadministration of griseofulvin, penicillins, or tetracyclines with OCs may decrease the pharmacologic effects of the OCs, possibly because of altered steroid gut metabolism secondary to changes in the intestinal flora. Menstrual irregularities (eg, spotting, BTB) and pregnancy may occur. An alternate or additional form of birth control may be advisable during concomitant use. OCs and troleandomycin may be associated with an increased risk of intrahepatic cholestasis.
Antidepressants Azole antifungals (eg, ketoconazole) Cimetidine Diltiazem Grapefruit juice Macrolides (eg, erythromycin) Verapamil	Contraceptives, hormonal	↑	Plasma levels of dienogest may be increased.
Aprepitant Barbiturates Bosentan Carbamazepine Felbamate Griseofulvin HIV protease inhibitors Hydantoins[b] Modafinil Oxcarbazepine Phenytoin Rifamycins Rufinamide St. John's wort Topiramate	Contraceptives, hormonal	↓	These agents may increase the hepatic metabolism of the OCs via hepatic microsomal enzyme induction, possibly resulting in decreased effectiveness of the OC; menstrual irregularities (eg, spotting, BTB) and pregnancy may occur. An alternate or additional form of birth control may be advisable during concomitant use.
Atorvastatin	Contraceptives, hormonal	↑	Coadministration increased AUC values for norethindrone and ethinyl estradiol ≈ 30% and 20%, respectively.
Fluconazole	Contraceptives, hormonal	↔	The therapeutic efficacy of oral contraceptives may be decreased while the blood levels of ethinyl estradiol and norethindrone are increased. Consider an alternate form of birth control.
Thiazolidinediones (eg, pioglitazone)	Contraceptives, hormonal	↓	Coadministration may decrease serum concentrations of hormonal contraceptives. Alternative forms of birth control may be advisable.
Tranexamic acid	Contraceptives, hormonal		The risk of hormonal contraceptive related thrombotic events may be increased.
Contraceptives, hormonal	Anticoagulants	↔	Because hormonal contraceptives can increase levels of certain circulating clotting factors and reduce antithrombin III levels, therapeutic efficacy of the anticoagulants may be decreased by hormonal contraceptives. However, both an increased and decreased effect has occurred.
Contraceptives, hormonal	Antidepressants, tricyclic Beta-blockers Caffeine Corticosteroids Theophyllines	↑	The hepatic metabolism of these agents may be decreased by hormonal contraceptives, resulting in increased therapeutic effects or toxicity.
Contraceptives, hormonal	Benzodiazepines	↑↓	Hormonal contraceptives may increase the clearance of the benzodiazepines that undergo glucuronidation (eg, lorazepam, oxazepam, temazepam) because of increased metabolism. Combination hormonal contraceptives with alprazolam, chlordiazepoxide, diazepam, and triazolam may inhibit hepatic mixed-function oxidases leading to a decrease in benzodiazepine oxidation rate (may prolong the half-life of benzodiazepines).
Contraceptives, hormonal	Corticosteroids	↑	Pharmacologic effects of corticosteroids may be increased. Monitor for signs of corticosteroid toxicity (Cushingoid face, weight gain) and reduce the dose if necessary.
Contraceptives, hormonal	Cyclosporine	↑	Hormonal contraceptives may inhibit the metabolism of cyclosporine, increasing the risk of toxicity. Avoid this combination if possible. If given together, monitor cyclosporine concentrations, as well as renal and hepatic function. Adjust cyclosporine dose as indicated.
Contraceptives, hormonal	Lamotrigine	↓	Hormonal contraceptives may increase lamotrigine metabolism, therefore decreasing the therapeutic effect.
Contraceptives, hormonal	Selegiline	↑	Coadministration may increase selegiline concentrations because of inhibition of its metabolism.
Contraceptives, hormonal	Valproic acid	↓	Plasma concentrations and pharmacodynamic effects of valproic acid may be decreased. Monitor valproic acid concentrations and clinical effects. Adjust the dosage as needed.

[a] ↑ = object drug increased; ↓ = object drug decreased; ↑↓ = object drug both increased and decreased; ↔ = undetermined clinical effect.
[b] Pharmacologic effects of the hydantoins also may be altered.

➤*Drug/Lab test interactions:* Estrogen-containing OCs may cause the following alterations in serum, plasma, or blood, unless specified otherwise.

CONTRACEPTIVES, ORAL

Increased – Factors I (prothrombin), VII, VIII, IX, X; fibrinogen; norepinephrine-induced platelet aggregation; thyroid-binding globulin (TBG), leading to increased total thyroid hormone (as measured by protein bound iodine, T_4 by column or radioimmunoassay); corticosteroid levels; triglycerides and phospholipids; aldosterone; amylase; gamma-glutamyltranspeptidase; iron-binding capacity; sex-hormone-binding globulins are increased and result in elevated levels of total circulating sex steroids (combination) and corticoids; transferrin; prolactin; renin activity; vitamin A.

Decreased – Antithrombin III; free T_3 resin uptake; response to metyrapone test; folate; glucose tolerance; albumin; cholinesterase; haptoglobin; tissue plasminogen activator; zinc; vitamin B_{12}; sex-hormone-binding globulin, thyroxine caused by decrease in thyroid-binding globulin (progestin-only).

Adverse Reactions

Serious – Arterial thromboembolism; cerebral hemorrhage; cerebral thrombosis; coronary thrombosis; focal nodular hyperplasia of the liver; gallbladder disease; hepatic adenomas or benign liver tumors; hypertension; mesenteric thrombosis; MI; pulmonary embolism; ruptured cyst; thrombophlebitis and venous thrombosis with or without embolism; uterine leiomyoma. See Warnings/Precautions for more information.

➤*CNS:* Dizziness; headache; mental depression; migraine.

➤*Dermatologic:* Melasma (may persist); rash (allergic).

➤*Endocrine:* Breast pain, tenderness, enlargement, secretion; diminution in lactation when given immediately postpartum.

➤*GI:* Abdominal cramps; bloating; cholestatic jaundice; nausea and vomiting (occurring in approximately 10% to 30% of patients during the first cycle, less common with low doses, and the majority resolve in 3 months).

➤*GU:* Amenorrhea during and after treatment; BTB (the majority, more than 80%, resolve in 3 months), spotting, change in menstrual flow; change in cervical erosion and secretions; invasive cervical cancer; temporary infertility after discontinuation; vaginal candidiasis.

➤*Ophthalmic:* Changes in corneal curvature (steepening); contact lens intolerance; neuro-ocular lesions (eg, retinal thrombosis, optic neuritis).

➤*Miscellaneous:* Edema; reduced carbohydrate tolerance; weight change (increase or decrease); prevalence of cervical chlamydia trachomatis may be increased; hirsutism (rare).

The following associations have been neither confirmed nor refuted: acne; acute hepatitis; anemia; Budd-Chiarri syndrome; cataracts; cerebrovascular disease with mitral valve prolapse; changes in appetite; changes in libido; colitis; colonic Crohn disease; cystitis-like syndrome; dizziness; EEG abnormalities; endometrial, cervical, and breast carcinoma (conflicting data; see Warnings/Precautions); erythema multiforme; erythema nodosum; fatigue; gingivitis; headache; hemolytic uremic syndrome; hemorrhagic eruption; herpes gestationis; hirsutism; itching; loss of scalp hair; lupus erythematosus or lupus-like syndromes; malignant hypertension; malignant melanoma; nervousness; pancreatitis; porphyria; photosensitivity;pituitary tumors; premenstrual syndrome; pulmonary embolism; renal function impairment; rhinitis; sickle cell disease; vaginitis.

➤*Emergency contraceptives:* The most common adverse events in the clinical trial for women receiving emergency contraceptives include the following: abdominal pain/cramps; breast tenderness; diarrhea; dizziness; fatigue; headache; menstrual irregularities; nausea; vomiting.

Overdosage

Serious ill effects have not been reported following acute overdosage of OCs in young children. Overdosage may cause nausea. Withdrawal bleeding may occur in females.

Patient Information

Patient package insert available with product.

To achieve maximum contraceptive effectiveness, inform the patient to take OCs exactly as directed at intervals not exceeding 24 hours, preferably at the same time each day, including throughout all bleeding episodes.Inform the patient to take tablets regularly with a meal or at bedtime. Efficacy depends on strict adherence to the dosage schedule. Missing a pill can cause spotting or light bleeding; the patient may be a little sick to her stomach on the days she takes the missed pill with her regularly scheduled pill. For missed doses, see Administration and Dosage.

Advise the patient to use a backup method (eg, condoms, spermicides) for the following 48 hours whenever a progestin-only OC is taken at least 3 hours late.

If pregnancy is terminated within the first 12 weeks, instruct the patient to start OCs immediately or within 7 days. If pregnancy is terminated after 12 weeks, instruct the patient to start OCs after 2 weeks.

OCs may cause spotting or BTB during the first few months of therapy; if bleeding occurs in more than 1 cycle or lasts more than a few days, advise the patient to notify the health care provider.

Advise the patient to inform the health care provider of prolonged episodes of bleeding, amenorrhea, or severe abdominal pain.

Advise the patient to use an additional method of birth control until after the first week of administration in the initial cycle or for the entire cycle if vomiting or diarrhea occurs.

Inform patients that OCs do not protect against HIV infection and other STDs.

In case of severe vomiting or diarrhea, absorption may not be complete and additional contraceptive measures should be taken. If vomiting or diarrhea occur within 3 to 4 hours after taking OC tablet, this can be regarded as a missed tablet.

MONOPHASIC CONTRACEPTIVES — ORAL

	Product & Distributor	Estrogen (mcg)	Progestin (mg)	How Supplied
Rx	**Necon 1/50** (Watson)	50 mg mestranol	1 norethindrone	Lactose. (WATSON 510). Lt. blue. In 21s and 28s. With 7 white inert tablets (WATSON P) in the 28s.
Rx	**Norinyl 1 + 50** (Watson)			Lactose. (Watson 265). White. In *Wallette* 28s. With 7 orange inert tablets (Watson P1).
Rx	**Ortho-Novum 1/50** (Ortho-McNeil)			Lactose. (Ortho 150). Yellow. In *Dialpak* 28s. With 7 green inert tablets.
Rx	**Ovcon-50** (Warner Chilcott)	50 ethinyl estradiol	1 norethindrone	Lactose. (MJ 584). Yellow. In 28s. With 7 green, capsule shape inert tablets (MJ 850).
Rx	**Zovia 1/50E** (Watson)		1 ethynodiol diacetate	Lactose. (WATSON 384). Pink. In 21s and 28s. With 7 white inert tablets (WATSON P) in the 28s.
Rx	**Ovral** (Wyeth-Ayerst)		0.5 norgestrel	Lactose. (WYETH 56). White. In *Pilpak* 21s and 28s. With 7 pink inert tablets (WYETH 445) in the 28s.
Rx	**Ogestrel 0.5/50** (Watson)			Lactose. (Watson 848). White. In 28s. With 7 peach inert tablets (Watson P1).

MONOPHASIC CONTRACEPTIVES — ORAL

	Product & Distributor	Estrogen (mcg)	Progestin (mg)	How Supplied
Rx	**Necon 1/35** (Watson)	35 ethinyl estradiol	1 norethindrone	Lactose. (WATSON 508). Dk. yellow. In 28s. With 7 white inert tablets (WATSON P).
Rx	**Norinyl 1 + 35** (Watson)			Lactose. (WATSON 259). Yellow-green. In *Wallette* 28s. With 7 orange inert tablets (WATSON P1).
Rx	**Nortrel 1/35** (Barr)			Lactose. (b 949). Yellow. In 21s and 28s. With 7 white inert tablets (b 944) in the 28s.
Rx	**Ortho-Novum 1/35** (Ortho-McNeil)			Lactose. (Ortho 135). Peach. In *Dialpak* and *Veridate* 28s. With 7 green inert tablets (Ortho).
Rx	**Brevicon** (Watson)		0.5 norethindrone	Lactose. (Watson 254). Blue. In *Wallette* 28s. With 7 orange inert tablets (Watson P1).
Rx	**Modicon** (Ortho-McNeil)			Lactose. (Ortho 535). White. In *Dialpak* and *Veridate* 28s. With 7 green inert tablets (Ortho).
Rx	**Necon 0.5/35** (Watson)			Lactose. (WATSON 507). Lt. yellow. In 21s and 28s. With 7 white inert tablets (WATSON P) in the 28s.
Rx	**Nortrel 0.5/35** (Barr)			Lactose. (b 941). Lt. yellow. In 21s and 28s. With 7 white inert tablets (b 944) in the 28s.
Rx	**Ovcon-35** (Warner Chilcott)		0.4 norethindrone	Lactose. (MJ 583). Peach. With 7 green capsule shape inert tablets (MJ 850). In 28s.
Rx	**Femcon Fe** (Warner Chilcott)			Chewable tablets. Lactose, maltodextrin, sucralose. (WIC 581). Spearmint flavor. In 21s. With 7 brown inert tablets (75 mg ferrous fumarate). Compressionable sugar. (PD 622).
Rx	**Balziva** (Barr Laboratories)			Lactose. (b 735). Lt. peach. In 28s. With 7 white inert tablets. Lactose. (b 944).
Rx	**Zenchent** (Watson)			Lactose. (wc 580). Lt. peach. In 28s. With 7 white inert tablets. Lactose. (wc 781). Capsule shape.
Rx	**MonoNessa** (Watson)		0.25 norgestimate	(Watson 526). Blue. In 28s.
Rx	**Previfem** (Qualitest)			Lactose. (b 987). Blue. In 28s. With 7 white inert tablets. (b 143).
Rx	**Ortho-Cyclen** (Ortho-McNeil)			Lactose. (Ortho 250). Blue. In *Dialpak* and *Veridate* 28s. With 7 green inert tablets.
Rx	**Sprintec** (Barr)			Lactose. (b 987). Blue. In 28s. With 7 white inert tablets (b 143).
Rx	**Kelnor 1/35** (Barr)		1 ethynodiol diacetate	Lt. yellow. In 28s. With 7 white inert tablets.
Rx	**Zovia 1/35E** (Watson)			Lactose. (WATSON 383). Lt. pink. In 21s and 28s. With 7 white inert tablets (WATSON P) in the 28s.
Rx	**Ocella** (Barr Labs)	30 ethinyl estradiol	3 drospirenone	Lactose. Yellow, round. Film-coated. In blister pack 28s, with 7 white inert tablets.
Rx	**Safyral** (Bayer)			Ethinyl estradiol as betadex clathrate. Lactose, levomefolate calcium 0.451 mg, PEG. (Y+). Orange, round. Film-coated. In 21s. With 7 lt. orange tablets (levomefolate calcium 0.451 mg). Lactose, PEG. (M+).
Rx	**Yasmin** (Bayer)			Lactose. Yellow. Film-coated. In blister pack 28s. With 7 white inert film-coated tablets.
Rx	**Junel 21 Day 1.5/30** (Barr)		1.5 norethindrone acetate	Lactose, sugar. Pink. In 21s.
Rx	**Junel Fe 1.5/30** (Barr)			Pink. In 28s. With 7 brown tablets (75 mg ferrous fumarate per tablet).
Rx	**Loestrin 21 1.5/30** (Teva)			Lactose, sugar. Green. In 21s.
Rx	**Loestrin Fe 1.5/30** (Teva)			Lactose, sugar (active tablets), sucrose (inert tablets). Green. In 28s. With 7 brown tablets (75 mg ferrous fumarate per tablet).
Rx	**Microgestin Fe 1.5/30** (Watson)			Lactose. (WATSON 631). Green. In 28s. With 7 brown tablets (75 mg ferrous fumarate per tablet; WATSON 632).
Rx	**Cryselle** (Barr)		0.3 norgestrel	White. (dp 543). In 21s and 28s. With 7 lt. green inert tablets (dp 331).
Rx	**Lo/Ovral** (Akrimax Pharmaceuticals)			Lactose. (Wyeth 78). White. In *Pilpak* 21s and 28s. With 7 pink inert tablets (Wyeth 486) in the 28s.
Rx	**Low-Ogestrel** (Watson)			Lactose. (WATSON 847). White. In 28s. With 7 peach inert tablets (WATSON P1).
Rx	**Apri** (Barr)		0.15 desogestrel	Lactose. (dp 575). Rose. In blister card 28s. With 7 white inert tablets (dp 570).
Rx	**Desogen** (Organon)			Lactose. (Organon T_5R). White. In 28s. With 7 green inert tablets (Organon K_2H).
Rx	**Ortho-Cept** (Ortho-McNeil)			Lactose. Orange. In *Dialpak* and *Veridate* 28s. With 7 green inert tablets.
Rx	**Reclipsen** (Watson)			Lactose. (WATSON 954). White. In 28s, including 7 green, inert tablets (WATSON P).
Rx	**Jolessa**[a] (Barr)		0.15 levonorgestrel	Lactose. (b 992). Film-coated. Pink. In 91s. With 7 white, inert tablets. Lactose. (b 208).
Rx	**Levora** (Watson)			Lactose. (15/30 WATSON). White. In 28s. With 7 peach inert tablets (WATSON P1).
Rx	**Nordette-28** (Barr/Duramed)			Lactose. (WYETH 75). Lt. orange. In 28s. With 7 pink inert tablets (WYETH 486).
Rx	**Portia** (Barr)			Lactose. (b 992). Pink. Film-coated. In 21s and 28s. With 7 white inert tablets (b 208) in the 28s.
Rx	**Quasense**[a] (Watson Pharma)			Lactose. (WATSON 966). In 91s. With 7 peach inert tablets. Lactose. (WATSON P1).
Rx	**Seasonale**[a] (Duramed)			Lactose. (S 62). Pink. Film-coated. In 91s with 7 white inert tablets (S 197).

Contraceptive Hormones

MONOPHASIC CONTRACEPTIVES — ORAL

	Product & Distributor	Estrogen (mcg)	Progestin (mg)	How Supplied
Rx	**Beyaz** (Bayer Health-care)	20 ethinyl estradiol	3 drospirenone	0.451 mg Levomefolate calcium, lactose, PEG. (Z+). Pink, round. Film-coated. In 24s. With 4 lt. orange tablets.
Rx	**Gianvi** (Teva)			Lactose, PEG, polysorbate 80. (b 257). Pink, round. Film-coated. In 24s. With 4 white, round, inert tablets. Film-coated. (b 208). In blister pack 28s.
Rx	**YAZ**[b] (Bayer)			Lactose. (DS). Lt. pink, hexagon. Film-coated. In 24s. With 4 white, hexagon, inert tablets (DP). In blister pack 28s.
Rx	**Lybrel**[c] (Wyeth)		0.09 levonorgestrel	Lactose. (W 1117). Yellow. Film-coated. In 28s.
Rx	**Alesse** (Wyeth-Ayerst)		0.1 levonorgestrel	Lactose. (W 912). Pink. In 28s. With 7 lt. green inert tablets (W 650).
Rx	**Aviane** (Barr)			Lactose. (dp 016). Orange. In 28s. With 7 lt. green inert tablets (dp 519).
Rx	**Lessina** (Barr)			Lactose. (b 965). Pink. Film-coated. In 21s and 28s. With 7 white inert tablets (b 208) in the 28s.
Rx	**Lutera** (Watson)			Lactose. (WATSON 949). White. In 28s. With 7 peach inert tablets (WATSON P1).
Rx	**Sronyx** (Watson Pharma)			Lactose. (WATSON 967). In 28s. With 7 peach inert tablets. Lactose. (WATSON P1).
Rx	**Junel 21 Day 1/20** (Barr)		1 norethindrone acetate	Lactose, sugar. Lt. yellow. In 21s.
Rx	**Junel Fe 1/20** (Barr)			Lt. yellow. In 28s. With 7 brown tablets (75 mg ferrous fumarate per tablet).
Rx	**Loestrin 24 Fe**[d] (Warner Chilcott)			Sugar, lactose. (P-D 915). White. In 28s. With 4 brown tablets (75 mg ferrous fumarate per tablet).
Rx	**Loestrin 21 1/20** (Teva)			Lactose, sugar. White. In 21s.
Rx	**Loestrin Fe 1/20** (Teva)			Lactose, sugar (active tablets), sucrose (inert tablets). White. In 28s. With 7 brown tablets (75 mg ferrous fumarate per tablet).
Rx	**Microgestin Fe 1/20** (Watson)			Lactose. (WATSON 630). White. In 28s. With 7 brown tablets (75 mg ferrous fumarate per tablet; WATSON 632).
Rx	**Solia** (Prasco)	30 ethinyl estradiol	0.15 desogestrel	Lactose. 21 white tablets (T_5R Prasco). In blister card 28s. With 7 green inert tablets (K_2H Prasco).

[a] Take 1 active tablet per day for 84 consecutive days, followed by 7 days of inert tablets.
[b] Take 1 lt. pink (active) tablet per day for 24 consecutive days, followed by 1 white (inert) tablet daily for 4 days.
[c] Take 1 tablet daily without any tablet-free interval. Take tablets at the same time each day.
[d] Take 1 white (active) tablet per day for 24 days, followed by 1 brown (inert) tablet for 4 days.

MONOPHASIC CONTRACEPTIVES, — ORAL

For complete and comparative prescribing information, refer to the Oral Contraceptives group monograph. The combination therapy products are listed in order of decreasing estrogen content.

BIPHASIC CONTRACEPTIVES — ORAL

	Product	*Phase 1*	*Phase 2*	How Supplied
Rx	**Azurette** (Watson)	0.15 desogestrel 20 mcg ethinyl estradiol (21 white tablets)	10 mcg ethinyl estradiol (5 lt. blue tablets)	Lactose. White, round. (WATSON 942). In blister pack 21s with 2 round, green inert tablets. (WATSON P).
Rx	**Kariva** (Barr)	0.15 desogestrel 20 mcg ethinyl estradiol (21 white tablets)	10 mcg ethinyl estradiol (5 lt. blue tablets)	Lactose. White = (021). Round. In 21s. Lt. blue = (022). Round. In 5s. With 2 round light green inert tablets (331).
Rx	**Mircette** (Duramed)	0.15 desogestrel 20 mcg ethinyl estradiol (21 white tablets)	10 mcg ethinyl estradiol (5 yellow tablets)	Lactose. White = (dp 021). Round. In 21s. Yellow = (dp 022). Round. In 5s. With 2 round light green inert tablets (dp 331).
Rx	**LoSeasonique** (Teva)	0.1 mg levonorgestrel 0.02 mg ethinyl estradiol (84 orange tablets)	0.01 mg ethinyl estradiol (7 yellow tablets)	Lactose. Orange, round = (b 28). In 84s. Lactose, PEG. Yellow = (b 556). In 7s.
Rx	**Seasonique** (Duramed)	0.15 mg levonorgestrel 30 mcg ethinyl estradiol (84 lt. blue-green tablets)	10 mcg ethinyl estradiol (7 yellow tablets)	Lactose. Lt. blue-green = (B 555). Film-coated. In 84s. Yellow = (B 556). Film-coated. In 7s.
Rx	**Necon 10/11** (Watson)	0.5 mg norethindrone, 35 mcg ethinyl estradiol (10 lt. yellow tablets)	1 mg norethindrone, 35 mcg ethinyl estradiol (11 dk. yellow tablets)	Lactose. Lt. yellow = (WATSON 507). Dk. yellow = (WATSON 508). In 28s with 7 white inert tablets (WATSON P).
Rx	**Ortho-Novum 10/11** (Ortho-McNeil)	0.5 mg norethindrone, 35 mcg ethinyl estradiol (10 white tablets)	1 mg norethindrone, 35 mcg ethinyl estradiol (11 peach tablets)	Lactose. White = (Ortho 535). Peach = (Ortho 135). In *Dialpak* 28s. With 7 green inert tablets (Ortho).

BIPHASIC CONTRACEPTIVES ORAL

For complete and comparative prescribing information, refer to the Oral Contraceptives group monograph. The combination therapy products are listed in order of decreasing estrogen content.

TRIPHASIC CONTRACEPTIVES — ORAL

	Product	*Phase 1*	*Phase 2*	*Phase 3*	How Supplied
Rx	**Tri-Norinyl** (Watson)	0.5 mg norethindrone, 35 mcg ethinyl estradiol (7 blue tablets)	1 mg norethindrone, 35 mcg ethinyl estradiol (9 yellow-green tablets)	0.5 mg norethindrone, 35 mcg ethinyl estradiol (5 blue tablets)	Lactose. Blue = (Watson 254). Yellow-green = (Watson 259). In *Wallette* 28s. With 7 orange inert tablets (Watson P1).
Rx	**Aranelle** (Barr)	0.5 mg norethindrone, 35 mcg ethinyl estradiol (7 lt. yellow tablets)	1 mg norethindrone, 35 mcg ethinyl estradiol (9 white tablets)	0.5 mg norethindrone, 35 mcg ethinyl estradiol (5 lt. yellow tablets)	Lactose. Lt. yellow = (b 341). White = (b 342). Peach = (b 343). Beveled. In 28s. With 7 peach inert tablets.
Rx	**Leena** (Watson)	0.5 mg norethindrone, 35 mcg ethinyl estradiol (7 lt. blue tablets)	1 mg norethindrone, 35 mcg ethinyl estradiol (9 lt. yellow-green tablets)	0.5 mg norethindrone, 35 mcg ethinyl estradiol (5 lt. blue tablets)	Lactose. Lt. blue = (Watson 243). Lt yellow-green = (Watson 244). Peach = (Watson P1). In 28s. With 7 orange inert tablets.
Rx	**Necon 7/7/7** (Watson)	0.5 mg norethindrone, 35 mcg ethinyl estradiol (7 white tablets)	0.75 mg norethindrone, 35 mcg ethinyl estradiol (7 lt. peach tablets)	1 mg norethindrone, 35 mcg ethinyl estradiol (7 peach tablets)	In 28s. With 7 green inert tablets.
Rx	**Ortho-Novum 7/7/7** (Ortho-McNeil)				Lactose. White = (Ortho 535). Lt. peach = (Ortho 75). Peach = (Ortho 135). In *Dialpak* and *Veridate* 28s. With 7 green inert tablets (Ortho).
Rx	**Enpresse** (Barr)	0.05 mg levonorgestrel, 30 mcg ethinyl estradiol (6 pink tablets)	0.075 mg levonorgestrel, 40 mcg ethinyl estradiol (5 white tablets)	0.125 mg levonorgestrel, 30 mcg ethinyl estradiol (10 orange tablets)	Lactose. Pink = (dp 510). White = (dp 511). Orange = (dp 512). In 28s. With 7 lt. green inert tablets (dp 519).

Contraceptive Hormones

TRIPHASIC CONTRACEPTIVES — ORAL

	Product	Phase 1	Phase 2	Phase 3	How Supplied
Rx	**Triphasil** (Wyeth Labs)	0.05 mg levonorgestrel, 30 mcg ethinyl estradiol (6 brown tablets)	0.075 mg levonorgestrel, 40 mcg ethinyl estradiol (5 white tablets)	0.125 mg levonorgestrel, 30 mcg ethinyl estradiol (10 lt. yellow tablets)	Lactose. Brown = (W 641). White = (W 642). Lt. yellow = (W 643). In 21s and 28s. With 7 lt. green inert tablets (W 650) in the 28s.
Rx	**Trivora** (Watson)	0.05 mg levonorgestrel, 30 mcg ethinyl estradiol (6 blue tablets)	0.075 mg levonorgestrel, 40 mcg ethinyl estradiol (5 white tablets)	0.125 mg levonorgestrel, 30 mcg ethinyl estradiol (10 pink tablets)	Lactose. Blue, white, and pink tablets. In 28s. With 7 peach inert tablets (WATSON P1).
Rx	**Cyclessa** (Organon)	0.1 mg desogestrel, 25 mcg ethinyl estradiol (7 lt. yellow tablets)	0.125 mg desogestrel, 25 mcg ethinyl estradiol (7 orange tablets)	0.15 mg desogestrel, 25 mcg ethinyl estradiol (7 red tablets)	Lactose, talc. Lt. yellow = (T_0R Organon). Orange = (T_6R Organon). Red = (T_1R Organon). In 28s. With 7 green inert tablets (K_2H Organon).
Rx	**Cesia** (Prasco)				Lactose, talc (lt. yellow, orange, green). Lt. yellow = (T_0R Organon). Orange = (T_6R Organon). Red = (T_1R Organon). Green = (K_2H Organon). With 7 green inert tablets. In 28s.
Rx	**Velivet** (Barr)	0.1 mg desogestrel, 25 mcg ethinyl estradiol (7 beige tablets)	0.125 mg desogestrel, 25 mcg ethinyl estradiol (7 orange tablets)	0.15 mg desogestrel, 25 mcg ethinyl estradiol (7 pink tablets)	With 7 white inert tablets. (b 334). In 28s.
Rx	**Caziant** (Watson Labs)	0.1 mg desogestrel, 25 mcg ethinyl estradiol (7 white tablets)	0.125 mg desogestrel, 25 mcg ethinyl estradiol (7 lt. blue tablets)	0.15 mg desogestrel, 25 mcg ethinyl estradiol (7 blue tablets)	Lactose. White, round = (WATSON 960). Lt. blue, round = (WATSON 961). Blue, round = (WATSON 962). In 28-day blister card with recyclable dispenser. With 7 green inert tablets (WATSON P).
Rx	**Ortho Tri-Cyclen** (Ortho-McNeil)	0.18 mg norgestimate, 35 mcg ethinyl estradiol (7 white tablets)	0.215 mg norgestimate, 35 mcg ethinyl estradiol (7 lt. blue tablets)	0.25 mg norgestimate, 35 mcg ethinyl estradiol (7 blue tablets)	Lactose. White= (Ortho 180). Lt. blue = (Ortho 215). Blue = (Ortho 250). In *Dialpak* and *Veridate* 28s. With 7 green inert tablets.
Rx	**Tri-Previfem** (Qualitest)				Lactose. White = (746). Lt. blue = (747). Blue = (748). In 28s. With 7 teal inert tablets.
Rx	**TriNessa** (Watson)				With 7 green inert tablets. In 28s.
Rx	**Tri-Sprintec** (Barr)	0.18 mg norgestimate, 35 mcg ethinyl estradiol (7 gray tablets)	0.215 mg norgestimate, 35 mcg ethinyl estradiol (7 lt. blue tablets)	0.25 mg norgestimate, 35 mcg ethinyl estradiol (7 blue tablets)	Lactose. Gray = (b 985). Lt. blue = (b 986). Blue = (b 987). White = (b 143). With 7 white inert tablets. In 28s.
Rx	**Ortho Tri-Cyclen Lo** (Ortho-McNeil)	0.18 mg norgestimate, 25 mcg ethinyl estradiol (7 white tablets)	0.215 mg norgestimate, 25 mcg ethinyl estradiol (7 lt. blue tablets)	0.25 mg norgestimate, 25 mcg ethinyl estradiol (7 dk. blue tablets)	Talc (green inert tablets), lactose. White = (O-M 180). Lt. blue = (O-M 215). Dk. blue = (O-M 250). In *Dialpak* and *Veridate* 28s. With 7 green inert tablets.
Rx	**Tilia Fe** (Watson)	1 mg norethindrone acetate, 20 mcg ethinyl estradiol (5 white triangular tablets)	1 mg norethindrone acetate, 30 mcg ethinyl estradiol (7 white square tablets)	1 mg norethindrone acetate, 35 mcg ethinyl estradiol (9 white round tablets)	Lactose. In 28s. With 7 brown tablets (75 mg ferrous fumarate per tablet).
Rx	**Tri-Legest** (Barr Labs)	1 mg norethindrone acetate, 20 mcg ethinyl estradiol (5 lt. pink tablets)	1 mg norethindrone acetate, 30 mcg ethinyl estradiol (7 lt. yellow tablets)	1 mg norethindrone acetate, 35 mcg ethinyl estradiol (9 lt. blue tablets)	Lactose. Pink = (b 711). Yellow = (b 712). Blue = (b 713). In 21s.
Rx	**Estrostep Fe** (Warner Chilcott)	1 mg norethindrone acetate, 20 mcg ethinyl estradiol (5 triangular tablets)	1 mg norethindrone acetate, 30 mcg ethinyl estradiol (7 square tablets)	1 mg norethindrone acetate, 35 mcg ethinyl estradiol (9 round tablets)	Lactose (white), sucrose (brown). White. In 28s. With 7 brown tablets (75 mg ferrous fumarate per tablet).
Rx	**Tri-Legest Fe** (Barr Labs)	1 mg norethindrone acetate, 20 mcg ethinyl estradiol (5 lt. pink tablets)	1 mg norethindrone acetate, 30 mcg ethinyl estradiol (7 lt. yellow tablets)	1 mg norethindrone acetate, 35 mcg ethinyl estradiol (9 lt. blue tablets)	Lactose. With 7 brown tablets (75 mg ferrous fumarate per tablet). Pink = (b 711). Yellow = (b 712). Blue = (b 713). Brown = (b 711). In 28s.

TRIPHASIC CONTRACEPTIVES, ORAL

For complete and comparative prescribing information, refer to the Oral Contraceptives group monograph. The combination therapy products are listed in order of decreasing estrogen content.

4-PHASIC CONTRACEPTIVES, — ORAL

	Product	Phase 1	Phase 2	Phase 3	Phase 4	How Supplied
Rx	**Natazia** (Bayer HealthCare Pharmaceuticals)	3 mg estradiol valerate (2 dark-yellow tablets)	2 mg estradiol valerate 2 mg dienogest (5 medium-red tablets)	2 mg estradiol valerate 3 mg dienogest (17 light-yellow tablets)	1 mg estradiol valerate (2 dark-red tablets)	Lactose. Round. Film-coated. Dark-yellow = (DD). Medium-red = (DJ). Light-yellow = (DH). Dark-red = (DN).In 28s with 2 white inert tablets (DT).

4-PHASIC CONTRACEPTIVES — ORAL

For complete and comparative prescribing information, refer to the Oral Contraceptives group monograph. The combination therapy products are listed in order of decreasing estrogen content.

Administration and Dosage

➤*Adults:*

Contraception – 1 tablet daily at the same time every day. Start on the first day of the menstrual cycle.

Missed doses:

• *One tablet* – If 1 tablet is missed for more than 12 hours during days 1 to 17, the missed tablet should be taken immediately and the next tablet at the usual time (2 tablets may have to be taken in 1 day). If 1 tablet is missed for more than 12 hours in days 18 to 24, no more tablets should be taken from the current blister pack and it should be discarded. Take the day 1 tablet from a new blister pack. Back-up contraception should be used for the next 9 days in both situations.

If 1 tablet is missed for more than 12 hours in days 25 to 28, the missed tablet should be taken immediately and the next tablet at the usual time (2 tablets may have to be taken in 1 day). No back-up contraception is needed.

Continue to take 1 tablet each day at the same time for the rest of the cycle.

• *Two tablets* – If 2 tablets in a row are missed during days 1 to 17, the missed tablets should not be taken; the tablet for the day on which the missed doses are noticed should be taken. If 2 tablets in a row are missed during days 17 to 25, no more tablets should be taken from the current blister pack and it should be discarded. Take the day 3 tablet from a new blister pack. Back-up contraception should be used for 9 days in both situations.

If 2 tablets in a row are missed in days 25 to 28, no more tablets should be taken from the current blister pack and it should be discarded. A new blister pack should be started that day or on the day a new pack would usually be started. No back-up contraception is needed.

Continue to take 1 tablet each day at the same time for the rest of the cycle.

➤*Administration:* Tablets should not be skipped or intake delayed by more than 12 hours.

PROGESTIN-ONLY PRODUCTS

Rx	**Norethindrone** (Glenmark Pharmaceuticals)	**Tablets; oral:** 0.35 mg norethindrone	Lactose. (305 G). Lt. yellow, round. In 28s.
Rx	**Camila** (Barr)		Lactose. (b 715). Lt. pink. In 28s.
Rx	**Errin** (Barr)		Lactose. (b 344). Yellow. In 28s.
Rx	**Heather** (Glenmark Generics)		Lactose. (303 G). Pale yellow. In 28s.
Rx	**Jolivette** (Watson)		Lactose. (WATSON 892). Green. In 28s.
Rx	**Nor-QD** (Watson)		Lactose. Yellow. In 28s.
Rx	**Nora-BE** (Watson)		Lactose. (Watson 629). White. In 28s.
Rx	**Ortho Micronor** (Ortho-McNeil)		Lactose. Green. In *Dialpak* 28s.

NORETHINDRONE — ORAL

For complete and comparative prescribing information, refer to the Oral Contraceptives class monograph.

Indications

➤*Contraception:* Progestin-only oral contraceptives (OCs) are indicated for the prevention of pregnancy.

Administration and Dosage

➤*Adults:*

Contraception –

Usual dosage: One tablet is taken every day, at the same time. Administration is continuous, with no interruption between pill packs.

Missed dose: If a dose is more than 3 hours late or 1 or more doses are missed, take the missed dose as soon as remembered, then take the next dose at the regular time, and use a backup method of contraception (eg, condom and/or spermicide) each time there is sexual intercourse for the next 48 hours.

➤*Children:* Use of this product before menarche is not indicated.

Contraception – See Adults for dosing.

➤*Hepatic function impairment:* Contraindicated in patients with acute liver disease.

➤*Administration:* If GI upset occurs, administer with food.

➤*Storage/Stability:* Store at controlled room temperature 25°C (77°F); excursions permitted to 15° to 30°C (59° to 86°F).

LEVONORGESTREL (EMERGENCY CONTRACEPTIVES)

otc[a]	**Levonorgestrel** (Perrigo Pharmaceuticals)	**Tablets; oral:** 0.75 mg	Lactose. (L840). White to off-white, round. In UD 2s.
otc[a]	**Next Choice** (Watson Laboratories)		Lactose. (475 WATSON). Peach, round. In UD 2s.
otc[b]	**Plan B** (Duramed)		Lactose. (INOR). White, round. In UD 2s.
otc[a]	**Plan B One-Step** (Duramed)	**Tablets; oral:** 1.5 mg	Lactose. (G00). White, round. In 1s.

[a] *Next Choice, Plan B One-Step,* and **levonorgestrel** 0.75 mg are approved for over-the-counter status for women ≥ 17 years of age. They are available by prescription only for women < 17 years of age.

[b] *Plan B* is approved for over-the-counter status for women ≥ 18 years of age. It is available by prescription only for women ≤ 17 years of age.

LEVONORGESTREL — ORAL

Indications

➤*Emergency contraception:* To prevent pregnancy after known or suspected contraceptive failure or unprotected intercourse. Emergency contraceptives (like all oral contraceptives) do not protect against infection with HIV (the virus that causes AIDS) and other sexually transmitted diseases.

Administration and Dosage

➤*General dosing considerations:* Efficacy is better if levonorgestrel is taken as directed as soon as possible after unprotected intercourse.

Levonorgestrel can be used at any time during the menstrual cycle.

➤*Adults:*

Emergency contraceptive –

Next Choice and *Plan B*: One tablet should be taken within 72 hours after unprotected intercourse. The second tablet should be taken 12 hours after the first dose.

Plan B One-Step: Take as soon as possible within 72 hours after unprotected intercourse or a known or suspected contraceptive failure.

➤*Children:*

Emergency contraceptive – See Adults for dosing.

➤*Administration:*

Plan B – The user should be instructed that if she vomits within 1 hour of taking either dose of medication, she should contact her health care provider to discuss whether to repeat that dose.

Next Choice and *Plan B One-Step* – If vomiting occurs within 2 hours of taking the tablet, consider repeating the dose.

➤*Storage/Stability:*

Plan B – Store at 25°C (77°F); excursions are permitted between 15° and 30°C (59° and 86°F).

Next Choice and *Plan B One-Step* – Store at 20° to 25°C (68° to 77°F).

Actions

➤*Pharmacology:* Emergency contraceptives are not effective if the woman is already pregnant. Levonorgestrel is believed to act as an emergency contraceptive principally by preventing ovulation or fertilization (by altering tubal transport of sperm and/or ova). In addition, it may inhibit implantation (by altering the endometrium). It is not effective once the process of implantation has begun.

➤*Pharmacokinetics:*

***Plan B* and *Next Choice* Pharmacokinetic Parameters**[a]

	Mean (± SD)					
	C_{max} (ng/mL)	T_{max} (h)	CL (L/h)	V_d (L)	t½ (h)	$AUC_{0-\infty}$ (ng/mL/h)
Levonorgestrel 0.75 mg (n = 16)	14.1±7.7	1.6±0.7	7.7±2.7	260	24.4±5.3	123.1±50.1

[a] SD = standard deviation; C_{max} = maximum plasma concentration; T_{max} = time to C_{max}; CL = clearance; Vol = volume of distribution; t½ = half-life; AUC = area under the curve.

***Plan B One-Step* Pharmacokinetic Parameters**

	Mean (± SD)				
	C_{max} (ng/mL)	AUC_t (ng•h/mL)[a]	AUC_{inf} (ng•h/mL)[a]	T_{max} (h)[b]	t½ (h)
Levonorgestrel 1.5 mg (n = 30)	19.1 (9.7)	294.8 (208.8)	307.5 (218.5)	1.7 (1 to 4)	27.5 (5.6)

[a] N = 29.
[b] Median (range).

Absorption – No specific investigation of the absolute bioavailability of levonorgestrel in humans has been conducted. However, literature indicates that levonorgestrel is rapidly and completely absorbed after oral administration (bioavailability about 100%) and is not subject to first pass metabolism.

Distribution –

Plan B: Levonorgestrel in serum is primarily protein bound. Approximately 50% is bound to albumin and 47.5% is bound to sex hormone–binding globulin (SHBG).

Plan B One-Step and *Next Choice*: The apparent volume of distribution of levonorgestrel is reported to be approximately 1.8 L/kg. It is about 97.5% to 99% protein-bound, principally to SHBG and, to a lesser extent, serum albumin.

Metabolism –

Plan B: Following a single oral dosage, levonorgestrel does not appear to be extensively metabolized by the liver. The primary metabolites are 3 alpha, 5 beta- and 3 alpha, 5 alpha-tetrahydrolevonorgestrel with 16 beta-hydroxynorgestrel also identified. Together these account for less than 10% of parent plasma levels. Urinary metabolites hydroxylated at the 2 alpha and 16 beta positions have also been identified. Small amounts of the metabolites are present in plasma as sulfate and glucuronide conjugates.

Plan B One-Step and *Next Choice*: Following absorption, levonorgestrel is conjugated at the 17 beta-OH position to form sulfate conjugates and, to a lesser extent, glucuronide conjugates in plasma. Significant amounts of conjugated and unconjugated 3 alpha, 5 beta-tetrahydrolevonorgestrel are also

LEVONORGESTREL — ORAL

present in plasma, along with much smaller amounts of 3 alpha, 5 alpha-tetrahydrolevonorgestrel and 16 beta hydroxylevonorgestrel. Levonorgestrel and its phase I metabolites are excreted primarily as glucuronide conjugates. Metabolic clearance rates may differ among individuals by serveral-fold, and this may account in part for the wide variation observed in levonorgestrel concentrations among users.

Excretion –

Plan B: The elimination half-life of levonorgestrel following single dose administration as *Plan B* (0.75 mg) is 24.4 ± 5.3 hours. Excretion following single-dose administration as emergency contraception is unknown, but based on chronic, low-dose contraceptive use, levonorgestrel and its metabolites are primarily excreted in the urine, with smaller amounts recovered in the feces.

Plan B One-Step and *Next Choice*: About 45% of levonorgestrel and its metabolites are excreted in the urine and about 32% are excreted in feces, mostly as glucuronide conjugates.

Special populations –

Race: No formal studies have evaluated the effect of race. However, clinical trials demonstrated a higher pregnancy rate in the Chinese population with *Plan B*, *Next Choice*, and the Yuzpe regimen (another form of emergency contraception consisting of 2 doses of ethinyl estradiol 0.1 mg + levonorgestrel 0.5 mg). There was a nonstatistically significant increased rate of pregnancy among Chinese women in the *Plan B One-Step* trial. The reason for this apparent increase in the pregnancy rate of emergency contraceptives in Chinese women is unknown.

Contraindications

Known or suspected pregnancy; hypersensitivity to any component of the product.

Warnings/Precautions

➤*Contraceptive use:* Levonorgestrel is not recommended for routine use as a contraceptive.

➤*Effects on menses:* Menstrual bleeding patterns are often irregular among women using progestin-only oral contraceptives and in clinical studies of levonorgestrel for postcoital and emergency contraceptive use. Some women may experience spotting a few days after taking levonorgestrel. At the time of expected menses, approximately 75% of women using levonorgestrel had vaginal bleeding similar to their normal menses, 12% to 13% bled more than usual, and 12% bled less than usual. The majority of women (87%) had their next menstrual period at the expected time or within ± 7 days, while 13% had a delay of more than 7 days beyond the anticipated onset of menses. If there is a delay in the onset of menses beyond 1 week, consider the possibility of pregnancy.

➤*Ectopic pregnancy:* Ectopic pregnancies account for approximately 2% of reported pregnancies. Up to 10% of pregnancies reported in clinical studies of routine use of progestin-only contraceptives are ectopic. Consider a history of ectopic pregnancy a contraindication of using the emergency contraceptive method. However, be alert to the possibility of an ectopic pregnancy in women who become pregnant or complain of lower abdominal pain after taking levonorgestrel.

➤*Sexually transmitted diseases:* Levonorgestrel, like progestin-only contraceptives, does not protect against HIV infection (AIDS) and other sexually transmitted diseases.

➤*Carbohydrate metabolism:* The effects of levonorgestrel on carbohydrate metabolism are unknown. Some users of progestin-only oral contraceptives may experience slight deterioration in glucose tolerance, with increases in plasma insulin; however, women with diabetes mellitus who use progestin-only oral contraceptives do not generally experience changes in their insulin requirements. Nonetheless, monitor diabetic women while they are taking levonorgestrel.

➤*Pregnancy: Category X.* Many studies have found no effects on fetal development associated with long-term use of contraceptive doses of oral progestins. The few studies of infant growth and development that have been conducted with progestin-only oral contraceptives have not demonstrated significant adverse effects. Levonorgestrel is not effective in terminating an existing pregnancy.

➤*Lactation:* Small amounts of progestin pass into the breast milk of women taking progestin-only oral contraceptives for long-term contraception, resulting in steroid levels in infant plasma of 1% to 6% of the levels of maternal plasma. However, no adverse effects caused by progestin-only oral contraceptives have been found on breast-feeding performance, either in the quality or quantity of the milk, or on the health, growth, or development of the infant. Isolated postmarketing cases of decreased milk production have been reported. The American Academy of Pediatrics classifies levonorgestrel as usually compatible with breast-feeding.

➤*Children:* Use of levonorgestrel emergency contraception before menarche is not indicated.

➤*Elderly:* This product is not intended for use in postmenopausal women.

➤*Monitoring:* A physical examination is not required prior to prescribing levonorgestrel. However, a follow-up physical or pelvic examination is recommended if there is any doubt concerning the general health or pregnancy status of any woman after taking levonorgestrel. Monitor diabetic women while taking levonorgestrel.

Drug Interactions

➤*CYP3A4 inducers:* Drugs or herbal products that induce enzymes, including CYP3A4, that metabolize progestins may decrease the plasma concentrations of progestins, and may decrease the effectiveness of progestin-only oral contraceptives. Some drugs or herbal products that may decrease the effectiveness of progestin-only oral contraceptives include: barbiturates, bosentan, carbamazepine, felbamate, griseofulvin, oxcarbazepine, phenytoin, rifampin, St. John's wort, and topiramate.

➤*Protease inhibitors/non-nucleoside reverse transcriptase inhibitors:* Significant changes (increase or decrease) in the plasma levels of the progestin have been noted in some cases of coadministration with HIV protease inhibitors or with non-nucleoside reverse transcriptase inhibitors.

Adverse Reactions

➤*Plan B* and *Next Choice*:

Common adverse reactions –

***Plan B* and *Next Choice* Adverse Reactions (≥ 5%)**	
Adverse reactions	Levonorgestrel (n = 977)
Miscellaneous	
Dizziness	11.2%
CNS	
Fatigue	16.9%
Headache	16.8%
GI	
Abdominal pain	17.6%
Diarrhea	5%
Nausea	23.1%
Vomiting	5.6%
GU	
Breast tenderness	10.7%
Heavier menstrual bleeding	13.8%
Lighter menstrual bleeding	12.5%
Other complaints	9.7%

➤*Plan B One-Step*:

Most common adverse reactions –

***Plan B One-Step* Adverse Reactions (> 4%)**	
Adverse reactions	Levonorgestrel (n = 1,359)
CNS	
Dizziness	9.6%
Fatigue	13.3%
Headache	10.3%
GI	
Lower abdominal pain	13.3%
Nausea	13.7%
GU	
Breast tenderness	8.2%
Delay of menses (> 7 days)	4.5%
Heavier menstrual bleeding	30.9%

➤*Postmarketing:*

CNS – Dizziness, fatigue, headache.

GI – Abdominal pain, nausea, vomiting.

GU – Dysmenorrhea, irregular menstruation, oligomenorrhea, pelvic pain.

Overdosage

There are no data on overdosage of levonorgestrel; although, the common adverse reaction of nausea and its associated vomiting may be anticipated.

ULIPRISTAL ACETATE (EMERGENCY CONTRACEPTIVE)

Rx	ella (Watson Pharma)	**Tablets; oral:** 30 mg	Lactose. (ella/ella). White to off-white, round and curved. In UD 1s.

ULIPRISTAL ACETATE — ORAL

Indications

➤*Emergency contraceptive:* For prevention of pregnancy following unprotected intercourse or a known or suspected contraceptive failure. Ulipristal is not intended for routine use as a contraceptive.

Administration and Dosage

➤*General dosing considerations:* Ulipristal can be taken at any time during the menstrual cycle.

➤*Adults:*

Emergency contraceptive – 1 tablet orally as soon as possible within 120 hours (5 days) after unprotected intercourse or a known or suspected contraceptive failure.

➤*Children:*

Emergency contraceptive – Use before menarche is not indicated. (See Adults for dosing.)

➤*Administration:* May be taken with or without food.

If vomiting occurs within 3 hours of ulipristal intake, consider repeating the dose.

➤*Storage/Stability:* Store at 20° to 25°C (68° to 77°F). Keep the blister in the outer carton in order to protect from light.

Actions

➤*Pharmacology:* Ulipristal is a selective progesterone receptor modulator with antagonistic and partial agonistic effects (a progesterone agonist/antagonist) at the progesterone receptor. It binds the human progesterone receptor and prevents progesterone from occupying its receptor.

When taken immediately before ovulation is to occur, ulipristal postpones follicular rupture. Therefore, the likely primary mechanism of action of ulipristal for emergency contraception is inhibition or delay of ovulation; however, alterations to the endometrium that may affect implantation may also contribute to efficacy.

➤*Pharmacokinetics:*

Ulipristal Pharmacokinetic Parameters[a]

Pharmacokinetic parameter	Mean (± SD)				
	C_{max} (ng/mL)	AUC_{0-t} (ng•h/mL)	$AUC_{0-\infty}$ (ng•h/mL)	T_{max} (h)[b]	t½ (h)
Ulipristal	176 (89)	548 (259)	556 (260)	0.9 (0.5 to 2)	32 (6.3)
Monodemethyl-ulipristal acetate	69 (26)	240 (59)	246 (59)	1 (0.8 to 2)	27 (6.9)

[a] C_{max} = maximum concentration; AUC_{0-t} = area under the curve from time 0 to time of last determinable concentration; $AUC_{0-\infty}$ = area under the curve from time 0 to infinity; T_{max} = time to maximum concentration; t½ = elimination half-life.
[b] Median (range).

Absorption – Following a single-dose administration of ulipristal in 20 women under fasting conditions, maximum plasma concentrations of ulipristal and the active metabolite, monodemethyl-ulipristal, were 176 and 69 ng/mL and were reached at 0.9 and 1 hour, respectively.

Effect of food: Administration of ulipristal together with a high-fat breakfast resulted in approximately 40% to 45% lower mean C_{max}, a delayed T_{max} (from a median of 0.75 to 3 hours) and 20% to 25% higher mean $AUC_{0-\infty}$ of ulipristal and monodemethyl-ulipristal acetate compared with administration in the fasting state. These differences are not expected to impair the efficacy or safety of ulipristal to a clinically significant extent; therefore, ulipristal can be taken with or without food.

Distribution – Ulipristal is highly bound (more than 94%) to plasma proteins, including high-density lipoprotein, alpha-l-acid glycoprotein, and albumin.

Metabolism – Ulipristal is metabolized to mono-demethylated and di-demethylated metabolites. In vitro data indicate that this is predominantly mediated by CYP3A4. The mono-demethylated metabolite is pharmacologically active.

Excretion – The terminal half-life of ulipristal in plasma following a single 30 mg dose is estimated to be 32.4 ± 6.3 hours.

Special populations –

Renal function impairment: No studies have been conducted to evaluate the effect of renal disease on the disposition of the ulipristal.

Hepatic function impairment: No studies have been conducted to evaluate the effect of hepatic disease on the disposition of ulipristal.

Contraindications

Known or suspected pregnancy.

Warnings/Precautions

➤*Existing pregnancy:* Ulipristal is not indicated for termination of an existing pregnancy. Exclude pregnancy before prescribing ulipristal. If pregnancy cannot be excluded on the basis of history and/or physical examination, perform pregnancy testing. A follow-up physical or pelvic examination is recommended if there is any doubt concerning the general health or pregnancy status of any woman after taking ulipristal.

➤*Ectopic pregnancy:* A history of ectopic pregnancy is not a contraindication to use of this emergency contraceptive method. Consider the possibility of ectopic pregnancy in women who become pregnant or complain of lower abdominal pain after taking ulipristal. A follow-up physical or pelvic examination is recommended if there is any doubt concerning the general health or pregnancy status of any woman after taking ulipristal.

➤*Repeated use:* Ulipristal is for occasional use as an emergency contraceptive. It should not replace a regular method of contraception. Repeated use of ulipristal within the same menstrual cycle is not recommended, as safety and efficacy of repeat use within the same cycle has not been evaluated.

➤*Fertility following use:* A rapid return of fertility is likely following treatment with ulipristal for emergency contraception; therefore, routine contraception should be continued or initiated as soon as possible following use of ulipristal to ensure ongoing prevention of pregnancy. Though there are no data about use of ulipristal with regular hormonal contraceptives, due to its high affinity binding to the progesterone receptor, use of ulipristal may reduce the contraceptive action of regular hormonal contraceptive methods. Therefore, after use of ulipristal, a reliable barrier method of contraception should be used with subsequent acts of intercourse that occur in that same menstrual cycle.

➤*Menstrual cycle effects:* After ulipristal intake, menses sometimes occur earlier or later than expected by a few days. In clinical trials, cycle length was increased by a mean of 2.5 days but returned to normal in the subsequent cycle. Seven percent of subjects reported menses occurring more than 7 days earlier than expected, and 19% reported a delay of more than 7 days. If there is a delay in the onset of expected menses beyond 1 week, rule out pregnancy.

Nine percent of women studied reported intermenstrual bleeding after use of ulipristal.

➤*Sexually transmitted infections/HIV:* Ulipristal does not protect against HIV infection (AIDS) or other sexually transmitted infections.

➤*Pregnancy: Category X.* Use of ulipristal is contraindicated during an existing or suspected pregnancy.

There are no adequate and well-controlled studies in pregnant women. The risks to a fetus when ulipristal is administered to a pregnant woman are unknown. If this drug is inadvertently used during pregnancy, apprise the patient of the potential hazard to the fetus.

Administration of ulipristal to pregnant monkeys for 4 days during the first trimester caused pregnancy termination in 2 of 5 animals at daily drug exposures 3 times the human exposure based on BSA.

➤*Lactation:* It is not known if ulipristal is excreted in human milk. However, ulipristal is detected in milk of lactating rats. Because many drugs are excreted in human milk, risk to the breast-fed child cannot be excluded. Use of ulipristal by breast-feeding women is not recommended.

➤*Children:* Safety and efficacy have been established in women of reproductive age. Safety and efficacy are expected to be the same for postpubertal adolescents younger than 18 years and for users 18 years of age and older. Use before menarche is not indicated.

➤*Elderly:* This product is not intended for use in postmenopausal women.

➤*Monitoring:* A follow-up physical or pelvic examination is recommended if there is any doubt concerning the general health or pregnancy status of any woman after taking ulipristal. Evaluate patients who complain of lower abdominal pain after taking ulipristal for the possibility of ectopic pregnancy.

Drug Interactions

Ulipristal Drug Interactions

Precipitant drug	Object drug[a]		Description
CYP3A4 inducers (eg, barbiturates, bosentan, carbamazepine, felbamate, griseofulvin, oxcarbazepine, phenytoin, rifampin, St. John's wort, topiramate)	Ulipristal	⬇	Ulipristal plasma concentration and pharmacologic effects may be decreased. Monitor the clinical response and adjust the ulipristal dose as needed.
CYP3A4 inhibitors (eg, itraconazole, ketoconazole)	Ulipristal	⬆	Ulipristal plasma concentrations may be elevated, increasing the pharmacologic effects and risk of adverse reactions. Monitor the clinical response and adjust the ulipristal dose as needed.

[a] ⬆ = object drug increased; ⬇ = object drug decreased.

ULIPRISTAL ACETATE — ORAL

➤*Drug/Food interactions:* Administration of ulipristal with a high-fat meal decreased the C_{max} approximately 40% to 45%, increased the AUC 20% to 25%, and delayed the T_{max} from a median of 0.75 hours to 3 hours compared with giving ulipristal in the fasting state. These changes are not expected to impair the safety and efficacy of ulipristal. Therefore, ulipristal can be taken without regard to food.

Adverse Reactions

➤*Adverse reactions (at least 5%):*

Ulipristal Adverse Reactions (≥ 5%)

Adverse reactions	Open-label study (N = 1,533)	Single-blind comparative study (N = 1,104)
CNS		
Dizziness	5%	5%
Fatigue	6%	6%
Headache	18%	19%
GI		
Abdominal and upper abdominal pain	15%	8%
Nausea	12%	13%
Miscellaneous		
Dysmenorrhea	7%	13%

➤*Postmarketing:*

Dermatologic – Acne.

Patient Information

Instruct patients to take ulipristal as soon as possible and not more than 120 hours after unprotected intercourse or a known or suspected contraceptive failure.

Advise patients not to take ulipristal if they know or suspect they are pregnant and that ulipristal is not indicated for termination of an existing pregnancy.

Advise patients to contact their health care provider immediately if they vomit within 3 hours of taking the tablet, to discuss whether to take another tablet.

Advise patients to seek medical attention if they experience severe lower abdominal pain 3 to 5 weeks after taking ulipristal, in order to be evaluated for an ectopic pregnancy.

Advise patients to contact their health care provider and consider the possibility of pregnancy if their period is delayed after taking ulipristal by more than 1 week beyond the date it was expected.

Advise patients not to use ulipristal as routine contraception, or to use it repeatedly in the same menstrual cycle.

Advise patients that ulipristal may reduce the contraceptive action of regular hormonal contraceptive methods and to use a reliable barrier method of contraception after using ulipristal, for any subsequent acts of intercourse that occur in that same menstrual cycle.

Inform patients that ulipristal does not protect against HIV infection (AIDS) and other sexually transmitted diseases/infections.

Advise patients not to use ulipristal if they are breast-feeding.

NORELGESTROMIN/ETHINYL ESTRADIOL — TRANSDERMAL SYSTEM

	Product	Surface Area (cm^2)	Total Content (per patch)	How Supplied
Rx	**Ortho Evra** (Ortho-McNeil)	20	Norelgestromin 6 mg/ ethinyl estradiol 0.75 mg	In cycles (3 patches) and single patches.

NORELGESTROMIN/ETHINYL ESTRADIOL — TRANSDERMAL SYSTEM

WARNING

Cigarette smoking and serious cardiovascular risks – Cigarette smoking increases the risk of serious cardiovascular events from hormonal contraceptive use. This risk increases with age, particularly in women older than 35 years, and with the number of cigarettes smoked. For this reason, hormonal contraceptives, including norelgestromin/ethinyl estradiol, should not be used by women who are older than 35 years and smoke.

Risk of venous thromboembolism – The risk of venous thromboembolism (VTE) among women aged 15 to 44 years who used the contraceptive patch compared with women who used oral contraceptives containing 30 to 35 mcg of ethinyl estradiol and either levonorgestrel or norgestimate was assessed in 4 US case-control studies using electronic health care claims data. The odds ratios ranged from 1.2 to 2.2; one of the studies found a statistically significant increased risk of VTE for current users of the contraceptive patch.

Hormone exposure – The pharmacokinetic profile for the contraceptive patch is different from the pharmacokinetic profile for oral contraceptives in that it has higher steady-state concentrations and lower peak concentrations. Area under the curve (AUC) and average concentration at steady state for ethinyl estradiol are approximately 60% higher in women using the contraceptive patch compared with women using an oral contraceptive containing ethinyl estradiol 35 mcg. In contrast, peak concentrations for ethinyl estradiol are approximately 25% lower in women using the contraceptive patch. It is not known whether there are changes in the risk of serious adverse events based on the differences in pharmacokinetic profiles of ethinyl estradiol in women using the contraceptive patch compared with women using oral contraceptives containing ethinyl estradiol 30 to 35 mcg. Increased estrogen exposure may increase the risk of adverse events, including venous thromboembolism.

Indications

➤*Contraception:* For prevention of pregnancy.

Administration and Dosage

➤*General dosing considerations:* This system uses a 28-day (4-week) cycle.

Given the nature of the transdermal application, dose delivery should be unaffected by vomiting.

➤*Adults:*

Contraception –

Usual dosage: Apply 1 patch each week for 3 weeks (21 days total), followed by 1 week that is patch free (week 4). Withdrawal bleeding is expected during this time. Each new patch should be applied on the same day of the week ("patch change day"), and only 1 patch should be worn at a time.

On the day after week 4 ends, a new 4-week cycle is started by applying a new patch. Under no circumstances should there be more than a 7-day patch-free interval between dosing cycles.

Starting the patch: If the woman is starting the patch for the first time, she should wait until the day she begins her menstrual period. Either a first day start or Sunday start may be chosen. The day she applies her first patch will be day 1. Her "patch change day" will be on this day every week.

• *First day start* – For first day start, the woman should apply her first patch during the first 24 hours of her menstrual period.

If therapy starts after day 1 of the menstrual cycle, a nonhormonal backup contraceptive (eg, condoms, spermicide, diaphragm) should be used concurrently for the first 7 consecutive days of the first treatment cycle.

• *Sunday start* – For Sunday start, the woman should apply her first patch on the first Sunday after her menstrual period starts. She must use backup contraception for the first week of her first cycle.

If the menstrual period begins on a Sunday, the first patch should be applied on that day and no backup contraception is needed.

➤*Children:* Safety and efficacy are expected to be the same for postpubertal adolescents younger than 16 years and for those 16 years and older. Use of this product before menarche is not indicated.

➤*Switching from an oral contraceptive:* Treatment with the contraceptive patch should begin on the first day of withdrawal bleeding. If there is no withdrawal bleeding within 5 days of the last active (hormone-containing) tablet, pregnancy must be ruled out. If therapy starts later than the first day of withdrawal bleeding, a nonhormonal contraceptive should be used concurrently for 7 days. If more than 7 days elapse after taking the last active oral contraceptive tablet, the possibility of ovulation and conception should be considered.

➤*Use after childbirth:* Women who elect not to breast-feed should start contraceptive therapy with the contraceptive patch no sooner than 4 weeks after childbirth. If a woman begins using the patch postpartum and has not yet had a period, the possibility of ovulation and conception occurring prior to use of the patch should be considered, and she should be instructed to use an additional method of contraception (eg, condoms, diaphragm, spermicide) for the first 7 days.

➤*Use after abortion or miscarriage:* After an abortion or miscarriage that occurs in the first trimester, the patch may be started immediately. An additional method of contraception is not needed if the patch is started immediately. If use of the patch is not started within 5 days following a first trimester abortion, the woman should follow the instructions for a woman starting the patch for the first time. In the meantime, she should be advised to use a nonhormonal contraceptive method. Ovulation may occur within 10 days after an abortion or miscarriage.

The patch should be started no earlier than 4 weeks after a second trimester abortion or miscarriage. When the patch is used postpartum or postabortion, the increased risk of thromboembolic disease must be considered.

➤*Breakthrough bleeding or spotting:* In the event of breakthrough bleeding or spotting (bleeding that occurs on the days that the patch is worn), continue treatment. If breakthrough bleeding persists longer than a few cycles, a cause other than the patch should be considered.

In the event of no withdrawal bleeding (bleeding that should occur during the patch-free week), treatment should be resumed on the next scheduled change day. If the patch has been used correctly, the absence of withdrawal bleeding is not necessarily an indication of pregnancy. Nevertheless, the pos-

NORELGESTROMIN/ETHINYL ESTRADIOL — TRANSDERMAL SYSTEM

sibility of pregnancy should be considered, especially if absence of withdrawal bleeding occurs in 2 consecutive cycles. Discontinue the patch if pregnancy is confirmed.

➤*Missed menstrual period:* If the woman has not adhered to the prescribed schedule, the possibility of pregnancy should be considered at the time of the first missed period. Discontinue hormonal contraceptive use if pregnancy is confirmed.

If the woman has adhered to the prescribed regimen and misses 1 period, she should continue using her contraceptive patches.

If the woman has adhered to the prescribed regimen and misses 2 consecutive periods, pregnancy should be ruled out. Discontinue use of the patch if pregnancy is confirmed.

➤*Application:* Apply the patch to clean, dry, intact, healthy skin on the buttock, abdomen, upper outer arm, or upper torso in a place where it will not be rubbed by tight clothing. The patch should not be placed on skin that is red, irritated, or cut, nor should it be placed on the breasts.

To prevent interference with the adhesive properties of the patch, no makeup, creams, lotions, powders, or other topical products should be applied to the skin area where the patch is or will be placed.

Patch changes may occur at any time on the change day. Apply each new patch to a new spot on the skin to help avoid irritation, although they may be kept within the same anatomic area.

➤*Application directions:* The foil pouch is opened by tearing it along the edge using the fingers. The foil pouch should be peeled apart and opened flat. A corner of the patch should be grasped firmly and gently removed from the foil pouch.

The woman should be instructed to use her fingernail to lift one corner of the patch and peel the patch and the plastic liner off the foil liner. Sometimes patches can stick to the inside of the pouch; the woman should be careful not to accidentally remove the clear liner as she removes the patch.

Half of the clear protective liner is to be peeled away. The woman should avoid touching the sticky surface of the patch.

The sticky surface of the patch is applied to the skin and the other half of the liner is removed. The woman should press down firmly on the patch with the palm of her hand for 10 seconds, making sure that the edges stick well. She should check her patch every day to make sure it is sticking.

The patch is worn for 7 days (1 week). On the "patch change day," day 8, the used patch is removed and a new one is applied immediately. The used patch still contains some active hormones. Used patches should not be flushed down the toilet.

A new patch is applied for week 2 (on day 8) and again for week 3 (on day 15) on the usual "patch change day." Patch changes may occur at any time on the "change day." Each new patch should be applied to a new spot on the skin to help avoid irritation, although they may be kept within the same anatomic area.

Week 4 is patch free (day 22 through day 28), thus completing the 4-week contraceptive cycle. Bleeding is expected to begin during this time.

The next 4-week cycle is started by applying a new patch on the usual "patch change day," the day after day 28, no matter when the menstrual period begins or ends.

Under no circumstances should there be more than a 7-day patch-free interval between patch cycles.

➤*Patch is partially or completely detached:* If a patch becomes partially or completely detached and remains detached, insufficient drug delivery occurs.

For less than 1 day (up to 24 hours) – The woman should try to reapply it to the same place or replace it with a new patch immediately. No backup contraception is needed. The woman's "patch change day" will remain the same.

For more than 1 day (24 hours or more) or if the woman is not sure how long the patch has been detached – The woman may not be protected from pregnancy. She should stop the current contraceptive cycle and start a new cycle immediately by applying a new patch. There is now a new "day 1" and a new "patch change day." Backup contraception (eg, condoms, spermicide, diaphragm) must be used for the first week of the new cycle.

A patch should not be reapplied if it is no longer sticky, if it has become stuck to itself or another surface, if it has other material stuck to it, or if it has previously become loose or fallen off. If a patch cannot be reapplied, a new patch should be applied immediately. Supplemental adhesives or wraps should not be used to hold the patch in place.

➤*Forgetting to change the patch:*

At the start of any patch cycle (week 1/day 1) – The woman may not be protected from pregnancy. She should apply the first patch of her new cycle as soon as she remembers. There is now a new "patch change day" and a new "day 1." The woman must use backup contraception (eg, condoms, spermicide, diaphragm) for the first week of the new cycle.

In the middle of the patch cycle (week 2/day 8 or week 3/day 15) –

For 1 or 2 days (up to 48 hours): The woman should apply a new patch immediately. The next patch should be applied on the usual "patch change day." No backup contraception is needed.

For more than 2 days (48 hours or more): The woman may not be protected from pregnancy. She should stop the current contraceptive cycle and start a new 4-week cycle immediately by putting on a new patch. There is now a new "patch change day" and a new "day 1." The woman must use backup contraception for 1 week.

At the end of the patch cycle (week 4/day 22) – If the woman forgets to remove her patch, she should take it off as soon as she remembers. The next cycle should be started on the usual "patch change day," which is the day after day 28. No backup contraception is needed.

Under no circumstances should there be more than a 7-day patch-free interval between cycles. If there are more than 7 patch-free days, the woman may not be protected from pregnancy, and backup contraception (eg, condoms, spermicide, diaphragm) must be used for 7 days. As with combined oral contraceptives, the risk of ovulation increases with each day beyond the recommended drug-free period. If intercourse has occurred during an extended patch-free interval, the possibility of fertilization should be considered.

➤*Changing the "patch change day":* If the woman wishes to change her "patch change day," she should complete her current cycle, removing the third patch on the correct day. During the patch-free week, she may select an earlier "patch change day" by applying a new patch on the desired day. In no case should there be more than 7 consecutive patch-free days.

➤*Skin irritation:* If patch use results in uncomfortable irritation, the patch may be removed and a new patch may be applied to a different location until the next change day. Only 1 patch should be worn at a time.

➤*Discontinuation of therapy:* Breakthrough bleeding, spotting, and amenorrhea are frequent reasons for patients discontinuing hormonal contraceptives. In case of breakthrough bleeding, as in all cases of irregular bleeding from the vagina, nonfunctional causes should be considered. In case of undiagnosed persistent or recurrent abnormal bleeding from the vagina, adequate diagnostic measures are indicated to rule out pregnancy or malignancy. If pathology has been excluded, time or a change to another method of contraception may solve the problem.

➤*Administration:* The patch should not be cut, damaged, or altered in any way. If the patch is cut, damaged, or altered in size, contraceptive efficacy may be impaired.

➤*Storage/Stability:* Store at 25°C (77°F); excursions are permitted between 15° and 30°C (59° and 86°F). Store patches in their protective pouches. Apply immediately upon removal from the protective pouch. Do not store in the refrigerator or freezer. Used patches still contain some active hormones. The sticky sides of the patch should be folded together and the folded patch placed in a sturdy container, preferably with a child-resistant cap, and the container thrown in the trash. Used patches should not be flushed down the toilet.

Actions

➤*Pharmacology:* Norelgestromin is the active progestin largely responsible for the progestational activity that occurs in women following application of norelgestromin/ethinyl estradiol transdermal patch. Norelgestromin is also the primary active metabolite produced following oral administration of norgestimate.

Combination oral contraceptives act by suppression of gonadotropins. Although the primary mechanism of this action is inhibition of ovulation, other alterations include changes in the cervical mucus (which increases the difficulty of sperm entry into the uterus) and the endometrium (which reduces the likelihood of implantation).

Receptor and human sex hormone–binding globulin (SHBG) binding studies, as well as studies in animals and humans, have shown that norgestimate and norelgestromin exhibit high progestational activity with minimal intrinsic androgenicity. Transdermally administered norelgestromin, in combination with ethinyl estradiol, does not counteract the estrogen-induced increases in SHBG, resulting in lower levels of free testosterone in serum compared with baseline.

One clinical trial assessed the return of hypothalamic-pituitary-ovarian axis function after therapy and found that follicle-stimulating hormone, luteinizing hormone, and estradiol mean values, although suppressed during therapy, returned to near baseline values during 6 weeks posttherapy.

➤*Pharmacokinetics:*

Absorption – Following a single application of the contraceptive patch, norelgestromin and ethinyl estradiol reach a plateau by approximately 48 hours. Pooled data from the 3 clinical studies have demonstrated that steady state is reached within 2 weeks of application. The steady-state concentration (C_{ss}) ranged from 0.305 to 1.53 ng/mL for norelgestromin and from 11.2 to 137 pg/mL for ethinyl estradiol.

Absorption of norelgestromin and ethinyl estradiol following application of the contraceptive patch to the buttock, upper outer arm, abdomen, and upper torso (excluding breast) was examined. While absorption from the abdomen was slightly lower than from other sites, absorption from these anatomic sites was considered to be therapeutically equivalent.

In multiple-dose studies, area under the curve ($AUC_{0\text{-}168}$) for norelgestromin and ethinyl estradiol was found to increase over time. In a 3-cycle study, these pharmacokinetic parameters reached steady-state conditions during cycle 3. Upon removal of the patch, serum levels of ethinyl estradiol and norelgestromin reach very low or nonmeasurable levels within 3 days.

NORELGESTROMIN/ETHINYL ESTRADIOL — TRANSDERMAL SYSTEM

Mean (% CV) Pharmacokinetic Parameters Following 3 Consecutive Cycles of Norelgestromin/Ethinyl Estradiol Transdermal Patch Wear on the Buttock[a]

Analyte	Parameter	Cycle 1 Week 1	Cycle 3 Week 1	Cycle 3 Week 2	Cycle 3 Week 3
Norelgestromin	C_{ss} (ng/mL)	0.7 (39.4)	0.7 (41.8)	0.8 (28.7)	0.7 (45.3)
	AUC_{0-168} (ng•h/mL)	107 (44.2)	105 (43.2)	132 (43.4)	120 (43.9)
	half-life (h)	NC	NC	NC	32.1 (40.3)
Ethinyl estradiol	C_{ss} (pg/mL)	46.4 (38.5)	47.6 (36.4)	59 (42.5)	49.6 (54.4)
	AUC_{0-168} (pg•h/mL)	6,796 (39.3)	7,160 (40.4)	10,054 (41.8)	8,840 (58.6)
	half-life (h)	NC	NC	NC	21 (43.2)

[a] % CV is percent of coefficient of variation = 100 (standard deviation/mean); NC = not calculated.

The absorption of norelgestromin and ethinyl estradiol following application of the contraceptive patch was studied under conditions encountered in a health club (sauna, whirlpool, and treadmill) and in a cold water bath. The results indicated that for norelgestromin there were no significant treatment effects on C_{ss} or AUC when compared with normal wear. For ethinyl estradiol, increased exposures were observed caused by sauna, whirlpool, and treadmill. There was no significant effect of cold water on these parameters.

Results from a study of consecutive patch wear for 7 days and 10 days indicated that serum concentrations of norelgestromin and ethinyl estradiol dropped slightly during the first 6 hours after the patch replacement, and recovered within 12 hours. By day 10 of patch administration, both norelgestromin and ethinyl estradiol concentrations had decreased by approximately 25% when compared with day 7 concentrations.

Patch adhesion: In the clinical trials with norelgestromin/ethinyl estradiol transdermal patches, approximately 2% of the cumulative number of patches completely detached. The proportion of subjects with at least 1 patch that completely detached ranged from 2% to 6%, with a reduction from cycle 1 (6%) to cycle 13 (2%). For instructions on how to manage detachment of patches, refer to Administration and Dosage.

Distribution – Norelgestromin and norgestrel (a serum metabolite of norelgestromin) are highly bound (more than 97%) to serum proteins. Norelgestromin is bound to albumin and not to SHBG, while norgestrel is bound primarily to SHBG, which limits its biologic activity. Ethinyl estradiol is extensively bound to serum albumin and induces an increase in the serum concentration of SHBG.

Metabolism – Because the patch is applied transdermally, first-pass metabolism (via the GI tract and/or liver) of norelgestromin and ethinyl estradiol that would be expected with oral administration is avoided. Hepatic metabolism of norelgestromin occurs, and metabolites include norgestrel, which is highly bound to SHBG, and various hydroxylated and conjugated metabolites. Ethinyl estradiol is also metabolized to various hydroxylated products and their glucuronide and sulfate conjugates.

Excretion – Following removal of patches, the elimination kinetics of norelgestromin and ethinyl estradiol were consistent for all studies with half-life values of approximately 28 and 17 hours, respectively. The metabolites of norelgestromin and ethinyl estradiol are eliminated by renal and fecal pathways.

Special populations –

Hepatic function impairment: Steroid hormones may be poorly metabolized in patients with impaired liver function.

Age/Body weight/Body surface area/Race: The effects of age, body weight, body surface area (BSA), and race on the pharmacokinetics of norelgestromin and ethinyl estradiol were evaluated in 230 healthy women from 9 pharmacokinetic studies of single 7-day applications of norelgestromin/ethinyl estradiol transdermal patch. For norelgestromin and ethinyl estradiol, increasing age, body weight, and BSA each were associated with slight decreases in C_{ss} and AUC values. However, only a small fraction (10% to 25%) of the overall variability in the pharmacokinetics of norelgestromin and ethinyl estradiol following application of the patch may be associated with any or all of the previous demographic parameters.

Obesity: With respect to weight, 5 of the 15 pregnancies reported with norelgestromin/ethinyl estradiol transdermal patch use were among women with a baseline body weight of at least 198 lb (90 kg), which constituted less than 3% of the study population. The greater proportion of pregnancies among women at or above 198 lb was statistically significant and suggests that the norelgestromin/ethinyl estradiol transdermal patch may be less effective in these women.

Contraindications

Thrombophlebitis; thromboembolic disorders; history of deep vein thrombophlebitis or thromboembolic disorders; known thrombophilic conditions; cerebrovascular or coronary artery disease (current or history); valvular heart disease with complications; persistent blood pressure values of 160 mm Hg or higher systolic or 100 mg Hg or higher diastolic; diabetes with vascular involvement; headaches with focal neurological symptoms; major surgery with prolonged immobilization; known or suspected carcinoma of the breast or personal history of breast cancer; carcinoma of the endometrium or other known or suspected estrogen-dependent neoplasia; undiagnosed abnormal genital bleeding; cholestatic jaundice of pregnancy or jaundice with prior hormonal contraceptive use; acute or chronic hepatocellular disease with abnormal liver function; hepatic adenomas or carcinomas; known or suspected pregnancy; hypersensitivity to any component of the product.

Warnings/Precautions

➤*Smoking:* See the Warning box for more information.

➤*Hormone exposure:* See the Warning box for more information.

➤*Special risk patients:* The use of combination hormonal contraceptives is associated with increased risks of several serious conditions, including myocardial infarction (MI), thromboembolism, stroke, hepatic neoplasia, and gallbladder disease, although the risk of serious morbidity or mortality is very small in healthy women without underlyng risk factors. The risk of morbidity and mortality increases significantly in the presence of other underlying risk factors, such as hypertension, hyperlipidemias, obesity, and diabetes.

➤*Thromboembolic disorders and other vascular problems:*

Thromboembolism – An increased risk of thromboembolic and thrombotic disease associated with the use of hormonal contraceptives is well established. Case-control studies have found the relative risk of users compared with nonusers to be 3 for the first episode of superficial venous thrombosis, 4 to 11 for deep vein thrombosis or pulmonary embolism, and 1.5 to 6 for women with predisposing conditions for venous thromboembolic disease. Cohort studies have shown the relative risk to be somewhat lower; approximately 3 for new cases and approximately 4.5 for new cases requiring hospitalization. The risk of thromboembolic disease associated with hormonal contraceptives is not related to length of use and disappears after hormonal contraceptive use is stopped. A 2- to 4-fold increase in relative risk of postoperative thromboembolic complications has been reported with the use of hormonal contraceptives. The relative risk of venous thrombosis in women who have predisposing conditions is twice that of women without such medical conditions. If feasible, discontinue hormonal contraceptives at least 4 weeks prior to and for 2 weeks after elective surgery of a type associated with an increase in risk of thromboembolism and during and following prolonged immobilization. Because the immediate postpartum period is also associated with an increased risk of thromboembolism, start hormonal contraceptives no earlier than 4 weeks after delivery in women who elect not to breast-feed.

In 3 large clinical trials (n = 3,330 with 1,704 women-years of exposure), 1 case of nonfatal pulmonary embolism occurred during norelgestromin/ethinyl estradiol transdermal patch use, and 1 case of postoperative nonfatal pulmonary embolism was also reported with use of the patch.

As with any combination hormonal contraceptives, be alert to the earliest manifestations of thrombotic disorders (thrombophlebitis, venous thromboembolism including pulmonary embolism, cerebrovascular disorders, and retinal thrombosis). Discontinue norelgestromin/ethinyl estradiol transdermal patch use immediately if any of these occur or are suspected.

Myocardial infarction – An increased risk of MI has been attributed to hormonal contraceptive use. This risk is primarily in smokers or women with other underlying risk factors of coronary artery disease (eg, hypertension, hypercholesterolemia, morbid obesity, diabetes). The relative risk of heart attack for current hormonal contraceptive users has been estimated to be 2 to 6 compared with nonusers. The risk is very low in patients younger than 30 years.

Hormonal contraceptives may compound the effects of well-known risk factors (eg, hypertension, diabetes, hyperlipidemias, age, obesity). In particular, some progestins are known to decrease high-density lipoprotein (HDL) cholesterol and cause glucose intolerance, while estrogens may create a state of hyperinsulinism. Hormonal contraceptives have been shown to increase blood pressure among some users. Similar effects on risk factors have been associated with an increased risk of heart disease. Use hormonal contraceptives, including norelgestromin/ethinyl estradiol transdermal patch, with caution in women with cardiovascular disease risk factors.

Norgestimate and norelgestromin have minimal androgenic activity. There is some evidence that the risk of MI associated with hormonal contraceptives is lower when the progestin has minimal androgenic activity than when the activity is greater.

Smoking: Smoking in combination with oral contraceptive use has been shown to contribute substantially to the incidence of MI in women in their mid-30s and older, with smoking accounting for the majority of excess cases. Mortality rates associated with circulatory disease have been shown to increase substantially in smokers, especially in those 35 years of age and older among women who use oral contraceptives.

Cerebrovascular diseases – Hormonal contraceptives have been shown to increase the relative and attributable risks of cerebrovascular events (thrombotic and hemorrhagic strokes), although, generally, the risk is greatest among hypertensive women older than 35 years who also smoke. Hypertension was found to be a risk factor of users and nonusers for both types of strokes, and smoking interacted to increase the risk of stroke.

In a large study, the relative risk of thrombotic strokes has been shown to range from 3 for normotensive users to 14 for users with severe hypertension. The relative risk of hemorrhagic stroke is reported to be 1.2 for nonsmokers who used hormonal contraceptives, 2.6 for smokers who did not use hormonal contraceptives, 7.6 for smokers who used hormonal contraceptives, 1.8 for normotensive users, and 25.7 for users with severe hypertension. The attributable risk is also greater in older women.

NORELGESTROMIN/ETHINYL ESTRADIOL — TRANSDERMAL SYSTEM

Dose-related risk of vascular disease – A positive association has been observed between the amount of estrogen and progestin in hormonal contraceptives and the risk of vascular disease. A decline in serum HDL has been reported with many progestational agents. A decline in serum HDL has been associated with an increased incidence of ischemic heart disease. Because estrogens increase HDL cholesterol, the net effect of a hormonal contraceptive depends on a balance achieved between doses of estrogen and progestin and the activity of the progestin used in the contraceptives. Consider the activity and amount of both hormones in the choice of a hormonal contraceptive.

Persistence of risk of vascular disease – Two studies have shown persistence of risk of vascular disease for ever-users of combination hormonal contraceptives. In a study in the United States, the risk of developing MI after discontinuing combination hormonal contraceptives persists for at least 9 years for women 40 to 49 years of age who had used combination hormonal contraceptives for at least 5 years, but this increased risk was not demonstrated in other age groups. In another study in Great Britain, the risk of developing cerebrovascular disease persisted for at least 6 years after discontinuation of combination hormonal contraceptives, although excess risk was very small. However, both studies were performed with combination hormonal contraceptive formulations containing at least 50 mcg of estrogens.

➤*Mortality:* One study gathered data from a variety of sources that have estimated the mortality rate associated with different methods of contraception at different ages. These estimates include the combined risk of death associated with contraceptive methods plus the risk attributable to pregnancy in the event of method failure. Each method of contraception has its specific benefits and risks. The study concluded that with the exception of combination oral contraceptive users 35 years and older who smoke, and 40 years and older who do not smoke, mortality associated with all methods of birth control is low and below that associated with childbirth.

The observation of a possible increase in risk of mortality with age for combination oral contraceptive users is based on data gathered in the 1970s but not reported until 1983. Current clinical recommendation involves the use of lower estrogen dose formulations and careful consideration of risk factors. In 1989, the Fertility and Maternal Health Drugs Advisory Committee was asked to review the use of combination hormonal contraceptives in women 40 years and older. The committee concluded that although cardiovascular disease risks may be increased with combination hormonal contraceptive use after 40 years of age in healthy nonsmoking women (even with the newer low-dose formulations), there are also greater potential health risks associated with pregnancy in older women and with the alternative surgical and medical procedures that may be necessary if such women do not have access to effective and acceptable means of contraception. The committee recommended that the benefits of low-dose combination hormonal contraceptive use by healthy nonsmoking women older than 40 years may outweigh the possible risks.

Although the data are mainly obtained with oral contraceptives, this is likely to apply to the contraceptive patch as well. Women of all ages who use combination hormonal contraceptives should use the lowest possible dose formulation that is effective and meets their needs.

➤*Carcinoma:* Numerous epidemiologic studies give conflicting reports on the relationship between breast cancer and combination oral contraceptive use. The risk of having breast cancer diagnosed may be slightly increased among current and recent users of combination oral contraceptives. However, this excess risk appears to decrease over time after combination oral contraceptive discontinuation, and by 10 years after cessation the increased risk disappears. Some studies report an increased risk with duration of use, while other studies do not, and no consistent relationships have been found with dose or type of steroid. Some studies have found a small increase in risk for women who first use combination oral contraceptives before 20 years of age. Most studies show a similar pattern of risk with combination oral contraceptive use regardless of a woman's reproductive history or her family breast cancer history.

In addition, breast cancers diagnosed in current or ever oral contraceptive users may be less clinically advanced than in never-users.

Women who currently have or have had breast cancer should not use hormonal contraceptives because breast cancer is usually a hormonally sensitive tumor.

Some studies suggest that combination oral contraceptive use has been associated with an increase in the risk of cervical intraepithelial neoplasia in some populations of women. However, there continues to be controversy about the extent to which such findings may be because of differences in sexual behavior and other factors.

In spite of many studies of the relationship between oral contraceptive use and breast and cervical cancers, a cause-and-effect relationship has not been established. It is not known whether the norelgestromin/ethinyl estradiol transdermal contraceptive patch is distinct from oral contraceptives with regard to the previous statements.

➤*Hepatic neoplasia:* Benign hepatic adenomas are associated with hormonal contraceptive use, although the incidence of benign tumors is rare in the United States. Indirect calculations have estimated the attributable risk to be in the range of 3.3 cases per 100,000 for users, a risk that increases after 4 or more years of use, especially with hormonal contraceptives containing estrogen 50 mcg or more. Rupture of benign hepatic adenomas may cause death through intra-abdominal hemorrhage.

Studies from Britain and the United States have shown an increased risk of developing hepatocellular carcinoma in long-term (8 years or more) oral contraceptive users. However, these cancers are extremely rare in the United States, and the attributable risk (the excess incidence) of liver cancers in oral contraceptive users approaches less than one per million users. It is unknown whether the norelgestromin/ethinyl estradiol transdermal patch is distinct from oral contraceptives in this regard.

➤*Ocular lesions:* There have been clinical case reports of retinal thrombosis associated with the use of hormonal contraceptives. Discontinue the contraceptive patch if there is unexplained partial or complete loss of vision, onset of proptosis or diplopia, papilledema, or retinal vascular lesions. Undertake appropriate diagnostic and therapeutic measures immediately.

➤*Gallbladder disease:* Earlier studies have reported an increased lifetime relative risk of gallbladder surgery in users of hormonal contraceptives and estrogens. However, more recent studies have shown that the relative risk of developing gallbladder disease among hormonal contraceptive users may be minimal. The recent findings of minimal risk may be related to the use of hormonal contraceptive formulations containing lower hormonal doses of estrogens and progestins.

Combination hormonal contraceptives, such as the norelgestromin/ethinyl estradiol transdermal contraceptive patch, may worsen existing gallbladder disease and may accelerate the development of this disease in previously asymptomatic women. Women with a history of combination hormonal contraceptive–related cholestasis are more likely to have the condition recur with subsequent combination hormonal contraceptive use.

➤*Glucose tolerance:* Hormonal contraceptives have been shown to cause a decrease in glucose tolerance in some users. However, in nondiabetic women, combination hormonal contraceptives appear to have no effect on fasting blood glucose. Carefully monitor prediabetic and diabetic women in particular while taking combination hormonal contraceptives, such as norelgestromin/ethinyl estradiol transdermal patch.

In clinical trials with oral contraceptives containing ethinyl estradiol and norgestimate, there were no clinically significant changes in fasting blood glucose levels. There were no clinically significant changes in glucose levels over 24 cycles of use. Moreover, glucose tolerance tests showed no clinically significant changes from baseline to cycles 3, 12, and 24. In a 6-cycle clinical trial with norelgestromin/ethinyl estradiol transdermal patch, there were no clinically significant changes in fasting blood glucose from baseline to end of treatment.

➤*Lipid effects:* A small proportion of women will have persistent hypertriglyceridemia while taking hormonal contraceptives. As discussed earlier, changes in serum triglycerides and lipoprotein levels have been reported in hormonal contraceptive users.

Closely follow women who are being treated for hyperlipidemias if they elect to use the norelgestromin/ethinyl estradiol transdermal patch. Some progestins may elevate low-density lipoprotein (LDL) levels and may render the control of hyperlipidemias more difficult.

➤*Elevated blood pressure:* Do not start women with significant hypertension on hormonal contraception. Encourage women with a history of hypertension or hypertension-related diseases or renal disease to use another method of contraception. If women elect to use the norelgestromin/ethinyl estradiol transdermal patch, monitor them closely, and discontinue the patch if a clinically significant elevation of blood pressure (at least 160 mm Hg systolic or at least 100 mg Hg diastolic) occurs and cannot be adequately controlled. In general, switch women who develop hypertension during hormonal contraceptive therapy to a nonhormonal contraceptive. If other contraceptive methods are not suitable, hormonal contraceptive therapy may continue combined with antihypertensive therapy. Regular monitoring of blood pressure throughout hormonal contraceptive therapy is recommended. For most women, elevated blood pressure will return to normal after stopping hormonal contraceptives, and there is no difference in the occurrence of hypertension between former users and never-users.

An increase in blood pressure has been reported in women taking hormonal contraceptives, and this increase is more likely in older hormonal contraceptive users and with extended duration of use. Data from the Royal College of General Practitioners and subsequent randomized trials have shown that the incidence of hypertension increases with increasing progestational activity.

➤*Headaches:* The onset or exacerbation of migraine headache or the development of headache with a new pattern that is recurrent, persistent, or severe requires discontinuation of the norelgestromin/ethinyl estradiol transdermal patch and evaluation of the cause.

➤*Bleeding irregularities and patterns:* Breakthrough bleeding and spotting are sometimes encountered in women using the contraceptive patch. Consider nonhormonal causes and take adequate diagnostic measures to rule out malignancy, other pathology, or pregnancy in the event of breakthrough bleeding, as in the case of any abnormal vaginal bleeding. If pathology has been excluded, time or a change to another contraceptive product may resolve the bleeding. In the event of amenorrhea, rule out pregnancy before initiating use of the contraceptive patch.

Some women may encounter amenorrhea or oligomenorrhea after discontinuation of hormonal contraceptive use, especially when such a condition was preexistent.

In the clinical trials, most women started their withdrawal bleeding on the fourth day of the drug-free interval, and the median duration of withdrawal bleeding was 5 to 6 days. On average, 26% of women per cycle had 7 or more total days of bleeding and/or spotting (this includes both withdrawal flow and breakthrough bleeding and/or spotting).

➤*Sexually transmitted diseases:* Counsel patients that this product does not protect against HIV infection (AIDS) and other sexually transmitted diseases.

NORELGESTROMIN/ETHINYL ESTRADIOL — TRANSDERMAL SYSTEM

➤*Body weight 90 kg (198 lb) or more:* Results of clinical trials suggest that the contraceptive patch may be less effective in women with a body weight of 90 kg (198 lb) or more than in women with lower body weights.

If considering norelgestromin/ethinyl estradiol transdermal patch for women at or above 198 lb, discuss the patient's individual needs in choosing the most appropriate contraceptive option.

➤*Physical examination follow-up:* It is good medical practice for women using the contraceptive patch, as for all women, to have annual medical evaluations and physical examinations. However, the physical examination may be deferred until after initiation of hormonal contraceptives if requested by the woman and judged appropriate by the clinician. The physical examination should include special reference to blood pressure, breasts, abdomen, and pelvic organs, including cervical cytology, and relevant laboratory tests. In case of undiagnosed, persistent, or recurrent abnormal vaginal bleeding, conduct appropriate measures to rule out malignancy or other pathology. Monitor women with a strong family history of breast cancer or who have breast nodules with particular care.

➤*Hepatic effects:* If jaundice develops in any woman using the norelgestromin/ethinyl estradiol transdermal patch, discontinue the medication.

➤*Fluid retention:* Steroid hormones such as those in the contraceptive patch may cause some degree of fluid retention. Prescribe this product with caution, and only with careful monitoring, in patients with conditions that might be aggravated by fluid retention.

➤*Depression:* Women who become significantly depressed while using combination hormonal contraceptives, such as the contraceptive patch, should stop the medication and use another method of contraception in an attempt to determine whether the symptom is drug related. Carefully observe women with a history of depression, and discontinue the product if significant depression occurs.

➤*Contact lenses:* Contact lens wearers who develop visual changes or changes in lens tolerance should be assessed by an ophthalmologist.

➤*Patch adhesion:* Experience with more than 70,000 norelgestromin/ethinyl estradiol transdermal patches worn for contraception for 6 to 13 cycles showed that 4.7% of patches were replaced because they either fell off (1.8%) or were partly detached (2.9%). Similarly, in a small study of patch wear under conditions of physical exertion and variable temperature and humidity, less than 2% of patches were replaced for complete or partial detachment.

If the norelgestromin/ethinyl estradiol transdermal patch becomes partially or completely detached and remains detached, insufficient drug delivery occurs. Do not reapply a patch if it is no longer sticky, if it has become stuck to itself or another surface, if it has other material stuck to it, or if it has become loose or fallen off before. If a patch cannot be reapplied, apply a new patch immediately. Do not use supplemental adhesives or wraps to hold the norelgestromin/ethinyl estradiol transdermal patch in place.

If a patch is partially or completely detached for more than 1 day (24 hours or more) or if the woman is not sure how long the patch has been detached, she may not be protected from pregnancy. She should stop the current contraceptive cycle and start a new cycle immediately by applying a new patch. Backup contraception, such as condoms, spermicide, or diaphragm, must be used for the first week of the new cycle.

➤*Hepatic function impairment:* The hormones in the patch may be poorly metabolized in women with liver function impairment.

➤*Pregnancy: Category X.* The contraceptive patch is contraindicated in known or suspected pregnancy. Norelgestromin was tested for its reproductive toxicity in a rabbit developmental toxicity study by the subcutaneous route of administration. Doses of 0, 1, 2, 4, and 6 mg/kg body weight, which gave systemic exposure of approximately 25 to 125 times the human exposure with the contraceptive patch, were administered daily on gestation days 7 through 19. Malformations reported were paw hyperflexion at 4 and 6 mg/kg and paw hyperextension and cleft palate at 6 mg/kg.

Ectopic pregnancy – Ectopic as well as intrauterine pregnancy may occur in contraceptive failures.

Risks of use before or during early pregnancy – Extensive epidemiologic studies have revealed no increased risk of birth defects in women who have used oral contraceptives prior to pregnancy. Studies also do not indicate a teratogenic effect, particularly in so far as cardiac anomalies and limb reduction defects are concerned, when oral contraceptives are taken inadvertently during early pregnancy.

Do not use combination hormonal contraceptives, such as the contraceptive patch, to induce withdrawal bleeding as a test for pregnancy. Do not use the contraceptive patch during pregnancy to treat threatened or habitual abortion. It is recommended that pregnancy be ruled out for any patient who has missed 2 consecutive periods. If the patient has not adhered to the prescribed schedule for the use of the contraceptive patch, consider the possibility of pregnancy at the time of the first missed period. Discontinue hormonal contraceptive use if pregnancy is confirmed.

➤*Lactation:* The effects of the contraceptive patch in breast-feeding mothers have not been evaluated and are unknown. Small amounts of combination hormonal contraceptive steroids have been identified in the milk of breast-feeding mothers, and a few adverse effects on the child have been reported, including jaundice and breast enlargement. In addition, combination hormonal contraceptives given in the postpartum period may interfere with lactation by decreasing the quantity and quality of breast milk. Long-term follow-up of infants whose mothers used combination hormonal contraceptives while breast-feeding has shown no deleterious effects. However, advise the breast-feeding mother not to use the contraceptive patch, but to use other forms of contraception until she has completely weaned her child.

➤*Children:* Safety and efficacy of the contraceptive patch have been established in women of reproductive age. Safety and efficacy are expected to be the same for postpubertal adolescents younger than 16 years of age and for users 16 years of age and older. Use of this product before menarche is not indicated.

➤*Elderly:* This product has not been studied in women older than 65 years and is not indicated in this population.

➤*Monitoring:* Closely monitor blood pressure; blood glucose in prediabetic and diabetic women; women with a history of depression; women with conditions that might be aggravated by fluid retention; women with a family history of breast cancer or who have breast nodules; and women with hyperlipidemias. Annual medical evaluations and physical examinations are recommended.

Drug Interactions

➤*Cytochrome P450 system:* Advise women taking norelgestromin/ethinyl estradiol who take a drug or herbal product that induces enzymes, including CYP3A4, that metabolize norelgestromin/ethinyl estradiol to use additional contraception or a different method of contraception. Drugs or herbal products that induce such enzymes may decrease the plasma concentration and effectiveness of norelgestromin/ethinyl estradiol or increase breakthrough bleeding.

Contraceptive Patch Drug Interactions

Precipitant drug	Object drug[a]		Description
Acetaminophen	Norelgestromin/ Ethinyl estradiol	↑	Ethinyl estradiol plasma concentrations may be increased. If estrogen-related adverse effects occur, consider coadministration of acetaminophen as a possible cause. Acetaminophen plasma concentrations may be reduced, decreasing the pharmacologic effect. However, the effect on acetaminophen is not likely to be clinically important.
Norelgestromin/ Ethinyl estradiol	Acetaminophen	↓	
Aprepitant	Norelgestromin/ Ethinyl estradiol	↓	Aprepitant may increase the metabolism of norelgestromin/ ethinyl estradiol, decreasing the effectiveness or increasing breakthrough bleeding. Advise women to use additional contraception or a different (nonhormonal) method of contraception.
Ascorbic acid	Norelgestromin/ Ethinyl estradiol	↑	Ethinyl estradiol plasma concentrations may be increased. If estrogen-related adverse effects occur, consider coadministration of ascorbic acid as a possible cause.
Azole antifungal agents (eg, itraconazole, ketoconazole)	Norelgestromin/ Ethinyl estradiol	↓↑	Pharmacologic effects of norelgestromin/ethinyl estradiol may be decreased by azole antifungal agents. Breakthrough bleeding and pregnancy may occur. Advise women to use additional contraception or a different (nonhormonal) method of contraception. In addition, ethinyl estradiol concentrations may be elevated.
Barbiturates (eg, phenobarbital)	Norelgestromin/ Ethinyl estradiol	↓	Barbiturates may increase the metabolism of norelgestromin/ ethinyl estradiol, decreasing the effectiveness or increasing breakthrough bleeding. Advise women to use additional contraception or a different (nonhormonal) method of contraception.
Bosentan	Norelgestromin/ Ethinyl estradiol	↓	Bosentan may increase the metabolism of norelgestromin/ ethinyl estradiol, decreasing the effectiveness or increasing breakthrough bleeding. Advise women to use additional contraception or a different (nonhormonal) method of contraception.

NORELGESTROMIN/ETHINYL ESTRADIOL — TRANSDERMAL SYSTEM

Contraceptive Patch Drug Interactions

Precipitant drug	Object drug[a]		Description
Carbamazepine	Norelgestromin/ Ethinyl estradiol	↓	Carbamazepine may increase the metabolism of norelgestromin/ ethinyl estradiol, decreasing the effectiveness or increasing breakthrough bleeding. Advise women to use additional contraception or a different (nonhormonal) method of contraception.
Efavirenz	Norelgestromin/ Ethinyl estradiol	↓	Efavirenz may increase the metabolism of norelgestromin/ ethinyl estradiol, decreasing the effectiveness or increasing breakthrough bleeding. A higher dose of norelgestromin/ethinyl estradiol may be needed during coadministration of efavirenz. If norelgestromin/ethinyl estradiol is being used for contraception, instruct women to always use a barrier method of contraception in addition to hormonal contraception.
Felbamate	Norelgestromin/ Ethinyl estradiol	↓	Felbamate may increase the metabolism of norelgestromin/ ethinyl estradiol, decreasing the effectiveness or increasing breakthrough bleeding. Advise women to use additional contraception or a different (nonhormonal) method of contraception.
Griseofulvin	Norelgestromin/ Ethinyl estradiol	↓	Griseofulvin may increase the metabolism of norelgestromin/ ethinyl estradiol, decreasing the effectiveness or increasing breakthrough bleeding. Advise women to use additional contraception or a different (nonhormonal) method of contraception.
HMG-CoA reductase inhibitors (eg, atorvastatin, rosuvastatin)	Norelgestromin/ Ethinyl estradiol	↑	Ethinyl estradiol plasma concentrations may be increased. If estrogen-related adverse effects occur, consider coadministration of the HMG-CoA reductase inhibitor as a possible cause.
Hydantoins (eg, phenytoin)	Norelgestromin/ Ethinyl estradiol	↓	Hydantoins may increase the metabolism of norelgestromin/ ethinyl estradiol, decreasing the effectiveness or increasing breakthrough bleeding. Advise women to use additional contraception or a different (nonhormonal) method of contraception.
Modafinil	Norelgestromin/ Ethinyl estradiol	↓	Modafinil may increase the metabolism of norelgestromin/ ethinyl estradiol, decreasing the effectiveness or increasing breakthrough bleeding. Alternative or concomitant methods of contraception are recommended for patients treated with modafinil and for 1 month after discontinuing modafinil.
Nevirapine	Norelgestromin/ Ethinyl estradiol	↓	Nevirapine may increase the metabolism of norelgestromin/ ethinyl estradiol, decreasing the effectiveness or increasing breakthrough bleeding. Advise women to use additional contraception or a different (nonhormonal) method of contraception.
Oxcarbazepine	Norelgestromin/ Ethinyl estradiol	↓	Oxcarbazepine may increase the metabolism of norelgestromin/ ethinyl estradiol, decreasing the effectiveness or increasing breakthrough bleeding. Advise women to use additional contraception or a different (nonhormonal) method of contraception.

Contraceptive Patch Drug Interactions

Precipitant drug	Object drug[a]		Description
Protease inhibitors (eg, indinavir, ritonavir)	Norelgestromin/ Ethinyl estradiol	↓↑	Protease inhibitors may increase or decrease norelgestromin/ ethinyl estradiol plasma concentrations. Advise women to use additional contraception or a different (nonhormonal) method of contraception.
Rifamycins (eg, rifampin)	Norelgestromin/ Ethinyl estradiol	↓	Rifamycins may increase the metabolism of norelgestromin/ ethinyl estradiol, decreasing the effectiveness or increasing breakthrough bleeding. Advise women to use additional contraception or a different (nonhormonal) method of contraception.
Rufinamide	Norelgestromin/ Ethinyl estradiol	↓	Rufinamide may increase the metabolism of norelgestromin/ ethinyl estradiol, decreasing the effectiveness or increasing breakthrough bleeding. Advise women to use additional contraception or a different (nonhormonal) method of contraception.
Smoking	Norelgestromin/ Ethinyl estradiol	↑	Cigarette smoking increases the risk of serious cardiovascular adverse effects from norelgestromin/ethinyl estradiol use. The risk increases with age and heavy smoking (15 or more cigarettes/day). Advise women who use norelgestromin/ethinyl estradiol to avoid smoking.
St. John's wort	Norelgestromin/ Ethinyl estradiol	↓	St. John's wort may increase the metabolism of norelgestromin/ ethinyl estradiol, decreasing the effectiveness or increasing breakthrough bleeding. Advise women to use additional contraception or a different (nonhormonal) method of contraception.
Topiramate	Norelgestromin/ Ethinyl estradiol	↓	Topiramate may increase the metabolism of norelgestromin/ ethinyl estradiol, decreasing the effectiveness or increasing breakthrough bleeding. Advise women to use additional contraception or a different (nonhormonal) method of contraception.
Voriconazole	Norelgestromin/ Ethinyl estradiol	↑	Ethinyl estradiol plasma concentrations may be increased. If estrogen-related adverse effects occur, consider coadministration of voriconazole as a possible cause.
Norelgestromin/ Ethinyl estradiol	Benzodiazepines (eg, diazepam, temazepam)	↑↓	Plasma concentrations of benzodiazepines that undergo glucuronidation (eg, lorazepam, oxazepam, temazepam) may be reduced, decreasing the pharmacologic effect. Plasma concentrations of benzodiazepines that undergo oxidation (eg, diazepam, midazolam, triazolam) may be increased and their effect prolonged. Monitor the patient's response to the benzodiazepine and adjust the benzodiazepine dose as needed.
Norelgestromin/ Ethinyl estradiol	Beta-blockers (eg, propranolol)	↑	Beta-blocker plasma concentrations may be increased because of inhibition of first-pass metabolism. Monitor the patient and adjust the beta-blocker dose as needed.

NORELGESTROMIN/ETHINYL ESTRADIOL — TRANSDERMAL SYSTEM

Contraceptive Patch Drug Interactions

Precipitant drug	Object drug[a]		Description
Norelgestromin/ Ethinyl estradiol	Clofibrate	↓	Clofibrate plasma concentrations may be reduced, decreasing the pharmacologic effects. If control of serum lipoprotein concentrations is lost during coadministration of norelgestromin/ethinyl estradiol, consider discontinuing norelgestromin/ethinyl estradiol or increasing the clofibrate dose.
Norelgestromin/ Ethinyl estradiol	Corticosteroids (eg, prednisolone)	↑	Corticosteroid plasma concentrations may be increased because of inhibition of metabolism. Risk of corticosteroid adverse reactions may be increased. Monitor the patient and adjust the corticosteroid dose as needed.
Norelgestromin/ Ethinyl estradiol	Cyclosporine	↑	Cyclosporine plasma concentrations may be increased because of inhibition of metabolism. Risk of cyclosporine toxicity may be increased. Monitor cyclosporine concentration and for cyclosporine toxicity. Adjust the cyclosporine dose as needed.
Norelgestromin/ Ethinyl estradiol	Lamotrigine	↓	Lamotrigine plasma concentrations may be decreased, reducing seizure control. Monitor lamotrigine concentrations and the patient response. Adjust the lamotrigine dose as needed.
Norelgestromin/ Ethinyl estradiol	Morphine	↓	Morphine plasma concentrations may be decreased, reducing the pharmacologic effect. Monitor the patient's response to morphine analgesia. Adjust the morphine dose as needed or use an alternative analgesic.
Norelgestromin/ Ethinyl estradiol	Salicylates (eg, aspirin)	↓	Salicylate plasma concentrations may be decreased, reducing the pharmacologic effect. Monitor the patient's response to salicylate analgesia. Adjust the salicylate dose as needed.
Norelgestromin/ Ethinyl estradiol	Theophyllines (eg, aminophylline)	↑	Theophylline plasma concentrations may be increased because of inhibition of metabolism. Risk of theophylline adverse reactions may be increased. Monitor theophylline concentrations and the patient for signs of theophylline toxicity. Adjust the theophylline dose as needed.
Norelgestromin/ Ethinyl estradiol	Valproic acid	↓	Valproic acid plasma concentrations may be decreased, increasing the risk of seizures. Monitor valproic acid concentrations and the patient's clinical response. Adjust the valproic acid dose as needed.

[a] ↑ = object drug increased; ↓ = object drug decreased; ↑↓ = object drug both increased and decreased.

➤*Drug/Lab test interactions:* The following certain endocrine and liver function tests and blood components may be affected by hormonal contraceptives:

- increased prothrombin and factors VII, VIII, IX, and X; decreased antithrombin III; increased norepinephrine-induced platelet aggregability.
- increased thyroid-binding globulin (TBG) leading to increased circulating total thyroid hormone as measured by protein-bound iodine, T4 by column or by radioimmunoassay. Free T3 resin uptake is decreased, reflecting the elevated TBG, free T4 concentration is unaltered.
- other binding proteins may be elevated in serum.
- sex hormone–binding globulins are increased and result in elevated levels of total circulating endogenous sex steroids and corticoids; however, free or biologically active levels either decrease or remain unchanged.
- triglycerides may be increased and levels of various other lipids and lipoproteins may be affected.
- glucose tolerance may be decreased.
- serum folate levels may be depressed by norelgestromin/ethinyl estradiol therapy, which may be clinically important if a woman becomes pregnant shortly after discontinuing norelgestromin/ethinyl estradiol.

➤*Drug/Food interactions:* Grapefruit ingestion may increase ethinyl estradiol plasma concentrations.

Adverse Reactions

➤*Common adverse reactions:* Adverse reactions commonly reported by users of combination hormonal contraceptives are breast tenderness, headache, irregular uterine bleeding, and nausea.

The most common adverse reactions reported during clinical trials were abdominal pain, application-site disorder, breast symptoms, dysmenorrhea, headache, and nausea.

➤*Discontinuation of therapy:* The most common reactions leading to discontinuation were application-site reaction, breast symptoms (including breast discomfort, engorgement, and pain), emotional lability, headache, and nausea and/or vomiting.

➤*Adverse reactions (2.5% or more):*

Norelgestromin/Ethinyl Estradiol Transdermal Patch Adverse Reactions (≥ 2.5%)

Adverse reaction	Norelgestromin/Ethinyl estradiol contraceptive patch (n = 3,322)
CNS	
Dizziness	3.3%
Fatigue	2.6%
Headache	21%
Migraine	2.7%
Mood, affect, and anxiety disorders[a]	6.3%
Dermatologic	
Acne	2.9%
Application-site disorder[a]	17.1%
Pruritus	2.5%
GI	
Abdominal pain[a]	8.1%
Diarrhea	4.2%
Nausea	16.6%
Vomiting	5.1%
GU	
Breast symptoms[a]	22.4%
Dysmenorrhea	7.8%
Vaginal bleeding and menstrual disorders[a]	6.4%
Vaginal yeast infection[a]	3.9%
Miscellaneous	
Weight increased	2.7%

[a] Represents a bundle of similar terms.

➤*Other adverse reactions (less than 2.5%):*

Cardiovascular – Blood pressure increased, pulmonary embolism.

CNS – Insomnia, libido decreased, libido increased, malaise.

Dermatologic – Chloasma, dermatitis contact, erythema, skin irritation.

GU – Galactorrhea, genital discharge, premenstrual syndrome, uterine spasm, vaginal discharge, vulvovaginal dryness.

Metabolic/Nutritional – Fluid retention (represents a bundle of similar terms), lipid disorders (represents a bundle of similar terms).

Miscellaneous – Abdominal distension, cholecystitis, muscle spasms.

➤*Postmarketing:*

Cardiovascular – Arterial thrombosis (represents a bundle of similar terms), cerebrovascular accident (represents a bundle of similar terms), deep vein thrombosis (represents a bundle of similar terms), hemorrhage intracranial (represents a bundle of similar terms); hypertension, hypertensive crisis, myocardial infarction (represents a bundle of similar terms), pulmonary embolism (represents a bundle of similar terms), thrombosis (represents a bundle of similar terms).

CNS – Anger, dysgeusia, emotional disorder, frustration, irritability, migraine with aura.

Dermatologic – Alopecia, eczema, erythema multiforme, erythema nodosum, photosensitivity reaction, pruritus, generalized rash (represents a bundle of similar terms), seborrheic dermatitis, skin reaction, urticaria.

Endocrine – Blood glucose abnormal, blood glucose decreased, hyperglycemia, insulin resistance.

NORELGESTROMIN/ETHINYL ESTRADIOL — TRANSDERMAL SYSTEM

GU – Breast cancer (represents a bundle of similar terms), breast mass, cervical dysplasia, cervix carcinoma, fibroadenoma of breast, menstrual disorder (represents a bundle of similar terms), suppressed lactation, uterine leiomyoma.

Hepatic – Cholelithiasis, cholestasis, hepatic adenoma, hepatic lesion, hepatic neoplasm, jaundice cholestatic.

Metabolic/Nutritional – Blood cholesterol abnormal, LDL increased.

Special senses – Contact lens intolerance or complication.

Miscellaneous – Allergic reaction (represents a bundle of similar terms), application-site reactions (represents a bundle of similar terms), colitis, edema (represents a bundle of similar terms).

Overdosage

➤*Symptoms:* Serious ill effects have not been reported following accidental ingestion of large doses of hormonal contraceptives. Overdosage may cause nausea and vomiting and withdrawal bleeding in women. Given the nature and design of the contraceptive patch, it is unlikely that overdosage will occur. Serious ill effects have not been reported following acute ingestion of large doses of oral contraceptives by young children.

➤*Treatment:* In case of suspected overdose, remove all contraceptive patches and give symptomatic treatment.

Patient Information

Counsel women that the contraceptive patch does not protect against HIV infection (AIDS) or other sexually transmitted diseases.

Advise women that every new patch must be applied on the same day of each week and to only wear 1 patch at a time.

Instruct women to apply the patch to clean, dry, intact healthy skin on the buttock, abdomen, upper outer arm, or upper torso. Instruct women not to place the patch on skin that is red, irritated, or cut, or on the breasts.

If any of these adverse reactions occur while using the patch, instruct patients to call their health care provider immediately: sharp chest pain, coughing of blood, sudden shortness of breath (indicating a possible clot in the lung); pain in the calf (indicating a possible clot in the leg); crushing chest pain or tightness in the chest (indicating a possible heart attack); sudden severe headache or vomiting, dizziness or fainting, disturbances of vision or speech, weakness or numbness in an arm or leg (indicating a possible stroke); sudden partial or complete loss of vision (indicating a possible clot in the eye); breast lumps (indicating possible breast cancer or fibrocystic disease of the breast); severe pain or tenderness in the stomach area (indicating a possibly ruptured liver tumor); severe problems with sleeping, weakness, lack of energy, fatigue, or change in mood (possibly indicating severe depression); jaundice or a yellowing of the skin or eyes accompanied frequently by fever, fatigue, loss of appetite, dark-colored urine, or light-colored bowel movements (indicating possible liver problems).

Inform patients who use hormonal contraceptives that there is a slight increased risk of increased blood pressure, gallbladder problems, or rare cancerous or noncancerous liver tumors.

Skin irritation, redness, or rash may occur at the site of application. If this occurs, the patch may be removed and a new patch may be applied to a new location until the next patch change day. Single replacement patches are available from pharmacies.

Irregular bleeding may occur during the first few months of contraceptive patch use, but also may occur after patients have been using the contraceptive patch for some time. If the bleeding occurs in more than a few cycles or lasts for more than a few days, instruct patients to talk with their health care provider.

Advise women who smoke to quit because the risk of serious cardiovascular adverse effects is increased.

Advise women that contact lens wearers who develop vision changes or changes in lens tolerance should be assessed by an ophthalmologist.

ETONOGESTREL/ETHINYL ESTRADIOL — VAGINAL RING

	Product and Distributor	Release Rate	Total Content	How Supplied
Rx	**NuvaRing** (Organon)	Etonogestrel 0.12 mg, Ethinyl estradiol 0.015 mg per day	Etonogestrel 11.7 mg Ethinyl estradiol 2.7 mg	In single-use 1s and 3s.

ETONOGESTREL/ETHINYL ESTRADIOL — VAGINAL RING

WARNING

Cigarette smoking increases the risk of serious cardiovascular adverse reactions from combination oral contraceptive use. This risk increases with age and heavy smoking (at least 15 cigarettes daily) and is quite marked in women older than 35 years of age. Strongly advise women who use combination hormonal contraceptives, including the contraceptive vaginal ring, not to smoke.

Indications

➤*Contraception:* For the prevention of pregnancy.

Administration and Dosage

➤*General dosing considerations:* Rule out pregnancy before inserting the etonogestrel/ethinyl estradiol vaginal ring.

To prevent loss of contraceptive efficacy, women should not deviate from the recommended regimen. The contraceptive vaginal ring should be left in the vagina for a continuous period of 3 weeks.

Timing of initial placement of the vaginal ring varies and is determined by the patients recent history. (See Usual dosage.)

Extra contraceptive measures may be needed in the event of ring-free intervals or prolonged use of the ring. (See Deviations from Recommended Regimen.)

➤*Adults:*

Contraception –

Usual dosage: One etonogestrel/ethinyl estradiol vaginal ring is inserted in the vagina. (See Initial dosage.)

This ring is to remain in place continuously for 3 weeks. It is removed for a 1-week break, during which a withdrawal bleed usually occurs. A new ring is inserted 1 week after the last ring was removed on the same day of the week as it was inserted in the previous cycle. The withdrawal bleed usually starts on day 2 to 3 after removal of the ring and may not have finished before the next ring is inserted. In order to maintain contraceptive effectiveness, insert the new ring 1 week after the previous one was removed even if menstrual bleeding has not finished. (See Deviations from Recommended Regimen in case of inadvertent removal or prolonged ring-free interval.)

Initial dosage: Consider the possibility of ovulation and conception prior to the first use of the contraceptive vaginal ring. Timing of initial placement of the vaginal ring varies and is determined by the patient's recent history as follows:

• *No preceding hormonal contraceptive use in the preceding cycle* – Insert the contraceptive vaginal ring on the first day of the woman's cycle (ie, the first day of her menstrual bleeding). The contraceptive vaginal ring may also be started on days 2 to 5 of the woman's cycle, but in this case a barrier method, such as male condoms or spermicide, is recommended for the first 7 days of contraceptive vaginal ring use in the first cycle.

• *Changing from a combined hormonal contraceptive* – The woman may switch from her previous combined hormonal contraceptive on any day, but at the latest on the day following the usual hormone-free interval, if she has been using her hormonal method consistently and correctly or if it is reasonably certain that she is not pregnant.

• *Changing from a progestin-only method (minipill, implant, or injection) or from a progestogen-releasing intrauterine system* – The woman may switch on any day from the minipill. She should switch from an implant or the intrauterine system on the day of its removal from an injectable on the day when the next injection would be due. In all of these cases, the woman should use an additional barrier method, such as a male condom or spermicide, for the first 7 days.

• *Following complete first-trimester abortion* – The patient may start using the contraceptive vaginal ring within the first 5 days following a complete first-trimester abortion and does not need to use an additional method of contraception. If use of the contraceptive vaginal ring is not started within 5 days following a first-trimester abortion, the patient should follow the instructions for no preceding hormonal contraceptive use in the preceding cycle. In the meantime, advise the patient to use a nonhormonal contraceptive method.

• *Following delivery or second-trimester abortion* – Initiate the use of the contraceptive vaginal ring 4 weeks postpartum in women who elect not to breast-feed. Advise women who are breast-feeding not to use the contraceptive vaginal ring but to use other forms of contraception until the child is weaned. Initiate use of the contraceptive vaginal ring 4 weeks after a second-trimester abortion. When the contraceptive vaginal ring is used postpartum or postabortion, consider the increased risk of thromboembolic disease (see Contraindications, Warnings/Precautions). If the patient begins using the contraceptive vaginal ring postpartum, instruct the patient to use an additional method of contraception (eg, male condoms, spermicide) for the first 7 days. If she has not yet had a period, the possibility of ovulation and conception occurring prior to initiation of the contraceptive vaginal ring should be considered.

➤*Children:*

16 years of age and older (or postpubertal adolescents younger than 16 years of age) – See Adults for dosing.

➤*Hepatic function impairment:* If jaundice develops in any woman using the contraceptive vaginal ring, discontinue the medication. The hormones in the contraceptive vaginal ring may be poorly metabolized in women with liver function impairment.

➤*Deviations from Recommended Regimen:*

Inadvertent removal, expulsion, or prolonged ring-free interval –

Ring-free interval of less than 3 hours: If the contraceptive vaginal ring is accidentally expelled and is left outside of the vagina for less than 3 hours, contraceptive efficacy is not reduced. The contraceptive vaginal ring can be rinsed with cool to lukewarm (not hot) water and reinserted as soon as possible, at the latest within 3 hours. If the contraceptive vaginal ring is lost, a new vaginal ring should be inserted and the regimen should be continued without alteration.

ETONOGESTREL/ETHINYL ESTRADIOL — VAGINAL RING

Ring-free interval of more than 3 hours: If the ring has been out of the vagina for more than 3 hours, contraceptive effectiveness may be reduced.

• *During weeks 1 and 2* – Reinsert the ring as soon as she remembers. A barrier method, such as condoms or spermicides, must be used until the ring has been used continuously for 7 days.

• *During week 3* – Discard that ring. One of the following 2 options should be chosen:

1.) Insert a new ring immediately. Inserting a new ring will start the next 3-week use period. The woman may not experience a withdrawal bleed from her previous cycle. However, breakthrough spotting or bleeding may occur.
2.) Have a withdrawal bleeding and insert a new ring no later than 7 days (7 × 24 hours) from the time the previous ring was removed or expelled. This option should only be chosen if the ring was used continuously for the preceding 7 days.

A barrier method such as condoms or spermicides must be used until the new ring has been used continuously for 7 days.

Ring-free interval of more than 1 week: Consider the possibility of pregnancy if the ring-free interval has been extended beyond 1 week. Use an additional method of contraception (eg, male condoms, spermicide) until the contraceptive vaginal ring has been used continuously for 7 days.

Prolonged use: If the contraceptive vaginal ring has been left in place for up to 1 extra week (up to 4 weeks total), the woman will remain protected. Remove the contraceptive vaginal ring and insert a new ring after a 1-week ring-free interval.

If the contraceptive vaginal ring has been left in place for longer than 4 weeks, pregnancy should be ruled out, and an additional method of contraception, such as male condoms or spermicide, must be used until a new contraceptive vaginal ring has been used continuously for 7 days.

Missed menstrual period: If the patient has not adhered to the prescribed regimen (the contraceptive vaginal ring has been out of the vagina for more than 3 hours or the preceding ring-free interval was extended beyond 1 week), consider the possibility of pregnancy at the time of the first missed period and discontinue the use of the contraceptive vaginal ring if pregnancy is confirmed.

Rule out pregnancy if the patient has adhered to the prescribed regimen and misses 2 consecutive periods.

Rule out pregnancy if the patient has retained 1 contraceptive vaginal ring for more than 4 weeks.

➤*Administration:*

Insertion – The user can choose the insertion position that is most comfortable for her, for example standing with one leg up, squatting, or lying down. The ring is to be compressed and inserted into the vagina. The exact position of the contraceptive vaginal ring inside the vagina is not critical for its function. The vaginal ring must be inserted on the appropriate day and left in place for 3 consecutive weeks.

Removal – The ring is removed 3 weeks later on the same day of the week as it was inserted and at about the same time. Remove the vaginal ring by hooking the index finger under the forward rim or by grasping the rim between the index and middle finger and pulling it out. The used ring should be placed in the sachet (foil pouch) and discarded in a waste receptacle out of the reach of children and pets (do not flush in toilet).

➤*Storage/Stability:* Prior to dispensing to the user, store refrigerated at 2° to 8°C (36° to 46°F).

After dispensing to the user, the contraceptive vaginal ring can be stored for up to 4 months at 15° to 30°C (59° to 86°F). Avoid storing the contraceptive vaginal ring in direct sunlight or at temperatures above 30°C (86°F). When the contraceptive vaginal ring is dispensed to the user, place an expiration date on the label. The date should not be more than 4 months from the date it was dispensed or the expiration date, whichever comes first.

Actions

➤*Pharmacology:* The contraceptive vaginal ring is a nonbiodegradable, flexible, transparent, colorless to almost colorless combination contraceptive vaginal ring containing 2 active components: a progestin, etonogestrel and an estrogen, ethinyl estradiol. Combination hormonal contraceptives act by suppression of gonadotropins. Although the primary effect of this action is inhibition of ovulation, other alterations include changes in the cervical mucus (which increase the difficulty of sperm entry into the uterus) and the endometrium (which reduce the likelihood of implantation).

Receptor-binding studies, as well as studies in animals, have shown that etonogestrel, the biologically active metabolite of desogestrel, combines high progestational activity with low intrinsic androgenicity. The relevance of this latter finding in humans is unknown.

➤*Pharmacokinetics:*

Absorption – Etonogestrel released by the vaginal ring is rapidly absorbed. Bioavailability of etonogestrel after vaginal administration is approximately 100%.

Ethinyl estradiol released by the vaginal ring is rapidly absorbed. Bioavailability of ethinyl estradiol after vaginal administration is approximately 56%, which is comparable with that of oral administration of ethinyl estradiol. The serum etonogestrel and ethinyl estradiol concentrations observed during 3 weeks of vaginal ring use are summarized in the following table.

Mean (SD[a]) Serum Etonogestrel and Ethinyl Estradiol Vaginal Ring Concentrations (n = 16)

Hormone	1 week	2 weeks	3 weeks
Etonogestrel (pg/mL)	1,578 (408)	1,476 (362)	1,374 (328)
Ethinyl estradiol (pg/mL)	19.1 (4.5)	18.3 (4.3)	17.6 (4.3)

[a] SD = standard deviation.

The pharmacokinetic parameters of etonogestrel and ethinyl estradiol were determined during 1 cycle of contraceptive vaginal ring use in 16 healthy women and are summarized in the following table.

Mean (SD) Pharmacokinetic Parameters of Etonogestrel/Ethinyl Estradiol Vaginal Ring (n = 16)

Hormone	C_{max} [a] (pg/mL)	T_{max} [b] (h)	$t_{½}$ [c] (h)	Apparent clearance (L/h)
Etonogestrel	1,716 (445)	200.3 (69.6)	29.3 (6.1)	3.4 (0.8)
Ethinyl estradiol	34.7 (17.5)	59.3 (67.5)	44.7 (28.8)	34.8 (11.6)

[a] C_{max} = maximum serum concentration.
[b] T_{max} = time at which maximum serum drug concentration occurs.
[c] $t_{½}$ = elimination half-life, calculated by $0.693/K_{elim}$.

Distribution – Etonogestrel is approximately 32% bound to sex hormone–binding globulin (SHBG) and approximately 66% bound to albumin in blood.

Ethinyl estradiol is highly but not specifically bound to serum albumin (approximately 98.5%) and induces an increase in the serum concentrations of SHBG.

Metabolism – In vitro data show that etonogestrel and ethinyl estradiol are metabolized in liver microsomes by the CYP-450 3A4 isoenzyme. Ethinyl estradiol is primarily metabolized by aromatic hydroxylation, but a wide variety of hydroxylated and methylated metabolites are formed. These are present as free metabolites and as sulfate and glucuronide conjugates. The hydroxylated ethinyl estradiol metabolites have weak estrogenic activity. The biological activity of etonogestrel metabolites is unknown.

Excretion – Etonogestrel and ethinyl estradiol are primarily eliminated in urine, bile, and feces.

Special populations

Hepatic function impairment: Steroid hormones may be poorly metabolized in women with impaired liver function.

Contraindications

Thrombophlebitis or thromboembolic disorders; a past history of deep vein thrombophlebitis or thromboembolic disorders; cerebral vascular or coronary artery disease (current or history); valvular heart disease with thrombogenic complications; severe hypertension; diabetes with vascular involvement; headaches with focal neurological symptoms; major surgery with prolonged immobility; known or suspected carcinoma of the breast or personal history of breast cancer; carcinoma of the endometrium or other known or suspected estrogen-dependent neoplasia; undiagnosed abnormal genital bleeding; cholestatic jaundice of pregnancy or jaundice with prior hormonal contraceptive use; hepatic tumors (benign or malignant); active liver disease; known or suspected pregnancy; heavy smoking (at least 15 cigarettes daily) and older than 35 years of age; hypersensitivity to any of the components of the contraceptive vaginal ring.

Warnings/Precautions

➤*Risk of oral contraceptive use:* The use of oral contraceptives is associated with increased risks of several serious conditions, including venous and arterial thrombotic and thromboembolic events (eg, myocardial infarction [MI], thromboembolism, stroke), hepatic neoplasia, gallbladder disease, and hypertension, although the risk of serious morbidity or mortality is very small in healthy women without underlying risk factors. The risk of morbidity and mortality increases significantly in the presence of other underlying risk factors, such as certain inherited thrombophilias, hypertension, hyperlipidemias, obesity, and diabetes.

➤*Thromboembolic disorders and other vascular problems:*

Thromboembolism – An increased risk of thromboembolic and thrombotic disease associated with the use of oral contraceptives is well established. Case control studies have found the relative risk of users compared with non-users to be 3 for the first episode of superficial venous thrombosis, 4 to 11 for deep vein thrombosis or pulmonary embolism, and 1.5 to 6 for women with predisposing conditions for venous thromboembolic disease. Cohort studies have shown the relative risk to be somewhat lower, approximately 3 for new cases and approximately 4.5 for new cases requiring hospitalization. The risk of thromboembolic disease associated with hormonal contraceptives is not related to length of use and disappears after pill use is stopped.

Several epidemiology studies indicate that third-generation oral contraceptives, including those containing desogestrel (etonogestrel, the progestin in the vaginal ring, is the biologically active metabolite of desogestrel), are associated with a higher risk of venous thromboembolism than certain second-generation oral contraceptives. In general, these studies indicate an approximately 2-fold increased risk, which corresponds to an additional 1 to 2 cases of venous thromboembolism per 10,000 women-years of use. However, data from additional studies have not shown this 2-fold increase in risk. It is unknown if the vaginal ring has a different risk of venous thromboembolism than second-generation oral contraceptives.

ETONOGESTREL/ETHINYL ESTRADIOL — VAGINAL RING

A 2- to 4-fold increase in relative risk of postoperative thromboembolic complications has been reported with the use of oral contraceptives. The relative risk of venous thrombosis in women who have predisposing conditions is twice that of women without such medical conditions. If feasible, discontinue the use of combination hormonal contraceptives, including the vaginal ring, for at least 4 weeks prior to and for 2 weeks after elective surgery of a type associated with increased risk of thromboembolism and during and following prolonged immobilization. Because the immediate postpartum period is also associated with an increased risk of thromboembolism, start combination hormonal contraceptives (eg, vaginal ring) no earlier than 4 weeks after delivery in women who elect not to breast-feed.

Be alert to the earliest manifestations of thrombotic disorders (thrombophlebitis, pulmonary embolism, cerebrovascular disorders, and retinal thrombosis). Should any of these occur or be suspected, immediately discontinue use of the vaginal ring.

MI – An increased risk of MI has been attributed to oral contraceptive use. The risk is primarily in smokers or women with other underlying risk factors for coronary artery disease (eg, hypertension, hypercholesterolemia, morbid obesity, diabetes). The relative risk of heart attack for current combination oral contraceptive users has been estimated to be 2 to 6. The risk is very low in women younger than 30 years of age.

Oral contraceptives may compound the effects of well-known risk factors (eg, hypertension, diabetes, hyperlipidemias, age, obesity). In particular, some progestogens are known to decrease high-density lipoprotein (HDL) cholesterol and cause glucose intolerance, while estrogens may create a state of hyperinsulinism. Oral contraceptives have been shown to increase blood pressure among users. Similar effects on risk factors have been associated with an increased risk of heart disease. Use the contraceptive vaginal ring with caution in women with cardiovascular disease risk factors.

Smoking: Smoking in combination with oral contraceptive use has been shown to contribute substantially to the incidence of MI in women in their mid-30s and older, with smoking accounting for the majority of excess cases. Mortality rates associated with circulatory disease have been shown to increase substantially in smokers older than 35 years of age and nonsmokers older than 40 years of age among women who use oral contraceptives (see the following table).

Circulatory Disease Mortality Rates Per 100,000 Woman-Years by Age, Smoking Status, and Combination Oral Contraceptive Use

Age (years)	Ever-users nonsmokers	Ever-users smokers	Controls nonsmokers	Controls smokers
15 to 24	0	10.5	0	0
25 to 34	4.4	14.2	2.7	4.2
35 to 44	21.5	63.4	6.4	15.2
45+	52.4	206.7	11.4	27.9

Cerebrovascular diseases – Oral contraceptives have been shown to increase the relative and attributable risks of cerebrovascular events (thrombotic and hemorrhagic strokes), although, in general, the risk is highest among older (older than 35 years of age), hypertensive women who also smoke. Hypertension was found to be a risk factor for users and non-users for both types of strokes, while smoking interacted to increase the risk for hemorrhagic strokes.

In a large study, the relative risk of thrombotic strokes ranged from 3 for normotensive users to 14 for users with severe hypertension. The relative risk of hemorrhagic stroke is reported to be 1.2 for nonsmokers who used oral contraceptives, 2.6 for smokers who did not use oral contraceptives, 7.6 for smokers who used oral contraceptives, 1.8 for normotensive users, and 25.7 for users with severe hypertension. The attributable risk is also greater in older women. Oral contraceptives also increase the risk for stroke in women with other underlying risk factors, such as certain inherited or acquired thrombophilias, hyperlipidemias, and obesity. Women with migraine (particularly migraine with aura) who take combination oral contraceptives may have an increased risk of stroke.

Dose-related risk – A positive association has been observed between the amount of estrogen and progestogen in oral contraceptives and the risk of vascular disease. A decline in serum HDL has been reported with many progestational agents. A decline in serum HDL has been associated with an increased incidence of ischemic heart disease. Because estrogens increase HDL cholesterol, the net effect of an oral contraceptive depends on a balance achieved between doses of estrogen and progestogen and the nature and absolute amount of progestogens used in the contraceptives. Consider the activity and amount of both hormones in the choice of a hormonal contraceptive.

Minimizing exposure to estrogen and progestogen is in keeping with good principles of therapeutics. For any particular estrogen/progestogen combination, prescribe the dosage regimen that contains the least amount of estrogen and progestogen that is compatible with a low failure rate and the needs of the individual patient. Start new acceptors of hormonal contraceptive agents on a product containing the lowest hormone content that provides satisfactory results in the individual.

Persistence of risk – There are 2 studies that have shown persistence of risk of vascular disease for ever-users of oral contraceptives. In a study in the United States, the risk of developing MI after discontinuing oral contraceptives persists for at least 9 years for women 40 to 49 years of age who had used oral contraceptives for at least 5 years, but this increased risk was not demonstrated in other age groups. In another study in Great Britain, the risk of developing cerebrovascular disease persisted for at least 6 years after discontinuation of oral contraceptives, although excess risk was very small. However, both studies were performed with oral contraceptive formulations containing at least 50 mcg of estrogen.

It is unknown whether the contraceptive vaginal ring is distinct from combination oral contraceptives with regard to the occurrence of venous or arterial thrombosis.

➤*Mortality:* One study gathered data from a variety of sources that have estimated the mortality rate associated with different methods of contraception at different ages. These estimates include the combined risk of death associated with contraceptive methods plus the risk attributable to pregnancy in the event of method failure. Each method of contraception has its specific benefits and risks. The study concluded that with the exception of oral contraceptive users at least 35 years of age who smoke and at least 40 years of age who do not smoke, mortality associated with all methods of birth control is low and below that associated with childbirth.

The observation of a possible increase in risk of mortality with age for oral contraceptive users is based on data gathered in the 1970s but not reported until 1983. However, current clinical practice involves the use of lower estrogen-dose formulations combined with careful restriction of hormonal contraceptive use to women who do not have the various risk factors listed in this labeling.

Because of these changes in practice and because of limited new data that suggest the risk of cardiovascular disease with the use of oral contraceptives may now be less than previously observed, the Fertility and Maternal Health Drugs Advisory Committee was asked to review the topic in 1989. The Committee concluded that although cardiovascular disease risks may be increased with oral contraceptive use after age 40 in healthy nonsmoking women (even with the newer low-dose formulations), there are also greater potential health risks associated with pregnancy in older women and with the alternative surgical and medical procedures that may be necessary if such women do not have access to effective and acceptable means of contraception. Therefore, the Committee recommended that the benefits of low-dose oral contraceptive use by healthy nonsmoking women older than 40 years of age may outweigh the possible risks. Older women, as all women who take hormonal contraceptives, should take the lowest possible dose formulation that is effective and meets the individual patient's needs.

➤*Carcinoma:* Numerous epidemiologic studies have been performed on the incidence of breast, endometrial, ovarian, and cervical cancer in women using combination oral contraceptives.

Although the risk of having breast cancer diagnosed may be slightly increased among current users of oral contraceptives (relative risk, 1.24), this excess risk decreases over time after oral contraceptive discontinuation, and by 10 years after cessation, the increased risk disappears. The risk does not increase with duration of use, and no relationships have been found with dose or type of steroid. The patterns of risk are also similar regardless of a woman's reproductive history or her family breast cancer history. The subgroup for whom risk has been found to be significantly elevated is women who first used oral contraceptives before age 20, but because breast cancer is so rare at these young ages, the number of cases attributable to this early oral contraceptive use is extremely small.

Breast cancers diagnosed in current or previous oral contraceptive users tend to be less clinically advanced than in never-users.

Women who currently have or have had breast cancer should not use hormonal contraceptives because breast cancer is usually a hormonal-sensitive tumor.

Some studies suggest that combination oral contraceptive use has been associated with an increase in the risk of cervical intraepithelial neoplasia in some populations of women. However, there continues to be controversy about the extent to which such findings may be caused by differences in sexual behavior and other factors.

In spite of many studies of the relationship between oral contraceptive use and breast and cervical cancers, a cause-and-effect relationship has not been established.

It is unknown whether the contraceptive vaginal ring is distinct from oral contraceptives with regard to the previous statements.

➤*Hepatic neoplasia:* Benign hepatic adenomas are associated with oral contraceptive use, although the incidence of benign tumors is rare in the United States. Indirect calculations have estimated the attributable risk to be in the range of 3.3 cases per 100,000 for users, a risk that increases after at least 4 years of use. Rupture of rare, benign, hepatic adenomas may cause death through intra-abdominal hemorrhage.

Studies from Great Britain have shown an increased risk of developing hepatocellular carcinoma in long-term (more than 8 years) oral contraceptive users. However, these cancers are extremely rare in the United States and the attributable risk (the excess incidence) of liver cancers in oral contraceptive users approaches less than 1 per million users. It is unknown whether the contraceptive vaginal ring is distinct from oral contraceptives in this regard.

➤*Ocular lesions:* There have been clinical case reports of retinal thrombosis associated with the use of oral contraceptives. Discontinue use of the contraceptive vaginal ring if there is unexplained partial or complete loss of vision, onset of proptosis or diplopia, papilledema, or retinal vascular lesions. Undertake appropriate diagnostic and therapeutic measures immediately.

➤*Gallbladder disease:* Combination hormonal contraceptives (eg, contraceptive vaginal ring) may worsen existing gallbladder disease and may accelerate the development of this disease in previously asymptomatic women. Women with a history of combination hormonal contraceptive-

ETONOGESTREL/ETHINYL ESTRADIOL — VAGINAL RING

related cholestasis are more likely to have the condition recur with subsequent combination hormonal contraceptive use.

➤*Glucose tolerance:* Hormonal contraceptives have been shown to cause a decrease in glucose tolerance in some users. However, in nondiabetic women, combination hormonal contraceptives appear to have no effect on fasting blood glucose. Carefully observe prediabetic and diabetic women while taking combination hormonal contraceptives (eg, contraceptive vaginal ring). In a clinical study involving 37 contraceptive vaginal ring–treated subjects, glucose tolerance tests showed no clinically significant changes in serum glucose levels from baseline to cycle 6.

➤*Carbohydrate and lipid effects:* A small proportion of women will have persistent hypertriglyceridemia while using hormonal contraceptives. Changes in serum triglycerides and lipoprotein levels have been reported in combination hormonal contraceptive users.

In women with familial defects of lipoprotein metabolism receiving estrogen-containing preparations, there have been case reports of significant elevations of plasma triglycerides leading to pancreatitis.

Closely follow women who are being treated for hyperlipidemias if they elect to use the contraceptive vaginal ring. Some progestogens may elevate low-density lipoprotein levels and may render the control of hyperlipidemias more difficult.

➤*Elevated blood pressure:* Do not start women with severe hypertension on hormonal contraceptives. An increase in blood pressure has been reported in women taking hormonal contraceptives; this increase is more likely in older oral contraceptive users and with continued use. Data from the Royal College of General Practitioners and subsequent randomized trials have shown that the incidence of hypertension increases with increasing concentrations of progestogens. Encourage women with a history of hypertension or hypertension-related diseases, or renal disease to use another method of contraception. Closely monitor these women if they elect to use the contraceptive vaginal ring. Discontinue use of the contraceptive vaginal ring if significant elevation of blood pressure occurs. For most women, elevated blood pressure will return to normal after stopping hormonal contraceptives, and there is no difference in the occurrence of hypertension between former and never users.

➤*Headache:* The onset or exacerbation of migraine or development of headache with a new pattern that is recurrent, persistent, or severe requires discontinuation of the contraceptive vaginal ring and evaluation of the cause.

➤*Bleeding irregularities and patterns:* Breakthrough bleeding and spotting are sometimes encountered in women using the contraceptive vaginal ring. If abnormal bleeding persists or is severe while using the contraceptive vaginal ring, investigate to rule out the possibility of organic pathology or pregnancy and institute appropriate treatment when necessary. Rule out pregnancy in the event of amenorrhea.

Bleeding patterns were evaluated in 3 large clinical studies. In the US-Canadian study (n = 1,177), the percentages of subjects with breakthrough bleeding/spotting ranged from 7.2% to 11.7% during cycles 1 to 13. In the 2 non-US studies, the percentages of subjects with breakthrough bleeding/spotting ranged from 2.6% to 6.4% (study 1, n = 1,145 European and Israeli subjects) and from 2% to 8.7% (study 2, n = 512 European and South American subjects). In these 3 studies, the percentages of women who did not have withdrawal bleeding in a given cycle ranged from 0.3% to 3.8%.

Some women may encounter amenorrhea or oligomenorrhea after discontinuing use of the contraceptive vaginal ring, especially when a condition was preexistent.

➤*Sexually transmitted diseases:* Counsel patients that this product does not protect against HIV infection (AIDS) and other sexually transmitted diseases.

➤*Physical examination and follow-up:* It is routine medical practice for women using the contraceptive vaginal ring, as for all women, to have an annual medical evaluation, including physical examination and relevant laboratory tests. The physical examination should include special reference to blood pressure, breasts, abdomen, pelvic organs, and vagina (including cervical cytology). In case of undiagnosed, persistent, or recurrent abnormal vaginal bleeding, conduct appropriate measures to rule out malignancy. Monitor women with a family history of breast cancer or who have breast nodules with particular care.

➤*Hepatic function impairment:* If jaundice develops in any woman using the contraceptive vaginal ring, discontinue the medication. The hormones in the contraceptive vaginal ring may be poorly metabolized in women with liver function impairment.

➤*Fluid retention:* Steroid hormones like those in the contraceptive vaginal ring may cause some degree of fluid retention. Prescribe this product with caution, and only with careful monitoring, in patients with conditions that might be aggravated by fluid retention.

➤*Depression:* Women who become significantly depressed while taking hormonal contraceptives should stop the medication and use another method of contraception in an attempt to determine whether the symptom is drug-related. Carefully observe women with a history of depression and discontinue the product if depression recurs to a serious degree.

➤*Tampon use:* On rare occasions, the contraceptive vaginal ring may be expelled while removing a tampon. Pharmacokinetic data show that the use of tampons has no effect on the systemic absorption of the hormones released by the contraceptive vaginal ring.

➤*Toxic shock syndrome (TSS):* Cases of TSS have been associated with tampons and certain barrier contraceptives. Very rare cases of TSS have been reported by contraceptive vaginal ring users; in some cases, the women were also using tampons. No causal relationship between the use of the contraceptive vaginal ring and TSS has been established. If a patient exhibits signs or symptoms of TSS, the possibility of this diagnosis should not be excluded; initiate appropriate medical evaluation and treatment.

➤*Contact lenses:* Contact lens wearers who develop visual changes or changes in lens tolerance should be assessed by an ophthalmologist.

➤*Vaginal use:* The contraceptive vaginal ring may not be suitable for women with conditions that make the vagina more susceptible to vaginal irritation or ulceration. Vaginal/cervical erosion or ulceration in women using the vaginal contraceptive ring has been rarely reported. In some cases, the ring adhered to vaginal tissue, necessitating removal by a health care provider. Some women are aware of the ring at random times during the 21 days of use or during intercourse. During intercourse, some sexual partners may feel the contraceptive vaginal ring in the vagina. However, clinical studies revealed that 90% of couples did not find this to be a problem.

The contraceptive vaginal ring may interfere with the correct placement and position of a diaphragm. Therefore, a diaphragm is not recommended as a backup method with contraceptive vaginal ring use.

➤*Urinary bladder insertion:* There have been rare reports of inadvertent insertions of the contraceptive vaginal ring into the urinary bladder, which required cystoscopic removal. Health care providers should assess for ring insertion into the urinary bladder in contraceptive vaginal ring users who present with persistent urinary symptoms and are unable to locate the ring.

➤*Expulsion:* The contraceptive vaginal ring can be accidentally expelled, for example, while removing a tampon, during intercourse, or with straining during a bowel movement. The contraceptive vaginal ring should be left in the vagina for a continuous period of 3 weeks. If the ring is accidentally expelled and is left outside of the vagina for less than 3 hours, contraceptive efficacy is not reduced. The contraceptive vaginal ring can be rinsed with cool to lukewarm (not hot) water and reinserted as soon as possible, at the latest within 3 hours. If the contraceptive vaginal ring is lost, insert a new vaginal ring and continue the regimen without alteration.

If the contraceptive vaginal ring is out of the vagina for more than 3 continuous hours – During weeks 1 and 2: If the contraceptive vaginal ring has been out of the vagina for more than 3 continuous hours during the first or second week of use, contraceptive efficacy may be reduced. The woman should reinsert the ring as soon as she remembers. A barrier method such as condoms or spermicides must be used until the ring has been used continuously for 7 days.

During week 3: If the contraceptive vaginal ring has been out of the vagina for more than 3 continuous hours during the third week of the 3-week use period, the woman should discard that ring. One of the following 2 options should be chosen:

1.) Insert a new ring immediately. Inserting a new ring will start the next 3-week use period. The woman may not experience a withdrawal bleed from her previous cycle. However, breakthrough spotting or bleeding may occur.
2.) Have a withdrawal bleeding and insert a new ring no later than 7 days (7 × 24 hours) from the time the previous ring was removed or expelled. This option should only be chosen if the ring was used continuously for the preceding 7 days.

A barrier method such as condoms or spermicides must be used until the new ring has been used continuously for 7 days.

➤*Disconnected ring:* There have been reported cases of the contraceptive vaginal ring disconnecting at the weld joint. This is not expected to affect the contraceptive effectiveness of the contraceptive vaginal ring. In the event of a disconnected ring, vaginal discomfort or expulsion (slipping out) is more likely to occur. If a women discovers that her contraceptive vaginal ring has disconnected, she should discard the ring and replace it with a new ring.

➤*Pregnancy: Category X.* The contraceptive vaginal ring is contraindicated in known or suspected pregnancy. Extensive epidemiologic studies have revealed no increased risk of birth defects in women who have used oral contraceptives prior to pregnancy. Studies also do not suggest a teratogenic effect, particularly where cardiac anomalies and limb reduction defects are concerned, when oral contraceptives are taken inadvertently during early pregnancy.

Combination hormonal contraceptives, such as the contraceptive vaginal ring, should not be used to induce withdrawal bleeding as a test for pregnancy. Do not use the vaginal ring during pregnancy to treat threatened or habitual abortion. It is recommended that for any woman who has not adhered to the prescribed regimen for use of the vaginal ring and has missed a menstrual period or 2 consecutive periods, pregnancy should be ruled out.

Teratology studies have been performed in rats and rabbits using the oral route of administration at doses of up to 130 and 260 times, respectively, the human contraceptive vaginal ring dose (based on body surface area) and have revealed no evidence of harm to the fetus caused by etonogestrel.

Ectopic pregnancy – Ectopic as well as intrauterine pregnancy may occur in contraceptive failures.

➤*Lactation:* The effects of the contraceptive vaginal ring in breast-feeding mothers have not been evaluated and are unknown. Small amounts of contraceptive steroids have been identified in the milk of breast-feeding mothers and a few adverse effects on the child have been reported, including jaundice and breast enlargement. In addition, contraceptive steroids given in the postpartum period may interfere with lactation by decreasing the quantity and quality of breast milk. Long-term follow-up of children whose

ETONOGESTREL/ETHINYL ESTRADIOL — VAGINAL RING

mothers used combination hormonal contraceptives while breast-feeding has shown no deleterious effects in infants. However, advise women who are breast-feeding not to use the contraceptive vaginal ring but to use other forms of contraception until the child is weaned.

➤*Children:* Safety and efficacy of the contraceptive vaginal ring have been established in women of reproductive age. Safety and efficacy are expected to be the same for postpubertal adolescents younger than 16 years of age and for users 16 years of age and older. Use of this product before menarche is not indicated.

➤*Monitoring:* Closely monitor blood pressure in women with a history of hypertension or hypertension-related diseases or renal disease. Monitor women with a family history of breast cancer or who have breast nodules with particular care. Closely follow women who are being treated for hyperlipidemias. Carefully monitor patients with conditions that might be aggravated by fluid retention. Monitor patients with a history of depression and discontinue the product if depression recurs to a serious degree.

Drug Interactions

Most drug interactions are based on oral contraceptives.

Contraceptive Vaginal Ring Drug Interactions

Precipitant drug	Object drug[a]		Description
Acetaminophen	Contraceptives, hormonal	↑	Ethinyl estradiol plasma levels may increase, whereas acetaminophen plasma concentrations may decrease.
Contraceptives, hormonal	Acetaminophen	↓	
Antibiotics	Contraceptives, hormonal	↓	Coadministration of griseofulvin, penicillins, or tetracyclines with hormonal contraceptives may decrease the pharmacologic effects of the hormonal contraceptive, possibly because of altered steroid gut metabolism secondary to changes in the intestinal flora. Menstrual irregularities (eg, spotting, breakthrough bleeding) and pregnancy may occur. An alternate or additional form of birth control may be advisable during concomitant use. Hormonal contraceptives and troleandomycin may be associated with an increased risk of intrahepatic cholestasis.
Ascorbic acid	Contraceptives, hormonal	↑	Ethinyl estradiol plasma levels may increase.
Atorvastatin	Contraceptives, hormonal	↑	Ethinyl estradiol AUC may increase by approximately 20%.
Barbiturates (eg, phenobarbital), bosentan, carbamazepine, felbamate, hydantoins (eg, phenytoin),[b] modafinil, nevirapine, oxcarbazepine, phenylbutazone, primidone, rifamycins (eg, rifampin), topiramate	Contraceptives, hormonal	↓	These agents may increase the hepatic metabolism of the contraceptive steroids via hepatic microsomal enzyme induction, possibly resulting in decreased effectiveness, menstrual irregularities (eg, spotting, breakthrough bleeding), and pregnancy. An alternate or additional form of birth control may be advisable during concomitant use.
CYP3A4 inhibitors (eg, itraconazole, ketoconazole)	Contraceptives, hormonal	↑	An increase in plasma hormone levels may occur.
Miconazole	Etonogestrel/ ethinyl estradiol vaginal ring	↑	Vaginally administered miconazole increased serum concentrations of etonogestrel and ethinyl estradiol by up to 40%.
Protease inhibitors (eg, nelfinavir, ritonavir, saquinavir)	Contraceptives, hormonal	↓	Increased metabolism of the hormonal contraceptive is suspected, resulting in a loss of effectiveness of the hormonal contraceptive. An alternate or additional form of birth control may be advisable during concomitant use.
St. John's wort	Contraceptives, hormonal	↓	St. John's wort may induce hepatic enzymes and P-glycoprotein transporter and may reduce the effectiveness of contraceptive steroids. This may also result in breakthrough bleeding.
Contraceptives, hormonal	Antidepressants, tricyclic (eg, amitriptyline), beta-blockers (eg, metoprolol), caffeine, corticosteroids (eg, prednisolone), theophyllines	↑↓	Hormone contraceptives may increase the clearance of temazepam. The hepatic metabolism of these agents may be decreased by hormonal contraceptives, resulting in increased therapeutic effects or toxicity.
Contraceptives, hormonal	Benzodiazepines (eg, alprazolam, chlordiazepoxide, diazepam, temazepam)	↑	Coadministration of combination hormonal contraceptives and certain benzodiazepines (eg, alprazolam, chlordiazepoxide, diazepam) that undergo oxidation may result in a prolongation of the benzodiazepine half-life. Observe closely.
Contraceptives, hormonal	Cyclosporine, selegiline	↑	Increased plasma concentrations of cyclosporine and selegiline have been reported with coadministration of hormonal contraceptives.
Contraceptives, hormonal	Clofibrate acid, morphine, salicylic acid, temazepam	↓	Increased clearance of these agents has been noted when administered with hormonal contraceptives.
Contraceptives, hormonal	Lamotrigine, valproic acid	↓	Hormonal contraceptives may increase the metabolism of lamotrigine and valproic acid; adjust the dose of lamotrigine and valproic acid as needed.

[a] ↑ = object drug increased; ↓ = object drug decreased; ↑↓ = object drug both increased and decreased.
[b] Pharmacologic effects of the hydantoins also may be altered.

➤*Drug/Lab test interactions:* Certain endocrine and liver function tests and blood components may be affected by hormonal contraceptives:

Increased – Prothrombin and factors VII, VIII, IX, and X; norepinephrine-induced platelet aggregability; thyroid-binding globulin leading to increased circulating total thyroid hormone as measured by protein-bound iodine (PBI), T4 by column or by radioimmunoassay. Other binding proteins may be elevated in serum. Sex hormone binding globulins are increased and result in elevated levels of total circulating sex steroids; however, free or biologically active levels either decrease or remain unchanged. Triglycerides may be increased and levels of various other lipids and lipoproteins may be affected.

Decreased – Antithrombin III, free T3 resin uptake, glucose tolerance. Serum folate levels may be depressed by oral contraceptive therapy. This may be of clinical significance if a woman becomes pregnant shortly after discontinuing the contraceptive vaginal ring.

Adverse Reactions

➤*Most common:* The most common adverse reactions reported by 5% to 14% of women using the contraceptive vaginal ring in clinical trials (n = 2,501) were the following: headache, nausea, sinusitis, upper respiratory tract infection, vaginal secretion, vaginitis, and weight gain.

➤*Discontinuation:* The most frequent system-organ class adverse reactions leading to discontinuation in 1% to 2.5% of women using the contraceptive vaginal ring in the trials included the following: device-related events (eg, coital problems, device expulsion, foreign body sensation), emotional lability, headache, vaginal symptoms (discomfort/vaginal secretion/vaginitis), and weight gain.

➤*Adverse reactions associated with other combination hormonal contraceptives:* The following adverse reactions have been associated with the use of combination hormonal contraceptives. These are also likely to apply to combination vaginal hormonal contraceptives such as the contraceptive vaginal ring.

Serious – Arterial thromboembolism; cerebral hemorrhage; cerebral thrombosis; gallbladder disease; hepatic adenomas or benign liver tumors; hypertension; mesenteric thrombosis; MI; pulmonary embolism; retinal thrombosis; thrombophlebitis and venous thrombosis with or without embolism.

CNS – Exacerbation of chorea, migraine, mood changes (including depression).

Dermatologic – Melasma/chloasma (which may persist).

GI – GI symptoms (eg, abdominal pain, bloating, cramps), nausea, vomiting.

GU – Amenorrhea, breakthrough bleeding, breast changes (enlargement, pain, secretion, tenderness), change in cervical ectropion and secretion, change in menstrual flow, possible diminution in lactation when given immediately postpartum, spotting, temporary infertility after discontinuation of treatment, vaginitis (including candidiasis).

Hypersensitivity – Anaphylactic/anaphylactoid reactions, including angioedema, severe reactions with respiratory and circulatory symptoms, and urticaria; rash (allergic).

Metabolic – Changes in weight or appetite (increase or decrease), edema/fluid retention.

Ophthalmic – Change in corneal curvature (steepening), intolerance to contact lenses.

Miscellaneous – Aggravation of varicose veins, cholestatic jaundice, decrease in serum folate levels, edema, exacerbation of porphyria, exacerbation of systemic lupus erythematosus.

➤*Other adverse reactions (combination hormonal contraceptives):* The following additional adverse reactions have been reported in users of combination hormonal contraceptives, and a causal association has been neither confirmed nor refuted.

CNS – Dizziness, headache, nervousness.

ETONOGESTREL/ETHINYL ESTRADIOL — VAGINAL RING

Dermatologic – Acne, erythema multiforme, erythema nodosum, hirsutism, loss of scalp hair.

GI – Colitis.

GU – Changes in libido, cystitis-like syndrome, dysmenorrhea, hemolytic uremic syndrome, premenstrual syndrome, renal function impairment.

Miscellaneous – Budd-Chiari syndrome; cataracts; hemorrhagic eruption; optic neuritis, which may lead to partial or complete loss of vision; pancreatitis.

Overdosage

➤*Symptoms:* Overdosage of combination hormonal contraceptives may cause nausea, vomiting, vaginal bleeding, or other menstrual irregularities. Given the nature and design of the contraceptive vaginal ring, it is unlikely that overdosage will occur. If the contraceptive vaginal ring is broken, it does not release a higher dose of hormones. Serious ill effects have not been reported following acute ingestion of large doses of oral contraceptives by young children.

➤*Treatment:* There are no antidotes and further treatment should be symptomatic.

Patient Information

Instruct the patient regarding the proper use of the contraceptive vaginal ring.

Counsel patients that this product does not protect against HIV infection (AIDS) and other sexually transmitted diseases.

Inform patients that if the contraceptive vaginal ring slips out of the vagina and it has been out for less than 3 hours, they should still be protected from pregnancy. The contraceptive vaginal ring can be rinsed with cool to lukewarm (not hot) water and reinserted as soon as possible, at the latest within 3 hours of removal or expulsion (slipping out).

Advise patients to call their health care provider right away if they experience any of the following symptoms:

- sharp chest pain, coughing blood, or sudden shortness of breath (possible clot in the lung)
- pain in the calf (back of lower leg; possible clot in the leg)
- crushing chest pain or heaviness in the chest (possible heart attack)
- sudden severe headache or vomiting, dizziness, or fainting; problems with vision or speech; weakness or numbness in an arm or leg (possible stroke)
- sudden partial or complete loss of vision (possible clot in the eye)
- yellowing of the skin or whites of the eyes (jaundice), especially with fever, tiredness, loss of appetite, dark-colored urine, or light-colored bowel movements (possible liver problems)
- severe pain, swelling, or tenderness in the abdomen (gallbladder or liver problems)
- breast lumps (possible breast cancer or benign breast disease)
- irregular vaginal bleeding or spotting that happens in at least 1 menstrual cycle or lasts for more than a few days
- swelling (edema) of the fingers or ankles
- difficulty in sleeping, weakness, lack of energy, fatigue, or a change in mood (possible severe depression).

ETONOGESTREL

Rx	**Implanon** (Organon)	**Implant:** 68 mg	Preloaded needle with disposable applicator.[a]

[a] Each etonogestrel implant rod consists of an EVA copolymer core containing 68 mg of synthetic progestin etonogestrel surrounded by an EVA copolymer skin.

ETONOGESTREL — IMPLANT

Indications

➤*Contraception:* For the prevention of pregnancy.

➤*Off-label uses:* Male contraceptive agent.

Administration and Dosage

➤*General dosing considerations:* Rule out pregnancy before inserting the etonogestrel implant.

The etonogestrel implant is a long-acting (up to 3 years), reversible contraceptive method to be inserted and removed by a trained healthcare provider (See Administration).

Timing of insertion depends on the patient's recent history (See Usual Dosage).

➤*Adults:*

Contraception –

Usual dosage: One etonogestrel implant inserted subdermally (See Initial Dosage for timing of insertion).

Initial dosage:

- *Timing of insertion depends on the patient's recent history as follows* –

  No preceding hormonal contraceptive use in the past month: Counting the first day of menstruation as day 1, the etonogestrel implant must be inserted between days 1 through 5, even if the woman is still bleeding.

  Switching from a combination hormonal contraceptive: The etonogestrel implant may be inserted
  - any time within 7 days after the last active (estrogen plus progestin) oral contraceptive tablet.
  - any time during the 7-day ring-free period of *NuvaRing* (etonogestrel/ethinyl estradiol vaginal ring).
  - any time during the 7-day patch-free period of a transdermal contraceptive system.

  Switching from a progestin-only method: There are several types of progestin-only methods. The etonogestrel implant insertion must be performed as follows
  - any day of the month when switching from a progestin-only pill. Do not skip any days between the last pill and insertion of the etonogestrel implant.
  - on the same day as contraceptive implant removal.
  - on the same day as removal of a progestin-containing intrauterine device (IUD).
  - on the day when the next contraceptive injection would be due.

Following a first trimester abortion: The etonogestrel implant may be inserted immediately following a complete, first trimester abortion. If the etonogestrel implant is not inserted within 5 days following a first trimester abortion, follow the instructions under "No preceding hormonal contraceptive use in the past month."

Following delivery or a second trimester abortion: The etonogestrel implant may be inserted between 21 to 28 days postpartum if not exclusively breast-feeding or between 21 to 28 days following a second trimester abortion. If more than 4 weeks have elapsed, pregnancy should be excluded, and the patient should use a nonhormonal method of birth control during the first 7 days after the insertion. If the patient is exclusively breast-feeding, insert the etonogestrel implant after the fourth postpartum week.

Duration of therapy: The etonogestrel implant must be removed by the end of the third year and may be replaced by a new implant at the time of removal if continued contraceptive protection is desired.

➤*Administration:* Insert the etonogestrel implant subdermally in the inner side of the upper arm (nondominant arm) about 6 to 8 cm (2½ to 3 inches) above the elbow crease overlying the groove between the biceps and the triceps.

If inserted as recommended, backup contraception is not necessary. If deviating from the recommended timing of insertion, rule out pregnancy and use backup nonhormonal contraception for 7 days after etonogestrel implant insertion.

➤*Storage/Stability:* Store the etonogestrel implant at 25°C (77°F); excursions are permitted between 15° and 30°C (59° and 86°F). Protect from light. Avoid storing in direct sunlight or at temperatures above 30°C (86°F).

Actions

➤*Pharmacology:* The contraceptive effect of the etonogestrel implant is achieved by several mechanisms that include suppression of ovulation, increased viscosity of the cervical mucus, and alterations in the endometrium.

➤*Pharmacokinetics:*

Absorption – After subdermal insertion of etonogestrel implant, etonogestrel is released into the circulation and is approximately 100% bioavailable. The mean peak serum concentrations in 3 pharmacokinetic studies ranged between 781 and 894 pg/mL and were reached within the first few weeks after insertion. The mean serum etonogestrel concentration decreases gradually over time, declining to 192 to 261 pg/mL at 12 months (n = 41), 154 to 194 pg/mL at 24 months (n = 35), and 156 to 177 pg/mL at 36 months (n = 17).

Distribution – The apparent volume of distribution averages about 201 L. Etonogestrel is approximately 32% bound to sex hormone-binding globulin (SHBG) and 66% bound to albumin in blood.

Metabolism – In vitro data show that etonogestrel is metabolized in liver microsomes by the CYP-450 3A*4* isoenzyme. The biological activity of etonogestrel metabolites is unknown.

Excretion – The elimination half-life of etonogestrel is approximately 25 hours. Excretion of etonogestrel and its metabolites, either as free steroid or as conjugates, is mainly in urine and to a lesser extent in feces. After removal of the etonogestrel implant, etonogestrel concentrations decreased below sensitivity of the assay by 1 week.

Special populations –

Hepatic function impairment: No formal studies were conducted to evaluate the effect of hepatic disease on the pharmacokinetics of the etonogestrel implant. However, etonogestrel is metabolized by the liver; therefore, use in patients with active liver disease is contraindicated.

Overweight women: The efficacy of the etonogestrel implant in overweight women has not been defined because women who weighed more than 130% of their ideal body weight were not studied. However, serum concentrations of etonogestrel are inversely related to body weight and decrease with time after insertion. It is therefore possible that, with time, the etonogestrel implant may be less effective in overweight women, especially in the presence of other factors that decrease etonogestrel concentrations, such as concomitant use of hepatic enzyme inducers.

ETONOGESTREL — IMPLANT

Contraindications

Do not use the etonogestrel implant in women who have known or suspected pregnancy, current or past history of thrombosis or thromboembolic disorders, hepatic tumors (benign or malignant) or active liver disease, undiagnosed abnormal genital bleeding, known or suspected carcinoma of the breast or personal history of breast cancer, or hypersensitivity to any of the components of the etonogestrel implant.

Warnings/Precautions

➤*Experience with etonogestrel implant:*

Complications of insertion and removal – Insert the etonogestrel implant subdermally so that it is palpable after insertion. Failure to insert the etonogestrel implant properly may go unnoticed unless the implant is palpated immediately after insertion. Deep insertions may lead to difficult or impossible removals. Failure to remove the etonogestrel implant may result in infertility, ectopic pregnancy, or inability to stop a drug-related adverse reaction. Undetected failure to insert the etonogestrel implant may lead to an unintended pregnancy.

Deep insertions may result in the need for a surgical procedure in an operating room in order to remove the etonogestrel implant. Any of the possible complications of surgery may occur. In postmarketing use, there have been cases of failure to localize and remove the implant, probably because of deep insertion. There has been 1 case of an intravascular insertion reported postmarketing which led to inability to remove the implant.

If infection develops at the insertion site, start suitable treatment. If infection persists, remove the etonogestrel implant. Incomplete insertions or infections may lead to expulsion.

Ectopic pregnancies – Be alert to the possibility of an ectopic pregnancy among patients using the etonogestrel implant who become pregnant or complain of lower abdominal pain. Although ectopic pregnancies should be uncommon among patients using the etonogestrel implant, a pregnancy that occurs in a patient using the etonogestrel implant may be more likely to be ectopic than a pregnancy occurring in a patient using no contraception.

Bleeding irregularities – Patients who use the etonogestrel implant are likely to have changes in their vaginal bleeding patterns that are often unpredictable. These may include changes in bleeding frequency or duration, or amenorrhea. Counsel patients regularly regarding unpredictable bleeding irregularities so that they know what to expect. Evaluate abnormal bleeding as needed to exclude pathologic conditions or pregnancy.

In clinical trials, bleeding changes were the single most common reason for stopping treatment with the etonogestrel implant (11.1%, or 105/942 patients using the etonogestrel implant). Most patients stopped treatment with the etonogestrel implant because of irregular bleeding (10.8%), but some stopped because of amenorrhea (0.3%). In these studies, patients using the etonogestrel implant had an average of 17.7 days of bleeding or spotting every 90 days (based on 3,315 intervals of 90 days recorded by 780 patients). The percentages of patients having 0, 1 to 7, 8 to 21, or more than 21 days of spotting or bleeding over a 90-day interval while using the etonogestrel implant are shown in the following table.

Etonogestrel Implant Patients With Spotting or Bleeding

Total days of spotting or bleeding	Treatment days 91 to 180 (n = 566)	Treatment days 270 to 360 (n = 554)	Treatment days 640 to 730 (n = 547)
0	19%	24%	17%
1 to 7	15%	13%	12%
8 to 21	30%	30%	37%
> 21	36%	33%	35%

Bleeding patterns observed with use of the etonogestrel implant for up to 2 years and the proportion of 90-day intervals with these bleeding patterns are summarized in the following table.

Bleeding Patterns Using the Etonogestrel Implant During the First 2 Years[a]

Bleeding patterns	Definitions	%[b]
Infrequent	< 3 bleeding and/or spotting episodes in 90 days (excluding amenorrhea)	33.6%
Amenorrhea	No bleeding and/or spotting in 90 days	22.2%
Prolonged	Any bleeding and/or spotting episode lasting more than 14 days in 90 days	17.7%
Frequent	> 5 bleeding and/or spotting episodes in 90 days	6.7%

[a] Based on 3,315 recording periods of 90 days' duration in 780 women, excluding the first 90 days after implant insertion.
[b] % = Percentage of 90-day intervals with this pattern.

Interaction with antiepileptic and other drugs – The etonogestrel implant is not recommended for women who chronically take drugs that are potent hepatic enzyme inducers because etonogestrel levels may be substantially reduced in these women.

Ovarian cysts – If follicular development occurs, atresia of the follicle is sometimes delayed, and the follicle may continue to grow beyond the size it would attain in a normal cycle. Generally, these enlarged follicles disappear spontaneously. Rarely, they can require surgery.

Thrombosis – There have been postmarketing reports of serious thromboembolic events, including cases of pulmonary emboli (some fatal) and strokes, in patients using the etonogestrel implant. Remove the etonogestrel implant in the event of a thrombosis. Consider removal of the etonogestrel implant in case of long-term immobilization due to surgery or illness. Inform women with a history of thromboembolic disorders of the possibility of recurrence.

➤*Experience with combination (progestin plus estrogen) oral contraceptives:*

Thromboembolic disorders and other vascular problems – Epidemiological investigations have associated the use of combination hormonal contraceptives with an increased incidence of venous thromboembolism, deep venous thrombosis, retinal vein thrombosis, and pulmonary embolism. The use of combination hormonal contraceptives is associated with increased risks of several serious conditions, including myocardial infarction, thromboembolism, and stroke, although the risk of serious morbidity or mortality is very small in healthy women without underlying risk factors. The risk increases significantly in the presence of other underlying risk factors such as hypertension, hyperlipidemias, obesity, and diabetes.

Cigarette smoking – Cigarette smoking increases the risk of serious cardiovascular adverse reactions from the use of combination hormonal contraceptives. This risk increases with age and with heavy smoking (15 or more cigarettes per day) and is quite marked in women older than 35 years of age who smoke. While this is believed to be an estrogen-related effect, it is not known whether a similar risk exists with progestin-only methods. However, advise patients not to smoke.

Elevated blood pressure – An increase in blood pressure has been reported in women taking combination hormonal contraceptives, and this increase is more likely with continued use and with older patients. Studies have shown that the incidence of hypertension increases with increasing concentrations of progestins.

Discourage women with a history of hypertension-related diseases or renal disease from using hormonal contraceptives. If women with hypertension elect to use hormonal contraceptives, monitor them closely. If sustained hypertension develops during the use of hormonal contraceptives, or if a significant increase in blood pressure does not respond adequately to antihypertensive therapy, discontinue hormonal contraceptives.

For most women, elevated blood pressure will return to normal after stopping hormonal contraceptives, and there is no difference in the occurrence of hypertension between those who have used and those who have never used hormonal contraceptives.

Carcinoma of the breast and reproductive organs – Women with breast cancer should not use hormonal contraceptives because breast cancer may be hormonally sensitive.

The risk of having breast cancer diagnosed may be slightly increased among current and recent users of combination oral contraceptives. However, after combination oral contraceptive discontinuation, this excess risk appears to decrease over time, and, within 10 years after cessation, the increased risk disappears. Some studies report an increased risk with duration of use while other studies do not, and no consistent relationships have been found with dose or type of steroid. Some studies have found a small increase in risk for women who first used combination oral contraceptives before 20 years of age. Most studies show a similar pattern of risk with combination oral contraceptive use regardless of a woman's reproductive history or her family breast cancer history.

In addition, breast cancers diagnosed in women who are using or have ever used oral contraceptives may be less clinically advanced than in those who have never used oral contraceptives.

Some studies suggest that oral contraceptive use has been associated with an increase in the risk of cervical intraepithelial neoplasia in some populations of women. However, there continues to be controversy about the extent to which such findings may be due to differences in sexual behavior and other factors.

Hepatic neoplasia – Benign hepatic adenomas have been associated with the use of combination oral contraceptives, although the incidence of benign tumors is rare in the United States. Indirect calculations have estimated the attributable risk to be in the range of 3.3 cases/100,000 for oral contraceptive users, a risk that increases after 4 or more years of use. Rupture of benign hepatic adenomas may cause death through intra-abdominal hemorrhage.

Gallbladder disease – Earlier studies have reported an increased lifetime relative risk of gallbladder surgery in users of combination oral contraceptives and estrogens. More recent studies, however, have shown that the relative risk of developing gallbladder disease among combination oral contraceptive users may be minimal. The recent findings of minimal risk may be related to the use of combination oral contraceptive formulations containing lower doses of estrogens and progestins.

➤*Carbohydrate and lipid metabolic effects:* The etonogestrel implant may induce mild insulin resistance and small changes in glucose concentrations of unknown clinical significance. Carefully observe women with diabetes or impaired glucose tolerance while using the etonogestrel implant.

Closely follow women who are being treated for hyperlipidemias if they elect to use hormonal contraceptives. Some progestins may elevate low-density lipoprotein levels and may render the control of hyperlipidemias more difficult.

➤*Contact lenses:* Contact lens wearers who develop visual changes or changes in lens tolerance should be assessed by an ophthalmologist.

ETONOGESTREL — IMPLANT

➤*Depression:* Carefully observe women with a history of depression. Consider removing the etonogestrel implant in patients who become significantly depressed.

➤*Fluid retention:* Steroid contraceptives may cause some degree of fluid retention. Prescribe steroid contraceptives with caution and only with careful monitoring in patients with conditions that might be aggravated by fluid retention. It is unknown if the etonogestrel implant causes fluid retention.

➤*Liver function:* If jaundice develops in any patient using the etonogestrel implant, remove the etonogestrel implant. The hormone in the etonogestrel implant may be poorly metabolized in patients with impaired liver function.

➤*Physical examination and follow-up:* Perform a complete medical evaluation, including history and physical examination and relevant laboratory tests, prior to etonogestrel implant insertion or reinsertion. It is good medical practice for patients using the etonogestrel implant to have regular physical examinations. In case of undiagnosed, persistent, or recurrent abnormal vaginal bleeding, conduct appropriate measures to rule out malignancy. Monitor women who have a family history of breast cancer or who have breast nodules with particular care.

➤*Return to ovulation:* In clinical trials, pregnancies occurred as early as during the first week after removal of the etonogestrel implant. Therefore, a patient should restart contraception immediately after removal of the etonogestrel implant if she still needs to prevent pregnancy.

➤*Sexually transmitted diseases:* This product does not protect against infection from HIV or other sexually transmitted diseases.

➤*Weight gain:* In clinical studies, mean weight gain in US etonogestrel implant users was 2.8 pounds after 1 year and 3.7 pounds after 2 years. How much of the weight gain was related to the etonogestrel implant is unknown. In studies, 2.3% of etonogestrel implant users reported weight gain as the reason for having the etonogestrel implant removed.

➤*Pregnancy: Category X.* The etonogestrel implant is not indicated for use during pregnancy.

Pregnancy must be excluded before inserting the etonogestrel implant.

Remove the etonogestrel implant if maintaining a pregnancy.

➤*Lactation:* Based on limited data, the etonogestrel implant may be used during lactation after the fourth postpartum week. Use of the etonogestrel implant before the fourth postpartum week has not been studied.

Small amounts of etonogestrel are excreted in breast milk. During the first months after etonogestrel implant insertion, when maternal blood levels of etonogestrel are highest, about 100 ng of etonogestrel may be ingested by the child per day based on an average daily milk ingestion of 658 mL. Based on daily milk ingestion of 150 mL/kg, the mean daily infant etonogestrel dose 1 month after insertion of the etonogestrel implant is about 2.2% of the weight-adjusted maternal daily dose, or about 0.2% of the estimated absolute maternal daily dose. The health of breast-fed infants whose mothers began using the etonogestrel implant during the fourth to eighth week postpartum (n = 38) was evaluated in a comparative study with infants of mothers using a nonhormonal IUD (n = 33). They were breast-fed for a mean duration of 14 months and followed up to 36 months of age. No significant effects and no differences between the groups were observed on the physical and psychomotor development of these infants. No differences between groups in the production or quality of breast milk were detected.

Discuss both hormonal and nonhormonal contraceptive options, as steroids may not be the initial choice for these patients.

➤*Children:* Safety and efficacy of the etonogestrel implant have been established in women of reproductive age. Safety and efficacy are expected to be the same for postpubertal adolescents. However, no clinical studies have been conducted in women younger than 18 years of age. Use of this product before menarche is not indicated.

➤*Elderly:* This product has not been studied in women older than 65 years of age and is not indicated in this population.

Drug Interactions

Etonogestrel Implant Drug Interactions

Precipitant Drug	Object drug[a]		Description
Anticonvulsants (eg, carbamazepine, oxcarbazepine, topiramate)	Etonogestrel	⬇	Anticonvulsants may increase hepatic metabolism of contraceptives, leading to a decrease in efficacy and possible unintended pregnancy.
Antifungals (eg, griseofulvin, ketoconazole, itraconazole)	Etonogestrel	⬇	Contraceptive efficacy may be reduced when hormonal contraceptives are coadministered with griseofulvin. Inhibitors of hepatic enzymes such as itraconazole and ketoconazole may increase plasma hormone levels.
Barbiturates (eg, butalbital, phenobarbital, secobarbital)	Etonogestrel	⬇	Barbituates induce progestin metabolism (CYP3A4) and increase sex hormone-binding globulin synthesis, reducing progestin concentrations.
Hydantoins (eg, fosphenytoin, phenytoin)	Etonogestrel	⬇	Hydantoins induce progestin metabolism (CYP3A4) and increase sex hormone-binding globulin synthesis, reducing progestin concentrations.
Protease inhibitors (eg, atazanavir, ritonavir)	Etonogestrel	⬇⬆	Significant changes (increase and decrease) in the mean AUC of progestin have been noted when hormonal contraceptives are coadministered with protease inhibitors.
Rifamycins (eg, rifampin, rifabutin)	Etonogestrel	⬇	Rifamycins may induce the metabolism of progestin (CYP3A4), leading to decreased efficacy of hormonal contraceptives.
St. John's wort	Etonogestrel	⬇	St. John's wort may induce hepatic enzymes and P-glycoprotein transporter and may reduce the efficacy of contraceptive steroids.
Etonogestrel	Lamotrigine	⬇	Hormonal contraceptives may increase lamotrigine metabolism, decreasing the therapeutic effect.
Etonogestrel	Selegiline	⬆	Hormonal contraceptives may inhibit the metabolism of selegiline, causing a loss of selective inhibition of monoamine oxidase type B and increasing the risk of adverse reactions.

[a] ⬆ = object drug increased; ⬇ = object drug decreased.

➤*Drug/Lab test interactions:* The following endocrine tests may be affected by etonogestrel implant use: SHGB concentrations may be decreased for the first 6 months after etonogestrel implant insertion followed by a gradual recovery; thyroxine concentrations may initially be slightly decreased followed by gradual recovery to baseline.

Adverse Reactions

In clinical trials including 942 subjects, bleeding irregularities were the most common adverse reactions causing discontinuation of the etonogestrel implant.

Etonogestrel Implant Adverse Reactions Leading to Discontinuation

Adverse reaction	All studies (N = 942)
CNS	
Depression[a]	1%
Emotional lability[b]	2.3%
Headache	1.6%
Dermatologic	
Acne	1.3%
GU	
Bleeding irregularities[c]	11%
Miscellaneous	
Weight increase	2.3%

[a] Among US subjects, 2.4% experienced depression that led to discontinuation.
[b] Among US subjects, 6.1% experienced emotional lability that lead to discontinuation.
[c] Includes frequent, heavy, prolonged, spotting, and other patterns of irregularity.

Adverse reactions that were reported by more than 5% of subjects in clinical trials appear in the following table.

Etonogestrel Implant Adverse Reactions (> 5%)[a]

Adverse reaction	All studies (N = 942)
CNS	
Depression	5.5%
Dizziness	7.2%
Emotional lability	6.5%
Headache	24.9%
Nervousness	5.6%
Dermatologic	
Acne	13.5%
GI	
Abdominal pain	10.9%
Nausea	6.4%
GU	
Breast pain	12.8%
Dysmenorrhea	7.2%
Leukorrhea	9.6%
Vaginitis	14.5%
Musculoskeletal	
Back pain	6.8%
Respiratory	
Pharyngitis	10.5%

ETONOGESTREL — IMPLANT

Etonogestrel Implant Adverse Reactions (> 5%)[a]	
Adverse reaction	All studies (N = 942)
Sinusitis	5.6%
Upper respiratory tract infection	12.6%
Miscellaneous	
Influenza-like symptoms	7.6%
Insertion site pain	5.2%
Pain	5.6%
Weight increase	13.7%

[a] List may include adverse reactions associated with, but unrelated to, etonogestrel implant use.

➤*Other adverse reactions:* Other less common adverse reactions reported in less than 5% of subjects in clinical trials include:

Cardiovascular – Hot flushes, hypertension, vein varicose.

CNS – Anxiety, asthenia, crying abnormal, fatigue, hypesthesia, insomnia, libido decreased, migraine, somnolence.

Dermatologic – Alopecia, pruritus, rash.

GI – Anorexia, appetite increased, constipation, diarrhea, dyspepsia, flatulence, gastritis, vomiting.

GU – Breast discharge, breast enlargement, breast fibroadenosis, cervical smear test positive, dysuria, lactation nonpuerperal, ovarian cyst, pelvic cramping, premenstrual tension, pruritus genital, sexual function abnormal, vaginal discomfort.

Musculoskeletal – Arthralgia, myalgia, skeletal pain.

Respiratory – Asthma, coughing, otitis media, rhinitis.

Miscellaneous – Allergic reaction, edema, edema generalized, fever, injection site reaction, vision abnormal, weight decrease.

Hypertrichosis has also been reported with use of progestin-only contraceptives.

Implant site complications were reported by 3.6% of subjects during any of the assessments in clinical trials. Pain was the most frequent implant site complication reported during and/or after insertion, occurring in 2.9% of subjects. Additionally, hematoma, redness, and swelling were reported by 0.1%, 0.3%, and 0.3% of patients, respectively.

Overdosage

Insertion of multiple rods has been reported. Overdosage may result if more than 1 etonogestrel implant rod is in place. In case of suspected overdose, remove the implant. It is important to remove the etonogestrel implant rod or other contraceptive implant(s) before inserting a new implant rod.

Patient Information

Counsel patients that the etonogestrel implant does not protect against infection from HIV or other sexually transmitted diseases.

The most common side effect of the etonogestrel implant is a change in menstrual periods. Counsel patients to expect their menstrual period to be irregular and unpredictable throughout the time they are using the etonogestrel implant. Warn patients that they may have more bleeding, less bleeding, or no bleeding, that the time between periods may vary, and in between periods they may have spotting.

Tell patients that they must have the etonogestrel implant removed after 3 years and that, if they want to continue using the etonogestrel implant, a health care provider can put a new etonogestrel implant under their skin after taking out the old one.

Patients should not use the etonogestrel implant if they:

- are pregnant or think they may be pregnant
- have, or have had serious blood clots, such as blood clots in their legs (deep venous thrombosis), lungs (pulmonary embolism), eyes (retinal thrombosis), heart (heart attack), or head (stroke)
- have unexplained vaginal bleeding
- have liver disease
- have breast cancer, now or in the past
- are allergic to anything in the etonogestrel implant.

Advise patients to tell their health care provider if they have or have ever had any of the conditions previously listed. Their health care provider can suggest another method of birth control In addition, advise patients to talk to their health care provider about using the etonogestrel implant if they have or had:

- diabetes
- high cholesterol or triglycerides
- headaches
- seizures or epilepsy
- gallbladder or kidney disease
- depression
- high blood pressure
- an allergic reaction to anesthetics or antiseptics. These medicines will be used when the etonogestrel implant is inserted into the arm.

Counsel patients that the timing of insertion is important. Depending on a patient's history, she may need to:

- have a pregnancy test before insertion;
- schedule the insertion at a specific time of your cycle (for example, within the first days of her regular menstrual bleeding); or
- use a backup method of birth control, such as condoms, for 7 days after etonogestrel implant insertion

Both the patient and the health care provider should check that the etonogestrel implant is in the arm by feeling the etonogestrel implant.

If the patient and the health care provider cannot feel the etonogestrel implant, advise the patient to use a nonhormonal birth control method such as condoms until the health care provider confirms that the etonogestrel implant is in place. The patient may need special tests to check that the etonogestrel implant is in place or to help find the etonogestrel implant when it is time to take it out.

Tell patients to review and sign a consent form prior to inserting the etonogestrel implant. Give them a user card to keep at home with their health records. Fill out the insertion and removal dates. Instruct patients to keep track of the removal date and schedule an appointment for removal with their health care provider on or before the removal date.

The insertion site is covered with 2 bandages. Instruct patients to leave the top bandage on for 24 hours and to keep the smaller bandage dry, clean, and in place for 3 to 5 days.

Advise patients to have checkups as advised by their health care provider.

The risk of thrombosis is increased in women who smoke. Advise patients who smoke to quit.

Advise patients to tell their health care provider at least 4 weeks before if they are going to have surgery or will need to be on bed rest. Inform patients that there is an increased risk of getting thrombosis during surgery or bed rest.

Inform patients that a few women who use birth control that contains hormones may get high blood pressure, gallbladder problems, or rare cancerous or noncancerous liver tumors.

Advise patients to call their health care provider right away if they get any of the following symptoms. They may be signs of a serious problem.

- sharp chest pain, coughing blood, or sudden shortness of breath (possible clot in the lung)
- persistent pain in the calf (back of lower leg) (possible clot in the leg)
- crushing chest pain or heaviness in the chest (possible heart attack)
- sudden severe headache or vomiting, dizziness or fainting, problems with vision or speech, weakness, or numbness in an arm or leg (possible stroke)
- sudden partial or complete blindness (possible clot in the eye)
- yellowing of the skin or whites of the eyes (jaundice), especially with fever, tiredness, loss of appetite, dark colored urine, or light colored bowel movements (possible liver problems)
- severe pain, swelling, or tenderness in the abdomen (possibly indicating an ectopic pregnancy, a ruptured or twisted ovarian follicle, or gallbladder or liver problems)
- breast lumps
- difficulty in sleeping, weakness, lack of energy, tiredness, or sadness (possible severe depression)
- heavy vaginal bleeding

LEVONORGESTREL

Rx	**Mirena** (Bayer HealthCare)	**Intrauterine device:** 52 mg[a]	1 T-shaped device covered by a silicone membrane with inserter.

[a] Releases ≈ 20 mcg of levonorgestrel per day

LEVONORGESTREL-RELEASING — INTRAUTERINE DEVICE

Indications

➤*Contraception:* For intrauterine contraception for up to 5 years.

➤*Heavy menstrual bleeding:* For the treatment of heavy menstrual bleeding in women who choose to use intrauterine contraception as their method of contraception.

➤*General information:* The intrauterine system is recommended for women who have had at least 1 child. The system should be replaced after 5 years if continued use is desired.

Administration and Dosage

➤*General dosing considerations:* If the intrauterine system is removed midcycle and the patient has had intercourse within the preceding week, she is at risk of pregnancy unless a new system is inserted immediately following removal.

Patients should be reexamined and evaluated 4 to 12 weeks after insertion and once a year thereafter, or more frequently if clinically indicated.

LEVONORGESTREL-RELEASING — INTRAUTERINE DEVICE

➤*Adults:* See manufacturer's prescribing information for insertion and removal instructions.

Contraception – With the provided inserter, insert system into the uterine cavity within 7 days of the onset of menstruation or immediately after first trimester abortion by carefully following the insertion instructions. The system should not remain in the uterus after 5 years. It can be replaced by a new intrauterine system at any time during the menstrual cycle.

Heavy menstrual bleeding – See Contraception for dosing.

➤*Children:* Use of the intrauterine system before menarche is not indicated.

➤*Discontinuation of therapy:* If a patient with regular cycles wants to start a different birth control method, remove the intrauterine system during the first 7 days of the menstrual cycle and start the new method.

If a patient with irregular cycles or amenorrhea wants to start a different birth control method, or if the health care provider removes the intrauterine system after the seventh day of the menstrual cycle, start the new method at least 7 days before removal.

➤*Storage/Stability:* Store at 25°C (77°F); excursions are permitted between 15° and 30°C (59° and 86°F). Insert before the end of the month shown on the label.

Actions

➤*Pharmacology:* The local mechanism by which continuously released levonorgestrel enhances contraceptive effectiveness of the intrauterine system has not been conclusively demonstrated. Studies of the intrauterine system prototypes have suggested several mechanisms that prevent pregnancy: thickening of cervical mucus preventing passage of sperm into the uterus, inhibition of sperm capacitation or survival, and alteration of the endometrium.

➤*Pharmacokinetics:*

Absorption – Low doses of levonorgestrel are administered into the uterine cavity with the intrauterine delivery system. Initially, levonorgestrel is released at a rate of approximately 20 mcg/day. This rate decreases progressively to half that value after 5 years. A stable serum concentration, without peaks and troughs, of levonorgestrel of 150 to 200 pg/mL occurs after the first few weeks following insertion of the intrauterine system. Levonorgestrel concentrations after long-term use of 12, 24, and 60 months were 180 ± 66 pg/mL, 192 ± 140 pg/mL, and 159 ± 59 pg/mL, respectively.

Distribution – The apparent volume of distribution of levonorgestrel is reported to be approximately 1.8 L/kg. It is approximately 97.5% to 99% protein-bound, principally to sex hormone binding globulin, and to a lesser extent, serum albumin.

Metabolism – Following absorption, levonorgestrel is conjugated at the 17-beta-OH position to form sulfate conjugates and to a lesser extent, glucuronide conjugates in serum. Significant amounts of conjugated and unconjugated 3-alpha, 5-beta-tetrahydrolevonorgestrel are also present in serum, along with much smaller amounts of 3-alpha, 5-alpha-tetrahydrolevonorgestrel, and 16-beta-hydroxylevonorgestrel. Levonorgestrel and its phase 1 metabolites are excreted primarily as glucuronide conjugates. Metabolic clearance rates may differ among individuals by several-fold, and this may partially account for wide individual variations in levonorgestrel concentrations seen in individuals using levonorgestrel-containing contraceptive products.

Excretion – Approximately 45% of levonorgestrel and its metabolites are excreted in the urine, and approximately 32% are excreted in feces, mostly as glucuronide conjugates. The elimination half-life of levonorgestrel after daily oral doses is approximately 17 hours.

Contraindications

Pregnancy or suspicion of pregnancy; congenital or acquired uterine anomaly, including fibroids if they distort the uterine cavity; acute pelvic inflammatory disease (PID) or a history of PID, unless there has been a subsequent intrauterine pregnancy; postpartum endometritis or infected abortion in the past 3 months; known or suspected uterine or cervical neoplasia, or unresolved, abnormal Papanicolaou test; genital bleeding of unknown etiology; untreated acute cervicitis or vaginitis, including bacterial vaginosis or other lower genital tract infections until infection is controlled; acute liver disease or liver tumor (benign or malignant); conditions associated with increased susceptibility to pelvic infections; a previously inserted intrauterine device that has not been removed; hypersensitivity to any component of this product; known or suspected carcinoma of the breast.

Warnings/Precautions

➤*Ectopic pregnancy:* Evaluate women who become pregnant while using the intrauterine system for ectopic pregnancy. Up to half of pregnancies that occur with the intrauterine system in place are ectopic. The incidence of ectopic pregnancy in clinical trials that excluded women with risk factors for ectopic pregnancy was approximately 0.1% per year.

Tell women who choose the intrauterine system about the risks of ectopic pregnancy, including the loss of fertility. Teach them to recognize and report to their health care provider promptly any symptoms of ectopic pregnancy. Women with a history of ectopic pregnancy, tubal surgery, or pelvic infection carry a higher risk of ectopic pregnancy.

➤*Intrauterine pregnancy:* If pregnancy should occur with the intrauterine system in place, the intrauterine system should be removed. Removal or manipulation of the intrauterine system may result in pregnancy loss. In the event of an intrauterine pregnancy with the intrauterine system, consider the following:

Septic abortion – In patients becoming pregnant with an intrauterine device in place, septic abortion, with septicemia, septic shock, and death, may occur.

Continuation of pregnancy – If a woman becomes pregnant with a intrauterine system in place and if the intrauterine system cannot be removed or the woman chooses not to have it removed, warn the patient that failure to remove the intrauterine system increases the risk of miscarriage, sepsis, premature labor, and premature delivery. Follow the patient closely and advise her to immediately report any flu-like symptoms, fever, chills, cramping, pain, bleeding, vaginal discharge, or leakage of fluid.

Long-term effects and congenital anomalies: When pregnancy continues with the intrauterine system in place, long-term effects on the offspring are unknown. As of September 2006, 390 live births out of an estimated 9.9 million levonorgestrel-releasing intrauterine system users had been reported. Congenital anomalies in live births have occurred infrequently. No clear trend towards specific anomalies has been observed. Because of the intrauterine administration of levonorgestrel and local exposure of the fetus to the hormone, the possibility of teratogenicity following exposure to the intrauterine system cannot be excluded. Some observational data support a small increased risk of masculinization of the external genitalia of the female fetus following exposure to progestins at doses greater than those currently used for oral contraception. Whether these data apply to the intrauterine system is unknown.

➤*Sepsis:* As of September 2006, 9 cases of group A streptococcal (GAS) sepsis out of an estimated 9.9 million levonorgestrel-releasing intrauterine system users had been reported. In some cases, severe pain occurred within hours of insertion followed by sepsis within days. Because death from GAS sepsis is more likely if treatment is delayed, it is important to be aware of these rare but serious infections. Aseptic technique during insertion of the intrauterine system is essential. GAS sepsis may also occur postpartum, after surgery, and from wounds.

➤*Pelvic inflammatory disease:* The intrauterine system is contraindicated in the presence of known or suspected PID or in women with a history of PID, unless there has been a subsequent intrauterine pregnancy. Use of intrauterine devices has been associated with an increased risk of PID. The highest risk of PID occurs shortly after insertion (usually within the first 20 days thereafter). A decision to use the intrauterine system must include consideration of the risks of PID.

PID is often associated with sexually transmitted diseases (STDs), and the intrauterine system does not protect against STDs. The risk of PID is greater for women who have multiple sexual partners, and also for women whose sexual partner(s) have multiple sexual partners. Women who have ever had PID are at increased risk for a recurrence or reinfection.

All women who choose the intrauterine system must be informed prior to insertion about the possibility of PID, and that PID can cause tubal damage leading to ectopic pregnancy or infertility, or in infrequent cases can necessitate hysterectomy, or can cause death. Patients must be taught to recognize and promptly report any symptoms of PID to their health care provider. These symptoms include development of menstrual disorders (prolonged or heavy bleeding), unusual vaginal discharge, abdominal or pelvic pain or tenderness, dyspareunia, chills, and fever.

PID may be asymptomatic, but can still result in tubal damage and its sequelae.

➤*Irregular bleeding and amenorrhea:* The intrauterine system can alter the bleeding pattern and result in spotting, irregular bleeding, heavy bleeding, oligomenorrhea, and amenorrhea. During the first 3 to 6 months of intrauterine system use, the number of bleeding and spotting days may be increased, and bleeding patterns may be irregular. Thereafter, the number of bleeding and spotting days usually decreases, but bleeding may remain irregular. If bleeding irregularities develop during prolonged treatment, take appropriate diagnostic measures to rule out endometrial pathology.

Amenorrhea develops in approximately 20% of intrauterine system users by 1 year. Consider the possibility of pregnancy if menstruation does not occur within 6 weeks of the onset of previous menstruation. Once pregnancy has been excluded, repeated pregnancy tests are not necessary in amenorrheic women unless indicated by other signs of pregnancy or by pelvic pain.

In most women with heavy menstrual bleeding, the number of bleeding and spotting days may also increase during the initial months of therapy but usually decrease with continued use; the volume of blood loss per cycle progressively becomes reduced.

➤*Embedment:* Embedment of the intrauterine system in the myometrium may occur. Embedment may decrease contraceptive effectiveness and result in pregnancy. Remove an embedded intrauterine system. Embedment can result in difficult removal and, in some cases, surgical removal may be necessary.

➤*Perforation:* Perforation or penetration of the uterine wall or cervix may occur during insertion, although the perforation may not be detected until later. If perforation occurs, pregnancy may result. The intrauterine system must be located and removed; surgery may be required. Delayed detection of perforation may result in migration outside the uterine cavity, adhesions, peritonitis, intestinal perforations, intestinal obstruction, abscesses, and erosion of adjacent viscera.

The risk of perforation may be increased in breast-feeding women, women with fixed retroverted uteri, and during the postpartum period. To decrease the risk of perforation postpartum, delay intrauterine system insertion a minimum of 6 weeks after delivery or until uterine involution is compete. If involution is substantially delayed, consider waiting until 12 weeks postpartum. Inserting the intrauterine system immediately after first trimester

LEVONORGESTREL-RELEASING — INTRAUTERINE DEVICE

abortion is not known to increase the risk of perforation, but delay insertion after second trimester abortion until uterine involution is complete.

➤*Expulsion:* Partial or complete expulsion of the intrauterine system may occur. Symptoms of the partial or complete expulsion of any intrauterine device may include bleeding or pain. However, the system can be expelled from the uterine cavity without the woman noticing it, resulting in the loss of contraceptive protection. Partial expulsion may decrease the effectiveness of the intrauterine system. As menstrual flow typically decreases after the first 3 to 6 months of intrauterine system use, an increase of menstrual flow may be indicative of an expulsion. If expulsion has occurred, the intrauterine system may be replaced within 7 days of a menstrual period after pregnancy has been ruled out.

➤*Ovarian cysts:* Because the contraceptive effect of the intrauterine system is mainly due to its local effect, ovulatory cycles with follicular rupture usually occur in women of fertile age using the intrauterine system. Sometimes atresia of the follicle is delayed, and the follicle may continue to grow. Enlarged follicles have been diagnosed in approximately 12% of the subjects using the intrauterine system. Most of these follicles are asymptomatic, although some may be accompanied by pelvic pain or dyspareunia. In most cases, the enlarged follicles disappear spontaneously during 2 to 3 months of observation. Evaluate persistent enlarged follicles. Surgical intervention is not usually required.

➤*Breast cancer:* Women who currently have or have had breast cancer, or have a suspicion of breast cancer, should not use hormonal contraception because breast cancer is a hormone-sensitive tumor.

Spontaneous reports of breast cancer have been received during postmarketing experience with the intrauterine system.

➤*Patient evaluation:* Obtain a complete medical and social history, including that of the partner, to determine conditions that might influence the selection of an intrauterine device for contraception. Give special attention to ascertaining whether the woman is at increased risk of infection (eg, leukemia, AIDS, intravenous drug use), or has a history of PID unless there has been a subsequent intrauterine pregnancy. The intrauterine system is contraindicated in these women.

A physical examination should include a pelvic examination, a Papanicolaou test, examination of the breasts, and appropriate tests for any other forms of genital or other STDs, such as gonorrhea and chlamydia laboratory evaluations, if indicated. Postpone the use of the intrauterine system in patients with vaginitis or cervicitis until proper treatment has eradicated the infection and until it has been shown that the cervicitis is not due to gonorrhea or chlamydia.

Irregular bleeding may mask symptoms and signs of endometrial polyps or cancer. Because irregular bleeding/spotting is common during the first months of intrauterine system use, exclude endometrial pathology prior to the insertion of the intrauterine system in women with persistent or uncharacteristic bleeding. If unexplained bleeding irregularities develop during the prolonged use of the intrauterine system, take appropriate diagnostic measures.

The health care provider should determine that the patient is not pregnant. The possibility of insertion of an intrauterine system in the presence of an existing undetermined pregnancy is reduced if insertion is performed within 7 days of the onset of a menstrual period. The intrauterine system can be replaced by a new system at any time in the cycle. The intrauterine system can be inserted immediately after first trimester abortion.

➤*Postpartum:* Do not insert the intrauterine system until 6 weeks postpartum or until involution of the uterus is complete to reduce the incidence of perforation and expulsion. If involution is substantially delayed, consider waiting until 12 weeks postpartum.

➤*Valvular/Congenital heart disease:* Patients with certain types of valvular or congenital heart disease and surgically constructed systemic-pulmonary shunts are at increased risk of infective endocarditis. Use of a intrauterine system in these patients may represent a potential source of septic emboli. Treat patients with known congenital heart disease who may be at increased risk with appropriate antibiotics at the time of insertion and removal.

➤*Special risk patients:* Monitor patients requiring long-term corticosteroid therapy or insulin for diabetes with special care for infection.

Use the intrauterine system with caution in patients who have coagulopathy or are receiving anticoagulants; in patients with marked increase of blood pressure; in patients with severe arterial disease, such as stroke or myocardial infarction; and in patients with migraine, focal migraine with asymmetrical visual loss, or other symptoms indicating transient cerebral ischemia, or an exceptionally severe headache.

➤*Neurovascular episodes:* If the patient develops decreased pulse, perspiration, or pallor, have her remain supine until these signs resolve. Insertion may be associated with some pain and/or bleeding. Syncope, bradycardia, or other neurovascular episodes may occur during insertion of the intrauterine system, especially in patients with a predisposition to these conditions or cervical stenosis.

➤*Pregnancy during use:* In the event a pregnancy is confirmed during intrauterine system use, take the following steps: determine whether pregnancy is ectopic and take appropriate measures if it is; inform the patient of the risks of leaving the intrauterine system in place or removing it during pregnancy, and of the lack of data on long-term effects on the offspring of women who have had the system in place during conception or gestation; if possible, remove the intrauterine system after the patient has been warned of the risks of removal. If removal is difficult, counsel and offer the patient pregnancy termination; if the intrauterine system is left in place, closely follow the patient's course.

➤*Sexually transmitted diseases:* If the patient's relationship ceases to be mutually monogamous, or if her partner becomes HIV positive or acquires an STD, instruct the patient to report this change to her health care provider immediately. Strongly recommend the use of a barrier method as a partial protection against acquiring STDs. Consider removal of the intrauterine system.

➤*Removal of the intrauterine system:* Remove the intrauterine system for the following medical reasons: new-onset menorrhagia and/or metrorrhagia producing anemia, STDs, pelvic infection, endometritis, symptomatic genital actinomycosis, intractable pelvic pain, severe dyspareunia, pregnancy, endometrial or cervical malignancy, and/or uterine or cervical perforation.

Also consider the removal of the intrauterine system if any of the following conditions arise for the first time: migraine or focal migraine with asymmetrical visual loss or other symptoms indicating transient cerebral ischemia, exceptionally severe headache, jaundice, marked increase of blood pressure, and/or severe arterial disease, such as stroke or myocardial infarction.

Removal may be associated with pain and/or bleeding or neurovascular episodes.

➤*Glucose tolerance:* Levonorgestrel may affect glucose tolerance; therefore, monitor the blood glucose concentration in diabetic users of the intrauterine system.

➤*Pregnancy: Category X.* See Contraindications for more information.

➤*Lactation:* Numerous studies indicate that levonorgestrel does not adversely affect the quality of breast milk, supply of breast milk, or duration of lactation. Small amounts of progestins pass into the breast milk of breastfeeding mothers, resulting in detectable steroid levels in infant plasma.

➤*Children:* Use of the intrauterine system before menarche is not indicated.

➤*Monitoring:* Reexamine and evaluate patients 4 to 12 weeks after insertion and once a year thereafter, or more frequently if clinically indicated. Promptly examine users with complaints of pain, odorous discharge, unexplained bleeding, fever, genital lesions, or sores. Consider the possibility of ectopic pregnancy in the case of lower abdominal pain, especially in association with missed periods or if an amenorrheic woman starts bleeding. Monitor blood glucose concentration in diabetic users of the intrauterine system.

Monitor patients requiring long-term corticosteroid therapy or insulin for diabetes with special care for infection.

Drug Interactions

Levonorgestrel Intrauterine System Drug Interactions

Precipitant drug	Object drug[a]		Description
Anticonvulsants (eg, barbiturates [eg, phenobarbital], carbamazepine, felbamate, hydantoins [eg, phenytoin], oxcarbazepine, rufinamide, topiramate)	Levonorgestrel	⬇	Plasma concentrations and pharmacologic effects of levonorgestrel may be decreased. Monitor the clinical response. Instruct patients to use alternative or additional nonhormonal methods of contraception during coadministration of these agents. Plasma concentrations and pharmacologic effects of levonorgestrel may be decreased. An alternative or nonhormonal method of birth control is recommended when topiramate is used for epilepsy at dosages greater than 200 mg/day.
Aprepitant	Levonorgestrel	⬇	Plasma concentrations and pharmacologic effects of levonorgestrel may be decreased. Instruct patients to use alternative or additional nonhormonal methods of contraception during and for 1 month following the last aprepitant dose.
Azole antifungal agents (eg, fluconazole, ketoconazole)	Levonorgestrel	⬇	Hormonal contraceptive failure has been reported. Monitor the clinical response. Instruct patients to use alternative or additional nonhormonal methods of contraception.

LEVONORGESTREL-RELEASING — INTRAUTERINE DEVICE

Levonorgestrel Intrauterine System Drug Interactions			
Precipitant drug	Object drug[a]		Description
Bosentan	Levonorgestrel	⬇	Plasma concentrations and pharmacologic effects of levonorgestrel may be decreased. Monitor the clinical response. Instruct patients to use alternative or additional nonhormonal methods of contraception during coadministration of these agents.
Griseofulvin	Levonorgestrel	⬇	Plasma concentrations and pharmacologic effects of levonorgestrel may be decreased. Monitor the clinical response. Instruct patients to use alternative or additional nonhormonal methods of contraception during coadministration of these agents.
Modafinil	Levonorgestrel	⬇	Plasma concentrations and pharmacologic effects of levonorgestrel may be decreased. Instruct patients to use alternative or additional nonhormonal methods of contraception during and for 1 month following the last modafinil dose.
Nonnucleoside reverse transcriptase inhibitors (eg, efavirenz, nevirapine)	Levonorgestrel	⬇	Levonorgestrel concentrations may be decreased. Monitor the clinical response. Instruct patients to use alternative or additional nonhormonal methods of contraception during coadministration of these agents.
Protease inhibitors (eg, atazanavir, ritonavir)	Levonorgestrel	⬆⬇	Levonorgestrel concentrations may be increased (eg, atazanavir) or decreased (eg, nelfinavir). Monitor the clinical response. Instruct patients to use alternative or additional nonhormonal methods of contraception during coadministration of these agents.
Rifamycins (eg, rifampin)	Levonorgestrel	⬇	Plasma concentrations and pharmacologic effects of levonorgestrel may be decreased. Avoid concurrent use. If coadministration cannot be avoided, instruct patients to use alternative or additional nonhormonal methods of contraception.
St. John's wort	Levonorgestrel	⬇	Plasma concentrations and pharmacologic effects of levonorgestrel may be decreased. Coadministration is not recommended. If coadministration cannot be avoided, instruct patients to use alternative or additional nonhormonal methods of contraception.
Levonorgestrel	Cyclosporine	⬆	Cyclosporine concentrations may be elevated, increasing the risk of toxicity. Monitor cyclosporine concentrations as well as hepatic and renal function. Adjust the cyclosporine dose as needed.
Levonorgestrel	Lamotrigine	⬇	Lamotrigine concentrations may be reduced, decreasing the efficacy. Monitor the clinical response and adjust the lamotrigine dose as needed.
Levonorgestrel	Selegiline	⬆	Selegiline concentrations may be elevated, increasing the risk of adverse reactions. Monitor the clinical response and adjust the selegiline dose as needed.

[a] ⬆ = object drug increased; ⬇ = object drug decreased; ⬆⬇ = object drug both increased and decreased

Adverse Reactions

➤*CNS:* Headache/migraine (7.7%); depressed/altered mood (6.4); decreased libido, nervousness (less than 5%).

➤*Dermatologic:* Acne (7.2%); alopecia, hirsutism, skin disorders including eczema, pruritus, rash, and urticaria (less than 5%).

➤*GI:* Abdominal pain/pelvic pain (12.8%); abdominal distension, nausea, weight increased (less than 5%).

➤*GU:* Uterine/vaginal bleeding/alterations (51.9%); amenorrhea (23.9%); intermenstrual bleeding and spotting (23.4%); ovarian cysts (12%); menorrhagia (6.3%); breast pain/tenderness, vaginal discharge, intrauterine device expulsion (4.9%); cervicitis/Papanicolaou test normal/class II, dysmenorrhea, vulvovaginitis, dyspareunia (less than 5%).

➤*Miscellaneous:* Anemia, back pain, edema, hypertension (less than 5%).

➤*Postmarketing:*

Miscellaneous – Device breakage and angioedema.

Patient Information

Advise patients that the intrauterine system is used to prevent pregnancy. It does not protect against HIV infection (AIDS) and other STDs.

Advise patients that the intrauterine system is a hormone-releasing system placed in the uterus to prevent pregnancy for up to 5 years.

Advise patients that they must have the intrauterine system removed after 5 years, but their health care provider can insert a new system then if they choose to continue using it.

Advise patients that they may become pregnant as soon as the intrauterine system is removed. Approximately 80% of women who want to become pregnant will become pregnant some time in the first year after the intrauterine system is removed.

Advise patients to call their health care provider right away if they think they are pregnant. If they get pregnant while using the intrauterine system, they may have an ectopic pregnancy. This means that the pregnancy is not in the uterus. Unusual vaginal bleeding or abdominal pain may be a sign of ectopic pregnancy.

Inform patients that the intrauterine system may come out by itself. This is called expulsion. The patient may become pregnant if the system comes out. The patient should use a backup birth control method, such as condoms, and call their health care provider if they notice that the system has come out.

Inform patients to call their health care provider if they think they are pregnant; have pelvic pain or pain during sex; have unusual vaginal discharge or genital sores; have unexplained fever; might have been exposed to STDs; cannot feel the system's threads; develop very severe or migraine headaches; have yellowing of the skin or whites of the eyes (these may be signs of liver problems); have a stroke or heart attack; have severe or prolonged vaginal bleeding; miss a menstrual period; or if their partner becomes HIV positive.

Prior to insertion, give the patient the patient information booklet. Give her the opportunity to read the information and discuss fully any questions she may have concerning the intrauterine system, as well as other methods of contraception and therapies for heavy menstrual bleeding. Also, inform the patient that the prescribing information is available to her upon request.

Inform the patient that irregular or prolonged bleeding and spotting and/or cramps may occur during the first few weeks after insertion. If her symptoms continue or are severe, she should report them to her health care provider.

Instruct the patient on how to check after her menstrual period to make certain that the threads still protrude from the cervix and caution her not to pull on the threads and displace the intrauterine system. Inform her that there is no contraceptive protection if the intrauterine system is displaced or expelled.

Contraceptive Hormones

MEDROXYPROGESTERONE CONTRACEPTIVE — INJECTION

Rx	**depo-subQ provera 104** (Pfizer)	**Injection:** 104 mg (160 mg/mL)	In 0.65 mL prefilled single-use syringes.[a]
Rx	**Medroxyprogesterone Acetate** (Various, eg, Greenstone, Sicor)	**Injection:** 150 mg/mL	In 1 mL vials.
Rx	**Depo-Provera** (Pharmacia Corp)		In 1 mL vials.[b]
Rx	**Depo-Provera** (Pharmacia Corp)	**Injection:** 400 mg/mL	In 2.5 and 10 mL vials and 1 mL *U-ject.*[c]

[a] With methylparaben 1.04 mg, propylparaben 0.098 mg, sodium chloride 5.2 mg, polyethylene glycol 18.688 mg, polysorbate 80 1.95 mg, monobasic sodium phosphate 0.451, dibasic sodium phosphate 0.382 mg, methionine 0.975 mg, povidone 3.25 mg, and possibly sodium hydroxide and/or hydrochloric acid.

[b] With 28.9 mg PEG 3350, 2.41 mg polysorbate 80, 8.68 mg sodium chloride, 1.37 mg methylparaben and 0.15 mg propylparaben.

[c] With polyethylene glycol 3350, sodium sulfate anhydrous, myristyl-gamma-picolinium Cl.

MEDROXYPROGESTERONE ACETATE — INJECTION

WARNING

Contraceptive injection – Patients should be counseled that this product does not protect against HIV infection (AIDS) or other sexually transmitted diseases.

Indications

➤*Endometrial/Renal carcinoma (400 mg/mL):* Adjunctive therapy and palliative treatment of inoperable, recurrent, and metastatic endometrial or renal carcinoma.

➤*Contraception (104 mg subcutaneous and 150 mg/mL IM):* Medroxyprogesterone acetate contraceptive injection is indicated only for the prevention of pregnancy. To ensure that medroxyprogesterone acetate contraceptive injection is not administered inadvertently to a pregnant woman, the first injection must be given only during the first 5 days of a normal menstrual period; only within the first 5 days postpartum if not breastfeeding, and if exclusively breast-feeding; only at the sixth postpartum week. The efficacy of medroxyprogesterone acetate contraceptive injection depends on adherence to the recommended dosage schedule. It is a long-term injectable contraceptive in women when administered at 3-month (13-week) intervals. Dosage does not need to be adjusted for body weight.

Administration and Dosage

➤*General dosing considerations:* The efficacy of medroxyprogesterone acetate as a contraceptive injection depends on adherence to the dosage schedule of administration.

➤*Adults:*

Contraception –

Usual dosage:

• *Intramuscular (IM) injection* – 150 mg every 3 months (13 weeks) administered by deep, IM injection in the gluteal or deltoid muscle.

To ensure the patient is not pregnant at the time of the first injection, the first injection must be given only during the first 5 days of a normal menstrual period; only within the first 5 days postpartum if not breastfeeding; and, if exclusively breast-feeding, only at the sixth postpartum week. If the time interval between injections is greater than 13 weeks, the health care provider should determine that the patient is not pregnant before administering the drug.

• *Subcutaneous injection* – 104 mg every 3 months (12 to 14 weeks) administered subcutaneously into the anterior thigh or abdomen.

Conversion: When switching from other contraceptive methods, give medroxyprogesterone in a manner than ensures continuous contraceptive coverage. For example, patients switching from combined (estrogen plus progestin) contraceptives should have their first injection within 7 days after the last day of using that method (7 days after taking the last active pill, removing the patch or ring). Similarly, contraceptive coverage will be maintained in switching from IM (150 mg) to subcutaneous (104 mg) provided the next injection is given within the prescribed dosing period for the IM (150 mg).

Endometrial carcinoma – Medroxyprogesterone acetate is not recommended as primary therapy, but as adjunctive and palliative treatment in advanced inoperable cases, including those with recurrent or metastatic disease.

Initial dosage: 400 to 1,000 mg IM weekly.

Maintenance dosage: If improvement is noted within a few weeks or months and the disease appears stabilized, it may be possible to maintain improvement with as little as 400 mg monthly.

Renal carcinoma – See Endometrial carcinoma.

➤*Renal function impairment:* Because progestational drugs may cause some degree of fluid retention, conditions that might be influenced by this condition, such as renal dysfunction, require careful observation.

➤*Preparation for administration:*

150mg/ml vial and prefilled syringe – Both the 1 mL vial and the 1 mL prefilled syringe of medroxyprogesterone acetate contraceptive injection should be vigorously shaken just before use to ensure that the dose being administered represents a uniform suspension.

➤*Administration:*

Contraception –

150 mg/ml vial and prefilled syringe: The suspension is intended for IM administration only.

104 mg/ml: The suspension is intended for subcutaneous administration only.

Endometrial/Renal carcinoma – Using the 400 mg/mL suspension, administer IM only.

Multidose use – When multidose vials are used for endometrial or renal carcinoma, special care to prevent contamination of the contents is essential. Although initially sterile, any multidose use of vials may lead to contamination unless strict aseptic technique is observed.

➤*Storage/Stability:* Store at 20° to 25°C (68° to 77°F).

Actions

➤*Pharmacology:*

400 mg/mL – Medroxyprogesterone acetate, administered parenterally in the recommended doses to women with adequate endogenous estrogen, transforms proliferative endometrium into secretory endometrium.

Medroxyprogesterone acetate inhibits (in the usual dose range) the secretion of pituitary gonadotropin which, in turn, prevents follicular maturation and ovulation.

Because of its prolonged action and the resulting difficulty in predicting the time of withdrawal bleeding following injection, medroxyprogesterone acetate is not recommended in secondary amenorrhea or dysfunctional uterine bleeding. In these conditions, oral therapy is recommended.

150 mg/mL – Medroxyprogesterone acetate contraceptive injection, when administered at the recommended dose to women every 3 months, inhibits the secretion of gonadotropins which, in turn, prevents follicular maturation and ovulation and results in endometrial thinning. These actions produce its contraceptive effect.

➤*Pharmacokinetics:*

Absorption – Following a single IM dose of medroxyprogesterone acetate contraceptive injection 150 mg, medroxyprogesterone acetate concentrations, measured by an extracted radioimmunoassay procedure, increase by approximately 3 weeks to reach peak plasma concentrations of 1 to 7 ng/mL. The levels then decreased exponentially until they become undetectable (less than 100 pg/mL) between 120 to 200 days following injection.

Metabolism – Using an unextracted radioimmunoassay procedure for the assay of medroxyprogesterone acetate in serum, the apparent half-life for medroxyprogesterone acetate following IM administration of medroxyprogesterone acetate contraceptive injection is approximately 50 days.

Women with lower body weights conceive sooner than women with higher body weights after discontinuing medroxyprogesterone acetate contraceptive injection.

Contraindications

Known or suspected pregnancy or as a diagnostic test for pregnancy; undiagnosed vaginal bleeding; known or suspected malignancy of breast; active thrombophlebitis, or current or past history of thromboembolic disorders, or cerebral vascular disease; liver dysfunction or disease; known sensitivity to medroxyprogesterone acetate or any of its other ingredients.

Warnings/Precautions

➤*Thromboembolic disorders:* The physician should be alert to the earliest manifestations of thrombotic disorder (thrombophlebitis, cerebrovascular disorder, pulmonary embolism, and retinal thrombosis). Should any of these occur or be suspected, the drug should not be readministered.

➤*Ocular disorders:* Medication should be discontinued pending examination if there is a sudden partial or complete loss of vision, or if there is a sudden onset of proptosis, diplopia, or migraine. If examination reveals papilledema or retinal vascular lesions, medication should not be readministered.

➤*400 mg/mL:*

Multi-dose use – Multi-dose use of medroxyprogesterone acetate sterile aqueous suspension from a single vial requires special care to avoid contamination. Although initially sterile, any multi-dose use of vials may lead to contamination unless strict aseptic technique is observed.

➤*150 mg/mL:*

Bleeding irregularities – Most women using medroxyprogesterone acetate contraceptive injection experience disruption of menstrual bleeding patterns. Altered menstrual bleeding patterns include irregular or unpredictable bleeding or spotting, or rarely, heavy or continuous bleeding. If abnormal bleeding persists or is severe, appropriate investigation should be instituted to rule out the possibility of organic pathology, and appropriate treatment should be instituted when necessary.

As women continue using medroxyprogesterone acetate contraceptive injection, fewer experience irregular bleeding and more experience amenorrhea. By month 12, amenorrhea was reported by 55% of women, and by month 24, amenorrhea was reported by 68% of women using medroxyprogesterone acetate contraceptive injection.

MEDROXYPROGESTERONE ACETATE — INJECTION

Bone mineral density changes – Use of medroxyprogesterone acetate contraceptive injection may be considered among the risk factors for development of osteoporosis. The rate of bone loss is greatest in the early years of use and then subsequently approaches the normal rate of age-related fall.

➤*History/Physical exam:* It is good medical practice for all women to have annual history and physical examinations, including women using medroxyprogesterone acetate injection. The physical examination, however, may be deferred until after initiation of medroxyprogesterone acetate injection if requested by the woman and judged appropriate by the clinician. The physical examination should include special reference to blood pressure, breasts, abdomen and pelvic organs, including cervical cytology and relevant laboratory tests. In case of undiagnosed, persistent or recurrent abnormal vaginal bleeding, appropriate measures should be conducted to rule out malignancy. Women with strong family histories of breast cancer or who have breast nodules should be monitored with particular care.

➤*Fluid retention:* Because progestational drugs may cause some degree of fluid retention, conditions which might be influenced by this condition, such as epilepsy, migraine, asthma, cardiac or renal dysfunction, require careful observation.

➤*400 mg/mL:*

Vaginal bleeding – In cases of breakthrough bleeding, as in all cases of irregular bleeding per vaginum, nonfunctional causes should be borne in mind and adequate diagnostic measures undertaken.

Masking of climacteric – The age of the patient constitutes no absolute limiting factor although treatment with progestin may mask the onset of the climacteric.

Use with estrogen – Studies of the addition of a progestin product to an estrogen replacement regimen for 7 or more days of a cycle of estrogen administration have reported a lowered incidence of endometrial hyperplasia. Morphological and biochemical studies of endometria suggest that 10 to 13 days of a progestin are needed to provide maximal maturation of the endometrium and to eliminate any hyperplastic changes. Whether this will provide protection from endometrial carcinoma has not been clearly established.

There are possible risks which may be associated with the inclusion of progestin in estrogen replacement regimen, including adverse effects on carbohydrate and lipid metabolism. The dosage used may be important in minimizing these adverse effects.

A decrease in glucose tolerance has been observed in a small percentage of patients on estrogen-progestin combination treatment. The mechanism of this decrease is obscure. For this reason, diabetic patients should be carefully observed while receiving such therapy.

Prolonged use – The effect of prolonged use of medroxyprogesterone acetate injection at the recommended doses on pituitary, ovarian, adrenal, hepatic, and uterine function is not known.

Multi-dose use – When multi-dose vials are used, special care to prevent contamination of the contents is essential. There is some evidence that benzalkonium chloride is not an adequate antiseptic for sterilizing medroxyprogesterone acetate injection multi-dose vials. A povidone-iodine solution or similar product is recommended to cleanse the vial top prior to aspiration of contents.

➤*150 mg/mL:*

Weight changes – There is a tendency for women to gain weight while on therapy with medroxyprogesterone acetate contraceptive injection. From an initial average body weight of 136 lbs, women who completed 1 year of therapy with medroxyprogesterone acetate contraceptive injection gained an average of 5.4 lbs. Women who completed 2 years of therapy gained an average of 8.1 lbs.

Women who completed 4 years gained an average of 13.8 lbs. Women who completed 6 years gained an average of 16.5 lbs. Two percent (2%) of women withdrew from a large-scale clinical trial because of excessive weight gain.

Return of fertility – Medroxyprogesterone acetate contraceptive injection has a prolonged contraceptive effect. In a large US study of women who discontinued use of medroxyprogesterone acetate contraceptive injection to become pregnant, data are available for 61% of them. Based on Life-Table analysis of these data, it is expected that 68% of women who do become pregnant may conceive within 12 months, 83% may conceive within 15 months, and 93% may conceive within 18 months from the last injection. The median time to conception for those who do conceive is 10 months following the last injection with a range of 4 to 31 months, and is unrelated to the duration of use. No data are available for 39% of the patients who discontinued medroxyprogesterone acetate contraceptive injection to become pregnant and who were lost to follow-up or changed their minds.

Convulsions – There have been a few reported cases of convulsions in patients who were treated with medroxyprogesterone acetate contraceptive injection. Association with drug use or preexisting conditions is not clear.

Carbohydrate metabolism – A decrease in glucose tolerance has been observed in some patients on medroxyprogesterone acetate contraceptive injection treatment. The mechanism of this decrease is obscure. For this reason, diabetic patients should be carefully observed while receiving such therapy.

Liver function – If jaundice develops, consideration should be given to not readministering the drug.

Protection against sexually transmitted diseases – Patients should be counseled that this product does not protect against HIV infection (AIDS) and other sexually transmitted diseases.

➤*Depression:* Patients who have a history of psychic depression should be carefully observed and the drug not be readministered if the depression recurs.

➤*Hypersensitivity reactions:*

Anaphylaxis and anaphylactoid reaction – Anaphylaxis and anaphylactoid reaction have been reported with the use of medroxyprogesterone acetate contraceptive injection. If an anaphylactic reaction occurs, appropriate therapy should be instituted. Serious anaphylactic reactions require emergency medical treatment.

➤*Pregnancy: Category X.* The use of progestational drugs during the first 4 months of pregnancy is not recommended. Progestational agents have been used beginning with the first trimester of pregnancy in attempts to prevent abortion, but there is no evidence that such use is effective. Furthermore, the use of progestational agents, with their uterine-relaxant properties, in patients with fertilized defective ova may cause a delay in spontaneous abortion.

Several reports suggest an association between intrauterine exposure to progestational drugs in the first trimester of pregnancy and genital abnormalities in male and female fetuses. The risk of hypospadias (5 to 8 per 1,000 male births in the general population) may be approximately doubled with exposure to these drugs. There are insufficient data to quantify the risk to exposed female fetuses, but insofar as some of these drugs induce mild virilization of the external genitalia of the female fetus, and because of the increased association of hypospadias in the male fetus, it is prudent to avoid the use of these drugs during the first trimester of pregnancy.

If the patient is exposed to medroxyprogesterone acetate injection during the first 4 months of pregnancy, or if she becomes pregnant while taking this drug, she should be apprised of the potential risks to the fetus.

150 mg/mL –

Unexpected pregnancies: To ensure that medroxyprogesterone acetate contraceptive injection is not administered inadvertently to a pregnant woman, the first injection must be given only during the first 5 days of a normal menstrual period; only within the first 5 days postpartum if not breast feeding, and if exclusively breastfeeding, only at the sixth postpartum week.

Neonates from unexpected pregnancies that occur 1 to 2 months after injection of medroxyprogesterone acetate contraceptive injection may be at an increased risk of low birth weight, which, in turn, is associated with an increased risk of neonatal death. The attributable risk is low because such pregnancies are uncommon.

A significant increase in incidence of polysyndactyly and chromosomal anomalies was observed among infants of users of medroxyprogesterone acetate contraceptive injection, the former being most pronounced in women younger than 30 years of age. The unrelated nature of these defects, the lack of confirmation from other studies, the distant preconceptual exposure to medroxyprogesterone acetate contraceptive injection, and the chance effects due to multiple statistical comparisons, make a causal association unlikely.

Neonates exposed to medroxyprogesterone acetate in utero and followed to adolescence, showed no evidence of any adverse effects on their health including their physical, intellectual, sexual, or social development.

Ectopic pregnancy: Healthcare providers should be alert to the possibility of an ectopic pregnancy among women using medroxyprogesterone acetate contraceptive injection who become pregnant or complain of severe abdominal pain.

➤*Lactation:* Detectable amounts of drug have been identified in the milk of mothers receiving progestational drugs. The effect of this on the nursing infant has not been determined.

In nursing mothers treated with medroxyprogesterone acetate contraceptive injection, milk composition, quality, and amount are not adversely affected. Neonates and infants exposed to medroxyprogesterone from breast milk have been studied for developmental and behavioral effects through puberty. No adverse effects have been noted.

➤*Children:* Safety and efficacy in children have not been established.

Drug Interactions

Aminoglutethimide administered concomitantly with medroxyprogesterone acetate injection may significantly depress the serum concentrations of medroxyprogesterone acetate. Medroxyprogesterone acetate users should be warned of the possibility of decreased efficacy with the use of this or any related drugs.

➤*Drug/Lab test interactions:* The pathologist should be advised of progestin therapy when relevant specimens are submitted. The following laboratory tests may be affected by progestins, including medroxyprogesterone acetate injection:

- Plasma and urinary steroid levels are decreased (eg, progesterone, estradiol, pregnanediol, testosterone, cortisol).
- Gonadotropin levels are decreased.
- Sex-hormone binding globulin concentrations are decreased.
- Protein bound iodine and butanol extractable protein bound iodine may increase. T_3 uptake values may decrease.
- Coagulation test values for prothrombin (Factor II), and Factors VII, VIII, IX, and X may increase.
- Sulfobromophthalein and other liver function test values may be increased.
- The effects of medroxyprogesterone acetate on lipid metabolism are inconsistent. Both increases and decreases in total cholesterol, triglycerides, low-density lipoprotein (LDL) cholesterol, and high-density lipoprotein (HDL) cholesterol have been observed in studies.

MEDROXYPROGESTERONE ACETATE — INJECTION

Adverse Reactions

➤*400 mg/mL:* Several reports suggest an association between intrauterine exposure to progestational drugs in the first trimester of pregnancy and genital abnormalities in male and female fetuses. The risk of hypospadias (5 to 8 per 1,000 male births in the general population) may be approximately doubled with exposure to these drugs. There are insufficient data to quantify the risk to exposed female fetuses, but insofar as some of these drugs induce mild virilization of the external genitalia of the female fetus, and because of the increased association of hypospadias in the male fetus, it is prudent to avoid the use of these drugs during the first trimester of pregnancy.

CNS – Dizziness, headache, insomnia, mental depression, nervousness.

Dermatologic – Skin sensitivity reactions consisting of urticaria, pruritus, edema, and generalized rash; acne, alopecia, and hirsutism.

Rash (allergic) with and without pruritus.

GU – Breakthrough bleeding, spotting, change in menstrual flow, amenorrhea, changes in cervical erosion and cervical secretions, breast tenderness and galactorrhea.

Hepatic – Cholestatic jaundice, including neonatal jaundice.

Hypersensitivity – Anaphylactoid reactions and anaphylaxis.

Metabolic – Change in weight (increase or decrease).

Miscellaneous – Edema, pyrexia, fatigue, nausea, somnolence.

In a few instances there have been undesirable sequelae at the site of injection, such as residual lump, change in skin color, or sterile abscess. A statistically significant association has been demonstrated between use of estrogen-progestin combination drugs and pulmonary embolism and cerebral thrombosis and embolism. For this reason, patients on progestin therapy should be carefully observed. There is also evidence suggestive of an association with neuro-ocular lesions (eg, retinal thrombosis and optic neuritis).

The following adverse reactions have been observed in patients receiving estrogen-progestin combination drugs – Rise in blood pressure in susceptible individuals, premenstrual syndrome, changes in libido, changes in appetite, cystitis-like syndrome, headache, nervousness, fatigue, backache, hirsutism, loss of scalp hair, erythema multiforme, erythema nodosum, hemorrhagic eruption, itching, dizziness.

Lab test abnormalities – The following laboratory results may be altered by the use of estrogen-progestin combination drugs: Increased sulfobromophthalein retention and other hepatic function tests; coagulation tests: Increase in prothrombin factors VII, VIII, IX, and X; metyrapone test; pregnanediol determinations; thyroid function: Increase in PBI, and butanol extractable protein bound iodine and decrease in T_3 uptake values.

➤*150 mg/mL:* In the largest clinical trial with medroxyprogesterone acetate contraceptive injection, with more than 3,900 women, who were treated for up to 7 years, reported the following adverse reactions, which may or may not be related to the use of medroxyprogesterone acetate contraceptive injection.

Adverse reactions reported by more than 5% of subjects using medroxyprogesterone acetate contraceptive injection – Menstrual irregularities (bleeding or amenorrhea, or both), abdominal pain or discomfort, weight changes, dizziness, headache, asthenia (weakness or fatigue), nervousness.

Adverse reactions reported by 1% to 5% of subjects using medroxyprogesterone acetate contraceptive injection – Decreased libido or anorgasmia, pelvic pain, backache, breast pain, leg cramps, no hair growth or alopecia, depression, bloating, nausea, rash, insomnia, edema, leukorrhea, hot flashes, acne, arthralgia, vaginitis.

Events reported by fewer than 1% of subjects using medroxyprogesterone acetate contraceptive injection – Galactorrhea, melasma, chloasma, convulsions, changes in appetite, gastrointestinal disturbances, jaundice, genitourinary infections, vaginal cysts, dyspareunia, paresthesia, chest pain, pulmonary embolus, allergic reactions, anemia, drowsiness, syncope, dyspnea and asthma, tachycardia, fever, excessive sweating and body odor, dry skin, chills, increased libido, excessive thirst, hoarseness, pain at injection site, blood dyscrasia, rectal bleeding, changes in breast size, breast lumps or nipple bleeding, axillary swelling, breast cancer, prevention of lactation, sensation of pregnancy, lack of return to fertility, paralysis, facial palsy, scleroderma, osteoporosis, uterine hyperplasia, cervical cancer, varicose veins, dysmenorrhea, hirsutism, unexpected pregnancy, thrombophlebitis, deep vein thrombosis.

In addition, voluntary reports have been received of anaphylaxis and anaphylactoid reaction with use of medroxyprogesterone acetate contraceptive injection.

CLOMIPHENE CITRATE

Rx	**Clomiphene Citrate** (Various, eg, Lemmon)	**Tablets:** 50 mg	In 10s and 30s.
Rx	**Clomid** (Aventis Pharm.)		(Clomid 50). White, scored. In 30s.
Rx	**Milophene** (Milex)		(M50). White, scored. In 30s.
Rx	**Serophene** (Serono)		(S). White, scored. In 10s and 30s.

CLOMIPHENE CITRATE — ORAL

Indications

➤*Treatment of ovulatory failure:* Clomiphene citrate is indicated for the treatment of ovulatory dysfunction in women desiring pregnancy. Impediments to achieving pregnancy must be excluded or adequately treated before beginning clomiphene citrate therapy. Those patients most likely to achieve success with clomiphene therapy include patients with polycystic ovary syndrome, amenorrhea-galactorrhea syndrome, psychogenic amenorrhea, post-oral-contraceptive amenorrhea, and certain cases of secondary amenorrhea of undetermined etiology.

➤*Off-label uses:*

Male infertility – [5] = Poor documentation. Initial data from limited controlled trials do not support clomiphene citrate as an effective treatment for idiopathic male infertility. Indirect measures of improved fertility were often present, such as increased testosterone, follicle-stimulating hormone, or luteinizing hormone levels; however, the clinical end point of achieving pregnancy was not increased with clomiphene therapy.

Administration and Dosage

➤*General dosing considerations:* The patient should be evaluated carefully to exclude pregnancy, ovarian enlargement, or ovarian cyst formation between each treatment cycle.

➤*Adults:*

Ovulatory failure –

Initial dosage: 50 mg daily (1 tablet) for 5 days.

If progestin-induced bleeding is planned, or if spontaneous uterine bleeding occurs prior to therapy, the regimen of 50 mg daily for 5 days should be started on or about the fifth day of the cycle. Therapy may be started at any time in patients who have had no recent uterine bleeding. When ovulation occurs at this dosage, there is no advantage to increasing the dose in subsequent cycles of treatment.

Dosage adjustment: The dose should be increased only in those patients who do not ovulate in response to cyclic clomiphene citrate 50 mg.

A low dosage or duration of treatment course is especially recommended if unusual sensitivity to pituitary gonadotropin is suspected, such as in patients with polycystic ovary syndrome.

Duration of therapy: Long-term cyclic therapy is not recommended beyond a total of approximately 6 cycles.

Second course of therapy: If ovulation does not appear to occur after the first course of therapy, a second course of 100 mg daily (two 50 mg tablets given as a single daily dose) for 5 days should be given.

This course may be started as early as 30 days after the previous course after precautions are taken to exclude the presence of pregnancy. Increasing the dosage or duration of therapy beyond 100 mg/day for 5 days is not recommended.

Third course of therapy: The majority of patients who are going to ovulate will do so after the first course of therapy. If ovulation does not occur after 3 courses of therapy, further treatment with clomiphene is not recommended and the patient should be reevaluated. If 3 ovulatory responses occur but pregnancy has not been achieved, further treatment is not recommended. If menses does not occur after an ovulatory response, the patient should be reevaluated.

➤*Storage/Stability:* Store tablets at controlled room temperature (15° to 30°C; 59° to 86°F). Protect from heat, light, and excessive humidity. Store in closed containers.

Actions

➤*Pharmacology:*

Action – Clomiphene citrate is a drug of considerable pharmacologic potency. With careful selection and proper management of the patient, clomiphene citrate has been demonstrated to be a useful therapy for the anovulatory patient desiring pregnancy.

Clomiphene citrate is capable of interacting with estrogen-receptor-containing tissues, including the hypothalamus, pituitary, ovary, endometrium, vagina, and cervix. It may compete with estrogen for estrogen-receptor-binding sites and may delay replenishment of intracellular estrogen receptors. These endocrine events culminate in a preovulatory gonadotropin surge and subsequent follicular rupture.

The first endocrine event in response to a course of clomiphene therapy is an increase in the release of pituitary gonadotropins. This initiates steroidogenesis and folliculogenesis, resulting in growth of the ovarian follicle and an increase in the circulating level of estradiol. Following ovulation, plasma progesterone and estradiol rise and fall as they would in a normal ovulatory cycle.

CLOMIPHENE CITRATE — ORAL

Available data suggest that both the estrogenic and antiestrogenic properties of clomiphene may participate in the initiation of ovulation. The 2 clomiphene isomers have been found to have mixed estrogenic and antiestrogenic effects, which may vary from one species to another. Some data suggest that zuclomiphene has greater estrogenic activity than enclomiphene.

Although there is no evidence of a "carryover effect" of clomiphene citrate, spontaneous ovulatory menses have been noted in some patients after clomiphene citrate therapy.

➤*Pharmacokinetics:* Based on early studies with ^{14}C-labeled clomiphene citrate, the drug was shown to be readily absorbed orally in humans and excreted principally in the feces. Cumulative urinary and fecal excretion of the ^{14}C averaged about 50% of the oral dose and 37% of an IV dose after 5 days. Mean urinary excretion was approximately 8% with fecal excretion of about 42%.

Some ^{14}C label was still present in the feces 6 weeks after administration. Subsequent single-dose studies in healthy volunteers showed that zuclomiphene (cis) has a longer half-life than enclomiphene (trans). Detectable levels of zuclomiphene persisted for greater than 1 month in these subjects. This may be suggestive of stereo-specific enterohepatic recycling or sequestering of the zuclomiphene. Thus, it is possible that some active drug may remain in the body during early pregnancy in women who conceive in the menstrual cycle during clomiphene citrate therapy.

Contraindications

➤*Hypersensitivity:* Clomiphene citrate is contraindicated in patients with a known hypersensitivity or allergy to clomiphene citrate or to any of its ingredients.

➤*Pregnancy:* See Warnings/Precautions for more information.

➤*Liver disease:* Clomiphene citrate therapy is contraindicated in patients with liver disease or a history of liver dysfunction.

➤*Abnormal uterine bleeding:* Clomiphene citrate is contraindicated in patients with abnormal uterine bleeding of undetermined origin.

➤*Ovarian cysts:* Clomiphene citrate is contraindicated in patients with ovarian cysts or enlargement not due to polycystic ovarian syndrome.

➤*Other:* Clomiphene citrate is contraindicated in patients with uncontrolled thyroid or adrenal dysfunction or in the presence of an organic intracranial lesion such as pituitary tumor.

Warnings/Precautions

➤*Ophthalmologic effects:* Patients should be advised that blurring or other visual symptoms such as spots or flashes (scintillating scotomata) may occasionally occur during therapy with clomiphene citrate. These visual symptoms increase in incidence with increasing total dose or therapy duration and generally disappear within a few days or weeks after clomiphene citrate is discontinued. Patients should be warned that these visual symptoms may render such activities as driving a car or operating machinery more hazardous than usual, particularly under conditions of variable lighting.

These visual symptoms appear to be due to intensification and prolongation of afterimages. Symptoms often first appear or are accentuated with exposure to a brightly lit environment. While measured visual acuity usually has not been affected, a study patient taking clomiphene citrate 200 mg daily developed visual blurring on the seventh day of treatment, which progressed to severe diminution of visual acuity by the day 10. No other abnormality was found, and the visual acuity returned to normal on the third day after treatment was stopped.

Ophthalmologically definable scotomata and retinal cell function (electroretinographic) changes have also been reported. A patient treated during clinical studies developed phosphenes and scotomata during prolonged clomiphene citrate administration, which disappeared by day 32 after stopping therapy.

Postmarketing surveillance of adverse events has also revealed other visual signs and symptoms during clomiphene citrate therapy (eg, abnormal accommodation, cataract, eye pain, macular edema, optic neuritis, photopsia, posterior vitreous detachment, retinal hemorrhage, retinal thrombosis, retinal vascular spasm, temporary loss of vision). While the etiology of these visual symptoms is not yet understood, patients with any visual symptoms should discontinue treatment and have a complete ophthalmological evaluation carried out promptly.

➤*Ovarian hyperstimulation syndrome:* The ovarian hyperstimulation syndrome (OHSS) has been reported to occur in patients receiving clomiphene citrate therapy for ovulation induction. In some cases, OHSS occurred following cyclic use of clomiphene citrate therapy or when clomiphene citrate was used in combination with gonadotropins. Transient liver function test abnormalities suggestive of hepatic dysfunction, which may be accompanied by morphologic changes on liver biopsy, have been reported in association with OHSS.

OHSS is a medical event distinct from uncomplicated ovarian enlargement. The clinical signs of this syndrome in severe cases can include gross ovarian enlargement, gastrointestinal symptoms, ascites, dyspnea, oliguria, and pleural effusion. In addition, the following symptoms have been reported in association with this syndrome: Pericardial effusion, anasarca, hydrothorax, acute abdomen, hypotension, renal failure, pulmonary edema, intraperitoneal and ovarian hemorrhage, deep venous thrombosis, torsion of the ovary, and acute respiratory distress.

The early warning signs of OHSS are abdominal pain and distention, nausea, vomiting, diarrhea, and weight gain. Elevated urinary steroid levels, varying degrees of electrolyte imbalance, hypovolemia, hemoconcentration, and hypoproteinemia may occur. Death caused by hypovolemic shock, hemoconcentration, or thromboembolism has occurred. Because of fragility of enlarged ovaries in severe cases, abdominal and pelvic examination should be performed very cautiously. If conception results, rapid progression to the severe form of the syndrome may occur.

To minimize the hazard associated with occasional abnormal ovarian enlargement associated with clomiphene citrate therapy, the lowest dose consistent with expected clinical results should be used. Maximal enlargement of the ovary, whether physiologic or abnormal, may not occur until several days after discontinuation of the recommended dose of clomiphene citrate. Some patients with polycystic ovary syndrome who are unusually sensitive to gonadotropin may have an exaggerated response to usual doses of clomiphene citrate. Therefore, patients with polycystic ovary syndrome should be started on the lowest recommended dose and shortest treatment duration for the first course of therapy.

If enlargement of the ovary occurs, additional clomiphene citrate therapy should not be given until the ovaries have returned to pretreatment size, and the dosage or duration of the next course should be reduced. Ovarian enlargement and cyst formation associated with clomiphene citrate therapy usually regress spontaneously within a few days or weeks after discontinuing treatment. The potential benefit of subsequent clomiphene citrate therapy in these cases should exceed the risk. Unless surgical indication for laparotomy exists, such cystic enlargement should always be managed conservatively.

A causal relationship between ovarian hyperstimulation and ovarian cancer has not been determined. However, because a correlation between ovarian cancer and nulliparity, infertility, and age has been suggested, if ovarian cysts do not regress spontaneously, a thorough evaluation should be performed to rule out the presence of ovarian neoplasia.

➤*Diagnosis prior to therapy:* Careful attention should be given to the selection of candidates for clomiphene citrate therapy. Pelvic examination is necessary prior to clomiphene citrate treatment and before each subsequent course.

➤*Drug abuse and dependence:* Tolerance, abuse, or dependence with clomiphene citrate has not been reported.

➤*Hazardous tasks:* Patients should be advised that blurring or other visual symptoms such as spots or flashes (scintillating scotomata) may occasionally occur during therapy with clomiphene citrate. These visual symptoms increase in incidence with increasing total dose or therapy duration and generally disappear within a few days or weeks after clomiphene citrate is discontinued. Patients should be warned that these visual symptoms may render such activities as driving a car or operating machinery more hazardous than usual, particularly under conditions of variable lighting.

➤*Pregnancy:* *Category X.* Clomiphene citrate should not be administered during pregnancy. Clomiphene citrate may cause fetal harm in animals (see Animal Fetotoxicity, below). Although no causative evidence of a deleterious effect of clomiphene citrate therapy on the human fetus has been established, there have been reports of birth anomalies which, during clinical studies, occurred at an incidence within the range reported for the general population.

To avoid inadvertent clomiphene citrate administration during early pregnancy, appropriate tests should be utilized during each treatment cycle to determine whether ovulation occurs. The patient should be evaluated carefully to exclude pregnancy, ovarian enlargement, or ovarian cyst formation between each treatment cycle. The next course of clomiphene citrate therapy should be delayed until these conditions have been excluded.

Fetal/neonatal anomalies and mortality – The following fetal abnormalities have been reported subsequent to pregnancies following ovulation induction therapy with clomiphene citrate during clinical trials. Each of the following fetal abnormalities were reported at a rate of less than 1% (experiences are listed in order of decreasing frequency): Congenital heart lesions, Down's syndrome, club foot, congenital gut lesions, hypospadias, microcephaly, harelip and cleft palate, congenital hip, hemangioma, undescended testicles, polydactyly, conjoined twins and teratomatous malformation, patent ductus arteriosus, amaurosis, arteriovenous fistula, inguinal hernia, umbilical hernia, syndactyly, pectus excavatum, myopathy, dermoid cyst of scalp, omphalocele, spina bifida occulta, ichthyosis, and persistent linqual frenulum. Neonatal death and fetal death/stillbirth in infants with birth defects have also been reported at a rate of less than 1%. The overall incidence of reported birth anomalies from pregnancies associated with maternal clomiphene citrate ingestion during clinical studies was within the range of that reported for the general population.

In addition, reports of birth anomalies have been received during postmarketing surveillance of clomiphene citrate (eg, delayed development; abnormal bone development including skeletal malformations of the skull, face, nasal passages, jaw, hand, limb [ectromelia, including amelia, hemimella, and phocomelia], foot, and joints; tissue malformations including imperforate anus, tracheoesophageal fistula, diaphragmatic hernia, renal agenesis and dysgenesis, and malformations of the eye and lens [cataract], ear, lung, heart [ventricular septal defect and tetralogy of Fallot], and genitalia; as well as dwarfism, deafness, mental retardation, chromosomal disorders, and neural tube defects [including anencephaly]).

Animal fetotoxicity – Oral administration of clomiphene citrate to pregnant rats during organogenesis at doses of 1 to 2 mg/kg/day resulted in hydramnion and weak, edematous fetuses with wavy ribs and other temporary bone changes. Doses of 8 mg/kg/day or more also caused increased resorptions and dead fetuses, dystocia, and delayed parturition, and 40 mg/kg/day resulted in increased maternal mortality. Single doses of 50 mg/kg caused fetal cataracts, while 200 mg/kg caused cleft palate.

CLOMIPHENE CITRATE — ORAL

Following injection of clomiphene citrate 2 mg/kg to mice and rats during pregnancy, the offspring exhibited metaplastic changes of the reproductive tract. Newborn mice and rats injected during the first few days of life also developed metaplastic changes in uterine and vaginal mucosa, as well as premature vaginal opening and anovulatory ovaries. These findings are similar to the abnormal reproductive behavior and sterility described with other estrogens and antiestrogens.

In rabbits, some temporary bone alterations were seen in fetuses from dams given oral doses of 20 or 40 mg/kg/day during pregnancy, but not following 8 mg/kg/day. No permanent malformations were observed in those studies. Also, rhesus monkeys given oral doses of 1.5 to 4.5 mg/kg/day for various periods during pregnancy did not have any abnormal offspring.

➤*Lactation:* It is not known whether clomiphene citrate is excreted in human milk. Because many drugs are excreted in human milk, caution should be exercised if clomiphene citrate is administered to a breast-feeding woman. In some patients, clomiphene citrate may reduce lactation.

Drug Interactions

Drug interactions with clomiphene citrate have not been documented.

Adverse Reactions

➤*Clinical trial adverse reactions:* Clomiphene citrate, at recommended dosages, is generally well tolerated. Adverse reactions usually have been mild and transient, and most have disappeared promptly after treatment has been discontinued. Adverse reactions reported in patients treated with clomiphene citrate during clinical studies are shown in the following table:

Incidence of Adverse Reactions in Clomiphene Citrate Clinical Studies (Reactions Greater Than 1%) (n = 8,029)[a]

Adverse reaction	%
Ovarian enlargement	13.6%
Vasomotor flushes	10.4%
Abdominal/pelvic discomfort/distention/bloating	5.5%
Nausea/vomiting	2.2%
Breast discomfort	2.1%
Visual symptoms (blurred vision, lights, floater, waves, unspecified visual complaints, photophobia, diplopia, scotomata, phosphenes	1.5%
Headache	1.3%
Abnormal uterine bleeding (intermenstrual spotting, menorrhagia)	1.3%

[a] Includes 498 patients whose reports may have been duplicated in the event totals and could not be distinguished as such. Also, excludes 47 patients who did not report symptom data.

The following adverse reactions have been reported in less than 1% of patients in clinical trials: Acute abdomen, appetite increase, constipation, dermatitis or rash, depression, diarrhea, dizziness, fatigue, hair loss/dry hair, increased urinary frequency/volume, insomnia, light-headedness, nervous tension, vaginal dryness, vertigo, weight gain/loss.

Patients on prolonged clomiphene citrate therapy may show elevated serum levels of desmosterol. This is most likely due to a direct interference with cholesterol synthesis. However, the serum sterols in patients receiving the recommended dose of clomiphene citrate are not significantly altered. Ovarian cancer has been infrequently reported in patients who have received fertility drugs. Infertility is a primary risk factor for ovarian cancer; however, epidemiology data suggest that prolonged use of clomiphene may increase the risk of a borderline or invasive ovarian tumor.

➤*Postmarketing adverse reactions:* The following adverse experiences were reported spontaneously with clomiphene citrate. The cause and effect relationship of the listed events to the administration of clomiphene citrate is not known.

Cardiovascular – Arrhythmia, chest pain, edema, hypertension, palpitation, phlebitis, pulmonary embolism, shortness of breath, tachycardia, thrombophlebitis.

CNS – Migraine headache, paresthesia, seizure, stroke, syncope.

Dermatologic – Acne, allergic reaction, erythema, erythema multiforme, erythema nodosum, hypertrichosis, pruritus.

GU – Endometriosis, ovarian cyst (ovarian enlargement or cysts could, as such, be complicated by adnexal torsion), ovarian hemorrhage, tubal pregnancy, uterine hemorrhage.

Hepatic – Transaminases increased, hepatitis.

Musculoskeletal – Arthralgia, back pain, myalgia.

Ophthalmic – Abnormal accommodation, cataract, eye pain, macular edema, optic neuritis, photopsia, posterior vitreous detachment, retinal hemorrhage, retinal thrombosis, retinal vascular spasm, temporary loss of vision.

Psychiatric – Anxiety, irritability, mood changes, psychosis.

Miscellaneous – Fever, tinnitus, weakness, leukocytosis, thyroid disorder.

Neoplasms: Liver (hepatic hemangiosarcoma, liver cell adenoma, hepatocellular carcinoma); breast (fibrocystic disease, breast carcinoma); endometrium (endometrial carcinoma); nervous system (astrocytoma, pituitary tumor, prolactinoma, neurofibromatosis, glioblastoma multiforme, brain abscess); ovary (luteoma of pregnancy, dermoid cyst of the ovary, ovarian carcinoma); trophoblastic (hydatiform mole, choriocarcinoma); miscellaneous (melanoma, myeloma, perianal cysts, renal cell carcinoma, Hodgkin's lymphoma, tongue carcinoma, bladder carcinoma); and neoplasms of offspring (neuroectodermal tumor, thyroid tumor, hepatoblastoma, lymphocytic leukemia).

Fetal/neonatal anomalies: The following fetal neonatal abnormalities have also been reported during postmarketing surveillance: Delayed development; abnormal bone development including skeletal malformations of the skull, face, nasal passages, jaw, hand, limb (ectromelia including amelia, hemimella, and phocomelia), foot, and joints; tissue malformations including imperforate anus, tracheoesophageal fistula, diaphragmatic hernia, renal agenesis and dysgenesis, and malformations of the eye and lens (cataract), ear, lung, heart (ventricular septal defect and tetralogy of Fallot), and genitalia; as well as dwarfism, deafness, mental retardation, chromosomal disorders, and neural tube defects (including anencephaly).

Overdosage

➤*Oral LD_{50}:* The acute oral LD_{50} of clomiphene citrate is 1,700 mg/kg in mice and 5,750 mg/kg in rats. The toxic dose in humans is not known.

➤*Symptoms:* Toxic effects accompanying acute overdosage of clomiphene citrate have not been reported. Signs and symptoms of overdosage as a result of the use of more than the recommended dose during clomiphene citrate therapy include nausea, vomiting, vasomotor flushes, visual blurring, spots or flashes, scotomata, ovarian enlargement with pelvic or abdominal pain. Clomiphene citrate is contraindicated in patients with ovarian cysts or enlargement not caused by polycystic ovarian syndrome.

➤*Treatment:* In the event of overdose, appropriate supportive measures should be employed in addition to gastrointestinal decontamination.

Dialysis – It is not known if clomiphene citrate is dialyzable.

Patient Information

The purpose and risks of clomiphene citrate therapy should be presented to the patient before starting treatment. It should be emphasized that the goal of clomiphene citrate therapy is ovulation for subsequent pregnancy. The physician should counsel the patient with special regard to the following potential risks:

➤*Visual symptoms:* Advise that blurring or other visual symptoms occasionally may occur during or shortly after clomiphene citrate therapy. Warn patients that visual symptoms may render such activities as driving a car or operating machinery more hazardous than usual, particularly under conditions of variable lighting.

The patient should be instructed to inform the physician whenever any unusual visual symptoms occur. If the patient has any visual symptoms, treatment should be discontinued and complete ophthalmologic evaluation performed.

➤*Abdominal/pelvic pain or distention:* Ovarian enlargement may occur during or shortly after therapy with clomiphene citrate. To minimize the risks associated with ovarian enlargement, the patient should be instructed to inform the physician of any abdominal or pelvic pain, weight gain, discomfort, or distention after taking clomiphene citrate.

➤*Multiple pregnancy:* Inform the patient that there is an increased chance of multiple pregnancy, including bilateral tubal pregnancy and coexisting tubal and intrauterine pregnancy, when conception occurs in relation to clomiphene citrate therapy. The potential complications and hazards of multiple pregnancy should be explained.

➤*Pregnancy wastage and birth anomalies:* The physician should explain the assumed risk of any pregnancy, whether ovulation is induced with the aid of clomiphene citrate or occurs naturally. The patient should be informed of the greater risks associated with certain characteristics or conditions of any pregnant woman (eg, age of female and male partner, history of spontaneous abortions, Rh genotype, abnormal menstrual history, infertility history, organic heart disease, diabetes, exposure to infectious agents such as rubella, familial history of birth anomaly, that may be pertinent to the patient for whom clomiphene citrate is being considered). Based upon the evaluation of the patient, genetic counseling may be indicated.

The overall incidence of reported birth anomalies from pregnancies associated with maternal clomiphene citrate ingestion during the investigational studies was within the range of that reported in published references for the general population. Clomiphene citrate should not be administered during pregnancy. During clinical investigation, the experience from patients with known pregnancy outcome shows a spontaneous abortion rate of 20.4% and stillbirth rate of 1%.

GONADOTROPINS
FOLLITROPINS

Indications

➤*Ovulation induction:* For the induction of ovulation and pregnancy in anovulatory infertile patients in whom the cause of infertility is functional and not caused by primary ovarian failure.

Refer to individual product monographs for specific indications.

➤*Follicle stimulation:* To stimulate the development of multiple follicles in ovulatory patients undergoing Assisted Reproductive Technologies (ART), eg, in vitro fertilization.

Actions

➤*Pharmacology:* **Urofollitropin** is a preparation of highly purified follicle-stimulating hormone (FSH) extracted from the urine of postmenopausal women. **Follitropin alfa** and **follitropin beta** are human FSH preparations of recombinant DNA origin. Follitropins stimulate ovarian follicular growth in women who do not have primary ovarian failure. FSH is required for normal follicular growth, maturation and gonadal steroid production. In the female, the level of FSH is critical for the onset and duration of follicular development, and consequently for the timing and number of follicles reaching maturity. In order to affect ovulation in the absence of endogenous LH surge, human chorionic gonadotropin (hCG) must be given following the administration of urofollitropin, follitropin alfa and beta when clinical and laboratory assessment of the patient indicate that sufficient follicular maturation has occurred.

➤*Pharmacokinetics:*

Absorption/Distribution – Follitropins have absorption-rate limited pharmacokinetics; the absorption rate following IM or subcutaneous administration is slower than the elimination rate. Bioavailability ranges from approximately 66% to 78% depending on the agent. Following a single IM or subcutaneous dose, AUCs are similar for all agents and C_{max} is similar for urofollitropin and follitropin alfa; however, the C_{max} for follitropin beta differs with respect to IM or subcutaneous administration (approximately 6.86 versus approximately 5.41 units/L, respectively).

Following multiple IM or subcutaneous doses, steady-state plasma levels are reached within 4 to 5 days. Peak follitropin alfa plasma levels were 6 to 12 units/L following 150 U/day administered subcutaneous for 7 days; follitropin beta peak levels, following 75, 150 or 225 units either subcutaneous or IM for 7 days, were approximately 4.3 or 4.65, 8.51 or 9.46, and 13.92 or 11.3 units/L, respectively.

Metabolism/Excretion – Total clearance of follitropin alfa following IV administration was 0.6 L/hr; data is lacking regarding clearance for the other two agents. Following multiple dosing, the terminal half-life for follitropin alfa (IM) and beta (subcutaneous) were approximately 30 hours.

Special populations –

Obesity: Body weight, measured as kg or as body mass index (BMI), was shown to influence the absorption rate and thus the AUC of follitropin alfa and beta. Increased body weight or BMI was associated with a decrease in the rate of follitropin absorption and a significantly smaller AUC. Clearance, however was essentially the same on a per kg basis.

Select Pharmacokinetic Parameters of Follitropins Following Subcutaneous (IM) Administration

	Mean T_{max} (hrs)	Mean elimination t½ (hrs)[a]	Mean V_d (L)
Follitropin alfa	16 (25)	24 and 32[b]	10
Follitropin beta	(27)	(≈ 30)	8
Urofollitropin	15 (10)	-	-

[a] This value increases with body mass index.
[b] In healthy and ART patients, respectively.

Contraindications

High levels of FSH indicating primary ovarian failure; uncontrolled thyroid or adrenal dysfunction; the presence of any cause of infertility other than anovulation; tumor of the ovary, breast, uterus, hypothalamus or pituitary gland; abnormal vaginal bleeding of undetermined origin; ovarian cysts or enlargement not due to polycystic ovary syndrome; hypersensitivity to the product or any of its components; pregnancy (see Warnings).

Warnings/Precautions

➤*Administration:* These medications should only be used by physicians who are thoroughly familiar with infertility problems and their management. It is a potent gonadotropic substance capable of causing mild to severe adverse reactions. To minimize risks, use only at the lowest effective dose. Monitor ovarian response with serum estradiol and vaginal ultrasound on a regular basis.

➤*Overstimulation of the ovary:*

Ovarian enlargement – Mild to moderate uncomplicated ovarian enlargement, which may be accompanied by abdominal distention or abdominal pain, occurs in approximately 20% of those treated with urofollitropin and hCG, and generally regresses without treatment within 2 or 3 weeks.

Ovarian Hyperstimulation Syndrome (OHSS) – The hyperstimulation syndrome is characterized by severe ovarian enlargement, abdominal pain/distention, nausea, vomiting, diarrhea, dyspnea and oliguria, and may be accompanied by ascites, pleural effusion, hypovolemia, electrolyte imbalance, hemoperitoneum and thromboembolic events. OHSS occurred in 6% of patients in trials.

If hyperstimulation occurs, stop treatment and hospitalize the patient. This syndrome develops rapidly within 24 hours to several days and generally occurs during the 7 to 10 days immediately following treatment. Hemoconcentration associated with fluid loss into the abdominal cavity has occurred and should be assessed in the following manner: 1) Fluid intake and output, 2) weight, 3) hematocrit, 4) serum and urinary electrolytes, 5) urine specific gravity, 6) BUN and creatinine and 7) abdominal girth. Perform these determinations daily or more often if the need arises. Treatment is primarily symptomatic and consists of bed rest, fluid and electrolyte replacement and analgesics. The ascitic, pleural and pericardial fluids should never be removed because of the potential danger of injury.

Hemoperitoneum from ruptured ovarian cysts is usually the result of pelvic examination. If this does occur, and if bleeding becomes such that surgery is required, design the surgical treatment to control bleeding and retain as much ovarian tissue as possible.

Intercourse should be prohibited in patients in whom significant ovarian enlargement occurs after ovulation because of the danger of hemoperitoneum resulting from ruptured ovarian cysts.

➤*Pulmonary and vascular complications:* Serious pulmonary conditions (eg, atelectasis, acute respiratory distress syndrome and exacerbation of asthma) have been reported. In addition, thromboembolic events both in association with, and separate from OHSS have been reported. Intravascular thrombosis and embolism can result in reduced blood flow to critical organs or the extremities. Sequelae of such events have included venous thrombophlebitis, pulmonary embolism, pulmonary infarction, cerebral vascular occlusion (stroke) and arterial occlusion resulting in loss of limb. In rare cases, pulmonary complications and thromboembolic events have resulted in death.

➤*Multiple births:* Reports of multiple pregnancies have been associated with these medications, including triplet and quintuplet gestations. Multiple births have occurred with **urofollitropin** (20.8%), **follitropin alfa** (12.3%) and **follotropin beta** (8%). Advise the patient of the potential risk of multiple births before starting treatment.

➤*Selection of patients:* Give careful attention to diagnosis in candidates for therapy. Before treatment is instituted:

1.) Perform a thorough gynecologic and endocrinologic evaluation including a hysterosalpingogram (to rule out uterine and tubal pathology) and documentation of anovulation by review of patient history, physical examination, determining serum hormonal levels as indicated and optionally performing an endometrial biopsy. Patients with tubal pathology should receive the drug only if enrolled in an in vitro fertilization program.
2.) Exclude primary ovarian failure by the determination of gonadotropin levels.
3.) Make careful examination to rule out early pregnancy.
4.) Patients in late reproductive life have a greater predilection to endometrial carcinoma and a higher incidence of anovulatory disorders. Perform a thorough diagnostic evaluation in patients who demonstrate abnormal uterine bleeding or other signs of endometrial abnormalities before starting therapy.
5.) Evaluate partner's fertility potential.

➤*Ovulation confirmation:* Treatment results in follicular growth and maturation to effect ovulation in the absence of an endogenous LH surge. HCG is given following the administration of urofollitropin and follitropin alfa and beta when clinical assessment indicates sufficient follicular maturation has occurred. This is indirectly estimated by the estrogenic effect upon the target organs. With serum or urinary estrogen determinations and ultrasonography, the estrogenic effect is an acceptable means for monitoring the growth and development of follicles, timing hCG administration and minimizing the risk of hyperstimulation. Clinically confirm ovulation, with the exception of pregnancy, by indirect indices of progesterone production. The indices most generally used are a rise in basal body temperature, increase in serum progesterone and menstruation following the shift in basal body temperature.

Other clinical parameters that may have potential use for monitoring urofollitropin therapy include changes in the vaginal cytology and appearance and volume of the cervical mucus.

➤*Pregnancy: Category X.* Contraindicated in pregnancy.

➤*Lactation:* It is not known if this drug is excreted in breast milk. Exercise caution if administering to a nursing mother.

➤*Children:* Safety and efficacy in pediatric patients have not been established, although this drug is not intended for use in children.

➤*Monitoring:* Monitor sufficient follicular maturation. This may be directly estimated by sonographic visualization of the ovaries and endometrial lining or measuring serum estradiol levels. The combination of both ultrasonography and measurement of estradiol levels is useful for monitoring the growth and development of follicles and timing hCG administration, as well as minimizing the risk of OHSS and multiple gestations.

The clinical evaluation of estrogenic activity (changes in vaginal cytology and changes in appearance and volume of cervical mucus) provides an indirect estimate of the estrogenic effect upon the target organs, and therefore it should only be used adjunctively with more direct estimates of follicular development (eg, ultrasonography and serum estradiol determinations).

GONADOTROPINS FOLLITROPINS

The clinical confirmation of ovulation is obtained by direct and indirect indices of progesterone production. The indices most generally used are as follows: 1) a rise in basal body temperature, 2) increase in serum progesterone, and 3) menstruation following the shift in basal body temperature.

When used in conjunction with indices of progesterone production, sonographic visualization of the ovaries will assist if ovulation has occurred. Sonographic evidence of ovulation may include the following: 1) fluid in the cul-de-sac, 2) follicle showing marked decrease in size, and 3) collapsed follicle.

Adverse Reactions

The following adverse reactions are listed in decreasing order of potential severity: Pulmonary and vascular complications (see Warnings); OHSS (see Warnings); adnexal torsion (as a complication of ovarian enlargement); mild to moderate ovarian enlargement; abdominal pain; sensitivity to urofollitropin (febrile reactions which may be accompanied by chills, musculoskeletal aches, joint pains, malaise, headache and fatigue have occurred. It is not clear whether or not these were pyrogenic responses or possible allergic reactions); ovarian cysts; GI symptoms (nausea, vomiting, diarrhea, abdominal cramps, bloating); pain, rash, swelling or irritation at the site of injection; breast tenderness; headache; dermatological symptoms (dry skin, body rash, hair loss, hives); hemoperitoneum has been reported during menotropins therapy and, therefore, may also occur during follitropin therapy.

The following adverse events have been reported in women treated with gonadotropins: Pulmonary and vascular complications (see Warnings), hemoperitoneum, adnexal torsion (as a complication of ovarian enlargement, abdominal pain), dizziness, tachycardia, dyspnea, tachypnea, febrile reactions, flu-like symptoms including fever, chills, musculoskeletal aches, joint pains, nausea, headache and malaise, ovarian cysts; gastrointestinal symptoms (nausea, vomiting, diarrhea, abdominal cramps, bloating); pain, rash, swelling or irritation at the site of injection; breast tenderness and dermatological symptoms (dry skin, body rash, hair loss and hives).

Overdosage

Aside from possible ovarian hyperstimulation and multiple gestations (see Warnings), little is known concerning the consequences of acute overdosage.

Patient Information

Prior to therapy, inform patients of the following: Duration of treatment and monitoring required; possible adverse reactions; risk of multiple births.

GONADOTROPINS UROFOLLITROPIN

Rx	**Bravelle** (Ferring)	**Powder for injection, lyophilized:** 75 units FSH activity[a]	In vials[b] with 2 mL vials NaCl as diluent.

[a] Contains up to 2% luteinizing hormone (LH) activity.

[b] With lactose monohydrate 23 mg.

UROFOLLITROPIN — INJECTION

For complete and comparative prescribing information, refer to the Follitropins group monograph.

Indications

➤*Ovulation induction:* In conjunction with human chorionic gonadotropin (hCG) for ovulation induction in patients who previously have received pituitary suppression.

➤*Multifollicular development during ART:* In conjunction with hCG for multiple follicular development (controlled ovarian stimulation) during assisted reproductive technologies (ART) cycles in patients who have previously received pituitary suppression.

Administration and Dosage

➤*General dosing considerations:* The dose to stimulate development of ovarian follicles must be individualized for each patient. Use the lowest dose consistent with achieving good results based on clinical experience and reported clinical data.

➤*Adults:*

Ovulation induction –

Maximum dose: 450 units/day.

Initial dosage: 150 units/day subcutaneous or IM for the first 5 days of treatment in patients who have received gonadotropin-releasing hormone (GnRH) agonist or antagonist pituitary suppression.

Dosage adjustment: Based on clinical monitoring (including serum estradiol levels and vaginal ultrasound results), adjust subsequent dosing according to individual patient response. Do not make adjustments in dose more frequently than once every 2 days and do not exceed more than 75 to 150 units per adjustment.

Duration of therapy: Dosing beyond 12 days is not recommended.

Concomitant therapy: If patient response is appropriate, give human chorionic gonadotropin (hCG) (5,000 to 10,000 units) 1day following the last dose of urofollitropin. Withhold the hCG if the serum estradiol is greater than 2,000 pg/mL, if the ovaries are abnormally enlarged, or if abdominal pain occurs, and advise the patient to refrain from intercourse. These precautions may reduce the risk of ovarian hyperstimulation syndrome (OHSS) and multiple gestations. Follow patients closely for at least 2 weeks after hCG administration. If there is inadequate follicle development or ovulation without subsequent pregnancy, the course of treatment may be repeated.

Encourage the couple to have intercourse daily, beginning on the day prior to the administration of hCG until ovulation becomes apparent from indices employed for the determination of progestational activity. In the light of the foregoing indices and parameters mentioned, it should become obvious that unless a health care provider is willing to devote considerable time to these patients and be familiar with and conduct the necessary laboratory studies, urofollitropin should not be used.

ART –

Maximum dose: 450 units/day.

Initial dosage: 225 units daily subcutaneously for the first 5 days for patients undergoing in vitro fertilization (IVF) and donor egg patients who have received GnRH agonist or antagonist pituitary suppression.

Dosage adjustment: Based on clinical monitoring (including serum estradiol levels and vaginal ultrasound results) subsequent dosing should be adjusted according to individual patient response. Adjustments in dose should not be made more frequently than once every 2 days and should not exceed more than 75 to 150 units per adjustment.

Duration of therapy: Dosing beyond 12 days is not recommended.

Concomitant therapy: Once adequate follicular development is evident, hCG (5,000 to 10,000units) should be administered to induce final follicular maturation in preparation for oocyte retrieval. The administration of hCG must be withheld in cases where the ovaries are abnormally enlarged on the last day of therapy to reduce the chance of developing OHSS.

➤*Preparation for administration:* Inject 1 mL of sterile saline for injection into the vial of urofollitropin. Do not shake, but gently swirl until the solution is clear. Urofollitropin dissolves immediately. Check the liquid in the container; if it is not clear or contains particles, do not use it.

For patients requiring a single injection from multiple vials of urofollitropin, up to 6 vials can be reconstituted with 1 mL of sterile saline for injection. This can be accomplished by reconstituting a single vial as described previously; then, draw the entire contents of the first vial into a syringe and inject the contents into a second vial of lyophilized urofollitropin. Gently swirl the second vial, once again checking to make sure the solution is clear and free of particles. This step can be repeated with 4 additional vials for a total of up to 6 vials of lyophilized urofollitropin into 1 mL of diluent.

➤*Administration:* May be administered by IM or subcutaneous injection depending on indication. Immediately administer the reconstituted solution. The recommended sites for subcutaneous injection are either side of the lower abdomen in alternating fashion. Injection into the thigh is not recommended.

➤*Storage/Stability:* Store at 3° to 25°C (37° to 77°F). Protect from light. Use immediately after reconstitution. Discard unused material.

GONDOTROPINS FOLLITROPIN ALFA

Rx	**Gonal-f** (Serono)	**Powder for injection, lyophilized:** 82 units FSH activity (to deliver 75 units)	30 mg sucrose. In 1 and 10 single-dose vials with sterile water for injection as diluent.
		600 units FSH activity (to deliver 450 units)	30 mg sucrose. In 1 multi-dose vial with prefilled syringe of bacteriostatic water[a] for injection as diluent and 6 syringes.
		1,200 units FSH activity (to deliver 1,050 units)	30 mg sucrose. In 1, 5, and 10 multi-dose vials with prefilled syringes of bacteriostatic water[a] for injection as diluent.
Rx	**Gonal-f RFF Pen** (Serono)	**Injection:** 415 units FSH activity (to deliver ≥ 300 units/0.5 mL)	In prefilled pens[b] with needles.
		568 units FSH activity (to deliver ≥ 450 units/0.75 mL)	
		1,026 units FSH activity (to deliver ≥ 900 units/1.5 mL)	

[a] With 0.9% benzyl alcohol.

[b] With 60 mg/mL sucrose, 3.0 mg/mL m-cresol, 1.1 mg/mL disodium hydrogen phosphate, 0.45 mg/mL sodium dihydrogen phosphate monohydrate, 0.1 mg//mL methionine, 0.1 mg/mL poloxamer 188.

FOLLITROPIN ALFA — INJECTION

For complete and comparative prescribing information, refer to the Follitropins group monograph.

Indications

➤*Ovulation induction:* For the induction of ovulation and pregnancy in oligo-anovulatory infertile patients in whom the cause of infertility is functional and not primary ovarian failure.

➤*Multifollicular development during assisted reproductive technology (ART):* To stimulate the development of multiple follicles in ovulatory patients participating in an ART program (eg, in vitro fertilization).

➤*Male infertility (except prefilled pen):* For the induction of spermatogenesis in men with primary and secondary hypogonadotropic hypogonadism in whom the cause of infertility is not primary testicular failure.

Administration and Dosage

➤*Adults:*

Ovulation induction –

Usual dosage: Individualize initial dose in subsequent cycles for each patient based on response in the preceding cycle. As in the initial cycle, 5,000 units of hCG must be given 1 day after the last dose of follitropin alfa to complete follicular development and induce ovulation. Follow the precautions to minimize the chances of developing ovarian hyperstimulation syndrome (OHSS) (see Discontinuation of Therapy).

Use the lowest dose consistent with the expectation of good results. Over the course of treatment, doses of follitropin alfa may range up to 300 units/day depending on patient response. Give until adequate follicular development is indicated by serum estradiol and vaginal ultrasonography. A response is generally evident after 5 to 7 days. Base subsequent monitoring intervals on patient response.

Encourage the couple to have intercourse daily, beginning on the day prior to hCG administration until ovulation becomes apparent. Take care to ensure insemination.

Maximum dose: Doses larger than 300 units/day of follicle stimulating hormone (FSH) are not routinely recommended.

Initial dosage: The initial dose for the first cycle is 75 units/day subcutaneously. An incremental adjustment in dose of up to 37.5 units may be considered after 14 days. Further dose increases of the same magnitude can be made, if necessary, every 7 days.

Duration of therapy: Do not exceed a treatment duration of 35 days unless an estradiol rise indicates imminent follicular development.

Concomitant therapy: To complete follicular development and effect ovulation in the absence of an endogenous luteinizing hormone surge, give 5,000 units of hCG 1 day after the last dose of follitropin alfa. Withhold hCG if the serum estradiol is greater than 2,000 pg/mL.

Discontinuation of therapy: If the ovaries are abnormally enlarged or abdominal pain occurs, discontinue follitropin alfa treatment, do not administer hCG, and advise the patient not to have intercourse; this may reduce the chance of developing OHSS and, should spontaneous ovulation occur, reduce the chance of multiple gestations. Conduct a follow-up visit in the luteal phase.

Male infertility (except prefilled pen) –

Usual dosage: The dose of follitropin alfa to induce spermatogenesis must be individualized for each patient. Use the lowest dose of follitropin alfa that induces spermatogenesis.

Prior to concomitant therapy with follitropin alfa and hCG, pretreatment with hCG alone (1,000 to 2,250 units 2 to 3 times per week) is required. Continue treatment for a period sufficient to achieve serum testosterone levels within the normal range. Such pretreatment may require 3 to 6 months, and the dose of hCG may need to be increased to achieve normal testosterone levels.

After normal serum testosterone levels are reached, the recommended dose of follitropin alfa is 150 units administered subcutaneously 3 times per week with hCG (see Concomitant Therapy).

Maximum dose: If azoospermia persists, the dose may be increased to a maximum of 300 units 3 times per week.

Duration of therapy: Follitropin alfa may need to be administered for up to 18 months to achieve adequate spermatogenesis.

Concomitant therapy: Give follitropin alfa in conjunction with hCG. The recommended dose of hCG is 1,000 units (or the dose required to maintain serum testosterone levels within the normal range) 3 times per week.

Multifollicular development during ART –

Usual dosage: In patients younger than 35 years of age undergoing ART, whose endogenous gonadotropin levels are suppressed, initiate follitropin alfa prefilled pens at a dose of 150 units/day. In patients 35 years of age and older undergoing ART, whose endogenous gonadotropin levels are suppressed, initiate follitropin alfa prefilled pens at a dose of 225 units/day. Continue treatment until adequate follicular development is indicated as determined by ultrasound in combination with measurement of serum estradiol levels.

Maximum dose: Doses of more than 450 units/day are not recommended.

Initial dosage: Initiate in the early follicular phase (cycle day 2 or 3) at a dose of 150 units/day until sufficient follicular development is attained.

Dosage adjustment: Consider dose adjustments after 5 days based on the patient's response; adjust subsequent dosage no more frequently than every 3 to 5 days and by no more than 75 to 150 units additionally at each adjustment.

Duration of therapy: In most cases, therapy should not exceed 10 days.

Concomitant therapy: Once adequate follicular development is evident, administer hCG (5,000 to 10,000 units) to induce final follicular maturation in preparation for oocyte retrieval. Withhold hCG in cases in which the ovaries are abnormally enlarged on the last day of therapy to reduce the risk of developing OHSS.

➤*Preparation for administration:*

Reconstitution –

Single-dose amps: Dissolve contents of 1 or more amps in 0.5 to 1 mL of sterile water for injection (concentration should not exceed 225 units per 0.5 mL) and immediately give subcutaneously. Discard unused reconstituted material.

Multidose vials: Dissolve the contents of 1 multidose vial (1,200 units) with the contents of 1 prefilled syringe (2 mL) containing bacteriostatic water for injection (benzyl alcohol 0.9%). Resulting concentration will be 600 units/mL. Following reconstitution as directed, product will deliver approximately 1,050 units of FSH. Instruct patients to use the accompanying syringes calibrated in FSH units for administration.

➤*Administration:* For subcutaneous administration only. Individualize dosage.

➤*Storage/Stability:*

Single-dose vials – Store vials in the refrigerator or at room temperature (2° to 25°C [36° to 77°F]). Protect from light. Use immediately after reconstitution. Discard unused material.

Multidose vials – Store multidose vials in the refrigerator or at room temperature until reconstituted (25°C [77°F]). Following reconstitution, refrigerate (2° to 8°C [36° to 46°F]) or store at room temperature (2° to 25°C [36° to 77°F]). Protect from light. Discard unused reconstituted solution after 28 days.

Prefilled pens – Store prefilled pens in the refrigerator (2° to 8°C [36° to 46°F]) until dispensed. Upon dispensing, refrigerate pen (2° to 8°C [36° to 46°F]) or store at room temperature (2° to 25°C [36° to 77°F]) for up to 1 month or until the expiration date, whichever occurs first. After the first injection, store pen in the refrigerator (2° to 8°C [36° to 46°F]) or at room temperature (2° to 25°C [36° to 77°F]) for up to 28 days. Protect from light. Do not freeze. Discard unused material after 28 days.

MENOTROPINS
FOLLITROPIN BETA

Rx	**Follistim** AQ Cartridge (Organon)	**Injection:** 175 units per 0.21 mL (delivering 150 units FSH[a] activity)	Benzyl alcohol 10 mg/mL, sucrose 50 mg/mL. In cartridges with *BD micro-fine* pen needles.
		350 units per 0.42 mL (delivering 300 units FSH activity)	Benzyl alcohol 10 mg/mL, sucrose 50 mg/mL. In cartridges with *BD micro-fine* pen needles.
		650 units per 0.78 mL (delivering 600 units FSH activity)	Benzyl alcohol 10 mg/mL, sucrose 50 mg/mL. In cartridges with *BD micro-fine* pen needles.
		975 units per 1.17 mL (delivering 900 units FSH activity)	Benzyl alcohol 10 mg/mL, sucrose 50 mg/mL. In cartridges with *BD micro-fine* pen needles.
	Follistim AQ (Organon)	**Injection:** 75 units per 0.5 mL	Sucrose 25 mg, sodium 7.35 mg. In single-use vials.
		150 units per 0.5 mL	Sucrose 25 mg, sodium 7.35 mg. In single-use vials.

[a] FSH = follicle-stimulating hormone.

FOLLITROPIN BETA — INJECTION

For complete and comparative prescribing information, refer to the Follitropin group monograph.

Indications

➤*Follicle stimulation:* For the development of multiple follicles in ovulatory patients participating in an assisted reproductive technology (ART) program.

➤*OI:* For the induction of ovulation and pregnancy in anovulatory infertile patients in whom the cause of infertility is functional and not due to primary ovarian failure.

Administration and Dosage

➤*Adults:*

Follicle stimulation during assisted reproductive technology –

Maximum dose:

• *Single-use vial* – The maximum individualized daily dose of follitropin beta used in clinical studies is 600 units.

Initial dosage:

• *Cartridge* – Follitropin beta 150 to 225 units or lower is recommended for at least the first 5 days of treatment. Generally, if a starting dose of lyophilized gonadotropin 150 to 225 units is used, then consider using a lower starting dose of follitropin beta. (See Dose Conversion Table.)

• *Single-use vial* – Follitropin beta 150 to 225 units for at least the first 4 days of treatment.

Maintenance dosage: For follitropin beta, consider lower maintenance doses for each patient.

• *Single-use vial* – In clinical studies with responding patients, it was shown that daily maintenance doses ranging from 75 to 300 units for 6 to 12 days are sufficient, although longer treatment may be necessary. However, in patients that were low or poor responders, maintenance doses of 375 to 600 units were administered according to individual response. This later category comprised approximately 10% of the women evaluated during clinical studies.

Dosage adjustment: After the initial dosage, adjust the dose for the individual patient based upon her ovarian response.

Concomitant therapy: During treatment with follitropin beta, when a sufficient number of follicles of adequate size are present, the final maturation of the follicles is induced by administering human chorionic gonadotropin (hCG) at a dose of 5,000 to 10,000 units. Oocyte (egg) retrieval is performed 34 to 36 hours later. The administration of hCG must be withheld in cases where the ovaries are abnormally enlarged on the last day of treatment with follitropin beta. This will reduce the chance of developing ovarian hyperstimulation syndrome (OHSS).

Ovulation induction – For ovulation induction (OI), encourage the couple to have intercourse daily, beginning on the day prior to the administration of hCG and until ovulation becomes apparent from the indices employed for the determination of progestational activity. Take care to ensure insemination.

Usual dosage:

• *Cartridge* – A starting dose of follitropin beta 75 units or lower is recommended for at least the first 7 days of treatment, with dose adjustments at weekly intervals based on patient response. If a starting dose of lyophilized gonadotropin 75 units generally is used, then consider using a lower starting dose of follitropin beta. (See Dose Conversion Table.)

• *Single-use vial* – In studies using follitropin beta, a stepwise, gradually-increasing dosing scheme was used. The starting dose was 75 units of follitropin beta for up to 14 days. The dose was then increased by 37.5 units of follitropin at weekly intervals until follicular growth and/or serum estradiol levels indicated an adequate response.

Maximum dose:

• *Single-use vial* – The maximum individualized daily dose of follitropin beta that has been safely used for OI in patients during clinical trials is 300 units.

Concomitant therapy: Continue treatment until ultrasonic visualizations and/or serum estradiol determinations indicate preovulatory conditions equivalent to or greater than those of the normal individual, followed by hCG 5,000 to 10,000 units. If the ovaries are abnormally enlarged on the last day of treatment with follitropin beta therapy, hCG must be withheld during this course of treatment; this will reduce the chances of developing OHSS.

➤*Dose conversion of follitropin beta administered with the Follistim Pen*: Consider a lower starting dose for gonadotropin stimulation and dose adjustments during gonadotropin stimulation for each patient. For that purpose, the following dose conversion table might be a useful reference.

Follitropin Beta Administered with the *Follistim Pen* Dose Conversion Table[a]

Lyophilized recombinant FSH dosing in ampules or vials, using conventional syringe	Follitropin beta dosing with the *Follistim Pen*
75 units	50 units
150 units	125 units
225 units	175 units
300 units	250 units
375 units	300 units
450 units	375 units

[a] Each value represents an 18% difference rounded to the nearest 25-unit increment.

Follitropin beta is delivered by the *Follistim Pen*, which accurately delivers the dose to which it is set. In a clinical bioavailability study that compared administration of the dissolved lyophilized follitropin beta preparation using a conventional syringe with needle and a ready-to-use follitropin beta solution in a cartridge injected with the pen device, it was shown that the pen device delivered, on average, an 18% higher amount of follitropin beta.

This difference is because of the accurate dosing obtained with the *Follistim Pen* compared with a conventional syringe. This 18% difference corresponds to a similar difference in serum FSH concentrations caused by differences between the anticipated and the actual volume of follitropin beta injected with the conventional syringe.

The net deliverable doses of 150, 300, 600, and 900 units are based upon a maximum of 2 injections of 75 units (for 150 units), 4 injections of 75 units (for 300 units), 6 injections of 100 units (for 600 units), and 9 injections of 100 units (for 900 units).

➤*Administration:*

Cartridges – Administer only as a subcutaneous injection.

Single-use vial – Administer as a subcutaneous or intramuscular injection.

➤*Admixture compatibility:* Do not add or combine other drugs into the follitropin beta cartridge. Do not mix follitropin beta with any other medicines in the same vial or syringe.

➤*Storage/Stability:*

Cartridges – Refrigerate at 2° to 8°C (36° to 46°F) until dispensed. Upon dispensing, the product may be stored by the patient at 2° to 8°C (36° to 46°F) until the expiration date or at 25°C (77°F) for 3 months or until expiration date, whichever occurs first. Once the rubber stopper of the follitropin beta cartridge has been pierced by a needle, the product can only be stored for a maximum of 28 days at 2° to 25°C (36° to 77°F). Protect from light. Do not freeze.

Single-use vial – Refrigerate at 2° to 8°C (36° to 46°F) until dispensed. Upon dispensing, the product may be stored by the patient at 2° to 8°C (36° to 46°F) until the expiration date or at or below 25°C (77°F) for 3 months or until expiration date, whichever occurs first. Protect from light; keep container in carton. Do not freeze.

GONADOTROPINS
MENOTROPINS

Rx	**Menopur** (Ferring)	**Powder or pellet for injection, lyophilized:** 75 units FSH activity, 75 units LH activity	In vials with diluent.
Rx	**Repronex** (Ferring)		In vials with diluent.
Rx	**Repronex** (Ferring)	**Powder or pellet for injection, lyophilized:** 150 units FSH activity, 150 units LH activity	In vials with diluent.

MENOTROPINS — INJECTION

Indications

➤*Menopur*: Menotropins, administered subcutaneously, are indicated for the development of multiple follicles and pregnancy in the ovulatory patients participating in the assisted reproductive technology (ART) program.

➤*Repronex*: Menotropins, in conjunction with human chorionic gonadotropin (hCG), is indicated for multiple follicular development (controlled ovarian stimulation) and ovulation induction in patients who have previously received pituitary suppression.

➤*Off-label uses:* Treatment of male infertility caused by hypogonadotropic hypogonadism when used in conjunction with hCG.

Administration and Dosage

➤*Adults:*

Development of multiple follicles and pregnancy in ovulatory patients (Menopur and Repronex) – For patients participating in the assisted reproductive technologies (ART) program.

Maximum dose: The maximum daily dose of menotropins given should not exceed 450 units.

Initial dosage: 225 units for patients who have received gonadotropin-releasing hormone (GnRH) agonist pituitary suppression.

Dosage adjustment: Based on clinical monitoring (including serum estradiol levels and vaginal ultrasound results), subsequent dosing, following initial dosage, should be adjusted according to individual patient response.

MENOTROPINS — INJECTION

Adjustments in dose should not be made more frequently than once every 2 days and should not exceed more than 75 to 150 units/adjustment for *Repronex* or 150 units/adjustment for *Menopur*.

Duration of therapy: Dosing beyond 12 days for *Repronex* and 20 days for *Menopur* is not recommended.

Concomitant therapy: Once adequate follicular development is evident, hCG (5,000 to 10,000 units) should be administered to induce final follicular maturation in preparation for oocyte retrieval. The administration of hCG must be withheld in cases in which the ovaries are abnormally enlarged on the last day of therapy. This should reduce the chance of developing Ovarian Hyperstimulation Syndrome (OHSS).

Infertile patients with oligoanovulation (Repronex only) – The dose of menotropins to stimulate development of ovarian follicles must be individualized for each patient. The lowest dose consistent with achieving good results based on clinical experience and reported clinical data should be used.

Maximum dose: The maximum daily dose of menotropins should not exceed 450 units.

Initial dosage: 150 units daily for the first 5 days of treatment for patients who have received GnRH agonist or antagonist pituitary suppression.

Dosage adjustment: Based on clinical monitoring (including serum estradiol levels and vaginal ultrasound results) subsequent dosing, following initial dosage, should be adjusted according to individual patient response.

Adjustments in dose should not be made more frequently than once every 2 days and should not exceed more than 75 to 150 units/adjustment.

Duration of therapy: Dosing beyond 12 days is not recommended.

Concomitant therapy: If patient response to menotropins is appropriate, hCG (5,000 to 10,000 units) should be given 1 day following the last dose of menotropins. The hCG should be withheld if the serum estradiol is more than 2,000 pg/mL, the ovaries are abnormally enlarged, or abdominal pain occurs, and the patient should be advised to refrain from intercourse. These precautions may reduce the risk of OHSS and multiple gestation.

Patients should be followed closely for at least 2 weeks after hCG administration. If there is inadequate follicle development or ovulation without subsequent pregnancy, the course of treatment with menotropins may be repeated.

The couple should be encouraged to have intercourse daily, beginning on the day prior to the administration of hCG until ovulation becomes apparent from the indices employed for the determination of progestational activity. In the light of the foregoing indices and parameters mentioned, it should become obvious that, unless a health care provider is willing to devote considerable time to these patients and be familiar with and conduct the necessary laboratory studies, menotropins should not be used.

➤*Preparation for administration:*

Menopur – Dissolve the contents of 1 to 6 vials of menotropins in 1 mL of sterile saline and administer subcutaneously immediately.

Repronex – Dissolve the contents of 1 to 6 vials of menotropins in 1 to 2 mL of sterile saline and administer subcutaneously or intramuscularly immediately.

➤*Administration:* The lower abdomen (alternating sides) should be used for subcutaneous administration.

Use immediately after reconstitution. Any unused reconstituted material should be discarded.

➤*Storage/Stability:* Lyophilized powder may be stored refrigerated or at room temperature (3° to 25°C; 37° to 77°F). Protect from light.

Actions

➤*Pharmacology:* Menotropins administered for 7 to 20 days with *Menopur* or 7 to 12 days with *Repronex* produces ovarian follicular growth and maturation in women who do not have primary ovarian failure. In order to produce final follicular maturation and ovulation in the absence of an endogenous LH surge, hCG must be administered following menotropin treatment at a time when patient monitoring indicates sufficient follicular development has occurred.

➤*Pharmacokinetics:*

Absorption/Distribution – Human tissue or organ distribution of FSH and LH have not been studied for menotropins.

Menopur: The subcutaneous route of administration trends toward greater bioavailability than the IM route for single and multiple doses of menotropins.

Two open-label, randomized, controlled trials were conducted to assess the pharmacokinetics of menotropins. Study 2003-02 compared single doses of subcutaneous administration of the US and European formulations of menotropins in 57 healthy, premenopausal women who had undergone pituitary suppression. The study established that the 2 formulations are bioequivalent. Study 2000-03 assessed single and multiple doses of menotropins administered subcutaneously and IM in a 3-phase, crossover design in 33 healthy, premenopausal women who had undergone pituitary suppression. The primary pharmacokinetic end points were FSH AUC and C_{max} values. The results are summarized in the following table.

Mean (± SD) FSH Pharmacokinetic Parameters Following Menotropins Administration (Study 2000-03)

Pharmacokinetic parameters	Single dose (225 units)		Multiple dose (225 units × 1 day, then 150 units × 6 days)	
	Subcutaneous	IM	Subcutaneous	IM
C_{max} (milliunits/mL)	8.5 (2.5)	7.8 (2.4)	15 (3.6)	12.5 (2.3)
T_{max} (h)	17.9 (5.8)	27.5 (25.4)	8 (3)	9 (7)
AUC[a] (milliunits•h/mL)	726.2 (243)	656.1 (233.7)	622.7 (153)	546.2 (91.2)

[a] Single dose C_{max} AUC_{120} and multiple dose $C_{max_{ss}}$, AUC_{ss}.

Repronex: The geometric mean of FSH maximum plasma drug concentration (C_{max}) and area under the curve ($AUC_{0-\infty}$) upon single-dose subcutaneous administration of menotropins is 5.62 milliunits/mL and 385.2 milliunits•h/mL, respectively; the corresponding geometric median of FSH time to maximum concentration (T_{max}) is 12 hours. The geometric mean of FSH C_{max} and $AUC_{0-\infty}$ upon single-dose IM administration of menotropins is 4.15 milliunits/mL and 320.1 milliunits•h/mL, respectively; the corresponding geometric median of FSH T_{max} is 18 hours.

Single doses of menotropins 300 units were administered subcutaneously and IM in a 2-period, crossover study to 16 healthy women while their endogenous FSH and LH were being suppressed. Serum FSH concentrations were determined. Based on the ratio of FSH C_{max} and $AUC_{0-\infty}$, subcutaneous and IM administration of menotropins are not bioequivalent. Compared with IM administration, the subcutaneous administration of menotropins results in an increase of FSH C_{max} and $AUC_{0-\infty}$ by 35% and 20%, respectively.

Based on 2 subjects who received either the highest subcutaneous or IM menotropins dose, FSH pharmacokinetics appears to be linear up to menotropins 450 units. The mean accumulation factors for FSH upon 6 doses of subcutaneous or IM menotropins 150 to 450 units/day are 1.6 and 1.4, respectively. Upon 6 doses of subcutaneous or IM menotropins 150 units/day, the observed serum FSH concentrations range from 1.7 to 15.9 milliunits/mL and 0.5 to 10.1 milliunits/mL, respectively. The FSH pharmacokinetic parameters from population modeling for these 2 studies are given in the following table.

FSH Pharmacokinetic Parameters[a] Upon Menotropins Administration

FSH parameter	Single dose[b]		Multiple dose[c]	
	Subcutaneous	IM	Subcutaneous	IM
$K_a(h^{-1})$	0.128 (42.1)	0.117 (21.3)	0.076 (46.3)	0.064 (63.2)
Cl/F[d] (L/h)	0.77 (17.1)	0.94 (6.9)	1.11 (39.5)	1.44 (43.5)
V/F[e] (L)	39.37 (14.1)	57.68 (11.4)	23.09 (8.3)	23.5 (2.5)

[a] Mean (coefficient of variation [CV]%).
[b] *Menogon* (European formulation of menotropins).
[c] *Repronex.*
[d] Cl/F = apparent plasma clearance.
[e] V/F = apparent volume of distribution.

Metabolism/Excretion – Metabolism of FSH and LH have not been studied for menotropins in humans.

Menopur: The elimination half-lives for FSH in the multiple-dose phase were similar (11 to 13 hours) for *Menopur* subcutaneous and *Menopur* IM.

Repronex: The mean elimination half-lives of FSH upon single-dose subcutaneous and IM administration of *Repronex* are 53.7 and 59.2 hours, respectively.

Contraindications

Menotropins are contraindicated in women who have: a high FSH level indicating primary ovarian failure; uncontrolled thyroid and adrenal dysfunction; an organic intracranial lesion, such as a pituitary tumor; the presence of any cause of infertility other than anovulation, unless they are candidates for IVF (*Repronex* only); sex hormone-dependent tumors of the reproductive tract and accessory organs (*Menopur* only); abnormal uterine bleeding of undetermined origin; ovarian cysts or enlargement not caused by polycystic ovary syndrome; prior hypersensitivity to menotropins; menotropins is not indicated in women who are pregnant. There are limited human data on the effects of menotropins when administered during pregnancy.

Warnings/Precautions

➤*Administration:* Menotropins should only be used by health care providers who are thoroughly familiar with infertility problems. It is a potent gonadotropic substance capable of causing OHSS in women with or without pulmonary or vascular complications and mild to severe adverse reactions in women. Gonadotropin therapy requires a certain time commitment by health care providers and supportive health professionals, and its use requires the availability of appropriate monitoring facilities.

➤*Overstimulation of the ovary during menotropins therapy:*

Ovarian enlargement – Mild to moderate uncomplicated ovarian enlargement, which may be accompanied by abdominal distension and/or abdominal pain, occurs in approximately 5% to 10% of women treated with menotropins and hCG and generally regresses without treatment within 2 or 3 weeks. The lowest dose consistent with expectation of good results and careful monitoring of ovarian response can further minimize the risk of overstimulation.

MENOTROPINS — INJECTION

To minimize the hazard associated with the occasional abnormal ovarian enlargement that may occur with menotropins and hCG therapy, use the lowest dose consistent with expectation of good results. Careful monitoring of ovarian response can further minimize the risk of overstimulation.

If the ovaries are abnormally enlarged on the last day of menotropins therapy, do not administer hCG in this course of treatment; this will reduce the chances of development of the OHSS.

OHSS – OHSS is a medical event distinct from uncomplicated ovarian enlargement. OHSS may progress rapidly to become a serious medical event. It is characterized by an apparent dramatic increase in vascular permeability that can result in a rapid accumulation of fluid in the peritoneal cavity, thorax, and, potentially, the pericardium. The early warning signs of development of OHSS are severe pelvic pain, nausea, vomiting, and weight gain. The following symptomatology has been seen with cases of OHSS: abdominal pain; abdominal distension; GI symptoms including nausea, vomiting, and diarrhea; severe ovarian enlargement; weight gain; dyspnea; and oliguria. Clinical evaluation may reveal hypovolemia, hemoconcentration, electrolyte imbalances, ascites, hemoperitoneum, pleural effusions, hydrothorax, acute pulmonary distress, and thromboembolic events. Transient liver function test abnormalities suggestive of hepatic dysfunction, which may be accompanied by morphologic changes on liver biopsy, have been reported in association with the OHSS.

In the IVF clinical study, 0399E, OHSS occurred in 7.2% of 373 menotropin-treated women.

OHSS occurred in 3 of 125 (2.4%) of *Repronex*-treated women during ART clinical studies. None of these cases was classified as severe. In OI clinical studies, 4 of 72 (5.5%) of *Repronex*-treated women developed OHSS and 1 of these cases was classified as severe (1.4%). Cases of OHSS are more common, severe, and protracted if pregnancy occurs. OHSS develops rapidly; therefore, follow patients for at least 2 weeks after hCG administration. Most often, OHSS occurs after treatment has been discontinued and reaches its maximum at about 7 to 10 days following treatment. Usually, OHSS resolves spontaneously with the onset of menses. If there is evidence that OHSS may be developing prior to hCG administration, withhold the hCG.

If severe OHSS occurs, stop treatment and hospitalize the patient.

Consult a health care provider experienced in the management of the syndrome or fluid and electrolyte imbalances.

Repronex: Treatment is primarily symptomatic, consisting of bed rest, fluid and electrolyte management, and analgesics if needed. The phenomenon of hemoconcentration associated with fluid loss into the peritoneal cavity, pleural cavity, and the pericardial cavity has occurred and should be thoroughly assessed in the following manner:

- Fluid intake and output
- Weight
- Hematocrit
- Serum and urinary electrolytes
- Urine specific gravity
- Serum urea nitrogen (BUN) and creatinine
- Abdominal girthThese determinations are to be performed daily or more often if the need arises.

With OHSS there is an increased risk of injury to the ovary. Do not remove the ascitic, pleural, and pericardial fluid unless absolutely necessary to relieve symptoms such as pulmonary distress or cardiac tamponade. Avoid pelvic examination, which may cause rupture of an ovarian cyst and may result in hemoperitoneum. If this does occur, and if bleeding becomes such that surgery is required, design the surgical treatment to control bleeding and to retain as much ovarian tissue as possible. Intercourse is prohibited in patients in whom significant ovarian enlargement occurs after ovulation because of the danger of hemoperitoneum resulting from ruptured ovarian cysts.

- *Management of OHSS* – The management of OHSS may be divided into 3 phases: acute, chronic, and resolution. Because the use of diuretics can accentuate the diminished intravascular volume, avoid diuretics except in the late phase of resolution as described in the following section.

Acute phase: During the acute phase, design management to prevent hemoconcentration due to loss of intravascular volume to the third space and to minimize the risk of thromboembolic phenomena and kidney damage. Treatment is designed to normalize electrolytes while maintaining an acceptable but somewhat reduced intravascular volume. Full correction of the intravascular volume deficit may lead to an unacceptable increase in the amount of third space fluid accumulation. Management includes administration of limited intravenous (IV) fluids, electrolytes, and human serum albumin. Monitoring for the development of hyperkalemia is recommended.

Chronic phase: After stabilizing the patient during the acute phase, limit excessive fluid accumulation in the third space by instituting severe potassium, sodium, and fluid restriction.

Resolution phase: A fall in hematocrit and an increasing urinary output without an increased intake are observed due to the return of third space fluid to the intravascular compartment. Peripheral and/or pulmonary edema may result if the kidneys are unable to excrete third-space fluid as rapidly as it is mobilized. Diuretics may be indicated during the resolution phase if necessary to combat pulmonary edema.

➤*Multiple pregnancies:*

Menopur – In the clinical trial, multiple pregnancy, as diagnosed by ultrasound, occurred in 35.3% (n = 30) of 85 total pregnancies.

Advise the patient and her partner of the potential risk of multiple births before starting treatment.

Repronex – Multiple pregnancies have occurred following treatment with IM and subcutaneous menotropins. In a clinical trial for ovulation induction in which menotropins IM and menotropins subcutaneous were directly compared, the rates of multiple pregnancies were as follows. Of the 4 clinical pregnancies with menotropins IM, 2 were single and 2 were multiple pregnancies. Both multiple pregnancies were triplet pregnancies. Of the 6 clinical pregnancies with menotropins subcutaneous, 3 were single and 3 were multiple pregnancies. The 3 multiple pregnancies included 1 twin pregnancy and 2 quadruplet pregnancies.

In a clinical trial of IVF patients in which menotropins IM and menotropins subcutaneous were directly compared, the rates of multiple pregnancies were as follows. Of the 24 continuing pregnancies on menotropins IM, 14 were single and 10 were multiple pregnancies. The 10 multiple pregnancies included 3 triplet and 7 twin pregnancies. Of the 29 continuing pregnancies on subcutaneous menotropins, 14 were single and 15 were multiple pregnancies. The 15 multiple pregnancies included 3 quadruplet, 3 triplet, and 9 twin pregnancies. Advise the patient and her partner of the potential risk of multiple births before starting treatment.

➤*Pulmonary and vascular complications:* Serious pulmonary conditions (eg, atelectasis, acute respiratory distress syndrome) have been reported. In addition, thromboembolic events in association with, and separate from, the OHSS have been reported following menotropins therapy. Intravascular thrombosis and embolism, which may originate in venous or arterial vessels, can result in reduced blood flow to critical organs or the extremities. Sequelae of such events have included venous thrombophlebitis, pulmonary embolism, pulmonary infarction, cerebral vascular occlusion (stroke), and arterial occlusion resulting in loss of limb. In rare cases, pulmonary complications and/or thromboembolic events have resulted in death.

➤*Diagnosis:* Give careful attention to a diagnosis of infertility in the selection of candidates for menotropins therapy.

➤*Hypersensitivity reactions:* Hypersensitivity/anaphylactic reactions associated with menotropins administration have been reported in some patients. These reactions presented as generalized urticaria, facial edema, angioneurotic edema, or dyspnea suggestive of laryngeal edema. The relationship of these symptoms to uncharacterized urinary proteins is uncertain.

➤*Pregnancy: Category X.* Menotropins are not indicated in women who are pregnant. There are limited human data on the effects of menotropins when administered during pregnancy.

With menotropin therapy, congenital abnormalities have been reported. One infant was shown to have multiple congenital anomalies consisting of aplasia of the sigmoid colon, cecovesicle fistula, bifid scrotum, meningocele, bilateral internal tibial torsion, and right metatarsus adductus. Other reported anomalies include imperforate anus, congenital heart lesions, supernumerary digits, hypospadias, exstrophy of the bladder, Down syndrome, and hydrocephalus. The incidence of congenital abnormalities does not exceed that found in the general population.

➤*Lactation:* It is not known whether this drug is excreted in human milk. Because many drugs are excreted in human milk, exercise caution if administering menotropins to a breast-feeding woman.

➤*Children:* Safety and efficacy in pediatric patients have not been established.

➤*Monitoring:*

Treatment for induction of ovulation – The combination of estradiol levels and ultrasonography are useful for monitoring the growth and development of follicles, timing hCG administration, and minimizing the risk of the OHSS and multiple gestation.

The clinical confirmation of ovulation, is determined by the following:

- A rise in basal body temperature.
- Increase in serum progesterone.
- Menstruation following the shift in basal body temperature.

When used in conjunction with indices of progesterone production, sonographic visualization of the ovaries will assist in determining if ovulation has occurred. Sonographic evidence of ovulation may include the following:

- Fluid in the cul-de-sac.
- Ovarian stigmata.
- Collapsed follicle.

Because of the subjectivity of the various tests for the determination of follicular maturation and ovulation, it cannot be overemphasized that the health care provider should choose tests with which he/she is thoroughly familiar.

Drug Interactions

No drug/drug interaction studies have been conducted for menotropins in humans.

Adverse Reactions

➤*Menopur*: The safety of menotropins was examined in 3 clinical studies that enrolled a total of 575 patients receiving menotropins in the IVF and OI studies. All adverse reactions (without regard to causality assessment) occurring at an incidence of at least 2% in women treated with menotropins are listed in the following table.

MENOTROPINS — INJECTION

Menopur (IM and Subcutaneous) Adverse Reactions in Women Undergoing IVF and OI (≥ 2%)

Adverse reactions	IVF[a] (n = 499)	OI[b] (n = 76)
CNS		
Dizziness	13 (2.6%)	0 (0%)
Headache	170 (34.1%)	12 (15.8%)
Migraine	12 (2.4%)	0 (0%)
GI		
Abdomen enlarged	12 (2.4%)	0 (0%)
Abdominal cramps	30 (6%)	5 (6.6%)
Abdominal fullness	16 (3.2%)	7 (9.2%)
Abdominal pain	88 (17.6%)	7 (9.2%)
Constipation	8 (1.6%)	0 (0%)
Diarrhea	14 (2.8%)	2 (2.6%)
Nausea	60 (12%)	6 (7.9%)
Vomiting	21 (4.2%)	2 (2.6%)
GU		
Breast tenderness	9 (1.8%)	2 (2.6%)
Hot flash	3 (0.6%)	2 (2.6%)
Menstrual disorder	16 (3.2%)	0 (0%)
OHSS	19 (3.8%)	10 (13.2%)
Pelvic cramps	0 (0%)	3 (3.9%)
Pelvic discomfort	2 (0.4%)	2 (2.6%)
Postretrieval pain	32 (6.4%)	0 (0%)
Uterine spasm	8 (1.6%)	3 (3.9%)
Respiratory		
Cough increased	8 (1.6%)	2 (2.6%)
Respiratory disorder	29 (5.8%)	3 (3.9%)
Miscellaneous		
Back pain	16 (3.2%)	0 (0%)
Elevated estradiol	12 (2.4%)	0 (0%)
Flu syndrome	13 (2.6%)	1 (1.3%)
Flushing	12 (2.4%)	0 (0%)
Injection site pain	27 (5.4%)	0 (0%)
Injection site reaction	48 (9.6%)	9 (11.8%)
Malaise	14 (2.8%)	2 (2.6%)
Pain	16 (3.2%)	2 (2.6%)

[a] Includes IM and subcutaneous subjects from protocols MFK/IVF/0399E and *Menopur* 2000-02.
[b] Includes IM and subcutaneous subjects from protocol *Menopur* 2000-01.

➤*Repronex*: The following adverse reactions, reported during menotropins therapy, are listed in decreasing order of potential severity:
- Pulmonary and vascular complications
- OHSS
- Hemoperitoneum
- Adnexal torsion (as a complication of ovarian enlargement)
- Mild-to-moderate ovarian enlargement
- Ovarian cysts
- Abdominal pain
- Sensitivity to menotropins. (Febrile reactions suggestive of allergic response have been reported following the administration of menotropins. Flu-like symptoms including fever, chills, musculoskeletal aches, joint pains, nausea, headaches, and malaise also have been reported.)
- GI symptoms (nausea, vomiting, diarrhea, abdominal cramps, bloating)
- Pain, rash, swelling, or irritation at the site of injection
- Body rashes
- Dizziness, dyspnea, tachycardia, tachypnea

The following medical events have been reported subsequent to pregnancies resulting from menotropins therapy: ectopic pregnancy, congenital abnormalities.

There have been infrequent reports of ovarian neoplasms, both benign and malignant, in women who have undergone multiple-drug regimens for ovulation induction; however, a causal relationship has not been established.

Adverse reactions occurring in at least 1% of patients exposed to menotropins IM or menotropins subcutaneous are described in the following table:

***Repronex* Adverse Reactions (≥ 1%)**

Adverse reactions	Menotropins IM (n = 101)	Menotropins subcutaneous (n = 96)
GI		
Abdominal cramping	7 (6.9%)	5 (5.2%)
Abdominal pain	5 (5%)	7 (7.3%)
Diarrhea	0 (0%)	2 (2.1%)
Enlarged abdomen	6 (6%)	2 (2.1%)
Nausea	4 (4%)	7 (7.3%)
Vomiting	0 (0%)	3 (3.1%)
GU		
Breast tenderness	2 (2%)	2 (2.1%)
Ectopic pregnancy	1 (1%)	1 (1%)
OHSS	2 (2%)	5 (5.2%)
Ovarian disease	3 (3%)	8 (8.3%)
Pelvic pain	3 (3%)	1 (1%)
Vaginal hemorrhage	8 (7.9%)	3 (3.1%)
Local		
Injection site edema	1 (1%)	8 (8.3%)[a]
Injection site reaction	2 (2%)	8 (8.3%)[a]
Miscellaneous		
Dyspnea	1 (1%)	2 (2.1%)
Headache	6 (6%)	5 (5.2%)
Infection	1 (1%)	0 (0%)

[a] Fisher exact/chi-square tests (significant for *Repronex* subcutaneous vs *Repronex* IM).

Overdosage

Aside from possible ovarian hyperstimulation, little is known concerning the consequences of acute overdosage with menotropins.

Patient Information

Prior to therapy, inform patients of the duration of treatment and the monitoring of their condition that will be required. Also discuss possible adverse reactions and the risk of multiple births.

GONADOTROPINS
LUTROPIN ALFA

Rx	**Luveris** (Serono)	**Powder for injection, lyophilized:** 82.5 units/vial	48 mg sucrose. In single-dose vials. Delivers 75 units lutropin alfa after reconstitution.

LUTROPIN ALFA — INJECTION

Indications

➤*Follicle stimulation:* Lutropin alfa coadministered with follitropin alfa (*Gonal-F*) is indicated for stimulation of follicular development in infertile, hypogonadotropic, hypogonadal women with profound luteinizing hormone (LH) deficiency (LH less than 1.2 units/L). A definitive effect on pregnancy in this population has not been demonstrated. The safety and efficacy of concomitant administration of lutropin alfa with any other preparation of recombinant human follicle stimulating hormone (FSH) or urinary human FSH is unknown.

Administration and Dosage

➤*General dosing considerations:* Encourage the couple to have intercourse daily, beginning on the day prior to hCG administration until ovulation becomes apparent in the indices used for the determination of progestational activity.

In light of the indices and parameters mentioned, it should become obvious that, unless a health care provider is willing to devote considerable time to these patients and be familiar with and conduct the necessary laboratory studies, he/she should not prescribe lutropin alfa.

➤*Adults:*

Follicle stimulation –

Initial dosage: 75 units lutropin alfa SQ coadministered with follitropin alfa in the initial treatment cycle. (See Concomitant therapy.)

Maintenance dosage: Individualize doses administered in subsequent cycles for each patient based on her response in the preceding cycle. Doses of follitropin alfa greater than 225 units daily are not routinely recommended.

As in the initial cycle, human chorionic gonadotropin (hCG) must be given to complete follicular development and induce ovulation. Follow the precautions described to minimize the chance of developing ovarian hyperstimulation syndrome. (See Discontinuation of therapy.)

Duration of therapy: Administer lutropin alfa and follitropin alfa daily until adequate follicular development is indicated by ovary ultrasonography

LUTROPIN ALFA — INJECTION

and serum estradiol. Treatment duration should not normally exceed 14 days unless signs of imminent follicular development are present.

Concomitant therapy: Coadminister with follitropin alfa 75 to 150 units SQ as 2 separate injections.

To complete follicular development and effect ovulation in the absence of an endogenous LH surge, give hCG 1 day after the last dose of lutropin alfa and follitropin alfa. Withhold treatment with hCG if the ovaries are abnormally enlarged or if excessive estradiol production has occurred.

Discontinuation of therapy: If the ovaries are abnormally enlarged or abdominal pain occurs, discontinue treatment with lutropin alfa and follitropin alfa and do not administer hCG. Advise the patient not to have intercourse; this may reduce the chances of developing ovarian hyperstimulation syndrome and, should spontaneous ovulation occur, reduce the chances of multiple gestation. Conduct a follow-up visit in the luteal phase.

➤*Preparation for administration:* Dissolve the contents of 1 vial of lutropin alfa in 1 mL sterile water for injection. Reconstitute and administer follitropin alfa as directed in the prescriber labeling for this product.

Mix gently. Do not shake.

➤*Administration:* For subcutaneous use only.

Administer entire contents of each vial subcutaneously as separate injections. For single use. Use immediately after reconstitution. Discard any unused reconstituted material.

Lutropin alfa and follitropin alfa may be self-administered by the patient. Follow the directions below for reconstituting and injecting as separate injections of lutropin alfa and follitropin alfa.

Instructions for self-administration –

Step 1: Prepare the vials: Wash hands thoroughly with soap and water. Begin by opening the cartons of lutropin alfa. Remove the plastic flip-tops from the vial of lutropin alfa powder and the vial of diluent provided with lutropin alfa. After removing the plastic flip-tops, wipe the rubber stoppers with alcohol. Do not touch the rubber stoppers after they are wiped.

Step 2: Withdraw the water into the syringe: Carefully remove the needle cover. Do not touch the needle or allow the needle to touch any surface. After removing the needle cover, draw air into the syringe by slowly pulling back the plunger to the 1 mL mark. Place the vial of diluent on a hard, flat surface. Carefully insert the needle through the rubber stopper into the vial with the sterile water (diluent). Gently inject the air into the vial (the injected air creates pressure, which makes withdrawing the solution easier). Without removing the needle, turn the vial upside down and withdraw all of the water into the syringe, making sure the tip of the needle remains in the water. Remove the needle from the vial.

Step 3: Inject the water into the lutropin alfa vial: Place the vial containing the lutropin alfa powder on a hard, flat surface. Insert the needle through the rubber stopper into the vial. Keep the syringe in a straight, upright position as you insert it through the center of the rubber stopper, or it may be difficult to depress the plunger. After inserting the needle, slowly inject the sterile water (diluent) by depressing the plunger on the syringe into the vial of lutropin alfa powder.

Step 4: Gently dissolve the lutropin alfa powder: Leaving the needle in the vial, gently rotate the vial between your fingers until all of the powder is dissolved. Do not shake. Check that the solution is clear and colorless. Do not use if the solution is cloudy, discolored, or contains particles.

Step 5: Withdraw the lutropin alfa solution from the vial: Without removing the needle, turn the vial upside down and withdraw all of the lutropin alfa solution into the syringe. Make sure the tip of the needle remains in the solution by slowly backing the needle out of the vial to withdraw as much of the solution as possible. Next, remove the needle from the vial.

Step 6: Replace needle and remove air bubbles in the syringe: Recap the syringe needle and twist the cap and needle off of syringe. Twist a new needle onto the end of the syringe and carefully remove the cap of the needle. To remove any air bubbles in the syringe, point the needle up and gently tap the syringe. When all the bubbles float to the top, slightly push the plunger until a small drop or two of solution begins to appear from the tip of the needle.

Step 7: Recap the syringe needle: Recap the syringe needle. Do not touch the needle or allow the needle to touch any surface. Carefully lay the syringe down on a flat, clean surface.

Step 8: Carefully clean the injection site: Suitable injection sites on the stomach (a few inches above or below the navel) will be advised by your fertility specialist. Occasionally, your fertility specialist may suggest an alternative site. Make yourself comfortable by sitting or lying down. Carefully clean the injection site with an alcohol wipe and allow it to air-dry.

Step 9: Administer the injection: Remove the needle cap from the syringe needle. Hold the syringe like a pencil. With the other hand, pinch the skin together. Using a dart-like motion, insert the needle at a 45° to 90° angle (just under the skin) into the pad of tissue as shown or as directed by your health care provider.

Do not inject into a vein. Release the hand pinching the skin and depress the plunger in a slow, steady motion until all the medication is injected.

Step 10: Gently withdraw the needle: Withdraw the needle.

Step 11: Storage and clean up: Discard the used needle and syringe into your safety container. Place gauze over the injection site. If any bleeding occurs, apply gentle pressure. If bleeding does not stop within a few minutes, place a clean piece of gauze over the injection site and cover it with an adhesive bandage. Remember that the injection materials must be kept sterile and cannot be reused.

➤*Storage/Stability:* Vials may be refrigerated or stored at room temperature (2° to 25°C; 36° to 77°F). Protect from light. Store in original package.

Actions

➤*Pharmacology:* The physicochemical, immunological, and biological activities of lutropin alfa are comparable with those of human pituitary LH. In the ovaries during the follicular phase, LH stimulates theca cells to secrete androgens that will be used as the substrate by granulosa cell aromatase enzyme to produce estradiol, supporting FSH-induced follicular development. Lutropin alfa is administered concomitantly with follitropin alfa to stimulate development of a potentially competent follicle and to indirectly prepare the reproductive tract for implantation and pregnancy.

➤*Pharmacokinetics:*

Absorption/Distribution – Following subcutaneous administration of lutropin alfa, maximum serum concentration is reached after approximately 4 to 16 hours. The mean absolute bioavailability of lutropin alfa following a single subcutaneous injection (at a much higher dose to allow proper quantification [10,000 units]) to healthy women is 56 ± 23%, supported by an immunoassay method. There were no statistical differences between the intramuscular and subcutaneous routes of administration for C_{max}, T_{max}, or bioavailability.

Following an IV dose of 300 units of lutropin alfa, a rapid distribution phase ($t_{½λ1}$ of approximately 1 hour) and a terminal half-life ($t_{½}$) of approximately 11 hours were observed for r-hLH. The steady state volume of distribution (V_{ss}) was approximately 10 L. Mean residence time (MRT) was approximately 6 hours.

When given by IV administration, lutropin alfa demonstrates linear pharmacokinetics over the 300 to 40,000 units dose range. Following a 75 unit dose, the concentration range is too small to allow proper quantification of the pharmacokinetic parameters. The disposition of r-hLH is adequately described by a biexponential model.

Following administration of lutropin alfa 150 units, r-hLH pharmacokinetics are described in the following table.

Pharmacokinetic Parameters[a] (mean ± SD) of r-hLH After Single-Dose Subcutaneous Administration of Lutropin Alfa in Pituitary Desensitized Healthy Female Volunteers

Parameter[a]	Lutropin alfa 150 units subcutaneous
C_{max} (units/L)	1.1 ± 0.3
T_{max} (h)[b]	6 (3 to 9)
AUC (h•units/L)	44 ± 44
$T_{½}$ (h)	14 ± 8

[a] C_{max}: peak concentration; T_{max}: time of C_{max}; AUC: total area under the curve; $t_{½}$: elimination half-life
[b] Median (range).

Metabolism/Excretion – Following subcutaneous administration of lutropin alfa, r-hLH is eliminated from the body with a mean terminal half-life of about 18 hours. Total body clearance is approximately 2 to 3 L/h with less than 5% of the dose being excreted unchanged renally.

Following subcutaneous administration, the terminal half-life is slightly longer than after IV administration. Upon repeated daily administration, a modest accumulation takes place (accumulation ratio of 1.6 ± 0.8).

Contraindications

Lutropin alfa is contraindicated in women who exhibit the following: prior hypersensitivity to hLH preparations or one of their excipients; primary ovarian failure; uncontrolled thyroid or adrenal dysfunction; uncontrolled organic intracranial lesion such as a pituitary tumor; abnormal uterine bleeding of undetermined origin; ovarian cyst or enlargement of undetermined origin; sex hormone dependent tumors of the reproductive tract and accessory organs; pregnancy.

Warnings/Precautions

➤*Administration:* Gonadotropins, including lutropin alfa, should only be used by health care providers who are thoroughly familiar with infertility problems and their management. Like other gonadotropin products, lutropin alfa is a potent gonadotropic substance capable of contributing to the development of ovarian hyperstimulation syndrome in women with or without pulmonary or vascular complications. Gonadotropin therapy requires a certain time commitment by health care providers, and requires the availability of appropriate monitoring facilities. Safe and effective use of lutropin alfa requires monitoring of ovarian response with serum estradiol and ovary ultrasound on a regular basis.

➤*Overstimulation of the ovary:*

Ovarian enlargement – Mild to moderate uncomplicated ovarian enlargement, which may be accompanied by abdominal distension and/or abdominal pain, may occur in patients treated with gonadotropins (such as lutropin alfa). These conditions generally regress without treatment within 2 or 3 weeks. Careful monitoring of ovarian response can further minimize the risk of overstimulation.

If the ovaries are abnormally enlarged on the last day of therapy with lutropin alfa and follitropin alfa, do not administer hCG in this course of therapy. This will reduce the risk of development of ovarian hyperstimulation syndrome.

Ovarian hyperstimulation syndrome – Ovarian hyperstimulation syndrome is a medical event distinct from uncomplicated ovarian enlargement. Severe ovarian hyperstimulation syndrome may progress rapidly (within 24 hours to several days) to become a serious medical event. It is characterized by an apparent dramatic increase in vascular permeability which can result in a rapid accumulation of fluid in the peritoneal cavity,

LUTROPIN ALFA — INJECTION

thorax, and potentially, the pericardium. The early warning signs of development of ovarian hyperstimulation syndrome are severe pelvic pain, nausea, vomiting, and weight gain. The following symptomatology has been seen with cases of ovarian hyperstimulation syndrome: abdominal pain, abdominal distension, GI symptoms (eg, nausea, vomiting, diarrhea), severe ovarian enlargement, weight gain, dyspnea, and oliguria. Clinical evaluation may reveal hypovolemia, hemoconcentration, electrolyte imbalances, ascites, hemoperitoneum, pleural effusions, hydrothorax, acute pulmonary distress, and thromboembolic events. Transient liver function test abnormalities that are suggestive of hepatic dysfunction have been reported in association with ovarian hyperstimulation syndrome. These liver function test abnormalities may be accompanied by morphological changes on liver biopsy.

In hypogonadotropic hypogonadal women with profound LH and FSH deficiency from 5 clinical trials, 4 cases of ovarian hyperstimulation syndrome were reported in 4 of 70 (5.7%) patients treated with lutropin alfa 75 units and follitropin alfa and 1 case was reported in 1 of 31 (3.2%) patients treated with follitropin alfa alone. Among women treated with any dose of lutropin alfa in these studies, 5 of 96 (5.2%) patients reported 6 cases of ovarian hyperstimulation syndrome after treatment with lutropin alfa and follitropin alfa.

Ovarian hyperstimulation syndrome may be more severe and more protracted if pregnancy occurs. Ovarian hyperstimulation syndrome develops rapidly; therefore, follow patients for at least 2 weeks after hCG administration. Most often, ovarian hyperstimulation syndrome occurs after treatment has been discontinued and reaches its maximum severity at 7 to 10 days following treatment. Usually, ovarian hyperstimulation syndrome resolves spontaneously with the onset of menses. If there is evidence that ovarian hyperstimulation syndrome may be developing prior to hCG administration, hCG must be withheld.

If severe ovarian hyperstimulation syndrome occurs, stop treatment with gonadotropins and hospitalize the patient.

Consult a health care provider experienced in the management of this syndrome or in the management of fluid and electrolyte imbalances.

➤*Multiple births:* Advise patients of the potential risk of multiple births before starting treatment.

➤*Pulmonary and vascular complications:* As with other gonadotropin products, a potential for the occurrence of arterial thromboembolism exists.

➤*General:* Give careful attention to the diagnosis of infertility in candidates for lutropin alfa therapy.

➤*Pregnancy: Category X.* When administered to rats during the late period of pregnancy, dosages of 10 units/kg/day and higher were also shown to affect the postnatal survival and growth of the newborns. There was no evidence of teratogenic effect in either rats or rabbits. Lutropin alfa is contraindicated in women who are pregnant and may cause fetal harm when administered to a pregnant woman. Reproductive toxicity studies performed in female rats and rabbits showed that lutropin alfa at doses of 10 units/kg/day and greater caused an increase in preimplantation and postimplantation losses.

➤*Lactation:* It is not known if this drug is excreted in human milk. Because many drugs are excreted in human milk, exercise caution if lutropin alfa is administered to a nursing woman.

➤*Children:* Lutropin alfa is not indicated in pediatric patients. Safety and efficacy in pediatric patients have not been established.

➤*Monitoring:* In most instances, treatment of women with LH and FSH results only in follicular recruitment and development. In the absence of an endogenous LH surge, hCG is given when monitoring of the patient indicates that sufficient follicular development has occurred. This may be estimated by ultrasound alone or in combination with measurement of serum estradiol levels. The combination of both ultrasound and serum estradiol measurement are useful for monitoring the development of follicles, for timing of the ovulatory trigger, as well as for detecting ovarian enlargement and minimizing the risk of the ovarian hyperstimulation syndrome and multiple gestation. It is recommended that the number of growing follicles be confirmed using ultrasonography because serum estrogens do not give an indication of the size or number of follicles.

With the exception of confirmation of pregnancy, the clinical confirmation of ovulation is obtained by direct and indirect indices of progesterone production. The indices most generally used are as follows:

1.) A rise in basal body temperature
2.) Increase in serum progesterone
3.) Menstruation following a shift in basal body temperature

When used in conjunction with the indices of progesterone production, sonographic visualization of the ovaries will assist in determining if ovulation has occurred. Sonographic evidence of ovulation may include the following:

1.) Fluid in the cul-de-sac
2.) Ovarian stigmata
3.) Collapsed follicle
4.) Secretory endometrium

Accurate interpretation of the indices of ovulation require a health care provider who is experienced in the interpretation of these tests.

Drug Interactions

There are no pharmacokinetic interactions with follitropin alfa when administered simultaneously with lutropin alfa. No drug-drug interaction studies have been conducted with lutropin alfa.

Adverse Reactions

The safety of lutropin alfa was examined in 6 clinical studies that treated 170 infertile women with HH of whom 152 received lutropin alfa and follitropin alfa in 283 treatment cycles. Adverse reactions reported by at least 2% of patients (regardless of causality) treated with any dose of lutropin alfa (25, 75, 150, or 225 units) are listed in the following table.

Lutropin Alfa & Follitropin Alfa Adverse Reactions Reported in ≥ 2% Patients in All Cycles in All HH Patients in Studies 6253, 6905,[a] 7798,[b] 8297,[c] 21008, and 21415

Adverse reactions	Lutropin alfa 0 units and follitropin alfa patients (n = 43) n (%)	Lutropin alfa 75 units and follitropin alfa patients (n = 118) n (%)	All doses of lutropin alfa and follitropin alfa patients (n = 152) n (%)
Patients with events	20 (46.5%)	50 (42.4%)	72 (47.4%)
CNS			
Headache	2 (4.7%)	12 (10.2%)	15 (9.9%)
GI			
Abdominal pain	5 (11.6%)	6 (5.1%)	13 (8.6%)
Constipation	0	3 (2.5%)	3 (2%)
Diarrhea	1 (2.3%)	3 (2.5%)	3 (2%)
Flatulence	3 (7%)	5 (4.2%)	6 (3.9%)
Nausea	0	8 (6.8%)	11 (7.2%)
GU			
Breast pain (female)	4 (9.3%)	6 (5.1%)	9 (5.9%)
Dysmenorrhea	1 (2.3%)	2 (1.7%)	4 (2.6%)
Ovarian cyst	4 (9.3%)	6 (5.1%)	8 (5.3%)
Ovarian disorder	0	2 (1.7%)	3 (2%)
Ovarian hyperstimulation	1 (2.3%)	7 (5.9%)	9 (5.9%)
Miscellaneous			
Fatigue	0	3 (2.5%)	5 (3.3%)
Injection site reaction	2 (4.7%)	4 (3.4%)	6 (3.9%)
Pain	3 (7%)	3 (2.5%)	6 (3.9)
Upper respiratory tract infection	2 (4.7%)	1 (0.8%)	3 (2%)

[a] Study 6905 was a randomized, open-label, dose-finding study to assess the safety and efficacy of lutropin alfa administered with follitropin alfa 150 units for induction of follicular development in HH women.
[b] Study 7798 was an uncontrolled, multicenter, dose-finding study to assess the safety and efficacy of lutropin alfa administered with follitropin alfa 150 units for induction of follicular development in LH and FSH deficient anovulatory women in Germany.
[c] Study 8297 was an uncontrolled, multicenter, dose-finding study to assess the safety and efficacy of lutropin alfa administered with follitropin alfa 150 units for induction of follicular development in HH women in Spain.

The following medical events have been reported subsequent to pregnancies resulting from administration of gonadotropins for ovulation induction in controlled clinical studies:

- Spontaneous abortion
- Ectopic pregnancy
- Premature labor
- Postpartum fever
- Congenital abnormalities

There is no evidence that use of any gonadotropin drug product for treatment of infertility is associated with an increased risk of congenital malformations.

The following adverse reactions have been previously reported during menotropin therapy:

- Pulmonary and vascular complications
- Adnexal torsion (as a complication of ovarian enlargement)
- Mild to moderate ovarian enlargement
- Hemoperitoneum

There have been infrequent reports of ovarian neoplasms, both benign and malignant, in women who have undergone multiple drug regimens for ovulation induction; however, a causal relationship has not been established.

Overdosage

Aside from possible ovarian hyperstimulation and multiple gestations, there is no information on the consequences of overdosage with lutropin alfa.

Patient Information

Prior to therapy with lutropin alfa, inform patients of the duration of treatment and monitoring of their condition that will be required. Also discuss the risks of ovarian hyperstimulation syndrome and multiple births and other possible adverse reactions.

HUMAN CHORIONIC GONADOTROPIN

Rx	**Chorionic Gonadotropin** (Various, eg, Goldline)	**Powder for Injection**: 5,000 units/vial with 10 mL diluent (to make 500 units/mL)	In 10 mL vials.
Rx	**Profasi** (Serono)		In 10 ml vials.[2]
Rx	**Chorionic Gonadotropin** (Various, eg, Goldline)	**Powder for Injection**: 10,000 units/vial with 10 mL diluent (to make 1,000 units/mL)	In 10 mL vials.
Rx	**Choron 10** (Forest)		In 10 mL vials.[2]
Rx	**Novarel** (Ferring)		In 10 mL vials.[2]
Rx	**Pregnyl** (Organon)		In 10 mL vials.[3]
Rx	**Profasi** (Serono)		In 10 mL vials.[2]
Rx	**Chorionic Gonadotropin** (Various, eg, Goldline)	**Powder for Injection**: 20,000 units/vial with 10 mL diluent (to make 2,000 units/mL)	In 10 mL vials.

[1] With benzyl alcohol, less than 0.2% phenol and lactose.
[2] With mannitol and 0.9% benzyl alcohol.
[3] With 0.9% benzyl alcohol.

HUMAN CHORIONIC GONADOTROPIN — INJECTION

WARNING

Human chorionic gonadotropin (hCG) has no known effect on fat mobilization, appetite, sense of hunger or body-fat distribution. Human chorionic gonadotropin (hCG) has not been demonstrated to be effective adjunctive therapy in the treatment of obesity. There is no substantial evidence that it increases weight loss beyond that resulting from caloric restriction, that it causes a more attractive or "normal" distribution of fat or that it decreases the hunger and discomfort associated with calorie-restricted diets.

Indications

➤*Prepubertal cryptorchidism:* Prepubertal cryptorchidism not caused by anatomic obstruction. In general, chorionic gonadotropin is thought to induce testicular descent in situations when descent would have occurred at puberty. Chorionic gonadotropin thus may help to predict whether or not orchiopexy will be needed in the future. Although, in some cases, descent following chorionic gonadotropin administration is permanent, in most cases the response is temporary. Therapy is usually instituted between the ages of 4 and 9.

➤*Hypogonadism:* Selected cases of hypogonadotropic hypogonadism (hypogonadism secondary to a pituitary deficiency) in males.

➤*Ovulation induction:* Induction of ovulation and pregnancy in the anovulatory, infertile woman in whom the cause of anovulation is secondary and not caused by primary ovarian failure, and who has been appropriately pretreated with human menotropins.

Administration and Dosage

➤*General dosing considerations:* For intramuscular (IM) use only. The dosage regimen to be used will depend upon the indication for use, the age and weight of the patient, and the physician's preference. The following regimens have been advocated by various authorities.

➤*Adults:*

Induction of ovulation and pregnancy – Induction of ovulation and pregnancy in the anovulatory, infertile woman in whom the cause of anovulation is secondary and not caused by primary ovarian failure and who has been appropriately pretreated with human menotropins.

Regimen 1: 5,000 to 10,000 units IM 1 day after the last dose of menotropins. A dosage of 10,000 units is recommended in the labeling for menotropins.

Selected cases of male hypogonadism secondary to pituitary failure –

Regimen 1: 500 to 1,000 units IM 3 times a week for 3 weeks, followed by the same dose twice a week for 3 weeks.

Regimen 2: 4,000 units IM 3 times weekly for 6 to 9 months, after which the dosage may be reduced to 2,000 units 3 times weekly for an additional 3 months.

➤*Children:*

Prepubertal cryptorchidism not caused by anatomical obstruction – Therapy is usually instituted between the ages of 4 and 9.

4 years of age and older:

- *Regimen 1* – 4,000 units IM 3 times weekly for 3 weeks.
- *Regimen 2* – 5,000 units IM every second day for 4 injections.
- *Regimen 3* – 15 injections of 500 to 1,000 units IM over a period of 6 weeks.
- *Regimen 4* – 500 units IM 3 times weekly for 4 to 6 weeks. If this course of treatment is not successful, another is begun 1 month later, giving 1,000 units/injection.

Selected cases of male hypogonadism secondary to pituitary failure – See Adults for dosing.

➤*Renal function impairment:* Because androgens may cause fluid retention, chorionic gonadotropin should be used with caution in patients with renal disease.

➤*Preparation for administration:*

Reconstitution (2-vial package) – Withdraw sterile air from lyophilized vial and inject into diluent vial. Remove 10 mL from diluent vial and add to lyophilized vial; agitate gently until solution is complete.

➤*Storage/Stability:* Store dry product at 15° to 30°C (59° to 86°F). After reconstitution, refrigerate the product at 2° to 8°C (36° to 46°F) and use within 30 days.

Actions

➤*Pharmacology:* The action of hCG is virtually identical to that of pituitary LH, although hCG appears to have a small degree of FSH activity as well. It stimulates production of gonadal steroid hormones by stimulating the interstitial cells (Leydig cells) of the testis to produce androgens and the corpus luteum of the ovary to produce progesterone. Androgen stimulation in the male leads to the development of secondary sex characteristics and may stimulate testicular descent when no anatomical impediment to descent is present. This descent is usually reversible when hCG is discontinued. During the normal menstrual cycle, LH participates with FSH in the development and maturation of the normal ovarian follicle, and the midcycle LH surge triggers ovulation. hCG can substitute for LH in this function.

During a normal pregnancy, hCG secreted by the placenta maintains the corpus luteum after LH secretion decreases, supporting continued secretion of estrogen and progesterone, and preventing menstruation. Human chorionic gonadotropin has no known effect on fat mobilization, appetite or sense of hunger, or body-fat distribution.

➤*Pharmacokinetics:*

Absorption/Distribution – Following IM injection, a detectable rise in serum hCG levels is seen in 2 hours; peak levels are reached in 6 hours and remain at this level for 36 hours. Human chorionic gonadotropin levels begin to decline at 48 hours and approach baseline (undetectable) levels at 72 hours.

Contraindications

Precocious puberty; prostatic carcinoma or other androgen-dependent neoplasia; prior allergic reaction to chorionic gonadotropin.

Warnings/Precautions

➤*Administration:* Human chorionic gonadotropin should be used in conjunction with human menopausal gonadotropins only by physicians experienced with infertility problems who are familiar with the criteria for patient selection and the contraindications, warnings, precautions, and adverse reactions described in the monograph for menotropins. The principal serious adverse reactions during this use are as follows: Ovarian hyperstimulation, a syndrome of sudden ovarian enlargement; ascites with or without pain, or pleural effusion; enlargement of preexisting ovarian cysts or rupture of ovarian cysts with resultant hemoperitonum; multiple births; and arterial thromboembolism.

➤*Benzyl alcohol:* The diluent used for reconstitution contains benzyl alcohol. Benzyl alcohol has been reported to be associated with a fatal "gasping syndrome" in premature infants.

➤*Precocious puberty:* Induction of androgen secretion by hCG may induce precocious puberty in patients treated for cryptorchidism. Therapy should be discontinued if signs of precocious puberty occur.

➤*Special risk:* Since androgens may cause fluid retention, chorionic gonadotropin should be used with caution in patients with epilepsy, migraine, asthma, cardiac or renal disease.

➤*Pregnancy: Category X.* Human chorionic gonadotropin is contraindicated in pregnant women. Combined hCG/PMS therapy has been noted to induce high incidences of external congenital anomalies in the offspring of mice, in a dose-dependent manner. The potential extrapolation to humans has not been determined.

Chorionic gonadotropin may cause fetal harm when administered to a pregnant woman. Defects of forelimbs and central nervous system and alterations in sex ratio have been reported in mice receiving combined gonadotropin and chorionic gonadotropin therapy in dosages to induce superovulation. Multiple ovulations with resulting plural gestations (mostly twins) have been reported to occur in approximately 20% of pregnancies when conception has followed chorionic gonadotropin therapy.

➤*Lactation:* It is not known whether chorionic gonadotropin is excreted in human milk. Because many drugs are excreted in human milk, caution should be exercised when hCG is administered to a nursing woman.

➤*Children:* Safety and efficacy in pediatric patients younger than 4 years of age have not been established.

HUMAN CHORIONIC GONADOTROPIN — INJECTION

The diluent used for reconstitution contains benzyl alcohol. Benzyl alcohol has been reported to be associated with a fatal "gasping syndrome" in premature infants.

➤*Monitoring:* In adult males and females, the following hormone levels may be monitored depending on the nature of the diagnostic and therapeutic purpose: Testosterone, dihydrotestosterone, 17β-estradiol, 17β-hydroxyprogesterone, progesterone, androstenedione. In prepubertal males, testosterone and dihydrotestosterone should be followed.

Drug Interactions

➤*Drug/Lab test interactions:* Human chorionic gonadotropin can cross-react in the radio-immunoassay of gonadotropins, especially LH. Each individual laboratory should establish the degree of cross-reactivity with their gonadotropin assay. Physicians should make the laboratory aware of patients on hCG if gonadotropin levels are requested.

Adverse Reactions

➤*Cardiovascular:* Arterial thromboembolism.

➤*CNS:* Headache; irritability; restlessness; depression; fatigue; aggressive behavior.

➤*GU:* Precocious puberty; gynecomastia; ovarian hyperstimulation syndrome; enlargement of preexisting ovarian cysts and possible rupture; phallic or testicular enlargement; growth of pubic hair; signs or symptoms of androgen excess. There have been rare reports of ovarian malignancy

➤*Hypersensitivity:* Hypersensitivity reactions both localized and systemic in nature, including erythema, urticaria, rash, angioedema, dyspnea, and shortness of breath, have been reported. The relationship of these allergic-like events to the polypeptide hormone or the diluent containing benzyl alcohol is not clear.

➤*Local:* Pain at the site of injection.

➤*Miscellaneous:* Edema.

Overdosage

➤*Symptoms:* There is no experience to date with deliberate overdosage of chorionic gonadotropin.

➤*Treatment:* Treatment must be symptomatic and supportive.

CHORIOGONADOTROPIN ALFA

Rx	**Ovidrel** (Serono)	**Injection:** 250 mcg/0.5 mL	28.1 mg mannitol, 505 mcg 85% O-phosphoric acid. In single-dose prefilled syringes.

CHORIOGONADOTROPIN ALFA — INJECTION

Indications

➤*Final follicular maturation:* Choriogonadotropin alfa for injection is indicated for the induction of final follicular maturation and early luteinization in infertile women who have undergone pituitary desensitization and who have been appropriately pretreated with follicle-stimulating hormones (FSH) as part of an assisted reproductive technology (ART) program such as in vitro fertilization and embryo transfer.

➤*Ovulation induction:* Choriogonadotropin alfa is also indicated for the induction of ovulation (OI) and pregnancy in anovulatory infertile patients in whom the cause of infertility is functional and not caused by primary ovarian failure.

Administration and Dosage

➤*General dosing considerations:* Do not administer choriogonadotropin alfa until adequate follicular development is indicated by serum estradiol and vaginal ultrasonography. Withhold administration in situations in which there is an excessive ovarian response, as evidenced by multiple follicular development, clinically significant ovarian enlargement or excessive estradiol production.

➤*Adults:*

Final follicular maturation – 250 mcg subcutaneous 1 day following the last dose of the follicle-stimulating agent.

Ovulation induction – See Final Follicular Maturation for dosing.

➤*Preparation for administration:* Choriogonadotropin alfa is intended for a single subcutaneous injection and should be administered following reconstitution with 1 mL of sterile water for injection. Any unused reconstituted material should be discarded.

➤*Administration:* For subcutaneous use only.

Choriogonadotropin alfa may be self-administered by the patient.

➤*Storage/Stability:* The choriogonadotropin alfa prefilled syringe must be stored at 2° to 8°C (36° to 46°F) before being dispensed to the patient. Patient may store the prefilled syringe at no more than 25°C (77°F) for up to 30 days prior to administration. Protect from light.

Actions

➤*Pharmacology:* The physicochemical, immunological, and biological activities of r-hCG are comparable with those of placental and human pregnancy u-hCG. Choriogonadotropin alfa stimulates late follicular maturation and resumption of oocyte meiosis, and initiates rupture of the preovulatory ovarian follicle. Choriogonadotropin alfa, the active component of choriogonadotropin alfa, is an analogue of LH and binds to the LH/hCG receptor of the granulosa and theca cells of the ovary to effect these changes in the absence of an endogenous LH surge. In pregnancy, hCG, secreted by the placenta, maintains the viability of the corpus luteum to provide the continued secretion of estrogen and progesterone necessary to support the first trimester of pregnancy. Choriogonadotropin alfa is administered when monitoring of the patient indicates that sufficient follicular development has occurred in response to FSH treatment for ovulation induction.

In women on oral contraception after an initial latency period, choriogonadotropin alfa induced a clear increase in androstenedione serum levels by 24 hours after dosing. Pharmacodynamic studies in females determined that the relationship of choriogonadotropin alfa pharmacokinetics to pharmacologic effect of choriogonadotropin alfa are complex and vary with the pharmacodynamic marker examined. In general, pharmacologic effects are not proportional to exposure and in some cases appear to be near maximal at a 250 mcg dose.

➤*Pharmacokinetics:* Pharmacokinetic parameter estimates following subcutaneous administration of choriogonadotropin alfa 250 mcg to women are presented in the following table.

In the following table, C_{max} is the peak concentration (above baseline), T_{max} is the time of C_{max}, AUC is the total area under the curve, $t_{½}$ is the elimination half-life, and F is bioavailability.

Pharmacokinetic Parameters (Mean ± SD) of r-hCG After Single Dosing in Healthy Women

Parameter	Choriogonadotropin alfa 250 mcg subcutaneously
C_{max} (units/L)	121 ± 44
T_{max} (h)[a]	24 (12 to 24)
AUC (h•IU/L)	7,701 ± 2,101
$T_{½}$ (h)	29 ± 6
F	0.4 ± 0.1

[a] Median (range).

Absorption – When given by intravenous (IV) administration, the pharmacokinetic profile of choriogonadotropin alfa followed a biexponential model and was linear over a range of 25 to 1,000 mcg.

Following subcutaneous administration of choriogonadotropin alfa 250 mcg, maximum serum concentration (121 ± 44 units/L) is reached after approximately 12 to 24 hours. The mean absolute bioavailability of choriogonadotropin alfa following a single subcutaneous injection to healthy female volunteers is approximately 40%.

Distribution – Following IV administration of choriogonadotropin alfa 250 mcg to healthy down-regulated women, the serum profile of hCG is described by a 2-compartment model with an initial half-life of 4.5 ± 0.5 hours. The volume of the central compartment is 3 ± 0.5 L and the steady state volume of distribution is 5.9 ± 1 L.

Metabolism/Excretion – Following subcutaneous administration of choriogonadotropin alfa, hCG is eliminated from the body with a mean terminal half-life of approximately 29 ± 6 hours. After IV administration of choriogonadotropin alfa 250 mcg to healthy down-regulated women, the mean terminal half-life is 26.5 ± 2.5 hours, and the total body clearance is 0.29 ± 0.04 L/hr. One-tenth of the dose is excreted in the urine.

Prefilled syringe –

Bioequivalence of formulations: Choriogonadotropin alfa prefilled syringe has been determined to be bioequivalent to choriogonadotropin alfa for injection based on the statistical evaluation of AUC and C_{max}. A summary of the choriogonadotropin alfa prefilled syringe pharmacokinetic parameters is presented in the following table.

Summary of Choriogonadotropin Alfa Prefilled Syringe Pharmacokinetic Parameters

	Parameter				
	C_{max} (milliunits/mL)	AUC_{last} (milliunits•h/mL)	AUC (milliunits•h/mL)	$AUC_{extrapolated}$ (%)	T_{max} (h)
Mean (min-max)	125 (68-294)	10,050 (5,646-14,850)	10,350 (5,800-15,100)	2.85 (1.08-6.27)	20 (9-48)

Contraindications

Choriogonadotropin alfa for injection is contraindicated in women who exhibit any of the following: prior hypersensitivity to hCG preparations or one of their excipients, primary ovarian failure, uncontrolled thyroid or adrenal dysfunction, an uncontrolled organic intracranial lesion such as a pituitary tumor, abnormal uterine bleeding of undetermined origin, ovarian cyst or enlargement of undetermined origin, sex hormone-dependent tumors of the reproductive tract and accessory organs, pregnancy.

CHORIOGONADOTROPIN ALFA — INJECTION

Warnings/Precautions

➤*Administration:* Gonadotropins, including choriogonadotropin alfa, should only be used by health care providers who are thoroughly familiar with infertility problems and their management. Like other hCG products, choriogonadotropin alfa is a potent gonadotropic substance capable of causing ovarian hyperstimulation syndrome in women with or without pulmonary or vascular complications. Gonadotropin therapy requires a certain time commitment by health care providers, and requires the availability of appropriate monitoring facilities. Safe and effective induction of ovulation and use of choriogonadotropin alfa in women requires monitoring of ovarian response with serum estradiol and transvaginal ultrasound on a regular basis.

➤*Overstimulation of the ovary following hCG therapy:*

Ovarian enlargement – Mild to moderate uncomplicated ovarian enlargement which may be accompanied by abdominal distention or abdominal pain may occur in patients treated with FSH and hCG, and generally regresses without treatment within 2 or 3 weeks. Careful monitoring of ovarian response can further minimize the risk of overstimulation.

If the ovaries are abnormally enlarged on the last day of FSH therapy, do not administer choriogonadotropin alfa in this course of therapy. This will reduce the risk of development of ovarian hyperstimulation syndrome.

Ovarian hyperstimulation syndrome – Ovarian hyperstimulation syndrome is a medical event distinct from uncomplicated ovarian enlargement. Severe ovarian hyperstimulation syndrome may progress rapidly (within 24 hours to several days) to become a serious medical event. It is characterized by an apparent dramatic increase in vascular permeability which can result in a rapid accumulation of fluid in the peritoneal cavity, thorax, and potentially, the pericardium. The early warning signs of development of ovarian hyperstimulation syndrome are severe pelvic pain, nausea, vomiting, and weight gain. The following symptomatology has been seen with cases of ovarian hyperstimulation syndrome: abdominal pain, abdominal distension, GI symptoms including nausea, vomiting and diarrhea, severe ovarian enlargement, weight gain, dyspnea, and oliguria. Clinical evaluation may reveal hypovolemia, hemoconcentration, electrolyte imbalances, ascites, hemoperitoneum, pleural effusions, hydrothorax, acute pulmonary distress, and thromboembolic events. Transient liver function test abnormalities suggestive of hepatic dysfunction, which may be accompanied by morphologic changes on liver biopsy, have been reported in association with ovarian hyperstimulation syndrome.

Ovarian hyperstimulation syndrome occurred in 4 of 236 (1.7%) patients treated with choriogonadotropin alfa 250 mcg during clinical trials for ART and 3 of 99 (3%) patients treated in the OI trial. ovarian hyperstimulation syndrome occurred in 8 of 89 (9%) patients who received choriogonadotropin alfa 500 mcg. Two patients treated with choriogonadotropin alfa 500 mcg developed severe ovarian hyperstimulation syndrome.

Ovarian hyperstimulation syndrome may be more severe and more protracted if pregnancy occurs. Ovarian hyperstimulation syndrome develops rapidly; therefore, patients should be followed for at least 2 weeks after hCG administration. Most often, ovarian hyperstimulation syndrome occurs after treatment has been discontinued and reaches its maximum at about 7 to 10 days following treatment. Usually, ovarian hyperstimulation syndrome resolves spontaneously with the onset of menses. If there is evidence that ovarian hyperstimulation syndrome may be developing prior to hCG administration, the hCG must be withheld.

If severe ovarian hyperstimulation syndrome occurs, stop treatment with gonadotropins and hospitalize the patient.

Consult a health care provider experienced in the management of this syndrome, or who is experienced in the management of fluid and electrolyte imbalances should be consulted.

➤*Multiple births:* As with other hCG products, reports of multiple births have been associated with choriogonadotropin alfa treatment. In ART, the risk of multiple births correlates to the number of embryos transferred. Multiple births occurred in 17 of 55 live deliveries (30.9%) experienced by women receiving choriogonadotropin alfa 250 mcg in the ART studies. In the ovulation induction clinical trial, 2 of 15 live deliveries (13.3%) were associated with multiple births in women receiving choriogonadotropin alfa. Advise the patient of the potential risk of multiple births before starting treatment.

➤*Pulmonary and vascular complications:* As with other hCG products, a potential for the occurrence of arterial thromboembolism exists.

➤*Pregnancy: Category X.* Fetal death and impaired parturition were observed in pregnant rats given a dose of choriogonadotropin alfa (25 mcg/day) equivalent to 6 times the maximum human dose of 250 mcg based on body surface area or for prefilled syringe of choriogonadotropin alfa: u-hCG (500 units) equivalent to 3 times the maximum human dose of 10,000 USP, based on body surface area.

➤*Lactation:* It is not known whether this drug is excreted in human milk. Because many drugs are excreted in human milk, exercise caution if hCG is administered to a breast-feeding woman.

➤*Children:* Safety and efficacy in children have not been established.

➤*Lab test abnormalities:* After the exclusion of preexisting conditions, elevations in ALT were found in 10 (3%) of 335 patients receiving choriogonadotropin alfa 250 mcg, 9 (10%) of 89 patients receiving choriogonadotropin alfa 500 mcg, and in 16 (4.8%) of 328 patients receiving u-hCG. The elevations ranged up to 1.2 times the upper limit of normal. The clinical significance of these findings is not known.

In most instances, treatment of women with FSH results only in follicular recruitment and development. In the absence of an endogenous LH surge, hCG is given when monitoring of the patient indicates that sufficient follicular development has occurred. This may be estimated by ultrasound alone or in combination with measurement of serum estradiol levels. The combination of both ultrasound and serum estradiol measurement are useful for monitoring the development of follicles, timing of the ovulatory trigger, as well as detecting ovarian enlargement and minimizing the risk of the ovarian hyperstimulation syndrome and multiple gestation. It is recommended that the number of growing follicles be confirmed using ultrasonography because serum estrogens do not give an indication of the size or number of follicles.

Human chorionic gonadotropins can crossreact in the radioimmunoassay of gonadotropins, especially luteinizing hormone. Each individual laboratory should establish the degree of crossreactivity with their gonadotropin assay. Make the laboratory aware of patients on hCG if gonadotropin levels are requested.

The clinical confirmation of ovulation, with the exception of pregnancy, is obtained by direct and indirect indices of progesterone production. The indices most generally used are as follows: a rise in basal body temperature, increase in serum progesterone, menstruation following a shift in basal body temperature.

When used in conjunction with the indices of progesterone production, sonographic visualization of the ovaries will assist in determining if ovulation has occurred. Sonographic evidence of ovulation may include the following: fluid in the cul-de-sac, ovarian stigmata, collapsed follicle, secretory endometrium.

Accurate interpretation of the indices of ovulation require a health care provider who is experienced in the interpretation of these tests.

➤*Monitoring:* Careful attention should be given to the diagnosis of infertility in candidates for hCG therapy.

Drug Interactions

No drug-drug interaction studies have been conducted.

➤*Drug/Lab test interactions:* Administration of choriogonadotropin alfa may interfere with the interpretation of pregnancy tests.

Adverse Reactions

The safety of choriogonadotropin alfa was examined in 4 clinical studies that treated 752 patients, of whom 335 received choriogonadotropin alfa 250 mcg following follicular recruitment with gonadotropins. When patients enrolled in 4 clinical studies (3 in ART and 1 in OI) were injected subcutaneously with either choriogonadotropin alfa or an approved u-hCG, 14.6 % (49 of 335 patients) in the choriogonadotropin alfa 250 mcg group experienced application site disorders, compared to 28% (92 of 328 patients) in the approved u-hCG group. Adverse reactions reported for choriogonadotropin alfa 250 mcg occurring in at least 2% of patients (regardless of causality) are listed in the following tables. The first table shows the 3 ART studies, and the second table shows the single OI study.

Incidence of Adverse Reactions of r-hCG in ART (Studies 7648, 7927, 9073)

Adverse reactions	Choriogonadotropin alfa 250 mcg (n = 236); incidence rate, % (n)
At least 1 adverse reaction	33.1% (78)
Abdominal pain	4.2% (10)
Application site disorders	14% (33)
Injection site bruising	4.7% (11)
Injection site pain	7.6% (18)
GI system disorders	8.5% (20)
Nausea	3.4% (8)
Postoperative pain	4.7% (11)
Secondary terms (postoperative pain)	4.7% (11)
Vomiting	2.5% (6)

Adverse reactions not listed in the above table that occurred in less than 2% of patients treated with choriogonadotropin alfa 250 mcg whether or not considered causally related to choriogonadotropin alfa, included the following: injection site inflammation and reaction; flatulence; diarrhea; hiccup; ectopic pregnancy; breast pain; intermenstrual bleeding; vaginal hemorrhage; cervical lesion; leukorrhea; ovarian hyperstimulation; uterine disorders; vaginitis; vaginal discomfort; body pain; back pain; fever; dizziness; headache; hot flashes; malaise; paresthesias; rash; emotional lability; insomnia; upper respiratory tract infection; cough; dysuria; urinary tract infection; urinary incontinence; albuminuria; cardiac arrhythmia; genital moniliasis; genital herpes; leukocytosis; heart murmur; cervical carcinoma.

Incidence of Adverse Reactions of r-hCG in Ovulation Induction (Study 8209)

Adverse reactions	Choriogonadotropin alfa 250 mcg (n = 236); incidence rate, % (n)
At least 1 adverse event	26.2% (26)
Abdominal pain	3% (3)
Application site disorders	16.2% (16)
GI system disorders	4% (4)

CHORIOGONADOTROPIN ALFA — INJECTION

Incidence of Adverse Reactions of r-hCG in Ovulation Induction (Study 8209)	
Adverse reactions	Choriogonadotropin alfa 250 mcg (n = 236); incidence rate, % (n)
Injection site bruising	3% (3)
Injection site inflammation	2% (2)
Injection site pain	8.1% (8)
Injection site reaction	3% (3)
Ovarian cyst	3% (3)
Ovarian hyperstimulation	3% (3)
Reproductive disorders, female	7.1% (7)

Additional adverse reactions not listed in the preceding table that occurred in less than 2% of patients treated with choriogonadotropin alfa 250 mcg, whether or not considered causally related to choriogonadotropin alfa, included the following: breast pain; flatulence; abdominal enlargement; pharyngitis; upper respiratory tract infection; hyperglycemia; pruritus.

The following medical events have been reported subsequent to pregnancies resulting from hCG therapy in controlled clinical studies: spontaneous abortion; ectopic pregnancy; premature labor; postpartum fever; congenital abnormalities.

Of 125 clinical pregnancies reported following treatment with FSH and choriogonadotropin alfa 250 or 500 mcg, 3 were associated with a congenital anomaly of the fetus or newborn. Among patients receiving choriogonadotropin alfa 250 mcg, cranial malformation was detected in the fetus of 1 woman and a chromosomal abnormality (47, XXX) in another. These events were judged by the investigators to be of unlikely or unknown relation to treatment. These 3 events represent an incidence of major congenital malformations of 2.4%, which is consistent with the reported rate for pregnancies resulting from natural or assisted conception. In a woman who received choriogonadotropin alfa 500 mcg, 1 birth in a set of triplets was associated with Down syndrome and atrial septal defect. This event was considered to be unrelated to the study drug.

The following adverse reactions have been previously reported during menotropin therapy: pulmonary and vascular complications; adnexal torsion (as a complication of ovarian enlargement); mild to moderate ovarian enlargement; hemoperitoneum.

There have been infrequent reports of ovarian neoplasms, both benign and malignant, in women who have undergone multiple drug regimens for ovulation induction; however, a causal relationship has not been established.

Patient Information

Prior to therapy with hCG, inform patients of the duration of treatment and monitoring of their condition that will be required. Also discuss the risks of ovarian hyperstimulation syndrome and multiple births in women and other possible adverse reactions.

NAFARELIN ACETATE

Rx	**Synarel** (Pfizer U.S.)	**Solution; intranasal:** 2 mg/mL	As nafarelin acetate. In 10 mL bottle with metered spray pump (delivers approximately 200 mcg/spray).[a]

[a] With benzalkonium chloride, glacial acetic acid and sorbitol.

NAFARELIN ACETATE — NASAL

Indications

➤*Endometriosis:* Nafarelin acetate is indicated for management of endometriosis, including pain relief and reduction of endometriotic lesions. Experience with nafarelin acetate for the management of endometriosis has been limited to women 18 years of age and older treated for 6 months.

➤*Central precocious puberty:* Nafarelin acetate is indicated for treatment of central precocious puberty (CPP) (gonadotropin-dependent precocious puberty) in children of both sexes.

Administration and Dosage

➤*Adults:*

Endometriosis –

Usual dosage: 400 mcg daily. This is achieved by one spray (200 mcg) into one nostril in the morning and one spray into the other nostril in the evening. Treatment should be started between days 2 and 4 of the menstrual cycle.

Dosage titration: In an occasional patient, the 400 mcg daily dose may not produce amenorrhea. For these patients with persistent regular menstruation after 2 months of treatment, increase to 800 mcg daily. The 800 mcg dose is administered as one spray into each nostril in the morning (a total of 2 sprays) and again in the evening.

Duration of therapy: 6 months. Re-treatment cannot be recommended since safety data for re-treatment are not available. If the symptoms of endometriosis recur after a course of therapy, and further treatment with nafarelin is contemplated, it is recommended that bone density be assessed before re-treatment begins to ensure that values are within normal limits.

➤*Children:*

Central precocious puberty –

Usual dosage: 1,600 mcg daily. This is achieved by 2 sprays (400 mcg) into each nostril in the morning (4 sprays) and 2 sprays into each nostril in the evening (4 sprays), a total of 8 sprays daily. If well tolerated, treatment should continue until resumption of puberty is desired.

Dosage titration: Increase to 1,800 mcg daily if adequate suppression cannot be achieved at 1,600 mcg/day. This is achieved by 3 sprays (600 mcg) into alternating nostrils 3 times a day, a total of 9 sprays per day.

➤*Concomitant therapy with nasal decongestants:* If the use of a nasal decongestant for rhinitis is necessary during treatment with nafarelin, the decongestant should not be used until at least 2 hours following dosing with nafarelin.

➤*Administration:* Administer intranasally with metered-spray pump. The patient's head should be tilted back slightly, and 30 seconds should elapse between sprays. Sneezing during or immediately after dosing with nafarelin should be avoided, if possible because this may impair drug absorption.

➤*Storage/Stability:* Store upright at 25°C (77°F); excursions permitted to 15° to 30°C (59° to 86°F). Protect from light.

Actions

➤*Pharmacology:* Nafarelin acetate is a potent agonistic analog of gonadotropin-releasing hormone (GnRH). At the onset of administration, nafarelin stimulates the release of the pituitary gonadotropins, LH and FSH, resulting in a temporary increase of ovarian steroidogenesis. Repeated dosing abolishes the stimulatory effect on the pituitary gland. Twice-daily administration leads to decreased secretion of gonadal steroids by about 4 weeks; consequently, tissues and functions that depend on gonadal steroids for their maintenance become quiescent.

Contraindications

Hypersensitivity to GnRH, GnRH agonist analogs or any of the excipients in nafarelin acetate; undiagnosed abnormal vaginal bleeding; use in women who are breast feeding (see Lactation); use in pregnancy or in women who may become pregnant while receiving the drug.

Warnings/Precautions

➤*Central Precocious Puberty:* The diagnosis of central precocious puberty (CPP) must be established before treatment is initiated. Regular monitoring of CPP patients is needed to assess both patient response as well as compliance. This is particularly important during the first 6 to 8 weeks of treatment to assure that suppression of pituitary-gonadal function is rapid. Testing may include LH response to GnRH stimulation and circulating gonadal sex steroid levels. Assessment of growth velocity and bone age velocity should begin within 3 to 6 months of treatment initiation.

Some patients may not show suppression of the pituitary-gonadal axis by clinical and/or biochemical parameters. This may be due to lack of compliance with the recommended treatment regimen and may be rectified by recommending that the dosing be done by caregivers. If compliance problems are excluded, the possibility of gonadotropin independent sexual precocity should be reconsidered and appropriate examinations should be conducted. If compliance problems are excluded and if gonadotropin independent sexual precocity is not present, the dose of nafarelin acetate may be increased to 1800 mcg/day administered as 600 mcg 3 times daily.

➤*Ovarian cysts:* As with other drugs that stimulate the release of gonadotropins or that induce ovulation, ovarian cysts have been reported to occur in the first two months of therapy with nafarelin acetate. Many, but not all, of these events occurred in patients with polycystic ovarian disease. These cystic enlargements may resolve spontaneously, generally by about 4 to 6 weeks of therapy, but in some cases may require discontinuation of drug and/or surgical intervention. The relevance, if any, of such events in children is unknown.

➤*Pregnancy: Category X.* Safe use of nafarelin acetate in pregnancy has not been established clinically. Before starting treatment with nafarelin acetate, pregnancy must be excluded.

When used regularly at the recommended dose, nafarelin acetate usually inhibits ovulation and stops menstruation. Contraception is not insured, however, by taking nafarelin acetate, particularly if patients miss successive doses. Therefore, patients should use nonhormonal methods of contraception. Patients should be advised to see their physician if they believe they may be pregnant. If a patient becomes pregnant during treatment, the drug must be discontinued and the patient must be apprised of the potential risk to the fetus.

Teratogenic – (See Contraindications.) Intramuscular nafarelin acetate was administered to rats during the period of organogenesis at 0.4, 1.6, and 6.4 mcg/kg/day (about 0.5, 2, and 7 times the maximum recommended human intranasal dose based on the relative bioavailability by the two routes of administration). An increase in major fetal abnormalities was observed in 4/80 fetuses at the highest dose. A similar, repeat study at the

NAFARELIN ACETATE — NASAL

same doses in rats and studies in mice and rabbits at doses up to 600 mcg/kg/day and 0.18 mcg/kg/day, respectively, failed to demonstrate an increase in fetal abnormalities after administration during the period of organogenesis. In rats and rabbits, there was a dose-related increase in fetal mortality and a decrease in fetal weight with the highest dose.

➤*Lactation:* It is not known whether nafarelin acetate is excreted in human milk. Because many drugs are excreted in human milk, and because the effects of nafarelin acetate on lactation and/or the breastfed child have not been determined, nafarelin acetate should not be used by nursing mothers.

➤*Children:* Safety and efficacy of nafarelin acetate for endometriosis in patients younger than 18 years of age have not been established.

Drug Interactions

No pharmacokinetic-based drug-drug interaction studies have been conducted with nafarelin acetate. However, because nafarelin acetate is a peptide that is primarily degraded by peptidase and not by cytochrome P-450 enzymes, and the drug is only about 80% bound to plasma proteins at 4°C (39.2°F), drug interactions would not be expected to occur.

➤*Drug/Lab test interactions:* Administration of nafarelin acetate in therapeutic doses results in suppression of the pituitary-gonadal system. Normal function is usually restored within 4 to 8 weeks after treatment is discontinued. Therefore, diagnostic tests of pituitary gonadotropic and gonadal functions conducted during treatment and up to 4 to 8 weeks after discontinuation of therapy with nafarelin acetate may be misleading.

Adverse Reactions

➤*Endometriosis:* In formal clinical trials of 1,509 healthy adult patients, symptoms suggestive of drug sensitivity, such as shortness of breath, chest pain, urticaria, rash and pruritus occurred in 3 patients (approximately 0.2%).

As would be expected with a drug which lowers serum estradiol levels, the most frequently reported adverse reactions were those related to hypoestrogenism.

In addition, less than 1% of patients experienced paresthesia, palpitations, chloasma, maculopapular rash, eye pain, asthenia, lactation, breast engorgement, and arthralgia.

Lab test abnormalities –

Plasma enzymes: During clinical trials with nafarelin acetate, regular laboratory monitoring revealed that APT and AST levels were more than twice the upper limit of normal in only one patient each. There was no other clinical or laboratory evidence of abnormal liver function and levels returned to normal in both patients after treatment was stopped.

Lipids: At enrollment, 9% of the patients in the group taking nafarelin acetate 400 mcg/day and 2% of the patients in the danazol group had total cholesterol values above 250 mg/dL. These patients also had cholesterol values above 250 mg/dL at the end of treatment.

Of those patients whose pretreatment cholesterol values were below 250 mg/dL, 6% in the group treated with nafarelin acetate and 18% in the danazol group, had post-treatment values above 250 mg/dL.

The mean (± SEM) pretreatment values for total cholesterol from all patients were 191.8 (4.3) mg/dL in the group treated with nafarelin acetate and 193.1 (4.6) mg/dL in the danazol group. At the end of treatment, the mean values for total cholesterol from all patients were 204.5 (4.8) mg/dL in the group treated with nafarelin acetate and 207.7 (5.1) mg/dL in the danazol group. These increases from the pretreatment values were statistically significant (p less than 0.05) in both groups.

Triglycerides were increased above the upper limit of 150 mg/dL in 12% of the patients who received nafarelin acetate and in 7% of the patients who received danazol.

At the end of treatment, no patients receiving nafarelin acetate had abnormally low HDL cholesterol fractions (less than 30 mg/dL) compared with 43% of patients receiving danazol. None of the patients receiving nafarelin acetate had abnormally high LDL cholesterol fractions (greater than 190 mg/dL) compared with 15% of those receiving danazol. There was no increase in the LDL/HDL ratio in patients receiving nafarelin acetate, but there was approximately a 2-fold increase in the LDL/HDL ratio in patients receiving danazol.

Other changes: In comparative studies, the following changes were seen in ≈ 10% to 15% of patients. Treatment with nafarelin acetate was associated with elevations of plasma phosphorus and eosinophil counts, and decreases in serum calcium and WBC counts. Danazol therapy was associated with an increase of hematocrit and WBC.

Musculoskeletal –

Changes in bone density: After 6 months of treatment with nafarelin acetate, vertebral trabecular bone density and total vertebral bone mass, measured by quantitative computed tomography (QCT), decreased by an average of 8.7% and 4.3%, respectively, compared to pretreatment levels. There was partial recovery of bone density in the post-treatment period; the average trabecular bone density and total bone mass were 4.9% and 3.3% less than the pretreatment levels, respectively. Total vertebral bone mass, measured by dual photon absorptiometry (DPA), decreased by a mean of 5.9% at the end of treatment.

After six months treatment with nafarelin acetate, bone mass as measured by dual x-ray bone densitometry (DEXA), decreased 3.2%. Mean total vertebral mass, re-examined by DEXA six months after completion of treatment, was 1.4% below pretreatment. There was little, if any, decrease in the mineral content in compact bone of the distal radius and second metacarpal. Use of nafarelin acetate for longer than the recommended 6 months or in the presence of other known risk factors for decreased bone mineral content may cause additional bone loss.

➤*Central precocious puberty:* In clinical trials of 155 pediatric patients, 2.6% reported symptoms suggestive of drug sensitivity, such as shortness of breath, chest pain, urticaria, rash, and pruritus.

In these 155 patients treated for an average of 41 months and as long as 80 months (6.7 years), adverse events most frequently reported (more than 3% of patients) consisted largely of episodes occurring during the first 6 weeks of treatment as a result of the transient stimulatory action of nafarelin upon the pituitary-gonadal axis:

- acne (10%)
- transient breast enlargement (8%)
- vaginal bleeding (8%)
- emotional lability (6%)
- transient increase in pubic hair (5%)
- body odor (4%)
- seborrhea (3%)

Hot flashes, common in adult women treated for endometriosis, occurred in only 3% of treated children and were transient. Other adverse reactions thought to be drug-related, and occurring in more than 3% of patients were rhinitis (5%) and white or brownish vaginal discharge (3%). Approximately 3% of patients withdrew from clinical trials due to adverse events.

In one male patient with concomitant congenital adrenal hyperplasia, and who had discontinued treatment 8 months previously to resume puberty, adrenal rest tumors were found in the left testis. Relationship to nafarelin acetate is unlikely.

Regular examinations of the pituitary gland by magnetic resonance imaging (MRI) or computer assisted tomography (CT) of children during long-term nafarelin therapy as well as during the post-treatment period has occasionally revealed changes in the shape and size of the pituitary gland. These changes include asymmetry and enlargement of the pituitary gland, and a pituitary microadenoma has been suspected in a few children. The relationship of these findings to nafarelin acetate is not known.

Overdosage

In experimental animals, a single subcutaneous administration of up to 60 times the recommended human dose (on a mcg/kg basis, not adjusted for bioavailability) had no adverse effects. At present, there is no clinical evidence of adverse effects following overdosage of GnRH analogs.

Based on studies in monkeys, nafarelin acetate is not absorbed after oral administration.

GANIRELIX ACETATE

Rx	**Ganirelix Acetate** (Organon)	**Injection:** 250 mcg per 0.5 mL	In 1 mL prefilled, disposable syringes. In 1s.

GANIRELIX ACETATE — INJECTION

Indications

➤*Infertility treatment:* For the inhibition of premature luteinizing hormone (LH) surges in women undergoing controlled ovarian hyperstimulation.

Administration and Dosage

➤*Adults:*

Infertility treatment –

Usual dosage: After initiating follicle-stimulating hormone (FSH) therapy on day 2 or 3 of the cycle, ganirelix 250 mcg may be administered subcutaneously once daily during the early- to mid-follicular phase. By taking advantage of endogenous pituitary FSH secretion, the requirement for exogenously administered FSH may be reduced.

Concomitant therapy: When a sufficient number of follicles of adequate size are present, as assessed by ultrasound, final maturation of follicles is induced by administering hCG. Withhold the administration of hCG in cases where the ovaries are abnormally enlarged on the last day of FSH therapy to reduce the chance of developing ovarian hyperstimulation syndrome (OHSS).

Discontinuation of therapy: Continue treatment with ganirelix daily until the day of chorionic gonadotropin (hCG) administration.

➤*Administration:* Ganirelix is intended for subcutaneous administration only. The most convenient sites for subcutaneous injection are in the abdomen around the navel or upper thigh.

Use the sterile, prefilled syringe only once and dispose of it properly.

➤*Storage / Stability:* Store at 25°C (77°F). Protect from light.

Actions

➤*Pharmacology:* Ganirelix is a synthetic decapeptide with high antagonistic activity against naturally occurring gonadotropin-releasing hormone (GnRH). Ganirelix is derived from native GnRH with substitutions of amino acids at positions 1, 2, 3, 6, 8, and 10.

GANIRELIX ACETATE — INJECTION

The pulsatile release of GnRH stimulates the synthesis and secretion of LH and FSH. Ganirelix acts by competitively blocking the GnRH receptors on the pituitary gonadotroph and subsequent transduction pathway. It induces a rapid, reversible suppression of gonadotropin secretion. The suppression of pituitary LH secretion by ganirelix is more pronounced than that of FSH. An initial release of endogenous gonadotropins has not been detected with ganirelix, which is consistent with an antagonist effect. Upon discontinuation of ganirelix, pituitary LH and FSH levels are fully recovered within 48 hours.

➤*Pharmacokinetics:* The pharmacokinetic parameters of single and multiple injections of ganirelix in healthy adult females are summarized in the following table. Steady-state serum concentrations are reached after 3 days of treatment. The pharmacokinetics of ganirelix are dose-proportional in the dose range of 125 to 500 mcg.

Mean Pharmacokinetic Parameters of Ganirelix	
Absorption	
Mean absolute bioavailability	91.1%[a]
C_{max}	14.8 ng/ml[a], 11.2 ng/ml[b]
T_{max}	1.1[a,b]
Distribution	
Vd	43.7 L[c], 76.5 L[b]
Protein binding	81.9%
Metabolism	
Metabolites	1 to 4 peptide and 1 to 6 peptide
Excretion	
Site	feces (75.1%)[d,e], urine (22.1%)[d,f]
Elimination t½	12.8 h[a], 16.2 h[b]
Clearance	2.4 L/h[c], 3.3[b]

[a] Based on single-dose administration of 250 mcg subcutaneously.
[b] Based on multiple-dose administration of 250 mcg daily subcutaneous × 7 days.
[c] Based on single-dose administration of 250 mcg IV.
[d] Recovered over 288 hours following single-dose administration of 1 mg IV.
[e] Fecal excretion plateaus 192 hours after dosing.
[f] Urinary excretion is complete in 24 hours.

Contraindications

Hypersensitivity to ganirelix, any of its components, GnRH, or any other GnRH analog; known or suspected pregnancy (see Warnings).

Warnings/Precautions

➤*Latex allergy:* The packaging of this product contains natural rubber latex, which may cause allergic reactions.

➤*Hypersensitivity reactions:* Caution is advised in patients with hypersensitivity to GnRH. Carefully monitor these patients after the first injection. Refer to the Management of Acute Hypersensitivity Reactions. Anaphylactic reactions or ganirelix antibody formation have not been reported in clinical trials.

➤*Pregnancy: Category X.* Ganirelix is contraindicated in pregnant women. When administered from day 7 to near term to pregnant rats and rabbits at doses 10 and 30 mcg/day (approximately 0.4 to 3.2 times the human dose based on body surface area) or more, ganirelix increased the incidence of litter resorption. There was no increase in fetal abnormalities.

The effects on fetal resorption are logical consequences of the alteration in hormonal levels brought about by the antigonadotrophic properties of this drug and could result in fetal loss in humans. Therefore, do not use this drug in pregnant women.

Ganirelix should be prescribed by physicians who are experienced in infertility treatment. Before starting treatment with ganirelix, exclude pregnancy. Safe use of ganirelix during pregnancy has not been established.

Congenital anomalies – Ongoing clinical follow-up studies of 283 newborns of women administered ganirelix were reviewed. There were 3 neonates with major congenital anomalies and 18 neonates with minor congenital anomalies. The major congenital anomalies were the following: Hydrocephalus/Meningocele, omphalocele, and Beckwith-Wiedemann syndrome. The minor congenital anomalies were the following: Nevus, skin tags, sacral sinus, hemangioma, torticollis/asymmetric skull, talipes, supernumerary digit finger, hip subluxation, torticollis/high palate, occiput/abnormal hand crease, hernia unbilicalis, hernia inguinalis, hydrocele, undescended testes, and hydronephrosis. The causal relationship between these congenital anomalies and ganirelix is unknown. Multiple factors, genetic, and others (including, but not limited to intracytoplasmatic sperm injection [ICSI], in vitro fertilization [IVF], gonadotropins, progesterone) may confound assisted reproductive technology (ART) procedures.

➤*Lactation:* It is not known whether this drug is excreted in breast milk. Ganirelix should not be used by breast-feeding women.

Drug Interactions

➤*Gonadotropins:* Because ganirelix can suppress the secretion of pituitary gonadotropins, dose adjustments of exogenous gonadotropins may be necessary when used during controlled ovarian hyperstimulation.

Adverse Reactions

In clinical studies, treatment duration ranged from 1 to 14 days. The following table represents adverse events from the first day of ganirelix administration until confirmation of pregnancy by ultrasound at an incidence of at least 1% in ganirelix-treated subjects without regard to causality.

Ganirelix Adverse Reactions (≥ 1%)	
Adverse reaction	Ganirelix (n = 794)
Abdominal pain (gynecological)	4.8%
Death, fetal	3.7%
Headache	3%
Ovarian hyperstimulation syndrome	2.4%
Vaginal bleeding	1.8%
Injection site reaction	1.1%
Nausea	1.1%
Abdominal pain (GI)	1%

➤*Lab test abnormalities:* A neutrophil count at least 8.3 ($\times 10^9$/L) was noted in 11.9% (16.8 $\times 10^9$/L or less) of all subjects in the clinical trials. In addition, downward shifts within the ganirelix group were observed for hematocrit and total bilirubin. The clinical significance of these findings was not determined.

Patient Information

Prior to therapy with ganirelix, inform patients of the duration of treatment and monitoring procedures that will be required. Discuss the risk of possible adverse reactions (see Adverse Reactions). Do not prescribe ganirelix if the patient is pregnant.

CETRORELIX ACETATE

Rx	**Cetrotide** (Serono)	**Injection:** 0.25 mg	In trays containing 1 vial of 0.26 to 0.27 mg cetrorelix acetate, 1 mL syringe of sterile water for injection, a 20-gauge needle, a 27-gauge needle, and alcohol swabs. In 1s and 7s.
		3 mg	In trays containing 1 vial of 3.12 to 3.24 mg cetrorelix acetate, a 3 mL syringe of sterile water for injection, a 20-gauge needle, a 27-gauge needle, and alcohol swabs. In 1s.

CETRORELIX ACETATE — INJECTION

Indications

➤*Infertility treatment:* Cetrorelix is indicated for the inhibition of premature luteinizing hormone (LH) surges in women undergoing controlled ovarian stimulation.

Administration and Dosage

➤*Adults:*

Infertility treatment –

Usual dosage: Start ovarian stimulation therapy with gonadotropins (follicle-stimulating hormone [FSH], human menopausal gonadotropin [HMG]) on cycle day 2 or 3. Adjust the dose of gonadotropins according to individual response.

Cetrorelix may be administered subcutaneously once daily (0.25 mg dose) or once (3 mg dose) during the early- to midfollicular phase.

When assessment by ultrasound shows a sufficient number of follicles of adequate size, administer human chorionic gonadotropin (hCG) to induce ovulation and final maturation of the oocytes. No hCG should be administered if the ovaries show an excessive response to the treatment with gonadotropins to reduce the chance of developing ovarian hyperstimulation syndrome (OHSS).

• *Single-dose cetrorelix regimen* – Administer cetrorelix 3 mg subcutaneously when the serum estradiol level is indicative of an appropriate stimulation response, usually on stimulation day 7 (range, day 5 to 9).

If hCG has not been administered within 4 days after injection of cetrorelix 3 mg, administer cetrorelix 0.25 mg subcutaneously once daily until the day of hCG administration.

• *Multiple-dose cetrorelix regimen* – Administer cetrorelix 0.25 mg subcutaneously on stimulation day 5 (morning or evening) or day 6 (morning) and continue daily until the day of hCG administration.

➤*Administration:* Cetrorelix 0.25 and 3 mg can be administered by the patient after appropriate instructions by her health care provider.

➤*Storage/Stability:* Store cetrorelix in a cool, dry place protected from excess moisture and heat. Store cetrorelix 3 mg at 25°C (77°F). Excursions are permitted to 15° to 30°C (59° to 86°F). Store cetrorelix 0.25 mg in the refrigerator at 2° to 8°C (36° to 46°F). Keep the packaged tray in the outer carton in order to protect it from light.

Use immediately after preparation. Discard unused material.

Actions

➤*Pharmacology:* GnRH induces the production and release of LH and follicle-stimulating hormone (FSH) from the gonadotrophic cells of the ante-

CETRORELIX ACETATE — INJECTION

rior pituitary. Because of a positive estradiol (E_2) feedback at midcycle, GnRH liberation is enhanced, resulting in an LH surge. This LH surge induces the ovulation of the dominant follicle, resumption of oocyte meiosis and, subsequently, luteinization, as indicated by rising progesterone levels.

Cetrorelix competes with natural GnRH for binding to membrane receptors on pituitary cells and thus controls the release of LH and FSH in a dose-dependent manner. The onset of LH suppression is approximately 1 hour with the 3 mg dose and 2 hours with the 0.25 mg dose. This suppression is maintained by continuous treatment, and there is a more pronounced effect on LH than on FSH. An initial release of endogenous gonadotropins has not been detected with cetrorelix, which is consistent with an antagonist effect.

The effects of cetrorelix on LH and FSH are reversible after discontinuation of treatment. In women, cetrorelix delays the LH surge and, consequently, ovulation in a dose-dependent fashion. FSH levels are not affected at the doses used during controlled ovarian stimulation. Following a single 3 mg dose of cetrorelix, duration of action of at least 4 days has been established. A dose of cetrorelix 0.25 mg every 24 hours has been shown to maintain the effect.

➤*Pharmacokinetics:* The pharmacokinetic parameters of single and multiple doses of cetrorelix in adult healthy women are summarized in the following table.

Pharmacokinetic Parameters of Cetrorelix Following 3 mg Single or 0.25 mg Single and Multiple (Daily for 14 Days) Subcutaneous Administration

Parameter	Single dose 3 mg (n = 12)	Single dose 0.25 mg (n = 12)	Multiple dose 0.25 mg (n = 12)
T_{max}[a,b] (h)	1.5 (0.5 to 2)	1 (0.5 to 1.5)	1 (0.5 to 2)
$T_{1/2}$[a,c] (h)	62.8 (38.2 to 108)	5 (2.4 to 48.8)	20.6 (4.1 to 179.3)
C_{max}[d] (ng/mL)	28.5 (22.5 to 36.2)	4.97 (4.17 to 5.92)	6.42 (5.18 to 7.96)
AUC[e] (ng•h/mL)	536 (451 to 636)	31.4 (23.4 to 42)	44.5 (36.7 to 54.2)
CL[f,g] (mL/min•kg)	1.28[h]		
Vz[f,i] (L/kg)	1.16[h]		

[a] Geometric mean (95% CI_{ln}), arithmetic mean.
[b] T_{max} = Time to reach observed maximum plasma concentration.
[c] $T_{1/2}$ = Elimination half-life.
[d] C_{max} = Maximum plasma concentration; multiple dose $C_{ss, max}$.
[e] AUC = Area under the curve; single dose $AUC_{0-\infty}$ multiple dose AUC_{Υ}.
[f] Geometric mean (95% CI_{ln}), median (minimum to maximum).
[g] CL = Total plasma clearance.
[h] Based on IV administration (n = 6, separate study 0013).
[i] V_z = Volume of distribution.

Absorption – Cetrorelix is rapidly absorbed following subcutaneous injection, maximal plasma concentrations being achieved approximately 1 to 2 hours after administration. The mean absolute bioavailability of cetrorelix following subcutaneous administration to healthy women is 85%.

Distribution – The volume of distribution of cetrorelix following a single IV dose of 3 mg is about 1 L/kg. In vitro protein binding to human plasma is 86%.

Cetrorelix concentrations in follicular fluid and plasma were similar on the day of oocyte pick-up in patients undergoing controlled ovarian stimulation. Following subcutaneous administration of cetrorelix 0.25 and 3 mg, plasma concentrations of cetrorelix were below or in the range of the lower limit of quantitation on the day of oocyte pick-up and embryo transfer.

Metabolism – After subcutaneous administration of cetrorelix 10 mg to women and men, cetrorelix and small amounts of (1 to 9), (1 to 7), (1 to 6), and (1 to 4) peptides were found in bile samples over 24 hours.

In in vitro studies, cetrorelix was stable against phase I- and phase II-metabolism. Cetrorelix was transformed by peptidases, and the (1 to 4) peptide was the predominant metabolite.

Excretion – Following subcutaneous administration of cetrorelix 10 mg to men and women, only unchanged cetrorelix was detected in urine. In 24 hours, cetrorelix and small amounts of the (1 to 9), (1 to 7), (1 to 6), and (1 to 4) peptides were found in bile samples. Two percent to 4% of the dose was eliminated in the urine as unchanged cetrorelix, while 5% to 10% was eliminated as cetrorelix and the 4 metabolites in bile. Therefore, only 7% to 14% of the total dose was recovered as unchanged cetrorelix and metabolites in urine and bile up to 24 hours. The remaining portion of the dose may not have been recovered since bile and urine were not collected for a longer period of time.

Contraindications

Hypersensitivity to cetrorelix acetate, extrinsic peptide hormones, or mannitol; known hypersensitivity to GnRH or any other GnRH analogs; known or suspected pregnancy, and lactation; severe renal impairment.

Warnings/Precautions

➤*Hypersensitivity reactions:* Caution is advised in patients with hypersensitivity to GnRH. Carefully monitor these patients after the first injection. A severe anaphylactic reaction associated with cough, rash, and hypotension was observed in 1 patient after 7 months of treatment with 10 mg/day cetrorelix in a study for an indication unrelated to infertility.

➤*Special risk:* Take special care in women with signs and symptoms of active allergic conditions or known history of allergic predisposition. Treatment with cetrorelix is not advised in women with severe allergic conditions.

➤*Pregnancy: Category X.* Cetrorelix is contraindicated in pregnant women.

Cetrorelix should be prescribed by health care providers who are experienced in fertility treatment. Before starting treatment with cetrorelix acetate, pregnancy must be excluded.

When administered to rats for the first 7 days of pregnancy, cetrorelix did not affect the development of the implanted conceptus at doses up to 38 mcg/kg (approximately 1 times the recommended human therapeutic dose based on body surface area). However, a dose of 139 mcg/kg (approximately 4 times the human dose) resulted in a resorption rate and a postimplantation loss of 100%.

When administered from day 6 to near term to pregnant rats and rabbits, very early resorptions and total implantation losses were seen in rats at doses from 4.6 mcg/kg (0.2 times the human dose) and in rabbits at doses from 6.8 mcg/kg (0.4 times the human dose). In animals that maintained their pregnancies, there was no increase in the incidence of fetal abnormalities.

The fetal resorption observed in animals is a logical consequence of the alteration in hormonal levels effected by the antigonadotrophic properties of cetrorelix acetate, which could result in fetal loss in humans as well. Therefore, do not use this drug in pregnant women.

Congenital anomalies – Clinical follow-up studies of 316 newborns of women administered cetrorelix were reviewed. One infant of a set of twin neonates was found to have anencephaly at birth and died after 4 days. The other twin was healthy. Developmental findings from ongoing baby follow-up included a child with a ventricular septal defect and another child with bilateral congenital glaucoma.

Four pregnancies that resulted in therapeutic abortion in phase 2 and phase 3 controlled ovarian stimulation studies had major anomalies (diaphragmatic hernia, trisomy 21, Klinefelter syndrome, polymalformation, and trisomy 18). In 3 of these 4 cases, intracytoplasmic sperm injection (ICSI) was the fertilization method employed; in the fourth case, in vitro fertilization (IVF) was the method employed.

The minor congenital anomalies reported include supernumerary nipple, bilateral strabismus, imperforate hymen, congenital nevi, hemangiomata, and QT syndrome.

The casual relationship between the reported anomalies and cetrorelix is unknown. Multiple factors, genetic and others (including, but not limited to ICSI, IVF, gonadotropins, and progesterone), make causal attribution difficult to study.

➤*Lactation:* It is not known whether cetrorelix is excreted in human milk. Because many drugs are excreted in human milk, and because the effects of cetrorelix on lactation or the breastfed child have not been determined, do not use cetrorelix acetate in nursing mothers.

➤*Elderly:* Cetrorelix is not intended to be used in subjects aged 65 years of age and older.

➤*Lab test abnormalities:* After the exclusion of preexisting conditions, enzyme elevations (ALT, AST, GGT, alkaline phosphatase) were found in 1% to 2% of patients receiving cetrorelix during controlled ovarian stimulation. The elevations ranged up to 3 times the upper limit of normal. The clinical significance of these findings was not determined.

During stimulation with human menopausal gonadotropin, cetrorelix had no notable effects on hormone levels aside from inhibition of LH surges.

➤*Monitoring:* Caution is advised in patients with hypersensitivity to GnRH. Carefully monitor these patients after the first injection. A severe anaphylactic reaction associated with cough, rash, and hypotension was observed in 1 patient after 7 months of treatment with cetrorelix 10 mg daily in a study for an indication unrelated to infertility.

Drug Interactions

No formal drug interaction studies have been performed with cetrorelix.

Adverse Reactions

The safety of cetrorelix in 949 patients undergoing controlled ovarian stimulation in clinical studies was evaluated. Women were between 19 and 40 years of age (mean age, 32). Ninety-four percent of them were white patients. Cetrorelix was given in doses ranging from 0.1 to 5 mg as a single or multiple dose.

The following table shows systemic adverse reactions, reported in clinical studies without regard to causality, from the beginning of cetrorelix treatment until confirmation of pregnancy by ultrasound at an incidence greater than or equal to 1% in cetrorelix-treated subjects undergoing COS.

Adverse Reactions in Cetrorelix-Treated Subjects (≥ 1%)

Adverse reaction	Cetrorelix for Injection (n = 949) % (n)
Nausea	1.3% (12)
Headache	1.1% (10)
Ovarian hyperstimulation syndrome[a]	3.5% (33)

[a] Intensity moderate or severe, or WHO grade 2 or 3, respectively.

Local site reactions (eg, redness, erythema, bruising, itching, swelling, pruritus) were reported. Usually they were of a transient nature, mild intensity,

CETRORELIX ACETATE — INJECTION

and short duration. During postmarketing surveillance, rare cases of hypersensitivity reactions including anaphylactoid reactions have been reported.

Two stillbirths were reported in phase 3 studies of cetrorelix.

Overdosage

There have been no reports of overdosage with 0.25 or 3 mg cetrorelix in humans. Single doses up to 120 mg cetrorelix have been well tolerated in patients treated for other indications without signs of overdosage.

Patient Information

Prior to therapy with cetrorelix, inform patients of the duration of treatment and monitoring procedures that will be required. Discuss the risk of possible adverse reactions. Cetrorelix should not be prescribed if a patient is pregnant.

DEGARELIX

Rx	**Firmagon** (Ferring)	**Injection, lyophilized powder for solution:** 80 mg	As degarelix acetate. Mannitol 200 mg. In vials.
		120 mg	As degarelix acetate. Mannitol 150 mg. In vials.

DEGARELIX ACETATE — INJECTION

Indications

➤*Advanced prostate cancer:* For treatment of patients with advanced prostate cancer.

Administration and Dosage

➤*General dosing considerations:* Degarelix is for subcutaneous administration only and is not to be administered intravenously (IV).

Caution should be exercised in handling and preparing the solution of degarelix. Several guidelines on proper handling and disposal of anticancer drugs have been published.

➤*Adults:*

Advanced prostate cancer –

Initial dosage: 240 mg subcutaneous injection (given as 2 injections of 120 mg at a concentration of 40 mg/mL).

Maintenance dosage: 80 mg subcutaneous injection (at a concentration of 20 mg/mL) every 28 days. The first maintenance dose should be given 28 days after the starting dose.

➤*Preparation for administration:* Degarelix is supplied as a powder to be reconstituted with sterile water for injection. The reconstitution procedure needs to be followed carefully. Administration of other concentrations is not recommended.

Instructions for proper use –

- Gloves should be worn during preparation and administration.
- Reconstituted drug must be administered within 1 hour after addition of sterile water for injection.
- Keep the vial vertical at all times.
- Do not shake the vials.
- Follow aseptic technique.

Degarelix 120 mg vial: The treatment initiation pack contains 2 vials of degarelix 120 mg that must be prepared for 2 subcutaneous injections. Hence, the following instructions need to be repeated a second time.

Prepare degarelix 120 mg for reconstitution by gathering the following:

- 6 mL of sterile water for injection; do not use bacteriostatic water for injection
- 2 reconstitution needles (21 G/2 inch)
- 2 administration needles for subcutaneous injection (27 G/1¼ inch)
- 2 injection syringes (5 mL).

1.) Draw up 3 mL of sterile water for injection with a reconstitution needle (21 G/2 in).
2.) Inject the sterile water for injection slowly into the degarelix 120 mg vial. To keep the product and syringe sterile, do not remove the syringe and the needle.
3.) Keeping the vial in an upright position, swirl it very gently until the liquid looks clear and is without undissolved powder or particles. If the powder adheres to the vial over the liquid surface, the vial can be tilted slightly to dissolve powder. Avoid shaking to prevent foam formation. A ring of small air bubbles on the surface of the liquid is acceptable. The reconstitution procedure may take up to 15 minutes.
4.) Tilt the vial slightly and keep the needle in the lowest part of the vial. Withdraw 3 mL of degarelix 120 mg without turning the vial upside down.
5.) Exchange the reconstitution needle with the administration needle for deep subcutaneous injection (27 G/1¼ in). Remove any air bubbles.
6.) Inject 3 mL of degarelix 120 mg subcutaneously immediately after reconstitution. Grasp the skin of the abdomen, elevate the subcutaneous tissue. Insert the needle deeply at an angle of not less than 45 degrees. Gently pull back the plunger to check if blood is aspirated. If blood appears in the syringe, the reconstituted product can no longer be used. Discontinue the procedure and discard the syringe and the needle (reconstitute a new dose for the patient).
7.) Repeat reconstitution procedure for the second dose. Choose a different injection site and inject 3 mL.

Degarelix 80 mg vial: The treatment maintenance pack contains 1 vial of degarelix 80 mg that must be prepared for subcutaneous injection.

Prepare degarelix 80 mg for reconstitution by gathering the following:

- 4.2 mL of sterile water for injection; do not use bacteriostatic water for injection
- 1 reconstitution needle (21 G/2 in)
- 1 administration needle for subcutaneous injection (27 G/1¼ in)
- 1 injection syringe (5 mL).

1.) Draw up 4.2 mL of sterile water for injection with the reconstitution needle (21 G/2 in).
2.) Inject the sterile water for injection slowly into the degarelix 80 mg vial. To keep the product and syringe sterile, do not remove the syringe and the needle.
3.) Keeping the vial in an upright position, swirl it very gently until the liquid looks clear and is without undissolved powder or particles. If the powder adheres to the vial over the liquid surface, the vial can be tilted slightly to dissolve powder. Avoid shaking to prevent foam formation. A ring of small air bubbles on the surface of the liquid is acceptable. The reconstitution procedure may take up to 15 minutes.
4.) Tilt the vial slightly and keep the needle in the lowest part of the vial. Withdraw 4 mL of degarelix 80 mg without turning the vial upside down.
5.) Exchange the reconstitution needle with the administration needle for deep subcutaneous injection (27 G/1¼ in). Remove any air bubbles.
6.) Inject 4 mL of degarelix 80 mg subcutaneously immediately after reconstitution. Grasp the skin of the abdomen, elevate the subcutaneous tissue. Insert the needle deeply at an angle of not less than 45 degrees. Gently pull back the plunger to check if blood is aspirated. If blood appears in the syringe, the reconstituted product can no longer be used. Discontinue the procedure and discard the syringe and the needle (reconstitute a new dose for the patient).

➤*Administration:* Degarelix is for subcutaneous administration only and is not to be administered IV.

Administer as a subcutaneous injection in the abdominal region. As with other drugs administered by subcutaneous injection, the injection site should vary periodically. Injections should be given in areas of the abdomen that will not be exposed to pressure (eg, not close to the waistband or belt, not close to the ribs).

➤*Storage/Stability:* Store at 25°C (77°F); excursions are permitted between 15° and 30°C (59° and 86°F). Reconstituted drug must be administered within 1 hour after addition of sterile water for injection.

Handling and disposal – Caution should be exercised in handling and preparing the solution of degarelix. Several guidelines on proper handling and disposal of anticancer drugs have been published. To minimize the risk of dermal exposure, always wear impervious gloves when handling degarelix. If degarelix solution contacts the skin, immediately wash the skin thoroughly with soap and water. If degarelix contacts mucous membranes, the membranes should be flushed immediately and thoroughly with water.

Actions

➤*Pharmacology:* Degarelix is a gonadotropin-releasing hormone (GnRH) receptor antagonist. It binds reversibly to the pituitary GnRH receptors, thereby reducing the release of gonadotropins and, consequently, testosterone.

Pharmacodynamics – A single dose of degarelix 240 mg causes a decrease in the plasma concentrations of luteinizing hormone and follicle-stimulating hormone, and, subsequently, testosterone.

Degarelix is effective in achieving and maintaining testosterone suppression below the castration level of 50 ng/dL.

➤*Pharmacokinetics:*

Absorption – Degarelix forms a depot upon subcutaneous administration, from which degarelix is released to the circulation. Following administration of degarelix 240 mg at a product concentration of 40 mg/mL, the mean maximal drug concentration (C_{max}) was 26.2 ng/mL (coefficient of variation [CV], 83%) and the mean area under the curve was 1,054 ng•day/mL (CV, 35%). Typically, C_{max} occurred within 2 days after subcutaneous administration. In patients with prostate cancer at a product concentration of 40 mg/mL, the pharmacokinetics of degarelix were linear over a dose range of 120 to 240 mg. The pharmacokinetic behavior of the drug is strongly influenced by its concentration in the injection solution.

Distribution – The volume of distribution of degarelix after IV (more than 1 L/kg) or subcutaneous administration (more than 1,000 L) indicates that degarelix is distributed throughout total body water. In vitro plasma protein binding of degarelix is estimated to be approximately 90%.

Metabolism – Degarelix is subject to peptide hydrolysis during the passage of the hepatobiliary system and is mainly excreted as peptide fragments in the feces. No quantitatively significant metabolites were detected in plasma samples after subcutaneous administration. In vitro studies have shown that degarelix is not a substrate, inducer, or inhibitor of the cytochrome P-450 (CYP-450) or P-glycoprotein transporter systems.

Excretion – Following subcutaneous administration of degarelix 240 mg at a concentration of 40 mg/mL to patients with prostate cancer, degarelix is eliminated in a biphasic fashion, with a median terminal half-life of approxi-

DEGARELIX ACETATE — INJECTION

mately 53 days. The long half-life after subcutaneous administration is a consequence of a very slow release of degarelix from the degarelix depot formed at the injection site(s). Approximately 20% to 30% of a given dose of degarelix was renally excreted, suggesting that approximately 70% to 80% is excreted via the hepatobiliary system in humans. Following subcutaneous administration of degarelix to patients with prostate cancer, the clearance is approximately 9 L/h.

Contraindications

Known hypersensitivity to degarelix or to any of the product components; women who are or may become pregnant.

Warnings/Precautions

➤*QT/QTc interval effects:* Long-term androgen-deprivation therapy prolongs the QT interval. Consider whether the benefits of androgen-deprivation therapy outweigh the potential risks in patients with congenital long QT syndrome, electrolyte abnormalities, or congestive heart failure, and in patients taking class IA (eg, procainamide, quinidine) or class III (eg, amiodarone, sotalol) antiarrhythmic medications.

In the randomized, active-controlled trial comparing degarelix with leuprolide, periodic electrocardiograms were performed. Seven patients, 3 (less than 1%) in the pooled degarelix group and 4 (2%) patients in the leuprolide 7.5 mg group, had a QTcF of 500 msec or more. From baseline to end of study, the median change for degarelix was 12.3 msec and for leuprolide was 16.7 msec.

➤*Immunogenicity:* Anti-degarelix antibody development has been observed in 10% of patients after treatment with degarelix for 1 year. There is no indication that the efficacy or safety of degarelix treatment is affected by antibody formation.

➤*Renal function impairment:* Data on patients with moderate or severe renal impairment is limited; therefore, use degarelix with caution in patients with CrCl less than 50 mL/min.

➤*Hepatic function impairment:* Because hepatic impairment can lower degarelix exposure, it is recommended that, in patients with hepatic impairment, testosterone concentrations are monitored on a monthly basis until medical castration is achieved. Once medical castration is achieved, consider an every-other-month testosterone monitoring approach.

Patients with severe hepatic dysfunction have not been studied; caution is therefore warranted in this group.

➤*Pregnancy: Category X.* Degarelix can cause fetal harm when administered to a pregnant woman. If this drug is used during pregnancy, or if the patient becomes pregnant while taking this drug, apprise the patient of the potential hazard to the fetus. Advise women who are or may become pregnant to not take degarelix.

When degarelix was given to rabbits during early organogenesis at dosages of 0.002 mg/kg/day (about 0.02% of the clinical loading dose on a mg/m^2 basis), there was an increase in early postimplantation loss. Degarelix given to rabbits during mid and late organogenesis at dosages of 0.006 mg/kg/day (about 0.05% of the clinical loading dose on a mg/m^2 basis) caused embryo/fetal lethality and abortion. When degarelix was given to female rats during early organogenesis, at dosages of 0.0045 mg/kg/day (about 0.036% of the clinical loading dose on a mg/m^2 basis), there was an increase in early postimplantation loss. When degarelix was given to female rats during mid and late organogenesis, at dosages of 0.045 mg/kg/day (about 0.36% of the clinical loading dose on a mg/m^2 basis), there was an increase in the number of minor skeletal abnormalities and variants.

➤*Lactation:* Degarelix is not indicated for use in women, and is contraindicated in women who are or who may become pregnant. It is not known whether this drug is excreted in human milk. Because many drugs are excreted in human milk and because of the potential for serious adverse reactions in breast-feeding infants from degarelix, decide whether to discontinue breast-feeding or the drug, taking into account the importance of the drug to the mother.

➤*Children:* Safety and effectiveness in children have not been established.

➤*Elderly:* No overall differences in safety or effectiveness were observed between these subjects and younger subjects, but greater sensitivity of some older individuals cannot be ruled out.

➤*Lab test abnormalities:* Therapy with degarelix results in suppression of the pituitary gonadal system. Results of diagnostic tests of the pituitary gonadotropic and gonadal functions conducted during and after degarelix may be affected.

➤*Monitoring:* In patients with hepatic impairment, monitor testosterone concentrations on a monthly basis until medical castration is achieved. Once medical castration is achieved, consider an every-other-month testosterone monitoring approach.

Monitor concentrations of prostate-specific antigen (PSA) periodically. If PSA increases, measure serum concentrations of testosterone.

Drug Interactions

An additive effect of degarelix with other drugs that prolong the QT interval cannot be excluded. The following drugs may prolong the QT interval and increase the risk of life-threatening cardiac arrhythmias, including torsades de pointes: antiarrhythmic agents (eg, amiodarone, bretylium, disopyramide, dofetilide, procainamide, quinidine, sotalol), arsenic trioxide, chlorpromazine, cisapride, dolasetron, droperidol, mefloquine, mesoridazine, moxifloxacin, pentamidine, pimozide, tacrolimus, thioridazine, ziprasidone. For a more complete list of drugs that may prolong the QT interval, see the appendix "Drug-Induced Prolongation of the QT Interval and Torsades de Pointes."

Adverse Reactions

For more information on QT interval prolongation, see the Warnings/Precautions section.

➤*Most common adverse reactions:* The most commonly observed adverse reactions during degarelix therapy included injection-site reactions (eg, pain, erythema, swelling, induration), hot flashes, increased weight, fatigue, and increases in serum levels of transaminases and gammaglutamyltransferase (GGT). The majority of the adverse reactions were grade 1 or 2, with grade 3/4 adverse reaction incidences of 1% or less.

Degarelix Adverse Reactions (≥ 5%)			
	Degarelix 240/160 mg (subcutaneous) (n = 202)	Degarelix 240/80 mg (subcutaneous) (n = 207)	Leuprolide 7.5 mg (IM) (n = 201)
Percentage of subjects with adverse reactions	83%	79%	78%
CNS			
Chills	4%	5%	0%
Fatigue	6%	3%	6%
Cardiovascular			
Hot flash	26%	26%	21%
Hypertension	7%	6%	4%
Musculoskeletal			
Arthralgia	4%	5%	9%
Back pain	6%	6%	8%
Miscellaneous			
Constipation	3%	5%	5%
Increases in transaminases and GGT	10%	10%	5%
Injection-site adverse events	44%	35%	< 1%
Urinary tract infection	2%	5%	9%
Weight increase	11%	9%	12%

➤*Local:* The most frequently reported adverse reactions at the injection sites were pain (28%), erythema (17%), swelling (6%), induration (4%), and nodule (3%). These adverse reactions were mostly transient, of mild to moderate intensity, occurred primarily with the starting dose, and led to few discontinuations (less than 1%). Grade 3 injection-site reactions occurred in 2% or less of patients receiving degarelix.

➤*Other adverse reactions:*

CNS – Asthenia, dizziness, fever, headache, insomnia (1% to 5%).

GI – Nausea (1% to 5%); diarrhea (at least 1%).

GU – Erectile dysfunction, gynecomastia, testicular atrophy (at least 1%).

Miscellaneous – Hyperhydrosis, night sweats (at least 1%).

Decreased bone density has been reported in the medical literature in men who have had orchiectomy or who have been treated with a GnRH agonist. It can be anticipated that long periods of medical castration in men will result in decreased bone density.

➤*Lab test abnormalities:* Hepatic laboratory abnormalities were primarily grade 1 or 2 and were generally reversible. Grade 3 hepatic laboratory abnormalities occurred in less than 1% of patients.

Overdosage

➤*Treatment:* There have been no reports of overdose with degarelix. In the case of overdose, however, discontinue degarelix, treat the patient symptomatically, and institute supportive measures.

Patient Information

Inform patient of the possible adverse reactions of androgen-deprivation therapy, including hot flashes, flushing of the skin, increased weight, decreased sex drive, and difficulties with erectile function. Possible adverse reactions related to therapy with degarelix include redness, swelling, and itching at the injection site; these are usually mild, self-limiting, and decrease within 3 days.

Anabolic steroids are classified as a *c-iii* controlled substance under the anabolic steroids act of 1990.

Indications

➤*Males:* For replacement therapy in hypogonadism associated with a deficiency or absence of endogenous testosterone.

Primary hypogonadism (congenital or acquired) – Testicular failure because of cryptorchidism, bilateral torsion, orchitis, vanishing testis syndrome or orchidectomy, Klinefelter syndrome, chemotherapy, or toxic damage from alcohol or heavy metals. These men usually have low serum testosterone levels and gonadotropins (FSH, LH) above the normal range.

Hypogonadotropic hypogonadism (congenital or acquired) – Idiopathic gonadotropin- or luteinizing hormone-releasing hormone (LHRH) deficiency or pituitary-hypothalamic injury from tumors, trauma, or radiation.

If the above conditions occur prior to puberty, androgen replacement therapy is needed for development of secondary sexual characteristics. Prolonged treatment is required to maintain sexual characteristics in these and other males who develop testosterone deficiency after puberty. However, appropriate adrenal cortical and thyroid hormone replacement therapy are still necessary and are of primary importance.

Delayed puberty – To stimulate puberty in carefully selected males with clearly delayed puberty. These patients usually have a familial pattern of delayed puberty that is not secondary to a pathological disorder; puberty is expected to occur spontaneously at a relatively late date. Brief occasional treatment with conservative doses may be justified if these patients do not respond to psychological support. Discuss the potential adverse effect on bone maturation with the patient and parents prior to androgen administration. To assess the effect of treatment on the epiphyseal centers, obtain an x-ray of the hand and wrist to determine bone age every 6 months.

➤*Females:*

Metastatic cancer – May be used secondarily in women with advancing inoperable metastatic (skeletal) mammary cancer who are 1 to 5 years postmenopausal. Primary goals of therapy include ablation of the ovaries. This treatment has been used in premenopausal women with breast cancer who have benefited from oophorectomy and have a hormone-responsive tumor.

Actions

➤*Pharmacology:* Testosterone, produced by the Leydig cells of the testis, is the primary male androgen.

In many tissues, the activity of testosterone appears to depend on reduction to dihydrotestosterone, which binds to cytosol receptor proteins. The steroid-receptor complex is transported to the nucleus where it initiates transcription events and cellular changes related to androgen action.

Endogenous androgens are responsible for the normal growth and development of the male sex organs and for maintenance of secondary sex characteristics. These effects include the growth and maturation of the prostate, seminal vesicles, penis, and scrotum; the development of male hair distribution, such as facial, pubic, chest, and axillary hair; laryngeal enlargement; vocal cord thickening; alterations in body musculature and fat distribution. These drugs also cause retention of nitrogen, sodium, potassium, phosphorus, and decreased urinary excretion of calcium. Androgens have been reported to increase protein anabolism and decrease protein catabolism. Nitrogen balance is improved only when there is sufficient intake of calories and protein.

Androgens are responsible for the growth spurt of adolescence and for the termination of linear growth by fusion of the epiphyseal growth centers. In children, exogenous androgens accelerate linear growth rates but may cause a disproportionate advancement in bone maturation. Use over long periods may result in fusion of the epiphyseal growth centers and termination of the growth process. Androgens have been reported to stimulate production of red blood cells by enhancing production of the erythropoietic stimulating factor.

During administration of exogenous androgens, endogenous testosterone release is inhibited through feedback inhibition of pituitary luteinizing hormone (LH). Large doses of exogenous androgens may suppress spermatogenesis through feedback inhibition of pituitary follicle-stimulating hormone (FSH).

➤*Pharmacokinetics:*

Absorption –

Oral: Testosterone is metabolized by the gut and 44% is cleared by the liver in the first pass. Doses as high as 400 mg daily are needed to achieve clinically effective blood levels for full replacement therapy. The synthetic androgen, **methyltestosterone**, is less extensively metabolized by the liver and has a longer half-life. It is more suitable than testosterone for oral administration.

IM: Testosterone esters are less polar than free testosterone. Testosterone esters in oil injected IM are absorbed slowly from the lipid phase; thus, **testosterone cypionate** and **enanthate** can be given at intervals of 2 to 4 weeks. Suspensions of testosterone or its esters in aqueous media may cause local irritation and the rate of absorption is not always uniform.

Topical gel: In a study with the dose of topical testosterone gel 10 g (to deliver testosterone 100 mg), all patients showed an increase in serum testosterone within 30 minutes, and 8 of 9 patients had a serum testosterone concentration within the normal range by 4 hours after the initial application. Absorption of testosterone into the blood continues for the entire 24-hour dosing interval. Serum concentrations approximate the steady-state level by the end of the first 24 hours and are at steady state by the second or third day of dosing.

When the topical gel treatment is discontinued after achieving steady state, serum testosterone levels remain in the normal range for 24 to 48 hours but return to their pretreatment levels by the fifth day after the last application.

Transdermal system:

• *Testoderm* – Following placement of *Testoderm* on scrotal skin, the serum testosterone concentration rises to a maximum at 2 to 4 hours and returns toward baseline within approximately 2 hours after system removal. Serum levels reach a plateau at 3 to 4 weeks. The testosterone levels achieved with *Testoderm* generally are within the range for normal men.

Scrotal skin is at least 5 times more permeable to testosterone than other skin sites. *Testoderm* and *Testoderm with Adhesive* will not produce adequate serum testosterone concentration if applied to nongenital skin.

• *Testoderm TTS* – The 3 recommended skin sites (arm, back, and upper buttocks) are interchangeable based on equivalent testosterone $AUC_{(0-27)}$ values.

• *Androderm* – Following application to nonscrotal skin, testosterone is continuously absorbed during the 24-hour dosing period. Daily application at approximately 10 p.m. results in a serum testosterone concentration profile that mimics the normal circadian variation observed in healthy young men. Maximum concentrations occur in the early morning hours with minimum concentrations in the evening. Normal range morning serum testosterone concentrations are reached during the first day of dosing. There is no accumulation of testosterone during continuous treatment.

Distribution – Testosterone in plasma is approximately 98% bound to a specific testosterone-estradiol-binding globulin. Generally, the amount of binding globulin will determine the percentage of free and bound testosterone; the free testosterone concentration will determine its half-life.

Metabolism/Excretion – There are considerable variations in the reported half-life of testosterone, ranging from 10 to 100 minutes. The half-life of **testosterone cypionate** IM is approximately 8 days; for oral **fluoxymesterone**, it is approximately 9.2 hours; **methyltestosterone** undergoes less extensive first-pass hepatic metabolism than testosterone following oral administration and has a longer half-life. Inactivation of testosterone occurs primarily in the liver. About 90% of a testosterone dose is excreted in the urine as conjugates of testosterone and its metabolites; about 6% of a dose is excreted in the feces.

Contraindications

Patients with serious cardiac, hepatic, or renal diseases; hypersensitivity to the drug or any components of the products; in men with carcinomas of the breast or known or suspected carcinoma of the prostate; women (*Testoderm*); pregnancy.

Pregnant women should avoid skin contact with *AndroGel* application sites in men. Testosterone may cause fetal harm. In the event that unwashed or unclothed skin to which *AndroGel* has been applied does come in direct contact with the skin of a pregnant woman, wash the general area of contact on the woman with soap and water as soon as possible. In vitro studies show that residual testosterone is removed from the skin surface by washing with soap and water.

Warnings/Precautions

➤*Hepatic effects:* Prolonged use of high doses of androgens has been associated with the development of potentially life-threatening peliosis hepatis, hepatic neoplasms, cholestatic hepatitis, jaundice, and hepatocellular carcinoma. Long-term therapy with **testosterone enanthate**, which elevates blood levels for prolonged periods, has produced multiple hepatic adenomas. Testosterone is not known to produce these adverse effects.

Cholestatic hepatitis and jaundice occur with **fluoxymesterone** and **methyltestosterone** at relatively low doses. If cholestatic hepatitis with jaundice appears with use of any androgen, or if liver function tests become abnormal, discontinue the androgen and determine the etiology. Drug-induced jaundice is reversible when the medication is discontinued.

➤*Athletic performance:* Although the anabolic steroids are generally the agents that are abused for enhancement of athletic performance, these agents also have been used for such purposes. However, these drugs are not safe and effective for this use and have a potential risk of serious side effects.

➤*Sleep apnea:* The treatment of hypogonadal men with testosterone esters may potentiate sleep apnea in some patients, especially those with risk factors such as obesity or chronic lung diseases.

➤*Breast cancer:* In patients with breast cancer, androgen therapy may cause hypercalcemia by stimulating osteolysis. If hypercalcemia occurs, discontinue the drug.

➤*Oligospermia:* Oligospermia and reduced ejaculatory volume may occur after prolonged administration or excessive dosage.

➤*Edema:* Edema, with or without congestive heart failure, may be a serious complication in patients with preexisting cardiac, renal, or hepatic disease. In addition to discontinuation of the drug, diuretic therapy may be required.

➤*Gynecomastia:* Gynecomastia frequently develops and occasionally persists in patients being treated for hypogonadism.

➤*Bone maturation:* Use cautiously in healthy males with delayed puberty. Monitor bone maturation by assessing bone age of the wrist and hand every 6 months.

➤*Product interchange:* Do not use **testosterone cypionate** interchangeably with **testosterone propionate** because of differences in duration of action.

➤*Virilization:* Observe women for signs of virilization (eg, deepening voice, hirsutism, acne, clitoromegaly, menstrual irregularities). Discontinue therapy at the time of evidence of mild virilism to prevent irreversible virilization. Virilization is usual following high-dose androgens. Some virilization should be tolerated during treatment for breast carcinoma.

Virilization of female partners has been reported with use of topical testosterone. Percutaneous creams leave as much as 90 mg residual testosterone on the skin. The results from one study indicated that, after removal of a *Testoderm* system, the potential for transfer of testosterone to a sexual partner was 6 mg, 1/45th the daily endogenous testosterone production by the female body. *Testoderm TTS* has an occlusive backing that prevents the partner from coming in contact with the active material in the system. If a *Testoderm TTS* system is inadvertently transferred to a female partner, remove it immediately and wash the contacted skin. Changes in body hair distribution or significant increases in acne of the female partner should be brought to the attention of a physician.

➤*Pellets:* Pellet implantation is much less flexible for dosage adjustment than is oral administration or IM injection of oil solutions or aqueous suspensions. Therefore, take great care when estimating the amount of testosterone needed. In the face of complications where the effects of testosterone should be discontinued, the pellets would have to be removed. In addition, there are times when the pellets may slough out. This accident is usually traceable to superficial implantation or to neglect in regard to aseptic precautions.

➤*Hypercholesterolemia:* Serum cholesterol may be altered during therapy.

➤*Tartrazine sensitivity:* Some of these products contain tartrazine, which may cause allergic-type reactions (including bronchial asthma) in susceptible individuals. Although the incidence of tartrazine sensitivity in the general population is low, it is frequently seen in patients who also have aspirin hypersensitivity. Specific products containing tartrazine are identified in the product listings.

➤*Special risk:* Patients with benign prostatic hypertrophy may develop acute urethral obstruction. Priapism or excessive sexual stimulation may develop. Oligospermia may occur after prolonged administration or excessive dosage. If any of these effects appear, stop administration. If restarted, use a lower dosage. Avoid stimulation to the point of increasing nervous, mental, and physical activities beyond the patient's cardiovascular capacity.

➤*Pregnancy:* Category X. Androgens are contraindicated in women who are or who may become pregnant; androgens may cause fetal harm. Androgens cause virilization of the external genitalia of the female fetus (eg, clitoromegaly, abnormal vaginal development, fusion of genital folds to form a scrotal-like structure). The degree of masculinization is related to the amount of drug given and the age of the fetus. Masculinization is most likely to occur in the female fetus when androgens are given in the first trimester. If the patient becomes pregnant while taking these drugs, apprise her of the potential hazards to the fetus.

➤*Lactation:* It is not known whether androgens are excreted in breast milk. Decide whether to discontinue nursing or to discontinue the drug, taking into account the importance of the drug to the mother. Testosterone transdermal systems and testosterone gel are not indicated for women and must not be used in women.

➤*Children:* Use androgens cautiously in children; the drugs should only be given by specialists who are aware of the adverse effects on bone maturation.

Androgens may accelerate bone maturation without producing compensatory gain in linear growth. This adverse effect may result in compromised adult stature. The younger the child, the greater the risk of compromising final mature height.

Safety and efficacy of *Testoderm* and *Androgel* products in children have not been established.

Benzyl alcohol – Benzyl alcohol-containing products have been associated with a fatal "gasping syndrome" in premature infants. Refer to product listings.

➤*Elderly:* Elderly men, or men in general, treated with androgens may be at an increased risk of developing prostatic hypertrophy, prostatic carcinoma, and prostatic hyperplasia.

Per the Beers list, **methyltestosterone** has the potential for prostatic hypertrophy and cardiac problems. Methyltestosterone is also considered a high risk medication for the elderly according to the Centers of Medicare and Medicaid Services.

➤*Monitoring:* Frequently determine urine and serum calcium levels during the course of therapy in women with disseminated breast carcinoma.

Periodically check liver function, prostate specific antigen, cholesterol, and high-density lipoprotein. To ensure proper dosing, measure serum testosterone concentrations.

Make periodic (every 6 months) x-ray examinations of bone age during treatment of prepubertal males to determine the rate of bone maturation and the effects of androgen therapy on the epiphyseal centers.

Check hemoglobin and hematocrit periodically for polycythemia in patients who are receiving high doses of androgens or who are receiving long-term administration.

Drug Interactions

Androgens Drug Interactions			
Precipitant drug	Object drug[a]		Description
Fluoxymesterone, Methyltestosterone	Anticoagulants	⬆	The anticoagulant effect may be potentiated by 17-alkyl testosterone derivatives (eg, fluoxymesterone, methyltestosterone). Although the non-17-alkylated agent (testosterone) appears safer, at least 1 case report described a similar interaction. Avoid the combination with 17-alkyl derivatives if possible.
Androgens	Oxyphenbutazone	⬆	Coadministration of oxyphenbutazone and androgens may result in elevated serum levels of oxyphenbutazone.
Androgens	Insulin	⬇	In diabetic patients, the metabolic effects of androgens may decrease blood glucose and, therefore, insulin requirements.
Testosterone	Propranolol	⬇	In a pharmacokinetic study of an injectable testosterone product, administration of testosterone cypionate led to an increased clearance of propranolol in the majority of men tested.
Testosterone	Corticosteroids, ACTH	⬆	The coadministration of testosterone with ACTH or corticosteroids may enhance edema formation; thus, administer these drugs cautiously, particularly in patients with cardiac or hepatic disease.
Methyltestosterone	Cyclosporine	⬆	Increased cyclosporine blood concentrations with possible toxicity (eg, nephrotoxicity) may occur. Consider monitoring serum bilirubin, serum creatinine, and cyclosporine concentrations in patients receiving cyclosporine and methyltestosterone concurrently. Adjust the doses as needed.

[a] ⬆ = Object drug increased. ⬇ = Object drug decreased.

➤*Drug/Lab test interactions:*

Thyroid function tests – Decreased levels of thyroxine-binding globulin, resulting in decreased total T_4 serum levels and increased resin uptake of T_3 and T_4. Free thyroid hormone levels remain unchanged, and there is no clinical evidence of thyroid dysfunction.

Adverse Reactions

Women –

Most common: Amenorrhea and other menstrual irregularities; inhibition of gonadotropin secretion and virilization, including deepening voice and clitoral enlargement. The latter usually is not reversible after androgens are discontinued. When administered to a pregnant woman, androgens cause virilization of external genitalia of the female fetus.

Androgen Adverse Reactions[a] (%)					
Adverse reaction	Oral	Injection	Transdermal	Implant	Topical (5 to 10 g dose)
Cardiovascular					
CHF	—	—	1	—	—
Hypertension	—	—	< 1	—	< 3
Tachycardia	—	—	< 1	—	—
Stroke	—	—	2	—	—
Deep vein phlebitis	—	—	1	—	—
Peripheral edema	—	—	—	—	1.4 to 3.1
Vasodilation	—	—	—	—	< 1
Peripheral vascular disease	—	—	< 1	—	—
CNS					
Headache	✓	✓	1 to 6	✓	< 4
Pain	—	—	2	—	—
Asthenia	—	—	2	—	< 3
Libido increased	✓	✓	1	✓	—
Memory loss	—	—	1	—	—
Nervousness/Anxiety	✓	✓	< 1	✓	< 3
Depression	✓	✓	< 3	✓	< 1
Dizziness/Vertigo	—	—	1 to 6	—	< 1
Dry mouth	—	—	< 1	—	—

Androgen Adverse Reactions[a] (%)					
Adverse reaction	Oral	Injection	Transdermal	Implant	Topical (5 to 10 g dose)
Insomnia	—	—	< 1	—	—
Libido decreased	✓	✓	< 1	✓	1 to 3
Personality disorder	—	—	< 1	—	—
CNS stimulation	—	—	< 1	—	—
Generalized paresthesia	✓	✓	< 1	✓	< 1
Emotional lability	—	—	—	—	< 3
Amnesia	—	—	—	—	< 1
Hostility	—	—	—	—	< 1
Fatigue	—	—	< 1	—	—
Confusion	—	—	< 1	—	—
Thinking abnormalities	—	—	< 1	—	—
Dermatologic					
Application site itching	—	—	7 to 12	—	—
Application site erythema	—	—	3 to 7	—	—
Application site discomfort	—	—	4	—	—
Application site irritation	—	—	2	—	—
Pruritus	—	—	2 to 37	—	—
Burning sensation	—	—	3	—	—
Rash	—	—	1 to 2	—	—
Acne	✓	✓	1 to 4	✓	2.8 to 12.5
Alopecia	—	—	< 1	—	< 1
Male pattern baldness	✓	✓	—	✓	—
Hirsutism	✓	✓	< 1	✓	< 1
Other application site reactions	—	—	< 6	—	3.1 to 10
Injection site pain/inflammation	—	✓	—	✓	—
Burn-like blister under system	—	—	12	—	—
Seborrhea	—	✓	—	—	—
Discolored hair	—	—	—	—	< 1
Dry skin	—	—	—	—	< 1
GI					
Abdominal pain	—	—	< 1	—	—
Diarrhea	—	—	< 1	—	—
Nausea	✓	✓	< 1	✓	—
Cholestatic jaundice	✓	✓	—	✓	—
Abnormal liver function tests	✓	✓	1	✓	—
Hepatocellular neoplasms	✓	✓	—	✓	—
Peliosis hepatis	✓	✓	—	✓	—
GI bleeding	—	—	2	—	—
Increased appetite	—	—	< 1	—	—
Stomatitis	—	—	✓	—	—
GU					
Abnormal ejaculation	—	—	< 1	—	—
Breast pain/tenderness	—	—	1 to 3	—	1 to 3
Dysuria	—	—	<	—	—
UTI/Prostatitis	—	—	1 to 4	—	—
Impaired urination	—	—	< 1	—	< 2.8
Frequent erections	✓	✓	—	✓	—
Prolonged erection	✓	✓	—	✓	—
Oligospermia	✓	✓	—	✓	—
Scrotal cellulitis	—	—	1	—	—
BPH	—	—	1	—	—
Rectal mucosal lesion over prostate	—	—	1	—	—
Hematuria/Bladder cancer	—	—	1	—	—
Papilloma on scrotum	—	—	1	—	—
Prostate disorder	—	—	< 5	—	2.8 to 18.8[b]
Testes disorder	—	—	< 1	—	< 3
Penis disorder	—	—	< 1	—	< 1
Pelvic pain	—	—	< 1	—	—
Incontinence	—	—	< 1	—	—
Gynecomastia	✓	✓	1 to 5	✓	< 3
Hematologic					
Suppression of clotting factors	✓	✓	—	✓	—
Polycythemia	✓	✓	—	✓	—
Metabolic/Nutritional					
Hyperglycemia	—	—	< 1	—	—
Hyperlipidemia	—	—	< 1	—	—
Hyponatremia	—	—	< 1	—	—
Electrolyte imbalance	✓	✓	—	✓	—
Increased serum cholesterol	✓	✓	—	✓	—
Abnormal lab tests[c]	—	—	—	—	4.2 to 6.3
Musculoskeletal					
Myalgia	—	—	2	—	—
Back pain	—	—	< 1	—	—
Arthralgia	—	—	< 1	—	—
Miscellaneous					
Accidental injury	—	—	2	—	—
Flu syndrome	—	—	1	—	—
Infection	—	—	< 1	—	—
Anaphylaxis	✓	✓	—	✓	—
Accelerated growth	—	—	< 1	—	—
Bronchitis	—	—	< 1	—	—
Papillary dilation	—	—	1	—	—
Sweating	—	—	—	—	< 1

– = No data.
✓ = Reported, incidence not listed.
[a] Data pooled from separate studies and are not necessarily comparable.
[b] Including prostate enlargement, BPH, elevated PSA results, new diagnosis of prostate cancer.
[c] Including abnormal hemoglobin, hematocrit, triglycerides, serum lipids, potassium, glucose, creatinine, bilirubin, liver function tests.

Overdosage

There is one report of acute overdosage by injection of testosterone enanthate: Testosterone levels of up to 11,400 ng/dL were implicated in a cerebrovascular accident.

Patient Information

Oral tablets may cause GI upset.

Notify physician if nausea, vomiting, swelling of the ankles (edema), too frequent or persistent erections of the penis, changes in skin color, and breathing disturbances, including those associated with sleep, occur.

➤*Women:* Notify physician if hoarseness, deepening of the voice, increases in facial hair, acne, or menstrual irregularities occur.

Advise male adolescent patients receiving androgens for delayed puberty to have bone development checked every 6 months.

TESTOSTERONE ENANTHATE (IN OIL)

c-iii	**Testosterone Enanthate** (Paddock Laboratories)	**Injection, solution:** 200 mg per mL	In 5 mL multidose vials.[a]
c-iii	**Delatestryl** (Indevus Pharmaceutical)		In 5 mL multidose vials.[a]

[a] In sesame oil with 5 mg chlorobutanol.

TESTOSTERONE ENANTHATE — INJECTION

For complete and comparative prescribing information, refer to the Androgens group monograph.

Indications

➤*Males:* Testosterone enanthate injection is indicated for replacement therapy in conditions associated with a deficiency or absence of endogenous testosterone.

Primary hypogonadism (congenital or acquired) – Testicular failure due to cryptorchidism; bilateral torsion, orchitis, vanishing testis syndrome, or orchidectomy.

Hypogonadotropic hypogonadism (congenital or acquired) –Idiopathic gonadotropin or luteinizing hormone-releasing hormone (LHRH) deficiency, or pituitary-hypothalamic injury from tumors, trauma, or radiation.

(Appropriate adrenal cortical and thyroid hormone replacement therapy are still necessary, however, and are actually of primary importance.)

If the above conditions occur prior to puberty, androgen replacement therapy will be needed during the adolescent years for development of secondary sexual characteristics. Prolonged androgen treatment will be required to maintain sexual characteristics in these and other males who develop testosterone deficiency after puberty.

Delayed puberty – Testosterone enanthate injection may be used to stimulate puberty in carefully selected males with clearly delayed puberty. These patients usually have a familial pattern of delayed puberty that is not secondary to a pathological disorder; puberty is expected to occur spontaneously at a relatively late date. Brief treatment with conservative doses may occasionally be justified in these patients if they do not respond to psycho-

TESTOSTERONE ENANTHATE — INJECTION

logical support. The potential adverse effect on bone maturation should be discussed with the patient and parents prior to androgen administration. An x-ray of the hand and wrist to determine bone age should be obtained every 6 months to assess the effect of treatment on the epiphyseal centers (see Warnings/Precautions).

➤*Females:*

Metastatic mammary cancer – Testosterone enanthate injection may be used secondarily in women with advancing inoperable metastatic (skeletal) mammary cancer who are 1 to 5 years postmenopausal. Primary goals of therapy in these women include ablation of the ovaries. Other methods of counteracting estrogen activity are adrenalectomy, hypophysectomy, or antiestrogen therapy. This treatment has also been used in premenopausal women with breast cancer who have benefited from oophorectomy and are considered to have a hormone-responsive tumor. Judgment concerning androgen therapy should be made by an oncologist with expertise in this field.

Administration and Dosage

➤*General dosing considerations:* Dosage and duration of therapy will depend on age, sex, diagnosis, patient's response to treatment, and appearance of adverse effects.

In general, total doses above 400 mg monthly are not required because of the prolonged action of the preparation. Injections more frequently than every 2 weeks are rarely indicated.

Women with metastatic breast carcinoma must be followed closely because androgen therapy occasionally appears to accelerate the disease.

➤*Adults:*

Metastatic mammary cancer in females – 200 to 400 mg every 2 to 4 weeks.

Testosterone replacement therapy in males – 50 to 400 mg every 2 to 4 weeks.

➤*Children:*

Delayed puberty in males – 50 to 200 mg every 2 to 4 weeks for a limited duration (for example, 4 to 6 months).

Various dosage regimens for delayed puberty have been used; some call for lower dosages initially with gradual increases as puberty progresses, with or without a decrease to maintenance levels. Other regimens call for higher dosage to induce pubertal changes and lower dosage for maintenance after puberty. The chronological and skeletal ages must be taken into consideration, both in determining the initial dose and in adjusting the dose. X-rays should be taken at appropriate intervals to determine the amount of bone maturation and skeletal development.

➤*Preparation for administration:* Warming and rotating the syringe unit or vial between the palms of the hands will redissolve any crystals that may have formed during storage at low temperatures. Use of a wet needle or wet syringe may cause the solution to become cloudy; however this does not affect the potency of the material.

Unimatic single-dose syringe – Screw the threaded tip of the plunger rod clockwise into the cartridge plunger, and push forward a few millimeters to break any friction between the cartridge plunger and syringe barrel. Remove the needle guard, hold the syringe erect, and push plunger forward until a drop appears at tip of needle and all of the air is evacuated. Following the usual aspiration procedure, complete the injection. Destroy the needle and syringe immediately after use.

➤*Administration:* Care should be taken to inject the preparation deeply into the gluteal muscle following the usual precautions for IM administration.

➤*Storage/Stability:* Store at room temperature.

TESTOSTERONE CYPIONATE (IN OIL)

c-iii	**Testosterone Cypionate** (Sandoz)	**Injection; solution**: 100 mg/mL	In 10 mL vials.[a]
c-iii	**Depo-Testosterone** (Pfizer)		In 10 mL vials.[a]
c-iii	**Testosterone Cypionate** (Various, eg, Sandoz, Watson)	**Injection; solution**: 200 mg/mL	Benzyl alcohol, cotton seed oil. In 1 and 10 mL vials.
c-iii	**Depo-Testosterone** (Pfizer)		In 1 and 10 mL vials.[b]

[a] In cottonseed oil 736 mg with benzyl benzoate 0.1 mL and benzyl alcohol 9.45 mg.

[b] In cottonseed oil 560 mg with benzyl benzoate 0.2 mL and benzyl alcohol 9.45 mg.

TESTOSTERONE CYPIONATE — INJECTION

For complete and comparative prescribing information, refer to the Androgens group monograph.

Indications

➤*Replacement therapy:* Testosterone cypionate sterile solution is indicated for replacement therapy in the male in conditions associated with symptoms of deficiency or absence of endogenous testosterone.

Primary hypogonadism (congenital or acquired) – Primary hypogonadism (congenital or acquired)-testicular failure caused by cryptorchidism, bilateral torsion, orchitis, vanishing testis syndrome; or orchidectomy.

Hypogonadotropic hypogonadism (congenital or acquired) – Hypogonadotropic hypogonadism (congenital or acquired)-idiopathic gonadotropin or LHRH deficiency, or pituitary-hypothalamic injury from tumors, trauma, or radiation.

Administration and Dosage

➤*General dosing considerations:* Testosterone cypionate should not be used interchangeably with testosterone propionate because of differences in duration of action.

The suggested dosage varies depending on the age, sex, and diagnosis of the individual patient.

Various dosage regimens have been used to induce pubertal changes in hypogonadal males; some experts have advocated lower dosages initially, gradually increasing the dose as puberty progresses, with or without a decrease to maintenance levels. Other experts emphasize that higher dosages are needed to induce pubertal changes and lower dosages can be used for maintenance after puberty. The chronological and skeletal ages must be taken into consideration, both in determining the initial dose and in adjusting the dose.

➤*Adults:*

Testosterone replacement therapy in males –

Usual dosage: 50 to 400 mg every 2 to 4 weeks.

Dosage adjustment: Dosage is adjusted according to the patient's response and the appearance of adverse reactions.

➤*Children:*

Testosterone replacement therapy in males – See Adults for dosing in children 12 years of age and older.

➤*Renal function impairment:* Contraindicated in patients with serious renal disease.

➤*Hepatic function impairment:* Contraindicated in patients with serious hepatic disease.

➤*Preparation for administration:* Warming and shaking the vial should redissolve any crystals that may have formed during storage at temperatures lower than recommended.

➤*Administration:* For intramuscular (IM) use only. IM injections should be given deep in the gluteal muscle. It should not be given intravenously.

➤*Storage/Stability:* Store at 20° to 25°C (68° to 77°F). Protect from light.

TESTOSTERONE PELLETS

c-iii	**Testopel** (Slate Pharmaceuticals)	**Implant; subcutaneous**: 75 mg	1 pellet per vial. In 3s, 10s, and 100s.

TESTOSTERONE — IMPLANT

For complete and comparative prescribing information, refer to the Androgens group monograph.

Indications

➤*Replacement therapy:* For replacement therapy in conditions associated with a deficiency or absence of endogenous testosterone.

Primary hypogonadism (congenital or acquired) – For testicular failure caused by cryptorchidism, bilateral torsion, orchitis, vanishing testis syndrome, or orchidectomy.

Hypogonadotropic hypogonadism (congenital or acquired) –Idiopathic gonadotropin or luteinizing hormone-releasing hormone deficiency, or pituitary-hypothalamic injury from tumors, trauma, or radiation.

If primary or hypogonadotropic hypogonadism occur prior to puberty, androgen replacement therapy will be needed during the adolescent years for development of secondary sexual characteristics. Prolonged androgen treatment will be required to maintain sexual characteristics in these and other males who develop testosterone deficiency after puberty.

Delayed puberty – To stimulate puberty in carefully selected males with clearly delayed puberty. These patients usually have a familial pattern of delayed puberty that is not secondary to a pathological disorder; puberty is expected to occur spontaneously at a relatively late date. Brief treatment with conservative doses may occasionally be justified in these patients if they do not respond to psychological support.

Discuss the potential adverse reaction on bone maturation with the patient and parents prior to androgen administration. Obtain an x-ray of the hand and wrist every 6 months to determine bone age and assess the effect of treatment on the epiphyseal centers.

TESTOSTERONE — IMPLANT

Administration and Dosage

➤*General dosing considerations:* The suggested dosage for androgens varies depending on the age and diagnosis of the individual patient. Dosage is adjusted according to the patient's response and the appearance of adverse reactions.

Pellet implantation is much less flexible for dosage adjustment compared with oral administration or intramuscular injection of oil solutions or aqueous suspensions. Therefore, great care should be used when estimating the amount of testosterone needed. (See Determination of dose.)

➤*Adults:*

Testosterone replacement therapy in males – 150 to 450 mg subcutaneous every 3 to 6 months.

➤*Children:*

Delayed puberty in males – Dosages used in delayed puberty generally are in the lower range of those listed for replacement therapy and are used for a limited duration (eg, 4 to 6 months).

Various dosage regimens have been used to induce pubertal changes in hypogonadal males; some experts have advocated lower dosages initially, gradually increasing the dose as puberty progresses, with or without a decrease to maintenance levels. Other experts emphasize that higher dosages are needed to induce pubertal changes and lower dosages can be used for maintenance after puberty. The chronological and skeletal ages must be taken into consideration while determining the initial dose and in adjusting the dose.

➤*Determination of dose:* The number of pellets to be implanted depends upon the minimal daily requirement of testosterone propionate determined by a gradual reduction of the amount administered parenterally. The usual ratio is as follows: implant two 75 mg pellets for each 25 mg of testosterone propionate required weekly. Thus, when a patient requires injections of 75 mg/week, it is usually necessary to implant 450 mg (6 pellets). With required injections of 50 mg/week, implantation of 300 mg (4 pellets) may suffice for approximately 3 months. With lower requirements by injection, correspondingly lower amounts may be implanted. It has been found that approximately ⅓ of the material is absorbed in the first month, ¼ in the second month, and ⅙ in the third month. Adequate effect of the pellets ordinarily continues for 3 to 4 months, sometimes as long as 6 months.

➤*Discontinuation of therapy:* In the face of complications in which the effects of testosterone should be discontinued, the pellets would have to be removed. In addition, there are times when the pellets may slough out. This accident is usually traceable to superficial implantation or to neglect in regard to aseptic precautions.

➤*Preparation for administration:*

Implanter kit – The implanter kit must be sterilized prior to use. The implanter kit may be sterilized by steam in an autoclave at 121°C (250°F) for a minimum of 15 minutes.

Preparation of skin – The skin is cleaned with an accepted antiseptic preparation and then anesthetized with 2 to 3 mL of local anaesthetic. Some health care providers use an epinephrine solution to ensure minimal capillary bleeding.

➤*Administration:* The pellets are fat-soluble and implanted subcutaneously. In most men, an area on the anterior abdominal wall is selected 1 inch medial to the anterior superior iliac spine, avoiding previous scars. An area on either buttocks may be chosen so that implantation is made beneath the external gluteus muscle.

The clinically indicated pellets are placed in a sterile tray. The *Bardani* implanter with stylet (solid tube with pointed end) in place is inserted parallel to the inguinal ligament and directed subcutaneously to the depth of the bolt (about 5 cm). When the stylet is removed, the pellets are placed in the groove of the implanter with the sterilized tissue forceps. The sterilized tray should be held beneath the implanter as the pellets are inserted, in case one is dropped inadvertently. A pellet that falls into the sterilized tray may be replaced, but a pellet that becomes contaminated must be discarded because it cannot be resterilized. The plunger (solid tube with blunt end) is then inserted and the pellets are eased into the fatty tissues. The implanter is removed and a dry dressing is given to the patient to apply with pressure for a few minutes. Cover the puncture site with an adhesive bandage.

➤*Storage / Stability:* Store in a cool place.

TESTOSTERONE — TRANSDERMAL

c-iii	**AndroGel** (Abbott)	**Gel; topical:** 1.62% (20.25 mg)	Ethyl alcohol. In metered multiple-dose pumps (60 metered 1.25 g doses)
c-iii	**AndroGel** (Abbott)	**Gel; topical:** 1% (50 mg)	Ethanol 67%. In 30 unit-dose packets (in 2.5 g [25 mg] or 5 g [50 mg] gel) or 75 g metered multiple-dose pumps (60 metered 1.25 g doses).
c-iii	**Testim** (Auxilium)		Ethanol 74%, glycerin, polyethylene glycol. In 30 unit-dose tubes (50 mg testosterone).
c-iii	**Fortesta** (Endo)	**Gel; topical:** 10 mg per 0.5 g	Ethanol, propylene glycol. In 60 g metered-dose pumps (120 metered 10 mg doses).
c-iii	**Axiron** (Lilly)	**Solution; topical:** 30 mg per 1.5 mL	Ethanol, isopropyl alcohol. In 110 mL metered-dose pumps with applicator (60 metered 30 mg doses)
c-iii	**Androderm** (Watson Pharma)	**Patch; transdermal:** 12.2 mg (total testosterone content)	2.5 mg per 24 h release rate; 37 cm^2 contact surface area. In 60s.
		24.3 mg (total testosterone content)	5 mg per 24 h release rate; 44 cm^2 contact surface area. In 30s.

TESTOSTERONE — TRANSDERMAL PATCH

For complete and comparative prescribing information, refer to the Androgens group monograph.

Indications

➤*Replacement therapy:* Testosterone transdermal system is indicated for testosterone replacement therapy in adult males for conditions associated with a deficiency or absence of endogenous testosterone.

➤*Primary hypogonadism (congenital or acquired):* Testicular failure due to cryptorchidism, bilateral torsion, orchitis, vanishing testis syndrome, orchidectomy, Klinefelter syndrome, chemotherapy, or toxic damage from alcohol or heavy metals. These men usually have low serum testosterone levels and gonadotropins (follicle-stimulating hormone [FSH], luteinizing hormone [LH]) above the normal range.

➤*Hypogonadotropic hypogonadism (congenital or acquired):* Idiopathic gonadotropin or luteinizing hormone-releasing hormone (LHRH) deficiency or pituitary-hypothalamic injury from tumors, trauma, or radiation. These men have low serum testosterone concentrations without associated elevation in gonadotropins.

Administration and Dosage

➤*Adults:*

Testosterone deficiency –

Initial dosage: 5 mg/day (one testosterone 5 mg transdermal system or 2 testosterone 2.5 mg transdermal systems) applied nightly for 24 hours.

Dosage adjustment: To ensure proper dosing, measure the morning serum testosterone concentration following system application the previous evening. If the serum concentration is outside the normal range, repeat sampling with assurance of proper system adhesion as well as appropriate application time. Confirmed serum concentrations outside the normal range may require increasing the daily dose to 7.5 mg (ie, one 5 mg and one 2.5 mg system or three 2.5 mg systems) or decreasing the daily dose to 2.5 mg (one 2.5 mg system), maintaining nightly application.

Nonvirilized patients: Testosterone therapy for nonvirilized patients may be initiated with one 2.5 mg/day system applied nightly.

➤*Skin irritation:* Mild skin irritation may be ameliorated by treatment of the affected skin with over-the-counter topical hydrocortisone cream applied after system removal.

Applying a small amount of triamcinolone acetonide 0.1% cream to the skin under the central drug reservoir of the testosterone transdermal system has been shown to reduce the incidence and severity of skin irritation. The administration of triamcinolone acetonide 0.1% cream does not significantly alter transdermal absorption of testosterone from the system. Do not use ointment formulations for pretreatment as they may significantly reduce testosterone absorption.

➤*Administration:* Apply the system immediately after opening the pouch and removing the protective release liner. The adhesive side of the testosterone transdermal system should be applied to a clean, dry area of the skin on the back, abdomen, upper arms, or thighs. Press the system firmly in place, making sure there is good contact with the skin, especially around the edges. Avoid application over bony prominences or on a part of the body that may be subject to prolonged pressure during sleep or sitting (eg, deltoid region of the upper arm, greater trochanter of the femur, ischial tuberosity). Do not apply to the scrotum. Rotate the sites of application, with an interval of 7 days between applications to the same site. The area selected should not be oily, damaged, or irritated.

➤*Storage / Stability:* Store at room temperature, 15° to 30°C (59° to 86°F). Apply to skin immediately upon removal from the protective pouch. Do not store outside the pouch provided. Do not use damaged systems. The drug reservoir may burst from excessive pressure or heat.

TESTOSTERONE — TRANSDERMAL MISCELLANEOUS

For complete and comparative prescribing information, refer to the Androgens class monograph.

WARNING

Virilization has been reported in children who were secondarily exposed to transdermal testosterone.

Children should avoid contact with unwashed or unclothed application sites in men using transdermal testosterone.

Advise patients to strictly adhere to recommended instructions for use.

Indications

Transdermal testosterone is indicated for testosterone replacement therapy in adult men for conditions associated with a deficiency or absence of endogenous testosterone:

➤*Primary hypogonadism (congenital or acquired):* Testicular failure caused by cryptorchidism, bilateral torsion, orchitis, vanishing testis syndrome, orchiectomy, Klinefelter syndrome, chemotherapy, or toxic damage from alcohol or heavy metals.

These men usually have low serum testosterone levels and gonadotropins (follicle-stimulating hormone [FSH], luteinizing hormone [LH]) above the normal range.

➤*Hypogonadotropic hypogonadism (congenital or acquired):* Idiopathic gonadotropin or luteinizing hormone–releasing hormone (LHRH) deficiency or pituitary-hypothalamic injury from tumors, trauma, or radiation.

These men have low serum testosterone concentrations but have gonadotropins in the normal or low range.

Administration and Dosage

➤*General dosing considerations:* Transdermal testosterone is for replacement therapy in adult men for conditions associated with a deficiency or absence of endogenous testosterone.

➤*Adults:*

Primary hypogonadism (congenital or acquired) –

Gel:

• *AndroGel 1%, Testim* –

Initial dosage: 5 g of testosterone 1% gel (to deliver testosterone 50 mg) applied once daily (preferably in the morning) to clean, dry, intact skin of the shoulders and/or upper arms. *AndroGel 1%* may also be applied to the abdomen.

Dosage adjustment: Measure serum testosterone levels 14 days after initiation of therapy to ensure proper dosing. If the serum testosterone concentration is below the normal range, or if the desired clinical response is not achieved, the dose may be increased from 5 to 7.5 g (*AndroGel 1%*) or 5 to 10 g (*Testim*) and from 7.5 to 10 g (*AndroGel 1%*).

If the serum testosterone concentration exceeds the normal range, the daily dose may be decreased.

Discontinuation of therapy: If the serum testosterone concentration consistently exceeds the normal range at a daily dose of 5 g, therapy should be discontinued.

• *AndroGel 1.62%* –

Initial dosage: 40.5 mg of testosterone (2 pump actuation) applied topically once daily in the morning to the shoulders and upper arms.

Dosage adjustment: The dose can be adjusted between a minimum of 20.25 mg of testosterone (1 pump actuation) and a maximum of 81 mg of testosterone (4 pump actuations). To ensure proper dosing, the dose should be titrated based on the pre-dose morning serum testosterone concentration from a single blood draw at approximately 14 and 28 days after starting treatment or following dose adjustment. In addition, serum testosterone concentration should be assessed periodically thereafter.

***AndroGel* 1.62% Dose Adjustment Criteria**[a]

Pre-dose monitoring total serum testosterone concentration	Dose titration
> 750 ng/dL	Decrease daily dose by 20.25 mg (1 pump actuation)
≥ 350 and ≤ 750 ng/dL	No change; continue on current dose
< 350 ng/dL	Increase daily dose by 20.25 mg (1 pump actuation)

[a] The application-site and dose of *AndroGel* 1.62% are not interchangeable with other transdermal testosterone products.

• *Fortesta* –

Initial dosage: 40 mg (4 pump actuations) applied once daily to the thighs in the morning.

Dosage titration: To ensure proper dosing, the dose should be titrated based on the serum testosterone concentration from a single blood draw 2 hours after applying testosterone and at approximately 14 days and 35 days after starting treatment or following dose adjustment. In addition, serum testosterone concentration should be assessed periodically thereafter.

Dosage adjustment: The dose can be adjusted between a minimum of 10 mg of testosterone and a maximum of 70 mg of testosterone.

Transdermal Testosterone (*Fortesta*) Dosage Adjustments[a]

Total serum testosterone concentration 2 hours after testosterone application	Dose titration
≥ 2,500 ng/dL	Decrease daily dose by 20 mg (2 pump actuations)
≥ 1,250 and < 2,500 ng/dL	Decrease daily dose by 10 mg (1 pump actuation)
≥ 500 and < 1,250 ng/dL	No change; continue on current dose
< 500 ng/dL	Increase daily dose by 10 mg (1 pump actuation)

[a] The application site and dose of testosterone are not interchangeable with other topical testosterone products.

Solution:

• *Initial dosage* – 60 mg of testosterone (2 pump actuations) applied once daily.

• *Dosage adjustment* – Serum testosterone concentrations should be measured after initiation of therapy to ensure that the desired concentrations (300 to 1,050 ng/dL) are achieved. The testosterone topical solution dose can be adjusted based on the serum testosterone concentration from a single blood draw 2 to 8 hours after application and at least 14 days after starting treatment or following dose adjustment.

If the measured serum testosterone concentration is below 300 ng/dL, the daily testosterone dose may be increased from 60 mg (2 pump actuations) to 90 mg (3 pump actuations) or from 90 to 120 mg (4 pump actuations). If the serum testosterone concentration exceeds 1,050 ng/dL, the daily testosterone dose should be decreased from 60 mg (2 pump actuations) to 30 mg (1 pump actuation).

• *Discontinuation of therapy* – If the serum testosterone concentration consistently exceeds 1,050 ng/dL at the lowest daily dose of 30 mg (1 pump actuation), therapy should be discontinued.

Hypogonadotrophic hypogonadism (congenital or acquired) – See Primary Hypogonadism (Congenital or Acquired) for dosing.

➤*Administration:*

Gel – Strict adherence to the following precautions is advised in order to minimize the potential for secondary exposure to testosterone from testosterone-treated skin.

• Children and women should avoid contact with the unclothed or unwashed application sites on the skin of men using testosterone gel.
• Patients should wash their hands immediately with soap and water after application of testosterone gel.
• Patients should cover the application site(s) with clothing (eg, a T-shirt, shorts of sufficient length, pants) after the gel has dried.
• Prior to any situation in which skin-to-skin contact with the application site is anticipated, patients should wash the application site thoroughly with soap and water to remove any testosterone residue.
• In the event that unwashed or unclothed skin to which testosterone gel has been applied comes in direct contact with the skin of another person, the general area of contact on the other person should be washed with soap and water as soon as possible.

AndroGel 1%, AndroGel 1.62%, Testim: Upon opening the packet(s) or tube, the entire contents should be squeezed into the palm of the hand and immediately apply it to the application sites. Alternatively, for *Androgel 1%*, patients may squeeze a portion of the gel from the packet into the palm of the hand and apply to application sites. Repeat until entire contents have been applied. Apply once daily (preferably in the morning) to clean, dry, intact skin of the shoulders and/or upper arms (areas of application should be limited to the area that will be covered by the patient's short-sleeve T-shirt). *AndroGel 1%* may also be applied to the abdomen; however, do not apply *AndroGel 1.62%* or *Testim* to the abdomen. Do not apply the gel to the genitals. Allow application sites to dry for a few minutes prior to dressing. Wash hands with soap and water after application. Cover the application sites with clothing after gel has dried.

• *AndroGel 1%* multidose pump – Patients should be instructed to prime the pump before using it for the first time by fully depressing the pump mechanism (actuation) 3 times and discarding this portion of the product to ensure precise dose delivery. After the priming procedure, patients should completely depress the pump 1 time (actuation) for every 1.25 g of product required to achieve the daily prescribed dosage. The product may be delivered directly into the palm of the hand and then applied to the desired application sites, either 1 pump actuation at a time or upon completion of all pump actuations required for the daily dose. Alternatively, the product can be applied directly to the application sites. Application directly to the sites may prevent loss of product that may occur during transfer from the palm of the hand onto the application sites.

The following table has specific dosing guidelines for adult men when the 75 g *AndroGel 1%* pump is used.

***AndroGel* 1% Dosing Guidelines for Using the Multidose Pump**

Prescribed daily dose	Number of pump actuations in 75 g pump
5 g	4 (once daily)
7.5 g	6 (once daily)
10 g	8 (once daily)

TESTOSTERONE — TRANSDERMAL MISCELLANEOUS

• *AndroGel* 1.62% – *AndroGel* 1.62% should be spread across the maximum surface area directed in the following table.

AndroGel 1.62% Application Sites			
		Pump actuations per upper arm and shoulder	
Total dose of testosterone	Total pump actuations	Upper arm and shoulder number 1	Upper arm and shoulder number 2
20.25 mg	1	1	0
40.5 mg	2	1	1
60.75 mg	3	2	1
81 mg	4	2	2

The patient should avoid swimming or showering or washing the administration site for a minimum of 2 hours after application.

To obtain a full first dose, it is necessary to prime the canister pump. To do so, with the canister in the upright position, slowly and fully depress the (actuator) 3 times. Safely discard the gel from the first 3 actuations. It is only necessary to prime the pump before the first dose.

After the priming procedure, fully depress the actuator once for every 20.25 mg of *AndroGel* 1.62%. *AndroGel* 1.62% should be delivered directly into the palm of the hand and then applied to the application sites. Alternatively, *AndroGel* 1.62% can be applied directly to the application sites.

• *Testim* – In order to prevent transfer to another person, clothing should be worn to cover the application sites. If direct skin-to-skin contact with another person is anticipated, the application sites must be washed thoroughly with soap and water.

In order to maintain serum testosterone levels in the normal range, the sites of application should not be washed for at least 2 hours after application.

Fortesta: Apply directly to clean, dry, intact skin of the front and inner thighs. Only apply to the front and inner thighs (area of application should be limited to the area that will be covered by the patient's shorts or pants). Do not apply to the genitals or other parts of the body. Patients should be instructed to use 1 finger to gently rub testosterone evenly onto the front and inner thigh as directed in the following table.

Testosterone Gel (*Fortesta*) Application Guidelines			
		Pump actuations per thigh	
Total dose of testosterone	Total pump actuations	Thigh #1	Thigh #2
10 mg	1	1	0
20 mg	2	1	1
30 mg	3	2	1
40 mg	4	2	2
50 mg	5	3	2
60 mg	6	3	3
70 mg	7	4	3

Once the application site is dry, the site should be covered with clothing. Wash hands thoroughly with soap and water. Avoid applying the gel to the thigh adjacent to the scrotum. Avoid fire, flames, or smoking until the gel has dried because alcohol-based products, including testosterone, are flammable.

The patient should avoid swimming or showering or washing the administration site for a minimum of 2 hours after application.

To obtain a full first dose, it is necessary to prime the canister pump. To do so, with the canister in the upright position, slowly and fully depress the actuator 8 times. The first 3 actuations may result in no discharge of gel. Safely discard the gel from the first 8 actuations. It is only necessary to prime the pump before the first dose.

Solution – The application site and dose of testosterone topical solution are not interchangeable with other topical testosterone products.

Apply to the axilla, preferably at the same time each morning, to clean, dry, intact skin. Do not apply to other parts of the body, including to the scrotum, penis, abdomen, shoulders, or upper arms. After applying the solution, the application site should be allowed to dry completely prior to dressing. Avoid fire, flames, or smoking until the solution has dried because alcohol-based products, including testosterone topical solution, are flammable.

Apply to the axilla using an applicator. When using testosterone topical solution for the first time, the pump should be primed by depressing the pump 3 times; discarding any product dispensed directly into a basin, sink, or toilet; and then washing the liquid away thoroughly. This priming should be done only prior to the first use of each pump. After priming, patients should completely depress the pump 1 time (1 pump actuation) to dispense 30 mg of testosterone. To dispense the solution, position the nozzle over the applicator cup and carefully depress the pump fully once. Ensure that the liquid is directed into the cup. The cup should be filled with no more than 30 mg (1 pump actuation) of testosterone. Dosing that requires greater than 1 pump actuation must be applied in increments of 30 mg as is shown in the following table.

Keeping the applicator upright, patients should place it up into the axilla and wipe steadily down and up into the axilla. If the solution drips or runs, it can be wiped back up with the applicator cup. The solution should not be rubbed into the skin with fingers or hand. The process is then repeated with application of 30 mg of testosterone (1 pump actuation) to the other axilla to achieve a total of 60 mg of testosterone applied. For patients prescribed the 90 mg dose of testosterone, the procedure is the same, but 3 applications are required. To dose 120 mg of testosterone, 4 applications are required, alternating left and right for each application as shown in the following table. When repeat application to the same axilla is required, the axilla should be allowed to dry completely before more testosterone topical solution is applied.

After use, the applicator should be rinsed under room temperature, running water and then patted dry with a tissue. The applicator and cap are then replaced on the bottle for storage.

When deodorants or antiperspirants are used as part of a regular program for personal hygiene, they should not interfere with the efficacy of testosterone topical solution in treating hypogonadism. If patients use an antiperspirant or deodorant (stick or roll-on), it should be applied prior to the application of testosterone topical solution to avoid contamination of the stick or roll-on product.

Patients should be advised to avoid swimming or washing the application site until 2 hours following application of testosterone topical solution.

To reduce the likelihood of interpersonal transfer of testosterone, the application site should always be washed prior to any skin-to-skin contact regardless of the length of time since application.

Testosterone Topical Solution Application Technique		
Daily prescribed dose of testosterone	Number of pump actuations	Application
30 mg	1 (once daily)	Apply once to one axilla only (left OR right).
60 mg	2 (once daily)	Apply once to the left axilla and then apply once to the right axilla.
90 mg	3 (once daily)	Apply once to the left and once to the right axilla, wait for the product to dry, and then apply once again to the left OR right axilla.
120 mg	4 (once daily)	Apply once to the left and once to the right axilla, wait for the product to dry, and then apply once again to the left AND once to the right axilla.

Hands should be washed thoroughly with soap and water after application.

Strict adherence to the following precautions is advised in order to minimize the potential for secondary exposure to testosterone from testosterone topical solution–treated skin.

- Children and women should avoid contact with the unclothed or unwashed application sites on the skin of men using testosterone topical solution.
- *AndroGel* 1.62% should only be applied to the upper arms and shoulders. The area of application should be limited to the area that will be covered by a short-sleeve shirt.
- Patients should wash their hands immediately with soap and water after application of testosterone topical solution.
- Patients should cover the application site(s) with clothing (eg, a T-shirt) after the solution has dried.
- Prior to any situation in which direct skin-to-skin contact is anticipated, patients should wash the application site thoroughly with soap and water to remove any testosterone residue.
- In the event that unwashed or unclothed skin to which testosterone topical solution has been applied comes in direct contact with the skin of another person, the general area of contact on the other person should be washed with soap and water as soon as possible.

While interpersonal testosterone transfer can occur with a T-shirt on, it has been shown that transfer can be substantially reduced by wearing a T-shirt and the majority of residual testosterone is removed from the skin surface by washing with soap and water.

➤*Storage/Stability:* Store at room temperature, 25°C (77°F); excursions are permitted to 15° to 30°C (59° to 86°F). Do not freeze.

TESTOSTERONE — BUCCAL

Rx	**Striant** (Columbia)	**Buccal system:** 30 mg testosterone	Lactose. In blister packs of 10 systems.

TESTOSTERONE — BUCCAL

For complete and comparative prescribing information, refer to the Androgens group monograph.

Indications

➤*Replacement therapy:* Testosterone buccal system is indicated for replacement therapy in men for conditions associated with a deficiency or absence of endogenous testosterone:

Hypogonadotropic hypogonadism (congenital or acquired) – Idiopathic gonadotropin or luteinizing hormone-releasing hormone (LHRH) deficiency, or pituitary-hypothalamic injury from tumors, trauma, or radiation. These patients have low serum testosterone levels but have gonadotropins in the normal or low range.

Primary hypogonadism (congenital or acquired) – Testicular failure caused by cryptorchidism, bilateral torsion, orchitis, vanishing testis syndrome, orchidectomy, Klinefelter syndrome, chemotherapy, or toxic damage from alcohol or heavy metals. These men usually have low serum testosterone levels and gonadotropins (follicle-stimulating hormone [FSH], luteinizing hormone [LH]) above the normal range.

Administration and Dosage

➤*Adults:*

Testosterone replacement therapy in males – 1 buccal system (30 mg) to the gum region twice daily, morning and evening (approximately 12 hours apart).

➤*Administration:* Place the buccal system in a comfortable position just above the incisor tooth (on either side of the mouth). Upon opening the packet, place the rounded side surface of the buccal system against the gum and hold it firmly in place with a finger over the lip and against the product for 30 seconds to ensure adhesion. The buccal system is designed to stay in position until removed. If the buccal system fails to properly adhere to the gum or falls off during the 12-hour dosing interval, remove the old buccal system and apply a new one. If the buccal system falls out of position within 4 hours prior to the next dose, apply a new buccal system and leave it in place until the time of next regularly scheduled dosing. With each application, rotate the buccal system to alternate sides of the mouth.

Take care to avoid dislodging the buccal system. Check to see if buccal system is in place following toothbrushing, use of mouthwash, and consumption of food or alcoholic/nonalcoholic beverages. Do not chew or swallow the buccal system. To remove the buccal system, gently slide it downward from the gum towards the tooth to avoid scratching the gum.

➤*Storage/Stability:* Store at 20° to 25°C (68° to 77°F). Protect from heat and moisture. Damaged blister packages should not be used. Dispose of discarded buccal systems in household trash in a manner that prevents accidental application or ingestion by children or pets.

METHYLTESTOSTERONE

c-iii	**Methyltestosterone** (Various, eg, Global)	**Tablets:** 10 mg	In 100s.
c-iii	**Methitest** (Global)		Lactose, sugar. (7037). White, scored. In 100s.
c-iii	**Methyltestosterone** (Various, eg, Global)	**Tablets:** 25 mg	In 100s.
c-iii	**Methyltestosterone** (Various, eg, Global)	**Tablets (buccal):** 10 mg	In 100s.
c-iii	**Android** (Valeant)	**Capsules:** 10 mg	(ICN 0901). Red. In 100s.
c-iii	**Testred** (Valeant)		(ICN 0901). Red. In 100s.
c-iii	**Virilon** (Star)		(Virilon 10 mg). Black and clear. In 100s and 1000s.

METHYLTESTOSTERONE — ORAL

For complete and comparative prescribing information, refer to the Androgens group monograph.

Indications

➤*Males:* Methyltestosterone is indicated for replacement therapy in conditions associated with a deficiency or absence of endogenous testosterone.

Primary hypogonadism (congenital or acquired) – Primary hypogonadism (congenital or acquired)—testicular failure caused by cryptorchidism, bilateral torsion, orchitis, vanishing testis syndrome; or orchidectomy.

Hypogonadotropic hypogonadism (congenital or acquired) – Hypogonadotropic hypogonadism (congenital or acquired) idiopathic gonadotropin or LHRH deficiency, or pituitary hypothalamic injury from tumors, trauma, or radiation. If the above conditions occur prior to puberty, androgen replacement therapy will be needed during the adolescent years to development of secondary sexual characteristics. Prolonged androgen treatment will be required to maintain sexual characteristics in these and other males who develop testosterone deficiency after puberty.

Delayed puberty – Androgens may be used to stimulate puberty in carefully selected males with clearly delayed puberty. These patients usually have a familial pattern of delayed puberty that is not secondary to a pathological disorder; puberty is expected to occur spontaneously at a relatively late date. Brief treatment with conservative doses may occasionally be justified in these patients if they do not respond to psychological support. The potential adverse effect on bone maturation should be discussed with the patient and parents prior to androgen administration. An x-ray of the hand and wrist to determine bone age should be obtained every 6 months to assess the effect of treatment on the epiphyseal centers (see Warnings).

➤*Females:*

Metastatic mammary cancer – Methyltestosterone may be used secondarily in women with advancing inoperable metastatic (skeletal) mammary cancer who are 1 to 5 years postmenopausal. Primary goals of therapy in these women include ablation of the ovaries. Other methods of counteracting estrogen activity are adrenalectomy, hypophysectomy, or antiestrogen therapy. This treatment has also been used in premenopausal women with breast cancer who have benefited from oophorectomy and are considered to have a hormone responsive tumor. Judgment concerning androgen therapy should be made by an oncologist with expertise in this field.

Administration and Dosage

➤*General dosing considerations:* Dosage must be strictly individualized. The suggested dose for androgens varies depending on the age, sex, and diagnosis of the individual patient. Methyltestosterone dosage is adjusted according to the patient's response and the appearance of adverse reactions.

➤*Adults:*

Men –

Hypogonadotropic hypogonadism (congenital or acquired):

- *Usual dosage* – 10 to 50 mg orally administered daily.

Primary hypogonadism (congenital or acquired): See Hypogonadotropic hypogonadism (congenital or acquired) for dosing.

Women –

Metastatic mammary cancer: Women with metastatic breast carcinoma must be followed closely because androgen therapy occasionally appears to accelerate the disease. Thus, many experts prefer to use the shorter-acting androgen preparations rather than those with prolonged activity for treating breast carcinoma, particularly during the early stages of androgen therapy.

- *Usual dosage* – 50 to 200 mg orally administered daily.

➤*Children:* Androgen therapy should be used very cautiously in children and only by specialists who are aware of the adverse effects on bone maturation. Skeletal maturation must be monitored every 6 months by an x-ray of hand or wrist.

Androgen treatment may accelerate bone maturation without producing compensatory gain in linear growth. The younger the child, the greater the risk is of compromising final mature height.

Delayed puberty in males – Various dosage recommendations have been used to induce pubertal changes in hypogonadal males. Some experts have advocated lower dosages initially, gradually increasing the dose as puberty progresses, with or without a decrease to maintenance levels. Other experts emphasize that higher dosages are needed to induce pubertal changes, and lower dosages can be used for maintenance after puberty. The chronological and skeletal ages must be taken into consideration, both in determining the initial dose and in adjusting the dose.

Usual dosage: 10 to 50 mg administered orally daily.

Duration of therapy: Dosages used in delayed puberty generally are in the lower ranges of those given, and for a limited duration (eg, 4 to 6 months).

Hypogonadotropic hypogonadism (congenital or acquired) in males – See Adults for dosing.

Primary hypogonadism (congenital or acquired) in males – See Adults for dosing.

➤*Elderly:* Elderly patients treated with androgens may be at an increased risk for the development of prostatic hypertrophy and prostatic carcinoma.

Priapism or excessive sexual stimulation may develop. Males, especially elderly men, may become overstimulated.

Per the Beers list, methyltestoterone has the potential for prostatic hypertrophy and cardiac problems.

Methyltestosterone is also considered a high-risk medication for elderly patients according to the Centers of Medicare and Medicaid Services.

Androgens

METHYLTESTOSTERONE — ORAL

➤*Preparation for administration:* Methyltestoterone is a hormonal agent and is considered a teratogen. Follow safe handling procedures when preparing, administering, or dispensing methyltestoterone. See Sample Policy: Preparing and Reconstituting Hazardous Drugs and Sample Policy: Safe Handling of Hazardous Drugs or refer to your institution-specific protocol.

➤*Storage/Stability:* Store between 15° and 30°C (59° and 83°F).

FLUOXYMESTERONE

c-iii	**Fluoxymesterone** (Various, eg, Major, Rosemont, United)	**Tablets**: 10 mg	In 100s.
c-iii	**Androxy** (Upsher-Smith)		Lactose. (832 86). Green, scored. In 100s.

FLUOXYMESTERONE — ORAL

For complete and comparative prescribing information, refer to the Androgens group monograph.

Indications

➤*Men:*

Replacement therapy – Fluoxymesterone is indicated in conditions associated with symptoms of deficiency or absence of endogenous testosterone.

Primary hypogonadism (congenital or acquired): Fluoxymesterone is indicated for testicular failure due to cryptorchidism, bilateral torsion, orchitis, vanishing testis syndrome, or orchidectomy.

Hypogonadotropic hypogonadism (congenital or acquired): Fluoxymesterone is indicated in idiopathic gonadotropin or LHRH deficiency, or pituitary-hypothalamic injury from tumors, trauma, or radiation.

Delayed puberty – Fluoxymesterone is indicated for delayed puberty provided it has been definitely established as such, and is not just a familial trait.

➤*Women:*

Metastatic mammary cancer – Fluoxymesterone tablets may be used secondarily in women with advancing inoperable metastatic (skeletal) mammary cancer who are 1 to 5 years postmenopausal. This treatment has been used in premenopausal women with breast cancer who have benefited from oophorectomy and are considered to have a hormone-responsive tumor. Judgment concerning androgen therapy should be made by an oncologist with expertise in this field.

➤*Off-label uses:* Palliative treatment of androgen-responsive, recurrent breast cancer in premenopausal women after oophorectomy.

Administration and Dosage

➤*General dosing considerations:* Dosage and duration of therapy will depend on age, sex, diagnosis, patient's response to treatment, and appearance of adverse effects.

Androgen therapy should be used very cautiously in children and only by specialists aware of the adverse effects on bone maturation. Skeletal maturation must be monitored every 6 months by an x-ray of the hand and wrist.

➤*Adults:*

Male hypogonadism –

Usual dosage: 5 to 20 mg daily as replacement therapy (for eunuchism).

Initial dosage: It is usually preferable to start therapy at a higher level within the range (eg, 10 mg) with subsequent adjustment as required.

Metastatic mammary cancer in women –

Usual dosage: 10 to 40 mg daily in divided doses.

Duration of therapy: Treatment should be continued for 3 months or more. Patients must be followed closely because androgen therapy occasionally appears to accelerate the disease.

Hormone therapy is adjunctive to and not a replacement for conventional therapy. Duration of therapy will depend on the response of the condition and the appearance of adverse reactions.

➤*Children:*

Male delayed puberty –

Usual dosage: 2.5 to 20 mg daily; generally in the lower range of 2.5 to 10 mg daily and for a limited duration (eg, 4 to 6 months). X-rays should be taken at appropriate intervals to determine the amount of bone maturation and skeletal development.

➤*Renal function impairment:* Fluoxymesterone is contraindicated in patients with serious renal disease.

➤*Hepatic function impairment:* Fluoxymesterone is contraindicated in patients with serious hepatic disease.

➤*Preparation for administration:* Fluoxymesterone is a hormonal agent and is considered a teratogen and potential mutagen. Follow safe handling procedures when preparing, administering, or dispensing fluoxymesterone.

➤*Administration:* May be given as a single daily dose or in divided doses.

➤*Storage/Stability:* Store at 20° to 25°C (68° to 77°F).

SEX HORMONES

DANAZOL

Rx	**Danazol** (Various, eg, Barr)	**Capsules**: 50 mg	In 100s.
		100 mg	In 100s.
		200 mg	In 60s, 100s, and 500s.

DANAZOL — ORAL

WARNING

Use of danazol in pregnancy is contraindicated. A sensitive test (eg, beta subunit test if available) capable of determining early pregnancy is recommended immediately prior to start of therapy. Additionally, a nonhormonal method of contraception should be used during therapy. If a patient becomes pregnant while taking danazol, discontinue administration of the drug and apprise the patient of the potential risk to the fetus.

Thromboembolism, thrombotic and thrombophlebitic events, including sagittal sinus thrombosis and life-threatening or fatal strokes have been reported.

Experience with long-term therapy with danazol is limited. Peliosis hepatis and benign hepatic adenoma have been observed with long-term use. Peliosis hepatis and hepatic adenoma may be silent until complicated by acute, potentially life-threatening intra-abdominal hemorrhage. Therefore, alert the physician to this possibility. Attempts should be made to determine the lowest dose that will provide adequate protection (see Warnings).

Danazol has been associated with several cases of benign intracranial hypertension also known as pseudotumor cerebri. Early signs and symptoms of benign intracranial hypertension include papilledema, headache, nausea and vomiting, and visual disturbances. Screen patients with these symptoms for papilledema and, if present, advise the patients to discontinue danazol immediately and refer them to a neurologist for further diagnosis and care.

Indications

➤*Endometriosis:* For the treatment of endometriosis amenable to hormonal management.

➤*Fibrocystic breast disease:* Most cases of symptomatic fibrocystic breast disease may be treated by simple measures (eg, padded bras, analgesics). Pain and tenderness may be severe enough to warrant suppression of ovarian function. Danazol is usually effective in decreasing nodularity, pain, and tenderness, but it considerably alters hormone levels. Recurrence of symptoms is very common after cessation of therapy.

➤*Hereditary angioedema:* For the prevention of attacks of angioedema (eg, cutaneous, abdominal, laryngeal) in men and women.

➤*Off-label uses:*

Autoimmune hemolytic anemia – [4] = Insufficient documentation. Danazol therapy in conjunction with corticosteroids has shown promising results in treating autoimmune hemolytic anemia (AIHA) in a small number of case series/case reports. Patients dependent on corticosteroids were able to decrease or discontinue the corticosteroids after responding to the addition of danazol. Patients with refractory AIHA and splenectomy also showed favorable response to danazol. Hepatic and androgenic adverse effects may be of concern with danazol therapy. Controlled trials are needed to confirm the safety and efficacy of danazol in treating AIHA.

Gynecomastia – [2] = Fair documentation. Danazol was effective in treating gynecomastia in men (16 to 50 years of age) in a randomized, controlled study and had varying results in a number of case series. Weight gain was the most significant adverse effect noted.

Idiopathic thrombocytopenic purpura – [2] = Fair documentation. Danazol in conjunction with corticosteroids has shown a partial response in the secondary treatment of chronic refractory idiopathic thrombocytopenic purpura (ITP) in a small number of case series and case reports; however, very few patients have shown complete response. Patients dependent on corticosteroids were able to decrease or discontinue the corticosteroids after responding to the addition of danazol. Guidelines include danazol as an option for second-line treatment.

DANAZOL — ORAL

Lupus-associated thrombocytopenia – [4] = Insufficient documentation. Based on evidence from case series and case reports, danazol was observed to be safe and effective in treating systemic lupus erythematosus-associated thrombocytopenia. Danazol therapy was effective in patients with or without splenectomy. When used in conjunction with corticosteroids, danazol therapy allowed the tapering or discontinuation of corticosteroids.

Precocious puberty – [5] = Poor documentation. Danazol halted the progression of breast development and stopped menstrual bleeding in girls with precocious puberty. However, in most cases, danazol failed to stop and possibly accelerated the progression of bone age, one of the main reasons for initiating therapy. Continuous, uninterrupted therapy is required to suppress the continuation of pubertal development.

Other possible off-label uses – Danazol has been used to treat menorrhagia.

Administration and Dosage

➤*General dosing considerations:* For treatment of endometriosis and fibrocystic breast disease, begin therapy during menstruation or make sure the patient is not pregnant.

Individualize dosage.

➤*Adults:*

Endometriosis –

Initial dosage: For mild cases, give 200 to 400 mg in 2 divided doses. In moderate to severe disease, or in patients infertile because of endometriosis, administer 800 mg daily in 2 divided doses to best achieve amenorrhea and rapid response to painful symptoms.

Dosage titration: Downward titration to a dose sufficient to maintain amenorrhea may be considered, depending upon response.

Duration of therapy: Continue therapy uninterrupted for 3 to 6 months; may extend to 9 months. If symptoms recur after termination, treatment can be reinstituted.

Fibrocystic breast disease –

Usual dosage: 100 to 400 mg daily in 2 divided doses. A nonhormonal method of contraception is recommended when danazol is administered at this dose because ovulation may not be suppressed.

Duration of therapy: Breast pain and tenderness are usually relieved by the first month and eliminated in 2 to 3 months; elimination of nodularity requires 4 to 6 months of uninterrupted therapy. Approximately 50% of patients may have recurring symptoms within 1 year; treatment may be reinstituted.

Hereditary angioedema –

Initial dosage: 200 mg 2 or 3 times daily.

Dosage adjustment: After a favorable initial response, determine continuing dosage by decreasing the dosage by 50% or less at intervals of at least 1 to 3 months if frequency of attacks prior to treatment dictates. If an attack occurs, increase dosage by 200 mg daily or less. During the dose-adjusting phase, monitor response closely, particularly if patient has a history of airway involvement.

Off-label dosing –

Autoimmune hemolytic anemia: [4] = Insufficient documentation. Danazol 200 mg orally 3 to 4 times daily, usually in conjunction with a corticosteroid. Once hemolysis is under control, give maintenance therapy of 200 to 400 mg/day and taper the corticosteroid. Initial dosages in studies ranged from 600 to 800 mg/day, with maintenance therapy ranging from 200 to 600 mg/day. Duration of danazol therapy ranged from several weeks to 7.6 years (91 months).

Gynecomastia: [2] = Fair documentation. 200 to 400 mg/day in 2 to 4 divided doses for 3 to 6 months. In some men, the initial danazol dosage was 300 mg/day in 3 divided doses for 4 to 6 weeks, then increased to 600 to 800 mg/day in 3 divided doses for 4 to 6 months, then reduced to 200 to 300 mg/day for 4 to 6 months, and then stopped. In some adolescents, the initial dosage was 200 to 300 mg/day in 2 to 3 divided doses for 3 to 4 months, and then reduced to a maintenance dosage of 200 mg/day for 4 to 6 months.

Idiopathic thrombocytopenic purpura: [2] = Fair documentation. 200 mg given 2 to 4 times daily, in conjunction with prednisone 1 mg/kg/day. Danazol may need to be given for 3 to 6 months before it is abandoned for alternative second-line therapy. Patients who respond should receive danazol at full dose for at least 1 year and then be tapered off by reducing 50 mg/day every 4 months.

Lupus-associated thrombocytopenia: [4] = Insufficient documentation. Initial dosage of 50 mg/day and increased up to 1,200 mg/day, depending on response, adverse effects, and concomitant drug therapy.

Maintenance dosages ranged from 200 to 400 mg/day. Duration of danazol therapy ranged from 2 to 42 months.

➤*Children:*

Off-label dosing –

Gynecomastia: [2] = Fair documentation. See Adults for adolescent dosing.

➤*Storage/Stability:* Store at controlled room temperature, 15° to 30°C (59° to 86°F).

Actions

➤*Pharmacology:* A synthetic androgen derived from ethisterone, danazol suppresses the pituitary-ovarian axis by inhibiting the output of pituitary gonadotropins. It also has weak, androgenic activity. Danazol depresses the output of both follicle-stimulating hormone (FSH) and luteinizing hormone (LH). Evidence suggests direct inhibitory effect at gonadal sites and a binding of danazol to receptors of gonadal steroids at target organs. In addition, danazol has been shown to significantly decrease IgG, IgM, and IgA levels, as well as phospholipid and IgG isotope autoantibodies in patients with endometriosis and associated elevations of autoantibodies. Generally, the pituitary suppressive action is reversible. Ovulation and cyclic bleeding usually return within 60 to 90 days after therapy is discontinued.

Endometriosis – In the treatment of endometriosis, danazol alters the normal and ectopic endometrial tissue so that it becomes inactive and atrophic. Complete resolution of endometrial lesions occurs in the majority of cases. Changes in vaginal cytology and cervical mucus reflect the suppressive effect of danazol on the pituitary-ovarian axis.

Hereditary angioedema – Danazol prevents attacks of the disease characterized by episodic edema of the abdominal viscera, extremities, face, and airway that may be disabling and, if the airway is involved, fatal. In addition, danazol partially or completely corrects the primary biochemical abnormality of hereditary angioedema. It increases the levels of the deficient C1 esterase inhibitor, thereby increasing the serum levels of the C4 component of the complement system.

➤*Pharmacokinetics:* Blood levels of danazol do not increase proportionately with increases in dose. When the dose is doubled, plasma levels increase only approximately 35% to 40%.

Contraindications

Undiagnosed abnormal genital bleeding; markedly impaired hepatic, renal, or cardiac function.

Pregnancy and lactation.

Patients with porphyria. Danazol can induce aminolevulinate acid (ALA) synthetase activity and hence porphyrin metabolism.

Warnings/Precautions

➤*Thrombotic events:* Thromboembolism, thrombotic and thrombophlebitic events including sagittal sinus thrombosis and life-threatening or fatal strokes have been reported.

➤*Hepatic effects:* Experience with long-term therapy with danazol is limited. Peliosis hepatis and benign hepatic adenoma have been observed with long-term use. Peliosis hepatis and hepatic adenoma may be silent until complicated by acute, potentially life-threatening intra-abdominal hemorrhage. Therefore, alert the physician to this possibility. Make attempts to determine the lowest dose that will provide adequate protection. If the drug was begun at a time of exacerbation of hereditary angioneurotic edema because of trauma, stress, or other cause, consider periodic attempts to decrease or withdraw therapy.

➤*Intracranial hypertension:* Danazol has been associated with several cases of benign intracranial hypertension (also known as pseudotumor cerebri). Early signs and symptoms of benign intracranial hypertension include papilledema, headache, nausea and vomiting, and visual disturbances. Screen patients with these symptoms for papilledema and, if present, advise the patients to discontinue danazol immediately and refer them to a neurologist for further diagnosis and care.

➤*Lipoprotein alterations:* A temporary alteration of lipoproteins in the form of decreased high density lipoproteins (HDL) and possibly increased low density lipoproteins (LDL) has been reported during danazol therapy. These alterations may be marked, and prescribers should consider the potential impact on the risk of atherosclerosis and coronary artery disease in accordance with the potential benefit of the therapy to the patient.

➤*Long-term experience:* Long-term experience with danazol is limited. Long-term therapy with other steroids alkylated at the 17 position has been associated with serious toxicity (eg, cholestatic jaundice, peliosis hepatis). Similar toxicity may develop after long-term danazol. Determine the lowest dose that will provide adequate protection. If the drug was begun for exacerbation of angioneurotic edema because of trauma, stress, or another cause, consider decreasing or withdrawing therapy periodically.

➤*Androgenic effects:* Androgenic effects may not be reversible even when the drug is discontinued. Watch patients closely for signs of virilization.

➤*Porphyria:* Danazol administration has been reported to cause exacerbation of the manifestations of acute intermittent porphyria.

➤*Pregnancy:* *Category X.* Use of danazol in pregnancy is contraindicated. A sensitive test (eg, beta subunit test if available) capable of determining early pregnancy is recommended immediately prior to start of therapy. Additionally, a nonhormonal method of contraception should be used during therapy. If a patient becomes pregnant while taking danazol, discontinue administration of the drug and apprise the patient of the potential risk to the fetus. Exposure to danazol in utero may result in androgenic effects on the female fetus; reports of clitoral hypertrophy, labial fusion, urogenital sinus defect, vaginal atresia, and ambiguous genitalia have been received.

In rabbits, the administration of danazol on days 6 to 18 of gestation at doses of at least 60 mg/kg daily (2 to 4 times the human dose) resulted in inhibition of fetal development.

➤*Lactation:* Breast-feeding is contraindicated in patients taking danazol.

➤*Children:* Safety and efficacy in children have not been established.

➤*Monitoring:*

Fluid retention – Conditions influenced by edema (eg, epilepsy, migraine, cardiac or renal dysfunction) require careful observation.

Hepatic dysfunction – Hepatic dysfunction has been reported manifested by modest increases in serum transaminase levels; perform periodic liver function tests.

Lipoproteins – Monitor HDL and LDL periodically.

DANAZOL — ORAL

Semen – Semen should be checked for volume, viscosity, sperm count, and motility.

Drug Interactions

Danazol Drug Interactions			
Precipitant drug	Object drug[a]		Description
Danazol	Carbamazepine	↑	Therapy with danazol may cause an increase in carbamazepine levels in patients taking both drugs.
Danazol	Cyclosporine	↑	Increased cyclosporine blood concentrations with possible toxicity (eg, nephrotoxicity) has occurred. Monitor serum bilirubin, serum creatinine, and cyclosporine concentrations in patients receiving concomitant therapy. Adjust doses of drugs as needed.
Danazol	Warfarin	↑	Prolongation of prothrombin time has been reported with concomitant use.

[a] ↑ = Object drug increased.

➤*Drug/Lab test interactions:* Danazol treatment may interfere with laboratory determinations of testosterone, androstenedione, and dehydroepiandrosterone.

Abnormalities in laboratory tests may occur during therapy with danazol including the following: CPK, glucose tolerance, glucagon, thyroid-binding globulin, sex hormone-binding globulin, other plasma proteins, lipids, and lipoproteins.

Adverse Reactions

Androgenic – Acne; edema; mild hirsutism; changes in the voice (eg, hoarseness, sore throat, instability, deepening of pitch); oily skin or hair; weight gain; seborrhea; hair loss; clitoral hypertrophy (rare).

➤*GU:* Menstrual disturbances including spotting; alteration of the timing of the cycle; amenorrhea. Although cyclical bleeding and ovulation usually return within 60 to 90 days after discontinuation of therapy with danazol, persistent amenorrhea has occasionally been reported. In the male, a modest reduction in spermatogenesis may occur during treatment. Abnormalities in semen volume, viscosity, sperm count, and motility may occur with long-term therapy.

Hypoestrogenic – Flushing; sweating; vaginal dryness/irritation; reduction in breast size; nervousness; emotional lability.

➤*Hepatic:* Dysfunction (elevated serum enzymes or jaundice) has been reported in patients receiving at least 400 mg daily. It is recommended that patients receiving danazol be monitored for hepatic dysfunction by laboratory tests and clinical observation. Serious hepatic toxicity, including cholestatic jaundice, peliosis hepatis, and hepatic adenoma has been reported.

➤*The following have been reported, but the causal relationship is not confirmed:*

CNS – Dizziness; headache; nervousness; emotional lability; fainting; weakness; Guillain-Barré syndrome; sleep disorders; fatigue; tremor; paresthesia; visual disturbances; anxiety; depression and changes in appetite; benign intracranial hypertension, convulsions (rare).

Dermatologic – Rashes (eg, maculopapular, vesicular, papular, purpuric, petechial); sun sensitivity, Stevens-Johnson syndrome (rare).

GI – Gastroenteritis; nausea; vomiting; constipation; pancreatitis (rare).

GU – Hematuria; prolonged posttherapy amenorrhea.

Hematologic – Increase in red cell and platelet count; reversible erythrocytosis, leukocytosis, or polycythemia; eosinophilia; leukopenia; thrombocytopenia.

Hypersensitivity – Urticaria, pruritus; nasal congestion (rare).

Musculoskeletal – Muscle cramps or spasms; pains; joint pain; joint lock-up; joint swelling; pain in back, neck, or extremities; carpal tunnel syndrome (rare, may be secondary to fluid retention).

Miscellaneous – Change in libido; elevated blood pressure; chills; increased insulin requirements in diabetic patients; cataracts, bleeding gums, fever, pelvic pain, nipple discharge, malignant liver tumors (after long-term use) (rare).

Patient Information

Notify physician if masculinizing effects occur (eg, abnormal growth of facial or other fine body hair, deepening of the voice).

Use nonhormonal contraceptive measures during therapy. Discontinue use if pregnancy is suspected.

Androgen Hormone Inhibitor

FINASTERIDE

Rx	**Propecia** (Merck)	**Tablets:** 1 mg	Lactose. (P Propecia). Tan, octagonal. Film-coated. In unit-of-use 30s, and *ProPAK* carton of 3 unit-of-use bottles of 30.
Rx	**Finasteride** (Teva)	**Tablets:** 5 mg	Lactose. (X 5825). Lt. blue. Film-coated. In 30s, 100s, and 500s.
Rx	**Proscar** (Merck)		Lactose. (MSD 72 Proscar). Blue, apple shape. Film-coated. In 1,000s, unit-of-use 30s and 100s, and UD 100s.

FINASTERIDE — ORAL

Indications

➤*Androgenetic alopecia (Propecia only):* Finasteride is indicated for the treatment of male pattern hair loss (androgenetic alopecia) in men only. Safety and efficacy were demonstrated in men between 18 to 41 years of age with mild to moderate hair loss of the vertex and anterior mid-scalp area. Efficacy in bitemporal recession has not been established.

➤*Benign prostatic hyperplasia (BPH) (Proscar only):* Finasteride is indicated for the treatment of symptomatic BPH in men with an enlarged prostate to improve symptoms, reduce the risk of acute urinary retention, and reduce the risk of the need for surgery including transurethral resection of the prostate (TURP) and prostatectomy.

Finasteride administered in combination with the alpha-blocker doxazosin is indicated to reduce the risk of symptomatic progression of BPH (a confirmed greater than or equal to 4-point increase in AUA symptom score).

➤*Off-label uses:*

Acne vulgaris – [5] = Poor documentation. Because finasteride is a type II selective 5-alpha reductase inhibitor, and because the type II isoenzyme is not located in the skin, its usefulness in the treatment of acne is predicted to be minimal. The limited clinical data evaluating its safety and efficacy for the treatment of acne show no benefit. Guidelines from the American Academy of Dermatology note that finasteride has not been shown to be effective for the treatment of acne.

Chronic pelvic pain syndrome – [2] = Fair documentation. In 3 small trials, finasteride improved symptoms of chronic pelvic pain syndrome when compared with placebo and saw palmetto. However, further studies are needed to compare finasteride with other treatments for chronic pelvic pain syndrome, including antibiotics and alpha-blockers.

Hirsutism (idiopathic) in women – [4] = Insufficient documentation. Guidelines primarily based on expert consensus recommend the use of finasteride in combination with an oral contraceptive for the treatment of polycystic ovary syndrome (PCOS)-related hirsutism. Trials in patients with PCOS and idiopathic hirsutism, which have been small and not well designed, have demonstrated benefit.

Hirsutism (PCOS-related) in women – [1] = Good documentation. Guidelines primarily based on expert consensus recommend the use of finasteride in combination with an oral contraceptive for the treatment of PCOS-related hirsutism.

Prostate cancer prevention – [1] = Good documentation. No widely established decision model has been developed to determine what men should receive chemoprevention with a 5-alpha reductase inhibitor, such as finasteride. The role of finasteride in the chemoprevention of prostate cancer was delineated in guidelines from the American Society of Clinical Oncology and the American Urological Association. The guideline authors recommend only that a discussion of benefits and risks of using 5-alpha reductase inhibitors for prevention of prostate cancer is warranted in men with a prostate-specific antigen (PSA) no greater than 3 who are regularly screened with PSA or are anticipating undergoing annual PSA screening for early detection of prostate cancer; they do not mandate that men in any subgroup be treated.

Tourette syndrome – [4] = Insufficient documentation. The use of finasteride to treat Tourette syndrome has been limited to one case report. The data suggest that this drug may be a useful alternative in patients with refractory disease, but larger controlled trials are needed to determine the optimal dosage schedule and to verify results.

Other possible off-label uses – Possible treatment of prostate cancer.

Administration and Dosage

➤*Adults:*

Androgenetic alopecia (Propecia only) –

Usual dosage: 1 mg orally once a day.

Duration of therapy: In general, daily use for 3 months or more is necessary before benefit is observed. Continued use is recommended to sustain benefit, which should be re-evaluated periodically. Withdrawal of treatment leads to reversal of effect within 12 months.

Benign prostatic hyperplasia (BPH) (Proscar only) –

Usual dosage: 5 mg orally once a day.

Concomitant therapy: Finasteride can be administered alone or in combination with the alpha-blocker doxazosin.

Androgen Hormone Inhibitor

FINASTERIDE — ORAL

Off-label dosing –

Chronic pelvic pain syndrome: [2] = Fair documentation. 5 mg daily.

Hirsutism (idiopathic) in women: [4] = Insufficient documentation. 2.5 to 5 mg daily as monotherapy or in combination therapy.

Hirsutism (PCOS-related) in women: [1] = Good documentation. 2.5 to 5 mg daily as monotherapy or in combination therapy.

Prostate cancer prevention: [1] = Good documentation. 5 mg orally once daily. Use of 5-alpha reductase inhibitors as primary prevention for prostate cancer has been evaluated for up to 7 years.

Tourette syndrome: [4] = Insufficient documentation. Oral dosing of 5 mg daily for 28 weeks.

➤*Administration:* Finasteride may be administered with or without meals.

Finasteride is a hormonal agent and is considered a potential teratogen. Follow safe handling procedures when preparing, administering, or dispensing finasteride.

➤*Storage/Stability:* Store at 15° to 30°C (59° to 86°F). Protect from moisture and light.

Actions

➤*Pharmacology:*

Propecia – Finasteride is a competitive and specific inhibitor of Type II 5α-reductase, an intracellular enzyme that converts the androgen testosterone into DHT. Two distinct isozymes are found in mice, rats, monkeys, and humans: Type I and II. Each of these isozymes is differentially expressed in tissues and developmental stages. In humans, Type I 5α-reductase is predominant in the sebaceous glands of most regions of skin, including scalp, and liver. Type I 5α-reductase is responsible for approximately one-third of circulating DHT. The Type II 5α-reductase isozyme is primarily found in prostate, seminal vesicles, epididymides, and hair follicles as well as liver, and is responsible for two-thirds of circulating DHT.

In humans, the mechanism of action of finasteride is based on its preferential inhibition of the Type II isozyme. Using native tissues (scalp and prostate), in vitro binding studies examining the potential of finasteride to inhibit either isozyme revealed a 100-fold selectivity for the human Type II 5α-reductase over Type I isozyme (IC_{50} = 500 and 4.2 nM for Type I and II, respectively). For both isozymes, the inhibition by finasteride is accompanied by reduction of the inhibitor to dihydrofinasteride and adduct formation with NADP+. The turnover for the enzyme complex is slow ($t_{½}$ approximately 30 days for the Type II enzyme complex and 14 days for the Type I complex).

Finasteride has no affinity for the androgen receptor and has no androgenic, antiandrogenic, estrogenic, antiestrogenic, or progestational effects. Inhibition of Type II 5α-reductase blocks the peripheral conversion of testosterone to DHT, resulting in significant decreases in serum and tissue DHT concentrations. Finasteride produces a rapid reduction in serum DHT concentration, reaching 65% suppression within 24 hours of oral dosing with a 1 mg tablet.

In men with male pattern hair loss (androgenetic alopecia), the balding scalp contains miniaturized hair follicles and increased amounts of DHT compared with hairy scalp. Administration of finasteride decreases scalp and serum DHT concentrations in these men. The relative contributions of these reductions to the treatment effect of finasteride have not been defined. By this mechanism, finasteride appears to interrupt a key factor in the development of androgenetic alopecia in those patients genetically predisposed.

A 48-week, placebo-controlled study designed to assess by phototrichogram the effect of finasteride 1 mg on total and actively growing (anagen) scalp hairs in vertex baldness enrolled 212 men with androgenetic alopecia. At baseline and 48 weeks, total and anagen hair counts were obtained in a 1 cm^2 target area of the scalp. Men treated with finasteride 1 mg showed increases from baseline in total and anagen hair counts of 7 hairs and 18 hairs, respectively, whereas men treated with placebo had decreases of 10 hairs and 9 hairs, respectively. These changes in hair counts resulted in a between-group difference of 17 hairs in total hair count (*P* less than 0.001) and 27 hairs in anagen hair count (*P* less than 0.001), and an improvement in the proportion of anagen hairs from 62% at baseline to 68% for men treated with finasteride.

Finasteride had no effect on circulating levels of cortisol, thyroid-stimulating hormone, or thyroxine, nor did it affect the plasma lipid profile (eg, total cholesterol, low-density lipoproteins, high-density lipoproteins and triglycerides) or bone mineral density. In studies with finasteride, no clinically meaningful changes in luteinizing hormone (LH) or follicle-stimulating hormone (FSH) were detected. In healthy volunteers, treatment with finasteride did not alter the response of LH and FSH to gonadotropin-releasing hormone, indicating that the hypothalamic-pituitary-testicular axis was not affected. Mean circulating levels of testosterone and estradiol were increased by approximately 15% as compared to baseline in the first year of treatment, but these levels were within the physiologic range.

Proscar – The development and enlargement of the prostate gland is dependent on the potent androgen, 5α-dihydrotestosterone (DHT). Type II 5α-reductase metabolizes testosterone to DHT in the prostate gland, liver and skin. DHT induces androgenic effects by binding to androgen receptors in the cell nuclei of these organs.

Finasteride is a competitive and specific inhibitor of Type II 5α-reductase with which it slowly forms a stable enzyme complex. Turnover from this complex is extremely slow ($t_{½}$ approximately 30 days). This has been demonstrated both in vivo and in vitro. Finasteride has no affinity for the androgen receptor.

In man, the 5α-reduced steroid metabolites in blood and urine are decreased after administration of finasteride. In man, a single 5 mg oral dose of finasteride produces a rapid reduction in serum DHT concentration, with the maximum effect observed 8 hours after the first dose. The suppression of DHT is maintained throughout the 24-hour dosing interval and with continued treatment. Daily dosing of finasteride at 5 mg/day for up to 4 years has been shown to reduce the serum DHT concentration by approximately 70%. The median circulating level of testosterone increased by approximately 10% to 20% but remained within the physiologic range.

Adult males with genetically inherited Type II 5α-reductase deficiency also have decreased levels of DHT. Except for the associated urogenital defects present at birth, no other clinical abnormalities related to Type II 5α-reductase deficiency have been observed in these individuals. These individuals have a small prostate gland throughout life and do not develop BPH.

In patients with BPH treated with finasteride (1 to 100 mg/day) for 7 to 10 days prior to prostatectomy, an approximate 80% lower DHT content was measured in prostatic tissue removed at surgery, compared to placebo; testosterone tissue concentration was increased up to 10 times over pretreatment levels, relative to placebo. Intraprostatic content of prostate-specific antigen (PSA) also was decreased.

In healthy men treated with finasteride for 14 days, discontinuation of therapy resulted in a return of DHT levels to pretreatment levels in approximately 2 weeks. In patients treated for 3 months, prostate volume, which declined by approximately 20%, returned to close to baseline value after approximately 3 months of discontinuation of therapy.

➤*Pharmacokinetics:*

Finasteride Pharmacokinetic Parameters in Healthy Young Subjects (n = 15)

Parameter	Mean (± SD)
Bioavailability	63% (34% to 108%)[a]
Clearance (mL/min)	165 (55)
Volume of distribution (L)	76 (14)
Half-life (hours)	6.2 (2.1)

[a] Range.

Noncompartmental Pharmacokinetic Parameters After Multiple Doses of Finasteride 5 mg/day in Older Men

Parameter	Mean (± SD)	
	45 to 60 years of age (n = 12)	≥ 70 years of age (n = 12)
AUC (ng•hr/mL)	389 (98)	463 (186)
Peak concentration (ng/mL)	46.2 (8.7)	48.4 (14.7)
Time to peak (hours)	1.8 (0.7)	1.8 (0.6)
Half-life (hours)[a]	6 (1.5)	8.2 (2.5)

[a] First-dose values; all other parameters are last-dose values.

Absorption –

Propecia: In a study in 15 healthy men, the mean bioavailability of finasteride 1 mg tablets was 65% (range, 26% to 170%), based on the ratio of AUC relative to a 5 mg IV dose infused over 60 minutes. Following IV infusion, mean plasma clearance was 165 mL/min (range, 70 to 279 mL/min) and mean steady-state volume of distribution was 76 L (range, 44 to 96 L). In a separate study, the bioavailability of finasteride was not affected by food.

There is a slow accumulation phase for finasteride after multiple dosing. At steady state following dosing with 1 mg/day, maximum finasteride plasma concentration averaged 9.2 ng/mL (range, 4.9 to 13.7 ng/mL) and was reached 1 to 2 hours postdose; $AUC_{(0-24\ h)}$ was 53 ng•h/mL (range, 20 to 154 ng•h/mL) and mean terminal half-life of elimination was 4.8 hours (range, 3.3 to 13.4 hours).

Semen levels have been measured in 35 men taking finasteride 1 mg daily for 6 weeks. In 60% (21 of 35) of the samples, finasteride levels were undetectable. The mean finasteride level was 0.26 ng/mL and the highest level measured was 1.52 ng/mL. Using this highest semen level measured and assuming 100% absorption from a 5 mL ejaculate daily, human exposure through vaginal absorption would be up to 7.6 ng daily, which is 750 times lower than the exposure from the no-effect dose for developmental abnormalities in rhesus monkeys. The in utero effects of finasteride exposure during the period of embryonic and fetal development were evaluated in the rhesus monkey (gestation days 20 to 100), a species more predictive of human development than rats or rabbits. IV administration of finasteride to pregnant monkeys at doses as high as 800 ng daily (at least 60 to 120 times the highest estimated exposure of pregnant women to finasteride from semen of men taking 5 mg daily) resulted in no abnormalities in male fetuses. In confirmation of the relevance of the rhesus model for human fetal development, oral administration of a very high dose of finasteride (2 mg/kg daily; 20 times the recommended human dose of 5 mg daily or approximately 1 to 2 million times the highest estimated exposure to finasteride from semen of men taking 5 mg daily) to pregnant monkeys resulted in external genital abnormalities in male fetuses. No other abnormalities were observed in male fetuses and no finasteride-related abnormalities were observed in female fetuses at any dose.

FINASTERIDE — ORAL

Proscar: In a study of 15 healthy young subjects, the mean bioavailability of finasteride 5 mg tablets was 63% (range, 34% to 108%), based on the ratio of area under the curve (AUC) relative to an IV reference dose. Maximum finasteride plasma concentration averaged 37 ng/mL (range, 27 to 49 ng/mL) and was reached 1 to 2 hours postdose. Bioavailability of finasteride was not affected by food.

Distribution – Mean steady-state volume of distribution was 76 L (range, 44 to 96 L). Approximately 90% of circulating finasteride is bound to plasma proteins. There is a slow accumulation phase for finasteride after multiple dosing. After dosing with 5 mg/day of finasteride for 17 days, plasma concentrations of finasteride were 47% and 54% higher than after the first dose in men 45 to 60 years old (n = 12) and greater than or equal to 70 years old (n = 12), respectively. Mean trough concentrations after 17 days of dosing were 6.2 ng/mL (range, 2.4 to 9.8 ng/mL) and 8.1 ng/mL (range, 1.8 to 19.7 ng/mL), respectively, in the 2 age groups. Although steady state was not reached in this study, mean trough plasma concentration in another study in patients with BPH (mean age, 65 years) receiving 5 mg/day was 9.4 ng/mL (range, 7.1 to 13.3 ng/mL; n = 22) after over a year of dosing.

Finasteride has been shown to cross the blood brain barrier but does not appear to distribute preferentially to the CSF.

In 2 studies of healthy subjects (n = 69) receiving finasteride 5 mg/day for 6 to 24 weeks, finasteride concentrations in semen ranged from undetectable (less than 0.1 ng/mL) to 10.54 ng/mL. In an earlier study using a less sensitive assay, finasteride concentrations in the semen of 16 subjects receiving finasteride 5 mg/day ranged from undetectable (less than 1 ng/mL) to 21 ng/mL. Thus, based on a 5 mL ejaculate volume, the amount of finasteride in semen was estimated to be 50- to 100-fold less than the dose of finasteride (5 mcg) that had no effect on circulating DHT levels in men.

Metabolism – Finasteride is extensively metabolized in the liver, primarily via the cytochrome P-450 3A4 enzyme subfamily. Two metabolites, the t-butyl side chain monohydroxylated and monocarboxylic acid metabolites, have been identified that possess no more than 20% of the 5α-reductase inhibitory activity of finasteride.

Excretion –

Propecia: Following an oral dose of ^{14}C-finasteride in man, a mean of 39% (range, 32% to 46%) of the dose was excreted in the urine in the form of metabolites; 57% (range, 51% to 64%) was excreted in the feces. The major compound isolated from urine was the monocarboxylic acid metabolite; virtually no unchanged drug was recovered. The t-butyl side chain monohydroxylated metabolite has been isolated from plasma. These metabolites possessed no more than 20% of the 5 α-reductase inhibitory activity of finasteride.

Proscar: In healthy young subjects (n = 15), mean plasma clearance of finasteride was 165 mL/min (range, 70 to 279 mL/min) and mean elimination half-life in plasma was 6 hours (range, 3 to 16 hours). Following an oral dose of ^{14}C-finasteride in man (n = 6), a mean of 39% (range, 32% to 46%) of the dose was excreted in the urine in the form of metabolites; 57% (range, 51% to 64%) was excreted in the feces.

The mean terminal half-life of finasteride in subjects greater than or equal to 70 years of age was approximately 8 hours (range, 6 to 15 hours; n = 12), compared with 6 hours (range, 4 to 12 hours; n = 12) in subjects 45 to 60 years of age. As a result, mean $AUC_{(0-24\ hr)}$ after 17 days of dosing was 15% higher in subjects greater than or equal to 70 years of age than in subjects 45 to 60 years of age (P = 0.02).

Contraindications

Finasteride use is contraindicated in women when they are or may potentially be pregnant. Because of the ability of Type II 5α-reductase inhibitors to inhibit the conversion of testosterone to DHT, finasteride may cause abnormalities of the external genitalia of a male fetus of a pregnant woman who receives finasteride. If this drug is used during pregnancy, or if pregnancy occurs while taking this drug, apprise the pregnant woman of the potential hazard to the male fetus. In female rats, low doses of finasteride administered during pregnancy have produced abnormalities of the external genitalia in male offspring.

Finasteride is contraindicated for hypersensitivity to any component of this medication.

Warnings/Precautions

➤*Exposure of women/risk to male fetus:* Finasteride is not indicated for use in pediatric patients or women. Women should not handle crushed or broken finasteride tablets when they are pregnant or may potentially be pregnant because of the possibility of absorption of finasteride and the subsequent potential risk to a male fetus. Finasteride tablets are coated and will prevent contact with the active ingredient during normal handling, provided that the tablets have not been broken or crushed.

➤*Proscar*:

Effects on PSA and prostate cancer detection – No clinical benefit has been demonstrated in patients with prostate cancer treated with finasteride. Patients with BPH and elevated PSA were monitored in controlled clinical studies with serial PSAs and prostate biopsies. In these studies, finasteride did not appear to alter the rate of prostate cancer detection. The overall incidence of prostate cancer was not significantly different in patients treated with finasteride or placebo.

Finasteride causes a decrease in serum PSA levels by approximately 50% in patients with BPH, even in the presence of prostate cancer. This decrease is predictable over the entire range of PSA values, although it may vary in individual patients. Analysis of PSA data from over 3,000 patients in PLESS confirmed that in typical patients treated with finasteride for 6 months or more, PSA values should be doubled for comparison with normal ranges in untreated men. This adjustment preserves the sensitivity and specificity of the PSA assay and maintains its ability to detect prostate cancer.

Carefully evaluate any sustained increases in PSA levels while on finasteride, including consideration of noncompliance to therapy with finasteride.

Percent free PSA (free to total PSA ratio) is not significantly decreased by finasteride. The ratio of free to total PSA remains constant even under the influence of finasteride. If clinicians elect to use percent free PSA as an aid in the detection of prostate cancer in men undergoing finasteride therapy, no adjustment to its value appears necessary.

➤*Hepatic function impairment:* Use caution in the administration of finasteride in patients with liver function abnormalities, as finasteride is metabolized extensively in the liver.

➤*Pregnancy: Category X.* Finasteride is not indicated for use in women. Administration of finasteride to pregnant rats at doses ranging from 100 mcg/kg/day to 100 mg/kg/day (1 to 1,000 times the maximum recommended human dose of 5 mg/day) resulted in dose-dependent development of hypospadias in 3.6% to 100% of male offspring. Pregnant rats produced male offspring with decreased prostatic and seminal vesicular weights, delayed preputial separation, and transient nipple development when given finasteride at greater than or equal to 30 mcg/kg/day (greater than or equal to 0.3 times the maximum recommended human dose of 5 mg/day) and decreased anogenital distance when given finasteride at greater than or equal to 3 mcg/kg/day (greater than or equal to 0.03 times the maximum recommended human dose of 5 mg/day). The critical period during which these effects can be induced in male rats has been defined to be days 16 to 17 of gestation. The changes described above are expected pharmacological effects of drugs belonging to the class of Type II 5α-reductase inhibitors and are similar to those reported in male infants with a genetic deficiency of Type II 5α-reductase. No abnormalities were observed in female offspring exposed to any dose of finasteride in utero.

The in utero effects of finasteride exposure during the period of embryonic and fetal development were evaluated in the rhesus monkey (gestation days 20 to 100), a species more predictive of human development than rats or rabbits. IV administration of finasteride to pregnant monkeys at doses as high as 800 ng/day (at least 60 to 120 times the highest estimated exposure of pregnant women to finasteride from semen of men taking 5 mg/day) resulted in no abnormalities in male fetuses. In confirmation of the relevance of the rhesus model for human fetal development, oral administration of a very high dose of finasteride (2 mg/kg/day; 20 times the recommended human dose of 5 mg/day or approximately 1 to 2 million times the highest estimated exposure to finasteride from semen of men taking 5 mg/day) to pregnant monkeys resulted in external genital abnormalities in male fetuses. No other abnormalities were observed in male fetuses and no finasteride-related abnormalities were observed in female fetuses at any dose.

➤*Lactation:* Finasteride is not indicated for use in women. It is not known whether finasteride is excreted in human milk.

➤*Children:* Finasteride is not indicated for use in pediatric patients. Safety and efficacy in children have not been established.

➤*Elderly:*

5 mg – Of the total number of subjects included in PLESS, 1,480 and 105 subjects were 65 years of age and older and 75 years of age and older, respectively. No overall differences in safety or effectiveness were observed between these subjects and younger subjects, and other reported clinical experience has not identified differences in responses between the elderly and younger patients. No dosage adjustment is necessary in the elderly.

➤*Monitoring:*

Proscar – Prior to initiating therapy with finasteride for BPH, perform appropriate evaluation to identify other conditions such as infection, prostate cancer, stricture disease, hypotonic bladder or other neurogenic disorders that might mimic BPH.

Carefully monitor patients with large residual urinary volume or severely diminished urinary flow for obstructive uropathy. These patients may not be candidates for finasteride therapy for BPH.

Drug Interactions

No drug interactions of clinical importance have been identified. Finasteride does not appear to affect the cytochrome P450-linked drug metabolizing enzyme system. Compounds that have been tested in man include antipyrine, digoxin, propranolol, theophylline, and warfarin, and no interactions were found.

➤*Other concomitant therapy:* Although specific interaction studies were not performed, finasteride doses of 1 mg or more were concomitantly used in clinical studies with acetaminophen, α-blockers, analgesics, angiotensin-converting enzyme (ACE) inhibitors, anticonvulsants, benzodiazepines, beta blockers, calcium-channel blockers, cardiac nitrates, diuretics, H_2 antagonists, HMG-CoA reductase inhibitors, prostaglandin synthetase inhibitors (NSAIDs), and quinolone anti-infectives without evidence of clinically significant adverse interactions.

➤*Drug/Lab test interactions:*

Propecia – In clinical studies with finasteride 1 mg in men 18 to 41 years of age, the mean value of serum prostate-specific antigen (PSA) decreased from 0.7 ng/mL at baseline to 0.5 ng/mL at month 12. When finasteride is used in older men who have benign prostatic hyperplasia (BPH), PSA levels are decreased by approximately 50%. Until further information is gathered in men older than 41 years of age without BPH, consider doubling the PSA level in men undergoing this test and taking finasteride.

Proscar – In patients with BPH, finasteride has no effect on circulating levels of cortisol, estradiol, prolactin, thyroid-stimulating hormone, or thy-

FINASTERIDE — ORAL

roxine. No clinically meaningful effect was observed on the plasma lipid profile (ie, total cholesterol, low density lipoproteins, high density lipoproteins, and triglycerides) or bone mineral density. Increases of about 10% were observed in luteinizing hormone (LH) and follicle-stimulating hormone (FSH) in patients receiving finasteride, but levels remained within the normal range. In healthy volunteers, treatment with finasteride did not alter the response of LH and FSH to gonadotropin-releasing hormone indicating that the hypothalamic-pituitary-testicular axis was not affected.

Treatment with finasteride for 24 weeks to evaluate semen parameters in healthy male volunteers revealed no clinically meaningful effects on sperm concentration, mobility, morphology, or pH. A 0.6 mL (22.1%) median decrease in ejaculate volume with a concomitant reduction in total sperm per ejaculate, was observed. These parameters remained within the normal range and were reversible upon discontinuation of therapy with an average time to return to baseline of 84 weeks.

Adverse Reactions

Finasteride is generally well tolerated; adverse effects usually have been mild and transient.

➤*Propecia:*

Clinical studies for finasteride 1 mg in the treatment of male pattern hair loss – In controlled clinical trials for finasteride of 12-month duration, 1.4% of the patients were discontinued due to adverse experiences that were considered to be possibly, probably or definitely drug-related (1.6% for placebo); 1.2% of patients on finasteride and 0.9% of patients on placebo discontinued therapy because of a drug-related sexual adverse experience. The following clinical adverse reactions were reported as possibly, probably or definitely drug-related in greater than or equal to 1% of patients treated for 12 months with finasteride or placebo, respectively: Decreased libido (1.8%, 1.3%), erectile dysfunction (1.3%, 0.7%) and ejaculation disorder (1.2%, 0.7%; primarily decreased volume of ejaculate [0.8%, 0.4%]). Integrated analysis of clinical adverse experiences showed that during treatment with finasteride, 36 (3.8%) of 945 men had reported 1 or more of these adverse experiences as compared to 20 (2.1%) of 934 men treated with placebo ($P = 0.04$). Resolution occurred in all men who discontinued therapy with finasteride because of these side effects and in most of those who continued therapy. The incidence of each of the above side effects decreased to less than or equal to 0.3% by the fifth year of treatment with finasteride.

In a study of finasteride 1 mg daily in healthy men, a median decrease in ejaculate volume of 0.3 mL (−11%) compared with 0.2 mL (−8%) for placebo was observed after 48 weeks of treatment. Two other studies showed that finasteride at 5 times the dosage of finasteride (5 mg daily) produced significant median decreases of approximately 0.5 mL (−25%) compared with placebo in ejaculate volume but this was reversible after discontinuation of treatment.

In the clinical studies with finasteride, the incidences for breast tenderness and enlargement, hypersensitivity reactions, and testicular pain in finasteride-treated patients were not different from those in patients treated with placebo.

Postmarketing experience for finasteride 1 mg – Breast tenderness and enlargement; hypersensitivity reactions including rash, pruritus, urticaria, and swelling of the lips and face; and testicular pain.

Controlled clinical trials and long-term open extension studies for finasteride 5 mg in the treatment of benign prostatic hyperplasia – In controlled clinical trials for finasteride 5 mg of 12-month duration, 1.3% of the patients were discontinued due to adverse experiences that were considered to be possibly, probably, or definitely drug-related (0.9% for placebo); only 1 patient on finasteride 5 mg (0.2%) and 1 patient on placebo (0.2%) discontinued therapy because of a drug-related sexual adverse experience.

The following clinical adverse reactions were reported as possibly, probably or definitely drug-related in greater than or equal to 1% of patients treated for 12 months with finasteride or placebo, respectively: erectile dysfunction (3.7%, 1.1%), decreased libido (3.3%, 1.6%), and decreased volume of ejaculate (2.8%, 0.9%). The adverse experience profiles for patients treated with finasteride 1 mg/day for 12 months and those maintained on finasteride for 24 to 48 months were similar to that observed in the 12-month controlled studies with finasteride. Sexual adverse experiences resolved with continued treatment in over 60% of patients who reported them.

The relationship between long-term use of finasteride and male breast neoplasia is currently unknown. During a 4- to 6-year placebo- and comparator-controlled study that enrolled 3,047 men, there were 4 cases of breast cancer in men treated with finasteride but no cases in men not treated with finasteride. In another 4-year, placebo-controlled study that enrolled 3,040 men, there were 2 cases of breast cancer in placebo-treated men, but no cases were reported in men treated with finasteride. In a 7-year placebo-controlled trial that enrolled 18,882 healthy men, 9,060 had prostate needle biopsy data available for analysis. In the finasteride group, 280 (6.4%) men had prostate cancer with Gleason scores of 7 to 10 detected on needle biopsy vs 237 (5.1%) men in the placebo group. Of the total cases of prostate cancer diagnosed in this study, approximately 98% were classified as intracapsular (stage T1 or T2). The clinical significance of these findings is unknown.

➤*Proscar:*

Four-year placebo-controlled study – In PLESS, 1,524 patients treated with finasteride and 1,516 patients treated with placebo were evaluated for safety over a period of 4 years. The most frequently reported adverse reactions were related to sexual function. 3.7% (57 patients) treated with finasteride and 2.1% (32 patients) treated with placebo discontinued therapy as a result of adverse reactions related to sexual function, which are the most frequently reported adverse reactions.

The table below presents the only clinical adverse reactions considered possibly, probably or definitely drug related by the investigator, for which the incidence on finasteride was greater than or equal to 1% and greater than placebo over the 4 years of the study. In years 2 to 4 of the study, there was no significant difference between treatment groups in the incidences of impotence, decreased libido and ejaculation disorder, which are the most frequently reported adverse reactions.

Most Frequently Reported Drug-Related Finasteride Adverse Reactions

Adverse reaction	Year 1		Years 2, 3, and 4[a]	
	Finasteride	Placebo	Finasteride	Placebo
Breast enlargement	0.5%	0.1%	1.8%	1.1%
Breast tenderness	0.4%	0.1%	0.7%	0.3%
Decreased libido	6.4%	3.4%	2.6%	2.6%
Decreased volume of ejaculate	3.7%	0.8%	1.5%	0.5%
Ejaculation disorder	0.8%	0.1%	0.2%	0.1%
Impotence	8.1%	3.7%	5.1%	5.1%
Rash	0.5%	0.2%	0.5%	0.1%

[a] Combined years 2 to 4.N = 1,524 and 1,516, finasteride vs placebo, respectively.

Phase 3 studies and 5-year open extensions – The adverse experience profile in the 1-year, placebo-controlled, Phase 3 studies, the 5-year open extensions, and PLESS were similar.

Medical Therapy of Prostatic Symptoms (MTOPS) Study: The incidence rates of drug-related adverse experiences reported by greater than or equal to 2% of patients in any treatment group in the MTOPS Study are listed in the following table.

The individual adverse effects which occurred more frequently in the combination group compared to either drug alone were asthenia, postural hypotension, peripheral edema, dizziness, decreased libido, rhinitis, abnormal ejaculation, impotence, and abnormal sexual function (see table below). Of these, the incidence of abnormal ejaculation in patients receiving combination therapy was comparable to the sum of the incidences of this adverse experience reported for the 2 monotherapies.

Combination therapy with finasteride and doxazosin was associated with no new clinical adverse experience.

Four patients in MTOPS reported the adverse experience breast cancer. Three of these patients were on finasteride only and 1 was on combination therapy. (See the following table.)

Finasteride and Doxazosin Drug-Related Adverse Events in MTOPS (Incidence of ≥ 2% in 1 or More Treatment Groups)

Adverse experience	Placebo (n = 737) (%)	Doxazosin 4 mg or 8 mg (n = 756) (%)	Finasteride (n = 768) (%)	Combination (n = 786) (%)
Cardiovascular				
Hypotension	0.7%	3.4%	1.2%	1.5%
Postural hypotension	8%	16.7%	9.1%	17.8%
CNS				
Dizziness	8.1%	17.7%	7.4%	23.2%
Libido decreased	5.7%	7%	10%	11.6%
Somnolence	1.5%	3.7%	1.7%	3.1%
GU				
Abnormal ejaculation	2.3%	4.5%	7.2%	14.1%
Gynecomastia	0.7%	1.1%	2.2%	1.5%
Impotence	12.2%	14.4%	18.5%	22.6%
Abnormal sexual function	0.9%	2%	2.5%	3.1%
Metabolic/Nutritional				
Peripheral edema	0.9%	2.6%	1.3%	3.3%
Respiratory				
Dyspnea	0.7%	2.1%	0.7%	1.9%
Rhinitis	0.5%	1.3%	1%	2.4%
Miscellaneous				
Asthenia	7.1%	15.7%	5.3%	16.8%
Headache	2.3%	4.1%	2%	2.3%

The MTOPS Study was not specifically designed to make statistical comparisons between groups for reported adverse experiences. In addition, direct comparisons of safety data between the MTOPS study and previous studies of the single agents may not be appropriate based upon differences in patient population, dosage or dose regimen, and other procedural and study design elements.

Long-term data: There is no evidence of increased adverse experiences with increased duration of treatment with finasteride. New reports of drug-related sexual adverse experiences decreased with duration of therapy.

FINASTERIDE — ORAL

During the 4- to 6-year placebo- and comparator-controlled MTOPS study that enrolled 3,047 men, there were 4 cases of breast cancer in men treated with finasteride but no cases in men not treated with finasteride. During the 4-year, placebo-controlled PLESS study that enrolled 3,040 men, there were 2 cases of breast cancer in placebo-treated men, but no cases were reported in men treated with finasteride. The relationship between long-term use of finasteride and male breast neoplasia is currently unknown.

In a 7-year placebo-controlled trial that enrolled 18,882 healthy men, 9,060 had prostate needle biopsy data available for analysis. In the finasteride group, 280 (6.4%) men had prostate cancer with Gleason scores of 7 to 10 detected on needle biopsy vs 237 (5.1%) men in the placebo group. Of the total cases of prostate cancer diagnosed in this study, approximately 98% were classified as intracapsular (stage T1 or T2). The clinical significance of these findings is unknown.

Postmarketing experience – The following additional adverse reactions have been reported in postmarketing experience: Hypersensitivity reactions, including pruritus, urticaria, and swelling of the lips and face, and testicular pain.

Overdosage

In clinical studies, single doses of finasteride up to 400 mg and multiple doses of finasteride up to 80 mg/day for 3 months did not result in adverse reactions. Until further experience is obtained, no specific treatment for an overdose with finasteride can be recommended.

Significant lethality was observed in male and female mice at single oral doses of 1,500 mg/m^2 (500 mg/kg) and in female and male rats at single oral doses of 2,360 mg/m^2 (400 mg/kg) and 5,900 mg/m^2 (1,000 mg/kg), respectively.

Patient Information

Finasteride is for use by men only.

Women should not handle crushed or broken finasteride tablets when they are pregnant or may potentially be pregnant because of the possibility of absorption of finasteride and the subsequent potential risk to a male fetus. Finasteride tablets are coated and will prevent contact with the active ingredient during normal handling, provided that the tablets have not been broken or crushed. Impotence and decreased libido may occur in patients treated with finasteride.

Instruct patients to read the patient package insert before starting therapy with finasteride and to reread it each time the prescription is renewed so that they are aware of current information for patients regarding finasteride.

Instruct patients to promptly report any changes in their breasts such as lumps, pain, or nipple discharge. Breast changes including breast enlargement, tenderness, and neoplasm have been reported.

DUTASTERIDE

Rx	**Avodart** (GlaxoSmithKline)	**Capsule, softgel; oral:** 0.5 mg	Butylated hydroxytoluene. (GX CE2). Opaque yellow, oblong. In 30s and 90s.

DUTASTERIDE — ORAL

Indications

➤*Benign prostatic hyperplasia:*

Monotherapy – Symptomatic benign prostatic hyperplasia (BPH) in men with an enlarged prostate to improve symptoms, reduce the risk of acute urinary retention, and reduce the risk of the need for BPH-related surgery.

Combination therapy – Symptomatic BPH in men with an enlarged prostate in combination with the alpha-blocker tamsulosin.

➤*Off-label uses:*

Prostate cancer prevention – [1] = Good documentation. No widely established decision model has been developed to determine which men should receive chemoprevention with a 5-alpha reductase inhibitor, such as dutasteride. The role of dutasteride in the chemoprevention of prostate cancer was delineated in guidelines from the American Society of Clinical Oncology and the American Urological Association. The guideline authors recommend only that a discussion of benefits and risks of using 5-alpha reductase inhibitors for prevention of prostate cancer is warranted in men with a prostate-specific antigen (PSA) no greater than 3 who are regularly screened for PSA or are anticipating undergoing annual PSA screening for early detection of prostate cancer; they do not mandate that men in any subgroup be treated.

Administration and Dosage

➤*Adults:*

Benign prostatic hyperplasia –

Monotherapy: 0.5 mg orally once daily.

Combination therapy: Dutasteride 0.5 mg once daily and tamsulosin 0.4 mg once daily.

Off-label dosing –

Prostate cancer prevention: [1] = Good documentation. 0.5 mg orally once daily. Use of 5-alpha reductase inhibitors as primary prevention for prostate cancer has been evaluated for up to 7 years.

➤*Preparation for administration:* Dutasteride is a hormonal agent and is also considered a teratogen. Follow safe handling procedures when preparing, administering, or dispensing dutasteride.

Dutasteride is absorbed through the skin. Dutasteride should not be handled by women who are pregnant or who may become pregnant because of the potential for absorption of dutasteride and the subsequent potential risk to a developing male fetus. If contact is made with a leaking capsule, the contact area should be washed immediately with soap and water.

➤*Administration:* May administer with or without food. The capsules should be swallowed whole and not chewed or opened, because contact with the capsule contents may result in irritation of the oropharyngeal mucosa.

➤*Storage/Stability:* Store at 25°C (77°F); excursions are permitted between 15° and 30°C (59° and 86°F).

Actions

➤*Pharmacology:* Dutasteride is a synthetic 4-azasteroid compound that inhibits the conversion of testosterone to 5 alpha-dihydrotestosterone (DHT). DHT is the androgen primarily responsible for the initial development and subsequent enlargement of the prostate gland. Testosterone is converted to DHT by the enzyme 5 alpha-reductase, which exists as 2 isoforms, type 1 and type 2. The type 2 isoenzyme is primarily active in the reproductive tissues, while the type 1 isoenzyme is also responsible for testosterone conversion in the skin and liver.

Dutasteride is a competitive and specific inhibitor of both type 1 and type 2 5 alpha-reductase isoenzymes, with which it forms a stable enzyme complex. Dissociation from this complex has been evaluated under in vitro and in vivo conditions and is extremely slow.

Pharmacodynamics –

Effect on 5 alpha-DHT and testosterone: The maximum effect of daily doses of dutasteride on the reduction of DHT is dose dependent and is observed within 1 to 2 weeks. After 1 and 2 weeks of daily dosing with dutasteride 0.5 mg, median serum DHT concentrations were reduced 85% and 90%, respectively. In patients with BPH who were treated with dutasteride 0.5 mg/day for 4 years, the median decrease in serum DHT was 94% at 1 year, 93% at 2 years, and 95% at both 3 and 4 years. The median increase in serum testosterone was 19% at both 1 and 2 years, 26% at 3 years, and 22% at 4 years, but the mean and median levels remained within the physiologic range.

In patients with BPH treated with dutasteride 5 mg/day or placebo for up to 12 weeks prior to transurethral resection of the prostate, mean DHT concentrations in prostatic tissue were significantly lower in the dutasteride group compared with placebo (784 and 5,793 pg/g, respectively; $P < 0.001$). Mean prostatic tissue concentrations of testosterone were significantly higher in the dutasteride group compared with placebo (2,073 and 93 pg/g, respectively; $P < 0.001$).

Effects on other hormones: Statistically significant, baseline-adjusted mean increases compared with placebo were observed for total testosterone at 8 weeks (97.1 ng/dL; $P < 0.003$) and thyroid-stimulating hormone (TSH) at 52 weeks (0.4 microunits/mL; $P < 0.05$). The median percentage changes from baseline within the dutasteride group were 17.9% for testosterone at 8 weeks and 12.4% for TSH at 52 weeks. After stopping dutasteride for 24 weeks, the mean levels of testosterone and TSH had returned to baseline in the group of subjects with available data at the visit. In patients with BPH treated with dutasteride in a large, randomized, double-blind, placebo-controlled study, there was a median percent increase in luteinizing hormone of 12% at 6 months and 19% at both 12 and 24 months.

➤*Pharmacokinetics:*

Absorption – Following administration of a single 0.5 mg dose, time to peak serum concentrations of dutasteride occurs within 2 to 3 hours. Absolute bioavailability in 5 healthy subjects is approximately 60% (range, 40% to 94%).

The average steady-state serum dutasteride concentration was 40 ng/mL following 0.5 mg/day for 1 year. Following daily dosing, dutasteride serum concentrations achieve 65% of steady-state concentration after 1 month and approximately 90% after 3 months.

Distribution – Pharmacokinetic data following single and repeat oral doses show that dutasteride has a large volume of distribution (300 to 500 L). Dutasteride is highly bound to plasma albumin (99%) and alpha-1 acid glycoprotein (96.6%).

In a study of healthy subjects (N = 26) receiving dutasteride 0.5 mg/day for 12 months, semen dutasteride concentrations averaged 3.4 ng/mL (range, 0.4 to 14 ng/mL) at 12 months and, similar to serum, achieved steady-state concentrations at 6 months. On average, at 12 months, 11.5% of serum dutasteride concentrations partitioned into semen.

Metabolism – Dutasteride is extensively metabolized in humans. In vitro studies showed that dutasteride is metabolized by the CYP3A4 and CYP3A5 isoenzymes. Both of these isoenzymes produced the 4′-hydroxydutasteride, 6-hydroxydutasteride, and 6,4′-dihydroxydutasteride metabolites. In addition, the 15-hydroxydutasteride metabolite was formed by CYP3A4.

In human serum, following dosing to steady state, unchanged dutasteride, 3 major metabolites (4′-hydroxydutasteride, 1,2-dihydrodutasteride, and

DUTASTERIDE — ORAL

6-hydroxydutasteride), and 2 minor metabolites (6,4′-dihydroxydutasteride and 15-hydroxydutasteride), as assessed by mass spectrometric response, have been detected. The absolute stereochemistry of the hydroxyl additions in the 6 and 15 positions is not known. In vitro, 4′-hydroxydutasteride and 1, 2-dihydrodutasteride metabolites are much less potent than dutasteride against both isoforms of human 5 alpha-reductase. The activity of 6 beta-hydroxydutasteride is comparable with that of dutasteride.

Excretion – Dutasteride and its metabolites were excreted mainly in the feces. As a percent of dose, there was approximately 5% unchanged dutasteride (approximately 1% to 15%) and 40% as dutasteride-related metabolites (approximately 2% to 90%). Only trace amounts of unchanged dutasteride were found in the urine (less than 1%). Therefore, on average, the dose unaccounted for approximated 55% (range, 5% to 97%).

The terminal elimination half-life of dutasteride is approximately 5 weeks at steady state. Because of the long half-life of dutasteride, serum concentrations remain detectable (more than 0.1 ng/mL) for up to 4 to 6 months after discontinuation of treatment.

Special populations –

Hepatic function impairment: See Warnings/Precautions for more information.

Gender: Dutasteride is contraindicated in pregnancy and women of childbearing potential and is not indicated for use in other women. The pharmacokinetics of dutasteride in women have not been studied.

Contraindications

Pregnancy; women of childbearing potential; children; patients with previously demonstrated, clinically significant hypersensitivity (eg, serious skin reactions, angioedema) to dutasteride or other 5 alpha-reductase inhibitors.

Warnings/Precautions

➤*Exposure of women/risk to male fetus:* Dutasteride should not be handled by a woman who is pregnant or who may become pregnant. Dutasteride is absorbed through the skin and could result in unintended fetal exposure. If a woman who is pregnant or who may become pregnant comes in contact with leaking capsules, wash the contact area immediately with soap and water.

➤*Other urological diseases:* Lower urinary tract symptoms of BPH can be indicative of other urological diseases, including prostate cancer. Assess patients to rule out prostate cancer and other urological diseases prior to treatment with dutasteride and periodically thereafter. Patients with a large residual urinary volume and/or severely diminished urinary flow many not be good candidates for 5 alpha-reductase inhibitor therapy; monitor carefully for obstructive uropathy.

➤*Prostate effects:* Dutasteride reduces total serum PSA concentration by approximately 40% following 3 months of treatment and by 50% following 6, 12, and 24 months of treatment. This decrease is predictable over the entire range of PSA values, although it may vary in individual patients. Therefore, for interpretation of serial PSAs in a man taking dutasteride, establish a new baseline PSA concentration after 3 to 6 months of treatment and use this new value to assess potentially cancer-related changes in PSA. To interpret an isolated PSA value in a man treated with dutasteride for 6 months or more, double the PSA value for comparison with normal values in untreated men. Any confirmed increases in PSA levels from nadir while on dutasteride may signal the presence of prostate cancer; carefully evaluate, even if those values are still within the normal range for men not taking a 5 alpha-reductase inhibitor.

The free-to-total PSA ratio (percent free PSA) remains constant at month 12, even under the influence of dutasteride. If health care providers elect to use percent free PSA as an aid in the detection of prostate cancer in men receiving dutasteride, no adjustment to its value appears necessary.

Coadministration of tamsulosin with dutasteride resulted in similar changes to total PSA as dutasteride monotherapy.

➤*Blood donation:* Men being treated with dutasteride should not donate blood until at least 6 months have passed following their last dose. The purpose of this deferred period is to prevent administration of dutasteride to a pregnant female transfusion recipient.

➤*Reproductive effects:* The effects of dutasteride 0.5 mg/day on semen characteristics were evaluated in healthy volunteers 18 to 52 years of age (dutasteride, n = 27; placebo, n = 23) throughout 52 weeks of treatment and 24 weeks of posttreatment follow-up. At 52 weeks, the mean percent reduction from baseline in total sperm count, semen volume, and sperm motility were 23%, 26%, and 18%, respectively, in the dutasteride group when adjusted for changes from baseline in the placebo group. Sperm concentration and sperm morphology were unaffected. After 24 weeks of follow-up, the mean percent change in total sperm count in the dutasteride group remained 23% lower than baseline. While mean values for all semen parameters at all time points remained within the normal ranges and did not meet predefined criteria for a clinically significant change (30%), 2 subjects in the dutasteride group had decreases in sperm count of more than 90% from baseline at 52 weeks, with partial recovery at the 24-week follow-up. The clinical significance of dutasteride's effect on semen characteristics for an individual patient's fertility is not known.

➤*Hepatic function impairment:* The effect of hepatic impairment on dutasteride pharmacokinetics has not been studied. Because dutasteride is extensively metabolized, exposure could be higher in hepatically impaired patients. However, in a clinical study in which 60 subjects received 5 mg (10 times the therapeutic dose) daily for 24 weeks, no additional adverse reactions were observed compared with those observed at the therapeutic dose of 0.5 mg.

➤*Pregnancy: Category X.* Dutasteride is contraindicated for use in women of childbearing potential and during pregnancy. Dutasteride is a 5 alpha-reductase inhibitor that prevents conversion of testosterone to DHT, a hormone necessary for normal development of male genitalia. In animal reproduction and developmental toxicity studies, dutasteride inhibited normal development of external genitalia in male fetuses. Therefore, dutasteride may cause fetal harm when administered to a pregnant woman. If dutasteride is used during pregnancy or if the patient becomes pregnant while taking dutasteride, apprise the patient of the potential hazard to the fetus.

Abnormalities in the genitalia of male fetuses are an expected physiological consequence of inhibition of the conversion of testosterone to 5 alpha-DHT by 5 alpha-reductase inhibitors. These results are similar to observations in male infants with genetic 5 alpha-reductase deficiency. Dutasteride is absorbed through the skin. To avoid potential fetal exposure, instruct women who are pregnant or may become pregnant not to handle dutasteride capsules. If contact is made with leaking capsules, wash the contact area immediately with soap and water. Dutasteride is secreted into male semen. The highest measured semen concentration of dutasteride in treated men was 14 ng/mL. Assuming exposure of a 50 kg woman to 5 mL of semen and 100% absorption, the woman's dutasteride concentration would be approximately 0.175 ng/mL. This concentration is more than 100 times less than concentrations producing abnormalities of male genitalia in animal studies. Dutasteride is highly protein bound in human semen (more than 96%), which may reduce the amount of dutasteride available for vaginal absorption.

In an IV embryofetal development study in the rhesus monkey (12 per group), administration of dutasteride at 400, 780, 1,325, or 2,010 ng/day on gestation days 20 to 100 did not adversely affect development of male external genitalia.

Reduction of fetal adrenal weights, reduction in fetal prostate weights, and increases in fetal ovarian and testis weights were observed in monkeys treated with the highest dose. Based on the highest measured semen concentration of dutasteride in treated men (14 ng/mL), these doses represent 0.8 to 16 times, based on blood levels of parent drug (32 to 186 times based on an ng/kg daily dose), the potential maximum exposure of a 50 kg woman to 5 mL of semen daily from a dutasteride-treated man, assuming 100% absorption.

In an embryofetal development study in female rats, oral administration of dutasteride at dosages of 0.05, 2.5, 12.5, and 30 mg/kg/day resulted in feminization of male fetuses (decreased anogenital distance) and male offspring (nipple development, hypospadias, and distended preputial glands) at all doses (0.07- to 111-fold the expected male clinical exposure). An increase in stillborn pups was observed at 30 mg/kg/day (111 times the maximum recommended human dose), and reduced fetal body weight was observed at doses of 2.5 mg/kg/day or more (15- to 111-fold the expected clinical exposure). Increased incidences of skeletal variations considered to be delays in ossification associated with reduced body weight were observed at dosages of 12.5 and 30 mg/kg/day (56- to 111-fold the expected clinical exposure).

In an oral pre- and postnatal development study in rats, dutasteride doses of 0.05, 2.5, 12.5, or 30 mg/kg/day were administered. Unequivocal evidence of feminization of the genitalia (ie, decreased anogenital distance, increased incidence of hypospadias, nipple development) of F1 generation male offspring occurred at doses of 2.5 mg/kg/day or more (14- to 90-fold the expected clinical exposure in men). At a daily dosage of 0.05 mg/kg/day (0.05-fold the expected clinical exposure), evidence of feminization was limited to a small but statistically significant decrease in anogenital distance. Dosages of 2.5 to 30 mg/kg/day resulted in prolonged gestation in the parental females and a decrease in time to vaginal patency for female offspring and decreased prostate and seminal vesicle weights in male offspring. Effects on newborn startle response were noted at dosages of 12.5 mg/kg/day or more. Increased stillbirths were noted at 30 mg/kg/day.

In the rabbit embryofetal study, doses of 30, 100, and 200 mg/kg (28- to 93-fold the expected clinical exposure in men) were administered orally on days 7 to 29 of pregnancy to encompass the late period of external genitalia development. Histological evaluation of the genital papilla of fetuses revealed evidence of feminization of the male fetus at all doses. A second embryofetal study in rabbits at doses of 0.05, 0.4, 3, and 30 mg/kg/day (0.3- to 53-fold the expected clinical exposure) also produced evidence of feminization of the genitalia in male fetuses at all doses. It is not known whether rabbits or rhesus monkeys produce any of the major human metabolites.

➤*Lactation:* Do not use dutasteride in breast-feeding women. It is not known whether dutasteride is excreted in human milk.

➤*Children:* Dutasteride is contraindicated for use in children. Safety and effectiveness in children have not been established.

➤*Monitoring:* Assess patients to rule out other urological diseases prior to treatment with dutasteride and periodically thereafter. Carefully monitor patients with a large residual urinary volume and/or severely diminished urinary flow.

Perform digital rectal examinations, as well as other evaluations for prostate cancer, on patients with BPH prior to initiating therapy with dutasteride and periodically thereafter.

Establish a new baseline PSA concentration after 3 to 6 months of treatment, and use this new value to assess potentially cancer-related changes in PSA. To interpret an isolated PSA value in a man treated with dutasteride for 6 months or more, double the PSA value for comparison with normal values in untreated men.

DUTASTERIDE — ORAL

Drug Interactions

Dutasteride Drug Interactions			
Precipitant drug	Object drug[a]		Description
Calcium channel antagonists (eg, diltiazem, verapamil)	Dutasteride	↑	A decrease in the clearance of dutasteride was noted when coadministered with CYP3A4 inhibitors verapamil and diltiazem. The change in dutasteride exposure was not considered clinically important. No dosage adjustment is recommended.
CYP3A4 inhibitors (eg, cimetidine, ciprofloxacin, ketoconazole, ritonavir, troleandomycin)	Dutasteride	↑	Blood concentrations of dutasteride may increase in the presence of potent, long-term CYP3A inhibitors. Coadminister with caution.
Tamsulosin	Dutasteride	↑	With treatment over a 2-year period, drug-related ejaculation disorders occurred in 9% of subjects receiving dutasteride and tamsulosin combination therapy compared with 2% or 3% with dutasteride or tamsulosin monotherapy, respectively. However, dutasteride combination therapy with tamsulosin is indicated for the treatment of symptomatic benign prostatic hyperplasia.

[a] ↑ = object drug increased.

➤*Drug/Lab test interactions:* Dutasteride reduces total serum PSA concentrations. The decrease is predictable over the entire range of PSA values, although it may vary in individual patients. Therefore, for interpretation of serial PSA values in a man taking dutasteride, establish a new baseline PSA concentration after 3 to 6 months of treatment. Use this new value to assess potentially cancer-related PSA changes.

➤*Drug/Food interactions:* When dutasteride is taken with food, the dutasteride maximum drug concentration is reduced 10% to 15%. This reduction is not considered to be clinically important. Dutasteride may be taken with or without food.

Adverse Reactions

➤*Monotherapy:*

Most common adverse reactions – The most common adverse reactions reported in subjects receiving dutasteride were impotence, decreased libido, breast disorders (including breast enlargement and tenderness), and ejaculation disorders.

Discontinuation – Study withdrawal because of adverse reactions occurred in 4% of subjects receiving dutasteride and 3% of subjects receiving placebo. The most common adverse reaction leading to study withdrawal was impotence (1%).

Adverse reactions (1% or more) –

Dutasteride Adverse Reactions (≥ 1%)				
	Adverse reaction time of onset			
Reproductive adverse reactions	Months 0 to 6 Dutasteride (n = 2,167); Placebo (n = 2,158)	Months 7 to 12 Dutasteride (n = 1,901); Placebo (n = 1,922)	Months 13 to 18 Dutasteride (n = 1,725); Placebo (n = 1,714)	Months 19 to 24 Dutasteride (n = 1,605); Placebo (n =1,555)
Impotence				
Dutasteride	4.7%	1.4%	1%	0.8%
Placebo	1.7%	1.5%	0.5%	0.9%
Decreased libido				
Dutasteride	3%	0.7%	0.3%	0.3%
Placebo	1.4%	0.6%	0.2%	0.1%
Ejaculation disorder				
Dutasteride	1.4%	0.5%	0.5%	0.1%
Placebo	0.5%	0.3%	0.1%	0%
Breast disorders[a]				
Dutasteride	0.5%	0.8%	1.1%	0.6%
Placebo	0.2%	0.3%	0.3%	0.1%

[a] Includes breast tenderness and breast enlargement.

➤*Combination with alpha-blocker therapy (CombAT):*

Most common adverse reactions – The most common adverse reactions reported in subjects receiving combination therapy (dutasteride plus tamsulosin) were breast disorders (including breast enlargement and tenderness), decreased libido, dizziness, ejaculation disorders, and impotence. Over 2 years of treatment, drug-related ejaculation disorder occurred more frequently in subjects receiving combination therapy (9%) compared with dutasteride (2%) or tamsulosin (3%) as monotherapy.

Discontinuation – Study withdrawal because of adverse reactions occurred in 5% of subjects receiving combination therapy (dutasteride plus tamsulosin) and 3% of subjects receiving dutasteride or tamsulosin as monotherapy. The most common adverse reaction leading to study withdrawal in subjects receiving combination therapy was impotence (1%).

Adverse reactions (1% or more) –

Dutasteride Combined With Tamsulosin Adverse Reactions (≥ 1%)				
	Adverse reaction time of onset			
Reproductive adverse reactions	Months 0 to 6 Combination[a] (n = 1,610) Dutasteride (n = 1,623) Tamsulosin (n = 1,611)	Months 7 to 12 Combination[a] (n = 1,524) Dutasteride (n = 1,547) Tamsulosin (n = 1,542)	Months 13 to 18 Combination[a] (n = 1,424) Dutasteride (n = 1,457) Tamsulosin (n = 1,468)	Months 19 to 24 Combination[a] (n = 1,345) Dutasteride (n = 1,378) Tamsulosin (n = 1,363)
Impotence				
Combination[a]	5.5%	1.2%	0.8%	0.3%
Dutasteride	3.9%	1.2%	0.6%	0.7%
Tamsulosin	2.7%	0.8%	0.4%	0.4%
Decreased libido				
Combination[a]	4.5%	0.9%	0.4%	< 0.1%
Dutasteride	3.3%	0.6%	0.7%	0.2%
Tamsulosin	1.9%	0.6%	0.4%	0.2%
Ejaculation disorders				
Combination[a]	7.6%	1.6%	0.4%	< 0.1%
Dutasteride	1.1%	0.6%	0.1%	0.1%
Tamsulosin	2.2%	0.5%	0.4%	0.1%
Breast disorders[b]				
Combination[a]	1%	1.1%	0.7%	0.3%
Dutasteride	0.9%	1%	0.8%	0.5%
Tamsulosin	0.4%	0.4%	0.2%	0.1%
Dizziness				
Combination[a]	1.1%	0.4%	0.2%	0%
Dutasteride	0.4%	0.2%	< 0.1%	< 0.1%
Tamsulosin	0.9%	0.5%	0.3%	0.1%

[a] Combination = dutasteride 0.5 mg once daily plus tamsulosin 0.4 mg once daily.
[b] Includes breast tenderness and breast enlargement.

Cardiac failure – In CombAT, after 4 years of treatment, the incidence of the composite term cardiac failure in the combination therapy group (0.7%) was higher than in either monotherapy group: dutasteride, 0.1% and tamsulosin, 0.6%. Composite cardiac failure was also examined in a separate 4-year, placebo-controlled trial evaluating dutasteride in men at risk of development of prostate cancer. The incidence of cardiac failure in subjects taking dutasteride was 0.6% compared with 0.4% in subjects on placebo. A majority of subjects with cardiac failure in both studies had comorbidities associated with an increased risk of cardiac failure. Therefore, the clinical significance of the numerical imbalances in cardiac failure is unknown. No causal relationship between dutasteride, alone or in combination with tamsulosin, and cardiac failure has been established. No imbalance was observed in the incidence of overall cardiovascular adverse reactions in either study.

➤*Postmarketing:*

Hypersensitivity – Hypersensitivity reactions, including angioedema, localized edema, pruritus, rash, serious skin reactions, and urticaria.

Overdosage

➤*Symptoms:* In volunteer studies, single doses of dutasteride of up to 40 mg (80 times the therapeutic dose) for 7 days have been administered without significant safety concerns. In a clinical study, daily doses of 5 mg (10 times the therapeutic dose) were administered to 60 subjects for 6 months with no additional adverse reactions to those seen at therapeutic doses of 0.5 mg.

➤*Treatment:* There is no specific antidote for dutasteride. Therefore, in cases of suspected overdosage, give symptomatic and supportive treatment as appropriate, taking the long half-life of dutasteride into consideration.

Patient Information

Inform patients that dutasteride capsules should not be handled by a woman who is pregnant or who may become pregnant because of the potential for absorption of dutasteride and the subsequent potential risk to a developing male fetus. Dutasteride is absorbed through the skin and could result in unintended fetal exposure. If a pregnant woman or woman of child-

Androgen Hormone Inhibitor

DUTASTERIDE — ORAL

bearing potential comes in contact with leaking dutasteride capsules, wash the contact area immediately with soap and water.

Inform men treated with dutasteride to not donate blood until at least 6 months following their last dose to prevent pregnant women from receiving dutasteride through blood transfusion. Serum levels of dutasteride are detectable for 4 to 6 months after treatment ends.

BENIGN PROSTATIC HYPERPLASIA (BPH) COMBINATIONS

Rx	**Jalyn** (GlaxoSmithKline)	**Capsules; oral:** dutasteride 0.5 mg/tamsulosin hydrochloride 0.4 mg	Glycerin. (GS 7CZ). Brown and orange. In 30s and 90s.

DUTASTERIDE/TAMSULOSIN HYDROCHLORIDE — ORAL

For complete and comparative prescribing information, refer to the dutasteride monograph and Alpha-1-Adrenergic Blockers class monograph.

Indications

➤*Benign prostatic hyperplasia:* For the treatment of symptomatic benign prostatic hyperplasia in men with an enlarged prostate.

Administration and Dosage

➤*Adults:*

Benign prostatic hyperplasia –

Usual dosage: 1 capsule once daily approximately 30 minutes after the same meal each day.

Concomitant therapy: Dutasteride/tamsulosin should not be used in combination with strong inhibitors of CYP3A4 (eg, ketoconazole).

➤*Administration:* The capsules should be swallowed whole and not chewed or opened. Contact with the contents of the capsule may result in irritation of the oropharyngeal mucosa.

Safe handling – Dutasteride is absorbed through the skin. Capsules should not be handled by women who are pregnant or who may become pregnant because of the potential for absorption of dutasteride and the subsequent potential risk to a developing male fetus.

➤*Storage/Stability:* Store at 25°C (77°F); excursions are permitted to 15° to 30°C (59° to 86°F). Capsules may become deformed and/or discolored if kept at high temperatures.

Anabolic Steroids

Effective February 27, 1991, these agents were switched to a ***c-iii*** status by the Drug Enforcement Administration (DEA) because of their abuse potential.

WARNING

Peliosis hepatis – Peliosis hepatis, a condition in which liver and, sometimes, splenic tissue is replaced with blood-filled cysts, has occurred in patients receiving androgenic anabolic steroids. These cysts are sometimes present with minimal hepatic dysfunction and have been associated with liver failure. Often, they are not recognized until life-threatening liver failure or intra-abdominal hemorrhage develops. Withdrawal of drug usually results in complete disappearance of lesions.

Liver cell tumors – Most often these tumors are benign and androgen-dependent, but fatal malignant tumors have occurred. Withdrawal of drug often results in regression or cessation of tumor progression. However, hepatic tumors associated with androgens or anabolic steroids are much more vascular than other hepatic tumors and may be silent until life-threatening, intra-abdominal hemorrhage develops.

Blood lipid changes – Blood lipid changes associated with increased risk of atherosclerosis are seen in patients treated with androgens and anabolic steroids. These changes include decreased high-density lipoprotein (HDL) and, sometimes, increased low-density lipoprotein (LDL). The changes may be very marked and could have a serious impact on the risk of atherosclerosis and coronary artery disease (CAD).

Indications

➤*Anemia (oxymetholone only):* For the treatment of anemias caused by deficient red cell production; acquired or congenital aplastic anemias, myelofibrosis, and/or hypoplastic anemias caused by the administration of myelotoxic drugs often respond.

➤*Anemia of renal insufficiency (nandrolone only):* For the management of the anemia of renal insufficiency. This drug increases hemoglobin and red cell mass. Surgically induced anephric patients have been reported to be less responsive.

➤*Bone pain (oxandrolone only):* For the relief of bone pain frequently accompanying osteoporosis.

➤*Protein catabolism (oxandrolone only):* To offset the protein catabolism associated with prolonged administration of corticosteroids.

➤*Weight gain (oxandrolone only):* Adjunctive therapy to promote weight gain after weight loss following extensive surgery, chronic infections, or severe trauma, and in some patients who, without definite pathophysiologic reasons, fail to gain or maintain normal weight.

➤*Off-label uses:*

Nandrolone and oxymetholone – HIV-associated wasting.

Oxandrolone – Catabolic illnesses, such as alcoholic liver disease and burn injury. The following have been designated orphan drug status: short stature associated with Turner syndrome, HIV-associated wasting, constitutional delay of growth and puberty; moderate/severe acute alcoholic hepatitis in the presence of moderate protein calorie malnutrition, Duchenne and Becker muscular dystrophy.

Actions

➤*Pharmacology:* Anabolic steroids are synthetic derivatives of testosterone. Certain clinical effects and adverse reactions demonstrate the androgenic properties of this class of drugs. Complete dissociation of anabolic and androgenic effects has not been achieved. Therefore, the actions of anabolic steroids are similar to those of male sex hormones, with the possibility of causing serious disturbances of growth and sexual development if given to young children. Anabolic steroids suppress the gonadotropic functions of the pituitary gland and may exert a direct effect upon the testis.

During exogenous administration of anabolic androgens, endogenous testosterone release is inhibited through inhibition of pituitary luteinizing hormone (LH). At large doses, spermatogenesis may be suppressed through feedback inhibition of pituitary follicle-stimulating hormone (FSH).

Anabolic steroids have been reported to increase LDL and decrease HDL. These changes revert to normal on discontinuation of treatment.

Nitrogen balance is improved with anabolic agents but only when there is sufficient intake of calories and protein. Whether this positive nitrogen balance is of primary benefit in the utilization of protein-building dietary substances has not been established. **Oxymetholone** enhances the production and urinary excretion of erythropoietin in patients with anemias caused by bone marrow failure and often stimulates erythropoiesis in anemias caused by deficient red cell production.

➤*Pharmacokinetics:* The pharmacokinetics of **nandrolone** (given as single 50 to 150 mg intramuscular [IM] doses) were studied in healthy young men. The mean T_{max} was found to be 2 to 3 days after injection, and the C_{max} ranged from 2.14 ng/mL (50 mg group) to 5.16 ng/mL (150 mg group). The mean elimination half-life was 7.1 days, 11.7 days, and 11.8 days for the 50 mg, 100 mg, and 150 mg groups, respectively. Nandrolone is metabolized to 2 metabolites that can be detected in the urine.

After oral administration, **oxandrolone** is well absorbed, with T_{max} occurring in approximately 1 hour, and approximately 95% is protein bound. Oxandrolone is relatively resistant to metabolism by the liver, and approximately 28% is excreted unchanged in the urine. Plasma levels decline in a biphasic manner; the distribution half-life is approximately 30 minutes, and the elimination half-life is approximately 9 hours.

Based on the structurally similar testosterone, it is assumed that **oxymetholone** is absorbed completely after oral administration. Oxymetholone undergoes both phase I and phase II metabolism. Along with other various metabolites, approximately 5% of oxymetholone has been recovered in the urine as glucuronic acid conjugates.

Contraindications

Known or suspected carcinoma of the prostate or breast in men; carcinoma of the breast in women with hypercalcemia (androgenic anabolic steroids may stimulate osteolytic resorption of bones); pregnancy (see Warnings); nephrosis or the nephrotic phase of nephritis; hypersensitivity to any component of the product; hypercalcemia (**oxandrolone** only); severe hepatic dysfunction (**oxymetholone** only).

Warnings/Precautions

➤*Peliosis hepatis:* Peliosis hepatis, a condition in which liver and sometimes splenic tissue is replaced with blood-filled cysts, has occurred in patients receiving androgenic anabolic steroids. These cysts are sometimes present with minimal hepatic dysfunction and have been associated with liver failure. Often, they are not recognized until life-threatening liver failure or intra-abdominal hemorrhage develops. Withdrawal of drug usually results in complete disappearance of lesions.

➤*Hepatitis:* Cholestatic hepatitis and jaundice occur with 17-alpha-alkylated androgens at relatively low doses. Clinical jaundice may be painless, with or without pruritus. It also may be associated with acute hepatic enlargement and right upper quadrant pain, which has been mistaken for acute (surgical) obstruction of the bile duct. If cholestatic hepatitis with jaundice appears or if liver function tests become abnormal, discontinue drug therapy and determine the etiology. Drug-induced jaundice is usually reversible when the medication is discontinued. Continued therapy has been associated with hepatic coma and death. Because of the hepatoxicity associated with drug administration, periodic liver function tests are recommended.

➤*Liver cell tumors:* See the Warning box for more information.

➤*Blood lipid changes:* Blood lipid changes associated with increased risk of atherosclerosis are seen in patients treated with androgens and anabolic steroids. These changes include decreased HDL and, sometimes, increased LDL. The changes may be very marked and could have a serious impact on the risk of atherosclerosis and CAD.

➤*Hypercalcemia:* In patients with breast cancer, anabolic steroids may cause hypercalcemia by stimulating osteolysis. Hypercalcemia may develop spontaneously and as a result of androgen therapy in women with disseminated breast carcinoma. Discontinue therapy if hypercalcemia occurs.

➤*Edema:* Edema, with or without congestive heart failure, may be a serious complication in patients with preexisting cardiac, renal, or hepatic disease. Coadministration with adrenal steroids or corticotropin may increase the edema. This is generally controllable with appropriate diuretics and/or digitalis therapy.

➤*Athletic performance:* Anabolic steroids have not been shown to be safe and effective for the enhancement of athletic ability. Because of the potential risk of serious adverse health effects, do not use this drug for such purpose.

➤*Virilization:* Observe women for signs of virilization (deepening of the voice, hirsutism, acne, and clitoromegaly). To prevent irreversible change, drug therapy must be discontinued when mild virilism is first detected. Virilization is usual following androgenic anabolic steroid use at high doses. Some virilizing changes in women are irreversible, even after prompt discontinuance of therapy, and are not prevented by coadministration of estrogens. Menstrual irregularities, including amenorrhea, also may occur.

➤*Leukemia:* Leukemia has been observed in patients with aplastic anemia treated with **oxymetholone**. The role, if any, of oxymetholone is unclear because malignant transformation has been seen in patients with blood dyscrasias, and leukemia has been reported in patients with aplastic anemia who have not been treated with oxymetholone.

➤*Benzyl alcohol:* Benzyl alcohol has been associated with a fatal "gasping syndrome" in premature infants. Refer to product listings.

➤*Special risk:* Because serum cholesterol may increase during therapy, use caution when administering these agents to patients with a history of myocardial infarction or CAD.

The insulin or oral hypoglycemic dosage may need to be adjusted in diabetic patients who receive anabolic steroids. Anabolic steroids have been shown to alter fasting blood sugar and glucose tolerance tests.

➤*Drug abuse and dependence:* Anabolic steroids are classified as a schedule III controlled substance under the Anabolic Steroids Control Act of 1990.

➤*Pregnancy: Category X.* Because of possible masculinization of the fetus, the use of anabolic steroids is contraindicated in pregnancy. **Oxandrolone** has been shown to cause embryotoxicity, fetotoxicity, infertility, and masculinization of the female animal offspring when given in doses 9 times the human dose. **Oxymetholone** can cause fetal harm when administered to pregnant women. It is contraindicated in women who are or may become pregnant. If a patient becomes pregnant while taking the drug, apprise her of the potential hazard to the fetus.

Fertility impairment – Oligospermia in men and amenorrhea in women are potential adverse effects of treatment with **oxymetholone**.

➤*Lactation:* It is not known whether anabolic steroids are excreted in human milk. Because of the potential for serious adverse reactions in breast-feeding infants, decide whether to discontinue breast-feeding or to discontinue the drug, taking into account the importance of the drug to the mother. Women who take **oxymetholone** should stop breast-feeding.

➤*Children:* Anabolic steroids may accelerate epiphyseal maturation more rapidly than linear growth in children, and the effect may continue for 6 months after the drug has been stopped. The younger the child the greater the risk of compromising final mature height. Therefore, monitor therapy by x-ray studies (eg, left wrist and hand) at 6-month intervals in order to avoid the risk of compromising the adult height. Use anabolic/androgenic steroids very cautiously in children and only by specialists who are aware of their effects on bone maturation. The safety and efficacy of **nandrolone** in children with metastatic breast cancer (rarely found) has not been established.

➤*Elderly:* Elderly men treated with androgenic anabolic steroids may be at an increased risk for the development of prostate hypertrophy and prostatic carcinoma. In general, exercise caution in dose selection for an elderly patient, usually starting at the low end of the dosing range, reflecting the greater frequency of decreased hepatic, renal, or cardiac function, and concomitant disease or other drug therapy.

➤*Lab test abnormalities:* Anabolic steroids may cause suppression of clotting factors II, V, VII, and X and an increase in prothrombin time.

Oxymetholone has been shown to decrease 17-ketosteroid excretion (see Adverse Reactions).

➤*Monitoring:* Because of the hepatotoxicity associated with the use of 17-alpha-alkylated anabolic steroids, obtain liver function tests periodically.

Periodically determine serum lipids and HDL-cholesterol.

Periodically check hemoglobin and hematocrit for polycythemia in patients who are receiving high doses of anabolic steroids. Because iron deficiency anemia has been observed in some patients treated with **oxymetholone**, periodic determination of the serum iron and iron binding capacity is recommended. If iron deficiency anemia is detected, treat appropriately with supplementary iron.

Women – Women with disseminated breast carcinoma should have frequent determination of urine and serum calcium levels during the course of therapy.

Children – Perform periodic (every 6 months) x-ray examinations of bone age during treatment of prepubertal patients to determine the rate of bone maturation and the effects of androgenic anabolic steroid therapy on the epiphyseal centers.

Drug Interactions

Anabolic Steroids Drug Interactions

Precipitant drug	Object drug[a]		Description
Anabolic steroids	Anticoagulants, oral	↑	The anticoagulant effects may be potentiated by anabolic steroids. Unexpected large increases in the international normalized ratio (INR) or the prothrombin time (PT) may occur. Monitor closely and adjust anticoagulant dose as needed.
Anabolic steroids — Oxandrolone	Hypoglycemic agents, oral	↑	Oxandrolone may inhibit the metabolism of oral hypoglycemic agents.

[a] ↑ = Object drug increased.

➤*Drug/Lab test interactions:* Anabolic steroids may decrease levels of thyroxine-binding globulin, resulting in decreased total T_4 serum levels and increased resin uptake of T_3 and T_4. Free thyroid hormone levels remain unchanged. Altered tests usually persist for 2 to 3 weeks after stopping anabolic steroid therapy. In addition, a decrease in protein-bound iodine (PBI) and radioactive iodine uptake may occur.

Anabolic steroids have been shown to alter fasting blood sugar and glucose tolerance tests.

Adverse Reactions

Anabolic Steroids Adverse Reactions

Adverse reactions	Nandrolone	Oxandrolone	Oxymetholone
CNS			
Depression	X[a]	X	
Excitation	X	X	X
Habituation	X	X	
Insomnia	X	X	X
Dermatologic			
Acne	X	X	X
Hirsutism/male-pattern baldness (women)	X	X	X
Male-pattern hair loss (postpubertal men)			X
GI			
Diarrhea	X		X
Nausea	X		X
Vomiting	X		X
GU			
Gynecomastia	X	X	X
Increased or decreased libido	X	X	X
Men (prepubertal):			
Increased frequency of erections	X	X	X
Phallic enlargement	X	X	X
Men (postpubertal):			
Bladder irritability	X	X	X
Chronic priapism	X	X	X
Decreased seminal volume			X
Epididymitis	X	X	X
Impotence	X	X	X
Inhibition of testicular function	X	X	X
Oligospermia	X	X	X
Testicular atrophy	X	X	X
Women:			
Clitoral enlargement	X	X	X
Menstrual irregularities	X	X	X
Hematologic			
Iron-deficiency anemia			X
Leukemia[b]			X
Hepatic			
Cholestatic jaundice with, rarely, hepatic necrosis and death[b]		X	X
Hepatocellular neoplasms[c]	X	X	X
Peliosis hepatis[c]	X	X	X
Metabolic			
Decreased glucose tolerance	X	X	X
Edema	X	X	X
Retention of serum electrolytes (ie, sodium, chloride, potassium, phosphate, calcium)	X	X	X
Musculoskeletal			
Muscle cramp			X
Premature closure of epiphyses in children[c]	X	X	X

Anabolic Steroids Adverse Reactions			
Adverse reactions	Nandrolone	Oxandrolone	Oxymetholone
Miscellaneous			
Chills			X
Deepening of the voice (women)	X	X	X
Inhibition of gonadotropin secretion		X	

[a] X = incidence not reported.
[b] See Precautions.
[c] See Warnings.

➤*Lab test abnormalities:* Reversible changes in liver function tests, including increased bromsulfophthalein retention and increases in serum bilirubin, AST, and alkaline phosphatase (see Precautions).

Increased serum levels of LDL and decreased HDL, increased creatine and creatinine excretion, and increased serum levels of creatinine phosphokinase.

Overdosage

➤*Symptoms:* No symptoms or signs associated with overdosage have been reported. It is possible that sodium and water retention may occur. The oral LD_{50} of **oxandrolone** in mice and dogs is greater than 5,000 mg/kg.

➤*Treatment:* No specific antidote is known, but gastric lavage may be used.

Patient Information

Instruct patients to immediately report any use of warfarin and any bleeding.

Instruct patients to also report any of the following side effects: ankle swelling, changes in skin color, nausea, vomiting.

Men: Instruct patients to report appearance or aggravation of acne and too frequent or persistent erections of the penis.

Women: Instruct patients to also report acne, changes in menstrual periods, hoarseness, or more facial hair.

OXYMETHOLONE

c-iii	**Anadrol-50** (Alaven)	**Tablets; oral:** 50 mg	Lactose. (0055 Alaven). Scored. In 100s.

OXYMETHOLONE — ORAL

For complete prescribing information, refer to the Anabolic Steroids group monograph.

WARNING

Peliosis hepatis – Peliosis hepatis, a condition in which liver and, sometimes, splenic tissue is replaced with blood-filled cysts, has occurred in patients receiving androgenic anabolic steroids. These cysts are sometimes present with minimal hepatic dysfunction and have been associated with liver failure. Often, they are not recognized until life-threatening liver failure or intra-abdominal hemorrhage develops. Withdrawal of drug usually results in complete disappearance of lesions.

Liver cell tumors – Most often these tumors are benign and androgen-dependent, but fatal malignant tumors have occurred. Withdrawal of drug often results in regression or cessation of tumor progression. However, hepatic tumors associated with androgens or anabolic steroids are much more vascular than other hepatic tumors and may be silent until life-threatening, intra-abdominal hemorrhage develops.

Blood lipid changes – Blood lipid changes associated with increased risk of atherosclerosis are seen in patients treated with androgens and anabolic steroids. These changes include decreased high-density lipoprotein (HDL) and, sometimes, increased low-density lipoprotein (LDL). The changes may be very marked and could have a serious impact on the risk of atherosclerosis and coronary artery disease.

Indications

➤*Anemia:* For the treatment of anemias caused by deficient red cell production. Acquired or congenital aplastic anemias, myelofibrosis, and/or hypoplastic anemias caused by the administration of myelotoxic drugs often respond.

Oxymetholone should not replace other supportive measures, such as transfusion; correction of iron, folic acid, vitamin B_{12}, or pyridoxine deficiency; antibacterial therapy; and the appropriate use of corticosteroids.

➤*Off-label uses:* HIV-associated wasting.

Administration and Dosage

➤*General dosing considerations:* Following remission, some patients may be maintained without the drug, while others may be maintained on an established lower daily dose. Continuous maintenance is usually necessary in patients with congenital aplastic anemia.

➤*Adults:*

Anemia – 1 to 5 mg/kg daily. The usual effective dosage is 1 to 2 mg/kg daily, but higher dosages may be required. Response often is not immediate; give a minimum trial of 3 to 6 months.

➤*Children:*

Anemia – See Adults for dosing.

➤*Renal function impairment:* Contraindicated in patients with nephrosis or patients in the nephrotic phase of nephritis.

➤*Hepatic function impairment:* Contraindicated in patients with severe hepatic dysfunction.

➤*Storage / Stability:* Store at 20° to 25°C (68° to 77°F); excursions permitted to 15° to 30°C (59° to 86°F).

OXANDROLONE

c-iii	**Oxandrolone** (Sandoz)	**Tablets; oral:** 2.5 mg	Lactose. In 100s and 1,000s.
c-iii	**Oxandrin** (Savient)		Lactose. (BTG 11). White, oval, scored. In 100s.
c-iii	**Oxandrolone** (Sandoz)	**Tablets; oral:** 10 mg	Lactose. In 100s and 1,000s.
c-iii	**Oxandrin** (Savient)		Lactose. (BTG 10). White, capsule shape. In 60s.

OXANDROLONE — ORAL

For complete prescribing information, refer to the Anabolic Steroids group monograph.

WARNING

Peliosis hepatis – Peliosis hepatis, a condition in which liver and, sometimes, splenic tissue is replaced with blood-filled cysts, has occurred in patients receiving androgenic anabolic steroids. These cysts are sometimes present with minimal hepatic dysfunction and have been associated with liver failure. Often, they are not recognized until life-threatening liver failure or intra-abdominal hemorrhage develops. Withdrawal of drug usually results in complete disappearance of lesions.

Liver cell tumors – Most often these tumors are benign and androgen-dependent, but fatal malignant tumors have occurred. Withdrawal of drug often results in regression or cessation of tumor progression. However, hepatic tumors associated with androgens or anabolic steroids are much more vascular than other hepatic tumors and may be silent until life-threatening, intra-abdominal hemorrhage develops.

Blood lipid changes – Blood lipid changes associated with increased risk of atherosclerosis are seen in patients treated with androgens and anabolic steroids. These changes include decreased high-density lipoprotein (HDL) and, sometimes, increased low-density lipoprotein (LDL). The changes may be very marked and could have a serious impact on the risk of atherosclerosis and coronary artery disease.

Indications

➤*Bone pain:* For the relief of the bone pain frequently accompanying osteoporosis.

➤*Protein catabolism:* To offset the protein catabolism associated with prolonged administration of corticosteroids.

➤*Weight gain:* Adjunctive therapy to promote weight gain after weight loss following extensive surgery, chronic infections, or severe trauma, and in some patients who, without definite pathophysiologic reasons, fail to gain or maintain normal weight.

➤*Off-label uses:* Catabolic illnesses, such as alcoholic liver disease and burn injury.

Orphan drug designation – Short stature associated with Turner syndrome, HIV-associated wasting, constitutional delay of growth and puberty, moderate/severe acute alcoholic hepatitis in the presence of moderate protein calorie malnutrition, Duchenne and Becker muscular dystrophy.

Administration and Dosage

➤*Adults:*

Bone pain –

Usual dosage: 2.5 to 20 mg daily in 2 to 4 divided doses. A daily dose of as little as 2.5 mg or as much as 20 mg may be required to achieve the desired response.

Duration of therapy: A course of therapy of 2 to 4 weeks is usually adequate. This may be repeated intermittently as indicated.

OXANDROLONE — ORAL

Protein catabolism – See Bone pain for dosing.

Weight gain – See Bone pain for dosing.

➤*Children:*

Bone pain –

Usual dosage: Total daily dose is 0.1 mg/kg or less.

Duration of therapy: This may be repeated intermittently as indicated.

Protein catabolism – See Bone pain for dosing.

Weight gain – See Bone pain for dosing.

➤*Renal function impairment:* Contraindicated in nephrosis or nephrotic phase of nephritis.

➤*Administration:* Take each dose without regard to meals, but take with food if stomach upset occurs.

➤*Storage/Stability:* Store at 15° to 25°C (59° to 77°F).

UTERINE-ACTIVE AGENTS

MIFEPRISTONE

Rx[a]	**Mifeprex** (Danco Labs)	**Tablets:** 200 mg	(MF). Lt. yellow, cylindrical, biconvex. In single-dose blister packets containing 3 tablets.

[a] Mifepristone will be supplied only to licensed physicians who sign and return a Prescriber's Agreement.

MIFEPRISTONE — ORAL

WARNING

Serious and sometimes fatal infections and bleeding occur very rarely following spontaneous, surgical, and medical abortions, including following mifepristone use. No causal relationship between the use of mifepristone and misoprostol and these reactions has been established. Before prescribing mifepristone, inform the patient about the risk of these serious events and discuss the Medication Guide and the Patient Agreement. Ensure that the patient knows whom to call and what to do, including going to an emergency room, if none of the provided contacts are reachable, if she experiences sustained fever, severe abdominal pain, prolonged heavy bleeding, or syncope, or if she experiences abdominal pain or discomfort or general malaise (including weakness, nausea, vomiting, or diarrhea) more than 24 hours after taking misoprostol.

Atypical infection – Patients with serious bacterial infections (eg, *Clostridium sordelli*) and sepsis can present without fever, bacteremia, or significant findings on pelvic examination following an abortion. Very rarely, deaths have been reported in patients who presented without fever, with or without abdominal pain, but with leukocytosis with a marked left shift, tachycardia, hemoconcentration, and general malaise. A high index of suspicion is needed to rule out serious infection and sepsis.

Bleeding – Prolonged heavy bleeding may be a sign of incomplete abortion or other complications, and prompt medical or surgical intervention may be needed. Advise patients to seek immediate medical attention if they experience prolonged heavy vaginal bleeding.

Advise patients to take their *Medication Guide* with them if they visit an emergency room or another health care provider who did not prescribe mifepristone, so that provider will be aware that the patient is undergoing a medical abortion.

Indications

➤*Termination of intrauterine pregnancy:* Mifepristone is indicated for the medical termination of intrauterine pregnancy through 49 days of pregnancy. For purposes of this treatment, pregnancy is dated from the first day of the last menstrual period in a presumed 28-day cycle with ovulation occurring at mid-cycle. The duration of pregnancy may be determined from menstrual history and by clinical examination. Use ultrasonographic scan if the duration of pregnancy is uncertain, or if ectopic pregnancy is suspected.

➤*General indications:* Pregnancy termination by surgery is recommended in cases when mifepristone and misoprostol fail to cause termination of intrauterine pregnancy because of the risk of fetal malformation resulting from the treatment.

➤*Off-label uses:* Emergency contraception; uterine leiomyomata.

Administration and Dosage

➤*General dosing considerations:* Mifepristone may be administered only in a clinic, medical office, or hospital, by or under the supervision of a physician able to assess the gestational age of an embryo and to diagnose ectopic pregnancies. Mifepristone will be supplied only to licensed physicians who sign and return a Prescriber's Agreement. Mifepristone is a prescription drug, although it will not be available to the public through licensed pharmacies.

Physicians must be able to provide surgical intervention in cases of incomplete abortion or severe bleeding, or have made plans to provide such care through others, and be able to ensure patient access to medical facilities equipped to provide blood transfusions and resuscitation, if necessary.

Patients must read the Medication Guide and read and sign the Patient Agreement before administration.

Give the patient instructions on what to do if significant discomfort, excessive vaginal bleeding, or other adverse reactions occur and a phone number to call if she has questions following the administration of the misoprostol. In addition, provide the name and phone number of the physician who will be handling emergencies for the patient.

➤*Adults:*

Termination of intrauterine pregnancy –

Day 1: Three mifepristone 200 mg tablets (600 mg) are taken in a single dose.

Day 3:

• *Usual dosage* – Two misoprostol 200 mcg tablets (400 mcg), unless abortion has occurred and has been confirmed by clinical examination or ultrasonographic scan.

• *Concomitant therapy* – During the period immediately following the administration of misoprostol, the patient may need medication for cramps or GI symptoms (eg, diarrhea, nausea, vomiting).

Day 14: Patients will return for a follow-up visit approximately 14 days after the administration of mifepristone. This visit is very important to confirm by clinical examination or ultrasonographic scan that a complete termination of pregnancy has occurred. Patients who have an ongoing pregnancy at this visit have a risk of fetal malformation resulting from the treatment. Surgical termination is recommended to manage medical abortion treatment failures.

➤*Administration:* Remove any intrauterine device (IUD) before treatment with mifepristone begins. Take mifepristone and misoprostol orally.

➤*Storage/Stability:* Store at 25°C (77°F); excursions are permitted to 15° to 30°C (59° to 86°F).

Actions

➤*Pharmacology:* The antiprogestational activity of mifepristone results from competitive interaction with progesterone at progesterone-receptor sites. Based on studies with various oral doses in several animal species (mouse, rat, rabbit, and monkey), the compound inhibits the activity of endogenous or exogenous progesterone. The termination of pregnancy results.

Doses greater than or equal to mifepristone 1 mg/kg have been shown to antagonize the endometrial and myometrial effects of progesterone in women. During pregnancy, the compound sensitizes the myometrium to the contraction-inducing activity of prostaglandins.

Mifepristone also exhibits antiglucocorticoid and weak antiandrogenic activity. The activity of the glucocorticoid dexamethasone in rats was inhibited following doses of mifepristone 10 to 25 mg/kg. Doses of 4.5 mg/kg or greater in humans resulted in a compensatory elevation of adrenocorticotropic hormone (ACTH) and cortisol. Antiandrogenic activity was observed in rats following repeated administration of doses from 10 to 100 mg/kg.

➤*Pharmacokinetics:*

Absorption – Following oral administration of a single dose of 600 mg, mifepristone is rapidly absorbed, with a peak plasma concentration of 1.98 mg/L occurring approximately 90 minutes after ingestion. The absolute bioavailability of a 20 mg oral dose is 69%.

Distribution – Mifepristone is 98% bound to plasma proteins, albumin, and α-1-acid glycoprotein. Binding to the latter protein is saturable, and the drug displays nonlinear kinetics with respect to plasma concentration and clearance.

Metabolism – Metabolism of mifepristone is primarily via pathways involving N-demethylation and terminal hydroxylation of the 17-propynyl chain. In vitro studies have shown that cytochrome P-450 3A4 is primarily responsible for the metabolism. The 3 major metabolites identified in humans are

1.) RU 42 633, the most widely found in plasma, which is the N-monodemethylated metabolite;

2.) RU 42 848, which results from the loss of 2 methyl groups from the 4-dimethylaminophenyl in position 11β; and

3.) RU 42 698, which results from terminal hydroxylation of the 17-propynyl chain.

Excretion – Following a distribution phase, elimination of mifepristone is slow at first (50% eliminated between 12 and 72 hours) and then becomes more rapid with a terminal elimination half-life of 18 hours. By 11 days after a 600 mg dose of tritiated compound, 83% of the drug has been accounted for by the feces and 9% by the urine. Serum levels are undetectable by 11 days.

Contraindications

Administration of mifepristone and misoprostol for the termination of pregnancy (the "treatment procedure") is contraindicated in patients with any one of the following conditions: confirmed or suspected ectopic pregnancy or undiagnosed adnexal mass (the treatment procedure will not be effective to terminate an ectopic pregnancy); IUD in place; chronic adrenal failure; concurrent long-term corticosteroid therapy; history of allergy to mifepristone,

MIFEPRISTONE — ORAL

misoprostol, or other prostaglandin; hemorrhagic disorders or concurrent anticoagulant therapy; inherited porphyrias.

➤*Access to medical care:* Because it is important to have access to appropriate medical care if an emergency develops, the treatment procedure is contraindicated if a patient does not have adequate access to medical facilities equipped to provide emergency treatment of incomplete abortion, blood transfusions, and emergency resuscitation during the period from the first visit until discharged by the administering health care provider.

Mifepristone also should not be used by any patient who may be unable to understand the effects of the treatment procedure or to comply with its regimen. Instruct patients to review the *Medication Guide* and the *Patient Agreement* provided with mifepristone carefully and give them a copy of the product label for their review. Patients should discuss their understanding of these materials with their health care providers, and retain the *Medication Guide* for later reference.

Warnings/Precautions

➤*Vaginal bleeding:* Vaginal bleeding occurs in almost all patients during a medical abortion. Prolonged heavy bleeding (soaking through 2 thick full-size sanitary pads per hour for 2 consecutive hours) may be a sign of incomplete abortion or other complications, and prompt medical or surgical intervention may be needed to prevent the development of hypovolemic shock. Counsel patients to seek immediate medical attention if they experience prolonged heavy vaginal bleeding following a medical abortion.

➤*Infection:* As with other types of abortion, cases of serious bacterial infection, including very rare cases of fatal septic shock, have been reported following the use of mifepristone. No causal relationship between these events and the use of mifepristone and misoprostol has been established. Physicians evaluating a patient who is undergoing a medical abortion should be alert to the possibility of this rare event. In particular, a sustained fever of 38°C (100.4°F) or higher, severe abdominal pain, or pelvic tenderness in the days after a medical abortion may be an indication of infection. Atypical presentations of serious infection and sepsis, without fever, severe abdominal pain, or pelvic tenderness, but with significant leukocytosis, tachycardia, or hemoconcentration can occur.

A high index of suspicion is needed to rule out sepsis (eg, *C. sordelli* if a patients reports abdominal pain or discomfort or general malaise (including weakness, nausea, vomiting, or diarrhea) more than 24 hours after taking misoprostol. Very rarely, deaths have been reported in patients who presented without fever, with or without abdominal pain, but with leukocytosis with a marked left shift, tachycardia, hemoconcentration, and general malaise. These deaths occurred in women who used vaginally administered misoprostol, but no causal relationship between vaginal misoprostol use and an increased risk of infection or death has been established. *C. sordelli* infections also have been reported very rarely following childbirth (vaginal delivery and caesarian section), and in other gynecologic and nongynecologic conditions.

➤*Pregnancy termination confirmation:* Schedule patients to return for a follow-up visit at approximately 14 days after administration of mifepristone to confirm that the pregnancy is completely terminated and to assess the degree of bleeding. Termination can be confirmed by clinical examination or ultrasonographic scan. Lack of bleeding following treatment, however, usually indicates failure; prolonged or heavy bleeding is not proof of a complete abortion. Manage medical abortion failures with surgical termination. Advise the patient whether you will provide such care or will refer her to another provider as part of counseling prior to prescribing mifepristone.

➤*Ectopic pregnancy:* Mifepristone is contraindicated in patients with a confirmed or suspected ectopic pregnancy since mifepristone is not effective for terminating these pregnancies. Remain alert to the possibility that a patient who is undergoing a medical abortion could have an undiagnosed ectopic pregnancy since some of the expected symptoms of a medical abortion may be similar to those of a ruptured ectopic pregnancy. The presence of an ectopic pregnancy may have been missed, even if the patient underwent ultrasonography prior to being prescribed mifepristone.

➤*Administration:* Mifepristone is available only in single-dose packaging. Administration must be under the supervision of a qualified physician. Mifepristone may be administered only in a clinic, medical office, or hospital, by or under the supervision of a physician able to assess the gestational age of an embryo and to diagnose ectopic pregnancies. Physicians must also be able to provide surgical intervention in cases of incomplete abortion or severe bleeding, or have made plans to provide such care through others, and be able to ensure patient access to medical facilities equipped to provide blood transfusions and resuscitation, if necessary.

➤*Rhesus immunization:* The use of mifepristone is assumed to require the same preventive measures as those taken prior to and during surgical abortion to prevent rhesus immunization.

➤*Effectiveness:* Although there is no clinical evidence, the effectiveness of mifepristone may be lower if misoprostol is administered more than 2 days after mifepristone administration.

➤*Special risk:* There are no data on the safety and efficacy of mifepristone in women with chronic medical conditions such as cardiovascular, hypertensive, hepatic, respiratory, or renal disease; type 1 diabetes mellitus; severe anemia; or heavy smoking. Treat women who are older than 35 years of age and who also smoke 10 or more cigarettes per day with caution because such patients were generally excluded from clinical trials of mifepristone.

➤*Pregnancy: Category X.* Mifepristone is indicated for use in the termination of pregnancy (through 49 days of pregnancy) and has no other approved indication for use during pregnancy.

Human data – As of September 2000, over 620,000 women in Europe have taken mifepristone in combination with a prostaglandin to terminate pregnancy. Among these 620,000 women, about 415,000 have received mifepristone together with misoprostol. As of May 2000, a total of 82 cases have been reported in which women with ongoing pregnancies after using mifepristone alone or mifepristone followed by misoprostol declined to have a surgical procedure at that time. These cases are summarized in the following table.

Pregnancies Not Terminated by Surgical Abortion at the End of Mifepristone Alone or Mifepristone-Misoprostol Treatment[a]

	Mifepristone alone (n = 42)	Mifepristone –Misoprostol (n = 40)	Total (n = 82)
Subsequently had surgical abortion	3	7	10
No abnormalities detected	2	7	9
Abnormalities detected (sirenomelia, cleft palate)	1	0	1
Subsequently resulted in live birth	13	13	26
No abnormalities detected at birth	13	13	26
Abnormalities detected at birth	0	0	0
Other/Unknown	26	20	46

[a] Reported cases as of May 2000.

Prostaglandins: Several reports in the literature indicate that prostaglandins, including misoprostol, may have teratogenic effects in human beings. Skull defects, cranial nerve palsies, delayed growth and psychomotor development, facial malformation, and limb defects have all been reported after first trimester exposure.

Animal data – Teratology studies in mice, rats, and rabbits at doses of 0.25 to 4 mg/kg (less than 1/100 to approximately 1/3 the human exposure level based on body surface area) were carried out. Because of the antiprogestational activity of mifepristone, fetal losses were much higher than in control animals. Skull deformities were detected in rabbit studies at approximately 1/6 the human exposure, although no teratogenic effects of mifepristone have been observed to date in rats or mice. These deformities were most likely due to the mechanical effects of uterine contractions resulting from decreased progesterone levels.

Nonteratogenic – The indication for use of mifepristone in conjunction with misoprostol is for the termination of pregnancy through 49 days' duration of pregnancy (as dated from the first day of the last menstrual period). These drugs together disrupt pregnancy by causing decidual necrosis, myometrial contractions, and cervical softening, leading to the expulsion of the products of conception.

➤*Lactation:* It is not known whether mifepristone is excreted in human milk. Many hormones with a similar chemical structure, however, are excreted in breast milk. Because the effects of mifepristone on infants are unknown, breast-feeding women should consult with their health care provider to decide if they should discard their breast milk for a few days following administration of the medications.

➤*Children:* Safety and efficacy in children have not been established.

➤*Lab test abnormalities:* Decreases in hemoglobin concentration, hematocrit, and red blood cell count occur in some women who bleed heavily. Hemoglobin decreases of more than 2 g/dL occurred in 5.5% of subjects during the French clinical trials of mifepristone and misoprostol.

Clinically significant changes in serum enzyme (alanine aminotransferase [ALT], aspartate aminotransferase [AST], alkaline phosphatase, gamma-glutamyltransferase [GT]) activities were rarely reported.

➤*Monitoring:* Clinical examination is necessary to confirm the complete termination of pregnancy after the treatment procedure. Changes in quantitative human chorionic gonadotropin (hCG) levels will not be decisive until at least 10 days after the administration of mifepristone. A continuing pregnancy can be confirmed by ultrasonographic scan.

The existence of debris in the uterus following the treatment procedure will not necessarily require surgery for its removal.

MIFEPRISTONE — ORAL

Drug Interactions

➤*CYP-450 system:*

Mifepristone Drug Interactions			
Precipitant Drug	Object Drug[a]		Description
CYP3A4 inducers (eg, rifampin, dexamethasone, St. John's wort, phenytoin, phenobarbital, carbamazepine)	Mifepristone	⬇	Induction of mifepristone metabolism may occur, resulting in lower serum levels.
CYP3A4 inhibitors (eg, ketoconazole, itraconazole, erythromycin, grape fruit juice)	Mifepristone	⬆	Mifepristone's metabolism may be inhibited, resulting in increased serum levels.

[a] ⬆ = Object drug increased. ⬇ = Object drug decreased.

Adverse Reactions

The treatment procedure is designed to induce the vaginal bleeding and uterine cramping necessary to produce an abortion. Nearly all of the women who receive mifepristone and misoprostol will report adverse reactions, and many can be expected to report more than 1 such reaction. About 90% of patients report adverse reactions following administration of misoprostol on day 3 of the treatment procedure. Those adverse reactions that occurred with a frequency greater than 1% in the US and French trials are shown in the following table.

Vaginal bleeding and cramping are expected consequences of the action of mifepristone as used in the treatment procedure. Following administration of mifepristone and misoprostol in the French clinical studies, 80% to 90% of women reported bleeding more heavily than they do during a heavy menstrual period. Women also typically experienced abdominal pain, including uterine cramping. Other commonly reported side effects were nausea, vomiting, and diarrhea. Some adverse reactions reported during the 4 hours following administration of misoprostol were judged by women as being more severe than others. The percentage of women who considered any particular adverse reaction as severe ranged from 2% to 35% in the US and French trials. After the third day of the treatment procedure, the number of reports of adverse reactions declined progressively in the French trials, so that by day 14, reports were rare except for reports of bleeding and spotting.

Mifepristone and Misoprostol Adverse Reactions (> 1%)		
Adverse reaction	US trials	French trials
CNS		
Anxiety	2%	NA[a]
Dizziness	12%	1%
Fainting	NA	2%
Fatigue	10%	NA
Headache	31%	2%
Insomnia	3%	NA
Syncope	1%	NA
GI		
Abdominal pain (cramping)	96%	NA
Diarrhea	20%	12%
Dyspepsia	3%	NA
Nausea	61%	43%
Vomiting	26%	18%
GU		
Endometritis/salpingitis/ pelvic inflammatory disease	1%	NA
Leukorrhea	2%	NA
Pelvic pain	NA	2%
Uterine cramping	NA	83%
Uterine hemorrhage	5%	NA
Vaginitis	3%	NA
Hematologic		
Anemia	2%	NA
Decrease in hemoglobin 2 g/dL	NA	6%
Miscellaneous		
Asthenia	2%	1%
Back pain	9%	NA
Fever	4%	NA
Leg pain	2%	NA
Rigors (chills/shaking)	3%	NA
Sinusitis	2%	NA
Viral infections	4%	NA

[a] NA: Not applicable

➤*Postmarketing:*

Cardiovascular – Hypotension (including orthostatic), shortness of breath, tachycardia (including racing pulse, heart palpitations, heart pounding).

CNS – Light-headedness, loss of consciousness.

Hypersensitivity – Allergic reaction (including rash, hives, itching).

Miscellaneous – Postabortal infection (including endomyometritis, parametritis), ruptured ectopic pregnancy.

Overdosage

No serious adverse reactions were reported in tolerance studies in healthy nonpregnant women and healthy men where mifepristone was administered in single doses greater than 3-fold that recommended for termination of pregnancy. If a patient ingests a massive overdose, observe her closely for signs of adrenal failure.

Patient Information

Fully advise patients of the treatment procedure and its effects. Give patients a copy of the *Medication Guide* and the *Patient Agreement*. (Additional copies of the *Medication Guide* and the *Patient Agreement* are available by contacting Danco Laboratories at 1-877-432-7596.) Advise patients to review both the *Medication Guide* and the *Patient Agreement*, and give them the opportunity to discuss them and obtain answers to any questions they may have prior to receiving mifepristone. Advise patients to take their *Medication Guide* with them if they visit an emergency room or another health care provider who did not prescribe mifepristone, so that provider will be aware that the patient is undergoing a medical abortion.

Each patient must understand:

- the necessity of completing the treatment schedule, including a follow-up visit approximately 14 days after taking mifepristone;
- that vaginal bleeding and uterine cramping probably will occur;
- that prolonged heavy vaginal bleeding is not proof of a complete abortion;
- that if the treatment fails, there is a risk of fetal malformation;
- that medical abortion treatment failures are managed by surgical termination; and
- the steps to take in an emergency situation, including precise instructions and a telephone number that she can call if she has any problems or concerns.

Another pregnancy can occur following termination of pregnancy and before resumption of normal menses. Contraception can be initiated as soon as the termination of the pregnancy has been confirmed, or before the woman resumes sexual intercourse.

Patient information is included with each package of mifepristone.

CARBOPROST TROMETHAMINE

Rx	**Hemabate** (Pharmacia & Upjohn)	**Injection:** carboprost 250 mcg and tromethamine 83 mcg/mL	Sodium chloride 9 mg, benzyl alcohol 9.45 mg. In 1 mL amps.[a]

[a] With 9.45% benzyl alcohol and sodium chloride 9 mg/mL.

CARBOPROST TROMETHAMINE — INJECTION

Indications

➤*Abortion:* For aborting pregnancy between week 13 and 20 of gestation as calculated from the first day of the last normal menstrual period and in the following conditions related to second trimester abortion:

1.) Failure of expulsion of the fetus during the course of treatment by another method;
2.) Premature rupture of membranes in intrauterine methods with loss of drug and insufficient or absent uterine activity;
3.) Requirement of a repeat intrauterine instillation of drug for expulsion of the fetus;
4.) Inadvertent or spontaneous rupture of membranes in the presence of a previable fetus and absence of adequate activity for expulsion.

➤*Postpartum uterine hemorrhage:* For the treatment of postpartum hemorrhage due to uterine atony that has not responded to conventional methods of management. Prior treatment should include the use of intravenously administered oxytocin, manipulative techniques such as uterine massage and, unless contraindicated, intramuscular ergot preparations. Studies have shown that, in such cases, the use of carboprost tromethamine has resulted in satisfactory control of hemorrhage, although it is unclear whether or not ongoing or delayed effects of previously administered ecbolic agents have contributed to the outcome. In a high proportion of cases,

CARBOPROST TROMETHAMINE — INJECTION

carboprost tromethamine used in this manner has resulted in the cessation of life-threatening bleeding and the avoidance of emergency surgical intervention.

Administration and Dosage

➤*Adults:*

Abortion –

Maximum dose: The total dose administered of carboprost tromethamine should not exceed 12 mg.

Test dose: An optional test dose of 100 mcg (0.4 mL) may be administered initially. The dose may be increased to 500 mcg (2 mL) if uterine contractility is judged to be inadequate after several doses of 250 mcg (1 mL).

Initial dosage: 1 mL of carboprost tromethamine sterile solution (containing the equivalent of carboprost 250 mcg) is to be administered deep in the muscle with a tuberculin syringe.

Maintenance dosage: Subsequent doses of 250 mcg should be administered at 1.5- to 3.5-hour intervals depending on uterine response.

Duration of therapy: Continuous administration of the drug for more than 2 days is not recommended.

Refractory postpartum uterine bleeding –

Maximum dose: The total dose of carboprost tromethamine should not exceed 2 mg (8 doses).

Initial dosage: 250 mcg of carboprost tromethamine sterile solution (1 mL of carboprost tromethamine) is to be given deep, intramuscularly.

Maintenance dosage: The need for additional injections and the interval at which these should be given can be determined only by the attending physicians as dictated by the course of clinical events.

➤*Storage/Stability:* Carboprost tromethamine must be refrigerated at 2° to 8° C (36° to 46° F).

DINOPROSTONE (Prostaglandin E_2; PGE_2)

Rx	**Prepidil** (Upjohn)	**Gel:** 0.5 mg	In 3 g (2.5 mL) syringes[a] with 2 shielded catheters (10 and 20 mm tip).
Rx	**Cervidil** (Forest)	**Vaginal insert:** 10 mg	In 1s.
Rx	**Prostin E2** (Pharmacia & Upjohn)	**Vaginal suppositories:** 20 mg	In containers of 1 each.

[a] With colloidal silicon dioxide NF 240 mg and triacetin 2,760 mg, USP.

DINOPROSTONE — VAGINAL

WARNING

Dinoprostone, as with other potent oxytocic agents, should be used only with strict adherence to recommended dosages. Dinoprostone should be used by medically trained personnel in a hospital which can provide immediate intensive care and acute surgical facilities.

Indications

➤*Vaginal suppository:* For the termination of pregnancy from the 12th through the 20th gestational week as calculated from the first day of the last normal menstrual period.

For evacuation of the uterine contents in the management of missed abortion or intrauterine fetal death up to 28 weeks of gestational age as calculated from the first day of the last normal menstrual period.

Management of nonmetastatic gestational trophoblastic disease (benign hydatidiform mole).

➤*Cervical gel and vaginal insert:* For the initiation or continuation of cervical ripening in patients at or near term in whom there is a medical or obstetrical indication for the induction of labor.

Administration and Dosage

➤*Adults:*

Abortion (vaginal suppository only) –

Usual dosage: 20 mg suppository inserted high into the vagina. Additional intravaginal administration of each subsequent suppository should be at 3- to 5-hour intervals until abortion occurs. Within the previously recommended intervals, administration time should be determined by abortifacient progress, uterine contractility response, and by patient tolerance.

Duration of therapy: Continuous administration of the drug for more than 2 days is not recommended.

Cervical ripening (cervical gel and vaginal insert only) –

Cervical gel:

• *Usual dosage* – 0.5 mg (1 syringe applicator). If there is no cervical/uterine response to the initial dose, repeat dosing with 0.5 mg, with a dosing interval of 6 hours.

• *Maximum dose* – The maximum recommended cumulative dose for a 24-hour period is 1.5 mg (7.5 mL).

• *Concomitant therapy* – If the desired response is obtained from dinoprostone cervical gel, the recommended interval before giving intravenous oxytocin is 6 to 12 hours.

Vaginal insert:

• *Usual dosage* – 10 mg, designed to be released at approximately 0.3 mg/hour over a 12-hour period.

• *Discontinuation of therapy* – The insert should be removed upon onset of active labor or 12 hours after insertion.

➤*Preparation for administration:*

Cervical gel – Dinoprostone cervical gel should be brought to room temperature (15° to 30°C; 59° to 86°F) just prior to administration. Do not force the warming process by using a water bath or other source of external heat (eg, microwave oven).

To prepare the product for use, remove the peel-off seal from the end of the syringe. Then remove the protective end cap (to serve as plunger extension) and insert the protective end cap into the plunger stopper assembly in the barrel of syringe. Choose the appropriate length shielded catheter (10 or 20 mm) and aseptically remove the sterile shielded catheter from the package. Careful vaginal examination will reveal the degree of effacement that will regulate the size of the shielded endocervical catheter to be used. That is, the 20 mm endocervical catheter should be used if no effacement is present, and the 10 mm catheter should be used if the cervix is 50% effaced. Firmly attach the catheter hub to the syringe tip as evidenced by a distinct click. Fill the catheter with sterile gel by pushing the plunger assembly to expel air from the catheter prior to administration to the patient.

➤*Administration:* Use caution in handling this product to prevent contact with skin. Wash hands thoroughly with soap and water after administration.

Vaginal suppository – Remove foil before use. A suppository containing dinoprostone 20 mg should be inserted high into the vagina. The patient should remain in the supine position for 10 minutes following insertion.

Cervical gel – To properly administer the product, the patient should be in a dorsal position with the cervix visualized using a speculum. Using sterile technique, introduce the gel with the catheter provided into the cervical canal just below the level of the internal os. Administer the contents of the syringe by gentle expulsion and then remove the catheter. The gel is easily extrudable from the syringe. Use the contents of 1 syringe for 1 patient only. No attempt should be made to administer the small amount of gel remaining in the catheter. The syringe, catheter, and any unused package contents should be discarded after use. Following administration of dinoprostone cervical gel, the patient should remain in the supine position for at least 15 to 30 minutes to minimize leakage from the cervical canal.

Vaginal insert – One dinoprostone vaginal insert is placed transversely in the posterior fornix of the vagina immediately after removal from its foil package. The insertion of the vaginal insert does not require sterile conditions. The vaginal insert must not be used without its retrieval system. There is no need for previous warming of the product. A minimal amount of water-miscible lubricant may be used to assist in insertion of dinoprostone vaginal insert. Care should be taken not to permit excess contact or coating with the lubricant and thus prevent optimal swelling and release of dinoprostone from the vaginal insert. Patients should remain in the supine position for 2 hours following insertion, but thereafter may be ambulatory.

➤*Storage/Stability:*

Vaginal suppository – Store in a freezer not above −20°C (−4°F) but bring to room temperature just prior to use.

Cervical gel – Dinoprostone cervical gel has a shelf life of 24 months when stored under continuous refrigeration (2° to 8°C; 36° to 46°F).

Vaginal insert – Store in a freezer between −20° and −10°C (−4° and 14°F). Dinoprostone vaginal insert is packed in foil and is stable when stored in a freezer for a period of 3 years. Vaginal inserts exposed to high humidity will absorb moisture from the air and thereby alter the release characteristics of dinoprostone. Once used, the vaginal insert should be discarded.

Actions

➤*Pharmacology:*

Dinoprostone vaginal suppository – Dinoprostone vaginal suppository administered intravaginally stimulates the myometrium of the gravid uterus to contract in a manner that is similar to the contractions seen in the term uterus during labor. Whether or not this action results from a direct effect of dinoprostone on the myometrium has not been determined with certainty at this time. Nonetheless, the myometrial contractions induced by the vaginal administration of dinoprostone are sufficient to produce evacuation of the products of conception from the uterus in the majority of cases.

Dinoprostone is also capable of stimulating the smooth muscle of the gastrointestinal tract of man. This activity may be responsible for the vomiting or diarrhea that is not uncommon when dinoprostone is used to terminate pregnancy.

In laboratory animals, and also in man, large doses of dinoprostone can lower blood pressure, probably as a consequence of its effect on the smooth muscle of the vascular system. With the doses of dinoprostone used for terminating pregnancy this effect has not been clinically significant. In laboratory animals, and also in man, dinoprostone can elevate body temperature. With the clinical doses of dinoprostone used for the termination of pregnancy some patients do exhibit temperature increases.

Dinoprostone cervical gel – Dinoprostone cervical gel administered endocervically may stimulate the myometrium of the gravid uterus to contract in a manner similar to contractions seen in the term uterus during labor. Whether or not this action results from a direct effect of dinoprostone

DINOPROSTONE — VAGINAL

on the myometrium has not been determined. Dinoprostone is also capable of stimulating smooth muscle of the gastrointestinal tract in humans. This activity may be responsible for the vomiting or diarrhea that is occasionally seen when dinoprostone is used for preinduction cervical ripening.

In laboratory animals, and also in humans, large doses of dinoprostone can lower blood pressure, probably as a result of its effect on smooth muscle of the vascular system. With the doses of dinoprostone used for cervical ripening this effect has not been seen. In laboratory animals, and also in humans, dinoprostone can elevate body temperature; however, with the dosing used for cervical ripening this effect has not been seen.

In addition to an oxytocic effect, there is evidence suggesting that this agent has a local cervical effect in initiating softening, effacement, and dilation. These changes, referred to as cervical ripening, occur spontaneously as the normal pregnancy progresses toward term and allow evacuation of uterine contents by decreasing cervical resistance at the same time that myometrial activity increases. While not completely understood, biochemical changes within the cervix during natural cervical ripening are similar to those following PGE_2-induced ripening. Further, it has been shown that these changes can take place independent of myometrial activity; however, it is quite likely that PGE_2 administered endocervically produces effacement and softening by combined contraction-inducing and cervical-ripening properties. There is evidence to suggest that the changes that take place within the cervix are due to collagen degradation resulting from collagenase secretion as a response, at least in part, to PGE_2.

Using an unvalidated assay, the following information was determined. When dinoprostone cervical gel was administered endocervically to women undergoing preinduction ripening, results from measurement of plasma levels of the metabolite 13,14-dihydro-15-keto-PGE_2 (DHK-PGE_2) showed that PGE_2 was relatively rapidly absorbed and the T_{max} was 0.5 to 0.75 hours. Plasma mean C_{max} for gel-treated subjects was 433 ± 51 pg/mL versus 137 ± 24 pg/mL for untreated controls. In those subjects in which a clinical response was observed, mean C_{max} was 484 ± 57 pg/mL versus 213 ± 69 pg/mL in nonresponders and 219 ± 92 pg/mL in control subjects who had positive clinical progression toward normal labor. These elevated levels in gel-treated subjects appear to be largely a result of absorption of PGE_2 from the gel rather than from endogenous sources.

PGE_2 is completely metabolized in humans. PGE_2 is extensively metabolized in the lungs, and the resulting metabolites are further metabolized in the liver and kidney. The major route of elimination of the products of PGE_2 metabolism is the kidneys.

Dinoprostone vaginal insert – Dinoprostone (PGE_2) is a naturally occurring biomolecule. It is found in low concentrations in most tissues of the body and functions as a local hormone. As with any local hormone, it is very rapidly metabolized in the tissues of synthesis (the half-life estimated to be 2.5 to 5 minutes). The rate limiting step for inactivation is regulated by the enzyme 15-hydroxyprostaglandin dehydrogenase (PGDH). Any PGE_2 that escapes local inactivation is rapidly cleared to the extent of 95% on the first pass through the pulmonary circulation.

In pregnancy, PGE_2 is secreted continuously by the fetal membranes and placenta and plays an important role in the final events leading to the initiation of labor. It is known that PGE_2 stimulates the production of PGF_2(alpha) which in turn sensitizes the myometrium to endogenous or exogenously administrated oxytocin. Although PGE_2 is capable of initiating uterine contractions and may interact with oxytocin to increase uterine contractility, the available evidence indicates that, in the concentrations found during the early part of labor, PGE_2 plays an important role in cervical ripening without affecting uterine contractions. This distinction serves as the basis for considering cervical ripening and induction of labor, usually by the use of oxytocin, as two separate processes.

PGE_2 plays an important role in the complex set of biochemical and structural alterations involved in cervical ripening. Cervical ripening involves a marked relaxation of the cervical smooth muscle fibers of the uterine cervix which must be transformed from a rigid structure to a softened, yielding and dilated configuration to allow passage of the fetus through the birth canal. This process involves activation of the enzyme collagenase, which is responsible for digestion of some of the structural collagen network of the cervix. This is associated with a concomitant increase in the amount of hydrophilic glycosaminoglycan, hyaluronic acid, and a decrease in dermatan sulfate. Failure of the cervix to undergo these natural physiologic changes, usually assessed by the method described by Bishop, prior to the onset of effective uterine contractions, results in an unfavorable outcome for successful vaginal delivery and may result in fetal compromise. It is estimated that in approximately 5% of pregnancies the cervix does not ripen normally. In an additional 10% to 11% of pregnancies, labor must be induced for medical or obstetric reasons prior to the time of cervical ripening.

The delivery rate of PGE_2 in vivo is about 0.3 mg/hour over a period of 12 hours. The controlled release of PGE_2 from the hydrogel insert is an attempt to provide sufficient quantities of PGE_2 to the local receptors to satisfy hormonal requirements. In the majority of patients, these local effects are manifested by changes in the consistency, dilatation and effacement of the cervix as measured by the Bishop score. Although some patients experience uterine hyperstimulation as a result of direct PGE_2- or PGF_2(alpha)-mediated sensitization of the myometrium to oxytocin, systemic effects of PGE_2 are rarely encountered. The insert is fitted with a biocompatible retrieval system which facilitates removal at the conclusion of therapy or in the event of an adverse reaction.

No correlation could be established between PGE_2 release and plasma concentrations of PGEm. The relative contributions of endogenously and exogenously released PGE_2 to the plasma levels of the metabolite PGEm could not be determined. Moreover, it is uncertain as to whether the measured concentrations of PGEm reflect the natural progression of PGEm concentrations in blood as birth approaches or to what extent the measured concentrations following PGE_2 administration represent an increase over basal levels that might be measured in control patients.

Contraindications

➤*Dinoprostone vaginal suppository:* Hypersensitivity to dinoprostone; acute pelvic inflammatory disease; patients with active cardiac, pulmonary, renal, or hepatic disease.

➤*Dinoprostone cervical gel:* Endocervically administered dinoprostone cervical gel is not recommended for the following: Patients in whom oxytocic drugs are generally contraindicated or where prolonged contractions of the uterus are considered inappropriate, such as cases with a history of cesarean section or major uterine surgery, cases in which cephalopelvic disproportion is present, cases in which there is a history of difficult labor and/or traumatic delivery, grand multiparae with 6 or more previous term pregnancies cases with non-vertex presentation, cases with hyperactive or hypertonic uterine patterns, cases of fetal distress where delivery is not imminent, and in obstetric emergencies where the benefit-to-risk ratio for either the fetus or the mother favors surgical intervention; patients with hypersensitivity to prostaglandins or constituents of the gel; patients with placenta previa or unexplained vaginal bleeding during this pregnancy; patients for whom vaginal delivery is not indicated, such as vasa previa or active herpes genitalia.

➤*Dinoprostone vaginal insert:* Patients with known hypersensitivity to prostaglandins; patients in whom there is clinical suspicion or definite evidence of fetal distress where delivery is not imminent; patients with unexplained vaginal bleeding during this pregnancy; patients in whom there is evidence or strong suspicion of marked cephalopelvic disproportion; patients already receiving intravenous oxytocic drugs; pultipara with 6 or more previous term pregnancies; patients in whom oxytocic drugs are contraindicated; when prolonged contraction of the uterus may be detrimental to fetal safety or uterine integrity (previous cesarean section or major uterine surgery).

Warnings/Precautions

➤*General information:* Dinoprostone does not appear to directly affect the fetoplacental unit. Therefore, the possibility does exist that the previable fetus aborted by dinoprostone could exhibit transient life signs.

Dinoprostone is not indicated if the fetus in utero has reached the stage of viability. Dinoprostone should not be considered a feticidal agent.

Evidence from animal studies has suggested that certain prostaglandins may have some teratogenic potential. Therefore, any failed pregnancy termination with dinoprostone should be completed by some other means.

➤*Dinoprostone vaginal suppository:* Animal studies lasting several weeks at high doses have shown that prostaglandins of the E and F series can induce proliferation of bone. Such effects have also been noted in newborn infants who have received prostaglandin E_1 during prolonged treatment. There is no evidence that short-term administration of dinoprostone vaginal suppository can cause similar bone effects.

As in spontaneous abortion, where the process is sometimes incomplete, abortion induced by dinoprostone may sometimes be incomplete. In such cases, other measures should be taken to ensure complete abortion.

In patients with a history of asthma, hypo- or hypertension, cardiovascular disease, renal disease, hepatic disease, anemia, jaundice, diabetes or history of epilepsy, dinoprostone should be used with caution.

Dinoprostone administered by the vaginal route should be used with caution in the presence of cervicitis, infected endocervical lesions, or acute vaginitis.

As with any oxytocic agent, dinoprostone should be used with caution in patients with compromised (scarred) uteri.

Dinoprostone vaginal therapy is associated with transient pyrexia that may be due to its effect on hypothalamic thermoregulation. In the patients studied, temperature elevations in excess of 1.1°C (2°F) were observed in approximately one-half of the patients on the recommended dosage regimen. In all cases, temperature returned to normal on discontinuation of therapy. Differentiation of post-abortion endometritis from drug-induced temperature elevations is difficult, but with increasing clinical exposure and experience with PGE_2 vaginal therapy the distinctions become more obviously apparent and are summarized below:

Apparent distinctions between endometritis pyrexia and PGE_2-induced pyrexia are compared below.

Time of onset – Endometritis pyrexia (38° C or higher) typically occurs on the third post-abortional day, while PGE_2-induced pyrexia typically occurs within 15 to 45 minutes of suppository administration.

Duration – Untreated endometritis pyrexia and infection continue and may give rise to other infective pelvic pathology. PGE_2-induced pyrexia elevations revert to pretreatment levels within 2 to 6 hours after discontinuation of therapy or removal of the suppository from the vagina without any other treatment.

Retention – In patients experiencing endometritis pyrexia, products of conception are often retained in the cervical os or uterine cavity. In PGE_2-induced pyrexia, elevation occurs irrespective of any retained tissue.

Histology – In patients experiencing endometritis pyrexia, the endometrium may show evidence of inflammatory lymphocytic infiltration with areas of necrotic or hemorrhagic tissue. In PGE_2-induced pyrexia, although the endometrial stroma may be edematous and vascular, there is relative absence of inflammatory reaction.

DINOPROSTONE — VAGINAL

The uterus – In patients experiencing endometritis pyrexia, the uterus often remains boggy and soft with tenderness over the fundus and pain on moving the cervix on bimanual examination. PGE_2-induced pyrexia is characterized by normal uterine involution without tenderness.

Discharge – Endometritis pyrexia is often associated with foul-smelling lochia and leukorrhea, while lochia are normal in PGE_2-induced pyrexia.

Cervical culture – The culture of pathological organisms from the cervix or uterine cavity after abortion does not, of itself, warrant the diagnosis of septic abortion in the absence of clinical evidence of sepsis. It is not uncommon to culture pathogens from cases of recent abortion not clinically infected. Persistent positive culture with clear clinical signs of infection are significant in the differential diagnosis.

Blood count – Leukocytosis and differential white cell counts are not of major clinical importance in distinguishing between the 2 conditions, since total WBCs may be increased as a result of infection and transient leukocytosis may also be drug induced.

In the absence of clinical or bacteriological evidence of intrauterine infection, supportive therapy for drug induced fevers includes the forcing of fluids. As all PGE_2-induced fevers have been found to be transient or self-limiting, it is doubtful if any simple empirical measures for temperature reduction are indicated.

Laboratory tests – When a pregnancy diagnosed as missed abortion is electively interrupted with intravaginal administration of dinoprostone, confirmation of intrauterine fetal death should be obtained in respect to a negative pregnancy test for chorionic gonadotropic activity (UCG test or equivalent). When a pregnancy with late fetal intrauterine death is interrupted with intravaginal administration of dinoprostone, confirmation of intrauterine fetal death should be obtained prior to treatment.

➤*Dinoprostone cervical gel:* During use, uterine activity, fetal status, and character of the cervix (dilation and effacement) should be carefully monitored either by auscultation or electronic fetal monitoring to detect possible evidence of undesired responses (eg, hypertonus, sustained uterine contractility, or fetal distress). In cases where there is a history of hypertonic uterine contractility or tetanic uterine contractions, it is recommended that uterine activity and the state of the fetus should be continuously monitored. The possibility of uterine rupture should be borne in mind when high-tone myometrial contractions are sustained. Feto-pelvic relationships should be carefully evaluated before use of dinoprostone cervical gel (see Contraindications).

Caution should be exercised in administration of dinoprostone cervical gel in patients with asthma or history of asthma, glaucoma or raised intraocular pressure.

Caution should be taken so as not to administer dinoprostone cervical gel above the level of the internal os. Careful vaginal examination will reveal the degree of effacement which will regulate the size of the shielded endocervical catheter to be used. That is, the 20 mm endocervical catheter should be used if no effacement is present, and the 10 mm catheter should be used if the cervix is 50% effaced. Placement of dinoprostone cervical gel into the extra-amniotic space has been associated with uterine hyperstimulation.

As dinoprostone cervical gel is extensively metabolized in the lung, liver, and kidney, and the major route of elimination is the kidney, dinoprostone cervical gel should be used with caution in patients with renal and hepatic dysfunction.

Patients with ruptured membranes – Caution should be exercised in the administration of dinoprostone cervical gel in patients with ruptured membranes. The safety of use of dinoprostone cervical gel in these patients has not been determined.

➤*Dinoprostone vaginal insert:* Because prostaglandins potentiate the effect of oxytocin, dinoprostone vaginal insert must be removed before oxytocin administration is initiated and the patient's uterine activity carefully monitored for uterine hyperstimulation. If uterine hyperstimulation is encountered or if labor commences, the vaginal insert should be removed. Dinoprostone vaginal insert should also be removed prior to amniotomy.

Caution should be exercised in the administration of dinoprostone vaginal insert for cervical ripening in patients with ruptured membranes, in cases of non-vertex, or non-singleton presentation, and in patients with a history of previous uterine hypertony, glaucoma, or a history of childhood asthma, even though there have been no asthma attacks in adulthood.

Uterine activity, fetal status and the progression of cervical dilatation and effacement should be carefully monitored whenever the dinoprostone vaginal insert is in place. Any evidence of uterine hyperstimulation, sustained uterine contractions, fetal distress, or other fetal or maternal adverse reactions, should be a cause for consideration of removal of the insert.

➤*Pregnancy: Category C.*

Dinoprostone vaginal suppository – Animal studies do not indicate that dinoprostone is teratogenic, however, it has been shown to be embryotoxic in rats and rabbits and any dose which produces increased uterine tone could put the embryo or fetus at risk.

Dinoprostone cervical gel and vaginal insert – Prostaglandin E_2 produced an increase in skeletal anomalies in rats and rabbits. No effect would be expected clinically, when used as indicated, because dinoprostone cervical gel is administered after the period of organogenesis. Dinoprostone cervical gel has been shown to be embryotoxic in rats and rabbits, and any dose that produces sustained increased uterine tone could put the embryo or fetus at risk (see Warnings/Precautions).

➤*Lactation:* It is unknown if dinoprostone is excreted in human milk. The use of dinoprostone for cervical ripening during delivery is generally brief and probably does not impact the production of milk hours or days later.

➤*Children:* Safety and efficacy in children have not been established.

Drug Interactions

Dinoprostone may augment the activity of other oxytocic drugs. Concomitant use with other oxytocic agents is not recommended.

➤*Dinoprostone cervical gel:* For the sequential use of oxytocin following dinoprostone cervical gel administration, a dosing interval of 6 to 12 hours is recommended.

➤*Dinoprostone vaginal insert:* A dosing interval of at least 30 minutes is recommended for the sequential use of oxytocin following the removal of the dinoprostone vaginal insert. No other drug interactions have been identified.

Adverse Reactions

➤*Dinoprostone vaginal suppository:* The most frequent adverse reactions observed with the use of dinoprostone for abortion are related to its contractile effect on smooth muscle.

In the patients studied, ≈ ⅔ experienced vomiting, ½ temperature elevations, ⅖ diarrhea, ⅓ some nausea, ⅒ headache, and ⅒ shivering and chills.

In addition, ≈ ⅒ of the patients studied exhibited transient diastolic blood pressure decreases of > 20 mmHg.

Two cases of myocardial infarction following the use of dinoprostone have been reported in patients with a history of cardiovascular disease.

It is not known whether these events were related to the administration of dinoprostone.

Adverse effects in decreasing order of their frequency, observed with the use of dinoprostone, not all of which are clearly drug related include: Vomiting; diarrhea; nausea; fever; headache; chills or shivering; backache; joint inflammation or pain, new or exacerbated; flushing or hot flashes; dizziness; arthralgia; vaginal pain; chest pain; dyspnea; endometritis; syncope or fainting sensation; vaginitis or vulvitis; weakness; muscular cramp or pain; tightness in chest; nocturnal leg cramps; uterine rupture; breast tenderness; blurred vision; coughing; rash; myalgia; stiff neck; dehydration; tremor; paresthesia; hearing impairment; urine retention; pharyngitis; laryngitis; diaphoresis; eye pain; wheezing; cardiac arrhythmia; skin discoloration; vaginismus; tension.

➤*Dinoprostone cervical gel:* Dinoprostone cervical gel is generally well-tolerated. In controlled trials, in which 1,731 women were entered, the following events were reported at an occurrence of at least 1%:

Dinoprostone Cervical Gel Adverse Reactions

	Dinoprostone cervical gel (n = 884)		Control[a] (n = 847)	
Adverse reaction	n	%	n	%
Maternal				
Uterine contractile abnormality	58	6.6%	34	4%
Any GI effect	50	5.7%	22	2.6%
Back pain	27	3.1%	0	0%
Warm feeling in vagina	13	1.5%	0	0%
Fever	12	1.4%	10	1.2%
Fetal				
Any fetal heart rate abnormality	150	17%	123	14.5%
Bradycardia	36	4.1%	26	3.1%
Deceleration, late	25	2.8%	18	2.1%
Deceleration, variable	38	4.3%	29	3.4%
Deceleration, unspecified	19	2.1%	19	2.2%

[a] Placebo gel or no treatment.

In addition, in other trials amnionitis and intrauterine fetal sepsis have been associated with extra-amniotic intrauterine administration of PGE_2. Uterine rupture has been reported in association with the use of dinoprostone cervical gel intracervically. Additional events reported in the literature, associated by the authors with the use of dinoprostone cervical gel, included premature rupture of membranes, fetal depression (1 min Apgar less than 7), and fetal acidosis (umbilical artery pH less than 7.15).

➤*Dinoprostone vaginal insert:* Dinoprostone vaginal insert is well tolerated. In placebo-controlled trials in which 658 women were entered and 320 received active therapy (218 without retrieval system, 102 with retrieval system), the following events were reported.

DINOPROSTONE — VAGINAL

Total Dinoprostone Vaginal Insert Drug-Related Adverse Reactions				
	Controlled studies[a]		Study 101-801[b]	
Adverse reactions	Active (n = 320)	Placebo (n = 338)	Active (n = 102)	Placebo (n = 104)
Uterine hyperstimulation with fetal distress	2.8%	0.3%	2.9%	0%
Uterine hyperstimulation without fetal distress	4.7%	0%	2%	0%
Fetal distress without uterine hyperstimulation	3.8%	1.2%	2.9%	1%

[a] Controlled studies (with and without retrieval system).
[b] Controlled study (with retrieval system).

Drug related fever, nausea, vomiting, diarrhea, and abdominal pain were noted in less than 1% of patients who received dinoprostone vaginal insert.

In Study 101-801 (with the retrieval system) cases of hyperstimulation reversed within 2 to 13 minutes of removal of the product. Tocolytics were required in 1 of the 5 cases.

In cases of fetal distress, when product removal was thought advisable there was a return to normal rhythm and no neonatal sequelae.

Five minute Apgar scores were 7 or above in 98.2% (646/658) of studied neonates whose mothers received dinoprostone vaginal insert. In a report of a 3 year pediatric follow-up study in 121 infants, 51 of whose mothers received dinoprostone vaginal insert, there were no deleterious effects on physical examination or psychomotor evaluation.

Overdosage

➤*Dinoprostone cervical gel:* Overdosage with dinoprostone cervical gel may be expressed by uterine hypercontractility and uterine hypertonus. Because of the transient nature of PGE_2 -induced myometrial hyperstimulation, nonspecific, conservative management was found to be effective in the vast majority of the cases; ie, maternal position change and administration of oxygen to the mother. Beta-adrenergic drugs may be used as a treatment of hyperstimulation following the administration of PGE_2 for cervical ripening.

➤*Dinoprostone vaginal insert:* Dinoprostone vaginal insert is used as a single dosage in a single application. Overdosage is usually manifested by uterine hyperstimulation which may be accompanied by fetal distress and is responsive to removal of the insert. Other treatment must be symptomatic since, to date, clinical experience with prostaglandin antagonists is insufficient. The use of beta-adrenergic agents should be considered in the event of undesirable increased uterine activity.

OXYTOCIN

Rx	**Oxytocin** (Various, eg, APP)	**Injection, solution:** 10 units/mL	In 3 and 10 mL vials.
Rx	**Pitocin** (JHP Pharmaceuticals)		In 1 mL amps[a], 10 mL multiple dose vial.[a]

[a] With 0.5% chlorobutanol.

OXYTOCIN — INJECTION

WARNING

Oxytocin is indicated for the medical, rather than the elective, induction of labor. Available data and information are inadequate to define the benefit-to-risk considerations in the use of oxytocin for elective induction.

Indications

➤*Antepartum:* For the initiation or improvement of uterine contractions, when this is desirable and considered suitable for reasons of fetal or maternal concern, in order to achieve vaginal delivery. It is indicated for patients with a medical indication for the initiation of labor such as Rh problems, maternal diabetes, preeclampsia at or near term, when delivery is in the best interest of mother and fetus, or when membranes are ruptured prematurely and delivery is indicated; stimulation or reinforcement of labor, as in selected cases of uterine inertia; adjunctive therapy for the management of inevitable or incomplete abortion. In the first trimester, curettage generally is considered primary therapy. In second trimester abortion, oxytocin infusion often is successful in emptying the uterus. However, other means of therapy may be required in such cases.

➤*Postpartum:* To produce uterine contractions during the third stage of labor and to control postpartum bleeding or hemorrhage.

Administration and Dosage

➤*Adults:*

Incomplete or inevitable abortion – IV infusion of oxytocin 10 units with 500 mL physiologic saline solution or 5% dextrose in physiologic saline solution infused at a rate of 10 to 20 milliunits (20 to 40 drops) per minute. Do not exceed 30 units in a 12-hour period because of the risk of water intoxication.

Induction or stimulation of labor – Start an IV infusion of nonoxytocin-containing solution. Use physiologic electrolyte solution, except under unusual circumstances.

Initial dosage: Up to 0.5 to 2 milliunits/min.

Dosage titration: Gradually increase the dose in increments of no more than 1 to 2 milliunits/min at 30- to 60-minute intervals until a contraction pattern has been established that is similar to normal labor.

Maintenance dosage: Infusion rates up to 6 milliunits/min give the same oxytocin levels that are found in spontaneous labor. At term, give higher infusion rates with great care; rates exceeding 9 to 10 milliunits/min rarely are required. Before term, when the sensitivity of the uterus is lower because of a lower concentration of oxytocin receptors, a higher infusion rate may be required.

Discontinuation of therapy: Discontinue the oxytocin infusion immediately in the event of uterine hyperactivity or fetal distress. Administer oxygen to the mother, who preferably should be put in a lateral position. Immediately evaluate the condition of the mother and fetus; take appropriate steps. If uterine contractions become too powerful, the infusion can be stopped abruptly; oxytocic stimulation of the uterine musculature will soon wane.

Postpartum uterine bleeding –

IV infusion: Add 10 to 40 units (maximum, 40 units) to 1,000 mL of a nonhydrating diluent and run at a rate necessary to control uterine atony.

Intramuscular: Administer 10 units intramuscular (IM) after delivery of the placenta.

➤*Preparation for administration:*

Reconstitution – Add oxytocin 1 mL (10 units) to 1,000 mL of 0.9% aqueous sodium chloride or Ringer's lactate. The solution contains 10 milliunits/mL (0.01 units/mL). Use a constant infusion pump to accurately control the rate of infusion.

Incomplete or inevitable abortion – Add oxytocin 10 units with 500 mL of physiologic saline solution or 5% dextrose in physiologic saline solution.

Postpartum uterine bleeding – Add 10 to 40 units (maximum, 40 units) to 1,000 mL of a nonhydrating diluent.

➤*Administration:*

Incomplete or inevitable abortion – Give by IV infusion at a rate of 10 to 20 milliunits (20 to 40 drops) per minute.

Induction or stimulation of labor – IV infusion (drip method) is the only acceptable method of parenteral administration for the induction or stimulation of labor. Accurate control of the rate of infusion flow is essential. An infusion pump or other device and frequent monitoring of strength, frequency, and duration of contractions, resting uterine tone, and fetal heart rate are necessary for the safe administration of oxytocin for the induction or stimulation of labor.

Postpartum uterine bleeding – Give by IV infusion or IM.

➤*Storage/Stability:*

Pitocin – Store at 2° to 8°C (36° to 46°F); may be held at 15° to 25°C (59° to 77°F) for up to 30 days. Discard after holding at 15° to 25°C (59° to 77°F).

Oxytocin – Store at controlled room temperature 15° to 30°C (59° to 86°F).

Actions

➤*Pharmacology:* Oxytocin acts on the smooth muscle of the uterus to stimulate contractions; response depends on the uterine threshold of excitability. It exerts a selective action on the smooth musculature of the uterus, particularly toward the end of pregnancy, during labor, and immediately following delivery. Oxytocin stimulates rhythmic contractions of the uterus, increases the frequency of existing contractions, and raises the tone of the uterine musculature.

➤*Pharmacokinetics:*

Absorption/Distribution – Oxytocin is distributed throughout the extracellular fluid. Small amounts of the drug probably reach the fetal circulation. Following IV administration, uterine response occurs almost immediately and subsides within 1 hour. Following IM injection, uterine response occurs within 3 to 5 minutes and persists for 2 to 3 hours.

Metabolism/Excretion – The plasma half-life is approximately 1 to 6 minutes, which is decreased in late pregnancy and lactation. Rapid removal from the plasma is accomplished mainly by the kidney and liver. Only small amounts are excreted in urine unchanged.

Contraindications

Significant cephalopelvic disproportion; unfavorable fetal positions or presentations that are undeliverable without conversion prior to delivery (eg, transverse lies); in obstetrical emergencies where the benefit-to-risk ratio for the fetus or the mother favors surgical intervention; cases of fetal distress where delivery is not imminent; prolonged use in uterine inertia or severe toxemia; hypertonic or hyperactive uterine patterns; where adequate uterine activity fails to achieve satisfactory progress; induction or augmentation of labor where vaginal delivery is contraindicated, such as invasive cervical carcinoma, active herpes genitalis, cord presentation or prolapse, total placenta previa, and vasa previa; hypersensitivity to the drug.

OXYTOCIN — INJECTION

Warnings/Precautions

➤*IV use:* When given for induction or augmentation of uterine activity, administer oxytocin only by the IV route and with adequate medical supervision in hospital. All patients receiving IV oxytocin must be under continuous observation by trained personnel who have a thorough knowledge of the drug and are qualified to identify complications.

➤*Special risk patients:* Except in unusual circumstances, do not administer oxytocin in the following conditions: fetal distress; hydramnios; partial placenta previa; prematurity; borderline cephalopelvic disproportion and any condition in which there is a predisposition for uterine rupture, such as previous major surgery on the cervix or uterus including cesarean section; overdistention of the uterus; grand multiparity; history of uterine sepsis or traumatic delivery; invasive cervical carcinoma. Weigh the potential benefits oxytocin can provide in a given case against rare but definite potential for the drug to produce hypertonicity or tetanic spasm.

➤*Maternal deaths:* Maternal deaths caused by hypertensive episodes, subarachnoid hemorrhage, or rupture of the uterus and fetal deaths caused by various causes have been associated with the use of parenteral oxytocic drugs for induction of labor or for augmentation in the first and second stages of labor.

➤*Uterine contractions:* When properly administered, oxytocin stimulates uterine contractions comparable with those in normal labor. Overstimulation of the uterus can be hazardous to the mother and fetus. Even with proper administration and adequate supervision, hypertonic contractions can occur in patients whose uteri are hypersensitive to oxytocin. Consider this fact in exercising judgment regarding patient selection.

➤*Water intoxication:* Oxytocin has an intrinsic antidiuretic effect, acting to increase water reabsorption from the glomerular filtrate. Consider the possibility of water intoxication, particularly when oxytocin is administered by continuous infusion and the patient is receiving fluids by mouth. Severe water intoxication with convulsions and coma has occurred and is associated with a slow infusion over a 24-hour period. Maternal death caused by oxytocin-induced water intoxication has been reported.

➤*Existent labor:* When oxytocin is used for induction or reinforcement of already existent labor, carefully select patients. Consider pelvic adequacy and maternal and fetal conditions before use of the drug.

➤*Pregnancy:* Category C. There are no known indications for use in the first and second trimester of pregnancy other than in relation to spontaneous or induced abortion. Oxytocin is not expected to present a risk of fetal abnormalities when used as indicated (see Adverse Reactions in the fetus).

➤*Lactation:* It is not known whether this drug is excreted in human milk. Because many drugs are excreted in human milk, exercise caution when administering to a nursing mother.

➤*Children:* Oxytocin is not intended for use in children.

➤*Monitoring:* During the induction or stimulation of labor, monitor fetal heart rate, resting uterine tone, and the frequency, duration, and force of contraction. Keep in mind the possibility of increased blood and afibrinogenemia when administering the drug. Monitor for signs of water intoxication (eg, drowsiness, listlessness, confusion, headache, anuria).

Electronic fetal monitoring provides the best means for early detection of overdosage (see Overdosage). However, keep in mind that only intrauterine pressure recording can accurately measure the intrauterine pressure during contractions. A fetal scalp electrode provides a more dependable recording of the fetal heart rate than any external monitoring system.

Drug Interactions

➤*QT prolongation:* An additive effect of oxytocin with other drugs that prolong the QT interval cannot be excluded. The following drugs may prolong the QT interval and increase the risk of life-threatening cardiac arrhythmias, including torsades de pointes: Antiarrhythmic agents (eg, amiodarone, bretylium, disopyramide, dofetilide, procainamide, quinidine, and sotalol), arsenic trioxide, chlorpromazine, cisapride, dolasetron, droperidol, mefloquine, mesoridazine, moxifloxacin, pentamidine, pimozide, tacrolimus, thioridazine, and ziprasidone. For a more complete list of drugs that may prolong the QT interval, see the appendix, Drug-Induced Prolongation of the QT Interval and Torsades de Pointes.

➤*Cyclopropane anesthesia:* Cyclopropane anesthesia may modify oxytocin's cardiovascular effects, producing unexpected results such as hypotension. Maternal sinus bradycardia with abnormal atrioventricular rhythms also has been noted when oxytocin was used concomitantly with cyclopropane anesthesia.

➤*Sympathomimetics:* If used concurrently with oxytocic drugs, the pressor effect of the sympathomimetics may be increased, possibly resulting in postpartum hypertension.

➤*Vasoconstrictors/caudal block anesthesia:* Severe hypertension occurred when oxytocin was given 3 to 4 hours following prophylactic administration of a vasoconstrictor in conjunction with caudal block anesthesia.

Adverse Reactions

➤*Maternal:*

Cardiovascular – Cardiac arrhythmia, hypertensive episodes, premature ventricular contractions.

GI – Nausea, vomiting.

GU – Pelvic hematoma, postpartum hemorrhage; rupture of the uterus, spasm, tetanic contraction, or uterine hypertonicity may occur from excessive dosage or hypersensitivity to the drug.

Miscellaneous – Anaphylactic reaction, fatal afibrinogenemia, subarachnoid hemorrhage; severe water intoxication with convulsions, coma, and death have been reported.

➤*Fetal or neonate (caused by induced uterine motility):*

Cardiovascular – Bradycardia, premature ventricular contractions, and other arrhythmias.

CNS – Permanent CNS or brain damage, neonatal seizures.

Miscellaneous – Fetal death, low Apgar scores at 5 minutes, neonatal jaundice, neonatal retinal hemorrhage.

Overdosage

➤*Symptoms:* Overdosage depends essentially on uterine hyperactivity, whether or not caused by hypersensitivity to this agent. Hyperstimulation with strong (hypertonic) or prolonged (tetanic) contractions or a resting tone of at least 15 to 20 mm H_2O between contractions can lead to tumultuous labor, uterine rupture, cervical and vaginal lacerations, postpartum hemorrhage, uteroplacental hypoperfusion, and variable deceleration of fetal heart, fetal hypoxia, hypercapnia, perinatal hepatic necrosis, or death. Water intoxication with convulsions, which is caused by the inherent antidiuretic effect of oxytocin, is a serious complication that may occur if large doses (40 to 50 milliunits/min) are infused for long periods.

➤*Treatment:* To treat, discontinue drug, restrict fluid intake, initiate diuresis, administer IV hypertonic saline solution, correct electrolyte imbalance, control convulsions, and provide supportive therapy.

ERGONOVINE MALEATE

Rx	**Ergotrate** (Pharmacist Pharmaceutical LLC)	**Tablets:** 0.2 mg	Mannitol. (HPS). White. In 100s, 500s, and 1,000s.

ERGONOVINE MALEATE — ORAL

Indications

➤*Postpartum/postabortal hemorrhage:* For the prevention and treatment of postpartum and postabortal hemorrhage caused by uterine atony.

➤*Off-label uses:* Oxytocin challenge test.

Administration and Dosage

➤*General dosing considerations:* The immediate postpartum dose of ergonovine is usually 0.2 mg. It is ordinarily administered parenterally.

➤*Adults:*

Postpartum/Postabortal hemorrhage –

Usual dosage: To minimize late postpartum bleeding, 1 or 2 tablets may be given orally 2 to 4 times daily (every 6 to 12 hours) until the danger of uterine atony has passed (usually 48 hours). Severe cramping is evidence of effectiveness but may justify reduction in dosage.

Duration of therapy: Usually 48 hours (until the danger of uterine atony has passed).

➤*Administration:* Tablets also may be administered sublingually.

➤*Storage/Stability:* Store at 15° to 30°C (59° to 86°F).

Actions

➤*Pharmacology:* Within 6 to 15 minutes, ergonovine produces a firm tetanic contraction of the postpartum uterus that, in the course of about 90 minutes, gradually changes to a series of clonic contractions that persist for another 90 minutes or more.

Contraindications

Induction of labor and in cases of threatened spontaneous abortion; do not administer to those patients who have shown allergic or idiosyncratic reactions to it.

Warnings/Precautions

➤*Duration:* As is the case with all ergot preparations, avoid prolonged use of ergonovine. Discontinue ergonovine if symptoms of ergotism appear.

➤*Vaginal bleeding:* Observe the character and amount of vaginal bleeding.

➤*Calcium deficiency:* Hypocalcemia may affect patient response to the drug. If the patient is not also taking digitalis, cautious administration of calcium gluconate IV may produce the desired oxytocic action.

ERGONOVINE MALEATE — ORAL

➤*Special risk:* Use ergonovine cautiously in patients with hypertension, heart disease, venoatrial shunts, mitral-valve stenosis, obliterative vascular disease, sepsis, or hepatic or renal impairment.

➤*Pregnancy:* Category X.

Uterine effects – All oxytocic agents are potentially dangerous. Mothers and infants have been injured, and some have died because of their injudicious use. Hyperstimulation of the uterus during labor may lead to uterine tetany and marked impairment of the uteroplacental blood flow, uterine rupture, cervical and perineal lacerations, amniotic fluid embolism, and trauma to the infant (eg, hypoxia, intracranial hemorrhage). Because of hazards that result from overdosage, oxytocic agents must be administered under conditions of meticulous observation.

Labor and delivery – Because of the high uterine tone produced, ergonovine is not recommended for routine use prior to the delivery of the placenta unless the operator is versed in the technique described by Davis and others and has adequate facilities and personnel at his disposal.

➤*Lactation:* Ergonovine given in the immediate postpartum period lowers serum basal prolactin and possibly suckling-induced prolactin increases. It also appears to decrease the rate of breast-feeding. Ergonovine is probably best avoided in mothers who wish to nurse, relying instead on suckling-induced oxytocin release to hasten uterine involution. The prolactin level in a mother with established lactation may not affect her ability to breast-feed.

➤*Monitoring:* Monitor blood pressure, pulse, and uterine response. Note sudden changes in vital signs or frequent periods of uterine relaxation.

Adverse Reactions

Nausea and vomiting may occur, but they are uncommon. Allergic phenomena, including shock, have been reported. Ergotism has also been reported. Elevation of blood pressure (sometimes extreme) may appear in a small percentage of patients, most frequently in association with regional anesthesia (caudal or spinal), previous administration of a vasoconstrictor, and the IV route of administration of the oxytocic. The mechanism of such hypertension is obscure because it may occur in the absence of anesthesia, vasoconstrictors, and oxytocics. These elevations are no more frequent with ergonovine than with other oxytocics. They usually subside promptly following IV administration of 15 mg chlorpromazine.

Overdosage

➤*Symptoms:* The principal manifestations of serious overdosage are convulsions and gangrene. Symptoms of overdosage include the following: vomiting, diarrhea, dizziness, rise or fall in blood pressure, weak pulse, dyspnea, loss of consciousness, numbness and coldness of the extremities, tingling, pain in the chest, gangrene of the fingers and toes, and hypercoagulability.

➤*Treatment:* Treat convulsions. Control hypercoagulability by the administration of heparin, and maintain blood-clotting time at approximately 3 times the normal. Give a vasodilator such as tolazine as an antidote; the rate of administration may be controlled by monitoring pulse rate and blood pressure. For emergency measures, delay absorption of ingested ergonovine by giving tap water, milk, or activated charcoal and then removing by gastric lavage or emesis followed by catharsis. Gangrene will require surgical amputation.

METHYLERGONOVINE MALEATE

Rx	**Methergine** (Sandoz)	**Tablets; oral:** 0.2 mg	Lactose, FD&C Blue No.1, parabens, sucrose. (78-54 SANDOZ). Orchid, round. In 100s.
Rx	**Methylergonovine** (PharmaForce)	**Injection, solution:** 0.2 mg/mL	In 1 mL vials.
Rx	**Methergine** (Sandoz)		In 1 mL ampuls.

METHYLERGONOVINE MALEATE — ORAL

Indications

➤*Uterine contractions/bleeding:* For routine management after delivery of the placenta; postpartum atony and hemorrhage; subinvolution. Under full obstetric supervision, it may be given in the second stage of labor following delivery of the anterior shoulder.

Administration and Dosage

➤*General dosing considerations:* Under full obstetric supervision, methylergonovine maleate may be given in the second stage of labor following delivery of the anterior shoulder.

➤*Adults:*

Uterine bleeding – 1 tablet (0.2 mg) 3 or 4 times daily in the puerperium for a maximum of 1 week.

Uterine contractions – See Uterine bleeding.

Subinvolution – See Uterine bleeding.

➤*Storage/Stability:* Store tablets below 25°C (77°F) in a tight, light-resistant container.

Actions

➤*Pharmacology:* Methylergonovine maleate acts directly on the smooth muscle of the uterus and increases the tone, rate, and amplitude of rhythmic contractions. Thus, it induces a rapid and sustained tetanic uterotonic effect which shortens the third stage of labor and reduces blood loss. The onset of action after oral administration is 5 to 10 minutes.

➤*Pharmacokinetics:*

Absorption/Distribution – The bioavailability after oral administration was reported to be about 60%, with no accumulation after repeated doses.

Bioavailability studies conducted in fasting, healthy female volunteers have shown that oral absorption of a 0.2 mg methylergonovine tablet was fairly rapid, with a mean peak plasma concentration of 3,243 ± 1,308 pg/mL observed at 1.12 ± 0.82 hours. The extent of absorption of the tablet, based upon methylergonovine plasma concentrations, was found to be equivalent to that of the IM solution given orally, and the extent of oral absorption of the IM solution was proportional to the dose following administration of 0.1, 0.2, and 0.4 mg. The volume of distribution (Vd_{ss}/F) of methylergonovine was calculated to be 56.1 ± 17 L, and the plasma clearance (CLp/F) was calculated to be 14.4 ± 4.5 L/hr. A delayed GI absorption (t_{max} about 3 hours) of methylergonovine maleate tablet might be observed in postpartum women during continuous treatment with this oxytocic agent.

Metabolism/Excretion – Ergot alkaloids are mostly eliminated by hepatic metabolism and excretion, and the decrease in bioavailability following oral administration is probably a result of first-pass metabolism in the liver.

The plasma level decline was biphasic with a mean elimination half-life of 3.39 hours (range, 1.5 to 12.7 hours).

Contraindications

Certain ergot alkaloid drugs (eg, dihydroergotamine, ergotamine) are contraindicated for concomitant use with potent CYP3A4 inhibitors (eg, protease inhibitors, macrolide antibiotics, azole antifungals) because of the risk of vasospasm leading to cerebral ischemia and/or ischemia of the extremities. Although there have been no reports of such interactions with methylergonovine alone, potent CYP3A4 inhibitors should not be used concomitantly with methylergonovine.

Hypertension, toxemia, pregnancy, and hypersensitivity.

Warnings/Precautions

➤*CYP3A4 inhibitors (eg, macrolide antibiotics and protease inhibitors):* There have been rare reports of serious adverse events in connection with the coadministration of certain ergot alkaloid drugs (eg, dihydroergotamine and ergotamine) and potent CYP3A4 inhibitors, resulting in vasospasm leading to cerebral ischemia and/or ischemia of the extremities. Although there have been no reports of such interactions with methylergonovine alone, potent CYP3A4 inhibitors should not be coadministered with methylergonovine.

➤*Special risk:* Exercise caution should be in the presence of sepsis, obliterative vascular disease, hepatic or renal involvement. Also use with caution during the second stage of labor. The necessity for manual removal of a retained placenta should occur only rarely with proper technique and adequate allowance of time for its spontaneous separation.

➤*Pregnancy:* Category C. Animal reproductive studies have not been conducted with methylergonovine maleate. It is also not known whether methylergonovine maleate can cause fetal harm or can affect reproductive capacity. Use of methylergonovine maleate is contraindicated during pregnancy because of its uterotonic effects.

Labor and delivery – The uterotonic effect of methylergonovine maleate is utilized after delivery to assist involution and decrease hemorrhage, shortening the third stage of labor.

➤*Lactation:* Methylergonovine maleate may be administered orally for a maximum of 1 week postpartum to control uterine bleeding. Recommended dosage is 1 tablet (0.2 mg) 3 or 4 times daily. At this dosage level, a small quantity of drug appears in mothers' milk. Caution should be exercised when methylergonovine maleate is administered to a nursing woman.

➤*Children:* Safety and efficacy in children patients have not been established.

Drug Interactions

➤*CYP3A4 inhibitors:* Methylergonovine should not be coadministered with potent CYP3A4 inhibitors. Examples of some of the more potent CYP3A4 inhibitors include macrolide antibiotics (eg, clarithromycin, erythromycin, troleandomycin), HIV protease or reverse transcriptase inhibitors (eg, delavirdine, indinavir, nelfinavir, ritonavir) or azole antifungals (eg, ketoconazole, itraconazole, voriconazole). Less potent CYP3A4 inhibitors should be administered with caution. Less potent inhibitors include saquinavir, nefazodone, fluconazole, grapefruit juice, fluoxetine, fluvoxamine, zileuton, and clotrimazole. These lists are not exhaustive, and the prescriber should consider the effects on CYP3A4 of other agents being considered for concomitant use with methylergonovine (see Warnings).

➤*Vasoconstrictors/Ergot alkaloids:* Exercise caution when methylergonovine maleate is used concurrently with other vasoconstrictors or ergot alkaloids.

METHYLERGONOVINE MALEATE — ORAL

Adverse Reactions

The most common adverse reaction is hypertension associated in several cases with seizure or headache. Hypotension has also been reported. Nausea and vomiting have occurred occasionally. Rarely observed reactions have included, in order of severity: acute myocardial infarction, transient chest pains, dyspnea, hematuria, thrombophlebitis, water intoxication, hallucinations, leg cramps, dizziness, tinnitus, nasal congestion, diarrhea, diaphoresis, palpitation, and foul taste.

There have been rare isolated reports of anaphylaxis, without a proven causal relationship to the drug product.

Overdosage

Because reports of overdosage with methylergonovine maleate are infrequent, the lethal dose in humans has not been established. The oral LD_{50} (in mg/kg) for the mouse is 187, the rat, 93, and the rabbit, 4.5. Several cases of accidental methylergonovine maleate injection in newborn infants have been reported, and, in such cases, 0.2 mg represents an overdose of great magnitude. However, recovery occurred in all but 1 case following a period of respiratory depression, hypothermia, hypertonicity with jerking movements, and, in 1 case, a single convulsion.

Also, several children 1 to 3 years of age have accidentally ingested up to 10 tablets (2 mg) with no apparent ill effects. A postpartum patient took 4 tablets at 1 time in error and reported paresthesias and clamminess as her only symptoms.

➤*Symptoms:* Symptoms of acute overdose may include the following: abdominal pain, nausea, numbness, tingling of the extremities, vomiting, rise in blood pressure, in severe cases followed by coma, convulsions, hypotension, hypothermia, and respiratory depression.

➤*Treatment:* Treatment of acute overdosage is symptomatic and includes the following usual procedures of: removal of offending drug by inducing emesis, gastric lavage, catharsis, and supportive diuresis; maintenance of adequate pulmonary ventilation, especially if convulsions or coma develop; correction of hypotension with pressor drugs as needed; control of convulsions with standard anticonvulsant agents; control of peripheral vasospasm with warmth to the extremities if needed.

METHYLERGONOVINE MALEATE — INJECTION

Indications

➤*Uterine contractions/bleeding:* For routine management after delivery of the placenta; postpartum atony and hemorrhage; subinvolution. Under full obstetric supervision, it may be given in the second stage of labor following delivery of the anterior shoulder.

Administration and Dosage

➤*Adults:*

Uterine contractions/bleeding –

Usual dosage:

• *Intramuscular* – 1 mL (0.2 mg) after delivery of the anterior shoulder, after delivery of the placenta, or during the puerperium. May be repeated as required, at intervals of 2 to 4 hours.

• *Intravenous* – Dosage is the same as intramuscular (IM). This drug should not be administered intravenously (IV) routinely because of the possibility of inducing sudden hypertensive and cerebrovascular accidents.

If IV administration is considered essential as a lifesaving measure, methylergonovine maleate should be given slowly over a period of no less than 60 seconds with careful monitoring of blood pressure. Intra-arterial or periarterial injection should be strictly avoided.

➤*Administration:* Administer only if solution is clear and colorless.

➤*Storage/Stability:*

Ampuls – Store in refrigerator, 2° to 8°C (36° to 46°F). Protect from light.

Actions

➤*Pharmacology:* Methylergonovine maleate injection acts directly on the smooth muscle of the uterus and increases the tone, rate, and amplitude of rhythmic contractions. Thus, it induces a rapid and sustained tetanic uterotonic effect which shortens the third stage of labor and reduces blood loss. The onset of action after IV administration is immediate; after IM administration, it is 2 to 5 minutes.

➤*Pharmacokinetics:*

Absorption/Distribution – Pharmacokinetic studies following an IV injection have shown that methylergonovine is rapidly distributed from plasma to peripheral tissues within 2 to 3 minutes or less. During delivery, with IM injection, bioavailability increased to 78%.

For a 0.2 mg IM injection, a mean peak plasma concentration of 5,918 ± 1,952 pg/mL was observed at 0.41 ± 0.21 hours. When given IM, the extent of absorption of methylergonovine maleate solution was about 25% greater than the tablet. The volume of distribution (Vd_{ss}/F) of methylergonovine was calculated to be 56.1 ± 17 L, and the plasma clearance (CLp/F) was calculated to be 14.4 ± 4.5 L/hr.

Metabolism/Excretion – The plasma level decline was biphasic with a mean elimination half-life of 3.39 hours (range 1.5 to 12.7 hours). Ergot alkaloids are mostly eliminated by hepatic metabolism and excretion, and the decrease in bioavailability following oral administration is probably a result of first-pass metabolism in the liver.

Contraindications

Certain ergot alkaloid drugs (eg, dihydroergotamine and ergotamine) are contraindicated for concomitant use with potent CYP3A4 inhibitors (eg, protease inhibitors, macrolide antibiotics, azole antifungals) because of the risk of vasospasm leading to cerebral ischemia and/or ischemia of the extremities. Although there have been no reports of such interactions with methylergonovine alone, potent CYP3A4 inhibitors should not be used concomitantly with methylergonovine.

Hypertension; toxemia; pregnancy; and hypersensitivity.

Warnings/Precautions

➤*Administration:* This drug should not be administered IV routinely because of the possibility of inducing sudden hypertensive and cerebrovascular accidents. If IV administration is considered essential as a lifesaving measure, methylergonovine maleate should be given slowly over a period of no less than 60 seconds with careful monitoring of blood pressure. Intra-arterial or periarterial injection should be strictly avoided.

➤*CYP3A4 inhibitors (eg, macrolide antibiotics and protease inhibitors):* There have been rare reports of serious adverse events in connection with the coadministration of certain ergot alkaloid drugs (eg, dihydroergotamine and ergotamine) and potent CYP3A4 inhibitors, resulting in vasospasm leading to cerebral ischemia and/or ischemia of the extremities. Although there have been no reports of such interactions with methylergonovine alone, potent CYP3A4 inhibitors should not be coadministered with methylergonovine.

➤*Special risk:* Exercised caution in the presence of sepsis, obliterative vascular disease, hepatic or renal involvement. Also use with caution during the second stage of labor. The necessity for manual removal of a retained placenta should occur only rarely with proper technique and adequate allowance of time for its spontaneous separation.

➤*Pregnancy:* *Category C.* Animal reproductive studies have not been conducted with methylergonovine maleate. It is also not known whether methylergonovine maleate can cause fetal harm or can affect reproductive capacity. Use of methylergonovine maleate is contraindicated during pregnancy because of its uterotonic effects.

Labor and delivery – The uterotonic effect of methylergonovine maleate is utilized after delivery to assist involution and decrease hemorrhage, shortening the third stage of labor.

➤*Lactation:* Methylergonovine maleate may be administered orally for a maximum of 1 week postpartum to control uterine bleeding. Recommended dosage is 1 tablet (0.2 mg) 3 or 4 times daily. At this dosage level a small quantity of drug appears in mothers' milk. Caution should be exercised when methylergonovine maleate is administered to a nursing woman.

➤*Children:* Safety and efficacy in children have not been established.

Drug Interactions

➤*CYP3A4 inhibitors:* Methylergonovine should not be coadministered with potent CYP3A4 inhibitors. Examples of some of the more potent CYP3A4 inhibitors include macrolide antibiotics (eg, clarithromycin, erythromycin, troleandomycin), HIV protease or reverse transcriptase inhibitors (eg, delavirdine, indinavir, nelfinavir, ritonavir) or azole antifungals (eg, itraconazole, ketoconazole, voriconazole). Less potent CYP3A4 inhibitors should be administered with caution. Less potent inhibitors include saquinavir, nefazodone, fluconazole, grapefruit juice, fluoxetine, fluvoxamine, zileuton, and clotrimazole. These lists are not exhaustive, and the prescriber should consider the effects on CYP3A4 of other agents being considered for concomitant use with methylergonovine (see Warnings).

➤*Vasoconstrictors/Ergo alkaloids:* Exercise caution when methylergonovine maleate injection is used concurrently with other vasoconstrictors or ergot alkaloids.

Adverse Reactions

The most common adverse reaction is hypertension associated in several cases with seizure or headache. Hypotension has also been reported. Nausea and vomiting have occurred occasionally. Rarely observed reactions have included, in order of severity: Acute myocardial infarction, transient chest pains, dyspnea, hematuria, thrombophlebitis, water intoxication, hallucinations, leg cramps, dizziness, tinnitus, nasal congestion, diarrhea, diaphoresis, palpitation, and foul taste.

There have been rare, isolated reports of anaphylaxis, without a proven causal relationship to the drug product.

Overdosage

Because reports of overdosage with methylergonovine maleate are infrequent, the lethal dose in humans has not been established. The oral LD_{50} (in mg/kg) for the mouse is 187, the rat, 93, and the rabbit, 4.5. Several cases of accidental methylergonovine maleate injection in newborn infants have been reported, and, in such cases, 0.2 mg represents an overdose of great magnitude. However, recovery occurred in all but 1 case following a period of respiratory depression, hypothermia, hypertonicity with jerking movements, and, in 1 case, a single convulsion.

Also, several children 1 to 3 years of age have accidentally ingested up to 10 tablets (2 mg) with no apparent ill effects. A postpartum patient took 4 tablets at 1 time in error, and reported paresthesias and clamminess as her only symptoms.

METHYLERGONOVINE MALEATE — INJECTION

➤*Symptoms:* Symptoms of acute overdose may include the following: nausea, vomiting, abdominal pain, numbness, tingling of the extremities, rise in blood pressure, in severe cases followed by hypotension, respiratory depression, hypothermia, convulsions, and coma.

➤*Treatment:* Treatment of acute overdosage is symptomatic and includes the usual procedures of the following: removal of offending drug by inducing emesis, gastric lavage, catharsis, and supportive diuresis; maintenance of adequate pulmonary ventilation, especially if convulsions or coma develop; correction of hypotension with pressor drugs as needed; control of convulsions with standard anticonvulsant agents; control of peripheral vasospasm with warmth to the extremities if needed.

BISPHOSPHONATES

Indications

➤*Glucocorticoid-induced osteoporosis (alendronate, risedronate immediate release, zoledronic acid):* For the prevention and treatment of glucocorticoid-induced osteoporosis in men and women who are either initiating or continuing systemic glucocorticoid treatment for chronic diseases.

➤*Heterotopic ossification (etidronate):* Prevention and treatment of heterotopic ossification following total hip replacement or caused by spinal injury.

➤*Hypercalcemia of malignancy :* For the treatment of hypercalcemia of malignancy (HCM) (**zoledronic acid**); in conjunction with adequate hydration (eg, saline hydration, with or without loop diuretics) for the treatment of moderate or severe hypercalcemia associated with malignancy with or without bone metastases (**pamidronate**; patients with epidermoid or non-epidermoid tumors respond to pamidronate).

➤*Multiple myeloma and bone metastases of solid tumors (zoledronic acid):* For the treatment of patients with multiple myeloma and patients with documented bone metastases from solid tumors in conjunction with standard antineoplastic therapy. Prostate cancer should have progressed after treatment with at least 1 hormonal therapy.

➤*Osteolytic bone metastases / lesions (pamidronate):* In conjunction with standard antineoplastic therapy for the treatment of osteolytic bone metastases of breast cancer and osteolytic lesions of multiple myeloma.

➤*Osteoporosis in men (alendronate, risedronate immediate release, zoledronic acid):* To increase bone mass in men with osteoporosis.

➤*Osteoporosis in postmenopausal women (alendronate, oral ibandronate, risedronate, zoledronic acid):* For the treatment and prevention of osteoporosis in postmenopausal women. Intravenous (IV) **ibandronate** and **risedronate** delayed release are indicated for treatment only.

➤*Paget disease (osteitis deformans):* For treatment of patients with Paget disease of bone having alkaline phosphatase at least 2 times the upper limit of normal (ULN), or those who are symptomatic or at risk for future complications from their disease (**alendronate**, **tiludronate**, **zoledronic acid**); treatment of symptomatic Paget disease (**etidronate**); treatment of moderate to severe Paget disease (**pamidronate**, **risedronate** immediate release).

➤*Off-label uses:* Refer to individual monographs for further information.

Bone metastases –
Ibandronate: [1] = Good documentation.

Hypercalcemia of malignancy –
Alendronate: [5] = Poor documentation.
Ibandronate: [2] = Fair documentation.
Risedronate: [5] = Poor documentation.

Hyperparathyroidism –
Pamidronate: [2] = Fair documentation.

Hypervitaminosis D (infants / children) –
Alendronate: [4] = Insufficient documentation.

Immobilization-related hypercalcemia –
Pamidronate: [2] = Fair documentation.

Multiple myeloma –
Ibandronate: [5] = Poor documentation.

Primary hyperparathyroidism –
Risedronate: [4] = Insufficient documentation.

Osteogenesis imperfecta –
Alendronate (adults): [2] = Fair documentation.
Alendronate (children): [2] = Fair documentation.

Osteopenia in androgen-deprived prostate cancer patients –
Zoledronic acid: [1] = Good documentation.

Osteopenia in estrogen-deprived breast cancer patients –
Zoledronic acid: [1] = Good documentation.

Osteoporosis with spinal cord injury –
Alendronate: [4] = Insufficient documentation.
Etidronate: [4] = Insufficient documentation.
Pamidronate: [4] = Insufficient documentation.
Tiludronate: [4] = Insufficient documentation.

Postoperative knee arthroplasty –
Alendronate: [2] = Fair documentation.

Prevention of glucocorticoid-induced osteoporosis –
Pamidronate: [2] = Fair documentation.

Prevention of postrenal transplant bone loss –
Ibandronate: [1] = Good documentation.
Zoledronic acid: [4] = Insufficient documentation.

Other possible off-label uses –
Etidronate: Prevention of corticosteroid-induced osteoporosis.
Ibandronate: Prevention and treatment of metastatic bone disease in breast cancer.
Pamidronate: Postmenopausal osteoporosis; reduce bone pain in patients with prostatic carcinoma.

Actions

➤*Pharmacology:* **Etidronate**, **tiludronate**, **pamidronate**, **risedronate**, **ibandronate**, **alendronate**, and **zoledronic acid** are bisphosphonates that act primarily on the bone. Their major pharmacologic action is the inhibition of normal and abnormal bone resorption. Secondarily, etidronate reduces bone formation because formation is coupled to resorption; pamidronate inhibits bone resorption, apparently without inhibiting bone formation and mineralization. Alendronate shows preferential localization to sites of bone resorption, specifically under osteoclasts. The osteoclasts adhere normally to the bone surface but lack the ruffled border that is indicative of active resorption. Alendronate does not interfere with osteoclast recruitment or attachment, but it does inhibit osteoclast activity. Tiludronate disodium appears to inhibit osteoclasts through at least 2 mechanisms: disruption of the cytoskeletal ring structure, possibly by inhibition of protein-tyrosine-phosphatase, thus leading to detachment of osteoclasts from the bone surface and the inhibition of the osteoclastic proton pump. Ibandronate also inhibits osteoclast activity, reducing the elevated rate of bone turnover leading to, on average, a net gain of bone mass.

Reduction of abnormal bone resorption is responsible for therapeutic benefit in hypercalcemia. The exact mechanism(s) is not fully understood, but may be related to inhibition of hydroxyapatite crystal dissolution or its action on bone-resorbing cells. Pamidronate inhibits accelerated bone resorption resulting from osteoclast hyperactivity induced by various tumors in animals. The number of osteoclasts in active bone turnover sites is substantially reduced after etidronate. Etidronate also can inhibit formation and growth of hydroxyapatite crystals and their amorphous precursors at concentrations in excess of those required to inhibit crystal dissolution.

Alendronate – As a result of bone resorption inhibition, asymptomatic reductions in serum calcium and phosphate concentrations are seen after treatment with alendronate. In long-term studies, reductions from baseline in serum calcium (approximately 2%) and phosphate (approximately 4% to 6%) were seen the first month after initiation of alendronate 10 mg, but no further decreases were seen for the 5-year duration of the studies. The reduction in serum phosphate may reflect not only the positive bone mineral balance caused by alendronate but also a decrease in renal phosphate reabsorption. Alendronate decreases the rate of bone resorption directly, leading to an indirect decrease in bone formation.

In Paget disease, alendronate 40 mg once daily for 6 months produced highly significant decreases in serum alkaline phosphatase as well as in urinary markers of bone collagen degradation. As a result of the inhibition of bone resorption, alendronate induced generally mild, transient, and asymptomatic decreases in serum calcium and phosphate.

Etidronate – Etidronate does not appear to alter renal tubular reabsorption of calcium and does not affect hypercalcemia in patients with hyperparathyroidism in which increased calcium reabsorption may be a factor in hypercalcemia. Hyperphosphatemia has been observed with oral etidronate, usually with dosages of 10 to 20 mg/kg/day; no adverse effects have been noted, and it is not a contraindication. It is apparently caused by drug-related increased phosphate tubular reabsorption by the kidneys. Serum phosphate levels generally return to normal 2 to 4 weeks after therapy.

In Paget disease, etidronate slows accelerated bone turnover (resorption and accretion) in pagetic lesions and to a lesser extent, in normal bone. Reduced bone turnover is often accompanied by symptomatic improvement, including reduced bone pain. Incidence of pagetic fractures may decrease, and elevated cardiac output and other vascular disorders improve.

Ibandronate – Treatment with ibandronate 2.5 mg daily resulted in decreases in biochemical markers of bone turnover, including urinary C-terminal telopeptide of type 1 collagen (uCTX) and serum osteocalcin, to levels similar to those in premenopausal women. Changes in markers of bone formation were observed later than changes in resorption markers, as expected, because of the coupled nature of bone resorption and formation. Treatment with ibandronate 2.5 mg daily decreased levels of uCTX within 1 month of starting treatment and decreased levels of osteocalcin within 3 months.

Pamidronate – Pamidronate therapy has decreased serum phosphate levels, presumably caused by decreased release of phosphate from bone and increased renal excretion as parathyroid hormone levels (usually suppressed in HCM) return toward normal. Phosphate therapy was administered in 30% of patients; levels usually returned to normal within 7 to 10 days.

Urinary calcium/creatinine and urinary hydroxyproline/creatinine ratios decrease and usually return to normal or below after treatment. The changes occur within the first week after treatment, as do decreases in serum calcium levels.

Risedronate – In pagetic patients treated with risedronate 30 mg/day for 2 months, bone turnover returned to normal in a majority of patients, as evidenced by significant reductions in serum alkaline phosphatase, a marker of bone formation, and in urinary hydroxyproline/creatinine and deoxypyridinoline/creatinine, markers of bone resorption. Radiographic structural changes of bone lesions, especially improvement of a majority of lesions with an osteolytic front in weightbearing bones, also were observed. In addition, histomorphometric data provide further support that risedronate decreases the extent of osteolysis in the appendicular and axial skeleton. Osteolytic lesions in the lower extremities improved or were unchanged in 15 of 16 (94%) assessed patients; 9 of 16 (56%) patients showed clear improvement in osteolytic lesions. No evidence of new fractures was observed.

Tiludronate – In pagetic patients treated with tiludronate 400 mg/day for 3 months, changes in urinary hydroxyproline, a biochemical marker of bone resorption and in serum alkaline phosphatase, a marker of bone formation, indicate a reduction toward normal in the rate of bone turnover. In addition, reduced numbers of osteoclasts by histomorphometric analysis and radiological improvement of lytic lesions indicate that tiludronate can suppress the pagetic disease process.

Zoledronic acid – In vitro, zoledronic acid inhibits osteoclastic activity and induces osteoclast apoptosis. Zoledronic acid also blocks the osteoclastic resorption of mineralized bone and cartilage through its binding to bone. Zoledronic acid inhibits the increased osteoclastic activity and skeletal calcium release induced by various stimulatory factors released by tumors.

➤*Pharmacokinetics:*

Alendronate – There is no evidence that alendronate is metabolized. Relative to an IV reference dose, mean oral bioavailability in women was 0.64% for 5 to 70 mg doses after an overnight fast and 2 hours before a standardized breakfast. Oral bioavailability of the 10 mg tablet in men (0.59%) was similar to that in women given after an overnight fast and 2 hours before breakfast. In 49 postmenopausal women, bioavailability was decreased by approximately 40% when 10 mg was given 30 minutes or 1 hour before a standardized breakfast compared with dosing 2 hours before eating. Bioavailability was negligible whether alendronate was given with or up to 2 hours after a standardized breakfast. Concomitant coffee or orange juice reduced bioavailability by approximately 60%. Mean steady-state volume of distribution (exclusive of bone) is at least 28 L. Protein binding in plasma is approximately 78%. After a single IV dose, approximately 50% was excreted in the urine with little or none recovered in the feces. After a single 10 mg IV dose, renal clearance was 71 mL/min; systemic clearance did not exceed 200 mL/min. Plasma levels fell by more than 95% within 6 hours after IV administration. The terminal half-life is estimated to exceed 10 years, probably reflecting alendronate release from the skeleton. Based on the above, it is estimated that after 10 years of 10 mg/day orally, the amount of alendronate released daily from the skeleton is approximately 25% of that absorbed from the GI tract.

Etidronate – Etidronate is not metabolized. The amount of drug absorbed after an oral dose is approximately 3%. In healthy subjects, the plasma half-life of etidronate, based on noncompartmental pharmacokinetics, is 1 to 6 hours. Within 24 hours, about 50% of the absorbed dose is excreted in urine; the remainder is distributed to bone compartments from which it is slowly eliminated. Animal studies have yielded bone clearance estimates of up to 165 days. In humans, the residence time on bone may vary due to factors such as specific metabolic condition and bone type. Unabsorbed drug is excreted intact in feces. Preclinical studies indicate etidronate disodium does not cross the blood-brain barrier.

Ibandronate – The absorption of oral ibandronate occurs in the upper GI tract. Following oral dosing, the time to maximum observed plasma ibandronate concentrations ranged from 0.5 to 2 hours (median, 1 hour) in fasted healthy postmenopausal women. The mean oral bioavailability of ibandronate 2.5 mg was approximately 0.6% compared with IV dosing. After absorption, ibandronate either binds rapidly to bone or is excreted into urine. In humans, the apparent terminal volume of distribution is at least 90 L, and the amount of dose removed from the circulation via the bone is estimated to be 40% to 50% of the circulating dose. In vitro protein binding in human serum was 99.5% to 90.9% over an ibandronate concentration range of 2 to 10 ng/mL in 1 study and approximately 85.7% over a concentration range of 0.5 to 10 ng/mL in another study. Ibandronate dose not undergo hepatic metabolism. The portion of ibandronate that is not removed from the circulation via bone absorption is eliminated unchanged by the kidney (approximately 50% to 60% of the absorbed dose). Unabsorbed ibandronate is eliminated unchanged in the feces. The observed apparent terminal half-life for the ibandronate 150 mg tablet upon oral administration to healthy postmenopausal women ranges from 37 to 157 hours. Total clearance of ibandronate is low, with average values in the range of 84 to 160 mL/min.

Pamidronate – Cancer patients (n = 24) who had minimal or no bony involvement were given an IV infusion of pamidronate 30, 60, or 90 mg of over 4 hours and pamidronate 90 mg over 24 hours. The mean ± standard deviation (SD) body retention of pamidronate was calculated to be 54% ± 16% of the dose over 120 hours.

Pamidronate is not metabolized and is exclusively eliminated by renal excretion. After administration of pamidronate 30, 60, and 90 mg over 4 hours and pamidronate 90 mg over 24 hours, an overall mean ± SD of 46% ± 16% of the drug was excreted unchanged in the urine within 120 hours. Cumulative urinary excretion was linearly related to dose. The mean ± SD elimination half-life is 28 ± 7 hours. Mean ± SD total and renal clearances of pamidronate were 107 ± 50 mL/min and 49 ± 28 mL/min, respectively. The rate of elimination from bone has not been determined.

After IV administration in rats, approximately 50% to 60% was rapidly adsorbed by bone and slowly eliminated by the kidneys. In rats given 10 mg/kg bolus injections, approximately 30% of the compound was found in the liver shortly after administration and was then redistributed to bone or eliminated by the kidneys over 24 to 48 hours. The drug was rapidly cleared from circulation and taken up mainly by bones, liver, spleen, teeth, and tracheal cartilage. Bone uptake occurred preferentially in areas of high bone turnover. The terminal phase of elimination half-life in bone was approximately 300 days.

Risedronate – Like other bisphosphonates, no evidence supports systemic metabolism of risedronate. Absorption is relatively rapid (time to maximal concentration [T_{max}] of approximately 1 hour for immediate release and 3 hours for delayed release) and is independent of dose. Mean oral bioavailability is 0.63%. Dosing for the immediate-release tablet either 30 minutes prior to breakfast or 2 hours after dinner reduces the extent of absorption by 55% compared with the fasting state. Dosing 1 hour prior to breakfast reduces the extent of absorption by 30% compared with dosing in the fasting state. The bioavailability of delayed-release risedronate 35 mg decreased by approximately 30% when administered immediately after a high-fat breakfast compared with administration in the morning 4 hours before a meal.

Animal studies indicate that approximately 60% of the dose is distributed to bone, with the remainder excreted in the urine. The mean steady-state volume of distribution is 13.8 L/kg; plasma protein binding is approximately 24%.

Approximately 50% of the absorbed dose is excreted in urine within 24 hours, and 85% of an IV dose is recovered in the urine over 28 days. Mean renal clearance is 105 mL/min and mean total clearance is 122 mL/min, with the difference primarily reflecting nonrenal clearance or clearance caused by adsorption to bone. The renal clearance is not concentration dependent, and there is a linear relationship between renal clearance and creatinine clearance. Unabsorbed drug is eliminated unchanged in feces. The terminal exponential half-life was 561 hours.

Tiludronate – In animals, tiludronic acid undergoes little, if any, metabolism. In vitro, tiludronic acid is not metabolized in human liver microsomes and hepatocytes.

Relative to IV reference dose, the mean oral bioavailability of tiludronate disodium in healthy men was 6% after an oral dose equivalent to 400 mg of tiludronic acid administered after an overnight fast and 4 hours before a standard breakfast. Bioavailability is reduced by food.

After administration of a single dose equivalent to 400 mg of tiludronic acid to healthy men, tiludronic acid was rapidly absorbed, with peak plasma concentrations of approximately 3 mg/L occurring within 2 hours. In pagetic patients, after repeated administration of doses equivalent to 400 mg/day of tiludronic acid (2 hours before or 2 hours after a meal) for durations of 12 days to 12 weeks, average plasma concentrations of tiludronic acid occurring between 1 and 2 hours after dosing ranged between 1 and 4.6 mg/L.

After oral administration of doses equivalent to 400 mg/day of tiludronic acid to nonpagetic patients with osteoarthrosis, the steady state in bone was not reached after 30 days of dosing. At plasma concentrations between 1 and 10 mg/L, tiludronic acid was approximately 90% bound to human serum protein (mainly albumin).

The principal route of elimination of tiludronic acid is in the urine. After IV administration to healthy volunteers, approximately 60% of the dose was excreted in the urine as tiludronic acid within 13 days. Renal clearance is dose independent and is approximately 10 mL/min in healthy subjects. In pagetic patients treated with doses equivalent to 400 mg/day of tiludronic acid for 12 days, the mean apparent plasma elimination half-life was approximately 150 hours. The elimination rate from human bone is unknown.

Zoledronic acid – Single or multiple (every 28 days) 5- or 15-minute infusions of zoledronic acid 2, 4, 8, or 16 mg were given to 64 patients with cancer and bone metastases. The postinfusion decline of zoledronic acid concentrations in plasma was consistent with a triphasic process, showing a rapid decrease from peak concentrations at end of infusion to less than 1% of maximal plasma concentration (C_{max}) 24 hours postinfusion with population half-lives of $t_{½alpha}$ 0.24 hours and $t_{½beta}$ 1.87 hours for the early disposition phases of the drug. the terminal elimination phase of the postinfusion, and a terminal elimination half-life $t_{½gamma}$ of 146 hours. The AUC_{0-24h} of zoledronic acid was dose proportional from 2 to 16 mg. The accumulation of zoledronic acid measured over 3 cycles was low, with mean AUC_{0-24h} rations for cycles 2 and 3 versus 1 of 1.13 ± 0.3 and 1.16 ± 0.36, respectively.

In vitro and ex vivo studies showed low affinity of zoledronic acid for cellular components of human blood. In vitro mean zoledronic acid protein binding in human plasma ranged from 28% at 200 ng/mL to 53% at 50 ng/mL.

Less than 3% of the administered IV dose was found in the feces, with the balance recovered in the urine or taken up by bone, indicating that the drug is eliminated intact via the kidney. Less than 3% of the administered IV dose was found in the feces, with the balance recovered in the urine or taken up by bone, indicating that the drug is eliminated intact via the kidney.

Special populations –

Renal function impairment: The pharmacokinetics of **pamidronate** were studied in cancer patients (n = 19) with normal and varying degrees of renal impairment. Given the recommended dose (90 mg infused over 4 hours), excessive accumulation of pamidronate in renally impaired patients is not anticipated if pamidronate is administered on a monthly basis. **Ibandronate** is not recommended in patients with severe renal impairment (CrCl less than 30 mL/min).

Following a single dose of ibandronate 0.5 mg IV, patients with creatinine clearance (CrCl) 40 to 70 mL/min had 55% higher exposure (area under the curve [AUC_∞]) than the exposure observed in subjects with CrCl greater than 90 mL/min. Patients with CrCl less than 30 mL/min had greater than a 2-fold increase in exposure compared with exposure for healthy subjects.

Compared with patients with healthy renal function (CrCl of at least 80 mL/min; n = 37), patients with mild renal impairment (CrCl of 50 to 80 mL/min; n = 15) showed an average increase in **zoledronic acid** (*Reclast*) plasma AUC of 15%, whereas patients with moderate renal impairment (CrCl of 30 to 50 mL/min; n = 11) showed an average increase in plasma AUC of 43%. No dosage adjustment is required in patients with a CrCl of at least 35 m/min. Zoledronic acid (*Reclast*) is not recommended for patients with severe renal impairment (CrCl of less than 35 mL/min) because of a lack of adequate clinical experience in this population.

Dose adjustments are recommended for zoledronic acid (*Zometa*) in patients with reduced renal function (mild to moderate impairment).

Risedronate is not recommended for patients with severe renal impairment (CrCl less than 30 mL/min).

Contraindications

Hypersensitivity to bisphosphonates or any component of the products; hypocalcemia (**alendronate**, **ibandronate**, **risedronate**, **zoledronic acid**, see Warnings/Precautions); abnormalities of the esophagus that delay esophageal emptying such as stricture or achalasia (**alendronate**, **etidronate**, **oral ibandronate**, **risedronate**); inability to stand or sit upright for at least 30 minutes (**alendronate**, **risedronate**); inability to stand or sit upright for at least 60 minutes (oral ibandronate); clinically overt osteomalacia (**etidronate**); increased risk of aspiration (**alendronate** solution).

Warnings/Precautions

➤*GI irritation/disorders:* Bisphosphonates cause local irritation of the upper GI mucosa. Instruct patients to alert their health care provider to any signs or symptoms signaling a possible esophageal reaction and instruct patients to discontinue bisphosphonates and seek medical attention if they develop dysphagia, odynophagia, retrosternal pain, or new or worsening heartburn.

The risk of severe esophageal adverse experiences appears to be greater in patients who lie down after taking bisphosphonates or who fail to swallow it with a full glass (6 to 8 oz) of water, or who continue to take bisphosphonates after developing symptoms suggestive of esophageal irritation. Therefore, it is very important that the full dosing instructions are provided to and understood by the patient. In patients who cannot comply with dosing instructions because of mental disability, use bisphosphonate therapy under appropriate supervision.

Because of possible irritant effects of bisphosphonates on the upper GI mucosa and a potential for worsening of the underlying disease, use caution when bisphosphonates are given to patients with active upper GI problems (eg, dysphagia, esophageal diseases, gastritis, duodenitis, ulcers). **Etidronate** therapy has been withheld from patients with enterocolitis because diarrhea is seen in some patients, particularly at higher doses.

➤*Osteoporosis (alendronate):* Consider causes of osteoporosis other than estrogen deficiency and aging; consider glucocorticoid use.

➤*Paget disease (etidronate):* Response to therapy may be slow and continue for months after treatment discontinuation. Do not increase dosage prematurely. Do not initiate retreatment until after at least a 90-day drug-free interval.

➤*Jaw osteonecrosis:* Osteonecrosis, primarily in the jaw, has been reported in patients treated with bisphosphonates. Most cases have been in cancer patients undergoing dental procedures, but some have occurred in patients with postmenopausal osteoporosis or other diagnoses. Known risk factors for osteonecrosis include a diagnosis of cancer, concomitant therapies (eg, chemotherapy, radiotherapy, corticosteroids), and comorbid disorders (eg, anemia, coagulopathy, infection, preexisting dental disease). Most reported cases have been in patients treated with bisphosphonates IV, but some have been in patients treated orally.

For patients who develop osteonecrosis of the jaw while receiving bisphosphonate therapy, dental surgery may exacerbate the condition. For patients requiring dental procedures, there are no data available to suggest whether discontinuation of bisphosphonate treatment reduces the risk of osteonecrosis of the jaw. Clinical judgment of the treating health care provider should guide the management plan of each patient based on individual benefit/risk assessment.

➤*Femoral fractures:* Atypical, low-energy, or low trauma fractures of the femoral shaft have been reported in bisphosphonate-treated patients. These fractures can occur anywhere in the femoral shaft from just below the lesser trochanter to above the supracondylar flare and are transverse or short oblique in orientation without evidence of comminution. Causality has not been established as these fractures also occur in osteoporotic patients who have not been treated with bisphosphonates.

Atypical femur fractures most commonly occur with minimal or no trauma to the affected area. They may be bilateral and many patients report prodromal pain in the affected area, usually presenting as dull, aching thigh pain, weeks to months before a complete fracture occurs. A number of reports note that patients were also receiving treatment with glucocorticoids (eg, prednisone) at the time of fracture.

Suspect any patient with a history of bisphosphonate exposure who presents with thigh or groin pain of having an atypical fracture and evaluate to rule out an incomplete femur fracture. Assess patients presenting with an atypical femur fracture for symptoms and signs of fracture in the contralateral limb. Consider interruption of bisphosphonate therapy, pending a risk/benefit assessment, on an individual basis.

➤*Musculoskeletal pain:* In postmarketing experience, severe and occasionally incapacitating bone, joint, and/or muscle pain has been reported in patients taking bisphosphonates that are approved for the prevention and treatment of osteoporosis. However, such reports have been infrequent. Most of the patients were postmenopausal women. The time to onset of symptoms varied from 1 day to several months after starting the drug. Most patients had relief of symptoms after stopping. A subset had recurrence of symptoms when rechallenged with the same drug or another bisphosphonate.

➤*Renal toxicity:* Treatment with IV bisphosphonates has been associated with renal toxicity manifested as deterioration in renal function (ie, increased serum creatinine) and, in rare cases, acute renal failure. The risk of serious renal toxicity with other IV bisphosphonates appears to be inversely related to the rate of drug administration.

➤*Asthma (zoledronic acid):* While not observed in clinical trials with zoledronic acid, administration of other bisphosphonates has been associated with bronchoconstriction in aspirin-sensitive asthmatic patients. Use zoledronic acid with caution in patients with aspirin-sensitive asthma.

➤*Glucocorticoid-induced osteoporosis:* Before initiating treatment for the treatment and prevention of glucocorticoid-induced osteoporosis, ascertain the sex steroid hormonal status of both men and women and consider appropriate replacement.

➤*Hypercalcemia:* Carefully monitor standard hypercalcemia-related metabolic parameters, such as serum levels of calcium, phosphate, and magnesium, as well as serum creatinine, following initiation of therapy with **zoledronic acid**. Patients with HCM must be adequately rehydrated prior to administration of zoledronic acid. Do not use loop diuretics until the patient is adequately rehydrated; use with caution in combination with zoledronic acid in order to avoid hypocalcemia. Use zoledronic acid with caution with other nephrotoxic drugs.

➤*Concomitant use with estrogen/hormone replacement therapy (alendronate):* Two clinical studies have shown that the degree of suppression of bone turnover (as assessed by mineralizing surface) was significantly greater with the combination than with either component alone. The safety and tolerability profile of the combination was consistent with those individual treatments.

➤*Nutrition:* Maintain adequate nutrition, particularly an adequate intake of calcium and vitamin D when taking oral **etidronate**, **ibandronate**, **risedronate**, and **alendronate**.

➤*Osteoid:* Oral **etidronate** suppresses bone turnover and may retard mineralization of osteoid laid down during the bone accretion process. These effects are dose- and time-dependent. Osteoid, which may accumulate noticeably at dosages of 10 to 20 mg/kg/day, mineralizes normally after therapy. In patients with fractures, especially of long bones, it may be advisable to delay or interrupt treatment until callus is evident.

➤*Fracture:* In patients with Paget disease, treatment regimens of oral **etidronate** exceeding the recommended daily maximum dose of 20 mg/kg or continuous administration for periods longer than 6 months may be associated with osteomalacia and an increased risk of fracture.

Long bones predominantly affected by lytic lesions, particularly in those patients unresponsive to therapy, may be especially prone to fracture. Radiographically and biochemically monitor patients with predominantly lytic lesions to permit termination of etidronate in those patients unresponsive to treatment.

➤*Hypocalcemia:* Ibandronate IV may cause a transient decrease in serum calcium values. Hypocalcemia has occurred with **pamidronate** (5% to 12%) and **ibandronate** therapy. Rare cases of symptomatic hypocalcemia (including tetany) occurred during pamidronate treatment. If hypocalcemia occurs, consider short-term calcium therapy.

Hypocalcemia must be corrected before therapy initiation with **alendronate**, **risedronate**, **zoledronic acid**. Also effectively treat other disturbances of mineral metabolism (eg, vitamin D deficiency). Presumably because of the effects of alendronate, ibandronate, and risedronate on increasing bone mineral, small asymptomatic decreases in serum calcium and phosphate may occur, especially in patients with Paget disease, in whom the pretreatment rate of bone turnover may be greatly elevated and in patients receiving glucocorticoids, in whom calcium absorption may be decreased. Ensure adequate calcium and vitamin D intake to provide for these enhanced needs.

➤*Renal function impairment:*

Alendronate – Although no clinical information is available, it is likely that alendronate elimination via the kidney will be reduced in impaired renal function. Therefore, somewhat greater accumulation of alendronate in bone might be expected in impaired renal function. No dosage adjustment is necessary in mild to moderate renal insufficiency (CrCl 35 to 60 mL/min). Alendronate use is not recommended in more severe renal insufficiency (CrCl less than 35 mL/min).

Etidronate – Dosage should be reduced when reductions in glomerular filtration rates are present. Monitor patients with renal impairment.

Ibandronate – Ibandronate is not recommended for use in patients with severe renal impairment (CrCl less than 30 mL/min).

Pamidronate – Bisphosphonates, including pamidronate, have been associated with renal toxicity manifested as deterioration of renal function and potential renal failure.

Because of the risk of clinically significant deterioration in renal function, which may progress to renal failure, single doses of pamidronate should not exceed 90 mg (see Administration and Dosage for appropriate infusion durations).

Pamidronate has not been tested in patients who have class Dc renal impairment (creatinine greater than 5 mg/dL) and has been tested in few multiple myeloma patients with serum creatinine 3 mg/dL or more. For the treatment of bone metastases, the use of pamidronate in patients with severe renal impairment is not recommended. In other indications, clinical judgement should determine whether the potential benefit outweighs the potential risk in such patients.

Risedronate – Risedronate is not recommended for patients with severe renal impairment (CrCl less than 30 mL/min). No dosage adjustment is needed when CrCl is greater than 30 mL/min.

Tiludronate – Tiludronate is not recommended for patients with severe renal failure (CrCl less than 30 mL/min). The plasma elimination half-life is longer.

Zoledronic acid – Because of the risk of clinically significant deterioration in renal function, which may progress to renal failure, single doses of zoledronic acid should not exceed 4 mg, and the duration of infusion should be no less than 15 minutes. Because safety and pharmacokinetic data are limited in patients with severe renal impairment, zoledronic acid treatment is not recommended in patients with bone metastases with severe renal impairment (in the clinical trials, patients with serum creatinine greater than 3 mg/dL were excluded). Consider zoledronic acid treatment in patients with HCM only after evaluating the risks and benefits of treatment (in the clinical trials, patients with serum creatinine greater than 400 mcmol/L or greater than 4.5 mg/dL were excluded).

In clinical trials, the risk for renal function deterioration (defined as an increase in serum creatinine) was significantly increased in patients who received zoledronic acid over 5 minutes compared with patients who received the same dose over 15 minutes. In addition, the risk for renal function deterioration and renal failure was significantly increased in patients who received zoledronic acid 8 mg, even when given over 15 minutes. While this risk is reduced with the zoledronic acid 4 mg dose administered over 15 minutes, deterioration in renal function can still occur. Risk factors for this deterioration include elevated baseline creatinine and multiple cycles of treatment with the bisphosphonate. Patients who receive zoledronic acid should have serum creatinine assessed prior to each treatment.

➤*Pregnancy:*

Category D. –

Pamidronate: Bolus IV studies conducted in rats and rabbits determined that pamidronate produces maternal toxicity and embryo/fetal effects when given during organogenesis at doses of 0.6 to 8.3 times the highest recommended human dose for a single IV infusion. Because it has been shown that pamidronate can cross the placenta in rats and has produced marked maternal and nonteratogenic embryo/fetal effects in rats and rabbits, do not give to women during pregnancy.

There are no adequate and well-controlled studies in pregnant women. If the patient becomes pregnant while taking this drug, apprise the patient of the potential harm to the fetus. Advise women of childbearing potential to avoid becoming pregnant.

Zoledronic acid: There are no studies in pregnant women using zoledronic acid. If the patient becomes pregnant while taking this drug, apprise the patient of the potential harm to the fetus. Advise women of childbearing potential to avoid becoming pregnant.

Do not use zoledronic acid during pregnancy. It may cause fetal harm when administered to a pregnant woman. In reproductive studies in pregnant rats, subcutaneous doses equivalent to 2.4 or 4.8 times the human systemic exposure (IV dose of 4 mg based on an AUC comparison) resulted in pre- and postimplantation losses, decreases in viable fetuses, and fetal skeletal, visceral, and external malformations.

Category C. –

Alendronate: There are no studies in pregnant women. Use alendronate during pregnancy only if the potential benefit justifies the risk to the mother and fetus.

Reproduction studies in rats showed decreased postimplantation survival at 2 mg/kg/day and decreased body weight gain in healthy pups at 1 mg/kg/day. Sites of incomplete fetal ossification were statistically significantly increased in rats beginning at 10 mg/kg/day in vertebral (cervical, thoracic, and lumbar), skull, and sternebral bones. Both total and ionized calcium decreased in pregnant rats at 15 mg/kg/day (3.9 times a 40 mg human daily dose based on surface area, mg/m^2), resulting in delays and failures of delivery. Protracted parturition because of maternal hypocalcemia occurred in rats at doses as low as 0.5 mg/kg/day (0.13 times a 40 mg human daily dose based on surface area [mg/m^2]) when rats were treated from before mating through gestation. Maternotoxicity (late pregnancy deaths) occurred in rats treated with alendronate 15 mg/kg/day for varying periods of time; these deaths were lessened but not eliminated by treatment cessation. Calcium could not ameliorate hypocalcemia or prevent maternal and neonatal deaths caused by delay in delivery; IV calcium supplementation prevented maternal but not fetal deaths.

Etidronate: There are no adequate and well-controlled studies in pregnant women. Use only when clearly needed and when the potential benefits outweigh potential hazards to the fetus. Etidronate has caused skeletal abnormalities in rats when given at oral dose levels of 300 mg/kg (15 to 60 times the human dose). Other effects on the offspring (including decreased live births) occur at dosages that cause significant toxicity in the parent generation and are 25 to 200 times the human dose. The skeletal effects are thought to be the result of the pharmacological effects of the drug on bone.

Ibandronate: There are no adequate and well-controlled studies in pregnant women. It is not known if ibandronate crosses the human placenta. Use ibandronate during pregnancy only if the potential benefit justifies the potential risk to the mother and fetus.

In pregnant rabbits treated orally with ibandronate during gestation at doses 8 times or more the recommended human daily oral dose of 2.5 mg and 4 times or more the recommended human once-monthly oral dose of 150 mg, dose-related maternal mortality was observed in all treatment groups. The deaths occurred prior to parturition and were associated with lung edema and hemorrhage.

Studies conducted in rats determined that ibandronate produces fetal toxicity when given during organogenesis at oral dosages of 9 to 13 times the highest recommended once-monthly human oral dosage of 150 mg. Rabbits given 19 times the recommended human IV dose during the period of organogenesis experienced increased maternal mortality, reduced maternal body weight gain, decreased litter size, and decreased fetal weight.

Risedronate: There are no adequate and well-controlled studies in pregnant women. Use during pregnancy only if the potential benefit justifies the potential risk to the fetus.

Survival of neonates was decreased in rats treated during gestation with oral doses of 16 mg/kg/day or more (approximately 5.2 times the 30 mg/day human dose based on surface area [mg/m^2]). Body weight was decreased in neonates from dams treated with 80 mg/kg (approximately 26 times the 30 mg/day human dose based on surface area [mg/m^2]). In rats treated during gestation, the number of fetuses exhibiting incomplete ossification of sternebrae or skull was statistically significantly increased at 7.1 mg/kg/day (approximately 2.3 times the 30 mg/day human dose based on surface area [mg/m^2]).

Tiludronate: There are no adequate and well-controlled studies in pregnant women. Use tiludronate during pregnancy only if the potential benefit justifies the potential risk to the fetus.

In rabbits at dosages of 42 and 130 mg/kg/day (2 and 5 times the 400 mg/day human dosage based on body surface area), there was dose-related scoliosis, likely attributable to the pharmacologic properties of tiludronate. Mice receiving 375 mg/kg/day (7 times the 400 mg/day human dosage based on body surface area [mg/m^2]) showed slight maternal toxicity. Maternal toxicity also was observed in rats dosed at 375 mg/kg/day (10 times the 400 mg/day human dosage).

➤*Lactation:* It is not known whether these drugs are excreted in breast milk. Exercise caution when administering **alendronate**, **etidronate**, **ibandronate**, **tiludronate**, **risedronate**, **pamidronate**, or **zoledronic acid** to a breast-feeding mother. Because zoledronic acid binds to bone long-term, do not administer to a breast-feeding woman. Because the amount of **ibandronate** absorbed by a breast-feeding infant should be clinically significant, breast-feeding is probably compatible with **ibandronate**.

➤*Children:* Safety and efficacy for use in children have not been established with most bisphosphonates (in children younger than 18 years of age for **risedronate**).

Zoledronic acid is not indicated for use in children.

Children have been treated with oral **etidronate** at doses recommended for adults to prevent heterotopic ossifications or soft tissue calcifications. A rachitic syndrome has been reported infrequently at dosages of 10 mg/kg/day or more and for prolonged periods approaching or exceeding 1 year. The epiphyseal radiologic changes associated with retarded mineralization of new osteoid and cartilage, and occasional symptoms reported, have been reversible when medication is discontinued.

➤*Monitoring:* Assess serum creatinine in patients who receive **pamidronate** prior to each treatment. Patients treated with pamidronate for bone metastases should have the dose withheld if renal function has deteriorated. Carefully monitor standard hypercalcemia-related metabolic parameters, such as serum levels of calcium, phosphate, magnesium, and potassium following pamidronate and **zoledronic acid** initiation. Asymptomatic hypophosphatemia (16%), hypomagnesemia (11%), hypokalemia (7%), and hypocalcemia (5% to 12%) have occurred. Also, closely monitor electrolytes, creatinine, complete blood cell count, differential, and hematocrit/hemoglobin. Carefully monitor patients who have preexisting anemia, leukopenia, or thrombocytopenia in the first 2 weeks following treatment.

Monitor patient for esophageal adverse reactions, such as dysphagia, odynophagia, retrosternal pain, and new or worsening heartburn. Monitor patients for signs and symptoms of incapacitating bone, joint, and/or muscle pain.

Drug Interactions

Bisphosphonate Drug Interactions			
Precipitant drug	Object drug[a]		Description
Aminoglycosides	Bisphosphonates (Zoledronic acid)	⬆	Caution is advised when bisphosphonates are administered with aminoglycosides because these agents may have an additive effect to lower serum calcium levels for prolonged periods.
Aspirin	Tiludronate	⬇	Aspirin may decrease the bioavailability of tiludronate by up to 50% when taken 2 hours after tiludronate.
Calcium supplements, antacids	Alendronate, Etidronate, Ibandronate, Risedronate, Tiludronate, Ibandronate	⬇	Products containing calcium and other multivalent cations interfere with alendronate, ibandronate, risedronate, and etidronate absorption. The bioavailability of tiludronate is decreased by 80% by calcium when administered at the same time and 60% by some aluminum- or magnesium-containing antacids when administered 1 hour before tiludronate.
Indomethacin	Tiludronate	⬆	The bioavailability of tiludronate is increased 2- to 4-fold by indomethacin, but is not significantly altered by coadministration of diclofenac.
Loop diuretics	Zoledronic acid	⬆	Use caution when zoledronic acid is used in combination with loop diuretics because of an increased risk of hypocalcemia.
Ranitidine	Alendronate	⬆	IV ranitidine doubled alendronate bioavailability. The clinical significance is unknown.
Alendronate	Aspirin	⬆	The risk of upper GI adverse effects associated with aspirin increased with alendronate dosages > 10 mg/day.
Etidronate	Warfarin	⬆	There have been isolated reports of patients experiencing increases in their prothrombin times when etidronate was added to warfarin therapy. Patients receiving warfarin should have their prothrombin time monitored.
Aluminum and/or magnesium supplements/ antacids	Risedronate	⬇	Products containing aluminum and/or magnesium supplements and aluminum and/or magnesium-containing antacids may decrease risedronate absorption. Administer risedronate at least 30 minutes before an aluminum and/or magnesium antacid is taken.

[a] ⬆ = object drug increased; ⬇ = object drug decreased.

➤*Drug/Lab test interactions:* Bisphosphonates are known to interfere with the use of bone-imaging agents.

➤*Drug/Food interactions:* In 1 study, bioavailability of **alendronate** was decreased by 40% when alendronate 10 mg was given 30 minutes or 1 hour before breakfast versus 2 hours before, and bioavailability was negligible when alendronate was given with or 2 hours after breakfast. Concomitant coffee or orange juice reduced bioavailability by 60%. Advise patients to take alendronate in the morning at least 30 minutes before the first meal, beverage, or medication.

Absorption of **etidronate** may be reduced by foods. Take on an empty stomach 2 hours before a meal.

Food or beverages, other than water, decrease the extent of **ibandronate** absorption. Administered with a standard breakfast reduces bioavailability approximately 90%, compared with ingestion in fasting individuals.

In single-dose studies, bioavailability of **tiludronate** was reduced by 90% when an oral dose equivalent to 400 mg of tiludronic acid was administered with or 2 hours after a standard breakfast compared with the same dose administered after an overnight fast and 4 hours before a standard breakfast.

Mean oral bioavailability of **risedronate** immediate release is decreased when given with food. Take at least 30 minutes before the first food or drink of the day other than water. Take risedronate delayed release in the morning immediately following breakfast.

Mean oral bioavailability of ibandronate is decreased by 90% when given with food. Take at least 60 minutes before the first food or drink (other than water) of the day or before taking any oral medications or supplementation, including calcium, antacids, or vitamins.

Adverse Reactions

Adverse reactions	Bisphosphonate Adverse Reactions (%)[a]																
	Pamidronate				Alendronate		Tiludronate	Risedronate				Zoledronic acid		Ibandronate			
	Osteolytic bone metastases of breast cancer and osteolytic lesions of multiple myeloma (average of 3 trials) 90 mg (n = 572)[b]	Hypercalcemia of malignancy study comparing these 3 dose regimens			Osteoporosis in postmenopausal women 10 mg/day[c] (n = 196)	Fracture intervention trial[d] (n = 3,236)	Pagetic patients 400 mg/day (n = 75)	Pagetic patients 30 mg/day x 2 months (n = 61)[e]	Postmenopausal osteoporosis trials 5 mg (n = 1,613)	Osteoporosis study in postmenopausal women comparing these 2 doseforms		Hypercalcemia of malignancy 4 mg (n = 86)	Combined multiple myeloma and bone metastases of solid tumor trials 4 mg (n = 1099)	Dosing IV administration study comparing these 2 doseforms		Osteoporosis study in postmenopausal women comparing these 2 doseforms	
		60 mg over 4 h (n = 23)	60 mg over 24 h (n = 73)	90 mg over 24 h (n = 17)						5 mg/day (immediate release) (n = 307)	35 mg/wk (delayed release) (n = 307)			2.5 mg/day (oral) (n = 465)	3 mg every 3 months (IV) (n = 469)	2.5 mg/day (n = 395)	150 mg/ month (n = 396)
Cardiovascular																	
Angina pectoris	—	—	—	—	—	—	—	—	2.5%	—	—	—	—	—	—	—	—
Atrial fibrillation	—	—	—	6%	—	—	—	—	—	—	—	—	—	—	—	—	—
Atrial flutter	—	—	1%	—	—	—	—	—	—	—	—	—	—	—	—	—	—
Cardiac failure	—	—	1%	—	—	—	—	—	—	—	—	—	—	—	—	—	—
Cardiovascular disorder	—	—	—	—	—	—	—	—	2.5%	—	—	—	—	—	—	—	—
Chest pain	—	—	—	—	—	—	2.7%	6.6%	5%	—	—	—	—	—	—	—	—
Hypertension	—	—	—	6%	—	—	—	—	10.5%	—	—	—	—	7.1%	5.3%	7.3%	6.3%
Hypotension	—	—	—	—	—	—	—	—	—	—	—	10.5%	—	—	—	—	—
Syncope	—	—	—	6%	—	—	—	—	—	—	—	—	—	—	—	—	—
Tachycardia	—	—	—	6%	—	—	—	—	—	—	—	—	—	—	—	—	—
Vasodilation	—	—	—	—	—	—	—	—	—	—	—	—	—	—	—	—	—
CNS																	
Agitation	—	—	—	—	—	—	—	—	—	—	—	12.8%	—	—	—	—	—
Anxiety	14.3%	—	—	—	—	—	—	—	—	—	—	14%	9%	—	—	—	—
Asthenia	22.2%	—	—	—	—	—	—	—	5.4%	3.5%	5.4%	—	21%	—	—	—	—
Confusion	—	—	—	—	—	—	—	—	—	—	—	12.8%	—	—	—	—	—
Convulsions	—	—	—	—	—	—	—	—	—	—	—	—	—	—	—	—	—
Depression	—	—	—	—	—	—	—	—	6.8%	—	—	—	12%	2.2%	1.3%	—	—
Dizziness	—	—	—	—	—	—	4%	6.6%	7.1%	3.3%	2.6%	—	14%	2.8%	1.9%	1%	2.3%
Fatigue	37.2%	—	—	12%	—	—	—	—	—	—	—	—	36%	1.1%	2.8%	—	—
Headache	26.2%	—	—	—	2.6%	0.2%	6.7%	18%	9.9%	4.9%	2.6%	—	18%	2.6%	3.6%	4.1%	3.3%
Hypertonia	—	—	—	—	—	—	—	—	—	—	—	—	—	—	—	—	—
Hypesthesia	—	—	—	—	—	—	—	—	—	—	—	—	10%	—	—	—	—
Insomnia	22.2%	—	1%	—	—	—	—	—	5%	—	—	15.1%	14%	2.6%	1.1%	0.8%	2%
Neuralgia	—	—	—	—	—	—	—	—	—	—	—	—	—	—	—	—	—
Paresthesia	—	—	—	—	—	—	4%	—	—	—	—	—	12%	—	—	—	—
Psychosis	—	4%	—	—	—	—	—	—	—	—	—	—	—	—	—	—	—
Rigors	—	—	—	—	—	—	—	—	—	—	—	—	10%	—	—	—	—
Somnolence	—	—	1%	6%	—	—	—	—	—	—	—	—	—	—	—	—	—
Vertigo	—	—	—	—	—	—	—	—	—	—	—	—	—	—	—	—	—
Dermatologic																	
Alopecia	—	—	—	—	—	—	—	—	—	—	—	—	11%	—	—	—	—
Dermatitis	—	—	—	—	—	—	—	—	—	—	—	—	10%	—	—	—	—
Pruritus	—	—	-	—	—	—	—	—	—	—	—	—	—	—	—	—	—
Rash	—	—	—	—	—	—	2.7%	11.5%	7.9%	—	—	—	—	2.8%	2.3%	1.3%	2.3%
Skin carcinoma	—	—	—	—	—	—	—	—	—	—	—	—	—	—	—	—	—

Adverse reactions	Bisphosphonate Adverse Reactions (%)[a] Pamidronate: Osteolytic bone metastases of breast cancer and osteolytic lesions of multiple myeloma (average of 3 trials) 90 mg (n = 572)[b]	Pamidronate: Hypercalcemia of malignancy study comparing these 3 dose regimens: 60 mg over 4 h (n = 23)	Pamidronate: Hypercalcemia of malignancy study comparing these 3 dose regimens: 60 mg over 24 h (n = 73)	Pamidronate: Hypercalcemia of malignancy study comparing these 3 dose regimens: 90 mg over 24 h (n = 17)	Alendronate: Osteoporosis in postmenopausal women 10 mg/day[c] (n = 196)	Alendronate: Fracture intervention trial[d] (n = 3,236)	Tiludronate: Pagetic patients 400 mg/day (n = 75)	Risedronate: Pagetic patients 30 mg/day × 2 months (n = 61)[e]	Risedronate: Postmenopausal osteoporosis trials 5 mg (n = 1,613)	Risedronate: Osteoporosis study in postmenopausal women comparing these 2 doseforms: 5 mg/day (immediate release) (n = 307)	Risedronate: Osteoporosis study in postmenopausal women comparing these 2 doseforms: 35 mg/wk (delayed release) (n = 307)	Zoledronic acid: Hypercalcemia of malignancy 4 mg (n = 86)	Zoledronic acid: Combined multiple myeloma and bone metastases of solid tumor trials 4 mg (n = 1099)	Ibandronate: Dosing IV administration study comparing these 2 doseforms: 2.5 mg/day (oral) (n = 465)	Ibandronate: Dosing IV administration study comparing these 2 doseforms: 3 mg every 3 months (IV) (n = 469)	Ibandronate: Osteoporosis study in postmenopausal women comparing these 2 doseforms: 2.5 mg/day (n = 395)	Ibandronate: Osteoporosis study in postmenopausal women comparing these 2 doseforms: 150 mg/month (n = 396)
Skin disorder	—	—	—	—	—	—	2.7%	—	—	—	—	—	—	—	—	—	—
GI																	
Abdominal pain	22.6%	—	1%	—	6.6%	1.5%	—	11.5%	12.2%	2.9%	5.2%	16.3%	12%	5.6%	5.1%	5.3%	7.8%
Abdominal distension	—	—	—	—	1%	—	—	—	—	—	—	—	—	—	—	—	—
Acid regurgitation	—	—	—	—	2%	1.1%	—	—	—	—	—	—	—	—	—	—	—
Anorexia	26%	4%	1%	12%	—	—	—	—	—	—	—	9.3%	20%	—	—	—	—
Appetite decreased	—	—	—	—	—	—	—	—	—	—	—	—	11%	—	—	—	—
Belching	—	—	—	—	—	—	—	—	—	—	—	—	—	—	—	—	—
Colitis	—	—	—	—	—	—	—	—	—	—	—	—	—	—	—	—	—
Constipation	33.2%	4%	—	6%	3.1%	0%	—	6.6%	12.9%	2.9%	4.9%	26.7%	28%	4.1%	3.4%	2.5%	4%
Diarrhea	28.5%	—	1%	—	3.1%	0.6%	9.3%	19.7%	10.8%	4.9%	8.8%	17.4%	22%	2.4%	2.8%	4.1%	5.1%
Dry mouth	—	—	—	—	—	—	—	—	—	—	—	—	—	—	—	—	—
Dyspepsia	22.6%	4%	—	—	3.6%	1.1%	5.3%	—	10.8%	3.9%	3.9%	—	—	4.3%	3.6%	7.1%	5.6%
Dysphasia	—	—	—	—	1%	0.1%	—	—	—	—	—	—	—	—	—	—	—
Esophageal ulcer	—	—	—	—	1.5%	0.1%	—	—	—	—	—	—	—	—	—	—	—
Flatulence	—	—	—	—	2.6%	0.2%	2.7%	—	—	—	—	—	—	—	—	—	—
Gastritis	—	—	—	—	0.5%	0.6%	—	—	2.7%	1%	1%	—	—	2.2%	1.9%	—	—
Gastroenteritis	—	—	—	—	—	—	—	—	—	—	—	—	—	3.4%	1.5%	—	—
GI disorder	—	—	—	—	—	—	—	—	—	—	—	—	—	—	—	—	—
GI hemorrhage	—	—	—	6%	—	—	—	—	—	—	—	—	—	—	—	—	—
Nausea	53.5%	4%	—	18%	3.6%	1.1%	9.3%	9.8%	10.5%	3.9%	3.6%	29.1%	43%	4.3%	2.1%	4.8%	5.1%
Rectal disorder	—	—	—	—	—	—	—	—	—	—	—	—	—	—	—	—	—
Stomatitis	—	—	1%	—	—	—	—	—	—	—	—	—	—	—	—	—	—
Tooth disorder	—	—	—	—	—	—	2.7%	—	—	—	—	—	—	—	—	—	—
Vomiting	35.7%	4%	—	—	1%	0.2%	4%	—	—	1.6%	4.9%	14%	30%	—	—	—	—
Weight decreased	—	—	—	—	—	—	—	—	—	—	—	—	13%	—	—	—	—
GU																	
Cystitis	—	—	—	—	—	—	—	—	—	—	—	—	—	3.4%	1.9%	—	—
Urinary tract infection	18.5%	—	—	—	—	—	—	—	11.1%	—	—	14%	11%	3.2%	2.6%	1.8%	2.3%
Hemic/Lymphatic																	
Anemia	42.5%	—	—	6%	—	—	—	—	—	—	—	22.1%	29%	—	—	—	—
Ecchymosis	—	—	—	—	—	—	—	—	—	—	—	—	—	—	—	—	—
Granulocytopenia	19.8%	—	—	—	—	—	—	—	—	—	—	—	—	—	—	—	—
Leukopenia	—	4%	—	—	—	—	—	—	—	—	—	—	—	—	—	—	—
Neutropenia	—	—	1%	—	—	—	—	—	—	—	—	—	11%	—	—	—	—
Thrombocytopenia	14%	—	1%	—	—	—	—	—	—	—	—	—	—	—	—	—	—
Lab abnormalities														—	—	—	—
Abnormal hepatic function	—	—	—	—	—	—	—	—	—	—	—	—	—	—	—	—	—
Hypocalcemia	3.3%	—	1%	12%	—	—	—	—	—	—	—	—	—	—	—	—	—

Bisphosphonate Adverse Reactions (%)[a]

Adverse reactions	Pamidronate				Alendronate		Tiludronate	Risedronate				Zoledronic acid		Ibandronate			
	Osteolytic bone metastases of breast cancer and osteolytic lesions of multiple myeloma (average of 3 trials) 90 mg (n = 572)[b]	Hypercalcemia of malignancy study comparing these 3 dose regimens			Osteoporosis in postmenopausal women 10 mg/day[c] (n = 196)	Fracture intervention trial[d] (n = 3,236)	Pagetic patients 400 mg/day (n = 75)	Pagetic patients 30 mg/day x 2 months (n = 61)[e]	Postmenopausal osteoporosis trials 5 mg (n = 1,613)	Osteoporosis study in postmenopausal women comparing these 2 doseforms		Hypercalcemia of malignancy 4 mg (n = 86)	Combined multiple myeloma and bone metastases of solid tumor trials 4 mg (n = 1099)	Dosing IV administration study comparing these 2 doseforms		Osteoporosis study in postmenopausal women comparing these 2 doseforms	
		60 mg over 4 h (n = 23)	60 mg over 24 h (n = 73)	90 mg over 24 h (n = 17)						5 mg/day (immediate release) (n = 307)	35 mg/wk (delayed release) (n = 307)			2.5 mg/day (oral) (n = 465)	3 mg every 3 months (IV) (n = 469)	2.5 mg/day (n = 395)	150 mg/month (n = 396)
Hypokalemia	10.5%	4%	4%	18%	—	—	—	—	—	—	—	11.6%	—	—	—	—	—
Hypomagnesemia	4.4%	4%	10%	12%	—	—	—	—	—	—	—	10.5%	—	—	—	—	—
Hypophosphatemia	1.7%	—	9%	18%	—	—	—	—	—	—	—	12.8%	—	—	—	—	—
Serum creatinine	18.5%	—	—	—	—	—	—	—	—	—	—	—	—	—	—	—	—
Musculoskeletal																	
Arthralgia	13.6%	—	—	—	—	—	2.7%	32.8%	23.7%	7.8%	6.8%	—	18%	8.6%	9.6%	3.5%	5.6%
Arthritis	—	—	—	—	—	—	—	—	9.6%	—	—	—	—	—	—	—	—
Arthrosis	—	—	—	—	—	—	2.7%	—	—	—	—	—	—	—	—	—	—
Back pain	—	—	—	—	—	—	8%	—	28%	5.9%	6.8%	—	10%	7.5%	7%	4.3%	4.5%
Bone disorder	—	—	—	—	—	—	—	—	—	—	—	—	—	—	—	—	—
Bone fracture	—	—	—	—	—	—	—	—	—	—	—	—	—	—	—	—	—
Bone/skeletal pain	66.8%	—	—	—	4.1%	0.4%	—	—	5.3%	1.6%	2%	11.6%	53%	—	—	—	—
Bursitis	—	—	—	—	—	—	—	—	—	—	—	—	—	—	—	—	—
Joint disorder	—	—	—	—	—	—	—	—	7%	—	—	—	—	—	—	—	—
Leg/Muscle cramps	—	—	—	—	—	0.2%	—	—	—	—	—	—	—	—	—	2%	1.8%
Myalgia	26%	—	1%	—	—	—	—	—	6.7%	1%	1.3%	—	21%	0.9%	2.8%	0.8%	2%
Myasthenia	—	—	—	—	—	—	—	—	—	—	—	—	—	—	—	—	—
Neck pain	—	—	—	—	—	—	—	—	5.4%	—	—	—	—	—	—	—	—
Tendon disorder	—	—	—	—	—	—	—	—	—	—	—	—	—	—	—	—	—
Respiratory																	
Bronchitis	—	—	—	—	—	—	—	—	10%	4.2%	3.9%	—	—	2.8%	2.1%	3.5%	2.5%
Coughing	25.7%	—	—	—	—	—	2.7%	—	—	—	—	11.6%	19%	—	—	—	—
Dyspnea	30.4%	—	—	—	—	—	—	—	—	—	—	22.1%	24%	—	—	—	—
Pharyngitis	—	—	—	—	—	—	2.7%	—	6%	—	—	—	—	—	—	—	—
Pleural effusion	10.7	—	—	—	—	—	—	—	—	—	—	—	—	—	—	—	—
Pneumonia	—	—	—	—	—	—	—	—	—	—	—	—	—	—	—	—	—
Rales	—	—	—	6%	—	—	—	—	—	—	—	—	—	—	—	—	—
Rhinitis	—	—	—	6%	—	—	5.3%	—	6.2%	—	—	—	—	—	—	—	—
Sinusitis	15.6%	—	—	—	—	—	5.3%	—	8.7%	—	—	—	—	—	—	—	—
Upper respiratory infection	24.1%	—	3%	—	—	—	5.3%	—	—	2.6%	3.6%	—	8%	2.8%	1.1%	2%	2%
Special senses																	
Amblyopia	—	—	—	—	—	—	—	—	—	—	—	—	—	—	—	—	—
Cataract	—	—	—	—	—	—	2.7%	—	—	—	—	—	—	—	—	—	—
Conjunctivitis	—	—	—	—	—	—	2.7%	—	6.5%	—	—	—	—	—	—	—	—
Dry eye	—	—	—	—	—	—	—	—	—	—	—	—	—	—	—	—	—
Glaucoma	—	—	—	—	—	—	2.7%	—	—	—	—	—	—	—	—	—	—
Nasopharyngitis	—	—	—	—	—	—	—	—	—	—	—	—	—	6%	3.4%	4.3%	3.5%
Otitis media	—	—	—	—	—	—	—	—	—	—	—	—	—	—	—	—	—
Taste perversion	—	—	—	—	0.5%	0.1%	—	—	—	—	—	—	—	—	—	—	—

Bisphosphonate Adverse Reactions (%)[a]

Adverse reactions	Pamidronate: Osteolytic bone metastases of breast cancer and osteolytic lesions of multiple myeloma (average of 3 trials) 90 mg (n = 572)[b]	Pamidronate: Hypercalcemia of malignancy study comparing these 3 dose regimens: 60 mg over 4 h (n = 23)	Pamidronate: Hypercalcemia of malignancy study comparing these 3 dose regimens: 60 mg over 24 h (n = 73)	Pamidronate: Hypercalcemia of malignancy study comparing these 3 dose regimens: 90 mg over 24 h (n = 17)	Alendronate: Osteoporosis in postmenopausal women 10 mg/day[c] (n = 196)	Alendronate: Fracture intervention trial[d] (n = 3,236)	Tiludronate: Pagetic patients 400 mg/day (n = 75)	Risedronate: Pagetic patients 30 mg/day × 2 months (n = 61)[e]	Risedronate: Postmenopausal osteoporosis trials 5 mg (n = 1,613)	Risedronate: Osteoporosis study in postmenopausal women comparing these 2 doseforms: 5 mg/day (immediate release) (n = 307)	Risedronate: Osteoporosis study in postmenopausal women comparing these 2 doseforms: 35 mg/wk (delayed release) (n = 307)	Zoledronic acid: Hypercalcemia of malignancy 4 mg (n = 86)	Zoledronic acid: Combined multiple myeloma and bone metastases of solid tumor trials 4 mg (n = 1099)	Ibandronate: Dosing IV administration study comparing these 2 doseforms: 2.5 mg/day (oral) (n = 465)	Ibandronate: Dosing IV administration study comparing these 2 doseforms: 3 mg every 3 months (IV) (n = 469)	Ibandronate: Osteoporosis study in postmenopausal women comparing these 2 doseforms: 2.5 mg/day (n = 395)	Ibandronate: Osteoporosis study in postmenopausal women comparing these 2 doseforms: 150 mg/month (n = 396)
Tinnitus	—	—	—	—	—	—	—	—	—	—	—	—	—	—	—	—	—
Miscellaneous																	
Accidental injury	—	—	—	—	—	—	4%	—	3.8%	—	—	—	—	—	—	—	—
Allergic reaction	—	—	—	—	—	—	—	—	—	—	—	—	—	—	—	—	—
Cancer progression	—	—	—	—	—	—	—	—	—	—	—	16.3%	—	—	—	—	—
Dehydration	—	—	—	—	—	—	—	—	—	—	—	—	12%	—	—	—	—
Edema/Peripheral edema	—	—	1%	—	—	—	2.7%	8.2%	7.7%	—	—	—	19%	—	—	—	—
Fever	38.5%	26%	19%	18%	—	—	—	—	—	—	—	44.2%	30%	—	—	—	—
Fluid overload	—	—	—	—	—	—	—	—	—	—	—	—	—	—	—	—	—
Hernia	—	—	—	—	—	—	—	—	—	—	—	—	—	—	—	—	—
Hypercholesterolemia	—	—	—	—	—	—	—	—	—	—	—	—	—	4.3%	1.5%	—	—
Hyperparathyroidism	—	—	—	—	—	—	2.7%	—	—	—	—	—	—	—	—	—	—
Hypothyroidism	—	—	—	6%	—	—	—	—	—	—	—	—	—	—	—	—	—
Infection	—	—	—	—	—	—	2.7%	—	31.1%	—		—	—	—	—	—	—
Influenza	—	—	—	—	—	—	—	—	—	6.2%	7.2%	—	—	8%	4.7%	3.8%	4%
Influenza-like symptoms	—	—	—	—	—	—	4%	9.8%	10.5%	—	—	—	—	1.1%	4.9%	0.8%	3.3%
Infusion-site reaction	—	—	4%	18%	—	—	—	—	—	—	—	—	—	—	—	—	—
Localized osteoarthritis	—	—	—	—	—	—	—	—	—	—	—	—	—	2.4%	1.5%	1.3%	3%
Metastases	20.5%	—	—	—	—	—	—	—	—	—	—	—	—	—	—	—	—
Moniliasis	—	—	—	6%	—	—	—	—	—	—	—	11.6%	—	—	—	—	—
Neoplasm	—	—	—	—	—	—	—	—	—	—	—	—	15%	—	—	—	—
Overdose	—	—	—	—	—	—	—	—	—	—	—	—	—	—	—	—	—
Pain	14.3%	—	—	—	—	—	21.3%	—	14.1%	—	—	—	—	—	—	—	—
Vitamin D deficiency	—	—	—	—	—	—	2.7%	—	—	—	—	—	—	—	—	—	—
Uremia	—	4%	—	—	—	—	—	—	—	—	—	—	—	—	—	—	—

— = no data.
[a] Data are pooled from separate studies and are not necessarily comparable.
[b] Most of these adverse experiences may have been related to the underlying disease state or cancer therapy.
[c] 10 mg/day for 3 years.
[d] 5 mg/day for 2 years and 10 mg/day for either 1 or 2 additional years.
[e] Considered to be possibly or probably causally related in ≥ 1 patient.

➤*Alendronate:*

Osteoporosis in postmenopausal women – One patient treated with 10 mg/day who had a history of peptic ulcer disease and gastrectomy and was taking concomitant aspirin developed an anastomotic ulcer with mild hemorrhage, which was considered drug related. Aspirin and alendronate were discontinued and the patient recovered.

Other: Rash, erythema (rare).

Alendronate Adverse Reactions in Osteoporosis Treatment Studies in Postmenopausal Women (≥ 1%)		
Adverse reactions	Alendronate 70 mg once weekly (n = 519)	Alendronate 10 mg/day (n = 370)
GI		
Abdominal distension	1%	1.4%
Abdominal pain	3.7%	3%
Acid regurgitation	1.9%	2.4%
Constipation	0.8%	1.6%
Dyspepsia	2.7%	2.2%
Flatulence	0.4%	1.6%
Gastric ulcer	0%	1.1%
Gastritis	0.2%	1.1%
Nausea	1.9%	2.4%
Musculoskeletal		
Muscle cramp	0.2%	1.1%
Musculoskeletal (bone, muscle, joint) pain	2.9%	3.2%

Alendronate Adverse Reactions in an Osteoporosis Study in Men (≥ 2%)		
Adverse reactions	Alendronate 10 mg/day (n = 146)	Placebo (n = 95)
GI		
Abdominal pain	2.1%	1.1%
Acid regurgitation	4.1%	3.2%
Dyspepsia	3.4%	0%
Flatulence	4.1%	1.1%
Nausea	2.1%	0%

Alendronate Adverse Reactions in Osteoporosis Prevention Studies in Postmenopausal Women (≥ 1%)				
	2- and 3-year studies		1-year study	
Adverse reactions	Alendronate 5 mg/day (n = 642)	Placebo (n = 648)	Alendronate 5 mg/day (n = 361)	Alendronate 35 mg once weekly (n = 362)
GI				
Abdominal distension	0.2%	0.3%	1.4%	1.1%
Abdominal pain	1.7%	3.4%	4.2%	2.2%
Acid regurgitation	1.4%	2.5%	4.2%	4.7%
Constipation	0.9%	0.5%	1.7%	0.3%
Diarrhea	1.1%	1.7%	1.1%	0.6%
Dyspepsia	1.9%	1.4%	2.2%	1.7%
Nausea	1.4%	1.4%	2.5%	1.4%
Musculoskeletal				
Musculoskeletal (bone, muscle, or joint) pain	0.8%	0.9%	1.9%	2.2%

Alendronate Adverse Reactions in 1-Year Studies in Glucocorticoid-Treated Patients (≥ 1%)			
Adverse reactions	Alendronate 10 mg/day (n = 157)	Alendronate 5 mg/day (n = 161)	Placebo (n = 159)
CNS			
Headache	0.6%	0%	1.3%
GI			
Abdominal pain	3.2%	1.9%	0%
Acid regurgitation	2.5%	1.9%	1.3%
Constipation	1.3%	0.6%	0%
Diarrhea	0%	0%	1.3%
Melena	1.3%	0%	0%
Nausea	0.6%	1.2%	0.6%

Paget disease: In clinical studies in osteoporosis and Paget disease in patients taking 40 mg/day for 3 to 12 months, the adverse experiences were similar to those in the 10 mg/day osteoporosis study. However, there was an increased incidence of upper GI adverse reactions in the 40 mg/day group (17.7% of the patients taking alendronate vs 10.2% receiving placebo). One case of esophagitis and 2 cases of gastritis resulted in treatment discontinuation.

Musculoskeletal pain, which also occurs with other bisphosphonates, occurred in approximately 6% of patients treated with alendronate 40 mg/day versus approximately 1% taking placebo, rarely resulting in discontinuation. Discontinuation caused by any adverse reaction occurred in 6.4% of patients with Paget disease treated with alendronate 40 mg/day versus 2.4% of placebo-treated patients.

Lab test abnormalities – In double-blind, multicenter, controlled studies, asymptomatic, mild, and transient decreases in serum calcium and phosphate occurred in approximately 18% and 10%, respectively, of patients taking alendronate versus approximately 12% and 3% of those taking placebo. However, the incidence of decreases in serum calcium to less than 8 mg/dL (2 mM) and serum phosphate to at least 2 mg/dL (0.65 mM) were similar in both treatment groups.

Postmarketing: Hypersensitivity reactions including urticaria and rarely angioedema; esophagitis; esophageal erosions; esophageal ulcers, rarely esophageal stricture or perforation; oropharyngeal ulceration; gastric or duodenal ulcers, some severe and with complications; rash (occasionally with photosensitivity); uveitis (rare).

➤*Etidronate:* The incidence of GI complaints (diarrhea, nausea) is the same at 5 mg/kg/day as for placebo (approximately 6.7%). At 10 to 20 mg/kg/day, the incidence may increase to 20% or 30%. These complaints are often alleviated by dividing the total daily dose.

Paget disease – Increased or recurrent bone pain at pagetic sites or the onset of pain at previously asymptomatic sites has occurred. At 5 mg/kg/day, approximately 10% (vs 6.7% with placebo) report these phenomena. At higher doses, the incidence rises to approximately 20%. When the therapy continues, pain resolves in some patients but persists in others.

Postmarketing – Other adverse events that have been reported and were thought to be possibly related to etidronate disodium include the following: alopecia; arthropathies, including arthralgia and arthritis; bone fracture; esophagitis; glossitis; hypersensitivity reactions, including angioedema, follicular eruption, macular rash, maculopapular rash, pruritus, a single case of Stevens-Johnson syndrome, and urticaria; neuropsychiatric events, including amnesia, confusion, depression, and hallucination; osteomalacia; and paresthesias.

In patients receiving etidronate disodium, there have been rare reports of agranulocytosis, pancytopenia, and a report of leukopenia with recurrence on rechallenge. In addition, there have been rare reports of exacerbation of asthma. Exacerbation of existing peptic ulcer disease has been reported in a few patients. In 1 patient, perforation also occurred. In osteoporosis clinical trials, arthralgia, gastritis, headache, and leg cramps occurred at a significantly greater incidence in patients who received etidronate compared with those who received placebo.

➤*Ibandronate:*

Acute phase reaction–like events – Symptoms consistent with acute phase reactions have been reported with bisphosphonate use. Over the 2 years of the study, the overall incidence of acute phase reaction symptoms was 3% in the **ibandronate** 2.5 mg daily group and 9% in the **ibandronate** 150 mg monthly group. These incidence rates are based on the reporting of any of 33 acute phase reaction–like symptoms within 3 days of the monthly dosing and lasting 7 days or less. Influenza-like illness was reported in no patients in the **ibandronate** 2.5 mg daily group and 2% in the **ibandronate** 150 mg monthly group.

Injection-site reactions – Local reactions at the injection site, such as redness or swelling, were observed infrequently, but at a higher incidence in patients treated with **ibandronate** 3 mg injection every 3 months (less than 2%) than in patients treated with placebo injections (less than 1%). In most cases, the reaction was of mild to moderate severity.

Special senses – Bisphosphonates may be associated with ocular inflammation such as uveitis and scleritis. In some cases, these reactions did not resolve until the bisphosphonate was discontinued.

Postmarketing –

Hypersensitivity: Anaphylaxis, angioedema, bronchospasm, rash.

Musculoskeletal: Bone, joint, or muscle pain (musculoskeletal pain) described as severe or incapacitating.

Miscellaneous: Hypocalcemia and osteonecrosis of the jaw.

➤*Pamidronate:*

Hypercalcemia of malignancy – Transient mild elevation of temperature by at least 1°C was noted 24 to 48 hours after administration in 34% of patients. In trials, patients treated with pamidronate (60 or 90 mg over 24 hours) developed electrolyte abnormalities more frequently.

Drug-related local soft tissue symptoms (redness, swelling, or induration, and pain on palpation) at the site of catheter insertion were most common in patients treated with 90 mg.

Rare cases of uveitis, iritis, scleritis, and episcleritis have occurred, including 1 case of scleritis and 1 case of uveitis upon separate rechallenges.

Five of 231 patients (2%) had seizures; 2 had preexisting seizure disorders. None of the seizures were considered to be drug-related. However, a possible relationship cannot be ruled out.

Other reactions in at least 15% of patients included the following: anorexia, constipation, fluid overload, generalized/abdominal/bone pain, hypertension, nausea, urinary tract infection, and vomiting.

Lab test abnormalities: Anemia, hypokalemia, hypomagnesemia, hypophosphatemia.

Paget disease: Transient mild elevation of temperature more than 1°C above pretreatment baseline was noted within 48 hours after completion of treatment in 21% of patients treated with 90 mg. Drug-related musculoskeletal pain and CNS symptoms (eg, dizziness, headache, increased sweating, paresthesia) were more common with Paget disease than with HCM treated with the same 90 mg dose.

Adverse experiences considered to be related to trial drug that occurred in at least 5% of patients with Paget disease treated with 90 mg of pamidronate in 2 US clinical trials were back pain, bone pain, fever, and nausea.

Other adverse reactions are as follows: hypertension, arthrosis, bone pain, headache (10%).

Osteolytic bone metastases of breast cancer and osteolytic lesions of multiple myeloma – In patients with multiple myeloma, there were 5 pamidronate-related serious and unexpected adverse experiences. Four of these were reported during the 12-month extension of the multiple myeloma trial. Three of the reports were of worsening renal function developing in patients with progressive multiple myeloma or multiple myeloma-associated amyloidosis. The fourth report was the adult respiratory distress syndrome developing in a patient recovering from pneumonia and acute gangrenous cholecystitis. One pamidronate-treated patient experienced an allergic reaction characterized by swollen and itchy eyes, runny nose, and scratchy throat within 24 hours after the sixth infusion.

In the breast cancer trials, there were 4 pamidronate-related adverse experiences, all moderate in severity, that caused a patient to discontinue participation in the trial. One was because of interstitial pneumonitis, another because of malaise and dyspnea. One pamidronate patient discontinued the trial because of asymptomatic hypocalcemia. Another pamidronate patient discontinued therapy because of severe bone pain after each infusion, which the investigator felt was trial drug related.

Postmarketing – Rare instances of allergic manifestations have been reported, including hypotension, dyspnea, or angioedema, and very rarely, anaphylactic shock.

➤*Tiludronate:* Adverse events associated with tiludronate usually have been mild and generally have not required discontinuation of therapy. Of patients receiving tiludronate 400 mg and placebo, 1.3% and 5.4%, respectively, discontinued therapy because of a clinical adverse reaction.

The most frequently occurring adverse reaction in patients who received tiludronate 400 mg/day were in the GI system: diarrhea (9.3%), nausea (9.3%), and dyspepsia (5.3%).

Paget disease – The following reactions occurred in at least 1% of patients.

CNS: Anxiety, involuntary muscle contractions, nervousness, vertigo.

Dermatologic: Increased sweating, pruritus, Stevens-Johnson–type syndrome (rare).

GI: Abdominal pain, constipation, dry mouth, gastritis.

Miscellaneous: Anorexia, asthenia, bronchitis, fatigue, flushing, hypertension, insomnia, pathological fracture, somnolence, syncope, urinary tract infection.

➤*Risedronate:* Duodenitis and glossitis have been reported uncommonly (0.1% to 1%). There have been rare reports of abnormal liver function tests (less than 0.1%).

Ophthalmic – Three patients who received risedronate 30 mg/day experienced acute iritis in 1 supportive study. All 3 patients recovered from their events. All patients were effectively treated with topical steroids.

Acute phase reactions – Symptoms consistent with acute phase reaction have been reported with bisphosphonate use. The overall incidence of acute phase reaction was 3.6% of patients on risedronate 5 mg daily and 7.6% of patients on risedronate 75 mg 2 consecutive days per month. These incidence rates are based on reporting of any of 33 acute phase reaction–like symptoms within 5 days of the first dose. Fever or influenza-like illness with onset within the same period were reported by 0% of patients on risedronate 5 mg daily and 0.6% of patients on risedronate 75 mg 2 consecutive days per month.

Lab test abnormalities – Asymptomatic and small decreases were observed in serum calcium and phosphorus levels. Overall, mean decreases of 0.8% in serum calcium and of 2.7% in phosphorus were observed at 6 months in patients receiving risedronate. Throughout the phase 3 studies, serum calcium levels below 8 mg/dL were observed in 18 patients, 9 (0.5%) in each treatment arm (risedronate and placebo). Serum phosphorus levels below 2 mg/dL were observed in 14 patients, 11 (0.6%) treated with risedronate and 3 (0.2%) treated with placebo.

Postmarketing –

GI: Events involving upper GI irritation, such as esophagitis and esophageal or gastric ulcers, have been reported.

Hypersensitivity: Hypersensitivity and skin reactions have been reported rarely, including angioedema, generalized rash, and bullous skin reactions, some severe.

Musculoskeletal: Bone, joint, or muscle pain, described as severe or incapacitating, have been reported rarely.

Special senses: Reactions of eye inflammation, including iritis and uveitis, have been reported rarely.

Miscellaneous: Osteonecrosis of the jaw has been reported rarely.

➤*Zoledronic acid:*

Hypercalcemia of malignancy – IV administration has been most commonly associated with fever. Occasionally, patients experience a flu-like syndrome consisting of fever, chills, bone pain or arthralgias, and myalgias. GI reactions, such as nausea and vomiting, have been reported following IV infusion. Local reactions at the infusion site, such as redness or swelling, were observed infrequently. In most cases, no specific treatment is required and the symptoms subside after 24 to 48 hours. Rare cases of rash, pruritus, chest pain, conjunctivitis, and hypomagnesemia have been reported.

Other adverse reactions 5% to less than 10% include the following: arthralgias, asthenia, chest pain, dehydration, dysphagia, granulocytopenia, headache, hypocalcemia, leg edema, metastases, mucositis, nonspecific infection, pancytopenia, pleural effusion, somnolence, thrombocytopenia.

Lab test abnormalities:

Zoledronic Acid vs. Pamidronate: Grade 3 to 4 Laboratory Abnormalities in Clinical Trials for Hypercalcemia of Malignancy

	Grade 3				Grade 4			
	Zoledronic acid 4 mg		Pamidronate 90 mg		Zoledronic acid 4 mg		Pamidronate 90 mg	
Laboratory parameter	n/N	%	n/N	%	n/N	%	n/N	%
Serum creatinine[a]	2/86	2.3	3/100	3	0/86	—	1/100	1
Hypocalcemia[b]	1/86	1.2	2/100	2	0/86	—	0/100	—
Hypophosphatemia[c]	36/70	51.4	27/81	33.3	1/70	1.4	4/81	4.9
Hypomagnesemia[d]	0/71	—	0/84	—	0/71	—	1/84	1.2

[a] Grade 3: > 3 times the ULN; grade 4: > 6 times the ULN.
[b] Grade 3: < 7 mg/dL; grade 4: < 6 mg/dL.
[c] Grade 3: < 2 mg/dL; grade 4: < 1 mg/dL.
[d] Grade 3: < 0.8 mEq/L; grade 4: < 0.5 mEq/L.

Multiple myeloma and bone metastases of solid tumors –

Lab test abnormalities:

Zoledronic Acid vs. Pamidronate: Grade 3 Laboratory Abnormalities in Clinical Trials in Patients With Bone Metastases

	Zoledronic acid 4 mg		Pamidronate 90 mg		Placebo	
Laboratory parameter	n/N	%	n/N	%	n/N	%
Serum creatinine[a]	7/529	1.3	4/268	1.5	2/241	0.8
Hypocalcemia[b]	7/1,041	0.7	4/610	0.7	0/415	—
Hypophosphatemia[c]	96/1,041	9.2	40/611	6.6	13/415	3.1
Hypermagnesemia[d]	19/1,039	1.8	3/609	0.5	8/415	1.9
Hypomagnesemia[e]	0/1,039	—	0/609	—	1/415	0.2

[a] Grade 3: > 3 times the ULN; grade 4: > 6 times the ULN. Serum creatinine data for all patients randomized after the 15-minute infusion amendment.
[b] Grade 3: < 7 mg/dL; grade 4: < 6 mg/dL.
[c] Grade 3: < 2 mg/dL; grade 4: < 1 mg/dL.
[d] Grade 3: > 3 mEq/L; grade 4: > 8 mEq/L.
[e] Grade 3: < 0.9 mEq/L; grade 4: < 0.7 mEq/L.

Zoledronic Acid vs. Pamidronate: Grade 4 Laboratory Abnormalities in Clinical Trials in Patients With Bone Metastases

	Zoledronic acid 4 mg		Pamidronate 90 mg		Placebo	
Laboratory parameter	n/N	%	n/N	%	n/N	%
Serum creatinine[a]	2/529	0.4	1/268	0.4	0/241	—
Hypocalcemia[b]	6/1,041	0.6	2/610	0.3	1/415	0.2
Hypophosphatemia[c]	6/1,041	0.6	0/611	—	1/415	0.2
Hypermagnesemia[d]	0/1,039	—	0/609	—	2/415	0.5
Hypomagnesemia[e]	2/1,039	0.2	2/609	0.3	0/415	—

[a] Grade 3: > 3 times the ULN; grade 4: > 6 times the ULN. Serum creatinine data for all patients randomized after the 15-minute infusion amendment.
[b] Grade 3: < 7 mg/dL; grade 4: < 6 mg/dL.
[c] Grade 3: < 2 mg/dL; grade 4: < 1 mg/dL.
[d] Grade 3: > 3 mEq/L; grade 4: > 8 mEq/L.
[e] Grade 3: < 0.9 mEq/L; grade 4: < 0.7 mEq/L.

Renal: In the bone metastases trials, renal deterioration was defined as an increase of 0.5 mg/dL for patients with normal baseline creatinine (less than 1.4 mg/dL) or an increase of 1 mg/dL for patients with an abnormal baseline creatinine (greater than 1.4 mg/dL). The percentage of patients with renal function deterioration who were randomized following the 15-minute zoledronic acid 4 mg infusion amendment were as follows:

Multiple myeloma and breast cancer: normal (9.3%), abnormal (3.8%), total (8.8%)

Solid tumors: normal (11%), abnormal (9.1%), total (10.9%)

Prostate cancer: normal (12.2%), abnormal (40%), total (15.2%)

Overdosage

➤*Alendronate and ibandronate:* Hypocalcemia, hypophosphatemia, and upper GI adverse events (eg, upset stomach, heartburn, esophagitis, gastritis, ulcer) may result from overdosage. Consider the administration of milk or antacids to bind alendronate. Dialysis would not be beneficial.

➤*Etidronate:* Clinical experience with etidronate overdosage is extremely limited. Decreases in serum calcium following substantial overdosage may be expected in some patients. Signs and symptoms of hypocalcemia also may occur and some patients may develop vomiting. In 1 event, an 18-year-old female who ingested an estimated single dose of 4,000 to 6,000 mg (67 to 100 mg/kg) was mildly hypocalcemic (7.52 mg/dL) and experienced paresthesia of the fingers. Some patients may develop vomiting and expel the drug. Orally administered etidronate disodium may cause hematologic abnormalities in some patients. Etidronate disodium suppresses bone turnover and may retard mineralization of osteoid laid down during the bone accretion process.

Gastric lavage may remove unabsorbed drug. Standard procedures for treating hypocalcemia, including the administration of calcium IV, would be expected to restore physiologic amounts of ionized calcium and relieve signs and symptoms of hypocalcemia. Such treatment has been effective.

➤*Ibandronate:* Oral overdosage may result in hypocalcemia, hypophosphatemia, and upper GI adverse reactions, such as upset stomach, dyspepsia, esophagitis, gastritis, or ulcer.

No specific information is available on the treatment of overdosage with **ibandronate**. Give milk or antacids to bind **ibandronate**. Because of the risk of esophageal irritation, do not induce vomiting. The patient should remain fully upright. Dialysis would not be beneficial.

➤*Pamidronate:* There have been several cases of drug maladministration of IV pamidronate in hypercalcemia patients with total doses of 225 to 300 mg given over 2.5 to 4 days. All patients survived but experienced hypocalcemia requiring IV or oral calcium.

One obese woman (95 kg) who was treated with pamidronate 285 mg/day for 3 days experienced high fever (39.5°C [102°F]), hypotension, and transient taste perversion noted approximately 6 hours after the first infusion. Fever and hypotension were rapidly corrected with steroids.

If overdosage occurs, symptomatic hypocalcemia also could result; treat such patients with short-term IV calcium.

➤*Risedronate:* Decreases in serum calcium following substantial overdose may be expected in some patients. Signs and symptoms of hypocalcemia also may occur in some of these patients.

Gastric lavage may remove unabsorbed drug. Administration of milk or antacids to chelate risedronate may be helpful. Standard procedures that are effective for treating hypocalcemia, including IV administration of calcium, would be expected to restore physiologic amounts of ionized calcium and to relieve signs and symptoms of hypocalcemia.

➤*Tiludronate:* Hypocalcemia is a potential consequence of tiludronate overdose. In 1 patient with HCM, IV administration of high doses of tiludronate (800 mg/day total dose, 6 mg/kg/day for 2 days) was associated with acute renal failure and death.

No specific information is available on the treatment of overdose with tiludronate. Dialysis would not be beneficial. Standard medical practices may be used to manage renal insufficiency or hypocalcemia if signs of these develop.

➤*Zoledronic acid:* Overdosage may cause clinically significant hypocalcemia, hypophosphatemia, and hypomagnesemia. Clinically relevant reductions in serum levels of calcium, phosphorus, and magnesium should be corrected by IV administration of calcium gluconate, potassium or sodium phosphate, and magnesium sulfate, respectively.

Patient Information

Bisphosphonates may cause GI upset (eg, nausea, diarrhea).

➤*Alendronate:* Instruct patients that the expected benefits of alendronate only may be obtained when each tablet is taken with plain water first thing in the morning and at least 30 minutes before the first food, beverage, or medication of the day. Also instruct them that waiting more than 30 minutes will improve alendronate absorption. Even dosing with orange juice or coffee markedly reduces the absorption of alendronate.

Instruct patients to take alendronate with a full glass of water (6 to 8 oz [180 to 240 mL]) and not to lie down for at least 30 minutes and until after the first food of the day following administration to facilitate delivery to the stomach and reduce the potential for esophageal irritation.

Patients should not chew or suck on the tablet because of a potential for oropharyngeal ulceration. Specifically instruct patients not to take alendronate at bedtime or before arising for the day. Inform patients that failure to follow these instructions may increase their risk of esophageal problems. Instruct patients that if they develop symptoms of esophageal disease (eg, difficulty or pain upon swallowing, retrosternal pain, new or worsening heartburn) they should stop taking alendronate and consult their health care provider.

Instruct patients that if they miss a dose of once-weekly alendronate they should take 1 tablet on the morning after they remember. They should not take 2 tablets on the same day but should return to taking 1 tablet once a week as originally scheduled on their chosen day.

Instruct patients to take supplemental calcium and vitamin D if dietary intake is inadequate. Consider weightbearing exercise along with the modification of certain behavioral factors, such as excessive cigarette smoking or alcohol consumption, if these factors exist.

It is likely that calcium supplements, antacids, and some oral medications will interfere with absorption of alendronate. Therefore, patients must wait at least 30 minutes after taking alendronate before taking any other oral medications.

➤*Etidronate:* Take on an empty stomach 2 hours before or after meals, including vitamin and mineral supplements or antacids, which are high in metals such as calcium, iron, magnesium, or aluminum.

➤*Ibandronate:* Advise patients to take **ibandronate** at least 60 minutes before the first food or drink (other than water) of the day and before taking any oral medications containing multivalent cations (including antacids, supplements, or vitamins).

To facilitate delivery to the stomach, and thus reduce the potential for esophageal irritation, advise patients to swallow **ibandronate** tablets whole with a full glass of plain water (180 to 240 mL [6 to 8 oz]) while standing or sitting in an upright position. Advise patients not to lie down for 60 minutes after taking ibandronate.

Advise patients to only drink plain water with ibandronate. Please note that some mineral waters may have a higher concentration of calcium and therefore should not be used.

Advise patients not to chew or suck the tablets because of a potential for oropharyngeal ulceration.

Advise patients to take the ibandronate 150 mg tablet on the same date each month (ie, the patient's ibandronate day).

If the once-monthly dose is missed, and the patient's next scheduled ibandronate day is more than 7 days away, instruct the patient to take 1 ibandronate 150 mg tablet in the morning following the date that it is remembered. If the patient's next scheduled ibandronate day is only 1 to 7 days away, the patient must wait until their next scheduled ibandronate day to take their tablet. Advise the patient to then return to taking 1 ibandronate 150 mg tablet every month in the morning of their chosen day, according to their original schedule.

Patients should receive supplemental calcium and vitamin D if dietary intake is inadequate. Advise patients to delay intake of supplemental calcium and vitamin D for at least 60 minutes following oral administration of ibandronate, in order to maximize absorption of ibandronate.

Instruct patients to discontinue ibandronate and seek medical attention if they develop symptoms of esophageal irritation (eg, new or worsening dysphagia, pain on swallowing, retrosternal pain, heartburn).

➤*Risedronate:* Instruct patients that if they miss a dose of risedronate 35 mg once weekly (immediate and delayed release), they should take 1 tablet on the morning after they remember and return to taking 1 tablet once weekly, as originally scheduled on their chosen day. Instruct patients not to take 2 tablets on the same day.

If the dose of risedronate 150 mg once a month is missed and the next month's scheduled dose is more than 7 days away, instruct the patient to take the missed tablet on the morning after the day it is remembered. Instruct patients to then return to taking their risedronate 150 mg once a month, as originally scheduled. Instruct patients not to take more than one 150 mg tablet within 7 days. If the dose of risedronate 150 mg once a month is missed and the next month's scheduled dose is within 7 days, instruct patients to wait until their next month's scheduled dose and then continue taking risedronate 150 mg once a month, as originally scheduled.

Inform patients to pay particular attention to the dosing instructions because clinical benefits may be compromised by failure to take the drug according to instructions. Take risedronate immediate release at least 30 minutes before the first food or drink of the day other than water. Instruct patients to take risedronate delayed release immediately following breakfast and not under fasting conditions.

In order to facilitate delivery to the stomach and minimize the possibility of esophageal irritation, instruct patients to take risedronate in an upright position, sitting or standing, with a full glass (6 to 8 oz [180 to 240 mL]) of plain water and to avoid lying down for 30 minutes after taking this medication. Advise patients to take supplemental calcium and vitamin D if dietary intake is inadequate (see Warnings/Precautions). Calcium, magnesium or aluminum supplements, or antacids may interfere with the absorption of risedronate; instruct patients to take them at a different time of the day as with food. Instruct patients not to chew or suck on tablets because of potential for oropharyngeal irritation.

Inform patients not to chew, cut, or crush risedronate delayed-release tablets.

Instruct patients that if they develop symptoms of esophageal disease (eg, difficulty or pain upon swallowing; retrosternal pain; severe, persistent, or worsening heartburn) to consult their health care provider before continuing risedronate.

Advise patients to consider weightbearing exercise along with the modification of certain behavioral factors, such as excessive cigarette smoking or alcohol consumption, if these factors exist.

➤*Tiludronate:* Take tiludronate with 6 to 8 oz (180 to 240 mL) of plain water. Do not take within 2 hours of food. Maintain adequate vitamin D and calcium intake. Do not take calcium supplements, aspirin, and indomethacin within 2 hours before or after tiludronate. If needed, take aluminum- or magnesium-containing antacids at least 2 hours after tiludronate.

➤*Zoledronic acid:* Inform patients of the importance of getting blood tests (serum creatinine) during the course of their zoledronic acid therapy.

Advise patients of the importance of good dental hygiene and to have a dental examination prior to treatment with zoledronic acid and also to avoid invasive dental procedures during treatment.

Adequate calcium and vitamin D intake is important in women with osteoporosis, and the current recommended daily intake for calcium is 1,200 mg and for vitamin D is 800 to 1,000 units daily. Advise patients of the importance of calcium and vitamin D supplementation in maintaining serum calcium levels.

It is strongly recommended that patients with Paget disease take calcium in divided doses (eg, 2 to 4 times a day), for a total of 1,500 mg/day of calcium, to prevent low blood calcium levels. This is especially important for the 2 weeks after getting zoledronic acid.

Advise patients with multiple myeloma and bone metastasis of solid tumors to take an oral calcium supplement of 500 mg and multiple vitamin containing vitamin D 400 units daily.

On the day of treatment, instruct patients to eat and drink normally, which includes drinking at least 2 glasses of fluid, such as water, within a few hours prior to the zoledronic acid infusion, as directed by their health care provider.

Advise patients of the most common adverse reactions of therapy, including abdominal pain, aggravated malignant neoplasm, anemia, anorexia, arthralgia, back pain, bone pain, constipation, cough, decreased weight, diarrhea, dizziness, dyspnea, fatigue, headache, insomnia, lower limb edema, myalgia, nausea, paresthesia, pyrexia, vomiting, and weakness.

Inform patients that there have been reports, primarily in patients treated with bisphosphonates for other illnesses, of persistent pain and/or nonhealing sore of the mouth or jaw. Instruct patients who experience these symptoms to tell their health care provider or dentist.

ALENDRONATE SODIUM

Rx	**Alendronate Sodium** (Teva)	**Tablets; oral:** 5 mg	As 6.53 mg alendronate monosodium salt trihydrate. (93 5140). In 30s and 100s.
Rx	**Fosamax** (Merck)		Lactose. (MRK 925). White. In unit-of-use 30s and 100s.
Rx	**Alendronate Sodium** (Teva)	**Tablets; oral:** 10 mg	As 13.05 mg alendronate monosodium salt trihydrate. 93 5141). In 30s and 100s.
Rx	**Fosamax** (Merck)		Lactose. (MRK 936). White, oval. In 1,000s, unit-of-use 30s and 100s, *Uniblister* cards of 31, and UD 100s.
Rx	**Alendronate Sodium** (Teva)	**Tablets; oral:** 35 mg	As 45.68 mg alendronate monosodium salt trihydrate. 93 5172). Pillow-shaped. In blister pack 4s and UD 20s.
Rx	**Fosamax** (Merck)		Lactose. (77). White, oval. In unit-of-use 4s and UD 20s.
Rx	**Alendronate Sodium** (Teva)	**Tablets; oral:** 40 mg	As 52.21 mg alendronate monosodium salt trihydrate. 93 5142). Oval. In 30s.
Rx	**Fosamax** (Merck)		Lactose. (MRK 212/Fosamax). White, triangular. In unit-of-use 30s.
Rx	**Alendronate Sodium** Various, eg, (Teva, Barr Labs)	**Tablets; oral:** 70 mg	As 91.37 mg alendronate monosodium salt trihydrate. In 20s, blister pack 4s and UD 20s.
Rx	**Fosamax** (Merck)		Lactose. (31). White, oval. In unit-of-use 4s and UD 20s.
Rx	**Fosamax** (Merck)	**Oral solution; oral:** 70 mg (as base)	Saccharin, parabens. Raspberry flavor. In 75 mL.

ALENDRONATE SODIUM — ORAL

For complete and comparative prescribing information, refer to the Bisphosphonates group monograph.

Indications

➤*Glucocorticoid-induced osteoporosis:* For the treatment of glucocorticoid-induced osteoporosis in men and women receiving glucocorticoids in a daily dosage equivalent to prednisone 7.5 mg or greater and who have low bone mineral density. Patients treated with glucocorticoids should receive adequate amounts of calcium and vitamin D.

➤*Osteoporosis in men:* As a treatment to increase bone mass in men with osteoporosis.

➤*Osteoporosis in postmenopausal women:* For the treatment and prevention of osteoporosis in postmenopausal women.

➤*Paget disease of bone:* For the treatment of Paget disease of bone in men and women. Treatment is indicated in patients with Paget disease of bone having alkaline phosphatase at least 2 times the upper limit of normal, those who are symptomatic, or those at risk for future complications from their disease.

➤*Off-label uses:*

Hypercalcemia of malignancy – [5] = Poor documentation. Limited data from studies indicate that intravenous (IV) alendronate may have a beneficial role in the management of hypercalcemia in patients with cancer. However, no studies have been performed using oral alendronate. Because oral alendronate has extremely poor bioavailability, rational use of alendronate cannot be established from the study results using IV alendronate.

Hypervitaminosis D (infants/children) – [4] = Insufficient documentation. Case reports describe the use of oral alendronate to effectively manage hypervitaminosis D in infants and children, although to date, these data have been reported in fewer than 10 patients.

Osteogenesis imperfecta – Initial data suggest that oral alendronate is equally as safe and effective as intravenous (IV) bisphosphonates and is a practical alternative. It is likely a more cost-effective alternative when compared with IV therapy.

Osteogenesis imperfecta (adults): [2] = Fair documentation.

Osteogenesis imperfecta (children/adolescents): [2] = Fair documentation.

Osteoporosis with spinal cord injury – [4] = Insufficient documentation. The bisphosphonates (eg, alendronate, etidronate, pamidronate, tiludronate) used to date in a limited number of acute spinal cord injury patients have all produced trends in reducing bone loss.

Postoperative knee arthroplasty – [2] = Fair documentation. Alendronate has been evaluated for the prevention of bone mineral density (BMD) loss after knee arthroplasty in 3 controlled studies that included more than 150 patients. Alendronate has been shown to effectively attenuate bone loss or improve BMD after knee arthroplasty; however, benefits appear short-lived after discontinuation of therapy.

Administration and Dosage

➤*Adults:*

Glucocorticoid-induced osteoporosis – 5 mg once daily. For postmenopausal women not receiving estrogen, the dosage is 10 mg once daily.

Osteoporosis in men – 70 mg once weekly (as one 70 mg tablet or 1 bottle of 70 mg oral solution) or 10 mg once daily.

Osteoporosis in postmenopausal women –

Prevention: One 35 mg tablet once weekly or 5 mg once daily.

Treatment: 70 mg once weekly (as one 70 mg tablet or 1 bottle of 70 mg oral solution) or 10 mg once daily.

Paget disease of bone –

Usual dosage: 40 mg once a day for 6 months.

Retreatment: Retreatment with alendronate may be considered following a 6-month posttreatment evaluation period in patients who have relapsed, based on increases in serum alkaline phosphatase, which should be measured periodically. Retreatment also may be considered in those who failed to normalize their serum alkaline phosphatase.

Off-label dosing –

Osteogenesis imperfecta (adults): [2] = Fair documentation. 10 mg once daily.

Osteoporosis with spinal cord injury: [4] = Insufficient documentation. 10 mg/day. Concurrent therapy with vitamin D and calcium carbonate.

Postoperative knee arthroplasty: [2] = Fair documentation. 10 mg once daily beginning after knee arthroplasty. Alendronate has been studied in this setting for a maximum of 1 year, but longer-term therapy may be required to sustain the benefits of therapy.

➤*Renal function impairment:* Alendronate is not recommended for patients with more severe renal function impairment (CrCl less than 35 mL/min) because of lack of experience.

➤*Concomitant therapy:* Patients should receive supplemental calcium and vitamin D if dietary intake is inadequate.

➤*Administration:* Alendronate must be taken at least 30 minutes before the first food, beverage, or medication of the day with plain water only. Waiting less than 30 minutes or taking alendronate with food, beverages (other than plain water), or other medications will lessen the effect of alendronate by decreasing its absorption into the body.

Alendronate should only be taken upon arising for the day. To facilitate delivery to the stomach and reduce the potential for esophageal irritation, an alendronate tablet should be swallowed with a full glass of water (180 to 240 mL). To facilitate gastric emptying, alendronate oral solution should be followed by at least 60 mL (one-fourth cup) of water. Patients should not lie down for at least 30 minutes and until after their first food of the day. Alendronate should not be taken at bedtime or before arising for the day. Failure to follow these instructions may increase the risk of esophageal adverse reactions.

➤*Storage/Stability:*

Tablets – Store in a well-closed container at room temperature, 15° to 30°C (59° to 86°F).

Oral solution – Store at 25°C (77°F); excursions are permitted to 15° to 30°C (59° to 86°F). Do not freeze.

ETIDRONATE DISODIUM

Rx	**Etidronate Disodium** (Mylan)	**Tablets; oral:** 200 mg	In 60s.
Rx	**Etidronate Disodium** (Mylan)	**Tablets; oral:** 400 mg	In 60s.
Rx	**Didronel** (Warner Chillcot)		(N E 406). White, scored, capsule-shape. In 60s.

ETIDRONATE DISODIUM — ORAL

For complete prescribing information, refer to the Bisphosphonates class monograph.

Indications

➤*Heterotopic ossification:* For the prevention and treatment of heterotopic ossification following total hip replacement or caused by spinal cord injury.

➤*Paget disease:* For the treatment of symptomatic Paget disease of bone.

The effects of etidronate treatment in patients with asymptomatic Paget disease have not been studied. However, etidronate treatment of such patients may be warranted if extensive involvement threatens irreversible neurologic damage, major joints, or major weight-bearing bones.

➤*General information:* Etidronate is not approved for the treatment of osteoporosis.

ETIDRONATE DISODIUM — ORAL

➤*Off-label uses:*

Osteoporosis with spinal cord injury – [4] = Insufficient documentation. The bisphosphonates used to date in a limited number of patients with acute spinal cord injury (eg, alendronate, etidronate, pamidronate, tiludronate) all have produced trends in reducing bone loss. However, larger controlled trials are needed to determine which agent may be preferred to optimize dosing regimens and define active rehabilitation protocols. (See Administration and Dosage.)

Other possible off-label uses – For the prevention and treatment of corticosteroid-induced osteoporosis.

Administration and Dosage

➤*Adults:*

Heterotopic ossification –

Spinal cord injury:

• *Usual dosage* – 20 mg/kg/day for 2 weeks, followed by 10 mg/kg/day for 10 weeks. Institute therapy as soon as medically feasible following the injury, preferably prior to evidence of heterotopic ossification.

• *Duration of therapy* – The total treatment period is 12 weeks.

Total hip replacement:

• *Usual dosage* – 20 mg/kg/day for 1 month before and 3 months after surgery.

• *Duration of therapy* – The total treatment period is 4 months.

Paget disease –

Maximum dose: Dosages higher than 20 mg/kg/day are not recommended.

Initial dosage: 5 to 10 mg/kg/day (not to exceed 6 months) or 11 to 20 mg/kg/day (not to exceed 3 months). Reserve dosages higher than 10 mg/kg/day for use when lower dosages are ineffective, or when there is an overriding need to suppress rapid bone turnover (especially when there is an irreversible neurologic damage is possible) or to reduce elevated cardiac output.

• *Re-treatment* – Initiate only after an etidronate-free period of at least 90 days and when there is biochemical, symptomatic, or other evidence of active disease process. Monitor patients every 3 to 6 months, although some patients may go drug-free for extended periods. Re-treatment regimens are the same as for initial treatment. For most patients, the original dose will be adequate for re-treatment. If not, consider increasing the dose within the recommended guidelines.

Off-label dosing –

Osteoporosis with spinal cord injury: [4] = Insufficient documentation. 800 mg daily for 2 weeks in a 15-week cycle. Two cycles administered.

➤*Elderly:* Because elderly patients are more likely to have decreased renal function, care should be taken when prescribing this drug therapy.

➤*Renal function impairment:* Etidronate dosage should be reduced when reductions in glomerular filtration rates are present. Patients with renal impairment should be closely monitored.

➤*Administration:* Administer as a single oral dose. However, if GI discomfort occurs, the dose may be divided.

Etidronate tablets should be swallowed with a full glass (6 to 8 oz) of water. Patients should not lie down after taking the medication.

To maximize absorption, patients should avoid taking the following within 2 hours of dosing: food, especially items high in calcium, such as milk or milk products; vitamins with mineral supplements or antacids high in metals (eg, aluminum, calcium, iron, magnesium).

➤*Storage/Stability:* Store at 20°C to 25°C (68°F to 77°F); excursions permitted to between 15°C and 30°C (59°F and 86°F). Avoid excessive heat (above 40°C [104°F]). Dispense in a tight, light-resistant container.

TILUDRONATE

Rx	**Skelid** (Sanofi-Aventis)	**Tablets; oral:** 200 mg	Equiv. to tiludronate disodium 240 mg. Lactose. (S.W 200). White, round. In UD 56s.

TILUDRONATE DISODIUM — ORAL

For complete and comparative prescribing information, refer to the Bisphosphonates class monograph.

Indications

➤*Paget disease:* For treatment of Paget disease of bone (osteitis deformans).

➤*Off-label uses:*

Osteoporosis with spinal cord injury – [4] = Insufficient documentation. The bisphosphonates (eg, alendronate, etidronate, pamidronate, tiludronate) used in a limited number of acute spinal cord injury patients all have reduced bone loss. However, larger, controlled trials are needed to determine which agent is preferred to optimize dosing regimens and define active rehabilitation protocols. (See Administration and Dosage.)

Administration and Dosage

➤*General dosing considerations:* Following therapy, allow an interval of 3 months to assess the response. Specific data regarding retreatment are limited, although results from uncontrolled studies indicate favorable biochemical improvement similar to initial tiludronate treatment.

➤*Adults:*

Paget disease –

Usual dosage: 400 mg once daily with 6 to 8 ounces of plain water for 3 months.

Concomitant therapy: Maintain adequate vitamin D and calcium intake.

Off-label dosing –

Osteoporosis with spinal cord injury: [4] = Insufficient documentation. 200 or 400 mg/day for 3 months.

➤*Renal function impairment:* Not recommended for patients with severe renal failure (ie, creatinine clearance [CrCl] less than 30 mL/min).

➤*Administration:* Administer with 6 to 8 ounces of plain water. Do not take within 2 hours of consuming food. Beverages other than plain water (including mineral water), food, and some medications are likely to reduce the absorption of tiludronate. Do not take calcium or mineral supplements, aspirin, or indomethacin within 2 hours before or 2 hours after tiludronate. Take aluminum- or magnesium-containing antacids at least 2 hours after taking tiludronate.

Patients should not lie down for at least 30 minutes after taking this medication. In patients who cannot comply with dosing instructions because of mental or physical disability, therapy with tiludronate should be used under appropriate supervision.

➤*Storage/Stability:* Store at 25°C (77°F); excursions are permitted to 15° to 30°C (59° to 86°F). Do not remove tablets from the foil strips until they are to be used.

RISEDRONATE SODIUM

Rx	**Actonel** (Warner Chilcott)	**Tablets; oral:** 5 mg	Lactose, PEG. (RSN 5 mg). Yellow, oval. Film-coated. In 30s.
		30 mg	Lactose, PEG. (RSN 30 mg). White, oval. Film-coated. In 30s.
		35 mg	Lactose, PEG. (RSN 35 mg). Orange, oval. Film-coated. In UD 4s and 12s.
		150 mg	PEG. (RSN 150 mg). Blue, oval. Film-coated. In UD 1s and 3s.
Rx	**Atelvia** (Warner Chilcott)	**Tablets, delayed-release; oral:** 35 mg	Edetate disodium. (EC 35). Yellow, oval. In UD 4s.

RISEDRONATE SODIUM — ORAL

For complete and comparative prescribing information, refer to the Bisphosphonates class monograph.

Indications

➤*Glucocorticoid-induced osteoporosis (immediate release only):* For the treatment and prevention of glucocorticoid-induced osteoporosis in men and women who are initiating or continuing systemic glucocorticoid treatment (daily dose of prednisone 7.5 mg or more or equivalent) for chronic diseases.

➤*Osteoporosis in men (immediate release only):* To increase bone mass in men with osteoporosis.

➤*Osteoporosis in postmenopausal women:*

Immediate release – For the treatment and prevention of osteoporosis in postmenopausal women.

In postmenopausal women with osteoporosis, risedronate reduces the incidence of vertebral fractures and a composite end point of nonvertebral osteoporosis-related fractures.

Delayed release – For the treatment of osteoporosis in postmenopausal women.

➤*Paget disease (immediate release only):* For treatment of Paget disease of bone in men and women.

➤*Off-label uses:*

Hypercalcemia of malignancy – [5] = Poor documentation. Experience with the use of risedronate for the treatment of tumor-induced hypercalcemia is limited to a single patient. In the same study in which successful reversal of hypercalcemia by risedronate was reported in 1 patient, another patient developed tumor-induced hypercalcemia during ongoing risedronate therapy. Risedronate is not recommended for the treatment of tumor-induced hypercalcemia.

Primary hyperparathyroidism – [4] = Insufficient documentation. Data available on the use of risedronate for primary hyperparathyroidism are limited by small sample size, short treatment period, and use of surrogate markers of bone health. Alendronate, another second-generation bisphosphonate related to risedronate, has been studied more extensively.

RISEDRONATE SODIUM — ORAL

These 2 compounds share a common mechanism of action and are likely to produce highly similar effects in the treatment of primary hyperparathyroidism. Although short-term treatment with risedronate normalized the serum calcium concentrations for some patients with mild primary hyperparathyroidism, changes in calcium levels or serum parathyroid hormone (PTH) have not been observed in studies of alendronate with larger patient sample sizes and longer follow-up times. Alendronate therapy has been shown to improve bone mineral density (BMD) in patients with primary hyperparathyroidism. Further studies are needed to determine if risedronate also has a beneficial effect on BMD and to evaluate its long-term safety. In particular, the clinical significance of the enhanced serum calcium increase after oral calcium dosing remains unclear.

Administration and Dosage

➤*Adults:*

Glucocorticoid-induced osteoporosis (immediate release only) – 5 mg daily.

Osteoporosis in men (immediate release only) – 35 mg once per week.

Osteoporosis in postmenopausal women –

Immediate release: 5 mg daily or 35 mg once per week or 75 mg taken on 2 consecutive days for a total of 2 tablets (150 mg) per month, or 150 mg once a month.

Delayed release: 35 mg once per week.

Paget disease (immediate release only) –

Usual dosage: 30 mg daily for 2 months.

Re-treatment: Consider re-treatment (following a posttreatment observation of at least 2 months) if relapse occurs or if treatment fails to normalize serum alkaline phosphatase. For re-treatment, the dose and duration of therapy are the same as for initial treatment.

Off-label dosing –

Primary hyperparathyroidism: [4] = Insufficient documentation. 20 or 40 mg orally once daily given 2 hours before breakfast. The study reviewed had a duration of 7 days; however, ongoing therapy would likely be required.

➤*Renal function impairment:* Risedronate is not recommended for use in patients with severe renal function impairment (creatinine clearance [CrCl] less than 30 mL/min).

➤*Hepatic function impairment:* Dosage adjustment is unlikely to be needed in patients with hepatic impairment.

➤*Concomitant therapy:* Patients should receive supplemental calcium and vitamin D if dietary intake is inadequate. In clinical studies with immediate-release risedronate, patients were given calcium (elemental) 500 to 1,000 mg/day with or without vitamin D (up to 1,000 units/day). Calcium supplements; calcium-, aluminum-, and magnesium-containing medications; laxatives; and iron preparations may interfere with the absorption of risedronate and should be taken at a different time of the day.

➤*Administration:*

Immediate release – Risedronate should be taken at least 30 minutes before the first food or drink of the day other than water. To facilitate delivery to the stomach, patients should take risedronate while in an upright position with a full glass of plain water (6 to 8 oz). Patients should not lie down for 30 minutes after taking this medication. Tablets should not be chewed or allowed to melt or dissolve in the mouth because of the potential for oropharyngeal irritation.

Delayed release – Delayed-release risedronate should be taken in the morning immediately following breakfast.

When compared with immediate-release risedronate, treatment with delayed-release risedronate resulted in a significantly higher incidence of abdominal pain when administered before breakfast under fasting conditions. Delayed-release risedronate should be taken immediately following breakfast and not under fasting conditions.

To facilitate delivery to the stomach, delayed-release risedronate should be swallowed whole while the patient is in an upright position and with at least 4 oz of plain water. Tablets should not be chewed, cut, or crushed. Patients should not lie down for 30 minutes after taking the medication.

➤*Storage/Stability:* Store at 20° to 25°C (68° to 77°F).

ZOLEDRONIC ACID

Rx	**Zometa** (Novartis)	**Injection, solution, concentrate:** 4 mg per 5 mL	Mannitol 220 mg. In 5 mL single-dose vials.
Rx	**Reclast** (Novartis)	**Injection, solution:** 5 mg per 100 mL	Mannitol 4,950 mg. In 100 mL ready-to-use bottles.

ZOLEDRONIC ACID — INJECTION

For complete and comparative prescribing information, refer to the Bisphosphonates class monograph.

Indications

➤*Reclast:*

Glucocorticoid-induced osteoporosis – For the treatment and prevention of glucocorticoid-induced osteoporosis in men and women who are initiating or continuing systemic glucocorticoids in a daily dosage equivalent to 7.5 mg or more of prednisone and who are expected to remain on glucocorticoids for at least 12 months.

Osteoporosis in men – To increase bone mass in men with osteoporosis.

Paget disease of bone – For the treatment of Paget disease of bone in men and women.

Prevention of osteoporosis in postmenopausal women – For prevention of osteoporosis in postmenopausal women.

Postmenopausal osteoporosis – For treatment and prevention of osteoporosis in postmenopausal women.

➤*Zometa:*

Hypercalcemia of malignancy – For the treatment of hypercalcemia of malignancy.

Multiple myeloma and bone metastases from solid tumors – For the treatment of patients with multiple myeloma and patients with documented bone metastases from solid tumors, in conjunction with standard antineoplastic therapy. Prostate cancer should have progressed after treatment with at least 1 hormonal therapy.

➤*Off-label uses:*

Osteopenia in androgen-deprived prostate cancer patients – [1] = Good documentation. National Comprehensive Cancer Network 2008 evidence-based guidelines recommend alendronate or zoledronic acid for prevention of osteopenia secondary to androgen deprivation therapy in prostate cancer patients. In placebo-controlled trials, zoledronic acid has led to improvement in bone mineral density (BMD) scans and decreases in biomarkers for bone turnover. Larger, controlled trials may be needed to determine optimal dosing and adverse events.

Osteopenia in estrogen-deprived breast cancer patients – [1] = Good documentation. Data from 3 controlled trials enrolling more than 1,000 women with breast cancer show that the addition of zoledronic acid when starting estrogen-depleting hormonal therapy preserves BMD. Patients receiving treatment regimens without zoledronic acid or in whom the addition of this agent is delayed may lose more bone mass, which leads to an increased risk of fractures.

Prevention of postrenal transplant bone loss – [4] = Insufficient documentation. Therapy with zoledronic acid after kidney transplantation may provide short-term benefits in increasing the calcium content of cancellous bone. This initial therapy after transplantation was not shown to provide long-term effects and was not superior to placebo after 3 years posttransplant. Additional studies with a larger sample size must be completed to determine whether there is a benefit with zoledronic acid therapy following kidney transplantation.

Administration and Dosage

➤*General dosing considerations:* Patients must be appropriately hydrated prior to administration of zoledronic acid.

Reclast – Administration of acetaminophen following zoledronic acid administration may reduce the incidence of acute-phase reaction symptoms.

➤*Adults:*

Reclast – The following recommended doses of zoledronic acid are for patients with a creatine clearance (CrCl) of 35 mL/min or more.

Glucocorticoid-induced osteoporosis:

• *Usual dosage* – A single 5 mg infusion once a year given intravenously (IV) over no less than 15 minutes.

• *Concomitant therapy* – Patients must be adequately supplemented with calcium and vitamin D if dietary intake is not sufficient. An average of at least 1,200 mg of calcium and 800 to 1,000 units of vitamin D daily is recommended.

Osteoporosis in men:

• *Usual dosage* – A single 5 mg infusion once a year given IV over no less than 15 minutes.

• *Concomitant therapy* – See Glucocorticoid-Induced Osteoporosis for dosing.

Patients must be adequately supplemented with calcium and vitamin D if dietary intake is not sufficient. An average of 1,200 mg of calcium and 800 to 1,000 units of vitamin D daily is recommended.

Paget disease of bone:

• *Usual dosage* – 5 mg infusion given IV at a constant rate over no less than 15 minutes.

• *Concomitant therapy* – To reduce the risk of hypocalcemia, all patients should receive elemental calcium 1,500 mg daily in divided doses (750 mg 2 times a day or 500 mg 3 times a day) and vitamin D 800 units daily, particularly in the 2 weeks following zoledronic acid administration. Instruct all patients on the importance of calcium and vitamin D supplementation in maintaining serum calcium levels and on the symptoms of hypocalcemia.

• *Rechallenge* – After a single treatment with zoledronic acid in Paget disease, an extended remission period is observed. Specific re-treatment data are not available. However, re-treatment with zoledronic acid may be considered in patients who have relapsed based on increases in serum alkaline phosphatase, in those patients who failed to achieve normalization of their serum alkaline phosphatase, or in those patients with symptoms, as dictated by medical practice.

Prevention of osteoporosis in postmenopausal women:

• *Usual dosage* – 5 mg infusion given IV once every 2 years over no less than 15 minutes.

• *Concomitant therapy* – See Glucocorticoid-Induced Osteoporosis for dosing.

ZOLEDRONIC ACID — INJECTION

Postmenopausal osteoporosis:

• *Usual dosage* – A single 5 mg infusion once a year given IV over no less than 15 minutes.

• *Concomitant therapy* – See Glucocorticoid-Induced Osteoporosis for dosing.

Zometa –

Hypercalcemia of malignancy: Consider the severity and the symptoms of tumor-induced hypercalcemia when considering use of zoledronic acid.

• *Usual dosage* – 4 mg dose must be given as a single-dose IV infusion over no less than 15 minutes. Patients who receive zoledronic acid should have serum creatinine assessed prior to each treatment.

• *Maximum dose* – 4 mg dose IV (albumin-corrected serum calcium is at least 12 mg/dL [3 mmol/L]).

• *Rechallenge* – Re-treatment with 4 mg may be considered if serum calcium does not return to normal or remain normal after initial treatment. It is recommended that a minimum of 7 days elapse before re-treatment to allow for full response to the initial dose. Renal function must be carefully monitored in all patients receiving zoledronic acid, and serum creatinine must be assessed prior to re-treatment with zoledronic acid.

• *Hydration* – Adequately rehydrate patients prior to administration of zoledronic acid. Promptly initiate vigorous saline hydration, an integral part of hypercalcemia therapy, and make an attempt to restore the urine output to approximately 2 L/day throughout treatment. Mild or asymptomatic hypercalcemia may be treated with conservative measures (ie, saline hydration with or without loop diuretics). Adequately hydrate patients throughout treatment, but overhydration, especially in those patients who have cardiac failure, must be avoided. Do not employ diuretic therapy prior to correction of hypovolemia.

Multiple myeloma and metastatic bone lesions of solid tumors:

• *Usual dosage* – 4 mg infused over no less than 15 minutes every 3 or 4 weeks for patients with CrCl more than 60 mL/min. The optimal duration of therapy is not known.

• *Concomitant therapy* – Administer patients an oral calcium supplement of 500 mg and a multiple vitamin containing vitamin D 400 units daily.

Off-label dosing –

Osteopenia in androgen-deprived prostate cancer patients: [1] = Good documentation. 4 mg IV infusion administered over 15 minutes given intermittently every 3 months or once yearly for the duration of 1 year.

Osteopenia in estrogen-deprived breast cancer patients: [1] = Good documentation. 4 mg infused IV over 15 minutes every 6 months for up to 5 years.

Prevention of postrenal transplant bone loss: [4] = Insufficient documentation. 4 mg infused IV over 15 minutes at week 2 and month 3 after engraftment.

➤*Renal function impairment:*

Reclast – The recommended dose in patients with a CrCl of 35 mL/min or more is zoledronic acid 5 mg infused over no less than 15 minutes at a constant infusion rate. Zoledronic acid is not recommended for use in patients with severe renal impairment (CrCl less than 35 mL/min).

Zometa –

Multiple myeloma and bone metastases from solid tumors:

Recommended Zoledronic Acid Dose for Patients With Mild to Moderate Renal Impairment	
Baseline CrCl (mL/min)	Zoledronic acid recommended dose[a]
> 60	4 mg
50 to 60	3.5 mg

Recommended Zoledronic Acid Dose for Patients With Mild to Moderate Renal Impairment	
Baseline CrCl (mL/min)	Zoledronic acid recommended dose[a]
40 to 49	3.3 mg
30 to 39	3 mg

[a] Doses calculated assuming target area under the curve (AUC) of 0.66 mg•h/L (CrCl = 75 mL/min).

During treatment, measure serum creatinine before each zoledronic acid dose and withhold treatment for renal deterioration.

In the clinical studies, zoledronic acid treatment was resumed only when the creatinine returned to within 10% of the baseline value. Reinitiate zoledronic acid at the same dose as that prior to treatment interruption.

➤*Preparation for administration:*

Zometa – Vials of zoledronic acid concentrate for infusion contain overfill, allowing for the withdrawal of 5 mL of concentrate (equivalent to zoledronic acid 4 mg). Dilute this concentrate immediately in 100 mL of sterile sodium chloride 0.9% or dextrose 5% injection. To avoid inadvertent injection, do not store undiluted concentrate in a syringe.

Reduced doses for patients with a baseline CrCl of 60 mL/min or less: Withdraw an appropriate volume of the zoledronic acid 5 mL concentrate as needed: 4.4 mL for 3.5 mg dose; 4.1 mL for 3.3 mg dose; 3.8 mL for 3 mg dose.

The withdrawn concentrate must be diluted in 100 mL of sterile sodium chloride 0.9% or dextrose 5% injection.

➤*Administration:* Patients must be appropriately hydrated prior to administration of zoledronic acid.

Reclast – The infusion time must not be less than 15 minutes given over a constant infusion rate.

Zoledronic acid for infusion must not be allowed to come in contact with any calcium- or other divalent cation–containing solutions, and should be administered as a single IV solution through a separate vented infusion line. Administration of acetaminophen following zoledronic acid administration may reduce the incidence of acute-phase reaction symptoms.

Zometa – Because of the risk of clinically significant deterioration in renal function, which may progress to renal failure, single doses of zoledronic acid should not exceed 4 mg, and the duration of infusion should be no less than 15 minutes. In the trials and in postmarketing experience, renal deterioration, progression to renal failure, and dialysis have occurred in patients, including those treated with the approved dose of 4 mg infused over 15 minutes. There have been instances of this occurring after the initial zoledronic acid dose.

➤*Admixture compatibility:* Zoledronic acid must not be mixed with calcium- or other divalent cation–containing infusion solutions, such as Ringer's lactate solution, and should be administered as a single IV solution in a line separate from all other drugs.

➤*Storage/Stability:*

Reclast – Store at 25°C (77°F); excursions are permitted between 15° and 30°C (59° and 86°F). After opening, the solution is stable for 24 hours at 2° to 8°C (36° to 46°F). If refrigerated, allow the refrigerated solution to reach room temperature before administration.

Zometa – Store at 25°C (77°F); excursions are permitted between 15° and 30°C (59° and 86°F).

If not used immediately after dilution with infusion media, refrigerate the solution at 2° to 8°C (36° to 46°F) for microbiological integrity. Then equilibrate the refrigerated solution to room temperature prior to administration. The total time between dilution, storage in the refrigerator, and end of administration must not exceed 24 hours.

IBANDRONATE

Rx	**Boniva** (Roche)	**Tablets; oral:** 150 mg	As ibandronate sodium 168.75 mg. Lactose. (BNVA 150). White, oblong. Film-coated. In UD 1s.
		Injection, solution: 1 mg/mL	As ibandronate sodium 3.375 mg. In single-use, prefilled syringe.

IBANDRONATE SODIUM — ORAL

For complete and comparative prescribing information, refer to the Bisphosphonates class monograph.

Indications

➤*Postmenopausal osteoporosis:* For the treatment and prevention of osteoporosis in postmenopausal women.

➤*Off-label uses:*

Bone metastases – [1] = Good documentation. Ibandronate was not commercially available in the United States when the American Society of Clinical Oncology (ASCO) guidelines were published on the use of bisphosphonates for breast cancer patients with bone health issues; therefore, the guidelines made no recommendations regarding the use of ibandronate in the management of bone metastases. Initial data from the controlled and noncontrolled trials suggest that once-daily treatment with oral ibandronate is a safe and effective treatment for metastatic bone disease from breast and colorectal cancer. It offers additional benefits of tolerability and convenience relative to intravenous (IV) bisphosphonate therapy. IV ibandronate is also effective in reducing skeletal complications related to metastatic bone disease.

Multiple myeloma – [5] = Poor documentation. The preferred agents for the treatment of skeletal complications resulting from multiple myeloma in the United States are IV pamidronate and zoledronic acid. The use of these drugs is endorsed by ASCO guidelines, which also state that no conclusions can be drawn regarding the comparative utility of ibandronate until the results of head-to-head comparative studies are available. In contrast to the established efficacy of pamidronate and zoledronic acid, Canadian guidelines specifically recommend against the use of ibandronate in this setting because a lack of therapeutic benefit.

Administration and Dosage

➤*Adults:*

Postmenopausal osteoporosis –

Usual dosage: 150 mg tablet taken once monthly on the same date each month (ie, the patient's ibandronate day).

Missed doses: If the dose is missed and the patient's next scheduled ibandronate day is more than 7 days away, instruct the patient to take one ibandronate 150 mg tablet in the morning following the date that it is remembered. The patient then should return to taking one ibandronate 150 mg tablet every month in the morning of their chosen day, according to the original schedule.

The patient must not take two 150 mg tablets within the same week. If the dose is missed, and the patient's next scheduled dose is only 1 to 7 days away, the patient must wait until their next scheduled ibandronate day to

IBANDRONATE SODIUM — ORAL

take the tablet. The patient should then return to taking one ibandronate 150 mg tablet every month in the morning of their chosen day, according to the original schedule.

Off-label dosing –

Bone metastases: [1] = Good documentation. 20 or 50 mg orally once daily for up to 96 weeks.

➤*Renal function impairment:* Not recommended for use in patients with severe renal impairment (creatinine clearance [CrCl] less than 30 mL/min).

➤*Administration:* Swallow tablet whole with a full glass of plain water (180 to 240 mL) while standing or sitting in an upright position. Do not chew or suck the tablets because of the potential for oropharyngeal ulceration. Take at least 60 minutes before the first food or drink (other than water) of the day or before taking any oral medication or supplementation, including calcium, antacids, or vitamins. Patients should not eat, drink anything except water, or take other medications for at least 60 minutes after taking ibandronate. Patients should not lie down for 60 minutes after taking ibandronate.

➤*Storage/Stability:* Store at 25°C (77°F); excursions are permitted between 15° and 30°C (59° and 86°F).

IBANDRONATE SODIUM — INJECTION

For complete and comparative prescribing information, refer to the Bisphosphonates class monograph.

Indications

➤*Postmenopausal osteoporosis:* For the treatment of osteoporosis in postmenopausal women.

➤*Off-label uses:*

Bone metastases – [1] = Good documentation. Ibandronate was not commercially available in the United States when American Society of Clinical Oncology (ASCO) guidelines were published on the use of bisphosphonates for breast cancer patients with bone health issues; therefore, the guidelines made no recommendations regarding the use of ibandronate in the management of bone metastases. Initial data from the controlled and noncontrolled trials suggest that once-daily treatment with oral ibandronate is a safe and effective treatment for metastatic bone disease from breast and colorectal cancer. It offers additional benefits of tolerability and convenience relative to intravenous (IV) bisphosphonate therapy. IV ibandronate is also effective in reducing skeletal complications related to metastatic bone disease.

Hypercalcemia of malignancy – [2] = Fair documentation. Data from high-quality, controlled clinical trials indicate that IV ibandronate has a beneficial role in the management of hypercalcemia in cancer patients. This medication is approved by the European Union and is used in more than 50 countries to treat hypercalcemia of malignancy; however, it is not Food and Drug Administration–approved in the United States for this indication.

Multiple myeloma – [5] = Poor documentation. The preferred agents for the treatment of skeletal complications resulting from multiple myeloma in the United States are IV pamidronate and zoledronic acid. The use of these drugs is endorsed by ASCO guidelines, which also state that no conclusion can be drawn regarding the comparative utility of ibandronate until the results of head-to-head comparative studies are available. In contrast to the established efficacy of pamidronate and zoledronic acid, Canadian guidelines specifically recommend against the use of ibandronate in this setting because a lack of therapeutic benefit.

Prevention of postrenal transplant bone loss – [1] = Good documentation. In the only well-controlled trial conducted, 4 doses of ibandronate at 3-month intervals were effective for preventing progression of posttransplant BMD losses. Although there was a documented reduction in spinal deformities with ibandronate use, larger trials are needed to show a significant difference in other clinically relevant outcomes such as fracture rates. The association between ibandronate use and reduced incidence of rejection merits further study.

Administration and Dosage

➤*Adults:*

Postmenopausal osteoporosis –

Usual dosage: 3 mg IV every 3 months administered over a period of 15 to 30 seconds.

Concomitant therapy: Patients must receive supplemental calcium and vitamin D.

Missed doses – If the dose is missed, administer the injection as soon as it can be rescheduled. Thereafter, schedule injections every 3 months from the date of the last injection. Do not administer more frequently than once every 3 months.

Off-label dosing –

Bone metastases: [1] = Good documentation. 2 mg IV bolus or 6 mg IV infusion over 1 to 2 hours given every 3 to 4 weeks for up to 2 years.

Hypercalcemia of malignancy: [2] = Fair documentation. 2 to 6 mg as a single IV infusion over 15 minutes to 4 hours every 4 weeks. Additional infusions of up to 6 mg total (including the initial dose) may be administered if albumin-corrected serum calcium has not normalized by day 4 after the initial infusion.

Prevention of postrenal transplant bone loss: [1] = Good documentation. 1 mg as an IV bolus immediately before kidney transplant and 2 mg as an IV bolus at 3, 6, and 9 months after kidney transplant.

➤*Renal function impairment:* Not recommended for use in patients with severe renal impairment or patients with serum creatinine greater than 200 mcmol/L (2.3 mg/dL) or creatinine clearance (CrCl) (measured or estimated) less than 30 mL/min.

➤*Administration:* Ibandronate must only be administered IV using the enclosed needle. Take care not to administer ibandronate intra-arterially or paravenously because this could lead to tissue damage.

➤*Admixture compatibility:* Ibandronate must not be mixed with calcium-containing solutions or other IV-administered drugs.

➤*Storage/Stability:* Store at 25°C (77°F); excursions between 15° and 30°C (59° and 86°F) are permitted. Discard unused portion.

PAMIDRONATE DISODIUM

Rx	**Pamidronate Disodium** (Sandoz)	**Powder for injection, lyophilized:** 30 mg	470 mg mannitol. In vials.
Rx	**Aredia** (Novartis)		470 mg mannitol. In vials.
Rx	**Pamidronate Disodium** (Sandoz)	**Powder for injection, lyophilized:** 90 mg	375 mg mannitol. In vials.
Rx	**Aredia** (Novartis)		375 mg mannitol. In vials.
Rx	**Pamidronate Disodium** (Various, eg, American Pharm Partners, Faulding)	**Injection:** 3 mg/mL	May contain mannitol. In 10 mL vials.
Rx	**Pamidronate Disodium** (Faulding)	**Injection:** 6 mg/mL	400 mg mannitol. In 10 mL vials.
Rx	**Pamidronate Disodium** (Various, eg, American Pharm Partners, Faulding)	**Injection:** 9 mg/mL	May contain mannitol. In 10 mL vials.

PAMIDRONATE DISODIUM — INJECTION

For complete and comparative prescribing information, refer to the Bisphosphonates group monograph.

Indications

➤*Hypercalcemia of malignancy:* Pamidronate, in conjunction with adequate hydration, is indicated for the treatment of moderate or severe hypercalcemia associated with malignancy, with or without bone metastases. Patients who have either epidermoid or nonepidermoid tumors respond to treatment with pamidronate. Initiate vigorous saline hydration, an integral part of hypercalcemia therapy, promptly and attempt to restore the urine output to about 2 L/day throughout treatment. Mild or asymptomatic hypercalcemia may be treated with conservative measures (ie, saline hydration, with or without loop diuretics). Patients should be hydrated adequately throughout the treatment, but overhydration, especially in those patients who have cardiac failure, must be avoided. Do not employ diuretic therapy prior to correction of hypovolemia. The safety and efficacy of pamidronate in the treatment of hypercalcemia associated with hyperparathyroidism or with other nontumor-related conditions have not been established.

➤*Paget disease:* Pamidronate is indicated for the treatment of patients with moderate to severe Paget disease of bone. The effectiveness of pamidronate was demonstrated primarily in patients with serum alkaline phosphatase greater than or equal to 3 times the upper limit of normal. Pamidronate therapy in patients with Paget disease has been effective in reducing serum alkaline phosphatase and urinary hydroxyproline levels by greater than or equal to 50% in at least 50% of patients, and by greater than or equal to 30% in at least 80% of patients. Pamidronate therapy has also been effective in reducing these biochemical markers in patients with Paget disease who failed to respond, or no longer responded to, other treatments.

➤*Osteolytic bone metastases of breast cancer and osteolytic lesions of multiple myeloma:* Pamidronate is indicated, in conjunction with standard antineoplastic therapy, for the treatment of osteolytic bone metastases of breast cancer and osteolytic lesions of multiple myeloma. The pamidronate treatment effect appeared to be smaller in the study of breast cancer patients receiving hormonal therapy than in the study of those receiving chemotherapy; however, overall evidence of clinical benefit has been demonstrated.

PAMIDRONATE DISODIUM — INJECTION

➤*Off-label uses:*

Hyperparathyroidism – [2] = Fair documentation. The definitive treatment for primary hyperparathyroidism is parathyroidectomy; however, pamidronate may be useful in patients who are not candidates for surgery, who refuse surgery, or who would benefit from a delay in surgery. Pamidronate is not curative, and doses must be repeated to control hypercalcemia. In patients with secondary hyperparathyroidism, pamidronate may help control hypercalcemia and allow for more aggressive use of calcitriol.

Immobilization-related hypercalcemia – [2] = Fair documentation. Pamidronate appears to be safe and effective for the treatment of immobilization-related hypercalcemia according to limited data from a small, noncontrolled study and case reports. Normocalcemia was achieved within 1 week of pamidronate administration for most patients. Larger, randomized, controlled studies are needed to identify the optimal dose and safety of pamidronate for this use.

Osteoporosis with spinal cord injury – [4] = Insufficient documentation. The bisphosphonates (eg, alendronate, etidronate, pamidronate, tiludronate) used to date in a limited number of acute spinal cord injury patients all have demonstrated an effect in reducing bone loss. Larger controlled trials are needed to determine which agent may be preferred and to optimize dosing regimens and define active rehabilitation protocols.

Prevention of glucocorticoid-induced osteoporosis – [2] = Fair documentation. Intravenous (IV) pamidronate was effective at preventing glucocorticoid-induced osteoporosis of the hip and spine. Repeated IV administration showed increased efficacy over single-dose administration in markers of bone formation. Further study in larger, controlled trials is needed to confirm these findings.

Other possible off-label uses – Postmenopausal osteoporosis; reduction of bone pain in patients with prostatic carcinoma.

Administration and Dosage

➤*General dosing considerations:* There must be strict adherence to the IV administration recommendations in order to decrease the risk of deterioration in renal function.

Vigorous saline hydration alone may be sufficient for treating mild, asymptomatic hypercalcemia. In hypercalcemia associated with hematologic malignancies, the use of glucocorticoid therapy may be helpful.

➤*Adults:*

Hypercalcemia of malignancy – Consider the severity and the symptoms of hypercalcemia.

Maximum dose: Single doses should not exceed 90 mg.

Single dose:

• *Moderate hypercalcemia (corrected serum calcium: 12 to 13.5 mg/dL)* – 60 to 90 mg IV infusion over at least 2 to 24 hours. Longer infusions (ie, greater than 2 hours) may reduce the risk for renal toxicity, particularly in patients with preexisting renal insufficiency.

• *Severe hypercalcemia (corrected serum calcium: greater than 13.5 mg/dL)* – 90 mg IV infusion over 2 to 24 hours. Longer infusions (ie, greater than 2 hours) may reduce the risk for renal toxicity, particularly in patients with preexisting renal insufficiency.

Concomitant therapy: Patients should be hydrated adequately throughout the treatment. Avoid overhydration in patients who have potential for cardiac failure.

Re-treatment:

Re-treatment in patients who show complete or partial response initially may be carried out if serum calcium does not return to normal or remain normal after initial treatment. It is recommended that a minimum of 7 days elapse before re-treatment, to allow for full response to the initial dose. The dose and manner of re-treatment is identical to that of the initial therapy.

Osteolytic bone lesions of multiple myeloma –

Usual dosage: 90 mg administered as a 4-hour infusion given on a monthly basis.

Maximum dose: Single doses should not exceed 90 mg.

Duration of therapy: The optimal duration of therapy is not yet known; however, in a study of patients with myeloma, final analysis after 21 months demonstrated overall benefits.

Concomitant therapy: Give patients with marked Bence-Jones proteinuria and dehydration adequate hydration prior to infusion.

Osteolytic bone metastases of breast cancer –

Usual dosage: 90 mg administered over a 2-hour infusion given every 3 to 4 weeks.

Maximum dose: Single doses should not exceed 90 mg.

Duration of therapy: The optimal duration of therapy is not known; however, in 2 breast cancer studies, final analyses performed after 24 months of therapy demonstrated overall benefits.

Concomitant therapy: Frequently used with doxorubicin, fluorouracil, cyclophosphamide, methotrexate, mitoxantrone, vinblastine, dexamethasone, prednisone, melphalan, vincristine, megesterol, and tamoxifen. It has been given less frequently with etoposide, cisplatin, cytarabine, paclitaxel, and aminoglutethimide.

Paget disease –

Usual dosage: 30 mg/day, administered as a 4-hour infusion on 3 consecutive days for a total dose of 90 mg.

Maximum dose: Single doses should not exceed 90 mg.

Re-treatment:

When clinically indicated, patients should be re-treated at the dose of initial therapy.

Off-label dosing –

Hyperparathyroidism: [2] = Fair documentation. 15 to 90 mg per dose as an IV infusion. Additional doses may be given when hypercalcemia recurs or on a set schedule of every 1 or 2 months. Pamidronate has been used for up to 1 year in an open-label study.

Immobilization-related hypercalcemia: [2] = Fair documentation. 10 to 90 mg administered as a single IV infusion. May be repeated if necessary to maintain normal calcium levels.

Osteoporosis with spinal cord injury: [4] = Insufficient documentation. 30 mg infusions (7.5 mg/h for 4 hours) every 4 weeks for 6 cycles.

Prevention of glucocorticoid-induced osteoporosis: [2] = Fair documentation. Initial dose of 90 mg IV, followed by 30 mg IV every 3 months.

➤*Renal function impairment:* Because pamidronate is excreted primarily by the kidney, the risk of adverse reactions may be increased in patients with impaired renal function. In patients receiving pamidronate for bone metastases and who have evidence of renal function deterioration, the drug should be withheld until renal function returns to baseline. Pamidronate has not been tested in patients with class Dc renal function impairment (creatinine above 5 mg/dL). Ensure that serum creatinine is assessed before each dose of pamidronate.

➤*Preparation for administration:* Reconstitute by adding 10 mL of sterile water for injection to each vial, resulting in a solution of 30 mg per 10 mL or 90 mg per 10 mL. Further dilution is required.

Hypercalcemia of malignancy – Dilute the recommended dose in 1,000 mL of sterile sodium chloride 0.45% or 0.9%, or dextrose 5% injection.

Osteolytic bone lesions of multiple myeloma – Dilute the recommended dose in 500 mL of sterile sodium chloride 0.45% or 0.9%, or dextrose 5% injection.

Osteolytic bone metastases of breast cancer – Dilute the recommended dose in 250 mL of sterile sodium chloride 0.45% or 0.9% or dextrose 5% injection.

Paget disease – Dilute the recommended dose in 500 mL of sterile sodium chloride 0.45% or 0.9%, or dextrose 5% injection.

➤*Administration:* Administer in a single IV solution and line separate from all other drugs.

Hypercalcemia of malignancy – Administer the 60 and 90 mg doses as an IV infusion over at least 2 to 24 hours.

Osteolytic bone lesions of multiple myeloma – Administer the 90 mg doses over a 4-hour period on a monthly basis.

Osteolytic bone metastases of breast cancer – Administer the 90 mg doses over a 2-hour period every 3 to 4 weeks.

Paget disease – Administer the 30 mg doses over a 4-hour period on 3 consecutive days.

➤*Admixture compatibility:* Do not mix with calcium-containing infusion solutions, such as Ringer solution.

➤*Storage/Stability:* Do not store unopened vials above 30°C (86°F). Pamidronate reconstituted with sterile water may be stored under refrigeration at 2° to 8°C (36° to 46°F) for up to 24 hours. Diluted solution for infusion is stable for up to 24 hours at room temperature.

BISPHOSPHONATE COMBINATIONS

Rx	**Actonel with Calcium** (Warner Chilcott)	**Tablets; oral**[a]: 35 mg risedronate, 1,250 mg calcium carbonate	Lactose. 4 **Actonel** tablets: (RSN 35 mg). Orange, oval. Film-coated. 24 calcium carbonate tablets: (NE 2). Lt. blue, oval. Film-coated. In 28-day course, blister package.
Rx	**Fosamax Plus D** (Merck)	**Tablets; oral**[b]: 70 mg alendronate/70 mcg vitamin D_3	Lactose, sucrose. (710). Capsule shape. In unit-of-use blisters of 4, and UD 20s.
		Tablets; oral[c]: 70 mg alendronate/140 mcg vitamin D_3	Lactose, sucrose. (270). Rectangle shape. In unit-of-use blisters of 4, and UD 20s.

[a] Equivalent to 500 mg elemental calcium.
[b] Equivalent to 2,800 units of vitamin D.
[c] Equivalent to 5,600 units of vitamin D.

BISPHOSPHONATE COMBINATIONS — ORAL

For complete prescribing information, refer to the Bisphosphonates class monograph and the Vitamin D monograph.

Indications

➤*Osteoporosis in men (Fosamax Plus D* only): For the treatment of osteoporosis in men by increasing bone mass.

➤*Osteoporosis in postmenopausal women:*

Prevention (Actonel with Calcium only) – Consider in postmenopausal women who are at risk of developing osteoporosis and for whom the desired clinical outcome is to maintain bone mass and to reduce the risk of fracture.

Treatment – For the treatment of osteoporosis in postmenopausal women by increasing bone mass and reducing the incidence of fractures, including those of the hip and spine (vertebral compression fractures).

Administration and Dosage

➤*General dosing considerations:* Causes of osteoporosis other than estrogen deficiency, aging, and glucocorticoid use should be considered.

➤*Adults:*

Prevention of osteoporosis in postmenopausal women –

Risedronate / Calcium: One risedronate 35 mg tablet taken once a week (day 1 of the 7-day treatment cycle) and 1 calcium 1,250 mg tablet (elemental calcium 500 mg) taken with food daily on each of the remaining 6 days (days 2 through 7 of the 7-day treatment cycle).

Treatment of osteoporosis in postmenopausal women –

Alendronate / Vitamin D_3: Alendronate 70 mg/vitamin D_3 2,800 units or alendronate 70 mg/vitamin D_3 5,600 units once weekly.

Risedronate / Calcium: See Prevention of osteoporosis in postmenopausal women.

Treatment of osteoporosis in men –

Alendronate / Vitamin D_3: Alendronate 70 mg/vitamin D_3 2,800 units or alendronate 70 mg/vitamin D_3 5,600 units once weekly.

➤*Renal function impairment:*

Alendronate / Vitamin D_3 – Alendronate/vitamin D_3 is not recommended for patients with more severe renal function impairment (creatinine clearance [CrCl] less than 35 mL/min) due to lack of experience.

Risedronate / Calcium – Risedronate/calcium is not recommended for patients with severe renal function impairment (CrCl less than 30 mL/min).

➤*Calcium / Vitamin D supplementation:* Patients should receive supplemental calcium if dietary intake is inadequate. The recommended total (diet and otherwise) daily calcium intake in postmenopausal women is elemental calcium 1,200 mg.

The recommended intake of vitamin D is 400 to 800 units daily. Alendronate 70 mg/vitamin D_3 2,800 units and alendronate 70 mg/vitamin D_3 5,600 units are intended to provide 7 days' worth of vitamin D 400 and 800 units daily in a single, once-weekly dose, respectively.

Patients at increased risk for vitamin D insufficiency (eg, those in nursing homes, those who are chronically ill or older than 70 years of age) may need vitamin D supplementation in addition to that provided in alendronate/vitamin D_3. Patients with GI malabsorption syndromes may require higher doses of vitamin D supplementation; measurement of 25-hydroxyvitamin D should be considered.

➤*Administration:* Must be taken at least 30 minutes before the first food, beverage, or medication of the day with plain water only. Other beverages (including mineral water), food, and some medications (including those containing calcium, aluminum, and magnesium) are likely to reduce the absorption of alendronate or risedronate. Waiting less than 30 minutes, or taking alendronate/cholecalciferol with food, beverages (other than plain water), or other medications will lessen the effect of alendronate by decreasing its absorption into the body.

To facilitate delivery to the stomach and thus reduce the potential for esophageal irritation, advise the patient to swallow the tablets with a full glass of water (6 to 8 ounces) upon arising for the day. Patients should not lie down for at least 30 minutes and until after their first food of the day. Instruct the patient not to take alendronate/cholecalciferol at bedtime or before arising for the day. Failure to follow these instructions may increase the risk of esophageal adverse experiences.

Calcium – If patients need calcium in excess of that provided by risedronate with calcium, this should be taken with food at a separate time of day.

➤*Storage / Stability:* Store at 20° to 25°C (68° to 77°F); excursions between 15° and 30°C (59° and 86°F) are permitted. Protect from moisture and light.

Fosamax Plus D (unit-of-use blister and unit dose packages) – Store tablets in original blister package until used.

ANTIDIABETIC AGENTS

Insulin

	Insulin Products							
Generic name	Insulin aspart	Insulin detemir	Insulin glargine	Insulin glulisine	Insulin isophane	Insulin isophane and regular	Insulin lispro	Insulin regular
Trade name	**Novolog** **Novolog Mix 70/30**	**Levemir**	**Lantus**	**Apidra**	**Humulin N** **Novolin N**	**Humulin 70/30** **Novolin 70/30**	**Humalog** **Humalog Mix 50/50** **Humalog Mix 75/25**	**Humulin R** **Novolin R**
Classification	Rapid acting	Long acting	Long acting	Rapid acting	Intermediate acting	Intermediate acting	**Humalog**: Rapid acting **Humalog Mix**: Rapid/Intermediate acting	Short acting
Compatibility	**Novolog**: May be mixed with NPH for subcutaneous use only; **Novolog** must be drawn into the syringe first. May also be diluted in sodium chloride 0.9% for IV[a] use. **Novolog 70/30**: Do not mix with any other insulins.	Do not mix or dilute with any other insulin.	Do not mix or dilute with any other insulin.	May be mixed with NPH for subcutaneous use only. **Apidra** must be drawn into the syringe first. May also be diluted only with sodium chloride 0.9% for IV use.	May be mixed with regular human insulin. **Humulin N** must be drawn into the syringe first.	Do not mix or dilute with any other insulin	**Humalog**: May be mixed longer-acting insulins. **Humalog** must be drawn into the syringe first. Vials may be diluted with sterile diluent to a concentration of 1:10 or 1:2. **Humalog Mix**: Do not mix or dilute with any other insulins.	May be mixed with longer-acting insulin; insulin regular must be drawn into the syringe first.
Route	**Novolog**: subcutaneous, IV, pump **Novolog 70/30** : subcutaneous	Subcutaneous	Subcutaneous	Subcutaneous, IV, pump	Subcutaneous	Subcutaneous	**Humalog**: subcutaneous, pump, IV **Humalog Mix** : subcutaneous	IV, subcutaneous, pump
Color	**Novolog**: clear **Novolog 70/30**: cloudy	Clear	Clear	Clear	Cloudy	Cloudy	**Humalog**: clear **Humalog Mix**: cloudy	Clear
Storage/ Stability	**Novolog**: Store in refrigerator. Do not freeze. May also be stored at room temperature for 28 days. *Penfill* cartridges and *Flexpen* prefilled syringes should be stored below 30°C (85°F) for up to 28 days while in use. Protect from excessive heat and sunlight. Vials being used are stable up to 28 days when kept in the refrigerator or at room temperature. **NovoLog** in the pump reservoir should be discarded after 48 h. **NovoLog** prepared in infusion bags is stable at room temperature for 24 h. **Novolog 70/30**: Store in the refrigerator. Do not freeze. Vials and pens may also be stored at room temperature for up to 28 and 14 days, respectively. Store *Flexpens* in-use at room temperature (< 86°F) and dispose after 14 days.	Store at 2° to 8° C (36° to 46° F). Do not freeze. Vials in use may be stored in the refrigerator or at room temperature for up to 42 days. Avoid direct heat and sunlight. *Flexpens* in use may be stored for up to 42 days at room temperature only and must not be stored with the needle in place.	Store in the refrigerator. Do not freeze. May also store at room temperature for 28 days. Vials and cartridges that are being used may be stored in the refrigerator or at room temperature for 28 days. Cartridges in the *OptiClik* device and *Solostar* pens that are in use should be kept at room temperature only and discarded after 28 days.	Store in the refrigerator. Do not freeze. May also store at room temperature for 28 days. Opened vials may be stored in the refrigerator or at room temperature and must be discarded after 28 days. Opened cartridge and *SoloStar* must be stored at room temperature and discarded after 28 days. **Apidra** in the reservoir pumps should be discarded after 48 h. IV preparations are stable for 48 h at room temperature.	Store in the refrigerator. Do not freeze. Vials in-use may be stored in the refrigerator or at room temperature and away from heat and light for up to 28 days. **Humulin N** pens in-use must be kept at room temperature and discarded after 14 days.	Store in the refrigerator. Do not freeze. Pens in-use should be stored at room temperature and away from direct sunlight and heat and discarded 10 days after first use.	**Humalog**: Store at 2° to 8°C (36° to 46°F). Do not freeze. Unopened **Humalog** may also be stored at room temperature for 28 days. Vials in-use may be stored in the refrigerator or at room temperature. Discard open vials after 28 days. Protect from heat and light. *D-TRON* and *D-TRON* plus pump cartridges should be discarded 7 days after opening. **Humalog** in an external pump reservoir should be discarded every 48 h. Diluted **Humalog** may remain in patient use for 28 days when stored at 5°C (42°F) and for 14 days when stored at 30°C (86°F). **Humalog Mix**: Store in the refrigerator. Do not freeze. May also be stored at room temperature for 28 days. Store pens unopened or in-use at room temperature and discard after 10 days. Vials in-use may be stored in the refrigerator or at room temperature. Discard open vials after 28 days.	Store in a refrigerator. Do not freeze. Opened vials may be kept in the refrigerator or at room temperature. Discard after 28 days. Keep away from direct sunlight and heat.

Insulin Products								
Generic name	Insulin aspart	Insulin detemir	Insulin glargine	Insulin glulisine	Insulin isophane	Insulin isophane and regular	Insulin lispro	Insulin regular
Trade name	**Novolog** **Novolog Mix 70/30**	**Levemir**	**Lantus**	**Apidra**	**Humulin N** **Novolin N**	**Humulin 70/30** **Novolin 70/30**	**Humalog** **Humalog Mix 50/50** **Humalog Mix 75/25**	**Humulin R** **Novolin R**
Administration	**NovoLog**: Administer within 5 to 10 min before a meal. Generally administer with an intermediate or long-acting insulin. **Novolog 70/30**: Administer within 30 min before a meal.	*Once daily dosing*: Administer with evening meal or at bedtime. *Twice daily dosing*: Evening dose may be administered with evening meal, at bedtime, or 12 h after morning dose.	Once daily dosing can be administered at any time of the day, but must be administered at the same time every day. Type 1 diabetes patients must use **Lantus** with a short-acting insulin.	Administer within 15 min before a meal or within 20 min after starting a meal. Generally administer with an intermediate or long-acting insulin.	Individualized dosing schedule.	Administer 30 to 60 min before a meal.	**Humalog**: Administer within 15 min before or immediately after eating if dosed as a meal-time insulin. Type 1 diabetics should use with a longer-acting insulin. **Humalog Mix**: Must be administered within 15 min before a meal.	Administer 30 to 60 min before a meal.

[a] IV = intravenous.

Indications

Insulin Indications								
Indication	Insulin aspart	Insulin detemir	Insulin glargine	Insulin glulisine	Insulin isophane	Insulin isophane and regular	Insulin lispro	Insulin regular
Diabetes mellitus	✓	✓	✓	✓	✓	✓	✓	✓
Gestational diabetes					✓	✓		✓
Hyperkalemia								✓
Hyperosmolar hyperglycemic state								✓
Immunologic insulin resistance					✓			✓
Injection-site lipodystrophy					✓			✓
Insulin resistance								✓[a]
Local insulin allergy					✓			✓
Severe ketoacidosis or diabetic coma								✓
Temporary use (eg, surgery, acute stress)					✓			✓

[a] Concentrated insulin regular only.

Administration and Dosage

➤*Preparation and administration:* The number and size of daily doses, time of administration, and diet and exercise require continuous medical supervision. Dosage adjustment may be necessary when changing types of insulin, particularly when changing from single-peak to the more purified animal or human insulins.

For insulin suspensions, ensure uniform dispersion by rolling the vial gently between hands. Avoid vigorous shaking that may result in the formation of air bubbles or foam. Regular insulin, insulin glargine, and insulin glulisine should be a clear solution.

Injection site – Administer maintenance doses subcutaneously. Rotate administration sites to prevent lipodystrophy. A general rule is not to administer within 1 inch of the same site for 1 month. The rate of absorption is more rapid when the injection is in the abdomen (possibly greater than 50% faster), followed by the upper arm, thigh, and buttocks. Therefore, it may be best to rotate sites within an area rather than rotating areas. Give regular insulin IV or IM in severe ketoacidosis or diabetic coma.

➤*Dosage guidelines:* Individualize doses and monitor patients with diabetes mellitus closely; the following dosage guidelines may be considered.

Children and adults – 0.5 to 1 unit/kg/day.

Insulin timing: Give insulin lispro within 15 minutes before a meal. Human regular insulin is best given 30 to 60 minutes before a meal. Give insulin glargine once daily subcutaneously at bedtime. Give insulin glulisine within 15 minutes before a meal or within 20 minutes after starting a meal. Give insulin aspart within 15 minutes before a meal. Give insulin detemir subcutaneously either once daily with the evening meal or at bedtime, and if used twice daily, give with the second dose either with the evening meal, at bedtime, or 12 hours after the morning dose.

Insulin requirements may be altered during intercurrent conditions such as illness, emotional disturbances, or stress.

Adjust doses to achieve premeal and bedtime blood glucose levels of 80 to 140 mg/dL (100 to 200 mg/dL in children younger than 5 years of age).

➤*Insulin mixtures:* When mixing 2 types of insulin, always draw clear regular insulin into the syringe first. Patients stabilized on mixtures should have a consistent response if the mixing is standardized. An unexpected response is most likely to occur when switching from separate injections to the use of mixture or vice versa. To avoid dosage error, do not alter order of mixing insulins or change model or brand of syringe or needle. Each type of insulin used must be of the same concentration (units/mL).

Isophane insulin (NPH)/regular mixtures of insulin are now available from the manufacturer in premixed formulations of 70% NPH and 30% regular. A 50/50 combination also is available. NPH/regular combinations of insulin are stable and are absorbed as if injected separately. In mixtures of regular and lente insulins, binding is detectable 5 minutes to 24 hours after mixing. If the regular/lente mixtures are not administered within the first 5 minutes after mixing, the effect of the regular insulin is diminished. The excess zinc binds with the regular and forms a lente-type insulin. Thus, it is critical that mixtures of regular with the lente insulins be mixed and injected immediately.

These mixtures remain stable for 1 month at room temperature or for 3 months refrigerated. These mixtures also can be stored in prefilled plastic or glass syringes for 1 week to possibly 14 days under refrigeration. Keep filled syringes in a vertical or oblique position with the needle pointing upward to avoid plugging problems. Prior to injection, pull back the plunger and tip the syringe back and forth, slightly agitating to remix the insulins. Check for normal appearance.

Semilente, ultralente, and lente insulins may be mixed in any ratio; they are chemically identical and differ only in size and structure of insulin particles. These mixtures are stable 1 month at room temperature or 3 months under refrigeration.

Long-acting insulins (detemir and glargine) should not be mixed or diluted with any other insulin preparations.

If insulin glulisine is mixed with NPH human insulin, draw insulin glulisine into the syringe first. Make the injection immediately after mixing. Do not mix insulin glulisine with insulin preparations other than NPH. When it is used in a pump, do not mix insulin glulisine with other insulins or with a diluent.

➤*Insulin adsorption:* Insulin adsorption into plastic IV infusion sets reportedly has removed up to 80% of a dose, but 20% to 30% is more common. The percent adsorbed is inversely proportional to insulin concentration; it takes place within 30 to 60 minutes. Because this phenomenon cannot be predicted accurately, patient monitoring is essential.

➤*Concomitant sulfonylurea therapy:* Insulin and oral sulfonylurea coadministration has been used with some success in type 2 diabetic patients who are difficult to control with diet and sulfonylurea therapy alone.

➤*Storage/Stability:* Proper storage is critical. Insulin preparations are generally stable if stored at room temperature (and not exposed to extreme temperatures or direct sunlight) for 1 month. Always store extra bottles in the refrigerator; do not freeze.

Insulin prefilled in plastic or glass syringes is stable for 28 days under refrigeration. Insulin lispro must be mixed immediately before injection.

Actions

➤*Pharmacology:* Insulin lowers blood glucose levels by stimulating peripheral glucose uptake, especially by skeletal muscle and fat, and by inhibiting hepatic glucose production. Insulin inhibits lipolysis in the adipocyte, inhibits proteolysis, and enhances protein synthesis. Insulin, secreted by the beta cells of the pancreas, is the principal hormone required for proper glucose use in normal metabolic processes. It is composed of 2 amino acid chains, A (acidic) and B (basic), joined together by disulfide linkages.

Insulin Amino Acids[a]							
	A-chain position			B-chain position			
Source/Types	A8	A10	A21	B28	B29	B30	B31 and B32
Human	Thr	Ile	Asn	Pro	Lys	Thr	–
Glargine	Thr	Ile	Gly	Pro	Lys	Thr	Arg
Aspart	Thr	Ile	Asn	Aspartic acid	Lys	Thr	–
Lispro	Thr	Ile	Asn	Lys	Pro	Thr	–
Glulisine	Thr	Ile	Asn	Pro	Glu	Thr	–
Detemir	Thr	Ile	Asn	Pro	Lys + C14 fatty acid chain	–	–

[a] Arg = arginine, Asn = asparagine, Gly = glycine, Ile = isoleucine, Lys = lysine, Pro = proline, Thr = threonine, Glu = glutamine.

Insulin aspart – Produced by recombinant DNA technology utilizing *Saccharomyces cerevisiae* (baker's yeast) as the production organism.

Insulin detemir – Produced by a process that includes expression of recombinant DNA in *S. cerevisiae* followed by chemical modification.

Insulin glargine, insulin glulisine – Produced by recombinant DNA technology utilizing a nonpathogenic laboratory strain of *Escherichia coli* (K12).

Insulin isophane, insulin lispro, insulin regular – Synthesized in a special nondisease-producing laboratory strain of *E. coli* bacteria that has been genetically altered.

➤*Pharmacokinetics:*

Insulin Pharmacokinetics

Insulin preparation	Bioavailability	C_{max}	Onset	Peak	Duration of action	Volume of distribution	Binding to plasma proteins	Half-life
Insulin aspart		82 microunits/mL	0.25 h	1 to 3 h	3 to 5 h		< 10%	81 min
Insulin detemir	60%		3 to 8 h	None	5.7 to 23.2 h	0.1 L/kg	> 98%	5 to 7 h
Insulin glargine			1.1 h	None	Up to 24 h			
Insulin glulisine	≈ 70%	83 to 84 microunits/mL	5 to 15 min	1 h	< 5 h	13 L		IV: 13 min. Subcutaneous: 42 min
Insulin isophane			1 to 1.5 h	4 to 12 h	14.5 h			
Insulin lispro	55% to 77%		0.25 h	0.5 to 4 h	Up to 24 h	0.26 to 0.36 L/kg		Subcutaneous: 1h IV: 26 min
Insulin regular		41 to 50 microunits/mL	0.5 to 1 h	1 to 5 h	4 to 12 h (24 h for the U-500)	0.26 to 0.36 L/kg		IV: 17 min. Subcutaneous: 86 to 141 min

Special populations –

Renal function impairment: Increased circulating levels of insulin in patients with renal failure. Dose adjustments may be necessary.

Hepatic function impairment: Increased circulating levels of insulin in patients with hepatic failure. Dose adjustments may be necessary.

Elderly: Higher **insulin detemir** area under the curve (AUC) levels up to 35%.

Children: Slightly higher **insulin detemir** AUC and C_{max} in children by 10% and 24%, respectively.

Race: **Insulin glulisine**, **insulin lispro**, and **insulin regular** have a greater initial exposure in Japanese patients compared with white patients, although total exposures were similar.

Contraindications

During episodes of hypoglycemia and in patients sensitive to any ingredient of the product(s).

Warnings/Precautions

➤*Antibody production:* All insulin products can elicit the formation of insulin antibodies. The presence of such insulin antibodies may increase or decrease the efficacy of insulin and may require adjustment of the insulin dose. Increases in anti-insulin antibodies are observed more frequently with **insulin aspart** than with **insulin regular**.

➤*Changing insulins:* Change insulins cautiously and under medical supervision. Changes in purity, strength, brand, or type may require dosage adjustment. Effects of each insulin product will vary between individual patients and at different times in the same individual patient based on site of injection, blood supply, temperature, and physical activity. Teach patients using insulin to self monitor blood glucose levels and keep daily records of results. Concomitant oral antidiabetic treatment may need to be adjusted.

➤*Diabetic ketoacidosis:* Diabetic ketoacidosis, a potentially life-threatening condition, requires prompt diagnosis and treatment. Diabetic ketoacidosis may result from eating significantly more than meal plan suggests, stress, illness or infection, inadequate dosing or insulin omission or may develop slowly after a long period of insulin control. Treat with fluids, correction of acidosis and hypotension, and low-dose regular insulin intramuscular (IM) or IV infusion. The symptoms of diabetic ketoacidosis usually come on gradually over a period of hours or days, and include a drowsy feeling, flushed face, thirst, or loss of appetite. Severe, sustained hyperglycemia may result in diabetic coma and death.

➤*Diet:* Patients must follow a prescribed diet and exercise regularly. Determine the time, number, and amount of individual doses and distribution of food among the meals of the day. Do not change this regimen unless prescribed otherwise.

➤*Exercise:* Exercising may cause the body's insulin requirements to decrease during and after the activity. The effects of insulin may also be increased, particularly if the area the insulin was injected was involved in the exercise routine.

➤*Hyperthyroidism/Hypothyroidism:* Hyperthyroidism may cause an increase in the renal clearance of insulin. Therefore, patients may need more insulin to control their diabetes. Hypothyroidism may delay insulin turnover, requiring less insulin to control diabetes.

➤*Hypoglycemia:* Hypoglycemia is the most common adverse effect of insulin therapy. The first signs/symptoms of hypoglycemia may appear suddenly. Early warning symptoms of hypoglycemia (eg, cold sweat, fatigue, shakiness, rapid heartbeat) may be different or less pronounced under certain conditions, such as long duration of diabetes, diabetic nerve disease, use of medications such as beta-blockers, or intensified diabetes control. Such situations may result in severe hypoglycemia (and possibly loss of consciousness, convulsions, temporary or permanent impairment of brain function or death) prior to patients' awareness of hypoglycemia. Rapid changes in serum glucose levels may induce symptoms of hypoglycemia in patients with diabetes, regardless of the glucose value.

➤*Hypokalemia:* All insulin products cause a shift in potassium from the extracellular to intracellular space, possibly leading to hypokalemia that, if left untreated, may cause respiratory paralysis, ventricular arrhythmia, and death. Use caution in patients who may be at risk for hypokalemia (ie, patients using potassium-lowering medications, patients taking medications sensitive to serum potassium concentrations, and patients receiving IV insulin).

➤*Insulin resistance:* Insulin resistance occurs rarely. Insulin resistant patients require more than 200 units of insulin/day for more than 2 days in the absence of ketoacidosis or acute infection. Sometimes, the resistance is due to high levels of IgG antibodies to insulin. Insulin resistance also may occur in obese patients, patients with acanthosis nigricans, ketoacidosis, endocrinopathies, and patients with insulin receptor defects; insulin resistance during infection may be caused by a postreceptor defect. Hyperglycemia may be managed by changing the insulin. Corticosteroids (prednisone 60 to 100 mg/day) may be given if changing the insulin is not effective. Corticosteroids may decrease IgG production or decrease insulin binding to the antibody. Closely monitor for signs of hyperglycemia and for adverse effects of high-dose corticosteroids. Highly concentrated insulin (U-500) also may be given to insulin-resistant patients. Use caution to avoid hypoglycemia. Some type 2 patients with insulin resistance have been treated with a combination of a sulfonylurea plus insulin.

➤*Intercurrent conditions:* Insulin requirements may be altered during intercurrent condition, such as illness (especially nausea and vomiting), emotional disturbances, or other stresses.

➤*Lipodystrophy:*

Lipoatrophy – Lipoatrophy is the breakdown of adipose tissue at the insulin injection site, causing a depression in the skin and possibly delaying insulin absorption. It may be the result of an immune response or when less pure insulins are administered. Injection of human insulins into the site over a 2- to 4-week period may result in subcutaneous fat accumulation.

Lipohypertrophy – Lipohypertrophy is the result of repeated insulin injection into the same site. It is the accumulation of subcutaneous fat, and it may interfere with insulin absorption from the site. This condition may be avoided by rotating the injection site.

➤*Sodium retention/edema:* Insulin may cause sodium retention and edema, particularly if previously poor metabolic control is improved by intensified insulin therapy.

➤*Weight gain:* May occur with insulin therapy and has been attributed to the anabolic effects of insulin and the decrease in glucosuria.

➤*Travel:* Dosing may need to change if traveling across more than 2 time zones.

➤*Hypersensitivity reactions:* Severe, life-threatening, generalized allergy, including anaphylaxis, may occur with any insulin product. Systemic reactions are less common and may present as a rash, pruritus, shortness of breath, wheezing, sweating, a drop in blood pressure, rapid pulse, bronchospasm, shock, angioedema, or anaphylaxis, which may be life-threatening. Occasionally, redness, swelling, and itching at the injection site may develop. These local reactions usually resolve in a few days to a few weeks, but in some cases, a change in the type of insulin may be considered.

Insulin aspart, insulin glulisine – Localized reactions and generalized myalgias have been reported with the use of protamine and metacresol/cresol as an injectable excipient.

➤*Renal/Hepatic function impairment:* Dose requirements for insulin may be reduced in patients with renal and/or hepatic impairment. Some studies with human insulin have shown increased circulating levels of insulin in patients with renal and/or hepatic failure. Careful glucose monitoring and dose adjustments of insulin may be necessary in patients with renal dysfunction and/or hepatic dysfunction.

Insulin glargine – Due to its long duration of action, insulin glargine is not recommended during periods of rapidly declining renal and/or hepatic function because of risk for prolonged hypoglycemia.

➤*Pregnancy: Category B* (**insulin aspart, insulin regular, insulin lispro**); *Category C* (**insulin aspart 70/30, insulin detemir, insulin glargine, insulin glulisine**). Pregnancy may make diabetes management more difficult. Because it is a very large molecule, insulin probably does not cross the placenta. However, there may be endogenous carrier proteins that allow passage of insulin to the embryo early in gestation. Insulin is the drug of choice for diabetes control in pregnancy. Keep patients under close medical supervision. Rigid control of serum glucose and avoidance of ketoacidosis are desired throughout pregnancy. It is essential for patients with diabetes or a history of gestational diabetes to maintain good metabolic control before conception and throughout pregnancy. Insulin requirements usually fall during the first trimester, increase during the second and third trimester, and rapidly decline after delivery. There are no well-controlled clinical studies of the use of insulin in pregnant women. Per Briggs *Drugs in Pregnancy and Lactation*, insulin is classified as compatible with pregnancy.

Insulin aspart – Insulin aspart caused pre- and postimplantation losses and visceral/skeletal abnormalities in rats at a dosage of 200 units/kg/day (approximately 32 times the human subcutaneous dosage of 1 unit/kg/day, based on unit/body surface area [BSA]) and in rabbits at a dosage of 10 units/kg/day (approximately 3 times the human subcutaneous dosage of 1 unit/kg/day, based on unit/BSA). The effects are probably secondary to maternal hypoglycemia at high doses.

Insulin detemir – Insulin detemir caused visceral anomalies in rat litters at dosages of 150 and 300 nmol/kg/day when given before mating, during mating, and throughout pregnancy. At dosages up to 900 nmol/kg/day given to rabbits during organogenesis caused increased incidence of fetal gall bladder abnormalities such as, small, bilobed, bifurcated and missing gall bladder. Insulin detemir probably should be avoided in gestation until human pregnancy experience is available. As with all insulins, the primary concern is severe maternal hypoglycemia.

Insulin glargine – Insulin glargine was given to female rats before mating, during mating, and throughout pregnancy at dosages up to 0.36 mg/kg/day, which is approximately 7 times the recommended human subcutaneous starting dosage of 10 units/day (0.008 mg/kg/day), based on mg/m^2. In rabbits, dosages of 0.072 mg/kg/day, which is approximately 2 times the recommended human subcutaneous starting dosage of 10 units/day (0.008 mg/kg/day) based on mg/m^2, were administered during organogenesis. In rabbits, 5 fetuses from 2 litters of the high-dose group exhibited dilation of the cerebral ventricles. Use this drug during pregnancy only if clearly needed.

Insulin glulisine – Insulin glulisine was given to female rabbits throughout pregnancy at subcutaneous dosages up to 1.5 units/kg/day (dosage resulting in an exposure 0.5 times the average human dose, based on BSA comparison). Adverse effects on embryo-fetal development were only seen at maternal toxic dose levels inducing hypoglycemia. Increased incidence of postimplantation losses and skeletal defects were observed at a dosage level of 1.5 units/kg once daily that also caused mortality in dams. A slight increased incidence of postimplantation losses was seen at the next lower dosage level of 0.5 units/kg once daily (dosage resulting in an exposure 0.2 times the average human dose, based on BSA comparison), which also was associated with severe hypoglycemia, but there were no defects at that dose. Use this drug during pregnancy only if the potential benefit justifies the potential risk to the fetus.

Insulin lispro, insulin regular – Use this drug in pregnancy only if the potential benefit justifies the potential risk to the fetus.

Fertility impairment –

Insulin glargine: In a combined fertility and prenatal and postnatal study in male and female rats at subcutaneous dosages of insulin glargine up to 0.36 mg/kg/day, which is approximately 7 times the recommended human subcutaneous starting dosage of 10 units/day (0.008 mg/kg/day), based on mg/m^2, maternal toxicity caused by dose-dependent hypoglycemia, including some deaths, was observed. Consequently, a reduction of the rearing rate occurred in the high-dose group only.

➤*Lactation:* Insulin is destroyed in the GI tract when administered orally and, therefore, would not be expected to be absorbed intact by the breast-feeding infant. However, inadequate or excessive insulin treatment of diabetic mothers inhibits milk production. Lactating women may require adjustments in insulin dose and diet. It is unknown whether insulin aspart, insulin detemir, insulin glargine, insulin lispro, or insulin glulisine are excreted in significant amounts in breast milk. Exercise caution when these insulins are administered to a breast-feeding woman. In general, mothers with diabetes using insulin may breast-feed their infants.

➤*Children:*

Insulin aspart – Approved for use in children for subcutaneous daily injections and for subcutaneous continuous infusion by external insulin pump.

Insulin lispro mix and insulin aspart 70/30 – Safety and efficacy have not been established.

Insulin detemir – Approved for use in children with type 1 diabetes.

Insulin glargine – Safety and efficacy have not been established in children younger than 6 years of age. **Insulin glargine** has not been studied in children with type 2 diabetes.

Insulin regular – There are no special precautions relating to the use of this insulin formulation in children.

Insulin glulisine – Safety and efficacy have not been established in children younger than 4 years of age. **Insulin glulisine** has not been studied in children with type 2 diabetes.

Insulin lispro – Clinical studies have been performed in children using **insulin lispro**.

➤*Elderly:* Conservatively administer initial dosing, dosing increments, and maintenance dosing to avoid hypoglycemic reactions. Hypoglycemia may be difficult to recognize in elderly patients.

➤*Monitoring:* Frequent monitoring of blood glucose is required. Periodically monitor hemoglobin A_{1c} (HbA_{1c}), as well as urine glucose, glycohemoglobin, and urine ketones when warranted. When insulin is administered IV, closely monitor glucose and potassium levels to avoid potentially fatal hypoglycemia and hypokalemia.

Drug Interactions

Drugs That Decrease the Hypoglycemic Effect of Insulin	
Acetazolamide	Epinephrine
AIDS antivirals	Estrogens
Albuterol	Ethacrynic acid
Alcohol	Glucagon
Antipsychotic medications, atypical (eg, olanzapine, clozapine)	Isoniazid
Asparaginase	Lithium salts
Beta-blockers	Morphine sulfate
Calcitonin	Niacin
Clonidine	Nicotine
Contraceptives, hormonal	Phenothiazines (eg, fluphenazine)
Corticosteroids	Phenytoin
Cyclophosphamide	Progestogens (eg, oral contraceptives)
Danazol	Protease inhibitors (eg, indinavir)
Dextrothyroxine	Somatropin
Diazoxide	Terbutaline
Diltiazem	Thiazide diuretics
Diuretics	Thyroid hormones
Dobutamine	

Drugs That Increase the Hypoglycemic Effect of Insulin	
ACE inhibitors[a]	MAOIs[a] (eg, phenelzine)
Alcohol	Mebendazole
Anabolic steroids	Lithium salts
Angiotensin II receptor blocking agents	Panax ginseng
Antidiabetic products, oral	Pentamidine[d]
Beta-blockers[b,c]	Pentoxifylline
Calcium	Phenylbutazone
Chloroquine	Pramlintide
Clofibrate	Propoxyphene
Clonidine[c]	Pyridoxine
Disopyramide	Reserpine[c]
Fenfluramine	Salicylates (eg, aspirin)
Fenugreek	Somatostatin analog (eg, octreotide)
Fibrates	Sulfinpyrazone
Fluoxetine	Sulfonamides
Guanethidine[c]	Tetracyclines

[a] ACE = angiotensin-converting enzyme. MAOI = monoamine oxidase inhibitors.
[b] Nonselective beta-blockers may delay recovery from hypoglycemic episodes and mask their signs/symptoms. Cardioselective agents may be alternatives.
[c] The signs of hypoglycemia may be reduced or absent in patients taking sympatholytic agents such as beta-blockers, clonidine, guanethidine, and reserpine.
[d] May sometimes be followed by hyperglycemia.

Adverse Reactions

➤*Insulin initiation and intensification of glucose control:* Intensification or rapid improvement in glucose control has been associated with a transitory, reversible ophthalmologic refraction disorder, worsening of diabetic retinopathy, and acute painful peripheral neuropathy. However, long-term glycemic control decreases the risk of diabetic retinopathy and neuropathy.

Insulin Adverse Reactions[a]							
Adverse reactions	Insulin aspart	Insulin detemir	Insulin glargine	Insulin glulisine	Insulin isophane	Insulin lispro	Insulin regular
CNS							
Depression			10.5%		9.7%		
Headache			10.3%	6.9%	9.3%		11.2%
Hypoglycemic seizure				6.1%			4.7%
Local							
Allergic reaction	✔[b]	✔	✔	4.3%	✔	✔	✔
Infusion-site reaction	13.3%			10.3%			
Injection-site reaction	7%	✔	✔		✔	✔	✔
Insulin allergy	✔	✔	✔	✔	✔	✔	✔
Lipodystrophy	✔	✔	✔	✔	✔	✔	✔
Pruritus	7%	✔	✔	✔	✔	✔	✔
Rash	7%	✔	✔	✔	✔	✔	✔
Metabolic/Nutritional							
Hypoglycemia	✔	✔	23%	16.2%	28.6%	19.3%	10.1%
Hypokalemia	✔	✔	✔	✔	✔	✔	✔
Peripheral edema	✔	✔	20%	7.5%	22.7%	✔	7.8%
Weight gain	✔	✔	✔	✔	✔	✔	✔
Musculoskeletal							
Arthralgia			14.2%	5.9%	16.1%		6.3%
Back pain			12.8%		12.3%		
Pain in extremity			13%		13.1%		
Respiratory							
Bronchitis			15.2%		14.1%		
Cough			12.1%		7.4%		
Nasopharyngitis				10.6%			9.5%
Upper respiratory tract infection			29%	10.5%	33.6%		10.8%
Special senses							
Cataract			18.1%		15.9%		
Pharyngitis			7.5%		8.6%		
Retinal vascular disorder			5.8%		7.4%		
Retinopathy			✔		✔		
Rhinitis			5.2%		5.1%		
Sinusitis			18.5%		17.9%		
Miscellaneous							
Accidental injury			5.7%		6.4%		
Antibody production	✔	✔	✔	✔	✔	✔	✔
Diarrhea			10.7%		10.3%		
Elevated alkaline phosphatase	✔						
Hypertension			19.6%	3.9%	18.9%		5.3%
Infection			13.8%		17.7%		
Influenza			18.7%	6.2%	19.5%		4.2%
Urinary tract infection			10.7%		10.1%		

[a] Data are pooled from separate trials and are not necessarily comparable.

[b] ✔ = occurs; incidence unknown.

Overdosage

➤*Symptoms:* Hypoglycemia. Hypokalemia may occur, especially after IV use.

➤*Treatment:* Mild episodes of hypoglycemia can be treated with oral glucose or carbohydrates. Adjustments in drug dosage, meal patterns, or exercise may be needed. More severe episodes with coma, seizure, or neurologic impairment may be treated with IM/subcutaneous glucagon or concentrated IV glucose. Sustained carbohydrate intake and observation may be necessary because hypoglycemia may recur after apparent clinical recovery.

Patient Information

Advise patients to use the same type and brand of syringe to avoid dosage errors.

Advise patients to rotate sites to prevent lipodystrophy.

Advise patients to not change the order of mixing insulins (if applicable) or change the brand, strength, type, species, or dose without discussing with their health care provider.

Inform patients that insulin requirements may change in patients who become ill, especially with vomiting or fever and during stress or emotional disturbances.

Advise patients to see their dentist twice yearly and to see an ophthalmologist regularly.

Advise patients to adhere to prescribed diet and exercise program.

Inform patients that periodic measurement of glycosylated hemoglobin is recommended for the monitoring of long-term glycemic control.

Advise patients to wear diabetic identification (*Medic-Alert*) so appropriate treatment can be given if complications occur away from home.

Advise patients to monitor blood glucose and urine for glucose and ketones as prescribed and to monitor blood pressure regularly.

Advise patients to inform their health care provider if they are pregnant or are contemplating pregnancy.

Inform patients that insulin stored at room temperature will be less painful to inject compared with that stored in the refrigerator, and patients will need to allow refrigerated insulin to come to room temperature prior to injection.

Advise patients to notify their health care provider right away if their urine test is positive for ketones (acetone) or if they have any of these symptoms (eg, drowsy feeling, flushed face, thirst and loss of appetite, fast or heavy breathing, rapid pulse).

Inform patients using subcutaneous insulin infusion pumps that they must have alternate insulin therapy available in case of pump failure.

Inform all insulin receiving patients of the symptoms of hypoglycemia and carry a form of easily consumable glucose (such as regular glucose tablets).

INSULIN REGULAR

otc	**Humulin R** (Lilly)	**Injection, solution**: 100 units/mL human insulin (rDNA)	In 10 mL vials.
otc	**Novolin R** (Novo Nordisk)		In 10 mL vials.
Rx	**Humulin R Regular U-500 (Concentrated)** (Lilly)	**Injection, solution, concentrate**: 500 units/mL (rDNA origin)	In 20 mL vials.[a]

[a] With 2.5 mg m-cresol and 16 mg glycerin per mL.

INSULIN REGULAR (HUMAN) — INJECTION

For complete and comparative prescribing information, refer to the Insulin group monograph.

Indications

➤*Type 1 diabetes mellitus (formerly known as insulin-dependent diabetes mellitus; IDDM):* Diabetes mellitus type 1.

➤*Type 2 diabetes mellitus (formerly known as non-insulin-dependent diabetes mellitus; NIDDM):* Diabetes mellitus type 2 that cannot be properly controlled by diet, exercise (physical activity), and weight control.

➤*Hyperkalemia:* Infusion of glucose and insulin produces a shift of potassium into cells and lowers serum potassium levels.

➤*Severe ketoacidosis/diabetic coma:* Regular human insulin may be given intravenously (IV) or intramuscularly (IM) for rapid effect in severe ketoacidosis or diabetic coma.

➤*Highly purified (single component) and human insulin:* Local insulin allergy, immunologic insulin resistance, injection site lipodystrophy; temporary insulin use (eg, surgery, acute stress, type 2 diabetes, gestational diabetes mellitus); newly diagnosed patients with diabetes.

➤*Hyperosmolar hyperglycemic state (HHS) [formerly known as hyperglycemic hyperosmolar nonketotic coma (HHNC)]:* Regular human insulin may be given IV or IM for rapid effect in patients with type 2 diabetes experiencing hyperosmolar hyperglycemic state (HHS).

Administration and Dosage

➤*Adults:*

Diabetes –

Usual dosage: 0.5 to 1 units/kg/day.

Dosage adjustment: Adjust doses to achieve premeal plasma glucose 90 to 130 mg/dL and peak postprandial plasma and bedtime glucose of less than 180 mg/dL. Insulin requirements may be altered during intercurrent conditions such as illness, emotional disturbances, or stress.

➤*Children:* See Adults for dosing for children older than 12 years of age.

➤*Elderly:* The initial dosing, dosing increments, and maintenance dosing should be conservative to avoid hypoglycemic reactions. Hypoglycemia may be difficult to recognize in the elderly.

➤*Renal function impairment:* Some studies with human insulin have shown increased circulating levels of insulin in patients with renal failure. Careful glucose monitoring and dose adjustments of insulin may be necessary in patients with renal dysfunction. Insulin requirements may be reduced in patients with renal impairment.

➤*Hepatic function impairment:* Some studies with human insulin have shown increased circulating levels of insulin in patients with hepatic failure. Careful glucose monitoring and dose adjustments of insulin may be necessary in patients with hepatic dysfunction.

➤*Preparation for administration:* Regular human insulin is not a suspension and therefore light shaking or rolling between the hands is not necessary. Avoid vigorous shaking that may result in the formation of air bubbles or foam. Regular human insulin should be a clear, colorless solution.

Keep filled syringes in a vertical or oblique position with the needle pointing upward to avoid plugging problems. Prior to injection, pull back the plunger and tip the syringe back and forth, slightly agitating to remix the insulins. Check for normal appearance.

Mixing insulins – When mixing other types of insulin with regular human insulin, always draw clear regular insulin into syringe first. Patients stabilized on mixtures should have a consistent response if the mixing is standardized. An unexpected response is most likely to occur when switching from separate injections to use of mixture or vice versa. To avoid dosage error, do not alter order of mixing insulins or change model or brand of syringe or needle. Each different type of insulin used must be of the same concentration (units/mL). Regular buffered insulin should not be mixed with other insulins due to the added phosphate buffer.

In mixtures of regular human and lente insulins, binding is detectable 5 minutes to 24 hours after mixing. If the regular/lente mixtures are not administered within the first 5 minutes after mixing, the effect of the regular insulin is diminished. The excess zinc binds with the regular and forms a lente-type insulin. Thus, it is critical that mixtures of regular with the lente insulins be mixed and injected immediately.

➤*Administration:* Administer maintenance doses subcutaneously 30 to 60 minutes before a meal. Give regular insulin IV or IM in severe ketoacidosis or diabetic coma.

Rotate administration sites to prevent lipodystrophy. A general rule is to not administer within 1 inch of the same site for 1 month. The rate of absorption is more rapid when the injection is in the abdomen (possibly greater than 50% faster), followed by the upper arm, thigh, and buttocks. Therefore, it may be best to rotate sites within an area rather than rotating areas.

➤*Admixture compatibility:* Insulin adsorption into plastic IV infusion sets has reportedly removed up to 80% of a dose, but 20% to 30% is more common. Percent adsorbed is inversely proportional to insulin concentration; it takes place within 30 to 60 minutes. Because this phenomenon cannot be accurately predicted, patient monitoring is essential.

➤*Storage/Stability:* Insulin preparations being used are generally stable if stored at room temperature (and not exposed to extreme temperatures or direct sunlight) for 1 month. Always store extra bottles in the refrigerator; do not freeze. Insulin prefilled in plastic or glass syringes is stable for 28 days under refrigeration. The insulin mixtures remain stable for 1 month at room temperature or for 3 months refrigerated. These mixtures can also be stored in prefilled plastic or glass syringes for 1 week to possibly 14 days under refrigeration.

INSULIN REGULAR CONCENTRATE (rDNA ORIGIN) — INJECTION

For complete prescribing information, refer to the Insulin group monograph.

Indications

➤*Insulin resistance:* Treatment of diabetic patients with marked insulin resistance (requirements greater than 200 units/day), because a large dose may be administered subcutaneously in a reasonable volume.

Administration and Dosage

➤*General dosing considerations:* Concentrated insulin injection is not modified by any agent that might prolong its action. It frequently has a duration similar to repository insulin; a single dose demonstrates activity for 24 hours. This has been credited to the high concentration of the preparation.

➤*Adults:*

Insulin resistance –

Usual dosage: Closely observe every patient exhibiting insulin resistance who requires concentrated insulin for diabetic control until appropriate dosing is established. Response will vary among patients. Most patients will show a "tolerance" to insulin, so that minor dosage variations will not cause untoward symptoms of insulin shock. Some may require only 1 dose daily; others may require 2 or 3 injections per day.

Duration of therapy: Insulin resistance is frequently self-limited; after several weeks or months of high dosage, responsiveness may be regained and dosage reduced.

➤*Children:* See Adults for dosing for children 12 years of age and older.

➤*Elderly:* The initial dosing, dosing increments, and maintenance dosing should be conservative to avoid hypoglycemic reactions. Hypoglycemia may be difficult to recognize in the elderly.

➤*Renal function impairment:* Some studies with human insulin have shown increased circulating levels of insulin in patients with renal failure. Careful glucose monitoring and dose adjustments of insulin may be necessary in patients with renal dysfunction. Insulin requirements may be reduced in patients with renal impairment.

➤*Hepatic function impairment:* Some studies with human insulin have shown increased circulating levels of insulin in patients with hepatic failure. Careful glucose monitoring and dose adjustments of insulin may be necessary in patients with hepatic dysfunction.

➤*Preparation for administration:* Use a tuberculin-type or insulin syringe for dosage measurement. Do not use if it is not water-clear. Discoloration, turbidity, or unusual viscosity indicates deterioration or contamination.

➤*Administration:* Administer subcutaneously. Do not inject intramuscularly (IM) or intravenously (IV). It is inadvisable to inject concentrated insulin intravenously because of possible inadvertent overdosage.

Dosage variations are frequent in the insulin-resistant patient because the individual is unresponsive to the pharmacologic effect of the insulin. Nevertheless, encourage accuracy of measurement because of the potential danger of the preparations. Inadvertent overdose may result in irreversible insulin shock. Serious consequences may result if not used under constant medical supervision.

➤*Admixture compatibility:* Regular insulin concentrate should not be mixed with other insulin formulations.

➤*Storage/Stability:* Keep in a cold place, preferably in a refrigerator. Do not freeze.

INSULIN ISOPHANE (NPH)

Insulin combined with protamine and zinc.

otc	**Humulin N** (Lilly)	**Injection (suspension):** 100 units/mL human insulin (rDNA)	In 5 × 3 mL disposable pen insulin delivery devices, and 10 mL vials.
otc	**Novolin N** (Novo Nordisk)		In 10 mL vials.

INSULIN ISOPHANE — INJECTION

For complete and comparative prescribing information, refer to the Insulin group monograph.

INSULIN ISOPHANE AND REGULAR

Provides rapid activity (onset 30 minutes) with a duration of up to 24 hours.

otc	**Humulin 70/30** (Lilly)	**Injection (suspension):** 100 units/mL human insulin (rDNA)	70% isophane insulin (NPH) and 30% insulin injection (regular). In 5 × 3 mL disposable pen insulin delivery devices, and 10 mL vials.
otc	**Novolin 70/30** (Novo Nordisk)		70% isophane insulin (NPH) and 30% insulin injection (regular). In 10 mL vials.
otc	**Humulin 50/50** (Lilly)	**Injection (suspension):** 100 units/mL human insulin (rDNA)	50% isophane insulin (NPH) and 50% insulin injection (regular). In 10 mL vials.

INSULIN ISOPHANE AND REGULAR — INJECTION

For complete and comparative prescribing information, refer to the Insulin group monograph.

INSULIN LISPRO

Rx	**Humalog** (Lilly)	**Injection, solution:** insulin lispro (human) 100 units/mL	In 10 mL vials, 5 × 1.5 mL and 5 × 3 mL cartridges, and 5 × 3 mL disposable pen insulin delivery devices.
Rx	**Humalog Mix 50/50** (Lilly)	**Injection, suspension:** insulin lispro (human) 100 units/mL[b]	Metacresol 2.20 mg/mL, protamine sulfate 0.19 mg/mL. In 10 mL vials and 5 × 3 mL disposable pen and *KwikPen* insulin delivery devices.
Rx	**Humalog Mix 75/25** (Lilly)	**Injection, suspension:** insulin lispro (human) 100 units/mL[a]	Protamine sulfate 0.28 mg/mL. In 10 mL vials and 5 × 3 mL disposable pen insulin delivery devices.

[a] Contains 75% insulin lispro protamine (rDNA origin) suspension and 25% insulin lispro (rDNA origin) injection.

[b] Contains 50% insulin lispro protamine (rDNA origin) suspension and 50% insulin lispro (rDNA origin) injection.

INSULIN LISPRO — INJECTION

For complete and comparative prescribing information, refer to the Insulin group monograph.

Indications

➤*Diabetes:* Insulin lispro is an insulin analog that is indicated in the treatment of patients with diabetes mellitus for the control of hyperglycemia. Insulin lispro has a more rapid onset and a shorter duration of action than human regular insulin. Therefore, in patients with type 1 diabetes, insulin lispro should be used in regimens that include a longer-acting insulin. However, in patients with type 2 diabetes, insulin lispro may be used without a longer-acting insulin when used in combination therapy with sulfonylurea agents.

Administration and Dosage

➤*General dosing considerations:* In patients with type 1 diabetes, insulin lispro should be used in regimens that include a longer-acting insulin. In patients with type 2 diabetes, insulin lispro may be used without a longer-acting insulin when used in combination therapy with sulfonylurea agents.

➤*Adults:*

Diabetes –

Concomitant insulin therapy: To achieve optimal glucose control, the amount of longer-acting insulin being given may need to be adjusted when using insulin lispro.

Conversion to insulin lispro: An adjustment of dose or schedule of basal insulin may be needed when a patient changes from other insulins to insulin lispro, particularly to prevent pre-meal hyperglycemia.

➤*Children:* Adjustment of basal insulin may be required. To improve accuracy in dosing in children, a diluent may be used.

See Adults for dosing.

➤*Renal function impairment:* The requirements for insulin may be reduced in patients with renal impairment. Careful glucose monitoring and dosage adjustment may be necessary in patients with renal dysfunction.

➤*Hepatic function impairment:* Although impaired hepatic function does not affect the absorption or disposition of insulin lispro, careful glucose monitoring and dose adjustments of insulin, including insulin lispro, may be necessary.

➤*Preparation for administration:* If the solution is cloudy, contains particulate matter, is thickened, or is discolored, the contents must not be injected.

➤*Administration:* Insulin lispro is intended for subcutaneous administration. When used as a meal-time insulin, insulin lispro should be given within 15 minutes before or immediately after a meal.

The rate of insulin absorption and consequently the onset of activity is known to be affected by the site of injection, exercise, and other variables. Insulin lispro was absorbed at a consistently faster rate than human regular insulin in healthy male volunteers given 0.2 units/kg human regular insulin or insulin lispro at abdominal, deltoid, or femoral sites, the 3 sites often used by patients with diabetes. When not mixed in the same syringe with other insulins, insulin lispro maintains its rapid onset of action and has less variability in its onset of action among injection sites compared with human regular insulin. After abdominal administration, insulin lispro concentrations are higher than those following deltoid or thigh injections. Also, the duration of action of insulin lispro is slightly shorter following abdominal injection, compared with deltoid and femoral injections.

As with all insulin preparations, the time course of action of insulin lispro may vary considerably in different individuals or within the same individual.

➤*Admixture compatibility:* Insulin lispro may be diluted with sterile diluent for insulin lispro, *Humulin N*, *Humulin 50/50*, *Humulin 70/30*, and *NPH Iletin* to a concentration of 1:10 (equivalent to U-10) or 1:2 (equivalent to U-50).

➤*Storage/Stability:* Insulin lispro should be stored in a refrigerator (2° to 8°C [36° to 46°F]), but not in the freezer. If refrigeration is impossible, the vial or cartridge of insulin lispro in use can be unrefrigerated for up to 28 days, as long as it is kept as cool as possible (not greater than 30°C [86°F]). Unrefrigerated vials and cartridges must be used within this time period or be discarded. Unrefrigerated (below 30°C [86°F]) pens and *KwikPens* must be used within 10 days or be discarded. Protect from direct heat and light. Do not use insulin lispro if it has been frozen.

Diluted insulin lispro may remain in patient use for 28 days when stored at 5°C (41°F) and for 14 days when stored at 30°C (86°F).

INSULIN ASPART

Rx	**NovoLog** (Novo Nordisk)	**Injection, solution:** insulin aspart 100 units/mL	With metacresol 1.72 mg/mL. In 10 mL vials, 3 mL *PenFill* cartridges, and 3 mL *FlexPen* prefilled syringes.
Rx	**Novolog Mix 70/30** (Novo Nordisk)	**Injection, solution:** insulin aspart 100 units/mL[a]	In 10 mL vials and 3 mL *FlexPen* prefilled syringes.

[a] Contains 70% insulin aspart protamine (rDNA origin) suspension and 30% insulin aspart (rDNA origin) injection.

INSULIN ASPART (rDNA ORIGIN) — INJECTION

For complete and comparative prescribing information, refer to the Insulin group monograph.

Indications

➤*Diabetes mellitus:* For the treatment of diabetes mellitus for the control of hyperglycemia.

Administration and Dosage

➤*Adults:*

Diabetes mellitus –

NovoLog:

• *Usual dosage* – 0.5 and 1 unit/kg/day. When used in a meal-related subcutaneous injection treatment regimen, 50% to 70% of total insulin requirements may be provided by *NovoLog* and the remainder by an intermediate- or long-acting insulin. Because of *NovoLog*'s comparatively rapid onset and short duration of glucose-lowering activity, some patients may require more basal insulin and more total insulin to prevent premeal hyperglycemia when using *NovoLog* than when using human regular insulin.

• *Concomitant therapy* – Insulin aspart should generally be used in regimens with an intermediate- or long-acting insulin.

NovoLog Mix 70/30 : Fixed ratio insulins are typically dosed on a twice-daily basis (ie, before breakfast and supper), with each dose intended to cover 2 meals or a meal and snack. The absorption rate of *NovoLog Mix 70/30* from the subcutaneous tissue allows dosing within 15 minutes of meal initiation.

➤*Children:*

Diabetes mellitus –

NovoLog:

• *Subcutaneous daily injections* –

2 years of age and older: See Adults.

• *Subcutaneous continuous infusion by external insulin pump* –

4 years of age and older: See Adults.

NovoLog Mix 70/30: Safety and efficacy of *NovoLog Mix 70/30* in children have not been established.

➤*Renal function impairment:* The dose requirements for insulin may be reduced in patients with renal impairment.

➤*Hepatic function impairment:* The dose requirements for insulin aspart may be reduced in patients with hepatic impairment.

➤*Preparation for administration:* Do not use *NovoLog* if it has become viscous (thickened) or cloudy; use it only if it is clear and colorless.

NovoLog Mix 70/30 suspension should be visually inspected and resuspended immediately before use. The resuspended *NovoLog Mix 70/30* must appear uniformly white and cloudy.

➤*Administration:*

NovoLog – Injection and infusion sites should be rotated within the same region to reduce the risk of lipodystrophy.

Subcutaneous injection: Insulin aspart should be administered by subcutaneous injection in the abdominal region, buttocks, thigh, or upper arm. Because insulin aspart has a more rapid onset and a shorter duration of activity than human regular insulin, it should be injected immediately (within 5 to 10 minutes) before a meal.

Continuous subcutaneous insulin infusion by external pump: Insulin aspart can also be infused subcutaneously by an external insulin pump. Diluted insulin should not be used in external insulin pumps. Because *NovoLog* has a more rapid onset and a shorter duration of activity than human regular insulin, premeal boluses of *NovoLog* should be infused immediately (within 5 to 10 minutes) before a meal. The initial programming of the external insulin infusion pump should be based on the total daily insulin dose of the previous regimen. Although there is significant interpatient variability, approximately 50% of the total dose is usually given as meal-related boluses of *NovoLog* and the remainder is given as a basal infusion. Change the insulin aspart in the reservoir, the infusion sets, and the infusion set insertion site at least every 48 hours.

Intravenous (IV) use: NovoLog can be administered IV under medical supervision for glycemic control with close monitoring of blood glucose and potassium levels to avoid hypoglycemia and hypokalemia. For IV use, *NovoLog* should be used at concentrations from 0.05 to 1 unit/mL in infusion systems using polypropylene infusion bags.

NovoLog Mix 70/30 – *NovoLog Mix 70/30* is intended only for subcutaneous injection (into the abdominal wall, thigh, or upper arm). *NovoLog Mix 70/30* should not be administered IV.

FlexPen prefilled syringes: Before use, roll the disposable *NovoLog Mix 70/30 FlexPen* prefilled syringe between the palms 10 times. Thereafter, turn the disposable *NovoLog Mix 70/30 FlexPen* prefilled syringe upside down so that the glass ball moves from one end of the reservoir to the other. Do this at least 10 times. The rolling and turning procedure must be repeated until the suspension appears uniformly white and cloudy. Inject immediately. Before each subsequent injection, turn the disposable *NovoLog Mix 70/30 FlexPen* prefilled syringe upside down so that the glass ball moves from one end of the reservoir to the other at least 10 times and until the suspension appears uniformly white and cloudy. Inject immediately. After use, needles on the disposable *NovoLog Mix 70/30 FlexPen* prefilled syringes should not be recapped.

Vial: Resuspend immediately before use. Roll the vial gently 10 times in your hands to mix it.

➤*Admixture compatibility:* Insulin aspart may be diluted with insulin-diluting medium for *NovoLog* for subcutaneous injection. Diluting 1 part insulin aspart to 9 parts diluent will yield a concentration one-tenth that of insulin aspart (equivalent to U-10). Diluting 1 part insulin aspart to 1 part diluent will yield a concentration one-half that of insulin aspart (equivalent to U-50).

NovoLog has been shown to be stable in infusion fluids such as sodium chloride 0.9%.

Mixing insulins – Mixing insulin aspart with neutral protamine Hagedorn (NPH) human insulin immediately before injection attenuates the peak concentration of insulin aspart, without significantly affecting the time to peak concentration or total bioavailability of insulin aspart. If insulin aspart is mixed with NPH human insulin, insulin aspart should be drawn into the syringe first. The injection should be made immediately after mixing. Mixtures should not be administered IV.

NovoLog Mix 70/30 should not be mixed with any other insulin product.

Continuous subcutaneous insulin infusion by external pump – When used in external subcutaneous infusion pumps for insulin, insulin aspart should not be mixed with any other insulins or diluent.

➤*Storage/Stability:* Unpunctured vials, *PenFill* cartridges, and *FlexPen* prefilled syringes can be used until the expiration date printed on the label if they are stored in a refrigerator. Keep unused vials, *PenFill* cartridges, and *FlexPen* prefilled syringes in the carton so they will stay clean and protected from light. Keep away from direct heat and sunlight.

NovoLog – Unused insulin aspart should be stored in the refrigerator between 2° and 8°C (36° and 46°F). Do not store in the freezer or directly adjacent to the refrigerator cooling element. Do not freeze insulin aspart and do not use insulin aspart if it has been frozen. Insulin aspart should not be drawn into a syringe and stored for later use.

Vials: After initial use, a vial may be kept at temperatures below 30°C (86°F) for up to 28 days. Opened vials may be refrigerated.

PenFill cartridges or *NovoLog FlexPen* prefilled syringes: Once a cartridge or a *NovoLog FlexPen* prefilled syringe is punctured, it should be kept at temperatures below 30°C (86°F) for up to 28 days. Do not store in the refrigerator. Always remove the needle after each injection and store the 3 mL *PenFill* cartridge delivery device or *NovoLog FlexPen* prefilled syringe without a needle attached. This prevents contamination and/or infection or leakage of insulin and will ensure accurate dosing. Always use a new needle for each injection to prevent contamination.

Pump: Insulin aspart in the pump reservoir should be discarded after at least every 48 hours of use or after exposure to temperatures that exceed 37°C (98.6°F).

Diluted NovoLog: Insulin aspart diluted with insulin diluting medium for *NovoLog* to a concentration equivalent to U-10 or U-50 may remain in patient use at temperatures below 30°C (86°F) for 28 days.

NovoLog in infusion fluids: Infusion bags prepared as previously indicated are stable at room temperature for 24 hours. Some insulin will be initially adsorbed to the material of the infusion bag.

NovoLog Mix 70/30 –

Vials: The vials should be stored in a refrigerator, not in a freezer. If refrigeration is not possible, the bottle in use can be kept unrefrigerated at room temperature below 30°C (86°F) for up to 28 days as long as it is kept as cool as possible.

FlexPen prefilled syringes: Once a *NovoLog Mix 70/30 FlexPen* prefilled syringe is punctured, it may be used for up to 14 days if it is kept at room temperature below 30°C (86°F). Do not store in the refrigerator.

INSULIN GLARGINE (rDNA ORIGIN)

Rx	**Lantus** (Sanofi-Aventis)	**Injection:** 100 units/mL (rDNA origin)	In 10 mL vials and 3 mL cartridge system for use with *OptiClik.*

INSULIN GLARGINE (rDNA ORIGIN) — INJECTION

For complete and comparative prescribing information, refer to the Insulin group monograph.

Indications

➤*Diabetes:* Once-daily subcutaneous administration for the treatment of adults and children with type 1 diabetes mellitus or adults with type 2 diabetes mellitus who require basal (long-acting) insulin for the control of hyperglycemia.

Insulin glargine is not the insulin of choice for the treatment of diabetic ketoacidosis. Short-acting intravenous (IV) insulin is the preferred treatment.

Administration and Dosage

➤*General dosing considerations:* A program of close metabolic monitoring under medical supervision is recommended.

➤*Adults:*

Diabetes –

Initial dosage: In a clinical study with insulin-naive patients with type 2 diabetes already treated with oral antidiabetic drugs, insulin glargine was started at an average dose of 10 units once daily and subsequently adjusted according to the patient's need.

INSULIN GLARGINE (rDNA ORIGIN) — INJECTION

Maintenance dosage: 2 to 100 units total daily dose.

Dosage adjustment: Dose adjustment of insulin glargine and other insulins or oral antidiabetic drugs may be required; for example, if the patient's timing of dosing, weight or lifestyle changes, or other circumstances arise that increase susceptibility to hypoglycemia or hyperglycemia. The dose also may have to be adjusted during intercurrent illness.

Conversion from other insulins: If changing from a treatment regimen with an intermediate- or long-acting insulin to a regimen with insulin glargine, the amount and timing of short-acting insulin, fast-acting insulin analog, or the dose of any oral antidiabetic drug may need to be adjusted.

The amount and timing of short- or fast-acting insulin analog may need to be adjusted. This is particularly true for patients with acquired antibodies to human insulin needing high insulin doses and occurs with all insulin analogs.

➤*Children:* See Adults for dosing for children 6 years of age and older.

➤*Elderly:* In elderly patients with diabetes, the initial dosing, dose increments, and maintenance dosage should be conservative to avoid hypoglycemic reactions. Hypoglycemia may be difficult to recognize in the elderly.

➤*Preparation for administration:* Use only if clear and colorless with no visible particles. The syringes must not contain any other medicinal product or residue. If *OptiClik*, the insulin delivery devise for insulin glargine, malfunctions, insulin glargine may be drawn from the cartridge system into a U-100 syringe and injected.

➤*Administration:* Administer subcutaneously once daily at the same time every day. Administer the dose at any time during the day.

Insulin glargine is not intended for IV administration. The prolonged duration of activity is dependent on injection into subcutaneous tissue. IV administration of the usual subcutaneous dose could result in severe hypoglycemia.

As with all insulins, injection sites within an injection area (abdomen, deltoid, or thigh) must be rotated from one injection to the next. The rate of absorption and, consequently, the onset and duration of action may be affected by exercise and other variables.

➤*Admixture compatibility:* Insulin glargine must not be diluted or mixed with any other insulin or solution. If insulin glargine is diluted or mixed, the solution may become cloudy and the pharmacokinetic/pharmacodynamic profile (eg, onset of action, time to peak effect) of insulin glargine and/or the mixed insulin may be altered in an unpredictable manner.

➤*Storage/Stability:* Store unopened insulin glargine vials and cartridges at 2° to 8°C (36° to 46°F). Do not store insulin glargine in the freezer or allow it to freeze. Discard if it has been frozen. If refrigeration is not possible, the open vial in use can be kept unrefrigerated for up to 28 days away from direct heat and light, as long as the temperature is not above 30°C (86°F). Opened vials, whether or not refrigerated, must be used within a 28-day period or they must be discarded.

Do not refrigerate the opened (in-use) cartridge system in *OptiClik*. Keep the opened cartridge system at room temperature below 30°C (86°F), away from direct heat and light. Discard the opened cartridge system in *OptiClik* that has been kept at room temperature after 28 days. Do not store *OptiClik*, with or without cartridge system, in a refrigerator at any time.

INSULIN GLULISINE

Rx	**Apidra** (Sanofi-Aventis)	**Injection:** 100 units/mL (rDNA origin)	Metacresol 3.15 mg/mL. In 10 mL vials and 3 mL cartridges for use with *OptiClik*.

INSULIN GLULISINE (rDNA ORIGIN) — INJECTION

For complete prescribing information, refer to the Insulin class monograph.

Indications

➤*Diabetes mellitus:* Indicated to improve glycemic control in adults and children with diabetes mellitus.

Administration and Dosage

➤*General dosing considerations:* Insulin glulisine is a recombinant insulin analog that has been shown to be equipotent to human insulin. One unit of insulin glulisine has the same glucose-lowering effect as 1 unit of regular human insulin when given intravenously (IV). When given subcutaneously, insulin glulisine has a more rapid onset of action and shorter duration of action than regular human insulin.

The dosage of insulin glulisine should be individualized.

Blood glucose monitoring is essential in all patients receiving insulin therapy.

Insulin requirements may be altered during stress, major illness, or with changes in exercise, meal patterns, or coadministered drugs.

➤*Adults:*

Diabetes mellitus –

Subcutaneous: 0.5 to 1 unit/kg/day administered 15 minutes before a meal or within 20 minutes of starting a meal. The total daily insulin requirement may vary.

Intravenous (IV): 0.05 to 1 unit/mL infused IV in sodium chloride 0.9% using polyvinyl chloride (PVC) infusion bags.

Continuous subcutaneous infusion pump: The dosage of insulin glulisine should be individualized.

➤*Children:*

Diabetes mellitus –

4 years of age and older: See Adults for dosing.

➤*Administration:*

Subcutaneous – Insulin glulisine should be administered by subcutaneous injection in the abdominal wall, thigh, or upper arm. Injection sites should be rotated within the same region (abdomen, thigh, or upper arm) from one injection to the next to reduce the risk of lipodystrophy.

Insulin glulisine given by subcutaneous injection should generally be used in regimens with intermediate- or long-acting insulin.

After subcutaneous administration, insulin glulisine has a more rapid onset and shorter duration of action than regular human insulin.

Insulin glulisine should be given within 15 minutes before a meal or within 20 minutes after the start of a meal.

If insulin glulisine is mixed with neutral protamine Hagedorn (NPH) human insulin, insulin glulisine should be drawn into the syringe first. Inject the mixture right away.

Continuous subcutaneous infusion (insulin pump) – Insulin glulisine may be administered by continuous subcutaneous infusion in the abdominal wall. Infusion sites should be rotated within the same region to reduce the risk of lipodystrophy.

The initial programming of the external insulin infusion pump should be based on the total daily insulin dose of the previous regimen.

Based on studies which have shown loss of the preservative, metacresol, and insulin degradation, insulin glulisine in the reservoir should be changed at least every 48 hours.

IV – IV administration of insulin glulisine may be administered under only strict medical supervision with close monitoring of blood glucose and potassium levels to avoid hypoglycemia and hypokalemia.

The glucose-lowering activities of insulin glulisine and of regular human insulin are equipotent when administered by the IV route.

For IV use, insulin glulisine should be used at concentrations of insulin glulisine 0.05 units/mL to 1 unit/mL in infusion systems with the infusion fluid, sterile sodium chloride 0.9% solution, using PVC bags.

Do not administer insulin mixtures IV.

➤*Admixture compatibility:* Insulin glulisine is not compatible with dextrose solution and Ringer's lactate solution and, therefore, cannot be used with these solution fluids. The use of insulin glulisine with other solutions has not been studied and is not recommended.

Subcutaneous – Insulin glulisine for subcutaneous injection should not be mixed with insulin preparations other than NPH insulin. If insulin glulisine is mixed with NPH insulin, insulin glulisine should be drawn into the syringe first. Injection should occur immediately after mixing.

Continuous subcutaneous infusion (infusion pump) – Insulin glulisine should not be mixed with other insulins or with a diluent when used in a pump.

IV – Insulin glulisine for IV administration should not be diluted with solutions other than sodium chloride 0.9% (normal saline).

Do not mix insulin glulisine with other insulins for IV administration.

➤*Storage/Stability:*

Unopened vial/cartridge system – Store in a refrigerator, 2° to 8°C (36° to 46°F). Protect from light. Do not store insulin glulisine in the freezer; do not allow it to freeze. Discard if it has been frozen.

Unopened vials/cartridge systems not stored in a refrigerator must be used within 28 days.

Open (in-use) vial – Opened vials, whether or not refrigerated, must be used within 28 days. If refrigeration is not possible, the open vial in use can be kept unrefrigerated for up to 28 days away from direct heat and light, as long as the temperature is not greater than 25°C (77°F).

Open (in-use) cartridge system – Do not refrigerate the opened (in-use) cartridge system inserted in *OptiClik*, but keep below 25°C (77°F) and away from direct heat and light. The opened (in-use) cartridge system must be discarded after 28 days. Do not store *OptiClik*, with or without cartridge system, in a refrigerator at any time.

Infusion sets and bags – Discard the infusion sets (eg, catheters, reservoirs, tubing) and the insulin glulisine in the reservoir after no more than 48 hours of use or after exposure to temperatures that exceed 37°C (98.6°F).

Infusion bags are stable at room temperature for 48 hours.

INSULIN DETEMIR

Rx	**Levemir** (Novo Nordisk)	**Injection:** 100 units/mL (rDNA origin)	In 3 mL *Penfill* cartridges and 10 mL vials.

INSULIN DETEMIR — INJECTION

Indications

➤*Diabetes:* For once- or twice-daily subcutaneous administration for the treatment of adult and pediatric patients with type 1 diabetes mellitus or adult patients with type 2 diabetes mellitus who require basal (long-acting) insulin for the control of hyperglycemia.

Administration and Dosage

➤*General dosing considerations:* Close glucose monitoring is recommended during the transition and in the initial weeks thereafter.

➤*Adults:*

Diabetes –

Initial dosage: 0.1 to 0.2 units/kg once daily in the evening or 10 units once or twice daily in insulin-naive patients with type 2 diabetes who are inadequately controlled on oral antidiabetic drugs.

Dosage adjustment: Adjust the dose of insulin detemir according to blood glucose measurements.

Conversion: Dose and timing of concurrent short-acting insulins or other concomitant antidiabetic treatment may need to be adjusted.

• *Basal bolus patients –* For patients with type 1 or type 2 diabetes on basal-bolus treatment, changing the basal insulin to insulin detemir can be done on a unit-to-unit basis. The dose of insulin detemir should then be adjusted to achieve glycemic targets. In some patients with type 2 diabetes, more insulin detemir may be required than neutral protamine Hagedorn (NPH) insulin. In a clinical study, the mean dose at end of treatment was 0.77 units/kg for insulin detemir and 0.52 units/kg for NPH human insulin.

• *Basal insulin only patients –* For patients currently receiving only basal insulin, changing the basal insulin to insulin detemir may be done on a unit-to-unit basis.

➤*Children:* See Adults for dosing.

➤*Elderly:* In elderly patients with diabetes, the initial dosing, dose increments, and maintenance dosage should be conservative to avoid hypoglycemic reactions. Hypoglycemia may be difficult to recognize in the elderly.

➤*Renal function impairment:* As with other insulins, the requirements for insulin detemir may need to be adjusted in patients with renal impairment.

➤*Hepatic function impairment:* As with other insulins, the requirements for insulin detemir may need to be adjusted in patients with hepatic impairment.

➤*Administration:* Administer by subcutaneous injection in the thigh, abdominal wall, or upper arm. Injection sites should be rotated within the same region. As with all insulins, the duration of action will vary according to the dose, injection site, blood flow, temperature, and level of physical activity.

Administer insulin detemir once or twice daily. For patients treated with insulin detemir once daily, administer the dose with the evening meal or at bedtime. For patients who require twice-daily dosing for effective blood glucose control, administer the evening dose with the evening meal, at bedtime, or 12 hours after the morning dose.

➤*Admixture compatibility:* Do not mix or dilute insulin detemir with any other insulin preparations.

➤*Storage/Stability:* Store unused insulin detemir between 2° and 8°C (36° and 46°F). Do not freeze. Do not use insulin detemir if it has been frozen.

Vials – After initial use, store vials in a refrigerator, never in a freezer. If refrigeration is not possible, the in-use vial can be kept unrefrigerated at room temperature, below 30°C (86°F), for up to 42 days, as long as it is kept as cool as possible and away from direct heat and light.

Unpunctured vials can be used until the expiration date printed on the label if they are stored in a refrigerator. Keep unused vials in the carton so they will stay clean and protected from light.

Cartridges and prefilled syringe cartridges – After initial use, a cartridge or prefilled syringe may be used for up to 42 days if it is kept at room temperature, below 30°C (86°F). In-use cartridges and prefilled syringes must not be stored in a refrigerator or with the needle in place. Keep all cartridges and prefilled syringes away from direct heat and sunlight.

Not in-use (unopened) cartridges and prefilled syringes can be used until the expiration date printed on the label if they are stored in a refrigerator. Keep unused cartridges and prefilled syringes in the carton so they will stay clean and protected from light.

Indications

➤*Type 2 diabetes:* As an adjunct to diet and exercise to lower the blood glucose in patients with type 2 diabetes mellitus (non-insulin-dependent) whose hyperglycemia cannot be controlled by diet and exercise alone.

➤*Off-label uses:* **Chlorpropamide** in doses of 200 to 500 mg/day has been used in the treatment of diabetes insipidus.

Sulfonylureas have been used as temporary adjuncts to insulin therapy in selected type 2 diabetes patients to improve diabetes control (see Administration and Dosage).

Administration and Dosage

➤*Institution of therapy:* Individualize therapy. Selection of an individual agent is influenced by the drug's potency, duration of action, metabolism, adverse reactions, patient's lack of response to other oral agents, and the patient's personal preference.

Monitor patient's blood glucose periodically to determine the minimum effective dose for the patient; to detect primary failure (ie, inadequate lowering of blood glucose at the maximum recommended dose of medication); and to detect secondary failure (ie, loss of adequate blood glucose response after an initial period of effectiveness). Glycosylated hemoglobin levels are also valuable in monitoring the patient's response to therapy.

➤*Short-term use:* Short-term administration of sulfonylureas may be sufficient during periods of transient loss of control in patients usually well controlled on diet.

➤*Transfer from other hypoglycemic agents:*

Sulfonylureas – When transferring patients from 1 oral hypoglycemic agent to another, no transitional period and no initial or priming dose is necessary. However, when transferring patients from **chlorpropamide**, exercise particular care during the first 2 weeks because the prolonged retention of chlorpropamide in the body and subsequent overlapping drug effects may provoke hypoglycemia. See specific guidelines for each agent in the individual Administration and Dosage sections.

Insulin – During insulin withdrawal period, test urine for glucose and ketones 3 times daily and report results to physician daily. For specific guidelines for each individual sulfonylurea, refer to the Administration and Dosage section for each agent.

General clinical characteristics which favor successful sulfonylureas monotherapy following insulin withdrawal include the following:

- Onset of diabetes at at least 35 years of age
- Obese or normal body weight
- Duration of diabetes less than 10 years
- Absence of ketoacidosis
- Fasting serum glucose 200 mg/dL or less
- Postprandial blood glucose values less than 250 mg/dL
- Insulin requirement less than 40 units/day
- Absence of renal or hepatic dysfunction

➤*Elderly patients:* Elderly patients may be particularly sensitive to these agents; therefore, start with a lower initial dose before breakfast, and check blood and urine glucoseduring the first 24 hours of therapy. If control is satisfactory, continue or gradually increase dose. If there is a tendency toward hypoglycemia, reduce dose or discontinue the drug.

➤*Acute complications:* During the course of intercurrent complications (eg, ketoacidosis, severe trauma, major surgery, infections, severe diarrhea, nausea, vomiting), supportive therapy with insulin may be necessary. Continue or withdraw sulfonylurea therapy while insulin is used. Insulin is indispensable in managing acute complications; carefully instruct all diabetes patients in its use.

➤*Combination insulin therapy:* Concurrent administration of insulin and an oral sulfonylurea (generally **glipizide** or **glyburide**) has been used with some success in type 2 diabetes patients who are difficult to control with diet and sulfonylurea therapy alone. One proposed method is referred to as the BIDS system: Bedtime Insulin (usually NPH) in combination with a Daytime (morning only or morning and evening) Sulfonylurea, usually glyburide.

Actions

➤*Pharmacology:* The sulfonylurea hypoglycemic agents are sulfonamide derivatives but are devoid of antibacterial activity. These agents are divided into 2 groups: First generation (**acetohexamide**, **chlorpropamide**, **tolazamide**, **tolbutamide**) and second generation (**glipizide**, **glyburide**, **glimepiride**). They are used as adjuncts to diet and exercise in the treatment of type 2 diabetes, previously known as non-insulin-dependent diabetes mellitus (NIDDM). Type 2 diabetes has also been referred to as adult-onset or maturity-onset diabetes and ketosis-resistant diabetes.

Type 2 diabetes not only leads to hyperglycemia but affects several organ systems resulting in dyslipidemia, hypertension, central obesity, and accelerated atherosclerosis. This multisystem disorder, also known as the insulin resistance syndrome, contributes to high rates of morbidity and mortality that are usually manifestations of coronary artery and cerebrovascular disease. Other factors influencing premature death in these patients are the duration of diabetes, lack of glycemic control, and other cardiovascular risk factors such as smoking and physical inactivity.

Type 2 diabetes is characterized by insulin resistance, impaired insulin secretion, and overproduction of hepatic glucose. Evidence suggests that insulin resistance is the predominant factor preceding the onset of hyperglycemia. During the transition from impaired glucose tolerance to frank disease, basal hepatic glucose production rates increase, insulin resistance becomes more severe (which may be partly due to acquired conditions such as age, obesity, and an inactive lifestyle), and beta-cell function decreases affecting insulin secretory ability.

By binding to the plasma membrane of functional beta-cells in the pancreatic islets, sulfonylureas cause a decrease in potassium (K+) permeability and membrane depolarization which, in turn, leads to an increase in intracellular calcium ions and subsequent exocytosis of insulin-containing secretory granules. This process is also stimulated by glucose and other insulin-releasing fuels; however, sulfonylureas increase insulin secretion at stimulatory levels lower than that required for glucose suggesting that they enhance beta-cell response rather than change beta-cell sensitivity to glucose. The role of extrapancreatic effects of sulfonylureas in the treatment of hyperglycemia are of questionable clinical significance with the possible exception of glimepiride, which has demonstrated increased sensitivity of peripheral tissues to insulin.

Other pharmacologic activity includes: Potentiation of the effect of antidiuretic hormone (ADH); tolazamide, acetohexamide, glyburide, and glipizide may produce a mild diuresis; acetohexamide has significant uricosuric activity;chlorpropamide can cause flushing (a disulfiram-like reaction) in some patients who consume alcohol.

➤*Pharmacokinetics:* The sulfonylureas are well absorbed after oral administration. All sulfonylureas except **glipizide** can be taken with food; absorption of glipizide is delayed by food. **Tolbutamide**, **glyburide**, and glipizide are more effective when taken approximately 30 minutes before a meal. **Tolazamide** is absorbed more slowly than the other sulfonylureas. They are metabolized in the liver to active and inactive metabolites and excreted primarily in the urine. The hypoglycemic effects of sulfonylureas may be prolonged in severe liver disease caused by decreased metabolism.

Although the mechanisms of action and maximal hypoglycemic effects are similar, the second and first generation sulfonylureas differ. Second generation compounds possess a more nonpolar or lipophilic side chain. Therapeutically effective doses and serum concentrations of the second generation sulfonylureas are lower, due to their higher intrinsic potency. All sulfonylureas are strongly bound to plasma proteins, primarily albumin. Protein binding of the first generation sulfonylureas is ionic; that of the second generation agents is predominantly nonionic. The clinical therapeutic significance of this difference is unknown; however, because they are bound to albumin by ionic bindings, the first generation agents may be more likely to be displaced by drugs that competitively bind to proteins (eg, warfarin). Displacement of sulfonylurea agents from protein would result in greater hypoglycemic response (see Drug Interactions).

Differences exist among the sulfonylureas in the duration of hypoglycemic effects (see following table). Tolbutamide is short-acting because it is rapidly metabolized to an inactive metabolite; it may be useful in patients with kidney disease. The active metabolite of acetohexamide is 2.5 times as potent as the parent compound. Because the metabolite is excreted in the urine, the duration of action of **acetohexamide** is prolonged in renal disease. Tolazamide has 2 active metabolites which are less potent than the parent compound. The renal elimination of chlorpropamide may be sensitive to changes in urinary pH; urinary alkalinization increases its excretion in the urine. When the urine pH is less than 6, urinary excretion decreases and hepatic metabolism is the primary route of elimination. The half-life of **chlorpropamide** is prolonged in renal disease.

Major Pharmacokinetic Parameters of the Sulfonylureas

Sulfonylureas	Approximate equivalent doses (mg)	Doses/ day	Serum t½ (h)	Onset (h)	Duration (h)	Renal excretion (%)	Active metabolites
First generation							
Acetohexamide	500 to 750	1 to 2	≈ 6 to 8 (parent drug + metabolite)	1	12 to 24	100	Yes
Chlorpropamide	250 to 375	1	36	1	24 to 60	100	Yes
Tolazamide	250 to 375	1 to 2	7	4 to 6	12 to 24	100	Yes
Tolbutamide	1,000 to 1,500	2 to 3	4.5 to 6.5	1	6 to 12	100	No
Second generation							
Glipizide	10	1 to 2	2 to 4	1 to 3	10 to 24	80 to 85	No
Glyburide, Nonmicronized	5	1 to 2	10	2 to 4	16 to 24	50	Yes[a]
Micronized	3	1 to 2	≈ 4	1	12 to 24	50	Yes[a]
Glimepiride	NA[b]	1	≈ 9	2 to 3	24	60	Yes

[a] Weakly active.
[b] Not applicable.

Contraindications

Hypersensitivity to sulfonylureas ; diabetes complicated by ketoacidosis, with or without coma; sole therapy of type 1 (insulin-dependent) diabetes mellitus; diabetes when complicated by pregnancy.

Warnings/Precautions

➤*Cardiovascular risk:* The administration of oral hypoglycemic drugs has been associated with increased cardiovascular mortality as compared with treatment with diet alone or diet plus insulin. Despite controversy regarding its interpretation, this warning is based on the study conducted by the University Group Diabetes Program (UGDP). This long-term prospective clinical trial involving 823 patients evaluated the effectiveness of glucose-lowering drugs in preventing or delaying vascular complications in patients with non-insulin-dependent diabetes. (*Diabetes* 1970;19]:747-830.)

Patients treated for 5 to 8 years with diet plus **tolbutamide** (1.5 g/day) had a rate of cardiovascular mortality approximately 2.5 times that of patients treated with diet alone. A significant increase in total mortality was not observed. Consider this for other sulfonylureas as well.

Sulfonylurea binding to ATP-dependent K+ channels has been shown to inhibit the response to ischemia, potentially delaying the recovery of contractile function and increasing infarct size during a MI. However, prevention of channel opening during ischemia could reduce the occurrence of ventricular fibrillation during ischemia. Inform the patient of potential risks, advantages, and alternative modes of therapy.

➤*Bioavailability:* Micronized **glyburide** 3 mg tablets provide serum concentrations that are *not* bioequivalent to those from the conventional formulation (nonmicronized) 5 mg tablets. Therefore, retitrate patients when transferring patients from any hypoglycemic agent to micronized glyburide.

➤*Diet and exercise:* Diet and exercise remain the primary considerations of diabetic patient management. Caloric restriction and weight loss are essential in the obese diabetic patient. These drugs are an adjunct to, not a substitute for, dietary regulation. Also, loss of blood glucose control on diet alone may be transient, thus requiring only short-term sulfonylurea therapy. Identify cardiovascular risk factors and take corrective measures where possible.

➤*Hypoglycemia:* All sulfonylureas may produce severe hypoglycemia. Proper patient selection, dosage, and instructions are important to avoid hypoglycemic episodes. Renal or hepatic insufficiency may elevate drug blood levels, and the latter may also diminish gluconeogenic capacity, both of which increase the risk of serious hypoglycemic reactions. Elderly, debilitated, or malnourished patients, and those with adrenal or pituitary insufficiency are particularly susceptible to the hypoglycemic action of glucose-lowering drugs. Hypoglycemia may be difficult to recognize in the elderly and in patients taking β-adrenergic blocking drugs. Hypoglycemia is more likely to occur when caloric intake is deficient, after severe or prolonged exercise, when alcohol is ingested, or when more than 1 glucose-lowering drug is used.

Because of the long half-life of **chlorpropamide**, patients who become hypoglycemic during therapy require careful supervision of the dose and frequent feedings for at least 3 to 5 days. Hospitalization and IV glucose may be necessary.

➤*Asymptomatic patients:* Controlling blood glucose in type 2 diabetes with sulfonylureas has not been definitely established to be effective in preventing the long-term cardiovascular or neural complications of diabetes.

➤*Loss of blood glucose control:* When a patient stabilized on any diabetic regimen is exposed to stress such as fever, trauma, infection, or surgery, a loss of control may occur. At such times, it may be necessary to discontinue the drug and give insulin.

The effectiveness of any oral hypoglycemic in lowering blood glucose to a desired level decreases in many patients over time (secondary failure); this may be due to progression of the severity of the diabetes or to diminished drug responsiveness. Adequately adjust dose and assess adherence to diet before classifying a patient as a secondary failure. Primary failure occurs when the drug is ineffective in a patient when first given. Certain patients who demonstrate an inadequate response or true primary or secondary failure to 1 sulfonylurea may benefit from a transfer to another sulfonylurea.

➤*Disulfiram-like syndrome:* A sulfonylurea-induced facial flushing reaction may occur when some sulfonylureas are administered with alcohol. This syndrome is characterized by facial flushing and occasional breathlessness but without the nausea, vomiting, and hypotension seen with a true alcohol-disulfiram reaction. The facial flushing reaction occurs in approximately 33% of type 2 diabetes patients taking **chlorpropamide** and alcohol. It is uncertain whether **glyburide** and **glipizide** can cause the facial flushing reaction.

➤*Syndrome of inappropriate secretion of antidiuretic hormone (SIADH):* Water retention and dilutional hyponatremia have occurred after administration of sulfonylureas to type 2 diabetes patients, especially those with CHF or hepatic cirrhosis. The drugs stimulate antidiuretic hormone (ADH) release, augmenting hypothalamic-pituitary release of ADH. The result is excessive water retention, hyponatremia, low serum osmolality, and high urine osmolality.

Glipizide, **acetohexamide**, **tolazamide**, and **glyburide** are mildly diuretic.

➤*Renal/Hepatic function impairment:* Oral hypoglycemic agents are metabolized in the liver. The drugs and most of their metabolites are excreted by the kidneys. Hepatic impairment may result in inadequate release of glucose in response to hypoglycemia. Renal impairment may cause decreased elimination of sulfonylureas leading to accumulation producing hypoglycemia. Therefore, use these agents with caution in type 2 diabetes patients with renal or hepatic impairment, and monitor renal and liver function frequently.

➤*Pregnancy:* (*Category C* – **glyburide** (per Briggs' Drugs in Pregnancy and Lactation; *Diabeta*), glipizide, tolazamide, chlorpropamide, tolbutamide, glimepiride. *Category B* – glyburide (per manufacturer's prescribing information). Sulfonylureas (except **glyburide**) are teratogenic in animals. There are no adequate studies in pregnant women. Use only if clearly needed. In general, avoid sulfonylureas in pregnancy; they will not provide good control in patients who cannot be controlled by diet alone.

Because abnormal blood glucose levels during pregnancy may be associated with a higher incidence of congenital abnormalities, insulin is recommended to maintain blood glucose levels as close to normal as possible. However, fetal mortality and major congenital anomalies generally occur 3 to 4 times more often in offspring of diabetic mothers.

Labor and delivery – Prolonged severe hypoglycemia (4 to 10 days) has occurred in neonates born to mothers on a sulfonylurea at the time of delivery. This has been reported more frequently with agents with prolonged half-lives. If used during pregnancy, discontinue at least 2 days to 4 weeks before expected delivery date.

➤*Lactation:* **Chlorpropamide** and **tolbutamide** are excreted in breast milk. A chlorpropamide breast milk concentration of 5 mcg/ml has been detected following a 500 mg dose (normal peak blood level after 250 mg is 30 mcg/ml). It is not known if other sulfonylureas are excreted in breast milk. Because of the potential for hypoglycemia in nursing infants, decide whether to discontinue nursing or the drug.

➤*Children:* Safety and efficacy in children have not been established.

➤*Elderly:* In elderly, debilitated, or malnourished patients, and patients with impaired renal or hepatic function, the initial and maintenance dosing should be conservative to avoid hypoglycemic reactions.

Per the Beers list, chlorpropamide has a prolonged half-life in elderly patients and could cause prolonged hypoglycemia. Additionally, it is the only oral hypoglycemic agent that causes SIADH. Chlorpropamide is also considered a high risk medication for the elderly according to the Centers of Medicare and Medicaid Services.

➤*Monitoring:* Keep patients under continuous medical supervision. During the initial test period, the patient should communicate with the physician daily, and report at least weekly for the first month for physical examination and evaluation of diabetes control. After the first month, examine at monthly intervals or as indicated. Uncooperative individuals may be unsuitable for treatment with oral agents.

During the transitional period, test the urine for glucose and acetone at least 3 times daily and have the results reviewed by a physician frequently. Measurement of glycosylated hemoglobin (HbA1c) is also recommended. It is important that patients be taught to correctly and frequently self-monitor blood glucose.

Hyperglycemia is a major risk factor in the development of diabetic complications. Maintaining blood glucose levels helps prevent the progression of nephropathy, neuropathy, and retinopathy. Hyperglycemia is also associated with the risk factors of atherosclerosis.

Treatment Goals for Type 2 Diabetes Mellitus

Patient population	Average preprandial glucose (mg/dl)	HbA1c[a](%)
ADA general recommendations[b]	80-120	< 7
Healthy, relatively young	80-120	< 8
Elderly and patients with serious medical conditions	100-140	< 9

[a] Glycosylated hemoglobin.
[b] American Diabetes Association 1999 Clinical Practice Recommendations.

Drug Interactions

Sulfonylurea Drug Interactions

Precipitant drug	Object drug[a]		Description
Androgens Anticoagulants Azole antifungals Chloramphenicol Clofibrate Fenfluramine Fluconazole Gemfibrozil Histamine H_2 antagonists Magnesium salts Methyldopa MAO inhibitors Probenecid Salicylates Sulfinpyrazone Sulfonamides Tricyclic antidepressants Urinary acidifiers	Sulfonylureas	⬆	The hypoglycemic effect of sulfonylureas may be enhanced because of various mechanisms (eg, decreased hepatic metabolism, inhibition of renal excretion, displacement from protein-binding sites, decreased blood glucose, alteration of carbohydrate metabolism). Monitor blood glucose carefully upon initiation, cessation, or changes in therapy with any of these agents.
Beta blockers Calcium channel blockers Cholestyramine Corticosteroids Diazoxide Estrogens Hydantoins Isoniazid Nicotinic acid Oral contraceptives Phenothiazines Rifampin Sympathomimetics Thiazide diuretics Thyroid agents Urinary alkalinizers	Sulfonylureas	⬇	The hypoglycemic effect of sulfonylureas may be decreased because of various mechanisms (eg, increased hepatic metabolism, decreased insulin release, increased renal excretion).
Charcoal	Sulfonylureas	⬇	Charcoal can reduce the absorption of sulfonylureas; depending on the clinical situation, this will reduce their efficacy or toxicity.
Ciprofloxacin	Glyburide	⬆	A possible interaction between glyburide and ciprofloxacin has been reported, resulting in a potentiation of the hypoglycemic action.
Ethanol	Sulfonylureas	⬌	Ethanol may prolong but not augment glipizide-induced reductions in blood glucose. Chronic ethanol use may decrease the half-life of tolbutamide. Ethanol ingestion by patients taking chlorpropamide may result in a disulfiram-like reaction (see Precautions).
Chlorpropamide	Barbiturates	⬆	Animal studies suggest that the action of barbiturates may be prolonged by therapy with chlorpropamide; coadminister with caution.
Glyburide	Anticoagulants	⬆ ⬇	Possible interactions between glyburide and coumarin derivatives have been reported that may either potentiate or weaken the effects of coumarin derivatives.
Sulfonylureas	Digitalis glycosides	⬆	Concurrent administration may result in increased digitalis serum levels.

[a] ⬆ = Object drug increased. ⬇ = Object drug decreased. ⬌ = Undetermined clinical effect.

➤*Drug/Lab test interactions:* A metabolite of **tolbutamide** in the urine may give a false-positive reaction for albumin if measured by the acidification-after-boiling test, which causes the metabolite to precipitate. There is no interference with the sulfosalicylic acid test.

➤*Drug/Food interactions:* Absorption of **glipizide** is delayed by approximately 40 minutes when taken with food; the drug is more effective when given approximately 30 minutes before a meal. The other sulfonylureas may be taken with food.

Adverse Reactions

Hypoglycemia – See Precautions.

➤*CNS:* Drowsiness; asthenia; nervousness; tremor; pain; insomnia; anxiety; depression; hypesthesia; chills; hypertonia; confusion; somnolence; abnormal gait; decreased libido; migraine; anorexia; arthralgia; myalgia; fatigue; weakness; paresthesia; dizziness; vertigo; malaise; headache (infrequent).

➤*Dermatologic:* Allergic skin reactions; eczema; pruritus; erythema multiforme; urticaria; morbilliform or maculopapular eruptions; lichenoid reactions; rash; sweating; exfoliative dermatitis. These may be transient and may disappear despite continued use of the drug; if skin reactions persist, discontinue the drug. Porphyria cutanea tarda; photosensitivity reactions.

➤*Endocrine:* Reactions identical to the syndrome of inappropriate secretion of antidiuretic hormone (SIADH). (See Precautions.)

➤*GI:* GI disturbances (eg, nausea, epigastric fullness, heartburn) are the most common reactions. They tend to be dose-related and may disappear when dosage is reduced. Diarrhea; taste alteration (tolbutamide); GI pain; constipation; gastralgia; dyspepsia; vomiting; hunger; proctocolitis; flatulence; cholestatic jaundice (rare, discontinue the drug if this occurs).

➤*Hematologic:* Leukopenia; thrombocytopenia (which may present as purpura); aplastic anemia; agranulocytosis; hemolytic anemia; pancytopenia; hepatic porphyria; eosinophilia.

➤*Miscellaneous:* Disulfiram-like reactions (see Precautions); tinnitus; fatigue; rhinitis; hepatic porphyria; hyponatremia; blurred vision; polyuria; trace blood in stool; thirst; edema; arrhythmia; flushing; hypertension; pharyngitis; eye pain; conjunctivitis; retinal hemorrhage; dysuria; hepatitis; dyspnea; leg cramps; syncope; vasculitis.

➤*Lab test abnormalities:* Elevated liver function tests; occasional mild-to-moderate elevations in BUN, creatinine, AST, LDH, alkaline phosphatase.

Overdosage

➤*Symptoms:* Overdosage can produce hypoglycemia. In order of general appearance, the signs and symptoms associated with hypoglycemia include: Tingling of lips and tongue; nausea; vomiting; mild epigastric pain diminished cerebral function (lethargy, yawning, confusion, agitation, nervousness); increased sympathetic activity (tachycardia, sweating, tremor, hunger) and ultimately, convulsions, stupor, coma, and death.

➤*Treatment:* Treat mild hypoglycemia without loss of consciousness or neurologic findings aggressively with oral glucose and adjustments in drug dosage or meal patterns. Continue close monitoring until the patient is stabilized. Severe hypoglycemic reactions occur infrequently, but require immediate hospitalization. If hypoglycemic coma is suspected, rapidly inject concentrated (50%) dextrose IV. Follow by a continuous infusion of more dilute (10%) dextrose at a rate that will maintain the blood glucose at a level more than 100 mg/dl. Closely monitor for a minimum of 24 to 48 hours because hypoglycemia may recur after apparent clinical recovery. Because of the long half-life of **chlorpropamide**, patients who become hypoglycemic from this drug require close supervision for a minimum of 3 to 5 days.

In 1 patient with renal failure on hemodialysis, charcoal hemoperfusion shortened the half-life of chlorpropamide following an overdose. Charcoal administration also reduces the absorption of the sulfonylureas and may reduce their toxicity.

Patient Information

Patients must receive full and complete instructions about the nature of diabetes. Strict adherence to prescribed diet, an exercise program, personal hygiene, and avoidance of infection are essential. It is important to teach patients to self-monitor blood glucose.

Do not discontinue medication except on the advice of a physician.

May cause GI upset; may be taken with food. Take **glipizide** approximately 30 minutes before a meal to increase effectiveness.

Advise patients to avoid alcohol; lack of blood sugar control may occur. Flushing has been reported with **chlorpropamide**.

Monitor urine for glucose and ketones as prescribed; monitor blood glucose as prescribed.

➤*Notify physician:* Notify physician if any of the following occurs:

Hypoglycemia – Fatigue, excessive hunger, profuse sweating, numbness of extremities.

Hyperglycemia – Excessive thirst or urination, urinary glucose, or ketones.

Other – Fever, sore throat, rash, unusual bruising or bleeding.

CHLORPROPAMIDE

Rx	**Chlorpropamide** (Various, eg, Sidmak)	**Tablets:** 100 mg	In 100s, 500s, 1,000s, and UD 100s and 600s.
Rx	**Chlorpropamide** (Various, eg, Major, Goldline, Sidmak, UDL)	**Tablets:** 250 mg	In 100s, 250s, 500s, 1,000s, and UD 100s and UD 600s.

CHLORPROPAMIDE — ORAL

For complete prescribing information, refer to the Sulfonylureas group monograph.

Indications

➤*Type 2 diabetes:* As an adjunct to diet to lower the blood glucose in patients with type 2 diabetes mellitus whose hyperglycemia cannot be controlled by diet alone.

Administration and Dosage

➤*Adults:*

Type 2 diabetes –

Maximum dose: Maintenance doses above 750 mg daily should be avoided.

Initial dosage: The mild to moderately severe, middle-aged, stable patient with type 2 diabetes should be started on 250 mg orally daily. In debilitated or malnourished patients, the initial dosing should be conservative to avoid hypoglycemic reactions.

Dosage titration: Five to 7 days after the initial therapy, the blood level of chlorpropamide reaches a plateau. Dosage may subsequently be adjusted upward or downward by increments of not more than 50 to 125 mg at intervals of 3 to 5 days to obtain optimal control. More frequent adjustments are usually undesirable.

Maintenance dosage: Most moderately severe, middle-aged, stable patients with type 2 diabetes are controlled by approximately 250 mg daily. Many investigators have found that some milder patients with diabetes do well on daily doses of 100 mg or less. Many of the more severe patients with diabetes may require 500 mg daily for adequate control. Patients who do not respond completely to 500 mg daily will usually not respond to higher doses. Maintenance doses above 750 mg daily should be avoided.

Conversion:

• *Transfer from other oral hypoglycemics* – No transition period is necessary when transferring patients from other oral hypoglycemic agents to chlorpropamide. The other agent may be discontinued abruptly and chlorpropamide started at once. In prescribing chlorpropamide, consideration must be given to its greater potency.

• *Transfer from insulin* – Many mild to moderately severe, middle-aged, stable patients with type 2 diabetes receiving insulin can be placed directly on the oral drug and their insulin abruptly discontinued.

For patients requiring more than 40 units of insulin daily, therapy with chlorpropamide may be initiated with a 50% reduction in insulin for the first few days, with subsequent further reductions dependent upon the response.

Hypoglycemia: During the initial period of therapy with chlorpropamide, hypoglycemic reactions may occasionally occur, particularly during the transition from insulin to the oral drug. Hypoglycemia within 24 hours after withdrawal of the intermediate or long-acting types of insulin will usually prove to be the result of insulin carryover and not primarily due to the effect of chlorpropamide.

Monitoring: During the insulin withdrawal period, the patient should test his or her urine for sugar and ketone bodies at least 3 times daily and report the results frequently to his or her health care provider. If they are abnormal, the health care provider should be notified immediately. In some cases, it may be advisable to consider hospitalization during the transition period.

➤*Elderly:* Older patients should be started on smaller amounts of chlorpropamide, in the range of 100 to 125 mg daily. Maintenance dosing should be conservative to avoid hypoglycemic reactions.

➤*Renal function impairment:* In patients with impaired renal function, the initial and maintenance dosing should be conservative to avoid hypoglycemic reactions.

➤*Hepatic function impairment:* In patients with impaired hepatic function, the initial and maintenance dosing should be conservative to avoid hypoglycemic reactions.

➤*Administration:* The total daily dosage is generally taken at a single time each morning with breakfast.

Occasionally cases of GI intolerance may be relieved by dividing the daily dosage.

Short-term administration of chlorpropamide may be sufficient during periods of transient loss of control in patients usually controlled well on diet.

➤*Storage/Stability:* Store below 30°C (86°F).

TOLAZAMIDE

Rx	**Tolazamide** (Various, eg, Zenith Goldline)	**Tablets:** 100 mg	In 100s and 250s.
Rx	**Tolazamide** (Various, eg, Mylan, Zenith Goldline)	**Tablets:** 250 mg	In 100s, 200s, 500s, and 1,000s.
		500 mg	In 100s, 250s, and 500s.

TOLAZAMIDE — ORAL

For complete prescribing information, refer to the Sulfonylureas group monograph.

Indications

➤*Type 2 diabetes:* As an adjunct to diet to lower the blood glucose in patients with type 2 diabetes (non-insulin dependent diabetes mellitus) whose hyperglycemia cannot be satisfactorily controlled by diet alone.

In initiating treatment for type 2 diabetes, diet should be emphasized as the primary form of treatment. Caloric restriction and weight loss are essential in the obese diabetic patient. Proper dietary management alone may be effective in controlling the blood glucose and symptoms of hyperglycemia. The importance of regular physical activity should also be stressed and cardiovascular risk factors should be identified and corrective measures taken where possible.

If this treatment program fails to reduce symptoms and/or blood glucose, the use of an oral sulfonylurea or insulin should be considered. Use of tolazamide must be viewed by both the physician and patient as a treatment in addition to diet and not as a substitute for diet or as a convenient mechanism for avoiding dietary restraint. Furthermore, loss of blood glucose con-

TOLAZAMIDE — ORAL

trol on diet alone may be transient thus requiring only short-term administration of tolazamide.

During maintenance programs, tolazamide should be discontinued if satisfactory lowering of blood glucose is no longer achieved. Judgments should be based on regular clinical and laboratory evaluations.

In considering the use of tolazamide in asymptomatic patients, it should be recognized that controlling the blood glucose in type 2 diabetes has not been definitely established to be effective in preventing the long-term cardiovascular or neural complications of diabetes.

Administration and Dosage

➤*General dosing considerations:* Failure to follow an appropriate dosage regimen may precipitate hypoglycemia. Hypoglycemia is more likely to occur when caloric intake is deficient, after severe or prolonged exercise, when alcohol is ingested, or when more than one glucose-lowering drug is used.

Short-term administration may be sufficient during periods of transient loss of control in patients usually controlled well on diet.

➤*Adults:*

Type 2 diabetes –

Usual dosage: 100 to 1,000 mg/day.

Maximum dose: 1,000 mg/day.

Initial dosage: 100 to 250 mg daily with breakfast or the first main meal.

- *Fasting blood glucose less than 200 mg/dL* – 100 mg/day.
- *Fasting blood glucose more than 200 mg/dL* – 250 mg/day.
- *Malnourished or underweight patients, elderly patients, or patients not eating properly* – 100 mg/day.

Dosage titration: Adjust dose in increments of 100 to 250 mg at weekly intervals based on the patient's blood glucose response.

Maintenance dosage: 250 to 500 mg/day. Once-daily therapy is usually satisfactory. Doses of up to 500 mg/day should be given as a single dose in the morning. 500 mg once daily is as effective as 250 mg twice daily. When a dose of more than 500 mg/day is required, the dose may be divided and given twice daily.

➤*Elderly:* The initial and maintenance dosing should be conservative to avoid hypoglycemic reactions. Elderly patients are particularly susceptible to the hypoglycemic action of glucose-lowering drugs. Hypoglycemia may be difficult to recognize in elderly patients.

➤*Renal function impairment:* The initial and maintenance dosing should be conservative to avoid hypoglycemic reactions. Renal insufficiency may cause elevated blood levels of tolazamide.

➤*Hepatic function impairment:* The initial and maintenance dosing should be conservative to avoid hypoglycemic reactions. Hepatic insufficiency may cause elevated blood levels of tolazamide and may also diminish gluconeogenic capacity, both of which increase the risk of serious hypoglycemic reactions.

➤*Conversion:* Transfer of patients from other oral antidiabetes regimens to tolazamide should be done conservatively. When transferring patients from oral hypoglycemic agents other than chlorpropamide to tolazamide, no transition period or initial or priming dose is necessary.

Tolbutamide – If receiving less than 1 g/day, begin at tolazamide 100 mg/day. If receiving 1 g or more daily, initiate at tolazamide 250 mg/day as a single dose.

Chlorpropamide – Chlorpropamide 250 mg may be considered to provide approximately the same degree of blood glucose control as tolazamide 250 mg. The patient should be observed carefully for hypoglycemia during the transition period from chlorpropamide to tolazamide (1 to 2 weeks) because of the prolonged retention of chlorpropamide in the body and the possibility of a subsequent overlapping drug effect.

Acetohexamide – Tolazamide 100 mg may be considered to provide approximately the same degree of blood glucose control as acetohexamide 250 mg.

Insulin – Some type 2 diabetic patients who have been treated only with insulin may respond satisfactorily to therapy with tolazamide. The dosage of tolazamide should be adjusted weekly (or more often in the group previously requiring more than 40 units of insulin). During this conversion period when both insulin and tolazamide are being used, hypoglycemia may rarely occur. During insulin withdrawal, patients should test their urine for glucose and acetone at least 3 times daily and report results to their health care provider. The appearance of persistent acetonuria with glycosuria indicates that the patient is a patient with type 1 diabetes who requires insulin therapy.

Insulin dosage of less than 20 units: Initiate tolazamide at 100 mg/day.

Insulin dosage of 21 to 40 units: Initiate tolazamide at 250 mg/day.

Insulin dosage more than 40 units: The insulin dosage should be decreased by 50% and initiate tolazamide 250 mg/day.

➤*Special risk patients:* Debilitated or malnourished patients and those with adrenal or pituitary insufficiency are particularly susceptible to the hypoglycemic action of glucose-lowering drugs. The initial and maintenance dosing should be conservative to avoid hypoglycemic reactions. Hypoglycemia may be difficult to recognize in people who are taking beta-adrenergic–blocking drugs.

➤*Administration:* Administer with food once or twice a day.

➤*Storage/Stability:* Store at 20° to 25°C (68° to 77°F).

TOLBUTAMIDE

Rx	**Tolbutamide** (Various, eg, Zenith Goldline, Mylan)	**Tablets:** 500 mg	In 100s and 500s.

TOLBUTAMIDE — ORAL

For complete prescribing information, refer to the Sulfonylureas group monograph.

Indications

➤*Type 2 diabetes:* As an adjunct to diet to lower the blood glucose in patients with type 2 diabetes whose hyperglycemia cannot be satisfactorily controlled by diet alone. In initiating treatment for type 2 diabetes, diet should be emphasized as the primary form of treatment. Caloric restriction and weight loss are essential in the obese diabetic patient. Proper dietary management alone may be effective in controlling the blood glucose and symptoms of hyperglycemia. The importance of regular physical activity should also be stressed, and cardiovascular risk factors should be identified and corrective measures taken where possible.

Administration and Dosage

➤*General dosing considerations:* Failure to follow an appropriate dosage regimen may precipitate hypoglycemia. Hypoglycemia is more likely to occur when caloric intake is deficient, after severe or prolonged exercise, when alcohol is ingested, or when more than 1 glucose-lowering drug is used.

Short-term administration of tolbutamide may be sufficient during periods of transient loss of control in patients usually controlled well on diet.

➤*Adults:*

Type 2 diabetes –

Maximum dose: 3 g/day.

Initial dosage: 1 to 2 g daily.

Maintenance dosage: 0.25 to 3 g daily either in the morning or in divided doses. The divided dose system is preferred by some clinicians from the standpoint of digestive tolerance. Maintenance doses above 2 g are seldom required.

Dosage adjustment: This may be increased or decreased depending on individual patient response.

➤*Elderly:* Elderly patients are particularly susceptible to the hypoglycemic action of glucose-lowering drugs. The initial and maintenance dosing should be conservative to avoid hypoglycemic reactions. Hypoglycemia may be difficult to recognize in elderly patients.

➤*Renal function impairment:* Renal insufficiency may cause elevated blood levels of tolbutamide and increase the risk of serious hypoglycemic reactions. The initial and maintenance dosing should be conservative to avoid hypoglycemic reactions.

➤*Hepatic function impairment:* Hepatic insufficiency may cause elevated blood levels of tolbutamide and may also diminish gluconeogenic capacity, both of which increase the risk of serious hypoglycemic reactions. The initial and maintenance dosing should be conservative to avoid hypoglycemic reactions.

➤*Conversion:* Transfer of patients from other oral antidiabetes regimens to tolbutamide should be done conservatively. When transferring patients from oral hypoglycemic agents other than chlorpropamide to tolbutamide, no transition period and no initial or priming doses are necessary.

Chlorpropamide – Particular care should be exercised during the first 2 weeks because of the prolonged retention of chlorpropamide in the body and the possibility that subsequent overlapping drug effects might provoke hypoglycemia.

Insulin – During this conversion period when both insulin and tolbutamide are being used, hypoglycemia may rarely occur. During insulin withdrawal, patients should test their urine for glucose and acetone at least 3 times daily and report results to their health care provider. The appearance of persistent acetonuria with glycosuria indicates that the patient is a patient with type 1 diabetes who requires insulin therapy.

Insulin dosage of less than 20 units: Initiate tolbutamide and discontinue insulin abruptly.

Insulin dosage between 20 and 40 units: Initiate tolbutamide with a concurrent 30% to 50% reduction in insulin dose, with further daily reduction of the insulin when response to tolbutamide is observed.

Insulin dosage more than 40 units: Initiate tolbutamide in conjunction with a 20% reduction in insulin dose the first day, with further careful reduction of insulin as response is observed. Occasionally, conversion to tolbutamide in the hospital may be advisable in candidates who require more than 40 units of insulin daily.

➤*Special risk patients:* In debilitated or malnourished patients and those with adrenal or pituitary insufficiency, the initial and maintenance dosing should be conservative to avoid hypoglycemic reactions. Hypoglycemia may be difficult to recognize in people who are taking beta-adrenergic–blocking drugs.

➤*Administration:* Administer with food either in the morning or in divided doses through the day.

➤*Storage/Stability:* Store at 15° to 30°C (59° to 86°F).

GLIPIZIDE

Rx	**Glipizide** (Various, eg, Endo, Mylan, UDL, Watson, Zenith Goldline)	**Tablets:** 5 mg	In 100s, 500s, 1,000s, and UD 100s.
Rx	**Glucotrol** (Pfizer)		Lactose. (Pfizer 411). Dye free. White, scored. Diamond shape. In 100s, 500s, and UD 100s.
Rx	**Glipizide** (Various, eg, Endo, Mylan, UDL, Watson, Zenith Goldline)	**Tablets:** 10 mg	In 100s, 500s, 1,000s, and UD 100s.
Rx	**Glucotrol** (Pfizer)		Lactose. (Pfizer 412). Dye free. White, diamond shape, scored. In 100s, 500s, and UD 100s.
Rx	**Glipizide Extended-Release** (Andrx Pharmaceuticals)	**Tablets, extended release:** 2.5 mg	(871). Blue. In 30s.
Rx	**Glucotrol XL** (Pfizer)		(Glucotrol XL 2.5). Blue. In 30s.
Rx	**Glipizide Extended-Release** (Various, eg, Andrx Pharmaceuticals, Watson)	**Tablets, extended release:** 5 mg	In 100s and 500s.
Rx	**Glucotrol XL** (Pfizer)		(Glucotrol XL 5). White. In 100s and 500s.
Rx	**Glipizide Extended-Release** (Various, eg, Andrx Pharmaceuticals, Watson)	**Tablets, extended release:** 10 mg	In 100s and 500s.
Rx	**Glucotrol XL** (Pfizer)		(GLUCOTROL XL 10). White. In 100s and 500s.

GLIPIZIDE — ORAL

For complete prescribing information, refer to the Sulfonylureas group monograph.

Indications

➤*Type 2 diabetes:* As an adjunct to diet for the control of hyperglycemia and its associated symptomatology in patients with type 2 diabetes formerly known as non-insulin-dependent diabetes mellitus (NIDDM) or maturity-onset diabetes, after an adequate trial of dietary therapy has proved unsatisfactory. Glipizide is indicated when diet alone has been unsuccessful in correcting hyperglycemia, but even after the introduction of the drug in the patient's regimen, dietary measures should continue to be considered as important. In 12-week, well-controlled studies, there was a maximal average net reduction in hemoglobin A_{1c} (HbA_{1c}) of 1.7% in absolute units between placebo-treated and glipizide-treated patients.

Administration and Dosage

➤*General dosing considerations:* Short-term administration of glipizide tablets may be sufficient during periods of transient loss of control in patients usually controlled on diet.

All sulfonylurea drugs are capable of producing severe hypoglycemia. Proper patient selection, dosage, and instructions are important to avoid hypoglycemic episodes. Therapy with a combination of glucose-lowering agents may increase the potential for hypoglycemia.

➤*Adults:*

Type 2 diabetes –

Extended-release:

• *Maximum dose* – 20 mg/day.

• *Initial dosage* – 5 mg/day, given with breakfast.

• *Dosage titration* – Dosage adjustment should be based on laboratory measures of glycemic control. While fasting blood glucose levels generally reach steady state following initiation of or change in glipizide dosage, a single fasting glucose determination may not accurately reflect the response to therapy. In most cases, HbA_{1c} level, measured at 3-month intervals, is the preferred means of monitoring response to therapy.

HbA_{1c} should be measured as glipizide therapy is initiated and repeated approximately 3 months later. If the result of this test suggests that glycemic control over the preceding 3 months was inadequate, the dose may be increased. Subsequent dosage adjustments should be made on the basis of HbA_{1c} levels measured at 3-month intervals. If no improvement is seen after 3 months of therapy with a higher dose, the previous dose should be resumed. Decisions which utilize fasting blood glucose to adjust glipizide therapy should be based on at least 2 or more similar, consecutive values obtained 7 days or more after the previous dose adjustment.

• *Maintenance dosage* – 5 to 10 mg once daily. Some patients may require up to 20 mg/day.

• *Conversion* – Patients receiving immediate-release glipizide may be switched safely to glipizide extended-release tablets once-a-day at the nearest equivalent total daily dose. Patients may also be titrated to the appropriate dose of glipizide extended-release starting with 5 mg once daily. The decision to switch to the nearest equivalent dose or to titrate should be based on clinical judgment.

Immediate-release:

• *Maximum dose* – 15 mg (single dose); 40 mg (total daily dose).

• *Initial dosage* – 5 mg, given before breakfast.

• *Dosage titration* – Dosage adjustments should ordinarily be in increments of 2.5 to 5 mg, as determined by blood glucose response. At least several days should elapse between titration steps. If response to a single dose is not satisfactory, dividing that dose may prove effective. Doses above 15 mg should ordinarily be divided and given before meals of adequate caloric content.

• *Maintenance dosage* – Some patients may be effectively controlled on a once-a-day regimen, while others show better response with divided dosing.

➤*Elderly:* The initial dosage should be 2.5 mg/day (immediate-release) or 5 mg/day (extended-release).

➤*Renal function impairment:* Renal insufficiency may affect the disposition of glipizide which increases the risk of serious hypoglycemic reactions. The initial and maintenance dosing should be conservative to avoid hypoglycemic reactions.

➤*Hepatic function impairment:* Hepatic insufficiency may affect the disposition of glipizide and may also diminish gluconeogenic capacity, both of which increase the risk of serious hypoglycemic reactions. The initial and maintenance dosing should be conservative to avoid hypoglycemic reactions.

The initial dosage should be 2.5 mg/day (immediate-release).

➤*Debilitated or malnourished patients or patients with adrenal or pituitary insufficiency:* Debilitated or malnourished patients are particularly susceptible to the hypoglycemic action of glucose-lowering drugs; the initial and maintenance dosing should be conservative to avoid hypoglycemic reactions.

➤*Concomitant oral hypoglycemic therapy:* When glipizide is used in combination with other oral blood glucose-lowering agents, the second agent should be added at the lowest recommended dose, and patients should be observed carefully. Titration of the added oral agent should be based on clinical judgment.

When adding glipizide extended-release tablets to other blood glucose-lowering agents, glipizide can be initiated at 5 mg. Those patients who may be more sensitive to hypoglycemic drugs may be started at a lower dose. Titration should be based on clinical judgment.

➤*Conversion from other sulfonylureas:* As with other sulfonylurea-class hypoglycemics, no transition period is necessary when transferring patients to glipizide extended- or immediate-release tablets. Patients should be observed carefully (1 to 2 weeks) for hypoglycemia when being transferred from longer half-life sulfonylureas (eg, chlorpropamide) to glipizide due to potential overlapping of drug effect.

➤*Conversion to or from insulin therapy:* As with other sulfonylurea-class hypoglycemics, many patients with stable type 2 diabetes receiving insulin may be transferred safely to treatment with glipizide. When transferring patients from insulin to glipizide, the following general guidelines should be considered:

- For patients whose daily insulin requirement is less than or equal to 20 units, insulin may be discontinued and glipizide therapy may begin at usual dosages. Several days should elapse between titration steps.
- For patients whose daily insulin requirement is greater than 20 units, the insulin dose should be reduced by 50%, and glipizide therapy may begin at usual dosages. Subsequent reductions in insulin dosage should depend on individual patient response. Several days should elapse between titration steps.
- During the insulin withdrawal period, the patient should test urine samples for sugar and ketone bodies at least 3 times daily. Patients should be instructed to contact the prescriber immediately if these tests are abnormal. In some cases, especially when the patient has been receiving greater than 40 units of insulin daily, it may be advisable to consider hospitalization during the transition period.

GLIPIZIDE — ORAL

➤*Administration:*

Extended-release – Give with breakfast.

Immediate-release – Give approximately 30 minutes before a meal to achieve the greatest reduction in postprandial hyperglycemia.

➤*Storage/Stability:*

Extended-release – Protect from moisture and humidity and store at controlled room temperature, 15° to 30°C (59° to 86°F).

Immediate-release – Store below 30°C (86°F).

GLIMEPIRIDE

Rx	**Glimepiride** (Various, eg, Dr. Reddy's, Par, Perrigo, Teva)	**Tablets; oral:** 1 mg	May contain lactose. In 30s, 100s, 500s, and 1,000s.
Rx	**Amaryl** (Sanofi-Aventis)		Lactose. (AMA RYL). Pink, scored. Oblong. In 100s.
Rx	**Glimepiride** (Various, eg, Dr. Reddy's, Par, Perrigo, Teva)	**Tablets; oral:** 2 mg	May contain lactose. In 30s, 100s, 500s, 1,000s, and UD 100s.
Rx	**Amaryl** (Sanofi-Aventis)		Lactose. (AMA RYL). Green, scored. Oblong. In 100s and UD 100s.
Rx	**Glimepiride** (Various, eg, Dr. Reddy's, Par, Perrigo, Teva)	**Tablets; oral:** 4 mg	May contain lactose. In 30s, 100s, 250s, 500s, 1,000s, and UD 100s.
Rx	**Amaryl** (Sanofi-Aventis)		Lactose. (AMA RYL). Blue, scored. Oblong. In 100s and UD 100s.

GLIMEPIRIDE — ORAL

For complete prescribing information, refer to the Sulfonylureas group monograph.

Indications

➤*Type 2 diabetes mellitus:* As an adjunct to diet and exercise to lower the blood glucose in patients with type 2 diabetes mellitus (formerly known as non-insulin–dependent diabetes mellitus) whose hyperglycemia cannot be controlled by diet and exercise alone.

Administration and Dosage

➤*General dosing considerations:* Failure to follow an appropriate dosage regimen may precipitate hypoglycemia.

Short-term administration of glimepiride may be sufficient during periods of transient loss of control in patients usually controlled well on diet and exercise.

➤*Adults:*

Type 2 diabetes mellitus –

Maximum dose: 8 mg once daily.

Initial dosage: 1 to 2 mg once daily, administered with breakfast or the first main meal. The maximum starting dose should be no more than 2 mg.

Dosage titration: After reaching a dose of 2 mg, dosage increases should be made in increments of no more than 2 mg at 1- to 2-week intervals based on the patient's blood glucose response.

Maintenance dosage: 1 to 4 mg once daily.

Concomitant therapy:

• *With metformin* – If patients do not respond adequately to the maximal dose of glimepiride monotherapy, the addition of metformin may be considered. The desired control of blood glucose may be obtained by adjusting the dose of each drug. However, attempts should be made to identify the minimum effective dose of each drug to achieve this goal. With concomitant therapy, the risk of hypoglycemia associated with glimepiride therapy continues and may be increased. Appropriate precautions should be taken.

• *With insulin* – Combination therapy with glimepiride and insulin may also be used in secondary failure patients. The fasting glucose level for instituting combination therapy is in the range of more than 150 mg/dL in plasma or serum, depending on the patient. The recommended glimepiride dosage is 8 mg once daily administered with the first main meal. After starting with low-dose insulin, upward adjustments of insulin can be done approximately weekly as guided by frequent measurements of fasting blood glucose.

➤*Elderly:* The initial dosing, dose increments, and maintenance dosage should be conservative to avoid hypoglycemic reactions. Patients should be started at 1 mg once daily and titrated carefully.

➤*Renal function impairment:* The initial dosing, dose increments, and maintenance dosage should be conservative to avoid hypoglycemic reactions. Patients should be started at 1 mg once daily and titrated carefully.

➤*Hepatic function impairment:* The initial dosing, dose increments, and maintenance dosage should be conservative to avoid hypoglycemic reactions. Patients should be started at 1 mg once daily and titrated carefully.

➤*Debilitated or malnourished patients, or patients with adrenal or pituitary insufficiency:* The initial dosing, dose increments, and maintenance dosage should be conservative to avoid hypoglycemic reactions. Patients should be started at 1 mg once daily and titrated carefully.

➤*Conversion from other oral hypoglycemic agents:* As with other sulfonylurea hypoglycemic agents, no transition period is necessary when transferring patients to glimepiride. Patients should be observed carefully (1 to 2 weeks) for hypoglycemia when being transferred from longer half-life sulfonylureas (eg, chlorpropamide) to glimepiride because of the potential overlapping of drug effect.

➤*Storage/Stability:* Store between 15° and 30°C (59° and 86°F). Dispense in well-closed containers with safety closures.

GLYBURIDE (Glibenclamide)

Rx	**Glyburide** (Various, eg, Copley, Geneva, Greenstone, Novopharm)	**Tablets; oral:** 1.25 mg	In 50s, 100s, and 500s.
Rx	**DiaBeta** (sanofi-aventis)		(Diaβ). Peach, capsule-shaped, scored. In 50s.
Rx	**Glyburide** (Various, eg, Copley, Mova, Novopharm)	**Tablets, micronized; oral:** 1.5 mg	In 100s, 500s, 1,000s, and UD 100s.
Rx	**Glynase PresTab** (Pharmacia & Upjohn)		Lactose. (GLYNASE 1.5/PT PT). White, scored. Oval. In 100s and UD 100s.
Rx	**Glyburide** (Various, eg, Copley, Geneva, Greenstone, Novopharm, UDL)	**Tablets; oral:** 2.5 mg	In 90s, 100s, 500s, 1,000s, UD 100s, and blister pack 25s, 100s, and 600s.
Rx	**DiaBeta** (sanofi-aventis)		(Diaβ). Pink, capsule-shaped, scored. In 100s and 500s.
Rx	**Glyburide** (Various, eg, Copley, Mova, Novopharm)	**Tablets, micronized; oral:** 3 mg	In 100s, 500s, 1,000s, and UD 100s.
Rx	**Glynase PresTab** (Pharmacia & Upjohn)		Lactose. (GLYNASE 3/PT PT). Blue, scored. Oval. In 100s, 500s, 1,000s, and UD 100s.
Rx	**Glyburide** (Various, eg, Mova)	**Tablets, micronized; oral:** 4.5 mg	In 100s, 500s, and 1,000s.
Rx	**Glyburide** (Various, eg, Copley, Geneva, Greenstone, Novopharm, UDL)	**Tablets; oral:** 5 mg	In 90s, 100s, 500s, 1,000s, UD 100s, and blister pack 25s, 100s, and 600s.
Rx	**DiaBeta** (sanofi-aventis)		(Diaβ). Green, capsule-shaped, scored. In 100s, 500s, and 1,000s.
Rx	**Glyburide** (Various, eg, Mova, Novopharm)	**Tablets, micronized; oral:** 6 mg	In 100s, 500s, and 1,000s.
Rx	**Glynase PresTab** (Pharmacia & Upjohn)		Lactose. (GLYNASE 6/PT PT) . Yellow, scored. Oval. In 100s and 500s.

GLYBURIDE — ORAL

For complete prescribing information, refer to the Sulfonylureas class monograph.

Indications

➤*Type 2 diabetes:* Indicated as an adjunct to diet and exercise to improve glycemic control in adults with type 2 diabetes mellitus.

Administration and Dosage

➤*General dosing considerations:* Short-term administration of glyburide may be sufficient during periods of transient loss of control in patients usually controlled well on diet.

➤*Adults:*

Type 2 diabetes –

Micronized tablets:

- *Maximum dose* – 12 mg/day.
- *Initial dosage* – 1.5 to 3 mg daily administered with breakfast or the first main meal. Those patients who may be more sensitive to hypoglycemic drugs should be started at 0.75 mg daily.
- *Dosage titration* – Dosage increases should be made in increments of no more than 1.5 mg at weekly intervals based upon the patient's blood glucose response.
- *Maintenance dosage* – 0.75 to 12 mg daily given as a single dose or in divided doses. Once-daily therapy is usually satisfactory. Some patients, particularly those receiving more than 6 mg daily, may have a more satisfactory response with twice-daily dosing.

Non-micronized tablets:

- *Maximum dose* – 20 mg/day.
- *Initial dosage* – 2.5 to 5 mg daily administered with breakfast or the first main meal. Those patients who may be more sensitive to hypoglycemic drugs should be started at 1.25 mg daily.
- *Dosage titration* – Dosage increases should be made in increments of no more than 2.5 mg at weekly intervals based upon the patient's blood glucose response.
- *Maintenance dosage* – 1.25 to 20 mg daily given as a single dose or in divided doses. Once-daily therapy is usually satisfactory, based upon usual meal patterns and a 10-hour half-life of glyburide. Some patients, particularly those receiving more than 10 mg daily, may have a more satisfactory response with twice-daily dosing.

➤*Elderly:* The initial and maintenance dosing should be conservative to avoid hypoglycemic reactions. The initial dosage should be 1.25 mg/day (non-micronized tablets) or 0.75 mg/day (micronized tablets).

➤*Renal function impairment:* The initial and maintenance dosing should be conservative to avoid hypoglycemic reactions. The initial dosage should be 1.25 mg/day (non-micronized tablets) or 0.75 mg/day (micronized tablets).

➤*Hepatic function impairment:* The initial and maintenance dosing should be conservative to avoid hypoglycemic reactions. The initial dosage should be 1.25 mg/day (non-micronized tablets) or 0.75 mg/day (micronized tablets).

➤*Debilitated or malnourished patients or patients with adrenal or pituitary insufficiency:* The initial and maintenance dosing should be conservative to avoid hypoglycemic reactions. The initial dosage should be 1.25 mg/day (non-micronized tablets) or 0.75 mg/day (micronized tablets).

➤*Concomitant glyburide and metformin therapy:* Glyburide should be added gradually to the dosing regimen of patients who have not responded to the maximum dose of metformin monotherapy after 4 weeks. With concomitant therapy, the desired control of blood glucose may be obtained by adjusting the dose of each drug. However, attempts should be made to identify the optimal dose of each drug needed to achieve this goal. The risk of hypoglycemia associated with sulfonylurea therapy continues and may be increased. Appropriate precautions should be taken.

➤*Conversion from other sulfonylureas:* Patients should be retitrated when transferred from non-micronized tablets or other oral hypoglycemic agents to micronized tablets. Transfer of patients from other oral antidiabetic regimens to glyburide should be done conservatively, and the initial daily dose should be 2.5 to 5 mg of non-micronized tablets or 1.5 to 3 mg of micronized tablets. Although patients may be transferred from the maximum dose of other sulfonylureas, the maximum starting dose should be 5 mg of non-micronized tablets or 3 mg of micronized tablets.

A maintenance dose of 5 mg of non-micronized tablets or 3 mg of micronized tablets provides approximately the same degree of blood glucose control as chlorpropamide 250 to 375 mg, tolazamide 250 to 375 mg, acetohexamide 500 to 750 mg, or tolbutamide 1,000 to 1,500 mg.

When transferring patients from oral hypoglycemic agents other than chlorpropamide to glyburide, no transition period and no initial or priming dose are necessary. When transferring patients from chlorpropamide, particular care should be exercised during the first 2 weeks because the prolonged retention of chlorpropamide in the body and subsequent overlapping drug effects may provoke hypoglycemia.

➤*Conversion from insulin:* If the insulin dosage is less than 20 units daily, substitution of 2.5 to 5 mg of non-micronized tablets or 1.5 to 3 mg of micronized tablets as a single daily dose may be tried. If the insulin dosage is between 20 and 40 units daily, the patient may be placed directly on 5 mg non-micronized tablets or 3 mg micronized tablets as a single daily dose. If the insulin dosage is more than 40 units daily, a transition period is required for conversion to glyburide. These patients may be started on a daily dose of 5 mg non-micronized tablets or 3 mg micronized tablets concomitantly with a 50% reduction in insulin dosage. Progressive withdrawal of insulin and increase of glyburide in increments of 1.25 to 2.5 mg every 2 to 10 days for non-micronized tablets or 0.75 to 1.5 mg every 2 to 10 days for micronized tablets is then carried out. During this conversion period when both insulin and glyburide are being used, hypoglycemia may rarely occur.

➤*Administration:* Administer with breakfast or the first main meal.

➤*Storage/Stability:* Store at 25°C (77°F). Excursions are permitted between 15° and 30°C (59° and 86°F).

Alpha-Glucosidase Inhibitors

ACARBOSE

Rx	**Acarbose** (Various, eg, Cobalt, Roxane)	**Tablets, oral:** 25 mg	In 100s and UD 100s.
Rx	**Precose** (Bayer Pharmaceuticals)		(PRECOSE 25). White to yellow. In 100s.
Rx	**Acarbose** (Various, eg, Cobalt, Roxane)	**Tablets, oral:** 50 mg	In 100s and UD 100s.
Rx	**Precose** (Bayer Pharmaceuticals)		(PRECOSE 50). White to yellow. In 100s and UD 100s.
Rx	**Acarbose** (Various, eg, Cobalt, Roxane)	**Tablets, oral:** 100 mg	In 100s.
Rx	**Precose** (Bayer Pharmaceuticals)		(PRECOSE 100). White to yellow. In 100s and UD 100s.

ACARBOSE — ORAL

Indications

➤*Type 2 diabetes:* Monotherapy as an adjunct to diet to lower blood glucose in patients with type 2 diabetes mellitus whose hyperglycemia cannot be managed on diet alone. Acarbose may also be used in combination with a sulfonylurea when diet plus either acarbose or a sulfonylurea do not result in adequate glycemic control. Also, acarbose may be used in combination with insulin or metformin. The effect of acarbose to enhance glycemic control is additive to that of sulfonylureas, insulin, or metformin when used in combination, presumably because its mechanism of action is different.

Administration and Dosage

➤*General dosing considerations:* There is no fixed dosage regimen for the management of diabetes mellitus with acarbose or any other pharmacologic agent. Dosage of acarbose must be individualized on the basis of both effectiveness and tolerance while not exceeding the maximum recommended dose.

Acarbose should be started at a low dose, with gradual dose escalation as described in the following, both to reduce GI adverse effects and to permit identification of the minimum dose required for adequate glycemic control of the patient.

During treatment initiation and dose titration, 1-hour postprandial plasma glucose may be used to determine the therapeutic response to acarbose and identify the minimum effective dose for the patient. Thereafter, glycosylated hemoglobin should be measured at intervals of approximately 3 months. The therapeutic goal should be to decrease both postprandial plasma glucose and glycosylated hemoglobin levels to normal or near normal by using the lowest effective dose of acarbose, either as monotherapy or in combination with sulfonylureas, insulin, or metformin.

➤*Adults:*

Type 2 diabetes mellitus –

Maximum dose:

- *60 kg or less* – 50 mg 3 times daily.
- *More than 60 kg* – 100 mg 3 times daily.

Initial dosage: 25 mg given orally 3 times daily at the start (with the first bite) of each main meal. However, some patients may benefit from more gradual dose titration to minimize GI adverse effects. This may be achieved by initiating treatment at 25 mg once per day and subsequently increasing the frequency of administration to achieve 25 mg 3 times daily.

Dosage titration: Once a 25 mg 3 times daily dosage regimen is reached, dosage of acarbose should be adjusted at 4- to 8-week intervals based on 1-hour postprandial glucose or glycosylated hemoglobin levels, and on tolerance. The dosage can be increased from 25 mg 3 times daily to 50 mg 3 times

ACARBOSE — ORAL

daily. Some patients may benefit from further increasing the dosage to 100 mg 3 times daily. The maintenance dose ranges from 50 mg 3 times daily to 100 mg 3 times daily. However, because patients with low body weight may be at increased risk for elevated serum transaminases, only patients with body weight greater than 60 kg should be considered for dose titration higher than 50 mg 3 times daily. If no further reduction in postprandial glucose or glycosylated hemoglobin levels is observed with titration to 100 mg 3 times daily, consideration should be given to lowering the dose. Once an effective and tolerated dosage is established, it should be maintained.

Concomitant therapy: Sulfonylurea agents or insulin may cause hypoglycemia. Acarbose, given in combination with a sulfonylurea or insulin, will cause a further lowering of blood glucose and may increase the potential for hypoglycemia. If hypoglycemia occurs, appropriate adjustments in the dosage of these agents should be made.

➤*Administration:* Acarbose should be taken 3 times daily at the start (with the first bite) of each main meal.

➤*Storage/Stability:* Do not store above 25°C (77°F). Protect from moisture. For bottles, keep container tightly closed.

Actions

➤*Pharmacology:* Acarbose is a complex oligosaccharide that delays the digestion of ingested carbohydrates, thereby resulting in a smaller rise in blood glucose concentration following meals. As a consequence of plasma glucose reduction, acarbose reduces levels of glycosylated hemoglobin in patients with type 2 diabetes mellitus. Systemic nonenzymatic protein glycosylation, as reflected by levels of glycosylated hemoglobin, is a function of average blood glucose concentration over time.

In contrast to sulfonylureas, acarbose does not enhance insulin secretion. The antihyperglycemic action of acarbose results from a competitive, reversible inhibition of pancreatic alpha-amylase and membrane-bound intestinal alpha-glucoside hydrolase enzymes. Pancreatic alpha-amylase hydrolyzes complex starches to oligosaccharides in the lumen of the small intestine, while the membrane-bound intestinal alpha-glucosidases hydrolyze oligosaccharides, trisaccharides, and disaccharides to glucose and other monosaccharides in the brush border of the small intestine. In diabetic patients, this enzyme inhibition results in a delayed glucose absorption and a lowering of postprandial hyperglycemia.

Because its mechanism of action is different, the effect of acarbose to enhance glycemic control is additive to that of sulfonylureas, insulin or metformin when used in combination. In addition, acarbose diminishes the insulinotropic and weight-increasing effects of sulfonylureas.

Acarbose has no inhibitory activity against lactase and consequently would not be expected to induce lactose intolerance.

➤*Pharmacokinetics:*

Absorption – In a study of 6 healthy men, less than 2% of an oral dose of acarbose was absorbed as active drug, while approximately 35% of total radioactivity from a ^{14}C-labeled oral dose was absorbed. An average of 51% of an oral dose was excreted in the feces as unabsorbed drug-related radioactivity within 96 hours of ingestion. Because acarbose acts locally within the gastrointestinal tract, this low systemic bioavailability of parent compound is therapeutically desired. Following oral dosing of healthy volunteers with ^{14}C-labeled acarbose, peak plasma concentrations of radioactivity were attained 14 to 24 hours after dosing, while peak plasma concentrations of active drug were attained at approximately 1 hour. The delayed absorption of acarbose-related radioactivity reflects the absorption of metabolites that may be formed by either intestinal bacteria or intestinal enzymatic hydrolysis.

Metabolism – Acarbose is metabolized exclusively within the GI tract, principally by intestinal bacteria, but also by digestive enzymes. A fraction of these metabolites (approximately 34% of the dose) was absorbed and subsequently excreted in the urine. At least 13 metabolites have been separated chromatographically from urine specimens. The major metabolites have been identified as 4-methylpyrogallol derivatives (ie, sulfate, methyl, glucuronide conjugates). One metabolite (formed by cleavage of a glucose molecule from acarbose) also has alpha-glucosidase inhibitory activity. This metabolite, together with the parent compound, recovered from the urine, accounts for less than 2% of the total administered dose.

Excretion – The fraction of acarbose that is absorbed as intact drug is almost completely excreted by the kidneys. When acarbose was given intravenously, 89% of the dose was recovered in the urine as active drug within 48 hours. In contrast, less than 2% of an oral dose was recovered in the urine as active (ie, parent compound and active metabolite) drug. This is consistent with the low bioavailability of the parent drug. The plasma elimination half-life of acarbose activity is approximately 2 hours in healthy volunteers. Consequently, drug accumulation does not occur with 3 times a day oral dosing.

Contraindications

Hypersensitivity to the drug; diabetic ketoacidosis or cirrhosis; inflammatory bowel disease; colonic ulceration; partial intestinal obstruction; patients predisposed to intestinal obstruction. In addition, acarbose is contraindicated in patients who have chronic intestinal diseases associated with marked disorders of digestion or absorption and in patients who have conditions that may deteriorate as a result of increased gas formation in the intestine.

Warnings/Precautions

➤*Calcium/vitamin B_6:* Low serum calcium and low plasma vitamin B_6 levels were associated with acarbose therapy but were thought to be either spurious or of no clinical significance.

➤*Hematocrit:* Small reductions in hematocrit occurred more often in acarbose-treated patients than in placebo-treated patients but were not associated with reductions in hemoglobin.

➤*Hypoglycemia:* Because of its mechanism of action, acarbose when administered alone should not cause hypoglycemia in the fasted or postprandial state. Sulfonylurea agents or insulin may cause hypoglycemia. Because acarbose given in combination with a sulfonylurea or insulin will cause a further lowering of blood glucose, it may increase the potential for hypoglycemia. Hypoglycemia does not occur in patients receiving metformin alone under usual circumstances of use, and no increased incidence of hypoglycemia was observed in patients when acarbose was added to metformin therapy. Oral glucose (dextrose), whose absorption is not inhibited by acarbose, should be used instead of sucrose (cane sugar) in the treatment of mild to moderate hypoglycemia. Sucrose, whose hydrolysis to glucose and fructose is inhibited by acarbose, is unsuitable for the rapid correction of hypoglycemia. Severe hypoglycemia may require the use of either intravenous glucose infusion or glucagon injection.

➤*Loss of control of blood glucose:* When diabetic patients are exposed to stress such as fever, trauma, infection, or surgery, a temporary loss of control of blood glucose may occur. At such times, temporary insulin therapy may be necessary.

➤*Renal function impairment:* Plasma concentrations of acarbose in renally impaired volunteers were proportionally increased relative to the degree of renal dysfunction. Long-term clinical trials in diabetic patients with significant renal dysfunction (serum creatinine greater than 2 mg/dL) have not been conducted. Therefore, treatment of these patients with acarbose is not recommended.

➤*Pregnancy:* Category B.

Teratogenic – The safety of acarbose in pregnant women has not been established. In rabbits, reduced maternal body weight gain, probably the result of the pharmacodynamic activity of high doses of acarbose in the intestines, may have been responsible for a slight increase in the number of embryonic losses. However, rabbits given 160 mg/kg acarbose (corresponding to 10 times the dose in man, based on body surface area) showed no evidence of embryotoxicity and there was no evidence of teratogenicity at a dose 32 times the dose in man (based on body surface area). There are, however, no adequate and well-controlled studies of acarbose in pregnant women. Because animal reproduction studies are not always predictive of the human response, this drug should be used during pregnancy only if clearly needed. Because current information strongly suggests that abnormal blood glucose levels during pregnancy are associated with a higher incidence of congenital anomalies as well as increased neonatal morbidity and mortality, most experts recommend that insulin be used during pregnancy to maintain blood glucose levels as close to normal as possible.

➤*Lactation:* A small amount of radioactivity has been found in the milk of lactating rats after administration of radiolabeled acarbose. It is not known whether this drug is excreted in human milk. Because many drugs are excreted in human milk, acarbose should not be administered to a nursing woman.

➤*Children:* Safety and efficacy of acarbose in pediatric patients have not been established.

➤*Elderly:* Of the total number of subjects in clinical studies of acarbose in the United States, 27% were greater than or equal to 65 years of age, while 4% were greater than or equal to 75 years of age. No overall differences in safety and effectiveness were observed between these subjects and younger subjects. The mean steady-state area under the curve (AUC) and maximum concentrations of acarbose were approximately 1.5 times higher in elderly compared to young volunteers; however, these differences were not statistically significant.

➤*Lab test abnormalities:* In long-term studies (up to 12 months, and including acarbose doses up to 300 mg 3 times daily) conducted in the United States, treatment-emergent elevations of serum transaminases (AST and/or ALT) above the upper limit of normal (ULN), greater than 1.8 times the ULN, and greater than 3 times the ULN occurred in 14%, 6%, and 3%, respectively, of acarbose-treated patients as compared to 7%, 2%, and 1%, respectively, of placebo-treated patients. Although these differences between treatments were statistically significant, these elevations were asymptomatic, reversible, more common in females, and, in general, were not associated with other evidence of liver dysfunction. In addition, these serum transaminase elevations appeared to be dose related. In US studies including acarbose doses up to the maximum approved dose of 100 mg 3 times daily, treatment-emergent elevations of AST and/or ALT at any level of severity were similar between acarbose-treated patients and placebo-treated patients ($P \geq 0.496$).

In approximately 3 million patient-years of international postmarketing experience with acarbose, 62 cases of serum transaminase elevations greater than 500 units/L (29 of which were associated with jaundice) have been reported. Forty-one of these 62 patients received treatment with 100 mg 3 times daily or greater and 33 of 45 patients for whom weight was reported weighed less than 60 kg. In the 59 cases where follow-up was recorded, hepatic abnormalities improved or resolved upon discontinuation of acarbose in 55 and were unchanged in 2. A few cases of fulminant hepatitis with fatal outcome have been reported; the relationship to acarbose is unclear.

➤*Monitoring:* Therapeutic response to acarbose should be monitored by periodic blood glucose tests. Measurement of glycosylated hemoglobin levels is recommended for the monitoring of long-term glycemic control.

Acarbose, particularly at doses in excess of 50 mg 3 times daily, may give rise to elevations of serum transaminases and, in rare instances, hyperbili-

ACARBOSE — ORAL

rubinemia. It is recommended that serum transaminase levels be checked every 3 months during the first year of treatment with acarbose and periodically thereafter. If elevated transaminases are observed, a reduction in dosage or withdrawal of therapy may be indicated, particularly if the elevations persist.

Drug Interactions

Acarbose Oral Drug Interactions			
Precipitant drug	Object drug[a]		Description
Acarbose	Digoxin	⬇	Serum digoxin concentrations may be reduced, decreasing the therapeutic effects.
Digestive enzymes (eg, amylase, pancreatin)	Acarbose	⬇	Effect of acarbose may be reduced. Do not use concomitantly.
Intestinal absorbents (eg, charcoal)	Acarbose	⬇	Effect of acarbose may be reduced. Do not use concomitantly.

[a] ⬇ = Object drug decreased.

Certain drugs tend to produce hyperglycemia and may lead to loss of blood glucose control. These drugs include the thiazides and other diuretics, corticosteroids, phenothiazines, thyroid products, estrogens, oral contraceptives, phenytoin, nicotinic acid, sympathomimetics, calcium channel-blocking drugs, and isoniazid. When such drugs are administered to a patient receiving acarbose, the patient should be closely observed for loss of blood glucose control. When such drugs are withdrawn from patients receiving acarbose in combination with sulfonylureas or insulin, patients should be observed closely for any evidence of hypoglycemia.

Adverse Reactions

➤*GI:* GI symptoms are the most common reactions to acarbose. In US placebo-controlled trials, the incidences of abdominal pain, diarrhea, and flatulence were 19%, 31%, and 74%, respectively, in 1255 patients treated with acarbose 50 to 300 mg 3 times daily, whereas the corresponding incidences were 9%, 12%, and 29% in 999 placebo-treated patients. In a 1-year safety study, during which patients kept diaries of GI symptoms, abdominal pain and diarrhea tended to return to pretreatment levels over time, and the frequency and intensity of flatulence tended to abate with time. The increased gastrointestinal tract symptoms in patients treated with acarbose are a manifestation of the mechanism of action of acarbose and are related to the presence of undigested carbohydrate in the lower GI tract. Rarely, these GI events may be severe and might be confused with paralytic ileus.

➤*Hypersensitivity:* Rarely, hypersensitive skin reactions such as rash may occur.

➤*Lab test abnormalities:* Elevated serum transaminase levels, small reductions in hematocrit occurred more often in acarbose-treated patients than in placebo-treated patients but were not associated with reductions in hemoglobin. Low serum calcium and low plasma vitamin B_6 levels were associated with acarbose therapy but are thought to be either spurious or of no clinical significance.

➤*Miscellaneous:* Edema in rare instances edema has been reported.

Overdosage

Unlike sulfonylureas or insulin, an overdose of acarbose will not result in hypoglycemia. An overdose may result in transient increases in flatulence, diarrhea, and abdominal discomfort which shortly subside.

Patient Information

Patients should be told to take acarbose orally 3 times a day at the start (with the first bite) of each main meal. It is important that patients continue to adhere to dietary instructions, a regular exercise program, and regular testing of urine or blood glucose.

Acarbose itself does not cause hypoglycemia even when administered to patients in the fasted state. Sulfonylurea drugs and insulin, however, can lower blood sugar levels enough to cause symptoms or sometimes life-threatening hypoglycemia. Because acarbose given in combination with a sulfonylurea or insulin will cause a further lowering of blood sugar, it may increase the hypoglycemic potential of these agents. Hypoglycemia does not occur in patients receiving metformin alone under usual circumstances of use, and no increased incidence of hypoglycemia was observed in patients when acarbose was added to metformin therapy. The risk of hypoglycemia, its symptoms and treatment, and conditions that predispose to its development should be well understood by patients and responsible family members. Because acarbose prevents the breakdown of table sugar, patients should have a readily available source of glucose (dextrose, D-glucose) to treat symptoms of low blood sugar when taking acarbose in combination with a sulfonylurea or insulin.

If side effects occur with acarbose, they usually develop during the first few weeks of therapy. They are most commonly mild-to-moderate gastrointestinal effects, such as flatulence, diarrhea, or abdominal discomfort, and generally diminish in frequency and intensity with time.

MIGLITOL

Rx	**Glyset** (Pfizer)	**Tablets:** 25 mg	(GLYSET 25). White. In 100s.
		50 mg	(GLYSET 50). White. In 100s.
		100 mg	(GLYSET 100). White. In 100s.

MIGLITOL — ORAL

Indications

➤*Type 2 diabetes:* Monotherapy as an adjunct to diet to improve glycemic control in patients with type 2 diabetes whose hyperglycemia cannot be managed with diet alone. Miglitol may also be used in combination with a sulfonylurea when diet plus either miglitol or a sulfonylurea alone do not result in adequate glycemic control. The effect of miglitol to enhance glycemic control is additive to that of sulfonylureas when used in combination, presumably because its mechanism of action is different.

Administration and Dosage

➤*General dosing considerations:* The therapeutic goal should be to decrease both postprandial plasma glucose and glycosylated hemoglobin levels to normal or near normal by using the lowest effective dose of miglitol, either as monotherapy or in combination with a sulfonylurea.

There is no fixed dosage regimen for the management of diabetes mellitus with miglitol tablets or any other pharmacologic agent. Dosage of miglitol must be individualized on the basis of both effectiveness and tolerance while not exceeding the maximum recommended dosage.

➤*Adults:*

Type 2 diabetes –

Maximum dose: 100 mg 3 times daily.

Initial dosage: 25 mg 3 times daily at the start (with the first bite) of each main meal. However, some patients may benefit by starting at 25 mg once daily to minimize GI adverse reactions and gradually increasing the frequency of administration to 3 times daily.

Dosage titration: Gradually titrate upward to allow adaptation to potential GI adverse reactions. After 4 to 8 weeks of the 25 mg 3 times daily regimen, increase to 50 mg 3 times daily for approximately 3 months, following which a glycosylated hemoglobin level should be measured to assess therapeutic response. If, at that time, the glycosylated hemoglobin level is not satisfactory, the dosage may be further increased to 100 mg 3 times daily, the maximum recommended dosage.

Maintenance dosage: 50 mg 3 times daily, although some patients may benefit from increasing the dose to 100 mg 3 times daily. If no further reduction in postprandial glucose or glycosylated hemoglobin levels is observed with titration to 100 mg 3 times daily, consideration should be given to lowering the dose. Once an effective and tolerated dosage is established, it should be maintained.

Concomitant therapy:
Miglitol given in combination with a sulfonylurea will cause a further lowering of blood glucose and may increase the risk of hypoglycemia because of the additive effects of the 2 agents. If hypoglycemia occurs, appropriate adjustments in the dosage of these agents should be made.

➤*Renal function impairment:* Not recommended if serum creatinine is more than 2mg/dL.

➤*Monitoring:* During treatment initiation and dose titration, 1-hour postprandial plasma glucose may be used to determine the therapeutic response to miglitol and identify the minimum effective dose for the patient. Thereafter, glycosylated hemoglobin should be measured at intervals of approximately 3 months.

➤*Administration:* Take 3 times daily at the start (with the first bite) of each main meal.

➤*Storage/Stability:* Store at 25°C (77°F); excursions permitted to 15° to 30°C (59° to 86°F).

Actions

➤*Pharmacology:* Miglitol is a desoxynojirimycin derivative that delays the digestion of ingested carbohydrates, thereby resulting in a smaller rise in blood glucose concentration following meals. As a consequence of plasma glucose reduction, miglitol tablets reduce levels of glycosylated hemoglobin in patients with type 2 diabetes mellitus. Systemic nonenzymatic protein glycosylation, as reflected by levels of glycosylated hemoglobin, is a function of average blood glucose concentration over time.

In contrast to sulfonylureas, miglitol does not enhance insulin secretion. The antihyperglycemic action of miglitol results from a reversible inhibition of membrane-bound intestinal α-glucoside hydrolase enzymes. Membrane-bound intestinal α-glucosidases hydrolyze oligosaccharides and disaccharides to glucose and other monosaccharides in the brush border of the small intestine. In diabetic patients, this enzyme inhibition results in delayed glucose absorption and lowering of postprandial hyperglycemia.

Because its mechanism of action is different, the effect of miglitol to enhance glycemic control is additive to that of sulfonylureas when used in combination. In addition, miglitol diminishes the insulinotropic and weight-increasing effects of sulfonylureas. Miglitol has minor inhibitory activity

MIGLITOL — ORAL

against lactase and consequently, at the recommended doses, would not be expected to induce lactose intolerance.

➤*Pharmacokinetics:*

Absorption – Absorption of miglitol is saturable at high doses; a dose of 25 mg is completely absorbed, whereas a dose of 100 mg is only 50% to 70% absorbed. For all doses, peak concentrations are reached in 2 to 3 hours. There is no evidence that systemic absorption of miglitol contributes to its therapeutic effect.

Distribution – The protein binding of miglitol is negligible (less than 4%). Miglitol has a volume of distribution of 0.18 L/kg, consistent with distribution primarily into the extracellular fluid.

Metabolism – Miglitol is not metabolized in man or in any animal species studied. No metabolites have been detected in plasma, urine, or feces, indicating a lack of either systemic or presystemic metabolism.

Excretion – Miglitol is eliminated by renal excretion as unchanged drug. Thus, following a 25 mg dose, over 95% of the dose is recovered in the urine within 24 hours. At higher doses, the cumulative recovery of drug from urine is somewhat lower due to the incomplete bioavailability. The elimination half-life of miglitol from plasma is approximately 2 hours.

Special populations –

Renal function impairment: Because miglitol is excreted primarily by the kidneys, accumulation of miglitol is expected in patients with renal impairment. Patients with creatinine clearance less than 25 mL/min taking 25 mg 3 times daily exhibited a more than 2-fold increase in miglitol plasma levels as compared to subjects with creatinine clearance more than 60 mL/min. Dosage adjustment to correct the increased plasma concentrations is not feasible because miglitol acts locally. Little information is available on the safety of miglitol in patients with creatinine clearance less than 25 mL/min.

Contraindications

Diabetic ketoacidosis; inflammatory bowel disease, colonic ulceration, or partial intestinal obstruction, and in patients predisposed to intestinal obstruction; chronic intestinal diseases associated with marked disorders of digestion or absorption, or with conditions that may deteriorate as a result of increased gas formation in the intestine; hypersensitivity to the drug or any of its components.

Warnings/Precautions

➤*Hypoglycemia:* Because of its mechanism of action, miglitol when administered alone should not cause hypoglycemia in the fasted or postprandial state. Sulfonylurea agents may cause hypoglycemia. Because miglitol tablets given in combination with a sulfonylurea will cause a further lowering of blood glucose, it may increase the hypoglycemic potential of the sulfonylurea, although this was not observed in clinical trials. Oral glucose (dextrose), whose absorption is not delayed by miglitol, should be used instead of sucrose (cane sugar) in the treatment of mild-to-moderate hypoglycemia. Sucrose, whose hydrolysis to glucose and fructose is inhibited by miglitol, is unsuitable for the rapid correction of hypoglycemia. Severe hypoglycemia may require the use of either IV glucose infusion or glucagon injection.

➤*Loss of control of blood glucose:* When diabetic patients are exposed to stress such as fever, trauma, infection, or surgery, a temporary loss of control of blood glucose may occur. At such times, temporary insulin therapy may be necessary.

➤*Renal function impairment:* Plasma concentrations of miglitol in renally impaired volunteers were proportionally increased relative to the degree of renal dysfunction. Long-term clinical trials in diabetic patients with significant renal dysfunction (serum creatinine more than 2 mg/dL) have not been conducted. Therefore, treatment of these patients with miglitol is not recommended.

➤*Pregnancy: Category B.*

Teratogenic – The safety of miglitol in pregnant women has not been established. Developmental toxicology studies have been performed in rats at doses of 50, 150 and 450 mg/kg, corresponding to levels of approximately 1.5, 4, and 12 times the maximum recommended human exposure based on body surface area. In rabbits, doses of 10, 45, and 200 mg/kg corresponding to levels of approximately 0.5, 3, and 10 times the human exposure were examined. These studies revealed no evidence of fetal malformations attributable to miglitol. Doses of miglitol up to 4 and 3 times the human dose (based on body surface area), for rats and rabbits, respectively, did not reveal evidence of impaired fertility or harm to the fetus. The highest doses tested in these studies, 450 mg/kg in the rat and 200 mg/kg in the rabbit promoted maternal or fetal toxicity. Fetotoxicity was indicated by a slight but significant reduction in fetal weight in the rat study and slight reduction in fetal weight, delayed ossification of the fetal skeleton and increase in the percentage of non-viable fetuses in the rabbit study. In the peri- and postnatal study in rats, the NOAEL (no observed adverse effect level) was 100 mg/kg (corresponding to approximately 4 times the exposure to humans, based on body surface area). An increase in stillborn progeny was noted at the high dose (300 mg/kg) in the rat peri- and postnatal study, but not at the high dose (450 mg/kg) in the delivery segment of the rat developmental toxicity study. Otherwise, there was no adverse effect on survival, growth, development, behavior, or fertility in either the rat developmental toxicity or peri-postnatal studies. There are, however, no adequate and well-controlled studies in pregnant women. Because animal reproduction studies are not always predictive of human response, this drug should be used during pregnancy only if clearly needed.

➤*Lactation:* Miglitol has been shown to be excreted in human milk to a very small degree. Total excretion into milk accounted for 0.02% of a 100 mg maternal dose. The estimated exposure to a nursing infant is approximately 0.4% of the maternal dose. Although the levels of miglitol reached in human milk are exceedingly low, it is recommended that miglitol not be administered to a nursing woman.

➤*Children:* Safety and efficacy of miglitol in children have not been established.

➤*Monitoring:* Therapeutic response to miglitol may be monitored by periodic blood glucose tests. Measurement of glycosylated hemoglobin level is recommended for the monitoring of long-term glycemic control.

Drug Interactions

Miglitol Oral Drug Interactions

Precipitant	Object drug[a]		Description
Miglitol	Digoxin	⬇	Coadministration may reduce the average plasma concentrations of digoxin by 19% to 28%. In 1 study in diabetic patients under treatment with digoxin, plasma digoxin concentrations were not altered when coadministered with miglitol 100 mg 3 times/day × 14 days.
Miglitol	Glyburide	⬇	Decreased AUC and C_{max} values for glyburide occurred when coadministered with miglitol. These differences were not statistically significant.
Miglitol	Metformin	⬇	Mean AUC and C_{max} values for metformin were 12% to 13% lower when the volunteers were given miglitol as compared with placebo, but this difference was not statistically significant.
Miglitol	Propranolol	⬇	Miglitol may significantly reduce the bioavailability of propranolol by 40%.
Miglitol	Ranitidine	⬇	Miglitol may significantly reduce the bioavailability of ranitidine by 60%.
Digestive enzymes (eg, amylase, pancreatin)	Miglitol	⬇	Digestive enzyme preparations may reduce the effect of miglitol. Do not take concomitantly.
Intestinal adsorbents (eg, charcoal)	Miglitol	⬇	Intestinal adsorbents may reduce the effect of miglitol. Do not take concomitantly.

[a] ⬇ = Object drug decreased.

Several studies investigated the possible interaction between miglitol and glyburide. In 6 healthy volunteers given a single dose of 5 mg glyburide on a background of 6 days treatment with miglitol (50 mg 3 times daily for 4 days followed by 100 mg 3 times daily for 2 days) or placebo, the mean C_{max} and AUC values for glyburide were 17% and 25% lower, respectively, when glyburide was given with miglitol. In a study in diabetic patients in which the effects of adding miglitol 100 mg 3 times daily × 7 days or placebo to a background regimen of 3.5 mg glyburide daily were investigated, the mean AUC value for glyburide was 18% lower in the group treated with miglitol, although this difference was not statistically significant. Further information on a potential interaction with glyburide was obtained from one of the large US clinical trials (study 7) in which patients were dosed with either miglitol or placebo on a background of glyburide 10 mg twice daily. At the 6-month and 1-year clinic visits, patients taking concomitant miglitol 100 mg 3 times daily exhibited mean C_{max} values for glyburide that were 16% and 8% lower, respectively, compared to patients taking glyburide alone. However, these differences were not statistically significant. Thus, although there was a trend toward lower AUC and C_{max} values for glyburide when coadministered with miglitol, no definitive statement regarding a potential interaction can be made based on the foregoing 3 studies.

In 12 healthy males, concomitantly administered antacid did not influence the pharmacokinetics of miglitol.

Adverse Reactions

➤*Dermatologic:* Skin rash was reported in 4.3% of patients treated with miglitol compared to 2.4% of placebo-treated patients. Rashes were generally transient, and most were assessed as unrelated to miglitol by physician-investigators.

➤*GI:* GI symptoms are the most common reactions to miglitol tablets. In US placebo-controlled trials, the incidences of abdominal pain, diarrhea, and flatulence were 11.7%, 28.7%, and 41.5%, respectively in 962 patients treated with miglitol 25 to 100 mg 3 times daily, whereas the corresponding incidences were 4.7%, 10%, and 12% in 603 placebo-treated patients. The incidence of diarrhea and abdominal pain tended to diminish considerably with continued treatment.

➤*Lab test abnormalities:* Low serum iron occurred more often in patients treated with miglitol (9.2%) than in placebo-treated patients (4.2%) but did

Alpha-Glucosidase Inhibitors

MIGLITOL — ORAL

not persist in the majority of cases and was not associated with reductions in hemoglobin or changes in other hematologic indices.

Overdosage

➤*Symptoms:* Unlike sulfonylureas or insulin, an overdose of miglitol tablets will not result in hypoglycemia. An overdose may result in transient increases in flatulence, diarrhea, and abdominal discomfort. Because of the lack of extra-intestinal effects seen with miglitol, no serious systemic reactions are expected in the event of an overdose.

Amylin Analog

PRAMLINTIDE ACETATE

Rx	**Symlin** (Amylin Pharmaceuticals, Inc.)	**Injection, solution:** 0.6 mg/mL	In 5 mL vials.
		1 mg/mL	In 1.5 and 2.7 mL multidose pen-injectors.

PRAMLINTIDE ACETATE — INJECTION

WARNING

Pramlintide is used with insulin and has been associated with an increased risk of insulin-induced severe hypoglycemia, particularly in patients with type 1 diabetes. When severe hypoglycemia associated with pramlintide use occurs, it is seen within 3 hours following a pramlintide injection. If severe hypoglycemia occurs while operating a motor vehicle, heavy machinery, or while engaging in other high-risk activities, serious injuries may occur. Appropriate patient selection, careful patient instruction, and insulin dose adjustments are critical elements for reducing this risk.

Indications

➤*Type 1 diabetes mellitus:* As an adjunct treatment in patients who use mealtime insulin therapy and who have failed to achieve desired glucose control despite optimal insulin therapy.

➤*Type 2 diabetes mellitus:* As an adjunct treatment in patients who use mealtime insulin therapy and who have failed to achieve desired glucose control despite optimal insulin therapy, with or without a concurrent sulfonylurea agent and/or metformin.

Administration and Dosage

➤*General dosing considerations:* Pramlintide dosage differs depending on whether the patient has type 2 or type 1 diabetes mellitus (see the following). When initiating therapy with pramlintide, initial insulin dose reduction is required in all patients (both type 2 and type 1 diabetes mellitus) to reduce the risk of insulin-induced hypoglycemia. Because this reduction in insulin may lead to glucose elevations, monitor patients at regular intervals to assess pramlintide tolerability and the effect on blood glucose so that individualized insulin adjustments may be initiated.

If pramlintide therapy is discontinued for any reason (eg, surgery, illness), follow the same initiation protocol when pramlintide therapy is reinstituted.

➤*Adults:*

Type 1 diabetes mellitus – Initiate pramlintide at a dose of 15 mcg and titrate at 15 mcg increments to a maintenance dose of 30 or 60 mcg, as tolerated. Instruct patients to:

- Initiate pramlintide at a starting dose of 15 mcg subcutaneously immediately prior to major meals.
- Reduce preprandial, rapid-acting or short-acting, insulin dosages, including fixed-mix insulins (eg, 70/30) by 50%.
- Frequently monitor blood glucose, including before and after meals and at bedtime.
- Increase the pramlintide dose to the next increment (30, 45, or 60 mcg) when no clinically significant nausea has occurred for at least 3 days. Only make pramlintide dose adjustments as directed by the health care provider. If significant nausea persists at the 45 or 60 mcg dose level, decrease the pramlintide dose to 30 mcg. If the 30 mcg dose is not tolerated, consider discontinuation of pramlintide therapy.
- Adjust insulin doses to optimize glycemic control once the target dose of pramlintide is achieved and nausea, if experienced, has subsided. Only make insulin dose adjustments as directed by the health care provider.
- Contact a health care provider skilled in the use of insulin to review pramlintide and insulin dose adjustments at least once weekly until a target dose of pramlintide is achieved, pramlintide is well-tolerated, and blood glucose concentrations are stable.

After a maintenance dose of pramlintide is achieved, instruct patients to:

- Adjust insulin doses to optimize glycemic control once the target dose of pramlintide is achieved and nausea, if experienced, has subsided. Only make insulin dose adjustments as directed by a health care provider.
- Contact a health care provider in the event of recurrent nausea or hypoglycemia. View an increased frequency of mild to moderate hypoglycemia as a warning sign of increased risk for severe hypoglycemia.

Type 2 diabetes mellitus, insulin-dependent – Initiate pramlintide at a dose of 60 mcg and increase to a dose of 120 mcg, as tolerated. Instruct patients to:

- Initiate pramlintide at 60 mcg subcutaneously immediately prior to major meals.
- Reduce preprandial, rapid-acting or short-acting, insulin dosages, including fixed-mix insulins (eg, 70/30) by 50%.
- Monitor blood glucose frequently, including before and after meals and at bedtime.
- Increase the dose to pramlintide 120 mcg when no clinically significant nausea has occurred for 3 to 7 days. Make pramlintide dose adjustments only as directed by a health care provider. If significant nausea persists at the 120 mcg dose, decrease the dose to pramlintide 60 mcg.
- Adjust insulin doses to optimize glycemic control once the target dose of pramlintide is achieved and nausea, if experienced, has subsided. Make insulin dose adjustments only as directed by the health care provider.
- Contact a health care provider skilled in the use of insulin to review pramlintide and insulin dose adjustments at least once weekly until a target dose of pramlintide is achieved, pramlintide is well-tolerated, and blood glucose concentrations are stable.

After a maintenance dose of pramlintide is achieved, instruct patients to:

- Adjust insulin doses to optimize glycemic control once the target dose of pramlintide is achieved and nausea, if experienced, has subsided. Only make insulin dose adjustments as directed by a health care provider.
- Contact a health care provider in the event of recurrent nausea or hypoglycemia. View an increased frequency of mild to moderate hypoglycemia as a warning sign of increased risk for severe hypoglycemia.

➤*Monitoring:* Monitor blood glucose levels frequently, including before and after meals and at bedtime.

➤*Discontinuation of therapy:* Discontinue pramlintide therapy if any of the following occurs:

- recurrent unexplained hypoglycemia that requires medical assistance,
- persistent clinically significant nausea,
- noncompliance with self-monitoring of blood glucose concentrations,
- noncompliance with insulin dose adjustments,
- noncompliance with scheduled health care provider contacts or recommended clinic visits.

➤*Administration:* Administer subcutaneously immediately prior to each major meal (at least 250 kcal or containing at least 30 g of carbohydrate).

Pramlintide should be at room temperature before injection to reduce potential injection-site reactions. Administer each pramlintide dose subcutaneously into the abdomen or thigh (administration into the arm is not recommended because of variable absorption). Rotate injection sites so that the same site is not used repeatedly. The injection site selected should also be distinct from the site chosen for any concomitant insulin injection.

Always administer pramlintide and insulin as separate injections. Do not mix pramlintide with any type of insulin. If dose is missed, wait until the next scheduled dose and administer the usual amount.

Vials – To administer pramlintide from vials, use a U-100 insulin syringe (preferably a 0.3 mL [0.3 cc] size) for optimal accuracy. If using a syringe calibrated for use with U-100 insulin, use the following chart to measure the microgram dosage in unit increments. Always use separate, new syringes and needles to give pramlintide injections.

Pramlintide Dose Conversion to Insulin Unit Equivalents

Pramlintide dosage prescribed (mcg)	Increment using a U-100 syringe (units)	Volume (cc or mL)
15	2.5	0.025
30	5	0.05
45	7.5	0.075
60	10	0.1
120	20	0.2

➤*Admixture compatibility:* Do not mix pramlintide with any type of insulin.

➤*Storage/Stability:* Store unopened (not in-use) pramlintide in a refrigerator at 2° to 8°C (36° to 46°F). Store opened (in-use) pramlintide in a refrigerator or up to 30°C (86°F) and use within 30 days. Protect from light. Do not freeze.

Actions

➤*Pharmacology:* Amylin is co-located with insulin in secretory granules and co-secreted with insulin by pancreatic beta cells in response to food intake. Amylin and insulin show similar fasting and postprandial patterns in healthy individuals.

Amylin affects the rate of postprandial glucose appearance through a variety of mechanisms. Amylin slows gastric emptying (ie, the rate at which food

PRAMLINTIDE ACETATE — INJECTION

is released from the stomach to the small intestine) without altering the overall absorption of nutrients. In addition, amylin suppresses glucagon secretion (not normalized by insulin alone), which leads to suppression of endogenous glucose output from the liver. Amylin also regulates food intake caused by centrally-mediated modulation of appetite.

In patients with insulin-using type 2 or type 1 diabetes, the pancreatic beta cells are dysfunctional or damaged, resulting in reduced secretion of insulin and amylin in response to food.

Pramlintide, by acting as an amylinomimetic agent, has the following effects: 1) modulation of gastric emptying; 2) prevention of the postprandial rise in plasma glucagon; and 3) satiety leading to decreased caloric intake and potential weight loss.

Gastric emptying – The gastric-emptying rate is an important determinant of the postprandial rise in plasma glucose. Pramlintide slows the rate at which food is released from the stomach to the small intestine after a meal, and, thus, it reduces the initial postprandial increase in plasma glucose. This effect lasts for approximately 3 hours after pramlintide administration. Pramlintide does not alter the net absorption of ingested carbohydrate or other nutrients.

Postprandial glucagon secretion – In patients with diabetes, glucagon concentrations are abnormally elevated during the postprandial period, contributing to hyperglycemia. Pramlintide has been shown to decrease postprandial glucagon concentrations in insulin-using patients with diabetes.

Satiety – Pramlintide administered prior to a meal has been shown to reduce total caloric intake. This effect appears to be independent of the nausea that may accompany pramlintide treatment.

Pharmacodynamics – In clinical studies in patients with insulin-using type 2 and type 1 diabetes, pramlintide administration resulted in a reduction in mean postprandial glucose concentrations, reduced glucose fluctuations, and reduced food intake. Pramlintide doses differ for insulin-using type 2 and type 1 patients.

➤*Pharmacokinetics:*

Absorption – The absolute bioavailability of a single subcutaneous dose of pramlintide is approximately 30% to 40%. Subcutaneous administration of different doses of pramlintide into the abdominal area or thigh of healthy subjects resulted in dose-proportionate maximum plasma concentrations (C_{max}) and overall exposure (expressed as area under the plasma concentration curve or [AUC]) (see the following table).

Mean Pharmacokinetic Parameters Following Administration of Single Subcutaneous Doses of Pramlintide

Subcutaneous dose (mcg)	$AUC_{(0-\infty)}$ (pmol*min/L)	C_{max} (pmol/L)	T_{max} (min)	Elimination $t_{1/2}$ (min)
30	3,750	39	21	55
60	6,778	79	20	49
90	8,507	102	19	51
120	11,970	147	21	48

Injection of pramlintide into the arm showed higher exposure with greater variability compared with exposure after injection of pramlintide into the abdominal area or thigh.

There was no strong correlation between the degree of adiposity as assessed by body mass index (BMI) or skin fold thickness measurements and relative bioavailability. Injections administered with 6 and 12.7 mm needles yielded similar bioavailability.

Distribution – Pramlintide does not bind extensively to blood cells or albumin (approximately 40% of the drug is unbound in plasma), and thus pramlintide's pharmacokinetics should be insensitive to changes in binding sites.

Metabolism/Excretion – In healthy subjects, the half-life of pramlintide is approximately 48 minutes. Pramlintide is metabolized primarily by the kidneys. Des-lys[1] pramlintide (2-37 pramlintide), the primary metabolite, has a similar half-life and is biologically active both in vitro and in vivo in rats. AUC values are relatively constant with repeat dosing, indicating no bioaccumulation.

Reduction in postprandial glucose concentrations – Pramlintide administered subcutaneously immediately prior to a meal reduced plasma glucose concentrations after the meal when used with regular insulin or rapid-acting insulin analogs. This reduction in postprandial glucose decreased the amount of short-acting insulin required and limited glucose fluctuations based upon 24-hour glucose monitoring. When rapid-acting analog insulins were used, plasma glucose concentrations tended to rise during the interval between 150 minutes following pramlintide injection and the next meal.

Reduced food intake – A single, subcutaneous dose of pramlintide 120 mcg (type 2 diabetes) or 30 mcg (type 1 diabetes) administered 1 hour prior to an unlimited buffet meal was associated with reductions in total caloric intake (placebo-subtracted mean changes of approximately 23% and 21%, respectively), which occurred without decreases in meal duration.

Contraindications

Hypersensitivity to pramlintide or any of its components, including metacresol; a confirmed diagnosis of gastroparesis; hypoglycemia unawareness.

Warnings/Precautions

➤*Patient selection:* Proper patient selection is critical to safe and effective use of pramlintide.

Before initiation of therapy, review the patient's HbA_{1c}, recent blood glucose monitoring data, history of insulin-induced hypoglycemia, current insulin regimen, and body weight. Only consider pramlintide therapy in patients with insulin-using type 2 or type 1 diabetes who have failed to achieve adequate glycemic control despite individualized insulin management and who are receiving ongoing care under the guidance of a health care professional skilled in the use of insulin and supported by the services of diabetes educator(s).

Do not consider patients meeting any of the following criteria for pramlintide therapy: poor compliance with current insulin regimen; poor compliance with prescribed self-blood glucose monitoring; have an HbA_{1c} greater than 9%; recurrent severe hypoglycemia requiring assistance during the past 6 months; presence of hypoglycemia unawareness; confirmed diagnosis of gastroparesis; require the use of drugs that stimulate GI motility; pediatric patients.

➤*Hypoglycemia:* Pramlintide alone does not cause hypoglycemia. However, pramlintide is indicated to be coadministered with insulin therapy, and, in this setting, pramlintide increases the risk of insulin-induced severe hypoglycemia, particularly in patients with type 1 diabetes. Severe hypoglycemia associated with pramlintide occurs within the first 3 hours following a pramlintide injection. If severe hypoglycemia occurs while operating a motor vehicle, heavy machinery, or while engaging in other high-risk activities, serious injuries may occur. Therefore, when introducing pramlintide therapy, take appropriate precautions to avoid increasing the risk for insulin-induced severe hypoglycemia. These precautions include frequent pre- and post-meal glucose monitoring combined with an initial 50% reduction in pre-meal doses of short-acting insulin.

Symptoms of hypoglycemia may include hunger, headache, sweating, tremor, irritability, or difficulty concentrating. Rapid reductions in blood glucose concentrations may induce such symptoms regardless of glucose values. More severe symptoms of hypoglycemia include loss of consciousness, coma, or seizure.

Early warning symptoms of hypoglycemia may be different or less pronounced under certain conditions, such as long duration of diabetes; diabetic nerve disease; use of medications such as beta-blockers, clonidine, guanethidine, or reserpine; or intensified diabetes control.

Clinical studies employing a controlled hypoglycemic challenge have demonstrated that pramlintide does not alter the counter-regulatory hormonal response to insulin-induced hypoglycemia. Likewise, in pramlintide-treated patients, the perception of hypoglycemic symptoms was not altered with plasma glucose concentrations as low as 45 mg/dL.

Drugs that increase the susceptibility to hypoglycemia – The addition of any antihyperglycemic agent (eg, pramlintide) to an existing regimen of 1 or more antihyperglycemic agents (eg, insulin, sulfonylurea) or to other agents that may increase the risk of hypoglycemia may necessitate further insulin dose adjustments and particularly close monitoring of blood glucose.

The following are examples of substances that may increase the blood glucose-lowering effect and susceptibility to hypoglycemia: oral antidiabetic products, angiotensin-converting enzyme (ACE) inhibitors, disopyramide, fibrates, fluoxetine, monoamine oxidase (MAO) inhibitors, pentoxifylline, propoxyphene, salicylates, and sulfonamide antibiotics.

➤*Hypersensitivity reactions:*

Local – Patients may experience redness, swelling, or itching at the site of injection. These minor reactions usually resolve within a few days to a few weeks. In some instances, these reactions may be related to factors other than pramlintide, such as irritants in a skin-cleansing agent or improper injection technique.

Systemic – In controlled clinical trials up to 12 months, potential systemic allergic reactions were reported in 65 (5%) of type 2 patients and 59 (5%) of type 1 pramlintide-treated patients. Similar reactions were reported by 18 (4%) and 28 (5%) of placebo-treated type 2 and type 1 patients, respectively. No patient receiving pramlintide was withdrawn from a trial because of a potential systemic allergic reaction.

➤*Hazardous tasks:* Severe hypoglycemia associated with pramlintide occurs within the first 3 hours following a pramlintide injection. If severe hypoglycemia occurs while operating a motor vehicle, heavy machinery, or while engaging in other high-risk activities, serious injuries may occur. Therefore, when introducing pramlintide therapy, take appropriate precautions to avoid increasing the risk for insulin-induced severe hypoglycemia. These precautions include frequent pre- and post-meal glucose monitoring combined with an initial 50% reduction in pre-meal doses of short-acting insulin.

➤*Pregnancy: Category C.* No adequate and well-controlled studies have been conducted in pregnant women. Studies in perfused human placenta indicate that pramlintide has low potential to cross the maternal/fetal placental barrier. Embryofetal toxicity studies with pramlintide have been performed in rats and rabbits. Increases in congenital abnormalities (neural tube defect, cleft palate, exencephaly) were observed in fetuses of rats treated during organogenesis with 0.3 and 1 mg/kg/day (10 and 47 times the exposure resulting from the maximum recommended human dose based on AUC, respectively). Administration of doses up to 0.3 mg/kg/day pramlintide (9 times maximum recommended dose based on AUC) to pregnant rabbits had no adverse effects in embryofetal development; however, animal reproduction studies are not always predictive of human response. Only use pramlintide during pregnancy if it is determined by the health care provider that the potential benefit justifies the potential risk to the fetus.

PRAMLINTIDE ACETATE — INJECTION

➤*Lactation:* It is unknown whether pramlintide is excreted in human milk. Many drugs, including peptide drugs, are excreted in human milk. Therefore, administer pramlintide to nursing women only if it is determined by the health care provider that the potential benefit outweighs the potential risk to the infant.

➤*Children:* Safety and efficacy in children have not been established.

➤*Elderly:* Pramlintide has been studied in patients ranging in age from 15 to 84 years of age, including 539 patients 65 years of age or older. The change in HbA_{1c} values and hypoglycemia frequencies did not differ by age, but greater sensitivity in some older individuals cannot be ruled out. Thus, carefully manage pramlintide and insulin regimens to obviate an increased risk of severe hypoglycemia.

➤*Monitoring:* Monitor blood glucose frequently, including pre- and post-meals and at bedtime.

Drug Interactions

➤*Drugs that alter GI motility/absorption:* Because of its effects on gastric emptying, do not consider pramlintide therapy for patients taking drugs that alter GI motility (eg, anticholinergic agents such as atropine) and agents that slow the intestinal absorption of nutrients (eg, alpha-glucosidase inhibitors). Patients using these drugs have not been studied in clinical trials.

➤*Pramlintide delays absorption of concomitantly administered drugs:* Pramlintide has the potential to delay the absorption of coadministered oral medications. When the rapid onset of an orally coadministered agent is a critical determinant of effectiveness (eg, analgesics), administer the agent at least 1 hour prior to or 2 hours after pramlintide injection.

Adverse Reactions

Adverse reactions (excluding hypoglycemia) commonly associated with pramlintide when coadministered with a fixed dose of insulin in the long-term, placebo-controlled trials in insulin-using type 2 diabetic patients and type 1 diabetic patients are presented in the table below and the following table, respectively. The same adverse reactions were also shown in the open-label clinical practice study, which employed flexible insulin dosing.

Pramlintide Adverse Reactions (≥ 5% and Incidence Greater Than Placebo) in Patients with Insulin-using Type 2 Diabetes

	Long-term, placebo-controlled studies		Open-label, clinical practice study
Adverse reactions	Placebo + Insulin (N = 284)	Pramlintide + Insulin (N = 292)	Pramlintide + Insulin (N = 166)
CNS			
Dizziness	11 (4%)	17 (6%)	3 (2%)
Fatigue	11 (4%)	20 (7%)	5 (3%)
Headache	19 (7%)	39 (13%)	8 (5%)
GI			
Abdominal pain	19 (7%)	23 (8%)	3 (2%)
Anorexia	5 (2%)	27 (9%)	1 (< 1%)
Nausea	34 (12%)	81 (28%)	53 (30%)
Vomiting	12 (4%)	24 (8%)	13 (7%)
Respiratory			
Coughing	12 (4%)	18 (6%)	4 (2%)
Pharyngitis	7 (2%)	15 (5%)	6 (3%)

Pramlintide Adverse Reactions (≥ 5% and Incidence Greater than Placebo) in Patients with Type 1 Diabetes

	Long-term, placebo-controlled studies		Open-label, clinical practice study
Adverse reactions	Placebo + insulin (N = 538)	Pramlintide + insulin (N = 716)	Pramlintide + insulin (N = 265)
CNS			
Dizziness	21 (4%)	34 (5%)	5 (2%)
Fatigue	22 (4%)	51 (7%)	12 (4.5%)
GI			
Anorexia	12 (2%)	122 (17%)	0 (0%)
Nausea	92 (17%)	342 (48%)	98 (37%)
Vomiting	36 (7%)	82 (11%)	18 (7%)
Miscellaneous			
Allergic reaction	28 (5%)	41 (6%)	1 (< 1%)
Arthralgia	27 (5%)	51 (7%)	6 (2%)
Inflicted injury	55 (10%)	97 (14%)	20 (8%)

GI – Most adverse events were GI in nature. In patients with type 2 or type 1 diabetes, the incidence of nausea was higher at the beginning of pramlintide treatment and decreased with time in most patients. The incidence and severity of nausea are reduced when pramlintide is gradually titrated to the recommended doses.

➤*Severe hypoglycemia:* Pramlintide alone (without the coadministration of insulin) does not cause hypoglycemia. However, pramlintide is indicated as an adjunct treatment in patients who use mealtime insulin therapy, and coadministration of pramlintide with insulin may increase the risk of insulin-induced hypoglycemia, particularly in patients with type 1 diabetes. The incidence of severe hypoglycemia during the pramlintide clinical development program is summarized in the following tables.

Severe Hypoglycemia in Patients With Type 2 Diabetes Treated with Insulin and Pramlintide

	Long-term, placebo-controlled studies (no insulin dose-reduction during initiation)				Open-label, clinical practice study (insulin dose-reduction during initiation)	
	Placebo + Insulin		Pramlintide + Insulin		Pramlintide + Insulin	
Severe hypoglycemia	0 to 3 months (n = 284)	> 3 to 6 months (n = 251)	0 to 3 months (n = 292)	> 3 to 6 months (n = 255)	0 to 3 months (n = 166)	> 3 to 6 months (n = 150)
Patient-ascertained [a]						
Reaction rate (reaction rate/ patient year)	0.24	0.13	0.45	0.39	0.05	0.03
Incidence (%)	2.1%	2.4%	8.2%	4.7%	0.6%	0.7%
Medically assisted [b]						
Reaction rate (reaction rate/ patient year)	0.06	0.07	0.09	0.02	0.05	0.03
Incidence (%)	0.7%	1.2%	1.7%	0.4%	0.6%	0.7%

[a] Patient-ascertained severe hypoglycemia: Requiring the assistance of another individual (including aid in ingestion of oral carbohydrate), and/or requiring the administration of glucagon injection, IV glucose, or other medical intervention.

[b] Medically assisted severe hypoglycemia: Requiring glucagon, IV glucose, hospitalization, paramedic assistance, emergency room visit, and/or assessed as a serious adverse event (SAE) by the investigator.

Severe Hypoglycemia in Patients With Type 1 Diabetes Treated with Insulin and Pramlintide

	Long-term, placebo-controlled studies (no insulin dose-reduction during initiation)				Open-label, clinical practice study (insulin dose-reduction during initiation)	
	Placebo + Insulin		Pramlintide + Insulin		Pramlintide + Insulin	
Severe hypoglycemia	0 to 3 months (n = 538)	> 3 to 6 months (n = 470)	0 to 3 months (n = 716)	> 3 to 6 months (n = 576)	0 to 3 months (n = 265)	> 3 to 6 months (n = 213)
Patient-ascertained [a]						
Reaction rate (reaction rate/ patient year)	1.33	1.06	1.55	0.82	0.29	0.16
Incidence (%)	10.8	8.7	16.8	11.1	5.7	3.8
Medically assisted [b]						
Reaction rate (reaction rate/ patient year)	0.19	0.24	0.50	0.27	0.1	0.04
Incidence (%)	3.3	4.3	7.3	5.2	2.3	0.9

[a] Patient-ascertained severe hypoglycemia: Requiring the assistance of another individual (including aid in ingestion of oral carbohydrate); and/or requiring the administration of glucagon injection, IV glucose, or other medical intervention.

[b] Medically assisted severe hypoglycemia: Requiring glucagon, IV glucose, hospitalization, paramedic assistance, emergency room visit, and/or assessed as an SAE by the investigator.

Overdosage

➤*Symptoms:* Single doses of pramlintide 10 mg (83 times the maximum dose of 120 mcg) were administered to 3 healthy volunteers. Severe nausea was reported in all 3 individuals and was associated with vomiting, diarrhea, vasodilatation, and dizziness. No hypoglycemia was reported.

➤*Treatment:* Pramlintide has a short half-life and, in the case of overdose, supportive measures are indicated.

Patient Information

Inform patients of the potential risks and advantages of pramlintide therapy. Also inform patients about self-management practices including glucose monitoring, proper injection technique, timing of dosing, and proper storage of pramlintide. In addition, advise patients of the importance of adherence to meal planning, physical activity, recognition and management of hypoglycemia and hyperglycemia, and assessment of diabetes complications. Refer patients to the pramlintide Medication Guide for additional information.

Instruct patients on handling of special situations such as intercurrent conditions (illness or stress), an inadequate or omitted insulin dose, inadvertent administration of increased insulin or pramlintide dose, inadequate food intake, or missed meals.

Amylin Analog

PRAMLINTIDE ACETATE — INJECTION

Always administer pramlintide and insulin as separate injections and never mix the injections.

Advise women with diabetes to inform their health care provider if they are pregnant or planning to become pregnant.

Glucagon-like Peptide 1 Receptor Agonist

EXENATIDE

Rx	**Byetta** (Amylin Pharmaceuticals)	**Injection, solution:** 250 mcg/mL	Mannitol, metacresol 2.2 mg. In 1.2[a] and 2.4[b] mL prefilled pens (60 doses).

[a] Provides 5 mcg per dose.

[b] Provides 10 mcg per dose.

EXENATIDE — INJECTION

Indications

➤*Type 2 diabetes mellitus:* As adjunctive therapy to diet and exercise to improve glycemic control in adult patients with type 2 diabetes mellitus.

Administration and Dosage

➤*Adults:*

Type 2 diabetes mellitus –

Initial dosage: 5 mcg subcutaneously twice daily at any time within the 60-minute period before the morning and evening meals (or before the 2 main meals of the day, approximately 6 hours or more apart). Initiation with 5 mcg reduces the incidence and severity of GI adverse effects.

Maintenance dosage: Based on clinical response, the dosage of exenatide can be increased to 10 mcg twice daily after 1 month of therapy.

➤*Renal function impairment:* Use caution when escalating doses of exenatide from 5 to 10 mcg in patients with moderate renal impairment (creatinine clearance [CrCl] 30 to 50 mL/min).

Exenatide is not recommended for use in patients with end-stage renal disease (ESRD) or severe renal impairment (CrCl less than 30 mL/min) and should be used with caution in patients with renal transplantation.

➤*Administration:* Each dose should be administered as a subcutaneous injection in the thigh, abdomen, or upper arm.

Exenatide should not be administered after a meal.

Exenatide pens are not to be shared with other patients.

➤*Storage/Stability:* Prior to the first use, refrigerate at 2° to 8°C (36° to 46°F). After the first use, exenatide can be kept at a temperature not to exceed 25°C (77°F). Do not freeze. Do not use exenatide if it has been frozen; protect from light. Discard 30 days after first use, even if some drug remains in the pen.

Actions

➤*Pharmacology:* Incretins, such as glucagonlike peptide-1 (GLP-1), enhance glucose-dependent insulin secretion and exhibit other antihyperglycemic actions following their release into the circulation from the gut. Exenatide is a GLP-1 receptor agonist that enhances glucose-dependent insulin secretion by the pancreatic beta cell, suppresses inappropriately elevated glucagon secretion, and slows gastric emptying.

The amino acid sequence of exenatide partially overlaps that of human GLP-1. Exenatide has been shown to bind and activate the known human GLP-1 receptor in vitro. This leads to an increase in both glucose-dependent synthesis of insulin and in vivo secretion of insulin from pancreatic beta cells by mechanisms involving cyclic adenosine monophosphate and/or other intracellular signaling pathways. Exenatide promotes insulin release from pancreatic beta cells in the presence of elevated glucose concentrations.

➤*Pharmacokinetics:*

Absorption – After subcutaneous administration to patients with type 2 diabetes, exenatide reaches median peak plasma concentrations in 2.1 hours. Mean peak exenatide concentration (C_{max}) was 211 pg/mL and overall mean area under the curve ($AUC_{0-\infty}$) was 1,036 pg•h/mL following subcutaneous administration of exenatide 10 mcg. Exenatide exposure (AUC) increased proportionally over the therapeutic dose range of 5 to 10 mcg. The C_{max} values increased less than proportionally over the same range. Similar exposure is achieved with subcutaneous administration of exenatide in the abdomen, thigh, or upper arm.

Distribution – The mean apparent volume of distribution of exenatide after subcutaneous administration of a single dose is 28.3 L.

Metabolism/Excretion – Nonclinical studies have shown that exenatide is predominantly eliminated by glomerular filtration with subsequent proteolytic degradation. The mean apparent clearance of exenatide in humans is 9.1 L/h and the mean terminal half-life is 2.4 hours. These pharmacokinetic characteristics of exenatide are independent of the dose. In most individuals, exenatide concentrations are measurable for approximately 10 hours postdose.

Special populations –

Renal function impairment: In patients with ESRD receiving dialysis, mean exenatide exposure increased by 3.37-fold compared with that of patients with healthy renal function.

Contraindications

Hypersensitivity to exenatide or any of its components.

Warnings/Precautions

➤*Acute pancreatitis:* Based on postmarketing data, exenatide has been associated with acute pancreatitis, including fatal and nonfatal hemorrhagic or necrotizing pancreatitis. After initiation of exenatide and after dose increases, observe patients carefully for signs and symptoms of pancreatitis (including persistent, severe abdominal pain, sometimes radiating to the back, which may or may not be accompanied by vomiting). If pancreatitis is suspected, promptly discontinue exenatide and initiate appropriate management. If pancreatitis is confirmed, exenatide should not be restarted. Consider antidiabetic therapies other than exenatide in patients with a history of pancreatitis.

➤*Renal effects:* There have been postmarketing reports of altered renal function, including increased serum creatinine, renal impairment, worsened chronic renal failure, and acute renal failure, sometimes requiring hemodialysis or kidney transplantation. Some of these events occurred in patients receiving 1 or more pharmacologic agents known to affect renal function or hydration status, such as angiotensin-converting enzyme inhibitors, nonsteroidal anti-inflammatory drugs, or diuretics. Some events occurred in patients who had been experiencing nausea, vomiting, or diarrhea, with or without dehydration. Reversibility of altered renal function has been observed in many cases with supportive treatment and discontinuation of potentially causative agents, including exenatide. Exenatide has not been found to be directly nephrotoxic in preclinical or clinical studies.

➤*GI disease:* Exenatide has not been studied in patients with severe GI disease, including gastroparesis. Its use is commonly associated with GI adverse reactions, including nausea, vomiting, and diarrhea. Therefore, the use of exenatide is not recommended in patients with severe GI disease.

➤*Insulin:* Exenatide is not a substitute for insulin. Do not use exenatide in patients with type 1 diabetes or for the treatment of diabetic ketoacidosis.

➤*Immunogenicity:* Consistent with the potentially immunogenic properties of protein and peptide pharmaceuticals, patients may develop antibodies to exenatide following treatment with exenatide.

In a small proportion of patients, the formation of antiexenatide antibodies at high titers could result in failure to achieve adequate improvement in glycemic control. If there is worsening of glycemic control or failure to achieve targeted glycemic control, consider alternative antidiabetic therapy.

➤*Hypersensitivity reactions:* There have been postmarketing reports of serious hypersensitivity reactions (eg, anaphylaxis, angioedema) in patients treated with exenatide. If a hypersensitivity reaction occurs, instruct the patient to discontinue exenatide and other suspect medications and promptly seek medical advice.

➤*Renal function impairment:* Do not use in patients with severe renal impairment (CrCl less than 30 mL/min) or ESRD, and use with caution in patients with renal transplantation. In patients with ESRD receiving dialysis, single doses of exenatide 5 mcg were not well tolerated because of GI adverse reactions. Because exenatide may induce nausea and vomiting with transient hypovolemia, treatment may worsen renal function. Apply or use caution when initiating or escalating doses of exenatide from 5 to 10 mcg in patients with moderate renal impairment (CrCl 30 to 50 mL/min).

➤*Hepatic function impairment:* No pharmacokinetic study has been performed in patients with a diagnosis of acute or chronic hepatic impairment. Because exenatide is cleared primarily by the kidney, hepatic dysfunction is not expected to affect blood concentrations of exenatide.

➤*Pregnancy: Category C.* There are no adequate and well-controlled studies in pregnant women. In animal studies, exenatide caused cleft palate, irregular skeletal ossification, and an increased number of neonatal deaths. Use exenatide during pregnancy only if the potential benefit justifies the potential risk to the fetus.

In pregnant mice given subcutaneous dosages of 6, 68, 460, or 760 mcg/kg/day from gestation day 6 through 15 (organogenesis), cleft palate (some with holes), irregular skeletal ossification of rib and skull bones, and reduced fetal and neonatal growth were observed at 6 mcg/day, a systemic exposure 3 times the human exposure resulting from the maximum recommended dosage of 20 mcg/kg/day, based on AUC.

In pregnant rabbits given subcutaneous dosages of 0.2, 2, 22, 156, or 260 mcg/kg/day from gestation day 6 through 18 (organogenesis), irregular skeletal ossifications were observed at 2 mcg/kg/day, a systemic exposure 12 times the human exposure resulting from the maximum recommended dosage of 20 mcg/day, based on AUC.

In pregnant mice given subcutaneous dosages of 6, 68, or 760 mcg/kg/day from gestation day 6 through lactation day 20 (weaning), an increased number of neonatal deaths was observed on postpartum days 2 to 4 in dams given 6 mcg/kg/day, a systemic exposure 3 times the human exposure resulting from the maximum recommended dosage of 20 mcg/day, based on AUC.

Pregnancy registry – The manufacturer maintains a pregnancy registry to monitor pregnancy outcomes of women exposed to exenatide during pregnancy. Health care providers are encouraged to register patients by calling 1-800-633-9081.

➤*Lactation:* It is not known whether exenatide is excreted in human milk. Many drugs are excreted in human milk. Because of the potential for clinically significant adverse reactions in breast-feeding infants from exenatide,

EXENATIDE — INJECTION

decide whether to discontinue breast-feeding or the drug, taking into account these potential risks against the glycemic benefits to the lactating woman. Studies in lactating mice have demonstrated that exenatide is present at low concentrations in milk (2.5% or less of the concentration in maternal plasma following subcutaneous dosing). The high molecular weight (approximately 4,187) and short elimination half-life (2.4 hours) suggest that little of the peptide amide will be excreted into breast milk. Exercise caution when administering exenatide to a breast-feeding woman.

➤*Children:* Safety and efficacy of exenatide have not been established in children.

➤*Monitoring:* Monitor glycemic control and international normalized ratio (INR) in patients who are also taking warfarin.

Monitor patients for signs and symptoms of hypersensitivity reactions and pancreatitis.

Drug Interactions

Exenatide Drug Interactions			
Precipitant drug	Object drug[a]		Description
Exenatide	Acetaminophen	⬇	When coadministered, acetaminophen AUC and C_{max} may be decreased and T_{max}[b] increased. Give acetaminophen at least 1 hour before or 4 hours after exenatide injection.
Exenatide	Digoxin	⬇	Coadministration of repeated doses of exenatide decreased digoxin C_{max} 17% and delayed T_{max} approximately 2.5 hours. Monitor the clinical response of the patient. If an interaction is suspected, adjust the digoxin dose as needed.
Exenatide	Lovastatin	⬇	Lovastatin AUC and C_{max} were decreased approximately 40% and 28%, respectively, and the T_{max} was delayed approximately 4 hours when coadministered with exenatide. Monitor the clinical response of the patient. If an interaction is suspected, adjust the lovastatin dose as needed.
Exenatide	Oral antibiotics, oral contraceptives	⬇	The effect of exenatide to slow gastric emptying may reduce the extent and rate of oral medications that require rapid GI absorption. Advise patients to take oral antibiotics and oral contraceptives at least 1 hour before exenatide.
Exenatide	Other hypoglycemic agents (eg, meglitinides [eg, repaglinide], sulfonylureas [eg, glimepiride])	⬆	The risk of hypoglycemia may be increased. Closely monitor blood glucose concentrations when exenatide is started or stopped in patients receiving other hypoglycemic agents. Reinforce patient instructions for hypoglycemic management, especially in patients receiving a sulfonylurea.
Exenatide	Warfarin	⬆	Exenatide may lead to increased INR and possibly increased bleeding when coadministered with warfarin. Monitor PT[c] times more frequently after starting or changing the dose of exenatide. Once a stable PT time is established, monitor PT times at intervals usually recommended for patients taking warfarin.

[a] ⬇ = object drug decreased; ⬆ = object drug increased.
[b] T_{max} = time to reach maximum concentration.
[c] PT = prothrombin time.

➤*Drug/Food interactions:* Do not administer exenatide after a meal; administer exenatide 60 minutes before the 2 main meals of the day, approximately 6 hours or more apart.

Adverse Reactions

Exenatide Hypoglycemia Incidence as Monotherapy or With Concomitant Antidiabetic Therapy[a,b]			
	Exenatide 5 mcg twice daily	Exenatide 10 mcg twice daily	Placebo twice daily
Monotherapy (24 weeks)			
n	77	78	77
% overall	5.2%	3.8%	1.3%
Rate (episode/patient-year)	0.21	0.52	0.03
% severe	0%	0%	0%
With metformin (30 weeks)			
n	110	113	113
% overall	4.5%	5.3%	5.3%
Rate (episode/patient-year)	0.13	0.12	0.12
% severe	0%	0%	0%
With a sulfonylurea (30 weeks)			
n	125	129	123
% overall	14.4%	35.7%	3.3%
Rate (episode/patient-year)	0.64	1.61	0.07
% severe	0%	0%	0%
With metformin and a sulfonylurea (30 weeks)			
n	245	241	247
% overall	19.2%	27.8%	12.6%
Rate (episode/patient-year)	0.78	1.71	0.58
% severe	0.4%	0%	0%
With a thiazolidinedione (16 weeks)			
n	—[c]	121	112
% overall	—	10.7%	7.1%
Rate (episode/patient-year)	—	0.98	0.56
% severe	—	0%	0%

[a] For the 30-week trials, a hypoglycemic episode was recorded if the patient reported symptoms consistent with hypoglycemia and was recorded as severe if the subject required the assistance of another person to treat the event. For the other trials, a hypoglycemic episode was recorded if a patient reported signs or symptoms of hypoglycemia or had a blood glucose value consistent with hypoglycemia regardless of associated symptoms or treatment and was recorded as severe if the subject required the assistance of another person to treat the event. The requirement for assistance had to be accompanied by a blood glucose measurement of less than 50 mg/dL or prompt recovery after administration of oral carbohydrate.
[b] n = The number of intent-to-treat subjects in each treatment group.
[c] Dose not studied.

➤*Monotherapy:*

Exenatide Adverse Reactions (≥ 2%) Excluding Hypoglycemia[a]		
Adverse reaction	All exenatide twice daily (n = 155)	Placebo twice daily (n = 77)
Dyspepsia	3%	0%
Nausea	8%	0%
Vomiting	4%	0%

[a] In a 24-week, placebo-controlled trial.

Adverse reactions reported in at least 1% to less than 2% of patients receiving exenatide and reported more frequently than with placebo included decreased appetite, diarrhea, and dizziness. The most frequently reported adverse reaction associated with exenatide, nausea, occurred in a dose-dependent fashion.

Discontinuation of therapy – Two of the 155 patients treated with exenatide withdrew because of adverse reactions of headache and nausea. No placebo-treated patients withdrew because of adverse reactions.

➤*Use with metformin and/or a sulfonylurea:*

Exenatide Adverse Reactions (≥ 2%) Excluding Hypoglycemia[a]		
Adverse reaction	All exenatide twice daily (n = 963)	Placebo twice daily (n = 483)
CNS		
Asthenia	4%	2%
Dizziness	9%	6%
Feeling jittery	9%	4%
Headache	9%	6%
GI		
Diarrhea	13%	6%
Dyspepsia	6%	3%

EXENATIDE — INJECTION

Exenatide Adverse Reactions (≥ 2%) Excluding Hypoglycemia[a]		
Adverse reaction	All exenatide twice daily (n = 963)	Placebo twice daily (n = 483)
Gastroesophageal reflux disease	3%	1%
Nausea	44%	18%
Vomiting	13%	4%
Miscellaneous		
Hyperhidrosis	3%	1%

[a] In three 30-week, placebo-controlled clinical trials.

Adverse reactions reported in at least 1% and less than 2% of patients receiving exenatide and reported more frequently than with placebo included decreased appetite.

Discontinuation of therapy – The most common adverse reactions leading to withdrawal for exenatide-treated patients were nausea (3%) and vomiting (1%). For placebo-treated patients, less than 1% withdrew because of nausea and 0% withdrew because of vomiting.

➤*Use with a thiazolidinedione with or without metformin:*

Exenatide Adverse Reactions (≥ 2%) Excluding Hypoglycemia[a]		
Adverse reaction	All exenatide twice daily (n = 121)	Placebo (n = 112)
Gastroesophageal reflux disease	3%	0%
Diarrhea	6%	3%
Dyspepsia	7%	1%
Nausea	40%	15%
Vomiting	13%	1%

[a] In a 16-week, placebo-controlled trial. Adverse reactions reported in greater than or equal to 1% to less than 2% of patients receiving exenatide and reported more frequently than with placebo included decreased appetite. Chills (n = 4) and injection-site reactions (n = 2) occurred only in exenatide-treated patients. The 2 patients who reported injection-site reaction had high titers of antibodies to exenatide.

Serious adverse reactions – Two serious adverse reactions, chest pain and chronic hypersensitivity pneumonitis, were reported in the exenatide arm. No serious adverse reactions were reported in the placebo arm.

Discontinuation of therapy: The most common adverse reactions leading to withdrawal for exenatide-treated patients were nausea (9%) and vomiting (5%). For placebo-treated patients, less than 1% withdrew because of nausea.

➤*Postmarketing:*

GI – Abdominal distention, abdominal pain, acute pancreatitis, constipation, eructation, flatulence, hemorrhagic and necrotizing pancreatitis sometimes resulting in death; nausea, vomiting, and/or diarrhea resulting in dehydration.

Hypersensitivity – Anaphylactic reaction, angioedema, generalized pruritus and/or urticaria, macular or papular rash.

Renal – Altered renal function, including increased serum creatinine, renal impairment, worsened chronic renal failure or acute renal failure (sometimes requiring hemodialysis), kidney transplant and kidney transplant dysfunction.

Miscellaneous – Dysgeusia, injection-site reactions, INR increased with concomitant warfarin use (some reports associated with bleeding), somnolence.

Overdosage

➤*Symptoms:* In a clinical study of exenatide, 3 patients with type 2 diabetes each experienced a single overdose of 100 mcg subcutaneously (10 times the maximum recommended dose). Effects of the overdoses included severe nausea, severe vomiting, and rapidly declining blood glucose concentrations. One of the 3 patients experienced severe hypoglycemia requiring parenteral glucose administration. The 3 patients recovered without complication.

➤*Treatment:* In the event of overdose, initiate appropriate supportive treatment according to the patient's clinical signs and symptoms.

Patient Information

Inform patients of the potential risks and benefits of exenatide and of alternative modes of therapy. Also, fully inform patients about self-management practices, including the importance of proper storage of exenatide, injection technique, timing of dosage of exenatide as well as concomitant oral drugs, adherence to meal planning, regular physical activity, periodic blood glucose monitoring and glycosylated hemoglobin (HbA_{1c}) testing, recognition and management of hypoglycemia and hyperglycemia, and assessment for diabetes complications.

Advise patients to inform their health care provider if they are pregnant or intend to become pregnant.

Instruct patients to administer each dose of exenatide as a subcutaneous injection in the thigh, abdomen, or upper arm at any time within the 60-minute period before the morning and evening meals (or before the 2 main meals of the day, approximately 6 or more hours apart). Do not administer exenatide after a meal. If a dose is missed, resume the treatment regimen as prescribed with the next scheduled dose.

Advise patients that the risk of hypoglycemia is increased when exenatide is used in combination with an agent that induces hypoglycemia, such as a sulfonylurea. Explain to the patient the symptoms, treatment, and conditions that predispose development of hypoglycemia. While the patient's usual instructions for hypoglycemia management do not need to be changed, review these instructions and reinforce them when initiating exenatide therapy, particularly when coadministered with a sulfonylurea.

Advise patients that treatment with exenatide may result in a reduction in appetite, food intake, and/or body weight, and that there is no need to modify the dosing regimen because of such effects. Treatment with exenatide may also result in nausea, particularly upon initiation of therapy.

Inform patients that persistent, severe abdominal pain that may radiate to the back and that may or may not be accompanied by vomiting is the hallmark symptom of acute pancreatitis. Instruct patients to promptly discontinue exenatide and contact their health care provider if persistent, severe abdominal pain occurs.

Inform patients treated with exenatide of the potential risk for worsening renal function and about associated signs and symptoms of renal dysfunction, as well as the possibility of dialysis as a medical intervention if renal failure occurs.

Inform patients that serious hypersensitivity reactions have been reported during postmarketing use of exenatide. If symptoms of hypersensitivity reactions occur, patients must stop taking exenatide and seek medical advice promptly.

Advise patients to read the Medication Guide and the pen user manual before starting exenatide therapy and to review them each time the prescription is refilled. Instruct the patient on proper use and storage of the pen, emphasizing how and when to set up a new pen and noting that only one setup step is necessary at initial use. Advise patients not to share the pen and needles.

Inform patients that pen needles are not included with the pen and must be purchased separately. Advise patients which needle length and gauge to use.

LIRAGLUTIDE

Rx	**Victoza** (Novo Nordisk)	**Injection, solution:** 6 mg/mL	In 3 mL prefilled, multidose pens.[a]

[a] Also contains propylene glycol 14 mg and phenol 5.5 mg.

LIRAGLUTIDE — INJECTION

WARNING

Thyroid C-cell tumor risk – Liraglutide causes dose-dependent and treatment-duration–dependent thyroid C-cell tumors at clinically relevant exposures in both genders of rats and mice. It is unknown whether liraglutide causes thyroid C-cell tumors, including medullary thyroid carcinoma, in humans, as human relevance could not be ruled out by clinical or nonclinical studies. Liraglutide is contraindicated in patients with a personal or family history of medullary thyroid carcinoma and in patients with multiple endocrine neoplasia syndrome type 2 (MEN2). Based on the findings in rodents, monitoring with serum calcitonin or thyroid ultrasound was performed during clinical trials, but this may have increased the number of unnecessary thyroid surgeries. It is unknown whether monitoring with serum calcitonin or thyroid ultrasound will mitigate human risk of thyroid C-cell tumors. Counsel patients regarding the risk and symptoms of thyroid tumors.

Indications

➤*Type 2 diabetes mellitus:* As an adjunct to diet and exercise to improve glycemic control in adults with type 2 diabetes mellitus.

➤*Important limitations of use:* Because of the uncertain relevance of the rodent thyroid C-cell tumor findings to humans, prescribe liraglutide only to patients for whom the potential benefits are considered to outweigh the potential risk. Liraglutide is not recommended as first-line therapy for patients who have inadequate glycemic control on diet and exercise.

The concurrent use of liraglutide and insulin has not been studied.

Administration and Dosage

➤*General dosing considerations:* The 0.6 mg dose is a starting dose intended to reduce GI symptoms during initial titration and is not effective for glycemic control.

➤*Adults:*

Type 2 diabetes mellitus –

Initial dosage: 0.6 mg subcutaneously per day for 1 week.

Dosage titration: After 1 week at 0.6 mg/day subcutaneously, the dose should be increased to 1.2 mg. If the 1.2 mg dose does not result in acceptable glycemic control, the dose can be increased to 1.8 mg.

Concomitant therapy: When initiating liraglutide, consider reducing the dose of administered insulin secretagogues (such as sulfonylureas) to reduce the risk of hypoglycemia.

LIRAGLUTIDE — INJECTION

➤*Administration:* Liraglutide can be administered once daily at any time of day, independently of meals, and can be injected subcutaneously in the abdomen, thigh, or upper arm. The injection site and timing can be changed without dose adjustment.

➤*Storage / Stability:* Prior to first use, store liraglutide in a refrigerator between 2° and 8°C (36° and 46°F). Do not store in the freezer or directly adjacent to the refrigerator cooling element. Do not freeze liraglutide and do not use if it has been frozen.

After initial use of the liraglutide pen, the pen can be stored for 30 days at 15° to 30°C (59° to 86°F) or in a refrigerator (2° to 8°C [36° to 46°F]). Keep the pen cap on when not in use. Protect from excessive heat and sunlight. Always remove and safely discard the needle after each injection and store the liraglutide pen without an injection needle attached. This will reduce the potential for contamination, infection, and leakage, while also ensuring dosing accuracy.

Liraglutide Pen Recommended Storage Conditions		
Prior to first use	After first use	
Refrigerated 2° to 8°C (36° to 46°F)	Room temperature 15° to 30°C (59° to 86°F)	Refrigerated 2° to 8°C (36° to 46°F)
Until expiration date	30 days	

Actions

➤*Pharmacology:* Liraglutide is an acylated glucagonlike peptide 1 (GLP-1) receptor agonist with 97% amino acid sequence homology to endogenous human GLP-1(7-37). GLP-1(7-37) represents less than 20% of total circulating endogenous GLP-1. Like GLP-1(7-37), liraglutide activates the GLP-1 receptor, a membrane-bound cell-surface receptor coupled to adenylyl cyclase by the stimulatory G-protein, Gs, in pancreatic beta cells. Liraglutide increases intracellular cyclic AMP (cAMP), leading to insulin release in the presence of elevated glucose concentrations. This insulin secretion subsides as blood glucose concentrations decrease and approach euglycemia. Liraglutide also decreases glucagon secretion in a glucose-dependent manner. The mechanism of blood-glucose lowering also involves a delay in gastric emptying.

GLP-1(7-37) has a half-life of 1.5 to 2 minutes because of degradation by the ubiquitous endogenous enzymes, dipeptidyl peptidase IV (DPPIV) and neutral endopeptidases (NEP). Unlike native GLP-1, liraglutide is stable against metabolic degradation by both peptidases and has a plasma half-life of 13 hours after subcutaneous administration. The pharmacokinetic profile of liraglutide, which makes it suitable for once-daily administration, is a result of self-association that delays absorption, plasma protein binding, and stability against metabolic degradation by DPPIV and NEP.

Pharmacodynamics – Liraglutide's pharmacodynamic profile is consistent with its pharmacokinetic profile observed after single subcutaneous administration, as liraglutide lowered fasting, premeal, and postprandial glucose throughout the day.

Fasting and postprandial glucose were measured before and for up to 5 hours after a standardized meal after treatment to steady state with liraglutide 0.6, 1.2, and 1.8 mg, or placebo. Compared with placebo, the postprandial plasma glucose area under the time curve ($AUC_{0\text{-}300min}$) was 35% lower after liraglutide 1.2 mg and 38% lower after liraglutide 1.8 mg.

Glucagon secretion: Liraglutide lowered blood glucose by stimulating insulin secretion and lowering glucagon secretion. A single dose of liraglutide 7.5 mcg/kg (approximately 0.7 mg) did not impair glucagon response to low glucose concentrations.

Gastric emptying: Liraglutide causes a delay of gastric emptying, thereby reducing the rate at which postprandial glucose appears in the circulation.

➤*Pharmacokinetics:*

Absorption – Following subcutaneous administration, maximum concentrations of liraglutide are achieved at 8 to 12 hours postdosing. The mean peak (C_{max}) and total (AUC) exposures of liraglutide were 35 ng/mL and 960 ng•h /mL, respectively, for a subcutaneous single dose of 0.6 mg. After subcutaneous single-dose administrations, C_{max} and AUC of liraglutide increased proportionally over the therapeutic dose range of 0.6 to 1.8 mg. At 1.8 mg of liraglutide, the average steady-state concentration of liraglutide over 24 hours was approximately 128 ng/mL. $AUC_{0-\infty}$ was equivalent between the upper arm and abdomen, and between the upper arm and thigh. $AUC_{0-\infty}$ from the thigh was 22% lower than that from the abdomen. However, liraglutide exposures were considered comparable among these 3 subcutaneous injection sites. Absolute bioavailability of liraglutide following subcutaneous administration is approximately 55%.

Distribution – The mean apparent volume of distribution after subcutaneous administration of liraglutide 0.6 mg is approximately 13 L. The mean volume of distribution after intravenous (IV) administration of liraglutide is 0.07 L/kg. Liraglutide is extensively bound to plasma protein (more than 98%).

Metabolism – During the initial 24 hours following administration of a single [^{3}H]-liraglutide dose to healthy subjects, the major component in plasma was intact liraglutide. Liraglutide is endogenously metabolized in a similar manner to large proteins without a specific organ as a major route of elimination.

Excretion – Following a [^{3}H]-liraglutide dose, intact liraglutide was not detected in urine or feces. Only a minor part of the administered radioactivity was excreted as liraglutide-related metabolites in urine or feces (6% and 5%, respectively). The majority of urine and feces radioactivity was excreted during the first 6 to 8 days. The mean apparent clearance following subcutaneous administration of a single dose of liraglutide is approximately 1.2 L/h with an elimination half-life of approximately 13 hours, making liraglutide suitable for once-daily administration.

Special populations –

Renal function impairment: Compared with healthy subjects, liraglutide AUC in mild, moderate, and severe renal impairment, and in end-stage renal disease was on average 35%, 19%, 29%, and 30% lower, respectively.

Hepatic function impairment: Compared with healthy subjects, liraglutide AUC in subjects with mild, moderate, and severe hepatic impairment was on average 11%, 14%, and 42% lower, respectively.

Gender: Based on the results of population pharmacokinetic analyses, women have a 34% lower weight-adjusted clearance of liraglutide compared with men.

Body weight: Body weight significantly affects the pharmacokinetics of liraglutide based on results of population pharmacokinetic analyses. The exposure of liraglutide decreases with an increase in baseline body weight. However, the doses of liraglutide 1.2 and 1.8 mg daily provided adequate systemic exposures over the body weight range of 40 to 160 kg evaluated in the clinical trials. Liraglutide was not studied in patients with body weight more than 160 kg.

Contraindications

Patients with a personal or family history of medullary thyroid carcinoma or in patients with MEN2.

Warnings/Precautions

➤*Thyroid C-cell tumors:* Liraglutide causes dose-dependent and treatment-duration–dependent thyroid C-cell tumors (adenomas and/or carcinomas) at clinically relevant exposures in both genders of rats and mice. Malignant thyroid C-cell carcinomas were detected in rats and mice. A statistically significant increase in cancer was observed in rats receiving liraglutide at 8 times the clinical exposure compared with controls. It is unknown whether liraglutide will cause thyroid C-cell tumors, including medullary thyroid carcinoma, in humans, as the human relevance of liraglutide-induced rodent thyroid C-cell tumors could not be determined by clinical or nonclinical studies.

In the clinical trials, there have been 4 reported cases of thyroid C-cell hyperplasia among liraglutide-treated patients and 1 case in a comparator-treated patient (1.3 vs 0.6 cases per 1,000 patient-years). One additional case of thyroid C-cell hyperplasia in a liraglutide-treated patient and 1 case of medullary thyroid carcinoma in a comparator-treated patient have subsequently been reported. This comparator-treated patient with medullary thyroid carcinoma had pretreatment serum calcitonin concentrations more than 1,000 ng/L, suggesting preexisting disease. All of these cases were diagnosed after thyroidectomy, which was prompted by abnormal results on routine, protocol-specified measurements of serum calcitonin. Four of the 5 liraglutide-treated patients had elevated calcitonin concentrations at baseline and throughout the trial. One liraglutide and one non-liraglutide–treated patient developed elevated calcitonin concentrations while on treatment.

Calcitonin, a biological marker of medullary thyroid carcinoma, was measured throughout the clinical development program. The serum calcitonin assay used in the liraglutide clinical trials had a lower limit of quantification (LLOQ) of 0.7 ng/L, and the upper limit of the reference range was 5 ng/L for women and 8.4 ng/L for men. At weeks 26 and 52 in the clinical trials, adjusted mean serum calcitonin concentrations were higher in liraglutide-treated patients compared with placebo-treated patients but not compared with patients receiving active comparator. At these timepoints, the adjusted mean serum calcitonin values (approximately 1 ng/L) were just above the LLOQ, with between-group differences in adjusted mean serum calcitonin values of approximately 0.1 ng/L or less. Among patients with pretreatment serum calcitonin below the upper limit of the reference range, shifts to above the upper limit of the reference range that persisted in subsequent measurements occurred most frequently among patients treated with liraglutide 1.8 mg/day. In trials with on-treatment serum calcitonin measurements out to 5 to 6 months, 1.9% of patients treated with liraglutide 1.8 mg/day developed new and persistent calcitonin elevations above the upper limit of the reference range compared with 0.8% to 1.1% of patients treated with control medication or the 0.6 and 1.2 mg doses of liraglutide. In trials with on-treatment serum calcitonin measurements out to 12 months, 1.3% of patients treated with liraglutide 1.8 mg/day had new and persistent elevations of calcitonin from below or within the reference range to above the upper limit of the reference range, compared with 0.6%, 0%, and 1% of patients treated with liraglutide 1.2 mg, placebo, and active control, respectively. Otherwise, liraglutide did not produce consistent dose-dependent or time-dependent increases in serum calcitonin.

Patients with medullary thyroid carcinoma usually have calcitonin values more than 50 ng/L. In liraglutide clinical trials, among patients with pretreatment serum calcitonin less than 50 ng/L, one liraglutide-treated patient and no comparator-treated patients developed serum calcitonin more than 50 ng/L. The liraglutide-treated patient who developed serum calcitonin more than 50 ng/L had an elevated pretreatment serum calcitonin of 10.7 ng/L that increased to 30.7 ng/L at week 12 and 53.5 ng/L at the end of the 6-month trial. Follow-up serum calcitonin was 22.3 ng/L more than 2.5 years after the last dose of liraglutide. The largest increase in serum calcitonin in a comparator-treated patient was seen with glimepiride in a patient whose serum calcitonin increased from 19.3 ng/L at baseline to 44.8 ng/L at week 65 and 38.1 ng/L at week 104. Among patients who began with serum calcitonin less than 20 ng/L, calcitonin elevations to more than 20 ng/L occurred in 0.7% of liraglutide-treated patients, 0.3% of placebo-treated patients, and 0.5% of active-comparator–treated patients, with an incidence of 1.1% among patients treated with 1.8 mg/day of liraglutide. The clinical significance of these findings is unknown.

LIRAGLUTIDE — INJECTION

Counsel patients regarding the risk for medullary thyroid carcinoma and the symptoms of thyroid tumors (eg, a mass in the neck, dysphagia, dyspnea or persistent hoarseness). It is unknown whether monitoring with serum calcitonin or thyroid ultrasound will mitigate the potential risk of medullary thyroid carcinoma, and such monitoring may increase the risk of unnecessary procedures because of low test specificity for serum calcitonin and a high background incidence of thyroid disease. Patients with thyroid nodules noted on physical examination or neck imaging obtained for other reasons should be referred to an endocrinologist for further evaluation. Although routine monitoring of serum calcitonin is of uncertain value in patients treated with liraglutide, if serum calcitonin is measured and found to be elevated, the patient should be referred to an endocrinologist for further evaluation.

➤*Pancreatitis:* In clinical trials of liraglutide, there were 7 cases of pancreatitis among liraglutide-treated patients and 1 case among comparator-treated patients (2.2 vs 0.6 cases per 1,000 patient-years). Five cases with liraglutide were reported as acute pancreatitis and 2 cases with liraglutide were reported as chronic pancreatitis. In 1 case in a liraglutide-treated patient, pancreatitis with necrosis was observed and led to death; however, clinical causality could not be established. One additional case of pancreatitis has subsequently been reported in a liraglutide-treated patient. Some patients had other risk factors for pancreatitis, such as a history of cholelithiasis or alcohol abuse. There are no conclusive data establishing a risk of pancreatitis with liraglutide treatment. After initiation of liraglutide and after dose increases, observe patients carefully for signs and symptoms of pancreatitis (including persistent severe abdominal pain sometimes radiating to the back and that may or may not be accompanied by vomiting). If pancreatitis is suspected, promptly discontinue liraglutide and other potentially suspect medications, perform confirmatory tests, and initiate appropriate management. If pancreatitis is confirmed, liraglutide should not be restarted. Use with caution in patients with a history of pancreatitis.

➤*Macrovascular outcomes:* There have been no clinical studies establishing conclusive evidence of macrovascular risk reduction with liraglutide or any other antidiabetic drug.

➤*Insulin:* Liraglutide is not a substitute for insulin. Do not use liraglutide in patients with type 1 diabetes mellitus or for the treatment of diabetic ketoacidosis because it would not be effective in these settings.

➤*Gastroparesis:* Liraglutide slows gastric emptying. Liraglutide has not been studied in patients with preexisting gastroparesis.

➤*Immunogenicity:* Consistent with the potentially immunogenic properties of protein and peptide pharmaceuticals, patients treated with liraglutide may develop anti-liraglutide antibodies. Approximately 50% to 70% of liraglutide-treated patients in the 5 clinical trials of 26 weeks duration or longer were tested for the presence of anti-liraglutide antibodies at the end of treatment. Low titers (concentrations not requiring dilution of serum) of anti-liraglutide antibodies were detected in 8.6% of these liraglutide-treated patients. Sampling was not performed uniformly across all patients in the clinical trials, and this may have resulted in an underestimate of the actual percentage of patients who developed antibodies. Cross-reacting anti-liraglutide antibodies to native GLP-1 occurred in 6.9% of the liraglutide-treated patients in the 52-week monotherapy trial and in 4.8% of the liraglutide-treated patients in the 26-week add-on combination therapy trials. These cross-reacting antibodies were not tested for neutralizing effects against native GLP-1, and thus the potential for clinically significant neutralization of native GLP-1 was not assessed. Antibodies that had a neutralizing effect on liraglutide in an in vitro assay occurred in 2.3% of the liraglutide-treated patients in the 52-week monotherapy trial and in 1% of the liraglutide-treated patients in the 26-week add-on combination therapy trials.

Among liraglutide-treated patients who developed anti-liraglutide antibodies, the most common category of adverse reactions was infections, which occurred among 40% of these patients compared with 36%, 34%, and 35% of antibody-negative liraglutide-treated, placebo-treated, and active-control-treated patients, respectively. The specific infections that occurred with greater frequency among liraglutide-treated antibody-positive patients were primarily nonserious upper respiratory tract infections, which occurred among 11% of liraglutide-treated antibody-positive patients; and among 7%, 7%, and 5% of antibody-negative liraglutide-treated, placebo-treated, and active-control-treated patients, respectively. Among liraglutide-treated antibody-negative patients, the most common category of adverse reactions was that of GI events, which occurred in 43%, 18%, and 19% of antibody-negative liraglutide-treated, placebo-treated, and active-control-treated patients, respectively. Antibody formation was not associated with reduced efficacy of liraglutide when comparing mean HbA_{1c} of all antibody-positive and all antibody-negative patients. However, the 3 patients with the highest titers of anti-liraglutide antibodies had no reduction in HbA_{1c} with liraglutide treatment.

In clinical trials of liraglutide, reactions from a composite of adverse reactions potentially related to immunogenicity (eg, urticaria, angioedema) occurred among 0.8% of liraglutide-treated patients and among 0.4% of comparator-treated patients. Urticaria accounted for approximately one-half of the reactions in this composite for liraglutide-treated patients. Patients who developed anti-liraglutide antibodies were not more likely to develop reactions from the immunogenicity events composite than were patients who did not develop anti-liraglutide antibodies.

➤*Renal function impairment:* There is limited experience in patients with mild, moderate, and severe renal impairment, including end-stage renal disease. Therefore, use liraglutide with caution in this patient population. No dose adjustment of liraglutide is recommended for patients with renal impairment.

➤*Hepatic function impairment:* There is limited experience in patients with mild, moderate, or severe hepatic impairment. Therefore, use liraglutide with caution in this patient population. No dose adjustment of liraglutide is recommended for patients with hepatic impairment.

➤*Pregnancy: Category C.* There are no adequate and well-controlled studies of liraglutide in pregnant women. Use liraglutide during pregnancy only if the potential benefit justifies the potential risk to the fetus.

Liraglutide has been shown to be teratogenic in rats at or above 0.8 times the human systemic exposures resulting from the maximum recommended human dose (MRHD) of 1.8 mg/day based on plasma AUC. Liraglutide has been shown to cause reduced growth and increased total major abnormalities in rabbits at systemic exposures below human exposure at the MRHD based on plasma AUC.

Female rats given subcutaneous dosages of liraglutide 0.1, 0.25, and 1 mg/kg/day beginning 2 weeks before mating through gestation day 17 had estimated systemic exposures 0.8, 3, and 11 times the human exposure at the MRHD based on plasma AUC comparison. The number of early embryonic deaths in the 1 mg/kg/day group increased slightly. Fetal abnormalities and variations in kidneys and blood vessels, irregular ossification of the skull, and a more complete state of ossification occurred at all doses. Mottled liver and minimally kinked ribs occurred at the highest dose. The incidence of fetal malformations in liraglutide-treated groups exceeding concurrent and historical controls were misshapen oropharynx and/or narrowed opening into larynx at 0.1 mg/kg/day and umbilical hernia at 0.1 and 0.25 mg/kg/day.

Pregnant rabbits given subcutaneous dosages of liraglutide 0.01, 0.025, and 0.05 mg/kg/day from gestation day 6 through day 18 inclusive, had estimated systemic exposures less than the human exposure at the MRHD of 1.8 mg/day at all dosages based on plasma AUC. Liraglutide decreased fetal weight and dose-dependently increased the incidence of total major fetal abnormalities at all doses. The incidence of malformations exceeded concurrent and historical controls at 0.01 mg/kg/day (kidneys, scapula), at least 0.01 mg/kg/day (eyes, forelimb), 0.025 mg/kg/day (brain, tail, and sacral vertebrae; major blood vessels and heart; umbilicus), at least 0.025 mg/kg/day (sternum), and at 0.05 mg/kg/day (parietal bones, major blood vessels). Irregular ossification and/or skeletal abnormalities occurred in the skull and jaw, vertebrae and ribs, sternum, pelvis, tail, and scapula; and dose-dependent minor skeletal variations were observed. Visceral abnormalities occurred in blood vessels, lung, liver, and esophagus. Bilobed or bifurcated gallbladder was seen in all treatment groups, but not in the control group.

In pregnant female rats given subcutaneous dosages of liraglutide 0.1, 0.25, and 1 mg/kg/day from gestation day 6 through weaning or termination of nursing on lactation day 24, estimated systemic exposures were 0.8, 3, and 11 times human exposure at the MRHD of 1.8 mg/day based on plasma AUC. A slight delay in parturition was observed in the majority of treated rats. Group mean body weight of neonatal rats from liraglutide-treated dams was lower than neonatal rats from control group dams. Bloody scabs and agitated behavior occurred in male rats descended from dams treated with liraglutide 1 mg/kg/day. Group mean body weight from birth to postpartum day 14 trended lower in F_2 generation rats descended from liraglutide-treated rats compared with F_2 generation rats descended from controls, but differences did not reach statistical significance for any group.

➤*Lactation:* It is not known whether liraglutide is excreted in human milk. Because many drugs are excreted in human milk and because of the potential for tumorigenicity shown for liraglutide in animal studies, decide whether to discontinue breast-feeding or liraglutide, taking into account the importance of the drug to the mother. In lactating rats, liraglutide was excreted unchanged in milk at concentrations approximately 50% of maternal plasma concentrations.

➤*Children:* Safety and effectiveness of liraglutide have not been established in children. Liraglutide is not recommended for use in children.

➤*Elderly:* No overall differences in safety or effectiveness were observed between these patients and younger patients, but greater sensitivity of some older individuals cannot be ruled out.

➤*Monitoring:* Periodically measure blood glucose and HbA_{1c} with a goal of decreasing these levels toward the normal range.

Although routine monitoring of serum calcitonin is of uncertain value in patients treated with liraglutide, if serum calcitonin is measured and found to be elevated, refer the patient to an endocrinologist for further evaluation.

After initiation of liraglutide and after dose increases, observe patients carefully for signs and symptoms of pancreatitis (including persistent severe abdominal pain, sometimes radiating to the back that may or may not be accompanied by vomiting).

Drug Interactions

➤*Oral medications:* Liraglutide causes a delay of gastric emptying, and thereby has the potential to impact the absorption of administered oral medications. Exercise caution when oral medications are coadministered with liraglutide.

Liraglutide Drug Interactions

Precipitant drug	Object drug[a]		Description
Antidiabetic agents (eg, sulfonylureas)	Liraglutide	↑	The risk of hypoglycemia may be increased when used with other antidiabetic agents. A lower dose of the antidiabetic may be needed.
Liraglutide	Antidiabetic agents (eg, sulfonylureas)		

LIRAGLUTIDE — INJECTION

Liraglutide Drug Interactions

Precipitant drug	Object drug[a]		Description
Liraglutide	Acetaminophen	⬇	When coadministered, acetaminophen C_{max} was decreased by 31% and T_{max}[b] was delayed up to 15 minutes; overall AUC was unchanged.
Liraglutide	Atorvastatin	⬇	Coadministration of liraglutide decreased atorvastatin C_{max} 38% and T_{max} was delayed 1 to 3 hours; overall AUC was unchanged.
Liraglutide	Digoxin	⬇	Coadministration of liraglutide decreased digoxin AUC 16%, C_{max} 31%, and delayed T_{max} approximately 1 to 1.5 hours.
Liraglutide	Griseofulvin	⬆	Griseofulvin C_{max} increased by 37%, while T_{max} and overall AUC did not change.

[a] ⬇ = object drug decreased; ⬆ = object drug increased.
[b] T_{max} = time of maximal concentration.

Adverse Reactions

➤*Discontinuation:* The incidence of withdrawal because of adverse reactions was 7.8% for liraglutide-treated patients and 3.4% for comparator-treated patients in the 5 controlled trials of 26 weeks duration or longer. This difference was driven by withdrawals because of GI adverse reactions, which occurred in 5% of liraglutide-treated patients and 0.5% of comparator-treated patients. The most common adverse reactions leading to withdrawal for liraglutide-treated patients were nausea (2.8% vs 0% for comparator) and vomiting (1.5% vs 0.1% for comparator). Withdrawal because of GI adverse reactions mainly occurred during the first 2 to 3 months of the trials.

➤*Adverse reactions (5% or more):*

Liraglutide vs Glimepiride Adverse Reactions (≥ 5%)

Adverse reactions	Liraglutide (n = 497)	Glimepiride (n = 248)
CNS		
Dizziness	5.8%	5.2%
Headache	9.1%	9.3%
GI		
Constipation	9.9%	4.8%
Diarrhea	17.1%	8.9%
Nausea	28.4%	8.5%
Vomiting	10.9%	3.6%
Respiratory		
Nasopharyngitis	5.2%	5.2%
Sinusitis	5.6%	6.0%
Upper respiratory tract infection	9.5%	5.6%
Miscellaneous		
Back pain	5%	4.4%
Hypertension	3%	6%
Influenza	7.4%	3.6%
Urinary tract infection	6%	4%

Liraglutide Adverse Reactions (≥ 5%) 26-Week Combination Therapy Trials

Adverse reactions	Liraglutide + metformin (n = 724)	Placebo + metformin (n = 121)	Glimepiride + metformin (n = 242)
Add-on to metformin trial			
CNS			
Headache	9%	6.6%	9.5%
GI			
Diarrhea	10.9%	4.1%	3.7%
Nausea	15.2%	4.1%	3.3%
Vomiting	6.5%	0.8%	0.4%
Add-on to glimepiride trial			
	Liraglutide + glimepiride (n = 695)	Placebo + glimepiride (n = 114)	Rosiglitazone + glimepiride (n = 231)
GI			
Constipation	5.3%	0.9%	1.7%
Diarrhea	7.2%	1.8%	2.2%
Dyspepsia	5.2%	0.9%	2.6%
Nausea	7.5%	1.8%	2.6%
Add-on to metformin + glimepiride			
	Liraglutide 1.8 mg + metformin + glimepiride (n = 230)	Placebo + metformin + glimepiride (n = 114)	Insulin glargine + metformin + glimepiride (n = 232)
CNS			
Headache	9.6%	7.9%	5.6%
GI			
Diarrhea	10%	5.3%	1.3%
Dyspepsia	6.5%	0.9%	1.7%
Nausea	13.9%	3.5%	1.3%
Vomiting	6.5%	3.5%	0.4%
Add-on to metformin + rosiglitazone			
	Liraglutide + metformin + rosiglitazone (n = 355)	Placebo + metformin + rosiglitazone (n = 175)	—
CNS			
Fatigue	5.1%	1.7%	—
Headache	8.2%	4.6%	—
GI			
Anorexia	9%	0%	—
Constipation	5.1%	1.1%	—
Decreased appetite	9.3%	1.1%	—
Diarrhea	14.1%	6.3%	—
Nausea	34.6%	8.6%	—
Vomiting	12.4%	2.9%	—

➤*GI:* In the 5 clinical trials of 26 weeks duration or longer, GI adverse reactions were reported in 41% of liraglutide-treated patients and were dose-related. GI adverse reactions occurred in 17% of comparator-treated patients. Reactions that occurred more commonly among liraglutide-treated patients included nausea, vomiting, diarrhea, dyspepsia, and constipation. In clinical trials of 26 weeks duration or longer, the percentage of patients who reported nausea declined over time. Approximately 13% of liraglutide-treated patients and 2% of comparator-treated patients reported nausea during the first 2 weeks of treatment.

➤*Local:* Injection-site reactions (eg, erythema, injection-site rash) were reported in approximately 2% of liraglutide-treated patients in the 5 clinical trials of at least 26 weeks duration. Less than 0.2% of liraglutide-treated patients discontinued because of injection-site reactions.

➤*Papillary thyroid carcinoma:* In clinical trials of liraglutide, there were 6 reported cases of papillary thyroid carcinoma in patients treated with liraglutide and 1 case in a comparator-treated patient (1.9 vs 0.6 cases per 1,000 patient-years). Most of these papillary thyroid carcinomas were less than 1 cm in greatest diameter and were diagnosed in surgical pathology specimens after thyroidectomy prompted by findings on protocol-specified screening with serum calcitonin or thyroid ultrasound.

➤*Hypoglycemia:* In the clinical trials of at least 26 weeks duration, hypoglycemia requiring the assistance of another person for treatment occurred in 7 liraglutide-treated patients (2.6 cases per 1,000 patient-years) and in no comparator-treated patients. Six of these 7 patients treated with liraglutide were also taking a sulfonylurea. One other patient was taking liraglutide in combination with metformin but had another likely explanation for the hypoglycemia (this event occurred during hospitalization and after insulin infusion). Two additional cases of hypoglycemia requiring the assistance of another person for treatment have subsequently been reported in patients who were not taking a concomitant sulfonylurea. Both patients were receiving liraglutide, one as monotherapy and the other in combination with metformin. Both patients had another likely explanation for the hypoglycemia (one received insulin during a frequently-sampled IV glucose tolerance test, and the other had intracranial hemorrhage and uncertain food intake).

LIRAGLUTIDE — INJECTION

Incidence (%) and Rate (Episodes/Patient-Year) of Hypoglycemia in the Liraglutide 52-Week Monotherapy Trial and in the 26-Week Combination Therapy Trials

	Liraglutide treatment	Active comparator	Placebo comparator
Monotherapy	Liraglutide (n = 497)	Glimepiride (n = 248)	None
Patient not able to self-treat	0	0	—
Patient able to self-treat	9.7 (0.24)	25 (1.66)	—
Not classified	1.2 (0.03)	2.4 (0.04)	—
Add-on to metformin	Liraglutide + metformin (n = 724)	Glimepiride + metformin (n = 242)	Placebo + metformin (n = 121)
Patient not able to self-treat	0.1 (0.001)	0	0
Patient able to self-treat	3.6 (0.05)	22.3 (0.87)	2.5 (0.06)
Add-on to glimepiride	Liraglutide + glimepiride (n = 695)	Rosiglitazone + glimepiride (n = 231)	Placebo + glimepiride (n = 114)
Patient not able to self-treat	0.1 (0.003)	0	0
Patient able to self-treat	7.5 (0.38)	4.3 (0.12)	2.6 (0.17)
Not classified	0.9 (0.05)	0.9 (0.02)	0
Add-on to metformin + rosiglitazone	Liraglutide + metformin + rosiglitazone (n = 355)	None	Placebo + metformin + rosiglitazone (n = 175)
Patient not able to self-treat	0	—	0
Patient able to self-treat	7.9 (0.49)	—	4.6 (0.15)
Not classified	0.6 (0.01)	—	1.1 (0.03)
Add-on to metformin + glimepiride	Liraglutide + metformin + glimepiride (n = 230)	Insulin glargine + metformin + glimepiride (n = 232)	Placebo + metformin + glimepiride (n = 114)
Patient not able to self-treat	2.2 (0.06)	0	0
Patient able to self-treat	27.4 (1.16)	28.9 (1.29)	16.7 (0.95)
Not classified	0	1.7 (0.04)	0

➤*Malignant neoplasm:* In a pooled analysis of clinical trials, the incidence rate (per 1,000 patient-years) for malignant neoplasms (based on investigator-reported events, medical history, pathology reports, and surgical reports from both blinded and open-label study periods) was 10.9 for liraglutide, 6.3 for placebo, and 7.2 for active comparator. After excluding papillary thyroid carcinoma events, no particular cancer cell type predominated. Seven malignant neoplasm events were reported beyond 1 year of exposure to study medication, 6 events among liraglutide-treated patients (4 colon, 1 prostate, and 1 nasopharyngeal), no events with placebo, and 1 event with active comparator (colon). Causality has not been established.

➤*Lab test abnormalities:* In the 5 clinical trials of at least 26 weeks duration, mildly elevated serum bilirubin concentrations (elevations to no more than twice the upper limit of the reference range) occurred in 4% of liraglutide-treated patients, 2.1% of placebo-treated patients, and 3.5% of active-comparator-treated patients. This finding was not accompanied by abnormalities in other liver tests. The significance of this isolated finding is unknown.

Overdosage

➤*Symptoms:* In a clinical trial, 1 patient with type 2 diabetes experienced a single overdose of subcutaneous liraglutide 17.4 mg (10 times the maximum recommended dose). Effects of the overdose included severe nausea and vomiting requiring hospitalization. No hypoglycemia was reported. The patient recovered without complications.

➤*Treatment:* In the event of overdosage, initiate appropriate supportive treatment according to the patient's clinical signs and symptoms.

Patient Information

Inform patients that liraglutide causes benign and malignant thyroid C-cell tumors in mice and rats and that the human relevance of this finding is unknown. Counsel patients to report symptoms of thyroid tumors (eg, a lump in the neck, dysphagia, persistent hoarseness or dyspnea) to their health care provider.

Inform patients that persistent severe abdominal pain that may radiate to the back and that may (or may not) be accompanied by vomiting is the hallmark symptom of acute pancreatitis. Instruct patients to discontinue liraglutide promptly and to contact their health care provider if persistent severe abdominal pain occurs.

Counsel patients that they should never share a liraglutide pen with another person, even if the needle is changed. Sharing of the pen between patients may pose a risk of transmission of infection.

Inform patients of the potential risks and benefits of liraglutide and of alternative modes of therapy. Also inform patients about the importance of adherence to dietary instructions, regular physical activity, periodic blood glucose monitoring and HbA_{1c} testing, recognition and management of hypoglycemia and hyperglycemia, and assessment for diabetes complications. During periods of stress, such as fever, trauma, infection, or surgery, medication requirements may change; advise patients to seek medical advice promptly.

Advise patients that the most common side effects of liraglutide are headache, nausea, and diarrhea. Nausea is most common when first starting liraglutide, but decreases over time in the majority of patients and does not typically require discontinuation of liraglutide.

Instruct patients to inform their health care provider or pharmacist if they develop any unusual symptom or if any known symptom persists or worsens.

Inform patients that response to all diabetic therapies should be monitored by periodic measurements of blood glucose and HbA_{1c} levels, with a goal of decreasing these levels toward the normal range. HbA_{1c} is especially useful for evaluating long-term glycemic control.

SAXAGLIPTIN

Rx	**Onglyza** (Bristol-Myers Squibb)	**Tablets; oral:** 2.5 mg	Equiv. to saxagliptin hydrochloride 2.79 mg. Lactose. (2.5 4214). Pale to lt. yellow, round, biconvex. Film-coated. In 30s and 90s.
		5 mg	Equiv. to saxagliptin hydrochloride 5.58 mg. Lactose. (5 4215). Pink, round, biconvex. Film-coated. In 30s, 90s, 500s, and UD 100s.

SAXAGLIPTIN HYDROCHLORIDE — ORAL

Indications

➤*Type 2 diabetes mellitus:* As an adjunct to diet and exercise to improve glycemic control in adults with type 2 diabetes mellitus in multiple clinical settings.

Administration and Dosage

➤*General dosing considerations:* Reduced doses are required in patients with renal impairment. (See Renal Function Impairment.)

Reduced doses are required during coadministration with strong CYP3A4/5 inhibitors. (See Strong CYP3A4/5 Inhibitors.)

➤*Adults:*

Type 2 diabetes mellitus – 2.5 or 5 mg once daily.

➤*Elderly:* Because elderly patients are more likely to have decreased renal function, take care in dose selection based on renal function.

➤*Renal function impairment:*

Moderate or severe renal impairment (creatinine clearance 50 mL/min or less) – 2.5 mg once daily.

End-stage renal disease requiring hemodialysis – 2.5 mg once daily after hemodialysis.

➤*Strong CYP3A4/5 inhibitors:* The dosage of saxagliptin is 2.5 mg once daily when coadministered with CYP3A4/5 inhibitors (eg, ketoconazole, atazanavir, clarithromycin, indinavir, itraconazole, nefazodone, nelfinavir, ritonavir, saquinavir, telithromycin).

➤*Administration:* Instruct patients to take without regard to meals.

➤*Storage/Stability:* Store at 20° to 25°C (68° to 77°F); excursions are permitted between 15° and 30°C (59° and 86°F).

Actions

➤*Pharmacology:* Increased concentrations of the incretin hormones, such as glucagonlike peptide-1 (GLP-1) and glucose-dependent insulinotropic polypeptide (GIP) are released into the bloodstream from the small intestine in response to meals. These hormones cause insulin release from the pancreatic beta cells in a glucose-dependent manner, but are inactivated by the DPP4 enzyme within minutes. GLP-1 also lowers glucagon secretion from pancreatic alpha cells, reducing hepatic glucose production. In patients with type 2 diabetes, concentrations of GLP-1 are reduced but the insulin response to GLP-1 is preserved. Saxagliptin is a competitive DPP4 inhibitor that slows the inactivation of the incretin hormones, thereby increasing their bloodstream concentrations and reducing fasting and postprandial glucose concentrations in a glucose-dependent manner in patients with type 2 diabetes mellitus.

Pharmacodynamics – In patients with type 2 diabetes mellitus, administration of saxagliptin inhibits DPP4 enzyme activity for a 24-hour period. After an oral glucose load or a meal, this DPP4 inhibition resulted in a 2- to 3-fold increase in circulating levels of active GLP-1 and GIP, decreased glucagon concentrations, and increased glucose-dependent insulin secretion

SAXAGLIPTIN HYDROCHLORIDE — ORAL

from pancreatic beta cells. The rise in insulin and decrease in glucagon were associated with lower fasting glucose concentrations and reduced glucose excursion following an oral glucose load or a meal.

➤*Pharmacokinetics:*

Absorption – Following a 5 mg single oral dose of saxagliptin to healthy subjects, the mean plasma AUC values for saxagliptin and its active metabolite were 78 and 214 ng•h/mL, respectively. The corresponding plasma C_{max} values were 24 and 47 ng/mL, respectively. The average variability (percent coefficient of variation) for AUC and C_{max} for both saxagliptin and its active metabolite was less than 25%.

The median time to maximum concentration (T_{max}) following the 5 mg once-daily dose was 2 hours for saxagliptin and 4 hours for its active metabolite.

Effect of food: Administration with a high-fat meal resulted in an increase in T_{max} of saxagliptin by approximately 20 minutes compared with fasted conditions. There was a 27% increase in the AUC of saxagliptin when given with a meal compared with fasted conditions. Saxagliptin may be administered with or without food.

Distribution – The in vitro protein binding of saxagliptin and its active metabolite in human serum is negligible. Therefore, changes in blood protein levels in various disease states (eg, renal or hepatic impairment) are not expected to alter the disposition of saxagliptin.

Metabolism – The metabolism of saxagliptin is primarily mediated by CYP3A4/5. The major metabolite of saxagliptin is also a DPP4 inhibitor, which is one-half as potent as saxagliptin. Therefore, strong CYP3A4/5 inhibitors and inducers will alter the pharmacokinetics of saxagliptin and its active metabolite.

Excretion – Saxagliptin is eliminated by both renal and hepatic pathways. Following a single 50 mg dose of ^{14}C-saxagliptin, 24%, 36%, and 75% of the dose was excreted in the urine as saxagliptin, its active metabolite, and total radioactivity, respectively. The average renal clearance of saxagliptin (approximately 230 mL/min) was greater than the average estimated glomerular filtration rate (approximately 120 mL/min), suggesting some active renal excretion. A total of 22% of the administered radioactivity was recovered in feces, representing the fraction of the saxagliptin dose excreted in bile and/or unabsorbed drug from the GI tract. Following a single oral dose of saxagliptin 5 mg to healthy subjects, the mean plasma terminal half-life for saxagliptin and its active metabolite was 2.5 and 3.1 hours, respectively.

Special populations –

Renal function impairment: In subjects with moderate or severe renal impairment, the AUC values of saxagliptin and its active metabolite were up to 2.1- and 4.5-fold higher, respectively, than AUC values in subjects with healthy renal function. To achieve plasma exposures of saxagliptin and its active metabolite similar to those in patients with healthy renal function, the recommended dosage is 2.5 mg once daily in patients with moderate and severe renal impairment, as well as in patients with end-stage renal disease requiring hemodialysis. Saxagliptin is removed by hemodialysis.

Hepatic function impairment: In subjects with hepatic impairment (Child-Pugh classes A, B, and C), mean C_{max} and AUC of saxagliptin were up to 8% and 77% higher, respectively, compared with healthy matched controls following administration of a single dose of saxagliptin 10 mg. The corresponding C_{max} and AUC of the active metabolite were up to 59% and 33% lower, respectively, compared with healthy matched controls.

Elderly: Elderly subjects (65 to 80 years of age) had 23% and 59% higher geometric mean C_{max} and geometric mean AUC values, respectively, for saxagliptin than younger subjects (18 to 40 years of age). Differences in active metabolite pharmacokinetics between elderly and younger subjects generally reflected the differences observed in saxagliptin pharmacokinetics. The difference between the pharmacokinetics of saxagliptin and the active metabolite in younger and elderly subjects is likely caused by multiple factors, including declining renal function and metabolic capacity with increasing age.

Contraindications

None known.

Warnings/Precautions

➤*Pregnancy: Category B.* There are no adequate and well-controlled studies in pregnant women. Because animal reproduction studies are not always predictive of human response, use saxagliptin, like other antidiabetic medications, during pregnancy only if clearly needed.

Saxagliptin was not teratogenic at any dose tested when administered to pregnant rats and rabbits during periods of organogenesis. Incomplete ossification of the pelvis, a form of developmental delay, occurred in rats at a dose of 240 mg/kg, or approximately 1,503 and 66 times human exposure to saxagliptin and the active metabolite, respectively, at the maximum recommended human dose (MRHD) of 5 mg. Maternal toxicity and reduced fetal body weights were observed at 7,986 and 328 times the human exposure at the MRHD for saxagliptin and the active metabolite, respectively. Minor skeletal variations in rabbits occurred at a maternally toxic dose of 200 mg/kg, or approximately 1,432 and 992 times the MRHD. When administered to rats in combination with metformin, saxagliptin was not teratogenic nor embryolethal at exposures 21 times the saxagliptin MRHD. Combination administration of metformin with a higher dose of saxagliptin (109 times the saxagliptin MRHD) was associated with craniorachischisis (a rare neural tube defect characterized by incomplete closure of the skull and spinal column) in 2 fetuses from a single dam. Metformin exposures in each combination were 4 times the human exposure of 2,000 mg daily.

Saxagliptin administered to female rats from gestation day 6 to lactation day 20 resulted in decreased body weights in male and female offspring only at maternally toxic doses (exposures greater than or equal to 1,629 and 53 times saxagliptin and its active metabolite at the MRHD). No functional or behavioral toxicity was observed in offspring of rats administered saxagliptin at any dose.

Saxagliptin crosses the placenta following dosing in pregnant rats.

➤*Lactation:* Saxagliptin is secreted in the milk of lactating rats at approximately a 1:1 ratio with plasma drug concentrations. It is not known whether saxagliptin is secreted in human milk. The molecular weight of the parent compound (about 315 for the nonhydrated form), lipophilic properties, lack of plasma protein binding, and terminal half-lives (2.5 hours for saxagliptin and 3.1 hours for the active metabolite) suggest that saxagliptin and its metabolite will be excreted into breast milk. Because many drugs are secreted in human milk, exercise caution when saxagliptin is administered to a breast-feeding woman.

➤*Children:* Safety and effectiveness of saxagliptin in children have not been established.

➤*Elderly:* Saxagliptin and its active metabolite are eliminated in part by the kidney. Because elderly patients are more likely to have decreased renal function, take care in dose selection in elderly patients based on renal function.

➤*Monitoring:* Assessment of renal function is recommended prior to initiation of saxagliptin and periodically thereafter. Periodically measure blood glucose and glycosylated hemoglobin (HbA_{1c}), with a goal of decreasing these levels toward the normal range. When clinically indicated, such as in settings of unusual or prolonged infection, measure lymphocyte count.

Drug Interactions

➤*Cytochrome P-450 system:* Saxagliptin metabolism is primarily mediated by CYP3A4 and CYP3A5. The major metabolite of saxagliptin is one-half as potent as saxagliptin. Therefore, strong CYP3A4/5 inhibitors and inducers will alter the pharmacokinetics of saxagliptin and its active metabolite. Drugs that induce these enzyme systems may increase saxagliptin metabolism, decreasing saxagliptin plasma concentrations and efficacy. Drugs that inhibit these enzyme systems may interfere with saxagliptin metabolism, elevating saxagliptin plasma concentrations and increasing the pharmacologic effects and risk of adverse reactions. Monitoring the patient's clinical response and making the appropriate adjustments in dose is important in minimizing the risk of a drug interaction.

Saxagliptin Drug Interactions

Precipitant drug	Object drug[a]		Description
Aluminum hydroxide + magnesium hydroxide + simethicone	Saxagliptin	↓	Coadministration of a single dose of saxagliptin 10 mg and liquid aluminum hydroxide/magnesium hydroxide/simethicone decreased the C_{max} of saxagliptin 26% but did not alter the AUC.
CYP3A4/5 inducers (eg, rifampin)	Saxagliptin	↓	Exposure to saxagliptin may be decreased. Coadministration of a single dose of saxagliptin 5 mg and rifampin (600 mg daily at steady state) decreased the saxagliptin C_{max} and AUC 53% and 76%, respectively. There was a corresponding 39% increase in the C_{max} of saxagliptin active metabolite but no significant change in the AUC. However, dosage adjustment is not recommended. Monitor the clinical response of the patient. If an interaction is suspected, adjust the saxagliptin dose as needed.
Famotidine	Saxagliptin	↑	Coadministration of a single dose of saxagliptin 10 mg 3 hours after a single dose of famotidine 40 mg increased the saxagliptin C_{max} 14% but did not alter the AUC.
Glyburide	Saxagliptin	↑	Coadministration of a single dose of saxagliptin 10 mg and glyburide 5 mg increased the saxagliptin C_{max} 8% but did not alter the AUC. Similarly, C_{max} of glyburide increased 16% but the AUC was unchanged.
Saxagliptin	Glyburide		
Metformin	Saxagliptin	↓	Coadministration of a single dose of saxagliptin and metformin decreased the C_{max} by 21% of saxagliptin but did not alter the AUC.

SAXAGLIPTIN HYDROCHLORIDE — ORAL

Saxagliptin Drug Interactions			
Precipitant drug	Object drug[a]		Description
Moderate CYP3A4/5 inhibitors (eg, amprenavir, aprepitant, diltiazem, erythromycin, fluconazole, fosamprenavir, verapamil)	Saxagliptin	↑	Exposure to saxagliptin will be increased. However, dosage adjustment is not recommended. Monitor the clinical response of the patient. If an interaction is suspected, adjust the saxagliptin dose as needed.
Simvastatin	Saxagliptin	↑	Coadministration of multiple daily doses of saxagliptin 10 mg and simvastatin 40 mg increased the saxagliptin C_{max} 21% but did not alter the AUC.
Strong CYP3A4/5 inhibitors (eg, atazanavir, clarithromycin, indinavir, itraconazole, ketoconazole, nefazodone, nelfinavir, ritonavir, saquinavir, telithromycin)	Saxagliptin	↑	Coadministration of a single dose of saxagliptin and ketoconazole (at steady state) increased the saxagliptin C_{max} 62% and the AUC 2.5-fold. The C_{max} and AUC of the active metabolite of saxagliptin decreased 95% and 91%, respectively. Similar increases in saxagliptin are anticipated with other strong CYP3A4/5 inhibitors. The dose of saxagliptin should be limited to 2.5 mg when administered with a strong CYP3A4/5 inhibitor. Monitor the clinical response of the patient.
Saxagliptin	Antidiabetic agents (eg, sulfonylureas)	↑	The risk of hypoglycemia may be increased when used with other antidiabetic agents. A lower dose of the antidiabetic may be needed.
Saxagliptin	Diltiazem	↑	Coadministration of a single dose of saxagliptin 10 mg and diltiazem (360 mg long-acting formulation at steady state) increased the diltiazem C_{max} 16% but did not alter the AUC.
Saxagliptin	Ketoconazole	↓	Coadministration of a single dose of saxagliptin and ketoconazole (at steady state) decreased the ketoconazole C_{max} and AUC 16% and 13%, respectively.
Saxagliptin	Pioglitazone	↑	Coadministration of a single dose of saxagliptin 10 mg and pioglitazone 45 mg increased the pioglitazone C_{max} 14% but did not alter the AUC.

[a] ↑ = object drug increased; ↓ = object drug decreased.

➤*Drug/Food interactions:* High-fat meals increase saxagliptin T_{max} approximately 20 minutes compared with fasting. Compared with fasting, giving saxagliptin with a meal increases the AUC by 27%. Saxagliptin may be administered without regard to food. Grapefruit juice increases exposure to saxagliptin; however, dosage adjustment is not recommended.

Adverse Reactions

➤*Monotherapy and add-on combination therapy:*

Discontinuation – Discontinuation of therapy because of adverse reactions occurred in 2.2%, 3.3%, and 1.8% of patients receiving saxagliptin 2.5 mg, saxagliptin 5 mg, and placebo, respectively.

The most common adverse reactions (reported in at least 2 patients treated with saxagliptin 2.5 mg or at least 2 patients treated with saxagliptin 5 mg) associated with premature discontinuation of therapy included lymphopenia (0.1% and 0.5% vs 0%, respectively), rash (0.2% and 0.3% vs 0.3%), blood creatinine increased (0.3% and 0% vs 0%), and blood creatine phosphokinase increased (0.1% and 0.2% vs 0%).

Common adverse reactions –

Saxagliptin Adverse Reactions (≥ 5%)[a]		
Adverse reaction	Saxagliptin 5 mg (n = 882)	Placebo (n = 799)
Headache	6.5%	5.9%
Upper respiratory tract infection	7.7%	7.6%
Urinary tract infection	6.8%	6.1%

[a] The 5 placebo-controlled trials include 2 monotherapy trials and 1 add-on combination therapy trial with each of the following: metformin, thiazolidinedione, or glyburide. The table shows 24-week data regardless of glycemic rescue.

Other adverse reactions – In this pooled analysis, adverse reactions that were reported in at least 2% of patients treated with saxagliptin 2.5 mg or saxagliptin 5 mg and at least 1% more frequently compared with placebo included: sinusitis (2.9% and 2.6% vs 1.6%, respectively), abdominal pain (2.4% and 1.7% vs 0.5%), gastroenteritis (1.9% and 2.3% vs 0.9%), and vomiting (2.2% and 2.3% vs 1.3%).

In the add-on to thiazolidinedione trial, the incidence of peripheral edema was higher for saxagliptin 5 mg versus placebo (8.1% and 4.3%, respectively). The incidence of peripheral edema for saxagliptin 2.5 mg was 3.1%. None of the reported adverse reactions of peripheral edema resulted in study drug discontinuation. Rates of peripheral edema for saxagliptin 2.5 mg and saxagliptin 5 mg versus placebo were 3.6% and 2% versus 3% given as monotherapy, 2.1% and 2.1% versus 2.2% given as add-on therapy to metformin, and 2.4% and 1.2% versus 2.2% given as add-on therapy to glyburide.

The incidence rate of fractures was 1 and 0.6 per 100 patient-years, respectively, for saxagliptin (pooled analysis of 2.5 mg, 5 mg, and 10 mg) and placebo. The incidence rate of fracture reactions in patients who received saxagliptin did not increase over time. Causality has not been established and nonclinical studies have not demonstrated adverse effects of saxagliptin on bone.

A reaction of thrombocytopenia, consistent with a diagnosis of idiopathic thrombocytopenic purpura, was observed in the clinical program. The relationship of this reaction to saxagliptin is not known.

Saxagliptin coadministered with metformin in treatment-naive patients –

Saxagliptin and Metformin Adverse Reactions in Treatment-Naive Patients (≥ 5%)		
Adverse reactions	Saxagliptin 5 mg + metformin[a] (n = 320)	Metformin[a] (n = 328)
Headache	7.5%	5.2%
Nasopharyngitis	6.9%	4%

[a] Metformin was initiated at a starting dosage of 500 mg daily and titrated up to a maximum of 2,000 mg daily.

➤*Hypoglycemia:* Adverse reactions of hypoglycemia were based on all reports of hypoglycemia; a concurrent glucose measurement was not required. In the add-on to glyburide study, the overall incidence of reported hypoglycemia was higher for saxagliptin 2.5 and 5 mg (13.3% and 14.6%) versus placebo (10.1%). The incidence of confirmed hypoglycemia in this study, defined as symptoms of hypoglycemia accompanied by a fingerstick glucose value of 50 mg/dL or less, was 2.4% and 0.8% for saxagliptin 2.5 and 5 mg and 0.7% for placebo. The incidence of reported hypoglycemia for saxagliptin 2.5 and 5 mg versus placebo given as monotherapy was 4% and 5.6% versus 4.1%, respectively, 7.8% and 5.8% versus 5% given as add-on therapy to metformin, and 4.1% and 2.7% versus 3.8% given as add-on therapy to thiazolidinedione. The incidence of reported hypoglycemia was 3.4% in treatment-naive patients given saxagliptin 5 mg plus metformin and 4% in patients given metformin alone.

➤*Hypersensitivity reactions:* Hypersensitivity-related reactions, such as urticaria and facial edema, in the 5-study pooled analysis up to week 24 were reported in 1.5%, 1.5%, and 0.4% of patients who received saxagliptin 2.5 mg, saxagliptin 5 mg, and placebo, respectively. None of these reactions in patients who received saxagliptin required hospitalization or were reported as life-threatening by the investigators. One saxagliptin-treated patient in this pooled analysis discontinued because of generalized urticaria and facial edema.

➤*Laboratory tests:*

Absolute lymphocyte counts – There was a dose-related mean decrease in absolute lymphocyte count observed with saxagliptin. From a baseline mean absolute lymphocyte count of approximately 2,200 cells/mcL, mean decreases of approximately 100 and 120 cells/mcL with saxagliptin 5 and 10 mg, respectively, relative to placebo were observed at 24 weeks in a pooled analysis of 5 placebo-controlled clinical studies. Similar effects were observed when saxagliptin 5 mg was given in initial combination with metformin compared with metformin alone. There was no difference observed for saxagliptin 2.5 mg relative to placebo. The proportion of patients who were reported to have a lymphocyte count of 750 cells/mcL or less was 0.5%, 1.5%, 1.4%, and 0.4% in the saxagliptin 2.5, 5, and 10 mg and placebo groups, respectively. In most patients, recurrence was not observed with repeated exposure to saxagliptin, although some patients had recurrent decreases upon rechallenge that led to discontinuation of saxagliptin. The decreases in lymphocyte count were not associated with clinically relevant adverse reactions.

The clinical significance of this decreases in lymphocyte count relative to placebo is not known. When clinically indicated, such as in settings of

SAXAGLIPTIN HYDROCHLORIDE — ORAL

unusual or prolonged infection, measure lymphocyte count. The effect of saxagliptin on lymphocyte counts in patients with lymphocyte abnormalities (eg, HIV) is unknown.

Overdosage

➤*Treatment:* In the event of an overdose, appropriate supportive treatment should be initiated as dictated by the patient's clinical status. Saxagliptin and its active metabolite are removed by hemodialysis (23% of dose over 4 hours).

Patient Information

Instruct patients to read the patient package insert before starting saxagliptin therapy and to reread it each time the prescription is renewed.

Inform patients of the potential risks and benefits of saxagliptin and of alternative modes of therapy. Also inform patients about the importance of adherence to dietary instructions, regular physical activity, periodic blood glucose monitoring and HbA_{1c} testing, recognition and management of hypoglycemia and hyperglycemia, and assessment of diabetes complications.

Advise patients to seek medical advice promptly during periods of stress, such as fever, trauma, infection, or surgery, because medication requirements may change.

Instruct patients to inform their health care provider or pharmacist if they develop any unusual symptom or if any existing symptom persists or worsens.

Inform patients that response to all diabetic therapies will be monitored by periodic measurements of blood glucose and HbA_{1c}, with a goal of decreasing these levels toward the normal range. HbA_{1c} is especially useful for evaluating long-term glycemic control.

Inform patients of the potential need to adjust their dose based on changes in renal function tests over time.

SITAGLIPTIN

Rx	**Januvia** (Merck)	**Tablets; oral:** 25 mg	Equiv. to sitagliptin phosphate 32.13 mg. (221). Pink, round. Film-coated. In 30s, 90s, and UD 100s.
		50 mg	Equiv. to sitagliptin phosphate 64.25 mg. (112). Lt. beige, round. Film-coated. In 30s, 90s, and UD 100s.
		100 mg	Equiv. to sitagliptin phosphate 128.5 mg. (277). Beige, round. Film-coated. In 30s, 90s, 500s, 1,000s, and UD 100s.

SITAGLIPTIN PHOSPHATE — ORAL

Indications

➤*Type 2 diabetes mellitus:* As an adjunct to diet and exercise to improve glycemic control in adults with type 2 diabetes mellitus as monotherapy or combination therapy.

Administration and Dosage

➤*Adults:*

Type 2 diabetes mellitus –

Usual dosage: 100 mg once daily.

Concomitant therapy: When used in combination with a sulfonylurea, a lower dose of the sulfonylurea may be required to reduce the risk of hypoglycemia.

➤*Renal function impairment:*

Sitagliptin Dosage in Patients With Renal Impairment

$CrCl^a$ or serum creatinine	Dose
Moderate renal impairment (CrCl ≥ 30 to < 50 mL/min) approximate serum creatinine levels (mg/dL): men, > 1.7 to ≤ 3; women, > 1.5 to ≤ 2.5	50 mg once daily
Severe renal impairment or ESRD[a] requiring hemodialysis or peritoneal dialysis[b] (CrCl < 30 mL/min) approximate serum creatinine levels (mg/dL): men, > 3; women, > 2.5; or on dialysis	25 mg once daily

[a] CrCl = creatinine clearance; ESRD = end-stage renal disease.
[b] May be administered without regard to the timing of hemodialysis.

➤*Administration:* Take orally with or without food.

➤*Storage/Stability:* Store at 20° to 25°C (68° to 77°F); excursions are permitted between 15° and 30°C (59° and 86°F).

Actions

➤*Pharmacology:* Sitagliptin is a dipeptidyl peptidase-4 (DPP-4) inhibitor that is believed to exert its actions in patients with type 2 diabetes by slowing the inactivation of incretin hormones. Concentrations of the active intact hormones are increased by sitagliptin, thereby increasing and prolonging the action of these hormones. Incretin hormones, including glucagonlike peptide 1 (GLP-1) and glucose-dependent insulinotropic polypeptide (GIP), are released by the intestine throughout the day, and levels are increased in response to a meal. These hormones are rapidly inactivated by the enzyme DPP-4. The incretins are part of an endogenous system involved in the physiologic regulation of glucose homeostasis. When blood glucose concentrations are normal or elevated, GLP-1 and GIP increase insulin synthesis and release from pancreatic beta cells by intracellular signaling pathways involving cyclic adenosine monophosphate. GLP-1 also lowers glucagon secretion from pancreatic alpha cells, leading to reduced hepatic glucose production. By increasing and prolonging active incretin levels, sitagliptin increases insulin release and decreases glucagon levels in the circulation in a glucose-dependent manner. Sitagliptin demonstrates selectivity for DPP-4, and does not inhibit DPP-8 or DPP-9 activity in vitro at concentrations approximating those from therapeutic doses.

➤*Pharmacokinetics:*

Absorption – After oral administration of a 100 mg dose to healthy patients, sitagliptin was rapidly absorbed, with peak plasma concentration (C_{max}) occurring 1 to 4 hours postdose. Plasma area under the curve (AUC) of sitagliptin increased in a dose-proportional manner. The absolute bioavailability of sitagliptin is approximately 87%. Following a single oral 100 mg dose to healthy volunteers, mean plasma AUC of sitagliptin was 8.52 mcM•h, maximum effective C_{max} was 950 nM. Plasma AUC of sitagliptin increased approximately 14% following 100 mg doses at steady state compared with the first dose. The intra- and intersubject coefficients of variation for sitagliptin AUC were small (5.8% and 15.1%, respectively).

Distribution – The mean volume of distribution at steady state following a single 100 mg intravenous dose of sitagliptin to healthy patients is approximately 198 L. The fraction of sitagliptin reversibly bound to plasma proteins is low (38%).

Metabolism – Following a [^{14}C] sitagliptin oral dose, approximately 16% of the radioactivity was excreted as metabolites of sitagliptin. Six metabolites were detected at trace levels and are not expected to contribute to the plasma DPP-4 inhibitory activity of sitagliptin. In vitro studies indicated that the primary enzyme responsible for the limited metabolism of sitagliptin was CYP3A4, with contribution from CYP2C8.

Excretion – Approximately 79% of sitagliptin is excreted unchanged in the urine, with metabolism being a minor pathway of elimination.

Following administration of an oral [^{14}C]sitagliptin dose to healthy patients, approximately 100% of the administered radioactivity was eliminated in feces (13%) or urine (87%) within 1 week of dosing. The apparent terminal half-life following a 100 mg oral dose of sitagliptin was approximately 12.4 hours and renal clearance was approximately 350 mL/min.

Elimination of sitagliptin occurs primarily via renal excretion and involves active tubular secretion. Sitagliptin is a substrate for human organic anion transporter-3, which may be involved in the renal elimination of sitagliptin. The clinical relevance of human organic anion transporter-3 in sitagliptin transport has not been established. Sitagliptin is also a substrate of P-glycoprotein, which may also be involved in mediating the renal elimination of sitagliptin.

Special populations –

Renal function impairment: Compared with healthy control patients, an approximate 1.1- to 1.6-fold increase in plasma AUC of sitagliptin was observed in patients with mild renal impairment. Because increases of this magnitude are not clinically relevant, dosage adjustment in patients with mild renal impairment is not necessary. Plasma AUC levels of sitagliptin were increased approximately 2- and 4-fold in patients with moderate and severe renal impairment, including patients with ESRD on hemodialysis, respectively. Sitagliptin was modestly removed by hemodialysis (13.5% over a 3- to 4-hour hemodialysis session starting 4 hours postdose). To achieve plasma concentrations of sitagliptin similar to those in patients with healthy renal function, lower dosages are recommended in patients with moderate and severe renal impairment, as well as in patients with ESRD requiring hemodialysis.

Elderly: Elderly patients (65 to 80 years of age) had approximately 19% higher plasma concentrations of sitagliptin compared with younger patients.

Contraindications

History of a serious hypersensitivity reaction to sitagliptin, such as anaphylaxis or angioedema.

Warnings/Precautions

➤*Pancreatitis:* There have been postmarketing reports of acute pancreatitis, including fatal and nonfatal hemorrhagic or necrotizing pancreatitis, in patients taking sitagliptin. After initiation of sitagliptin, carefully observe patients for signs and symptoms of pancreatitis. If pancreatitis is suspected, promptly discontinue sitagliptin and initiate appropriate management. It is unknown whether patients with a history of pancreatitis are at increased risk of the development of pancreatitis while using sitagliptin.

➤*Hypersensitivity reactions:* There have been postmarketing reports of serious hypersensitivity reactions in patients treated with sitagliptin. These reactions include anaphylaxis, angioedema, and exfoliative skin conditions, including Stevens-Johnson syndrome. Because these reactions are reported voluntarily from a population of uncertain size, it is generally not possible to reliably estimate their frequency or establish a causal relationship to drug exposure. Onset of these reactions occurred within the first 3 months after initiation of treatment with sitagliptin, with some reports occurring after

SITAGLIPTIN PHOSPHATE — ORAL

the first dose. If a hypersensitivity reaction is suspected, discontinue sitagliptin, assess for other potential causes for the reaction, and institute alternative treatment for diabetes.

➤*Renal function impairment:* See Administration and Dosage and Actions for more information.

➤*Pregnancy: Category B.* There are no adequate and well-controlled studies in pregnant women. Because animal reproduction studies are not always predictive of human response, only use this drug during pregnancy if clearly needed.

Placental transfer of sitagliptin administered to pregnant rats was approximately 45% at 2 hours and 80% at 24 hours postdose. Placental transfer of sitagliptin administered to pregnant rabbits was approximately 66% at 2 hours and 30% at 24 hours.

Sitagliptin administered to pregnant female rats and rabbits from gestation days 6 to 20 (organogenesis) was not teratogenic at oral doses of up to 250 mg/kg (rats) and 125 mg/kg (rabbits), or approximately 30 and 20 times, respectively, human exposure at the MRHD of 100 mg/day based on AUC comparisons. Higher doses increased the incidence of rib malformations in offspring at 1,000 mg/kg, or approximately 100 times the human exposure at the MRHD.

Pregnancy registry – The manufacturer maintains a registry to monitor the pregnancy outcomes of women exposed to sitagliptin while pregnant. Health care providers are encouraged to report any prenatal exposure to sitagliptin by calling the pregnancy registry at 1-800-986-8999.

➤*Lactation:* Sitagliptin is secreted in the milk of lactating rats at a milk-to-plasma ratio of 4:1. It is not known whether sitagliptin is excreted in human milk. Because many drugs are excreted in human milk, exercise caution when sitagliptin is administered to a breast-feeding woman.

➤*Children:* Safety and efficacy of sitagliptin in children younger than 18 years of age have not been established.

➤*Elderly:* This drug is known to be substantially excreted by the kidneys. Because elderly patients are more likely to have decreased renal function, take care in dose selection in the elderly; it may be useful to assess renal function in these patients prior to initiating dosing and periodically thereafter.

➤*Monitoring:* Periodically monitor blood glucose and glycosylated hemoglobin (HbA_{1c}). Assessment of renal function is recommended prior to initiation of sitagliptin and periodically thereafter. Observe patients carefully for signs and symptoms of pancreatitis.

Drug Interactions

Sitagliptin Drug Interactions

Precipitant drug	Object drug[a]		Description
Cyclosporine	Sitagliptin	↑	Coadministration of a single oral dose of sitagliptin 100 mg and a single oral dose of cyclosporine 600 mg increased the AUC and C_{max} of sitagliptin 29% and 68%, respectively. These modest changes in sitagliptin pharmacokinetics are not considered clinically meaningful.
Sitagliptin	Digoxin	↑	Coadministration of oral digoxin 0.25 mg and sitagliptin 100 mg daily for 10 days increased the digoxin AUC and C_{max} 11% and 18%, respectively. These changes are minimal and no digoxin dosage adjustment is recommended.
Sitagliptin	Sulfonylureas (eg, tolbutamide)	↑	A lower dose of the sulfonylurea may be needed to reduce the risk of hypoglycemia.

[a] ↑ = object drug increased.

Adverse Reactions

➤*Adverse reactions (5% or more):*

Sitagliptin Adverse Reactions (≥ 5%)[a]

Adverse reactions	Sitagliptin 100 mg (n = 443)	Placebo (n = 363)
Nasopharyngitis	5.2%	3.3%
	Sitagliptin 100 mg + pioglitazone (n = 175)	Placebo + pioglitazone (n = 178)
Headache	5.1%	3.9%
Upper respiratory tract infection	6.3%	3.4%
	Sitagliptin 100 mg + glimepiride (± metformin) (n = 222)	Placebo + glimepiride (± metformin) (n = 219)
Headache	5.9%	2.3%
Hypoglycemia	12.2%	1.8%
Nasopharyngitis	6.3%	4.6%

[a] Intent-to-treat (ITT) population.

➤*Combination therapy with metformin:* In the study of patients receiving sitagliptin as add-on combination therapy with metformin, there were no adverse reactions reported regardless of investigator assessment of causality in 5% or more of patients and more commonly than in patients given placebo.

In an additional 24-week, placebo-controlled factorial study of initial therapy with sitagliptin in combination with metformin, the incidence of hypoglycemia was 0.6% in patients given placebo, 0.6% in patients given sitagliptin alone, 0.8% in patients given metformin alone, and 1.6% in patients given sitagliptin in combination with metformin.

Sitagliptin and Metformin Adverse Reactions (≥ 5%)[a]

Adverse reactions	Sitagliptin 100 mg daily (n = 179)	Metformin 500 or 1,000 mg twice daily[b] (n = 364)[b]	Sitagliptin 50 mg twice daily + metformin 500 or 1,000 mg twice daily[b] (n = 372)[b]	Placebo (n = 176)
Headache	1.1%	3.8%	5.9%	2.8%
Upper respiratory tract infection	4.5%	5.2%	6.2%	5.1%

[a] ITT population.
[b] Data pooled for the patients given the lower and higher doses of metformin.

➤*Lab test abnormalities:* In a 12-week study of 91 patients with chronic renal impairment, 37 patients with moderate renal impairment were randomized to sitagliptin 50 mg daily, while 14 patients with the same magnitude of renal impairment were randomized to placebo. Mean standard error increases in serum creatinine were observed in patients treated with sitagliptin (0.12 mg/dL [0.04]) and in patients treated with placebo (0.07 mg/dL [0.07]). The clinical significance of this added increase in serum creatinine relative to placebo is not known.

➤*Postmarketing:*

Hypersensitivity – Anaphylaxis; angioedema; cutaneous vasculitis; exfoliative skin conditions, including Stevens-Johnson syndrome; rash; urticaria.

Hepatic – Acute pancreatitis, including fatal and nonfatal hemorrhagic and necrotizing pancreatitis; hepatic enzyme elevations.

Overdosage

➤*Symptoms:* During controlled clinical trials in healthy patients, single doses of sitagliptin of up to 800 mg were administered. Maximal mean increases in QTc of 8 msec were observed in 1 study at a dose of sitagliptin 800 mg, a mean effect that is not considered clinically important. There is no experience with doses above 800 mg in humans.

➤*Treatment:* In the event of an overdose, it is reasonable to employ the usual supportive measures (eg, remove unabsorbed material from the GI tract, employ clinical monitoring including an ECG), and institute supportive therapy as dictated by the patient's clinical status.

Sitagliptin is modestly dialyzable. In clinical studies, approximately 13.5% of the dose was removed over a 3- to 4-hour hemodialysis session. Prolonged hemodialysis may be considered if clinically appropriate. It is not known if sitagliptin is dialyzable by peritoneal dialysis.

Patient Information

Inform patients of the potential risks and benefits of sitagliptin and of alternative modes of therapy. Also inform patients about the importance of adherence to dietary instructions, regular physical activity, periodic blood glucose monitoring and HbA_{1c} testing, recognition and management of hypoglycemia and hyperglycemia, and assessment for diabetes complications. During periods of stress, such as fever, trauma, infection, or surgery, medication requirements may change; advise patients to seek medical advice promptly.

Inform patients that acute pancreatitis has been reported during postmarketing use of sitagliptin. Inform patients that severe, persistent abdominal pain, sometimes radiating to the back, which may or may not be accompanied by vomiting, is the hallmark symptom of acute pancreatitis. Instruct patients to promptly discontinue sitagliptin and contact their health care provider if persistent severe abdominal pain occurs.

Inform patients that allergic reactions have been reported during postmarketing use of sitagliptin. If symptoms of allergic reactions (including rash, hives, and swelling of the face, lips, tongue, and throat that may cause difficulty breathing or swallowing) occur, patients must stop taking sitagliptin and seek medical advice promptly.

Inform patients that response to all diabetic therapies will be monitored by periodic measurements of blood glucose and HbA_{1c} levels, with a goal of decreasing these levels towards the healthy range. HbA_{1c} is especially useful for evaluating long-term glycemic control. Inform patients of the potential need to adjust the dose based on changes in renal function tests over time.

Dipeptidyl Peptidase-4 Inhibitor

LINAGLIPTIN

Rx	**Tradjenta** (Boehringer Ingelheim)	**Tablets; oral:** 5 mg	Mannitol. (D5). Lt red, round. Film-coated. In 30s, 90s, 1,000s, and UD 100s.

LINAGLIPTIN — ORAL

Indications

➤*Type 2 diabetes mellitus:*

Monotherapy and combination therapy – Linagliptin tablets are indicated as an adjunct to diet and exercise to improve glycemic control in adults with type 2 diabetes mellitus.

Important limitations of use – Linagliptin should not be used in patients with type 1 diabetes or for the treatment of diabetic ketoacidosis, as it would not be effective in these settings.

Linagliptin has not been studied in combination with insulin.

Administration and Dosage

➤*Adults:*

Type 2 diabetes mellitus –

Usual dosage: 5 mg once daily.

Concomitant therapy: When linagliptin is used in combination with an insulin secretagogue (eg, sulfonylurea), a lower dose of the insulin secretagogue may be required to reduce the risk of hypoglycemia.

➤*Children:* Safety and effectiveness have not been established.

➤*Administration:* Linagliptin tablets can be taken with or without food.

➤*Storage/Stability:* Store at 25°C (77°F); excursions permitted to 15° to 30°C (59° to 86°F).

Actions

➤*Pharmacology:*

Mechanism of action – Linagliptin is an inhibitor of DPP-4, an enzyme that degrades the incretin hormones glucagon-like peptide-1 (GLP-1) and glucose-dependent insulinotropic polypeptide (GIP). Thus, linagliptin increases the concentrations of active incretin hormones, stimulating the release of insulin in a glucose-dependent manner and decreasing the levels of glucagon in the circulation. Both incretin hormones are involved in the physiological regulation of glucose homeostasis. Incretin hormones are secreted at a low basal level throughout the day and levels rise immediately after meal intake. GLP-1 and GIP increase insulin biosynthesis and secretion from pancreatic beta cells in the presence of normal and elevated blood glucose levels. Furthermore, GLP-1 also reduces glucagon secretion from pancreatic alpha cells, resulting in a reduction in hepatic glucose output.

Pharmacodynamics – Linagliptin binds to DPP-4 in a reversible manner and thus increases the concentrations of incretin hormones. Linagliptin glucose-dependently increases insulin secretion and lowers glucagon secretion thus resulting in a better regulation of the glucose homeostasis. Linagliptin binds selectively to DPP-4 and selectively inhibits DPP-4 but not DPP-8 or DPP-9 activity in vitro at concentrations approximating therapeutic exposures.

Cardiac electrophysiology: In a randomized, placebo-controlled, active-comparator, 4-way crossover study, 36 healthy subjects were administered a single oral dose of linagliptin 5 mg, linagliptin 100 mg (20 times the recommended dose), moxifloxacin, and placebo. No increase in QTc was observed with either the recommended dose of 5 mg or the 100 mg dose. At the 100-mg dose, peak linagliptin plasma concentrations were approximately 38-fold higher than the peak concentrations following a 5 mg dose.

➤*Pharmacokinetics:* The pharmacokinetics of linagliptin has been characterized in healthy subjects and patients with type 2 diabetes. After oral administration of a single 5-mg dose to healthy subjects, peak plasma concentrations of linagliptin occurred at approximately 1.5 hours post dose (T_{max}); the mean plasma area under the curve (AUC) was 139 nmol•h/L and maximum concentration (C_{max}) was 8.9 nmol/L.

Plasma concentrations of linagliptin decline in at least a biphasic manner with a long terminal half-life (more than 100 hours), related to the saturable binding of linagliptin to DPP-4. The prolonged elimination phase does not contribute to the accumulation of the drug. The effective half-life for accumulation of linagliptin, as determined from oral administration of multiple doses of linagliptin 5 mg, is approximately 12 hours. After once-daily dosing, steady-state plasma concentrations of linagliptin 5 mg are reached by the third dose, and C_{max} and AUC increased by a factor of 1.3 at steady state compared with the first dose. The intra-subject and inter-subject coefficients of variation for linagliptin AUC were small (12.6% and 28.5%, respectively). Plasma AUC of linagliptin increased in a less than dose proportional manner in the dose range of 1 to 10 mg. The pharmacokinetics of linagliptin is similar in healthy subjects and in patients with type 2 diabetes.

Absorption – The absolute bioavailability of linagliptin is approximately 30%. High-fat meal reduced C_{max} by 15% and increased AUC by 4%; this effect is not clinically relevant. Linagliptin may be administered with or without food.

Distribution – The mean apparent volume of distribution at steady state following a single intravenous dose of linagliptin 5 mg to healthy subjects is approximately 1110 L, indicating that linagliptin extensively distributes to the tissues. Plasma protein binding of linagliptin is concentration-dependent, decreasing from about 99% at 1 nmol/L to 75%-89% at 30 nmol/L or more, reflecting saturation of binding to DPP-4 with increasing concentration of linagliptin. At high concentrations, where DPP-4 is fully saturated, 70% to 80% of linagliptin remains bound to plasma proteins and 20% to 30% is unbound in plasma. Plasma binding is not altered in patients with renal or hepatic impairment.

Metabolism – Following oral administration, the majority (about 90%) of linagliptin is excreted unchanged, indicating that metabolism represents a minor elimination pathway. A small fraction of absorbed linagliptin is metabolized to a pharmacologically inactive metabolite, which shows a steady-state exposure of 13.3% relative to linagliptin.

Excretion – Following administration of an oral [^{14}C]-linagliptin dose to healthy subjects, approximately 85% of the administered radioactivity was eliminated via the enterohepatic system (80%) or urine (5%) within 4 days of dosing. Renal clearance at steady state was approximately 70 mL/min.

Special populations –

Renal function impairment: An open-label pharmacokinetic study evaluated the pharmacokinetics of linagliptin 5 mg in male and female patients with varying degrees of chronic renal impairment. The study included 6 healthy subjects with normal renal function (creatinine clearance [CrCl] 80 mL/min or higher), 6 patients with mild renal impairment (CrCl 50 to less than 80 mL/min), 6 patients with moderate renal impairment (CrCl 30 to less than 50 mL/min), 10 patients with type 2 diabetes mellitus and severe renal impairment (CrCl less than 30 mL/min), and 11 patients with type 2 diabetes mellitus and normal renal function. Creatinine clearance was measured by 24-hour urinary creatinine clearance measurements or estimated from serum creatinine based on the Cockcroft-Gault formula.

Under steady-state conditions, linagliptin exposure in patients with mild renal impairment was comparable to healthy subjects.

In patients with moderate renal impairment under steady-state conditions, mean exposure of linagliptin increased ($AUC_{tau,ss}$ by 71% and C_{max} by 46%) compared with healthy subjects. This increase was not associated with a prolonged accumulation half-life, terminal half-life, or an increased accumulation factor. Renal excretion of linagliptin was below 5% of the administered dose and was not affected by decreased renal function.

Patients with type 2 diabetes mellitus and severe renal impairment showed steady-state exposure approximately 40% higher than that of patients with type 2 diabetes mellitus and normal renal function (increase in $AUC_{tau,ss}$ by 42% and C_{max} by 35%). For both type 2 diabetes mellitus groups, renal excretion was below 7% of the administered dose.

Results of this study, supported by results of population pharmacokinetic analyses, indicate that no dose adjustment is recommended in patients with renal impairment.

Hepatic function impairment: In patients with mild hepatic impairment (Child-Pugh class A) steady-state exposure ($AUC_{tau,ss}$) of linagliptin was approximately 25% lower and $C_{max,ss}$ was approximately 36% lower than in healthy subjects. In patients with moderate hepatic impairment (Child-Pugh class B), AUC^{ss} of linagliptin was about 14% lower and $C_{max,ss}$ was approximately 8% lower than in healthy subjects. Patients with severe hepatic impairment (Child-Pugh class C) had comparable exposure of linagliptin in terms of AUC_{0-24} and approximately 23% lower C_{max} compared with healthy subjects. Reductions in the pharmacokinetic parameters seen in patients with hepatic impairment did not result in reductions in DPP-4 inhibition. No dose adjustment of linagliptin is necessary in patients with hepatic impairment.

Elderly: No dose adjustment is recommended based on age, as age did not have a clinically meaningful impact on the pharmacokinetics of linagliptin based on a population pharmacokinetic analysis.

Children: Studies characterizing the pharmacokinetics of linagliptin in pediatric patients have not yet been performed.

Gender: No dose adjustment is necessary based on gender. Gender had no clinically meaningful effect on the pharmacokinetics of linagliptin based on a population pharmacokinetic analysis.

Race: No dose adjustment is necessary based on race. Race had no clinically meaningful effect on the pharmacokinetics of linagliptin based on available pharmacokinetic data, including subjects of White, Hispanic, Black, and Asian racial groups.

Body Mass Index (BMI)/Weight: No dose adjustment is necessary based on BMI/weight. BMI/weight had no clinically meaningful effect on the pharmacokinetics of linagliptin based on a population pharmacokinetic analysis.

Contraindications

Linagliptin is contraindicated in patients with a history of a hypersensitivity reaction to linagliptin, such as urticaria, angioedema, or bronchial hyperreactivity.

Warnings/Precautions

➤*Use with medications known to cause hypoglycemia:* Insulin secretagogues are known to cause hypoglycemia. The use of linagliptin in combination with an insulin secretagogue (e.g., sulfonylurea) was associated with a higher rate of hypoglycemia compared with placebo in a clinical trial. Therefore, a lower dose of the insulin secretagogue may be required to reduce the risk of hypoglycemia when used in combination with linagliptin.

➤*Macrovascular outcomes:* There have been no clinical studies establishing conclusive evidence of macrovascular risk reduction with linagliptin tablets or any other antidiabetic drug.

➤*Renal function impairment:* No dose adjustment is recommended for patients with renal impairment.

➤*Hepatic function impairment:* No dose adjustment is recommended for patients with hepatic impairment.

LINAGLIPTIN — ORAL

➤*Pregnancy: Category B.* Reproduction studies have been performed in rats and rabbits. There are, however, no adequate and well-controlled studies in pregnant women. Because animal reproduction studies are not always predictive of human response, this drug should be used during pregnancy only if clearly needed.

Linagliptin administered during the period of organogenesis was not teratogenic at doses up to 30 mg/kg in the rat and 150 mg/kg in the rabbit, or approximately 49 and 1943 times the clinical dose based on AUC exposure. Doses of linagliptin causing maternal toxicity in the rat and the rabbit also caused developmental delays in skeletal ossification and slightly increased embryofetal loss in rat (1,000 times the clinical dose) and increased fetal resorptions and visceral and skeletal variations in the rabbit (1943 times the clinical dose).

Linagliptin administered to female rats from gestation day 6 to lactation day 21 resulted in decreased body weight and delays in physical and behavioral development in male and female offspring at maternally toxic doses (exposures more than 1,000 times the clinical dose). No functional, behavioral, or reproductive toxicity was observed in offspring of rats exposed to 49 times the clinical dose.

Linagliptin crossed the placenta into the fetus following oral dosing in pregnant rats and rabbits.

➤*Lactation:* Available animal data have shown excretion of linagliptin in milk at a milk-to-plasma ratio of 4:1. It is not known whether this drug is excreted in human milk. Because many drugs are excreted in human milk, caution should be exercised when linagliptin is administered to a nursing woman.

➤*Children:* Safety and effectiveness of linagliptin in pediatric patients have not been established.

➤*Elderly:* Of the total number of patients (n= 4,040) in clinical studies of linagliptin, 1,085 patients were 65 years and over, while 131 patients were 75 years and over. No overall differences in safety or effectiveness were observed between patients 65 years and over and younger patients. While this and other reported clinical experience have not identified differences in response between the elderly and younger patients, greater sensitivity of some older individuals cannot be ruled out. No dose adjustment is recommended in this population.

Drug Interactions

➤*Inducers of P-glycoprotein or CYP3A4 enzymes:* Rifampin decreased linagliptin exposure suggesting that the efficacy of linagliptin may be reduced when administered in combination with a strong P-gp or CYP 3A4 inducer. Therefore, use of alternative treatments is strongly recommended when linagliptin is to be administered with P-gp or CYP 3A4 inducer.

➤*In vitro assessment of drug interactions:* Linagliptin is a weak to moderate inhibitor of CYP isozyme CYP3A4, but does not inhibit other CYP isozymes and is not an inducer of CYP isozymes, including CYP1A2, 2A6, 2B6, 2C8, 2C9, 2C19, 2D6, 2E1, and 4A11.

Linagliptin is P-glycoprotein (P-gp) substrate, and inhibits P-gp mediated transport of digoxin at high concentrations. Based on these results and in vivo drug interaction studies, linagliptin is considered unlikely to cause interactions with other P-gp substrates at therapeutic concentrations.

➤*In vivo assessment of drug interactions:* Inducers of CYP3A4 or P-gp (eg, rifampin) decrease exposure to linagliptin to subtherapeutic and likely ineffective concentrations. For patients requiring use of such drugs, an alternative to linagliptin is strongly recommended. In vivo studies indicated evidence of a low propensity for causing drug interaction with substrates of CYYP3A4, CYP2C9, CYP2C8, P-gp and organic cationic transporter (OCT). No dose adjustments of linagliptin is recommended based on results of the described pharmacokinetic studies.

Effect of Coadministered Drugs on Systemic Exposure of Linagliptin

Coadministered drug	Dosing of coadministered drug[a]	Dosing of linagliptin[a]	Geometric mean ratio (ratio with/without coadminstered drug) No effect = 1: AUC[b]	C_{max}
Metformin	850 mg 3 times daily	10 mg once daily	1.2	1.03
Glyburide	1.75 mg[c]	5 mg once daily	1.02	1.01
Pioglitazone	45 mg once daily	10 mg once daily	1.13	1.07
Ritonavir	200 mg twice daily	5 mg[c]	2.01	2.96
Rifampin	600 mg once daily	5 mg once daily	0.6	0.56

[a] Multiple dose (steady state) unless otherwise noted.
[b] AUC = area under the curve; $AUC_{0\ to\ 24\ hours}$ for single dose treatments and $AUC = AUC_{tau}$ for multiple dose treatments.
[c] Single dose.

Effect of Linagliptin on Systemic Exposure of Coadministered Drugs[a]

Coadministered drug	Dosing of coadministered drug[b]	Dosing of linagliptin[b]		Geometric mean ratio (ratio with/without coadminstered drug) No effect = 1: AUC[c]	C_{max}
Metformin	850 mg three times daily	10 mg once daily	metformin	1.01	0.89
Glyburide	1.75 mg[d]	5 mg once daily	glyburide	0.86	0.86
Pioglitazone	45 mg once daily	10 mg once daily	pioglitazone	0.94	0.86
			metabolite M-III	0.98	0.96
			metabolite M-IV	1.04	1.05
Digoxin	0.25 mg once daily	5 mg once daily	digoxin	1.02	0.94
Simvastatin	40 mg once daily	10 mg once daily	simvastatin	1.34	1.1
			simvastatin acid	1.33	1.21
Warfarin	10 mg[d]	5 mg once daily	R-warfarin	0.99	1
			S-warfarin	1.03	1.01
			INR	0.93[e]	1.04[e]
			PT	1.03[e]	1.15[e]
Ethinylestradiol and levonorgestrel	ethinylestradiol 0.03 mg and levonorgestrel 0.15 mg once daily	5 mg once daily	ethinylestradiol	1.01	1.08
			levonorgestrel	1.09	1.13

[a] INR = international normalized ratio; PT = prothrombin time.
[b] Multiple dose (steady state) unless otherwise noted.
[c] $AUC = AUC_{inf}$ for single dose treatments and $AUC = AUC_{tau}$ for multiple dose treatments.
[d] Single dose.
[e] $AUC = AUC_{0\text{-}168}$ and $C_{max} = E_{max}$ for pharmacodynamic endpoints.

Adverse Reactions

➤*Clinical trials experience:* Because clinical trials are conducted under widely varying conditions, adverse reaction rates observed in the clinical trials of a drug cannot be directly compared to rates in the clinical trials of another drug and may not reflect the rates observed in practice.

The safety of linagliptin has been evaluated in over 4,000 patients with type 2 diabetes in clinical trials, including 12 placebo-controlled studies and 1 active-controlled study with glimepiride.

Linagliptin 5 mg once daily was studied as monotherapy in two placebo-controlled trials of 18- and 24-weeks duration. Five placebo-controlled trials investigated linagliptin in combination with other oral anti-glycemic agents: two with metformin (12- and 24-weeks treatment duration); one with a sulfonylurea (18-weeks treatment duration); one with metformin and sulfonylurea (24-week treatment duration); and one with pioglitazone (24-week treatment duration). In placebo-controlled clinical trials, adverse reactions that occurred in 5% or more of patients receiving linagliptin (n = 2,566) and more commonly than in patients given placebo (n = 1,183) included nasopharyngitis (5.8% vs 5.5%). Adverse reactions reported in 2% or more of patients treated with linagliptin 5 mg daily as monotherapy or in combination with pioglitazone, sulfonylurea, or metformin and at least 2-fold more commonly than in patients treated with placebo are shown in Table 1.

LINAGLIPTIN — ORAL

Table 1 Adverse Reactions Reported in ≥ 2% of Patients Treated with Linagliptin and at Least 2-Fold Greater than with Placebo in Placebo-Controlled Clinical Studies of Linagliptin Monotherapy or Combination Therapy[a]

–	Monotherapy n (%)[b]		Combination with Metformin[c] n (%)		Combination with SU n (%)		Combination with Metformin + SU n (%)		Combination with Pioglitazone n (%)	
	Linagliptin n = 765	Placebo n = 458	Linagliptin n = 590	Placebo n = 248	Linagliptin n = 161	Placebo n = 84	Linagliptin n = 791	Placebo n = 263	Linagliptin n = 259	Placebo n = 130
Nasopharyngitis					7 (4.3)	1 (1.2)				
Hyperlipidemia									7 (2.7)	1 (0.8)
Cough							19 (2.4)	3 (1.1)		
Hypertriglyceridemia[d]					4 (2.4)	0 (0.0)				
Weight increased									6 (2.3)	1 (0.8)

[a] SU = sulfonylurea.
[b] Pooled data from 7 studies.
[c] Pooled data from 2 studies.
[d] Includes reports of hypertriglyceridemia (n = 2; 1.2%) and blood triglycerides increased (n = 2; 1.2%).

Following 52 weeks treatment in a controlled study comparing linagliptin with glimepiride in which all patients were also receiving metformin, adverse reactions reported in 5% or more patients treated with linagliptin (n = 776) and more frequently than in patients treated with a sulfonylurea (n = 775) were arthralgia (5.7% vs 3.5%), back pain (6.4% vs 5.2%), and headache (5.7% vs 4.2%).

Other adverse reactions reported in clinical studies with treatment of linagliptin were hypersensitivity (e.g., urticaria, angioedema, localized skin exfoliation, or bronchial hyperreactivity), and myalgia. In the clinical trial program, pancreatitis was reported in 8 of 4,687 patients (4,311 patient years of exposure) while being treated with linagliptin compared with 0 of 1,183 patients (433 patient years of exposure) treated with placebo. Three additional cases of pancreatitis were reported following the last administered dose of linagliptin.

➤*Hypoglycemia:* In the placebo-controlled studies, 195 (7.6%) of the total 2,566 patients treated with linagliptin 5 mg reported hypoglycemia compared to 49 patients (4.1%) of 1,183 placebo treated patients. The incidence of hypoglycemia was similar to placebo when linagliptin was administered as monotherapy or in combination with metformin, or with pioglitazone. When linagliptin was administered in combination with metformin and a sulfonylurea, 181 of 791 (22.9%) of patients reported hypoglycemia compared with 39 of 263 (14.8%) of patients administered placebo in combination with metformin and a sulfonylurea.

➤*Lab test abnormalities:* Changes in laboratory findings were similar in patients treated with linagliptin 5 mg compared to patients treated with placebo. Changes in laboratory values that occurred more frequently in the linagliptin group and at least 1% more than in the placebo group were increases in uric acid (1.3% in the placebo group, 2.7 % in the linagliptin group). No clinically meaningful changes in vital signs were observed in patients treated with linagliptin.

Overdosage

➤*Treatment:* During controlled clinical trials in healthy subjects, with single doses of up to 600 mg of linagliptin (equivalent to 120 times the recommended daily dose) there were no dose related clinical adverse drug reactions. There is no experience with doses above 600 mg in humans.

In the event of an overdose, contact the Poison Control Center. It is also reasonable to employ the usual supportive measures, e.g., remove unabsorbed material from the gastrointestinal tract, employ clinical monitoring, and institute supportive treatment as dictated by the patient's clinical status. Linagliptin is not expected to be eliminated to a therapeutically significant degree by hemodialysis or peritoneal dialysis.

Patient Information

See FDA-Approved Patient Labeling.

Inform patients of the potential risks and benefits of linagliptin and of alternative modes of therapy. Also inform patients about the importance of adherence to dietary instructions, regular physical activity, periodic blood glucose monitoring and A_{1C} testing, recognition and management of hypoglycemia and hyperglycemia, and assessment for diabetes complications. Advise patients to seek medical advice promptly during periods of stress such as fever, trauma, infection, or surgery, as medication requirements may change.

Instruct patients to take linagliptin only as prescribed. If a dose is missed, advise patients not to double their next dose.

Instruct patients to read the Patient Information before starting linagliptin therapy and to reread it each time the prescription is renewed.

Instruct patients to inform their doctor or pharmacist if they develop any unusual symptom, or if any known symptom persists or worsens.

Inform patients that response to all diabetic therapies should be monitored by periodic measurements of blood glucose and A_{1C} levels, with a goal of decreasing these levels toward the normal range. A_{1C} monitoring is especially useful for evaluating long-term glycemic control.

METFORMIN HYDROCHLORIDE

Rx	**Metformin Hydrochloride** (Various, eg, Teva, Watson)	**Tablets; oral:** 500 mg	In 100s, 500s, 1,000s, 2,000s, and UD 100s.
Rx	**Glucophage** (Bristol-Myers Squibb)		(BMS 6060 500). White to off-white, round. Film-coated. In 100s and 500s.
Rx	**Metformin Hydrochloride** (Various, eg, Teva, Watson)	**Tablets; oral:** 850 mg	In 100s, 500s, 1,000s, and UD 100s.
Rx	**Glucophage** (Bristol-Myers Squibb)		(BMS 6070 850). White to off-white, round. Film-coated. In 100s.
Rx	**Metformin Hydrochloride** (Various, eg, Teva, Watson)	**Tablets; oral:** 1,000 mg	In 100s, 500s, 1,000s, and UD 100s.
Rx	**Glucophage** (Bristol-Myers Squibb)		(BMS 6071 1000). White, oval, bisected. Film-coated. In 100s.
Rx	**Metformin Hydrochloride** (Various, eg, Teva, Watson)	**Tablets, extended-release; oral:** 500 mg	In 100s, 500s, and 1,000s.
Rx	**Fortamet** (First Horizon)		PEG. (574). White, biconvex. Film-coated. In 60s.
Rx	**Glucophage XR** (Bristol-Myers Squibb)		(BMS 6063 500). White to off-white, capsule shape. In 100s.
Rx	**Glumetza** (Depomed)		(GMZ 500). Blue, oval. Film-coated. In 100s.
Rx	**Metformin Hydrochloride** (Various, eg, Teva, Watson)	**Tablets, extended-release; oral:** 750 mg	In 100s, 500s, and 1,000s.
Rx	**Glucophage XR** (Bristol-Myers Squibb)		(BMS 6064 750). Pale red, capsule shape. In 100s.
Rx	**Glumetza** (Depomed)	**Tablets, extended-release; oral:** 1,000 mg	Polyvinyl alcohol, PEG. (M1000). White, oval. Film-coated. In 90s.
Rx	**Fortamet** (First Horizon)		PEG. (575). White, biconvex. Film-coated. In 60s.
Rx	**Riomet** (Ranbaxy)	**Solution; oral:** 500 mg per 5 mL	Saccharin, xylitol. Cherry flavor. In 118 and 473 mL.

METFORMIN HYDROCHLORIDE — ORAL

WARNING

Lactic acidosis – Lactic acidosis is a rare but serious metabolic complication that can occur because of metformin accumulation during treatment with metformin; when it occurs, it is fatal in approximately 50% of cases. Lactic acidosis may also occur in association with a number of pathophysiologic conditions, including diabetes mellitus and whenever there is significant tissue hypoperfusion and hypoxemia. Lactic acidosis is characterized by elevated blood lactate levels (5 mmol/L or more), decreased blood pH, electrolyte disturbances with an increased anion gap, and an increased lactate/pyruvate ratio. When metformin is implicated as the cause of lactic acidosis, metformin plasma levels of 5 mcg/mL or more are generally found.

The reported incidence of lactic acidosis in patients receiving metformin is very low (approximately 0.03 cases per 1,000 patient-years, with approximately 0.015 fatal cases per 1,000 patient-years). In more than 20,000 patient-years' exposure to metformin in clinical trials, there were no reports of lactic acidosis. Reported cases have occurred primarily in diabetic patients with significant renal function impairment, including intrinsic renal disease and renal hypoperfusion, often in the setting of multiple concomitant medical/surgical problems and multiple concomitant medications. Patients with congestive heart failure (CHF) requiring pharmacologic management, in particular those with unstable or acute CHF who are at risk of hypoperfusion and hypoxemia, are at increased risk of lactic acidosis. The risk of lactic acidosis increases with the degree of renal dysfunction and the patient's age. Therefore, the risk of lactic acidosis may be significantly decreased by regular monitoring of renal function in patients taking metformin and by use of the minimum effective dose of metformin. In particular, accompany treatment of elderly patients with careful monitoring of renal function. Do not initiate metformin treatment in patients 80 years of age and older unless measurement of creatinine clearance (CrCl) demonstrates that renal function is not reduced because these patients are more susceptible to developing lactic acidosis. In addition, promptly withhold metformin in the presence of any condition associated with hypoxemia, dehydration, or sepsis. Because hepatic function impairment may significantly limit the ability to clear lactate, generally avoid using metformin in patients with clinical or laboratory evidence of hepatic disease. Caution patients against excessive alcohol intake, either acute or chronic, when taking metformin because alcohol potentiates the effects of metformin on lactate metabolism. In addition, temporarily discontinue metformin prior to any intravascular radiocontrast study and for any surgical procedure.

The onset of lactic acidosis is often subtle and accompanied only by nonspecific symptoms such as malaise, myalgias, respiratory distress, increasing somnolence, and nonspecific abdominal distress. There may be associated hypothermia, hypotension, and resistant bradyarrhythmias with more marked acidosis. The patient and the patient's health care provider must be aware of the possible importance of such symptoms. Instruct patients to notify their health care provider immediately if these symptoms occur. Withdraw metformin until the situation is clarified. Serum electrolytes, ketones, blood glucose, and, if indicated, blood pH, lactate levels, and even blood metformin levels may be useful. Once a patient is stabilized on any dose level of metformin, GI symptoms, which are common during initiation of therapy, are unlikely to be drug related. Later occurrence of GI symptoms could be caused by lactic acidosis or other serious disease.

Levels of fasting venous plasma lactate above the upper limit of normal (ULN) but less than 5 mmol/L in patients taking metformin do not necessarily indicate impending lactic acidosis and may be explained by other mechanisms, such as poorly controlled diabetes or obesity, vigorous physical activity, or technical problems in sample handling.

Suspect lactic acidosis in any diabetic patient with metabolic acidosis lacking evidence of ketoacidosis (ketonuria and ketonemia).

Lactic acidosis is a medical emergency that must be treated in a hospital setting. In a patient with lactic acidosis who is taking metformin, immediately discontinue the drug and promptly institute general supportive measures. Because metformin is dialyzable (with a clearance of up to 170 mL/min under good hemodynamic conditions), prompt hemodialysis is recommended to correct the acidosis and remove the accumulated metformin. Such management often results in prompt reversal of symptoms and recovery.

Indications

➤*Type 2 diabetes:*

Monotherapy – As an adjunct to diet and exercise to improve glycemic control in patients with type 2 diabetes. Metformin immediate-release tablets and solution are indicated in patients 10 years of age and older. Metformin extended-release (ER) tablets are indicated in adults.

Combination therapy – Metformin may be used concomitantly with a sulfonylurea or insulin to improve glycemic control in adults.

➤*Off-label uses:*

Antipsychotic-induced weight gain – [4] = Insufficient documentation. Preliminary data with metformin in other disease states suggest a possible relationship with this drug and weight loss. Limited data are available for reducing weight gain associated with antipsychotics and currently offer inconsistent results. (See Administration and Dosage.)

Polycystic ovary syndrome – [1] = Good documentation. Metformin has been shown to improve insulin sensitivity, retard progression of type 2 diabetes in patients with impaired glucose tolerance, improve menstrual cyclicity and ovulation, and decrease androgen levels. These characteristics make metformin a commonly used drug for polycystic ovary syndrome. The effects of metformin in early pregnancy are unknown, although it appears to be safe. (See Administration and Dosage.)

Administration and Dosage

➤*General dosing considerations:* There is no fixed dose regimen for the management of hyperglycemia in patients with type 2 diabetes with metformin or any other pharmacologic agent. Dosage of metformin must be individualized on the basis of efficacy and tolerance, while not exceeding the maximum recommended daily doses.

Short-term administration of metformin may be sufficient during periods of transient loss of control in patients usually well controlled on diet alone.

➤*Adults:*

Type 2 diabetes – In general, clinically significant responses are not seen at dosages below 1,500 mg/day. However, a lower recommended starting dose and gradually increased dosage is advised to minimize GI symptoms and to permit identification of the minimum dose required for adequate glycemic control of the patient.

Immediate-release tablets / solution –

Maximum dose: 2,550 mg/day (25.5 mL/day).

Initial dosage: The usual starting dosage is 500 mg (5 mL) twice daily or 850 mg (8.5 mL) once daily, given with meals.

Dosage titration: Make dosage increases in increments of 500 mg (5 mL) weekly or 850 mg (8.5 mL) every 2 weeks, up to a total of 2,000 mg/day (20 mL per day), given in divided doses. Patients also can be titrated from 500 mg (5 mL) twice daily to 850 mg (8.5 mL) twice daily after 2 weeks. Doses above 2,000 mg (20 mL) may be better tolerated given 3 times a day with meals.

ER tablets –

Maximum dose: 2,000 mg once daily (2,500 mg for *Fortamet*).

Initial dosage: The usual starting dosage is 500 mg (1,000 mg for *Glumetza* and *Fortamet*) once daily with the evening meal.

Dosage titration: Make dosage increases in increments of 500 mg weekly, up to a maximum of 2,000 mg once daily (2,500 mg for *Fortamet*) with the evening meal. If glycemic control is not achieved on 2,000 mg once daily, consider a trial of 1,000 mg twice daily. If higher doses of metformin are required, use metformin immediate-release tablets at total daily doses of up to 2,550 mg administered in divided daily doses.

Off-label dosing –

Antipsychotic-induced weight gain: [4] = Insufficient documentation. 500 to 2,550 mg daily in adults, administered in 3 divided doses for 8 weeks.

Polycystic ovary syndrome: [1] = Good documentation. Used as monotherapy or as part of a combination at oral dosages ranging from 1,500 to 2,000 mg daily in divided doses.

➤*Children:*

Type 2 diabetes –

Immediate-release tablets / solution:

- *10 years of age and older* –
  - *Maximum dose:* 2,000 mg/day (20 mL/day).
  - *Initial dosage:* 500 mg (5 mL) twice a day, given with meals.
  - *Dosage titration:* Make dosage increases in increments of 500 mg (5 mL) weekly up to a maximum of 2,000 mg/day (20 mL), given in divided doses.
- *Younger than 10 years of age* – Safety and effectiveness have not been established.

ER tablets: Safety and effectiveness have not been established.

Off-label dosing –

Antipsychotic-induced weight gain: [4] = Insufficient documentation. In children 10 years of age and older, 500 mg 3 times daily for 8 to 12 weeks.

➤*Elderly:* The initial and maintenance dosing of metformin should be conservative in patients with advanced age because of the potential for decreased renal function in this population. Base any dosage adjustment on a careful assessment of renal function. Generally, do not titrate elderly, debilitated, and malnourished patients to the maximum dose of metformin.

➤*Renal function impairment:* Because metformin can accumulate to toxic levels in patients with renal function impairment, administration of metformin is contraindicated in these patients.

➤*Hepatic function impairment:* Because hepatic function impairment has been associated with some cases of lactic acidosis, generally avoid metformin in patients with clinical or laboratory evidence of hepatic disease.

➤*Debilitated or malnourished patients:* Debilitated or malnourished patients should not be titrated to the maximum dose of metformin.

➤*Conversion from immediate-release to ER tablets:* Results of a randomized trial suggest that patients receiving metformin immediate-release treatment may be safely switched to metformin ER treatment once daily at the same total daily dose, up to 2,000 mg once daily (2,500 mg for *Fortamet*). Following a switch from metformin immediate-release to ER tablets, closely monitor glycemic control and make dosage adjustments accordingly.

➤*Transfer from other antidiabetic therapy:* When transferring patients from standard oral hypoglycemic agents other than chlorpropamide to metformin, generally, no transition period is necessary. When transferring patients from chlorpropamide, exercise care during the first 2 weeks because of the prolonged retention of chlorpropamide in the body, leading to overlapping drug effects and possible hypoglycemia.

METFORMIN HYDROCHLORIDE — ORAL

➤*Concomitant metformin and oral sulfonylurea therapy in adults:* If a patient has not responded to 4 weeks of the maximum dose of metformin monotherapy, give consideration to gradual addition of an oral sulfonylurea while continuing metformin at the maximum dose, even if prior primary or secondary failure to a sulfonylurea has occurred. Clinical and pharmacokinetic drug-drug interaction data are currently available only for metformin plus glyburide.

With concomitant metformin and sulfonylurea therapy, the desired control of blood glucose may be obtained by adjusting the dose of each drug. Make attempts to identify the minimum effective dose of each drug to achieve this goal. With concomitant metformin and sulfonylurea therapy, the risk of hypoglycemia associated with sulfonylurea therapy continues and may be increased. Take appropriate precautions.

If a patient has not satisfactorily responded to 1 to 3 months of concomitant therapy with the maximum doses of metformin and an oral sulfonylurea, consider therapeutic alternatives, including switching to insulin with or without metformin.

➤*Concomitant insulin therapy:* Continue the current insulin dose upon initiation of metformin therapy. Initiate metformin therapy at 500 mg once daily in patients on insulin therapy. For patients not responding adequately, increase the dose of metformin by 500 mg after approximately 1 week and by 500 mg every week thereafter until adequate glycemic control is achieved. The maximum recommended daily dose is 2,500 mg for metformin immediate-release tablets and solution and 2,000 mg for metformin ER tablets (2,500 mg for *Fortamet*). It is recommended that the insulin dose be decreased 10% to 25% when FPG concentrations decrease to less than 120 mg/dL in patients receiving concomitant insulin and metformin. Individualize further adjustment based on glucose-lowering response.

➤*Administration:*

Immediate-release tablets/solution – Give immediate-release tablets and solution in divided doses with meals. Start metformin at a low dose, with gradual dose escalation to reduce GI adverse reactions and to permit identification of the minimum dose required for adequate glycemic control of the patient.

ER – Metformin ER tablets must be swallowed whole and never split, crushed, or chewed. Occasionally, the inactive ingredients of the 500 mg ER tablets will be eliminated in the feces as a soft, hydrated mass, while the 1,000 mg ER tablets will leave an insoluble shell.

Administer *Fortamet* with a full glass of water once daily with the evening meal.

➤*Storage/Stability:*

Tablets (immediate-release and ER) – Store at 20° to 25°C (68° to 77°F); excursions are permitted between 15° and 30°C (59° and 86°F). Dispense in light-resistant containers. Keep tightly closed (protect from moisture). Protect from light. Avoid excessive heat and humidity.

Solution – Store at controlled room temperature, 15° to 30°C (59° to 86°F).

Actions

➤*Pharmacology:* Metformin is an antihyperglycemic agent that improves glucose tolerance in patients with type 2 diabetes, lowering basal and postprandial glucose (PPG). Its pharmacologic mechanisms of action are different from other classes of oral antihyperglycemic agents. Metformin decreases hepatic glucose production, decreases intestinal absorption of glucose, and improves insulin sensitivity by increasing peripheral glucose uptake and utilization. Unlike sulfonylureas, metformin does not produce hypoglycemia in patients with type 2 diabetes or healthy subjects, except in special circumstances (eg, when caloric intake is deficient, when strenuous exercise is not compensated by caloric supplementation, during concomitant use with other glucose-lowering agents [such as sulfonylureas and insulin] or ethanol), and does not cause hyperinsulinemia. With metformin therapy, insulin secretion remains unchanged, while fasting insulin levels and daylong plasma insulin response may actually decrease.

➤*Pharmacokinetics:*

Absorption –

Tablets (immediate-release and ER): The absolute bioavailability of a metformin immediate-release 500 mg tablet given under fasting conditions is approximately 50% to 60%. Studies using single oral doses of metformin immediate-release 500 to 1,500 mg, and 850 to 2,550 mg, indicate that there is a lack of dose proportionality with increasing doses, which is caused by decreased absorption rather than an alteration in elimination.

Following a single oral dose of metformin ER, C_{max} is achieved with a median value of 7 hours and a range of 4 to 8 hours. Peak plasma levels are approximately 20% lower compared with the same dose of metformin immediate-release; however, the extent of absorption (as measured by area under the curve [AUC]) is similar to metformin immediate-release.

At steady state, the AUC and C_{max} are less than dose proportional for metformin ER within the range of 500 to 2,000 mg administered once daily. Peak plasma levels are approximately 0.6, 1.1, 1.4, and 1.8 mcg/mL for 500, 1,000, 1,500, and 2,000 mg once-daily doses, respectively. The extent of metformin absorption (as measured by AUC) from metformin ER at a 2,000 mg once-daily dose is similar to the same total daily dose administered as metformin immediate release 1,000 mg twice daily. After repeated administration of metformin ER, metformin did not accumulate in plasma.

Within-subject variability in C_{max} and AUC of metformin from metformin ER is comparable with that from metformin immediate-release.

• *Effect of food* – Food decreases the extent and slightly delays the absorption of metformin immediate-release, as shown by an approximately 40% lower mean peak plasma concentration, a 25% lower AUC, and a 35-minute prolongation of T_{max} following administration of a single metformin 850 mg tablet with food, compared with the same tablet strength administered while fasting. The clinical relevance of these decreases is unknown.

Although the extent of metformin absorption (as measured by AUC) from metformin ER increased approximately 50% when given with food, there was no effect of food on C_{max} and T_{max} of metformin. Both high- and low-fat meals had the same effect on the pharmacokinetics of metformin ER.

Fortamet: The appearance of metformin in plasma from a *Fortamet* ER tablet is slower and more prolonged compared with metformin immediate-release.

In a multiple-dose, crossover study, 23 patients with type 2 diabetes mellitus were administered either *Fortamet* 2,000 mg once daily (after dinner) or metformin immediate-release 1,000 mg twice daily (after breakfast and after dinner). After 4 weeks of treatment, steady-state pharmacokinetic parameters (AUC, T_{max}, and C_{max}) were evaluated.

Fortamet vs Metformin Immediate-Release Steady-State Pharmacokinetic Parameters at 4 Weeks

Pharmacokinetic parameters (mean ± SD[a])	*Fortamet* 2,000 mg (administered once daily after dinner)	Metformin immediate-release 2,000 mg (1,000 mg twice daily)
AUC_{0-24h} (ng•h/mL)	26,811 ± 7,055	27,371 ± 5,781
T_{max} (h)	6 (3 to 10)	3 (1 to 8)
C_{max} (ng/mL)	2,849 ± 797	1,820 ± 370

[a] SD = standard deviation.

In 4 single-dose studies and 1 multiple-dose study, the bioavailability of *Fortamet* 2,000 mg given once daily in the evening under fed conditions (as measured by AUC) was similar to the same total daily dose administered as metformin immediate-release 1,000 mg given twice daily. The geometric mean ratios (*Fortamet*/metformin immediate-release) of AUC_{0-24h}, AUC_{0-72h}, and $AUC_{0-\infty}$ for these 5 studies ranged from 0.96 to 1.08.

In a single-dose, 4-period replicate crossover design study comparing 2 *Fortamet* 500 mg tablets to 1 *Fortamet* 1,000 mg tablet administered in the evening with food to 29 healthy men, 2 *Fortamet* 500 mg tablets were found to be equivalent to 1 *Fortamet* 1,000 mg tablet.

In a study carried out with *Fortamet*, there was a dose-associated increase in metformin exposure over 24 hours following oral administration of 1,000, 1,500, 2,000, and 2,500 mg.

• *Effect of food* – In 3 studies with *Fortamet* using different treatment regimens (2,000 mg after dinner; 1,000 mg after breakfast and after dinner; and 2,500 mg after dinner), the pharmacokinetics of metformin as measured by AUC appeared linear following multiple-dose administration.

The extent of metformin absorption (as measured by AUC) from *Fortamet* increased by approximately 60% when given with food. When *Fortamet* was administered with food, C_{max} was increased by approximately 30% and T_{max} was more prolonged compared with the fasting state (6.1 vs 4 hours).

Glumetza: The following pharmacokinetic studies were performed with the 500 mg dosage form. Following a single oral dose of *Glumetza* 1,000 mg (two 500 mg tablets) after a meal, the T_{max} is achieved at approximately 7 to 8 hours. In both single- and multiple-dose studies in healthy subjects, once-daily 1,000 mg (two 500 mg tablets) dosing provides equivalent systemic exposure, as measured by AUC, and up to 35% higher C_{max}, of metformin relative to the immediate-release given as 500 mg twice daily. *Glumetza* must be administered immediately after a meal to maximize therapeutic benefit.

Summary of _Glumetza_ Pharmacokinetic Parameters After One-Day Dosing

Pharmacokinetic parameters	*Glumetza* two 500 mg tablets	*Glumetza* one 500 mg tablet twice daily	Glucophage one 500 mg tablet twice daily
AUC_{0-36} (ng•h/mL)	14,182 ± 2,415	15,260 ± 3,496	15,342 ± 3,398
C_{max} (ng/mL)	1,301.4 ± 285.7	811.9 ± 173.7	959.1 ± 204
T_{max} (h)	7.5 ± 1.2	7.1 ± 1.2	4.2 ± 1.6

Single oral doses of *Glumetza* 500 to 2,500 mg resulted in a less than proportional increase in both AUC and C_{max}. The mean C_{max} values were 473 ± 145, 868 ± 223, 1,171 ± 297, and 1,630 ± 399 ng/mL for single doses of 500, 1,000, 1,500, and 2,500 mg, respectively. For AUC, the mean values were 3,501 ± 796, 6,705 ± 1,918, 9,299 ± 2,833, and 14,161 ± 4,432 ng•h/mL for single doses of 500, 1,000, 1,500, and 2,500 mg, respectively.

• *Effect of food* – Low- and high-fat meals increased the systemic exposure (as measured by AUC) from *Glumetza* by approximately 38% and 73%, respectively, relative to fasting. Both meals prolonged metformin T_{max} by approximately 3 hours, but C_{max} was not affected.

• *Bioequivalence* – In a 2-way, single-dose, crossover study in healthy volunteers, the 1,000 mg tablet was found to be bioequivalent to two 500 mg tablets under fed conditions based on equivalent C_{max} and AUCs for the 2 formulations.

METFORMIN HYDROCHLORIDE — ORAL

Mean (± SD) Pharmacokinetic Parameters for *Glumetza* 1,000 mg Tablet and *Glumetza* 2 × 500 mg Tablets		
Pharmacokinetic parameters	*Glumetza* 1,000 mg tablet	*Glumetza* 2 × 500 mg tablets
AUC_{0-t} (ng•h/mL)	11,706 ± 2,520	12,408 ± 2,581
$AUC_{0-\infty}$ (ng•h/mL)	11,907 ± 2,521	12,599 ± 2,616
C_{max} (ng/mL)	1,238 ± 271	1,116 ± 254

Solution: Two pharmacokinetic studies have been performed in healthy volunteers to evaluate the bioavailability of metformin solution in comparison with the commercially available metformin tablets under fasting and fed conditions (studies 1 and 2). A third pharmacokinetic study (study 3) assessed effects of food on absorption of metformin solution.

The rate and extent of absorption with metformin solution was found to be comparable with that of metformin tablets under fasting or fed conditions.

Studies using single oral doses of metformin 500 to 1,500 mg and 850 to 2,550 mg tablet formulations indicate that there is a lack of dose proportionality with increasing doses, which is caused by decreased absorption rather than an alteration in elimination.

• *Effect of food* – The food-effect study (study 3) assessed the effects of a high-fat/high-calorie meal and low-fat/low-calorie meal on the bioavailability of metformin solution in comparison with administration in the fasted state in healthy volunteers. The extent of absorption was increased 21% and 17% with the low-fat/low-calorie meal and the high-fat/high-calorie meal, respectively, compared with the administration in the fasted state. The rate and extent of absorption with high-fat/high-calorie and low-fat/low-calorie meals were similar. The mean T_{max} was 2.5 hours under fasting conditions compared with 3.9 hours with both low-fat/low-calorie and high-fat/high-calorie meals.

Distribution – The apparent volume of distribution (V/F) of metformin following single oral doses of metformin immediate-release 850 mg averaged 654 ± 358 L. Metformin is negligibly bound to plasma proteins, in contrast to sulfonylureas, which are more than 90% protein bound. Metformin partitions into erythrocytes, most likely as a function of time. At usual clinical doses and dosing schedules of metformin, steady-state plasma concentrations of metformin are reached within 24 to 48 hours and are generally 1 mcg/mL or less. During controlled clinical trials of metformin, maximum metformin plasma levels did not exceed 5 mcg/mL, even at maximum doses.

Metabolism/Excretion – Intravenous (IV) single-dose studies in healthy subjects demonstrate that metformin is excreted unchanged in the urine and does not undergo hepatic metabolism (no metabolites have been identified in humans) nor biliary excretion. Renal clearance is approximately 3.5 times greater than CrCl, which indicates that tubular secretion is the major route of metformin elimination. Following oral administration, approximately 90% of the absorbed drug is eliminated via the renal route within the first 24 hours, with a plasma elimination half-life of approximately 6.2 hours. In blood, the elimination half-life is approximately 17.6 hours, suggesting that the erythrocyte mass may be a compartment of distribution.

Fortamet: In healthy, nondiabetic adults (N = 18) receiving *Fortamet* 2,500 mg once-daily, the percent of the metformin dose excreted in urine over 24 hours was 40.9% and the renal clearance was 542 ± 310 mL/min. After repeated administration of *Fortamet*, there is little or no accumulation of metformin in plasma, with most of the drug being eliminated via renal excretion over a 24-hour dosing interval. The half-life was 5.4 hours for *Fortamet*.

Special populations –

Renal function impairment: In patients with decreased renal function (based on measured CrCl), the plasma and blood half-life of metformin are prolonged, and the renal clearance is decreased in proportion to the decrease in CrCl. Because metformin can accumulate to toxic levels in patients with renal function impairment, administration of metformin is contraindicated in these patients.

• *Glumetza* – In patients with mild and moderate renal failure (based on measured CrCl), the oral and renal clearance of metformin were decreased by 33% and 50% and 16% and 53%, respectively. Metformin peak and systemic exposure were significantly greater in patients with renal failure relative to healthy volunteers with healthy renal function. There was a rank-order correlation of metformin AUC and C_{max} with degree of renal failure.

Elderly: Limited data from controlled pharmacokinetic studies of metformin in healthy elderly subjects suggest that total plasma clearance of metformin is decreased, the half-life is prolonged, and C_{max} is increased compared with healthy younger subjects. From these data, it appears that the change in metformin pharmacokinetics with aging is primarily accounted for by a change in renal function. Do not initiate metformin treatment in patients 80 years of age and older unless measurement of CrCl demonstrates that renal function is not reduced.

Gender:

• *Glumetza* – In the pharmacokinetic studies in healthy volunteers, there were no important differences between male and female subjects with respect to metformin AUC (males = 268, females = 293) and half-life (males = 229, females = 260). However, C_{max} for metformin were somewhat higher in women (female/male C_{max} ratio, 1.4). The gender differences for C_{max} are unlikely to be clinically important.

Race:

• *Glumetza* – The data suggest a trend towards higher metformin C_{max} and AUC values for metformin obtained in Asian subjects when compared with white, Hispanic, and black subjects. The difference between the Asian and white groups is unlikely to be clinically important.

Contraindications

Renal disease or renal function impairment (eg, as suggested by serum creatinine levels of 1.5 mg/dL or more [men] and 1.4 mg/dL or more [women], or abnormal CrCl) that also may result from conditions such as cardiovascular collapse (shock), acute myocardial infarction (MI), and septicemia; known hypersensitivity to metformin ; acute or chronic metabolic acidosis, including diabetic ketoacidosis, with or without coma. Treat diabetic ketoacidosis with insulin.

Temporarily discontinue metformin in patients undergoing radiologic studies involving intravascular administration of iodinated contrast materials because use of such products may result in acute alteration of renal function.

Warnings/Precautions

➤*Lactic acidosis:* See the Warning box for more information.

➤*Iodinated contrast materials:* Radiologic studies involving the use of intravascular iodinated contrast materials (ie, IV urogram, IV cholangiography, angiography, and computed tomography [CT] scans with intravascular contrast materials) can lead to acute alteration of renal function and have been associated with lactic acidosis in patients receiving metformin. Therefore, in patients in whom any such study is planned, temporarily discontinue metformin at the time of or prior to the procedure and withhold for 48 hours subsequent to the procedure; reinstitute only after renal function has been reevaluated and found to be normal.

➤*Hypoxic states:* Cardiovascular collapse (shock) from whatever cause, acute CHF, acute MI, and other conditions characterized by hypoxemia have been associated with lactic acidosis and also may cause prerenal azotemia. When such events occur in patients on metformin therapy, promptly discontinue the drug.

➤*Surgical procedures:* Temporarily suspend metformin therapy for any surgical procedure (except minor procedures not associated with restricted intake of food and fluids), and do not restart until the patient's oral intake has resumed and renal function has been evaluated and found to be normal.

➤*Vitamin B_{12} levels:* In controlled clinical trials of metformin of 29 weeks' duration, a decrease to subnormal levels of previously normal serum vitamin B_{12} levels, without clinical manifestations, was observed in approximately 7% of patients. Such a decrease, possibly caused by interference with B_{12} absorption from the B_{12}-intrinsic factor complex, is, however, very rarely associated with anemia and appears to be rapidly reversible with discontinuation of metformin or vitamin B_{12} supplementation. Measurement of hematologic parameters on an annual basis is advised in patients receiving metformin, and any apparent abnormalities should be appropriately investigated and managed.

Certain individuals (those with inadequate vitamin B_{12} or calcium intake or absorption) appear to be predisposed to developing subnormal vitamin B_{12} levels. In these patients, routine serum vitamin B_{12} measurements at 2- to 3-year intervals may be useful.

➤*Change in clinical status:* Promptly evaluate patients with type 2 diabetes previously well controlled on metformin who develop laboratory abnormalities or clinical illness (especially vague and poorly defined illness) for evidence of ketoacidosis or lactic acidosis. Evaluation should include serum electrolytes and ketones, blood glucose, and, if indicated, blood pH, lactate, pyruvate, and metformin levels. If acidosis of either form occurs, discontinue metformin immediately and initiate other appropriate corrective measures.

➤*Hypoglycemia:* Hypoglycemia does not occur in patients receiving metformin alone under usual circumstances of use but could occur when caloric intake is deficient, when strenuous exercise is not compensated by caloric supplementation, or during concomitant use with other glucose-lowering agents (eg, sulfonylureas and insulin) or ethanol.

Elderly, debilitated, or malnourished patients, and those with adrenal or pituitary insufficiency or alcohol intoxication are particularly susceptible to hypoglycemic effects. Hypoglycemia may be difficult to recognize in elderly patients and in people who are taking beta-adrenergic–blocking drugs.

➤*Loss of control of blood glucose:* When a patient stabilized on any diabetic regimen is exposed to stress (eg, fever, trauma, infection, surgery), a temporary loss of glycemic control may occur. At such times, it may be necessary to withhold metformin and temporarily administer insulin. Metformin may be reinstituted after the acute episode is resolved.

The effectiveness of oral antidiabetic drugs in lowering blood glucose to a targeted level decreases in many patients over a period of time. This phenomenon, which may be caused by progression of the underlying disease or diminished responsiveness to the drug, is known as secondary failure, to distinguish it from primary failure in which the drug is ineffective during initial therapy. Should secondary failure occur with either metformin or sulfonylurea monotherapy, combined therapy with metformin and a sulfonylurea may result in a response. Should secondary failure occur with combined metformin/sulfonylurea therapy, it may be necessary to consider therapeutic alternatives, including initiation of insulin therapy.

➤*Renal function impairment:* Metformin is contraindicated in patients with renal disease or renal function impairment (eg, as suggested by serum creatinine levels of 1.5 mg/dL or more [men] and 1.4 mg/dL [women], or as abnormal CrCl) that also may result from conditions such as cardiovascular collapse (shock), acute MI, and septicemia.

Metformin is known to be substantially excreted by the kidney, and the risk of metformin accumulation and lactic acidosis increases with the degree of impairment of renal function. Thus, patients with serum creatinine levels above the ULN for their age should not receive metformin. In patients with

METFORMIN HYDROCHLORIDE — ORAL

advanced age, titrate metformin carefully to establish the minimum dose for adequate glycemic effect because aging is associated with reduced renal function. In elderly patients, particularly those 80 years of age and older, monitor renal function regularly and, generally, do not titrate metformin to the maximum dose.

Concomitant medication(s) that may affect renal function or result in significant hemodynamic change or may interfere with the disposition of metformin, such as cationic drugs that are eliminated by renal tubular secretion, should be used with caution.

➤*Hepatic function impairment:* Because hepatic function impairment has been associated with some cases of lactic acidosis, generally avoid metformin in patients with clinical or laboratory evidence of hepatic disease.

➤*Pregnancy: Category B.*

Teratogenic – Recent information strongly suggests that abnormal blood glucose levels during pregnancy are associated with a higher incidence of congenital abnormalities. Most experts recommend that insulin be used during pregnancy to maintain blood glucose levels as close to normal as possible. There are no adequate and well-controlled studies in pregnant women with metformin. Because animal reproduction studies are not always predictive of human response, do not use metformin during pregnancy unless clearly needed.

➤*Lactation:* Studies in lactating rats show that metformin is excreted into milk and reaches levels comparable with those in plasma. Consistent with its molecular weight (approximately 166), metformin is considered to be excreted into breast milk. Because the potential for hypoglycemia or other serious adverse reactions in breast-fed infants may exist, decide whether to discontinue breast-feeding or the drug, taking into account the importance of the drug to the mother. If metformin is discontinued, and if diet alone is inadequate for controlling blood glucose, consider insulin therapy.

➤*Children:*

Immediate-release tablets / solution – The safety and effectiveness of metformin for the treatment of type 2 diabetes have been established in children 10 to 16 years of age (studies have not been conducted in children younger than 10 years of age). Use of metformin in this age group is supported by evidence from adequate and well-controlled studies of metformin in adults with additional data from a controlled clinical study in children 10 to 16 years of age with type 2 diabetes, which demonstrated a similar response in glycemic control to that seen in adults. In this study, adverse reactions were similar to those described in adults. A maximum daily dose of 2,000 mg is recommended.

ER tablets – Safety and efficacy of metformin ER tablets in children have not been established.

➤*Elderly:* Do not initiate metformin therapy in patients 80 years of age and older, unless measurement of CrCl demonstrates that renal function is not reduced, because these patients are more susceptible to developing lactic acidosis.

In general, dose selection for an elderly patient should be cautious, usually starting at the low end of the dosing range, reflecting the greater frequency of decreased hepatic, renal, or cardiac function, and of concomitant disease or other drug therapy.

Metformin is known to be substantially excreted by the kidney; because the risk of serious adverse reactions to the drug is greater in patients with renal function impairment, only use metformin in patients with healthy renal function. Because aging is associated with reduced renal function, use metformin with caution as age increases. Take care in dose selection, and base dose on careful and regular monitoring of renal function. Generally, do not titrate elderly patients to the maximum dose of metformin.

➤*Monitoring:* Before initiation of metformin therapy and at least annually thereafter, assess renal function and verify as healthy. In patients in whom development of renal function impairment is anticipated, assess renal function more frequently and discontinue metformin if evidence of renal function impairment is present.

Monitor response to all diabetic therapies by periodic assessments of FPG and HbA_{1c} levels, with a goal of decreasing these levels toward the normal range. During initial dose titration, fasting glucose can be used to determine the therapeutic response. Thereafter, monitor both glucose and HbA_{1c} every 3 months. Measurements of HbA_{1c} may be especially useful for evaluating long-term control. Monitoring of blood glucose and HbA_{1c} also will permit detection of primary failure (ie, inadequate lowering of blood glucose at the maximum recommended dose of medication) and secondary failure (ie, loss of an adequate blood glucose–lowering response after an initial period of efficacy).

Perform initial and periodic monitoring of hematologic parameters (eg, hemoglobin/hematocrit and red blood cell indices) and renal function (serum creatinine) at least on an annual basis. While megaloblastic anemia has rarely been seen with metformin therapy, if this is suspected, exclude vitamin B_{12} deficiency.

Drug Interactions

Metformin Drug Interactions

Precipitant drug	Object drug[a]		Description
Alcohol	Metformin	⬆	Alcohol potentiates the effect of metformin on lactate metabolism. Warn patients against excessive alcohol intake, acute or chronic, while receiving metformin.
Calcium channel blockers Corticosteroids Estrogens Hormonal contraceptives Isoniazid Nicotinic acid Phenothiazines Phenytoin Sympathomimetics Thiazide diuretics Thyroid agents	Metformin	⬇	Certain drugs tend to produce hyperglycemia and may lead to loss of glycemic control. When such drugs are withdrawn from a patient receiving metformin, closely observe the patient for hypoglycemia.
Cationic drugs (eg, amiloride, cephalexin, digoxin, morphine, procainamide, quinidine, quinine, ranitidine, triamterene, trimethoprim, vancomycin)	Metformin	⬆	Cationic drugs that are eliminated by renal tubular secretion theoretically have the potential for interaction with metformin by competing for common renal tubular transport systems. Although such interactions remain theoretical, careful patient monitoring and dose adjustment of metformin and/or the interfering drug are recommended in patients who are taking cationic medications excreted via the proximal renal tubular secretory system.
Cimetidine	Metformin	⬆	Cimetidine caused a 60% increase in peak metformin plasma concentrations and a 40% increase in AUC.
Furosemide	Metformin	⬆	Furosemide increased the metformin plasma and blood C_{max} 22% and blood AUC 15%, without any significant change in metformin renal clearance. When administered with metformin, the C_{max} and AUC of furosemide were 31% and 12% smaller, respectively, than when administered alone, and the terminal half-life was decreased 32%, without any significant change in furosemide renal clearance.
Metformin	Furosemide	⬇	
Iodinated contrast material	Metformin	⬆	Parenteral contrast studies with iodinated materials can lead to acute renal failure and have been associated with lactic acidosis in patients receiving metformin. Therefore, in patients in whom any such study is planned, temporarily discontinue metformin at the time of or prior to the procedure and withhold for 48 hours subsequent to the procedure; reinstitute only after renal function has been reevaluated and found to be normal.
Nifedipine	Metformin	⬆	Coadministration increased plasma metformin C_{max} and AUC 20% and 9%, respectively, and increased the amount excreted in the urine. Nifedipine appears to enhance the absorption of metformin.
Rofecoxib	Metformin	⬆	Plasma concentrations and pharmacologic effects of metformin may be increased by rofecoxib.

METFORMIN HYDROCHLORIDE — ORAL

Metformin Drug Interactions			
Precipitant drug	Object drug[a]		Description
Metformin	Glyburide	↔	Following coadministration of single doses, decreases in glyburide AUC and C_{max} were observed but were highly variable; the clinical significance of this interaction is uncertain.

[a] ↑ = object drug increased; ↓ = object drug decreased; ↔ = undetermined clinical effect.

➤*Drug/Food interactions:* Food decreases the extent and slightly delays the absorption of metformin, as shown by an approximately 40% lower mean C_{max}, a 25% lower AUC, and a 35-minute prolongation of T_{max} following administration of a single metformin 850 mg tablet with food, compared with the same tablet strength administered fasting. The clinical relevance of these decreases is unknown.

Although the extent of metformin absorption (as measured by AUC) from metformin ER increased approximately 50% when given with food, there was no effect of food on C_{max} and T_{max} of metformin. Both high- and low-fat meals had the same effect on the pharmacokinetics of metformin ER.

The extent of metformin absorption (as measured by AUC) from *Fortamet* increased by approximately 60% when given with food. When *Fortamet* was administered with food, C_{max} was increased by approximately 30%, and T_{max} was more prolonged compared with the fasting state (6.1 vs 4 hours).

Low- and high-fat meals increased the systemic exposure (as measured by AUC) from *Glumetza* by approximately 38% and 73%, respectively, relative to fasting. Both meals prolonged metformin T_{max} by approximately 3 hours, but C_{max} was not affected.

Adverse Reactions

➤*Immediate-release tablets/solution:*

Metformin Immediate-Release Tablets and Solution Adverse Reactions (> 5%) (Monotherapy Study)[a]		
Adverse reaction	Metformin (n = 141)	Placebo (n = 145)
CNS		
Asthenia	9.2%	5.5%
Headache	5.7%	4.8%
GI		
Abdominal discomfort	6.4%	4.8%
Diarrhea	53.2%	11.7%
Flatulence	12.1%	5.5%
Indigestion	7.1%	4.1%
Nausea/Vomiting	25.5%	8.3%

[a] Reactions that were more common in metformin- than placebo-treated patients.

Diarrhea led to discontinuation of study medication in 6% of patients treated with metformin.

Other adverse reactions (1% to 5%) – Additionally, the following adverse reactions were reported in between 1% and 5% of metformin patients and were more commonly reported with metformin than placebo:

CNS: Chills, light-headedness.

Dermatologic: Flushing, nail disorder, rash, sweating increased.

GI: Abnormal stools, taste disorder.

Miscellaneous: Chest discomfort, dyspnea, flu syndrome, hypoglycemia, myalgia, palpitation.

➤*Metformin ER:*

Glucophage XR –

Glucophage XR Adverse Reactions (> 5%)[a]		
Adverse reaction	Metformin ER (n = 781)	Placebo (n = 195)
GI		
Diarrhea	9.6%	2.6%
Nausea/Vomiting	6.5%	1.5%

[a] Reactions that were more common in patients treated with metformin ER tablets than with placebo.

Diarrhea led to discontinuation of study medication in 0.6% of patients treated with metformin ER tablets.

Other adverse reactions (1% to 5%): Additionally, the following adverse reactions were reported in at least 1% to 5% of metformin ER–treated patients and were more commonly reported with metformin ER tablets than placebo:

• *CNS* – Dizziness, headache.
• *GI* – Abdomen distention, abdominal pain, constipation, dyspepsia/heartburn, flatulence.
• *Miscellaneous* – Taste disturbance, upper respiratory tract infection.

Fortamet –

Fortamet Adverse Reactions (> 5%)		
Adverse reaction	*Fortamet* (n = 424)	Metformin immediate-release (n = 430)
CNS		
Headache	4.7%	5.1%
GI		
Diarrhea	16.7%	11.9%
Dyspepsia	4.2%	5.1%
Nausea	8.5%	7.4%
Respiratory		
Rhinitis	4.2%	5.6%
Miscellaneous		
Accidental injury	7.3%	5.6%
Infection	20.5%	20.9%

The most frequent adverse reactions thought to be related to *Fortamet* were abdominal pain, diarrhea, dyspepsia, flatulence, and nausea. The frequency of dyspepsia was 4.2% in the *Fortamet* group, compared with 5.1% in the metformin immediate-release group; the frequency of flatulence was 3.5% in the *Fortamet* group, compared with 3.7% in the metformin immediate-release group; and the frequency of abdominal pain was 3.3% in the *Fortamet* group, compared with 4.4% in the metformin immediate-release group.

In the controlled studies, 4.7% of patients treated with *Fortamet* and 4.9% of patients treated with metformin immediate-release were discontinued because of adverse reactions.

Glumetza –

In the 24-week, active-controlled monotherapy trial, serious adverse reactions were reported in 3.6% (19/528) of the *Glumetza*-treated patients compared with 2.9% (5/174) of the patients treated with metformin immediate-release. During the 6-month, open-label, uncontrolled extension trial, an additional 10 (4%) *Glumetza*-treated patients reported a serious adverse reaction. In the add-on to sulfonylurea study, a serious adverse reaction was reported in 2.1% (9/431) of the *Glumetza* plus glyburide-treated patients compared with 1.4% (2/144) of the placebo plus glyburide-treated patients. When the data from all clinical trials were combined, the most frequently (incidence at least 0.5%) reported serious adverse reactions classified by system organ class were GI disorders (1% of *Glumetza*-treated patients compared with 0% of patients not treated with *Glumetza*) and cardiac disorders (0.4% of *Glumetza*-treated patients compared with 0.5% of patients not treated with *Glumetza*). Only 2 serious adverse reactions (unstable angina [n = 2]) were reported in more than 1 *Glumetza*-treated patient.

In the placebo-controlled study, patients receiving background glyburide therapy were randomized to receive add-on treatment of either 1 of 3 different regimens of *Glumetza* or placebo. In total, 431 patients received *Glumetza* plus sulfonylurea, and 144 patients received placebo plus sulfonylurea. Adverse reactions reported in more than 5% of patients treated with *Glumetza* that were more common in the combined *Glumetza* plus sulfonylurea group than in the placebo plus sulfonylurea group are shown in the following table.

In 0.7% of patients treated with *Glumetza* plus sulfonylurea, diarrhea was responsible for discontinuation of study medication compared with zero in the placebo plus sulfonylurea group.

Glumetza Adverse Reactions (> 5%)[a]		
Adverse reaction	*Glumetza* + sulfonylurea (n = 431)	Placebo + sulfonylurea (n = 144)
GI		
Diarrhea	12.5%	5.6%
Nausea	6.7%	4.2%
Miscellaneous		
Hypoglycemia	13.7%	4.9%

[a] Adverse reactions that were more common in *Glumetza*-treated patients than in placebo-treated patients.

Other adverse reactions (1% to 5%): In the same study, the following adverse reactions were reported by 1% to 5% of patients for the combined *Glumetza* plus a sulfonylurea group, and these reactions occurred more commonly in *Glumetza*-treated patients than in placebo-treated patients.

• *CNS* – Asthenia, dizziness, hypoasthesia, sinus headache, tremor.
• *GI* – Abdominal distension, abdominal pain, dyspepsia, flatulence, gastroenteritis viral, loose stools, toothache, upper abdominal pain, vomiting.
• *Musculoskeletal* – Muscle cramp, muscle strain, myalgia, pain in limb.
• *Respiratory* – Nasal congestion, seasonal allergy.
• *Miscellaneous* – Chest pain, contusion, ear pain, fungal infection, hypertension, tonsillitis, tooth abscess.

Overdosage

➤*Symptoms:* Overdose of metformin has occurred, including ingestion of amounts of more than 50 g. Hypoglycemia was reported in approximately 10% of cases, but no causal association with metformin has been established. Lactic acidosis has been reported in approximately 32% of metformin overdose cases. In other metformin clinical trials, hypoglycemia has not

METFORMIN HYDROCHLORIDE — ORAL

been seen, even with ingestion of up to 85 g of metformin, although lactic acidosis has occurred in such circumstances.

Glumetza – No cases of overdose were reported during *Glumetza* clinical trials. It would be expected that adverse reactions of a more intense character, including epigastric discomfort, nausea, and vomiting followed by diarrhea, drowsiness, weakness, dizziness, malaise, and headache, might be seen. Should these symptoms persist, lactic acidosis should be excluded. Discontinue the drug and institute proper supportive therapy.

➤*Treatment:* Metformin is dialyzable, with a clearance of up to 170 mL/min under good hemodynamic conditions. Therefore, hemodialysis may be useful for removal of accumulated drug from patients in whom metformin overdosage is suspected.

Patient Information

Inform patients of the potential risks and benefits of metformin and of alternative modes of therapy. Also inform patients about the importance of adherence to dietary instructions, a regular exercise program, and regular testing of blood glucose, HbA_{1c}, renal function, and hematologic parameters.

Explain to patients the risks of lactic acidosis, its symptoms, and conditions that predispose to its development. Advise patients to discontinue metformin immediately and to promptly notify their health care provider if unexplained hyperventilation, myalgia, malaise, unusual somnolence, or other nonspecific symptoms occur. Once a patient is stabilized on any dose level of metformin, GI symptoms, which are common during initiation of metformin therapy, are unlikely to be drug related. Later occurrence of GI symptoms could be caused by lactic acidosis or other serious disease.

Counsel patients against excessive alcohol intake, either acute or chronic, while receiving metformin.

Metformin alone does not usually cause hypoglycemia, although it may occur when metformin is used in conjunction with oral sulfonylureas and insulin. When initiating combination therapy, explain to patients and responsible family members the risks of hypoglycemia, its symptoms and treatment, and conditions that predispose to its development.

Inform patients that metformin ER tablets must be swallowed whole and not crushed or chewed, and that the inactive ingredients may occasionally be eliminated in the feces as a soft mass that may resemble the original tablet.

REPAGLINIDE

Rx	**Prandin** (Novo Nordisk)	**Tablets:** 0.5 mg	White. In 100s, 500s, and 1,000s.
		1 mg	Yellow. In 100s, 500s, and 1,000s.
		2 mg	Peach. In 100s, 500s, and 1,000s.

REPAGLINIDE — ORAL

Indications

➤*Type 2 diabetes mellitus:* As an adjunct to diet and exercise to lower the blood glucose in patients with type 2 diabetes mellitus (non-insulin-dependent diabetes mellitus [NIDDM]) whose hyperglycemia cannot be controlled satisfactorily by diet and exercise alone.

Repaglinide is also indicated for combination therapy use (with metformin or thiazolidinediones) to lower blood glucose in patients whose hyperglycemia cannot be controlled by diet and exercise plus monotherapy with any of the following agents: Metformin, sulfonylureas, repaglinide, or thiazolidinediones. If glucose control has not been achieved after a suitable trial of combination therapy, give consideration to discontinuing these drugs and using insulin. Base judgments on regular clinical and laboratory evaluations.

Administration and Dosage

➤*General dosing considerations:* The patient's blood glucose should be monitored periodically to determine the minimum effective dose for the patient, to detect primary failure (ie, inadequate lowering of blood glucose at the maximum recommended dose of medication), and to detect secondary failure (ie, loss of an adequate blood glucose-lowering response after an initial period of effectiveness).

Long-term efficacy should be monitored by measurement of HbA_{1c} levels approximately every 3 months.

Failure to follow an appropriate dosage regimen may precipitate hypoglycemia or hyperglycemia.

Short-term administration may be sufficient during periods of transient loss of control in patients usually well controlled on diet.

➤*Adults:*

Type 2 diabetes –

Usual dosage: 0.5 mg to 4 mg taken with meals.

Maximum dose: 16 mg daily.

Initial dosage:

• *Patients not previously treated or whose HbA_{1c} is less than 8%* – 0.5 mg with each meal preprandially.

• *Patients previously treated or whose HbA_{1c} is 8% or more* – 1 or 2 mg with each meal preprandially.

Dosage adjustment: Dosing adjustments should be determined by blood glucose response, usually fasting blood glucose. Postprandial glucose levels testing may be clinically helpful in patients whose premeal blood glucose levels are satisfactory but whose overall glycemic control (HbA_{1c}) is inadequate. The preprandial dose should be doubled up to 4 mg with each meal until satisfactory blood glucose response is achieved. At least 1 week should elapse to assess response after each dose adjustment.

Concomitant therapy: If monotherapy does not result in adequate glycemic control, metformin or a thiazolidinedione may be added. If metformin or thiazolidinedione monotherapy does not provide adequate control, repaglinide may be added. The starting dose and dose adjustments for repaglinide combination therapy are the same as for repaglinide monotherapy. The dose of each drug should be carefully adjusted to determine the minimal dose required to achieve the desired pharmacologic effect. Failure to do so could result in an increase in the incidence of hypoglycemic episodes. Appropriate monitoring of FPG and HbA_{1c} measurements should be used to ensure that the patient is not subjected to excessive drug exposure or increased probability of secondary drug failure. When hypoglycemia occurs in patients taking a combination of repaglinide and a thiazolidinedione or repaglinide and metformin, the dose of repaglinide should be reduced.

Conversion: When repaglinide is used to replace therapy with other oral hypoglycemic agents, repaglinide may be started on the day after the final dose is given. Patients should then be observed carefully for hypoglycemia due to potential overlapping of drug effects. When transferred from longer half-life sulfonylurea agents (eg, chlorpropamide) to repaglinide, close monitoring may be indicated for up to 1 week or longer.

➤*Elderly:* Elderly may be more susceptible to the hypoglycemic action of repaglinide. Hypoglycemia may be difficult to recognize in elderly patients.

➤*Renal function impairment:* Initiate therapy with a 0.5 mg dose in patients with severe renal impairment; subsequently, titrate patients carefully.

➤*Hepatic function impairment:* Use cautiously. Utilize longer intervals between dose adjustments to allow full assessment of response.

➤*Special risk patients:* Debilitated or malnourished patients and patients with adrenal or pituitary insufficiency may be particularly susceptible to the hypoglycemic action of glucose-lowering drugs.

➤*Administration:* Doses are usually taken within 15 minutes of the meal, but time may vary from immediately preceding the meal to as long as 30 minutes before the meal. May be dosed preprandially 2, 3, or 4 times a day in response to changes in the patient's meal pattern.

➤*Storage / Stability:* Do not store above 25°C (77°F). Protect from moisture.

Actions

➤*Pharmacology:* Repaglinide lowers blood glucose levels by stimulating the release of insulin from the pancreas. This action is dependent upon functioning beta cells in the pancreatic islets. Insulin release is glucose-dependent and diminishes at low glucose concentrations.

Repaglinide closes ATP-dependent potassium channels in the beta-cell membrane by binding at characterizable sites. This potassium channel blockade depolarizes the beta-cell, which leads to an opening of calcium channels. The resulting increased calcium influx induces insulin secretion. The ion channel mechanism is highly tissue-selective, with low affinity for heart and skeletal muscle.

➤*Pharmacokinetics:* The pharmacokinetic parameters of repaglinide obtained from a single-dose, crossover study in healthy subjects and from a multiple-dose, parallel, dose-proportionality (0.5, 1, 2, and 4 mg) study in patients with type 2 diabetes are summarized in the following table:

Repaglinide Pharmacokinetic Parameters in Diabetic and Healthy Subjects

Parameter	Patients with Type 2 Diabetes[a]
Dose	$AUC_{0-24\ h}$ (mean ± SD) (ng/mL•h):
0.5 mg	68.9 ± 154.4
1 mg	125.8 ± 129.8
2 mg	152.4 ± 89.6
4 mg	447.4 ± 211.3
Dose	$C_{max\ 0-5\ h}$ (mean ± SD) (ng/mL):
0.5 mg	9.8 ± 10.2
1 mg	18.3 ± 9.1
2 mg	26 ± 13
4 mg	65.8 ± 30.1
Dose	$T_{max\ 0-5\ h}$ means (SD)
0.5 to 4 mg	1 to 1.4 (0.3 to 0.5) h

REPAGLINIDE — ORAL

Repaglinide Pharmacokinetic Parameters in Diabetic and Healthy Subjects

Parameter	Patients with Type 2 Diabetes[a]
Dose	t½ (Ind Range)
0.5 to 4 mg	1 to 1.4 (0.4 to 8) h
Parameter	Healthy subjects
CL[b] based on IV	38 ± 16 L/h
V_{ss}[c] based on IV	31 ± 12 L
AbsBio[d]	56 ± 9%

[a] Dosed preprandially with 3 meals.
[b] CL = total body clearance.
[c] V_{ss} = volume of distribution at steady-state.
[d] AbsBio = absolute bioavailability.

These data indicate that repaglinide did not accumulate in serum. Clearance of oral repaglinide did not change over the 0.5 to 4 mg dose range, indicating a linear relationship between dose and plasma drug levels.

Variability of exposure – Repaglinide AUC after multiple doses of 0.25 to 4 mg with each meal varies over a wide range. The intra-individual and interindividual coefficients of variation were 36% and 69%, respectively. AUC over the therapeutic dose range included 69 to 1005 ng/mL•h, but AUC exposure up to 5417 ng/mL•h was reached in dose escalation studies without apparent adverse consequences.

Absorption – After oral administration, repaglinide is rapidly and completely absorbed from the GI tract. After single and multiple oral doses in healthy subjects or in patients, peak plasma drug levels (C_{max}) occur within 1 hour (t_{max}). Repaglinide is rapidly eliminated from the blood stream with a half-life of approximately 1 hour. The mean absolute bioavailability is 56%. When repaglinide was given with food, the mean T_{max} was not changed, but the mean C_{max} and AUC (area under the time/plasma concentration curve) were decreased 20% and 12.4%, respectively.

Distribution – After IV dosing in healthy subjects, the volume of distribution at steady state (V_{ss}) was 31 L, and the total body clearance (CL) was 38L/h. Protein binding and binding to human serum albumin was greater than 98%.

Metabolism – Repaglinide is completely metabolized by oxidative biotransformation and direct conjugation with glucuronic acid after either an IV or oral dose. The major metabolites are an oxidized dicarboxylic acid (M2), the aromatic amine (M1), and the acyl glucuronide (M7). The cytochrome P450 enzyme system, specifically 3A4, has been shown to be involved in the N-dealkylation of repaglinide to M2 and the further oxidation to M1. Metabolites do not contribute to the glucose-lowering effect of repaglinide.

Excretion – Within 96 hours after dosing with ^{14}C-repaglinide as a single, oral dose, approximately 90% of the radiolabel was recovered in the feces and approximately 8% in the urine. Only 0.1% of the dose is cleared in the urine as parent compound. The major metabolite (M2) accounted for 60% of the administered dose. Less than 2% of parent drug was recovered in feces.

Special populations –

Renal function impairment: Single-dose and steady-state pharmacokinetics of repaglinide were compared between patients with type 2 diabetes and healthy renal function (Ccr greater than 80 mL/min), mild-to-moderate renal function impairment (Ccr = 40 to 80 mL/min), and severe renal function impairment (Ccr = 20 to 40 mL/min). Both AUC and C_{max} of repaglinide were similar in patients with normal and mild to moderately impaired renal function (mean values 56.7 ng/mL•h vs 57.2 ng/mL•h and 37.5 ng/mL vs 37.7 ng/mL, respectively.) Patients with severely reduced renal function had elevated mean AUC and C_{max} values (98 ng/mL•h and 50.7 ng/mL, respectively), but this study showed only a weak correlation between repaglinide levels and creatinine clearance. Initial dose adjustment does not appear to be necessary for patients with mild-to-moderate renal dysfunction. However, initiate patients with type 2 diabetes who have severe renal function impairment with the repaglinide 0.5 mg dose; subsequently, titrate patients carefully. Studies were not conducted in patients with creatinine clearances below 20 mL/min or patients with renal failure requiring hemodialysis.

Hepatic function impairment: A single-dose, open-label study was conducted in 12 healthy subjects and 12 patients with chronic liver disease (CLD) classified by Child-Pugh scale and caffeine clearance. Patients with moderate-to-severe impairment of liver function had higher and more prolonged serum concentrations of both total and unbound repaglinide than healthy subjects (healthy AUC, 91.6 ng/mL•h; CLD patients AUC, 368.9 ng/mL•h; healthy C_{max}, 46.7 ng/mL; CLD patients C_{max}, 105.4 ng/mL). AUC was statistically correlated with caffeine clearance. No difference in glucose profiles was observed across patient groups. Patients with impaired liver function may be exposed to higher concentrations of repaglinide and its associated metabolites than would patients with normal liver function receiving usual doses. Therefore, use repaglinide cautiously in patients with impaired liver function. Utilize longer intervals between dose adjustments to allow full assessment of response.

Gender: A comparison of pharmacokinetics in males and females showed the AUC over the 0.5 to 4 mg dose range to be 15% to 70% higher in females with type 2 diabetes. This difference was not reflected in the frequency of hypoglycemic episodes (male: 16%; female: 17%) or other adverse events. With respect to gender, no change in general dosage recommendation is indicated since dosage for each patient should be individualized to achieve optimal clinical response.

Contraindications

Type 1 diabetes; known hypersensitivity to the drug or its inactive ingredients; diabetic ketoacidosis, with or without coma. Treat this condition with insulin.

Warnings/Precautions

➤*Use with insulin:* Repaglinide is not indicated for use in combination with NPH-insulin.

➤*Hypoglycemia:* All oral blood glucose-lowering drugs are capable of producing hypoglycemia. Proper patient selection, dosage, and instructions to the patients are important to avoid hypoglycemic episodes. Hepatic insufficiency may cause elevated repaglinide blood levels and may diminish gluconeogenic capacity, both of which increase the risk of serious hypoglycemia. Elderly, debilitated, or malnourished patients, and those with adrenal, pituitary, hepatic insufficiency or severe renal insufficiency are particularly susceptible to the hypoglycemic action of glucose-lowering drugs.

Hypoglycemia may be difficult to recognize in the elderly and in people taking beta-adrenergic-blocking drugs. Hypoglycemia is more likely to occur when caloric intake is deficient, after severe or prolonged exercise, when alcohol is ingested, or when more than 1 glucose-lowering drug is used.

The frequency of hypoglycemia is greater in patients with type 2 diabetes who have not been previously treated with oral blood glucose-lowering drugs (naive) or whose HbA_{1c} is less than 8%. Administer repaglinide with meals to lessen the risk of hypoglycemia.

➤*Secondary failure:* When a patient stabilized on any diabetic regimen is exposed to stress such as fever, trauma, infection, or surgery, a loss of glycemic control may occur. At such times, it may be necessary to discontinue repaglinide and administer insulin. The effectiveness of any hypoglycemic drug in lowering blood glucose to a desired level decreases in many patients over a period of time, which may be due to progression of the severity of diabetes or to diminished responsiveness to the drug. This phenomenon is known as secondary failure, to distinguish it from primary failure in which the drug is ineffective in an individual patient when the drug is first given. Adequate adjustment of dose and adherence to diet should be assessed before classifying a patient as a secondary failure.

➤*Hepatic function impairment:* Patients with impaired liver function may be exposed to higher concentrations of repaglinide and its associated metabolites than would patients with normal liver function receiving usual doses. Therefore, use repaglinide cautiously in patients with impaired liver function. Utilize longer intervals between dose adjustments to allow full assessment of response.

➤*Pregnancy: Category C.*

Teratogenic – Safety in pregnant women has not been established. Because animal reproduction studies are not always predictive of human response, use repaglinide during pregnancy only if it is clearly needed.

Nonteratogenic – Offspring of rat dams exposed to repaglinide at 15 times clinical exposure on a mg/m^2 basis during days 17 to 22 of gestation and during lactation developed nonteratogenic skeletal deformities consisting of shortening, thickening, and bending of the humerus during the postnatal period. This effect was not seen at doses up to 2.5 times clinical exposure (on a mg/m^2 basis) on days 1 to 22 of pregnancy or at higher doses given during days 1 to 16 of pregnancy. Relevant human exposure has not occurred to date and therefore the safety of repaglinide administration throughout pregnancy or lactation cannot be established.

➤*Lactation:* In rat reproduction studies, measurable levels of repaglinide were detected in the breast milk of the dams and lowered blood glucose levels were observed in the pups. Cross fostering studies indicated that skeletal changes could be induced in control pups nursed by treated dams, although this occurred to a lesser degree than those pups treated in utero. Although it is not known whether repaglinide is excreted in human milk some oral agents are known to be excreted by this route. Because the potential for hypoglycemia in nursing infants may exist, and because of the effects on nursing animals, a decision should be made as to whether repaglinide should be discontinued in nursing mothers, or if mothers should discontinue nursing. If repaglinide is discontinued and if diet alone is inadequate for controlling blood glucose, consider insulin therapy.

➤*Children:* No studies have been performed in children.

➤*Monitoring:* Monitor response to all diabetic therapies by periodic measurements of fasting blood glucose and glycosylated hemoglobin levels with a goal of decreasing these levels towards the normal range. During dose adjustment, fasting glucose can be used to determine the therapeutic response. Thereafter, monitor both glucose and glycosylated hemoglobin. Glycosylated hemoglobin may be especially useful for evaluating long-term glycemic control. Postprandial glucose level testing may be clinically helpful in patients whose premeal blood glucose levels are satisfactory but whose overall glycemic control (HbA_{1c}) is inadequate.

Drug Interactions

➤*CYP-450 inhibitors:* In vitro data indicate that repaglinide metabolism may be inhibited by antifungal agents like ketoconazole and miconazole, and antibacterial agents like erythromycin (cytochrome P-450 enzyme system 3A4 inhibitors).

➤*CYP-450 inducers:* Drugs that induce the cytochrome P-450 enzyme system 3A4 may increase repaglinide metabolism; such drugs include troglitazone, rifampin, barbiturates, and carbamazepine.

REPAGLINIDE — ORAL

Repaglinide Drug Interactions			
Precipitant drug	Object drug[a]		Description
Beta blockers Chloramphenicol, Coumarins, MAOIs, NSAIDs, Probenecid, Salicylates, Sulfonamide	Repaglinide	↑	The action of repaglinide may be potentiated by certain drugs, including those highly protein bound. Observe for hypoglycemia and loss of glycemic control.
Calcium channel blockers Corticosteroids, Estrogens, Isoniazid, Nicotinic acid, Oral contraceptives, Phenothiazines, Phenytoin, Sympathomimetics, Thiazides and other diuretics, Thyroid products	Repaglinide	↓	Certain drugs tend to produce hyperglycemia and may lead to loss of glycemic control. Observe closely.
CYP 4503A4 inhibitors (eg, ketoconazole, miconazole, clarithromycin)	Repaglinide	↑	Coadministration may increase repaglinide plasma levels because of inhibition of its metabolism. Monitor blood glucose and adjust repaglinide dose as needed.
CYP 4503A4 inducers (eg, rifampin, barbiturates, carbamazepine)	Repaglinide	↓	Coadministration may decrease repaglinide plasma levels because of induction of its metabolism. Monitor blood glucose and adjust repaglinide dose as needed.
Gemfibrozil	Repaglinide	↑	Concomitant use may result in enhanced and prolonged blood glucose-lowering effects of repaglinide. Use caution in patients already on repaglinide. Monitor blood glucose levels. Repaglinide dose adjustment may be needed.
Gemfibrozil and Itraconazole	Repaglinide	↑	Gemfibrozil and itraconazole have a synergistic metabolic inhibitory effect on repaglinide. Therefore, patients taking repaglinide and gemfibrozil should not take itraconazole.
Levonorgestrel and ethinyl estradiol	Repaglinide	↑	Coadministration of a combination tablet of 0.15 mg levonorgestrel and 0.03 mg ethinyl estradiol administered once daily for 21 days with 2 mg repaglinide administered 3 times/day on days 1 to 4 and a single dose on day 5 resulted in 20% increases in repaglinide, levonorgestrel, and ethinyl estradiol C_{max}. Ethinyl estradiol AUC parameters were increased by 20%, while repaglinide and levonorgestrel AUC values remained unchanged.
Repaglinide	Levonorgestrel and ethinyl estradiol		
Simvastatin	Repaglinide	↑	Coadministration of 20 mg simvastatin and a single dose of 2 mg repaglinide (after 4 days of once-daily 20 mg simvastatin and 2 mg repaglinide 3 times/day) resulted in a 26% increase in repaglinide C_{max}.

[a] ↑ = Object drug increased. ↓ = Object drug decreased.

➤*Drug/Food interactions:* When given with food, mean C_{max} and AUC of repaglinide were decreased 20% and 12.4%, respectively. Administer repaglinide before meals.

Adverse Reactions

Repaglinide has been administered to 2,931 individuals during clinical trials. Approximately 1,500 of these individuals with type 2 diabetes have been treated for at least 3 months, 1,000 for at least 6 months and 800 for at least 1 year. The majority of these individuals (1,228) received repaglinide in 1 of five 1-year, active-controlled trials. The comparator drugs in these 1-year trials were oral sulfonylurea drugs including glyburide and glipizide. Over 1 year, 13% of repaglinide patients were discontinued because of adverse reactions vs 14% of sulfonylurea patients. The most common adverse events leading to withdrawal were hyperglycemia, hypoglycemia, and related symptoms. Mild or moderate hypoglycemia occurred in 16% of repaglinide patients, 20% of glyburide patients, and 19% of glipizide patients.

The table below lists common adverse reactions for repaglinide patients compared to both placebo (in trials 12 to 24 weeks duration) and to glyburide and glipizide in 1-year trials. The adverse-event profile of repaglinide was generally comparable to that for sulfonylurea drugs.

Repaglinide Adverse Reactions (%)[a]				
Adverse reaction	Repaglinide (n = 352)	Placebo (n = 108)	Repaglinide (n = 1,228)	Sulfonylurea (n = 498)
	Placebo-controlled studies		Active-controlled studies	
CNS				
Headache	11%	10%	9%	8%
Paresthesia	3%	3%	2%	1%
GI				
Constipation	3%	2%	2%	3%
Diarrhea	5%	2%	4%	6%
Dyspepsia	2%	2%	4%	2%
Nausea	5%	5%	3%	2%
Vomiting	3%	3%	2%	1%
Musculoskeletal				
Arthralgia	6%	3%	3%	4%
Back pain	5%	4%	6%	7%
Respiratory				
Bronchitis	2%	1%	6%	7%
Rhinitis	3%	3%	7%	8%
Sinusitis	6%	2%	3%	4%
Upper respiratory tract infection	16%	8%	10%	10%
Miscellaneous				
Allergy	2%	0%	1%	< 1%
Chest pain	3%	1%	2%	1%
Hypoglycemia	31%[b]	7%	16%	20%
Tooth disorder	2%	0%	< 1%	< 1%
Urinary tract infection	2%	1%	3%	3%

[a] Events greater than or equal to 2% for the repaglinide group in the placebo-controlled studies and events occurring as often or more often than those in the placebo group.

[b] In a double-blind, placebo-controlled, 3 months' dose-titration study, repaglinide or placebo doses for each patient were increased weekly from 0.25 mg through 0.5, 1, and 2 mg, to a maximum of 4 mg, until an FPG level less than 160 mg/dL was achieved or the maximum dose reached. The dose that achieved the targeted control or the maximum dose was continued to end of study. FPG and 2-hour PPG increased in patients receiving placebo and decreased in patients treated with repaglinide. Differences between the repaglinide- and placebo-treated groups were −61 mg/dL (FPG) and −104 mg/dL (PPG). The between-group change in HbA_{1c}, which reflects long-term glycemic control, was 1.7% units.

➤*Hypoglycemia:* All oral blood glucose-lowering drugs are capable of producing hypoglycemia. Proper patient selection, dosage, and instructions to the patients are important to avoid hypoglycemic episodes.

Severe hypoglycemic reactions with coma, seizure, or other neurological impairment occur infrequently, but constitute medical emergencies requiring immediate hospitalization.

➤*Cardiovascular:* Cardiovascular events also occur commonly in patients with type 2 diabetes. In 1-year comparator trials, the incidence of individual events was not greater than 1% except for chest pain (1.8%) and angina (1.8%). The individual incidence of other cardiovascular events (hypertension, abnormal EKG, myocardial infarction, arrhythmias, and palpitations) was less than or equal to 1% and not different for repaglinide and the comparator drugs.

The incidence of total serious cardiovascular adverse events added together, including ischemia, was slightly higher for repaglinide (4%) than for sulfonylurea drugs (3%) in controlled comparator clinical trials. In 1-year controlled trials, repaglinide treatment was not associated with excess mortality rates when compared with rates observed with other oral hypoglycemic agent therapies.

Serious Repaglinide Cardiovascular Reactions (%)		
Adverse reaction	Repaglinide (n = 1,228)	Sulfonylurea[a] (n = 498)
Serious CV reactions	4%	3%
Cardiac ischemic reactions	2%	2%
Deaths caused by CV reactions	0.5%	0.4%

[a] Glyburide and glipizide.

Seven controlled clinical trials included repaglinide combination therapy with NPH-insulin (n = 431), insulin formulations alone (n = 388) or other

REPAGLINIDE — ORAL

combinations (sulfonylurea plus NPH-insulin or repaglinide plus metformin) (n = 120). There were 6 serious adverse events of myocardial ischemia in patients treated with repaglinide plus NPH-insulin from 2 studies, and 1 event in patients using insulin formulations alone from another study.

Infrequent adverse reactions (less than 1%) – Less common adverse clinical or laboratory events observed in clinical trials included elevated liver enzymes, thrombocytopenia, leukopenia, and anaphylactoid reactions (1 patient).

Combination therapy with thiazolidinediones – During 24-week treatment clinical trials of repaglinide-rosiglitazone or repaglinide-pioglitazone combination therapy (a total of 250 patients in combination therapy), hypoglycemia (blood glucose less than 50 mg/dL) occurred in 7% of combination therapy patients in comparison with 7% for repaglinide monotherapy, and 2% for thiazolidinedione monotherapy.

Peripheral edema was reported in 12 out of 250 repaglinide-thiazolidinedione combination therapy patients and 3 out of 124 thiazolidinedione monotherapy patients, with no cases reported in these trials for repaglinide monotherapy. When corrected for dropout rates of the treatment groups, the percentage of patients having events of peripheral edema per 24 weeks of treatment were 5% for repaglinide-thiazolidinedione combination therapy, and 4% for thiazolidinedione monotherapy. There were reports in 2 of 250 patients (0.8%) treated with repaglinide-thiazolidinedione therapy of episodes of edema with congestive heart failure. Both patients had a history of coronary artery disease and recovered after treatment with diuretic agents. No comparable cases in the monotherapy treatment groups were reported.

Mean change in weight from baseline was +4.9 kg for repaglinide-thiazolidinedione therapy. There were no patients on repaglinide-thiazolidinedione combination therapy who had elevations of liver transaminases (defined as 3 times the upper limit of normal levels).

➤*Postmarketing:* Although no causal relationship has been established, postmarketing experience includes reports of the following rare adverse reactions: Alopecia, hemolytic anemia, pancreatitis, Stevens-Johnson syndrome, and severe hepatic dysfunction.

Overdosage

➤*Symptoms:* In a clinical trial, patients received increasing doses of repaglinide up to 80 mg a day for 14 days. There were few adverse effects other than those associated with the intended effect of lowering blood glucose. Hypoglycemia did not occur when meals were given with these high doses.

➤*Treatment:* Treat hypoglycemic symptoms without loss of consciousness or neurologic findings aggressively with oral glucose and adjustments in drug dosage and/or meal patterns. Close monitoring may continue until the physician is assured that the patient is out of danger. Closely monitor patients for a minimum of 24 to 48 hours, since hypoglycemia may recur after apparent clinical recovery. There is no evidence that repaglinide is dialyzable using hemodialysis.

Severe hypoglycemic reactions with coma, seizure, or other neurological impairment occur infrequently, but constitute medical emergencies requiring immediate hospitalization. If hypoglycemic coma is diagnosed or suspected, the patient should be given a rapid intravenous injection of concentrated (50%) glucose solution. This should be followed by a continuous infusion of more dilute (10%) glucose solution at a rate that will maintain the blood glucose at a level above 100 mg/dL.

Patient Information

Inform patients of the potential risks and advantages of repaglinide and of alternative modes of therapy. Also inform them about the importance of adherence to dietary instructions, of a regular exercise program, and of regular testing of blood glucose and HbA_{1c}. Explain the risks of hypoglycemia, its symptoms and treatment, and its conditions that predispose to its development and concomitant administration of other glucose-lowering drugs to patients and responsible family members. Also explain primary and secondary failure.

Instruct patients to take repaglinide before meals (2, 3, or 4 times a day preprandially). Doses are usually taken within 15 minutes of the meal but time may vary from immediately preceding the meal to as long as 30 minutes before the meal. Instruct patients who skip a meal (or add an extra meal) to skip (or add) a dose for that meal.

NATEGLINIDE

Rx	**Nateglinide** (Par Pharmaceutical)	**Tablets; oral:** 60 mg	Lactose. (P 984). Pink, round. In UD 30s.
Rx	**Starlix** (Novartis)		Lactose. (STARLIX 60). Pink, round. In 100s.
Rx	**Nateglinide** (Par Pharmaceutical)	**Tablets; oral:** 120 mg	Lactose. (P 985). Orange, oval. In UD 30s.
Rx	**Starlix** (Novartis)		Lactose. (STARLIX 120). Yellow, oval. In 100s.

NATEGLINIDE — ORAL

Indications

➤*Type 2 diabetes mellitus:* For the treatment of adults with type 2 diabetes mellitus as an adjunct to diet and exercise to improve glycemic control.

Administration and Dosage

➤*Adults:*

Type 2 diabetes mellitus –

Usual dosage: 120 mg 3 times daily before meals. The 60 mg dose may be used in patients who are near goal glycosylated hemoglobin (HbA_{1C}) when treatment is initiated.

Concomitant therapy: May be taken in combination with metformin or a thiazolidinedione.

➤*Administration:* Take orally 1 to 30 minutes prior to meals. If a meal is skipped, the dose should be skipped to reduce the risk of hypoglycemia.

➤*Storage/Stability:* Store at 25°C (77°F); excursions are permitted between 15° and 30°C (59° and 86°F).

Actions

➤*Pharmacology:* Nateglinide is an amino-acid derivative that lowers blood glucose levels by stimulating insulin secretion from the pancreas. This action is dependent upon functioning beta cells in the pancreatic islets. Nateglinide interacts with the ATP-sensitive potassium ($K+_{ATP}$) channel on pancreatic beta cells. The subsequent depolarization of the beta cell opens the calcium channel, producing calcium influx and insulin secretion. The extent of insulin release is glucose dependent and diminishes at low glucose levels. Nateglinide is highly tissue selective with low affinity for heart and skeletal muscle.

Pharmacodynamics – Nateglinide is rapidly absorbed and stimulates pancreatic insulin secretion within 20 minutes of oral administration. When nateglinide is dosed 3 times daily before meals, there is a rapid rise in plasma insulin, with peak levels approximately 1 hour after dosing and a fall to baseline by 4 hours after dosing.

In a double-blind, controlled clinical trial in which nateglinide was administered before each of 3 meals, plasma glucose levels were determined over a 12-hour daytime period after 7 weeks of treatment. Nateglinide was administered 10 minutes before meals. The meals were based on standard diabetic weight maintenance menus with the total caloric content based on each subject's height. Nateglinide produced statistically significant decreases in fasting and postprandial glycemia compared with placebo.

➤*Pharmacokinetics:*

Absorption – Following oral administration immediately prior to a meal, nateglinide is rapidly absorbed with mean peak plasma drug concentrations (C_{max}) generally occurring within 1 hour (T_{max}) after dosing. When administered to patients with type 2 diabetes over the dosage range 60 to 240 mg 3 times a day for 1 week, nateglinide demonstrated linear pharmacokinetics for both area under the time/plasma concentration curve (AUC) and C_{max}. T_{max} was also found to be independent of dose in this patient population. Absolute bioavailability is estimated to be approximately 73%. When given with or after meals, the extent of nateglinide absorption (AUC) remains unaffected. However, there is a delay in the rate of absorption characterized by a decrease in C_{max} and a delay in time to peak plasma concentration (T_{max}). Plasma profiles are characterized by multiple plasma concentration peaks when nateglinide is administered under fasting conditions. This effect is diminished when nateglinide is taken prior to a meal.

Distribution – Based on data following IV administration of nateglinide, the steady-state volume of distribution of nateglinide is estimated to be approximately 10 L in healthy subjects. Nateglinide is extensively bound (98%) to serum proteins, primarily serum albumin, and to a lesser extent α_1 acid glycoprotein. The extent of serum protein binding is independent of drug concentration over the test range of 0.1 to 10 mcg/mL.

Metabolism – Nateglinide is metabolized by the mixed-function oxidase system prior to elimination. The major routes of metabolism are hydroxylation followed by glucuronide conjugation. The major metabolites are less potent antidiabetic agents than nateglinide. The isoprene minor metabolite possesses potency similar to that of the parent compound nateglinide.

In vitro data demonstrate that nateglinide is predominantly metabolized by cytochrome P450 isoenzymes CYP2C9 (70%) and CYP3A4 (30%).

Excretion – Nateglinide and its metabolites are rapidly and completely eliminated following oral administration. Within 6 hours after dosing, approximately 75% of the administered ^{14}C-nateglinide was recovered in the urine. Eighty-three percent (83%) of the ^{14}C-nateglinide was excreted in the urine with an additional 10% eliminated in the feces. Approximately 16% of the ^{14}C-nateglinide was excreted in the urine as parent compound. In all studies of healthy volunteers and patients with type 2 diabetes, nateglinide plasma concentrations declined rapidly with an average elimination half-life of approximately 1.5 hours. Consistent with this short elimination half-life, there was no apparent accumulation of nateglinide upon multiple dosing of up to 240 mg 3 times daily for 7 days.

Special populations –

Renal function impairment: Compared to healthy matched subjects, patients with type 2 diabetes and moderate to severe renal insufficiency (creatinine clearance [Ccr] 15 to 50 mL/min) not on dialysis displayed similar apparent clearance, AUC, and C_{max}. Patients with type 2 diabetes and renal failure on dialysis exhibited reduced overall drug exposure. However, hemodialysis patients also experienced reductions in plasma protein binding compared with the matched healthy volunteers.

Hepatic function impairment: The peak and total exposure of nateglinide in nondiabetic subjects with mild hepatic insufficiency were increased by

NATEGLINIDE — ORAL

30% compared with matched healthy subjects. Use nateglinide with caution in patients with chronic liver disease.

Contraindications

Known hypersensitivity to the drug or its inactive ingredients; type 1 diabetes; diabetic ketoacidosis. This condition should be treated with insulin.

Warnings/Precautions

➤*Hypoglycemia:* All oral blood glucose-lowering drugs that are absorbed systemically are capable of producing hypoglycemia. The frequency of hypoglycemia is related to the severity of the diabetes, the level of glycemic control, and other patient characteristics. Geriatric patients, malnourished patients, and those with adrenal or pituitary insufficiency or severe renal impairment are more susceptible to the glucose-lowering effect of these treatments. The risk of hypoglycemia may be increased by strenuous physical exercise, ingestion of alcohol, insufficient caloric intake on an acute or chronic basis, or combinations with other oral antidiabetic agents. Hypoglycemia may be difficult to recognize in patients with autonomic neuropathy or those who use beta blockers. Administer nateglinide prior to meals to reduce the risk of hypoglycemia. Patients who skip meals should also skip their scheduled dose of nateglinide to reduce the risk of hypoglycemia.

➤*Loss of glycemic control:* Transient loss of glycemic control may occur with fever, infection, trauma, or surgery. Insulin therapy may be needed instead of nateglinide therapy at such times. Secondary failure, or reduced effectiveness of nateglinide over a period of time, may occur.

➤*Hepatic function impairment:* Use nateglinide with caution in patients with moderate to severe liver disease because such patients have not been studied.

➤*Pregnancy: Category C.* In the rabbit, embryonic development was adversely affected and the incidence of gallbladder agenesis or small gallbladder was increased at a dose of 500 mg/kg (approximately 40 times the human therapeutic exposure with a recommended nateglinide dose of 120 mg, 3 times daily before meals). There are no adequate and well-controlled studies in pregnant women. Do not use nateglinide during pregnancy.

➤*Lactation:* Studies in lactating rats showed that nateglinide is excreted in the milk; the $AUC_{0\text{-}48hr}$ ratio in milk to plasma was approximately 1:4. During the peri- and postnatal period, body weights were lower in offspring of rats administered nateglinide at 1,000 mg/kg (approximately 60 times the human therapeutic exposure with a recommended nateglinide dose of 120 mg, 3 times daily before meals). It is not known whether nateglinide is excreted in human milk. Because many drugs are excreted in human milk, do not administer nateglinide to a nursing woman.

➤*Children:* The safety and efficacy of nateglinide in pediatric patients have not been established.

➤*Elderly:* No differences were observed in safety or efficacy of nateglinide between patients 65 years of age or older, and those younger than 65 years of age. However, greater sensitivity of some older individuals to nateglinide therapy cannot be ruled out.

➤*Monitoring:* Periodically assess response to therapies with glucose values and HbA_{1C} levels.

Drug Interactions

➤*Cytochrome P450:* In vitro metabolism studies indicate that nateglinide is predominantly metabolized by the cytochrome P450 isozyme CYP2C9 (70%) and to a lesser extent CYP3A4 (30%). Nateglinide is a potential inhibitor of the CYP2C9 isoenzyme in vivo as indicated by its ability to inhibit the in vitro metabolism of tolbutamide. Inhibition of CYP3A4 metabolic reactions was not detected in in vitro experiments.

Nateglinide Drug Interactions

Precipitant drug	Object drug[a]		Description
Beta-adrenergic blockers, nonselective MAOIs NSAIDS Salicylates	Nateglinide	⬆	These drugs may potentiate the hypoglycemic effects of nateglinide and other oral antidiabetic agents. Closely monitor blood glucose when these agents are started or stopped.
Corticosteroids Sympathomimetics Thiazides Thyroid products	Nateglinide	⬇	These agents may reduce the hypoglycemic action of nateglinide and other oral antidiabetic agents. Closely monitor blood glucose when these agents are started or stopped.
Rifamycins (eg, rifampin)	Nateglinide	⬇	Nateglinide plasma concentrations and pharmacologic effects may be decreased with coadministration. Closely monitor blood glucose levels when starting and stopping rifamycin therapy and adjust nateglinide dose as necessary.

[a] ⬆ = Object drug increased. ⬇ = Object drug decreased.

➤*Drug/Food interactions:* Peak plasma levels were significantly reduced when nateglinide was administered 10 minutes prior to a liquid meal.

Adverse Reactions

Hypoglycemia was relatively uncommon in all treatment arms of the clinical trials. Only 0.3% of nateglinide patients discontinued due to hypoglycemia. GI symptoms, especially diarrhea and nausea, were no more common in patients using the combination of nateglinide and metformin than in patients receiving metformin alone. Likewise, peripheral edema was no more common in patients using the combination of nateglinide and rosiglitazone than in patients receiving rosiglitazone alone. The following table lists events that occurred more frequently in nateglinide patients than in placebo patients in controlled clinical trials.

Common Nateglinide Adverse Reactions in Monotherapy Trials (≥ 2%)

Adverse reaction	Placebo (n = 458)	Nateglinide (n = 1,441)
Preferred term		
Accidental trauma	1.7%	2.9%
Arthropathy	2.2%	3.3%
Back pain	3.7%	4%
Bronchitis	2.6%	2.7%
Coughing	2.2%	2.4%
Diarrhea	3.1%	3.2%
Dizziness	2.2%	3.6%
Flu symptoms	2.6%	3.6%
Hypoglycemia	0.4%	2.4%
Upper respiratory tract infection	8.1%	10.5%

During postmarketing experience, rare cases of hypersensitivity reactions such as rash, itching, and urticaria have been reported.

➤*Lab test abnormalities:*

Uric acid – There were increases in mean uric acid levels for patients treated with nateglinide alone, nateglinide in combination with metformin, metformin alone, and glyburide alone. The respective differences from placebo were 0.29 mg/dL, 0.45 mg/dL, 0.28 mg/dL, and 0.19 mg/dL. The clinical significance of these findings is unknown.

Overdosage

➤*Symptoms:* In a clinical study in patients with type 2 diabetes, nateglinide was administered in increasing doses up to 720 mg daily for 7 days and there were no clinically significant adverse events reported. There have been no instances of overdose with nateglinide in clinical trials. However, an overdose may result in an exaggerated glucose-lowering effect with the development of hypoglycemic symptoms.

➤*Treatment:* Treat hypoglycemic symptoms without loss of consciousness or neurological findings with oral glucose and adjustments in dosage or meal patterns. Treat severe hypoglycemic reactions with coma, seizure, or other neurological symptoms with IV glucose. As nateglinide is highly protein bound, dialysis is not an efficient means of removing it from the blood.

Patient Information

Inform patients of the potential risks and benefits of nateglinide and of alternative modes of therapy. Explain the risks and management of hypoglycemia. Instruct patients to take nateglinide 1 to 30 minutes before ingesting a meal, but to skip their scheduled dose if they skip the meal so that the risk of hypoglycemia will be reduced. Discuss drug interactions with patients. Inform patients of potential drug-drug interactions with nateglinide.

WARNING

Thiazolidinediones cause or exacerbate congestive heart failure (CHF) in some patients. After initiation and dose increases, observe patients carefully for signs and symptoms of heart failure (including excessive, rapid weight gain, dyspnea, and/or edema). If these signs/symptoms develop, manage the heart failure according to current standards of care. Furthermore, consider discontinuation or dose reduction of the thiazolidinedione.

Thiazolidinediones are not recommended for patients with symptomatic heart failure. Initiation of thiazolidinediones in patients with New York Heart Association (NYHA) class III or IV heart failure is contraindicated.

A meta-analysis of 52 clinical studies (mean duration, 6 months; 16,995 total patients), most of which compared **rosiglitazone** with placebo, showed rosiglitazone to be associated with an increased risk of myocardial infarction (MI). Three other studies (mean duration, 46 months; 14,067 total patients) comparing rosiglitazone to other approved oral antidiabetic agents or placebo showed a statistically nonsignificant increased risk of MI, and a statistically nonsignificant decreased risk of death. There have been no clinical trials directly comparing cardiovascular risk of rosiglitazone and pioglitazone, but on a separate trial, pioglitazone (when compared with placebo) did show an increased risk of MI or death. In their entirety, the available data on the risk of myocardial ischemia are inconclusive.

Indications

Thiazolidinedione Indications

Indication	Pioglitazone	Rosiglitazone
FDA-approved uses		
Type 2 diabetes monotherapy	X	X
Type 2 diabetes combination therapy with a sulfonylurea	X	X
Type 2 diabetes combination therapy with metformin	X	X
Type 2 diabetes combination therapy with insulin	X	
Type 2 diabetes combination therapy with metformin and a sulfonylurea		X
Off-label uses		
Polycystic ovary syndrome	X[a]	X[a]
Prevention of in-stent restenosis	X[b]	X[b]

[a] Good documentation.
[b] Safety concerns.

➤*Off-label uses:*

Polycystic ovary syndrome –

Pioglitazone: [1] = Good documentation.

Rosiglitazone: [1] = Good documentation.

Prevention of in-stent restenosis –

Pioglitazone: [3] = Safety concerns.

Rosiglitazone: [3] = Safety concerns.

Actions

➤*Pharmacology:* **Pioglitazone** and **rosiglitazone**, members of the thiazolidinedione class of antidiabetic agents, improve glycemic control by improving sensitivity to insulin in muscle and adipose tissue and inhibiting hepatic gluconeogenesis. They depend on the presence of insulin for their mechanism of action. Thiazolidinediones are highly selective and potent agonists for the peroxisome proliferator-activated receptor-gamma (PPAR-gamma). PPAR receptors are found in adipose tissue, skeletal muscle, and the liver. Activation of PPAR-gamma nuclear receptors regulates the transcription of insulin-responsive genes involved in the control of glucose production, transport, and utilization, and participates in the regulation of fatty acid metabolism.

➤*Pharmacokinetics:*

Thiazolidinediones Pharmacokinetics[a]

Parameters	Pioglitazone	Rosiglitazone
Absorption		
Bioavailability	—	99%
$AUC_{0\text{-}inf}$[b]	—	1 mg[c]: 358 ng•h/mL 2 mg[c]: 733 ng•h/mL 8 mg[c]: 2,971 ng•h/mL 8 mg[d]: 2,890 ng•h/mL
C_{max}[b]	—	1 mg[c]: 76 ng/mL 2 mg[c]: 156 ng/mL 8 mg[c]: 598 ng/mL 8 mg[d]: 432 ng/mL
T_{max}	2 h	1 h
Food effect	Delay in T_{max} (3 to 4 h)	28% decrease in C_{max} and delay in T_{max} (1.75 h)
Distribution		
Volume of distribution	≈ 0.63 L/kg[b]	17.6 L
Protein binding	> 99%	≈ 99.8%
Metabolism		
Mechanism	Hydroxylation, oxidation, CYP2C8, CYP3A4, CYP1A1	N-demethylation, hydroxylation, conjugation with sulfate and glucuronic acid CYP2C8, CYP2C9 (minor)
Active metabolites	MII[e], MIII[f], MIV[e]	
Excretion		
Site	Urine (15% to 30%), feces	Urine (64%), feces (23%)
Elimination half-life	Pioglitazone: 3 to 7 h Total pioglitazone: 16 to 24 h	3 to 4 h
Oral clearance	5 to 7 L/h	1 mg[c]: 3.03 L/h 2 mg[c]: 2.89 L/h 8 mg[c]: 2.85 L/h 8 mg[d]: 2.97 L/h

[a] AUC = area under the curve; C_{max} = maximal drug concentration; T_{max} = time to maximal concentration.
[b] Following single oral doses.
[c] In the fasting state.
[d] In the fed state.
[e] Hydroxy derivatives of pioglitazone.
[f] Keto derivative of pioglitazone.

Special populations –

Hepatic function impairment: Patients with impaired hepatic function (Child-Pugh class B/C) have approximately 45% reduction in **pioglitazone** and total pioglitazone mean peak concentrations. Unbound oral clearance of **rosiglitazone** was significantly lower in patients with moderate to severe liver disease (Child-Pugh class B/C). As a result, unbound rosiglitazone C_{max} and $AUC_{0\text{-}inf}$ were increased 2- and 3-fold, respectively. Elimination half-life for rosiglitazone is about 2 hours longer in patients with liver disease. Do not initiate pioglitazone or rosiglitazone if the patient exhibits clinical evidence of active liver disease or serum transaminase levels (ALT more than 2.5 times the upper limit of normal [ULN]).

Gender: The mean **pioglitazone** C_{max} and AUC values were increased 20% to 60% in women. Mean oral clearance of **rosiglitazone** in women was approximately 6% lower compared with men.

Obesity: Both oral clearance and oral steady-state volume of distribution were shown to increase with increases in body weight.

Contraindications

Initiation in patients with established NYHA class III or IV heart failure; known hypersensitivity to **pioglitazone**, **rosiglitazone**, or any of their components.

Warnings/Precautions

➤*Cardiac effects:* Thiazolidinediones, alone or in combination with other antidiabetic agents, can cause fluid retention, which may exacerbate or lead to heart failure. Observe patients for signs and symptoms of heart failure. If these signs and symptoms develop, manage the heart failure according to current standards of care. Furthermore, consider discontinuation or dose reduction of the thiazolidinedione.

Initiation of thiazolidinediones in patients with established NYHA class III or IV heart failure is contraindicated. **Rosiglitazone** is not recommended in patients with symptomatic heart failure. Initiation of rosiglitazone is not recommended for patients experiencing an acute coronary event; consider discontinuation of rosiglitazone during this acute phase. Initiate **pioglitazone** at the lowest approved dose if it is prescribed for patients with systolic heart failure (NYHA class II). If subsequent dose escalation is necessary, increase dose gradually only after several months of treatment with careful monitoring for weight gain, edema, or signs or symptoms of CHF exacerbation.

➤*Type 1 diabetes:* Thiazolidinediones are active only in the presence of insulin. Therefore, do not use thiazolidinediones in patients with type 1 diabetes or for the treatment of diabetes ketoacidosis.

➤*Hypoglycemia:* Patients receiving thiazolidinediones in combination with oral hypoglycemics (eg, sulfonylureas) may be at risk for hypoglycemia; reduction in the dose of the concomitant agent may be necessary. Perform periodic fasting blood glucose and hemoglobin$_{1c}$ (HbA_{1c}) measurements to monitor therapeutic response.

➤*Edema:* Use with caution in patients with edema. Because thiazolidinediones can cause fluid retention, which can exacerbate or lead to CHF, use with caution in patients at risk for heart failure; monitor patients at risk for heart failure for signs and symptoms of heart failure.

➤*Weight gain:* Dose-related weight gain was seen with thiazolidinediones alone and in combination with other hypoglycemic agents. The mechanism of weight gain is unclear but probably involves a combination of fluid retention and fat accumulation. Assess patients who experience unusual rapid increases in weight for fluid accumulation and volume-related events (eg, CHF, excessive edema).

➤*Hepatotoxicity:* It is recommended that patients treated with thiazolidinediones undergo periodic monitoring of liver enzymes. Check liver enzymes prior to the initiation of therapy and periodically thereafter. Do not initiate therapy in patients with increased baseline liver enzyme levels (ALT more than 2.5 times the ULN). Evaluate patients with mildly elevated liver enzymes (ALT levels 2.5 times the ULN or less) at baseline or during therapy to determine the cause of the liver enzyme elevation. Proceed with caution in the initiation or continuation of therapy in patients with mild liver enzyme elevations and include appropriate close clinical follow-up, including more frequent liver enzyme monitoring, to determine if the liver enzyme elevations resolve or worsen. If, at any time, ALT levels increase to more than 3 times the ULN in patients on therapy, recheck liver enzyme levels as soon as possible. If ALT levels remain more than 3 times the ULN or if the patient is jaundice, discontinue therapy.

If any patient develops symptoms suggestive of hepatic dysfunction (eg, abdominal pain, anorexia, dark urine, fatigue, unexplained nausea, vomiting), check liver enzymes. Guide the decision of whether to continue the patient on therapy by clinical judgement and laboratory evaluations. If jaundice is observed, discontinue therapy.

➤*Macular edema:* Macular edema has been reported in postmarketing experience. Some patients present with blurred vision or decreased visual acuity, but some patients appear to have been diagnosed on routine ophthalmologic examination. Most patients had peripheral edema at the time macular edema was diagnosed. Some patients had improvement in their macular edema after discontinuation of therapy. Patients with diabetes should have regular eye exams by an ophthalmologist, per the Standards of Care of the American Diabetes Association. Additionally, promptly refer any diabetic patient who reports any kind of visual symptom to an ophthalmologist, regardless of the patient's underlying medications or other physical findings.

➤*Fractures:* An increased incidence of bone fractures was noted in women taking thiazolidinediones. This increased incidence was noted after the first year of treatment and persisted during the course of the studies. The majority of fractures in women who received **pioglitazone** were nonvertebral fractures of the lower limb and distal upper limb. The majority of fractures in women who received **rosiglitazone** occurred in the upper arm, hand, and foot. These sites of fracture are different from those usually associated with postmenopausal osteoporosis. Consider the risk of fracture in the care of patients, especially women, and assess and maintain bone health according to current standards of care.

➤*Hematologic:* Mean decreases in hemoglobin and hematocrit were observed during thiazolidinedione therapy. The observed changes may be related to the increased plasma volume observed with treatment and have not been associated with any significant hematologic clinical effects.

➤*Ovulation:* Therapy with thiazolidinediones may result in ovulation in some premenopausal anovulatory women. As a result, these patients may be at an increased risk for pregnancy while taking thiazolidinediones. Thus, recommend adequate contraception in premenopausal women.

➤*Pregnancy: Category C.* **Rosiglitazone** has been reported to cross the human placenta and be detectable in fetal tissue. The molecular weight of the parent compound of **pioglitazone** (about 393 for the hydrochloride salt) is low enough that transfer to the fetus should be expected. There are no adequate and well-controlled studies in pregnant women. Use pioglitazone during pregnancy only if the potential benefit justifies the potential risk to the fetus. Do not use rosiglitazone during pregnancy.

Because current information strongly suggests that abnormal blood glucose levels during pregnancy are associated with a higher incidence of congenital anomalies, as well as increased neonatal morbidity and mortality, most experts recommend that insulin be used during pregnancy to maintain blood glucose levels as close to normal as possible.

➤*Lactation:* It is not known whether **pioglitazone** or **rosiglitazone** are secreted in human milk. The molecular weight of pioglitazone (about 393 for the hydrochloride salt) is low enough that secretion in breast milk should be expected. The molecular weight of the free base of rosiglitazone (about 357) and the long elimination half-life (103 to 158 hours) suggest that excretion in breast milk should be expected. Because many drugs are excreted in human milk, do not administer thiazolidinediones to a breast-feeding woman.

➤*Children:* Safety and effectiveness in children have not been established.

➤*Monitoring:* Perform fasting plasma glucose and HbA_{1c} measurements periodically to monitor glycemic control and the therapeutic response.

Liver enzyme monitoring is recommended prior to initiation of therapy and periodically thereafter.

After initiation or with dose increase, carefully monitor patients for adverse reactions related to fluid retention, weight gain, or signs and symptoms of CHF exacerbation.

Instruct patients with diabetes to have regular eye exams by an ophthalmologist.

Drug Interactions

Thiazolidinediones Drug Interactions

Precipitant drug	Object drug[a]		Description
Atorvastatin	Thiazolidinediones Pioglitazone	↓	Concurrent use for 7 days resulted in a decrease in pioglitazone and atorvastatin serum concentrations.
Thiazolidinediones Pioglitazone	Atorvastatin		
CYP2C8 inducers (eg, rifampin)	Thiazolidinediones	↓	Coadministration may decrease thiazolidinedione concentrations, possibly resulting in decreased glycemic control.
CYP2C8 inhibitors (eg, gemfibrozil, ketoconazole, trimethoprim)	Thiazolidinediones	↑	Coadministration may increase thiazolidinedione plasma concentrations, increasing hypoglycemic and other adverse reactions.
Gatifloxacin	Thiazolidinediones Pioglitazone	↑	Severe and persistent hypoglycemia may occur. Avoid concomitant use.
Gemfibrozil	Thiazolidinediones Pioglitazone	↑	Coadministration resulted in an increase in pioglitazone AUC of 226%.
Insulin	Thiazolidinediones Pioglitazone Rosiglitazone	↑	During coadministration, the incidence of edema may be increased. Possible additive or synergistic pharmacologic effects may occur.
Thiazolidinediones Pioglitazone Rosiglitazone	Insulin		
Thiazolidinediones Pioglitazone	Contraceptives, hormonal (eg, ethinyl estradiol)	↓	Coadministration resulted in an 11% and 11% to 14% decrease in ethinyl estradiol $AUC_{(0\text{-}24\ h)}$ and C_{max}, respectively. The clinical significance of this is unknown.
Thiazolidinediones Rosiglitazone	Glyburide	↓	Repeat dosages of rosiglitazone 8 mg once daily for 8 days caused a 30% decrease in glyburide AUC and C_{max}.
Thiazolidinediones Pioglitazone	Midazolam	↓	Coadministration resulted in a 26% reduction in midazolam C_{max} and AUC.
Thiazolidinediones Rosiglitazone	Nevirapine	↓	Based on 1 small study, rosiglitazone may reduce nevirapine plasma concentrations.
Thiazolidinediones Pioglitazone	Nifedipine	↓	Concurrent use of pioglitazone and nifedipine extended-release resulted in a decrease in nifedipine concentrations. The clinical significance is unknown.
Thiazolidinediones Rosiglitazone	Nitrates (eg, nitroglycerin)	↔	A greater increased risk of myocardial ischemia was observed with concurrent therapy. Coadministration is not recommended.

[a] ↑ = object drug increased; ↓ = object drug decreased; ↔ = undetermined clinical effect.

➤*Drug/Food interactions:* Food slightly delays **pioglitazone** time to peak serum concentrations to 3 to 4 hours but does not alter the extent of absorption.

Adverse Reactions

Thiazolidinediones Adverse Reactions[a]

Adverse reactions	Pioglitazone (n = 606)	Rosiglitazone (n = 2,526)
CNS		
Fatigue	—	3.6%
Headache	9.1%	17%
GI		
Diarrhea	—	2.3%
Tooth disorder	5.3%	—

Thiazolidinediones Adverse Reactions[a]		
Adverse reactions	Pioglitazone (n = 606)	Rosiglitazone (n = 2,526)
Metabolic		
Aggravated diabetes mellitus	5.1%	—
Hyperglycemia	—	3.9%
Hypoglycemia	—	0.6%
Respiratory		
Pharyngitis	5.1%	—
Sinusitis	6.3%	3.2%
Upper respiratory tract infection	13.2%	9.9%
Miscellaneous		
Anemia	—	1.9%
Back pain	—	4%
Edema	4.8%	4.8%
Injury	—	7.6%
Myalgia	5.4%	—

[a] Data are pooled from separate studies and are not necessarily comparable.

➤*Other adverse reactions:*

Miscellaneous – Fractures (9%); nausea (4%); arthralgia, hypertension, nasopharyngitis (3%; **rosiglitazone** only).

➤*Lab test abnormalities:*

Pioglitazone – Decreased alkaline phosphatase, AST, gamma-glutamyl transferase, hematocrit, hemoglobin, triglycerides; increased ALT, creatine phosphokinase, high-density lipoprotein (HDL).

Rosiglitazone – Decreased free fatty acids, hematocrit, hemoglobin, white blood cells; increased ALT, bilirubin, HDL, low-density lipoprotein, total cholesterol.

➤*Postmarketing:*

Cardiovascular – CHF, pleural effusions and pulmonary edema with or without a fatal outcome.

Hepatic – Elevated hepatic enzymes to 3 or more times the ULN, hepatic failure with and without fatal outcome; hepatitis.

Hypersensitivity – Anaphylactic reaction; angioedema, pruritus, rash, Steven-Johnson syndrome, urticaria.

Miscellaneous – New onset or worsening diabetic macular edema with decreased visual acuity.

Overdosage

➤*Treatment:* Initiate appropriate supportive treatment according to patient's clinical signs and symptoms.

Patient Information

Advise patients to read the Medication Guide before starting therapy and with each refill.

Pioglitazone and **rosiglitazone** may be taken with or without meals. If the dose is missed at the usual meal, it may be taken at the next meal. If the dose is missed on 1 day, the dose should not be doubled the following day.

Inform patients that results of a set of clinical studies suggest that treatment with rosiglitazone is associated with an increased risk for MI, especially in patients taking insulin. Inform patients that rosiglitazone is not recommended for patients who are taking insulin.

Management of type 2 diabetes should include diet control. Caloric restriction, weight loss, and exercise are essential for the proper treatment of the diabetic patient because they help improve insulin sensitivity. This is important not only in the primary treatment of type 2 diabetes but in maintaining the efficacy of drug therapy.

Inform patients that it is important for them to adhere to dietary instructions and to have blood glucose and glycosylated hemoglobin tested regularly. During periods of stress (eg, fever, infection, surgery, trauma), medication requirements may change, and patients should seek the advice of their health care provider.

Inform patients that blood will be drawn to check their liver function prior to the start of therapy and periodically thereafter.

When using combination therapy with insulin or an oral hypoglycemic agent, explain the risks of hypoglycemia, its symptoms, treatment, and predisposing conditions to patients and their family members.

Instruct patients who experience an unusually rapid increase in weight or edema or who develop shortness of breath or other symptoms of heart failure while on therapy to immediately report these symptoms to their health care provider.

Instruct patients to immediately report any signs or symptoms of hepatic dysfunction (eg, abdominal pain, anorexia, dark urine, fatigue, jaundice, nausea, vomiting) to their health care provider.

Advise patients that it can take 2 weeks of **rosiglitazone** therapy to see a reduction in blood glucose and 2 to 3 months to see full effect.

Advise premenopausal women that thiazolidinedione therapy may result in ovulation in some anovulatory women. Recommend adequate contraception in premenopausal women.

Advise patients that thiazolidinedione therapy is not recommended for patients with symptomatic heart failure.

ROSIGLITAZONE

Rx **Avandia** (GlaxoSmithKline)	**Tablets; oral:** 2 mg	As rosiglitazone maleate. Lactose, PEG. (SB 2). Pink, pentagonal. Film-coated. In 60s.
	4 mg	As rosiglitazone maleate. Lactose, PEG. (SB 4). Orange, pentagonal. Film-coated. In 30s.
	8 mg	As rosiglitazone maleate. Lactose, PEG. (SB 8). Red-brown, pentagonal. Film-coated. In 30s and 90s.

ROSIGLITAZONE MALEATE — ORAL

For complete and comparative prescribing information, refer to the Thiazolidinediones class monograph.

WARNING

Thiazolidinediones, including rosiglitazone, cause or exacerbate congestive heart failure (CHF) in some patients. After initiation of rosiglitazone and after dose increases, observe patients carefully for signs and symptoms of heart failure (including excessive, rapid weight gain; dyspnea; and/or edema). If these signs and symptoms develop, manage the heart failure according to current standards of care. Furthermore, consider discontinuation or dose reduction of rosiglitazone.

Rosiglitazone is not recommended in patients with symptomatic heart failure. Initiation of rosiglitazone in patients with established New York Heart Association (NYHA) class III or IV heart failure is contraindicated.

A meta-analysis of 52 clinical trials (mean duration, 6 months; 16,995 total patients), most of which compared rosiglitazone with placebo, showed rosiglitazone to be associated with a statistically significant increased risk of myocardial infarction (MI). Three other trials (mean duration, 46 months; 14,067 total patients) comparing rosiglitazone with some other approved oral antidiabetic agents or placebo showed a statistically nonsignificant increased risk of MI and a statistically nonsignificant decreased risk of death. There have been no clinical trials directly comparing the cardiovascular risk of rosiglitazone and pioglitazone, another thiazolidinedione, but in a separate trial, pioglitazone (when compared with placebo) did not show an increased risk of MI or death.

Indications

➤*Type 2 diabetes:* As an adjunct to diet and exercise to improve glycemic control in adults with type 2 diabetes mellitus who either are already taking rosiglitazone or are not already taking rosiglitazone and are unable to achieve adequate glycemic control on other diabetes medications, and in consultation with their health care provider, have decided not to take pioglitazone for medical reasons.

➤*Off-label uses:*

Polycystic ovary syndrome – [1] = Good documentation. Although only small studies evaluating the use of thiazolidinediones in polycystic ovary syndrome (PCOS) have been conducted, the results appear to show benefit. The American College of Obstetricians and Gynecologists and American Association of Clinical Endocrinologists present conflicting assessments on rosiglitazone's use as a treatment option to restore ovulation and fertility in women with PCOS.

Prevention of in-stent restenosis – [3] = Safety concerns. Multiple trials confirm that rosiglitazone is effective in reducing the risk of repeat target vessel revascularization in patients with type 2 diabetes following coronary stent implantation. Rosiglitazone's safety profile is of concern, and, if used, regularly monitor patients.

Administration and Dosage

➤*Adults:*

Type 2 diabetes –

Maximum dose: 8 mg/day.

Initial dosage: 4 mg as a single dose once daily or in 2 divided doses.

Dosage adjustment: Increase dosage to 8 mg daily for patients who respond inadequately following 8 to 12 weeks of treatment, as determined by reduction in fasting plasma glucose (FPG). Increases in the dose of rosiglitazone should be accompanied by careful monitoring for adverse reactions related to fluid retention.

Concomitant therapy: Patients receiving rosiglitazone in combination with other hypoglycemic agents may be at risk for hypoglycemia, and a reduction in the dose of concomitant agent may be necessary.

ROSIGLITAZONE MALEATE — ORAL

Off-label dosing –

Polycystic ovary syndrome: [1] = Good documentation. As monotherapy or in combination therapy at an oral dosage of 2 to 8 mg daily in 1 to 2 divided doses.

Prevention of in-stent restenosis: [3] = Safety concerns. 4 to 8 mg orally daily for 6 months as monotherapy or as part of a combination regimen.

➤*Renal function impairment:* Because metformin is contraindicated in patients with renal impairment, coadministration of metformin and rosiglitazone is contraindicated in these patients.

➤*Hepatic function impairment:* Therapy with rosiglitazone should not be initiated if the patient exhibits clinical evidence of active liver disease or increased serum transaminase levels (ALT more than 2.5 times the upper limit of normal [ULN] at start of therapy).

➤*Administration:* May be taken with or without food.

➤*Storage/Stability:* Store at 25°C (77°F); excursions are permitted between 15° and 30°C (59° and 86°F).

PIOGLITAZONE

Rx	**Actos** (Takeda Pharmaceuticals America)	**Tablets; oral:** 15 mg	As pioglitazone hydrochloride. Lactose. (ACTOS 15). White to off-white. In 30s, 90s, and 500s.
		30 mg	As pioglitazone hydrochloride. Lactose. (ACTOS 30). White to off-white. In 30s, 90s, and 500s.
		45 mg	As pioglitazone hydrochloride. Lactose. (ACTOS 45). White to off-white. In 30s, 90s, and 500s.

PIOGLITAZONE HYDROCHLORIDE — ORAL

For complete and comparative prescribing information, refer to the Thiazolidinediones group monograph.

WARNING

Congestive heart failure (CHF) – Thiazolidinediones, including pioglitazone, cause or exacerbate CHF in some patients. After initiation of pioglitazone, and after dose increases, observe patients carefully for signs and symptoms of heart failure (including excessive, rapid weight gain, dyspnea, and/or edema). If these signs and symptoms develop, manage the heart failure according to the current standards of care. Furthermore, discontinuation or dose reduction of pioglitazone must be considered.

Pioglitazone is not recommended in patients with symptomatic heart failure. Initiation of pioglitazone in patients with established New York Heart Association (NYHA) class III or IV heart failure is contraindicated.

Indications

➤*Type 2 diabetes:* Monotherapy as an adjunct to diet and exercise to improve glycemic control in patients with type 2 diabetes.

Also indicated for use in combination with a sulfonylurea, metformin, or insulin when diet and exercise plus the single agent do not result in adequate glycemic control.

➤*Off-label uses:*

Polycystic ovary syndrome – [1] = Good documentation. Although only small studies evaluating the use of thiazolidinediones in polycystic ovary syndrome (PCOS) have been conducted, the results appear to show benefit. American College of Obstetricians and Gynecologists and American Association of Clinical Endocrinologists present conflicting assessments of the medication's use as a treatment option to restore ovulation and fertility in women with PCOS. (See Administration and Dosage.)

Prevention of in-stent restenosis – [3] = Safety concerns. Multiple trials confirm that pioglitazone is effective in reducing the risk of repeat target vessel revascularization in patients with type 2 diabetes following coronary stent implantation. Pioglitazone's safety profile is of concern, and, if used, patients taking it should be monitored regularly.

Administration and Dosage

➤*General dosing considerations:* After initiation of pioglitazone or with dose increase, patients should be carefully monitored for adverse reactions related to fluid retention.

➤*Adults:*

Type 2 diabetes –

Maximum dose: 45 mg/day (monotherapy or combination therapy).

Initial dosage: 15 or 30 mg once daily.

Dosage titration: For patients who respond inadequately to the initial dose of pioglitazone (as monotherapy), the dose can be increased in increments up to 45 mg once daily. Consider combination therapy for patients not responding adequately to monotherapy.

Concomitant therapy:

- *Sulfonylureas –* Initiate pioglitazone at 15 or 30 mg once daily. Continue the current sulfonylurea upon initiation of pioglitazone therapy. Decrease the dose of the sulfonylurea if the patient reports hypoglycemia.
- *Metformin –* Initiate pioglitazone at 15 or 30 mg once daily. Continue the current metformin dose upon initiation of pioglitazone therapy. It is unlikely that the dose of metformin will require adjustment because of hypoglycemia during combination therapy with pioglitazone.
- *Insulin –* Initiate pioglitazone at 15 or 30 mg once daily. Continue the current insulin dose upon initiation of pioglitazone therapy. Decrease the insulin dose by 10% to 25% if the patient reports hypoglycemia or if plasma glucose concentrations decrease to less than 100 mg/dL. Individualize further adjustments based on glucose-lowering response.

Off-label dosing –

Polycystic ovary syndrome: [1] = Good documentation. Use as monotherapy or in combination therapy at a single oral dose of 15 to 30 mg daily, without regard to meals.

Prevention of in-stent restenosis: [3] = Safety concerns. 30 mg orally daily for 6 months as monotherapy or as part of a combination regimen.

➤*Hepatic function impairment:* Do not initiate pioglitazone therapy if the patient exhibits clinical evidence of active liver disease or increased serum transaminase levels (ALT more than 2.5 times the upper limit of normal [ULN]) at the start of therapy. Liver enzyme monitoring is recommended in all patients prior to initiation of therapy with pioglitazone and periodically thereafter.

➤*Administration:* Pioglitazone should be taken once daily without regard to meals.

➤*Storage/Stability:* Store at 25°C (77°F); excursions are permitted to 15° to 30°C (59° to 86°F). Keep the container tightly closed, and protect it from moisture and humidity.

GLYBURIDE/METFORMIN HYDROCHLORIDE

Rx	**Glyburide/Metformin Hydrochloride** (PAR)	**Tablets; oral:** 1.25 mg/250 mg	(6057). Pale yellow, capsule shape. Film-coated. In 100s.
Rx	**Glucovance** (Bristol-Myers Squibb)		(BMS 6072). Pale yellow, capsule shape. Film-coated. In 100s.
Rx	**Glyburide/Metformin Hydrochloride** (PAR)	**Tablets; oral:** 2.5 mg/500 mg	(6058). Pale orange, capsule shape. Film-coated. In 100s.
Rx	**Glucovance** (Bristol-Myers Squibb)		(BMS 6073). Pale orange, capsule shape. Film-coated. In 100s.
Rx	**Glyburide/Metformin Hydrochloride** (PAR)	**Tablets; oral:** 5 mg/500 mg	(6059). Yellow, capsule shape. Film-coated. In 100s.
Rx	**Glucovance** (Bristol-Myers Squibb)		(BMS 6074). Yellow, capsule shape. Film-coated. In 100s.

GLYBURIDE/METFORMIN HYDROCHLORIDE — ORAL

For complete and comparative prescribing information, refer to the Sulfonylureas group monograph and the Metformin and Rosiglitazone individual monographs.

WARNING

Lactic acidosis – Lactic acidosis is a rare, but serious, metabolic complication that can occur because of metformin accumulation during treatment with glyburide/metformin; when it occurs, it is fatal in approximately 50% of cases. Lactic acidosis may also occur in association with a number of pathophysiologic conditions, including diabetes mellitus, and whenever there is significant tissue hypoperfusion and hypoxemia. Lactic acidosis is characterized by elevated blood lactate levels (more than 5 mmol/L), decreased blood pH, electrolyte disturbances with an increased anion gap, and an increased lactate/pyruvate ratio. When metformin is implicated as the cause of lactic acidosis, metformin plasma levels of more than 5 mcg/mL are generally found.

The reported incidence of lactic acidosis in patients receiving metformin hydrochloride is very low (approximately 0.03 cases per 1,000 patient-years, with approximately 0.015 fatal cases per 1,000 patient-years). In more than 20,000 patient-years' exposure to metformin in clinical trials, there were no reports of lactic acidosis. Reported cases have occurred primarily in diabetic patients with significant renal function impairment, including both intrinsic renal disease and renal hypoperfusion, often in the setting of multiple concomitant medical/surgical problems and multiple concomitant medications. Patients with congestive heart failure requiring pharmacologic management, in particular those with unstable or acute congestive heart failure who are at risk of hypoperfusion and hypoxemia, are at increased risk of lactic acidosis. The risk of lactic acidosis increases with the degree of renal function impairment and the patient's age. The risk of lactic acidosis may, therefore, be significantly decreased by regular monitoring of renal function in patients taking metformin and use of the minimum effective dose of metformin. In particular, accompany the treatment of elderly patients with careful monitoring of renal function. Do not initiate glyburide/metformin treatment in patients 80 years of age and older unless measurement of creatinine clearance (CrCl) demonstrates that renal function is not reduced because these patients are more susceptible to developing lactic acidosis. In addition, promptly withhold glyburide/metformin in the presence of any condition associated with dehydration, hypoxemia, or sepsis. Because hepatic function impairment may significantly limit the ability to clear lactate, generally avoid glyburide/metformin in patients with clinical or laboratory evidence of hepatic disease. Caution patients against excessive alcohol intake, acute or chronic, when taking glyburide/metformin because alcohol potentiates the effects of metformin on lactate metabolism. In addition, temporarily discontinue glyburide/metformin prior to any intravascular radiocontrast study and for any surgical procedure.

The onset of lactic acidosis often is subtle and accompanied only by nonspecific symptoms, such as increasing somnolence, malaise, myalgias, nonspecific abdominal distress, and respiratory distress. There may be associated hypotension, hypothermia, and resistant bradyarrhythmias with more marked acidosis. The patient and the patient's health care provider must be aware of the possible importance of such symptoms. Instruct the patient to notify their health care provider immediately if symptoms occur. Withdraw glyburide/metformin until the situation is clarified. Serum electrolytes, ketones, blood glucose, and, if indicated, blood pH, lactate levels, and even blood metformin levels may be useful. Once a patient is stabilized on any dose level of glyburide/metformin, GI symptoms, which are common during initiation of therapy with metformin, are unlikely to be drug related. Later occurrence of GI symptoms could be caused by lactic acidosis or other serious disease.

Levels of fasting venous plasma lactate above the upper limit of normal but less than 5 mmol/L in patients taking glyburide/metformin do not necessarily indicate impending lactic acidosis and may be explainable by other mechanisms, such as poorly controlled diabetes or obesity, vigorous physical activity, or technical problems in sample handling.

Suspect lactic acidosis in any diabetic patient with metabolic acidosis lacking evidence of ketoacidosis (eg, ketonemia, ketonuria).

Lactic acidosis is a medical emergency that must be treated in a hospital setting. In a patient with lactic acidosis who is taking glyburide/metformin, immediately discontinue the drug and institute general supportive measures promptly. Because metformin is dialyzable (with a clearance of up to 170 mL/min under good hemodynamic conditions), prompt hemodialysis is recommended to correct the acidosis and remove accumulated metformin. Such management often results in prompt reversal of symptoms and recovery.

Indications

➤*Type 2 diabetes (initial therapy):* As initial therapy, as an adjunct to diet and exercise, to improve glycemic control in patients with type 2 diabetes whose hyperglycemia cannot be satisfactorily managed with diet and exercise alone.

➤*Type 2 diabetes (second-line therapy):* As second-line therapy when diet, exercise, and initial treatment with a sulfonylurea or metformin do not result in adequate glycemic control in patients with type 2 diabetes. For patients requiring additional therapy, a thiazolidinedione may be added to glyburide/metformin to achieve additional glycemic control.

Administration and Dosage

➤*General dosing considerations:* Glyburide/metformin should be initiated at a low dose, with gradual dose escalation, in order to avoid hypoglycemia (largely caused by glyburide), reduce GI adverse reactions (largely due to metformin), and permit determination of the minimum effective dose for adequate control of blood glucose for the individual patient.

With initial treatment and during dose titration, appropriate blood glucose monitoring should be used to determine the therapeutic response to glyburide/metformin and to identify the minimum effective dose for the patient.

➤*Adults:*

Type 2 diabetes (initial therapy) –

Initial dosage: 1.25 mg/250 mg once or twice daily with meals. In patients with a baseline HbA_{1c} of more than 9% or an FPG of more than 200 mg/dL, a starting dosage of glyburide/metformin 1.25 mg/250 mg twice daily with the morning and evening meals may be used. Glyburide 5 mg/metformin 500 mg should not be used as initial therapy because of an increased risk of hypoglycemia.

Dosage titration: Dosage increases should be made in increments of 1.25 mg/250 mg/day every 2 weeks, up to the minimum effective dose necessary to achieve adequate control of blood glucose.

Type 2 diabetes (second-line therapy) –

Maximum dose: Glyburide 20 mg/metformin 2,000 mg.

Initial dosage: 2.5 mg/500 mg or 5 mg/500 mg twice daily with meals. In order to avoid hypoglycemia, the starting dose of glyburide/metformin should not exceed the daily doses of glyburide or metformin already being taken.

Dosage titration: The daily dose should be titrated in increments of no more than 5 mg/500 mg, up to the minimum effective dose to achieve adequate control of blood glucose.

➤*Elderly:* The initial and maintenance dosing of glyburide/metformin should be conservative in patients with advanced age because of the potential for decreased renal function in this population. Any dosage adjustment requires a careful assessment of renal function. In elderly patients, particularly those 80 years of age and older, do not titrate glyburide/metformin to the maximum dose.

➤*Renal function impairment:* Glyburide/metformin is contraindicated in patients with renal disease or renal impairment (eg, as suggested by serum creatinine levels of 1.5 mg/dL or more [men], 1.4 mg/dL or more [women], or abnormal CrCl). Do not give glyburide/metformin to patients with serum creatinine levels above the ULN for their age.

➤*Hepatic function impairment:* Because hepatic function impairment has been associated with some cases of lactic acidosis, generally avoid glyburide/metformin in patients with clinical or laboratory evidence of hepatic disease.

➤*Debilitated or malnourished patients:* Debilitated or malnourished patients should not be titrated to the maximum dose to avoid the risk of hypoglycemia.

➤*Concomitant therapy with thiazolidinediones:* For patients not adequately controlled on glyburide/metformin, a thiazolidinedione can be added to glyburide/metformin therapy. When a thiazolidinedione is added to glyburide/metformin therapy, the current dose of glyburide/metformin can be continued, and the thiazolidinedione can be initiated at its recommended starting dose. For patients needing additional glycemic control, the dose of the thiazolidinedione can be increased based on its recommended titration schedule. The increased glycemic control attainable with glyburide/metformin plus a thiazolidinedione may increase the potential for hypoglycemia at any time of day. In patients who develop hypoglycemia when receiving glyburide/metformin and a thiazolidinedione, consideration should be given to reducing the dose of the glyburide component of glyburide/metformin. As clinically warranted, adjustment of the dosages of the other components of the antidiabetic regimen should also be considered.

➤*Administration:* Give glyburide/metformin with meals.

➤*Storage / Stability:* Store at temperatures up to 25°C (77°F).

GLIPIZIDE/METFORMIN HYDROCHLORIDE

Rx	**Glipizide/Metformin Hydrochloride** (Various, eg, Barr, Mylan)	**Tablets; oral:** glipizide 2.5 mg/ metformin 250 mg	In 100s.
Rx	**Metaglip** (Bristol-Myers Squibb)		(BMS 6081). Pink, oval. Film-coated. In 100s.
Rx	**Glipizide/Metformin Hydrochloride** (Various, eg, Barr, Mylan)	**Tablets; oral:** glipizide 2.5 mg/ metformin 500 mg	In 100s.
Rx	**Glipizide/Metformin Hydrochloride** (Various, eg, Barr, Mylan)	**Tablets; oral:** glipizide 5 mg/ metformin 500 mg	In 100s.

GLIPIZIDE/METFORMIN HYDROCHLORIDE — ORAL

For complete and comparative prescribing information, refer to the Sulfonylureas group monograph and the Metformin Hydrochloride monograph.

WARNING

Lactic acidosis – Lactic acidosis is a rare, but serious, metabolic complication that can occur because of metformin accumulation during treatment with glipizide/metformin; when it occurs, it is fatal in approximately 50% of cases. Lactic acidosis may also occur in association with a number of pathophysiologic conditions, including diabetes mellitus, and whenever there is significant tissue hypoperfusion and hypoxemia. Lactic acidosis is characterized by elevated blood lactate levels (more than 5 mmol/L), decreased blood pH, electrolyte disturbances with an increased anion gap, and an increased lactate/pyruvate ratio. When metformin is implicated as the cause of lactic acidosis, metformin plasma levels of more than 5 mcg/mL are generally found.

The reported incidence of lactic acidosis in patients receiving metformin is very low (approximately 0.03 cases per 1,000 patient-years, with approximately 0.015 fatal cases per 1,000 patient-years). In more than 20,000 patient-years of exposure to metformin in clinical trials, there were no reports of lactic acidosis. Reported cases have occurred primarily in diabetic patients with significant renal function impairment, including both intrinsic renal disease and renal hypoperfusion, often in the setting of multiple concomitant medical/surgical problems and multiple concomitant medications. Patients with congestive heart failure (CHF) requiring pharmacologic management, in particular those with unstable or acute CHF who are at risk of hypoperfusion and hypoxemia, are at increased risk of lactic acidosis. The risk of lactic acidosis increases with the degree of renal function impairment and the patient's age. The risk of lactic acidosis may, therefore, be significantly decreased by regular monitoring of renal function in patients taking metformin and the use of the minimum effective dose of metformin. In particular, accompany the treatment of elderly patients with careful monitoring of renal function. Do not initiate glipizide/metformin treatment in patients 80 years of age and older unless measurement of creatinine clearance (CrCl) demonstrates that renal function is not reduced, because these patients are more susceptible to developing lactic acidosis. In addition, promptly withhold glipizide/metformin in the presence of any condition associated with dehydration, hypoxemia, or sepsis. Because hepatic function impairment may significantly limit the ability to clear lactate, generally avoid glipizide/metformin in patients with clinical or laboratory evidence of hepatic disease. Caution patients against excessive alcohol intake, acute or chronic, when taking glipizide/metformin, because alcohol potentiates the effects of metformin on lactate metabolism. In addition, temporarily discontinue glipizide/metformin prior to any intravascular radiocontrast study and for any surgical procedure.

The onset of lactic acidosis is often subtle and accompanied only by nonspecific symptoms, such as increasing somnolence, malaise, myalgia, nonspecific abdominal distress, and respiratory distress. There may be associated hypotension, hypothermia, and resistant bradyarrhythmias with more marked acidosis. The patient and the patient's health care provider must be aware of the possible importance of such symptoms. Instruct the patient to notify their health care provider immediately if symptoms occur. Withdraw glipizide/metformin until the situation is clarified. Serum electrolytes, ketones, blood glucose, and, if indicated, blood pH, lactate levels, and even blood metformin levels may be useful. Once a patient is stabilized on any dose level of glipizide/metformin, GI symptoms, which are common during initiation of therapy with metformin, are unlikely to be drug-related. Later occurrence of GI symptoms could be caused by lactic acidosis or other serious disease.

Levels of fasting venous plasma lactate above the upper limit of normal (ULN) but less than 5 mmol/L in patients taking glipizide/metformin do not necessarily indicate impending lactic acidosis and may be explainable by other mechanisms, such as poorly controlled diabetes or obesity, vigorous physical activity, or technical problems in sample handling.

Suspect lactic acidosis in any diabetic patient with metabolic acidosis lacking evidence of ketoacidosis (eg, ketonemia, ketonuria).

Lactic acidosis is a medical emergency that must be treated in a hospital setting. In a patient with lactic acidosis who is taking glipizide/metformin, discontinue the drug immediately and institute general supportive measures promptly. Because metformin is dialyzable (with a clearance of up to 170 mL/min under good hemodynamic conditions), prompt hemodialysis is recommended to correct the acidosis and remove the accumulated metformin. Such management often results in prompt reversal of symptoms and recovery.

Indications

➤*Type 2 diabetes:* As an adjunct to diet and exercise to improve glycemic control in patients with type 2 diabetes mellitus.

Administration and Dosage

➤*General dosing considerations:* Dosage must be individualized on the basis of effectiveness and tolerance. Glipizide/metformin should be given with meals and initiated at a low dose, with gradual dose escalation as described in the following information, in order to avoid hypoglycemia (largely caused by glipizide), reduce GI adverse reactions (largely caused by metformin), and permit determination of the minimum effective dose for adequate control of blood glucose in the individual patient.

➤*Adults:*

Type 2 diabetes –

Patients with inadequate glycemic control on diet and exercise alone:

• *Maximum dose* – In clinical trials of glipizide/metformin as initial therapy, there was no experience with total daily doses of more than glipizide 10 mg/metformin 2,000 mg per day in divided doses.

• *Initial dosage* – Glipizide 2.5 mg/metformin 250 mg once a day with a meal.

For patients whose fasting plasma glucose (FPG) is 280 to 320 mg/dL, a starting dosage of glipizide 2.5 mg/metformin 500 mg twice daily should be considered. The efficacy of glipizide/metformin in patients whose FPG exceeds 320 mg/dL has not been established.

• *Dosage titration* – Dosage increases to achieve adequate glycemic control should be made in increments of 1 tablet per day every 2 weeks, up to a maximum of glipizide 10 mg/metformin 1,000 mg or glipizide 10 mg/ metformin 2,000 mg/day given in divided doses.

Patients with inadequate glycemic control on a sulfonylurea and/or metformin:

• *Maximum dose* – Glipizide 20 mg/metformin 2,000 mg per day in divided doses.

• *Initial dosage* – Glipizide 2.5 mg/metformin 500 mg or glipizide 5 mg/metformin 500 mg twice daily with the morning and evening meals.

In order to avoid hypoglycemia, the starting dose of glipizide/metformin should not exceed the daily doses of glipizide or metformin already being taken.

• *Dosage titration* – The daily dose should be titrated in increments of no more than glipizide 5 mg/metformin 500 mg up to the minimum effective dose to achieve adequate control of blood glucose, or to a maximum dose of glipizide 20 mg/metformin 2,000 mg per day.

• *Conversion* – No studies have been performed specifically examining the safety and efficacy of switching to glipizide/metformin therapy in patients taking concomitant glipizide (or other sulfonylurea) plus metformin. Changes in glycemic control may occur in such patients, with either hyperglycemia or hypoglycemia possible.

Patients previously treated with combination therapy of glipizide (or another sulfonylurea) plus metformin may be switched to glipizide 2.5 mg/metformin 500 mg or glipizide 5 mg/metformin 500 mg; the starting dose should not exceed the daily dose of glipizide (or equivalent dose of another sulfonylurea) and metformin already being taken. The decision to switch to the nearest equivalent dose or titrate should be based on clinical judgment. Patients should be monitored closely for signs and symptoms of hypoglycemia following such a switch or any change in therapy of type 2 diabetes, and the dose of glipizide/metformin should be titrated as previously described to achieve adequate control of blood glucose.

➤*Elderly:* The initial and maintenance dosing should be conservative in patients with advanced age because of the potential for renal function impairment in this population. Any dosage adjustment requires a careful assessment of renal function. Monitoring of renal function is necessary to aid in prevention of metformin-associated lactic acidosis, particularly in elderly patients. Generally, elderly, debilitated, and malnourished patients should not be titrated to the maximum dose to avoid the risk of hypoglycemia.

➤*Renal function impairment:* The metabolism and excretion of glipizide may be slowed in patients with renal function impairment. If hypoglycemia should occur in such patients, it may be prolonged; institute appropriate management.

Metformin is known to be substantially excreted by the kidney, and the risk of metformin accumulation and lactic acidosis increases with the degree of renal function impairment. Thus, patients with serum creatinine levels above the upper limit of normal for their age should not receive glipizide/ metformin. In patients with advanced age, carefully titrate glipizide/ metformin to establish the minimum dose for adequate glycemic effect because aging is associated with reduced renal function. In elderly patients, particularly those 80 years of age and older, monitor renal function regularly and, generally, do not titrate glipizide/metformin to the maximum dose. Before initiation of glipizide/metformin therapy and at least annually thereafter, assess renal function and verify as normal. In patients in whom development of renal function impairment is anticipated, assess renal function more frequently and discontinue glipizide/metformin if evidence of renal function impairment is present.

GLIPIZIDE/METFORMIN HYDROCHLORIDE — ORAL

Use with caution concomitant medication(s) that may affect renal function, result in significant hemodynamic change, or interfere with the disposition of metformin, such as cationic drugs that are eliminated by renal tubular secretion.

➤*Hepatic function impairment:* The metabolism and excretion of glipizide may be slowed in patients with hepatic function impairment. If hypoglycemia should occur in such patients, it may be prolonged; institute appropriate management.

Because hepatic function impairment has been associated with some cases of lactic acidosis, generally avoid glipizide/metformin in patients with clinical or laboratory evidence of hepatic disease.

➤*Therapeutic drug monitoring:* With initial treatment and during dose titration, appropriate blood glucose monitoring should be used to determine the therapeutic response to glipizide/metformin and to identify the minimum effective dose for the patient. Thereafter, glycosylated hemoglobin (HbA_{1c}) should be measured at intervals of approximately 3 months to assess the effectiveness of therapy. The therapeutic goal in all patients with type 2 diabetes is to decrease FPG, postprandial plasma glucose, and HbA_{1c} to normal or as near normal as possible. Ideally, the response to therapy should be evaluated using HbA_{1c}, which is a better indicator of long-term glycemic control than FPG alone.

Any change in therapy of type 2 diabetes should be undertaken with care and appropriate monitoring.

➤*Administration:* Administer with meals.

➤*Storage/Stability:* Store at 20° to 25°C (68° to 77°F); excursions are permitted to 15° to 30°C (59° to 86°F).

ROSIGLITAZONE/METFORMIN HYDROCHLORIDE

Rx	**Avandamet** (GlaxoSmithKline)	**Tablets; oral:** rosiglitazone 2 mg/ metformin hydrochloride 500 mg	As rosiglitazone maleate. Lactose, PEG (gsk 2/500). Pale pink, oval. Film-coated. In 60s.
		rosiglitazone 2 mg/metformin hydrochloride 1,000 mg	As rosiglitazone maleate. Lactose, PEG (gsk 2/1,000). Yellow, oval. Film-coated. In 60s.
		rosiglitazone 4 mg/metformin hydrochloride 500 mg	As rosiglitazone maleate. Lactose, PEG (gsk 4/500). Orange, oval. Film-coated. In 60s.
		rosiglitazone 4 mg/metformin hydrochloride 1,000 mg	As rosiglitazone maleate. Lactose, PEG (gsk 4/1,000). Pink, oval. Film-coated. In 60s.

ROSIGLITAZONE MALEATE/METFORMIN HYDROCHLORIDE — ORAL

For complete and comparative prescribing information, refer to the Thiazolidinediones class monograph and the Metformin monograph.

WARNING

Congestive heart failure and myocardial ischemia – Thiazolidinediones, including rosiglitazone, cause or exacerbate congestive heart failure (CHF) in some patients. After initiation of rosiglitazone/metformin, and after dose increases, observe patients carefully for signs and symptoms of heart failure (including excessive, rapid weight gain, dyspnea, and/or edema). If these signs and symptoms develop, the heart failure should be managed according to the current standards of care. Furthermore, it is important to consider discontinuation or dose reduction of rosiglitazone/ metformin.

Rosiglitazone/metformin is not recommended in patients with symptomatic heart failure. Initiation of rosiglitazone/metformin in patients with established New York Heart Association (NYHA) class III or IV heart failure is contraindicated.

A meta-analysis of 52 clinical studies (mean duration, 6 months; 16,995 total patients), most of which compared rosiglitazone with placebo, showed rosiglitazone to be associated with an increased risk of myocardial infarction (MI). Three other studies (mean duration, 46 months; 14,067 total patients) comparing rosiglitazone with some other approved oral antidiabetic agents or placebo showed a statistically nonsignificant increased risk of MI, and a statistically nonsignificant decreased risk of death. There have been no clinical trials directly comparing cardiovascular risk of rosiglitazone and pioglitazone, another thiazolidinedione, but in a separate trial, pioglitazone (when compared with placebo) did not show an increased risk of MI or death.

Lactic acidosis – Lactic acidosis is a rare but serious metabolic complication that can occur because of metformin accumulation. The risk increases with conditions, such as sepsis, dehydration, excess alcohol intake, hepatic insufficiency, renal impairment, and acute CHF.

Symptoms include malaise, myalgias, respiratory distress, increasing somnolence, and nonspecific abdominal distress. Laboratory abnormalities include low pH, increased anion gap, and elevated blood lactate.

If acidosis is suspected, discontinue rosiglitazone/metformin and hospitalize the patient immediately.

Indications

➤*Type 2 diabetes:* As an adjunct to diet and exercise to improve glycemic control when treatment with both rosiglitazone and metformin therapy is appropriate in adults with type 2 diabetes mellitus who are already taking rosiglitazone or are not already taking rosiglitazone, but are unable to achieve glycemic control on other diabetes medications and, in consultation with their health care provider, have decided not to take pioglitazone or pioglitazone-containing products for medical reasons.

Administration and Dosage

➤*Adults:*

Type 2 diabetes –

Maximum dose: Rosiglitazone 8 mg/metformin 2,000 mg per day.

Initial dosage: All patients should start the rosiglitazone component of rosiglitazone/metformin at the lowest recommended dose.

Dosage titration: Perform gradual dose escalation with careful monitoring for adverse reactions related to fluid retention. This reduces GI adverse reactions (largely due to metformin) and permits determination of the minimum effective dose for the individual patient.

Give sufficient time to assess adequacy of therapeutic response. Fasting plasma glucose (FPG) should be used to initially determine the therapeutic response to rosiglitazone/metformin. If additional glycemic control is needed, the daily dose of rosiglitazone/metformin may be increased by increments of rosiglitazone 4 mg and/or metformin 500 mg.

After an increase in metformin dosage, dose titration is recommended if patients are not adequately controlled after 1 to 2 weeks. After an increase in rosiglitazone dosage, dose titration is recommended if patients are not adequately controlled after 8 to 12 weeks.

➤*Elderly:* The initial and maintenance dose should be conservative in elderly patients because of the potential for decreased renal function in this population. Generally, elderly patients should not be titrated to the maximum dose.

➤*Renal function impairment:* Any dosage adjustment should be based on a careful assessment of renal function. Monitoring of renal function is necessary to aid in prevention of metformin-associated lactic acidosis, particularly in elderly patients.

➤*Hepatic function impairment:* Liver enzyme monitoring is recommended in all patients prior to initiation of therapy. Therapy should not be initiated if the patient exhibits clinical evidence of active liver disease or increased serum transaminase levels (ALT greater than 2.5 times the upper limit of normal [ULN] at start of therapy).

➤*Debilitated/Malnourished patients:* Generally, debilitated and malnourished patients should not be titrated to the maximum dose.

➤*Administration:* Administer in divided doses with meals.

➤*Storage/Stability:* Store at 25°C (77°F); excursions are permitted between 15° and 30°C (59° and 86°F).

PIOGLITAZONE/METFORMIN HYDROCHLORIDE

Rx	**ActoPlus Met** (Takeda)	**Tablets; oral:** pioglitazone 15 mg/ metformin hydrochloride 500 mg	As pioglitazone hydrochloride. PEG. (4833M 15/500). White to off-white, oblong. Film-coated. In 60s and 180s.
		pioglitazone 15 mg/metformin hydrochloride 850 mg	As pioglitazone hydrochloride. PEG. (4833M 15/850). White to off-white, oblong. Film-coated. In 60s and 180s.
Rx	**ActoPlus Met XR** (Takeda)	**Tablets, extended-release; oral:** pioglitazone 15 mg/extended-release metformin hydrochloride 1,000 mg	As pioglitazone hydrochloride. Lactose, PEG. (4833X 15/1000). White to off-white, round. Film-coated. In 30s, 60s, and 90s.
		pioglitazone 30 mg/extended-release metformin hydrochloride 1,000 mg	As pioglitazone hydrochloride. Lactose, PEG. (4833X 30/1000). White to off-white, round. Film-coated. In 30s, 60s, and 90s.

PIOGLITAZONE HYDROCHLORIDE/METFORMIN HYDROCHLORIDE — ORAL

WARNING

Congestive heart failure – Thiazolidinediones, including pioglitazone, which is a component of pioglitazone/metformin, cause or exacerbate congestive heart failure (CHF) in some patients. After initiation of pioglitazone/metformin, and after dose increases, observe patients carefully for signs and symptoms of heart failure (including excessive, rapid weight gain, dyspnea, and/or edema). If these signs and symptoms develop, manage the heart failure according to the current standards of care. Furthermore, consider discontinuation or dose reduction of pioglitazone/metformin.

Pioglitazone/metformin is not recommended in patients with symptomatic heart failure. Initiation of pioglitazone/metformin in patients with established New York Heart Association (NYHA) class III or IV heart failure is contraindicated.

Lactic acidosis – Lactic acidosis is a rare but serious complication that can occur because of metformin accumulation. The risk increases with conditions such as sepsis, dehydration, excess alcohol intake, hepatic insufficiency, renal impairment, and acute congestive heart failure. The onset is often subtle, accompanied only by nonspecific symptoms such as malaise, myalgias, respiratory distress, increasing somnolence, and nonspecific abdominal distress. Laboratory abnormalities include low pH, increased anion gap, and elevated blood lactate. If acidosis is suspected, pioglitazone/metformin should be discontinued and the patient hospitalized immediately.

Indications

➤*Type 2 diabetes:* As an adjunct to diet and exercise to improve glycemic control in adults with type 2 diabetes mellitus who are already treated with pioglitazone and metformin or who have inadequate glycemic control on pioglitazone alone or metformin alone.

Management of type 2 diabetes should also include nutritional counseling, weight reduction as needed, and exercise. These efforts are important not only in the primary treatment of type 2 diabetes, but also to maintain the efficacy of drug therapy. Prior to initiation or escalation of oral antidiabetic therapy in patients with type 2 diabetes mellitus, secondary causes of poor glycemic control (eg, infection) should be investigated and treated.

Administration and Dosage

➤*General dosing considerations:* The use of pioglitazone/metformin in the management of type 2 diabetes should be individualized on the basis of effectiveness and tolerability.

The starting doses of pioglitazone/metformin should be based on the patient's current regimen of pioglitazone and/or metformin and the starting doses of these 2 drugs. The usual starting dosage of pioglitazone is 15 to 30 mg/day. The usual starting dosage of metformin is 850 to 1,000 mg/day.

To reduce the GI side effects associated with metformin, pioglitazone/metformin should be administered with a meal.

After initiation of pioglitazone/metformin, or with dose increase, patients should be carefully monitored for adverse events related to fluid retention.

The dose of pioglitazone/metformin should be gradually titrated as needed, based on the adequacy of the therapeutic response.

Sufficient time should be given to assess adequacy of therapeutic response. Ideally, the response to therapy should be evaluated using hemoglobin A_{1c} (HbA_{1c}), which is a better indicator of long-term glycemic control than fasting plasma glucose (FPG) alone. HbA_{1c} reflects glycemia over the previous 2 to 3 months. In clinical use, it is recommended that patients be treated with pioglitazone/metformin for a period of time adequate to evaluate change in HbA_{1c} (8 to 12 weeks), unless glycemic control as measured by FPG deteriorates.

➤*Adults:*

Type 2 diabetes –

Maximum dose:

- *Immediate-release* – Pioglitazone 45 mg/metformin 2,550 mg per day.
- *Extended-release* – Pioglitazone 45 mg/ER metformin 2,000 mg per day.

Initial dosage: Selecting the starting dose of pioglitazone/metformin should be based on the patient's current regimen of pioglitazone and/or metformin.

- *Immediate-release* – Pioglitazone 15 mg/metformin 500 mg or pioglitazone 15 mg/metformin 850 mg once or twice daily with food.
- *Extended-release* – Pioglitazone 15 mg/ER metformin 1,000 mg or pioglitazone 30 mg/ER metformin 1,000 mg once daily with the evening meal.

➤*Elderly:* The initial and maintenance dosing of pioglitazone/metformin should be conservative in patients with advanced age because of the potential for decreased renal function in this population. Any dosage adjustment should be based on a careful assessment of renal function. Generally, elderly, debilitated, and malnourished patients should not be titrated to the maximum dose of pioglitazone/metformin.

➤*Renal function impairment:* Monitoring of renal function is necessary to aid in prevention of metformin-associated lactic acidosis, particularly in elderly patients. Metformin is substantially excreted by the kidney. Pioglitazone/metformin should only be used in patients with normal renal function. Any dosage adjustment in pioglitazone/metformin should be based on careful assessment of renal function.

➤*Hepatic function impairment:* Therapy with pioglitazone/metformin should not be initiated if the patient exhibits clinical evidence of active liver disease or increased serum transaminase levels (ALT greater than 2.5 times the upper limit of normal [ULN]) at start of therapy. Liver enzyme monitoring is recommended in all patients prior to initiation of therapy with pioglitazone/metformin and periodically thereafter.

➤*Administration:* Pioglitazone/metformin should be given in divided daily doses with meals to reduce the GI adverse reactions associated with metformin.

Pioglitazone/ER metformin must be swallowed whole and not chewed, cut, or crushed. Inform patients that the inactive ingredients may occasionally be eliminated in the feces as a soft mass that may resemble the original tablet.

➤*Storage/Stability:* Store at 25°C (77°F); excursions are permitted to 15° to 30°C (59° to 86°F). Keep the container tightly closed, and avoid excessive heat and humidity.

PIOGLITAZONE/GLIMEPIRIDE

Rx	**Duetact** (Takeda Pharmaceuticals America)	**Tablets; oral:** pioglitazone 30 mg/glimepiride 2 mg	As pioglitazone hydrochloride. Lactose. (4833G 30/2). White to off-white. Round. In 30s and 90s.
		pioglitazone 30 mg/glimepiride 4 mg	As pioglitazone hydrochloride. Lactose. (4833G 30/4). White to off-white. Round. In 30s and 90s.

PIOGLITAZONE HYDROCHLORIDE/GLIMEPIRIDE — ORAL

For complete and comparative prescribing information, refer to the Thiazolidinediones class monograph and Sulfonylureas class monograph.

WARNING

Congestive heart failure – Thiazolidinediones, including pioglitazone, which is a component of pioglitazone/glimepiride, cause or exacerbate congestive heart failure (CHF) in some patients. After initiation of pioglitazone/glimepiride, observe patients carefully for signs and symptoms of heart failure (including excessive, rapid weight gain, dyspnea, and/or edema). If these signs and symptoms develop, manage the heart failure according to the current standards of care. Furthermore, consider discontinuation of pioglitazone/glimepiride.

Pioglitazone/glimepiride is not recommended in patients with symptomatic heart failure. Initiation of pioglitazone/glimepiride in patients with established New York Heart Association (NYHA) class III or IV heart failure is contraindicated.

Indications

➤*Type 2 diabetes:* As an adjunct to diet and exercise to improve glycemic control in adults with type 2 diabetes mellitus who are already treated with a thiazolidinedione and a sulfonylurea, or who have inadequate glycemic control on a thiazolidinedione alone or sulfonylurea alone.

Administration and Dosage

➤*General dosing considerations:* The use of antihyperglycemic therapy in the management of type 2 diabetes should be individualized on the basis of effectiveness and tolerability. Failure to follow an appropriate dosage regimen may precipitate hypoglycemia.

The selection of the starting dose of pioglitazone/glimepiride should be based on the patient's current regimen of pioglitazone and/or sulfonylurea. Patients who may be more sensitive to antihyperglycemic drugs should be monitored carefully during dose adjustment. After initiation of pioglitazone/glimepiride, patients should be carefully monitored for adverse events related to fluid retention.

Pioglitazone/glimepiride should not be given more than once daily at any of the tablet strengths.

During initiation of pioglitazone/glimepiride therapy and any subsequent dosage adjustment, patients should be observed carefully for hypoglycemia.

➤*Adults:*

Type 2 diabetes –

Maximum dose: Pioglitazone 45 mg/glimepiride 8 mg per day.

Patients currently on glimepiride monotherapy: Based on the usual starting dosage of pioglitazone (15 or 30 mg daily), pioglitazone/glimepiride may be initiated at 30 mg/2 mg or 30 mg/4 mg tablet strengths once daily and adjusted after assessing adequacy of therapeutic response.

Patients currently on pioglitazone monotherapy: Based on the usual starting dose of glimepiride (1 or 2 mg once daily) and pioglitazone 15 or 30 mg, pioglitazone/glimepiride may be initiated at 30 mg/2 mg once daily and adjusted after assessing adequacy of therapeutic response.

Patients switching from combination therapy of pioglitazone plus glimepiride as separate tablets: Pioglitazone/glimepiride may be initiated with 30 mg/2 mg or 30 mg/4 mg tablet strengths based on the dose of pioglitazone

PIOGLITAZONE HYDROCHLORIDE/GLIMEPIRIDE — ORAL

and glimepiride already being taken. Patients who are not controlled with pioglitazone 15 mg in combination with glimepiride should be carefully monitored when switched to pioglitazone/glimepiride.

Patients currently on a different sulfonylurea monotherapy or switching from combination therapy of pioglitazone plus a different sulfonylurea (eg, glyburide, glipizide, chlorpropamide, tolbutamide, acetohexamide): No exact dosage relationship exists between glimepiride and other sulfonylurea agents. Therefore, based on the maximum starting dose of glimepiride 2 mg, pioglitazone/glimepiride should be limited initially to a starting dosage of 30 mg/2 mg once daily and adjusted after assessing adequacy of therapeutic response.

Any change in diabetic therapy should be undertaken with care and appropriate monitoring, because changes in glycemic control can occur. Patients should be observed carefully for hypoglycemia (for 1 to 2 weeks) when being transferred to pioglitazone/glimepiride, especially from longer half-life sulfonylureas (eg, chlorpropamide), because of potential overlapping of drug effect.

Sufficient time should be given to assess adequacy of therapeutic response. Ideally, the response to therapy should be evaluated using hemoglobin A_{1c} (HbA_{1c}), which is a better indicator of long-term glycemic control than fasting plasma glucose (FPG) alone. HbA_{1c} reflects glycemia over the past 2 to 3 months. In clinical use, it is recommended that patients be treated with pioglitazone/glimepiride for a period of time adequate to evaluate change in HbA_{1c} (8 to 12 weeks), unless glycemic control, as measured by FPG, deteriorates.

➤*Elderly:* The initial dosing, dose increments, and maintenance dosage should be conservative to avoid hypoglycemic reactions. The initial dose should be started at glimepiride 1 mg prior to prescribing pioglitazone/glimepiride.

➤*Renal function impairment:* The initial dosing, dose increments, and maintenance dosage should be conservative to avoid hypoglycemic reactions. The initial dose should be started at glimepiride 1 mg prior to prescribing pioglitazone/glimepiride.

➤*Hepatic function impairment:* The initial dosing, dose increments, and maintenance dosage should be conservative to avoid hypoglycemic reactions. The initial dose should be started at glimepiride 1 mg prior to prescribing pioglitazone/glimepiride.

Therapy with pioglitazone/glimepiride should not be initiated if the patient exhibits clinical evidence of active liver disease or increased serum transaminase levels (ALT more than 2.5 times the upper limit of normal [ULN]) at start of therapy. Liver enzyme monitoring is recommended in all patients prior to initiation of therapy with pioglitazone/glimepiride and periodically thereafter.

➤*Debilitated or malnourished patients:* The initial dosing, dose increments, and maintenance dosage of pioglitazone/glimepiride should be conservative to avoid hypoglycemic reactions. These patients should be started at glimepiride 1 mg prior to prescribing pioglitazone/glimepiride.

➤*Congestive heart failure and hypertension:* The lowest approved dose of pioglitazone/glimepiride therapy should be prescribed to patients with type 2 diabetes and systolic dysfunction only after titration from 15 to 30 mg of pioglitazone has been safely tolerated. If subsequent dose adjustment is necessary, patients should be carefully monitored for weight gain, edema, or signs and symptoms of CHF exacerbation.

➤*Administration:* Administer once daily with the first main meal.

➤*Storage/Stability:* Store at 25°C (77°F); excursions are permitted between 15° and 30°C (59° and 86°F). Keep the container tightly closed and protect it from moisture and humidity.

ROSIGLITAZONE/GLIMEPIRIDE

Rx	**Avandaryl** (GlaxoSmithKline)	**Tablets; oral:** rosiglitazone 4 mg/glimepiride 1 mg	As rosiglitazone maleate. Lactose, PEG. (gsk 4/1). Yellow, rounded triangle. In 30s.
		rosiglitazone 4 mg/glimepiride 2 mg	As rosiglitazone maleate. Lactose, PEG. (gsk 4/2). Orange, rounded triangle. In 30s.
		rosiglitazone 4 mg/glimepiride 4 mg	As rosiglitazone maleate. Lactose, PEG. (gsk 4/4). Pink, rounded triangle. In 30s.
		rosiglitazone 8 mg/glimepiride 2 mg	As rosiglitazone maleate. Lactose, PEG. (gsk 8/2). Pale pink, rounded triangle. In 30s.
		rosiglitazone 8 mg/glimepiride 4 mg	As rosiglitazone maleate. Lactose, PEG. (gsk 8/4). Red, rounded triangle. In 30s.

ROSIGLITAZONE MALEATE/GLIMEPIRIDE — ORAL

For complete and comparative prescribing information, refer to the Thiazolidinediones class monograph, the Rosiglitazone monograph, the Sulfonylurea class monograph, and the Glimepiride monograph.

WARNING

For complete and comparative prescribing information, refer to the Thiazolidinediones class monograph, the Rosiglitazone monograph, Sulfonylurea class monograph, and the Glimepiride monograph.

Congestive heart failure and myocardial infarction – Thiazolidinediones, including rosiglitazone, cause or exacerbate congestive heart failure (CHF) in some patients. After initiation of rosiglitazone/glimepiride and after dose increases, observe patients carefully for signs and symptoms of heart failure, including excessive, rapid weight gain, dyspnea, and/or edema. If these signs and symptoms develop, manage the heart failure according to the current standards of care. Furthermore, discontinuation or dose reduction of rosiglitazone/glimepiride must be considered.

Rosiglitazone/glimepiride is not recommended in patients with symptomatic heart failure. Initiation of rosiglitazone/glimepiride in patients with established New York Heart Association (NYHA) class III or IV heart failure is contraindicated.

A meta-analysis of 52 clinical trials (mean duration, 6 months; 16,995 total patients), most of which compared rosiglitazone with placebo, showed rosiglitazone to be associated with an increased risk of myocardial infarction (MI). Three other trials (mean duration, 46 months; 14,067 total patients), comparing rosiglitazone with some other approved oral antidiabetic agents or placebo, showed a statistically nonsignificant increased risk of MI, and a statistically nonsignificant decreased risk of death. There have been no clinical trials directly comparing cardiovascular risk of rosiglitazone and pioglitazone (another thiazolidinedione), but in a separate trial, pioglitazone (when compared with placebo) did not show an increased risk of MI or death.

Indications

➤*Type 2 diabetes:* As an adjunct to diet and exercise to improve glycemic control when treatment with both rosiglitazone/glimepiride is appropriate in adults with type 2 diabetes mellitus who either are already taking rosiglitazone or are not already taking rosiglitazone and are unable to achieve glycemic control taking other diabetes medications, and, in consultation with their health care provider, have decided not to take pioglitazone or pioglitazone-containing products for medical reasons.

Administration and Dosage

➤*Adults:*

Type 2 diabetes –

Maximum dose: Rosiglitazone 8 mg/glimepiride 4 mg per day.

Initial dosage: Rosiglitazone 4 mg/glimepiride 1 mg once daily with the first meal of the day. For patients already treated with a sulfonylurea or thiazolidinedione, a starting dose of rosiglitazone 4 mg/glimepiride 2 mg may be considered.

Dosage titration: Individualize dose increases according to the glycemic response of the patient. If hypoglycemia occurs during up titration of the dose or while maintained on therapy, a dosage reduction of the glimepiride component of rosiglitazone/glimepiride may be considered.

Conversion:

• *Rosiglitazone monotherapy to rosiglitazone/glimepiride –* To switch to rosiglitazone/glimepiride for adults currently treated with rosiglitazone, dose titration of the glimepiride component of rosiglitazone/glimepiride is recommended if the patient is not adequately controlled after 1 to 2 weeks. The glimepiride component may be increased in no more than 2 mg increments. After an increase in the dosage of the glimepiride component, dose titration of rosiglitazone/glimepiride is recommended if patients are not adequately controlled after 1 to 2 weeks.

• *Sulfonylurea monotherapy to rosiglitazone/glimepiride –* For patients currently treated with sulfonylurea and switched to rosiglitazone/glimepiride, it may take 2 weeks to see a reduction in blood glucose and 2 to 3 months to see the full effect of the rosiglitazone component. Therefore, dose titration of the rosiglitazone component of rosiglitazone/glimepiride is recommended if patients are not adequately controlled after 8 to 12 weeks. Patients should be observed carefully (1 to 2 weeks) for hypoglycemia when being transferred from longer half-life sulfonylureas (eg, chlorpropamide) to rosiglitazone/glimepiride because of the potential overlapping of drug effect. After an increase in the dosage of the rosiglitazone component, dose titration of rosiglitazone/glimepiride is recommended if the patient is not adequately controlled after 2 to 3 months.

➤*Elderly:* A starting dose of rosiglitazone 4 mg/glimepiride 1 mg followed by appropriate dose titration is recommended.

➤*Hepatic function impairment:* See Elderly for dosing.

Do not initiate therapy with rosiglitazone/glimepiride if the patient exhibits clinical evidence of active liver disease or increased serum transaminase levels (ALT greater than 2.5 times the upper limit of normal [ULN]) at baseline. (See Warnings/Precautions for more information.)

➤*Special risk patients:* See Elderly for dosing.

➤*Discontinuation of therapy:* If at any time ALT levels increase to more than 3 times the ULN in patients on therapy with rosiglitazone/glimepiride, liver enzyme levels should be rechecked as soon as possible. If ALT levels remain more than 3 times the ULN or if jaundice is observed, therapy with rosiglitazone/glimepiride should be discontinued.

➤*Administration:* Give with the first meal of the day.

➤*Storage/Stability:* Store at 25°C (77°F); excursions are permitted between 15° and 30°C (59° and 86°F). Protect from light.

SITAGLIPTIN/METFORMIN HYDROCHLORIDE

Rx	Janumet (Merck)	**Tablets; oral:** sitagliptin 50 mg/metformin hydrochloride 500 mg	Equiv. to sitagliptin phosphate 64.25 mg. (575). Lt. pink, capsule shape. Film-coated. In 60s, 180s, 1,000s, and UD 50s.
		sitagliptin 50 mg/metformin hydrochloride 1,000 mg	Equiv. to sitagliptin phosphate 64.25 mg. (577). Red, capsule shape. Film-coated. In 60s, 180s, 1,000s, and UD 50s.

SITAGLIPTIN PHOSPHATE/METFORMIN HYDROCHLORIDE — ORAL

For complete and comparative prescribing information, refer to the individual monographs for Sitagliptin Phosphate and Metformin Hydrochloride.

WARNING

Lactic acidosis – Lactic acidosis is a rare but serious complication that can occur because of metformin accumulation. The risk increases with conditions such as sepsis, dehydration, excess alcohol intake, hepatic insufficiency, renal impairment, and acute congestive heart failure.

The onset is often subtle, accompanied only by nonspecific symptoms such as malaise, myalgias, respiratory distress, increasing somnolence, and nonspecific abdominal distress.

Laboratory abnormalities include low pH, increased anion gap, and elevated blood lactate.

If acidosis is suspected, discontinue sitagliptin/metformin and hospitalize the patient immediately.

Indications

➤*Type 2 diabetes mellitus:* As an adjunct to diet and exercise to improve glycemic control in adults with type 2 diabetes mellitus when treatment with both sitagliptin and metformin is appropriate.

Administration and Dosage

➤*General dosing considerations:* Base the starting dose of sitagliptin/metformin on the patient's current regimen. Individualize the dosage on the basis of the patient's current regimen, efficacy, and tolerability.

➤*Adults:*

Type 2 diabetes mellitus –

Patients inadequately controlled with diet and exercise alone:

- *Initial dosage* – Sitagliptin 50 mg/metformin 500 mg twice daily.
- *Dosage titration* – Patients with inadequate glycemic control on the initial dosage can be titrated up to sitagliptin 50 mg/metformin 1,000 mg twice daily.

Patients inadequately controlled on metformin monotherapy –

Initial dosage: The usual starting dosage of sitagliptin/metformin should be equal to a 100 mg total daily dose (50 mg twice daily) of sitagliptin plus the dose of metformin already being taken. For patients taking metformin 850 mg twice daily, the recommended starting dosage is sitagliptin 50 mg/metformin 1,000 mg twice daily.

Patients inadequately controlled on sitagliptin monotherapy –

Initial dosage: Sitagliptin 50 mg/metformin 500 mg twice daily.

Dosage titration: Patients may be titrated up to sitagliptin 50 mg/metformin 1,000 mg twice daily.

Patients taking a sitagliptin monotherapy dose adjusted for renal impairment should not be switched to sitagliptin/metformin.

Patients switching from sitagliptin coadministered with metformin – Sitagliptin/metformin may be initiated at the dose of sitagliptin and metformin already being taken.

Patients inadequately controlled on dual combination therapy with any 2 of the following antihyperglycemic agents: sitagliptin, metformin, or a sulfonylurea –

Initial dosage: The usual starting dose of sitagliptin/metformin should provide sitagliptin dosed as 50 mg twice daily (100 mg total daily dose). In determining the starting dose of the metformin component, consider the patient's level of glycemic control and current dose (if any) of metformin. Patients currently on or initiating a sulfonylurea may require lower sulfonylurea doses to reduce the risk of hypoglycemia.

Dosage titration: Consider gradual dose escalation to reduce GI adverse reactions associated with metformin.

➤*Elderly:* Use sitagliptin/metformin with caution as age increases. Take care in dose selection and base it on careful and regular monitoring of renal function. Do not initiate metformin treatment in patients 80 years of age and older unless measurement of creatinine clearance (CrCl) demonstrates that renal function is not reduced because these patients are more susceptible to developing lactic acidosis.

➤*Renal function impairment:* The risk of metformin accumulation and lactic acidosis increases with the degree of renal impairment. Sitagliptin/metformin is contraindicated in patients with renal disease or renal impairment (eg, as suggested by serum creatinine levels at least 1.5 mg/dL in men or at least 1.4 mg/dL in women, or abnormal CrCl that may also result from other conditions).

➤*Hepatic function impairment:* Because hepatic impairment has been associated with some cases of lactic acidosis, generally avoid giving sitagliptin/metformin to patients with clinical or laboratory evidence of hepatic disease.

➤*Administration:* Administer twice daily with meals.

➤*Storage/Stability:* Store at 20° to 25°C (68° to 77°F); excursions are permitted between 15° and 30°C (59° and 86°F).

SAXAGLIPTIN/METFORMIN HYDROCHLORIDE

Rx	Kombiglyze XR (Bristol-Myers Squibb)	**Tablets, extended-release; oral:** saxagliptin 5 mg/metformin hydrochloride extended-release 500 mg	Equiv. to saxagliptin hydrochloride 5.58 mg. (5/500 4221). Light brown to brown, capsule-shaped. Film-coated. In 30s.
		saxagliptin 2.5 mg/metformin hydrochloride extended-release 1,000 mg	Equiv. to saxagliptin hydrochloride 2.79 mg. (2.5/1000 4222). Pale yellow to light yellow, capsule-shaped. Film-coated. In 60s and 500s.
		saxagliptin 5 mg/metformin hydrochloride extended-release 1,000 mg	Equiv. to saxagliptin hydrochloride 5.58 mg. (5/1000 4223). Pink, capsule-shaped. Film-coated. In 30s, 90s, and 500s.

SAXAGLIPTIN HYDROCHLORIDE/METFORMIN HYDROCHLORIDE — ORAL

WARNING

Lactic acidosis – Lactic acidosis is a rare, but serious, complication that can occur due to metformin accumulation. The risk increases with conditions such as sepsis, dehydration, excess alcohol intake, hepatic impairment, renal impairment, and acute congestive heart failure.

The onset of lactic acidosis is often subtle, accompanied only by nonspecific symptoms such as malaise, myalgias, respiratory distress, increasing somnolence, and nonspecific abdominal distress.

Laboratory abnormalities include low pH, increased anion gap, and elevated blood lactate.

If acidosis is suspected, discontinue saxagliptin/metformin extended-release (ER) and immediately hospitalize the patient.

Indications

➤*Type 2 diabetes mellitus:* As an adjunct to diet and exercise to improve glycemic control in adults with type 2 diabetes mellitus when treatment with both saxagliptin and metformin is appropriate.

Administration and Dosage

➤*Adults:*

Type 2 diabetes mellitus –

Usual dosage:

- *Patients who need saxagliptin 2.5 mg in combination with metformin* – Saxagliptin 2.5 mg/metformin ER 1,000 mg once daily. Patients who need saxagliptin 2.5 mg who are either metformin naive or who require a dose of metformin higher than 1,000 mg should use the individual components.
- *Patients who need saxagliptin 5 mg who are not currently treated with metformin* – Saxagliptin 5 mg/metformin ER 500 mg once daily with gradual dose escalation to reduce the GI adverse effects due to metformin.
- *Patients treated with metformin* – The dose of saxagliptin/metformin ER should provide metformin at the dose already being taken or the nearest therapeutically appropriate dose.

Maximum dose: Saxagliptin 5 mg/metformin ER 2,000 mg daily.

Concomitant therapy:

- *Strong CYP3A4/5 inhibitors* – When coadministered with strong cytochrome P450 3A4/5 (CYP3A4/5) inhibitors (eg, atazanavir, clarithromycin, indinavir, itraconazole, ketoconazole, nefazodone, nelfinavir, ritonavir, saquinavir, telithromycin), limit the dosage to saxagliptin 2.5 mg/metformin ER 1,000 mg once daily.

➤*Renal function impairment:* Contraindicated in patients with renal impairment.

➤*Hepatic function impairment:* Not recommended in patients with hepatic impairment.

➤*Administration:* Administer once daily with the evening meal, with gradual dose titration to reduce the GI adverse effects associated with metformin. Advise patients to swallow tablets whole and never crush, cut, or chew the tablets.

➤*Storage/Stability:* Store at 20° to 25°C (68° to 77°F); excursions are permitted between 15° and 30°C (59° and 86°F).

REPAGLINIDE/METFORMIN HYDROCHLORIDE

Rx	**PrandiMet** (Novo Nordisk A/S)	**Tablets; oral:** repaglinide 1 mg/metformin hydrochloride 500 mg	PEG, sorbitol. (1/500). Yellow, oval. In 20s and 100s.
		repaglinide 2 mg/metformin hydrochloride 500 mg	PEG, sorbitol. (2/500). Pink, oval. In 20s and 100s.

REPAGLINIDE/METFORMIN HYDROCHLORIDE — ORAL

WARNING

Lactic acidosis – Lactic acidosis is a rare but serious complication that can occur because of metformin accumulation. The risk increases with conditions such as sepsis, dehydration, excess alcohol intake, hepatic impairment, renal impairment, and acute congestive heart failure (CHF).

The onset of lactic acidosis is often subtle and accompanied only by nonspecific symptoms, such as malaise, myalgia, respiratory distress, increasing somnolence, and nonspecific abdominal distress.

Laboratory abnormalities include low pH, increased anion gap, and elevated blood lactate.

If acidosis is suspected, discontinue repaglinide/metformin and hospitalize the patient immediately.

Indications

➤*Type 2 diabetes:* As an adjunct to diet and exercise to improve glycemic control in adults with type 2 diabetes mellitus who are already treated with a meglitinide and metformin, or who have inadequate glycemic control on a meglitinide alone or metformin alone.

Administration and Dosage

➤*General dosing considerations:* Blood glucose monitoring should be performed to determine the therapeutic response to repaglinide/metformin.

➤*Adults:*

Type 2 diabetes –

Maximum dose: Repaglinide 10 mg/metformin 2,500 mg daily; repaglinide 4 mg/metformin 1,000 mg as a single dose per meal.

Patients currently using repaglinide and metformin concomitantly: Repaglinide/metformin can be initiated at the dose of repaglinide and metformin similar to, but not exceeding, the patient's current doses, then may be titrated to the maximum daily dose as necessary to achieve targeted glycemic control.

Patients inadequately controlled with metformin monotherapy: Start with repaglinide 1 mg/metformin 500 mg administered twice daily with meals, with gradual dose escalation (based on glycemic response) to reduce the risk of hypoglycemia with repaglinide.

Patients inadequately controlled with meglitinide monotherapy: Start with 500 mg of the metformin component of repaglinide/metformin twice daily, with gradual dose escalation (based on glycemic response) to reduce GI adverse reactions associated with metformin.

➤*Renal function impairment:* Do not use in patients with renal impairment.

➤*Hepatic function impairment:* Avoid use in patients with hepatic impairment.

➤*Administration:* Administer 2 to 3 times daily within 15 minutes prior to the meal, but the timing can vary from immediately preceding the meal up to 30 minutes before the meal. Patients who skip a meal should be instructed to skip the dose for that meal.

➤*Storage/Stability:* Do not store at temperatures higher than 25°C (77°F). Protect from moisture.

GLUCOSE ELEVATING AGENTS

GLUCAGON (rDNA ORIGIN)

Rx	**GlucaGen HypoKit** (Novo Nordisk)	**Injection, lyophilized powder for solution:** 1 mg (1 unit)	Lactose 107 mg. In 1 unit vial with disposable syringes with 1 mL diluent.
Rx	**GlucaGen Diagnostic Kit** (Bedford)		Lactose 107 mg. In 1 unit vials with 1 mL diluent.
Rx	**Glucagon Emergency Kit** (Eli Lilly)		Lactose 49 mg. In vials with 1 mL syringe diluent.[a]

[a] With glycerin 12 mg/mL.

GLUCAGON (rDNA ORIGIN) — INJECTION

Indications

➤*Diagnostic aid:* As a diagnostic aid during radiologic examinations to temporarily inhibit movement of the GI tract. Glucagon is as effective for this examination as anticholinergic drugs. However, the addition of an anticholinergic agent may result in increased adverse reactions. Because glucagon depletes glycogen stores, give the patient oral carbohydrates as soon as the procedure is completed, if this is compatible with the diagnostic procedure applied.

➤*Hypoglycemia:* To treat severe hypoglycemic reactions that may occur in patients with diabetes mellitus treated with insulin.

➤*Off-label uses:* For the management of beta-blocker and calcium channel blocker overdoses; as an alternative agent for the treatment of an anaphylactic reaction.

Administration and Dosage

➤*General dosing considerations:* Glucagon must be administered by medical personnel.

Because glucagon depletes glycogen stores, the patient, especially children or adolescents, should be given supplemental carbohydrates as soon as he or she awakens and is able to swallow. Medical evaluation is recommended for all patients who experience severe hypoglycemia.

When glucagon is used as a diagnostic aid and when the diagnostic procedure is over, give oral carbohydrate to restore the liver glycogen and prevent occurrence of secondary hypoglycemia.

When used for severe hypoglycemia, emergency assistance should be sought if the patient fails to respond immediately after subcutaneous or intramuscular (IM) injection of glucagon. The glucagon injection may be repeated using a new kit while waiting for emergency assistance. Intravenous (IV) glucose must be administered if the patient fails to respond to glucagon.

➤*Adults:*

Diagnostic aid –

Usual dosage:

- *Relaxation of the stomach, duodenal bulb, duodenum, and small bowel* – 0.2 to 0.5 mg IV or 1 mg IM.
- *Relaxation of the colon* – 0.5 to 0.75 mg IV or 1 to 2 mg IM.

Hypoglycemia (GlucaGen HypoKit and *Glucagon Emergency Kit)* – Inject 1 mL subcutaneously, IM, or IV.

➤*Children:*

Severe hypoglycemia – See also Off-Label Dosing.

Usual dosage:

- *GlucaGen –*
  - *More than 25 kg or older than 6 to 8 years of age and weight is unknown:* See Adults.
  - *Less than 25 kg or younger than 6 to 8 years of age and weight is unknown:* 0.5 mL subcutaneously, IM, or IV.
- *Glucagon Emergency Kit –*
  - *More than 20 kg or older than 6 to 8 years of age:* See Adults.
  - *Less than 20 kg:* 0.5 mg subcutaneously, IM, or IV every 20 minutes as needed. Glucagon has been given 0.02 to 0.03 mg/kg every 20 minutes as needed.

Off-label dosing –

Severe hypoglycemia:

- *Usual dose* – 0.2 mg/kg subcutaneously, IM, or IV push.
- *Maximum dose* – 1 mg.
- *Continuous infusion* – Initiate with 10 to 20 mcg/kg per hour (0.5 to 1 mg/day).

➤*Elderly:* Exercise caution when glucagon is used to inhibit GI motility in elderly patients with known cardiac disease.

➤*Preparation for administration:*

Reconstitution – Shake the vial gently until powder is completely dissolved and no particles remain in the fluid. The reconstituted fluid should be clear and of water-like consistency. The reconstituted glucagon gives a concentration of approximately 1 mg/mL of glucagon. The reconstituted glucagon should be used immediately after reconstitution. Discard any unused portion.

Vial with prefilled syringe (kit): Using the supplied prefilled syringe, carefully insert the needle through the rubber stopper of the vial containing glucagon powder and inject all the liquid from the syringe into the vial.

Vial with supplied vial of sterile water: Glucagon should be reconstituted with 1 mL of sterile water for reconstitution (if supplied) or 1 mL of sterile water for injection. Draw up all of the sterile water for reconstitution with the syringe and inject into the glucagon vial.

➤*Administration:* For subcutaneous, IM, or IV administration.

➤*Storage/Stability:*

Before reconstitution – Avoid freezing and protect from light. The *GlucaGen* package may be stored up to 24 months. Store between 20° and 25°C

GLUCAGON (rDNA ORIGIN) — INJECTION

(68° and 77°F), prior to reconstitution. Glucagon should not be used after the expiration date on the vials. Glucagon does not contain preservatives and is for single use only.

After reconstitution – Reconstituted glucagon should be used immediately. Discard any unused portion. If the solution shows any sign of gel formation or particles, it should be discarded.

Actions

➤*Pharmacology:*

Antihypoglycemic action – Glucagon induces liver glycogen breakdown, releasing glucose from the liver. Blood glucose concentration rises within 10 minutes of injection and maximal concentrations are attained at approximately a half hour after injection. Hepatic stores of glycogen are necessary for glucagon to produce an antihypoglycemic effect.

GI motility inhibition – Extrahepatic effects of glucagon include relaxation of the smooth muscle of the stomach, duodenum, small bowel, and colon.

Hypoglycemia – Blood glucose concentration rises within 10 minutes of injection and maximal concentrations are attained at approximately 30 minutes after injection. The duration of hyperglycemic action after IV or IM injection is 60 to 90 minutes.

Pharmacodynamic Properties of Glucagon

Route of administration	Dose[a]	Time of maximal glucose concentration[b]	Time of onset of action for GI smooth muscle relaxation	Duration of smooth muscle relaxation
IV	0.25 to 0.5 mg (0.25 to 0.5 units)	5 to 20 min	45 seconds	9 to 17 min
	2 mg (2 units)	5 to 20 min	45 seconds	22 to 25 min
IM	1 mg (1 unit)	30 min	8 to 10 min	12 to 27 min
	2 mg (2 units)	30 min	4 to 7 min	21 to 32 min

[a] The usual diagnostic dose for relaxation of the stomach, duodenal bulb, duodenum, and small bowel is 0.2 to 0.5 mg IV or 1 mg IM. The usual dose to relax the colon is 0.5 to 0.75 mg IV and 1 to 2 mg IM.

[b] The time of maximal glucose concentration for glucagon administered subcutaneously is 30 to 45 minutes.

➤*Pharmacokinetics:* IM injection of glucagon resulted in a mean maximal concentration (C_{max}) (coefficient of variation %) of 1,686 pg/mL (43%) and median time to C_{max} of 12.5 minutes. The mean apparent half-life of 45 minutes after IM injection probably reflects prolonged absorption from the injection site. Glucagon is degraded in the liver, kidney, and plasma.

Contraindications

Known hypersensitivity to glucagon or any constituent in the product; patients with pheochromocytoma or insulinoma.

Warnings/Precautions

➤*Pheochromocytoma/insulinoma:* Administer glucagon cautiously to patients suspected of having pheochromocytoma, insulinoma, or both. Secondary hypoglycemia may occur and should be countered by adequate carbohydrate intake following glucagon treatment. In patients with insulinoma, IV administration of glucagon may produce an initial increase in blood glucose; however, because of glucagon's hyperglycemic effect the insulinoma may release insulin and cause subsequent hypoglycemia. Give a patient developing symptoms of hypoglycemia after a dose of glucagon glucose orally, IV, or by gavage, whichever is most appropriate.

Glucagon may release catecholamines from pheochromocytomas and is contraindicated in patients with this condition. In the presence of pheochromocytoma, glucagon can cause the tumor to release catecholamines, which may result in a sudden and marked increase in blood pressure. If a patient develops a sudden increase in blood pressure, 5 to 10 mg of phentolamine mesylate may be administered IV in an attempt to control the blood pressure.

➤*Hypersensitivity reactions:* Allergic reactions may occur and include generalized rash, urticaria, and, in rare cases, anaphylactic shock with breathing difficulties, and hypotension. The anaphylactic reactions have generally occurred in association with endoscopic examination during which patients often received other agents, including contrast media and local anesthetics. Give the patients standard treatment for anaphylaxis, including an injection of epinephrine, if they encounter respiratory difficulties after glucagon injection.

➤*Special risk:* In order for glucagon treatment to reverse hypoglycemia, adequate amounts of glucose must be stored in the liver (as glycogen). Therefore, use glucagon with caution in patients with conditions such as prolonged fasting, starvation, adrenal insufficiency, or chronic hypoglycemia because these conditions result in low levels of releasable glucose in the liver and an inadequate reversal of hypoglycemia by glucagon treatment. Observe caution when glucagon is used in diabetic patients or in elderly patients with known cardiac disease to inhibit GI motility.

➤*Pregnancy: Category B.* There are no adequate and well-controlled studies in pregnant women. Because animal reproduction studies are not always predictive of human response, use this drug during pregnancy only if clearly needed.

➤*Lactation:* It is not known whether this drug is excreted in human milk. Because many drugs are excreted in human milk, exercise caution when glucagon is administered to a breast-feeding woman.

No clinical studies have been performed in breast-feeding mothers; however, glucagon is a peptide and intact glucagon is not absorbed from the GI tract. Therefore, even if the infant ingested glucagon it would be unlikely to have any effect on the infant. Additionally, glucagon has a short plasma half-life, limiting the amount available to the child.

➤*Children:* The use of glucagon in children has been reported to be safe and effective for the treatment of hypoglycemia.

Safety and efficacy of glucagon as a diagnostic aid in children have not been established.

➤*Elderly:* In general, dose selection for an elderly patient should be cautious, usually starting at the low end of the dosing range, reflecting the greater frequency of decreased hepatic, renal, or cardiac function, and of concomitant disease or other drug therapy.

Observe caution when glucagon is used to inhibit GI motility in elderly patients with known cardiac disease.

➤*Monitoring:* Obtain blood glucose measurements to follow the patient with hypoglycemia until the patient is asymptomatic.

Adverse Reactions

Severe adverse reactions are very rare, although nausea and vomiting may occur occasionally, especially with doses above 1 mg or with rapid injection (less than 1 minute). Adverse reactions indicating toxicity of glucagon have not been reported.

➤*Cardiovascular:* Hypotension has been reported up to 2 hours after administration in patients receiving glucagon as premedication for upper GI endoscopy procedures. Glucagon exerts positive inotropic and chronotropic effect and may, therefore, cause tachycardia and hypertension. A transient increase in both blood pressure and pulse rate may occur following the administration of glucagon. Patients taking beta-blockers might be expected to have a greater increase in both pulse and blood pressure, an increase that will be transient because of glucagon's short half-life. The increase in blood pressure and pulse rate may require therapy in patients with pheochromocytoma or coronary artery disease.

➤*Hypersensitivity:* Allergic reactions may occur in rare cases.

Overdosage

➤*Symptoms:* There have been no reports of overdosage with glucagon. It is expected, if overdosage did occur, that the patient may experience nausea, vomiting, diarrhea, inhibition of GI tract motility, or an increase in blood pressure and pulse rate. Patients taking beta-blockers might be expected to have a greater increase in both pulse and blood pressure, an increase that will be transient because of glucagon's short half-life. In case of suspected overdosing, the serum potassium may decrease; monitor and correct if needed.

When glucagon was given in large doses to patients with cardiac disease, investigators reported a positive inotropic effect. These investigators administered glucagon in doses of 0.5 to 16 mg/h by continuous infusion for periods of 5 to 166 hours. Total doses ranged from 25 to 996 mg, and an infant 21 months of age received approximately 8.25 mg in 165 hours. Adverse reactions included nausea, vomiting, and decreased serum potassium concentration. Serum potassium concentration could be maintained within normal limits with supplemental potassium.

Because glucagon is a polypeptide, it would be rapidly destroyed in the GI tract if it were to be accidentally ingested.

The IV and subcutaneous median lethal dose (LD_{50}) for glucagon in rats and mice ranges from 100 to greater than 200 mg/kg of body weight.

➤*Treatment:* Standard symptomatic treatment may be undertaken if overdosage occurs. In view of the extremely short half-life of glucagon and its prompt destruction and excretion, the treatment of overdosage is symptomatic, primarily for nausea, vomiting, and possible hypokalemia.An increase in blood pressure and pulse rate may require therapy in patients with pheochromocytoma or coronary artery disease. If the patient develops a dramatic increase in blood pressure, 5 to 10 mg of phentolamine mesylate has been shown to be effective in lowering blood pressure for the short time that control would be needed. Forced diuresis, peritoneal dialysis, hemodialysis, or charcoal hemoperfusion have not been established as beneficial for an overdose of glucagon, but such procedures are unlikely to provide any benefit given the short half-life and nature of the symptoms of overdose.

Patient Information

Refer patients and family members to the patient information leaflet for instructions describing the method of preparing and injecting glucagon. Advise the patient and family members to become familiar with the technique of preparing glucagon before an emergency arises. To prevent severe hypoglycemia, inform patients and family members of the symptoms of mild hypoglycemia and how to treat it appropriately. Inform family members to arouse the patient as quickly as possible because prolonged hypoglycemia may result in damage to the CNS. Advise patients to inform their health care provider when hypoglycemic reactions occur so that the treatment regimen may be adjusted if necessary.

GLUCAGON (rDNA ORIGIN) — INJECTION

Inform patients and family members of the following measures to prevent hypoglycemic reactions due to insulin:

1.) Reasonable uniformity from day to day with regard to diet, insulin, and exercise
2.) Careful adjustment of the insulin program so that the type (or types) of insulin, dose, and time (or times) of administration are suited to the individual patient
3.) Frequent testing of the blood or urine for glucose, so that a change in insulin requirements can be foreseen
4.) Routine carrying of sugar, candy, or other readily absorbable carbohydrate by the patient so that it may be taken at the first warning of an oncoming reaction

Glucagon or IV glucose should awaken the patient sufficiently so that oral carbohydrates may be taken.

Allergic reactions may occur rarely and include generalized rash, anaphylactic shock, breathing difficulties, and hypotension (low blood pressure).

A few people may be allergic to glucagon or to one of the inactive ingredients in glucagon, or may experience rapid heartbeat for a short while.

Keep the kit out of the reach of children.

Glucagon is only of benefit in hypoglycemia (low blood sugar) when the liver has sufficient glucose (in the form of glycogen) to release. For that reason, glucagon has little or no effect if you are fasting or if you are suffering from adrenal insufficiency, chronic hypoglycemia, or alcohol-induced hypoglycemia. Remember glucagon has the opposite effect of insulin. If the glucagon solution shows any sign of gel formation or particles, discard it.

The vial has a protective cap. You must remove the plastic cap to inject the water and reconstitute the freeze-dried glucagon. If the cap is loose or missing when you buy the package, return it to your local pharmacy.

Glucagon is a hormone that is always present in humans. Glucagon is intended for infrequent use during acute, severe hypoglycemic attacks, and may be used during pregnancy.

Breast-feeding following treatment with glucagon for your hypoglycemic attack should not put your baby at risk. Glucagon does not stay very long in the body. Also, because glucagon is a protein, even if your baby ingested glucagon, it would be unlikely to have any effect because it would be digested.

DIAZOXIDE

Rx	**Proglycem** (Ivax)	**Capsules:** 50 mg	(BNP 6000). Orange and clear. In 100s.
		Oral Suspension: 50 mg	7.25% alcohol, parabens, sorbitol. Chocolate-mint flavor. In 30 mL calibrated dropper.

DIAZOXIDE — ORAL

Indications

➤*Hypoglycemia:* Oral diazoxide is useful in the management of hypoglycemia due to hyperinsulinism associated with the following conditions:

➤*Adults:* Inoperable islet cell adenoma or carcinoma, or extrapancreatic malignancy.

➤*Infants and children:* Leucine sensitivity, islet cell hyperplasia, nesidioblastosis, extrapancreatic malignancy, islet cell adenoma, or adenomatosis. Diazoxide may be used preoperatively as a temporary measure, and postoperatively, if hypoglycemia persists.

➤*General information:* When other specific medical therapy or surgical management either has been unsuccessful or is not feasible, treatment with diazoxide should be considered.

Administration and Dosage

➤*General dosing considerations:* Patients should be under close clinical observation when treatment with diazoxide is initiated. (See Monitoring).

The dosage of diazoxide must be individualized based on the severity of the hypoglycemic condition, and the blood glucose level and clinical response of the patient.

➤*Adults:*

Hypoglycemia due to hyperinsulinism –

Usual dosage: 3 to 8 mg/kg, divided into 2 or 3 equal doses every 8 or 12 hours. In certain instances, patients with refractory hypoglycemia may require higher dosages.

Initial dosage: Ordinarily, an appropriate starting dosage is 3 mg/kg/day, divided into 3 equal doses every 8 hours. Thus, an average adult would receive a starting dosage of approximately 200 mg daily.

Dosage adjustment: The dosage should be adjusted until the desired clinical and laboratory effects are produced with the least amount of the drug.

➤*Children:* Special care should be taken to assure accuracy of dosage in infants and young children.

Hypoglycemia due to hyperinsulinism – See Adults for dosing for children 12 months of age and older.

11 months of age and younger (newborns/infants):

• *Usual dosage* – 8 to 15 mg/kg divided into 2 or 3 equal doses every 8 to 12 hours.

• *Initial dosage* – An appropriate starting dosage is 10 mg/kg/day, divided into 3 equal doses every 8 hours.

• *Dosage adjustment* – See Adults.

➤*Renal function impairment:* Because the plasma half-life of diazoxide is prolonged in patients with impaired renal function, a reduced dosage should be considered. Serum electrolyte levels should also be evaluated for such patients.

➤*Monitoring:* The clinical response and blood glucose level should be carefully monitored until the patient's condition has stabilized satisfactory; in most instances, this may be accomplished in several days.

➤*Discontinuation of therapy:* If administration of diazoxide is not effective after 2 or 3 weeks, the drug should be discontinued.

➤*Administration:* Shake oral suspension well before each use.

➤*Storage/Stability:* Store diazoxide capsules and suspension between 2° and 30°C (36° and 86°F). Protect from light. Store in carton until contents are used. Store in light resistant container.

Actions

➤*Pharmacology:* Diazoxide administered orally produces a prompt dose-related increase in blood glucose level, due primarily to an inhibition of insulin release from the pancreas, and also to an extrapancreatic effect.

The hyperglycemic effect begins within an hour and generally lasts no more than 8 hours in the presence of normal renal function.

Diazoxide decreases the excretion of sodium and water, resulting in fluid retention which may be clinically significant.

The hypotensive effect of diazoxide on blood pressure is usually not marked with the oral preparation. This contrasts with the intravenous preparation of diazoxide.

Other pharmacologic actions of diazoxide include increased pulse rate; increased serum uric acid levels due to decreased excretion; increased serum levels of free fatty acids' decreased chloride excretion; decreased para-aminohippuric acid; (PAH) clearance with no appreciable effect on glomerular filtration rate.

The concomitant administration of a benzothiazide diuretic may intensify the hyperglycemic and hyperuricemic effects of diazoxide. In the presence of hypokalemia, hyperglycemic effects are also potentiated.

Diazoxide-induced hyperglycemia is reversed by the administration of insulin or tolbutamide. The inhibition of insulin release by diazoxide is antagonized by alpha-adrenergic blocking agents.

Animal pharmacology or toxicology – Oral diazoxide in the mouse, rat, rabbit, dog, pig, and monkey produces a rapid and transient rise in blood glucose levels. In dogs, increased blood glucose is accompanied by increased free fatty acids, lactate, and pyruvate in the serum. In mice, a marked decrease in liver glycogen and an increase in the blood urea nitrogen level occur.

In acute toxicity studies the LD_{50} for oral diazoxide suspension is greater than 5000 mg/kg in the rat, greater than 522 mg/kg in the neonatal rat, between 1900 and 2572 mg/kg in the mouse, and 219 mg/kg in the guinea pig. Although the oral LD_{50} was not determined in the dog, a dosage of up to 500 mg/kg was well tolerated.

In subacute oral toxicity studies, diazoxide at 400 mg/kg in the rat produced growth retardation, edema, increases in liver and kidney weights, and adrenal hypertrophy. Daily dosages up to 1080 mg/kg for 3 months produced hyperglycemia, an increase in liver weight and an increase in mortality. In dogs given oral diazoxide at approximately 40 mg/kg/day for 1 month, no biologically significant gross or microscopic abnormalities were observed. Cataracts, attributed to markedly disturbed carbohydrate metabolism, have been observed in a few dogs given repeated daily doses of oral or intravenous diazoxide. The lenticular changes resembled those which occur experimentally in animals with increased blood glucose levels. In chronic toxicity studies, rats given a daily dose of 200 mg/kg diazoxide for 52 weeks had a decrease in weight gain and an increase in heart, liver, adrenal and thyroid weights. Mortality in drug-treated and control groups was not different. Dogs treated with diazoxide at dosages of 50, 100, and 200 mg/kg/day for 82 weeks had higher blood glucose levels than controls. Mild bone marrow stimulation and increased pancreas weights were evident in the drug-treated dogs, several developed inguinal hernias, 1 had a testicular seminoma, and another had a mass near the penis. Two females had inguinal mammary swellings. The etiology of these changes was not established. There was no difference in mortality between drug-treated and control groups. In a second chronic oral toxicity study, dogs given milled diazoxide at 50, 100, and 200 mg/kg/day had anorexia and severe weight loss, causing death in a few. Hematologic, biochemical and histologic examination did not indicate any cause of death other than inanition. After 1 year of treatment, there is no evidence of herniation or tissue swelling in any of the dogs.

When diazoxide was administered at high dosages concomitantly with either chlorothiazide to rats or trichlormethiazide to dogs, increased toxicity was observed in rats, the combination was nephrotoxic; epithelial hyperplasia was observed in the collecting tubules. In dogs, a diabetic syndrome was produced which resulted in ketosis and death. Neither of the drugs given alone produced these effects.

Although the data are inconclusive, reproduction and teratology studies in several species of animals indicate that diazoxide, when administered dur-

DIAZOXIDE — ORAL

ing the critical period of embryo formation, may interfere with normal fetal development, possibly through altered glucose metabolism. Parturition was occasionally prolonged in animals treated at term. Intravenous administration of diazoxide to pregnant sheep, goats, and swine produced in the fetus an appreciable increase in blood glucose level and degeneration of the beta cells of the Islets of Langerhans. The reversibility of these effects was not studied.

➤*Pharmacokinetics:* Diazoxide is extensively bound (more than 90%) to serum proteins, and is excreted in the kidneys. The plasma half-life following IV administration is 28 ± 8.3 hours. Limited data on oral administration revealed a half-life of 24 and 36 hours in 2 adults. In 4 children aged 4 months to 6 years, the plasma half-life varied from 9.5 to 24 hours on long-term oral administration. The half-life may be prolonged following overdosage, and in patients with impaired renal function.

Contraindications

The use of diazoxide for functional hypoglycemia is contraindicated. The drug should not be used in patients hypersensitive to diazoxide or to other thiazides unless the potential benefits outweigh the possible risks.

Warnings/Precautions

➤*Fluid retention:* The antidiuretic property of diazoxide may lead to significant fluid retention, which in patients with compromised cardiac reserve, may precipitate congestive heart failure. The fluid retention will respond to conventional therapy with diuretics.

➤*Thiazides:* It should be noted that concomitantly administered thiazides may potentiate the hyperglycemic and hyperuricemic actions of diazoxide.

➤*Ketoacidosis/nonketotic hyperosmolar coma:* Ketoacidosis and nonketotic hyperosmolar coma have been reported in patients treated with recommended doses of diazoxide usually during intercurrent illness. Prompt recognition and treatment are essential, and prolonged surveillance following the acute episode is necessary because of the long drug half-life of approximately 30 hours. The occurrence of these serious events may be reduced by careful education of patients regarding the need for monitoring the urine for sugar and ketones and for prompt reporting of abnormal findings and unusual symptoms to the physician.

➤*Cataracts:* Transient cataracts occurred in association with hyperosmolar coma in an infant, and subsided on correction of the hyperosmolarity. Cataracts have been observed in several animals receiving daily doses of intravenous or oral diazoxide.

➤*Renal function impairment:* Since the plasma half-life of diazoxide is prolonged in patients with impaired renal function, a reduced dosage should be considered. Serum electrolyte levels should also be evaluated for such patients.

➤*Special risk:* The effects of diazoxide on the hematopoietic system and the level of serum uric acid should be kept in mind; the latter should be considered particularly in patients with hyperuricemia or a history of gout.

In some patients, higher blood levels have been observed with the oral suspension than with the capsule formulation of diazoxide. Dosage should be adjusted as necessary in individual patients if changed from one formulation to the other.

The antihypertensive effect of other drugs may be enhanced by diazoxide, and this should be kept in mind when administering it concomitantly with antihypertensive agents.

Because of the protein binding, administration of diazoxide with coumarin or its derivatives may require reduction in the dosage of the anticoagulant, although there has been no reported evidence of excessive anticoagulant effect. In addition, diazoxide may possibly displace bilirubin from albumin; this should be kept in mind particularly when treating newborns with increased bilirubinemia.

➤*Pregnancy: Category C.* Reproduction studies using the oral preparation in rats have revealed increased fetal resorptions and delayed parturition, as well as fetal skeletal anomalies; evidence of skeletal and cardiac teratogenic effects in rabbits has been noted with intravenous administration. The drug has also been demonstrated to cross the placental barrier in animals and to cause degeneration of the fetal pancreatic beta cells. Since there are no adequate data on fetal effects of this drug when given to pregnant women, safety in pregnancy has not been established. When the use of diazoxide is considered, the indications should be limited to those approved for adults, and the potential benefits to the mother must be weighed against possible harmful effects to the fetus.

Nonteratogenic – Diazoxide crosses the placental barrier and appears in cord blood. When given to the mother prior to delivery of the infant, the drug may produce fetal or neonatal hyperbilirubinemia, thrombocytopenia, altered carbohydrate metabolism, and possibly other side effects that have occurred in adults.

Alopecia and hypertrichosis lanuginosa have occurred in infants whose mothers received oral diazoxide during the last 19 to 60 days of pregnancy.

Labor and delivery – Since intravenous administration of the drug during labor may cause cessation of uterine contractions, and administration of oxytocic agents may be required to reinstate labor, caution is advised in administering diazoxide at that time.

➤*Lactation:* Information is not available concerning the passage of diazoxide in breast milk. Because many drugs are excreted in human milk and because of the potential for adverse reactions from diazoxide in nursing infants, a decision should be made whether to discontinue nursing or to discontinue the drug, taking into account the importance of the drug to the mother.

➤*Children:* The development of abnormal facial features in 4 children treated chronically (greater than 4 years of age) with diazoxide for hypoglycemia hyperinsulinism in the same clinic has been reported.

Infants and children – Oral diazoxide is useful in the management of hypoglycemia due to hyperinsulinism associated with the following conditions: Leucine sensitivity, islet cell hyperplasia, nesidioblastosis, extrapancreatic malignancy, islet cell adenoma, or adenomatosis. Diazoxide may be used preoperatively as a temporary measure, and postoperatively, if hypoglycemia persists.

➤*Monitoring:* Treatment with diazoxide should be initiated under close clinical supervision, with careful monitoring of blood glucose and clinical response until the patient's condition has stabilized. This usually requires several days. If not effective in 2 to 3 weeks, the drug should be discontinued.

Prolonged treatment requires regular monitoring of the urine for sugar and ketones, especially under stress conditions, with prompt reporting of any abnormalities to the physician. Additionally, blood sugar levels should be monitored periodically by the physician to determine the need for dose adjustment.

Laboratory tests – The following procedures may be especially important in patient monitoring (not necessarily inclusive); blood glucose determinations (recommended at periodic intervals in patients taking diazoxide orally for treatment of hypoglycemia, until stabilized); blood urea nitrogen (BUN) determinations and creatinine clearance determinations; hematocrit determinations; platelet count determinations; total and differential leukocyte counts; serum aspartate aminotransferase (AST) level determinations; serum uric acid level determinations; and urine testing for glucose and ketones (in patients being treated with diazoxide for hypoglycemia, semi-quantitative estimation of sugar and ketones in serum performed by the patient and reported to the physician provides frequent and relatively inexpensive monitoring of the condition).

Drug Interactions

Since diazoxide is highly bound to serum proteins, it may displace other substances which are also bound to protein, such as bilirubin or coumarin and its derivatives, resulting in higher blood levels of these substances. Concomitant administration of oral diazoxide and diphenylhydantoin may result in a loss of seizure control. These potential interactions must be considered when administering diazoxide capsules or suspension.

The concomitant administration of thiazides or other commonly used diuretics may potentiate the hyperglycemic and hyperuricemic effects of diazoxide.

➤*Drug/Lab test interactions:* The hyperglycemic and hyperuricemic effects of diazoxide preclude proper assessment of these metabolic states. Increased renin secretion, IgG concentrations and decreased cortisol secretions have also been noted. Diazoxide inhibits glucagon-stimulated insulin release and causes a false-negative insulin response to glucagon.

Adverse Reactions

➤*Frequent and serious adverse reactions:* Sodium and fluid retention is most common in young infants and in adults and may precipitate congestive heart failure in patients with compromised cardiac reserve. It usually responds to diuretic therapy.

➤*Infrequent but serious adverse reactions:* Diabetic ketoacidosis and hyperosmolar nonketotic coma may develop very rapidly. Conventional therapy with insulin and restoration of fluid and electrolyte balance is usually effective if instituted promptly. Prolonged surveillance is essential in view of the long half-life of diazoxide.

➤*Other frequent adverse reactions:* Hirsutism of the lanugo type, mainly on the forehead, back and limbs, occurs most commonly in children and women and may be cosmetically unacceptable. It subsides on discontinuation of the drug.

Hyperglycemia or glycosuria may require reduction in dosage in order to avoid progression to ketoacidosis or hyperosmolar coma.

Gastrointestinal intolerance may include anorexia, nausea, vomiting, abdominal pain, ileus, diarrhea, and transient loss of taste. Tachycardia, palpitations, and increased levels of serum uric acid are common.

Thrombocytopenia with or without purpura may require discontinuation of the drug. Neutropenia is transient, is not associated with increased susceptibility to infection, and ordinarily does not require discontinuation of the drug. Skin rash, headache, weakness, and malaise may also occur.

➤*Other observed adverse reactions:*

Cardiovascular – Hypotension occurs occasionally, which may be augmented by thiazide diuretics given concurrently. A few cases of transient hypertension, for which no explanation is apparent, have been noted. Chest pain has been reported rarely.

CNS – Anxiety, dizziness, insomnia, polyneuritis, paresthesia, pruritus, extrapyramidal signs.

Hematologic – Eosinophilia, decreased hemoglobin/hematocrit, excessive bleeding, decreased IgG.

Hepatic – Increased AST, alkaline phosphatase.

Musculoskeletal – Monilial dermatitis, herpes, advance in bone age, loss of scalp hair.

Ophthalmic – Transient cataracts, subconjunctival hemorrhage, ring scotoma, blurred vision, diplopia, lacrimation.

DIAZOXIDE — ORAL

Renal – Azotemia, decreased creatinine clearance, reversible nephrotic syndrome, decreased urinary output, hematuria, albuminuria.

Miscellaneous – Fever, lymphadenopathy, gout acute pancreatitis/pancreatic necrosis, galactorrhea, enlargement of lump in breast.

Overdosage

➤*Treatment:* An overdosage of diazoxide causes marked hyperglycemia which may be associated with ketoacidosis. It will respond to prompt insulin administration and restoration of fluid and electrolyte balance. Because of the drug's long half-life (approximately 30 hours), the symptoms of overdosage require prolonged surveillance for periods up to 7 days until the blood sugar level stabilizes within the normal range. One investigator reported successful lowering of diazoxide blood levels by peritoneal dialysis in 1 patient and by hemodialysis in another.

Patient Information

During treatment with diazoxide, the patient should be advised to consult regularly with the physician and to cooperate in the periodic monitoring of his or her condition by laboratory tests.

➤*The patient should be advised:*

- To take the drug on a regular schedule as prescribed, not to skip doses, and not to take extra doses.
- Not to use this drug with other medications unless this is done with the physician's advice.
- Not to allow anyone else to take this medication.
- To follow dietary instructions.
- To report promptly any adverse effects (ie, increased urinary frequency, increased thirst, fruity breath odor).
- To report pregnancy or to discuss plans for pregnancy.

GLUCOSE

otc	**Glutose** (Paddock)	**Gel:** Liquid glucose (40% dextrose)	Dye free. In 80 g bottle and 25 g tube.
otc	**Insta-Glucose** (ICN)		Cherry flavor. In UD 30.8 g tubes.
otc	**Insulin Reaction** (Sherwood)		Lime flavor. In UD 25 g tubes.
otc	**Dex4 Glucose** (Can-Am Care)	**Tablets:** Glucose	Lemon, orange, raspberry and grape flavors. In 10s and 50s.
otc	**BD Glucose** (Becton Dickinson)	**Tablets, chewable:** 5 g	In 36s.

GLUCOSE — ORAL

Refer to parenteral dextrose (d-glucose) in Nutrients and Nutritional Agents which is also used in the treatment of acute hypoglycemia.

Indications

➤*Hypoglycemia:* Management of hypoglycemia.

Administration and Dosage

➤*General dosing considerations:* Glucose is not absorbed from the buccal cavity; it must be swallowed to be effective. While swallowing reflexes may be preserved in the unconscious patient, the lack of normal gag reflexes may lead to aspiration. When possible, use other methods of treating hypoglycemia in unconscious patients.

➤*Adults:*

Management of hypoglycemia – Administer 10 to 20 g orally; repeat in 10 minutes if necessary. Response should occur in 10 minutes.

➤*Children:*

Management of hypoglycemia –

2 years of age and older: See Adults for dosing.

Younger than 2 years of age: Do not give to children younger than 2 years of age, unless directed by a health care provider.

Actions

➤*Pharmacology:* Glucose, a monosaccharide, is absorbed from the intestine after administration and then used, distributed and stored by the tissues. Direct absorption takes place, resulting in a rapid increased blood glucose concentration. Therefore, it is effective in small doses; no evidence of toxicity has been reported. Glucose provides 4 cal/g.

Warnings/Precautions

➤*Pregnancy: Category: Undetermined.* Consult a health care provider before using in pregnant women.

➤*Lactation:* Consult a health care provider before using in breast-feeding women.

Adverse Reactions

Isolated reports of nausea, which also may occur with hypoglycemia.

ADRENOCORTICAL STEROIDS

Corticotropin (ACTH)

Indications

➤*ACTH and cosyntropin:* For diagnostic testing of adrenocortical function and in the screening of patients presumed to have adrenocortical insufficiency. Cosyntropin is less allergenic than the exogenous ACTH preparations.

➤*ACTH:* Corticotropin has limited therapeutic value in conditions responsive to corticosteroid therapy; in such cases, corticosteroid therapy is the treatment of choice. Repository corticotropin may be used in the following disorders:

Allergic states – Control of severe or incapacitating allergic conditions intractable to adequate trials of conventional treatment: Seasonal or perennial allergic rhinitis; bronchial asthma; contact dermatitis; atopic dermatitis; serum sickness.

Collagen diseases – During an exacerbation or as maintenance therapy in selected cases of systemic lupus erythematosus; systemic dermatomyositis (polymyositis); acute rheumatic carditis.

Dermatologic diseases – Pemphigus; bullous dermatitis herpetiformis; severe erythema multiforme (Stevens-Johnson syndrome); exfoliative dermatitis; severe psoriasis; severe seborrheic dermatitis; mycosis fungoides.

Edematous state – To induce a diuresis or a remission of proteinuria in the nephrotic syndrome without uremia of the idiopathic type or that due to lupus erythematosus.

Endocrine disorders – Nonsuppurative thyroiditis; hypercalcemia associated with cancer.

GI diseases – To tide the patient over a critical period of the disease in ulcerative colitis and regional enteritis.

Hematologic disorders – Acquired (autoimmune) hemolytic anemia; secondary thrombocytopenia in adults; erythroblastopenia (RBC anemia); congenital (erythroid) hypoplastic anemia.

Neoplastic disease – For palliative management of leukemias and lymphomas in adults and acute leukemia of childhood.

Nervous system diseases – Acute exacerbations of multiple sclerosis.

Ophthalmic diseases – Severe acute and chronic allergic and inflammatory processes involving the eye and its adnexa such as the following: Allergic conjunctivitis; keratitis; herpes zoster ophthalmicus; iritis and iridocyclitis; diffuse posterior uveitis and choroiditis; optic neuritis; sympathetic ophthalmia; chorioretinitis; anterior segment inflammation; allergic corneal marginal ulcers.

Rheumatic disorders – As adjunctive therapy for short-term administration (to tide the patient over an acute episode or exacerbation) in the following: Psoriatic arthritis; rheumatoid arthritis, including juvenile rheumatoid arthritis (selected cases may require low-dose maintenance therapy); ankylosing spondylitis; acute and subacute bursitis; acute nonspecific tenosynovitis; acute gouty arthritis; post-traumatic arthritis; synovitis of osteoarthritis; epicondylitis.

Respiratory diseases – Symptomatic sarcoidosis; Loeffler syndrome not manageable by other means; berylliosis; fulminating or disseminated pulmonary tuberculosis when used concurrently with antituberculous chemotherapy; aspiration pneumonitis.

Miscellaneous – Tuberculous meningitis with subarachnoid block or impending block when accompanied by antituberculous chemotherapy; trichinosis with neurologic or myocardial involvement.

➤*Off-label uses:* Treatment of infantile spasms.

Actions

➤*Pharmacology:* ACTH stimulates the adrenal cortex to secrete cortisol, corticosterone, aldosterone, and a number of weakly androgenic substances. Although ACTH does stimulate secretion of aldosterone, the rate is relatively independent. Prolonged administration of large doses of ACTH induces hyperplasia and hypertrophy of the adrenal cortex and continuous high output of cortisol, corticosterone, and weak androgens. The release of ACTH is under the influence of the nervous system via the corticotropin regulatory hormone released from the hypothalamus and by a negative corticosteroid feedback mechanism. Elevated plasma cortisol suppresses ACTH release.

Cosyntropin is a synthetic peptide corresponding to the amino acid residues 1 to 24 of human ACTH, which exhibits the full corticosteroidogenic activity of natural ACTH. A dose of 0.25 mg cosyntropin is pharmacologically equivalent to 25 units of natural ACTH. Cosyntropin is less allergenic than natural ACTH.

➤*Pharmacokinetics:* ACTH rapidly disappears from the circulation following its IV administration; in humans, the plasma half-life is about 15 minutes. The maximal effects of a trophic hormone on a target organ are achieved when optimal amounts of hormone are acting continuously. Thus, a fixed dose of ACTH will demonstrate a linear increase in adrenocortical secretion with increasing duration for the infusion.

Contraindications

➤*Repository corticotropin:* Scleroderma; osteoporosis; systemic fungal infections; ocular herpes simplex; recent surgery; history of or presence of peptic ulcer; congestive heart failure (CHF); hypertension; sensitivity to porcine proteins; IV administration. Treatment of conditions accompanied by primary adrenocortical insufficiency or adrenocortical hyperfunction.

➤*Cosyntropin:* Previous adverse reaction to drug.

Warnings/Precautions

➤*Do not administer:* Do not administer until adrenal responsiveness has been verified with the route of administration (IM or subcutaneous) that will be used during treatment. A rise in urinary and plasma corticosteroid values provides direct evidence of a stimulatory effect.

➤*Chronic administration:* Chronic administration may lead to irreversible adverse effects. ACTH may suppress signs and symptoms of chronic disease without altering the natural course of the disease. Since complications with corticotropin use are dependent on the dose and duration of treatment, a risk to benefit decision must be made in each case.

➤*Ocular effects:* Prolonged use increases the risk of hypersensitivity reactions and may produce posterior subcapsular cataracts and glaucoma with possible damage to the optic nerve.

➤*Stress:* Although the action of ACTH is similar to that of exogenous adrenocortical steroids, the quantity of adrenocorticoid secreted may be variable. In patients who receive prolonged corticotropin therapy, use additional rapidly acting corticosteroids before, during, and after an unusually stressful situation.

➤*Infection:* ACTH may mask signs of infection including fungal or viral eye infections that may appear during its use. There may be decreased resistance and inability to localize infection. When infection is present, administer appropriate anti-infective therapy.

Tuberculosis – Observe patients with latent tuberculosis. During prolonged ACTH therapy, administer chemoprophylaxis.

➤*Immunosuppression:* Perform immunization procedures with caution, especially when high doses are administered, because of the possible hazards of neurological complications and lack of antibody response. While on corticotropin therapy, patients should not be vaccinated against smallpox.

➤*Blood pressure and electrolytes:* Corticotropin can elevate blood pressure, cause salt and water retention, and increase potassium and calcium excretion. Dietary salt restriction and potassium supplementation may be necessary.

➤*Hypersensitivity:* Cosyntropin exhibits slight immunologic activity, does not contain animal protein, and is less risky to use than natural ACTH. Patients known to be sensitized to natural ACTH with markedly positive skin tests will, with few exceptions, react negatively when tested intradermally with *Cortrosyn*. Most patients with a history of a previous hypersensitivity reaction to natural ACTH or a pre-existing allergic disease will tolerate cosyntropin; however, hypersensitivity reactions are possible. Refer to Management of Acute Hypersensitivity Reactions.

➤*Concomitant therapy:* Because maximal corticotropin stimulation of the adrenals may be limited during the first few days of treatment, administer other drugs when an immediate therapeutic effect is desirable.

Administer for treatment only when disease is intractable to nonsteroid treatment.

➤*Use the lowest possible dose:* Use the lowest possible dose to control the condition, and when reduction in dosage is possible, it should be gradual.

➤*Adrenocortical insufficiency:* Suppression of the pituitary adrenal axis occurs following prolonged therapy, which may be slow in returning to normal. Protect patients from the stress of trauma or surgery by the use of corticosteroids during the period of stress.

➤*Hypothyroidism and cirrhosis:* An enhanced effect of corticotropin may occur.

➤*Multiple sclerosis:* Although ACTH may speed the resolution of acute exacerbations of multiple sclerosis, it does not affect the ultimate outcome or natural course of the disease. Relatively high doses of ACTH are necessary to demonstrate a significant effect.

➤*Acute gouty arthritis:* Limit treatment of acute gouty arthritis to a few days. Since rebound attacks may occur when corticotropin is discontinued, administer conventional concomitant therapy during corticotropin treatment and for several days after it is stopped.

➤*Mental disturbances:* Psychic symptoms may appear, or pre-existing symptoms may be enhanced. These may range from mood alteration to a psychotic state.

➤*Secondary disease:* Patients with a secondary disease may have that disease worsened. Use with caution in patients with diabetes, diverticulitis, renal insufficiency, and myasthenia gravis.

➤*Pregnancy: Category C.* ACTH has embryocidal effects. Use in pregnancy only when clearly needed and when potential benefits outweigh potential hazards to the fetus.

➤*Lactation:* It is not known whether this drug is excreted in breast milk. Because of the potential for serious adverse reactions in breast-feeding infants from ACTH, decide whether to discontinue breast-feeding or to discontinue the drug.

➤*Children:* Prolonged use of corticotropin in children will inhibit skeletal growth. If use is necessary, give intermittently and carefully observe the child.

Drug Interactions

Corticotropin (ACTH) Drug Interactions

Precipitant drug	Object drug[a]		Description
Corticotropin, Cosyntropin	Anticholinesterases	⬇	Corticosteroids antagonize the effects of anticholinesterases in myasthenia gravis.
Corticotropin, Cosyntropin	Aspirin	⬇	Corticosteroids will reduce serum salicylate levels and may decrease their effectiveness. Use aspirin cautiously in conjunction with corticotropin in hypoprothrombinemia.
Corticotropin, Cosyntropin	Diuretics	⬆	Corticotropin may accentuate the electrolyte loss associated with diuretic therapy.
Barbiturates	Corticotropin, Cosyntropin	⬇	Decreased pharmacologic effects of the corticosteroid may be observed. Avoid this combination if possible. Monitor closely. Increases in the corticosteroid dosage may be required.
Hydantoins (eg, phenytoin)	Corticotropin, Cosyntropin	⬇	Decreased corticosteroid effects may occur. Phenytoin levels may be reduced. Monitor phenytoin levels and adjust dose of either agent if needed.
Corticotropin, Cosyntropin	Hydantoins (eg, phenytoin)		

[a] ⬆ = Object drug increased. ⬇ = Object drug decreased.

Adverse Reactions

➤*Cardiovascular:* Hypertension; CHF; necrotizing angiitis; bradycardia; tachycardia.

➤*CNS:* Convulsions; vertigo; headache; increased intracranial pressure with papilledema (pseudotumor cerebri), usually after treatment.

➤*Dermatologic:* Impaired wound healing; petechiae and ecchymoses; increased sweating; hyperpigmentation; thin fragile skin; facial erythema; acne; suppression of skin test reactions; rash.

➤*Endocrine:* Menstrual irregularities; suppression of growth in children; hirsutism; development of Cushingoid state; manifestations of latent diabetes mellitus; decreased carbohydrate tolerance; increased requirements for insulin or oral hypoglycemic agents in diabetics; secondary adrenocortical and pituitary unresponsiveness, especially during stress.

➤*GI:* Pancreatitis; ulcerative esophagitis; abdominal distention; peptic ulcer with possible perforation and hemorrhage.

➤*Hypersensitivity:* Allergic reactions may manifest as dizziness, nausea, vomiting, shock, and skin reactions. A rare hypersensitivity reaction usually associated with pre-existing allergic disease and/or a previous reaction to natural ACTH is possible. Symptoms may include slight whealing with splotchy erythema at the injection site. There have been rare reports of anaphylactic reaction.

➤*Metabolic:* Negative nitrogen balance caused by protein catabolism; sodium and fluid retention; potassium and calcium loss; hypokalemic alkalosis; peripheral edema.

➤*Musculoskeletal:* Muscle weakness; steroid myopathy; loss of muscle mass; osteoporosis; vertebral compression fractures; pathologic fracture of long bones; aseptic necrosis of femoral and humeral heads.

➤*Ophthalmic:* Posterior subcapsular cataracts; increased intraocular pressure; glaucoma with possible damage to optic nerve; exophthalmos.

➤*Miscellaneous:* Abscess; prolonged use of ACTH may result in antibody production and subsequent loss of the stimulatory effect.

Overdosage

An acute overdose would present no different adverse reactions.

Patient Information

ACTH may mask signs of infection. There may be decreased resistance and inability to localize infection.

Diabetics may have increased requirements for insulin or oral hypoglycemics.

Notify physician if marked fluid retention, muscle weakness, abdominal pain, seizures, or headache occurs.

REPOSITORY CORTICOTROPIN

Rx	**H.P. Acthar Gel** (Questcor)	**Repository injection:** 80 units/mL	In 5 mL multidose vials.[a]

[a] With 16% gelatin.

REPOSITORY CORTICOTROPIN — INJECTION

For complete and comparative prescribing information, refer to the Corticotropin group monograph.

Indications

➤*Diagnostic agent:* For diagnostic testing of adrenocortical function.

➤*Conditions responsive to corticosteroids:* Repository corticotropin injection has limited therapeutic value in those conditions responsive to corticosteroid therapy; in such cases, corticosteroid therapy is considered to be the treatment of choice. Repository corticotropin injection may be employed in the following disorders:

➤*Endocrine disorders:* Nonsuppurative thyroiditis; hypercalcemia associated with cancer.

➤*Nervous system diseases:* Acute exacerbations of multiple sclerosis.

➤*Rheumatic disorders:* As adjunctive therapy for short-term administration (to tide the patient over an acute episode or exacerbation) in the following: Psoriatic arthritis; rheumatoid arthritis, including juvenile rheumatoid arthritis (selected cases may require low-dose maintenance therapy); ankylosing spondylitis; acute and subacute bursitis; acute nonspecific tenosynovitis; acute gouty arthritis; posttraumatic arthritis; synovitis of osteoarthritis; epicondylitis.

➤*Collagen diseases:* During an exacerbation or as maintenance therapy in selected cases of the following: Systemic lupus erythematosus; systemic dermatomyositis (polymyositis); acute rheumatic carditis.

➤*Dermatologic diseases:* Pemphigus; bullous dermatitis herpetiformis; severe erythema multiforme (Stevens-Johnson syndrome); exfoliative dermatitis; severe psoriasis; severe seborrheic dermatitis; mycosis fungoides.

➤*Allergic states:* Control of severe or incapacitating allergic conditions intractable to adequate trials of conventional treatment, such as the following: Seasonal or perennial allergic rhinitis; bronchial asthma; contact dermatitis; atopic dermatitis; serum sickness.

➤*Ophthalmic diseases:* Severe acute and chronic allergic and inflammatory processes involving the eye and its adnexa, such as the following: Allergic conjunctivitis; keratitis; herpes zoster ophthalmicus; iritis and iridocyclitis; diffuse posterior uveitis and choroiditis; optic neuritis; sympathetic ophthalmia; chorioretinitis; anterior segment inflammation; allergic corneal marginal ulcers.

➤*Respiratory diseases:* Symptomatic sarcoidosis; Loeffler syndrome not manageable by other means; berylliosis; fulminating or disseminated pulmonary tuberculosis when used concurrently with antituberculous chemotherapy; aspiration pneumonitis.

➤*Hematologic disorders:* Acquired (autoimmune) hemolytic anemia; secondary thrombocytopenia in adults; erythro-blastopenia (RBC anemia); congenital (erythroid) hypoplastic anemia.

➤*Neoplastic diseases:* For palliative management of leukemias and lymphomas in adults or acute leukemia of childhood.

➤*Edematous state:* To induce a diuresis or a remission of proteinuria in the nephrotic syndrome without uremia of the idiopathic type or that due to lupus erythematosus.

➤*GI diseases:* To tide the patient over a critical period of the disease in ulcerative colitis or regional enteritis.

➤*Miscellaneous:* Tuberculous meningitis with subarachnoid block or impending block when used concurrently with appropriate antituberculous chemotherapy; trichinosis with neurologic or myocardial involvement.

➤*Off-label uses:* Treatment of infantile spasms.

Administration and Dosage

➤*General dosing considerations:* Repository corticotropin should not be administered for treatment until adrenal responsiveness has been verified with the route of administration that will be utilized during treatment, IM or subcutaneous (see Test Dose).

Frequency and dose of the drug should be determined by considering severity of the disease, plasma and urine corticosteroid levels, and the initial response of the patient. Only gradual change in dosage schedules should be attempted after full drug effects have become apparent. Use the lowest dose for the shortest period of time to accomplish the therapeutic goal.

➤*Adults:*

All approved uses except multiple sclerosis –

Usual dosage: 40 to 80 units given IM or subcutaneously every 24 to 72 hours. The chronic administration of more than 40 units daily may be associated with uncontrollable adverse reactions.

Dosage adjustment: When reduction in dosage is indicated, this should be done gradually by either reducing the amount of each injection, administering injections at longer intervals, or by a combination of both of the above. During reduction of dosage, careful consideration should be given to the disease being treated, the general medical conditions of the patient, and the duration over which corticotropin was administered.

Multiple sclerosis – 80 to 120 units IM daily for 2 to 3 weeks.

➤*Children:* Prolonged use in children will inhibit skeletal growth. If use is necessary, repository corticotropin should be given intermittently and the child observed carefully.

➤*Test dose:* Standard tests for verification of adrenal responsiveness to corticotropin may utilize as much as 80 units as a single injection or 1 or more injections of a lesser dosage. Verification tests should be performed prior to treatment with corticotropins. The test should utilize the route(s) of administration proposed for treatment.

➤*Preparation for administration:* Warm to room temperature before using. Do not overpressurize the vial prior to withdrawing the product.

➤*Administration:* For IM or subcutaneous use depending on indication. IV administration is contraindicated.

➤*Storage/Stability:* Store between 2° and 8°C (36° and 46°F).

COSYNTROPIN

Rx	**Cosyntropin** (Sandoz)	**Injection, solution:** 0.25 mg/mL	Preservative free. In 1 mL single-dose vials.[b]
Rx	**Cortrosyn** (Amphastar)	**Powder for Injection, lyophilized:** 0.25 mg	In single-dose vials[a] with diluent.

[a] With 10 mg mannitol.

[b] With 10 mg mannitol, 6.4 mg sodium chloride.

COSYNTROPIN — INJECTION

For complete and comparative prescribing information, refer to the Corticotropin group monograph.

Indications

➤*Diagnostic agent:* For use as a diagnostic agent in the screening of patients presumed to have adrenocortical insufficiency. Because of its rapid effect on the adrenal cortex it may be utilized to perform a 30-minute test of adrenal function (plasma cortisol response) as an office or outpatient procedure, using only 2 venipunctures.

Administration and Dosage

➤*Adults:*

Diagnostic agent for adrenocortical insufficiency –

Usual dosage:

- *Cortrosyn* – 0.25 to 0.75 mg intramuscularly (IM) or intravenously (IV).
- *Cosyntropin (by Sandoz)* – 0.25 to 0.75 mg IV.

Alternative dosage: 0.25 mg as an IV infusion at 40 mcg/h over 6 h to provide a greater stimulus to the adrenal glands.

➤*Children:*

Diagnostic agent for adrenocortical insufficiency –

Older than 2 years of age: See Adults for dosing for children older than 2 years of age.

2 years of age and younger:

- *Cortrosyn* – 0.125 mg IM or IV.
- *Cosyntropin (by Sandoz)* – 0.125 mg IV.

➤*Measurement of adrenal response:* Adrenal response may be measured in the usual manner by determining urinary steroid excretion before and after treatment or by measuring plasma cortisol levels before and at the end of the infusion. The latter is preferable because the urinary steroid excretion does not always accurately reflect the adrenal or plasma cortisol response to ACTH.

Another method for a rapid screening test of adrenal function has also been suggested. A control blood sample of 6 to 7 mL is collected in a heparinized tube. A second blood sample is collected exactly 30 minutes after administration. Both blood samples should be refrigerated until sent to the laboratory for determination of the plasma cortisol response by some appropriate method. If it is not possible to send them to the laboratory or perform the fluorimetric procedure within 12 hours, then the plasma should be separated and refrigerated or frozen according to need.

The test may be performed at any time during the day, but because of the physiological diurnal variation of plasma cortisol, the criteria listed by Wood cannot apply. It has been shown that basal plasma cortisol levels and the post cosyntropin increment exhibit diurnal changes. However, the 30-minute plasma cortisol level remains unchanged throughout the day so that only this single criterion should be used.

Plasma cortisol levels usually peak about 45 to 60 minutes after an injection of cosyntropin and some prefer the 60-minute interval for testing for this reason. While it is true that the 60-minute values are usually higher than the 30-minute values, the difference may not be significant enough in most cases to outweigh the disadvantage of a longer testing period. If the 60-minute test period is used, the criterion for a normal response is an approximate doubling of the basal plasma cortisol value.

Corticotropin (ACTH)

COSYNTROPIN — INJECTION

➤*Interpretation of cortisol levels:* The usual normal response in most cases is an approximate doubling of the basal level, provided that the basal level does not exceed the normal range. Many patients with normal adrenal function, however, do not respond to the expected degree so that the following criteria have been established to denote a normal response:

1.) The control plasma cortisol level should exceed 5 mcg/100 mL.
2.) The 30-minute level should show an increment of at least 7 mcg/100 mL above the basal level.
3.) The 30-minute level should exceed 18 mcg/100 mL. Comparable figures have been reported by others. These criteria also apply when the drug is injected IV in 2 to 5 mL of saline over a 2-minute period.

In patients with a raised plasma bilirubin or in patients in whom the plasma contains free hemoglobin, falsely high fluorescence measurements will result.

➤*Concomitant therapy:* Patients taking inadvertent doses of cortisone or hydrocortisone on the test day and patients taking spironolactone or women taking drugs that contain estrogen may exhibit abnormally high basal plasma cortisol levels. A paradoxical response may be noted in the former group, as seen in a decrease in plasma cortisol values following a stimulating dose of cosyntropin. In the latter group, only a normal incremental response is to be expected. Patients receiving cortisone, hydrocortisone, or spironolactone should omit their pretest doses on the day selected for testing.

➤*Preparation for administration:*

IM – Reconstitute 0.25 mg of *Cortrosyn* in solvent (ampul of 1 mL of 0.9% sodium chloride injection) and inject IM.

IV – For IV administration, reconstitute cosyntropin with 2 to 5 mL of 0.9% sodium chloride injection. For administration as an IV infusion, cosyntropin 0.25 mg may be added to glucose or saline solutions.

➤*Administration:* Cosyntropin can be injected IV over a 2-minute period. When given as an IV infusion, give at a rate of approximately 40 mcg per hour over a 6-hour period.

Cosyntropin (by Sandoz) – Do not administer IM; may be administered as a direct IV injection or as an IV infusion.

Cortrosyn – May be administered IM or as a direct IV injection.

➤*Admixture compatibility:* Cosyntropin should not be added to blood or plasma, as it is apt to be inactivated by enzymes.

➤*Storage/Stability:*

Cosyntropin (by Sandoz) – Store refrigerated between 2° and 8°C (36° and 46°F). Protect from light. Protect from freezing.

Cortrosyn – Store at 15° to 30°C (59° to 86°F).

Glucocorticoids

Indications

➤*Allergic states:* Control ofsevere or incapacitating allergic conditions intractable to conventional treatment in serum sickness and drug hypersensitivity reactions.

Parenteral therapy is indicated for urticarial transfusion reactions and acute noninfectious laryngeal edema (epinephrine is the first drug of choice).

➤*Collagen diseases:* For exacerbation or maintenance therapy in selected cases of systemic lupus erythematosus, acute rheumatic carditis or systemic dermatomyositis (polymyositis).

➤*Dermatologic diseases:* Pemphigus; bullous dermatitis herpetiformis; severe erythema multiforme (Stevens-Johnson syndrome); mycosis fungoides; severe psoriasis; angioedema or urticaria; exfoliative, severe seborrheic, contact, or atopic dermatitis.

➤*Edematous states:* To induce diuresis or remission of proteinuria in the nephrotic syndrome (without uremia) of the idiopathic type or that are caused by lupus erythematosus.

➤*Endocrine disorders:* Primary or secondary adrenal cortical insufficiency (hydrocortisone or cortisone is the drug of choice; synthetic analogs may be used in conjunction with mineralocorticoids; in infancy, mineralocorticoid supplementation is important); congenital adrenal hyperplasia; nonsuppurative thyroiditis; hypercalcemia associated with cancer.

Parenteral – Acute adrenal cortical insufficiency (hydrocortisone or cortisone is drug of choice); preoperatively or in serious trauma or illness with known adrenal insufficiency or when adrenal cortical reserve is doubtful; shock unresponsive to conventional therapy if adrenal cortical insufficiency exists or is suspected.

➤*GI diseases:* To tide the patient over a critical period of the disease in ulcerative colitis, regional enteritis (Crohn's disease), and intractable sprue.

➤*Hematologic disorders:* Idiopathic thrombocytopenic purpura and secondary thrombocytopenia in adults (IV only; IM use is contraindicated); acquired (autoimmune) hemolytic anemia; erythroblastopenia (RBC anemia); congenital (erythroid) hypoplastic anemia.

➤*Intra-articular or soft tissue administration:* Short-term adjunctive therapy (to tide the patient over an acute episode) in synovitis of osteoarthritis; rheumatoid arthritis; acute and subacute bursitis; acute gouty arthritis; epicondylitis; acute nonspecific tenosynovitis; post-traumatic osteoarthritis.

➤*Intralesional administration:* Keloids; localized hypertrophic, infiltrated, inflammatory lesions of lichen planus, psoriatic plaques, granuloma annulare, lichen simplex chronicus (neurodermatitis); discoid lupus erythematosus; necrobiosis lipoidica diabeticorum; alopecia areata. May be useful in cystic tumors of an aponeurosis or tendon (ganglia).

➤*Neoplastic diseases:* For palliative management of leukemias and lymphomas in adults and acute leukemia of childhood.

➤*Nervous system:* Acute exacerbations of multiple sclerosis (see Precautions).

➤*Ophthalmic:* Severe acute and chronic allergic and inflammatory processes involving the eye and its adnexa such as in the following: Allergic conjunctivitis; keratitis; allergic corneal marginal ulcers; herpes zoster ophthalmicus; iritis and iridocyclitis; chorioretinitis; diffuse posterior uveitis and choroiditis; optic neuritis; sympathetic ophthalmia and anterior segment inflammation.

➤*Respiratory diseases:* Symptomatic sarcoidosis; bronchial asthma (including status asthmaticus); Loeffler's syndrome not manageable by other means; berylliosis; fulminating or disseminated pulmonary tuberculosis when accompanied by appropriate antituberculous chemotherapy; aspiration pneumonitis; seasonal or perennial allergic rhinitis.

➤*Rheumatic disorders:* Adjunctive therapy for short-term use (acute episode or exacerbation) in the following: Ankylosing spondylitis; acute and subacute bursitis; acute nonspecific tenosynovitis; acute gouty arthritis; psoriatic arthritis; rheumatoid arthritis, including juvenile (selected cases may require low-dose maintenance therapy); post-traumatic osteoarthritis; synovitis of osteoarthritis; epicondylitis.

➤*Miscellaneous:* Tuberculous meningitis with subarachnoid block or impending block when accompanied by appropriate antituberculous chemotherapy; in trichinosis with neurologic or myocardial involvement.

➤*Dexamethasone:* Dexamethasone also is indicated for testing of adrenal cortical hyperfunction; cerebral edema associated with primary or metastatic brain tumor, craniotomy, or head injury.

➤*Triamcinolone:* Triamcinolone also is indicated for the treatment of pulmonary emphysema where bronchospasm or bronchial edema plays a significant role, and diffuse interstitial pulmonary fibrosis (Hamman-Rich syndrome); in conjunction with diuretic agents to induce a diuresis in refractory CHF and in cirrhosis of the liver with refractory ascites; and for postoperative dental inflammatory reactions.

➤*Off-label uses:* Refer to individual monographs for further information.

Glucocorticoid Unlabeled Uses

Use	Drug/Comment
Antiemetic	Dexamethasone most common, 16 to 20 mg
Bacterial meningitis	Dexamethasone 0.15 mg/kg q 6 h; to decrease incidence of hearing loss
Bronchopulmonary dysplasia in preterm infants	Dexamethasone 0.5 mg/kg, then taper.
COPD	Prednisone 30 to 60 mg/day for 1 to 2 weeks, then taper
Depression, diagnosis of	Dexamethasone 1 mg
Duchenne's muscular dystrophy	Prednisone 0.75 to 1.5 mg/kg/day; to improve strength and function
Graves ophthalmopathy	Prednisone 60 mg/day, taper to 20 mg/day
Hepatitis, severe alcoholic	Methylprednisolone 32 mg/day; to reduce mortality
Hirsutism	Dexamethasone 0.5 to 1 mg/day
Respiratory distress syndrome	Prevention in premature neonates (betamethasone most common); adults, methylprednisolone 30 mg/kg (controversial)
Septic shock	Methylprednisolone 30 mg/kg IV most common (very controversial)
Spinal cord injury, acute	Methylprednisolone IV within 8 hrs of injury; to improve neurologic function
Tuberculous pleurisy	Prednisolone 0.75 mg/kg/day, then taper; concurrently w/antituberculous therapy

Eosinophilic esophagitis –

Budesonide: [2] = Fair documentation.

Prednisone: [3] = Safety concerns.

Juvenile idiopathic arthritis –

Betamethasone sodium phosphate/betamethasone acetate (intra-articular): [4] = Insufficient documentation.

Methylprednisolone (injection) (pulse therapy): [4] = Insufficient documentation.

Methylprednosolone (intra-articular): [4] = Insufficient documentation.

Triamcinolone acetonide (intra-articular): [2] = Fair documentation.

Triamcinolone hexacetonide (intra-articular): [2] = Fair documentation.

Nausea and vomiting of pregnancy –

Methylprednisolone (oral and injection): [3] = Safety concerns.

Postherpetic neuralgia –
Methylprednisolone (epidural): [5] = Poor documentation.
Methylprednisolone (intrathecal): [4] = Insufficient documentation.
Methylprednisolone (iontophoretic): [4] = Insufficient documentation.
Triamcinolone (intralesional): [5] = Poor documentation.

Prevention of altitude sickness –
Dexamethasone: [2] = Fair documentation.

Treatment of migraine (adults) –
Dexamethasone (injection): [4] = Insufficient documentation.

Other possible off-label uses –
Dexamethasone: For the treatment of nonrheumatic carditis; mixed connective tissue disease; polyarteritis nodosa; relapsing polychondritis; vasculitis; severe eczema; pemphigoid; localized cutaneous sarcoid; sarcoidosis; hemolysis; prevention of nausea and vomiting associated with chemotherapy, especially cisplatin-containing regimens; breast and prostatic carcinoma; adjunct treatment for fever caused by malignant neoplasm; adjunct treatment for brain neoplasm; multiple myeloma; myasthenia gravis; cerebral ischemia; cerebri pseudomotor; desquamative gingivitis; oral lesions associated with corticosteroid responsive disorder; recurrent aphthous stomatitis; pericarditis; nasal polyps; croup; acute and chronic asthmatic bronchitis; noncardiogenic pulmonary edema; airway-obstructing hemangioma in infants; acute calcium pyrophosphate deposition disease; Reiter disease; rheumatic fever; organ transplant rejection.

Methylprednisolone: Prevention of nausea and vomiting associated with chemotherapy, especially cisplatin-containing regimens; prevention and treatment of acute graft-versus-host disease following bone marrow transplantation.

Administration and Dosage

➤*Administration:* The maximal activity of the adrenal cortex is between 2 and 8 am, and it is minimal between 4 pm and midnight. Exogenous corticosteroids suppress adrenocortical activity the least when given at the time of maximal activity (am). Therefore, administer glucocorticoids in the morning prior to 9 am. When large doses are given, administer antacids between meals to help prevent peptic ulcers.

➤*Initiation of therapy:* The initial dosage depends on the specific disease entity being treated. Maintain or adjust the initial dosage until a satisfactory response is noted. If after a reasonable period of time there is a lack of satisfactory clinical response, discontinue the drug and transfer the patient to other appropriate therapy. It should be emphasized that dosage requirements are variable and must be individualized. For infants and children, the recommended dosage should be governed by the same considerations rather than by strict adherence to the ratio indicated by age or body weight.

➤*Maintenance therapy:* After a favorable response is observed, determine the maintenance dosage by decreasing the initial dosage in small amounts at intervals until the lowest dosage that will maintain an adequate clinical response is reached. Constant monitoring of drug dosage is required. Situations that may make dosage adjustments necessary are changes in the disease process, the patient's individual drug responsiveness, and the effect of patient exposure to stress; in this latter situation it may be necessary to increase the dosage for a period of time consistent with the patient's condition.

➤*Withdrawal of therapy:* If, after long-term therapy, the drug is to be stopped, it must be withdrawn gradually. If spontaneous remission occurs in a chronic condition, discontinue treatment gradually. Continued supervision of the patient after discontinuation of corticosteroids is essential, because there may be a sudden reappearance of severe manifestations of the disease.

➤*Alternate-day therapy:* Alternate day therapy is a dosing regimen in which twice the usual daily dose is administered every other morning. The purpose is to provide the patient requiring long-term treatment with the beneficial effects of corticosteroids while minimizing pituitary-adrenal suppression, the cushingoid state, withdrawal symptoms, and growth suppression in children. The benefits of alternate-day therapy are only achieved by using the intermediate-acting agents.

The rationale for this treatment schedule is based on 2 major premises: a) The therapeutic effect of intermediate-acting corticosteroids persists longer than their physical presence and metabolic effects; b) administration of the corticosteroid every other morning allows for reestablishment of a more normal hypothalamic-pituitary-adrenal (HPA) activity on the off-steroid day. Keep the following in mind when considering alternate day therapy:

1.) Benefits of alternate day therapy do not encourage indiscriminate steroid use.
2.) Alternate day therapy is primarily designed for patients in whom long-term corticosteroid therapy is anticipated.
3.) In less severe disease processes, it may be possible to initiate treatment with alternate day therapy. More severe disease states usually require daily divided high-dose therapy for initial control. Continue initial suppressive dose until satisfactory clinical response is obtained, usually 4 to 10 days in the case of many allergic and collagen diseases. Keep the period of initial suppressive dose as brief as possible, particularly when alternate day therapy is intended. Once control is established, 2 courses are available: a) Change to alternate day therapy, then gradually reduce the amount of corticosteroid given every other day, or b) reduce daily corticosteroid dose to the lowest effective level as rapidly as possible, then change over to an alternate day schedule. Theoretically, course a) may be preferable.
4.) Because of the advantages of alternate day therapy, it may be desirable to try patients on this form of therapy who have been on daily corticosteroids for long periods of time (eg, patients with rheumatoid arthritis). Because these patients may already have a suppressed HPA axis, establishing them on alternate day therapy may be difficult and not always successful; however, it is recommended that such regular attempts be made. It may be helpful to triple or even quadruple the daily maintenance dose and administer this every other day rather than just doubling the daily dose if difficulty is encountered. Once the patient is controlled, attempt to reduce this dose to a minimum.
5.) Long-acting corticosteroids (eg, **dexamethasone**, **betamethasone**), because of their prolonged suppressive effect on adrenal activity, are not recommended for alternate day therapy.
6.) It is important to individualize therapy. Complete control of symptoms will not be possible in all patients. An explanation of the benefits of alternate day therapy will help the patient to understand and tolerate the possible flare-up in symptoms that may occur in the latter part of the off-steroid day. Other therapy to relieve symptoms may be added or increased at this time if needed.
7.) In the event of an acute flare-up of the disease process, it may be necessary to return to a full suppressive daily corticosteroid dose for control. Once control is established, alternate day therapy may be reinstituted.

➤*Intra-articular injection:* Dose depends on the joint size and varies with the severity of the condition. In chronic cases, injections may be repeated at intervals of 1 to 5 or more weeks, depending upon the degree of relief obtained from the initial injection. Injection must be made into the synovial space. Do not inject unstable joints. Repeated intra-articular injection may result in joint instability. X-ray follow-up is suggested in selected cases to detect deterioration.

Suitable sites – Suitable sites for injection are the knee, ankle, wrist, elbow, shoulder, hip, and phalangeal joints. Because difficulty is frequently encountered in entering the hip joint, avoid any large blood vessels in the area. Joints not suitable for injection are those that are anatomically inaccessible and devoid of synovial space, such as the spinal joints and the sacroiliac joints. Treatment failures frequently result from failure to enter the joint space; little or no benefit follows injection into surrounding tissue. If failures occur when injections into the synovial spaces are certain, as determined by aspiration of fluid, repeated injections are usually of no benefit. Local therapy does not alter the underlying disease process; whenever possible, employ comprehensive therapy, including physiotherapy and orthopedic correction (see Precautions).

➤*Miscellaneous (tendinitis, epicondylitis, ganglion):* In the treatment of conditions such as tendinitis or tenosynovitis, inject into the tendon sheath rather than into the substance of the tendon. When treating conditions such as epicondylitis, outline the area of greatest tenderness and infiltrate the drug into the area. For ganglia of the tendon sheaths, inject the drug directly into the cyst. In many cases, a single injection markedly decreases size of the cystic tumor and may effect disappearance. The dose varies with the condition being treated. In recurrent or chronic conditions, repeated injections may be needed.

➤*Injections for local effect in dermatologic conditions:* Avoid injection of sufficient material to cause blanching because this may be followed by a small slough. One to four injections are usually employed. Intervals between injections vary with the type of lesion being treated and duration of improvement produced by initial injection.

Actions

➤*Pharmacology:* The naturally occurring adrenocortical steroids have both anti-inflammatory (glucocorticoid) and salt-retaining (mineralocorticoid) properties. Glucocorticoids cause profound and varied metabolic effects. In addition, they modify the body's immune responses to diverse stimuli.

These compounds, including **hydrocortisone** (cortisol) and **cortisone**, are used as replacement therapy in adrenocortical deficiency states and may be used for their anti-inflammatory effects. The synthetic steroid compounds **prednisone**, **prednisolone**, and **fludrocortisone** also have glucocorticoid and mineralocorticoid activity. Prednisone and prednisolone are used primarily for their glucocorticoid effects.

In addition, a group of synthetic compounds with marked glucocorticoid activity are distinguished by the absence of any significant salt-retaining activity. These include **triamcinolone**, **dexamethasone**, **methylprednisolone**, and **betamethasone**. These agents are used for their potent anti-inflammatory effects.

The following table summarizes the approximate dosage equivalencies (based on glucocorticoid properties) of the various glucocorticoid preparations and several of their pharmacokinetic parameters. The half-life values refer to the intrinsic activity of each agent; insoluble salts of these drugs are used as repository injections and have sustained effects because of delayed absorption from the injection site.

Glucocorticoid Equivalencies, Potencies, and Half-Life

Glucocorticoid	Equivalent potency dose (mg)[a]	Anti-inflammatory potency[a]	Sodium-retaining potency	Half-life plasma (min)
Short-acting				
Cortisone	25	0.8	2	30
Hydrocortisone	20	1	2	80-118

Glucocorticoid Equivalencies, Potencies, and Half-Life				
Glucocorticoid	Equivalent potency dose (mg)[a]	Anti-inflammatory potency[a]	Sodium-retaining potency	Half-life plasma (min)
Intermediate-acting				
Prednisone	5	4	1	60
Prednisolone	5	4	1	115-212
Triamcinolone	4	5	0	200+
Methylprednisolone	4	5	0	78-188
Long-acting				
Dexamethasone	0.75	20-30	0	110-210
Betamethasone	0.6-0.75	20-30	0	300+

[a] When converting doses, use only equivalent potency column, not anti-inflammatory potency column.

➤*Pharmacokinetics:*

Absorption – **Hydrocortisone** and most of its congeners are readily absorbed from the GI tract; greatly altered onsets and durations are usually achieved with injections of suspensions and esters.

Distribution – **Hydrocortisone** is reversibly bound to corticosteroid-binding globulin (CBG or transcortin) and corticosteroid binding albumin (CBA). Exogenous glucocorticoids are bound to these proteins to a significantly lesser degree. In hypoproteinemic or dysproteinemic states, the total endogenous hydrocortisone levels are decreased. Conversely, with increased CBG (pregnancy, estrogen therapy), the total plasma hydrocortisone levels are elevated. These alterations are not of clinical significance because it is the unbound fraction of the hormone that is metabolically active. However, the administration of exogenous glucocorticoids to patients with altered protein-binding capacities will result in significant differences in glucocorticoid pharmacological effects.

Metabolism/Excretion – Hydrocortisone is metabolized by the liver, which is the rate-limiting step in its clearance. The metabolism and excretion of the synthetic glucocorticoids generally parallel hydrocortisone. Induction of hepatic enzymes will increase the metabolic clearance of hydrocortisone and the synthetic glucocorticoids. About 1% of its usual daily production, or about 200 mcg unchanged hormone is excreted in urine daily. Renal clearance is increased when plasma levels are increased. **Prednisone** is inactive and must be metabolized to **prednisolone**.

Contraindications

Systemic fungal infections; hypersensitivity to the drug; IM use in idiopathic thrombocytopenic purpura; administration of live virus vaccines (eg, smallpox) in patients receiving immunosuppressive corticosteroid doses (see Warnings).

Warnings/Precautions

➤*Infections:* Corticosteroids may mask signs of infection, and new infections may appear during their use. There may be decreased resistance and inability of the host defense mechanisms to prevent dissemination of the infection. If an infection occurs during therapy, it should be promptly controlled by suitable antimicrobial therapy.

Tuberculosis – Restrict use in active tuberculosis to cases of fulminating or disseminated disease in which the corticosteroid is used for disease management with appropriate chemotherapy. If corticosteroids are indicated in latent tuberculosis or tuberculin reactivity, observe closely; disease reactivation may occur. During prolonged corticosteroid use, these patients should receive chemoprophylaxis.

Fungal – Corticosteroids may exacerbate systemic fungal infections; do not use in such infections, except to control drug reactions caused by amphotericin B. Concomitant use of amphotericin B and **hydrocortisone** has been followed by cardiac enlargement and CHF.

Amebiasis – Corticosteroids may activate latent amebiasis. Rule out amebiasis before giving to a patient who has been in the tropics or has unexplained diarrhea.

Cerebral malaria – A double-blind trial has shown corticosteroid use is associated with prolongation of coma and a higher incidence of pneumonia and GI bleeding.

➤*Hepatitis:* Although advocated for use in chronic active hepatitis, corticosteroids may be harmful in chronic active hepatitis positive for hepatitis B surface antigen.

➤*Ocular effects:* Prolonged use may produce posterior subcapsular cataracts, glaucoma with possible damage to the optic nerves, and may enhance the establishment of secondary ocular infections due to fungi or viruses. Use cautiously in ocular herpes simplex because of possible corneal perforation.

➤*Fluid and electrolyte balance:* Average and large doses of **hydrocortisone** or **cortisone** can cause elevation of blood pressure, salt and water retention, and increased excretion of potassium. These effects are less likely to occur with the synthetic derivatives except when used in large doses. Dietary salt restriction and potassium supplementation may be necessary. All corticosteroids increase calcium excretion.

➤*Peptic ulcer:* The relationship between peptic ulceration and glucocorticoid therapy is unclear. Patients who appear to be at risk are those being treated for nephrotic syndrome or liver disease or who are comatose post-craniotomy. Other predisposing factors include a total **prednisone** intake exceeding 1 g, a history of ulcer disease, concomitant use of known gastric irritants (as in arthritic patients), and stress. It may be desirable to use prophylactic antacids pending clarification of the relationship.

➤*Immunosuppression:* During therapy, do not use live virus vaccines (eg, smallpox). Do not immunize patients who are receiving corticosteroids, especially high doses, because of possible hazards of neurological complications and a lack of antibody response. This does not apply to patients receiving corticosteroids as replacement therapy. Corticosteroids may suppress reactions to skin tests.

➤*Adrenal suppression:* Prolonged therapy of pharmacologic doses may lead to hypothalamic-pituitary-adrenal suppression. The degree of adrenal suppression varies with the dosage, relative glucocorticoid activity, biological half-life and duration of glucocorticoid therapy within each individual. Adrenal suppression may be minimized by the use of intermediate-acting glucocorticoids (**prednisone**, **prednisolone**, **methylprednisolone**) on an alternate day schedule (see Administration and Dosage).

Withdrawal of therapy – Following prolonged therapy, abrupt discontinuation may result in a withdrawal syndrome without evidence of adrenal insufficiency. To minimize morbidity associated with adrenal insufficiency, discontinue exogenous corticosteroid therapy gradually. During withdrawal therapy, increased supplementation may be necessary during times of stress. Symptoms of adrenal insufficiency as a result of too rapid withdrawal include the following: Nausea; fatigue; anorexia; dyspnea; hypotension; hypoglycemia; myalgia; fever; malaise; arthralgia; dizziness; desquamation of skin; fainting. Continued supervision after therapy termination is essential; severe disease manifestations may reappear suddenly.

➤*Stress:* In patients receiving or recently withdrawn from corticosteroid therapy subjected to unusual stress, increased dosage of rapidly acting corticosteroids is indicated before, during, and after stressful situations, except in patients on high-dose therapy. Relative adrenocortical insufficiency may persist for months after therapy ends; in any stress situation occurring during that period, reinstitute therapy. Because mineralocorticoid secretion may be impaired, administer salt or a mineralocorticoid concurrently.

➤*Cardiovascular:* Reports suggest an apparent association between corticosteroid use and left ventricular free wall rupture after a recent myocardial infarction. Use with great caution in these patients.

➤*Use the lowest possible dose:* Make a benefit/risk decision in each individual case as to the size of the dose, duration of treatment, and the use of daily or intermittent therapy because complications of treatment are dependent on these factors.

➤*Use with caution in:*

GI – Nonspecific ulcerative colitis if there is a probability of impending perforation, abscess or other pyogenic infection; diverticulitis; fresh intestinal anastomoses; active or latent peptic ulcer (see Warnings).

Cardiovascular – Hypertension; CHF; thromboembolitic tendencies; thrombophlebitis.

Miscellaneous – Osteoporosis; exanthema; Cushing syndrome; antibiotic-resistant infections; convulsive disorders; metastatic carcinoma; myasthenia gravis; vaccinia; varicella; diabetes mellitus; hypothyroidism, cirrhosis (enhanced effect of corticosteroids).

➤*Steroid psychosis:* Steroid psychosis is characterized by a delirious or toxic psychosis with clouded sensorium. Other symptoms may include euphoria, insomnia, mood swings, personality changes, and severe depression. The onset of symptoms usually occurs within 15 to 30 days. Predisposing factors include doses more than 40 mg **prednisone** equivalent, female predominance, and, possibly, a family history of psychiatric illness. A patient history of psychiatric problems does not correlate well with predisposition to steroid-induced psychosis. Incidence appears to correlate with dose. One study of 718 patients treated with prednisone revealed less than or equal to 40 mg/day = 1.3%; 41 to 80 mg/day = 4.6%; greater than or equal to 80 mg/day = 18.4%. If the steroids cannot be discontinued, psychotropic medication is effective.

➤*Multiple sclerosis:* Although corticosteroids are effective in speeding the resolution of acute exacerbations of multiple sclerosis, they do not affect the ultimate outcome or natural history of the disease. Relatively high doses of corticosteroids are necessary to demonstrate a significant effect.

➤*Repository injections:* To minimize the likelihood and severity of atrophy, do not inject subcutaneous, avoid injection into the deltoid, and avoid repeated IM injections into the same site, if possible. Repository injections are not recommended as initial therapy in acute situations.

➤*Local injections:* Intra-articular injection may produce systemic and local effects. A marked increase in pain accompanied by local swelling, further restriction of joint motion, fever, and malaise is suggestive of septic arthritis. Appropriate examination of any joint fluid present is necessary. If a diagnosis of sepsis is confirmed, institute appropriate antimicrobial therapy. Avoid local injection into an infected site and into unstable joints.

Strongly impress patients with the importance of not overusing joints in which symptomatic benefit has been obtained as long as the inflammatory process remains active. Frequent intra-articular injection may damage joint tissues.

Avoid overdistention of the joint capsule and deposition of steroid along the needle track in intra-articular injection, as it may lead to subcutaneous atrophy. While crystals of adrenal steroids in the dermis suppress inflammatory reactions, their presence may cause disintegration of the cellular elements and physiochemical changes in the ground substance of the connective tissue.

The resultant dermal or subdermal changes may form depressions in the skin at the injection site; the degree will vary with the amount of adrenal steroid injection. Regeneration is usually complete within a few months or after all crystals of the adrenal steroid have been absorbed. In order to minimize the incidence of dermal and subdermal atrophy, exercise care not to exceed recommended doses in injections. Make multiple small injections into the area of the lesion whenever possible.

➤*Hypersensitivity reactions:* Anaphylactoid reactions have occurred rarely with corticosteroid therapy; take precautionary measures, especially in patients with a history of allergies. Refer to Management of Acute Hypersensitivity Reactions.

➤*Tartrazine sensitivity:* Some of these products contain tartrazine, which may cause allergic-type reactions (including bronchial asthma) in susceptible individuals. Although the incidence of tartrazine sensitivity in the general population is low, it is frequently seen in patients who also have aspirin hypersensitivity. Specific products containing tartrazine are identified in the product listings.

➤*Sulfite sensitivity:* Some of these products contain sulfites which may cause severe allergic reactions in certain susceptible individuals, particularly asthmatics. Anaphylactoid and hypersensitivity reactions have occurred. Do not use in patients allergic to sulfites. Products containing sulfites are identified in product listings.

➤*Renal function impairment:* Edema may occur in the presence of renal disease with a fixed or decreased glomerular filtration rate. Use with caution in renal insufficiency, acute glomerulonephritis, and chronic nephritis.

➤*Pregnancy:* (*Category C* - **methylprednisolone, prednisolone sodium phosphate** [per manufacturer's prescribing information] **betamethasone, cortisone, dexamethasone, hydrocortisone, prednisolone, prednisone** [per Briggs' Drugs in Pregnancy and Lactation]), (*Category D* if used in the first trimester [per Briggs' Drugs in Pregnancy and Lactation]. Corticosteroids cross the placenta (**prednisone** has the poorest transport). In animal studies, large doses of cortisol administered early in pregnancy produced cleft palate, stillborn fetuses, and decreased fetal size. Chronic maternal ingestion during the first trimester has shown a 1% incidence of cleft palate in humans. If used in pregnancy, or in women of childbearing potential, weigh benefits against the potential hazards to the mother and fetus. Carefully observe infants born of mothers who have received substantial corticosteroid doses during pregnancy for signs of hypoadrenalism.

➤*Lactation:* Corticosteroids appear in breast milk and could suppress growth, interfere with endogenous corticosteroid production or cause other unwanted effects in the nursing infant. Advise mothers taking pharmacologic corticosteroid doses not to nurse. However, several studies suggest that amounts excreted in breast milk are negligible with **prednisone** or **prednisolone** doses ≤ 20 mg/day or **methylprednisolone** doses ≤ 8 mg/day, and large doses for short periods may not harm the infant. Alternatives to consider include waiting 3 to 4 hours after the dose before breastfeeding and using prednisolone rather than prednisone (resulting in a lower corticosteroid dose to the infant).

➤*Children:* Carefully observe growth and development of infants and children on prolonged corticosteroid therapy.

Benzyl alcohol – Some of these products contain benzyl alcohol, which has been associated with a fatal "gasping syndrome" in premature infants.

➤*Elderly:* Consider the risk/benefit factors of steroid use. Consider lower doses because of body changes caused by aging (ie, diminution of muscle mass and plasma volume). Monitor blood pressure, blood glucose and electrolytes at least every 6 months.

➤*Monitoring:* Observe patients for weight increase, edema, hypertension, and excessive potassium excretion, as well as for less obvious signs of adrenocortical steroid-induced untoward effects. Monitor for a negative nitrogen balance due to protein catabolism. A liberal protein intake is essential during prolonged therapy. Evaluate blood pressure and body weight, and do routine laboratory studies, including 2-hour postprandial blood glucose and serum potassium and a chest x-ray at regular intervals during prolonged therapy. Upper GI x-rays are desirable in patients with known or suspected peptic ulcer disease or significant dyspepsia or in patients complaining of gastric distress. Observe growth and development of infants and children on prolonged therapy.

Drug Interactions

Corticosteroid Drug Interactions

Precipitant drug	Object drug[a]		Description
Aminoglutethimide	Dexamethasone	↓	Possible loss of dexamethasone-induced adrenal suppression.
Barbiturates	Corticosteroids	↓	Decreased pharmacologic effects of the corticosteroid may be observed.
Cholestyramine	Hydrocortisone	↓	The hydrocortisone AUC may be decreased.
Contraceptives, oral	Corticosteroids	↑	Corticosteroid half-life and concentration may be increased and clearance decreased.
Ephedrine	Dexamethasone	↓	A decreased half-life and increased clearance of dexamethasone may occur.
Estrogens	Corticosteroids	↑	Corticosteroid clearance may be decreased.

Corticosteroid Drug Interactions

Precipitant drug	Object drug[a]		Description
Hydantoins	Corticosteroids	↓	Corticosteroid clearance may be increased, resulting in reduced therapeutic effects.
Ketoconazole	Corticosteroids	↑	Corticosteroid clearance may be decreased and the AUC increased.
Macrolide antibiotics	Methylprednisolone	↑	Significant decrease in methylprednisolone clearance may require a decrease in methylprednisolone dose and the dosing interval.
Rifampin	Corticosteroids	↓	Corticosteroid clearance may be increased, resulting in decreased therapeutic effects.
Corticosteroids	Anticholinesterases	↓	Anticholinesterase effects may be antagonized in myasthenia gravis.
Corticosteroids	Anticoagulants, oral	↔	Anticoagulant dose requirements may be reduced. Conversely, corticosteroids may oppose the anticoagulant action.
Corticosteroids	Cyclosporine	↑	Although this combination is therapeutically beneficial for organ transplants, toxicity may be enhanced.
Corticosteroids	Digitalis glycosides	↑	Coadministration may enhance the possibility of digitalis toxicity associated with hypokalemia.
Corticosteroids	Isoniazid	↓	Isoniazid serum concentrations may be decreased.
Corticosteroids	Nondepolarizing muscle relaxants	↔	Corticosteroids may potentiate, counteract, or have no effect on the neuromuscular blocking action.
Corticosteroids	Potassium-depleting agents (eg, diuretics)	↑	Observe patients for hypokalemia.
Corticosteroids	Salicylates	↓	Corticosteroids will reduce serum salicylate levels and may decrease their effectiveness.
Corticosteroids	Somatrem	↓	Growth-promoting effect of somatrem may be inhibited.
Corticosteroids	Theophyllines	↔	Alterations in the pharmacologic activity of either agent may occur.
Theophyllines	Corticosteroids	↔	Alterations in the pharmacologic activity of either agent may occur.

[a] ↑ = Object drug increased. ↓ = Object drug decreased. ↔ = Undetermined clinical effect.

➤*Drug/Lab test interactions:* Urine glucose and serum cholesterol levels may increase.

Decreased serum levels of potassium, triiodothyronine (T_3), and a minimal decrease of thyroxine (T_4) may occur. Thyroid I^{131} uptake may be decreased. False-negative results with the nitroblue-tetrazolium test for bacterial infection may occur. **Dexamethasone**, given for cerebral edema, may alter the results of a brain scan (decreased uptake of radioactive material).

Adverse Reactions

Parenteral therapy – Rare instances of blindness associated with intralesional therapy around the face and head; hyperpigmentation or hypopigmentation; subcutaneous and cutaneous atrophy; sterile abscess; Charcot-like arthropathy; burning or tingling, especially in the perineal area (after IV injection); scarring, induration, inflammation, paresthesia, occasional irritation at the injection site or occasional brief increase in joint discomfort; transient or delayed pain or soreness; muscle twitching, ataxia, hiccoughs and nystagmus (low incidence following injection); anaphylactic reactions with or without circulatory collapse; cardiac arrest; bronchospasm; arachnoiditis after intrathecal use; foreign body granulomatous reactions involving the synovium with repeated injections.

Intra-articular: Osteonecrosis; tendon rupture; infection; skin atrophy; postinjection flare; hypersensitivity; facial flushing. Systemic reactions may also occur.

Intraspinal: Meningitis (tuberculous, bacterial, cryptococcal, aseptic, chemical); adhesive arachnoiditis; conus medullaris syndrome.

➤*Cardiovascular:* Thromboembolism or fat embolism; thrombophlebitis; necrotizing angiitis; cardiac arrhythmias or ECG changes caused by potassium deficiency; syncopal episodes; aggravation of hypertension; myocardial rupture following recent MI (see Warnings). There are reports of cardiac arrhythmias, fatal arrest, or circulatory collapse following the rapid administration of large IV doses of **methylprednisolone** (0.5 to 1 g in less than 10 to 120 minutes) (see Electrolyte Disturbance).

➤*CNS:* Convulsions; increased intracranial pressure with papilledema (pseudotumor cerebri), usually after stopping treatment; vertigo; headache;

neuritis/paresthesias; aggravation of pre-existing psychiatric conditions; steroid psychoses (see Precautions).

➤*Dermatologic:* Impaired wound healing; thin fragile skin; petechiae and ecchymoses; erythema; lupus erythematosus-like lesions; suppression of skin test reactions; subcutaneous fat atrophy; purpura; striae; hirsutism; acneiform eruptions; other cutaneous reactions such as allergic dermatitis; urticaria; angioneurotic edema; perineal irritation.

➤*Endocrine:* Amenorrhea, postmenopausal bleeding and other menstrual irregularities; development of cushingoid state (eg, moonface, buffalo hump, supraclavicular fat pad enlargement, central obesity); suppression of growth in children; secondary adrenocortical and pituitary unresponsiveness, particularly in times of stress (eg, trauma, surgery, illness); increased sweating; decreased carbohydrate tolerance; hyperglycemia; glycosuria; increased insulin or sulfonylurea requirements in diabetics; manifestations of latent diabetes mellitus; negative nitrogen balance caused by protein catabolism; hirsutism.

➤*Electrolyte disturbance:* Sodium and fluid retention; hypokalemia; hypokalemic alkalosis; metabolic alkalosis; hypocalcemia; CHF in susceptible patients; hypotension or shock-like reactions; hypertension (see Warnings).

➤*GI:* Pancreatitis; abdominal distension; ulcerative esophagitis; nausea; vomiting; increased appetite and weight gain; peptic ulcer with perforation and hemorrhage (see Warnings); perforation of the small and large bowel, particularly in inflammatory bowel disease.

➤*Musculoskeletal:* Muscle weakness; steroid myopathy; muscle mass loss; tendon rupture; osteoporosis; aseptic necrosis of femoral and humeral heads (1% to 37%); spontaneous fractures, including vertebral compression fractures and pathologic fracture of long bones.

➤*Ophthalmic:* Posterior subcapsular cataracts; increased IOP; glaucoma; exophthalmos.

➤*Miscellaneous:* Anaphylactoid/hypersensitivity reactions, aggravation/masking of infections (see Warnings); malaise; leukocytosis (including neonates receiving dexamethasone via maternal injection); fatigue; insomnia; increased or decreased motility and number of spermatozoa.

Overdosage

➤*Symptoms:* There are 2 categories of toxic effects from therapeutic use of glucocorticoids:

Acute adrenal insufficiency – Acute adrenal insufficiency caused by too rapid corticosteroid withdrawal after long-term use, resulting in fever, myalgia, arthralgia, malaise, anorexia, nausea, skin desquamation, orthostatic hypotension, dizziness, fainting, dyspnea, and hypoglycemia.

Cushingoid changes – Cushingoid changes from continued use of large doses resulting in moonface, central obesity, striae, hirsutism, acne, ecchymoses, hypertension, osteoporosis, myopathy, sexual dysfunction, diabetes, hyperlipidemia, peptic ulcer, increased susceptibility to infection and electrolyte and fluid imbalance. Reports of acute toxicity or death are rare.

➤*Treatment:* Recovery of normal adrenal and pituitary function may require up to 9 months. Gradually taper the steroid under the supervision of a physician. Frequent lab tests are necessary. Supplementation is required during periods of stress (eg, illness, surgery, injury). Eventually reduce to the lowest dose that will control the symptoms or discontinue the corticosteroid completely. For large, acute overdoses, treatment includes gastric lavage or emesis and usual supportive measures. Refer to General Management of Acute Overdosage.

Patient Information

May cause GI upset; take with meals or snacks. Take single daily or alternate day doses in the morning prior to 9 a.m. Take multiple doses at evenly spaced intervals throughout the day.

Patients on chronic steroid therapy should wear or carry identification to that effect.

Notify physician if unusual weight gain, swelling of the lower extremities, muscle weakness, black tarry stools, vomiting of blood, puffing of the face, menstrual irregularities, prolonged sore throat, fever, cold, or infection occurs.

Signs of adrenal insufficiency include fatigue, anorexia, nausea, vomiting, diarrhea, weight loss, weakness, dizziness, and low blood sugar. Notify physician promptly if these symptoms occur following dosage reduction or withdrawal of therapy.

➤*High-dose or long-term therapy:* Avoid abrupt withdrawal of therapy.

BETAMETHASONE

Rx	Celestone (Schering)	**Solution:** **Oral:** 0.6 mg per 5 mL	Alcohol. Sorbitol, sugar. In 118 mL. Cherry flavor.

BETAMETHASONE — ORAL

For complete and comparative prescribing information, refer to the Glucocorticoids class monograph.

Indications

➤*Endocrine disorders:* Primary or secondary adrenocortical insufficiency (hydrocortisone or cortisone is the first choice; synthetic analogs may be used in conjunction with mineralocorticoid where applicable; in infancy mineralocorticoid supplementation is of particular importance); congenital adrenal hyperplasia; nonsuppurative thyroiditis; hypercalcemia associated with cancer.

➤*Rheumatic disorders:* As adjunctive therapy for short-term administration (to tide the patient over an acute episode or exacerbation) in: psoriatic arthritis; rheumatoid arthritis (selected cases may require low-dose maintenance therapy); ankylosing spondylitis; acute and subacute bursitis; acute nonspecific tenosynovitis; acute gouty arthritis; post-traumatic osteoarthritis; synovitis of osteoarthritis; epicondylitis.

➤*Collagen diseases:* During an exacerbation or as maintenance therapy in selected cases of: systemic lupus erythematosus, acute rheumatic carditis.

➤*Dermatologic diseases:* Pemphigus, bullous dermatitis herpetiformis, severe erythema multiforme (Stevens-Johnson syndrome), exfoliative dermatitis, mycosis fungoides, severe psoriasis, severe seborrheic dermatitis.

➤*Allergic states:* Control of severe or incapacitating allergic conditions intractable to adequate trials of conventional treatment: seasonal or perennial allergic rhinitis, serum sickness, bronchia asthma, contact dermatitis, atopic dermatitis, drug hypersensitivity reactions.

➤*Ophthalmic disease:* Severe acute and chronic allergic and inflammatory processes involving the eye and its adnexa, such as: allergic conjunctivitis, keratitis, allergic corneal marginal ulcers, herpes zoster ophthalmicus, iritis and iridocyclitis, chorioretinitis, anterior segment inflammation, diffuse posterior uveitis and choroiditis, optic neuritis, sympathetic ophthalmia.

➤*Respiratory diseases:* Symptomatic sarcoidosis, Loeffler's syndrome not manageable by other means, berylliosis, fulminating or disseminated pulmonary tuberculosis when used concurrently with appropriate antituberculous chemotherapy, aspiration pneumonitis.

➤*Hematologic disorders:* Idiopathic thrombocytopenic purpura in adults, secondary thrombocytopenia in adults, acquired (autoimmune) hemolytic anemia, erythroblastopenia (RBC anemia), congenital (erythroid) hypoplastic anemia.

➤*Neoplastic diseases:* For palliative management of leukemias and lymphomas in adults, acute leukemia of childhood.

➤*Edematous states:* To induce a diuresis or remission of proteinuria in the nephrotic syndrome, without uremia, of the idiopathic type or that due to lupus erythematosus.

➤*GI diseases:* To tide the patient over a critical period of the disease in: ulcerative colitis, regional enteritis.

➤*Miscellaneous:* Tuberculous meningitis with subarachnoid block or impending block when used concurrently with appropriate antituberculous chemotherapy, trichinosis with neurologic or myocardial involvement.

Administration and Dosage

➤*General dosing considerations:* Individualize dosage.

➤*Adults:*

Anti-inflammatory / immunosuppressive / endocrine disorders – For more details on specific uses, see Indications.

Initial dosage: 0.6 to 7.2 mg/day.

➤*Children:* Growth and development of infants and children on prolonged corticosteroid therapy should be carefully followed.

Anti-inflammatory / immunosuppressive / endocrine disorders – See Adults for dosing.

➤*Storage / Stability:* Store between 2° and 30°C (36° and 86°F). Protect from excessive moisture.

Warnings/Precautions

➤*Pregnancy: Category C. Category D* if used in first trimester (per Briggs' *Drugs in Pregnancy and Lactation*). Betamethasone crosses the placenta to the fetus. Because adequate human reproduction studies have not been done with corticosteroids, the use of these drugs in pregnancy, or women of childbearing potential requires that the possible benefits of the drug be weighted against the potential hazards to the mother and embryo or fetus. Infants born of mothers who have received substantial doses of corticosteroids during pregnancy should be carefully observed for signs of hypoadrenalism.

➤*Lactation:* The molecular weight of betamethasone is low enough that excretion into milk should be expected. The use of betamethasone in breastfeeding mothers requires that the possible benefits of the drug be weighed against the potential hazards to the mother and embryo or fetus.

BETAMETHASONE SODIUM PHOSPHATE/BETAMETHASONE ACETATE

Rx	Celestone Soluspan (Schering)	Injection: 3 mg betamethasone acetate and 3 mg betamethasone (as sodium phosphate)/mL suspension	In 5 mL multidose vials.[a]

[a] With EDTA and benzalkonium chloride.

BETAMETHASONE SODIUM PHOSPHATE/BETAMETHASONE ACETATE — INJECTION

For complete and comparative prescribing information, refer to the Glucocorticoids group monograph.

Administration and Dosage

➤*General dosing considerations:* Dosage requirements are variable and must be individualized on the basis of the disease under treatment and the response of the patient.

➤*Adults:*

Anti-inflammatory/immunosuppressive/endocrine disorders – For more details on specific uses, see Indications.

Initial dosage: 0.5 to 9 mg/day. In situations of less severity, lower doses will generally suffice, while in selected patients higher initial doses may be required. The initial dosage should be maintained or adjusted until a satisfactory response is noted. If, after a reasonable period of time, there is a lack of satisfactory clinical response, betamethasone sodium phosphate/betamethasone acetate should be discontinued and the patient transferred to other appropriate therapy.

Maintenance dosage: After a favorable response is noted, the proper maintenance dosage should be determined by decreasing the initial drug dosage in small decrements at appropriate time intervals until the lowest dosage that will maintain an adequate clinical response is reached.

Dosage adjustment: It should be kept in mind that constant monitoring is needed in regard to drug dosage. Included in the situations which may make dosage adjustments necessary are changes in clinical status secondary to remissions or exacerbations in the disease process, the patient's individual drug responsiveness, and the effect of patient exposure to stressful situations not directly related to the disease entity under treatment. In this latter situation, it may be necessary to increase the dosage of betamethasone sodium phosphate/betamethasone acetate for a period of time consistent with the patient's condition.

Discontinuation of therapy: If, after long-term therapy, the drug is to be stopped, it is recommended that it be withdrawn gradually rather than abruptly.

Conversion from oral therapy: Usually the parenteral dosage ranges are 1/3 to 1/2 the oral dose given every 12 hours. However, in certain overwhelming, acute, life-threatening situations, administration in dosages exceeding the usual dosages may be justified and may be in multiples of the oral dosages.

Bursitis –

Initial dosage: In acute subdeltoid, subacromial, olecranon, and prepatellar bursitis, 1 intrabursal injection of 1 mL betamethasone sodium phosphate/betamethasone acetate can relieve pain and restore full range of movement.

Maintenance dosage: Several intrabursal injections of corticosteroids are usually required in recurrent acute bursitis and in acute exacerbations of chronic bursitis. Partial relief of pain and some increase in mobility can be expected in both conditions after 1 or 2 injections.

Chronic bursitis may be treated with reduced dosage once the acute condition is controlled.

Dermatologic conditions –

Usual dosage: In intralesional treatment, 0.2 mL/cm^2 is injected intradermally (not subcutaneously).

Maximum dose: A total of no more than 1 mL at weekly intervals is recommended.

Disorders of the foot –

Bursitis: 0.25 to 0.5 mL when under the heloma durum or the heloma molle, 0.5 mL when under the calcaneal spur, and 0.5 mL when over the hallux rigidus or the digiti quinti varus, at intervals of 3 days to a week.

Tenosynovitis (periostitis of cuboid): 0.5 mL at intervals of 3 days to a week.

Acute gouty arthritis: 0.5 to 1 mL, at intervals of 3 days to a week.

Tenosynovitis, peritendinitis – In tenosynovitis and tendinitis, 3 or 4 local injections at intervals of 1 to 2 weeks between injections are given in most cases. Injections should be made into the affected tendon sheaths, rather than into the tendons themselves. In ganglions of joint capsules and tendon sheaths, an injection of 0.5 mL directly into the ganglion cysts has produced marked reduction in the size of the lesions.

Rheumatoid arthritis and osteoarthritis –

Usual dosage: Following intra-articular administration of 0.5 to 2 mL, relief of pain, soreness, and stiffness may be experienced. Duration of relief varies widely in both diseases.

Initial dosage:

- *Very large joints (eg, hip)* – 1 to 2 mL for intra-articular injection.
- *Large joints (eg, ankle, knee, shoulder)* – 1 mL.
- *Medium joints (eg, elbow, wrist)* – 0.5 to 1 mL.
- *Small joints (eg, metacarpophalangeal, interphalangeal, sternoclavicular)* – 0.25 to 0.5 mL.

Concomitant therapy: A portion of the administered dose of betamethasone sodium phosphate/betamethasone acetate is absorbed systemically following intra-articular injection. In patients being treated concomitantly with oral or parenteral corticosteroids, especially those receiving large doses, the systemic absorption of the drug should be considered in determining intra-articular dosage.

➤*Children:* Growth and development of infants and children on prolonged corticosteroid therapy should be carefully followed. See Adults for dosing.

➤*Preparation for administration:* Shake well before using.

Coadministration with a local anesthetic – If coadministration of a local anesthetic is desired, betamethasone sodium phosphate/betamethasone acetate injectable suspension may be mixed with 1% or 2% lidocaine hydrochloride, using the formulations which do not contain parabens. Similar local anesthetics may also be used. Diluents containing methylparaben, propylparaben, or phenol should be avoided since these compounds may cause flocculation of the steroid. The required dose of betamethasone sodium phosphate/betamethasone acetate is first withdrawn from the vial into the syringe. The local anesthetic is then drawn in, and the syringe shaken briefly. Do not inject local anesthetics into the vial of betamethasone sodium phosphate/betamethasone acetate.

➤*Administration:*

Disorders of the foot – A tuberculin syringe with a 25-gauge, ¾-inch needle is suitable for most injections into the foot.

Intra-articular injection – Intra-articular injection is well tolerated in joints and periarticular tissues. There is virtually no pain on injection, and the "secondary flare" that sometimes occurs a few hours after intra-articular injection of corticosteroids has not been reported with betamethasone sodium phosphate/betamethasone acetate.

Using sterile technique, a 20- to 24-gauge needle on an empty syringe is inserted into the synovial cavity and a few drops of synovial fluid are withdrawn to confirm that the needle is in the joint. The aspirating syringe is replaced by a syringe containing betamethasone sodium phosphate/betamethasone acetate, and injection is then made into the joint.

Intradermal injection – Intralesional treatment should use a tuberculin syringe with a 25-gauge, ½-inch needle. Care should be taken to deposit a uniform depot of medication intradermally.

➤*Storage/Stability:* Store between 2° and 25°C (36° and 77°F). Protect from light.

BUDESONIDE

Rx	Entocort EC (Prometheus)	Capsules: 3 mg budesonide (micronized)	Sugar spheres. (ENTOCORT EC 3 mg). Lt. gray/pink. In 100s.

BUDESONIDE — ORAL

For complete and comparative prescribing information, refer to the Glucocorticoids group monograph.

Indications

➤*Crohn disease:* For the treatment of mild to moderate active Crohn disease involving the ileum or the ascending colon and the maintenance of clinical remission of mild to moderate Crohn disease involving the ileum and/or the ascending colon for up to 3 months.

➤*Off-label uses:*

Eosinophilic esophagitis (children) – [2] = Fair documentation. American Gastroenterological Association Institute and North American Society for Pediatric Gastroenterology, Hepatology and Nutrition guidelines recommend budesonide slurry, especially for younger or developmentally disabled children who might have difficulty using a metered-dose inhaler, as an alternative steroid administration method.

Administration and Dosage

➤*Adults:*

Crohn disease –

Short-term therapy: 9 mg once daily in the morning for up to 8 weeks. Repeated 8-week courses can be given for recurring episodes of active disease.

Maintenance dosage: Following an 8-week course(s) of treatment for active disease and once the patient's symptoms are controlled (Crohn Disease Activity Index [CDAI] less than 150), budesonide 6 mg is recommended once daily for maintenance of clinical remission up to 3 months. If symptom control is still maintained at 3 months, an attempt to taper to complete cessation is recommended.

Concomitant therapy: If coadministration with ketoconazole or any other CYP3A4 inhibitor is indicated, patients should be closely monitored for increased signs and/or symptoms of hypercorticism. Reduction in the dose of budesonide should be considered.

BUDESONIDE — ORAL

Switching from prednisolone: Because prednisolone should not be stopped abruptly, tapering should begin concomitantly with initiating budesonide treatment.

➤*Children:*

Off-label dosing –

Eosinophilic esophagitis (children): [2] = Fair documentation.

• *Usual dose* – 1 to 2 mg as a viscous slurry each day, divided into 2 doses, for 3 to 4 months before repeat endoscopy.

Patients were instructed to avoid ingesting any solid or liquid food for 30 minutes after budesonide administration.

See Preparation for Administration for compounding information.

• *Initial dosage –*

Older than 10 years of age: 1 mg twice daily.

Younger than 10 years of age: 500 mcg twice daily, but may be increased to 1 mg twice daily if no response is observed.

➤*Hepatic function impairment:* Patients with moderate to severe liver disease should be monitored for increased signs or symptoms of hypercorticism. Reducing the dose of budesonide should be considered in these patients.

➤*Preparation for administration:*

Extemporaneous compounding – Viscous budesonide was made by mixing a 0.5 mg *Pulmicort Respule* with sucralose 5 g to provide a final volume of 8 to 12 mL.

➤*Administration:* Budesonide should be swallowed whole and not chewed or broken.

➤*Storage/Stability:* Store at 25°C (77°F); excursions permitted to 15° to 30°C (59° to 86°F). Keep container tightly closed.

CORTISONE

Rx	**Cortisone Acetate** (Various, eg, Ivax, Major)	**Tablets:** 25 mg	In 8s, 100s, 500s, 1000s, and UD 100s.

CORTISONE ACETATE — ORAL

For complete and comparative prescribing information, refer to the Glucocorticoids group monograph.

Indications

➤*Allergic states:* Control of severe or incapacitating allergic conditions intractable to adequate trials of conventional treatment: Seasonal or perennial allergic rhinitis; bronchial asthma; contact dermatitis; atopic dermatitis; serum sickness; drug hypersensitivity reactions.

➤*Collagen diseases:* During an exacerbation or as maintenance therapy in selected cases of: Systemic lupus erythematosus; acute rheumatic carditis; systemic dermatomyositis (polymyositis).

➤*Dermatologic diseases:* Pemphigus; bullous dermatitis herpetiformis; severe erythema multiforme (Stevens-Johnson syndrome); exfoliative dermatitis; mycosis fungoides; severe psoriasis; severe seborrheic dermatitis.

➤*Edematous states:* To induce a diuresis of remission or proteinuria in the nephrotic syndrome, without uremia, of the idiopathic type or that caused by lupus erythematosus.

➤*Endocrine disorders:* Primary or secondary adrenocortical insufficiency (hydrocortisone or cortisone is the first choice; synthetic analogs may be used in conjunction with mineralocorticoids where applicable; in infancy mineralocorticoid supplementation is of particular importance). Congenital adrenal hyperplasia; nonsuppurative thyroiditis; hypercalcemia associated with cancer.

➤*Gastrointestinal diseases:* To tide the patient over a critical period of the disease in: ulcerative colitis; regional enteritis.

➤*Hematologic disorders:* Idiopathic thrombocytopenic purpura in adults; secondary thrombocytopenia in adults; acquired (autoimmune) hemolytic anemia; erythroblastopenia (RBC anemia); congenital (erythroid) hypoplastic anemia.

➤*Neoplastic diseases:* For palliative management of: leukemias and lymphomas in adults; acute leukemia of childhood.

➤*Ophthalmic diseases:* Severe acute and chronic allergic and inflammatory processes involving the eye and its adnexa, such as: allergic conjunctivitis; keratitis; allergic corneal marginal ulcers; herpes zoster ophthalmicus; iritis and iridocyclitis; chorioretinitis; anterior segment inflammation; diffuse posterior uveitis and choroiditis; optic neuritis; sympathetic ophthalmia.

➤*Respiratory diseases:* Symptomatic sarcoidosis; Loeffler syndrome not manageable by other means; berylliosis; fulminating or disseminated pulmonary tuberculosis when used concurrently with appropriate antituberculosis chemotherapy; aspiration pneumonitis.

➤*Rheumatic disorders:* As adjunctive therapy for short-term administration (to tide the patient over an acute episode or exacerbation) in: Psoriatic arthritis; rheumatoid arthritis (RA), including juvenile RA (selected cases may require low-dose maintenance therapy); ankylosing spondylitis; acute and subacute bursitis; acute nonspecific tenosynovitis; acute gouty arthritis; posttraumatic osteoarthritis; synovitis of osteoarthritis; epicondylitis.

➤*Miscellaneous:* Tuberculous meningitis with subarachnoid block or impending block when used concurrently with appropriate antituberculous chemotherapy; trichinosis with neurologic or myocardial involvement.

➤*Off-label uses:* For the treatment of acute nonrheumatic carditis; pemphigoid; hemolysis; as an adjunct treatment for brain neoplasm; myasthenia gravis; desquamative gingivitis; recurrent aphthous stomatitis; pericarditis; acute or chronic asthmatic bronchitis; chronic obstructive pulmonary disease; noncardiogenic pulmonary edema; airway obstructing hemangioma in infants; status asthmaticus; rheumatic fever; acute calcium pyrophosphate deposition disease; shock; Reiter disease, prophylaxis and treatment of organ transplant rejection; oral lesions associated with corticosteroid responsive disorders; multiple myeloma; fever caused by malignant neoplasm; malignant neoplasm of the breast and prostate; severe eczema; mixed connective tissue disease; polyarteritis nodosa; relapsing polychondritis; vasculitis.

Administration and Dosage

➤*General dosing considerations:* Dosage requirements are variable and must be individualized based on disease and response of patient.

➤*Adults:*

Anti-inflammatory/immunosuppressive/endocrine disorders – For more details on specific uses, see Indications.

Initial dosage: 25 to 300 mg/day (oral). In less severe diseases, lower doses may suffice.

Maintenance dosage: Decrease initial dosage in small amounts to the lowest dosage that maintains an adequate clinical response.

Dosage adjustment: Changes in clinical status resulting from remissions or exacerbations of the disease, individual drug responsiveness, and the effect of stress (ie, surgery, infection, trauma) may require dosage adjustment. During stress it may be necessary to temporarily increase the dose.

Discontinuation of therapy: If the drug is to be stopped after more than a few days of treatment, it usually should be withdrawn gradually.

➤*Children:* Growth and development of infants and children on prolonged corticosteroid therapy should be carefully observed. See Adults for dosing.

➤*Elderly:* Consider the risk/benefit factors of steroid use. Consider lower doses because of body changes caused by aging (ie, diminution of muscle mass, plasma volume).

➤*Storage/Stability:* Store at controlled room temperature 15° to 30°C (59° to 86°F). Protect from light and moisture.

Dispense in a tight, light-resistant container using a child-resistant closure.

DEXAMETHASONE

Rx	**Dexamethasone** (Various, eg, Par)	**Tablets; oral:** 0.25 mg	In 100s and 1000s.
Rx	**Dexamethasone** (Various, eg, Ivax, Roxane, Par)	**Tablets; oral:** 0.5 mg	In 100s, 1000s, and UD 100s.
Rx	**Dexamethasone** (Various, eg, Ivax, Roxane, Par)	**Tablets; oral:** 0.75 mg	In 100s, 500s, 1000s, and UD 100s.
Rx	**Dexamethasone** (Roxane)	**Tablets; oral:** 1 mg	(54 489). Yellow, scored. In 100s and UD 100s.
Rx	**Dexamethasone** (Various, eg, Ivax, Roxane, Par)	**Tablets; oral:** 1.5 mg	In 50s, 100s, 500s, 1000s, and UD 100s.
Rx	**DexPak 6 Day TaperPak** (ECR)		Lactose. (ECR 86). Pink, pentagonal, scored. 6-day pack. In 21s.
Rx	**DexPak 13 Day TaperPak** (ECR)		Lactose. (54/943). Pink, scored. 13-day pack. In 51s.
Rx	**DexPak Jr. 10 Day TaperPak** (ECR)		Lactose. (54/943). Pink, scored. 10-day pack. In 35s.
Rx	**DexPak Taperpack** (ECR)		(54/943). Pink, scored. In 51s.
Rx	**Zema-Pak 10 Day** (Macoven Pharmaceuticals)		Lactose, sucrose. (54/943). Pink, round, scored. In 35s.
Rx	**Zema-Pak 13 Day** (Macoven Pharmaceuticals)		Lactose, sucrose. (54/943). Pink, round, scored. In 51s.
Rx	**Dexamethasone** (Roxane)	**Tablets; oral:** 2 mg	(54 662). White, scored. In 100s and UD 100s.
Rx	**Dexamethasone** (Various, eg, Ivax, Roxane, Par)	**Tablets; oral:** 4 mg	In 50s, 100s, 500s, 1000s, and UD 100s.

DEXAMETHASONE

Rx	**Dexamethasone** (Various, eg, Roxane, Par)	**Tablets; oral:** 6 mg	In 50s, 100s, and UD 100s.
Rx	**Dexamethasone** (Various, eg, Ivax)	**Elixir; oral:** 0.5 mg per 5 mL	May contain alcohol. In 100 and 237 mL.
Rx	**Baycadron** (Wockhardt)		Alcohol 5.1%, benzoic acid 0.1%, sugar. Raspberry flavor. In 237 mL.
Rx sf	**Dexamethasone** (Various, eg, Roxane, Morton Groves)	**Solution; oral:** 0.5 mg per 5 mL	May contain sorbitol. In 500 mL and UD 5 and 20 mL, and 237 mL.
Rx	**Dexamethasone Intensol** (Roxane)	**Solution, concentrate; oral:** 1 mg per mL	30% alcohol. In 30 mL w/dropper.

DEXAMETHASONE — ORAL

For complete and comparative prescribing information, refer to the Glucocorticoids group monograph.

Indications

➤*Allergic states:* Control of severe or incapacitating allergic conditions intractable to adequate trials of conventional treatment: seasonal or perennial allergic rhinitis, bronchial asthma, contact dermatitis, atopic dermatitis, serum sickness, drug hypersensitivity reactions.

➤*Collagen diseases:* During an exacerbation or as maintenance therapy in selected cases of systemic lupus erythematosus or acute rheumatic carditis.

➤*Dermatologic diseases:* Pemphigus; bullous dermatitis herpetiformis; severe erythema multiforme (Stevens-Johnson syndrome); exfoliative erythroderma; mycosis fungoides; severe psoriasis; severe seborrheic dermatitis.

➤*Diagnostic testing:* Adrenocortical hyperfunction.

➤*Edematous states:* To induce a diuresis or remission of proteinuria in the nephrotic syndrome, without uremia, of the idiopathic type or that because of lupus erythematosus.

➤*Endocrine disorders:* Primary or secondary adrenocortical insufficiency (hydrocortisone or cortisone is the first choice; synthetic analogs may be used in conjunction with mineralocorticoids where applicable; in infancy, mineralocorticoid supplementation is of particular importance); congenital adrenal hyperplasia; nonsuppurative thyroiditis; hypercalcemia associated with cancer.

➤*GI diseases:* To tide the patient over a critical period of the disease in ulcerative colitis or regional enteritis.

➤*Hematologic disorders:* Idiopathic thrombocytopenic purpura in adults; selected cases of secondary thrombocytopenia; acquired (autoimmune) hemolytic anemia; pure red cell aplasia; congenital (erythroid) hypoplastic anemia (Diamond Blackfan anemia).

➤*Neoplastic diseases:* For palliative management of leukemias and lymphomas.

➤*Nervous system:* Acute exacerbations of multiple sclerosis; cerebral edema associated with primary or metastatic brain tumor, craniotomy, or head injury.

➤*Ophthalmic diseases:* Severe acute and chronic allergic and inflammatory processes involving the eye and its adnexa such as allergic conjunctivitis; keratitis; allergic corneal marginal ulcers; herpes zoster ophthalmicus; iritis and iridocyclitis; chorioretinitis; anterior segment inflammation; diffuse posterior uveitis and choroiditis; optic neuritis; sympathetic ophthalmia; temporal arteritis; uveitis; ocular inflammatory conditions unresponsive to topical corticosteroids.

➤*Renal diseases:* To induce a diuresis or remission of proteinuria in idiopathic nephrotic syndrome or that due to lupus erythematosus.

➤*Respiratory diseases:* Symptomatic sarcoidosis; Loeffler syndrome not manageable by other means; berylliosis; fulminating or disseminated pulmonary tuberculosis when used concurrently with appropriate antituberculous chemotherapy; aspiration pneumonitis; idiopathic eosinophilic pneumonias.

➤*Rheumatic disorders:* As adjunctive therapy for short-term administration (to tide the patient over an acute episode or exacerbation) in psoriatic arthritis; rheumatoid arthritis (RA), including juvenile RA (selected cases may require low-dose maintenance therapy); acute rheumatic carditis; ankylosing spondylitis; acute and subacute bursitis; acute nonspecific tenosynovitis; acute gouty arthritis; posttraumatic osteoarthritis; synovitis of osteoarthritis; epicondylitis. For the treatment of dermatomyositis, polymyositis, and systemic lupus erythematosus.

➤*Miscellaneous:* Tuberculous meningitis with subarachnoid block or impending block when used with appropriate antituberculous chemotherapy; trichinosis with neurologic or myocardial involvement.

➤*Off-label uses:*

Prevention of altitude sickness – [2] = Fair documentation. Because of the potential for rebound and other adverse effects, Canadian guidelines for altitude sickness recommend that dexamethasone be reserved for patients who are intolerant of or allergic to acetazolamide. Dexamethasone might also be useful for patients who climb regularly and have previously experienced high altitude sickness despite acetazolamide, or as an adjunct to acetazolamide in cases of forced, rapid ascent to high altitude. The optimal duration of treatment is unclear, and some small studies have reported rebound symptoms after dexamethasone discontinuation. (See Administration and Dosage.)

Other possible off-label uses – For the treatment of nonrheumatic carditis; mixed connective tissue disease; polyarteritis nodosa; relapsing polychondritis; vasculitis; diagnosis of endogenous depression; severe eczema; pemphigoid; localized cutaneous sarcoid; sarcoidosis; hemolysis; prevention of nausea and vomiting associated with chemotherapy, especially cisplatin-containing regimens; breast and prostatic carcinoma; adjunct treatment for fever caused by malignant neoplasm; adjunct treatment for brain neoplasm; multiple myeloma; myasthenia gravis; cerebral ischemia; cerebri pseudomotor; desquamative gingivitis; oral lesions associated with corticosteroid responsive disorder; recurrent aphthous stomatitis; pericarditis; nasal polyps; croup; acute and chronic asthmatic bronchitis; noncardiogenic pulmonary edema; airway-obstructing hemangioma in infants; respiratory distress syndrome; acute calcium pyrophosphate deposition disease; Reiter disease; rheumatic fever; organ transplant rejection; adjunctive treatment for bacterial meningitis; for reducing the risk of chronic lung disease (CLD) by facilitating extubation and improving lung function in high-risk infants.

Administration and Dosage

➤*General dosing considerations:* Dosage requirements are variable and must be individualized based on disease and response of patient.

➤*Adults:*

Anti-inflammatory/immunosuppressive/endocrine disorders – For more details on specific uses, see Indications.

Initial dosage: 0.75 to 9 mg/day, depending on the specific disease entity being treated. In situations of less severity, lower doses will generally suffice; while in selected patients, higher initial doses may be required. The initial dosage should be maintained or adjusted until a satisfactory response is noted. If, after a reasonable period of time, there is a lack of satisfactory clinical response, dexamethasone should be discontinued and the patient transferred to other appropriate therapy.

Maintenance dosage: Decrease initial dosage in small decrements at appropriate time intervals until the lowest dosage that maintains an adequate clinical response is reached. If the drug is to be stopped after more than a few days of treatment, it usually should be withdrawn gradually.

Dosage adjustment: Changes in clinical status resulting from remissions or exacerbations of the disease, individual drug responsiveness, and the effect of stress (ie, surgery, infection, trauma). During stress it may be necessary to increase the dose temporarily.

Discontinuation of therapy: If, after long-term therapy, the drug is to be stopped, it is recommended that it be withdrawn gradually, rather than abruptly.

Acute, self-limited allergic disorders or acute exacerbations of chronic allergic disorders – The following dosage schedule combining parenteral (dexamethasone sodium phosphate 4 mg/mL injection) and oral therapy (0.75 mg tablets) is suggested.

First day, 1 or 2 mL intramuscularly (IM); second and third day, four 0.75 mg tablets in 2 divided doses; fourth day, two 0.75 mg tablets in 2 divided doses; fifth and sixth day, one 0.75 mg tablet; seventh day, no treatment; eighth day, follow-up visit.

Multiple sclerosis – In the treatment of acute exacerbations of multiple sclerosis, daily doses of dexamethasone 30 mg for a week followed by 4 to 12 mg every other day for 1 month have been shown to be effective.

Palliative management of recurrent or inoperable brain tumors – 2 mg 2 or 3 times/day for maintenance therapy.

Suppression tests –

For Cushing syndrome: Give 1 mg at 11 pm. Draw blood for plasma cortisol determination at 8 am the following morning. For greater accuracy, give 0.5 mg orally every 6 hours for 48 hours. Collect 24-hour urine to determine 17-hydroxycorticosteroid excretion.

Test to distinguish Cushing syndrome because of pituitary adrenocorticotropic hormone excess from Cushing syndrome because of other causes: Give 2 mg orally every 6 hours for 48 hours. Collect 24-hour urine to determine 17-hydroxycorticosteroid excretion.

Off-label dosing –

Prevention of altitude sickness: [2] = Fair documentation. 4 mg every 8 to 12 hours, beginning 12 to 24 hours before ascent and continuing for 48 hours or until the time of descent.

➤*Children:* Carefully follow growth and development of children on prolonged corticosteroid therapy.

Anti-inflammatory/immunosuppressive/endocrine disorders – For more details on specific uses, see Indications.

Initial dosage: The range of initial doses is 0.02 to 0.3 mg/kg/day in 3 or 4 divided doses (0.6 to 9 mg/m^2 body surface area [BSA]/day). (See also Off-Label Dosing.)

Maintenance dosage: See Adults.
Dosage adjustment: See Adults.
Discontinuation of therapy: See Adults.

DEXAMETHASONE — ORAL

Off-label dosing –

Anti-inflammatory disorders: 0.08 to 0.3 mg/kg/day in divided doses every 6 to 12 hours.

Prevention of chronic lung disease: AAP does not recommend the use in the prevention or treatment in low birth weight infants; AAP strongly discourages the routine systemic use.

• *Infants between 7 and 14 days of age* – 0.075 mg/kg every 12 hours for 3 days, 0.05 mg/kg every 12 hours for 3 days, 0.025 mg/kg every 12 hours for 2 days, and 0.01 mg/kg every 12 hours for 2 days. Begin after day 7 but before day 14 of life. Do not give with indomethacin.

Croup: 0.6 mg/kg/dose for 1 dose.

➤*Equivalents of various corticosteroids:* The following are the equivalent milligram dosages of various glucocorticoids: dexamethasone 1.5 mg, betamethasone 1.5 mg, paramethasone 4 mg, methylprednisolone or triamcinolone 8 mg, prednisolone or prednisone 10 mg, hydrocortisone 40 mg, and cortisone 50 mg.

These dose relationships apply only to oral or intravenous administration of these compounds. When these substances or their derivatives are injected IM or into joint spaces, their relative properties may be greatly altered.

➤*Administration:*

Intensol – Recommend mixing with liquids, such as water, juices, soda or soda-like beverages, or semi-solid foods, such as applesauce and puddings. Use the provided calibrated dropper to administer the prescribed amount of *Intensol* into a liquid or semi-solid food. Stir gently for a few seconds. The entire amount of the liquid or food should be consumed immediately; do not store for future use.

➤*Storage/Stability:*

Tablets – Store at controlled room temperature, 68° to 77°F (20° to 25°C).

Oral solution – Store at 68° to 77°F (20° to 25°C). Do not freeze. Do not use if solution contains a precipitate. Dispense calibrated dropper with oral solution concentrate.

Elixir – Store at controlled room temperature. Keep tightly closed and avoid freezing.

DEXAMETHASONE SODIUM PHOSPHATE

Rx	**Dexamethasone Sodium Phosphate** (Various)	**Injection:** 4 mg/mL dexamethasone phosphate (as sodium phosphate) solution	In 1, 5, 10 and 30 mL vials, 1 mL disp. syringe and 1 mL fill in 2 mL vials.
Rx	**Dexamethasone Sodium Phosphate** (Various)	**Injection:** 10 mg/mL dexamethasone phosphate (as sodium phosphate) solution	In 1 and 10 mL vials and 1 mL disp. syringe.

DEXAMETHASONE SODIUM PHOSPHATE — INJECTION

For complete and comparative prescribing information, refer to the Glucocorticoids group monograph.

Administration and Dosage

➤*General dosing considerations:* Dosage requirements are variable and must be individualized on the basis of the disease and the response of the patient.

When the IV route of administration is used, dosage usually should be the same as the oral dosage. However, in certain overwhelming, acute, life-threatening situations, administration in dosages exceeding the usual dosages may be justified and may be in multiples of the oral dosages.

The slower rate of absorption by intramuscular (IM) administration should be recognized.

➤*Adults:*

Acute allergic disorders – In acute, self-limited allergic disorders or acute exacerbations of chronic allergic disorders, the following dosage schedule combining parenteral and oral therapy is suggested.

Dexamethasone sodium phosphate injection, 4 mg/mL: First day, 1 or 2 mL (4 or 8 mg) IM.

Dexamethasone tablets, 0.75 mg: Second and third days, 4 tablets in 2 divided doses each day; fourth day, 2 tablets in 2 divided doses; fifth and sixth days, 1 tablet each day; seventh day, no treatment; eighth day, follow-up visit.

This schedule is designed to ensure adequate therapy during acute episodes, while minimizing the risk of overdosage in chronic cases

Anti-inflammatory/immunosuppressive/endocrine disorders – For more details on specific uses, see Indications.

Intra-articular, intralesional, and soft tissue injection: Intra-articular, intralesional, and soft tissue injections are generally employed when the affected joints or areas are limited to 1 or 2 sites. Dosage and frequency of injection varies depending on the condition and the site of injection.

• *Usual dosage* – 0.2 to 6 mg. The frequency usually ranges from once every 3 to 5 days to once every 2 to 3 weeks. Frequent intra-articular injection may result in damage to joint tissues.

Following are some of the usual single doses.

Dexamethasone Sodium Phosphate Dosages

Site of injection	Amount of dexamethasone phosphate (mg)
Large joints (eg, knee)	2 to 4
Small joints (eg, interphalangeal, temporomandibular)	0.8 to 1
Bursae	2 to 3
Tendon sheaths	0.4 to 1
Soft tissue infiltration	2 to 6
Ganglia	1 to 2

• *Concomitant therapy* – Dexamethasone sodium phosphate injection is particularly recommended for use in conjunction with 1 of the less soluble, longer-acting steroids for intra-articular and soft tissue injection.

IV and IM injection:

• *Initial dosage* – 0.5 to 9 mg a day IV or IM, depending on the disease being treated. In less severe diseases, doses lower than 0.5 mg may suffice, while in severe diseases, doses higher than 9 mg may be required. The initial dosage should be maintained or adjusted until the patient's response is satisfactory. If a satisfactory clinical response does not occur after a reasonable period of time, discontinue dexamethasone injection and transfer the patient to other therapy.

• *Maintenance dosage* – After a favorable initial response, the proper maintenance dosage should be determined by decreasing the initial dosage in small amounts to the lowest dosage that maintains an adequate clinical response. Patients should be observed closely for signs that might require dosage adjustment, including changes in clinical status resulting from remissions or exacerbations of the disease, individual drug responsiveness, and the effect of stress (eg, surgery, infection, trauma). During stress, it may be necessary to increase dosage temporarily.

• *Discontinuation of therapy* – If the drug is to be stopped after more than a few days of treatment, it usually should be withdrawn gradually.

Cerebral edema –

Initial dosage: 10 mg IV followed by 4 mg every 6 hours IM until the symptoms of cerebral edema subside. Response is usually noted within 12 to 24 hours and dosage may be reduced after 2 to 4 days and gradually discontinued over a period of 5 to 7 days.

Maintenance dosage: For palliative management of patients with recurrent or inoperable brain tumors, maintenance therapy with 2 mg 2 or 3 times a day may be effective.

Shock – There is a tendency in current medical practice to use high (pharmacologic) doses of corticosteroids for the treatment of unresponsive shock.

Although adverse reactions associated with high-dose, short-term corticosteroid therapy are uncommon, peptic ulceration may occur.

Usual dosage: The following dosages of dexamethasone sodium phosphate injection have been suggested.

Dexamethasone Sodium Phosphate Dosage

Author	Dosage
Cavanagh	3 mg/kg of body weight per 24 hours by constant IV infusion after an initial IV injection of 20 mg
Dietzman	2 to 6 mg/kg of body weight as a single IV injection
Frank	40 mg initially followed by repeat IV injection every 4 to 6 hours while shock persists
Oaks	40 mg initially followed by repeat IV injection every 2 to 6 hours while shock persists
Schumer	1 mg/kg of body weight as a single IV injection

Duration of therapy: Administration of high-dose corticosteroid therapy should be continued only until the patient's condition has stabilized and usually not longer than 48 to 72 hours.

Off-label dosing –

Treatment of migraine (adults): [4] = Insufficient documentation. A single dose of dexamethasone 8 to 20 mg administered by slow IV injection.

➤*Children:* Growth and development of infants and children on prolonged corticosteroid therapy should be carefully observed. See Adults for dosing.

➤*Administration:* Dexamethasone sodium phosphate 4 mg/mL injection is for IV, IM, intra-articular, intralesional, and soft tissue injection.

Dexamethasone sodium phosphate 10 mg/mL injection is for IV and IM injection only.

Dexamethasone sodium phosphate injection can be given directly from the vial or added to sodium chloride injection or dextrose injection and admin-

DEXAMETHASONE SODIUM PHOSPHATE — INJECTION

istered by IV drip. Solutions used for IV administration or further dilution of this product should be preservative-free when used in neonates, especially premature infants.

➤*Storage/Stability:* Store at 25°C (77°F), with excursions permitted between 15° and 30°C (59° and 86°F). The product is sensitive to heat. Do not autoclave. Protect from freezing and light. Store container in carton until contents have been used. Because infusion solutions generally do not contain preservatives, mixtures should be used within 24 hours.

HYDROCORTISONE (Cortisol)

Rx	**Hydrocortisone** (Various, eg, Glades, Qualitest)	**Tablets; oral:** 5 mg	May contain lactose. In 10s, 50s, 100s, 1,000s.
Rx	**Cortef** (Upjohn)		(Cortef 5). White, scored. In 50s.
Rx	**Hydrocortisone** (Major)	**Tablets; oral:** 10 mg	In 100s.
Rx	**Cortef** (Upjohn)		(Cortef 10). White, scored. In 100s.
Rx	**Hydrocortisone** (Various, eg, Major, Moore, URL)	**Tablets; oral:** 20 mg	In 100s.
Rx	**Cortef** (Upjohn)		(Cortef 20). White, scored. In 100s.

HYDROCORTISONE — ORAL

For complete and comparative prescribing information, refer to the Glucocorticoids group monograph.

Administration and Dosage

➤*General dosing considerations:* Dosage requirements are variable and must be individualized on the basis of the disease and the response of the patient.

➤*Adults:*

All approved uses –

Initial dosage: 20 to 240 mg daily. In less severe diseases doses less than 20 mg may suffice, while in severe diseases doses more than 240 mg may be required. The initial dosage should be maintained or adjusted until the patient's response is satisfactory. If satisfactory clinical response does not occur after a reasonable period of time, discontinue hydrocortisone tablets and transfer the patient to other therapy.

Maintenance dosage: Determined by decreasing the initial dosage in small amounts to the lowest dosage that maintains an adequate clinical response.

• *Multiple sclerosis* – In treatment of acute exacerbations of multiple sclerosis, daily doses of 200 mg of prednisolone for a week followed by 80 mg every other day for 1 month have been shown to be effective (20 mg of hydrocortisone is equivalent to 5 mg of prednisolone).

Dosage adjustment: Observe patients closely for signs that might require dosage adjustment, including changes in clinical status resulting from remissions or exacerbations of the disease, individual drug responsiveness, and the effect of stress (eg, surgery, infection, trauma). During stress it may be necessary to increase dosage temporarily.

Discontinuation of therapy: If the drug is to be stopped after more than a few days of treatment, it usually should be withdrawn gradually.

➤*Children:*

Off-label dosing –

Adrenal insufficiency: 9 to 12 mg/m² daily.

• *Congenital adrenal hyperplasia* – 25 mg/m² daily.

• *Physiologic replacement* – 7 to 18 mg/m² daily divided in 2 to 3 doses.

• *Stress dose* – 75 mg/m² daily by mouth divided in 3 to 4 doses.

Anti-inflammatory/immunosuppressive:

• *Preadolescence* – 2.5 to 10 mg/kg daily divided in 3 to 4 doses.

• *Adolescence* – 15 to 240 mg twice daily.

Physiologic replacement: 7 to 18 mg/m² daily divided in 2 to 3 doses.

➤*Storage/Stability:* Store at 20° to 25°C (68° to 77°F).

HYDROCORTISONE SODIUM SUCCINATE

Rx	**A-Hydrocort** (Hospira)	**Injection, powder for solution:** 100 mg per vial	In 2 mL *Univials* and fliptop vials.
Rx	**Solu-Cortef** (Pfizer)		Preservative free. In vials and 2 mL single-dose *Act-O-Vials*.
Rx	**A-Hydrocort** (Hospira)	**Injection, powder for solution:** 250 mg per vial	In 2 mL *Univials* and fliptop vials.
Rx	**Solu-Cortef** (Pfizer)		Preservative free. In 2 mL single-dose *Act-O-Vials*.
Rx	**A-Hydrocort** (Hospira)	**Injection, powder for solution:** 500 mg per vial	In 4 mL *Univials* and fliptop vials.
Rx	**Solu-Cortef** (Pfizer)		Preservative free. In 4 mL single-dose *Act-O-Vials*.
Rx	**A-Hydrocort** (Hospira)	**Injection, powder for solution:** 1,000 mg per vial	In 8 mL *Univials* and fliptop vials.
Rx	**Solu-Cortef** (Pfizer)		Preservative free. In 8 mL single-dose *Act-O-Vials*

HYDROCORTISONE SODIUM SUCCINATE — INJECTION

For complete prescribing information, refer to the Glucocorticoids group monograph.

Administration and Dosage

➤*General dosing considerations:* Patients subjected to severe stress following corticosteroid therapy should be observed closely for signs and symptoms of adrenocortical insufficiency.

Corticoid therapy is an adjunct to, and not a replacement for, conventional therapy.

Although adverse effects associated with high-dose, short-term corticoid therapy are uncommon, peptic ulceration may occur. Prophylactic antacid therapy may be indicated.

When high-dose hydrocortisone therapy must be continued beyond 48 to 72 hours, hypernatremia may occur. Under such circumstances it may be desirable to replace hydrocortisone sodium succinate with a corticoid such as methylprednisolone sodium succinate which causes little or no sodium retention.

Following the initial emergency period, consideration should be given to employing a longer-acting injectable preparation or an oral preparation.

Patients subjected to severe stress following corticosteroid therapy should be observed closely for signs and symptoms of adrenocortical insufficiency.

➤*Adults:*

All approved uses –

Initial dosage: 100 to 500 mg IV over a period of 30 seconds (eg, 100 mg) to 10 minutes (eg, at least 500 mg), depending on the severity of the condition. May repeat every 2, 4, or 6 hours as indicated by the patient's response and clinical condition.

Duration of therapy: In general, high-dose corticosteroid therapy should be continued only until the patient's condition has stabilized, usually not beyond 48 to 72 hours.

➤*Children:* While the dose may be reduced for infants and children, it is governed more by the severity of the condition and response of the patient than by age or body weight but should not be less than 25 mg daily.

The use of hydrocortisone sodium succinate injection is contraindicated in premature infants because the 100, 250, 500, and 1,000 mg *Act-O-Vial* system contains benzyl alcohol.

Off-label dosing –

Acute adrenal crisis:

• *1 to 12 years of age* – 50 to 100 mg IV bolus followed by 50 mg/m² daily by continuous IV drip or divided every 3 to 4 hours. Alternatively, 1 to 2 mg/kg IV bolus followed by 150 to 250 mg/kg daily divided every 6 to 8 hours.

• *1 month to younger than 1 year of age* – 25 mg IV bolus followed by 50 mg/m² daily by continuous IV drip or divided every 3 to 4 hours. Alternatively, 1 to 2 mg/kg IV bolus followed by 25 to 150 mg/kg daily divided every 6 to 8 hours.

Adrenal insufficiency:

• *Glucocorticoid maintenance –*

Congenital adrenal hyperplasia: 12.5 mg/m² IV or IM daily. Alternatively, 1 to 2 mg/kg followed by 2 mg/kg every 8 hours. Oral therapy is usual; resume oral therapy when possible.

Pure adrenal insufficiency: 7 to 12 mg/m²/day in 2 or 3 doses or 0.25 to 0.35 mg/kg IM daily.

Mineralocorticoid maintenance: 50 mg/m²/day IV.

Stress dose:

• *Stress* – 20 to 50 mg/m²/day IV or IM as a continuous drip or divided every 3 to 6 hours.

• *Surgery or severe illness* – 50 to 100 mg/m²/day IV.

Anti-inflammatory/immunosuppressive therapy:

• *Usual dose* – 1 to 5 mg/kg/day or 30 to 150 mg/m² given once a day or every 12 hours.

• *Maximum dose* – 2 g daily.

Chorioamnionitis exposed extremely low birth weight infants:

• *Initial dosage* – 0.5 mg/kg/dose IV every 12 hours for 12 days.

• *Maintenance dosage* – 0.25 mg/kg IV every 12 hours for 3 days.

Cystic fibrosis: 10 mg/kg/day divided every 6 hours for 10 days added to standard treatment for lower respiratory illness.

Hypoglycemia:

HYDROCORTISONE SODIUM SUCCINATE — INJECTION

• *Neonates* – 5 mg/kg/day divided every 12 hours. Use preservative-free formulation.

Hypotension:

• *Neonates* – 2 to 6 mg/kg/day divided every 6, 12, or 24 hours depending on response. Use preservative-free formulation.

➤*Preparation for administration:* For IV or IM injection, prepare solution by aseptically adding not more than 2 mL of bacteriostatic water for injection or bacteriostatic sodium chloride injection to the contents of 1 vial. For IV infusion, first prepare solution by adding not more than 2 mL of bacteriostatic water for injection to the vial; this solution may then be added to 100 to 1,000 mL of the following: dextrose 5% in water (or isotonic saline solution or dextrose 5% in isotonic saline solution if patient is not on sodium restriction).

Directions for using the Act-o-Vial system –

1.) Press down on plastic activator to force diluent into the lower compartment.
2.) Gently agitate solution.
3.) Remove plastic tab covering center of stopper.
4.) Sterilize top of stopper with a suitable germicide.
5.) Insert needle squarely through center of stopper until tip is just visible. Invert vial and withdraw dose.

Further dilution is not necessary for IV or IM injection. For IV infusion, first prepare *Act-O-Vial*solution as just described. The 100 mg solution may then be added to 100 to 1,000 mL of dextrose 5% in water (or isotonic saline solution or dextrose 5% in isotonic saline solution if patient is not on sodium restriction). The 250 mg solution may be added to 250 to 1,000 mL, the 500 mg solution may be added to 500 to 1,000 mL and the 1,000 mg solution to 1,000 mL of the same diluents. In cases where administration of a small volume of fluid is desirable, 100 mg to 3,000 mg of hydrocortisone sodium succinate injection may be added to 50 mL of the above diluents. The resulting solutions are stable for at least 4 hours and may be administered either directly or by IV piggyback.

When reconstituted as directed, pHs of the solutions range from 7 to 8 and the tonicities are: 100 mg *Act-O-Vial*, 0.36 osmolar; 250 mg *Act-O-Vial*, 500 mg *Act-O-Vial*, and the 1,000 mg *Act-O-Vial*, 0.57 osmolar, (isotonic saline = 0.28 osmolar.)

➤*Administration:* Administer by IV injection, IV infusion, or IM injection, the preferred method for initial emergency use being IV injection. Following the initial emergency period, consideration should be given to employing a longer-acting injectable preparation or an oral preparation.

➤*Storage/Stability:* Store unreconstituted product at 20° to 25°C (68° to 77°F).

Store solution at 20° to 25°C (68° to 77°F) and protect from light. Use solution only if it is clear. Unused solution should be discarded after 3 days.

METHYLPREDNISOLONE

Rx	**Medrol** (Upjohn)	**Tablets; oral:** 2 mg	Lactose, sucrose. (MEDROL 2). Pink, scored. Elliptical. In 100s.
Rx	**Methylprednisolone** (Various, eg, Geneva, Major, Moore, Parmed)	**Tablets; oral:** 4 mg	In 21s, 100s, and unit-of-use 21s.
Rx	**Medrol** (Upjohn)		Lactose, sucrose. White, scored. Elliptical. In 30s, 100s, and UD 100s.
Rx	**Methylprednisolone** (Various, eg, Cadista)	**Tablets; oral:** 8 mg	May contain lactose. (TL 002). White, oval, scored. In 25s.
Rx	**Medrol** (Upjohn)		Lactose, sucrose. Peach, scored. Elliptical. In 25s.
Rx	**Methylprednisolone** (Various, eg, URL)	**Tablets; oral:** 16 mg	May contain lactose. In 50s.
Rx	**Medrol** (Upjohn)		Lactose, sucrose. White, scored. Elliptical. In 50s and ADT Pak 14s.
Rx	**Medrol** (Upjohn)	**Tablets; oral:** 24 mg	Lactose, sucrose. Tartrazine. Yellow, scored. Elliptical. In 25s.
Rx	**Methylprednisolone** (Cadista)	**Tablets; oral:** 32 mg	Lactose. (TL 015). Oval, scored. In 25s.
Rx	**Medrol** (Upjohn)		Lactose and sucrose. Peach, scored. Elliptical. In 25s.

METHYLPREDNISOLONE — ORAL

For complete and comparative prescribing information, refer to the Glucocorticoids group monograph.

Administration and Dosage

➤*Adults:*

Anti-inflammatory/immunosuppresive –

Initial dosage: 4 to 48 mg daily, depending on the specific disease entity being treated. In situations of less severity, lower doses will generally suffice, while in selected patients higher initial doses may be required. The initial dosage should be maintained or adjusted until a satisfactory response is noted. If, after a reasonable period of time, there is a lack of satisfactory clinical response, methylprednisolone should be discontinued and the patient transferred to other appropriate therapy.

Maintenance dosage: After a favorable response is noted, the proper maintenance dosage should be determined by decreasing the initial drug dosage in small decrements at appropriate time intervals until the lowest dosage that will maintain an adequate clinical response is reached. Constant monitoring is needed in regard to drug dosage. Included in the situations in which dosage adjustments may become necessary are changes in clinical status secondary to remissions or exacerbations in the disease process, the patient's individual drug responsiveness, and the effect of patient exposure to stressful situations not directly related to the disease entity under treatment; in this latter situation, it may be necessary to increase the dosage of methylprednisolone for a period of time consistent with the patient's condition.

• *Multiple sclerosis* – In the treatment of acute exacerbation of multiple sclerosis, daily doses of prednisolone 200 mg for a week followed by 80 mg every other day for 1 month have been shown to be effective (methylprednisolone 4 mg is equivalent to prednisolone 5 mg).

Discontinuation of therapy: If, after long-term therapy, the drug is stopped, it is recommended that the drug be withdrawn gradually rather than abruptly.

Alternate-day therapy: Alternate-day therapy is a corticosteroid dosing regimen in which twice the usual daily dose of corticoid is administered every other morning. The purpose of this mode of therapy is to provide the patient requiring long-term pharmacologic dose treatment with the beneficial effects of corticoids, while minimizing certain undesirable effects, including pituitary-adrenal suppression, the cushingoid state, corticoid withdrawal symptoms, and growth suppression in children.

➤*Children:* Growth and development of infants and children on prolonged corticosteroid therapy should be carefully observed.

See Adults for dosing.

➤*Storage/Stability:* Store at controlled room temperature, 20° to 25°C (68° to 77°F).

METHYLPREDNISOLONE ACETATE

Rx	**Depo-Medrol** (Pharmacia and Upjohn)	**Injection, suspension:** 20 mg/mL	In 5 mL vials.[a]
Rx	**Methylprednisolone Acetate** (Various, eg, Sandoz, Teva)	**Injection, suspension:** 40 mg/mL	In 5 and 10 ml vials.
Rx	**Depo-Medrol** (Pharmacia and Upjohn)		In 5 and 10 mL vials.[a]
Rx	**Methylprednisolone Acetate** (Various, eg, Sandoz, Teva)	**Injection, suspension:** 80 mg/mL	In 5 mL vials.
Rx	**Depo-Medrol** (Pharmacia and Upjohn)		In 5 mL vials.[a]

[a] With benzyl alcohol, PEG, polysorbate 80, and sodium phosphate.

METHYLPREDNISOLONE ACETATE — INJECTION

For complete and comparative prescribing information, refer to the Glucocorticoids class monograph.

Indications

➤*Intramuscular administration:*

Allergic – Control of severe or incapacitating allergic conditions intractable to adequate trials of conventional treatment in asthma, atopic dermatitis, contact dermatitis, drug hypersensitivity reactions, seasonal or perennial allergic rhinitis, serum sickness, and/or transfusion reactions.

CNS – Acute exacerbations of multiple sclerosis; cerebral edema associated with primary or metastatic brain tumor or craniotomy.

Dermatologic – Treatment of bullous dermatitis herpetiformis, exfoliative erythroderma, mycosis fungoides, pemphigus, and/or severe erythema multiforme (Stevens-Johnson syndrome).

Endocrine – Treatment of primary or secondary adrenocortical insufficiency (hydrocortisone or cortisone is the drug of choice; synthetic analogs may be used in conjunction with mineralocorticoids when applicable; in infancy, mineralocorticoid supplementation is of particular importance), congenital adrenal hyperplasia, hypercalcemia associated with cancer, and/or nonsuppurative thyroiditis.

GI – To tide the patient over a critical period of the disease in regional enteritis (systemic therapy) and/or ulcerative colitis.

Hematologic – Treatment of acquired (autoimmune) hemolytic anemia, congenital (erythroid) hypoplastic anemia (Diamond blackfan anemia), pure red cell aplasia, and/or select cases of secondary thrombocytopenia.

Neoplastic – For palliative management of leukemias and lymphomas.

Ophthalmic – Treatment of sympathetic ophthalmia, temporal arteritis, and/or uveitis and ocular inflammatory conditions unresponsive to topical corticosteroids.

Renal – To induce diuresis or remission of proteinuria in idiopathic nephrotic syndrome, or that due to lupus erythematosus.

Respiratory – Treatment of berylliosis, symptomatic sarcoidosis, fulminating or disseminated pulmonary tuberculosis when used concurrently with appropriate antituberculous chemotherapy, idiopathic eosinophilic pneumonias, and/orsymptomatic sarcoidosis.

Rheumatic – As adjunctive therapy for short-term administration (to tide the patient over an acute episode or exacerbation) in acute gouty arthritis, acute rheumatic carditis, ankylosing spondylitis, psoriatic arthritis, and/or rheumatoid arthritis, including juvenile rheumatoid arthritis (selected cases may require low-dose maintenance therapy); for the treatment of dermatomyositis, polymyositis, and/or systemic lupus erythematosus.

Miscellaneous – Treatment of trichinosis with neurologic or myocardial involvement; and/or tuberculous meningitis with subarachnoid block or impending block when used concurrently with appropriate antituberculous chemotherapy.

➤*Intra-articular or soft tissue administration:* As adjunctive therapy for short-term administration (to tide the patient over an acute episode or exacerbation) in acute gouty arthritis, acute and subacute bursitis, acute nonspecific tenosynovitis, epicondylitis, rheumatoid arthritis, and/or synovitis of osteoarthritis.

➤*Intralesional administration:* For intralesional use in alopecia areata, discoid lupus erythematosus, keloids, localized hypertrophic, infiltrated, inflammatory lesions of granuloma annulare, lichen planus, lichen simplex chronicus (neurodermatitis), and psoriatic plaques, necrobiosis lipoidica diabeticorum. Methylprednisolone acetate also may be useful in cystic tumor of an aponeurosis or tendon (ganglia).

➤*Off-label uses:*

Juvenile idiopathic arthritis (intra-articular) – [4] = Insufficient documentation. Data evaluating the safety and efficacy of methylprednisolone acetate intra-articular injections for the treatment of juvenile idiopathic arthritis (JIA) are limited and indicate that it is less effective than alternative agents. Intra-articular injections of corticosteroids are now generally considered to be a standard of care for JIA for select patient groups (uncomplicated monoarticular disease, oligoarticular disease), with data supporting triamcinolone hexacetonide as the preferred product because of its longer duration of effect. Currently, there are no national guidelines for the management of JIA.

Administration and Dosage

➤*General dosing considerations:* Exercise care not to exceed recommended dosages to minimize the incidence of dermal atrophy.

If a rapid hormonal effect of maximum intensity is required, the intravenous (IV) administration of highly soluble methylprednisolone sodium succinate is indicated.

➤*Adults:*

Anti-inflammatory / immunosuppressive / endocrine disorders – For more details on specific uses, see Indications.

Usual dosage:

• *Intra-articular* – In recurrent or long-term cases, injections may be repeated at intervals ranging from 1 to 5 or more weeks, depending on the degree of relief obtained from the initial injection.

Large joint (knees, ankles, shoulders): 20 to 80 mg.

Medium joint (elbows, wrists): 10 to 40 mg.

Small joint (metacarpophalangeal, interphalangeal, sternoclavicular, acromioclavicular): 4 to 10 mg.

Tendinous or bursal structures: 4 to 30 mg.

• *Intralesional* – 20 to 60 mg injected into the lesion. It may be necessary to distribute doses ranging from 20 to 40 mg by repeated local injections in the case of large lesions. One to 4 injections are usually employed, the intervals between injections varying with the type of lesion being treated and the duration of improvement produced by the initial injection.

• *Intramuscular* –

Acute severe dermatitis because of poison ivy: 80 to 120 mg single dose; relief may result within 8 to 12 hours.

Adrenogenital syndrome: 40 mg single dose every 2 weeks.

Allergic rhinitis: 80 to 120 mg; relief may result within 6 hours and persist for several days to 3 weeks.

Asthma: 80 to 120 mg; relief may result within 6 to 48 hours and persist for several days to 2 weeks.

Long-term contact dermatitis: Repeated injections at 5- to 10-day intervals may be necessary.

Dermatologic lesions: 40 to 120 mg at weekly intervals for 1 to 4 weeks.

Multiple sclerosis: 160 mg daily for 1 week followed by 64 mg every other day for 1 month.

Rheumatoid arthritis: 40 to 120 mg weekly.

Seborrheic dermatitis: 80 mg weekly.

Initial dosage: 4 to 120 mg.

Maintenance dosage: After a favorable response is noted, the proper maintenance dose should be determined by decreasing the initial drug dosage in small increments at appropriate time intervals until the lowest dosage that will maintain an adequate clinical response is reached.

Dosage adjustment: Situations that may make dosage adjustments necessary are changes in clinical status secondary to remissions or exacerbations in the disease process, the patient's individual drug responsiveness, and the effect of patient exposure to stressful situations not directly related to the disease entity under treatment. In this latter situation, it may be necessary to increase the dosage for a period of time consistent with the patient's condition.

Conversion: When employed as a temporary substitute for oral therapy, a single intramuscular (IM) injection during each 24-hour period of a dose of the suspension equal to the total daily oral dose of methylprednisolone is usually sufficient. When a prolonged effect is desired, the weekly dose may be calculated by multiplying the daily oral dose by 7 and given as a single IM injection.

Discontinuation of therapy: If the drug is to be stopped after long-term therapy, it is recommended that it be withdrawn gradually rather than abruptly.

➤*Children:*

Anti-inflammatory / immunosuppressive / endocrine disorders – For more details on specific uses, see Indications.

Initial dosage: 0.11 to 1.6 mg/kg/day IM.

Off-label dosing –

Anti-inflammatory / immunosuppressive / endocrine disorders: 0.5 to 1.7 mg/kg/day IM divided 2 to 4 times a day.

Asthma exacerbations:

• *13 years of age and older* – 40 to 80 mg/day IM divided every 12 to 24 hours or 120 to 180 mg/day IM divided 3 to 4 times a day for 2 days, then 60 to 80 mg/day in 2 divided doses.

• *12 years of age and younger* –

Usual dosage: 1 mg/kg/day IM divided 2 times a day or 1 mg/kg IM every 6 hours for 2 days, then 1 to 2 mg/kg/day IM divided twice daily.

Maximum dose: 60 mg/day.

Juvenile idiopathic arthritis (intra-articular): [4] = Insufficient documentation. 1 to 1.5 mg/kg per joint, administered by inta-articular injections.

Outpatient asthma exacerbation burst therapy:

• *13 years of age and older* – 240 mg IM single dose.

• *12 years of age and younger* –

Maximum dose: 240 mg IM.

Single dose: 7.5 mg/kg IM.

➤*Administration:* Do not use intrathecally; reports of severe medical events have occurred. Take precautions against injection or leakage into the dermis.

Intra-articular – It is recommended that the anatomy of the joint involved be reviewed before attempting intra-articular injection. To obtain the full anti-inflammatory effect, it is important that the injection be made into the synovial space. Employing the same sterile technique as for a lumbar puncture, a sterile 20- to 24-gauge needle (on a dry syringe) is quickly inserted into the synovial cavity. Procaine infiltration is elective. The aspiration of only a few drops of joint fluid proves the joint space has been entered by the needle. The injection site for each joint is determined by that location where the synovial cavity is most superficial and most free of large vessels and nerves. With the needle in place, the aspirating syringe is removed and replaced by a second syringe containing the desired amount of methylprednisolone. The plunger is then pulled outward slightly to aspirate synovial fluid and to make sure the needle is still in the synovial space. After injection, the joint is moved gently a few times to aid mixing of the synovial fluid and the suspension. The site is covered with a small sterile dressing.

Suitable sites for intra-articular injection are the knee, ankle, wrist, elbow, shoulder, phalangeal, and hip joints. Because difficulty is not infrequently encountered in entering the hip joint, precautions should be taken to avoid any large blood vessels in the area. Joints not suitable for injection are those that are anatomically inaccessible such as the spinal joints and those like the sacroiliac joints that are devoid of synovial space. Treatment failures are

METHYLPREDNISOLONE ACETATE — INJECTION

most frequently the result of failure to enter the joint space. Little or no benefit follows injection into surrounding tissue. If failures occur when injections into the synovial spaces are certain, as determined by aspiration of fluid, repeated injections are usually futile.

Bursitis: The area around the injection site is prepared in a sterile way and a wheal at the site made with procaine 1%. A 20- to 24-gauge needle attached to a dry syringe is inserted into the bursa and the fluid aspirated. The needle is left in place and the aspirating syringe changed for a small syringe containing the desired dose. After injection, the needle is withdrawn and a small dressing applied.

Ganglion, tendinitis, epicondylitis: Care should be taken, following application of a suitable antiseptic to the overlying skin, to inject the suspension into the tendon sheath rather than into the substance of the tendon. The tendon may be readily palpated when placed on a stretch. When treating conditions such as epicondylitis, the area of greatest tenderness should be outlined carefully and the suspension infiltrated into the area. For ganglia of the tendon sheaths, the suspension is injected directly into the cyst. In many cases, a single injection causes a marked decrease in the size of the cystic tumor and may effect disappearance. The usual sterile precautions should be observed with each injection.

Intralesional – Following cleansing with an appropriate antiseptic such as alcohol 70%, the suspension is injected into the lesion. Make multiple small injections into the area of the lesion whenever possible. Care should be taken to avoid injection of sufficient material to cause blanching because this may be followed by a small slough.

Intramuscular – Avoid injection into the deltoid muscle because of a high incidence of subcutaneous atrophy. Exercise care not to exceed recommended dosages in order to minimize the incidence of subdermal atrophy. Take precautions against injection or leakage into the dermis.

➤*Admixture compatibility:* Because of possible physical incompatibilities, methylprednisolone should not be diluted or mixed with other solutions.

➤*Storage/Stability:* Store at 20° to 25°C (68° to 77°F). These products may be sensitive to heat. Do not autoclave when it is desirable to sterilize the outside of the vial.

METHYLPREDNISOLONE SODIUM SUCCINATE

Rx	**Methylprednisolone Sodium Succinate** (Various)	**Powder for injection:** 40 mg/vial	In 1 and 3 mL vials.
Rx	**A-Methapred** (Hospira)		In 1 mL *Univial.*[a]
Rx	**Solu-Medrol** (Pfizer)		In 1 mL *Act-O-Vial.*[a]
Rx	**Methylprednisolone Sodium Succinate** (Various)	**Powder for injection:** 125 mg/vial	In 2 and 5 mL vials.
Rx	**A-Methapred** (Hospira)		In 2 mL *Univial.*[b]
Rx	**Solu-Medrol** (Pfizer)		In 2 mL *Act-O-Vial.*[b]
Rx	**Methylprednisolone Sodium Succinate** (Various)	**Powder for injection:** 500 mg/vial	In 1, 4 and 20 mL vials.
Rx	**Solu-Medrol** (Pfizer)		In 8 mL vials and 8 mL vials w/diluent.[c]
Rx	**Methylprednisolone Sodium Succinate** (Various)	**Powder for Injection:** 1 g/vial	In 1, 8 and 50 mL vials.
Rx	**Solu-Medrol** (Pfizer)		In 1 g vials, 1 g vials w/diluent and 8 mL *Act-O-Vial.*[d]
Rx	**Solu-Medrol** (Pfizer)	**Powder for Injection:** 2 g/vial	In 2 g vials w/diluent.

[a] With sodium phosphate anhydrous (1.6 mg monobasic, 17.5 mg dibasic), 25 mg lactose and 9 mg benzyl alcohol.
[b] With sodium phosphate anhydrous (1.6 mg monobasic, 17.4 mg dibasic), approximately 18 mg benzyl alcohol.
[c] With sodium phosphate anhydrous (6.4 mg monobasic, 69.6 mg dibasic). May contain 36 to 70.2 mg benzyl alcohol.
[d] With sodium phosphate anhydrous (12.8 mg monobasic, 139.2 mg dibasic). May contain 66.8 to 141 mg benzyl alcohol.

METHYLPREDNISOLONE SODIUM SUCCINATE — INJECTION

For complete and comparative prescribing information, refer to the Glucocorticoids group monograph.

Administration and Dosage

➤*Adults:*

Anti-inflammatory/immunosuppressive –

Initial dosage: 10 to 40 mg IV over a period of several minutes. The larger doses may be required for short-term management of severe, acute conditions. Subsequent doses may be given IV or IM at intervals dictated by the patient's response and clinical condition. Corticoid therapy is an adjunct to, and not replacement for conventional therapy.

• *Multiple sclerosis* – In the treatment of acute exacerbations of multiple sclerosis, daily doses of prednisolone 200 mg for a week followed by 80 mg every other day for 1 month have been shown to be effective (methylprednisolone 4 mg is equivalent to prednisolone 5 mg).

Discontinuation of therapy: Dosage must be decreased or discontinued gradually when the drug has been administered for more than a few days. If a period of spontaneous remission occurs in a chronic condition, treatment should be discontinued.

High-dose therapy:

• *Usual dosage* – 30 mg/kg administered IV over at least 30 minutes. This dose may be repeated every 4 to 6 hours for 48 hours. In general, high-dose corticosteroid therapy should be continued only until the patient's condition has stabilized, usually not beyond 48 to 72 hours.

• *Concomitant therapy* – Although adverse reactions associated with high-dose, short-term corticoid therapy are uncommon, peptic ulceration may occur. Prophylactic antacid therapy may be indicated.

Off-label dosing –

Nausea and vomiting of pregnancy: [3] = Safety concerns. 16 mg intravenously (IV) every 8 hours for 3 days. Patients with no response after 3 days are unlikely to benefit and should have therapy discontinued. In patients who do respond, the dose should be tapered over 2 weeks. For recurrent nausea and vomiting, the lowest effective dose may be resumed, but the total duration of therapy should be limited to 6 weeks.

➤*Children:* Growth and development of infants and children on prolonged corticosteroid therapy should be carefully observed.

Use in premature infants is contraindicated because some of the products and the accompanying diluent may contain benzyl alcohol. Benzyl alcohol has been reported to be associated with a fatal gasping syndrome in premature infants.

Usual dosage – Dosage may be reduced for infants and children but should be governed more by the severity of the condition and response of the patient than by age or size. It should not be less than 0.5 mg/kg every 24 hours. See Adults for more information.

Off-label dosing –

Juvenile idiopathic arthritis (pulse therapy): [4] = Insufficient documentation.

• *6 months to 15 years of age* – Methylprednisolone pulse therapy was given in various dosing regimens, to a maximum of 1 g per dose.

➤*Monitoring:* Routine laboratory studies, such as urinalysis, 2-hour postprandial blood sugar, determination of blood pressure and body weight, and a chest x-ray should be made at regular intervals during prolonged therapy. Upper GI x-rays are desirable in patients with an ulcer history or significant dyspepsia.

➤*Preparation for administration:* Prepare solutions for IV or IM injection as directed. To prepare solutions for IV infusion, first prepare the solution for injection as directed. This solution may then be added to indicated amounts of 5% dextrose in water, isotonic saline solution, or 5% dextrose in isotonic saline solution.

Act-O-Vial system – Use only the accompanying diluent or bacteriostatic water for injection with benzyl alcohol when reconstituting methylprednisolone sodium succinate. Use within 48 hours after mixing.

➤*Administration:* May be administered by IV or IM injection or by IV infusion; the preferred method for initial emergency use is IV injection. The desired dose may be administered IV over a period of several minutes. If desired, the medication may be administered in diluted solutions by adding water for injection or other suitable diluent (see Preparation for Administration) to the *Act-O-Vial* and withdrawing the indicated dose.

➤*Storage/Stability:* Protect from light. Store powder at controlled room temperature, 20° to 25°C (68° to 77°F).

Store reconstituted solution at controlled room temperature, 20° to 25°C (68° to 77°F). Use solution within 48 hours after mixing.

PREDNISOLONE

Rx	**Prednisolone** (Various, eg, Geneva, Major, Moore, Roxane, Schein)	**Tablets; oral:** 5 mg	In 100s, 1,000s, and 5,000s.
Rx	**Millipred** (Laser Pharmaceuticals)		Lactose. (DAN DAN 5059). Peach, round, scored. In 100s and 1,000s.
Rx	**Orapred ODT** (Sciele)	**Tablets, orally disintegrating; oral:** 10 mg	Equiv. to prednisolone sodium phosphate 13.4 mg. Mannitol, sucralose, sucrose. (ORA 10). Grape flavor. In 48s.
		15 mg	Equiv. to prednisolone sodium phosphate 20.2 mg. Mannitol, sucralose, sucrose. (ORA 15). Grape flavor. In 48s.
		30 mg	Equiv. to prednisolone sodium phosphate 40.3 mg. Mannitol, sucralose, sucrose. (ORA 30). Grape flavor. In 48s.
Rx	**Prelone** (Aero)	**Syrup; oral:** 15 mg per 5 mL	5% alcohol. Saccharin, sucrose. Cherry flavor. In 240 mL.
Rx	**Prednisolone** (Various, eg, WE Pharmaceuticals)	**Syrup; oral:** 15 mg per 5 mL	Sucrose. In 240 and 480 mL.
Rx	**Prednisolone Sodium Phosphate** (Various, eg, Air Pharma, Ethex, Morton, Upstate Pharma)	**Solution; oral:** 5 mg per 5 mL	Equiv. to prednisolone sodium phosphate 6.7 mg per 5 mL. In 120 mL.
Rx	**Pediapred** (Celltech Pharmaceuticals)		Equiv. to prednisolone sodium phosphate 6.7 mg per 5 mL. Dye free. EDTA, methylparaben, sorbitol. Raspberry flavor. In 120 mL.
Rx	**Millipred** (Laser Pharmaceuticals)	**Solution; oral:** 10 mg per 5 mL	Equiv to prednisolone sodium phosphate 13.4 mg. Dye free. Edetate disodium, corn syrup, glycerin, methylparaben, saccharin. Grape flavor. In 237 mL.
Rx	**Prednisolone Sodium Phosphate** (Various, eg, Ethex, Hi-Tech, Morton, Pharmaceutical Associates)	**Solution; oral:** 15 mg per 5 mL	Equiv. to prednisolone sodium phosphate 20.2 mg. In 237 mL.
Rx	**AsmalPred Plus** (Tiber Labs)		Equiv. to prednisolone sodium phosphate 20.2 mg. Alcohol 1.8%, glycerin, sodium benzoate, sorbitol, sucrose. Grape flavor. In 237 mL.
Rx	**Orapred** (Sciele)		Equiv. to prednisolone sodium phosphate 20.2 mg. Dye free. Alcohol 2%, fructose, monoammonium glycyrrhizinate, sorbitol. Grape flavor. In 20 and 237 mL.
Rx	**Veripred 20** (Hawthorn Pharmaceuticals)	**Solution; oral:** 20 mg per 5 mL	Equiv. to prednisolone sodium phosphate 26.9 mg. Corn syrup, edetate disodium, methylparaben, saccharin. Grape flavor. In 237 mL.
Rx	**Flo-Pred** (Taro Pharmaceuticals)	**Suspension; oral:** 15 mg per 5 mL	Equiv. to prednisolone acetate 16.7 mg. Sorbitol, sucralose, EDTA, butylparaben. Cherry flavor. In 120 mL.

PREDNISOLONE — ORAL

For complete and comparative prescribing information, refer to the Glucocorticoids group monograph.

Administration and Dosage

➤*General dosing considerations:* Dosage should be individualized according to the severity of the disease and the response of the patient. For infants and children, the recommended dosage should be governed by the same considerations rather than strict adherence to the ratio indicated by age or body weight. It should be kept in mind that constant monitoring is needed in regard to drug dosage.

The severity, prognosis, expected duration of the disease, and the reaction of the patient to medication are primary factors in determining dosage.

The lowest possible dose should be used to control the condition under treatment, and when reduction in dosage is possible, the reduction should be gradual.

Prednisolone must be tapered prior to discontinuation. (See Discontinuation of Therapy.)

Hormone therapy is an adjunct to and not a replacement for conventional therapy.

➤*Adults:*

Anti-inflammatory/immunosuppressive/endocrine disorders – For more details on specific uses, see Indications.

Initial dosage: 5 to 60 mg per day, depending on the specific disease entity being treated. In situations of less severity, lower doses will generally suffice, while in selected patients, higher initial doses may be required. The initial dosage should be maintained or adjusted until a satisfactory response is noted.

Maintenance dosage: After a favorable response is noted, the proper maintenance dosage should be determined by decreasing the initial drug dosage in small decrements at appropriate time intervals until the lowest dosage that will maintain an adequate clinical response is reached.

Dosage adjustment: Included in the situations that may make dosage adjustments necessary are changes in clinical status secondary to remissions or exacerbations in the disease process, the patient's individual drug responsiveness, and the effect of patient exposure to stressful situations not directly related to the disease entity under treatment. In this latter situation, it may be necessary to increase the dosage for a period of time consistent with the patient's condition.

➤*Children:*

Anti-inflammatory/immunosuppressive/endocrine disorders – For more details on specific uses, see Indications.

Initial dosage: 0.14 to 2 mg/kg/day in 3 or 4 divided doses (4 to 60 mg/m^2/day). In situations of less severity, lower doses will generally suffice, while in selected patients, higher initial doses may be required. The initial dosage should be maintained or adjusted until a satisfactory response is noted.

Maintenance dosage: After a favorable response is noted, the proper maintenance dosage should be determined by decreasing the initial drug dosage in small decrements at appropriate time intervals until the lowest dosage that will maintain an adequate clinical response is reached.

Dosage adjustment: Included in the situations that may make dosage adjustments necessary are changes in clinical status secondary to remissions or exacerbations in the disease process, the patient's individual drug responsiveness, and the effect of patient exposure to stressful situations not directly related to the disease entity under treatment. In this latter situation, it may be necessary to increase the dosage for a period of time consistent with the patient's condition.

Off-label dosing –

Acute asthma:

- *Usual dose* – 2 mg/kg/day in 1 to 2 divided doses for 3 to 7 days.
- *Maximum dose* – 80 mg/day.

Physiologic replacement: 2.5 to 3.5 mg/m^2/day in 2 divided doses.

➤*Alternate-day therapy:* Alternate-day therapy is a corticosteroid dosing regimen in which twice the usual daily dose of corticoid is administered every other morning. The purpose of this mode of therapy is to provide the patient requiring long-term pharmacologic dose treatment with the beneficial effects of corticoids while minimizing certain undesirable effects, including pituitary-adrenal suppression, the cushingoid state, corticoid withdrawal symptoms, and growth suppression in children.

➤*Discontinuation of therapy:* Dosage should be decreased or discontinued gradually when the drug has been administered for more than a few days. If after a reasonable period of time there is a lack of satisfactory clinical response, prednisolone should be discontinued and the patient transferred to other appropriate therapy. If a period of spontaneous remission occurs in a chronic condition, treatment should be discontinued. If after long-term therapy the drug is to be stopped, it is recommended that it be withdrawn gradually rather than abruptly.

PREDNISOLONE — ORAL

➤*Administration:* Take with meals or snacks to avoid GI irritation. Dispense syrup with suitable calibrated measuring device to ensure proper measuring of dose.

➤*Storage/Stability:* Store at 15° to 30°C (59° to 86°F). Do not refrigerate syrup. Protect from light.

PREDNISOLONE ACETATE — ORAL

For complete and comparative prescribing information, refer to the Glucocorticoids group monograph.

Indications

➤*Allergic conditions:* Control of severe or incapacitating allergic conditions intractable to adequate trials of conventional treatment in adults and children with the following: atopic dermatitis, drug hypersensitivity reactions, seasonal or perennial allergic rhinitis, serum sickness.

➤*CNS conditions:* Acute exacerbations of multiple sclerosis; cerebral edema associated with primary or metastatic brain tumor, craniotomy, or head injury.

➤*Dermatologic diseases:* Bullous dermatitis herpetiformis, contact dermatitis, exfoliative erythroderma, mycosis fungoides, pemphigus, severe erythema multiforme (Stevens-Johnson syndrome).

➤*Endocrine conditions:* Congenital adrenal hyperplasia, hypercalcemia of malignancy, nonsuppurative thyroiditis, primary or secondary adrenocortical insufficiency (hydrocortisone or cortisone is the first choice; synthetic analogs may be used in conjunction with mineralocorticoids where applicable).

➤*GI diseases:* During acute episodes in Crohn's disease and ulcerative colitis.

➤*Hematologic diseases:* Acquired (autoimmune) hemolytic anemia, Diamond-Blackfan anemia, idiopathic thrombocytopenic purpura in adults, pure red cell aplasia, secondary thrombocytopenia in adults.

➤*Infectious diseases:* Trichinosis with neurologic or myocardial involvement, tuberculous meningitis with subarachnoid block or impending block used concurrently with appropriate antituberculous chemotherapy.

➤*Neoplastic conditions:* For the treatment of acute leukemia and aggressive lymphomas.

➤*Ophthalmic conditions:* Sympathetic ophthalmia, uveitis and ocular inflammatory conditions unresponsive to topical steroids.

➤*Organ transplantation:* Acute or chronic solid organ rejection.

➤*Pulmonary diseases:* Acute exacerbations of chronic obstructive pulmonary disease, allergic bronchopulmonary aspergillosis, aspiration pneumonitis, asthma, fulminating or disseminated pulmonary tuberculosis when used concurrently with appropriate chemotherapy, hypersensitivity pneumonitis, idiopathic bronchiolitis obliterans with organizing pneumonia, idiopathic eosinophilic pneumonias, idiopathic pulmonary fibrosis, pneumocystis carinii pneumonia (PCP) associated with hypoxemia occurring in an HIV-positive individual who is also under treatment with appropriate anti-PCP antibiotics, symptomatic sarcoidosis.

➤*Renal conditions:* To induce a diuresis or remission of proteinuria in nephrotic syndrome, without uremia, of the idiopathic type or that caused by lupus erythematosus.

➤*Rheumatologic conditions:* As adjunctive therapy for short-term administration (to tide the patient over an acute episode or exacerbation) in acute gouty arthritis.

During an exacerbation or as maintenance therapy in selected cases of the following: ankylosing spondylitis; dermatomyositis/polymyositis; polymyalgia rheumatica; psoriatic arthritis; relapsing polychondritis; rheumatoid arthritis, including juvenile rheumatoid arthritis (selected cases may require low-dose maintenance therapy); Sjogren syndrome; systemic lupus erythematosus; vasculitis.

Administration and Dosage

➤*General dosing considerations:* Dosage should be individualized according to the severity of the disease and the response of the patient. For children, the recommended dosage should be governed by the same considerations rather than strict adherence to the ratio indicated by age or body weight. It should be kept in mind that constant monitoring is needed with regards to drug dosage.

In order to minimize the potential growth effects of corticosteroids, titrate children to the lowest effective dose.

Prednisolone must be tapered prior to discontinuation. (See Discontinuation of therapy.)

➤*Adults:*

Anti-inflammatory/immunosuppressive/endocrine disorders – For more details on specific uses, see Indications.

Initial dosage: 5 to 60 mg/day, depending on the specific disease entity being treated. In situations of less severity, lower doses will generally suffice, while in selected patients, higher initial doses may be required. The initial dosage should be maintained or adjusted until a satisfactory response is noted.

Maintenance dosage: After a favorable response is noted, the proper maintenance dosage should be determined by decreasing the initial drug dosage in small decrements at appropriate time intervals until the lowest dosage that will maintain an adequate clinical response is reached.

Dosage adjustment: Included in the situations that may make dosage adjustments necessary are changes in clinical status secondary to remissions or exacerbations in the disease process, the patient's individual drug responsiveness, and the effect of patient exposure to stressful situations not directly related to the disease entity under treatment. In this latter situation, it may be necessary to increase the dosage of prednisolone for a period of time consistent with the patient's condition.

Multiple sclerosis – 200 mg daily followed by 80 mg every other day for 1 month.

➤*Children:*

Anti-inflammatory/immunosuppressive/endocrine disorders – For more details on specific uses, see Indications.

Initial dosage: 0.14 to 2 mg/kg/day in 3 or 4 divided doses (4 to 60 mg/m^2/day).

Maintenance dosage: After a favorable response is noted, the proper maintenance dosage should be determined by decreasing the initial drug dosage in small decrements at appropriate time intervals until the lowest dosage that will maintain an adequate clinical response is reached.

Dosage adjustment: Included in the situations that may make dosage adjustments necessary are changes in clinical status secondary to remissions or exacerbations in the disease process, the patient's individual drug responsiveness, and the effect of patient exposure to stressful situations not directly related to the disease entity under treatment. In this latter situation, it may be necessary to increase the dosage of prednisolone for a period of time consistent with the patient's condition.

Asthma – 1 to 2 mg/kg/day in single or divided doses. It is further recommended that short-course or burst therapy be continued until the child achieves a peak expiratory flow rate of 80% of his or her personal best or symptoms resolve. This usually requires 3 to 10 days of treatment, although it may take longer. There is no evidence that tapering the dose after improvement will prevent a relapse. (See also Off-Label Uses.)

Nephrotic syndrome – 60 mg/m^2/day given in 3 divided doses for 4 weeks, followed by 4 weeks of single-dose alternate-day therapy at 40 mg/m^2/day.

Off-label dosing –

Acute asthma:

- *Usual dose* – 2 mg/kg/day in 1 to 2 divided doses for 3 to 7 days.
- *Maximum dose* – 80 mg/day.

Physiologic replacement: 2.5 to 3.5 mg/m^2/day in 2 divided doses.

➤*Monitoring:* Blood pressure, body weight, routine laboratory studies (including 2-hour postprandial blood glucose and serum potassium), and a chest x-ray should be obtained at regular intervals during prolonged therapy. Upper GI x-rays are desirable in patients with known or suspected peptic ulcer disease.

➤*Discontinuation of therapy:* If a period of spontaneous remission occurs in a chronic condition, treatment should be discontinued. If, after a reasonable period of time, there is a lack of satisfactory clinical response, prednisolone should be discontinued and the patient transferred to other appropriate therapy. If, after long-term therapy, the drug is to be stopped, it is recommended that it be withdrawn gradually rather than abruptly.

➤*Administration:* Take with meals or snacks to avoid GI irritation. Dispense suspension with suitable calibrated measuring device to ensure proper measuring of dose.

➤*Storage/Stability:* Store between 20° and 25°C (68° and 77°F). Dispense in the original container. Do not transfer the bottle contents to other containers to prevent loss of the viscous formulation. Do not refrigerate.

PREDNISOLONE SODIUM PHOSPHATE — ORAL

For complete and comparative prescribing information, refer to the Glucocorticoids group monograph.

Indications

➤*Allergic states:* Control of severe or incapacitating allergic conditions intractable to adequate trials of conventional treatment in adults and children with seasonal or perennial allergic rhinitis, asthma, atopic dermatitis, contact dermatitis, drug hypersensitivity reactions, and serum sickness.

➤*Dermatologic diseases:* Bullous dermatitis herpetiformis, exfoliative erythroderma, pemphigus, mycosis fungoides, severe erythema multiforme (Stevens-Johnson syndrome).

➤*Edematous states:* To induce diuresis or remission of proteinuria in nephrotic syndrome in adults with lupus erythematosus and in adults and children with idiopathic nephrotic syndrome without uremia.

➤*Endocrine disorders:* Congenital adrenal hyperplasia, hypercalcemia associated with cancer, nonsuppurative thyroiditis, primary or secondary adrenocortical insufficiency (hydrocortisone or cortisone is the first choice; synthetic analogs may be used in conjunction with mineralocorticoids where applicable; in infancy, mineralocorticoid supplementation is of particular importance).

➤*GI diseases:* To tide the patient over a critical period of the disease in regional enteritis or ulcerative colitis.

PREDNISOLONE SODIUM PHOSPHATE — ORAL

➤*Hematologic disorders:* Acquired (autoimmune) hemolytic anemia, Diamond-Blackfan anemia, idiopathic thrombocytopenic purpura in adults, pure red cell aplasia, and selected cases of secondary thrombocytopenia.

➤*Neoplastic diseases:* For the treatment of acute leukemia and aggressive lymphomas in adults and children.

➤*Nervous system:* Acute exacerbations of multiple sclerosis.

➤*Ophthalmic diseases:* Sympathetic ophthalmia, temporal arteritis, and uveitis and ocular inflammatory conditions unresponsive to topical corticosteroids.

➤*Respiratory diseases:* Acute exacerbations of chronic obstructive pulmonary disease (COPD); asthma (distinct from allergic asthma); fulminating or disseminated pulmonary tuberculosis when used concurrently with appropriate antituberculous chemotherapy; hypersensitivity pneumonitis; idiopathic eosinophilic pneumonias; idiopathic pulmonary fibrosis; *Pneumocystis carinii* pneumonia (PCP) associated with hypoxemia occurring in an HIV-positive individual who is also under treatment with appropriate anti-PCP antibiotics; and symptomatic sarcoidosis. Studies support the efficacy of systemic corticosteroids for the treatment of the following conditions: allergic bronchopulmonary aspergillosis and idiopathic bronchiolitis obliterans with organizing pneumonia.

➤*Rheumatic disorders:* As adjunctive therapy for short-term administration (to tide the patient over an acute episode or exacerbation) in the following: acute and subacute bursitis; acute gouty arthritis; acute nonspecific tenosynovitis; ankylosing spondylitis; epicondylitis; psoriatic arthritis; and rheumatoid arthritis, including juvenile rheumatoid arthritis (selected cases may require low-dose maintenance therapy). For the treatment of certain cases of dermatomyositis (polymyositis), polymyalgia rheumatica, relapsing polychondritis, Sjogren syndrome, systemic lupus erythematosus, and vasculitis.

➤*Miscellaneous:* Acute or chronic solid organ rejection (with or without other agents); trichinosis with neurologic or myocardial involvement; tuberculous meningitis with subarachnoid block or impending block; tuberculosis with enlarged mediastinal lymph nodes causing respiratory difficulty; and tuberculosis with pleural or pericardial effusion (use appropriate antituberculous chemotherapy concurrently when treating any tuberculosis complications).

Administration and Dosage

➤*General dosing considerations:* It should be emphasized that dosage requirements are variable and must be individualized on the basis of the disease under treatment and the response of the patient. It should be kept in mind that constant monitoring is needed in regard to drug dosage.

Use the lowest possible dose of corticosteroid to control the condition under treatment; when reduction in dosage is possible, the reduction should be gradual. In order to minimize the potential growth effects of corticosteroids, titrate children to the lowest effective dose.

Prednisolone needs to be tapered prior to discontinuation. (See Discontinuation of therapy.)

➤*Adults:*

Anti-inflammatory/immunosuppressive/endocrine disorders – For more details on specific uses, see Indications.

Initial dosage: 5 to 60 mg/day (as base) oral solution or 10 to 60 mg/day (as base) orally disintegrating tablets (ODT). In situations of less severity, lower doses will generally suffice, while in selected patients, higher initial doses may be required. The initial dosage should be maintained or adjusted until a satisfactory response is noted.

Maintenance dosage: After a favorable response is noted, the proper maintenance dosage should be determined by decreasing the initial drug dosage in small decrements at appropriate time intervals until the lowest dosage that will maintain an adequate clinical response is reached.

Dosage adjustment: Included in the situations that may make dosage adjustments necessary are changes in clinical status secondary to remissions or exacerbations in the disease process, the patient's individual drug responsiveness, and the effect of patient exposure to stressful situations not directly related to the disease entity under treatment; in this latter situation, it may be necessary to increase the dosage of prednisolone for a period of time consistent with the patient's condition.

Multiple sclerosis – 200 mg daily for a week followed by 80 mg every other day for 1 month has been shown to be effective.

➤*Children:*

Anti-inflammatory/immunosuppressive/endocrine disorders – For more details on specific uses, see Indications.

Initial dosage: 0.14 to 2 mg/kg/day in 3 or 4 divided doses (4 to 60 mg/m^2 body surface area/day). In situations of less severity, lower doses will generally suffice, while in selected patients, higher initial doses may be required. The initial dosage should be maintained or adjusted until a satisfactory response is noted.

Maintenance dosage: After a favorable response is noted, the proper maintenance dosage should be determined by decreasing the initial drug dosage in small decrements at appropriate time intervals until the lowest dosage that will maintain an adequate clinical response is reached.

Dosage adjustment: Included in the situations that may make dosage adjustments necessary are changes in clinical status secondary to remissions or exacerbations in the disease process, the patient's individual drug responsiveness, and the effect of patient exposure to stressful situations not directly related to the disease entity under treatment; in this latter situation, it may be necessary to increase the dosage of prednisolone for a period of time consistent with the patient's condition.

Asthma – 1 to 2 mg/kg/day in single or divided doses. A short-course, or burst, therapy should be continued until a child achieves a peak expiratory flow rate of 80% of his or her personal best or until symptoms resolve. This usually requires 3 to 10 days of treatment, although it can take longer.

Nephrotic syndrome – 60 mg/m^2/day given in 3 divided doses for 4 weeks, followed by 4 weeks of single-dose, alternate-day therapy at 40 mg/m^2/day.

Off-label dosing –

Acute asthma:

- *Usual dose* – 2 mg/kg/day in 1 to 2 divided doses for 3 to 7 days.
- *Maximum dose* – 80 mg/day.

Physiologic replacement: 2.5 to 3.5 mg/m^2/day in 2 divided doses.

➤*Discontinuation of therapy:* If after a reasonable period of time there is a lack of satisfactory clinical response, prednisolone should be discontinued and the patient placed on other appropriate therapy. If after long-term therapy the drug is to be stopped, it is recommended that it be withdrawn gradually rather than abruptly.

➤*Administration:* Take with meals or snacks to avoid GI irritation. Dispense syrup with suitable calibrated measuring device to ensure proper measuring of dose.

ODT – Do not break or use partial prednisolone ODT. Patients should be instructed not to remove the tablet from the blister pack until just prior to dosing. The blister pack should then be peeled open and the ODT placed on the tongue, where tablets may be swallowed whole like any conventional tablet or allowed to dissolve in the mouth with or without the assistance of water. ODT dosage forms are friable and are not intended to be cut, split, or broken.

Use an appropriate formulation of prednisolone if indicated dose cannot be obtained using ODT. This may become important in the treatment of conditions that require tapering doses that cannot be adequately accommodated by ODT (eg, tapering the dose below 10 mg).

➤*Storage/Stability:*

ODT – Store at 20° to 25°C (68° to 77°F). Protect from moisture.

Oral solutions – Store 5 mg per 5 mL at 4° to 25°C (39° to 77°F). May be refrigerated. Store 15 mg per 5 mL at 2° and 8°C (36° and 48°F). Dispense in tight, light-resistant glass or polyethylene terphthalate plastic containers.

PREDNISONE

Rx	**Prednisone** (Roxane)	**Tablets:** 1 mg	Lactose. (54 092). White, scored. In 100s, 1,000s, and UD 100s.
Rx	**Prednisone** (Roxane)	**Tablets:** 2.5 mg	Lactose. (54 339). White, scored. In 100s and UD 100s.
Rx	**Prednisone** (Various, eg, Barr, Geneva, Lannett, Major, Parmed, Roxane)	**Tablets:** 5 mg	In 100s, 500s, 1,000s, 5,000s, and UD 100s.
Rx	**Prednisone** (Various, eg, Barr, Geneva, Major, Parmed, Roxane)	**Tablets:** 10 mg	In 100s, 500s, 1,000s, and UD 100s.
Rx	**Prednisone** (Various, eg, Barr, Geneva, Lannett, Major, Parmed, Roxane)	**Tablets:** 20 mg	In 100s, 500s, 1,000s, and UD 100s.
Rx	**Prednisone** (Various, eg, Geneva, Major, Roxane)	**Tablets:** 50 mg	In 100s and UD 100s.
Rx	**Prednisone** (Roxane)	**Oral Solution:** 5 mg per 5 mL	5% alcohol, EDTA, fructose, saccharin. In 120 and 500 mL and UD 5 mL.
Rx	**Prednisone Intensol Concentrate** (Roxane)	**Oral Solution:** 5 mg/mL	30% alcohol. In 30 mL w/calibrated dropper.

PREDNISONE — ORAL

For complete and comparative prescribing information, refer to the Glucocorticoids group monograph.

Administration and Dosage

➤*General dosing considerations:* Dosage of prednisone should be individualized according to the severity, prognosis, expected duration of the disease, and the reaction of the patient to medication. For infants and children, the recommended dosage should be governed by the same considerations rather than strict adherence to the ratio indicated by age or body weight.

➤*Adults:*

Anti-inflammatory/immunosuppressive/endocrine disorders –

Initial dosage: 5 to 60 mg/day depending on the specific disease entity being treated. In situations of less severity lower doses will generally suffice while in selected patients higher initial doses may be required. The initial dosage should be maintained or adjusted until a satisfactory response is noted. If after a reasonable period of time there is a lack of satisfactory clinical response, prednisone should be discontinued and the patient transferred to other appropriate therapy.

Maintenance dosage: After a favorable response is noted, the proper maintenance dosage should be determined by decreasing the initial drug dosage in small decrements at appropriate time intervals until the lowest dosage which will maintain an adequate clinical response is reached. It should be kept in mind that constant monitoring is needed in regard to drug dosage. Included in the situations which may make dosage adjustments necessary are changes in clinical status secondary to remissions or exacerbations in the disease process, the patient's individual drug responsiveness, and the effect of patient exposure to stressful situations not directly related to the disease entity under treatment; in this latter situation it may be necessary to increase the dosage of prednisone for a period of time consistent with the patient's condition.

• *Multiple sclerosis* – In the treatment of acute exacerbation of multiple sclerosis, daily doses of prednisone 200 mg for a week followed by 80 mg every other day for 1 month have been shown to be effective. (Dosage range is the same for prednisone and prednisolone.)

Discontinuation of therapy: The dosage should be decreased or discontinued gradually when the drug has been administered for more than a few days. If a period of spontaneous remission occurs in a chronic condition, treatment should be discontinued.

Alternate day therapy (ADT): ADT is a corticosteroid dosing regimen in which twice the usual daily dose of corticoid is administered every other morning. The purpose of this mode of therapy is to provide the patient requiring long-term pharmacologic dose treatment with the beneficial effects of corticoids while minimizing certain undesirable effects, including pituitary-adrenal suppression, the Cushingoid state, corticoid withdrawal symptoms, and growth suppression in children.

Off-label dosing –

Eosinophilic esophagitis: [3] = Safety concerns. The recommended dosage is 1 to 2 mg/kg/day orally, up to a maximum of 60 mg/day, until urgent symptom relief is achieved. A gradual dose reduction similar to that used for patients with inflammatory bowel disease was recommended.

➤*Children:* Growth and development of infants and children on prolonged corticosteroid therapy should be carefully observed.

Anti-inflammatory/immunosuppressive/endocrine disorders – For more details on specific uses, see Indications.

Initial dosage: 5 to 60 mg/day depending on the specific disease entity being treated. In situations of less severity lower doses will generally suffice while in selected patients higher initial doses may be required. The initial dosage should be maintained or adjusted until a satisfactory response is noted. If after a reasonable period of time there is a lack of satisfactory clinical response, prednisone should be discontinued and the patient transferred to other appropriate therapy.

Maintenance dosage: After a favorable response is noted, the proper maintenance dosage should be determined by decreasing the initial drug dosage in small decrements at appropriate time intervals until the lowest dosage which will maintain an adequate clinical response is reached. It should be kept in mind that constant monitoring is needed in regard to drug dosage. Included in the situations which may make dosage adjustments necessary are changes in clinical status secondary to remissions or exacerbations in the disease process, the patient's individual drug responsiveness, and the effect of patient exposure to stressful situations not directly related to the disease entity under treatment; in this latter situation it may be necessary to increase the dosage of prednisone for a period of time consistent with the patient's condition.

• *Multiple sclerosis* – In the treatment of acute exacerbation of multiple sclerosis, daily doses of prednisone 200 mg for a week followed by 80 mg every other day for 1 month have been shown to be effective. (Dosage range is the same for prednisone and prednisolone.)

Discontinuation of therapy: The dosage should be decreased or discontinued gradually when the drug has been administered for more than a few days. If a period of spontaneous remission occurs in a chronic condition, treatment should be discontinued.

Alternate day therapy (ADT): ADT is a corticosteroid dosing regimen in which twice the usual daily dose of corticoid is administered every other morning. The purpose of this mode of therapy is to provide the patient requiring long-term pharmacologic dose treatment with the beneficial effects of corticoids while minimizing certain undesirable effects, including pituitary-adrenal suppression, the Cushingoid state, corticoid withdrawal symptoms, and growth suppression in children.

See Adults for more information.

Off-label dosing –

Anti-inflammatory/immunosuppressive disorders: 0.5 to 2 mg/kg/day divided into 1 to 2 doses/day.

Acute asthma:

• *Usual dose* – 2 mg/kg/day in divided doses 1 to 2 times/day for 3 to 7 days.
• *Maximum dose* – 80 mg/day.

Asthma exacerbations:

• *13 years of age and older* – 40 to 80 mg/day divided into 1 to 2 doses/day.
• *12 years of age and younger –*
  Usual dosage: 1 mg/kg/day divided into 2 doses per day.
  Maximum dose: 60 mg/day.

Eosinophilic esophagitis: [3] = Safety concerns. The recommended dosage is 1 to 2 mg/kg/day orally, up to a maximum of 60 mg/day, until urgent symptom relief is achieved. A gradual dose reduction similar to that used for patients with inflammatory bowel disease was recommended.

Outpatients asthma exacerbation burst therapy:

• *13 years of age and older* – 40 to 60 mg/day in divided doses 1 to 2 times/day for 5 to 10 days.
• *12 years of age and younger –*
  Usual dosage: 1 to 2 mg/kg/day divided 1 to 2 doses/day for 3 to 10 days.
  Maximum dose: 60 mg/day.

Nephrotic syndrome:

• *Maximum dose* – 80 mg/day.
• *Initial dosage* – 2 mg/kg/day.
• *Dosage adjustment* – Adjust dose according to patient response.

➤*Storage/Stability:* Store at controlled room temperature 15° to 30°C (59° to 86°F).

TRIAMCINOLONE ACETONIDE

Rx	**Triamcinolone Acetonide** (Sandoz)	**Injection, suspension**: 10 mg/mL	Benzyl alcohol 0.9%. In 5 mL multidose vials.[a]
Rx	**Kenalog-10** (Bristol-Myers Squibb)		Benzyl alcohol 0.9%. In 5 mL vials.[a]
Rx	**Kenalog-40** (Bristol-Myers Squibb)	**Injection, suspension**: 40 mg/mL	Benzyl alcohol 0.9%. In 1, 5, and 10 mL vials.[a]
Rx	**Trivaris** (Allergan)	**Injection, gel suspension**: 80 mg/mL	Preservative free. Sodium hyaluronate 2.3%. In single-use glass syringe.

[a] Exposure to excessive amounts of benzyl alcohol has been associated with toxicity, particularly in neonates.

TRIAMCINOLONE ACETONIDE — INJECTION

For complete and comparative prescribing information, refer to the Glucocorticoids class monograph.

Indications

➤*Intra-articular or soft tissue administration:* As adjunctive therapy for short-term administration (to tide the patient over an acute episode or exacerbation) in acute gouty arthritis, acute and subacute bursitis, acute nonspecific tenosynovitis, epicondylitis, rheumatoid arthritis, or synovitis of osteoarthritis.

➤*Intralesional (Kenalog-10* injection *only):* For treatment of alopecia areata; discoid lupus erythematosus; keloids; localized hypertrophic, infiltrated, inflammatory lesions of granuloma annulare, lichen planus, lichen simplex chronicus (neurodermatitis), and psoriatic plaques; and necrobiosis lipoidica diabeticorum. May also be useful in cystic tumors of an aponeurosis or tendon (ganglia).

➤*Intramuscular:*

Kenalog-40 and *Trivaris* only –

Infeasibility of oral therapy: When oral therapy is not feasible use as follows:

• *Allergic states* – Control of severe or incapacitating allergic conditions intractable to adequate trials of conventional treatment in asthma, atopic dermatitis, contact dermatitis, drug hypersensitivity reactions, perennial or seasonal allergic rhinitis, serum sickness, or transfusion reactions.

• *Dermatologic diseases* – Bullous dermatitis herpetiformis, exfoliative erythroderma, mycosis fungoides, pemphigus, or severe erythema multiforme (Stevens-Johnson syndrome).

• *Endocrine disorders* – Primary or secondary adrenocortical insufficiency (hydrocortisone or cortisone is the drug of choice; synthetic analogs may be used in conjunction with mineralocorticoids when applicable; in

TRIAMCINOLONE ACETONIDE — INJECTION

infancy, mineralocorticoid supplementation is of particular importance), congenital adrenal hyperplasia, hypercalcemia associated with cancer, or nonsuppurative thyroiditis.

• *GI diseases* – To tide the patient over a critical period of disease in regional enteritis and ulcerative colitis.

• *Hematologic disorders* – Acquired (autoimmune) hemolytic anemia, Diamond-Blackfan anemia, pure red cell aplasia, selected cases of secondary thrombocytopenia.

• *Neoplastic diseases* – For palliative management of leukemias and lymphomas.

• *Nervous system* – Acute exacerbations of multiple sclerosis; cerebral edema associated with primary or metastatic brain tumor, craniotomy, or head injury.

• *Ophthalmic diseases* – Sympathetic ophthalmia, temporal arteritis, uveitis, and ocular inflammatory conditions unresponsive to topical corticosteroids.

• *Renal diseases* – To induce diuresis or remission of proteinuria in idiopathic nephrotic syndrome or that caused by lupus erythematosus.

• *Respiratory diseases* – Berylliosis, fulminating or disseminated pulmonary tuberculosis when used concurrently with appropriate antituberculous chemotherapy, idiopathic eosinophilic pneumonias, symptomatic sarcoidosis.

• *Rheumatic disorders* – As adjunctive therapy for short-term administration (to tide the patient over an acute episode or exacerbation) in acute gouty arthritis; acute rheumatic carditis; ankylosing spondylitis; psoriatic arthritis; rheumatoid arthritis, including juvenile rheumatoid arthritis (selected cases may require low-dose maintenance therapy). For the treatment of dermatomyositis, polymyositis, and systemic lupus erythematosus.

• *Miscellaneous* – Trichinosis with neurologic or myocardial involvement, tuberculous meningitis with subarachnoid block or impending block when used with appropriate antituberculous chemotherapy.

➤*Off-label uses:*

Juvenile idiopathic arthritis – [2] = Fair documentation. Data evaluating the safety and efficacy of triamcinolone acetonide intra-articular injections for the treatment of juvenile idiopathic arthritis (JIA) are more limited than data available for the hexacetonide salt of triamcinolone, but the results are consistently favorable. Data support use of the hexacetonide salt of triamcinolone over the acetonide salt because of its longer duration of effect. Intra-articular injections of corticosteroids are now generally considered standard care for JIA for select patient groups (uncomplicated monoarticular disease, oligoarticular disease).

Postherpetic neuralgia – [5] = Poor documentation. Results from the one noncontrolled trial conducted in the 1970s showed some benefit with intralesional triamcinolone for patients with postherpetic neuralgia (PHN). However, there were safety issues, including some significant systemic effects. The American Academy of Neurology clinical practice guidelines state that the efficacy of intralesional triamcinolone for the treatment of PHN is unproven (level U, single class intravenous [IV] study). Based on the lack of good data and the safety concerns, avoid routine use.

Administration and Dosage

➤*General dosing considerations:* Use the lowest possible dose of the corticosteroid to control the condition under treatment. When reduction in dosage is possible, the reduction should be gradual. (See Maintenance Dosage.)

➤*Adults:*

Intra-articular – For more details on specific uses, see Indications.

Kenalog-10:

• *Usual dosage* – A single local injection is frequently sufficient, but several injections may be needed for adequate relief of symptoms. Single injections into several joints, up to a total of 20 mg or more, have been given.

• *Initial dosage* – May vary from 2.5 to 5 mg for smaller joints and from 5 to 15 mg for larger joints, depending on the specific disease entity being treated.

Kenalog-40:

• *Usual dosage* – A single local injection is frequently sufficient, but several injections may be needed for adequate relief of symptoms. Single injections into several joints, up to a total of 80 mg or more, have been given.

• *Initial dosage* – May vary from 2.5 to 5 mg for smaller joints and from 5 to 15 mg for larger joints, depending on the specific disease entity being treated. Doses up to 10 mg for smaller areas and up to 40 mg for larger areas have usually been sufficient.

Trivaris:

• *Initial dosage* – May vary from 2.5 to 100 mg, depending on the specific disease entity being treated.

• *Dosage adjustment* – In certain overwhelming, acute, life-threatening situations, administration in dosages exceeding the usual dosages may be justified and may be in multiples of the oral dosages.

Intralesional – For more details on specific uses, see Indications.

Kenalog-10 only:

• *Initial dosage* – Dose per injection site will vary depending on the specific disease entity and lesion being treated.

Multiple sites separated by 1 cm or more may be injected, keeping in mind that the greater the total volume employed, the more corticosteroid becomes available for systemic absorption and systemic effects. Such injections may be repeated, if necessary, at weekly or less frequent intervals.

Intramuscular – For more details on specific uses, see Indications. *Kenalog-10* is not approved for intramuscular (IM) administration.

Kenalog-40 and *Trivaris*:

• *Initial dosage* – The suggested initial dose is 60 mg, injected deeply into the gluteal muscle. Atrophy of subcutaneous fat may occur if the injection is not properly given.

• *Dosage adjustment* – Dosage is usually adjusted within the range of 40 to 80 mg, depending upon patient response and duration of relief. However, some patients may be well controlled on doses as low as 20 mg or less. In certain overwhelming, acute, life-threatening situations, administration in dosages exceeding the usual dosages may be justified and may be in multiples of the oral dosages.

• *Acute exacerbations of multiple sclerosis* – 160 mg daily for a week, followed by 64 mg every other day for 1 month.

• *Hay fever or pollen asthma* – Patients with hay fever or pollen asthma who are not responding to pollen administration and other conventional therapy may obtain a remission of symptoms lasting throughout the pollen season after a single injection of 40 to 100 mg.

Off-label dosing –

➤*Children:*

Intra-articular – For more details on specific uses, see Indications.

Kenalog-10 only:

• *Usual dosage* – A single local injection is frequently sufficient, but several injections may be needed for adequate relief of symptoms. Single injections into several joints, up to a total of 20 mg or more, have been given.

• *Initial dosage* – May vary from 2.5 to 5 mg for smaller joints and from 5 to 15 mg for larger joints, depending on the specific disease entity being treated.

Intralesional – For more details on specific uses, see Indications.

Kenalog-10 only:

• *Initial dosage* – Dose per injection site will vary depending on the specific disease entity and lesion being treated.

Multiple sites separated by 1 cm or more may be injected, keeping in mind that the greater the total volume employed, the more corticosteroid becomes available for systemic absorption and systemic effects. Such injections may be repeated, if necessary, at weekly or less frequent intervals.

Intramuscular – For more details on specific uses, see Indications. *Kenalog-10* is not approved for IM administration.

Kenalog-40 and *Trivaris* only:

• *Initial dosage* – May vary depending on the specific disease entity being treated. The range of initial dosages is 0.11 to 1.6 mg/kg/day in 3 or 4 divided doses (3.2 to 48 mg/m^2 body surface area per day).

Off-label dosing –

Juvenile idiopathic arthritis: [2] = Fair documentation.

• *2 years of age and older* – 0.5 to 1 mg/kg, depending on the joint size, administered as intra-articular injections.

➤*Dosage adjustment:* Situations that may make dosage adjustments necessary are changes in clinical status secondary to remissions or exacerbations in the disease process, the patient's individual drug responsiveness, and the effect of patient exposure to stressful situations not directly related to the disease entity under treatment. In this latter situation, it may be necessary to increase the dosage of the corticosteroid for a period of time consistent with the patient's condition.

➤*Dosage equivalents:* For the purpose of comparison, the following is the equivalent mg dosage of the various glucocorticoids:

Equivalent Dosage of the Various Glucocorticoids[a]	
Betamethasone	0.75 mg
Cortisone	25 mg
Dexamethasone	0.75 mg
Hydrocortisone	20 mg
Methylprednisolone	4 mg
Paramethasone	2 mg
Prednisolone	5 mg
Prednisone	5 mg
Triamcinolone	4 mg

[a] These dose relationships apply only to oral or IV administration of these compounds. When these substances or their derivatives are injected IM or into joint spaces, their relative properties may be greatly altered.

➤*Maintenance dosage:* After a favorable response is noted, the proper maintenance dosage should be determined by decreasing the initial drug dosage in small decrements at appropriate time intervals until the lowest dosage that will maintain an adequate clinical response is reached.

In order to minimize the potential growth effects of corticosteroids, titrate children to the lowest effective dose.

➤*Duration of therapy:* Because complications of treatment with glucocorticoids are dependent on the size of the dose and the duration of treatment, a risk/benefit decision must be made in each individual case as to dose and duration of treatment, and as to whether daily or intermittent therapy should be used.

➤*Discontinuation of therapy:* If after long-term therapy the drug is to be stopped, it is recommended that it be withdrawn gradually rather than abruptly.

➤*Preparation for administration:*

Kenalog-10 and *Kenalog-40* – The vial should be shaken before use to ensure a uniform suspension. Prior to withdrawal, the suspension should be

TRIAMCINOLONE ACETONIDE — INJECTION

inspected for clumping or granular appearance (agglomeration). An agglomerated product results from exposure to freezing temperatures and should not be used. After withdrawal, triamcinolone injection should be injected without delay to prevent settling in the syringe.

Trivaris – Always allow the prefilled glass syringe to sit at room temperature for at least 30 minutes before the procedure.

➤*Administration:*

Trivaris – Each syringe should only be used for a single treatment. Multiple injections may be required to reach the recommended dose.

Intra-articular – Prior use of a local anesthetic may often be desirable. Care should be taken with this kind of injection, particularly in the deltoid region, to avoid injecting the suspension into the tissues surrounding the site, because this may lead to tissue atrophy.

Joints: The usual intra-articular injection technique should be followed. If an excessive amount of synovial fluid is present in the joint, some, but not all, should be aspirated to aid in the relief of pain and to prevent undue dilution of the steroid.

Acute nonspecific tenosynovitis: Care should be taken to ensure that the injection of triamcinolone is made into the tendon sheath rather than the tendon substance. Epicondylitis may be treated by infiltrating the preparation into the area of greatest tenderness.

Intralesional (Kenalog-10 only) – For treatment of dermal lesions, triamcinolone should be injected directly into the lesion (ie, intradermally, subcutaneously). For accuracy of dosage measurement and ease of administration, it is preferable to employ a tuberculin syringe and a small-bore needle (23 to 25 gauge). Ethyl chloride spray may be used to alleviate the discomfort of the injection.

Intramuscular – The injection should be made deeply into the gluteal muscle. A minimum needle length of 1.5 inches is recommended. In obese patients, a longer needle may be required. Use alternative site for subsequent injections. Because of the significantly higher incidence of local atrophy when the material is injected into the deltoid area, avoid this injection site in favor of the gluteal area.

➤*Storage/Stability:*

Kenalog-10 and *Kenalog-40* – Store at 20° to 25°C (68° to 77°F). Avoid freezing and protect from light. Triamcinolone injection, like many other steroid formulations, is sensitive to heat. Therefore, it should not be autoclaved when it is desirable to sterilize the exterior of the vial.

Trivaris – Keep refrigerated at 2° to 8°C (36° to 46°F) until use. Avoid freezing and protect from light.

TRIAMCINOLONE HEXACETONIDE

Rx	**Aristospan Intralesional** (Sandoz)	**Injection, suspension:** 5 mg/mL	In 5 mL vials.[a]
Rx	**Aristospan Intra-articular** (Sandoz)	**Injection, suspension:** 20 mg/mL	In 1 and 5 mL vials.[a]

[a] With polysorbate 80, sorbitol, and benzyl alcohol.

For complete and comparative prescribing information, refer to the Glucocorticoids class monograph.

TRIAMCINOLONE HEXACETONIDE — INTRALESIONAL

Indications

➤*Dermatologic diseases:* For the treatment of alopecia areata; discoid lupus erythematosus; keloids; localized hypertrophic, infiltrated, inflammatory lesions of granuloma annulare, lichen planus, lichen simplex chronicus (neurodermatitis), and psoriatic plaques; necrobiosis lipoidica diabeticorum; and cystic tumors of an aponeurosis or tendon (ganglia).

➤*Off-label uses:*

Postherpetic neuralgia – [5] = Poor documentation. Results from the one noncontrolled trial conducted in the 1970s showed some benefit with intralesional triamcinolone for patients with postherpetic neuralgia (PHN). However, there were safety issues, including some significant systemic effects. American Academy of Neurology clinical practice guidelines state that the efficacy of intralesional triamcinolone for the treatment of PHN is unproven (level U, single class 4 study). Based on the lack of good data and the safety concerns, routine use should be avoided.

Administration and Dosage

➤*General dosing considerations:* This product contains benzyl alcohol; do not use in newborns.

➤*Adults:*

Dermatologic diseases –

Usual dosage: Average dose is up to 0.5 mg per square inch of affected skin injected intralesionally or sublesionally. The frequency of subsequent injections is best determined by the clinical response. In certain overwhelming, acute, life-threatening situations, administration in dosages exceeding the usual dosages may be justified and may be in multiples of the oral dosages.

Initial dosage: 2 to 48 mg/day injected intralesionally or sublesionally.

Maintenance dosage: After a favorable response is noted, determine the proper maintenance dosage by decreasing the initial drug dosage in small decrements at appropriate time intervals until the lowest dosage that will maintain an adequate clinical response is reached.

Off-label dosing –

Postherpetic neuralgia: Use is not recommended. 2 mg/mL at a typical dosage of 60 mg daily was injected subcutaneously into the site of pain; injections were repeated daily until desired results were obtained. In the study reviewed, the average number of injections was 12 per patient (range, 1 to 48).

➤*Children:*

Dermatologic diseases –

30 days of age and older:

• *Usual dosage* – In certain overwhelming, acute, life-threatening situations, administration in dosages exceeding the usual dosages may be justified and may be in multiples of the oral dosages.

• *Initial dosage* – 0.11 to 1.6 mg/kg/day injected intralesionally or sublesionally in 3 or 4 divided doses (3.2 to 48 mg/m^2 body surface area/day).

• *Maintenance dosage* – After a favorable response is noted, determine the proper maintenance dosage by decreasing the initial drug dosage in small decrements at appropriate time intervals until the lowest dosage that will maintain an adequate clinical response is reached.

➤*Dosage adjustment:* When reduction in dosage is possible, the reduction must be gradual. Situations that may make dosage adjustments necessary are changes in clinical status secondary to remissions or exacerbations in the disease process, the patient's individual drug responsiveness, and the effect of patient exposure to stressful situations not directly related to the disease entity under treatment. In this latter situation, it may be necessary to increase the dosage of the corticosteroid for a period of time consistent with the patient's condition.

Increased dosage of rapidly acting corticosteroids is indicated in patients on corticosteroid therapy subjected to any unusual stress before, during, and after the stressful situation.

➤*Discontinuation of therapy:* If, after long-term therapy, the drug is to be stopped, it is recommended that it be withdrawn gradually rather than abruptly.

➤*Preparation for administration:* Triamcinolone may be mixed with lidocaine 1% or 2%, using the formulations that do not contain parabens. Similar local anesthetics may also be used. These dilutions will retain full potency for 1 week, but exercise care to avoid contamination of the vial's contents and discard the dilutions after 7 days.

Triamcinolone may also be diluted, if desired, with dextrose and sodium chloride injection (dextrose 5% and 10%), sodium chloride injection, or sterile water for injection.

The optimum dilution (ie, 1:1, 1:2, 1:4) should be determined by the nature of the lesion, its size, the depth of injection, the volume needed, and location of the lesion. In general, perform more superficial injections with greater dilution. Certain conditions, such as keloids, require a less diluted suspension, such as 5 mg/mL, with variation in dose and dilution as dictated by the condition of the individual patient. Subsequent dosage, dilution, and frequency of injections are best judged by the clinical response.

Gently agitate the syringe to achieve uniform suspension before use. Because this product has been designed for ease of administration, a small-bore needle (not smaller than 24 gauge) may be used.

➤*Administration:* For intralesional administration; not for IV use. Injection of a steroid into an infected site is to be avoided. Strict aseptic administration technique is mandatory. Topical ethylchloride spray may be used locally before injection.

A lesser initial dosage range of triamcinolone may produce the desired effect when the drug is administered to provide a localized concentration. The site of the injection and the volume of the injection should be considered carefully when triamcinolone is administered for this purpose.

➤*Admixture compatibility:*

Compatibility – Triamcinolone may be mixed with lidocaine 1% or 2%, using the formulations that do not contain parabens. Similar local anesthetics may also be used. Triamcinolone may also be diluted, if desired, with dextrose and sodium chloride injection (dextrose 5% and 10%), sodium chloride injection, or sterile water for injection.

Incompatibility – Diluents containing methylparaben, propylparaben, phenol, etc, should be avoided because these compounds may cause flocculation of the steroid.

➤*Storage/Stability:* Store at 20° to 25°C (68° to 77°F). Protect from light. Do not freeze. Diluted solutions of triamcinolone will retain full potency for 1 week; discard the dilutions after 7 days. This product, like many other steroid formulations, is sensitive to heat. Therefore, do not autoclave when it is desirable to sterilize the exterior of the vial.

TRIAMCINOLONE HEXACETONIDE — INTRA-ARTICULAR

For complete and comparative prescribing information, refer to the Glucocorticoids class monograph.

Indications

➤*Adjunctive therapy:* As adjunctive therapy for short-term administration (to tide the patient over an acute episode or exacerbation) in acute gouty arthritis, acute and subacute bursitis, acute nonspecific tenosynovitis, epicondylitis, rheumatoid arthritis (RA), or synovitis of osteoarthritis.

➤*Off-label uses:*

Juvenile idiopathic arthritis – [2] = Fair documentation. Data evaluating the safety and efficacy of triamcinolone hexacetonide intra-articular injections for the treatment of juvenile idiopathic arthritis (JIA) date back many years and consistently show favorable results. Intra-articular injections of corticosteroids are now generally considered standard care for JIA for select patient groups (uncomplicated monoarticular disease, oligoarticular disease), with data supporting triamcinolone hexacetonide as the preferred product because of its longer duration of effect.

Administration and Dosage

➤*General dosing considerations:* This product contains benzyl alcohol; do not use in newborns.

Intra-articular injection may result in damage to joint tissues.

➤*Adults:*

Adjunctive therapy –

Usual dosage: 2 to 20 mg (0.1 to 1 mL). The dose depends on the size of the joint to be injected, the degree of inflammation, and the amount of fluid present. In general, large joints (eg, hip, knee, shoulder) require 10 to 20 mg. For small joints (eg, interphalangeal, metacarpophalangeal), 2 to 6 mg may be employed. The usual frequency of injection into a single joint is every 3 or 4 weeks; injection more frequently than that is generally not advisable

In certain overwhelming, acute, life-threatening situations, administration in dosages exceeding the usual dosages may be justified and may be in multiples of the oral dosages.

Maintenance dosage: After a favorable response is noted, the proper maintenance dosage should be determined by decreasing the initial drug dosage in small decrements at appropriate time intervals to the lowest dosage that will maintain an adequate clinical response is reached.

➤*Children:*

Adjunctive therapy –

30 days of age and older:

• *Usual dosage* – The dose depends on the size of the joint to be injected, the degree of inflammation, and the amount of fluid present. The usual frequency of injection into a single joint is every 3 or 4 weeks; injection more frequently than that is generally not advisable

In certain overwhelming, acute, life-threatening situations, administration in dosages exceeding the usual dosages may be justified and may be in multiples of the oral dosages.

• *Initial dosage* – 0.11 to 1.6 mg/kg/day in 3 or 4 divided doses (3.2 to 48 mg/m² body surface area/day).

• *Maintenance dosage* – After a favorable response is noted, the proper maintenance dosage should be determined by decreasing the initial drug dosage in small decrements at appropriate time intervals to the lowest dosage that will maintain an adequate clinical response is reached.

Off-label dosing –

Juvenile idiopathic arthritis: [2] = Fair documentation. Intra-articular injections were given as fixed doses (20 to 40 mg per joint) or weight-based doses (typically 1 mg/kg; maximum dose, 60 mg). Larger joints (eg, knee) usually received 40 mg doses and smaller joints (eg, elbow, ankle) received smaller doses (20 mg). A review of the literature suggests doses of 1 mg/kg for larger joints (hips, knees, shoulders) and 0.5 mg/kg for smaller joints (elbows, wrists, ankles).

➤*Dosage adjustment:* When reduction in dosage is possible, the reduction should be gradual. Situations that may make dosage adjustments necessary are changes in clinical status secondary to remissions or exacerbations in the disease process, the patient's individual drug responsiveness, and the effect of patient exposure to stressful situations not directly related to the disease entity under treatment. In this latter situation, it may be necessary to increase the dosage of the corticosteroid for a period of time consistent with the patient's condition.

Increased dosage of rapidly acting corticosteroids is indicated in patients on corticosteroid therapy subjected to any unusual stress before, during, and after the stressful situation.

➤*Discontinuation of therapy:* If after long-term therapy the drug is to be stopped it is recommended that it be withdrawn gradually rather than abruptly.

➤*Preparation for administration:* Triamcinolone may be mixed with lidocaine hydrochloride 1% or 2%, using the formulations that do not contain parabens. Similar local anesthetics may also be used. These dilutions will retain full potency for 1 week, but care should be exercised to avoid contamination of the vials contents, and the dilutions should be discarded after 7 days.

When the amount of synovial fluid is increased, aspiration may be performed before administering triamcinolone. The syringe should be gently agitated to achieve uniform suspension before use. Because this product has been designed for ease of administration, a small-bore needle (not smaller than 24 gauge) may be used.

➤*Administration:* For intra-articular use; not for IV use. Injection of a steroid into an infected site is to be avoided. Local injection of a steroid into a previously infected joint is not usually recommended. Corticosteroid injection into unstable joints is generally not recommended. Strict aseptic administration technique is mandatory. Topical ethylchloride spray may be used locally before injection.

To avoid possible joint destruction from repeated use of intra-articular corticosteroids, injection should be as infrequent as possible, consistent with adequate patient care. Attention should be paid to avoiding deposition of drug along the needle path, which might produce atrophy.

Appropriate examination of any joint fluid present is necessary to exclude a septic process.

A marked increase in pain accompanied by local swelling, further restriction of joint motion, fever, and malaise are suggestive of septic arthritis. If this complication occurs and the diagnosis of sepsis is confirmed, institute appropriate antimicrobial therapy.

These dose relationships apply only to oral or IV administration of these compounds. When these substances or their derivatives are injected IM or into joint spaces, their relative properties may be greatly altered.

➤*Admixture compatibility:*

Compatibility – Triamcinolone may be mixed with lidocaine hydrochloride 1% or 2%, using the formulations that do not contain parabens. Similar local anesthetics may also be used.

Incompatibility – Diluents containing methylparaben, propylparaben, or phenol should be avoided because these compounds may cause flocculation of the steroid.

➤*Storage/Stability:* Store at 20° to 25°C (68° to 77°F). Protect from light. Do not freeze. Diluted solutions of triamcinolone will retain full potency for 1 week; discard the dilutions after 7 days. This product, like many other steroid formulations, is sensitive to heat. Therefore, do not autoclave triamcinolone when it is desirable to sterilize the exterior of the vial.

Mineralocorticoids

FLUDROCORTISONE ACETATE

Rx	**Fludrocortisone Acetate** (Various, eg, Global)	**Tablets:** 0.1 mg	In 100s.
Rx	**Florinef Acetate** (Monarch)		Lactose. (429). White, scored. In 100s.

FLUDROCORTISONE ACETATE — ORAL

Indications

➤*Addison disease/Adrenogenital syndrome:* Partial replacement therapy for primary and secondary adrenocortical insufficiency in Addison disease and for the treatment of salt-losing adrenogenital syndrome.

➤*Off-label uses:* Fludrocortisone has been used in the management of symptomatic orthostatic hypotension.

Fludrocortisone has been used in children for the treatment of Addison disease/adrenogenital syndrome and congenital adrenal hyperplasia.

Administration and Dosage

➤*General dosing considerations:* Dosage depends on the severity of the disease and the response of the patient. Continually monitor patients for signs that indicate dosage adjustment is necessary, such as remissions or exacerbations of the disease and stress (surgery, infection, trauma).

Use the lowest possible dose of corticosteroid to control the condition being treated. Make a gradual reduction in dosage when possible. Adverse reactions to corticosteroids may be produced by too-rapid withdrawal or by continued use of large doses.

➤*Adults:*

Addison disease –

Usual dosage: 0.1 mg/day (range, 0.1 mg 3times weekly to 0.2 mg/day).

Dosage adjustment: Reduce the dose to 0.05 mg/day if transient hypertension develops as a consequence of therapy.

Concomitant therapy: Administration in conjunction with cortisone (10 to 37.5 mg/day in divided doses) or hydrocortisone (10 to 30 mg/day in divided doses) is preferable. In Addison disease, the combination of fludrocortisone acetate tablets with a glucocorticoid such as hydrocortisone or cortisone provides substitution therapy approximating normal adrenal activity with minimal risks of unwanted effects.

Salt-losing adrenogenital syndrome – 0.1 to 0.2 mg/day.

➤*Storage/Stability:* Store at room temperature; avoid excessive heat.

FLUDROCORTISONE ACETATE — ORAL

Actions

➤*Pharmacology:* Fludrocortisone is a synthetic, adrenocortical steroid with potent mineralocorticoid properties and high glucocorticoid activity; it is used only for its mineralocorticoid effects.

The physiological action of fludrocortisone is similar to that of hydrocortisone. However, the effects of fludrocortison, particularly on electrolyte balance, but also on carbohydrate metabolism, are considerably heightened and prolonged. Mineralocorticoids act on the renal distal tubules to enhance the reabsorption of sodium. They increase urinary excretion of both potassium and hydrogen ions. The consequence of these 3 primary effects together with similar actions on cation transport in other tissues appears to account for the spectrum of physiological activities characteristic of mineralocorticoids.

In small oral doses, fludrocortisone produces marked sodium retention and increased urinary potassium excretion. It also causes a rise in blood pressure, apparently because of these effects on electrolyte levels. In larger doses, fludrocortisone inhibits endogenous adrenal cortical secretion, thymic activity, and pituitary corticotropin excretion, promotes the deposition of liver glycogen, and, unless protein intake is adequate, induces negative nitrogen balance.

➤*Pharmacokinetics:* Plasma half-life is approximately 3.5 hours; biological half-life ranges from 18 to 36 hours.

Contraindications

Hypersensitivity to fludrocortisone; systemic fungal infections.

Warnings/Precautions

➤*Sodium retention:* Because of its marked effect on sodium retention, the use of fludrocortisone in the treatment of conditions other than those indicated is not advised.

➤*Infections:* Corticosteroids may mask some signs of infection, and new infections may appear during their use. There may be decreased resistance and inability to localize infection when corticosteroids are used. If an infection occurs during fludrocortisone acetate therapy, it should be controlled promptly by suitable antimicrobial therapy.

Tuberculosis – Restrict the use of fludrocortisone acetate tablets in patients with active tuberculosis to cases of fulminating or disseminated tuberculosis in which the corticosteroid is used for the management of the disease in conjunction with an appropriate antituberculous regimen. If corticosteroids are indicated in patients with latent tuberculosis or tuberculin reactivity, close observation is necessary because reactivation of the disease may occur. During prolonged corticosteroid therapy, these patients should receive chemoprophylaxis.

Children – Children who are on immunosuppressant drugs are more susceptible to infections than healthy children. Chicken pox and measles, for example, can have a more serious or even fatal course in children on immunosuppressant corticosteroids. In such children, or in adults who have not had these diseases, take particular care to avoid exposure. If exposed, therapy with varicella zoster immune globulin or pooled IV immunoglobulin, as appropriate, may be indicated. If chicken pox develops, consider treatment with antiviral agents.

➤*Ocular effects:* Prolonged use of corticosteroids may produce posterior subcapsular cataracts and glaucoma with possible damage to the optic nerves and may enhance the establishment of secondary ocular infections caused by fungi or viruses.

Use corticosteroids cautiously in patients with ocular herpes simplex because of possible corneal perforation.

➤*Adrenal insufficiency:* To avoid drug-induced adrenal insufficiency, supportive dosage may be required in times of stress (eg, trauma, surgery, severe illness), both during treatment with fludrocortisone and for a year afterwards.

➤*Fluid and electrolyte balance:* Average and large doses of hydrocortisone or cortisone can cause elevation of blood pressure, retention of salt and water, and increased excretion of potassium. These effects are less likely to occur with the synthetic derivatives except when they are used in large doses. However, because fludrocortisone is a potent mineralocorticoid, carefully monitor the dosage and salt intake in order to avoid the development of hypertension, edema, or weight gain. Periodic checking of serum electrolyte levels is advisable during prolonged therapy; dietary salt restriction and potassium supplementation may be necessary. All corticosteroids increase calcium excretion.

➤*Vaccinations:* Do not vaccinate patients against smallpox while they are on corticosteroid therapy. Do not undertake other immunization procedures in patients who are on corticosteroids, especially high doses because of possible hazards of neurological complications and a lack of antibody response.

➤*Use with caution:*

GI – Use corticosteroids with caution in patients with nonspecific ulcerative colitis if there is a probability of impending perforation, abscess, or other pyogenic infection and in patients with diverticulitis, fresh intestinal anastomoses, or active or latent peptic ulcer.

Miscellaneous – There is an enhanced corticosteroid effect in patients with hypothyroidism and cirrhosis. Use with caution in patients with renal insufficiency, hypertension, osteoporosis, and myasthenia gravis.

➤*Psychiatric effects:* Psychic derangements may appear when corticosteroids are used. These may range from euphoria, insomnia, mood swings, personality changes, and severe depression to frank psychotic manifestations. Corticosteroids also may aggravate existing emotional instability or psychotic tendencies.

➤*Pregnancy: Category C.* Adequate animal reproduction studies have not been conducted with fludrocortisone acetate. However, many corticosteroids have been shown to be teratogenic in laboratory animals at low doses. Teratogenicity of these agents in humans has not been demonstrated. It is not known whether fludrocortisone acetate can cause fetal harm when administered to a pregnant woman or can affect reproduction capacity. Give fludrocortisone acetate to a pregnant woman only if clearly needed.

Carefully observe infants born of mothers who have received substantial doses of fludrocortisone acetate during pregnancy for signs of hypoadrenalism.

➤*Lactation:* Corticosteroids are found in the breast milk of lactating women. Exercise caution when administering these drugs to nursing women.

➤*Children:* Safety and efficacy in children have not been established. Monitor growth and development of infants and children on prolonged therapy.

➤*Monitoring:* Regularly monitor patients for blood pressure and serum electrolyte determinations.

Drug Interactions

Fludrocortisone Drug Interactions

Precipitant drug	Object drug[a]		Description
Anabolic steroids	Fludrocortisone	↑	Concurrent use may enhance the tendency toward edema. Use with caution, especially in patients with hepatic or cardiac disease.
Barbiturates Hydantoins Rifamycins	Fludrocortisone	↓	Fludrocortisone hepatic metabolism may be increased, resulting in decreased therapeutic effects.
Estrogens	Fludrocortisone	↑	Corticosteroid metabolism may be decreased.
Fludrocortisone	Amphotericin B Potassium-depleting diuretics	↑	Coadministration may enhance hypokalemia. Check serum potassium levels at frequent intervals. Use potassium supplements if necessary.
Fludrocortisone	Anticholinesterases	↓	Although fludrocortisone is not used to treat myasthenia gravis, corticosteroids may antagonize the effects of anticholinesterases in myasthenia gravis.
Fludrocortisone	Anticoagulants, oral	↑↓	Anticoagulant dose requirements may be reduced. Conversely, corticosteroids may oppose the anticoagulant action. Monitor prothrombin time and adjust dose accordingly.
Fludrocortisone	Antidiabetic agents (oral agents and insulin)	↓	Antidiabetic effect may be decreased. Monitor for signs of hyperglycemia; adjust dose of antidiabetic agent if necessary.
Fludrocortisone	Digitalis glycosides	↑	Coadministration may enhance the possibility of arrhythmias or digitalis toxicity associated with hypokalemia. Monitor serum potassium levels and use potassium supplements if necessary.
Fludrocortisone	Nondepolarizing muscle relaxants	↓	Corticosteroids may decrease the actions of the nondepolarizing muscle relaxants.
Fludrocortisone	Salicylates	↑↓	Corticosteroids will reduce serum salicylate levels and may decrease their effectiveness. Coadministration also may increase the ulcerogenic effects of each.
Fludrocortisone	Vaccines	↑↓	Concurrent use may increase neurological complications and decrease antibody response (see Warnings).

[a] ↑ = Object increased. ↓ = Object decreased.

➤*Drug/Lab test interactions:* Corticosteroids may affect the nitrobluetetrazollum test for bacterial infection and produce false-negative results.

Adverse Reactions

Most adverse reactions are caused by fludrocortisone's mineralocorticoid activity (retention of sodium and water). When fludrocortisone is used in the small dosages recommended, the glucocorticoid side effects often seen with cortisone and its derivatives are not usually a problem; however, keep in

FLUDROCORTISONE ACETATE — ORAL

mind the following untoward effects, particularly when fludrocortisone is used over a prolonged period of time or in conjunction with cortisone or a similar glucocorticoid.

➤*Cardiovascular:* Hypertension; CHF; cardiac enlargement.

➤*CNS:* Convulsions; increased intracranial pressure with papilledema (pseudotumor cerebri), usually after treatment; vertigo; headache; severe mental disturbances.

➤*Dermatologic:* Allergic skin rash; maculopapular rash; urticaria; impaired wound healing; thin, fragile skin; bruising; petechiae and ecchymoses; facial erythema; increased sweating; subcutaneous fat atrophy; purpura; striae; hyperpigmentation of skin and nails; hirsutism; acneiform eruptions; hives. Reactions to skin tests may be suppressed.

➤*Endocrine:* Menstrual irregularities; development of the cushingoid state; suppression of growth in children; secondary adrenocortical and pituitary unresponsiveness, particularly in times of stress (eg, trauma, surgery, illness); decreased carbohydrate tolerance; manifestations of latent diabetes mellitus; increased requirements for insulin or oral hypoglycemic agents in diabetics.

➤*GI:* Peptic ulcer with possible perforation and hemorrhage; pancreatitis; abdominal distention; ulcerative esophagitis.

➤*Metabolic:* Hyperglycemia; glycosuria; negative nitrogen balance caused by protein catabolism; potassium loss; edema; hypokalemic alkalosis.

➤*Musculoskeletal:* Muscle weakness; steroid myopathy; loss of muscle mass; osteoporosis; vertebral compression fractures; aseptic necrosis of femoral and humeral heads; pathologic fracture of long bones; spontaneous fractures.

➤*Ophthalmic:* Posterior subcapsular cataracts; increased intraocular pressure; glaucoma; exophthalmos.

➤*Miscellaneous:* Necrotizing angiitis; thrombophlebitis; aggravation or masking of infections; insomnia; syncopal episodes; anaphylactoid reactions.

Overdosage

➤*Symptoms:* Hypertension; edema; hypokalemia; excessive weight gain; increase in heart size.

➤*Treatment:* Discontinue the drug; symptoms usually subside within several days. Resume subsequent treatment with reduced doses. Muscular weakness may develop because of excessive potassium loss; treat with potassium supplements. Monitor blood pressure and serum electrolytes regularly.

Patient Information

Notify physician if dizziness, severe or continuing headaches, swelling of feet or lower legs, or unusual weight gain occurs.

Warn patients who are on immunosuppressant doses of corticosteroids to avoid exposure to chicken pox or measles and, if exposed, to obtain medical advice.

Advise the patient to use the medicine only as directed, to take a missed dose as soon as possible, unless it is almost time for the next dose, and not to double the next dose.

PARATHYROID HORMONE

TERIPARATIDE, rDNA origin

Rx	**Forteo** (Eli Lilly)	**Injection, solution:** 250 mcg/mL[a]	In 2.4 mL prefilled pen that delivers teriparatide 20 mcg per dose.

[a] With mannitol 45.4 mg and metacresol 3 mg.

TERIPARATIDE — INJECTION

WARNING

Potential risk of osteosarcoma – In male and female rats, teriparatide caused an increase in the incidence of osteosarcoma (a malignant bone tumor) that was dependent on dose and treatment duration. The effect was observed at systemic exposures to teriparatide ranging from 3 to 60 times the exposure in humans given a 20 mcg dose. Because of the uncertain relevance of the rat osteosarcoma finding to humans, prescribe teriparatide only to patients for whom the potential benefits are considered to outweigh the potential risk. Teriparatide should not be prescribed for patients who are at increased baseline risk for osteosarcoma (eg, those with Paget disease of bone or unexplained elevations of alkaline phosphatase, children and young adult patients with open epiphyses, or patients with prior external beam or implant radiation therapy involving the skeleton).

Indications

➤*Glucocorticoid-induced osteoporosis:* Treatment of men and women with osteoporosis associated with sustained systemic glucocorticoid therapy (daily dosage equivalent to prednisone 5 mg or more) at high risk for fracture.

➤*Osteoporosis in men:* To increase bone mass in men with primary or hypogonadal osteoporosis who are at high risk for fracture.

➤*Osteoporosis in postmenopausal women:* For the treatment of postmenopausal women with osteoporosis who are at high risk for fracture.

Administration and Dosage

➤*Adults:*

Osteoporosis –

Usual dosage: 20 mcg subcutaneously once a day.

Duration of therapy: Use of the drug for more than 2 years is not recommended.

➤*Administration:* Teriparatide should be administered as a subcutaneous injection into the thigh or abdominal wall. Teriparatide should be administered initially under circumstances in which the patient can sit or lie down if symptoms of orthostatic hypotension occur.

➤*Storage/Stability:* Store at 2° to 8°C (36° to 46°F). Recap the delivery device when not in use to protect the cartridge from physical damage and light. During the use period, time out of the refrigerator should be minimized; the dose may be delivered immediately following removal from the refrigerator. Do not freeze. Do not use teriparatide if it has been frozen.

Each teriparatide delivery device can be used for up to 28 days after the first injection. After the 28-day use period, discard the teriparatide delivery device, even if it still contains some unused solution.

Actions

➤*Pharmacology:* Endogenous 84-amino-acid parathyroid hormone (PTH) is the primary regulator of calcium and phosphate metabolism in bone and kidney. Physiological actions of PTH include regulation of bone metabolism, renal tubular reabsorption of calcium and phosphate, and intestinal calcium absorption. The biological actions of PTH and teriparatide are mediated through binding to specific high-affinity cell-surface receptors. Teriparatide and the 34 N-terminal amino acids of PTH bind to these receptors with the same affinity and have the same physiological actions on bone and kidney. Teriparatide is not expected to accumulate in bone or other tissues.

The skeletal effects of teriparatide depend upon the pattern of systemic exposure. Once-daily administration of teriparatide stimulates new bone formation on trabecular and cortical (periosteal and/or endosteal) bone surfaces by preferential stimulation of osteoblastic activity over osteoclastic activity. In monkey studies, teriparatide improved trabecular microarchitecture and increased bone mass and strength by stimulating new bone formation in cancellous and cortical bone. In humans, the anabolic effects of teriparatide are manifest as an increase in skeletal mass, an increase in markers of bone formation and resorption, and an increase in bone strength. By contrast, continuous excess of endogenous PTH, as occurs in hyperparathyroidism, may be detrimental to the skeleton because bone resorption may be stimulated more than bone formation.

➤*Pharmacokinetics:*

Absorption/Distribution – Teriparatide is absorbed after subcutaneous injection; the absolute bioavailability is approximately 95% based on pooled data from 20, 40, and 80 mcg doses. The rates of absorption and elimination are rapid. The peptide reaches peak serum concentrations approximately 30 minutes after subcutaneous injection of a 20 mcg dose and declines to nonquantifiable concentrations within 3 hours.

Volume of distribution, following intravenous (IV) injection, is approximately 0.12 L/kg. Intersubject variability in systemic clearance and volume of distribution is 25% to 50%.

Metabolism/Excretion – No metabolism or excretion studies have been performed with teriparatide. However, the mechanisms of metabolism and elimination of PTH(1-34) and intact PTH have been extensively described in published literature. Peripheral metabolism of PTH is believed to occur by nonspecific enzymatic mechanisms in the liver followed by excretion via the kidneys. Systemic clearance of teriparatide (approximately 62 L/h in women and 94 L/h in men) exceeds the rate of normal liver plasma flow, consistent with hepatic and extrahepatic clearance. The half-life of teriparatide in serum is 5 minutes when administered by IV injection and approximately 1 hour when administered by subcutaneous injection. The longer half-life following subcutaneous administration reflects the time required for absorption from the injection site.

Special populations –

Renal function impairment: In 5 patients with severe renal impairment (creatinine clearance [CrCl] less than 30 mL/min), the area under the curve (AUC) and half-life of teriparatide were increased by 73% and 77%, respectively. Maximum serum concentration (C_{max}) of teriparatide was not increased.

Gender: Although systemic exposure to teriparatide was approximately 20% to 30% lower in men than women, the recommended dosage for both genders is 20 mcg/day.

TERIPARATIDE — INJECTION

Contraindications

Hypersensitivity (eg, anaphylaxis, angioedema) to teriparatide or any of its excipients.

Warnings/Precautions

➤*Osteosarcoma:* See the Warning box for more information.

Encourage patients to enroll in the voluntary teriparatide patient registry, which is designed to collect information about any potential risk of osteosarcoma in patients who have taken teriparatide. Enrollment information can be obtained by calling 1-866-382-6813, or by visiting http://www.forteoregistry.rti.org.

➤*Long-term therapy:* See Administration and Dosage for more information.

➤*Urolithiasis or preexisting hypercalciuria:* In clinical trials, the frequency of urolithiasis was similar in patients treated with teriparatide and placebo; however, teriparatide has not been studied in patients with active urolithiasis. If active urolithiasis or preexisting hypercalciuria are suspected, consider measurement of urinary calcium excretion. Use teriparatide with caution in patients with active or recent urolithiasis because of the potential to exacerbate this condition.

➤*Orthostatic hypotension:* Administer teriparatide initially under circumstances in which the patient can sit or lie down if symptoms of orthostatic hypotension occur. In short-term clinical pharmacology studies with teriparatide, transient episodes of symptomatic orthostatic hypotension were observed in 5% of patients. Typically, an event began within 4 hours of dosing and spontaneously resolved within a few minutes to a few hours. When transient orthostatic hypotension occurred, it happened within the first several doses, it was relieved by placing the person in a reclining position, and it did not preclude continued treatment.

➤*Immunogenicity:* In a large clinical trial, antibodies that cross-reacted with teriparatide were detected in 3% of women receiving teriparatide. Generally, antibodies were first detected following 12 months of treatment and diminished after withdrawal of therapy. There was no evidence of hypersensitivity reactions or allergic reactions among these patients. Antibody formation did not appear to have effects on serum calcium or bone mineral density (BMD) response.

➤*Renal function impairment:* See Actions for more information.

➤*Special risk:* Do not treat patients with teriparatide if they have bone metastases, a history of skeletal malignancies, or metabolic bone diseases other than osteoporosis.

Teriparatide has not been studied in patients with preexisting hypercalcemia. Do not treat these patients with teriparatide because of the possibility of exacerbating hypercalcemia. Do not treat patients known to have an underlying hypercalcemic disorder, such as primary hyperparathyroidism, with teriparatide.

➤*Pregnancy: Category C.* There are no adequate and well-controlled studies of teriparatide in pregnant women. Use teriparatide during pregnancy only if the potential benefit justifies the potential risk to the fetus.

In animal studies, pregnant mice received teriparatide during organogenesis at subcutaneous doses 8 to 267 times the human dose. At doses 60 or more times the human dose, the fetuses showed an increased incidence of skeletal deviations or variations (eg, interrupted rib, extra vertebra or rib). When pregnant rats received subcutaneous teriparatide during organogenesis at doses 16 to 540 times the human dose, the fetuses showed no abnormal findings.

In a perinatal/postnatal study, pregnant rats received subcutaneous teriparatide from organogenesis through lactation. Mild growth retardation occurred in female offspring at doses 120 times the human dose or more (based on surface area, mcg/m^2). Mild growth retardation in male offspring and reduced motor activity in male and female offspring occurred at maternal doses 540 times the human dose. There were no developmental or reproductive effects in mice or rats at doses 8 or 16 times the human dose, respectively.

Exposure multiples were normalized based on body surface area (mcg/m^2). Actual animal doses: mice (30 to 1,000 mcg/kg/day); rats (30 to 1,000 mcg/kg/day).

➤*Lactation:* It is not known whether teriparatide is excreted in human milk. Given the high molecular weight and low oral bioavailability of teriparatide, it is unlikely to cross into breast milk or be absorbed by the breastfeeding infant. Because of the potential for tumorigenicity shown for teriparatide in animal studies, make a decision to discontinue breastfeeding or the drug, taking into account the importance of the drug to the mother.

➤*Children:* The safety and efficacy of teriparatide have not been established in children.

See the Warning box for more information.

➤*Elderly:* Reported clinical experience has not identified differences in responses between elderly and younger patients, but greater sensitivity of some older individuals cannot be ruled out.

➤*Monitoring:* Monitor serum calcium and phosphorus as needed. If active urolithiasis or preexisting hypercalciuria are suspected, consider measurement of urinary calcium excretion.

Drug Interactions

Teriparatide Drug Interactions

Precipitant drug	Object drug[a]		Description
Loop diuretic (eg, furosemide)	Teriparatide	↑	In a study of 9 healthy subjects and 17 patients with mild, moderate, or severe renal insufficiency (CrCl 13 to 72 mL/min), coadministration of IV furosemide (20 to 100 mg) with teriparatide 40 mcg resulted in small increases in the serum calcium (2%) and 24-hour urine calcium (37%) responses to teriparatide that did not appear to be clinically important.
Thiazide diuretics (eg, hydrochlorothiazide)	Teriparatide	↓	In a study of 20 healthy subjects, the coadministration of hydrochlorothiazide 25 mg with teriparatide did not affect the serum calcium response to teriparatide 40 mcg. The 24-hour urine excretion of calcium was reduced by a clinically unimportant amount (15%). The effect of giving a higher dose of hydrochlorothiazide with teriparatide on serum calcium levels has not been studied.
Teriparatide	Digoxin	↑	Hypercalcemia may predispose patients to digitalis toxicity. Because teriparatide transiently increases serum calcium (4 to 6 hours postdose), use teriparatide with caution in patients taking digoxin.

[a] ↑ = object drug increased; ↓= object drug decreased.

Adverse Reactions

➤*Osteoporosis in men and postmenopausal women:*

Mortality – The incidence of all-cause mortality was 1% in the teriparatide group and 1% in the placebo group.

Serious adverse reactions – The incidence of serious adverse reactions was 16% in teriparatide patients and 19% in placebo patients.

Discontinuation – Early discontinuation because of adverse reactions occurred in 7% of teriparatide patients and 6% of placebo patients.

Teriparatide Adverse Reactions in Men and Postmenopausal Women With Osteoporosis (≥ 2%)[a]

Adverse reaction	Teriparatide (n = 691)	Placebo (n = 691)
Cardiovascular		
Angina pectoris	2.5%	1.6%
Hypertension	7.1%	6.8%
Syncope	2.6%	1.4%
CNS		
Asthenia	8.7%	6.8%
Depression	4.1%	2.7%
Dizziness	8%	5.4%
Headache	7.5%	7.4%
Insomnia	4.3%	3.6%
Vertigo	3.8%	2.7%
Dermatologic		
Rash	4.9%	4.5%
Sweating	2.2%	1.7%
GI		
Constipation	5.4%	4.5%
Diarrhea	5.1%	4.6%
Dyspepsia	5.2%	4.1%
GI disorder	2.3%	2%
Nausea	8.5%	6.7%
Tooth disorder	2%	1.3%
Vomiting	3%	2.3%
Musculoskeletal		
Arthralgia	10.1%	8.4%
Leg cramps	2.6%	1.3%

TERIPARATIDE — INJECTION

Teriparatide Adverse Reactions in Men and Postmenopausal Women With Osteoporosis (≥ 2%)[a]

Adverse reaction	Teriparatide (n = 691)	Placebo (n = 691)
Respiratory		
Dyspnea	3.6%	2.6%
Increased cough	6.4%	5.5%
Pharyngitis	5.5%	4.8%
Pneumonia	3.9%	3.3%
Rhinitis	9.6%	8.8%
Miscellaneous		
Neck pain	3%	2.7%
Pain	21.3%	20.5%

[a] Adverse reactions are shown without attribution of causality.

➤*Glucocorticoid-induced osteoporosis:*

Mortality – The incidence of all-cause mortality was 4% in the teriparatide group and 6% in the active control group.

Serious adverse reactions – The incidence of serious adverse reactions was 21% in teriparatide patients and 18% in active control patients and included pneumonia (3% teriparatide, 1% active control).

Discontinuation – Early discontinuation because of adverse reactions occurred in 15% of teriparatide patients and 12% of active control patients and included dizziness (2% teriparatide, 0% active control).

Adverse reactions –
CNS: Insomnia (5%, 1%), anxiety (4%, 1%).
GI: Nausea (14%, 7%), gastritis (7%, 3%).
Respiratory: Dyspnea (6%, 3%), pneumonia (6%, 3%).
Miscellaneous: Herpes zoster (3%, 1%).

➤*Lab test abnormalities:*

Serum calcium – Teriparatide transiently increases serum calcium, with the maximal effect observed at approximately 4 to 6 hours postdose. Serum calcium measured at least 16 hours postdose was not different from pretreatment levels. In clinical trials, the frequency of at least 1 episode of transient hypercalcemia in the 4 to 6 hours after teriparatide administration was increased from 2% of women and none of the men treated with placebo to 11% of women and 6% of men treated with teriparatide. The number of patients treated with teriparatide whose transient hypercalcemia was verified on consecutive measurements was 3% of women and 1% of men.

Urinary calcium – Teriparatide increases urinary calcium excretion, but the frequency of hypercalciuria in clinical trials was similar for patients treated with teriparatide and placebo.

Uric acid – Teriparatide increases serum uric acid concentrations. In clinical trials, 3% of teriparatide patients had serum uric acid concentrations above the upper limit of normal (ULN) compared with 1% of placebo patients; however, the hyperuricemia did not result in an increase in gout, arthralgia, or urolithiasis.

➤*Postmarketing:*

Hypersensitivity – Anaphylactic reactions, angioedema, drug hypersensitivity, urticaria (temporally, but not necessarily causally, related to teriparatide).

Local – Injection-site reactions, including injection-site pain, swelling, and bruising (temporally, but not necessarily causally, related to teriparatide).

Respiratory – Acute dyspnea, chest pain (temporally, but not necessarily causally, related to teriparatide).

Miscellaneous – Bone turnover, hypercalcemia great than 13 mg/dL, osteosarcoma, hyperuricemia, muscle spasms of the leg or back, oro-facial edema (temporally, but not necessarily causally, related to teriparatide).

Overdosage

➤*Symptoms:* The effects of overdose that might be expected include a delayed hypercalcemic effect and risk of orthostatic hypotension. Nausea, vomiting, dizziness, and headache might also occur.

In postmarketing spontaneous reports, there have been cases of medication errors in which the entire contents (up to 800 mcg) of the teriparatide delivery device (pen) have been administered as a single dose. Transient events reported have included nausea, weakness/lethargy, and hypotension. In some cases, no adverse events occurred as a result of the overdose. No fatalities associated with overdose have been reported.

➤*Treatment:* There is no specific antidote for teriparatide. Treatment of suspected overdose includes discontinuation of teriparatide, monitoring of serum calcium and phosphorus, and implementation of appropriate supportive measures, such as hydration.

Patient Information

Advise patients to read the Medication Guide and delivery device user manual before starting therapy with teriparatide and reread them each time the prescription is renewed. Patients need to understand and follow the instructions in the teriparatide delivery device user manual. Failure to do so may result in inaccurate dosing.

Inform patients that in rats, teriparatide caused an increase in the incidence of osteosarcoma (a malignant bone tumor) that was dependent on dose and treatment duration. Encourage patients to enroll in the voluntary teriparatide patient registry, which is designed to collect information about any potential risk of osteosarcoma in patients who have taken teriparatide. Enrollment information can be obtained by calling 1-866-382-6813 or by visiting http://www.forteoregistry.rti.org.

Administer teriparatide initially under circumstances where the patient can immediately sit or lie down if symptoms occur. Instruct patients that if they feel light-headed or have palpitations after the injection, they should sit or lie down until the symptoms resolve. If symptoms persist or worsen, instruct patients to consult a health care provider before continuing treatment.

Although symptomatic hypercalcemia was not observed in clinical trials, instruct patients to contact a health care provider if they develop persistent symptoms of hypercalcemia (ie, constipation, lethargy, muscle weakness, nausea, vomiting).

Instruct patients and caregivers who administer teriparatide on how to properly use the delivery device and properly dispose of needles, and instruct them not to share their delivery device with other patients. Instruct patients to not transfer the contents of the delivery device to a syringe.

Instruct patients that each teriparatide delivery device can be used for up to 28 days, including the first injection from the delivery device. Advise patients to discard the teriparatide delivery device after the 28-day use period, even if it still contains some unused solution.

Inform patients regarding the roles of supplemental calcium or vitamin D, weight-bearing exercise, and modification of certain behavioral factors, such as cigarette smoking or alcohol consumption.

THYROID DRUGS

Thyroid Hormones

Synthetic derivatives include levothyroxine (T_4), liothyronine (T_3), and liotrix (a 4 to 1 mixture of T_4 and T_3).

WARNING

Drugs with thyroid hormone activity, alone or with other therapeutic agents, have been used for the treatment of obesity. In euthyroid patients, doses within the range of daily hormonal requirements are ineffective for weight reduction. Larger doses may produce serious or even life-threatening manifestations of toxicity, particularly when given in association with sympathomimetic amines such as those used for their anorectic effects.

Indications

➤*Hypothyroidism:* As replacement or supplemental therapy in hypothyroidism of any etiology, except transient hypothyroidism during the recovery phase of subacute thyroiditis. Specific indications include the following: Cretinism, myxedema, and ordinary hypothyroidism; primary hypothyroidism resulting from functional deficiency, primary atrophy, partial or total absence of thyroid gland, or the effects of surgery, radiation, or drugs, with or without the presence of goiter; secondary (pituitary) or tertiary (hypothalamic) hypothyroidism.

➤*Pituitary TSH suppressants:* In the prevention or treatment of various types of euthyroid goiters, including thyroid nodules, subacute or chronic lymphocytic thyroiditis (Hashimoto), and multinodular goiter and in the management of thyroid cancer (except liothyronine).

➤*Diagnostic use (except levothyroxine):* Diagnostic use in suppression tests to differentiate suspected mild hyperthyroidism or thyroid gland autonomy.

➤*Myxedema coma/precoma (injection only):* For the treatment of myxedema coma/precoma.

➤*Off-label uses:*

Hypothyroidism: once- weekly administration –
Levothyroxine: [4] = Insufficient documentation.

Other possible off-label uses – Thyroid hormones have been used to treat obesity; however, they are ineffective and should not be used for this condition (see Warnings).

Administration and Dosage

Individualize dosage. Determine patient response by clinical judgment in conjunction with laboratory findings.

Generally, institute thyroid therapy at relatively low doses and slowly increase in small increments until the desired response is obtained. Administer thyroid as a single daily dose, preferably before breakfast.

➤*Treatment of choice:* Treatment of choice for hypothyroidism is levothyroxine (T_4) under most circumstances because of its predictable potency and prolonged half-life.

➤*Thyroid cancer:* Exogenous thyroid hormone may produce regression of metastases from follicular and papillary carcinoma of the thyroid and is used as ancillary therapy of these conditions with radioactive iodine. Larger doses than those used for replacement therapy are required. Medullary thyroid carcinoma usually is unresponsive.

➤*Laboratory tests:* Laboratory tests useful in the diagnosis and evaluation of thyroid function are listed in the following table, indicating the alterations noted in various thyroid disorders.

Laboratory Tests for Diagnosis and Evaluation of Thyroid Function

↑ = Increased; ↓ = Decreased; N = Normal; X = Contraindicated	Pregnancy	Primary hypothyroidism	Secondary hypothyroidism	Hyperthyroidism	T_3 thyrotoxicosis	Normal values
Free T_4 (unbound)	N	↓	↓	↑	N	12 to 32 pmol/L
Total T_4	↑	↓	↓	↑	N	55 to 160 nmol/L
T_3	↑	↓	↓	↑	↑	0.6 to 3.1 nmol/L
RAIU[a]	X	↓	-	↑	–	5% to 30%
Free thyroxine index (FT_4I)	N	↓	↓	↑	-	6.5 to 12.5[b] 1.3 to 3.9[c]
TSH[a]	N	↑	N/↓	↓	↓	0.4 to 4.2 milliunit/L

[a] RAIU = radioactive iodine uptake; TSH = thyroid-stimulating hormone
[b] T_4 uptake method
[c] $TT_4 \times RT_3U$ method

➤*Dosage equivalents of thyroid products:* In changing from one thyroid product to another, the following dosage equivalents may be used. However, these equivalents are only estimates; each patient still may require fine dosage adjustments.

Approximate Dosage Equivalents of Thyroid Products[a]

Preparation	Composition ratio T_4	Composition ratio T_3	Dosage equivalents
Thyroid desiccated	4	1	≈ 60 to 65 mg (1 grain)
Levothyroxine	1	0	≈ 50 to 60 mcg (range, 50 to 100 mcg)
Liothyronine	0	1	≈ 25 mcg (range, 15 to 37.5 mcg)
Liotrix	4	1	≈ 1 grain (12.5 mcg T_3/50 mcg T_4)

[a] References may vary in dosage equivalent recommendations.

Actions

➤*Pharmacology:* Thyroid hormones include natural and synthetic derivatives. The natural product, desiccated thyroid, is derived from beef or pork. The US Pharmacopeia (USP) has standardized the total iodine content of natural preparations. Thyroid USP contains not less than 0.17% and not more than 0.23% iodine. Iodine content is only an indirect indicator of true hormonal biologic activity.

Physiological effects – The mechanisms by which thyroid hormones exert their physiologic action are not well understood. It is believed that most of their effects are exerted through control of DNA transcription and protein synthesis. These hormones enhance oxygen consumption by most tissues of the body and increase the basal metabolic rate and metabolism of carbohydrates, lipids, and proteins in the body. Thyroid hormones exert a profound influence on every organ system and are particularly important in CNS development. The physiological actions of thyroid hormones are produced predominantly by T_3, the majority of which (approximately 80%) is derived from T_4 by deiodination in peripheral tissues.

Regulation of thyroid secretion: Thyroid hormone synthesis and secretion are controlled by thyrotropin (thyroid-stimulating hormone; TSH) secreted by the anterior pituitary. TSH secretion is, in turn, controlled by a feedback mechanism effected by thyroid hormones and thyrotropin-releasing hormone (TRH), a tripeptide of hypothalamic origin. Endogenous thyroid hormone secretion is suppressed when exogenous thyroid hormones are given to euthyroid individuals in excess of the normal gland's secretion.

The normal thyroid gland contains, per gram of gland, approximately 200 mcg of T_4 and 15 mcg of T_3. The ratio of these 2 hormones in the circulation does not represent the ratio in the thyroid gland because about 80% of peripheral T_3 comes from monodeiodination of T_4. Peripheral monodeiodination of T_4 also results in the formation of reverse triiodothyronine (rT_3), which is calorigenically inactive.

Low triiodothyronine syndrome – The T_3 level is low in the fetus and newborn, in the elderly, and in cases of chronic caloric deprivation, hepatic cirrhosis, renal failure, surgical stress, and chronic illnesses.

➤*Pharmacokinetics:*

Absorption – Absorption of orally administered T_4 varies from 40% to 80% of the administered dose. T_4 absorption is increased by fasting and decreased in malabsorption syndromes and by certain foods, such as soybean infant formula. Dietary fiber decreases bioavailability of T_4. Absorption also may decrease with age. In addition, many drugs and foods affect T_4 absorption. In 4 hours, T_3 is approximately 95% absorbed. The hormones in natural preparations are absorbed in a manner similar to the synthetic hormones.

Distribution – More than 99% of circulating hormones are bound to serum proteins, including thyroxine-binding globulin (TBG) and thyroxine-binding prealbumin (TBPA) and albumin (TBA), whose capacities and affinities vary for the hormones. The higher affinity of T_4 for TBG and TBPA as compared with T_3 partially explains the higher serum levels and longer half-life of T_4. Both protein-bound hormones exist in reverse equilibrium with minute amounts of free hormone, the latter accounting for the metabolic activity.

Metabolism – Approximately 80% of T_3 comes from monodeiodination of T_4. Deiodination of T_4 occurs at a number of sites, including liver, kidney, and other tissues. The conjugated hormone, in the form of glucuronide or sulfate, is found in the bile and gut where it may complete an enterohepatic circulation. Of T_4 metabolized daily, 80% to 85% is deiodinated to yield equal amounts of T_3 and reverse T_3 (rT_3). T_3 and rT_3 are further deiodinated to diiodothyronine.

Excretion – Thyroid hormones are primarily eliminated by the kidneys. A portion of the conjugated hormone reaches the colon unchanged and is eliminated in the feces. Approximately 20% of T_4 is eliminated in the stool. Urinary excretion of T_4 decreases with age.

Various Pharmacokinetic Parameters of Thyroid Hormones

Hormone	Ratio in thyroglobulin	Biologic potency	Half-life (days)	Protein binding (%)[a]
Levothyroxine (T_4)	10 to 20	1	6 to 7[b]	99+
Liothyronine (T_3)	1	4	≤ 2.5	99+

[a] Includes TBG, TBPA, and TBA.
[b] 3 to 4 days in hyperthyroidism, 9 to 10 days in hypothyroidism.

Contraindications

In patients with diagnosed but uncorrected adrenal cortical insufficiency; untreated thyrotoxicosis; hypersensitivity to active or extraneous constituents.

Levothyroxine is contraindicated in patients with untreated subclinical thyrotoxicosis (suppressed serum TSH level with normal T_3 and T_4 levels) and in patients with acute MI.

Concomitant use of *Triostat* and artificial rewarming of patients is contraindicated.

Warnings/Precautions

➤*Obesity:* Obesity has been treated with thyroid hormones. In euthyroid patients, hormonal replacement doses are ineffective for weight reduction. Larger doses may produce serious or even life-threatening toxicity, particularly when given with sympathomimetic amines such as anorexiants.

➤*Infertility:* Thyroid hormone therapy is unjustified for the treatment of male or female infertility unless the condition is accompanied by hypothyroidism.

➤*Cardiovascular disease:* Use great caution when the integrity of the cardiovascular system, particularly the coronary arteries, is suspected. This includes patients with angina pectoris or the elderly, in whom there is a greater likelihood of occult cardiac disease. In these patients, initiate therapy with low doses. When, in such patients, a euthyroid state only can be reached at the expense of an aggravation of the cardiovascular disease, reduce thyroid hormone dosage.

Overtreatment with levothyroxine sodium may have adverse cardiovascular effects such as an increase in heart rate, cardiac wall thickness, and cardiac contractility and may precipitate angina or arrhythmias. During surgical procedures, closely monitor patients with coronary artery disease who are receiving levothyroxine therapy because the possibility of precipitating cardiac arrhythmias may be greater in those treated with levothyroxine. Concomitant administration of levothyroxine and sympathomimetic agents to patients with coronary artery disease may precipitate coronary insufficiency.

➤*Endocrine disorders:* Thyroid hormone therapy in patients with concomitant diabetes mellitus or insipidus or adrenal cortical insufficiency (Addison disease) exacerbates the intensity of their symptoms. Appropriate adjustments in the therapy of these concomitant endocrine diseases are required.

Autoimmune polyglandular syndrome – Occasionally, chronic autoimmune thyroiditis may occur in association with other autoimmune disorders, such as adrenal insufficiency, pernicious anemia, and insulin-dependent diabetes mellitus. Treat patients with concomitant adrenal insufficiency with replacement glucocorticoids prior to initiation of treatment. Failure to do so may precipitate an acute adrenal crisis when thyroid hormone therapy is initiated because of increased metabolic clearance of glucocorticoids by thyroid hormone. Patients with diabetes mellitus may require upward adjustments of their antidiabetic therapeutic regimens.

In patients with secondary or tertiary hypothyroidism, consider additional hypothalamic/pituitary hormone deficiencies and, if diagnosed, treat.

➤*Nontoxic diffuse goiter or nodular thyroid disease:* Exercise caution when administering levothyroxine to patients with nontoxic diffuse goiter or nodular thyroid disease in order to prevent precipitation of thyrotoxicosis. If the serum TSH is already suppressed, do not administer levothyroxine.

➤*Severe and prolonged hypothyroidism:* Severe and prolonged hypothyroidism can lead to a decreased level of adrenocortical activity commensurate with the lowered metabolic state. When thyroid replacement therapy is administered, the metabolism increases at a greater rate than adrenocortical activity, which can precipitate adrenocortical insufficiency. Therefore, in severe and prolonged hypothyroidism, supplemental adrenocortical steroids may be necessary.

➤*Morphologic hypogonadism and nephrosis:* Rule out morphologic hypogonadism and nephrosis prior to initiating therapy. If hypopituitarism is present, the adrenal deficiency must be corrected prior to starting the drug.

➤*Myxedema:* Patients with myxedema are particularly sensitive to thyroid preparations. Start dosage at a very low level and increase gradually, as acute changes may precipitate adverse cardiovascular events. Myxedema coma therapy requires simultaneous administration of glucocorticoids.

➤*Hyperthyroid effects:* In rare instances, the administration of thyroid hormone may precipitate a hyperthyroid state or may aggravate existing hyperthyroidism.

➤*Decreased bone mineral density:* In women, long-term levothyroxine therapy has been associated with increased bone resorption, thereby decreasing bone mineral density, especially in postmenopausal women on greater than replacement doses or in women who are receiving suppressive doses of levothyroxine. The increased bone resorption may be associated with increased serum levels and urinary excretion of calcium and phosphorus, elevations in bone alkaline phosphatase, and suppressed serum parathyroid hormone levels. Therefore, it is recommended that patients receiving levothyroxine be given the minimum dose necessary to achieve the desired clinical and biochemical response.

➤*Pregnancy: Category A.* Thyroid hormones cross the placental barrier to some extent, as evidenced by levels in cord blood of athyreotic fetuses being approximately one-third maternal levels. Transfer of thyroid hormone from the mother to the fetus, however, may not be adequate to prevent in utero hypothyroidism. Clinical experience does not indicate any adverse effect on the fetus when thyroid hormones are administered to a pregnant woman. Do not discontinue thyroid replacement therapy in hypothyroid women during pregnancy.

➤*Lactation:* Minimal amounts of thyroid hormones are excreted in breast milk. Thyroid is not associated with serious adverse reactions. However, exercise caution when thyroid is administered to a nursing woman.

➤*Children:* There is limited experience with liothyronine sodium injection in the pediatric population. Safety and efficacy in pediatric patients have not been established.

Congenital hypothyroidism – Pregnant women provide little or no thyroid hormone to the fetus. The incidence of congenital hypothyroidism is relatively high (1:4,000) and the hypothyroid fetus would not benefit from the small amounts of hormone crossing the placenta. Routine determinations of serum T_4 and/or TSH are strongly advised in neonates in view of the deleterious effects of thyroid deficiency on growth and development.

Initiate treatment immediately upon diagnosis, and maintain for life, unless transient hypothyroidism is suspected; in this case, therapy may be interrupted for 2 to 8 weeks after 3 years of age to reassess the condition. Cessation of therapy is justified in patients who have maintained a normal TSH during those 2 to 8 weeks.

In infants, excessive doses of thyroid hormone preparations may produce craniosynostosis and may adversely affect the tempo of brain maturation and accelerate the bone age with resultant premature closure of the epiphyses and compromised adult stature.

In children, partial loss of hair may be experienced in the first few months of thyroid therapy; this usually is a transient phenomenon that results in later recovery.

➤*Elderly:* Per the Beers list, desiccated thyroid use in elderly may be inappropriate because of the concerns about cardiac effects. Safer alternatives are available.

➤*Monitoring:* Treatment of patients with thyroid hormones requires the periodic assessment of thyroid status by means of appropriate laboratory tests. The TSH suppression test can be used to test the effectiveness of any thyroid preparation, keeping in mind the relative insensitivity of the infant pituitary to the negative feedback effect of thyroid hormones. Serum T_4 levels can be used to test the effectiveness of all thyroid medications except T_3. When the total serum T_4 is low but TSH is normal, a test specific to assess unbound (free) T_4 levels is warranted.

The frequency of TSH monitoring during levothyroxine dose titration depends on the clinical situation, but it is generally recommended at 6- to 8-week intervals until normalization. For patients who have recently initiated levothyroxine therapy and whose serum TSH has normalized or in patients who have had their dosage or brand of levothyroxine changed, measure the serum TSH concentration after 8 to 12 weeks. When the optimum replacement dose has been attained, clinical (physical examination) and biochemical monitoring may be performed every 6 to 12 months, depending on the clinical situation, and whenever there is a change in the patient's status.

The recommended frequency of monitoring of TSH and total or free T_4 in children is as follows: At 2 and 4 weeks after initiation of treatment; every 1 to 2 months during the first year of life; every 2 to 3 months between 1 and 3 years of age; and every 3 to 12 months thereafter until growth is completed. It is recommended that TSH and T_4 levels and a physical examination, if indicated, be performed 2 weeks after any change in levothyroxine dosage.

Specific measurements of T_4 and T_3 by competitive protein binding or radioimmunoassay are not influenced by blood levels of organic or inorganic iodine and have essentially replaced older tests (ie, PBI, BEI, T_4 by column) (see Administration and Dosage).

Persistent clinical and laboratory evidence of hypothyroidism in spite of adequate dosage replacement indicates poor patient compliance, poor absorption, excessive fecal loss, or inactivity of the preparation. Intracellular resistance to thyroid hormone is rare.

Drug Interactions

Thyroid Hormone Drug Interactions

Precipitant drug	Object drug[a]		Description
Amiodarone Glucocorticoids (eg, dexamethasone ≥ 4 mg/day) Propylthiouracil	Thyroid hormones	↓	Concurrent use may decrease the peripheral conversion of T_4 to T_3, leading to decreased T_3 levels. However, serum T_4 levels are usually normal but occasionally may be slightly elevated.
Antacids (aluminum and magnesium hydroxides) Bile acid sequestrants (cholestyramine, colestipol) Calcium carbonate Iron salts Sodium polystyrene sulfonate Simethicone Sucralfate	Thyroid hormones	↓	Concurrent use may reduce the efficacy of the thyroid hormone because of possible binding in the GI tract, preventing absorption. Separate administration by at least 4 hours.
Beta-blockers (eg, propranolol> 160 mg/day)	Thyroid hormones	↓	Concurrent use may decrease the peripheral conversion of T_4 to T_3, leading to decreased T_3 levels. However, serum T_4 levels usually are normal but occasionally may be slightly elevated.
Thyroid hormones	Beta-blockers		The actions of particular beta blockers may be impaired when the hypothyroid patient is converted to the euthyroid state.
Carbamazepine Hydantoins Phenobarbital Rifamycins	Thyroid hormones	↓	Hepatic degradation of levothyroxine may increase, resulting in increased levothyroxine requirements.
Estrogens, oral contraceptives	Thyroid hormones	↓	Estrogens increase TBG and may therefore decrease the response to thyroid hormone therapy in patients with a nonfunctioning thyroid gland. An increased thyroid dose may be needed.
Furosemide (> 80 mg IV) Heparin Hydantoins NSAIDs Salicylates (> 2 g/day)	Thyroid hormones	↔	Administration of these agents with levothyroxine results in an initial transient increase in FT_4. Continued administration results in a decrease in serum T_4 and normal FT_4 and TSH; therefore, patients are clinically euthyroid.
Selective serotonin reuptake inhibitors (eg, sertraline)	Thyroid hormones	↓	Administration of sertraline in patients stabilized on levothyroxine may result in increased levothyroxine requirements.
Tricyclic antidepressants Tetracyclic antidepressants	Thyroid hormones	↑	Concurrent use of tricyclic/tetracyclic antidepressants and levothyroxine may increase the therapeutic and toxic effects of both drugs, possibly because of increased receptor sensitivity to catecholamines. Toxic effects may include increased risk of cardiac arrhythmias and CNS stimulation.
Thyroid hormones	Tricyclic antidepressants Tetracyclic antidepressants		
Thyroid hormones	Anticoagulants	↑	The anticoagulant action is increased; a decreased dose may be necessary.
Thyroid hormones	Antidiabetic agents Biguanides Meglitinides Sulfonylureas Thiazolidinediones Insulin	↓	Initiating thyroid hormones may cause increases in insulin or oral hypoglycemic requirements. Monitor closely.

Thyroid Hormone Drug Interactions			
Precipitant drug	Object drug[a]		Description
Thyroid hormones	Digitalis glycosides	⬇	Serum digitalis glycoside levels are reduced in hyperthyroidism or when the hypothyroid patient is converted to the euthyroid state. Therapeutic effects of digitalis glycosides may be reduced.
Thyroid hormones	Growth hormones (somatrem, somatropin)	⬆	Excessive use of thyroid hormones with growth hormones may accelerate epiphyseal closure. However, untreated hypothyroidism may interfere with growth response to growth hormone.
Thyroid hormones	Ketamine	⬆	Concurrent use may produce marked hypertension and tachycardia. Administer with caution.
Thyroid hormones	Radiographic agents	⬇	Thyroid hormones may reduce the uptake of ^{123}I, ^{131}I, ^{99m}TC.
Thyroid hormones	Sympathomimetics	⬆	Concurrent use may increase the effects of either agent. Thyroid hormones may increase the risk of coronary insufficiency when sympathomimetics are given to patients with coronary artery disease. Use with caution.
Sympathomimetics	Thyroid hormones		
Thyroid hormones	Theophyllines	⬆	Decreased theophylline clearance can be expected in hypothyroid patients; clearance returns to normal when euthyroid state is achieved.

[a] ⬆ = Object drug increased ⬇ = Object drug decreased
⟷ = Undetermined clinical effect.

➤*Drug/Lab test interactions:* Consider changes in TBG concentration when interpreting T_4 and T_3 values. In such cases, measure the unbound (free) hormone and/or free T_4 index (FT_4I). Pregnancy, infectious hepatitis, estrogens, estrogen-containing oral contraceptives, and acute intermittent porphyria increase TBG concentrations. Decreases in TBG concentrations are observed in nephrosis, severe hypoproteinemia, severe liver disease, and acromegaly, and after androgen or corticosteroid therapy. Familial hyper- or hypothyroxine binding globulinemias have been described. The incidence of TBG deficiency approximates 1 in 9,000.

Medicinal or dietary iodine interferes with all in vivo tests of radioiodine uptake, producing low uptakes that may not reflect a true decrease in hormone synthesis.

Cytokines: Interferon-α and interleukin-2 – Therapy with interferon-α has been associated with the development of antithyroid microsomal antibodies in 20% of patients and some have transient hypothyroidism, hyperthyroidism, or both. Patients who have antithyroid antibodies before treatment are at higher risk of thyroid dysfunction during treatment. Interleukin-2 has been associated with transient painless thyroiditis in 20% of patients. Interferon-β and -γ have not been reported to cause thyroid dysfunction.

Drugs That May Reduce TSH Secretion	
Dopamine/Dopamine agonists Glucocorticoids Octreotide	Use of these agents may result in a transient reduction in TSH secretion when administered at the following doses: Dopamine (≥ 1 mcg/kg/min); glucocorticoids (hydrocortisone ≥ 100 mg/day or equivalent); octreotide (> 100 mcg/day).

Drugs That May Decrease Thyroid Hormone Secretion	
Aminoglutethimide Amiodarone Iodide (including iodine-containing radiographic contrast agents) Lithium Methimazole Propylthiouracil Sulfonamides Tolbutamide	Long-term lithium therapy can result in goiter in up to 50% of patients and in subclinical or overt hypothyroidism, each in up to 20% of patients. Oral cholecystographic agents and amiodarone slowly are excreted, producing more prolonged hypothyroidism than parenterally administered iodinated contrast agents. Long-term aminoglutethimide therapy may minimally decrease T_4 and T_3 levels and increase TSH, although all values remain within normal limits in most patients.

Drugs That May Increase Thyroid Hormone Secretion	
Amiodarone Iodide (including iodine-containing radiographic contrast agents)	Iodide and drugs that contain pharmacologic amounts of iodide may cause hyperthyroidism in euthyroid patients with Grave disease previously treated with antithyroid drugs or in euthyroid patients with thyroid autonomy (eg, multinodular goiter or hyperfunctioning thyroid adenoma). Hyperthyroidism may develop over several weeks and may persist for several months after therapy discontinuation. Amiodarone may induce hyperthyroidism by causing thyroiditis.

Drugs That May Alter Serum TBG Concentration	
Drugs that may increase serum TBG concentration	Drugs that may decrease serum TBG concentration
Estrogen-containing oral contraceptives Estrogens (oral) Heroin/Methadone 5-Fluorouracil Mitotane Tamoxifen	Androgens/Anabolic steroids Asparaginase Glucocorticoids Slow-release nicotinic acid

Drugs Associated with Thyroid Hormone and/or TSH Level Alterations by Various Mechanisms	
Chloral hydrate	Nitroprusside
Diazepam	Para-aminosalicylate sodium
Ethionamide	Perphenazine
Lovastatin	Resorcinol (excessive topical use)
Metoclopramide	Thiazide diuretics
6-Mercaptopurine	

➤*Drug/Food interactions:* Consumption of certain foods may affect levothyroxine absorption, thereby necessitating adjustments in dosing. Soybean flour (infant formula), cotton seed meal, walnuts, and dietary fiber may bind and decrease the absorption of levothyroxine from the GI tract.

Adverse Reactions

Adverse reactions other than those indicating hyperthyroidism caused by therapeutic overdosage, initially or during the maintenance period, are rare. Symptoms of overdosage include the following:

➤*Cardiovascular:* Palpitations; tachycardia; arrhythmias; angina; cardiac arrest; increased pulse and blood pressure; CHF; MI.

➤*CNS:* Tremors; headache; nervousness; insomnia; hyperactivity; anxiety, irritability; emotional lability; seizures (rare).

➤*GI:* Diarrhea; vomiting; abdominal cramps.

➤*Hypersensitivity:* Allergic skin reactions (rare). Hypersensitivity reactions to inactive ingredients have occurred in patients treated with thyroid hormone products. These include the following: Urticaria, pruritus, skin rash, flushing, angioedema, various GI symptoms (eg, abdominal pain, nausea, vomiting, diarrhea), fever, arthralgia, serum sickness, and wheezing. Hypersensitivity to levothyroxine itself is not known to occur.

➤*Miscellaneous:* Weight loss; fatigue; increased appetite; menstrual irregularities; excessive sweating; heat intolerance; fever; muscle weakness; dyspnea; hair loss; flushing; decreased bone mineral density; impaired fertility; increase in liver function tests.

Pseudotumor cerebri and slipped capital femoral epiphysis have been reported in children receiving levothyroxine therapy. Overtreatment may result in craniosynostosis in infants and premature closure of the epiphyses in children with resultant compromised adult height.

Liothyronine injection only – Hypotension; phlebitis; twitching.

Overdosage

➤*Acute massive overdosage:* Large doses of antithyroid drugs (eg, methimazole, propylthiouracil) followed in 1 to 2 hours by large doses of iodine may be given to inhibit synthesis and release of thyroid hormones. Glucocorticoids may be given to inhibit the conversion of T_4 to T_3. Because T_4 is highly protein bound, very little drug will be removed by dialysis. Treatment is aimed at reducing GI absorption of the drug and counteracting central and peripheral effects, mainly those of increased sympathetic activity. Refer to General Management of Acute Overdosage. Cardiac glycosides may be indicated if CHF develops. Control fever, hypoglycemia, or fluid loss, if needed. Antiadrenergic agents, particularly propranolol (1 to 3 mg IV over 10 minutes or 80 to 160 mg orally per day), have been used to treat increased sympathetic activity.

➤*Symptoms:* Chronic excessive dosage will produce signs and symptoms of hyperthyroidism (eg, headache, irritability, nervousness, tremor, sweating, increased bowel motility, menstrual irregularities). Angina pectoris, arrhythmia, tachycardia, acute MI, or CHF may be induced or aggravated. In addition, confusion and disorientation may occur. Cerebral embolism, shock, coma, and death have been reported. Seizures have occurred in a child ingesting approximately 18 to 20 mg levothyroxine. Symptoms may not necessarily be evident or may not appear until several days after ingestion of levothyroxine sodium. Massive overdosage may result in symptoms resembling thyroid storm.

➤*Treatment:* Reduce dosage or temporarily discontinue therapy. Reinstitute treatment at a lower dosage. In healthy individuals, normal hypothalamic-pituitary-thyroid axis function is restored in 6 to 8 weeks after thyroid suppression.

Patient Information

Replacement therapy is to be taken for life, except in cases of transient hypothyroidism, usually associated with thyroiditis, and in those receiving a trial of the drug.

Take as a single daily dose, preferably at least 30 minutes before breakfast.

➤*Brand interchange:* Inform patients not to change from one brand of this drug to another without consulting their pharmacist or physician. Products manufactured by different companies may not be equally effective.

Inform patients not to discontinue medication except on the advice of a physician.

Instruct patients to notify their physician if the following symptoms occur: Rapid or irregular heartbeat, chest pain, shortness of breath, leg cramps, headache, nervousness, irritability, sleeplessness, tremors, change in appetite, weight gain or loss, vomiting, diarrhea, excessive sweating, heat intolerance, fever, changes in menstrual periods, hives or skin rash, or any other unusual medical event.

Children my experience partial hair loss in the first few months of therapy, but this is usually a transient phenomenon that results in later recovery.

Not for use as primary or adjunctive therapy in a weight-control program.

Advise patients to notify their physician if they become pregnant while taking thyroid hormones; their dose may need to be changed.

THYROID DESICCATED (Porcine-Derived)

Rx	**Armour Thyroid** (Forest)	**Tablets; oral**: 15 mg (¼ gr)[a]	Dextrose. (A TC). Lt. tan. In 100s.
Rx	**Nature-Throid** (RLC Labs)	**Tablets; oral:**16.25 mg (¼ gr)[a]	Lactose, PEG 400. In 100s and 990s Polybags.
Rx	**Westhroid** (RLC Labs)		Lactose. In 30s, 60s, 90s, 100s, 990s, 1,000s, and 1,008s.
Rx	**Armour Thyroid** (Forest)	**Tablets; oral**: 30 mg (½ gr)[a]	Dextrose. (A TD). Lt. tan. In 100s, 1,000s, 50,000s and UD 100s.
Rx	**NP Thyroid** (Acella Pharmaceuticals)		Dextrose, maltodextrin, mineral oil. (329). Lt. tan, round. In 100s.
Rx	**Nature-Throid** (RLC Labs)	**Tablets; oral**: 32.4 mg (½ gr)[a]	In 100s.
Rx	**Westhroid** (RLC Labs)	**Tablets; oral**: 32.5 mg (½ gr)[a]	In 100s.
Rx	**Thyroid USP** (Various, eg, URL)		In 100s and 1,000s.
Rx	**Nature Throid** (RLC Labs)	**Tablets; oral**: 48.75 mg (¾ gr)[a]	Lactose. In 30s, 60s, 90s, 100s, 990s, 1,000s, and 1,008s.
Rx	**Westhroid** (RLC Labs)		Lactose. In 30s, 60s, 90s, 100s, 990s, 1,000s, and 1,008s.
Rx	**Armour Thyroid** (Forest)	**Tablets; oral**: 60 mg (1 gr)[a]	Dextrose. (A TE). Lt. tan. In 100s, 1,000s, 5000s, 50,000s, and UD 100s.
Rx	**NP Thyroid** (Acella Pharmaceuticals)		Dextrose, maltodextrin, mineral oil. (330). Lt. tan, round. In 100s.
Rx	**Nature-Throid** (RLC Labs)	**Tablets; oral**: 64.8 mg (1 gr)[a]	In 100s.
Rx	**Westhroid** (RLC Labs)	**Tablets; oral**: 65 mg (1 gr)[a]	In 100s.
Rx	**Thyroid USP** (Various, eg, URL)		In 100s and 1,000s.
Rx	**Nature Throid** (RLC Labs)	**Tablets; oral**: 81.25 mg (1 ¼ gr)[a]	Lactose. In 30s, 60s, 90s, 100s, 990s, 1,000s, and 1,008s.
Rx	**Westhroid** (RLC Labs)		Lactose. In 30s, 60s, 90s, 100s, 990s, 1,000s, and 1,008s.
Rx	**Armour Thyroid** (Forest)	**Tablets; oral**: 90 mg (1½ gr)[a]	Dextrose. (A TJ). Lt. tan. In 100s.
Rx	**NP Thyroid** (Acella Pharmaceuticals)		Dextrose, maltodextrin, mineral oil. (331). Lt. tan, round. In 100s.
Rx	**Nature Throid** (RLC Labs)	**Tablets; oral**: 97.5 mg (1 ½ gr)[a]	Lactose. In 30s, 60s, 90s, 100s, 990s, 1,000s, and 1,008s.
Rx	**Westhroid** (RLC Labs)		Lactose. In 30s, 60s, 90s, 100s, 990s, 1,000s, and 1,008s.
Rx	**Nature Throid** (RLC Labs)	**Tablets; oral**: 113.75 mg (1 ¾ gr)[a]	Lactose. In 30s, 60s, 90s, 100s, 990s, 1,000s, and 1,008s.
Rx	**Westhroid** (RLC Labs)		Lactose. In 30s, 60s, 90s, 100s, 990s, 1,000s, and 1,008s.
Rx	**Armour Thyroid** (Forest)	**Tablets; oral**: 120 mg (2 gr)[a]	Dextrose. (A TF). Lt. tan. In 100s, 1,000s, 50,000s, and UD 100s.
Rx	**Nature-Throid** (RLC Labs)	**Tablets; oral**: 129.6 mg (2 gr)[a]	In 100s.
Rx	**Westhroid** (RLC Labs)	**Tablets; oral**: 130 mg (2 gr)[a]	In 100s.
Rx	**Thyroid USP** (Various, eg, URL)		In 100s and 1,000s.
Rx	**Nature Throid** (RLC Labs)	**Tablets; oral**: 146.25 mg (2 ¼ gr)[a]	Lactose. In 30s, 60s, 90s, 100s, 990s, 1,000s, and 1,008s.
Rx	**Westhroid** (RLC Labs)		Lactose. In 30s, 60s, 90s, 100s, 990s, 1,000s, and 1,008s.
Rx	**Nature Throid** (RLC Labs)	**Tablets; oral**: 162.5 mg (2 ½ gr)[a]	Lactose. In 30s, 60s, 90s, 100s, 990s, 1,000s, and 1,008s.
Rx	**Westhroid** (RLC Labs)		Lactose. In 30s, 60s, 90s, 100s, 990s, 1,000s, and 1,008s.
Rx	**Armour Thyroid** (Forest)	**Tablets; oral**: 180 mg (3 gr)[a]	Dextrose. (A TG). Lt. tan, scored. In 100s and 1,000s.
Rx	**Nature-Throid** (RLC Labs)	**Tablets; oral**: 194.4 mg (3 gr)[a]	In 100s.
Rx	**Westhroid** (RLC Labs)		In 100s.
Rx	**Thyroid USP** (Various, eg, URL)	**Tablets; oral**: 195 mg (3 gr)[a]	In 100s and 1,000s.
Rx	**Armour Thyroid** (Forest)	**Tablets**: 240 mg (4 gr)[a]	Dextrose. (A TH). Lt. tan. In 100s.
Rx	**Nature Throid** (RLC Labs)	**Tablets; oral**: 260 (4 gr)[a]	Lactose. In 30s, 60s, 90s, 100s, 990s, 1,000s, and 1,008s.
Rx	**Westhroid** (RLC Labs)		Lactose. In 30s, 60s, 90s, 100s, 990s, 1,000s, and 1,008s.
Rx	**Armour Thyroid** (Forest)	**Tablets; oral**: 300 mg (5 gr)[a]	Dextrose. (A TI). Lt. tan, scored. In 100s.
Rx	**Nature Throid** (RLC Labs)	**Tablets; oral**: 325 mg (5 gr)[a]	Lactose. In 30s, 60s, 90s, 100s, 990s, 1,000s, and 1,008s.
Rx	**Westhroid** (RLC Labs)		Lactose. In 30s, 60s, 90s, 100s, 990s, 1,000s, and 1,008s.

THYROID DESICCATED (Porcine-Derived)

Rx	**Bio-Throid** (Bio-Tech)	**Capsules; oral**: 7.5 mg (⅛ gr)[a]	In 100s and 1,000s.
		15 mg (¼ gr)[a]	In 100s and 1,000s.
		30 mg (½ gr)[a]	In 100s and 1,000s.
		60 mg (1 gr)[a]	In 100s and 1,000s.
		90 mg (1½ gr)[a]	In 100s and 1,000s.
		120 mg (2 gr)[a]	In 100s and 1,000s.
		150 mg (2½ gr)[a]	In 100s and 1,000s.
		180 mg (3 gr)[a]	In 100s and 1,000s.
		240 mg (4 gr)[a]	In 100s and 1,000s.

[a] The amounts given in grains are according to the respective manufacturers. The exact equivalent is: 1 gr = 64.8 mg.

THYROID DESICCATED — ORAL

For complete prescribing information, refer to the Thyroid Drugs group monograph.

WARNING

Drugs with thyroid hormone activity, alone or with other therapeutic agents, have been used for the treatment of obesity. In euthyroid patients, doses within the range of daily hormonal requirements are ineffective for weight reduction. Larger doses may produce serious or even life-threatening manifestations of toxicity, particularly when given in association with sympathomimetic amines such as those used for their anorectic effects.

Indications

➤*Hypothyroidism:* As replacement or supplemental therapy in patients with hypothyroidism of any etiology, except transient hypothyroidism during the recovery phase of subacute thyroiditis. This category includes cretinism, myxedema, and ordinary hypothyroidism in patients of any age (children, adults, the elderly), or state (including pregnancy); primary hypothyroidism resulting from functional deficiency, primary atrophy, partial or total absence of thyroid gland, or the effects of surgery, radiation, or drugs, with or without the presence of goiter; and secondary (pituitary) or tertiary (hypothalamic) hypothyroidism.

➤*Pituitary thyroid stimulating hormone (TSH) suppression:* As pituitary TSH suppressants in the prevention or treatment of various types of euthyroid goiters, including thyroid nodules, subacute or chronic lymphocytic thyroiditis (Hashimoto), and multinodular goiter and in the management of thyroid cancer.

➤*Diagnostic agent:* As diagnostic agents in suppression tests to differentiate suspected mild hyperthyroidism or thyroid gland autonomy.

Administration and Dosage

➤*Adults:*

Diagnostic agent – 1.56 mcg/kg of body weight per day given for 7 to 10 days. These doses usually yield normal serum T_4 and T_3 levels and lack of response to TSH.

Hypothyroidism –
Initial dosage: 30 mg/day. Use 15 mg/day in patients with long-standing myxedema, particularly if cardiovascular impairment is suspected.
Dosage titration: Increase with increments of 15 mg every 2 to 3 weeks. Reduce dosage if angina occurs.
Maintenance dosage: 60 to 120 mg/day; failure to respond to 180 mg doses suggests lack of compliance or malabsorption. Adequate therapy usually results in normal TSH and T_4 levels after 2 to 3 weeks of therapy.
Dosage adjustment: Readjust dosage within the first 4 weeks of therapy after proper clinical and laboratory evaluations.

Thyroid cancer – Requires larger amounts than those used for replacement therapy.

➤*Children:*

Congenital hypothyroidism – In infants, institute therapy with full doses as soon as diagnosis is made.

Thyroid Desiccated Dosage for Children With Congenital Hypothyroidism

Age	Dose per day	Daily dose per kg
0 to 6 mo	7.5 to 30 mg	2.4 to 6 mg
6 to 12 mo	30 to 45 mg	3.6 to 4.8 mg
1 to 5 y	45 to 60 mg	3 to 3.6 mg
6 to 12 y	60 to 90 mg	2.4 to 3 mg
> 12 y	> 90 mg	1.2 to 1.8 mg

➤*Elderly:* Initiate therapy in low doses (15 to 30 mg).

➤*Storage/Stability:* Store at 15° to 30°C (59° to 86°F).

LEVOTHYROXINE SODIUM (T_4; L-thyroxine)

Rx	**Levothyroxine Sodium** (Various, eg, Mylan, Sandoz)	**Tablets**: 25 mcg (0.025 mg)	In 100s.
Rx	**Levothroid** (Forest)		(25). Orange, caplet shape. In 100s and 1,000s.
Rx	**Levoxyl** (Jones Pharma)		(25). Orange, oval. In 100s and 1,000s.
Rx	**Synthroid** (Abbott)		Sugar, lactose. (SYNTHROID 25). Orange, scored. In 100s and 1,000s.
Rx	**Thyro-Tabs** (Lloyd[a])		(25). Orange, capsule shape. In 100s and 1,000s.
Rx	**Unithroid Direct** (Lannett)		Lactose. (JS 513). Peach. In 100s, 1,000s, and blister pack 84s.
Rx	**Levothyroxine Sodium** (Various, eg, Mylan, Sandoz)	**Tablets**: 50 mcg (0.05 mg)	In 100s.
Rx	**Levothroid** (Forest)		(50). White, caplet shape. In 100s and 1,000s.
Rx	**Levoxyl** (Jones Pharma)		(50). White, oval. In 100s and 1,000s.
Rx	**Synthroid** (Abbott)		Sugar, lactose. (SYNTHROID 50). White, scored. In 100s, 1,000s, and UD 100s.
Rx	**Thyro-Tabs** (Lloyd[a])		(50). White, capsule shape. In 100s and 1,000s.
Rx	**Unithroid Direct** (Lannett)		Lactose. (JS 514). In 100s, 1,000s, and blister pack 84s.
Rx	**Levothyroxine Sodium** (Various, eg, Mylan, Sandoz)	**Tablets**: 75 mcg (0.075 mg)	In 100s.
Rx	**Levothroid** (Forest)		(75) Violet, caplet shape. In 100s and 1,000s.
Rx	**Levoxyl** (Jones Pharma)		(75). Purple, oval. In 100s and 1,000s.
Rx	**Synthroid** (Abbott)		Sugar, lactose. (SYNTHROID 75). Violet, scored. In 100s, 1,000s, and UD 100s.
Rx	**Thyro-Tabs** (Lloyd[a])		(75). Violet, capsule shape. In 100s and 1,000s.
Rx	**Unithroid Direct** (Lannett)		Lactose. (JS 515). Purple. In 100s, 1,000s, and blister pack 84s.

LEVOTHYROXINE SODIUM (T_4; L-thyroxine)

Rx	**Levothyroxine Sodium** (Various, eg, Mylan, Sandoz)	**Tablets**: 88 mcg (0.088 mg)	In 100s.
Rx	**Levothroid** (Forest)		(88). Mint green, caplet shape. In 100s and 1,000s.
Rx	**Levoxyl** (Jones Pharma)		(88). Olive, oval. In 100s, 1,000s, and UD 100s.
Rx	**Synthroid** (Abbott)		Sugar, lactose. (SYNTHROID 88). Olive, scored. In 100s and 1,000s.
Rx	**Thyro-Tabs** (Lloyd[a])		(88). Rose, capsule shape. In 100s and 1,000s.
Rx	**Unithroid Direct** (Lannett)		Lactose. (JS 561). Olive, scored. In 100s, 1,000s, and blister packs 84s.
Rx	**Levothyroxine Sodium** (Various, eg, Mylan, Sandoz)	**Tablets**: 100 mcg (0.1 mg)	In 100s.
Rx	**Levothroid** (Forest)		(100). Yellow, caplet shape. In 100s and 1,000s.
Rx	**Levoxyl** (Jones Pharma)		(100). Yellow, oval. In 100s and 1,000s.
Rx	**Synthroid** (Abbott)		Sugar, lactose. (SYNTHROID 100). Yellow, scored. In 100s, 1,000s, and UD 100s.
Rx	**Thyro-Tabs** (Lloyd[a])		(100). Yellow, capsule shape. In 100s and 1,000s.
Rx	**Unithroid Direct** (Lannett)		Lactose. (JS 516). Yellow. In 100s, 1,000s, and blister pack 84s.
Rx	**Levothyroxine Sodium** (Various, eg, Mylan, Sandoz)	**Tablets**: 112 mcg (0.112 mg)	In 100s.
Rx	**Levothroid** (Forest)		(112). Rose, caplet shape. In 100s and 1,000s.
Rx	**Levoxyl** (Jones Pharma)		(112). Rose, oval. In 100s, 1,000s, and UD 100s.
Rx	**Synthroid** (Abbott)		Sugar, lactose. (SYNTHROID 112). Rose, scored. In 100s and 1,000s.
Rx	**Thyro-Tabs** (Lloyd[a])		(112). Mint green, capsule shape. In 100s and 1,000s.
Rx	**Unithroid Direct** (Lannett)		Lactose.. (JS 562). Rose, scored. In 100s, 1,000s, and blister packs 84s.
Rx	**Levothyroxine Sodium** (Various, eg, Mylan, Sandoz)	**Tablets**: 125 mcg (0.125 mg)	In 100s.
Rx	**Levothroid** (Forest)		(125). Brown, caplet shape. In 100s and 1,000s.
Rx	**Levoxyl** (Jones Pharma)		(125). Brown, oval. In 100s and 1,000s.
Rx	**Synthroid** (Abbott)		Sugar, lactose. (SYNTHROID 125). Brown, scored. In 100s, 1,000s, and UD 100s.
Rx	**Thyro-Tabs** (Lloyd[a])		(125). Brown, capsule shape. In 100s and 1,000s.
Rx	**Unithroid Direct** (Lannett)		Lactose. (JS 519). Tan. In 100s, 1,000,s and blister packs 84s.
Rx	**Levothyroxine Sodium** (Sandoz)	**Tablets**: 137 mcg (0.137 mg)	(GG 137). Turquoise, scored, capsule shape. In 100s.
Rx	**Levoxyl** (Jones Pharma)		(137). Dk blue, oval. In 100s, 1,000s, and UD 100s.
Rx	**Synthroid** (Abbott)		Sugar, lactose. (SYNTHROID 137). Turquoise, scored. In 100s and 1,000s.
Rx	**Levothyroxine Sodium** (Various, eg, Mylan, Sandoz)	**Tablets**: 150 mcg (0.15 mg)	In 100s.
Rx	**Levothroid** (Forest)		(150). Blue, caplet shape. In 100s and 1,000s.
Rx	**Levoxyl** (Jones Pharma)		(150). Blue, oval. In 100s and 1,000s.
Rx	**Synthroid** (Abbott)		Sugar, lactose. (SYNTHROID 150). Blue, scored. In 100s, 1,000s, and UD 100s.
Rx	**Thyro-Tabs** (Lloyd[a])		(150). Blue, capsule shape. In 100s and 1,000s.
Rx	**Unithroid Direct** (Lannett)		Lactose. (JS 520). Blue, scored. In 100s, 1,000s, and blister pack 84s.
Rx	**Levothyroxine Sodium** (Various, eg, Mylan, Sandoz)	**Tablets**: 175 mcg (0.175 mg)	In 100s.
Rx	**Levothroid** (Forest)		(175). Lilac, caplet shape. In 100s and 1,000s.
Rx	**Levoxyl** (Jones Pharma)		(175). Turquoise, oval. In 100s, 1,000s, and UD 100s.
Rx	**Synthroid** (Abbott)		Sugar, lactose. (SYNTHROID 175). Lilac, scored. In 100s and 1,000s.
Rx	**Thyro-Tabs** (Lloyd[a])		(175). Lilac, capsule shape. In 100s and 1,000s.
Rx	**Unithroid Direct** (Lannett)		Lactose. (JS 563). Lilac. In 100s, 1,000s, and blister packs 84s.
Rx	**Levothyroxine Sodium** (Various, eg, Mylan, Sandoz)	**Tablets**: 200 mcg (0.2 mg)	In 100s.
Rx	**Levothroid** (Forest)		(200). Pink, caplet shape. In 100s and 1,000s.
Rx	**Levoxyl** (Jones Pharma)		(200). Pink, oval. In 100s and 1,000s.
Rx	**Synthroid** (Abbott)		Sugar, lactose. (SYNTHROID 200). Pink, scored. In 100s, 1,000s, and UD 100s.
Rx	**Thyro-Tabs** (Lloyd[a])		(200). Pink, capsule shape. In 100s and 1,000s.
Rx	**Unithroid Direct** (Lannett)		Lactose. (JS 522). Pink. In 100s, 1,000s, and blister packs 84s.
Rx	**Levothyroxine Sodium** (Various, eg, Mylan, Sandoz)	**Tablets**: 300 mcg (0.3 mg)	In 100s.
Rx	**Levothroid** (Forest)		(300). Green, caplet shape. In 100s and 1,000s.
Rx	**Levoxyl** (Jones Pharma)		(300). Green, oval. In 100s, 1,000s, and UD 100s.
Rx	**Synthroid** (Abbott)		Sugar, lactose. (SYNTHROID 300). Green, scored. In 100s and 1,000s.
Rx	**Thyro-Tabs** (Lloyd[a])		(300). Green, capsule shape. In 100s and 1,000s.
Rx	**Unithroid Direct** (Lannett)		Lactose. (JS 523). Green, scored. In 100s, 1,000, and blister packs 84s.

LEVOTHYROXINE SODIUM (T_4; L-thyroxine)

Rx	**Tirosint** (Akrimax)	**Capsules, liquid-filled; oral:** 13 mcg (0.013 mg)	Amber, round. In blister 56s.
		25 mcg (0.025 mg)	Amber, round. In blister 56s.
		50 mcg (0.05 mg)	Amber, round. In blister 56s.
		75 mcg (0.075 mg)	Amber, round. In blister 56s.
		88 mcg (0.088 mg)	Amber, round. In blister 56s.
		100 mcg (0.1 mg)	Amber, round. In blister 56s.
		112 mcg (0.112 mg)	Amber, round. In blister 56s.
		125 mcg (0.125 mg)	Amber, round. In blister 56s.
		137 mcg (0.137 mg)	Amber, round. In blister 56s.
		150 mcg (0.15 mg)	Amber, round. In blister 56s.
Rx	**Levothyroxine Sodium** (Various, eg, Bedford, McGuff)	**Powder for injection, lyophilized:** 200 mcg (0.2 mg)	In 10 mL vials.
		500 mcg (0.5 mg)	In 10 mL vials.

[a] Lloyd, Inc., PO Box 130, Shenandoah, IA 51601; (800) 831-0004.

LEVOTHYROXINE SODIUM — ORAL

For complete and comparative prescribing information, refer to the Thyroid Hormones group monograph.

WARNING

Do not use thyroid hormones, including levothyroxine, either alone or with other therapeutic agents, for the treatment of obesity or for weight loss. In euthyroid patients, doses within the range of daily hormonal requirements are ineffective for weight reduction. Larger doses may produce serious or even life-threatening manifestations of toxicity, particularly when given in association with sympathomimetic amines such as those used for their anorectic effects.

Indications

➤*Hypothyroidism:* As replacement or supplemental therapy in congenital or acquired hypothyroidism of any etiology, except transient hypothyroidism during the recovery phase of subacute thyroiditis. Specific indications include primary (thyroidal), secondary (pituitary), and tertiary (hypothalamic) hypothyroidism and subclinical hypothyroidism. Primary hypothyroidism may result from functional deficiency, primary atrophy, partial or total congenital absence of the thyroid gland, or from the effects of surgery, radiation, or drugs, with or without the presence of goiter.

➤*Pituitary thyrotropin-stimulating hormone (TSH) suppression:* In the prevention or treatment of various types of euthyroid goiters, including thyroid nodules, subacute or chronic lymphocytic thyroiditis (Hashimoto thyroiditis), multinodular goiter and as an adjunct to surgery and radioiodine therapy in the management of thyrotropin-dependent well-differentiated thyroid cancer.

➤*Off-label uses:*

Hypothyroidism: once-weekly administration – [4] = Insufficient documentation. Initial data regarding the use of a single weekly dose of thyroxine show that it appears to be as effective as daily dosing in maintaining biochemical euthyroidism and may be useful in combating noncompliance with a daily regimen. However, the exact dose has not been clearly established, with 1 small study suggesting that a slightly larger dose than 7 times the normal daily dose might be needed. Larger, controlled trials are needed.

Administration and Dosage

➤*General dosing considerations:* Because of the long half-life of levothyroxine, the peak therapeutic effect at a given dose may not be attained for 4 to 6 weeks.

Therapy may begin at full replacement doses in otherwise healthy individuals who are at low risk of coronary artery disease.

➤*Adults:*

Hypothyroidism –

Usual dosage: The average full replacement dosage is approximately 1.7 mcg/kg/day (0.0017 mg/kg/day) (eg, 100 to 125 mcg/day for a 70 kg adult). Dosages greater than 200 mcg/day (0.2 mg/day) are seldom required. An inadequate response to daily dosages of 300 mcg/day (0.3 mg/day) or more is rare and may indicate poor compliance, malabsorption, or drug interactions.

Severe hypothyroidism: Initial dosage is 12.5 to 25 mcg/day (0.0125 to 0.025 mg/day) with increases of 25 mcg/day (0.025 mg/day) every 2 to 4 weeks, accompanied by clinical and laboratory assessment, until the TSH level is normalized.

Secondary (pituitary) or tertiary (hypothalamic) hypothyroidism: Titrate the dose until the patient is clinically euthyroid and the serum-free T_4 level is restored to the upper half of the normal range.

Subclinical hypothyroidism: If this condition is treated, a lower dose (eg, 1 mcg/kg/day [0.001 mg/kg/day]) than that used for full replacement may be adequate to normalize the serum TSH level. Monitor patients who are not treated yearly for changes in clinical status and thyroid laboratory parameters.

TSH suppression in well-differentiated thyroid cancer and thyroid nodules – The target level for TSH suppression in these conditions has not been established with controlled studies. In addition, the efficacy of TSH suppression for benign nodular disease is controversial. Therefore, individualize the dose of levothyroxine used for TSH suppression based on the specific disease and the patient being treated.

Well-differentiated (papillary and follicular) thyroid cancer: Levothyroxine is used as an adjunct to surgery and radioiodine therapy. Generally, TSH is suppressed to less than 0.1 milliunit/L, and this usually requires a dosage greater than 2 mcg/kg/day (0.002 mg/kg/day). However, in patients with high-risk tumors, the target level for TSH suppression may be less than 0.01 milliunit/L.

Benign nodules and nontoxic multinodular goiter: TSH is generally suppressed to a higher target (eg, 0.1 to 0.5 milliunit/L for nodules and 0.5 to 1 milliunit/L for multinodular goiter) than that used for the treatment of thyroid cancer. Levothyroxine is contraindicated if the serum TSH is already suppressed because of the risk of precipitating overt thyrotoxicosis. If the serum TSH level is not suppressed, use levothyroxine with caution in conjunction with careful monitoring of thyroid function for evidence of hyperthyroidism and clinical monitoring for potentially associated adverse cardiovascular signs and symptoms of hyperthyroidism.

Off-label dosing –

Hypothyroidism: once-weekly administration: [4] = Insufficient documentation. Weekly administration of 7 times the daily dose of thyroxine. In case reports, approximately 2 to 4 times the daily dose was given once weekly.

➤*Children:* Hyperactivity in an older child can be minimized if the starting dose is one-fourth of the recommended full replacement dose, and the dose is then increased on a weekly basis by an amount equal to one-fourth the full-recommended replacement dose until the full recommended replacement dose is reached.

Delays in diagnosis and institution of therapy may have deleterious effects on the child's intellectual and physical growth and development.

Hypothyroidism – In general, institute levothyroxine therapy at full replacement doses as soon as possible with the recommended dose per body weight decreasing with age.

Levothyroxine Oral Dosing Guidelines for Children With Hypothyroidism

Age	Daily dosage per kg body weight[a]
0 to 3 months	10 to 15 mcg/kg/day (0.01 to 0.015 mg/kg/day)[b]
3 to 6 months	8 to 10 mcg/kg/day (0.008 to 0.01 mg/kg/day)
6 to 12 months	6 to 8 mcg/kg/day (0.006 to 0.008 mg/kg/day)
1 to 5 years	5 to 6 mcg/kg/day (0.005 to 0.006 mg/kg/day)
6 to 12 years	4 to 5 mcg/kg/day (0.004 to 0.005 mg/kg/day)
> 12 years but growth and puberty incomplete	2 to 3 mcg/kg/day (0.002 to 0.003 mg/kg/day)
Growth and puberty complete	1.7 mcg/kg/day (0.0017 mg/kg/day)

[a] Adjust the dosage based on clinical response and laboratory parameters.
[b] Levothyroxine has been given as 8 to 10 mcg/kg/day in children 0 to 6 months of age.

Newborns:

- *Usual dosage* – 37.5 to 50 mcg/day for an average term infant.
- *Initial dosage* – 10 to 15 mcg/kg/day (0.01 to 0.015 mg/kg/day). Consider a lower starting dosage (eg, 25 mcg/day [0.025 mg/day]) in infants at risk for cardiac failure. In infants with very low (less than 5 mcg/dL) or undetectable serum T_4 concentrations, the recommended initial starting dosage is 50 mcg/day (0.05 mg/day).
- *Dosage titration* – Increase the dose in 4 to 6 weeks as needed based on clinical and laboratory response to treatment. Adjust doses in 12.5 mcg increments.

Chronic or severe hypothyroidism:

- *Initial dosage* – 25 mcg/day (0.025 mg/day).

LEVOTHYROXINE SODIUM — ORAL

• *Dosage titration* – Increments of 25 mcg (0.025 mg) every 2 to 4 weeks until the desired effect is achieved.

➤*Elderly:* For most patients older than 50 years of age, an initial starting dosage of 25 to 50 mcg/day (0.025 to 0.05 mg/day) is recommended, with gradual increments in dose at 6- to 8-week intervals, as needed.

The recommended starting dosage in elderly patients with cardiac disease is 12.5 to 25 mcg/day (0.0125 to 0.025 mg/day), with gradual dose increments at 4- to 6-week intervals. The levothyroxine dose is generally adjusted in 12.5 to 25 mcg (0.0125 to 0.025 mg) increments until the patient with primary hypothyroidism is clinically euthyroid and the serum TSH has normalized.

Elderly patients may require less than 1 mcg/kg/day (0.001 mg/kg/day) for treatment of hypothyroidism.

Because of the increased prevalence of cardiovascular disease among the elderly, do not initiate levothyroxine therapy at the full replacement dose or at lower doses than those recommended in younger individuals or in patients without cardiac disease. If cardiac symptoms develop or worsen, reduce the dose or withhold the dose for 1 week and then cautiously restart at a lower dose.

➤*Patients with underlying cardiovascular disease:* For patients younger than 50 years of age with underlying cardiac disease, an initial starting dosage of 25 to 50 mcg/day (0.025 to 0.05 mg/day) levothyroxine is recommended, with gradual increments in dose at 6- to 8-week intervals, as needed.

➤*Pregnancy:* Pregnancy may increase levothyroxine requirements.

➤*Myxedema coma:* Myxedema coma is a life-threatening emergency characterized by poor circulation and hypometabolism, and may result in unpredictable absorption of levothyroxine from the GI tract. Therefore, oral thyroid hormone drug products are not recommended to treat this condition. Administer thyroid hormone products formulated for IV administration.

➤*Monitoring:*

Adults – In patients with primary (thyroidal) hypothyroidism, serum TSH levels (using a sensitive assay) alone may be used to monitor therapy. The frequency of TSH monitoring during dose titration depends on the clinical situation, but it is generally recommended at 6- to 8-week intervals until normalization. For patients who have recently initiated therapy and whose serum TSH has normalized or in patients who have had their dosage or brand of levothyroxine changed, measure the serum TSH concentration after 8 to 12 weeks. When the optimum replacement dose has been attained, clinical (physical examination) and biochemical monitoring may be performed every 6 to 12 months, depending on the clinical situation, and whenever there is a change in the patient's status. It is recommended that a physical examination and a serum TSH measurement be performed at least annually in patients receiving levothyroxine.

Children – In patients with congenital hypothyroidism, assess the adequacy of replacement therapy by measuring both serum TSH (using a sensitive assay) and total or free T_4. During the first 3 years of life, the serum total or free T_4 should be maintained at all times in the upper half of the normal range. While the aim of therapy is to also normalize the serum TSH level, this is not always possible in a small percentage of patients, particularly in the first few months of therapy. TSH may not normalize because of a resetting of the pituitary-thyroid feedback threshold as a result of in utero hypothyroidism. Failure of the serum T_4 to increase into the upper half of the normal range within 2 weeks of initiation of therapy or of the serum TSH to decrease below 20 milliunits/L within 4 weeks should alert the health care provider to the possibility that the child is not receiving adequate therapy. Make careful inquiry regarding compliance, dose of medication administered, and method of administration prior to raising the dose of levothyroxine.

The recommended frequency of monitoring of TSH and total or free T_4 in children is as follows: at 2 and 4 weeks after the initiation of treatment; every 1 to 2 months during the first year of life; every 2 to 3 months between 1 and 3 years of age; and every 3 to 12 months thereafter until growth is completed. More frequent intervals of monitoring may be necessary if poor compliance is suspected or abnormal values are obtained. It is recommended that TSH and T_4 levels, and a physical examination, if indicated, be performed 2 weeks after any change in levothyroxine dosage. Perform routine clinical examination, including assessment of mental and physical growth and development, and bone maturation, at regular intervals.

Secondary (pituitary) and tertiary (hypothalamic) hypothyroidism – Assess adequacy of therapy by measuring serum free T_4 levels, which should be maintained in the upper half of the normal range in these patients.

➤*Administration:* Administer as a single daily dose and instruct patient to take in the morning on an empty stomach, at least 30 minutes to 1 hour before breakfast. Levothyroxine should be taken at least 4 hours apart from drugs that are known to interfere with its absorption (eg, aluminum- and magnesium-containing antacids; hydroxides, such as simethicone; bile acid sequestrants [cholestyramine and colestipol]; calcium carbonate; cation exchange resins [kayexalate]; ferrous sulfate; sucralfate).

Levothyroxine may be administered to infants and children who cannot swallow intact tablets by crushing the tablet and suspending the freshly crushed tablet in a small amount (5 to 10 mL or 1 to 2 teaspoons) of water. This suspension can be administered by spoon or dropper. Do not store the suspension. Do not use foods that decrease absorption of levothyroxine for administering levothyroxine tablets. Soybean flour (infant formula), cotton seed meal, walnuts, and dietary fiber may bind and decrease the absorption of levothyroxine from the GI tract.

➤*Storage/Stability:* Store at 20° to 25°C (68° to 77°F); excursions permitted between 15° and 30°C (59° and 86°F). Protect levothyroxine tablets from light and moisture and dispense in tight, light-resistant containers with child-resistant closure.

LEVOTHYROXINE SODIUM — INJECTION

For complete and comparative prescribing information, refer to the Thyroid Hormones group monograph.

WARNING

Drugs with thyroid hormone activity, alone or together with other therapeutic agents, have been used for the treatment of obesity. In euthyroid patients, doses within the range of daily hormonal requirements are ineffective for weight reduction. Larger doses may produce serious or even life-threatening manifestations of toxicity, particularly when given in association with sympathomimetic amines such as those used for their anorectic effects.

Indications

➤*Hypothyroidism:* As specific replacement therapy for reduced or absent thyroid function of any etiology. Levothyroxine sodium can be used IV whenever a rapid onset of effect is critical, and either IV or IM in hypothyroid patients whenever the oral route is precluded for long periods of time.

Administration and Dosage

➤*General dosing considerations:* The age and general physical condition of the patient and the severity and duration of hypothyroid symptoms determine the starting dosage and the rate of incremental dosage increase leading to a final maintenance dosage. Clearly it is the health care provider's judgment of the severity of the disease and closer observation of patient response that determine the rate and extent of dosage increase.

➤*Adults:*

Hypothyroidism –

Initial dosage: Approximately one-half of the previously established oral dosage of levothyroxine tablets given IV or IM.

Maintenance dosage: 50 to 100 mcg/day (0.05 to 0.1 mg/day) IV or IM. Close observation of the patient, with individual adjustment of the dosage as needed, is recommended.

Myxedema coma or stupor without concomitant severe heart disease: 200 to 500 mcg (0.2 to 0.5 mg) IV as a solution containing 100 mcg/mL (0.1 mg/mL). Although the patient may show evidence of increased responsivity within 6 to 8 hours, full therapeutic effect may not be evident until the following day. An additional 100 to 300 mcg (0.1 to 0.3 mg) or more may be given on the second day if evidence of significant and progressive improvements has not occurred. Levothyroxine produces a predictable increase in the reservoir level of hormone with a 7-day half-life. This usually precludes the need for multiple injections, but continued daily administration of lesser amounts parenterally should be maintained until the patient is fully capable of accepting a daily oral dose.

Myxedema coma or stupor with concomitant severe heart disease: The sudden administration of such large doses of levothyroxine IV is clearly not without its cardiovascular risks. Under such circumstances, IV therapy should not be undertaken without weighing the alternative risks of the myxedema coma and the cardiovascular disease. Clinical judgment in this situation may dictate smaller IV doses of levothyroxine.

➤*Children:* See Adults for dosing.

In infants and children, there is great urgency to achieve full thyroid replacement because of the critical importance of thyroid hormone in sustaining growth and maturation. Despite the smaller body size, the dosage needed to sustain a full rate of growth, development and general thriving is higher in the child than in the adult.

Off-label dosing –

Hypothyroidism:

• *Initial dosage* – 5 to 8 mcg/kg IV once daily.

➤*Monitoring:* Measurements of normal blood levels of thyroxine in patients on oral replacement regimens frequently coincide with clinical impressions of normal thyroid status, higher than normal levels occur occasionally and should not be considered evidence of overdosage. In all cases, clinical impressions of the well-being of the patient take precedence over laboratory determination of appropriate individual dosage.

Optimal maintenance levels should be adjusted individually to obtain normal serum T_3, T_4, free T_4, index and thyroid-stimulating hormone (TSH) values after several weeks of therapy for hypothyroidism. The patient's clinical status is most important and some patents may be clinically euthyroid with individual laboratory values that are not within normal range (ie, elevated total T_4 with normal T_3). An exception may be seen in congenital hypothyroidism where elevated serum TSH values may persist for the first 2 to 3 years of life despite normalization of free T_4 measurements. In such cases, it generally is recommended that maintenance of normal serum-free T_4 values alone should be considered therapeutically sufficient.

➤*Preparation for administration:* Reconstitute the lyophilized levothyroxine by aseptically adding 5 mL of sodium chloride 0.9% injection only. Shake vial to ensure complete mixing. Use immediately after reconstitution. Discard any unused portion.

➤*Administration:* Administer IM or IV.

LEVOTHYROXINE SODIUM — INJECTION

➤*Admixture compatibility:* Levothyroxine is compatible with sodium chloride 0.9% injection only. Do not add to other IV fluids.

➤*Storage/Stability:* Store dry product at controlled room temperature 15° to 30°C (59° to 86°F). Protect from light.

LIOTHYRONINE SODIUM (T_3)

Rx	**Liothyronine Sodium** (Various, eg, Mylan, Paddock)	**Tablets; oral:** 5 mcg	May contain sucrose. In 100s and 1,000s.
Rx	**Cytomel** (Monarch)		Sucrose. (JMI D14). White. In 100s.
Rx	**Liothyronine Sodium** (Various, eg, Mylan, Paddock)	**Tablets; oral:** 25 mcg	May contain sucrose. In 100s and 1,000s.
Rx	**Cytomel** (Monarch		Sucrose. (JMI D16). White, scored. In 100s.
Rx	**Liothyronine Sodium** (Various, eg, Mylan, Paddock)	**Tablets; oral:** 50 mcg	May contain sucrose. In 100s and 1,000s.
Rx	**Cytomel** (Monarch		Sucrose. (JMI D17). White, scored. In 100s.
Rx	**Liothyronine Sodium** (X-Gen)	**Injection, solution:** 10 mcg/mL	Alcohol 6.8%, ammonia 2.19 mg. In 1 mL vials.
Rx	**Triostat** (JHP Pharmaceuticals)		In 1 mL vials.[a]

[a] With 6.8% alcohol, 2.19 mg ammonia (as ammonium hydroxide) per mL.

LIOTHYRONINE SODIUM — ORAL

For complete and comparative prescribing information, refer to the Thyroid Hormones group monograph.

Indications

➤*Thyroid disorders:* As replacement or supplemental therapy in patients with hypothyroidism of any etiology, except transient hypothyroidism during the recovery phase of subacute thyroiditis. This category includes cretinism, myxedema and ordinary hypothyroidism in patients of any age (pediatric patients, adults, the elderly), or state (including pregnancy); primary hypothyroidism resulting from functional deficiency, primary atrophy, partial or total absence of thyroid gland, or the effects of surgery, radiation, or drugs, with or without the presence of goiter; and secondary (pituitary) or tertiary (hypothalamic) hypothyroidism (see Warnings/Precautions). As pituitary thyroid-stimulating hormone (TSH) suppressants, in the prevention or treatment of various types of euthyroid goiters, including thyroid nodules, subacute or chronic lymphocytic thyroiditis (Hashimoto's) and multinodular goiter. As diagnostic agents in suppression tests to differentiate suspected mild hyperthyroidism or thyroid gland autonomy.

➤*General information:* Liothyronine sodium tablets can be used in patients allergic to desiccated thyroid or thyroid extract derived from pork or beef.

Administration and Dosage

➤*General dosing considerations:* The dosage of thyroid hormones is determined by the indication and must in every case be individualized.

The rapid onset and dissipation of action of liothyronine sodium (T_3), as compared with levothyroxine sodium (T_4), has led some clinicians to prefer its use in patients who might be more susceptible to the untoward effects of thyroid medication. However, the wide swings in serum T_3 levels that follow its administration, and the possibility of more pronounced cardiovascular adverse reactions, tend to counterbalance the stated advantages.

Liothyronine sodium tablets may be used in preference to levothyroxine (T_4) during radioisotope scanning procedures, because induction of hypothyroidism in those cases is more abrupt and can be of shorter duration. It may also be preferred when impairment of peripheral conversion of T_4 to T_3 is suspected.

➤*Adults:*

Mild hypothyroidism –
Initial dosage: 25 mcg daily.
Maintenance dosage: 25 to 75 mcg daily.
Dosage adjustment: Daily dosage may be increased by up to 25 mcg every 1 or 2 weeks.

Myxedema –
Initial dosage: 5 mcg daily.
Maintenance dosage: 50 to 100 mcg daily.
Dosage adjustment: The initial dosage may be increased by 5 to 10 mcg daily every 1 or 2 weeks. When 25 mcg daily is reached, dosage may be increased by 5 to 25 mcg every 1 or 2 weeks until a satisfactory therapeutic response is attained.

Myxedema coma – Myxedema coma is usually precipitated in the hypothyroid patient of long standing by intercurrent illness or drugs such as sedatives and anesthetics and should be considered a medical emergency.

An IV preparation of liothyronine sodium is marketed for use in myxedema coma/precoma.

Simple (nontoxic) goiter –
Initial dosage: 5 mcg daily.
Maintenance dosage: 75 mcg daily.
Dosage adjustment: The initial dosage may be increased by 5 to 10 mcg daily every 1 to 2 weeks. When 25 mcg daily is reached, dosage may be increased every week or two by 12.5 or 25 mcg.
Conversion to liothyronine: When switching a patient to liothyronine sodium tablets from thyroid, L-thyroxine, or thyroglobulin, discontinue the other medication, initiate liothyronine sodium at a low dosage, and increase gradually according to the patient's response.

When selecting a starting dosage, bear in mind that this drug has a rapid onset of action, and that residual effects of the other thyroid preparation may persist for the first several weeks of therapy.

Thyroid-suppression therapy – Liothyronine sodium tablets are given in doses of 75 to 100 mcg/day for 7 days, and radioactive iodine uptake is determined before and after administration of the hormone. If thyroid function is under normal control, the radioiodine uptake will drop significantly after treatment.

Liothyronine sodium tablets should be administered cautiously to patients in whom there is a strong suspicion of thyroid-gland autonomy, in view of the fact that the exogenous hormone effects will be additive to the endogenous source.

➤*Children:*

Congenital hypothyroidism –
Initial dosage: 5 mcg daily.
Maintenance dosage: Infants a few months old may require only 20 mcg daily for maintenance. At 1 year of age, 50 mcg daily may be required. If children are older than 3 years of age, full adult dosage may be necessary.
Dosage adjustment: Increase the initial dosage with a 5 mcg increment every 3 to 4 days until the desired response is achieved.
Duration of therapy: Treatment should be initiated immediately upon diagnosis and maintained for life, unless transient hypothyroidism is suspected, in which case, therapy may be interrupted for 2 to 8 weeks after the age of 3 years to reassess the condition. Cessation of therapy is justified in patients who have maintained a normal thyroid-stimulating hormone during those 2 to 8 weeks.

➤*Elderly:* In the elderly or in pediatric patients, therapy should be started with 5 mcg daily and increased only by 5 mcg increments at the recommended intervals.

This drug is known to be substantially excreted by the kidney, and the risk of toxic reactions to this drug may be greater in patients with impaired renal function. Because elderly patients are more likely to have decreased renal function, care should be taken in dose selection, and it may be useful to monitor renal function.

➤*Administration:* Liothyronine sodium tablets are intended for oral administration; once-a-day dosage is recommended. Although liothyronine sodium has a rapid cutoff, its metabolic effects persist for a few days following discontinuance.

➤*Storage/Stability:* Store between 15° and 30°C (59° and 86°F).

LIOTHYRONINE SODIUM — INJECTION

For complete and comparative prescribing information, refer to the Thyroid Hormones group monograph.

Indications

➤*Myxedema coma/precoma:* Treatment of myxedema coma/precoma.

➤*General information:* Liothyronine sodium injection can be used in patients allergic to desiccated thyroid or thyroid extract derived from pork or beef.

Administration and Dosage

➤*General dosing considerations:* Myxedema coma is usually precipitated in the hypothyroid patient of long standing by intercurrent illness or drugs such as sedatives and anesthetics and should be considered a medical emergency.

Therapy should be directed at the correction of electrolyte disturbances, possible infection, or other intercurrent illness in addition to the administration of IV liothyronine (T_3).

Prompt administration of an adequate dose of IV liothyronine (T_3) is important in determining clinical outcome.

LIOTHYRONINE SODIUM — INJECTION

Oral therapy should be resumed as soon as the clinical situation has been stabilized and the patient is able to take oral medication. (See Conversion.)

➤*Adults:*

Myxedema coma/precoma –

Usual dosage: Doses of at least 65 mcg/day in the initial days of treatment have been shown to decrease mortality in myxedema case reports. However, there is limited clinical experience at total daily doses above 100 mcg.

Normally at least 4 hours should be allowed between doses to adequately assess therapeutic response, and no more than 12 hours should elapse between doses to avoid fluctuations in hormone levels.

Initial dosage: An initial IV liothyronine sodium injection dose ranging from 25 to 50 mcg is recommended in the emergency treatment of myxedema coma/precoma in adults. In patients with known or suspected cardiovascular disease, an initial dose of 10 to 20 mcg is suggested.

Dosage adjustment: Caution should be exercised in adjusting the dose because of the potential of large changes to precipitate adverse cardiovascular events.

Concomitant therapy: Simultaneous glucocorticosteroids are required.

Conversion: When switching a patient to liothyronine sodium tablets from liothyronine sodium injection, discontinue liothyronine sodium injection, initiate oral therapy at a low dosage, and increase gradually according to the patient's response.

If levothyroxine rather than liothyronine sodium is used in initiating oral therapy, the physician should bear in mind that there is a delay of several days in the onset of levothyroxine activity and that IV therapy should be discontinued gradually.

➤*Elderly:* Dosage reduction may be required in elderly patients with renal impairment. (See Renal function impairment.)

➤*Renal function impairment:* This drug is known to be substantially excreted by the kidney, and the risk of toxic reactions to this drug may be greater in patients with impaired renal function.

Because elderly patients are more likely to have decreased renal function, care should be taken in dose selection, and it may be useful to monitor renal function.

➤*Therapeutic drug monitoring:* Serum T_3 and thyroid-stimulating hormone levels should be monitored to assess dosage adequacy and biologic effectiveness.

➤*Administration:* Liothyronine sodium injection (T_3) is for IV administration only. It should not be given IM or subcutaneously.

➤*Storage/Stability:* Store between 2° and 8°C (35° and 46°F).

LIOTRIX

	Product and distributor	Tablet strength (grain)	Content (mcg)[a] T_3	Content (mcg)[a] T_4	Thyroid equivalent (mg)	How supplied
Rx	**Thyrolar** (Forest)	¼	3.1	12.5	15	Lactose. (YC). Violet/White. Two-layered. In 100s.
		½	6.25	25	30	Lactose. (YD). Peach/White. Two-layered. In 100s.
		1	12.5	50	60	Lactose. (YE). Pink/White. Two-layered. In 100s.
		2	25	100	120	Lactose. (YF). Green/White. Two-layered. In 100s.
		3	37.5	150	180	Lactose. (YH). Yellow/White. Two-layered. In 100s.

[a] Liothyronine sodium (T_3) is approximately 4 times as potent as levothyroxine (T_4) on a microgram-for-microgram basis.

LIOTRIX — ORAL

For complete prescribing information, refer to the Thyroid Hormones group monograph.

WARNING

Drugs with thyroid hormone activity, alone or with other therapeutic agents have been used for the treatment of obesity. In euthyroid patients, doses within the range of daily hormonal requirements are ineffective for weight reduction. Larger doses may produce serious or even life-threatening manifestations of toxicity, particularly when given in association with sympathomimetic amines such as those used for their anorectic effects.

Indications

➤*Hypothyroidism:* As replacement or supplemental therapy in patients with hypothyroidism of any etiology, except transient hypothyroidism during the recovery phase of subacute thyroiditis. This category includes cretinism, myxedema, and ordinary hypothyroidism in patients of any age (children, adults, the elderly), or state (including pregnancy); primary hypothyroidism resulting from functional deficiency, primary atrophy, partial or total absence of thyroid gland, or the effects of surgery, radiation, or drugs, with or without the presence of goiter; and secondary (pituitary) or tertiary (hypothalamic) hypothyroidism.

➤*Pituitary thyroid stimulating hormone (TSH) suppression:* As pituitary TSH suppressants in the prevention or treatment of various types of euthyroid goiters, including thyroid nodules, subacute or chronic lymphocytic thyroiditis (Hashimoto), and multinodular goiter and in the management of thyroid cancer.

➤*Diagnostic agent:* As diagnostic agents in suppression tests to differentiate suspected mild hyperthyroidism or thyroid gland autonomy.

Administration and Dosage

➤*General dosing considerations:*

Dosage equivalents – Each liotrix 60 mg tablet will usually replace approximately 60 to 65 mg (1 grain) of desiccated thyroid.

Optimal dosage is determined by patient's clinical response and laboratory findings.

➤*Adults:*

Diagnostic agent – The usual suppressive dose of T_4 is 1.56 mcg/kg of body weight per day given for 7 to 10 days. These doses usually yield normal serum T_4 and T_3 levels and lack of response to TSH.

Hypothyroidism –

Initial dosage: Initiate therapy using low doses with increments that depend on cardiovascular status.

Usual starting dose is 1 tablet of *Thyrolar ½* daily with increments of 1 tablet of *Thyrolar ¼* every 2 to 3 weeks. A lower starting dose, 1 tablet *Thyrolar ¼* daily, is recommended in patients with long-standing myxedema, particularly if cardiovascular impairment is suspected, in which case extreme caution is recommended.

Maintenance dosage: Most patients require 1 tablet *Thyrolar 1* to 1 tablet *Thyrolar 2* per day; failure to respond to 1 tablet *Thyrolar 3* suggests lack of compliance or malabsorption.

Maintenance dosages of 1 tablet *Thyrolar 1* to 1 tablet of *Thyrolar 2* per day usually result in normal serum levothyroxine and triiodothyronine levels. Adequate therapy usually results in normal TSH and T_4 levels after 2 to 3 weeks of therapy.

Dosage adjustment: Adjust dosage within the first 4 weeks of therapy after proper clinical and laboratory evaluations, including serum levels of T_4 bound and free and TSH.

Reduce dosage if angina occurs.

Thyroid cancer – Larger amounts of thyroid hormone than those used for replacement therapy are required. Medullary carcinoma of the thyroid is usually unresponsive to this therapy.

➤*Children:*

Congenital hypothyroidism –

Usual dosage: Follow recommendations in the following table. In infants with congenital hypothyroidism, institute therapy with full doses as soon as diagnosis is made.

Liotrix Pediatric Dosage for Congenital Hypothyroidism

Age	Dose per day in mcg T_3/T_4	to	T_3/T_4
0 to 6 mo	3.1/12.5	to	6.25/25
6 to 12 mo	6.25/25	to	9.35/37.5
1 to 5 y	9.35/37.5	to	12.5/50
6 to 12 y	12.5/50	to	18.75/75
Over 12 y			> 18.75/75

Duration of therapy: Treatment should be initiated immediately upon diagnosis and maintained for life, unless transient hypothyroidism is suspected; in which case, therapy may be interrupted for 2 to 8 weeks after 3 years of age to reassess the condition.

Discontinuation of therapy: Cessation of therapy is justified in patients who have maintained a normal TSH for 2 to 8 weeks following therapy interruption because of transient hypothyroidism. In infants, excessive doses of thyroid hormone preparations may produce craniosynostosis.

➤*Elderly:* In patients with angina pectoris or the elderly, in whom there is a greater likelihood of occult cardiac disease, initiate therapy with low doses (1 tablet of *Thyrolar ¼* or *Thyrolar ½*).

➤*Storage/Stability:* Store at cold temperature between 2° and 8°C (36° and 46°F) in a tight, light-resistant container.

IODINE PRODUCTS

otc	**ThyroSafe** (Recip)	**Tablets; oral:** potassium iodide 65 mg	Lactose. White, round, scored. In 10s and 20s.
otc	**Iosat** (Anbex)	**Tablets; oral:** potassium iodide 130 mg	(IOSAT). White, round, scored. In 14s.
Rx	**Strong Iodine Solution (Lugol's Solution)** (Various, eg, Lannett)	**Solution; oral:** iodine 5% (50 mg/mL)/potassium iodide 10% (100 mg/mL)	In 120 mL, 437 mL, and gal.
otc	**ThyroShield** (Fleming)	**Solution; oral:** potassium iodide 65 mg/mL	Parabens, saccharin, sucrose. Black-raspberry flavor. In 30 mL.
Rx	**Potassium Iodide** (Various, eg, Balan, Goldline, Harber)	**Solution; oral:** potassium iodide 1 g/mL	In 30 and 240 mL and pt.
Rx sf	**Potassium Iodide** (Roxane)		In 30 and 240 mL.
Rx	**SSKI** (Upsher-Smith)		In 30 and 240 mL.
Rx	**Pima** (Fleming)	**Syrup; oral:** potassium iodide 325 mg per 5 mL	Sugar. Black-raspberry flavor. In pt and gal.

IODINE PRODUCTS — ORAL

WARNING

Potassium iodide should only be used during nuclear radiation emergency when recommended by public officials. In a nuclear radiation emergency, radioactive iodine could be released into the air. Potassium iodide protects only the thyroid gland from uptake or radioactive iodine. Therefore, potassium iodide should be used along with other emergency measures recommended by public officials.

Potassium iodide for nuclear radiation emergency should not be taken more than once every 24 hours. Higher amounts of potassium iodide will not provide additional benefits and may increase the chances of adverse effects. Potassium iodide should not be used in patients who are allergic to iodine.

Indications

➤*Hyperthyroidism (strong iodine solution):* Used adjunctively with an antithyroid drug in hyperthyroid patients in preparation for thyroidectomy and to treat thyrotoxic crisis or neonatal thyrotoxicosis.

Strong iodine solution may be used alone, but more frequently is used after the hyperthyroidism is controlled by an antithyroid drug. Optimal control of hyperthyroidism is achieved if antithyroid drugs are first given alone.

➤*Nuclear radiation emergency (Iosat, ThyroSafe, ThyroShield):* Thyroid blocking in a nuclear radiation emergency.

➤*General information:* For use of potassium iodide as an expectorant and for other respiratory tract conditions, see the Potassium Iodide (Expectorant) monograph.

➤*Off-label uses:* Potassium iodide (60 mg 3 times daily) has been used effectively in a limited number of patients for Sweet syndrome (acute febrile neutrophilic dermatosis) in combination with a potent topical steroid, as an alternative to systemic corticosteroids.

Also effective for the treatment of lymphocutaneous sporotrichosis (a dimorphic fungus that typically infects the skin and lymphatic system).

Administration and Dosage

➤*General dosing considerations:* To prepare hyperthyroid patients for thyroidectomy, administer for 10 days prior to surgery.

Patients with both a nodular thyroid condition such as multinodular goiter with heart disease should not take potassium iodide for nuclear radiation emergency . Patients with other thyroid conditions may take potassium iodide as previously directed, but a health care provider should be consulted if potassium iodide is administered for more than a few days.

➤*Adults:*

Dietary reference intake for iodine – Refer to Dietary Reference Intakes of Vitamins and Minerals table.

Hyperthyroidism –

Strong iodine solution: See also Off-Label Dosing recommendations.
- *Usual dose* – 0.3 mL 3 times daily.
- *Dose range* – 0.1 to 0.9 mL daily.

Nuclear radiation emergency –

Iosat, ThyroSafe, and *ThyroShield*:
- *Usual dose* – 130 mg every 24 hours.
- *Maximum dose* – More than 1 dose in 24 hours should not be taken.
- *Pregnant or breast-feeding women* – Pregnant or breast-feeding women should take as directed as previously described and call a health care provider as soon as possible. Repeat dosing should be avoided. Women who are pregnant or breast-feeding should be checked by a doctor if repeat dosing is necessary. Although these precautions should be taken, the benefits of short-term use of potassium iodide to block uptake of radioactive iodine by thyroid gland far exceed its chances of adverse effects.

Off-label dosing –

Thyroid storm:
- *Strong iodine solution* – 4 to 8 drops every 6 to 8 hours, started at least 1 hour after a thionamide.

Thyrotoxicosis:
- *Strong iodine solution* – 3 to 5 drops daily (assuming 20 drops per mL and a concentration of 8 mg per drop).

➤*Children:*

Dietary reference intake for iodine – Refer to Dietary Reference Intakes of Vitamins and Minerals table.

Hyperthyroidism –

Strong iodine solution: See also Off-Label Dosing Recommendations. See Adults for dosing.

Nuclear radiation emergency –

Iosat, ThyroSafe, and *ThyroShield:*
- *Usual dose* –
  - *12 to 18 years of age and at least 150 lb:* 130 mg every 24 hours.
  - *12 to 18 years of age and less than 150 lb:* 65 mg every 24 hours.
  - *Older than 3 years to 12 years of age:* 65 mg every 24 hours.
  - *Older than 1 month to 3 years of age:* 32.5 mg every 24 hours.
  - *Infants from birth to 1 month of age:* 16.25 mg every 24 hours.

Administer as previously described and call a health care provider as soon as possible. Repeat dosing should be avoided. Thyroid function should be checked in infants younger than 1 month of age who take potassium iodide. Although these precautions should be taken, the benefits of short-term use of potassium iodide to block uptake of radioactive iodine by the thyroid gland far exceed the chances of adverse effects.
- *Maximum dose* – Do not administer more than 1 dose in 24 hours.

Off-label dosing –

Neonatal Graves disease:
- *Strong iodine solution* – 1 drop every 8 hours.

Thyroid storm:
- *Strong iodine solution* – See Adults for dosing.

Thyrotoxicosis:
- *Strong iodine solution* – See Adults for dosing.

➤*Preparation for administration:*

Potassium iodide liquid mixture – Tablets can be crushed and mixed in many liquids. To take the tablet in liquid solution, use the following dosing directions.

Put one tablet into a small bowl and grind it into a fine powder using the back of a metal teaspoon against the inside of the bowl. The powder should not have any large pieces.

Add 4 teaspoons of water to the crushed potassium iodide powder in the bowl and mix until the potassium iodide powder is dissolved in the water.

Take the potassium iodide water mixture solution and mix it with 4 teaspoons of low-fat white or chocolate milk, orange juice, flat soda, raspberry syrup, or infant formula.

The potassium iodide liquid mixture will keep for up to 7 days in the refrigerator. It is recommended that the potassium iodide liquid mixtures be prepared weekly. Throw away unused portions.

➤*Administration:* Dilute strong iodine solution in water or juice prior to administration.

Potassium iodide tablets may be administered whole or crushed.

Potassium iodide liquid mixture – The amount of potassium iodide in the drink when mixed as previously described is 16.25 mg/tsp for the 130 mg tablet (*Iostat*) and 8.125 mg/tsp for the 65 mg tablet (*ThyroSafe*). The number of teaspoons of the drink to administer depends on the child's age as described in the following table.

Potassium Iodide Liquid Mixture Administration Guide

Age	Amount of potassium iodide liquid mixture to administer	
	Iostat	*ThyroSafe*
Older than 12 years to 18 years of age and weight less than 150 lb	65 mg	65 mg
Older than 3 years to 12 years of age	65 mg	65 mg
Older than 1 month to 3 years of age	32.5 mg	32.5 mg
0 to 1 month	16.25 mg	16.25 mg

Note: This is the amount to give children for one single dose in teaspoonfuls (not tablespoonfuls).

IODINE PRODUCTS — ORAL

➤*Storage/Stability:*

ThyroShield – Store at 25°C (77°F); excursions permitted to 15° to 30°C (59° to 86°F). Protect from light.

Iosat and *ThyroSafe* – Store at 20° to 25°C (68° to 77°F). Keep dry and foil intact.

Actions

➤*Pharmacology:* An adequate intake of iodine is necessary for normal thyroid function and the synthesis of thyroid hormones.

Elemental iodine (from the diet or as medication) is reduced in the GI tract and enters the circulation in the form of iodide, which is actively transported and concentrated by the thyroid gland. Hormone synthesis requires the oxidation of iodide and iodination of tyrosyl residues in thyroglobulin to form iodotyrosine precursors. These precursors undergo a "coupling reaction" to yield the active thyroid hormones T_3 and T_4. High concentrations of iodide greatly influence iodine metabolism by the thyroid gland. Large doses of iodides can inhibit T_4 and T_3 synthesis and rapidly inhibit proteolysis of colloid and the release of T_4 and T_3 into the bloodstream.

The effects of iodides are evident within 24 hours; maximum effects are attained after 10 to 15 days of continuous therapy. If administered chronically, therapeutic effects may persist for up to 6 weeks after the crisis has abated.

Contraindications

Hypersensitivity to iodine.

➤*Strong iodine solution:* Active tuberculosis.

➤*Iosat*, *ThyroSafe*, and *ThyroShield*: Dermatitis herpetiformis; hypocomplementemic vasculitis; nodular thyroid disease with heart disease.

Warnings/Precautions

➤*Pregnancy:* Category D (potassium iodide). Iodides readily cross the placenta and may cause hypothyroidism and goiter in the fetus or newborn when used long-term or close to term; short-term use (eg, 10 days) may not carry this risk. Administer to pregnant women only if clearly needed.

➤*Lactation:* Iodide is excreted in breast milk; however, the significance to the infant is not known. According to the American Academy of Pediatrics, these agents are not contraindicated in breast-feeding.

Drug Interactions

➤*Lithium carbonate:* Lithium carbonate and iodide preparations may have synergistic hypothyroid activity; concomitant use may result in hypothyroidism.

Adverse Reactions

Possible adverse effects of potassium iodide include: skin rashes; swelling of the salivary glands; "iodism" (metallic taste, burning mouth and throat, sore teeth and gums, symptoms of a head cold and sometimes stomach upset, nausea, vomiting, and diarrhea); allergic reactions (ie, fever and joint pains; swelling of parts of the face and body; trouble breathing, speaking or swallowing; severe shortness of breath requiring immediate medical attention). Overactivity or underactivity of the thyroid gland or enlargement of the thyroid gland (goiter) may occur rarely.

Overdosage

➤*Acute poisoning:*

Symptoms – Iodine is corrosive, and toxic symptoms are mainly the result of local GI tract irritation. Gastroenteritis, abdominal pain and diarrhea (sometimes bloody) may be seen. Fatalities may occur from circulatory collapse caused by shock, corrosive gastritis or asphyxiation from swelling of the glottis or larynx.

Treatment – Gastric lavage with a soluble starch solution (15 g cornstarch or flour in 500 mL water) is recommended for removing iodine from the stomach. A 1% oral solution of sodium thiosulfate is a specific antidote, as it will reduce iodine to iodide. Milk may help relieve gastric irritation. Correct fluid and electrolyte imbalance, and treat shock if necessary.

➤*Chronic poisoning:* Discontinue use of iodine or iodides. High sodium chloride intake will speed recovery. For iodism characterized by skin or mucous membrane reactions, give cortisone or equivalent corticosteroid 25 to 100 mg every 6 hours orally until symptoms abate.

Patient Information

➤*Strong iodine solution:* Dilute with water or fruit juice to improve taste.

Advise patients to discontinue use and notify healthy care provider if fever; skin rash; metallic taste; swelling of the mouth, tongue or throat; burning of the mouth and throat; sore gums and teeth; head cold symptoms; trouble breathing, speaking, or swallowing; severe GI distress or enlargement of the thyroid gland (goiter) occurs.

POTASSIUM IODIDE (EXPECTORANT) — ORAL

Indications

➤*Expectorant:* As an expectorant in the treatment of chronic pulmonary diseases where tenacious mucus complicates the problem. These include bronchial asthma, chronic bronchitis, bronchiectasis, pulmonary emphysema, and sinus congestion.

➤*Off-label uses:* Potassium iodide (60 mg 3 times daily) has been used effectively in a limited number of patients for Sweet syndrome (acute febrile neutrophilic dermatosis) in combination with a potent topical steroid, as an alternative to systemic corticosteroids.

Thyroid storm or thyrotoxicosis. (See Administration and Dosage.)

Administration and Dosage

➤*General dosing considerations:* Use no longer than necessary to produce the desired effect.

➤*Adults:*

Expectorant –

Pima: 5 to 10 mL 3 times daily.

SSKI:

- *Usual dosage* – 0.3 mL (300 mg) to 0.6 mL (600 mg) 3 or 4 times a day.
- *Maximum dose* – Do not take more than 12 times a day.

Off-label dosing –

Thyroid storm:

- *SSKI* – 5 drops orally every 6 hours, started at least 1 hour after a thionamide.

Thyrotoxicosis:

- *SSKI* – 1 drop orally daily. Another reference suggests 3 to 10 drops orally daily for patients with Graves disease. Administer for 7 to 14 days preoperatively if using to prepare a patient for thyroid surgery.

➤*Children:*

Expectorant –

Pima:

- *Older than 3 years of age* – 5 mL 3 times daily.
- *Younger than 3 years of age* – 2.5 mL 3 times daily.

Off-label dosing –

Thyrotoxicosis:

- *SSKI* – 50 to 250 mg (approximately 1 to 5 drops) orally 3 times daily.

➤*Preparation for administration:* When exposed to cold temperatures, crystallization may occur, but on warming and shaking, the crystals will redissolve. If the solution turns brownish-yellow in color, it should be discarded. Dilute each dose of *SSKI* in one glassful of water, fruit juice, or milk.

➤*Administration:* Take each dose with at least 120 to 240 mL of water. To minimize gastric irritation, take with food or milk.

➤*Storage/Stability:* Store at 25°C (77°F). Excursions permitted between 15° and 30°C (59° and 86°F). Protect from heat, light, and moisture.

Actions

➤*Pharmacology:* Potassium iodide enhances the secretion of respiratory fluids, thus decreasing mucus viscosity.

Warnings/Precautions

➤*Hypersensitivity reactions:* Patients who are hyperthyroid or who may be sensitive to iodides may temporarily develop iodine-induced swelling of a lymph or salivary gland. Other adverse events in iodide-sensitive patients may include GI upset, metallic taste, minor skin eruptions, nausea, vomiting.

➤*Pregnancy:* Category D per Briggs' *Drugs in Pregnancy and Lactation*.

➤*Lactation:* Potassium iodide is excreted in breast milk (per Briggs' *Drugs in Pregnancy and Lactation*).

WARNING

Propylthiouracil –

Hepatotoxicity: Severe liver injury and acute liver failure, in some cases fatal, have been reported in patients treated with propylthiouracil. These reports of hepatic reactions include cases requiring liver transplantation in adults and children. Reserve propylthiouracil for patients who cannot tolerate methimazole and in whom radioactive iodine therapy or surgery are not appropriate treatments for the management of hyperthyroidism.

Pregnancy: Because of the risk of fetal abnormalities associated with methimazole, propylthiouracil may be the treatment of choice when an antithyroid drug is indicated during or just prior to the first trimester of pregnancy.

Indications

➤*Hyperthyroidism:* Long-term therapy may lead to disease remission. Also used to ameliorate hyperthyroidism in preparation for subtotal thyroidectomy or radioactive iodine therapy.

Reserve propylthiouracil for patients who are intolerant of methimazole and for whom surgery or radioactive iodine therapy is not an appropriate treatment regimen.

Propylthiouracil and methimazole are also used when thyroidectomy is contraindicated or not advisable.

➤*Off-label uses:* Propylthiouracil (300 mg/day) may be useful in reducing mortality caused by alcoholic liver disease by reducing the hepatic hypermetabolic state induced by alcohol.

Administration and Dosage

In one study, the rate of remission and time to relapse of Graves disease was significantly increased when antithyroid therapy was given for a prolonged duration (18 months) versus short-term (6 months) treatment. However, the monitoring of thyroid-stimulating antibody values may be a useful guide for shortening the duration of treatment in some patients.

One small study reported that single and divided daily doses of methimazole were equally effective in hyperthyroid patients. Traditionally administered in divided doses, it was suggested that a single daily dose would be effective because methimazole is present in the thyroid for 20 hours and is active for 40 hours despite a serum half-life of 6 to 13 hours. Further study is needed.

Actions

➤*Pharmacology:* Propylthiouracil and methimazole inhibit the synthesis of thyroid hormones and, thus, are effective in the treatment of hyperthyroidism. They do not inactivate existing thyroxine (T_4) and triiodothyronine (T_3), which are stored in the thyroid or which circulate in the blood, nor do they interfere with the effectiveness of exogenous thyroid hormones. Propylthiouracil partially inhibits the peripheral conversion of T_4 to T_3.

Both drugs are concentrated in the thyroid gland. Pharmacokinetic data are summarized in the following table:

Various Pharmacokinetic Parameters of Antithyroid Agents

Antithyroid agent	Bioavailability	Protein binding	Transplacental passage	Breast milk levels (M:P)[a]	Half-life	Excreted in urine
Propylthiouracil	80% to 95%	75% to 80%	Low	Low (0.1)	1 to 2 h	< 35%
Methimazole	80% to 95%	0%	High	High (1)	6 to 13 h	< 10%

[a] Approximate milk:plasma ratio.

Contraindications

Hypersensitivity to antithyroid drugs; breast-feeding mothers (methimazole).

Warnings/Precautions

➤*Hepatic effects:* Liver injury resulting in liver failure, liver transplantation, or death has been reported with propylthiouracil therapy in adults and children. No cases of liver failure have been reported with the use of methimazole in children. Propylthiouracil is not recommended in children except when methimazole is not well tolerated and surgery or radioactive iodine therapy are not appropriate.

Cases of livery injury, including liver failure and death, have been reported in women treated with propylthiouracil during pregnancy. Use of an alternative antithyroid medication (eg, methimazole) may be advisable following the first trimester.

Instruct patients to report any symptoms of hepatic dysfunction (eg, anorexia, pruritis, right upper quadrant pain), particularly during the first 6 months of therapy. If these symptoms occur, discontinue propylthiouracil immediately and obtain liver function tests and ALT and AST levels. Routine monitoring of liver function and hepatocellular integrity is not expected to decrease the risk of sever liver injury because of the rapid and unpredictable onset.

➤*Hematologic effects:* Agranulocytosis is a potentially life-threatening adverse effect of therapy. Instruct patients to report any symptoms of agranulocytosis, such as hay fever, sore throat, skin eruptions, fever, headache, or general malaise. In such cases, take white blood cell (WBC) and differential counts to determine whether agranulocytosis has developed. Exercise particular care with patients receiving additional drugs known to cause agranulocytosis. Leukopenia, thrombocytopenia, and aplastic anemia (pancytopenia) may also occur. Discontinue the drug in the presence of agranulocytosis, aplastic anemia, hepatitis, fever, or exfoliative dermatitis. Monitor the patient's bone marrow function.

One report recommends routine monitoring of the WBC count for at least the first 3 months of therapy, thereby potentially detecting agranulocytosis prior to becoming evident by infection.

➤*Hemorrhagic effects:* Because propylthiouracil may cause hypoprothrombinemia and bleeding, monitor prothrombin time during therapy, especially before surgical procedures.

➤*Hypothyroidism:* Propylthiouracil can cause hypothyroidism, necessitating routine monitoring of thyroid-stimulating hormone and free T_4 levels, with adjustments in dose to maintain a euthyroid state.

➤*Pregnancy:* Category D. These agents, used judiciously, are effective drugs in hyperthyroidism complicated by pregnancy. Because they readily cross the placenta and can induce goiter and even cretinism in the developing fetus, it is important that a sufficient, but not excessive, dose be given. In many pregnant women, thyroid dysfunction diminishes as the pregnancy proceeds, thus making a reduction of dose possible. In some instances, these products can be withdrawn 2 or 3 weeks before delivery. Propylthiouracil can cause fetal harm when administered to a pregnant woman. Approximately 10% will develop neonatal goiter. However, if an antithyroid agent is needed, propylthiouracil is preferred because it is less likely than methimazole to cross the placenta and induce fetal/neonatal complications (eg, aplasia cutis). Given the potential maternal adverse effects of propylthiouracil (eg, hepatotoxicity), it may be preferable to switch from propylthiouracil to methimazole for the second and third trimesters.

➤*Lactation:* Methimazole is contraindicated in breast-feeding women. Propylthiouracil is transferred to breast milk to a small extent; therefore, it is likely to result in clinically insignificant doses to the breast-feeding infant. The mean amount of propylthiouracil excreted during 4 hours after a 400 mg dose was 0.025% of the administered dose.

➤*Children:* Postmarketing reports of severe liver injury, including hepatic failure requiring liver transplantation or resulting in death, have been reported in children. No such reports have been observed with methimazole. Propylthiouracil is not recommended in children except when methimazole is not well tolerated and surgery or radioactive iodine therapy are not appropriate.

➤*Monitoring:* Monitor thyroid function tests periodically during therapy. Once clinical evidence of hyperthyroidism has resolved, the finding of an elevated serum thyroid-stimulating hormone indicates to use a lower maintenance dose of propylthiouracil.

Drug Interactions

➤*Anticoagulants:* The activity of oral anticoagulants may be potentiated by the anti–vitamin K activity attributed to propylthiouracil.

Adverse Reactions

Adverse reactions probably occur in less than 1% of patients.

➤*CNS:* CNS stimulation, depression, drowsiness, headache, neuritis, neuropathies, paresthesias, vertigo.

➤*Dermatologic:* Erythema nodosum; exfoliative dermatitis; lupus-like syndrome, including splenomegaly and vasculitis; pruritus; skin pigmentation; skin rash; skin ulcers; urticaria.

➤*GI:* Epigastric distress, loss of taste, nausea and vomiting, sialadenopathy.

➤*Hematologic:* Aplastic anemia, hypoprothrombinemia and bleeding, inhibition of myelopoiesis (agranulocytosis, granulocytopenia, and thrombocytopenia), periarteritis. Approximately 10% of patients with untreated hyperthyroidism have leukopenia (WBC count less than 4,000/mm^3), often with relative granulocytopenia.

➤*Hepatic:* Hepatitis; jaundice (may persist for several weeks after discontinuance); liver injury resulting in hepatitis, liver failure, a need for liver transplantation, or death (propylthiouracil).

➤*Renal:* Glomerulonephritis, nephritis.

➤*Respiratory:* Alveolar hemorrhage, interstitial pneumonitis, pulmonary infiltrates.

➤*Miscellaneous:* Abnormal hair loss, antineutrophil cytoplasmic antibody–positive vasculitis that may include rapidly progressive glomerulonephritis sometimes leading to acute renal failure, arthralgia, drug fever, edema, insulin autoimmune syndrome (may result in hypoglycemic coma), leukocytoclastic vasculitis, lymphadenopathy, myalgia.

Overdosage

➤*Symptoms:* Arthralgia, edema, epigastric distress, fever, headache, nausea, pancytopenia, pruritus, vomiting. Agranulocytosis is the most serious effect. Rarely, CNS depression or stimulation, exfoliative dermatitis, hepatitis, or neuropathies may occur.

➤*Treatment:* Protect the patient's airway and support ventilation and perfusion. Meticulously monitor and maintain, within acceptable limits, the patient's vital signs, blood gases, and serum electrolytes. Monitor the patient's bone marrow function. Refer to General Management of Acute Overdosage.

Patient Information

Advise patients to take at regular intervals around the clock (usually every 8 hours).

Advise patients to notify health care provider if the following symptoms occur: headache, fever, rash, sore throat, unusual bleeding or bruising, yellowing of the skin, or vomiting.

PROPYLTHIOURACIL (PTU)

Rx	**Propylthiouracil** (Various, eg, DAVA)	**Tablets; oral:** 50 mg	In 100s and 1,000s. May contain sodium benzoate.

PROPYLTHIOURACIL — ORAL

For complete prescribing information, refer to the Antithyroid Agents class monograph.

WARNING

Hepatotoxicity – Severe liver injury and acute liver failure, in some cases fatal, have been reported in patients treated with propylthiouracil. These reports of hepatic reactions include cases requiring liver transplantation in adults and children.

Reserve propylthiouracil for patients who can not tolerate methimazole and in whom radioactive iodine therapy or surgery are not appropriate treatments for the management of hyperthyroidism.

Pregnancy – Because of the risk of fetal abnormalities associated with methimazole, propylthiouracil may be the treatment of choice when an antithyroid drug is indicated during or just prior to the first trimester of pregnancy.

Indications

➤*Hyperthyroidism:* Patients with Graves disease with hyperthyroidism or toxic multinodular goiter who are intolerant of methimazole and for whom surgery or radioactive iodine therapy is not an appropriate treatment regimen; to ameliorate symptoms of hyperthyroidism in preparation for subtotal thyroidectomy or radioactive iodine therapy in patients who are intolerant of methimazole.

➤*Off-label uses:* Propylthiouracil 300 mg/day may be useful in reducing mortality caused by alcoholic liver disease by reducing the hepatic hypermetabolic state induced by alcohol.

Administration and Dosage

➤*Adults:*

Hyperthyroidism –

Initial dosage: 300 mg daily in 3 equal doses every 8 hours. In patients with severe hyperthyroidism, very large goiters, or both, the initial dosage may be increased to 400 mg daily; an occasional patient will require 600 to 900 mg daily initially.

Maintenance dosage: 100 to 150 mg daily in divided doses every 8 hours.

➤*Children:* Propylthiouracil is generally not recommended for use in children, except in rare instances in which other alternative therapies are not appropriate options.

Hyperthyroidism – See also Off-label Dosing.

6 years of age and older:

- *Initial dosage* – 50 mg daily in divided doses every 8 hours.
- *Maintenance dosage* – Carefully titrate dosage upward based on clinical response and evaluation of thyroid-stimulating hormone (TSH) and free thyroxine (T4) levels. Cases of severe liver injury have been reported with dosages as low as 50 mg/day; however, most cases were associated with dosages of 300 mg/day or higher.

Off-label dosing –

Hyperthyroidism:

- *Older than 10 years of age –*
  Initial dosage: 150 to 300 mg/day in divided doses every 8 hours or 5 to 7 mg/kg/day divided every 8 hours.
  Maintenance dosage: ⅓ to ⅔ the initial dosage divided every 8 to 12 hours when the patient is euthyroid (usually after 2 months).
- *6 to 10 years of age –*
  Initial dosage: 50 to 150 mg/day divided every 8 hours or 5 to 7 mg/kg/day divided every 8 hours.
  Maintenance dosage: ⅓ to ⅔ the initial dosage divided every 8 to 12 hours when the patient is euthyroid (usually after 2 months).
- *Infants and children younger than 6 years of age –*
  Initial dosage: 5 to 7 mg/kg/day divided every 8 hours.
  Maintenance dosage: ⅓ to ⅔ the initial dosage divided every 8 to 12 hours when the patient is euthyroid (usually after 2 months).
- *Neonates* – 5 to 10 mg/kg/day divided every 8 hours.

➤*Administration:* Administer with meals to minimize GI irritation.

➤*Storage/Stability:* Store at 15° to 30°C (59° to 86°F).

METHIMAZOLE

Rx	**Methimazole** (Par Pharm)	**Tablets; oral:** 5 mg	Lactose. (EM/5). White to off-white. In 100s.
Rx	**Northyx** (Centrix Pharmaceutical)		Lactose. (M5). Scored. In 100s.
Rx	**Tapazole** (Monarch)		Lactose. (J94). White to off white, scored. In 100s.
Rx	**Methimazole** (Par Pharm)	**Tablets; oral:** 10 mg	Lactose. (EM/10). White to off-white. In 100s.
Rx	**Northyx** (Centrix Pharmaceutical)		Lactose. (M10). Scored. In 100s.
Rx	**Tapazole** (Monarch)		Lactose. (J95). White to off white, scored. In 100s.
Rx	**Northyx** (Centrix Pharmaceutical)	**Tablets; oral:** 15 mg	Lactose. (M15). Scored. In 100s.
		20 mg	Lactose. (M20). Scored. In 100s.

METHIMAZOLE — ORAL

For complete prescribing information, refer to the Antithyroid Agents group monograph.

Indications

➤*Hyperthyroidism:* Medical treatment of hyperthyroidism. Long-term therapy may lead to remission of the disease. Methimazole may be used to ameliorate hyperthyroidism in preparation for subtotal thyroidectomy or radioactive iodine therapy. Methimazole also is used when thyroidectomy is contraindicated or not advisable.

Administration and Dosage

➤*Adults:*

Hyperthyroidism –

Initial dosage:

- *Mild hyperthyroidism* – 15 mg daily divided into 3 doses and given at 8-hour intervals.
- *Moderate to severe hyperthyroidism* – 30 to 40 mg daily divided into 3 doses and given at 8-hour intervals.
- *Severe hyperthyroidism* – 60 mg daily divided into 3 doses and given at 8-hour intervals.

Maintenance dosage: 5 to 15 mg daily.

➤*Children:*

Hyperthyroidism –

Initial dosage: 0.4 mg/kg of body weight divided into 3 doses and given at 8-hour intervals. (See Off-label dosing.)

Maintenance dosage: The maintenance dosage is approximately one half of the initial dose.

Off-label dosing –

Hyperthyroidism:

- *Maximum dose* – 30 mg/day.
- *Initial dosage* – 0.4 to 0.7 mg/kg/day or 15 to 20 mg/m²/day in 3 divided doses given every 8 hours.
- *Maintenance dosage* – ⅓ to ⅔ of the initial dosage in 3 divided doses given every 8 hours.

➤*Storage/Stability:* Store at 15° to 30°C (59° to 86°F).

SODIUM IODIDE I 131

For Sodium Iodide I 131 prescribing information, see the monograph in the Antineoplastics Chapter.

MECASERMIN (rDNA ORIGIN)

Rx	**Increlex** (Tercica)	**Injection:** 10 mg/mL	In 4 mL multiple dose vials.[a]

[a] Each vial contains 9 mg/mL benzyl alcohol, 5.84 mg/mL sodium chloride, 2 mg/mL polysorbate 20, and 0.5 M acetate.

MECASERMIN (rDNA ORIGIN) — INJECTION

Indications

➤*Growth failure:* For the long-term treatment of growth failure in children with severe primary insulin-like growth factor-1 (IGF-1) deficiency (primary IGFD) or with growth hormone (GH) gene deletion who have developed neutralizing antibodies to GH. Severe primary IGFD is defined by:

- height standard deviation score less than or equal to −3,
- basal IGF-1 standard deviation score less than or equal to −3, and
- normal or elevated GH.

Severe primary IGFD includes patients with mutations in the GH receptor (GHR), post-GHR signaling pathway, and IGF-1 gene defects; they are not GH deficient; therefore, they cannot be expected to respond adequately to exogenous GH treatment.

Mecasermin is not intended for use in subjects with secondary forms of IGF-1 deficiency, such as GH deficiency, malnutrition, hypothyroidism, or chronic treatment with pharmacologic doses of anti-inflammatory steroids. Correct thyroid and nutritional deficiencies before initiating mecasermin treatment

Mecasermin is not a substitute for GH treatment.

Administration and Dosage

➤*General dosing considerations:* The dosage of mecasermin should be individualized for each patient.

Preprandial glucose monitoring should be considered at treatment initiation and until a well-tolerated dose is established. If frequent symptoms of hypoglycemia or severe hypoglycemia occur, preprandial glucose monitoring should continue.

➤*Children:*

2 years of age and older –

Growth failure:

- *Maximum dose* – 0.12 mg/kg given twice daily.
- *Initial dosage* – 0.04 to 0.08 mg/kg (40 to 80 mcg/kg) twice daily by subcutaneous injection, shortly before or after (approximately 20 minutes) a meal or snack.
- *Dosage titration* – If well-tolerated for at least 1 week, the dose may be increased by 0.04 mg/kg per dose, to the maximum dose of 0.12 mg/kg given twice daily.
- *Dosage adjustment* – If hypoglycemia occurs with recommended doses, despite adequate food intake, the dose should be reduced.

➤*Administration:* Mecasermin should be administered subcutaneously shortly before or after (approximately 20 minutes) a meal or snack. If the patient is unable to eat shortly before or after a dose for any reason, that dose of mecasermin should be withheld. Subsequent doses of mecasermin should never be increased to make up for 1 or more omitted doses.

Injection sites should be rotated to a different site with each injection.

Mecasermin should be administered using sterile disposable syringes and needles. The syringes should be of small enough volume that the prescribed dose can be withdrawn from the vial with reasonable accuracy.

Vial contents should be clear without particulate matter. If the solution is cloudy or contains particulate matter, the contents must not be injected.

➤*Storage/Stability:*

Before opening – Vials of mecasermin are stable when refrigerated (2° to 8°C [35° to 46°F]). Avoid freezing the vials of mecasermin. Protect from direct light.

After opening – Vials of mecasermin are stable for 30 days after initial vial entry when stored at 2° to 8°C (35° to 46°F). Avoid freezing vials of mecasermin. Protect from direct light. Keep refrigerated and use within 30 days of initial vial entry. Remaining unused material should be discarded.

Actions

➤*Pharmacology:* IGF-1 is the principal hormonal mediator of statural growth. Under normal circumstances, GH binds to its receptor in the liver and other tissues, and stimulates the synthesis/secretion of IGF-1. In target tissues, the type 1 IGF-1 receptor, which is homologous to the insulin receptor, is activated by IGF-1, leading to intracellular signaling, which stimulates multiple processes leading to statural growth. The metabolic actions of IGF-1 are, in part, directed at stimulating the uptake of glucose, fatty acids, and amino acids so that metabolism supports growing tissues.

The following actions have been demonstrated for endogenous human IGF-1:

Tissue growth – 1) Skeletal growth occurs at the cartilage growth plates of the epiphyses of bones where stem cells divide to produce new cartilage cells or chondrocytes. The growth of chondrocytes is under the control of IGF-1 and GH. The chondrocytes become calcified so that new bone is formed, allowing the length of the bones to increase. This results in skeletal growth until the cartilage growth plates fuse at the end of puberty. 2) Cell growth: IGF-1 receptors are present on most types of cells and tissues. IGF-1 has mitogenic activities that lead to an increased number of cells in the body. 3) Organ growth: Treatment of IGF-1 deficient rats with rhIGF-1 results in whole body and organ growth.

Carbohydrate metabolism – IGF-1 suppresses hepatic glucose production and stimulates peripheral glucose utilization and therefore has a hypoglycemic potential. IGF-1 has inhibitory effects on insulin secretion.

➤*Pharmacokinetics:*

Absorption – While the bioavailability of rhIGF-1 after subcutaneous administration in healthy subjects has been reported to be close to 100%, the absolute bioavailability of mecasermin given subcutaneously to subjects with primary IGFD has not been determined.

Distribution – In blood, IGF-1 is bound to 6 IGF binding proteins, with greater than 80% bound as a complex with IGF binding protein 3 (IGFBP-3) and an acid-labile subunit. IGFBP-3 is greatly reduced in subjects with severe primary IGFD, resulting in increased clearance of IGF-1 in these subjects relative to healthy subjects. The total IGF-1 volume of distribution after subcutaneous administration in subjects with severe primary IGFD is estimated to be 0.257 (0.073) L/kg at an mecasermin dose of 0.045 mg/kg, and is estimated to increase as the dose of mecasermin increases.

Metabolism – Both the liver and the kidney have been shown to metabolize IGF-1.

Excretion – The mean terminal half-life after single subcutaneous administration of mecasermin 0.12 mg/kg in pediatric subjects with severe primary IGFD is estimated to be 5.8 hours. Clearance of mecasermin is inversely proportional to IGFBP-3 levels and clearance is estimated to be 0.04 L/h/kg at IGFBP-3 three mcg/mL.

Summary of Mecasermin Single-Dose Pharmacokinetic Parameters[a] in Children[b] with Severe Primary IGFD (0.12 mg/kg SC[c])

	C_{max}[d] (ng/mL)	T_{max}[e] (h)	AUC_{0-8}[f] (h•ng/mL)	$T_{½}$[g] (h)	Vd/F[h] (L/kg)	CL/F[i] (L/h/kg)
n	3	3	3	3	12[j]	12[j]
Mean	234	2	2,932	5.8	0.257	0.0424
CV%[k]	23	0	50	64	28	38

[a] Pharmacokinetic parameters based on baseline adjusted plasma concentrations.
[b] Male/female data combined, ages 12 to 22 years.
[c] SC = subcutaneous injection.
[d] C_{max} = maximum concentration.
[e] T_{max} = time of maximum concentration.
[f] AUC_{0-8} = area under the curve.
[g] $t_{½}$ = half-life.
[h] Vd/F = volume of distribution.
[i] CL/F = systemic clearance.
[j] Data represents 3 subjects each at doses 0.015, 0.03, 0.06, and 0.12 mg/kg SC.
[k] CV% = coefficient of variation in %.

Contraindications

Do not use mecasermin for growth promotion in patients with closed epiphyses.

Contraindicated in the presence of active or suspected neoplasia; discontinue therapy if evidence of neoplasia develops.

Intravenous (IV) administration of mecasermin is contraindicated.

Mecasermin should not be used by patients who are allergic to mecasermin (IGF-1) or any of the inactive ingredients in mecasermin.

Warnings/Precautions

➤*Benzyl alcohol:* Mecasermin contains benzyl alcohol as a preservative. Benzyl alcohol as a preservative has been associated with neurologic toxicity in neonates.

➤*Experienced health care providers:* Treatment with mecasermin should be directed by health care providers who are experienced in the diagnosis and management of patients with growth disorders.

➤*Hypoglycemic effects:* Administer mecasermin shortly before or after a meal or snack, because it has insulin-like hypoglycemic effects. Pay special attention to small children because their oral intake may not be consistent. Do not administer mecasermin when the meal or snack is omitted. Never increase the dose of mecasermin to make up for 1 or more omitted doses. Initiate mecasermin therapy at a low dose and increase the dose only if no hypoglycemia episodes have occurred after at least 7 days of dosing. If severe hypoglycemia or persistent hypoglycemia occurs on treatment despite adequate food intake, consider mecasermin dose reduction.

➤*High-risk activities:* Patients should avoid engaging in any high-risk activities (eg, driving) within 2 to 3 hours after dosing, particularly at the initiation of mecasermin treatment, until a well-tolerated dose of mecasermin has been established.

➤*Lymphoid tissue hypertrophy:* Lymphoid tissue (eg, tonsillar) hypertrophy associated with complications, such as snoring, sleep apnea, and chronic middle-ear effusions, have been reported with the use of mecasermin. Patients should have periodic examinations to rule out such potential complications and receive appropriate treatment if necessary.

MECASERMIN (rDNA ORIGIN) — INJECTION

➤*Intracranial hypertension (IH):* IH with papilledema, visual changes, headache, nausea, and/or vomiting have been reported in patients treated with mecasermin, as they have been reported with therapeutic GH administration. IH-associated signs and symptoms resolved after interruption of dosing. Funduscopic examination is recommended at the initiation and periodically during the course of mecasermin therapy.

➤*Protein reaction:* As with any exogenous protein administration, local or systemic allergic reactions may occur. Inform parents and patients that such reactions are possible and that if an allergic reaction occurs, treatment should be interrupted and prompt medical attention sought.

➤*Hypersensitivity reactions:* If sensitivity to mecasermin occurs, discontinue treatment.

➤*Pregnancy: Category C.* Embryo-fetal toxicity studies were conducted in Sprague Dawley rats with dosages of 1, 4, and 16 mg/kg/day, and in New Zealand White rabbits with dosages of 0.125, 0.5, and 2 mg/kg/day administered IV. No embryo-fetal developmental abnormalities were observed in rats with dosages up to 16 mg/kg/day (20 times the MRHD based on body surface area [BSA] comparison). In the rabbit study, the no-observed-adverse-effect-level (NOAEL) for maternal toxicity was 2 mg/kg (8 times the MRHD based on BSA) and the NOAEL for fetal toxicity was 0.5 mg/kg (2 times the MRHD based on BSA). Mecasermin displayed no teratogenicity at doses up to 2 mg/kg (8 times the MRHD based on BSA).

The effects of mecasermin on the fetus have not been studied. Therefore, there is insufficient medical information to determine whether there are significant risks to a fetus.

➤*Lactation:* It is not known whether this drug is excreted in human milk. Because many drugs are excreted in human milk, exercise caution when mecasermin is administered to a breast-feeding woman.

➤*Children:* Mecasermin has not been studied in children younger than 2 years of age or in adults.

➤*Monitoring:* Consider preprandial glucose monitoring at treatment initiation and until a well-tolerated dose is established. If frequent symptoms of hypoglycemia or severe hypoglycemia occur, continue preprandial glucose monitoring.

Thickening of the soft tissues of the face was observed in several patients and should be monitored during mecasermin treatment.

Slipped capital femoral epiphysis and progression of scoliosis can occur in patients who experience rapid growth. These conditions and other symptoms and signs known to be associated with GH treatment in general should be monitored during mecasermin treatment.

Drug Interactions

None known.

Adverse Reactions

As with all protein pharmaceuticals, some patients may develop antibodies to mecasermin. Anti-IGF-1 antibodies were present at 1 or more of the periodic assessments in 14 of 23 children with primary IGFD treated for 2 years. However, no clinical consequences of these antibodies were observed (eg, allergic reactions, attenuation of growth).

In clinical studies of 71 subjects with primary IGFD treated for a mean duration of 3.9 years and representing 274 subject-years, no subjects withdrew from any clinical study because of adverse reactions. Adverse reactions considered related to mecasermin treatment that occurred in 5% or more of these study participants are listed by organ class.

➤*Cardiovascular:* Cardiac murmur.

➤*CNS:* Convulsions, dizziness, headache.

➤*GI:* Vomiting.

➤*Hematologic/Lymphatic:* Thymus hypertrophy.

➤*Metabolic/Nutritional:* Hypoglycemia.

➤*Musculoskeletal:* Arthralgia, pain in extremity.

➤*Respiratory:* Snoring, tonsillar hypertrophy.

➤*Special senses:* Abnormal tympanometry, ear pain, ear tube insertion, fluid in middle ear, hypoacusis, otitis media, serous otitis media.

➤*Miscellaneous:* Bruising, lipohypertrophy.

➤*Hypoglycemia:* Hypoglycemia was reported by 30 subjects (42%) at least once during their course of therapy. Most cases of hypoglycemia were mild or moderate in severity. Five subjects had severe hypoglycemia (requiring assistance and treatment) on 1 or more occasion and 4 subjects experienced hypoglycemic seizures/loss of consciousness on 1 or more occasion. Of the 30 subjects reporting hypoglycemia, 14 (47%) had a history of hypoglycemia prior to treatment. The frequency of hypoglycemia was highest in the first month of treatment, and episodes were more frequent in younger children. Symptomatic hypoglycemia was generally avoided when a meal or snack was consumed either shortly (ie, 20 minutes) before or after the administration of mecasermin.

➤*Lymphoid tissue hypertrophy:* Tonsillar hypertrophy was noted in 11 (15%) subjects in the first 1 to 2 years of therapy with lesser tonsillar growth in subsequent years. Tonsillectomy or tonsillectomy/adenoidectomy was performed in 7 subjects; 3 of these had obstructive sleep apnea, which resolved after the procedure in all 3 cases.

➤*Intracranial hypertension:* Intracranial hypertension occurred in 3 subjects. In 2 subjects the events resolved without interruption of mecasermin treatment. Mecasermin treatment was discontinued in the third subject and resumed later at a lower dose without recurrence.

➤*Miscellaneous:* Mild elevations in the serum AST and lactate dehydrogenase (LDH) were found in a significant proportion of patients before and during treatment and no rise in levels of these serum enzymes led to treatment discontinuation. ALT elevations were occasionally noted during treatment. Renal and splenic lengths (measured by ultrasound) increased rapidly on mecasermin treatment during the first years of therapy. This lengthening slowed down subsequently; though in some patients, renal and/or splenic length reached or surpassed the 95th percentile. Renal function (as defined by serum creatinine and calculated creatinine clearance) was normal in all patients, irrespective of renal growth. Elevations in cholesterol and triglycerides to above the upper limit of normal were observed before and during treatment. Echocardiographic evidence of cardiomegaly/valvulopathy was observed in a few individuals without associated clinical symptoms. Because of underlying disease and the lack of control group, the relation of the cardiac changes to drug treatment cannot be assessed.

Thickening of the soft tissues of the face was observed in several patients and should be monitored during mecasermin treatment.

Overdosage

There is no clinical experience with overdosage of mecasermin.

➤*Symptoms:* Based on known pharmacological effects, acute overdosage would be predicted to lead to hypoglycemia. Long-term overdosage may result in signs and symptoms of acromegaly.

➤*Treatment:* Treatment of acute overdose of mecasermin should be directed at reversing hypoglycemia. Oral glucose or food should be consumed. If the overdose results in loss of consciousness, IV glucose or parenteral glucagon may be required to reverse the hypoglycemic effects.

Patient Information

Instruct patients and/or their parents in the safe administration of mecasermin. Give mecasermin shortly before or after (20 minutes on either side of) a meal or snack. Mecasermin should not be administered when the meal or snack is omitted. Never increase the dose of mecasermin to make up for 1 or more omitted doses. Initiate mecasermin therapy at a low dose and increase the dose only if no hypoglycemia episodes have occurred after at least 7 days of dosing. If severe hypoglycemia or persistent hypoglycemia occurs on treatment despite adequate food intake, consider mecasermin dose reduction. Educate patients and caregivers on how to recognize the signs and symptoms of hypoglycemia.

Thoroughly instruct patients and/or parents in the importance of proper needle disposal. Use a puncture-resistant container for the disposal of used needles and/or syringes (consistent with applicable state requirements). Do not reuse needles and syringes.

GROWTH HORMONE RELEASING FACTOR

TESAMORELIN

Rx	**Egrifta** (EMD Serono)	**Injection, lyophilized powder for solution:** 1 mg	Equiv. to tesamorelin acetate 1.1 mg. Preservative free. Mannitol 50 mg. In single-use vials.

TESAMORELIN ACETATE — INJECTION

Indications

➤*Lipodystrophy in HIV-infected patients:* For the reduction of excess abdominal fat in HIV-infected patients with lipodystrophy.

Administration and Dosage

➤*Adults:*

Lipodystrophy in HIV-infected patients – 2 mg subcutaneously once a day.

➤*Preparation for administration:* Insert 2.2 mL of sterile water into the tesamorelin vial. Push the plunger in slowly on a slight angle so water goes down the inside of the tesamorelin vial instead of directly onto the powder to avoid foaming. While keeping the syringe with the needle attached in the vial and the vial upright, roll the vial gently for 30 seconds, until the sterile water and tesamorelin powder are well mixed. Do not shake the vial. Remove all of the liquid inside the vial (2.2 mL).

Place the 1½ inch 18-gauge mixing needle with its protective cap in place onto the syringe. Insert the needle into the second tesamorelin vial. Push the plunger in slowly on a slight angle so that the water goes down the inside of the wall instead of directly into the powder to avoid foaming. Keeping the syringe in the vial and the vial upright, roll the vial gently for 30 seconds until the water and powder are mixed well. Do not shake. Remove all the liquid inside the vial (2.2 mL).

TESAMORELIN ACETATE — INJECTION

➤*Administration:* Administer by subcutaneous injection in the abdomen immediately after reconstitution. Injection sites should be rotated to different areas of the abdomen. Do not inject into scar tissue, bruises, or the navel.

➤*Storage/Stability:* Store unreconstituted tesamorelin vials between 2° and 8°C (36° and 46°F). Store the diluent, syringes, and needles between 20° and 25°C (68° and 77°F). Protect from light and keep in the original box until time of use. The reconstituted solution should be discarded if not used immediately. Do not freeze or refrigerate the reconstituted solution.

Actions

➤*Pharmacology:* Tesamorelin, an analog of human growth hormone-releasing factor (GRF), also known as growth hormone-releasing hormone (GHRH), is a hypothalamic peptide that acts on the pituitary somatotroph cells to stimulate the synthesis and pulsatile release of endogenous growth hormone (GH), which is both anabolic and lipolytic. GH exerts its effects by interacting with specific receptors on a variety of target cells, including chondrocytes, osteoblasts, myocytes, hepatocytes, and adipocytes, resulting in a host of pharmacodynamic effects. Some, but not all, of these effects are primarily mediated by insulin-like growth factor 1 (IGF-1) produced in the liver and in peripheral tissues. In vitro, tesamorelin binds and stimulates human GRF receptors with similar potency as the endogenous GRF.

➤*Pharmacokinetics:*

Absorption – The absolute bioavailability of tesamorelin after subcutaneous administration of a 2 mg dose was determined to be less than 4% in healthy adult subjects.

The mean values (coefficient of variation [CV]) of the extent of absorption (area under the curve [AUC]) for tesamorelin were 634.6 (72.4) and 852.8 (91.9) pg•h/mL in healthy subjects and HIV-infected patients, respectively, after a single subcutaneous administration of a tesamorelin 2 mg dose. The mean (CV) peak tesamorelin concentration (C_{max}) values were 2,874.6 (43.9) pg/mL in healthy subjects and 2,822.3 (48.9) pg/mL in HIV-infected patients. The median time to peak plasma tesamorelin concentration (T_{max}) was 0.15 h in both populations.

Distribution – The mean volume of distribution (± standard deviation [SD]) of tesamorelin following a single subcutaneous administration was 9.4 ± 3.1 L/kg in healthy subjects and 10.5 ± 6.1 L/kg in HIV-infected patients.

Excretion – Mean elimination half-life of tesamorelin was 26 and 38 minutes in healthy subjects and HIV-infected patients, respectively, after subcutaneous administration for 14 consecutive days.

Contraindications

Disruption of the hypothalamic-pituitary axis due to hypophysectomy, hypopituitarism, pituitary tumor/surgery, head irradiation, or head trauma; active malignancy (newly diagnosed or recurrent); known hypersensitivity to tesamorelin and/or mannitol; pregnancy.

Warnings/Precautions

➤*Neoplasms:* Tesamorelin induces the release of endogenous GH, a known growth factor. Thus, do not treat patients who have active malignancy with tesamorelin. Any preexisting malignancy should be inactive and its treatment complete prior to instituting therapy with tesamorelin.

For patients with a history of nonmalignant neoplasms, initiate tesamorelin after careful evaluation of the potential benefit of treatment. For patients with a history of treated and stable malignancies, initiate tesamorelin only after careful evaluation of the potential benefit of treatment relative to the risk of re-activation of the underlying malignancy.

In addition, consider carefully the decision to start treatment with tesamorelin based on the increased background risk of malignancies in HIV-positive patients.

➤*Elevated IGF-1:* Tesamorelin stimulates GH production and increases serum IGF-1. Given that IGF-1 is a growth factor and the effect of prolonged elevations in IGF-1 levels on the development or progression of malignancies is unknown, monitor IGF-1 levels closely. Give careful consideration to discontinuing tesamorelin in patients with persistent elevations of IGF-1 levels (eg, more than 3 SD scores), particularly if the efficacy response is not robust (eg, based on visceral adipose tissue changes measured by waist circumference or computed tomography [CT] scan).

➤*Fluid retention:* Fluid retention may occur during tesamorelin therapy and is thought to be related to the induction of GH secretion. It manifests as increased tissue turgor and musculoskeletal discomfort resulting in a variety of adverse reactions (eg, arthralgia, carpal tunnel syndrome, edema) that are either transient or resolve with discontinuation of treatment.

➤*Glucose intolerance:* Tesamorelin may result in glucose intolerance. During the phase 3 clinical trials, the percentages of patients with elevated glycosylated hemoglobin (HbA_{1c}) levels (6.5% or more) from baseline to week 26 were 4.5% and 1.3% in the tesamorelin and placebo groups, respectively. An increased risk of developing diabetes with tesamorelin (HbA_{1c} level of 6.5% or more) relative to placebo was observed (intent-to-treat hazard odds ratio of 3.3 (confidence interval [CI], 1.4 to 9.6). Therefore, carefully evaluate glucose status prior to initiating tesamorelin. In addition, monitor all patients treated with tesamorelin periodically for changes in glucose metabolism to diagnose those who develop impaired glucose tolerance or diabetes. Diabetes is a known cardiovascular risk factor and patients who develop glucose intolerance have an elevated risk of developing diabetes. Exercise caution in treating HIV-positive patients with lipodystrophy with tesamorelin if they develop glucose intolerance or diabetes, and give careful consideration to discontinuing tesamorelin treatment in patients who do not show a clear efficacy response as judged by the degree of reduction in visceral adipose tissue by waist circumference of CT scan measurements.

Because tesamorelin increases IGF-1, monitor patients with diabetes who are receiving ongoing treatment with tesamorelin at regular intervals for potential development or worsening of retinopathy.

➤*Injection-site reactions:* Tesamorelin treatment may cause injection-site reactions, including injection-site erythema, pruritus, pain, irritation, and bruising. The incidence of injection-site reactions was 24.5% in tesamorelin-treated patients and 14.4% in placebo-treated patients during the first 26 weeks of treatment in the phase 3 clinical trials. For patients who continued tesamorelin for an additional 26 weeks, the incidence of injection-site reactions was 6.1%. In order to reduce the incidence of injection-site reactions, it is recommended to rotate the site of injection to different areas of the abdomen.

➤*Acute critical illness:* Increased mortality in patients with acute critical illness due to complications following open heart surgery, abdominal surgery, multiple accidental trauma, or those with acute respiratory failure has been reported after treatment with pharmacologic amounts of GH. Tesamorelin has not been studied in patients with acute critical illness. Because tesamorelin stimulates GH production, give careful consideration to discontinuing tesamorelin in critically ill patients.

➤*Immunogenicity:* As with all therapeutic proteins and peptides, there is a potential for in vivo development of anti-tesamorelin antibodies. In the combined phase 3 clinical trials, anti-tesamorelin immune globulin G (IgG) antibodies were detected in 49.5% of patients treated with tesamorelin for 26 weeks and 47.4% of patients who received tesamorelin for 52 weeks. In the subset of patients with hypersensitivity reactions, antitesamorelin IgG antibodies were detected in 85.2%. Crossreactivity to endogenous GHRH was observed in approximately 60% of patients who developed antitesamorelin antibodies. Patients with and without antitesamorelin IgG antibodies had similar mean reductions in visceral adipose tissue (VAT) and IGF-1 response, suggesting that the presence of antibodies did not alter the efficacy of tesamorelin. In a group of patients who had antibodies to tesamorelin after 26 weeks of treatment (56%) and were reassessed 6 months later after stopping tesamorelin treatment, 18% were still antibody positive.

Neutralizing antibodies to tesamorelin and GHRH were detected in vitro at week 52 in 10% and 5% of tesamorelin-treated patients, respectively. They did not appear to have an impact on efficacy, as evidenced by comparable changes in VAT and IGF-1 levels in patients with or without in vitro neutralizing antibodies.

➤*Hypersensitivity reactions:* Hypersensitivity reactions may occur in patients treated with tesamorelin. Hypersensitivity reactions occurred in 3.6% of patients with HIV-associated lipodystrophy treated with tesamorelin in the phase 3 clinical trials. These reactions included pruritus, erythema, flushing, urticaria, and other rash. In cases of suspected hypersensitivity reactions, advise patients to seek prompt medical attention and discontinue treatment with tesamorelin immediately.

➤*Pregnancy: Category X.* Tesamorelin is contraindicated in pregnant women. During pregnancy, VAT increases due to normal metabolic and hormonal changes. Modifying this physiologic change of pregnancy with tesamorelin offers no known benefit and could result in fetal harm. Tesamorelin administration to rats during organogenesis and lactation resulted in hydrocephaly in offspring at a dose of approximately 2 and 4 times the clinical dose, respectively, based on measured drug exposure (AUC). If pregnancy occurs, discontinue tesamorelin. If this drug is used during pregnancy, or if the patient becomes pregnant while taking this drug, apprise the patient of the potential hazard to the fetus.

Tesamorelin administration to rats during organogenesis and lactation produced hydrocephaly in offspring at a dose of approximately 2 and 4 times the clinical dose, respectively, based on measured drug exposure (AUC). Actual animal dose was 1.2 mg/kg. During organogenesis, lower doses approximately 0.1 to 1 times the clinical dose caused delayed skull ossification in rats. Actual animal doses were 0.1 to 0.6 mg/kg. No adverse developmental effects occurred in rabbits using doses up to approximately 500 times the clinical dose.

➤*Lactation:* The Centers for Disease Control and Prevention recommend that HIV-infected mothers in the United States not breast-feed their infants to avoid risking postnatal transmission of HIV-1 infection. It is not known whether tesamorelin is excreted in human milk. Because of the potential for HIV-1 infection transmission and serious adverse reactions in breast-feeding infants, instruct mothers receiving tesamorelin not to breast-feed.

➤*Children:* Safety and effectiveness in children have not been established. Do not use tesamorelin in children with open epiphyses, because excess GH and IGF-1 may result in linear growth acceleration and excessive growth.

➤*Monitoring:* Monitor efficacy of treatment as judged by the degree of reduction in VAT measured by waist circumference or CT scan. Monitor IGF-1 levels closely. Evaluate glucose status prior to initiating therapy. Monitor patients periodically for changes in glucose metabolism. Monitor patients with diabetes at regular intervals for the development or worsening of diabetic retinopathy.

Drug Interactions

➤*Growth hormone:* GH is known to inhibit 11-beta-hydroxysteroid dehydrogenase type 1 (11-beta-HSD 1), a microsomal enzyme required for conversion of cortisone to its active metabolite, cortisol, in hepatic and adipose tissue. Because tesamorelin stimulates GH production, patients receiving glucocorticoid replacement for previously diagnosed hypoadrenalism may require an increase in maintenance or stress doses following initiation of tesamorelin, particularly patients treated with cortisone acetate and pred-

TESAMORELIN ACETATE — INJECTION

nisone because conversion of these drugs to their biologically active metabolites is dependent on activity of 11-beta-HSD 1.

Tesamorelin Drug Interactions

Precipitant Drug	Object Drug		Description
Tesamorelin	Ritonavir	↓	In healthy subjects, administration of multiple doses of tesamorelin 2 mg with ritonavir decreased the ritonavir AUC and C_{max} 9% and 11%, respectively. These changes are not likely to be clinically important.
Tesamorelin	Simvastatin	↑↓	In healthy subjects, coadministration of tesamorelin with simvastatin decreased the extent of simvastatin absorption 8% and increased the rate of absorption 5%. For simvastatin acid, the extent and rate of absorption decreased 15% and 1%, respectively. These changes are not likely to be clinically important.

[a] ↑ = object drug increased; ↑↓ = object drug both increased and decreased.

Adverse Reactions

➤*Most common adverse reactions:* The most commonly reported adverse reactions are hypersensitivity (eg, rash, urticaria) reactions due to the effect of GH (eg, arthralgia, carpal tunnel syndrome, extremity pain, hyperglycemia, peripheral edema), and injection-site reactions (injection-site erythema, irritation, pruritus, pain, urticaria, swelling, hemorrhage).

➤*Discontinuation:* During the first 26 weeks of treatment (main phase), discontinuations as a result of adverse reactions occurred in 9.6% of patients receiving tesamorelin and 6.8% of patients receiving placebo. Apart from patients with hypersensitivity reactions identified during the studies and who were discontinued per protocol (2.2%), the most common reasons for discontinuation of tesamorelin treatment were local injection-site reactions (4.6%) and adverse reactions due to the effect of GH (4.2%).

During the following 26 weeks of treatment (extension phase), discontinuations as a result of adverse reactions occurred in 2.4% of patients in the T-T group (patients treated with tesamorelin for weeks 0 to 26 and with tesamorelin for week 26 to 52) and 5.2% of patients in the T-P group (patients treated with tesamorelin for weeks 0 to 26 and with placebo for weeks 26 to 52).

➤*Adverse reactions in the first 26 weeks of therapy (1% or more):*

Tesamorelin Adverse Reactions in the First 26 Weeks of Therapy (≥ 1%)

Adverse reactions	Tesamorelin (n = 543)	Placebo (n = 263)
Cardiovascular		
Hypertension	1.3%	0.8%
Palpitations	1.1%	0.4%
CNS		
Depression	2%	1.5%
Hypesthesia	4.2%	1.5%
Night sweats	1.1%	0.4%
Paresthesia	4.8%	2.3%
Pruritus	2.4%	1.1%
Rash	3.7%	1.5%
GI		
Abdominal pain upper	1.1%	0.4%
Dyspepsia	1.7%	0.8%
Nausea	4.4%	3.8%
Vomiting	2.6%	0%
Local		
Injection-site erythema	8.5%	2.7%
Injection-site hemorrhage	1.7%	0.4%
Injection-site irritation	2.9%	1.1%
Injection-site pain	4.1%	3%
Injection-site pruritus	7.6%	0.8%
Injection-site rash	1.1%	0%
Injection-site reaction	1.3%	0.8%
Injection-site swelling	1.5%	0.4%
Injection-site urticaria	1.7%	0.4%
Musculoskeletal		
Arthralgia	13.3%	11%
Carpal tunnel syndrome	1.5%	0%
Joint stiffness	1.5%	0.8%
Joint swelling	1.1%	0%
Muscle spasms	1.1%	0.8%
Muscle strain	1.1%	0%
Musculoskeletal pain	1.8%	0.8%
Musculoskeletal stiffness	1.7%	0.4%
Myalgia	5.5%	1.9%
Pain in extremity	6.1%	4.6%
Miscellaneous		
Blood creatine phosphokinase increased	1.5%	0.4%
Chest pain	1.1%	0.8%
Edema peripheral	6.1%	2.3%
Pain	1.7%	1.1%

Glucose – In the tesamorelin phase 3 clinical trials, mean baseline (week 0) HbA_{1c} was 5.26% among patients in the tesamorelin group and 5.28% among those in the placebo group. At week 26, mean HbA_{1c} was higher among patients treated with tesamorelin compared with placebo (5.39% vs 5.28% for tesamorelin and placebo groups, respectively; mean treatment difference of 0.12%; $P = 0.0004$). Patients receiving tesamorelin had an increased risk of developing diabetes (HbA_{1c} level 6.5% or more) compared with placebo (4.5% vs 1.3%), with a hazard ratio of 3.3 (CI, 1.4 to 9.6).

➤*Adverse reactions in weeks 26 to 52 of therapy (1% or more):*

Tesamorelin Adverse Reactions in Weeks 26 to 52 of Therapy (≥ 1%)

Adverse reactions	Tesamorelin (n = 246)	Placebo (n = 135)
CNS		
Depression	1.6%	0.7%
Hypesthesia	1.6%	0.7%
Insomnia	1.2%	0%
Neuropathy peripheral	1.6%	1.5%
Paresthesia	1.6%	1.5%
Dermatologic		
Hot flush	1.2%	0.7%
Night sweats	1.2%	0%
Pruritus	1.2%	0.7%
Urticaria	1.2%	0%
Local		
Injection-site erythema	1.2%	0%
Injection-site pruritus	2%	0%
Musculoskeletal		
Myalgia	1.2%	0%
Pain in extremity	3.3%	0.7%
Miscellaneous		
Edema peripheral	2%	0%
Hypertension	1.6%	1.5%
Vomiting	2%	0.7%

Overdosage

No data are available on overdosage.

Patient Information

Advise patients that treatment may cause symptoms consistent with fluid retention, including edema, arthralgia, and carpal tunnel syndrome. These reactions are either transient or resolve with discontinuation of treatment.

Advise patients that hypersensitivity reactions (eg, rash, urticaria) may occur during treatment. Advise patients to seek prompt medical attention and to immediately discontinue treatment with tesamorelin.

Advise patients of possible injection-site reactions, including injection-site erythema, pruritus, pain, irritation, and bruising. To reduce the incidence of injection-site reactions, advise patients to rotate the site of injection.

Counsel patients that they must never share a syringe with another person, even if the needle is changed. Sharing of syringes or needles between patients may pose a risk of transmission of infection.

Advise women to discontinue tesamorelin if pregnancy occurs, because the drug offers no known benefit to pregnant women and could result in fetal harm.

Because of the potential for HIV-1 infection transmission and serious adverse reactions in breast-feeding infants, instruct mothers receiving tesamorelin not to breast-feed.

SOMATROPIN

Rx	**Genotropin Miniquick** (Pfizer)	**Injection, lyophilized powder for solution**: 0.2 mg (≈ 0.6 units)/ cartridge	Preservative free. With glycine 0.23 mg, mannitol 1.14 mg in the front chamber; mannitol 12.6 mg in 0.275 mL of water for injection in the back chamber. In single-use syringe device with 2-chamber cartridge. In 7s.
		0.4 mg (≈ 1.2 units)/cartridge	
		0.6 mg (≈ 1.8 units)/cartridge	
		0.8 mg (≈ 2.4 units)/cartridge	
		1 mg (≈ 3 units)/cartridge	
		1.2 mg (≈ 3.6 units)/cartridge	
		1.4 mg (≈ 4.2 units)/cartridge	
Rx	**Omnitrope** (Sandoz)	**Injection, lyophilized powder for solution**: 1.5 mg (≈ 4.5 units)/ vial	With glycine 27.6 mg. In vials with diluent (sterile water for injection).
Rx	**Genotropin Miniquick** (Pfizer)	**Injection, lyophilized powder for solution**: 1.6 mg (≈ 4.8 mg)/ cartridge	Preservative free. With glycine 0.23 mg, mannitol 1.14 mg in the front chamber; mannitol 12.6 mg in 0.275 mL of water for injection in the back chamber. In single-use syringe device with 2-chamber cartridge. In 7s.
		1.8 mg (≈ 5.4 units)/cartridge	
		2 mg (≈ 6 units)/cartridge	
Rx	**Serostim** (Serono)	**Injection, lyophilized powder for solution**: 4 mg (≈ 12 units)/vial	With sucrose 27.3 mg. In single-use vials with diluent.
Rx	**Humatrope** (Eli Lilly)	**Injection, lyophilized powder for solution**: 5 mg (≈ 15 units)/vial	With mannitol 25 mg, glycine 5 mg. In vials with 5 mL of diluent (metacresol 0.3% as a preservative and glycerin 1.7%).
Rx	**Nutropin** (Genentech)		With mannitol 45 mg, glycine 1.7 mg. In vials with multidose vial of diluent (bacteriostatic water for injection [benzyl alcohol 0.9% preserved]).
Rx	**Saizen** (Serono)		With sucrose 34.2 mg. In vials with 10 mL of diluent (bacteriostatic water for injection [benzyl alcohol 0.9%]).
Rx	**Serostim** (Serono)		With sucrose 34.2 mg. In single-use vials with diluent.
Rx	**Tev-Tropin** (Gate)		With mannitol 30 mg. In vials with diluent (bacteriostatic sodium chloride 0.9% for injection with benzyl alcohol 0.9%).
Rx	**Genotropin** (Pfizer)	**Injection, lyophilized powder for solution**: 5.8 mg (≈ 17.4 units)/ cartridge	With glycine 2.2 mg, mannitol 1.8 mg in front chamber; metacresol 0.3% and mannitol 45 mg in 1.14 mL of water for injection. In 1s and 5s.
Rx	**Omnitrope** (Sandoz)	**Injection, lyophilized powder for solution**: 5.8 mg/vial	With glycine 27.6 mg. In vials with diluent (bacteriostatic water for injection containing benzyl alcohol 1.5% as a preservative).
Rx	**Serostim** (Serono)	**Injection, lyophilized powder for solution**: 6 mg (≈ 18 units)/vial	With sucrose 41 mg. In single-use vials with diluent.
Rx	**HumatroPen** (Eli Lilly)	**Injection, lyophilized powder for solution**: 6 mg (18 units)/ cartridge	With mannitol 18 mg, glycine 6 mg. In cartridges with prefilled syringe of diluent (metacresol 0.3% as a preservative and glycerin 1.7%).
Rx	**Saizen** (Serono)	**Injection, lyophilized powder for solution**: 8.8 mg (≈ 26.4 units)/ vial	With sucrose 60.2 mg. In vials with diluent (bacteriostatic water for injection [benzyl alcohol preserved]). Also available in *click.easy* cartridges with bacteriostatic water for injection (metacresol 0.3%).
Rx	**Serostim** (Serono)		With sucrose 60.2 mg. In multidose vials with diluent (bacteriostatic water for injection [benzyl alcohol preserved]).
Rx	**Nutropin** (Genentech)	**Injection, lyophilized powder for solution**: 10 mg (≈ 30 units)/vial	With mannitol 90 mg, glycine 3.4 mg. In vials with multidose vial of diluent (bacteriostatic water for injection [benzyl alcohol 0.9% preserved]).
Rx	**HumatroPen** (Eli Lilly)	**Injection, lyophilized powder for solution**: 12 mg (36 units)/ cartridge	With mannitol 36 mg, glycine 12 mg. In cartridges with prefilled syringe of diluent (metacresol 0.3% as preservative, glycerin 0.29%).
Rx	**Genotropin** (Pfizer)	**Injection, lyophilized powder for solution**: 13.8 mg (≈ 41.4 units)/ cartridge	With glycine 2.3 mg, mannitol 14 mg in front chamber; metacresol 0.3% and mannitol 32 mg in 1.13 mL water for injection in rear chamber. In 1s and 5s.
Rx	**HumatroPen** (Eli Lilly)	**Injection, lyophilized powder for solution**: 24 mg (72 units)/ cartridge	With mannitol 72 mg, glycine 24 mg. In cartridges with prefilled syringe of diluent (metacresol 0.3% as a preservative, glycerin 0.29%).
Rx	**Zorbtive** (Serono)	**Injection, powder for solution**: 8.8 mg (≈ 26.4 units)/vial	With sucrose 60.19 mg, phosphoric acid 2.05 mg. In multidose vials with bacteriostatic water for injection as diluent (benzyl alcohol 0.9%).
Rx	**Norditropin** (Novo Nordisk)	**Injection, solution**: 5 mg per 1.5 mL	With histidine 1 mg, poloxamer 188 (4.5 mg), phenol 4.5 mg, mannitol 60 mg. In *NordiFlex* prefilled pens, and in cartridges to be administered using the *NordiPen* delivery system.
Rx	**Omnitrope** (Sandoz)		With poloxamer 188 (3 mg), mannitol 52.5 mg, benzyl alcohol. In cartridges.
Rx	**Accretropin** (Cangene)	**Injection, solution**: 5 mg (15 units)/mL	With sodium chloride 0.75%, phenol 0.34% (as preservative). In multidose vials.
Rx	**Nutropin AQ NuSpin 5** (Genentech)	**Injection, solution**: 5 mg (≈ 15 units)/mL	With sodium chloride 17.4 mg, phenol 5 mg, polysorbate 20 (4 mg), sodium citrate 10 mM. In multidose prefilled injection devices.
Rx	**Norditropin** (Novo Nordisk)	**Injection, solution**: 10 mg per 1.5 mL	With histidine 1 mg, poloxamer 188 (4.5 mg), phenol 4.5 mg, mannitol 60 mg. In *NordiFlex* prefilled pens.
Rx	**Omnitrope** (Sandoz)		With glycine 27.75 mg, phenol 4.5 mg, poloxamer 188 (3 mg). In cartridges.

SOMATROPIN

Rx	**Nutropin AQ** (Genentech)	**Injection, solution**: 10 mg (≈ 30 units)/vial or cartridge	With sodium chloride 17.4 mg, phenol 5 mg, polysorbate 20 (4 mg), sodium citrate 10 mM. In 2 mL vials and pen cartridges.
Rx	**Nutropin AQ NuSpin 10** (Genentech)		With sodium chloride 17.4 mg, phenol 5 mg, polysorbate 20 (4 mg), sodium citrate 10 mM. In multidose prefilled injection devices.
Rx	**Norditropin** (Novo Nordisk)	**Injection, solution**: 15 mg per 1.5 mL	With histidine 1.7 mg, poloxamer 188 (4.5 mg), phenol 4.5 mg, mannitol 58 mg. In *NordiFlex* prefilled pen, and in cartridges to be administered using the *NordiPen* delivery system.
Rx	**Nutropin AQ** (Genentech)	**Injection, solution**: 20 mg (≈ 60 units)/cartridge	With sodium chloride 17.4 mg, phenol 5 mg, polysorbate 20 (4 mg), sodium citrate 10 mM. In 2 mL pen cartridges.
Rx	**Nutropin AQ NuSpin 20** (Genentech)		With sodium chloride 17.4 mg, phenol 5 mg, polysorbate 20 (4 mg), sodium citrate 10 mM. In multidose prefilled injection devices.
Rx	**Norditropin** (Novo Nordisk)	**Injection, solution**: 30 mg per 3 mL	With histidine 3.3 mg, poloxamer 188 (9 mg), phenol 9 mg, mannitol 117 mg. In *NordiFlex* prefilled pens.

SOMATROPIN — INJECTION

Indications

➤*Growth failure associated with chronic renal insufficiency (Nutropin and Nutropin AQ)*: Growth failure associated with chronic renal insufficiency up to the time of renal transplantation. *Nutropin* and *Nutropin AQ* therapy should be used in conjunction with optimal management of chronic renal insufficiency.

➤*Growth failure associated with Noonan syndrome (Norditropin)*: For the treatment of children with short stature associated with Noonan syndrome.

➤*Growth failure associated with Prader-Willi syndrome (Genotropin)*: For children who have growth failure caused by Prader-Willi syndrome. The diagnosis of Prader-Willi syndrome should be confirmed by appropriate genetic testing.

➤*Growth failure associated with Turner syndrome (Accretropin, Genotropin, Humatrope, HumatroPen, Norditropin, Nutropin,* and *Nutropin AQ)*: For the treatment of growth failure associated with Turner syndrome in patients who have open epiphyses.

➤*Growth failure in children (Accretropin, Genotropin, Humatrope, HumatroPen, Norditropin, Nutropin, Nutropin AQ, Omnitrope, Saizen,* and *Tev-Tropin)*: For children who have growth failure caused by an inadequate secretion of endogenous growth hormone.

For children born small for gestational age (SGA) who fail to manifest catch-up growth by 2 years of age (*Genotropin*).

For the treatment of children with short stature born SGA with no catch-up growth by 2 to 4 years of age (*Humatrope* and *Norditropin*).

➤*Growth hormone deficiency in adults (Genotropin, Humatrope, HumatroPen, Norditropin, Nutropin, Nutropin AQ, Omnitrope,* and *Saizen)*: For the replacement of endogenous growth hormone in adults with growth hormone deficiency (GHD) who meet either of the following 2 criteria:

Adult-onset – Patients who have GHD, either alone or associated with multiple hormone deficiencies (hypopituitarism), as a result of pituitary disease, hypothalamic disease, surgery, radiation, or trauma.

Childhood-onset – Patients who were GHD during childhood as a result of congenital, genetic, acquired, or idiopathic causes.

In general, confirmation of the diagnosis of adult GHD in both groups usually requires an appropriate growth hormone stimulation test. However, confirmatory testing may not be required in patients with congenital/genetic GHD or multiple pituitary hormone deficiencies caused by organic disease.

Other causes of short stature in children should be excluded.

➤*Idiopathic short stature (Genotropin, Humatrope, HumatroPen, Nutropin,* and *Nutropin AQ)*: For the long-term treatment of idiopathic short stature (also called non–growth hormone deficient short stature, defined by height standard deviation score [SDS] less than or equal to −2.25) associated with growth rates unlikely to permit attainment of adult height in the normal range in children whose epiphyses are not closed and for whom diagnostic evaluation excludes other causes associated with short stature that should be observed or treated by other means.

➤*Short bowel syndrome (Zorbtive)*: For the treatment of short bowel syndrome in patients receiving specialized nutritional support.

Zorbtive therapy should be used in conjunction with optimal management of short bowel syndrome.

Specialized nutritional support may consist of a high-carbohydrate, low-fat diet adjusted for individual patient requirements and preferences. Nutritional supplements may be added according to the discretion of the treating health care provider. Optimal management of short bowel syndrome may include dietary adjustments, enteral feedings, parenteral nutrition, and fluid and micronutrient supplements, as needed.

➤*Short stature homeobox–containing gene deficiency (Humatrope* and *HumatroPen)*: For the treatment of short stature or growth failure in children with short stature homeobox (SHOX)–deficiency whose epiphyses are not closed.

➤*Wasting or cachexia associated with HIV (Serostim)*: For the treatment of patients with HIV with wasting or cachexia to increase lean body mass (LBM) and body weight, and improve physical endurance. Concomitant antiretroviral therapy is necessary.

➤*Off-label uses:*

Lipodystrophy (HIV related) – [4] = Insufficient documentation. Results from 2 small, prospective, open trials suggest that recombinant growth hormone may be effective in the treatment of HIV-related lipodystrophy; however, it appears that the benefit of the drug is seriously limited by the high incidence of adverse effects. Tolerability may be improved with lower doses.

Administration and Dosage

➤*General dosing considerations:* Dosage of somatropin must be adjusted for the individual patient.

Response to growth hormone therapy in children tends to decrease with time. However, in children, failure to increase growth rate, particularly during the first year of therapy, suggests the need for close assessment of compliance and evaluation of other causes of growth failure, such as hypothyroidism, undernutrition, and advanced bone age.

➤*Adults:*

Growth hormone deficiency in adults – Clinical response, adverse reactions, and determination of age- and gender-adjusted serum insulin-like growth factor 1 (IGF-1) levels may be used as guidance in dose titration.

Maintenance dosages may vary considerably from person to person.

Genotropin and *Omnitrope*:

- *Maximum dose* – 0.08 mg/kg/week.
- *Initial dosage* – Not more than 0.04 mg/kg/week, given in 7 divided daily subcutaneous injections.
- *Dosage adjustment* – The dose may be increased at 4- to 8-week intervals, according to the individual patient requirements, to a maximum of 0.08 mg/kg/week.
- *Alternative dosage* – Starting dosage of approximately 0.2 mg/day (range, 0.15 to 0.3 mg/day) may be used without consideration of body weight. This dose can be increased gradually every 1 to 2 months by increments of approximately 0.1 to 0.2 mg/day, according to individual patient requirements based on the clinical response and serum IGF-1 concentrations. During therapy, the dose should be decreased if required by the occurrence of adverse events and/or serum IGF-1 levels above the age- and gender-specific normal range. Maintenance dosages vary considerably from person to person.

Humatrope and *HumatroPen*:

- *Maximum dose* – 0.0125 mg/kg/day.
- *Initial dosage* – Not more than 0.006 mg/kg, given as a daily subcutaneous injection.
- *Dosage adjustment* – The dosage may be increased according to individual patient requirements to a maximum of 0.0125 mg/kg/day.
- *Alternative dosage* – Based on published consensus guidelines, a starting dosage of approximately 0.2 mg/day (range, 0.15 to 0.3 mg/day) may be used without consideration of body weight. This dosage can be increased gradually every 1 to 2 months by increments of approximately 0.1 to 0.2 mg/day, according to individual patient requirements based on the clinical response and serum IGF-1 concentrations. The dose should be decreased as necessary on the basis of adverse events and/or serum IGF-1 concentrations above the age- and gender-specific normal range. Maintenance dosages vary considerably from person to person, and between male and female patients.

Norditropin:

- *Maximum dose* – 0.016 mg/kg/day.
- *Initial dosage* – Not more than 0.004 mg/kg/day by subcutaneous injection.
- *Dosage adjustment* – The dosage may be increased to not more than 0.016 mg/kg/day after approximately 6 weeks, according to individual patient requirements.
- *Alternative dosage* – A starting dosage of approximately 0.2 mg/day (range, 0.15 to 0.3 mg/day) may be used without consideration of body weight. This dosage can be increased gradually every 1 to 2 months by increments of approximately 0.1 to 0.2 mg/day, according to individual patient requirements based on the clinical response and serum IGF-1 concentra-

SOMATROPIN — INJECTION

tions. The dose should be decreased if required by the occurrence of adverse events and/or serum IGF-1 concentrations above the age- and gender-specific normal range. Maintenance dosages vary considerably from person to person.

Nutropin and *Nutropin AQ*:

• *Maximum dose* – 0.025 mg/kg/day in patients younger than 35 years of age; 0.0125 mg/kg/day in patients older than 35 years of age.

• *Initial dosage* – Not more than 0.006 mg/kg, given as a daily subcutaneous injection.

• *Dosage adjustment* – The dosage may be increased according to individual requirements to a maximum of 0.025 mg/kg/day in patients younger than 35 years of age and to a maximum of 0.0125 mg/kg/day in patients older than 35 years of age.

• *Alternative dosage* – A starting dosage of approximately 0.2 mg/day (range, 0.15 to 0.3 mg/day) may be used without consideration of body weight. This dosage can be increased gradually every 1 to 2 months by increments of approximately 0.1 to 0.2 mg/day, according to individual patient requirements based on the clinical response and serum IGF-1 concentrations. The dose should be decreased if required by the occurrence of adverse events and/or serum IGF-1 concentrations above the age- and gender-specific normal range. Maintenance dosages vary considerably from person to person.

Saizen:

• *Maximum dose* – 0.01 mg/kg/day.

• *Initial dosage* – Not more than 0.005 mg/kg, given as a daily subcutaneous injection.

• *Dosage adjustment* – The dosage may be increased to not more than 0.01 mg/kg/day after 4 weeks, according to individual patient requirements.

• *Alternative dosage* – A starting dosage of approximately 0.2 mg/day (range, 0.15 to 0.3 mg/day) may be used without consideration of body weight. This dosage can be increased gradually every 1 to 2 months by increments of approximately 0.1 to 0.2 mg/day, according to individual patient requirements, based on the clinical response and serum IGF-1 concentrations. During therapy, the dose should be decreased if required by the occurrence of adverse reactions and/or serum IGF-1 levels above the age- and gender-specific normal range. Maintenance dosages vary considerably from person to person.

Short bowel syndrome –

Zorbtive:

• *Usual dosage* – Approximately 0.1 mg/kg/day subcutaneously, to a maximum of 8 mg daily. Injections should be administered daily for 4 weeks. Injection sites should be rotated.

• *Maximum dose* – 8 mg/day.

• *Dosage adjustment* – Patients and health care providers should monitor for adverse reactions. Treat moderate fluid retention and arthralgias symptomatically or reduce by 50% of the original dose.

Discontinue for up to 5 days for severe toxicities. Upon resolution of symptoms, resume at 50% of the original dose.

• *Concomitant therapy* – Changes to concomitant medications should be avoided.

• *Discontinuation of therapy* – Permanently discontinue treatment if severe toxicity recurs or does not disappear within 5 days.

Wasting or cachexia associated with HIV –

Serostim:

• *Maximum dose* – 6 mg/day.

• *Initial dosage* – 0.1 mg/kg/day subcutaneously (up to 6 mg). It should be administered subcutaneously daily at bedtime according to the following dosage recommendations:

***Serostim* Dosing Recommendations**

Weight range	Dose
> 55 kg (> 121 lb)	6 mg[a] subcutaneously daily
45 to 55 kg (99 to 121 lb)	5 mg[a] subcutaneously daily
35 to 45 kg (75 to 99 lb)	4 mg[a] subcutaneously daily
< 35 kg (< 75 lb)	0.1 mg/kg subcutaneously daily

[a] Based on an approximate daily dose of 0.1 mg/kg.

• *Maintenance dosage* – Most of the effect of *Serostim* on work output and LBM was apparent after 12 weeks of treatment. The effect was maintained during an additional 12 weeks of therapy.

• *Alternative dosage* – Treatment with *Serostim* 0.1 mg/kg every other day was associated with fewer adverse reactions and resulted in a similar improvement in work output, compared with *Serostim* 0.1 mg/kg/day. Therefore, a starting dosage of *Serostim* 0.1 mg/kg every other day should be considered in patients with an increased risk for adverse reactions related to recombinant human growth hormone (rhGH) therapy (ie, glucose intolerance). In general, dose reductions (ie, reducing the total daily dose or the number of doses per week) should be considered for adverse reactions potentially related to rhGH therapy that are unresponsive to symptom-directed treatment.

Off-label dosing –

Lipodystrophy (HIV related): [4] = Insufficient documentation. rhGH was administered as 6 mg nightly for 24 weeks, followed by a 12-week washout, then administered as 4 mg every other day. In another study, rhGH was administered as 6 mg daily for 12 weeks.

➤*Children:*

Growth failure in children – Serum IGF-1 levels may be useful during dose titration. Response to somatropin therapy in children tends to decrease with time. However, in children, the failure to increase growth rate, particularly during the first year of therapy, indicates the need for close assessment of compliance and evaluation for other causes of growth failure, such as hypothyroidism, undernutrition, advanced bone age, and antibodies to rhGH.

Therapy should not be continued if epiphyseal fusion has occurred.

Accretropin: 0.18 to 0.3 mg/kg (0.9 units/kg) per week, divided into equal daily doses given 6 or 7 times per week subcutaneously.

Genotropin: For children with growth hormone deficiency, the dosage is 0.16 to 0.24 mg/kg/week divided into 6 or 7 daily subcutaneous injections.

For children born SGA, the dosage is 0.48 mg/kg/week divided into 6 or 7 subcutaneous injections.

Humatrope and *HumatroPen*: For children with GHD, the subcutaneous dosage is 0.026 to 0.043 mg/kg/day (0.18 to 0.3 mg/kg/week divided into 6 or 7 daily subcutaneous injections).

For children born SGA, the subcutaneous dosage is up to 0.067 mg/kg/day (0.47 mg/kg/week divided into 6 or 7 daily subcutaneous injections). Recent literature has recommended initial treatment with larger doses of somatropin (eg, 0.067 mg/kg/day), especially in very short children (ie, height SDS greater than −3), and/or older pubertal children, and that a reduction in dosage (eg, gradually towards 0.033 mg/kg/day) should be considered if substantial catch-up growth is observed during the first few years of therapy. On the other hand, in younger SGA children (eg, approximately younger than 4 years of age who respond the best in general) with less severe short stature (ie, baseline height SDS values between −2 and −3), consideration should be given to initiating treatment at a lower dose (eg, 0.033 mg/kg/day), and titrating the dose as needed over time. In all children, clinicians should carefully monitor the growth response, and adjust the somatropin dose as necessary.

Norditropin: For children with GHD, 0.024 to 0.034 mg/kg/day, 6 to 7 times a week by subcutaneous injection.

For children with short stature born SGA with no catch-up growth by 2 to 4 years of age, a dosage of up to 0.067 mg/kg/day is recommended. Initial treatment with larger doses of somatropin (eg, 0.067 mg/kg/day) is recommended, especially in very short children (ie, height standard deviation score [HSDS] less than −3) and/or older/early pubertal children; a reduction in dosage (eg, gradually toward 0.033 mg/kg/day) should be considered if substantial growth is observed during the first few years of therapy. On the other hand, in younger SGA children (eg, younger than 4 years of age) who generally respond best, with less severe short stature (ie, baseline HSDS values between −2 and −3), consideration should be given to initiating treatment at a lower dose (eg, 0.033 mg/kg/day), and titrating the dose as needed over time. In all children, carefully monitor the growth response and adjust the rhGH dose as necessary.

Nutropin and *Nutropin AQ*: Up to 0.3 mg/kg/week, divided into daily subcutaneous injections. In pubertal patients, up to 0.7 mg/kg/week divided into daily injections may be used.

Omnitrope: 0.16 to 0.24 mg/kg/week, divided into 6 or 7 daily subcutaneous doses.

Saizen: 0.06 mg/kg (approximately 0.18 units/kg), administered 3 times per week by subcutaneous or intramuscular (IM) injection.

Tev-Tropin: Up to 0.1 mg/kg (0.3 units/kg) administered 3 times per week by subcutaneous injection is recommended. Subcutaneous injection of more than 1 mL of reconstituted solution is not recommended.

Discontinuation of therapy: Therapy should not be continued if epiphyseal fusion has occurred.

Growth failure associated with chronic renal insufficiency –

Nutropin and *Nutropin AQ*:

• *Usual dosage* – Up to 0.35 mg/kg/week, divided into daily subcutaneous injections.

• *Discontinuation of therapy* – Therapy may be continued up to the time of renal transplantation.

• *Hemodialysis patients* – Hemodialysis patients should receive their injection at night just prior to going to sleep or at least 3 to 4 hours after hemodialysis to prevent hematoma formation caused by heparin.

• *Chronic cycling peritoneal dialysis patients* – These patients should receive their injection in the morning after completing dialysis.

• *Chronic ambulatory peritoneal dialysis patients* – These patients should receive their injection in the evening at the time of the overnight exchange.

Growth failure associated with Noonan syndrome –

Not all patients with Noonan syndrome have short stature; some will achieve normal height without treatment. Therefore, prior to initiating *Norditropin* for a patient with Noonan syndrome, establish that the patient does have short stature.

Norditropin: Up to 0.066 mg/kg/day by subcutaneous injection.

Growth failure associated with Prader-Willi syndrome –

Genotropin: 0.24 mg/kg/week, divided into 6 or 7 subcutaneous injections.

Growth failure associated with Turner syndrome –

Accretropin: 0.36 mg/kg/week, divided into equal daily doses given 6 or 7 times per week subcutaneously.

Genotropin: 0.33 mg/kg/week, divided into 6 or 7 subcutaneous injections.

Humatrope and *HumatroPen*: Up to 0.054 mg/kg/day (0.375 mg/kg/week divided into 6 or 7 daily subcutaneous injections).

Norditropin: Up to 0.067 mg/kg/day by subcutaneous injection.

Nutropin and *Nutropin AQ*: Up to 0.375 mg/kg/week, divided into equal daily doses given 3 to 7 times per week subcutaneously.

Idiopathic short stature –

Genotropin: Up to 0.47 mg/kg/week, divided into 6 or 7 subcutaneous injections.

Humatrope and *HumatroPen*: Up to 0.053 mg/kg/day (0.37 mg/kg/week divided into 6 or 7 daily subcutaneous injections).

SOMATROPIN — INJECTION

Nutropin and *Nutropin AQ*: Up to 0.3 mg/kg/week divided into daily subcutaneous injections.

Short stature homeobox–containing gene –

Humatrope and *HumatroPen*: 0.05 mg/kg/day (0.35 mg/kg/week divided into 6 or 7 daily subcutaneous injections).

➤*Elderly:* Elderly patients may be more sensitive to the action of somatropin and may be more prone to develop adverse reactions. Consider a lower starting dose and smaller dose increments for older patients.

➤*Renal function impairment:*

Nutropin and *Nutropin AQ* – In order to optimize therapy for children with growth failure associated with chronic renal insufficiency who require dialysis, the following guidelines for injection schedule are recommended:

Hemodialysis patients: These patients should receive their injection at night just prior to going to sleep or at least 3 to 4 hours after hemodialysis to prevent hematoma formation caused by heparin.

Chronic cycling peritoneal dialysis patients: These patients should receive their injection in the morning after completing dialysis.

Chronic ambulatory peritoneal dialysis patients: These patients should receive their injection in the evening at the time of the overnight exchange.

➤*Obese patients:* Obese individuals are more likely to manifest adverse reactions when treated with a weight-based regimen.

➤*Gender:* In order to reach the defined treatment goal, estrogen-replete women may need higher doses than men. Oral estrogen administration may increase the dose requirements in women.

➤*Preparation for administration:* To reconstitute vials, inject the diluent into the vial by aiming the stream of liquid against the glass wall. Swirl the vial with a gentle rotary motion until the contents are dissolved completely. Do not shake. Because somatropin is a protein, shaking may cause denaturation of the protein, resulting in a cloudy solution.

If the solution is cloudy or contains particulate matter, the contents must not be injected. However, occasionally after refrigeration, some cloudiness may occur. This is not unusual for proteins like growth hormone. Allow the product to warm to room temperature. If cloudiness persists or particulate matter is noted, the contents must not be used (*Accretropin*, *Tev-Tropin*, and *Zorbtive*).

When administering to newborns, reconstitute with sterile isotonic sodium chloride solution for injection. Do not use bacteriostatic isotonic sodium chloride solution because it contains benzyl alcohol as a preservative, which has been associated with toxicity in newborns.

For multiuse vials, approximately 10% mechanical loss can be associated with reconstitution and administration.

Genotropin – *Genotropin* is supplied in a 2-chamber cartridge, with the lyophilized powder in the front chamber and a diluent in the rear chamber. A reconstitution device is used to mix the diluent and powder.

Serostim – Each vial of 4, 5, or 6 mg is reconstituted with 0.5 to 1 mL of sterile water for injection. Each 8.8 mg vial is reconstituted with 1 to 2 mL of bacteriostatic water for injection (benzyl alcohol 0.9% preserved).

Humatrope – Each 5 mg vial should be reconstituted with 1.5 to 5 mL of diluent for *Humatrope*. Each cartridge should only be reconstituted using the diluent syringe that accompanies the cartridge and should not be reconstituted with the diluent for *Humatrope* provided with the vials.

Nutropin – After the dose has been determined, reconstitute as follows: each 5 mg vial should be reconstituted with 1 to 5 mL of bacteriostatic water for injection (benzyl alcohol preserved); or each 10 mg vial should be reconstituted with 1 to 10 mL of bacteriostatic water for injection (benzyl alcohol preserved).

Omnitrope – Each cartridge must be inserted into its corresponding *Omnitrope* Pen 5 or *Omnitrope* Pen 10 delivery system.

Saizen – Reconstitute each vial as follows: 5 mg vial with 1 to 3 mL of bacteriostatic water for injection (benzyl alcohol preserved); 8.8 mg vial with 2 to 3 mL of bacteriostatic water for injection (benzyl alcohol preserved).

Tev-Tropin – Reconstitute with 1 to 5 mL of bacteriostatic sodium chloride 0.9% for injection (benzyl alcohol preserved).

Zorbtive – Each 8.8 mg vial is reconstituted in 1 to 2 mL of bacteriostatic water for injection (benzyl alcohol 0.9%).

➤*Administration:*

Accretropin – *Accretropin* should not be injected intravenously (IV).

Genotropin and *Omnitrope* – *Genotropin* and *Omnitrope* may be given subcutaneously in the thigh, buttocks, or abdomen; the site of subcutaneous injections should be rotated daily to help prevent lipoatrophy. *Genotropin* and *Omnitrope* must not be injected IV.

Norditropin – Injection sites must be rotated to avoid lipoatrophy. The cartridges must be administered using the *NordiPen* delivery systems. Each cartridge size has a corresponding, color-coded pen that is graduated to deliver the appropriate dose based on the concentration of *Norditropin* in the cartridge.

Serostim – *Serostim* 4, 5, or 6 mg single-use vials should be administered to patients requiring 4, 5, or 6 mg daily, respectively, as shown in the weight-based dosing table. Serostim 8.8 mg multi-use vials should be administered as per the weight-based dosing table. Do not inject *Serostim* if the reconstituted product is cloudy immediately after reconstitution or after refrigeration (2° to 8°C; 36° to 46°F) for up to 14 days. Injection sites should be rotated.

Humatrope, *HumatroPen*, *Nutropin*, *Nutropin AQ*, *Saizen*, and *Tev-Tropin* – It is recommended that these products be administered using sterile, disposable syringes and needles. The syringes should be of small enough volume that the prescribed dose can be drawn from the vial with reasonable accuracy.

Zorbtive – A standard insulin-type subcutaneous syringe is recommended for administration.

➤*Storage/Stability:*

Accretropin – Store vials in the refrigerator, 2° to 8°C (36° to 46°F). Avoid freezing and shaking. Once opened, vials may be stored up to 14 days when refrigerated at 2° to 8°C (36° to 46°F). Discard 14 days after first use. Protect from light.

Genotropin – Except as noted in the following, store *Genotropin* lyophilized powder under refrigeration at 2° to 8°C (36° to 46°F). Do not freeze. Protect from light.

The 5.8 and 13.8 mg cartridges contain a diluent with a preservative. Thus, after reconstitution, they may be refrigerated for up to 28 days.

Genotropin Miniquick should be refrigerated prior to dispensing but may be stored at or below 25°C (77°F) for up to 3 months after dispensing. The diluent has no preservative. After reconstitution, *Genotropin Miniquick* may be refrigerated for up to 24 hours before use. *Genotropin Miniquick* should be used only once and then discarded.

Humatrope – Avoid freezing the diluent and reconstituted vials and cartridges.

Vials:

- *Before reconstitution* – Vials and diluent are stable when refrigerated at 2° to 8°C (36° to 46°F).
- *After reconstitution* – Vials are stable for up to 14 days when reconstituted with diluent for *Humatrope* or bacteriostatic water for injection and refrigerated at 2° to 8°C (36° to 46°F).
- *After reconstitution with sterile water* – Use only 1 dose per vial and discard the unused portion. If the solution is not used immediately, it must be refrigerated at 2° to 8°C (36° to 46°F) and used within 24 hours.

Cartridges:

- *Before reconstitution* – Cartridges and diluent are stable when refrigerated at 2° to 8°C (36° to 46°F).
- *After reconstitution* – Cartridges are stable for up to 28 days when reconstituted with diluent for *Humatrope* and refrigerated at 2° to 8°C (36° to 46°F). Store the injection device without the needle attached.

Norditropin – Refrigerate unused *Norditropin* cartridges at 2° to 8°C (36° to 46°F). Do not freeze. Avoid direct light.

Cartridges 5 mg per 1.5 mL: After a *Norditropin* cartridge (5 mg per 1.5 mL) has been inserted into the *NordiPen* delivery system, it may be stored in the pen in the refrigerator (2° to 8°C; 36° to 46°F) and used within 4 weeks or stored for up to 3 weeks at not more than 25°C (77°F). Discard unused portion.

Cartridges 15 mg per 1.5 mL: After a *Norditropin* cartridge (15 mg per 1.5 mL) has been inserted into its *NordiPen* delivery system, it must be stored in the pen in the refrigerator (2° to 8°C; 36° to 46°F) and used within 4 weeks. Discard unused portion after 4 weeks.

Prefilled pens: Unused *Norditropin NordiFlex* prefilled pens must be refrigerated at 2° to 8°C (36° to 46°F). Do not freeze. Avoid direct light.

- *5 mg per 1.5 mL and 10 mg per 1.5 mL* – After the initial injection, a *Norditropin NordiFlex* (5 mg per 1.5 mL or 10 mg per 1.5 mL) prefilled pen may be refrigerated (2° to 8°C; 36° to 46°F) and used within 4 weeks or stored for up to 3 weeks at not more than 25°C (77°F). Discard unused portion.
- *15 mg per 1.5 mL and 30 mg per 3 mL* – After the initial injection, a *Norditropin NordiFlex* (15 mg per 1.5 mL or 30 mg per 3 mL) prefilled pen must be refrigerated at 2° to 8°C (36° to 46°F) and used within 4 weeks. Discard unused portion after 4 weeks.

***Norditropin* Prefilled Pen Storage Options**			
Norditropin product formulation	Before use	In-use (after first injection)	
	Storage requirement	Storage option 1 (refrigeration)	Storage option 2 (room temperature)
5 mg	2° to 8°C (36° to 46°F) until expiration date	2° to 8°C (36° to 46°F) for 4 weeks	Up to 25°C (77°F) for 3 weeks
10 mg			
15 mg			Does not apply
30 mg			

Nutropin –

Before reconstitution: Nutropin and diluent must be stored at 2° to 8°C (36° to 46°F) under refrigeration. Avoid freezing.

After reconstitution: Vial contents are stable for 14 days when reconstituted with bacteriostatic water for injection (benzyl alcohol preserved) and stored at 2° to 8°C (36° to 46°F) under refrigeration. Avoid freezing.

Nutropin AQ – Vial, cartridge, and *NuSpin* contents are stable for 28 days after initial use refrigerated at 2° to 8°C (36° to 46°F). Avoid freezing. *Nutropin AQ* is light-sensitive. When not in use, store *Nutropin AQ* under refrigeration and protect from light.

Omnitrope – Refrigerate at 2° to 8°C (36° to 46°F). Do not freeze. *Omnitrope* is light-sensitive; store in carton.

Omnitrope cartridges: After the first use, keep the cartridge in the pen and refrigerate at 2° to 8°C (36° to 46°F) for a maximum of 21 days (5 mg per 1.5 mL) or 28 days (10 mg per 1.5 mL).

SOMATROPIN — INJECTION

Omnitrope 1.5 mg vials: *Omnitrope* 1.5 mg is supplied with diluent without preservative. After reconstitution, the vial may be refrigerated for up to 24 hours. Use once and discard any remaining solution.

Omnitrope 5.8 mg vials: *Omnitrope* 5.8 mg is supplied with a diluent containing benzyl alcohol as a preservative. After reconstitution, use the contents of the vial within 3 weeks. After the first injection, the vial should be stored in the carton in a refrigerator at 2° to 8°C (36° to 46°F).

Saizen –

Before reconstitution: Store at room temperature (15° to 30°C [59° to 86°F]).

After reconstitution: Saizen 5 and 8.8 mg vials reconstituted with bacteriostatic water for injection (benzyl alcohol 0.9%) provided should be refrigerated (2° to 8°C [36° to 46°F]) for up to 14 days. *Saizen* 8.8 mg *click-easy* cartridge reconstituted with the bacteriostatic water for injection (metacresol 0.3%) provided should be refrigerated (2° to 8°C [36° to 46°F]) for up to 21 days. Avoid freezing.

Serostim –

Before reconstitution: Store vials and diluent at room temperature (15° to 30°C [59° to 86°F]).

After reconstitution with sterile water for injection: Immediately use the reconstituted solution and discard any unused portion.

After reconstitution with bacteriostatic water for injection (benzyl alcohol 0.9%): Refrigerate the reconstituted solution at 2° to 8°C (36° to 46°F) for up to 14 days. Avoid freezing.

Tev-Tropin –

Before reconstitution: Refrigerate vials at 2° to 8°C (36° to 46°F).

After reconstitution: Vials are stable for up to 14 days when reconstituted with bacteriostatic sodium chloride 0.9% and refrigerated at 2° to 8°C (36° to 46°F). Do not freeze.

Zorbtive –

Before reconstitution: Store at room temperature (15° to 30°C [59° to 86°F]).

After reconstitution with bacteriostatic water for injection (benzyl alcohol 0.9%): Refrigerate the reconstituted solution at 2° to 8°C (36° to 46°F) for up to 14 days. Avoid freezing.

Actions

➤*Pharmacology:* In vitro, preclinical, and clinical tests have demonstrated that somatropins are therapeutically equivalent to hGH of pituitary origin and achieve similar pharmacokinetic profiles in healthy adults. In children who have GHD, Prader-Willi syndrome, or who were born with SGA, patients with CRI, or patients with Turner syndrome, treatment with somatropin stimulated linear growth and normalized concentrations of IGF-1.

In adults, treatment with somatropin results in reduced fat mass, increased LBM, metabolic alterations that include beneficial changes in lipid metabolism, and normalization of IGF-1 concentrations.

Short bowel syndrome (Zorbtive) – Intestinal mucosa contains receptors for growth hormone and for IGF-1, which is known to mediate many of the cellular actions of growth hormone. Thus, the actions of growth hormone on the gut may be direct or mediated via the local or systemic production of IGF-1.

In human clinical studies, the administration of growth hormone enhanced the transmucosal transport of water, electrolytes, and nutrients.

Pharmacodynamics –

Tissue growth:

• *Skeletal growth* – Somatropin stimulates skeletal growth in children with GHD, Prader-Willi syndrome, SGA, Turner syndrome, or CRI. The measurable increase in body length after administration of somatropin results from an effect on the epiphyseal plates of long bones. Concentrations of IGF-1, which may play a role in skeletal growth, are generally low in the serum of children with GHD, Prader-Willi syndrome, or SGA, but tend to increase during treatment with somatropin. Elevations in mean serum alkaline phosphatase concentration also have been seen.

• *Cell growth* – It has been shown that there are fewer skeletal muscle cells in short-statured children who lack endogenous growth hormone as compared with the healthy pediatric population. Treatment with somatropin results in an increase in the number and size of muscle cells.

• *Organ growth* – Growth hormone influences the size of internal organs, including kidneys, and increases red cell mass.

Protein metabolism: Linear growth is facilitated in part by growth hormone–stimulated cellular protein synthesis. This synthesis and growth are reflected by nitrogen retention, which can be quantitated by observing the decline in urinary nitrogen excretion and blood urea nitrogen following the initiation of somatropin therapy.

Carbohydrate metabolism: Children with hypopituitarism sometimes experience fasting hypoglycemia that is improved by treatment with somatropin. Large doses of growth hormone may impair glucose tolerance. Although the precise mechanism of the diabetogenic effect of somatropin is not known, it is attributed to blocking the action of insulin rather than blocking insulin secretion. Insulin levels in serum actually increase as somatropin levels increase. Administration of hGH to healthy adults and patients with GHD results in increases in mean serum fasting and postprandial insulin levels, although mean values remain in the normal range. In addition, mean fasting and postprandial glucose and hemoglobin A_{1c} levels remain in the normal range.

Untreated patients with CRI and Turner syndrome have an increased incidence of glucose intolerance. Administration of hGH to adults or children resulted in increases in mean serum fasting and postprandial insulin levels although mean values remained in the normal range. In addition, mean fasting and postprandial glucose and hemoglobin A_{1c} levels remained in the normal range.

Lipid metabolism: In GHD patients, administration of somatropin has resulted in lipid mobilization, reduction in body fat stores, and increased plasma fatty acids.

Somatropin stimulates intracellular lipolysis, and administration of somatropin leads to an increase in plasma free fatty acids and triglycerides. Untreated GHD is associated with increased body fat stores, including increased abdominal visceral and subcutaneous adipose tissue. Treatment of GHD patients with somatropin results in a general reduction of fat stores, and decreased serum levels of low-density lipoprotein (LDL) cholesterol.

Mineral metabolism: Somatropin induces retention of sodium, potassium, and phosphorus. Serum concentrations of inorganic phosphate are increased in patients with GHD after therapy with somatropin. Serum calcium is not significantly altered by somatropin. Growth hormone could increase calciuria. Although calcium excretion in the urine is increased, there is a simultaneous increase in calcium absorption from the intestine. Negative calcium balance, however, may occasionally occur during somatropin treatment. Sodium retention also occurs.

Connective tissue metabolism: Somatropin stimulates the synthesis of chondroitin sulfate and collagen, and increases the urinary excretion of hydroxyproline.

Body composition: Adult GHD patients treated with somatropin at the recommended adult dose demonstrate a decrease in fat mass and an increase in LBM. When these alterations are coupled with the increase in total body water, the overall effect of somatropin is to modify body composition, an effect that is maintained with continued treatment.

Physical performance: Cycle ergometry work output and treadmill performance were examined in separate 12-week, placebo-controlled trials. In both studies, work output improved significantly in the group receiving *Serostim* 0.1 mg/kg/day subcutaneously versus placebo. Isometric muscle performance, as measured by grip strength dynamometry, declined, probably as a result of a transient increase in tissue turgor known to occur with *Serostim* therapy.

➤*Pharmacokinetics:*

Absorption –

Genotropin: Following a 0.03 mg/kg subcutaneous injection in the thigh of *Genotropin* 1.3 mg/mL to adult GHD patients, approximately 80% of the dose was systemically available as compared with that available following IV dosing. Results were comparable in men and women. Similar bioavailability has been observed in healthy adult men. In healthy adult men, following an subcutaneous injection in the thigh of 0.03 mg/kg, the extent of absorption (area under the curve [AUC]) of a concentration of *Genotropin* 5.3 mg/mL was 35% greater than that for *Genotropin* 1.3 mg/mL. The mean (± standard deviation [SD]) peak serum levels (maximal drug concentration [C_{max}]) were 23 (± 9.4) ng/mL and 17.4 (± 9.2) ng/mL, respectively. In a similar study involving pediatric GHD patients, *Genotropin* 5.3 mg/mL yielded a mean AUC that was 17% greater than that for *Genotropin* 1.3 mg/mL. The mean C_{max} levels were 21 ng/mL and 16.3 ng/mL, respectively. Adult GHD patients received 2 single subcutaneous doses of *Genotropin* 0.03 mg/kg at a concentration of 1.3 mg/mL, with a 1- to 4-week washout period between injections. Mean C_{max} levels were 12.4 ng/mL (first injection) and 12.2 ng/mL (second injection), achieved at approximately 6 hours after dosing. There are no data on the bioequivalence between the 12 mg/mL formulation and either the 1.3 mg/mL or the 5.3 mg/mL formulations.

Humatrope: The absolute bioavailability of *Humatrope* is 75% and 63% after subcutaneous and IM administration, respectively.

Norditropin: An 180-minute IV infusion of *Norditropin* (33 ng/kg/min) was given to 9 patients with GHD. A mean (± SD) hGH steady-state serum level of approximately 23.1 (± 15) ng/mL was reached at 150 minutes and a mean clearance rate of approximately 2.3 (± 1.8) mL/min/kg or 139 (± 105) mL/min for hGH was obtained. Following infusion, serum hGH levels had a biexponential decay with a terminal elimination half-life ($t_{½}$) of approximately 21.1 (± 5.1) minutes.

In a study conducted in 18 adult GHD patients, where an subcutaneous dose of 0.024 mg/kg or 3 units/m^2 was given in the thigh, the mean (± SD) C_{max} values of 13.8 (± 5.8) and 17.1 (± 10) ng/mL were obtained for the *Norditropin* 4 and 8 mg vials, respectively, at approximately 4 to 5 hours postdose. The mean apparent terminal $t_{½}$ values were estimated to be approximately 7 to 10 hours. However, the absolute bioavailability for *Norditropin* after the subcutaneous route of administration is not known.

• *Bioequivalency* – *Norditropin* cartridge formulation is bioequivalent to *Norditropin* vial formulation.

Nutropin and *Nutropin AQ*: The absolute bioavailability of *Nutropin* and *Nutropin AQ* after subcutaneous administration in healthy adult men is 81 ± 20%. The mean terminal $t_{½}$ after subcutaneous administration is significantly longer than that seen after IV administration (2.1 ± 0.43 hours vs 19.5 ± 3.1 minutes), indicating that the subcutaneous absorption of the compound is slow and rate-limiting.

• *Bioequivalency* – *Nutropin* has been determined to be bioequivalent to *Nutropin AQ* based on the statistical evaluation of AUC and C_{max}.

Omnitrope: Following a subcutaneous injection of a single dose of 5 mg in healthy men and women, the C_{max} and time of maximal concentration (T_{max}) values were 72 ± 28 mcg/L and 4 ± 2 hours, respectively. There are no pharmacokinetic data from patients with GHD.

• *Bioequivalency* – The aqueous *Omnitrope* cartridge is bioequivalent to the lyophilized *Omnitrope* formulation.

Saizen: The absolute bioavailability of rhGH after subcutaneous administration ranges between 70% and 90%.

Serostim and *Zorbtive*: The absolute bioavailability of *Serostim* and *Zorbtive* after subcutaneous administration of a formulation not equivalent to the marketed formulation was determined to be 70% to 90%. The $t_{½}$ (mean ± SD) after subcutaneous administration is significantly longer than that seen after IV administration in healthy men down-regulated with somatostatin (3.94 ± 3.44 hours vs 0.58 ± 0.08 hours), indicating that the subcutaneous absorption of the clinically tested formulation of the compound is slow and rate-limiting.

Tev-Tropin: After a subcutaneous injection of *Tev-Tropin* 0.1 mg/kg to the forearm, the mean peak serum concentration (± SD) was 80 (± 50) ng/mL, which occurred approximately 7 hours postinjection, and the apparent elimination t½ was approximately 2.7 hours. Compared with IV administration, the extent of systemic availability from subcutaneous administration was approximately 70%.

Distribution –

Genotropin: The mean volume of distribution of *Genotropin* following administration to adults with GHD was estimated to be 1.3 (± 0.8) L/kg.

Humatrope: The volume of distribution of *Humatrope* after IV injection is about 0.07 L/kg.

Nutropin and *Nutropin AQ*: Animal studies with *Nutropin* and *Nutropin AQ* showed that growth hormone localizes to highly perfused organs, particularly the liver and kidney. The volume of distribution at steady state for *Nutropin* and *Nutropin AQ* in healthy men is about 50 mL/kg body weight, approximating the serum volume.

Omnitrope: The mean volume of distribution following administration to healthy adults was estimated to be 1.4 L/kg.

Saizen, *Serostim*, and *Zorbtive*: The steady-state volume of distribution (mean ± SD) following IV administration of *Serostim* and *Zorbtive* in healthy volunteers is 12 ± 1.08 L.

Metabolism – The metabolic fate of somatropin involves classical protein catabolism in the liver and kidneys. In renal cells, at least a portion of the breakdown products is returned to the systemic circulation.

Nutropin and *Nutropin AQ*: Animal studies suggest that the kidney is the dominant organ of clearance. Growth hormone is filtered at the glomerulus and reabsorbed in the proximal tubules. It is then cleaved within renal cells into its constituent amino acids, which return to the systemic circulation.

Excretion –

Accretropin: The mean t½ of subcutaneously administered *Accretropin* is 3.63 hours.

Genotropin: The mean terminal t½ of IV *Genotropin* in healthy adults is 0.4 hours; however, subcutaneously administered *Genotropin* has a t½ of 3 hours in adults with GHD. The observed difference is caused by slow absorption from the subcutaneous injection site.

The mean clearance of subcutaneously administered *Genotropin* in 16 adult GHD patients was 0.3 (± 0.11) L/kg/h.

Humatrope: In healthy volunteers, mean clearance is 0.14 L/h/kg. The mean t½ of IV *Humatrope* is 0.36 hours, whereas subcutaneously and intramuscularly administered *Humatrope* have mean half-lives of 3.8 and 4.9 hours, respectively. The longer t½ observed after subcutaneous or IM administration is caused by slow absorption from the injection site. Urinary excretion of intact *Humatrope* has not been measured. Small amounts of somatropin have been detected in the urine of children following replacement therapy.

Nutropin and *Nutropin AQ* : The mean terminal t½ after IV administration of rhGH in healthy men is estimated to be 19.5 ± 3.1 minutes. Clearance of rhGH after IV administration in healthy adults and children is reported to be in the range of 116 to 174 mL/kg/h.

Omnitrope: The mean clearance of subcutaneously administered *Omnitrope* in healthy adults was 0.14 (± 0.04) L/h•kg. The mean terminal t½ of *Omnitrope* after subcutaneous administration in healthy adults is 2.8 hours.

Saizen: The mean t½ of IV somatropin in healthy men is 0.6 hours, whereas subcutaneously and IM administered somatropin has a t½ of 1.75 and 3.4 hours, respectively. The longer t½ observed after subcutaneous or IM administration is caused by slow absorption from the injection site.

The mean clearance of IV administered rhGH in 6 healthy men was 14.6 ± 2.8 L/h.

Serostim and *Zorbtive*: The t½ (mean ± SD) in 9 patients with HIV-associated wasting with an average weight of 56.7 ± 6.8 kg, given a fixed dose of rhGH 6 mg subcutaneously, was 4.28 ± 2.15 hours. The renal clearance of rhGH after subcutaneous administration in 9 patients with HIV-associated wasting was 0.0015 ± 0.0037 L/h. No significant accumulation of rhGH appears to occur after 6 weeks of dosing as indicated.

Tev-Tropin: Following IV administration of *Tev-Tropin* 0.1 mg/kg, the elimination t½ was about 0.42 hours (approximately 25 minutes) and the mean plasma clearance (± SD) was 133 (± 16) mL/min in healthy men.

Special populations –

Renal function impairment:

• *Nutropin* and *Nutropin AQ* – Children and adults with CRI and end-stage renal disease tend to have decreased clearance compared with healthy subjects. In a study with 6 children 7 to 11 years of age, the clearance of *Nutropin* was reduced 21.5% and 22.6% after the IV infusion and subcutaneous injection, respectively, of *Nutropin* 0.05 mg/kg compared with healthy adults. Endogenous growth hormone production may also increase in some individuals with end-stage renal disease. However, no rhGH accumulation has been reported in children with CRI or end-stage renal disease dosed with current regimens.

• *Saizen* – Children and adults with CRI tend to have decreased clearance of rhGH as compared with healthy individuals.

• *Serostim* and *Zorbtive* – It has been reported that individuals with CRI tend to have decreased rhGH clearance compared with healthy individuals, but there are no data on *Serostim* and *Zorbtive* use in the presence of renal insufficiency.

Hepatic function impairment: A reduction in rhGH clearance has been noted in patients with severe liver dysfunction. The clinical significance of this decrease is unknown.

Gender:

• *Omnitrope* – No gender studies have been performed in children; however, following a subcutaneous injection of *Omnitrope* 5 mg (around 0.07 mg/kg) to healthy adult volunteers, gender has no effect on some pharmacokinetic parameters of *Omnitrope* (C_{max} and T_{max}). However, statistical differences were observed for some pharmacokinetic parameters (AUC, volume of distribution during the terminal phase, plasma clearance) of *Omnitrope* and between men and women, which can be explained by differences in body weight.

• *Serostim* and *Zorbtive* – Biomedical literature indicates that a gender-related difference in the mean clearance of rhGH could exist (clearance of rhGH in men greater than clearance of rhGH in women). However, no gender-based analysis is available in healthy volunteers or patients infected with HIV or SBS.

Pharmacokinetic parameters –

Accretropin:

Accretropin Pharmacokinetic Parameters in Healthy Patients[a]					
	$AUC_{(0\text{-}t)}$ [b] (ng•h/mL)	$AUC_{(0\text{-}inf)}$ [c] (ng•h/mL)	C_{max} (ng/mL)	T_{max} [d] (h)	t½ (h)
mean ± SD	238.09 ± 44.11	255.31 ± 43.03	29.49 ± 8.32	3.5 (2 to 6)	3.63 ± 1.33

[a] 4 mg dose administered subcutaneously.
[b] $AUC_{(0\text{-}t)}$ = AUC until 24 hours after administration.
[c] $AUC_{(0\text{-}inf)}$ = AUC to infinity.
[d] T_{max} = given as the median value with range.

Genotropin:

Genotropin Mean Subcutaneous Pharmacokinetic Parameters in Adults With GHD					
	Bioavailability (%) (n = 15)	T_{max} (h) (n = 16)	CL/F[a] (L/h × kg) (n = 16)	V_{ss}/F[b] (L/kg) (n = 16)	Terminal t½ (h) (n = 16)
Mean	80.5	5.9	0.3	1.3	3
(± SD)	c	(± 1.65)	(± 0.11)	(± 0.8)	(± 1.44)
95% CI[d]	70.5 to 92.1	5 to 6.7	0.2 to 0.4	0.9 to 1.8	2.2 to 3.7

[a] CL/F = plasma clearance.
[b] Vss/F = volume of distribution at steady state after non-IV administration.
[c] The absolute bioavailability was estimated under the assumption that the log-transformed data follow a normal distribution. The mean and standard deviation of the log-transformed data were mean = 0.22 (± 0.241).
[d] CI = confidence interval.

Humatrope:

Summary of Somatropin Parameters in the Healthy Population					
	C_{max} (ng/mL)	t½ (h)	$AUC_{0\text{-}\infty}$ (ng•h/mL)	Cls[a] (L/kg•h)	Vβ[b] (L/kg)
0.02 mg (0.05 units[c])/kg administered IV					
Mean	415	0.363	156	0.135	0.0703
SD	75	0.053	33	0.029	0.0173
0.1 mg (0.27 units[c])/kg administered IM					
Mean	53.2	4.93	495	0.215	1.55
SD	25.9	2.66	106	0.047	0.91
0.1 mg (0.27 units[c])/kg administered subcutaneously					
Mean	63.3	3.81	585	0.179	0.957
SD	18.2	1.4	90	0.028	0.301

[a] Cls = systemic clearance.
[b] Vβ = volume of distribution during terminal phase.
[c] Based on previous International Standard of 2.7 units = 1 mg.

Nutropin and *Nutropin AQ*:

Summary of *Nutropin* Pharmacokinetic Parameters in Healthy Men 0.1 mg (Approximately 0.3 units[a])/kg Subcutaneous					
	C_{max} (mcg/L)	T_{max} (h)	t½ (h)	$AUC_{0\text{-}\infty}$ (mcg•h/L)	CL/F_{sc} [b] mL/(h•kg)
Nutropin					
Mean[c]	67.2	6.2	2.1	643	158
CV%[d]	29	37	20	12	12
Nutropin AQ					
Mean[c]	71.1	3.9	2.3	677	150
CV%[d]	17	56	18	13	13

[a] Based on current International Standard of 3 units = 1 mg.
[b] F_{sc} = subcutaneous bioavailability (not determined).
[c] n = 36
[d] CV = coefficient of variation.

Contraindications

Hypersensitivity to somatropin, growth hormone, or any of the excipients in the products. Do not use somatropin for growth promotion in children with closed epiphyses; in patients with active proliferative, preproliferative, or severe nonproliferative diabetic retinopathy; hypersensitivity to growth hormone; evidence of active malignancy. Antimalignancy treatment must be

SOMATROPIN — INJECTION

complete with evidence of remission prior to the institution of therapy. Discontinue somatropin if there is evidence of recurrent activity. Because GHD may be an early sign of the presence of a pituitary tumor (or, rarely, other brain tumors), rule out the presence of such tumors prior to initiation of treatment. Do not use somatropin in patients with any evidence of progression or recurrence of an underlying intracranial tumor. Discontinue therapy with somatropin if there is evidence of recurrent tumor growth.

Do not initiate growth hormone to treat patients with acute critical illness caused by complications following open-heart or abdominal surgery or multiple accidental trauma, or to treat patients having acute respiratory failure. Two placebo-controlled clinical trials in non-GHD adults (n = 522) with these conditions revealed a significant increase in mortality (41.9% vs 19.3%) among somatropin-treated patients (doses 5.3 to 8 mg/day) compared with those receiving placebo.

Somatropin injection, when reconstituted with bacteriostatic water for injection (benzyl alcohol 0.9 %), should not be used in patients with a known sensitivity to benzyl alcohol.

➤*Humatrope*: Patients with a known sensitivity to metacresol or glycerin should not receive *Humatrope* reconstituted with the supplied diluent.

➤*Genotropin*, *Humatrope*, *Norditropin*, *Nutropin*, *Nutropin AQ*, *Omnitrope*, *Saizen*, and *Tev-Tropin*: Contraindicated in patients with Prader-Willi syndrome who are severely obese or have severe respiratory impairment.

Unless patients with Prader-Willi syndrome also have a diagnosis of GHD, *Humatrope*, *Norditropin*, *Nutropin*, *Nutropin AQ*, *Omnitrope*, *Saizen*, and *Tev-Tropin* are not indicated for the treatment of children who have growth failure caused by genetically confirmed Prader-Willi syndrome.

Warnings/Precautions

➤*Benzyl alcohol:* Benzyl alcohol as a preservative in bacteriostatic water for injection has been associated with toxicity in newborns. When administering to newborns, use sterile water for injection. When reconstituted in this manner, immediately use the reconstituted solution and discard any unused solution. Do not use *Omnitrope* in premature infants or newborns.

➤*Critical illness:* Do not initiate growth hormone in patients with acute critical illness caused by complications following open-heart or abdominal surgery, multiple accidental trauma, or acute respiratory failure. The safety of continuing growth hormone treatment in patients receiving replacement doses for approved indications who concurrently develop these illnesses has not been established. Therefore, weigh the potential benefit of treatment continuation with growth hormone in patients developing acute critical illnesses against the potential risk.

➤*Prader-Willi syndrome in children:* There have been reports of fatalities after initiating somatropin therapy in children with Prader-Willi syndrome who had 1 or more of the following risk factors: severe obesity, history of upper airway obstructions or sleep apnea, or unidentified respiratory infection. Male patients with 1 or more of these factors may be at greater risk than female patients. Patients with Prader-Willi syndrome should be evaluated for signs of upper airway obstruction and sleep apnea before initiation of treatment with somatropin. If during somatropin treatment patients show signs of upper airway obstruction (including onset of or increased snoring) and/or new onset of sleep apnea, interrupt treatment. All patients with Prader-Willi syndrome treated with somatropin should also have effective weight control and be monitored for signs of respiratory infection, which should be diagnosed as early as possible and treated aggressively.

Unless patients with Prader-Willi syndrome also have a diagnosis of GHD, *Humatrope*, *Norditropin*, *Nutropin*, *Nutropin AQ*, *Saizen*, and/or *Tev-Tropin* are not indicated in the treatment of children who have growth failure caused by genetically confirmed Prader-Willi syndrome.

➤*Neoplasms/Malignancies:* Routinely examine patients with preexisting tumors or GHD secondary to an intracranial lesion for progression or recurrence of the underlying disease process. In children, the literature has revealed no relationship between somatropin replacement therapy and CNS tumor recurrence or new extracranial tumors. However, in childhood cancer survivors, an increased risk of a second neoplasm has been reported in patients treated with somatropin after their first neoplasm. Intracranial tumors, in particular meningiomas, in patients treated with radiation to the head for their first neoplasm were the most common of these second neoplasms. In adults, it is unknown whether there is any relationship between somatropin replacement therapy and CNS tumor recurrence.

➤*Glucose intolerance/diabetes:* The use of somatropin has been associated with cases of new-onset impaired glucose intolerance, new-onset type 2 diabetes mellitus, and exacerbation of preexisting diabetes mellitus. Some patients developed diabetic ketoacidosis and diabetic coma. In some patients, these conditions improved when somatropin was discontinued, while in others the glucose intolerance persisted.

Treatment with somatropin may decrease insulin sensitivity, particularly at higher doses in susceptible patients. As a result, previously undiagnosed impaired glucose tolerance and overt diabetes mellitus may be unmasked during somatropin treatment. Therefore, monitor glucose levels in all patients treated with somatropin, especially in those with risk factors for diabetes mellitus, such as obesity (including obese patients with Prader-Willi syndrome), Turner syndrome, or a family history of diabetes mellitus. Closely monitor patients with preexisting type 1 or type 2 diabetes mellitus or impaired glucose tolerance during somatropin therapy. The doses of antihyperglycemic drugs (insulin or oral agents) may require adjustment when somatropin therapy is instituted in these patients.

➤*Intracranial hypertension:* Intracranial hypertension with papilledema, visual changes, headache, nausea, and/or vomiting has been reported in a small number of patients treated with somatropin products. Symptoms usually occurred within the first 8 weeks after the initiation of somatropin therapy. In all reported cases, intracranial hypertension-associated signs and symptoms rapidly resolved after cessation of therapy or a reduction in the somatropin dose. Routinely perform funduscopic examination before initiating treatment with somatropin to exclude preexisting papilledema, and periodically during the course of somatropin therapy. If papilledema is observed by funduscopy during somatropin treatment, discontinue treatment. If somatropin-induced intracranial hypertension is diagnosed, treatment with somatropin can be restarted at a lower dose after intracranial hypertension-associated signs and symptoms have resolved. Patients with Turner syndrome, CRI, and Prader-Willi syndrome may be at increased risk for the development of intracranial hypertension.

➤*Fluid retention:* Fluid retention during somatropin replacement therapy in adults may frequently occur. Clinical manifestations of fluid retention are usually transient and dose dependent.

➤*Hypothyroidism:* Undiagnosed/untreated hypothyroidism may prevent an optimal response to somatropin, in particular, the growth response in children. Patients with Turner syndrome have an inherently increased risk of developing autoimmune thyroid disease and primary hypothyroidism. In patients with GHD, central (secondary) hypothyroidism may first become evident or worsen during somatropin treatment. Therefore, perform periodic thyroid function tests in patients treated with somatropin and initiate or appropriately adjust thyroid hormone replacement therapy when indicated. In patients with hypopituitarism (multiple hormone deficiencies), closely monitor standard hormonal replacement therapy when somatropin therapy is administered.

➤*Slipped capital femoral epiphyses:* Slipped capital femoral epiphyses may occur more frequently in patients with endocrine disorders, including pediatric GHD and Turner syndrome, or in patients undergoing rapid growth. Carefully evaluate any child with the onset of a limp or complaints of hip or knee pain during somatropin therapy.

➤*Renal osteodystrophy:* Periodically examine children with growth failure secondary to CRI for evidence of progression of renal osteodystrophy. Slipped capital femoral epiphyses or avascular necrosis of the femoral head may be seen in children with advanced renal osteodystrophy, and it is uncertain whether these problems are affected by somatropin therapy. Obtain x-rays of the hip prior to initiating somatropin therapy in CRI patients. Health care providers and parents should be alert to the development of a limp or complaints of hip or knee pain in CRI patients treated with *Nutropin AQ*.

➤*Progression of preexisting scoliosis:* Progression of scoliosis can occur in patients who experience rapid growth. Because somatropin increases growth rate, monitor patients with a history of scoliosis who are treated with somatropin for progression of scoliosis. However, somatropin has not been shown to increase the occurrence of scoliosis. Skeletal abnormalities, including scoliosis, are commonly seen in untreated Turner syndrome patients. Scoliosis is also commonly seen in untreated patients with Prader-Willi syndrome. Be alert to these abnormalities that may manifest during somatropin therapy.

➤*Otitis media and cardiovascular disorders in patients with Turner syndrome:* Carefully evaluate patients with Turner syndrome for otitis media and other ear disorders because these patients have an increased risk of ear or hearing disorders. Somatropin treatment may increase the occurrence of otitis media in patients with Tuner syndrome. In addition, closely monitor patients with Turner syndrome for cardiovascular disorders (eg, stroke, aortic aneurysm/dissection, hypertension) as these patients are also at risk for these conditions.

➤*Tissue atrophy:* When somatropin is administered subcutaneously at the same site over a long period of time, tissue atrophy may result. This can be avoided by rotating the injection site.

➤*Swelling/Pain (Serostim* and *Zorbtive):* Increased tissue turgor (swelling, particularly in the hands and feet) and musculoskeletal discomfort (pain, swelling, and/or stiffness) may occur during treatment with *Serostim* or *Zorbtive*, but may resolve spontaneously, with analgesic therapy, or after reducing the frequency of dosing.

➤*Carpal tunnel syndrome (Serostim* and *Zorbtive)*: Carpal tunnel syndrome may occur during treatment with *Serostim* or *Zorbtive*. If the symptoms of carpal tunnel syndrome do not resolve by decreasing the doses or frequency of *Serostim* or *Zorbtive*, it is recommended that treatment be discontinued.

➤*Pancreatitis (Serostim* and *Zorbtive)*: rhGH has been associated with acute pancreatitis.

➤*Experienced health care provider:* Treatment with growth hormone preparations should be directed by health care providers who are experienced in the diagnosis and management of patients with GHD, Prader-Willi syndrome, Turner syndrome, and those who were born SGA, idiopathic short stature, or chronic renal insufficiency.

Serostim therapy should be carried out under the regular guidance of a health care provider who is experienced in the diagnosis and management of HIV infection. Inadequate nutritional intake, malabsorption, and hypogonadism, which are common in individuals with HIV infection and may contribute to catabolism and weight loss, should be diagnosed and treated.

➤*Confirmation of childhood-onset GHD in adults:* Reevaluate patients with epiphyseal closure who were treated with growth hormone replacement therapy in childhood before continuing somatropin therapy at the reduced dose level recommended for GHD adults.

SOMATROPIN — INJECTION

➤*Concomitant antiretroviral treatment (Serostim):* In some experimental systems, rhGH has been shown to potentiate HIV replication in vitro at concentrations ranging from 50 to 250 ng/mL. There was no increase in virus production when the antiretroviral agents zidovudine, didanosine, or lamivudine were added to the culture medium. Additional in vitro studies have shown that rhGH does not interfere with the antiviral activity of zalcitabine or stavudine.

In the controlled clinical trials, no significant growth hormone-associated increase in viral burden was observed. However, the protocol required all participants to be on concomitant antiretroviral therapy for the duration of the study. In view of the potential for acceleration of virus replication, it is recommended that HIV patients be maintained on antiretroviral therapy for the duration of *Serostim* treatment.

➤*Hypersensitivity reactions:* As with any protein, local or systemic allergic reactions may occur. Parents/patients should be informed that such reactions are possible and that prompt medical attention should be sought if allergic reactions occur. Do not use *Humatrope* cartridges if the patient is allergic to metacresol or glycerin.

Genotropin contains metacresol as a preservative and should not be used by patients with a known sensitivity to this preservative.

➤*Renal function impairment:* No studies have been completed evaluating somatropin in patients who have received renal transplants. Currently, treatment of patients with functioning renal allografts is not indicated.

Children and adults with CRI tend to have decreased clearance of rhGH as compared with healthy patients.

In a study with 6 children 7 to 11 years of age, the clearance of *Nutropin* was reduced 21.5% and 22.6% after the IV infusion and subcutaneous injection, respectively, of 0.05 mg/kg of *Nutropin* compared with healthy adults. Endogenous growth hormone production may also increase in some individuals with end-stage renal disease. However, no rhGH accumulation has been reported in children with CRI or end-stage renal disease dosed with current regimens.

➤*Hepatic function impairment:* A reduction in rhGH clearance has been noted in patients with severe liver function impairment. However, the clinical significance of this in patients with SBS or GHD, or patients who are HIV-positive is unknown.

➤*Pregnancy: Category B* (*Genotropin, Omnitrope, Saizen, Serostim,* and *Zorbtive*).

Category C (*Accretropin, Humatrope, Norditropin, Nutropin, Nutropin AQ,* and *Tev-Tropin*).

Animal reproduction studies have not been conducted with somatropin (except with *Genotropin* and *Zorbtive*). It is not known whether somatropin can cause fetal harm when administered to a pregnant woman or can affect reproductive capacity. Only give somatropin to a pregnant woman if clearly needed.

Genotropin – In rats receiving subcutaneous doses during gametogenesis and for up to 7 days of pregnancy, 3.3 mg/kg/day produced anestrus or extended estrus cycles in females and fewer and less motile sperm in males. When given to pregnant female rats (days 1 to 7 of gestation) at a dose of 3.3 mg/kg/day, a very slight increase in fetal deaths was observed. At a dose of 1 mg/kg/day, rats showed slightly extended estrus cycles.

In perinatal and postnatal studies in rats, somatropin doses of 0.3, 1, and 3.3 mg/kg/day produced growth-promoting effects in the dams but not in the fetuses.

Zorbtive – Reproduction studies have been performed in rats and rabbits. Doses up to 5 to 10 times the human dose, based on body surface area, have revealed no evidence of impaired fertility or harm to the fetus.

➤*Lactation:* It is not known whether somatropin is excreted in human milk. Because many drugs are excreted in human milk, exercise caution when administering to a breast-feeding woman.

Genotropin – At the highest dose, young rats showed increase weight gain during suckling, but the effect was not apparent by 10 weeks of age.

➤*Children:* Benzyl alcohol as a preservative in bacteriostatic water for injection has been associated with toxicity in newborns. When administering to newborns, use sterile water for injection. When reconstituted in this manner, immediately use the reconstituted solution and discard any unused solution. Do not use *Omnitrope* in premature babies or newborns.

There are no formal studies in children with SBS (*Zorbtive*).

In 2 small studies, 11 children with HIV-associated failure to thrive were treated subcutaneously with hGH. In 1 study, 5 children (range, 6 to 17 years of age) were treated with 0.04 mg/kg/day for 26 weeks. In a second study, 6 children (range, 8 to 14 years of age) were treated with 0.07 mg/kg/day for 4 weeks. Treatment appeared to be well tolerated in both studies. The preliminary data collected on a limited number of patients with HIV-associated failure to thrive appear to be consistent with safety observations in growth hormone-treated adults with AIDS wasting.

➤*Elderly:* The safety and effectiveness of somatropin in patients 65 years of age and older have not been evaluated in clinical studies. Elderly patients may be more sensitive to the action of somatropin and may be more prone to develop adverse reactions. Consider a lower starting dose and smaller dose increments for older patients.

➤*Lab test abnormalities:* Serum levels of inorganic phosphorus, alkaline phosphatase, parathyroid hormone, and IGF-1 may increase after somatropin therapy.

➤*Monitoring:* Give patients periodic thyroid function tests and initiate or appropriately adjust thyroid hormone replacement therapy when indicated.

In patients with hypopituitarism (multiple hormone deficiencies), closely monitor standard hormonal replacement therapy when somatropin therapy is administered.

Carefully monitor patients for any malignant transformation of skin lesions.

Monitor glucose levels in all patients treated with somatropin, especially in those with risk factors for diabetes mellitus, such as obesity (including obese patients with Prader-Willi syndrome), Turner syndrome, or a family history of diabetes mellitus. Closely monitor patients with preexisting type 1 or 2 diabetes mellitus or impaired glucose tolerance during somatropin therapy.

All patients with Prader-Willi syndrome treated with somatropin also should have effective weight control; monitor for signs of respiratory infection, which should be diagnosed as early as possible and treated aggressively.

Because somatropin increases growth rate, monitor patients with a history of scoliosis who are treated with somatropin for progression of scoliosis.

Drug Interactions

Somatropin Drug Interactions

Precipitant drug	Object drug[a]		Description
Estrogens, oral	Somatropin	⬇	In adult women on oral estrogen replacement, a larger somatropin dose may be required to achieve the defined treatment goal.
Glucocorticoids (ie, cortisol, cortisone, prednisone)	Somatropin	⬇	Somatropin inhibits 11β-hydroxysteroid dehydrogenase type 1 (11 βHSD-1) in adipose/hepatic tissue and may significantly impact the metabolism of cortisol and cortisone. Excessive glucocorticoid therapy may attenuate the growth-promoting effects of somatropin in children.
Somatropin	Glucocorticoids (ie, cortisol, cortisone, prednisone)		
Somatropin	CYP-450 substrates (eg, anticonvulsants, corticosteroids, cyclosporine, sex steroids)	⬇	Limited published data indicate that somatropin treatment increases CYP-450 mediated clearance in man.
Somatropin	Insulin or oral antihyperglycemic agents	⬇	Treatment with somatropin may decrease insulin sensitivity, particularly at higher doses in susceptible patients. The doses of antihyperglycemic drugs (insulin or oral agents) may require adjustment when somatropin therapy is instituted in these patients.

[a] ⬇ = object drug decreased.

Adverse Reactions

➤*Leukemia:* Leukemia has been reported in a small number of GHD patients treated with growth hormone. It is uncertain whether this increased risk is related to the pathology of GHD itself, growth hormone therapy, or other associated treatments such as radiation therapy for intracranial tumors. On the basis of current evidence, experts cannot conclude that growth hormone therapy is responsible for these occurrences. The risk to GHD, CRI, or Turner syndrome patients, if any, remains to be established.

➤*Accretropin:* As with all protein pharmaceuticals, some patients may develop antibodies to the protein. In more than 3 years of *Accretropin* therapy, no patient with the GHD or Turner syndrome developed anti-GH antibodies with binding capacities greater than 0.67 mg/L, which is below the threshold at which attenuation of growth velocity has been observed. Anti-GH antibody titers peaked by 6 to 12 months and remained stable or declined subsequently. Anti-*Escherichia coli* antibody titers increased slightly during *Accretropin* treatment. No growth attenuation was noted in any patient who developed anti-hGH or anti-*E. coli* antibodies.

GHD children – In the clinical study conducted in children with GHD, injection-site reactions (includes the following: bruising, edema, erythema, hemorrhage, pain, pruritus, rash, swelling) were the most frequent treatment-related adverse reactions reported in 50% of patients. Other treatment-related adverse reactions (as assessed by the investigators) with a frequency of 3% or more were fatigue, headache, nausea, and scoliosis. One patient with preexisting type 1 diabetes required adjustment of the insulin dose under observation.

Turner syndrome patients – In the clinical study conducted in children with Turner syndrome, the only treatment-related adverse event (as assessed by the investigators) that occurred in 3% or more of patients was injection-site reaction (includes the following: erythema, edema, pain, pruritus), which occurred in 32% of patients .

➤*Genotropin:* As with all protein drugs, a small number of patients may develop antibodies to the protein. Growth hormone antibody with binding lower than 2 mg/L has not been associated with growth attenuation. In some

SOMATROPIN — INJECTION

cases, when binding capacity is greater than 2 mg/L, interference with growth response has been observed.

In 419 children evaluated in clinical studies with *Genotropin*, 244 had been treated previously with *Genotropin* or other growth hormone preparations and 175 had received no previous growth hormone therapy. Antibodies to growth hormone (anti-hGH antibodies) were present in 6 previously treated patients at baseline. Three of the 6 became negative for anti-hGH antibodies during 6 to 12 months of treatment with *Genotropin*. Of the remaining 413 patients, 8 (1.9%) developed detectable anti-hGH antibodies during treatment with *Genotropin*; none had an antibody-binding capacity greater than 2 mg/L. There was no evidence that the growth response to *Genotropin* was affected in these antibody-positive patients.

Children with GHD – In clinical studies with *Genotropin* in pediatric GHD patients, the following adverse reactions were reported infrequently: injection-site reactions, including pain or burning associated with the injection, bleeding, fibrosis, inflammation, nodules, pigmentation, or rash; headache; hematuria; hypothyroidism; lipoatrophy; and mild hyperglycemia.

Children with Prader-Willi syndrome – In 2 clinical studies with *Genotropin* in children with Prader-Willi syndrome, the following drug-related reactions were reported: aggressiveness, arthralgia, benign intracranial hypertension, edema, hair loss, headache, and myalgia.

Children with SGA – In clinical studies of 273 children born SGA treated with *Genotropin*, the following clinically significant reactions were reported: mild transient hyperglycemia, 1 patient with benign intracranial hypertension, 2 patients with central precocious puberty, 2 patients with jaw prominence, and several patients with aggravation of preexisting scoliosis, injection-site reactions, and self-limited progression of pigmented nevi. Anti-hGH antibodies were not detected in any of the patients treated with *Genotropin*.

Children with Turner syndrome – In 2 clinical trials with *Genotropin* in children with Turner syndrome, the most frequently reported adverse reactions were joint pain, respiratory illnesses (influenza, otitis, sinusitis, tonsillitis), and urinary tract infection. The only treatment-related adverse reaction that occurred in more than 1 patient was joint pain.

Adults with GHD –

The following table displays the adverse reactions reported by 5% or more of adult GHD patients in clinical trials after various durations of treatment with *Genotropin*. Also presented are the corresponding incidence rates of these adverse reactions in placebo patients during the 6-month, double-blind portion of the clinical trials.

Genotropin Adverse Reactions in Adults With GHD (≥ 5%)

Adverse reaction	Double-blind phase		Open-label phase *Genotropin*		
	Placebo 0 to 6 mo (n = 572)	*Genotropin* 0 to 6 mo (n = 573)	6 to 12 mo (n = 504)	12 to 18 mo (n = 63)	18 to 24 mo (n = 60)
CNS					
Headache	7.7%	9.9%	6.2%	0%	0%
Paresthesia	1.9%	9.6%[a]	2.2%	3.2%	0%
Musculoskeletal					
Arthralgia	4.2%	17.3%[a]	6.9%	6.3%	3.3%
Myalgia	1.6%	4.9%[a]	2%	4.8%	6.7%
Stiffness of extremities	1.6%	7.9%[a]	2.4%	1.6%	0%
Respiratory					
Upper respiratory tract infection	14.5%	15.5%	13.1%	15.9%	13.3%
Miscellaneous					
Back pain	4.4%	2.8%	3.4%	4.8%	5%
Edema, peripheral	2.6%	10.8%[a]	3%	0%	0%
Fatigue	3.8%	5.8%	4.6%	6.3%	1.7%
Pain, extremities	5.9%	14.7%[a]	6.7%	1.6%	3.3%
Swelling, peripheral	5.1%	17.5%[a]	5.6%	0%	1.7%

[a] Increased significantly when compared with placebo, $P \leq 0.025$: Fisher's exact test (one-sided).

In expanded posttrial extension studies, diabetes mellitus developed in 12 of 3,031 (0.4%) patients during treatment with *Genotropin*. All 12 patients had predisposing factors (eg, elevated glycated hemoglobin levels or marked obesity) prior to receiving *Genotropin*. Of the 3,031 patients receiving *Genotropin*, 61 (2%) developed symptoms of carpal tunnel syndrome, which lessened after dosage reduction or treatment interruption (52) or surgery (9). Other adverse reactions that have been reported include generalized edema and hypesthesia.

➤*Humatrope*:

Children with GHD – As with all protein pharmaceuticals, a small percentage of patients may develop antibodies to the protein. During the first 6 months of *Humatrope* therapy in 314 naive patients, only 1.6% developed specific antibodies to *Humatrope* (binding capacity greater that or equal to 0.02 mg/L). None had antibody concentrations that exceeded 2 mg/L. Throughout 8 years of this same study, 2 (0.6%) patients had binding capacity greater than 2 mg/L. Neither patient demonstrated a decrease in growth velocity at or near the time of increased antibody production. It has been reported that growth attenuation from pituitary-derived growth hormone may occur when antibody concentrations are greater than 1.5 mg/L.

In addition to an evaluation of compliance with the treatment program and of thyroid status, testing for antibodies to hGH should be carried out in any patient who fails to respond to therapy.

In studies with GHD children, injection-site pain was reported infrequently. A mild and transient edema, which appeared in 2.5% of patients, was observed early during the course of treatment.

Turner syndrome patients – In a randomized, concurrent controlled trial, there was a statistically significant increase in the occurrence of otitis media (43% vs 26%), ear disorders (18% vs 5%), and surgical procedures (45% vs 27%) in patients receiving *Humatrope* compared with untreated control patients. Other adverse reactions of special interest to Turner syndrome patients were not significantly different between treatment groups. A similar increase in otitis media was observed in an 18-month, placebo-controlled trial (see following table).

***Humatrope* Treatment-Emergent Reactions of Special Interest in Turner Syndrome**

Adverse reaction	Treatment group		
	Humatrope[a] (n = 74)	Untreated[b] (n = 62)	Significance
Dermatological			
Increased nevi[c]	10.8%	3.2%	NS[d]
Metabolic			
Hyperglycemia	0%	0%	NS
Special senses			
Conjunctival edema	0%	1.6%	NS
Ear disorders	17.6%	4.8%	$P \leq 0.05$
Otitis media	43.2%	25.8%	$P \leq 0.05$
Miscellaneous			
Bone disorder	8.1%	11.3%	NS
Facial edema	1.4%	0%	NS
Hyperthyroidism	13.5%	8.1%	NS
Lymphedema	0%	0%	NS
Nonspecific edema	2.7%	1.6%	NS
Peripheral edema	6.8%	1.6%	NS
Surgical procedure	44.6%	27.4%	$P \leq 0.05$

[a] Dose = 0.3 mg/kg/wk.
[b] Open label study.
[c] Includes any nevi coded to the following preferred terms: melanosis, skin hypertrophy, or skin benign neoplasm.
[d] NS = not significant.

Patients with idiopathic short stature – In the placebo-controlled study, the adverse reactions associated with *Humatrope* therapy were similar to those observed in other pediatric populations treated with *Humatrope* (see the following table). Mean serum glucose level did not change during *Humatrope* treatment. Mean fasting serum insulin levels increased 10% in the *Humatrope* treatment group at the end of treatment relative to baseline values but remained within the normal reference range. For the same duration of treatment the mean fasting serum insulin levels decreased 2% in the placebo group. The incidence of above-range values for glucose, insulin, and glycosylated hemoglobin were similar in the growth hormone– and placebo-treated groups. No patient developed diabetes mellitus. Consistent with the known mechanism of growth hormone action, *Humatrope*-treated patients had greater mean increases, relative to baseline, in serum IGF-1 than placebo-treated patients at each study observation. However, there was no significant difference between the *Humatrope* and placebo treatment groups in the proportion of patients who had at least 1 serum IGF-1 concentration more than 2 SD above the age- and gender-appropriate mean (*Humatrope*, 9 of 35 patients [26%]; placebo, 7 of 28 patients [25%]).

***Humatrope* Adverse Reactions in Patients With Idiopathic Short Stature**

Adverse reaction	Treatment group	
	Humatrope	Placebo
Total number of patients	37	31
Cardiovascular		
Hypertension	2.7%	0%
GU		
Gynecomastia	5.4%	3.2%
Musculoskeletal		
Aching joints	0%	3.2%
Arthralgia	10.8%	3.2%
Arthrosis	10.8%	6.5%
Hip pain	2.7%	0%
Myalgia	24.3%	12.9%
Scoliosis	18.9%	12.9%

SOMATROPIN — INJECTION

Humatrope Adverse Reactions in Patients With Idiopathic Short Stature		
	Treatment group	
Adverse reaction	*Humatrope*	Placebo
Special senses		
Otitis media	16.2%	6.5%
Miscellaneous		
Hyperlipidemia	8.1%	3.2%
Hypothyroidism	0%	6.5%

The adverse reactions observed in the dose-response study (239 patients treated for 2 years) did not indicate a pattern suggestive of a growth hormone dose effect. Among *Humatrope* dose groups, mean fasting blood glucose, mean glycosylated hemoglobin, and the incidence of elevated fasting blood glucose concentrations were similar. One patient developed abnormalities of carbohydrate metabolism (glucose intolerance and high serum glycosylated hemoglobin) on treatment.

Patients with SHOX deficiency – Clinically significant adverse reactions (adverse reactions previously observed in association with growth hormone treatment in general) were assessed prospectively during the 2-year, randomized, open-label study; those observed are presented in the following table. In both treatment groups, the mean fasting plasma glucose concentration at the end of the first year was similar to the baseline value and remained in the normal range. No patient developed diabetes mellitus or had an above normal value for fasting plasma glucose at the end of 1 year of treatment. During the 2-year study period, the proportion of patients who had at least 1 IGF-1 concentration greater than 2 SD above the age- and gender-appropriate mean was 10 of 27 (37%) for the *Humatrope*-treated group versus 0 of 24 (0%) patients for the untreated group. The proportion of patients who had at least 1 IGFBP-3 concentration greater than 2 SD above the age and gender appropriate mean was 16 of 27 (59.3%) for the *Humatrope*-treated group versus 7 of 24 (29.2%) for the untreated group.

Humatrope Adverse Reactions[a,b] in Patients With SHOX Deficiency		
	Treatment group	
Adverse reactions	Untreated (n = 25)	*Humatrope* (n = 27)
Patients with ≥ 1 event	2	5
Dermatologic		
Excessive number of cutaneous nevi	0%	7.4%
GU		
Gynecomastia[c]	0%	8.3%
Musculoskeletal		
Arthralgia	8%	11.1%
Scoliosis	0%	3.7%

[a] All reactions were nonserious.
[b] Reactions are included only if reported for a greater number of *Humatrope*-treated than untreated patients.
[c] Percentage calculated for male patients only (1 of 12).

Adult patients – In clinical studies in which high doses of *Humatrope* were administered to healthy adult volunteers, the following reactions occurred infrequently: glucosuria, headache, localized muscle pain, mild hyperglycemia, and weakness.

In the first 6 months of controlled, blinded trials during which patients received *Humatrope* or placebo, adult-onset GHD adults who received *Humatrope* experienced a statistically significant increase in edema (*Humatrope* 17.3% vs placebo 4.4%, $P = 0.043$) and peripheral edema (11.5% vs 0%, respectively, $P = 0.017$). In patients with adult-onset GHD, edema, muscle pain, joint disorder, and joint pain were reported early in therapy and tended to be transient or responsive to dosage titration.

Two of 113 adult-onset patients developed carpal tunnel syndrome after beginning maintenance therapy without a low dose (0.00625 mg/kg/day) lead-in phase. Symptoms abated in these patients after dosage reduction.

All treatment-emergent adverse reactions with greater than or equal to 5% overall incidence during 12 or 18 months of replacement therapy with *Humatrope* are shown in the following table (adult-onset patients and childhood-onset patients).

Adult patients treated with *Humatrope* who had been diagnosed with GHD in childhood reported adverse reactions less frequently than those with adult-onset GHD.

Humatrope Adverse Reactions (≥ 5%) in Adult-Onset GHD Patients		
Adverse reaction	18 months exposure (placebo [6 months]/ *Humatrope* [12 months]) (n = 46)	18 months *Humatrope* exposure (n = 52)
Cardiovascular		
Hypertension	4.3%	7.7%
CNS		
Headache	10.9%	7.7%
Paresthesia	13%	17.3%
Dermatologic		
Acne	0%	5.8%
Musculoskeletal		
Arthralgia	15.2%	17.3%
Joint disorder	2.2%	5.8%
Myalgia	13%	13.5%
Miscellaneous		
Back pain	10.9%	9.6%
Edema[a]	15.2%	21.2%
Flu syndrome	6.5%	3.9%
Pain	13%	13.5%
Peripheral edema[b]	17.4%	11.5%
Rhinitis	10.9%	13.5%
Surgical procedure	2.2%	5.8%

[a] $P = 0.04$ as compared with placebo (6 months).
[b] $P = 0.02$ as compared with placebo (6 months).

Humatrope Adverse Reactions (≥ 5%) in Childhood-Onset GHD Patients		
Adverse reaction	18 months exposure (placebo [6 months]/ *Humatrope* [12 months]) (n = 35)	18 months *Humatrope* exposure (n = 32)
CNS		
Asthenia	2.9%	6.3%
Headache	11.4%	9.4%
Hypesthesia	0%	6.3%
GI		
Gastritis	5.7%	0%
Hepatic		
ALT increased	5.7%	6.3%
AST increased[a]	5.7%	12.5%
Musculoskeletal		
Myalgia	5.7%	6.3%
Respiratory		
Cough increased	0%	6.3%
Pharyngitis	14.3%	3.1%
Respiratory tract disorder	5.7%	3.1%
Rhinitis	5.7%	6.3%
Miscellaneous		
Edema	8.6%	6.3%
Flu syndrome	22.9%	15.6%
Pain	8.6%	6.3%

[a] $P = 0.03$ as compared with placebo (6 months).

Other adverse drug reactions that have been reported in growth hormone-treated patients include the following:

Dermatologic – Increased growth of preexisting nevi (rare). Carefully monitor patients for malignant transformation.

Musculoskeletal – Carpal tunnel syndrome (rare).

Miscellaneous – Infrequent, mild, and transient peripheral or generalized edema; gynecomastia; pancreatitis (rare).

➤*Norditropin*:

Most serious and/or most frequently observed adverse reactions – This list presents the most serious (a) and/or most frequently observed (b) adverse reactions during treatment with somatropin:

- (a) sudden death in children with Prader-Willi syndrome with risk factors including severe obesity, history of upper airway obstruction or sleep apnea, and unidentified respiratory infection
- (a) intracranial tumors, in particular meningiomas, in teenagers/young adults treated with radiation to the head as children for a first neoplasm and somatropin
- (a,b) glucose intolerance including impaired glucose tolerance/impaired fasting glucose and overt diabetes mellitus
- (a) intracranial hypertension
- (a) significant diabetic retinopathy
- (a) slipped capital femoral epiphysis in children

SOMATROPIN — INJECTION

- (a) progression of preexisting scoliosis in children
- (b) fluid retention manifested by edema, arthralgia, myalgia, nerve compression syndromes including carpal tunnel syndrome/paresthesias
- (b) unmasking of latent central hypothyroidism
- (b) injection-site reactions/rashes and lipoatrophy (as well as rare generalized hypersensitivity reactions).

GHD children – As with all protein drugs, a small percentage of patients may develop antibodies to the protein. Growth hormone antibody with binding capacity lower than 2 mg/L has not been associated with growth attenuation. In some cases, when binding capacity is greater than 2 mg/L, interference with growth response has been observed. In clinical trials, patients receiving *Norditropin* for up to 12 months have been tested for induction of antibodies and 0 of 358 patients developed antibodies with binding capacities more than 2 mg/L. Among these patients, 165 had previously been treated with other preparations of growth hormone and 193 were previously untreated naive patients.

Children with Noonan syndrome – *Norditropin* was studied in a 2-year prospective, randomized, parallel-dose group trial in 21 children 3 to 14 years of age with Noonan syndrome. Doses were 0.033 and 0.066 mg/kg/day. After the initial 2-year randomized trial, children continued *Norditropin* treatment until final height was achieved; randomized dose groups were not maintained. Final height and adverse reaction data were later collected retrospectively from 18 children; total follow-up was 11 years. An additional 6 children were not randomized but followed the protocol and are included in this assessment of adverse reactions.

Based on the mean dose per treatment group, no significant difference in the incidence of adverse reactions was seen between the 2 groups. The most frequent adverse reactions were the common infections of childhood, including upper respiratory tract infection, gastroenteritis, ear infection, and influenza. Cardiac disorder was the system organ class with the second most adverse reactions reported. However, congenital heart disease is an inherent component of Noonan syndrome, and there was no evidence of somatropin-induced ventricular hypertrophy or exacerbation of preexisting ventricular hypertrophy (as judged by echocardiography) during this study. Children who had baseline cardiac disease judged to be significant enough to potentially affect growth were excluded from the study; therefore, the safety of *Norditropin* in children with Noonan syndrome and significant cardiac disease is not known. Among children who received 0.033 mg/kg/day, there was 1 adverse reaction of scoliosis; among children who received 0.066 mg/kg/day, there were 4 adverse reactions of scoliosis. Mean serum IGF-1 SDS levels did not exceed +1 in response to somatropin treatment. The mean serum IGF-1 level was low at baseline and normalized during treatment.

Children with Turner syndrome – In 2 clinical studies in which children with Turner syndrome were treated with various doses of *Norditropin*until final height, the most frequently reported adverse reactions were common childhood diseases including influenza-like illness, otitis media, upper respiratory tract infection, otitis externa, gastroenteritis, and eczema. Otitis media adverse reactions in study 1 were most frequent in the highest dose groups (86.4% in the 0.045 to 0.067 to 0.089 mg/kg/day group vs 78.3% in the 0.045 to 0.067 mg/kg/day group vs 69.6% in the 0.045 mg/kg/day group), suggesting a possible dose-response relationship. Of note, approximately 40% to 50% of these otitis media adverse reactions were designated as serious. No patients in either study developed clearcut overt diabetes mellitus; however, in study 1, impaired fasting glucose at month 48 was more frequent in patients in the 0.045 to 0.067 mg/kg/day group (n = 4 of 18) compared with the 0.045 mg/kg/day group (n = 1 of 20). Transient episodes of fasting blood sugars between 100 and 126 mg/dL, and, on occasion, exceeding 126 mg/dL, also occurred more often with larger doses of *Norditropin* in both studies. Three patients withdrew from the 2 high-dose groups in study 1 because of concern about excessive growth of hands or feet. In addition, in study 1, exacerbation of preexisting scoliosis was designated a serious adverse reaction in 2 patients in the 0.045 mg/kg/day group.

GHD adults – Adverse reactions with an incidence of at least 5% occurring in patients with adult-onset GHD during the 6-month placebo-controlled portion of the largest of the 6 adult GHD *Norditropin* trials are presented in the following table. Peripheral edema, other types of edema, arthralgia, myalgia, and paresthesia were common in the *Norditropin*-treated patients and reported much more frequently than in the placebo group. These types of adverse reactions are thought to be related to the fluid accumulating effects of somatropin. In general, these adverse reactions were mild and transient in nature. During the placebo-controlled portion of this study, approximately 5% of patients without preexisting diabetes mellitus treated with *Norditropin* were diagnosed with overt type 2 diabetes mellitus compared with none in the placebo group. Antigrowth hormone antibodies were not detected.

Of note, the doses of *Norditropin* employed during this study (completed in the mid-1990s) were substantially larger than those currently recommended by the Growth Hormone Research Society, and more than likely, resulted in a greater than expected incidence of fluid retention– and glucose intolerance–related adverse reactions. A similar incidence and pattern of adverse reactions were observed during the other 3 placebo-controlled, adult-onset GHD trials and during the 2 placebo-controlled childhood-onset GHD trials.

Norditropin Adverse Reactions (≥ 5%) in Adult-Onset GHD Patients

Adverse reaction	*Norditropin* (n = 53)	Placebo (n = 52)
Cardiovascular		
Hypertension	8%	2%
CNS		
Headache	9%	6%
Paresthesia	11%	6%
GI		
Gastroenteritis	8%	8%
Musculoskeletal		
Arthralgia	19%	15%
Myalgia	15%	8%
Skeletal pain	11%	2%
Respiratory		
Bronchitis	9%	0%
Laryngitis	6%	6%
Miscellaneous		
Edema	25%	0%
Flu-like symptoms	8%	4%
Glucose tolerance abnormal	6%	2%
Increased sweating	8%	2%
Infection (nonviral)	13%	8%
Leg edema	15%	4%
Other nonclassifiable disorders (excludes accidental injury)	8%	6%
Peripheral edema	42%	8%

The adverse reaction pattern observed during the open-label phase of the study was similar to the one presented above.

Postmarketing – The adverse reactions reported during postmarketing surveillance do not differ from those listed/discussed in the previous children and adult sections.

The following additional adverse reactions have been observed during the appropriate use of somatropin: headaches (children and adults), gynecomastia (children), and pancreatitis (children).

➤*Nutropin* and *Nutropin AQ*: As with all protein pharmaceuticals, a small percentage of patients may develop antibodies to the protein. Growth hormone antibody–binding capacities below 2 mg/L have not been associated with growth attenuation. In some cases when binding capacity exceeds 2 mg/L, growth attenuation has been observed. In clinical studies of children that were treated with *Nutropin* for the first time, 0 of 107 GHD patients, 0 of 125 CRI patients, 0 of 112 Turner syndrome, and 0 of 117 idiopathic short stature patients screened for antibody production developed antibodies with binding capacities greater than or equal to 2 mg/L at 6 months. In a clinical study of patients who were treated with *Nutropin AQ* for the first time, 0 of 38 GHD patients screened for antibody production for up to 15 months developed antibodies with binding capacities of 2 mg/L or more.

Additional short-term immunologic and renal function studies were carried out in a group of patients with CRI after approximately 1 year of treatment to detect other potential adverse reactions of antibodies to growth hormone. Testing included measurements of C1q, C3, C4, rheumatoid factor, creatinine, creatinine clearance, and blood urea nitrogen. No adverse reactions of growth hormone antibodies were noted.

In addition to an evaluation of compliance with the prescribed treatment program and thyroid status, test for antibodies to growth hormone in any patient who fails to respond to therapy.

In a postmarketing surveillance study, the National Cooperation Growth Study, the pattern of adverse reactions in more than 8,000 patients with idiopathic short stature was consistent with the known safety profile of growth hormone, and no new safety signals attribute to growth hormone were identified. The frequency of protocol-defined targeted adverse reactions is described in the following table.

Nutropin and _Nutropin AQ_ Adverse Reactions in Patients With Idiopathic Short Stature (Postmarketing Study)

Adverse reactions	N = 8,018
Any adverse reaction/targeted adverse reactions	1.3%
Cardiovascular	
Intracranial hypertension	0%
CNS	
CNS tumor	0%
Endocrine	
Diabetes mellitus	0.1%
GU	
Gynecomastia	0.1%

SOMATROPIN — INJECTION

Nutropin and *Nutropin AQ* Adverse Reactions in Patients With Idiopathic Short Stature (Postmarketing Study)	
Adverse reactions	N = 8,018
Musculoskeletal	
Abnormal bone or other growth	0%
Arthralgia or arthritis	0.1%
Carpal tunnel syndrome	0%
Fracture	0%
New-onset or progression of scoliosis	0.2%
New or recurrent slipped capital femoral epiphyses or avascular necrosis[a]	0%
Miscellaneous	
Any new-onset or recurring tumor (benign)	0.1%
Cancer, neoplasm (new-onset or recurrence)	0%
Edema	0.1%
Injection-site reaction	0.3%

[a] Data obtained with several rhGH products (*Nutropin* and *Nutropin AQ*)

Injection-site discomfort has been reported. This is more commonly observed in children switched from another growth hormone product to *Nutropin AQ*. Experience with *Nutropin AQ* in adults is limited.

In studies in patients treated with *Nutropin*, injection-site pain was reported infrequently.

Other adverse drug reactions that have been reported in growth hormone–treated patients include the following:

Dermatologic – Increased growth of preexisting nevi (rare); monitor patients for malignant transformation.

Musculoskeletal – Arthralgias; carpal tunnel syndrome. In GHD adults, arthralgias and other joint disorders were reported in 27% of growth hormone–treated patients and 15% of placebo-treated patients.

Miscellaneous – Mild, transient peripheral edema; gynecomastia; pancreatitis (rare). In GHD adults, edema or peripheral edema was reported in 41% of growth hormone–treated patients and 25% of placebo-treated patients.

➤*Omnitrope*:

Most serious and/or most frequently observed adverse reactions – This list presents the most serious (a) and/or most frequently observed (b) adverse reactions during treatment with somatropin:

- (a) sudden death in children with Prader-Willi syndrome with risk factors including severe obesity, history of upper airway obstruction or sleep apnea, and unidentified respiratory infection
- (a) intracranial tumors, in particular meningiomas, in teenagers/young adults treated with radiation to the head as children for a first neoplasm and somatropin
- (a, b) glucose intolerance including impaired glucose tolerance/impaired fasting glucose and overt diabetes mellitus
- (a) intracranial hypertension
- (a) significant diabetic retinopathy
- (a) slipped capital femoral epiphysis in children
- (a) progression of preexisting scoliosis in children
- (b) fluid retention manifested by edema, arthralgia, myalgia, nerve compression syndromes including carpal tunnel syndrome/paresthesias
- (b) unmasking of latent central hypothyroidism
- (b) injection-site reactions/rashes and lipoatrophy (as well as rare generalized hypersensitivity reactions).

GHD children – As with all protein drugs, a small number of patients may develop antibodies to the protein. Growth hormone antibody with binding capacity less than 2 mg/L has not been associated with growth attenuation. In some cases when binding capacity is more than 2 mg/L, interference with growth response has been observed.

The following reactions were observed during clinical studies with *Omnitrope* cartridge conducted in children with GHD.

Omnitrope Cartridge Adverse Reactions in Children With GHD (≥ 5%)	
Adverse reaction	N = 86
Elevated glycosylated hemoglobin	14%
Eosinophilia	12%
Hematoma	9%

The following reactions were observed during the *Omnitrope* injection clinical studies conducted in children with GHD.

Omnitrope Injection Adverse Reactions in Children With GHD (≥ 5%)	
Adverse reaction	N = 44
CNS	
Headache	7%
Endocrine	
Elevated glycosylated hemoglobin	14%
Hematologic	
Eosinophilia	11%
Hematoma	9%
Metabolic	
Hypertriglyceridemia	5%
Miscellaneous	
Hypothyroidism	16%
Leg pain	5%

GHD adults – In clinical trials with somatropin in GHD adults, the majority of the adverse reactions consisted of mild to moderate symptoms of fluid retention, including peripheral swelling, arthralgia, pain and stiffness of the extremities, peripheral edema, myalgia, paresthesia, and hypesthesia. These reactions were reported early during therapy and tended to be transient and/or responsive to dosage reduction.

Postmarketing – Headaches (children and adults), gynecomastia (children), pancreatitis (children).

➤*Saizen*:

GHD children – As with all protein pharmaceuticals, a small percentage of patients may develop antibodies to the protein. Antigrowth hormone antibody capacities less than 2 mg/L have not been associated with growth attenuation. In some cases when binding capacity exceeds 2 mg/L, growth attenuation has been described. In clinical studies with *Saizen* involving 280 patients (204 naive and 76 transfer patients), 1 patient at 6 months of therapy developed antigrowth hormone antibodies with binding capacities greater than 2 mg/L. Despite the high-binding capacity, these antibodies were not growth attenuating. The patient was subsequently shown to have an hGH-N gene defect. Thus, conduct genetic analysis in any patient in whom antigrowth hormone antibodies with high-binding capacities occur. No antibodies against proteins of the host cells were detected in the sera of patients treated up to 5 years. Test any patient with well-documented GHD who fails to respond to therapy for antibodies to hGH and for thyroid status.

In clinical studies in which *Saizen* was administered to GHD children, the following reactions were infrequently seen: local reactions at the injection site (eg, numbness, pain, redness, swelling), hypoglycemia, hypothyroidism, seizures, exacerbation of preexisting psoriasis, and disturbances in fluid balance.

GHD adults – During the 6-month placebo-controlled study, adverse reactions were reported in 56 (93.3%) patients in the somatropin-treated group and 42 (76.4%) patients in the placebo-treated group. Adverse reactions with an incidence of 5% or more in *Saizen*-treated patients, which were more frequent in *Saizen*-treated patients compared with placebo-treated patients, are listed in the following table. Arthralgia, myalgia, peripheral edema, other types of edema, carpal tunnel syndrome, paraesthesia, and hypesthesia were common in the somatropin-treated patients and reported more frequently than in the placebo group. These types of adverse reactions are thought to be related to the fluid accumulating effects of somatropin. During the placebo-controlled portion of the study, approximately 10% of patients without preexisting diabetes mellitus or impaired glucose tolerance treated with somatropin manifested mild but persistent abnormalities of glucose tolerance, compared with none in the placebo group. During the open-label phase of the study, approximately 10% of patients treated with somatropin required a small upward adjustment of thyroid hormone replacement therapy for preexisting central hypothyroidism; 1 patient was newly diagnosed with central hypothyroidism. In addition, during the open-label phase of the study, when all patients were being treated with somatropin, 2 patients with preexisting central hypoadrenalism required upward titration of hydrocortisone maintenance therapy that was considered to be suboptimal (unrelated to intercurrent stress, surgery, or disease), and 1 patient was diagnosed de novo with central adrenal insufficiency after 6 months of somatropin treatment. Antigrowth hormone antibodies were not detected.

Saizen Adverse Reactions (≥ 5%)		
Adverse reactions	*Saizen*-treated (n = 60)	Placebo (n = 55)
CNS		
Depression	5%	0%
Dizziness	6.7%	5.5%
Headache	18.3%	14.5%
Hypesthesia	6.7%	0%
Insomnia	5%	0%
Paresthesia	6.7%	1.8%
GI		
Nausea	5%	3.6%
Musculoskeletal		
Arthralgia	23.3%	12.7%
Carpal tunnel syndrome	5%	1.8%
Myalgia	8.3%	3.6%
Skeletal pain	5%	1.8%

SOMATROPIN — INJECTION

Saizen Adverse Reactions (≥ 5%)		
Adverse reactions	*Saizen*-treated (n = 60)	Placebo (n = 55)
Respiratory		
Rhinitis	8.3%	3.6%
Upper respiratory tract infection	6.7%	3.6%
Miscellaneous		
Back pain	10%	9.1%
Chest pain	5%	0%
Edema dependent	5%	3.6%
Edema generalized	5%	0%
Edema peripheral	15%	3.7%
Hypothyroidism	5%	0%
Influenza-like symptoms	15%	5.5%

The adverse reaction pattern during the open-label phase of the study was similar to the one previously presented.

➤*Serostim*: In the 12-week, placebo-controlled clinical trial, 2,510 patients were treated with *Serostim*. The most common adverse reactions judged to be associated with *Serostim* were musculoskeletal discomfort and increased tissue turgor (swelling, particularly of the hands or feet), and were more frequently observed when *Serostim* 0.1 mg/kg was administered on a daily basis (see the following table). These symptoms were generally rated by investigators as mild to moderate in severity and often subsided with continued treatment or dose reduction. Approximately 23% of patients receiving *Serostim* 0.1 mg/kg/day and 11% of patients receiving 0.1 mg/kg every other day required dose reductions. Discontinuations as a result of adverse reactions occurred in 10.3% of patients receiving *Serostim* 0.1 mg/kg/day and 6.6% of patients receiving 0.1 mg/kg every other day. The most common reasons for dose reduction and/or drug discontinuation were arthralgia, myalgia, edema, carpal tunnel syndrome, elevated glucose levels, and elevated triglyceride levels.

Clinical adverse reactions which occurred during the first 12 weeks of study in at least 5% of the patients in any 1 of the 3 treatment groups are listed in the following table by treatment group, without regard to causality assessment.

Serostim Adverse Reactions			
Adverse reaction	Placebo (n = 247)	*Serostim* 0.1 mg/kg every other day (n = 257)	*Serostim* 0.1 mg/kg/day (n = 253)
CNS			
Headache	9.3%	10.1%	12.6%
Hypesthesia	2.4%	1.6%	5.1%
Insomnia	6.1%	3.9%	5.9%
Paresthesia	4.5%	7.4%	7.9%
GI			
Diarrhea	10.1%	10.1%	5.5%
Nausea	4.9%	5.4%	9.1%
GU			
Gynecomastia	0.4%	3.5%	5.5%
Musculoskeletal			
Arthralgia	11.3%	24.5%	36.4%
Arthrosis	3.6%	7.8%	10.7%
Myalgia	11.7%	17.9%	30.4%
Respiratory			
Bronchitis	5.3%	2.3%	4.7%
Rhinitis	6.5%	5.1%	4%
Upper respiratory tract infection	5.7%	4.3%	3.6%
Miscellaneous			
Edema generalized	1.2%	1.2%	5.9%
Edema peripheral	2.8%	11.3%	26.1%
Fatigue	4.5%	3.5%	5.1%

Adverse reactions that occurred in 1% to less than 5% of study participants receiving *Serostim* during the 12-week, placebo-controlled clinical trial 2 are listed as follows by body system. The list of adverse reactions has been compiled regardless of causal relationship to *Serostim*.

Cardiovascular – Hypertension, tachycardia.

CNS – Anxiety, depression, dizziness, hypertonia, peripheral neuropathy, somnolence.

Dermatologic – Folliculitis, maculopapular rash, rash, verruca.

GI – Abdominal pain, anorexia, constipation, dyspepsia, gastroenteritis, vomiting.

GU – Renal calculus, urinary tract infection.

Hematologic/Lymphatic – Lymphadenopathy.

Metabolic/Nutritional – Hyperglycemia, hypertriglyceridemia.

Musculoskeletal – Arthropathy, back pain, musculoskeletal pain.

Ophthalmic – Conjunctivitis.

Respiratory – Coughing, pharyngitis, pneumonia, sinusitis.

Miscellaneous – Accident (not otherwise specified), asthenia, carpal tunnel syndrome, chest pain, dependent edema, edema/face edema, fever, flu-like symptoms, herpes simplex, leg pain, male breast neoplasm, moniliasis, night sweats, pain, periorbital edema, rigors, viral infection. During the 12-week, placebo-controlled portion of clinical trial 2, the incidence of hyperglycemia reported as an adverse reaction was 3.6% for the placebo group, 1.9% for the 0.1 mg/kg every other day group, and 3.2% for the 0.1 mg/kg/day group. One case of diabetes mellitus was noted in the 0.1 mg/kg/day group during the first 12 weeks of therapy. In addition, during the extension phase of clinical trial 2, two patients converted from placebo to full-dose *Serostim* and 1 patient converted from placebo to half-dose *Serostim* were discontinued because of the development of diabetes mellitus.

Postmarketing – During postmarketing surveillance, cases of new-onset impaired glucose intolerance, new-onset type 2 diabetes mellitus, and exacerbation of preexisting diabetes mellitus have been reported in patients receiving *Serostim*. Some patients developed diabetic ketoacidosis and diabetic coma. In some patients, these conditions improved when *Serostim* was discontinued, while in others the glucose intolerance persisted. Some patients necessitated initiation or adjustment of antidiabetic treatment while on *Serostim*.

➤*Tev-Tropin*: Using a double-antibody immunoassay, no antibodies to growth hormone could be detected in a group of 164 naive and previously treated clinical trial patients after treatment with *Tev-Tropin* for up to 40 months. However, using the less specific polyethylene glycol precipitation immunoassay, 27 of the 164 patient group were tested after treatment with *Tev-Tropin* for 4 to 6 months and antibodies to growth hormone were detected in 2 (7.4%) patients. The binding capacity of the antibodies from the 2 antibody positive patients was not determined.

None of the patients with antigrowth hormone antibodies in the clinical studies experienced decreased linear growth response to *Tev-Tropin* or any other associated adverse reaction. Growth hormone antibody binding capacities below 2 mg/L have not been associated with growth attenuation. In some cases, when binding capacity exceeds 2 mg/L, growth attenuation has been observed.

In studies of GHD children, headaches occurred infrequently. Injection-site reactions (eg, bruise, pain) occurred in 8 of the 164 treated patients.

➤*Zorbtive*: The following table summarizes the number of subjects by system-organ class who experienced an adverse reaction during the 4-week treatment period of the phase 3 SBS study. To be listed in the table, an adverse reaction must have occurred in more than 10% of subjects in any treatment group.

Zorbtive Adverse Reactions During 4-Week Treatment Period[a]			
Adverse reaction	SOD [GLN] (n = 9)	rhGH + SOD (n = 16)	rhGH + SOD[GLN] (n = 16)
Total number of subjects with at least 1 adverse reaction	89%	100%	100%
CNS			
Depression	22%	0%	0%
Dizziness	0%	6%	13%
Headache	11%	6%	6%
Hypesthesia	11%	6%	6%
Psychiatric disorders	22%	6%	0%
Dermatologic			
Nail disorder	11%	0%	0%
Pruritus	11%	0%	6%
Rash	0%	6%	13%
Sweating increased	0%	13%	0%
GI			
Abdominal pain	11%	25%	13%
Flatulence	22%	25%	25%
Hemorrhoids	11%	6%	0%
Mouth dry	11%	6%	0%
Nausea	0%	13%	31%
Tenesmus	33%	6%	19%
Vomiting	11%	19%	19%

SOMATROPIN — INJECTION

Zorbtive Adverse Reactions During 4-Week Treatment Period[a]			
Adverse reaction	SOD [GLN] (n = 9)	rhGH + SOD (n = 16)	rhGH + SOD[GLN] (n = 16)
Total number of subjects with at least 1 adverse reaction	89%	100%	100%
GU			
Breast pain (female)	11%	6%	0%
GU, female	11%	13%	0%
Pyelonephritis	11%	0%	0%
Local			
Injection-site pain	0%	31%	0%
Injection-site reaction	11%	19%	25%
Metabolic/Nutritional			
Dehydration	11%	19%	0%
Thirst	11%	0%	0%
Musculoskeletal			
Arthralgia	0%	44%	31%
Myalgia	11%	13%	0%
Respiratory			
Rhinitis	11%	0%	19%
Special senses			
Ear or hearing symptoms	0%	0%	13%
Miscellaneous			
Abdomen enlarged	11%	0%	0%
Allergic reaction	11%	0%	0%
Back pain	11%	6%	0%
Chest pain	0%	19%	0%
Edema, facial	0%	50%	44%
Edema, generalized	0%	13%	0%
Edema, peripheral	11%	69%	81%
Fever	22%	0%	6%
Flu-like disorder	11%	0%	6%
Infection	33%	0%	6%
Infection bacterial	11%	19%	0%
Infection viral	0%	6%	13%
Malaise	0%	13%	0%
Moniliasis	0%	13%	0%
Pain	11%	19%	6%
Resistance mechanism disorders	44%	38%	19%
Rigors (chills)	11%	0%	0%

[a] SOD[GLN] = specialized oral diet supplemented with glutamine; rhGH + SOD = hGH plus specialized oral diet; rhGH + SOD[GLN] = hGH plus specialized oral diet supplemented with glutamine.

The following table summarizes the number of subjects by system-organ class who experienced an adverse reaction during the 12-week follow-up period of the phase 3 SBS study. To be listed in the table, an adverse reaction must have occurred in more than 10% of subjects in any treatment group.

Zorbtive Adverse Reactions: 12-Week Follow-Up Period			
Adverse reactions	SOD[GLN] (n = 9)	rhGH + SOD (n = 15)	rhGH + SOD[GLN] (n = 16)
Total number of subjects with at least 1 adverse reaction	78%	80%	81%
Cardiovascular			
Vascular disorder	11%	0%	0%
CNS			
Depression	11%	0%	0%
Insomnia	11%	0%	0%
Dermatologic			
Application-site disorders	11%	0%	0%
Injection-site reaction	11%	0%	0%
Rash	11%	7%	0%
GI			
Abdominal pain	0%	20%	6%
Constipation	11%	0%	0%
Crohn disease aggravated	11%	0%	0%
Gastric ulcer	11%	0%	0%
GI fistula	11%	0%	0%
Nausea	22%	20%	0%
Pancreatitis	11%	0%	6%
Tenesmus	11%	0%	19%
Vomiting	0%	13%	19%
GU			
Pyelonephritis	11%	0%	0%
Renal calculus	11%	0%	0%
Vaginal fungal infection	11%	0%	0%
Musculoskeletal			
Arthralgia	0%	13%	13%
Respiratory			
Laryngitis	11%	0%	0%
Pharyngitis	11%	0%	0%
Rhinitis	0%	7%	19%
Miscellaneous			
Fatigue	0%	13%	0%
Fever	11%	13%	6%
Hepatic function impaired	11%	0%	0%
Infection	11%	7%	13%
Infection, bacterial	33%	0%	13%
Infection, viral	11%	20%	6%
Resistance mechanism disorders	56%	40%	31%
Sepsis	0%	20%	6%

Adverse reactions that occurred in 1% to less than 10% of study participants receiving *Zorbtive* in the placebo-controlled clinical efficacy trial are listed by body system. The list of adverse reactions has been compiled regardless of causal relationship to *Zorbtive*.

Cardiovascular – Tachycardia, vasodilation.

CNS – Insomnia, paresthesia, phantom pain, visual field defect.

Dermatologic – Alopecia, bullous eruption, increased sweating, skin disorder.

GI – Melena, mouth disorder, rectal hemorrhage, steatorrhea.

GU – Abnormal urine, dysuria, urinary tract infection.
Female: Breast enlargement, vaginal fungal infection.

Hematologic – Prothrombin decrease, purpura.

Local – Inflammation at injection sites, reaction pain.

Metabolic/Nutritional – Hypomagnesemia.

Musculoskeletal – Arthritis, arthropathy, bursitis, cramps.

Respiratory – Bronchospasm, dyspnea, pharyngitis, respiratory tract disorder, respiratory tract infection.

Miscellaneous – Edema, fungal infection, periorbital edema.

The safety profile of patients receiving *Zorbtive* with glutamine was similar to the safety profile of patients receiving *Zorbtive* without glutamine. During the baseline period, 88% of patients receiving *Zorbtive* with glutamine, 88% of patients receiving *Zorbtive* without glutamine, and 78% of patients receiving placebo with glutamine reported baseline signs and symptoms. During the treatment period, 100% of patients receiving *Zorbtive* with and without glutamine reported at least 1 adverse reaction; however, 89% of patients receiving placebo with glutamine reported at least 1 adverse reaction. During the follow-up period, 81% of patients receiving *Zorbtive* with glutamine, 80% of patients receiving *Zorbtive* without glutamine, and 78% of patients receiving placebo with glutamine experienced at least 1 adverse reaction. Comparison of the number of serious adverse reactions before and during treatment demonstrates that this subject population experiences numerous baseline signs and symptoms and adverse reactions caused by their underlying conditions and parenteral nutrition complications. Four (25%) subjects receiving *Zorbtive* without glutamine and 1 (11%) subject in receiving placebo with glutamine experienced at least 1 serious adverse reaction during the treatment period (*Zorbtive* without glutamine: chest pain, fungal infection, pharyngitis, purpura; placebo with glutamine: hemorrhoids). None of the subjects receiving *Zorbtive* with glutamine experienced serious adverse

SOMATROPIN — INJECTION

reactions during the treatment period. During the follow-up period, 3 (19%) subjects receiving *Zorbtive* with glutamine, 5 (33%) subjects receiving *Zorbtive* without glutamine, and 3 (33%) subjects receiving placebo with glutamine experienced at least 1 serious adverse reaction. There were no deaths in this study.

Overdosage

➤*Symptoms:* The recommended dosage of any somatropin (rDNA origin) formulation should not be exceeded. Acute overdosage could lead to fluid retention. Additionally, acute overdosage could initially lead to hypoglycemia and subsequently to hyperglycemia. Glucose intolerance can occur with overdosage. Long-term overdosage could result in signs and symptoms of gigantism and/or acromegaly, consistent with the known effects of excess growth hormone.

Patient Information

Inform patients being treated with growth hormone or their parents of the potential benefits and risks associated with treatment. Provide instructions on appropriate use, including a review of the contents of the patient information insert. This information is intended to aid in the safe and effective administration of the medication. It is not a disclosure of all possible adverse or intended effects.

If home use is prescribed, thoroughly instruct patients or parents in the importance of proper needle disposal. A puncture-resistant container should be used for the disposal of used needles or syringes (consistent with applicable state requirements). Needles and syringes must not be reused.

Inform patients that allergic reactions are possible and to seek prompt medical attention if an allergic reaction occurs.

Instruct patients to rotate injection sites to avoid localized tissue atrophy.

Instruct patients to contact their health care provider if they experience any adverse reactions or discomfort during treatment with somatropin.

Provide patients and caregivers who will administer somatropin in medically unsupervised situations with appropriate training and instruction on the proper use of somatropin from the health care provider or other suitably qualified health care professional.

POSTERIOR PITUITARY HORMONES

VASOPRESSIN (8-Arginine-Vasopressin)

Rx	**Vasopressin** (Various, eg, American Pharmaceutical Partners, American Regent)	**Injection:** 20 pressor units/mL	0.5% chlorobutanol. In 0.5, 1, and 10 mL vials.
Rx	**Pitressin Synthetic** (JHP Pharm)		0.5% chlorobutanol. In 1 mL vials.

VASOPRESSIN — INJECTION

Indications

For prevention and treatment of postoperative abdominal distention, in abdominal roentgenography to dispel interfering gas shadows, and in diabetes insipidus.

➤*Off-label uses:*

Esophageal varices – [2] = Fair documentation. Use of vasopressin for the treatment of esophageal variceal hemorrhage is limited by its adverse effects. Current practice guidelines recommend treatment with either somastatin or a somastatin analogue for 3 to 5 days after diagnosis. Vasopressin is recommended if other agents are unavailable. To minimize adverse effects, vasopressin should be given at the lowest effective dose for no more than 24 hours and in combination with nitroglycerin.

Traumatic brain injury – [4] = Insufficient documentation. One low-quality, noncontrolled trial suggested a possible benefit of vasopressin therapy in patients with traumatic brain injury (TBI), but a better quality study found no effect of therapy. Because of a lack of evidence of efficacy, vasopressin was not recommended by the Neurobehavioral Guidelines Working Group for improving learning and memory in patients with TBI.

Other possible off-label uses – For the treatment of pulseless cardiac arrest, 1 dose of vasopressin (40 units intravenously or intraosseously) may replace either the first or second dose of epinephrine.

Vasopressin has also been used for the hemodynamic support of septic shock and vasodilatory shock due to systemic inflammatory response syndrome. For patients with refractory shock despite fluid resuscitation and conventional vasopressors, vasopressin has been given at an infusion rate of 0.01 to 0.04 units/minute.

Administration and Dosage

➤*General dosing considerations:* It is desirable to administer a dose not much larger than is just sufficient to elicit the desired physiologic response. Excessive doses may cause undesirable adverse effects (blanching of the skin, abdominal cramps, nausea), which, though not serious, may alarm the patient. (See Administration.)

➤*Adults:*

Abdominal distention – Vasopressin used in this manner will frequently prevent or relieve postoperative distention. These recommendations also apply to distention complicating pneumonia or other acute toxemias.

Initial dosage: 5 units (0.25 mL) intramuscularly (IM) at 3- or 4-hour intervals.

Dosage titration: Increase to 10 units (0.5 mL) IM at subsequent injections, if necessary.

Abdominal roentgenography – 2 injections of 10 units (0.5 mL) administered subcutaneously or IM 2 hours and 30 minutes, respectively, before films are exposed. Many roentgenologists advise giving an enema prior to the first dose of vasopressin.

Diabetes insipidus –

Injection: 5 to 10 units (0.25 to 0.5 mL) subcutaneously or IM repeated 2 or 3 times daily, as needed.

Intranasal: Dosage and interval between treatments must be determined for each patient.

Off-label dosing –

Esophageal varices: [2] = Fair documentation. Continuous intravenous (IV) infusion of 0.2 to 0.4 units/min titrated to a maximum of 0.8 units/min with a maximum duration of 24 hours.

Traumatic brain injury: [4] = Insufficient documentation. 8 to 16 international units/day intranasally in a single dose or 2 divided doses.

➤*Children:* Dosage to be reduced proportionately for children.

➤*Administration:* May be administered IM, subcutaneously, or intranasally depending on indication. Adverse effects, such as blanching of skin, abdominal cramps, and nausea, may be reduced by drinking 1 or 2 glasses of water at the time of vasopressin administration. For diabetes insipidus, may be administered intranasally on cotton pledgets, by nasal spray, or by dropper.

➤*Extravasation:* Extravasation resulting in severe tissue damage may occur during administration of vasopressin. If signs or symptoms of extravasation occur, stop the infusion immediately. If possible, withdraw 3 to 5 mL of blood to remove some of the drug. Remove the infusion needle. Delineate the infiltrated area on the patient's skin with a felt-tip marker. Elevate for 48 hours above heart level using a sling or stockinette dressing with an observation window cut in the dressing. Avoid pressure or friction. Do not rub area. Observe for signs of increased erythema, pain, or skin necrosis. If increased symptoms occur, consult a plastic surgeon. Ensure that no medication is given distally to extravasation site. After 48 hours, encourage the patient to use the extremity normally to promote full range of motion.

➤*Storage/Stability:* Store between 15° and 25°C (59° and 77°F). Do not freeze.

Actions

➤*Pharmacology:* The antidiuretic action of vasopressin is ascribed to increasing reabsorption of water by the renal tubules.

Vasopressin can cause contraction of smooth muscle of the gastrointestinal tract and of all parts of the vascular bed, especially the capillaries, small arterioles, and venules with less effect on the smooth musculature of the large veins. The direct effect on the contractile elements is neither antagonized by adrenergic blocking agents nor prevented by vascular denervation.

➤*Pharmacokinetics:* Following subcutaneous or intramuscular administration of vasopressin injection, the duration of antidiuretic activity is variable but effects are usually maintained for 2 to 8 hours.

The majority of a dose of vasopressin is metabolized and rapidly destroyed in the liver and kidneys. Vasopressin has a plasma half-life of about 10 to 20 minutes. Approximately 5% of a subcutaneous dose of vasopressin is excreted in urine unchanged after 4 hours.

Contraindications

Anaphylaxis or hypersensitivity to the drug or its components.

Warnings/Precautions

➤*Vascular disease:* This drug should not be used in patients with vascular disease, especially disease of the coronary arteries, except with extreme caution. In such patients, even small doses may precipitate anginal pain, and with larger doses, the possibility of myocardial infarction should be considered.

➤*Water intoxication:* Vasopressin may produce water intoxication. The early signs of drowsiness, listlessness, and headaches should be recognized to prevent terminal coma and convulsions.

➤*Chronic nephritis:* Chronic nephritis with nitrogen retention contraindicates the use of vasopressin until reasonable nitrogen blood levels have been attained.

➤*Extravasation:* See Administration and Dosage for more information.

➤*Special risk:* Vasopressin should be used cautiously in the presence of epilepsy, migraine, asthma, heart failure, or any state in which a rapid addition to extracellular water may produce hazard for an already overburdened system.

➤*Pregnancy:* *Category C* per manufacturer's prescribing information. *Category B* per Briggs' *Drugs in Pregnancy and Lactation*. Animal reproduction studies have not been conducted with vasopressin. It is also not known

VASOPRESSIN — INJECTION

whether vasopressin can cause fetal harm when administered to a pregnant woman or can affect reproduction capacity. Vasopressin should be given to a pregnant woman only if clearly needed.

Labor and delivery – Doses of vasopressin sufficient for an antidiuretic effect are not likely to produce tonic uterine contractions that could be deleterious to the fetus or threaten the continuation of the pregnancy.

➤*Lactation:* Exercised caution when vasopressin is administered to a breast-feeding woman.

➤*Monitoring:* Electrocardiograms (ECG) and fluid and electrolyte status determinations are recommended at periodic intervals during therapy.

Drug Interactions

➤*QT prolongation:* An additive effect of vasopressin with other drugs that prolong the QT interval cannot be excluded. The following drugs may prolong the QT interval and increase the risk of life-threatening cardiac arrhythmias, including torsades de pointes: Antiarrhythmic agents (eg, amiodarone, bretylium, disopyramide, dofetilide, procainamide, quinidine, and sotalol), arsenic trioxide, chlorpromazine, cisapride, dolasetron, droperidol, mefloquine, mesoridazine, moxifloxacin, pentamidine, pimozide, tacrolimus, thioridazine, and ziprasidone. For a more complete list of drugs that may prolong the QT interval, see the appendix, Drug-Induced Prolongation of the QT Interval and Torsades de Pointes.

The following drugs may potentiate the antidiuretic effect of vasopressin when used concurrently: carbamazepine, chlorpropamide, clofibrate, urea, fludrocortisone, tricyclic antidepressants.

The following drugs may decrease the antidiuretic effect of vasopressin when used concurrently: demeclocycline, norepinephrine, lithium, heparin, alcohol.

Ganglionic blocking agents may produce a marked increase in sensitivity to the pressor effects of vasopressin.

Adverse Reactions

Local or systemic allergic reactions may occur in hypersensitive individuals. The following side effects have been reported following the administration of vasopressin.

➤*Cardiovascular:* Cardiac arrest; circumoral pallor; arrhythmias; decreased cardiac output; angina; myocardial ischemia; peripheral vasoconstriction; and gangrene.

➤*CNS:* Tremor; vertigo; "pounding" in head.

➤*Dermatologic:* Sweating; urticaria; cutaneous gangrene.

➤*GI:* Abdominal cramps; nausea; vomiting; passage of gas.

➤*Hypersensitivity:* Anaphylaxis (cardiac arrest and/or shock) has been observed shortly after injection of vasopressin.

➤*Respiratory:* Bronchial constriction.

Overdosage

Water intoxication may be treated with water restriction and temporary withdrawal of vasopressin until polyuria occurs. Severe water intoxication may require osmotic diuresis with mannitol, hypertonic dextrose, or urea alone or with furosemide.

Patient Information

Side effects such as blanching of skin, abdominal cramps, and nausea may be reduced by taking 1 or 2 glasses of water at the time of vasopressin administration. These side effects are usually not serious and probably will disappear within a few minutes.

DESMOPRESSIN ACETATE (1-Deamino-8-D-Arginine Vasopressin)

Rx	**Desmopressin Acetate** (Various, eg, Apotex, Barr, Teva)	**Tablets; oral:** 0.1 mg	May contain lactose. In 100s.
Rx	**DDAVP** (Sanofi-Aventis)		Lactose. (0.1 36 AV). In 100s.
Rx	**Desmopressin Acetate** (Various, eg, Apotex, Barr, Teva)	**Tablets; oral:** 0.2 mg	May contain lactose. In 100s.
Rx	**DDAVP** (Sanofi-Aventis)		Lactose. (0.2 37 AV). In 100s.
Rx	**Desmopressin Acetate** (Various, eg, Apotex, Bausch & Lomb)	**Spray, solution; intranasal:** 0.1 mg/mL	10 mcg/spray. In 5 mL (50 sprays) bottle or 2.5 mL rhinal tube delivery system (2 rhinal tube applicators per carton).
Rx	**DDAVP** (Sanofi-Aventis)		10 mcg spray. In 5 mL (50 sprays) bottle or 2.5 mL rhinal tube delivery system (2 rhinal tube applicators per carton).
Rx	**Stimate** (CSL Behring)	**Spray, solution; intranasal:** 1.5 mg/mL	150 mcg/spray. In 2.5 mL (25 sprays) bottle.
Rx	**Desmopressin Acetate** (Various, eg, Ferring, Hospira, Sicor)	**Injection, solution:** 4 mcg/mL	1 mL single-dose amps and 10 mL multidose vials.
Rx	**DDAVP** (Sanofi-Aventis)		In 1 mL single-dose amps and 10 mL multidose vials.[a]

[a] With chlorobutanol 5 mg/mL.

DESMOPRESSIN ACETATE — ORAL

Indications

➤*Central diabetes insipidus:* As antidiuretic replacement therapy in the management of central diabetes insipidus and for the management of the temporary polyuria and polydipsia following head trauma or surgery in the pituitary region.

➤*Primary nocturnal enuresis:* For the management of primary nocturnal enuresis. Desmopressin may be used alone or as an adjunct to behavioral conditioning or other nonpharmacologic intervention.

Administration and Dosage

➤*General dosing considerations:* Response should be estimated by 2 parameters: adequate duration of sleep and adequate, not excessive, water turnover.

During the initial dose titration period, patients should be observed closely and appropriate safety parameters measured to ensure adequate response. Patients should be monitored at regular intervals during the course of therapy to ensure adequate antidiuretic response.

➤*Adults:*

Central diabetes insipidus –

Usual dosage: Most patients in clinical trials found that the optimal dosage range is 0.1 to 0.8 mg daily, administered in divided doses.

Maximum dose: 1.2 mg/day.

Initial dosage: 0.05 mg (half of the 0.1 mg tablet) 2 times a day.

Dosage adjustment: Total daily dosage should be increased or decreased in the range of 0.1 to 1.2 mg divided into 2 or 3 daily doses as needed to obtain adequate antidiuresis. Each dose should be separately adjusted for an adequate diurnal rhythm of water turnover. Modifications in dosage regimen should be implemented as necessary to ensure adequate water turnover.

Conversion: Patients previously on intranasal therapy should begin tablet therapy 12 hours after the last intranasal dose.

➤*Children:*

Central diabetes insipidus –

4 years of age and older: See Adults for dosing.

Younger than 4 years of age: See Off-label dosing.

Primary nocturnal enuresis –

6 years of age and older:

- *Maximum dose* – 0.6 mg at bedtime.
- *Initial dosage* – 0.2 mg at bedtime.
- *Dosage titration* – The dose may be titrated up to 0.6 mg to achieve the desired response.
- *Conversion* – Patients previously on intranasal can begin tablet therapy the night following (24 hours after) the last intranasal dose.

Off-label dosing –

Central diabetes insipidus:

- *Younger than 4 years of age* –

Usual dosage: 0.1 to 0.8 mg/day.

Initial dosage: 0.05 mg (half of the 0.1 mg tablet) 2 times a day.

Dosage adjustment: Adjust dose to effect.

➤*Renal function impairment:* Contraindicated in moderate to severe renal impairment (creatinine clearance [CrCl] below 50 mL/min).

➤*Administration:* Administer with or without food. Fluid restriction should be observed.

Primary nocturnal enuresis – Fluid intake should be limited to a minimum from 1 hour before administration until the next morning or at least 8 hours after administration.

➤*Storage/Stability:* Store at controlled room temperature (20° to 25°C [68° to 77°F]). Avoid exposure to excessive heat or light.

Actions

➤*Pharmacology:* Desmopressin is a synthetic analog of the natural pituitary hormone arginine vasopressin, an antidiuretic hormone affecting renal water conservation.

The use of desmopressin in patients with central diabetes insipidus will result in a reduction in urinary output with an accompanying increase in urine osmolality. These effects usually will allow resumption of a more normal lifestyle, with a decrease in urinary frequency and nocturia.

DESMOPRESSIN ACETATE — ORAL

➤*Pharmacokinetics:*

Absorption – The bioavailability of desmopressin tablets is approximately 5% compared with intranasal desmopressin, and approximately 0.16% compared with intravenous (IV) desmopressin. The time to reach maximum plasma desmopressin levels ranged from 0.9 to 1.5 hours following oral or intranasal administration, respectively. Following administration of desmopressin tablets, the onset of antidiuretic effect occurs approximately 1 hour, and it reaches a maximum at approximately 4 to 7 hours based on the measurement of increased urine osmolality.

Excretion – Desmopressin is mainly excreted in the urine.

The plasma half-life of desmopressin followed a monoexponential time course with half-life values of 1.5 to 2.5 hours, which was independent of dose.

Special populations –

Renal function impairment: A pharmacokinetic study conducted in healthy volunteers and patients with mild, moderate, or severe renal function impairment (N = 24; 6 subjects in each group) receiving single dose desmopressin (2 mcg) injection demonstrated a difference in desmopressin terminal half-life. Terminal half-life significantly increased from 3 hours in healthy patients to 9 hours in patients with severe renal function impairment.

Contraindications

Hypersensitivity to desmopressin or to any of the components of desmopressin tablets; moderate to severe renal function impairment (defined as creatinine clearance [CrCl] below 50 mL/min); hyponatremia or a history of hyponatremia.

Warnings/Precautions

➤*Hyponatremia:* Very rare cases of hyponatremia have been reported from worldwide postmarketing experience in patients treated with desmopressin, a potent antidiuretic that may lead to water intoxication and/or hyponatremia when administered. Unless properly diagnosed and treated, hyponatremia can be fatal; therefore, fluid restriction is recommended and should be discussed with the patient and/or guardian. Careful medical supervision is required.

In particular, in very young and elderly patients, adjust fluid intake downward to decrease the potential occurrence of water intoxication and hyponatremia. Observe all patients receiving desmopressin for the following signs and symptoms associated with hyponatremia: headache, nausea/vomiting, decreased serum sodium, weight gain, restlessness, fatigue, lethargy, disorientation, depressed reflexes, loss of appetite, irritability, muscles weakness, muscle spasms or cramps, and abnormal mental status (eg, hallucinations, decreased consciousness, confusion). Severe symptoms may include 1 or a combination of the following: seizure, coma, and/or respiratory arrest. Pay particular attention to the possibility of the rare occurrence of an extreme decrease in plasma osmolality that may result in seizures that could lead to coma.

Use desmopressin with caution in patients with habitual or psychogenic polydipsia who may be more likely to drink excessive amounts of water, putting them at greater risk of hyponatremia.

➤*Hypersensitivity reactions:* Rare severe allergic reactions have been reported with desmopressin. Anaphylaxis has rarely been reported with IV and intranasal administration of desmopressin, but not with tablets.

➤*Special risk:* Use desmopressin with caution in patients with conditions associated with fluid and electrolyte imbalance, such as cystic fibrosis, heart failure, and renal disorders, since these patients are prone to hyponatremia. Although this effect has not been observed when single oral doses of up to 0.6 mg have been administered, use this drug with caution in patients with coronary artery insufficiency and/or hypertensive cardiovascular disease because of a possible rise in blood pressure.

➤*Pregnancy:* Category B.

There are no adequate and well-controlled studies in pregnant women. Because animal studies are not always predictive of human response, use this drug during pregnancy only if clearly needed.

➤*Lactation:* There have been no controlled studies in breast-feeding mothers; however, patients receiving desmopressin for diabetes insipidus have been reported to breast-feed without apparent problems in the infant. A single study in postpartum women demonstrated a marked change in plasma, but little if any change in assayable desmopressin in breast milk following an intranasal dose of 0.01 mg.

It is not known whether the drug is excreted in human milk. Because many drugs are excreted in human milk, exercise caution when desmopressin is administered to breast-feeding mothers.

➤*Children:*

Central diabetes insipidus – Desmopressin tablets have been used safely in children 4 years of age and older with diabetes insipidus for periods of 44 months or less. In younger children, the dose must be individually adjusted in order to prevent an excessive decrease in plasma osmolality leading to hyponatremia and possible convulsions; start dosing at 0.05 mg (half of the 0.1 mg tablet). Use of desmopressin in children requires careful fluid intake restrictions to prevent possible hyponatremia and water intoxication.

Primary nocturnal enuresis – Desmopressin tablets have been safely used in children 6 years of age or older with primary nocturnal enuresis for 6 months or less. Some patients respond to a dose of 0.2 mg; however, increasing responses are seen at doses of 0.4 and 0.6 mg. No increase in the frequency or severity of adverse reactions or decrease in efficacy was seen with an increased dose or duration. Individually adjust the dose to achieve the best results. Interrupt treatment with desmopressin for primary nocturnal enuresis during acute intercurrent illness characterized by fluid and/or electrolyte imbalance (eg, systemic infections, fever, recurrent vomiting, diarrhea) or under conditions of extremely hot weather, during vigorous exercise, or other conditions associated with increased water intake.

➤*Elderly:* In general, use caution in dose selection for an elderly patient, usually starting at the low end of the dosing range, reflecting the greater frequency of decreased hepatic, renal, or cardiac function, and of concomitant disease or other drug therapy.

This drug is known to be substantially excreted in the kidney, and the risk of toxic reactions to this drug may be greater in patients with impaired renal function. Because elderly patients are more likely to have decreased renal function, use caution when making dose selection, and it may be useful to monitor renal function. Desmopressin is contraindicated in patients with moderate to severe renal function impairment (defined as CrCl less than 50 mL/min).

Use of desmopressin in elderly patients requires careful fluid intake restrictions to prevent possible hyponatremia and water intoxication.

➤*Monitoring:* Monitor patients at regular intervals during the course of therapy to ensure adequate antidiuretic response. Monitor fluid intake and observe patients for signs and symptoms of hyponatremia.

Laboratory tests for monitoring the patient with central diabetes insipidus or postsurgical or head trauma–related polyuria and polydipsia include urine volume and osmolality. In some cases, measurements of plasma osmolality may be useful.

Drug Interactions

➤*Pressor agents:* Although the pressor activity of desmopressin is very low compared with its antidiuretic activity, use large doses of desmopressin with other pressor agents only with careful patient monitoring.

Desmopressin Drug Interactions

Precipitant drug	Object drug[a]		Description
Carbamazepine	Desmopressin	↑	Coadministration may increase the risk of water intoxication with hyponatremia. Use with caution.
Chlorpromazine	Desmopressin	↑	Coadministration may increase the risk of water intoxication with hyponatremia. Use with caution.
Lamotrigine	Desmopressin	↑	Coadministration may increase the risk of water intoxication with hyponatremia. Use with caution.
NSAIDs[b] (eg, naproxen)	Desmopressin	↑	Coadministration may increase the risk of water intoxication with hyponatremia. Use with caution.
Opiate analgesics (eg, methadone)	Desmopressin	↑	Coadministration may increase the risk of water intoxication with hyponatremia. Use with caution.
SSRIs[b] (eg, fluoxetine)	Desmopressin	↑	Coadministration may increase the risk of water intoxication with hyponatremia. Use with caution.
TCAs[b] (eg, amitriptyline)	Desmopressin	↑	Coadministration may increase the risk of water intoxication with hyponatremia. Use with caution.

[a] ↑ = object drug increased.
[b] NSAIDs = nonsteroidal anti-inflammatory drugs; SSRIs = selective serotonin reuptake inhibitors; TCAs = tricyclic antidepressants.

Adverse Reactions

➤*CNS:* The only adverse reaction occurring in at least 3% of patients with primary nocturnal enuresis in controlled clinical trials with desmopressin that was probably, possibly, or remotely related to study drug was headache (4% desmopressin, 3% placebo). Abnormal thinking was also reported (relationship to desmopressin not established).

➤*Hepatic:* In long-term clinical studies in which patients with diabetes insipidus were followed for periods of 44 months or less of desmopressin tablet therapy, transient increases in AST of 1.5 or less times the upper limit of normal were occasionally observed. Elevated AST returned to the normal range despite continued use of desmopressin tablets.

➤*Miscellaneous:* Diarrhea and edema-weight gain has been reported (relationship to desmopressin not established).

➤*Intranasal / Injection:* Infrequently, large doses of the intranasal formulations of desmopressin and desmopressin injection have produced transient headache, nausea, flushing, and mild abdominal cramps. These symptoms have disappeared with reduction in dosage.

➤*Postmarketing:* There have been rare reports of hyponatremic convulsions associated with concomitant use with the following medications: oxybutynin and imipramine.

Overdosage

➤*Symptoms:* Signs of overdose may include confusion, drowsiness, continuing headache, problems with passing urine, and rapid weight gain caused by fluid retention.

DESMOPRESSIN ACETATE — ORAL

➤*Treatment:* In case of overdose, reduce the dose, decrease the frequency of administration, or withdraw the drug according to the severity of the condition. There is no known specific antidote for desmopressin. Observe the patient and treat with appropriate symptomatic therapy.

Patient Information

Advise patient and/or guardian that desmopressin therapy requires careful fluid intake restriction to prevent possible hyponatremia and water intoxication.

Advise patient that treatment with desmopressin for primary nocturnal enuresis should be interrupted during acute intercurrent illness characterized by fluid and/or electrolyte imbalance (eg, systemic infections, fever, recurrent vomiting or diarrhea) or under conditions of extremely hot weather, during vigorous exercise, or other conditions associated with increased water intake.

DESMOPRESSIN ACETATE — INTRANASAL

Indications

➤*Central diabetes insipidus (DDAVP only):* As antidiuretic replacement therapy in the management of central cranial diabetes insipidus and for the management of temporary polyuria and polydipsia following head trauma or surgery in the pituitary region. It is ineffective for the treatment of nephrogenic diabetes insipidus.

➤*Hemophilia A (Stimate only):* For patients with hemophilia A with factor VIII coagulant activity levels more than 5%. Desmopressin will also stop bleeding in patients with hemophilia A with episodes of spontaneous or trauma-induced injuries, such as hemarthroses, intramuscular (IM) hematomas, or mucosal bleeding.

➤*von Willebrand disease (type 1) (Stimate only):* For patients with mild to moderate classic von Willebrand disease (type 1) with factor VIII levels more than 5%. Desmopressin will also stop bleeding in patients with mild to moderate von Willebrand disease with episodes of spontaneous or trauma-induced injuries such as hemarthroses, IM hematomas, mucosal bleeding, or menorrhagia.

➤*Off-label uses:* Treatment of chronic autonomic failure (eg, nocturnal polyuria, overnight weight loss, morning postural hypotension).

Administration and Dosage

➤*General dosing considerations:* Fluid restriction should be observed.

Response should be estimated by 2 parameters: adequate duration of sleep and adequate, not excessive, water turnover. Patients with nasal congestion and blockage have often responded well to desmopressin.

➤*Adults:*

DDAVP –

Central diabetes insipidus:

• *Usual dosage* – 10 to 40 mcg daily, either as a single dose or divided into 2 or 3 doses.

• *Dosage adjustment* – The morning and evening doses should be adjusted separately for an adequate diurnal rhythm of water turnover.

Stimate –

Hemophilia A:

• *Usual dosage* – 1 spray (150 mcg) per nostril, to provide a total dose of 300 mcg.

Patients weighing less than 50 kg: 150 mcg administered as a single spray.

• *Test dose* – Before the initial therapeutic administration, establish that the patient shows an appropriate change in coagulation profile following a test dose of intranasal administration.

• *Repeat dose* – The necessity for repeat administration or use of any blood products for hemostasis should be determined by laboratory response as well as the clinical condition of the patient. The tendency toward tachyphylaxis (lessening of response) with repeated administration given more frequently than every 48 hours should be considered in treating each patient.

von Willebrand disease (type I): See Hemophilia A for dosing.

➤*Children:*

DDAVP –

Central diabetes insipidus:

• *13 years of age and older* – See Adults for dosing.

• *3 months to 12 years of age* – 5 to 30 mcg daily, either as a single dose or divided into 2 doses.

Stimate –

Hemophilia A:

• *11 months of age and older* – See Adults for dosing.

von Willebrand disease (type I):

• *11 months of age and older* – See Adults for dosing.

➤*Renal function impairment:* Contraindicated in moderate to severe renal impairment (CrCl less than 50 mL/min).

➤*Preparation for administration:*

DDAVP nasal spray – The spray pump must be primed prior to the first use. To prime the pump, press down 4 times. The bottle will deliver 10 mcg of drug per spray.

Stimate – The spray pump must be primed prior to the first use. To prime the pump, press down 4 times.

➤*Administration:* For intranasal use only. For intranasal administration, ensure that nasal passages are intact, clean, and free of obstruction before administration of drug. Only use in patients where orally administered formulations are not feasible.

DDAVP nasal spray – Do not use the nasal spray in children requiring less than 0.1 mL (10 mcg) per dose.

DDAVP rhinal tube – Administered into the nose through a soft, flexible plastic rhinal tube with 4 graduation marks, measuring 0.2, 0.15, 0.1, and 0.05 mL. Draw solution up into this tube and insert into nostril. Place opposite end of tube in mouth and blow into tube to deliver medication.

Stimate – Administer by nasal insufflation. If used preoperatively, it should be administered 2 hours prior to the scheduled procedure.

➤*Storage/Stability:*

DDAVP nasal spray – Store upright at 20° to 25°C. Discard after 50 sprays because thereafter, the amount delivered per spray may be substantially less than 10 mcg.

DDAVP rhinal tube – Store at 2° to 8°C. When traveling, product will maintain stability for 3 weeks when stored at 20° to 25°C.

Stimate – Store at 2° to 8°C. When traveling, product will maintain stability for 3 weeks when stored at 20° to 25°C. The bottle should be discarded after 25 doses because thereafter, the amount delivered per spray may be substantially less than 150 mcg.

Actions

➤*Pharmacology:* Desmopressin is a synthetic analog of the natural pituitary hormone arginine vasopressin, an antidiuretic hormone affecting renal water conservation.

The use of desmopressin in patients with an established diagnosis of central diabetes insipidus will result in a reduction in urinary output, with an increase in urine osmolality and a decrease in plasma osmolality. This will allow the resumption of a more normal life-style with a decrease in urinary frequency and nocturia.

Desmopressin has been shown to be more potent than arginine vasopressin in increasing plasma levels of factor VIII activity in patients with hemophilia and von Willebrand disease type I.

➤*Pharmacokinetics:*

Absorption – Dose-response studies were performed in healthy persons using doses of 150 to 450 mcg, administered as 1 to 3 sprays. The response to desmopressin is dose-related, with maximal plasma levels of 150% to 250% of initial concentrations achieved for both factor VIII and von Willebrand factor. The increase is rapid and evident within 30 minutes, reaching a maximum at approximately 1.5 hours.

Desmopressin is absorbed rapidly from the nasal mucosa. The bioavailability of desmopressin when administered by the intranasal route as a 1.5 mg/mL solution is between 3.3% and 4.1%. Plasma concentrations of desmopressin were maximal approximately 40 to 45 minutes after intranasal dosing.

Excretion – Desmopressin is mainly excreted in the urine. The half-life of desmopressin is between 3.3 and 3.5 hours over the 150 to 450 mcg range of intranasal doses. Desmopressin exhibits a biphasic elimination profile with half-lives of 7.8 and 75.5 minutes for the initial and terminal phases, respectively, compared with lysine vasopressin, another form of the hormone used in this condition, which has initial and terminal phase half-lives of 2.5 and 14.5 minutes, respectively. As a result, intranasal desmopressin provides a prompt onset of antidiuretic action with a long duration after each administration.

Special populations –

Renal function impairment: A pharmacokinetic study conducted in healthy volunteers and patients with mild, moderate, and severe renal function impairment (N = 24; 6 subjects in each group) receiving a single-dose desmopressin (2 mcg) injection demonstrated a difference in desmopressin terminal half-life. Terminal half-life significantly increased from 3 hours in healthy patients to 9 hours in patients with severe renal function impairment.

Contraindications

Hypersensitivity to desmopressin or to any of the components of the nasal spray; moderate to severe renal function impairment (defined as creatinine clearance [CrCl] less than 50 mL/min); hyponatremia or a history of hyponatremia.

Warnings/Precautions

➤*Administration:* For intranasal use only. Only use in patients where orally administered formulations are not feasible.

➤*Hyponatremia:* Very rare cases of hyponatremia have been reported from worldwide postmarketing experience in patients treated with desmopressin. Desmopressin is a potent antidiuretic that, when administered, may lead to water intoxication and/or hyponatremia. Unless properly diagnosed and treated, hyponatremia can be fatal. Therefore, fluid restriction is recommended and should be discussed with the patient and/or guardian. Careful medical supervision is required.

DESMOPRESSIN ACETATE — INTRANASAL

When desmopressin is administered, in particular to children and elderly patients, adjust fluid intake downward in an effort to decrease the potential occurrence of water intoxication and hyponatremia with accompanying signs and symptoms (eg, headache, nausea/vomiting, decreased serum sodium, weight gain, restlessness, fatigue, lethargy, disorientation, depressed reflexes, loss of appetite, irritability, muscle weakness, muscle spasms or cramps, and abnormal mental status [eg, hallucinations, decreased consciousness, confusion]). Severe symptoms may include 1 or a combination of the following: seizure, coma, and/or respiratory arrest. Pay particular attention to the possibility of the rare occurrence of an extreme decrease in plasma osmolarity that may result in seizures, which could lead to coma.

Caution patients who do not have need of antidiuretic hormone for its antidiuretic effect, in particular those who are young or elderly, to ingest only enough fluid to satisfy thirst, in order to decrease the potential occurrence of water intoxication and hyponatremia.

Use desmopressin with caution in patients with habitual or psychogenic polydipsia who may be more likely to drink excessive amounts of water, putting them at greater risk of hyponatremia.

➤*von Willebrand disease (type IIB):* Do not use desmopressin to treat patients with von Willebrand disease type IIB because platelet aggregation may be induced.

➤*Cardiovascular effects:* Intranasal desmopressin has infrequently produced changes in blood pressure, causing either a slight elevation in blood pressure, which disappeared with reduction in dose, or a transient fall in blood pressure and a compensatory increase in heart rate. Use the drug with caution in patients with coronary artery insufficiency and/or hypertensive cardiovascular disease.

There have been rare reports of thrombotic events (thrombosis, acute cerebrovascular thrombosis, acute myocardial infarction [MI]) following desmopressin injection in patients predisposed to thrombus formation. No causality has been determined; however, use desmopressin with caution in these patients.

➤*Nasal mucosa changes:* Because desmopressin is used intranasally, changes in the nasal mucosa, such as scarring, edema, or other disease that may cause erratic, unreliable absorption, can occur. In these cases, discontinue desmopressin until the nasal problems resolve. For such situations, consider desmopressin injection.

➤*Change in response:* There are reports of an occasional change in response with time, usually more than 6 months. Some patients may show a decreased responsiveness, others a shortened duration of effect. There is no evidence this effect is caused by the development of binding antibodies but may be because of a local inactivation of the peptide.

➤*Hypersensitivity reactions:* Severe allergic reactions have been reported rarely. Fatal anaphylaxis has been reported in one patient who received desmopressin injection. It is not known whether antibodies to desmopressin are produced after repeated administration.

➤*Special risk:* Use desmopressin with caution in patients with conditions associated with fluid and electrolyte imbalance, such as cystic fibrosis, heart failure, and renal disorders, because these patients are prone to hyponatremia.

➤*Pregnancy: Category B.* There are no adequate and well-controlled studies in pregnant women. Only use this drug during pregnancy only if clearly needed.

➤*Lactation:* There have been no controlled studies in breast-feeding mothers; however, patients receiving desmopressin for diabetes insipidus have been reported to breast-feed without apparent problems in the infant. A single study in postpartum women demonstrated a marked change in plasma, but little if any change in assayable desmopressin in breast milk following an intranasal dose of 10 mcg. It is not known whether this drug is excreted in human milk. Because many drugs are excreted in human milk, exercise caution when desmopressin is administered to a breast-feeding woman.

➤*Children:*

Hemophilia A / von Willebrand disease – Use in infants and children will require careful fluid intake restriction to prevent possible hyponatremia and water intoxication. Do not use desmopressin in infants younger than 11 months of age in the treatment of hemophilia A or von Willebrand disease; safety and effectiveness in children between 11 months and 12 years of age has been demonstrated.

Central cranial diabetes insipidus – Desmopressin has been used in children with diabetes insipidus. Use in infants and children will require careful fluid intake restriction to prevent possible hyponatremia and water intoxication. The dose must be individually adjusted to the patient with attention in the very young to the danger of an extreme decrease in plasma osmolality with resulting convulsions. Start doses at 0.05 mL or less.

Because the spray cannot deliver less than 0.1 mL (10 mcg), administer smaller doses using the rhinal tube delivery system. Do not use the nasal spray in children requiring less than 0.1 mL (10 mcg) per dose.

➤*Elderly:* Clinical studies did not include sufficient numbers of subjects 65 years of age and older to determine whether they respond differently than younger subjects. However, other postmarketing experience has reported the occurrence of hyponatremia with the use of desmopressin and fluid overload.

Other reported clinical experience has not identified differences in responses between elderly subjects and younger subjects. In general, use caution when making dose selection for an elderly patient, usually starting at the low end of the dosing range, reflecting the greater frequency of decreased hepatic, renal, or cardiac function, and of concomitant disease or drug therapy.

This drug is known to be especially excreted in the kidney, and the risk of toxic reactions to this drug may be greater in patients with impaired renal function. Because elderly patients are more likely to have decreased renal function, take care in dose selection and it may be useful to monitor renal function. Desmopressin is contraindicated in patients with moderate to severe renal function impairment (defined as a CrCl lower than 50 mL/min).

In elderly patients, adjust fluid intake downward in an effort to decrease the potential occurrence of water intoxication and hyponatremia. Pay particular attention to the possibility of the rare occurrence of an extreme decrease in plasma osmolarity that may result in seizures, which could lead to coma.

Caution patients who do not have need of antidiuretic hormone for its antidiuretic effect to ingest only enough fluid to satisfy thirst in an effort to decrease the potential occurrence of water intoxication and hyponatremia.

As for all patients, ensure dosing for elderly patients is appropriate to their overall situation.

➤*Monitoring:* Monitor patients at regular intervals during the course of therapy to ensure adequate antidiuretic response. Monitor fluid intake and observe patients for signs and symptoms of hyponatremia.

Laboratory tests for assessing the status of patients with hemophilia A include levels of factor VIII coagulant, factor VIII antigen, and factor VIII ristocetin cofactor (von Willebrand factor), as well as activated partial thromboplastin time. Determine factor VIII coagulant activity before giving desmopressin for hemostasis. If factor VIII coagulant activity is present at less than 5% of normal, do not rely on desmopressin.

Check bleeding time and factor VIII coagulant activity, factor VIII ristocetin cofactor activity, and factor VIII von Willebrand factor antigen after initial administration and periodically to ensure adequate levels have been achieved in patients with von Willebrand disease. The skin bleeding time may be helpful in following these patients.

Laboratory tests for following the patient with central diabetes insipidus or postsurgical or head trauma–related polyuria and polydipsia include urine volume and osmolality. In some cases, plasma osmolality measurements may be required.

Drug Interactions

➤*Pressor agents:* Although the pressor activity of intranasal desmopressin acetate is very low compared with the antidiuretic activity, only use large doses of desmopressin with other pressor agents with careful patient monitoring.

Desmopressin Drug Interactions

Precipitant drug	Object drug[a]		Description
Carbamazepine	Desmopressin	↑	Coadministration may increase the risk of water intoxication with hyponatremia. Use with caution.
Chlorpromazine	Desmopressin	↑	Coadministration may increase the risk of water intoxication with hyponatremia. Use with caution.
Lamotrigine	Desmopressin	↑	Coadministration may increase the risk of water intoxication with hyponatremia. Use with caution.
NSAIDs[b] (eg, naproxen)	Desmopressin	↑	Coadministration may increase the risk of water intoxication with hyponatremia. Use with caution.
Opiate analgesics (eg, methadone)	Desmopressin	↑	Coadministration may increase the risk of water intoxication with hyponatremia. Use with caution.
SSRIs[b] (eg, fluoxetine)	Desmopressin	↑	Coadministration may increase the risk of water intoxication with hyponatremia. Use with caution.
TCAs[b] (eg, amitriptyline)	Desmopressin	↑	Coadministration may increase the risk of water intoxication with hyponatremia. Use with caution.

[a] ↑ = object drug increased.
[b] NSAIDs = nonsteroidal anti-inflammatory drugs; SSRIs = selective serotonin reuptake inhibitors; TCAs = tricyclic antidepressants.

Adverse Reactions

➤*Infrequent adverse reactions:* Infrequently, high dosages of intranasal desmopressin have produced transient headache and nausea. Nasal congestion, rhinitis, and flushing have also been reported occasionally along with mild abdominal cramps. These symptoms disappeared with reduction in dosage. Nosebleed, sore throat, cough, and upper respiratory tract infections have also been reported. In addition to those previously listed, the following adverse reactions have also been reported in clinical trials with *Stimate*: agitation, balanitis, chest pain, chills, dizziness, dyspepsia, edema, insomnia, itchy or light-sensitive eyes, pain, palpitations, somnolence, tachycardia, vomiting, warm feeling.

DESMOPRESSIN ACETATE — INTRANASAL

Desmopressin Intranasal Adverse Reactions			
Adverse reaction	Placebo (n = 59)	Desmopressin 20 mcg (n = 60)	Desmopressin 40 mcg (n = 61)
CNS			
Asthenia	0%	0%	2%
Depression	2%	0%	0%
Dizziness	0%	0%	3%
Headache	0%	2%	5%
GI			
Abdominal pain	0%	2%	2%
GI disorder	0%	2%	0%
Nausea	0%	0%	2%
Respiratory			
Epistaxis	2%	3%	0%
Nostril pain	0%	2%	0%
Rhinitis	2%	8%	3%
Special senses			
Conjunctivitis	0%	2%	0%
Edema eyes	0%	2%	0%
Lacrimation disorder	0%	0%	2%
Miscellaneous			
Chills	0%	0%	2%

➤*Postmarketing:* There have been rare reports of hyponatremic convulsions associated with concomitant use with the following medications: oxybutynin and imipramine.

Overdosage

➤*Symptoms:* Signs of overdose may include confusion, drowsiness, continuing headache, problems with passing urine, and rapid weight gain because of fluid retention.

➤*Treatment:* In cases of overdosage, reduce the dose, decrease the frequency of administration, or withdraw the drug according to the severity of the condition. There is no known specific antidote for desmopressin.

Patient Information

Inform patients that *Stimate* accurately delivers 25 doses of 150 mcg each and to discard any solution remaining after 25 doses because the amount delivered thereafter may be substantially less than 150 mcg of desmopressin. No attempt should be made to transfer remaining solution to another bottle. Instruct patients to carefully read the accompanying directions on the use of the spray pump before use.

Advise patients that if bleeding is not controlled to contact their health care provider.

Ensure that administration in children is under adult supervision in order to control the dose intake.

Inform patients that *DDAVP* nasal spray accurately delivers 50 doses of 10 mcg each and to discard any solution remaining after 50 doses since thereafter the amount delivered may be substantially less than 10 mcg of desmopressin. No attempt should be made to transfer remaining solution to another bottle. Instruct patients to carefully read the accompanying directions on the use of the spray pump before use.

Advise patients to adjust fluid intake downward based on discussion with their health care provider.

DESMOPRESSIN ACETATE — INJECTION

Indications

➤*Central diabetes insipidus:* As antidiuretic replacement therapy in the management of central (cranial) diabetes insipidus and for the management of the temporary polyuria and polydipsia following head trauma or surgery in the pituitary region.

➤*Hemophilia A:* For patients with hemophilia A with factor VIII coagulant activity levels more than 5%. Desmopressin will often maintain hemostasis in patients with hemophilia A during surgical procedures and postoperatively when administered 30 minutes prior to the scheduled procedure. Desmopressin will also stop bleeding in hemophilia A patients with episodes of spontaneous or trauma-induced injuries, such as hemarthroses, intramuscular (IM) hematomas, or mucosal bleeding.

➤*von Willebrand disease (type I):* For patients with mild to moderate classic von Willebrand disease (type I) with factor VIII levels more than 5%. Desmopressin will often maintain hemostasis in patients with mild to moderate von Willebrand disease during surgical procedures and postoperatively when administered 30 minutes prior to the scheduled procedure. Desmopressin will usually stop bleeding in mild to moderate von Willebrand patients with episodes of spontaneous or trauma-induced injuries, such as hemarthroses, IM hematomas, or mucosal bleeding.

Administration and Dosage

➤*General dosing considerations:* Fluid intake should be observed.

➤*Adults:*

Central diabetes insipidus –

Usual dosage: 0.5 to 1 mL (2 to 4 mcg) IV or subcutaneously, usually in 2 divided doses.

Maximum dose: 4 mcg daily.

Dosage adjustment: Desmopressin dosage must be determined for each patient and adjusted according to the pattern of response. The morning and evening doses should be separately adjusted for an adequate diurnal rhythm of water turnover.

Conversion: For patients who have been controlled on intranasal desmopressin and who must be switched to the injection form, either because of poor intranasal absorption or because of the need for surgery, the comparable antidiuretic dose of the injection is about one-tenth of the intranasal dose.

Response to therapy: Response should be estimated by 2 parameters: adequate duration of sleep and adequate, not excessive, water turnover. Fluid intake should be observed.

Hemophilia A –

Usual dosage: 0.3 mcg/kg body weight IV, diluted in sterile physiological saline and infused slowly over 15 to 30 minutes.

Blood pressure and pulse should be monitored during infusion. If desmopressin is used preoperatively, it should be administered 30 minutes prior to the scheduled procedure.

Repeat doses: The necessity for repeat administration of desmopressin or use of any blood products for hemostasis should be determined by laboratory response, as well as the clinical condition of the patient. The tendency toward tachyphylaxis (lessening of response) with repeated administration given more frequently than every 48 hours should be considered in treating each patient.

von Willebrand disease (type I) – See Hemophilia A for dosing.

➤*Children:*

Central diabetes insipidus –

12 years of age and older: See Adults for dosing for children 12 years of age and older.

Hemophilia A –

3 months of age and older: See Adults for dosing for children 3 months of age and older.

von Willebrand disease (type I) –

3 months of age and older: See Adults for dosing for children 3 months of age and older.

➤*Renal function impairment:* Desmopressin is contraindicated in patients with moderate to severe renal impairment (CrCl less than 50 mL/min).

➤*Preparation for administration:*

Hemophilia A or von Willebrand disease (type 1) – In adults and children weighing more than 10 kg, 50 mL of diluent is recommended; in children weighing 10 kg or less, 10 mL of diluent is recommended.

Other formulations – Desmopressin is also available as an intranasal preparation; however, this route of administration can be compromised by a variety of factors that can make nasal insufflation ineffective or inappropriate. These include poor intranasal absorption, nasal congestion and blockage, nasal discharge, atrophy of nasal mucosa, and severe atrophic rhinitis. Intranasal delivery may be inappropriate where there is an impaired level of consciousness. In addition, cranial surgical procedures, such as transsphenoidal hypophysectomy, create situations where an alternative route of administration is needed, as in cases of nasal packing or recovery from surgery.

➤*Storage/Stability:* Store refrigerated at 2° to 8°C (36° to 46°F).

Actions

➤*Pharmacology:* Desmopressin is a synthetic analog of the natural pituitary hormone arginine vasopressin, an antidiuretic hormone affecting renal water conservation. Desmopressin has been shown to be more potent than arginine vasopressin in increasing plasma levels of factor VIII activity in patients with hemophilia and von Willebrand disease type I.

➤*Pharmacokinetics:*

Absorption – Dose-response studies were performed in healthy persons using doses of 0.1 to 0.4 mcg/kg body weight infused over a 10-minute period. Maximal dose response occurred at 0.3 to 0.4 mcg/kg. The response to desmopressin of factor VIII activity and plasminogen activator is dose-related, with maximal plasma levels of 300% to 400% of initial concentrations obtained after infusion of 0.4 mcg/kg body weight. The increase is rapid and evident within 30 minutes, reaching a maximum at a point ranging from 90 minutes to 2 hours. The factor VIII–related antigen and ristocetin cofactor activity were also increased to a smaller degree, but still were dose-dependent.

Excretion – Desmopressin is mainly excreted in the urine. The biphasic half-lives of desmopressin were 7.8 and 75.5 minutes for the fast and slow phases, respectively, compared with 2.5 and 14.5 minutes for lysine vasopressin, another form of the hormone. As a result, desmopressin provides a prompt onset of antidiuretic action with a long duration after each administration.

DESMOPRESSIN ACETATE — INJECTION

Special populations –

Renal function impairment: A pharmacokinetic study conducted in healthy volunteers and patients with mild, moderate, and severe renal function impairment (N = 24; 6 subjects in each group) receiving a single-dose desmopressin (2 mcg) injection demonstrated a difference in desmopressin terminal half-life. Terminal half-life significantly increased from 3 hours in healthy patients to 9 hours in patients with severe renal function impairment.

Contraindications

Known hypersensitivity to desmopressin or to any of the components of the injection; moderate to severe renal function impairment (creatinine clearance [CrCl] below 50 mL/min); hyponatremia or a history of hyponatremia.

Warnings/Precautions

➤*Hyponatremia:* Very rare cases of hyponatremia have been reported from worldwide postmarketing experience in patients treated with desmopressin, a potent antidiuretic that, when administered, may lead to water intoxication and/or hyponatremia. Unless properly diagnosed and treated, hyponatremia can be fatal. Therefore, fluid restriction is recommended and should be discussed with the patient and/or guardian. Careful medical supervision is required.

When desmopressin is administered to patients who do not have need of antidiuretic hormone for its antidiuretic effect, in particular in children and elderly patients, adjust fluid intake downward to decrease the potential occurrence of water intoxication and hyponatremia. Observe all patients receiving desmopressin injection therapy for the following signs or symptoms associated with hyponatremia: headache, nausea/vomiting, decreased serum sodium, weight gain, restlessness, fatigue, lethargy, disorientation, depressed reflexes, loss of appetite, irritability, muscle weakness, muscle spasms or cramps, and abnormal mental status such as hallucinations, decreased consciousness and confusion. Severe symptoms may include 1 or a combination of the following: seizure, coma, and/or respiratory arrest. Pay particular attention to the possibility of the rare occurrence of an extreme decrease in plasma osmolality that may result in seizures, which could lead to coma.

Use desmopressin with caution in patients with habitual or psychogenic polydipsia who may be more likely to drink excessive amounts of water, putting them at greater risk of hyponatremia.

➤*von Willebrand disease (type IIB):* Do not use desmopressin to treat patients with von Willebrand disease type IIB because platelet aggregation may be induced.

➤*Cardiovascular effects:* Desmopressin has infrequently produced changes in blood pressure, causing either a slight elevation in blood pressure or a transient fall in blood pressure and a compensatory increase in heart rate. Use the drug with caution in patients with coronary artery insufficiency and/or hypertensive cardiovascular disease.

There have been rare reports of thrombotic events following desmopressin in patients predisposed to thrombus formation. No causality has been determined; however, use the drug with caution in these patients.

➤*Hypersensitivity reactions:* Severe allergic reactions have been rarely reported. Anaphylaxis has been rarely reported with IV desmopressin, including isolated cases of fatal anaphylaxis with IV desmopressin. It is not known whether antibodies to desmopressin are produced after repeated injections.

➤*Special risk:* Use desmopressin with caution in patients with conditions associated with fluid and electrolyte imbalance, such as cystic fibrosis, heart failure, and renal disorders, because these patients are prone to hyponatremia.

➤*Pregnancy: Category B.* There are no adequate and well-controlled studies in pregnant women. Because animal reproduction studies are not always predictive of human response, use this drug during pregnancy only if clearly needed.

➤*Lactation:* There have been no controlled studies in breast-feeding mothers; however, patients receiving desmopressin for diabetes insipidus have been reported to breast-feed without apparent problems in the infant. A single study in postpartum women demonstrated a marked change in plasma, but little if any change in assayable desmopressin in breast milk following an intranasal dose of 10 mcg. It is not known whether this drug is excreted in human milk. Because many drugs are excreted in human milk, exercise caution when desmopressin is administered to a breast-feeding woman.

➤*Children:* Do not use desmopressin in infants younger than 3 months of age in the treatment of hemophilia A or von Willebrand disease; safety and efficacy in children younger than 12 years of age with diabetes insipidus have not been established.

Use in infants and children will require careful fluid intake restriction to prevent possible hyponatremia and water intoxication. Discuss fluid restriction with the patient and/or guardian.

➤*Elderly:* In general, use caution in dose selection, usually starting at the low end of the dosing range, reflecting the greater frequency of decreased hepatic, renal, or cardiac function, and of concomitant disease or other drug therapy.

This drug is known to be substantially excreted by the kidney, and the risk of toxic reactions to this drug may be greater in patients with renal function impairment. Because elderly patients are more likely to have decreased renal function, take care in dose selection; it may be useful to monitor renal function. Desmopressin is contraindicated in patients with moderate to severe renal function impairment (defined as CrCl less than 50 mL/min).

Use of desmopressin in elderly patients will require careful fluid intake restrictions to prevent possible hyponatremia and water intoxication.

➤*Monitoring:* Monitor patient at regular intervals during the course of therapy to ensure adequate antidiuretic response. Monitor fluid intake and observe patient for signs and symptoms of hyponatremia. Monitor blood pressure and pulse during infusion.

Laboratory tests for assessing the status of patients with hemophilia A include levels of factor VIII coagulant, factor VIII antigen, and factor VIII ristocetin cofactor (von Willebrand factor), as well as activated partial thromboplastin time. Determine factor VIII coagulant activity before giving desmopressin for hemostasis. If factor VIII coagulant activity is present at less than 5% of normal, do not rely on desmopressin.

Laboratory tests for assessing the status of patients with von Willebrand disease include levels of factor VIII coagulant activity, factor VIII ristocetin cofactor activity, and factor VIII von Willebrand factor antigen. The skin bleeding time may be helpful in following these patients.

Laboratory tests for monitoring the patient with central diabetes insipidus include urine volume and osmolality. In some cases, plasma osmolality may be required.

Drug Interactions

➤*Pressor agents:* Although the pressor activity of desmopressin is very low compared with the antidiuretic activity, the use of doses as large as 0.3 mcg/kg of desmopressin with other pressor agents should only be done with careful patient monitoring.

Desmopressin Drug Interactions

Precipitant drug	Object drug[a]		Description
Carbamazepine	Desmopressin	↑	Coadministration may increase the risk of water intoxication. Use with caution.
Chlorpromazine	Desmopressin	↑	Coadministration may increase the risk of water intoxication. Use with caution.
Lamotrigine	Desmopressin	↑	Coadministration may increase the risk of water intoxication. Use with caution.
NSAIDs[b] (eg, naproxen)	Desmopressin	↑	Coadministration may increase the risk of water intoxication. Use with caution.
Opiate analgesics (eg, methadone)	Desmopressin	↑	Coadministration may increase the risk of water intoxication. Use with caution.
SSRIs[b] (eg, fluoxetine)	Desmopressin	↑	Coadministration may increase the risk of water intoxication. Use with caution.
TCAs[b] (eg, amitriptyline)	Desmopressin	↑	Coadministration may increase the risk of water intoxication. Use with caution.

[a] ↑ = object drug increased.
[b] NSAIDs = nonsteroidal anti-inflammatory drugs; SSRIs = selective serotonin reuptake inhibitors; TCAs = tricyclic antidepressants.

Adverse Reactions

➤*Cardiovascular:* Desmopressin has infrequently produced changes in blood pressure, causing either a slight elevation or a transient fall and a compensatory increase in heart rate.

➤*Dermatologic:* Occasional facial flushing has been reported with the administration of desmopressin.

➤*Hypersensitivity:* Severe allergic reactions, including anaphylaxis, have rarely been reported with desmopressin.

➤*Local:* Occasionally, injection of desmopressin has produced local burning pain, erythema, or swelling.

➤*Miscellaneous:* Infrequently, desmopressin has produced mild abdominal cramps, nausea, transient headache, and vulval pain. These symptoms disappeared with reduction in dosage.

➤*Postmarketing:* There have been rare reports of thrombotic events (acute cerebrovascular thrombosis, acute myocardial infarction) following desmopressin injection in patients predisposed to thrombus formation and rare reports of hyponatremic convulsions associated with concomitant use with the following medications: oxybutynin and imipramine.

Overdosage

➤*Symptoms:* Signs of overdose may include confusion, drowsiness, continuing headache, problems with passing urine, and rapid weight gain caused by fluid retention.

➤*Treatment:* There is no known specific antidote for desmopressin. In case of overdosage, reduce the dosage, decrease the frequency of administration, or withdraw the drug according to the severity of the condition.

Patient Information

Advise the patient and/or guardian that desmopressin therapy requires careful fluid intake restriction to prevent possible hyponatremia and water intoxication.

TOLVAPTAN

Rx	Samsca (Otsuka)	Tablets; oral: 15 mg	Lactose. OTSUKA 15. Blue, triangular. In UD 10s.
		30 mg	Lactose. OTSUKA 30. Blue, round. In UD 10s.

TOLVAPTAN — ORAL

WARNING

Initiation of therapy – Initiate and reinitiate tolvaptan in patients only in a hospital where serum sodium can be closely monitored.

Monitor serum sodium – Too rapid correction of hyponatremia (eg, more than 12 mEq/L per 24 hours) can cause osmotic demyelination, resulting in dysarthria, mutism, dysphagia, lethargy, affective changes, spastic quadriparesis, seizures, coma, and death. In susceptible patients, including those with severe malnutrition, alcoholism, or advanced liver disease, slower rates of correction may be advisable.

Indications

➤*Hypervolemic and euvolemic hyponatremia:* For the treatment of clinically significant Hypervolemic and euvolemic hyponatremia (serum sodium of less than 125 mEq/L or less marked hyponatremia that is symptomatic and has resisted correction with fluid restriction), including patients with heart failure, cirrhosis, and syndrome of inappropriate antidiuretic hormone (SIADH).

Important limitations – Patients requiring intervention to raise serum sodium urgently to prevent or to treat serious neurological symptoms should not be treated with tolvaptan.

It has not been established that raising serum sodium with tolvaptan provides a symptomatic benefit to patients.

Administration and Dosage

➤*Maximum dose:* 60 mg daily.

➤*General dosing considerations:* Patients should be in a hospital for initiation and reinitiation of therapy to evaluate the therapeutic response and because too rapid correction of hyponatremia can cause osmotic demyelination, resulting in dysarthria, mutism, dysphagia, lethargy, affective changes, spastic quadriparesis, seizures, coma, and death.

Avoid fluid restriction during the first 24 hours of therapy. Patients receiving tolvaptan should be advised that they can continue ingestion of fluid in response to thirst.

➤*Adults:*

Hypervolemic and euvolemic hyponatremia –

Maximum dose: 60 mg once daily.

Initial dosage: 15 mg administered once daily without regard to meals.

Dosage titration: After at least 24 hours, increase the dosage to 30 mg once daily to a maximum of 60 mg once daily, as needed to achieve the desired level of serum sodium.

Concomitant therapy:

• *CYP3A4 inhibitors* – Tolvaptan is metabolized by cytochrome P450 3A (CYP3A), and use with strong CYP3A inhibitors causes a marked (5-fold) increase in exposure. Avoid coadministration with moderate CYP3A inhibitors; use with strong CYP3A inhibitors is contraindicated.

• *CYP3A5 inducers* – Coadministration of tolvaptan with potent CYP3A inducers (eg, rifampin) reduces tolvaptan plasma concentrations by 85%. Patient response should be monitored and the dose adjusted accordingly.

• *P-glycoprotein inhibitors* – Tolvaptan is a substrate of P-glycoprotein. Coadministration of tolvaptan with inhibitors of P-glycoprotein (eg, cyclosporine) may necessitate a decrease in tolvaptan dose.

➤*Therapeutic drug monitoring:* During initiation and titration, frequently monitor for changes in serum electrolytes and volume.

➤*Discontinuation of therapy:* Following discontinuation from tolvaptan, patients should be advised to resume fluid restriction and should be monitored for changes in serum sodium and volume status.

➤*Storage/Stability:* Store at 25° (77°F); excursions are permitted between 15° and 30°C (59° and 86°F).

Actions

➤*Pharmacology:* Tolvaptan is a selective vasopressin V_2-receptor antagonist with an affinity for the V_2-receptor that is 1.8 times that of native arginine vasopressin (AVP). Tolvaptan affinity for the V_2-receptor is 29 times greater than for the V_{1a}-receptor. When taken orally, 15 to 60 mg doses of tolvaptan antagonize the effect of vasopressin and cause an increase in urine water excretion that results in an increase in free water clearance (aquaresis), a decrease in urine osmolality, and a resulting increase in serum sodium concentrations. Urinary excretion of sodium and potassium and plasma potassium concentrations are not significantly changed. Tolvaptan metabolites have no or weak antagonist activity for human V_2-receptors compared with tolvaptan.

Plasma concentrations of native AVP may increase (average, 2 to 9 pg/mL) with tolvaptan administration.

Pharmacodynamics – In healthy subjects receiving a single dose of tolvaptan 60 mg, the onset of the aquaretic and sodium increasing effects occurs within 2 to 4 hours postdose. A peak effect of approximately 6 mEq increase in serum sodium and approximately 9 mL/min increase in urine excretion rate is observed between 4 and 8 hours postdose; thus, the pharmacological activity lags behind the plasma concentrations of tolvaptan. Approximately 60% of the peak effect on serum sodium is sustained at 24 hours postdose, but the urinary excretion rate is no longer elevated by that time. Doses higher than tolvaptan 60 mg do not increase aquaresis or serum sodium further. The effects of tolvaptan in the recommended dosage range of 15 to 60 mg once daily appear to be limited to aquaresis and the resulting increase in sodium concentration.

In a parallel-arm, double-blind (for tolvaptan and placebo), placebo- and positive-controlled, multiple-dose study of the effect of tolvaptan on the QTc interval, 172 healthy subjects were randomized to tolvaptan 30 mg, tolvaptan 300 mg, placebo, or moxifloxacin 400 mg once daily. At both the 30 and 300 mg doses, no significant effect of administering tolvaptan on the QTc interval was detected on day 1 and 5. At the 300 mg dose, peak tolvaptan plasma concentrations were approximately 4-fold higher than the peak concentrations following a 30 mg dose. Moxifloxacin increased the QT interval by 12 msec at 2 hours after dosing on day 1 and 17 msec at 1 hour after dosing on day 5, indicating that the study was adequately designed and conducted to detect tolvaptan's effect on the QT interval, had an effect been present.

➤*Pharmacokinetics:*

Absorption/Distribution – In healthy subjects, the pharmacokinetics of tolvaptan after single doses of up to 480 mg and multiple dosages of up to 300 mg once daily have been examined. Area under the curve (AUC) increases proportionally with dose; however, after administration of doses of 60 mg or more, maximal drug concentration [C_{max}] increases less than proportionally with dose. The pharmacokinetic properties of tolvaptan are stereospecific, with a steady-state ratio of the S-(-) to the R-(+) enantiomer of about 3. The absolute bioavailability of tolvaptan is unknown. At least 40% of the dose is absorbed as tolvaptan or metabolites. Peak concentrations of tolvaptan are observed between 2 and 4 hours postdose. Tolvaptan is highly plasma protein bound (99%) and distributed into an apparent volume of distribution of approximately 3 L/kg.

Food effects: Food does not impact the bioavailability of tolvaptan.

Metabolism/Excretion – In vitro data indicate that tolvaptan is a substrate and inhibitor of P-glycoprotein. Tolvaptan is eliminated entirely by nonrenal routes and mainly, if not exclusively, metabolized by CYP3A. After oral dosing, clearance is approximately 4 mL/min/kg and the terminal phase half-life is approximately 12 hours. The accumulation factor of tolvaptan with the once-daily regimen is 1.3 and the trough concentrations amount to 16% or less of the peak concentrations, suggesting a dominant half-life somewhat shorter than 12 hours. There is marked intersubject variation in peak and average exposure to tolvaptan with a percent coefficient of variation ranging between 30% and 60%.

Special populations –

Renal function impairment: Exposure and response to tolvaptan in subjects with creatinine clearance (CrCl) ranging between 10 and 79 mL/min and patients with normal renal function are not different.

Hepatic function impairment: Moderate or severe hepatic impairment or congestive heart failure decrease the clearance and increase the volume of distribution of tolvaptan, but the respective changes are not clinically relevant.

Hyponatremia: In patients with hyponatremia of any origin, the clearance of tolvaptan is reduced to approximately 2 mL/min/kg.

Contraindications

➤*Urgent need to raise serum sodium acutely:* Tolvaptan has not been studied in a setting of urgent need to raise serum sodium acutely.

➤*Inability of the patient to sense or appropriately respond to thirst* : Patients who are unable to autoregulate fluid balance are at substantially increased risk of incurring an overly rapid correction of serum sodium, hypernatremia, and hypovolemia.

➤*Hypovolemic hyponatremia:* Risks associated with worsening hypovolemia, including complications such as hypotension and renal failure, outweigh possible benefits.

➤*Concomitant use of strong CYP3A inhibitors:* Ketoconazole 200 mg administered with tolvaptan increased tolvaptan exposure by 5-fold. Larger doses would be expected to produce larger increases in tolvaptan exposure. There is no adequate experience to define the dose adjustment that would be needed to allow safe use of tolvaptan with strong CYP3A inhibitors such as clarithromycin, ketoconazole, itraconazole, ritonavir, indinavir, nelfinavir, saquinavir, nefazodone, and telithromycin.

➤*Patients who are anuric:* In patients unable to make urine, no clinical benefit can be expected.

Warnings/Precautions

➤*Rapid correction of serum sodium:* Osmotic demyelination syndrome is a risk associated with too rapid correction of hyponatremia (eg, more than 12 mEq/L per 24 hours). Osmotic demyelination results in dysarthria, mutism, dysphagia, lethargy, affective changes, spastic quadriparesis, seizures, coma, or death. In susceptible patients including those with severe malnutrition, alcoholism, or advanced liver disease, slower rates of correction may be advisable. In controlled clinical trials in which tolvaptan was administered in titrated dosages starting at 15 mg once daily, 7% of tolvaptan-treated subjects with a serum sodium less than 130 mEq/L had an increase

TOLVAPTAN — ORAL

in serum sodium greater than 8 mEq/L at approximately 8 hours and 2% had an increase greater than 12 mEq/L at 24 hours. Approximately 1% of placebo-treated subjects with a serum sodium less than 130 mEq/L had a rise greater than 8 mEq/L at 8 hours, and no patient had a rise greater than 12 mEq/L per 24 hours. None of the patients in these studies had evidence of osmotic demyelination syndrome or related neurological sequelae, but such complications have been reported following too-rapid correction of serum sodium. Monitor patients treated with tolvaptan to assess serum sodium concentrations and neurologic status, especially during initiation and after titration. Subjects with SIADH or very low baseline serum sodium concentrations may be at greater risk for too-rapid correction of serum sodium. In patients receiving tolvaptan who develop a too-rapid rise in serum sodium, discontinue or interrupt treatment with tolvaptan, and consider administration of hypotonic fluid. Fluid restriction during the first 24 hours of therapy with tolvaptan may increase the likelihood of overly rapid correction of serum sodium and should generally be avoided. (See Black Box Warning.)

➤*Patients with cirrhosis:* In patients with cirrhosis treated with tolvaptan in hyponatremia trials, GI bleeding was reported in 6 of 63 (10%) tolvaptan-treated patients and 1 of 57 (2%) placebo-treated patients. Use tolvaptan in patients with cirrhosis only when the need to treat outweighs this risk.

➤*Dehydration and hypovolemia:* Tolvaptan therapy induces copious aquaresis, which is normally partially offset by fluid intake. Dehydration and hypovolemia can occur, especially in potentially volume-depleted patients receiving diuretics or those who are fluid restricted. In multiple-dose, placebo-controlled trials in which 607 hyponatremic patients were treated with tolvaptan, the incidence of dehydration was 3.3% for tolvaptan and 1.5% for placebo-treated patients. In patients receiving tolvaptan who develop medically significant signs or symptoms of hypovolemia, interrupt or discontinue tolvaptan therapy and provide supportive care with careful management of vital signs, fluid balance, and electrolytes. Fluid restriction during therapy with tolvaptan may increase the risk of dehydration and hypovolemia. Patients receiving tolvaptan should continue ingestion of fluid in response to thirst.

➤*Coadministration with hypertonic saline:* There is no experience with concomitant use of tolvaptan and hypertonic saline. Concomitant use with hypertonic saline is not recommended.

➤*Hyperkalemia:* Treatment with tolvaptan is associated with an acute reduction of the extracellular fluid volume that could result in increased serum potassium. Monitor serum potassium levels after initiation of tolvaptan treatment in patients with a serum potassium greater than 5 mEq/L and in those who are receiving drugs known to increase serum potassium levels.

➤*Patients with congestive heart failure:* The exposure to tolvaptan in patients with congestive heart failure is not clinically relevantly increased. No dose adjustment is necessary.

➤*Renal function impairment:* Exposure and response to tolvaptan are similar in patients with a CrCl of 10 to 79 mL/min and in patients without renal impairment. No dose adjustment is necessary. Exposure and response to tolvaptan in patients with a CrCl of less than 10 mL/min or in patients on long-term dialysis have not been studied. No benefit can be expected in patients who are anuric.

➤*Hepatic function impairment:* Moderate and severe hepatic impairment do not affect exposure to tolvaptan to a clinically relevant extent. No dose adjustment of tolvaptan is necessary.

➤*Pregnancy: Category C.* There are no adequate and well-controlled studies of tolvaptan use in pregnant women. In animal studies, cleft palate, brachymelia, microphthalmia, skeletal malformations, decreased fetal weight, delayed fetal ossification, and embryo-fetal death occurred. Use tolvaptan during pregnancy only if the potential benefit justifies the potential risk to the fetus.

In pregnant rats, oral administration of tolvaptan at 10, 100, and 1,000 mg/kg/day during organogenesis was associated with a reduction in maternal body weight gain and food consumption at 100 and 1,000 mg/kg/day, and reduced fetal weight and delayed ossification of fetuses at 1,000 mg/kg/day (162 times the maximum recommended human dose [MRHD] on a body surface area [BSA] basis). Oral administration of tolvaptan at 100, 300, and 1,000 mg/kg/day to pregnant rabbits during organogenesis was associated with reductions in maternal body weight gain and food consumption at all doses, and abortions at mid- and high-doses. At 1,000 mg/kg/day (324 times the MRHD), increased incidences of embryo-fetal death, fetal microphthalmia, open eyelids, cleft palate, brachymelia, and skeletal malformations were observed.

In embryo-fetal development studies, pregnant rats and rabbits received oral tolvaptan during organogenesis. Rats received 2 to 162 times the MRHD of tolvaptan (on a BSA basis). Reduced fetal weights and delayed fetal ossification occurred at 162 times the MRHD. Signs of maternal toxicity (reduction in body weight gain and food consumption) occurred at 16 and 162 times the MRHD. When pregnant rabbits received oral tolvaptan at 32 to 324 times the MRHD (on a BSA basis), there were reductions in maternal body weight gain and food consumption at all doses, and increased abortions at the mid and high doses (approximately 97 and 324 times the MRHD). At 324 times the MRHD, there were increased rates of embryo-fetal death, fetal microphthalmia, open eyelids, cleft palate, brachymelia, and skeletal malformations.

➤*Lactation:* It is not known whether tolvaptan is excreted into human milk. Tolvaptan is excreted into the milk of lactating rats. Because many drugs are excreted into human milk and because of the potential for serious adverse reactions in breast-feeding infants from tolvaptan, make a decision to discontinue breast-feeding or tolvaptan, taking into consideration the importance of tolvaptan to the mother.

➤*Children:* Safety and effectiveness of tolvaptan in children have not been established.

➤*Elderly:* Of the total number of hyponatremic subjects treated with tolvaptan in clinical studies, 42% were 65 years of age and older, while 19% were 75 years of age and older. Increasing age has no effect on tolvaptan plasma concentrations.

➤*Monitoring:* Frequently monitor for changes in serum electrolytes and volume. Assess serum sodium concentrations and neurologic status, especially during initiation and titration. Monitor serum potassium levels after initiation of tolvaptan treatment in patients with a serum potassium greater than 5 mEq/L and in those who are receiving drugs known to increase serum potassium levels.

Drug Interactions

Tolvaptan Drug Interactions

Precipitant drug	Object drug[a]		Description
Aprepitant	Tolvaptan	↑	CYP3A inhibitors may increase the plasma concentration of tolvaptan. Adjust the dose of tolvaptan as needed.
Azole antifungals (eg, itraconazole, ketoconazole)	Tolvaptan	↑	Ketoconazole increased tolvaptan exposure by 5-fold. Coadministration is contraindicated.
Barbiturates	Tolvaptan	↓	CYP3A inducers may reduce the plasma concentration of tolvaptan. Adjust the dose of tolvaptan as needed.
Calcium channel blockers (eg, diltiazem, verapamil)	Tolvaptan	↑	CYP3A inhibitors may increase the plasma concentration of tolvaptan. Adjust the dose of tolvaptan as needed.
Carbamazepine	Tolvaptan	↓	CYP3A inducers may reduce the plasma concentration of tolvaptan. Adjust the dose of tolvaptan as needed.
Erythromycins (eg, clarithromycin)	Tolvaptan	↑	Clarithromycin may increase tolvaptan plasma levels by up to 5-fold. Coadministration is contraindicated. Use erythromycin with caution; adjust dose as needed.
Nefazodone	Tolvaptan	↑	CYP3A inhibitors may increase tolvaptan plasma levels by up to 5-fold. Coadministration is contraindicated.
P-glycoprotein inhibitors (eg, cyclosporine)	Tolvaptan	↑	Reduction in the tolvaptan dose may be required with coadministration.
Phenytoin	Tolvaptan	↓	CYP3A inducers may reduce the plasma concentration of tolvaptan. Adjust the dose of tolvaptan as needed.
Protease inhibitors (eg, indinavir, nelfinavir, ritonavir)	Tolvaptan	↑	CYP3A inhibitors may increase tolvaptan plasma levels by up to 5-fold. Coadministration is contraindicated.
Rifamycins (eg, rifampin)	Tolvaptan	↓	CYP3A inducers may reduce the plasma concentration of tolvaptan. Adjust the dose of tolvaptan as needed.
St. John's wort	Tolvaptan	↓	CYP3A inducers may reduce the plasma concentration of tolvaptan. Adjust the dose of tolvaptan as needed.
Telithromycin	Tolvaptan	↑	CYP3A inhibitors may increase tolvaptan plasma levels by up to 5-fold. Coadministration is contraindicated.
Tolvaptan	Angiotensin-converting enzyme inhibitors	↑	Coadministration may increase the hyperkalemic effects of both agents.
Tolvaptan	Angiotensin receptor blockers	↑	Coadministration may increase the hyperkalemic effects of both agents.
Tolvaptan	Digoxin	↑	Tolvaptan coadministration resulted in a 1.3-fold increase in digoxin exposure.

TOLVAPTAN — ORAL

Tolvaptan Drug Interactions

Precipitant drug	Object drug[a]		Description
Tolvaptan	Lovastatin	↑	Coadministration increased lovastatin and its metabolites by 1.4- and 1.3-fold, respectively.
Tolvaptan	Potassium-sparing diuretics	↑	Coadministration may increase the hyperkalemic effects of both agents.

[a] ↑ = object drug increased; ↓ = object drug decreased.

➤*Drug/Food interactions:* Coadministration with grapefruit juice results in a 1.8-fold increase in exposure to tolvaptan.

Adverse Reactions

➤*Clinical trials experience:* In multiple-dose, placebo-controlled trials, 607 patients with hyponatremia (serum sodium of less than 135 mEq/L) were treated with tolvaptan. The patients were a mean of 62 years of age; 70% of patients were men and 82% were white. One hundred eighty-nine tolvaptan-treated patients had a serum sodium of less than 130 mEq/L, and 52 patients had a serum sodium of less than 125 mEq/L. Hyponatremia was attributed to cirrhosis in 17% of patients, heart failure in 68%, and SIADH/other in 16%. Of these patients, 223 were treated with the recommended dose titration (15 mg titrated to 60 mg as needed to raise serum sodium).

Overall, over 4,000 patients have been treated with oral doses of tolvaptan in open-label or placebo-controlled clinical trials. Approximately 650 of these patients had hyponatremia; approximately 219 of these patients with hyponatremia were treated with tolvaptan for 6 months or more.

The most common adverse reactions (incidence at least 5% more than placebo) seen in two 30-day, double-blind, placebo-controlled hyponatremia trials in which tolvaptan was administered in titrated dosages (15 to 60 mg once daily) were asthenia, constipation, dry mouth, hyperglycemia, pollakiuria or polyuria, and thirst. In these trials, 10% (23/223) of tolvaptan-treated patients discontinued treatment because of an adverse reaction, compared with 12% (26/220) of placebo-treated patients; no adverse reaction resulting in discontinuation of trial medication occurred at an incidence of more than 1% in tolvaptan-treated patients.

Adverse reactions reported in tolvaptan-treated patients with hyponatremia (serum sodium of less than 135 mEq/L) and at a rate at least 2% greater than placebo-treated patients in two 30-day, double-blind, placebo-controlled trials. In these studies, 223 patients were exposed to tolvaptan (starting dose 15 mg, titrated to 30 and 60 mg as needed to raise serum sodium). Adverse reactions resulting in death in these trials were 6% in tolvaptan-treated patients and 6% in placebo-treated patients.

Tolvaptan Adverse Reactions (> 2%)

Adverse reactions	Tolvaptan 15 to 60 mg/day (n = 223)	Placebo (n = 220)
GI		
Anorexia[a]	4%	1%
Constipation	7%	2%
Dry mouth	13%	4%
Metabolism/Nutritional		
Hyperglycemia[b]	6%	1%
Thirst[c]	16%	5%
Miscellaneous		
Asthenia	9%	4%
Pollakiuria or polyuria[d]	11%	3%
Pyrexia	4%	1%

[a] Includes decreased appetite.
[b] Includes diabetes mellitus.
[c] Includes polydipsia.
[d] Includes urine output increased, micturition urgency, nocturia.

In a subgroup of patients with hyponatremia (N = 475, serum sodium of less than 135 mEq/L) enrolled in a double-blind, placebo-controlled trial (mean duration of treatment, 9 months) of patients with worsening heart failure, the following adverse reactions occurred in tolvaptan-treated patients at a rate at least 2% greater than placebo: mortality (42% tolvaptan, 38% placebo), nausea (21% tolvaptan, 16% placebo), thirst (12% tolvaptan, 2% placebo), dry mouth (7% tolvaptan, 2% placebo), and polyuria or pollakiuria (4% tolvaptan, 1% placebo).

Adverse reactions in less than 2% – The following adverse reactions occurred in less than 2% of patients with hyponatremia treated with tolvaptan and at a rate greater than placebo in double-blind, placebo-controlled trials (n = 607 tolvaptan; n = 518 placebo) or in less than 2% of patients in an uncontrolled trial of patients with hyponatremia (n = 111) and are not mentioned elsewhere in the label.

Cardiovascular – Cerebrovascular accident, deep vein thrombosis, disseminated intravascular coagulation, intracardiac thrombus, ventricular fibrillation.

GU – Urethral hemorrhage, vaginal hemorrhage.

Respiratory – Pulmonary embolism, respiratory failure.

Miscellaneous – Diabetic ketoacidosis, ischemic colitis, prothrombin time prolonged, rhabdomyolysis.

Overdosage

➤*Symptoms:* Single oral doses of up to 480 mg and multiple doses of up to 300 mg once daily for 5 days have been well tolerated in studies of healthy subjects. There is no specific antidote for tolvaptan intoxication. The signs and symptoms of an acute overdose can be anticipated to be those of excessive pharmacologic effect: a rise in serum sodium concentration, dehydration/hypovolemia, polyuria, and thirst.

The oral median lethal dose of tolvaptan in rats and dogs is greater than 2,000 mg/kg. No mortality was observed in rats or dogs following single oral doses of 2,000 mg/kg (maximum feasible dose). A single oral dose of 2,000 mg/kg was lethal in mice, and symptoms of toxicity in affected mice included decreased locomotor activity, staggering gait, tremor, and hypothermia.

➤*Treatment:* If overdose occurs, estimation of the severity of poisoning is an important first step. Obtain a thorough history and details of overdose and perform a physical examination.

Consider the possibility of multi-drug involvement. Involve symptomatic and supportive care in treatment, with respiratory, electrocardiogram (ECG), and blood pressure monitoring, and water/electrolyte supplements as needed. A profuse and prolonged aquaresis should be anticipated, which, if not matched by oral fluid ingestion, should be replaced with intravenous hypotonic fluids, while closely monitoring electrolytes and fluid balance.

Begin ECG monitoring immediately and continue until ECG parameters are within normal ranges. Dialysis may not be effective in removing tolvaptan because of its high binding affinity for human plasma protein (greater than 99%). Continue close medical supervision and monitoring until the patient recovers.

Patient Information

As a part of patient counseling, health care providers must review the tolvaptan Medication Guide with every patient.

Advise patients to inform their health care provider if they are taking or plan to take any prescription or nonprescription drugs because there is a potential for interactions.

Advise patients to inform their health care provider if they use strong (eg, ketoconazole, itraconazole, clarithromycin, telithromycin, nelfinavir, saquinavir, indinavir, ritonavir) or moderate CYP3A inhibitors (eg, aprepitant, erythromycin, diltiazem, verapamil, fluconazole) or P-glycoprotein inhibitors (eg, cyclosporine).

Advise patients not to breast-feed an infant if they are taking tolvaptan.

CONIVAPTAN HYDROCHLORIDE

Rx	**Vaprisol** (Astellas Pharma)	**Injection, solution, concentrate**: 5 mg/mL	Propylene glycol 1.2 g, ethanol 0.4 g. In 4 mL amps.
Rx	**Vaprisol Premixed in Dextrose 5%** (Astellas Pharma)	**Injection, solution:** 0.2 mg/mL	Dextrose 5 g. In 100 mL single-use *Intravia* plastic container.

CONIVAPTAN HYDROCHLORIDE — INJECTION

Indications

➤*Euvolemic and hypervolemic hyponatremia:* For the treatment of euvolemic and hypervolemic hyponatremia in hospitalized patients.

Administration and Dosage

➤*General dosing considerations:* For intravenous (IV) use only. For use in hospitalized patients only.

Conivaptan ampule should be diluted only with dextrose 5% injection (see Preparation for Administration).

➤*Adults:*

Euvolemic and hypervolemic hyponatremia –

Usual dosage: The loading dose should be followed by conivaptan 20 mg administered as a continuous IV infusion throughout a 24-hour period. Following the initial day of treatment, conivaptan is to be administered for an additional 1 to 3 days in a continuous infusion of 20 mg/day.

Maximum dose: The maximum daily dosage of conivaptan (after the loading dose) is 40 mg/day.

Loading dose: Begin with a loading dose of 20 mg IV administered throughout a 30-minute period.

CONIVAPTAN HYDROCHLORIDE — INJECTION

Dosage titration: If serum sodium is not rising at the desired rate, conivaptan may be titrated upward to a dosage of 40 mg/day, again administered as a continuous IV infusion.

Dosage adjustment: For patients who develop an undesirably rapid rate of rise of serum sodium, conivaptan should be discontinued, and serum sodium and neurologic status should be carefully monitored. If the serum sodium continues to rise, conivaptan should not be resumed. If hyponatremia persists or recurs and the patient has had no evidence of neurologic sequelae of rapid rise in serum sodium, conivaptan may be resumed at a reduced dose.

For patients who develop hypovolemia or hypotension while receiving conivaptan, conivaptan should be discontinued, and volume status and vital signs should be frequently monitored. Once the patient is again euvolemic and is no longer hypotensive, conivaptan may be resumed at a reduced dose if the patient remains hyponatremic.

Duration of therapy: The total duration of infusion of conivaptan (after the loading dose) should not exceed 4 days.

Monitoring: Frequently monitor serum sodium and volume status. An overly rapid rise in serum sodium (greater than 12 mEq/L per 24 hours) may result in serious neurologic sequelae.

➤*Elderly:* In general, the adverse reaction profile in elderly patients was similar to that seen in the general study population.

➤*Preparation for administration:*

Ampule –

Loading dose: Withdraw 4 mL (20 mg) of conivaptan and add to an infusion bag containing dextrose 5% injection 100 mL. Gently invert the bag several times to ensure complete mixing of the solution.

Continuous infusion: To prepare a continuous IV infusion containing conivaptan 20 mg, withdraw 4 mL (20 mg) from a single ampule of conivaptan and dilute into an IV bag containing 250 mL of dextrose 5% injection. Gently invert the bag several times to ensure complete mixing of the solution.

To prepare a continuous IV infusion containing conivaptan 40 mg, withdraw 4 mL (20 mg) from each of 2 ampules of conivaptan (8 mL [40 mg] of conivaptan) and dilute into an IV bag containing 250 mL of dextrose 5% injection. Gently invert the bag several times to ensure complete mixing of the solution.

Conivaptan premixed – Supplied in single-use, 100 mL flexible plastic containers containing a sterile, premixed dilute, ready-to-use, nonpyrogenic solution of conivaptan hydrochloride 0.2 mg/mL (20 mg per 100 mL) in dextrose 5%. No further dilution of this preparation is necessary.

Do not remove container from overwrap until ready to use. The overwrap is a moisture and light barrier. The inner container maintains the sterility of the product.

Tear overwrap down the side at the slit and remove solution from container. Some opacity of the plastic caused by moisture absorption during the sterilization process may be observed. This is normal and does not affect the solution quality or safety. The opacity will diminish gradually. After removing overwrap, check for minute leaks by squeezing the inner container firmly. If leaks are found, discard solution, as sterility may be impaired.

Suspend container from eyelet support and remove protector from outlet port at bottom of container. Attach administration set and refer to complete directions accompanying set.

➤*Administration:* For IV use only. For use in hospitalized patients only. Administer conivaptan through large veins and change the infusion site every 24 hours to minimize the risk of vascular irritation.

Ampule –

Loading dose: The contents of the IV bag should be administered during a 30-minute period.

Continuous infusion: The contents of the IV bag should be administered during a 24-hour period.

Conivaptan premixed –

Loading dose: Administer conivaptan 20 mg per 100 mL flexible plastic container over 30 minutes.

Continuous infusion: For patients requiring conivaptan 20 mg/day, administer one 20 mg per 100 mL flexible plastic container over 24 hours.

For patients requiring conivaptan 40 mg/day, administer 2 consecutive 20 mg per 100 mL flexible plastic containers over 24 hours. Because the flexible container is for single use only, any unused portion should be discarded.

Do not use plastic containers in series connections. Such use could result in air embolism because of residual air being drawn from the primary container before administration of the fluid from the secondary container is completed.

➤*Admixture compatibility:* Conivaptan ampule is compatible with dextrose 5% and should be diluted only with dextrose 5% injection.

Conivaptan ampule should not be mixed or administered with Ringer's lactate injection or sodium chloride 0.9% injection. Compatibility with other drugs has not been studied; therefore, conivaptan should not be combined with any other product in the same IV line or container.

➤*Storage/Stability:*

Ampule – Store at 25°C (77°F); excursions are permitted to 15° to 30°C (59° to 86°F). Do not store below 15°C (59°F). Store ampules in their cardboard container and protect from light until ready for use.

The conivaptan ampule is for single use only. Discard unused contents of the ampule. Use the diluted solution of conivaptan immediately and complete administration within 24 hours of mixing.

Conivaptan premixed – Store at 25°C (77°F); however, brief exposure up to 40°C (104°F) does not adversely affect the product. Avoid excessive heat. Protect from freezing. Protect from light until ready to use.

Actions

➤*Pharmacology:* Conivaptan is a dual arginine vasopressin (AVP) antagonist with nanomolar affinity for human V_{1A} and V_2 receptors in vitro. The level of AVP in circulating blood is critical for the regulation of water and electrolyte balance and is usually elevated in both euvolemic and hypervolemic hyponatremia. The AVP effect is mediated through V_2 receptors, which are functionally coupled to aquaporin channels in the apical membrane of the collecting ducts of the kidney. These receptors help to maintain plasma osmolality within the normal range. The predominant pharmacodynamic effect of conivaptan in the treatment of hyponatremia is through its V_2 antagonism of AVP in the renal collecting ducts, an effect that results in aquaresis, or excretion of free water. The pharmacodynamic effects of conivaptan include increased free water excretion (ie, effective water clearance), generally accompanied by increased net fluid loss, increased urine output, and decreased urine osmolality.

➤*Pharmacokinetics:* In an open-label safety and efficacy study, the pharmacokinetics of conivaptan were characterized in hypervolemic or euvolemic hyponatremia patients (20 to 92 years of age) receiving conivaptan 20 mg as a loading dose (infused during a 30-minute period), followed by a continuous infusion of 20 or 40 mg/day for 4 days.

The pharmacokinetic parameters are summarized in the following table.

Conivaptan Pharmacokinetic Parameters		
Parameter	Conivaptan 20 mg/day IV	Conivaptan 40 mg/day IV
Conivaptan concentration at the end of loading dose (ng/mL, at 0.5 h)		
N[a]	31	170
Median (range)	659.4 (144.5 to 1,587.6)	679.5 (0 to 1,910.8)
Conivaptan concentration at the end of infusion (ng/mL, at 96 hours)		
N[a]	30	172
Median (range)	117.6 (4.9 to 938.3)	215.7 (2.1 to 1,999.3)
Elimination half-life (h)		
N[b]	8	8
Median (range)	5.3 (3.3 to 9.3)	8.1 (4.1 to 22.5)
Clearance (L/h)		
N[b]	8	8
Median (range)	16.1 (7.2 to 37.6)	8.73 (2.1 to 20.9)

[a] Number from the rich and the sparse pharmacokinetic sampling.
[b] Number from the rich pharmacokinetic sampling.

Absorption/Distribution – The pharmacokinetics of conivaptan have been characterized in healthy subjects, special populations, and patients following both oral and IV dosing regimens. The pharmacokinetics of conivaptan following IV infusion (40 to 80 mg/day) and oral administration are nonlinear, and inhibition by conivaptan of its own metabolism seems to be the major factor for the nonlinearity. The intersubject variability of conivaptan pharmacokinetics is high (94% coefficient of variation in clearance).

The pharmacokinetics of conivaptan and its metabolites were characterized in healthy men administered conivaptan 20 mg as a loading dose (infused during a 30-minute period), followed by a continuous infusion of 40 mg/day for 3 days. Mean maximum drug concentration (C_{max}) for conivaptan was 619 ng/mL and occurred at the end of the loading dose. Plasma concentrations reached a minimum at approximately 12 hours after the start of the loading dose, then gradually increased throughout the duration of the infusion to a mean concentration of 188 ng/mL at the end of the infusion.

Conivaptan is extensively bound to human plasma proteins, being 99% bound over the concentration range of approximately 10 to 1,000 ng/mL.

Metabolism/Excretion – CYP3A4 was identified as the sole cytochrome P450 (CYP-450) isozyme responsible for the metabolism of conivaptan. Four metabolites have been identified. The pharmacological activity of the metabolites at V_{1A} and V_2 receptors ranged from approximately 3% to 50% and 50% to 100% that of conivaptan, respectively. The combined exposure of the metabolites following IV administration of conivaptan is approximately 7% that of conivaptan and, therefore, their contribution to the clinical effect of conivaptan is minimal.

After IV (10 mg) or oral (20 mg) administration of conivaptan in a mass balance study, approximately 83% of the dose was excreted in feces as total radioactivity and 12% in urine throughout several days of collection. During the first 24 hours after dosing, approximately 1% of the IV dose was excreted in urine as intact conivaptan.

The mean terminal elimination half-life after conivaptan infusion was 5 hours, and the mean clearance was 15.2 L/h.

Special populations –

Renal function impairment: The effect of renal function impairment on the elimination of conivaptan after IV administration has not been evaluated. However, following administration of oral conivaptan, the area under the curve (AUC) for conivaptan was up to 80% higher in patients with renal function impairment (creatinine clearance [CrCl] less than 60 mL/min/1.73 m²) compared with those with healthy renal function. IV conivaptan resulted in higher conivaptan exposure than oral conivaptan in study subjects without renal function impairment. Exercise caution when administering conivaptan to patients with renal function impairment.

CONIVAPTAN HYDROCHLORIDE — INJECTION

Hepatic function impairment: The effect of hepatic function impairment (including ascites, cirrhosis, or portal hypertension) on the elimination of conivaptan after IV administration has not been systemically evaluated. However, increased systemic exposures after administration of oral conivaptan (up to a mean 2.8-fold increase) have been seen in patients with stable cirrhosis and moderate hepatic function impairment. IV conivaptan resulted in higher conivaptan exposure than did oral conivaptan in study subjects without hepatic function impairment. Exercise caution when administering conivaptan to patients with hepatic function impairment.

Elderly: Following a single oral dose of conivaptan (15, 30, or 60 mg), drug exposure (AUC) in elderly men and women (65 to 90 years of age) compared with that seen in younger men was similar for the 15 and 30 mg doses but increased nearly 2-fold at the 60 mg dose.

Contraindications

Hypovolemic hyponatremia; coadministration with potent CYP3A4 inhibitors such as ketoconazole, itraconazole, clarithromycin, ritonavir, and indinavir; patients with known allergy to corn or corn products (conivaptan premixed).

Warnings/Precautions

➤*Congestive heart failure:* Conivaptan is not indicated for the treatment of patients with congestive heart failure (CHF). Only use conivaptan for the treatment of hyponatremia in patients with underlying heart failure when the expected clinical benefit of raising serum sodium outweighs the increased risk of adverse reactions for heart failure patients.

The number of heart failure patients with hypervolemic hyponatremia who have been treated with IV conivaptan is too small to establish safety in patients with underlying CHF (see Adverse Reactions).

➤*Rapid correction of serum sodium:* An overly rapid increase in serum sodium concentration (greater than 12 mEq/L per 24 hours) may result in serious sequelae. In controlled clinical trials of conivaptan, approximately 9% of patients who received conivaptan in dosages of 20 to 40 mg/day IV met laboratory criteria for overly rapid correction of serum sodium, but none of these patients had permanent neurologic sequelae. Although not observed in the clinical studies with conivaptan, osmotic demyelination syndrome has been reported following rapid correction of low serum sodium concentrations.

See Administration and Dosage for more information.

➤*Injection-site reactions:* Conivaptan may cause significant injection-site reactions, even with proper dilution and infusion rates. Conivaptan must only be administered when properly prepared and diluted via large veins; rotate the infusion sites every 24 hours.

➤*Renal function impairment:* See Actions for more information.

➤*Hepatic function impairment:* See Actions for more information.

➤*Pregnancy: Category C.* Conivaptan has been shown to have adverse effects on the fetus when given to animals during pregnancy at systemic exposures less than those achieved at a therapeutic dose based on AUC comparisons. There are no adequate and well-controlled studies in pregnant women. Use conivaptan during pregnancy only if the potential benefit justifies the potential risk to the fetus. Apprise the patient of the potential hazard to the fetus.

Conivaptan crosses the placenta and is found in fetal tissue in rats. Fetal tissue levels were less than 10% of maternal plasma concentrations, while placental levels were 2.2-fold higher than maternal plasma concentrations, indicating that conivaptan can be transferred to the fetus. Conivaptan that is taken up by fetal tissue is slowly cleared, suggesting that fetal accumulation is possible. Milk levels were up to 3 times higher than maternal plasma levels following an IV dose of 1 mg/kg (systemic exposures less than therapeutic based on AUC comparisons).

Labor and delivery – The effect of conivaptan on labor and delivery in humans has not been studied. Conivaptan delayed delivery in rats dosed orally at 10 mg/kg/day by oral gavage (systemic exposures equivalent to the therapeutic dose based on AUC comparisons). Administration of conivaptan 2.5 mg/kg/day IV increased peripartum pup mortality (systemic exposures were less than the therapeutic dose based on AUC comparisons). These effects may be associated with conivaptan activity on oxytocin receptors in rats. The relevance to humans is unclear.

➤*Lactation:* It is not known whether conivaptan is excreted in human milk. Because many drugs are excreted in human milk, exercise caution when conivaptan is administered to a breast-feeding woman. The molecular weight (approximately 499 for the free base) and the administration of a continuous IV over several days suggest that the drug will be excreted into milk. Conivaptan is excreted in milk and detected in neonates when given by IV administration to lactating rats. Milk levels of conivaptan in rats reached maximal levels at 1 hour postdose following IV administrations and were up to 3 times greater than maternal plasma levels. Administration of conivaptan at 2.5 mg/kg/day IV increased peripartum pup mortality (systemic exposures were less than the therapeutic dose based on AUC comparisons).

➤*Children:* The safety and efficacy of conivaptan in children have not been studied.

➤*Monitoring:* Patients receiving conivaptan must have frequent monitoring of serum sodium, neurologic status, and volume status. An overly rapid rise in serum sodium (greater than 12 mEq/L in 24 hours) may result in serious sequelae. Monitor vital signs and volume status frequently in patients who develop hypovolemia or hypotension during therapy.

Drug Interactions

➤*CYP-450 system:* Conivaptan is a substrate of CYP3A4. Coadministration of conivaptan with CYP3A4 inhibitors could lead to an increase in conivaptan concentrations. The consequences of increased conivaptan concentrations are unknown. Concomitant use of conivaptan with potent CYP3A4 inhibitors (eg, ketoconazole, itraconazole, clarithromycin, ritonavir, indinavir) is contraindicated.

Conivaptan is a potent inhibitor of CYP3A4. Conivaptan may increase plasma concentrations of coadministered drugs that are primarily metabolized by CYP3A4. Monitor concomitant use of conivaptan with drugs that are primarily metabolized by CYP3A4 or avoid the combination. If a clinical decision is made to discontinue concomitant medications at recommended doses, allow an appropriate amount of time (at least 24 hours) following the end of conivaptan administration before resuming these medications.

Conivaptan Drug Interactions

Precipitant drug	Object drug[a]		Description
CYP3A4 inhibitors (eg, clarithromycin, indinavir, itraconazole, ketoconazole, ritonavir)	Conivaptan	↑	Because conivaptan is a substrate of CYP3A4, coadministration of itraconazole, ketoconazole, clarithromycin, indinavir, and/or ritonavir may increase conivaptan plasma concentrations. Coadministration of conivaptan and these agents is contraindicated.
Conivaptan	CYP3A4 substrates (eg, amlodipine, atorvastatin, covastatin, midazolam, simvastatin)	↑	Conivaptan is a potent CYP3A4 inhibitor and may increase plasma concentrations of coadministered drugs that are primarily metabolized by CYP3A4.
Conivaptan	Digoxin	↑	Coadministration of conivaptan and digoxin resulted in a 30% reduction in clearance and a 79% and 43% increase in digoxin C_{max} and AUC values, respectively.

[a] ↑ = object drug increased.

Adverse Reactions

Conivaptan Adverse Reactions (≥ 5%)[a,b]

Adverse reactions	Placebo (n = 69)	20 mg (n = 37)	40 mg (n = 315)
Cardiovascular			
Atrial fibrillation	0%	5%	2%
ECG ST segment depression	0%	5%	0%
Hypertension NOS	0%	8%	6%
Hypotension NOS	3%	8%	5%
Orthostatic hypotension	0%	14%	6%
CNS			
Confusional state	3%	0%	5%
Headache	3%	8%	10%
Insomnia	0%	5%	4%
GI			
Constipation	3%	8%	6%
Diarrhea NOS	0%	0%	7%
Nausea	4%	3%	5%
Postprocedural diarrhea	0%	5%	0%
Thirst	1%	3%	6%
Vomiting	0%	5%	7%
Local			
Infusion-site erythema	0%	0%	6%
Infusion-site pain	1%	0%	5%
Infusion-site phlebitis	1%	51%	32%
Infusion-site reaction	0%	22%	19%
Metabolic/Nutritional			
Hypokalemia	3%	22%	10%
Hypomagnesemia	0%	5%	2%
Hyponatremia	1%	8%	6%
Respiratory			
Pharyngolaryngeal pain	4%	5%	1%
Pneumonia	0%	5%	2%

CONIVAPTAN HYDROCHLORIDE — INJECTION

Conivaptan Adverse Reactions (≥ 5%)[a,b]			
Adverse reactions	Placebo (n = 69)	20 mg (n = 37)	40 mg (n = 315)
Miscellaneous			
Anemia NOS	3%	5%	6%
Peripheral edema	1%	3%	8%
Pruritus	0%	5%	1%
Pyrexia	0%	11%	5%
Urinary tract infection NOS	3%	5%	4%

[a] Adapted from the Medical Dictionary for Regulatory Activities version 6.0.
[b] ECG = electrocardiogram; NOS = not otherwise specified.

➤*Infusion-site reactions:* The most common adverse reactions reported with conivaptan administration were infusion-site reactions. In studies in patients and healthy volunteers, infusion-site reactions occurred in 73% and 63% of subjects treated with conivaptan 20 and 40 mg/day, respectively, compared with 4% in the placebo group. Infusion-site reactions were the most common type of adverse reaction leading to the discontinuation of conivaptan. Discontinuations from treatment because of infusion-site reactions were more common among conivaptan-treated patients (3%) than placebo-treated patients (0%). Some serious infusion-site reactions did occur.

Although a dosage of 80 mg/day IV was also studied, it was associated with a higher incidence of infusion-site reactions and a higher rate of discontinuation because of adverse reactions than the conivaptan 40 mg/day IV dose. The maximum daily dosage of conivaptan (after the loading dose) is 40 mg/day.

➤*Congestive heart failure:* In clinical trials in which IV conivaptan was administered to 79 hypervolemic hyponatremic patients with underlying heart failure and IV placebo was administered to 10 patients, adverse cardiac failure events, atrial dysrhythmias, and sepsis occurred more frequently among patients treated with conivaptan (32%, 5%, and 8%, respectively) than among patients treated with placebo (20%, 0%, and 0%, respectively). The number of heart failure patients with hypervolemic hyponatremia who have been treated with IV conivaptan is too small to establish safety in this specific population. Only use conivaptan in patients with underlying heart failure when the expected clinical benefit of raising serum sodium outweighs the risk of adverse reactions.

In 10 phase 2/pilot heart failure studies, conivaptan did not show statistically significant improvement for heart failure outcomes, including such measures as length of hospital stay, changes in categorized physical findings of heart failure, change in ejection fraction, change in exercise tolerance, change in functional status, or change in heart failure symptoms, compared with placebo. In these studies, the changes in the physical findings and heart failure symptoms were no worse in the conivaptan-treated group (n = 818) compared with the placebo group (n = 290).

Overdosage

➤*Symptoms:* Although no data on overdosage in humans are available, conivaptan has been administered as a 20 mg loading dose on day 1, followed by continuous infusion of 80 mg/day for 4 days in patients with hyponatremia and up to 120 mg/day for 2 days in patients with CHF. No new toxicities were identified at these higher doses, but adverse reactions related to the pharmacologic activity of conivaptan (eg, hypotension, thirst) occurred more frequently at these higher doses.

➤*Treatment:* In case of overdose, based on expected exaggerated pharmacological activity, symptomatic treatment with frequent monitoring of vital signs and close observation of the patient is recommended.

Patient Information

This medicine may cause dizziness, light-headedness, or fainting. Advise patients to not drive, operate machinery, or do anything else that could be dangerous until they know how they react to this medicine.

This medicine may cause harm to the fetus. If the patient may be pregnant, discuss the benefits and risks of using this medicine during pregnancy. It is not known if this medicine is found in breast milk. Advise patients to check with their health care provider if they are or will be breast-feeding while using this medicine and to discuss any possible risks to the baby.

SOMATOSTATIN ANALOGS

OCTREOTIDE

Rx	**Octreotide Acetate** (Abraxis, APP, Bedford, Sun Pharm)	**Injection, solution**: 50 mcg/mL (0.05 mg/mL)	As octreotide acetate. In 1 mL single-dose vials.
Rx	**Sandostatin** (Novartis)		As octreotide acetate. In 1 mL amps.
Rx	**Octreotide Acetate** (Abraxis, APP, Bedford, Sun Pharm)	**Injection, solution**: 100 mcg/mL (0.1 mg/mL)	As octreotide acetate. In 1 mL single-dose vials.
Rx	**Sandostatin** (Novartis)		As octreotide acetate. In 1 mL amps.
Rx	**Octreotide Acetate** (Abraxis, APP, Bedford, Sun Pharm)	**Injection, solution**: 200 mcg/mL (0.2 mg/mL)	As octreotide acetate. In 5 mL multidose vials.
Rx	**Sandostatin** (Novartis)		As octreotide acetate. In 5 mL multidose vials.
Rx	**Octreotide Acetate** (Abraxis, APP, Bedford, Sun Pharm)	**Injection, solution**:500 mcg/mL (0.5 mg/mL)	As octreotide acetate. In 1 mL single-dose vials.
Rx	**Sandostatin** (Novartis)		As octreotide acetate. In 1 mL amps.
Rx	**Octreotide Acetate** (Abraxis, APP, Bedford, Sun Pharm)	**Injection, solution**: 1,000 mcg/mL (1 mg/mL)	As octreotide acetate. In 5 mL multidose vials.
Rx	**Sandostatin** (Novartis)		As octreotide acetate. In 5 mL multidose vials.
Rx	**Sandostatin LAR Depot** (Novartis)	**Injection, powder for suspension**: 10 mg per 5 mL	Equivalent to octreotide acetate 11.2 mg. In single-use kits.
		20 mg per 5 mL	Equivalent to octreotide acetate 22.4 mg. In single-use kits.
		30 mg per 5 mL	Equivalent to octreotide acetate 33.6 mg. In single-use kits.

OCTREOTIDE ACETATE — INJECTION

Indications

➤*Acromegaly:* To reduce blood levels of growth hormone (GH) and insulin-like growth factor 1 (IGF-1) (somatomedin C) in acromegaly patients who have had inadequate response to or cannot be treated with surgical resection, pituitary irradiation, and bromocriptine mesylate at maximally tolerated doses (solution); for long-term maintenance therapy in acromegalic patients who have had an inadequate response to surgery and/or radiotherapy, or for whom surgery and/or radiotherapy is not an option (suspension).

➤*Carcinoid tumors:* For the symptomatic treatment of patients with metastatic carcinoid tumors where it suppresses or inhibits the severe diarrhea and flushing episodes associated with the disease (solution); for long-term treatment of the severe diarrhea and flushing episodes associated with metastatic carcinoid tumors (suspension).

➤*Vasoactive intestinal peptide tumors (VIPomas):* For the treatment of the profuse watery diarrhea associated with VIP-secreting tumors (solution); for long-term treatment of the profuse watery diarrhea associated with VIP-secreting tumor (suspension).

➤*Off-label uses:*

Chemotherapy-induced diarrhea – [2] = Fair documentation. Initial data from 3 small, randomized, comparative trials showed a beneficial role of octreotide. The case series showed improvement in chemotherapy-induced diarrhea (CID) with octreotide. Larger trials with longer follow-up periods are necessary to prove octreotide's role in the treatment of CID.

Dumping syndrome – [1] = Good documentation. Subcutaneous octreotide has been shown to be effective in the short-term treatment of dumping syndrome and is recommended as second-line treatment of chronic secretory diarrhea associated with dumping syndrome. Octreotide therapy is not recommended in the long-term treatment of dumping syndrome because of lack of efficacy and adverse effects. Long-acting release octreotide was effective, but subcutaneous octreotide was more effective in treating severe cases of dumping syndrome.

Gastrointestinal fistula – [4] = Insufficient documentation. Data are conflicting on whether or not octreotide decreases fistula output, increases the rate of fistula closure, decreases length of hospital stay, or decreases cost. More data are required before octreotide can be recommended.

Irritable bowel syndrome – [5] = Poor documentation. In short-term controlled studies, octreotide appeared to be effective in prolonging mouth-to-cecum transit time, inhibiting response to rectal distention, and increasing discomfort thresholds in patients with irritable bowel syndrome (IBS); however, in the only long-term study performed, octreotide was no more effective than placebo in improving IBS symptoms such as abdominal pain, fecal frequency, and other GI symptoms (eg, flatulence, bloating, urgency). In addition, long-term use of octreotide has been associated with serious adverse effects. Because octreotide has not demonstrated long-term efficacy

OCTREOTIDE ACETATE — INJECTION

in improving IBS symptoms and has significant safety concerns associated with its use, it is not recommended for the treatment of IBS.

Orthostatic hypotension – [1] = Good documentation. The use of octreotide is possibly effective in the treatment of orthostatic hypotension according to the European Federation of Neurological Societies (EFNS) evidence-based guidelines. As stated in the guidelines, fludrocortisone should be implemented as a first-line therapy, with midodrine as one of the second-line agents of choice. The combination of octreotide and midodrine, however, has been shown to be more effective at controlling orthostatic hypotension than either agent alone. It is important to note that these therapies may not treat the primary cause of orthostatic hypotension because the autonomic nervous system basis of the disorder may have to be further addressed.

Pancreatic endocrine tumors – [1] = Good documentation. National Comprehensive Cancer Network (NCCN) guidelines suggest that octreotide may be useful in the treatment of metastatic and/or stage IV neuroendocrine tumors, specifically islet cell tumors, as an adjunct in the management of associated clinical symptoms.

Reversal of carcinoid crisis – [4] = Insufficient documentation. Octreotide is commonly used for managing carcinoid syndrome and has been reported in case reports to safely and successfully reverse carcinoid crisis also.

Variceal bleeding – Dosages ranged from 25 to 50 mcg/h via continuous infusion. Duration is from 18 hours to 5 days.

Other possible off-label uses –

Diarrheal states: Because octreotide prolongs intestinal transit time, it is beneficial in relieving diarrhea associated with a variety of conditions, including AIDS-related diarrhea (100 to 500 mcg subcutaneously 2 times daily); idiopathic secretory diarrhea; short bowel (ileostomy) syndrome (intravenous [IV] infusion of 25 mcg/h or subcutaneously 50 mcg twice daily); diabetes; pancreatic cholera syndrome; diarrhea caused by radiation in cancer patients (50 to 100 mcg subcutaneously 3 times daily for 1 to 3 days).

Irritable bowel syndrome: 100 mcg single dose to 125 mcg subcutaneously twice daily.

Pancreatic fistula: To reduce output from pancreatic fistula. Dosages range from 50 to 200 mcg every 8 hours.

Variceal bleeding: Dosage ranges from 25 to 50 mcg/h via continuous infusion. Duration is from 18 hours to 5 days. Other uses for which octreotide may be beneficial to include pancreatitis; pancreatic surgery; glucagonoma; insulinoma; gastrinoma (Zollinger-Ellison syndrome); intestinal obstruction; local radiotherapy; chronic pain management; antineoplastic therapy; decreased insulin requirements in diabetes mellitus; thyrotropin- and thyroid-stimulating hormone–secreting tumors.

Administration and Dosage

➤*Adults:*

Solution –

Acromegaly:

- *Usual dosage* – 100 mcg 3 times daily subcutaneously or IV, but some patients require up to 500 mcg 3 times daily for maximum effectiveness.
- *Initial dosage* – 50 mcg 3 times daily subcutaneously or IV.
- *Dosage titration* – IGF-1 (somatomedin C) levels every 2 weeks can be used to guide titration. Alternatively, multiple GH levels at 0 to 8 hours after octreotide administration permit more rapid titration of dose. The goal is to achieve GH levels less than 5 ng/mL or IGF-1 (somatomedin C) levels less than 1.9 units/mL in men and less than 2.2 units/mL in women.
- *Discontinuation of therapy* – Octreotide should be withdrawn yearly for approximately 4 weeks from patients who have received irradiation to assess disease activity. If GH or IGF-1 (somatomedin C) levels increase and signs and symptoms recur, octreotide therapy may be resumed.
- *Monitoring* – IGF-1 (somatomedin C) or GH levels should be reevaluated at 6 month intervals.

Carcinoid tumors:

- *Initial dosage* – 100 to 600 mcg/day in 2 to 4 divided doses subcutaneously or IV during the first 2 weeks.
- *Maintenance dosage* – Median dose is 450 mcg/day; range, 50 to 1,500 mcg/day.

VIPomas:

- *Initial dosage* – 200 to 300 mcg/day in 2 to 4 divided doses subcutaneously or IV during the first 2 weeks (range, 150 to 750 mcg/day).
- *Maintenance dosage* – Doses more than 450 mcg/day are usually not required.

Suspension – Octreotide suspension is indicated in patients in whom initial treatment with octreotide solution has been shown to be effective and tolerated for at least 2 weeks.

Acromegaly (patients currently receiving solution):

- *Maximum dose* – 40 mg.
- *Initial dosage* – 20 mg IM intragluteally at 4-week intervals for 3 months.
- *Dosage adjustment* – After initial 3 months:

  GH 2.5 ng/mL or less, IGF-1 normal, and clinical symptoms controlled : Maintain dosage at 20 mg every 4 weeks.

  GH more than 2.5 ng/mL, IGF-1 elevated, and/or clinical symptoms uncontrolled: Increase dosage to 30 mg every 4 weeks.

  GH 1 ng/mL or less, IGF-1 normal, and clinical symptoms controlled: Reduce dosage to 10 mg every 4 weeks.

  GH, IGF-1, and symptoms are not adequately controlled at a dose of 30 mg: Increase to 40 mg every 4 weeks.

- *Discontinuation of therapy* – In patients who have received pituitary irradiation, octreotide suspension should be withdrawn yearly for approximately 8 weeks to assess disease activity. If GH or IGF-1 levels increase and signs and symptoms recur, octreotide suspension therapy may be resumed.

Carcinoid tumors (patients currently receiving solution):

- *Maximum dose* – 30 mg.
- *Initial dosage* – 20 mg IM intragluteally at 4-week intervals for 2 months. Because of the need for serum octreotide to reach therapeutically effective levels following initial injection of octreotide suspension, carcinoid tumor patients should continue to receive octreotide solution subcutaneously for at least 2 weeks in the same dosage they were taking before the switch. Failure to continue subcutaneous injections for this period may result in exacerbation of symptoms. Some patients may require 3 or 4 weeks of such therapy.
- *Dosage adjustment* – After initial 2 months:

  Symptoms adequately controlled: Dose reduction to 10 mg every 4 weeks for a trial period. If symptoms recur, the dosage should then be increased to 20 mg every 4 weeks.

  Symptoms not adequately controlled: 30 mg every 4 weeks.

- *Exacerbation of symptoms* – Despite good overall control of symptoms, patients with carcinoid tumors often experience periodic exacerbation of symptoms (regardless of whether they are being maintained on octreotide solution or suspension). During these periods, they may be given octreotide solution subcutaneously for a few days at the dosage they were receiving prior to the switch to octreotide suspension. When symptoms are again controlled, the octreotide solution can be discontinued.

VIPomas (patients currently receiving solution): See Carcinoid tumors.

Off-label dosing –

Chemotherapy-induced diarrhea: [2] = Fair documentation. Octreotide 0.1 to 0.5 mg subcutaneously 2 to 3 times a day or 0.15 up to 2.4 mg IV in 24 hours. In 1 case series, intramuscular long-acting (LAR) octreotide 20 to 40 mg per month was used. Duration of octreotide therapy ranged from 1 day to 1 month.

Dumping syndrome: [1] = Good documentation. 50 to 100 mcg subcutaneously 1 to 3 times a day before meals (range, 25 to 600 mcg/day) or IM depot long-acting release octreotide 10 to 20 mg/month. Octreotide therapy has been documented for as long as 17 years' duration.

Gastrointestinal fistula: [4] = Insufficient documentation. 75 to 100 mcg subcutaneously 3 times daily (or every 8 hours) for 2 to 12 days.

Orthostatic hypotension: [1] = Good documentation. 25 to 50 mcg administered subcutaneously 30 minutes prior to a meal.

Pancreatic endocrine tumors: [1] = Good documentation. 25 to 50 mcg administered subcutaneously 30 minutes prior to a meal.

Reversal of carcinoid crisis: [4] = Insufficient documentation. IV doses of octreotide 100 to 200 mcg have been reported. Subsequent continuous infusions have been administered in some cases.

Variceal bleeding: Dosage ranges from 25 to 50 mcg/h via continuous infusion. Duration is from 18 hours to 5 days.

➤*Children:*

Off-label dosing –

GI and endocrine indications:

Octreotide Pediatric Off-Label Dosage Recommendations

Indication	Pediatric dosage[a]
Chylothorax/ Chyloperitoneum	0.3 to 2 mcg/kg/h by continuous IV infusion initially; gradually increase until effect is seen. 10 mcg/kg/day subcutaneous divided 3 times daily; increase by 5 to 10 mcg/kg/day at 2- to 3-day intervals until effect is seen (up to 20 to 40 mcg/kg/day).
Diarrhea	13 to 200 mcg/day subcutaneous or IV divided 2 times daily. 1.4 to 20 mcg/kg/day divided every 12 h or continuous infusion 1 mcg/kg/h increased by 0.3 mcg/kg/dose every 3 days has been used.
Excessive growth hormone secretion	Adolescents: 500 to 1,500 mcg/day divided 2 to 3 times daily. Children: 300 to 600 mcg/day divided 3 times daily. Continuous subcutaneous infusion with the majority of the total daily dose given overnight has been found to be better than subcutaneous or depot injection.
Fistula closure	Children: 50 to 300 mcg/day subcutaneously divided 2 to 3 times daily. Start at the low end of range and increase gradually. Neonates: 1.4 mcg/kg/day subcutaneous divided 2 times daily; gradually increase to 5 mcg/kg/day subcutaneous divided 2 times daily.

OCTREOTIDE ACETATE — INJECTION

Octreotide Pediatric Off-Label Dosage Recommendations	
Indication	Pediatric dosage[a]
GI bleeding	1 to 2 mcg/kg bolus, followed by 1 mcg/kg/h IV infusion or 3 mcg/kg/day IV divided every 8 hours. Continuous infusion can be increased every 8 hours if needed. Taper dose by 50% every 12 h when no active bleeding for 24 h, and can be stopped when dose is 25% of initial dose. For chronic GI bleeding, 4 to 8 mcg/kg/day subcutaneous has been given with concurrent iron therapy.
Hyperinsulinemia	Initial doses of 2 to 10 mcg/kg/day subcutaneous in 2 to 6 doses. Titrated up to 40 mcg/kg/day based on glucose concentrations. Total daily dose may be given subcutaneous in divided doses or continuous infusion via a subcutaneous or IV infusion pump.
Hypoglycemia of infancy	Initial doses of 2 to 10 mcg/kg/day subcutaneous in 2 to 6 doses. Titrated up to 40 mcg/kg/day based on glucose concentrations. Total daily dose may be given subcutaneous in divided doses or continuous infusion via a subcutaneous or IV infusion pump.
Increased GI output	13 to 200 mcg/day subcutaneous or IV divided 2 times daily. 1.4 to 20 mcg/kg/day divided every 12 h or continuous infusion 1 mcg/kg/h increased by 0.3 mcg/kg/dose every 3 days has been used.
Pancreatic tumors	A 10-year-old received 1.5 mcg/kg/h IV for pancreatic pseudocyst. A 15-month-old received 2 mcg/kg subcutaneous every 6 hours increased up to 20 mcg/kg for recurrent pancreatitis and ascites.
Pancreatitis	A 10-year-old received 1.5 mcg/kg/h IV for pancreatic pseudocyst. A 15-month-old received 2 mcg/kg subcutaneous every 6 hours increased up to 20 mcg/kg for recurrent pancreatitis and ascites.
Sulfonylurea poisoning	25 mcg IV, subcutaneous, or continuous infusion once or 2 mcg/kg/day subcutaneous divided every 12 h.
Tall stature	Adolescents: 500 to 1,500 mcg/day divided 2 to 3 times daily. Children: 300 to 600 mcg/day divided 3 times daily. Continuous subcutaneous infusion with the majority of the total daily dose given overnight has been found to be better than subcutaneous or depot injection.

[a] Phelps SJ, Hak EB, Crill CM, eds. *Teddy Bear Book: Pediatric Injectable Drugs*. 8th ed. Bethseda, MD: American Society of Health-System Pharmacists; 2007.

➤*Renal function impairment:* In patients with renal failure requiring dialysis, the starting dosage of octreotide suspension should be 10 mg every 4 weeks. In other patients with renal function impairment, the starting dosage should be similar to a nonrenal patient (ie, 20 mg every 4 weeks). (See Warnings/Precautions.)

➤*Hepatic function impairment:* In patients with established cirrhosis of the liver, the starting dosage should be 10 mg every 4 weeks. (See Warnings/Precautions.)

➤*Preparation for administration:*

Solution – Octreotide is stable in sterile isotonic saline solutions or sterile solutions of dextrose 5% in water for 24 hours. It may be diluted in volumes of 50 to 200 mL.

Suspension – Closely follow the mixing instructions included in the packaging. Octreotide must be administered immediately after mixing.

➤*Administration:*

Solution – Administer subcutaneously or IV. Subcutaneous injection is the usual route of administration. Solution may be infused IV over 15 to 30 minutes or administered by IV push over 3 minutes. In emergency situations (eg, carcinoid crisis), it may be given by rapid bolus. Pain with subcutaneous administration may be reduced by using the smallest volume that will deliver the desired dose. Multiple subcutaneous injections at the same site within short periods of time should be avoided. Sites should be rotated in a systematic manner.

Suspension – Do not directly inject diluent without preparing suspension. Octreotide suspension should be administered intragluteally at 4-week intervals. Deltoid injections are to be avoided because of significant discomfort at the injection site when given in that area. Octreotide suspension should never be administered by the IV or subcutaneous routes. Injection site should be rotated in a systematic manner to avoid irritation.

➤*Admixture compatibility:* Octreotide solution is not compatible in total parenteral nutrition (TPN) solutions because of the formation of a glycosyl octreotide conjugate, which may decrease the efficacy of the product.

➤*Storage/Stability:* For prolonged storage, store at 2° to 8°C (36° to 46°F), and protect from light until time of use.

Solution – At 20° to 30°C (70° to 86°F), octreotide solution is stable for 14 days if protected from light. The solution can be allowed to come to room temperature prior to administration. Do not warm artificially. After initial use, discard multiple dose vials within 14 days. Open ampules just prior to administration and discard the unused portion.

Suspension – Octreotide suspension kit should remain at room temperature for 30 to 60 minutes prior to preparation. However, after preparation, the drug suspension must be administered immediately.

Actions

➤*Pharmacology:* Octreotide exerts pharmacologic actions similar to the natural hormone somatostatin. It is an even more potent inhibitor of GH, glucagon, and insulin than somatostatin. Like somatostatin, it also suppresses luteinizing hormone (LH) response to gonadotropin-releasing hormone (GnRH), decreases splanchnic blood flow, and inhibits release of serotonin, gastrin, vasoactive intestinal peptide (VIP), secretin, motilin, and pancreatic polypeptide.

By virtue of these pharmacological actions, octreotide has been used to treat the symptoms associated with metastatic carcinoid tumors (flushing and diarrhea), and VIP-secreting adenomas (watery diarrhea).

➤*Pharmacokinetics:*

Absorption –

Solution: Octreotide solution is absorbed rapidly and completely from the injection site. Peak concentrations of 5.2 ng/mL (100 mcg dose) were reached 0.4 hours after dosing. Using a specific radioimmunoassay, IV and subcutaneous doses were found to be bioequivalent. Peak concentrations and area under the curve (AUC) values were dose proportional after IV single doses of up to 200 mcg and subcutaneous single doses of up to 500 mcg, and after subcutaneous multiple dosages of up to 500 mcg 3 times daily (1,500 mcg/day). Clearance was reduced by about 66% suggesting nonlinear kinetics of the drug at daily doses of 600 mcg/day compared with 150 mcg/day. The relative decrease in clearance with doses above 600 mcg/day is not defined.

In patients with acromegaly, the pharmacokinetics differ somewhat from those in healthy volunteers. A mean peak concentration of 2.8 ng/mL (100 mcg dose) was reached in 0.7 hours after subcutaneous dosing.

Suspension: After a single IM injection of the octreotide suspension long-acting depot dosage form in healthy volunteer subjects, the serum octreotide concentration reached a transient initial peak of approximately 0.03 ng/mL/mg within 1 hour after administration progressively declining over the following 3 to 5 days to a nadir of less than 0.01 ng/mL/mg, then slowly increasing and reaching a plateau about 2 to 3 weeks postinjection. Plateau concentrations were maintained over a period of nearly 2 to 3 weeks, showing dose-proportional peak concentrations of approximately 0.07 ng/mL/mg. After approximately 6 weeks postinjection, octreotide concentration slowly decreased to less than 0.01 ng/mL/mg by weeks 12 to 13, concomitant with the terminal degradation phase of the polymer matrix of the dosage form. The relative bioavailability of the long-acting–release octreotide suspension compared with immediate-release octreotide solution given subcutaneously was 60% to 63%.

In patients with acromegaly, the octreotide concentrations after single doses of octreotide 10, 20, and 30 mg suspension were dose proportional. The transient day-1 peak, amounting to 0.3, 0.8, and 1.3 ng/mL, respectively, was followed by plateau concentrations of 0.5, 1.3, and 2 ng/mL, respectively, achieved approximately 3 weeks postinjection. These plateau concentrations were maintained for nearly 2 weeks.

Following multiple doses of octreotide suspension given every 4 weeks, steady-state octreotide serum concentrations were achieved after the third injection. Concentrations were dose proportional and higher by a factor of approximately 1.6 to 2 compared with the concentrations after a single dose. The steady-state concentrations were 1.2 and 2.1 ng/mL, respectively, at trough and 1.6 and 2.6 ng/mL, respectively, at peak with 20 and 30 mg octreotide suspension given every 4 weeks. No accumulation of octreotide beyond that expected from the overlapping release profiles occurred over a duration of up to 28-monthly injections of octreotide suspension.

With the octreotide suspension long-acting depot formulation administered IM every 4 weeks, the peak-to-trough variation in octreotide concentrations ranged from 44% to 68%, compared with the 163% to 209% variation encountered with the daily subcutaneous 3 times daily regimen of octreotide solution.

In patients with carcinoid tumors, the mean octreotide concentrations after 6 doses of octreotide 10, 20, and 30 mg suspension administered by IM injection every 4 weeks were 1.2, 2.5, and 4.2 ng/mL, respectively. Concentrations were dose proportional and steady-state concentrations were reached after 2 injections of 20 and 30 mg and after 3 injections of 10 mg.

Distribution – In healthy volunteers, the distribution of octreotide solution from plasma was rapid (terminal half-life [$t\alpha_{1/2}$] = 0.2 h), the volume of distribution (V_{dss}) was estimated to be 13.6 L, and the total body clearance ranged from 7 to 10 L/h.

In patients with acromegaly, the V_{dss} was estimated to be 21.6 ± 8.5 L and the total body clearance was increased to 18 L/h. The mean percent of the drug bound was 41.2%.

OCTREOTIDE ACETATE — INJECTION

In blood, the distribution into the erythrocytes was found to be negligible and approximately 65% was bound in the plasma in a concentration-independent manner. Binding was mainly to lipoprotein and, to a lesser extent, to albumin.

Metabolism/Excretion – The elimination of octreotide from plasma had an apparent half-life of 1.7 to 1.9 hours compared with 1 to 3 minutes with the natural hormone somatostatin. The duration of action of octreotide solution is variable, but extends up to 12 hours depending upon the type of tumor, necessitating multiple daily dosing with this immediate-release dosage form. About 32% of the dose is excreted unchanged into the urine.

In patients with acromegaly, the total body clearance was increased to 18 L/h. The disposition and elimination half-lives were similar to healthy patients.

Special populations –

Renal function impairment: In patients with renal function impairment, the elimination of octreotide solution from plasma was prolonged and total body clearance reduced. In mild renal function impairment (creatinine clearance [CrCl] 40 to 60 mL/min), octreotide solution $t_{1/2}$ was 2.4 hours and total body clearance was 8.8 L/h. In moderate renal function impairment (CrCl 10 to 39 mL/min), $t_{1/2}$ was 3 hours and total body clearance was 7.3 L/h. In severe renal function impairment not requiring dialysis (CrCl less than 10 mL/min), $t_{1/2}$ was 3.1 hours and total body clearance was 7.6 L/h.

In patients with severe renal failure requiring dialysis, total body clearance was reduced to about half that found in healthy subjects (from approximately 10 to 4.5 L/h).

Hepatic function impairment: Patients with liver cirrhosis showed prolonged elimination of drug, with octreotide solution $t_{1/2}$ increasing to 3.7 hours and total body clearance decreasing to 5.9 L/h, whereas patients with fatty liver disease showed $t_{1/2}$ increased to 3.4 hours and total body clearance of 8.2 L/h. In healthy subjects, octreotide solution half-life is 1.9 h and the clearance is 8.3 L/h, which is comparable with the clearance in fatty liver patients.

Elderly: In an elderly population, dose adjustments may be necessary because of a significant increase in the half-life (46%) and a significant decrease in the clearance (26%) of the drug.

Children: In children with hypothalamic obesity, the mean octreotide concentration after 6 doses of octreotide 40 mg suspension administered by IM injection every 4 weeks was approximately 3 ng/mL. Steady-state concentration was achieved after 3 injections of a 40 mg dose.

Contraindications

Sensitivity to this drug or any of its components.

Warnings/Precautions

➤*Gallbladder effects:* Single doses have been shown to inhibit gallbladder contractility and decrease bile secretion in healthy volunteers. In clinical trials with octreotide solution (primarily patients with acromegaly or psoriasis) in patients who had not previously received octreotide, the incidence of biliary tract abnormalities was 63% (gallstones, 27%; sludge without stones, 24%; biliary duct dilatation, 12%). The incidence of stones or sludge in patients who received octreotide solution for at least 12 months was 52%. Less than 2% of patients treated with octreotide solution for 1 month or less developed gallstones. The incidence of gallstones did not appear to be related to age, sex, or dose. Like patients without gallbladder abnormalities, the majority of patients developing gallbladder abnormalities on ultrasound had GI symptoms. The symptoms were not specific for gallbladder disease. A few patients developed acute cholecystitis, ascending cholangitis, biliary obstruction, cholestatic hepatitis, or pancreatitis during octreotide solution therapy or following its withdrawal. One patient developed ascending cholangitis during octreotide solution therapy and died.

➤*Blood glucose effects:* Octreotide alters the balance between the counter-regulatory hormones, insulin, glucagon, and GH, which may result in hypoglycemia or hyperglycemia. However, the incidence of these adverse reactions during long-term therapy was determined vigorously only in acromegaly patients who, because of their underlying disease or the subsequent treatment they receive, are at an increased risk for the development of diabetes mellitus. Although the degree to which these abnormalities are related to octreotide therapy is not clear, new abnormalities of glycemic control developed during octreotide therapy and are described in the following sections.

The hypoglycemia or hyperglycemia that occurs during octreotide therapy is usually mild, but may result in overt diabetes mellitus or necessitate dose changes in insulin or other hypoglycemic agents. Hypoglycemia and hyperglycemia occurred on octreotide solution in 3% and 16% of acromegalic patients, respectively. Severe hyperglycemia, subsequent pneumonia, and death following initiation of octreotide therapy was reported in 1 patient with no history of hyperglycemia.

In patients with concomitant type I diabetes mellitus, octreotide solution and suspension are likely to affect glucose regulation, and insulin requirements may be reduced. Symptomatic hypoglycemia, which may be severe, has been reported in these patients. In patients without diabetes and patients with type II diabetes with partially intact insulin reserves, octreotide solution or suspension administration may result in decreases in plasma insulin levels and hyperglycemia. It is therefore recommended that glucose tolerance and antidiabetic treatment be periodically monitored during therapy with these drugs.

➤*Thyroid effects:* In acromegalic patients, 12% developed biochemical hypothyroidism only, 8% developed goiter, and 4% required initiation of thyroid replacement therapy while receiving octreotide solution. Baseline and periodic assessment of thyroid function (TSH, total and/or free T_4) is recommended during chronic therapy. Octreotide suppresses the secretion of TSH, which may result in hypothyroidism.

➤*Cardiovascular effects:* Cardiac conduction abnormalities have occurred during treatment with octreotide.

In both acromegalic and carcinoid syndrome patients, bradycardia, arrhythmias, and conduction abnormalities have been reported during octreotide therapy. Other electrocardiogram (ECG) changes, such as QT prolongation, axis shifts, early repolarization, low voltage, R/S transition, early R wave progression, and nonspecific ST-T wave changes, were observed. These ECG changes are not uncommon in acromegalic patients. The relationship of these reactions to octreotide is not established because many of these patients have underlying cardiac disease. Dose adjustments in drugs such as beta-blockers that have bradycardia effects may be necessary. In one acromegalic patient with severe congestive heart failure (CHF), initiation of octreotide solution therapy resulted in worsening of CHF with improvement when the drug was discontinued. Confirmation of a drug effect was obtained with a positive rechallenge.

➤*Nutritional effects:* Octreotide may alter absorption of dietary fats. Depressed vitamin B_{12} levels and abnormal Schilling tests have been observed in some patients receiving octreotide therapy, and monitoring of vitamin B_{12} levels is recommended during therapy with octreotide.

Octreotide has been investigated for the reduction of excessive fluid loss from the GI tract in patients with conditions producing such a loss. If such patients are receiving total parenteral nutrition (TPN), serum zinc may rise excessively when the fluid loss is reversed. Periodically monitor zinc levels in patients on TPN and octreotide.

➤*Pancreatitis:* Several cases of pancreatitis have been reported in patients receiving octreotide solution therapy.

➤*Immunogenicity:* Studies to date have shown that antibodies to octreotide develop in up to 25% of patients treated with octreotide. These antibodies do not influence the degree of efficacy response to octreotide; however, in 2 acromegalic patients who received octreotide solution, the duration of GH suppression following each injection was about twice as long as in patients without antibodies. It has not been determined whether octreotide antibodies will also prolong the duration of GH suppression in patients being treated with octreotide suspension.

➤*Renal function impairment:* In patients with severe renal failure requiring dialysis, the half-life of octreotide may be increased, necessitating adjustment of the maintenance dosage.

In patients with renal failure requiring dialysis, the starting dose of octreotide suspension should be 10 mg. Up-titrate the dose based on clinical response and speed of response as deemed necessary by the health care provider. In patients with mild, moderate, or severe renal function impairment, there is no need to adjust the starting dose of octreotide. Adjust the maintenance dose thereafter based on clinical response and tolerability as in non-renal patients.

➤*Pregnancy: Category B.* There are no adequate and well-controlled studies in pregnant women. Reproduction studies have been performed in rats and rabbits at doses of up to 16 times the highest recommended human dose and have revealed no evidence of harm to the fetus due to octreotide. However, because animal reproduction studies are not always predictive of human response, use this drug during pregnancy only if clearly needed.

➤*Lactation:* It is not known whether this drug is excreted in human milk. Because many drugs are excreted in milk, exercise caution when octreotide is administered to a breast-feeding woman.

➤*Children:*

Solution – Experience with octreotide solution in children is limited. Although formal controlled clinical trials have not been performed to evaluate safety and effectiveness in this age group, there are reports of 49 cases in the literature of neonates and infants with congenital hyperinsulinism (also called familial hyperinsulinism, persistent hyperinsulinemic hypoglycemia of infancy, or nesidioblastosis) who have received octreotide solution as an inhibitor of insulin release. The following efficacy and safety information is derived from these 49 patients.

Octreotide solution has been used to stabilize plasma glucose levels prior to pancreatectomy and to treat recurrent postoperative hypoglycemia. Although most use of octreotide in this setting is short-term, a few reports in the literature have documented longer-term therapy in children (2.2 to 5.5 years). Octreotide is an alternative medical treatment to diazoxide for control of hypoglycemia in this disorder. Of 31 children who received octreotide solution as prescribed for congenital hyperinsulinism and for which long-term follow-up was available, octreotide obviated the need for surgery in 3 (10%) patients and was replaced by diazoxide in 4 (13%) patients because of uncontrolled hypoglycemia. Although the remainder of these patients required surgery, there have been a few reports in the literature of patients who have responded to octreotide after failing treatment with surgery and/or diazoxide. Doses of 3 to 40 mcg/kg/day have been used. At these doses, the majority of adverse reactions were GI and included diarrhea, steatorrhea, vomiting, and abdominal distention, each reported in 22% to 35% (n = 11 to 17) of patients. However, they were generally short-lived, with resolution of vomiting and distention in 2 to 4 days, and diarrhea/steatorrhea within 2 to 4 weeks. Steatorrhea was controlled in most patients with pancreatic enzyme supplements. Poor growth was reported in 37% (n = 7) of patients who received octreotide solution for 1 to 4.33 years. It was associated with low serum GH or IGF-1 levels in 4 out of 6 patients in whom these parameters were measured. Catch-up growth occurred in 3 out of 3 patients who were followed after octreotide solution was discontinued. Poor weight gain was reported in 32% (n = 6) of patients. Tachyphylaxis was reported in 35% (n = 17) of patients. Asymptomatic gallstones with sludge

OCTREOTIDE ACETATE — INJECTION

was reported in 1 infant after 1 year of therapy and was treated with ursodeoxycholic acid. There has been a single report of an infant with nesidioblastosis who experienced a seizure thought to be independent of octreotide solution therapy. A single death has been reported in a 16-month-old male with enterocutaneous fistula who developed sudden abdominal pain and increased nasogastric drainage and expired 8 hours after receiving a single 100 mcg subcutaneous dose of octreotide solution.

Suspension – The efficacy and safety of octreotide suspension were examined in a randomized, double-blind, placebo-controlled 6-month study in 60 children 6 to 17 years of age with hypothalamic obesity resulting from cranial insult. Mean body mass index increased 0.1 kg/m^2 in octreotide suspension–treated subjects compared with 0.0 kg/m^2 in saline control–treated subjects. Diarrhea occurred in 11 of 30 (37%) patients treated with octreotide suspension. No unexpected adverse reactions were observed. However, with octreotide 40 mg suspension once a month, the incidence of new cholelithiasis in this pediatric population (33%) was higher than that seen in other adult indications such as acromegaly (22%) or malignant carcinoid syndrome (24%), where octreotide suspension was 10 to 30 mg once a month.

➤*Elderly:* Dose selection for an elderly patient should be cautious, usually starting at the low end of the dosing range, reflecting the greater frequency of decreased hepatic, renal, or cardiac function, and of concomitant disease or other drug therapy.

➤*Monitoring:* GH-secreting tumors may sometimes expand and cause serious complications (eg, visual field defects). Therefore, carefully monitor all patients with these tumors.

Baseline and periodic assessment of thyroid function (TSH, total or free T_4) and vitamin B_{12} levels is recommended during chronic therapy. Periodically monitor zinc levels in patients on TPN and octreotide. Monitor blood glucose tolerance periodically during treatment.

Laboratory tests that may be helpful as biochemical markers in determining and following patient response depend on the specific tumor. Based on diagnosis, measurement of the following substances may be useful in monitoring the progress of therapy:

Acromegaly – GH, IGF-1 (somatomedin C). Responsiveness to octreotide solution may be evaluated by determining GH levels at 1 to 4 hour intervals for 8 to 12 hours postdose. Alternatively, a single measurement of IGF-1 (somatomedin C) level may be made 2 weeks after drug initiation or dosage change.

Carcinoid – 5-HIAA (urinary 5-hydroxyindole acetic acid), plasma serotonin, plasma Substance P.

VIPoma – VIP. Perform baseline and periodic total and/or free T_4 measurements during chronic therapy.

Drug Interactions

➤*QT prolongation:* An additive effect of octreotide with other drugs that prolong the QT interval cannot be excluded. The following drugs may prolong the QT interval and increase the risk of life-threatening cardiac arrhythmias, including torsades de pointes: Antiarrhythmic agents (eg, amiodarone, bretylium, disopyramide, dofetilide, procainamide, quinidine, and sotalol), arsenic trioxide, chlorpromazine, cisapride, dolasetron, droperidol, mefloquine, mesoridazine, moxifloxacin, pentamidine, pimozide, tacrolimus, thioridazine, and ziprasidone. For a more complete list of drugs that may prolong the QT interval, see the appendix, Drug-Induced Prolongation of the QT Interval and Torsades de Pointes.

➤*CYP-450 system:* Limited published data indicate that somatostatin analogs may decrease the metabolic clearance of compounds known to be metabolized by CYP-450 enzymes, which may be due to the suppression of growth hormone. Because it cannot be excluded that octreotide may have this effect, use other drugs mainly metabolized by CYP3A4 and that have a low therapeutic index (eg, quinidine, terfenadine) with caution.

Octreotide has been associated with alterations in nutrient absorption, so it may have an effect on absorption of orally administered drugs. Patients receiving calcium channel blockers or agents to control fluid and electrolyte balance may require dose adjustments of these therapeutic agents.

➤*Insulin/Oral hypoglycemic drugs:* Octreotide inhibits the secretion of insulin and glucagon. Therefore, monitor blood glucose levels when octreotide treatment is initiated or when the dose is altered and adjust antidiabetic treatment accordingly.

Octreotide Drug Interactions

Precipitant drug	Object drug[a]		Description
Octreotide	Beta-blockers (eg, propranolol)	↑	Coadministration may have an additive effect on the reduction of heart rate associated with octreotide. Dose adjustment of beta-blocker may be necessary.
Octreotide	Bromocriptine	↑	Coadministration may increase the availability of bromocriptine.
Octreotide	Cyclosporine	↓	Coadministration may decrease blood levels of cyclosporine and result in transplant rejection.
Octreotide	CYP3A4 metabolism (eg, quinidine, terfenadine[b])	↑	Octreotide may decrease the metabolic clearance of drugs known to be metabolized by CYP-450 enzymes, which have a low therapeutic index, such as quinidine and terfenadine. Use with caution and consider dose reductions of the coadministered medications.

[a] ↑ = object drug increased; ↓ = object drug decreased.
[b] No longer marketed in the United States.

➤*Drug/Food interactions:* Octreotide may alter absorption of dietary fats in some patients.

Adverse Reactions

➤*Solution:*

Cardiovascular – In acromegalic patients, sinus bradycardia (less than 50 bpm) developed in 25%, conduction abnormalities occurred in 10%, and arrhythmias developed in 9% of patients during octreotide solution therapy.

Chest pain, CHF, hypertension, hypertensive reaction, ischemia, orthostatic blood pressure decrease, palpitations, shortness of breath, tachycardia, thrombophlebitis (less than 1%).

CNS – Headache (6%); dizziness (5%); depression, fatigue, weakness (1% to 4%); amnesia, anxiety, Bell palsy, hearing loss, increased intraocular pressure, libido decrease, neuritis, paranoia, pituitary apoplexy, seizure, syncope, tremor, vertigo (less than 1%).

Dermatologic – Bruise, flushing, hair loss, pruritus (1% to 4%); basal cell carcinoma, cellulitis, petechiae, rash, urticaria (less than 1%).

Endocrine – Hypoglycemia and hyperglycemia occurred in 3% and 16% of acromegalic patients, respectively, but only in approximately 1.5% of other patients. Symptoms of hypoglycemia were noted in approximately 2% of patients.

In acromegalics, biochemical hypothyroidism alone occurred in 12% while goiter occurred in 6% during octreotide solution therapy. In patients without acromegaly, hypothyroidism has only been reported in several isolated patients, and goiter has not been reported.

Diabetes insipidus, hypoadrenalism (less than 1%).

GI – Abdominal discomfort, diarrhea, loose stools, and nausea were each seen in 34% to 61% of acromegalic patients in US studies, although only 2.6% of the patients discontinued therapy because of these symptoms. These symptoms were seen in 5% to 10% of patients with other disorders.

The frequency of these symptoms was not dose related, but abdominal discomfort and diarrhea generally resolved more quickly in patients treated with 300 mcg/day than in those treated with 750 mcg/day. Abdominal distention, abnormal stools, constipation, flatulence, and vomiting were each seen in less than 10% of patients.

Appendicitis, gallbladder polyp, gastric/peptic ulcer, GI bleeding, hemorrhoids, (less than 1%).

Gallbladder abnormalities, especially stones or biliary sludge, frequently develop in patients on chronic octreotide solution therapy.

In rare instances, GI adverse reactions may resemble acute intestinal obstruction, with progressive abdominal distention, abdominal tenderness, guarding, and severe epigastric pain.

GU – Pollakiuria urinary tract infection (1% to 4%); amenorrhea, galactorrhea, gynecomastia, hematuria, nephrolithiasis, oligomenorrhea, polymenorrhea, vaginitis (less than 1%).

Hematologic – Anemia, epistaxis, iron deficiency (less than 1%).

Hepatic – Hepatitis, increased liver enzymes, jaundice (less than 1%).

Hypersensitivity – Anaphylactoid reactions, including anaphylactoid shock, have been reported in several patients receiving octreotide solution.

Musculoskeletal – Backache, joint pain (1% to 4%); arthritis, joint effusion, muscle pain, Raynaud phenomenon (less than 1%).

Respiratory – Pneumonia, pulmonary nodule, status asthmaticus (less than 1%).

Special senses – Blurred vision, visual disturbances (1% to 4%); otitis (less than 1%).

Miscellaneous – Pain on injection (7.7%); cold symptoms, edema, fat malabsorption, flu symptoms, injection-site hematoma (1% to 4%); allergic reaction, increased creatine kinase (CK), weight loss (less than 1%). Pancreatitis was also observed.

Immunogenicity – Evaluation of 20 patients treated for at least 6 months has failed to demonstrate titers of antibodies exceeding background levels. However, antibody titers to octreotide solution were subsequently reported in 3 patients and resulted in prolonged duration of drug action in 2 patients.

OCTREOTIDE ACETATE — INJECTION

➤*Suspension:*

Acromegaly –

Octreotide Adverse Reactions (≥ 10%) in Acromegalic Patients	
Adverse reaction	Subjects with adverse reactions 10 mg/20 mg/30 mg (n = 261)
CNS	
Dizziness	11.5%
Fatigue	11.1%
Headache	15.3%
GI	
Abdominal pain	28.7%
Constipation	17.6%
Diarrhea	35.6%
Flatulence	25.3%
Miscellaneous	
Anemia	15.3%
Cholelithiasis	13.4%
Hypertension	12.6%
Influenza-like symptoms	19.9%
Injection-site pain	13.8%

Gallbladder abnormalities: Single doses of octreotide solution have been shown to inhibit gallbladder contractility and decrease bile secretion in healthy volunteers. In clinical trials with octreotide solution (primarily patients with acromegaly or psoriasis) in patients who had not previously received octreotide, the incidence of biliary tract abnormalities was 63% (gallstones, 27%; sludge without stones, 24%; biliary duct dilatation, 12%). The incidence of stones or sludge in patients who received octreotide solution for 12 months or longer was 52%. The incidence of gallbladder abnormalities did not appear to be related to age, sex, or dose, but was related to duration of exposure.

In clinical trials, 52% of acromegalic patients, most of whom received octreotide suspension for 12 months or longer, developed new biliary abnormalities, including gallstones, microlithiasis, sediment, sludge, and dilatation. The incidence of new cholelithiasis was 22%, of which 7% were microstones.

Across all trials, a few patients developed acute cholecystitis, ascending cholangitis, biliary obstruction, cholestatic hepatitis, or pancreatitis during octreotide solution therapy or following its withdrawal. One patient developed ascending cholangitis during octreotide solution therapy and died. Despite the high incidence of new gallstones in patients receiving octreotide, 1% of patients developed acute symptoms requiring cholecystectomy.

Cardiovascular: In acromegalic patients, sinus bradycardia (fewer than 50 bpm) developed in 25%, conduction abnormalities occurred in 10%, and arrhythmias developed in 9% of patients during octreotide solution therapy. The relationship of these reactions to octreotide is not established because many of these patients have underlying cardiac disease.

Endocrine: In acromegalic patients treated with either octreotide solution or suspension, hypoglycemia occurred in approximately 2%, and hyperglycemia in approximately 15% of patients.

In acromegalic patients receiving octreotide solution, 12% developed biochemical hypothyroidism, 8% developed goiter, and 4% required initiation of thyroid replacement therapy while receiving octreotide solution. In acromegalic patients treated with octreotide suspension, hypothyroidism was reported as an adverse reaction in 2% and goiter in 2%. Two patients receiving octreotide suspension required initiation of thyroid hormone replacement therapy.

GI: The most common symptoms are GI. The overall incidence of the most frequent of these symptoms in clinical trials of acromegalic patients treated for approximately 1 to 4 years is shown in the following table.

Octreotide Common GI Adverse Reactions in Acromegalic Patients		
GI adverse reactions	Octreotide solution (n = 114)	Octreotide suspension (n = 261)
Abdominal pain or discomfort	43.9%	29.1%
Constipation	8.8%	18.8%
Diarrhea	57.9%	36.4%
Flatulence	13.2%	25.7%
Nausea	29.8%	10.3%
Vomiting	4.4%	6.5%

Only 2.6% of the patients on octreotide solution in US clinical trials discontinued therapy because of these symptoms. No acromegalic patient receiving octreotide suspension discontinued therapy for a GI reaction.

In patients receiving octreotide suspension, the incidence of diarrhea was dose related. Diarrhea, abdominal pain, and nausea developed primarily during the first month of treatment with octreotide suspension. Thereafter, new cases of these reactions were uncommon. The vast majority of these reactions were mild to moderate in severity.

In rare instances, GI adverse reactions may resemble acute intestinal obstruction, with progressive abdominal distention, severe epigastric pain, abdominal tenderness, and guarding.

Dyspepsia, steatorrhea, discoloration of feces, and tenesmus were reported in 4% to 6% of patients.

In a clinical trial of carcinoid syndrome, nausea, abdominal pain, and flatulence were reported in 27% to 38% and constipation or vomiting in 15% to 21% of patients treated with octreotide suspension. Diarrhea was reported as an adverse reaction in 14% of patients, but because most of the patients had diarrhea as a symptom of carcinoid syndrome, it is difficult to assess the actual incidence of drug-related diarrhea.

Local: Pain on injection, which is generally mild to moderate and short-lived (usually about 1 hour), is dose related, being reported by 2%, 9%, and 11% of acromegalic patients receiving doses of 10, 20, and 30 mg, respectively, of octreotide suspension. In carcinoid patients, where a diary was kept, pain at the injection site was reported by about 20% to 25% at a 10 mg dose and about 30% to 50% at the 20 and 30 mg dose.

Carcinoid and VIPomas –

Octreotide Adverse Reactions (≥ 15%) of Carcinoid Tumor and VIPoma Patients				
	(N = 93)			
Adverse reaction	Solution (n = 26)	10 mg suspension (n = 22)	20 mg suspension (n = 20)	30 mg suspension (n = 25)
CNS				
Dizziness	15.4%	18.2%	20%	20%
Fatigue	11.5%	31.8%	10%	8%
Headache	19.2%	18.2%	30%	16%
Dermatologic				
Pruritus	0%	18.2%	0%	0%
Rash	3.8%	0%	15%	0%
GI				
Abdominal pain	30.8%	35.4%	10%	20%
Flatulence	11.5%	9.1%	10%	16%
Nausea	30.8%	40.9%	30%	24%
Vomiting	11.5%	0%	0%	16%
Musculoskeletal				
Arthropathy	19.2%	9.1%	15%	8%
Back pain	26.9%	27.3%	10%	8%
Musculoskeletal pain	15.4%	0%	5%	0%
Myalgia	0%	18.2%	5%	4%
Respiratory				
Sinusitis	15.4%	0%	5%	12%
Upper respiratory tract infection	23.1%	18.2%	10%	12%
Miscellaneous				
Generalized pain	15.4%	9.1%	15%	4%

Cardiovascular: Electrocardiograms were performed only in carcinoid patients receiving octreotide suspension. In carcinoid syndrome patients, sinus bradycardia developed in 19%, conduction abnormalities occurred in 9%, and arrhythmias developed in 3%. The relationship of these reactions to octreotide is not established because many of these patients have underlying cardiac disease.

GI: In clinical trials, 62% of malignant carcinoid patients who received octreotide suspension for up to 18 months developed new biliary abnormalities, including jaundice, gallstones, sludge, and dilatation. New gallstones occurred in a total of 24% of patients.

Endocrine: In carcinoid patients, hypoglycemia occurred in 4% and hyperglycemia in 27% of patients treated with octreotide suspension.

In carcinoid patients, hypothyroidism has only been reported in isolated patients and goiter has not been reported.

Miscellaneous: Other clinically significant adverse reactions (relationship to drug not established) in acromegalic and/or carcinoid syndrome patients receiving octreotide suspension were malignant hyperpyrexia, cerebral vascular disorder, rectal bleeding, ascites, pulmonary embolism, pneumonia, and pleural effusion.

➤*Postmarketing (suspension):*

Octreotide Postmarketing Adverse Reactions (≥ 10%)		
Adverse reaction	Octreotide suspension (n = 76)	Surgery (n = 64)
GI		
Abdominal pain	25%	3.1%
Abdominal pain, upper	10.5%	0%
Diarrhea	47.4%	3.1%
Nausea	15.8%	7.8%

OCTREOTIDE ACETATE — INJECTION

Octreotide Postmarketing Adverse Reactions (≥ 10%)		
Adverse reaction	Octreotide suspension (n = 76)	Surgery (n = 64)
Miscellaneous		
Alopecia	13.2%	7.8%
Cholelithiasis	38.2%	4.7%
Epistaxis	0%	10.9%
Headache	10.5%	9.4%
Injection-site pain	11.8%	0%

Cardiovascular – Aneurysm; arterial thrombosis of the arm; atrial fibrillation; cardiac arrest; myocardial infarction has been observed, mainly in patients with CV risk factors; orthostatic hypotension; Raynaud syndrome.

CNS – Aphasia, Bell palsy, convulsions, hemiparesis, intracranial hemorrhage, migraines, paranoia, paresis, suicide attempt.

Dermatologic – Petechiae, urticaria.

Endocrine – Diabetes insipidus, diabetes mellitus, hypoadrenalism has been reported in some reports in patients 18 months of age and younger, pituitary apoplexy.

GI – Abdomen enlarged, appendicitis, gallbladder polyp, GI hemorrhage, intestinal obstruction, pancreatitis, peptic/gastric ulcer.

GU – Breast carcinoma, galactorrhea, gynecomastia, hematuria, libido decrease.

Hematologic/Lymphatic – Pancytopenia, retinal vein thrombosis, thrombocytopenia.

Hepatic – Fatty liver, hepatitis, increased liver enzymes.

Lab test abnormalities – CK increased, creatinine increased.

Musculoskeletal – Arthritis, joint effusion.

Renal – Renal failure, renal function impairment.

Respiratory – Pneumothorax aggravated, pulmonary hypertension, pulmonary nodule, status asthmaticus.

Special senses – Deafness, glaucoma, scotoma, visual field defect.

Miscellaneous – Anaphylactoid reactions, including anaphylactic shock; cellulitis; facial edema; generalized edema.

Overdosage

➤*Symptoms:* No frank overdose has occurred in any patient to date. Octreotide solution given in IV bolus doses of 1 mg (1,000 mcg) to healthy volunteers did not result in serious ill effects, nor did doses of 30 mg (30,000 mcg) given IV over 20 minutes and of 120 mg (120,000 mcg) given IV over 8 hours to research patients. Doses of 2.5 mg (2,500 mcg) of octreotide solution subcutaneously have, however, caused hypoglycemia, flushing, dizziness, and nausea.

➤*Treatment:* Up-to-date information about the treatment of overdose can often be obtained from a certified Regional Poison Control Center. The American Association of Poison Control Centers' phone number is 1-800-222-1222.

Patient Information

Give patients and other persons who may administer octreotide careful instruction in sterile subcutaneous injection technique.

Advise patients to adhere closely to their scheduled return visits.

LANREOTIDE

Rx	**Somatuline Depot** (Tercica)	**Injection, solution, extended-release:** 60 mg per 0.2 mL	Equiv. to lanreotide acetate 79.8 mg. In single-use, prefilled syringes.
		90 mg per 0.3 mL	Equiv. to lanreotide acetate 116.4 mg. In single-use, prefilled syringes.
		120 mg per 0.5 mL	Equiv. to lanreotide acetate 155.5 mg. In single-use, prefilled syringes.

LANREOTIDE ACETATE — INJECTION

Indications

➤*Acromegaly:* For the long-term treatment of acromegalic patients who have had an inadequate response to surgery and/or radiotherapy, or for whom surgery and/or radiotherapy is not an option.

Administration and Dosage

➤*Adults:*

Acromegaly –

Initial dosage: 90 mg subcutaneously at 4-week intervals for 3 months.

Dosage adjustment: After 3 months, the dosage may be adjusted as follows:

Lanreotide Dosage Adjustment Recommendations	
GH[a] levels (ng/mL)	Lanreotide dosage adjustment
GH > 1 to ≤ 2.5 ng/mL, IGF-1 normal, and clinical symptoms controlled	Maintain dosage at 90 mg every 4 weeks.
GH > 2.5 ng/mL, IGF-1 elevated, and/or clinical symptoms uncontrolled	Increase dosage to 120 mg every 4 weeks.
GH ≤ 1 ng/mL, IGF-1 normal, and clinical symptoms controlled	Reduce dosage to 60 mg every 4 weeks.

[a] GH = growth hormone.

Thereafter, the dose should be adjusted according to the response of the patient, as judged by a reduction in serum GH and/or IGF-1 levels, and/or changes in symptoms of acromegaly.

Patients who are controlled on lanreotide 60 or 90 mg may be considered for an extended dosing interval of lanreotide 120 mg every 6 or 8 weeks. GH and IGF-1 levels should be obtained 6 weeks after this change in dosing regimen to evaluate persistence of patient response.

Continued monitoring of patient response with dose adjustments for biochemical and clinical symptom control, as necessary, is recommended.

➤*Renal function impairment:*

Moderate to severe renal impairment – Initially, 60 mg subcutaneously at 4-week intervals for 3 months, followed by dose adjustment as previously described. Caution should be exercised when considering these patients for an extended dosing interval of lanreotide 120 mg every 6 or 8 weeks.

➤*Hepatic function impairment:*

Moderate to severe hepatic impairment – Initially, 60 mg subcutaneously at 4-week intervals for 3 months, followed by dose adjustment as previously described. Caution should be exercised when considering these patients for an extended dosing interval of lanreotide 120 mg every 6 or 8 weeks.

➤*Preparation for administration:* Thirty minutes prior to the injection, remove the sealed pouch of lanreotide from the refrigerator and allow it to come to room temperature.

➤*Administration:* Lanreotide is for deep subcutaneous injection in the superior external quadrant of the buttock. The skin should not be folded, and the needle should be rapidly inserted perpendicular to the skin and to its full length. The injection site should alternate between the right and left side.

➤*Storage/Stability:* Store in a refrigerator at 2° to 8°C (36° to 46°F) and protect from light in the original package. Keep the pouch sealed until injection.

Actions

➤*Pharmacology:* Lanreotide is a synthetic cyclical octapeptide analog of the natural hormone somatostatin. The mechanism of action of lanreotide is believed to be similar to that of natural somatostatin.

Pharmacodynamics – Lanreotide has a high affinity for human somatostatin receptors (SSTR) 2 and 5 and a reduced binding affinity for human SSTR1, 3, and 4. Activity at human SSTR2 and 5 is the primary mechanism believed to be responsible for GH inhibition. Like somatostatin, lanreotide is an inhibitor of various endocrine, neuroendocrine, exocrine, and paracrine functions.

The primary pharmacodynamic effect of lanreotide is a reduction of GH and/or IGF-1 levels, enabling normalization of levels in acromegalic patients. In acromegalic patients, lanreotide reduces GH levels in a dose-dependent way. After a single injection of lanreotide, plasma GH levels fall rapidly and are maintained for at least 28 days.

➤*Pharmacokinetics:*

Absorption/Distribution – After a single deep subcutaneous injection, the mean absolute bioavailability of lanreotide in healthy subjects was 73.4%, 69%, and 78.4% for the 60, 90, and 120 mg doses, respectively. Mean maximum effective plasma concentration (C_{max}) values ranged from 4.3 to 8.4 ng/mL during the first day. Single-dose linearity was demonstrated with respect to area under the curve (AUC) and C_{max}, and showed high intersubject variability.

In a repeat-dose administration pharmacokinetics study in acromegalic patients, rapid initial release was seen, giving peak levels during the first day after administration. At doses of lanreotide between 60 and 120 mg, linear pharmacokinetics were observed in acromegalic patients. At steady state, mean C_{max} values were 3.8 ± 0.5 ng/mL, 5.7 ± 1.7 ng/mL, and 7.7 ± 2.5 ng/mL, increasing linearly with dose. The mean accumulation ratio index was 2.7, which is in line with the range of values for the half-life of lanreotide. The steady-state trough serum lanreotide concentrations in patients receiving lanreotide every 28 days were 1.8 ± 0.3 ng/mL, 2.5 ± 0.9 ng/mL, and 3.8 ± 1 ng/mL at 60, 90, and 120 mg doses, respectively. A limited initial burst effect and a low peak to trough fluctuation (81% to 108%) of the serum concentration at the plateau was observed.

Pharmacokinetic data from studies evaluating extended dosing use of lanreotide 120 mg demonstrated mean steady state, minimum concentration values between 1.6 and 2.3 ng/mL for the 8- and 6-week treatment interval, respectively.

LANREOTIDE ACETATE — INJECTION

Excretion – In studies evaluating excretion, less than 5% of lanreotide was excreted in urine and less than 0.5% was recovered unchanged in feces, indicative of some biliary excretion.

Lanreotide showed sustained release with a half-life of 23 to 30 days. Mean serum concentrations were more than 1 ng/mL throughout 28 days at 90 and 120 mg and more than 0.9 ng/mL with 60 mg.

Special populations –

Renal function impairment: Lanreotide has not been studied in patients with mild, moderate, or severe renal impairment. The pharmacokinetics of lanreotide in renally impaired subjects were evaluated after IV administration of lanreotide immediate-release formulation at 7 mcg/kg dose. Subjects with end-stage renal disease requiring dialysis showed an approximate 2-fold decrease in total serum clearance of lanreotide, with a consequent 2-fold increase in half-life and AUC.

See Administration and Dosage for more information.

Hepatic function impairment: The pharmacokinetics of lanreotide in hepatically impaired subjects were evaluated after IV administration of immediate-release lanreotide at a 7 mcg/kg dose. In subjects with moderate to severe hepatic impairment, a 30% reduction in lanreotide clearance was observed.

See Administration and Dosage for more information.

Elderly: The pharmacokinetics of lanreotide in elderly subjects were evaluated after IV administration of immediate-release lanreotide at a 7 mcg/kg dose. Studies in healthy elderly subjects showed an 85% increase in half-life and a 65% increase in mean residence time of lanreotide compared with those seen in healthy, younger subjects.

Contraindications

None well documented.

Warnings/Precautions

➤*Cholelithiasis and gallbladder sludge:* Lanreotide may reduce gallbladder motility and lead to gallstone formation; therefore, patients treated with lanreotide may need to be monitored periodically.

➤*Hyperglycemia and hypoglycemia:* Pharmacological studies in animals and humans show that lanreotide, like somatostatin and other somatostatin analogs, inhibits the secretion of insulin and glucagon. Hence, patients treated with lanreotide may experience hypoglycemia or hyperglycemia. Monitor blood glucose levels when lanreotide treatment is initiated or when the dose is altered, and adjust antidiabetic treatment accordingly.

➤*Thyroid function abnormalities:* Slight decreases in thyroid function have occurred during treatment with lanreotide in acromegalic patients, although clinical hypothyroidism is rare (less than 1%). Thyroid function tests are recommended when clinically indicated.

➤*Cardiovascular abnormalities:* The most common overall cardiac adverse reactions observed in 3 pooled lanreotide cardiac studies in patients with acromegaly were sinus bradycardia (5.5%), bradycardia (2.8%), and hypertension (5.6%).

In patients without underlying cardiac disease, lanreotide may lead to a decrease in heart rate without necessarily reaching the threshold of bradycardia. In patients suffering from cardiac disorders prior to lanreotide treatment, sinus bradycardia may occur. Take care when initiating treatment with lanreotide in patients with bradycardia.

➤*Renal function impairment:* See Administration and Dosage for more information.

➤*Hepatic function impairment:* See Administration and Dosage for more information.

➤*Pregnancy:* Category C. Lanreotide has been shown to have an embryocidal effect in rats and rabbits. There are no adequate and well-controlled studies in pregnant women. Use lanreotide during pregnancy only if the potential benefit justifies the potential risk to the fetus.

Reproductive studies in pregnant rats given 30 mg/kg by subcutaneous injection every 2 weeks (5 times the human dose based on body surface area [BSA] comparisons) resulted in decreased embryo/fetal survival. Studies in pregnant rabbits given subcutaneous injections of 0.45 mg/kg/day (2 times the human therapeutic exposures at the maximum recommended dose of 120 mg, based on comparisons of relative BSA) show decreased fetal survival and increased fetal skeletal/soft tissue abnormalities.

➤*Lactation:* It is not known whether lanreotide is excreted in human milk. Many drugs are excreted in human milk. Because of serious adverse reactions in animals and the potential for adverse reactions in breastfeeding infants from lanreotide, make a decision whether to discontinue breastfeeding or the drug, taking into account the importance of the drug to the mother.

➤*Children:* Safety and efficacy in children have not been established.

➤*Monitoring:* Periodically monitor serum GH and IGF-1 levels; they are useful markers of the disease and the efficacy of treatment.

Periodically monitor gallbladder motility and thyroid function.

Monitor blood glucose levels when lanreotide treatment is initiated or when the dose is altered.

Drug Interactions

Lanreotide Drug Interactions

Precipitant drug	Object drug[a]		Description
Beta-blockers (eg, atenolol, propranolol)	Lanreotide	⬆	Coadministration with drugs such as beta-blockers may have an additive effect on the reduction of heart rate associated with lanreotide. Dose adjustments of concomitant medication may be necessary.
Lanreotide	Beta-blockers (eg, atenolol, propranolol)		
Lanreotide	Bromocriptine	⬆	Coadministration may increase the availability of bromocriptine. Clinical monitoring is warranted. If an interaction is suspected, adjust the bromocriptine dose as needed.
Lanreotide	Cyclosporine	⬇	Coadministration of cyclosporine with lanreotide may decrease the relative bioavailability of cyclosporine and, therefore, may necessitate adjustment of the cyclosporine dose to maintain therapeutic levels.
Lanreotide	CYP3A4 metabolism (eg, quinidine)	⬆	Lanreotide may decrease the metabolic clearance of drugs known to be metabolized by CYP-450[b] enzymes, which have a low therapeutic index, such as quinidine. Use with caution and consider dose reductions of the coadministered medications.
Lanreotide	Insulin, oral hypoglycemic agents	⬇	Lanreotide inhibits the secretion of insulin and glucagon. Monitor blood glucose concentrations when lanreotide treatment is started or when the dose is altered. Adjust antidiabetic treatment accordingly.

[a] ⬆ = object drug increased; ⬇ = object drug decreased.
[b] CYP-450 = cytochrome P450.

Adverse Reactions

➤*Common adverse reactions:* The most commonly reported adverse reactions reported by more than 5% of patients who received lanreotide (N = 416) in the overall pooled safety studies in acromegaly patients were cholelithiasis, GI disorders (eg, abdominal pain, constipation, diarrhea, flatulence, loose stools, nausea, vomiting), and injection-site reactions.

➤*Adverse reactions (more than 5%):*

Lanreotide Adverse Reactions (> 5%)[a]

	Fixed-dose phase double-blind + single-blind (weeks 0 to 20)				Placebo-controlled, double-blind phase (weeks 0 to 4)	
Adverse reactions	Lanreotide overall (n = 83)	Lanreotide 60 mg (n = 34)	Lanreotide 90 mg (n = 36)	Lanreotide 120 mg (n = 37)	Lanreotide overall (n = 107)	Placebo (n = 25)
Cardiovascular	10%	21%	6%	14%	13%	0%
Bradycardia	8%	18%	6%	5%	9%	0%
GI	36%	35%	58%	73%	56%	4%
Abdominal pain	7%	9%	17%	19%	15%	4%
Diarrhea	31%	26%	42%	65%	45%	0%
Flatulence	6%	0%	8%	14%	7%	0%
Hematologic	7%	6%	14%	5%	8%	0%
Anemia	7%	6%	14%	5%	8%	0%
Hepatic	4%	26%	19%	11%	19%	4%
Cholelithiasis	2%	15%	17%	8%	13%	0%
Local[b]	6%	9%	11%	22%	14%	0%
Metabolic/Nutritional	16%	24%	25%	11%	20%	12%
Weight decrease	8%	9%	11%	5%	8%	0%

[a] A patient is counted only once for each body system and adverse reaction.
[b] Includes injection-site mass/pain/reaction/inflammation.

LANREOTIDE ACETATE — INJECTION

➤*Long-term studies:*

Lanreotide Adverse Reactions in Long-Term Studies (> 5%)[a]		
Adverse reactions	Studies 1 and 2 (n = 170)	Overall pooled data (N = 416)
Any adverse reaction	92%	86%
CNS	20%	19%
Headache	5%	7%
GI	71%	57%
Abdominal pain	20%	19%
Constipation	5%	8%
Diarrhea	48%	37%
Flatulence	7%	7%
Loose stools	9%	6%
Nausea	9%	11%
Vomiting	5%	7%
Hepatic	31%	24%
Cholelithiasis	27%	20%
Local	30%	22%
Injection-site pain/mass/ induration/nodule/pruritus	17%	9%
Musculoskeletal	26%	17%
Arthralgia	10%	7%

[a] Patients with elevated GH and IGF-1 levels were either naive to somatostatin analog therapy or had undergone a 3-month washout.

➤*Additional adverse reactions in long term studies:*

Cardiovascular – Sinus bradycardia occurred in 7% of patients in pooled studies 1 and 2 and in 3% of patients in the overall pooled studies.Hypertension occurred in 7% of patients in pooled studies 1 and 2 and in 5% of patients in the overall pooled studies.

➤*Cardiovascular:* In the pooled clinical studies, sinus bradycardia (3.1%) was the most frequently observed heart rate and rhythm disorder. All other cardiac adverse drug reactions were observed in less than 1% of patients. The relationship of these reactions to lanreotide could not be established because many of these patients had underlying cardiac disease.

A comparative echocardiography study of lanreotide and another somatostatin analog demonstrated no difference in the development of new or worsening valvular regurgitation between the 2 treatments over 1 year. The occurrence of clinically significant mitral regurgitation (ie, moderate or severe in intensity) or of clinically significant aortic regurgitation (ie, at least mild in intensity) was low in both groups of patients throughout the study.

➤*GI:* In the pooled clinical studies of lanreotide, a variety of GI reactions occurred, the majority of which were mild to moderate in severity. One percent of acromegalic patients treated with lanreotide in the pooled clinical studies discontinued treatment because of GI reactions.

Pancreatitis was reported in less than 1% of patients.

In clinical studies involving 416 acromegalic patients treated with lanreotide, cholelithiasis and gallbladder sludge were reported in 20% of patients. Among 167 acromegalic patients treated with lanreotide who underwent routine evaluation with gallbladder ultrasound, 17.4% had gallstones at baseline. New cholelithiasis was reported in 12% of patients. Cholelithiasis may be related to dose or duration of exposure.

➤*Hematologic:* Anemia occurred in 7% of patients in the pooled studies 1 and 2 and in 3% of patients in the overall pooled studies.

➤*Local:* In the pooled clinical studies, injection-site pain (4.1%) and injection-site mass (1.7%) were the most frequently reported local adverse drug reactions that occurred with the administration of lanreotide. In a specific analysis, 4.8% of patients presented indurations at the injection site. Injection-site adverse reactions were more commonly reported soon after the start of treatment and were less commonly reported as treatment continued. Such adverse reactions were usually mild or moderate but did lead to withdrawal from clinical studies in 2 subjects.

➤*Metabolic:* In the clinical studies in acromegalic patients treated with lanreotide, adverse reactions of dysglycemia (eg, diabetes, hyperglycemia, hypoglycemia) were reported by 14% of patients and were considered related to study drug in 7% of patients.

➤*Immunogenicity:* Laboratory investigations of acromegalic patients treated with lanreotide in clinical studies show that the percentage of patients with putative antibodies at any time point after treatment is low (less than 1% to 4% of patients in specific studies whose antibodies were tested). The antibodies did not appear to affect the efficacy or safety of lanreotide.

➤*Postmarketing:*

GI – GI disorders (eg, abdominal pain, diarrhea), pancreatitis.

Miscellaneous – General disordersand administration-site conditions (eg, injection-site reactions)

Overdosage

➤*Treatment:* If overdose occurs, symptomatic management is indicated.

Patient Information

Advise patients to inform their health care provider or pharmacist if they develop any unusual symptoms or if any known symptom persists or worsens.

Advise patients that a response to lanreotide should be monitored by periodic measurements of GH and IGF-1 levels, with a goal of decreasing these levels to the normal range.

PEGVISOMANT

PEGVISOMANT

Rx	Somavert (Pfizer)	Injection, lyophilized powder for solution: 10 mg (as protein)/vial	Mannitol 36 mg. In single-dose vials with diluent.
		15 mg (as protein)/vial	Mannitol 36 mg. In single-dose vials with diluent.
		20 mg (as protein)/vial	Mannitol 36 mg. In single-dose vials with diluent.

PEGVISOMANT — INJECTION

Indications

➤*Acromegaly:* For the treatment of acromegaly in patients who have had an inadequate response to surgery and/or radiation therapy and/or other medical therapies, or for whom these therapies are not appropriate. The goal of treatment is to normalize serum insulin-like growth factor-I (IGF-I) levels.

Administration and Dosage

➤*Adults:*

Acromegaly –

Maximum dose: 30 mg daily maintenance dose.

Loading dose: 40 mg subcutaneously under physician supervision.

Maintenance dosage: 10 mg subcutaneously daily.

Dosage adjustment: Serum IGF-I concentrations should be measured every 4 to 6 weeks, at which time the dosage should be adjusted in 5 mg increments if IGF-I levels are still elevated (or 5 mg decrements if IGF-I levels have decreased below the normal range). While the goals of therapy are to achieve (and then maintain) serum IGF-I concentrations within the age-adjusted normal range and to alleviate the signs and symptoms of acromegaly, titration of dosing should be based on IGF-I levels. It is unknown whether patients who remain symptomatic while achieving normalized IGF-I levels would benefit from increased dosing.

➤*Hepatic function impairment:* Assess liver enzymes prior to starting therapy. Do not start therapy if liver enzymes are greater than 3 times the upper limit of normal (ULN) until a comprehensive workup establishes the cause of the patient's liver dysfunction. If the decision is to treat, liver function tests and clinical symptoms should be monitored very closely.

➤*Preparation for administration:* To prepare the solution, withdraw 1 mL of the provided sterile water for injection and inject it into the vial, aiming the stream of liquid against the glass wall. Hold the vial between the palms of both hands and gently roll it to dissolve the powder. Do not shake the vial, as this may cause denaturation. Discard the diluent vial containing the remaining water for injection. After reconstitution, each vial contains 10, 15, or 20 mg of pegvisomant protein in 1 mL of solution.

➤*Administration:* For subcutaneous administration only. Not for intradermal, intramuscular, or intravenous (IV) administration. Rotate injection sites (eg, thigh, abdomen, upper arm). Give new injections at least 1 inch from old site and never into areas where the skin is tender, bruised, red, or hard. Only 1 dose should be administered from each vial. Administer within 6 hours after reconstitution.

➤*Storage/Stability:* Store vials at 2° to 8°C (36° to 46°F). Protect from freezing. After reconstitution, administer within 6 hours.

Actions

➤*Pharmacology:* Pegvisomant selectively binds to growth hormone (GH) receptors on cell surfaces, where it blocks the binding of endogenous GH, and thus interferes with GH signal transduction. Inhibition of GH action results in decreased serum concentrations of insulin-like growth factor-I (IGF-I), as well as other GH-responsive serum proteins, including IGF binding protein-3 (IGFBP-3), and the acid-labile subunit (ALS).

PEGVISOMANT — INJECTION

➤*Pharmacokinetics:*

Absorption – Following subcutaneous administration, peak serum pegvisomant concentrations are not generally attained until 33 to 77 hours after administration. The mean extent of absorption of a 20 mg subcutaneous dose was 57%, relative to a 10 mg IV dose.

Distribution – The mean apparent volume of distribution of pegvisomant is 7 L (12% coefficient of variation), suggesting that pegvisomant does not distribute extensively into tissues. After a single subcutaneous administration, exposure (C_{max}, AUC) to pegvisomant increases disproportionately with increasing dose. Mean ± SEM serum pegvisomant concentrations after 12 weeks of therapy with daily doses of 10, 15, and 20 mg were 6,600 ± 1330; 16,000 ± 2,200; and 27,000 ± 3,100 ng/mL, respectively.

Metabolism/Excretion – The pegvisomant molecule contains covalently bound polyethylene glycol polymers in order to reduce the clearance rate. Clearance of pegvisomant following multiple doses is lower than seen following a single dose. The mean total body systemic clearance of pegvisomant following multiple doses is estimated to range between 36 to 28 mL/h for subcutaneous doses ranging from 10 to 20 mg/day, respectively. Clearance of pegvisomant was found to increase with body weight. Pegvisomant is eliminated from serum with a mean half-life of approximately 6 days following either single or multiple doses. Less than 1% of administered drug is recovered in the urine over 96 hours. The elimination route of pegvisomant has not been studied in humans.

Contraindications

Hypersensitivity to pegvisomant or any of its components. The stopper on the vial of pegvisomant contains latex.

Warnings/Precautions

➤*Tumor growth:* Tumors that secrete growth hormone (GH) may expand and cause serious complications. Therefore, all patients with these tumors, including those who are receiving pegvisomant, should be carefully monitored with periodic imaging scans of the sella turcica. During clinical studies of pegvisomant, 2 patients manifested progressive tumor growth. Both patients had, at baseline, large globular tumors impinging on the optic chiasm, which had been relatively resistant to previous antiacromegalic therapies. Overall, mean tumor size was unchanged during the course of treatment with pegvisomant in the clinical studies.

➤*Glucose metabolism:* GH opposes the effects of insulin on carbohydrate metabolism by decreasing insulin sensitivity; thus, glucose tolerance may increase in some patients treated with pegvisomant. Although none of the acromegalic patients with diabetes mellitus who were treated with pegvisomant during the clinical studies had clinically relevant hypoglycemia, these patients should be carefully monitored and doses of antidiabetic drugs reduced as necessary.

➤*GH deficiency:* A state of functional GH deficiency may result from administration of pegvisomant, despite the presence of elevated serum GH levels. Therefore, during treatment with pegvisomant, patients should be carefully observed for the clinical signs and symptoms of a GH-deficient state, and serum IGF-I concentrations should be monitored and maintained within the age-adjusted normal range (by adjustment of the dose of pegvisomant).

➤*Pregnancy:* Category B. At the 10 mg/kg/day dose (10 times the maximum human therapeutic dose based on body surface area), a reproducible, slight increase in post-implantation loss was observed in both studies. There are no adequate and well-controlled studies in pregnant women. Because animal reproduction studies are not always predictive of human responses, pegvisomant should be used during pregnancy only if clearly needed.

➤*Lactation:* It is not known whether pegvisomant is excreted in human milk. Because many drugs are excreted in milk, caution should be exercised when pegvisomant is administered to a breast-feeding woman.

➤*Children:* The safety and efficacy of pegvisomant in children have not been established.

➤*Elderly:* Clinical studies of pegvisomant did not include sufficient numbers of subjects 65 years of age and older to determine whether they respond differently from younger subjects. In general, dose selection for an elderly patient should be cautious, usually starting at the low end of the dosing range, reflecting the greater frequency of decreased hepatic, renal, or cardiac function, and of concomitant disease or other drug therapy.

➤*Lab test abnormalities:*

Liver tests – Recommendations for monitoring LTs are stated above.

IGF-I levels – Treatment with pegvisomant should be evaluated by monitoring serum IGF-I concentrations 4 to 6 weeks after therapy is initiated or any dose adjustments are made and at least every 6 months after IGF-I levels have normalized. The goals of treatment should be to maintain a patient's serum IGF-I concentration within the age-adjusted normal range and to control the signs and symptoms of acromegaly.

GH levels – Pegvisomant interferes with the measurement of serum GH concentrations by commercially available GH assays. Furthermore, even when accurately determined, GH levels usually increase during therapy with pegvisomant. Therefore, treatment with pegvisomant should not be adjusted based on serum GH concentrations.

➤*Monitoring:*

Liver tests (LTs) – Elevations of serum concentrations of alanine aminotransferase (ALT) and aspartate aminotransferase (AST) greater than 10 times the ULN were reported in 2 patients (0.8%) exposed to pegvisomant during premarketing clinical studies. One patient was rechallenged with pegvisomant, and the recurrence of elevated transaminase levels suggested a probable causal relationship between administration of the drug and the elevation in liver enzymes. A liver biopsy performed on the second patient was consistent with chronic hepatitis of unknown etiology. In both patients, the transaminase elevations normalized after discontinuation of the drug.

During the premarketing clinical studies, the incidence of elevations in ALT greater than 3 times but less than or equal to 10 times the ULN in patients treated with pegvisomant and placebo were 1.2% and 2.1%, respectively.

Elevations in ALT and AST levels were not associated with increased levels of serum total bilirubin (TBIL) and alkaline phosphatase (ALP), with the exception of 2 patients with minimal associated increases in ALP levels (ie, less than 3 times ULN). The transaminase elevations did not appear to be related to the dose of pegvisomant administered, generally occurred within 4 to 12 weeks of initiation of therapy, and were not associated with any identifiable biochemical, phenotypic, or genetic predictors.

Baseline serum ALT, AST, TBIL, and ALP levels should be obtained prior to initiating therapy with pegvisomant. The following table lists recommendations regarding initiation of treatment with pegvisomant, based on the results of these liver tests (LTs).

Initiation of Pegvisomant Treatment Based on Liver Test Results

Baseline LT levels	Recommendations
Normal	May treat with pegvisomant. Monitor LTs at monthly intervals during the first 6 months of treatment, quarterly for the next 6 months, and then biannually for the next year.
Elevated, but ≤ 3 × ULN	May treat with pegvisomant; however, monitor LTs monthly for at least 1 year after initiation of therapy and then biannually for the next year.
> 3 × ULN	Do not treat with pegvisomant until a comprehensive workup establishes the cause of the patient's liver dysfunction. Determine if cholelithiasis or choledocholithiasis is present, particularly in patients with a history of prior therapy with somatostatin analogs. Based on the workup, consider initiation of therapy with pegvisomant. If the decision is to treat, LTs and clinical symptoms should be monitored very closely.

If a patient develops LT elevations, or any other signs or symptoms of liver dysfunction while receiving pegvisomant, the following patient management is recommended (see following table).

Continuation of Treatment with Pegvisomant Based on Results of Liver Tests

LT levels and clinical signs/symptoms	Recommendations
≥ 3, but < 5 × ULN (without signs/symptoms of hepatitis or other liver injury, or increase in serum TBIL)	May continue therapy with pegvisomant. However, monitor LTs weekly to determine if further increases occur (see below). In addition, perform a comprehensive hepatic workup to discern if an alternative cause of liver dysfunction is present.
≥ 5 × ULN, or transaminase elevations ≥ 3 × ULN associated with any increase in serum TBIL (with or without signs/symptoms of hepatitis or other liver injury)	Discontinue pegvisomant immediately. Perform a comprehensive hepatic workup, including serial LTs, to determine if and when serum levels return to normal. If LTsv normalize (regardless of whether an alternative cause of the liver dysfunction is discovered), consider cautious reinitiation of therapy with pegvisomant, with frequent LT monitoring.
Signs or symptoms suggestive of hepatitis or other liver injury (eg, jaundice, bilirubinuria, fatigue, nausea, vomiting, right upper quadrant pain, ascites, unexplained edema, easy bruisability)	Immediately perform a comprehensive hepatic workup. If liver injury is confirmed, the drug should be discontinued.

Drug Interactions

➤*Insulin/Oral hypoglycemic agents:* Acromegalic patients with diabetes mellitus being treated with insulin or oral hypoglycemic agents may

PEGVISOMANT — INJECTION

require dose reductions of these therapeutic agents after the initiation of therapy with pegvisomant.

➤*Opioids:* In clinical studies, patients on opioids often needed higher serum pegvisomant concentrations to achieve appropriate IGF-I suppression compared with patients not receiving opioids. The mechanism of this interaction is not known.

➤*Drug/Lab test interactions:* Pegvisomant has significant structural similarity to GH, which causes it to cross-react in commercially available GH assays. Because serum concentrations of pegvisomant at therapeutically effective doses are generally 100 to 1,000 times higher than endogenous serum GH levels seen in patients with acromegaly, commercially available GH assays will overestimate true GH levels. Treatment with pegvisomant should therefore not be monitored or adjusted based on serum GH concentrations reported from these assays. Instead, monitoring and dose adjustments should only be based on serum IGF-I levels.

Adverse Reactions

➤*Laboratory changes:* See Warnings/Precautions for more information. Nine acromegalic patients (9.6%) withdrew from premarketing clinical studies because of adverse reactions, including 2 patients with marked transaminase elevations, 1 patient with lipohypertrophy at the injection sites, and 1 patient with substantial weight gain. The majority of reported adverse reactions were of mild to moderate intensity and limited duration. Most adverse reactions did not appear to be dose dependent.

Pegvisomant Adverse Reactions in Acromegaly Patients in a 12-week placebo-controlled study[a]

Adverse reaction	Pegvisomant 10 mg/day (n = 26)	Pegvisomant 15 mg/day (n = 26)	Pegvisomant 20 mg/day (n = 28)	Placebo (n = 32)
Cardiovascular				
Hypertension	0	2 (8%)	0	0
CNS				
Dizziness	2 (8%)	1 (4%)	1 (4%)	2 (6%)
Paresthesia	0	0	2 (7%)	2 (6%)
GI				
Abnormal liver function tests	3 (12%)	1 (4%)	1 (4%)	1 (3%)
Diarrhea	1 (4%)	0	4 (14%)	1 (3%)
Nausea	0	2 (8%)	4 (14%)	1 (3%)
Metabolic/nutritional				
Peripheral edema	2 (8%)	0	1 (4%)	0
Respiratory				
Sinusitis	2 (8%)	0	1 (4%)	1 (3%)

Pegvisomant Adverse Reactions in Acromegaly Patients in a 12-week placebo-controlled study[a]

Adverse reaction	Pegvisomant 10 mg/day (n = 26)	Pegvisomant 15 mg/day (n = 26)	Pegvisomant 20 mg/day (n = 28)	Placebo (n = 32)
Miscellaneous				
Infection[b]	6 (23%)	0	0	2 (6%)
Pain	2 (8%)	1 (4%)	4 (14%)	2 (6%)
Injection site reaction	2 (8%)	1 (4%)	3 (11%)	0
Accidental injury	2 (8%)	1 (4%)	0	1 (3%)
Back pain	2 (8%)	0	1 (4%)	1 (3%)
Flu syndrome	1 (4%)	3 (12%)	2 (7%)	0
Chest pain	1 (4%)	2 (8%)	0	0

[a] Table includes only those reactions that were reported in at least 2 patients and at a higher incidence in patients treated with pegvisomant than in patients treated with placebo.

[b] The 6 reactions coded as "infection" in the group treated with pegvisomant 10 mg were reported as cold symptoms (3), upper respiratory tract infection (1), blister (1), and ear infection (1). The 2 reactions in the placebo group were reported as cold symptoms (1) and chest infection (1).

➤*Immunogenicity:* In premarketing clinical studies, approximately 17% of the patients developed low titer, non-neutralizing anti-GH antibodies. Although the presence of these antibodies did not appear to impact the efficacy of pegvisomant, the long-term clinical significance of these antibodies is not known. No assay for anti-pegvisomant antibodies is commercially available for patients receiving pegvisomant.

Overdosage

➤*Symptoms:* In 1 reported incident of acute overdose with pegvisomant during premarketing clinical studies, a patient self-administered 80 mg/day for 7 days. The patient experienced a slight increase in fatigue, had no other complaints, and demonstrated no significant clinical laboratory abnormalities.

➤*Treatment:* Administration of pegvisomant should be discontinued and not resumed until IGF-I levels return to within or above the normal range.

Patient Information

Patients and any other persons who may administer pegvisomant should be carefully instructed by a healthcare professional on how to properly reconstitute and inject the product.

Patients should be informed about the need for serial monitoring of LTs, and told to immediately discontinue therapy and contact their physicians if they become jaundiced. In addition, patients should be made aware that serial IGF-I levels will need to be obtained to allow their physician to properly adjust the dose of pegvisomant.

LARONIDASE

Rx	**Aldurazyme** (Genzyme)	**Injection, solution, concentrate**: 2.9 mg per 5 mL	Preservative free. In 5 mL single-use vials.[a]

[a] Contains albumin (human) 0.1% after dilution. Also contains 43.9 mg of sodium chloride, 63.5 mg of sodium phosphate monobasic monohydrate, 10.7 mg of sodium phosphate dibasic heptahydrate, and 0.05 mg of polysorbate 80.

LARONIDASE — INJECTION

WARNING

Risk of anaphylaxis – Life-threatening anaphylactic reactions have been observed in some patients during laronidase infusions. Therefore, ensure that appropriate medical support is readily available when laronidase is administered. Patients with compromised respiratory function or acute respiratory disease may be at risk of serious acute exacerbation of their respiratory compromise because of infusion reactions, and may require additional monitoring.

Indications

➤*Mucopolysaccharidosis I:* For patients with Hurler and Hurler-Scheie forms of mucopolysaccharidosis I and for patients with the Scheie form who have moderate to severe symptoms. The risks and benefits of treating mildly affected patients with the Scheie form have not been established.

Administration and Dosage

April 30, 2003.

➤*General dosing considerations:* Pretreatment with antipyretics and/or antihistamines is recommended 60 minutes prior to the start of the infusion.

➤*Adults:*

Mucopolysaccharidosis I –

Usual dosage: 0.58 mg/kg once weekly as an intravenous (IV) infusion.

The total volume of the infusion is determined by the patient's body weight and should be delivered over approximately 3 to 4 hours. Patients with a body weight of 20 kg or less should receive a total volume of 100 mL. Patients with a body weight of more than 20 kg should receive a total volume of 250 mL.

Dosage titration: The initial infusion rate of 10 mcg/kg/h may be incrementally increased every 15 minutes during the first hour, as tolerated, until a maximum infusion rate of 200 mcg/kg/h is reached. The maximum rate should then be maintained for the remainder of the infusion (2 to 3 hours). (See Laronidase Infusion Rate tables for infusion rate titration).

Laronidase Infusion Rate for Patients Weighing 20 kg or Less

Total volume of laronidase infusion = 100 mL	
2 mL/h × 15 min (10 mcg/kg/h)	Obtain vital signs; if stable, then increase rate to:
4 mL/h × 15 min (20 mcg/kg/h)	Obtain vital signs; if stable, then increase the rate to:
8 mL/h × 15 min (50 mcg/kg/h)	Obtain vital signs; if stable, then increase the rate to:
16 mL/h × 15 min (100 mcg/kg/h)	Obtain vital signs; if stable, then increase the rate to:
32 mL/h × approximately 3 h (200 mcg/kg/h)	For the remainder of the infusion.

Laronidase Infusion Rate for Patients Weighing More Than 20 kg

Total volume of laronidase infusion = 250 mL	
5 mL/h × 15 min (10 mcg/kg/h)	Obtain vital signs; if stable, then increase the rate to:
10 mL/h × 15 min (20 mcg/kg/h)	Obtain vital signs; if stable, then increase the rate to:

LARONIDASE — INJECTION

Laronidase Infusion Rate for Patients Weighing More Than 20 kg	
Total volume of laronidase infusion = 250 mL	
20 mL/h × 15 min (50 mcg/kg/h)	Obtain vital signs; if stable, then increase the rate to:
40 mL/h × 15 min (100 mcg/kg/h)	Obtain vital signs; if stable, then increase the rate to:
80 mL/h × approximately 3 h (200 mcg/kg/h)	For the remainder of the infusion.

➤*Children:*

5 years of age and older –

Mucopolysaccharidosis I: See Adults for dosing.

➤*Preparation for administration:* Each vial of laronidase provides laronidase 2.9 mg in 5 mL of solution and is intended for single use only. Do not use the vial more than 1 time.

The concentrated solution for infusion must be diluted with albumin (human) 0.1% in sodium chloride 0.9% injection using aseptic techniques.

Laronidase should be prepared using polyvinyl chloride (PVC) containers and administered with a PVC infusion set equipped with an in-line, low protein–binding 0.2 micrometer filter. There is no information on the compatibility of diluted laronidase with glass containers.

1.) Determine the number of vials to be diluted based on the individual patient's weight and the recommended dose of 0.58 mg/kg (patient's weight [kg] × 1 mL/kg of laronidase = total # mL of laronidase, then total # of mL of laronidase ÷ 5 mL per vial = total # of vials). Round up to the nearest whole vial. Remove the required number of vials from the refrigerator to allow them to reach room temperature. Do not heat or microwave vials.
2.) Before withdrawing laronidase from the vial, visually inspect each vial for particulate matter and discoloration. The laronidase solution should be clear to slightly opalescent and colorless to pale yellow. A few translucent particles may be present. Do not use if the solution is discolored or if there is particulate matter in the solution.
3.) Determine the total volume of the infusion to be used based on the patient's body weight. The total final volume should be 100 mL (if weight is 20 kg or less) or 250 mL (if weight is more than 20 kg).
4.) Prepare an infusion bag of albumin (human) 0.1% in sodium chloride 0.9% injection. Remove and discard a volume of sodium chloride 0.9% injection equal to the volume of albumin (human) to be added to the infusion bag. Add the appropriate volume of albumin (human) to the infusion bag, and gently rotate the infusion bag to ensure proper distribution of the albumin (see the following table).
5.) Withdraw and discard a volume of the albumin (human) 0.1% in sodium chloride 0.9% injection from the infusion bag that is equal to the volume of laronidase concentrate to be added.
6.) Slowly withdraw the calculated volume of laronidase from the appropriate number of vials using caution to avoid excessive agitation. Do not use a filter needle because this may cause agitation. Agitation may denature laronidase, rendering it biologically inactive.
7.) Slowly add the laronidase solution to the albumin (human) 0.1% in sodium chloride 0.9% injection using care to avoid agitation of the solutions. Do not use a filter needle.
8.) Gently rotate the infusion bag to ensure proper distribution of laronidase. Do not shake the solution.

Albumin Addition by Laronidase Volume		
Total volume of laronidase infusion	Volume of albumin (human) 5% to be added	Volume of albumin (human) 25% to be added
100 mL	2 mL	0.4 mL
250 mL	5 mL	1 mL

➤*Administration:* Administer once weekly as an intravenous (IV) infusion.

Administer with a PVC infusion set equipped with an in-line, low protein-binding 0.2 micrometer filter.

➤*Admixture compatibility:* Laronidase must not be mixed with other medicinal products in the same infusion.

➤*Storage/Stability:* Store laronidase under refrigeration, at 2° to 8°C (36° to 46°F).

The diluted solution should be used immediately. If immediate use is not possible, the diluted solution should be refrigerated at 2° to 8°C (36° to 46°F). The in-use storage should not be longer than 36 hours from the time of preparation to completion of administration. Room temperature storage of diluted solution is not recommended.

Actions

➤*Pharmacology:* Mucopolysaccharide storage disorders are caused by the deficiency of specific lysosomal enzymes required for the catabolism of glycosaminoglycans (GAG).

Mucopolysaccharidosis I is characterized by the deficiency of α-L-iduronidase, a lysosomal hydrolase that catalyses the hydrolysis of terminal α-L-iduronic acid residues of dermatan sulfate and heparan sulfate. Reduced or absent α-L-iduronidase activity results in the accumulation of the GAG substrates, dermatan sulfate, and heparan sulfate throughout the body, and leads to widespread cellular, tissue, and organ dysfunction.

The rationale of laronidase therapy in mucopolysaccharidosis I is to provide exogenous enzyme for uptake into lysosomes and to increase the catabolism of GAG. Laronidase uptake by cells into lysosomes is most likely mediated by the mannose-6-phosphate–terminated oligosaccharide chains of laronidase binding to specific mannose-6-phosphate receptors.

➤*Pharmacokinetics:*

Absorption/Distribution – The pharmacokinetics of laronidase were evaluated in 12 patients with mucopolysaccharidosis I who received laronidase 0.58 mg/kg as a 4-hour infusion. After weeks 1, 12, and 26 of weekly infusions, the mean maximum plasma concentrations ranged from 1.2 to 1.7 mcg/mL for the 3 time points. The mean area under the plasma concentration-time curve (AUC_∞) ranged from 4.5 to 6.9 mcg•h/mL. The mean volume of distribution ranged from 0.24 to 0.6 L/kg.

Excretion – Mean plasma clearance ranged from 1.7 to 2.7 mL/min/kg, and the mean elimination half-life ranged from 1.5 to 3.6 hours.

Most patients who received once-weekly infusions of laronidase developed antibodies to laronidase by week 12. Between weeks 1 and 12, increases in plasma clearance of laronidase that appeared to be proportional to the antibody titer were observed in some patients. At week 26, plasma clearance of laronidase was comparable with that at week 1, in spite of the continued and, in some cases, increased titers of antibodies.

Contraindications

None known.

Warnings/Precautions

➤*Pretreatment:* Ensure that patients receive antipyretics and/or antihistamines prior to infusion. If an infusion reaction occurs, regardless of pretreatment, decreasing the infusion rate, temporarily stopping the infusion, and/or administration of additional antipyretics and/or antihistamines may ameliorate the symptoms. If severe hypersensitivity or anaphylactic reactions occur, immediately discontinue the infusion of laronidase and initiate appropriate treatment. Exercise caution if epinephrine is being considered for use in patients with mucopolysaccharidosis I because of the increased prevalence of coronary artery disease.

➤*Immunogenicity:* In clinical studies, 50 of 55 (91%) patients treated with laronidase were positive for antibodies to laronidase. The clinical significance of antibodies to laronidase, including the potential for product neutralization, is not known.

The data reflect the percentage of patients whose test results were considered positive for antibodies to laronidase using an enzyme-linked immunosorbent assay (ELISA) for laronidase-specific immunoglobulin (Ig) G–binding antibodies, and are highly dependent on the sensitivity and specificity of the assay. Additionally, the observed incidence of antibodies in an assay may be influenced by several factors, including sample handling, timing of sample collection, concomitant medications, and underlying disease. For these reasons, comparison of the incidence of antibodies to laronidase with the incidence of antibodies to other products may be misleading.

Four patients in the controlled study who experienced severe infusion-related reactions were tested for laronidase-specific IgE antibodies and complement activation. IgE testing was performed by ELISA, and complement activation was measured by the Quidel enzyme immunoassay. One of the 4 patients had an anaphylactic reaction consisting of urticaria and airway obstruction and tested positive for both laronidase-specific IgE-binding antibodies and complement activation.

➤*Hypersensitivity reactions:* Life-threatening anaphylactic reactions have been observed in some patients during or up to 3 hours after laronidase infusions. Reactions have included respiratory failure, respiratory distress, stridor, tachypnea, bronchospasm, airway obstruction, hypoxia, hypotension, bradycardia, and urticaria. Interventions have included resuscitation, mechanical ventilatory support, emergency tracheotomy, hospitalization, and treatment with inhaled beta-adrenergic agonists, epinephrine, and IV corticosteroids.

In clinical trials and postmarketing safety experience with laronidase, approximately 1% of patients experienced severe or serious allergic reactions. In patients with mucopolysaccharidosis I, preexisting upper airway obstruction may have contributed to the severity of some reactions. Because of the potential for severe allergic reactions, ensure that appropriate medical support is readily available when laronidase is administered. Because of the potential for recurrent reactions, some patients who experience initial severe reactions may require prolonged observation.

Patients with an acute illness at the time of laronidase infusion appear to be at greater risk for infusion-related reactions. Carefully consider the patient's clinical status prior to administration of laronidase. One patient with acute bronchitis and hypoxia experienced increased tachypnea during the first laronidase infusion that resolved without intervention. The patient's respiratory symptoms returned within 30 minutes of completing the infusion and responded to bronchodilator therapy. Approximately 6 hours after the infusion, the patient experienced coughing, then respiratory arrest, and died.

Consider the risks and benefits of readministering laronidase following a severe hypersensitivity or anaphylactic reaction. Exercise extreme care, with appropriate resuscitation measures available, if the decision is made to readminister the product.

➤*Pregnancy: Category B.* There are no adequate and well-controlled studies in pregnant women. Because animal reproduction studies are not always predictive of human response, use laronidase during pregnancy only if clearly needed.

LARONIDASE — INJECTION

➤*Lactation:* It is not known whether laronidase is excreted in human milk. Because many drugs are excreted in human milk, exercise caution when laronidase is administered to a breast-feeding woman.

➤*Children:* Patients younger than 5 years of age were not included in the clinical studies because of inability to comply with efficacy outcome assessments. It is not known if children younger than 5 years of age respond differently from older children.

Drug Interactions

None known.

Adverse Reactions

➤*Serious adverse reactions:* The most serious adverse reactions reported with laronidase during clinical trials and the postmarketing period were anaphylactic and allergic reactions.

➤*Most common adverse reactions:* The most common adverse reactions associated with laronidase treatment during clinical studies were upper respiratory tract infection, rash, and injection-site reaction.

Laronidase Adverse Reactions

Adverse reaction	Placebo (n = 23)	Laronidase (n = 22)
Cardiovascular		
Dependent edema	0%	9%
Hypotension	0%	9%
Vein disorder	4%	14%
CNS		
Hyperreflexia	0%	14%
Paresthesia	4%	14%
Local		
Injection-site pain	0%	9%
Injection-site reaction	9%	18%
Miscellaneous		
Abscess	0%	9%
Bilirubinemia	0%	9%
Chest pain	0%	9%
Corneal opacity	0%	9%
Facial edema	0%	9%
Rash	22%	36%
Thrombocytopenia	0%	9%
Upper respiratory tract infection	17%	32%

➤*Infusion-related reactions:* In clinical studies, the most common adverse reactions requiring intervention were infusion-related reactions reported in 32% (7/22) of patients treated with laronidase. The most common infusion-related reactions were flushing, fever, headache, and rash. Flushing occurred in 23% (5/22) of patients receiving laronidase; the other reactions were less frequent. Infusion-related reactions were not significantly different between the laronidase treatment group and the placebo group who received infusions of diluent and all components of laronidase except the laronidase enzyme. All reactions were mild to moderate in severity. The frequency of infusion-related reactions decreased with continued use during the open-label extended use period. Less common Infusion-related reactions included cough, bronchospasm, dyspnea, urticaria, angioedema and pruritus. Most infusion-related reactions requiring intervention were ameliorated with slowing of the infusion rate, temporarily stopping the infusion, and/or administering additional antipyretics and/or antihistamines.

➤*Postmarketing:* In postmarketing experience with laronidase, severe and serious infusion-related reactions have been reported, some of which were life-threatening. The most frequently reported adverse reactions (using Medical Dictionary for Regulatory Activities terminology) included chills, vomiting, nausea, arthralgia, diarrhea, tachycardia, abdominal pain, increased blood pressure, and decreased oxygen saturation.

Patient Information

Inform patients that a registry for mucopolysaccharidosis I patients has been established in order to better understand the variability and progression of mucopolysaccharidosis I disease, and to continue to monitor and evaluate treatments. Encourage patients to participate, and advise them that their participation may involve long-term follow-up. Information regarding the registry program may be found at http://www.MPSIregistry.com or by calling 800-745-4447.

GALSULFASE

Rx	**Naglazyme** (BioMarin)	**Solution for Injection:** 1 mg/mL (expressed as protein content)	Preservative-free. In 5 mL single-use vials.[a]

[a] Contains sodium chloride 43.8 mg, sodium phosphate monobasic monohydrate 6.2 mg, sodium phosphate dibasic heptahydrate 1.34 mg, and polysorbate 0.25 mg 80.

GALSULFASE — INJECTION

Indications

➤*Mucopolysaccharidosis VI:* For patients with mucopolysaccharidosis VI (MPS VI; Maroteaux-Lamy syndrome). Galsulfase has been shown to improve walking and stair-climbing capacity.

Administration and Dosage

➤*General dosing considerations:* Galsulfase concentrated solution for infusion must be diluted before use. (See Preparation for Administration.)

➤*Adults:*

Mucopolysaccharidosis VI –

Younger than 29 years of age: The majority of individuals in the clinical studies were pediatric patients.

• *Usual dosage* – 1 mg/kg of body weight administered once weekly as an IV infusion.

• *Pretreatment* – Pretreatment with antihistamines with or without antipyretics is recommended 30 to 60 minutes prior to the start of the infusion.

➤*Children:*

Mucopolysaccharidosis VI –

5 years of age and older: See Adults for dosing.

➤*Preparation for administration:* The concentrated solution for infusion must be diluted in 0.9% sodium chloride injection to a final volume of 250 mL. Galsulfase should be prepared using polyvinyl chloride (PVC) containers. There is no information on the compatibility of diluted galsulfase with glass containers.

Use aseptic technique.

1.) Determine the number of vials to be diluted based on the individual patient's weight and the recommended dose of 1 mg/kg:

Patient's weight (kg) × 1 mL/kg of galsulfase = Total mL of galsulfase

Total mL of galsulfase ÷ 5 mL per vial = Total number of vials

Round to the nearest whole vial. Remove the required number of vials from the refrigerator to allow them to reach room temperature. Do not allow vials to remain at room temperature longer than 24 hours prior to dilution. Do not heat or microwave vials.

2.) Before withdrawing the galsulfase from the vial, visually inspect each vial for particulate matter and discoloration. The galsulfase solution should be clear to slightly opalescent and colorless to pale yellow. A few translucent particles may be present. Do not use if the solution is discolored or if there is particulate matter in the solution.

3.) From a 250 mL infusion bag of 0.9% sodium chloride injection, withdraw and discard a volume equal to the volume of galsulfase to be added. If using a 100 mL infusion bag, this is not necessary.

4.) Slowly withdraw the calculated volume of galsulfase from the appropriate number of vials using caution to avoid excessive agitation. Do not use a filter needle because this may cause agitation. Agitation may denature galsulfase, rendering it biologically inactive.

5.) Slowly add the galsulfase solution to the 0.9% sodium chloride injection, using care to avoid agitation of the solutions. Do not use a filter needle.

6.) Gently rotate the infusion bag to ensure proper distribution of galsulfase. Do not shake the solution.

➤*Administration:* Galsulfase should be diluted in 0.9% sodium chloride injection and delivered by controlled IV infusion using an infusion pump. Administer with a PVC infusion set equipped with an in-line, low-proteinbinding 0.2 mcm filter.

The total volume of the infusion should be delivered over no less than 4 hours.

The initial infusion rate should be 6 mL/h for the first hour. If the infusion is well tolerated, the rate of infusion may be increased to 80 mL/h for the remaining 3 hours. The infusion time can be extended up to 20 hours if infusion reactions occur.

For patients 20 kg or less who are susceptible to fluid volume overload, consider diluting galsulfase in a volume of 100 mL. The infusion rate (mL/min) should be decreased so that the total infusion duration remains no less than 4 hours.

GALSULFASE — INJECTION

➤*Admixture compatibility:* Galsulfase must not be infused with other products in the infusion tubing. The compatibility of galsulfase in solution with other products has not been evaluated.

➤*Storage/Stability:* Store galsulfase under refrigeration at 2° to 8°C (36° to 46°F). Do not freeze or shake. The diluted solution should be used immediately. If immediate use is not possible, the diluted solution should be stored refrigerated at 2° to 8°C (36° to 46°F). Storage after dilution should not exceed 48 hours from the time of preparation to completion of administration. Room temperature storage of diluted solution, other than during infusion, is not recommended.

Galsulfase does not contain preservatives; therefore, after dilution with saline in the infusion bags, any unused product or waste material should be discarded and disposed of in accordance with local requirements.

Actions

➤*Pharmacology:* Mucopolysaccharide storage disorders are caused by the deficiency of specific lysosomal enzymes required for the catabolism of GAG. MPS VI is characterized by the absence or marked reduction in N-acetylgalactosamine 4-sulfatase. The sulfatase activity deficiency results in the accumulation of the GAG substrate dermatan sulfate, throughout the body. This accumulation leads to widespread cellular, tissue, and organ dysfunction. Galsulfase is intended to provide an exogenous enzyme that will be taken up into lysosomes and increase the catabolism of GAG. Galsulfase uptake by cells into lysosomes is most likely mediated by the binding of mannose-phosphate-terminated oligosaccharide chains of galsulfase to specific mannose-6-phosphate receptors.

➤*Pharmacokinetics:* The pharmacokinetic parameters of galsulfase were evaluated in 13 patients with MPS VI who received 1 mg/kg of galsulfase as a 4-hour infusion weekly for 24 weeks. The pharmacokinetic parameters at week 1 and week 24 are shown in the following table.

Galsulfase Pharmacokinetic Parameters (Median, Range)

Pharmacokinetic parameter	Week 1	Week 24
C_{max} (mcg/mL)	0.8 (0.4 to 1.3)	1.5 (0.2 to 5.5)
AUC_{0-t} (h•mcg/mL)[a]	2.3 (1 to 3.5)	4.3 (0.3 to 14.2)
Volume of distribution (mL/kg)	103 (56 to 323)	69 (59 to 2,799)
CL (mL/kg/min)	7.2 (4.7 to 10.5)	3.7 (1.1 to 55.9)
Half-life (min)	9 (6 to 21)	26 (8 to 40)

[a] Area under the plasma galsulfase concentration-time curve from start of infusion to 60 minutes post infusion.

Nearly all patients who receive treatment with galsulfase develop antibodies to galsulfase. Of 30 patients with MPS VI who received weekly galsulfase infusions and had pharmacokinetics evaluated, 29 developed antibodies to galsulfase. Four patients with high antibody titers had decreases in plasma AUC between weeks 1 and 24. One patient with high antibody titers had an increase in plasma AUC between weeks 1 and 24.

Contraindications

None known.

Warnings/Precautions

➤*Infusion reactions:* Because of the potential for infusion reactions, give patients antihistamines with or without antipyretics prior to infusion. Despite routine pretreatment with antihistamines, infusion reactions, some severe, occurred in 30 of 55 patients treated with galsulfase. Severe symptoms included angioneurotic edema, hypotension, dyspnea, bronchospasm, respiratory distress, apnea, and urticaria. The most common symptoms of infusion reactions included fever, chills/rigors, headache, rash, and mild to moderate urticaria. Nausea, vomiting, elevated blood pressure, retrosternal pain, abdominal pain, malaise, and joint pain were also reported. Initial reactions were observed as late as week 55 of treatment.

Symptoms typically abated with slowing or temporary interruption of the infusion and administration of additional antihistamines, antipyretics, and, occasionally, corticosteroids. Most patients were able to complete their infusions. Subsequent infusions were managed with a slower rate of galsulfase administration, treatment with additional prophylactic antihistamines, and, in the event of a more severe reaction, treatment with prophylactic corticosteroids. Despite these measures, 13 of 30 patients had additional infusion reactions.

If severe infusion reactions occur, immediately discontinue the infusion of galsulfase and initiate appropriate treatment. Consider the risks and benefits of readministering galsulfase following a severe reaction.

No factors were identified that predisposed patients to infusion reactions. There was no association between severity of infusion reactions and titer of antigalsulfase antibodies.

➤*Sleep apnea:* Sleep apnea is common in MPS VI patients and antihistamine pretreatment may increase the risk of apneic episodes. Evaluation of airway patency should be considered prior to initiation of treatment. Patients using supplemental oxygen or continuous positive airway pressure (CPAP) during sleep should have these treatments readily available during infusion in the event of an infusion reaction, or extreme drowsiness/sleep induced by antihistamine use.

➤*Acute febrile or respiratory illness:* Consider delaying galsulfase infusions in patients who present with an acute febrile or respiratory illness.

➤*Immunogenicity:* Ninety-eight percent (53/54) of all patients treated with galsulfase developed antigalsulfase immunoglobulin G (IgG) antibodies. Initial evidence of antibody development typically appeared following 4 to 8 weeks of treatment. No association was observed between antibody development and urinary GAG levels.

Five patients with high antibody levels had observable differences in pharmacokinetic parameters. Antibodies from 1 patient were analyzed for neutralizing effect and showed evidence of in vitro inhibition of galsulfase activity. Because only 1 patient sample was analyzed for neutralizing activity, the effects of neutralizing antibodies are unclear.

The data reflect the percentage of patients whose test results were considered positive for antibodies to galsulfase using an enzyme-linked immunosorbent assay (ELISA) for galsulfase-specific IgG-binding antibodies, and are highly dependent on the sensitivity and specificity of the assay. Additionally, the observed incidence of antibodies in an assay may be influenced by several factors, including sample handling, timing of sample collection, concomitant medications, and underlying disease. For these reasons, comparison of the incidence of antibodies to galsulfase with the incidence of antibodies to other products may be misleading.

➤*Pregnancy: Category B.* There are no adequate and well-controlled studies in pregnant women. Because animal reproduction studies are not always predictive of human response, use this drug during pregnancy only if clearly needed.

See Patient Information for more information.

➤*Lactation:* It is not known whether galsulfase is excreted in human milk. Because many drugs are excreted in human milk, exercise caution when galsulfase is administered to a breast-feeding woman. Breast-feeding women are encouraged to participate in the clinical surveillance program.

➤*Children:* Safety and efficacy in patients younger than 5 years of age have not been evaluated.

Drug Interactions

No formal drug interaction studies have been conducted.

Adverse Reactions

The most frequent serious adverse reactions related to the use of galsulfase occurred during infusions and included urticaria of the face and neck, bronchospasm, respiratory distress, and apnea.

The most common adverse reactions observed in the clinical studies were headache, fever, arthralgia, vomiting, upper respiratory tract infections, abdominal pain, diarrhea, ear pain, cough, and otitis media.

The most common adverse reactions requiring interventions were infusion-related reactions.

Because clinical trials are conducted under widely varying conditions, the observed adverse reaction rates may not predict the rates observed in patients in clinical practice.

The following table enumerates adverse reactions that were reported during the 6-month placebo-controlled trial and occurred in at least 2 patients more in the reactions group than in the placebo group. Observed adverse reactions in the phase 1, phase 2, and open-label extension studies were not different in nature or severity.

Galsulfase Adverse Reactions

Adverse reaction	Galsulfase (n = 19)	Placebo (n = 20)
All	19 (100%)	20 (100%)
Cardiovascular		
Hypertension	2 (11%)	0
GI		
Abdominal pain	10 (53%)	6 (30%)
Gastroenteritis	2 (11%)	0
Respiratory		
Dyspnea	4 (21%)	2 (10%)
Nasal congestion	2 (11%)	0
Pharyngitis	3 (16%)	1 (5%)
Special senses		
Conjunctivitis	4 (21%)	0
Ear pain	8 (42%)	4 (20%)
Increased corneal opacification	2 (11%)	0
Miscellaneous		
Areflexia	2 (11%)	0
Chest pain	3 (16%)	1 (5%)
Face edema	2 (11%)	0
Malaise	2 (11%)	0
Pain	5 (26%)	1 (5%)
Rigors	4 (21%)	0
Umbilical hernia	2 (11%)	0

Overdosage

There is no experience with overdose of galsulfase.

GALSULFASE — INJECTION

Patient Information

Inform patients that a clinical surveillance program has been established in order to better understand the variability and progression of the disease in the population as a whole, and to monitor and evaluate long-term treatment effects of galsulfase. The clinical surveillance program will also monitor the effect of galsulfase on pregnant women and their offspring, and determine if galsulfase is excreted in breast milk. Encourage patients to participate and advise them that their participation is voluntary and may involve long-term follow-up. For more information, visit http://www.MPSVI.com or call 1-866-906-6100.

IDURSULFASE

Rx	**Elaprase** (Shire Human Genetic Therapies)	**Solution for injection:** 2 mg/mL[a]	Preservative free. In 5 mL single-use vials.[b]

[a] Concentrated solution must be diluted.
[b] Each vial contains an extractable volume of 3 mL with an idursulfase concentration of 2 mg/mL, providing 6 mg idursulfase, 24 mg sodium chloride, 6.75 mg sodium phosphate monobasic monohydrate, 2.97 mg sodium phosphate dibasic heptahydrate, and 0.66 mg polysorbate 20.

IDURSULFASE — INJECTION

WARNING

Hypersensitivity reactions – Anaphylactoid reactions, which may be life-threatening, have been observed in some patients during idursulfase infusions. Therefore, make appropriate medical support readily available when administering idursulfase. Patients with compromised respiratory function or acute respiratory disease may be at risk for serious acute exacerbation of their respiratory compromise because of infusion reactions and require additional monitoring.

Indications

➤*Hunter syndrome:* For patients with Hunter syndrome (mucopolysaccharidosis type II). Idursulfase has been shown to improve walking capacity in these patients.

Administration and Dosage

➤*General dosing considerations:* Idursulfase is a concentrated solution for intravenous (IV) infusion and must be diluted before administration. (See Preparation for Administration.)

➤*Adults:*

Hunter syndrome (mucopolysaccharidosis type II) – 0.5 mg/kg of body weight administered every week as an IV infusion.

➤*Children:*

Hunter syndrome (mucopolysaccharidosis type II) –

5 years of age and older: See Adults.

➤*Preparation for administration:* Idursulfase is a concentrated solution for IV infusion and must be diluted in 100 mL of sodium chloride 0.9% injection. Each vial of idursulfase contains a 2 mg/mL solution of idursulfase protein (6 mg) in an extractable volume of 3 mL and is for single use only.

Use aseptic techniques. Idursulfase should be prepared and administered by a health care provider.

1.) Determine the total volume of idursulfase to be administered and the number of vials needed based on the patient's weight and the recommended dose of 0.5 mg/kg. Round up to determine the number of whole vials needed from which to withdraw the calculated volume of idursulfase to be administered.

Patient's weight (kg) × 0.5 mg per kg of idursulfase ÷ 2 mg per mL = total # mL of idursulfase

Total # mL of idursulfase ÷ 3 mL per vial = total # of vials

2.) Perform a visual inspection of each vial. Idursulfase is a clear to slightly opalescent, colorless solution. Do not use if the solution in the vials is discolored or particulate matter is present. Idursulfase should not be shaken.
3.) Withdraw the calculated volume of idursulfase from the appropriate number of vials.
4.) Dilute the total calculated volume of idursulfase in 100 mL of sodium chloride 0.9% injection. Once the solution is diluted into normal saline in the infusion bag, mix gently but do not shake. Discard diluted solution if not administered or refrigerated within 8 hours of preparation. Diluted solution may be stored refrigerated for up to 48 hours.
5.) Idursulfase is supplied in single-use vials. Dispose of remaining idursulfase left in a vial after withdrawing the patient's calculated dose in accordance with local requirements.

➤*Administration:* Use of an infusion set equipped with a 0.2 mcm filter is recommended.

Infusion rate – The total volume of infusion may be administered over a period of 1 to 3 hours. Patients may require longer infusion times because of infusion reactions; however, infusion times should not exceed 8 hours. The initial infusion rate should be 8 mL/h for the first 15 minutes. If the infusion is well-tolerated, the rate may be increased by 8 mL/h increments at 15-minute intervals in order to administer the full volume within the desired period of time. However, at no time should the infusion rate exceed 100 mL/h. If infusion reactions occur, the infusion rate may be slowed and/or temporarily stopped, or discontinued for that visit, based on clinical judgment.

➤*Admixture compatibility:* Idursulfase should not be infused with other products in the infusion tubing.

➤*Storage/Stability:* Store idursulfase vials under refrigeration at 2° to 8°C (36° to 46°F) and protect from light. Do not freeze or shake.

This product contains no preservatives. Use the diluted solution immediately. If immediate use is not possible, the diluted solution can be stored refrigerated at 2° to 8°C (36° to 46°F) for up to 48 hours or must be administered within 8 hours if held at room temperature.

Actions

➤*Pharmacology:* Hunter syndrome is an X-linked recessive disease caused by insufficient levels of the lysosomal enzyme iduronate-2-sulfatase. This enzyme cleaves the terminal 2-*O*-sulfate moieties from the glycosaminoglycans (GAG) dermatan sulfate and heparin sulfate. Because of the missing or defective iduronate-2-sulfatase enzyme in patients with Hunter syndrome, GAG progressively accumulate in the lysosomes of a variety of cells, leading to cellular engorgement, organomegaly, tissue destruction, and organ system dysfunction.

Treatment of Hunter syndrome patients with idursulfase provides exogenous enzyme for uptake into cellular lysosomes. Mannose-6-phosphate (M6P) residues on the oligosaccharide chains allow specific binding of the enzyme to the M6P receptors on the cell surface, leading to cellular internalization of the enzyme, targeting to intracellular lysosomes, and subsequent catabolism of accumulated GAG.

➤*Pharmacokinetics:* The pharmacokinetic characteristics of idursulfase were evaluated in several studies in patients with Hunter syndrome. The serum concentration of idursulfase was quantified using an antigen-specific, enzyme-linked immunoabsorbent assay (ELISA). The area under the concentration-time curve (AUC) increased in a greater than dose proportional manner as the dose increased from 0.15 to 1.5 mg/kg following a single 1-hour infusion of idursulfase. The pharmacokinetic parameters at the recommended dosage regimen (idursulfase 0.5 mg/kg administered weekly as a 3-hour infusion) were determined at weeks 1 and 27 in 10 patients 7.7 to 27 years of age (see the following table). There were no apparent differences in pharmacokinetic parameter values between weeks 1 and 27.

Idursulfase Pharmacokinetic Parameters (Mean, Standard Deviation)

Pharmacokinetic parameter	Week 1	Week 27
C_{max} (mcg/mL)[a]	1.5 (0.6)	1.1 (0.3)
AUC (min•mcg/mL)	206 (87)	169 (55)
$t_{½}$ (min)[b]	44 (19)	48 (21)
Cl (mL/min/kg)[c]	3 (1.2)	3.4 (1)
V_{ss} (% BW)[d]	21 (8)	25 (9)

[a] C_{max} = maximum plasma concentration.
[b] $t_{½}$ = terminal half-life.
[c] Cl = clearance.
[d] V_{ss} = volume of distribution at steady state; BW = body weight.

Contraindications

None known.

Warnings/Precautions

➤*Hypersensitivity infusion reactions:* See the Warning box for more information.

Reactions have included distress, hypoxia, hypotension, angioedema, or seizure. In clinical trials with idursulfase, 16 of 108 patients (15%) experienced infusion reactions during 26 of 8,274 infusions (0.3%) that involved adverse reactions in at least 2 of the following 3 body systems: cutaneous, respiratory, or cardiovascular. Of these 16 patients, 11 experienced significant hypersensitivity reactions during 19 of 8,274 infusion (0.2%). One of the episodes occurred in a patient with a tracheotomy and severe airway disease who received an idursulfase infusion while he had a preexisting febrile illness, and then experienced respiratory distress, hypoxia, cyanosis, and seizure with loss of consciousness.

Because of the potential for severe infusion reactions, make appropriate medical support readily available when idursulfase is administered.

When severe infusion reactions occurred during clinical studies, subsequent infusions were managed by use of antihistamines and/or corticosteroids prior to or during infusions, a slower rate of idursulfase administration, and/or early discontinuation of the idursulfase infusion if serious symptoms developed. With these measures, no patient discontinued treatment permanently because of a hypersensitivity reaction.

IDURSULFASE — INJECTION

Patients with compromised respiratory function or acute respiratory disease may be at higher risk of life-threatening complications from infusion reactions. Consider delaying the idursulfase infusion in patients with concomitant acute respiratory and/or febrile illness.

If a severe infusion reaction occurs, immediately suspend the infusion of idursulfase and initiate appropriate treatment depending on the severity of the symptoms. Consider resuming the infusion at a slower rate or, if the reaction is serious enough to warrant it, discontinue the idursulfase infusion for that visit.

➤*Hunter Outcome Survey:* A Hunter Outcome Survey has been established to better understand the variability and progression of Hunter syndrome in the population as a whole, and to monitor and evaluate long-term treatment effects of idursulfase. Patients and their health care providers are encouraged to participate in this program. For more information, visit http://www.elaprase.com or call OnePath at 1-866-888-0660.

➤*Pregnancy: Category C.* Reproduction studies in pregnant female animals have not been conducted with idursulfase. It is not known whether idursulfase can cause fetal harm when administered to a pregnant woman or can affect reproduction capacity. Give idursulfase to pregnant women only if clearly needed.

➤*Lactation:* It is not known whether this product is excreted in breast milk. Because many drugs are excreted in breast milk, exercise caution when idursulfase is administered to a breast-feeding woman.

➤*Children:* Patients in the clinical studies were 5 years of age and older. Children, adolescents, and adults responded similarly to treatment with idursulfase. Safety and efficacy have not been established in children younger than 5 years of age.

Drug Interactions

No formal drug interactions studies have been conducted with idursulfase.

Adverse Reactions

The most common adverse reactions requiring intervention were infusion-related reactions.

In clinical studies, the most frequent serious adverse reactions related to the use of idursulfase were hypoxic episodes. Other notable serious adverse reactions that occurred in the idursulfase-treated patients but not in the placebo patients included 1 case each of the following: arthralgia, cardiac arrhythmia, cyanosis, infection, pulmonary embolism, and respiratory failure.

Adverse reactions were commonly reported in association with infusions. The most common infusion-related reactions were cutaneous reactions (erythema, pruritus, rash, and urticaria), fever, headache, and hypertension. The frequency of infusion-related reactions decreased over time with continued idursulfase treatment.

Because clinical trials are conducted under widely varying conditions, adverse reaction rates observed in the clinical trials of a product cannot be directly compared with rates in the clinical trials of another product and may not reflect the rates observed in practice.

The following table enumerates adverse reactions reported during the 53-week, placebo-controlled study that occurred in at least 10% of patients treated with idursulfase weekly administration and more frequently than in the placebo patients. The most common (more than 30%) adverse reactions were arthralgia, headache, and pyrexia.

Idursulfase Adverse Reactions (≥ 10%)

Adverse reaction	Idursulfase 0.5 mg/kg weekly (n = 32)	Placebo (n = 32)
Cardiovascular		
Atrial abnormality	4 (13%)	3 (9%)
Hypertension	8 (25%)	7 (22%)
CNS		
Anxiety, irritability	4 (13%)	1 (3%)
Headache	19 (59%)	14 (44%)
Dermatologic		
Abscess	5 (16%)	0
Pruritic rash	4 (13%)	0
Pruritus	9 (28%)	5 (16%)
Skin disorder[a]	4 (13%)	1 (3%)
Urticaria	5 (16%)	0
GI		
Dyspepsia	4 (13%)	0
Musculoskeletal		
Arthralgia	10 (31%)	9 (28%)
Chest wall musculoskeletal pain	5 (16%)	0
Musculoskeletal dysfunction[a]	5 (16%)	3 (9%)
Respiratory		
Wheezing	6 (19%)	5 (16%)
Special senses		
Visual disturbance	7 (22%)	2 (6%)
Miscellaneous		
Adverse reactions resulting from injury	4 (13%)	2 (6%)
Infusion site edema	4 (13%)	3 (9%)
Limb pain	9 (28%)	8 (25%)
Malaise	7 (22%)	6 (19%)
Pyrexia	20 (63%)	19 (59%)
Superficial injury	4 (13%)	3 (9%)

[a] Not otherwise specified.

➤*Immunogenicity:* Fifty-one percent (32/63) of patients in the weekly idursulfase treatment arm in the clinical study (53-week, placebo-controlled study with an open-label extension) developed anti-idursulfase IgG antibodies as assessed by ELISA or conformation specific antibody assay and confirmed by radioimmunoprecipitation assay (RIP). Sera from 4 out of 32 RIP confirmed anti-idursulfase antibody-positive patients were found to neutralize idursulfase activity in vitro. The incidence of antibodies that inhibit cellular uptake of idursulfase into cells is currently unknown, and the incidence of immunoglobulin E (IgE) antibodies to idursulfase is not known. Patients who developed IgG antibodies at any time had an increased incidence of infusion reactions, including hypersensitivity reactions. The reduction of urinary GAG excretion was less in patients in whom circulating anti-idursulfase antibodies were detected. The relationship between the presence of anti-idursulfase antibodies and clinical efficacy outcomes is unknown.

The data reflect the percentage of patients whose test results were positive for antibodies to idursulfase in specific assays and are highly dependent on the sensitivity and specificity of these assays. Additionally, the observed incidence of antibodies positivity in an assay may be influenced by several factors, including sample handling, timing of sample collection, concomitant medication, and underlying disease. For these reasons, comparison of the incidence of antibodies to idursulfase with the incidence of antibodies to other products may be misleading.

Overdosage

There is no experience with overdosage of idursulfase in humans. Single IV doses of idursulfase up to 20 mg/kg were not lethal in male rats and cynomolgus monkeys (approximately 6.5 and 13 times, respectively, of the recommended human dose based on body surface area), and there were no clinical signs of toxicity.

Patient Information

A Hunter Outcome Survey has been established to better understand the variability and progression of Hunter syndrome in the population as a whole, and to monitor and evaluate long-term treatment effects of idursulfase. Patients and their health care providers are encouraged to participate in this program. For more information, visit http://www.elaprase.com or call OnePath at 1-866-888-0660.

AGALSIDASE BETA

Rx	**Fabrazyme** (Genzyme)	**Powder for injection, lyophilized:** 5.5 mg (5 mg/mL when reconstituted)	Preservative free. In 5 mL single-use vials.[a]
		37 mg (5 mg/mL when reconstituted)	Preservative free. In 20 mL single-use vials.[b]

[a] Contains mannitol 33 mg, sodium phosphate monobasic monohydrate 3 mg, sodium phosphate dibasic heptahydrate 8.8 mg/vial.

[b] Contains mannitol 222 mg, sodium phosphate monobasic monohydrate 20.4 mg, sodium phosphate dibasic heptahydrate 59.2 mg/vial.

AGALSIDASE BETA — INJECTION

Indications

➤*Fabry disease:* For use in patients with Fabry disease. Agalsidase beta reduces globotriasylceramide (GL-3) deposition in capillary endothelium of the kidney and certain other cell types.

Administration and Dosage

➤*Adults:*

Fabry disease – 1 mg/kg body weight infused every 2 weeks as an IV infusion.

➤*Premedication:* Patients should receive antipyretics prior to infusion. If an infusion reaction occurs, regardless of pretreatment, decreasing the infusion rate, temporarily stopping the infusion, or administration of additional antipyretics, antihistamines or steroids may ameliorate the symptoms. Because of the potential for severe infusion reactions, appropriate medical support measures should be readily available when agalsidase beta is administered.

➤*Preparation for administration:* Shaking or agitation of this product should be avoided. Do not use filter needles during the preparation of the infusion.

Agalsidase beta vials and diluent should be allowed to reach room temperature prior to reconstitution (approximately 30 minutes).

Reconstitute each vial of agalsidase beta by slowly injecting 7.2 mL of sterile water for injection down the inside wall of each vial. Roll and tilt each vial gently. Each vial will yield a 5 mg/mL clear, colorless solution (total extractable amount per vial is 35 mg, 7 mL).

The reconstituted solution should be further diluted with 0.9% sodium chloride injection to a final total volume of 500 mL. Prior to adding the volume of reconstituted agalsidase beta required for the patient dose, remove an equal volume of 0.9% Sodium Chloride for Injection from the 500 mL infusion bag.

Slowly withdraw the reconstituted solution from each vial up to the total volume required for the patient dose. Inject the reconstituted agalsidase beta solution directly into the 0.9% sodium chloride solution. Do not inject in the airspace within the infusion bag. Discard any vial with unused reconstituted solution.

Gently invert infusion bag to mix the solution, avoiding vigorous shaking and agitation.

➤*Administration:* The initial IV infusion rate should be no more than 0.25 mg/min (15 mg/h). The infusion rate may be slowed in the event of infusion-associated reactions. After patient tolerance to the infusion is well established, the infusion rate may be increased in increments of 0.05 to 0.08 mg/min (increments of 3 to 5 mg/h) each subsequent infusion. Thirty-one (53%) of 58 patients have received infusions at rates of at least 33 mg/h.

Agalsidase beta should not be infused in the same intravenous line with other products.

The diluted solution may be filtered through an in-line low protein-binding 0.2 mcm filter during administration.

➤*Storage/Stability:* Store agalsidase beta under refrigeration between 2° to 8°C (36° to 46°F).

Reconstituted and diluted solutions of agalsidase beta should be used immediately. If immediate use is not possible, the reconstituted and diluted solution may be stored for up to 24 hours at 2° to 8°C (36° to 46°F).

Agalsidase beta does not contain any preservatives. Vials are for single-use only. Any unused product should be discarded.

Actions

➤*Pharmacology:* Fabry disease is an X-linked genetic disorder of glycosphingolipid metabolism. Deficiency of the lysosomal enzyme α-galactosidase A leads to progressive accumulation of glycosphingolipids, predominantly GL-3, in many body tissues, occurring over a period of years or decades. Clinical manifestations of Fabry disease include renal failure, cardiomyopathy, and cerebrovascular accidents. Accumulation of GL-3 in renal endothelial cells may play a role in renal failure.

Agalsidase beta is intended to provide an exogenous source of α-galactosidase A in Fabry disease patients. Preclinical and clinical studies evaluating a limited number of cell types indicate that agalsidase beta will catalyze the hydrolysis of glycosphingolipids including GL-3.

➤*Pharmacokinetics:* Plasma profiles of agalsidase beta were studied at 0.3, 1 and 3 mg/kg in 15 patients with Fabry disease. The area under the plasma concentration-time curve (AUC_{∞}) and the clearance did not increase proportionately with increasing doses, demonstrating that the enzyme follows nonlinear pharmacokinetics. Terminal half-life was dose independent with a range of 45 to 102 minutes.

In 11 patients with Fabry disease given 1 mg/kg agalsidase beta every 14 days for a total of 11 infusions, the pharmacokinetic responses following repeated dosing fell into 3 categories. In some patients, pharmacokinetic responses were maintained with repeated dosing, whereas in other patients, pharmacokinetic values decreased at infusion 7 relative to baseline and returned to baseline values by infusion 11. In the remaining patients, AUC declined and failed to return to baseline by infusion 11. In these patients, the average AUC was 25% of its initial level. Some patients with elevated titers of antibody to agalsidase were among those with decreased AUC. The development of antibodies to agalsidase did not influence half-life, but reduced both apparent C_{max} and AUC. The long-term consequence of antibody development to the pharmacokinetics of agalsidase has not been established.

Contraindications

No known contraindications.

Warnings/Precautions

➤*Infusion reactions:* Infusion reactions occurred in many patients treated with agalsidase beta. Some of the reactions were severe. Infusion reactions included fever, rigors, chest tightness, hypertension, hypotension, pruritus, myalgia, dyspnea, urticaria, abdominal pain, and headache. All patients were pretreated with acetaminophen and an antihistamine. Infusion reactions occurred in some patients after receiving antipyretics, antihistamines and oral steroids.

Patients should be given antipyretics prior to infusion. If an infusion reaction occurs, regardless of pretreatment, decreasing the infusion rate, temporarily stopping the infusion, or administration of additional antipyretics, antihistamines or steroids may ameliorate the symptoms. Because of the potential for severe infusion reactions, appropriate medical support measures should be readily available when agalsidase beta is administered.

➤*Cardiac function:* Patients with advanced Fabry disease may have compromised cardiac function, which may predispose them to a higher risk of severe complications from infusion reactions. Infusion reactions included fever, rigors, chest tightness, hypertension, hypotension, pruritus, myalgia, dyspnea, urticaria, abdominal pain, and headache. Patients with compromised cardiac function should be monitored closely if the decision is made to administer agalsidase beta.

➤*Immunogenetics:* Most patients develop IgG antibodies to agalsidase beta. Sixty-three (63) of 71 (89%) patients in the clinical studies treated with agalsidase beta have developed antibodies to agalsidase beta. Most patients who develop antibodies do so within the first 3 months of exposure. Some patients developed IgE or skin test reactivity specific to agalsidase beta. Physicians should consider testing for IgE in patients who experienced suspected allergic reactions and consider the risks and benefits of continued treatment in patients with antiagalsidase beta IgE.

➤*Pregnancy: Category B.* There are no adequate and well-controlled studies in pregnant women. Because animal reproduction studies are not always predictive of human response, this drug should be used during pregnancy only if clearly needed.

See Patient Information for more information.

Responses in women – Fabry disease is an X-linked genetic disorder. However, some heterozygous women will develop signs and symptoms of Fabry disease due to the variability of the X chromosome inactivation within cells. Generally, the rates of progression of organ impairment are slower than in male Fabry disease patients and severity of signs and symptoms is variable.

➤*Lactation:* It is not known whether agalsidase beta is excreted in human milk. Because many drugs are excreted in human milk, caution should be exercised when agalsidase beta is administered to a breast-feeding woman.

Nursing mothers should be encouraged to enroll in the Fabry registry (see Patient Information).

➤*Children:* The safety and efficacy of agalsidase beta in pediatric patients have not been established.

Drug Interactions

No drug interaction studies were performed.

Adverse Reactions

The most serious and most common adverse reactions reported with agalsidase beta are infusion reactions. Serious or frequently occurring infusion reactions consisted of 1 or more of the following: Tachycardia, hypertension, throat tightness, chest pain/tightness, dyspnea, fever, chills/rigors, abdominal pain, pruritus, urticaria, nausea, vomiting, lip or ear edema, and rash. Infusion reactions declined in frequency with continued use of agalsidase beta. However, serious infusion reactions may occur after extended durations of agalsidase beta treatment.

Other reported serious adverse events included stroke, pain, ataxia, bradycardia, cardiac arrhythmia, cardiac arrest, decreased cardiac output, vertigo, hypoacousia, and nephrotic syndrome. These adverse events also occur as manifestations of Fabry disease; an alteration in frequency or severity cannot be determined from the small numbers of patients studied.

The data described below reflect exposure of 29 patients to 1 mg/kg agalsidase beta every 2 weeks for 5 months in a placebo-controlled study. All 58

AGALSIDASE BETA — INJECTION

patients continued into an open-label extension study of agalsidase beta treatment for up to 30 additional months. An additional 28 patients received open-label treatment. All patients were treated with antipyretics and antihistamines prior to the infusions.

Because clinical trials are conducted under widely varying and controlled conditions, the observed adverse reaction rates may not predict the rates observed in patients in clinical practice.

The table below enumerates adverse events and selected laboratory abnormalities that occurred during the placebo-controlled trial in at least 2 patients more in the agalsidase beta group than was observed in the placebo group. Reported adverse events have been classified by organ system. Observed adverse events in the Phase ½ study and the open-label treatment period following the controlled study were not different in nature or severity.

Agalsidase Beta Adverse Reactions		
Adverse reaction	Placebo (n = 29)	Agalsidase beta (n = 29)
Cardiovascular		
Cardiomegaly	1 (3%)	3 (10%)
Hypertension	0	3 (10%)
Hypotension	2 (7%)	4 (14%)
Edema dependent	1 (3%)	6 (21%)
CNS		
Dizziness	2 (7%)	4 (14%)
Headache	11 (38%)	13 (45%)
Paraesthesia	2 (7%)	4 (14%)
Anxiety	5 (17%)	8 (28%)
Depression	1 (3%)	3 (10%)
GI		
Dyspepsia	1 (3%)	3 (10%)
Nausea	4 (14%)	8 (28%)
GU (male)		
Testicular pain	0	2 (7%)
Musculoskeletal		
Arthrosis	0	3 (10%)
Skeletal pain	0	6 (21%)
Respiratory		
Bronchitis	1 (3%)	3 (10%)
Bronchospasm	0	2 (7%)
Laryngitis	0	2 (7%)
Pharyngitis	2 (7%)	8 (28%)
Rhinitis	7 (24%)	11 (38%)
Sinusitis	0	2 (7%)
Miscellaneous		
Chest pain	3 (10%)	5 (17%)
Fever	5 (17%)	14 (48%)
Pain	3 (10%)	6 (21%)
Pallor	1 (3%)	4 (14%)
Rigors	4 (14%)	15 (52%)
Temperature change sensation	1 (3%)	5 (17%)

➤*Immunogenicity:* Sixty-three (63) of 71 (89%) patients in the clinical studies treated with agalsidase beta have developed antibodies to agalsidase beta. Most patients who develop antibodies do so within the first 3 months of exposure. Antibodies to agalsidase beta were purified from 15 patients with high antibodies titers (greater than or equal to 12,800) and studied for inhibition of in vitro enzyme activity. Under the conditions of this assay, most of these 15 patients had inhibition of in vitro enzyme activity ranging between 14% to 74% at 1 or more time points during the study. No general pattern was seen in individual patient reactivity over time. The clinical significance of binding or inhibitory antibodies to agalsidase beta is not known. In patients followed in the open-label study, reduction of GL-3 in plasma and GL-3 inclusions in superficial skin capillaries was maintained after antibodies formation.

The data reflect the percentage of patients whose test results were considered positive for antibodies to agalsidase beta using an ELISA and radioimmunoprecipitation (RIP) assay for antibodies. These results are highly dependent on the sensitivity and specificity of the assay. Additionally, the observed incidence of antibodies in an assay may be influenced by several factors including sample handling, timing of sample collection, concomitant medications, and underlying disease. For these reasons, comparison of the incidence of antibodies to agalsidase beta with the incidence of antibodies to other products may be misleading.

Overdosage

There have been no reports of overdose with agalsidase beta. In clinical trials, patients received doses up to 3 mg/kg body weight.

Patient Information

Patients should be informed that a registry has been established in order to better understand the variability and progression of Fabry disease in the population as a whole and in women, and to monitor and evaluate long-term treatment effects of agalsidase beta. The registry will also monitor the effect of agalsidase beta on pregnant women and their offspring, and determine if agalsidase beta is excreted in breast milk. Patients should be encouraged to participate and advised that their participation is voluntary and may involve long-term follow-up. For more information visit http://www.fabryregistry.com or call (800) 745-4447.

MIGLUSTAT

Rx	**Zavesca** (Actelion)	**Capsules:** 100 mg	Sodium starch glucollate. (OGT 918, 100). White, opaque. Gelatin. In 90s and blister card 18s.

MIGLUSTAT — ORAL

Indications

➤*Gaucher disease:* For the treatment of adult patients with mild to moderate type 1 Gaucher disease for whom enzyme replacement therapy is not a therapeutic option (eg, because of constraints such as allergy, hypersensitivity, or poor venous access).

Administration and Dosage

➤*Adults:*

Gaucher disease –

Usual dosage: 100 mg 3 times a day.

Dosage adjustment: It may be necessary to reduce the dose to 100 mg once or twice a day in some patients if adverse reactions, such as diarrhea or tremor, occur.

➤*Renal function impairment:*

Creatinine clearance 50 to 70 mL/min/1.73 m² – 100 mg twice per day.

Creatinine clearance of 30 to 50 mL/min/1.73 m² – 100 mg daily.

Creatinine clearance of less than 30 mL/min/1.73 m² – Not recommended.

➤*Administration:* Take orally at regular intervals.

➤*Storage/Stability:* Store at 20° to 25°C (68° to 77°F). Brief exposure to 15° to 30°C (59° to 86°F) permitted.

Actions

➤*Pharmacology:* Miglustat functions as a competitive and reversible inhibitor of the enzyme glucosylceramide synthase, the initial enzyme in a series of reactions which results in the synthesis of most glycosphingolipids. The goal of treatment with miglustat is to reduce the rate of glycosphingolipid biosynthesis so that the amount of glycosphingolipid substrate is reduced to a level which allows the residual activity of the deficient glucocerebrosidase enzyme to be more effective (substrate reduction therapy). In vitro and in vivo studies have shown that miglustat can reduce the synthesis of glucosylceramide-based glycosphingolipids. In clinical trials, miglustat improved liver and spleen volume, as well as hemoglobin concentration and platelet count.

➤*Pharmacokinetics:*

Absorption – After a 100 mg oral dose, the time to maximum observed plasma concentration of miglustat (t_{max}) ranged from 2 to 2.5 hours in Gaucher patients. Plasma concentrations show a biexponential decline, characterized by a short distribution phase and a longer elimination phase. The effective half-life of miglustat is approximately 6 to 7 hours, which predicts that steady-state will be achieved by 1.5 to 2 days following the start of 3 times daily dosing.

Miglustat, dosed at 50 and 100 mg in Gaucher patients, exhibits dose proportional pharmacokinetics. Miglustat's pharmacokinetics were not altered after repeated dosing 3 times daily for up to 12 months.

Coadministration of miglustat with food results in a decrease in the rate of absorption of miglustat (maximum serum concentration [C_{max}] was decreased by 36% and t_{max} delayed 2 hours) but has no statistically signifi-

MIGLUSTAT — ORAL

cant effect on the extent of absorption of miglustat (area under the plasma concentration curve [AUC] was decreased by 14%).

The mean oral bioavailability of a 100 mg miglustat capsule is about 97% relative to an oral solution administered under fasting conditions.

Distribution – Miglustat does not bind to plasma proteins. Mean apparent volume of distribution of miglustat is 83 to 105 L in Gaucher patients, indicating that miglustat distributes into extravascular tissues.

Excretion – The major route of excretion of miglustat is renal. Miglustat is excreted unchanged in the urine. Renal impairment has a significant effect on the pharmacokinetics of miglustat resulting in increased systemic exposure of miglustat in such patients. There is no evidence that miglustat is metabolized in humans.

Special populations –

Renal function impairment: Limited data in patients with Fabry disease and impaired renal function indicate that clearance (CL/F) of miglustat decreases with decreasing renal function. While the number of subjects with mild and moderate renal impairment was very small, the data suggest an approximate decrease in CL/F of 40% and 60%, respectively, in mild and moderate renal impairment, justifying the need to decrease the dosing of miglustat in such patients dependent upon creatinine clearance levels.

Data in severe renal impairment are limited to 2 patients with creatinine clearances in the range 18 to 29 mL/min and cannot be extrapolated below this range. These data suggest a decrease in CL/F by at least 70% in patients with severe renal impairment. Treatment with miglustat in patients with severe renal impairment is therefore not recommended.

Contraindications

Hypersensitivity to the active substance or any of the excipients; women who are or may become pregnant. If this drug is administered to a woman with reproductive potential, the patient should be apprised of the potential hazard to a fetus.

Warnings/Precautions

➤*Peripheral neuropathy:* Cases of peripheral neuropathy have been reported in patients treated with miglustat. All patients undergoing miglustat treatment should undergo baseline and repeat neurological evaluations at approximately 6-month intervals. Patients who develop symptoms such as numbness and tingling should have a careful re-assessment of the risk/benefit of miglustat therapy and cessation of treatment may be considered.

➤*Administration:* Therapy should be directed by physicians knowledgeable in the management of patients with Gaucher disease.

➤*Tremor:* Approximately 30% of patients have reported tremor or exacerbation of existing tremor on treatment. These tremors were described as an exaggerated physiological tremor of the hands. Tremor usually began within the first month of therapy and in many cases resolved between 1 to 3 months during treatment. Dose reduction may ameliorate the tremor (usually within days), but discontinuation with treatment may sometimes be required.

➤*Diarrhea and weight loss:* Diarrhea and weight loss were common in clinical studies of patients treated with miglustat; approximately 85% and up to 65% of treated patients, respectively, reported these conditions. Diarrhea appears to be the result of the disaccharidase inhibitory activity of miglustat, with a resultant osmotic diarrhea. It is unclear if weight loss results from the diarrhea and associated gastrointestinal complaints, a decrease in food intake, or a combination of these or other factors. The incidence of diarrhea was noted to decrease over time with continued miglustat treatment, and was noted to result in an increase in the use of antidiarrheal medications, most commonly loperamide. Patients may be instructed to avoid high carbohydrate content foods during treatment with miglustat if they present with diarrhea. The incidence of weight loss was most evident in the first 12 months of treatment.

➤*Male fertility:* Male patients should maintain reliable contraceptive methods while taking miglustat. Studies in the rat have shown that miglustat adversely affects spermatogenesis and sperm parameters, thereby reducing fertility. Until further information is available, it is advised that before seeking to conceive, male patients should cease miglustat and maintain reliable contraceptive methods for 3 months thereafter.

➤*Renal function impairment:* Miglustat is known to be substantially excreted by the kidney, and the risk of adverse reactions to this drug may be greater in patients with impaired renal function. The clearance of miglustat is decreased by 40% to 60% in patients with mild to moderate renal impairment, and up to 70% in patients with severe renal impairment. As a result of this, dose reductions are recommended for those patients with mild to moderate renal impairment, the reduction being dependent upon the level of their creatinine clearance adjustment. For those patients with severe renal impairment, treatment with miglustat is not recommended. Because elderly patients are more likely to have decreased renal function, care should be taken in dose selection, and it may be useful to monitor renal function.

➤*Pregnancy:* Category X. There are no adequate and well-controlled studies of miglustat in pregnant women. Miglustat should not be used during pregnancy.

Miglustat may cause fetal harm when administered to a pregnant woman. In female rats given miglustat by oral gavage at doses of 20, 60, 180 mg/kg/day beginning 14 days before mating and continuing through gestation day 17 (organogenesis), decreased live births including complete litter loss and decreased fetal weight was observed in the mid- and high-dose groups (systemic exposures greater than or equal to 2 times the human therapeutic systemic exposure based on body surface area comparison). In pregnant rats given miglustat by oral gavage at doses of 20, 60, 180 mg/kg/day from gestation day 6 through lactation (postpartum day 20), dystocia and delayed parturition were observed in the mid- and high-dose groups (systemic exposures greater than or equal to 2 times the human therapeutic systemic exposure, based on body surface area comparison). In addition, decreased live births and pup body weights were observed at greater than 20 mg/kg/day (systemic exposures less than the human therapeutic systemic exposure, based on body surface area comparison).

In pregnant rabbits given miglustat by oral gavage at doses of 15, 30, 45 mg/kg/day during gestation days 6 to 18 (organogenesis), maternal death and decreased body weight gain were observed at 15 mg/kg/day (systemic exposures less than the human therapeutic systemic exposure, based on body surface area comparisons).

Labor and delivery – Studies in pregnant rats exposed to miglustat during gestation through lactation are associated with dystocia and delayed parturition at systemic exposure 2 times the human therapeutic systemic exposure, based on body surface area comparisons.

➤*Lactation:* It is not known whether miglustat is excreted in human milk. Because many drugs are excreted in human milk and because of the potential for serious adverse reactions in nursing infants from miglustat, the drug should not be used in nursing mothers unless the potential benefit justifies the potential risk to the infant. A decision should be made whether to discontinue nursing or discontinue the drug, taking into account the importance of the drug to the lactating woman.

➤*Children:* The safety and efficacy of miglustat have not been evaluated in patients under the age of 18. Treatment with miglustat is associated with diarrhea and weight loss in approximately 85% and up to 65%, respectively, of adult patients. The effects of miglustat on growth and development in children have not been evaluated.

Drug Interactions

➤*Imiglucerase:* While coadministration of miglustat appeared to increase the clearance of imiglucerase by 70%, these results are not conclusive because of the small number of subjects studied and because patients took variable doses of imiglucerase. Combination therapy with imiglucerase and miglustat is not indicated.

Adverse Reactions

➤*Open-label uncontrolled monotherapy trials:* In 2 open-label, uncontrolled monotherapy trials in adult type 1 Gaucher disease patients treated with miglustat at a starting dose of 100 mg 3 times daily (dose range 100 to 200 mg 3 times daily) for 12 months in 28 patients [Study 1], or at a dose of 50 mg 3 times daily for 6 months in 18 patients [Study 2], GI events were observed in more than 80% of patients either at the outset of treatment, or intermittently during treatment. Diarrhea was observed in approximately 85% of patients. Weight loss has been observed in up to 65% of patients.

Miglustat Adverse Reactions in 2 Open-Label, Uncontrolled Monotherapy Trials (≥ 5%)

Adverse reactions	Study 1 (starting dose 100 mg 3 times daily) (n = 28)	Study 2 (50 mg 3 times daily) (n = 18)
CNS		
Dizziness	0%	11%
Headache	21%	22%
Leg cramps	4%	11%
Migraine	0%	6%
Paresthesia	7%	0%
Tremor	11%	11%
GI		
Abdominal pain	18%	50%
Anorexia	7%	0%
Bloating	0%	6%
Diarrhea	89%	89%
Dyspepsia	7%	0%
Epigastric pain not food-related	0%	6%
Flatulence	29%	44%
Nausea	14%	22%
Vomiting	4%	11%
GU, female		
Menstrual disorder	0%	6%
Hematologic		
Thrombocytopenia	7%	6%
Metabolic/Nutritional		
Weight decrease	39%	67%
Musculoskeletal		
Cramps	0%	11%
Ophthalmic		
Visual disturbance	0%	17%

MIGLUSTAT — ORAL

➤*Open-label active-controlled study:*

Miglustat Adverse Reactions in an Open-Label Active Controlled Study (≥ 5%)

Adverse reaction	Miglustat alone (n = 12)	Imiglucerase alone (n = 12)	Miglustat + imiglucerase (n = 12)
CNS			
Dizziness	8%	0%	25%
Gait unsteady	8%	0%	0%
Leg cramps	8%	0%	0%
Numbness localized	0%	0%	8%
Shaking	0%	0%	8%
Tremor	17%	0%	33%
GI			
Abdominal pain	67%	0%	58%
Constipation	8%	0%	25%
Diarrhea	100%	0%	83%
Dry mouth	8%	0%	0%
Flatulence	50%	0%	42%
Nausea	8%	0%	8%
GU, female			
Menstrual irregularity	0%	0%	8%
Metabolic/Nutritional			
Weight decrease	67%	0%	42%
Ophthalmic			
Eye abnormality	0%	0%	8%
Visual disturbance	0%	0%	8%
Psychiatric			
Appetite absent	0%	0%	8%
Jitteriness	0%	0%	8%
Memory loss	8%	0%	0%
Miscellaneous			
Abdominal distension	8%	0%	8%
Abdominal distension, gaseous	8%	0%	0%
Back pain	8%	0%	0%
Chills	0%	0%	8%
Heaviness in limbs	8%	0%	0%
Influenza-like symptoms	0%	0%	8%
Pain	0%	8%	8%
Pain legs	0%	0%	8%
Weakness, generalized	17%	0%	8%

Overdosage

In the clinical development program for miglustat, no patient experienced an overdose of study drug. However, miglustat has been administered at doses of up to 3,000 mg/day (approximately 10 times the recommended starting dose administered to Gaucher patients) for up to 6 months in human immunodeficiency virus (HIV)-positive patients. Adverse events observed in the HIV studies included granulocytopenia, dizziness, and paresthesia. Leukopenia and neutropenia have also been observed in a similar group of patients receiving 800 mg/day or above.

Patient Information

Patients should be informed of the potential risks and benefits of miglustat and of alternative modes of therapy. Patients should be advised that diarrhea, GI complaints, and weight loss are common side effects of miglustat therapy, and to adhere to dietary instructions. Patients should also be advised to promptly report any numbness, pain, or burning in the hands and feet, and the development of tremor or worsening in an existing tremor.

4-HYDROXYPHENYLPYRUVATE DIOXYGENASE INHIBITOR

NITISINONE

Rx	**Orfadin** (Rare Disease Therapeutics, Inc.)	**Capsules:** 2 mg	NTBC 2 mg. White. In 60s.
		5 mg	NTBC 5 mg. White. In 60s.
		10 mg	NTBC 10 mg. White. In 60s.

NITISINONE — ORAL

Indications

➤*Hereditary tyrosinemia type 1 (HT-1):* Adjunct to dietary reduction of tyrosine and phenylalanine in the treatment of HT-1.

Administration and Dosage

➤*General dosing considerations:* A nutritionist skilled in managing children with inborn errors of metabolism should be employed to design a low-protein diet deficient in tyrosine and phenylalanine.

Treatment should block the flux through the tyrosine degradation pathway at the level of 4-hydroxyphenylpyruvate dioxygenase. Treatment should lead to normalized porphyrin metabolism (ie, normal erythrocyte porphobilinogen synthase (PBG-S) activity and urine 5-aminolevulinic acid [5-ALA]). Succinylacetone should not be detectable in urine or plasma.

Monitoring – Since plasma nitisinone concentration, plasma succinylacetone, urine 5-ALA, and erythrocyte PBG-S activity are not routinely available, it is appropriate during regular monitoring to follow urine succinylacetone, liver function tests, alpha-fetoprotein, and serum tyrosine and phenylalanine levels. However, during initiation of therapy and acute exacerbations, it may be necessary to follow more closely all available biochemical parameters.

➤*Adults:*

Hereditary tyrosinemia type 1 –

Maximum dose: 2 mg/kg/day.

Initial dosage: 1 mg/kg/day divided for morning and evening administration.

Dosage adjustment: If the biochemical parameters (except plasma succinylacetone) are not normalized within 1 month after start of treatment, the dosage should be increased to 1.5 mg/kg/day. For plasma succinylacetone, it may take up to 3 months before the level is normalized after the start of treatment. A dosage of 2 mg/kg/day may be needed once liver function has improved.

➤*Children:*

Hereditary tyrosinemia type 1 – See Adults for dosing.

➤*Administration:* Take orally at least 1 hour before a meal. The total dose may be split unevenly as convenient in order to limit the total number of capsules given at each administration. For young children, capsules may be opened and the contents suspended in a small amount of water, formula, or applesauce immediately before use.

➤*Storage/Stability:* Store at 2° to 8° C (36° to 46° F).

Actions

➤*Pharmacology:* Nitisinone is a competitive inhibitor of 4-hydroxyphenylpyruvate dioxygenase, an enzyme upstream of fumarylacetoacetase (FAH) in the tyrosine catabolic pathway. By inhibiting the normal catabolism of tyrosine in patients with HT-1, nitisinone prevents the accumulation of the catabolic intermediates maleylacetoacetate and fumarylacetoacetate. In patients with HT-1, these catabolic intermediates are converted to the toxic metabolites succinylacetone and succinylacetoacetate, which are responsible for the observed liver and kidney toxicity. Succinylacetone can also inhibit the porphyrin synthesis pathway leading to the accumulation of 5-aminolevulinate, a neurotoxin responsible for the porphyric crises characteristic of HT-1.

Since nitisinone inhibits catabolism of tyrosine, use of this drug can result in elevated plasma levels of this amino acid. Treatment with nitisinone, therefore, requires restriction of the daily intake of tyrosine and phenylalanine to prevent the toxicity associated with elevated plasma levels of tyrosine.

➤*Pharmacokinetics:*

Absorption/Distribution – Nitisinone was greater than 90% bioavailable following oral administration of the labeled compound in rats and was distributed to different organs, particularly the liver and kidney, where radioactivity remained for 7 days after administration. The single-dose pharmacokinetics of nitisinone have been studied in 10 healthy male volunteers 19 to 39 years of age (median age, 32 years). Nitisinone, 1 mg/kg body weight, was administered as a capsule and a liquid. The median time for maximum plasma concentration was 3 hours for the capsule and 15 minutes for the liquid. The capsule and liquid formulation were found to be bioequivalent based on an analysis of area under the plasma concentration-time curve and maximum plasma concentration.

Metabolism – No information on the metabolism of nitisinone in humans is available.

Excretion – Nitisinone was biotransformed in rats and excreted via the urine.

The mean terminal plasma half-life of nitisinone in healthy male volunteers was 54 hours.

NITISINONE — ORAL

Contraindications

None known.

Warnings/Precautions

➤*High plasma tyrosine levels:* Inadequate restriction of tyrosine and phenylalanine intake can result in elevations in plasma tyrosine. Plasma tyrosine levels should be kept below 500 mcmol/L in order to avoid toxic effects to the eyes (corneal ulcers, corneal opacities, keratitis, conjunctivitis, eye pain, and photophobia), skin (painful hyperkeratotic plaques on the soles and palms), and nervous system (variable degrees of mental retardation and developmental delay). In most patients, eye symptoms were transient, lasting less than 1 week. Six patients had prolonged episodes lasting 16 to 672 days.

➤*Transient thrombocytopenia and leucopenia:* Patients treated with nitisinone and dietary restriction in clinical trials were observed to develop transient thrombocytopenia (3%), leucopenia (3%), or both (1.5%). One patient, who developed both leucopenia and thrombocytopenia, improved after the dose of nitisinone was decreased from 2 to 1 mg/kg. Another patient, who developed thrombocytopenia, had nitisinone stopped for 2 weeks, but platelet values continued to be low for 3 months and slowly returned to normal after 5 months. In all other patients, platelet values and white blood cell counts normalized gradually without documented change in nitisinone dose. No patients developed infections or bleeding as a result of the episodes of leucopenia and thrombocytopenia. Regularly monitor platelet and white blood cell counts during nitisinone therapy.

➤*Risk of porphyric crises, liver failure, and hepatic neoplasms:* Patients with HT-1 are at increased risk of developing porphyric crises, liver failure, or hepatic neoplasms requiring liver transplantation. These complications of HT-1 were observed in patients treated with nitisinone for a median of 22 months during the clinical trial (liver transplantation, 13%; liver failure, 7%; malignant hepatic neoplasms, 5%; benign hepatic neoplasms, 3%; porphyria, 0.5%). Regular liver monitoring by imaging (ultrasound, computerized tomography, magnetic resonance imaging) and laboratory tests, including serum alpha-fetoprotein concentration, is recommended. An increase in serum alpha-fetoprotein concentration may be a sign of inadequate treatment, but always evaluate patients with increasing alpha-fetoprotein or signs of nodules of the liver during treatment with nitisinone for hepatic malignancy.

➤*General ophthalmologic care:* Perform slit-lamp examination of the eyes before initiation of nitisinone treatment. Patients who develop photophobia, eye pain, or signs of inflammation such as redness, swelling, or burning of the eyes during treatment with nitisinone should undergo slit-lamp reexamination and immediate measurement of the plasma tyrosine concentration. Implement a more restricted diet if the plasma tyrosine level is above 500 mcmol/L. Do not adjust nitisinone dosage in order to lower the plasma tyrosine concentration because the HT-1 metabolic defect may result in deterioration of the patient's clinical condition.

➤*Pregnancy: Category C.* Adequate reproductive toxicity studies have not been conducted with nitisinone. It is not known if nitisinone can cause harm to the fetus if administered to pregnant women. Give nitisinone to a pregnant woman only if clearly needed.

In a single dose-group study in rats given 100 mg/kg/day (12 times the recommended clinical dose based on relative body surface area), reduced litter size, decreased pup weight at birth, and decreased survival of pups after birth were demonstrated.

➤*Lactation:* Although the exposure was not quantified, naive pups that were exposed to nitisinone via breast milk showed signs of ocular toxicity and lower body weight. This suggests that nitisinone is excreted via breast milk in rats. It is not known whether nitisinone is excreted in human milk. Because many drugs are excreted in human milk, exercise caution when nitisinone is administered to a breast-feeding woman.

➤*Children:* Nitisinone has been studied in patients ranging in age from birth to 21.7 years. The median age of enrollment in a study of 207 patients with HT-1 was 9 months.

➤*Elderly:* Clinical studies of nitisinone did not include any subjects 65 years of age or older to determine whether they respond differently from younger subjects. HT-1 is presently a disease of the pediatric population. In general, dose selection for an elderly patient should be cautious, usually starting at the low end of the dosing range, reflecting the greater frequency of decreased hepatic, renal, or cardiac function, and of concomitant disease or other drug therapy in this patient population.

➤*Lab test abnormalities:* Plasma nitisinone concentration, urine and plasma succinylacetone levels, urine 5-ALA levels, and erythrocyte PBG-S activity were used during clinical trials to guide drug dosage. The probability of recurrence of abnormal values of urine succinylacetone was 1% at a nitisinone concentration of 37 mcmol/L (95% confidence interval, 23 to 51 mcmol/L). Assays for plasma nitisinone concentration, plasma succinylacetone, urine 5-ALA, and erythrocyte PBG-S activity are not routinely available in the United States. However, urine succinylacetone levels can be used to guide drug dose adjustment.

Serum alpha-fetoprotein concentrations are generally markedly elevated at the time of diagnosis, and gradually decrease during the course of nitisinone treatment. Increases during therapy may be a sign of inadequate treatment. Promptly evaluate an exponential increase in serum alpha-fetoprotein concentration for potential liver neoplasia.

➤*Monitoring:* It is appropriate during regular monitoring to follow urine succinylacetone, liver function tests, alpha-fetoprotein, platelets, white blood cell counts, and serum tyrosine and phenylalanine levels. However, during the initiation of therapy and during acute exacerbations, it may be necessary to follow more closely all available biochemical parameters (eg, plasma nitisinone concentration, plasma succinylacetone levels, urine 5-ALA levels, and erythrocyte PBG-S activity). Regular liver monitoring by imaging (ultrasound, computerized tomography, magnetic resonance imaging) is recommended. Measure serum phosphate as a screening test for patients with renal involvement at risk for secondary hypophosphatemia and rickets. Perform slit-lamp examinations of the eyes before initiation of treatment and during any eye adverse reactions (eg, photophobia, eye pain, signs of inflammation).

Drug Interactions

No drug-drug interaction studies have been conducted with nitisinone.

Adverse Reactions

➤*Most frequent adverse reactions:* In a clinical trial of 207 patients treated with nitisinone for HT-1, the most frequent adverse reactions, regardless of causality assessment, occurred in the following organ systems:

Dermatologic – Alopecia, dry skin, exfoliative dermatitis, maculopapular rash, pruritus (1%).

Hematologic/Lymphatic – Leukopenia, thrombocytopenia (3%); epistaxis, porphyria (1%).

Hepatic – Hepatic neoplasm (8%); liver failure (7%).

Special senses – Conjunctivitis, corneal opacity, keratitis, photophobia (2%); blepharitis, cataracts, eye pain (1%).

➤*Adverse reactions occurring in less than 1% of patients:* Adverse reactions that occurred in less than 1% of the patients, regardless of causality assessment, are the following:

Cardiovascular – Cyanosis.

CNS – Brain tumor, encephalopathy, headache, hyperkinesia, nervousness, seizures, somnolence.

GI – Abdominal pain, diarrhea, enanthema, gastritis, gastroenteritis, GI hemorrhage, melena, tooth discoloration.

GU – Amenorrhea.

Hepatic – Elevated hepatic enzymes, hepatic function disorder, liver enlargement.

Metabolic/Nutritional – Dehydration, hypoglycemia, thirst.

Musculoskeletal – Pathologic fracture.

Respiratory – Bronchitis, respiratory insufficiency.

Miscellaneous – Death, infection, otitis, septicemia.

Overdosage

➤*Symptoms:* Accidental ingestion of this drug by individuals eating normal diets not restricted in tyrosine and phenylalanine will result in elevated tyrosine levels. In volunteers given a single 1 mg/kg dose of nitisinone, the plasma tyrosine level reached a maximum of 1,200 mcmol/L from 48 to 120 hours after dosing. After a washout period of 14 days, the mean value of plasma tyrosine was still 808 mcmol/L. Fasted follow-up samples obtained from volunteers several weeks later showed tyrosine values back to normal. Nitisinone was generally well tolerated in these studies. There were no reports of changes in vital signs or laboratory data of any clinical significance. One patient did report sensitivity to sunlight.

Tyrosinemia has been associated with toxicity to eyes, skin, and the nervous system.

➤*Treatment:* No information about specific treatment of overdose is available. Restriction of tyrosine and phenylalanine in the diet should limit toxicity associated with tyrosinemia. Monitor patients for potential adverse reactions.

Patient Information

Advise patients and their caregivers of the need to maintain dietary restriction of tyrosine and phenylalanine when taking nitisinone to treat HT-1.

Advise patients and their caregivers to promptly report unexplained eye symptoms, rash, jaundice, or excessive bleeding.

ALGLUCERASE

Rx	**Ceredase** (Genzyme Corporation)	**Solution for injection:** 80 units/mL	Preservative free. In 5 mL. With 1% albumin.

ALGLUCERASE — INJECTION

Indications

➤*Type 1 Gaucher disease:* For use as long-term enzyme replacement therapy for children, adolescents, and adults with a confirmed diagnosis of type 1 Gaucher disease who exhibit signs and symptoms that are severe enough to result in 1 or more of the following conditions: moderate to severe anemia, thrombocytopenia with bleeding tendency, bone disease, significant hepatomegaly, or splenomegaly.

➤*Off-label uses:* Alglucerase has received orphan drug designation for replacement therapy in types 2 and3 Gaucher disease.

Administration and Dosage

➤*General dosing considerations:* Dosage should be individualized for each patient.

➤*Adults:*

Type 1 Gaucher disease –

Usual dosage: Most data are available for the dosage of 60 units/kg every 2 weeks.

Initial dosage: 2.5 units/kg 3 times a week to 60 units/kg administered as frequently as once a week or as infrequently as every 4 weeks.

Disease severity may dictate that the drug be initiated with relatively high doses or relatively frequent administration.

Dosage adjustment: After patient response is well established, a reduction in dosage may be attempted for maintenance therapy. Progressive reductions can be made at intervals of 3 to 6 months while carefully monitoring response parameters.

Relatively low toxicity, combined with the extended time course of response, allows small dosage adjustments to be made occasionally to avoid discarding partially used bottles. Thus, the dosage administered in individual infusions may be slightly increased or decreased to fully utilize each bottle, as long as the monthly administered dosage remains substantially unaltered.

➤*Children:*

Type 1 Gaucher disease – See Adults for dosing for children 2 years of age and older.

➤*Preparation for administration:* Alglucerase should not be shaken.

On the day of use, the appropriate amount of alglucerase is diluted with sodium chloride 0.9% IV solution to a final volume not to exceed 200 mL. The use of an inline particulate filter is recommended for the infusion apparatus.

➤*Administration:* Alglucerase is administered by intravenous (IV) infusion over 1 to 2 hours.

➤*Storage/Stability:* Store at 2° to 8°C (36° to 46°F). Alglucerase, diluted to 100 to 200 mL, has been shown to be stable for up to 18 hours when stored at 2° to 8°C. Because alglucerase does not contain any preservative, after opening, bottles should not be stored for subsequent use.

Actions

➤*Pharmacology:* Alglucerase catalyzes the hydrolysis of the glycolipid glucocerebroside to glucose and ceramide as part of the normal degradation pathway for membrane lipids. Glucocerebroside is primarily derived from hematologic cell turnover. Gaucher disease is characterized by functional deficiency in β-glucocerebrosidase enzymatic activity and the resultant accumulation of lipid glucocerebroside in tissue macrophages, which become engorged and are termed Gaucher cells. Gaucher cells are typically found in the liver, spleen, and bone marrow, and, occasionally, in the lung, kidney, and intestine. Secondary hematologic sequelae include severe anemia and thrombocytopenia in addition to the characteristic progressive hepatosplenomegaly. Skeletal complications, including osteonecrosis and osteopenia with secondary pathological fractures, are a common feature of Gaucher disease.

➤*Pharmacokinetics:*

Absorption – Following an IV infusion of different doses of alglucerase (between 0.6 and 234 units/kg) over a 4-hour period, steady-state enzymatic activity was achieved by 60 minutes. Individual steady-state enzymatic activity and area under the curve of the activity increased linearly with the infused dose (0.6 to 121 units/kg).

Distribution – The volume of distribution ranged from 49.4 to 282.1 mL/kg. Within the dosage range of 0.6 to 121 units/kg, volume of distribution values appear to be independent of the infused dose.

Metabolism/Excretion – Following infusion termination, plasma enzymatic activity declined rapidly, with the elimination half-life ranging between 3.6 and 10.4 minutes. Plasma clearance of alglucerase, calculated from its plasma enzymatic activity, was variable and ranged between 6.34 and 25.39 mL/min/kg. Within the dosage range of 0.6 to 121 units/kg, elimination half-life and plasma clearance values appear to be independent of the infused dose.

Contraindications

None known.

Warnings/Precautions

➤*Antibodies:* Approximately 13% of patients treated clinically and tested to date have developed immunoglobulin (Ig) G antibodies to alglucerase during the first year of therapy. It appears that patients who will develop IgG antibodies are most likely to do so within 6 months of treatment and will rarely develop antibodies to alglucerase after 12 months of therapy. Approximately 25% of patients with detectable IgG antibodies experienced symptoms of hypersensitivity.

Thus, patients with antibodies to alglucerase are at a higher risk of hypersensitivity reactions. Conversely, not all patients with symptoms of hypersensitivity have detectable antibodies and further evaluation of their antibody isotypes and mechanisms is continuing. It is suggested that patients be monitored periodically for IgG antibody formation.

At present, if a patient experiences a reaction with symptoms suggestive of hypersensitivity, it is recommended that a serum sample for tryptase levels and complement activation be drawn within 2 hours of the reaction after appropriate treatment of the symptoms. Subsequent serum for testing antibody to alglucerase would be helpful. Decreased efficacy has been noted in less than 0.5% of treated patients due to antibodies to alglucerase.

➤*Pretreatment:* Pretreatment with antihistamines has allowed continued use of alglucerase in some patients.

➤*Transmission of viral disease:* Alglucerase is prepared from pooled human placental tissue that may contain the causative agents of some viral diseases. Manufacturing steps have been designed to reduce the risk of transmitting viral infectious agents. These steps have demonstrated in vitro inactivation of a panel of model viruses, including HIV-1. The risk of contamination from slowly acting or latent viruses, including the Creutzfeldt-Jacob disease agent, is believed to be remote but has not been tested. Accordingly, assess the benefits and the risks of treatment with this product prior to use.

➤*Hypersensitivity reactions:* Approach treatment with alglucerase with caution in patients who have exhibited symptoms of hypersensitivity to the product.

➤*Special risk:* Use alglucerase with caution in patients with androgen-sensitive malignancies (eg, prostate cancer) and patients with known prior allergies to hCG.

➤*Pregnancy: Category C.* Animal reproductive studies have not been conducted with alglucerase. It is also not known whether alglucerase can cause fetal harm when administered to a pregnant woman or affect reproductive capacity. Prescribe alglucerase to a pregnant woman only if clearly needed.

➤*Lactation:* Since alglucerase may be excreted in human milk, exercise caution when alglucerase is administered to a breast-feeding woman.

➤*Children:* The safety and efficacy of alglucerase have been established in patients between 2 and 16 years of age. Use of alglucerase in this age group is supported by evidence from adequate and well-controlled studies of alglucerase and imiglucerase in adults and children, with additional data obtained from the medical literature and from long-term postmarketing experience. Alglucerase has been administered to patients younger than 2 years of age; however, the safety and efficacy in patients younger than 2 years of age have not been established.

As hCG has been detected in alglucerase, be alert for signs of early virilization in male children younger than 10 years of age. One case of precocious puberty has been reported to date; however, because of the recent introduction of manufacturing steps designed to reduce the level of hCG in alglucerase, the likelihood of this occurrence is reduced.

➤*Monitoring:* Periodically monitor patients for IgG antibody formation.

A health care provider knowledgeable in the management of patients with Gaucher disease should direct therapy with alglucerase.

Drug Interactions

None known.

➤*Drug/Lab test interactions:* False-positive pregnancy tests have previously been reported, but because of the introduction of manufacturing steps designed to reduce the level of hCG in alglucerase, the likelihood of these occurrences is reduced.

Adverse Reactions

Experience in more than 1,000 patients treated with alglucerase has revealed a small number of adverse reactions. Some of these reactions were related to the route of administration, including discomfort, pruritus, burning and swelling, or sterile abscess at the site of venipuncture. The remaining experiences consisted of slight fever, chills, abdominal discomfort, nausea, or vomiting. None of these reactions were judged to require medical intervention.

➤*Hypersensitivity:* Symptoms suggestive of hypersensitivity have been noted in a limited number of patients. Onset of such symptoms has occurred during or shortly after infusions; these symptoms have included pruritus, flushing, urticaria/angioedema (a small number of patients have had upper airway involvement), chest discomfort, respiratory symptoms, nausea, and abdominal cramping. Hypotension has been reported to occur during a few

ALGLUCERASE — INJECTION

of these reactions. Pretreatment with antihistamines and a reduced rate of infusion have allowed continued use of alglucerase in most patients.

➤*Additional adverse reactions:*

CNS – Dysosmia, fatigue, headache, light-headedness, weakness.

GI – Diarrhea, oral ulcerations.

GU – Menstrual abnormalities and false-positive pregnancy tests have previously been reported, but because of the introduction of manufacturing steps designed to reduce the level of hCG in alglucerase, the likelihood of these occurrences is reduced.

Musculoskeletal – Backache.

Miscellaneous – Transient peripheral edema, vasomotor irritability, or hot flash.

Overdosage

No obvious toxicity was detected after single doses up to 234 units/kg. There is no experience with larger doses.

Patient Information

Advise patients that this medicine is usually administered as an injection at their health care provider's office, hospital, or clinic. If they are to use this medicine at home, advise patients to carefully follow the injection procedures taught by their health care provider.

Advise patients not to drive, operate machinery, or do anything else that could be dangerous until they know how they react to this medicine.

IMIGLUCERASE

IMIGLUCERASE

Rx	**Cerezyme** (Genzyme)	**Powder for injection, lyophilized:** 212 units (equiv. to a withdrawal dose of 200 units imiglucerase).	Preservative free. In vials.[a]
		424 units (equiv. to a withdrawal dose of 400 units imiglucerase).	Preservative free. In vials.[b]

[a] Contains mannitol 170 mg and sodium citrate 70 mg (trisodium citrate 52 mg, disodium hydrogen citrate 18 mg) per vial.

[b] Contains mannitol 340 mg and sodium citrate 140 mg (trisodium citrate 104 mg, disodium hydrogen citrate 36 mg) per vial.

IMIGLUCERASE — INJECTION

Indications

➤*Gaucher disease:* Imiglucerase is indicated for long-term enzyme replacement therapy for patients with a confirmed diagnosis of Type 1 Gaucher disease that results in 1 or more of the following conditions: anemia, bone disease, hepatomegaly or splenomegaly, and thrombocytopenia.

Administration and Dosage

➤*General dosing considerations:* Individualize dosage to each patient.

➤*Adults:*

Gaucher disease –

Usual dosage: 60 units/kg of body weight by IV infusion 3 times a week once every 2 weeks is the dosage for which the most data are available.

Disease severity may dictate initiation of treatment at a relatively high dose or relatively frequent administration.

Initial dosage: 2.5 units/kg to 60 units/kg of body weight by IV infusion 3 times a week once every 2 weeks.

Dosage adjustment: Make dosage adjustments on an individual basis; these may increase or decrease based on achievement of therapeutic goals as assessed by routine comprehensive evaluations of the patient's clinical manifestations.

➤*Children:*

Gaucher disease –

2 years of age and older: See Adults for dosing.

➤*Preparation for administration:* Imiglucerase vials must be reconstituted and promptly diluted before use.

Reconstitution – On the day of use, after the correct amount of imiglucerase to be administered to the patient has been determined, the appropriate number of vials are each reconstituted with sterile water for injection. The final concentrations and administration volumes are provided in the following table.

Final Imiglucerase Concentrations and Administration Volumes		
Parameter	200 unit vial	400 unit vial
Sterile water for reconstitution	5.1 mL	10.2 mL
Final volume of reconstituted product	5.3 mL	10.6 mL
Concentration after reconstitution	40 units/mL	40 units/mL
Withdrawal volume	5 mL	10 mL
Units of enzyme within final volume	200 units	400 units

A nominal 5 mL for the 200 unit vial (10 mL for the 400 unit vial) is withdrawn from each vial. Using aseptic technique, the appropriate amount of imiglucerase for each patient is diluted with sodium chloride 0.9% injection, to a final volume of 100 to 200 mL.

After reconstitution, visually inspect imiglucerase before use. As a protein solution, slight flocculation (described as thin translucent fibers) occasionally occurs after dilution. Do not use any vials exhibiting opaque particles discoloration.

➤*Administration:* Imiglucerase is administered by IV infusion over 1 to 2 hours. The diluted solution may be filtered through an in-line, low protein-binding 0.2 mcm filter during administration.

Relatively low toxicity, combined with the extended time course of response, allows small dosage adjustments to be made occasionally to avoid discarding partially used bottles. Thus, the dosage administered in individual infusions may be slightly increased or decreased to fully utilize each vial as long as the monthly administered dosage remains substantially unaltered.

➤*Storage/Stability:* Store at 2° to 8°C (36° to 46°F).

Because imiglucerase does not contain any preservative, promptly dilute vials after reconstitution. Do not store for subsequent use. Imiglucerase, after reconstitution, has been shown to be stable for up to 12 hours when stored at room temperature (25°C; 77°F) and at 2° to 8°C (36° to 46°F). Imiglucerase, when diluted, has been shown to be stable for up to 24 hours when stored at 2° to 8°C (36° to 46°F).

Actions

➤*Pharmacology:* Imiglucerase catalyzes the hydrolysis of glucocerebroside to glucose and ceramide. In clinical trials, imiglucerase improved anemia and thrombocytopenia, reduced spleen and liver size, and decreased cachexia to a degree similar to that observed with alglucerase.

➤*Pharmacokinetics:* During 1-hour IV infusions of 4 imiglucerase doses (7.5, 15, 30, 60 units/kg) for injection, steady-state enzymatic activity was achieved within 30 minutes. Following infusion, plasma enzymatic activity declined rapidly with a half-life ranging from 3.6 to 10.4 minutes. Plasma clearance ranged from 9.8 to 20.3 mL/min/kg, (mean ± SD, 14.5 ± 4 mL/min/kg). The volume of distribution corrected for weight ranged from 0.09 to 0.15 L/kg (0.12 ± 0.02 L/kg). These variables do not appear to be influenced by dose or duration of infusion. However, only 1 or 2 patients were studied at each dose level and infusion rate. The pharmacokinetics of imiglucerase do not appear to be different from placental-derived alglucerase.

In patients who developed IgG antibody to imiglucerase, an apparent effect on serum enzyme levels resulted in diminished volume of distribution and clearance and increased elimination half-life compared to patients without antibody.

Contraindications

There are no known contraindications to the use of imiglucerase. Carefully re-evaluate treatment with imiglucerase if there is significant clinical evidence of hypersensitivity to the product.

Warnings/Precautions

➤*Antibodies:* To date, approximately 15% of patients treated and tested have developed IgG antibody to imiglucerase for injection during the first year of therapy. Patients who developed IgG antibody largely did so within 6 months of treatment and rarely developed antibodies to imiglucerase for injection after 12 months of therapy. Approximately 46% of patients with detectable IgG antibodies experienced symptoms of hypersensitivity.

Patients with antibody to imiglucerase for injection have a higher risk of hypersensitivity reaction. Conversely, not all patients with symptoms of hypersensitivity have detectable IgG antibody. It is suggested that patients be monitored periodically for IgG antibody formation during the first year of treatment.

➤*Pulmonary hypertension and pneumonia:* In less than 1% of the patient population, pulmonary hypertension and pneumonia also have been observed during treatment with imiglucerase. Pulmonary hypertension and pneumonia are known complications of Gaucher disease, and have been observed in patients receiving and not receiving imiglucerase. No causal relationship with imiglucerase has been established. Evaluate patients with respiratory symptoms in the absence of fever for the presence of pulmonary hypertension.

Therapy with imiglucerase should be directed by health care providers knowledgeable in the management of patients with Gaucher disease.

➤*Prior treatment with alglucerase:* Caution may be advisable in administration of imiglucerase to patients previously treated with alglucerase and who have developed antibody to alglucerase or who have exhibited symptoms of hypersensitivity to alglucerase.

➤*Hypersensitivity reactions:* Cautiously approach treatment with imiglucerase in patients who have exhibited symptoms of hypersensitivity to the product.

Anaphylactoid reaction has been reported in less than 1% of the patient population. Cautiously conduct further treatment with imiglucerase. Most patients have successfully continued therapy after a reduction in rate of infusion and pretreatment with antihistamines and/or corticosteroids.

IMIGLUCERASE — INJECTION

➤*Pregnancy: Category C.* Animal reproduction studies have not been conducted with imiglucerase. It also is not known whether imiglucerase causes fetal harm when administered to a pregnant woman, or affects reproductive capacity. Do not administer imiglucerase during pregnancy except when the indication and need are clear and the potential benefit is judged by the health care provider to substantially justify the risk.

➤*Lactation:* It is not known whether this drug is excreted in human milk. Because many drugs are excreted in human milk, exercise caution when imiglucerase is administered to a nursing woman.

➤*Children:* The safety and efficacy of imiglucerase have been established in patients between 2 and 16 years of age. Use of imiglucerase in this age group is supported by evidence from adequate and well-controlled studies of imiglucerase and alglucerase in adults and pediatric patients, with additional data obtained from the medical literature and from long-term postmarketing experience. Imiglucerase has been administered to patients younger than 2 years of age, however, the safety and effectiveness in patients younger than 2 years of age have not been established.

Adverse Reactions

Experience in patients treated with imiglucerase has revealed that approximately 13.8% of patients experienced adverse events that were judged to be related to imiglucerase administration and occurred with an increase in frequency. Some of the adverse events were related to the route of administration. These include discomfort, pruritus, burning, swelling, or sterile abscess at the site of venipuncture. Each of these events were found to occur in less than 1% of the total patient population.

➤*Hypersensitivity:* Symptoms suggestive of hypersensitivity have been noted in approximately 6.6% of patients. Onset of such symptoms has occurred during or shortly after infusions; these symptoms include pruritus, flushing, urticaria, angioedema, chest discomfort, dyspnea, coughing, cyanosis, and hypotension. Anaphylactoid reaction also has been reported. Each of these events occurred in less than 1.5% of the total patient population. Pretreatment with antihistamines and/or corticosteroids and reduced rate of infusion have allowed continued use of imiglucerase in most patients.

➤*Miscellaneous:* Additional adverse reactions that have been reported in approximately 6.5% of patients treated with imiglucerase include nausea, abdominal pain, vomiting, diarrhea, rash, fatigue, headache, fever, dizziness, chills, backache, and tachycardia. Each of these events occurred in less than 1.5% of the total patient population.

Incidence rates cannot be calculated from the spontaneously reported adverse reactions in the postmarketing database. From this database, the most commonly reported adverse events in children (defined as 2 to 12 years of age) included dyspnea, fever, nausea, flushing, vomiting, and coughing, whereas in adolescents (12 to 16 years of age) and in adults (older than 16 years of age) the most commonly reported reactions included headache, pruritus, and rash.

In addition to the adverse reactions that have been observed in patients treated with imiglucerase, the following adverse reactions have been reported for this therapeutic class of drug: Transient peripheral edema and vomiting.

Overdosage

Experience with doses up to 240 units/kg every 2 weeks have been reported. At that dose there have been no reports of obvious toxicity.

VELAGLUCERASE ALFA

VELAGLUCERASE ALFA

Rx	**VPRIV** (Shire Human Genetic Therapies)	**Injection, lyophilized powder for solution:** 200 units	Preservative free. Sucrose 100 mg. In single-use vials.
		400 units	Preservative free. Sucrose 200 mg. In single-use vials.

VELAGLUCERASE ALFA — INJECTION

Indications

➤*Gaucher disease:* For long-term enzyme replacement therapy for children and adults with type 1 Gaucher disease.

Administration and Dosage

➤*General dosing considerations:* Pretreatment with antihistamines and/or corticosteroids may prevent subsequent reactions in cases in which symptomatic treatment was required.

➤*Adults:*

Gaucher disease –

Usual dosage: 60 units/kg every other week as a 60-minute intravenous (IV) infusion.

Dosage adjustment: Dosage adjustments can be made based on achievement and maintenance of each patient's therapeutic goals. Clinical studies have evaluated doses ranging from 15 to 60 units/kg every other week.

Conversion: Patients being treated with imiglucerase may be switched to velaglucerase alfa. Patients previously treated on a stable dose of imiglucerase are recommended to begin treatment with velaglucerase alfa at that same dose when they switch from imiglucerase to velaglucerase alfa.

➤*Children:*

Gaucher disease –

4 to 17 years of age: See Adults for dosing.

➤*Preparation for administration:*

Reconstitution –

Velaglucerase Alfa Reconstitution Instructions		
	200 units/vial	400 units/vial
Volume of sterile water for injection for reconstitution	2.2 mL	4.3 mL
Concentration after reconstitution	100 units/mL	100 units/mL
Withdrawal volume	2 mL	4 mL

Upon reconstitution, mix vials gently. Do not shake. Prior to further dilution, visually inspect the solution in the vials; the solution should be clear to slightly opalescent and colorless; do not use if the solution is discolored or if foreign particulate matter is present.

Dilution – Withdraw the calculated volume of drug from the appropriate number of vials and dilute the total volume required in 100 mL of sodium chloride 0.9% solution suitable for IV administration. Mix gently. Do not shake.

➤*Administration:* For IV infusion only over 60 minutes. The diluted solution should be filtered through an in-line, low protein-binding 0.2 mcm filter during administration.

➤*Admixture compatibility:* Velaglucerase alfa should not be infused with other products in the same infusion tubing because the compatibility in a solution with other products has not been evaluated.

➤*Storage/Stability:* Store at 2° to 8°C (36° to 46°F). Once reconstituted, the product should be used immediately. If immediate use is not possible, the reconstituted or diluted product may be stored for up to 24 hours at 2° to 8°C (36° to 46°F). The infusion should be completed within 24 hours of reconstitution of vials. Do not freeze. Protect from light. Discard any unused solution.

Actions

➤*Pharmacology:* Gaucher disease is an autosomal recessive disorder caused by mutations in the GBA gene, which results in a deficiency of the lysosomal enzyme beta-glucocerebrosidase. Glucocerebrosidase catalyzes the conversion of the sphingolipid glucocerebroside into glucose and ceramide. The enzymatic deficiency causes an accumulation of glucocerebroside primarily in the lysosomal compartment of macrophages, giving rise to foam cells or "Gaucher cells." In this lysosomal storage disorder, clinical features are reflective of the accumulation of Gaucher cells in the liver, spleen, bone marrow, and other organs. The accumulation of Gaucher cells in the liver and spleen leads to organomegaly. The presence of Gaucher cells in the bone marrow and spleen leads to clinically significant anemia and thrombocytopenia.

Velaglucerase alfa, a hydrolytic lysosomal glucocerebroside-specific enzyme, catalyzes the hydrolysis of glucocerebroside, reducing the amount of accumulated glucocerebroside.

➤*Pharmacokinetics:*

Distribution – The mean volume of distribution at steady state ranged from 82 to 108 mL/kg (8.2% to 10.8% of body weight).

Excretion – Serum velaglucerase alfa concentrations declined rapidly with a mean half-life of 11 to 12 minutes. The mean velaglucerase alfa clearance ranged from 6.72 to 7.56 mL/min/kg.

Contraindications

None well documented.

Warnings/Precautions

➤*Infusion-related reactions:* Infusion-related reactions were the most commonly observed adverse reactions in patients treated with velaglucerase alfa in clinical studies. The most commonly observed symptoms of infusion-related reactions were as follows: dizziness, fatigue/asthenia, headache, hypertension, hypotension, nausea, and pyrexia. Generally, the infusion-related reactions were mild and, in treatment-naive patients, onset occurred mostly during the first 6 months of treatment and tended to occur less frequently with time.

Base the management of infusion-related reactions on the severity of the reaction (eg, slowing the infusion rate; treatment with medications, such as antihistamines, antipyretics, and/or corticosteroids; and/or stopping and resuming treatment with increased infusion time).

Pretreatment with antihistamines and/or corticosteroids may prevent subsequent reactions in cases in which symptomatic treatment was required. Patients were not routinely premedicated prior to velaglucerase alfa infusion during clinical studies.

VELAGLUCERASE ALFA — INJECTION

➤*Immunogenicity:* As with all therapeutic proteins, there is a potential for immunogenicity. In clinical studies, 1 of 54 treatment-naive patients treated with velaglucerase alfa developed immunoglobulin G (IgG) class antibodies to velaglucerase alfa. In this patient, the antibodies were determined to be neutralizing in an in vitro assay, and no infusion-related reactions were reported.

It is unknown if the presence of IgG antibodies to velaglucerase alfa is associated with a higher risk of infusion reactions. Patients with an immune response to other enzyme replacement therapies who are switching to velaglucerase alfa should continue to be monitored for antibodies.

➤*Hypersensitivity reactions:* Hypersensitivity reactions have been reported in patients in clinical studies with velaglucerase alfa. As with any IV protein product, hypersensitivity reactions are possible; therefore, have appropriate medical support readily available when velaglucerase alfa is administered. If a severe reaction occurs, follow current medical standards for emergency treatment.

Approach treatment with velaglucerase alfa with caution in patients who have exhibited symptoms of hypersensitivity to the active ingredient or excipients in the drug product or to other enzyme replacement therapy.

➤*Pregnancy: Category B.*

There are no adequate and well-controlled studies in pregnant women. Because animal reproduction studies are not always predictive of human response, use velaglucerase alfa during pregnancy only if clearly needed.

➤*Lactation:* There are no data from studies in lactating women. It is not known whether this drug is excreted in human milk. Because many drugs are excreted in human milk, exercise caution when velaglucerase alfa is administered to a breast-feeding woman.

➤*Children:* The safety of velaglucerase alfa has not been established in children younger than 4 years of age.

➤*Elderly:* In general, cautiously approach dose selection for an elderly patient, considering potential comorbid conditions.

➤*Monitoring:* Monitor patients for infusion-related reactions and for signs and/or symptoms of hypersensitivity reactions.

Drug Interactions

None well documented.

Adverse Reactions

➤*Serious adverse reactions:* The most serious adverse reactions in patients treated with velaglucerase alfa were hypersensitivity reactions.

➤*Most common adverse reactions:*

Velaglucerase Alfa Adverse Reactions (≥ 10%)

Adverse reactions	Naive to ERT[a] (n = 54)	Switched from imiglucerase to velaglucerase alfa (n = 40)
CNS		
Asthenia/Fatigue	13%	12.5%
Dizziness	22.2%	7.5%
Headache	35.2%	30%

Velaglucerase Alfa Adverse Reactions (≥ 10%)

Adverse reactions	Naive to ERT[a] (n = 54)	Switched from imiglucerase to velaglucerase alfa (n = 40)
GI		
Abdominal pain	18.5%	15%
Nausea	5.6%	10%
Musculoskeletal		
Back pain	16.7%	17.5%
Joint pain (knee)	14.8%	7.5%
Miscellaneous		
Activated partial thromboplastin time prolonged	11.1%	5%
Infusion-related reaction[b]	51.9%	22.5%
Pyrexia	22.2%	12.5%
Upper respiratory tract infection	31.5%	30%

[a] ERT = enzyme replacement therapy.
[b] Denotes any reaction considered related to and occurring within up to 24 hours of velaglucerase alfa infusion.

➤*Less common adverse reactions:* Less common adverse reactions affecting more than 1 patient (more than 3% in the treatment-naive group and more than 2% in patients switched from imiglucerase to velaglucerase alfa treatment) were bone pain, flushing, hypertension, hypotension, rash, tachycardia, and urticaria.

➤*Children:* Adverse reactions more commonly seen in children compared with adult patients (more than 10% difference) are as follows: activated partial thromboplastin time prolonged, pyrexia, rash, and upper respiratory tract infection.

Patient Information

Inform patients that velaglucerase alfa will be administered under the supervision of a health care provider. Velaglucerase alfa is a treatment that is given IV every other week. The infusion typically takes up to 60 minutes.

Advise patients that velaglucerase alfa may cause hypersensitivity reactions or infusion-related reactions. Infusion-related reactions can usually be managed by slowing the infusion rate; treatment with medications such as antihistamines, antipyretics, and/or corticosteroids; and/or stopping and resuming treatment with increased infusion time. Pretreatment with antihistamines and/or corticosteroids may prevent subsequent reactions. Carefully reevaluate treatment with velaglucerase alfa in the presence of significant evidence of hypersensitivity to the product.

ALGLUCOSIDASE ALFA

Rx	**Myozyme** (Genzyme Corporation)	**Injection, lyophilized powder for solution:** 50 mg	Preservative free. Mannitol 210 mg, polysorbate 80 0.5 mg. In 20 mL single-use vials.
Rx	**Lumizyme** (Genzyme Corporation)		

ALGLUCOSIDASE ALFA — INJECTION

WARNING

Risk of hypersensitivity reactions – Life-threatening anaphylactic reactions, severe allergic reactions, and immune-mediated reactions have been observed in patients during alglucosidase alfa infusion.

Because of the potential for severe infusion reactions, appropriate medical support measures must be readily available when alglucosidase alfa is administered.

Risk of cardiorespiratory failure – Patients with compromised cardiac or respiratory function may be at risk of serious acute exacerbation of their cardiac or respiratory compromise due to infusion reactions and require additional monitoring.

Lumizyme – Because of the potential risk of rapid disease progression in patients younger than 8 years of age with Pompe disease, alglucosidase alfa is available only through a restricted distribution program called the *Lumizyme* Alglucosidase Alfa Control and Education (ACE) Program. Only health care providers and health care facilities enrolled in the program may prescribe, dispense, or administer alglucosidase alfa. Alglucosidase alfa may be administered only to patients who are enrolled in and meet all the conditions of the *Lumizyme* ACE Program. To enroll in the *Lumizyme* ACE Program, call 1-800-745-4447.

Indications

➤*Late-onset Pompe disease (Lumizyme):* For use in patients 8 years of age and older with late (noninfantile)–onset Pompe disease (acid alpha-glucosidase deficiency) who do not have evidence of cardiac hypertrophy.

➤*Pompe disease (Myozyme):* For use in patients with Pompe disease (acid alpha-glucosidase deficiency).

Myozyme has been shown to improve ventilator-free survival in patients with infantile-onset Pompe disease compared with an untreated historical control, whereas use of *Myozyme* in patients with other forms of Pompe disease has not been adequately studied to ensure safety and efficacy.

Administration and Dosage

➤*Adults:*

Pompe disease – 20 mg/kg body weight administered every 2 weeks as an intravenous (IV) infusion. The total volume of infusion is determined by the patient's body weight and should be administered over approximately 4 hours.

➤*Children:*

Pompe disease – See Adults for dosing.

ALGLUCOSIDASE ALFA — INJECTION

➤*Preparation for administration:* Do not use filter needles during preparation.

Determine the number of vials to be reconstituted based on the patient's weight and the recommended dose of 20 mg/kg. If the number of vials includes a fraction, round up to the next whole number.

Remove the required number of vials from the refrigerator and allow them to reach room temperature prior to reconstitution (approximately 30 minutes).

Reconstitute each alglucosidase alfa vial by slowly injecting 10.3 mL of sterile water for injection to the inside wall of each vial. Each vial will yield 5 mg/mL. The total extractable dose per vial is 50 mg per 10 mL. Avoid forceful impact of the water for injection on the powder and avoid foaming. This is done by slow drop-wise addition of the water for injection down the inside of the vial and not directly onto the lyophilized cake. Tilt and roll each vial gently. Do not invert, swirl, or shake. The reconstituted alglucosidase alfa solution should be protected from light.

Alglucosidase alfa should be diluted in sodium chloride 0.9% for injection immediately after reconstitution to a final alglucosidase concentration of 0.5 to 4 mg/mL. Add the reconstituted alglucosidase alfa solution slowly and directly into the sodium chloride solution. Slowly withdraw the reconstituted solution from each vial. Avoid foaming in the syringe. Remove airspace from the infusion bag to minimize particle formation caused by the sensitivity of alglucosidase alfa to air-liquid interfaces. Do not add directly into airspace that may remain within the infusion bag. Avoid foaming in the infusion bag. Gently invert or massage the infusion bag to mix. Do not shake.

➤*Administration:* The diluted solution should be filtered through a 0.2 mcm, low–protein-binding, in-line filter during administration to remove any visible particles.

Infusions should be administered in a step-wise manner using an infusion pump. The initial infusion rate should be no more than 1 mg/kg/h. After patient tolerance to the infusion rate is established, the infusion rate may be increased by 2 mg/kg/h every 30 minutes until a maximum rate of 7 mg/kg/h is reached. Vital signs should be obtained at the end of each step. If the patient is stable, alglucosidase alfa may be administered at the maximum rate of 7 mg/kg/h until the infusion is completed. The infusion rate may be slowed and/or temporarily stopped in the event of infusion reactions. See the following table for the infusion rate at each step, expressed as mL/h based on the recommended infusion volume by patient weight.

Alglucosidase Alfa Recommended Infusion Volumes and Rates

Patient weight range (kg)	Total infusion volume (mL)	Step 1 1 mg/kg/h (mL/h)	Step 2 3 mg/kg/h (mL/h)	Step 3 5 mg/kg/h (mL/h)	Step 4 7 mg/kg/h (mL/h)
1.25 to 10	50	3	8	13	18
10.1 to 20	100	5	15	25	35
20.1 to 30	150	8	23	38	53
30.1 to 35	200	10	30	50	70
35.1 to 50	250	13	38	63	88
50.1 to 60	300	15	45	75	105
60.1 to 100	500	25	75	125	175
100.1 to 120	600	30	90	150	210
120.1 to 140	700	35	105	175	245
140.1 to 160	800	40	120	200	280
160.1 to 180	900	45	135	225	315
180.1 to 200	1,000	50	150	250	350

➤*Admixture compatibility:* Alglucosidase alfa should not be infused in the same IV line with other products.

➤*Storage/Stability:* Refrigerate between 2° and 8°C (36° and 46°F). Do not use alglucosidase alfa after the expiration date on the vial. Alglucosidase alfa does not contain any preservatives. Vials are single-use only. Any unused product should be discarded.

The reconstituted and diluted solution should be administered without delay. If immediate use is not possible, the reconstituted and diluted solution is stable for up to 24 hours at 2° to 8°C (36° to 46°F). Storage of the reconstituted solution at room temperature is not recommended. The reconstituted and diluted alglucosidase alfa solution should be protected from light. Do not freeze or shake.

Actions

➤*Pharmacology:* Pompe disease (glycogenosis type 2, acid maltase deficiency, glycogen storage disease type II) is an inherited disorder of glycogen metabolism caused by the absence or marked deficiency of the lysosomal enzyme acid alpha-glucosidase.

In the infantile-onset form, Pompe disease results in intralysosomal accumulation of glycogen in various tissues, particularly cardiac and skeletal muscles and hepatic tissues, leading to the development of cardiomyopathy, progressive muscle weakness, and impairment of respiratory function.

In the juvenile- and adult-onset forms, intralysosomal accumulation of glycogen is limited primarily to skeletal muscle, resulting in progressive muscle weakness. Death in all forms is usually related to respiratory failure.

Alglucosidase alfa provides an exogenous source of acid alpha-glucosidase. Binding to mannose-6-phosphate receptors on the cell surface has been shown to occur via carbohydrate groups on the acid alpha-glucosidase molecule, after which it is internalized and transported into lysosomes, where it undergoes proteolytic cleavage that results in increased enzymatic activity. It then exerts enzymatic activity in cleaving glycogen.

➤*Pharmacokinetics:*

Myozyme – The pharmacokinetics of alglucosidase alfa were evaluated in 13 patients ranging from 1 to 7 months of age with infantile-onset Pompe disease who received alglucosidase alfa 20 mg/kg (as an approximate 4-hour infusion) or 40 mg/kg (as an approximate 6.5-hour infusion) every 2 weeks. The measurement of alglucosidase alfa plasma concentration was based on an activity assay using an artificial substrate. Systemic exposure was approximately dose proportional between the 20 and 40 mg/kg doses.

Pharmacokinetic Parameters (Mean ± SD) After Single IV Infusion of Alglucosidase Alfa[a]

Pharmacokinetic parameter	20 mg/kg (n = 5)	40 mg/kg (n = 8)
C_{max} (mcg/mL)	162 ± 31	276 ± 64
AUC_∞ (mcg-h/mL)	811 ± 141	1,781 ± 520
Clearance (mL/h/kg)	25 ± 4	24 ± 7
V_{ss} (mL/kg)	96 ± 16	119 ± 28
Half-life (h)	2.3 ± 0.4	2.9 ± 0.5

[a] SD = standard deviation; C_{max} = maximum effective plasma concentration; AUC_∞ = area under the curve; V_{ss} = apparent volume of distribution.

The pharmacokinetics of alglucosidase alfa were also evaluated in a separate trial in 14 patients ranging from 6 months to 3.5 years of age with Pompe disease who received alglucosidase alfa 20 mg/kg as an approximate 4-hour infusion every 2 weeks. The pharmacokinetic parameters were similar to those observed for the 20 mg/kg dose group in the trial of patients ranging from 1 to 7 months of age.

Lumizyme – The pharmacokinetics of alglucosidase alfa were studied in 32 late-onset patients with Pompe disease ranging from 21 to 70 years of age who received *Lumizyme* 20 mg/kg every other week in a randomized, double-blind, placebo-controlled study. The pharmacokinetics were not time-dependent for patients who did not develop high antibody titer/inhibitory antibody. Parameter values did not change across visits at weeks 0, 12, and 52.

Absorption –

Lumizyme: At week 52 of biweekly administration, the estimates of AUC (2,700 mcg•h/mL with 30.4% coefficient of variation [CV], n = 29) and C_{max} (372 mcg/mL with 22.7% CV, n = 29) were determined at steady state.

Excretion –

Lumizyme: Clearance was 601 mL/h (CV = 28.2%, n = 29) at steady state. The declining portion of the concentration-time profile of alglucosidase alfa appears biphasic within the observed sampling time. The half-life for the first phase is 2.4 hours with a between-subject variation of 10%. Concentrations of alglucosidase alfa were not sampled long enough to adequately determine the half-life for the second phase.

Special populations –

Antibody formation:

- *Myozyme* – Nineteen of 21 patients who received treatment with alglucosidase alfa and had pharmacokinetics and antibody titer data available at week 12 developed antibodies to alglucosidase alfa. Five patients with antibody titers of at least 12,800 at week 12 had an average increase in clearance of 50% (range, 5% to 90%) from weeks 1 to 12. The other 14 patients with antibody titers less than 12,800 at week 12 had similar average clearance values at weeks 1 and 12.
- *Lumizyme* – Higher mean clearance (42%) was observed at week 52 in 4 of 5 patients who tested positive for antibodies that inhibit the cellular uptake of enzyme. Pharmacokinetics in 4 of these 5 individuals over time indicated an increase in clearance with increase in immunoglobulin G (IgG) titer. Positive inhibitory antibody status correlated with higher IgG titers in patients who received alglucosidase alfa. The relationship between exposure and efficacy has not been defined.

Contraindications

None well documented.

Warnings/Precautions

➤*Immune-mediated reactions:* Severe cutaneous reactions have been reported with alglucosidase alfa, including ulcerative and necrotizing skin lesions. Systemic immune-mediated reactions, including possible type III immune complex–mediated reactions, have been observed with alglucosidase alfa. These reactions occurred several weeks to 3 years after initiation of alglucosidase alfa infusions. Skin biopsy in 1 patient demonstrated deposition of anti-rhGAA antibodies in the lesion. Another patient developed severe inflammatory arthropathy in association with fever and elevated erythrocyte sedimentation rate. Monitor patients for the development of systemic immune complex–mediated reactions involving skin and other organs while receiving alglucosidase alfa. If immune-mediated reactions occur, consider discontinuation of the administration of alglucosidase alfa and initiate appropriate medical treatment. Consider the risks and benefits of readministering alglucosidase alfa following an immune-mediated reaction. Some patients have successfully been rechallenged and have continued to receive alglucosidase alfa under close clinical supervision.

➤*Cardiorespiratory failure:* Patients with acute underlying respiratory illness or compromised cardiac and/or respiratory function may be at risk of

ALGLUCOSIDASE ALFA — INJECTION

serious exacerbation of their cardiac or respiratory compromise during infusions. Make appropriate medical support and monitoring measures readily available during alglucosidase alfa infusion; some patients may require prolonged observation times that should be based on the individual needs of the patient. Acute cardiorespiratory failure requiring intubation and inotropic support has been observed in a few infantile-onset patients with Pompe disease with underlying cardiac hypertrophy, possibly associated with fluid overload with IV administration of alglucosidase alfa.

➤*General/regional anesthesia:* Administration of general anesthesia can be complicated by the presence of severe cardiac and skeletal (including respiratory) muscle weakness. Cardiac arrhythmia, including ventricular fibrillation, ventricular tachycardia, and bradycardia, resulting in cardiac arrest or death or requiring cardiac resuscitation or defibrillation have been observed in infantile-onset patients with Pompe disease with cardiac hypertrophy associated with the use of general anesthesia for the placement of a central venous catheter intended for alglucosidase alfa infusion. Because Pompe disease is considered a neuromuscular disease, use caution when administering general anesthesia in patients with Pompe disease.

➤*Infusion reactions:* Infusion reactions occurred in 51% of patients treated with alglucosidase alfa in clinical studies. Some reactions were severe. Severe infusion reactions reported in more than 1 patient in clinical studies and the expanded access program included cyanosis, decreased oxygen saturation, fever, hypotension, and tachycardia. Other infusion reactions reported in more than 1 patient in clinical studies and the expanded access program included agitation, bronchospasm, cough, cyanosis, decreased oxygen saturation, erythema, face edema, feeling hot, fever, flushing, headache, hyperhidrosis, hypertension, hypotension, increased blood pressure, irritability, lacrimation increased, livedo reticularis, nausea, pallor, periorbital edema, pruritus, rash, restlessness, retching, rigors, tachycardia, tachypnea, tremor, urticaria, vomiting, and wheezing. Some patients were pretreated with antihistamines, antipyretics, and/or steroids. Infusion reactions occurred in some patients after receiving antipyretics, antihistamines, or steroids. Infusion reactions may occur at any time during or up to 2 hours after the infusion of alglucosidase alfa and are more likely with higher infusion rates.

Patients with advanced Pompe disease may have compromised cardiac and respiratory function, which may predispose them to a higher risk of severe complications from infusion reactions. Therefore, monitor these patients more closely during administration of alglucosidase alfa.

Patients may be treated with antipyretics and/or antihistamines prior to infusion. If an infusion reaction occurs, regardless of pretreatment, decreasing the infusion rate, temporarily stopping the infusion, and/or administration of antihistamines and/or antipyretics may ameliorate the symptoms. If severe infusion reactions occur, consider immediate discontinuation of the administration of alglucosidase alfa and initiate appropriate medical treatment. Severe reactions are generally managed with administration of antihistamines, corticosteroids, IV fluids, and/or oxygen, when clinically indicated. Because of the potential for severe infusion reactions, make appropriate medical support measures, including cardiopulmonary resuscitation equipment, readily available when administering alglucosidase alfa. Treat patients who have experienced infusion reactions with caution when readministering alglucosidase alfa.

➤*Concomitant illness:* Patients with an acute underlying illness at the time of alglucosidase alfa infusion appear to be at greater risk for infusion reactions. Give careful consideration to the patient's clinical status prior to administration of alglucosidase alfa.

➤*Immunogenicity:* As with all therapeutic proteins, there is potential for immunogenicity. The data reflect the percentage of patients whose test results were considered positive for antibodies to alglucosidase alfa using an enzyme-linked immunosorbent assay and confirmed by a radioimmunoprecipitation assay for alglucosidase alfa–specific IgG antibodies. The incidence of antibody formation is highly dependent on the sensitivity and specificity of the assay. Additionally, the observed incidence of antibody (including inhibitory antibody) positivity in an assay may be influenced by several factors, including assay methodology, sample handling, timing of sample collection, concomitant medications, and underlying disease. For these reasons, comparison of the incidence of antibodies to alglucosidase alfa with the incidence of antibodies to other products may be misleading.

Myozyme – The majority of patients (89%) in the 2 clinical trials tested positive for IgG antibodies to alglucosidase alfa. Most patients who develop antibodies do so within the first 3 months of exposure. There is evidence to suggest that patients developing sustained titers of at least 12,800 of anti-alglucosidase alfa antibodies may have a poorer clinical response to treatment or may lose motor function as antibody titers increase. Test patients who have been treated and experience a decrease in motor function for neutralization of enzyme uptake or activity. Five patients with antibody titers of at least 12,800 at week 12 had an average increase in clearance of 50% from week 1 to 12.

The effect of antibody development on the long-term efficacy of alglucosidase alfa is not fully understood. There is an observation that some patients who develop high and sustained antialglucosidase alfa antibody titers, including those who possess 2 null mutations, have a poorer clinical response.

Some IgG-positive patients in clinical trials and on commercial therapy who were evaluated for the presence of inhibitory antibodies tested positive for inhibition of enzyme activity and/or uptake in in vitro assays.

Infusion reactions were reported in 51% of patients treated with alglucosidase alfa in clinical studies and appear to be more common in antibody-positive patients: 8 of 15 patients with high antibody titers experienced infusion reactions, whereas none of 3 antibody-negative patients experienced infusion reactions.

Patients in clinical trials, expanded access programs, and on commercial therapy have undergone testing for alglucosidase alfa–specific immunoglobulin E (IgE) antibodies. Testing was performed for infusion reactions, especially moderate to severe or recurrent reactions, for which mast-cell activation was suspected. A small number of these patients tested positive for alglucosidase alfa–specific IgE-binding antibodies, some of whom experienced an anaphylactic reaction.

Lumizyme – In the randomized, double-blind, placebo-controlled study, all patients with available samples treated with alglucosidase alfa (N = 59, 100%) developed IgG antibodies to alglucosidase alfa. All patients who developed IgG antibodies did so within the first 3 months of exposure (median time to seroconversion, 4 weeks). There was no apparent association between mean or peak IgG antibody titers and the occurrence of adverse reactions.

Patients who developed IgG antibodies to alglucosidase alfa were also evaluated for inhibition of enzyme activity or cellular uptake of enzyme in in vitro assays. None of the 59 evaluable patients tested positive for inhibition of enzyme activity. Antibody titers for cellular uptake inhibition were present in 31% of patients by week 78. All other patients tested negative for inhibition of cellular uptake. Patients who were positive for uptake inhibition tended to have higher IgG titers than patients who tested negative for uptake inhibition. Among the 32 patients with evaluable pharmacokinetic samples, 5 patients tested positive for uptake inhibition at times corresponding to pharmacokinetic sampling times compared with other patients. The clearance values for 4 of these 5 patients were approximately 1.2- to 1.8-fold greater in the presence (week 52) compared with in the absence of inhibitory antibodies (week 0).

Patients in the clinical studies or in the postmarketing setting have undergone testing for alglucosidase alfa–specific IgE antibodies. Testing was performed in patients who experienced moderate to severe or recurrent infusion reactions, for which mast-cell activation was suspected.

Ten patients in the randomized, double-blind, placebo-controlled study underwent testing for alglucosidase alfa–specific IgE antibodies. Two of 10 patients evaluated tested positive for alglucosidase alfa–specific IgE-binding antibodies, both of whom experienced anaphylactic reactions. One patient who developed IgE antibodies discontinued the study following anaphylaxis.

A small number of alglucosidase alfa-treated patients in the postmarketing setting who were evaluated tested positive for presence of alglucosidase alfa–specific IgE antibodies. Some of these patients experienced anaphylaxis.

Some patients who tested positive for alglucosidase alfa–specific IgE antibodies were successfully rechallenged with alglucosidase alfa using a slower infusion rate at lower initial doses and have continued to receive treatment under close clinical supervision.

Patients who develop IgE antibodies to alglucosidase alfa appear to be at a higher risk for the occurrence of anaphylaxis and severe allergic reactions. Therefore, monitor these patients more closely during administration of alglucosidase alfa.

➤*Lumizyme distribution program: Lumizyme* is available only under a restricted distribution program called the *Lumizyme* ACE Program.

The purpose of the program is to ensure that the known risks of anaphylaxis and severe allergic reactions and the potential risks of severe cutaneous and systemic immune complex–mediated reactions associated with the use of alglucosidase alfa are communicated to patients, caregivers, and health care providers. In addition, the purpose of the program is to mitigate the potential risk of rapid disease progression in infantile-onset patients with Pompe disease and late (noninfantile)–onset patients with Pompe disease younger than 8 years of age for whom the safety and effectiveness of alglucosidase alfa have not been evaluated.

Under this program, only trained and certified health care providers and health care facilities enrolled in the program are able to prescribe, dispense, or administer *Lumizyme*, and only patients who are enrolled in and meet all the conditions of the *Lumizyme* ACE Program may receive *Lumizyme*.

For information about the ACE Program, call 1-800-745-4447.

➤*Hypersensitivity reactions:* If severe hypersensitivity or anaphylactic reactions occur, consider immediate discontinuation of the administration of alglucosidase alfa and initiate appropriate medical treatment. Severe reactions are generally managed with infusion interruption, administration of antihistamines, corticosteroids, IV fluids, and/or oxygen, when clinically indicated. In some cases of anaphylaxis, epinephrine has been administered. Because of the potential for severe infusion reactions, make appropriate medical support measures, including cardiopulmonary resuscitation equipment, readily available when administering alglucosidase alfa.

Consider the risks and benefits of readministering alglucosidase alfa following an anaphylactic or severe allergic reaction. Some patients have been rechallenged and have continued to receive alglucosidase alfa under close clinical supervision. Exercise extreme care, with appropriate resuscitation measures available, if the decision is made to readminister the product.

Myozyme – Life-threatening and severe allergic reactions have been reported in some patients during and within 3 hours after infusion. Reactions have included anaphylactic shock, cardiac arrest, respiratory distress, hypotension, bradycardia, hypoxia, bronchospasm, throat tightness, dyspnea, angioedema, and urticaria. Interventions have included cardiopulmonary resuscitation, mechanical ventilatory support, oxygen supplementation, IV fluids, hospitalization, treatment with inhaled beta-adrenergic agonists, epinephrine, and IV corticosteroids.

In clinical trials and postmarketing safety experience with alglucosidase alfa, approximately 1% of patients developed anaphylactic shock and/or cardiac arrest during alglucosidase alfa infusion that required life-support

ALGLUCOSIDASE ALFA — INJECTION

measures. In clinical trials and expanded access programs with alglucosidase alfa, approximately 14% of patients treated with alglucosidase alfa have developed allergic reactions that involved at least 2 of 3 body systems: the cutaneous, respiratory, or cardiovascular systems. These events included hypotension, cyanosis, hypertension, tachycardia, ventricular extrasystoles, bradycardia, pallor, flushing, nodal rhythm, peripheral coldness (cardiovascular); tachypnea, wheezing/bronchospasm, rales, throat tightness, hypoxia, dyspnea, cough, respiratory tract irritation, oxygen saturation decreased (respiratory); and angioedema, urticaria, rash, erythema, periorbital edema, pruritus, hyperhidrosis, cold sweat, and livedo reticularis (cutaneous).

Lumizyme – Anaphylaxis and severe allergic reactions have been observed in patients during and up to 3 hours after infusion. Some of the reactions were life-threatening and included anaphylactic shock, respiratory arrest, apnea, dyspnea, bradycardia, tachycardia, and hypotension. Other accompanying reactions included chest discomfort/pain, throat tightness, bronchospasm, wheezing, tachypnea, cyanosis, decreased oxygen saturation/hypoxia, convulsions, angioedema (including tongue or lip swelling, periorbital edema, and face edema), pruritus, rash, urticaria, hyperhidrosis, nausea, dizziness, hypertension, flushing/erythema, fever, pallor, peripheral coldness, feeling hot, restlessness, nervousness, headache, back pain, and paraesthesia. Some of these reactions were IgE-mediated.

➤*Pregnancy: Category B.* There are no adequate and well controlled studies in pregnant women. Because animal reproduction studies are not always predictive of human response, only use this drug during pregnancy if clearly needed. Encourage women of childbearing potential to enroll in the Pompe disease patient registry program.

Reproduction studies have been performed in pregnant mice at IV dosages up to 40 mg/kg/day (plasma AUC of 64.6 mg•min/mL, 0.4 times the human steady-state exposure at the recommended biweekly dose) and pregnant rabbits at IV dosages up to 40 mg/kg/day (plasma AUC of 85 mg•min/mL, 0.5 times the human steady-state exposure at the recommended biweekly dose) and have revealed no evidence of impaired fertility or harm to the fetus caused by alglucosidase alfa.

It is not known if alglucosidase alfa crosses the human placenta. The molecular weight (about 99,377 to 109,000) and the short plasma half-life suggest that little, if any, of the glycoprotein will cross to the embryo or fetus.

Untreated Pompe disease is a fatal condition with death usually related to respiratory failure. Therefore, if a woman requires alglucosidase alfa, do not withhold because of pregnancy.

➤*Lactation:* It is not known whether alglucosidase alfa is excreted in human milk. The molecular weight (about 99,377 to 109,000) and the short plasma half-life (2.3 to 2.9 hours) suggest that little, if any, of the glycoprotein will be excreted into breast milk. Because many drugs are excreted in human milk, exercise caution when administering alglucosidase alfa to a breast-feeding woman. Encourage breast-feeding women to participate in the Pompe disease registry program.

The indication for alglucosidase alfa implies that the mother would have received the enzyme during pregnancy. Untreated Pompe disease is a fatal condition with death usually related to respiratory failure. Therefore, if a woman requires alglucosidase alfa, do not withhold because of breast-feeding.

➤*Children:*

Myozyme – Children 1 month to 3.5 years of age at time of first infusion have been treated with *Myozyme* in clinical trials. Other open-label clinical trials of *Myozyme* have been performed in older children ranging from 2 to 16 years of age at the initiation of treatment (juvenile-onset Pompe disease); however, the risks and benefits of *Myozyme* treatment have not been established in the juvenile-onset Pompe disease population.

Lumizyme – *Lumizyme* is not for use in patients with infantile-onset Pompe disease or late (noninfantile)-onset Pompe disease who are younger than 8 years of age. The safety and effectiveness of *Lumizyme* in these patients have not been evaluated in clinical trials.

➤*Elderly:*

Myozyme – Clinical studies did not include any patients 65 years of age and older. It is not known whether they respond differently than younger patients.

Lumizyme – The randomized, double-blind, placebo-controlled study of *Lumizyme* did not include sufficient numbers (n = 4) of patients 65 years of age and older to determine whether they respond differently from younger patients.

➤*Monitoring:* Monitor patients for IgG antibody formation every 3 months for 2 years and then annually thereafter. Testing for IgG titers may also be considered if patients develop allergic or other immune-mediated reactions. There are currently no marketed tests for antibodies against alglucosidase alfa. Contact your local Genzyme representative or Genzyme Corporation at 1-800-745-4447 for information on testing and to obtain a sample collection box. Monitor patients for the development of systemic immune complex-mediated reactions involving skin and other organs while receiving alglucosidase alfa.

Patients who experience anaphylactic or allergic reactions may also be tested for IgE antibodies to alglucosidase alfa and other mediators of anaphylaxis.

Evaluate liver enzymes prior to the initiation of alglucosidase alfa treatment and periodically thereafter. Exercise care in interpreting these tests because AST and ALT levels may also be raised as a result of the muscle pathology in patients with Pompe disease.

Monitor vital signs at the end of each infusion rate increase.

Drug Interactions

No drug interaction studies have been performed.

Adverse Reactions

➤*Myozyme:*

Serious adverse reactions – The most serious adverse reactions reported with alglucosidase alfa were acute cardiorespiratory failure, cardiac arrest, and anaphylactic reactions. Acute cardiorespiratory failure, possibly associated with fluid overload, has been reported in infantile-onset patients with Pompe disease; preexisting cardiac hypertrophy likely contributed to the severity of the reaction. Anaphylactic reactions have been reported during and within 3 hours after alglucosidase alfa infusion.

Most common adverse reactions – The most common serious treatment-emergent adverse reactions (regardless of relationship) observed in clinical studies with alglucosidase alfa were catheter-related infection, fever, gastroenteritis, pneumonia, respiratory distress, respiratory failure, and respiratory syncytial virus infection.

The most common treatment-emergent adverse reactions (regardless of relationship) were cough, decreased oxygen saturation, diarrhea, fever, gastroenteritis, otitis media, pneumonia, rash, upper respiratory tract infection, and vomiting.

Infusion-related reactions – The most common adverse reactions requiring intervention were infusion reactions. Twenty (51%) of 39 patients treated with alglucosidase alfa in clinical studies developed infusion reactions during the infusion or during the 2 hours following infusion. The majority of these reactions were mild to moderate. Infusion reactions reported in more than 1 patient in clinical studies and the expanded access program included agitation, bronchospasm, cough, cyanosis, decreased oxygen saturation, erythema, face edema, feeling hot, fever, flushing, headache, hyperhidrosis, hypertension, hypotension, increased blood pressure, irritability, lacrimation increased, livedo reticularis, nausea, pallor, periorbital edema, pruritus, rash, retching, restlessness, rigors, tachycardia, tachypnea, tremor, urticaria, vomiting, and wheezing. Most infusion reactions requiring intervention were ameliorated with slowing of the infusion rate, temporarily stopping the infusion, and/or administration of antipyretics, antihistamines, or steroids.

Adverse reactions (at least 20%) –

Alglucosidase Alfa Adverse Reactions (≥ 20%)	
Adverse reactions	Alglucosidase alfa (n = 39)
Any adverse reaction	100%
Cardiovascular	62%
Bradycardia	21%
Flushing	21%
Tachycardia	23%
Vascular disorders	36%
Dermatologic	82%
Diaper dermatitis	36%
Rash	54%
Urticaria	21%
GI	82%
Constipation	23%
Diarrhea	62%
Gastroenteritis	41%
Gastroesophageal reflux disease	26%
Vomiting	49%
Hematologic/Lymphatic	44%
Anemia	31%
Respiratory	97%
Bronchiolitis	23%
Cough	46%
Pharyngitis	36%
Pneumonia	46%
Respiratory distress	33%
Respiratory failure	31%
Tachypnea	23%
Upper respiratory tract infection	44%
Special senses	
Ear infection	33%
Nasopharyngitis	23%
Otitis media	44%
Rhinorrhea	28%

ALGLUCOSIDASE ALFA — INJECTION

Alglucosidase Alfa Adverse Reactions (≥ 20%)	
Adverse reactions	Alglucosidase alfa (n = 39)
Miscellaneous	
Catheter-related infection	28%
General disorders and administration-site conditions	97%
Infections and infestations	95%
Injury, poisoning, and procedural complications	56%
Investigations	72%
Oral candidiasis	31%
Oxygen saturation decreased	41%
Postprocedural pain	26%
Pyrexia	92%

Juvenile-onset disease – Five additional juvenile-onset patients with Pompe disease were evaluated in a single-center, open-label, nonrandomized, uncontrolled clinical trial. Patients were 5 to 15 years of age, ambulatory (able to walk at least 10 meters in 6 minutes), and not receiving invasive ventilatory support at study entry. All 5 patients received treatment with alglucosidase alfa 20 mg/kg for 26 weeks. The most common treatment-emergent adverse reactions (regardless of causality) observed with alglucosidase alfa treatment in this study were headache, malaise, pharyngitis, rhinitis, and upper abdominal pain.

➤*Lumizyme*:

Discontinuation – Two patients receiving alglucosidase alfa discontinued the study because of anaphylactic reactions. A third patient in the alglucosidase alfa group died during the study because of brain stem ischemia secondary to thrombosis of a basilar aneurysm, which was considered unrelated to treatment.

Serious adverse reactions – Serious adverse reactions reported with alglucosidase alfa in the randomized, double-blind, placebo-controlled study included anaphylaxis. Anaphylactic reactions included angioedema, chest pain/discomfort, and throat tightness. One patient with a history of Wolff-Parkinson-White syndrome experienced a serious adverse reaction of supraventricular tachycardia. Other serious adverse events that occurred in a higher incidence in alglucosidase alfa-treated patients compared with placebo included coronary artery disease, dehydration, gastroenteritis, intervertebral disc protrusion, and pneumonia.

Infusion reactions – The most common adverse reactions observed were infusion reactions. Infusion reactions, defined as an adverse reaction occurring during the infusion or within 2 hours after completion of the infusion, that occurred in alglucosidase alfa–treated patients at an incidence of at least 5% compared with placebo in the controlled study included anaphylaxis, chest discomfort, diarrhea, dyspnea, fall, flushing/feeling hot, hypoacusis, neck pain, pain in extremity, pharyngolaryngeal pain, pruritus, rash/erythema, urticaria, and vomiting. Additional infusion reactions observed in other clinical trials and expanded access programs with alglucosidase alfa included agitation, cough, increased lacrimation, irritability, livedo reticularis, respiratory distress, retching, rigors, and tremor.

If an infusion reaction occurs, decreasing the infusion rate, temporarily stopping the infusion, and/or administration of antihistamines and/or antipyretics may ameliorate the symptoms. If severe infusion or allergic reactions occur, consider immediate discontinuation of the administration of alglucosidase alfa and initiate appropriate medical treatment. Severe infusion reactions are generally managed with infusion interruption, administration of antihistamines, corticosteroids, IV fluids, and/or oxygen when clinically indicated. In some cases of anaphylactic reactions, epinephrine was administered. Treat patients who have experienced infusion reactions with caution when they are readministered alglucosidase alfa.

Delayed-onset infusion reactions have also been observed with alglucosidase alfa infusion. Delayed-onset infusion reactions, defined as adverse reactions that occurred within 48 hours after completion of alglucosidase alfa infusion, occurred in alglucosidase alfa–treated patients at an incidence of at least 3% compared with placebo-treated patients in a controlled trial. Symptoms included dizziness, epistaxis, insomnia, malaise, muscle spasms, musculoskeletal pain, musculoskeletal stiffness, musculoskeletal weakness, neck pain, pharyngolaryngeal pain, procedural pain, and urticaria. Counsel patients about the possibility of delayed-onset infusion reactions and give proper follow-up instructions.

Adverse reactions (at least 5%) – The following table enumerates adverse reactions that occurred in *Lumizyme*-treated patients at an incidence of at least 5% compared with placebo-treated patients during the randomized, double-blind, placebo-controlled study.

Alglucosidase Alfa Adverse Reactions (≥ 5%)		
Adverse reactions	Alglucosidase alfa (n = 60)	Placebo (n = 30)
CNS		
Malaise	5%	0%
Somnolence	5%	0%
Tremor	6.7%	0%
Vertigo	6.7%	0%
Dermatological		
Hyperhidrosis	8.3%	0%
Pruritus	10%	3.3%
Urticaria	10%	0%
GI		
Constipation	10%	0%
Dyspepsia	8.3%	0%
Gastroenteritis	10%	3.3%
Vomiting	21.7%	10%
Musculoskeletal		
Muscle twitching	8.3%	3.3%
Musculoskeletal pain	36.7%	30%
Musculoskeletal stiffness or tightness	15%	6.7%
Respiratory		
Dyspnea, exertional	6.7%	0%
Epistaxis	5%	0%
Respiratory tract infection	5%	0%
Upper respiratory tract infection	18.3%	10%
Special senses		
Ear discomfort or pain	11.7%	6.7%
Hypoacusis	33.3%	23.3%
Vision blurred	5%	0%
Miscellaneous		
Anaphylaxis	6.7%	0%
Chest discomfort or pain	16.7%	6.7%
Hypokalemia	5%	0%
Infusion-site reactions	13.3%	0%
Lymphadenopathy	8.3%	0%
Nephrolithiasis	5%	0%
Pain	8.3%	3.3%
Peripheral edema	16.7%	10%
Procedural pain	15%	10%

➤*Postmarketing*:

Myozyme – In postmarketing experience with alglucosidase alfa, severe and serious infusion reactions have been reported, some of which were life-threatening, including anaphylactic shock. Acute cardiorespiratory failure, possibly associated with fluid overload, has been reported in infantile-onset patients with Pompe disease with preexisting hypertrophic cardiomyopathy. In addition to the infusion reactions reported in clinical trials and expanded access programs, the following infusion reactions have been reported in patients during postmarketing use of alglucosidase alfa: cardiac arrest, chest discomfort, chest pain, conjunctivitis, fatigue, muscle spasm, peripheral edema, and pharyngeal edema. Systemic and cutaneous immune-mediated reactions, including ulcerative and necrotizing skin lesions, have been reported.

Lumizyme – In postmarketing experience with alglucosidase alfa, deaths and serious adverse reactions have been reported, including anaphylaxis. Adverse reactions resulting in death reported in the postmarketing setting with alglucosidase alfa treatment included aortic dissection, cardiac failure, cardiorespiratory arrest, cerebrovascular accident, hemothorax, pneumothorax, respiratory failure, sepsis, and skin necrosis. The most frequently reported serious adverse reactions were infusion reactions. In addition to the infusion reactions reported in clinical trials, the following serious adverse events have been reported in at least 2 patients: bronchospasm, chest discomfort, chest pain, cyanosis, decreased oxygen saturation/hypoxia, dyspnea, erythema, flushing, hypersensitivity, hypertension, hypotension, lung infection, pharyngeal edema, respiratory failure, stridor, and tachycardia. One case of hyperparathyroidism has been reported.

Systemic and cutaneous immune-mediated reactions, including necrotizing skin lesions, have been reported in postmarketing safety experience with alglucosidase alfa.

Overdosage

There have been no reports of overdose with alglucosidase alfa. In clinical trials, patients received doses up to 40 mg/kg (*Myozyme*) or 20 mg/kg (*Lumizyme*) of body weight.

Patient Information

Inform patients and their caregivers that a registry for patients with Pompe disease has been established in order to better understand the variability and progression of Pompe disease and to continue to monitor and evaluate long-term treatment effects. The registry will also monitor the effect of

ALGLUCOSIDASE ALFA — INJECTION

alglucosidase alfa on pregnant women and their offspring. Encourage patients and their caregivers to participate and advise them that their participation may involve long-term follow-up. Information regarding the registry program may be found at http://www.pomperegistry.com or by calling 1-800-745-4447.

Inform patients and caregivers that *Lumizyme* is available only under a restricted distribution program called the *Lumizyme* ACE Program. The purpose of the program is to ensure that the known risks of anaphylaxis and severe allergic reactions and the potential risks of severe cutaneous and systemic immune complex-mediated reactions associated with the use of *Lumizyme* are communicated to patients, caregivers, and health care providers. In addition, the purpose of the program is to mitigate the potential risk of rapid disease progression in infantile-onset patients with Pompe disease and late (noninfantile)–onset patients with Pompe disease younger than 8 years of age for whom the safety and effectiveness of *Lumizyme* have not been evaluated. Inform patients and caregivers that only trained and certified health care providers and health care facilities enrolled in the program are able to prescribe, dispense, or administer *Lumizyme*, and that patients must be enrolled in and meet all the conditions of the *Lumizyme* ACE Program to receive *Lumizyme*.

Inform patients and caregivers that a common adverse reaction is infusion reaction. Infusion reactions may occur during or within 2 hours after completion of the infusion. Symptoms associated with infusion reactions include agitation, cough, diarrhea, dyspnea, fall and chest discomfort, flushing/feeling hot, hypoacusis, increased lacrimation, irritability, livedo reticularis, neck pain, pain in extremity, pharyngolaryngeal pain, pruritus, rash/erythema, respiratory distress, retching, rigors, tremor, urticaria, and vomiting.

CALCITONIN-SALMON

CALCITONIN-SALMON

Rx	**Miacalcin** (Novartis)	**Injection**: 200 units/mL	With phenol. In 2 mL vials.
Rx	**Calcitonin-Salmon** (Various, eg, Apotex, Sandoz)	**Solution; intranasal**: 200 units per 0.09 mL	In 3.7 mL glass bottle.
Rx	**Fortical** (Upsher-Smith)		Sodium chloride, benzyl alcohol, phenylethyl alcohol. In 3.7 mL metered-dose, glass bottle with pump.
Rx	**Miacalcin** (Novartis)		8.5 mg sodium chloride. In 2 mL metered-dose, glass bottle with pump.

CALCITONIN-SALMON — INJECTION

Indications

➤*Paget disease:* At the present time, effectiveness has been demonstrated principally in patients with moderate to severe disease characterized by polyostotic involvement with elevated serum alkaline phosphatase and urinary hydroxyproline excretion.

➤*Hypercalcemia:* For early treatment of hypercalcemic emergencies, along with other appropriate agents, when a rapid decrease in serum calcium is required, until more specific treatment of the underlying disease can be accomplished. It may also be added to existing therapeutic regimens for hypercalcemia such as intravenous fluids and furosemide, oral phosphate or corticosteroids, or other agents.

➤*Postmenopausal osteoporosis:* For the treatment of postmenopausal osteoporosis in females more than 5 years postmenopause with low bone mass relative to healthy premenopausal females. Calcitonin-salmon injection should be reserved for patients who refuse or cannot tolerate estrogens or in whom estrogens are contraindicated. Use of calcitonin-salmon injection is recommended in conjunction with adequate calcium and vitamin D intake to prevent the progressive loss of bone mass.

No evidence currently exists to indicate whether or not calcitonin-salmon decreases the risk of vertebral crush fractures or spinal deformity. A recent controlled study, which was discontinued prior to completion because of questions regarding its design and implementation, failed to demonstrate any benefit of salmon calcitonin on fracture rate. No adequate controlled trials have examined the effect of salmon calcitonin injection on vertebral bone mineral density beyond 1 year of treatment. Two (2) placebo-controlled studies with salmon calcitonin have shown an increase in total body calcium at 1 year, followed by a trend to decreasing total body calcium (still above baseline) at 2 years. The minimum effective dose of calcitonin-salmon for prevention of vertebral bone mineral density loss has not been established. It has been suggested that those postmenopausal patients having increased rates of bone turnover may be more likely to respond to antiresorptive agents such as calcitonin-salmon.

Administration and Dosage

➤*General dosing considerations:* For patients with suspected sensitivity to calcitonin, skin testing should be considered prior to treatment (see Skin Testing).

➤*Adults:*

Hypercalcemia –

Maximum dose: 8 units/kg every 6 hours.

Initial dosage: 4 units/kg body weight every 12 hours subcutaneously or intramuscularly (IM).

Dosage titration: If the response to the initial dose is not satisfactory after 1 or 2 days, the dose may be increased to 8 units/kg every 12 hours. If the response remains unsatisfactory after 2 more days, the dose may be further increased to a maximum of 8 units/kg every 6 hours.

Paget disease –

Initial dosage: 100 units (0.5 mL) per day subcutaneously (preferred for outpatient self-administration) or IM.

Maintenance dosage: In many patients, doses of 50 units (0.25 mL) per day or every other day are sufficient to maintain biochemical and clinical improvement. At the present time, however, there are insufficient data to determine whether this reduced dose will have the same effect as the higher dose on forming more normal bone structure. It appears preferable, therefore, to maintain the higher dose in any patient with serious deformity or neurological involvement.

Relapse: In any patient with a good response initially who later relapses, either clinically or biochemically, the possibility of antibody formation should be explored. The patient may be tested for antibodies by an appropriate specialized test or evaluated for the possibility of antibody formation by critical clinical evaluation.

Patient compliance should also be assessed in the event of relapse.

In patients who relapse, whether because of antibodies or for unexplained reasons, a dosage increase beyond 100 units/day does not usually appear to elicit an improved response.

Monitoring: Drug effect should be monitored by periodic measurement of serum alkaline phosphatase and 24-hour urinary hydroxyproline (if available) and evaluations of symptoms. A decrease toward normal of the biochemical abnormalities is usually seen, if it is going to occur, within the first few months. Bone pain may also decrease during that time. Improvement of neurologic lesions, when it occurs, requires a longer period of treatment, often more than 1 year.

Postmenopausal osteroporosis –

Usual dosage: The minimum effective dose of calcitonin-salmon for the prevention of vertebral bone mineral density loss has not been established. Data from a single 1-year, placebo-controlled study with calcitonin-salmon injection suggested that 100 units (subcutaneously or IM) every other day might be effective in preserving vertebral bone mineral density. Baseline and interval monitoring of biochemical markers of bone resorption/turnover (eg, fasting AM, second-voided urine hydroxyproline to creatinine ratio) and of bone mineral density may be useful in achieving the minimum effective dose.

Concomitant therapy: Patients should also receive supplemental calcium such as calcium carbonate 1.5 g daily and an adequate vitamin D intake (400 units daily). An adequate diet is also essential.

➤*Skin testing:* For patients with suspected sensitivity to calcitonin, skin testing should be considered prior to treatment. Prepare a dilution at 10 units/mL by withdrawing 0.05 mL of the 200 units/mL solution in a tuberculin syringe and filling it to 1 mL with sodium chloride injection. Mix well, discard 0.9 mL and inject intracutaneously 0.1 mL (approximately 1 unit) on the inner aspect of the forearm. Observe the injection site 15 minutes after injection. The appearance of more than mild erythema or wheal constitutes a positive response. Health care providers may wish to refer patients who require skin testing to an allergist.

➤*Administration:* If the volume to be injected exceeds 2 mL, IM injection is preferable and multiple sites of injection should be used.

➤*Storage / Stability:* Store in refrigerator between 2° and 8°C (36° and 46°F).

Actions

➤*Pharmacology:* Calcitonin acts primarily on bone, but direct renal effects and actions on the gastrointestinal tract are also recognized. Calcitonin-salmon appears to have actions essentially identical to calcitonins of mammalian origin, but its potency per mg is greater and it has a longer duration of action. The actions of calcitonin on bone and its role in normal human bone physiology are still incompletely understood.

Bone – Single injections of calcitonin cause a marked transient inhibition of the ongoing bone resorptive process. With prolonged use, there is a persistent, smaller decrease in the rate of bone resorption. Histologically, this is associated with a decreased number of osteoclasts and an apparent decrease in their resorptive activity. Decreased osteocytic resorption may also be involved. There is some evidence that initially bone formation may be augmented by calcitonin through increased osteoblastic activity. However, calcitonin will probably not induce a long-term increase in bone formation.

Animal studies indicate that endogenous calcitonin, primarily through its action on bone, participates with parathyroid hormone in the homeostatic regulation of blood calcium. Thus, high blood calcium levels cause increased secretion of calcitonin which, in turn, inhibits bone resorption. This reduces the transfer of calcium from bone to blood and tends to return blood calcium to the normal level. The importance of this process in humans has not been determined. In healthy adults, who have a relatively low rate of bone resorp-

CALCITONIN-SALMON — INJECTION

tion, the administration of exogenous calcitonin results in only a slight decrease in serum calcium. In healthy children and in patients with generalized Paget's disease, bone resorption is more rapid and decreases in serum calcium are more pronounced in response to calcitonin.

Paget disease of bone (osteitis deformans) –

Calcitonin-salmon, presumably by an initial blocking effect on bone resorption, causes a decreased rate of bone turnover with a resultant fall in the serum alkaline phosphatase and urinary hydroxyproline excretion in approximately ⅔ of patients treated. These biochemical changes appear to correspond to changes toward more normal bone, as evidenced by a small number of documented examples of:

1.) Radiologic regression of Pagetic lesions,
2.) Improvement of impaired auditory nerve and other neurologic function,
3.) Decreases (measured) in abnormally elevated cardiac output. These improvements occur extremely rarely, if ever, and spontaneously, and are not predictable (elevated cardiac output may disappear over a period of years when the disease slowly enters a sclerotic phase; in the cases treated with calcitonin, however, the decreases were seen in less than 1 year.)

Some patients with Paget disease who have good biochemical or symptomatic responses initially, later relapse. Suggested explanations have included the formation of neutralizing antibodies and the development of secondary hyperparathyroidism, but neither suggestion appears to explain adequately the majority of relapses.

Although the parathyroid hormone levels do appear to rise transiently during each hypocalcemic response to calcitonin, most investigators have been unable to demonstrate persistent hypersecretion of parathyroid hormone in patients treated chronically with calcitonin-salmon.

Circulating antibodies to calcitonin after 2 to 18 months of treatment have been reported in about half of the patients with Paget disease in whom antibody studies were done, but calcitonin treatment remained effective in many of these cases. Occasionally, patients with high antibody titers are found. These patients usually will have suffered a biochemical relapse of Paget disease and are unresponsive to the acute hypocalcemic effects of calcitonin.

Hypercalcemia – In clinical trials, calcitonin-salmon has been shown to lower the elevated serum calcium of patients with carcinoma (with or without demonstrated metastases), multiple myeloma or primary hyperparathyroidism (lesser response). Patients with higher values for serum calcium tend to show greater reduction during calcitonin therapy. The decrease in calcium occurs about 2 hours after the first injection and lasts for about 6 to 8 hours. Calcitonin-salmon given every 12 hours maintained a calcium lowering effect for about 5 to 8 days, the time period evaluated for most patients during the clinical studies. The average reduction of 8-hour post-injection serum calcium during this period was about 9%.

Kidney – Calcitonin increases the excretion of filtered phosphate, calcium, and sodium by decreasing their tubular reabsorption. In some patients, the inhibition of bone resorption by calcitonin is of such magnitude that the consequent reduction of filtered calcium load more than compensates for the decrease in tubular reabsorption of calcium. The result in these patients is a decrease rather than an increase in urinary calcium.

Transient increases in sodium and water excretion may occur after the initial injection of calcitonin. In most patients, these changes return to pretreatment levels with continued therapy.

GI tract – Increasing evidence indicates that calcitonin has significant actions on the gastrointestinal tract. Short-term administration results in marked transient decreases in the volume and acidity of gastric juice and in the volume and the trypsin and amylase content of pancreatic juice. Whether these effects continue to be elicited after each injection of calcitonin during chronic therapy has not been investigated.

➤*Pharmacokinetics:* Peak plasma concentration time for the injection is 16 to 25 minutes.

The metabolism of calcitonin-salmon has not yet been studied clinically. Information from animal studies with calcitonin-salmon and from clinical studies with calcitonins of porcine and human origin suggest that calcitonin-salmon is rapidly metabolized by conversion to smaller inactive fragments, primarily in the kidneys, but also in the blood and peripheral tissues. A small amount of unchanged hormone and its inactive metabolites are excreted in the urine.

It appears that calcitonin-salmon cannot cross the placental barrier and its passage to the cerebrospinal fluid or to breast milk has not been determined.

Contraindications

Clinical allergy to synthetic calcitonin-salmon.

Warnings/Precautions

➤*Hypocalcemic tetany:* The administration of calcitonin possibly could lead to hypocalcemic tetany under special circumstances although no cases have yet been reported. Provisions for parenteral calcium administration should be available during the first several administrations of calcitonin.

➤*Hypersensitivity reactions:* Because calcitonin is protein in nature, the possibility of a systemic allergic reaction exists. Administration of calcitonin-salmon has been reported in a few cases to cause serious allergic-type reactions (eg, bronchospasm, swelling of the tongue or throat, and anaphylactic shock), and in 1 case, death attributed to anaphylaxis. The usual provisions should be made for the emergency treatment of such a reaction should it occur. Allergic reactions should be differentiated from generalized flushing and hypotension.

➤*Pregnancy:* *Category C.*

Teratogenic – Calcitonin-salmon has been shown to cause a decrease in fetal birth weights in rabbits when given in doses 14 to 56 times the dose recommended for human use. Since calcitonin does not cross the placental barrier, this finding may be due to metabolic effects on the pregnant animal. There are no adequate and well-controlled studies in pregnant women. Calcitonin-salmon injection, synthetic should be used during pregnancy only if the potential benefit justifies the potential risk to the fetus.

➤*Lactation:* It is not known whether this drug is excreted in human milk. As a general rule, nursing should not be undertaken while a patient is on this drug because many drugs are excreted in human milk. Calcitonin has been shown to inhibit lactation in animals.

➤*Children:* Disorders of bone in children referred to as juvenile Paget disease have been reported rarely. The relationship of these disorders to adult Paget disease has not been established and experience with the use of calcitonin in these disorders is very limited. There is no adequate data to support the use of calcitonin-salmon injection, synthetic in children.

➤*Lab test abnormalities:* Periodic examinations of urine sediment of patients on chronic therapy are recommended.

Coarse granular casts and casts containing renal tubular epithelial cells were reported in young adult volunteers at bed rest who were given calcitonin-salmon to study the effect of immobilization on osteoporosis. There was no other evidence of renal abnormality and the urine sediment became normal after calcitonin was stopped. Urine sediment abnormalities have not been reported by other investigators.

Adverse Reactions

➤*Dermatologic:* Local inflammatory reactions at the site of subcutaneous or intramuscular injection have been reported in about 10% of patients. Flushing of face or hands occurred in about 2% to 5% of patients. Skin rashes and pruritus of the ear lobes have also been reported.

➤*GI:* Nausea with or without vomiting has been noted in about 10% of patients treated with calcitonin. It is most evident when treatment is first initiated and tends to decrease or disappear with continued administration.

➤*Miscellaneous:* Nocturia, feverish sensation, pain in the eyes, poor appetite, abdominal pain, edema of feet, and salty taste have been reported in patients treated with calcitonin-salmon. Administration of calcitonin-salmon has been reported in a few cases to cause serious allergic-type reactions (eg, bronchospasm, swelling of the tongue or throat, and anaphylactic shock), and in 1 case, death attributed to anaphylaxis. The usual provisions should be made for the emergency treatment of such a reaction should it occur. Allergic reactions should be differentiated from generalized flushing and hypotension.

Overdosage

A dose of 1,000 units subcutaneously may produce nausea and vomiting as the only adverse effects. Doses of 32 units/kg/day for 1 to 2 days demonstrate no other adverse effects.

Data on chronic high dose administration are insufficient to judge toxicity.

Patient Information

Careful instruction in sterile injection technique should be given to the patient, and to other persons who may administer calcitonin-salmon injection, synthetic.

CALCITONIN-SALMON — INTRANASAL

Indications

➤*Postmenopausal osteoporosis:* For the treatment of postmenopausal osteoporosis in females more than 5 years postmenopause with low bone mass relative to healthy premenopausal females. Reserve calcitonin-salmon nasal spray for patients who refuse or cannot tolerate estrogens or in whom estrogens are contraindicated. Use of calcitonin-salmon nasal spray is recommended in conjunction with an adequate calcium (at least 1,000 mg elemental calcium per day) and vitamin D (400 units/day) intake to retard the progressive loss of bone mass. An adequate diet is also essential. The evidence of efficacy is based on increases in spinal bone mineral density observed in clinical trials.

Administration and Dosage

➤*Adults:*

Postmenopausal osteoporosis – 1 spray (200 units) per day administered intranasally, alternating nostrils daily.

➤*Monitoring:* Drug effect may be monitored by periodic measurements of lumbar vertebral bone mass to document stabilization of bone loss or increases in bone density. Effects of calcitonin-salmon nasal spray on biochemical markers of bone turnover have not been consistently demonstrated in studies in postmenopausal osteoporosis. Therefore, do not utilize these parameters solely to determine clinical response to calcitonin-salmon nasal spray therapy in these patients.

➤*Preparation for administration:* Before the first dose and administration, bring calcitonin-salmon nasal spray to room temperature.

CALCITONIN-SALMON — INTRANASAL

To prime the pump, hold the bottle upright and depress the 2 white side arms of the pump toward the bottle until a full spray is produced. The pump is primed once the first full spray is emitted. Do not prime the pump before each daily dose.

➤*Administration:* To administer, carefully place the nozzle into the nostril with the head in the upright position, and firmly depress the pump toward the bottle.

➤*Storage/Stability:* Store unopened bottle(s) in refrigerator between 2° and 8°C (36° and 46°F). Protect from freezing.

Store bottle in use at room temperature between 15° and 30°C (59° and 86°F) in an upright position, for up to 35 days. Each bottle contains at least 30 doses.

Discard all unrefrigerated bottles after 30 days.

Actions

➤*Pharmacology:* Calcitonin acts primarily on bone, but direct renal effects and actions on the GI tract are also recognized. Calcitonin-salmon appears to have actions essentially identical to calcitonins of mammalian origin, but its potency per mg is greater and it has a longer duration of action.

The following information describing the clinical pharmacology of calcitonin has been derived from studies with injectable calcitonin. The mean bioavailability of calcitonin-salmon nasal spray is approximately 3% of that of injectable calcitonin in healthy subjects and, therefore, the conclusions concerning the clinical pharmacology of this preparation may be different.

The actions of calcitonin on bone and its role in normal human bone physiology are still not completely elucidated, although calcitonin receptors have been discovered in osteoclasts and osteoblasts.

Single injections of calcitonin cause a marked transient inhibition of the ongoing bone resorptive process. With prolonged use, there is a persistent, smaller decrease in the rate of bone resorption. Histologically, this is associated with a decreased number of osteoclasts and an apparent decrease in their resorptive activity. In vitro studies have shown that calcitonin-salmon causes inhibition of osteoclast function with loss of the ruffled osteoclast border responsible for resorption of bone. This activity resumes following removal of calcitonin-salmon from the test system. There is some evidence from the in vitro studies that bone formation may be augmented by calcitonin through increased osteoblastic activity.

Animal studies indicate that endogenous calcitonin, primarily through its action on bone, participates with parathyroid hormone in the homeostatic regulation of blood calcium. Thus, high blood calcium levels cause increased secretion of calcitonin that, in turn, inhibits bone resorption. This reduces the transfer of calcium from bone to blood and tends to return blood calcium towards the normal level. The importance of this process in humans has not been determined. In healthy adults who have a relatively low rate of bone resorption, the administration of exogenous calcitonin results in only a slight decrease in serum calcium in the limits of the normal range. In healthy children and in patients with Paget disease in whom bone resorption is more rapid, decreases in serum calcium are more pronounced in response to calcitonin.

Bone biopsy and radial bone mass studies at baseline and after 26 months of daily injectable calcitonin indicate that calcitonin therapy results in formation of normal bone.

Postmenopausal osteoporosis –

Calcitonin-salmon given by the intranasal route has been shown to increase spinal bone mass in postmenopausal women with established osteoporosis but not in early postmenopausal women.

Calcium homeostasis – In 2 clinical studies designed to evaluate the pharmacodynamic response to calcitonin-salmon nasal spray, administration of 100 to 1,600 units to healthy volunteers resulted in rapid and sustained small decreases (but still within the normal range) in both total serum calcium and serum ionized calcium. Single doses greater than 400 units did not produce any further biological response to the drug. The development of hypocalcemia has not been reported in studies in healthy volunteers or postmenopausal females.

Kidney – Studies with injectable calcitonin show increases in the excretion of filtered phosphate, calcium, and sodium by decreasing their tubular reabsorption. Comparable studies have not been carried out with calcitonin-salmon nasal spray.

GI tract – Some evidence from studies with injectable preparations suggest that calcitonin may have significant actions on the GI tract. Short-term administration of injectable calcitonin results in marked transient decreases in the volume and acidity of gastric juice and in the volume and the trypsin and amylase content of pancreatic juice. Whether these effects continue to be elicited after each injection of calcitonin during chronic therapy has not been investigated. These studies have not been conducted with calcitonin-salmon nasal spray.

➤*Pharmacokinetics:*

Absorption/Distribution – The data on bioavailability of calcitonin-salmon nasal spray obtained by various investigators using different methods show great variability. Calcitonin-salmon nasal spray is absorbed rapidly by the nasal mucosa. Peak plasma concentrations of drug appear 31 to 39 minutes after nasal administration compared with 16 to 25 minutes following parenteral dosing. In healthy volunteers approximately 3% (range, 0.3% to 30.6%) of a nasally administered dose is bioavailable compared with the same dose administered by intramuscular (IM) injection.

There is no accumulation of the drug on repeated nasal administration at 10-hour intervals for up to 15 days. Absorption of nasally administered calcitonin has not been studied in postmenopausal women.

Metabolism/Excretion – The half-life of elimination of calcitonin-salmon is calculated to be 43 minutes.

Animal studies suggest that calcitonin is rapidly converted to smaller inactive fragments, primarily in the kidneys but also in the blood and peripheral tissues. A small amount of unchanged hormone and its inactive metabolites are excreted in the urine.

Contraindications

Clinical allergies to calcitonin-salmon.

Warnings/Precautions

➤*Periodic nasal examinations:* Periodic nasal examinations with visualization of the nasal mucosa, turbinates, septum and mucosal blood vessel status are recommended.

➤*Nasal mucosal alterations:* The development of mucosal alterations or transient nasal conditions occurred in up to 9% of patients who received calcitonin-salmon nasal spray and in up to 12% of patients who received placebo nasal spray in studies in postmenopausal females. The majority of patients (approximately 90%) in whom nasal abnormalities were noted also reported nasally related complaints/symptoms as adverse reactions. Therefore, perform a nasal examination prior to start of treatment with nasal calcitonin and at any time nasal complaints occur.

In all postmenopausal patients treated with calcitonin-salmon nasal spray, the most commonly reported nasal adverse reactions included rhinitis (12%), epistaxis (3.5%), and sinusitis (2.3%). Smoking was shown not to have any contributory effect on the occurrence of nasal adverse events. One patient (0.3%) treated with calcitonin-salmon nasal spray who was receiving 400 units daily developed a small nasal wound. In clinical trials in another disorder (Paget disease), 2.8% of patients developed nasal ulcerations.

If severe ulceration of the nasal mucosa occurs, as indicated by ulcers greater than 1.5 mm in diameter or penetrating below the mucosa, or those associated with heavy bleeding, discontinue calcitonin-salmon nasal spray. Although smaller ulcers often heal without withdrawal of calcitonin-salmon nasal spray, discontinue medication temporarily until healing occurs.

➤*Hypersensitivity reactions:* Because calcitonin is a polypeptide, the possibility of a systemic allergic reaction exists. A few cases of allergic-type reactions have been reported in patients receiving calcitonin-salmon nasal spray, including 1 case of anaphylactic shock, which appears to have been caused by the preservative because the patient could tolerate injectable calcitonin-salmon without incident. With injectable calcitonin-salmon there have been a few reports of serious allergic-type reactions (eg, bronchospasm, swelling of the tongue or throat, anaphylactic shock, and in 1 case death attributed to anaphylaxis). Make the usual provisions for the emergency treatment of such a reaction if it should occur. Allergic reactions should be differentiated from generalized flushing and hypotension.

For patients with suspected sensitivity to calcitonin, consider skin testing prior to treatment utilizing a dilute, sterile solution of calcitonin-salmon synthetic injection. Health care providers may wish to refer patients who require skin testing to an allergist.

➤*Pregnancy: Category C.*

Teratogenic – Calcitonin-salmon has been shown to cause a decrease in fetal birth weights in rabbits when given by injection in doses 8 to 33 times the parenteral dose and 70 to 278 times the intranasal dose recommended for human use based on body surface area.

Because calcitonin does not cross the placental barrier, this finding may be due to metabolic effects on the pregnant animal. There are no adequate and well-controlled studies in pregnant women with calcitonin-salmon. Calcitonin-salmon nasal spray is not indicated for use in pregnancy.

➤*Lactation:* It is not known whether this drug is excreted in human milk. As a general rule, a patient should not breastfeed while on this drug because many drugs are excreted in human milk. Calcitonin has been shown to inhibit lactation in animals.

➤*Children:* There are no data to support the use of calcitonin-salmon nasal spray in children. Disorders of bone in children referred to as idiopathic juvenile osteoporosis have been reported rarely. The relationship of these disorders to postmenopausal osteoporosis has not been established and experience with the use of calcitonin in these disorders is very limited.

➤*Lab test abnormalities:* Urine sediment abnormalities have not been reported in ambulatory volunteers treated with calcitonin-salmon nasal spray. Coarse granular casts containing renal tubular epithelial cells were reported in young adult volunteers at bed rest who were given injectable calcitonin-salmon to study the effect of immobilization on osteoporosis. There was no evidence of renal abnormality, and the urine sediment became normal after calcitonin was stopped. Consider periodic examinations of urine sediment.

Drug Interactions

Currently, no drug interactions with calcitonin-salmon have been observed. The effects of prior use of diphosphonates in postmenopausal osteoporosis patients have not been assessed; however, in patients with Paget disease prior diphosphonate use appears to reduce the antiresorptive response to calcitonin-salmon nasal spray.

Adverse Reactions

The incidence of adverse reactions reported in studies involving postmenopausal osteoporotic patients chronically exposed to calcitonin-salmon nasal

CALCITONIN-SALMON — INTRANASAL

spray (n = 341) and to placebo nasal spray (n = 131) and reported in greater than 3% of calcitonin-salmon nasal spray-treated patients are presented in the following table. Most adverse reactions were mild to moderate in severity. Nasal adverse reactions were most common, with 70% mild, 25% moderate, and 5% severe in nature (placebo rates were 71% mild, 27% moderate, and 2% severe).

Calcitonin-Salmon Intranasal Adverse Reactions in Postmenopausal Patients Treated Chronically (≥ 3%)

Adverse reaction	Calcitonin-salmon nasal spray (n = 341)	Placebo (n = 131)
Arthralgia	3.8%	5.3%
Back pain	5%	2.3%
Epistaxis	3.5%	4.6%
Headache	3.2%	4.6%
Rhinitis	12%	6.9%
Symptom of nose[a]	10.6%	16%

[a] Symptom of nose includes nasal crusts, dryness, redness or erythema, nasal sores, irritation, itching, thick feeling, soreness, pallor, infection, stenosis, runny/blocked, small wound, bleeding wound, tenderness, uncomfortable feeling, and sore across bridge of nose.

In addition, the following adverse reactions were reported in fewer than 3% of patients during chronic therapy with calcitonin-salmon nasal spray. Adverse reactions reported in 1% to 3% of patients are identified. The remainder occurred in less than 1% of patients. Other than flushing, nausea, possible allergic reactions, and possible local irritative effects in the respiratory tract, a relationship to calcitonin-salmon nasal spray has not been established.

➤*Cardiovascular:* Angina pectoris (1% to 3%), bundle branch block (less than 1%), hypertension (1% to 3%), myocardial infarction (less than 1%), palpitation (less than 1%), tachycardia (less than 1%).

Vascular – Cerebrovascular accident (less than 1%), flushing (less than 1%), thrombophlebitis (less than 1%).

➤*CNS:* Agitation (less than 1%), dizziness (1% to 3%), migraine (less than 1%), neuralgia (less than 1%), paresthesia (1% to 3%), vertigo (less than 1%).

➤*Dermatologic:* Alopecia (less than 1%), eczema (less than 1%), erythematous rash (1% to 3%), increased sweating (less than 1%), pruritus (less than 1%), skin ulceration (less than 1%).

➤*Endocrine:* Goiter (less than 1%), hyperthyroidism (less than 1%).

➤*GI:* Abdominal pain (1% to 3%), constipation (1% to 3%), diarrhea (1% to 3%), dry mouth (less than 1%), dyspepsia (1% to 3%), flatulence (less than 1%), gastritis (less than 1%), increased appetite (less than 1%), nausea (1% to 3%), vomiting (less than 1%).

➤*Hematologic/Lymphatic:* Anemia (less than 1%), infection (1% to 3%), lymphadenopathy (1% to 3%).

➤*Hepatic:* Cholelithiasis (less than 1%), hepatitis (less than 1%).

➤*Metabolic:* Weight increase (less than 1%).

➤*Musculoskeletal:* Arthritis (less than 1%), arthrosis (1% to 3%), myalgia (1% to 3%), polymyalgia rheumatica (less than 1%), stiffness (less than 1%).

➤*Renal:* Cystitis (1% to 3%), hematuria (less than 1%), pyelonephritis (less than 1%), renal calculus (less than 1%).

➤*Ophthalmic:* Abnormal lacrimation (1% to 3%), blurred vision (less than 1%), conjunctivitis (1% to 3%), vitreous floater (less than 1%).

➤*Psychiatric:* Anorexia (less than 1%), anxiety (less than 1%), depression (1% to 3%); insomnia (less than 1%).

➤*Respiratory:* Bronchitis (less than 1%), bronchospasm (1% to 3%), coughing (less than 1%), dyspnea (less than 1%), pharyngitis (less than 1%), pneumonia (less than 1%), sinusitis (1% to 3%), upper respiratory tract infection (1% to 3%).

➤*Special senses:* Earache (less than 1%), hearing loss (less than 1%), parosmia (less than 1%), taste perversion (less than 1%), thirst (less than 1%), tinnitus (less than 1%).

➤*Miscellaneous:* Fatigue (1% to 3%), fever (less than 1%), influenza-like symptoms (1% to 3%), periorbital edema (less than 1%).

➤*Common adverse reactions associated with the use of injectable calcitonin-salmon vs calcitonin-salmon nasal spray:* Common adverse reactions associated with the use of injectable calcitonin-salmon occurred less frequently in patients treated with calcitonin-salmon nasal spray than in those patients treated with injectable calcitonin. Nausea, with or without vomiting, which occurred in 1.8% of patients treated with the nasal spray (and 1.5% of those receiving placebo nasal spray) occurs in about 10% of patients who take injectable calcitonin-salmon. Flushing, which occurred in less than 1% of patients treated with the nasal spray, occurs in 2% to 5% of patients treated with injectable calcitonin-salmon. Although the administered dosages of injectable and nasal spray calcitonin-salmon are comparable (50 to 100 units daily of injectable versus 200 units daily of nasal spray), the nasal dosage form has a mean bioavailability of about 3% (range 0.3% to 30.6%) and therefore provides less drug to the systemic circulation, possibly accounting for the decrease in frequency of adverse reactions.

Overdosage

No instances of overdose with calcitonin-salmon nasal spray have been reported and no serious adverse reactions have been associated with high doses. There is no known potential for drug abuse for calcitonin-salmon.

Single doses of calcitonin-salmon nasal spray up to 1,600 units, doses up to 800 units/day for 3 days and chronic administration of doses up to 600 units/day have been studied without serious adverse effects. A dose of 1,000 units of calcitonin-salmon injectable solution given subcutaneously may produce nausea and vomiting. A dose of calcitonin-salmon injectable solution of 32 units/kg/day for 1 or 2 days demonstrated no additional adverse effects.

There have been no reports of hypocalcemic tetany. However, the pharmacologic actions of calcitonin-salmon nasal spray suggest that this could occur in overdose. Therefore, provisions for parenteral administration of calcium should be available for the treatment of overdose.

Patient Information

Give careful instructions on pump assembly, priming of the pump, and nasal introduction of calcitonin-salmon nasal spray to the patient. Although instructions for patients are supplied with individual bottles, demonstrate procedures for use to each patient. Patients should notify their doctors if they develop significant nasal irritation.

Advise patients of the following:

- Store new, unassembled bottles in the refrigerator between 2° to 8°C (36° to 46°F).
- Protect the product from freezing.
- Before priming the pump and using a new bottle, allow it to reach room temperature.
- Store bottle in use at room temperature between 15° to 30°C (59° to 86°F) in an upright position, for up to 30 days. Each bottle contains at least 30 doses.

You should keep track of the number of doses used from the bottle. After 30 doses, each spray may not deliver the correct amount of medication, even if the bottle is not completely empty.

CALCIMIMETICS

CINACALCET

Rx	**Sensipar** (Amgen)	**Tablets; oral:** 30 mg	Equiv. to cinacalcet hydrochloride 33 mg. (AMG 30). Light green, oval. Film-coated. In 30s.
		60 mg	Equiv. to cinacalcet hydrochloride 66 mg. (AMG 60). Light green, oval. Film-coated. In 30s.
		90 mg	Equiv. to cinacalcet hydrochloride 99 mg. (AMG 90). Light green, oval. Film-coated. In 30s.

CINACALCET HYDROCHLORIDE — ORAL

Indications

➤*Hypercalcemia in parathyroid carcinoma:* For the treatment of hypercalcemia in patients with parathyroid carcinoma.

➤*Primary hyperparathyroidism:* For the treatment of severe hypercalcemia in patients with primary hyperparathyroidism who are unable to undergo parathyroidectomy.

➤*Secondary hyperparathyroidism:* For the treatment of secondary hyperparathyroidism in patients with chronic kidney disease on dialysis.

Administration and Dosage

➤*General dosing considerations:* Measure serum calcium, serum phosphorus, and intact parathyroid hormone (PTH) after initiation or dose adjustments of cinacalcet (see Warnings/Precautions).

➤*Adults:*

Hypercalcemia in parathyroid carcinoma –

Initial dosage: 30 mg twice daily.

Dosage titration: Titrate the dosage every 2 to 4 weeks through sequential dosages of 30 mg twice daily, 60 mg twice daily, 90 mg twice daily, and 90 mg 3 or 4 times daily as necessary to normalize serum calcium levels.

CINACALCET HYDROCHLORIDE — ORAL

Primary hyperparathyroidism – See Hypercalcemia in Parathyroid Carcinoma for dosing.

Secondary hyperparathyroidism –

Initial dosage: 30 mg once daily.

Dosage titration: Titrate no more frequently than every 2 to 4 weeks through sequential dosages of 30, 60, 90, 120, and 180 mg once daily to target intact PTH levels of 150 to 300 pg/mL. Serum intact PTH levels should be assessed no earlier then 12 hours after dosing.

During dose titration, monitor serum calcium levels frequently, and if levels decrease below the normal range, take appropriate steps to increase serum calcium levels, such as providing supplemental calcium, initiating or increasing the dose of calcium-based phosphate binder, initiating or increasing the dose of vitamin D sterols, or temporarily withholding treatment with cinacalcet.

Concomitant therapy: Cinacalcet can be used alone or in combination with vitamin D sterols and/or phosphate binders.

➤*Hypocalcemia:* If serum calcium falls below 8.4 mg/dL but remains above 7.5 mg/dL or if symptoms of hypocalcemia occur, use calcium-containing phosphate binders and/or vitamin D sterols to raise serum calcium. If serum calcium falls below 7.5 mg/dL or if symptoms of hypocalcemia persist and the dose of vitamin D cannot be increased, withhold administration of cinacalcet until serum calcium levels reach 8 mg/dL and/or symptoms of hypocalcemia have resolved. Reinitiate treatment using the next lowest dose of cinacalcet.

➤*Administration:* Tablets should be taken whole and should not be divided. Tablets should be taken with food or shortly after a meal.

➤*Storage/Stability:* Store at 25°C (77°F); excursions are permitted to 15° to 30°C (59° to 86°F).

Actions

➤*Pharmacology:* Cinacalcet is a calcimimetic agent that increases the sensitivity of the calcium-sensing receptor to activation by extracellular calcium. The calcium-sensing receptor on the surface of the chief cell of the parathyroid gland is the principal regulator of PTH synthesis and secretion. Cinacalcet directly lowers PTH levels by increasing the sensitivity of the calcium-sensing receptor to extracellular calcium. The reduction in PTH is associated with a concomitant decrease in serum calcium levels.

➤*Pharmacokinetics:*

Absorption/Distribution – After oral administration, C_{max} is achieved in approximately 2 to 6 hours. Steady-state drug levels are achieved within 7 days. The mean accumulation ratio is approximately 2 with once-daily oral administration. The median accumulation ratio is approximately 2 to 5 with twice-daily oral administration. The area under the curve (AUC) and C_{max} of cinacalcet increase proportionally over the dose range of 30 to 180 mg once daily. The volume of distribution is approximately 1,000 L, indicating extensive distribution. Cinacalcet is approximately 93% to 97% bound to plasma protein(s). The ratio of blood cinacalcet concentration to plasma cinacalcet concentration is 0.8 at a blood cinacalcet concentration of 10 ng/mL.

Effect of food: Cinacalcet C_{max} and $AUC_{(0\text{-}inf)}$ were increased 82% and 68%, respectively, when cinacalcet was administered with a high-fat meal compared with fasting. The C_{max} and $AUC_{(0\text{-}inf)}$ of cinacalcet were increased by 65% and 50%, respectively, when cinacalcet was administered with a low-fat meal compared with fasting.

Metabolism/Excretion – Cinacalcet is metabolized by multiple enzymes, primarily CYP3A4, CYP2D6, and CYP1A2. After administration of a 75 mg radiolabeled dose to healthy volunteers, cinacalcet was metabolized via oxidative N-dealkylation to hydrocinnamic acid and hydroxy-hydrocinnamic acid, which are further metabolized via beta-oxidation and glycine conjugation; the oxidative N-dealkylation process also generates metabolites that contain the naphthalene ring; and oxidation of the naphthalene ring on the parent drug to form dihydrodiols, which are further conjugated with glucuronic acid. The plasma concentrations of the major circulating metabolites, including the cinnamic acid derivatives and glucuronidated dihydrodiols, markedly exceed parent drug concentrations. The hydrocinnamic acid metabolite and glucuronide conjugates have minimal or no calcimimetic activity. Renal excretion of metabolites was the primary route of elimination of radioactivity.

After absorption, cinacalcet concentrations decline in a biphasic fashion, with a terminal half-life of 30 to 40 hours. Approximately 80% of the dose was recovered in the urine and 15% in the feces.

Special populations –

Hepatic function impairment: In patients with moderate and severe hepatic impairment (as indicated by the Child-Pugh method), cinacalcet exposures as defined by the $AUC_{(0\text{-}inf)}$ were 2.4 and 4.2 times higher, respectively, than those of healthy patients. The mean half-life of cinacalcet increased from 49 hours in healthy volunteers to 65 and 84 hours in patients with moderate and severe hepatic impairment, respectively. Protein binding of cinacalcet is not affected by impaired hepatic function.

Contraindications

Hypocalcemia.

Warnings/Precautions

➤*Hypocalcemia:* Cinacalcet lowers serum calcium. Cinacalcet treatment should not be initiated if serum calcium is less than the lower limit of the normal range.

Monitor patients carefully for the occurrence of hypocalcemia. Potential manifestations of hypocalcemia include convulsions, muscle cramping, myalgias, paresthesias, and tetany.

Measure serum calcium within 1 week after initiation or dose adjustment of cinacalcet. Once the maintenance dose has been established, measure serum calcium approximately monthly.

See Administration and Dosage for more information.

In the 26-week studies of patients with chronic kidney disease on dialysis, 66% of patients receiving cinacalcet compared with 25% of patients receiving placebo developed at least 1 serum calcium value less than 8.4 mg/dL. Less than 1% of patients in each group permanently discontinued study drug because of hypocalcemia.

Cinacalcet is not indicated for patients with chronic kidney disease not on dialysis. The long-term safety and efficacy of cinacalcet have not been established for patients with chronic kidney disease with secondary hyperparathyroidism not on dialysis. Clinical studies indicate that cinacalcet-treated chronic kidney disease patients not on dialysis have an increased risk of hypocalcemia compared with cinacalcet-treated chronic kidney disease patients on dialysis, which may be due to lower baseline calcium levels. In a phase 3 study of 32 weeks' duration and including 404 subjects with chronic kidney disease not on dialysis (302 cinacalcet, 102 placebo), in which the median dose for cinacalcet was 60 mg at the completion of the study, 80% of cinacalcet-treated patients experienced at least 1 serum calcium value less than 8.4 mg/dL compared with 5% of patients receiving placebo.

➤*Seizures:* In 3 clinical studies of patients with chronic kidney disease on dialysis, 5% of the patients in both the cinacalcet and placebo groups reported a history of seizure disorder at baseline. During the trials, seizures (primarily generalized or tonic-clonic) were observed in 1.4% of cinacalcet patients and 0.4% of placebo-treated patients. Five of the 9 cinacalcet patients had a history of a seizure disorder, and 2 patients were receiving antiseizure medication at the time of their seizure. Both placebo-treated patients had a history of seizure disorder and were receiving antiseizure medication at the time of their seizure. While the basis for the reported difference in seizure rate is not clear, the threshold for seizures is lowered by significant reductions in serum calcium levels. Therefore, closely monitor serum calcium levels in patients receiving cinacalcet, particularly in patients with a history of a seizure disorder.

➤*Cardiovascular effects:* In postmarketing safety surveillance, isolated, idiosyncratic cases of hypotension, arrhythmia, and/or worsening heart failure have been reported in patients with impaired cardiac function, in which a causal relationship to cinacalcet could not be completely excluded and may be mediated by reductions in serum calcium levels.

➤*Adynamic bone disease:* Adynamic bone disease may develop if intact PTH levels are suppressed below 100 pg/mL. One clinical study evaluated bone histomorphometry in patients treated with cinacalcet for 1 year. Three patients with mild hyperparathyroid bone disease at the beginning of the study developed adynamic bone disease during treatment with cinacalcet. Two of these patients had intact PTH levels below 100 pg/mL at multiple time points during the study. In the three 6-month, phase 3 studies conducted in chronic kidney disease patients on dialysis, 11% of patients treated with cinacalcet had mean intact PTH values below 100 pg/mL during the efficacy-assessment phase. If intact PTH levels decrease below 150 pg/mL in patients treated with cinacalcet, reduce the dose of cinacalcet and/or vitamin D sterols or discontinue therapy.

➤*Hepatic function impairment:* Cinacalcet exposure as assessed by $AUC_{(0\text{-}inf)}$ in patients with moderate and severe hepatic impairment were 2.4 and 4.2 times higher, respectively. Monitor serum calcium, serum phosphorus, and intact PTH levels closely throughout treatment in patients with moderate and severe hepatic impairment.

➤*Pregnancy: Category C.* There are no adequate and well-controlled studies in pregnant women. It is not known if cinacalcet crosses the human placenta. The molecular weight (about 358 for the free base) and long terminal half-life suggest that the drug will cross to the embryo and fetus. However, the extensive metabolism and high plasma protein binding should decrease the exposure to the parent drug. Use cinacalcet during pregnancy only if the potential benefit justifies the potential risk to the fetus.

In pregnant female rats given oral gavage dosages of 2, 25, and 50 mg/kg/day during gestation, no teratogenicity was observed at dosages of up to 50 mg/kg/day (exposure 4 times those resulting with a human oral dosage of 180 mg/day based on AUC comparison). Decreased fetal body weights were observed at all doses (less than 1 to 4 times a human oral dosage of 180 mg/day based on AUC comparison) in conjunction with maternal toxicity (decreased food consumption and body weight gain).

In pregnant female rabbits given oral gavage dosages of 2, 12, and 25 mg/kg/day during gestation, no adverse fetal effects were observed (exposures less than with a human oral dosage of 180 mg/day based on AUC comparisons). Reductions in maternal food consumption and body weight gain were seen at dosages of 12 and 25 mg/kg/day. Cinacalcet crosses the placental barrier in rabbits.

Higher dosages of 15 and 25 mg/kg/day (exposures 2 to 3 times a human oral dosage of 180 mg/day based on AUC comparisons) were accompanied by maternal signs of hypocalcemia (periparturient mortality and early postnatal pup loss), and reductions in postnatal maternal and pup body weight gain.

Pregnancy registry – Women who become pregnant during cinacalcet treatment are encouraged to enroll in Amgen's Pregnancy Surveillance Program. Patients or their health care providers should call 1-800-772-6436 to enroll.

➤*Lactation:* Studies in rats have shown that cinacalcet is excreted in the milk with a high milk-to-plasma ratio. It is not known whether this drug is excreted in human breast milk. The molecular weight (about 358 for the free base) and long terminal half-life (30 to 40 hours) suggest the drug will be

CINACALCET HYDROCHLORIDE — ORAL

excreted in breast milk. However, the extensive metabolism and high plasma protein binding (93% to 97%) should decrease the amount of parent drug in milk. Considering the data in rats, and because many drugs are excreted in human milk and there is a potential for clinically significant adverse reactions in infants who ingest cinacalcet, decide whether to discontinue breast-feeding or the drug, taking into account the importance of the drug to the breast-feeding woman.

➤*Children:* The safety and efficacy of cinacalcet in children have not been established.

➤*Monitoring:* Closely monitor serum calcium levels in patients receiving cinacalcet, particularly in patients with a history of seizure disorder. In patients with moderate and severe hepatic impairment, closely monitor intact PTH, serum phosphorus, and serum calcium concentrations throughout treatment with cinacalcet.

Secondary hyperparathyroidism – Measure serum calcium and serum phosphorus within 1 week, and measure intact PTH 1 to 4 weeks after initiation or dose adjustment of cinacalcet. Once the maintenance dose has been established, measure serum calcium and serum phosphorus approximately monthly and intact PTH every 1 to 3 months. Measurements of PTH during the cinacalcet trials were obtained using the Nichols intact PTH IRMA.

Hypercalcemia in parathyroid carcinoma or primary hyperparathyroidism – Measure serum calcium within 1 week after initiation or dose adjustment of cinacalcet. Once maintenance dose levels have been established, measure serum calcium every 2 months.

Drug Interactions

Cinacalcet Drug Interactions			
Precipitant drug	Object drug[a]		Description
CYP3A4 inhibitors (eg, erythromycin, itraconazole, ketoconazole)	Cinacalcet	↑	Cinacalcet plasma concentrations may be elevated, increasing the pharmacologic effects and adverse reactions. Dose adjustments of cinacalcet may be required; closely monitor PTH and serum calcium concentrations.
Cinacalcet	CYP2D6 substrates (eg, carvedilol, flecainide, metoprolol, thioridazine, tricyclic antidepressants [eg, amitriptyline, desipramine, nortriptyline])	↑	Cinacalcet is a strong inhibitor of CYP2D6; therefore, dose adjustments of concomitant medications that are predominantly metabolized by CYP2D6 and particularly those that have a narrow therapeutic index (eg, flecainide, tricyclic antidepressants) may be required.

[a] ↑ = object drug increased.

➤*Drug/Food Interaction:* See Actions for more information.

Adverse Reactions

➤*Secondary hyperparathyroidism:*

Most frequent adverse reactions – The most frequently reported reactions in the cinacalcet group were nausea, vomiting, and diarrhea.

Adverse reactions (5% or more) –

Cinacalcet Adverse Reactions in Secondary Hyperparathyroidism (≥ 5%)		
Adverse reactions[a]	Cinacalcet (n = 656)	Placebo (n = 470)
CNS		
Asthenia	7%	4%
Dizziness	10%	8%
GI		
Anorexia	6%	4%
Diarrhea	21%	20%
Nausea	31%	19%
Vomiting	27%	15%
Miscellaneous		
Access infection	5%	4%
Chest pain, noncardiac	6%	4%
Hypertension	7%	5%
Myalgia	15%	14%

[a] Included are reactions that were reported at a greater incidence in the cinacalcet group than in the placebo group.

➤*Hypercalcemia in parathyroid carcinoma and primary hyperparathyroidism:*

Discontinuation – Twenty percent of patients withdrew from the study because of adverse reactions.

Most frequent adverse reactions – The most frequent adverse reactions and the most frequent cause of withdrawal in this patient group were nausea and vomiting. Severe or prolonged cases of nausea and vomiting can lead to dehydration and worsening hypercalcemia, so careful monitoring of electrolytes is recommended in patients with these symptoms.

Mortality – Eight patients died during the study, 7 with parathyroid carcinoma (24%) and 1 (6%) with intractable primary hyperparathyroidism. Causes of death were cardiovascular (5 patients), multiorgan failure (1 patient), GI hemorrhage (1 patient), and metastatic carcinoma (1 patient). Adverse reactions of hypocalcemia were reported in 3 patients (7%).

Adverse reactions (10% or more) –

Cinacalcet Adverse Reactions (≥ 10%)[a]			
	Cinacalcet		
Adverse reactions	Parathyroid carcinoma (n = 29)	Intractable primary hyperparathyroidism (n = 17)	Total (n = 46)
Subjects reporting adverse reactions	97%	100%	98%
CNS			
Asthenia	17%	12%	15%
Depression	10%	18%	13%
Fatigue	21%	12%	17%
Headache	21%	0%	13%
Paresthesia	14%	29%	20%
GI			
Anorexia	21%	6%	15%
Constipation	10%	18%	13%
Nausea	66%	59%	63%
Vomiting	52%	35%	46%
Metabolic/Nutritional			
Dehydration	24%	0%	15%
Hypercalcemia	21%	12%	17%
Musculoskeletal			
Arthralgia	17%	6%	13%
Fracture	21%	12%	17%
Pain limb	10%	12%	11%
Miscellaneous			
Anemia	17%	6%	13%
Infection, upper respiratory tract	10%	12%	11%

[a] n = number of subjects receiving ≥ 1 dose of study drug.

➤*Lab test abnormalities:* In patients with end-stage renal disease, testosterone levels are often below the normal range. In a placebo-controlled trial in patients with chronic kidney disease on dialysis, there were reductions in total and free testosterone in men following 6 months of treatment with cinacalcet. Levels of total testosterone decreased by a median of 15.8% in the cinacalcet-treated patients and by 0.6% in the placebo-treated patients. Levels of free testosterone decreased by a median of 31.3% in the cinacalcet-treated patients and by 16.3% in the placebo-treated patients. The clinical significance of these reductions in serum testosterone is unknown.

➤*Postmarketing:*

Cardiovascular – Isolated, idiosyncratic cases of hypotension, worsening heart failure, and/or arrhythmia have been reported in cinacalcet-treated patients with impaired cardiac function.

Hypersensitivity – Hypersensitivity reactions (including angioedema and urticaria).

Miscellaneous – Diarrhea, myalgia, and rash.

Overdosage

➤*Symptoms:* Dosages titrated up to 300 mg once daily have been safely administered to patients on dialysis. Overdosage of cinacalcet may lead to hypocalcemia.

➤*Treatment:* In the event of overdosage, monitor patients for signs and symptoms of hypocalcemia and take appropriate measures to correct serum calcium levels. Because cinacalcet is highly protein bound, hemodialysis is not an effective treatment for overdosage of cinacalcet.

Patient Information

Advise patients to take with food or shortly after a meal. Advise patients to swallow tablets whole and not divide them.

Inform patients of the importance of regular blood tests, in order to monitor the safety and efficacy of cinacalcet therapy.

CINACALCET HYDROCHLORIDE — ORAL

Advise patients to report nausea, vomiting, and potential symptoms of hypocalcemia, including tingling/numbness of the skin, muscle pain, and muscle cramping.

Ask patients if they are taking medication to prevent seizures or have had seizures in the past, and advise them to report any seizure episodes while taking cinacalcet.

GALLIUM NITRATE

Rx	Ganite (Genta)	Injection: 25 mg/mL	Preservative free. In 20 mL single-dose vials.

GALLIUM NITRATE — INJECTION

WARNING

Concurrent use of gallium nitrate with other potentially nephrotoxic drugs (eg, aminoglycosides, amphotericin B) may increase the risk for developing severe renal insufficiency in patients with cancer-related hypercalcemia. If use of a potentially nephrotoxic drug is indicated during gallium nitrate therapy, gallium nitrate administration should be discontinued and it is recommended that hydration be continued for several days after administration of the potentially nephrotoxic drug. Serum creatinine and urine output should be closely monitored during and subsequent to this period. Gallium nitrate therapy should be discontinued if the serum creatinine level exceeds 2.5 mg/dL.

Indications

➤*Cancer-related hypercalcemia:* For the treatment of clearly symptomatic cancer-related hypercalcemia that has not responded to adequate hydration. In general, patients with a serum calcium (corrected for albumin) less than 12 mg/dL would not be expected to be symptomatic. Mild or asymptomatic hypercalcemia may be treated with conservative measures (ie, saline hydration, with or without diuretics). In the treatment of cancer-related hypercalcemia, it is important first to establish adequate hydration, preferably with intravenous saline, in order to increase the renal excretion of calcium and correct dehydration caused by hypercalcemia.

Administration and Dosage

➤*General dosing considerations:* Adequate hydration must be maintained throughout the treatment period, with careful attention to avoid overhydration in patients with compromised cardiovascular status.

➤*Adults:*

Cancer-related hypercalcemia –

Usual dosage: 200 mg/m^2 of body surface area daily for 5 consecutive days as an IV infusion over 24 hours.

Alternative dosage: In patients with mild hypercalcemia and few symptoms, a lower dosage of 100 mg/m^2/day for 5 days may be considered.

Discontinuation of therapy: If serum calcium levels are lowered into the normal range in less than 5 days, treatment may be discontinued early.

➤*Renal function impairment:* The use of gallium nitrate in patients with marked renal insufficiency (serum creatinine greater than 2.5 mg/dL) has not been systematically examined. If therapy is undertaken in patients with moderately impaired renal function (serum creatinine 2 to 2.5 mg/dL), frequent monitoring of the patients renal status is recommended. Treatment should be discontinued if the serum creatinine level exceeds 2.5 mg/dL.

➤*Preparation for administration:* The daily dose should be diluted, preferably in 1,000 mL of sodium chloride 0.9% injection or dextrose 5% injection, for administration as an IV infusion.

➤*Administration:* The daily dose must be administered as an IV infusion over 24 hours.

➤*Storage/Stability:* Store at 20° to 25°C (68° to 77°F). Contains no preservative. Discard unused portion.

When gallium nitrate is added to either sodium chloride 0.9% injection or dextrose 5% injection, it is stable for 48 hours at room temperature (15° to 30°C [59° to 86°F]) or for 7 days if stored under refrigeration (2° to 8°C [35.6° to 46.4°F]).

Actions

➤*Pharmacology:* Gallium nitrate exerts a hypocalcemic effect by inhibiting calcium resorption from bone, possibly by reducing increased bone turnover. Although in vitro and animal studies have been performed to investigate the mechanism of action of gallium nitrate, the precise mechanism for inhibiting calcium resorption has not been determined. No cytotoxic effects were observed on bone cells in drug-treated animals.

➤*Pharmacokinetics:*

Absorption/Distribution – Gallium nitrate was infused at a daily dose of 200 mg/m^2 for 5 (n = 2) or 7 (n = 10) consecutive days to 12 cancer patients. In most patients, apparent steady-state is achieved by 24 to 48 hours. The range of average steady-state plasma levels of gallium observed among 7 fully evaluable patients was between 1,134 and 2,399 ng/mL. The average plasma clearance of gallium (n = 7) following daily infusion of gallium nitrate at a dose of 200 mg/m^2 for 5 or 7 days was 0.15 L/hr/kg (range: 0.12 to 0.2 L/hr/kg). In 1 patient who received daily infusion doses of 100, 150, and 200 mg/m^2, the apparent steady-state levels of gallium did not increase proportionally with an increase in dose.

Metabolism/Excretion – Gallium nitrate is not metabolized either by the liver or the kidney and appears to be significantly excreted via the kidney. Urinary excretion data for a dose of 200 mg/m^2 has not been determined.

Contraindications

Severe renal impairment (serum creatinine greater than 2.5 mg/dL).

Warnings/Precautions

➤*Nephrotoxic drugs:* Combined use of gallium nitrate with other potentially nephrotoxic drugs (eg, aminoglycosides, amphotericin B) may increase the risk of developing renal insufficiency in patients with cancer-related hypercalcemia.

➤*Asymptomatic or mild to moderate hypocalcemia:* Asymptomatic or mild to moderate hypocalcemia (6.5 to 8 mg/dL, corrected for serum albumin) occurred in approximately 38% of patients treated with gallium nitrate in the controlled clinical trial. One patient exhibited a positive Chvostek's sign. If hypocalcemia occurs, gallium nitrate therapy should be stopped and short-term calcium therapy may be necessary.

➤*Renal function impairment:* The hypercalcemic state in cancer patients is commonly associated with impaired renal function. Abnormalities in renal function (elevated BUN and/or serum creatinine) have been observed in clinical trials with gallium nitrate. It is strongly recommended that serum creatinine be monitored during gallium nitrate therapy. Because patients with cancer-related hypercalcemia are frequently dehydrated, it is important that such patients be adequately hydrated with oral and/or intravenous fluids (preferably saline) and that a satisfactory urine output (a urine output of 2 L/day is recommended) be established before therapy with gallium nitrate is started. Adequate hydration should be maintained throughout the treatment period, with careful attention to avoid overhydration in patients with compromised cardiovascular status. Diuretic therapy should not be employed prior to correction of hypovolemia. Gallium nitrate therapy should be discontinued if the serum creatinine level exceeds 2.5 mg/dL.

The use of gallium nitrate in patients with marked renal insufficiency (serum creatinine greater than 2.5 mg/dL) has not been systematically examined. If therapy is undertaken in patients with moderately impaired renal function (serum creatinine 2 to 2.5 mg/dL), frequent monitoring of the patient's renal status is recommended. Treatment should be discontinued if the serum creatinine level exceeds 2.5 mg/dL.

➤*Pregnancy: Category C.* Animal reproduction studies have not been conducted with gallium nitrate. It is also not known whether gallium nitrate can cause fetal harm when administered to a pregnant woman or can affect reproductive capacity. Gallium nitrate should be administered to a pregnant woman only if clearly needed.

➤*Lactation:* It is not known whether gallium nitrate is excreted in human milk. Because of the potential for serious adverse reactions in nursing infants from gallium nitrate, a decision should be made whether to discontinue nursing or discontinue the drug, taking into account the importance of the drug to the mother.

➤*Children:* The safety and efficacy of gallium nitrate in children have not been established.

➤*Monitoring:* Renal function (serum creatinine and BUN) and serum calcium must be closely monitored during gallium nitrate therapy. In addition to baseline assessment, the suggested frequency of calcium and phosphorus determinations is daily and twice weekly, respectively. Gallium nitrate should be discontinued if the serum creatinine exceeds 2.5 mg/dL.

Drug Interactions

The concomitant use of highly nephrotoxic drugs in combination with gallium nitrate may increase the risk for development of renal insufficiency. Available information does not indicate any adverse interaction with diuretics such as furosemide. A symptom complex of dyspnea (associated with interstitial pneumonitis in some instances), mouth soreness, and asthenia has been reported in a small number of multiple myeloma patients receiving low dose (40 mg) gallium nitrate subcutaneously in addition to oral cyclophosphamide and prednisone. The serious nature of the underlying condition of these patients precludes a precise understanding of the relationship of these events to either gallium nitrate treatment alone or with cyclophosphamide.

Adverse Reactions

➤*Cardiovascular:* A decrease in mean systolic and diastolic blood pressure was observed several days after treatment with gallium nitrate in a controlled clinical trial. The decrease in blood pressure was asymptomatic and did not require specific treatment.

➤*Hematologic:* The use of very high doses of gallium nitrate (up to 1,400 mg/m^2) in treating patients for advanced cancer has been associated with anemia, and several patients have received red blood cell transfusions. Because of the serious nature of the underlying illness, it is uncertain that the anemia was caused by gallium nitrate.

➤*Metabolic:* Hypocalcemia may occur after gallium nitrate treatment.

GALLIUM NITRATE — INJECTION

Transient hypophosphatemia of mild-to-moderate degree may occur in up to 79% of hypercalcemic patients following treatment with gallium nitrate. In a controlled clinical trial, 33% of patients had at least 1 serum phosphorus measurement between 1.5 to 2.4 mg/dL, while 46% of patients had at least 1 serum phosphorus value less than 1.5 mg/dL. Patients who develop hypophosphatemia may require oral phosphorus therapy.

Decreased serum bicarbonate, possibly secondary to mild respiratory alkalosis was reported in 40% to 50% of cancer patients treated with gallium nitrate. The cause for this effect is not clear. This effect has been asymptomatic and has not required specific treatment.

➤*Renal:* Adverse renal effects, as demonstrated by rising BUN and creatinine, have been reported in about 12.5% of patients treated with gallium nitrate. In a controlled clinical trial of patients with cancer-related hypercalcemia, 2 patients receiving gallium nitrate and 1 patient receiving calcitonin developed acute renal failure. Due to the serious nature of the patients' underlying conditions, the relationship of these events to the drug was unclear. Gallium nitrate should not be administered to patients with serum creatinine greater than 2.5 mg/dL.

➤*Special senses:* In cancer chemotherapy trials, a small proportion (less than 1%) of patients treated with multiple high doses of gallium nitrate combined with other investigational anticancer drugs, have developed acute optic neuritis. While these patients were critically ill and had received multiple drugs, a reaction to high-dose gallium nitrate is possible. Most patients had full recovery; however, at least one case of permanent blindness has been reported. One patient with cancer-related hypercalcemia was reported to develop decreased hearing following gallium nitrate administration. Because of the patient's underlying condition and concurrent therapies, the relationship of this event to gallium nitrate administration is unclear. Tinnitus and partial loss of auditory acuity have been reported rarely (less than 1%) in patients who received high-dose gallium nitrate as anticancer treatment.

➤*Miscellaneous:* Other clinical events reported in association with gallium nitrate treatment for cancer as well as cancer-related hypercalcemia include nausea and/or vomiting, tachycardia, lethargy, confusion, dreams and hallucinations, diarrhea, constipation, lower extremity edema, hypothermia, fever, dyspnea, rales and rhonchi, anemia, leukopenia, paresthesia, skin rash, pleural effusion, and pulmonary infiltrates. Due to the serious nature of the underlying condition of these patients, the relationship of these events to therapy with gallium nitrate is unknown. A single case of encephalopathy followed rapidly by coma and death has been reported after treatment in a cancer chemotherapy trial with gallium nitrate 300 mg/m²/day for 7 days. Treatment with gallium nitrate other than as described in this monograph may be complicated by adverse events not listed.

Overdosage

➤*Symptoms:* Rapid intravenous infusion of gallium nitrate or use of doses higher than recommended (200 mg/m²) may cause nausea and vomiting and a substantially increased risk of renal insufficiency.

➤*Treatment:* In the event of overdosage, further drug administration should be discontinued, serum calcium should be monitored, and the patient should receive vigorous intravenous hydration, with or without diuretics, for 2 to 3 days. During this time period, renal function and urinary output should be carefully monitored so that fluid intake and output are balanced.

SODIUM PHENYLBUTYRATE

SODIUM PHENYLBUTYRATE

Rx	**Buphenyl** (Medicis)	**Tablets:** 500 mg	(UCY 500). Off-white, oval. In 250s and 500s.
		Powder: 3 g per 5 mL	In 500 mL bottles. Measurers provided.

SODIUM PHENYLBUTYRATE — ORAL

Indications

➤*Cycle disorders:* Adjunctive therapy in the chronic management of patients with urea cycle disorders involving deficiencies of carbamoyl phosphate synthetase (CPS), ornithine transcarbamoylase (OTC), or argininosuccinic acid synthetase (AAS). It is indicated in all patients with neonatal-onset deficiency (complete enzymatic deficiency, presenting within the first 28 days of life). It is also indicated in patients with late-onset disease (partial enzymatic deficiency, presenting after the first month of life) who have a history of hyperammonemic encephalopathy. It is important that the diagnosis be made early and treatment initiated immediately to improve survival. Any episode of acute hyperammonemia should be treated as a life-threatening emergency.

Administration and Dosage

➤*Adults:*

Cycle disorders –

Powder:

• *More than 20 kg* – 9.9 to 13 g/m²/day in equally divided doses, 4 to 6 times daily.

• *Less than 20 kg* – 450 to 600 mg/kg/day in equally divided doses, 4 to 6 times daily.

Tablets:

• *More than 20 kg* – 9.9 to 13 g/m²/day in equally divided doses 3 times daily.

• *Less than 20 kg* – 450 to 600 mg/kg/day in equally divided doses 3 times daily.

➤*Children:*

Cycle disorders –

Powder: See Adults for dosing.

Tablets:

• *More than 20 kg* – 9.9 to 13 g/m²/day in equally divided doses 3 times daily.

• *Less than 20 kg* – Not recommended.

➤*Administration:*

Powder – For oral use via mouth, gastrostomy or nasogastric tube only. Take in equally divided amounts with each meal or feeding, 4 to 6 times daily. Mix with food (solid or liquid). Avoid acidic beverages. Shake lightly before use.

Tablets – For oral use only. Take in equally divided amounts with each meal (eg, 3 times daily).

➤*Storage/Stability:* Store at 15° to 30°C (59° to 86°F).

Actions

➤*Pharmacology:* Sodium phenylbutyrate is a pro-drug and is rapidly metabolized to phenylacetate. Phenylacetate is a metabolically-active compound that conjugates with glutamine via acetylation to form phenylacetylglutamine. Phenylacetylglutamine is excreted then by the kidneys. On a molar basis, it is comparable to urea (each containing two moles of nitrogen). Therefore, phenylacetylglutamine provides an alternate vehicle for waste nitrogen excretion.

➤*Pharmacokinetics:*

Absorption – Peak plasma levels of phenylbutyrate occur within 1 hour after a single dose of 5 g sodium phenylbutyrate powder with a C_{max} of 195 mcg/ml and for the tablets, a C_{max} of 218 mcg/ml under fasting conditions. The effect of food on phenylbutyrate's absorption is unknown.

Excretion – A majority of the administered compound (approximately 80% to 100%) is excreted by the kidneys within 24 hours as the conjugation product, phenylacetylglutamine. For each gram of sodium phenylbutyrate administered, it is estimated that between 0.12 to 0.15 g of phenylacetylglutamine nitrogen is produced.

Following oral administration of 5 g, measurable plasma levels of phenylbutyrate and phenylacetate were detected 15 and 30 min after dosing, respectively, and phenylacetylglutamine was detected shortly thereafter. The pharmacokinetic parameters for phenylbutyrate for C_{max} (mcg/ml), T_{max} (hours) and elimination half-life were 195, 1 and 0.76 hours, respectively, and for phenylacetate 45.3, 3.55 and 1.29 hours, respectively. The major sites for metabolism are the liver and kidney.

In patients with urea cycle disorders, sodium phenylbutyrate decreases elevated plasma ammonia and glutamine levels. It increases waste nitrogen excretion in the form of phenylacetylglutamine.

Special populations –

Gender: The pharmacokinetic parameters, AUC and C_{max} for both plasma phenylbutyrate and phenylacetate were about 30% to 50% greater in women than in men.

Contraindications

Management of acute hyperammonemia, which is a medical emergency.

Warnings/Precautions

➤*Fluid retention:* Use with great care, if at all, in patients with CHF or severe renal insufficiency, and in clinical states in which there is sodium retention with edema.

➤*Preexisting neurologic impairment:* Reversal of preexisting neurologic impairment is not likely to occur with treatment, and neurologic deterioration may continue.

➤*Acute hyperammonemic encephalopathy:* Acute hyperammonemic encephalopathy recurred in the majority of patients.

➤*Long-term:* Sodium phenylbutyrate may be required life-long unless orthotopic liver transplantation is elected.

➤*Renal/Hepatic function impairment:* Sodium phenylbutyrate is metabolized in the liver and kidney, and phenylacetylglutamine is primarily excreted by the kidney. Use caution when administering the drug to patients with hepatic or renal insufficiency.

➤*Pregnancy: Category C.* It is not known whether sodium phenylbutyrate can cause fetal harm when administered to a pregnant woman or can affect reproduction capacity. Give sodium phenylbutyrate to a pregnant woman only if clearly needed.

➤*Lactation:* It is not known whether this drug is excreted in breast milk. Because many drugs are excreted in breast milk, exercise caution when administering sodium phenylbutyrate to a breast-feeding woman.

SODIUM PHENYLBUTYRATE — ORAL

➤*Children:* The use of tablets for neonates, infants, and children 20 kg or less is not recommended (see Administration and Dosage).

➤*Monitoring:* Maintain plasma levels of ammonia, arginine, branched-chain amino acids and serum proteins within normal limits, and maintain plasma glutamine at levels less than 1,000 mcmol/L. Periodically monitor serum drug levels of phenylbutyrate and its metabolites, phenylacetate, and phenylacetylglutamine.

Drug Interactions

Sodium Phenylbutyrate Drug Interactions

Precipitant drug	Object drug[a]		Description
Corticosteroids	Sodium phenylbutyrate	↓	Corticosteroids may cause the breakdown of body protein and increase plasma ammonia levels.
Haloperidol/ Valproate	Sodium phenylbutyrate	↓	Haloperidol/Valproate may cause hyperammonemia.
Probenecid	Sodium phenylbutyrate	↑	Probenecid is known to inhibit the renal transport of many organic compounds, including hippuric acid, and may affect renal excretion of the conjugation product of sodium phenylbutyrate, as well as its metabolite.

[a] ↑ = Object drug increased. ↓ = Object drug decreased.

Adverse Reactions

Amenorrhea/menstrual dysfunction (23%); decreased appetite (4%); body odor (probably caused by the metabolite phenylacetate), bad taste or taste aversion (3%).

Other adverse reactions reported in 2% or less of patients:

➤*Cardiovascular:* Arrhythmia, edema (one patient).

➤*CNS:* Depression, neurotoxicity (fatigue, light-headedness, and somnolence; less frequently, disorientation, dysgeusia, exacerbation of a preexisting neuropathy, headache, hypoacusis, and impaired memory). These adverse reactions were mainly mild in severity. The acute onset and reversibility when the phenylacetate infusion was discontinued suggest a drug effect.

➤*GI:* Abdominal pain, constipation, gastritis, nausea, vomiting, rectal bleeding, peptic ulcer disease, pancreatitis (one patient).

➤*Hematologic:* Aplastic anemia, ecchymosis (one patient).

➤*Miscellaneous:* Headache, renal tubular acidosis, rash, syncope, weight gain.

➤*Lab test abnormalities:*

Metabolic – Acidosis (14%); alkalosis, hyperchloremia (7%); hypophosphatemia (6%); hyperuricemia, hyperphosphatemia (2%); hypernatremia, hypokalemia (1%).

Nutritional – Hypoalbuminemia (11%); decreased total protein (3%).

Hepatic – Increased alkaline phosphatase (6%); increased liver transaminases (4%); hyperbilirubinemia (1%).

Hematologic – Anemia (9%); leukopenia, leukocytosis (4%); thrombocytopenia (3%); thrombocytosis (1%).

Overdosage

No adverse experiences have been reported involving overdoses of sodium phenylbutyrate in patients with urea cycle disorders.

➤*Treatment:* In the event of an overdose, discontinue the drug and institute supportive measures. Hemodialysis or peritoneal dialysis may be beneficial.

BETAINE ANHYDROUS

Rx	**Cystadane** (Rare Disease Therapeutics)	**Powder:** 1 g/1.7 mL	White, granular. In 180 g bottles.

BETAINE ANHYDROUS — ORAL

Indications

➤*Homocystinuria:* Betaine is indicated for the treatment of homocystinuria to decrease elevated homocysteine blood levels. Included within the category of homocystinuria are deficiencies or defects in: 1) Cystathionine beta-synthase (CBS); 2) 5,10–methylenetetrahydrofolate reductase (MTHFR); and 3) cobalamin cofactor metabolism (cbl).

Betaine has been administered concomitantly with vitamin B_6 (pyridoxine), vitamin B_{12} (cyanocobalamin) and folate.

Administration and Dosage

➤*Adults:*

Homocystinuria –

Usual dosage: 6 g/day administered orally in divided doses of 3 g twice daily.

Dosage titration: Dosage can be gradually increased until plasma homocysteine is undetectable or present only in small amounts. Dosages of up to 20 g/day have been necessary to control homocysteine levels in some patients.

➤*Children:*

Homocystinuria – See Adults for dosing for children 3 years of age and older.

Younger than 3 years of age:

- *Initial dosage* – 100 mg/kg/day.
- *Dosage titration* – Increase weekly by 100 mg/kg increments. Dosages of up to 20 g/day have been necessary to control homocysteine levels in some patients.

➤*Preparation for administration:* Measure prescribed amount with the measuring scoop provided (one level 1.7 mL scoop is equal to 1 g of betaine anhydrous powder) and then dissolve in 120 to 180 mL (4 to 6 oz) of water for immediate ingestion.

➤*Storage/Stability:* Store at room temperature, 15° to 30°C (59° to 86°F).

Actions

➤*Pharmacology:* Betaine acts as a methyl group donor in the remethylation of homocysteine to methionine in patients with homocystinuria. As a result, toxic blood levels of homocysteine are reduced in these patients, usually 20% to 30% or less of pre-treatment levels.

Elevated homocysteine blood levels are associated with clinical problems such as cardiovascular thrombosis, osteoporosis, skeletal abnormalities and optic lens dislocation. Plasma levels of homocysteine were decreased in nearly all patients treated with betaine. In observational studies without concurrent controls, clinical improvement was reported by physicians in approximately ¾ of patients taking betaine. Many of these patients were also taking other therapies such as vitamin B_6 (pyridoxine), vitamin B_{12} (cyanocobalamin) and folate with variable biochemical responses. In most cases, adding betaine resulted in a further reduction in homocysteine.

Betaine lowers plasma homocysteine levels in the three types of homocystinuria: Cystathionine beta-synthase (CBS) deficiency; 5,10–methylenetetrahydrofolate reductase (MTHFR) deficiency; and cobalamin cofactor metabolism (cbl) defect.

Betaine has also increased low plasma methionine and S-adenosylmethionine (SAM) levels in patients with MTHFR deficiency and cbl defect.

In CBS-deficient patients, large increases in methionine levels have been observed. However, the increased methionine levels do not appear to have been associated with adverse clinical consequences.

Betaine occurs naturally in the body. It is a metabolite of choline and is present in small amounts in foods (eg, beets, spinach, cereals and seafood).

➤*Pharmacokinetics:* The onset of action is within several days and a steady state in response to dosage is achieved within several weeks. Patients have taken betaine for many years without evidence of tolerance.

Warnings/Precautions

➤*Pregnancy: Category C.* It is not known whether betaine can cause fetal harm when administered to a pregnant woman or can affect reproductive capacity. Give to a pregnant woman only if clearly needed.

➤*Lactation:* It is not known whether betaine is excreted in breast milk. Its metabolic precursor, choline, occurs at high levels in breast milk. Exercise caution when administering to a nursing woman.

➤*Children:* The majority of case studies of homocystinuria patients treated wih betaine have been pediatric patients. The disorder, in its most severe form, can be manifested within the first months or years of life by lethargy, failure to thrive, developmental delays, seizures or optic lens displacement. Patients have been treated successfully without adverse effects within the first months or years of life with dosages greater than or equal to 6 g/day with resultant biochemical and clinical improvement. However, dosage titration may be preferable in pediatric patients (see Dosage and Administration).

Adverse Reactions

Betaine Anhydrous Adverse Reactions

Adverse reaction	n = 111
Nausea	2
GI distress	2
Diarrhea	1
Aspirated the powder	1
Caused odor	1
Questionable psychological changes	1
Unspecified problem	1

BETAINE ANHYDROUS — ORAL

Overdosage

In an acute toxicology study in rats, death frequently occurred at doses greater than or equal to 10,000 mg/kg.

Patient Information

Shake bottle lightly before removing cap.

Measure with the scoop provided.

One level scoop (1.7 ml) is equivalent to 1 g of betaine anhydrous powder. Measure the number of scoops your physician has prescribed.

Mix with 120 to 180 ml (4 to 6 oz) of water until completely dissolved, then drink immediately.

Always replace the cap tightly after using. Protect from moisture. Do not use if powder does not completely dissolve or gives a colored solution.

CYSTEAMINE BITARTRATE

CYSTEAMINE BITARTRATE

Rx	**Cystagon** (Mylan)	**Capsules:** 50 mg (as base)	(Cysta 50 Mylan). White. In 500s.
		150 mg (as base)	(Cystagon 150 Mylan). White. In 500s.

CYSTEAMINE BITARTRATE — ORAL

Indications

➤*Nephropathic cystinosis:* For the management of nephropathic cystinosis in children and adults.

Administration and Dosage

➤*General dosing considerations:* Cystinotic patients taking cysteamine hydrochloride or phosphocysteamine solutions may be transferred to equimolar doses of cysteamine bitartrate capsules.

Initiate therapy promptly once the diagnosis is confirmed (ie, increased white cell cystine).

➤*Adults:*

Nephropathic cystinosis –

Initial dosage: Start new patients on ¼ to ⅙ of the maintenance dose of cysteamine. The dose should then be raised gradually over 4 to 6 weeks to avoid intolerance.

Maintenance dosage: 2 g/day, in 4 divided doses. This dosage should be reached after 4 to 6 weeks of incremental dosage increases. The dose should be raised if the leukocyte cystine level remains more than 2 nmol/½ cystine/mg of protein.

➤*Children:*

Nephropathic cystinosis –

Children 12 years of age or older or over 110 lbs: See Adults for dosing.

Children younger than 12 years of age:

• *Initial dosage* – Start new patients on ¼ to ⅙ of the maintenance dose of cysteamine. The dose should then be raised gradually over 4 to 6 weeks to avoid intolerance.

• *Maintenance dosage* – The recommended cysteamine maintenance dosage for children younger than 12 years of age is 1.3 g/m^2/day of the free base, given in 4 divided doses.

➤*Tolerance:* When cysteamine is well-tolerated, the goal of therapy is to keep leukocyte cystine levels less than 1 nmol/½ cystine/mg of protein 5 to 6 hours following administration of cysteamine. Patients with poorer tolerability still receive significant benefit if white cell cystine levels are less than 2 nmol/½ cystine/mg of protein. The cysteamine dosage can be increased to a maximum of 1.95 g/m^2/day to achieve this level. The dosage of 1.95 g/m^2/day has been associated with an increased rate of withdrawal from treatment because of intolerance and an increased incidence of adverse reactions.

If cysteamine is poorly tolerated initially because of GI tract symptoms or transient skin rashes, temporarily stop therapy; reinstitute at a lower dose and gradually increase to the proper dose.

➤*Cystine measurements:* For new patients, obtain leukocyte cystine measurements 5 to 6 hours after dose administration once the maintenance dose is achieved. Patients being transferred from cysteamine hydrochloride or phosphocysteamine solutions to capsules should have their white cell cystine levels measured 2 weeks after the initial dose and every 3 months thereafter to assess optimal dosage as described previously.

➤*Concomitant therapy:* Cysteamine can be administered with electrolyte and mineral replacements necessary for management of Fanconi syndrome, as well as vitamin D and thyroid hormone.

➤*Administration:* Intact cysteamine capsules should not be administered to children younger than approximately 6 years of age because of the risk of aspiration. Cysteamine capsules may be administered to children younger than approximately 6 years of age by sprinkling the capsule contents over food.

➤*Storage/Stability:* Store at 20° to 25°C (68° to 77°F). Protect from light and moisture.

Actions

➤*Pharmacology:* Cysteamine is a cystine-depleting agent that lowers the cystine content of cells in patients with cystinosis, an inherited defect of lysosomal transport. Cysteamine is an aminothiol that participates within lysosomes in a thiol-disulfide interchange reaction converting cystine into cysteine and cysteine-cysteamine mixed disulfide, both of which can exit the lysosome in patients with cystinosis.

Pharmacodynamics – Because cysteamine hydrochloride has an unpleasant taste and odor, other formulations have been developed, including cysteamine bitartrate and phosphocysteamine, the phosphorothioester of cysteamine that is rapidly converted to cysteamine in the gut. Cysteamine bitartrate has been shown in a transfer study in 8 patients to maintain white cell cystine levels below 1 nmol/½ cystine/mg of protein when substituted for cysteamine hydrochloride or phosphocysteamine. Total cysteamine levels 2 and 6 hours postdose were higher after cysteamine bitartrate than for the solutions.

The pharmacodynamic response increased with the plasma cysteamine concentration. Maximum response occurred approximately 1.8 hours postdose with an average reduction of white cell cystine concentration of approximately 0.46 nmol/½ cystine/mg of protein and returning to baseline level 6 hours postdose. The apparent plasma clearance of cysteamine is 1.2 L/min.

➤*Pharmacokinetics:*

Absorption/Distribution – Following repeated oral administration of cysteamine bitartrate 225 to 550 mg, the mean time to peak plasma concentration occurred at about 1.4 hours postdose, with mean steady-state peak plasma concentration and area under the concentration-time curve of 2.6 mcg/mL and 6.3 mcg•h/mL, respectively. The apparent volume of distribution of cysteamine is 156 L.

Cysteamine was moderately bound to human plasma proteins, predominantly to albumin, with mean protein binding of about 52%. Plasma protein binding was independent of concentration over the concentration range achieved clinically with the recommended doses.

Contraindications

Hypersensitivity to cysteamine or penicillamine.

Warnings/Precautions

➤*Rash:* If a skin rash develops, withhold cysteamine until the rash clears. Cysteamine may be restarted at a lower dose under close supervision, then slowly titrated to the therapeutic dose. If a severe skin rash such as erythema multiforme bullosa or toxic epidermal necrolysis develops, do not readminister cysteamine.

➤*CNS effects:* CNS symptoms, such as seizures, lethargy, somnolence, depression, and encephalopathy, have been associated with cysteamine. If CNS symptoms develop, carefully evaluate the patient and adjust the dose as necessary. Neurological complications have been described in some cystinotic patients not on cysteamine treatment. This may be a manifestation of the primary disorder. Patients should not engage in hazardous activities until the effects of cysteamine on mental performance are known.

➤*GI effects:* GI ulceration and bleeding have been reported in patients receiving cysteamine bitartrate. Remain alert for signs of ulceration and bleeding; inform patients and/or guardians about the signs and symptoms of serious GI toxicity and what steps to take if they occur.

GI tract symptoms, including nausea, vomiting, anorexia, and abdominal pain, sometimes severe, have been associated with cysteamine. If these develop, therapy may have to be interrupted and the dose adjusted. A cysteamine dosage of 1.95 g/m^2/day (approximately 80 to 90 mg/kg/day) was associated with an increased number of withdrawals from treatment because of intolerance and an increased incidence of adverse reactions.

➤*Hazardous tasks:* Cysteamine may cause some people to become drowsy or less alert than they are normally. Make sure you know how you or your child (the patient) reacts to this medicine before doing anything that could be dangerous if not alert.

➤*Pregnancy: Category C.* Teratology studies have been performed in rats at oral dosages in a range of 37.5 to 150 mg/kg/day (about 0.2 to 0.7 times the recommended human maintenance dose on a body surface basis) and have revealed cysteamine bitartrate to be teratogenic and fetotoxic. Observed teratogenic findings were cleft palate, kyphosis, heart ventricular septal defects, microcephaly, and exencephaly. There are no adequate and well-controlled studies in pregnant women. Use cysteamine bitartrate during pregnancy only if the potential benefit justifies the potential risk to the fetus.

➤*Lactation:* It is not known whether cysteamine is excreted in human milk. Because many drugs are excreted in human milk and because of the manifested potential of cysteamine for developmental toxicity in suckling rat pups when it was administered to their lactating mothers at an oral dosage of 375 mg/kg/day (2,250 mg/m^2/day, 1.7 times the recommended human dose based on body surface area), decide whether to discontinue breast-feeding or the drug, taking into account the importance of the drug to the mother.

➤*Children:* The safety and efficacy of cysteamine bitartrate for cystinotic children have been established. Initiate cysteamine therapy as soon as the diagnosis of nephropathic cystinosis has been confirmed.

CYSTEAMINE BITARTRATE — ORAL

➤*Monitoring:* Cysteamine has occasionally been associated with reversible leukopenia and abnormal liver function studies. Therefore, monitor blood counts and liver function studies.

Leukocyte cystine measurements are useful to determine adequate dosage and compliance. When measured 5 to 6 hours after cysteamine administration, the goal should be a level less than 1 nmol/½ cystine/mg of protein. In some patients with poor tolerability for cysteamine, benefit may still be received with a white cell cystine level of less than 2 nmol/½ cystine/mg of protein. Measurements should be done every 3 months, or more frequently (eg, in 2 weeks then every 3 months) when patients are transferred from cysteamine hydrochloride or phosphocysteamine solutions to cysteamine bitartrate.

Follow patients for signs and symptoms of GI ulceration and bleeding, and inform patients and/or guardians of the importance of this follow-up.

Adverse Reactions

The most frequent adverse reactions seen involve the GI tract and CNS. These adverse reactions are especially prominent at the initiation of cysteamine therapy. Temporarily suspending treatment, then gradually reintroducing it may be effective in improving tolerance.

The most common adverse reactions (greater than 5%) were anorexia 31%, diarrhea 16%, fever 22%, lethargy 11%, rash 7%, and vomiting 35%.

➤*Discontinuation of drug:* Adverse reactions or intolerance leading to cessation of treatment occurred in 8% of patients in the US studies. Withdrawals because of intolerance, vomiting associated with medication, anorexia, lethargy, and fever appeared dose-related, occurring more frequently in those patients receiving 1.95 g/m²/day, as compared with 1.3 g/m²/day.

Adverse Reactions Leading to Cysteamine Withdrawal[a]

Adverse reaction	1.3 g/m²/day (n = 42)	1.95 g/m²/day (n = 51)
Anorexia	33%	51%
Diarrhea	31%	31%
Fever	28%	45%
Lethargy	17%	27%
Vomiting considered related to medicine	31%	67%

[a] Sudden deaths have been reported in this disease state.

➤*Less common adverse reactions:*

CNS – Abnormal thinking, ataxia, confusion, decreased hearing, depression, dizziness, emotional lability, encephalopathy, hallucinations, headache, hyperkinesia, jitteriness, nervousness, nightmares, seizures, somnolence, tremor.

GI – Abdominal pain, bad breath, constipation, duodenitis, dyspepsia, gastroenteritis, GI ulceration and bleeding, nausea.

GU – Interstitial nephritis, renal failure.

Miscellaneous – Abnormal liver function, anemia, dehydration, hypertension, leukopenia, urticaria.

Postmarketing – Postmarketing reports include 1 report of interstitial nephritis with early renal failure.

Overdosage

➤*Symptoms:* A single oral dose of cysteamine at 660 mg/kg was lethal to rats. Symptoms of acute toxicity were reduction of motor activity and generalized hemorrhage in the GI tract and kidneys.

Two cases of human overdosage have been reported. In 1 case, the patient immediately vomited the drug and did not develop any symptoms. The second incident involved an accidental ingestion of a 200 to 250 mg/kg dose by a healthy child 13 months of age. Vomiting and dehydration occurred. The child was hospitalized and fluids were administered. A full recovery was made.

➤*Treatment:* Should overdose occur, appropriately support the respiratory and cardiovascular systems. No specific antidote is known. Hemodialysis may be considered because cysteamine is poorly bound to plasma proteins. Refer to General Management of Acute Overdosage.

Patient Information

Inform the patient not to increase or decrease these medications without their health care provider's approval. There have been reports of unexpected deaths in children with cystinosis. Some of these children were receiving cysteamine/phosphocysteamine treatment for their cystinosis, while others were not.

Inform patients to not give capsules to children younger than approximately 6 years of age because they may not be able to swallow them and they may choke. For children younger than approximately 6 years of age, the capsule may be opened and the contents sprinkled on food or mixed in formula. Instruct patients to consult their health care provider for complete directions.

Medical treatment will include, in addition to cysteamine bitartrate, 1 or more supplements to replace important electrolytes lost through the kidneys. Instruct patients that it is important to take or give these supplements exactly as instructed.

Regular blood tests to measure the amount of cystine inside white blood cells are necessary to help determine the correct dose of cysteamine bitartrate. Arrange for the blood tests to be done. Inform patients that regular blood and urine tests to measure the levels of the body's important electrolytes are also necessary to correctly adjust the doses of these supplements.

Ulcers and bleeding in the digestive tract have occurred while taking this medicine. Explain to the patient and/or guardian the warning signs of these adverse reactions.

Inform patients that their health care provider may want to do certain tests to find out if unwanted effects are occurring. The tests are very important because serious adverse reactions, including ulcers or bleeding in the digestive tract, can occur.

CARGLUMIC ACID

Rx	**Carbaglu** (Accredo Health Group Inc)	**Tablets, dispersible; oral:** 200 mg.	(C). White, elongated, scored. In 5s and 60s.

CARGLUMIC ACID — ORAL

Indications

➤*Hyperammonemia:* Adjunctive therapy in the treatment of acute hyperammonemia and maintenance therapy of chronic hyperammonemia due to the deficiency of the hepatic enzyme N-acetylglutamate synthase (NAGS).

Administration and Dosage

➤*Adults:*

Hyperammonemia –

Initial dosage: 100 to 250 mg/kg/day divided into 2 to 4 doses (rounded to the nearest 100 mg) for acute hyperammonemia.

Dosage titration: Titrate dose based on individual patient plasma ammonia levels and clinical symptoms.

Maintenance dosage: Usually less than 100 mg/kg/day based on 22 patients in a retrospective case series. Titrate to target normal plasma ammonia level for age.

Concomitant therapy: Concomitant administration of other ammonia-lowering therapies is recommended.

➤*Children:*

Hyperammonemia – See Adults for dosing.

➤*Preparation for administration:*

Oral administration (adults) – Each 200 mg tablet should be dispersed in a minimum of 2.5 mL of water and taken immediately. Carglumic acid tablets do not dissolve completely in water and undissolved particles of the tablet may remain in the mixing container. To ensure complete delivery of the dose, the mixing container should be rinsed with additional volumes of water and the contents swallowed immediately. Use in other foods and liquids has not been studied clinically and is therefore not recommended.

Oral syringe (children) – For administration by oral syringe, mix each 200 mg tablet in 2.5 mL of water to yield a concentration of 80 mg/mL in a mixing container. Shake gently to allow for quick dispersal. Draw up the appropriate volume of dispersion in an oral syringe and administer immediately. Discard the unused portion. Refill the oral syringe with a minimum volume of water (1 to 2 mL) and administer immediately.

Nasogastric tube (adults) – For patients who have a nasogastric tube in place, administer by mixing each 200 mg tablet in a minimum of 2.5 mL of water. Shake gently to allow for quick dispersal. Administer the dispersion immediately through the nasogastric tube. Flush with additional water to clear the nasogastric tube.

Nasogastric tube (children) – For children who have a nasogastric tube in place, administer by mixing each 200 mg tablet in 2.5 mL of water to yield a concentration of 80 mg/mL in a mixing container. Shake gently to allow for quick dispersal. Draw up the appropriate volume of dispersion and administer immediately through a nasogastric tube. Discard the unused portion. Flush with additional water to clear the nasogastric tube.

➤*Administration:* The tablets should not be swallowed whole or crushed. Disperse tablets in water (minimum of 2.5 mL) immediately before use. The tablets may be administered orally or through a nasogastric tube.

Divide the total daily dose into 2 to 4 doses and administer immediately before meals or feedings.

Each divided dose should be rounded to the nearest 100 mg.

➤*Storage/Stability:* Before opening tablets, store refrigerated at 2° to 8°C (36° to 46°F).

After first opening the container, do not refrigerate or store above 30°C (86° F). Protect from moisture. Write the date of opening on the tablet container and discard 1 month after first opening.

CARGLUMIC ACID — ORAL

Actions

➤*Pharmacology:* Carglumic acid is a synthetic structural analogue of N-acetylglutamate (NAG), which is an essential allosteric activator of carbamoyl phosphate synthetase 1 (CPS 1) in liver mitochondria. CPS 1 is the first enzyme of the urea cycle, which converts ammonia into urea. NAG is the product of NAGS, a mitochondrial enzyme. Carglumic acid acts as a replacement for NAG in NAGS deficiency patients by activating CPS 1.

➤*Pharmacokinetics:*

Absorption – The median time to maximal plasma concentration (T_{max}) of carglumic acid was 3 hours (range, 2 to 4). Absolute bioavailability has not been determined.

Distribution – The apparent volume of distribution was 2,657 L (range, 1,616 to 5,797). Protein binding has not been determined.

Metabolism – A proportion of carglumic acid may be metabolized by the intestinal bacterial flora. The likely end product of carglumic acid metabolism is carbon dioxide, eliminated through the lungs.

Excretion – Median value for the terminal half-life was 5.6 hours (range, 4.3 to 9.5), the apparent total clearance was 5.7 L/min (range, 3 to 9.7), the renal clearance was 290 mL/min (range, 204 to 445), and the 24-hour urinary excretion was 4.5% of the dose (range, 3.5 to 7.5). Following administration of a single radiolabeled oral dose of 100 mg/kg of body weight, 9% of the dose was excreted unchanged in the urine, and up to 60% of the dose was excreted unchanged in the feces.

Contraindications

None well documented.

Warnings/Precautions

➤*Hyperammonemia:* Treat any episode of acute symptomatic hyperammonemia as a life-threatening emergency. Treatment of hyperammonemia may require dialysis, preferably hemodialysis, to remove a large burden of ammonia. Uncontrolled hyperammonemia can rapidly result in brain injury/damage or death, and prompt use of all therapies necessary to reduce plasma ammonia levels is essential. Coordinate management of hyperammonemia due to NAGS deficiency with medical personnel experienced in metabolic disorders. Ongoing monitoring of plasma ammonia levels, neurological status, laboratory tests, and clinical responses in patients receiving carglumic acid is crucial to assess patient response to treatment.

➤*Nutritional management:* During acute hyperammonemic episodes, protein restriction and hypercaloric intake is recommended to block ammonia-generating catabolic pathways. When plasma ammonia levels have normalized, protein intake can usually be increased with the goal of unrestricted protein intake.

➤*Pregnancy: Category C.* There are no adequate and well-controlled studies or available human data with carglumic acid in pregnant women.

Decreased survival and growth occurred in offspring born to animals that received carglumic acid at doses similar to the maximum recommended starting human dose during pregnancy and lactation. Because untreated NAGS deficiency results in irreversible neurologic damage and death, women with NAGS must remain on treatment throughout pregnancy. In embryofetal developmental toxicity studies, pregnant rats and rabbits received oral carglumic acid during organogenesis at doses up to 1.3 times the maximum recommended human starting dose based on body surface area (BSA) (mg/m^2). Actual dosages were 500 and 2,000 mg/kg/day (rats) and 250 and 1,000 mg/kg/day (rabbits). The high doses resulted in maternal toxicity in both rats and rabbits. No effects on embryofetal development were observed in either species.

In a peri- and postnatal developmental study, female rats received oral carglumic acid from organogenesis through day 21 postpartum at doses up to 1.3 times the maximum recommended starting human dose based on BSA (mg/m^2). Actual dosages were 500 and 2,000 mg/kg/day. A reduction in offspring survival was seen at the high dose, and a reduction in offspring growth was seen at both doses.

➤*Lactation:* It is not known whether carglumic acid is excreted in human milk. Carglumic acid is excreted in rat milk, and an increase in mortality and impairment of body weight gain occurred in neonatal rats nursed by mothers receiving carglumic acid. Because many drugs are excreted in human milk and because of the potential for serious adverse reactions in breast-feeding infants from carglumic acid, human milk-feeding is not recommended. Treatment is continuous and life-long for NAGS deficiency patients.

➤*Children:* The efficacy of carglumic acid for the treatment of hyperammonemia in patients with NAGS deficiency from birth to adulthood was evaluated in a retrospective review of the clinical course of 23 NAGS deficiency patients who all began carglumic acid treatment during infancy or childhood. There are no apparent differences in clinical response between adult and pediatric NAGS deficiency patients treated with carglumic acid; however, data are limited.

➤*Elderly:* Carglumic acid has not been studied in elderly patients. Therefore, the safety and effectiveness in elderly patients have not been established.

➤*Monitoring:* To assess patient response to treatment, ongoing monitoring of plasma ammonia levels, neurological status, laboratory tests, and clinical responses in patients is crucial.

Maintain plasma ammonia levels within normal range for age via individual dose adjustment.

Drug Interactions

None well documented.

Adverse Reactions

➤*Common adverse reactions:* The most common adverse reactions (occurring in at least 13% of patients), regardless of causality, are: vomiting, abdominal pain, pyrexia, tonsillitis, anemia, ear infection, diarrhea, nasopharyngitis, and headache.

Adverse reactions (occurring in 2 or more patients) –

Carglumic Acid Adverse Reactions (> 2 Patients)	
Adverse reactions	Carglumic acid (N = 23)
CNS	
Asthenia	9%
Headache	13%
Somnolence	9%
Dermatologic	
Hyperhidrosis	9%
Rash	9%
GI	
Abdominal pain	17%
Diarrhea	13%
Dysgeusia	9%
Vomiting	26%
Hematologic	
Anemia	13%
Hemoglobin decreased	13%
Metabolic/Nutrition	
Anorexia	9%
Weight decreased	9%
Respiratory	
Nasopharyngitis	13%
Pneumonia	9%
Tonsillitis	17%
Miscellaneous	
Ear infection	13%
Infection	13%
Influenza	9%
Pyrexia	17%

Overdosage

➤*Symptoms:* One patient treated with 650 mg/kg/day of carglumic acid developed symptoms characterized as a monosodium glutamate intoxication-like syndrome: tachycardia, profuse sweating, increased bronchial secretion, increased body temperature, and restlessness. These symptoms resolved upon reduction of dose.

Patient Information

Instruct patients that the tablets should not be swallowed whole or crushed and that each tablet should be dispersed in a minimum of 2.5 mL of water.

Inform patients that not all of the tablet will dissolve completely in water and undissolved particles of the tablet may remain in the mixing container. Instruct patients to rinse the mixing container with additional volumes of water and to swallow the contents immediately.

Inform patients of the proper storage of the tablets. Before opening the tablets, store them in a refrigerator and keep in a container tightly closed to protect from moisture. After the first opening of the container, do not refrigerate the tablets or store above 30°C (86°F). Write the date of opening on the tablet container and discard 1 month after first opening.

Inform patients that when plasma ammonia levels have normalized, that dietary protein intake can usually be increased with the goal of unrestricted protein intake.

Advise patients that breast-feeding is not recommended.

Inform patients that the most common adverse reactions are vomiting, abdominal pain, pyrexia, tonsillitis, anemia, ear infection, diarrhea, nasopharyngitis, and headache.

SODIUM BENZOATE AND SODIUM PHENYLACETATE

Rx	**Ammonul** (Ucyclyd Pharma)	**Injection:** sodium benzoate 100 mg and sodium phenylacetate 100 mg per mL	In 50 mL single-use vials.

SODIUM BENZOATE AND SODIUM PHENYLACETATE — INJECTION

Indications

➤*Hyperammonemia:* Adjunctive therapy for the treatment of acute hyperammonemia and associated encephalopathy in patients with deficiencies in enzymes of the urea cycle. In acute neonatal hyperammonemic coma, moderate to severe episodes of hyperammonemic encephalopathy, and episodes of hyperammonemia that fail to respond to an initial course of sodium phenylacetate and sodium benzoate therapy, hemodialysis is the most rapid and effective technique for removing ammonia. In such cases, the coadministration of sodium phenylacetate and sodium benzoate can help prevent the reaccumulation of ammonia by increasing waste nitrogen excretion.

Administration and Dosage

➤*General dosing considerations:* Start infusion as soon as the diagnosis of hyperammonemia is made. Administration of analogous oral drugs (eg, sodium phenylbutyrate) should be terminated prior to infusion.

Do not administer repeat loading doses because of prolonged phenylacetate plasma levels.

Hyperammonemic coma (regardless of cause) in the newborn infant should be treated aggressively while the specific diagnosis is pursued (see hyperammonemic infants).

Intravenous (IV) arginine is an essential component of therapy for patients with carbamyl phosphate synthetase (CPS), ornithine transcarbamylase (OTC), argininosuccinate synthetase (ASS), or argininosuccinate lyase (ASL) deficiency. Because a hyperchloremic acidosis may ensue after high-dose arginine administration, plasma levels of chloride and bicarbonate should be monitored and appropriate amounts of bicarbonate administered.

➤*Adults:*

Hyperammonemia due to carbamyl phosphate synthetase and ornithine transcarbamylase deficiency –

Patients weighing 0 to 20 kg:

• *Loading dose* – 2.5 mL/kg IV over 90 to 120 minutes (provides 250 mg/kg of sodium phenylacetate and sodium benzoate).

• *Maintenance dosage* – 2.5 mL/kg IV over 24 hours.

• *Concomitant therapy* – 2 mL/kg IV of arginine 10% injection (arginine 200 mg/kg).

Patients weighing over 20 kg:

• *Loading dose* – 55 mL/min^2 IV over 90 to 120 minutes (provides 5.5 g/m^2 of sodium phenylacetate and sodium benzoate).

• *Maintenance dosage* – 55 mL/min^2 IV over 24 hours.

• *Concomitant therapy* – 2 mL/kg IV of arginine 10% injection (arginine 200 mg/kg).

Hyperammonemia due to argininosuccinate synthetase and argininosuccinate lyase deficiency –

Patients weighing 0 to 20 kg:

• *Loading dose* – 2.5 mL/kg IV over 90 to 120 minutes (provides 250 mg/kg of sodium phenylacetate and sodium benzoate).

• *Maintenance dosage* – 2.5 mL/kg IV over 24 hours.

• *Concomitant therapy* – 6 mL/kg IV of arginine 10% injection (provides arginine 600 mg/kg).

Patients weighing over 20 kg:

• *Loading dose* – 55 mL/min^2 IV over 90 to 120 minutes (provides 5.5 g/m^2 of sodium phenylacetate and sodium benzoate).

• *Maintenance dosage* – 55 mL/min^2 IV over 24 hours.

• *Concomitant therapy* – 6 mL/kg IV of arginine 10% injection (provides arginine 600 mg/kg).

Patients suspected of having argininosuccinate synthetase deficiency: Patients suspected of having ASS should be infused with sodium phenylacetate and sodium benzoate and arginine 600 mg/kg as a loading dose over a 6-hour infusion period. If the patient is confirmed with ASS, then the loading-dose infusion is administered over 90 minutes.

➤*Children:*

Hyperammonemia due to carbamyl phosphate synthetase and ornithine transcarbamylase deficiency – See Adults for dosing.

Hyperammonemia due to argininosuccinate synthetase and argininosuccinate lyase deficiency – See Adults for dosing.

➤*Renal function impairment:*

Hemodialysis – All patients should be promptly hemodialyzed as the procedure of choice using the largest catheters consistent with the patient's size. A target blood flow of 150 mL/min/m^2 may be attained using a 7F catheter. (Ammonia clearance [mL/min] is similar to the blood flow rate [mL/min] through the dialyzer). Clearance of ammonia is approximately 10 times greater by hemodialysis than by peritoneal dialysis or hemofiltration. Exchange transfusion is ineffective in the management of hyperammonemia. Hemodialysis may be repeated until the plasma ammonia level is stable at normal or near normal levels.

➤*Caloric supplementation and protein restriction:* Treatment of hyperammonemia also requires caloric supplementation and restriction of dietary protein. Nonprotein calories should be supplied principally as glucose (8 to 10 mg/kg/min) with *Intralipid* added. Attempts should be made to maintain a caloric intake of more than 80 cal/kg/day.

➤*Conversion to oral treatment:* Once elevated ammonia levels have been reduced to the normal range, oral therapy, such as sodium phenylbutyrate, dietary management, and protein restrictions, should be started or reinitiated.

➤*Hyperammonemic infants:* Pending a specific diagnosis, IV arginine (6 mL/kg of arginine 10% injection over 90 minutes, followed by the same dose over 24 hours) should be given to hyperammonemic infants suspected of having a urea cycle disorder for 2 reasons: 1) infants with deficiencies in enzymes of the urea cycle (apart from arginase deficiency) are usually arginine deficient; 2) hyperammonemia in infants with ASS or ASL deficiency usually respond favorably to arginine administration. If deficiencies of ASS or ASL are excluded as diagnostic possibilities, the IV dose of arginine should be reduced to 2 mL/kg/day.

➤*Preparation for administration:* Dilute with sterile dextrose 10% injection to a volume of at least 25 mL/kg before administration. Do not administer undiluted product.

➤*Administration:* Administration must be through a central line. Do not administer by any other route. Administration through a peripheral line may cause burns. Administer IV as a loading dose infusion administered over 90 to 120 minutes, followed by an equivalent maintenance dose infusion administered over 24 hours. Maintenance infusions may be continued until elevated plasma ammonia levels have been normalized or the patient can tolerate oral nutrition and medications.

➤*Admixture compatibility:* No compatibility information is presently available except for arginine 10% injection, which may be mixed in the same container. Other infusion solutions and drug products should not be administered together. Solutions may be prepared in glass and polyvinyl chloride (PVC) containers.

➤*Storage/Stability:* Store at 25°C (77°F); excursions are permitted to 15° to 30°C (59° to 86°F). Diluted solutions are physically and chemically stable for up to 24 hours at room temperature and room lighting conditions.

Actions

➤*Pharmacology:* Sodium phenylacetate and sodium benzoate are metabolically active compounds that can serve as alternatives to urea for the excretion of waste nitrogen. It has been shown that phenylacetylglutamine and hippurate can serve as alternative vehicles to effectively reduce waste nitrogen levels in patients with deficiencies of urea cycle enzymes and, thus, attenuate the risk of ammonia and glutamine-induced neurotoxicity.

Pharmacodynamics – In patients with hyperammonemia caused by deficiencies in enzymes of the urea cycle, sodium phenylacetate and sodium benzoate has been shown to decrease elevated plasma ammonia levels and improve encephalopathy and survival outcome compared with historical controls. These effects are considered to be the result of reduction in nitrogen overload through glutamine and glycine scavenging by sodium phenylacetate and sodium benzoate in combination with appropriate dietary and other supportive measures.

➤*Pharmacokinetics:*

Absorption/Distribution – The pharmacokinetics of IV administered sodium phenylacetate and sodium benzoate were characterized in healthy adult volunteers. Benzoate and phenylacetate exhibited nonlinear kinetics. Following 90-minute IV infusion, mean area under the curve (AUC_{last}) for benzoate was 20.3, 114.9, 564.6, 562.8, and 1,599.1 mcg/mL after doses of 1, 2, 3.75, 4, and 5.5 g/m^2, respectively. The total clearance decreased from 5.19 to 3.62 L/h/m^2 at the 3.75 and 5.5 g/m^2 doses, respectively.

Similarly, phenylacetate exhibited nonlinear kinetics following the priming dose regimens. AUC_{last} was 175.6, 713.8, 2,040.6, 2,181.6, and 3,829.2 mcg•h/mL following doses of 1, 2, 3.75, 4, and 5.5 g/m^2, respectively. The total clearance decreased from 1.82 to 0.89 mcg•h/mL with increasing dose (3.75 and 4 g/m^2 , respectively).

During the sequence of 90-minute priming infusion followed by a 24-hour maintenance infusion, phenylacetate was detected in the plasma at the end of infusion (time to peak concentration [T_{max}] of 2 hours at 3.75 g/m^2), whereas benzoate concentrations declined rapidly (T_{max} of 1.5 hours at 3.75 g/m^2) and were undetectable at 14 and 26 hours following the 3.75 and 4 g/m^2 , dose, respectively.

Metabolism/Excretion – A difference in the metabolic rates for phenylacetate and benzoate was noted. The formation of hippurate from benzoate occurred more rapidly than that of phenylacetylglutamine from phenylacetate, and the rate of elimination for hippurate appeared to be more rapid than that of phenylacetylglutamine.

Phenylacetate conjugates with glutamine in the liver and kidneys to form phenylacetylglutamine, via acetylation. Phenylacetylglutamine is excreted by the kidneys via glomerular filtration and tubular secretion. The nitrogen content of phenylacetylglutamine per mole is identical to that of urea (both contain 2 moles of nitrogen). Similarly, preceded by acylation, benzoate conjugates with glycine to form hippuric acid, which is rapidly excreted by the kidneys by glomerular filtration and tubular secretion. One mole of hippuric acid contains 1 mole of waste nitrogen.

SODIUM BENZOATE AND SODIUM PHENYLACETATE — INJECTION

Special populations –

Renal function impairment: For effective sodium phenylacetate and sodium benzoate drug therapy, renal clearance of the drug metabolites and subsequently ammonia is required. Closely monitor patients with impaired renal function.

Gender:

Adult patients with advanced solid tumors: The pharmacokinetics of IV phenylacetate have been reported following administration to adult patients with advanced solid tumors. The decline in serum phenylacetate concentrations following a loading infusion of 150 mg/kg was consistent with saturable enzyme kinetics. Ninety-nine percent of administered phenylacetate was excreted as phenylacetylglutamine.

Contraindications

Hypersensitivity to sodium phenylacetate or sodium benzoate.

Warnings/Precautions

➤*Acute symptomatic hyperammonemia:* Treat any episode of acute symptomatic hyperammonemia as a life-threatening emergency. Treatment of hyperammonemia may require dialysis, preferably hemodialysis, to remove a large burden of ammonia. Uncontrolled hyperammonemia can rapidly result in brain damage or death, and prompt use of all therapies necessary to reduce ammonia levels is essential.

➤*Appropriate management of hyperammonemia:* Perform management of hyperammonemia caused by inborn errors of metabolism in coordination with medical personnel familiar with these diseases. The severity of the disorder may necessitate the use of hemodialysis combined with nutritional management and medical support. The multidisciplinary nature of the treatment usually requires the facilities of a tertiary or quaternary care center.

➤*Sodium:* Sodium phenylacetate and sodium benzoate contains 30.5 mg of sodium/mL of undiluted product. Use sodium phenylacetate and sodium benzoate with great care, if at all, in patients with congestive heart failure or severe renal insufficiency, and in clinical states in which there is sodium retention with edema. If an adverse reaction does occur, discontinue administration of sodium phenylacetate and sodium benzoate, evaluate the patient, and institute appropriate therapeutic countermeasures.

➤*Extravasation:* Bolus infusion flow rates are relatively high, especially for infants. Extravasation of sodium phenylacetate and sodium benzoate into the perivenous tissues may lead to skin necrosis. If extravasation is suspected, discontinue the infusion and resume at a different infusion site, if necessary. Standard treatment for extravasation can include aspiration of residual drug from the catheter, limb elevation, and intermittent cooling using cold packs. The infusion site must be monitored closely for possible infiltration during drug administration. Do not administer undiluted product.

➤*Nausea and vomiting:* Sodium phenylacetate and sodium benzoate infusion has been associated with nausea and vomiting. An antiemetic may be administered during sodium phenylacetate and sodium benzoate infusion.

➤*Loading doses:* Because of prolonged plasma levels achieved by phenylacetate in pharmacokinetic studies, do not administer repeat loading doses of sodium phenylacetate and sodium benzoate.

➤*Corticosteroids:* Use of corticosteroids may cause the breakdown of body protein and, thereby, potentially increase plasma ammonia levels in patients with impaired ability to form urea.

➤*Neurotoxicity:* Neurotoxicity was reported in cancer patients receiving IV phenylacetate, 250 to 300 mg/kg/day for 14 days, repeated at 4-week intervals. Manifestations were predominantly somnolence, fatigue, and light-headedness, with less frequent headaches, dysgeusia, hypoacusis, disorientation, impaired memory, and exacerbation of a preexisting neuropathy. These adverse reactions were mainly mild. The acute onset of symptoms upon initiation of treatment and reversibility of symptoms when the phenylacetate was discontinued suggest a drug effect.

➤*Renal/Hepatic function impairment:* Because sodium phenylacetate and sodium benzoate are metabolized in the liver and kidney, and because phenylacetylglutamine and hippurate are excreted primarily by the kidney, use caution when administering sodium phenylacetate and sodium benzoate to patients with hepatic or renal function impairment.

➤*Pregnancy:* *Category C.* Animal reproduction studies have not been conducted with sodium phenylacetate and sodium benzoate. It is not known whether sodium phenylacetate and sodium benzoate can cause fetal harm when administered to a pregnant woman or can affect reproduction capacity. Give sodium phenylacetate and sodium benzoate to a pregnant woman only if clearly needed.

➤*Lactation:* It is not known whether sodium phenylacetate, sodium benzoate, or their conjugation products are excreted in human milk. Because many drugs are excreted in human milk, exercise caution when sodium phenylacetate and sodium benzoate is administered to a breast-feeding woman.

➤*Children:* Sodium phenylacetate and sodium benzoate has been used as a treatment for acute hyperammonemia in pediatric patients, including patients in the early neonatal period.

➤*Monitoring:* During and after infusion of sodium phenylacetate and sodium benzoate, ongoing monitoring of neurological status, plasma ammonia levels, clinical laboratory values, and clinical responses are crucial to assess patient response to treatment. The need for other interventions to control hyperammonemia must be considered throughout the course of treatment. Patients with a large ammonia burden or who are not responsive to sodium phenylacetate and sodium benzoate administration require aggressive therapy including hemodialysis.

Because urine potassium loss is enhanced by the excretion of the nonreabsorbable anions, phenylacetylglutamine and hippurate, carefully monitor potassium levels and treat appropriately when necessary. Monitor serum electrolyte levels and maintain them within the normal range.

Because of structural similarities between phenylacetate and benzoate to salicylate, sodium phenylacetate and sodium benzoate may cause side effects typically associated with salicylate overdose, such as hyperventilation and metabolic acidosis. Perform blood chemistry profiles and frequent blood pH and pCO_2 monitoring.

Drug Interactions

Sodium Phenylacetate and Sodium Benzoate Drug Interactions

Precipitant drug	Object drug[a]		Description
Penicillin	Sodium phenylacetate/ sodium benzoate	⬇	Some antibiotics such as penicillin may compete with phenylacetylglutamine and hippurate for active secretion by renal tubules, which may affect the overall disposition of the infused drug.
Probenecid	Sodium phenylacetate/ sodium benzoate	⬇	Probenecid inhibits renal transport of aminohippuric acid and may affect renal excretion of phenylacetylglutamine.
Valproic acid	Sodium phenylacetate/ sodium benzoate	⬇	Valproic acid given to patients with UCDs may exacerbate the condition and antagonize the efficacy of sodium phenylacetate/ sodium benzoate.

[a] ⬇ = Object drug decreased.

Adverse Reactions

Sodium Phenylacetate and Benzoate Adverse Reactions (≥ 3%)

Adverse reaction	Patients (n = 316)
Patients with any adverse reaction	163 (52%)
Cardiovascular	
Cardiac disorders	28 (9%)
Hypotension NOS[a]	14 (4%)
Vascular disorders	19 (6%)
CNS	
Agitation	8 (3%)
Brain edema	17 (5%)
CNS disorders	71 (22%)
Coma	10 (3%)
Convulsions NOS	19 (6%)
Mental impairment NOS	18 (6%)
Psychiatric disorders	16 (5%)
Dermatologic	
Skin and subcutaneous tissue disorders	19 (6%)
GI	
Diarrhea NOS	10 (3%)
GI disorders	42 (13%)
Nausea	9 (3%)
Vomiting NOS	29 (12%)
GU	
Renal and urinary disorders	14 (4%)
Urinary tract infection NOS	9 (3%)
Hematologic/Lymphatic	35 (11%)
Anemia NOS	12 (4%)
Disseminated intravascular coagulation	11 (3%)
Metabolic/Nutritional	
Acidosis NOS	8 (3%)
Hyperammonemia	17 (5%)
Hyperglycemia NOS	22 (7%)
Hypocalcemia	8 (3%)
Hypokalemia	23 (7%)
Metabolic acidosis NOS	13 (4%)
Metabolism and nutrition disorders	67 (21%)

SODIUM BENZOATE AND SODIUM PHENYLACETATE — INJECTION

Sodium Phenylacetate and Benzoate Adverse Reactions (≥ 3%)	
Adverse reaction	Patients (n = 316)
Respiratory	
Respiratory distress	9 (3%)
Respiratory, thoracic and mediastinal disorders	47 (15%)
Miscellaneous	
General disorders and administration-site conditions	45 (14%)
Infections	39 (12%)
Injection-site reaction NOS	11 (3%)
Injury, poisoning, and procedural complications	12 (4%)
Investigations	32 (10%)
Pyrexia	17 (5%)

[a] Not otherwise specified.

➤*Clinically important adverse reactions:* Adverse reactions occurred most frequently in the following system organ classes: nervous system disorders (22% of patients), metabolism and nutrition disorders (21% of patients), and respiratory, thoracic, and mediastinal disorders (15% of patients). The most frequently reported adverse reactions were vomiting (9% of patients), hyperglycemia (7% of patients), hypokalemia (7% of patients), convulsions (6% of patients), and mental impairment (6% of patients).

Adverse reactions leading to discontinuation – Adverse reactions leading to study drug discontinuation occurred in 4% of patients. Metabolic acidosis and injection-site reactions each led to discontinuation in 2 patients (less than 1%). Adverse reactions leading to discontinuation in 1 patient included bradycardia, abdominal distension, injection-site extravasation, injection-site hemorrhage, blister, overdose, subdural hematoma, hyperammonemia, hypoglycemia, clonus, coma, increased intracranial pressure, hypercapnia, Kussmaul respiration, respiratory distress, respiratory failure, pruritus, and maculopapular rash.

➤*Less common adverse reactions that could represent drug-induced reactions or are characterized as severe:*

Cardiovascular – Atrial rupture, cardiac or cardiopulmonary arrest/failure, cardiac output decreased, cardiogenic shock, cardiomyopathy, hypertension, pericardial effusion, phlebothrombosis/thrombosis (less than 3%).

CNS – Acute psychosis, aggression, areflexia, ataxia, brain hemorrhage, brain infarction, cerebral atrophy, clonus, confusional state, depressed level of consciousness, encephalopathy, hallucinations, intracranial pressure increased, nerve paralysis, tremor (less than 3%).

Dermatologic – Alopecia, generalized pruritus, rash, urticaria (less than 3%).

GI – GI hemorrhage (less than 3%).

GU – Anuria, renal failure, urinary retention (less than 3%).

Hematologic – Blood carbon dioxide changes, blood pH increased, coagulopathy, pancytopenia, thrombocytopenia (less than 3%).

Hepatic – Cholestasis, hepatic artery stenosis, hepatic failure/hepatotoxicity, jaundice (less than 3%).

Metabolic/Nutritional – Alkalosis, blood glucose changes, dehydration, fluid overload/retention, hyperkalemia, hypernatremia, tetany (less than 3%).

Respiratory – Acute respiratory distress syndrome, pCO_2 changes, dyspnea, hypercapnia, hyperventilation, Kussmaul respiration, pneumonia aspiration, pneumothorax, pulmonary edema, pulmonary hemorrhage, respiratory acidosis or alkalosis, respiratory arrest/failure, respiratory rate increased (less than 3%).

Special senses – Blindness (less than 3%).

Miscellaneous – Acquired hemangioma, asthenia, brain death, brain herniation, chest pain, edema, flushing, hemorrhage, multiorgan failure, neoplasms (benign, malignant, and unspecified), sepsis/septic shock, subdural hematoma (less than 3%).

Overdosage

➤*Symptoms:* Overdosage has been reported during sodium phenylacetate and sodium benzoate treatment in urea cycle-deficient patients. All patients in the uncontrolled open-label study were to be treated at the same dose of sodium phenylacetate and sodium benzoate. However, some patients received more than the dose level specified in the protocol. In 16 of the 64 deaths, the patient received a known overdose of sodium phenylacetate and sodium benzoate. Causes of death in these patients included cardiorespiratory failure/arrest (6 patients), hyperammonemia (3 patients), increased intracranial pressure (2 patients), pneumonitis with septic shock and coagulopathy (1 patient), error in dialysis procedure (1 patient), respiratory failure (1 patient), intractable hypotension and probable sepsis (1 patient), and unknown (1 patient). Additionally, other signs of intoxication may include obtundation (in the absence of hyperammonemia), hyperventilation, a severe compensated metabolic acidosis, perhaps with a respiratory component, large anion gap, hypernatremia and hyperosmolarity, progressive encephalopathy, cardiovascular collapse, and death.

➤*Treatment:* In case of overdose of sodium phenylacetate and sodium benzoate, discontinue the drug and institute appropriate emergency medical monitoring and procedures. In severe cases, the latter may include hemodialysis (procedure of choice) or peritoneal dialysis (when hemodialysis is unavailable).

BROMOCRIPTINE MESYLATE

BROMOCRIPTINE MESYLATE

For complete and comparative prescribing information, see the Bromocriptine mesylate monograph in the Antiparkinson agents group monograph in the CNS chapter.

CABERGOLINE

CABERGOLINE

Rx	**Cabergoline** (Various, eg, Greenstone, Par)	**Tablets:** 0.5 mg	May contain lactose. In 8s.

CABERGOLINE — ORAL

Indications

➤*Hyperprolactinemic disorders:* For the treatment of hyperprolactinemic disorders, either idiopathic or caused by pituitary adenomas.

➤*Off-label uses:*

Restless legs syndrome – [3] = Safety concerns. Guidelines suggest that cabergoline is effective in the short-term management of moderate to severe restless legs syndrome (RLS), with possible effectiveness in long-term management as well. Comparative studies indicate that cabergoline is more effective than levodopa in reducing International RLS Severity Scale scores and less likely to cause augmentation. However, both guidelines and studies note that its use may be limited by the high incidence of adverse effects. Because heart valve disorders have been associated with other ergot-derived dopamine agonists (eg, bromocriptine, pergolide), guidelines also recommend cardiac monitoring during cabergoline treatment.

Administration and Dosage

➤*Adults:*

Hyperprolactinemic disorders –

Initial dosage: 0.25 mg orally twice a week.

Dosage titration: Increase by 0.25 mg twice weekly up to a dosage of 1 mg twice a week according to the patient's serum prolactin level. Dosage increases should not occur more rapidly than every 4 weeks, so that the physician can assess the patient's response to each dosage level.

Maintenance dosage: If the patient does not respond adequately, and no additional benefit is observed with higher doses, the lowest dose that achieved maximal response should be used and other therapeutic approaches considered.

Duration of therapy: After a normal serum prolactin level has been maintained for 6 months, cabergoline may be discontinued, with periodic monitoring of the serum prolactin level to determine whether or when treatment with cabergoline should be reinstituted. The durability of efficacy beyond 24 months of therapy with cabergoline has not been established.

Off-label dosing –

Restless legs syndrome: [3] = Safety concerns. 0.5 to 4 mg daily. In one study, doses were administered 3 hours prior to bedtime.

➤*Hepatic function impairment:* Because cabergoline is extensively metabolized by the liver, caution should be used, and careful monitoring exercised, when administering cabergoline to patients with hepatic impairment.

➤*Storage/Stability:* Store at controlled room temperature 20° to 25°C (68° to 77°F).

Actions

➤*Pharmacology:* The secretion of prolactin by the anterior pituitary is mainly under hypothalmic inhibitory control, likely exerted through release of dopamine by tuberoinfundibular neurons. Cabergoline is a long-acting dopamine receptor agonist with a high affinity for D_2 receptors. Results of in vitro studies demonstrate that cabergoline exerts a direct inhibitory effect on the secretion of prolactin by rat pituitary lactotrophs. Cabergoline decreased serum prolactin levels in reserpinized rats. Receptor-binding studies indicate that cabergoline has low affinity for dopamine D_1, α_1- and α_2-adrenergic, and 5-HT_1- and 5-HT_2-serotonin receptors.

Pharmacodynamics – Dose response with inhibition of plasma prolactin, onset of maximal effect, and duration of effect has been documented fol-

CABERGOLINE — ORAL

lowing single cabergoline doses to healthy volunteers (0.05 to 1.5 mg) and hyperprolactinemic patients (0.3 to 1 mg). In volunteers, prolactin inhibition was evident at doses greater than 0.2 mg, while doses greater than or equal to 0.5 mg caused maximal suppression in most subjects. Higher doses produce prolactin suppression in a greater proportion of subjects and with an earlier onset and longer duration of action. In 12 healthy volunteers, 0.5, 1, and 1.5 mg doses resulted in complete prolactin inhibition, with a maximum effect within 3 hours in 92% to 100% of subjects after the 1 and 1.5 mg doses compared with 50% of subjects after the 0.5 mg dose.

In hyperprolactinemic patients (n = 51), the maximal prolactin decrease after a 0.6 mg single dose of cabergoline was comparable to 2.5 mg bromocriptine; however, the duration of effect was markedly longer (14 days vs 24 hours). The time to maximal effect was shorter for bromocriptine than cabergoline (6 hours vs 48 hours).

In 72 healthy volunteers, single or multiple doses (up to 2 mg) of cabergoline resulted in selective inhibition of prolactin with no apparent effect on other anterior pituitary hormones (growth hormone, follicle-stimulating hormone, luteinizing hormone, advenocorticotropic hormone, and thyroid-stimulating hormone) or cortisol.

➤*Pharmacokinetics:*

Absorption – Following single oral doses of 0.5 mg to 1.5 mg given to 12 healthy adult volunteers, mean peak plasma levels of 30 to 70 picograms (pg)/mL of cabergoline were observed within 2 to 3 hours. Over the 0.5-to-7 mg dose range, cabergoline plasma levels appeared to be dose-proportional in 12 healthy adult volunteers and nine adult parkinsonian patients. A repeat-dose study in 12 healthy volunteers suggests that steady-state levels following a once-weekly dosing schedule are expected to be twofold to threefold higher than after a single dose. The absolute bioavailability of cabergoline is unknown. A significant fraction of the administered dose undergoes a first-pass effect. The elimination half-life of cabergoline estimated from urinary data of 12 healthy subjects ranged between 63 to 69 hours. The prolonged prolactin-lowering effect of cabergoline may be related to its slow elimination and long half-life.

Distribution – In animals, based on total radioactivity, cabergoline (and/or its metabolites) has shown extensive tissue distribution. Radioactivity in the pituitary exceeded that in plasma by greater than 100-fold and was eliminated with a half-life of approximately 60 hours. This finding is consistent with the long-lasting prolactin-lowering effect of the drug. Whole body autoradiography studies in pregnant rats showed no fetal uptake but high levels in the uterine wall. Significant radioactivity (parent plus metabolites) detected in the milk of lactating rats suggests a potential for exposure to nursing infants. The drug is extensively distributed throughout the body. Cabergoline is moderately bound (40% to 42%) to human plasma proteins in a concentration-independent manner. Concomitant dosing of highly protein-bound drugs is unlikely to affect its disposition.

Metabolism – In both animals and humans, cabergoline is extensively metabolized, predominately via hydrolysis of the acylurea bond or the urea moiety. Cytochrome P-450 mediated metabolism appears to be minimal. Cabergoline does not cause enzyme induction and/or inhibition in the rat. Hydrolysis of the acylurea or urea moiety abolishes the prolactin-lowering effect of cabergoline, and major metabolites identified thus far do not contribute to the therapeutic effect.

Excretion – After oral dosing of radioactive cabergoline to five healthy volunteers, approximately 22% and 60% of the dose was excreted within 20 days in the urine and feces, respectively. Less than 4% of the dose was excreted unchanged in the urine. Nonrenal and renal clearances for cabergoline are about 3.2 L/min and 0.08 L/min, respectively. Urinary excretion in hyperprolactinemic patients was similar.

Special populations –

Hepatic function impairment: In 12 patients with mild-to-moderate hepatic dysfunction (Child-Pugh score less than or equal to 10), no effect on mean cabergoline C_{max} or area under the plasma concentration curve (AUC) was observed. However, patients with severe insufficiency (Child-Pugh score greater than 10) show a substantial increase in the mean cabergoline C_{max} and AUC, and thus necessitate caution.

Contraindications

Uncontrolled hypertension; known hypersensitivity to ergot derivatives.

Warnings/Precautions

➤*Orthostatic hypotension:* Initial doses higher than 1 mg may produce orthostatic hypotension. Care should be exercised when administering cabergoline with other medications known to lower blood pressure.

➤*Postpartum lactation inhibition or suppression:* Cabergoline is not indicated for the inhibition or suppression of physiologic lactation. Use of bromocriptine, another dopamine agonist for this purpose, has been associated with cases of hypertension, stroke, and seizures.

➤*Hepatic function impairment:* Because cabergoline is extensively metabolized by the liver, caution should be used, and careful monitoring exercised, when administering cabergoline to patients with hepatic impairment.

➤*Pregnancy:* *Category B.*

Pregnancy-induced hypertension – Dopamine agonists in general should not be used in patients with pregnancy-induced hypertension, for example, preeclampsia and eclampsia, unless the potential benefit is judged to outweigh the possible risk.

Teratogenic – Reproduction studies have been performed with cabergoline in mice, rats, and rabbits administered by gavage.

(Multiples of the maximum recommended human dose in this section are calculated on a body surface area basis using total mg/m²/week for animals and mg/m²/week for a 50 kg human.)

There were maternotoxic effects but no teratogenic effects in mice given cabergoline at doses up to 8 mg/kg/day (approximately 55 times the maximum recommended human dose) during the period of organogenesis.

A dose of 0.012 mg/kg/day (approximately 1/7 the maximum recommended human dose) during the period of organogenesis in rats caused an increase in post-implantation embryofetal losses. These losses could be due to the prolactin inhibitory properties of cabergoline in rats. At daily doses of 0.5 mg/kg/day (approximately 19 times the maximum recommended human dose) during the period of organogenesis in the rabbit, cabergoline caused maternotoxicity characterized by a loss of body weight and decreased food consumption. Doses of 4 mg/kg/day (approximately 150 times the maximum recommended human dose) during the period of organogenesis in the rabbit caused an increased occurrence of various malformations. However, in another study in rabbits, no treatment-related malformations or embryofetotoxicity were observed at doses up to 8 mg/kg/day (approximately 300 times the maximum recommended human dose).

In rats, doses higher than 0.003 mg/kg/day (approximately 1/28 the maximum recommended human dose) from 6 days before parturition and throughout the lactation period inhibited growth and caused death of offspring due to decreased milk secretion.

There are, however, no adequate and well-controlled studies in pregnant women. Because animal reproduction studies are not always predictive of human response, this drug should be used during pregnancy only if clearly needed.

➤*Lactation:* It is not known whether this drug is excreted in human milk. Because many drugs are excreted in human milk and because of the potential for serious adverse reactions in nursing infants from cabergoline, a decision should be made whether to discontinue nursing or to discontinue the drug, taking into account the importance of the drug to the mother. Use of cabergoline for the inhibition or suppression of physiologic lactation is not recommended (see Precautions).

The prolactin-lowering action of cabergoline suggests that it will interfere with lactation. Due to this interference with lactation, cabergoline should not be given to women postpartum who are breastfeeding or who are planning to breastfeed.

➤*Children:* Safety and effectiveness of cabergoline in pediatric patients have not been established.

➤*Elderly:* In general, dose selection for an elderly patient should be cautious, usually starting at the low end of the dosing range, reflecting the greater frequency of decreased hepatic, renal, or cardiac function, and of concomitant disease or other drug therapy.

Drug Interactions

Cabergoline Drug Interactions

Precipitant drug	Object drug[a]		Description
Cabergoline	Antihypertensives	⬆	Additive hypotensive effects may occur when cabergoline is administered with other hypotensive medications. In addition, antihypertensive dosage adjustments may be necessary if antihypertensive medications are administered concurrently with cabergoline.
Dopamine (D_2) antagonists (eg, phenothiazines, butyrophenones, thioxanthenes or metoclopramide)	Cabergoline	⬇	Dopamine (D_2) antagonists may reduce the therapeutic effects of cabergoline. Do not administer with cabergoline.

[a] ⬆ = object drug increased; ⬇ = object drug decreased.

Adverse Reactions

In a 4-week, double-blind, placebo-controlled study, treatment consisted of placebo or cabergoline at fixed doses of 0.125, 0.5, 0.75, or 1 mg twice weekly. Doses were halved during the first week. Since a possible dose-related effect was observed for nausea only, the four cabergoline treatment groups have been combined.

Cabergoline Adverse Reactions During the 4-Week, Double-Blind, Placebo-Controlled Trial (≥ 1%)

Adverse reaction	Cabergoline 0.125 to 1 mg twice weekly (n = 168)	Placebo (n = 20)
CNS		
Depression	5 (3%)	1 (5%)
Dizziness	25 (15%)	1 (5%)
Headache	43 (26%)	5 (25%)
Nervousness	4 (2%)	0
Paresthesia	2 (1%)	0

CABERGOLINE — ORAL

Cabergoline Adverse Reactions During the 4-Week, Double-Blind, Placebo-Controlled Trial (≥ 1%)

Adverse reaction	Cabergoline 0.125 to 1 mg twice weekly (n = 168)	Placebo (n = 20)
Postural hypotension	6 (4%)	0
Somnolence	9 (5%)	1 (5%)
Vertigo	2 (1%)	0
GI		
Abdominal pain	9 (5%)	1 (5%)
Constipation	16 (10%)	0
Dyspepsia	4 (2%)	0
Nausea	45 (27%)	4 (20%)
Vomiting	4 (2%)	0
GU (female)		
Breast pain	2 (1%)	0
Dysmenorrhea	2 (1%)	0
Ophthalmic		
Abnormal vision	2 (1%)	0
Miscellaneous		
Asthenia	15 (9%)	2 (10%)
Fatigue	12 (7%)	0
Hot flashes	2 (1%)	1 (5%)

In the 8-week, double-blind period of the comparative trial with bromocriptine, cabergoline (at a dose of 0.5 mg twice weekly) was discontinued because of an adverse event in 4 of 221 patients (2%) while bromocriptine (at a dose of 2.5 mg twice a day) was discontinued in 14 of 231 patients (6%). The most common reasons for discontinuation from cabergoline were headache, nausea and vomiting (3, 2 and 2 patients respectively); the most common reasons for discontinuation from bromocriptine were nausea, vomiting, headache, and dizziness or vertigo (10, 3, 3, and 3 patients respectively).

Cabergoline Adverse Reactions During the 8-Week, Double-Blind Period of the Comparative Trial with Bromocriptine (≥ 1%)

Adverse reaction	Cabergoline (n = 221)	Bromocriptine (n = 231)
Cardiovascular		
Dependent edema	2 (1%)	1
Hot flashes	6 (3%)	3 (1%)
Hypotension	3 (1%)	4 (2%)
Palpitation	2 (1%)	5 (2%)
Dermatologic		
Acne	3 (1%)	0
Pruritus	2 (1%)	1
GI		
Abdominal pain	12 (5%)	19 (8%)
Constipation	15 (7%)	21 (9%)
Diarrhea	4 (2%)	7 (3%)
Dry mouth	5 (2%)	2 (1%)
Dyspepsia	11 (5%)	16 (7%)
Flatulence	4 (2%)	3 (1%)
Nausea	63 (29%)	100 (43%)
Throat irritation	2 (1%)	0
Toothache	2 (1%)	0
Vomiting	9 (4%)	16 (7%)
GU (female)		
Breast pain	5 (2%)	8 (3%)
Dysmenorrhea	2 (1%)	1

Cabergoline Adverse Reactions During the 8-Week, Double-Blind Period of the Comparative Trial with Bromocriptine (≥ 1%)

Adverse reaction	Cabergoline (n = 221)	Bromocriptine (n = 231)
CNS		
Anorexia	3 (1%)	3 (1%)
Anxiety	3 (1%)	3 (1%)
Depression	7 (3%)	5 (2%)
Headache	58 (26%)	62 (27%)
Dizziness	38 (17%)	42 (18%)
Impaired concentration	2 (1%)	1
Insomnia	3 (1%)	2 (1%)
Nervousness	2 (1%)	5 (2%)
Paresthesia	5 (2%)	6 (3%)
Somnolence	5 (2%)	5 (2%)
Vertigo	9 (4%)	10 (4%)
Musculoskeletal		
Arthralgia	2 (1%)	0
Pain	4 (2%)	6 (3%)
Ophthalmic		
Abnormal vision	2 (1%)	2 (1%)
Respiratory		
Rhinitis	2 (1%)	9 (4%)
Miscellaneous		
Asthenia	13 (6%)	15 (6%)
Fatigue	10 (5%)	18 (8%)
Influenza-like symptoms	2 (1%)	0
Malaise	2 (1%)	0
Periorbital edema	2 (1%)	2 (1%)
Peripheral edema	2 (1%)	1
Syncope	3 (1%)	3 (1%)

Other adverse reactions that were reported at an incidence of less than 1% in the overall clinical studies follow.

➤*Cardiovascular:* Hypotension, syncope, palpitations.

➤*CNS:* Somnolence, nervousness, paresthesia, insomnia, anxiety.

➤*Dermatologic:* Acne, pruritus.

➤*GI:* Dry mouth, flatulence, diarrhea, anorexia.

➤*GU:* Dysmenorrhea, increased libido.

➤*Metabolic/Nutritional:* Weight loss, weight gain.

➤*Respiratory:* Epistaxis, nasal stuffiness.

➤*Special senses:* Abnormal vision.

➤*Miscellaneous:* Facial edema, influenza-like symptoms, malaise. The safety of cabergoline has been evaluated in approximately 1,200 patients with Parkinson disease in controlled and uncontrolled studies at dosages of up to 11.5 mg/day which greatly exceeds the maximum recommended dosage of cabergoline for hyperprolactinemic disorders. In addition to the adverse reactions that occurred in the patients with hyperprolactinemic disorders, the most common adverse reactions in patients with Parkinson disease were dyskinesia, hallucinations, confusion, and peripheral edema. Heart failure, pleural effusion, pulmonary fibrosis, and gastric or duodenal ulcer occurred rarely. One case of constrictive pericarditis has been reported.

Overdosage

Overdosage might be expected to produce nasal congestion, syncope, or hallucinations. Measures to support blood pressure should be taken if necessary.

Patient Information

A patient should be instructed to notify her physician if she suspects she is pregnant, becomes pregnant, or intends to become pregnant during therapy. A pregnancy test should be done if there is any suspicion of pregnancy and continuation of treatment should be discussed with her physician.

AGENTS FOR GOUT

In addition to the agents in this section, sulindac and indomethacin (see Nonsteroidal Anti-inflammatory Agents monograph) are indicated for the treatment of gout. See also probenecid in the Uricosurics section.

Uricosurics

PROBENECID

Rx	**Probenecid** (Various, eg, Geneva, Moore, Parmed, Purepac, Schein, URL)	**Tablets:** 0.5 g	In 100s and 1,000s.

PROBENECID — ORAL

Indications

➤*Hyperuricemia:* For treatment of hyperuricemia associated with gout and gouty arthritis.

➤*Elevation/Prolongation of plasma levels of antibiotics:* As an adjunctive to therapy with penicillin, or with ampicillin, methicillin, oxacillin, cloxacillin, or nafcillin, for elevation and prolongation of plasma levels by whatever route the antibiotic is given.

Administration and Dosage

➤*General dosing considerations:* Therapy should not be started until the acute gouty attack has subsided. However, if an acute attack is precipitated during therapy, probenecid may be continued without changing the dosage, and full therapeutic dosage of colchicine, or other appropriate therapy, should be given to control the acute attack.

The PSP excretion test may be used to determine the effectiveness of probenecid in retarding penicillin excretion and maintaining therapeutic levels. The renal clearance of PSP is reduced to about one-fifth the normal rate when dosage of probenecid is adequate.

➤*Adults:*

Gout –

Usual dosage: 250 mg (½ tablet), twice a day for 1 week, followed by 500 mg (1 tablet) twice a day thereafter. Gastric intolerance may be indicative of overdosage and may be corrected by decreasing the dosage.

Maintenance dosage: Continue at the dosage that will maintain normal serum urate levels. When acute attacks have been absent for 6 months or more and serum urate levels remain within normal limits, the daily dosage may be decreased by 500 mg every 6 months. The maintenance dosage should not be reduced to the point where serum urate levels tend to rise.

Concomitant therapy: As uric acid tends to crystallize out of acid urine, a liberal fluid intake is recommended, as well as sufficient sodium bicarbonate (3,000 to 7,500 mg/day) or potassium citrate (7,500 mg/day) to maintain an alkaline urine. In these cases when alkali is administered, the acid-base balance of the patient should be watched. Alkalization of the urine is recommended until the serum urate level returns to normal limits and tophaceous deposits disappear (ie, during the period when urinary excretion of uric acid is at a high level). Thereafter, alkalization of the urine and the usual restriction of purine-producing goods may be somewhat relaxed.

In conjunction with penicillin therapy – 2,000 mg (4 tablets) daily in divided doses.

In conjunction with penicillin therapy for gonorrhea – Before treating gonococcal infections in patients with suspected primary to secondary syphilis, perform proper diagnostic procedures, including darkfield examinations. If concomitant syphilis is suspected, perform monthly serological tests for at least 4 months.

Probenecid and Penicillin Therapy for Gonorrhea[a]

Statement	Recommended regimens[b]	Remarks
Uncomplicated gonococcal infection in men and women (urethral, cervical, or rectal)	4.8 million units of aqueous procaine penicillin G[c] IM, in at least 2 doses injected at different sites at 1 visit, plus 1 g probenecid orally just before injections or 3.5 g of ampicillin [c]orally plus 1 g probenecid orally given simultaneously.	Follow-up: Obtain urethral and other appropriate cultures from men, and cervical, anal, and other appropriate cultures from women, 7 to 14 days after completion of treatment.
		Treatment of sexual partners: Persons with known recent exposure to gonorrhea should receive the same treatment as those known to have gonorrhea. Examination and treatment of male sex partners of persons with gonorrhea are essential because of the high prevalence of nonsymptomatic urethral gonococcal infection in such men.
Pharyngeal gonococcal infection in men and women	4.8 million units of aqueous procaine penicillin G[c] IM in at least 2 doses injected at different sites at 1 visit plus 1 g of probenecid just before injections.	Pharyngeal gonococcal infections may be more difficult to treat than anogenital gonorrhea. Posttreatment cultures are essential.
Uncomplicated gonorrhea in pregnant patients	4.8 million units of aqueous procaine penicillin G[c] IM in at least 2 doses injected at different sites at 1 visit, plus 1 g probenecid orally just before injections or 3.5 g ampicillin[c] orally plus 1 g probenecid orally given simultaneously	
Acute gonococcal salpingitis	Outpatients: Aqueous procaine penicillin G[c] or ampicillin[c] with probenecid as for gonorrhea in pregnancy, followed by ampicillin 500 mg[c] 4 times a day for 10 days.	Follow-up of patients with acute salpingitis is essential. All patients should receive repeat pelvic examinations and cultures for *Neisseria gonorrhoeae* after treatment.
	Hospitalized patients: See the detailed treatment recommendations in the CDC guidelines.	Examination and appropriate treatment of male sex partners are essential because of the high prevalence of nonsymptomatic urethral gonorrhea in such men.
Disseminated gonococcal infection (arthritis-dermatitis syndrome)	10 million units of aqueous crystalline penicillin G[c] IV a day for 3 days or until significant clinical improvement occurs. May be followed with ampicillin 500 mg[c] 4 times a day orally to complete 7 days of treatment or 3.5 g ampicillin[c] orally plus 1 g probenecid followed by ampicillin 500 mg[c] 4 times a day for at least 7 days.	

[a] Recommended by Venereal Disease Control Advisory Committee; Center for Disease Control, US Department of Health, Education, and Welfare, Public Health Service. (*MMWR*. 1974;23:341, 342, 347, 348.)

[b] See CDC recommendations for definition of regimens of choice, alternative regimens, treatment of hypersensitive patients, and other aspects of therapy.

[c] See package circulars of manufacturers for detailed information about contraindications, warnings, precautions, and adverse reactions.

➤*Children:*

15 years of age and older and weighing more than 50 kg – See Adults for dosing.

2 to 14 years of age and 50 kg or less:

• *In conjunction with penicillin therapy* –

Initial dosage: 25 mg/kg body weight (or 0.7 g/m^2 body surface).

Maintenance dosage: 40 mg/kg body weight (or 1.2 g/m^2 body surface) per day, divided into 4 doses.

• *In conjunction with penicillin therapy for gonorrhea* – Before treating gonococcal infections in patients with suspected primary to secondary syphilis, perform proper diagnostic procedures, including darkfield examinations. If concomitant syphilis is suspected, perform monthly serological tests for at least 4 months.

Probenecid and Penicillin Therapy for Gonorrhea[a]

Statement	Recommended regimens[b]	Remarks
Gonococcal infection in children	Uncomplicated vulvovaginitis and urethritis: Aqueous procaine penicillin G[c] 75,000 to 10,000 units/kg IM with probenecid 23 mg/kg orally.	See CDC recommendations for detailed information about prevention and treatment of neonatal gonococcal infection and gonococcal ophthalmia

[a] Recommended by Venereal Disease Control Advisory Committee; Center for Disease Control, US Department of Health, Education, and Welfare, Public Health Service. (*MMWR*. 1974;23:341, 342, 347, 348.)

[b] See CDC recommendations for definition of regimens of choice, alternative regimens, treatment of hypersensitive patients, and other aspects of therapy.

[c] See package circulars of manufacturers for detailed information abut contraindications, warnings, precautions, and adverse reactions.

➤*Elderly:* Dosage should be reduced in older patients in whom renal impairment may be present.

➤*Renal function impairment:* Probenecid has been used in patients with some renal impairment, but dosage requirements may be increased. Pro-

PROBENECID — ORAL

benecid may not be effective in chronic renal insufficiency, particularly when the glomerular filtration rate is 30 mL/min or less. Because of its mechanism of action, probenecid is not recommended in conjunction with penicillin in the presence of known renal impairment. A daily dosage of 1,000 mg may be adequate. However, if necessary, the daily dosage may be increased by 500 mg increments every 4 weeks within tolerance (and usually not above 2,000 mg/day) if symptoms of gouty arthritis are not controlled or the 24-hour urate excretion is not higher than 700 mg.

➤*Administration:* May cause GI upset and may be taken with food or antacids. Drink plenty of water, at least 6 to 8 full (8 oz) glasses daily, to prevent development of kidney stones.

➤*Storage/Stability:* Store at 15° to 30°C (59° to 86°F).

Actions

➤*Pharmacology:* Probenecid is a uricosuric and renal tubular-blocking agent. It inhibits the tubular reabsorption of urate, thus increasing the urinary excretion of uric acid and decreasing serum urate levels. Effective uricosuria reduces the miscible urate pool, retards urate deposition, and promotes resorption of urate deposits.

Probenecid inhibits the tubular secretion of penicillin and usually increases penicillin plasma levels by any route the antibiotic is given. A 2- to 4-fold elevation has been demonstrated for various penicillins.

Probenecid has also been reported to inhibit the renal transport of many other compounds including aminohippuric acid (PAH), aminosalicylic acid (PAS), dyphylline, indomethacin, sodium iodomethamate and related iodinated organic acids, 17-ketosteroids, pantothenic acid, phenolsulfonphthalein (PSP), sulfonamides, and sulfonylureas.

Probenecid decreases both hepatic and renal excretion of sulfobromophthalein (BSP). The tubular reabsorption of phosphorus is inhibited in hypoparathyroid but not in euparathyroid individuals.

Probenecid does not influence plasma concentrations of salicylates, nor the excretion of streptomycin, chloramphenicol, chlortetracycline, oxytetracycline or neomycin.

Contraindications

Hypersensitivity to probenecid; children younger than 2 years of age; blood dyscrasias or uric acid kidney stones.

Therapy with probenecid should not be started until an acute gouty attack has subsided.

Warnings/Precautions

➤*Exacerbation of gout:* Exacerbation of gout following therapy with probenecid may occur; in such cases colchicine or other appropriate therapy is advisable.

➤*Methotrexate:* See Drug Interactions for more information.

➤*Salicylates:* In patients on probenecid the use of salicylates in either small or large doses is contraindicated because it antagonizes the uricosuric action of probenecid.

The biphasic action of salicylates in the renal tubules accounts for the so-called "paradoxical effect" of uricosuric agents. In patients on probenecid who require a mild analgesic agent the use of acetaminophen rather than small doses of salicylates would be preferred.

➤*Alkalinization of urine:* Hematuria, renal colic, costovertebral pain, and formation of uric acid stones associated with the use of probenecid in gouty patients may be prevented by alkalization of the urine and liberal fluid intake. As uric acid tends to crystallize out of an acid urine, a liberal fluid intake is recommended, as well as sufficient sodium bicarbonate (3,000 to 7,500 mg/day), or potassium citrate (7,500 mg/day) to maintain an alkaline urine. In these cases when alkali is administered, the acid-base balance of the patient should be watched.

➤*Hypersensitivity reactions:* The appearance of hypersensitivity reactions requires cessation of therapy with probenecid.

➤*Renal function impairment:* Probenecid has been used in patients with some renal impairment, but dosage requirements may be increased. Probenecid may not be effective in chronic renal insufficiency particularly when the glomerular filtration rate is 30 mL/minute or less. Because of its mechanism of action, probenecid is not recommended in conjunction with a penicillin in the presence of known renal impairment.

➤*Special risk:* Use with caution in patients with a history of peptic ulcer.

➤*Pregnancy: Category C* per Briggs' *Drugs in Pregnancy and Lactation*. Probenecid crosses the placenta and appears in cord blood. It has been used during pregnancy without producing adverse effects in the fetus or in the infant. Use only when clearly needed and when potential benefits outweigh potential hazards to the fetus.

➤*Lactation:* Consistent with its molecular weight (about 286), probenecid is excreted into breast milk.

Drug Interactions

Probenecid Drug Interactions

Precipitant drug	Object drug[a]		Description
Probenecid	Acyclovir	⬆	Decreased acyclovir renal clearance and increased bioavailability following IV use may occur.
Probenecid	Allopurinol	⬆	A beneficial interaction; coadministration may increase the uric acid lowering effect.
Probenecid	Barbiturates	⬆	The anesthesia produced by thiopental may be extended or achieved at lower doses.
Probenecid	Benzodiazepines	⬆	A more rapid onset or more prolonged benzodiazepine effect may occur.
Probenecid	Clofibrate	⬆	Accumulation of clofibric acid (active metabolite of clofibrate) may occur, leading to higher steady-state serum concentrations.
Probenecid	Dapsone	⬆	Possible accumulation of dapsone and its metabolites.
Probenecid	Dyphylline	⬆	Increased half-life and decreased clearance of dyphylline may occur. This may be beneficial in extending the dyphylline dosing interval.
Probenecid	Methotrexate	⬆	Methotrexate's plasma levels, therapeutic effects and toxicity may be enhanced.
Probenecid	NSAIDs	⬆	NSAID plasma levels may be increased; toxicity may be enhanced.
Probenecid	Pantothenic acid	⬆	Renal transport of pantothenic acid may be inhibited; plasma levels may increase.
Probenecid	Penicillamine	⬆	Pharmacologic effects of penicillamine may be attenuated.
Probenecid	Rifampin	⬆	Renal transport of rifampin may be inhibited; plasma levels may increase.
Probenecid	Sulfonamides	⬆	Renal transport of sulfonamides may be inhibited; plasma levels may increase.
Probenecid	Sulfonylureas	⬆	Half-life of sulfonylureas may be increased.
Probenecid	Zidovudine	⬆	Increased zidovudine bioavailability may occur; cutaneous eruptions accompanied by systemic symptoms including malaise, myalgia or fever have occurred.
Salicylates	Probenecid	⬇	Coadministration may inhibit the uricosuric action of either drug alone.

[a] ⬆ = Object drug increased. ⬇ = Object drug decreased.

➤*Drug/Lab test interactions:*

Theophylline – Falsely high readings for theophylline have been reported in an in vitro study, using the Schack and Waxler technique, when therapeutic concentrations of theophylline and probenecid were added to human plasma. A reducing substance may appear in the urine of patients receiving probenecid. This disappears with discontinuance of therapy. Suspected glycosuria should be confirmed by using a test specific for glucose.

Adverse Reactions

Headache, GI symptoms (eg, anorexia, nausea, vomiting), urinary frequency, hypersensitivity reactions (including anaphylaxis, dermatitis, pruritus, and fever), sore gums, flushing, dizziness, and anemia have occurred.

In gouty patients, exacerbation of gout and uric acid stones with or without hematuria, renal colic, or costovertebral pain, have been observed.

Nephrotic syndrome, hepatic necrosis, and aplastic anemia occur rarely. Hemolytic anemia, which in some instances could be related to genetic deficiency of glucose-6-phosphate dehydrogenase in red blood cells, has been reported.

Patient Information

Avoid taking aspirin or other salicylates that antagonize the effects of probenecid.

Probenecid may cause GI upset and may be taken with food or antacids. If nausea, vomiting or loss of appetite persists, notify physician.

Drink plenty of water, at least 6 to 8 full (8 oz) glasses daily, to prevent development of kidney stones.

FEBUXOSTAT

Rx	**Uloric** (Takeda Pharmaceuticals America)	**Tablets; oral:** 40 mg	Lactose. (TAP 40). Lt. green to green, round. In 30s, 90s, 500s, and UD 100s.
		80 mg	Lactose. (TAP 80). Lt. green to green, teardrop shape. In 30s, 100s, 1,000s, and UD 100s.

FEBUXOSTAT — ORAL

Indications

➤*Hyperuricemia:* For the chronic management of hyperuricemia in patients with gout.

Administration and Dosage

➤*General dosing considerations:* Testing for the target serum uric acid (SUA) level of less than 6 mg/dL may be performed as early as 2 weeks after initiating febuxostat therapy.

If a gout flare occurs during febuxostat treatment, febuxostat need not be discontinued. The gout flare should be managed concurrently, as appropriate for the individual patient. (See Concomitant therapy.)

➤*Adults:*

Hyperuricemia –

Usual dosage: 40 or 80 mg once daily.

Initial dosage: 40 mg once daily.

Dosage adjustment: For patients who do not achieve a SUA level of less than 6 mg/dL after 2 weeks with 40 mg, febuxostat 80 mg is recommended.

Concomitant therapy: Gout flares may occur after initiation of febuxostat because of changing SUA levels, resulting in mobilization of urate from tissue deposits. Flare prophylaxis with a nonsteroidal anti-inflammatory drug (NSAID) or colchicine is recommended upon initiation of febuxostat. Prophylactic therapy may be beneficial for up to 6 months.

➤*Administration:* May be taken without regard to food or antacid use.

➤*Storage / Stability:* Store at 25°C (77°F); excursions are permitted to 15° to 30°C (59° to 86°F). Protect from light.

Actions

➤*Pharmacology:* Febuxostat, a xanthine oxidase inhibitor, achieves its therapeutic effect by decreasing SUA.

➤*Pharmacokinetics:*

Absorption – In healthy subjects, maximum plasma concentrations (C_{max}) and area under the curve (AUC) of febuxostat increased in a dose-proportional manner following single and multiple doses of 10 to 120 mg. There is no accumulation when therapeutic doses are administered every 24 hours. The absorption of radiolabeled febuxostat following oral dose administration was estimated to be at least 49% (based on total radioactivity recovered in urine). C_{max} of febuxostat occurred between 1 and 1.5 hours postdose. After multiple oral 40 and 80 mg once-daily doses, C_{max} is approximately 1.6 ± 0.6 mcg/mL (n = 30) and 2.6 ± 1.7 mcg/mL (n = 227), respectively. Absolute bioavailability of the febuxostat tablet has not been studied.

Effect of food: Following multiple 80 mg once-daily doses with a high-fat meal, there was a 49% decrease in C_{max} and an 18% decrease in AUC. However, no clinically significant change in the percent decrease in SUA concentration was observed (58% fed vs 51% fasting). Thus, febuxostat may be taken without regard to food.

Distribution – The mean apparent steady-state volume of distribution of febuxostat was approximately 50 L (coefficient variant approximately 40%). The plasma protein binding of febuxostat is approximately 99.2% (primarily to albumin) and is constant over the concentration range achieved with 40 and 80 mg doses.

Metabolism – Febuxostat is extensively metabolized by both conjugation via uridine diphosphate glucuronosyltransferase (UGT) enzymes, including UGT1A1, UGT1A3, UGT1A9, and UGT2B7, and oxidation via CYP-450 enzymes, including CYP1A2, 2C8 and 2C9, and non-P450 enzymes. The relative contribution of each enzyme isoform in the metabolism of febuxostat is not clear. The oxidation of the isobutyl side chain leads to the formation of 4 pharmacologically active hydroxy metabolites, all of which occur in plasma of humans at a much lower extent than febuxostat.

In urine and feces, acyl glucuronide metabolites of febuxostat (approximately 35% of the dose) and oxidative metabolites 67M-1 (approximately 10% of the dose), 67M-2 (approximately 11% of the dose), and 67M-4, a secondary metabolite from 67M-1 (approximately 14% of the dose), appeared to be the major metabolites of febuxostat in vivo.

Excretion – Febuxostat is eliminated by both hepatic and renal pathways. Following an 80 mg oral dose of ^{14}C-labeled febuxostat, approximately 49% of the dose was recovered in the urine as unchanged febuxostat (3%), the acyl glucuronide of the drug (30%), its known oxidative metabolites and their conjugates (13%), and other unknown metabolites (3%). In addition to the urinary excretion, approximately 45% of the dose was recovered in the feces as the unchanged febuxostat (12%), the acyl glucuronide of the drug (1%), its known oxidative metabolites and their conjugates (25%), and other unknown metabolites (7%).

The apparent mean terminal elimination half-life ($t_{½}$) of febuxostat was approximately 5 to 8 hours.

Special populations –

Renal function impairment: AUC and half-life of febuxostat increased in subjects with renal impairment compared with subjects with healthy renal function, but values were similar among 3 renal impairment groups. Mean febuxostat AUC values were up to 1.8 times higher in subjects with renal impairment compared with those with healthy renal function. Mean C_{max} and AUC values for 3 active metabolites increased up to 2- and 4-fold, respectively.

Hepatic function impairment: Following multiple febuxostat 80 mg doses in patients with mild (Child-Pugh class A) or moderate (Child-Pugh class B) hepatic impairment, an average of 20% to 30% increase was observed for both C_{max} and AUC_{24} (total and unbound) in hepatic impairment groups compared with subjects with healthy hepatic function.

Gender: Following multiple oral doses of febuxostat, the C_{max} and AUC_{24} of febuxostat were 30% and 14% higher in women than in men, respectively.

Contraindications

Concomitant therapy with azathioprine or mercaptopurine.

Warnings/Precautions

➤*Gout flare:* After initiation of febuxostat, an increase in gout flares is frequently observed. This increase is caused by reduction in SUA levels, resulting in mobilization of urate from tissue deposits.

In order to prevent gout flares when febuxostat is initiated, concurrent prophylactic treatment with an NSAID or colchicine is recommended.

➤*Cardiovascular events:* In the randomized, controlled studies, there was a higher rate of cardiovascular thromboembolic events (cardiovascular deaths, nonfatal myocardial infarctions (MIs), and nonfatal strokes) in patients treated with febuxostat (0.74 per 100 patient-years [95% confidence interval, 0.36 to 1.37]) than allopurinol (0.6 per 100 patient-years [95% confidence interval, 0.16 to 1.53]). A causal relationship with febuxostat has not been established. Monitor for signs and symptoms of MI and stroke.

➤*Liver enzyme elevations:* During randomized controlled studies, transaminase elevations greater than 3 times the upper limit of normal (ULN) were observed (AST: 2%, 2% and ALT: 3%, 2% in febuxostat- and allopurinol-treated patients, respectively). No dose-effect relationship for these transaminase elevations was noted. Laboratory assessment of liver function is recommended at, for example, 2 and 4 months following initiation of febuxostat, and periodically thereafter.

➤*Renal function impairment:* There are insufficient data in patients with severe renal impairment (CrCl less than 30 mL/min); therefore, exercise caution in these patients.

➤*Hepatic function impairment:* No studies have been conducted in patients with severe hepatic impairment (Child-Pugh class C); therefore, exercise caution in these patients.

➤*Special risk:* No studies have been conducted in patients with secondary hyperuricemia (including organ transplant recipients); febuxostat is not recommended for use in patients in whom the rate of urate formation is greatly increased (eg, malignant disease and its treatment, Lesch-Nyhan syndrome). The concentration of xanthine in urine could, in rare cases, rise sufficiently to allow deposition in the urinary tract.

➤*Pregnancy: Category C.* There are no adequate and well-controlled studies in pregnant women. Use febuxostat during pregnancy only if the potential benefit justifies the potential risk to the fetus.

Increased neonatal mortality and a reduction in the neonatal body weight gain were observed when pregnant rats were treated with oral doses of up to 48 mg/kg (40 times the human plasma exposure at 80 mg/day) during organogenesis and through lactation period.

➤*Lactation:* Febuxostat is excreted in the milk of rats. It is not known whether this drug is excreted in human milk. Because many drugs are excreted in human milk, exercise caution when febuxostat is administered to a breast-feeding woman.

➤*Children:* Safety and effectiveness in children younger than 18 years of age have not been established.

➤*Monitoring:* Monitor for signs and symptoms of MI and stroke.

Laboratory assessment of liver function is recommended at, for example, 2 and 4 months following initiation of febuxostat and periodically thereafter.

FEBUXOSTAT — ORAL

Drug Interactions

Febuxostat Drug Interactions

Precipitant drug	Object drug[a]		Description
Antacids (eg, aluminum, magnesium)	Febuxostat	↓	Concomitant ingestion of an antacid containing magnesium hydroxide and aluminum hydroxide with an 80 mg single dose of febuxostat has been shown to delay absorption of febuxostat (approximately 1 hour) and to cause a 31% decrease in C_{max} and 15% decrease in AUC_{∞}. Because AUC rather than C_{max} was related to drug effect, change observed in AUC was not considered clinically significant. Therefore, febuxostat may be taken without regard to antacid use.
Febuxostat	Didanosine	↑	Systemic exposures of didanosine are increased during coadministration. Concurrent use is contraindicated.
Febuxostat	Xanthine oxidase substrate drugs (eg, azathioprine, mercaptopurine, theophylline)	↑	Febuxostat is a xanthine oxidase inhibitor. Inhibition of xanthine oxidase by febuxostat may cause increased plasma concentrations of these drugs, leading to toxicity. Concurrent use with azathioprine or mercaptopurine is contraindicated. Use with caution when administering with theophylline.

[a] ↑ = object drug increased; ↓ = object drug decreased.

➤*Minimally or non-interacting drugs:* Based on drug interaction studies, febuxostat does not have clinically significant interactions with colchicine, naproxen, indomethacin, hydrochlorothiazide, warfarin, or desipramine. Febuxostat may be used concomitantly with these medications.

➤*Drug/Food interactions:* See Actions for more information.

Adverse Reactions

➤*Discontinuation of therapy:* The most common adverse reaction leading to discontinuation from therapy was liver function abnormalities in 1.8% of febuxostat 40 mg patients, 1.2% of febuxostat 80 mg patients, and 0.9% of allopurinol-treated subjects.

➤*Most common adverse reactions:*

Febuxostat Adverse Reactions (≥ 1%)

	Placebo	Febuxostat		Allopurinol[a]
Adverse reactions	(n = 134)	40 mg daily (n = 757)	80 mg daily (n = 1,279)	(n = 1,277)
Arthralgia	0%	1.1%	0.7%	0.7%
Liver function abnormalities	0.7%	6.6%	4.6%	4.2%
Nausea	0.7%	1.1%	1.3%	0.8%
Rash	0.7%	0.5%	1.6%	1.6%

[a] Of the subjects who received allopurinol, 10 received 100 mg, 145 received 200 mg, and 1,122 received 300 mg, based on level of renal impairment.

In addition, dizziness was reported in more than 1% of febuxostat-treated subjects, although not at a rate of more than 0.5% greater than placebo.

➤*Less common adverse reactions:*

Cardiovascular – Angina pectoris, atrial fibrillation/flutter, cardiac murmur, cerebrovascular accident, electrocardiogram abnormal, hypertension, hypotension, palpitations, sinus bradycardia, tachycardia, transient ischemic attack (less than 1%).

CNS – Agitation, altered taste, anxiety, balance disorder, depression, fatigue, gait disturbance, Guillain-Barré syndrome, headache, hemiparesis, hypoesthesia, hyposmia, insomnia, irritability, lacunar infarction, lethargy, libido decreased, mental impairment, migraine, nervousness, panic attack, paresthesia, personality change, somnolence, tremor (less than 1%).

Dermatologic – Alopecia, angioedema, dermatitis, dermographism, ecchymosis, eczema, hair color changes, hair growth abnormal, hyperhidrosis, peeling skin, petechiae, photosensitivity, pruritus, purpura, skin discoloration/altered pigmentation, skin lesion, skin odor abnormal, urticaria (less than 1%).

GI – Abdominal distention, abdominal pain, constipation, dry mouth, dyspepsia, flatulence, frequent stools, gastritis, gastroesophageal reflux disease, gastrointestinal discomfort, gingival pain, haematemesis, hematochezia, hyperchlorhydria, mouth ulceration, pancreatitis, peptic ulcer, vomiting (less than 1%).

GU – Breast pain, erectile dysfunction, gynecomastia, hematuria, incontinence, nephrolithiasis, pollakiuria, proteinuria, renal failure, renal insufficiency, urgency (less than 1%).

Hematologic/Lymphatic – Anemia, idiopathic thrombocytopenic purpura, leukocytosis/leukopenia, neutropenia, pancytopenia, splenomegaly, thrombocytopenia (less than 1%).

Hepatic – Cholelithiasis/cholecystitis, hepatic steatosis, hepatitis, hepatomegaly (less than 1%).

Metabolic/Nutritional – Anorexia, appetite decreased/increased, dehydration, diabetes mellitus, hypercholesterolemia, hyperglycemia, hyperlipidemia, hypertriglyceridemia, hypokalemia, weight decreased/increased (less than 1%).

Musculoskeletal – Arthritis, joint stiffness, joint swelling, muscle spasms/twitching/tightness/weakness, musculoskeletal pain/stiffness, myalgia (less than 1%).

Respiratory – Bronchitis, cough, dyspnea, epistaxis, nasal dryness, paranasal sinus hypersecretion, pharyngeal edema, respiratory tract congestion, sneezing, throat irritation, upper respiratory tract infection (less than 1%).

Special senses – Deafness, tinnitus, vertigo, vision blurred (less than 1%).

Miscellaneous – Asthenia, chest pain/discomfort, contusion, edema, feeling abnormal, flushing, herpes zoster, hot flush, hypersensitivity, influenza-like symptoms, mass, pain, thirst (less than 1%).

➤*Cardiovascular safety:* Cardiovascular events and deaths were adjudicated to one of the predefined end points from the Antiplatelet Trialists Collaborations (APTC) (cardiovascular death, nonfatal MI, and nonfatal stroke) in the randomized, controlled, and long-term extension studies. In the phase 3, randomized, controlled studies, the incidences of adjudicated APTC events per 100 patient-years of exposure were the following: placebo, 0 (95% confidence interval [CI], 0 to 6.16); febuxostat 40 mg, 0 (95% CI, 0 to 1.08); febuxostat 80 mg, 1.09 (95% CI, 0.44 to 2.24); and allopurinol, 0.6 (95% CI, 0.16 to 1.53).

In the long-term extension studies, the incidences of adjudicated APTC events were the following: febuxostat 80 mg, 0.97 (95% CI, 0.57 to 1.56), and allopurinol, 0.58 (95% CI, 0.02 to 3.24).

Overall, a higher rate of APTC events was observed in febuxostat-treated patients than in allopurinol-treated patients. A causal relationship with febuxostat has not been established. Monitor for signs and symptoms of MI and stroke.

➤*Lab test abnormalities:* Activated partial thromboplastin time prolonged, alkaline phosphatase increased, amylase increased, bicarbonate decreased, blood urea increased, cholesterol increased, coagulation test abnormal, creatine increased, creatine phosphokinase (CPK) increased, creatinine increased, electroencephalograph abnormal, glucose increased, hematocrit decreased, hemoglobin decreased, lactate dehydrogenase increased, low-density lipoprotein increased, lymphocyte count decreased, mean corpuscular volume increased, neutrophil count decreased, platelet count decreased, potassium increased, prostate-specific antigen increased, prothrombin time prolonged, red blood cell count decreased, serum urea nitrogen (BUN)/creatinine ratio increased, sodium increased, thyroid-stimulating hormone increased, triglycerides increased, urinary casts, urine output increased/decreased, urine positive for white blood cells and protein, white blood cell count increased/decreased (less than 1%).

Overdosage

➤*Treatment:* Manage patients with symptomatic and supportive care if there is an overdose.

Patient Information

Advise patients of the potential benefits and risks of febuxostat. Inform patients about the potential for gout flares, elevated liver enzymes, and adverse cardiovascular events after initiation of febuxostat therapy.

Consider concomitant prophylaxis with an NSAID or colchicine for gout flares.

Instruct patients to inform their health care provider if they develop a rash, chest pain, shortness of breath, or neurologic symptoms suggesting a stroke.

Instruct patients to inform their health care provider of any other medications they are currently taking with febuxostat, including nonprescription medications.

ALLOPURINOL

Rx	**Allopurinol** (Various, eg, Boots, Geneva, Major, Mylan, Parmed, Vangard)	**Tablets:** 100 mg	In 100s, 500s, 1,000s and UD 100s.
Rx	**Zyloprim** (Faro Pharmaceuticals, Inc.)		Lactose. (Zyloprim 100). White, scored. In 100s.
Rx	**Allopurinol** (Various, eg, Boots, Geneva, Major, Mylan, Parmed, Vangard)	**Tablets:** 300 mg	In 100s, 500s, 1,000s and UD 100s.
Rx	**Zyloprim** (Faro Pharmaceuticals, Inc.)		Lactose. (Zyloprim 300). Peach, scored. In 100s and 500s.

Xanthine Oxidase Inhibitors

ALLOPURINOL

Rx	**Allopurinol Sodium** (Bedford Labs)	**Powder for injection, lyophilized:** 500 mg	Preservative free. In 30 mL vials with rubber stoppers.
Rx	**Aloprim** (Nabi)		Preservative free. In 30 mL vials with rubber stoppers.

ALLOPURINOL — ORAL

For information on allopurinol injection, please refer to the Purine Analogs and Related Agents in the Antineoplastics chapter.

Indications

➤*General information:* This is not an innocuous drug. It is not recommended for the treatment of asymptomatic hyperuricemia.

Allopurinol reduces serum and urinary uric acid concentrations. Its use should be individualized for each patient and requires an understanding of its mode of action and pharmacokinetics.

➤*Gout:* The management of patients with signs and symptoms of primary or secondary gout (acute attacks, tophi, joint destruction, uric acid lithiasis, and/or nephropathy).

➤*Malignancies:* The management of patients with leukemia, lymphoma, and malignancies who are receiving cancer therapy that causes elevations of serum and urinary uric acid levels. Treatment with allopurinol should be discontinued when the potential for overproduction of uric acid is no longer present.

➤*Calcium oxalate calculi:* The management of patients with recurrent calcium oxalate calculi whose daily uric acid excretion exceeds 800 mg/day in male patients and 750 mg/day in female patients. Therapy in such patients should be carefully assessed initially and reassessed periodically to determine in each case that treatment is beneficial and that the benefits outweigh the risks.

➤*Off-label uses:*

Chagas disease – The efficacy of allopurinol in patients with Chagas disease (American trypanosomiasis) has revealed inconsistent results. Parasitological cure was noted with allopurinol in a large, controlled study of patients with chronic disease; however, a smaller efficacy study did not support this outcome. In head-to-head trials in patients with chronic Chagas disease, itraconazole was found to provide more protection than allopurinol against the development of new electrocardiogram (ECG) changes.

Chagas disease (adults): [4] = Insufficient documentation.

Chagas disease (children/adolescents): [4] = Insufficient documentation.

Prevention of acute pancreatitis – [4] = Insufficient documentation. Studies evaluating the efficacy of allopurinol for prevention of post-endoscopic retrograde cholangiopancreatography (ERCP) pancreatitis demonstrated conflicting results. To date, studies to treat pancreatitis with allopurinol have only been performed in animals or in patients with chronic pancreatitis. Therefore, more controlled studies in humans are needed.

Stomatitis – [2] = Fair documentation. The majority of trials have demonstrated a reduction in stomatitis severity and occurrence when allopurinol was used in concentrations of 5 mg/mL to as high as 16 mg/mL in adult patients receiving fluorouracil as monotherapy or in combination with other antineoplastics. Efficacy of allopurinol may be dose related, as studies utilizing weaker mouthwash concentrations (1 mg/mL) or shorter mouthwash durations tended to have no effect on pain and incidence of stomatitis. (See Administration and Dosage.)

Other possible off-label uses – Recent studies suggest a role for allopurinol in the prevention of ischemic reperfusion tissue damage; to reduce the incidence of perioperative mortality and postoperative arrhythmias in coronary artery bypass surgery patients (300 mg 12 and 1 hour before surgery); to reduce relapse rates of *H. pylori*—induced duodenal ulcers and treatment of hematemesis from NSAID-induced erosive gastritis (50 mg 4 times/day); to alleviate pain related to acute pancreatitis (50 mg 4 times/day, rectally); to ex vivo preservation and function of organs for liver and kidney transplantation by supplementing preservation solutions with allopurinol; and to reduce rejection episodes in adult cadaver renal transplant recipients by adding low-dose allopurinol 25 mg on alternate days to a triple immunosuppressive regimen of azathioprine/cyclosporine/prednisolone. Allopurinol 20 mg/kg for 15 days has been used successfully against *Leishmania* in the treatment of American cutaneous leishmaniasis and against *Trypanosoma cruzi*; for Chagas disease (600 to 900 mg/day for 60 days); and as an alternative for patients with epileptic seizures refractory to standard therapy (150 mg/day for children less than 20 kg, otherwise 300 mg/day).

Administration and Dosage

➤*Adults:*

Gout and hyperuricemia –

Usual dosage: 200 to 300 mg/day for patients with mild gout and 400 to 600 mg/day for those with moderately severe tophaceous gout. The minimal effective dosage is 100 to 200 mg daily.

The appropriate dosage may be administered in divided doses or as a single equivalent dose with the 300 mg tablet. Dosage requirements in excess of 300 mg should be administered in divided doses.

Maximum dose: 800 mg/day.

Dosage titration: To reduce the possibility of flare-up of acute gouty attacks, it is recommended that the patient start with a low dose of allopurinol (100 mg daily) and increase at weekly intervals by 100 mg until a serum uric acid level of 6 mg/dL or less is attained without exceeding the maximal recommended dosage.

Hyperuricosuria – Patients also may benefit from dietary changes, such as a reduction of animal protein, sodium, refined sugars, oxalate-rich foods, and excessive calcium intake, as well as an increase in oral fluids and dietary fiber.

Usual dosage: 200 to 300 mg/day in single or divided doses.

Dosage adjustment: Adjust dose up or down depending upon the resultant control of the hyperuricosuria based upon subsequent 24-hour urinary urate determination.

Prevention of uric acid nephropathy during vigorous therapy of neoplastic disease –

Usual dosage: 600 to 800 mg daily for 2 or 3 days with a high fluid intake. Otherwise similar considerations to the previous recommendations for treating patients with gout govern the regulation of dosage for maintenance purposes in secondary hyperuricemia.

Recurrent calcium oxalate stones – Patients also may benefit from dietary changes, such as a reduction of animal protein, sodium, refined sugars, oxalate-rich foods, and excessive calcium intake, as well as an increase in oral fluids and dietary fiber.

Usual dosage: 200 to 300 mg/day in single or divided doses.

Dosage adjustment: Adjust dose up or down depending upon the resultant control of the hyperuricosuria based upon subsequent 24-hour urinary urate determination.

Off-label dosing –

Chagas disease: [4] = Insufficient documentation. 8.5 mg/kg/day or 900 mg/day for 60 days.

Prevention of acute pancreatitis: [4] = Insufficient documentation. 200 to 600 mg given as a single dose 1 to 4 hours prior to ERCP or high-dose therapy of 600 mg given 15 hours and 3 hours prior to ERCP.

Stomatitis: [2] = Fair documentation. Several formulations and strengths (1% to 16%) of allopurinol have been used as 10 to 20 mL 4 to 6 times daily during and after fluorouracil administration. Contact time or mouthwash duration ranged from as little as a few seconds to 5 minutes. Most patients were instructed not to swallow the mouthwash.

➤*Children:*

Secondary hyperuricemia associated with malignancies –

Children 6 to 10 years of age:

- *Usual dosage* – 300 mg daily.
- *Dosage adjustment* – The response is evaluated after approximately 48 hours of therapy, and a dosage adjustment is made if necessary.
- *Alternative dosage* – 1 mg/kg/day divided every 6 hours, to a maximum of 600 mg/day. After 48 hours of treatment, titrate dose according to serum uric acid levels.

Children younger than 6 years of age:

- *Usual dosage* – 150 mg daily.
- *Dosage adjustment* – The response is evaluated after approximately 48 hours of therapy, and a dosage adjustment is made if necessary.
- *Alternative dosage* – 1 mg/kg/day divided every 6 hours, to a maximum of 600 mg/day. After 48 hours of treatment, titrate dose according to serum uric acid levels.

Off-label dosing –

Chagas disease: [4] = Insufficient documentation.

- *9 years of age and older* – 8.5 mg/kg/day for 60 days.

➤*Renal function impairment:* Because allopurinol and its metabolites are primarily eliminated by the kidneys, accumulation of the drug can occur in renal failure and the dose of allopurinol should consequently be reduced.

Dosage adjustment – According to the manufacturer's prescribing information, the dose of allopurinol in patients with renal function impairment should be adjusted based on the following recommendations.

Creatinine clearance (CrCl) 10 to 20 mL/min: 200 mg/day.

CrCl less than 10 mL/min: The daily dosage should not exceed 100 mg.

CrCl less than 3 mL/min: The interval between doses also may need to be lengthened.

Alternative dosage adjustment – An alternative dosing regimen is:

CrCl greater than 50 mL/min: 75% of usual daily dose.

CrCl 10 to 50 mL/min: 50% of usual daily dose.

CrCl less than 10 mL/min: 25% of usual daily dose.

Hemodialysis – Administer 50% supplemental dose after dialysis.

Continuous renal replacement therapy: Dose as CrCl 10 to 50 mL/min.

➤*Concomitant therapy:* While adjusting the dosage of allopurinol in patients who are being treated with colchicine and/or anti-inflammatory agents, it is wise to continue the latter therapy until serum uric acid has been normalized and there has been freedom from acute gouty attacks for several months.

➤*Serum uric acid levels:* Normal serum urate levels are usually achieved in 1 to 3 weeks. The upper limit of normal is about 7 mg/dL for men and postmenopausal women and 6 mg/dL for premenopausal women. Too much reliance should not be placed on a single serum uric acid determination because, for technical reasons, estimation of uric acid may be difficult. By selecting the appropriate dosage and, in certain patients, using uricosuric agents concurrently, it is possible to reduce serum uric acid to normal or, if desired, to as low as 2 to 3 mg/dL, and keep it there indefinitely.

ALLOPURINOL — ORAL

➤*Switching to allopurinol from a uricosuric agent:* In transferring a patient from a uricosuric agent to allopurinol, the dose of the uricosuric agent should be gradually reduced over a period of several weeks and the dose of allopurinol gradually increased to the required dose needed to maintain a normal serum uric acid level.

➤*Administration:* Allopurinol is generally better tolerated if taken following meals. A fluid intake sufficient to yield a daily urinary output of at least 2 liters and the maintenance of a neutral or, preferably, slightly alkaline urine is desirable.

➤*Storage / Stability:* Store at 15° to 25°C (59° to 77°F) in a dry place and protect from light.

Actions

➤*Pharmacology:* Allopurinol acts on purine catabolism, without disrupting the biosynthesis of purines. It reduces the production of uric acid by inhibiting the biochemical reactions immediately preceding its formation.

Allopurinol is a structural analog of the natural purine base, hypoxanthine. It is an inhibitor of xanthine oxidase, the enzyme responsible for the conversion of hypoxanthine to xanthine and of xanthine to uric acid, the end product of purine metabolism in man. Allopurinol is metabolized to the corresponding xanthine analog, oxipurinol (alloxanthine), which also is an inhibitor of xanthine oxidase.

It has been shown that reutilization of both hypoxanthine and xanthine for nucleotide and nucleic acid synthesis is markedly enhanced when their oxidations are inhibited by allopurinol and oxipurinol. This reutilization does not disrupt normal nucleic acid anabolism, however, because feedback inhibition is an integral part of purine biosynthesis. As a result of xanthine oxidase inhibition, the serum concentration of hypoxanthine plus xanthine in patients receiving allopurinol for treatment of hyperuricemia is usually in the range of 0.3 to 0.4 mg/dL compared with a normal level of approximately 0.15 mg/dL. A maximum of 0.9 mg/dL of these oxypurines has been reported when the serum urate was lowered to less than 2 mg/dL by high doses of allopurinol. These values are far below the saturation levels at which point their precipitation would be expected to occur (above 7 mg/dL).

Administration of allopurinol generally results in a fall in both serum and urinary uric acid within 2 to 3 days. The degree of this decrease can be manipulated almost at will since it is dose-dependent. A week or more of treatment with allopurinol may be required before its full effects are manifested; likewise, uric acid may return to pretreatment levels slowly (usually after a period of 7 to 10 days following cessation of therapy). This reflects primarily the accumulation and slow clearance of oxipurinol. In some patients a dramatic fall in urinary uric acid excretion may not occur, particularly in those with severe tophaceous gout. It has been postulated that this may be due to the mobilization of urate from tissue deposits as the serum uric acid level begins to fall.

The action of allopurinol differs from that of uricosuric agents, which lower the serum uric acid level by increasing urinary excretion of uric acid. Allopurinol reduces both the serum and urinary uric acid levels by inhibiting the formation of uric acid. The use of allopurinol to block the formation of urates avoids the hazard of increased renal excretion of uric acid posed by uricosuric drugs.

Allopurinol can substantially reduce serum and urinary uric acid levels in previously refractory patients even in the presence of renal damage serious enough to render uricosuric drugs virtually ineffective. Salicylates may be given conjointly for their antirheumatic effect without compromising the action of allopurinol. This is in contrast to the nullifying effect of salicylates on uricosuric drugs.

Allopurinol also inhibits the enzymatic oxidation of mercaptopurine, the sulfur-containing analog of hypoxanthine, to 6-thiouric acid. This oxidation, which is catalyzed by xanthine oxidase, inactivates mercaptopurine. Hence, the inhibition of such oxidation by allopurinol may result in as much as a 75% reduction in the therapeutic dose requirement of mercaptopurine when the two compounds are given together (see Drug Interactions).

➤*Pharmacokinetics:* The renal clearance of hypoxanthine and xanthine is at least 10 times greater than that of uric acid. The increased xanthine and hypoxanthine in the urine have not been accompanied by problems of nephrolithiasis. Xanthine crystalluria has been reported in only three patients. Two of the patients had Lesch-Nyhan syndrome, which is characterized by excessive uric acid production combined with a deficiency of the enzyme, hypoxanthineguanine phosphoribosyltransferase (HGPRTase). This enzyme is required for the conversion of hypoxanthine, xanthine, and guanine to their respective nucleotides. The third patient had lymphosarcoma and produced an extremely large amount of uric acid because of rapid cell lysis during chemotherapy.

Allopurinol is approximately 90% absorbed from the gastrointestinal tract. Peak plasma levels generally occur at 1.5 hours and 4.5 hours for allopurinol and oxipurinol, respectively, and after a single oral dose of 300 mg allopurinol, maximum plasma levels of about 3 mcg/mL of allopurinol and 6.5 mcg/mL of oxipurinol are produced.

Approximately 20% of the ingested allopurinol is excreted in the feces. Because of its rapid oxidation to oxipurinol and a renal clearance rate approximately that of glomerular filtration rate, allopurinol has a plasma half-life of about 1 to 2 hours. Oxipurinol, however, has a longer plasma half-life (approximately 15 hours) and therefore effective xanthine oxidase inhibition is maintained over a 24-hour period with single daily doses of allopurinol. Whereas allopurinol is cleared essentially by glomerular filtration, oxipurinol is reabsorbed in the kidney tubules in a manner similar to the reabsorption of uric acid.

The clearance of oxipurinol is increased by uricosuric drugs, and as a consequence, the addition of a uricosuric agent reduces to some degree the inhibition of xanthine oxidase by oxipurinol and increases to some degree the urinary excretion of uric acid. In practice, the net effect of such combined therapy may be useful in some patients in achieving minimum serum uric acid levels provided the total urinary uric acid load does not exceed the competence of the patient's renal function.

Contraindications

Patients who have developed a severe reaction to allopurinol should not be restarted on the drug.

Warnings/Precautions

➤*Concomitant medication:* See Drug Interactions for more information.

➤*Drowsiness:* Because of the occasional occurrence of drowsiness, patients should be alerted to the need for due precaution when engaging in activities where alertness is mandatory.

➤*Acute gout attacks:* An increase in acute attacks of gout has been reported during the early stages of administration of allopurinol, even when normal or subnormal serum uric acid levels have been attained. Accordingly, maintenance doses of colchicine generally should be given prophylactically when allopurinol is begun. In addition, it is recommended that the patient start with a low dose of allopurinol (100 mg daily) and increase at weekly intervals by 100 mg until a serum uric acid level of 6 mg/dl or less is attained but without exceeding the maximum recommended dose (800 mg per day). The use of colchicine or anti-inflammatory agents may be required to suppress gouty attacks in some cases. The attacks usually become shorter and less severe after several months of therapy. The mobilization of urates from tissue deposits which cause fluctuations in the serum uric acid levels may be a possible explanation for these episodes. Even with adequate therapy with allopurinol, it may require several months to deplete the uric acid pool sufficiently to achieve control of the acute attacks.

➤*Fluid intake:* A fluid intake sufficient to yield a daily urinary output of at least 2 liters and the maintenance of a neutral or, preferably, slightly alkaline urine are desirable to:

1.) avoid the theoretical possibility of formation of xanthine calculi under the influence of therapy with allopurinol; and
2.) help prevent renal precipitation of urates in patients receiving concomitant uricosuric agents.

➤*Bone marrow depression:* Bone marrow depression has been reported in patients receiving allopurinol, most of whom received concomitant drugs with the potential for causing this reaction. This has occurred as early as 6 weeks to as long as 6 years after the initiation of therapy of allopurinol. Rarely, a patient may develop varying degrees of bone marrow depression, affecting one or more cell lines, while receiving allopurinol alone.

➤*Hypersensitivity reactions:* Allopurinol should be discontinued at the first appearance of skin rash or other signs which may indicate an allergic reaction. In some instances a skin rash may be followed by more severe hypersensitivity reactions such as exfoliative, urticarial, and purpuric lesions, as well as Stevens-Johnson syndrome (erythema multiforme exudativum), and/or generalized vasculitis, irreversible hepatotoxicity, and, on rare occasions, death.

➤*Renal function impairment:* The occurrence of hypersensitivity reactions to allopurinol may be increased in patients with decreased renal function receiving thiazide diuretics and allopurinol concurrently. For this reason, in this clinical setting, such combinations should be administered with caution and patients should be observed closely.

Some patients with pre-existing renal disease or poor urate clearance have shown a rise in BUN during administration of allopurinol. Although the mechanism responsible for this has not been established, patients with impaired renal function should be carefully observed during the early stages of administration of allopurinol and the dosage decreased or the drug withdrawn if increased abnormalities in renal function appear and persist.

Renal failure in association with administration of allopurinol has been observed among patients with hyperuricemia secondary to neoplastic diseases. Concurrent conditions such as multiple myeloma and congestive myocardial disease were present among those patients whose renal dysfunction increased after allopurinol was begun. Renal failure is also frequently associated with gouty nephropathy and rarely with hypersensitivity reactions associated with allopurinol. Albuminuria has been observed among patients who developed clinical gout following chronic glomerulonephritis and chronic pyelonephritis.

Patients with decreased renal function require lower doses of allopurinol than those with normal renal function. Lower than recommended doses should be used to initiate therapy in any patients with decreased renal function and they should be observed closely during the early stages of administration of allopurinol. In patients with severely impaired renal function or decreased urate clearance, the half-life of oxipurinol in the plasma is greatly prolonged. Therefore, a dose of 100 mg per day or 300 mg twice a week, or perhaps less, may be sufficient to maintain adequate xanthine oxidase inhibition to reduce serum urate levels.

➤*Hepatic function impairment:* A few cases of reversible clinical hepatotoxicity have been noted in patients taking allopurinol, and in some patients, asymptomatic rises in serum alkaline phosphatase or serum transaminase have been observed. If anorexia, weight loss, or pruritus develop in patients on allopurinol, evaluation of liver function should be part of their diagnostic workup. In patients with pre-existing liver disease, periodic liver function tests are recommended during the early stages of therapy.

➤*Pregnancy: Category C.* Reproductive studies have been performed in rats and rabbits at doses up to twenty times the usual human dose (5 mg/

ALLOPURINOL — ORAL

kg/day), and it was concluded that there was no impaired fertility or harm to the fetus due to allopurinol. There is a published report of a study in pregnant mice given 50 or 100 mg/kg allopurinol intraperitoneally on gestation days 10 or 13. There were increased numbers of dead fetuses in dams given 100 mg/kg allopurinol but not in those given 50 mg/kg. There were increased numbers of external malformations in fetuses at both doses of allopurinol on gestation day 10 and increased numbers of skeletal malformations in fetuses at both doses on gestation day 13. It cannot be determined whether this represented a fetal effect or an effect secondary to maternal toxicity. There are, however, no adequate or well-controlled studies in pregnant women. Because animal reproduction studies are not always predictive of human response, this drug should be used during pregnancy only if clearly needed.

Experience with allopurinol during human pregnancy has been limited partly because women of reproductive age rarely require treatment with allopurinol. There are two unpublished reports and one published paper of women giving birth to normal offspring after receiving allopurinol during pregnancy.

➤*Lactation:* Allopurinol and oxipurinol have been found in the milk of a mother who was receiving allopurinol. Since the effect of allopurinol on the nursing infant is unknown, caution should be exercised when allopurinol is administered to a nursing woman.

➤*Children:* Allopurinol is rarely indicated for use in children with the exception of those with hyperuricemia secondary to malignancy or to certain rare inborn errors of purine metabolism (see Indications and Administration and Dosage).

➤*Monitoring:* The correct dosage and schedule for maintaining the serum uric acid within the normal range is best determined by using the serum uric acid as an index.

In patients with preexisting liver disease, periodic liver function tests are recommended during the early stages of therapy (see Warnings).

Allopurinol and its primary active metabolite, oxipurinol, are eliminated by the kidneys; therefore, changes in renal function have a profound effect on dosage. In patients with decreased renal function or who have concurrent illnesses which can affect renal function such as hypertension and diabetes mellitus, periodic laboratory parameters of renal function, particularly BUN and serum creatinine or creatinine clearance, should be performed and the patient's dosage of allopurinol reassessed.

The prothrombin time should be reassessed periodically in the patients receiving dicumarol who are given allopurinol.

Drug Interactions

➤*Mercaptopurine, azathioprine:* In patients receiving mercaptopurine or azathioprine, the concomitant administration of 300 to 600 mg of allopurinol per day will require a reduction in dose to approximately one third to one fourth of the usual dose of mercaptopurine or azathioprine. Subsequent adjustment of doses of mercaptopurine or azathioprine should be made on the basis of therapeutic response and the appearance of toxic effects.

➤*Thiazide diuretics:* The reports that the concomitant use of allopurinol and thiazide diuretics may contribute to the enhancement of allopurinol toxicity in some patients have been reviewed in an attempt to establish a cause-and-effect relationship and a mechanism of causation. Review of these case reports indicates that the patients were mainly receiving thiazide diuretics for hypertension and that tests to rule out decreased renal function secondary to hypertensive nephropathy were not often performed. In those patients in whom renal insufficiency was documented, however, the recommendation to lower the dose of allopurinol was not followed. Although a causal mechanism and a cause-and-effect relationship have not been established, current evidence suggests that renal function should be monitored in patients on thiazide diuretics and allopurinol even in the absence of renal failure, and dosage levels should be even more conservatively adjusted in those patients on such combined therapy if diminished renal function is detected.

➤*Cytotoxic agents:* Enhanced bone marrow suppression by cyclophosphamide and other cytotoxic agents has been reported among patients with neoplastic disease, except leukemia, in the presence of allopurinol. However, in a well-controlled study of patients with lymphoma on combination therapy, allopurinol did not increase the marrow toxicity of patients treated with cyclophosphamide, doxorubicin, bleomycin, procarbazine, and/or mechlorethamine.

Myelosuppressive effects of cyclophosphamide may be enhanced, possibly increasing the risk of bleeding or infection.

➤*Chlorpropamide:* Chlorpropamide's plasma half-life may be prolonged by allopurinol since allopurinol and chlorpropamide may compete for excretion in the renal tubule. The risk of hypoglycemia secondary to this mechanism may be increased if allopurinol and chlorpropamide are given concomitantly in the presence of renal insufficiency.

➤*Cyclosporine:* Rare reports indicate that cyclosporine levels may be increased during concomitant treatment with allopurinol. Monitoring of cyclosporine levels and possible adjustment of cyclosporine dosage should be considered when these drugs are coadministered.

Allopurinol Drug Interactions

Precipitant drug	Object drug[a]		Description
Allopurinol	Ampicillin, amoxicillin	↑	The rate of skin rash appears much higher with allopurinol coadministration than with either drug alone.
Allopurinol	Anticoagulants, oral	↑	Data are conflicting. The anticoagulant action of some agents may be enhanced, but probably not that of warfarin.
Allopurinol	Cyclophosphamide	↑	Myelosuppressive effects of cyclophosphamide may be enhanced, possibly increasing the risk of bleeding or infection.
Allopurinol	Theophyllines	↑	Theophylline clearance may be decreased with large allopurinol doses (600 mg/day) leading to increased plasma theophylline levels and possible toxicity.
Allopurinol	Thiopurines	↑	Clinically significant increases in pharmacologic and toxic effects of oral thiopurines have occurred.
ACE Inhibitors	Allopurinol	↑	There is possibly a higher risk of hypersensitivity reaction when these agents are coadministered than when each drug is administered alone.
Aluminum salts	Allopurinol	↓	Pharmacologic effects of allopurinol may be decreased.
Thiazide diuretics	Allopurinol	↑	Coadministration may increase the incidence of hypersensitivity reactions to allopurinol.
Uricosuric agents	Allopurinol	↓	Uricosuric agents that increase the excretion of urate are also likely to increase the excretion of oxipurinol and thus lower the degree of inhibition of xanthine oxidase.

[a] ↑ = Object drug increased. ↓ = Object drug decreased.

Adverse Reactions

Data upon which the following estimates of incidence of adverse reactions are made are derived from experiences reported in the literature, unpublished clinical trials and voluntary reports since marketing of allopurinol (allopurinol) began. Past experience suggested that the most frequent event following the initiation of allopurinol treatment was an increase in acute attacks of gout (average 6% in early studies). An analysis of current usage suggests that the incidence of acute gouty attacks has diminished to less than 1%. The explanation for this decrease has not been determined but may be due in part to initiating therapy more gradually (see Warnings and Administration and Dosage).

➤*Hypersensitivity:* The most frequent adverse reaction to allopurinol is skin rash. Skin reactions can be severe and sometimes fatal. Therefore, treatment with allopurinol should be discontinued immediately if a rash develops (see Warnings). Some patients with the most severe reaction also had fever, chills, arthralgias, cholestatic jaundice, eosinophilia and mild leukocytosis or leukopenia. Among 55 patients with gout treated with allopurinol for 3 to 34 months (average greater than 1 year) and followed prospectively, Rundles observed that 3% of patients developed a type of drug reaction which was predominantly a pruritic maculopapular skin eruption, sometimes scaly or exfoliative. However, with current usage, skin reactions have been observed less frequently than 1%. The explanation for this decrease is not obvious. The incidence of skin rash may be increased in the presence of renal insufficiency. The frequency of skin rash among patients receiving ampicillin or amoxicillin concurrently with allopurinol has been reported to be increased (see Drug Interactions).

➤*Most common adverse reactions probably causally related:* Early clinical studies and incidence rates from early clinical experience with allopurinol suggested that these adverse reactions were found to occur at a rate of greater than 1%. The most frequent event observed was acute attacks of gout following the initiation of therapy. Analyses of current usage suggest that the incidence of these adverse reactions is now less than 1%. The explanation for this decrease has not been determined, but it may be due to following recommended usage (see Adverse Reactions introduction, Indications, Warnings, and Administration and Dosage).

Dermatologic – Rash; maculopapular rash.

GI – Diarrhea; nausea; alkaline phosphatase increase; AST/ALT increase.

Metabolic/Nutritional – Acute attacks of gout.

➤*Incidence less than 1% probably causally related:*

Cardiovascular – Necrotizing angiitis; vasculitis.

CNS – Headache; peripheral neuropathy; neuritis; paresthesia; somnolence.

Dermatologic – Erythema multiforme exudativum (Stevens-Johnson syndrome); toxic epidermal necrolysis (Lyell's syndrome); hypersensitivity vasculitis; purpura; vesicular bullous dermatitis; exfoliative dermatitis; eczematoid dermatitis; pruritus; urticaria; alopecia; onycholysis; lichen planus.

ALLOPURINOL — ORAL

GI – Hyperbilirubinemia; vomiting; intermittent abdominal pain; gastritis; dyspepsia.

GU – Renal failure; uremia (see Warnings).

Hematologic – Thrombocytopenia; eosinophilia; leukocytosis; leukopenia.

Hepatic – Increased alkaline phosphatase, AST and ALT; hepatic necrosis; granulomatous hepatitis; hepatomegaly; cholestatic jaundice.

Musculoskeletal – Myopathy; arthralgias.

Respiratory – Epistaxis.

Special senses – Taste loss/perversion.

Miscellaneous – Ecchymosis; fever.

➤*Incidence less than 1% causal relationship unknown:*

Cardiovascular – Pericarditis; peripheral vascular disease; thrombophlebitis; bradycardia; vasodilation.

CNS – Optic neuritis; confusion; dizziness; vertigo; foot drop; decrease in libido; depression; amnesia; tinnitus; asthenia; insomnia.

Dermatologic – Furunculosis; facial edema; sweating; skin edema.

Endocrine – Infertility (male); hypercalcemia; gynecomastia (male).

GI – Hemorrhagic pancreatitis; GI bleeding; stomatitis; salivary gland swelling; hyperlipidemia; tongue edema; anorexia.

GU – Nephritis; impotence; primary hematuria; albuminuria.

Hematologic/Lymphatic – Aplastic anemia; agranulocytosis; eosinophilic fibrohistiocytic lesion of bone marrow; pancytopenia; prothrombin decrease; anemia; hemolytic anemia; reticulocytosis; lymphadenopathy; lymphocytosis.

Musculoskeletal – Myalgia.

Respiratory – Bronchospasm; asthma; pharyngitis; rhinitis.

Special senses – Cataracts; macular retinitis; iritis; conjunctivitis; amblyopia.

Miscellaneous – Malaise.

Overdosage

In the management of overdosage there is no specific antidote for allopurinol. There has been no clinical experience in the management of a patient who has taken massive amounts of allopurinol. Both allopurinol and oxipurinol are dialyzable; however, the usefulness of hemodialysis or peritoneal dialysis in the management of an overdose of allopurinol is unknown.

Patient Information

Allopurinol is better tolerated if taken with food or milk. A fluid intake, sufficient to yield a daily urinary output of at least 2 L and the maintenance of a neutral or, preferably slightly alkaline urine are desirable. Drink at least 10 to 12 (8 oz) glasses of fluids daily.

Discontinue allopurinol and to consult your doctor immediately at the first sign of a skin rash, painful urination, blood in the urine, irritation of the eyes, or swelling of the lips or mouth.

Continue drug therapy prescribed for gouty attacks since optimal benefit of allopurinol may be delayed for 2 to 6 weeks.

Increase fluid intake during therapy to prevent renal stones.

If a single dose of allopurinol is occasionally forgotten, there is no need to double the dose at the next scheduled time.

There may be certain risks associated with the concomitant use of allopurinol and dicumarol, sulfinpyrazone, mercaptopurine, azathioprine, ampicillin, amoxicillin, and thiazide diuretics, and patients should follow the instructions of their doctor.

Because of the occasional occurrence of drowsiness, patients should take precautions when engaging in activities where alertness is mandatory.

Patients may wish to take allopurinol after meals to minimize gastric irritation.

Use caution when taking large doses of vitamin C; urinary acidification with large doses of vitamin C may increase the possibility of kidney stone formation.

PEGLOTICASE

Rx	**Krystexxa** (Savient Pharmaceuticals Inc)	**Injection, solution, concentrate:** 8 mg/mL	As uricase protein (recombinant). In single-use 2 mL vials.

PEGLOTICASE — INJECTION

WARNING

Anaphylaxis and infusion reactions have been reported to occur during and after administration of pegloticase.

Anaphylaxis may occur with any infusion, including a first infusion, and generally manifests within 2 hours of the infusion. However, delayed-type hypersensitivity reactions have also been reported.

Pegloticase should be administered in health care settings by health care providers prepared to manage anaphylaxis and infusion reactions.

Patients should be premedicated with antihistamines and corticosteroids.

Patients should be closely monitored for anaphylaxis for an appropriate period of time after pegloticase administration.

Monitor serum uric acid levels prior to infusions and consider discontinuing treatment if levels increase to higher than 6 mg/dL, particularly when 2 consecutive levels higher than 6 mg/dL are observed.

Indications

➤*Gout:* For the treatment of long-term gout in adult patients refractory to conventional therapy.

Administration and Dosage

➤*Adults:*

Gout –

Usual dosage: 8 mg given as an intravenous (IV) infusion every 2 weeks.

Duration of therapy: The optimal treatment duration has not been established.

➤*Preparation for administration:* Use appropriate aseptic technique. Withdraw 1 mL of pegloticase from the vial into a sterile syringe. Discard any unused portion of product remaining in the 2 mL vial. Inject into a single 250 mL bag of sodium chloride 0.9% injection or sodium chloride 0.45% injection for IV infusion.

Invert the infusion bag containing the dilute solution a number of times to ensure thorough mixing. Do not shake.

Before administration, allow the diluted solution to reach room temperature. Pegloticase in a vial or in an IV infusion fluid should never be subjected to artificial heating (eg, hot water, microwave).

➤*Administration:* Administer by IV infusion over no less than 120 minutes via gravity feed, syringe-type pump, or infusion pump. Do not administer as an IV push or bolus.

Premedication – Patients should receive preinfusion medications (eg, antihistamines, corticosteroids) to minimize the risk of anaphylaxis and infusion reactions. Pegloticase should be administered in a health care setting by health care providers prepared to manage anaphylaxis and infusion reactions. Patients should be observed for an appropriate period of time after administration.

Infusion reactions – The risk of anaphylaxis and infusion reactions is higher in patients who have lost therapeutic response.

If an infusion reaction occurs during pegloticase administration, the infusion may be slowed, or stopped and restarted at a slower rate, at the discretion of the health care provider. Because the infusion reactions can occur after infusion completion, observation of patients for approximately 1 hour postinfusion should be considered.

➤*Admixture compatibility:* Dilute with sodium chloride 0.9% or sodium chloride 0.45% only; do not mix or dilute with other drugs.

➤*Storage/Stability:* Store vials in the carton and refrigerate between 2° to 8°C (36° to 46°F) at all times. Protect from light. Do not shake or freeze.

Pegloticase diluted in infusion bags is stable for 4 hours at 2° to 8°C (36° to 46°F) and at room temperature (20° to 25°C [68° to 77°F]). However, it is recommended that diluted solutions be refrigerated (not frozen), protected from light, and used within 4 hours of dilution.

Actions

➤*Pharmacology:* Pegloticase is a uric acid specific enzyme that is a recombinant uricase and achieves its therapeutic effect by catalyzing the oxidation of uric acid to allantoin, thereby lowering serum uric acid. Allantoin is an inert and water soluble purine metabolite. It is readily eliminated, primarily by renal excretion.

Pharmacodynamics – Approximately 24 hours following the first dose of pegloticase, the mean plasma uric acid level was 0.7 mg/dL for the pegloticase 8 mg every 2 weeks group. In comparison, the mean plasma uric acid level for the placebo group was 8.2 mg/dL.

In a single-dose, dose-ranging trial following 1-hour IV infusions of pegloticase 0.5, 1, 2, 4, 8, or 12 mg in 24 patients with symptomatic gout (n = 4 subjects/dose group), plasma uric acid decreased with increasing pegloticase dose or concentrations. The duration of plasma uric acid suppression appeared to be positively associated with pegloticase dose. Sustained decrease in plasma uric acid below the solubility concentration of 6 mg/dL for more than 300 hours was observed with doses of 8 and 12 mg.

➤*Pharmacokinetics:* Pegloticase levels were determined in serum based on measurements of uricase enzyme activity.

Significant covariates included in the model for determining clearance and volume of distribution were body surface area and anti-pegloticase antibodies.

PEGLOTICASE — INJECTION

Absorption – Following single IV infusions of pegloticase 0.5 to 12 mg in 23 patients with symptomatic gout, maximum serum concentrations of pegloticase increased in proportion to the dose administered.

Contraindications

Glucose-6-phosphate dehydrogenase (G6PD) deficiency.

Warnings/Precautions

➤*Infusion reactions:* During premarketing controlled clinical trials, infusion reactions were reported in 26% of patients treated with pegloticase 8 mg every 2 weeks and 41% of patients treated with pegloticase 8 mg every 4 weeks compared with 5% of patients treated with placebo. These infusion reactions occurred in patients pretreated with an oral antihistamine, IV corticosteroid, and/or acetaminophen. This pretreatment may have blunted or obscured symptoms or signs of infusion reactions, and, therefore, the reported frequency may be an underestimate.

See the Warning box for more information.

Infuse pegloticase slowly over no less than 120 minutes. In the event of an infusion reaction, slow or stop the infusion and restart at a slower rate.

The risk of infusion reactions is higher in patients whose uric acid level increases to higher than 6 mg/dL, particularly when 2 consecutive levels higher than 6 mg/dL are observed. Monitor serum uric acid levels prior to infusions and consider discontinuing treatment if levels increase higher than 6 mg/dL.

➤*Gout flares:* Gout flares may occur after initiation of pegloticase. An increase in gout flares is frequently observed upon initiation of antihyperuricemic therapy due to changing serum uric acid levels resulting in mobilization of urate from tissue deposits. Gout flare prophylaxis with a nonsteroidal anti-inflammatory drug (NSAID) or colchicine is recommended starting at least 1 week before initiation of pegloticase therapy and lasting at least 6 months, unless medically contraindicated or not tolerated. Pegloticase does not need to be discontinued because of a gout flare. Manage the gout flare concurrently as appropriate for the individual patient.

➤*Congestive heart failure:* Pegloticase has not been formally studied in patients with congestive heart failure, but some patients in the clinical trials experienced exacerbation. Exercise caution when using pegloticase in patients who have congestive heart failure, and monitor patients closely following infusion.

➤*Retreatment:* No controlled trial data are available on the safety and efficacy of re-treatment with pegloticase after stopping treatment for longer than 4 weeks. Because of the immunogenicity of pegloticase, patients receiving retreatment may be at increased risk of anaphylaxis and infusion reactions. Therefore, carefully monitor patients receiving re-treatment after a drug-free interval.

➤*G6PD deficiency:* It is recommended that patients at higher risk for G6PD deficiency (ie, patients of African or Mediterranean ancestry) be screened for G6PD deficiency before starting pegloticase. Pegloticase is contraindicated in patients with G6PD deficiency due to the risk of hemolysis and methemoglobinemia.

➤*Immunogenicity:* Anti-pegloticase antibodies developed in 92% of patients treated with pegloticase every 2 weeks and 28% for placebo. Anti–polyethylene glycol (PEG) antibodies were also detected in 42% of patients treated with pegloticase. A high anti-pegloticase antibody titer was associated with a failure to maintain pegloticase-induced normalization of uric acid. The impact of anti-PEG antibodies on patient response to other PEG-containing therapeutics is unknown.

There was a higher incidence of infusion reactions in patients with high anti-pegloticase antibody titer: 53% in the pegloticase every-2-weeks group compared with 6% in patients who had undetectable or low antibody titers.

➤*Hypersensitivity reactions:* During premarketing controlled clinical trials, anaphylaxis was reported in 6.5% of patients treated with pegloticase every 2 weeks, compared with none with placebo. Manifestations included wheezing, perioral or lingual edema, or hemodynamic instability, with or without rash or urticaria. Cases occurred in patients being pretreated with 1 or more doses of an oral antihistamine, an IV corticosteroid, and/or acetaminophen. This pretreatment may have blunted or obscured symptoms or signs of anaphylaxis and, therefore, the reported frequency may be an underestimate.

See the Warning box for more information.

Inform patients of the symptoms and signs of anaphylaxis and instruct them to seek immediate medical care if anaphylaxis occurs after discharge from the health care setting.

The risk of anaphylaxis is higher in patients whose uric acid level increases to higher than 6 mg/dL, particularly when 2 consecutive levels higher than 6 mg/dL are observed. Monitor serum uric acid levels prior to infusions and consider discontinuing treatment if levels increase higher than 6 mg/dL.

➤*Pregnancy: Category C.* A complete evaluation of the reproductive and developmental toxicity of pegloticase has not been completed. Adequate animal reproduction studies have not been conducted with pegloticase. It is not known whether pegloticase can cause fetal harm when administered to a pregnant woman or can affect reproductive capacity. There are no adequate and well-controlled studies in pregnant women. Pegloticase should be used during pregnancy only if clearly needed.

➤*Lactation:* It is not known whether this drug is excreted in human milk. Because many drugs are excreted in human milk and because of the potential for serious adverse reactions in breast-feeding infants, it is not recommended to administer pegloticase to a breast-feeding mother.

➤*Children:* The safety and effectiveness in children younger than 18 years of age have not been established.

➤*Elderly:* No overall differences in safety or effectiveness were observed between older and younger patients, but greater sensitivity of some older individuals cannot be ruled out. No dose adjustment is needed for patients 65 years of age and older.

➤*Monitoring:* Closely monitor patients for an appropriate period of time after administration of pegloticase for anaphylaxis.

Monitor serum uric acid levels prior to infusions and consider discontinuing treatment if levels increase to higher than 6 mg/dL, particularly when 2 consecutive levels higher than 6 mg/dL are observed.

Carefully monitor patients receiving retreatment after a drug-free interval because of an increased risk for anaphylaxis and infusion reactions.

Monitor heart failure patients closely following pegloticase infusion.

Drug Interactions

No drug interaction studies of pegloticase with other drugs have been conducted.

Adverse Reactions

➤*Most common serious adverse reactions:* The most commonly reported serious adverse reactions from premarketing controlled clinical trials were anaphylaxis, which occurred in 6.5% of patients treated with pegloticase 8 mg every 2 weeks compared with none with placebo; infusion reactions, which occurred in 26% of patients treated with pegloticase 8 mg every 2 weeks compared with 5% treated with placebo; and gout flares, which were more common during the first 3 months of treatment with pegloticase compared with placebo. All patients in premarketing controlled clinical trials were pretreated with an oral antihistamine, IV corticosteroid, and/or acetaminophen to prevent anaphylaxis and infusion reactions. Patients also received NSAIDs or colchicine or both for at least 7 days as gout flare prophylaxis before beginning pegloticase treatment.

➤*Adverse reactions (5% or more):*

Pegloticase Adverse Reactions (≥ 5%)		
Adverse reaction	Pegloticase 8 mg every 2 weeks (n = 85)[a]	Placebo (n = 43)
GI		
Constipation	6%	5%
Nausea	12%	2%
Vomiting	5%	2%
Miscellaneous		
Anaphylaxis	5%	0%
Chest pain	6%	2%
Contusion or ecchymosis[b]	11%	5%
Gout flare	77%	81%
Infusion reaction	26%	5%
Nasopharyngitis	7%	2%

[a] If the same subject in a given group had more than 1 adverse reaction occurrence in the same reaction category, the subject was counted only once.
[b] Most did not occur on the day of infusion and could be related to other factors (eg, concomitant medications relevant to contusion or ecchymosis, insulin-dependent diabetes mellitus).

Hypersensitivity – Diagnostic criteria of anaphylaxis were skin or mucosal tissue involvement, and, either airway compromise, and/or reduced blood pressure with or without associated symptoms, and a temporal relationship to pegloticase or placebo injection with no other identifiable cause. Using these clinical criteria, anaphylaxis was identified in 5.1% of patients studied in the clinical program of IV pegloticase. The frequency was 6.5% for the every 2-week dosing regimen and 4.8% for the 4-week dosing regimen of pegloticase. There were no cases of anaphylaxis in patients receiving placebo. Anaphylaxis generally occurred within 2 hours of treatment. This occurred with patients pretreated with an oral antihistamine, IV corticosteroid, and acetaminophen.

Infusion reactions – Infusion reactions occurred in 26% of patients in the 2-week dosing regimen group and 41% of patients in the 4-week dosing regimen group, compared with 5% of placebo-treated patients. Manifestations of these reactions included urticaria (10.6%), dyspnea (7.1%), chest discomfort (9.5%), chest pain (9.5%), erythema (9.5%), and pruritus (9.5%). These manifestations overlap with the symptoms of anaphylaxis, but did not occur together to satisfy the clinical criteria for diagnosing anaphylaxis. Infusion reactions are thought to result from release of various mediators, such as cytokines. Infusion reactions occurred at any time during a course of treatment, with approximately 3% occurring with the first infusion and approximately 91% occurring during the time of infusion. Some infusion reaction manifestations were reduced by slowing the rate of infusion or stopping the infusion and restarting at a slower rate. These infusion reactions occurred with all patients being pretreated with an oral antihistamine, IV corticosteroid, and acetaminophen.

Gout flares – Gout flares were common in the study patients before randomization to treatment, with patients experiencing an average of 10 flares in the preceding 18 months prior to study entry. During the controlled treatment period of pegloticase or placebo, the frequencies of gout flares were high in all treatment groups but more so during the first 3 months of peg-

PEGLOTICASE — INJECTION

loticase treatment, which seemed to decrease in the subsequent 3 months of treatment. The percentages of patients with any flare for the first 3 months were 74%, 81%, and 51%, for pegloticase 8 mg every 2 weeks, pegloticase 8 mg every 4 weeks, and placebo, respectively. The percentages of patients with any flare for the subsequent 3 months were 41%, 57%, and 67%, for pegloticase 8 mg every 2 weeks, pegloticase 8 mg every 4 weeks, and placebo, respectively. Patients received gout flare prophylaxis with colchicine and/or NSAIDs starting at least 1 week before receiving pegloticase.

➤*Cardiovascular:* Two cases of congestive heart failure exacerbation occurred during the trials in patients receiving pegloticase 8 mg every 2 weeks. No cases were reported in placebo-treated patients. Four subjects had exacerbations of preexisting congestive heart failure while receiving pegloticase 8 mg every 2 weeks during the open-label extension study.

Overdosage

➤*Symptoms:* No reports of overdosage with pegloticase have been reported. The maximum dose administered as a single IV dose is 12 mg as uricase protein.

➤*Treatment:* Monitor patients suspected of receiving an overdose, and initiate general supportive measures because no specific antidote has been identified.

Patient Information

Inform patients that anaphylaxis and infusion reactions can occur at any infusion while on therapy. Counsel patients on the importance of adhering to any prescribed medications to help prevent or lessen the severity of these reactions.

Educate patients on the signs and symptoms of anaphylaxis, including wheezing, perioral or lingual edema, hemodynamic instability, and rash or urticaria.

Educate patients on the most common signs and symptoms of an infusion reaction, including urticaria, erythema, dyspnea, flushing, chest discomfort, chest pain, and rash.

Advise patients to seek medical care immediately if they experience any symptoms of an allergic reaction during or at any time after the infusion of pegloticase.

Inform patients not to take pegloticase if they have a condition known as G6PD deficiency. Explain to patients that G6PD deficiency is more frequently found in individuals of African or Mediterranean ancestry and that they may be tested to determine if they have G6PD deficiency, unless already known.

Explain to patients that gout flares may initially increase when starting treatment with pegloticase, and that medications to help reduce flares may need to be taken regularly for the first few months after pegloticase is started. Advise patients not to stop pegloticase therapy if they have a flare.

COLCHICINE

Rx	**Colchicine** (Various, eg, Watson)	**Tablets; oral:** 0.6 mg (1/100 gr)	May contain lactose. In 30s, 60s, 100s, and 1,000s.
Rx	**Colcrys** (AR Scientific)		Lactose, PEG, polydextrose. (AR 374). Purple, capsule-shaped, scored. Film-coated. In 30s, 60s, 100s, 250s, 500s, and 1,000s.

COLCHICINE — ORAL

Indications

➤*Familial Mediterranean fever (Colcrys only):* For the treatment of familial Mediterranean fever in adults and children 4 years of age and older.

➤*Gout flares:* For the prophylaxis and the treatment of acute gout flares when taken at the first sign of a flare.

➤*Off-label uses:*

Behçet syndrome – [2] = Fair documentation. Data from controlled trials indicate that colchicine as monotherapy has benefits over placebo for treatment of arthritis in patients with Behçet syndrome. Other benefits, such as reduction in genital ulceration and erythema nodosum, were limited to women. Oral ulcerations and folliculitis were not improved. Cyclosporine was superior to colchicine for treatment of ocular manifestations, dermal lesions, and aphthous ulcers. Based on the reviewed information, colchicine alone may be useful for patients with milder disease without ocular involvement; however, more aggressive treatment with alternate or combination therapy may be necessary for more severe disease.

Hepatic cirrhosis – [5] = Poor documentation. Small, early studies of colchicine for the treatment of hepatic cirrhosis garnered favorable results and generated interest in the use of this therapy in which few options are available. Although some health care providers prescribe colchicine for hepatic cirrhosis, the weight of the evidence from larger, more recent, and better-controlled trials does not favor efficacy. A systematic review concluded that the use of colchicine was not warranted in this setting except in a controlled trial because of a lack of benefit and an association with adverse reactions.

Pericarditis (adults) – [2] = Fair documentation. The use of colchicine to prevent recurrences of pericarditis has most often been used as second-line therapy (after failure of nonsteroidal anti-inflammatory drugs [NSAIDs] and before corticosteroid initiation) and as third-line therapy (only after corticosteroid use). More recent studies have suggested that it may also be useful as initial therapy for recurrences, although the required duration of therapy is not known.

Pericarditis (children/adolescents) – [4] = Insufficient documentation. The incidence of pericarditis in children is low, which limits the spectrum of information available for this age group. In addition, available data in children are conflicting because of a lack of a good control of variables. Further controlled trials are required.

Prevention of postpericardiotomy syndrome – [5] = Poor documentation. The use of colchicine to prevent postpericardiotomy syndrome has been limited to 1 controlled trial, which showed no significant difference in efficacy when compared with placebo. Based on these data, this drug is not recommended after cardiac surgery to prevent postpericardiotomy syndrome. Larger, controlled trials are needed.

Primary amyloidosis – [5] = Poor documentation. There is no cure for amyloidosis, but varying drug regimens have been used to improve symptoms and extend life. Colchicine in combination with melphalan and prednisone was found to be more effective in prolonging life than colchicine alone; however, data do not support improved efficacy with the addition of colchicine. Larger, controlled studies are needed to further evaluate the use of colchicine for the treatment of primary amyloidosis.

Primary biliary cirrhosis – [5] = Poor documentation. Results from randomized clinical trials have not shown colchicine to be efficacious over placebo, ursodeoxycholic acid, or other drugs in the treatment of primary biliary cirrhosis. Alternative therapy options with more conclusive evidence of efficacy are available.

Other possible off-label uses – Scleroderma (1 mg/day). Sweet syndrome (0.5 mg 1 to 3 times daily).

Colchicine also has been used in the treatment of sarcoid arthritis, acute inflammatory calcific tendonitis, arthritis associated with erythema nodosum, leukemia, adenocarcinoma of the GI tract, and mycosis fungoides, and topically to treat intraurethral condyloma acuminata in men.

Administration and Dosage

➤*General dosing considerations:* *Colcrys* is the only Food and Drug Administration (FDA)–approved single-ingredient colchicine product.

Dosing adjustment may be required for patients with renal impairment. (See Renal Function Impairment.)

➤*Adults:*

Familial Mediterranean fever (Colcrys only) –

Usual dosage: 1.2 to 2.4 mg daily in 1 or 2 divided doses.

Dosage adjustment: Increase as needed in increments of 0.3 mg/day to a maximum recommended daily dose to control disease and as tolerated. If intolerable adverse effects develop, the dosage should be decreased in increments of 0.3 mg/day.

Prophylaxis of gout flares –

Usual dosage: 0.6 mg once or twice daily.

Maximum dose: 1.2 mg/day.

Alternative dosage: The following dosing information is based on product labeling from non–FDA-approved colchicine products.

- *Less than 1 attack per year* – 0.6 mg/day, 3 or 4 days a week.
- *More than 1 attack per year* – 0.6 mg daily. Severe cases may require 1.2 or 1.8 mg daily.
- *Surgical patients* – 0.6 mg 3 times daily for 3 days before and 3 days after surgery.

Treatment of gout flares –

Usual dosage: 1.2 mg at the first sign of the flare, followed by 0.6 mg 1 hour later. If also taking colchicine for prophylaxis of gout flares, wait 12 hours after taking the last dose for treatment of the flare, then resume prophylaxis dosage.

Maximum dose: 1.8 mg over a 1-hour period.

Alternative dosage: The following dosing information is based on product labeling from non–FDA-approved colchicine products.

Initial dosage is 0.6 to 1.2 mg at the first sign of the flare, followed by 0.6 mg every hour or 1.2 mg every 2 hours until pain is relieved or until diarrhea ensues. After the initial dose, it is sometimes sufficient to take 0.6 mg every 2 or 3 hours. The drug should be stopped if there is GI discomfort or diarrhea. Opiates may be needed to control diarrhea. The total amount of colchicine needed during an attack usually ranges from 4 to 8 mg. An interval of 3 days between colchicine courses is advised in order to minimize the possibility of cumulative toxicity.

If corticotropin (ACTH) is administered, it is recommended that colchicine also be given in dosages of at least 1 mg/day, and that colchicine be continued for a few days after the hormone is withdrawn.

Off-label dosing –

Behçet syndrome: [2] = Fair documentation. 1 to 2 mg/day in divided doses (eg, 0.5 or 0.6 mg 3 times daily) used as primary or adjunctive therapy. Medication is for prolonged treatment and was studied for 2 years in a major study.

Pericarditis (adults): [2] = Fair documentation.

- *Acute pericarditis* – Initial loading dosages ranged from 1 to 2 mg daily. Maintenance dosages were 0.5 to 1 mg daily for at least 3 months.
- *Recurrent pericarditis* – Initial loading dosages ranged from 1 to 3 mg daily. Maintenance dosages were 0.5 to 2 mg daily for at least 6 months.

COLCHICINE — ORAL

➤*Children:*

Familial Mediterranean fever (Colcrys only*)* –

13 years of age and older: See Adults for dosing.

6 to 12 years of age:

• *Usual dosage* – 0.9 to 1.8 mg daily in 1 or 2 divided doses.

• *Dosage adjustment* – Increase as needed in increments of 0.3 mg/day to a maximum daily recommended dose to control disease and as tolerated. If intolerable adverse effects develop, the dosage should be decreased in increments of 0.3 mg/day.

4 to 6 years of age:

• *Usual dosage* – 0.3 to 1.8 mg daily in 1 or 2 divided doses.

• *Dosage adjustment* – Increase as needed in increments of 0.3 mg/day to a maximum daily recommended dose to control disease and as tolerated. If intolerable adverse effects develop, the dosage should be decreased in increments of 0.3 mg/day.

Off-label dosing –

Pericarditis (children/adolescents): [4] = Insufficient documentation. Initial loading dosages ranged from 0.5 to 1.5 mg daily. Maintenance dosages ranged from 0.25 to 2 mg daily up to several months.

➤*Renal function impairment:*

Mild renal impairment (creatinine clearance [CrCl] of 50 to 80 mL/min) –

Familial Mediterranean fever: Dosage adjustment may be necessary. Monitor closely for adverse reactions.

Gout flares:

Treatment of gout flares is not recommended in patients with renal impairment who are receiving colchicine for prophylaxis.

Moderate renal impairment (CrCl of 30 to 50 mL/min) –

Familial Mediterranean fever: Dosage adjustment may be necessary. Monitor closely for adverse reactions.

Gout flares:

Treatment of gout flares is not recommended in patients with renal impairment who are receiving colchicine for prophylaxis.

Severe renal impairment (CrCl less than 30 mL/min) –

Familial Mediterranean fever: Start with 0.3 mg/day; any increase in dosage should be done with adequate monitoring of the patient for adverse reactions.

Gout flares: Treatment of gout flares is not recommended in patients with renal impairment who are receiving colchicine for prophylaxis.

• *Prophylaxis* – Initially, 0.3 mg/day. Any increase should be done with close monitoring.

• *Treatment* – Dosage adjustment is not required, but a treatment course should be repeated no more than once every 2 weeks. For patients requiring repeated courses, consider alternate therapy.

Dialysis –

Familial Mediterranean fever: Initial dosage should be 0.3 g/day. Dosing can be increased with close monitoring.

Gout flares: Treatment of gout flares is not recommended in patients with renal impairment who are receiving colchicine for prophylaxis.

• *Prophylaxis* – 0.3 mg twice a week with close monitoring.

• *Treatment* – Single dose of 0.6 mg. A treatment course should not be repeated more than once every 2 weeks.

Alternative dosing regimen –

Gout flares:

• *CrCl more than 50 mL/min* – 100% of usual daily dose.

• *CrCl of 10 to 50 mL/min* – 50% to 100% of usual daily dose.

• *CrCl less than 10 mL/min* – 25% of usual daily dose.

• *Peritoneal dialysis* – 25% of usual daily dose.

• *Continuous renal replacement therapy* – 50% to 100% of usual daily dose.

➤*Hepatic function impairment:*

Familial Mediterranean fever –

In patients with severe hepatic impairment, dosage reduction should be considered with careful monitoring as necessary.

Gout flares – Treatment of gout flares is not recommended in patients with hepatic impairment who are receiving colchicine for prophylaxis.

Prophylaxis:

Dosage adjustment should be considered in severe hepatic disease.

Treatment: Dosage adjustment is not required in patients with mild or moderate hepatic impairment, but monitor patient carefully.

In patients with severe hepatic impairment, carefully monitor and do not repeat the treatment course more than once every 2 weeks. For these patients requiring repeated courses, consideration should be given to alternate therapy.

➤*Concomitant therapy:* Coadministration of colchicine with P-glycoprotein inhibitors or strong CYP3A4 inhibitors in patients with renal or hepatic impairment is contraindicated. If patients are taking or have recently completed treatment with a strong or moderate CYP3A4 inhibitor or P-glycoprotein inhibitor within the prior 14 days, colchicine dosage adjustments are required.

Strong CYP3A4 inhibitors (eg, atazanavir, clarithromycin, indinavir, itraconazole, ketoconazole, nefazodone, nelfinavir, ritonavir, saquinavir, telithromycin) –

Familial Mediterranean fever: Maximum daily dose of 0.6 mg. May be given as 0.3 mg twice daily.

Gout flares:

• *Prophylaxis* – If taking 0.6 mg twice daily, decrease dosage to 0.3 mg once daily. If taking 0.6 mg once daily, decrease dosage to 0.3 mg every other day.

• *Treatment* – 0.6 mg as 1 dose at the first sign of attack, followed by 0.3 mg 1 hour later. Dose to be repeated no earlier than 3 days. Use is not recommended in patients receiving prophylactic dose of colchicine and a CYP3A4 inhibitor.

Moderate CYP3A4 inhibitors (amprenavir, aprepitant, diltiazem, erythromycin, fluconazole, fosamprenavir, grapefruit juice, verapamil) –

Familial Mediterranean fever: Maximum daily dose of 1.2 mg. May be given as 0.6 mg twice daily.

Gout flares:

• *Prophylaxis* – If taking 0.6 mg twice daily, decrease dosage to 0.3 mg twice daily. If taking 0.6 mg once daily, decrease dosage to 0.3 mg once daily.

• *Treatment* – 1.2 mg as 1 dose at the first sign of attack. Dose to be repeated no earlier than 3 days. Use is not recommended in patients receiving prophylactic dose of colchicine and CYP3A4 inhibitor.

P-glycoprotein inhibitors (eg, cyclosporine, ranolazine) –

Familial Mediterranean fever: Maximum daily dose of 0.6 mg. May be given as 0.3 mg twice daily.

Gout flares:

• *Prophylaxis* – If taking 0.6 mg twice daily, decrease dosage to 0.3 mg once daily. If taking 0.6 mg once daily, decrease dosage to 0.3 mg every other day.

• *Treatment* – 0.6 mg as 1 dose at the first sign of attack. Dose to be repeated no earlier than 3 days.

➤*Administration:* Administer orally without regard to meals.

➤*Storage/Stability:* Store at 20° to 25°C (68° to 77°F). Protect from light.

Actions

➤*Pharmacology:*

Gout – The exact mechanism of action of colchicine, an anti-inflammatory agent, in gout is not completely known, but it involves a reduction in lactic acid production by leukocytes, which results in a decrease in uric acid deposition and a reduction in phagocytosis, with abatement of the inflammatory response.

Colchicine is not an analgesic, though it relieves pain in acute attacks of gout. It is not a uricosuric agent and will not prevent progression of gout to chronic gouty arthritis. It does have a prophylactic, suppressive effect that helps to reduce the incidence of acute attacks and to relieve the residual pain and mild discomfort that patients with gout occasionally feel.

Familial Mediterranean fever – The mechanism by which colchicine exerts its beneficial effect in patients with familial Mediterranean fever has not been fully elucidated; however, recent data suggest that colchicine may interfere with the intracellular assembly of the inflammasome complex present in neutrophils and monocytes that mediates activation of interleukin-1 beta. Additionally, colchicine disrupts cytoskeletal functions through inhibition of beta-tubulin polymerization into microtubules, and, consequently, prevents the activation, degranulation, and migration of neutrophils.

➤*Pharmacokinetics:*

Colchicine Mean (% Coefficient of Variation) Pharmacokinetic Parameters[a]				
C_{max}	T_{max}[b]	Vd/F[c]	Cl/F[d]	Half-life
Colchicine 0.6 mg single dose (n = 13)				
2.5 ng/mL (28.7)	1.5 h (1 to 3)	341.5 L (54.4)	54.1 L/h (31)	
Colchicine 0.6 mg twice daily for 10 days (n = 13)				
3.6 ng/mL (23.7)	1.3 h (0.5 to 3)	1,150 L (18.7)	30.3 L/h (19)	26.6 h (16.3)

[a] C_{max} = peak plasma concentration; T_{max} = time to C_{max}; Vd = volume of distribution; Cl = clearance.
[b] T_{max} mean (range).
[c] Vd = Cl/Ke (calculated from mean values).
[d] Cl = dose/area under the curve (AUC) (calculated from mean values).

Absorption – In healthy adults, colchicine is rapidly absorbed when given orally, reaching a mean C_{max} of 2.5 ng/mL (range, 1.1 to 4.4 ng/mL) in 1 to 2 hours (range, 0.5 to 3 hours) after a single dose administered under fasting conditions. After 10 days on a regimen of 0.6 mg twice daily, C_{max} is 3.1 to 3.6 ng/mL (range, 1.6 to 6 ng/mL), occurring 1.3 to 1.4 hours postdose (range, 0.5 to 3 hours).

Following oral administration of colchicine 1.8 mg over 1 hour to healthy young adults under fasting conditions, colchicine appears to be readily absorbed, reaching mean C_{max} of 6.2 ng/mL at a median of 1.81 hours (range, 1 to 2.5 hours). Following administration of the nonrecommended high-dose regimen (4.8 mg over 6 hours), mean C_{max} was 6.8 ng/mL, at a median of 4.47 hours (range, 3.1 to 7.5 hours).

In some subjects, secondary colchicine peaks are seen, occurring between 3 and 36 hours postdose and ranging from 39% to 155% of the height of the initial peak. These observations are attributed to intestinal secretion and reabsorption and/or biliary recirculation. Absolute bioavailability is reported to be approximately 45%.

Effect of food: Administration of colchicine with food has no effect on the rate of colchicine absorption, but did decrease the extent of colchicine absorption by approximately 15%. This is without clinical significance.

Distribution – Large amounts of the drug and metabolites enter the intestinal tract in bile and intestinal secretions. High concentrations are found in the kidney, liver, and spleen. The mean apparent volume of distribution in healthy young volunteers was approximately 5 to 8 L/kg.

COLCHICINE — ORAL

Colchicine binding to serum protein is low (39% ± 5%), primarily to albumin regardless of concentration.

See the Pregnancy section in Warnings/Precautions for more information.

Metabolism – Colchicine is demethylated to 2 primary metabolites, 2-0-demethylcolchicine and 3-0-demethy1colchicine (2- and 3-DMC, respectively), and one minor metabolite, 10-O-demethy1colchicine (also known as colchiceine). In vitro studies using human liver microsomes have shown that CYP3A4 is involved in the metabolism of colchicine to 2- and 3-DMC. Plasma levels of these metabolites are minimal (less than 5% of the parent drug).

Excretion – Colchicine is significantly excreted in urine in healthy subjects. In healthy volunteers (n = 12), 40% to 65% of colchicine 1 mg administered orally was recovered unchanged in the urine. Enterohepatic recirculation and biliary excretion are also postulated to play a role in colchicine elimination. Following multiple oral doses (0.6 mg twice daily), the mean elimination half-lives in young healthy volunteers (mean age, 25 to 28 years) is 26.6 to 31.2 hours. Colchicine is a substrate of P-glycoprotein.

Special populations –

Renal function impairment: Patients with end-stage renal disease had 75% lower colchicine clearance (0.17 vs 0.73 L/h/kg) and prolonged plasma elimination half-life (18.8 vs 4.4 hours) as compared with familial Mediterranean fever and healthy renal function.

Hepatic function impairment: In some subjects with mild to moderate cirrhosis, the clearance of colchicine is significantly reduced and plasma half-life prolonged compared with healthy subjects. In subjects with primary biliary cirrhosis, no consistent trends were noted. No pharmacokinetic data are available for patients with severe hepatic impairment.

Elderly: Mean peak plasma levels and AUC of colchicine were 2 times higher in elderly subjects compared with young, healthy men; however, it is possible that the higher exposure in the elderly subjects was caused by decreased renal function.

Contraindications

Hypersensitivity to the drug; serious GI, renal, hepatic, or cardiac disorders; blood dyscrasias; coadministration with P-glycoprotein or strong CYP3A4 inhibitors in patients with renal or hepatic impairment (*Colcrys* only).

Warnings/Precautions

➤*Fatal overdose:* Fatal overdoses, both accidental and intentional, have been reported in adults and children who have ingested colchicine.

➤*Hematologic effects:* Myelosuppression, leukopenia, granulocytopenia, thrombocytopenia, pancytopenia, and aplastic anemia with colchicine used in therapeutic doses have been reported. Use with caution in patients with hematologic disorders.

➤*Neuromuscular toxicity:* Colchicine-induced neuromuscular toxicity and rhabdomyolysis have been reported with chronic treatment in therapeutic doses. Patients with renal dysfunction and elderly patients, even those with healthy renal and hepatic function, are at increased risk. Concomitant use of atorvastatin, simvastatin, pravastatin, fluvastatin, gemfibrozil, fenofibrate, fenofibric acid, or benzafibrate (themselves associated with myotoxicity), or cyclosporine may potentiate the development of myopathy. Once colchicine is stopped, the symptoms generally resolve within 1 week to several months.

➤*GI effects:* If nausea, vomiting, or diarrhea occurs, discontinue the drug.

➤*Renal function impairment:*

Prophylaxis of gout flares – For prophylaxis of gout flares in patients with mild (CrCl of 50 to 80 mL/min) to moderate (CrCl of 30 to 50 mL/min) renal impairment, adjustment of the recommended dosage is not required; however, monitor patients closely for adverse effects of colchicine. In patients with severe impairment, start the dosage at 0.3 mg/day and make any increase in dosage with close monitoring. For the prophylaxis of gout flares in patients undergoing dialysis, starting doses at 0.3 mg given twice a week with close monitoring.

Treatment of gout flares – For treatment of gout flares in patients with mild (CrCl of 50 to 80 mL/min) to moderate (CrCl of 30 to 50 mL/min) renal impairment, adjustment of the recommended dosage is not required; however, monitor patients closely for adverse effects of colchicine. In patients with severe impairment, while the dosage does not need to be adjusted for the treatment of gout flares, repeat a treatment course no more than once every 2 weeks. For patients with gout flares requiring repeated courses consider alternate therapy. For patients undergoing dialysis, reduce the total recommended dose for the treatment of gout flares to a single dose of 0.6 mg (1 tablet). For these patients, repeat the treatment course no more than once every 2 weeks.

Familial Mediterranean fever – Although pharmacokinetics of colchicine in patients with mild (CrCl of 50 to 80 mL/min) and moderate (CrCl of 30 to 50 mL/min) renal impairment is not known, monitor these patients closely for adverse effects of colchicine. Dosage reduction may be necessary. In patients with severe renal failure (CrCl less than 30 mL/minute) and end-stage renal disease requiring dialysis, colchicine may be started at the dosage of 0.3 mg/day. Any increase in dosage should be done with adequate monitoring of the patient for adverse effects of colchicine.

➤*Hepatic function impairment:*

Prophylaxis of gout flares – For prophylaxis of gout flares in patients with mild to moderate hepatic impairment, adjustment of the recommended dosage is not required; however, monitor patients closely for adverse effects of colchicine. Consider dosage reduction for the prophylaxis of gout flares in patients with severe hepatic impairment.

Treatment of gout flares – For treatment of gout flares in patients with mild to moderate hepatic impairment, adjustment of the recommended colchicine dosage is not required; however, monitor patients closely for adverse effects of colchicine. For the treatment of gout flares in patients with severe impairment, while the dosage does not need to be adjusted, repeat the treatment course no more than once every 2 weeks. For these patients, requiring repeated courses for the treatment of gout flares, consideration should be given to alternate therapy.

Familial Mediterranean fever – In patients with severe hepatic disease, consider dosage reduction with careful monitoring.

➤*Special risk:* Administer with caution to debilitated patients and to those with early manifestations of GI or cardiac disorders.

➤*Pregnancy:* Category C. Colchicine has been shown to be teratogenic in mice when given doses of 1.25 and 1.5 mg/kg and in hamsters when given 10 mg/kg. There are no adequate and well-controlled studies in pregnant women. Use colchicine during pregnancy only if the potential benefit justifies the potential risk to the fetus.

Colchicine crosses the human placenta (plasma levels in the fetus are reported to be approximately 15% of the maternal concentration). While not studied in the treatment of gout flares, data from a limited number of published studies found no evidence of an increased risk of miscarriage, stillbirth, or teratogenic effects among pregnant women using colchicine to treat familial Mediterranean fever. Although animal and developmental studies were not conducted with colchicine, published animal reproductive and developmental studies indicate that colchicine causes embryofetal toxicity, teratogenicity, and altered postnatal development at exposures within or above the clinical range.

Fertility impairment – Reproductive studies also reported abnormal sperm morphology and reduced sperm counts in males, and interference with sperm penetration, second meiotic division, and normal cleavage in females when exposed to colchicine.

➤*Lactation:* Colchicine is excreted into human milk. Limited information suggests that exclusively breast-fed infants receive less than 10% of the maternal weight-adjusted dose. While there are no published reports of adverse effects in breast-feeding infants of mothers taking colchicine, colchicine can affect GI cell renewal and permeability. Exercise caution and observe breast-feeding infants for adverse effects when colchicine is administered to a breast-feeding woman.

➤*Children:* The safety and efficacy of colchicine in children of all ages with familial Mediterranean fever has been evaluated in uncontrolled studies; however, dosing is approved only for children 4 years of age and older. There does not appear to be an adverse effect on growth in children with familial Mediterranean fever treated long-term with colchicine.

Gout is rare in children; safety and effectiveness of colchicine in children have not been established.

➤*Elderly:* In general, use caution in dose selection, usually starting at the low end of the dosing range, reflecting the greater frequency of decreased hepatic or renal function, and of concomitant disease or other drug therapy.

➤*Lab test abnormalities:* Colchicine therapy may cause elevated alkaline phosphatase and ALT. Decreased thrombocyte values may occur during therapy.

➤*Monitoring:* In patients receiving long-term therapy, perform periodic blood counts. Closely monitor patients with renal or hepatic impairment for adverse reactions.

Drug Interactions

Colchicine Drug Interactions

Precipitant drug	Object drug[a]		Description
Acidifying agents	Colchicine	⬇	The action of colchicine is inhibited by acidifying agents. Avoid coadministration.
Alkalinizing agents	Colchicine	⬆	The action of colchicine is potentiated by alkalinizing agents. Avoid coadministration.
Digoxin	Colchicine	⬆	The risk for myopathy or rhabdomyolysis may be increased. If coadministration cannot be avoided, monitor the patient for signs of any unexplained muscle pain, tenderness, or weakness. If colchicine toxicity is suspected, discontinue colchicine.
Colchicine	Digoxin		
Cyclosporine	Colchicine	⬆	The risk for myopathy or rhabdomyolysis may be increased. If coadministration cannot be avoided, monitor the patient for signs of any unexplained muscle pain, tenderness, or weakness. If colchicine toxicity is suspected, discontinue colchicine.
Colchicine	Cyclosporine		

COLCHICINE — ORAL

Colchicine Drug Interactions			
Precipitant drug	Object drug[a]		Description
Fibric acids (eg, fenofibrate, gemfibrozil)	Colchicine	↑	The risk for myopathy or rhabdomyolysis may be increased. If coadministration cannot be avoided, monitor the patient for signs of any unexplained muscle pain, tenderness, or weakness. If colchicine toxicity is suspected, discontinue colchicine.
Colchicine	Fibric acids (eg, fenofibrate, gemfibrozil)		
HMG-CoA reductase inhibitors (eg, atorvastatin, fluvastatin, pravastatin, simvastatin)	Colchicine	↑	The risk for myopathy or rhabdomyolysis may be increased. If coadministration cannot be avoided, monitor the patient for signs of any unexplained muscle pain, tenderness, or weakness. If colchicine toxicity is suspected, discontinue colchicine.
Colchicine	HMG-CoA reductase inhibitors (eg, atorvastatin, fluvastatin, pravastatin, simvastatin)		
Moderate CYP3A4 inhibitors (eg, aprepitant, diltiazem, erythromycin, fluconazole, fosamprenavir, verapamil)	Colchicine	↑	Colchicine plasma concentrations may be elevated, increasing the risk of toxicity (eg, myopathy). Coadminister with caution, starting at reduced colchicine doses and increased monitoring of creatine phosphokinase and for adverse reactions. If colchicine toxicity is suspected, discontinue colchicine.
P-glycoprotein inhibitors (eg, cyclosporine, ranolazine)	Colchicine	↑	Life-threatening and fatal drug interactions have been reported in patients receiving colchicine and a P-glycoprotein inhibitor. Coadministration of colchicine and a P-glycoprotein inhibitor to patients with renal or hepatic impairment is contraindicated. If treatment with a P-glycoprotein inhibitor is needed in patients with healthy renal and hepatic function, the colchicine dose may need to be reduced or withheld. If colchicine toxicity is suspected, discontinue colchicine.
Strong CYP3A4 inhibitors (eg, atazanavir, clarithromycin, indinavir, itraconazole, ketoconazole, nefazodone, nelfinavir, ritonavir, saquinavir, telithromycin, voriconazole)	Colchicine	↑	Life-threatening and fatal drug interactions have been reported in patients receiving colchicine and a strong CYP3A4 inhibitor. Coadministration of colchicine and a strong CYP3A4 inhibitor to patients with renal or hepatic impairment is contraindicated. If treatment with a strong CYP3A4 inhibitor is needed in patients with healthy renal and hepatic function, the colchicine dose may need to be reduced or withheld. If colchicine toxicity is suspected, discontinue colchicine.
Colchicine	CNS depressants	↑	Colchicine may increase sensitivity to the action of CNS depressants. Monitor the patient and adjust the CNS depressant dose as needed.
Colchicine	Sympathomimetics	↑	The action of sympathomimetics may be increased. Monitor the patient and adjust the sympathomimetic dose as needed.

[a] ↑ = object drug increased; ↓ = object drug decreased.

➤*Drug/Lab test interactions:* Colchicine may cause false-positive results when testing urine for red blood cell count or hemoglobin.

➤*Drug/Food interactions:* Colchicine plasma concentrations may be elevated by grapefruit juice ingestion, increasing the risk of toxicity (eg, myopathy). Patients taking colchicine should not consume grapefruit juice.

See Actions for more information.

Adverse Reactions

➤*Most common adverse reactions:*

Gout – The most common adverse reactions reported in the clinical trial with colchicine for the treatment of gout flares were diarrhea (23%) and pharyngolaryngeal pain (3%). Diarrhea was the most commonly reported adverse reaction in prophylaxis clinical trials.

Familial Mediterranean fever – GI adverse reactions are the most frequent adverse effects in patients initiating colchicine, usually presenting within 24 hours and occurring in up to 20% of patients given therapeutic doses. Typical symptoms include cramping, nausea, diarrhea, abdominal pain, and vomiting. These reactions should be viewed as dose-limiting if severe because they can herald the onset of more significant toxicity.

➤*Long-term use:* Bone marrow depression with aplastic anemia, agranulocytosis, or thrombocytopenia may occur in patients receiving long-term therapy. Peripheral neuritis, purpura, loss of hair, myopathy, and reversible azoospermia have also been reported.

➤*Gout:*

GI – In a randomized, double-blind, placebo-controlled trial in patients with a gout flare, GI adverse reactions occurred in 26% of patients using the recommended dose (1.8 mg over 1 hour) of colchicine compared with 77% of patients taking a nonrecommended high-dose (4.8 mg over 6 hours) of colchicine and 20% of patients taking placebo. Diarrhea was the most commonly reported drug related GI adverse reactions. Diarrhea was more likely to occur in patients taking the high-dose regimen than the low-dose regimen. Severe diarrhea occurred in 19% and vomiting occurred in 17% of patients taking the nonrecommended high-dose colchicine regimen, but it did not occur in the recommended low-dose regimen.

Diarrhea, nausea, and vomiting may occur, especially when maximal doses are necessary for a therapeutic effect. To avoid more serious toxicity, discontinue the drug when these symptoms appear, regardless of whether joint pain has been relieved.

Colchicine Adverse Reactions (≥ 2%)			
	Colchicine		
Adverse reactions	High-dose (n = 52)	Low-dose (n = 74)	Placebo (n = 59)
Patients with ≥ 1 drug-related treatment emergent adverse reaction	77%	37%	27%
CNS	2%	1.4%	3%
Fatigue	4%	1%	2%
Headache	2%	1%	3%
GI	77%	26%	20%
Abdominal discomfort	0%	0%	3%
Diarrhea	77%	23%	14%
Nausea	17%	4%	5%
Vomiting	17%	0%	0%
Metabolic/Nutritional	0%	4%	3%
Gout	0%	4%	2%
Miscellaneous			
General disorders and administration-site conditions	8%	1%	2%
Pharyngolaryngeal pain	2%	3%	0%
Respiratory thoracic mediastinal disorders	2%	3%	0%

➤*Dermatologic:* Dermatoses have been reported.

➤*Hypersensitivity:* Hypersensitivity reactions may occur infrequently.

➤*Postmarketing:*

CNS – Sensory motor neuropathy.

Dermatologic – Alopecia, maculopapular rash, purpura, rash.

GI – Abdominal cramping, abdominal pain, diarrhea, lactose intolerance, nausea, vomiting.

GU – Azoospermia, oligospermia.

Hematologic – Aplastic anemia, granulocytopenia, leukopenia, pancytopenia, thrombocytopenia.

Hepatic – Elevated ALT, elevated AST.

Musculoskeletal – Elevated creatine phosphokinase, muscle pain, muscle weakness, myopathy, myotonia, rhabdomyolysis.

Miscellaneous – Serious toxic manifestations include myelosuppression, disseminated intravascular coagulation, and injury to cells in the renal, hepatic, circulatory, and central nervous systems. These most often occur with excessive accumulation or overdosage.

Overdosage

➤*Symptoms:* The exact dose of colchicine that produces significant toxicity is unknown. Fatalities have occurred after ingestion of a dose as low as 7 mg over a 4-day period, while other patients have survived after ingesting than 60 mg. A review of 150 patients who overdosed on colchicine found that those who ingested less than 0.5 mg/kg survived and tended to have milder

COLCHICINE — ORAL

toxicities, such as GI symptoms, whereas those who took 0.5 to 0. 8 mg/kg had more severe reactions, such as myelosuppression. There was 100% mortality in those who ingested more than 0.8 mg/kg.

The first stage of acute colchicine toxicity typically begins with 24 hours of ingestion and includes GI symptoms, such as abdominal pain, nausea, vomiting, diarrhea, and significant fluid loss, leading to volume depletion. The diarrhea may be bloody because of hemorrhagic gastroenteritis. Burning sensations of the throat, stomach, and skin may be prominent symptoms. Peripheral leukocytosis may also be seen. Life-threatening complications occur during the second stage, which occurs 24 to 72 hours after drug administration, attributed to multiorgan failure and its consequences. Extensive vascular damage may result in shock. Kidney damage, evidenced by hematuria and oliguria, may occur. Muscular weakness may be marked, and ascending paralysis of the CNS may develop; the patient usually remains conscious. Delirium and convulsions may occur. Death is usually a result of respiratory depression and cardiovascular collapse. If the patient survives, recovery of multiorgan injury may be accompanied by rebound leukocytosis and alopecia starting about 1 week after the initial ingestion.

➤*Treatment:* Begin treatment of colchicine poisoning with gastric lavage and measures to prevent shock. Otherwise, treatment is symptomatic and supportive. Recent studies appear to support the use of hemodialysis or peritoneal dialysis as part of the treatment of acute overdosage in addition to gastric lavage. Symptomatic and supportive treatment may include atropine and morphine for the relief of abdominal pain, and artificial respiration with oxygen to combat respiratory distress. No specific antidote is known.

Patient Information

Advise patients to take colchicine every day as prescribed, even if they are feeling better. Advise patients not to alter the dosage or discontinue treatment without consulting with their health care provider. If a dose is missed for treatment of a gout flare when the patient is not being dosed for prophylaxis, advise the patient to take the missed dose as soon as possible; for treatment of a gout flare during prophylaxis, advise the patient to take the missed dose immediately, wait 12 hours, then resume the previous dosing schedule; for prophylaxis without treatment for a gout flare or for familial Mediterranean fever, advise the patient to take the missed dose as soon as possible and then return to the normal dosing schedule. However, if a dose is skipped, advise the patient not to double the next dose.

Inform patients that fatal overdoses, both accidental and intentional, have been reported in patients who have ingested colchicine.

Inform patients that bone marrow depression with agranulocytosis, aplastic anemia, and thrombocytopenia may occur.

Advise patients that many drugs or other substances may interact with colchicine and some interactions could be fatal. Instruct patients to report all current medications to their health care provider, and to check with their health care provider before starting any new medications, particularly antibiotics. Also advise patients to report the use of nonprescription medication or herbal products. Grapefruit and grapefruit juice may also interact; advise patients not to consume these during colchicine treatment.

Inform patients that muscle pain or weakness and tingling or numbness in the fingers or toes may occur with colchicine alone or when it is used with certain other drugs. Patients developing any of these signs or symptoms must discontinue colchicine and seek medical evaluation immediately.

Advise patients with gout to discontinue medication as soon as gout pain is relieved or at the first sign of nausea, vomiting, stomach pain, or diarrhea. If symptoms persist, notify the health care provider.

PROBENECID AND COLCHICINE

Rx	**Probenecid and Colchicine** (Various, eg, Ivax, Schein)	**Tablets:** 500 mg probenecid, 0.5 mg colchicine	In 100s and 1,000s.

PROBENECID AND COLCHICINE — ORAL

For complete and comparative prescribing information see the individual probenecid and colchicine monographs.

Indications

➤*Gouty arthritis:* For the treatment of chronic gouty arthritis when complicated by frequent, recurrent acute attacks of gout

Administration and Dosage

➤*General dosing considerations:* Do not start therapy until an acute gouty attack has subsided. However, if an acute attack is precipitated during therapy, probenecid and colchicine may be continued without changing the dosage and additional colchicine or other appropriate therapy given to control the acute attack.

➤*Adults:*

Chronic gouty arthritis –

Usual dosage: 1 tablet/day for 1 week followed by 1 tablet twice/day.

Dosage titration: If necessary, the daily dosage may be increased by 1 tablet at 4-week intervals as tolerated (usually not more than 4 tablets/day).

➤*Renal function impairment:* May not be effective in patients with chronic renal function impairment (creatinine clearance 30 mL/min or less); dose may need to be increased.

➤*Administration:* Administer with food if GI upset occurs. Maintain adequate fluid intake (at least eight 8 oz glasses of water/day).

➤*Storage/Stability:* Store at 15° to 30°C (59° to 86°F).

Warnings/Precautions

➤*Pregnancy: Category D* (colchicine). *Category C* (probenecid per Briggs' *Drugs in Pregnancy and Lactation*). Probenecid crosses the placental barrier and appears in cord blood. Colchicine can arrest cell division in animals and plants. In certain species of animals under certain conditions, colchicine has produced teratogenic effects. The possibility of such effects in humans also has been reported. Because of the colchicine component, probenecid and colchicine is contraindicated in pregnant patients. The use of any drug in women of childbearing potential requires that the anticipated benefit be weighed against the possible hazards.

➤*Lactation:* Consistent with its molecular weight (about 286), probenecid is excreted into breast milk.

Colchicine is excreted into breast milk. Because of the absence of infant toxicity observed during breast-feeding, the American Academy of Pediatrics classifies colchicine as compatible with breast-feeding.

EMERGENCY KITS

EMERGENCY KITS

Rx	**Cyanide Antidote Package** (Various, eg, Taylor)	Sodium nitrite, 300 mg in 10 mL (2 amps) Sodium thiosulfate, 12.5 g in 50 mL (2 vials) Amyl nitrite inhalant, 5 minim/0.3 mL (12 amps)	Also disposable syringes, stomach tube, tourniquet, and instructions.

EMERGENCY KITS

Indications

➤*Cyanide poisoning:* For treatment of cyanide poisoning.

Administration and Dosage

➤*General dosing considerations:* Personnel should acquire some skill in the proper method of administering the contents of this package prior to an emergency. Cyanide poisoning is rapidly fatal (See Administration).

Calculate the doses for children on a body surface area or on a weight basis with the dosage adjusted so that excessive methemoglobin is not formed.

➤*Adults:*

Cyanide poisoning –

Usual dosage:

1.) Instruct an assistant how to break an ampule of amyl nitrite, one at a time, in a handkerchief and hold it in front of the patient's mouth for 15 seconds, followed by a rest for 15 seconds. Then reapply until sodium nitrite can be administered. This interrupted schedule is important because continuous use of amyl nitrite may prevent adequate oxygenation.
2.) Discontinue amyl nitrite then administer 300 mg (10 mL of a 3% solution) sodium nitrite IV at the rate of 2.5 to 5 mL/min.
3.) Immediately after sodium nitrite, administer 12.5 g (50 mL of a 25% solution) sodium thiosulfate IV. The same needle and vein may be used.

Duration of therapy: Watch the patient closely for at least 24 to 48 hours. If signs of poisoning reappear, repeat the injection of both sodium nitrite and sodium thiosulfate, but each in 50% of the original dose. Even if the patient seems perfectly well, the medication may be given for prophylactic purposes 2 hours after the first injections.

EMERGENCY KITS

➤*Children:*

Cyanide poisoning –

Usual dosage:

1.) Instruct an assistant how to break an ampule of amyl nitrite, one at a time, in a handkerchief and hold it in front of the patient's mouth for 15 seconds, followed by a rest for 15 seconds. Then reapply until sodium nitrite can be administered. This interrupted schedule is important because continuous use of amyl nitrite may prevent adequate oxygenation.
2.) Discontinue amyl nitrite then administer 6 to 8 mL/m^2 (approximately 0.2 mL/kg body weight) sodium nitrite IV up to 10 mL, at the rate of 2.5 to 5 mL/min.
3.) Immediately after sodium nitrite, administer 7 g/m^2 of body surface area sodium thiosulfate IV, but dosage should not exceed 12.5 g. The same needle and vein may be used.

Duration of therapy: See Adults.

➤*Administration:* The prevention of death demands a quick diagnosis and the prompt use of specific antidotes. No valuable time should be lost. Even though the diagnosis is doubtful, institute the recommended therapy immediately.

If the poison was taken by mouth, perform gastric lavage as soon as possible, but this should not delay the treatments outlined above. Lavage may be done concurrently by a third person, health care provider or a nurse if one is available. One should take quick action without waiting for positive diagnostic tests.

If respiration has ceased but the pulse is palpable, apply artificial respiration at once. The purpose is not to revive, rather to keep the heart beating. Lay the gauze sponge or handkerchief containing the amyl nitrite over the patient's nose, for it may hasten the resumption of respiratory movements. When signs of breathing appear, promptly administer the emergency kit solutions as directed.

➤*Storage/Stability:* No storage info provided.

Warnings/Precautions

➤*Methemoglobinemia:* Both sodium nitrite and amyl nitrite in excessive doses induce dangerous methemoglobinemia and can cause death.

➤*Pregnancy: Category C* (amyl nitrite [per Briggs' *Drugs in Pregnancy and Lactation*]).

➤*Lactation:* Per Briggs' *Drugs in Pregnancy and Lactation*, amyl nitrite is probably compatible with breast-feeding.

➤*Children:* The amounts found in a single cyanide antidote package are not excessive for an adult. Calculate the doses for children on a surface area or on a weight basis with the dosage adjusted so that excessive methemoglobin is not formed.

DETOXIFICATION AGENTS

Various Detoxification Agents and Their Uses

Drug (trade name)	Toxic/Overdosed substance
Dimercaprol (*BAL In Oil*)	Arsenic, gold, mercury, lead
Deferoxamine mesylate (*Desferal*)	Iron
Dexrazoxane (*Zinecard*)	Doxorubicin-induced cardiomyopathy
Digoxin immune fab (*Digibind, Digifab*)	Digoxin, digitoxin
Edetate calcium disodium (*Calcium Disodium Versenate*)	Lead
Flumazenil (*Romazicon*)	Benzodiazepines
Fomepizole (*Antizol*)	Ethylene glycol, methanol
Mesna (*Mesnex*)	Ifosfamide-induced hemorrhagic cystitis
Methylene blue (Various)	Nitrites
Narcotic antagonists Naloxone (*Narcan*) Naltrexone (*ReVia*)	Opioids
Physostigmine salicylate (*Antilirium*)	Anticholinergics (including tricyclic antidepressants)
Pralidoxime Cl (*Protopam Cl*)	Organophosphates Anticholinesterases
Sodium thiosulfate (Various)	Cyanide
Succimer (*Chemet*)	Lead
Trientene (*Syprine*)	Copper
Other agents used additionally as antidotes:	
Acetylcysteine (*Mucomyst, Mucosil*)	Acetaminophen
Amyl nitrite, Na Nitrite, Na Thiosulfate (*Cyanide antidote kit*)	Cyanide
Anticholinesterases Pyridostigmine Br (*Mestinon, Regonol*) Neostigmine Br (*Prostigmin*) Edrophonium Cl (*Tensilon*)	Nondepolarizing muscle relaxants
Atropine (Various)	Cholinergic agents: Organophosphates, carbamates, pilocarpine, physostigmine, or choline esters.
Glucagon	Insulin-induced hypoglycemia, beta blockers
Hydroxocobalamin (Various)	Cyanide poisoning
Leucovorin calcium (*Wellcovorin*)	Folic acid antagonists (eg, methotrexate)
Protamine sulfate (Various)	Heparin
Pyridoxine	Isoniazid
Vitamin K_1 (Various)	Oral anticoagulants
Nonspecific therapy of overdoses include the following:	
Activated charcoal (Various) Cathartics Osmotic diuretics Polyethylene glycol electrolyte solution (*GoLYTELY*) Syrup of ipecac (Various) Urinary acidifiers Urinary alkalinizers	Nonspecific, supportive therapies of overdoses. See also General Management of Acute Overdosage.

Chelating Agents

TRIENTINE HYDROCHLORIDE

Rx	**Syprine** (Aton)	**Capsules; oral:** 250 mg	(SYPRINE/MSD 661). Light brown. In 100s.

TRIENTINE HYDROCHLORIDE — ORAL

Indications

➤*Wilson disease:* Treatment of patients with Wilson disease who are intolerant of penicillamine.

Administration and Dosage

➤*Adults:*

Wilson disease –

Maximum dose: 2,000 mg/day.

Initial dosage: 750 to 1,250 mg/day in divided doses 2, 3, or 4 times/day.

Dosage adjustment: Increase the daily dose only when the clinical response is not adequate or the concentration of free serum copper is persistently above 20 mcg/dL. Determine optimal long-term maintenance dosage at 6- to 12-month intervals.

➤*Children:*

Wilson disease –

See Adults for dosing for children 13 years of age and older.

12 years of age and younger:

• *Maximum dose* – 1,500 mg/day.

• *Initial dosage* – 500 to 750 mg/day in divided doses 2, 3, or 4 times/day.

• *Dosage adjustment* – Increase the daily dose only when the clinical response is not adequate or the concentration of free serum copper is persistently above 20 mcg/dL. Determine optimal long-term maintenance dosage at 6- to 12-month intervals.

➤*Administration:* Take on an empty stomach at least 1 hour before or 2 hours after meals and at least 1 hour apart from any other drug, food, or milk. Swallow the capsules whole and do not open or chew. Because of the potential for contact dermatitis, promptly wash any site of exposure to the capsule contents with water.

➤*Storage/Stability:* Store at 2° to 8°C (36° to 46°F).

Actions

➤*Pharmacology:* Wilson disease (hepatolenticular degeneration) is an inherited metabolic defect resulting in excess copper accumulation, possibly because the liver lacks the mechanism to excrete free copper into the bile. Hepatocytes store excess copper, but when their capacity is exceeded, copper is released into the blood and is taken up into extrahepatic sites. Treat this condition with a low copper diet and chelating agents that bind copper to facilitate its excretion from the body. Trientine is a chelating compound for removal of excess copper from the body.

Contraindications

Hypersensitivity to trientine.

TRIENTINE HYDROCHLORIDE — ORAL

Warnings/Precautions

➤*Not indicated for the following:* Not indicated for cystinuria; rheumatoid arthritis; biliary cirrhosis.

➤*Patient supervision:* Patients should remain under regular medical supervision throughout the period of drug administration.

➤*Iron deficiency anemia:* Closely monitor patients (especially women) for evidence of iron deficiency anemia.

➤*Hypersensitivity:* There are no reports of hypersensitivity in patients given trientine for Wilson disease. However, there have been reports of asthma, bronchitis, and dermatitis occurring after prolonged environmental exposure in workers who use trientine as a hardener of epoxy resins. Observe patients closely for signs of possible hypersensitivity. Refer to Management of Hypersensitivity Reactions.

➤*Pregnancy: Category C.* Trientine was teratogenic in rats at doses similar to the human dose. The frequencies of resorptions and fetal abnormalities, including hemorrhage and edema, increased while fetal copper levels decreased. There are no adequate and well-controlled studies in pregnant women. Use during pregnancy only when the potential benefits outweigh the potential hazards to the fetus.

➤*Lactation:* It is not known whether this drug is excreted in breast milk. Exercise caution when administering to a breast-feeding woman.

➤*Children:* Safety and efficacy for use in children have not been established. Trientine has been used clinically in children as young as 6 years of age with no reported adverse effects.

➤*Elderly:* In general, dose selection should be cautious, usually starting at the low end of the dosing range, reflecting the greater frequency of decreased hepatic, renal, or cardiac function, and of concomitant disease or other drug therapy.

➤*Monitoring:* The most reliable index for monitoring treatment is the determination of free copper in the serum, which equals the difference between quantitatively determined total copper and ceruloplasmin-copper. Adequately treated patients will usually have less than 10 mcg free copper/dL of serum.

Therapy may be monitored with a 24-hour urinary copper analysis periodically (ie, every 6 to 12 months). Urine must be collected in copper-free glassware. Because a low copper diet should keep copper absorption down to less than 1 mg/day, the patient probably will be in the desired state of negative copper balance if 0.5 to 1 mg of copper is present in a 24-hour collection of urine.

Drug Interactions

➤*Mineral supplements:* In general, do not give mineral supplements; they may block the absorption of trientine. However, iron deficiency may develop, especially in children and menstruating or pregnant women, or as a result of the low copper diet recommended for Wilson disease. If necessary, iron may be given in short courses, but because iron and trientine each inhibit absorption of the other, allow 2 hours to elapse between administration of trientine and iron.

➤*Drug/Food interactions:* It is important that trientene be taken on an empty stomach at least 1 hour before or 2 hours after meals and at least 1 hour apart from any other drug, food, or milk. This permits maximum absorption; also, coadministration may inactivate trientine by metal binding in the GI tract.

Adverse Reactions

Iron deficiency, systemic lupus erythematosus, dystonia, muscular spasm, and myasthenia gravis have occurred in patients with Wilson disease who were being treated with trientine.

Trientine is not indicated for treatment of biliary cirrhosis, but in 1 study of 4 patients treated with trientine for primary biliary cirrhosis, the following adverse reactions were reported: Heartburn; epigastric pain and tenderness; thickening, fissuring, and flaking of the skin; hypochromic microcytic anemia; acute gastritis; aphthoid ulcers; abdominal pain; melena; anorexia; malaise; cramps; muscle pain; weakness; rhabdomyolysis. A causal relationship to drug therapy could not be rejected or established.

Overdosage

There is a report of an adult woman who ingested trientine 30 g without apparent ill effects.

Patient Information

Take on an empty stomach at least 1 hour before or 2 hours after meals and at least 1 hour apart from any other drug, food, or milk.

Swallow capsules whole with water. Do not open or chew.

Because of the potential for contact dermatitis, promptly wash any site of exposure to the capsule contents with water.

Take temperature nightly for the first month of treatment, and report any symptoms such as fever or skin eruption.

SUCCIMER (DMSA)

Rx	**Chemet** (Ovation)	**Capsules:** 100 mg	Sucrose. (Chemet 100). White. In 100s.

SUCCIMER — ORAL

Indications

➤*Lead poisoning:* Succimer is indicated for the treatment of lead poisoning in pediatric patients with blood lead levels greater than 45 mcg/dL. Succimer is not indicated for prophylaxis of lead poisoning in a lead-containing environment; the use of succimer should always be accompanied by identification and removal of the source of the lead exposure.

➤*Off-label uses:* Succimer may be beneficial in the treatment of other heavy metal poisonings (eg, mercury, arsenic); further study is needed.

Administration and Dosage

➤*General dosing considerations:* All patients undergoing treatment should be adequately hydrated.

Identification of the source of lead in the pediatric patient's environment and its abatement are critical to a successful therapy outcome. Chelation therapy is not a substitute for preventing further exposure to lead and should not be used to permit continued exposure to lead.

➤*Children:*

Lead poisoning –

12 months of age and older:

• *Initial dosage* – 10 mg/kg or 350 mg/m² every 8 hours for 5 days. Initiation of therapy at higher doses is not recommended.

Succimer Pediatric Dosing

kg	Dose[a]	Number of capsules[a]
8 to 15	100 mg	1
16 to 23	200 mg	2
24 to 34	300 mg	3
35 to 44	400 mg	4
> 45	500 mg	5

[a] To be administered every 8 hours for 5 days, followed by dosing every 12 hours for 14 days.

• *Dosage adjustment* – Reduce frequency of administration to 10 mg/kg or 350 mg/m² every 12 hours (two-thirds of initial daily dosage) for an additional 14 days.

• *Duration of therapy* – 19 days.

• *Concomitant therapy* – Patients who have received calcium EDTA with or without dimercaprol may use succimer for subsequent treatment after an interval of 4 weeks. Data on the concomitant use of succimer with calcium EDTA with or without dimercaprol are not available, and such use is not recommended.

• *Repeat course* – Repeated courses may be necessary if indicated by weekly monitoring of blood lead concentration. A minimum of 2 weeks between courses is recommended unless blood lead levels indicate the need for more prompt treatment.

➤*Administration:* In young children who cannot swallow capsules, succimer can be administered by separating the capsule and sprinkling the medicated beads on a small amount of soft food or putting them in a spoon and following with fruit drink.

➤*Storage/Stability:* Store between 15° and 25°C (59° and 77°F) and avoid excessive heat.

Actions

➤*Pharmacology:* Succimer is a lead chelator; it forms water-soluble chelates and, consequently, increases the urinary excretion of lead.

➤*Pharmacokinetics:*

Absorption – In a study performed in healthy adult volunteers, after a single dose of ^{14}C-succimer at 16, 32, or 48 mg/kg, absorption was rapid but variable, with peak blood radioactivity levels between 1 and 2 hours.

Metabolism/Excretion – On average, 49% of the radiolabeled dose was excreted: 39% in the feces, 9% in the urine, and 1% as carbon dioxide from the lungs. Since fecal excretion probably represented nonabsorbed drug, most of the absorbed drug was excreted by the kidneys. The apparent elimination half-life of the radiolabeled material in the blood was approximately 2 days.

In other studies of healthy adult volunteers receiving a single oral dose of 10 mg/kg, the chemical analysis of succimer and its metabolites in the urine showed that succimer was rapidly and extensively metabolized. Approximately 25% of the administered dose was excreted in the urine, with the peak blood level and urinary excretion occurring between 2 and 4 hours. Of the total amount of drug eliminated in the urine, approximately 90% was eliminated in altered form as mixed succimer-cysteine disulfides; the remaining 10% was eliminated unchanged. The majority of mixed disulfides consisted of succimer in disulfide linkages with 2 molecules of L-cysteine, the remaining disulfides contained one L-cysteine per succimer molecule.

SUCCIMER — ORAL

Contraindications

Allergy to the drug.

Warnings/Precautions

➤*Lead exposure:* Succimer is not a substitute for effective abatement of lead exposure.

➤*Neutropenia:* Mild-to-moderate neutropenia has been observed in some patients receiving succimer. While a causal relationship to succimer has not been definitely established, neutropenia has been reported with other drugs in the same chemical class. A complete blood count with white blood cell differential and direct platelet counts should be obtained prior to and weekly during treatment with succimer. Therapy should either be withheld or discontinued if the absolute neutrophil count (ANC) is less than 1,200/mcL and the patient is followed closely to document recovery of the ANC to greater than 1,500/mcL or to the patient's baseline neutrophil count. There is limited experience with reexposure in patients who have developed neutropenia. Therefore, such patients should be rechallenged only if the benefit of succimer therapy clearly outweighs the potential risk of another episode of neutropenia and then only with careful patient monitoring.

Patients treated with succimer should be instructed to promptly report any signs of infection. If infection is suspected, the above laboratory tests should be conducted immediately.

➤*Rebound blood lead levels:* Elevated blood lead levels and associated symptoms may return rapidly after discontinuation of succimer because of redistribution of lead from bone stores to soft tissues and blood. After therapy, patients should be monitored for rebound of blood lead levels, by measuring blood lead levels at least once weekly until stable. However, the severity of lead intoxication (as measured by the initial blood lead level and the rate and degree of rebound of blood lead) should be used as a guide for more frequent blood lead monitoring.

➤*Repeated courses:* Clinical experience with repeated courses is limited. The safety of uninterrupted dosing longer than 3 weeks has not been established, and it is not recommended.

➤*Hypersensitivity reactions:* The possibility of allergic or other mucocutaneous reactions to the drug must be borne in mind on readministration (as well as during initial courses). Patients requiring repeated courses of succimer should be monitored during each treatment course. One patient experienced recurrent mucocutaneous vesicular eruptions of increasing severity affecting the oral mucosa, the external urethral meatus and the perianal area on the third, fourth, and fifth courses of the drug. The reaction resolved between courses and upon discontinuation of therapy.

➤*Renal function impairment:* All patients undergoing treatment should be adequately hydrated. Caution should be exercised in using succimer therapy in patients with compromised renal function. Limited data suggests that succimer is dialyzable, but that the lead chelates are not.

➤*Hepatic function impairment:* Transient mild elevations of serum transaminases have been observed in 6% to 10% of patients during the course of succimer therapy. Serum transaminases should be monitored before the start of therapy and at least weekly during therapy. Patients with histories of liver disease should be monitored closely. No data are available regarding the metabolism of succimer in patients with liver disease.

➤*Pregnancy: Category C.*

Teratogenic – Succimer has been shown to be teratogenic and fetotoxic in pregnant mice when given subcutaneously in a dose range of 410 to 1,640 mg/kg/day during the period of organogenesis. There are no adequate and well-controlled studies in pregnant women. Succimer should be used during pregnancy only if the potential benefit justifies the potential risk to the fetus.

➤*Lactation:* It is not known whether this drug is excreted in human milk. Because many drugs and heavy metals are excreted in human milk, nursing mothers requiring succimer therapy should be discouraged from breastfeeding their infants.

➤*Children:* Safety and efficacy in pediatric patients younger than 12 months of age have not been established.

➤*Monitoring:* The extent of clinical experience with succimer is limited. Therefore, patients should be carefully observed during treatment.

Neutropenia – See Warnings/Precautions for more information.

Drug Interactions

Succimer is not known to interact with other drugs, including iron supplements; interactions have not been systematically studied. Concomitant administration of succimer with other chelation therapy, such as calcium EDTA is not recommended.

➤*Drug/Lab test interactions:* Succimer may interfere with serum and urinary laboratory tests. In vitro studies have shown succimer to cause false-positive results for ketones in urine using nitroprusside reagents such as *Ketostix* and falsely decreased measurements of serum uric acid and CPK.

Adverse Reactions

Clinical experience with succimer has been limited. Consequently, the full spectrum and incidence of adverse reactions, including the possibility of hypersensitivity or idiosyncratic reactions, have not been determined. The most common events attributable to succimer (ie, GI symptoms, increases in serum transaminases), have been observed in approximately 10% of patients. Transient mild elevations of serum transaminases have been observed in 6% to 10% of patients during the course of succimer therapy. Rashes, some necessitating discontinuation of therapy, have been reported in approximately 4% of patients. If rash occurs, other causes (eg, measles) should be considered before ascribing the reaction to succimer.

Rechallenge with succimer may be considered if lead levels are high enough to warrant retreatment. One allergic mucocutaneous reaction has been reported on repeated administration of the drug. The patient experienced recurrent mucocutaneous vesicular eruptions of increasing severity affecting the oral mucosa, the external urethral meatus and the perianal area on the third, fourth, and fifth courses of the drug. Mild-to-moderate neutropenia has been observed in some patients receiving succimer. While a causal relationship to succimer has not been definitely established, neutropenia has been reported with other drugs in the same chemical class. The following information presents adverse events reported with the administration of succimer for the treatment of lead and other heavy metal intoxication.

Incidence of Adverse Reactions in Domestic Studies Regardless of Attribution or Succimer Dosage

	Pediatric patients (191)		Adults (134)	
	%	(n)	%	(n)
GI				
Nausea, vomiting, diarrhea, appetite loss, hemorrhoidal symptoms, loose stools, metallic taste in mouth	12%	23	20.9%	28
Metabolic				
Elevated ALT, AST, alkaline phosphatase, elevated serum cholesterol	4.2%	8	10.4%	14
CNS				
Drowsiness, dizziness, sensorimotor neuropathy, sleepiness, paresthesia	1%	2	12.7%	17
Dermatologic				
Papular rash, herpetic rash, rash, mucocutaneous eruptions, pruritus	2.6%	5	11.2%	15
Special senses				
Cloudy film in eye, ears plugged, otitis media, eyes watery	1%	2	3.7%	5
Respiratory				
Sore throat, rhinorrhea, nasal congestion, cough	3.7%	7	0.7%	1
GU				
Decreased urination, voiding difficulty, increased proteinuria	0%		3.7%	5
Cardiovascular				
Arrhythmia	0%		1.8%	2
Hematologic-lymphatic				
Mild-to-moderate neutropenia, increased platelet count, intermittent eosinophilia	0.5[a]	1	1.5[a]	2
Musculoskeletal				
Kneecap pain, leg pains	0%		3%	4
Miscellaneous				
Back pain, abdominal cramps, stomach pains, head pain, rib pain, chills, flank pain, fever, flu-like symptoms, heavy head/tired, head cold, headache, moniliasis	5.2%	10	15.7%	21

[a] Does not include neutropenia.

Overdosage

➤*Symptoms:* Doses of 2,300 mg/kg in the rat and 2,400 mg/kg in the mouse produced ataxia, convulsions, labored respiration, and frequently death. No case of overdosage has been reported in humans. Limited data indicate that succimer is dialyzable.

➤*Treatment:* In case of acute overdosage, induction of vomiting or gastric lavage followed by administration of an activated charcoal slurry and appropriate supportive therapy are recommended.

Patient Information

Patients should be instructed to maintain adequate fluid intake. If rash occurs, patients should consult their physicians. Patients should be instructed to promptly report any indication of infection, which may be a sign of neutropenia.

In young pediatric patients unable to swallow capsules, the contents of the capsule can be administered in a small amount of food. Administer by separating the capsule and sprinkling the medicated beads on a small amount of soft food or putting them in a spoon and following with a fruit drink.

DIMERCAPROL

Rx	**BAL In Oil** (Taylor)	**Injection:** 10% (100 mg/mL)	In peanut oil with 20% benzyl benzoate. In 3 mL amps.

DIMERCAPROL — INJECTION

Indications

➤*Poisoning:* Treatment of arsenic, gold, and mercury poisoning. It is indicated in acute lead poisoning when used concomitantly with edetate calcium disodium injection.

Dimercaprol injection is effective for use in acute poisoning by mercury salts if therapy is begun within 1 or 2 hours following ingestion. It is not very effective for chronic mercury poisoning.

Dimercaprol injection is of questionable value in poisoning caused by other heavy metals such as antimony and bismuth.

Administration and Dosage

➤*General dosing considerations:* Successful treatment depends on beginning injections at the earliest possible moment and on the use of adequate amounts at frequent intervals. Always use other supportive measures in conjunction with dimercaprol injection therapy.

➤*Adults:*

Acute lead encephalopathy –

Initial dosage: 4 mg/kg body weight IM alone in the first dose.

Maintenance dosage: Administer 4 mg/kg body weight IM thereafter at 4-hour intervals in combination with edetate calcium disodium injection at a separate site. For less severe poisoning, reduce the dose to 3 mg/kg after the first dose.

Duration of therapy: Maintain treatment for 2 to 7 days, depending on clinical response.

Acute mercury poisoning – 5 mg/kg initially, followed by 2.5 mg/kg 1 or 2 times daily for 10 days.

Arsenic or gold poisoning –

Mild poisoning: 2.5 mg/kg of body weight IM 4 times daily for 2 days, 2 times on the third day, and once daily thereafter for 10 days.

Severe poisoning: 3 mg/kg IM every 4 hours for 2 days, 4 times on the third day, then twice daily thereafter for 10 days.

➤*Children:* See Adults for dosing.

➤*Renal function impairment:* Discontinue dimercaprol injection or use only with extreme caution if acute renal insufficiency develops during therapy.

➤*Hepatic function impairment:* Dimercaprol injection is contraindicated in most instances of hepatic insufficiency, with the exception of post-arsenical jaundice.

➤*Administration:* Administer by deep IM injection only.

➤*Storage/Stability:* Store at 15° to 25°C (59° to 77°F).

Actions

➤*Pharmacology:* The sulfhydryl groups of dimercaprol form complexes with certain heavy metals, thus preventing or reversing the metallic binding of sulfhydryl-containing enzymes. The complex is excreted. The sustained presence of dimercaprol promotes continued excretion of the metallic poisons (arsenic, gold, and mercury). It is also used in combination with edetate calcium disodium injection to promote the excretion of lead.

Contraindications

Dimercaprol injection is contraindicated in most instances of hepatic insufficiency with the exception of postarsenical jaundice. Discontinue the drug or use only with extreme caution if acute renal insufficiency develops during therapy.

Do not use in iron, cadmium, or selenium poisoning, as the resulting dimercaprol-metal complexes are more toxic than the metal alone, especially to the kidneys.

Warnings/Precautions

➤*Injection site reaction:* There may be local pain at the site of the injection. A reaction apparently peculiar to children is fever which may persist during therapy. It occurs in approximately 30% of children. A transient reduction of the percentage of polymorphonuclear leukocytes may also be observed.

➤*Urinary alkalinization:* Urinary alkalinization is recommended because the dimercaprol-metal complex breaks down easily in an acid medium. Alkaline urine protects the kidney during therapy.

➤*G-6-PD deficiency:* Use with caution in these patients; hemolysis may occur.

➤*Renal function impairment:* Discontinue dimercaprol injection or use only with extreme caution if acute renal insufficiency develops during therapy.

➤*Hepatic function impairment:* Dimercaprol injection is contraindicated in most instances of hepatic insufficiency, with the exception of post-arsenical jaundice.

➤*Pregnancy: Category C.* Animal reproduction studies have not been conducted with dimercaprol injection. It is also not known whether dimercaprol injection can cause fetal harm when administered to a pregnant woman, or can affect reproduction capacity. Give dimercaprol injection to a pregnant woman only if clearly needed.

➤*Lactation:* It is not known whether this drug is excreted in human milk. However, because many drugs are excreted in human milk, exercise caution when administering dimercaprol injection to a breast-feeding woman.

Drug Interactions

➤*Iron:* Do not administer medicinal iron to patients under therapy with dimercaprol injection.

Adverse Reactions

One of the most consistent responses to dimercaprol injection is a rise in blood pressure accompanied by tachycardia. This rise is roughly proportional to the dose administered. Doses larger than those recommended may cause other transitory signs and symptoms in approximate order of frequency as follows: nausea and, in some instances, vomiting; headache; a burning sensation in the lips, mouth, and throat; a feeling of constriction, even pain, in the throat, chest, or hands; conjunctivitis, lacrimation, blepheral spasm, rhinorrhea, and salivation; tingling of the hands; a burning sensation in the penis; sweating of the forehead, hands, and other areas; abdominal pain; and occasional appearance of painful sterile abscesses. Many of the above symptoms are accompanied by a feeling of anxiety, weakness, and unrest and often are relieved by administration of antihistamine.

Overdosage

➤*Symptoms:* Dosage exceeding 5 mg/kg will usually be followed by vomiting, convulsions, and stupor, beginning within 30 minutes and subsiding within 6 hours following injection.

DEFEROXAMINE MESYLATE

Rx	**Deferoxamine Mesylate** (Hospira)	**Powder for injection, lyophilized:** 500 mg	In vials.
Rx	**Desferal** (Novartis)		In vials.
Rx	**Deferoxamine Mesylate** (Hospira)	**Powder for injection, lyophilized:** 2 g	In vials.
Rx	**Desferal** (Novartis)		In vials.

DEFEROXAMINE MESYLATE — INJECTION

Indications

➤*Acute iron intoxication:* An adjunct to standard treatment measures.

➤*Chronic iron overload:* Deferoxamine can promote iron excretion in patients with secondary iron overload from multiple transfusions (as may occur in the treatment of some chronic anemias, including thalassemia). Long-term therapy with deferoxamine slows hepatic iron accumulation; retards or eliminates hepatic fibrosis progression.

➤*Off-label uses:* In patients with chronic renal failure, deferoxamine has been used in the treatment of aluminum overload, commonly related to the use of aluminum-contaminated dialysate or ingestion of aluminum-containing phosphorous binding drugs.

Deferoxamine also has been used as a diagnostic test for iron storage disease in patients with normal renal function.

Administration and Dosage

➤*General dosing considerations:* Use IV administration for acute iron intoxication only in cardiovascular collapse and give by slow infusion.

Individualize dosage for treatment of chronic iron overload.

➤*Adults:*

Acute iron intoxication –

Intramuscularly:

- *Maximum dose* – Do not exceed 6 g/day.
- *Initial dosage* – 1 g, then 500 mg every 4 hours for 2 doses.
- *Maintenance dosage* – 500 mg every 4 to 12 hours based on clinical response.

Intravenously:

- *Maximum dose* – The total amount administered should not exceed 6 g/day.

DEFEROXAMINE MESYLATE — INJECTION

• *Initial dosage* – Administer an initial dose of 1 g at a rate not to exceed 15 mg/kg/h. This may be followed by 500 mg over 4 hours for 2 doses.

• *Maintenance dosage* – Depending on the clinical response, subsequent doses of 500 mg may be administered over 4 to 12 hours.

• *Duration of therapy* – As soon as possible, stop IV and give intramuscularly (IM).

Chronic iron overload –

Intramuscularly:

• *Usual dosage* – 500 mg to 1 g/day IM. Give an additional 2 g IV with, but separate from, each unit of blood. The rate of IV infusion must not exceed 15 mg/kg/h.

• *Maximum dose* – The total daily dose should not exceed 1 g in the absence of a transfusion, or 6 g even if 3 or more units of blood or packed red blood cells are transfused.

Subcutaneously: 1 to 2 g/day (20 to 40 mg/kg/day) over 8 to 24 hours with continuous mini-infusion pump. Individualize infusion duration.

➤*Children:*

Acute iron intoxication – See adults for dosing for children 3 years of age and older.

Chronic iron overload – See adults for dosing for children 3 years of age and older.

➤*Preparation for administration:* Deferoxamine is preferably dissolved by adding 5 mL sterile water for injection to each 500 mg vial or 20 mL sterile water for injection to each 2 g vial. The reconstituted deferoxamine solution is isotonic, clear, and colorless to slightly yellowish at the recommended concentration of 10%.

In clinical situations requiring a smaller volume of solution (eg, IM injection), deferoxamine may be dissolved by adding 2 mL sterile water for injection to each 500 mg vial or 8 mL sterile water for injection to each 2 g vial. This concentration may produce a stronger yellow colored solution. Completely dissolve the drug before the solution is withdrawn. Do not use turbid solutions.

Reconstituting deferoxamine in solvents or under conditions other than indicated may result in precipitation.

Deferoxamine reconstituted with sterile water for injection is for single use only.

The reconstituted solution is added to physiologic saline, glucose in water, or lactated Ringer's solution.

➤*Administration:* IM is the preferred route for the treatment of acute iron intoxication; use for all patients not in shock.

The rate of IV infusion should not exceed 15 mg/kg/h for the first 1 g administered. Subsequent IV dosing, if needed, must be at a slower rate, not to exceed 125 mg/h.

➤*Storage/Stability:* Do not store above 25°C (77°F).

Use the product immediately after reconstitution (commencement of treatment within 3 hours) for microbiological safety. When reconstitution is carried out under validated aseptic conditions (in a sterile laminar flow hood using aseptic technique), the product may be stored at room temperature for a maximum period of 24 hours before use. Do not refrigerate reconstituted solution.

Actions

➤*Pharmacology:* Deferoxamine chelates iron by forming a stable complex that prevents the iron from entering into further chemical reactions. It readily chelates iron from ferritin and hemosiderin but not readily from transferrin; it does not combine with the iron from cytochromes and hemoglobin. One hundred parts by weight can bind approximately 8.5 parts of ferric iron. Does not demonstrably increase electrolyte/trace metal excretion.

➤*Pharmacokinetics:* Deferoxamine is metabolized principally by plasma enzymes, but the pathways have not yet been defined. Iron chelate is excreted renally, giving urine a reddish color. Some is excreted in feces via bile. Elimination half-life is about 6 hours.

Contraindications

Severe renal disease or anuria.

Warnings/Precautions

➤*Primary hemochromatosis:* Deferoxamine is not indicated for the treatment of primary hemochromatosis because phlebotomy is the method of choice of removing excess iron in this disorder.

➤*Ocular and auditory disturbances:* Ocular and auditory disturbances have been reported when deferoxamine was administered over prolonged periods of time, at high doses, or in patients with low ferritin levels. The ocular disturbances observed have been blurring of vision; cataracts after prolonged administration in chronic iron overload; decreased visual acuity including visual loss, visual defects, scotoma; impaired peripheral, color, and night vision; optic neuritis, cataracts, corneal opacities, and retinal pigmentary abnormalities. The auditory abnormalities reported have been tinnitus and hearing loss including high frequency sensorineural hearing loss. In most cases, ocular and auditory disturbances were reversible upon immediate cessation of treatment.

Visual acuity tests, slit-lamp examinations, funduscopy, and audiometry are recommended periodically in patients treated for prolonged periods of time. Toxicity is more likely to be reversed if symptoms or test abnormalities are detected early.

➤*Acute respiratory distress syndrome:* Acute respiratory distress syndrome, also reported in children, has been described following treatment with excessively high IV doses in patients with acute iron intoxication or thalassemia.

➤*Infections:* Iron overload increases susceptibility of patients to *Yersinia enterocolitica* and *Yersinia pseudotuberculosis* infections. In some rare cases, treatment of deferoxamine has enhanced this susceptibility, resulting in generalized infections by providing this bacteria with a siderophore otherwise missing. In such cases, discontinue deferoxamine treatment until the infection is resolved.

In patients receiving deferoxamine, rare cases of mucormycosis, some with a fatal outcome, have been reported. If any of the suspected signs or symptoms occur, discontinue deferoxamine, carry out mycological tests, and institute appropriate treatment immediately.

➤*Aluminum overload:* In patients with aluminum-related encephalopathy, high doses of deferoxamine may exacerbate neurological dysfunction (seizures), probably owing to an acute increase in circulating aluminum. Deferoxamine may precipitate the onset of dialysis dementia. Treatment with deferoxamine in the presence of aluminum overload may result in decreased serum calcium and aggravation of hyperparathyroidism.

➤*Rapid infusion:* Flushing of the skin, urticaria, hypotension, and shock have occurred in a few patients with rapid IV injection. Therefore, give deferoxamine IM or by slow subcutaneous or IV infusion.

➤*Vitamin C use:* Patients with iron overload usually become vitamin C deficient, probably because iron oxidizes the vitamin. As an adjuvant to iron chelation therapy, vitamin C in doses up to 200 mg for adults may be given in divided doses, starting after an initial month of regular treatment with deferoxamine. Vitamin C increases availability of iron for chelation. In general, 50 mg/day suffices for children under 10 years of age and 100 mg/day for older children. Larger doses of vitamin C fail to produce any additional increase in excretion of iron complex.

In patients with severe chronic iron overload, impairment of cardiac function has been reported following concomitant treatment with deferoxamine and high doses of vitamin C (more than 500 mg/day in adults). The cardiac dysfunction was reversible when vitamin C was discontinued. Take the following precautions when vitamin C and deferoxamine are to be used concomitantly: a) do not give vitamin C supplements to patients with cardiac failure; b) start supplemental vitamin C only after an initial month of regular treatment with deferoxamine; c) give vitamin C only if the patient is receiving deferoxamine regularly, ideally soon after setting up the infusion pump; d) do not exceed the daily vitamin C dose of 200 mg in adults, given in divided doses; e) clinical monitoring of cardiac function is advisable during such combined therapy.

➤*Pregnancy:* *Category C* per manufacturer's prescribing information. *Category B* per Briggs' *Drugs in Pregnancy and Lactation*. Delayed ossification in mice and skeletal anomalies in rabbits were observed after deferoxamine was administered in daily doses up to 4.5 times the maximum daily human dose. No adverse effects were observed in similar studies in rats. There are no adequate and well-controlled studies in pregnant women. Use deferoxamine during pregnancy only if the potential benefit justifies the potential risk to the fetus.

➤*Lactation:* It is not known whether this drug is excreted in human milk. Exercise caution when deferoxamine is administered to a breast-feeding woman.

➤*Children:* Safety and efficacy in pediatric patients younger than 3 years of age have not been established. Iron mobilization by deferoxamine is relatively poor in patients younger than 3 years of age with relatively little iron overload. Ordinarily, do not give the drug to such patients unless significant iron mobilization (eg, 1 mg or more of iron/day) can be demonstrated.

High doses of deferoxamine and concomitant low ferritin levels also have been associated with growth retardation. After reduction of deferoxamine dose, growth velocity may partially resume to pretreatment rates.

Monitor children receiving deferoxamine for body weight and growth every 3 months.

Drug Interactions

Deferoxamine Drug Interactions			
Precipitant drug	Object drug[a]		Description
Deferoxamine	Gallium-67	⬇	Imaging results may be distorted because of the rapid urinary excretion of deferoxamine-bound gallium-67. Discontinue deferoxamine 48 hours prior to scintigraphy.
Deferoxamine	Prochlorperazine	⬆	Concurrent use may lead to temporary impairment of consciousness.

[a] ⬆ = Object drug increased. ⬇ = Object drug decreased.

Adverse Reactions

The following adverse reactions have been observed, but there are not enough data to support an estimate of their frequency.

➤*Cardiovascular:* Hypotension, shock, tachycardia.

DEFEROXAMINE MESYLATE — INJECTION

➤*CNS:* Neurological disturbances including dizziness, peripheral sensory, motor, or mixed neuropathy, paresthesias; exacerbation or precipitation of aluminum-related dialysis encephalopathy (see Precautions).

➤*GI:* Abdominal discomfort, diarrhea, nausea, vomiting.

➤*GU:* Dysuria, impaired renal function (see Contraindications); reddish urine (see Pharmacokinetics).

➤*Hematologic:* Blood dyscrasia (ie, cases of thrombocytopenia and/or leukopenia have been reported. A causal relationship has not been clearly established).

➤*Hypersensitivity:* Anaphylactic reaction with or without shock, angioedema, generalized rash, urticaria.

➤*Local:* Burning, crusting, erythema, eschar, induration, infiltration, local edema, localized irritation, pain, pruritus, swelling, vesicles, wheal formation. Injection site reactions may be associated with systemic allergic reactions.

➤*Musculoskeletal:* Leg cramps have occurred. Growth retardation and bone changes (eg, metaphyseal dysplasia) are common in chelated patients given doses above 60 mg/kg, especially those who begin iron chelation in the first 3 years of life. If doses are kept to 40 mg/kg or below, the risk may be reduced (see Warnings).

➤*Respiratory:* Acute respiratory distress syndrome (with dyspnea, cyanosis, and/or interstitial infiltrates) (see Warnings).

➤*Special senses:* High-frequency sensorineural hearing loss and/or tinnitus are uncommon if dosage guidelines are not exceeded and if dose is reduced when ferritin levels decline. Visual disturbances are rare if dosage guidelines are not exceeded. These may include decreased acuity, blurred vision, loss of vision, dyschromatopsia, night blindness, visual field defects, scotoma, retinopathy (pigmentary degeneration), optic neuritis, and cataracts (see Warnings).

➤*Miscellaneous:* Local injection site reactions may be accompanied by systemic reactions (eg, arthralgia, fever, headache, myalgia, nausea, vomiting, abdominal pain, asthma). Generalized rash has occurred very rarely.

Rare infections with *Yersinia* and mucormycosis have been reported in association with deferoxamine use (see Precautions).

Overdosage

➤*Symptoms:* Inadvertent administration of an overdose or inadvertent IV bolus administration/rapid IV infusion may be associated with hypotension, tachycardia, and GI disturbances; acute but transient loss of vision, aphasia, agitation, headache, nausea, pallor, CNS depression including coma, bradycardia, and acute renal failure have been reported.

➤*Treatment:* There is no specific antidote. Discontinue deferoxamine and undertake appropriate symptomatic measures. Deferoxamine is readily dialyzable.

Patient Information

Patients experiencing dizziness or other nervous system disturbances or impairment of vision or hearing should refrain from driving or operating potentially hazardous machines.

Inform patients that occasionally their urine may show a reddish discoloration.

EDETATE CALCIUM DISODIUM

Rx	**Calcium Disodium Versenate** (Graceway)	**Injection solution:** 200 mg/mL	In 5 mL amps.

EDETATE CALCIUM DISODIUM — INJECTION

WARNING

Edetate calcium disodium is capable of producing toxic effects that can be fatal. Lead encephalopathy is relatively rare in adults, but occurs more often in pediatric patients in whom it may be incipient and thus overlooked. The mortality rate in pediatric patients has been high. Patients with lead encephalopathy and cerebral edema may experience a lethal increase in intracranial pressure following intravenous (IV) infusion; the intramuscular (IM) route is preferred for these patients. In cases where the IV route is necessary, avoid rapid infusion. The dosage schedule should be followed and at no time should the recommended daily dose be exceeded.

Indications

➤*Lead poisoning:* Edetate calcium disodium is indicated for the reduction of blood levels and depot stores of lead in lead poisoning (acute and chronic) and lead encephalopathy, in both pediatric populations and adults. Chelation therapy should not replace effective measures to eliminate or reduce further exposure to lead.

Administration and Dosage

➤*Adults:*

Lead poisoning –

Usual dosage: 1,000 mg/m²/day given IV or IM to asymptomatic patients whose blood lead level is less than 70 mcg/dL but greater than 20 mcg/dL (World Health Organization recommended upper allowable level).

When used alone, regardless of method of administration, edetate calcium disodium should not be given at doses larger than those recommended.

Alternative dosage:

- *For adults with lead nephropathy –*
  - *Serum creatinine levels of 2 to 3 mg/dL:* 500 mg/m² every 24 hours for 5 days.
  - *Serum creatinine levels of 3 to 4 mg/dL:* 500 mg/m² every 48 hours for 3 doses.
  - *Serum creatinine levels above 4 mg/dL:* 500 mg/m² once weekly. These regimens may be repeated at 1-month intervals.

Duration of therapy: 5 days. Therapy is then interrupted for 2 to 4 days to allow redistribution of the lead and to prevent severe depletion of zinc and other essential metals. Two courses of treatment are usually employed; however, it depends on severity of the lead toxicity and the patient's tolerance of the drug.

Concomitant therapy: When the blood lead level is greater than 70 mcg/dL or clinical symptoms consistent with lead poisoning are present, it is recommended that edetate calcium disodium be used in conjunction with dimercaprol. Please consult published protocols and specialized references for dosage recommendations of combination therapy.

Discontinuation of therapy: Administration of edetate calcium disodium should be stopped whenever there is cessation of urine flow in order to avoid unduly high tissue levels of the drug.

➤*Children:*

Lead poisoning – The IM route is preferred by some for young pediatric patients. In cases where the IV route is necessary, avoid rapid infusion.

Usual dosage: See Adults.

Duration of therapy: See Adults.

Concomitant therapy: See Adults.

Discontinuation of therapy: See Adults.

➤*Renal function impairment:* Edetate calcium disodium must be used in reduced doses in patients with preexisting mild renal disease.

Edetate calcium disodium therapy must be stopped if anuria or severe oliguria develops.

➤*Hepatic function impairment:* Edetate calcium disodium should not be given to patients with hepatitis.

➤*Administration:* Edetate calcium disodium is equally effective whether administered IV or IM. The IM route is used for all patients with overt lead encephalopathy and this route is preferred by some for young pediatric patients.

Acutely ill individuals may be dehydrated from vomiting. Since edetate calcium disodium is excreted almost exclusively in the urine, it is very important to establish urine flow with IV fluid administration before the first dose of the chelating agent is given; however, excessive fluid must be avoided in patients with encephalopathy. Once urine flow is established, further IV fluid is restricted to basal water and electrolyte requirements. Administration of edetate calcium disodium should be stopped whenever there is cessation of urine flow in order to avoid unduly high tissue levels of the drug. Monitor urine outflow throughout therapy.

IV administration – Add the total daily dose of edetate calcium disodium (1,000 mg/m²/day) to 250 to 500 mL of 5% dextrose or 0.9% sodium chloride injection. The total daily dose should be infused over a period of 8 to 12 hours.

IM administration – The total daily dosage (1,000 mg/m²/day) should be divided into equal doses spaced 8 to 12 hours apart. Lidocaine or procaine should be added to the edetate calcium disodium injection to minimize pain at the injection site. The final lidocaine or procaine concentration of 5 mg/mL (0.5%) can be obtained as follows: 0.25 mL of lidocaine 10% solution per 5 mL (entire contents of ampule) concentrated edetate calcium disodium; 1 mL of 1% lidocaine or procaine solution per mL of concentrated edetate calcium disodium.

➤*Admixture compatibility:*

Admixture incompatibility – Edetate calcium disodium injection is incompatible with dextrose 10%, invert sugar 10% in sodium chloride 0.9%, lactate Ringer's, Ringer's, one-sixth molar sodium lactate injections, and with injectable amphotericin B and hydralazine hydrochloride.

➤*Storage/Stability:* Store at 15° to 30°C (59° to 86°F).

Actions

➤*Pharmacology:* The pharmacologic effects of edetate calcium disodium are due to the formation of chelates with divalent and trivalent metals. A stable chelate will form with any metal that has the ability to displace calcium from the molecule, a feature shared by lead, zinc, cadmium, manganese, iron, and mercury. The amounts of manganese and iron mobilized are not significant. Copper is not mobilized and mercury is unavailable for chelation because it is too tightly bound to body ligands or it is stored in inaccessible body compartments.

The primary source of lead chelated by edetate calcium disodium is from bone; subsequently, soft-tissue lead is redistributed to bone when chelation is stopped. There is also some reduction in kidney lead levels following chelation therapy. It has been shown in animals that following a single dose of edetate calcium disodium urinary lead output increases, blood lead concen-

EDETATE CALCIUM DISODIUM — INJECTION

tration decreases, but brain lead is significantly increased due to internal redistribution of lead (see Warnings). These data are in agreement with the recent results of others in experimental animals showing that after a 5 day course of treatment there is no net reduction in brain lead.

➤*Pharmacokinetics:*

Absorption – Edetate calcium disodium is poorly absorbed from the GI tract.

Distribution – In blood, all the drug is found in the plasma. Edetate calcium disodium does not appear to penetrate cells; it is distributed primarily in the extracellular fluid with only about 5% of the plasma concentration found in spinal fluid.

Metabolism – Almost none of the compound is metabolized.

Excretion – The half-life of edetate calcium disodium is 20 to 60 minutes. The excretion of calcium by the body is not increased following IV administration of edetate calcium disodium, but the excretion of zinc is considerably increased.

Edetate calcium disodium is excreted primarily by the kidney, with about 50% excreted in 1 hour and over 95% within 24 hours.

Contraindications

Edetate calcium disodium should not be given during periods of anuria, nor to patients with active renal disease or hepatitis.

Warnings/Precautions

➤*Renal effects:* Edetate calcium disodium may produce the same renal damage as lead poisoning, such as proteinuria and microscopic hematuria. Treatment-induced nephrotoxicity is dose-dependent and may be reduced by ensuring adequate diuresis before therapy begins. Urine flow must be monitored throughout therapy which must be stopped if anuria or severe oliguria develop. The proximal tubule hydropic degeneration usually recovers upon cessation of therapy. Edetate calcium disodium must be used in reduced doses in patients with preexisting mild renal disease. Patients should be monitored for cardiac rhythm irregularities and other ECG changes during IV therapy.

➤*Pregnancy: Category B.* One reproduction study was performed in rats at doses up to 13 times the human dose and revealed no evidence of impaired fertility or harm to the fetus caused by edetate calcium disodium. Another reproduction study performed in rats at doses up to about 25 to 40 times the human dose revealed evidence of fetal malformations caused by edetate calcium disodium, which were prevented by simultaneous supplementation of dietary zinc. There are, however, no adequate and well-controlled studies in pregnant women. Because animal reproduction studies are not always predictive of human response, this drug should be used during pregnancy only if clearly needed.

Labor and delivery – Edetate calcium disodium has no recognized use during labor and delivery, and its effects during these processes are unknown.

➤*Lactation:* It is not known whether this drug is excreted in human milk. Because many drugs are excreted in human milk, caution should be exercised when edetate calcium disodium is administered to a breast-feeding woman.

➤*Children:* Because lead poisoning occurs in pediatric populations and adults but is frequently more severe in pediatric patients, edetate calcium disodium is used in patients of all ages. The IM route is preferred by some for young pediatric patients. In cases where the IV route is necessary, avoid rapid infusion (see Warning Box). Urine flow must be monitored throughout therapy; edetate calcium disodium therapy must be stopped if anuria or severe oliguria develops. At no time should the recommended daily dosage be exceeded.

➤*Monitoring:* Urinalysis and urine sediment, renal and hepatic function and serum electrolyte levels should be checked before each course of therapy and then be monitored daily during therapy in severe cases, and in less serious cases after the second and fifth day of therapy. Therapy must be discontinued at the first sign of renal toxicity. The presence of large renal epithelial cells or increasing number of red blood cells in urinary sediment or greater proteinuria call for immediate stopping of edetate calcium disodium administration. Alkaline phosphatase values are frequently depressed (possibly due to decreased serum zinc levels), but return to normal within 48 hours after cessation of therapy. Elevated erythrocyte protoporphyrin levels (greater than 35 mcg/dL of whole blood) indicate the need to perform a venous blood lead determination. If the whole blood lead concentration is between 25 to 55 mcg/dL a mobilization test can be considered (see Administration and Dosage, Diagnostic test). An elevation of urinary coproporphyrin (adults, greater than 250 mcg/day; pediatric patients under 80 pounds, greater than 75 mcg/day) and elevation of urinary delta aminolevulinic acid (ALA) (adults, greater than 4 mg/day; pediatric patients, greater than 3 mg/ m^2/day) are associated with blood lead levels greater than 40 mcg/dL. Urinary coproporphyrin may be falsely negative in terminal patients and in severely iron-depleted pediatric patients who are not regenerating heme. In growing pediatric patients long bone x-rays showing lead lines and abdominal x-rays showing radioopaque material in the abdomen may be of help in estimating the level of exposure to lead.

Drug Interactions

Steroids enhance the renal toxicity of edetate calcium disodium in animals. Edetate calcium disodium interferes with the action of zinc insulin preparations by chelating the zinc.

Adverse Reactions

The following adverse reactions have been associated with the use of edetate calcium disodium:

➤*Allergic:* Histamine-like reactions (sneezing, nasal congestion, lacrimation), rash.

➤*Cardiovascular:* Hypotension, cardiac rhythm irregularities.

➤*CNS:* Tremors, headache, numbness, tingling.

➤*GI:* Cheilosis, nausea, vomiting, anorexia, excessive thirst.

➤*GU:* Glycosuria, proteinuria, microscopic hematuria and large epithelial cells in urinary sediment.

➤*Hematologic:* Transient bone marrow depression, anemia.

➤*Lab test abnormalities:* Mild increases in AST and ALT are common, and return to normal within 48 hours after cessation of therapy.

➤*Metabolic:* Zinc deficiency, hypercalcemia.

➤*Renal:* Acute necrosis of proximal tubules (which may result in fatal nephrosis), infrequent changes in distal tubules and glomeruli.

➤*Miscellaneous:* Pain at IM injection site, fever, chills, malaise, fatigue, myalgia, arthralgia.

Overdosage

➤*Symptoms:* Inadvertent administration of 5 times the recommended dose, infused IV over a 24-hour period, to an asymptomatic 16-month-old patient with a blood lead content of 56 mcg/dL did not cause any ill effects. Edetate calcium disodium can aggravate the symptoms of severe lead poisoning, therefore, most toxic effects (cerebral edema, renal tubular necrosis) appear to be associated with lead poisoning. Because of cerebral edema, a therapeutic dose may be lethal to an adult or a pediatric patient with lead encephalopathy. Higher dosage of edetate calcium disodium may produce a more severe zinc deficiency.

➤*Treatment:* Cerebral edema should be treated with repeated doses of mannitol. Steroids enhance the renal toxicity of edetate calcium disodium in animals and, therefore, are no longer recommended. Zinc levels must be monitored. Good urinary output must be maintained because diuresis will enhance drug elimination. It is not known if edetate calcium disodium is dialyzable.

Patient Information

Patients should be instructed to immediately inform their physician if urine output stops for a period of 12 hours.

PENTETATE ZINC TRISODIUM (Zn-DTPA)

Rx	**Pentetate Zinc Trisodium** (Akorn)	**Solution:** 200 mg/mL	In 5 mL single-use ampules.

PENTETATE ZINC TRISODIUM (Zn-DTPA) — INJECTION OR INHALATION

Indications

➤*Radiation contamination:* For treatment of individuals with known or suspected internal contamination with plutonium, americium, or curium to increase the rates of elimination.

Administration and Dosage

➤*General dosing considerations:* It is preferable to administer pentetate calcium trisodium, if available, as the initial dose during the first 24 hours after internal contamination because pentetate calcium trisodium is more effective than pentetate zinc trisodium during this time period. After 24 hours, pentetate zinc trisodium and pentetate calcium trisodium are equally effective.

Drink plenty of fluids and void frequently to promote dilution of the radioactive chelate in the urine and minimize radiation exposure directly to the bladder.

➤*Adults:*

Radiation contamination –

Initial dosage: A single 1 g dose IV.

Maintenance dosage: 1 g once daily IV.

➤*Children:*

Radiation contamination – See Adults for dosing for children 12 years of age and older.

11 years of age and younger:
- *Maximum dose* – 1 g/day.
- *Initial dosage* – A single 14 mg/kg dose IV, not to exceed 1 g.
- *Maintenance dosage* – 14 mg/kg once daily IV, not to exceed 1 g/day.

➤*Chelation treatment:* Chelation treatment is most effective if administered within the first 24 hours after internal contamination and should be started as soon as possible after suspected or known internal contamination. However, even when treatment cannot be started right away, give individuals chelation treatment as soon as it becomes available. Chelation treatment is still effective even after time has elapsed following internal contamina-

PENTETATE ZINC TRISODIUM (Zn-DTPA) — INJECTION OR INHALATION

tion; however, the chelating effects of pentetate zinc trisodium are greatest when the radiocontaminants are still circulating or are in interstitial fluids. The efficacy of chelation decreases with time following internal contamination as the radiocontaminants become sequestered in liver and bone.

➤*Concomitant therapy:* If internal contamination with radiocontaminants other than plutonium, americium, or curium, or unknown radiocontaminants is suspected, additional therapies may be needed (eg, Prussian blue, potassium iodide).

➤*Duration of therapy:* The duration of chelation treatment depends on the amount of internal contamination and individual response to treatment.

➤*Preparation for administration:*

IV – Dilute in 100 to 250 mL of dextrose 5% in water, lactated Ringer's solution, or normal saline.

Inhalation – Dilute for nebulization at a 1:1 ratio with sterile water or saline.

➤*Administration:*

IV – The IV route is recommended and should be used if the route of internal contamination is not known or if multiple routes of internal contamination are likely. Administer solution (1 g in 5 mL) either with a slow IV push over a period of 3 to 4 minutes or by IV infusion over 30 minutes (further dilution required).

Inhalation – In individuals whose internal contamination is only by inhalation, administer by nebulized inhalation as an alternative route of administration. The safety and efficacy of the nebulized route of administration have not been established in children. After nebulization, encourage individuals to avoid swallowing any expectorant. Some individuals may experience respiratory adverse reactions after inhalation therapy.

➤*Storage/Stability:* Store between 15° and 30°C (59° and 86°F).

Actions

➤*Pharmacology:* Pentetate zinc trisodium forms stable chelates with metal ions by exchanging zinc for a metal of greater binding capacity. The radioactive chelates are then excreted by glomerular filtration into the urine. In animal studies, pentetate zinc trisodium forms less stable chelates with uranium and neptunium in vivo, resulting in deposition of these elements in tissues, including the bone. Pentetate zinc trisodium treatments are not expected for uranium and neptunium. Radioactive iodine is not bound by pentetate trisodium.

The efficacy of chelation decreases with time after internal contamination because the transuranium elements become incorporated into the tissues. Give chelation treatment as soon as possible after known or suspected internal contamination with transuranium elements has occurred.

Pentetate zinc trisodium results in minimal depletion of magnesium and manganese.

➤*Pharmacokinetics:*

Absorption – Pentetate zinc trisodium is poorly absorbed in the GI tract. In animal studies, after oral administration, absorption was approximately 5%. In a US Registry of 18 patients who received a single inhaled or IV dose of 1 g, urine data indicate that the inhaled product was absorbed and resulted in a comparable elimination of the radiocontaminant. One study of 2 human subjects who received pentetate calcium trisodium with ^{14}C-DTPA by inhalation revealed approximately 20% absorption from the lungs. Human or animal bioavailability comparisons for pentetate zinc trisodium are not available after administration by inhalation and IV injection.

Distribution – Following IV administration, pentetate zinc trisodium is rapidly distributed throughout the extracellular fluid space. No significant amount of pentetate zinc trisodium penetrates into erythrocytes or other cells. No accumulation of pentetate zinc trisodium in specific organs has been observed. There is little or no binding of the chelating agent by the renal parenchyma.

Metabolism – pentetate zinc trisodium undergoes a minimal amount of metabolic change in the body.

Excretion – Pentetate zinc trisodium is cleared from the plasma in the first few hours after dosing through urinary excretion by glomerular filtration. Renal tubular excretion has not been documented. In stool samples, only a very small amount of radioactivity (less than 3%) was detected.

Special populations –

Renal function impairment: Both pentetate zinc trisodium and its radioactive chelates are excreted by glomerular filtration. Impaired renal function may decrease their rates of elimination and increase the serum half-life of pentetate zinc trisodium.

Contraindications

None known.

Warnings/Precautions

➤*Exacerbation of asthma:* Nebulized chelation therapy may be associated with exacerbation of asthma. Exercise caution when administering pentetate zinc trisodium by the inhalation route.

➤*Endogenous metal depletion:* Treatment over several months with pentetate zinc trisodium could lead to depletion of body stores of endogenous metals (eg, magnesium, manganese). Routinely monitor these elements and, if appropriate, provide mineral or vitamin-plus-mineral supplements.

➤*Unknown/multiple radiocontaminants:* When an individual is contaminated with multiple radiocontaminants, or when the radiocontaminants are unknown, additional therapies may be needed (eg, Prussian blue, potassium iodide).

➤*Collection of patient treatment data:* To develop long-term response data and information on the risk of developing late malignancy, provide detailed information on patient treatment to the manufacturer. These data should include a record of the radioactive body burden and bioassay results at defined time intervals, a description of measurement methods to facilitate analysis of data, and adverse reactions.

Refer questions regarding the use of pentetate zinc trisodium for the treatment of internal contamination with transuranium elements to the manufacturer.

➤*Pregnancy: Category B.* There are no human pregnancy outcome data from which to assess the risk of pentetate zinc trisodium exposure on fetal development. Reproduction studies have been performed in pregnant mice at doses up to 11.5 mmol/kg (31 times the recommended daily dose of 1 g based on body surface area [BSA] adjusted dose) and have revealed no evidence of impaired fertility or harm to the fetus. There was a slight reduction in the average birth weight. Treatment of pregnant women should begin and continue with pentetate zinc trisodium. Use during pregnancy only if clearly needed. Weigh the risk of toxicity from untreated internal radioactive contamination against the risk of pentetate zinc trisodium treatment.

➤*Lactation:* Studies to determine if pentetate zinc trisodium is excreted in breast milk have not been conducted. Radiocontaminants are known to be excreted in breast milk. Women with known or suspected internal contamination with radiocontaminants should not breastfeed, whether or not they are receiving chelation therapy. Take precautions when discarding breast milk.

➤*Children:* The safety and efficacy of pentetate zinc trisodium were established in the adult population and efficacy was extrapolated to the pediatric population for the IV route based on the comparability of pathophysiologic mechanisms. The dose is based on body size adjustment for an IV drug that is renally cleared. The safety and efficacy of the nebulized route of administration have not been established in the pediatric population.

➤*Monitoring:* Closely monitor serum electrolytes and essential metals during pentetate zinc trisodium treatment. Mineral or vitamin-plus-mineral supplements may be given as appropriate.

When possible, obtain baseline blood and urine samples (complete blood count [CBC] with differential, blood urea nitrogen [BUN], serum chemistries and electrolytes, urinalysis, and blood and urine radioassays) before initiating treatment.

To establish an elimination curve, obtain a quantitative baseline estimate of the total internalized transuranium elements and measures of radioactivity elimination by appropriate whole-body counting, bioassay (eg, biodosimetry), or fecal/urine sample whenever possible.

During treatment –

- Measure the radioactivity in blood, urine, and fecal samples weekly to monitor the radioactive contaminant elimination rate.
- Monitor CBC with differential, BUN, serum chemistries and electrolytes, and urinalysis measurements regularly.
- Record any adverse reactions from pentetate zinc trisodium.

Drug Interactions

None well documented.

Adverse Reactions

Overall, the presence or absence of adverse reactions was recorded in 310 of 646 individuals. Of these, 19 (6.1%) individuals reported at least 1 adverse reaction. The total number of recorded adverse reactions was 20. Of the 20 adverse reactions, 1 individual treated with pentetate zinc trisodium reported headache, light-headedness, and pelvic pain.

Two individuals experienced cough and/or wheezing with nebulized pentetate calcium trisodium therapy; however, there was no such report of such reactions with nebulized pentetate zinc trisodium.

Patient Information

In individuals with recent internal contamination with plutonium, americium, or curium, pentetate zinc trisodium treatment increases excretion of radioactivity in the urine. Take appropriate safety measures to minimize contamination of others.

When possible, use a toilet instead of a urinal, and flush several times after each use. Completely clean up spilled urine or feces and wash hands thoroughly. If blood or urine comes in contact with clothing or linens, wash them separately.

Drink plenty of fluids and void frequently.

If coughing occurs, carefully dispose of any expectorant. Avoid swallowing the expectorant if possible.

Parents and childcare givers should take extra precaution in handling the urine, feces, and expectorants of children to avoid any additional exposure to either the caregiver or to the child.

Breastfeeding mothers should take extra precaution in disposing of breast milk.

PENTETATE CALCIUM TRISODIUM (Ca-DTPA)

Rx	Pentetate Calcium Trisodium (Akorn)	Injection: 200 mg/mL	In 5 mL single-use ampules.

PENTETATE CALCIUM TRISODIUM (Ca-DTPA) — INJECTION OR INHALATION

Indications

➤*Internal contamination:* Pentetate calcium trisodium is indicated for treatment of individuals with known or suspected internal contamination with plutonium, americium, or curium to increase the rates of elimination.

Administration and Dosage

➤*General dosing considerations:* If additional chelation therapy is indicated after the initial dose, on the next day, it is preferable to switch to pentetate zinc trisodium if available because of the safety concerns associated with prolonged pentetate calcium trisodium use. If pentetate zinc trisodium is not available, treatment may continue with pentetate calcium trisodium; however, give mineral supplements containing zinc concomitantly, as appropriate.

Drink plenty of fluids and void frequently to promote dilution of the radioactive chelate in the urine and minimize radiation exposure directly to the bladder.

➤*Adults:*

Internal contamination –

Initial dosage: A single 1 g dose IV.

Maintenance dosage: 1 g once daily IV. (See General Dosing Considerations.)

➤*Children:*

Internal contamination – See Adults for dosing for children older than 12 years of age

11 years of age and younger:

- *Maximum dose* – 1g/day.
- *Initial dosage* – A single 14 mg/kg dose IV, not to exceed 1 g.
- *Maintenance dosage* – 14 mg/kg once a day IV.

➤*Chelation treatment:* Chelation treatment is most effective if administered within the first 24 hours after internal contamination. Start as soon as possible after suspected or known internal contamination. However, even when treatment cannot be started right away, give individuals chelation treatment as soon as it becomes available. Chelation treatment is effective even after time has elapsed following internal contamination; however, the chelating effects of pentetate are greatest when radiocontaminants are circulating or are in interstitial fluids. The efficacy of chelation decreases with time following internal contamination as the radiocontaminants become sequestered in liver and bone.

➤*Concomitant therapy:* If internal contamination with radiocontaminants other than plutonium, americium, or curium, or unknown radiocontaminants is suspected, additional therapies may be needed (eg, Prussian blue, potassium iodide).

➤*Duration of therapy:* The duration of chelation treatment depends on the amount of internal contamination and individual response to treatment.

➤*Preparation for administration:* To open the ampule, turn so that the point faces upward and break off the neck with a downward movement. The product may be filtered using a sterile filter if particles are seen subsequent to opening of the ampule.

IV infusion – Dilute in 100 to 250 mL of dextrose 5% in water, Ringer's lactate, or normal lactate.

Inhalation – Dilute pentetate for nebulization at a 1:1 ratio with sterile water or saline.

➤*Administration:*

IV – IV administration is recommended; use if the route of internal contamination is not known or if multiple routes of internal contamination are likely. Administer solution (1 g in 5 mL) either with a slow IV push over a period of 3 to 4 minutes or by IV infusion (further dilution required).

Inhalation – In individuals whose internal contamination is only by inhalation within the preceding 24 hours, pentetate can be administered by nebulized inhalation as an alternative route of administration. The safety and efficacy of the nebulized route of administration have not been established in children. After nebulization, encourage individuals to avoid swallowing any expectorant. Some individuals may experience respiratory adverse reactions after inhalation therapy.

➤*Storage/Stability:* Store between 15° to 30°C (59° to 86°F).

Actions

➤*Pharmacology:* Pentetate calcium trisodium forms stable chelates with metal ions by exchanging calcium for a metal of greater binding capacity. The radioactive chelates are then excreted by glomerular filtration into the urine. In animal studies, pentetate calcium trisodium forms less stable chelates with uranium and neptunium in vivo resulting in the deposition of these elements in tissues, including the bone. Pentetate calcium trisodium treatments are not expected to be effective for uranium and neptunium. Radioactive iodine is not bound by pentetate trisodium.

Literature and US Registry data in humans indicate that IV administration of pentetate calcium trisodium forms chelates with radioactive contaminants found in the circulation, interstitial fluid, and tissues.

When pentetate calcium trisodium is administered by inhalation within 24 hours of internal radioactive contamination, it can chelate transuranium elements. Expectoration is expected to decrease the amount of radioactive contaminant available for systemic absorption.

The efficacy of chelation decreases with time after internal contamination because the transuranium elements become incorporated into the tissues. Give chelation treatment as soon as possible after known or suspected internal contamination with transuranium elements has occurred.

➤*Pharmacokinetics:*

Absorption – Pentetate calcium trisodium is absorbed poorly in the GI tract. In animal studies, after oral administration, absorption was approximately 5%. In a US Registry of 18 patients who received a single inhaled or IV dose of 1 g, urine data indicate that the inhaled product was absorbed and resulted in a comparable elimination of the radiocontaminant. One study of 2 human subjects that received pentetate calcium trisodium with ^{14}C-DTPA by inhalation revealed approximately 20% absorption from the lungs. Human or animal bioavailability comparisons for pentetate calcium trisodium are not available after administration by inhalation and IV injection.

Distribution – Following IV administration, pentetate calcium trisodium is distributed rapidly throughout the extracellular fluid space. No significant amount of pentetate calcium trisodium penetrates into erythrocytes or other cells. No accumulation of pentetate calcium trisodium in specific organs has been observed. There is little or no binding of the chelating agent by the renal parenchyma.

Metabolism – Pentetate calcium trisodium undergoes a minimal amount of metabolic change in the body.

Studies in animals and humans showed that pentetate calcium trisodium binds endogenous metals of the body (ie, zinc, magnesium, manganese). In an animal study, high doses of pentetate calcium trisodium led to the loss of zinc and manganese mainly from the small intestine, skeleton, pancreas, and testes. Dosing over several days resulted in mobilization or binding of endogenous metals in exchange for calcium and a consequent impairment of metal-controlled or activated systems. The rate and amount of endogenous metal depletion increased with split daily dosing and with the length of treatment. Depletion of these endogenous metals can interfere with necessary mitotic cellular processes. Over longer time periods, depletion of zinc caused by pentetate calcium trisodium therapy may result in transient inhibition of a metalloenzyme-d-aminolevulinic acid dehydrase (ALAD) in the blood and suppressed hematopoiesis.

Excretion – Pentetate calcium trisodium is cleared from the plasma in the first few hours after dosing through urinary excretion by glomerular filtration. Renal tubular excretion has not been documented. In stool samples tested, only a very small amount of radioactivity (less than 3%) was detected.

The plasma retention up to 7 hours postdosing was expressed by the sum of 3 exponential components with average half-lives of 1.4, 14.5, and 94.4 minutes. The level of activity in the plasma was below the limit of detection 24 hours after injection. During the study, no detectable activity was exhaled or excreted in the feces. By 24 hours, cumulative urinary excretion was more than 99% of the injected dose.

Special populations –

Renal function impairment: Pentetate calcium trisodium and its radioactive chelates are excreted by glomerular filtration. Impaired renal function may decrease their rates of elimination and increase the serum half-life of pentetate calcium trisodium.

Contraindications

None known.

Warnings/Precautions

➤*Endogenous trace metal depletion:* Pentetate calcium trisodium is associated with depletion of endogenous trace metals (eg, zinc, magnesium, manganese). The magnitude of depletion increases with split daily dosing, increasing dose, and increased treatment duration. Only a single initial dose of pentetate calcium trisodium is recommended. If additional chelation therapy is indicated after the initial single dose of pentetate calcium trisodium, it is recommended that therapy be continued with pentetate zinc trisodium. If pentetate zinc trisodium is not available, chelation therapy may continue with pentetate calcium trisodium, but give mineral supplements containing zinc concomitantly, as appropriate.

➤*Asthma exacerbation:* Nebulized chelation therapy may be associated with exacerbation of asthma. Exercise caution when administering pentetate calcium trisodium by the inhalation route.

➤*Fluids:* Advise patients to drink plenty of fluids and void frequently to promote dilution of the radioactive chelate in the urine and minimize radiation exposure directly to the bladder.

➤*Internal contamination with other radiocontaminants:* If internal contamination with radiocontaminants other than plutonium, americium, or curium, or unknown radiocontaminants is suspected, additional therapies may be needed (eg, Prussian blue, potassium iodide).

➤*Collection of patient treatment data:* To develop long-term response data and information on the risk of developing late malignancy, provide detailed information on patient treatment to the manufacturer. In case additional forms are needed, please visit http://www.hameln-pharmaceuticals.com. These data should include a record of the radioactive

PENTETATE CALCIUM TRISODIUM (Ca-DTPA) — INJECTION OR INHALATION

body burden and bioassay results at defined time intervals, a description of measurement methods to facilitate analysis of data, and adverse reactions.

Refer questions regarding the use of pentetate calcium trisodium for the treatment of internal contamination with transuranium elements to the manufacturer.

➤*Special risk:*

Hemochromatosis – Use pentetate calcium trisodium with caution in individuals with severe hemochromatosis. Deaths have been reported in patients with severe hemochromatosis who received up to 4 times the recommended daily dose by IM injection for more than 1 day. Causal association with these events and the drug has not been established.

➤*Pregnancy: Category C.* There are no human pregnancy outcome data from which to assess the risk of pentetate calcium trisodium exposure on fetal development. Pentetate calcium trisodium is believed to be teratogenic based on animal data and because chelation therapy results in the depletion of body stores of zinc which is known to affect deoxyribonucleic acid (DNA) and ribonucleic acid (RNA) synthesis in humans.

In mice, pentetate calcium trisodium has been shown to be teratogenic and embryocidal following 5 daily injections of pentetate calcium trisodium 720 to 2,880 mcmol/kg (2 to 8 times the recommended daily human dose of 1 g based on body surface area [BSA] adjusted dose) given during any period of gestation. The frequency of gross malformations (eg, exencephaly, spina bifida, cleft palate) increased with dose, with higher susceptibility in early- and mid-gestation. Studies of 2 pregnant dogs given daily injections of pentetate calcium trisodium 30 mcmol/kg (approximately half the recommended daily human dose based on BSA) from implantation until parturition showed severe teratogenic effects (especially brain damage).

Multiple doses of pentetate calcium trisodium could result in an increased risk for adverse reproductive outcomes and, thus, are not recommended during pregnancy. Therefore, treatment of pregnant women should begin and continue with pentetate zinc trisodium, if available, except in cases of high internal radioactive contamination. In these cases, consider the risk of immediate and delayed radiation-induced toxicity to the mother and the fetus in comparison with the risk of pentetate calcium trisodium toxicity. Also, because pentetate calcium trisodium is more effective than pentetate zinc trisodium in the first 24 hours after internal contamination, it may be appropriate to use a single dose of pentetate calcium trisodium with vitamin or mineral supplements that contain zinc as the initial treatment.

➤*Lactation:* Studies to determine if pentetate calcium trisodium is excreted in breast milk have not been conducted. Radiocontaminants are known to be excreted in breast milk. Advise women with known or suspected internal contamination with radiocontaminants not to breast-feed, whether or not they are receiving chelation therapy. Take precautions when discarding breast milk.

➤*Children:* The safety and efficacy of pentetate calcium trisodium were established in the adult population, and efficacy was extrapolated to children for the IV route based on the comparability of pathophysiologic mechanisms. The dose is based on body size adjustment for an IV drug that is cleared renally. The safety and efficacy of the nebulized route of administration have not been established in the pediatric population.

➤*Monitoring:* When possible, obtain baseline blood and urine samples (complete blood cell counts [CBC] with differential, serum urea nitrogen, serum chemistries and electrolytes, urinalysis, and blood and urine radioassays) before initiating treatment.

Pentetate calcium trisodium must be given with very careful monitoring of serum zinc and CBC. When appropriate, administer vitamin or mineral supplements that contain zinc.

To establish an elimination curve, obtain a quantitative baseline estimate of the total internalized transuranium element(s) and measures of elimination of radioactivity by appropriate whole-body counting, bioassay (eg, biodosimetry), or fecal/urine sample whenever possible.

Monitoring during treatment –

Measure the radioactivity in blood, urine, and fecal samples weekly to monitor the radioactive contaminant elimination rate.

Monitor CBC with differential, serum urea nitrogen, serum chemistries and electrolytes, and urinalysis regularly. If the patient is receiving more than 1 dose of pentetate calcium trisodium, monitor these laboratory tests very carefully and consider mineral supplementation as appropriate.

Record any adverse reactions from pentetate calcium trisodium.

Drug Interactions

None well documented.

Adverse Reactions

Overall, the presence or absence of adverse reactions was recorded in 310 of 646 patients. Of these, 19 (6.1%) reported at least 1 adverse reaction. The total number of recorded adverse reactions was 20. Of the 20 adverse reactions, 18 occurred after treatment with pentetate calcium trisodium. Adverse reactions included allergic reaction, chest pain, dermatitis, diarrhea, headache, injection-site reactions, light-headedness, metallic taste, and nausea. Cough and/or wheezing were experienced by 2 individuals receiving nebulized pentetate calcium trisodium, 1 of whom had a history of asthma.

In the literature, prolonged treatment with pentetate calcium trisodium resulted in depletion of zinc, magnesium, manganese, and, possibly, metalloproteinases.

Overdosage

In previous clinical studies, 3 deaths were reported in patients with severe hemochromatosis who were treated with daily IM pentetate calcium trisodium dosed up to 4 g/day to reduce iron stores. One patient became comatose and died after receiving a total of pentetate calcium trisodium 14 g, and the other 2 died after 2 weeks of daily treatment. Causal association with these events and the drug has not been established.

Patient Information

Radioactive metals are known to be excreted in the urine, feces, and breast milk. In patients with recent internal contamination with plutonium, americium, or curium, pentetate calcium trisodium treatment increases excretion of radioactivity in the urine.

Take appropriate safety measures to minimize contamination of others. When possible, use a toilet instead of a urinal, and flush it several times after each use. Completely clean up spilled urine or feces and wash your hands thoroughly. If blood or urine comes in contact with clothing or linens, wash them separately.

Drink plenty of fluids and void frequently. If patients are coughing, carefully dispose of any expectorant. Avoid swallowing the expectorant if possible.

Parents and caregivers should take extra precaution in handling the urine, feces, and expectorants of children to avoid any additional exposure to either the caregiver or to the child. Breast-feeding mothers should take extra precaution in disposing of breast milk.

PRUSSIAN BLUE

Rx	**Radiogardase** (Heyltex Corporation)	**Capsules:** 0.5 g (blue powder in gelatin capsules)	In 30s.

PRUSSIAN BLUE — ORAL

Indications

➤*Internal contamination:* For the treatment of patients with known or suspected internal contamination with radioactive cesium and/or radioactive or non-radioactive thallium to increase their rates of elimination.

Administration and Dosage

➤*General dosing considerations:* Treatment should be initiated as soon as possible after contamination is suspected. Contamination should be verified as soon as possible. However, even when treatment cannot be started right away, patients should be given Prussian blue as soon as it becomes available. Treatment is still effective for radioactive cesium contamination, even after time has elapsed since exposure.

In patients who have contamination with multiple or unknown radioactive isotopes, additional decontamination and treatment procedures may be needed.

Manage the patient to minimize further injury and to stabilize before external decontamination. Establish if the patient suffers from a single or combined injury (eg, radiation, burns, trauma, chemical, biological) and whether the contaminant may be internalized. The route of entry of the radiation contaminant needs to be identified and recorded. The route of entry will determine other treatment methods needed (eg, wound debridement, stomach lavage if ingested). Patients need to be triaged based on their injuries and the level and type of contamination.

➤*Adults:*

Radioactive cesium (^{137}Cs) contamination –

Usual dosage: 3 g orally 3 times a day.

Dosage adjustment: When the internal radioactivity is substantially decreased, the dose may be decreased to 1 or 2 g 3 times daily to improve GI tolerance.

Duration of therapy: Treatment should continue for a minimum of 30 days, and then the patient should be reassessed for the amount of residual whole body radioactivity. The duration of treatment after exposure is dictated by the level of contamination and the judgment of the attending physician. Before, during, and after therapy, pertinent measurements for radioactivity should be made to help determine when to terminate treatment.

Thallium contamination –

Usual dosage: 3 g orally 3 times a day.

Concomitant therapy: In cases of severe thallium intoxication, additional types of elimination treatment may be necessary, such as induced emesis followed by gastric intubation and lavage, forced diuresis until urinary thallium excretion is less than 1 mg per 24 hours, charcoal hemoperfusion, which may be useful during the first 48 hours after thallium ingestion (biodistribution phase), and hemodialysis, which has been reported to be effective in thallium intoxication.

➤*Children:*

Radioactive cesium (^{137}Cs) contamination – See Adults for dosing for children 13 years of age and older.

2 to 12 years of age:

• *Usual dosage* – 1 g orally 3 times a day.

PRUSSIAN BLUE — ORAL

Thallium contamination – See Adults for dosing for children 13 years of age and older.

2 to 12 years of age:

- *Usual dosage* – 1 g orally 3 times a day.
- *Concomitant therapy* – In cases of severe thallium intoxication, additional types of elimination treatment may be necessary, such as induced emesis followed by gastric intubation and lavage, forced diuresis until urinary thallium excretion is less than 1 mg per 24 hours, charcoal hemoperfusion, which may be useful during the first 48 hours after thallium ingestion (biodistribution phase), and hemodialysis, which has been reported to be effective in thallium intoxication.

➤*Monitoring:*

Cesium contamination – A quantitative baseline of the internalized contamination of ^{137}Cs should be obtained by appropriate whole-body counting and/or bioassay (eg, biodosimetry) or feces/urine sample whenever possible to obtain an estimated internalized radiation contamination of ^{137}Cs and rate of measured elimination of radiation in the feces in order to establish an elimination curve. During treatment, the radioactivity counts in urine and fecal samples should be measured and recorded weekly to monitor the ^{137}Cs elimination rate, and the occurrence of any adverse reactions (eg, constipation, which can be treated by increasing the amount of fiber in the diet) should be noted.

Thallium contamination – Patients with thallium contamination should also have weekly complete blood counts (CBCs), serum chemistry, and electrolytes while under treatment. The response to other oral medications should be closely monitored.

➤*Handling and disposal:*

Cesium contamination – Health professionals should wear appropriate radiation-protective attire and follow procedures at all times. Protect health professionals who are handling patients from unnecessary radiation exposure and monitor health professionals and the area of operation for radiation levels using radiation detection, indication, and computation devices (RADIAC), or thermal luminescent devices (TLD). Control the spread of radiation contamination by establishing patient triage site, patient decontamination area, and a contaminated or dirty material dumpsite. Proper labeling, handling, and disposal of contaminated material needs to be established and followed.

Thallium contamination – There is no need for radiation safety precautions when treating patients contaminated with nonradioactive thallium. For both radioactive and nonradioactive thallium contamination, a quantitative baseline of the internalized thallium contamination should be ascertained by appropriate whole-body counting and/or bioassay whenever possible.

➤*Administration:* In patients who cannot tolerate swallowing large numbers of capsules, the capsules may be opened and mixed with bland food or liquid. This may result in blue discoloration of the mouth and teeth. Take with food to stimulate excretion of cesium or thallium.

➤*Storage/Stability:* Store in the dark at 25°C (77°F); excursions permitted to 15° to 30°C (59° to 86°F).

Actions

➤*Pharmacology:* Prussian blue insoluble ferric(III) hexacyanoferrate(II) is not absorbed through the intact GI wall after oral ingestion. Its clearance from the body depends on the GI tract transit time. Prussian blue insoluble acts by ion-exchange, adsorption, and mechanical trapping within the crystal structure and has a very high affinity for radioactive and non-radioactive cesium and thallium.

Prussian blue insoluble binds cesium and thallium isotopes in the GI tract after these isotopes are ingested or excreted in the bile by the liver, thereby reducing GI reabsorption (enterohepatic circulation). In studies of rats, pigs, and dogs that were internally contaminated with cesium and thallium, the presence of the insoluble complexes in the GI lumen changed the primary elimination route from the kidney to the feces and increased the rate of elimination of these 2 contaminants.

The rate of cesium and thallium elimination was proportional to the duration and dose of Prussian blue insoluble. A radioactive element has a constant rate of disintegration that is reflected by its physical half-life. The rate of element elimination from the body is reflected by its biologic half-life. The combined rate of radiation disintegration and rate of element elimination is reflected by the effective half-life.

Cesium-137 (^{137}Cs) has a physical half-life of 30 years, with a beta energy peak at 174 keV. After entry into the blood, it is distributed uniformly through all body tissues. Approximately 10% of cesium is eliminated rapidly with a biological half-life of 2 days, and 90% is eliminated more slowly, with a biological half-life of 110 days. Less than 1% of the cesium is retained with a longer biological half-life of about 500 days. Cesium follows the movement of potassium and is excreted into the intestine and reabsorbed from the gut into the blood, then to the bile, where it is excreted again into the gut (enterohepatic circulation). Without Prussian blue insoluble treatment, approximately 80% of cesium is excreted through the kidneys and approximately 20% in the feces. Because of cesium's long physical half-life, the rate of radiation elimination is similar to the rate of element elimination from the body.

Thallium-201 (^{201}Tl) has a physical half-life of 3 days with electron and photon emissions, with a gamma energy peak at 167.4 keV. After entry into the blood, thallium is distributed in the kidneys (3%) and all other organs (97%). Nonradioactive thallium, depending on the tissue, has a biological half-life of 8 to 10 days. Thallium also follows the movement of potassium and is excreted by the bile in enterohepatic recirculation. Without Prussian blue insoluble treatment, the fecal to urine excretion ratio of thallium is approximately 2:1.

Based on the mechanisms of action, Prussian blue insoluble may bind to other elements (eg, potassium), and cause electrolyte or other nutritional imbalances.

➤*Pharmacokinetics:*

Absorption – Absorption from multiple doses has not been studied. Food effect studies were not identified in the literature. In animal studies, Prussian blue insoluble was not significantly absorbed.

Excretion – In an animal study (pigs, N= 38), after a single dose of labeled Prussian blue insoluble 40 mg, 99% of the administered Prussian blue dose was excreted unchanged in feces. Food may increase the effectiveness of Prussian blue insoluble by stimulating bile secretion. Food is known to increase bile production and enterohepatic circulation. The increase in enterohepatic circulation may increase the amount of cesium and thallium in the GI lumen, and may increase the amounts available for binding with Prussian blue insoluble.

Special populations –

Renal function impairment:

Hepatic function impairment: Prussian blue insoluble may be less effective in patients with impaired liver function because of decreased excretion of cesium and thallium in the bile.

Contraindications

None known.

Warnings/Precautions

➤*Radiation toxicity:* Prussian blue insoluble is administered to decrease radiation exposure. It does not treat the complications of radiation exposure. Patients contaminated with high doses of ^{137}Cs may develop radiation toxicity, including bone marrow suppression with severe neutropenia and thrombocytopenia. Give supportive treatment for radiation toxicity symptoms concomitantly with Prussian blue insoluble treatment.

➤*Contamination with multiple radioactive elements:* In radiological emergencies, the type of elemental exposure may not be known. Prussian blue insoluble may not bind to all radioactive elements, and some radioactive elements may not undergo enterohepatic circulation, which is needed for Prussian blue insoluble binding and elimination. Patients contaminated with unknown or multiple radioactive elements may require treatment with other agents in addition to Prussian blue insoluble.

➤*GI effects:* GI Prussian blue insoluble may cause constipation. Decreased GI motility will slow the transit time of ^{137}Cs bound to Prussian blue insoluble in the GI tract and may increase the radiation absorbed dose to the GI mucosa. Constipation occurring during Prussian blue insoluble treatment may be treated with a fiber-based laxative and/or a high-fiber diet. Use Prussian blue insoluble with caution in patients with disorders associated with decreased GI motility.

➤*Special risk:* Exercise caution when treating patients with preexisting cardiac arrhythmias or electrolyte imbalances. Prussian blue insoluble may bind to some oral therapeutic drugs.

➤*Pregnancy: Category C.* Comprehensive animal reproductive studies have not been conducted with Prussian blue insoluble. Since Prussian blue insoluble is not absorbed from the GI tract, effects on the fetus are not expected. In 1 patient who became pregnant 3 years and 8 months after being treated with Prussian blue insoluble for internal contamination with ^{137}Cs (8 mCi), complications or birth defects were not identified in the literature report.

Cesium-137 is known to cross the human placenta. One patient, in Goiânia, was contaminated with 0.005 mCi ^{137}Cs during her fourth month of pregnancy. She was not treated with Prussian blue insoluble. At birth, the concentration of ^{137}Cs was the same in the mother and the infant. Thallium crosses the human placenta. Reported fetal effects in the reviewed literature include fetal death, failure to thrive, alopecia, or in some instances, outwardly normal development. The risk of toxicity from untreated radioactive cesium or thallium exposure is expected to be more than the reproductive toxicity risk of Prussian blue insoluble.

➤*Lactation:* Studies to determine if Prussian blue insoluble is excreted in human milk have not been conducted. Since Prussian blue insoluble is not absorbed from the GI tract, its excretion in milk is highly unlikely. However, cesium and thallium are transmitted from mother to infant in breast milk. Women internally contaminated with cesium or thallium should not breastfeed.

➤*Children:* The safety and efficacy of Prussian blue insoluble and its dosing for children were extrapolated from adult data and supported by pediatric patients who were internally contaminated with ^{137}Cs and treated with Prussian blue insoluble in the Goiânia accident.

Overall, 27 pediatric patients received Prussian blue insoluble in the range of 3 to 10 g/day in divided doses. Prussian blue insoluble treatment reduced the whole-body effective half-life of ^{137}Cs 46% in adolescents and 43% in children ranging from 4 to 12 years of age. In 12 patients for whom the rate of radiation elimination data are available, the rate was similar to that in adults treated with 3 g 3 times daily and in pediatric patients treated with 1 g 3 times daily. By body weight, the dose ranged from 0.32 g/kg in the 12-year-old patient (Prussian blue 10 g daily dose, 31 kg weight) to 0.21 g/kg in the 4-year-old patient (Prussian blue 3 g daily dose, 14 kg weight). Children 2 to 4 years of age are expected to have biliary and GI function that is comparable with the 4-year-old.

PRUSSIAN BLUE — ORAL

There are variations in the developmental maturity of the biliary system and GI tract of neonates and infants (0 to 2 years of age). The dose-related adverse effects of Prussian blue insoluble on an immature GI tract are not known. Dosing in infants and neonates has not been established.

➤*Monitoring:* Closely monitor serum electrolytes during Prussian blue insoluble treatment. Prussian blue insoluble may bind to some oral therapeutic drugs. As appropriate, monitor blood levels or clinical response to oral medications.

Patients should also have weekly CBC, serum chemistry, and electrolytes monitored while under treatment.

Drug Interactions

Binding to some therapeutic drugs and essential nutrients is possible. The literature contains anecdotal reports of asymptomatic hypokalemia and decreased bioavailability of oral tetracycline. Monitor the serum levels and/or clinical response to critical oral products.

Adverse Reactions

Deaths or serious or severe adverse reactions attributed to Prussian blue insoluble have not been reported.

➤*GI:* Constipation was reported in 10 of 42 patients in the Goiânia accident treated with Prussian blue insoluble. Severity of constipation was mild in 7 patients and moderate in 3 patients. Constipation was successfully treated with a high-fiber diet. Undefined gastric distress was reported in 3 patients treated with Prussian blue insoluble 20 g/day. In these patients, the dose was reduced to 10 g/day for continued treatment.

➤*Lab test abnormalities:* Prussian blue insoluble may bind to electrolytes found in the GI tract. Asymptomatic hypokalemia, with serum potassium levels of 2.5 to 2.9 (normal 3.5 to 5) was reported in 3 of 42 of patients on treatment with Prussian blue insoluble. Exercise caution when treating patients with preexisting cardiac arrhythmias or electrolyte imbalances.

Overdosage

➤*Symptoms:* The clinical effects of overdosing with Prussian blue insoluble are not known. Based on reported adverse reactions and mechanism of action, possible overdose symptoms may include obstipation, obstruction, or severe decrease in electrolytes.

Patient Information

Cesium-137 is excreted in the urine and feces. Take appropriate safety measures to minimize radiation exposure to others. When possible, a toilet should be used instead of a urinal, and it should be flushed several times after each use. Spilled urine or feces should be cleaned up completely, and patients should wash their hands thoroughly. If blood or urine gets onto clothing, such clothing should be washed separately.

Parents and child care givers should take extra precaution in handling the urine and feces of pediatric patients. Care is intended to prevent re-exposure to the adult and pediatric patient.

In patients with constipation, a fiber-based laxative and/or high-fiber diet is recommended during treatment with Prussian blue insoluble. Inform patients taking Prussian blue insoluble that their stools might be blue in color.

In patients who cannot swallow capsules, when the capsules are opened and the contents are mixed with food and eaten, the mouth and teeth might be colored blue.

DEFERASIROX

Rx	Exjade (Novartis)	Tablets for suspension, dispersible; oral: 125 mg	Lactose. (J 125/NVR). Off-white, round. In 30s.
		250 mg	Lactose. (J 250/NVR). Off-white, round. In 30s.
		500 mg	Lactose. (J 500/NVR). Off-white, round. In 30s.

DEFERASIROX — ORAL

WARNING

Renal or hepatic failure and/or GI hemorrhage – Deferasirox may cause renal impairment and failure, hepatic impairment and failure, and GI hemorrhage.

In some reported cases, these reactions were fatal. These reactions were more frequently observed in patients with advanced age, high-risk myelodysplastic syndromes, underlying renal or hepatic impairment, or low platelet counts (less than 50×10^9/L). Deferasirox therapy requires close patient monitoring, including measurement of the following:

- serum creatinine and/or creatinine clearance (CrCl) prior to initiation of therapy and monthly thereafter; monitor creatinine and/or CrCl weekly for the first month, then monthly thereafter in patients with underlying renal impairment or risk factors for renal impairment;
- serum transaminases and bilirubin prior to initiation of therapy, every 2 weeks during the first month, and monthly thereafter.

Indications

➤*Chronic iron overload:* For the treatment of chronic iron overload caused by blood transfusions (transfusional hemosiderosis) in patients 2 years of age and older.

Administration and Dosage

➤*General dosing considerations:* Prior to starting therapy, obtain baseline serum ferritin and iron levels. The risk for toxicity may be increased when deferasirox is given to patients with low iron burden or with serum ferritin levels that are only slightly elevated.

The safety and efficacy of deferasirox when administered with other iron chelation therapy have not been established.

The decision to remove accumulated iron should be individualized based on the anticipated clinical benefits and risks of deferasirox therapy. In patients who are in need of iron chelation therapy, it is recommended that therapy with deferasirox start when a patient has evidence of chronic iron overload, such as the transfusion of approximately 100 mL/kg of packed red blood cells (approximately 20 units for a 40 kg patient) and a serum ferritin level consistently greater than 1,000 mcg/L.

Deferasirox-treated patients experienced dose-dependent increases in serum creatinine. Consider dose reduction, interruption, or discontinuation of treatment for increases in serum creatinine (see Renal Function Impairment and Warnings/Precautions).

Doses (mg/kg/day) should be calculated to the nearest whole tablet.

➤*Adults:*

Chronic iron overload –

Maximum dose: Dosages greater than 40 mg/kg/day are not recommended.

Initial dosage: 20 mg/kg body weight daily.

Dosage adjustment:

After commencing initial therapy, monitor serum ferritin every month and adjust the dosage of deferasirox if necessary every 3 to 6 months based on serum ferritin trends. Make dose adjustments in increments of 5 or 10 mg/kg and tailor adjustments to the individual patient's response and therapeutic goals (maintenance or reduction of body iron burden). In patients not adequately controlled with doses of 30 mg/kg (eg, serum ferritin levels persistently above 2,500 mcg/L and not showing a decreasing trend over time), doses of up to 40 mg/kg may be considered. Doses greater than 40 mg/kg are not recommended. If the serum ferritin falls consistently below 500 mcg/L, consider temporarily interrupting therapy with deferasirox.

➤*Children:*

Chronic iron overload –

2 years of age and older: See Adults for dosing.

➤*Renal function impairment:*

Adults – Reduce the daily dose of deferasirox by 10 mg/kg if a rise in serum creatinine is more than 33% above the average of the pretreatment measurements seen at 2 consecutive visits and cannot be attributed to other causes.

Children – Reduce the dose by 10 mg/kg if serum creatinine levels rise above the age-appropriate upper limit of normal (ULN) at 2 consecutive visits.

➤*Concomitant therapy:* Concomitant use of UDP-glucuronosyltransferase (UGT) inducers or cholestyramine decreases deferasirox systemic exposure (AUC). Avoid the concomitant use of cholestyramine or potent UGT inducers (eg, rifampicin, phenobarbital, phenytoin, ritonavir) with deferasirox. If these agents must be coadministered together, consider increasing the initial dose of deferasirox to 30 mg/kg, and monitor serum ferritin levels and clinical responses for further dose modification.

➤*Administration:* Deferasirox should be taken once daily on an empty stomach at least 30 minutes before food, preferably at the same time each day. Tablets should not be chewed or swallowed whole.

Tablets should be completely dispersed by stirring in water, orange juice, or apple juice until a fine suspension is obtained. Doses of less than 1 g should be dispersed in 3.5 ounces of liquid and doses of 1 g or more should be dispersed in 7 ounces of liquid. After swallowing the suspension, resuspend any residue in a small volume of liquid and swallow.

Deferasirox should not be taken with aluminum-containing antacid products.

➤*Storage/Stability:* Store at 25°C (77°F); excursions are permitted to 15° to 30°C (59° to 86°F). Protect from moisture.

Actions

➤*Pharmacology:* Deferasirox is an orally active chelator that is selective for iron (as Fe^{3+}). It is a tridentate ligand that binds iron with high affinity in a 2:1 ratio. Although deferasirox has very low affinity for zinc and copper, there are variable decreases in the serum concentration of these trace metals after the administration of deferasirox. The clinical significance of these decreases is uncertain.

➤*Pharmacokinetics:*

Absorption – Deferasirox is absorbed following oral administration with median times to maximum plasma concentration (T_{max}) of approximately 1.5 to 4 hours. The maximum plasma concentration (C_{max}) and AUC of deferasirox increase approximately linearly with the dose after single administration and under steady-state conditions. Exposure to deferasirox increased by an accumulation factor of 1.3 to 2.3 after multiple doses. The

DEFERASIROX — ORAL

absolute bioavailability (AUC) of deferasirox tablets for oral suspension is 70% compared with an intravenous dose.

Effect of food: The bioavailability (AUC) of deferasirox was variably increased when taken with a meal.

Distribution – Deferasirox is highly protein bound (approximately 99%), almost exclusively to serum albumin. The percentage of deferasirox confined to the blood cells was 5% in humans. The volume of distribution at steady state of deferasirox is 14.37 ± 2.69 L in adults.

Metabolism – Glucuronidation is the main metabolic pathway for deferasirox, with subsequent biliary excretion. Deconjugation of glucuronidates in the intestine and subsequent reabsorption (enterohepatic recycling) is likely to occur. Deferasirox is mainly glucuronidated by UGT1A1 and to a lesser extent UGT1A3. Cytochrome P450 (CYP-450)–catalyzed (oxidative) metabolism of deferasirox appears to be minor in humans (approximately 8%). Deconjugation of glucuronide metabolites in the intestine and subsequent reabsorption (enterohepatic recycling) was confirmed in a healthy volunteer study in which the administration of cholestyramine 12 g twice daily (strongly binds to deferasirox and its conjugates) 4 and 10 hours after a single dose of deferasirox resulted in a 45% decrease in deferasirox exposure (AUC) by interfering with the enterohepatic recycling of deferasirox.

Excretion – Deferasirox and metabolites are primarily excreted in the feces (84% of the dose). Renal excretion of deferasirox and metabolites is minimal (8% of the administered dose). The mean terminal half-life ranged from 8 to 16 hours following oral administration.

Special populations –

Children: Following oral administration of single or multiple doses, systemic exposure of adolescents and children to deferasirox was less than in adults. In children younger than 6 years of age, systemic exposure was approximately 50% lower than in adults.

Gender: Women have a moderately lower apparent clearance (by 17.5%) of deferasirox compared with men.

Contraindications

CrCl less than 40 mL/min or serum creatinine greater than 2 times the age-appropriate ULN; poor performance status and high-risk myelodysplastic syndromes or advanced malignancies; platelet counts less than 50 × 10^9/L; known hypersensitivity to deferasirox or any component of deferasirox.

Warnings/Precautions

➤*Renal toxicity:* Acute renal failure, some with a fatal outcome and some requiring dialysis, has been reported following postmarketing use of deferasirox. Most of the fatalities occurred in patients with multiple comorbidities and who were in advanced stages of hematological disorders. Give particular attention to monitoring serum creatinine and/or CrCl in patients who are at increased risk of complications, have preexisting renal conditions, are elderly, have comorbid conditions, or are receiving medicinal products that depress renal function. Closely monitor the renal function of patients with CrCl between 40 and less than 60 mL/min, particularly in situations in which patients have additional risk factors that may further impair renal function such as concomitant medications, dehydration, or severe infections.

Assess serum creatinine and/or CrCl in duplicate before initiating therapy to establish a reliable pretreatment baseline because of variations in measurements. Monitor serum creatinine and/or CrCl monthly thereafter. Monitor patients with additional renal risk factors weekly during the first month after initiation or modification of therapy, and monitor monthly thereafter.

Consider dose reduction, interruption, or discontinuation of treatment for increases in serum creatinine. If there is a progressive increase in serum creatinine beyond the age-appropriate ULN, interrupt deferasirox therapy. Once the creatinine has returned to within normal range, reinitiate therapy with deferasirox at a lower dose, followed by a gradual dose escalation if the clinical benefit is expected to outweigh potential risks.

In clinical studies, for increases of serum creatinine on 2 consecutive measures (more than 33% in patients older than 15 years of age or more than 33% or more than the age-appropriate ULN in patients younger than 15 years of age), the daily dose of deferasirox was reduced by 10 mg/kg. Patients with baseline serum creatinine above the ULN were excluded from clinical studies.

Deferasirox-treated patients experienced dose-dependent increases in serum creatinine. These increases occurred at a greater frequency compared with deferoxamine-treated patients (38% vs 14%, respectively, in study 1, and 36% vs 22%, respectively, in study 3). Most of the creatinine elevations remained within the normal range. There have also been reports of renal tubulopathy in patients treated with deferasirox. The majority of these patients were children and adolescents with beta-thalassemia and serum ferritin levels less than 1,500 mcg/L.

➤*Hepatic effects:* In study 1, four patients discontinued deferasirox because of hepatic abnormalities (drug-induced hepatitis in 2 patients and increased serum transaminases in 2 additional patients). There have been postmarketing reports of hepatic failure, some with a fatal outcome, in patients treated with deferasirox. Most of these reactions occurred in patients older than 55 years of age. Most reports of hepatic failure involved patients with significant comorbidities, including liver cirrhosis and multi-organ failure. Monitor serum transaminases and bilirubin before the initiation of treatment, every 2 weeks during the first month, and monthly thereafter. Consider dosage modifications or interruption of treatment for severe or persistent elevations.

➤*GI effects:* Fatal GI hemorrhages, especially in elderly patients who had advanced hematologic malignancies and/or low platelet counts, have been reported. Nonfatal upper GI irritation, ulceration, and hemorrhage have been reported in patients, including children and adolescents, receiving deferasirox. Health care providers and patients should remain alert for signs and symptoms of GI ulceration and hemorrhage during deferasirox therapy, and promptly initiate additional evaluation and treatment if a serious GI adverse reaction is suspected. Use caution when administering deferasirox in combination with drugs that have ulcerogenic or hemorrhagic potential, such as nonsteroidal anti-inflammatory drugs (NSAIDs), corticosteroids, oral bisphosphonates, or anticoagulants.

➤*Cytopenias:* There have been postmarketing reports (spontaneous and from clinical trials) of cytopenias, including agranulocytosis, neutropenia, and thrombocytopenia, in patients treated with deferasirox, some with a fatal outcome. The relationship of these episodes to treatment with deferasirox is uncertain. Most of these patients had preexisting hematologic disorders that are frequently associated with bone marrow failure. In line with the standard clinical management of such hematological disorders, regularly monitor blood cell counts. Consider interruption of treatment with deferasirox in patients who develop unexplained cytopenia. Consider reintroduction with deferasirox once the cause of cytopenia has been elucidated.

➤*Rash:* Skin rashes may occur during deferasirox treatment. For rashes of mild to moderate severity, deferasirox may be continued without dosage adjustment because the rash often resolves spontaneously. In severe cases, deferasirox therapy may be interrupted. Consider reintroduction at a lower dose with escalation in combination with a short period of oral steroid administration. Erythema multiforme has been reported during deferasirox treatment.

➤*Comorbidities:* Clinical trials to demonstrate increased survival or to confirm clinical benefit have not been completed. Deferasirox decreased serum ferritin and liver iron concentration in clinical trials. Consider the importance of these factors, as well as individual patient factors and the prognosis associated with any underlying conditions, before initiation of deferasirox therapy.

In postmarketing experience, there have been reports of serious adverse reactions, some with a fatal outcome, in patients taking deferasirox therapy, predominantly when the drug was administered to patients with advanced age, complications from underlying conditions, or very advanced disease. Most of these deaths occurred within 6 months of deferasirox initiation and generally involved worsening of the underlying condition. The reports do not rule out the possibility that deferasirox may have contributed to the deaths.

➤*Special senses:* Auditory disturbances (eg, high-frequency hearing loss, decreased hearing) and ocular disturbances (eg, lens opacities, cataracts, elevations in intraocular pressure, retinal disorders) have been reported at a frequency of less than 1% with deferasirox therapy in the clinical studies. Auditory and ophthalmic testing (including slit lamp examinations and dilated fundoscopy) are recommended before starting deferasirox treatment and thereafter at regular intervals (every 12 months). If disturbances are noted, consider dose reduction or interruption of therapy.

➤*Hypersensitivity reactions:* Serious hypersensitivity reactions (eg, anaphylaxis, angioedema) have been reported in patients receiving deferasirox, with the onset of the reaction occurring in the majority of cases within the first month of treatment. If reactions are severe, discontinue deferasirox and institute appropriate medical intervention.

➤*Pregnancy:* *Category C* (per manufacturer's prescribing information); *Category B* (per Briggs' Drugs in Pregnancy and Lactation). There are no adequate and well-controlled studies with deferasirox in pregnant women. Administration of deferasirox to animals during pregnancy and lactation resulted in decreased offspring viability and an increase in renal anomalies in male offspring at exposures that were less than the recommended human exposure. Use deferasirox during pregnancy only if the potential benefit justifies the potential risk to the fetus. It is not known if deferasirox crosses the human placenta. The molecular weight (about 373) and long elimination half-life suggest that exposure of the embryo and/or fetus will occur, but the very high protein binding should limit the exposure.

In embryofetal development studies, pregnant rats and rabbits received oral deferasirox during the period of organogenesis at doses of up to 0.8 times the MRHD on a mg/m^2 basis (100 mg/kg/day in rats and 50 mg/kg/day in rabbits). These doses resulted in maternal toxicity, but no fetal harm was observed.

In prenatal and postnatal development study, pregnant rats received oral deferasirox daily from organogenesis through lactation day 20 at doses 0.08, 0.2, and 0.7 times the MRHD on a mg/m^2 basis (10, 30, and 90 mg/kg/day). Maternal toxicity, loss of litters, and decreased offspring viability occurred at 0.7 times the MRHD on a mg/m^2basis, and increases in renal anomalies in male offspring occurred at 0.2 times the MRHD on a mg/m^2 basis.

➤*Lactation:* It is not known whether deferasirox is excreted in human milk. Deferasirox and its metabolites were excreted in the breast milk of rats. The molecular weight (about 373) and long elimination half-life (8 to 16 hours) suggest that the drug also will be excreted into breast milk. Because many drugs are excreted in human milk and because of the potential for serious adverse reactions in breast-feeding infants from deferasirox and its metabolites, decide whether to discontinue the drug, taking into account the importance of the drug to the mother.

➤*Children:* Children 2 to younger than 6 years of age have a systemic exposure to deferasirox approximately 50% of that of adults. However, the safety and efficacy of deferasirox in children were similar to that of adult patients, and younger children responded similarly to older children. The recommended starting dose and dosing modification are the same for children and adults.

Growth and development were within normal limits in children followed for up to 5 years in clinical trials.

DEFERASIROX — ORAL

➤*Elderly:* In clinical trials, elderly patients experienced a higher frequency of adverse reactions than younger patients. Closely monitor elderly patients for early signs or symptoms of adverse reactions that may require a dose adjustment. Elderly patients are at an increased risk for deferasirox toxicity because of the greater frequency of decreased hepatic, renal, or cardiac function, and of concomitant disease or other drug therapy.

➤*Monitoring:* Measure serum ferritin monthly to assess response to therapy and to evaluate for the possibility of overchelation of iron. If the serum ferritin falls consistently below 500 mcg/L, consider temporarily interrupting therapy with deferasirox. In clinical studies, the correlation coefficient between the serum ferritin and liver iron concentration was 0.63. Therefore, changes in serum ferritin levels may not always reliably reflect changes in liver iron concentration.

Assess serum creatinine and/or creatinine clearance in duplicate before initiating therapy and monitor monthly thereafter. Monitor patients with additional renal risk factors weekly during the first month after initiation or modification of therapy; monitor monthly thereafter. Close monitoring of urine protein is also recommended. Monitor serum transaminases and bilirubin prior to initiation of therapy, every 2 weeks during the first month, and monthly thereafter. Auditory and ophthalmic testing (including slit lamp examinations and dilated funduscopy) are recommended before the start of deferasirox treatment and thereafter at regular intervals (every 12 months). Perform regular laboratory monitoring of blood cell counts.

Drug Interactions

Deferasirox Drug Interactions

Precipitant drug	Object drug[a]		Description
Aluminum-containing antacids (eg, aluminum hydroxide)	Deferasirox	↓	Deferasirox absorption may be decreased. The coadministration of deferasirox and aluminum-containing antacid preparations has not been formally studied. Although deferasirox has a lower affinity for aluminum than for iron, do not take deferasirox with aluminum-containing antacid preparations.
Anticoagulants (eg, warfarin)	Deferasirox	↑	The risk of hemorrhage may be increased as a result of additive adverse reactions. Use with caution. Monitor for signs and symptoms of hemorrhage. If serious bleeding occurs, initiate prompt evaluation and treatment.
Deferasirox	Anticoagulants (eg, warfarin)		
Biphosphonates, oral (eg, alendronate)	Deferasirox	↑	The risk of GI irritation and ulcers may be increased as a result of additive adverse reactions. Use with caution. Monitor for signs and symptoms of GI ulceration. If a serious GI adverse event occurs, initiate prompt evaluation and treatment.
Deferasirox	Biphosphonates, oral (eg, alendronate)		
Cholestyramine	Deferasirox	↓	Deferasirox efficacy may be decreased. In healthy volunteers, administration of cholestyramine after a single dose of deferasirox decreased deferasirox exposure (AUC) 45%. If coadministration of deferasirox and cholestyramine cannot be avoided, consider increasing the initial dose of deferasirox to 30 mg/kg. Monitor serum ferritin concentrations and the patient's clinical response for further dose modification.
Corticosteroids (eg, prednisone)	Deferasirox	↑	The risk of GI irritation and ulcers may be increased as a result of additive adverse reactions. Use with caution. Monitor for signs and symptoms of GI ulceration. If a serious GI adverse event occurs, initiate prompt evaluation and treatment.
Deferasirox	Corticosteroids (eg, prednisone)		
Iron-chelator therapies	Deferasirox	↔	Do not combine deferasirox with other iron chelator therapies because the safety of these combinations has not been established.

Deferasirox Drug Interactions

Precipitant drug	Object drug[a]		Description
NSAIDs (eg, ibuprofen)	Deferasirox	↑	The risk of GI irritation and ulcers may be increased as a result of additive adverse reactions. Use with caution. Monitor for signs and symptoms of GI ulceration. If a serious GI adverse event occurs, initiate prompt evaluation and treatment.
Deferasirox	NSAIDs (eg, ibuprofen)		
Potent UDP-UGT inducers (eg, phenobarbital, phenytoin, rifampin, ritonavir)	Deferasirox	↓	Deferasirox efficacy may be decreased. Coadministration of a single dose of deferasirox 30 mg/kg and rifampin 600 mg daily for 9 days decreased deferasirox systemic exposure (AUC) 44%. If coadministration of deferasirox and a potent UGT inducer cannot be avoided, consider increasing the initial dose of deferasirox to 30 mg/kg. Monitor serum ferritin concentrations and the patient's clinical response for further dose modification.
Deferasirox	Cyclosporine	↓	Cyclosporine concentrations may be reduced, decreasing the effectiveness. Use with caution. Monitor cyclosporine concentrations and observe the patient for signs of reduced immunosuppression. Adjust the cyclosporine dose as needed.
Deferasirox	Hormonal contraceptives	↓	Hormonal contraceptive concentrations may be reduced, decreasing the efficacy. Because hormonal contraceptive failure is possible, consider using an additional, nonhormonal contraceptive.
Deferasirox	Midazolam	↓	Coadministration of deferasirox and midazolam decreased midazolam C_{max} and AUC 23% and 17%, respectively. Use with caution. Monitor the response of the patient and adjust the midazolam dose as needed.
Deferasirox	Paclitaxel	↑	Paclitaxel plasma concentrations may be elevated, increasing the pharmacologic effect and risk of toxicity. Use with caution. Monitor the patient and adjust treatment as needed.
Deferasirox	Repaglinide	↑	Coadministration of repaglinide and deferasirox increased repaglinide systemic exposure to 2.3 of control and increased the C_{max} 62%. If deferasirox and repaglinide are coadministered, consider decreasing the dose of repaglinide. Carefully monitor blood glucose concentrations for further repaglinide dose modifications.
Deferasirox	Simvastatin	↓	Simvastatin concentrations may be reduced, decreasing the effectiveness. Use with caution. Monitor the response of the patient. If an interaction is suspected, adjust the simvastatin dose as needed.

[a] ↑ = object drug increased; ↓ = object drug decreased; ↔ = undetermined clinical effect.

➤*Drug/Food interactions:* The bioavailability (AUC) of deferasirox was variably increased when taken with a meal. Deferasirox should be taken on an empty stomach 30 minutes before eating.

Adverse Reactions

➤*Discontinuation:* In study 1, adverse reactions that led to discontinuations included abnormal liver function tests (2 patients) and drug-induced hepatitis (2 patients), skin rash, glycosuria/proteinuria, Henoch-Schönlein purpura, hyperactivity/insomnia, drug fever, and cataract (1 patient each).

In study 3, four additional patients discontinued deferasirox because of adverse reactions with a suspected relationship to study drug, including atypical tuberculosis, diarrhea, pancreatitis associated with gallstones, and skin rash.

DEFERASIROX — ORAL

➤*Adverse reactions (greater than 5%):* Abdominal pain, diarrhea, increases in serum creatinine, nausea, skin rashes, and vomiting were the most frequent adverse reactions reported with a suspected relationship to deferasirox. GI symptoms, increases in serum creatinine, and skin rash were dose-related.

Deferasirox Adverse Reactions (> 5%)[a]

	Study 1 (beta-thalassemia)		Study 3 (sickle cell disease)	
Adverse reactions	Deferasirox (n = 296)	Deferoxamine (n = 290)	Deferasirox (n = 132)	Deferoxamine (n = 63)
GI				
Abdominal pain[b]	21.3%	14.1%	28%	14.3%
Diarrhea	11.8%	7.2%	19.7%	4.8%
Nausea	10.5%	4.8%	22.7%	11.1%
Vomiting	10.1%	9.7%	21.2%	15.9%
Miscellaneous				
Creatinine increased[c]	11.1%	0%	6.8%	0%
Rash	8.4%	3.1%	10.6%	4.8%

[a] Adverse reaction frequencies are based on adverse reactions reported regardless of relationship to study drug.
[b] Includes abdominal pain, abdominal pain lower, and abdominal pain upper, which were reported as adverse reactions.
[c] Includes blood creatinine increased and blood creatinine abnormal, which were reported as adverse reactions. Also see the following table.

➤*Other adverse reactions:*

CNS – Anxiety, dizziness, fatigue, sleep disorder (0.1% to 1%).

Dermatologic – Erythema multiforme (0.01% to 0.1%); pigmentation disorder (0.1% to 1%).

GI – Cholelithiasis, duodenal ulcer (0.1% to 1%), esophagitis (0.01% to 0.1%), gastritis, gastric ulcer (including multiple ulcers), GI hemorrhage.

Special senses – Early cataract, hearing loss, maculopathy (0.1% to 1%); optic neuritis (0.01% to 0.1%).

Miscellaneous – Edema, pharyngolaryngeal pain, pyrexia, renal tubulopathy (Fanconi syndrome) (0.1% to 1%).

➤*Dose interruption/adjustment:* Adverse reactions that most frequently led to dose interruption or dosage adjustment were GI disorders, increased serum creatinine, increased serum transaminases, infections, and rash.

➤*Lab test abnormalities:* In study 1, 38% of patients treated with deferasirox had increases in serum creatinine more than 33% above baseline on 2 separate occasions. Eight percent of patients required dose reductions. Increases in serum creatinine appeared to be dose-related. Six percent of patients treated with deferasirox developed elevations in ALT levels more than 5 times the ULN at 2 consecutive visits. Of these, 2 patients had liver biopsy–proven drug-induced hepatitis and both discontinued deferasirox therapy. Two additional patients who did not have elevations in ALT more than 5 times the ULN discontinued deferasirox because of increased ALT. Increases in transaminases did not appear to be dose-related.

In study 3, a total of 36% of patients treated with deferasirox had increases in serum creatinine more than 33% above baseline on 2 separate occasions. Of the patients who experienced creatinine increases in study 3, eight deferasirox-treated patients required dose reductions. In this study, 5 patients in the deferasirox group developed elevations in ALT levels more than 5 times the upper limit of normal at 2 consecutive visits and 1 patient subsequently had deferasirox permanently discontinued.

Deferasirox Versus Deferoxamine Increases in Serum Creatinine or ALT

	Study 1 (beta-thalassemia)		Study 3 (sickle cell disease)	
Laboratory parameters	Deferasirox (n = 296)	Deferoxamine (n = 290)	Deferasirox (n = 132)	Deferoxamine (n = 63)
Serum creatinine				
Creatinine increase > 33% and < ULN at 2 consecutive postbaseline visits	38.2%	14.1%	36.4%	22.2%
Creatinine increase > 33% and > ULN at 2 consecutive postbaseline visits	2.4%	0.3%	2.3%	3.2%
ALT				
ALT > 5 × ULN at 2 postbaseline visits	8.4%	2.4%	1.5%	0%
ALT > 5 × ULN at 2 consecutive postbaseline visits	5.7%	1.7%	3.8%	0%

Proteinuria – In clinical studies, urine protein was measured monthly. Intermittent proteinuria (urine protein/creatinine ratio more than 0.6 mg/mg) occurred in 18.6% of deferasirox-treated patients compared with 7.2% of deferoxamine-treated patients in study 1. Although no patients were discontinued from deferasirox in clinical studies up to 1 year because of proteinuria, monthly monitoring is recommended. The mechanism and clinical significance of the proteinuria are uncertain.

➤*Postmarketing:*

Dermatologic – Skin and subcutaneous tissue disorders, including alopecia, leukocytoclastic, urticaria, and vasculitis.

Hypersensitivity – Hypersensitivity reactions (eg, anaphylaxis, angioedema).

Overdosage

➤*Symptoms:* Cases of overdose (2 to 3 times the prescribed dose for several weeks) have been reported. In 1 case, this resulted in hepatitis, which resolved without long-term consequences after a dose interruption. Single doses of up to 80 mg/kg in patients with iron-overloaded beta-thalassemia have been tolerated, with nausea and diarrhea noted. In healthy volunteers, single dosages of up to 40 mg/kg/day were tolerated.

➤*Treatment:* There is no specific antidote for deferasirox. In case of overdose, employ gastric lavage.

Patient Information

Advise patients to take deferasirox once daily on an empty stomach at least 30 minutes prior to food, preferably at the same time every day. Tablets should not be chewed or swallowed whole. Instruct patients to completely disperse the tablets first in water, orange juice, or apple juice, and drink the resulting suspension immediately. After swallowing the suspension, instruct patients to resuspend any residue in a small volume of the liquid and swallow.

Advise patients who experience diarrhea or vomiting to maintain adequate hydration.

Caution patients not to take aluminum-containing antacids and deferasirox simultaneously.

Because auditory and ocular disturbances have been reported with deferasirox, tell patients to have auditory and ophthalmic testing before starting deferasirox treatment and thereafter at regular intervals.

Advise patients experiencing dizziness to exercise caution when driving or operating machinery.

Caution patients about the potential for the development of GI ulcers or bleeding when taking deferasirox in combination with drugs that have ulcerogenic or hemorrhagic potential, such as NSAIDs, corticosteroids, oral bisphosphates, or anticoagulants.

Advise patients to carefully monitor glucose levels when repaglinide is used concomitantly with deferasirox.

Advise patients that blood tests will be performed because deferasirox may affect the kidneys, liver, or blood. The blood tests will be performed every month or more frequently if there is an increased risk of complications (eg, preexisting kidney condition, 65 years of age and older, multiple medical conditions, or taking medicine that affects the organs). There have been reports of severe kidney and liver problems, blood disorders, stomach bleeds, and death in patients taking deferasirox.

Inform patients to interrupt treatment of deferasirox if severe skin rashes occur. Serious allergic reactions (which include swelling of the throat) have been reported in patients taking deferasirox, usually within the first month of treatment. If reactions are severe, advise patients to stop taking deferasirox and contact their health care provider immediately.

HYDROXOCOBALAMIN

For complete and comparative prescribing information, refer to the Hydroxocobalamin monograph in the Nutrients and Nutritional Agents chapter.

SODIUM THIOSULFATE

Rx	**Sodium Thiosulfate** (American Regent)	**Injection:** 10% (100 mg/mL) (as pentahydrate)	Preservative-free. In 10 mL single-dose vials.
		25% (250 mg/mL) (as pentahydrate)	Preservative-free. In 50 mL single-dose vials.

SODIUM THIOSULFATE — INJECTION

Indications

➤*Cyanide poisoning:* Sodium thiosulfate is indicated for the treatment of cyanide poisoning.

➤*Off-label uses:*

Calciphylaxis – [4] = Insufficient documentation. Because of the limited experience with sodium thiosulfate for the treatment of calciphylaxis, its use cannot be routinely recommended over the conventional initial therapies of hemodialysis intensification with a low calcium dialysate, switches to non-calcium phosphate binders, wound care, and pain management. With the exception of 1 case of intraperitoneal administration in which the patient initially responded but ultimately experienced lesion progression, sepsis, and death, sodium thiosulfate treatment for calciphylaxis has been associated with rapid improvement in pain and resolution of or improvement in skin ulcers. Given the high mortality rate associated with calciphylaxis, sodium thiosulfate might be considered for patients who do not respond after an adequate trial of conventional therapy.

Cisplatin extravasation – [4] = Insufficient documentation. Although a variety of authors recommend use of sodium thiosulfate for cisplatin extravasation, these recommendations are based on extrapolation of results from mechlorethamine reports and on unpublished experiences. Treatment may be needed only if concentrated cisplatin was used, based on evidence that less concentrated solutions of cisplatin rarely produce toxicity upon extravasation. Sodium thiosulfate should be administered immediately after the cisplatin extravasation occurs.

Cisplatin-induced nephrotoxicity – [2] = Fair documentation. Sodium thiosulfate was shown to be safe and effective as a detoxifying agent for cisplatin overdose even when used with some delay. Intraperitoneal cisplatin with sodium thiosulfate protection has shown promise in patients with advanced ovarian cancer and minimal residual disease, but randomized, controlled trials are needed, and the benefits of intraperitoneal chemotherapy must be weighed against the associated adverse effects. One patient died from complications after surgical replacement of her peritoneal catheter. In another study, high-dose intraperitoneal cisplatin plus etoposide with sodium thiosulfate protection was associated with significant toxicities; treatment had to be prematurely stopped in 17 of 29 patients. With successful approaches to reducing cisplatin renal toxicity and administration of high-dose cisplatin, new dose-limiting toxicities have emerged such as myelosuppression, neurotoxicity, and ototoxicity. Methods that permit safe dose escalation are needed.

Administration and Dosage

➤*General dosing considerations:* Death from cyanide poisoning occurs rapidly. Delays in administering the antidote should be avoided.

➤*Adults:*

Cyanide poising –

Usual dosage: 12.5 g intravenously (IV) over approximately 10 minutes used alone or in combination with other cyanide antidotes.

Repeat dosage: Patients should be closely monitored for 24 to 48 hours for symptoms of cyanide poisoning to reappear. In the event symptoms return, sodium thiosulfate administration should be repeated at one-half the original dose.

Off-label dosing –

Calciphylaxis: [4] = Insufficient documentation. 25 g IV 3 times per week after dialysis for 6 weeks to 9 months. Other treatment regimens used in studies were 25 g every other day, 25 g twice per week, 20 g 3 times per week, 5 g 4 times per week, and 25 g every other day by the intraperitoneal route.

Cisplatin extravasation: [4] = Insufficient documentation. A ⅙ M solution is prepared by mixing 4 mL of sodium thiosulfate 10% with 6 mL of sterile water for injection and infiltrating into the affected area. A dose of 2 mL through the existing IV line for each 100 mg of cisplatin suspected to have extravasated has been suggested. Additional 0.1 mL injections clockwise around the area of extravasation may be administered, for a total dose of 1 mL, and repeated several times in the 3 to 4 hours after the extravasation incident.

Cisplatin-induced nephrotoxicity: [2] = Fair documentation. 4 g/m^2 as an IV bolus followed by 12 g/m^2 as an IV infusion over 6 hours.

➤*Children:*

Cyanide poising –

Usual dosage: 7 g/m^2 of body surface area IV over approximately 10 minutes used alone or in combination with other cyanide antidotes.

Maximum dose: 12.5 g/dosage.

Repeat dosage: Patients should be closely monitored for 24 to 48 hours for symptoms of cyanide poisoning to reappear. In the event symptoms return, sodium thiosulfate administration should be repeated at one-half the original dose.

Off-label dosing –

Cisplatin extravasation: [4] = Insufficient documentation. See Adults for dosing.

Cisplatin-induced nephrotoxicity: [2] = Fair documentation. In the case of accidental cisplatin overdose in a child 14 years of age, sodium thiosulfate was given IV as a 4 g/m^2 loading dose, followed by 2.7 g/m^2/day in 3 divided doses and continued until urinary platinum levels fell below 1 mcg/mL.

➤*Administration:* For slow IV use only.

➤*Storage/Stability:* Store at 15° to 30°C (59° to 86°F).

Actions

➤*Pharmacology:* Sodium thiosulfate is used as an antidote for cyanide poisoning. The primary mechanism of cyanide detoxification involves the conversion of cyanide to the thiocyanate ion, which is relatively nontoxic. This reaction involves the enzyme rhodanese (thiosulfate: cyanide sulfurtransferase) that is found in many body tissues, but with the major activity in the liver. The body has the capability to detoxify cyanide, however, the rhodanese enzyme system is slow to respond to large amounts of cyanide. The rhodanese enzyme reaction can be accelerated by supplying an exogenous source of sulfur. This is commonly accomplished by administering sodium thiosulfate. Sodium thiosulfate may be used alone or in combination with nitrite compounds such as amyl nitrite or sodium nitrite.

➤*Pharmacokinetics:* Following IV injection, sodium thiosulfate is distributed throughout the extracellular fluid and is excreted unchanged in the urine. The biological half-life is reported to be 0.65 hours.

Contraindications

None known.

Warnings/Precautions

➤*Hypovolemia:* Sodium thiosulfate is essentially nontoxic. However, studies conducted in dogs, with a constant infusion of sodium thiosulfate, showed hypovolemia that was considered to be caused by an osmotic diuretic effect of sodium thiosulfate.

➤*Pregnancy: Category C.* Animal reproduction studies have not been conducted with sodium thiosulfate. It is also not known whether sodium thiosulfate can cause fetal harm when administered to a pregnant woman or can affect reproduction capacity. Sodium thiosulfate should be given to a pregnant woman only if clearly needed.

➤*Lactation:* There are no information regarding sodium thiosulfate in breast-feeding women.

➤*Monitoring:* Patients should be closely monitored for 24 to 48 hours for symptoms of cyanide poisoning to reappear. In the event symptoms return, sodium thiosulfate administration should be repeated at one-half the original dose.

Adverse Reactions

None known.

SODIUM NITRITE

Rx	**Sodium Nitrite** (Hope)	**Injection:** 30 mg/mL	In 10 mL vials.

SODIUM NITRITE — INJECTION

Indications

➤*Cyanide poisoning:* For use with sodium thiosulfate injection and amyl nitrite inhalants in the treatment of cyanide poisoning.

➤*Off-label uses:* Hydrogen sulfide poisoning.

Administration and Dosage

➤*General dosing considerations:* Personnel should acquire some skill in the proper method of administering cyanide antidote medications prior to an emergency. Cyanide poisoning is rapidly fatal. The patient seldom survives many hours. The prevention of death demands a quick diagnosis and the

SODIUM NITRITE — INJECTION

prompt use of specific antidotes. No valuable time should be lost. Even though the diagnosis is doubtful, the therapy recommended should be instituted immediately.

Instruct an assistant how to break an ampule of amyl nitrite, 1 at a time, in a handkerchief and hold it in front of the patient's mouth for 15 seconds, followed by a rest for 15 seconds. Then reapply until sodium nitrite can be administered. This interrupted schedule is important because continuous use of amyl nitrite may prevent adequate oxygenation.

If the poison was taken by mouth, gastric lavage should be performed as soon as possible, but this should not delay the treatments outlined. Lavage may be done concurrently by a third person, a physician or a nurse, if one is available. One should take quick action without waiting for positive diagnostic tests.

If respiration has ceased but the pulse is palpable, artificial respiration should be applied at once. The purpose is not to revive, per se, but to keep the heart beating. The gauze sponge or handkerchief continuing the amyl nitrite should be laid over the patient's nose, for it may hasten the resumption of respiration movements. When signs of breathing appear, injections of sodium nitrite and sodium thiosulfate should be made promptly.

The doses for children should be calculated on a surface area or on a weight basis with the dosage adjusted so that excessive methemoglobulin is not formed.

➤*Adults:*

Cyanide poisoning –

Usual dosage: Discontinue amyl nitrite; administer 300 mg IV (10 mL of a 3% solution) at the rate of 2.5 to 5 mL/min. Immediately thereafter, inject 12.5 g (50 mL of a 25% solution) of sodium thiosulfate.

Repeat dosage: The patient should be watched closely for at least 24 to 48 hours. If signs of poisoning reappear, injection of both sodium nitrite and sodium thiosulfate should be repeated, but each in one-half of the original dose. Even if the patient seems perfectly well, the medication may be given for prophylactic purposes 2 hours after the first injections.

➤*Children:*

Cyanide poisoning –

Usual dosage: Discontinue amyl nitrite; administer 6 to 8 mL/m^2 (approximately 0.2 mL/kg of body weight) IV, not to exceed 300 mg (10 mL) at a rate of 2.5 to 5 mL/min. Immediately thereafter, inject 7 g/m^2 of body surface area of sodium thiosulfate, not to exceed 12.5 g.

Maximum dose: 300 mg/dosage.

Repeat dosage: The patient should be watched closely for at least 24 to 48 hours. If signs of poisoning reappear, injection of both sodium nitrite and sodium thiosulfate should be repeated, but each in one-half of the original dose. Even if the patient seems perfectly well, the medication may be given for prophylactic purposes 2 hours after the first injections.

➤*Administration:* For IV administration only. The same needle and vein may be used when administering sodium thiosulfate.

➤*Storage/Stability:* Store at 15° to 30°C (59° to 86°F).

Actions

➤*Pharmacology:* Sodium nitrite reacts with hemoglobin to form methemoglobin. The latter removes cyanide ions from various tissues and couples with them to become cyanmethemoglobin, which has relatively low toxicity. The function of sodium thiosulfate is to convert cyanide to thiocyanate, probably by an enzyme known as rhodanese. The combined mechanism may thus be expressed in a chemical manner:

- $NaNO_2$ + hemoglobin = methemoglobin.
- HCN + methemoglobin = cyanmethemoglobin.
- $Na_2S_2O_3$ + HCN + O = HSCN

The combination of sodium nitrite and sodium thiosulfate is effective therapy against cyanide and hydrocyanic acid poisoning. The 2 substances intravenously injected, 1 after the other (nitrite followed by the thiosulfate) are capable of detoxifying approximately 20 lethal doses of sodium cyanide in dogs and are effective even after respiration has stopped. As long as the heart is still beating, the chances of recovery by utilizing this method are good.

There is not only a summation but also a definite potentiation of action when the nitrite and the thiosulfate are administered together.

Warnings/Precautions

➤*Methemoglobinemia:* Both sodium nitrite and amyl nitrite in excessive doses induce dangerous methemoglobinemia and can cause death. The dosage recommended is not excessive for an adult. The doses for children should be calculated on a surface area or on a weight basis with the dosage adjusted so that excessive methemoglobulin is not formed.

If signs of excessive methemoglobulin develop (ie, blue skin and mucous membranes, vomiting, shock, and coma), 1% methylene blue solution should be given intravenously. A total dose of 1 to 2 mg/kg of body weight should be administered over a period of 5 to 10 minutes and should be repeated in 1 hour if necessary.

In addition, oxygen inhalation and transfusion of whole fresh blood should be considered.

➤*Pregnancy: Category: Undetermined.* There is no information regarding sodium nitrite in pregnant women.

➤*Lactation:* There is no information regarding sodium nitrite in breastfeeding women.

➤*Monitoring:* Nitrites produce significant vasodilation, and rapid administration may result in hypotension. Hypotension may be avoided or lessened by slow administration (eg, IV push over at least 5 minutes) or by diluting the dose in 50 to 100 mL of 5% dextrose in water or normal saline and beginning infusion as a slow drip then increasing to the most rapid rate tolerated. Frequently monitor blood pressure during treatment with sodium nitrite.

Adverse Reactions

Dizziness, flushing, headache, hypotension, methemoglobinemia, nausea, syncope, tachycardia, and vomiting may occur.

NALOXONE HYDROCHLORIDE

Rx	**Naloxone Hydrochloride** (Various, eg, Hospira, SoloPak)	**Injection:** 0.4 mg/mL	In 1 mL amps, 1 mL syringes and 1, 2 and 10 mL vials.
Rx	**Narcan** (DuPont Pharm.)		In 1 mL amps and 10 mL vials.[a]
Rx	**Naloxone Hydrochloride** (Various, eg, Hospira)	**Neonatal injection:** 0.02 mg/mL	In 2 ml vials.

[a] Available with or without parabens.

NALOXONE HYDROCHLORIDE — INJECTION

Indications

➤*Reversal of opioid effects:* For the complete or partial reversal of narcotic depression, including respiratory depression, induced by opioid including natural and synthetic narcotics, propoxyphene, methadone, nalbuphine, butorphanol and pentazocine.

➤*Opioid overdose:* For the diagnosis of suspected acute opioid overdosage.

➤*Off-label uses:*

Alzheimer disease – [5] = Poor documentation. Limited data suggest that naloxone does not have beneficial cognitive or behavioral effects in patients with Alzheimer disease.

Other possible off-label uses – Naloxone has been used to improve circulation in refractory shock. Naloxone has also been used for the reversal of alcoholic coma and in schizophrenia.

Administration and Dosage

➤*General dosing considerations:* Keep patients under continued surveillance and give repeat doses as necessary. Duration of action of some narcotics may exceed that of naloxone.

➤*Adults:*

Opioid overdose – Initial dose is 0.4 to 2 mg IV; may repeat IV at 2- to 3-minute intervals. IM or subcutaneous administration may be necessary if the IV route is not available. If no response is observed after 10 mg has been administered, question the diagnosis of narcotic-induced or partial narcotic-induced toxicity.

Postoperative opioid depression – Small doses are usually sufficient. Titrate dose according to the patient's response. Excessive dosage may result in significant reversal of analgesia and increase in blood pressure. Similarly, too rapid reversal may induce nausea, vomiting, sweating or circulatory stress.

Initial dosage: Inject in increments of 0.1 to 0.2 mg IV at 2 to 3 minute intervals to the desired degree of reversal (ie, adequate ventilation and alertness without significant pain or discomfort).

Repeat dose: Repeat doses may be required within 1- or 2-hour intervals depending on the amount, type (ie, short- or long-acting), and time interval since last administration. Supplemental IM doses have produced a longer lasting effect.

Off-label dosing –

➤*Children:*

One month of age and older –

Opioid overdose: Initial dose is 0.01 mg/kg IV; give a subsequent dose of 0.1 mg/kg if needed. If an IV route is not available, may be given IM or subcutaneously in divided doses. If necessary, dilute with sterile water for injection.

Postoperative opioid depression: Follow the recommendations and cautions under adult administration guidelines. For initial reversal of respiratory depression, inject in increments of 0.005 to 0.01 mg IV at 2- to 3-minute intervals to desired degree of reversal.

Neonates –

Opioid-induced depression: Initial dose is 0.01 mg/kg IV, IM, or subcutaneous; may be repeated in accordance with adult administration guidelines.

➤*Preparation for administration:* Dilute in normal saline or dextrose 5% solutions. The addition of 2 mg in 500 mL of either solution provides a concentration of 0.004 mg/mL.

NALOXONE HYDROCHLORIDE — INJECTION

➤*Administration:* Give IV, IM, or subcutaneously. The most rapid onset of action is achieved with IV use, which is recommended in emergency situations. Titrate the administration rate in accordance with the patient's response.

➤*Admixture compatibility:* Do not mix with preparations containing bisulfite, metabisulfite, long-chain or high molecular weight anions, or any solution having an alkaline pH. Do not add any drug or chemical agent unless its effect on the chemical and physical stability of the solution has first been established.

➤*Storage/Stability:* Store at 59°F to 86°F. Protect from light. Use diluted solution for infusion within 24 hours. Discard any unused infusion solution after 24 hours.

Actions

➤*Pharmacology:* The narcotic antagonist naloxone is clinically useful in the reversal of narcotic-induced respiratory depression. Naloxone, a pure narcotic antagonist, will precipitate abstinence syndrome in the presence of narcotic addiction. Because it is devoid of undesirable agonist properties, naloxone is preferred for reversal of narcotic-induced respiratory depression. Naloxone prevents or reverses opioid effects including respiratory depression, sedation and hypotension; it can reverse psychotomimetic and dysphoric effects of agonist-antagonists (eg, pentazocine).

The mechanism of action is not fully understood; evidence suggests that it antagonizes the opioid effects by competing for the same receptor sites. Naloxone is an essentially pure narcotic antagonist, ie, it does not possess "agonistic" or morphine-like properties.

Naloxone does not produce respiratory depression, psychotomimetic effects or pupillary constriction. In the absence of narcotics or agonistic effects of other narcotic antagonists, naloxone exhibits essentially no pharmacologic activity.

➤*Pharmacokinetics:*

Distribution – After parenteral use, naloxone is rapidly distributed in the body. Onset of action of IV naloxone is generally apparent within 2 min; it is only slightly less rapid when given subcutaneously or IM. Duration of action depends upon dose and route. IM use produces a more prolonged effect than IV use. The requirement for repeat doses will also depend upon amount, type and route of the narcotic being antagonized.

Metabolism – Naloxone is metabolized in the liver, primarily by glucuronide conjugation. It is excreted in the urine. The serum of half-life in adults ranged from 30 to 81 minutes (mean 64 ± 12 minutes); in neonates, 3.1 ± 0.5 hours.

Contraindications

Hypersensitivity to these agents.

Warnings/Precautions

➤*Drug dependence:* Administer cautiously to persons who are known or suspected to be physically dependent on opioids, including newborns of mothers with narcotic dependence. Reversal of narcotic effect will precipitate acute abstinence syndrome.

➤*Repeat administration:* The patient who has satisfactorily responded should be kept under continued surveillance. Administer repeated doses as necessary, because the duration of action of some narcotics may exceed that of the narcotic antagonist.

➤*Respiratory depression:* Not effective against respiratory depression due to nonopioid drugs. Reversal of buprenorphine-induced respiratory depression may be incomplete; if an incomplete response occurs, mechanically assist respiration.

➤*Other supportive therapy:* Maintain a free airway and provide artificial respiration, cardiac massage and vasopressor agents; employ when necessary to counteract acute narcotic overdosage.

➤*Cardiovascular effects:* Several instances of hypotension, hypertension, pulmonary edema, ventricular tachycardia and fibrillation have been reported in postoperative patients, most of whom had preexisting cardiovascular disorders or had received other drugs that may have similar adverse cardiovascular effects. A direct cause and effect relationship is not established; use caution in patients with pre-existing cardiac disease or who have received potentially cardiotoxic drugs.

➤*Pregnancy: Category B.* No adequate and well controlled studies in pregnant women. Use during pregnancy only when clearly needed.

➤*Lactation:* It is not known whether the drug is excreted in breast milk. Use caution when administering to a nursing woman.

Adverse Reactions

Abrupt reversal of narcotic depression may result in nausea, vomiting, sweating, tachycardia, increased blood pressure and tremulousness.

In postoperative patients, excessive dosage may result in excitement and significant reversal of analgesia, hypotension, hypertension, pulmonary edema and ventricular tachycardia and fibrillation. Seizures have been reported infrequently.

METHYLNALTREXONE BROMIDE

Rx	**Relistor** (Wyeth)	**Injection, solution:** 12 mg per 0.6 mL	Edetate calcium disodium 0.24 mg, glycine 0.18 mg. In single-use vials.

METHYLNALTREXONE BROMIDE — INJECTION

Indications

➤*Opioid-induced constipation:* For the treatment of opioid-induced constipation in patients with advanced illness who are receiving palliative care, when response to laxative therapy has not been sufficient.

Administration and Dosage

➤*Adults:*

Opioid-induced constipation –

Usual dosage:

Methylnaltrexone Dosage Recommendations

Weight	Injection volume	Dose[a]
< 38 kg	[b]	0.15 mg/kg
38 to < 62 kg	0.4 mL	8 mg
62 to 114 kg	0.6 mL	12 mg
> 114 kg	[a]	0.15 mg/kg

[a] The usual schedule is 1 dose every other day as needed, but no more frequently than 1 dose in a 24-hour period.

[b] The injection volume for these patients should be calculated by multiplying the patient weight in kilograms by 0.0075 and rounding up the volume to the nearest 0.1 mL.

➤*Renal function impairment:*

Severe renal impairment (creatinine clearance [CrCl] less than 30 mL/min) – Dose reduction by one-half is recommended.

➤*Administration:* Administer subcutaneously in the upper arm, abdomen, or thigh.

➤*Storage/Stability:* Store between 20° and 25°C (68° and 77°F); excursions are permitted between 15° and 30°C (59° and 86°F). Do not freeze. Protect from light. Once drawn into the syringe, if immediate administration is not possible, store at ambient room temperature and administer within 24 hours.

Actions

➤*Pharmacology:* Methylnaltrexone is a selective antagonist of opioid binding at the mu-opioid receptor. As a quaternary amine, the ability of methylnaltrexone to cross the blood-brain barrier is restricted. This allows methylnaltrexone to function as a peripherally acting mu-opioid receptor antagonist in tissues, such as the GI tract, thereby decreasing the constipating effects of opioids without impacting opioid-mediated analgesic effects on the CNS.

➤*Pharmacokinetics:*

Absorption – Methylnaltrexone is absorbed rapidly, with peak concentrations (C_{max}) achieved at approximately 0.5 hours.

Methylnaltrexone Pharmacokinetic Parameters Following Single Subcutaneous Doses

Parameter	0.15 mg/kg	0.3 mg/kg	0.5 mg/kg
C_{max} (ng/mL)[a]	117 (32.7)	239 (62.2)	392 (147.9)
T_{max}[b] (h)[c]	0.5 (0.25 to 0.75)	0.5 (0.25 to 0.75)	0.5 (0.25 to 0.75)
AUC_{24} (ng•h/mL)[ab]	175 (36.6)	362 (63.8)	582 (111.2)

[a] Expressed as mean (standard deviation [SD]).

[b] T_{max} = amount of time to reach C_{max}; AUC = area under the curve.

[c] Expressed as median (range).

Distribution – Methylnaltrexone undergoes moderate tissue distribution. The steady-state volume of distribution is approximately 1.1 L/kg. The fraction of methylnaltrexone bound to human plasma proteins is 11% to 15.3%, as determined by equilibrium dialysis.

Metabolism – In a mass balance study, approximately 60% of the administered radioactivity recovered with 5 distinct metabolites and none of the detected metabolites was in amounts of more than 6% of administered radioactivity. Conversion to methyl-6-naltrexol isomers (5% of total) and methylnaltrexone sulfate (1.3% of total) appear to be the primary pathways of metabolism. N-demethylation of methylnaltrexone to produce naltrexone is not significant.

Excretion – Methylnaltrexone is eliminated primarily as unchanged drug (85% of administered radioactivity). Approximately half of the dose is excreted in the urine and somewhat less in feces. The terminal half-life is approximately 8 hours.

Special populations –

Renal function impairment: In a study of volunteers with varying degrees of renal impairment receiving a single dose of methylnaltrexone 0.3 mg/kg, renal impairment had a marked effect on the renal excretion of methylnaltrexone. Severe renal impairment decreased the renal clearance of methyl-

METHYLNALTREXONE BROMIDE — INJECTION

naltrexone by 8- to 9-fold and resulted in a 2-fold increase in total methylnaltrexone exposure (AUC). C_{max} was not significantly changed. No studies were performed in patients with end-stage renal impairment requiring dialysis.

Contraindications

Known or suspected mechanical GI obstruction.

Warnings/Precautions

➤*Severe or persistent diarrhea:* If severe or persistent diarrhea occurs during treatment, advise patients to discontinue therapy with methylnaltrexone and consult their health care provider.

➤*Intestinal perforation:* Rare cases of GI perforation have been reported in advanced illness patients with conditions that may be associated with localized or diffuse reduction of structural integrity in the wall of the GI tract (ie, cancer, peptic ulcer, Ogilvie syndrome). Perforations have involved varying regions of the GI tract (eg, stomach, duodenum, colon).

Use with caution in patients with known or suspected lesions of the GI tract. Advise patients to discontinue therapy and promptly notify their health care provider if they develop severe, persistent, and/or worsening abdominal symptoms.

➤*Renal function impairment:* See Administration and Dosage for more information.

➤*Pregnancy: Category B.* There are no adequate and well-controlled studies in pregnant women. Because animal reproduction studies are not always predictive of human response, use methylnaltrexone during pregnancy only if clearly needed.

➤*Lactation:* Results from an animal study using [^{3}H]-labeled methylnaltrexone indicate that methylnaltrexone is excreted via the milk of lactating rats. It is not known whether this drug is excreted in human milk. The molecular weight (approximately 436), minimal plasma protein binding (less than 15%), and long elimination half-life (about 8 hours) suggest that the drug will be excreted into breast milk. Because many drugs are excreted in human milk, exercise caution when methylnaltrexone is administered to a breast-feeding woman.

➤*Children:* Safety and efficacy of methylnaltrexone have not been established in children.

Adverse Reactions

Methylnaltrexone Adverse Reactions[a]

Adverse reactions	Methylnaltrexone (n = 165)	Placebo (n = 123)
GI		
Abdominal pain	28.5%	9.8%
Diarrhea	5.5%	2.4%
Flatulence	13.3%	5.7%
Nausea	11.5%	4.9%
Miscellaneous		
Dizziness	7.3%	2.4%
Hyperhidrosis	6.7%	6.5%

[a] Doses: 0.075, 0.15, and 0.3 mg/kg/dose.

➤*Postmarketing:*

GI – Rare cases of GI perforation have been reported in advanced illness patients with conditions that may be associated with localized or diffuse reduction of structural integrity in the wall of the GI tract (eg, cancer, peptic ulcer, Ogilvie syndrome). Perforations have involved varying regions of the GI tract (eg, stomach, duodenum, colon).

Overdosage

➤*Symptoms:* A study of healthy volunteers noted orthostatic hypotension associated with a dose of 0.64 mg/kg administered as an intravenous (IV) bolus.

➤*Treatment:* In the event of overdose, employ the usual supportive measures (eg, clinical monitoring and supportive therapy as dictated by the patient's clinical status). Monitor signs or symptoms of orthostatic hypotension and initiate treatment as appropriate.

Patient Information

Instruct patients that the usual schedule is 1 dose every other day as needed, but no more frequently than 1 dose in a 24-hour period.

In approximately 30% of patients in clinical trials, laxation was reported within 30 minutes of a dose of methylnaltrexone; therefore, advise patients to be within close proximity to toilet facilities once the drug is administered.

Instruct patients not to continue taking methylnaltrexone if they experience severe or persistent diarrhea. Instruct patients that common adverse reactions of methylnaltrexone include transient abdominal pain, nausea, and vomiting.

Instruct patients not to continue taking methylnaltrexone and to promptly notify their health care provider if they experience severe, persistent, and/or worsening abdominal symptoms because these could be symptoms of intestinal perforation.

Instruct patients to discontinue methylnaltrexone if they stop taking their opioid pain medication.

NALTREXONE HYDROCHLORIDE

Rx	**Naltrexone Hydrochloride** (Various, eg, Barr, Eon, Mallinckrodt)	**Tablets; oral:** 50 mg	May contain lactose, PEG. In 30s, 100s, and 500s.
Rx	**ReVia** (Duramed)		Lactose, PEG. (ReVia b/275). Beige, round, scored. Film-coated. In 100s and UD 30s.
Rx	**Vivitrol** (Alkermes)	**Injection, powder for suspension, extended-release:** 380 mg	In single-use vials with 4 mL diluent, syringe, and needles.

NALTREXONE HYDROCHLORIDE — ORAL

WARNING

Hepatotoxicity – Naltrexone has the capacity to cause hepatocellular injury when given in excessive doses. Naltrexone is contraindicated in acute hepatitis or liver failure, and its use in patients with active liver disease must be carefully considered in light of its hepatotoxic effects. The margin of separation between the apparently safe dose of naltrexone and the dose causing hepatic injury appears to be only 5-fold or less. Naltrexone does not appear to be a hepatotoxin at the recommended doses. Warn patients of the risk of hepatic injury and advise them to stop the use of naltrexone and seek medical attention if they experience symptoms of acute hepatitis.

Indications

➤*Alcohol dependence:* For the treatment of alcohol dependence.

➤*Opioid dependence:* For the blockade of the effects of exogenously administered opioids.

➤*Off-label uses:*

Cholestatic pruritus (adults) – [2] = Fair documentation. Data from published trials suggest that oral naltrexone is effective in the management of cholestatic-related pruritus, with an onset of action as early as the first day in some patients. Guidelines recommend the use of this agent in patients who fail cholestyramine or rifampicin. The limiting factor to naltrexone use in the management of cholestatic pruritus is the possibility of an opioid-withdrawal–like reaction, which may be avoided by starting the drug at a lower dose and titrating upward.

Eating disorders – [4] = Insufficient documentation. At standard dosing, naltrexone has not consistently been superior to placebo, and significant safety issues arise with higher dosages. American Psychiatric Association guidelines recommend antidepressants as the initial treatment for patients with bulimia nervosa or binge-eating disorder.

Irritable bowel syndrome – [3] = Safety concerns. Initial data from 1 small, noncontrolled trial suggest that low-dose naltrexone may have a beneficial role in the management of irritable bowel syndrome (IBS) or symptoms of IBS in some patients.

Pathological gambling – [4] = Insufficient documentation. Data regarding the use of naltrexone for the treatment of pathological gambling are limited to 1 small, controlled trial and 2 case reports (fewer than 25 naltrexone-treated patients). These initial data are positive, suggesting beneficial effects of the drug in this patient population. However, data analysis in the clinical trial also suggested a high placebo response.

Posttraumatic stress disorder – [4] = Insufficient documentation. The use of naltrexone in the management of posttraumatic stress disorder is not recognized in national guidelines. Data from controlled and noncontrolled trials suggest that further studies are required to identify an optimal dose and most responsive candidates.

Prevention of spinal opioid–related pruritus – [4] = Insufficient documentation. Initial data suggest that naltrexone may be beneficial in the prevention of spinal opioid–related pruritus. These data are limited by small population, and further study in larger, controlled settings is needed.

Pruritus – [2] = Fair documentation. Because of the potential for withdrawal-type reactions, the utility of this agent may be limited to patients with severe pruritus who are refractory to traditional treatment.

NALTREXONE HYDROCHLORIDE — ORAL

Although most patients experience improvement in cholestatic pruritus–related symptoms with naltrexone, results are mixed in patients with uremic pruritus.

Smoking cessation – [5] = Poor documentation. Studies evaluating naltrexone as an aid in smoking cessation have produced inconsistent data. No randomized, placebo-controlled trials have shown a long-term benefit in using naltrexone to improve cessation rates or evidence that naltrexone is superior to Food and Drug Administration-approved first-line smoking cessation agents, such as bupropion and varenicline. With no evidence of clear benefit in this setting and with first-line alternatives available, naltrexone is not a rational therapeutic choice.

Uremic pruritus (adults) – [4] = Insufficient documentation. There are no guidelines that specifically address the treatment of uremic pruritus. Small, controlled trials have produced conflicting results regarding the efficacy of naltrexone in the management of uremic pruritus. Although a small subset of patients in one study showed marked improvement with naltrexone, it is not clear which patients would benefit from treatment. In addition, most trials have demonstrated a high incidence of adverse reactions. Until larger, controlled trials confirm its efficacy, naltrexone is not recommended for routine use or as first-line treatment in the management of uremic pruritus.

Other possible off-label uses – Naltrexone has been used in the treatment of postconcussional syndrome unresponsive to other treatments. To increase patient compliance, a subcutaneous implant is being studied.

Administration and Dosage

➤*General dosing considerations:* Do not initiate naltrexone therapy until the naloxone challenge is negative (see Naloxone Challenge Test).

Alcohol dependence – A patient is a candidate for treatment with naltrexone if the patient is willing to take medicine to help with alcohol dependence, the patient is opioid free for 7 to 10 days, the patient does not have severe or active liver or kidney problems (typical guidelines suggest liver function tests no greater than 3 times the upper limits of normal, and bilirubin normal), the patient is not allergic to naltrexone, and no other contraindications are present.

Opioid dependence – Treatment should not be attempted unless the patient has remained opioid free for at least 7 to 10 days. Self-reporting of abstinence from opioids in opioid addicts should be verified by analysis of the patient's urine for absence of opioids. The patient should not be manifesting withdrawal signs or reporting withdrawal symptoms.

If there is any question of occult opioid dependence, perform a naloxone challenge test. If signs of opioid withdrawal are still observed following naloxone challenge, treatment with naltrexone should not be attempted. The naloxone challenge can be repeated in 24 hours.

➤*Adults:*

Alcohol dependence –

Usual dosage: 50 mg once daily (see Alternative Dosage).

Duration of therapy: The placebo-controlled studies that demonstrated the efficacy of naltrexone as an adjunctive treatment of alcoholism used a dose regimen of naltrexone 50 mg once daily for up to 12 weeks. Other durations of therapy were not evaluated in these trials.

Opioid dependence –

Initial dosage: Initiate carefully at 25 mg.

Maintenance dosage: If no withdrawal signs occur after initiation, the patient may be started on 50 mg/day thereafter (see Alternative Dosage).

Off-label dosing –

Cholestatic pruritus (adults): [2] = Fair documentation. According to guidelines, oral naltrexone should be initiated at 12.5 mg (a quarter of a tablet) and increased by a quarter (12.5 mg) every 3 to 7 days until the pruritus is eliminated. Drug administration can be held or the dose kept constant if the patient exhibits signs of opiate-like withdrawal syndrome. A reduced dose may be required in patients with decompensated liver disease because metabolites can accumulate.

Dosages of 50 mg daily from 1 week up to 28 weeks have been used in published reports, which are higher dosages than recommended in guidelines.

Eating disorders: [4] = Insufficient documentation. 50 mg daily. Some data are available for higher dosages of 200 to 300 mg daily.

Irritable bowel syndrome: [3] = Safety concerns. 0.5 mg daily taken at bedtime for 4 weeks.

Pathological gambling: [4] = Insufficient documentation. 25 to 50 mg daily and titrate up to 100 to 250 mg daily.

Posttraumatic stress disorder: [4] = Insufficient documentation. Initiate at oral dosing of 50 mg daily for up to 12 weeks, or with gradual increases of increments of 50 mg every 2 days to up to 100 mg daily, and then increase, if tolerated, to 200 mg daily for a total duration of 2 weeks.

Prevention of spinal opioid–related pruritus: [4] = Insufficient documentation. Oral naltrexone 3 or 6 mg administered via oral solution in 10 mL volume administered at 60 minutes after intrathecal morphine postoperative dose.

Pruritus: [2] = Fair documentation. 50 mg daily.

Uremic pruritus (adults): [4] = Insufficient documentation. Administered orally as 50 mg daily for up to 4 weeks.

➤*Hepatic function impairment:* Naltrexone has the capacity to cause hepatocellular injury when given in excessive doses. Naltrexone is contraindicated in acute hepatitis or liver failure, and its use in patients with active liver disease must be carefully considered in light of its hepatotoxic effects.

➤*Naloxone challenge test:* Do not perform in a patient showing clinical signs or symptoms of opioid withdrawal, or in a patient whose urine contains opioids. Administer the test either by intravenous (IV) or subcutaneous routes. Individual patients, especially those with opioid dependence, may respond to lower doses of naloxone.

IV – Naloxone 0.2 mg; observe for 30 seconds for signs or symptoms of withdrawal. If no evidence of withdrawal is observed, inject naloxone 0.6 mg; observe for an additional 20 minutes. In some cases, naloxone 0.1 mg IV has produced a diagnostic response.

Subcutaneous – Naloxone 0.8 mg; observe for 20 minutes for signs or symptoms of withdrawal.

Interpretation of the challenge – Monitor vital signs and observe the patient for signs and symptoms of opioid withdrawal.

If signs or symptoms of withdrawal appear, the test is positive and no additional naloxone should be administered. If the test is positive do not initiate naltrexone therapy. Repeat the challenge in 24 hours. If the test is negative, naltrexone therapy may be started if no other contraindications are present. If there is any doubt about the result of the test, hold naltrexone and repeat the challenge in 24 hours.

➤*Alternative dosage:* Once the patient has been started on naltrexone, 50 mg every 24 hours will produce adequate clinical blockade of the actions of parenterally administered opioids (ie, this dose will block the effects of a heroin 25 mg IV challenge). A flexible approach to a dosing regimen may need to be employed in cases of supervised administration. Thus, patients may receive naltrexone 50 mg every weekday with a 100 mg dose on Saturday, 100 mg every other day, or 150 mg every third day. The degree of blockade produced by naltrexone may be reduced by these extended dosing intervals. There may be a higher risk of hepatocellular injury with single doses above 50 mg, and use of higher doses and extended dosing intervals should balance the possible risks against the probable benefits.

➤*Administration:* Administer orally without regard to meals but administer with food if GI upset occurs.

➤*Storage/Stability:* Store at 20° to 25°C (68° to 77°F).

Actions

➤*Pharmacology:*

Alcohol dependence – The mechanism of action of naltrexone in alcoholism is not understood; however, involvement of the endogenous opioid system is suggested by preclinical data. Naltrexone, a pure opioid receptor antagonist, competitively binds to such receptors and may block the effects of endogenous opioids. Opioid antagonists reduce alcohol consumption by animals, and naltrexone has been shown to reduce alcohol consumption in clinical studies.

Opioid dependence – Naltrexone markedly attenuates or completely blocks, reversibly, the subjective effects of IV-administered opioids by competitive binding (ie, analogous to competitive inhibition of enzymes) at opioid receptors. This makes the blockade produced potentially surmountable, but overcoming full naltrexone blockade by administration of very high doses of opiates has resulted in excessive symptoms of histamine release in experimental subjects. When coadministered with morphine, on a long-term basis, naltrexone blocks the physical dependence to morphine, heroin, and other opioids.

➤*Pharmacokinetics:*

Absorption – Following oral administration, naltrexone undergoes rapid and nearly complete absorption with approximately 96% of the dose absorbed from the GI tract. Peak plasma levels of both naltrexone and 6-beta-naltrexol occur within 1 hour of dosing.

Oral bioavailability estimates range from 5% to 40%. The activity of naltrexone is believed to be due to both parent and the 6-beta-naltrexol metabolite. Naltrexone and 6-beta-naltrexol are dose proportional in terms of area under the curve (AUC) and maximal drug concentration (C_{max}) over the range of 50 to 200 mg and do not accumulate after 100 mg daily doses.

Distribution – The volume of distribution for naltrexone following IV administration is estimated to be 1,350 L. In vitro tests with human plasma show naltrexone is 21% bound to plasma proteins over the therapeutic dose range.

Metabolism – Although well absorbed orally, naltrexone is subject to significant first-pass metabolism. The systemic clearance (after IV administration) of naltrexone is approximately 3.5 L/min, which exceeds liver blood flow (approximately 1.2 L/min). This suggests that naltrexone is a highly extracted drug (greater than 98% metabolized) and that extrahepatic sites of drug metabolism exist. The major metabolite of naltrexone is 6-beta-naltrexol. Two other minor metabolites are 2-hydroxy-3-methoxy-6-beta-naltrexol and 2-hydroxy-3-methyl-naltrexone. Naltrexone and its metabolites are also conjugated to form additional metabolic products.

Excretion – Both parent drug and metabolites are excreted primarily by the kidney (53% to 79% of the dose); however, urinary excretion of unchanged naltrexone accounts for less than 2% of an oral dose and fecal excretion is a minor elimination pathway. The mean elimination half-life values for naltrexone and 6-beta-naltrexol are 4 and 13 hours, respectively. The renal clearance for naltrexone ranges from 30 to 127 mL/min and suggests that renal elimination is primarily by glomerular filtration. In comparison, the renal clearance for 6-beta-naltrexol ranges from 230 to 369 mL/min, suggesting an additional renal tubular secretory mechanism. The urinary excretion of unchanged naltrexone accounts for less than 2% of an oral dose; urinary excretion of unchanged and conjugated 6-beta-naltrexol

NALTREXONE HYDROCHLORIDE — ORAL

accounts for 43% of an oral dose. The pharmacokinetic profile of naltrexone suggests that naltrexone and its metabolites may undergo enterohepatic recycling.

Special populations –

Hepatic function impairment: Naltrexone appears to have extrahepatic sites of drug metabolism. An increase in naltrexone AUC of approximately 5- and 10-fold in patients with compensated and decompensated liver cirrhosis, respectively, compared with subjects with normal liver function has been reported. These data also suggest that alterations in naltrexone bioavailability are related to liver disease severity. Adequate studies of naltrexone in patients with severe hepatic impairment have not been conducted.

Contraindications

Patients receiving opioid analgesics; patients currently dependent on opioids, including those currently maintained on opiate agonists (methadone or levo-alpha-acetyl-methadol); patients in acute opioid withdrawal; any individual who has failed the naloxone challenge test or who has a positive urine screen for opioids; any individual with acute hepatitis or liver failure; any individual with a history of sensitivity to naltrexone or any other components of this product.

Warnings/Precautions

➤*Hepatotoxicity:* Evidence of the hepatotoxic potential of naltrexone is derived primarily from a placebo-controlled study in which naltrexone was administered to obese subjects at a dose approximately 5-fold that recommended for the blockade of opiate receptors (300 mg/day). In that study, 5 of 26 naltrexone recipients developed elevations of serum transaminases (ie, peak ALT values ranging from a low of 121 to a high of 532; or 3 to 19 times their baseline values) after 3 to 8 weeks of treatment. Although the patients involved were generally clinically asymptomatic and the transaminase levels of all patients on whom follow-up was obtained returned to (or toward) baseline values in a matter of weeks, the lack of any transaminase elevations of similar magnitude in any of the 24 placebo patients in the same study is persuasive evidence that naltrexone is a direct (ie, not idiosyncratic) hepatotoxin.

This conclusion is also supported by evidence from other placebo-controlled studies in which exposure to naltrexone at doses above the amount recommended for the treatment of alcoholism or opiate blockade (50 mg/day) consistently produced more numerous and more significant elevations of serum transaminases than did placebo. Transaminase elevations in 3 of 9 patients with Alzheimer disease who received naltrexone (at dosages up to 300 mg/day) for 5 to 8 weeks in an open clinical trial have been reported.

Although no cases of hepatic failure due to naltrexone administration have ever been reported, health care providers are advised to consider this as a possible risk of treatment and to use the same care in prescribing naltrexone as they would other drugs with the potential for causing hepatic injury.

➤*Abstinence syndrome:* To prevent occurrence of an acute abstinence syndrome, or exacerbation of a preexisting subclinical abstinence syndrome, patients must be opioid free for a minimum of 7 to 10 days before starting naltrexone. Since the absence of an opioid drug in the urine is often not sufficient proof that a patient is opioid free, a naloxone challenge should be employed if the prescribing health care provider feels there is a risk of precipitating a withdrawal reaction following administration of naltrexone.

➤*Overcoming blockade:* While naltrexone is a potent antagonist with a prolonged pharmacologic effect (24 to 72 hours), the blockade produced by naltrexone is surmountable. This is useful in patients who may require analgesia, but poses a potential risk to individuals who attempt, on their own, to overcome the blockade by administering large amounts of exogenous opioids. Indeed, any attempt by a patient to overcome the antagonism by taking opioids is very dangerous and may lead to a fatal overdose. Injury may arise because the plasma concentration of exogenous opioids attained immediately following their acute administration may be sufficient to overcome the competitive receptor blockade. As a consequence, the patient may be in immediate danger of suffering life-endangering opioid intoxication (eg, respiratory arrest, circulatory collapse). Patients should be told of the serious consequences of trying to overcome the opiate blockage.

There is also the possibility that a patient who had been treated with naltrexone will respond to lower doses of opioids than previously used, particularly if taken in such a manner that high plasma concentrations remain in the body beyond the time that naltrexone exerts its therapeutic effects. This could result in potentially life-threatening opioid intoxication (eg, respiratory compromise or arrest, circulatory collapse). Patients should be aware that they may be more sensitive to lower doses of opioids after naltrexone treatment is discontinued.

➤*Rapid opiate detoxification programs:* Safe use of naltrexone in rapid opiate detoxification programs has not been established.

➤*Reversal of blockade:* In an emergency situation in patients receiving fully blocking doses of naltrexone, a suggested plan of management is regional analgesia, conscious sedation with a benzodiazepine, use of nonopioid analgesics or general anesthesia.

In a situation requiring opioid analgesia, the amount of opioid required may be greater than usual, and the resulting respiratory depression may be deeper and more prolonged.

A rapidly acting opioid analgesic that minimizes the duration of respiratory depression is preferred. Titrate amount of analgesic administered to the needs of the patient. Nonreceptor-mediated actions may occur and should be expected (eg, facial swelling, itching, generalized erythema, bronchoconstriction) presumably due to histamine release.

Irrespective of the drug chosen to reverse naltrexone blockade, the patient should be monitored closely by appropriately trained personnel in a setting equipped and staffed for cardiopulmonary resuscitation.

➤*Withdrawal:* Severe opioid withdrawal syndromes precipitated by the accidental ingestion of naltrexone have been reported in opioid-dependent individuals. Symptoms of withdrawal have usually appeared within 5 minutes of ingestion of naltrexone and have lasted for up to 48 hours. Mental status changes including confusion, somnolence, and visual hallucinations have occurred. Significant fluid losses from vomiting and diarrhea have required IV fluid administration. In all cases, patients were closely monitored, and therapy with nonopioid medications was tailored to meet individual requirements.

Use of naltrexone does not eliminate or diminish withdrawal symptoms. If naltrexone is initiated early in the abstinence process, it will not preclude the patient's experience of the full range of signs and symptoms that would be experienced if naltrexone had not been started. Numerous adverse events are known to be associated with withdrawal.

➤*Suicide:* The risk of suicide is known to be increased in patients with substance abuse with or without concomitant depression. This risk is not abated by treatment with naltrexone.

➤*Hypersensitivity reactions:* It is not known if there is any cross-sensitivity with naloxone or the phenanthrene-containing opioids.

➤*Renal function impairment:* Naltrexone and its primary metabolite are excreted primarily in the urine, and caution is recommended in administering the drug to patients with renal impairment.

➤*Hepatic function impairment:* Exercise caution when naltrexone is administered to patients with liver disease.

➤*Drug abuse and dependence:* Naltrexone is a pure opioid antagonist. It does not lead to physical or psychological dependence. Tolerance to the opioid antagonist effect is not known to occur.

➤*Pregnancy:* *Category C.* There are no adequate and well-controlled studies in pregnant women. The human placental transfer of naltrexone has not been studied, but the molecular weight of the drug (about 378) suggests that transfer to the embryo and fetus should be expected. Although naltrexone did not produce gross structural abnormalities in any of the animal studies, it did alter some opioid receptors in the brain that appeared to have long-lasting consequences. This potential for behavioral alteration in humans cannot be assessed because of the lack of data, but concern is warranted. Use naltrexone in pregnancy only when the potential benefit justifies the potential risk to the fetus.

Naltrexone increased the incidence of early fetal loss when administered to rats in oral dosages greater than or equal to 30 mg/kg/day (180 mg/m^2/day; 5 times the recommended therapeutic dose, based on body surface area [BSA]) and to rabbits at oral dosages greater than or equal to 60 mg/kg/day (720 mg/m^2/day; 18 times the recommended therapeutic dose, based on BSA).

➤*Lactation:* In animal studies, naltrexone and 6-beta-naltrexol were excreted in the milk of lactating rats dosed orally with naltrexone. Whether or not naltrexone is excreted in human milk is unknown. The molecular weight (about 378) is low enough that excretion into breast milk is expected. The effects of this exposure on a breast-fed infant are unknown, but there appears to be the potential for altering opioid receptors in the brain. In addition, based on studies in adults, baseline levels of some hormones of hypothalamic, pituitary, adrenal, and gonadal origin may also be altered. Because many drugs are excreted in human milk, exercise caution when naltrexone is administered to a breast-feeding woman.

➤*Children:* The safe use of naltrexone in patients younger than 18 years of age has not been established.

➤*Monitoring:* Evaluations using appropriate tests to detect liver injury are recommended at a frequency appropriate to the clinical situation and the dose of naltrexone.

Monitor for development of depression or suicidal thinking.

Drug Interactions

Naltrexone Drug Interactions

Precipitant drug	Object drug[a]		Description
Naltrexone	Opioid analgesics	⬇	The effects of the opioid analgesic may be reduced or attenuated, precipitating a severe opioid withdrawal syndrome. Naltrexone administration is contraindicated in patients receiving opioid analgesics or dependent on opioids, including patients maintained on opiate agonists (eg, methadone).
Naltrexone	Opioid-containing products	⬇	Patients taking naltrexone may not benefit from opioid-containing products, such as cough/cold and antidiarrheal preparations and opioid analgesics. The amount of opioid required may be greater than usual and the resulting respiratory depression may be deeper and more prolonged.

NALTREXONE HYDROCHLORIDE — ORAL

Naltrexone Drug Interactions			
Precipitant drug	Object drug[a]		Description
Naltrexone	Thioridazine	↑	Lethargy and somnolence have occurred with concurrent use. If an interaction is suspected, it may be necessary to discontinue naltrexone.

[a] ↑ = object drug increased; ↓ = object drug decreased.

➤*Drug/Lab test interactions:* Naltrexone may or may not interfere with enzymatic methods for detection of opioids, depending on the specificity of the test.

Adverse Reactions

➤*Hepatic effects:* While extensive clinical studies evaluating the use of naltrexone in detoxified, formerly opioid-dependent individuals failed to identify any single, serious untoward risk of naltrexone use, placebo-controlled studies employing up to 5-fold higher doses of naltrexone hydrochloride (up to 300 mg/day) than that recommended for use in opiate receptor blockade have shown that naltrexone causes hepatocellular injury in a substantial proportion of patients exposed at higher doses.

➤*Exacerbation of abstinence symptoms:* It is critical to recognize that naltrexone can precipitate or exacerbate abstinence signs and symptoms in any individual who is not completely free of exogenous opioids.

➤*Opioid withdrawal-like adverse reactions:* Studies in alcoholic populations and in volunteers in clinical pharmacology studies have suggested that a small fraction of patients may experience an opioid withdrawal-like symptom complex consisting of tearfulness, mild nausea, abdominal cramps, restlessness, bone pain or joint pain, myalgia, and nasal symptoms. This may represent the unmasking of occult opioid use, or it may represent symptoms attributable to naltrexone. A number of alternative dosing patterns have been recommended to try to reduce the frequency of these complaints.

➤*Alcohol dependence:* During 2 randomized, double-blind, placebo-controlled, 12-week trials to evaluate the efficacy of naltrexone as an adjunctive treatment of alcohol dependence, most patients tolerated naltrexone well. In these studies, a total of 93 patients received naltrexone at a dosage of 50 mg once daily. Five of these patients discontinued naltrexone because of nausea. No serious adverse events were reported during these 2 trials.

Adverse reactions (2% or more) –

CNS: Headache (7%), dizziness (4%), fatigue (4%), nervousness (4%), insomnia (3%), anxiety (2%), and somnolence (2%). Depression, suicidal ideation, and suicidal attempts have been reported in all groups when comparing naltrexone, placebo, or controls undergoing treatment for alcoholism.

GI: Nausea (10%), vomiting (3%).

➤*Opioid dependence:*

Adverse reactions (more than 10%) –

CNS: Anxiety, difficulty sleeping, headache, low energy, and nervousness.

GI: Abdominal pain/cramps, nausea, or vomiting.

Musculoskeletal: Joint and muscle pain.

Adverse reactions (less than 10%) –

CNS: Dizziness, feeling down, increased energy, irritability.

GI: Constipation, diarrhea, increased thirst, loss of appetite.

Miscellaneous: Chills, decreased potency, delayed ejaculation, and skin rash.

Adverse reactions (less than 1%) –

Cardiovascular: Edema, increased blood pressure, nonspecific electrocardiogram changes, palpitations, phlebitis, tachycardia.

CNS: Bad dreams, confusion, depression, disorientation, fatigue, hallucinations, head "pounding," nightmares, paranoia, restlessness, somnolence.

Dermatologic: Acne, alopecia, athlete's foot, cold sores , oily skin, pruritus.

GI: Diarrhea, dry mouth, excessive gas, hemorrhoids, increased appetite, ulcer, weight gain, weight loss.

GU: Increased frequency of urination, or discomfort during urination; increased or decreased sexual interest; inguinal pain.

Musculoskeletal: Painful shoulders, legs, or knees; tremors; twitching.

Respiratory: Cough, excess mucus or phlegm, heavy breathing, hoarseness, itching, nasal congestion, rhinorrhea, shortness of breath, sinus trouble, sneezing, sore throat.

Special senses: Aching eyes, blurred vision, "clogged" ears, earache, eyes burning, eyes strained, light sensitivity, nosebleeds, swollen eyes, tinnitus.

Miscellaneous: Cold feet, fever, "hot spells," "side" pains, swollen glands, yawning.

➤*Postmarketing:*

Cardiovascular – Changes in blood pressure, hot flushes, palpitations.

CNS – Abnormal thinking, agitation, anxiety, asthenia, confusion, dizziness, fatigue, euphoria, hallucinations, headache, hyperkinesia, insomnia, malaise, nervousness, somnolence, tremor.

Depression, suicide, attempted suicide, and suicidal ideation have been reported in the postmarketing experience with naltrexone used in the treatment of opioid dependence. No causal relationship has been demonstrated.

Dermatologic – Increased sweating, rash.

GI – Abdominal pain, anorexia, diarrhea, nausea, vomiting.

Hematologic – Idiopathic thrombocytopenic purpura was reported in 1 patient who may have been sensitized to naltrexone in a previous course of treatment with naltrexone. The condition cleared without sequelae after discontinuation of naltrexone and corticosteroid treatment.

Hepatic – Elevations in liver enzymes or bilirubin, hepatic function abnormalities, hepatitis.

Miscellaneous – Chest pain, dyspnea, myalgia, vision abnormalities.

Endogenous opioids have been theorized to contribute to a variety of conditions. In some individuals, the use of opioid antagonists has been associated with a change in baseline levels of some hypothalamic, pituitary, adrenal, or gonadal hormones. The clinical significance of such changes is not fully understood.

Adverse reactions, including withdrawal symptoms and death, have been reported with the use of naltrexone in ultra rapid opiate detoxification programs. The cause of death in these cases is not known.

Overdosage

➤*Symptoms:* There is limited clinical experience with naltrexone overdosage in humans. In 1 study, subjects who received naltrexone 800 mg daily for up to 1 week showed no evidence of toxicity.

➤*Treatment:* In view of the lack of actual experience in the treatment of naltrexone overdose, symptomatically treat patients in a closely supervised environment. Health care providers should contact a poison control center for the most up-to-date information.

Patient Information

Inform patients they have been prescribed naltrexone as part of the comprehensive treatment for alcoholism or drug dependence. Advise patients to carry identification to alert medical personnel to the fact that they are taking naltrexone. A naltrexone medication card may be obtained from their health care provider and can be used for this purpose. Advise patients to carry the identification card to help ensure that they can obtain adequate treatment in an emergency. If patients require medical treatment, advise them to tell their health care provider that they are receiving naltrexone therapy.

Advise patients to take naltrexone as directed by their health care provider. Advise patients that if they attempt to self-administer heroin or any other opiate drug in small doses while on naltrexone, they will not perceive any effect. Most importantly, however, if patients attempt to self-administer large doses of heroin or any other opioid (including methadone or levo-alpha-acetyl-methadol) while on naltrexone, they may die or sustain serious injury including coma.

Naltrexone is well tolerated in the recommended doses, but may cause liver injury when taken in excess or in persons who develop liver disease from other causes. If patients develop abdominal pain lasting more than a few days, white bowel movements, dark urine, or yellowing of the eyes, they should stop taking naltrexone immediately and see their health care provider as soon as possible.

NALTREXONE — INJECTION

WARNING

Hepatotoxicity – Naltrexone has the capacity to cause hepatocellular injury when given in excessive doses. Naltrexone is contraindicated in patients with acute hepatitis or liver failure, and its use in patients with acute liver disease must be carefully considered in light of its hepatotoxic effects. The margin of separation between the apparently safe dose of naltrexone and the dose causing hepatic injury appears to be only 5-fold or less. Naltrexone does not appear to be a hepatotoxin at the recommended doses. Warn patients of the risk of hepatic injury and advise them to seek medical attention if they experience symptoms of acute hepatitis. Discontinue use of naltrexone in the event of symptoms and/or signs of acute hepatitis.

Indications

➤*Alcohol dependence:* For the treatment of alcohol dependence in patients who are able to abstain from alcohol in an outpatient setting prior to initiation of treatment. Patients should not be actively drinking at the time of initial naltrexone administration.

➤*Opioid dependence:* For the prevention of relapse to opioid dependence, following opioid detoxification.

Administration and Dosage

➤*Adults:*

Alcohol dependence –

Usual dosage: 380 mg intramuscularly (IM) every 4 weeks or once a month.

Opioid dependence –

Usual dosage: 380 mg IM every 4 weeks or once a month.

➤*Hepatic function impairment:* Naltrexone can cause hepatocellular injury when given in excessive doses. Naltrexone is contraindicated in patients with acute hepatitis or liver failure, and its use in patients with acute liver disease must be carefully considered in light of its hepatotoxic effects.

➤*Preparation for administration:* Prior to preparation, allow the drug to reach room temperature (approximately 45 minutes). To ease mixing, firmly tap the vial on a hard surface and ensure the powder moves freely.

NALTREXONE — INJECTION

Remove flip-off caps from both vials. Do not use if flip-off caps are broken or missing. Wipe the vial tops with an alcohol swab. Place the 1-inch preparation needle on the syringe and withdraw 3.4 mL of the diluent from the diluent vial. Some diluent will remain in the diluent vial. Inject the 3.4 mL of diluent into the naltrexone vial. Mix the powder and diluent by vigorously shaking the vial for approximately 1 minute. Ensure that the dose is thoroughly suspended prior to proceeding to the next step. A properly mixed suspension will be milky white, will not contain any clumps, and will move freely down the walls of the vial.

Immediately after suspension, withdraw 4.2 mL of the suspension into the syringe using the same preparation needle. Select the appropriate needle for an IM injection based on patient's body habitus (1.5-inch *Terumo* needle, 2-inch *Needle-Pro* needle). Remove the preparation needle and replace with the appropriately selected administration needle for immediate use. Peel the blister pouch of the selected administration needle open halfway. Grasp sheath using the plastic pouch. Attach the luer connection to the syringe with an easy clockwise twisting motion. Seat the needle firmly on the needle protection device with a push and clockwise twist. Pull the sheath away from the needle; do not twist the sheath because it could result in loosening the needle. Prior to injecting, tap the syringe to release any air bubbles, then push gently on the plunger until 4 mL of the suspension remains in the syringe.

➤*Administration:* Administer as a deep IM gluteal injection, alternating buttocks for each subsequent injection, using the carton components provided. Inject in a smooth and continuous motion. Naltrexone must not be administered intravenously (IV) or subcutaneously.

➤*Storage/Stability:* Store at 2° to 8°C (36° to 46°F). Naltrexone can be stored at temperatures not exceeding 25°C (77°F) for no more than 7 days prior to administration. Do not expose the product to temperatures above 25°C (77°F). Do not freeze. Dispose of used and unused items in proper waste containers.

Actions

➤*Pharmacology:* Naltrexone is an opioid antagonist with highest affinity for the mu-opioid receptor. Naltrexone has little or no opioid agonist activity. Occupation of opioid receptors by naltrexone may block the effects of endogenous opioid peptides. It markedly attenuates or completely blocks, reversibly, the subjective effects of exogenous opioids. The neurobiological mechanisms responsible for the reduction in alcohol consumption observed in alcohol-dependent patients treated with naltrexone are not entirely understood. However, involvement of the endogenous opioid system is suggested by preclinical data.

Naltrexone blocks the effects of opioids by competitive binding at opioid receptors. This makes the blockade produced potentially surmountable, but overcoming full naltrexone blockade by administration of opioids may result in nonopioid receptor–mediated symptoms such as histamine release.

➤*Pharmacokinetics:*

Absorption – After IM injection, the naltrexone plasma concentration time profile is characterized by a transient initial peak, which occurs approximately 2 hours after injection, followed by a second peak observed approximately 2 to 3 days later. Beginning approximately 14 days after dosing, concentrations slowly decline, with measurable levels for greater than 1 month.

Maximum plasma concentration (C_{max}) and area under the curve (AUC) for naltrexone and 6-beta-naltrexol (the major metabolite) following naltrexone administration are dose proportional. Compared with daily oral dosing with naltrexone 50 mg over 28 days, total naltrexone exposure is 3- to 4-fold higher following administration of a single dose of naltrexone 380 mg. Steady state is reached at the end of the dosing interval following the first injection. There is minimal accumulation (less than 15%) of naltrexone or 6-beta-naltrexol upon repeat administration of naltrexone.

Distribution – In vitro data demonstrate that naltrexone plasma protein binding is low (21%).

Metabolism – Naltrexone is extensively metabolized in humans. Production of the primary metabolite, 6-beta-naltrexol, is mediated by dihydrodiol dehydrogenase, a cytosolic family of enzymes. The cytochrome P450 system is not involved in naltrexone metabolism. Two other minor metabolites are 2-hydroxy-3-methoxy-6-beta-naltrexol and 2-hydroxy-3-methoxy-naltrexone. Naltrexone and its metabolites are also conjugated to form glucuronide products.

Significantly less 6-beta-naltrexol is generated following IM administration of naltrexone than with administration of oral naltrexone because of a reduction in first-pass hepatic metabolism.

Excretion – Elimination of naltrexone and its metabolites occurs primarily via urine, with minimal excretion of unchanged naltrexone.

The elimination half-life of naltrexone following naltrexone administration is 5 to 10 days and is dependent on the erosion of the polymer. The elimination half-life of 6-beta-naltrexol following naltrexone administration is 5 to 10 days.

Contraindications

Patients with acute hepatitis or liver failure; patients receiving opioid analgesics; patients with current physiologic opioid dependence; patients in acute opiate withdrawal; any individual who has failed the naloxone challenge test or has a positive urine screen for opioids; patients who have previously exhibited hypersensitivity to naltrexone, polylactide-co-glycolide, carboxymethylcellulose, or any other components of the diluent.

Warnings/Precautions

➤*Hepatotoxicity:* See the Warning box for more information.

➤*Injection-site reactions:* Naltrexone injections may be followed by pain, tenderness, induration, swelling, erythema, bruising, or pruritus; however, in some cases, injection-site reactions may be very severe. In the clinical trials, 1 patient developed an area of induration that continued to enlarge after 4 weeks, with subsequent development of necrotic tissue that required surgical excision. In the postmarketing period, additional cases of injection-site reaction with features including induration, cellulitis, hematoma, abscess, sterile abscess, and necrosis have been reported. Some cases required surgical intervention, including debridement of necrotic tissue. Some cases resulted in significant scarring. The reported cases occurred primarily in women.

Naltrexone is administered as an IM gluteal injections and inadvertent subcutaneous injection of naltrexone may increase the likelihood of severe injection-site reactions. The needles provided in the carton are customized needles. Naltrexone must not be injected using any other needle. The needle lengths (either 1.5 or 2 inches) may not be adequate in every patient because of body habitus. Assess body habitus prior to each injection for each patient to ensure that the proper needle is selected and that the needle length is adequate for IM administration. Ensure that the naltrexone injection is given correctly, and consider alternate treatment for those patients whose body habitus precludes an IM gluteal injection with one of the provided needles.

Inform patients that any concerning injection-site reactions should be brought to the attention of the health care provider. Patients exhibiting signs of abscess, cellulitis, necrosis, or extensive swelling should be evaluated by a health care provider to determine if referral to a surgeon is warranted.

➤*Eosinophilic pneumonia:* In clinical trials with naltrexone, there was 1 diagnosed case and 1 suspected case of eosinophilic pneumonia. Both cases required hospitalization and resolved after treatment with antibiotics and corticosteroids. Similar cases have been reported in postmarketing use. If a person receiving naltrexone develops progressive dyspnea and hypoxemia, consider the diagnosis of eosinophilic pneumonia. Warn patients of the risk of eosinophilic pneumonia, and advise them to seek medical attention if they develop symptoms of pneumonia. Consider the possibility of eosinophilic pneumonia in patients who do not respond to antibiotics.

➤*Abstinence syndrome:* To prevent occurrence of an acute abstinence syndrome (withdrawal) in patients dependent on opioids, or exacerbation of a preexisting subclinical abstinence syndrome, opioid-dependent patients, including those being treated for alcohol dependence, must be opioid-free for a minimum of 7 to 10 days before starting naltrexone treatment. Because the absence of an opioid drug in the urine is often not sufficient proof that a patient is opioid free, employ a naloxone challenge test if the prescribing health care provider feels there is a risk of precipitating a withdrawal reaction following administration of naltrexone. Assess patients treated for alcohol dependence with naltrexone for underlying opioid dependence and for any recent use of opioids prior to initiation of treatment with naltrexone. Precipitated opioid withdrawal has been observed in alcohol-dependent patients in circumstances in which the prescriber had been unaware of the additional use of opioids or dependence on opioids.

➤*Overcoming blockade:* After opioid detoxification, patients are likely to have reduced tolerance to opioids. Although naltrexone blocks the effects of exogenous opioids for 28 days after administration, cases of opioid overdose with fatal outcomes have been reported in patients who use opioids at the end of a dosing interval or when missing a dose. Patients who have been treated with naltrexone may respond to lower doses of opioids than previously used. This could result in potentially life-threatening opioid intoxication (eg, respiratory compromise or arrest, circulatory collapse). Inform patients that they may be more sensitive to lower doses of opioids after naltrexone treatment is discontinued. Reduced tolerance is especially of concern at the end of a dosing interval, that is, near the end of the month after naltrexone was administered, or after a dose of naltrexone is missed. It is important that patients inform family members and the people closest to the patient of this increased sensitivity to opioids and the risk of overdose.

There is also the possibility that a patient who is treated with naltrexone could overcome the opioid blockade effect of naltrexone. Although naltrexone is a potent antagonist with a prolonged pharmacological effect, the blockade produced by naltrexone is surmountable. This poses a potential risk to individuals who attempt, on their own, to overcome the blockade by administering large amounts of exogenous opioids. Any attempt by patients to overcome the antagonism by taking opioids is very dangerous and may lead to fatal overdose. Injury may arise because the plasma concentration of exogenous opioids attained immediately following their acute administration may be sufficient to overcome the competitive receptor blockade. As a consequence, the patient may be in immediate danger of suffering life-endangering opioid intoxication (eg, circulatory collapse, respiratory arrest). Inform patients of the serious consequences of trying to overcome the opioid blockade.

➤*Depression and suicidality:*

Alcohol dependence – In controlled clinical trials of naltrexone administered to adults with alcohol dependence, adverse reactions of a suicidal nature (suicidal ideation, suicide attempts, completed suicides) were infrequent overall, but were more common in naltrexone-treated patients than in placebo-treated patients (1% vs 0%). In some cases, the suicidal thoughts or behavior occurred after study discontinuation, but were in the context of an episode of depression that began while the patient was on study drug. Two completed suicides occurred, both involving patients treated with naltrexone.

NALTREXONE — INJECTION

Depression-related events associated with premature discontinuation of study drug were also more common in naltrexone-treated patients (approximately 1%) than in placebo-treated patients (0%).

In the 24-week, placebo-controlled pivotal trial in 624 alcohol-dependent patients, adverse reactions involving depressed mood were reported by 10% of patients treated with naltrexone 380 mg, compared with 5% of patients treated with placebo injections.

Opioid dependence – In an open-label, long-term safety study conducted in the United States, adverse events of a suicidal nature (depressed mood, suicidal ideation, suicide attempt) were reported by 5% of opioid-dependent patients treated with naltrexone 380 mg and 10% of opioid-dependent patients treated with oral naltrexone. In the 24-week, placebo-controlled pivotal trial that was conducted in Russia in 250 opioid-dependent patients, adverse events involving depressed mood or suicidal thinking were not reported by any patient in either treatment group (naltrexone 380 mg or placebo).

➤*Hematologic effects:* As with any IM injection, administer naltrexone with caution to patients with thrombocytopenia or any coagulation disorder (eg, hemophilia, severe hepatic failure).

➤*Reversal of blockade:* In an emergency situation in patients receiving naltrexone, suggestions for pain management include regional analgesia or use of nonopioid analgesics. If opioid therapy is required as part of anesthesia or analgesia, patients should be continuously monitored in an anesthesia care setting by persons not involved in the conduct of the surgical or diagnostic procedure. The opioid therapy must be provided by individuals specifically trained in the use of anesthetic drugs and the management of the respiratory effects of potent opioids, specifically the establishment and maintenance of a patent airway and assisted ventilation.

Irrespective of the drug chosen to reverse naltrexone blockade, appropriately trained personnel should closely monitor patients in a setting equipped and staffed for cardiopulmonary resuscitation.

➤*Alcohol withdrawal:* Use of naltrexone does not eliminate nor diminish alcohol withdrawal symptoms.

➤*Hypersensitivity reactions:* Cases of urticaria, angioedema, and anaphylaxis have been observed with the use of naltrexone in the clinical trial setting and in postmarketing use. Warn patients of the risk of hypersensitivity reactions, including anaphylaxis. In the event of a hypersensitivity reaction, advise patients to seek immediate medical attention in a health care setting prepared to treat anaphylaxis. The patients should not receive any further treatment with naltrexone.

➤*Renal function impairment:* Because naltrexone and its primary metabolite are excreted primarily in the urine, caution is recommended in administering naltrexone to patients with moderate to severe renal function impairment.

➤*Pregnancy: Category C.* There are no adequate and well-controlled studies of naltrexone in pregnant women. The human placental transfer of naltrexone has not been studied, but the molecular weight of the drug (about 378) suggests that transfer to the embryo and fetus should be expected. Although naltrexone did not produce gross structural abnormalities in any of the animal studies, it did alter some opioid receptors in the brain that appeared to have long-lasting consequences. This potential for behavioral alteration in humans cannot be assessed because of the lack of data, but concern is warranted. Use naltrexone during pregnancy only if the potential benefit justifies the potential risk to the fetus.

Naltrexone increased the incidence of early fetal loss in rats administered 30 mg/kg/day or more (11 times the human exposure based on an $AUC_{(0\text{-}28d)}$ comparison) and rabbits administered 60 mg/kg/day or more (2 times the human exposure based on an $AUC_{(0\text{-}28d)}$ comparison).

➤*Lactation:* Transfer of naltrexone and 6-beta-naltrexol into human milk has been reported with oral naltrexone. The effects of this exposure on a breast-feeding infant are unknown, but there appears to be the potential for altering opioid receptors in the brain. In addition, based on studies in adults, baseline levels of some hormones of hypothalamic, pituitary, adrenal, and gonadal origin may also be altered. Because of the potential for tumorigenicity shown for naltrexone in animal studies, and because of the potential for serious adverse reactions in breast-feeding infants from naltrexone, make a decision whether to discontinue breast-feeding or the drug, taking into account the importance of the drug to the mother.

➤*Children:* The safety and efficacy of naltrexone have not been established in children.

➤*Monitoring:* Evaluations using appropriate tests to detect liver injury are recommended at a frequency appropriate to the clinical situation and the dose of naltrexone. Monitor for the development of depression or suicidal thinking.

Drug Interactions

Naltrexone Drug Interactions

Precipitant drug	Object drug[a]		Description
Naltrexone	Opioid analgesics	⬇	The effects of the opioid analgesic may be reduced or attenuated, precipitating a severe opioid withdrawal syndrome. Naltrexone administration is contraindicated in patients receiving opioid analgesics or dependent on opioids, including patients maintained on opiate agonists (eg, methadone).
Naltrexone	Opioid-containing products	⬇	Patients taking naltrexone may not benefit from opioid-containing products, such as cough/cold and antidiarrheal preparations and opioid analgesics. The amount of opioid required may be greater than usual and the resulting respiratory depression may be deeper and more prolonged.
Naltrexone	Thioridazine	⬆	Lethargy and somnolence have occurred with concurrent use. If an interaction is suspected, it may be necessary to discontinue naltrexone.

[a] ⬆ = object drug increased; ⬇ = object drug decreased.

➤*Drug/Lab test interactions:* Naltrexone may be cross-reactive with certain immunoassay methods for detecting drugs of abuse, specifically opioids, in the urine.

Adverse Reactions

➤*Serious adverse reactions:* Serious adverse reactions that may be associated with naltrexone therapy in clinical use include accidental opioid overdose and depression and suicidality, eosinophilic pneumonia, serious allergic reactions, severe injection-site reactions, unintended precipitation of opioid withdrawal.

➤*Frequent adverse reactions:*

Alcohol dependence – The adverse reactions seen most frequently in association with naltrexone therapy for alcohol dependence (ie, those occurring in at least 5% and at least twice as frequently with naltrexone than placebo) include anorexia, nausea, decreased appetite or other appetite disorders, dizziness or syncope, injection-site reactions (including induration, pruritis, nodules, and swelling), muscle cramps, somnolence or sedation, and vomiting.

Opioid dependence – The adverse reactions seen most frequently in association with naltrexone therapy in opioid-dependent patients (ie, those occurring in at least 3% and at least twice as frequently with naltrexone than placebo) were hepatic enzyme abnormalities, injection-site pain, insomnia, nasopharyngitis, and toothache.

➤*Alcohol dependence:*

Discontinuation – In controlled trials of 6 months or less in alcohol-dependent patients, 9% of alcohol-dependent patients treated with naltrexone discontinued treatment because of an adverse reaction, as compared with 7% of the alcohol-dependent patients treated with placebo. Adverse reactions in the naltrexone 380 mg group that led to more dropouts than in the placebo-treated group were injection-site reactions (3%), nausea (2%), pregnancy (1%), headache (1%), and suicide-related reactions (0.3%). In the placebo group, 1% of patients withdrew because of injection-site reactions, and 0% of patients withdrew because of the other adverse reactions.

Adverse reactions (5% or more) –

Naltrexone Adverse Reactions in Alcohol Dependence (≥ 5%)

Adverse reactions	Naltrexone 400 mg (n = 25)	Naltrexone 380 mg (n = 205)	Naltrexone 190 mg (n = 210)	All (n = 440)	Placebo (n = 214)
CNS					
Anxiety[a]	8%	12%	8%	10%	8%
Asthenic conditions[b]	12%	23%	19%	20%	12%
Depression	0%	8%	3%	5%	4%
Dizziness, syncope	16%	13%	13%	13%	4%
Headache[c]	36%	25%	16%	21%	18%
Insomnia, sleep disorder	8%	14%	13%	13%	12%
Somnolence, sedation	12%	4%	4%	5%	1%
Dermatologic					
Rash[d]	12%	6%	5%	6%	4%

NALTREXONE — INJECTION

Naltrexone Adverse Reactions in Alcohol Dependence (≥ 5%)					
Adverse reactions	Naltrexone 400 mg (n = 25)	Naltrexone 380 mg (n = 205)	Naltrexone 190 mg (n = 210)	All (n = 440)	Placebo (n = 214)
GI					
Abdominal pain[e]	16%	11%	11%	11%	8%
Diarrhea[f]	12%	13%	13%	13%	10%
Dry mouth	24%	5%	4%	5%	4%
Nausea	32%	33%	25%	29%	11%
Vomiting, NOS[g]	12%	14%	10%	12%	6%
Local					
Any injection-site reaction	88%	69%	58%	65%	50%
Injection-site ecchymosis	0%	7%	4%	5%	5%
Injection-site induration	28%	35%	25%	30%	8%
Injection-site pain	0%	17%	10%	13%	7%
Injection-site pruritus	0%	10%	6%	8%	0%
Injection-site tenderness	72%	45%	42%	45%	39%
Other injection-site reactions (primarily nodules, swelling)	32%	15%	8%	12%	4%
Musculoskeletal					
Arthralgia, arthritis, joint stiffness	4%	12%	6%	9%	5%
Back pain, back stiffness	4%	6%	7%	6%	5%
Muscle cramps[h]	0%	8%	2%	5%	1%
Miscellaneous					
Anorexia, appetite decreased NOS[g] appetite disorder NOS	20%	14%	6%	11%	3%
Pharyngitis[i]	0%	11%	17%	13%	11%

[a] Includes the preferred terms: anxiety (not elsewhere classified), aggravated anxiety, agitation, obsessive-compulsive disorder, panic attack, nervousness, posttraumatic stress.
[b] Includes the preferred terms: fatigue (these two comprise the majority of cases), lethargy, malaise, sluggishness.
[c] Includes the preferred terms: frequent headaches, headache NOS, migraine, sinus headache.
[d] Includes the preferred terms: heat rash, rash NOS, rash papular.
[e] Includes the preferred terms: abdominal pain NOS, lower abdominal pain, stomach discomfort, upper abdominal pain.
[f] Includes the preferred terms: diarrhea NOS, frequent bowel movements, GI upset, loose stools.
[g] NOS = Not otherwise specified.
[h] Includes the preferred terms: muscle cramps, rigidity, spasms, stiffness, tightness, twitching.
[i] Includes the preferred terms: nasopharyngitis, pharyngitis NOS, pharyngitis streptococcal.

➤*Opioid dependence:*

Discontinuation – In a controlled trial of 6 months, 2% of opioid-dependent patients treated with naltrexone discontinued treatment because of an adverse reaction, compared with 2% of the opioid-dependent patients treated with placebo.

Adverse reactions (2% or more) –

Naltrexone Adverse Reactions in Opioid Dependence (≥ 2%)		
Adverse reactions	Naltrexone 380 mg (n = 126)	Placebo (n = 124)
CNS		
Headache	3%	2%
Insomnia	6%	1%
Hepatic		
ALT increased	13%	6%
AST increased	10%	2%
GGT increased[a]	7%	3%
Miscellaneous		
Hypertension	5%	3%
Influenza	5%	4%
Injection-site pain	5%	1%
Nasopharyngitis	7%	2%
Toothache	4%	2%

[a] GGT = gamma-glutamyltransferase.

➤*Other adverse reactions:*

Cardiovascular – Angina pectoris, atrial fibrillation, congestive cardiac failure, coronary artery atherosclerosis, deep venous thrombosis, hot flushes, ischemic stroke, myocardial infarction, palpitations, pulmonary embolism, unstable angina.

CNS – Abnormal dreams, agitation, alcohol withdrawal syndrome, cerebral arterial aneurysm, chills, convulsions, delirium, disturbance in attention, dysgeusia, euphoric mood, irritability, lethargy, libido decreased, mental impairment, migraine, paresthesia.

Dermatologic – Increased sweating, night sweats, pruritus.

GI – Abdominal discomfort, colitis, constipation, flatulence, gastroenteritis, gastroesophageal reflux disease, GI hemorrhage, hemorrhoids, pancreatitis acute, paralytic ileus, perirectal abscess.

GU – Missed abortion, urinary tract infection.

Hematologic / Lymphatic – Lymphadenopathy (including cervical adenitis), white blood cell count increased.

Hepatic – Cholecystitis acute, cholelithiasis.

Hypersensitivity – Hypersensitivity reaction (including angioneurotic edema and urticaria), seasonal allergy.

Metabolic / Nutritional – Appetite increased, dehydration, heat exhaustion, hypercholesterolemia, weight decreased, weight increased.

Musculoskeletal – Joint stiffness, muscle spasms, myalgia, pain in limb, rigors.

Special senses – Conjunctivitis, vision blurred.

Respiratory – Bronchitis, chronic obstructive pulmonary disease, dyspnea, laryngitis, pharyngolaryngeal pain, pneumonia, sinusitis, sinus congestion, upper respiratory tract infection.

Miscellaneous – Advanced HIV disease in HIV-infected patients, chest pain, chest tightness, face edema, pyrexia, retinal artery occlusion.

➤*Lab test abnormalities:*

Hematological – In clinical trials, subjects on naltrexone had increases in eosinophil counts relative to subjects on placebo. With continued use of naltrexone, eosinophil counts returned to normal over a period of several months.

Naltrexone 380 mg was associated with a decrease in platelet count. In clinical trials, alcohol-dependent patients treated with naltrexone experienced a mean maximal decrease in platelet count of 17.8×10^3/mcL, compared with 2.6×10^3/mcL in placebo patients.

After 24 weeks of treatment, opioid-dependent patients treated with naltrexone experienced a mean maximal decrease in platelet count of 62.8×10^3/mcL, compared with 39.9×10^3/mcL in placebo patients. In randomized, controlled trials, naltrexone was not associated with an increase in bleeding-related adverse events.

Hepatic – In short-term controlled trials in alcohol-dependent patients, the incidence of AST elevations associated with naltrexone treatment was similar to that observed with oral naltrexone treatment (1.5% each) and slightly higher than that observed with placebo treatment (0.9%).

In the 6-month controlled trial conducted in opioid-dependent subjects, 89% had a baseline diagnosis of hepatitis C infection, and 41% had a baseline diagnosis of HIV infection. There were frequently observed elevated liver enzyme levels (ALT, AST, and GGT); these were more commonly reported as adverse events in the naltrexone 380 mg group than in the placebo group. Patients could not enroll in this trial if they had a baseline ALT or AST value that was more than 3 times the upper limit of normal. More patients treated with naltrexone in this study experienced treatment-emergent elevations in transaminases to more than 3 times the upper limit of normal than patients treated with placebo. Shifts to more than 3 times the upper limit of normal occurred in 20% of patients treated with naltrexone as compared with 13% of placebo patients. Shifts in values of AST to more than 3 times the upper limit were also more common in the naltrexone (14%) arm compared with the placebo (11%) arm. Opioid-dependent patients treated with naltrexone experienced a mean maximal increase from baseline ALT levels of 61 units/L compared with 48 units/L in placebo patients. Similarly for AST, opioid-dependent patients treated with naltrexone experienced a mean maximal increase from baseline AST levels of 40 units/L compared with 31 units/L in placebo patients.

Creatine phosphokinase – In short-term controlled trials in alcohol-dependent patients, more patients treated with naltrexone 380 mg (11%) and oral naltrexone (17%) shifted from normal creatine phosphokinase (CPK) levels before treatment to abnormal CPK levels at the end of the trials, compared with placebo patients (8%).

In open-label trials, 16% of patients dosed for more than 6 months had increases in CPK. For both the oral naltrexone and naltrexone 380 mg groups, CPK abnormalities were most frequently in the range of 1 to 2 times the upper limits of normal (ULN). However, there were reports of CPK abnormalities as high as 4 times ULN for the oral naltrexone group and 35 times ULN for the naltrexone 380 mg group. Overall, there were no dif-

NALTREXONE — INJECTION

ferences between the placebo and naltrexone (oral or injectable) groups with respect to the proportions of patients with a CPK value at least 3 times the ULN. No factors other than naltrexone exposure were associated with the CPK elevations.

More opioid-dependent patients treated with naltrexone 380 mg (39%) shifted from normal CPK levels before treatment to abnormal CPK levels during the study as compared with patients treated with placebo (32%). There were reports of CPK abnormalities as high as 41.8 × ULN for the placebo group, and 22.1 × ULN for the naltrexone 380 mg group.

➤*Postmarketing:*

Hypersensitivity – Hypersensitivity reactions including anaphylaxis have been reported.

Miscellaneous – Retinal artery occlusion after injection with another drug product containing polylactide-co-glycolide microspheres has been reported very rarely during postmarketing surveillance. This event has been reported in the presence of abnormal arteriovenous anastomosis. No cases of retinal artery occlusion have been reported during naltrexone clinical trials or postmarketing surveillance. Administer naltrexone by IM injection into the gluteal muscle, and take care to avoid inadvertent injection into a blood vessel.

Overdosage

➤*Symptoms:* There is limited experience with naltrexone overdose. Single doses of up to 784 mg were administered to 5 healthy subjects. There were no serious or severe adverse reactions. The most common reactions were injection-site reactions, nausea, abdominal pain, somnolence, and dizziness. There were no significant increases in hepatic enzymes.

➤*Treatment:* In the event of an overdose, initiate appropriate supportive treatment.

Patient Information

Advise families and caregivers of patients being treated with naltrexone of the need to monitor patients for the emergence of symptoms of depression or suicidality and to report such symptoms to the patient's health care provider.

Advise patients that a reaction at the site of naltrexone injection may occur. Reactions include pain, swelling, erythema, tenderness, induration, bruising, and pruritus. Serious injection-site reactions including necrosis may occur. Patients should receive their injection from a health care provider qualified to administer the injection. Advise patients to seek medical attention for worsening skin reactions.

Advise patients that they should be off all opioid-containing medicines (including methadone or buprenorphine) for 7 to 10 days before starting naltrexone in order to avoid precipitation of opioid withdrawal. Advise patients not to take naltrexone if they have any symptoms of opioid withdrawal. Advise patients with alcohol dependence that it is imperative to notify their health care provider of any recent use of opioids or any history of opioid dependence before starting naltrexone to avoid precipitation of opioid withdrawal.

Advise patients that if they previously used opioids, they may be more sensitive to lower doses of opioids after naltrexone treatment is discontinued. It is important that patients inform family members and the people closest to the patient of this increased sensitivity to opioids and the risk of overdose.

Advise patients that administration of large doses of heroin or any other opioid while on naltrexone may lead to serious injury, coma, or death. In addition, administration of previously tolerated doses of opioids at the end of the dosing interval or after missing a dose may lead to overdose.

Advise patients that because naltrexone can block the effects of opiates and opiate-like drugs, patients will not perceive any effect if they attempt to self-administer heroin or any other opioid drug in small doses while on naltrexone. Also, patients on naltrexone may not experience the same effects from opioid-containing analgesic, antidiarrheal, or antitussive medications.

Advise patients that naltrexone may cause liver injury in people who develop liver disease from other causes. Tell patients to immediately notify their health care provider if they develop symptoms and/or signs of liver disease.

Advise patients that they may experience depression while taking naltrexone. Inform family members and the people closest to the patient that they are taking naltrexone and to call their health care provider right away if they become depressed or experience symptoms of depression.

Advise patients not to take naltrexone if they are allergic to naltrexone or any of the microsphere or diluent components.

Advise patients that naltrexone may cause an allergic pneumonia. Advise patients to immediately notify their health care provider if they develop signs and symptoms of pneumonia, including dyspnea, coughing, or wheezing.

Advise patients to carry documentation to alert medical personnel to the fact that they are taking naltrexone. This will help to ensure that the patients obtain adequate medical treatment in an emergency.

Advise patients that they may experience nausea following the initial injection of naltrexone. These episodes of nausea tend to be mild and subside within a few days postinjection. Patients are less likely to experience nausea in subsequent injections. Advise patients that they may also experience tiredness, headache, vomiting, decreased appetite, painful joints, and muscle cramps.

Advise patients that because naltrexone is an IM injection and not an implanted device, once naltrexone is injected, it is not possible to remove it from the body.

Advise patients that naltrexone has been shown to treat alcohol dependence only when used as part of a treatment program that includes counseling and support.

Advise patients that dizziness may occur with naltrexone treatment, and to avoid driving or operating heavy machinery until they have determined how naltrexone affects them.

Advise patients to notify their health care provider if they become pregnant or intend to become pregnant during treatment with naltrexone; are breastfeeding; experience respiratory symptoms such as dyspnea, coughing, or wheezing when taking naltrexone; experience any allergic reactions when taking naltrexone; or experience other unusual or significant adverse reactions while taking naltrexone therapy.

FLUMAZENIL

Rx	**Flumazenil** (Various, American Pharmaceutical Partners, Bedford)	**Injection:** 0.1 mg/mL	Parabens, NaCl, EDTA. In 5 and 10 mL vials.
Rx	**Romazicon** (Hoffman-La Roche)		Parabens, EDTA. In 5 and 10 mL vials.

FLUMAZENIL — INJECTION

WARNING

The use of flumazenil has been associated with the occurrence of seizures.

These are most frequent in patients who have been on benzodiazepines for long-term sedation or in overdose cases where patients are showing signs of serious cyclic antidepressant overdose.

Practitioners should individualize the dosage of flumazenil and be prepared to manage seizures.

Indications

➤*Adult patients:* For the complete or partial reversal of the sedative effects of benzodiazepines in cases where general anesthesia has been induced or maintained with benzodiazepines, where sedation has been produced with benzodiazepines for diagnostic and therapeutic procedures, and for the management of benzodiazepine overdose.

➤*Pediatric patients (1 to 17 years of age):* Flumazenil is indicated for the reversal of conscious sedation induced with benzodiazepines.

➤*Off-label uses:*

Hepatic encephalopathy – [1] = Good documentation. According to American College of Gastroenterology guidelines, flumazenil may be used in patients with hepatic encephalopathy and suspected benzodiazepine use. Results from controlled trials have also shown its effectiveness in patients with cirrhosis who did not have benzodiazepine involvement.

Administration and Dosage

➤*Administration:* Flumazenil is recommended for intravenous use only. It is compatible with 5% dextrose in water, lactated ringer's and normal saline solutions. If flumazenil is drawn into a syringe or mixed with any of these solutions, it should be discarded after 24 hours. For optimum sterility, flumazenil should remain in the vial until just before use. As with all parenteral drug products, flumazenil should be inspected visually for particulate matter and discoloration prior to administration, whenever solution and container permit.

To minimize the likelihood of pain at the injection site, flumazenil should be administered through a freely running intravenous infusion into a large vein.

➤*Reversal of conscious sedation:*

Adult patients – For the reversal of the sedative effects of benzodiazepines administered for conscious sedation, the recommended initial dose of flumazenil is 0.2 mg (2 mL) administered intravenously over 15 seconds. If the desired level of consciousness is not obtained after waiting an additional 45 seconds, a further dose of 0.2 mg (2 mL) can be injected and repeated at 60-second intervals where necessary (up to a maximum of 4 additional times) to a maximum total dose of 1 mg (10 mL). The dosage should be individualized based on the patient's response, with most patients responding to doses of 0.6 mg to 1 mg (see Individualization of dosage).

In the event of resedation, repeated dose may be administered at 20-minute intervals as needed. For repeat treatment, no more than 1 mg (given as 0.2 mg/min) should be administered at any one time, and no more than 3 mg should be given in any 1 hour.

It is recommended that flumazenil be administered as the series of small injections described (not as a single bolus injection) to allow the practitioner to control the reversal of sedation to the approximate endpoint desired and to minimize the possibility of adverse effects (see Individualization of dosage).

FLUMAZENIL — INJECTION

Pediatric patients – For the reversal of the sedative effects of benzodiazepines administered for conscious sedation in pediatric patients, the recommended initial dose is 0.01 mg/kg (up to 0.2 mg) administered intravenously over 15 seconds. If the desired level of consciousness is not obtained after waiting an additional 45 seconds, further injections of 0.01 mg/kg (up to 0.2 mg) can be administered and repeated at 60-second intervals where necessary (up to a maximum of 4 additional times) to a maximum total dose of 0.05 mg/kg or 1 mg, whichever is lower. The dose should be individualized based on the patient's response. The mean total dose administered in the pediatric clinical trial of flumazenil was 0.65 mg (range, 0.08 mg to 1 mg). Approximately one-half of patients required the maximum of 5 injections.

Resedation occurred in 7 of 60 pediatric patients who were fully alert 10 minutes after the start of flumazenil administration. The safety and efficacy of repeated flumazenil administration in pediatric patients experiencing resedation have not been established.

It is recommended that flumazenil be administered as the series of small injections described (not as a single bolus injection) to allow the practitioner to control the reversal of sedation to the approximate endpoint desired and to minimize the possibility of adverse effects (see Individualization of dosage).

The safety and efficacy of flumazenil in the reversal of conscious sedation in pediatric patients below the age of 1 year have not been established.

➤*Reversal of general anesthesia in adult patients:* For the reversal of the sedative effects of benzodiazepines administered for general anesthesia, the recommended initial dose of flumazenil is 0.2 mg (2 mL) administered intravenously over 15 seconds. If the desired level of consciousness is not obtained after waiting an additional 45 seconds, a further dose of 0.2 mg (2 mL) can be injected and repeated at 60-second intervals where necessary (up to a maximum of 4 additional times) to a maximum total dose of 1 mg (10 mL). The dosage should be individualized based on the patient's response, with most patients responding to doses of 0.6 mg to 1 mg.

In the event of resedation, repeated doses may be administered at 20-minute intervals as needed. For repeat treatment, no more than 1 mg (given as 0.2 mg/min) should be administered at any one time, and no more than 3 mg should be given in any 1 hour.

It is recommended that flumazenil be administered as the series of small injections described (not as a single bolus injection) to allow the practitioner to control the reversal of sedation to the approximate endpoint desired and to minimize the possibility of adverse effects.

➤*Management of suspected benzodiazepine overdose in adult patients:* For initial management of a known or suspected benzodiazepine overdose, the recommended initial dose of flumazenil is 0.2 mg (2 mL) administered intravenously over 30 seconds. If the desired level of consciousness is not obtained after waiting 30 seconds, a further dose of 0.3 mg (3 mL) can be administered over another 30 seconds. Further doses of 0.5 mg (5 mL) can be administered over 30 seconds at 1-minute intervals up to a cumulative dose of 3 mg.

Do not rush the administration of flumazenil. Patients should have a secure airway and intravenous access before administration of the drug and be awakened gradually.

Most patients with a benzodiazepine overdose will respond to a cumulative dose of 1 mg to 3 mg of flumazenil, and doses beyond 3 mg do not reliably produce additional effects. On rare occasions, patients with a partial response at 3 mg may require additional titration up to a total dose of 5 mg (administered slowly in the same manner).

If a patient has not responded 5 minutes after receiving a cumulative dose of 5 mg of flumazenil, the major cause of sedation is likely not to be due to benzodiazepines, and additional flumazenil is likely to have no effect.

In the event of resedation, repeated doses may be given at 20-minute intervals if needed. For repeat treatment, no more than 1 mg (given as 0.5 mg/min) should be given at any one time and no more than 3 mg should be given in any one hour.

➤*Individualization of dosage:*

General principles – The serious adverse effects of flumazenil are related to the reversal of benzodiazepine effects. Using more than the minimally effective dose of flumazenil is tolerated by most patients but may complicate the management of patients who are physically dependent on benzodiazepines or patients who are depending on benzodiazepines for therapeutic effect (such as suppression of seizures in cyclic antidepressant overdose).

In high-risk patients, it is important to administer the smallest amount of flumazenil that is effective. The 1-minute wait between individual doses in the dose-titration recommended for general clinical populations may be too short for high-risk patients. This is because it takes 6 to 10 minutes for any single dose of flumazenil to reach full effects. Practitioners should slow the rate of administration of flumazenil administered to high-risk patients as recommended below.

Anesthesia and conscious sedation in adult patients – Flumazenil is well tolerated at the recommended doses in individuals who have no tolerance to (or dependence on) benzodiazepines. The recommended doses and titration rates in anesthesia and conscious sedation (0.2 mg to 1 mg given at 0.2 mg/min) are well tolerated in patients receiving the drug for reversal of a single benzodiazepine exposure in most clinical settings. The major risk will be resedation because the duration of effect of a long-acting (or large dose of a short-acting) benzodiazepine may exceed that of flumazenil. Resedation may be treated by giving a repeat dose at no less than 20-minute intervals. For repeat treatment, no more than 1 mg (at 0.2 mg/min doses) should be given at any one time and no more than 3 mg should be given in any 1 hour.

Overdose in adult patients – The risk of confusion, agitation, emotional lability and perceptual distortion with the doses recommended in patients with benzodiazepine overdose (3 mg to 5 mg administered as 0.5 mg/min) may be greater than that expected with lower doses and slower administration. The recommended doses represent a compromise between desirable slow awakening and the need for prompt response and a persistent effect in the overdose situation. If circumstances permit, the physician may elect to use the 0.2 mg/min titration rate to slowly awaken the patient over 5 to 10 minutes, which may help to reduce signs and symptoms on emergence.

Flumazenil has no effect in cases where benzodiazepines are not responsible for sedation. Once doses of 3 mg to 5 mg have been reached without clinical response, additional flumazenil is likely to have no effect.

Patients tolerant to benzodiazepines – Flumazenil may cause benzodiazepine withdrawal symptoms in individuals who have been taking benzodiazepines long enough to have some degree of tolerance. Patients who had been taking benzodiazepines prior to entry into the flumazenil trials who were given flumazenil in doses over 1 mg, experienced withdrawal-like events 2 to 5 times more frequently than patients who received less than 1 mg.

In patients who may have tolerance to benzodiazepines, as indicated by clinical history or by the need for larger than usual doses of benzodiazepines, slower titration rates of 0.1 mg/min and lower total doses may help reduce the frequency of emergent confusion and agitation. In such cases, special care must be taken to monitor the patients for resedation because of the lower doses of flumazenil used.

Patients physically dependent on benzodiazepines – Flumazenil is known to precipitate withdrawal seizures in patients who are physically dependent on benzodiazepines, even if such dependence was established in a relatively few days of high dose sedation in intensive care unit (ICU) environments. The risk of either seizures or resedation in such cases is high and patients have experienced seizures before regaining consciousness. Flumazenil should be used in such settings with extreme caution, since the use of flumazenil in this situation has not been studied and no information as to dose and rate of titration is available. Flumazenil should be used in such patients only if the potential benefits of using the drug outweigh the risks of precipitated seizures. Physicians are directed to the scientific literature for the most current information in this area.

➤*Off-label dosing:*

Hepatic encephalopathy – [1] = Good documentation. Intravenous (IV) 1 mg bolus.

➤*Storage/Stability:* Store at 25°C (77°F); excursions permitted to 15° to 30°C (59° to 86°F).

Actions

➤*Pharmacology:* Flumazenil, an imidazobenzodiazepine derivative, antagonizes the actions of benzodiazepines on the central nervous system. Flumazenil competitively inhibits the activity at the benzodiazepine recognition site on the GABA/benzodiazepine receptor complex. Flumazenil is a weak partial agonist in some animal models of activity, but has little or no agonist activity in man.

Flumazenil does not antagonize the central nervous system effects of drugs affecting GABA-ergic neurons by means other than the benzodiazepine receptor (including ethanol, barbiturates, or general anesthetics) and does not reverse the effects of opioids.

In animals pretreated with high doses of benzodiazepines over several weeks, flumazenil elicited symptoms of benzodiazepine withdrawal, including seizures. A similar effect was seen in adult human subjects.

Intravenous flumazenil has been shown to antagonize sedation, impairment of recall, psychomotor impairment and ventilatory depression produced by benzodiazepines in healthy human volunteers.

The duration and degree of reversal of benzodiazepine effects are related to the dose and plasma concentrations of flumazenil.

Generally, doses of approximately 0.1 mg to 0.2 mg (corresponding to peak plasma levels of 3 to 6 ng/mL) produce partial antagonism, whereas higher doses of 0.4 to 1 mg (peak plasma levels of 12 to 28 ng/mL) usually produce complete antagonism in patients who have received the usual sedating doses of benzodiazepines. The onset of reversal is usually evident within 1 to 2 minutes after the injection is completed. Eighty percent (80%) response will be reached within 3 minutes, with the peak effect occurring at 6 to 10 minutes. The duration and degree of reversal are related to the plasma concentration of the sedating benzodiazepine as well as the dose of flumazenil given.

In healthy volunteers, flumazenil did not alter intraocular pressure when given alone and reversed the decrease in intraocular pressure seen after administration of midazolam.

➤*Pharmacokinetics:*

Flumazenil Pharmacokinetic Parameters Following a 5-minute 1 mg Infusion	
Parameter	Mean (range)
C_{max}	24 ng/mL (38%; 11 to 43)
AUC	15 ng•h/mL (22%; 10 to 22)
V_{ss}	1 L/kg (24%; 0.8 to 1.6)
Cl	1 L/h/kg (20%; 0.7 to 1.4)
Half-life	54 min (21%; 41 to 79)

Absorption – After IV administration, plasma concentrations of flumazenil follow a 2-exponential decay model. The pharmacokinetics of flumazenil are dose-proportional up to 100 mg.

FLUMAZENIL — INJECTION

Food effects: Ingestion of food during an intravenous infusion of the drug results in a 50% increase in clearance, most likely due to the increased hepatic blood flow that accompanies a meal.

Distribution – Flumazenil is extensively distributed in the extravascular space with an initial distribution half-life of 4 to 11 minutes and a terminal half-life of 40 to 80 minutes. Peak concentrations of flumazenil are proportional to dose, with an apparent initial volume of distribution of 0.5 L/kg. The volume of distribution at steady-state is 0.9 to 1.1 L/kg. Flumazenil is a weak lipophilic base. Protein binding is approximately 50% and the drug shows no preferential partitioning into red blood cells. Albumin accounts for two-thirds of plasma protein binding.

Metabolism – Flumazenil is completely (99%) metabolized. Very little unchanged flumazenil (less than 1%) is found in the urine. The major metabolites of flumazenil identified in urine are the de-ethylated free acid and its glucuronide conjugate. In preclinical studies there was no evidence of pharmacologic activity exhibited by the de-ethylated free acid.

Excretion – Elimination of radiolabeled drug is essentially complete within 72 hours, with 90% to 95% of the radioactivity appearing in urine and 5% to 10% in the feces. Clearance of flumazenil occurs primarily by hepatic metabolism and is dependent on hepatic blood flow. In pharmacokinetic studies of healthy volunteers, total clearance ranged from 0.8 to 1 L/hr/kg.

Special populations –

Hepatic function impairment: For patients with moderate liver dysfunction, their mean total clearance is decreased to 40% to 60% and in patients with severe liver dysfunction, it is decreased to 25% of normal value, compared with age-matched healthy subjects. This results in a prolongation of the half-life to 1.3 hours in patients with moderate hepatic impairment and 2.4 hours in severely impaired patients. Caution should be exercised with initial and/or repeated dosing to patients with liver disease.

Children: The pharmacokinetics of flumazenil have been evaluated in 29 pediatric patients ranging in age from 1 to 17 years who had undergone minor surgical procedures. The average doses administered were 0.53 mg (0.044 mg/kg) in patients aged 1 to 5 years, 0.63 mg (0.02 mg/kg) in patients aged 6 to 12 years, and 0.8 mg (0.014 mg/kg) in patients aged 13 to 17 years. Compared to adults, the elimination half-life in pediatric patients was more variable, averaging 40 minutes (range: 20 to 75 minutes). Clearance and volume of distribution, normalized for body weight, were in the same range as those seen in adults, although more variability was seen in the pediatric patients.

Contraindications

Hypersensitivity to flumazenil or benzodiazepines; patients who have been given a benzodiazepine for control of a potentially life-threatening condition (eg, control of intracranial pressure or status epilepticus); patients who are showing signs of serious cyclic antidepressant overdose.

Warnings/Precautions

➤*Risk of seizures:* The reversal of benzodiazepine effects may be associated with the onset of seizures in certain high-risk populations. Possible risk factors for seizures include concurrent major sedative-hypnotic drug withdrawal, recent therapy with repeated doses of parenteral benzodiazepines, myoclonic jerking or seizure activity prior to flumazenil administration in overdose cases, or concurrent cyclic antidepressant poisoning.

Flumazenil is not recommended in cases of serious cyclic antidepressant poisoning, as manifested by motor abnormalities (twitching, rigidity, focal seizure), dysrhythmia (wide QRS, ventricular dysrhythmia, heart block), anticholinergic signs (mydriasis, dry mucosa, hypoperistalsis), and cardiovascular collapse at presentation. In such cases flumazenil should be withheld and the patient should be allowed to remain sedated (with ventilatory and circulatory support as needed) until the signs of antidepressant toxicity have subsided. Treatment with flumazenil has no known benefit to the seriously ill mixed-overdose patient other than reversing sedation and should not be used in cases where seizures (from any cause) are likely.

Most convulsions associated with flumazenil administration require treatment and have been successfully managed with benzodiazepines, phenytoin or barbiturates. Because of the presence of flumazenil, higher than usual doses of benzodiazepines may be required.

➤*Hypoventilation:* Patients who have received flumazenil for the reversal of benzodiazepine effects (after conscious sedation or general anesthesia) should be monitored for resedation, respiratory depression, or other residual benzodiazepine effects for an appropriate period (up to 120 minutes) based on the dose and duration of effect of the benzodiazepine employed.

This is because flumazenil has not been established in patients as an effective treatment for hypoventilation due to benzodiazepine administration. In healthy male volunteers, flumazenil is capable of reversing benzodiazepine-induced depression of the ventilatory responses to hypercapnia and hypoxia after a benzodiazepine alone. However, such depression may recur because the ventilatory effects of typical doses of flumazenil (1 mg or less) may wear off before the effects of many benzodiazepines. The effects of flumazenil on ventilatory response following sedation with a benzodiazepine in combination with an opioid are inconsistent and have not been adequately studied. The availability of flumazenil does not diminish the need for prompt detection of hypoventilation and the ability to effectively intervene by establishing an airway and assisting ventilation.

Overdose cases should always be monitored for resedation until the patients are stable and resedation is unlikely.

➤*Return of sedation:* Flumazenil may be expected to improve the alertness of patients recovering from a procedure involving sedation or anesthesia with benzodiazepines, but should not be substituted for an adequate period of postprocedure monitoring. The availability of flumazenil does not reduce the risks associated with the use of large doses of benzodiazepines for sedation.

Patients should be monitored for resedation, respiratory depression or other persistent or recurrent agonist effects for an adequate period of time after administration of flumazenil.

Resedation is least likely in cases where flumazenil is administered to reverse a low dose of a short-acting benzodiazepine (less than 10 mg midazolam). It is most likely in cases where a large single or cumulative dose of a benzodiazepine has been given in the course of a long procedure along with neuromuscular blocking agents and multiple anesthetic agents.

Profound resedation was observed in 1% to 3% of adult patients in the clinical studies. In clinical situations where resedation must be prevented in adult patients, physicians may wish to repeat the initial dose (up to 1 mg of flumazenil given at 0.2 mg/min) at 30 minutes and possibly again at 60 minutes. This dosage schedule, although not studied in clinical trials, was effective in preventing resedation in a pharmacologic study in normal volunteers.

The use of flumazenil to reverse the effects of benzodiazepines used for conscious sedation has been evaluated in 1 open-label clinical trial involving 107 pediatric patients between the ages of 1 and 17 years. This study suggested that pediatric patients who have become fully awake following treatment with flumazenil may experience a recurrence of sedation, especially younger patients (ages 1 to 5). Resedation was experienced in 7 of 60 patients who were fully alert 10 minutes after the start of flumazenil administration. No patient experienced a return to the baseline level of sedation. Mean time to resedation was 25 minutes (range, 19 to 50 minutes). The safety and effectiveness of repeated flumazenil administration in pediatric patients experiencing resedation have not been established.

➤*Use in the ICU:* Flumazenil should be used with caution in the ICU because of the increased risk of unrecognized benzodiazepine dependence in such settings. Flumazenil may produce convulsions in patients physically dependent on benzodiazepines.

Administration of flumazenil to diagnose benzodiazepine-induced sedation in the ICU is not recommended due to the risk of adverse events as described above. In addition, the prognostic significance of a patient's failure to respond to flumazenil in cases confounded by metabolic disorder, traumatic injury, drugs other than benzodiazepines, or any other reasons not associated with benzodiazepine receptor occupancy is unknown.

➤*Use in overdose:* Flumazenil is intended as an adjunct to, not as a substitute for, proper management of airway, assisted breathing, circulatory access and support, internal decontamination by lavage and charcoal, and adequate clinical evaluation.

Necessary measures should be instituted to secure airway, ventilation and intravenous access prior to administering flumazenil. Upon arousal, patients may attempt to withdraw endotracheal tubes or intravenous lines as the result of confusion and agitation following awakening.

➤*Neuromuscular blocking agents:* Flumazenil should not be used until the effects of neuromuscular blockade have been fully reversed.

➤*Psychiatric patients:* Flumazenil has been reported to provoke panic attacks in patients with a history of panic disorder.

➤*Pain on injection:* To minimize the likelihood of pain or inflammation at the injection site, flumazenil should be administered through a freely flowing intravenous infusion into a large vein. Local irritation may occur following extravasation into perivascular tissues.

➤*Respiratory disease:* The primary treatment of patients with serious lung disease who experience serious respiratory depression due to benzodiazepines should be appropriate ventilatory support rather than the administration of flumazenil. Flumazenil is capable of partially reversing benzodiazepine-induced alterations in ventilatory drive in healthy volunteers, but has not been shown to be clinically effective.

➤*Cardiovascular disease:* Flumazenil did not increase the work of the heart when used to reverse benzodiazepines in cardiac patients when given at a rate of 0.1 mg/min in total doses of less than 0.5 mg in studies reported in the clinical literature. Flumazenil alone had no significant effects on cardiovascular parameters when administered to patients with stable ischemic heart disease.

➤*Ambulatory patients:* The effects of flumazenil may wear off before a long-acting benzodiazepine is completely cleared from the body. In general, if a patient shows no signs of sedation within 2 hours after a 1 mg dose of flumazenil, serious resedation at a later time is unlikely. An adequate period of observation must be provided for any patient in whom either long-acting benzodiazepines (such as diazepam) or large doses of short-acting benzodiazepines (such as greater than 10 mg of midazolam) have been used.

➤*Head injury:* Flumazenil should be used with caution in patients with head injury as it may be capable of precipitating convulsions or altering cerebral blood flow in patients receiving benzodiazepines. It should be used only by practitioners prepared to manage such complications should they occur.

➤*Use in drug- and alcohol-dependent patients:* Flumazenil should be used with caution in patients with alcoholism and other drug dependencies due to the increased frequency of benzodiazepine tolerance and dependence observed in these patient populations.

Flumazenil is not recommended either as a treatment for benzodiazepine dependence or for the management of protracted benzodiazepine abstinence syndromes, as such use has not been studied.

The administration of flumazenil can precipitate benzodiazepine withdrawal in animals and man. This has been seen in healthy volunteers treated with

FLUMAZENIL — INJECTION

therapeutic doses of oral lorazepam for up to 2 weeks who exhibited effects such as hot flushes, agitation and tremor when treated with cumulative doses of up to 3 mg doses of flumazenil.

Similar adverse experiences suggestive of flumazenil precipitation of benzodiazepine withdrawal have occurred in some adult patients in clinical trials. Such patients had a short-lived syndrome characterized by dizziness, mild confusion, emotional lability, agitation (with signs and symptoms of anxiety), and mild sensory distortions. This response was dose-related, most common at doses above 1 mg, rarely required treatment other than reassurance and was usually short lived. When required (5 to 10 cases), these patients were successfully treated with usual doses of a barbiturate, a benzodiazepine, or other sedative drug.

Practitioners should assume that flumazenil administration may trigger dose-dependent withdrawal syndromes in patients with established physical dependence on benzodiazepines and may complicate the management of withdrawal syndromes for alcohol, barbiturates, and cross-tolerant sedatives.

➤*Hepatic function impairment:* The clearance of flumazenil is reduced to 40% to 60% of healthy in patients with mild to moderate hepatic disease and to 25% of normal in patients with severe hepatic dysfunction. While the dose of flumazenil used for initial reversal of benzodiazepine effects is not affected, repeat doses of the drug in liver disease should be reduced in size or frequency.

➤*Drug abuse and dependence:* Flumazenil acts as a benzodiazepine antagonist, blocks the effects of benzodiazepines in animals and man, antagonizes benzodiazepine reinforcement in animal models, produces dysphoria in healthy subjects, and has had no reported abuse in foreign marketing. Although flumazenil has a benzodiazepine-like structure it does not act as a benzodiazepine agonist in man and is not a controlled substance.

➤*Pregnancy: Category C.* There are no adequate and well-controlled studies of the use of flumazenil in pregnant women. Flumazenil should be used during pregnancy only if the potential benefit justifies the potential risk to the fetus.

Teratogenic –

In rabbits, embryocidal effects (as evidenced by increased preimplantation and postimplantation losses) were observed at 50 mg/kg or 200 times the human exposure from a maximum recommended intravenous dose of 5 mg. The no-effect dose of 15 mg/kg in rabbits represents 60 times the human exposure.

Nonteratogenic – An animal reproduction study was conducted in rats at oral dosages of 5, 25, and 125 mg/kg/day of flumazenil. Pup survival was decreased during the lactating period, pup liver weight at weaning was increased for the high-dose group (125 mg/kg/day) and incisor eruption and ear opening in the offspring were delayed; the delay in ear opening was associated with a delay in the appearance of the auditory startle response. No treatment-related adverse effects were noted for the other dose groups. Based on the available data from AUC, the effect level (125 mg/kg) represents 120 times the human exposure from 5 mg, the maximum recommended intravenous dose in humans. The no-effect level represents 24 times the human exposure from an intravenous dose of 5 mg.

Labor and delivery – The use of flumazenil to reverse the effects of benzodiazepines used during labor and delivery is not recommended because the effects of the drug in the newborn are unknown.

➤*Lactation:* Caution should be exercised when deciding to administer flumazenil to a breast-feeding woman because it is not known whether flumazenil is excreted in human milk.

➤*Children:* The safety and efficacy of flumazenil have been established in pediatric patients 1 year of age and older. Use of flumazenil in this age group is supported by evidence from adequate and well-controlled studies of flumazenil in adults with additional data from uncontrolled pediatric studies including 1 open-label trial.

The use of flumazenil to reverse the effects of benzodiazepines used for conscious sedation was evaluated in 1 uncontrolled clinical trial involving 107 pediatric patients between the ages of 1 and 17 years. At the doses used, flumazenil's safety was established in this population. Patients received up to 5 injections of 0.01 mg/kg flumazenil up to a maximum total dose of 1 mg at a rate not exceeding 0.2 mg/min.

Of 60 patients who were fully alert at 10 minutes, 7 experienced resedation. Resedation occurred between 19 and 50 minutes after the start of flumazenil administration. None of the patients experienced a return to the baseline level of sedation. All 7 patients were between the ages of 1 and 5 years. The types and frequency of adverse events noted in these pediatric patients were similar to those previously documented in clinical trials with flumazenil to reverse conscious sedation in adults. No patient experienced a serious adverse event attributable to flumazenil.

The safety and efficacy of flumazenil in the reversal of conscious sedation in pediatric patients below the age of 1 year have not been established.

The safety and efficacy of flumazenil have not been established in pediatric patients for reversal of the sedative effects of benzodiazepines used for induction of general anesthesia, for the management of overdose, or for the resuscitation of the newborn, as no well-controlled clinical studies have been performed to determine the risks, benefits, and dosages to be used. However, published anecdotal reports discussing the use of flumazenil in pediatric patients for these indications have reported similar safety profiles and dosing guidelines to those described for the reversal of conscious sedation.

The risks identified in the adult population with flumazenil use also apply to pediatric patients.

➤*Elderly:* Of the total number of subjects in clinical studies of flumazenil, 248 were 65 years and over. No overall differences in safety or effectiveness were observed between these subjects and younger subjects. Other reported clinical experience has not identified differences in responses between the elderly and younger patients, but greater sensitivity of some older individuals cannot be ruled out.

The pharmacokinetics of flumazenil have been studied in the elderly and are not significantly different from younger patients. Several studies of flumazenil in subjects over the age of 65 years and 1 study in subjects over the age of 80 years suggest that while the doses of benzodiazepine used to induce sedation should be reduced, ordinary doses of flumazenil may be used for reversal.

Drug Interactions

Interaction with central nervous system depressants other than benzodiazepines has not been specifically studied; however, no deleterious interactions were seen when flumazenil was administered after narcotics, inhalational anesthetics, muscle relaxants and muscle relaxant antagonists administered in conjunction with sedation or anesthesia. Particular caution is necessary when using flumazenil in cases of mixed drug overdose, since the toxic effects (such as convulsions and cardiac dysrhythmias) of other drugs taken in overdose (especially cyclic antidepressants) may emerge with the reversal of the benzodiazepine effect by flumazenil.

The use of flumazenil is not recommended in epileptic patients who have been receiving benzodiazepine treatment for a prolonged period. Although flumazenil exerts a slight intrinsic anticonvulsant effect, its abrupt suppression of the protective effect of a benzodiazepine agonist can give rise to convulsions in epileptic patients.

Flumazenil blocks the central effects of benzodiazepines by competitive interaction at the receptor level. The effects of nonbenzodiazepine agonists at benzodiazepine receptors, such as zopiclone, triazolopyridazines and others, are also blocked by flumazenil.

Adverse Reactions

Deaths have occurred in patients who received flumazenil in a variety of clinical settings. The majority of deaths occurred in patients with serious underlying disease or in patients who had ingested large amounts of nonbenzodiazepine drugs (usually cyclic antidepressants), as part of an overdose.

Serious adverse events have occurred in all clinical settings, and convulsions are the most common serious adverse events reported. Flumazenil administration has been associated with the onset of convulsions in patients who are relying on benzodiazepine effects to control seizures, are physically dependent on benzodiazepines, or who have ingested large doses of other drugs.

Two of the 446 patients who received flumazenil in controlled clinical trials for the management of a benzodiazepine overdose had cardiac dysrhythmias (1 ventricular tachycardia, 1 junctional tachycardia).

➤*Adverse events in clinical studies:* The following adverse reactions were considered to be related to flumazenil administration (both alone and for the reversal of benzodiazepine effects) and were reported in studies involving 1,875 individuals who received flumazenil in controlled trials. Adverse events most frequently associated with flumazenil alone were limited to dizziness, injection site pain, increased sweating, headache, and abnormal or blurred vision (3% to 9%). Observed percentage reported if greater than 9%.

Cardiovascular – Cutaneous vasodilation (sweating, flushing, hot flushes) (1% to 3%).

GI – Nausea and vomiting (11%).

CNS – Dizziness (vertigo, ataxia) (10%); agitation (anxiety, nervousness, dry mouth, tremor, palpitations, insomnia, dyspnea, hyperventilation) (3% to 9%), and emotional lability (crying abnormal, depersonalization, euphoria, increased tears, depression, dysphoria, paranoia) (1% to 3%).

Special senses – Abnormal vision (visual field defect, diplopia) and paresthesia (sensation abnormal, hypoesthesia).

Miscellaneous – Injection site pain (3% to 9%); fatigue (asthenia, malaise), headache, and injection site reaction (thrombophlebitis, skin abnormality, rash) (1% to 3%).

➤*Less than 1% incidence:* The following adverse events were observed infrequently (less than 1%) in the clinical studies, but were judged as probably related to flumazenil administration and/or reversal of benzodiazepine effects.

CNS – Confusion (difficulty concentrating, delirium), convulsions, and somnolence (stupor).

Special senses – Abnormal hearing (transient hearing impairment, hyperacusis, tinnitus).

➤*Less than 1% incidence; unknown relationship to flumazenil:* The following adverse events occurred with frequencies less than 1% in the clinical trials. Their relationship to flumazenil administration is unknown, but they are included as alerting information for the physician.

Not included in this list is operative site pain that occurred with the same frequency in patients receiving placebo as in patients receiving flumazenil for reversal of sedation following a surgical procedure.

Cardiovascular – Arrhythmia (atrial, nodal, ventricular extrasystoles), bradycardia, tachycardia, hypertension and chest pain.

CNS – Speech disorder (dysphonia, thick tongue).

Miscellaneous – Rigors, shivering, hiccup.

FLUMAZENIL — INJECTION

➤*Additional adverse reactions reported during postmarketing experience:* The following events have been reported during postapproval use of flumazenil.

CNS – Fear, panic attacks in patients with a history of panic disorders.

Miscellaneous – Withdrawal symptoms may occur following rapid injection of flumazenil in patients with long-term exposure to benzodiazepines.

Overdosage

➤*Symptoms:* Large intravenous doses of flumazenil, when administered to healthy volunteers in the absence of a benzodiazepine agonist, produced no serious adverse reactions, severe signs or symptoms, or clinically significant laboratory test abnormalities. In clinical studies, most adverse reactions to flumazenil were an extension of the pharmacologic effects of the drug in reversing benzodiazepine effects. Reversal with an excessively high dose of flumazenil may produce anxiety, agitation, increased muscle tone, hyperesthesia and possibly convulsions. Convulsions have been treated with barbiturates, benzodiazepines and phenytoin, generally with prompt resolution of the seizures.

The risk of confusion, agitation, emotional lability and perceptual distortion with the doses recommended in patients with benzodiazepine overdose (3 mg to 5 mg administered as 0.5 mg/min) may be greater than that expected with lower doses and slower administration. The recommended doses represent a compromise between desirable slow awakening and the need for prompt response and a persistent effect in the overdose situation. If circumstances permit, the physician may elect to use the 0.2 mg/min titration rate to slowly awaken the patient over 5 to 10 minutes, which may help to reduce signs and symptoms on emergence.

➤*Treatment:* Flumazenil has no effect in cases where benzodiazepines are not responsible for sedation. Once doses of 3 mg to 5 mg have been reached without clinical response, additional flumazenil is likely to have no effect.

Patient Information

Flumazenil does not consistently reverse amnesia. Patients cannot be expected to remember information told to them in the postprocedure period and instructions given to patients should be reinforced in writing or given to a responsible family member. Physicians are advised to discuss with patients or their guardians, both before surgery and at discharge, that although the patient may feel alert at the time of discharge, the effects of the benzodiazepine may recur. As a result, the patient should be instructed, preferably in writing, that their memory and judgment may be impaired and specifically advised about the following:

1.) Not to engage in any activities requiring complete alertness, and not to operate hazardous machinery or a motor vehicle during the first 24 hours after discharge, and it is certain no residual sedative effects of the benzodiazepine remain.
2.) Not to take any alcohol or nonprescription drugs during the first 24 hours after flumazenil administration or if the effects of the benzodiazepine persist.

PHYSOSTIGMINE SALICYLATE

Rx	**Physostigmine Salicylate** (Akorn)	**Injection, solution:** 1 mg/mL	With benzyl alcohol 2% and sodium metabisulfite 0.1%. In 2 mL ampules.

PHYSOSTIGMINE SALICYLATE — INJECTION

Indications

➤*Anticholinergic toxicity:* To reverse the effect upon the CNS, caused by clinical or toxic dosages of drugs capable of producing the anticholinergic syndrome.

Physostigmine should not be used to manage anticholinergic symptoms due to an overdosage of tricyclic antidepressants. It may cause cardiac toxicity, including bradycardia and asystole, and it may also precipitate seizures in tricyclic antidepressant–poisoned patients. Physostigmine should also not be used if a patient has QRS or QTc prolongation Consult with a medical toxicologist or poison control center regarding the use of physostigmine.

➤*Off-label uses:* Physostigmine has been used to treat delirium tremens and Alzheimer disease. It may also antagonize diazepam's CNS-depressant effects.

Administration and Dosage

➤*General dosing considerations:* In all cases of poisoning, the usual supportive measures should be undertaken.

Atropine should always be at hand because it is an antagonist and antidote for physostigmine.

➤*Adults:*

Anticholinergic toxicity – 1 to 2 mg intravenously (IV) over at least 5 minutes. May repeat dosage in 10 to 15 minutes if reversal of symptoms has not occurred or life-threatening signs, such as arrhythmia, convulsions, or coma occur. If anticholinergic symptoms initially resolve but clinical relapse occurs, additional doses may be needed.

Postanesthesia care – Administer 0.5 to 1 mg intramuscularly (IM) or IV. IV administration should be at a slow, controlled rate of not more than 1 mg per minute. Dosage may be repeated at intervals of 10 to 30 minutes if desired patient response is not obtained.

➤*Children:*

Anticholinergic toxicity –

Usual dosage: 0.02 mg/kg over at least 5 minutes. May repeat dosage in 10 to 15 minutes if reversal of symptoms has not occurred or life-threatening signs, such as arrhythmia, convulsions, or coma occur. If anticholinergic symptoms initially resolve but clinical relapse occurs, additional doses may be needed.

Maximum dose: 0.5 mg (single dose); 2 mg (total dose).

➤*Renal function impairment:* Dosage adjustment is not required.

➤*Discontinuation of therapy:* If excessive symptoms of salivation, emesis, urination, and defecation occur, terminate the use of physostigmine salicylate injection. If excessive sweating or nausea occur, reduce the dosage.

➤*Administration:* IV administration should be at a slow, controlled rate, no more than 1 mg per minute for adults and 0.5 mg per minute for children. Rapid administration can cause bradycardia, hypersalivation leading to respiratory difficulties, and possible convulsions. According to the prescribing information, physostigmine may also be administered IM.

➤*Storage/Stability:* Store at 15° to 25°C (59° to 77°F).

Actions

➤*Pharmacology:* Physostigmine is a reversible anticholinesterase which effectively increases the concentration of acetylcholine at the sites of cholinergic transmission. The action of acetylcholine is normally very transient because of its hydrolysis by the enzyme, acetylcholinesterase. Physostigmine inhibits the destructive action of acetylcholinesterase and thereby prolongs and exaggerates the effect of the acetylcholine.

Physostigmine can reverse both central and peripheral anticholinergia. The anticholinergic syndrome has both central and peripheral signs and symptoms. Central toxic effects include anxiety, delirium, disorientation, hallucinations, hyperactivity, and seizures. Severe poisoning may produce coma, medullary paralysis, and death. Peripheral toxicity is characterized by tachycardia, hyperpyrexia, mydriasis, vasodilation, urinary retention, diminution of GI motility, decrease of secretion in salivary and sweat glands, and loss of secretions in the pharynx, bronchi, and nasal passages.

➤*Pharmacokinetics:*

Absorption/Distribution – Physostigmine contains a tertiary amine and easily penetrates the blood brain barrier, while an anticholinesterase, such as neostigmine, which has a quaternary ammonium ion is not capable of crossing the barrier. Dramatic reversal of the effects of anticholinergic symptoms can be expected in minutes after the IV administration of physostigmine, if the diagnosis is correct and the patient has not suffered anoxia or other insult. The duration of action of physostigmine is relatively short, approximately 45 to 60 minutes.

Metabolism/Excretion – Physostigmine is rapidly hydrolyzed by cholinesterase. Plasma half-life is approximately 1 to 2 hours.

Contraindications

Physostigmine should not be used in the presence of asthma, gangrene, diabetes, cardiovascular disease, mechanical obstruction of the intestine or urogenital tract or any vagotonic state, and in patients receiving choline esters or depolarizing neuromuscular blocking agents (decamethonium, succinylcholine).

For postanesthesia, the concomitant use of atropine with physostigmine is not recommended because atropine antagonizes the action of physostigmine.

Warnings/Precautions

➤*Tricyclic antidepressant overdosage:* Physostigmine should not be used to manage anticholinergic symptoms due to an overdosage of tricyclic antidepressants. It may cause cardiac toxicity, including bradycardia and asystole, or precipitate seizures in tricyclic antidepressant–poisoned patients. Physostigmine should not be used if a patient has QRS or QTc prolongation. Consult with a medical toxicologist or poison control center regarding the use of physostigmine.

➤*Discontinuation:* If excessive symptoms of salivation, emesis, urination, and defecation occur, terminate the use of physostigmine. If excessive sweating or nausea occur, reduce the dosage.

➤*Administration:* IV administration should be at a slow, controlled rate, no more than 1 mg per minute. Rapid administration can cause bradycardia, hypersalivation leading to respiratory difficulties, and possible convulsions.

➤*Cholinergic crisis:* An overdose of physostigmine can cause a cholinergic crisis.

➤*Benzyl alcohol:* Benzyl alcohol, contained in this product as a preservative, has been associated with a fatal "gasping syndrome" in premature infants.

➤*Hypersensitivity reactions:* Because of the possibility of hypersensitivity in an occasional patient, atropine should always be at hand because it is an antagonist and antidote for physostigmine.

➤*Sulfite sensitivity:* Some of these products contain sodium-bisulfite, a sulfite that may cause allergic-type reactions including anaphylactic symptoms and life-threatening or less severe asthmatic episodes in certain susceptible people. The overall prevalence of sulfite sensitivity in the general population is unknown and probably low. Sulfite sensitivity is seen more frequently in asthmatic or atopic nonasthmatic people than in nonasthmatic people.

PHYSOSTIGMINE SALICYLATE — INJECTION

➤*Pregnancy: Category C.* Transient muscular weakness has been noted in neonates whose mothers were treated with other cholinesterase inhibitors for myasthenia gravis.

Safe use in pregnancy has not been established; therefore, use in pregnant women or women who may become pregnant requires that possible benefits be weighed against possible hazards to the mother and fetus. Physostigmine should be expected to cross the human placenta.

➤*Lactation:* Safety for use has not been established; therefore, use in breastfeeding women requires that possible benefits be weighed against possible hazards to the mother and child.

➤*Children:* Reserve for life-threatening situations only.

Drug Interactions

Physostigmine Drug Interactions

Precipitant drug	Object drug[a]		Description
Cholinergic agonists (eg, pilocarpine), depolarizing neuromuscular blocking agents, other anticholinesterase agents	Physostigmine	⬆	Additive effects are expected when physostigmine is administered with cholinergic agonists (eg, pilocarpine), depolarizing neuromuscular blocking agents, and other anticholinesterase agents.
Physostigmine	Cholinergic agonists (eg, pilocarpine), depolarizing neuromuscular blocking agents, other anticholinesterase agents		
Quinine derivatives	Physostigmine	⬇	Quinine derivatives may reverse the beneficial effects of physostigmine in the treatment of myasthenia gravis; avoid concurrent use.
Physostigmine	Drugs metabolized by plasma cholinesterases (eg, succinylcholine, cocaine, mivacurium)	⬆	When administered with physostigmine, the actions of drugs metabolized by plasma cholinesterases are expected to be prolonged.
Physostigmine	Valproic acid	⬆	Pharmacologic effects of valproic acid may be increased. Adjust valproic acid dosage as needed.
Physostigmine	Varicella live vaccine	⬆	Reye syndrome has been associated with salicylates (eg, physostigmine salicylate) in children and adolescents during a varicella infection. Avoid using salicylates for 6 weeks following vaccination with varicella live vaccine.

[a] ⬆ = object drug increased; ⬇ = object drug decreased.

Adverse Reactions

Nausea, vomiting, and salivation; can be offset by reducing dosage. Bradycardia and convulsions, if IV administration is too rapid.

Overdosage

➤*Symptoms:* Can cause a cholinergic crisis if overdosed.

➤*Treatment:* Appropriate antidote is atropine sulfate.

FOMEPIZOLE (4-Methylpyrazole; 4-MP)

Rx	**Fomepizole** (X-Gen Pharmaceuticals)	**Injection, concentrate:** 1 g/mL	Preservative-free. In 1.5 mL vials.
Rx	**Antizol** (Jazz Pharmaceuticals)		Preservative-free. In 1.5 mL vials.

FOMEPIZOLE (4-Methylpyrazole; 4-MP) — INJECTION

Indications

➤*Ethylene glycol or methanol poisoning:* As an antidote for ethylene glycol (antifreeze) and methanol poisoning or for use in suspected ethylene glycol or methanol ingestion, either alone or in combination with hemodialysis.

Administration and Dosage

➤*General dosing considerations:* If ethylene glycol or methanol poisoning is left untreated, the natural progression of the poisoning leads to accumulation of toxic metabolites, including glycolic and oxalic acids (ethylene glycol intoxication) and formic acid (methanol intoxication). These metabolites can induce metabolic acidosis, nausea/vomiting, seizures, stupor, coma, calcium oxaluria, acute tubular necrosis, blindness, and death.

The diagnosis of these poisonings may be difficult because ethylene glycol or methanol concentrations diminish in the blood as they are metabolized to their respective metabolites. Hence, frequently monitor both ethylene glycol and methanol concentrations and acid-base balance, as determined by serum electrolyte (anion gap) or arterial blood gas analysis, and use to guide treatment.

Treatment consists of blocking the formation of toxic metabolites using inhibitors of alcohol dehydrogenase, such as fomepizole, and correction of metabolic abnormalities. In patients with high ethylene glycol or methanol concentrations (at least 50 mg/dL), significant metabolic acidosis or renal failure, consider hemodialysis to remove ethylene glycol or methanol and the respective toxic metabolites of these alcohols.

Begin fomepizole treatment immediately upon suspicion of ethylene glycol or methanol ingestion based on patient history or anion gap metabolic acidosis, increased osmolar gap, visual disturbances, oxalate crystals in the urine or a documented serum ethylene glycol or methanol concentration of more than 20 mg/dL.

➤*Adults:*

Ethylene glycol poisoning –

Usual dosage: Administer a loading dose of 15 mg/kg, followed by doses of 10 mg/kg every 12 hours for 4 doses, then 15 mg/kg every 12 hours thereafter until ethylene glycol or methanol concentrations are undetectable or have been reduced to less than 20 mg/dL, and the patient is asymptomatic with normal pH. Administer all doses as a slow IV infusion over 30 minutes.

Loading dose: 15 mg/kg.

Methanol poisoning – See Ethylene Glycol poisoning for dosing.

➤*Renal function impairment:* Consider hemodialysis in addition to fomepizole in the case of renal failure, significant or worsening metabolic acidosis, or a measured ethylene glycol or methanol concentration of at least 50 mg/dL. Dialyze patients to correct metabolic abnormalities and to lower the ethylene glycol concentrations to less than 50 mg/dL.

Hemodialysis – Fomepizole is dialyzable; increase the frequency of dosing to every 4 hours during hemodialysis.

Fomepizole Dosing in Patients Requiring Hemodialysis

Parameters	Dosing Schedule
At beginning of hemodialysis	
< 6 h since last dose	Do not administer dose.
≥ 6 h since last dose	Administer next scheduled dose.
During hemodialysis	Every 4 h.
At end of hemodialysis	
< 1 h since last dose	Do not administer dose.
1 to 3 h since last dose	Administer ½ of next scheduled dose.
> 3 h since last dose	Administer next scheduled dose.
Maintenance dosing off hemodialysis	Administer next scheduled dose 12 h from last dose.

➤*Discontinuation of therapy:* Treatment with fomepizole may be discontinued when ethylene glycol or methanol concentrations are undetectable or have been reduced to less than 20 mg/dL, and the patient is asymptomatic with normal pH.

➤*Preparation for administration:* Using sterile technique, draw the appropriate dose of fomepizole from the vial with a syringe and inject into at least 100 mL of sterile sodium chloride 0.9% injection or dextrose 5% injection. Mix well. Infuse the entire contents of the resulting solution over 30 minutes.

Fomepizole solidifies at temperatures less than 25°C (77°F). If the fomepizole solution has become solid in the vial, liquefy by running the vial under warm water or by holding in the hand. Solidification does not affect the efficacy, safety, or stability of fomepizole.

➤*Administration:* Administer all doses as a slow IV infusion over 30 minutes.

Do not give fomepizole undiluted or by bolus injection.

➤*Storage/Stability:* Store at controlled room temperature, 20° to 25°C (68° to 77°F). Fomepizole diluted in sodium chloride 0.9% injection or dextrose 5% injection remains stable and sterile for at least 24 hours when stored refrigerated or at room temperature. Fomepizole does not contain a preservative. Therefore, maintain sterile conditions and after dilution, do not use after 24 hours. Solutions showing haziness, particulate matter, precipitate, discoloration, or leakage should not be used.

FOMEPIZOLE (4-Methylpyrazole; 4-MP) — INJECTION

Actions

➤*Pharmacology:* Fomepizole is a competitive inhibitor of alcohol dehydrogenase that catalyzes the oxidation of ethanol to acetaldehyde. Alcohol dehydrogenase also catalyzes the initial steps in the metabolism of ethylene glycol and methanol to their toxic metabolites.

Ethylene glycol is metabolized to glycoaldehyde, which undergoes subsequent sequential oxidations to yield glycolate, glyoxylate, and oxalate. Glycolate and oxalate are the metabolic by-products primarily responsible for the metabolic acidosis and renal damage seen in ethylene glycol toxicosis. The lethal dose of ethylene glycol is approximately 1.4 mL/kg.

Methanol, the main component of windshield wiper fluid, is slowly metabolized via alcohol dehydrogenase to formaldehyde with subsequent oxidation via formaldehyde dehydrogenase to yield formic acid. Formic acid is primarily responsible for the metabolic acidosis and visual disturbances (eg, decreased visual acuity and potential blindness) associated with methanol poisoning. A lethal dose of methanol in humans is approximately 1 to 2 mL/kg.

➤*Pharmacokinetics:*

Absorption / Distribution – After IV infusion, fomepizole rapidly distributes to total body water. The volume of distribution is between 0.6 and 1.02 L/kg. The plasma half-life varies with the dose, even in patients with normal renal function, and has not been calculated. The concentration of fomepizole at which alcohol dehydrogenase is inhibited by 50% in vitro is approximately 0.1 mcmol/L. Fomepizole concentrations in the range of 100 to 300 mcmol/L (8.6 to 24.6 mg/L) have been targeted to ensure adequate plasma concentrations for the effective inhibition of alcohol dehydrogenase.

In healthy volunteers, oral doses of fomepizole (10 to 20 mg/kg) significantly reduced the rate of elimination of moderate doses of ethanol, which is also metabolized through the action of alcohol dehydrogenase (see Drug Interactions.)

Metabolism / Excretion – Only 1% to 3.5% of the administered dose of fomepizole (7 to 20 mg/kg oral and IV) was excreted unchanged in the urine, indicating that metabolism is the major route of elimination. In humans, the primary metabolite of fomepizole is 4-carboxypyrazole (approximately 80% to 85% of administered dose), which is excreted in the urine. With multiple doses, fomepizole rapidly induces its own metabolism via the P-450 system, producing a significant increase in the elimination rate after approximately 30 to 40 hours. After enzyme induction, elimination follows first-order kinetics. Saturable elimination occurs at therapeutic blood concentrations (100 to 300 mcmol/L, 8.2 to 24.6 mg/L).

Contraindications

Documented serious hypersensitivity reaction to fomepizole or other pyrazoles.

Warnings/Precautions

➤*Administration:* Do not give fomepizole undiluted or by bolus injection. Venous irritation and phlebosclerosis occurred in 2 of 6 healthy volunteers given bolus injections (over 5 minutes) of fomepizole at a concentration of 25 mg/mL.

➤*Allergic reactions:* Minor allergic reactions (mild rash, eosinophilia) have been reported in a few patients receiving fomepizole (see Adverse Reactions). Therefore, monitor patients for signs of allergic reactions.

➤*Pregnancy: Category C.* It is not known whether fomepizole can cause fetal harm when administered to pregnant women or can affect reproduction capacity. Give to pregnant women only if clearly needed.

➤*Lactation:* It is not known whether this drug is excreted in breast milk. Exercise caution when fomepizole is administered to a breast-feeding woman.

➤*Children:* Safety and efficacy have not been established.

➤*Elderly:* Safety and effectiveness in elderly patients have not been established.

➤*Monitoring:* In addition to specific antidote treatment with fomepizole, patients intoxicated with ethylene glycol or methanol must be managed for metabolic acidosis, acute renal failure (ethylene glycol), adult respiratory distress syndrome, visual disturbances (methanol), and hypocalcemia. Fluid therapy and sodium bicarbonate administration are potential supportive therapies. In addition, potassium and calcium supplementation and oxygen administration are usually necessary. Hemodialysis is necessary in the anuric patient or in patients with severe metabolic acidosis or azotemia (see Administration and Dosage). Assess treatment success by frequent measurements of blood gases, pH, electrolytes, BUN, creatinine, and urinalysis, in addition to other laboratory tests as indicated by individual patient conditions. At frequent intervals throughout the treatment, patients poisoned with ethylene glycol should be monitored for ethylene glycol concentrations in serum and urine, and the presence of urinary oxalate crystals. Similarly, monitor serum methanol concentrations in patients poisoned with methanol.

Because acidosis and electrolyte imbalances can affect the cardiovascular system, perform electrocardiography. In the comatose patient, electroencephalography may also be required. In addition, monitor hepatic enzymes and WBC counts during treatment, as transient increases in serum transaminase concentrations and eosinophilia have been noted with repeated fomepizole dosing.

Drug Interactions

➤*Ethanol:* Oral doses of fomepizole (10 to 20 mg/kg), via alcohol dehydrogenase inhibition, significantly reduced the rate of elimination of ethanol (by approximately 40%) given to healthy volunteers in moderate doses. Similarly, ethanol decreased the rate of elimination of fomepizole (by approximately 50%) by the same mechanism.

Reciprocal interactions may occur with concomitant use of fomepizole and drugs that increase or inhibit the cytochrome P-450 system (eg, carbamazepine, cimetidine, ketoconazole, phenytoin), although this has not been studied.

Adverse Reactions

The most frequent adverse events reported as drug-related or unknown relationship to study drug in the 78 patients and 63 healthy volunteers who received fomepizole were headache (14%), nausea (11%), dizziness, increased drowsiness, and bad taste/metallic taste (6% each). Other adverse events reported in approximately 3% or less of those receiving fomepizole are listed below:

➤*Cardiovascular:* Sinus bradycardia/bradycardia; tachycardia; phlebitis; shock; hypotension; phlebosclerosis.

➤*CNS:* Seizure; vertigo; light-headedness; nystagmus; agitation; facial flush; anxiety; feeling of drunkenness; strange feeling; decreased environmental awareness.

➤*GI:* Vomiting; diarrhea; dyspepsia; decreased appetite; transient transaminitis; heartburn.

➤*Hematologic / Lymphatic:* Lymphangitis; eosinophilia/hypereosinophilia; disseminated intravascular coagulation; anemia.

➤*Respiratory:* Hiccups; pharyngitis.

➤*Special senses:* Abnormal smell; speech/visual disturbances; roar in ear; transient blurred vision.

➤*Miscellaneous:* Abdominal pain; fever; multiorgan system failure; pain during fomepizole injection; inflammation at injection site; anuria; lumbalgia/backache; hangover; rash; application site reaction.

Overdosage

Nausea, dizziness, and vertigo occurred in healthy volunteers receiving 50 and 100 mg/kg doses of fomepizole (at plasma concentrations of 290 to 520 mcmol/L, 23.8 to 42.6 mg/L). These doses are 3 to 6 times the recommended dose. This dose-dependent CNS effect was short-lived in most subjects and lasted up to 30 hours in 1 subject. Fomepizole is dialyzable, and hemodialysis may be useful in treating cases of overdosage.

ATROPINE/PRALIDOXIME CHLORIDE

Rx	**DuoDote** (Survival Technology)	**Injection, solution:** atropine 2.1 mg per 0.7 mL/ pralidoxime chloride 600 mg per 2 mL	Benzyl alcohol 40 mg. In single-use, dual chamber, prefilled auto-injectors.

ATROPINE/PRALIDOXIME CHLORIDE — INJECTION

Indications

➤*Organophosphorus poisoning:* For the treatment of poisoning by organophosphorus nerve agents and organophosphorus insecticides.

➤*General information:* Administer atropine/pralidoxime as soon as symptoms of organophosphorus poisoning appear (eg, usually tearing, excessive oral secretions, sneezing, muscle fasciculations).

Individuals should not rely solely upon atropine/pralidoxime to provide complete protection from chemical nerve agents and insecticide poisoning.

Administration and Dosage

➤*General dosing considerations:* The atropine/pralidoxime auto-injector is for intramuscular (IM) use only.

Three atropine/pralidoxime auto-injectors should be available for use in each patient (including emergency medical services personnel) at risk for organophosphorus poisoning, 1 for mild symptoms plus 2 more for severe symptoms.

Common symptoms of organophosphorus exposure are listed in the following paragraphs. Patients may not have all symptoms.

Mild symptoms – Mild symptoms of organophosphorus poisoning include blurred vision and miosis; excessive, unexplained teary eyes; excessive, unexplained runny nose; increased salivation such as sudden drooling; chest tightness or difficulty breathing; tremors throughout the body or muscular twitching; nausea and/or vomiting; unexplained wheezing, coughing, or increased airway secretions; acute onset of stomach cramps; and tachycardia or bradycardia.

Severe symptoms – Severe symptoms of organophosphorus poisoning include strange or confused behavior, severe difficulty breathing or copious secretions from lungs/airway, severe muscular twitching and general weakness, involuntary urination and defecation, convulsions, and unconsciousness.

➤*Adults:*

Organophosphorus poisoning –

Maximum dose: No more than 3 doses of atropine/pralidoxime should be administered unless definitive medical care (eg, hospitalization, respiratory support) is available.

ATROPINE/PRALIDOXIME CHLORIDE — INJECTION

Mild symptoms:

• *Initial dosage* – One atropine/pralidoxime injection into the midlateral thigh if the patient experiences 2 or more mild symptoms of nerve gas or insecticide exposure.

Emergency medical services personnel with mild symptoms may self-administer a single dose of atropine/pralidoxime.

Wait 10 to 15 minutes for atropine/pralidoxime to take effect. If after 10 to 15 minutes the patient does not develop any of the severe symptoms previously listed, no additional atropine/pralidoxime injections are recommended, but definitive medical care should ordinarily be sought immediately.

For emergency medical services personnel who have self-administered atropine/pralidoxime, an individual decision will need to be made to determine their capacity to continue to provide emergency care.

• *Repeat doses* – If at any time after the first dose the patient develops any of the severe symptoms, administer 2 additional atropine/pralidoxime injections in rapid succession and immediately seek definitive medical care.

Severe symptoms:

• *Usual dosage* – Administer 3 atropine/pralidoxime injections into the patient's midlateral thigh in rapid succession and immediately seek definitive medical care.

• *Concomitant therapy* – Emergency care of the severely poisoned individual should include removal of oral and bronchial secretions, maintenance of a patent airway, supplemental oxygen, and, if necessary, artificial ventilation.

An anticonvulsant, such as diazepam, may be administered to treat convulsions if suspected in the unconscious individual. The effects of nerve agents and some insecticides can mask the motor signs of a seizure.

• *Monitoring* – Close supervision of all severely poisoned patients is indicated for at least 48 to 72 hours.

➤*Storage/Stability:* Store at 25°C (77°F); excursions are permitted to 15° to 30°C (59° to 86°F). Contains no latex. Keep from freezing; protect from light.

Actions

➤*Pharmacology:*

Atropine – Atropine competitively blocks the effects of acetylcholine, including excess acetylcholine due to organophosphorus poisoning, at muscarinic cholinergic receptors on smooth muscle, cardiac muscle, and secretory gland cells, and in peripheral autonomic ganglia and the CNS.

Pralidoxime – Pralidoxime reactivates acetylcholinesterase that has been inactivated by phosphorylation because of an organophosphorus nerve agent or insecticide. However, pralidoxime does not reactivate acetylcholinesterase inactivated by all organophosphorus nerve agents (eg, soman). Reactivated acetylcholinesterase hydrolyzes excess acetylcholine resulting from organophosphorus poisoning to help restore impaired cholinergic neural function. Reactivation is clinically important because only a small proportion of active acetylcholinesterase is needed to maintain vital functions. Pralidoxime cannot reactivate phosphorylated acetylcholinesterases that have undergone a further chemical reaction known as "aging."

➤*Pharmacokinetics:*

Absorption/Distribution –

Atropine: Atropine is rapidly and well absorbed after IM administration. Atropine disappears rapidly from the blood and is distributed throughout the various body tissues and fluids. The maximum plasma concentration (C_{max}), time to C_{max} (T_{max}), and half-life of atropine given IM by atropine/pralidoxime delivery system were 13 ± 3 ng/mL, 31 ± 30 minutes, and 2.4 ± 0.3 hours, respectively. The protein binding of atropine is 14% to 22% in plasma.

Pralidoxime: Pralidoxime is rapidly absorbed after IM injection. The C_{max}, T_{max}, and half-life of pralidoxime following pralidoxime 600 mg given IM by atropine/pralidoxime delivery system were 7 ± 3 ng/mL, 28 ± 15 minutes, and 2 ± 1 hour, respectively. Pralidoxime distributes into tissues and is not appreciably bound to serum protein.

Metabolism/Excretion –

Atropine: In healthy volunteers, approximately 50% to 60% of intravenous (IV) atropine is excreted in the urine as unchanged drug with approximately 17% to 28% renally eliminated in the first 100 minutes. Noratropine, atropine N-oxide, tropic acid, and tropine are the reported metabolites in the urine. Much of the drug is destroyed by enzymatic hydrolysis, particularly in the liver. The half-life of IV atropine is 3 ± 0.9 hours in adults and 10 ± 7.3 hours in elderly patients 65 to 75 years of age.

Pralidoxime: In healthy volunteers, approximately 72% to 94% of IV pralidoxime is excreted unchanged in the urine, about 57% to 70% in the first 30 minutes, partly as metabolite. Pralidoxime is subject to active renal secretion, Elimination of pralidoxime can be reduced by the coadministration of organic bases such as thiamine, but not organic acids, and can be altered by urine pH.

Special populations –

Renal function impairment:

• *Atropine* – Patients with severe renal function impairment may eliminate atropine more slowly and might require smaller and/or less frequent doses after initial atropinization.

• *Pralidoxime* – Pralidoxime pharmacokinetics have not been evaluated in patients with renal function impairment. Since pralidoxime is primarily excreted in the urine, a decrease in renal function will result in increased blood levels of the drug. Consider dose reduction for patients with renal insufficiency.

Hepatic function impairment:

• *Atropine* – Atropine pharmacokinetics have not been evaluated in patients with hepatic function impairment. Patients with severe hepatic function impairment may eliminate atropine more slowly and might require smaller and/or less frequent doses after initial atropinization.

Gender:

• *Atropine* – Atropine/pralidoxime area under the curve (AUC_{0-inf}) and C_{max} values for atropine are 15% higher in women than men. The half-life of atropine is approximately 20 minutes shorter in women than men.

• *Pralidoxime* – A single atropine/pralidoxime injection produced a mean C_{max} for pralidoxime about 36% higher in women than men. T_{max} is 23 minutes in women and 32 minutes in men. Pralidoxime half-life in men and women are 153 and 107 minutes, respectively.

Contraindications

None known.

Warnings/Precautions

➤*Complete protection against exposure:* Individuals should not rely solely upon atropine and pralidoxime to provide complete protection from chemical nerve agents and insecticide poisoning.

Primary protection against exposure to chemical nerve agents and insecticide poisoning is the wearing of protective garments, including masks designed specifically for this use.

➤*Evacuation and decontamination procedures:* Evacuation and decontamination procedures should be undertaken as soon as possible. Medical personnel assisting evacuated victims of nerve agent poisoning should avoid contaminating themselves by exposure to the victim's clothing.

➤*Maximum dosage:* More than one dose of atropine/pralidoxime, to a maximum of 3 doses, may be necessary initially when symptoms are severe. No more than 3 doses should be administered unless definitive medical care (eg, hospitalization, respiratory support) is available.

➤*Cardiovascular effects:* Organophosphorus nerve agent poisoning often causes bradycardia but can be associated with a heart rate in the low, high, or normal range. Atropine increases heart rate and alleviates the bradycardia. In patients with recent myocardial infarction (MI) and/or severe coronary artery disease, there is a possibility that atropine-induced tachycardia may cause ischemia, extend or initiate myocardial infarcts, and stimulate ventricular ectopy and fibrillation. In patients without cardiac disease, atropine administration is associated with the rare occurrence of ventricular ectopy or ventricular tachycardia.

➤*Artificial respiration:* Severe difficulty in breathing after organophosphorus poisoning requires artificial respiration in addition to the use of atropine/pralidoxime.

➤*Heat injury:* A potential hazardous effect of atropine is inhibition of sweating, which, in a warm environment or with exercise, can lead to hyperthermia and heat injury.

➤*Symptoms from atropine/pralidoxime treatment:* The desperate condition of the organophosphorus-poisoned individual will generally mask such minor signs and symptoms of atropine and pralidoxime treatment as have been noted in normal subjects.

➤*Increased blood pressure:* Atropine/pralidoxime temporarily increases blood pressure, a known effect of pralidoxime. In a study of 24 healthy young adults administered a single dose of atropine and pralidoxime auto-injector IM (approximately 9 mg/kg of pralidoxime chloride), diastolic blood pressure increased from baseline by 11 ± 14 mm Hg (mean ± standard deviation), and systolic blood pressure increased by 16 ± 19 mm Hg, at 15 minutes postdose. Blood pressures remained elevated at these approximate levels through 1 hour postdose, began to decrease at 2 hours postdose, and were near predose baseline at 4 hours postdose. IV pralidoxime doses of 30 to 45 mg/kg can produce moderate to marked increases in diastolic and systolic blood pressure.

➤*Inadvertent injection:* The atropine/pralidoxime auto-injector should be administered by emergency medical services personnel to treat organophosphorus poisoning. However, an injection might be given by mistake to someone who is not poisoned.

Studies have been conducted to evaluate the effect of atropine and pralidoxime on individuals in the absence of poisoning.

Atropine 2 mg IM, roughly the equivalent of one atropine/pralidoxime auto-injector, when given to healthy men, is associated with minimal effects on visual, motor, and mental functions, though unsteadiness walking and difficulty concentrating may occur. Atropine reduces body sweating and increases body temperature, particularly with exercise and under hot conditions.

Atropine 4 mg IM, roughly the equivalent of 2 atropine/pralidoxime auto-injectors, when given to healthy men, is associated with impaired visual acuity, visual near point accommodation, logical reasoning, digital recall, learning, and cognitive reaction time. Ability to read is reduced or lost. Subjects are unsteady and need to concentrate on walking. These effects begin about 15 minutes to 1 hour or more postdose.

Atropine 6 mg IM, roughly the equivalent of 3 atropine/pralidoxime auto-injectors, when given to healthy men, is associated with the effects described above plus additional central effects including poor coordination, poor attention span, and visual hallucinations (colored flashes) in many subjects. Frank visual hallucinations, auditory hallucinations, disorientation, and ataxia occur in some subjects. Skilled and labor-intense tasks are performed more slowly and less efficiently. Decision making takes longer and is sometimes impaired.

ATROPINE/PRALIDOXIME CHLORIDE — INJECTION

It is unclear if the results of these studies can be extrapolated to other populations. In elderly patients and patients with comorbid conditions, the effects of atropine 2 mg or more on the ability to see, walk, and think properly are unstudied; effects may be greater in susceptible populations.

Patients who are mistakenly injected with atropine/pralidoxime should avoid potentially dangerous overheating, avoid vigorous physical activity, and seek medical attention as soon as feasible.

➤*Renal function impairment:* Because pralidoxime is excreted in the urine, a decrease in renal function will result in increased blood levels of the drug.

➤*Special risk:* When symptoms of poisoning are not severe, use atropine/pralidoxime with extreme caution in people with heart disease, arrhythmias, recent MI, severe narrow-angle glaucoma, pyloric stenosis, prostatic hypertrophy, significant renal insufficiency, chronic pulmonary disease, or hypersensitivity to any component of the product. Conventional systemic doses may precipitate acute glaucoma in susceptible individuals, convert partial pyloric stenosis into complete pyloric obstruction, precipitate urinary retention in individuals with prostatic hypertrophy, or cause inspiration of bronchial secretions and formation of dangerous viscid plugs in individuals with chronic lung disease.

Elderly patients and children may be more susceptible to the effects of atropine.

➤*Pregnancy: Category C.* Adequate animal reproduction studies have not been conducted with atropine, pralidoxime, or the combination. It is not known whether pralidoxime or atropine can cause fetal harm when administered to a pregnant woman or if they can affect reproductive capacity. Atropine readily crosses the placental barrier and enters the fetal circulation.

Use atropine/pralidoxime during pregnancy only if the potential benefit justifies the potential risk to the fetus.

➤*Lactation:* Atropine has been reported to be excreted in human milk. It is not known whether pralidoxime is excreted in human milk. Because many drugs are excreted in human milk, exercise caution when administering atropine/pralidoxime to a breast-feeding woman.

➤*Children:* Safety and efficacy of atropine/pralidoxime in children have not been established.

➤*Monitoring:* If organophosphorus poisoning is known or suspected, initiate treatment without waiting for confirmation of the diagnosis by laboratory tests. Red blood cell and plasma cholinesterase as well as urinary paranitrophenol measurements (in the case of parathion exposure) may be helpful in confirming the diagnosis and following the course of the illness. However, miosis, rhinorrhea, and/or airway symptoms caused by nerve agent vapor exposure may occur with normal cholinesterase levels. Also, normal red blood cell and plasma cholinesterase values vary widely by ethnic group, age, and whether the person is pregnant. A reduction in red blood cell cholinesterase concentration to below 50% or normal is strongly suggestive of organophosphorus ester poisoning.

Drug Interactions

Keep in mind the following precautions in the treatment of anticholinesterase poisoning, although they do not bear directly on the use of atropine and pralidoxime. Avoid morphine, theophylline, aminophylline, succinylcholine, reserpine, and phenothiazine-type tranquilizers in treated personnel with organophosphorus poisoning.

Atropine/Pralidoxime Drug Interactions			
Precipitant drug	Object drug[a]		Description
Pralidoxime	Atropine/ pralidoxime	↑	When atropine and pralidoxime are used together, pralidoxime may potentiate the effects of atropine. Signs of atropinization (eg, flushing, mydriasis, tachycardia, dryness of mouth and nose) may occur earlier than expected.
Atropine/ pralidoxime	Barbiturates	↑	Barbiturates are potentiated by anticholinesterases; therefore, use barbiturates cautiously in the treatment of convulsions.
Atropine/ pralidoxime	Mivacurium, succinylcholine	↓	Succinylcholine and mivacurium are metabolized by cholinesterases. Because pralidoxime reactivates cholinesterases, use of pralidoxime in organophosphorus poisoning may accelerate reversal of the neuromuscular-blocking effects of succinylcholine and mivacurium.

[a] ↑ = object drug increased; ↓ = object drug decreased.

Adverse Reactions

➤*Atropine:* The most common adverse reactions of atropine can be attributed to its antimuscarinic action. These include the adverse reactions listed in the following sections.

Larger or toxic doses may produce such central effects as restlessness, tremor, fatigue, locomotor difficulties, delirium followed by hallucinations, depression, and, ultimately, medullary paralysis and death. Large doses can also lead to circulatory collapse. In such cases, blood pressure declines and death due to respiratory failure may ensue following paralysis and coma.

Cardiovascular – Asystole, atrial fibrillation, atrial flutter, cardiac syncope, flushing, MI, palpitations, premature ventricular contractions, sinus tachycardia, tachycardia, ventricular fibrillation, ventricular flutter.

CNS – Confusion, dizziness, headache, loss of libido.

Dermatologic – Maculopapular rash, petechial rash, scarlatiniform.

GI – Abdominal distention, abdominal pain, constipation, dryness of the mouth, dysphagia, nausea and vomiting, paralytic ileus.

GU – Impotence, urinary hesitancy or retention.

Hypersensitivity – Hypersensitivity reactions will occasionally occur, are usually seen as skin rashes, and may progress to exfoliation. Anaphylactic reaction and laryngospasm are rare.

Ophthalmic – Acute angle closure glaucoma, blurred vision, dry eyes, photophobia.

Miscellaneous – Anhidrosis may produce heat intolerance and impairment of temperature regulation in a hot environment.

➤*Pralidoxime:* In several cases of organophosphorus poisoning, excitement and manic behavior have occurred immediately following recovery of consciousness, in either the presence of absence of pralidoxime administration. However, similar behavior has not been reported in subjects given pralidoxime in the absence of organophosphorus poisoning.

Cardiovascular – Increased systolic and diastolic blood pressure, tachycardia.

CNS – Dizziness, drowsiness, headache, impaired accommodation, muscular weakness.

Dermatologic – Decreased sweating when given parenterally to normal volunteers who have been exposed to anticholinesterase poisons, dry skin, rash.

GI – Dry mouth, emesis, nausea.

Lab test abnormalities – Elevations of AST and/or ALT enzyme levels were observed in 1 of 6 normal volunteers given pralidoxime 1,200 mg IM, and in 4 of 6 volunteers given 1,800 mg IM. Levels returned to normal in about 2 weeks. Transient elevations in creatine kinase were observed in all normal volunteers given the drug.

Ophthalmic – Blurred vision, diplopia.

Miscellaneous – Decreased renal function, hyperventilation.

➤*Atropine and pralidoxime:* When atropine and pralidoxime are used together, the signs of atropinization may occur earlier than might be expected when atropine is used alone. Muscle tightness and sometimes pain may occur at the injection site.

Overdosage

➤*Symptoms:*

Atropine – Manifestations of atropine overdose are dose-related and include flushing, dry skin and mucous membranes, tachycardia, widely dilated pupils that are poorly responsive to light, blurred vision, and fever (which can sometimes be dangerously elevated). Locomotor difficulties, disorientation, hallucinations, delirium, confusion, agitation, coma, and central depression can occur and may last 48 hours or longer. In instances of severe atropine intoxication, respiratory depression, coma, circulatory collapse, and death may occur.

The fatal dose of atropine is unknown. In the treatment of organophosphorus poisoning, doses as high as 1,000 mg have been given. The few deaths reported in adults were generally seen using typical clinical doses of atropine, often in the setting of bradycardia associated with an acute MI, or with larger doses, caused by overheating in a setting of vigorous physical activity in a hot environment.

Pralidoxime – It may be difficult to differentiate some of the adverse reactions caused by pralidoxime from those caused by organophosphorus poisoning. Symptoms of pralidoxime overdose may include dizziness, blurred vision, diplopia, headache, impaired accommodation, nausea, and slight tachycardia. Transient hypertension caused by pralidoxime may last several hours.

➤*Treatment:*

Atropine – For atropine overdose, administer supportive treatment. If respiration is depressed, artificial respiration with oxygen is necessary. Ice bags, a hypothermia blanket, or other methods of cooling may be required to reduce atropine-induced fever, especially in children. Catheterization may be necessary if urinary retention occurs. Because atropine elimination takes place through the kidney, urinary output must be maintained and increased if possible; IV fluids may be indicated. Because of atropine-induced photophobia, darken the room.

A short-acting barbiturate or diazepam may be needed to control marked excitement and convulsions. However, avoid large doses for sedation because central depressant action may coincide with the depression occurring late in severe atropine poisoning. Central stimulants are not recommended.

Physostigmine, given as an atropine antidote by slow IV injection of 1 to 4 mg (0.5 to 1 mg in children) rapidly abolishes delirium and coma caused by large doses of atropine. Because physostigmine has a short duration of action, the patient may again lapse into coma after 1 or 2 hours and require repeated doses. Neostigmine, pilocarpine, and methacholine are of little benefit because they do not penetrate the blood-brain barrier.

ATROPINE/PRALIDOXIME CHLORIDE — INJECTION

Pralidoxime – Pralidoxime-induced hypertension has been treated by administering phentolamine 5 mg IV, repeated if necessary because of phentolamine's short duration of action. In the absence of substantial clinical data regarding use of phentolamine to treat pralidoxime-induced hypertension, consider slow infusion to avoid precipitous corrections in blood pressure.

PRALIDOXIME CHLORIDE (2-PAM)

Rx	**Protopam Chloride** (Baxter)	**Injection, powder for solution**[a]: 1 g	In 20 mL single-use vials.

[a] Porous cake.

PRALIDOXIME CHLORIDE — INJECTION

Indications

➤*Anticholinesterase overdosage:* For the control of overdosage by anticholinesterase drugsused in the treatment of myasthenia gravis.

➤*Organophosphate poisoning:* As an antidote in the treatment of poisoning caused by pesticides and chemicals (eg, nerve agents) of the organophosphate class that have anticholinesterase activity.

Administration and Dosage

➤*General dosing considerations:* Pralidoxime must be administered with atropine when treating organophosphate poisoning (see Concomitant Therapy).

Pralidoxime is most effective if administered immediately after organophosphate poisoning. Generally, little is accomplished if the drug is given more than 36 hours after termination of exposure. When the poison has been ingested, however, exposure may continue for some time because of slow absorption from the lower bowel, and fatal relapses have been reported after initial improvement. In such cases, additional doses may be needed every 3 to 8 hours. In effect, the patient should be titrated with pralidoxime for as long as signs of poisoning recur. Close supervision of the patient is indicated for at least 48 to 72 hours.

➤*Adults:*

Anticholinesterase overdose – 1 to 2 g intravenous (IV) followed by increments of 250 mg every 5 minutes.

Organophosphate poisoning –

IV:

- *Initial dosage* – 1 to 2 g IV infusion. If this is not practical or if pulmonary edema is present, give by slow IV injection.
- *Additional doses* – After about 1 hour, a second dose of 1 to 2 g will be indicated if muscle weakness has not been relieved. Additional doses may be given every 10 to 12 hours if muscle weakness persists.

Intramuscular:

- *Mild symptoms* –

  Initial dosage: 600 mg intramuscular (IM). Wait 15 minutes.

  Additional doses: After 15 minutes, if symptoms persist, administer a second dose. If, after an additional 15 minutes, symptoms continue to persist, a third dose may be administered for a total cumulative dose of 1,800 mg. If at any time after the first dose the patient develops severe symptoms, administer 2 additional 600 mg doses in rapid succession for a total cumulative dose of 1,800 mg.
- *Severe symptoms* – Three 600 mg doses in rapid succession for a total dose of 1,800 mg.
- *Persistent symptoms* – If symptoms persist after administering the complete 1,800 mg regimen (3 injections of 600 mg each), the series may be repeated beginning approximately 1 hour after the last injection.

➤*Renal function impairment:* Reduce the dosage in the presence of renal insufficiency.

➤*Concomitant therapy:*

Organophosphate poisoning – Give atropine as soon as possible after hypoxemia is improved. Do not give atropine in the presence of significant hypoxia because of the risk of atropine-induced ventricular fibrillation. In adults, atropine may be given IV in doses of 2 to 4 mg. Repeat this at 5- to 10-minute intervals until full atropinization (secretions are inhibited) or signs of atropine toxicity appear (delirium, hyperthermia, muscle twitching). Maintain some degree of atropinization for at least 48 hours and until any depressed blood cholinesterase activity is reversed. After the effects of atropine become apparent, pralidoxime may be administered.

Use of morphine, theophylline, aminophylline, reserpine, and phenothiazine-type tranquilizers should be avoided. Prolonged paralysis has been reported in patients when succinylcholine is given with drugs having anticholinesterase activity; therefore, it should be used with caution.

➤*Dermal exposure:* If dermal exposure to an organophosphate has occurred, remove clothing and wash the hair and skin thoroughly with sodium bicarbonate or alcohol as soon as possible.

➤*Preparation for administration:*

IV infusion – Reconstitute a single 1 g vial by adding 20 mL of sterile water for injection, which results in a 50 mg/mL concentration. The solution should be further diluted with normal saline to achieve a concentration of 10 to 20 mg/mL (eg, 1 or 2 g in 100 mL).

IV injection – Reconstitute a single 1 g vial by adding 20 mL of sterile water for injection, which results in a 50 mg/mL concentration.

IM – Reconstitute a single pralidoxime 1 g vial by adding 3.3 mL of sterile water for injection, which results in an approximate concentration of 300 mg/mL.

➤*Administration:* Administer preferably by infusion. If infusion administration is not feasible, IM or IV injection should be used.

IV infusion – Administer slowly over 15 to 30 minutes by continuous or intermittent infusion. Too-rapid administration may result in temporary worsening of cholinergic manifestations (ie, tachycardia, cardiac arrest, laryngospasm, and muscle rigidity or paralysis). The intermittent infusion rate should not exceed 200 mg/min.

IV injection – Administer slowly over not less than 5 minutes.

IM – In children, administer in the anterolateral aspect of the thigh to avoid the nerve, artery, and vein, as well as the femur.

➤*Storage/Stability:* Store at 20° to 25°C (68° to 77°F); excursions are permitted between 15° and 30°C (59° and 86°F). Discard unused solution after a dose has been withdrawn.

Actions

➤*Pharmacology:* The principal action of pralidoxime is to reactivate cholinesterase (mainly outside of the CNS) that has been inactivated by phosphorylation caused by an organophosphate pesticide or related compound. The destruction of accumulated acetylcholine can then proceed, and neuromuscular junctions will again function normally. Pralidoxime also slows the process of aging of phosphorylated cholinesterase to a nonreactivatable form, and detoxifies certain organophosphates by direct chemical reaction. The drug has its most critical effect in relieving paralysis of the muscles of respiration. Because pralidoxime is less effective in relieving depression of the respiratory center, atropine is always required concomitantly to block the effect of accumulated acetylcholine at this site. Pralidoxime relieves muscarinic signs and symptoms (eg, salivation, bronchospasm), but this action is relatively unimportant because atropine is adequate for this purpose.

➤*Pharmacokinetics:*

Absorption/Distribution – In 1 study of healthy adult volunteers and patients self-poisoned with organophosphate compounds, a single IM injection of pralidoxime 1 g resulted in mean peak plasma levels (C_{max}) of 7.5 ± 1.7 mcg/mL and 9.9 ± 2.4 mcg/mL, respectively. Time to reach C_{max} in both groups was similar (34 minutes in healthy adults and 33 minutes in poisoned patients).

Some evidence suggests that a loading dose followed by continuous IV infusion of pralidoxime may maintain therapeutic levels for longer than short intermittent infusion therapy. In a crossover study of 7 healthy adults 18 to 50 years of age, a short IV infusion dose of 16 mg/kg over 30 minutes was compared with an IV loading dose of 4 mg/kg over 15 minutes followed by 3.2 mg/kg/h for 3.75 hours (for a total dose of 16 mg/kg). Results showed that the mean time during which plasma levels were maintained above 4 mcg/mL was prolonged in the volunteers who received a loading dose followed by continuous infusion compared with those who received short infusion therapy (257.5 ± 50.5 min vs 118 ± 52.1 min). Use of continuous IV infusion in adult patients with organophosphate poisoning has been described in several case reports, with and without loading doses. Infusion rates ranged from 400 to 600 mg/h. In 1 case, the blood levels were 11.6 to 13.7 mcg/mL when patients were given 400 mg/h over 5 days (measured at 5, 10, and 18 hours). In another case, following an initial loading dose of 1 g, blood levels were 11.79 mcg/mL when patients were given 500 mg/h, and 17.26 mcg/mL when patients were given 600 mg/h. In 2 other cases, blood levels were not measured.

Pralidoxime is distributed throughout the extracellular water; its apparent volume of distribution at steady state has been reported to range from 0.6 to 2.7 L/kg. It is not bound to plasma protein. Consequently, pralidoxime is relatively short-acting, and repeated doses may be needed, unless continuous IV infusion is selected. Simulations suggest that after a dose of 1 g given IV, concentrations fall below 4 mcg/mL in approximately 1.5 hours. Consider the short duration of action and the necessity for repeated doses, especially when there is any evidence of continuing absorption of the poison.

Excretion – The drug is rapidly excreted in the urine by renal tubular secretion, partly unchanged and partly as a metabolite produced by the liver. After IM administration of pralidoxime 1 g, the renal clearance has been reported to be 7.2 ± 2.9 mL/min/kg in healthy volunteers and 3.6 ± 1.5 mL/min/kg in organophosphate-poisoned patients. The apparent half-life of pralidoxime is 74 to 77 minutes. Mean half-life was approximately 3 hours in healthy volunteers and in patients self-poisoned with organophosphate compounds. The elimination half-life of pralidoxime was 4 hours.

Special populations –

Renal function impairment: Decreased renal function will result in increased blood levels of the drug.

Children: In 1 study of 11 organophosphate-poisoned children 0.8 to 18 years of age, an IV loading dose of pralidoxime 15 to 50 mg/kg (mean, 29 mg/kg) followed by a continuous infusion of 10 to 16 mg/kg/h (mean, 14 mg/kg/h) over 12 to 43 hours (mean, 27 ± 8 hours) resulted in an average steady-state plasma concentration of 22 mg/L (6.9 to 47.4 mg/L) and an average body clearance of 0.88 L/kg/h (0.28 to 2.2 L/kg/h). After the continuous infusion was discontinued, determinations of the apparent volume of distribution and half-life ranged from 1.7 to 13.8 L/kg and from 2.4 to 5.3 hours, respectively.

PRALIDOXIME CHLORIDE — INJECTION

Animal pharmacokinetics: Animal studies suggest that the minimum therapeutic concentration of pralidoxime in plasma is 4 mcg/mL; this level is reached in about 16 minutes after a single injection of pralidoxime 600 mg.

Contraindications

Hypersensitivity to the drug and other situations in which the risk of its use clearly outweighs possible benefit.

Warnings/Precautions

➤*Other poisoning:* Pralidoxime is not effective in the treatment of poisoning caused by phosphorus, inorganic phosphates, or organophosphates not having anticholinesterase activity, and is not indicated as an antidote for intoxication by pesticides of the carbamate class because it may increase the toxicity of carbaryl.

➤*General information:* Pralidoxime has been well tolerated in most cases, but it must be remembered that the desperate condition of the organophosphate-poisoned patient will generally mask such minor signs and symptoms as have been noted in healthy subjects.

➤*Administration:* See Administration and Dosage for more information.

➤*Myasthenia gravis:* Use pralidoxime with great caution in treating organophosphate overdosage in cases of myasthenia gravis because it may precipitate a myasthenic crisis.

➤*Renal function impairment:* See Administration and Dosage for more information.

➤*Pregnancy: Category C.*

Teratogenic – It is also not known whether pralidoxime can cause fetal harm when administered to a pregnant woman or can affect reproduction capacity. It is not known if pralidoxime crosses the human placenta to the embryo or fetus. Give pralidoxime to a pregnant woman only if clearly needed. Although the risk this agent represents in pregnancy cannot be assessed, the maternal benefit clearly outweighs any concern regarding embryo or fetal toxicity. Therefore, do not withhold pralidoxime because of pregnancy. Pralidoxime chloride is a quaternary ammonium compound, but the molecular weight of the free base (approximately 137) is low enough for passage across the placenta. The rapid elimination of the drug should mitigate this transfer. Animal reproduction studies have not been conducted with pralidoxime.

➤*Lactation:* It is not known whether this drug is excreted in human milk. Pralidoxime is a quaternary ammonium compound, but the molecular weight of the free base (approximately 137) is low enough for excretion into breast milk. The rapid elimination of the drug should mitigate this transfer into milk. Moreover, the emergency nature of its use suggests that breastfeeding is unlikely when it has been used. In any event, the maternal benefit is clear; withhold breast-feeding for at least 6 to 7 hours (about 5 half-lives) after a dose is given. Because many drugs are excreted in human milk, exercise caution when pralidoxime is administered to a breast-feeding woman.

➤*Children:* There are no adequate and well-controlled clinical trials that establish the effectiveness of pralidoxime in children. Efficacy has been extrapolated from the adult population and is supported by nonclinical studies, pharmacokinetic studies in adults, and experience in children.

➤*Monitoring:* Institute treatment of organophosphate poisoning without waiting for the results of laboratory tests. Red blood cell, plasma cholinesterase, and urinary paranitrophenol measurements (in the case of parathion exposure) may be helpful in confirming the diagnosis and following the course of the illness, although such tests may be normal in the face of clinically significant organophosphate poisoning. A reduction in red blood cell cholinesterase concentration to below 50% of normal has been seen only with organophosphate ester poisoning.

Drug Interactions

➤*Combination of atropine and pralidoxime:* When atropine and pralidoxime are used together, the signs of atropinization (flushing, mydriasis, tachycardia, dryness of the mouth and nose) may occur earlier than might be expected when atropine is used alone. This is especially true if the total dose of atropine has been large and the administration of pralidoxime has been delayed. Closely monitor the clinical response.

Keep the following precautions in mind during the treatment of anticholinesterase poisoning, although they do not bear directly on the use of pralidoxime: because barbiturates are potentiated by the anticholinesterases, use them cautiously in the treatment of convulsions; avoid morphine, theophylline, aminophylline, reserpine, and phenothiazine-type tranquilizers in patients with organophosphate poisoning. Prolonged paralysis has been reported in patients when succinylcholine is given with drugs having anticholinesterase activity; therefore, use it with caution.

Adverse Reactions

➤*Concomitant atropine therapy:* When atropine and pralidoxime are used together, the signs of atropinization may occur earlier than might be expected when atropine is used alone. This is especially true if the total dose of atropine has been large and the administration of pralidoxime has been delayed. Excitement and manic behavior immediately following recovery of consciousness have been reported in several cases; however, similar behavior has occurred in cases of organophosphate poisoning that were not treated with pralidoxime.

➤*Cardiovascular:* Increased systolic and diastolic blood pressure, tachycardia.

➤*CNS:* Dizziness, drowsiness, headache.

➤*Lab test abnormalities:* Elevations in AST and/or ALT enzyme levels were observed in 1 of 6 healthy volunteers given pralidoxime 1,200 mg IM, and in 4 of 6 volunteers given 1,800 mg IM. Levels returned to normal in about 2 weeks. Transient elevations in creatine phosphokinase were observed in all healthy volunteers given the drug.

➤*Local:* 40 to 60 minutes after IM injection, mild to moderate pain may be experienced at the site of injection.

➤*Special senses:* Blurred vision, diplopia, impaired accommodation.

➤*Miscellaneous:* Hyperventilation, muscular weakness, nausea.

Children – As in adults, cardiac arrest, laryngospasm, muscle rigidity or paralysis, and tachycardia have been reported following rapid IV injection. Apnea, convulsions, and muscle fasciculations have also been reported.

Overdosage

➤*Symptoms:* The following have been observed in healthy subjects only: blurred vision, diplopia, dizziness, headache, impaired accommodation, nausea, and slight tachycardia. During therapy, it has been difficult to differentiate adverse reactions caused by the drug from those caused by the effects of the poison.

➤*Treatment:* Administer artificial respiration and other supportive therapy as needed.

Patient Information

Advise patient, family, or caregiver that medication will be prepared and administered by a health care provider in a health care setting.

Advise patient, family, or caregiver to immediately report any of the following to health care provider: excessive salivation, injection-site reaction or pain, nausea, or vomiting.

DIGOXIN IMMUNE FAB (Ovine)

Rx	**Digibind** (GlaxoSmithKline)	**Powder for injection, lyophilized:** 38 mg/vial. Each vial will bind approximately 0.5 mg digoxin.	Sodium chloride 28 mg. Preservative free. In vials.
Rx	**DigiFab** (BTG International)	**Powder for injection, lyophilized:** 40 mg/vial. Each vial will bind approximately 0.5 mg digoxin.	Sodium acetate 2 mg. Preservative free. In vials.

DIGOXIN IMMUNE FAB (Ovine) — INJECTION

Indications

➤*Digoxin toxicity:* For the treatment of life-threatening or potentially life-threatening digoxin toxicity or overdose. *Digibind* also has been successfully used to treat life-threatening digitoxin (not available in the United States) overdose. Digoxin immune Fab is not indicated for milder cases of digitalis toxicity.

Clinical conditions requiring administration include the following:

- Known suicidal or accidental consumption of more than 10 mg of digoxin in previously healthy adults or 4 mg (or more than 0.1 mg/kg [*DigiFab*]) in previously healthy children, or ingestion causing steady-state serum concentrations greater than 10 ng/mL;
- chronic ingestions causing steady-state serum digoxin concentrations exceeding 6 ng/mL in adults or 4 ng/mL in children (*DigiFab*); and
- manifestions of life-threatening toxicity caused by digoxin overdose, including severe ventricular arrhythmias (eg, ventricular tachycardia or fibrillation), progressive bradycardia, and second or third degree heart block not responsive to atropine, serum potassium levels exceeding 5 mEq/L (*Digibind*) or 5.5 mEq/L in adults or 6 mEq/L in children (*DigiFab*) with rapidly progressive signs and symptoms of digoxin toxicity.

Administration and Dosage

➤*General dosing considerations:* The dosage of digoxin immune Fab varies according to the amount of digoxin or digitoxin to be neutralized.

In small children, it is important to monitor for volume overload.

Erroneous calculations may result from inaccurate estimates of the amount of digitalis ingested or absorbed or from nonsteady-state serum digitalis concentrations. Inaccurate serum digitalis concentration measurements are a possible source of error.

Dosage calculations are based on a steady-state volume of distribution of approximately 5 L/kg for digoxin (0.5 L/kg for digitoxin) to convert serum digitalis concentration to the amount of digitalis in the body. Many patients

DIGOXIN IMMUNE FAB (Ovine) — INJECTION

may require higher doses for complete neutralization. Ordinarily, round the doses up to the next whole vial.

Failure of the patient to respond to digoxin immune Fab should alert the physician to the possibility that the clinical problem may not be caused by digitalis toxicity.

➤*Adults:*

Digoxin or digitoxin toxicity/overdose –

Usual dosage:

• *Acute ingestion of unknown amount* – Twenty vials (760 mg of *Digibind* or 800 mg of *DigiFab*) are adequate to treat most life-threatening ingestions. In general, a large dose of digoxin immune Fab has a faster onset of effect, but may enhance the possibility of a febrile reaction. The physician may consider administering 10 vials, observing the patient's response, and following with an additional 10 vials if clinically indicated.

• *Acute ingestion of known amount* – Each vial will bind approximately 0.5 mg of digoxin (or digitoxin).

$$\text{Dose (in \# of vials)} = \frac{\text{Total digitalis body load (mg)}}{\text{0.5 mg of digitalis bound/vial}}$$

For toxicity from an acute ingestion, total body load in milligrams will be approximately equal to the amount ingested in milligrams for digoxin capsules or digitoxin, or the amount ingested in milligrams multiplied by 0.8 (to account for incomplete absorption) for digoxin tablets.

• *Calculations based on steady-state serum digoxin concentrations* –To estimate number of vials for adult patients for whom a steady-state serum digoxin concentration is known, use the following formula:

$$\text{Dose (in \# of vials)} = \frac{\text{(Serum digoxin concentration in ng/mL) (weight in kg)}}{100}$$

If in any case the dose estimated based on ingested amount differs substantially from that calculated based on the serum digoxin or digitoxin concentration, it may be preferable to use the higher dose estimate.

• *Calculations based on steady-state digitoxin concentrations* – The dosage of digoxin immune Fab for digitoxin toxicity can be approximated using the following formula:

$$\text{Dose (in \# of vials)} = \frac{\text{(Serum digitoxin concentration in ng/mL) (weight in kg)}}{1{,}000}$$

• *Toxicity during chronic therapy* – Six vials (228 mg [*Digibind*] or 240 mg [*DigiFab*]) are usually adequate to reverse most cases of toxicity. This dose can be used in patients who are in acute distress or for whom a serum digoxin or digitoxin concentration is not available.

Repeat dosage: If toxicity has not adequately reversed after several hours or appears to recur, readministration of *Digibind* at a dose guided by clinical judgment may be required. If a patient is in need of readministration of *DigiFab* because of recurrent toxicity, or to a new toxic episode that occurs soon after the first episode, measurement of free (unbound) serum digitalis concentrations should be considered because Fab may still be present in the body.

➤*Children:*

Digoxin or digitoxin toxicity/overdose – This agent has been used successfully in infants with no apparent adverse sequelae. Use of this drug in infants should be based on careful consideration of the benefits of the drug balanced against the potential risk involved.

Usual dosage:

• *Acute ingestion of unknown amount* – See Adults for dosing.

• *Acute ingestion of known amount* – See Adults for dosing.

• *Calculations based on steady-state serum digoxin concentrations* –
Digibind:

$$\text{Dose (in mg)} = \frac{\text{(Dose [in \# of vials])}}{\text{(38 mg/vial)}}$$

DigiFab:

$$\text{Dose (in mg)} = \frac{\text{(Dose [in \# of vials])}}{\text{(40 mg/vial)}}$$

• *Calculations based on steady-state digitoxin concentrations* – See Adults for dosing.

• *Toxicity during chronic therapy* –
Children 12 months of age and older and weighing more than 20 kg: See Adults for dosing.
Children younger than 12 months of age or weighing 20 kg or less: A single vial usually should suffice.

Repeat dosage: See Adults for dosing.

➤*Preparation for administration:* Dissolve the contents in each vial with 4 mL of sterile water for injection. Mix gently to give a protein concentration of 9.5 mg/mL (*Digibind*) or 10 mg/mL (*DigiFab*). Use reconstituted product promptly. If it is not used immediately, store at 2° to 8°C (36° to 46°F) for up to 4 hours. The reconstituted product may be diluted with sterile isotonic saline to a convenient volume.

Infants/children weighing 20 kg or less –

Digibind: Because infants and small children can have much smaller dosage requirements, reconstitute the 38 mg vial as directed and administer with a tuberculin syringe. For very small doses, dilute the reconstituted vial with sterile isotonic saline 34 mL to achieve 1 mg/mL concentration.

DigiFab: Because infants and small children can have much smaller dosage requirements, it is recommended that the 40 mg vial be reconstituted as directed and administered with a tuberculin syringe. For very small doses, a reconstituted vial can be diluted with 36 mL of sterile isotonic saline to achieve a 1 mg/mL concentration.

➤*Administration:* Administer IV slowly as an IV infusion over at least 30 minutes. If infusion rate-related reactions occur, stop the infusion and restart at a slower rate. If cardiac arrest is imminent, digoxin can be given as a bolus injection. With bolus injection, an increased incidence of infusion-related reactions may be expected.

It is recommended for *Digibind* to be infused through a 0.22 micron membrane filter to ensure no undissolved particulate matter is administered.

➤*Storage/Stability:* Refrigerate at 2° to 8°C (36° to 46°F) for up to 4 hours after reconstitution.

Digibind – Unreconstituted vials can be stored at up to 30°C (86°F) for a total of 30 days.

DigiFab – Do not freeze.

Actions

➤*Pharmacology:* Digoxin immune Fab (ovine) is antigen binding fragments (Fab) derived from specific antidigoxin antibodies produced in sheep. Production involves conjugation of digoxin as a hapten to human albumin. Sheep are immunized with this material to produce antibodies specific for the digoxin molecule. The antibody is papain digested, and digoxin-specific Fab fragments are isolated and purified.

Improvement in signs and symptoms of digitalis intoxication ordinarily begins in 30 minutes or less. Digoxin immune Fab binds molecules of digoxin, making them unavailable for binding at their site of action. The Fab fragment-digoxin complex accumulates in the blood and is excreted by the kidneys. The net effect is to shift the equilibrium away from binding of digoxin to its receptors in the body, thereby reversing its effects.

➤*Pharmacokinetics:* The pharmacokinetic profiles of Fab are similar for both products. The similar volumes of distribution (0.3 L/kg and 0.4 L/kg for *DigiFab* and *Digibind*, respectively) indicate considerable penetration from the circulation into the extracellular space and are consistent with previous reports of ovine Fab distribution, as are the elimination half-life values (15 and 23 hours for *DigiFab* and *Digibind*, respectively). The elimination half-life of 15 to 20 hours in patients with normal renal function appears to be increased up to 10-fold in patients with renal impairment, although volume of distribution remains unaffected.

Contraindications

None known.

Warnings/Precautions

➤*Allergy to papain or derivatives:* Patients with allergies to papain, chymopapain, other papaya extracts, or the pineapple enzyme bromelain may also be at risk for an allergic reaction to digoxin immune Fab. In addition, it has been noted in the literature that some dust mite allergens and some latex allergens share antigenic structures with papain and patients with these allergies may be allergic to papain. Do not administer digoxin immune Fab to patients with a known history of hypersensitivity to papaya or papain unless the benefits outweigh the risks and appropriate management for anaphylactic reactions is readily available.

➤*Skin testing:*

Digibind – Skin testing for allergy was performed during the clinical investigation of this agent. Only 1 patient developed erythema at the site of skin testing. The patient had no adverse reaction to systemic treatment. Allergy testing is not routinely required before treatment of life-threatening digitalis toxicity because it can delay urgently needed therapy.

Skin testing may be appropriate for high-risk individuals, especially patients with known allergies or those previously treated with digoxin immune Fab. The intradermal skin test can be performed by: 1) Diluting 0.1 mL of reconstituted drug (9.5 mg/mL) in 9.9 mL sterile isotonic saline; 2) injecting 0.1 mL of the 1:100 dilution (9.5 mcg) intradermally and observing for an urticarial wheal surrounded by a zone of erythema. Read the test at 20 minutes.

The scratch test procedure is performed by placing 1 drop of a 1:100 dilution on the skin and making a ¼-inch scratch through the drop with a needle. The area is inspected at 20 minutes for an urticarial wheal surrounded by erythema.

If skin testing causes a systemic reaction, apply a tourniquet above the site of testing and treat anaphylaxis. Avoid further administration of the drug unless its use is absolutely essential; in this case, pretreat the patient with corticosteroids and diphenhydramine and make preparations for treating anaphylaxis.

DigiFab – Skin testing has not proved useful in predicting allergic response to *Digibind*. Because of this and because it may delay urgently needed therapy, skin testing was not performed during the clinical studies of *DigiFab* and is not suggested prior to dosing with this product.

➤*Standard intoxication management:* Standard therapy for digitalis intoxication includes withdrawal of the drug, correction of electrolyte disturbances (especially hyperkalemia), acid-base imbalances, hypoxia, and treatment of cardiac arrhythmias. Massive digitalis intoxication can cause hyperkalemia; administration of potassium supplements in the setting of digitalis intoxication may be hazardous.

➤*Digoxin withdrawal:* In a few instances, the condition of those with low cardiac output states and CHF could have been exacerbated by withdrawal of the inotropic effects of digitalis. Patients with atrial fibrillation may develop a rapid ventricular response from withdrawal of the effects of digitalis on the AV node.

Patients with intrinsically poor cardiac function may deteriorate from withdrawal of digoxin. Additional support can be provided by use of IV inotropes

DIGOXIN IMMUNE FAB (Ovine) — INJECTION

(eg, dopamine or dobutamine) or vasodilators. With catecholamines, take care not to aggravate digitalis toxic rhythm disturbances. Do not use other types of digitalis glycosides. Redigitalization should be postponed if possible until the Fab fragments have been eliminated from the body; this may require several days. Patients with impaired renal function may require a week or longer.

➤*Immunogenicity:* Prior treatment with digoxin-specific ovine immune Fab carries a theoretical risk of sensitization to ovine serum protein and possible diminution of the efficacy of the drug due to the presence of human antibodies against ovine Fab. Human antibodies to ovine Fab have been reported in some patients receiving *Digibind*; however, to date, there have been no clinical reports of human antiovine immunoglobulin antibodies causing a reduction in binding of ovine digoxin immune Fab or neutralization response to ovine digoxin immune Fab.

➤*Hypersensitivity reactions:* Allergic reactions have occurred rarely, but consider the possibility of anaphylactic, hypersensitivity, or febrile reactions. If an anaphylactoid reaction occurs, discontinue the drug infusion and initiate appropriate therapy. The need for epinephrine should be balanced against its potential risk in the setting of digitalis toxicity. Refer to Management of Acute Hypersensitivity Reactions.

Patients with known allergies or allergies to sheep protein would be particularly at risk, as would individuals who have previously received antibodies or Fab fragments raised in sheep. Patients with a history of allergy, especially to antibiotics, appear to be at particular risk.

➤*Renal function impairment:* The elimination half-life in renal failure has not been clearly defined. Patients with renal dysfunction have been successfully treated with digoxin immune Fab. There is no evidence to suggest any difference between these patients and patients with normal renal function, but excretion of the Fab fragment-digoxin complex from the body is probably delayed. In patients who are functionally anephric, anticipate failure to clear the Fab fragment-digoxin complex from the blood by glomerular filtration and renal excretion. Whether this would lead to reintoxication by release of newly unbound digoxin into the blood is uncertain. Monitor such patients for a prolonged period for possible recurrence of digitalis toxicity. Monitoring of free (unbound) digoxin concentrations after the administration may be appropriate in order to establish recrudescent toxicity in renal failure patients.

➤*Pregnancy: Category C.* It is not known whether this agent can cause fetal harm or affect reproduction capacity. Use only if clearly needed.

➤*Lactation:* It is not known whether this drug is excreted in breast milk. Exercise caution when administering to a breast-feeding mother.

➤*Children:* This agent has been used successfully in infants with no apparent adverse sequelae. Use of this drug in infants should be based on careful consideration of the benefits of the drug balanced against the potential risk involved.

➤*Elderly:* Because elderly patients are more likely to have decreased renal function, it may be useful to monitor renal function and to observe for possible recurrence of toxicity.

➤*Monitoring:* Digoxin immune Fab will interfere with digitalis immunoassay measurements. The standard serum digoxin concentration measurement can be clinically misleading until the Fab fragment is eliminated from the body. Obtain digoxin serum concentrations before digoxin immune Fab or drug administration. These measurements may be difficult to interpret if drawn soon after the last digitalis dose, because at least 6 to 8 hours are required for equilibration of digoxin between serum and tissue. Closely monitor the patient, including temperature, blood pressure, ECG, and potassium concentration during and after drug administration. The total serum digoxin concentration may rise precipitously following administration, but this will be almost entirely bound to the Fab fragment.

Potassium – Severe digitalis intoxication can cause life-threatening elevation in serum potassium concentration by shifting potassium from inside to outside the cell. This can lead to increased renal excretion of potassium. These patients may have hyperkalemia with a total body deficit of potassium. When the effect of digitalis is reversed, potassium shifts back inside the cell with a resulting decline in serum potassium concentration. Hypokalemia may develop rapidly. Monitor serum potassium concentration repeatedly, especially over the first several hours after the drug is given, and cautiously give potassium supplementation when necessary.

Adverse Reactions

Exacerbation of low cardiac output and CHF; hypokalemia; allergic reactions (rarely); rapid ventricular response in patients with atrial fibrillation caused by digoxin withdrawal (see Precautions).

Patient Information

Advise patients to contact their physician immediately if they experience any signs and symptoms of delayed allergic reactions or serum sickness (eg, rash, pruritus, urticaria) after hospital discharge.

ACETYLCYSTEINE (N-Acetylcysteine)

Rx	**Acetylcysteine** (Various, eg, American Regent, Hospira, Roxane)	**Solution; oral:** 10%	Preservative free. May contain disodium edetate. In 4, 10, and 30 mL vials.
Rx	**Acetylcysteine** (Various, eg, American Regent, Hospira, Roxane)	**Solution, concentrate; oral:** 20%	Preservative free. May contain disodium edetate. In 4, 10, and 30 mL vials.
Rx	**Acetadote** (Cumberland)	**Injection, solution:** 20% (200 mg/mL)	Preservative free. 0.5 mg/mL disodium edetate. In 30 mL single-dose vials.

ACETYLCYSTEINE — ORAL

For information on use as a mucolytic, refer to the Acetylcysteine monograph in the Respiratory chapter.

Indications

➤*Acetaminophen overdose:* To prevent or lessen hepatic injury after ingestion of a potentially hepatotoxic quantity of acetaminophen.

It is essential to initiate treatment as soon as possible after the overdose and, in any case, within 24 hours of ingestion.

➤*Off-label uses:*

Blepharitis (chronic) – [4] = Insufficient documentation. Initial data from one small controlled trial suggest that acetylcysteine may be of benefit in patients with chronic blepharitis.

Prevention of contrast media nephrotoxicity – [2] = Fair documentation. The use of acetylcysteine in conjunction with saline hydration initially appeared beneficial as a preventive agent for radiocontrast-induced nephrotoxicity. Initial data suggested that this agent may be particularly useful for populations known to be at increased risk of contrast nephrotoxicity (eg, diabetes mellitus, reduced renal function). Recent data have been conflicting about the benefit of this agent, suggesting that it is no more effective than hydration alone in the prevention of radiocontrast nephropathy. However, it should be recognized that when used short term, the adverse reaction profile of this drug is minimal and inexpensive. The morbidity and mortality associated with contrast nephropathy, including prolonged hospitalization, are significant. Although additional larger controlled studies may clarify these issues and be more directive in identifying optimal candidates, until then, the use of this agent with hydration as a protectant for contrast nephrotoxicity may be observed in the clinical setting.

Helicobacter pylori infection – [4] = Insufficient documentation. The use of acetylcysteine as adjunctive therapy in the management of *Helicobacter pylori* infection has been published in one small, placebo-controlled trial suggesting an enhanced effect when compared with antibiotic/proton pump inhibitor therapy alone. Larger controlled trials are needed before this agent can be recommended for addition to current multidrug regimens.

Lung cancer prevention – [5] = Poor documentation. American College of Chest Physicians guidelines evaluated the use of acetylcysteine for chemoprevention of lung cancer. Acetylcysteine was not recommended for primary, secondary, or tertiary prevention of lung cancer.

Administration and Dosage

➤*General dosing considerations:* Immediately administer acetylcysteine if 24 hours or less have elapsed from the reported time of ingestion of an acetaminophen overdose. Do not await results of assay for acetaminophen level before initiating treatment.

Plasma or serum acetaminophen concentrations, determined as early as possible but no sooner than 4 hours following an acute overdose, are essential in assessing the potential risk of hepatotoxicity. If an assay for acetaminophen cannot be obtained, it is necessary to assume that the overdose is potentially toxic. Acetaminophen levels drawn less than 4 hours postingestion may be misleading. See Interpretation of Acetaminophen Assay for more information.

➤*Adults:*

Acetaminophen overdose –

Loading dose: 140 mg/kg.

Maintenance dosage: 70 mg/kg 4 hours after loading dose and at 4-hour intervals thereafter for 17 total doses.

Off-label dosing –

Blepharitis (chronic): [4] = Insufficient documentation. 100 mg orally 3 times daily for 8 weeks.

Prevention of contrast media nephrotoxicity: [2] = Fair documentation. The most common regimen used in studies was 4 doses of acetylcysteine administered orally as 600 mg twice daily, typically started the day prior to the procedure and continued through the day of contrast agent administration. Other regimens include 1 dose (600 mg) administered prior to catheterization and contrast administration and 3 doses administered after catheterization. Two studies employed higher oral dosages of 1,200 or 1,500 mg twice daily for 2 and 4 doses, respectively.

H. pylori infection: [4] = Insufficient documentation. 400 mg per 10 mL 3 times daily with clarithromycin (500 mg twice daily) and lansoprazole (30 mg twice daily) for 10 days.

➤*Children:*

Acetaminophen overdose – See Adults for dosing.

➤*Interpretation of acetaminophen assays:* When results of the plasma acetaminophen assay are available, refer to the Rumack-Matthew nomo-

ACETYLCYSTEINE — ORAL

gram to determine if the plasma concentration is in the potentially toxic range. Values above the line connecting 200 mcg/mL at 4 hours with 50 mcg/mL at 12 hours (probable line) are associated with a probability of hepatic toxicity if an antidote is not administered.

If the predetoxification plasma level is above the line connecting 150 mcg/mL at 4 hours with 37.5 mcg/mL at 12 hours (possible line), continue with maintenance doses of acetylcysteine. It is better to err on the safe side, and thus this line, defining possible toxicity, is plotted 25% below the line defining probable toxicity. If the predetoxification plasma level is below the line connecting 150 mcg/mL at 4 hours with 37.5 mcg/mL at 12 hours (possible line), there is minimal risk of hepatic toxicity, and acetylcysteine treatment may be discontinued.

➤*Discontinuation of therapy:* If predetoxification acetaminophen level is clearly in the nontoxic range and the acetaminophen overdose occurred at least 4 hours before the prodetoxification acetaminophen plasma assays, discontinue acetylcysteine. If predetoxification acetaminophen level was in the nontoxic range, but time of ingestion was unknown or less than 4 hours, obtain a second plasma level in order to decide whether or not the full 17-dose detoxification treatment is necessary.

➤*Preparation for administration:* Dilute the solution with diet cola or other diet soft drinks to a final concentration of 5%. If administered via gastric tube or Miller-Abbott tube, water may be used as the diluent. Take care to minimize contamination of the sterile solution. Use freshly prepared solutions. Dilute N-acetylcysteine to 5%. Dilute the proper dose of 10% N-acetylcysteine with 1 mL fluid per 1 mL of N-acetylcysteine.

20% solution –

20 kg or more:

Acetylcysteine 20% Oral Solution Dilution

Body weight	Acetylcysteine	Acetylcysteine 20%	Diluent	Total 5% solution
Loading dose				
100 to 109 kg	15 g	75 mL	225 mL	300 mL
90 to 99 kg	14 g	70 mL	210 mL	280 mL
80 to 89 kg	13 g	65 mL	195 mL	260 mL
70 to 79 kg	11 g	55 mL	165 mL	220 mL
60 to 69 kg	10 g	50 mL	150 mL	200 mL
50 to 59 kg	8 g	40 mL	120 mL	160 mL
40 to 49 kg	7 g	35 mL	105 mL	140 mL
30 to 39 kg	6 g	30 mL	90 mL	120 mL
20 to 29 kg	4 g	20 mL	60 mL	80 mL
Maintenance dosage				
100 to 109 kg	7.5 g	37 mL	113 mL	150 mL
90 to 99 kg	7 g	35 mL	105 mL	140 mL
80 to 89 kg	6.5 g	33 mL	97 mL	130 mL
70 to 79 kg	5.5 g	28 mL	82 mL	110 mL
60 to 69 kg	5 g	25 mL	75 mL	100 mL
50 to 59 kg	4 g	20 mL	60 mL	80 mL
40 to 49 kg	3.5 g	18 mL	52 mL	70 mL
30 to 39 kg	3 g	15 mL	45 mL	60 mL
20 to 29 kg	2 g	10 mL	30 mL	40 mL

19 kg or less: Calculate the dose of acetylcysteine. Each milliliter of acetylcysteine 20% contains 200 mg of acetylcysteine. Three milliliter of diluent are added to each milliliter of acetylcysteine 20%. Do not decrease the proportion of diluent.

10% solution – Dilute the proper dose of acetylcysteine 10% with 1 mL of diluent per 1 mL of acetylcysteine.

➤*Administration:* For oral administration. Not for parenteral injection.

The stomach should be emptied promptly by lavage. In the case of mixed drug overdose, activated charcoal may be indicated. However, if activated charcoal has been administered, lavage before administering acetylcysteine treatment.

If the patient vomits within 1 hour of administration, repeat the dose. If the patient persistently is unable to retain the orally administered acetylcysteine, administer by duodenal intubation.

➤*Storage/Stability:* Store unopened vials at 20° to 25°C (68° to 77°F); excursions are permitted to 15° to 30°C (59° to 86°F).

Use diluted solutions within 1 hour. Remaining undiluted solutions in opened vials can be stored under refrigeration for up to 96 hours.

Actions

➤*Pharmacology:* Acetylcysteine has been shown to reduce the extent of liver injury following acetaminophen overdose. Its effectiveness depends on early oral administration, with benefit seen principally in patients treated within 16 hours of the overdose. Acetylcysteine likely protects the liver by maintaining or restoring the glutathione levels or by acting as an alternate substrate for conjugation with, and thus detoxification of, the acetaminophen-reactive metabolite.

➤*Pharmacokinetics:*

Distribution – The steady-state volume of distribution and the protein binding for acetylcysteine were reported to be 0.47 L/kg and 83%, respectively.

Metabolism/Excretion – Acetylcysteine may form cysteine, disulfides, and conjugates in vivo (eg, N, N'-diacetylcysteine, N-acetylcysteine-cysteine, N-acetylcysteine-glutathione, N-acetylcysteine-protein). Based on published data, it was reported that after an oral dose of ^{35}S-acetylcysteine, approximately 22% of total radioactivity was excreted in urine after 24 hours. No metabolites were identified.

After a single intravenous (IV) dose of acetylcysteine, the plasma concentration of total acetylcysteine declined in a polyexponential decay manner with a mean terminal half-life of 5.6 hours. The mean clearance for acetylcysteine was reported to be 0.11 L/h/kg and renal clearance constituted approximately 30% of total clearance.

Special populations –

Renal function impairment: Pharmacokinetic information is not available.

Hepatic function impairment: After IV administration in subjects with severe liver damage (ie, cirrhosis caused by alcohol [with Child-Pugh score of 7 to 13]) or primary and/or secondary biliary cirrhosis (with Child-Pugh score of 5 to 7), mean half-life increased by 80%, while mean clearance decreased by 30% compared with control group.

Elderly: Adequate information on acetylcysteine pharmacokinetics in elderly patients is not available.

Children: The mean elimination half-life of acetylcysteine is longer in newborns (11 hours) than in adults (5.6 hours).

Gender: Adequate information is not available to assess if there are differences in pharmacokinetics between men and women.

Contraindications

None well documented.

Warnings/Precautions

➤*Urticaria:* Generalized urticaria has been observed rarely in patients receiving oral acetylcysteine for acetaminophen overdose. If this occurs or other allergic symptoms appear, discontinue treatment with acetylcysteine unless it is deemed essential and the allergic symptoms can be otherwise controlled.

➤*Encephalopathy:* If encephalopathy caused by hepatic failure becomes evident, discontinue acetylcysteine treatment to avoid further administration of nitrogenous substances. There are no data indicating that acetylcysteine influences hepatic failure, but this remains a theoretical possibility.

➤*Emesis:* Occasionally, severe and persistent vomiting occurs as a symptom of acute acetaminophen overdose. Treatment with oral acetylcysteine may aggravate the vomiting. Evaluate patients at risk of gastric hemorrhage (eg, esophageal varices, peptic ulcers) concerning the risk of upper GI hemorrhage vs the risk of developing hepatic toxicity; give acetylcysteine treatment accordingly. Dilution of the acetylcysteine minimizes the propensity of acetylcysteine to aggravate vomiting.

➤*Pregnancy: Category B.* There are no adequate and well-controlled studies in pregnant women. Consistent with its low molecular weight (approximately 163), acetylcysteine crosses the human placenta. Because animal reproduction studies may not always be predictive of human responses, use during pregnancy only if clearly needed. A 1999 report concluded that acetaminophen overdose in pregnant women should be managed the same way as in nonpregnant patients and that acetylcysteine therapy was protective to both the mother and the fetus. In 4 pregnant women with acetaminophen toxicity, acetylcysteine was administered at the time of delivery. Acetylcysteine was measurable in newborn circulation and cord blood of 3 viable infants following delivery and in cardiac blood of a fourth infant at autopsy (22 weeks gestational age who died 3 hours after birth). No adverse sequelae developed in the 3 viable infants. All mothers recovered and none of the infants had evidence of acetaminophen poisoning.

➤*Lactation:* It is not known whether this drug is excreted in human milk. The molecular weight of the drug (approximately 163) is low enough for excretion into breast milk. Because many drugs are excreted in human milk, exercise caution when administering acetylcysteine to a breast-feeding woman. Moreover, IV acetylcysteine has been administered directly to preterm neonates for therapeutic indications at doses far above those that would be obtained from milk, without causing toxicity.

➤*Monitoring:* On admission for suspected acetaminophen overdose, draw a serum blood sample at least 4 hours after ingestion to determine the acetaminophen level; this will serve as a basis for determining the need for acetylcysteine treatment. If the patient presents after 4 hours postingestion, immediately determine the serum acetaminophen sample.

Determine the AST, ALT, bilirubin, prothrombin time, creatinine, serum urea nitrogen (BUN), blood glucose, and electrolytes at baseline and daily in order to monitor hepatic and renal function and electrolyte and fluid balance.

Drug Interactions

None well documented.

Adverse Reactions

➤*Dermatologic:* Rash with or without mild fever has been observed rarely.

➤*GI:* Oral administration of acetylcysteine, especially in the large doses needed to treat acetaminophen overdose, may result in nausea, vomiting, and other GI symptoms.

Patient Information

Inform patients that occasionally severe and persistent vomiting may occur. Inform patients that generalized urticaria has occurred.

ACETYLCYSTEINE — INJECTION

For information on use as a mucolytic, refer to the Acetylcysteine monograph in the Respiratory chapter.

Indications

➤*Acetaminophen overdose:* To prevent or lessen hepatic injury after ingestion of a potentially hepatotoxic quantity of acetaminophen when administered intravenously (IV) within 8 to 10 hours of ingestion.

Administration and Dosage

➤*General dosing considerations:* Plasma or serum acetaminophen concentrations, determined as early as possible but no sooner than 4 hours following an acute overdose, are essential in assessing the potential risk of hepatotoxicity. If an assay for acetaminophen cannot be obtained, it is necessary to assume that the overdose is potentially toxic. Acetaminophen levels drawn less than 4 hours postingestion may be misleading.

With an extended-release preparation, an acetaminophen level drawn less than 8 hours postingestion may be misleading. Draw a second level at 4 to 6 hours after the initial level. If either falls above the toxicity line, initiate treatment.

Acetylcysteine may be withheld until acetaminophen assay results are available as long as initiation of treatment is not delayed beyond 8 hours postingestion. If more than 8 hours postingestion, start treatment immediately (see Interpretation of Acetaminophen Assay).

➤*Adults:*

Acetaminophen toxicity –

Usual dosage: 300 mg/kg IV over 21 hours.

Dosage titration:

- *Loading dose* – 150 mg/kg IV over 60 minutes.
- *Second dose* – 50 mg/kg IV over 4 hours.
- *Third dose* – 100 mg/kg IV over 16 hours.

➤*Interpretation of acetaminophen assay:* When results of the plasma acetaminophen assay are available, refer to the Rumack-Matthew nomogram to determine if the plasma concentration is in the potentially toxic range. Values above the line connecting 200 mcg/mL at 4 hours with 50 mcg/mL at 12 hours (probable line) are associated with a probability of hepatic toxicity if an antidote is not administered.

If the predetoxification plasma level is above the line connecting 150 mcg/mL at 4 hours with 37.5 mcg/mL at 12 hours (possible line), continue with maintenance doses of acetylcysteine. It is better to err on the safe side, and thus this line defining possible toxicity, is plotted 25% below the line, defining probable toxicity.

If the predetoxification plasma level is below the line connecting 150 mcg/mL at 4 hours with 37.5 mcg/mL at 12 hours (possible line), there is minimal risk of hepatic toxicity, and acetylcysteine treatment may be discontinued.

➤*Preparation for administration:*

Acetylcysteine Injection Preparation						
	Loading dose		Second dose		Third dose	
Body weight	Acetylcysteine 150 mg/kg over 60 minutes	Diluent	Acetylcysteine 50 mg/kg over 4 hours	Diluent	Acetylcysteine 100 mg/kg over 16 hours	Diluent
100 kg	75 mL	200 mL	25 mL	500 mL	50 mL	1,000 mL
90 kg	67.5 mL	200 mL	22.5 mL	500 mL	45 mL	1,000 mL
80 kg	60 mL	200 mL	20 mL	500 mL	40 mL	1,000 mL
70 kg	52.5 mL	200 mL	17.5 mL	500 mL	35 mL	1,000 mL
60 kg	45 mL	200 mL	15 mL	500 mL	30 mL	1,000 mL
50 kg	37.5 mL	200 mL	12.5 mL	500 mL	25 mL	1,000 mL
40 kg	30 mL	200 mL	10 mL	500 mL	20 mL	1,000 mL
30 kg	22.5 mL	100 mL	7.5 mL	250 mL	15 mL	500 mL
25 kg	18.75 mL	100 mL	6.25 mL	250 mL	12.5 mL	500 mL
20 kg	15 mL	60 mL	5 mL	140 mL	10 mL	280 mL
15 kg	11.25 mL	45 mL	3.75 mL	105 mL	7.5 mL	210 mL
10 kg	7.5 mL	30 mL	2.5 mL	70 mL	5 mL	140 mL

Fluid overload – In patients requiring fluid restriction, reduce the volume of diluent needed.

➤*Administration:* Administer loading dose IV over 60 minutes; administer second dose IV over 4 hours; administer third dose IV over 16 hours. Administer within 8 hours from acetaminophen ingestion for maximal protection against hepatic injury for patients whose serum acetaminophen levels fall above the "possible" toxicity line on the Rumack-Matthew nomogram (line connecting 150 mcg/mL at 4 hours with 50 mcg/mL at 12 hours). If the time of ingestion is unknown, or the serum acetaminophen level is not available, cannot be interpreted, or is not available within the 8-hour time interval from acetaminophen ingestion, acetylcysteine should be administered immediately if 24 hours or less have elapsed from the reported time of ingestion of an overdose of acetaminophen, regardless of the quantity reported to have been ingested.

The critical ingestion-treatment interval for maximal protection against severe hepatic injury is between 0 and 8 hours. Efficacy diminishes progressively after 8 hours, and treatment initiation between 15 and 24 hours postingestion of acetaminophen yields limited efficacy. However, it does not appear to worsen the condition of patients, and it should not be withheld because the reported time of ingestion may not be correct.

➤*Admixture compatibility:* Acetylcysteine is hyperosmolar and is compatible with dextrose 5%, isotonic sodium chloride 50% solution (sodium chloride 0.45% injection), and water for injection.

➤*Storage/Stability:* Store unopened vials at 20° to 25°C (68° to 77°F). Discard unused portion. If vial was previously opened, do not use for IV administration. The diluted solution is stable for 24 hours at controlled room temperature.

Actions

➤*Pharmacology:* Acetylcysteine has been shown to reduce the extent of liver injury following acetaminophen overdose. It is most effective when given early, with benefit seen principally in patients treated within 8 to 10 hours of the overdose. Acetylcysteine likely protects the liver by maintaining or restoring the glutathione levels, or by acting as an alternate substrate for conjugation with, and thus detoxification of, the reactive metabolite.

➤*Pharmacokinetics:*

Distribution – The steady-state volume of distribution (Vd_{ss}) and the protein binding for acetylcysteine were reported to be 0.47 L/kg and 83%, respectively.

Metabolism – Acetylcysteine may form cysteine, disulfides, and conjugates in vivo (N, N′-diacetylcysteine, N-acetylcysteine-cysteine, N-acetylcysteine-glutathione, N-acetylcysteine-protein).

Excretion – Based on published data, it was reported that after an oral dose of ^{35}S-acetylcysteine, about 22% of total radioactivity was excreted in urine after 24 hours. No metabolites were identified. After a single IV dose of acetylcysteine, the plasma concentration of total acetylcysteine declined in a poly-exponential decay manner with a mean terminal half-life of 5.6 hours. The mean clearance for acetylcysteine was reported to be 0.11 L/h/kg and renal clearance constituted about 30% of total clearance.

Special populations –

Hepatic function impairment: In subjects with severe liver damage (ie, cirrhosis caused by alcohol with Child-Pugh score of 7 to 13, or primary or secondary biliary cirrhosis with Child-Pugh score of 5 to 7), mean half-life increased by 80%, while mean clearance decreased by 30% compared with the control group.

Children: The mean elimination half-life of acetylcysteine is longer in newborns (11 hours) than in adults (5.6 hours).

Pregnancy: See the Pregnancy section in Warnings/Precautions for more information.

Contraindications

Previous anaphylactoid reactions to acetylcysteine.

Warnings/Precautions

➤*Asthma/Bronchospasm:* Use acetylcysteine with caution in patients with asthma, or when there is a history of bronchospasm.

➤*Fluid overload:* Adjust the total volume administered for patients less than 40 kg and for those requiring fluid restriction. To avoid fluid overload, reduce the volume of diluent as needed. If volume is not adjusted, fluid overload can occur, potentially resulting in hyponatremia, seizure, and death.

➤*Hypersensitivity reactions:* Serious anaphylactoid reactions, including death in a patient with asthma, have been reported. Acute flushing and erythema of the skin may occur. These reactions usually occur 30 to 60 minutes after initiating the infusion and often resolve spontaneously despite continued infusion of acetylcysteine. Anaphylactoid reactions (defined as the occurrence of an acute hypersensitivity reaction during acetylcysteine administration, including rash, hypotension, wheezing, and/or shortness of breath) have been observed in patients receiving acetylcysteine for acetaminophen overdose and occurred soon after initiation of the infusion. If a reaction to acetylcysteine involves more than simply flushing and erythema of the skin, treat it as an anaphylactoid reaction. This usually entails administering antihistaminic drugs as well as epinephrine in severe cases. In addition, the acetylcysteine infusion may be interrupted until treatment of the anaphylactoid symptoms has been initiated and then carefully restarted. If the anaphylactoid reaction returns upon reinitiation of treatment or increases in severity, discontinue acetylcysteine IV and consider alternative patient management.

➤*Pregnancy: Category B.* There are no adequate and well-controlled studies in pregnant women. Consistent with its low molecular weight (approximately 163), acetylcysteine crosses the human placenta. However, limited case reports of pregnant women exposed to acetylcysteine during various trimesters did not report any adverse maternal, fetal, or neonatal outcomes. A 1999 report concluded that acetaminophen overdose in pregnant women should be managed the same way as in nonpregnant patients and that acetylcysteine therapy is protective to both the mother and the fetus. In 4 pregnant women with acetaminophen toxicity, acetylcysteine was administered at the time of delivery. Acetylcysteine was measurable in newborn circulation and cord blood of 3 viable infants following delivery, and in cardiac blood of a fourth infant at autopsy (22 weeks gestational age who died 3 hours after birth). No adverse sequelae developed in the 3 viable infants. All mothers recovered; none of the infants had evidence of acetaminophen poisoning.

➤*Lactation:* It is not known whether this drug is excreted in human milk. The molecular weight of acetylcysteine (approximately 163) is low enough for excretion into breast milk. Because many drugs are excreted in human

ACETYLCYSTEINE — INJECTION

milk, exercise caution when acetylcysteine is administered to a breast-feeding woman. Based on the pharmacokinetics of acetylcysteine, it should be nearly completely cleared 30 hours after administration. Breast-feeding women may consider resuming nursing 30 hours after administration. Moreover, IV acetylcysteine has been administered directly to preterm neonates for therapeutic indications at doses far above those that would be obtained from milk, without causing toxicity.

➤*Children:* There are no adequate and well-controlled studies in children.

➤*Monitoring:* On admission for suspected acetaminophen overdose, draw a serum blood sample at least 4 hours after ingestion to determine the acetaminophen level; this will serve as a basis for determining the need for treatment with acetylcysteine. If the patient presents after 4 hours postingestion, determine the serum acetaminophen sample immediately.

Determine AST, ALT, bilirubin, prothrombin time, creatinine, serum urea nitrogen, blood glucose, and electrolytes at baseline and daily in order to monitor hepatic and renal function and electrolyte and fluid balance.

➤*Adverse reactions during the first 2 hours of administration:*

Acetylcysteine IV Adverse Reactions Occurring Within the First 2 Hours of Administration

Treatment group	15 minutes (n = 109)				60 minutes (n = 71)			
Cardiovascular	5%				3%			
Severity:	Unknown	Mild	Moderate	Severe	Unknown	Mild	Moderate	Severe
Tachycardia NOS[a]		4%	1%			3%		
Dermatologic	6%				7%			
Severity:	Unknown	Mild	Moderate	Severe	Unknown	Mild	Moderate	Severe
Flushing		1%	1%			3%	1%	
Pruritus		1%				3%		
Rash NOS		3%	2%			4%		
GI	15%				10%			
Severity:	Unknown	Mild	Moderate	Severe	Unknown	Mild	Moderate	Severe
Nausea	1%		6%			1%	1%	
Vomiting NOS		2%	10%			3%	6%	
Respiratory	2%				3%			
Severity:	Unknown	Mild	Moderate	Severe	Unknown	Mild	Moderate	Severe
Pharyngitis			1%					
Rhinorrhoea		1%						
Rhonchi						1%		
Throat tightness						1%		
Miscellaneous	20%				15%			
Severity:	Unknown	Mild	Moderate	Severe	Unknown	Mild	Moderate	Severe
Anaphylactoid reaction	2%	6%	10%	1%		6%	7%	1%
Immune system disorders	18%				14%			
Vascular disorders	2%				4%			

[a] NOS = not otherwise specified.

➤*Postmarketing:* The overall incidence of anaphylactoid reactions was 7.9% in adults and 9.5% in children.

Acetylcysteine Anaphylactoid Postmarketing Adverse Reactions

Anaphylactoid adverse reactions	Adults (n = 4,709)	Children (n = 1,905)
Anaphylaxis	0.1%	0.2%
Edema	1.6%	1.2%
Hypotension	0.1%	0.1%
Pruritus	4.3%	4.1%
Respiratory symptoms[a]	1.9%	2.2%
Urticaria/Facial flushing	6.1%	7.6%

[a] Respiratory symptoms are defined as presence of any of the following: cough, wheezing, stridor, shortness of breath, chest tightness, respiratory distress, or bronchospasm.

Drug Interactions

None well documented.

Adverse Reactions

➤*Most frequent adverse reactions:* In the literature, the most frequently reported adverse reactions attributed to acetylcysteine were rash, urticaria, and pruritus. The frequency of adverse reactions has been reported to be between 0.2% and 20.8%, and they most commonly occur during the initial loading dose of acetylcysteine.

➤*Anaphylactoid reactions:* Within the first 2 hours following acetylcysteine administration, 17% of patients developed an anaphylactoid reaction (18% in the 15-minute treatment group; 14% in the 60-minute treatment group).

Overdosage

➤*Animal toxicology:* Single IV doses of acetylcysteine at 1,000 mg/kg in mice, 2,445 mg/kg in rats, 1,500 mg/kg in guinea pigs, 1,200 mg/kg in rabbits, and 500 mg/kg in dogs were lethal. Symptoms of acute toxicity were ataxia, hypoactivity, labored respiration, cyanosis, loss of righting reflex, and convulsions.

Patient Information

Advise patients to report any history of sensitivity to acetylcysteine to their health care provider.

Advise patients to report any history of asthma to their health care provider.

Inform patients that serious anaphylactic reactions, including death in a patient with asthma, have been reported.

IPECAC SYRUP

otc	**Ipecac** (Various, eg, Roxane)	**Syrup**	1.5% to 1.75% alcohol. In 15 and 30 mL.
Rx	**Ipecac** (Various, eg, Paddock)	**Syrup**	2% alcohol. In 15 and 30 mL.

IPECAC — ORAL

Indications

➤*Overdose/Poisoning:* Treatment of drug overdose and in certain poisonings.

Administration and Dosage

➤*General dosing considerations:* Do not confuse ipecac syrup with ipecac fluid extract, which is 14 times stronger and has caused some deaths.

Do not use in unconscious persons (See Administration).

➤*Adults:*

Overdose/Poisoning –

Usual dosage: 15 to 30 mL followed by 3 to 4 glasses of water.

Repeat dosage: 15 mL once if vomiting does not occur within 20 to 30 minutes. If vomiting does not occur within 30 to 45 minutes after the second dose, perform gastric lavage.

➤*Children:*

Overdose/Poisoning –

13 years of age and older: See Adults for dosing.

1 to 12 years of age:

- *Usual dosage* – 15 mL followed by 1 to 2 glasses of water.
- *Repeat dosage* – See Adults for repeat dosage.

Younger than 1 year of age:

- *Usual dosage* – 5 to 10 mL, then ½ to 1 glass water. Should probably give only with medical supervision. There is controversy over giving to children younger than 1 year of age, although it appears to be safe and effective.

➤*Administration:* Ipecac syrup may not work on an empty stomach. Have patient sit upright with head forward before administering dose.

Do not administer milk with this product.

➤*Storage/Stability:* Keep tightly closed at 15° to 30°C (59° to 86°F).

Actions

➤*Pharmacology:* Ipecac produces vomiting by a local irritant effect on GI mucosa and a central medullary effect (stimulation of chemoreceptor trigger zone). The central effect is caused by emetine and cephaeline, the two alkaloids. An adequate dose causes vomiting within 30 min in more than 90% of patients (average time is less than 20 min).

Contraindications

Semiconscious or unconscious patients. Do not use if strychnine, corrosives such as alkalies and strong acids, or petroleum distillates have been ingested.

Warnings/Precautions

➤*Special risk: Keep out of reach of children.*

➤*Do not use:* Ordinarily this drug should not be used if strychnine, corrosives such as alkalies (lye) and strong acids, or petroleum distillates such as kerosene, gasoline, coal oil, fuel oil, paint thinner, or cleaning fluid have been ingested.

Do not use in unconscious persons.

➤*Administration:* Do not administer milk with this product.

➤*Syrup/Fluid extract:* Do not confuse ipecac syrup with ipecac fluid extract, which is 14 times stronger and has caused some deaths.

➤*Call an emergency room:* Call an emergency room, poison control center or physician before using; if vomiting does not occur within 30 to 45 minutes after the second dose, perform gastric lavage.

➤*Ipecac Syrup Abuse:* Ipecac syrup abuse may occur in bulimic and anorexic patients. It has been implicated as the causative factor of severe cardiomyopathies, and even death, in several persons with eating disorders who used it regularly to induce vomiting.

➤*Absorption:* Ipecac syrup can be cardiotoxic if not vomited and allowed to be absorbed. Absorption of emetine may occur and cause heart conduction disturbances, atrial fibrillation or fatal myocarditis.

➤*Pregnancy: Category C.* It is not known whether the drug can cause harm when administered to a pregnant woman. Minimal systemic absorption is expected when used as directed (see Administration and Dosage).

➤*Lactation:* It is not known whether ipecac alkaloids are excreted in breast milk. Exercise caution if ipecac syrup is used for treatment of a nursing woman.

Drug Interactions

➤*Activated charcoal:* Activated charcoal will absorb ipecac syrup. Do not give activated charcoal until after the patient has vomited, unless directed by a health professional.

Adverse Reactions

Reactions are generally not significant if the dose is not exceeded. Diarrhea (25% in children younger than 3 years of age); drowsiness (20% in children younger than 3 years of age); coughing or choking in association with emesis (less than 4%); mild CNS depression; GI upset (may last several hours after emesis).

Overdosage

➤*Symptoms:* Ipecac is cardiotoxic if absorbed and may cause cardiac conduction disturbances, bradycardia, atrial fibrillation, hypotension, or fatal myocarditis.

➤*Treatment:* Activated charcoal may be given to adsorb ipecac syrup; perform gastric lavage. Support cardiovascular system by symptomatic treatment.

Patient Information

Always consult a physician or poison control center in cases of accidental ingestion.

Give with adequate amounts of water; do not use milk or carbonated beverages. Do not exceed recommended dosage.

CHARCOAL

otc	**Charcoal Plus DS** (Kramer)	**Tablets; oral:** 250 mg	Sorbitol. In 120s.
otc	**Charcoal** (Various, eg, Nature's Bounty)	**Capsules; oral:** 260 mg	In 50s and 100s.
otc	**CharcoCaps** (Requa)		In 8s, 36s, and 100s.
otc	**Activated Charcoal** (Various)	**Powder; oral**	In 15, 30, 40, 120, and 240 g and UD 30 g.
otc	**Activated Charcoal** (Various)	**Liquid; oral:** 208 mg/mL	12.5 g with propylene glycol. In 60 mL bottle. 25 g with propylene glycol. In 120 mL bottle.
otc	**Actidose-Aqua** (Paddock)		Activated. 25 g in 120 mL suspension. 50 g in 240 mL suspension.
otc	**Actidose with Sorbitol** (Paddock)		Activated. 25 g in 120 mL suspension with sorbitol. 50 g in 240 mL suspension with sorbitol.
otc	**Liqui-Char** (Jones Medical)		Activated. 12.5 g in 60 mL bottle, 15 g in 75 mL bottle, 25 g in 120 mL squeeze container, 30 g in 120 mL squeeze container, 50 g in 240 mL squeeze container.
otc	**CharcoAid** (Requa)	**Suspension; oral:** 15 g	Activated. Sorbitol. In 120 mL.
		30 g	Activated. Sorbitol. In 150 mL.
otc	**CharcoAid 2000** (Requa)	**Liquid; oral:** 15 g	Activated. With and without sorbitol. In 120 mL.
		50 g	Activated. With and without sorbitol. In 240 mL.
		Granules; oral: 15 g	Activated. In 120 mL.

CHARCOAL — ORAL

Indications

➤*Charcoal:*

Intestinal gas/diarrhea/GI distress – For relief of intestinal gas, diarrhea and GI distress associated with indigestion and accompanying cramps or odor.

Pruritus associated with kidney dialysis treatment – For the prevention of nonspecific pruritus associated with dialysis treatment.

➤*Activated charcoal:*

Poisoning – For the emergency poison treatment of cases of acute toxic ingestion.

Administration and Dosage

➤*General dosing considerations:* Activated charcoal in a sorbitol base is not recommended for multiple-dose activated charcoal therapy because of excessive cathartic action.

➤*Adults:*

Charcoal –

Usual dosage: 500 to 520 mg after meals or at first sign of discomfort. Repeat as needed.

Maximum dose: 5 g daily.

Activated charcoal –

Poisoning:

• *Activated charcoal in a sorbitol base* – 50 to 60 g (or the contents of two 25 or 30 g containers).

• *Activated charcoal in an aqueous base* –

Usual dosage: 5 to 60 g.

The dosage should be from 8 to 10 times by volume greater than the amount of toxic substance ingested, if that factor is known. If the amount of toxic substance ingested is not known, the amount of activated charcoal in an aqueous base administered should be based upon the weight, size, and age of the patient.

Initial dosage: At least 20 to 30 g.

Repeat doses: After the first dose has been administered, additional activated charcoal may be given at the direction of the poison control center or the emergency room health care provider. However, no damage or harm will occur to the patient if a larger than minimal dosage is administered, as the charcoal is readily tolerated by the body and will be eliminated through the intestinal tract.

➤*Children:*

Charcoal –

3 years of age and older: See Adults for dosing.

Activated charcoal –

Poisoning:

• *Activated charcoal in a sorbitol base* – See Adults for dosing for children older than 12 years of age.

1 to 12 years of ageMore than 32 kg: 50 to 60 g.16 to 32 kg 25 to 30 g.

• *Activated charcoal in an aqueous base* – See Adults for dosing for children 1 year of age and older.

➤*Concomitant therapy:* The effectiveness of other medications that may be administered concurrently may be decreased because of the adsorption of the activated charcoal.

➤*Preparation for administration:*

Activated charcoal – When administering activated charcoal from a unit-dose bottle, stir thoroughly and shake vigorously the contents of the unit-dose container prior to administration. When administering activated charcoal from a unit-dose tube, knead and shake vigorously before using. Carefully cut tip.

➤*Administration:*

Charcoal – Take charcoal 2 hours before or 1 hour after other medication.

Activated charcoal –

First, check to ensure that the patient is breathing and remove food or dental work from the mouth so that adequate air can get to the lungs. If the patient is not breathing, administer artificial respiration because the air flow to the lungs must not be impeded. The patient should receive no drugs, coffee, alcohol, or carbonated beverages. The patient should be kept warm though not overheated.

When possible, activated charcoal should be administered promptly, preferably within 30 minutes following ingestion of the toxins. To delay treatment longer will permit time for the toxins to permeate the patient's body and so decrease the effectiveness of the charcoal's adsorptive action.

When administering activated charcoal from a unit-dose bottle, the patient should ingest its entire contents. If a substantial quantity of charcoal remains after administration, add water to the container, shake again, and readminister.

Administer activated charcoal from a unit-dose tube through a gastric tube or squeeze contents into a glass and have the patient drink contents.

➤*Admixture compatibility:* Milk, ice cream, or sherbet should not be mixed with the charcoal because it will decrease the adsorptive capacity of the activated charcoal.

➤*Storage/Stability:* Store in a tightly closed container. Premixed suspension can be stored for up to 1 year.

Actions

➤*Pharmacology:* Charcoal is an adsorbent, detoxicant, and soothing agent. It reduces the volume of intestinal gas and relieves related discomfort. Activated charcoal adsorbs the toxic substances ingested by forming an effective barrier between any remaining particulate material and the GI mucosa, thus inhibiting any GI absorption.

Activated charcoal in a sorbitol base – Sorbitol is hexahydric sugar alcohol that primarily serves as an osmotic cathartic. As a hyperosmotic, cathartic sorbitol produces a hygroscopic action resulting in increased water in the large intestines and increased intraluminal pressure which stimulates catharsis.

➤*Pharmacokinetics:*

Absorption – Testing of activated charcoal liquid indicates that the adsorption power of each size of the activated charcoal, when treated with 10% of the alkaloid strychnine sulfate (based on the quantity of charcoal per bottle [eg, 1.5 g of alkaloid to 15 g of charcoal]) is not less than 99%. Treatment of the product with dyes (methylene blue) produces similar results. The adsorptive properties of the activated charcoal liquid are slightly decreased during the shelf-life of the product but are still capable of adsorbing at least 99% of the substance tested.

Activated charcoal in a sorbitol base: Catharsis of activated charcoal in a sorbitol base generally occurs in an average of 1 to 1.5 hours and persists for 8 to 12 hours. The onset of action may be expected to be longer in patients who have ingested toxins that decrease bowel motility such as pharmacologic agents and plants with anticholinergic properties and drugs like narcotics.

Warnings/Precautions

➤*High dosage or prolonged use:* High dosage or prolonged use does not cause adverse effects or harm the patient's nutritional state.

➤*Diarrhea:* Do not use activated charcoal in a sorbitol base in any person known to have a rare autosomal recessive genetic intolerance to fructose or in patients who are known to be dehydrated. Activated charcoal in a sorbitol base may cause excessive diarrhea.

Because a profound cathartic effect may occur following use of this product, provide proper attention to the patient's fluid and electrolyte needs.

➤*Multiple doses:* Use activated charcoal in a sorbitol base cautiously in patients receiving multiple doses. If activated charcoal in a sorbitol base is used at each dosage interval, profound catharsis may develop, resulting in dehydration and even hypotension.

➤*Pregnancy:* *Category: Undetermined*. If pregnant, ask a health care provider before use.

➤*Lactation:* If breast-feeding, ask a health care provider before use.

➤*Children:* Do not use charcoal in children younger than 3 years of age. Do not use activated charcoal in children younger than 1 year of age.

Drug Interactions

Activated charcoal can adsorb drugs while they are in the GI tract. Therefore, take charcoal 2 hours before or 1 hour after other medication.

Charcoal Drug Interactions

Precipitant drug	Object drug[a]			Description
Charcoal	Acetaminophen Barbiturates Carbamazepine Digitoxin Digoxin Furosemide Glutethimide Hydantoins Methotrexate Nizatidine Phenothiazines	Phenylbutazones Propoxyphene Salicylates Sulfones Sulfonylureas Tetracyclines Theophyllines Tricyclic antidepressants Valproic acid	⬇	Charcoal can reduce absorption of these drugs and remove them from the systemic circulation, which may reduce the effectiveness of a given agent.

[a] ⬇ = object drug decreased.

Antidotes

CHARCOAL — ORAL

➤*Drug/Food interactions:* See Administration and Dosage for more information.

Adverse Reactions

➤*GI:* Activated charcoal will color stool black, which may be alarming to the patient, although it is medically insignificant.

Patient Information

Inform patients that their stools may be black for several days.

➤*Diarrhea:* Advise patients to consult their health care provider if diarrhea persists for more than 2 days or is accompanied by fever.

METHYLENE BLUE

Rx	**Methylene Blue** (Various, eg, Pasadena)	**Injection:** 10 mg/mL	In 1 and 10 mL amps.

METHYLENE BLUE — INJECTION

Indications

➤*Methemoglobinemia:* Drug-induced methemoglobinemia.

Administration and Dosage

➤*Adults:*

Drug-induced methemoglobinemia – 1 to 2 mg/kg intravenously (IV) very slowly over a period of several minutes.

➤*Children:*

Drug-induced methemoglobinemia – 1 to 2 mg/kg IV very slowly over a period of several minutes.

➤*Storage/Stability:* Store below 40°C (104°F), preferably between 15° and 30°C (59° and 86°F).

Actions

➤*Pharmacology:* Methylene blue will produce 2 opposite actions on hemoglobin. Low concentrations will convert methemoglobin to hemoglobin. High concentrations convert the ferrous iron of reduced hemoglobin to ferric iron which results in the formation of methemoglobin.

Contraindications

Intraspinal injection is contraindicated.

Warnings/Precautions

➤*Administration:* Methylene blue should not be given by subcutaneous or intrathecal injection.

➤*Additional methemoglobin:* Methylene blue must be injected IV very slowly over a period of several minutes to prevent local high concentration of the compound from producing additional methemoglobin. Do not exceed recommended dosage.

➤*Pregnancy:* *Category C* (per manufacturer prescribing information). *Category D* if injected intra-aminotically (per Briggs' *Drugs in Pregnancy and Lactation*).Safety for use in pregnancy has not been established. Use of methylene blue in women of childbearing potential requires that anticipated benefits be weighed against possible hazards.

➤*Lactation:* No human data is available in breast-feeding women; use is probably compatible.

Adverse Reactions

Large IV doses of methylene blue produce nausea, abdominal and precordial pain, dizziness, headache, profuse sweating, mental confusion and the formation of methemoglobin.

PHENYLKETONURIA AGENTS

SAPROPTERIN DIHYDROCHLORIDE

Rx	**Kuvan** (BioMarin Pharmaceutical Inc)	**Tablets; oral:** 100 mg	Equiv to sapropterin base 76.8 mg. D-mannitol. (177). Off-white to light-yellow. In 120s.

SAPROPTERIN DIHYDROCHLORIDE — ORAL

Indications

➤*Hyperphenylalaninemia:* To reduce blood phenylalanine (Phe) levels in patients with hyperphenylalaninemia caused by tetrahydrobiopterin (BH4)-responsive phenylketonuria.

Sapropterin is to be used in conjunction with a Phe-restricted diet.

Administration and Dosage

➤*General dosing considerations:*

Monitoring – Blood Phe levels should be checked after 1 week of treatment and periodically for up to a month. Frequent blood monitoring is recommended in children to ensure adequate blood Phe level control.

➤*Adults:*

Hyperphenylalaninemia –

Initial dosage: 10 mg/kg/day once daily.

Dosage titration: Response to therapy is determined by change in blood Phe following treatment. If blood Phe does not decrease from baseline at 10 mg/kg/day after a period of up to 1 month, the dose may be increased to 20 mg/kg/day. Patients whose blood Phe does not decrease after 1 month of treatment at 20 mg/kg/day are nonresponders, and treatment with should be discontinued in these patients.

Maintenance dosage: Once responsiveness has been established, the dose may be adjusted within the range of 5 to 20 mg/kg/day, according to response to therapy.

Missed dose: A missed dose should be taken as soon as possible, but 2 doses should not be taken on the same day.

➤*Children:*

Hyperphenylalaninemia – See Adults for dosing for children 4 years of age and older.

➤*Administration:* Administer orally with food to increase absorption, preferably at the same time each day. Tablets should be dissolved in 120 to 240 mL of water or apple juice and taken within 15 minutes of dissolution. It may take a few minutes for the tablets to dissolve. To make the tablets dissolve faster, stir or crush them. The tablets may not dissolve completely. Patients may see small pieces floating on top of the water or apple juice. This is normal and safe for patients to swallow. If after drinking the medicine patients still see pieces of the tablet, they can add more water or apple juice to make sure that they take all of the medicine.

➤*Storage/Stability:* Store at 20° to 25°C (68° to 77°F); excursions are allowed between 15° and 30°C (59° and 86°F). Protect from moisture.

Actions

➤*Pharmacology:* Sapropterin is a synthetic form of BH4, the cofactor for the enzyme phenylalanine hydroxylase (PAH). PAH hydroxylates Phe through an oxidative reaction to form tyrosine. In patients with phenylketonuria, PAH activity is absent or deficient. Treatment with BH4 can activate residual PAH enzyme, improve the normal oxidative metabolism of Phe, and decrease Phe levels in some patients.

Pharmacodynamics – In phenylketonuria patients who are responsive to BH4 treatment, blood Phe levels decrease within 24 hours after a single administration of sapropterin, although maximal effect on Phe level may take up to a month, depending on the patient. A single daily dose of sapropterin is adequate to maintain stable blood Phe levels over a 24-hour period. Twelve patients with blood Phe levels ranging from 516 to 986 mcmol/L (mean, 747 ± 153 mcmol/L) were assessed with 24-hour blood Phe level monitoring following a daily morning dose of 10 mg/kg/day. The blood Phe level remained stable during a 24-hour observation period. No substantial increases in blood Phe levels were observed following food intake throughout the 24-hour period.

Doses higher than 20 mg/kg/day have not been evaluated in clinical studies.

➤*Pharmacokinetics:*

Absorption – Studies in healthy volunteers have shown comparable absorption of sapropterin when tablets are dissolved in water or orange juice and taken under fasted conditions.

Food effects: Administration of dissolved tablets after a high-fat/high-calorie meal resulted in mean increases in maximum plasma concentration (C_{max}) of 84% and area under the curve (AUC) of 87% (dissolved in water). However, there was extensive variability in individual subject values for C_{max} and AUC across the different modes of administration and meal conditions. In the clinical trials of sapropterin, drug was administered in the morning as a dissolved tablet without regard to meals.

Excretion – The mean elimination half-life in phenylketonuria patients was approximately 6.7 hours (range, 3.9 to 17 hours), comparable with values seen in healthy subjects (range, 3 to 5.3 hours).

Contraindications

None known.

Warnings/Precautions

➤*Blood Phe levels:* Health care providers knowledgeable in the management of phenylketonuria should direct treatment with sapropterin. Prolonged elevations in blood Phe levels in patients with phenylketonuria can result in severe neurologic damage, including severe mental retardation, microcephaly, delayed speech, seizures, and behavioral abnormalities. This

SAPROPTERIN DIHYDROCHLORIDE — ORAL

may occur even if patients are taking sapropterin but not adequately controlling their blood Phe levels within recommended target range. Long-term studies of neurocognitive outcomes with sapropterin treatment have not been conducted. Conversely, prolonged levels of blood Phe that are too low have been associated with catabolism and protein breakdown. Active management of dietary Phe intake while taking sapropterin is required to ensure adequate Phe control and nutritional balance.

➤*Nonresponders to treatment:* Not all patients with phenylketonuria respond to treatment with sapropterin. In clinical trials, approximately 20% to 56% of phenylketonuria patients responded to treatment with sapropterin. Response to treatment cannot be predetermined by laboratory testing (eg, genetic testing), and can only be determined by a therapeutic trial of sapropterin.

➤*Phe-restricted diet:* Patients with phenylketonuria who are being treated with sapropterin should also be treated with a Phe-restricted diet. The initiation of sapropterin therapy does not eliminate the need for appropriate monitoring by trained professionals to ensure that blood Phe control is maintained in the context of ongoing dietary management.

➤*Hypersensitivity reactions:* Patients who have a known severe allergy to any of the components of sapropterin should not take this medicine. In clinical trials conducted with sapropterin, no severe allergic reactions were observed. Consider the risks and benefits of continued treatment with sapropterin in patients with mild to moderate allergic reactions (eg, rash).

➤*Renal function impairment:* Patients with renal function impairment have not been evaluated in clinical trials. Carefully monitor patients who have renal function impairment when they are receiving sapropterin.

➤*Hepatic function impairment:* Patients with hepatic function impairment have not been evaluated in clinical trials with sapropterin. Carefully monitor patients who have hepatic function impairment when they are receiving sapropterin because hepatic damage has been associated with impaired Phe metabolism.

➤*Pregnancy: Category C.* Women who are exposed to sapropterin during pregnancy are encouraged to enroll in the sapropterin patient registry.

Teratogenicity studies with sapropterin have been conducted in rats at oral doses of up to 400 mg/kg/day (about 3 times the maximum recommended human dose of 20 mg/kg/day, based on BSA) and in rabbits at oral doses of up to 600 mg/kg/day (about 10 times the maximum recommended human dose, based on BSA).

No clear evidence of teratogenic activity was found in either species; however, in the rabbit teratogenicity study, there was an increase (not statistically significant) in the incidence of holoprosencephaly at the 600 mg/kg/day dose compared with controls.

There are no adequate and well-controlled studies of sapropterin in pregnant women. Because animal reproduction studies are not always predictive of human response, use this drug during pregnancy only if clearly needed. A study of 468 pregnancies and 331 live births in phenylketonuria-affected women (Maternal Phenylketonuria Collaborative Study, Rouse 1997) has demonstrated that uncontrolled Phe levels higher than 600 mcmol/L are associated with a very high incidence of neurological, cardiac, facial dysmorphism, and growth anomalies. Good dietary control of Phe levels during pregnancy is essential in reducing the incidence of Phe-induced teratogenic effects.

➤*Lactation:* Sapropterin is excreted in the milk of intravenously, but not orally treated lactating rats. It is not known whether sapropterin is excreted in human milk. Because of the potential for serious adverse reactions in breast-feeding infants from sapropterin and because of the potential for tumorigenicity shown for sapropterin in the rat carcinogenicity study, decide whether to discontinue breast-feeding or the drug, taking into account the importance of the drug to the mother.

➤*Children:* Children with phenylketonuria, 4 to 16 years of age, have been treated with sapropterin in clinical studies. The safety and efficacy of sapropterin in children younger than 4 years of age have not been assessed in clinical studies. Frequent blood monitoring is recommended in children to ensure adequate blood Phe level control.

➤*Monitoring:* Carefully monitor patients with renal and/or hepatic function impairment. Frequent blood monitoring is recommended in children to ensure adequate blood Phe level control. Check blood Phe levels after 1 week of sapropterin treatment and periodically for up to a month to determine response. When sapropterin is used in combination with a Phe-restricted diet, monitor patients closely to ensure that blood Phe levels are not too low, and, if necessary, adjust the dose of sapropterin.

Drug Interactions

Sapropterin Drug Interactions

Precipitant drug	Object drug[a]		Description
Levodopa	Sapropterin	↑	Three patients with underlying neurologic disorders experienced convulsions, exacerbation of convulsions, overstimulation, or irritability during coadministration of levodopa and sapropterin. Use with caution.
Methotrexate	Sapropterin	↓	Use caution when administering drugs known to affect folate metabolism (eg, methotrexate) and their derivatives with sapropterin because these drugs can decrease BH4 levels by inhibiting the enzyme dihydropteridine reductase.
PDE5[b] inhibitors (eg, sildenafil, tadalafil, vardenafil)	Sapropterin	↑	Use caution when administering sapropterin with drugs that affect nitric oxide–mediated vasorelaxation (eg, sildenafil, tadalafil, vardenafil) because both sapropterin and PDE5 inhibitors may induce vasorelaxation and reduce blood pressure.
Sapropterin	PDE5 inhibitors (eg, sildenafil, tadalafil, vardenafil)		

[a] ↑ = object drug increased; ↓ = object drug decreased.
[b] PDE5 = phosphodiesterase type 5.

Adverse Reactions

The most serious adverse reactions during sapropterin administration (regardless of relationship to treatment) were gastritis, spinal cord injury, streptococcal infection, testicular carcinoma, and urinary tract infection. Mild to moderate neutropenia was noted during sapropterin administration in 24 (4%) of 579 patients. The most common (occurring in at least 4% of patients treated with sapropterin) across all studies (N = 579) were abdominal pain, diarrhea, headache, nausea, pharyngolaryngeal pain, upper respiratory tract infection, and vomiting.

The following data reflect exposure of 74 patients with phenylketonuria to sapropterin at doses of 10 to 20 mg/kg/day for 6 to 10 weeks in 2 double-blind, placebo-controlled clinical trials. The overall incidence of adverse reactions in patients receiving sapropterin was similar to that reported with patients receiving placebo.

Sapropterin Adverse Reactions (≥ 4%)

Adverse reaction	Sapropterin (n = 74)	Placebo (n = 59)
Any adverse reaction	64%	71%
Dermatologic		
Contusion	5%	2%
Rash	5%	7%
GI		
Abdominal pain	5%	8%
Diarrhea	8%	5%
Vomiting	8%	7%
Respiratory		
Cough	7%	5%
Nasal congestion	4%	0%
Pharyngolaryngeal pain	10%	2%
Rhinorrhea	11%	0%
Upper respiratory tract infection	12%	24%
Miscellaneous		
Headache	15%	14%
Pyrexia	7%	7%

➤*Adverse reactions for non-phenylketonuria indications:* Approximately 800 healthy volunteers and patients with disorders other than phenylketonuria, some of whom had underlying neurologic disorders or cardiovascular disease, have been administered a different formulation of the same active ingredient (sapropterin) in approximately 19 controlled and uncontrolled clinical trials. In these clinical trials, subjects were administered sapropterin at doses ranging from 1 to 20 mg/kg/day for lengths of exposure from 1 day to 2 years. Serious and severe adverse reactions (regardless of relationship) during sapropterin administration were convulsions, exacerbation of convulsions, dizziness, GI bleeding, headache, irritability, myocardial infarction, overstimulation, postprocedural bleeding, and respiratory failure. Common adverse reactions were agitation, arthralgia, dizziness, headache, peripheral edema, polyuria, and upper respiratory tract infection.

➤*Postmarketing:* The following adverse reactions have been identified during a 10-year postapproval safety surveillance program in Japan of another formulation of the same active ingredient (sapropterin). This safety surveillance program was conducted in 30 patients, 27 of whom had disorders other than phenylketonuria and had an underlying neurologic condition. The most common adverse reactions were convulsions and exacerbation of convulsions in 3 of the non-phenylketonuria patients, and increased gamma-glutamyltransferase in 2 of the non-phenylketonuria patients.

SAPROPTERIN DIHYDROCHLORIDE — ORAL

Overdosage

➤*Symptoms:* In the only reported overdosage with sapropterin, a patient participating in a 26-week study received a single dose of 4,500 mg (36 mg/kg), instead of 2,600 mg (20 mg/kg), in week 16. The patient reported mild headache and mild dizziness immediately after taking the dose; both symptoms resolved within 1 hour with no treatment intervention. Results from liver function laboratory tests obtained immediately following the event were within normal limits. The patient suspended therapy for 24 hours and then restarted sapropterin with no reports of abnormal signs or symptoms.

Patient Information

Inform patients that in order to determine response to treatment with sapropterin, the patient must be treated with sapropterin and evaluated for changes in blood Phe. Measure blood Phe levels and dietary Phe intake frequently.

Inform patients being treated with sapropterin to have frequent blood Phe measurements and nutritional counseling with their health care provider and other members of the health care team to ensure maintenance of blood Phe levels in the desirable range.

Advise patients that changes in dietary Phe intake can obscure the effect of sapropterin on blood Phe levels, and because not all patients will respond to treatment with sapropterin, all patients with phenylketonuria should be treated with a Phe-restricted diet in addition to treatment with sapropterin.

To determine if a patient responds to sapropterin therapy, patients must not modify their existing dietary Phe intake during the evaluation period in order to get an accurate assessment of the effect of sapropterin on blood Phe levels. Take baseline blood Phe measurements just prior to initiation of a sapropterin response test.

Advise patients to actively manage their dietary Phe intake using medical foods and natural sources of proteins to ensure blood Phe control and adequate nutritional balance.

Advise patients that prolonged high blood Phe levels are neurotoxic and lead to impairment of intelligence and other brain functions (such as attentiveness). Reduction of blood Phe levels through dietary control is an important determinant of long-term neurologic outcome in phenylketonuria patients, and reduction of blood Phe levels in patients with phenylketonuria has been shown to decrease the long-term risk of neurologic injury.

Inform patients that response to sapropterin treatment in phenylketonuria patients is variable. Not all patients responded to treatment with sapropterin in clinical trials, and the initiation of sapropterin treatment does not eliminate the need to monitor for adequate blood Phe control. Prolonged elevations in blood Phe levels can result in neurologic impairment. Conversely, some patients in clinical trials who were following Phe-restricted diets and received treatment with sapropterin experienced substantial reductions of blood Phe. Levels of blood Phe that are too low may be associated with catabolism and protein breakdown. Therefore, when sapropterin is used in combination with a Phe-restricted diet, monitor patients closely to ensure that blood Phe levels are not too low, and, if necessary, adjust the dose of sapropterin.

Inform patients that the most serious adverse reactions during sapropterin administration (regardless of relationship to treatment) were gastritis, spinal cord injury, streptococcal infection, testicular carcinoma, and urinary tract infection. The most common adverse reactions across all studies were headache, diarrhea, abdominal pain, upper respiratory tract infection, pharyngolaryngeal pain, vomiting, and nausea.

Inform patients that long-term studies of neurocognitive outcomes have not been conducted with sapropterin.

Advise patients that the manufacturer will establish a general disease registry for phenylketonuria patients and a pregnancy registry for women who are pregnant while receiving sapropterin treatment.

Cardiac Glycosides

DIGOXIN

Rx	**Digoxin** (Various, eg, UDL, West-Ward)	**Tablets; oral:** 125 mcg (0.125 mg)	In 100s, 1,000s, 5,000s, and UD 100s.
Rx	**Lanoxin** (GlaxoSmithKline)		Lactose. (Lanoxin Y3B). Yellow, scored. In 100s, 1,000s, and UD 100s.
Rx	**Digoxin** (Various, eg, UDL, West-Ward)	**Tablets; oral:** 250 mcg (0.25 mg)	In 100s, 1,000s, 5,000s, and UD 100s.
Rx	**Lanoxin** (GlaxoSmithKline)		Lactose. (Lanoxin X3A). White, scored. In 100s, 1000s, 5,000s and UD 100s.
Rx	**Digoxin**[a] (Various, eg, Roxane)	**Solution; oral:** 50 mcg/mL (0.05 mg/mL)	In 60 mL and UD 2.5 and 5 mL.
Rx	**Digoxin** (Various, eg, Baxter, Sandoz)	**Injection, solution:** 250 mcg/mL (0.25 mg/mL)	In 2 mL amps.[b]
Rx	**Digoxin** (Various, eg, Hospira)		In 1 and 2 mL *Tubex* or *Carpuject*.[b]
Rx	**Lanoxin** (GlaxoSmithKline)		In 2 mL amps.[b]
Rx	**Lanoxin** (GlaxoSmithKline)	**Injection, solution, pediatric:** 100 mcg/mL (0.1 mg/mL)	In 1 mL amps.[b]

[a] May contain 10% alcohol.

[b] May contain 40% propylene glycol and 10% alcohol.

DIGOXIN — ORAL

Indications

➤*Atrial fibrillation:* For the control of ventricular response rate in patients with chronic atrial fibrillation.

➤*Heart failure:* For the treatment of mild to moderate heart failure. Digoxin increases left ventricular ejection fraction (LVEF) and improves heart failure symptoms as evidenced by exercise capacity and heart failure–related hospitalizations and emergency care, while having no effect on mortality. Where possible, use digoxin with a diuretic and an angiotensin-converting enzyme (ACE) inhibitor, but an optimal order for starting these 3 drugs cannot be specified.

Administration and Dosage

➤*General dosing considerations:* Recommended dosages of digoxin may require considerable modification because of individual sensitivity of the patient to the drug, the presence of associated conditions, or the use of concurrent medications.

In selecting a dose of digoxin, consider the following factors:

1.) The body weight of the patient. Calculate doses based upon lean (ie, ideal) body weight.
2.) The patient's renal function, preferably evaluated on the basis of estimated creatinine clearance (CrCl).
3.) The patient's age. Infants and children require different doses of digoxin than adults. Also, advanced age may be indicative of diminished renal function, even in patients with healthy serum creatinine concentration (ie, below 1.5 mg/dL).
4.) Concomitant disease states, concurrent medications, or other factors likely to alter the pharmacokinetic or pharmacodynamic profile of digoxin.

Digitalization may be accomplished by either of 2 general approaches that vary in dosage and frequency of administration, but reach the same end point in terms of total amount of digoxin accumulated in the body.

1.) If rapid digitalization is considered medically appropriate, it may be achieved by administering a loading dose based upon projected peak digoxin body stores. Calculate maintenance dose as a percentage of the loading dose.
2.) Obtain more gradual digitalization by beginning an appropriate maintenance dose; this allows digoxin body stores to accumulate slowly. Steady-state serum digoxin concentrations will be achieved in approximately 5 half-lives of the drug for the individual patient. Depending upon the patient's renal function, this will take between 1 and 3 weeks.

➤*Adults:*

Atrial fibrillation – See also off-label dosing from the American College of Cardiology/American Heart Association (ACC/AHA) guidelines. The following information is according to the prescribing information.

Loading dose: Peak digoxin body stores larger than the 8 to 12 mcg/kg (0.008 to 0.012 mg/kg) required for most patients with heart failure and healthy sinus rhythm have been used for control of ventricular rate in patients with atrial fibrillation.

Maintenance dosage: Titrate doses of digoxin used for the treatment of chronic atrial fibrillation to the minimum dose that achieves the desired ventricular rate control without causing undesirable side effects. Data are not available to establish the appropriate resting or exercise target rates that should be achieved.

Heart failure – See also off-label dosing from the ACC/AHA guidelines. The following information is according to the prescribing information. However, ACC/AHA guidelines state that loading doses are not needed.

Rapid digitalization: Peak digoxin body stores of 8 to 12 mcg/kg (0.008 to 0.012 mg/kg) should provide therapeutic effect with minimum risk of toxicity. Administer the loading dose in several portions, with roughly half of the total given as the first dose. Additional fractions of this planned total dose may be given at 6- to 8-hour intervals, with careful assessment of clinical response before each additional dose. If the patient's clinical response necessitates a change from the calculated loading dose of digoxin, base calculation of the maintenance dose upon the amount actually given.

A single initial dose of 500 to 750 mcg (0.5 to 0.75 mg) of digoxin tablets usually produces a detectable effect in 0.5 to 2 hours, which becomes maximal in 2 to 6 hours. Give additional doses of 125 to 375 mcg (0.125 to 0.375 mg) cautiously at 6- to 8-hour intervals until clinical evidence of an adequate effect is noted. The usual amount of digoxin tablets that a 70 kg patient requires to achieve 8 to 12 mcg/kg (0.008 to 0.012 mg/kg) peak body stores is 750 to 1,250 mcg (0.75 to 1.25 mg).

Gradual digitalization:

• *Initial dosage* – Therapy is generally initiated at a dosage of 250 mcg (0.25 mg) once daily in patients younger than 70 years of age with good renal function, at a dosage of 125 mcg (0.125 mg) once daily in patients older than 70 years of age or with impaired renal function, and at a dosage of 62.5 mcg (0.0625 mg) once daily in patients with marked renal impairment.

• *Dosage titration* – Doses may be increased every 2 weeks according to clinical response. In controlled trials in patients with heart failure, the digoxin dose has been generally titrated according to the patient's age, lean body weight, and renal function.

• *Maintenance dosage* – Dosages have ranged from 125 to 500 mcg (0.125 to 0.5 mg) once daily.

Base the maintenance dose upon the percentage of the peak body stores lost each day through elimination. The following formula has had wide clinical use:

Maintenance dose = peak body stores (ie, loading dose) × % daily loss/100, where: % daily loss = 14 + (CrCl/5) (CrCl is creatinine clearance, corrected to 70 kg body weight or 1.73 m^2 body surface area).

Off-label dosing –

Atrial fibrillation:

• *Acute setting* – 125 to 375 mcg (0.125 to 0.375 mg) once daily, after initial load with digoxin intravenous (IV).

• *Nonacute setting* –

Loading dose: 500 mcg (0.5 mg) orally once daily. Onset of action is 2 days.

Maintenance dosage: 125 to 375 mcg (0.125 to 0.375 mg) once daily.

Heart failure:

• *Loading dose* – According to the ACC/AHA guidelines, there is no reason to use loading doses to initiate digoxin therapy in patients with heart failure.

• *Maintenance dosage* – 125 to 250 mcg (0.125 to 0.25 mg) once daily. The low end of the dosing range (125 mcg [0.125 mg] once daily or every other day) should be used initially if the patient has renal function impairment, low lean body mass, or is older than 70 years of age. Higher dosages (eg, 375 to 500 mcg [0.375 to 0.5 mg]) are not needed and are rarely used.

➤*Children:*

Heart failure – In general, divided daily dosing is recommended for infants and young children (younger than 10 years of age). In the newborn period, renal clearance of digoxin is diminished and suitable dosage adjustments must be observed. This is especially pronounced in the premature infant. Beyond the immediate newborn period, children generally require proportionally larger doses than adults on the basis of body weight or surface area. Children older than 10 years of age require adult dosages in proportion to their body weight. Some researchers have suggested that infants and young children tolerate slightly higher serum concentrations than adults.

Maintenance dosage: The following information is according to the prescribing information (see Off-Label Dosing for alternative dosages). Daily maintenance doses for each age group are given in the following table and should provide therapeutic effects with minimum risk of toxicity in most patients with heart failure and healthy sinus rhythm. These recommendations assume the presence of healthy renal function.

Digoxin Oral Daily Maintenance Doses in Children with Healthy Renal Function

Age	Daily maintenance dose
2 to 5 years	10 to 15 mcg/kg
5 to 10 years	7 to 10 mcg/kg
≥ 10 years	3 to 5 mcg/kg

In children with renal disease, carefully titrate digoxin dosing based upon desired clinical response.

DIGOXIN — ORAL

Off-label dosing –

11 years of age or older and less than 100 kg:

• *Initial dosage* – 5 to 7.5 mcg/kg initially, then 2.5 to 3.75 mcg/kg every 8 to 18 hours for 2 doses. Obtain ECG 6 hours after dose to assess for toxicity.

• *Maintenance dosage* – 2.5 to 5 mcg/kg once daily.

2 to 10 years of age:

• *Initial dosage* – 15 to 20 mcg/kg initially, then 7.5 to 10 mcg/kg every 8 to 18 hours for 2 doses. Obtain ECG 6 hours after dose to assess for toxicity.

• *Maintenance dosage* – 4 to 5 mcg/kg twice daily.

23 months and younger:

• *Initial dosage* – 20 to 25 mcg/kg initially, then 10 to 12.5 mcg/kg every 8 to 18 hours for 2 doses. Obtain ECG 6 hours after dose to assess for toxicity.

• *Maintenance dosage* – 5 to 6 mcg/kg twice daily.

Neonates, full term:

• *Initial dosage* – 15 mcg/kg initially, then 7.5 mcg/kg every 8 to 18 hours for 2 doses. Obtain ECG 6 hours after dose to assess for toxicity.

• *Maintenance dosage* – 4 to 5 mcg/kg twice daily.

• *Alternative dosage –*

49 weeks or older postmenstrual age: 50 mcg/kg/day divided into 3 doses as a loading dose, then 6 mcg/kg every 12 hours.

37 to 48 weeks postmenstrual age: 40 mcg/kg/day divided into 3 doses as a loading dose, then 5 mcg/kg every 12 hours.

Premature:

• *Initial dosage* – 10 mcg/kg initially, then 5 mcg/kg every 8 to 18 hours for 2 doses. Obtain ECG 6 hours after dose to assess for toxicity.

• *Maintenance dosage* – 2.5 mcg/kg twice daily.

• *Alternative dosage –*

30 to 36 weeks postmenstrual age: 25 mcg/kg/day divided into 3 doses as a loading dose, then 6 mcg/kg once daily.

29 weeks or younger postmenstrual age: 20 mcg/kg/day divided into 3 doses as a loading dose, then 5 mcg/kg once daily.

➤*Elderly:* Because elderly patients are more likely to have decreased renal function, take care in dose selection, which should be based on renal function.

Per the Beers list, digoxin should not exceed 0.125 mg/day, except when treating atrial arrhythmias.

➤*Renal function impairment:*

Loading dose – For rapid digitalization, projected peak body stores for patients with renal impairment should be conservative (ie, 6 to 10 mcg/kg).

Maintenance-dose – Digoxin is primarily excreted by the kidneys; therefore, patients with impaired renal function require smaller than usual maintenance doses of digoxin.

CrCl 10 to 50 mL/min: 25% to 75% of the normal dose or usual dose every 36 hours.

CrCl less than 10 mL/min or hemodialysis: 10% to 25% of the normal dose or usual dose every 48 hours.

➤*Conversion:* The difference in bioavailability between digoxin injection or digoxin solution or tablets must be considered when changing patients from one dosage form to another.

Comparisons of the Systemic Availability and Equivalent Doses for Preparations of Digoxin

Product	Absolute bioavailability	Equivalent doses (mcg)[a] among dosage forms			
Digoxin tablets	60% to 80%	62.5	125	250	500
Digoxin oral solution	70% to 85%	62.5	125	250	500
Digoxin injection/IV	100%	50	100	200	400

[a] For example, digoxin 125 mcg (0.125 mg) tablets equivalent to digoxin 125 mcg (0.125 mg) oral solution equivalent to digoxin 100 mcg (0.1 mg) injection/IV.

➤*Therapeutic drug monitoring:* In general, determine the dose of digoxin on clinical grounds. However, measurement of serum digoxin concentrations can be helpful in determining the adequacy of digoxin therapy and in assigning certain probabilities to the likelihood of digoxin intoxication. About two-thirds of adults considered adequately digitalized (without evidence of toxicity) have serum digoxin concentrations ranging from 0.8 to 2 ng/mL. However, digoxin may produce clinical benefits even at serum concentrations below this range. About two-thirds of adult patients with clinical toxicity have serum digoxin concentrations of more than 2 ng/mL. However, because one-third of patients with clinical toxicity have concentrations less than 2 ng/mL, values less than 2 ng/mL do not rule out the possibility that a certain sign or symptom is related to digoxin therapy. Rarely, there are patients who are unable to tolerate digoxin at serum concentrations less than 0.8 ng/mL. Consequently, always interpret the serum concentration of digoxin in the overall clinical context, and do not use an isolated measurement alone as the basis for increasing or decreasing the dose of the drug.

To allow adequate time for equilibration of digoxin between serum and tissue, perform sampling of serum concentrations just before the next scheduled dose of the drug. If this is not possible, perform sampling at least 6 to 8 hours after the last dose, regardless of the route of administration or the formulation used. On a once-daily dosing schedule, the concentration of digoxin will be 10% to 25% lower when sampled at 24 versus 8 hours, depending upon the patient's renal function. On a twice-daily dosing schedule, there will be only minor differences in serum digoxin concentrations whether sampling is done at 8 or 12 hours after a dose.

If a discrepancy exists between the reported serum concentration and the observed clinical response, consider the following possibilities:

1.) Analytical problems in the assay procedure.
2.) Inappropriate serum-sampling time.
3.) Administration of a digitalis glycoside other than digoxin.
4.) Conditions causing an alteration in the sensitivity of the patient to digoxin (eg, restrictive cardiomyopathy, constrictive pericarditis, amyloid heart disease, acute cor pulmonale). Patients with idiopathic hypertrophic subaortic stenosis may have worsening of the outflow obstruction because of the inotropic effects of digoxin.
5.) Serum digoxin concentration may decrease acutely during periods of exercise without any associated change in clinical efficacy because of increased binding of digoxin to skeletal muscle.

➤*Administration:*

Oral solution – The calibrated dropper supplied with each 60 mL bottle of digoxin oral solution is not appropriate to measure doses below 0.2 mL. Doses of less than 0.2 mL require appropriate methods or measuring devices designed to administer an accurate amount to the patient.

➤*Storage/Stability:* Store at 25°C (77°F); excursions are permitted between 15° and 30°C (59° and 86°F). Store in a dry place and protect from light.

Actions

➤*Pharmacology:* Digoxin inhibits sodium-potassium adenosine triphosphatase, an enzyme that regulates the quantity of sodium and potassium inside cells. Inhibition of the enzyme leads to an increase in the intracellular concentration of sodium and, thus (by stimulation of sodium-calcium exchange), an increase in the intracellular concentration of calcium. The beneficial effects of digoxin result from direct actions on cardiac muscle, as well as indirect actions on the cardiovascular system, mediated by effects on the autonomic nervous system.

Autonomic effects – The autonomic effects include the following:

1.) A vagomimetic action, which is responsible for the effects of digoxin on the sinoatrial and atrioventricular (AV) nodes.
2.) Baroreceptor sensitization, which results in increased afferent inhibitory activity and reduced activity of the sympathetic nervous system and renin-angiotensin system for any given increment in mean arterial pressure.

Pharmacologic consequences – The pharmacologic consequences of these direct and indirect effects are the following:

1.) An increase in the force and velocity of myocardial systolic contraction (positive inotropic action).
2.) A decrease in the degree of activation of the sympathetic nervous system and renin-angiotensin system (neurohormonal deactivating effect).
3.) Slowing of the heart rate and decreased conduction velocity through the AV node (vagomimetic effect).

The effects of digoxin in heart failure are mediated by its positive inotropic and neurohormonal, deactivating effects, whereas the effects of the drug in atrial arrhythmias are related to its vagomimetic actions. In high doses, digoxin increases sympathetic outflow from the CNS. This increase in sympathetic activity may be an important factor in digitalis toxicity.

Pharmacodynamics – The times to onset of pharmacologic effect and to peak effect of preparations of digoxin are shown in the following table.

Times to Onset of Pharmacologic Effect and to Peak Effect of Preparations of Digoxin

Product	Time to onset of effect[a]	Time to peak effect[a]
Digoxin tablets	0.5 to 2 h	2 to 6 h
Digoxin oral solution	0.5 to 2 h	2 to 6 h
Digoxin injection/IV	5 to 30 min[b]	1 to 4 h

[a] Documented for ventricular response rate in atrial fibrillation, inotropic effects and electrocardiographic effects.
[b] Depending upon rate of infusion.

Hemodynamic – Digoxin produces hemodynamic improvement in patients with heart failure. Short- and long-term therapy with the drug increases cardiac output and lowers pulmonary artery pressure, pulmonary capillary wedge pressure, and systemic vascular resistance. These hemodynamic effects are accompanied by an increase in the LVEF and a decrease in end-systolic and end-diastolic dimensions.

➤*Pharmacokinetics:*

Absorption –

Tablets: Following oral administration, peak serum concentrations of digoxin occur at 1 to 3 hours. Absorption of digoxin from digoxin tablets has been demonstrated to be 60% to 80% complete compared with an identical IV dose of digoxin. Comparisons of the systemic availability and equivalent doses for preparation of digoxin are shown in the following table.

Oral solution: Following oral administration, peak serum concentrations of digoxin occur at 30 to 90 minutes. In children and adult volunteers, absolute bioavailability of digoxin from the solution formulation is 70% to 85%, similar to that seen (in adults) with standard tablets (60% to 80%). Digoxin absorption may be affected by various concomitant therapy modulating gastric pH and P-glycoprotein.

Tablets and solution: Comparisons of the systemic availability and equivalent doses for oral preparations of digoxin are shown in the following table.

DIGOXIN — ORAL

In some patients, orally administered digoxin is converted to inactive reduction products (eg, dihydrodigoxin) by colonic bacteria in the gut. Data suggest that 1 in 10 patients treated with digoxin tablets will degrade 40% or more of the ingested dose. As a result, certain antibiotics may increase the absorption of digoxin in such patients. Although inactivation of these bacteria by antibiotics is rapid, the serum digoxin concentration will rise at a rate consistent with the elimination half-life of digoxin. The magnitude of rise in serum digoxin concentration relates to the extent of bacterial inactivation, and may be as much as 2-fold in some cases.

Effect of food: When digoxin tablets are taken after meals, the rate of absorption is slowed, but the total amount of digoxin absorbed is usually unchanged. When the solution is taken after meals, the peak serum concentrations increase by 20% and the total amount of digoxin absorbed increases by 43%, but the rate of digoxin absorption is unchanged. When taken with meals high in bran fiber, the amount absorbed from an oral dose may be reduced.

Distribution – Following drug administration, a 6- to 8-hour tissue-distribution phase is observed. This is followed by a much more gradual decline in the serum concentration of the drug, which is dependent on the elimination of digoxin from the body. The peak height and slope of the early portion (absorption/distribution phases) of the serum concentration-time curve are dependent upon the route of administration and the absorption characteristics of the formulation. Clinical evidence indicates that the early high serum concentrations do not reflect the concentration of digoxin at its site of action, but that with chronic use, the steady-state postdistribution serum concentrations are in equilibrium with tissue concentrations and correlate with pharmacologic effects. In individual patients, these postdistribution serum concentrations may be useful in evaluating therapeutic and toxic effects.

Digoxin is concentrated in tissues and, therefore, has a large apparent volume of distribution. Digoxin crosses both the blood-brain barrier and placenta. At delivery, the serum digoxin concentration in the newborn is similar to the serum concentration in the mother. Approximately 25% of digoxin in the plasma is bound to protein. Serum digoxin concentrations are not significantly altered by large changes in fat tissue weight, so that its distribution space correlates best with lean (ie, ideal) body weight, not total body weight.

Metabolism – Only a small percentage (16%) of a dose of digoxin is metabolized. The end metabolites, which include 3-beta-digoxigenin, 3-keto-digoxigenin, and their glucuronide and sulfate conjugates, are polar in nature and are postulated to be formed via hydrolysis, oxidation, and conjugation. The metabolism of digoxin is not dependent upon the cytochrome P450 (CYP-450) system, and digoxin is not known to induce or inhibit the CYP-450 system.

Excretion – Elimination of digoxin follows first-order kinetics (that is, the quantity of digoxin eliminated at any time is proportional to the total body content). Following (IV administration to healthy volunteers, 50% to 70% of a digoxin dose is excreted unchanged in the urine. Renal excretion of digoxin is proportional to glomerular filtration rate and is largely independent of urine flow. In healthy volunteers (with healthy renal function), digoxin has a half-life of 1.5 to 2 days. The half-life in anuric patients is prolonged to 3.5 to 5 days. Digoxin is not effectively removed from the body by dialysis, exchange transfusion, or during cardiopulmonary bypass because most of the drug is bound to tissue and does not circulate in the blood.

Special populations –

Renal function impairment: The clearance of digoxin can be primarily correlated with renal function as indicated by CrCl (see also Warnings/Precautions).

Elderly: Adjust the dose of digoxin in elderly patients based on renal function.

Children: For children with known or suspected renal dysfunction, consider lower starting doses combined with frequent monitoring of digoxin levels.

Gender: No clinically significant gender differences in digoxin pharmacokinetics have been reported.

Thyroid status: In hyperthyroidism, lower serum digoxin concentrations have been reported because of decreased absorption of digoxin. Patients with hypothyroidism may require smaller doses of digoxin because of the higher serum digoxin concentrations observed in such patients.

Malabsorption conditions: The absorption of digoxin is reduced in some malabsorption conditions.

Contraindications

Ventricular fibrillation; hypersensitivity to digoxin or to other digitalis preparations.

Warnings/Precautions

➤*Sinus node disease and AV block:* Because digoxin slows sinoatrial and AV conduction, the drug commonly prolongs the PR interval. The drug may cause severe sinus bradycardia or sinoatrial block in patients with preexisting sinus node disease and may cause advanced or complete heart block in patients with preexisting incomplete AV block. In such patients, consider the insertion of a pacemaker before treatment with digoxin.

➤*Accessory AV pathway (Wolff-Parkinson-White syndrome):* After IV digoxin therapy, some patients with paroxysmal atrial fibrillation or flutter and a coexisting accessory AV pathway have developed increased antegrade conduction across the accessory pathway bypassing the AV node, leading to a very rapid ventricular response or ventricular fibrillation. Unless conduction down the accessory pathway has been blocked (pharmacologically or by surgery), do not use digoxin in such patients. The treatment of paroxysmal supraventricular tachycardia in such patients is usually direct-current cardioversion.

➤*Preserved left ventricular systolic function:* Patients with certain disorders involving heart failure associated with preserved LVEF may be particularly susceptible to toxicity of the drug. Such disorders include restrictive cardiomyopathy, constrictive pericarditis, amyloid heart disease, and acute cor pulmonale. Patients with idiopathic hypertrophic subaortic stenosis may have worsening of the outflow obstruction because of the inotropic effects of digoxin.

➤*Renal function impairment:* Digoxin is primarily excreted by the kidneys; therefore, patients with impaired renal function require smaller than usual maintenance doses of digoxin. Because of the prolonged elimination half-life, a longer period of time is required to achieve an initial or new steady-state serum concentration in patients with renal impairment than in patients with healthy renal function. If appropriate care is not taken to reduce the dose of digoxin, such patients are at high risk for toxicity, and toxic effects will last longer in such patients than in patients with healthy renal function.

➤*Special risk:*

Electrolyte disorders – In patients with hypokalemia or hypomagnesemia, toxicity may occur despite serum digoxin concentrations less than 2 ng/mL, because potassium or magnesium depletion sensitizes the myocardium to digoxin. Therefore, it is desirable to maintain healthy serum potassium and magnesium concentrations in patients being treated with digoxin. Deficiencies of these electrolytes may result from diarrhea, malnutrition, or prolonged vomiting, as well as the use of the following drugs or procedures: amphotericin B, antacids, corticosteroids, dialysis, diuretics, and mechanical suction of GI secretions.

Hypercalcemia from any cause predisposes the patient to digitalis toxicity. Calcium, particularly when administered rapidly by the IV route, may produce serious arrhythmias in digitalized patients. On the other hand, hypocalcemia can nullify the effects of digoxin in humans; thus, digoxin may be ineffective until serum calcium is restored to healthy levels. These interactions are related to the fact that digoxin affects contractility and excitability of the heart in a manner similar to that of calcium.

Thyroid disorders and hypermetabolic states – Hypothyroidism may reduce the requirements for digoxin. Heart failure and/or atrial arrhythmias resulting from hypermetabolic or hyperdynamic states (eg, arteriovenous shunt, hyperthyroidism, hypoxia) are best treated by addressing the underlying condition. Atrial arrhythmias associated with hypermetabolic states are particularly resistant to digoxin treatment. Take care to avoid toxicity if digoxin is used.

Acute myocardial infarction – Use digoxin with caution in patients with acute myocardial infarction. The use of inotropic drugs in some patients in this setting may result in undesirable increases in myocardial oxygen demand and ischemia.

Electrical cardioversion – It may be desirable to reduce the dose of digoxin for 1 to 2 days prior to electrical cardioversion of atrial fibrillation to avoid the induction of ventricular arrhythmias, but consider the consequences of increasing the ventricular response if digoxin is withdrawn. If digitalis toxicity is suspected, delay elective cardioversion. If it is not prudent to delay cardioversion, select the lowest possible energy level to avoid provoking ventricular arrhythmias.

➤*Pregnancy:* Category C. Digoxin crosses the placenta. At delivery, the serum digoxin concentration in the newborn is similar to the serum concentration of the mother. Give digoxin to a pregnant woman only if clearly needed. Digoxin has been used for both maternal and fetal indications (eg, congestive heart failure and supraventricular tachycardia) during all stages of gestation without causing fetal harm. Direct administration of digoxin to the fetus by periodic intramuscular (IM) injections has been used to treat supraventricular tachycardia when indirect therapy via the mother failed to control arrhythmia.

➤*Lactation:* Studies have shown that digoxin concentrations in the mother's serum and milk are similar. Digoxin milk:plasma ratios have varied from 0.6 to 0.9. Although these amounts seem high, they represent very small amounts of digoxin because of significant maternal protein binding. The estimated exposure of a breast-feeding infant to digoxin via breast-feeding will be far below the usual infant maintenance dose. Therefore, this amount should have no pharmacologic effect on the infant. No adverse effects in the breast-feeding infant have been reported. Nevertheless, exercise caution when digoxin is administered to a breast-feeding woman. The American Academy of Pediatrics classified digoxin as compatible with breast-feeding.

➤*Children:* Newborn infants display considerable variability in their tolerance to digoxin. Premature and immature infants are particularly sensitive to the effects of digoxin. Reduce and individualize the dosage of the drug according to their degrees of maturity.

Digoxin increases myocardial contractility in children with congestive heart failure. There are no controlled, randomized studies of digoxin in children with atrial tachyarrhythmias.

➤*Elderly:* The majority of clinical experience gained with digoxin has been in the elderly population. This experience has not identified differences in response or adverse effects between the elderly and younger patients. However, this drug is known to be substantially excreted by the kidney, and the risk of toxic reactions to this drug may be greater in patients with impaired renal function. Because elderly patients are more likely to have decreased renal function, take care in dose selection, which should be based on renal function. It may be useful to monitor renal function.

DIGOXIN — ORAL

See Administration and Dosage for more information.

➤*Lab test abnormalities:* The use of therapeutic doses of digoxin may cause prolongation of the PR interval and depression of the ST segment on the ECG. Digoxin may produce false-positive ST-T changes on the electrocardiogram during exercise testing. These electrophysiologic effects reflect an expected effect of the drug and are not indicative of toxicity.

➤*Monitoring:* Patients receiving digoxin should have their serum electrolytes and renal functions (serum creatinine concentrations) assessed periodically; the frequency of assessments depends on the clinical setting.

See also Therapeutic Drug Monitoring in Administration & Dosage.

Assays of digoxin levels in serum are widely available. Digoxin levels in saliva do not correlate well with those in serum.

Drug Interactions

Because digoxin has a narrow therapeutic index, routine monitoring of the clinical response of the patient and digoxin serum concentrations for possible drug interactions is appropriate. Drug interactions occurring with drugs that have a narrow therapeutic index can be life-threatening or have serious clinical consequences.

➤*Digoxin clearance:* Numerous drugs may alter digoxin clearance. Itraconazole may reduce digoxin clearance, increasing digoxin serum concentrations and the risk of toxicity, while rifampin may decrease digoxin clearance by increasing non-renal clearance.

➤*GI motility:* By slowing GI motility, drugs (eg, diphenoxylate) may increase digoxin absorption. In contrast, drugs (eg, metoclopramide) that increase GI motility may decrease digoxin absorption.

➤*Digoxin reduction products:* In approximately 10% of the population, digoxin is metabolized to inactive metabolites (ie, digoxin reduction products [DRPs]) by bacteria in the lower GI tract. Certain antibiotics (eg, tetracycline) reverse this process by altering GI flora, allowing more digoxin to be absorbed and increasing the risk of toxicity.

➤*Renal function:* Coadminister digoxin with caution with any drug that may cause renal function impairment. A decrease in glomerular filtration or tubular secretion may decrease digoxin elimination

Digoxin Oral Drug Interactions

Precipitant drug	Object drug[a]		Description
Acarbose	Digoxin	⬇	Digoxin serum concentrations may be reduced, decreasing the efficacy. Monitor digoxin serum concentrations and adjust the digoxin dose as needed.
Albuterol	Digoxin	⬇	Digoxin serum concentrations may be reduced, decreasing the efficacy. Monitor digoxin serum concentrations and adjust the digoxin dose as needed.
Alprazolam	Digoxin	⬆	Digoxin serum concentrations may be elevated, particularly in elderly patients, increasing the risk of toxicity. Monitor digoxin serum concentrations and observe the patient for evidence of digoxin toxicity. Adjust the digoxin dosage accordingly.
Aluminum salts (eg, aluminum hydroxide, kaolin-pectin, magaldrate)	Digoxin	⬇	Digoxin serum concentrations may be reduced, decreasing the efficacy. Administer digoxin ≥ 2 hours before the aluminum salt.
Amiloride	Digoxin	⬇	Amiloride may attenuate the positive inotropic effect of digoxin. If an interaction is suspected, discontinue one or both drugs. Increasing the digoxin dose does not appear to overcome the effects of this interaction.
Aminoglycosides (eg, neomycin)	Digoxin	⬆⬇	Variable effects. Digoxin pharmacologic effects may be increased or decreased. Observe the clinical response of the patient and monitor digoxin serum concentrations. Adjust the digoxin dose as needed.
Amphotericin B	Digoxin	⬆	Amphotericin B-induced hypokalemia may increase the risk of digoxin toxicity.
Antiarrhythmic agents (ie, amiodarone, dronedarone, propafenone, quinidine)	Digoxin	⬆	Digoxin serum concentrations may be elevated, increasing the pharmacologic effects and risk of toxicity. Monitor digoxin serum concentrations and observe the patient for evidence of digoxin toxicity. Adjust the digoxin dose accordingly. On initiation of one of these antiarrhythmic agents, consider reducing the digoxin dose ≈ 50% or discontinue.
Anticholinergics (eg, diphenoxylate, propantheline)	Digoxin	⬆	Digoxin absorption may be increased because of a decrease in GI motility. The effects of this interaction are product specific.
Antineoplastics (ie, bleomycin, carmustine, cyclophosphamide, cytarabine, doxorubicin, methotrexate, vincristine)	Digoxin	⬇	Digoxin serum concentrations may be reduced, decreasing the efficacy. Monitor digoxin serum concentrations and adjust the digoxin dose as needed.
Azole antifungal agents (ie, itraconazole, ketoconazole)	Digoxin	⬆	According to case reports, concomitant use may elevate digoxin serum concentrations. Monitor the digoxin serum concentration and adjust the digoxin dose as needed.
Beta-blockers (eg, carvedilol)	Digoxin	⬆	Although beta-blockers and digoxin may be useful in combination to control atrial fibrillation, their additive effects on AV node conduction may result in advanced or complete heart block. In addition, carvedilol may elevate digoxin serum concentrations, increasing the risk of toxicity. Monitor cardiac function and digoxin serum concentrations. Adjust treatment as needed. Consider decreasing the digoxin dose ≈ 25% in children receiving carvedilol concurrently.
Bile acid sequestrants (ie, cholestyramine, colestipol)	Digoxin	⬇	The bile acid sequestrant may physically bind with digoxin, decreasing GI absorption and enterohepatic recycling. Separate the administration times of both drugs by as much as possible and monitor digoxin serum concentrations. Adjust the digoxin dose as needed.
Calcium	Digoxin	⬆	Calcium administered rapidly by the IV route may produce serious arrhythmias in digitalized patients.
Calcium channel blockers (eg, diltiazem, nifedipine, nisoldipine, verapamil)	Digoxin	⬆	Although calcium channel blockers and digoxin may be useful in combination to control atrial fibrillation, their additive effects on AV node conduction may result in advanced or complete heart block. Diltiazem, nisoldipine, and verapamil may increase digoxin concentrations, increasing the risk of toxicity. Verapamil may increase digoxin serum concentrations as much as 75% during the first week of therapy, increasing the risk of toxicity. Monitor digoxin serum concentrations when starting, stopping, or changing the dose of diltiazem or nifedipine, and adjust the digoxin dosage accordingly.

DIGOXIN — ORAL

Digoxin Oral Drug Interactions			
Precipitant drug	Object drug[a]		Description
Cyclosporine	Digoxin	↑	Digoxin serum concentrations may be elevated, increasing the pharmacologic effects and risk of toxicity. Monitor digoxin serum concentrations and observe the patient for evidence of digoxin toxicity. Adjust the digoxin dosage accordingly.
Epoprostenol	Digoxin	↑	Digoxin serum concentrations may be elevated after stating epoprostenol, which may be clinically important in patients prone to digoxin toxicity.
Ginseng	Digoxin	↑	Digoxin serum concentrations may be elevated, increasing the risk of toxicity. Monitor digoxin serum concentrations and observe the patient for evidence of digoxin toxicity; adjust the digoxin dosage accordingly.
Hydantoins (eg, phenytoin)	Digoxin	↑↓	Variable effects. Digoxin pharmacologic effects may be increased or decreased. Observe the clinical response of the patient and monitor digoxin serum concentration. Adjust the digoxin dose as needed.
Loop diuretics (eg, furosemide)	Digoxin	↑	Diuretic-induced electrolyte disturbances may predispose to digitalis-induced arrhythmias. Measure plasma levels of potassium and magnesium, and supplement low levels. Prevent further losses with dietary sodium restriction or potassium-sparing diuretics.
Macrolide and related antibiotics (eg, clarithromycin, erythromycin, telithromycin)	Digoxin	↑	Digoxin serum concentrations may be elevated, increasing the risk of toxicity. The effect of the interaction may persist for several weeks after stopping the antibiotic. Monitor digoxin serum concentrations and observe the patient for evidence of digoxin toxicity. Adjust the digoxin dose accordingly.
Metoclopramide	Digoxin	↓	Digoxin absorption may be decreased because of an increase in GI motility. The effects of this interaction are product specific.
Nefazodone	Digoxin	↑	Digoxin serum concentrations may be elevated, increasing the pharmacologic effects and risk of toxicity. Monitor digoxin serum concentrations and observe the patient for evidence of digoxin toxicity. Adjust the digoxin dosage accordingly.
Nonsteroidal anti-inflammatory (ie, diclofenac, ibuprofen, indomethacin)	Digoxin	↑	Digoxin serum concentrations may be elevated, increasing the toxic effects. The effect of ibuprofen on digoxin appears to be transient. Monitor digoxin serum concentrations and observe the patient for evidence of digoxin toxicity. Adjust the digoxin dose accordingly.
Penicillamine	Digoxin	↓	Digoxin serum concentrations may be reduced, decreasing the pharmacologic effects. Monitor digoxin serum concentrations and observe the clinical response of the patient. Adjust the digoxin dosage accordingly.

Digoxin Oral Drug Interactions			
Precipitant drug	Object drug[a]		Description
Protease inhibitors (eg, ritonavir, saquinavir)	Digoxin	↑	Certain protease inhibitors may elevate digoxin serum concentrations, increasing the pharmacologic effects and risk of toxicity. Monitor digoxin serum concentrations and observe the patient for evidence of digoxin toxicity. Adjust the digoxin dosage accordingly.
Proton pump inhibitors (eg, lansoprazole, omeprazole, rabeprazole)	Digoxin	↑↓	Omeprazole and rabeprazole may elevate digoxin serum concentrations, increasing the risk of toxicity. In contrast, lansoprazole and esomeprazole may decrease digoxin serum concentrations. Monitor digoxin serum concentrations and adjust the digoxin dose as needed.
Quinine	Digoxin	↑	Digoxin serum concentrations may be elevated, increasing the pharmacologic effects and risk of toxicity. Monitor digoxin serum concentrations and observe the patient for evidence of digoxin toxicity. Adjust the digoxin dosage accordingly.
Ranolazine	Digoxin	↑	Digoxin serum concentrations may be elevated 1.5-fold, increasing the pharmacologic effects and risk of toxicity. Monitor digoxin serum concentrations and observe the patient for evidence of digoxin toxicity. Adjust the digoxin dosage accordingly.
Rifamycins (eg, rifampin)	Digoxin	↓	Digoxin serum concentrations may be reduced, decreasing the efficacy, especially in patients with renal function impairment. Monitor digoxin serum concentrations and adjust the digoxin dose as needed.
Serotonin reuptake inhibitors (eg, fluoxetine, paroxetine, sertraline)	Digoxin	↑	Digoxin serum concentrations may be elevated, increasing the pharmacologic effects and risk of toxicity. Monitor digoxin serum concentrations and observe the patient for evidence of digoxin toxicity. Adjust the digoxin dosage accordingly.
Spironolactone	Digoxin	↑	Spironolactone may attenuate the positive inotropic effect of digoxin. Digoxin serum concentrations may be elevated. In addition, spironolactone may interfere with digoxin assay, resulting in falsely elevated levels. Monitor patients closely and be aware of potentially false concentrations.
St. John's wort	Digoxin	↓	Digoxin serum concentrations may be reduced because of induction of intestinal P-glycoprotein activity, decreasing digoxin efficacy. Monitor digoxin serum concentrations and adjust the digoxin dose as needed.
Succinylcholine	Digoxin	↑	Succinylcholine may cause a sudden extrusion of potassium from muscle cells, thereby causing arrhythmias in digitalized patients.
Sucralfate	Digoxin	↓	Digoxin serum concentrations may be reduced, decreasing the efficacy. Monitor digoxin serum concentrations. Separate the administration times by ≥ 2 hours.
Sulfasalazine	Digoxin	↓	Digoxin serum concentrations may be reduced, decreasing the efficacy. Monitor digoxin serum concentrations. If an interaction is suspected, it may be necessary to discontinue sulfasalazine.

DIGOXIN — ORAL

Digoxin Oral Drug Interactions			
Precipitant drug	Object drug[a]		Description
Sympathomimetics	Digoxin	↑	Concomitant use increases the risk of cardiac arrhythmias.
Telmisartan	Digoxin	↑	Digoxin peak and trough serum concentrations may be elevated ≈ 50% and 20%, respectively, increasing the risk of digoxin toxicity. Monitor digoxin serum concentrations and adjust the digoxin dosage accordingly.
Tetracyclines (eg, tetracycline)	Digoxin	↑	In ≈ 10% of patients, digoxin serum concentrations may be increased because of alterations in the GI flora, allowing more digoxin to be absorbed. The effect may persist for several months after stopping the tetracycline. The effects of this interaction are product specific.
Thiazide diuretics (eg, hydrochlorothiazide)	Digoxin	↑	Diuretic-induced electrolyte disturbances may predispose to digitalis-induced arrhythmias. Measure plasma levels of potassium and magnesium and supplement low levels. Prevent further losses with dietary sodium restriction or potassium-sparing diuretics.
Thioamines (eg, methimazole, propylthiouracil)	Digoxin	↑	Hyperthyroid patients may require a reduced dose of digoxin if they become euthyroid.
Thyroid hormones (eg, levothyroxine)	Digoxin	↓	Thyroid administration to a digitalized, hypothyroid patient may increase the dose requirement of digoxin.
Tramadol	Digoxin	↑	Postmarketing experience has revealed rare reports of digoxin toxicity during coadministration with tramadol.
Vasopressin receptor antagonists (eg, conivaptan)	Digoxin	↑	Digoxin serum concentrations may be elevated, increasing the pharmacologic effects and risk of toxicity. Observe the clinical response of the patient and monitor digoxin concentrations. Adjust the digoxin dose as needed.
Digoxin	Dofetilide	↑	Coadministration of digoxin and dofetilide has been associated with an increased rate of torsades de pointes compared with dofetilide alone.

[a] ↑ = object drug increased; ↓ = object drug decreased.

➤*Drug/Food interaction:* Food, especially high-fiber meals, may decrease digoxin absorption.

➤*Drug/Lab test interactions:* Endogenous substances of unknown composition (digoxin-like immunoreactive substances [DLIS]) can interfere with standard radioimmunoassays for digoxin. The interference most often causes results to be falsely positive or falsely elevated, but sometimes it causes results to falsely reduced. Some assays are more subject to these failings than others. A liquid chromatography-mass spectrometry-mass (LC/MS/MS) method is available that may provide a more accurate determination of plasma digoxin levels; however, clinical trials have not been conducted to determine its susceptibility to DLIS interference. DLIS are present in up to half of all neonates and in varying percentages of pregnant women, patients with hypertrophic cardiomyopathy, patients with renal or hepatic dysfunction, and other patients who are volume-expanded for any reason. The measured levels of DLIS (as digoxin equivalents) are usually low (0.2 to 0.4 ng/mL), but sometimes they reach levels that would be considered therapeutic or even toxic.

In some assays spironolactone may be falsely detected as digoxin, at levels up to 0.5 ng/mL. Some traditional Chinese medicines cause similar interference.

Spironolactone and DLIS are much more extensively protein-bound than digoxin. As a result, assays of free digoxin levels (which tend to be about 25% less than total levels, consistent with the usual extent of protein binding) are not affected by spironolactone or DLIS.

Adverse Reactions

In general, the adverse reactions of digoxin are dose dependent and occur at doses higher than those needed to achieve a therapeutic effect. Hence, adverse reactions are less common when digoxin is used within the recommended dose range or therapeutic serum concentration range and when there is careful attention to concurrent medications and conditions.

Because some patients may be particularly susceptible to side effects with digoxin, always select the dosage of the drug carefully and adjust as the clinical condition of the patient warrants. In the past, when high doses of digoxin were used and little attention was paid to clinical status or concurrent medications, adverse reactions to digoxin were more frequent and severe. Cardiac adverse reactions accounted for about one-half, GI disturbances for approximately one-fourth, and CNS and other toxicity for approximately one-fourth of these adverse reactions. However, available evidence suggests that the incidence and severity of digoxin toxicity has decreased substantially in recent years. In recent controlled clinical trials, in patients with predominantly mild to moderate heart failure, the incidence of adverse reactions was comparable in patients taking digoxin and in those taking placebo. In a large mortality trial, the incidence of hospitalization for suspected digoxin toxicity was 2% in patients taking digoxin compared with 0.9% in patients taking placebo. In this trial, the most common manifestations of digoxin toxicity included GI disturbances and cardiac disturbances; CNS manifestations were less common.

➤*Adults:*

Cardiovascular – Therapeutic doses of digoxin may cause heart block in patients with preexisting sinoatrial or AV conduction disorders; avoid heart block by adjusting the dose of digoxin. Consider prophylactic use of a cardiac pacemaker if the risk of heart block is considered unacceptable. High doses of digoxin may produce a variety of rhythm disturbances, such as first-degree, second-degree (Wenckebach), or third-degree heart block (including asystole); atrial tachycardia with block; AV dissociation; accelerated junctional (nodal) rhythm; unifocal or multiform ventricular premature contractions (especially bigeminy or trigeminy); ventricular tachycardia; and ventricular fibrillation. Digoxin produces PR prolongation and ST-segment depression, which should not by themselves be considered digoxin toxicity. Cardiac toxicity can also occur at therapeutic doses in patients who have conditions that may alter their sensitivity to digoxin. Such disorders include acute cor pulmonale, amyloid heart disease, constrictive pericarditis, and restrictive cardiomyopathy. Patients with idiopathic hypertrophic subaortic stenosis may have worsening of the outflow obstruction because of the inotropic effects of digoxin.

CNS – Digoxin can produce apathy, confusion, dizziness, headache, mental disturbances (eg, anxiety, depression, delirium, hallucination), visual disturbances (blurred or yellow vision), and weakness.

GI – Digoxin may cause anorexia, diarrhea, nausea, and vomiting. Rarely, the use of digoxin has been associated with abdominal pain, hemorrhagic necrosis of the intestines, and intestinal ischemia.

Miscellaneous – Gynecomastia has been occasionally observed following the prolonged use of digoxin. Thrombocytopenia and maculopapular rash and other skin reactions have been rarely observed. The following table summarizes the incidence of those adverse reactions previously listed for patients treated with digoxin tablets or placebo from 2 randomized, double-blind, placebo-controlled withdrawal trials. Patients in these trials were also receiving diuretics with or without ACE inhibitors. These patients had been stable on digoxin, and were randomized to digoxin or placebo. The results shown in the following table reflect the experience in patients following dosage titration with the use of serum digoxin concentrations and careful follow-up. These adverse reactions are consistent with results from a large, placebo-controlled mortality trial (DIG trial) wherein more than half the patients were not receiving digoxin prior to enrollment.

Digoxin Oral Adverse Reactions in 2 Parallel, Double-Blind, Placebo-Controlled Withdrawal Trials (Number of Patients Reporting)		
Adverse reactions	Digoxin (n = 123)	Placebo (n = 125)
Cardiovascular		
Heart arrest	1	1
Palpitation	1	4
Tachycardia	2	1
Ventricular extrasystole	1	1
CNS		
Dizziness	6	5
Headache	4	4
Mental disturbances	5	1
GI		
Abdominal pain	0	6
Anorexia	1	4
Diarrhea	4	1
Nausea	4	2
Vomiting	2	1
Miscellaneous		
Death	4	3
Rash	2	1

➤*Children:* The side effects of digoxin in infants and children differ from those seen in adults in several respects. Although digoxin may produce anorexia, CNS disturbances, diarrhea, nausea, and vomiting in young

DIGOXIN — ORAL

patients, these are rarely the initial symptoms of overdosage. Rather, the earliest and most frequent manifestation of excessive dosing with digoxin in infants and children is the appearance of cardiac arrhythmias, including sinus bradycardia. In children, the use of digoxin may produce any arrhythmia. The most common are conduction disturbances or supraventricular tachyarrhythmias, such as atrial tachycardia (with or without block) and junctional (nodal) tachycardia. Ventricular arrhythmias are less common. Sinus bradycardia may be a sign of impending digoxin intoxication, especially in infants, even in the absence of first-degree heart block. Assume that any arrhythmia or alteration in cardiac conduction that develops in a child taking digoxin is caused by digoxin, until further evaluation proves otherwise.

Visual disturbances (blurred or yellow vision), headache, weakness, apathy, and psychosis can occur. These may be difficult to recognize in infants and children. In 1 reported case, asymmetric chorea was seen at high digoxin levels and reappeared when similar levels were inadvertently reachieved.

Overdosage

➤*Symptoms:* Manifestations of life-threatening toxicity include ventricular tachycardia or ventricular fibrillation, progressive bradyarrhythmias, or heart block. The administration of more than 10 mg of digoxin in a previously healthy adult or more than 4 mg in a previously healthy child, or a steady-state serum concentration of more than 10 ng/mL often results in cardiac arrest.

➤*Treatment:* Temporarily discontinue digoxin until the adverse reaction resolves. Make every effort to correct factors that may contribute to the adverse reaction (eg, concurrent medications, electrolyte disturbances). Once the adverse reaction has resolved, therapy with digoxin may be reinstituted, following a careful reassessment of dose.

Withdrawal of digoxin may be all that is required to treat the adverse reaction. However, when the primary manifestation of digoxin overdosage is a cardiac arrhythmia, additional therapy may be needed.

If the rhythm disturbance is a symptomatic bradyarrhythmia or heart block, consider the reversal of toxicity with digoxin immune fab (ovine), use of atropine, or insertion of a temporary cardiac pacemaker. However, asymptomatic bradycardia or heart block related to digoxin may require only temporary withdrawal of the drug and cardiac monitoring of the patient.

If the rhythm disturbance is a ventricular arrhythmia, consider the correction of electrolyte disorders, particularly if hypokalemia or hypomagnesemia is present. Digoxin immune fab (ovine) is a specific antidote for digoxin and may be used to reverse potentially life-threatening ventricular arrhythmias caused by digoxin overdosage.

Make every effort to maintain the serum potassium concentration between 4 and 5.5 mmol/L. Potassium is usually administered orally, but when correction of the arrhythmia is urgent and the serum potassium concentration is low, potassium may be administered cautiously by the IV route. Monitor the ECG for any evidence of potassium toxicity (eg, peaking of T waves) and observe the effect on the arrhythmia. Potassium salts may be dangerous in patients who manifest bradycardia or heart block because of digoxin (unless primarily related to supraventricular tachycardia) and in the setting of massive digitalis overdosage.

Massive overdosage –

Ensure that patients with massive digitalis ingestion receive large doses of activated charcoal to prevent absorption and bind digoxin in the gut during enteroenteric recirculation. Gastric lavage may be indicated especially if ingestion has occurred within 30 minutes of the patient's presentation at the hospital. If a patient presents more than 2 hours after ingestion or already has toxic manifestations, it may be unsafe to attempt passage of a gastric tube, because such maneuvers may induce an acute vagal episode that can worsen digitalis-related arrhythmias.

Severe digitalis intoxication can cause a massive shift of potassium from inside to outside the cell, leading to life-threatening hyperkalemia. The administration of potassium supplements in the setting of massive intoxication may be hazardous and should be avoided. Hyperkalemia caused by massive digitalis toxicity is best treated with digoxin immune fab (ovine); initial treatment with glucose and insulin may also be required if hyperkalemia itself is acutely life-threatening.

Patient Information

Instruct patient to check with their health care provider before taking any new medication, including over-the-counter medications.

Instruct patients to contact their health care provider right away if they experience vision changes (eg, blurred or yellow vision); mental changes; severe nausea, vomiting, or diarrhea; stomach pain; or unusual weakness.

DIGOXIN — INJECTION

Indications

➤*Atrial fibrillation:* For the control of ventricular response rate in patients with chronic atrial fibrillation.

➤*Heart failure:* Treatment of mild to moderate heart failure. Digoxin increases left ventricular ejection fraction (LVEF) and improves heart failure symptoms as evidenced by exercise capacity and heart failure-related hospitalizations and emergency care, while having no effect on mortality. Where possible, use digoxin with a diuretic and an angiotensin-converting enzyme (ACE) inhibitor, but an optimal order for starting these 3 drugs cannot be specified.

Administration and Dosage

➤*General dosing considerations:* Intramuscular (IM) injection of digoxin is extremely painful and offers no advantages, unless other routes of administration are contraindicated.

Recommended dosages of digoxin may require considerable modification because of individual sensitivity of the patient to the drug, the presence of associated conditions, or the use of concurrent medications. It cannot be overemphasized that dosage guidelines are based upon average patient response and substantial individual variation can be expected. Accordingly, base ultimate dosage selection upon clinical assessment of the patient.

Use parenteral administration of digoxin only when the need for rapid digitalization is urgent or when the drug cannot be taken orally.

In selecting a dose of digoxin, consider the following factors:

1.) The body weight of the patient. Calculate doses based upon lean (ie, ideal) body weight.
2.) The patient's renal function, preferably evaluated on the basis of estimated creatinine clearance (CrCl).
3.) The patient's age. Infants and children require different doses of digoxin than adults. Also, advanced age may be indicative of diminished renal function, even in patients with healthy serum creatinine concentration (ie, less than 1.5 mg/dL).
4.) Concomitant disease states, concurrent medications, or other factors likely to alter the pharmacokinetic or pharmacodynamic profile of digoxin (eg, electrolyte disturbances, hypothyroidism, restrictive cardiomyopathy).

Accomplish digitalization by either of 2 general approaches that vary in dosage and frequency of administration, but reach the same end point in terms of total amount of digoxin body stores. Calculate maintenance dose as a percentage of the loading dose.

1.) If rapid digitalization is considered medically appropriate, achieve it by administering a loading dose based upon projected peak digoxin body stores. Calculate maintenance dose as a percentage of the loading dose.
2.) Obtain more gradual digitalization by beginning an appropriate maintenance dose, thus allowing digoxin body stores to accumulate slowly. Steady-state serum digoxin concentrations will be achieved in approximately 5 half-lives of the drug for the individual patient. Depending on the patient's renal function, this will take between 1 and 3 weeks.

➤*Adults:*

Atrial fibrillation – See also off-label dosing for recommendations from the American College of Cardiology/American Heart Association (ACC/AHA) guidelines. The following information is according to the prescribing information.

Loading dose: Peak digoxin body stores larger than the 8 to 12 mcg/kg (0.008 to 0.012 mg/kg) required for most patients with heart failure and healthy sinus rhythm have been used for control of ventricular rate in patients with atrial fibrillation.

Maintenance dosage: Titrate doses of digoxin used for the treatment of chronic atrial fibrillation to the minimum dose that achieves the desired ventricular rate control without causing undesirable side effects. Data are not available to establish the appropriate resting or exercise target rates that should be achieved.

Heart failure – See also off-label dosing for recommendations from the ACC/AHA guidelines. The following information is according to the prescribing information. ACC/AHA guidelines state that loading doses are not needed.

Rapid digitalization: Peak body stores of 8 to 12 mcg/kg (0.008 to 0.012 mg/kg) should provide therapeutic effect with minimum risk of toxicity. Administer the loading dose in several portions, with roughly half of the total given as the first dose. Additional fractions of this planned total dose may be given at 6- to 8-hour intervals, with careful assessment of clinical response before each additional dose. If the patient's clinical response necessitates a change from the calculated loading dose of digoxin, base the calculation of the maintenance dose upon the amount actually given.

A single initial intravenous (IV) dose of 400 to 600 mcg (0.4 to 0.6 mg) of digoxin injection usually produces a detectable effect in 5 to 30 minutes that becomes maximal in 1 to 4 hours. Additional doses of 100 to 300 mcg (0.1 to 0.3 mg) may be given cautiously at 6- to 8-hour intervals until clinical evidence of an adequate effect is noted. The usual amount of digoxin injection that a 70 kg patient requires to achieve 8 to 12 mcg/kg (0.008 to 0.012 mg/kg) peak body stores is 600 to 1,000 mcg (0.6 to 1 mg).

Gradual digitalization:

• *Initial dosage –* Therapy is generally initiated at a dose of 250 mcg (0.25 mg) once daily in patients younger than 70 years of age with good renal function, at a dose of 125 mcg (0.125 mg) once daily in patients older than 70 years of age or with impaired renal function, and at a dose of 62.5 mcg (0.0625 mg) in patients with marked renal impairment.

• *Dosage titration –* Increase doses every 2 weeks according to clinical response. The digoxin dose has been generally titrated according to the patient's age, lean body weight, and renal function.

• *Maintenance dosage –* Dosages have ranged from 125 to 500 mcg orally (0.125 to 0.5 mg once daily).

Base the maintenance dose upon the percentage of the peak body stores lost each day through elimination. The following formula has had wide clinical use.

Maintenance dose = Peak body stores (ie, loading dose) × % daily loss/100, where % daily loss = 14 + CrCl/5.

CrCl is corrected to 70 kg body weight or 1.73 m^2 body surface area.

DIGOXIN — INJECTION

Off-label dosing –

Atrial fibrillation:

• *Loading dose* – 250 mcg (0.25 mg) IV every 2 hours, up to 1,500 mcg (1.5 mg) total dose, in an acute setting.

• *Maintenance dosage* – 125 to 375 mcg (0.125 to 0.375 mg) IV or orally once daily.

Heart failure:

• *Loading dose* – According to the ACC/AHA guidelines, there is no reason to use loading doses to initiate digoxin therapy in patients with heart failure.

• *Maintenance dosage* – 125 to 250 mcg (0.125 to 0.25 mg) once daily. The low end of the dosing range (125 mcg [0.125 mg] once daily or every other day) should be used initially if the patient has renal function impairment, low lean body mass, or is older than 70 years of age. Higher dosages (eg, 375 to 500 mcg [0.375 to 0.5 mg]) are not needed and rarely used.

➤*Children:*

Heart failure – In general, divided daily dosing is recommended for infants and young children (younger than 10 years of age). In the newborn period, renal clearance of digoxin is diminished and suitable dosage adjustments must be observed. This is especially pronounced in the premature infant. Beyond the immediate newborn period, children generally require proportionally larger doses than adults on the basis of body weight or body surface area. Children older than 10 years of age require adult dosages in proportion to their body weight. Some researchers have suggested that infants and young children tolerate slightly higher serum concentrations than adults.

Rapid digitalization: Administer the loading dose in several portions, with roughly half of the total given as the first dose. Give additional fractions of this planned total dose at 4- to 8-hour intervals, with careful assessment of clinical response before each additional dose. If the patient's clinical response necessitates a change from the calculated loading dose of digoxin, base the calculation of the maintenance dose upon the amount actually given. Digitalizing doses for each age group (according to the prescribing information) are given in the following table and should provide therapeutic effect with minimum risk of toxicity in most patients with heart failure and healthy sinus rhythm (see also Off-Label Dosing for alternative dosages).

Gradual digitalization: More gradual digitalization can also be accomplished by beginning an appropriate maintenance dose. Daily maintenance doses for each age group (according to the prescribing information) are given in the following table and should provide therapeutic effect with minimum risk of toxicity in most patients with heart failure and healthy sinus rhythm (see also Off-Label Dosing for alternative dosages).

These dosages assume the presence of healthy renal function. In children with renal disease, digoxin dosing must be carefully titrated based on clinical response.

Usual Digitalizing and Maintenance Dosages for Digoxin Pediatric Injection in Children With Healthy Renal Function Based on Lean Body Weight

Age	IV digitalizing[a] dose (mcg/kg)	Daily IV maintenance dose[b] (mcg/kg)
Premature	15 to 25	20% to 30% of the IV digitalizing dose[c]
Full term	20 to 30	25% to 35% of the IV digitalizing dose[c]
1 to 24 months	30 to 50	
2 to 5 years	25 to 35	
5 to 10 years	15 to 30	
> 10 years	8 to 12	

[a] IV digitalizing doses are 80% of oral digitalizing doses.
[b] Divided daily dosing is recommended for children younger than 10 years of age.
[c] Projected or actual digitalizing dose providing clinical response.

It cannot be overemphasized that these pediatric dosage guidelines are based on average patient response and substantial individual variation can be expected. Accordingly, base ultimate dosage selection upon clinical assessment of the patient.

Off-label dosing –

11 years of age or older and less than 100 kg:

• *Maximum dose* – 1 mg loading dose.

• *Loading dose* – 4 to 6 mcg/kg IV/IM initially, then 2 to 3 mcg/kg every 8 to 18 hours for 2 doses. Obtain ECG 6 hours after dose to assess for toxicity.

• *Maintenance dosage* – 2 to 3 mcg/kg/day IV/IM divided into 1 to 2 doses.

2 to 10 years of age:

• *Maximum dose* – 1 mg loading dose.

• *Loading dose* – 10 to 17.5 mcg/kg IV/IM initially, then 5 to 8.75 mcg/kg every 8 to 18 hours for 2 doses. Obtain ECG 6 hours after dose to assess for toxicity.

• *Maintenance dosage* – 3 to 5 mcg/kg IV/IM twice daily.

23 months and younger:

• *Maximum dose* – 1 mg loading dose.

• *Loading dose* – 15 to 25 mcg/kg IV/IM initially, then 7.5 to 12.5 mcg/kg every 8 to 18 hours for 2 doses. Obtain ECG 6 hours after dose to assess for toxicity.

• *Maintenance dosage* – 3.75 to 6 mcg/kg IV/IM twice daily.

Neonates, full-term:

• *Maximum dose* – 1 mg loading dose.

• *Loading dose* – 5 to 15 mcg/kg IV/IM initially, then 2.5 to 7.5 mcg/kg every 8 to 18 hours for 2 doses. Obtain ECG 6 hours after dose to assess for toxicity.

• *Maintenance dosage* – 3 to 5 mcg/kg IV/IM twice daily.

• *Alternative dosage* –

49 weeks or older postmenstrual age: 40 mcg/kg/day IV divided into 3 doses as a loading dose, then 5 mcg/kg IV every 12 hours. Adjust dosage based on clinical response.

37 to 48 weeks postmenstrual age: 30 mcg/kg/day IV divided into 3 doses as a loading dose, then 4 mcg/kg IV every 12 hours. Adjust dosage based on clinical response.

Neonates, premature:

• *Maximum dose* – 1 mg loading dose.

• *Loading dose* – 7.5 to 15 mcg/kg initially, then 3.75 to 7.5 mcg/kg every 8 to 18 hours for 2 doses. Obtain ECG 6 hours after dose to assess for toxicity.

• *Maintenance dosage* – 1.5 to 5 mcg/kg twice daily.

• *Alternative dosage* –

30 to 36 weeks postmenstrual age: 20 mcg/kg/day IV divided into 3 doses as a loading dose, then 5 mcg/kg IV once daily. Adjust dosage based on clinical response.

29 weeks or younger postmenstrual age: 15 mcg/kg/day IV divided into 3 doses as a loading dose, then 4 mcg/kg IV once daily. Adjust dosage based on clinical response.

➤*Elderly:* Because elderly patients are more likely to have decreased renal function, take care in dose selection.

Per the Beers list, digoxin should not exceed 0.125 mg/day, except when treating atrial arrhythmias.

➤*Renal function impairment:* Digoxin is primarily excreted by the kidneys; therefore, patients with impaired renal function require smaller than usual maintenance doses of digoxin.

Loading dose – Because of altered digoxin distribution and elimination, projected peak body stores for patients with renal insufficiency should be conservative (ie, 6 to 10 mcg/kg [0.006 to 0.01 mg/kg]).

Maintenance dose –

CrCl 10 to 50 mL/min: 25% to 75% normal dose or usual dose every 36 hours.

CrCl less than 10 mL/min or hemodialysis: 10% to 25% normal dose or usual dose every 48 hours.

➤*Conversion:* Use digoxin injection to achieve rapid digitalization with conversion to an oral formulation of digoxin for maintenance therapy. Consider the differences in bioavailability between injectable digoxin or digoxin tablets and oral solution when changing patients from 1 dosage form to another.

Comparisons of the systemic availability and equivalent doses for preparations of digoxin are shown in the following table:

Comparisons of the Systemic Availability and Equivalent Doses for Preparation of Digoxin

Product	Absolute bioavailability	Equivalent doses (mcg)[a] among dosage forms			
Digoxin tablets	60% to 80%	62.5	125	250	500
Digoxin oral solution	70% to 85%	62.5	125	250	500
Digoxin injection/IV	100%	50	100	200	400

[a] For example, digoxin 125 mcg (0.125 mg) tablets equivalent to digoxin 125 mcg (0.125 mg) oral solution equivalent to 100 mcg (0.1 mg) digoxin injection.

➤*Therapeutic drug monitoring:* In general, determine the dose of digoxin used on clinical grounds. However, measurement of serum digoxin concentrations can be helpful in determining the adequacy of digoxin therapy and in assigning certain probabilities to the likelihood of digoxin intoxication. About two-thirds of adults considered adequately digitalized (without evidence of toxicity) have serum digoxin concentrations ranging from 0.8 to 2 ng/mL. However, digoxin may produce clinical benefits even at serum concentrations below this range. About two-thirds of adult patients with clinical toxicity have serum digoxin concentrations more than 2 ng/mL. However, since one-third of patients with clinical toxicity have concentrations less than 2 ng/mL, values below 2 ng/mL do not rule out the possibility that a certain sign or symptom is related to digoxin therapy. Rarely, there are patients who are unable to tolerate digoxin at serum concentrations below 0.8 ng/mL. Consequently, the serum concentration of digoxin should always be interpreted in the overall clinical context; do not use an isolated measurement alone as the basis for increasing or decreasing the dose of the drug.

To allow adequate time for equilibration of digoxin between serum and tissue, perform sampling of serum concentrations just before the next scheduled dose of the drug. If this is not possible, perform sampling at least 6 to 8 hours after the last dose, regardless of the route of administration or the formulation used. On a once-daily dosing schedule, the concentration of digoxin will be 10% to 25% lower when sampled at 24 versus 8 hours, depending upon the patient's renal function. On a twice-daily dosing schedule, there will be only minor differences in serum digoxin concentrations whether sampling is done at 8 or 12 hours after a dose.

If a discrepancy exists between the reported serum concentration and the observed clinical response, consider the following possibilities:

1.) Analytical problems in the assay procedure.
2.) Inappropriate serum sampling time.
3.) Administration of a digitalis glycoside other than digoxin.

DIGOXIN — INJECTION

4.) Conditions (eg, electrolyte disturbances, hypothyroidism, restrictive cardiomyopathy) causing an alteration in the patient's sensitivity to digoxin.
5.) Serum digoxin concentration may decrease acutely during periods of exercise without any associated change in clinical efficacy because of increased binding of digoxin to skeletal muscle.

➤*Preparation for administration:* Administer digoxin undiluted or diluted with a 4-fold or greater volume of sterile water for injection, sodium chloride 0.9% injection, or dextrose 5% injection. The use of less than a 4-fold volume of diluent could lead to precipitation of the digoxin. Immediate use of the diluted product is recommended.

➤*Administration:* IM injection can lead to severe pain at the injection site; thus, IV administration is preferred. If the drug must be administered by the IM route, inject it deeply into the muscle and follow with massage.

If tuberculin syringes are used to measure very small doses, one must be aware of the problem of inadvertent overadministration of digoxin. Do not flush the syringe with the parenteral solution after its contents are expelled into an indwelling vascular catheter.

Slow infusion of digoxin is preferable to bolus administration. Rapid infusion of digitalis glycosides has been shown to cause systemic and coronary arteriolar constriction, which may be clinically undesirable. Caution is thus advised, and digoxin should probably be administered over a period of 5 minutes or longer.

Adults – Do not inject more than 500 mcg (0.5 mg) (2 mL) into a single site.

Children – Do not inject more than 200 mcg (0.2 mg) (2 mL) into a single site.

➤*Admixture compatibility:* According to manufacturer's prescribing information, mixing of digoxin with other drugs in the same container or simultaneous administration in the same IV line is not recommended.

➤*Storage/Stability:* Store at 25°C (77°F); excursions are permitted between 15° and 30°C (59° and 86°F). Protect from light.

Actions

➤*Pharmacology:* Digoxin inhibits sodium-potassium adenosine triphosphatase (ATPase), an enzyme that regulates the quantity of sodium and potassium inside cells. Inhibition of the enzyme leads to an increase in the intracellular concentration of sodium and thus (by stimulation of sodium-calcium exchange) an increase in the intracellular concentration of calcium. The beneficial effects of digoxin result from direct actions on cardiac muscle, as well as indirect actions on the cardiovascular system mediated by effects on the autonomic nervous system.

Autonomic effects – The autonomic effects include the following:

1.) A vagomimetic action, which is responsible for the effects of digoxin on the sinoatrial and atrioventricular (AV) nodes.
2.) Baroreceptor sensitization, which results in increased afferent inhibitory activity and reduced activity of the sympathetic nervous system and renin-angiotensin system for any given increment in mean arterial pressure.

Pharmacologic consequences – The pharmacologic consequences of these direct and indirect effects are the following:

1.) An increase in the force and velocity of myocardial systolic contraction (positive inotropic action).
2.) A decrease in the degree of activation of the sympathetic nervous system and renin-angiotensin system (neurohormonal deactivating effect).
3.) Slowing of the heart rate and decreased conduction velocity through the AV node (vagomimetic effect).

The effects of digoxin in heart failure are mediated by its positive inotropic and neurohormonal deactivating effects, whereas the effects of the drug in atrial arrhythmias are related to its vagomimetic actions. In high doses, digoxin increases sympathetic outflow from the CNS. This increase in sympathetic activity may be an important factor in digitalis toxicity.

Pharmacodynamics – The following are times to onset of pharmacologic effect and peak effect of digoxin preparations.

Times to Onset of Pharmacologic Effect and to Peak Effect of Preparations of Digoxin

Product	Time to onset of effect[a]	Time to peak effect[a]
Digoxin tablets	0.5 to 2 hours	2 to 6 hours
Digoxin oral solution	0.5 to 2 hours	2 to 6 hours
Digoxin injection/IV	5 to 30 minutes[b]	1 to 4 hours

[a] Documented for ventricular response rate in atrial fibrillation, inotropic effects, and ECG changes.
[b] Depending upon rate of infusion.

Hemodynamic – Digoxin produces hemodynamic improvement in patients with heart failure. Short- and long-term therapy with the drug increases cardiac output and lowers pulmonary artery pressure, pulmonary capillary wedge pressure, and systemic vascular resistance. These hemodynamic effects are accompanied by an increase in the left ventricular ejection fraction (LVEF) and a decrease in end-systolic and end-diastolic dimensions.

➤*Pharmacokinetics:* The following data are from studies performed in adults, unless otherwise stated.

Distribution – Following drug administration, a 6- to 8-hour tissue distribution phase is observed. This is followed by a much more gradual decline in the serum concentration of the drug, which is dependent on the elimination of digoxin from the body. The peak height and slope of the early portion (absorption/distribution phases) of the serum concentration-time curve are dependent upon the route of administration and the absorption characteristics of the formulation. Clinical evidence indicates that the early high serum concentrations do not reflect the concentration of digoxin at its site of action, but that with chronic use, the steady-state postdistribution serum concentrations are in equilibrium with tissue concentrations and correlate with pharmacologic effects. In individual patients, these postdistribution serum concentrations may be useful in evaluating therapeutic and toxic effects.

Digoxin is concentrated in tissues and, therefore, has a large apparent volume of distribution. Digoxin crosses both the blood-brain barrier and the placenta. At delivery, the serum digoxin concentration in the newborn is similar to the serum concentration in the mother. Approximately 25% of digoxin in the plasma is bound to protein. Serum digoxin concentrations are not significantly altered by large changes in fat tissue weight, so that its distribution space correlates best with lean (ie, ideal) body weight, not total body weight.

Metabolism – Only a small percentage (16%) of a dose of digoxin is metabolized. The end metabolites, which include 3 beta-digoxigenin, 3-keto-digoxigenin, and their glucuronide and sulfate conjugates, are polar in nature and are postulated to be formed via hydrolysis, oxidation, and conjugation. The metabolism of digoxin is not dependent upon the cytochrome P450 (CYP-450) system, and digoxin is not known to induce or inhibit the CYP-450 system.

Excretion – Elimination of digoxin follows first-order kinetics (ie, the quantity of digoxin eliminated at any time is proportional to the total body content). Following IV administration to healthy volunteers, 50% to 70% of a digoxin dose is excreted unchanged in the urine. Renal excretion of digoxin is proportional to glomerular filtration rate and is largely independent of urine flow. In healthy volunteers with healthy renal function, digoxin has a half-life of 1.5 to 2 days. The half-life in anuric patients is prolonged to 3.5 to 5 days. Digoxin is not effectively removed from the body by dialysis, exchange transfusion, or during cardiopulmonary bypass because most of the drug is bound to tissue and does not circulate in the blood.

Special populations –

Renal function impairment: The clearance of digoxin can be primarily correlated with renal function as indicated by CrCl (see also Warnings/Precautions).

Contraindications

Ventricular fibrillation; hypersensitivity to digoxin or to other digitalis preparations.

Warnings/Precautions

➤*Sinus node disease and AV block:* Because digoxin slows sinoatrial and AV conduction, the drug commonly prolongs the PR interval. The drug may cause severe sinus bradycardia or sinoatrial block in patients with preexisting sinus node disease and may cause advanced or complete heart block in patients with preexisting incomplete AV block. In such patients, consider insertion of a pacemaker before treatment with digoxin.

➤*Accessory AV pathway (Wolff-Parkinson-White syndrome):* After IV digoxin therapy, some patients with paroxysmal atrial fibrillation or flutter and a coexisting accessory AV pathway have developed increased antegrade conduction across the accessory pathway bypassing the AV node, leading to a very rapid ventricular response or ventricular fibrillation. Unless conduction down the accessory pathway has been blocked (pharmacologically or by surgery), do not use digoxin in such patients. The treatment of paroxysmal supraventricular tachycardia in such patients is usually direct-current cardioversion.

➤*Preserved left ventricular systolic function:* Patients with certain disorders involving heart failure associated with preserved LVEF may be particularly susceptible to toxicity of the drug. Such disorders include restrictive cardiomyopathy, constrictive pericarditis, amyloid heart disease, and acute cor pulmonale. Patients with idiopathic hypertrophic subaortic stenosis may have worsening of the outflow obstruction because of the inotropic effects of digoxin.

➤*Renal function impairment:* Digoxin is primarily excreted by the kidneys; therefore, patients with impaired renal function require smaller than usual maintenance doses of digoxin. Because of the prolonged elimination half-life, a longer period of time is required to achieve an initial or new steady-state serum concentration in patients with renal impairment than in patients with healthy renal function. If appropriate care is not taken to reduce the dose of digoxin, such patients are at high risk for toxicity, and toxic effects will last longer in such patients than in patients with healthy renal function.

➤*Special risk:*

Electrolyte disorders – In patients with hypokalemia or hypomagnesemia, toxicity may occur despite serum digoxin concentrations less than 2 ng/mL, because potassium or magnesium depletion sensitizes the myocardium to digoxin. Therefore, it is desirable to maintain healthy serum potassium and magnesium concentrations in patients being treated with digoxin. Deficiencies of these electrolytes may result from malnutrition, diarrhea, or prolonged vomiting, as well as the use of the following drugs or procedures: amphotericin B, antacids, corticosteroids, dialysis, diuretics, and mechanical suction of GI secretions.

Hypercalcemia from any cause predisposes the patient to digitalis toxicity. Calcium, particularly when administered rapidly by the IV route, may produce serious arrhythmias in digitalized patients. On the other hand, hypocalcemia can nullify the effects of digoxin in humans; thus, digoxin may be ineffective until serum calcium is restored to healthy levels. These interac-

DIGOXIN — INJECTION

tions are related to the fact that digoxin affects contractility and excitability of the heart in a manner similar to that of calcium.

Thyroid disorders and hypermetabolic states – Hypothyroidism may reduce the requirements for digoxin. Heart failure and/or atrial arrhythmias resulting from hypermetabolic or hyperdynamic states (eg, arteriovenous shunt, hyperthyroidism, hypoxia) are best treated by addressing the underlying condition. Atrial arrhythmias associated with hypermetabolic states are particularly resistant to digoxin treatment. Take care to avoid toxicity if digoxin is used.

Acute myocardial infarction – Use digoxin with caution in patients with acute myocardial infarction. The use of inotropic drugs in some patients in this setting may result in undesirable increases in myocardial oxygen demand and ischemia.

Electrical cardioversion – It may be desirable to reduce the dose of digoxin for 1 to 2 days prior to electrical cardioversion of atrial fibrillation to avoid the induction of ventricular arrhythmias, but consider the consequences of increasing the ventricular response if digoxin is withdrawn. If digitalis toxicity is suspected, delay elective cardioversion. If it is not prudent to delay cardioversion, select the lowest possible energy level to avoid provoking ventricular arrhythmias.

➤*Pregnancy:* Category C. Digoxin crosses the placenta. At delivery, the serum digoxin concentration in the newborn is similar to the serum concentration in the mother. Give digoxin to a pregnant woman only if clearly needed. Digoxin has been used for both maternal and fetal indications (eg, congestive heart failure and supraventricular tachycardia) during all stages of gestation without causing fetal harm. Direct administration of digoxin to the fetus by periodic IM injections has been used to treat supraventricular tachycardia when indirect therapy via the mother failed to control the arrhythmia.

➤*Lactation:* Studies have shown that digoxin concentrations in the mother's serum and milk are similar. Digoxin milk:plasma ratios have varied from 0.6 to 0.9. Although these amounts seem high, they represent very small amounts of digoxin because of significant maternal protein binding. The estimated exposure of a breast-feeding infant to digoxin via breast-feeding will be far below the usual infant maintenance dose. Therefore, this amount should have no pharmacologic effect upon the infant. No adverse effects in the breast-feeding infant have been reported. Nevertheless, exercise caution when administering digoxin to a breast-feeding woman. The American Academy of Pediatrics classifies digoxin as compatible with breast-feeding.

➤*Children:* Newborn infants display considerable variability in their tolerance to digoxin. Premature and immature infants are particularly sensitive to the effects of digoxin, and the dosage of the drug must not only be reduced but must be individualized according to their degree of maturity.

➤*Elderly:* The majority of clinical experience gained with digoxin has been in the elderly population. This experience has not identified differences in response or adverse reactions between the elderly and younger patients. However, this drug is known to be substantially excreted by the kidney, and the risk of toxic reactions to this drug may be greater in patients with impaired renal function. Because elderly patients are more likely to have decreased renal function, take care in dose selection, which should be based on renal function; it may be useful to monitor renal function.

See Administration and Dosage for more information.

➤*Lab test abnormalities:* The use of therapeutic doses of digoxin may cause prolongation of the PR interval and depression of the ST segment on the ECG. Digoxin may produce false-positive ST-T changes on the ECG during exercise testing. These electrophysiologic effects reflect an expected effect of the drug and are not indicative of toxicity.

➤*Monitoring:* Patients receiving digoxin should have their serum electrolytes and renal function (serum creatinine concentrations) assessed periodically; the frequency of assessments will depend on the clinical setting

See also Therapeutic drug monitoring in Administration and Dosage.

Drug Interactions

Because digoxin has a narrow therapeutic index, routine monitoring of the clinical response of the patient and digoxin serum concentrations for possible drug interactions is appropriate. Drug interactions occurring with drugs that have a narrow therapeutic index can be life-threatening or have serious clinical consequences.

➤*Renal function:* Coadminister digoxin with caution with any drug that may cause renal function impairment. A decrease in glomerular filtration or tubular secretion may decrease digoxin elimination

Digoxin Injection Drug Interactions

Precipitant drug	Object drug[a]		Description
Acarbose	Digoxin	⬇	Digoxin serum concentrations may be reduced, decreasing the efficacy. Monitor digoxin serum concentrations and adjust the digoxin dose as needed.
Albuterol	Digoxin	⬇	Digoxin serum concentrations may be reduced, decreasing the efficacy. Monitor digoxin serum concentrations and adjust the digoxin dose as needed.
Alprazolam	Digoxin	⬆	Digoxin serum concentrations may be elevated, particularly in elderly patients, increasing the risk of toxicity. Monitor digoxin serum concentrations and observe the patient for evidence of digoxin toxicity. Adjust the digoxin dosage accordingly.
Amiloride	Digoxin	⬇	Amiloride may attenuate the positive inotropic effect of digoxin. If an interaction is suspected, discontinue one or both drugs. Increasing the digoxin dose does not appear to overcome the effects of this interaction.
Amphotericin B	Digoxin	⬆	Amphotericin B–induced hypokalemia may increase the risk of digoxin toxicity.
Antiarrhythmic agents (ie, amiodarone, dronedarone, propafenone, quinidine)	Digoxin	⬆	Digoxin serum concentrations may be elevated, increasing the pharmacologic effects and risk of toxicity. Monitor digoxin serum concentrations and observe the patient for evidence of digoxin toxicity. Adjust the digoxin dose accordingly. On initiation of one of these antiarrhythmic agents, reduce the digoxin dose ≈ 50% or discontinue.
Azole antifungal agents (ie, itraconazole, ketoconazole)	Digoxin	⬆	Digoxin serum concentrations may be elevated, increasing the pharmacologic effects and risk of toxicity. Monitor digoxin serum concentrations and observe the patient for evidence of digoxin toxicity. Adjust the digoxin dose accordingly.
Beta-blockers (eg, carvedilol)	Digoxin	⬆	Although beta-blockers and digoxin may be useful in combination to control atrial fibrillation, their additive effects on AV node conduction may result in advanced or complete heart block.
Calcium	Digoxin	⬆	Calcium administered rapidly by the IV route may produce serious arrhythmias in digitalized patients.
Calcium channel blockers (eg, diltiazem, nifedipine, nisoldipine, verapamil)	Digoxin	⬆	Although calcium channel blockers and digoxin may be useful in combination to control atrial fibrillation, their additive effects on AV node conduction may result in advanced or complete heart block. Diltiazem, nisoldipine, and verapamil may increase digoxin concentrations, increasing the risk of toxicity. Verapamil may increase digoxin serum concentrations as much as 75% during the first week of therapy, increasing the risk of toxicity. Monitor digoxin serum concentrations when starting, stopping, or changing the dose of diltiazem or nifedipine, and adjust the digoxin dosage accordingly.
Cyclosporine	Digoxin	⬆	Digoxin serum concentrations may be elevated, increasing the pharmacologic effects and risk of toxicity. Monitor digoxin serum concentrations and observe the patient for evidence of digoxin toxicity. Adjust the digoxin dosage accordingly.

DIGOXIN — INJECTION

Digoxin Injection Drug Interactions			
Precipitant drug	Object drug[a]		Description
Ginseng	Digoxin	↑	Digoxin serum concentrations may be elevated, increasing the risk of toxicity. Monitor digoxin serum concentrations and observe the patient for evidence of digoxin toxicity; adjust the digoxin dosage accordingly.
Hydantoins (eg, phenytoin)	Digoxin	↑↓	Variable effects. Digoxin pharmacologic effects may be increased or decreased. Observe the clinical response of the patient and monitor digoxin serum concentrations. Adjust the digoxin dose as needed.
Loop diuretics (eg, furosemide)	Digoxin	↑	Diuretic-induced electrolyte disturbances may predispose to digitalis-induced arrhythmias. Measure plasma levels of potassium and magnesium and supplement low levels. Prevent further losses with dietary sodium restriction or potassium-sparing diuretics.
Macrolide and related antibiotics (eg, clarithromycin, erythromycin, telithromycin)	Digoxin	↑	Digoxin serum concentrations may be elevated, increasing the risk of toxicity. The effect of the interaction may persist for several weeks after stopping the antibiotic. Monitor digoxin serum concentrations and observe the patient for evidence of digoxin toxicity. Adjust the digoxin dose accordingly.
Milnacipran	Digoxin	↑	The risk of adverse hemodynamic effects (eg, hypotension, tachycardia) may be increased. Avoid coadministration.
Nefazodone	Digoxin	↑	Digoxin serum concentrations may be elevated, increasing the pharmacologic effects and risk of toxicity. Monitor digoxin serum concentrations and observe the patient for evidence of digoxin toxicity. Adjust the digoxin dosage accordingly.
Nonsteroidal anti-inflammatory drugs (ie, diclofenac, ibuprofen, indomethacin)	Digoxin	↑	Digoxin serum concentrations may be elevated, increasing the toxic effects. The effect of ibuprofen on digoxin appears to be transient. Monitor digoxin serum concentrations and observe the patient for evidence of digoxin toxicity. Adjust the digoxin dose accordingly.
Penicillamine	Digoxin	↓	Digoxin serum concentrations may be reduced, decreasing the pharmacologic effects. Monitor digoxin serum concentrations and observe the clinical response of the patient. Adjust the digoxin dosage accordingly.
Protease inhibitors (eg, ritonavir, saquinavir)	Digoxin	↑	Certain protease inhibitors may elevate digoxin serum concentrations, increasing the pharmacologic effects and risk of toxicity. Monitor digoxin serum concentrations and observe the patient for evidence of digoxin toxicity. Adjust the digoxin dosage accordingly.
Quinine	Digoxin	↑	Digoxin serum concentrations may be elevated, increasing the pharmacologic effects and risk of toxicity. Monitor digoxin serum concentrations and observe the patient for evidence of digoxin toxicity. Adjust the digoxin dosage accordingly.

Digoxin Injection Drug Interactions			
Precipitant drug	Object drug[a]		Description
Ranolazine	Digoxin	↑	Digoxin serum concentrations may be elevated 1.5-fold, increasing the pharmacologic effects and risk of toxicity. Monitor digoxin serum concentrations and observe the patient for evidence of digoxin toxicity. Adjust the digoxin dosage accordingly.
Rifamycins (eg, rifampin)	Digoxin	↓	Digoxin serum concentrations may be reduced, decreasing the efficacy, especially in patients with renal function impairment. Monitor digoxin serum concentrations and adjust the digoxin dose as needed.
Serotonin reuptake inhibitors (eg, fluoxetine, paroxetine, sertraline)	Digoxin	↑	Digoxin serum concentrations may be elevated, increasing the pharmacologic effects and risk of toxicity. Monitor digoxin serum concentrations and observe the patient for evidence of digoxin toxicity. Adjust the digoxin dosage accordingly.
Spironolactone	Digoxin		Spironolactone may attenuate the positive inotropic effect of digoxin. Digoxin serum concentrations may be elevated. In addition, spironolactone may interfere with digoxin assay, resulting in falsely elevated levels. Monitor patients closely and be aware of potentially false concentrations.
Succinylcholine	Digoxin	↑	Succinylcholine may cause a sudden extrusion of potassium from muscle cells, thereby causing arrhythmias in digitalized patients.
Sympathomimetics	Digoxin	↑	Concomitant use increases the risk of cardiac arrhythmias.
Telmisartan	Digoxin	↑	Digoxin peak and trough serum concentrations may be elevated ≈ 50% and 20%, respectively, increasing the risk of digoxin toxicity. Monitor digoxin serum concentrations when starting, stopping, or changing the dose of telmisartan, and adjust the digoxin dosage accordingly.
Thiazide diuretics (eg, hydrochlorothiazide)	Digoxin	↑	Diuretic-induced electrolyte disturbances may predispose to digitalis-induced arrhythmias. Measure plasma levels of potassium and magnesium and supplement low levels. Prevent further losses with dietary sodium restriction or potassium-sparing diuretics.
Thioamines (eg, methimazole, propylthiouracil)	Digoxin	↑	Hyperthyroid patients may require a reduced dose of digoxin if they become euthyroid.
Thyroid hormones (eg, levothyroxine)	Digoxin	↓	Thyroid administration to a digitalized, hypothyroid patient may increase the dose requirement of digoxin.
Tramadol	Digoxin	↑	Postmarketing experience has revealed rare reports of digoxin toxicity during coadministration with tramadol.
Vasopressin receptor antagonists (eg, conivaptan)	Digoxin	↑	Digoxin serum concentrations may be elevated, increasing the pharmacologic effects and risk of toxicity. Observe the clinical response of the patient and monitor digoxin concentrations. Adjust the digoxin dose as needed.

DIGOXIN — INJECTION

Digoxin Injection Drug Interactions

Precipitant drug	Object drug[a]		Description
Digoxin	Dofetilide	↑	Coadministration of digoxin and dofetilide has been associated with an increased rate of torsades de pointes compared with dofetilide alone.

[a] ↑ = object drug increased; ↓ = object drug decreased.

Adverse Reactions

In general, the adverse reactions of digoxin are dose dependent and occur at doses higher than those needed to achieve a therapeutic effect. Hence, adverse reactions are less common when digoxin is used within the recommended dose range or therapeutic serum concentration range and when there is careful attention to concurrent medications and conditions.

Because some patients may be particularly susceptible to side effects with digoxin, always select the dosage of the drug carefully and adjust as the clinical condition of the patient warrants. In the past, when high doses of digoxin were used and little attention was paid to clinical status or concurrent medications, adverse reactions to digoxin were more frequent and severe. Cardiac adverse reactions accounted for about one-half, GI disturbances for about one-fourth, and CNS and other toxicityfor about one-fourth of these adverse reactions. However, available evidence suggests that the incidence and severity of digoxin toxicity has decreased substantially in recent years. In recent controlled clinical trials, in patients with predominantly mild to moderate heart failure, the incidence of adverse reactions was comparable in patients taking digoxin and in those taking placebo. In a large mortality trial, the incidence of hospitalization for suspected digoxin toxicity was 2% in patients taking digoxin tablets compared with 0.9% in patients taking placebo. In this trial, the most common manifestations of digoxin toxicity included GI disturbances and cardiac disturbances; CNS manifestations were less common.

See also the Digoxin Oral monograph for adverse reactions in patients treated with digoxin tablets.

➤*Adults:*

Cardiovascular – Therapeutic doses of digoxin may cause heart block in patients with preexisting sinoatrial or AV conduction disorders; heart block can be avoided by adjusting the dose of digoxin. Prophylactic use of a cardiac pacemaker may be considered if the risk of heart block is considered unacceptable. High doses of digoxin may produce a variety of rhythm disturbances, such as first-degree, second-degree (Wenckebach), or third-degree heart block (including asystole); atrial tachycardia with block; AV dissociation; accelerated junctional (nodal) rhythm; unifocal or multiform ventricular premature contractions (especially bigeminy or trigeminy); ventricular tachycardia; and ventricular fibrillation. Digoxin produces PR prolongation and ST-segment depression, which should not by themselves be considered digoxin toxicity. Cardiac toxicity can also occur at therapeutic doses in patients who have conditions that may alter their sensitivity to digoxin (eg, restrictive cardiomyopathy, electrolyte disturbances, hypothyroidism).

CNS – Digoxin can produce apathy, confusion, dizziness, headache, mental disturbances (eg, anxiety, delirium, depression, hallucination), visual disturbances (blurred or yellow vision), and weakness.

GI – Digoxin may cause anorexia, diarrhea, nausea, and vomiting. Rarely, the use of digoxin has been associated with abdominal pain, hemorrhagic necrosis of the intestines, and intestinal ischemia.

Miscellaneous – Gynecomastia has been occasionally observed following the prolonged use of digoxin. Thrombocytopenia and maculopapular rash and other skin reactions have been rarely observed.

➤*Children:* The adverse effects of digoxin in infants and children differ from those seen in adults in several respects. Although digoxin may produce anorexia, CNS disturbances, diarrhea, nausea, and vomiting in young patients, these are rarely the initial symptoms of overdosage. Rather, the earliest and most frequent manifestation of excessive dosing with digoxin in infants and children is the appearance of cardiac arrhythmias, including sinus bradycardia. In children, the use of digoxin may produce any arrhythmia. The most common are conduction disturbances or supraventricular tachyarrhythmias, such as atrial tachycardia (with or without block) and junctional (nodal) tachycardia. Ventricular arrhythmias are less common. Sinus bradycardia may be a sign of impending digoxin intoxication, especially in infants, even in the absence of first-degree heart block. Assume any arrhythmia or alteration in cardiac conduction that develops in a child taking digoxin to be caused by digoxin, until further evaluation proves otherwise.

Overdosage

➤*Symptoms:* Manifestations of life-threatening toxicity include ventricular tachycardia or ventricular fibrillation or progressive bradyarrhythmias or heart block. The administration of more than 10 mg of digoxin in a previously healthy adult, or more than 4 mg in a previously healthy child, or a steady-state serum concentration of more than 10 ng/mL often results in cardiac arrest.

➤*Treatment:* Temporarily discontinue digoxin until the adverse reaction resolves. Also make every effort to correct factors that may contribute to the adverse reaction (eg, electrolyte disturbances, concurrent medications). Once the adverse reaction has resolved, therapy with digoxin may be reinstituted, following a careful reassessment of dose.

Withdrawal of digoxin may be all that is required to treat the adverse reaction. However, when the primary manifestation of digoxin overdosage is a cardiac arrhythmia, additional therapy may be needed.

If the rhythm disturbance is a symptomatic bradyarrhythmia or heart block, consider the reversal of toxicity with digoxin immune fab (ovine), the use of atropine, or the insertion of a temporary cardiac pacemaker. However, asymptomatic bradycardia or heart block related to digoxin may require only temporary withdrawal of the drug and cardiac monitoring of the patient.

If the rhythm disturbance is a ventricular arrhythmia, consider the correction of electrolyte disorders, particularly if hypokalemia or hypomagnesemia is present. Digoxin immune fab (ovine) is a specific antidote for digoxin and may be used to reverse potentially life-threatening ventricular arrhythmias because of digoxin overdosage.

Make every effort to maintain the serum potassium concentration between 4 and 5.5 mmol/L. Potassium is usually administered orally, but when correction of the arrhythmia is urgent and the serum potassium concentration is low, potassium may be administered cautiously by the IV route. Monitor the ECG for any evidence of potassium toxicity (eg, peaking of T waves) and to observe the effect on the arrhythmia. Potassium salts may be dangerous in patients who manifest bradycardia or heart block because of digoxin (unless primarily related to supraventricular tachycardia) and in the setting of massive digitalis overdosage.

Massive overdosage – Ensure that patients with massive digitalis ingestion receive large doses of activated charcoal to prevent absorption and bind digoxin in the gut during enteroenteric recirculation. Gastric lavage may be indicated especially if ingestion has occurred within 30 minutes of the patient's presentation at the hospital. If a patient presents more than 2 hours after ingestion or already has toxic manifestations, it may be unsafe to attempt passage of a gastric tube because such maneuvers may induce an acute vagal episode that can worsen digitalis-related arrhythmias.

Severe digitalis intoxication can cause a massive shift of potassium from inside to outside the cell, leading to life-threatening hyperkalemia. Avoid the administration of potassium supplements in the setting of massive intoxication because it may be hazardous. Hyperkalemia caused by massive digitalis toxicity is best treated with digoxin immune fab (ovine); initial treatment with glucose and insulin may also be required if hyperkalemia itself is acutely life-threatening.

INAMRINONE LACTATE

Rx	**Inamrinone Lactate** (Abbott Hospital)	**Injection:** 5 mg/mL (as lactate)	In 20 mL amps.[a]

[a] With 0.25 mg/mL sodium metabisulfite.

INAMRINONE — INJECTION

Indications

➤*Congestive heart failure:* For the short-term management of congestive heart failure. Because of limited experience and the potential for serious adverse effects (such as thrombocytopenia, arrhythmia, hypotension, chest pain, hepatotoxicity, hypersensitivity reactions, and fever), inamrinone should be used only in patients who can be closely monitored and who have not responded adequately to digitalis, diuretics, or vasodilators. Experience with IV inamrinone in controlled trials does not extend beyond 48 hours of repeated boluses or continuous infusions.

Administration and Dosage

➤*General dosing considerations:* Monitoring central venous pressure (CVP) may be valuable in the assessment of hypotension and fluid balance management. Prior correction or adjustment of fluid/electrolytes is essential to obtain satisfactory response with inamrinone.

Patient improvement may be reflected by increases in cardiac output, reduction in pulmonary capillary wedge pressure, and such clinical responses as a lessening of dyspnea and an improvement in other symptoms of heart failure, such as orthopnea and fatigue.

The rate of administration and the duration of therapy should be adjusted according to the response of the patient. The physician may wish to reduce or titrate the infusion downward based on clinical responsiveness or untoward effects.

➤*Adults:*

Congestive heart failure –

Loading dose: Initiate therapy with a 0.75 mg/kg loading dose given slowly over 2 to 3 minutes. Based on clinical response, an additional loading dose of 0.75 mg/kg may be given 30 minutes after the initiation of therapy.

The following procedure is recommended for the administration of inamrinone injection.

INAMRINONE — INJECTION

Inamrinone Loading Dose Determination 0.75 mg/kg (Undiluted)										
	Patient weight (kg)									
	30	40	50	60	70	80	90	100	110	120
mL of undiluted inamrinone injection	4.5	6	7.5	9	10.5	12	13.5	15	16.5	18

Maintenance dosage: Continue therapy with a maintenance infusion between 5 and 10 mcg/kg/min. (See Administration.)

The above dosing regimens can be expected to place most patients' plasma concentration of inamrinone at approximately 3 mcg/mL. Increases in cardiac index show a linear relationship to plasma concentration of a range of 0.5 to 7 mcg/mL. No observations have been made at greater plasma concentrations.

➤*Children:* Safety and efficacy in children have not been established. In preterm infants, short-term use of inamrinone (5 mcg/kg/min) was effective in the management of CHF.

➤*Preparation for administration:* To prepare the 2.5 mg/mL concentration recommended for infusion, mix inamrinone with an equal volume of diluent (normal or half normal saline). For example, mix three 20 mL ampuls of inamrinone injection (3 × 20 mL = 60 mL) with 60 mL of diluent for a total volume of 120 mL of the final 2.5 mg/mL solution of inamrinone.

➤*Administration:* Inamrinone injection may be injected into running dextrose (glucose) infusions through a Y-connector or directly into the tubing where preferable.

Loading doses – Loading doses of inamrinone injection should be administered as supplied (undiluted). Administer loading doses slowly over 2 to 3 minutes.

Infusions – Infusions of inamrinone injection may be administered in normal, or half-normal saline solution to a concentration of 1 to 3 mg/mL. Diluted solutions should be used with 24 hours. Administer at a rate between 5 and 10 mcg/kg/min.

The rate of infusion usually ranges from 5 to 10 mcg/kg/min, such that the recommended total daily dose (including loading doses) does not exceed 10 mg/kg. A limited number of patients studied at higher doses support a dosage regimen up to 18 mg/kg/day for shortened durations of therapy.

The following infusion rate table may be used to ensure that the calculations are made correctly. To use the following table, the concentration of inamrinone infusion solution used must be 2.5 mg/mL (2,500 mcg/mL).

Inamrinone IV Infusion Rate (mL/h) Using 2.5 mg/mL Infusion Concentration										
	Patient weight (kg)									
Dosage	30	40	50	60	70	80	90	100	110	120
5 mcg/kg/min	4	5	6	7	8	10	11	12	13	14
7.5 mcg/kg/min	5	7	9	11	13	14	16	18	20	22
10 mcg/kg/min	7	10	12	14	17	19	22	24	26	29

Example: A 70 kg patient would require a loading dose of 10.5 mL of undiluted inamrinone. If the physician selects a dose of 7.5 mcg/kg/min for the infusion, the flow rate would be 13 mL/h at the 2.5 mg/mL concentration of inamrinone.

➤*Admixture compatibility:*

Incompatibility – A chemical interaction occurs slowly over a 24-hour period when the IV solution of inamrinone injection is mixed directly with dextrose (glucose)-containing solutions. Therefore, inamrinone injection should not be diluted with solutions that contain dextrose (glucose) prior to injection.

A chemical interaction occurs immediately, which is evidenced by the formation of a precipitate when furosemide is injected into an IV line of an infusion of inamrinone. Therefore, furosemide should not be administered in IV lines containing inamrinone.

➤*Storage/Stability:* Protect ampuls from light by retaining in carton until time of use. Store at 15° to 30°C (59° to 86°F).

Actions

➤*Pharmacology:* Inamrinone injection is a positive inotropic agent with vasodilator activity, different in structure and mode of action from either digitalis glycosides or catecholamines.

The mechanism of its inotropic and vasodilator effects has not been fully elucidated.

With respect to its inotropic effect, experimental evidence indicates that it is not a beta-adrenergic agonist. It inhibits myocardial cyclic adenosine monophosphate (c-AMP) phosphodiesterase activity and increases cellular levels of c-AMP. Unlike digitalis, it does not inhibit sodium-potassium adenosine triphosphatase activity.

With respect to its vasodilatory activity, inamrinone reduces afterload and preload by its direct relaxant effect on vascular smooth muscle.

➤*Pharmacokinetics:*

Distribution – Following IV bolus (1 to 2 minutes) injection of 0.68 to 1.2 mg/kg to healthy volunteers, inamrinone had a volume of distribution of 1.2 L/kg. Infants and children have a larger volume of distribution.

Inamrinone has been shown in 1 study to be 10% to 22% bound to human plasma protein by ultrafiltration in vitro, and in another study 35% to 49% bound by either ultrafiltration or equilibrium dialysis.

Metabolism/Excretion – Following a distributive phase half-life of about 4.6 minutes in plasma, had a mean apparent first-order terminal elimination half-life of about 3.6 hours. In patients with congestive heart failure receiving infusions of inamrinone the mean apparent first-order terminal elimination half-life was about 5.8 hours. Infants and children have a decreased elimination half-life.

The primary route of excretion in man is via the urine as both inamrinone and several metabolites (N-glycolyl, N-acetate, O-glucuronide and N-glucuronide). In healthy volunteers, approximately 63% of an oral dose of ^{14}C-labeled inamrinone was excreted in the urine over a 96-hour period. In the first 8 hours, 51% of the radioactivity in the urine was inamrinone with 5% as the N-acetate, 8% as the N-glycolate, and less than 5% for each glucuronide. Approximately 18% of the administered dose was excreted in the feces in 72 hours.

In a 24-hour nonradioactive IV study, 10% to 40% of the dose was excreted in urine as unchanged inamrinone with the N-acetyl metabolite representing less than 2% of the dose.

Special populations –

Children:

Congestive heart failure: In congestive heart failure patients, after a loading bolus dose, steady-state plasma levels of about 2.4 mcg/mL were able to be maintained by an infusion of 5 to 10 mcg/kg/min. In some congestive heart failure patients, with associated compromised renal and hepatic perfusion, it is possible that plasma levels of inamrinone may rise during the infusion period; therefore, in these patients, it may be necessary to monitor the hemodynamic response or drug level. The principal measures of patient response include cardiac index, pulmonary capillary wedge pressure, central venous pressure, and their relationship to plasma concentrations. Additionally, measurements of blood pressure, urine output, and body weight may prove useful, as may such clinical symptoms as orthopnea, dyspnea, and fatigue.

Contraindications

Hypersensitivity to inamrinone or bisulfites.

Warnings/Precautions

➤*Pulmonic and/or aortic valvular disease:* Inamrinone injection should not be used in patients with severe aortic or pulmonic valvular disease in lieu of surgical relief of the obstruction. Like other inotropic agents, it may aggravate outflow tract obstruction in hypertrophic subaortic stenosis.

➤*Fluid and electrolyte intake:* Patients who have received vigorous diuretic therapy may have insufficient cardiac-filling pressure to respond adequately to inamrinone injection, in which case, cautious liberalization of fluid and electrolyte intake may be indicated.

➤*Arrhythmias:* Supraventricular and ventricular arrhythmias have been observed in the very high-risk population treated. While inamrinone per se has not been shown to be arrhythmogenic, the potential for arrhythmia, present in congestive heart failure itself, may be increased by any drug or combination of drugs.

➤*Use in acute myocardial infarction:* No clinical trials have been carried out in patients in the acute phase of postmyocardial infarction. Therefore, inamrinone injection is not recommended in these cases.

➤*Sulfite sensitivity:* Some of these products contain sodium metabisulfite, a sulfite that may cause allergic-type reactions including anaphylactic symptoms and life-threatening or less severe asthmatic episodes in certain susceptible people. The overall prevalence of sulfite sensitivity in the general population is unknown and probably low. Sulfite sensitivity is seen more frequently in asthmatic than in nonasthmatic people.

➤*Pregnancy: Category C.* In New Zealand white rabbits, inamrinone has been shown to produce fetal skeletal and gross external malformations at oral doses of 16 and 50 mg/kg which were toxic for the rabbit. Studies in French Hy/Cr rabbits using oral doses up to 32 mg/kg/day did not confirm this finding. No malformations were seen in rats receiving inamrinone IV at the maximum dose used, 15 mg/kg/day (approximately the recommended daily IV dose for patients with congestive heart failure). There are no adequate and well-controlled studies in pregnant women. Inamrinone should be used during pregnancy only if the potential benefit justifies the potential risk to the fetus.

➤*Lactation:* Caution should be exercised when inamrinone is administered to nursing women, since it is not known whether it is excreted in human milk.

➤*Children:* Safety and efficacy in pediatric patients have not been established. In preterm infants, short-term use of inamrinone (5 mcg/kg/min) was effective in the management of CHF.

➤*Monitoring:* Fluid and electrolyte changes and renal function should be carefully monitored during inamrinone lactate therapy. Improvement in cardiac output with resultant diuresis may necessitate a reduction in the dose of diuretic. Potassium loss due to excessive diuresis may predispose digitalized patients to arrhythmias. Therefore, hypokalemia should be corrected by potassium supplementation in advance of or during inamrinone use.

During IV therapy with inamrinone injection, blood pressure and heart rate should be monitored and the rate of infusion slowed or stopped in patients showing excessive decreases in blood pressure.

INAMRINONE — INJECTION

Drug Interactions

In a relatively limited experience, no untoward clinical manifestations have been observed in patients in which inamrinone injection was used concurrently with the following drugs: Digitalis glycosides; lidocaine, quinidine; metoprolol, propranolol; hydralazine, prazosin; isosorbide dinitrate, nitroglycerin; chlorthalidone, ethacrynic acid, furosemide, hydrochlorothiazide, spironolactone; captopril; heparin, warfarin; potassium supplements; insulin; diazepam.

One case report of excessive hypotension has been reported when inamrinone was used concurrently with disopyramide.

Until additional experience is available, concurrent administration with disopyramide should be undertaken with caution.

Adverse Reactions

➤*Cardiovascular:* Cardiovascular adverse reactions reported with inamrinone injection include arrhythmia (3%) and hypotension (1.3%).

➤*GI:* GI adverse reactions reported with inamrinone injection during clinical use included nausea (1.7%), vomiting (0.9%), abdominal pain (0.4%), and anorexia (0.4%).

While GI side effects were seen infrequently with IV therapy, should severe or debilitating ones occur, the physician may wish to reduce dosage or discontinue the drug based on the usual benefit-to-risk considerations.

➤*Hematologic:*

Thrombocytopenia – IV inamrinone injection resulted in platelet count reductions to below 100,000/mm^3 or normal limits in 2.4% of the patients.

It is more common in patients receiving prolonged therapy. To date, in closely monitored clinical trials, in patients whose platelet counts were not allowed to remain depressed, no bleeding phenomena have been observed.

Platelet reduction is dose dependent and appears due to a decrease in platelet survival time. Several patients who developed thrombocytopenia while receiving inamrinone had bone marrow examinations which were normal. There is no evidence relating platelet reduction to immune response or to a platelet-activating factor.

Management of platelet count reductions – Asymptomatic platelet count reduction (to less than 150,000/mm^3) may be reversed within 1 week of a decrease in drug dosage. Further, with no change in drug dosage, the count may stabilize at lower than predrug levels without any clinical sequelae. Predrug platelet counts and frequent platelet counts during therapy are recommended to assist in decisions regarding dosage modifications.

If a platelet count less than 150,000/mm^3 occurs, the following actions may be considered:

- Maintain total daily dose unchanged, since in some cases counts have either stabilized or returned to pretreatment levels.
- Decrease total daily dose.
- Discontinue inamrinone if, in the clinical judgment of the physician, risk exceeds the potential benefit.

➤*Hepatic:* In dogs, at IV doses between 9 and 32 mg/kg/day, inamrinone showed dose-related hepatotoxicity manifested either as enzyme elevation or hepatic cell necrosis or both. Hepatotoxicity has been observed in man following long-term oral dosing and has been observed, in a limited experience (0.2%), following IV administration of inamrinone. There have also been rare reports of enzyme and bilirubin elevation and jaundice.

In clinical experience to date with IV administration, hepatotoxicity has been observed rarely. If acute marked alterations in liver enzymes occur together with clinical symptoms suggesting an idiosyncratic hypersensitivity reaction, inamrinone therapy should be promptly discontinued.

If less than marked enzyme alterations occur without clinical symptoms, these nonspecific changes should be evaluated on an individual basis. The clinician may wish to continue inamrinone, reduce dosage, or discontinue the drug based on the usual benefit/risk considerations.

➤*Hypersensitivity:* There have been reports of several apparent hypersensitivity reactions in patients treated with oral inamrinone for about 2 weeks. Signs and symptoms were variable but included pericarditis, pleuritis and ascites (1 case), myositis with interstitial shadowing on chest x-ray and elevated sedimentation rate (1 case) and vasculitis with nodular pulmonary densities, hypoxemia, and jaundice (1 case). The first patient died, not necessarily of the possible reaction, while the last two resolved with discontinuation of therapy. None of the cases were rechallenged so that attribution to inamrinone is not certain, but possible hypersensitivity reactions should be considered in any patient maintained for a prolonged period on inamrinone.

➤*Miscellaneous:* Additional adverse reactions observed in IV inamrinone clinical studies include fever (0.9%), chest pain (0.2%), and burning at the site of injection (0.2%).

Overdosage

➤*Symptoms:* A death has been reported with a massive accidental overdose (840 mg over 3 hours by initial bolus and infusion) of inamrinone, although causal relation is uncertain. Diligence should be exercised during product preparation and administration.

➤*Treatment:* Doses of inamrinone injection may produce hypotension because of its vasodilator effect. If this occurs, inamrinone administration should be reduced or discontinued. No specific antidote is known, but general measures for circulatory support should be taken.

MILRINONE LACTATE

Rx	Milrinone Lactate (Bedford)	Injection: 1 mg/mL	47 mg/mL dextrose. In 10, 20, and 50 mL single-dose vials.

MILRINONE LACTATE — INJECTION

Indications

➤*Acute decompensated heart failure:* For the short-term IV treatment of patients with acute decompensated heart failure.

Administration and Dosage

➤*General dosing considerations:* Administer milrinone lactate with a loading dose followed by a continuous infusion (maintenance dose).

When administering milrinone lactate by continuous infusion, it is advisable to use a calibrated electronic infusion device.

➤*Adults:*

Acute decompensated heart failure (short-term) –

Maximum dose: 1.13 mg/kg/day (maintenance dose).

Loading dose: 50 mcg/kg administered intravenously (IV) slowly over 10 minutes. The loading dose may be given undiluted, but diluting to a rounded total volume of 10 or 20 mL may simplify the visualization of the injection rate (see Preparation of administration).

Dosage titration: Dosage may be titrated to the maximum hemodynamic effect and should not exceed 1.13 mg/kg/day.

Maintenance dosage:

Milrinone Maintenance Dose

	Infusion rate	Total daily dose (24 hours)	
Minimum	0.375 mcg/kg/min	0.59 mg/kg	Administer as a continuous IV infusion.
Standard	0.5 mcg/kg/min	0.77 mg/kg	
Maximum	0.75 mcg/kg/min	1.13 mg/kg	

Duration of therapy: Duration of therapy should depend upon patient responsiveness.

➤*Renal function impairment:* Reductions in infusion rate may be necessary in patients with renal impairment. See the following table.

Milrinone Dosing in Renal Function Impairment

Creatinine clearance (mL/min/1.73 m^2)	Infusion rate (mcg/kg/min)
5	0.2
10	0.23
20	0.28
30	0.33
40	0.38
50	0.43

➤*Preparation for administration:*

Dilution – Dilute milrinone lactate drawn from vials prior to maintenance dose administration. The diluents that may be used are sodium chloride 0.45% injection, sodium chloride 0.9% injection, or dextrose 5% injection. The following table shows the volume of diluent in milliliters (mL) that must be used to achieve 200 mcg/mL concentration for infusion and the resultant total volumes.

Milrinone Dilution

Desired infusion concentration (mcg/mL)	Milrinone 1 mg/mL (mL)	Diluent (mL)	Total volume (mL)
200	10	40	50
200	20	80	100

The flexible container has a concentration of milrinone equivalent to 200 mcg /mL in dextrose 5% injection and is more convenient to use than dilutions prepared from the vials. To use the flexible container, tear the overwrap at the notch and remove the premixed solution container. Squeeze the container firmly to check for leaks. Discard the container if leaks are found since the sterility of the product could be affected. Do not add supplementary medication. To prepare the container for administration of milrinone lactate IV, use aseptic techniques.

MILRINONE LACTATE — INJECTION

➤*Admixture compatibility:* There is an immediate chemical interaction which is evidenced by the formation of a precipitate when furosemide is injected into an IV line of an infusion of milrinone lactate. Therefore, furosemide should not be administered in IV lines containing milrinone lactate.

➤*Storage/Stability:* Discard unused portion after initial use. Store at controlled room temperature 15° to 30°C (59° to 86°F). Avoid freezing. Exposure of pharmaceutical products to heat should be minimized. Avoid excessive heat. Protect from freezing. It is recommended that the flexible containers be stored at room temperature, 25°C (77°F); however, brief exposure up to 40°C (104°F) does not adversely affect the product.

Actions

➤*Pharmacology:* Milrinone lactate is a positive inotrope and vasodilator, with little chronotropic activity different in structure and mode of action from either the digitalis glycosides or catecholamines.

Milrinone lactate, at relevant inotropic and vasorelaxant concentrations, is a selective inhibitor of peak III cyclic adenosine monophosphate (cAMP) phosphodiesterase isozyme in cardiac and vascular muscle. This inhibitory action is consistent with cAMP-mediated increases in intracellular ionized calcium and contractile force in cardiac muscle, as well as with cAMP-dependent contractile protein phosphorylation and relaxation in vascular muscle. Additional experimental evidence also indicates that milrinone lactate is not a beta-adrenergic agonist nor does it inhibit sodium-potassium adenosine triphosphatase activity as do the digitalis glycosides.

Clinical studies in patients with congestive heart failure have shown that milrinone lactate produces dose- and plasma drug concentration-related increases in the maximum rate of increase of left ventricular pressure. Studies in healthy subjects have shown that milrinone lactate produces increases in the slope of the left ventricular pressure-dimension relationship, indicating a direct inotropic effect of the drug. Milrinone lactate also produces dose- and plasma concentration-related increases in forearm blood flow in patients with congestive heart failure, indicating a direct arterial vasodilator activity of the drug.

Both the inotropic and vasodilatory effects have been observed over the therapeutic range of plasma milrinone concentrations of 100 to 300 ng/mL.

In addition to increasing myocardial contractility, milrinone lactate improves diastolic function as evidenced by improvements in left ventricular diastolic relaxation.

Pharmacodynamics – In patients with heart failure due to depressed myocardial function, milrinone lactate produced a prompt dose- and plasma concentration-related increase in cardiac output and decreases in pulmonary capillary wedge pressure and vascular resistance, which were accompanied by mild-to-moderate increases in heart rate. Additionally, there is no increased effect on myocardial oxygen consumption. In uncontrolled studies, hemodynamic improvement during IV therapy with milrinone lactate was accompanied by clinical symptomatic improvement, but the ability of milrinone lactate to relieve symptoms has not been evaluated in controlled clinical trials. The great majority of patients experience improvements in hemodynamic function within 5 to 15 minutes of the initiation of therapy.

In studies in congestive heart failure patients, milrinone lactate, when administered as a loading injection followed by a maintenance infusion, produced significant mean initial increases in cardiac index of 25%, 38%, and 42% at dose regimens of 37.5 mcg/kg/0.375 mcg/kg/min, 50 mcg/kg/0.5 mcg/kg/min, and 75 mcg/kg/0.75 mcg/kg/min, respectively. Over the same range of loading injections and maintenance infusions, pulmonary capillary wedge pressure significantly decreased by 20%, 23%, and 36%, respectively, while systemic vascular resistance significantly decreased by 17%, 21%, and 37%. Mean arterial pressure fell by up to 5% at the 2 lower dose regimens, but by 17% at the highest dose. Patients evaluated for 48 hours maintained improvements in hemodynamic function, with no evidence of diminished response (tachyphylaxis). A smaller number of patients have received infusions of milrinone lactate for periods up to 72 hours without evidence of tachyphylaxis.

The duration of therapy should depend upon patient responsiveness. Patients have been maintained on infusions for up to 5 days.

Milrinone lactate has a favorable inotropic effect in fully digitalized patients without causing signs of glycoside toxicity. Theoretically, in cases of atrial flutter/fibrillation, it is possible that milrinone lactate may increase ventricular response rate because of its slight enhancement of AV node conduction. In these cases, digitalis should be considered prior to the institution of therapy with milrinone lactate.

Improvement in left ventricular function in patients with ischemic heart disease has been observed. The improvement has occurred without inducing symptoms or electrocardiographic signs of myocardial ischemia.

➤*Pharmacokinetics:*

Absorption/Distribution – The steady-state plasma milrinone concentrations after approximately 6 to 12 hours of unchanging maintenance infusion of 0.5 mcg/kg/min are approximately 200 ng/mL. Near maximum favorable effects of milrinone lactate on cardiac output and pulmonary capillary wedge pressure are seen at plasma milrinone concentrations in the 150 to 250 ng/mL range.

Following IV injections of 12.5 to 125 mcg/kg to congestive heart failure patients, milrinone lactate had a volume of distribution of 0.38 L/kg, a mean terminal elimination half-life of 2.3 hours, and a clearance of 0.13 L/kg/h. Following IV infusions of 0.2 to 0.7 mcg/kg/min to congestive heart failure patients, the drug had a volume of distribution of about 0.45 L/kg, a mean terminal elimination half-life of 2.4 hours, and a clearance of 0.14 L/kg/h. These pharmacokinetic parameters were not dose dependent, and the area under the plasma concentration versus time curve following injections was significantly dose dependent.

Milrinone lactate has been shown (by equilibrium dialysis) to be approximately 70% bound to human plasma protein.

Excretion – The primary route of excretion of milrinone lactate in man is via the urine. The major urinary excretions of orally administered milrinone lactate in man are milrinone (83%) and its 0-glucuronide metabolite (12%). Elimination in healthy subjects via the urine is rapid, with approximately 60% recovered within the first 2 hours following dosing and approximately 90% recovered within the first 8 hours following dosing. The mean renal clearance of milrinone lactate is approximately 0.3 L/min, indicative of active secretion.

Contraindications

Hypersensitivity to milrinone.

Warnings/Precautions

➤*Arrhythmias:* The use of milrinone has been associated with increased frequency of ventricular arrhythmias, including nonsustained ventricular tachycardia. Long-term oral use has been associated with an increased risk of sudden death. Hence, patients receiving milrinone lactate should be observed closely with the use of continuous electrocardiograph monitoring to allow the prompt detection and management of ventricular arrhythmias.

➤*Arrhythmias:* Supraventricular and ventricular arrhythmias have been observed in the high-risk population treated. In some patients, injections of milrinone lactate and oral milrinone lactate have been shown to increase ventricular ectopy, including nonsustained ventricular tachycardia. The potential for arrhythmia, present in congestive heart failure itself, may be increased by many drugs or combinations of drugs. Patients receiving milrinone lactate should be closely monitored during infusion.

Milrinone lactate produces a slight shortening of AV node conduction time, indicating a potential for an increased ventricular response rate in patients with atrial flutter/fibrillation which is not controlled with digitalis therapy.

➤*Special risk:*

Use in acute myocardial infarction – No clinical studies have been conducted in patients in the acute phase of post myocardial infarction. Until further clinical experience with this class of drugs is gained, milrinone lactate is not recommended in these patients. Milrinone lactate should not be used in patients with severe obstructive aortic or pulmonic valvular disease in lieu of surgical relief of the obstruction. Like other inotropic agents, it may aggravate outflow tract obstruction in hypertrophic subaortic stenosis.

➤*Pregnancy: Category C.* There are no adequate and well-controlled studies in pregnant women. Milrinone lactate should be used during pregnancy only if the potential benefit justifies the potential risk to the fetus.

➤*Lactation:* Caution should be exercised when milrinone lactate is administered to breast-feeding women, because it is not known whether it is excreted in human milk.

➤*Children:* Safety and efficacy in pediatric patients have not been established.

➤*Monitoring:* Patients receiving milrinone lactate should be observed closely with appropriate electrocardiographic equipment. The facility for immediate treatment of potential cardiac events, which may include life-threatening ventricular arrythmias, must be available. The majority of experience with IV milrinone lactate has been in patients receiving digoxin and diuretics. There is no experience in controlled trials with infusions of milrinone lactate for periods exceeding 48 hours.

Fluid and electrolyte changes and renal function should be carefully monitored during therapy with milrinone lactate. Improvement in cardiac output with resultant diuresis may necessitate a reduction in the dose of diuretic. Potassium loss due to excessive diuresis may predispose digitalized patients to arrhythmias. Therefore, hypokalemia should be corrected by potassium supplementation in advance of or during use of milrinone lactate.

During therapy with milrinone lactate, blood pressure and heart rate should be monitored and the rate of infusion slowed or stopped in patients showing excessive decreases in blood pressure.

If prior vigorous diuretic therapy is suspected to have caused significant decreases in cardiac filling pressure, milrinone lactate should be cautiously administered with monitoring of blood pressure, heart rate, and clinical symptomatology.

Adverse Reactions

➤*Cardiovascular:* In patients receiving milrinone lactate in phase II and III clinical trials, ventricular arrhythmias were reported in 12.1%: Ventricular ectopic activity, 8.5%; nonsustained ventricular tachycardia, 2.8%; sustained ventricular tachycardia, 1% and ventricular fibrillation, 0.2% (2 patients experienced more than 1 type of arrhythmia). Holter recordings demonstrated that in some patients injection of milrinone lactate increased ventricular ectopy, including nonsustained ventricular tachycardia. Life-threatening arrhythmias were infrequent, and, when present, have been associated with certain underlying factors such as preexisting arrhythmias, metabolic abnormalities (eg, hypokalemia), abnormal digoxin levels and catheter insertion. Milrinone lactate was not shown to be arrhythmogenic in an electrophysiology study. Supraventricular arrhythmias were reported in 3.8% of the patients receiving milrinone lactate. The incidence of both supraventricular and ventricular arrhythmias has not been related to the dose or plasma milrinone concentration.

Other cardiovascular adverse reactions include hypotension, 2.9% and angina/chest pain, 1.2%.

MILRINONE LACTATE — INJECTION

➤*CNS:* Headaches, usually mild to moderate in severity, have been reported in 2.9% of patients receiving milrinone lactate.

➤*Lab test abnormalities:* In the postmarketing experience, liver function test abnormalities have been reported.

➤*Miscellaneous:* Other adverse reactions reported, but not definitely related to the administration of milrinone lactate include hypokalemia, 0.6%; tremor, 0.4%; and thrombocytopenia, 0.4%.

Isolated spontaneous reports of bronchospasm have been received.

Overdosage

➤*Symptoms:* Doses of milrinone lactate may produce hypotension because of its vasodilator effect.

➤*Treatment:* If hypotension occurs, administration of milrinone lactate should be reduced or temporarily discontinued until the patient's condition stabilizes. No specific antidote is known, but general measures for circulatory support should be taken.

ANTIARRHYTHMIC AGENTS

Optimal therapy of cardiac arrhythmias requires documentation, accurate diagnosis and modification of precipitating causes, and if indicated, proper selection and use of antiarrhythmic drugs. Comprehensive information on individual agents is presented in the following monographs.

These drugs are classified according to their effects on the action potential of cardiac cells and their presumed mechanism of action. Although drugs within the same group are similar, that does not imply that another agent within the group would not be more effective or safer in an individual patient.

➤*Group I:* Local anesthetics or membrane-stabilizing agents that depress phase 0.

I*A (quinidine, procainamide, disopyramide)* – Depress phase 0 and prolong the action potential duration.

I*B (tocainide, lidocaine, phenytoin, mexiletine)* – Depress phase 0 slightly and may shorten the action potential duration. Although arrhythmia is not a labeled indication for phenytoin, it is commonly used in treatment of digitalis-induced arrhythmias.

I*C (flecainide, propafenone)* – Marked depression of phase 0. Slight effect on repolarization. Profound slowing of conduction.

Moricizine – A Group I agent that shares some of the characteristics of the Group IA, B and C agents.

➤*Group II (propranolol, esmolol, acebutolol):* Depress phase 4 depolarization.

➤*Group III (bretylium, amiodarone, sotalol):* Produce a prolongation of phase 3 (repolarization).

➤*Group IV (verapamil):* Depresses phase 4 depolarization and lengthen phases 1 and 2 of repolarization.

➤*Digitalis glycosides (digoxin):* Causes a decrease in maximal diastolic potential and action potential duration and increases the slope of phase 4 depolarization.

➤*Adenosine:* Adenosine slows conduction time through the AV node and can interrupt the reentry pathways through the AV node.

➤*Serum drug levels:* Some antiarrhythmic drugs (eg, quinidine) can produce toxic effects that can be easily confused with the symptoms for which the drug has been prescribed. Drug serum levels are important in evaluating toxic or subtherapeutic dosage regimens of most antiarrhythmic drugs. They also aid in monitoring active metabolites (eg, procainamide/NAPA), suspected drug interactions and subtherapeutic response due to drug failure, noncompliance, altered clearance or altered absorption.

➤*Proarrhythmic effects:* Antiarrhythmic agents may cause new or worsened arrhythmias. Such proarrhythmic effects range from an increase in frequency of PVCs to the development of more severe ventricular tachycardia, ventricular fibrillation or torsade de pointes (ie, tachycardia that is more sustained or more rapid), which may lead to death. It is often not possible to distinguish a proarrhythmic effect from the patient's underlying rhythm disorder. It is therefore essential that each patient be evaluated electrocardiographically and clinically prior to and during therapy to determine whether the response to the drug supports continued treatment.

➤*Cardiac arrhythmia suppression trial:* In the National Heart, Lung and Blood Institute's Cardiac Arrhythmia Suppression Trial (CAST), a long-term, multicenter, randomized, double-blind study in patients with asymptomatic non-life-threatening ventricular ectopy who had had a myocardial infarction (MI) more than 6 days but less than 2 years previously, and who demonstrated mild to moderate left ventricular dysfunction, an excessive mortality or nonfatal cardiac arrest rate was seen in patients treated with encainide or flecainide (56/730) compared with that seen in patients assigned to carefully matched placebo treated groups (22/725). This led to discontinuation of those two arms of the trial. In this study, the average duration of treatment with flecainide was 10 months.

The moricizine and placebo arms of the trial were continued in CAST II. In this randomized, double-blind trial, patients with asymptomatic non-life-threatening arrhythmias who had had an MI within 4 to 90 days and left ventricular ejection fraction less than or equal to 0.4 prior to enrollment were evaluated. The average duration of moricizine treatment was 18 months. The study was discontinued because there was no possibility of demonstrating a benefit toward improved survival with moricizine and because of an evolving adverse trend after long-term treatment.

The applicability of these results to other populations (eg, those without recent MI) and to other antiarrhythmic drugs is uncertain, but at present it is prudent (1) to consider any IC agent (especially one documented to provoke new serious arrhythmias) to have a similar risk and (2) to consider the risks of Class IC agents, coupled with the lack of any evidence of improved survival, generally unacceptable in patients without life-threatening ventricular arrhythmias, even if the patients are experiencing unpleasant, but not life-threatening symptoms or signs.

➤*Pharmacokinetics:* The information in the pharmacokinetics table with clinical data and observation can be a valuable tool. However, the information must be used rationally and the data obtained properly (ie, obtaining and analyzing serum level data) to be effective. See individual monographs for more detailed explanations.

Antiarrhythmic Electrophysiology/Electrocardiogram Effects

Antiarrhythmic		Electrophysiology[a]										ECG changes[a]				
		Automaticity		Conduction velocity			Refractory period									
Group	Drug	SA node	Ectopic pacemaker	Atrium	AV node	His-Purkinje	Atrium	AV node	His-Purkinje	Ventricle	Accessory pathways[b]	Heart rate	PR interval	QRS complex	QT$_c$ interval	JT interval
I	Moricizine[c]	0	↓	0	↓	↓	±	0	0	0-↑	↑	0-↑	↑	↑	0	↓
	Quinidine	±	↓	↓	±	↓	↑↑	0-↑[d]	↑↑	↑	↑	±	±	↑	↑	↑
	Procainamide	±	↓	↓	±	↓	↑	0-↑[d]	↑↑	↑	↑↑	±	±	↑	↑	↑
	Disopyramide	±	↓	↓	±	↓	↑↑	0-↑[d]	↑↑	↑	↑	±	±	↑	↑	↑
	Lidocaine	0	↓	—	0	0	0	±	±	±	↑-↓	0	0	0	0-↓	0
	Phenytoin	↓-0	↓	—	0	0	0	±	±	±	—	±	0-↓	0	↓	0
	Tocainide	0-↓	↓	0	0	0	↓	↓	±	↓	↑	0	0	0	0-↓	0
	Mexiletine	↓	↓	0	↓	0	0	±	↑	↑	↑	-	0	0	0	0
	Flecainide	↓	↓	↓↓	↓	↓↓	0	0	↑	↑	↑↑	0	↑[e]	↑↑[e]	0-↑[e]	0
	Propafenone	↓	↓	0	↓	↓	0	↑	↑	↑	↑	0	↑[e]	↑	0-↑[e]	0
II	Propranolol	↓	↓	±	↓	0-↓	±	↑	0	0	0-↑	↓	0-↑	0	0-↓	0
	Esmolol	↓	↓	±	↓	0-	±	↑	0	0	0-↑	↓	0-↑	0	0-↓	0
	Acebutolol	↓	↓	±	↓	0	±	↑	0	0	0-↑	↓	0-↑	0	0-↓	0
III	Bretylium	↑	↑	0	↑	0-↑	0	↓-↑[f]	↑	0-↑	±	↓	0	0	↑	↑
	Amiodarone	↓	↓	↓	↓	↓	↑	↑	↑	↑	↑	↓	↑	↑	↑↑	↑↑
	Sotalol[g]	↓	↓	0	↓	0	↑↑	↑↑	↑↑	↑↑	↑↑	↓	↑	0	↑↑	↑↑
IV	Verapamil	↓	↓	0	↓	0	0	↑	0	0	0	↓	↑	0	0	0

Antiarrhythmic Electrophysiology/Electrocardiogram Effects

Antiarrhythmic		Electrophysiology[a]										ECG changes[a]				
		Automaticity		Conduction velocity			Refractory period									
Group	Drug	SA node	Ectopic pacemaker	Atrium	AV node	His-Purkinje	Atrium	AV node	His-Purkinje	Ventricle	Accessory pathways[b]	Heart rate	PR interval	QRS complex	QT_c interval	JT interval
—	Digoxin	0-↓	↑	±	↓	0-↓	±	↑	0	↓	↓-↑	↓	↑	0	↓	↓
—	Adenosine	↓	↓	0	↓	0	0	↑	0	0	0	↑	↑	0	0	—

[a] These values assume therapeutic levels.
[b] Accessory pathways occur in Wolff-Parkinson-White syndrome (preexcitation phenomena) and possibly other abnormal conditions.
[c] Does not belong to any of the 3 subclasses (A, B or C), but does have some properties of each.
[d] Retrograde AV node RP↑; antegrade RP not affected.
[e] Dose-related increases.
[f] Due to a complex balance of direct and indirect autonomic effects.
[g] Has both Group II (beta blocking) and III properties; Class III effects are seen at doses more than 160 mg.

Antiarrhythmic Pharmacokinetics

Antiarrhythmic									
Group		Drug	Onset (h) (oral)[a]	Duration (h)	Half-life (h)	Protein binding (%)	Excreted unchanged (%)	Therapeutic serum level (mcg/mL)	Toxic serum levels (mcg/mL)
I	A	Moricizine	2	10 to 24	1.5 to 3.5[b]	95	< 1	Not applicable	—
		Quinidine	0.5	6 to 8	6 to 7	80 to 90	10 to 50	2 to 6	> 8
		Procainamide	0.5	3+	2.5 to 4.7	14 to 23	40 to 70	4 to 8	> 16
		Disopyramide	0.5	6 to 7	4 to 10	20 to 60[c]	40 to 60	2 to 8	> 9
	B	Lidocaine		0.25[d]	1 to 2	40 to 80	< 3	1.5 to 6	> 7
		Phenytoin	0.5-1	24+	22 to 36[e]	87 to 93	< 5	10 to 20	> 20
		Tocainide	—	—	11 to 15	10 to 20	28 to 55	4 to 10	> 10
		Mexiletine	—	—	10 to 12	50 to 60	10	0.5 to 2	> 2
	C	Flecainide	—	—	12 to 27	40	30	0.2 to 1	> 1
		Propafenone	—	—	2 to 10[f]	97	< 1	0.06 to 1	—
II		Propranolol	0.5	3 to 5	2 to 3	90 to 95	< 1	0.05 to 0.1	—
		Esmolol	< 5 min	very short	0.15	55	< 2	—	—
		Acebutolol	—	24 to 30	3 to 4	26	15 to 20	—	—
III		Bretylium	—	6 to 8	5 to 10	0 to 8	> 80	0.5 to 1.5	—
		Amiodarone	1 to 3 wks[g]	weeks to months	26 to 107 days	96	negligible	0.5 to 2.5	> 2.5
		Sotalol	—	—	12	0	100	—	—
IV		Verapamil	0.5	6	3 to 7	90	3 to 4	0.08 to 0.3	—
—		Digoxin	0.5 to 2	24+	30 to 40	20 to 25	60	0.5 to 2 ng/mL	> 2.5 ng/mL
—		Adenosine	(34 sec IV)	1 to 2 min	< 10 sec	—	0 (enters body pool)	Not applicable	—

[a] Within 1 to 5 minutes with IV use.
[b] Half-life may be reduced in patients after multiple dosing.
[c] Protein binding is concentration dependent.
[d] Very short after discontinuation of IV infusion.
[e] Half-life increases with increasing dosage.
[f] Half-life 10 to 32 hours in < 10% of patients (slow metabolizers).
[g] Onset of action may occur in 2 to 3 days.

IBUTILIDE FUMARATE

Rx	**Ibutilide Fumarate** (Bioniche Pharma Group)	**Injection, solution:** 0.1 mg/mL	Equiv. to 0.087 mg ibutilide. In 10 mL single-dose vials.
Rx	**Corvert** (Pharmacia & Upjohn)		Equiv. to 0.087 mg ibutilide. In 10 mL vials.

IBUTILIDE FUMARATE INJECTION

Refer to the general introductory discussion concerning Antiarrhythmic Agents.

WARNING

Life-threatening arrhythmias – Ibutilide fumarate can cause potentially fatal arrythmias, particularly sustained polymorphic ventricular tachycardia usually in association with QT prolongation (torsades de pointes), but sometimes without documented QT prolongation. In registration studies, these arrythmias, which require cardioversion, occurred in 1.7% of treated patients during or within a number of hours of using ibutilide fumarate.

These arrythmias can be reversed if treated promptly. It is essential that ibutilide be administered in a setting of continuous ECG monitoring and by personnel trained in identification and treatment of acute ventricular arrythmias, particularly polymorphic ventricular tachycardia. Patients with atrial fibrillation of more than 2 to 3 days' duration must be adequately anticoagulated, generally for at least 2 weeks.

Appropriate treatment environment –

Choice of patients: Patients with chronic atrial fibrillation have a strong tendency to revert after conversion to sinus rhythm and treatments to maintain sinus rhythm carry risks. Patients to be treated with ibutilide fumarate, therefore, should be carefully selected such that the expected benefits of maintaining sinus rhythm outweigh the immediate risks of ibutilide, and the risks of maintenance therapy, and are likely to offer an advantage compared with alternative management.

Indications

➤*Rapid conversion of atrial fibrillation or atrial flutter:* For the rapid conversion of atrial fibrillation or atrial flutter of recent onset to sinus rhythm. Patients with atrial arrhythmias of longer duration are less likely to respond to ibutilide fumarate. The effectiveness of ibutilide has not been determined in patients with arrhythmias of more than 90 days in duration.

Administration and Dosage

➤*Adults:*

Rapid conversion of atrial fibrillation or atrial flutter of recent onset to sinus rhythm –

Usual dosage: The recommended dose based on controlled trials is outlined below. Ibutilide infusion should be stopped as soon as the presenting arrhythmia is terminated or in the event of sustained or nonsustained ventricular tachycardia, or marked prolongation of QT or QTc.

IBUTILIDE FUMARATE — INJECTION

Recommended Dose of Ibutilide		
Patient weight	Initial infusion (over 10 minutes)	Second infusion
60 kg (132 lbs) or more	1 vial (1 mg ibutilide fumarate)	If the arrhythmia does not terminate within 10 minutes after the end of the initial infusion, a second 10-minute infusion of equal strength may be administered 10 minutes after completion of the first infusion.
Less than 60 kg (132 lbs)	0.1 mL/kg (0.01 mg/kg ibutilide fumarate)	

In a trial comparing ibutilide and sotalol, ibutilide fumarate 2 mg administered as a single infusion to patients weighing 60 kg or more was also effective in terminating atrial fibrillation or atrial flutter.

In the postcardiac surgery study, 1 or 2 IV infusions of 0.5 mg (0.005 mg/kg/dose for patients weighing less than 60 kg) was effective in terminating atrial fibrillation or atrial flutter.

➤*ECG monitoring:* Patients should be observed with continuous ECG monitoring for at least 4 hours following infusion or until QTc has returned to baseline. Longer monitoring is required if any arrhythmic activity is noted.

➤*Preparation for administration:* Ibutilide fumarate may be added to 0.9% sodium chloride injection or 5% dextrose injection before infusion. The contents of one 10 mL vial (0.1 mg/mL) may be added to a 50 mL infusion bag to form an ibutilide fumarate admixture of approximately 0.017 mg/mL.

➤*Administration:* Give by rapid IV therapy (duration less than or equal to 30 minutes).

Administer undiluted or diluted in 50 mL of diluent.

Skilled personnel and proper equipment, such as a cardioverter/defibrillator, and medication for treatment of sustained ventricular tachycardia, including polymorphic ventricular tachycardia, must be available during administration of ibutilide fumarate and subsequent monitoring of the patient.

➤*Admixture compatibility:* The following diluents are compatible with ibutilide fumarate injection (0.1 mg/mL): dextrose 5% injection and sodium chloride 0.9% injection.

The following IV solution containers are compatible with admixtures of ibutilide fumarate injection (0.1 mg/mL): polyvinyl chloride plastic bags and polyolefin bags.

➤*Storage/Stability:* Store at 20° to 25°C (68° to 77°F). Store vial in carton until used.

Admixtures of the product, with approved diluents, are chemically and physically stable for 24 hours at room temperature (15° to 30°C; 59° to 86°F) and for 48 hours at refrigerated temperatures (2° to 8°C; 36° to 46°F). Strict adherence to the use of aseptic technique during the preparation of the admixture is recommended in order to maintain sterility.

Actions

➤*Pharmacology:* Ibutilide fumarate injection prolongs action potential duration in isolated adult cardiac myocytes and increases both atrial and ventricular refractoriness in vivo (ie, class III electrophysiologic effects). Voltage clamp studies indicate that ibutilide fumarate, at nanomolar concentrations, delays repolarization by activation of a slow, inward current (predominantly sodium), rather than by blocking outward potassium currents, which is the mechanism by which most other class III antiarrhythmics act. These effects lead to prolongation of atrial and ventricular action potential duration and refractoriness, the predominant electrophysiologic properties of ibutilide fumarate in humans that are thought to be the basis for its antiarrhythmic effect.

➤*Pharmacokinetics:* The pharmacokinetics of ibutilide are linear with respect to the dose of ibutilide fumarate over the dose range of 0.01 mg/kg to 0.1 mg/kg. The enantiomers of ibutilide fumarate have pharmacokinetic properties similar to each other and to ibutilide fumarate.

Absorption/Distribution – After IV infusion, ibutilide plasma concentrations rapidly decrease in a multiexponential fashion. The pharmacokinetics of ibutilide are highly variable among subjects. Ibutilide has a high systemic plasma clearance that approximates liver blood flow (approximately 29 mL/min/kg), a large steady-state volume of distribution (approximately 11 L/kg) in healthy volunteers, and minimal (approximately 40%) protein binding. Ibutilide is also cleared rapidly and highly distributed in patients being treated for atrial flutter or atrial fibrillation.

The pharmacokinetics of ibutilide are linear with respect to the dose of ibutilide fumarate over the dose range of 0.01 mg/kg to 0.1 mg/kg. The enantiomers of ibutilide fumarate have pharmacokinetic properties similar to each other and to ibutilide fumarate.

Metabolism/Excretion – In healthy male volunteers, approximately 82% of a 0.01 mg/kg dose of ibutilide fumarate was excreted in the urine (approximately 7% of the dose as unchanged ibutilide) and the remainder (approximately 19%) was recovered in the feces. Ibutilide has a high systemic plasma clearance that approximates liver blood flow (approximately 29 mL/min/kg). The elimination half-life averages approximately 6 hours (range, 2 to 12 hours).

Eight metabolites of ibutilide were detected in metabolic profiling of urine. These metabolites are thought to be formed primarily by ω-oxidation followed by sequential β-oxidation of the heptyl side chain of ibutilide. Of the 8 metabolites, only the ω-hydroxy metabolite possesses class III electrophysiologic properties similar to that of ibutilide in an in vitro isolated rabbit myocardium model. The plasma concentrations of this active metabolite, however, are less than 10% of that of ibutilide.

Contraindications

Hypersensitivity to ibutilide or any of the other product components.

Warnings/Precautions

➤*Proarrhythmia:* Like other antiarrhythmic agents, ibutilide fumarate injection can induce or worsen ventricular arrhythmias in some patients. This may have potentially fatal consequences. Torsades de pointes, a polymorphic ventricular tachycardia that develops in the selling of a prolonged QT interval, may occur because of the effect ibutilide fumarate has on cardiac repolarization, but ibutilide fumarate can also cause polymorphic VT in the absence of excessive prolongation of the QT interval. In general, with drugs that prolong the QT interval, the risk of torsades de pointes is thought to increase progressively as the QT interval is prolonged and may be worsened with bradycardia, a varying heart rate, and hypokalemia. In clinical trials conducted in patients with atrial fibrillation and atrial flutter, those with QTc intervals more than 440 msec were not usually allowed to participate, and serum potassium had to be more than 4 mEq/L. Although change in QTc was dose dependent for ibutilide, there was no clear relationship between risk of serious proarrhythmia and dose in clinical studies, possibly due to the small number of events.

➤*Heart block:* Of the 9 (1.5%) ibutilide-treated patients with reports of reversible heart block, 5 had first-degree, 3 had second-degree, and 1 had complete heart block.

➤*Renal/Hepatic function impairment:* Patients with abnormal liver function should be monitored by telemetry for more than the 4-hour period generally recommended.

The safety, efficacy, and pharmacokinetics of ibutilide fumarate have not been established in patients with hepatic or renal dysfunction. However, it is unlikely that dosing adjustments would be necessary in patients with compromised renal or hepatic function based on the following considerations:

- Ibutilide fumarate is indicated for rapid IV therapy (duration less than or equal to 30 minutes) and is dosed to a known, well-defined pharmacologic action (termination of arrhythmia) or to a maximum of two 10-minute infusions.
- Less than 10% of the dose of ibutilide fumarate is excreted unchanged in the urine.
- Drug distribution appears to be one of the primary mechanisms responsible for termination of the pharmacologic effect. Nonetheless, patients with abnormal liver function should be monitored by telemetry for more than the 4–hour period generally recommended.

➤*Pregnancy: Category C.* Ibutilide administered orally was teratogenic (abnormalities included adactyly, interventricular septal defects, and scoliosis) and embryocidal in reproduction studies in rats. On a mg/m^2 basis, corrected for the 3% oral bioavailability, the no adverse effect dose (5 mg/kg/day given orally) was approximately the same as the maximum recommended human dose (MRHD); the teratogenic dose (20 mg/kg/day given orally) was approximately 4 times the MRHD on a mg/m^2 basis, or 16 times the MRHD on a mg/kg basis. Ibutilide fumarate should not be administered to a pregnant woman unless clinical benefit outweighs potential risk to the fetus.

➤*Lactation:* The excretion of ibutilide into breast milk has not been studied, accordingly, breast-feeding should be discouraged during therapy with ibutilide fumarate.

➤*Children:* Safety and efficacy of ibutilide in children younger than 18 years of age have not been established.

➤*Monitoring:* Observe patients with continuous ECG monitoring for at least 4 hours following infusion or until QTc has returned to baseline. Longer monitoring is required if any arrhythmic activity is noted. Skilled personnel and proper equipment, such as a cardioverter/defibrillator, and medication for treatment of sustained ventricular tachycardia, including polymorphic ventricular tachycardia, must be available during administration of ibutilide fumarate and subsequent monitoring of the patient.

Drug Interactions

➤*QT prolongation:* An additive effect of ibutilide with other drugs that prolong the QT interval cannot be excluded. The following drugs may prolong the QT interval and increase the risk of life-threatening cardiac arrhythmias, including torsade de pointes: Antiarrhythmic agents (eg, amiodarone, bretylium, disopyramide, dofetilide, procainamide, quinidine, and sotalol), arsenic trioxide, chlorpromazine, cisapride, dolasetron, droperidol, mefloquine, mesoridazine, moxifloxacin, pentamidine, pimozide, tacrolimus, thioridazine, and ziprasidone. For a more complete list of drugs that may prolong the QT interval, see the appendix, Drug-Induced Prolongation of the QT Interval and Torsade de Pointes.

➤*Digoxin:* Supraventricular arrhythmias may mask the cardiotoxicity associated with excessive digoxin levels. Therefore, it is advisable to be particularly cautious in patients whose plasma digoxin levels are above or suspected to be above the usual therapeutic range. Coadministration of digoxin did not have effects on either the safety or efficacy of ibutilide in the clinical trials.

Adverse Reactions

Ibutilide fumarate injection was generally well tolerated in clinical trials. Of the 586 patients with atrial fibrillation or atrial flutter who received ibutilide fumarate in phase 2 or 3 studies, 149 (25%) reported medical events related to the cardiovascular system, including sustained polymorphic ventricular tachycardia (1.7%) and nonsustained polymorphic ventricular tachycardia (2.7%).

IBUTILIDE FUMARATE — INJECTION

Other clinically important adverse events with an uncertain relationship to ibutilide fumarate include the following (0.2% represents 1 patient): Sustained monomorphic ventricular tachycardia (0.2%), nonsustained monomorphic ventricular tachycardia (4.9%), AV block (1.5%), bundle branch block (1.9%), ventricular extrasystoles (5.1%), supraventricular extrasystoles (0.9%), hypotension/postural hypotension (2%), bradycardia/sinus bradycardia (1.2%), nodal arrhythmia (0.7%), congestive heart failure (0.5%), tachycardia/sinus tachycardia/supraventricular tachycardia (2.7%), idioventricular rhythm (0.2%), syncope (0.3%), and renal failure (0.3%). The incidence of those events, except for syncope, was greater in the group treated with ibutilide fumarate than in the placebo group. Another adverse reaction that may be associated with the administration of ibutilide fumarate was nausea, which occurred with a frequency greater than 1% more in ibutilide-treated patients than those treated with placebo.

Ibutilide Treatment-Emergent Adverse Reactions (≥ 1% More Than Placebo)

Adverse reaction	Placebo patients (n = 127)		All ibutilide patients (n = 586)	
	n	%	n	%
Cardiovascular				
Ventricular extrasystoles	1	0.8%	30	5.1%
Nonsustained monomorphic VT	1	0.8%	29	4.9%
Nonsustained polymorphic VT	-	-	16	2.7%
Hypotension	2	1.6%	12	2%
Bundle branch block	-	-	11	1.9%
Sustained polymorphic VT	-	-	10	1.7%
AV block	1	0.8%	9	1.5%
Hypertension	-	-	7	1.2%
QT segment prolonged	-	-	7	1.2%
Bradycardia	1	0.8%	7	1%
Palpitation	1	0.8%	6	1%
Tachycardia	1	0.8%	16	2.7%
CNS				
Headache	4	3.1%	21	3.6%
GI				
Nausea	1	0.8%	11	1.9%

In the postcardiac surgery study, similar types of medical events were reported. In the 1 mg ibutilide fumarate treatment group (n = 70), 2 patients (2.9%) developed sustained polymorphic ventricular tachycardia and 2 other patients (2.9%) developed nonsustained polymorphic ventricular tachycardia. Polymorphic ventricular tachycardia was not reported in the 73 patients in the 0.5 mg dose group or in the 75 patients in the 0.25 mg dose group.

Overdosage

➤*Symptoms:*

Human experience – In the registration trials with ibutilide fumarate injection, 4 patients were unintentionally overdosed. The largest dose was 3.4 mg administered over 15 minutes. One patient (0.025 mg/kg) developed increased ventricular octopy and monomorphic ventricular tachycardia, another patient (0.032 mg/kg) developed AV block third-degree and nonsustained polymorphic VT, and 2 patients (0.038 and 0.02 mg/kg) had no medical event reports. Based on known pharmacology, the clinical effects of an overdosage with ibutilide could exaggerate the expected prolongation of repolarization seen at usual clinical doses.

➤*Treatment:* Medical events (eg, proarrhythmia, AV block) that occur after the overdosage should be treated with measures appropriate for that condition.

DRONEDARONE

Rx	**Multaq** (Sanofi-Aventis)	**Tablets; oral:** 400 mg	Lactose. (4142). White, oblong. Film-coated. In 60s, 180s, 500s, and UD 100s.

DRONEDARONE — ORAL

WARNING

Dronedarone is contraindicated in patients with New York Heart Association (NYHA) class IV heart failure or NYHA class II to III heart failure with a recent decompensation requiring hospitalization or referral to a specialized heart failure clinic.

In a placebo-controlled study in patients with severe heart failure requiring recent hospitalization or referral to a specialized heart failure clinic for worsening symptoms (the ANDROMEDA study), patients given dronedarone had a greater than 2-fold increase in mortality. Do not give such patients dronedarone.

Indications

➤*Paroxysmal or persistent atrial fibrillation or paroxysmal or persistent atrial flutter:* To reduce the risk of cardiovascular hospitalization in patients with paroxysmal or persistent atrial fibrillation or paroxysmal or persistent atrial flutter, with a recent episode of atrial fibrillation/atrial flutter and associated cardiovascular risk factors (ie, older than 70 years of age, hypertension, diabetes, prior cerebrovascular accident, left atrial diameter 50 mm or more or left ventricular ejection fraction [LVEF] less than 40%), who are in sinus rhythm or who will be cardioverted.

Administration and Dosage

➤*General dosing considerations:* Treatment with class I or III antiarrhythmics (eg, amiodarone, flecainide, propafenone, quinidine, disopyramide, dofetilide, sotalol) or drugs that are strong inhibitors of CYP3A4 (eg, ketoconazole) must be stopped before taking dronedarone.

➤*Adults:*

Paroxysmal or persistent atrial fibrillation or atrial flutter –
Usual dosage: 400 mg orally twice daily with morning and evening meals.

➤*Administration:* Take with morning and evening meals.

➤*Storage/Stability:* Store at 25°C (77°F); excursions are permitted to 15° to 30°C (59° to 86°F).

Actions

➤*Pharmacology:* The mechanism of action of dronedarone is unknown. Dronedarone has antiarrhythmic properties belonging to all 4 Vaughan-Williams classes, but the contribution of each of these activities to the clinical effect is unknown.

Pharmacodynamics –
Electrophysiological effects: Dronedarone exhibits properties of all 4 Vaughan-Williams antiarrhythmic classes, although it is unclear which of these are important in producing dronedarone's clinical effects. The effect of dronedarone on 12-lead electrocardiogram parameters (heart rate, PR, and QTc) was investigated in healthy subjects following repeated oral dosages of up to 1,600 mg once daily or 800 mg twice daily for 14 days and 1,600 mg twice daily for 10 days. In the dronedarone 400 mg twice daily group, there was no apparent effect on heart rate; a moderate heart rate lowering effect (about 4 bpm) was noted at 800 mg twice daily. There was a clear dose-dependent effect on PR interval, with an increase of +5 ms at 400 mg twice daily and up to +50 ms at 1,600 mg twice daily. There was a moderate dose-related effect on the QTc interval with an increase of +10 ms at 400 mg twice daily and up to +25 ms with 1,600 mg twice daily.

➤*Pharmacokinetics:*

Absorption – After oral administration in fed conditions, peak plasma concentrations of dronedarone and the main circulating active metabolite (N-debutyl metabolite) are reached within 3 to 6 hours. After repeated administration of 400 mg twice daily, steady state is reached within 4 to 8 days of treatment, and the mean accumulation ratio for dronedarone ranges from 2.6 to 4.5. The steady-state maximum drug concentration (C_{max}) and exposure of the main N-debutyl metabolite is similar to that of the parent compound. The pharmacokinetics of dronedarone and its N-debutyl metabolite deviate moderately from dose proportionality: a 2-fold increase in dose results in an approximate 2.5- to 3-fold increase with respect to C_{max} and area under the curve (AUC).

Effect of food: The bioavailability of dronedarone is increased by meals. Because of presystemic first-pass metabolism, the absolute bioavailability of dronedarone without food is low, about 4%. It increases to approximately 15% when dronedarone is administered with a high-fat meal.

Distribution – The in vitro plasma protein binding of dronedarone and its N-debutyl metabolite is greater than 98% and not saturable. Both compounds bind mainly to albumin. After intravenous (IV) administration, the volume of distribution at steady state is about 1,400 L.

Metabolism – Dronedarone is extensively metabolized, mainly by CYP3A. The initial metabolic pathway includes N-debutylation to form the active N-debutyl metabolite, oxidative deamination to form the inactive propanoic acid metabolite, and direct oxidation. The metabolites undergo further metabolism to yield over 30 uncharacterized metabolites. The N-debutyl metabolite exhibits pharmacodynamic activity but is 1/10 to 1/3 as potent as dronedarone.

Excretion – In a mass balance study with orally administered dronedarone (^{14}C-labeled), approximately 6% of the labeled dose was excreted in urine, mainly as metabolites (no unchanged compound excreted in urine), and 84% was excreted in feces, mainly as metabolites. Dronedarone and its N-debutyl active metabolite accounted for less than 15% of the resultant radioactivity in the plasma.

After IV administration, the plasma clearance of dronedarone ranges from 130 to 150 L/h. The elimination half-life of dronedarone ranges from 13 to 19 hours.

Special populations –
Hepatic function impairment: In subjects with moderate hepatic impairment, the mean dronedarone exposure increased by 1.3-fold relative to subjects with healthy hepatic function, and the mean exposure of the N-debutyl metabolite decreased by about 50%. Pharmacokinetic data were significantly more variable in subjects with moderate hepatic impairment. The

DRONEDARONE — ORAL

effect of severe hepatic impairment on the pharmacokinetics of dronedarone was not assessed. Dronedarone is contraindicated in severe hepatic impairment.

Gender: Dronedarone exposures are on average 30% higher in women than in men.

Race: Pharmacokinetic differences related to race were not formally assessed. However, based on a cross-study comparison following single dose administration (400 mg), Asian men (Japanese) have about a 2-fold higher exposure than white men. The pharmacokinetics of dronedarone in other races have not been assessed.

Contraindications

NYHA class IV heart failure or NYHA class II to III heart failure with a recent decompensation requiring hospitalization or referral to a specialized heart failure clinic; second-degree or third-degree atrioventricular (AV) block or sick sinus syndrome (except when used in conjunction with a functioning pacemaker); bradycardia less than 50 bpm; concomitant use of strong CYP3A inhibitors, such as ketoconazole, itraconazole, voriconazole, cyclosporine, telithromycin, clarithromycin, nefazodone, and ritonavir; concomitant use of drugs or herbal products that prolong the QT interval and might increase the risk of torsades de pointes, such as phenothiazine antipsychotics, tricyclic antidepressants, certain oral macrolide antibiotics, and class I and III antiarrhythmics; QTc Bazett interval 500 ms or more or PR interval more than 280 ms; severe hepatic impairment; pregnancy; breast-feeding mothers.

Warnings/Precautions

➤*Heart failure:* Advise patients to consult a health care provider if they develop signs or symptoms of heart failure, such as weight gain, dependent edema, or increasing shortness of breath. There are limited data available for atrial fibrillation/atrial flutter patients who develop worsening heart failure during treatment with dronedarone. If heart failure develops or worsens, consider the suspension or discontinuation of dronedarone.

➤*Concomitant use with potassium-depleting diuretics:* Hypokalemia or hypomagnesemia may occur with coadministration of potassium-depleting diuretics. Potassium levels should be within the normal range prior to administration of dronedarone and maintained in the normal range during administration of dronedarone.

➤*QT interval prolongation:* Dronedarone induces a moderate (average of about 10 ms, but much greater effects have been observed) QTc (Bazett) prolongation. If the QTc Bazett interval is 500 ms or more, stop dronedarone.

➤*Renal effects:* Serum creatinine levels increase by about 0.1 mg/dL following dronedarone treatment initiation. The elevation has a rapid onset, reaches a plateau after 7 days, and is reversible after discontinuation. If an increase in serum creatinine occurs and plateaus, use this increased value as the patient's new baseline. The change in creatinine levels has been shown to be the result of an inhibition of creatinine's tubular secretion, with no effect upon the glomerular filtration rate.

➤*Women of childbearing potential:* Premenopausal women who have not undergone a hysterectomy or oophorectomy must use effective contraception while using dronedarone. Dronedarone caused fetal harm in animal studies at doses equivalent to recommended human doses. Counsel women of childbearing potential regarding appropriate contraceptive choices, taking into consideration their underlying medical conditions and lifestyle preferences.

➤*Hepatic function impairment:* See Administration and Dosage for more information.

➤*Pregnancy: Category X.* Dronedarone may cause fetal harm when administered to a pregnant woman. Dronedarone is contraindicated in women who are or may become pregnant. If this drug is used during pregnancy or if the patient becomes pregnant while taking this drug, apprise the patient of the potential hazard to the fetus.

In animal studies, dronedarone was teratogenic in rats at the MRHD and in rabbits at half the MRHD. When pregnant rats received dronedarone at oral doses of the MRHD or more (on a mg/m^2 basis), fetuses had increased rates of external, visceral, and skeletal malformations (cranioschisis, cleft palate, incomplete evagination of pineal body, brachygnathia, partially fused carotid arteries, truncus arteriosus, abnormal lobation of the liver, partially duplicated inferior vena cava, brachydactyly, ectrodactylia, syndactylia, and anterior and/or posterior club feet). When pregnant rabbits received dronedarone at a dose approximately half the MRHD (on a mg/m^2 basis), fetuses had an increased rate of skeletal abnormalities (anomalous ribcage and vertebrae, pelvic asymmetry) at doses 20 mg/kg or more (the lowest dose tested and approximately half the MRHD on a mg/m^2 basis). Actual animal doses: rat (80 mg/kg/day or more); rabbit (20 mg/kg or more).

➤*Lactation:* It is not known whether dronedarone is excreted in human milk. Dronedarone is contraindicated in breast-feeding women. Because many drugs are excreted in human milk and because of the potential for serious adverse reactions in breast-feeding infants from dronedarone, make a decision whether to discontinue breast-feeding or the drug, taking into account the importance of the drug to the mother. Dronedarone and its metabolites are excreted in rat milk. During a pre- and postnatal study in rats, maternal dronedarone administration was associated with minor reduced body-weight gain in the offspring.

➤*Children:* Safety and efficacy in children younger than 18 years of age have not been established.

Drug Interactions

➤*QT prolongation:* An additive effect of dronedarone with other drugs that prolong the QT interval cannot be excluded. The following drugs may prolong the QT interval and increase the risk of life-threatening cardiac arrhythmias, including torsades de pointes: antiarrhythmic agents (eg, amiodarone, bretylium, disopyramide, dofetilide, procainamide, quinidine, sotalol), arsenic trioxide, chlorpromazine, cisapride, dolasetron, droperidol, mefloquine, mesoridazine, moxifloxacin, pentamidine, pimozide, tacrolimus, thioridazine, and ziprasidone. For a more complete list of drugs that may prolong the QT interval, see the appendix "Drug-Induced Prolongation of the QT Interval and Torsades de Pointes."

Dronedarone Drug Interactions[a]

Precipitant drug	Object drug[b]		Description
Beta-blockers (eg, metoprolol propranolol)	Dronedarone	↑	Bradycardia was more frequently observed when dronedarone was given with beta-blockers. Dronedarone may increase beta-blocker exposure. Give lower initial dose of beta-blockers and increase only after ECG verification of good tolerability.
Dronedarone	Beta-blockers (eg, metoprolol propranolol)		
Calcium channel blockers (eg, diltiazem, verapamil)	Dronedarone	↑	Increased dronedarone exposure may occur. Dronedarone may increase calcium channel blocker exposure. Give lower initial dose of calcium channel blockers and increase only after ECG verification of good tolerability.
Dronedarone	Calcium channel blockers (eg, diltiazem, verapamil)		
Class I and III antiarrhythmics (eg, amiodarone, disopyramide, dofetilide, flecainide, propafenone, quinidine, sotalol)	Dronedarone	↑	Contraindicated because of the potential risk of torsades de pointes–type ventricular tachycardia.
CYP3A inducers (eg, carbamazepine, phenobarbital, phenytoin, rifampin, St. John's wort)	Dronedarone	↓	Rifampin decreased dronedarone exposure by 80%. Avoid concomitant use.
CYP3A inhibitors (eg, cyclosporine, itraconazole, ketoconazole, macrolide antibiotics [eg, clarithromycin, telithromycin], nefazodone, ritonavir, voriconazole)	Dronedarone	↑	Concomitant use with strong CYP3A inhibitors is contraindicated. Repeated doses of ketoconazole resulted in a 17-fold increase in dronedarone exposure and a 9-fold increase in C_{max}.
Phenothiazine antipsychotics (eg, chlorpromazine, thioridazine)	Dronedarone	↑	Contraindicated because of the potential risk of torsades de pointes–type ventricular tachycardia.
TCAs (eg, amitriptyline)	Dronedarone	↑	Contraindicated because of the potential risk of torsades de pointes–type ventricular tachycardia. TCAs may have increased exposure upon coadministration with dronedarone.
Dronedarone	TCAs (eg, amitriptyline)		
Dronedarone	CYP2D6 (eg, SSRIs [fluoxetine]) and 3A substrates (eg, midazolam, pimozide, sirolimus, tacrolimus)	↑	Dronedarone may increase the plasma concentrations of these drugs when given. Dose adjustment may be needed.

DRONEDARONE — ORAL

Dronedarone Drug Interactions[a]			
Precipitant drug	Object drug[b]		Description
Dronedarone	P-glycoprotein substrates (eg, digoxin)	⬆	Increased P-glycoprotein substrate exposure may be expected. Digoxin can potentiate the electrophysiologic effects of dronedarone. Decrease digoxin dose by 50%, monitor serum levels closely, and observe for toxicity.
P-glycoprotein substrates (eg, digoxin)	Dronedarone		
Dronedarone	Simvastatin	⬆	Increased simvastatin and simvastatin acid exposure by 4- and 2-fold, respectively.
Dronedarone	Warfarin	⬆	Dronedarone may increase S-warfarin exposure. Monitor INR.

[a] ECG = electrocardiogram; SSRI = serotonin reuptake inhibitor; TCA = tricyclic antidepressant; INR = international normalized ratio.
[b] ⬆ = object drug increased; ⬇ = object drug decreased.

➤*Drug/Food interactions:* Grapefruit juice, a moderate inhibitor of CYP3A, resulted in a 3-fold increase in dronedarone exposure and a 2.5 fold increase in C_{max}. Therefore, instruct patients to avoid grapefruit beverages while taking dronedarone.

Adverse Reactions

➤*Discontinuation:* In clinical trials, premature discontinuation because of adverse reactions occurred in 11.8% of the dronedarone-treated patients and in 7.7% of the placebo-treated group. The most common reasons for discontinuation of therapy with dronedarone were GI disorders (3.2% vs 1.8% in the placebo group) and QT prolongation (1.5% vs 0.5% in the placebo group).

➤*Most frequent adverse reactions:*

Dronedarone Adverse Drug Reactions (≥ 1%)		
Adverse reaction	Dronedarone 400 mg twice daily (n = 3,282)	Placebo (n = 2,875)
GI		
Abdominal pain	4%	3%
Diarrhea	9%	6%
Dyspeptic signs and symptoms	2%	1%
Nausea	5%	3%
Vomiting	2%	1%
Miscellaneous		
Asthenic conditions	7%	5%

Dronedarone Adverse Drug Reactions (≥ 1%)		
Adverse reaction	Dronedarone 400 mg twice daily (n = 3,282)	Placebo (n = 2,875)
Bradycardia	3%	1%
Skin and subcutaneous tissue including rashes (generalized, macular, maculopapular, erythematous), pruritus, eczema, dermatitis, dermatitis allergic	5%	3%

➤*Other adverse reactions:* Dysgeusia, photosensitivity reaction (less than 1%).

➤*Lab test abnormalities:*

Dronedarone Laboratory/ECG Effects		
	Dronedarone 400 mg twice daily	Placebo
Serum creatinine increased ≥ 10% five days after treatment initiation	(n = 3,282) 51%	(n = 2,875) 21%
QTc Bazett prolonged (> 450 ms in men, > 470 ms in women)	(n = 2,701) 28%	(n = 2,237) 19%

Overdosage

➤*Treatment:* Monitor the patient's cardiac rhythm and blood pressure. Treatment should be supportive and based on symptoms. It is not known whether dronedarone or its metabolites can be removed by dialysis (hemodialysis, peritoneal dialysis, or hemofiltration). There is no specific antidote available.

Patient Information

Administer dronedarone with a meal. Warn patients not to take dronedarone with grapefruit juice.

If a dose is missed, instruct patients to take the next dose at the regularly scheduled time and not to double the dose.

Advise patients to consult a health care provider if they develop signs or symptoms of worsening heart failure such as acute weight gain, dependent edema, or increasing shortness of breath.

Advise patients to inform their health care provider of any history of heart failure, rhythm disturbance other than atrial fibrillation or flutter, or predisposing conditions such as uncorrected hypokalemia.

Dronedarone may interact with some drugs; therefore, advise patients to report to their health care provider the use of any other prescription, nonprescription medication, or herbal products, particularly St. John's wort.

Counsel women of childbearing potential regarding appropriate contraceptive choices, taking into consideration their underlying medical conditions and lifestyle preferences.

QUINIDINE

Quinidine gluconate contains 62% anhydrous quinidine alkaloid. Quinidine sulfate contains 83% anhydrous quinidine alkaloid.

Rx	**Quinidine Sulfate** (Mutual)	**Tablets; oral:** 100 mg	In 50s, 100s, 250s, 500s, and 1,000s.
Rx	**Quinidine Sulfate** (Various, eg, Danbury, Eon, Mutual)	**Tablets; oral:** 200 mg	In 50s, 100s, 250s, 500s, and 1000s.
Rx	**Quinidine Sulfate** (Various, eg, Danbury, Eon, Mutual)	**Tablets; oral:** 300 mg	In 50s, 100s, 250s, 500,s and 1000s.
Rx	**Quinidine Gluconate** (Various, eg, UDL Labs)	**Tablets, sustained-release:** 324 mg	In 100s, 250s, and 500s.
Rx	**Quinidine Sulfate** (Various, eg, Teva)	**Tablets, sustained-release; oral:** 300 mg	In 100s and 250s.
Rx	**Quinidine Gluconate** (Lilly)	**Injection:** 80 mg/mL (50 mg/mL quinidine)	In 10 mL multi-dose vials.[a]

[a] With 0.005% EDTA and 0.25% phenol.

QUINIDINE SULFATE — ORAL

For complete and comparative prescribing information, refer to the Quinidine group monograph.

QUINIDINE GLUCONATE — INJECTION

For complete and comparative prescribing information, refer to the Quinidine group monograph.

PROCAINAMIDE HYDROCHLORIDE

Rx	**Procainamide HCl** (Hospira)	**Injection solution:** 100 mg/mL	Methylparaben, sodium metabisulfite. In 10 mL multi-dose vials.
Rx	**Procainamide HCl** (Various, eg, Hospira)	**Injection solution:** 500 mg/mL	May contain methylparaben and sodium metabisulfite. In 2 mL vials.

[a] These extended-release tablets are dosed at 6-hour intervals.

[b] These extended-release tablets are dosed at 12-hour intervals.

PROCAINAMIDE HYDROCHLORIDE — INJECTION

WARNING

The prolonged administration of procainamide often leads to the development of a positive antinuclear antibody (ANA) test, with or without symptoms of a lupus erythematosus-like syndrome. If a positive ANA titer develops, the benefits versus risks of continued procainamide therapy should be assessed.

Mortality – In the National Heart, Lung and Blood Institute's Cardiac Arrhythmia Suppression Trial (CAST), a long-term, multicenter, randomized, double-blind study in patients with asymptomatic non-life-threatening ventricular arrhythmias who had myocardial infarction more than 6 days but less than 2 years previously, an excessive mortality or nonfatal cardiac arrest rate (7.7%) was seen in patients treated with encainide or flecainide compared with that seen in patients assigned to matched placebo-treated group (3%). The average duration of treatment with onoalnide or flocainide in this study was 10 months.

The applicability of the cast results to other populations (eg, those without recent myocardial infarctions) is uncertain. Considering the known proarrhythmic properties of procainamide and the lack of evidence of improved survival for any antiarrhythmic drug in patients without life-threatening arrhythmias, the use of procainamide as well as other antiarrhythmic agents should be reserved for patients with life-threatening ventricular arrhythmias.

Blood dyscrasias – Agranulocytosis, bone marrow depression, neutropenia, hypoplastic anemia and thrombocytopenia in patients receiving procainamide HCl have been reported at a rate of approximately 0.5%. Most of these patients received procainamide within the recommended dosage range. Fatalities have occurred (with approximately 20 to 25% mortality in reported cases of agranulocytosis). Since most of these events have been noted during the first 12 weeks of therapy, it is recommended that complete blood counts including white cell, differential and platelet counts be performed at weekly intervals for the first 3 months of therapy, and periodically thereafter. Complete blood counts should be performed promptly if the patient develops any signs of infection (such as fever, chills, sore throat or stomatitis), bruising or bleeding. If any of those hematologic disorders are identified, procainamide therapy should be discontinued. Blood counts usually return to normal within 1 month of discontinuation. Caution should be used in patients with preexisting marrow failure or cytopenia of any type.

Indications

➤*Ventricular arrhythmias:* For the treatment of documented ventricular arrhythmias, such as sustained ventricular tachycardia, that, in the judgment of the physician, are life-threatening. Because of the proarrhythmic effects of procainamide, its use with lesser arrhythmias is generally not recommended. Treatment of patients with asymptomatic ventricular premature contractions should be avoided.

➤*Off-label uses:*

Atrial fibrillation/flutter – Procainamide has been used to convert atrial fibrillation/flutter to sinus rhythm.

Use in children – The following doses of procainamide have been suggested:

IM: 20 to 30 mg/kg/day.

IV: Loading dose is 3 to 6 mg/kg infused over 5 minutes, not to exceed 100 mg/dose. Maintenance dose is 20 to 80 mcg/kg/min as continuous IV infusion; usual maximum is 2 g/day.

For the treatment of hemodynamically stable ventricular tachycardia in children, procainamide (loading dose of 15 mg/kg IV infused over 30 to 60 minutes) may be considered as an alternative agent to amiodarone.

Administration and Dosage

➤*General dosing considerations:* Intravenous (IV) therapy allows most rapid control of serious arrhythmias, including those following myocardial infarction; it should be carried out in circumstances where close observation and monitoring of the patient are possible, such as in hospital or emergency facilities. Intramuscular (IM) administration is less apt to produce temporary high plasma levels, but therapeutic plasma levels are not obtained as rapidly as with IV administration. Oral procainamide dosage forms are preferable for less urgent arrhythmias, as well as for long-term maintenance after initial parenteral PA therapy.

➤*Adults:*

Treatment of ventricular arrhythmias –

IM: IM administration may be used as an alternative to the oral route for patients with less threatening arrhythmias but who are nauseated or vomiting, who are ordered to receive nothing by mouth preoperatively, or who may have malabsorptive problems.

• *Initial dosage* – An initial daily dose of 50 mg/kg may be estimated. This amount should be divided into fractional doses of ⅛ to ¼ to be injected IM every 3 to 6 hours until oral therapy is possible. If more than 3 injections are given, the health care provider may wish to assess patient factors such as age and renal function (see the following), clinical response, and, if available, blood levels of PA and NAPA in adjusting further doses for that individual.

IV: IV administration of procainamide HCl injection should be done cautiously to avoid a possible hypotensive response. If the blood pressure falls 15 mm Hg or more, PA administration should be temporarily discontinued. Electrocardiographic (ECG) monitoring is advisable as well, both for observation of the progress and response of the arrhythmia under treatment, and for early detection of any tendency to excessive widening of the QRS complex, prolongation of the PR interval, or any signs of heart block. Parenteral therapy with PA should be limited to use in hospitals in which monitoring and intensive supportive care are available, or to emergency situations in which equivalent observation and treatment can be provided. Initial arrhythmia control, under blood pressure and ECG monitoring, may usually be accomplished safely within a half-hour by either of the 2 methods which follow.

Dilutions and Rates for IV Infusions[a]: Procainamide Injection

	Final concentration	Infusion volume[b]	Procainamide to be added	Infusion rate
Initial loading infusion	20 mg/mL	50 mL	1,000 mg	1 mL/min (for up to 25 to 30 min[a])
Maintenance infusion	2 mg/mL	500 mL	1,000 mg	1 mL/min to 3 mL/min
	or			
	4 mg/mL	250 mL	1,000 mg	0.5 mL/min to 1.5 mL/min
The maintenance infusion rates are calculated to deliver 2 mg to 6 mg/min, depending on body weight, renal elimination rate, and steady-state plasma level needed to maintain control of the arrhythmia. The 4 mg/mL maintenance concentration may be preferred if total infused volume must be limited.				

[a] All infusions should be made up to final volume with dextrose 5% injection.
[b] The flow rate of any IV procainamide infusion must be monitored closely to avoid transiently high plasma levels and possible hypotension.

• *Direct injection* – Direct injection into a vein or into tubing of an established infusion line should be done slowly at a rate not to exceed 50 mg/min. It is advisable to dilute the procainamide HCl 500 mg/mL concentration injection prior to IV injection to facilitate control of dosage rate. Doses of 100 mg may be administered every 5 minutes at this rate until the arrhythmia is suppressed or until 500 mg has been administered, after which it is advisable to wait 10 minutes or longer to allow for more distribution into tissues before resuming.

• *Loading infusion* –

Usual dosage: Alternatively, a loading infusion containing procainamide 20 mg/mL (1 g diluted to 50 mL with dextrose 5% injection) may be administered at a constant rate of 1 mL/min for 25 to 30 minutes to deliver 500 to 600 mg of PA. Some effects may be seen after infusion of the first 100 or 200 mg; it is unusual to require more than 600 mg to achieve satisfactory antiarrhythmic effects.

Maximum dose: The maximum advisable dosage to be given either by repeated bolus injections or such loading infusion is 1 g.

Maintenance dosage: To maintain therapeutic levels, a more dilute IV infusion at a concentration of 2 mg/mL is convenient (1 g procainamide injection in 500 mL of dextrose 5% injection), and may be administered at 1 mL/min to 3 mL/min. If daily total fluid intake must be limited, a 4 mg/mL concentration (1 g of procainamide HCl injection in 250 mL of dextrose 5% injection) administered at 0.5 mL/min to 1.5 mL/min will deliver an equivalent 2 mg to 6 mg/min. The amount needed in a given patient to maintain the therapeutic level should be assessed principally from the clinical response, and will depend upon the patient's weight and age, renal elimination, hepatic acetylation rate, and cardiac status, but should be adjusted for each patient based upon close observation. A maintenance infusion rate of 50 mcg/kg/min to a person with a healthy renal PA elimination half time of 3 hours may be expected to produce a plasma level of approximately 6.5 mcg/mL.

➤*Children:* Safety and effectiveness in children have not been established.

➤*Elderly:* Advancing age reduces the renal excretion of PA and NAPA independently of reductions in creatinine clearance; compared with healthy young adults, there is approximately 25% reduction at 50 years of age and 50% at 75 years of age. Because the principal route for elimination of PA and NAPA is renal excretion, reduced excretion will prolong the half-life of elimination and lower the dose rate needed to maintain therapeutic levels.

➤*Renal function impairment:* Because the principal route for elimination of PA and NAPA is renal excretion, reduced excretion will prolong the half-life of elimination and lower the dose rate needed to maintain therapeutic levels. See Warnings/Precautions.

➤*Discontinuation of therapy:* IV therapy should be terminated if persistent conduction disturbances or hypotension develop. As soon as the patient's basic cardiac rhythm appears to be stabilized, oral antiarrhythmic maintenance therapy is preferable, if indicated and possible. A period of about 3 to 4 hours (one half time for renal elimination, ordinarily) should elapse after the last IV dose before administering the first dose of oral procainamide.

➤*Preparation for administration:* Parenteral drug products should be examined visually for particulate matter and discoloration prior to administration. The solutions, which are clear and colorless initially, may develop a slight yellow color in time.

➤*Storage/Stability:* The solutions, which are clear and colorless initially, may develop a slight yellow color in time. This does not indicate a change

PROCAINAMIDE HYDROCHLORIDE — INJECTION

that should preclude its use, but a solution darker than slightly yellow, or discolored in any other way should not be used.

Store at controlled room temperature 15° to 30°C (59° to 86°F). Do not freeze.

Actions

➤*Pharmacology:* Procainamide (PA) increases the effective refractory period of the atria, and to a lesser extent the bundle of His-Purkinje system and ventricles of the heart. It reduces impulse conduction velocity in the atria, His-Purkinje fibers, and ventricular muscle, but has variable effects on the atrioventricular (AV) node, a direct slowing action and a weaker vagolytic effect which may speed AV conduction slightly. Myocardial excitability is reduced in the atria, Purkinje fibers, papillary muscles, and ventricles by an increase in the threshold for excitation, combined with inhibition of ectopic pacemaker activity by retardation of the slow phase of diastolic depolarization, thus decreasing automaticity especially in ectopic sites. Contractility of the undamaged heart is usually not affected by therapeutic concentrations, although slight reduction of cardiac output may occur, and may be significant in the presence of myocardial damage. Therapeutic levels of PA may exert vagolytic effects and produce slight acceleration of heart rate, while high or toxic concentrations may prolong AV conduction time or induce AV block, or even cause abnormal automaticity and spontaneous firing, by unknown mechanisms.

The electrocardiogram may reflect these effects by showing slight sinus tachycardia (due to the anticholinergic action) and widened QRS complexes and, less regularly, prolonged Q-T and P-R intervals (due to longer systole and slower conduction), as well as some decrease in QRS and T wave amplitude. These direct effects of PA on electrical activity, conduction, responsiveness, excitability and automaticity are characteristic of a Group 1A antiarrhythmic agent, the prototype for which is quinidine; PA effects are very similar. However, PA has weaker vagal blocking action than does quinidine, does not induce alpha-adrenergic blockade, and is less depressing to cardiac contractility.

➤*Pharmacokinetics:*

Absorption / Distribution – Following intramuscular injection, procainamide injection is rapidly absorbed into the bloodstream, and plasma levels peak in 15 to 60 minutes, considerably faster than the orally administered procainamide tablets or capsules which produce peak plasma levels in 90 to 120 minutes. Intravenous administration of procainamide can produce therapeutic procainamide levels within minutes after infusion is started. About 15% to 20% of PA is reversibly bound to plasma proteins, and considerable amounts are more slowly and reversibly bound to tissues of the heart, liver, lung, and kidney. The apparent volume of distribution eventually reaches about 2 L/kg body weight with a half-time of approximately 5 minutes. While PA has been shown in the dog to cross the blood-brain barrier, it did not concentrate in the brain at levels higher than in plasma. It is not known if PA crosses the placenta. Plasma estereses are far less active in hydrolysis of PA than of procaine.

Metabolism / Excretion – The half-time for elimination of PA is 3 to 4 hours in patients with normal renal function, but reduced creatinine clearance and advancing age each prolong the half-time of elimination of PA. A significant fraction of the circulating PA may be metabolized in hepatocytes to N-acetylprocainamide (NAPA), ranging from 16% to 21% of an administered dose in "slow-acetylators" to 24% to 33% in "fast-acetylators". Since NAPA also has significant antiarrhythmic activity and somewhat slower renal clearance than PA, both hepatic acetylation rate capability and renal function, as well as age, have significant effects on the effective biologic half-time of therapeutic action of administered PA and the NAPA derivative. Trace amounts may be excreted in the urine as free and conjugated p-aminobenzoic acid, 30% to 60% as unchanged PA, and 6% to 52% as the NAPA derivative. Both PA and NAPA are eliminated by active tubular secretion as well as by glomerular filtration. Action of PA on the central nervous system is not prominent, but high plasma concentrations may cause tremors. While therapeutic plasma levels for PA have been reported to be 3 mcg/mL to 10 mcg/mL, certain patients such as those with sustained ventricular tachycardia, may need higher levels for adequate control. This may justify the increased risk of toxicity. Plasma levels above 10 mcg/mL are increasingly associated with toxic findings, which are seen occasionally in the 10 mcg/mL to 12 mcg/mL range, more often in the 12 mcg/mL to 15 mcg/mL range, and commonly in patients with plasma levels greater than 15 mcg/mL. Where programmed ventricular stimulation has been used to evaluate efficacy of PA in preventing recurrent ventricular tachyarrhythmias, higher plasma levels (mean, 13.6 mcg/mL) of PA were found necessary for adequate control.

Contraindications

➤*Complete heart block:* Procainamide should not be administered to patients with complete heart block because of its effects in suppressing nodal or ventricular pacemakers and the hazard of asystole. It may be difficult to recognize complete heart block in patients with ventricular tachycardia, but if significant slowing of ventricular rate occurs during PA treatment without evidence of AV conduction appearing, PA should be stopped. In cases of second degree AV block or various types of hemiblock, PA should be avoided or discontinued because of the possibility of increased severity of block, unless the ventricular rate is controlled by an electrical pacemaker.

➤*Idiosyncratic hypersensitivity:* In patients sensitive to procaine or other ester-type local anesthetics, cross sensitivity to PA is unlikely. However, it should be borne in mind, and PA should not be used if it produces acute allergic dermatitis, asthma, or anaphylactic symptoms.

➤*Lupus erythematosus:* An established diagnosis of systemic lupus erythematous is a contraindication to PA therapy, since aggravation of symptoms is highly likely.

➤*Torsades de pointes:* In the unusual ventricular arrhythmia called "les torsades de pointes" (twistings of the points), characterized by alternation of 1 or more ventricular premature beats in the directions of the QRS complexes on ECG in persons with prolonged Q-T and often enhanced U waves, Group 1A antiarrhythmic drugs are contraindicated. Administration of PA in such cases may aggravate this special type of ventricular extrasystole or tachycardia instead of suppressing it.

Warnings/Precautions

➤*Mortality:* Considering the known proarrhythmic properties of procainamide and the lack of evidence of improved survival for any antiarrhythmic drug in patients without life-threatening arrhythmias, the use of procainamide as well as other antiarrhythmic agents should be reserved for patients with life-threatening ventricular arrhythmias.

➤*Blood dyscrasias:* Agranulocytosis, bone marrow depression, neutropenia, hypoplastic anemia and thrombocytopenia in patients receiving procainamide have been reported at a rate of approximately 0.5%. Most of these patients received procainamide within the recommended dosage range. Fatalities have occurred (with approximately 20 to 25% mortality in reported cases of agranulocytosis). Since most of these events have been noted during the first 12 weeks of therapy, it is recommended that complete blood counts including white cell, differential and platelet counts be performed at weekly intervals for the first 3 months of therapy, and periodically thereafter. Complete blood counts should be performed promptly if the patient develops any signs of infection (such as fever, chills, sore throat or stomatitis), bruising or bleeding. If any of those hematologic disorders are identified, procainamide therapy should be discontinued. Blood counts usually return to normal within 1 month of discontinuation. Caution should be used in patients with preexisting marrow failure or cytopenia of any type.

➤*Digitalis intoxication:* Caution should be exercised in the use of procainamide in arrhythmias associated with digitalis intoxication. Procainamide can suppress digitalis-induced arrhythmias; however, if there is concomitant marked disturbance of atrioventricular conduction, additional depression of conduction and ventricular asystole or fibrillation may result. Therefore, use of procainamide should be considered only if discontinuation of digitalis, and therapy with potassium, lidocaine, or phenytoin are ineffective.

➤*First degree heart block:* Caution should be exercised also if the patient exhibits or develops first degree heart block while taking PA, and dosage reduction is advised in such cases. If the block persists despite dosage reduction, continuation of PA administration must be evaluated on the basis of current benefit versus risk of increased heart block.

➤*Predigitalization for atrial flutter or fibrillation:* Patients with atrial flutter or fibrillation should be cardioverted or digitalized prior to PA administration to avoid enhancement of AV conduction which may result in ventricular rate acceleration beyond tolerable limits. Adequate digitalization reduces but does not eliminate the possibility of sudden increase in ventricular rate as the atrial rate is slowed by PA in these arrhythmias.

➤*Congestive heart failure:* For patients in congestive heart failure, and those with acute ischemic heart disease or cardiomyopathy, caution should be used in PA therapy, since even slight depression of myocardial contractility may further reduce cardiac output of the damaged heart.

➤*Concurrent use with other antiarrhythmic agents:* Concurrent use of PA with other Group 1A antiarrhythmic agents such as quinidine or disopyramide may produce enhanced prolongation of conduction or depression of contractility and hypotension, especially in patients with cardiac decompensation. Such use should be reserved for patients with serious arrhythmias unresponsive to a single drug and employed only if close observation is possible.

➤*Myasthenia gravis:* Patients with myasthenia gravis may show worsening of symptoms from PA due to its procaine-like effect on diminishing acetylcholine release at skeletal muscle motor nerve endings, so that PA administration may be hazardous without optimal adjustment of anticholinesterase medications and other precautions.

➤*Hypersensitivity reactions:* Immediately after initiation of PA therapy, patients should be closely observed for possible hypersensitivity reactions. In conversion of atrial fibrillation to normal sinus rhythm by any means, dislodgement of mural thrombi may lead to embolization, which should be kept in mind.

➤*Sulfite sensitivity:* Procainamide HCl injection contains sodium metabisulfite, a sulfite that may cause allergic-type reactions including anaphylactic symptoms and life-threatening or less severe asthmatic episodes in certain susceptible people. The overall prevalence of sulfite sensitivity in the general population is unknown and probably low. Sulfite sensitivity is seen more frequently in asthmatic than in nonasthmatic people.

➤*Renal function impairment:* Renal insufficiency may lead to accumulation of high plasma levels from conventional doses of PA, with effects similar to those of overdosage, unless dosage is adjusted for the individual patient. Progressive widening of the QRS complex, prolonged Q-T and P-R intervals, lowering of the R and T waves, as well as increasing A-V block, may be seen with doses which are excessive for a given patient. Increased ventricular extrasystoles or even ventricular tachycardia or fibrillation may occur. After intravenous administration but seldom after oral therapy, transient high plasma levels of PA may induce hypotension, affecting systolic

PROCAINAMIDE HYDROCHLORIDE — INJECTION

more than diastolic pressures, especially in hypertensive patients. Such high levels may also produce central nervous depression, tremor, and even respiratory depression.

➤*Special risk:*

Digitalis intoxication – Caution should be exercised in the use of procainamide in arrhythmias associated with digitalis intoxication. Procainamide can suppress digitalis-induced arrhythmias; however, if there is concomitant marked disturbance of atrioventricular conduction, additional depression of conduction and ventricular asystole or fibrillation may result. Therefore, use of procainamide should be considered only if discontinuation of digitalis, and therapy with potassium, lidocaine, or phenytoin are ineffective.

➤*Pregnancy:* Category C.

Teratogenic – Animal reproduction studies have not been conducted with PA. It also is not known whether PA can cause fetal harm when administered to a pregnant woman or can affect reproduction capacity. PA should be given to a pregnant woman only if clearly needed.

➤*Lactation:* Both PA and NAPA are excreted in human milk, and absorbed by the breast-feeding infant. Because of the potential for serious adverse reactions in nursing infants, a decision to discontinue breast-feeding or the drug should be made, taking into account the importance of the drug to the mother.

➤*Children:* Safety and effectiveness in pediatric patients have not been established.

➤*Monitoring:* Laboratory tests such as complete blood count (CBC), electrocardiogram, and serum creatinine or urea nitrogen may be indicated depending on the clinical situation, and periodic rechecking of the CBC and ANA may be helpful in early detection of untoward reactions.

Blood pressure and ECG monitoring – Blood pressure should be monitored with the patient supine during parenteral, especially intravenous, administration of PA. There is a possibility that relatively high, although transient plasma levels of PA may be attained and cause hypotension before the PA can be distributed from the plasma volume to its full apparent volume of distribution which is approximately 50 times greater. Therefore, caution should be exercised to avoid overly rapid administration of PA. If the blood pressure falls 15 mm Hg or more. PA administration should be temporarily discontinued. Electrocardiographic (ECG) monitoring is advisable as well, both for observation of the progress and response of the arrhythmia under treatment, and for early detection of any tendency to excessive widening of the QRS complex, prolongation of the P-R interval, or any signs of heart block. Parenteral therapy with PA should be limited to use in hospitals in which monitoring and intensive supportive care are available, or to emergency situations in which equivalent observation and treatment can be provided.

After achieving and maintaining therapeutic plasma concentrations and satisfactory electrocardiographic and clinical responses, continued frequent periodic monitoring of vital signs and electrocardiograms is advised. If evidence of QRS widening of more than 25% or marked prolongation of the Q-T interval occurs, concern for overdosage is appropriate, and interruption of the PA infusion is advisable if a 50% increase occurs. Elevated serum creatinine or urea nitrogen, reduced creatinine clearance or history of renal insufficiency, as well as use in older patients (over age 50), provide grounds to anticipate that less than the usual dosage or infusion rate may suffice, since the urinary elimination of PA and NAPA may be reduced, leading to gradual accumulation beyond normally predicted amounts. If facilities are available for measurement of plasma PA and NAPA, or acetylation capability, individual dose adjustment for optimal therapeutic levels may be easier, but close observation of clinical effectiveness is the most important criterion.

Drug Interactions

➤*QT prolongation:* An additive effect of procainamide with other drugs that prolong the QT interval cannot be excluded. The following drugs may prolong the QT interval and increase the risk of life-threatening cardiac arrhythmias, including torsade de pointes: Antiarrhythmic agents (eg, amiodarone, bretylium, disopyramide, dofetilide, quinidine, and sotalol), arsenic trioxide, chlorpromazine, cisapride, dolasetron, droperidol, mefloquine, mesoridazine, moxifloxacin, pentamidine, pimozide, tacrolimus, thioridazine, and ziprasidone. For a more complete list of drugs that may prolong the QT interval, see the appendix, Drug-Induced Prolongation of the QT Interval and Torsade de Pointes.

Procainamide Drug Interactions

Precipitant drug	Object drug[a]		Description
Amiodarone	Procainamide	↑	Amiodarone may increase procainamide serum concentrations. Monitor procainamide concentrations closely.
Anticholinergics	Procainamide	↑	Coadministration may produce additive antivagal effects on AV conduction. This effect is not as well documented for procainamide as for quinidine.
Antiarrhythmics	Procainamide	↑	Additive effects on the heart may occur with concurrent use of procainamide and other antiarrhythmics (eg, lidocaine, quinidine, disopyramide). Dosage reduction may be necessary (see Warnings). Quinidine also may increase procainamide and NAPA concentrations.
Cimetidine Ranitidine	Procainamide	↑	Cimetidine may increase procainamide serum concentrations because of decreased renal clearance. Avoid this combination, if possible. If cimetidine is necessary, then monitor procainamide concentrations closely and adjust the dose as needed. Large (> 300 mg/day) doses of ranitidine also may have this effect.
Ethanol	Procainamide	↔	The actions of procainamide could be altered, but because the main metabolite (NAPA) is also an antiarrhythmic, specific effects are unclear.
Propranolol	Procainamide	↑	One study showed that propranolol increased procainamide serum concentrations by decreasing the plasma clearance. Another study showed no changes in procainamide clearance.
Quinolones	Procainamide	↑	The risk of life-threatening cardiac arrhythmias, including torsades de pointes, may be increased when procainamide is given with sparfloxacin, gatifloxacin, or moxifloxacin. Sparfloxacin is contraindicated with class IA antiarrhythmics. Also, ofloxacin may increase procainamide concentrations. Monitor concentrations and adjust dose as indicated.
Thioridazine Ziprasidone	Procainamide	↑	Concurrent use may result in synergistic or additive prolongation of the QT_c interval and increase the risk for life-threatening cardiac arrhythmias, including torsades de pointes.
Trimethoprim	Procainamide	↑	Elevated procainamide and NAPA serum levels may occur, possibly resulting in increased pharmacologic effects. Monitor serum concentrations.
Procainamide	Neuromuscular blockers (eg, succinylcholine)	↑	Procainamide may potentiate the neuromuscular blockade produced by agents such as succinylcholine. A reduced dose of the neuromuscular blocker may be required.

[a] ↑ = Object drug increased. ↔ = Undetermined clinical effect.

➤*Drug/Lab test interactions:* Suprapharmacologic concentrations of lidocaine and meprobamate may inhibit fluorescence of PA and NAPA, and propranolol shows a native fluorescence close to the PA/NAPA peak wavelengths, so that tests which depend on fluorescence measurement may be affected.

Adverse Reactions

➤*Cardiovascular:* Hypotension and serious disturbances of cardiorhythm such as ventricular asystole or fibrillation are more common with intravenous administration of PA than with intramuscular administration. Because PA is a peripheral vasodilator in concentrations higher than the usual therapeutic range, transient high plasma levels which may occur especially during intravenous administration may produce temporary but at times severe lowering of blood pressure.

➤*CNS:* Dizziness or giddiness, weakness, mental depression and psychosis with hallucinations have been reported.

➤*Dermatologic:* Angioneurotic edema, urticaria, pruritus, flushing, and maculopapular rash have also occurred.

➤*GI:* Anorexia, nausea, vomiting, abdominal pain, bitter taste or diarrhea may occur in 3% to 4% of patients taking oral procainamide.

PROCAINAMIDE HYDROCHLORIDE — INJECTION

➤*Hematologic:* Neutropenia, thrombocytopenia, or hemolytic anemia may rarely be encountered. Agranulocytosis has occurred after repeated use of PA; and deaths have been reported.

➤*Hepatic:* Elevations of transaminase with and without elevations of alkaline phosphatase and bilirubin have been reported. Some patients have had clinical symptoms (eg, malaise, right upper quadrant pain). Deaths from liver failure have been reported.

➤*Miscellaneous:* A lupus erythematosus-like syndrome of arthralgia, pleural or abdominal pain, and sometimes arthritis, pleural effusion, pericarditis, fever, chills, myalgia, and possibly related hematologic or skin lesions (see below) is fairly common after prolonged PA administration, perhaps more often in patients who are slow acetylators.

While some series have reported less than 1 in 500, others have reported the syndrome in up to 30% of patients on long-term oral PA therapy. If discontinuation of PA does not reverse the lupoid symptoms, corticosteroid treatment may be effective.

Overdosage

➤*Symptoms:* Progressive widening of the QRS complex, prolonged QT and PR intervals, lowering of the R and T waves, as well as increasing A-V block, may be seen with doses which are excessive for a given patient. Increased ventricular extrasystoles or even ventricular tachycardia or fibrillation may occur. After intravenous administration but seldom after oral therapy, transient high plasma levels of PA may induce hypotension, affecting systolic more than diastolic pressures, especially in hypertensive patients. Such high levels may also produce central nervous depression, tremor, and even respiratory depression.

Plasma levels above 10 mcg/mL are increasingly associated with toxic findings, which are seen occasionally in the 10 mcg/mL to 12 mcg/mL range, more often in the 12 mcg/mL to 15 mcg/mL range, and commonly in patients with plasma levels greater than 15 mcg/mL.

➤*Treatment:* Treatment of overdosage or toxic manifestations includes general supportive measures, close observation, monitoring of vital signs and possibly intravenous pressor agents and mechanical cardiorespiratory support if available, PA and NAPA plasma levels may be helpful in assessing the potential degree of toxicity and response to therapy. Both PA and NAPA are removed from the circulation by hemodialysis but not peritoneal dialysis. No specific antidote for PA is known.

Patient Information

The patient should be encouraged to disclose any history of drug sensitivity, especially to procaine or other local anesthetic agents, or aspirin, and to report any history of kidney disease, congestive heart failure, myasthenia gravis, liver disease, or lupus erythematosus.

The patient should be counseled to report any symptoms of arthralgia, myalgia, fever, chills, skin rash, easy bruising, sore throat or sore mouth, infections, dark urine or icterus, wheezing, muscular weakness, chest or abdominal pain, palpitations, nausea, vomiting, anorexia, diarrhea, hallucinations, dizziness, or depression.

DISOPYRAMIDE

Rx	**Disopyramide Phosphate** (Various, eg, Geneva, Tava)	**Capsules:** 100 mg (as phosphate)	In 100s and 500s.
Rx	**Norpace** (Pharmacia)		Lactose. (SEARLE 2752 NORPACE 100 MG). White/Orange. In 100s and 1000s.
Rx	**Disopyramide Phosphate** (Various, eg, Geneva, Teva)	**Capsules:** 150 mg (as phosphate)	In 100s and 500s.
Rx	**Norpace** (Pharmacia)		Lactose. (SEARLE 2762 NORPACE 150 MG). Brown/Orange. In 100s and 1000s.
Rx	**Norpace CR** (Pharmacia)	**Capsules, extended-release:** 100 mg (as phosphate)	Sucrose. (SEARLE 2732 NORPACE CR 100 mg). White/Lt. green. In 100s, 500s, and UD 100s.
Rx	**Disopyramide Phosphate** (Various, eg, Ethex, Geneva)	**Capsules, extended-release:** 150 mg (as phosphate)	In 100s.
Rx	**Norpace CR** (Pharmacia)		Sucrose. (SEARLE 2742 NORPACE CR 150 mg). Brown/Lt. green. In 100s, 500s, and UD 100s.

DISOPYRAMIDE PHOSPHATE — ORAL

Refer to the general introductory discussion concerning Antiarrhythmic Agents.

WARNING

In the National Heart, Lung, and Blood Institute's Cardiac Arrhythmia Suppression Trial (CAST), a long-term, multicenter, randomized, double-blind study in patients with asymptomatic non-life-threatening ventricular arrhythmias who had an MI more than 6 days but less than 2 years previously, an excessive mortality or nonfatal cardiac arrest rate (7.7%) was seen in patients treated with encainide or flecainide compared with that seen in patients assigned to carefully matched placebo-treated groups (3%). The average duration of treatment with encainide or flecainide in this study was 10 months.

The applicability of the CAST results to other populations (eg, those without recent MI) is uncertain. Considering the known proarrhythmic properties of disopyramide and the lack of evidence of improved survival for any antiarrhythmic drug in patients without life-threatening arrhythmias, the use of disopyramide as well as other antiarrhythmic agents should be reserved for patients with life-threatening ventricular arrhythmias.

Indications

➤*Ventricular arrhythmias:* Treatment of documented ventricular arrhythmias (eg, sustained ventricular tachycardia) considered to be life-threatening.

➤*Off-label uses:* Disopyramide may be beneficial in the treatment of paroxysmal supraventricular tachycardia.

Administration and Dosage

➤*General dosing considerations:* Individualize dosage. Initiate treatment in the hospital.

Do not use the controlled-release form initially if rapid plasma levels are desired.

➤*Adults:*

Cardiomyopathy or possible cardiac decompensation –

Initial dosage: Do not administer a loading dose; limit the initial dosage to 100 mg immediate-release every 6 to 8 hours.

Dosage titration: Make subsequent dosage adjustments gradually.

Severe refractory ventricular tachycardia – A limited number of patients have tolerated up to 1,600 mg/day (400 mg every 6 hours), resulting in plasma levels of up to 9 mcg/mL. Hospitalize patients for close evaluation and continuous monitoring.

Ventricular arrhythmias –

Usual dosage: 400 to 800 mg/day given in divided doses. The recommended dosage for most adults is 600 mg/day given in divided doses. For patients weighing less than 50 kg (110 pounds), give 400 mg/day. Divide the total daily dose and administer every 6 hours in the immediate-release form or every 12 hours in the controlled-release form.

Loading dose: For rapid control of ventricular arrhythmia, give an initial loading dose of 300 mg immediate-release (200 mg for patients weighing less than 50 kg [110 lb]). Therapeutic effects are attained in 30 minutes to 3 hours.

Dosage adjustment: In the event of increased anticholinergic side effects, plasma levels of disopyramide should be monitored and the dose of the drug adjusted accordingly. A reduction of the dose by one-third, from the recommended 600 mg/day to 400 mg/day, would be reasonable, without changing the dosing interval.

Alternative dosage: If there is no response or no evidence of toxicity within 6 hours of the loading dose, 200 mg every 6 hours may be administered instead of the usual 150 mg. If there is no response within 48 hours, discontinue the drug or carefully monitor subsequent immediate-release doses of 250 or 300 mg every 6 hours.

➤*Children:*

Off-label dosing –

Ventricular arrhythmias: Divide daily dosage and administer equal doses every 6 hours or at intervals according to patient needs. Start dose titration at the lower end of the ranges provided:

Suggested Total Daily Disopyramide Dosage in Children[a]

Age (years)	Disopyramide (mg/kg/day)
< 1	10 to 30
1 to 4	10 to 20
4 to 12	10 to 15
12 to 18	6 to 15

[a] Prepare a 1 to 10 mg/mL suspension by adding contents of the immediate-release capsule to cherry syrup, NF. The resulting suspension, when refrigerated, is stable for 1 month; shake thoroughly before measuring dose. Dispense in an amber glass bottle. Do not use the controlled-release form to prepare the solution.

➤*Renal function impairment:* For patients with moderate renal insufficiency (CrCl more than 40 mL/min) the recommended dosage is 400 mg/day given in divided doses (either 100 mg every 6 hours for immediate-release or 200 mg every 12 hours for controlled-release).

In severe renal insufficiency (CrCl 40 mL/min or less), the recommended dosage is 100 mg of immediate-release form given at intervals shown in the

DISOPYRAMIDE PHOSPHATE — ORAL

following table, with or without an initial loading dose of 150 mg. The controlled-release form is not recommended for patients with severe renal insufficiency.

Disopyramide (Immediate-release) Dosage in Renal Impairment			
CrCl (mL/min)	Loading dose (mg)	Dose (mg)	Dosage interval (hours)
30 to 40	150	100	8
15 to 30	150	100	12
< 15	150	100	24

➤*Hepatic function impairment:* For patients with hepatic insufficiency, the recommended dosage is 400 mg/day given in divided doses (either 100 mg every 6 hours for immediate-release or 200 mg every 12 hours for controlled-release).

➤*Conversion:* Based on theoretical considerations, use the regular maintenance schedule, without a loading dose, 6 to 12 hours after the last dose of quinidine or 3 to 6 hours after the last dose of procainamide. Where withdrawal of quinidine or procainamide is likely to produce life-threatening arrhythmias, consider hospitalization.

When transferring from immediate- to controlled-release, start maintenance schedule of controlled-release 6 hours after the last dose of immediate-release.

➤*Therapeutic drug monitoring:* Closely monitor plasma levels and therapeutic response.

➤*Administration:* Divide the total daily dose and administer every 6 hours in the immediate-release form or every 12 hours in the controlled-release form.

Do not break or chew extended-release capsules.

➤*Storage/Stability:* Store at 25°C (77°F); excursions permitted between 15° and 30°C (59° and 86°F).

Actions

➤*Pharmacology:* Disopyramide is a class IA antiarrhythmic agent pharmacologically similar to, but chemically unrelated to, procainamide and quinidine. It decreases the rate of diastolic depolarization (phase 4), decreases the upstroke velocity (phase 0), increases the action potential duration of normal cardiac cells, and prolongs the refractory period (phases 2 and 3). It also decreases the disparity in refractoriness between infarcted and adjacent normally perfused myocardium and does not affect alpha- or beta-adrenergic receptors.

Anticholinergic activity – In vitro anticholinergic activity is approximately 0.06% that of atropine; the usual dose of 150 mg every 6 hours or 300 mg controlled release every 12 hours compares with approximately 0.4 to 0.6 mg of atropine.

Hemodynamic effects – At recommended oral doses, disopyramide rarely produces significant alterations of blood pressure in patients without congestive heart failure. With IV disopyramide (dosage form not available in US), either increases in systolic/diastolic or decreases in systolic blood pressure have occurred depending on the infusion rate and the patient population. IV disopyramide may cause cardiac depression with an approximate mean 10% reduction of cardiac output, which is more pronounced in patients with cardiac dysfunction.

➤*Pharmacokinetics:*

Absorption/Distribution – Following oral administration of immediate-release disopyramide, the drug is rapidly and almost completely (approximately 90%) absorbed. Peak plasma levels usually occur within 2 hours. Therapeutic plasma levels of disopyramide are 2 to 4 mcg/mL. Protein binding is concentration-dependent and varies from 50% to 65%; it is difficult to predict the concentration of the free drug when total drug is measured. After the oral administration of 200 mg disopyramide to 10 cardiac patients with borderline to moderate heart failure, the time to peak serum concentration of 2.3 ± 1.5 hours was increased, and the mean peak serum concentration of 4.8 ± 1.6 mcg/mL was higher than in healthy volunteers.

Immediate-release vs controlled-release: In a crossover study in healthy subjects, the bioavailability of the controlled-release form was similar to that from the immediate-release capsules. With a single 300 mg oral dose, peak disopyramide plasma concentrations of 3.23 ± 0.75 mcg/mL at 2.5 ± 2.3 hours were obtained with two 150 mg immediate-release capsules and 2.22 ± 0.47 mcg/mL at 4.9 ± 1.4 hours with two 150 mg controlled-release capsules. The elimination half-life was 8.31 ± 1.83 hours with the immediate-release capsules and 11.65 ± 4.72 hours with controlled-release capsules. The amount of disopyramide and MND excreted in the urine in 48 hours was 128 and 48 mg, respectively, with the immediate-release capsules and 112 and 33 mg, respectively, with controlled-release capsules.

Following multiple doses, steady-state plasma levels of between 2 and 4 mcg/mL were attained following either 150 mg every 6 hours with immediate-release capsules or 300 mg every 12 hours with controlled-release capsules.

Metabolism/Excretion – About 50% is excreted in the urine as the unchanged drug and 30% as metabolites (20% MND). The plasma concentration of MND is approximately one tenth that of disopyramide. The mean plasma half-life is 6.7 hours (range, 4 to 10 hours).

Special populations –

Renal function impairment: A preliminary report of 3 patients on long-term hemodialysis revealed a 45% to 72% reduction in disopyramide half-life during dialysis. In contrast, another study in patients on chronic hemodialysis demonstrated little difference in disopyramide half-life without dialysis (16.8 vs 16.1 hours). Resin and charcoal hemoperfusion were effective in rapidly decreasing disopyramide plasma levels in acute overdosage.

In impaired renal function (creatinine clearance [Ccr] less than 40 mL/min), half-life values ranged from 8 to 18 hours. Therefore, decrease the dose in renal failure to avoid drug accumulation. Altering urinary pH does not affect plasma half-life.

Contraindications

Cardiogenic shock; preexisting second- or third-degree AV block (if no pacemaker is present); congenital QT prolongation; hypersensitivity to disopyramide.

Warnings/Precautions

➤*Mortality:* Considering the known proarrhythmic properties of disopyramide and the lack of evidence of improved survival for any antiarrhythmic drug in patients without life-threatening arrhythmias, the use of disopyramide as well as other antiarrhythmic agents should be reserved for patients with life-threatening ventricular arrhythmias.

➤*Proarrhythmic effects:* Because of the proarrhythmic effects, use with lesser arrhythmias is generally not recommended.

➤*Asymptomatic ventricular premature contractions:* Avoid treatment of patients with this condition.

➤*Survival:* Antiarrhythmic drugs have not been shown to enhance survival in patients with ventricular arrhythmias.

➤*Negative inotropic properties:*

Heart failure/hypotension – May cause or aggravate CHF or produce severe hypotension, especially in patients with primary cardiomyopathy or inadequately compensated CHF. Do not use in patients with uncompensated or marginally compensated CHF or hypotension unless secondary to cardiac arrhythmia. Treat patients with a history of heart failure with careful attention to the maintenance of cardiac function, including optimal digitalization. If hypotension occurs or CHF worsens, discontinue use; restart at a lower dosage after adequate cardiac compensation has been established.

Do not give a loading dose to patients with myocarditis or other cardiomyopathy; closely monitor initial dosage and subsequent adjustments.

QRS widening – Although unusual, QRS widening (more than 25%) may occur; discontinue use in such cases.

QT_c prolongation – QT_c prolongation and worsening of the arrhythmia, including ventricular tachycardia and fibrillation, may occur. Patients who have QT prolongation in response to quinidine may be at particular risk. As with other Type IA antiarrhythmics, disopyramide has been associated with torsade de pointes. If QT prolongation more than 25% is observed and if ectopy continues, monitor closely and consider discontinuing the drug.

➤*Atrial tachyarrhythmias:* Digitalize patients with atrial flutter or fibrillation prior to administration to ensure that enhancement of AV conduction does not increase ventricular rate beyond acceptable limits.

➤*Conduction abnormalities:* Use caution in patients with sick sinus syndrome, Wolff-Parkinson-White (WPW), syndrome or bundle branch block.

➤*Heart block:* If first degree heart block develops, reduce dosage. If the block persists, drug continuation must depend upon the benefit compared to the risk of higher degrees of heart block. Development of second- or third-degree AV block or unifascicular, bifascicular, or trifascicular block requires discontinuation of therapy, unless ventricular rate is controlled by a ventricular pacemaker.

➤*Concomitant antiarrhythmic therapy:* Reserve concomitant use of disopyramide with other class IA or class IC antiarrhythmics or propranolol for life-threatening arrhythmias unresponsive to a single agent. Such use may produce serious negative inotropic effects or may excessively prolong conduction, particularly in patients with cardiac decompensation.

➤*Hypoglycemia:* Reported in rare instances. Monitor blood glucose levels in patients with CHF, chronic malnutrition, hepatic or renal disease, and in those taking drugs which could compromise normal glucoregulatory mechanisms in the absence of food (eg, beta-adrenoceptor blockers, alcohol).

➤*Anticholinergic activity:* Do not use in patients with urinary retention, glaucoma, or myasthenia gravis unless adequate overriding measures are taken. Urinary retention may occur in either sex, but males with benign prostatic hypertrophy are at particular risk. In patients with a family history of glaucoma, measure intraocular pressure before initiating therapy. Use with special care in patients with myasthenia gravis, because disopyramide could precipitate a myasthenic crisis.

➤*Potassium imbalance:* Disopyramide may be ineffective in *hypo*kalemia and its toxic effects may be enhanced in *hyper*kalemia. Correct any potassium deficit before instituting therapy.

➤*Renal function impairment:* Reduce dosage in impaired renal function. Carefully monitor ECG for prolongation of PR interval, evidence of QRS widening or other signs of overdosage. The controlled-release form is not recommended for patients with severe renal insufficiency (Ccr less than or equal to 40 mL/min).

➤*Hepatic function impairment:* Hepatic function impairment increases plasma half-life; therefore, reduce dosage in such patients. Carefully monitor the ECG. Patients with cardiac dysfunction have a higher potential for hepatic impairment.

➤*Pregnancy: Category C.* Disopyramide was associated with decreased numbers of implantation sites and decreased growth and survival of pups

DISOPYRAMIDE PHOSPHATE — ORAL

when administered to pregnant rats at 250 mg/kg/day (≥ 20 times the usual daily human dose), a level at which weight gain and food consumption of dams were also reduced. Increased resorption rates were reported in rabbits at 60 mg/kg/day (≥ 5 times the usual daily human dose). At a maternal concentration of 2.3 mg/L disopyramide, the fetal cord concentration is 0.9 mg/L. Well-controlled studies have not been performed in pregnant women and experience is limited. Use only when clearly needed and when the potential benefits outweigh the potential hazards to the fetus. Disopyramide has been found in human fetal blood. Disopyramide may stimulate contractions of the pregnant uterus.

➤*Lactation:* Disopyramide has been detected in breast milk at a concentration not exceeding that in maternal plasma. Therefore, decide whether to discontinue breast-feeding or to discontinue the drug taking into account the importance of the drug to the mother.

➤*Children:* Safety and efficacy have not been established.

➤*Elderly:* Per the Beers list, of all the antiarrhythmic drugs, disopyramide is the most potent negative inotrope and therefore may induce heart failure in elderly patients. It is also strongly anticholinergic. Other antiarrhythmic drugs should be used.

Drug Interactions

➤*CYP-450 system:* In vitro metabolic studies indicate that disopyramide is metabolized by CYP3A4; inhibitors of this system (eg, erythromycin, clarithromycin) may elevate plasma levels of disopyramide.

➤*QT prolongation:* An additive effect of disopyramide with other drugs that prolong the QT interval cannot be excluded. The following drugs may prolong the QT interval and increase the risk of life-threatening cardiac arrhythmias, including torsade de pointes: Antiarrhythmic agents (eg, amiodarone, bretylium, dofetilide, procainamide, quinidine, and sotalol), arsenic trioxide, chlorpromazine, cisapride, dolasetron, droperidol, mefloquine, mesoridazine, moxifloxacin, pentamidine, pimozide, tacrolimus, thioridazine, and ziprasidone. For a more complete list of drugs that may prolong the QT interval, see the appendix, Drug-Induced Prolongation of the QT Interval and Torsade de Pointes.

Disopyramide Drug Interactions

Precipitant drug	Object drug[a]		Description
Antiarrhythmics	Disopyramide	↑	Other antiarrhythmics (eg, procainamide, lidocaine) have been used with disopyramide; however, widening of the QRS complex or QT prolongation may occur.
Beta-blockers	Disopyramide	↔	This interaction is difficult to predict. Disopyramide clearance may be decreased; other adverse effects (eg, sinus bradycardia, hypotension) may occur. Others report no occurrence of synergistic or additive negative inotropic effects.
Cisapride	Disopyramide	↑	The risk of life-threatening cardiac arrhythmias, including torsades de pointes, may be increased due to possibly additive prolongation of the QT interval.
Disopyramide	Cisapride		
Clarithromycin Erythromycin	Disopyramide	↑	Increased disopyramide plasma levels may occur. Arrhythmias and increased QTc intervals have occurred.
Fluoroquinolones	Disopyramide	↑	The risk of life-threatening cardiac arrhythmias, including torsades de pointes, may be increased. Sparfloxacin is contraindicated and gatifloxacin, levofloxacin, and moxifloxacin should be avoided in patients receiving disopyramide.
Hydantoins	Disopyramide	↓	Disopyramide serum levels, half-life and bioavailability may be decreased; anticholinergic effects may be enhanced. Effects may persist for several days after hydantoin withdrawal.
Quinidine	Disopyramide	↑	Concurrent use may result in increased disopyramide serum levels and decreased quinidine levels. This may result in disopyramide toxicity or decreased response to quinidine.
Disopyramide	Quinidine	↓	
Rifampin	Disopyramide	↓	Disopyramide serum levels may be decreased.
Thioridazine Ziprasidone	Disopyramide	↑	The risk of life-threatening cardiac arrhythmias, including torsades de pointes, may be increased. Coadministration is contraindicated.
Verapamil	Disopyramide	↔	Until data on this interaction are available, it is recommended that disopyramide not be administered within 48 hours before or 24 hours after verapamil.
Disopyramide	Anticoagulants	↓	Decreased prothrombin time after disopyramide discontinuation may occur. However, this may be due to a hemodynamic effect and not an interaction.
Disopyramide	Digoxin	↑	Although serum digoxin levels may be increased, a clinically significant interaction appears unlikely. A beneficial interaction has also been suggested.

[a] ↑ = Object drug increased. ↓ = Object drug decreased. ↔ = Undetermined clinical effect.

Adverse Reactions

The most serious adverse reactions are hypotension and CHF. The most common reactions are anticholinergic and dose-dependent. These may be transitory, but may be persistent or severe. Urinary retention is the most serious anticholinergic effect.

➤*Cardiovascular:* Hypotension with or without CHF, increased CHF, edema, weight gain, cardiac conduction disturbances, shortness of breath, syncope, chest pain (1% to 3%); AV block (less than 1%). There have been reports of severe myocardial depression (with hypotension and an increase in venous pressure) and unexplained severe epigastric pain following standard oral doses.

➤*CNS:* Dizziness, fatigue, headache (3% to 9%); nervousness (1% to 3%); depression, insomnia (less than 1%); acute psychosis (rare, prompt reversal when therapy discontinued).

➤*Dermatologic:* Generalized rash, dermatoses, itching (1% to 3%).

➤*GI:* Dry mouth (32%); nausea, pain, bloating, gas (3% to 9%); anorexia, diarrhea, vomiting (1% to 3%); elevated liver enzymes (less than 1%); reversible cholestatic jaundice.

➤*GU:* Urinary hesitancy (14%); constipation (11%); urinary retention, frequency and urgency (3% to 9%); impotence (1% to 3%); dysuria, elevated creatinine (less than 1%).

➤*Hematologic:* Decreased hemoglobin, hematocrit (less than 1%); thrombocytopenia, reversible agranulocytosis (rare).

➤*Musculoskeletal:* Muscle weakness, malaise, aches/pain (3% to 9%);

➤*Special senses:* Blurred vision, dry nose, eyes and throat (3% to 9%).

➤*Miscellaneous:* Hypokalemia, elevated cholesterol and triglycerides (1% to 3%); numbness, tingling, elevated BUN (less than 1%); hypoglycemia; fever and respiratory difficulty; gynecomastia (rare); anaphylactoid reactions; lupus erythematosus symptoms (most cases occurred in patients who had been switched to disopyramide from procainamide after developing symptoms).

Overdosage

➤*Symptoms:* Overdose may be followed by apnea, loss of consciousness, cardiac arrhythmias, loss of spontaneous respiration and death. Toxic plasma levels produce excessive widening of the QRS complex and QT interval, worsening of CHF, hypotension, varying conduction disturbances, bradycardia, and finally, asystole. Anticholinergic effects may also be observed.

➤*Treatment:* Prompt, vigorous treatment is necessary even in the absence of symptoms. Such treatment may be lifesaving and may include gastric lavage followed by activated charcoal by mouth or stomach tube.

Administration of isoproterenol, dopamine, cardiac glycosides, diuretics, intra-aortic balloon counterpulsation, mechanical ventilation, hemodialysis or charcoal hemoperfusion may be used. Monitor ECG.

If progressive AV block develops, implement endocardial pacing. In case of impaired renal function, measures to increase the GFR may reduce the toxicity. Altering urinary pH does not affect plasma half-life or the amount of disopyramide excreted in the urine.

Anticholinergic effects can be reversed with neostigmine.

Refer also to General Management of Acute Overdosage.

Patient Information

May cause dry mouth, difficult urination, dizziness, breathing difficulty, constipation or blurred vision. Notify physician if symptoms persist, but do not discontinue unless instructed to do so by physician.

Do not break or chew extended-release capsules.

LIDOCAINE HYDROCHLORIDE

For complete prescribing information, see the Lidocaine Hydrochloride monograph in the CNS chapter.

FLECAINIDE ACETATE

Rx	**Flecainide** (Various, eg, Mylan, Par)	**Tablets; oral:** 50 mg	In 100s.
Rx	**Tambocor** (Graceway Pharmaceuticals)		(TR 50 3M). White. In 100s and UD 100s.
Rx	**Flecainide** (Various, eg, Mylan, Par)	**Tablets; oral:** 100 mg	In 100s.
Rx	**Tambocor** (Graceway Pharmaceuticals)		(TR 100 3M). White, scored. In 100s and UD 100s.
Rx	**Flecainide** (Various, eg, Mylan, Par)	**Tablets; oral:** 150 mg	In 100s.
Rx	**Tambocor** (Graceway Pharmaceuticals)		(TR 150 3M). White, scored. Oval. In 100s.

FLECAINIDE ACETATE — ORAL

Refer to the general introductory discussion concerning Antiarrhythmic Agents.

WARNING

Mortality – Flecainide was included in the National Heart Lung and Blood Institute's Cardiac Arrhythmia Suppression Trial (CAST), a long-term, multicenter, randomized, double-blind study in patients with asymptomatic non-life-threatening ventricular arrhythmias who had an MI more than 6 days but less than 2 years previously. An excessive mortality or non-fatal cardiac arrest rate was seen in patients treated with flecainide compared with that seen in patients assigned to a carefully matched placebo-treated group. This rate was 5.1% for flecainide and 2.3% for the matched placebo. The average duration of treatment with flecainide in this study was 10 months.

The applicability of the CAST results to other populations (eg, those without recent MI) is uncertain, but at present, it is prudent to consider the risks of Class IC agents (including flecainide), coupled with the lack of any evidence of improved survival, generally unacceptable in patients without life-threatening ventricular arrhythmias, even if the patients are experiencing unpleasant, but not life-threatening, symptoms or signs.

Ventricular proarrhythmic effects in patients with atrial fibrillation/flutter – A review of the world literature revealed reports of 568 patients treated with oral flecainide for paroxysmal atrial fibrillation/flutter (PAF). Ventricular tachycardia was experienced in 0.4% of these patients. Of 19 patients in the literature with chronic atrial fibrillation (CAF), 10.5% experienced ventricular tachycardia (VT) or ventricular fibrillation (VF). Flecainide is not recommended for use in patients with CAF. Case reports of ventricular proarrhythmic effects in patients treated with flecainide for atrial fibrillation/flutter have included increased premature ventricular contractions (PVCs), VT, VF, and death.

As with other Class I agents, patients treated with flecainide for atrial flutter have been reported with 1:1 atrioventricular conduction due to slowing the atrial rate. A paradoxical increase in the ventricular rate also may occur in patients with atrial fibrillation who receive flecainide. Concomitant negative chronotropic therapy such as digoxin or beta-blockers may lower the risk of this complication.

Indications

➤*Paroxysmal atrial fibrillation/flutter:* For the prevention of paroxysmal atrial fibrillation/flutter associated with disabling symptoms and paroxysmal supraventricular tachycardias (PSVT), including atrioventricular nodal reentrant tachycardia, atrioventricular reentrant tachycardia and other supraventricular tachycardias of unspecified mechanism associated with disabling symptoms in patients without structural heart disease.

➤*Ventricular arrhythmias:* Prevention of documented life-threatening ventricular arrhythmias, such as sustained ventricular tachycardia.

Administration and Dosage

➤*General dosing considerations:* For patients with sustained ventricular tachycardia, initiate therapy in the hospital and monitor rhythm.

Flecainide has a long half-life (12 to 27 hours). Steady-state plasma levels in normal renal and hepatic function may not be achieved until 3 to 5 days of therapy at a given dose. Therefore, do not increase dosage more frequently than once every 4 days, because optimal effect may not be achieved during the first 2 to 3 days of therapy.

Once the arrhythmia is controlled, it may be possible to reduce the dose, as necessary, to minimize side effects or effects on conduction.

An occasional patient not adequately controlled by (or intolerant of) a dose given at 12-hour intervals may be dosed at 8-hour intervals.

Use cautiously in patients with a history of CHF or myocardial dysfunction.

➤*Adults:*

Prevention of ventricular arrhythmias (eg, sustained ventricular tachycardia) –

Maximum dose: 400 mg/day.

Initial dosage: 100 mg every 12 hours.

Loading dose: A loading dose is not recommended. Use of higher initial doses and more rapid dosage adjustments have resulted in an increased incidence of proarrhythmic events and CHF, particularly during the first few days of dosing.

Dosage titration: Increase in 50 mg increments twice daily every 4 days until effective. Most patients do not require more than 150 mg every 12 hours (300 mg/day).

Concomitant therapy: When flecainide is given in the presence of amiodarone, reduce the usual flecainide dose by 50% and monitor the patient closely for adverse effects. Plasma level monitoring is strongly recommended to guide dosage with such combination therapy.

Prevention of paroxysmal atrial fibrillation/flutter (PAF) –

Initial dosage: 50 mg every 12 hours.

Dosage titration: Doses may be increased in increments of 50 mg twice daily every 4 days until efficacy is achieved.

Alternative dosage: A substantial increase in efficacy without a substantial increase in discontinuation for adverse experiences may be achieved by increasing the flecainide dose from 50 to 100 mg twice daily.

Concomitant therapy: See Prevention of ventricular arrhythmias-concomitant therapy.

Conversion: See Prevention of ventricular arrhythmias-conversion.

Prevention of paroxysmal supraventricular tachycardias (PSVT) –

Maximum dose: 300 mg/day.

Initial dosage: 50 mg every 12 hours.

Dosage titration: Doses may be increased in increments of 50 mg twice daily every 4 days until efficacy is achieved.

Concomitant therapy: See Prevention of ventricular arrhythmias-concomitant therapy.

Conversion: See Prevention of ventricular arrhythmias-conversion.

➤*Renal function impairment:*

Severe renal impairment ($CrCl$ 35 mL/min/1.73 m^2 or less) – The initial dosage is 100 mg once daily (or 50 mg twice daily). Frequent plasma level monitoring is required to guide dosage adjustments.

Less severe renal disease – The initial dosage is 100 mg every 12 hours. Increase dosage cautiously at intervals of more than 4 days, observing the patient closely for signs of adverse cardiac effects or other toxicity. It may take more than 4 days before a new steady-state plasma level is reached following a dosage change. Monitor plasma levels to guide dosage adjustments.

➤*Hepatic function impairment:* Because flecainide elimination from plasma can be markedly slower in patients with significant hepatic impairment, do not use in such patients unless the potential benefits outweigh the risks. If used, frequent and early plasma level monitoring is required to guide dosage; make dosage increases very cautiously when plasma levels have plateaued (after more than 4 days).

➤*Concomitant therapy:* When flecainide is given in the presence of amiodarone, reduce the usual flecainide dose by 50% and monitor the patient closely for adverse effects. Plasma level monitoring is strongly recommended to guide dosage with such combination therapy.

➤*Conversion to flecainide:* Theoretically, when transferring patients from another antiarrhythmic to flecainide, allow at least 2 to 4 plasma half-lives to elapse for the drug being discontinued before starting flecainide at the usual dosage. Consider hospitalization of patients in whom withdrawal of a previous antiarrhythmic is likely to produce life-threatening arrhythmias.

➤*Therapeutic drug monitoring:* Monitor trough plasma levels periodically, especially in patients with severe or moderate chronic renal failure or severe hepatic disease and CHF, as drug elimination may be slower. The majority of patients treated successfully had trough plasma levels between 0.2 and 1 mcg/mL. The probability of adverse experiences, especially cardiac, may increase with higher trough plasma levels, especially levels more than 1 mcg/mL.

➤*Storage/Stability:* Store at controlled room temperature 15° to 30°C (59° to 86°F) in a tight, light-resistant container.

Actions

➤*Pharmacology:* Flecainide has local anesthetic activity and belongs to the membrane stabilizing (Class I) group of antiarrhythmic agents; it has electrophysiologic effects characteristic of the IC class of antiarrhythmics.

Hemodynamic effects – Flecainide does not usually alter heart rate, although bradycardia and tachycardia have been reported occasionally.

Decreases in ejection fraction, consistent with a negative inotropic effect, have been observed after a single dose of 200 to 250 mg; both increases and decreases in ejection fraction have been encountered during multidose therapy at usual therapeutic doses.

➤*Pharmacokinetics:*

Absorption/Distribution – Oral absorption is nearly complete. Peak plasma levels are attained at about 3 hours (range, 1 to 6 hours). Flecainide does not undergo significant first-pass effect.

FLECAINIDE ACETATE — ORAL

The plasma half-life averages 20 hours (range, 12 to 27 hours) after multiple oral doses. Steady-state levels are approached in 3 to 5 days; once at steady-state, no accumulation occurs during chronic therapy. Over the usual therapeutic range, plasma levels are approximately proportional to dose.

In patients with congestive heart failure (CHF; NYHA class III), the rate of flecainide elimination from plasma (mean half-life, 19 hours) is moderately slower than for healthy subjects (mean half-life, 14 hours).

Plasma protein binding is about 40% and is independent of plasma drug level over the range of 0.015 to about 3.4 mcg/mL.

Metabolism / Excretion – In vitro metabolic studies have confirmed that cytochrome P450 2D6 is involved in the metabolism of flecainide. About 30% of a single oral dose (range, 10% to 50%) is excreted in urine unchanged. The two major urinary metabolites are meta-O-dealkylated flecainide (active, but ≈ ⅕ as potent) and the meta-O-dealkylated lactam (inactive). These two metabolites (primarily conjugated) account for most of the remaining portion of the dose. Several minor metabolites (≤ 3%) are also found in urine; 5% is excreted in feces.

Special populations –

Renal function impairment: Flecainide elimination depends on renal function. With increasing renal impairment, the extent of unchanged drug in urine is reduced and the half-life is prolonged. There is no simple relationship between creatinine clearance and the rate of flecainide elimination from plasma.

Hemodialysis removes only approximately 1% of an oral dose as unchanged flecainide.

Contraindications

Preexisting second- or third-degree AV block, right bundle branch block when associated with a left hemiblock (bifascicular block), unless a pacemaker is present to sustain the cardiac rhythm if complete heart block occurs; recent MI; presence of cardiogenic shock; hypersensitivity to the drug.

Warnings/Precautions

➤*Mortality:* Flecainide was included in the National Heart Lung and Blood Institute's Cardiac Arrhythmia Suppression Trial (CAST), a long-term multicenter, randomized, double-blind study in patients with asymptomatic non-life-threatening ventricular arrhythmias who had an MI more than 6 days, but less than 2 years previously. An excessive mortality or nonfatal cardiac arrest rate was seen in patients treated with flecainide compared with that seen in a carefully matched placebo-treated group. This rate was 16/315 (5.1%) for flecainide and 7/309 (2.3%) for its matched placebo. The average duration of treatment was 10 months.

As with other antiarrhythmics, there is no evidence that flecainide favorably affects survival or the incidence of sudden death.

➤*Ventricular proarrhythmic effects in patients with atrial fibrillation / flutter:* A review of the world literature revealed reports of 568 patients treated with oral flecainide for paroxysmal atrial fibrillation/flutter (PAF). Ventricular tachycardia was experienced in 0.4% (2/568) of these patients. Of 19 patients in the literature with chronic atrial fibrillation (CAF), 10.5% (2) experienced VT or VF. Flecainide is not recommended for use in patients with chronic atrial fibrillation. Case reports of ventricular proarrhythmic effects in patients treated with flecainide for atrial fibrillation/flutter have included increased PVCs, VT, VF and death.

As with other class I agents, patients treated with flecainide for atrial flutter have been reported with 1:1 atrioventricular conduction because of slowing the atrial rate. A paradoxical increase in the ventricular rate also may occur in patients with atrial fibrillation who receive flecainide. Concomitant negative chronotropic therapy such as digoxin or beta-blockers may lower the risk of this complication.

➤*Non-life-threatening ventricular arrhythmias:* The applicability of the CAST results to other populations (eg, those without recent infarction) is uncertain, but at present it is prudent to consider the risks of Class IC agents, coupled with the lack of any evidence of improved survival, generally unacceptable in patients whose ventricular arrhythmias are not life-threatening, even if the patients are experiencing unpleasant but not life-threatening symptoms or signs.

➤*Proarrhythmic effects:* Flecainide can cause new or worsened arrhythmias. Such proarrhythmic effects range from an increase in frequency of PVCs to the development of more severe ventricular tachycardia (eg, tachycardia that is more sustained or more resistant to conversion to sinus rhythm, with potentially fatal consequences. Three-fourths of proarrhythmic events were new or worsened ventricular tachyarrhythmias, the remainder being increased frequency of PVCs or new supraventricular arrhythmias.

The relatively high frequency of proarrhythmic events in patients with sustained ventricular tachycardia and serious underlying heart disease, and the need for titration and monitoring, requires that therapy of patients with sustained ventricular tachycardia be started in the hospital.

➤*Sick sinus syndrome:* Use only with extreme caution; the drug may cause sinus bradycardia, sinus pause or sinus arrest. The frequency probably increases with higher trough plasma levels, especially when they exceed 1 mcg/mL.

➤*Heart failure:* Flecainide has a negative inotropic effect and may cause or worsen CHF, particularly in patients with cardiomyopathy, preexisting severe heart failure (NYHA functional class III or IV) or low ejection fractions (< 30%). In patients with supraventricular arrhythmias, new or worsened CHF developed in 0.4% of patients. In patients with sustained ventricular tachycardia during a mean duration of 7.9 months of flecainide therapy, 6.3% developed new CHF. In patients with sustained ventricular tachycardia and a history of CHF in a mean duration of 5.4 months of therapy, 25.7% developed worsened CHF. Exacerbation of preexisting CHF occurred more commonly in studies including patients with Class III or IV failure than in studies which excluded such patients. Use cautiously in patients with a history of CHF or myocardial dysfunction. The initial dosage should be no more than 100 mg twice daily; monitor patients carefully. Give close attention to maintenance of cardiac function, including optimal digitalis, diuretic or other therapy. Where CHF has developed or worsened during treatment, the time of onset has ranged from a few hours to several months after starting therapy. Some patients who develop reduced myocardial function while on flecainide can continue with adjustment of digitalis or diuretics; others may require dosage reduction or discontinuation of flecainide. When feasible, monitor plasma flecainide levels. Keep trough plasma levels less than 0.7 to 1 mcg/mL.

➤*Cardiac conduction:* Flecainide slows cardiac conduction in most patients to produce dose-related increases in PR, QRS and QT intervals.

➤*Electrolyte disturbance:* Hypokalemia or hyperkalemia may alter the effects of Class I antiarrhythmic drugs. Correct preexisting hypokalemia or hyperkalemia before administration.

➤*Effects on pacemaker thresholds:* Flecainide increases endocardial pacing thresholds and may suppress ventricular escape rhythms. Effects are reversible if flecainide is discontinued. Use with caution in patients with permanent pacemakers or temporary pacing electrodes. Do not administer to patients with existing poor thresholds or nonprogrammable pacemakers unless suitable pacing rescue is available.

Determine the pacing threshold in patients with pacemakers prior to instituting therapy, after 1 week of administration and at regular intervals thereafter. Generally, threshold changes are within the range of multiprogrammable pacemakers, and a doubling of either voltage or pulse width is usually sufficient to regain capture.

➤*Urinary pH:* Flecainide elimination is altered by urinary pH; alkalinization (as may occur in rare conditions such as renal tubular acidosis or strict vegetarian diet) decreases, and acidification increases flecainide renal excretion. These alterations in pH (outside a range of pH 5 to 7) may produce toxic or subtherapeutic plasma levels.

➤*Hepatic function impairment:* Because flecainide elimination from plasma can be markedly slower in patients with significant hepatic impairment, do not use in such patients unless the potential benefits outweigh the risks. If used, frequent and early plasma level monitoring is required to guide dosage; make dosage increases very cautiously when plasma levels have plateaued (after more than 4 days).

➤*Pregnancy: Category C.* Flecainide had teratogenic and embryotoxic effects in one breed of rabbit when given in doses up to 35 mg/kg/day. There are no adequate and well controlled studies in pregnant women. Use during pregnancy only if potential benefits outweigh potential hazards to the fetus.

➤*Lactation:* Flecainide is excreted in breast milk in concentrations as high as 4 times (with average levels about 2.5 times) corresponding plasma levels; assuming a maternal plasma level at the top of the therapeutic range (1 mcg/mL), the calculated daily dose to a breast-feeding infant (assuming about 700 mL breast milk over 24 hours) would be less than 3 mg. Because of the drug's potential for serious adverse effects in infants, determine whether to discontinue nursing or discontinue the drug, taking into account the importance of the drug to the mother.

➤*Children:* Safety and efficacy for use in children younger than 18 years of age have not been established.

In pediatric patients with structural heart disease, flecainide has been associated with cardiac arrest and sudden death. Flecainide should be started in the hospital with rhythm monitoring. Any use of flecainide in children should be directly supervised by a cardiologist skilled in the treatment of arrhythmias in children.

➤*Elderly:* From age 20 to 80, plasma levels are only slightly higher with advancing age; flecainide elimination from plasma is somewhat slower in elderly subjects than in younger subjects. Patients up to age 80 and above have been safely treated with usual doses.

➤*Monitoring:* The majority of patients treated successfully had trough plasma levels between 0.2 and 1 mcg/mL. The probability of adverse experiences, especially cardiac, may increase with higher trough plasma levels, especially levels more than 1 mcg/mL. Monitor trough plasma levels periodically, especially in patients with severe or moderate chronic renal failure or severe hepatic disease and CHF, as drug elimination may be slower.

Drug Interactions

➤*CYP450 system:* Drugs that inhibit CYP2D6 (such as quinidine) may increase the plasma concentrations of flecainide in patients who are on chronic flecainide therapy, especially if these patients are extensive metabolizers.

➤*QT prolongation:* An additive effect of flecainide with other drugs that prolong the QT interval cannot be excluded. The following drugs may prolong the QT interval and increase the risk of life-threatening cardiac arrhythmias, including torsade de pointes: Antiarrhythmic agents (eg, amiodarone, bretylium, disopyramide, dofetilide, procainamide, quinidine, and sotalol), arsenic trioxide, chlorpromazine, cisapride, dolasetron, droperidol, mefloquine, mesoridazine, moxifloxacin, pentamidine, pimozide, tacrolimus, thioridazine, and ziprasidone. For a more complete list of drugs that may prolong the QT interval, see the appendix, Drug-Induced Prolongation of the QT Interval and Torsade de Pointes.

FLECAINIDE ACETATE — ORAL

Flecainide Drug Interactions			
Precipitant drug	Object drug[a]		Description
Amiodarone	Flecainide	↑	Flecainide plasma levels may be increased.
Cimetidine	Flecainide	↑	Flecainide plasma levels and half-life may be increased.
Cisapride	Flecainide	↑	The risk of life-threatening cardiac arrhythmias, including torsades de pointes, may be increased due to possibly additive prolongation of the QT interval.
Flecainide	Cisapride		
Disopyramide	Flecainide	↑	Disopyramide has negative inotropic properties; do not use with flecainide unless benefits outweigh risks.
Propranolol	Flecainide	↑	Flecainide and propranolol levels were increased in healthy subjects. Negative inotropic effects were additive; effects on PR interval were less than additive.
Flecainide	Propranolol	↑	
Ritonavir	Flecainide	↑	Coadministration may produce large increases in serum flecainide concentrations. Ritonavir is contraindicated in patients receiving flecainide.
Urinary acidifiers	Flecainide	↓	Alterations in urinary excretion and plasma elimination of flecainide occur with changes in urinary pH (acidic urine increases elimination and decreases bioavailability; alkaline urine decreases elimination and increases bioavailability).
Urinary alkalinizers	Flecainide	↑	
Verapamil	Flecainide	↑	Verapamil has negative inotropic properties; do not use with flecainide unless benefits outweigh risks.
Flecainide	Digoxin	↑	Digoxin's absorption, peak concentration and bioavailability may be increased.

[a] ↑ = Object drug increased. ↓ = Object drug decreased.

➤*Drug/Food interactions:* Milk may inhibit absorption in infants. A reduction in flecainide dosage should be considered when milk is removed from the diet of infants.

Adverse Reactions

Most frequent – Dizziness (18.9%), including light-headedness, faintness, unsteadiness and near syncope; dyspnea (10.3%); headache (9.6%); nausea (8.9%); fatigue (7.7%); palpitation (6.1%); chest pain (5.4%); asthenia (4.9%); tremor (4.7%); constipation (4.4%); edema (3.5%); abdominal pain (3.3%).

➤*Cardiovascular:* New or worsened arrhythmias; episodes of unresuscitatable VT or ventricular fibrillation (cardiac arrest); new or worsened CHF; second-degree (0.5%) or third-degree (0.4%) AV block; sinus bradycardia, sinus pause or sinus arrest (1.2%); tachycardia (1% to 3%); angina pectoris, bradycardia, hypertension, hypotension (less than 1%).

In post-MI patients with asymptomatic PVCs and nonsustained ventricular tachycardia, flecainide therapy was associated with a 5.1% rate of death and nonfatal cardiac arrest, compared with a 2.3% rate in a matched placebo group.

➤*CNS:* Hypesthesia, paresthesia, paresis, ataxia, flushing, increased sweating, vertigo, syncope, somnolence, tinnitus, anxiety, insomnia, depression, malaise (1% to 3%); twitching, weakness, convulsions, neuropathy, speech disorder, stupor, amnesia, confusion, euphoria, depersonalization, morbid dreams, apathy (less than 1%).

➤*Dermatologic:* Rash (1% to 3%); urticaria, exfoliative dermatitis, pruritus, alopecia (less than 1%).

➤*GI:* Vomiting, diarrhea, dyspepsia, anorexia (1% to 3%); flatulence, change in taste, dry mouth (less than 1%).

➤*GU:* Impotence, decreased libido, polyuria, urinary retention (less than 1%).

➤*Hematologic:* Leukopenia, thrombocytopenia (less than 1%).

➤*Ophthalmic:* Visual disturbances including blurred vision, difficulty in focusing, spots before eyes (15.9%); diplopia (1% to 3%); eye pain/irritation, photophobia, nystagmus (less than 1%).

➤*Miscellaneous:* Fever (1% to 3%); swollen lips, tongue and mouth, arthralgia, bronchospasm, myalgia (less than 1%).

Overdosage

➤*Symptoms:* Animal studies suggest that the following events might occur with overdosage: Lengthening of the PR interval; increase in the QRS duration, QT interval and amplitude of the T wave; reduction in heart rate and myocardial contractility; conduction disturbances; hypotension; death from respiratory failure or asystole.

➤*Treatment:* Treatment should be supportive and may include the following: Removal of unabsorbed drug from the GI tract (charcoal instillation appears to be effective in lowering flecainide plasma concentrations, even after an interval of 90 minutes from ingestion of flecainide); inotropic agents or cardiac stimulants such as dopamine, dobutamine or isoproterenol; mechanical ventilation; circulatory assists such as intra-aortic balloon pumping; transvenous pacing in the event of conduction block. Because of the drug's long plasma half-life (12 to 27 hours) and the possibility of nonlinear elimination kinetics at very high doses, these supportive treatments may need to be continued for extended periods of time. Since flecainide elimination is much slower when urine is very alkaline (pH $\geq$ 8), theoretically, acidification of urine to promote drug excretion may be beneficial in overdose cases with very alkaline urine. There is no evidence that acidification from normal urinary pH increases excretion. Hemodialysis is not effective. Refer to General Management of Acute Overdosage.

Patient Information

Take as prescribed; serious heart disturbances can result from missing doses, and serious side effects can result from increasing or decreasing doses without supervision.

MEXILETINE HYDROCHLORIDE

Rx	**Mexiletine Hydrochloride** (Various, eg, Teva)	**Capsules; oral:** 150 mg	In 30s, 60s, 90s, 100s, 120s, and 240s.
		200 mg	In 100s.
		250 mg	In 90s and 100s.
Rx	**Mexitil** (Boehringer Ingelheim)	**Capsules; oral:** 150 mg	(BI 66). Red and caramel. In 100s and UD 100s.
		200 mg	(BI 67). Red. In 100s and UD 100s.
		250 mg	(BI 68). Red and aqua. In 100s and UD 100s.

MEXILETINE HYDROCHLORIDE — ORAL

Refer to the general introductory discussion concerning Antiarrhythmic Agents.

Indications

➤*Ventricular arrhythmias:* For the treatment of documented ventricular arrhythmias, such as sustained ventricular tachycardia, that, in the judgment of the physician, are life-threatening. Because of the proarrhythmic effects of mexiletine, its use with lesser arrhythmias is generally not recommended. Treatment of patients with asymptomatic ventricular premature contractions should be avoided.

➤*General information:* Initiation of mexiletine treatment, as with other antiarrhythmic agents used to treat life-threatening arrhythmias, should be carried out in the hospital.

➤*Off-label uses:*

Diabetic neuropathy – [3] = Safety concerns. In guidelines for the management of diabetic neuropathy, mexiletine is either not included or is classified as level A/B for inefficacy or discrepant results. Because of significant safety issues associated with the use of mexiletine and a lack of consistent results in published data, other agents are recommended for the treatment of diabetic neuropathy.

Neuropathy (nondiabetic) – [5] = Poor documentation. Based on initial trials, mexiletine does not appear to be useful for treatment of neuropathic pain related to HIV or spinal cord injury. Initial beneficial results in a small number of patients with other neuropathic pain syndromes need to be validated by larger controlled trials.

Other possible off-label uses – The use of prophylactic mexiletine may significantly reduce the incidence of ventricular tachycardia and other ventricular arrhythmias in the acute phase of myocardial infarction. However, mortality may not be reduced.

Administration and Dosage

➤*General dosing considerations:* The dosage of mexiletine must be individualized on the basis of response and tolerance, both of which are dose related.

As with any antiarrhythmic drug, clinical and electrocardiographic evaluation (including Holter monitoring if necessary for evaluation) are needed to determine whether the desired antiarrhythmic effect has been obtained and to guide titration and dose adjustment.

MEXILETINE HYDROCHLORIDE — ORAL

➤*Adults:*

Ventricular arrhythmias –

Usual dosage: 200 to 300 mg given every 8 hours with food or antacid. If satisfactory response has not been achieved at 300 mg every 8 hours, and the patient tolerates mexiletine well, a dose of 400 mg every 8 hours may be tried.

Maximum dose: As the severity of CNS side effects increases with total daily dose, the dose should not exceed 1,200 mg/day.

Initial dosage: 200 mg every 8 hours when rapid control of arrhythmia is not essential.

Loading dose: 400 mg may be administered, followed by a 200 mg dose in 8 hours when rapid control of ventricular arrhythmia is essential. Onset of therapeutic effect is usually observed within 30 minutes to 2 hours.

Dosage adjustment: Dose may be adjusted in 50 or 100 mg increments up or down. A minimum of 2 to 3 days between dose adjustments is recommended.

Alternative dosage: Some patients responding to mexiletine may be transferred to a 12-hour dosage schedule to improve convenience and compliance. If adequate suppression is achieved on a mexiletine dose of 300 mg or less every 8 hours, the same total daily dose may be given in divided doses every 12 hours while monitoring carefully the degree of suppression of ventricular ectopy. This dose may be adjusted up to a maximum of 450 mg every 12 hours to achieve the desired response.

Off-label dosing –

Diabetic neuropathy: [3] = Safety concerns. Efficacy is evidenced by some clinical reports, but significant safety concerns (eg, adverse events or drug interactions) must be considered prior to use. Significant safety data have been identified by controlled or noncontrolled reports and/or Food and Drug Administration or manufacturer safety notifications (eg, black box warnings).

Initial dosage of 75 mg 3 times daily with slow titration up to 450 or 675 mg/day to avoid adverse effects. Maintenance dosages ranged from 150 to 675 mg/day administered in 3 divided doses.

➤*Renal function impairment:* In general, patients with renal failure will require the usual doses of mexiletine. Patients with severe liver disease, however, may require lower doses and must be monitored closely. Similarly, marked, right-sided congestive heart failure can reduce hepatic metabolism and reduce the needed dose. Plasma level may also be affected by certain concomitant drugs.

➤*Transferring to mexiletine:* The following dosage schedule, based on theoretical considerations rather than experimental data, is suggested for transferring patients from other Class I oral antiarrhythmic agents to mexiletine.

Mexiletine treatment may be initiated with a 200 mg dose, and titrated to response as described above, 6 to 12 hours after the last dose of quinidine sulfate, 3 to 6 hours after the last dose of procainamide, 6 to 12 hours after the last dose of disopyramide or 8 to 12 hours after the last dose of tocainide.

In patients in whom withdrawal of the previous antiarrhythmic agent is likely to produce life-threatening arrhythmias, hospitalization of the patient is recommended.

When transferring from lidocaine to mexiletine, the lidocaine infusion should be stopped when the first oral dose of mexiletine is administered. The infusion line should be left open until suppression of the arrhythmia appears to be satisfactorily maintained. Consideration should be given to the similarity of the adverse effects of lidocaine and mexiletine and the possibility that they may be additive.

➤*Administration:* Administration with food or antacid is recommended.

➤*Storage / Stability:* Store at 20° to 25°C (68° to 77°F).

Actions

➤*Pharmacology:* Mexiletine is a local anesthetic, antiarrhythmic agent, structurally similar to lidocaine, but orally active. In animal studies, mexiletine has been shown to be effective in the suppression of induced ventricular arrhythmias, including those induced by glycoside toxicity and coronary artery ligation. Mexiletine, like lidocaine, inhibits the inward sodium current, thus reducing the rate of rise of the action potential, Phase 0. Mexiletine decreased the effective refractory period (ERP) in Purkinje fibers. The decrease in ERP was of lesser magnitude than the decrease in action potential duration (APD), with a resulting increase in the ERP/APD ratio.

➤*Pharmacokinetics:*

Absorption – Mexiletine is well absorbed (approximately 90%) from the GI tract. Unlike lidocaine, its first-pass metabolism is low. Peak blood levels are reached in 2 to 3 hours.

The absorption rate of mexiletine is reduced in clinical situations such as acute myocardial infarction in which gastric emptying time is increased. Narcotics, atropine and magnesium-aluminum hydroxide have also been reported to slow the absorption of mexiletine. Metoclopramide has been reported to accelerate absorption.

Distribution – Mexiletine is 50% to 60% bound to plasma protein, with a volume of distribution of 5 to 7 L/kg.

Metabolism – Mexiletine is metabolized in the liver.

Several metabolites of mexiletine have shown minimal antiarrhythmic activity in animal models. The most active is the minor metabolite N-methylmexiletine, which is less than 20% as potent as mexiletine. The urinary excretion of N-methylmexiletine in man is less than 0.5%. Thus the therapeutic activity of mexiletine is due to the parent compound.

Excretion – Approximately 10% is excreted unchanged by the kidney. While urinary pH does not normally have much influence on elimination, marked changes in urinary pH influence the rate of excretion: acidification accelerates excretion, while alkalinization retards it.

In healthy subjects, the plasma elimination half-life of mexiletine is approximately 10 to 12 hours.

Mexiletine plasma levels of at least 0.5 mcg/mL are generally required for therapeutic response. An increase in the frequency of CNS adverse effects has been observed when plasma levels exceed 2 mcg/mL. Thus the therapeutic range is approximately 0.5 to 2 mcg/mL. Plasma levels within the therapeutic range can be attained with either 3 times daily or twice-daily dosing but peak to trough differences are greater with the latter regimen, creating the possibility of adverse effects at peak and arrhythmic escape at trough. Nevertheless, some patients may be transferred successfully to the twice-daily regimen. If adequate suppression is achieved on a mexiletine dose of 300 mg or less every 8 hours, the same total daily dose may be given in divided doses every 12 hours while monitoring carefully the degree of suppression of ventricular ectopy. This dose may be adjusted up to a maximum of 450 mg every 12 hours to achieve the desired response.

Special populations –

Renal function impairment: Consistent with the limited renal elimination of mexiletine, little change in the half-life has been detected in patients with reduced renal function. In 8 patients with creatinine clearance less than 10 mL/min, the mean plasma elimination half-life was 15.7 hours; in 7 patients with creatinine clearance between 11 to 40 mL/min, the mean half-life was 13.4 hours.

Hepatic function impairment: Hepatic impairment prolongs the elimination half-life of mexiletine. In 8 patients with moderate to severe liver disease, the mean half-life was approximately 25 hours.

Contraindications

Cardiogenic shock or preexisting second- or third-degree AV block (if no pacemaker is present).

Warnings/Precautions

➤*Mortality:* Considering the known proarrhythmic properties of mexiletine and the lack of evidence of improved survival for any antiarrhythmic drug in patients without life-threatening arrhythmias, the use of mexiletine as well as other antiarrhythmic agents should be reserved for patients with life-threatening ventricular arrhythmia.

➤*Proarrhythmia:* Like other antiarrhythmics, mexiletine can cause worsening of arrhythmias. This has been uncommon in patients with less serious arrhythmias (frequent premature beats or nonsustained ventricular tachycardia), but is of greater concern in patients with life-threatening arrhythmias such as sustained ventricular tachycardia. In patients with such arrhythmias subjected to programmed electrical stimulation or to exercise provocation, 10% to 15% of patients had exacerbation of the arrhythmia, a rate not greater than that of other agents.

➤*Urinary pH:* Concurrent drug therapy or dietary regimens which may markedly alter urinary pH should be avoided during mexiletine therapy. The minor fluctuations in urinary pH associated with normal diet do not affect the excretion of mexiletine.

➤*Blood dyscrasias:* Among 10,867 patients treated with mexiletine in the compassionate-use program, marked leukopenia (neutrophils less than 1,000/mm^3) or agranulocytosis were seen in 0.06%, and milder depressions of leukocytes were seen in 0.08%, and thrombocytopenia was observed in 0.16%. Many of these patients were seriously ill and receiving concomitant medications with known hematologic adverse effects. Rechallenge with mexiletine in several cases was negative. Marked leukopenia or agranulocytosis did not occur in any patient receiving mexiletine alone; 5 of the 6 cases of agranulocytosis were associated with procainamide (sustained-release preparations in 4) and 1 with vinblastine. If significant hematologic changes are observed, the patient should be evaluated carefully, and, if warranted, mexiletine should be discontinued. Blood counts usually return to normal within 1 month of discontinuation.

➤*Hepatic effects:*

Acute liver injury – In postmarketing experience, abnormal liver function tests have been reported some in the first few weeks of therapy with mexiletine. Most of these have been observed in the setting of congestive heart failure or ischemia, and their relationship to mexiletine has not been established.

AST elevation and liver injury – In 3-month controlled trials, elevations of AST greater than 3 times the upper limit of normal occurred in about 1% of both mexiletine-treated and control patients. Approximately 2% of patients in the mexiletine compassionate use program had elevations of AST greater than or equal to 3 times the upper limit of normal. These elevations frequently occurred in association with identifiable clinical events and therapeutic measures such as congestive heart failure, acute myocardial infarction, blood transfusions and other medications. These elevations were often asymptomatic and transient, usually not associated with elevated bilirubin levels and usually did not require discontinuation of therapy. Marked elevations of AST (greater than 1000 U/L) were seen before death in 4 patients with end-stage cardiac disease (severe congestive heart failure, cardiogenic shock).

Rare instances of severe liver injury, including hepatic necrosis, have been reported in association with mexiletine treatment. It is recommended that patients in whom an abnormal liver test has occurred, or who have signs or symptoms suggesting liver dysfunction, be evaluated carefully. If persistent or worsening elevation of hepatic enzymes is detected, consideration should be given to discontinuing therapy.

MEXILETINE HYDROCHLORIDE — ORAL

➤*Seizures:* Convulsions (seizures) did not occur in mexiletine controlled clinical trials. In the compassionate-use program, convulsions were reported in about 2 of 1,000 patients. Twenty-eight percent (28%) of these patients discontinued therapy. Convulsions were reported in patients with and without a history of seizures. Mexiletine should be used with caution in patients with known seizure disorder.

➤*Special risk:* If a ventricular pacemaker is operative, patients with second- or third-degree heart block may be treated with mexiletine if monitored continuously. A limited number of patients (45 of 475 in controlled clinical trials) with preexisting first-degree AV block were treated with mexiletine; none of these patients developed second- or third-degree AV block. Caution should be exercised when it is used in such patients or in patients with preexisting sinus node dysfunction or intraventricular conduction abnormalities.

Mexiletine should be used with caution in patients with hypotension and severe congestive heart failure because of the potential for aggravating these conditions.

➤*Pregnancy:* Category C.

Teratogenic – Reproduction studies performed with mexiletine in rats, mice and rabbits at doses up to 4 times the maximum human oral dose (24 mg/kg in a 50 kg patient) revealed no evidence of teratogenicity or impaired fertility but did show an increase in fetal resorption. There are no adequate and well-controlled studies in pregnant women; this drug should be used in pregnancy only if the potential benefit justifies the potential risk to the fetus.

➤*Lactation:* Mexiletine appears in human milk in concentrations similar to those observed in plasma. Therefore, if the use of mexiletine is deemed essential, an alternative method of infant feeding should be considered.

➤*Children:* Safety and efficacy in the pediatric population have not been established.

➤*Monitoring:* Because mexiletine is metabolized in the liver, and hepatic impairment has been reported to prolong the elimination half-life of mexiletine, patients with liver disease should be followed carefully while receiving mexiletine. The same caution should be observed in patients with hepatic dysfunction secondary to congestive heart failure.

Drug Interactions

➤*CYP-450 system:* Because mexiletine is a substrate for CYP2D6 and CYP1A2, inhibition or induction of either of these enzymes would be expected to alter mexiletine concentrations.

Mexiletine Drug Interactions

Precipitant drug	Object drug[a]		Description
Aluminum-Magnesium Hydroxide Atropine Narcotics	Mexiletine	↓	Mexiletine absorption may be slowed.
Cimetidine	Mexiletine	↔	Cimetidine may increase or decrease mexiletine plasma levels.
Fluvoxamine	Mexiletine	↑	The clearance of mexiletine was decreased by 38% following coadministration with fluvoxamine, a CYP1A2 inhibitor.
Hydantoins	Mexiletine	↓	Increased mexiletine clearance leading to lower steady-state plasma levels may occur.
Metoclopramide	Mexiletine	↑	Mexiletine absorption may be accelerated.
Propafenone	Mexiletine	↑	Mexiletine plasma concentrations may be elevated in extensive metabolizers due to propafenone inhibiting the metabolism (CYP2D6) of mexiletine. When mexiletine is initiated, slowly titrate the dose.
Rifampin	Mexiletine	↓	Increased mexiletine clearance leading to lower steady-state plasma levels may occur.
Urinary acidifiers	Mexiletine	↓	Renal clearance of mexiletine is related to urinary pH. In acidic urine, mexiletine clearance may be increased.
Urinary alkalinizers	Mexiletine	↑	Renal clearance of mexiletine is related to urinary pH. In alkaline urine, mexiletine clearance may be decreased.
Mexiletine	Caffeine	↑	Clearance of caffeine may be decreased by 50%

Mexiletine Drug Interactions

Precipitant drug	Object drug[a]		Description
Mexiletine	Theophylline	↑	Serum theophylline levels may be increased; increased pharmacologic and toxic effects may occur.

[a] ↑ = Object drug increased. ↓ = Object drug decreased. ↔ = Undetermined clinical effect.

Adverse Reactions

Mexiletine commonly produces reversible GI and nervous system adverse reactions but is otherwise well tolerated. Mexiletine has been evaluated in 483 patients in 1- and 3-month controlled studies and in over 10,000 patients in a large, compassionate-use program. Dosages in the controlled studies ranged from 600 to 1200 mg/day; some patients (8%) in the compassionate-use program were treated with higher daily doses (1600 to 3200 mg/day). In the 3-month controlled trials comparing mexiletine to quinidine, procainamide and disopyramide, the most frequent adverse reactions were upper GI distress (41%), light-headedness (10.5%), tremor (12.6%) and coordination difficulties (10.2%). Similar frequency and incidence were observed in the 1-month placebo-controlled trial. Although these reactions were generally not serious, and were dose related and reversible with a reduction in dosage, by taking the drug with food or antacid or by therapy discontinuation, they led to therapy discontinuation in 40% of patients in the controlled trials.

Adverse Reactions with Mexiletine vs Placebo in the 4-Week, Double-Blind Crossover Trial

Adverse reactions	Mexiletine (n = 53)	Placebo (n = 49)
Cardiovascular		
Palpitations	7.5%	10.2%
Chest pain	7.5%	4.1%
Increased ventricular arrhythmia/PVCs	1.9%	—
CNS		
Dizziness/light-headedness	26.4%	14.3%
Tremor	13.2%	—
Nervousness	11.3%	6.1%
Coordination difficulties	9.4%	—
Changes in sleep habits	7.5%	16.3%
Paresthesias/numbness	3.8%	2%
Weakness	1.9%	4.1%
Fatigue	1.9%	2%
Tinnitus	1.9%	4.1%
Confusion/Clouded sensorium	1.9%	2%
GI		
Nausea/vomiting/heartburn	39.6%	6.1%
Miscellaneous		
Blurred vision/visual disturbances	7.5%	2%
Dyspnea/respiratory	5.7%	10.2%
Headache	7.5%	6.1%
Nonspecific edema	3.8%	—
Rash	3.8%	2%

Adverse Reactions with Mexiletine vs Controls in the 12-week Double-Blind Trials (≥ 1%)

Adverse reactions	Mexiletine (n = 430)	Quinidine (n = 262)	Procainamide (n = 78)	Disopyramide (n = 69)
Cardiovascular				
Palpitations	4.3%	4.6%	1.3%	5.8%
Chest pain	2.6%	3.4%	1.3%	2.9%
Angina/angina-like pain	1.7%	1.9%	2.6%	2.9%
Increased ventricular arrhythmias/PVCs	1%	2.7%	2.6%	—
CNS				
Dizziness/light-headedness	18.9%	14.1%	14.1%	2.9%
Tremor	13.2%	2.3%	3.8%	1.4%
Coordination difficulties	9.7%	1.1%	1.3%	—
Changes in sleep habits	7.1%	2.7%	11.5%	8.7%
Weakness	5%	5.3%	7.7%	2.9%
Nervousness	5%	1.9%	6.4%	5.8%
Fatigue	3.8%	5.7%	5.1%	1.4%
Speech difficulties	2.6%	0.4%	—	—

MEXILETINE HYDROCHLORIDE — ORAL

Adverse Reactions with Mexiletine vs Controls in the 12-week Double-Blind Trials (≥ 1%)				
Adverse reactions	Mexiletine (n = 430)	Quinidine (n = 262)	Procainamide (n = 78)	Disopyramide (n = 69)
Confusion/ Clouded sensorium	2.6%		3.8%	
Paresthesias/ numbness	2.4%	2.3%	2.6%	—
Tinnitus	2.4%	1.5%	—	—
Depression	2.4%	1.1%	1.3%	1.4%
GI				
Nausea/ vomiting/ heartburn	39.3%	21.4%	33.3%	14.5%
Diarrhea	5.2%	33.2%	2.6%	8.7%
Constipation	4%	—	6.4%	11.6%
Changes in appetite	2.6%	1.9%	—	—
Abdominal pain/ cramps/ discomfort	1.2%	1.5%	—	1.4%
Miscellaneous				
Blurred vision/ Visual disturbances	5.7%	3.1%	5.1%	7.2%
Headache	5.7%	6.9%	7.7%	4.3%
Rash	4.2%	3.8%	10.3%	1.4%
Dyspnea/ respiratory	3.3%	3.1%	5.1%	2.9%
Dry mouth	2.8%	1.9%	5.1%	14.5%
Arthralgia	1.7%	2.3%	5.1%	1.4%
Fever	1.2%	3.1%	2.6%	—

➤*Less than 1%:* Syncope, edema, hot flashes, hypertension, short-term memory loss, loss of consciousness, other psychological changes, diaphoresis, urinary hesitancy/retention, malaise, impotence/decreased libido, pharyngitis, congestive heart failure.

➤*Treatment under compassionate-use circumstances:* An additional group of over 10,000 patients has been treated in a program allowing administration of mexiletine under compassionate-use circumstances. These patients were seriously ill, with the large majority on multiple drug therapy. Twenty-four percent (24%) of the patients continued in the program for 1 year or longer. Adverse reactions leading to therapy discontinuation occurred in 15% of patients (usually upper GI system or nervous system effects). In general, the more common adverse reactions were similar to those in the controlled trials. Less common adverse events possibly related to mexiletine use include the following:

Cardiovascular – Syncope and hypotension, each about 6 in 1000; bradycardia, about 4 in 1000; angina/angina-like pain, about 3 in 1000; edema, atrioventricular block/conduction disturbances and hot flashes, each about 2 in 1000; atrial arrhythmias, hypertension and cardiogenic shock, each about 1 in 1000.

CNS – Short-term memory loss, about 9 in 1000 patients; hallucinations and other psychological changes, each about 3 in 1000; psychosis and convulsions/seizures, each about 2 in 1000; loss of consciousness, about 6 in 10,000.

Dermatologic – Rare cases of exfoliative dermatitis and Stevens-Johnson syndrome with mexiletine treatment have been reported.

GI – Dysphagia, about 2 in 1000; peptic ulcer, about 8 in 10,000; upper GI bleeding, about 7 in 10,000; esophageal ulceration, about 1 in 10,000. Rare cases of severe hepatitis/acute hepatic necrosis.

Hematologic – Blood dyscrasias were not seen in the controlled trials but did occur among 10,867 patients treated with mexiletine in the compassionate-use program.

Myelofibrosis was reported in 2 patients in the compassionate-use program: 1 was receiving long-term thiotepa therapy, and the other had pretreatment myeloid abnormalities.

Lab test abnormalities – Abnormal liver function tests, about 5 in 1,000 patients; positive ANA and thrombocytopenia, each about 2 in 1,000; leukopenia (including neutropenia and agranulocytosis), about 1 in 1,000; myelofibrosis, about 2 in 10,000 patients.

Miscellaneous – Diaphoresis, about 6 in 1,000; altered taste, about 5 in 1,000; salivary changes, hair loss and impotence/decreased libido, each about 4 in 1000; malaise, about 3 in 1,000; urinary hesitancy/retention, each about 2 in 1,000; hiccups, dry skin, laryngeal and pharyngeal changes and changes in oral mucous membranes, each about 1 in 1,000; SLE syndrome, about 4 in 10,000.

➤*Postmarketing:* In postmarketing experience, there have been isolated, spontaneous reports of pulmonary changes including pulmonary fibrosis during mexiletine therapy with or without other drugs or diseases that are known to produce pulmonary toxicity. A causal relationship to mexiletine therapy has not been established. In addition, there have been isolated reports of exacerbation of congestive heart failure in patients with preexisting compromised ventricular function. There have been rare reports of pancreatitis associated with mexiletine treatment.

Overdosage

➤*Symptoms:* Clinical findings associated with mexiletine overdosage have included nausea, hypotension, sinus bradycardia, paresthesia, seizures, bundle branch block, AV heart block, asystole, ventricular tachyarrythmia, including ventricular fibrillation, cardiovascular collapse and coma. The lowest known dose in a fatality case was 4.4 g, with postmortem serum mexiletine level of 34 to 37 mcg/mL. Patients have recovered from ingestion of 4 to 18 g of mexiletine.

➤*Treatment:* There is no specific antidote for mexiletine. Management of mexiletine overdosage includes general supportive measures, close observation and monitoring of vital signs. In addition, the use of pharmacologic interventions (eg, pressor agents, atropine, anticonvulsants) or transvenous cardiac pacing is suggested, depending on the patient's clinical condition.

Patient Information

Take medication with food or an antacid.

Adverse effects such as nausea, vomiting, heartburn, diarrhea, constipation, dizziness, tremor, nervousness, coordination difficulties, changes in sleep habits, headache, visual disturbances, tingling/numbness, weakness, ringing in the ears and palpitations/chest pain may occur. Notify physician if they become bothersome.

Notify physician if signs of liver injury or blood cell damage occur, such as unexplained general tiredness, jaundice, fever or sore throat.

Avoid changes in diet that could drastically acidify or alkalinize the urine.

PROPAFENONE HYDROCHLORIDE

Rx	**Propafenone** (Various, eg, Watson)	**Tablets; oral:** 150 mg	In 100s and 500s.
Rx	**Rythmol** (GlaxoSmithKline)		(150). White, scored. Film coated. In 100s and UD 100s.
Rx	**Propafenone** (Various, eg, Watson)	**Tablets; oral:** 225 mg	In 100s and 500s.
Rx	**Rythmol** (GlaxoSmithKline)		(225). Tan, scored. Film coated. In 100s and UD 1000s.
Rx	**Propafenone** (Various, eg, Ethex, Mutual, URL)	**Tablets; oral:** 300 mg	In 100s.
Rx	**Propafenone** (Par)	**Capsules, extended-release; oral:** 225 mg	Lactose. (par/209). Peach, opaque. In 60s, 90s, 100s, 500s, and 1,000s.
Rx	**Rythmol SR** (GlaxoSmithKline)		(a 225). White. In 60s.
Rx	**Propafenone** (Par)	**Capsules, extended-release; oral:** 325 mg	Lactose. (par/210). Orange, opaque. In 60s, 90s, 100s, 500s, and 1,000s.
Rx	**Rythmol SR** (GlaxoSmithKline)		(a 325). White. In 60s.
Rx	**Propafenone** (Par)	**Capsules, extended-release; oral:** 425 mg	Lactose. (par/211). Red, opaque. In 60s, 90s, 100s, 500s, and 1,000s.
Rx	**Rythmol SR** (GlaxoSmithKline)		(a 425). White. In 60s.

PROPAFENONE HYDROCHLORIDE — ORAL

Refer to the general introductory discussion concerning Antiarrhythmic Agents.

WARNING

In the National Heart, Lung, and Blood Institute's Cardiac Arrhythmia Suppression Trial (CAST), a long-term, multicenter, randomized, double-blind study in patients with asymptomatic non-life-threatening ventricular arrhythmias who had an MI more than 6 days but less than 2 years previously, an increased rate of death or reversed cardiac arrest rate (7.7%) was seen in patients treated with encainide or flecainide (Class 1C antiarrhythmics) compared with that seen in patients assigned to placebo (3%). The average duration of treatment with encainide or flecainide in this study was 10 months.

The applicability of the CAST results to other populations (eg, those without recent MI) or other antiarrhythmic drugs is uncertain, but at present, it is prudent to consider any 1C antiarrhythmic to have a significant risk in patients with structural heart disease. Given the lack of any evidence that these drugs improve survival, antiarrhythmic agents should generally be avoided in patients with nonlife-threatening ventricular arrhythmias, even if the patients are experiencing unpleasant, but not life-threatening symptoms or signs.

Indications

➤*Atrial fibrillation/flutter:*

Immediate-release (IR) – To prolong the time to recurrence of paroxysmal atrial fibrillation/flutter associated with disabling symptoms in patients without structural heart disease.

Some patients with atrial flutter treated with propafenone have developed 1:1 conduction, producing an increase in ventricular rate. Concomitant treatment with drugs that increase the functional AV refractory period is recommended.

Extended-release (ER) – To prolong the time to recurrence of symptomatic atrial fibrillation in patients with structural heart disease.

➤*Paroxysmal supraventricular tachycardia (PSVT) (IR only):* To prolong the time to recurrence of PSVT associated with disabling symptoms in patients without structural heart disease.

➤*Ventricular arrhythmias (IR only):* For the treatment of ventricular arrhythmias, such as sustained ventricular tachycardia, that are life-threatening. Because of the proarrhythmic effects of propafenone, its use with lesser ventricular arrhythmias is not recommended, even if patients are symptomatic, and reserve any use of the drug for patients in whom the potential benefits outweigh the risks.

Propafenone, like other antiarrhythmic drugs, has not been shown to enhance survival in patients with ventricular or atrial arrhythmias.

Administration and Dosage

➤*Adults:*

Immediate release –

Atrial fibrillation/flutter:

- *Initial dosage* – 150 mg every 8 hours.
- *Dosage titration* – Dosage may be increased at a minimum of 3- to 4-day intervals to 225 mg every 8 hours and, if necessary, to 300 mg every 8 hours.
- *Dosage adjustment* – In those patients in whom significant widening of the QRS complex or second- or third-degree AV block occurs, consider dose reduction.

Paroxysmal supraventricular tachycardia: See Atrial fibrillation/flutter for dosing.

Ventricular arrhythmias: See Atrial fibrillation/flutter for dosing.

Extended release –

Atrial fibrillation/flutter:

- *Initial dosage* – 225 mg given every 12 hours.
- *Dosage titration* – Dosage may be increased at a minimum of 5-day intervals to 325 mg given every 12 hours. If additional therapeutic effect is needed, the dose may be increased to 425 mg every 12 hours.
- *Dosage adjustment* – In patients with hepatic impairment or having significant widening of the QRS complex or second- or third-degree AV block, dose reduction should be considered.

➤*Elderly:* Use with caution. Increase dose more gradually during initial treatment phase.

➤*Hepatic function impairment:* Use with caution. The dose in patients with severe liver dysfunction should be approximately 20% to 30% of the dose given to patients with healthy hepatic function.

➤*Special risk patients:* Patients with marked previous myocardial damage should increase dose more gradually during initial treatment phase.

➤*Administration:* The extended-release capsules can be taken with or without food. Do not crush or further divide the contents of the capsule.

➤*Storage/Stability:* Store at 25°C (77°F); excursions permitted between 15° and 30°C (59° and 86°F). Dispense in a tight, light-resistant container.

Actions

➤*Pharmacology:* Propafenone is a Class IC antiarrhythmic with local anesthetic effects and direct stabilizing action on myocardial membranes. Propafenone's electrophysiologic effect manifests itself in a reduction of upstroke velocity (Phase 0) of the monophasic action potential. In Purkinje fibers, and to a lesser extent myocardial fibers, propafenone reduces fast inward current carried by sodium ions. Diastolic excitability threshold is increased and effective refractory period prolonged. Propafenone reduces spontaneous automaticity and depresses triggered activity.

➤*Pharmacokinetics:*

Absorption/Distribution – Propafenone is nearly completely absorbed after oral administration with peak plasma levels occurring approximately 3.5 hours after administration in most individuals. It exhibits extensive first-pass metabolism resulting in a dose-dependent and dosage-form-dependent absolute bioavailability (eg, a 150 mg tablet had absolute bioavailability of 3.4%, a 300 mg tablet 10.6% and 300 mg solution 21.4%). Bioavailability increases further at doses above those recommended. Propafenone follows a nonlinear pharmacokinetic disposition presumably due to saturation of first-pass hepatic metabolism as the liver is exposed to higher concentrations of propafenone and shows a very high degree of interindividual variability. For example, for a threefold increase in daily dose from 300 to 900 mg/day, there is a tenfold increase in steady-state plasma concentration.

Metabolism/Excretion – There are two genetically determined patterns of propafenone metabolism. In more than 90% of patients, the drug is rapidly and extensively metabolized with an elimination half-life of 2 to 10 hours. These patients metabolize propafenone into two active metabolites: 5-hydroxypropafenone (formed by CYP2D6) and N-depropylpropafenone (formed by CYP3A4 and CYP1A2). In vitro, these metabolites have antiarrhythmic activity comparable to propafenone, but in man they both are usually present in concentrations less than 20% of propafenone. Nine additional metabolites have been identified, most in only trace amounts. The saturable hydroxylation pathway is responsible for the nonlinear pharmacokinetic disposition.

In fewer than 10% of patients, propafenone metabolism is slower because the 5-hydroxy metabolite is not formed or is minimally formed. The estimated propafenone elimination half-life ranges from 10 to 32 hours. In these patients, the N-depropylpropafenone is present in quantities comparable to the levels measured in extensive metabolizers. In slow metabolizers, propafenone pharmacokinetics are linear.

There are significant differences in plasma concentrations of propafenone in slow and extensive metabolizers, the former achieving concentrations 1.5 to 2 times those of the extensive metabolizers at daily doses of 675 to 900 mg/day. At low doses the differences are greater, with slow metabolizers attaining concentrations more than 5 times those of extensive metabolizers. Because the difference decreases at high doses and is mitigated by the lack of the active 5-hydroxy metabolite in the slow metabolizers, and because steady-state conditions are achieved after 4 to 5 days of dosing, the recommended dosing regimen is the same for all patients. Titrate dosage carefully with close attention to clinical and ECG evidence of toxicity. In addition, the beta-blocking action of propafenone appears to be enhanced in slow metabolizers.

Special populations –

Hepatic function impairment: Bioavailability increases and the clearance of propafenone is reduced and the elimination half-life increased in patients with significant hepatic dysfunction (see Warnings).

Contraindications

Uncontrolled CHF; cardiogenic shock; sinoatrial, AV and intraventricular disorders of impulse generation or conduction (eg, sick sinus node syndrome, AV block) in the absence of an artificial pacemaker; bradycardia; marked hypotension; bronchospastic disorders; manifest electrolyte imbalance; hypersensitivity to the drug.

Warnings/Precautions

➤*Mortality:* See the Warning box for more information.

➤*Proarrhythmic effects:* Propafenone, like other antiarrhythmic agents, may cause new or worsened arrhythmias. Such proarrhythmic effects range from an increase in frequency of PVCs to the development of more severe ventricular tachycardia, ventricular fibrillation or torsades de pointes (ie, tachycardia that is more sustained or more rapid), which may lead to fatal consequences. It may also worsen premature ventricular contractions or supraventricular arrhythmias, and it may prolong the QT interval. It is therefore essential that each patient be evaluated electrocardiographically and clinically prior to, and during therapy to determine whether response to propafenone supports continued use. Because propafenone prolongs the QRS interval in the electrocardiogram, changes in the QT interval are difficult to interpret.

➤*Non-life-threatening arrhythmias:* Use of propafenone is not recommended in patients with less severe ventricular arrhythmias, even if the patients are symptomatic.

➤*Survival:* There is no evidence from controlled trials that the use of propafenone favorably affects survival or the incidence of sudden death.

➤*Nonallergic bronchospasm (eg, chronic bronchitis, emphysema):* In general, these patients should not receive propafenone or other agents with beta-adrenergic blocking activity.

➤*Congestive heart failure (CHF):* New or worsened CHF has occurred in 3.7% of patients with ventricular arrhythmia; of those, 0.9% were probably or definitely related to propafenone. Of the patients with CHF probably related to propafenone, 80% had preexisting heart failure and 85% had coronary artery disease. CHF attributable to propafenone developed rarely (less than 0.2%) in patients who had no previous history of CHF.

As propafenone exerts both beta blockade and a (dose-related) negative inotropic effect on cardiac muscle, patients with CHF should be fully compen-

PROPAFENONE HYDROCHLORIDE — ORAL

sated before receiving propafenone. If CHF worsens, discontinue propafenone unless CHF is due to the cardiac arrhythmia and, if indicated, restart at a lower dosage only after adequate cardiac compensation has been established.

➤*Conduction disturbances:* Propafenone slows AV conduction and also causes first degree AV block. Average PR interval prolongation and increases in QRS duration are closely correlated with dosage increases and concomitant increases in propafenone plasma concentrations. The incidence of first-, second- and third-degree AV block observed in 2127 ventricular arrhythmia patients was 2.5%, 0.6% and 0.2%, respectively. Development of second- or third-degree AV block requires a reduction in dosage or discontinuation of propafenone. Bundle branch block (1.2%) and intraventricular conduction delay (1.1%) have occurred in patients receiving propafenone. Bradycardia has also occurred (1.5%). Experience in patients with sick sinus node syndrome is limited and these patients should not be treated with propafenone.

Propafenone should not be given to patients with atrioventricular and intraventricular conduction defects in the absence of a pacemaker (see Contraindications).

➤*Effects on pacemaker threshold:* Pacing and sensing thresholds of artificial pacemakers may be altered. Monitor and program pacemakers accordingly during therapy.

➤*Hematologic disturbances:* Agranulocytosis (fever, chills, weakness, and neutropenia) has been reported in patients receiving propafenone. Generally, the agranulocytosis occurred within the first 2 months of propafenone therapy and upon discontinuation of therapy, the white count usually normalized by 14 days. Unexplained fever and/or decrease in white cell count, particularly during the first 3 months of therapy, warrants consideration of possible agranulocytosis/granulocytopenia. Instruct patients to promptly report the development of any signs of infection such as fever, sore throat or chills.

➤*Elevated ANA titers:* Positive ANA titers have occurred. They have been reversible upon cessation of treatment and may disappear even with continued therapy. These laboratory findings were usually not associated with clinical symptoms, but there is one case of drug-induced lupus erythematosus (positive rechallenge); it resolved completely upon therapy discontinuation. Carefully evaluate patients who develop an abnormal ANA test and, if persistent or worsening elevation of ANA titers is detected, consider discontinuing therapy.

➤*Renal/Hepatic changes:* Renal changes have been observed in the rat following 6 months of oral administration of propafenone at doses of 180 and 360 mg/kg/day (2 to 4 times the maximum recommended human dose). Both inflammatory and noninflammatory changes in the renal tubules with accompanying interstitial nephritis were observed. These lesions were reversible in that they were not found in rats treated at these dosage levels and allowed to recover for 6 weeks. Fatty degenerative changes of the liver were found in rats following chronic administration of propafenone at dose levels 3 times the maximum recommended human dose.

➤*Neuromuscular dysfunction:* Exacerbation of myasthenia gravis has been reported during propafenone therapy.

➤*Renal function impairment:* A considerable percentage of propafenone metabolites (18.5% to 38% of the dose/48 hours) are excreted in the urine. Administer cautiously to patients with impaired renal function. Carefully monitor for signs of overdosage.

➤*Hepatic function impairment:* Propafenone is highly metabolized by the liver; administer cautiously to patients with impaired hepatic function. Severe liver dysfunction increases the bioavailability of propafenone to approximately 70%, compared to 3% to 40% for patients with normal liver function; the mean half-life is approximately 9 hours. The dose of propafenone should be approximately 20% to 30% of the dose given to patients with normal hepatic function. Carefully monitor for excessive pharmacological effects.

➤*Pregnancy: Category C.* Propafenone is embryotoxic in rabbits and rats when given in doses 3 and 6 times, respectively, the maximum recommended human dose. There are no adequate and well controlled studies in pregnant women. Use during pregnancy only if the potential benefit justifies the potential risk to the fetus.

➤*Lactation:* Propafenone is excreted in breast milk. Decide whether to discontinue nursing or to discontinue the drug, taking into account the importance of the drug to the mother.

➤*Children:* The safety and efficacy of propafenone in children have not been established.

➤*Elderly:* Because of the possible increased risk of impaired hepatic or renal function in this age group, use with caution. The effective dose may be lower in these patients.

Drug Interactions

➤*CYP-450 system:* Drugs that inhibit CYP2D6, CYP1A2, and CYP3A4 might lead to increased plasma levels of propafenone. When propafenone is administered with inhibitors of these enzymes, closely monitor patients and adjust dose accordingly.

➤*QT prolongation:* An additive effect of propafenone with other drugs that prolong the QT interval cannot be excluded. The following drugs may prolong the QT interval and increase the risk of life-threatening cardiac arrhythmias, including torsade de pointes: Antiarrhythmic agents (eg, amiodarone, bretylium, disopyramide, dofetilide, procainamide, quinidine, and sotalol), arsenic trioxide, chlorpromazine, cisapride, dolasetron, droperidol, mefloquine, mesoridazine, moxifloxacin, pentamidine, pimozide, tacrolimus, thioridazine, and ziprasidone. For a more complete list of drugs that may prolong the QT interval, see the appendix, Drug-Induced Prolongation of the QT Interval and Torsade de Pointes.

Propafenone Drug Interactions

Precipitant drug	Object drug[a]		Description
Anesthetics, local	Propafenone	⬆	Concurrent use (ie, during pacemaker implantations, surgery or dental use) may increase the risks of CNS side effects.
Cimetidine	Propafenone	⬆	The maximum propafenone concentration may be increased, possibly resulting in increased pharmacologic effects.
Cisapride	Propafenone	⬆	The risk of life-threatening cardiac arrhythmias, including torsades de pointes, may be increased due to possibly additive prolongation of the QT interval.
Propafenone	Cisapride		
Quinidine	Propafenone	⬆	Serum propafenone levels may be increased in rapid, extensive metabolizers of the drug, possibly increasing the pharmacologic effects.
Rifamycins	Propafenone	⬇	Increased propafenone clearance may occur, resulting in decreased plasma levels and a possible loss of therapeutic effect.
Ritonavir	Propafenone	⬆	Coadministration may produce large increases in serum propafenone concentrations. Ritonavir is contraindicated in patients receiving propafenone.
SSRIs (eg, fluoxetine)	Propafenone	⬆	Plasma propafenone levels may be elevated. Certain SSRIs may inhibit the metabolism (CYP2D6) of propafenone.
Propafenone	Anticoagulants	⬆	Increased warfarin plasma levels and prothrombin time may occur.
Propafenone	Beta-blockers	⬆	The plasma levels and pharmacologic effects of beta blockers metabolized by the liver may be increased.
Propafenone	Cyclosporine	⬆	Increased whole blood cyclosporine trough levels and decreased renal function may occur.
Propafenone	Desipramine	⬆	Coadministration may result in elevated serum desipramine levels.
Propafenone	Digoxin	⬆	Serum digoxin levels may be increased, resulting in toxicity.
Propafenone	Mexiletine	⬆	Mexiletine plasma concentrations may be elevated in extensive metabolizers due to propafenone inhibiting the metabolism (CYP2D6) of mexiletine.
Propafenone	Theophylline	⬆	Propafenone may increase theophylline concentrations, possibly resulting in toxicity.

[a] ⬆ = object drug increased; ⬇ = object drug decreased.

➤*Drug/Food interactions:* Although food increased the peak blood level and bioavailability of propafenone in a single dose study, food did not change bioavailability significantly during multiple dose administration.

Adverse Reactions

Propafenone Adverse Reactions (%)[a]

Adverse reaction	Incidence by total daily dose: 450 mg (n = 1430)	600 mg (n = 1337)	≥ 900 mg (n = 1333)	Total incidence (n = 2127)	% of patients who discontinued	Incidence vs placebo: Propafenone (n = 247)	Placebo (n = 111)
Cardiovascular							
Angina	1.7	2.1	3.2	4.6	0.5	1.2	—
Atrial fibrillation	0.7	0.7	0.5	1.2	0.4	—	—
AV block, first-degree	0.8	1.2	2.1	2.5	0.3	4.5	0.9

PROPAFENONE HYDROCHLORIDE — ORAL

Propafenone Adverse Reactions (%)[a]							
	Incidence by total daily dose					Incidence vs placebo	
Adverse reaction	450 mg (n = 1430)	600 mg (n = 1337)	≥ 900 mg (n = 1333)	Total incidence (n = 2127)	% of patients who discontinued	Propafenone (n = 247)	Placebo (n = 111)
AV block, second-degree	—	—	—	—	—	1.2	—
Bradycardia	0.5	0.8	1.1	1.5	0.5	—	—
Bundle branch block	0.3	0.7	1	1.2	0.5	1.2	—
Chest pain	0.5	0.7	1.4	1.8	0.2	—	—
CHF	0.8	2.2	2.6	3.7	1.4	—	—
Hypotension	0.1	0.5	1	1.1	0.4	—	—
Intraventricular conduction delay	0.2	0.7	0.9	1.1	0.1	4	—
Palpitations	0.6	1.6	2.6	3.4	0.5	2.4	0.9
Proarrhythmia	2	2.1	2.9	4.7	4.7	1.2	—
PVCs	0.6	0.6	1.1	1.5	0.1	—	—
QRS duration, increased	0.5	0.9	1.7	1.9	0.5	—	—
Syncope	0.8	1.3	1.4	2.2	0.7	—	—
Ventricular tachycardia	1.4	1.6	2.9	3.4	1.2	—	—
CNS							
Anorexia	0.5	0.7	1.6	1.7	0.4	1.6	0.9
Anxiety	0.7	0.5	0.9	1.5	0.6	2	1.8
Ataxia	0.3	0.6	1.5	1.6	0.2	—	—
Dizziness	3.6	6.6	11	12.5	2.4	6.5	5.4
Drowsiness	0.6	0.5	0.7	1.2	0.2	—	—
Fatigue	1.8	2.8	4.1	6	1	—	—
Headache	1.5	2.5	2.8	4.5	1	4.5	4.5
Insomnia	0.3	1.3	0.7	1.5	0.3	—	—
Loss of balance	—	—	—	—	—	1.2	—
Tremor	0.3	0.8	1.1	1.4	0.3	—	—
GI							
Abdominal pain/cramps	0.8	0.9	1.1	1.7	0.4	—	—
Constipation	2	4.1	5.3	7.2	0.5	4	—
Diarrhea	0.5	1.6	1.7	2.5	0.6	1.2	0.9
Dry mouth	0.9	1	1.4	2.4	0.2	2	0.9
Dyspepsia	1.3	1.7	2.5	3.4	0.9	—	—
Flatulence	0.3	0.7	0.9	1.2	0.1	1.2	—
Nausea/vomiting	2.4	6.1	8.9	10.7	3.4	2.8	0.9
Unusual taste	2.5	4.9	6.3	8.8	0.7	7.3	0.9
Other							
Blurred vision	0.6	2.4	3.1	3.8	0.8	2	0.9
Diaphoresis	0.6	0.4	1.1	1.4	0.3	—	—
Dyspnea	2.2	2.3	3.6	5.3	1.6	2	2.7
Edema	0.6	0.4	1	1.4	0.2	—	—
Pain, joints	0.2	0.4	0.9	1	0.1	—	—
Rash	0.6	1.4	1.9	2.6	0.8	—	—
Weakness	0.6	1.6	1.7	2.4	0.7	—	—

[a] Data are pooled from separate studies and are not necessarily comparable.

Adverse reactions occur most frequently in the GI, cardiovascular, and CNS. About 20% of patients discontinued treatment due to adverse reactions. The most common events were dizziness, unusual taste, first-degree AV block, intraventricular conduction delay, nausea or vomiting and constipation. Headache was common, but not increased compared to placebo.

The most common adverse reactions appeared to be dose-related, especially dizziness, nausea or vomiting, unusual taste, constipation and blurred vision. Some less common reactions may also have been dose-related, such as first degree AV block, CHF, dyspepsia and weakness.

In addition to the reactions listed in the table, the following adverse reactions were reported (< 1%) either in clinical trials or in marketing experience (causal relationship not determined).

➤*Cardiovascular:* Atrial flutter; AV dissociation; cardiac arrest; flushing; hot flashes; sick sinus syndrome; sinus pause or arrest; supraventricular tachycardia; prolongation of the PR and QRS intervals.

➤*CNS:* Abnormal dreams, speech or vision; apnea; coma; confusion; depression; memory loss; numbness; paresthesias; psychosis/mania; seizures (0.3%); tinnitus; unusual smell sensation; vertigo.

➤*GI:* Cholestasis (0.1%); elevated liver enzymes (alkaline phosphatase, serum transaminases) (0.2%); gastroenteritis, hepatitis (0.03%). A number of patients with liver abnormalities associated with propafenone therapy have been reported in postmarketing experience. Some appeared due to hepatocellular injury, some were cholestatic and some showed a mixed picture.

➤*Hematologic:* Agranulocytosis; anemia; bruising; granulocytopenia; increased bleeding time; leukopenia; purpura; thrombocytopenia.

➤*Miscellaneous:* Alopecia; eye irritation; hyponatremia/inappropriate ADH secretion; impotence; increased glucose; kidney failure; positive ANA (0.7%); lupus erythematosus; muscle cramps; muscle weakness; nephrotic syndrome; pain; pruritus.

Overdosage

➤*Symptoms:* The following symptoms are usually most severe within 3 hours of ingestion may include hypotension, somnolence, bradycardia, intra-atrial and intraventricular conduction disturbances, and rarely convulsions and high grade ventricular arrhythmias.

➤*Treatment:* Defibrillation as well as infusion of dopamine and isoproterenol have been effective in controlling rhythm and blood pressure. Convulsions have been alleviated with IV diazepam. General supportive measures such as ventilatory assistance and cardiopulmonary resuscitation may be necessary. Refer to General Management of Acute Overdosage. Hemodialysis does not appear to alter drug clearance.

Patient Information

Palpitations, chest pain, blurred or abnormal vision, or difficult breathing may occur. Notify the physician if these become bothersome.

Notify the physician if signs of infection develop such as fever, sore throat, chills or unusual bruising or bleeding.

Be aware of signs of overdosage or toxicity such as hypotension, excessive drowsiness, decreased heart rate or abnormal heartbeat.

AMIODARONE HYDROCHLORIDE

Rx	**Pacerone** (Upsher Smith)	**Tablets; oral:** 100 mg	Lactose. (P U-S 144). In 30s and UD 100s.
Rx	**Amiodarone Hydrochloride** (Various, eg, Eon Labs, Teva, Taro)	**Tablets; oral:** 200 mg	May contain lactose. In 60s, 100s, 250s, 500s, and UD 100s.
Rx	**Cordarone** (Wyeth-Ayerst)		Lactose. (C 200 WYETH 4188). Pink, scored, convex. In 60s.
Rx	**Pacerone** (Upsher Smith)		Lactose. (P_{200} U-S 0147). Pink, scored. In 60s, 90s, 500s, and UD 100s.
Rx	**Amiodarone Hydrochloride** (Taro)	**Tablets; oral:** 400 mg	May contain lactose. In 30s and UD 100s.
Rx	**Pacerone** (Upsher Smith)		Lactose. (P_{400} 01 45). Lt. yellow, oval, scored. In 30s, 100s, 500s, and UD 100s.
Rx	**Amiodarone Hydrochloride** (Various, eg, American Pharm Partners, Faulding)	**Injection, solution:** 50 mg/mL	May contain benzyl alcohol. In 3 and 9 mL single-dose vials, and 18 mL multiple-dose vials.
Rx	**Nexterone** (Prism Pharmaceuticals)		In 3, 10, and 30 mL single-dose vials, and 3 mL prefilled syringes.
Rx	**Nexterone** (Prism Pharmaceuticals)	**Injection, solution:** 1.5 mg/mL **Injection, solution:** 1.8 mg/mL	Premixed in dextrose. In 100 and 200 mL single-dose *Galaxy* containers.

AMIODARONE HYDROCHLORIDE — ORAL

Refer to the general introductory discussion concerning Antiarrhythmic Agents.

WARNING

Life-threatening arrhythmias – Amiodarone is intended for use only in patients with the indicated life-threatening arrhythmias because its use is accompanied by substantial toxicity.

Potentially fatal toxicities – Amiodarone has several potentially fatal toxicities, the most important of which is pulmonary toxicity (hypersensitivity pneumonitis or interstitial/alveolar pneumonitis) that has resulted in clinically manifest disease at rates as high as 10% to 17% in some series of patients with ventricular arrhythmias given doses of approximately 400 mg/day, and as abnormal diffusion capacity without symptoms in a much higher percentage of patients. Pulmonary toxicity has been fatal approximately 10% of the time. Liver injury is common with amiodarone, but is usually mild and evidenced only by abnormal liver enzymes. Overt liver disease can occur, however, and has been fatal in a few cases. Like other antiarrhythmics, amiodarone can exacerbate the arrhythmia (eg, by making the arrhythmia less well tolerated or more difficult to reverse). This has occurred in 2% to 5% of patients in various series, and significant heart block or sinus bradycardia has been seen in 2% to 5%. In most cases, all of these events should be manageable in the proper clinical setting. Although the frequency of such proarrhythmic events does not appear greater with amiodarone than with many other agents used in this population, the effects are prolonged when they occur.

High-risk patients – Even in patients at high risk of arrhythmic death in whom the toxicity of amiodarone is an acceptable risk, amiodarone poses major management problems that could be life-threatening in a population at risk of sudden death; therefore, make every effort to utilize alternative agents first.

The difficulty of using amiodarone effectively and safely poses a significant risk to patients. Patients with the indicated arrhythmias must be hospitalized while the loading dose of amiodarone is given, and a response generally requires at least 1 week, usually 2 weeks or more. Because absorption and elimination are variable, maintenance dose selection is difficult, and it is not unusual to require dosage decrease or discontinuation of treatment. In a retrospective survey of 192 patients with ventricular tachyarrhythmias, 84 patients required dose reduction and 18 required at least temporary discontinuation because of adverse reactions, and several series have reported 15% to 20% overall frequencies of discontinuation because of adverse reactions. The time at which a previously controlled life-threatening arrhythmia will recur after discontinuation or dose adjustment is unpredictable, ranging from weeks to months. The patient is obviously at great risk during this time and may need prolonged hospitalization. Attempts to substitute other antiarrhythmic agents when amiodarone must be stopped will be made difficult by the gradually, but unpredictably, changing amiodarone body burden. A similar problem exists when amiodarone is not effective; it still poses the risk of an interaction with whatever subsequent treatment is tried.

Indications

➤*Ventricular arrhythmias:* Because of its life-threatening adverse reactions and the substantial management difficulties associated with its use, amiodarone is indicated only for the treatment of the following documented, life-threatening recurrent ventricular arrhythmias when these have not responded to documented adequate doses of other available antiarrhythmics or when alternative agents could not be tolerated:

1.) recurrent ventricular fibrillation
2.) recurrent hemodynamically unstable ventricular tachycardia.

➤*Off-label uses:*

Atrioventricular nodal reentry tachycardia – [4] = Insufficient documentation. Amiodarone is a second-line therapeutic option for the treatment of atrioventricular (AV) nodal reentry tachycardia only in select adults based on expert opinion. Because of serious safety risks and weak efficacy data, amiodarone should be used only when other treatment options are inappropriate.

Conversion of atrial fibrillation to sinus rhythm – [2] = Fair documentation. Amiodarone is highly lipophilic and has a long half-life, which results in delayed onset of therapeutic effect. Serious safety issues limit its use. Amiodarone can serve as an alternative to other agents for patients without underlying cardiac disease, and it may be an appropriate first-line agent in patients with structural heart disease or congestive heart failure for whom other drug choices would be contraindicated. Consensus guidelines support the use of intravenous (IV) amiodarone for cardioversion of atrial fibrillation in adults.

Supraventricular tachycardia – Amiodarone is an effective therapeutic option with a variety of potential uses in the management of supraventricular tachycardia; however, safety risks limit its therapeutic use. In many cases, amiodarone is reserved for use in patients who have failed other therapies or who have structural heart disease, including left ventricular dysfunction.

Supraventricular tachycardia (adults): [3] = Safety concerns.

Supraventricular tachycardia (infants/children/adolescents): [2] = Fair documentation.

Other possible off-label uses – Postoperative conversion of atrial fibrillation and prevention of recurrence of symptomatic paroxysmal and persistent atrial fibrillation after cardioversion.

Administration and Dosage

➤*General dosing considerations:* Upon starting amiodarone therapy, attempt to gradually discontinue prior antiarrhythmic drugs (see Dosage Titration).

Because of the unique pharmacokinetic properties, difficult dosing schedule, and severity of adverse reactions if patients are improperly monitored, amiodarone should be administered only by health care providers who are experienced in the treatment of life-threatening arrhythmias, thoroughly familiar with the risks and benefits of amiodarone therapy, and who have access to laboratory facilities capable of adequately monitoring the efficacy and adverse reactions of treatment.

In order to ensure that an antiarrhythmic effect will be observed without waiting several months, loading doses are required. A uniform, optimal dosage schedule for administration of amiodarone has not been determined.

➤*Adults:*

Life-threatening ventricular arrhythmias (eg, ventricular fibrillation or hemodynamically unstable ventricular tachycardia) –

Loading dose: 800 to 1,600 mg/day are required for 1 to 3 weeks (occasionally longer) until initial therapeutic response occurs.

Close monitoring of the patient is indicated during the loading phase, particularly until the risk of recurrent ventricular tachycardia or fibrillation has abated. Because of the serious nature of the arrhythmia and the lack of predictable time course of effect, loading should be performed in a hospital setting. Elimination of recurrence of ventricular fibrillation and tachycardia usually occurs within 1 to 3 weeks, along with reduction in complex and total ventricular ectopic beats.

Dosage titration: Individual patient titration is suggested according to the following guidelines. Upon starting amiodarone therapy, attempt to gradually discontinue prior antiarrhythmic drugs. When adequate arrhythmia control is achieved or if adverse reactions become prominent, reduce the amiodarone dose to 600 to 800 mg/day for 1 month and then reduce to the maintenance dose.

Maintenance dosage: The maintenance dose is usually 400 mg/day or in patients with severe GI intolerance, 200 mg twice daily. Some patients may require larger maintenance doses of up to 600 mg/day and some can be controlled on lower doses.

Use the lowest effective dose to prevent the occurrence of adverse reactions. In all instances, the health care provider must be guided by the severity of the individual patient's arrhythmia and response to therapy.

In each patient, determine the chronic maintenance dose according to antiarrhythmic effect as assessed by symptoms, Holter recordings and/or programmed electrical stimulation (PES), and by patient tolerance.

Dosage adjustment: If adverse reactions become excessive, reduce the dose. When dosage adjustments are necessary, closely monitor the patient for an extended period of time because of the long and variable half-life of amiodarone and the difficulty in predicting the time required to attain a new steady-state level of drug.

Off-label dosing –

Atrioventricular nodal reentry tachycardia: [4] = Insufficient documentation. According to national guidelines for atrial fibrillation, the recommended IV dose of amiodarone is 150 mg over 10 minutes, followed by a maintenance dose of 0.5 to 1 mg/min. For long-term oral management in adults, the following schedule is recommended: 800 mg daily for 1 week, followed by 600 mg daily for 1 week, followed by 400 mg daily for 4 to 6 weeks, followed by maintenance therapy with 200 mg/day.

The largest reported experience with amiodarone used 5 mg/kg IV for acute termination of AV nodal reentry tachycardia, followed by daily oral maintenance therapy with 200 to 400 mg. Another small study reported starting dosages of 600 to 1,200 mg/day for the first 5 to 7 days, followed by maintenance dosing with an average of 245 mg/day.

In a case report, oral maintenance was initiated at 1,200 mg/day for 1 week, followed by 800 mg/day for 1 week, 600 mg/day for 1 week, and 400 mg/day thereafter.

Conversion of atrial fibrillation to sinus rhythm: [2] = Fair documentation.

• *Intravenous/Oral* – 5 to 7 mg/kg IV over 30 to 60 minutes, then 1.2 to 1.8 g/day as a continuous IV infusion or in divided oral doses until 10 g total, then 200 to 400 mg/day oral maintenance.

Supraventricular tachycardia (adults): [3] = Safety concerns.

• *Initial dosage* – 50 mg IV over 10 minutes, followed by 0.5 to 1 mg/min, then switched to oral maintenance dosing.

• *Maintenance dosage* – 800 mg daily orally for 1 week, followed by 600 mg daily for 1 week, followed by 400 mg daily for 4 to 6 weeks, followed by maintenance therapy with 200 mg/day.

➤*Children:*

Off-label dosing –

Supraventricular tachycardia (infants/children/adolescents): [3] = Safety concerns.

• *Initial dosage* – 5 mg/kg given IV over 1 hour, followed by 5 mg/kg/day for 47 hours.

• *Maintenance dosage* – 10 to 20 mg/kg/day for 7 to 10 days, followed by 3 to 20 mg/kg/day.

Life-threatening or drug-resistant refractory cardiac arrhythmias (eg, ventricular tachyarrhythmia, junctional ectopic tachycardia):

• *Children 1 year of age and older* –

Initial dosage: 10 to 15 mg/kg/day given once every 24 hours or in divided doses given every 12 hours. Continue treatment for 4 to 14 days and/or until adequate control is achieved.

AMIODARONE HYDROCHLORIDE — ORAL

Maintenance dosage: If initial treatment regimen is effective, decrease the dosage to 5 mg/kg/day given once every 24 hours or in divided doses given every 12 hours.

• *Children younger than 1 year of age –*

Initial dosage: 600 to 800 mg per 1.73 m^2 per day given once every 24 hours or in divided doses given every 12 hours. Continue treatment for 4 to 14 days and/or until adequate control is achieved.

Maintenance dosage: If initial treatment regimen is effective, decrease the dosage to 200 to 400 mg per 1.73 m^2 every 24 hours.

➤*Therapeutic drug monitoring:* The therapeutic plasma concentration is between 1 to 2.5 mg/L.

➤*Administration:* Administration of amiodarone in divided doses with meals is suggested for total daily doses of 1,000 mg or more or when GI intolerance occurs. Because of the food effect on absorption, administer amiodarone consistently with regard to meals.

➤*Storage/Stability:* Store at controlled room temperature, 20° to 25°C (68° to 77°F). Excursions are permitted to 15° to 30°C (59° to 86°F). Protect from light. Dispense in a light-resistant, tight container; keep tightly closed.

Actions

➤*Pharmacology:* In animals, amiodarone is effective in the prevention or suppression of experimentally induced arrhythmias. The antiarrhythmic effect of amiodarone may be due to at least 2 major properties:

1.) a prolongation of the myocardial cell-action potential duration and refractory period, and
2.) noncompetitive alpha- and beta-adrenergic inhibition.

Amiodarone prolongs the duration of the action potential of all cardiac fibers while causing minimal reduction of dV/dt (maximal upstroke velocity of the action potential). The refractory period is prolonged in all cardiac tissues. Amiodarone increases the cardiac refractory period without influencing resting membrane potential, except in automatic cells in which the slope of the prepotential is reduced, generally reducing automaticity. These electrophysiologic effects are reflected in a decreased sinus rate of 15% to 20%, increased PR and QT intervals of approximately 10%, the development of U-waves, and changes in T-wave contour. These changes should not require discontinuation of amiodarone, as they are evidence of its pharmacological action, although amiodarone can cause marked sinus bradycardia or sinus arrest and heart block. On rare occasions, QT prolongation has been associated with worsening of arrhythmia.

➤*Pharmacokinetics:*

Absorption – Following oral administration in humans, amiodarone is slowly and variably absorbed. The bioavailability of amiodarone is approximately 50%, but has varied between 35% and 65% in various studies. Maximum plasma concentrations are attained 3 to 7 hours after a single dose. Despite this, the onset of action may occur in 2 to 3 days but more commonly takes 1 to 3 weeks, even with loading doses. Plasma concentrations with chronic dosing at 100 to 600 mg/day are approximately dose proportional, with a mean 0.5 mg/L increase for each 100 mg/day. These means, however, include considerable individual variability.

Although electrophysiologic effects, such as prolongation of QTc, can be seen within hours after a parenteral dose of amiodarone, effects on abnormal rhythms are not seen before 2 to 3 days and usually require 1 to 3 weeks, even when a loading dose is used. There may be a continued increase in effect for longer periods still. There is evidence that the time to effect is shorter when a loading-dose regimen is used.

Food effects: See Drug Interactions for more information.

Distribution – Amiodarone has a very large but variable volume of distribution, averaging approximately 60 L/kg, because of extensive accumulation in various sites, especially adipose tissue and highly perfused organs, such as the liver, lung, and spleen. One major metabolite of amiodarone, desethylamiodarone, has been identified in humans; it accumulates to an even greater extent in almost all tissues.

Amiodarone and its metabolite have a limited transplacental transfer of approximately 10% to 50%. The parent drug and its metabolite have been detected in breast milk.

Amiodarone is highly protein bound (approximately 96%).

Metabolism – Desethylamiodarone is the major metabolite of amiodarone. No data are available on the activity of desethylamiodarone in humans, but in animals it has significant electrophysiologic and antiarrhythmic effects generally similar to amiodarone. Desethylamiodarone's precise role and contribution to the antiarrhythmic activity of oral amiodarone are not certain. The development of maximal ventricular class III effects after oral amiodarone administration in humans correlates more closely with desethylamiodarone accumulation over time than with amiodarone accumulation.

Amiodarone is metabolized to desethylamiodarone by the CYP-450 enzyme group, specifically CYP-450 3A4 (CYP-3A4) and CYP-2C8. The CYP-3A4 isoenzyme is present in both the liver and intestines.

Each amiodarone 200 mg tablet contains iodide 75 mg, which releases approximately 6 mg of iodide during the metabolism of the drug.

Excretion – Amiodarone is eliminated primarily by hepatic metabolism and biliary excretion and there is negligible excretion of amiodarone or desethylamiodarone in urine. Neither amiodarone nor desethylamiodarone is dialyzable. In clinical studies of 2 to 7 days, clearance of amiodarone after intravenous (IV) administration in patients with ventricular tachycardia and ventricular fibrillation ranged between 220 and 440 mL/h/kg.

Following single-dose administration in 12 healthy subjects, amiodarone exhibited multicompartmental pharmacokinetics, with a mean apparent plasma terminal elimination half-life of 58 days (range, 15 to 142 days) for amiodarone and 36 days (range, 14 to 75 days) for the active metabolite (desethylamiodarone). Following discontinuation of chronic oral therapy in patients, amiodarone has been shown to have a biphasic elimination with an initial one-half reduction of plasma levels after 2.5 to 10 days. A much slower terminal plasma-elimination phase shows a half-life of the parent compound ranging from 26 to 107 days, with a mean of approximately 53 days and most patients in the 40- to 55-day range. In the absence of a loading-dose period, steady-state plasma concentrations at constant oral dosing would therefore be reached between 130 and 535 days, with an average of 265 days. For the metabolite, the mean plasma elimination half-life was approximately 61 days. These data probably reflect an initial elimination of drug from well-perfused tissue (the 2.5- to 10-day half-life phase), followed by a terminal phase representing extremely slow elimination from poorly perfused tissue compartments such as fat.

The considerable intersubject variation in both phases of elimination, as well as uncertainty as to what compartment is critical to drug effect, requires attention to individual responses once arrhythmia control is achieved with loading doses because the correct maintenance dose is determined, in part, by the elimination rates. Base daily maintenance doses of amiodarone on individual patient requirements.

Consistent with the slow rate of elimination, antiarrhythmic effects persist for weeks or months after amiodarone is discontinued, but the time of recurrence is variable and unpredictable. In general, when the drug is resumed after recurrence of the arrhythmia, control is established relatively rapidly compared with the initial response, presumably because tissue stores were not wholly depleted at the time of recurrence.

Special populations –

Elderly: Healthy subjects older than 65 years of age show lower clearances (approximately 100 mL/h/kg) than younger subjects (approximately 150 mL/h/kg) and an increase in half-life ($t_{1/2}$) (from approximately 20 to 47 days).

• *Left ventricular dysfunction* – In patients with severe left ventricular dysfunction, the pharmacokinetics of amiodarone are not significantly altered but the terminal disposition $t_{1/2}$ of desethylamiodarone is prolonged.

Contraindications

Cardiogenic shock; severe sinus node dysfunction, causing marked sinus bradycardia; second- or third-degree AV block; when episodes of bradycardia have caused syncope (except when used in conjunction with a pacemaker); hypersensitivity to the drug or to any of its components, including iodine.

Warnings/Precautions

➤*Life-threatening arrhythmias:* See the Warning box for more information.

➤*Potentially fatal toxicities:* See the Warning box for more information.

➤*High-risk patients:* See the Warning box for more information.

➤*Mortality:* In the National Heart, Lung, and Blood Institute's Cardiac Arrhythmia Suppression Trial (CAST), a long-term, multicentered, randomized, double-blind study in patients with asymptomatic non–life-threatening ventricular arrhythmias who had myocardial infarctions more than 6 days but less than 2 years previously, an excessive mortality or nonfatal cardiac arrest rate was seen in patients treated with encainide or flecainide (56/730) compared with that seen in patients assigned to matched placebo-treated groups (22/725). The average duration of treatment with encainide or flecainide in this study was 10 months.

Amiodarone therapy was evaluated in 2 multicentered, randomized, double-blind, placebo-controlled trials involving 1,202 (Canadian Amiodarone Myocardial Infarction Arrhythmia Trial [CAMIAT]) and 1,486 (European Myocardial Infarction Amiodarone Trial [EMIAT]) post–myocardial infarction patients followed for up to 2 years. Patients in CAMIAT qualified with ventricular arrhythmias, and those randomized to amiodarone received weight- and response-adjusted doses of 200 to 400 mg/day. Patients in EMIAT qualified with ejection fraction of less than 40%, and those randomized to amiodarone received fixed doses of 200 mg/day. Both studies had weeks-long loading dose schedules. Intent-to-treat all-cause mortality results were as follows.

Intent-to-Treat All-Cause Mortality Results of Amiodarone Trials

	Placebo		Amiodarone		Relative risk	
	n	Deaths	n	Deaths		95% CI[a]
EMIAT	743	102	743	103	0.99	0.76 to 1.31
CAMIAT	596	68	606	57	0.88	0.58 to 1.16

[a] CI = confidence interval.

These data are consistent with the results of a pooled analysis of smaller, controlled studies involving patients with structural heart disease (including myocardial infarction).

➤*Pulmonary effects:*

Pulmonary toxicity – There have been postmarketing reports of acute-onset (days to weeks) pulmonary injury in patients treated with oral amiodarone with or without initial IV therapy. Findings have included pulmonary infiltrates and/or masses on bronchospasm, cough, dyspnea, fever, hemoptysis, hypoxia, wheezing, and x-ray. Some cases have progressed to respiratory failure and/or death.

Amiodarone may cause a clinical syndrome of cough and progressive dyspnea accompanied by functional, radiographic, gallium-scan, and pathological data consistent with pulmonary toxicity, the frequency of which varies from 2% to 7% in most published reports but is as high as 10% to 17% in some reports. Therefore, when amiodarone therapy is initiated, perform a

AMIODARONE HYDROCHLORIDE — ORAL

baseline chest x-ray and pulmonary-function tests, including diffusion capacity. The patient should return for a history, physical exam, and chest x-ray every 3 to 6 months.

In a patient receiving amiodarone, any new respiratory symptoms should suggest the possibility of pulmonary toxicity, and the history, physical exam, chest x-ray, and pulmonary function tests (with diffusion capacity) should be repeated and evaluated. A 15% decrease in diffusion capacity has a high sensitivity but only a moderate specificity for pulmonary toxicity; as the decrease in diffusion capacity approaches 30%, the sensitivity decreases but the specificity increases. A gallium scan also may be performed as part of the diagnostic workup.

Fatalities, secondary to pulmonary toxicity, have occurred in approximately 10% of cases. However, in patients with life-threatening arrhythmias, undertake discontinuation of amiodarone therapy because of suspected drug-induced pulmonary toxicity with caution, as the most common cause of death in these patients is sudden cardiac death. Therefore, make every effort to rule out other causes of respiratory impairment (ie, congestive heart failure [CHF] with Swan-Ganz catheterization if necessary, respiratory infection, pulmonary embolism, malignancy) before discontinuing amiodarone in these patients. In addition, bronchoalveolar lavage, transbronchial lung biopsy, and/or open lung biopsy may be necessary to confirm the diagnosis, especially in those cases in which no acceptable alternative therapy is available.

Pulmonary toxicity secondary to amiodarone seems to result from either indirect or direct toxicity as represented by hypersensitivity pneumonitis or interstitial/alveolar pneumonitis, respectively.

Patients with preexisting pulmonary disease have a poorer prognosis if pulmonary toxicity develops.

Hypersensitivity pneumonitis – Hypersensitivity pneumonitis usually appears earlier in the course of therapy, and rechallenging these patients with amiodarone results in a more rapid recurrence of greater severity.

Bronchoalveolar lavage is the procedure of choice to confirm this diagnosis, which can be made when a T suppressor/cytotoxic (CD8-positive) lymphocytosis is noted. Institute steroid therapy and discontinue amiodarone therapy in these patients.

If a diagnosis of amiodarone-induced hypersensitivity pneumonitis is made, discontinue amiodarone and institute treatment with steroids.

Interstitial / Alveolar pneumonitis – Interstitial/alveolar pneumonitis may result from the release of oxygen radicals and/or phospholipidosis and is characterized by findings of diffuse alveolar damage, interstitial pneumonitis, or fibrosis in lung biopsy specimens.

Phospholipidosis (foamy cells and foamy macrophages) due to inhibition of phospholipase will be present in most cases of amiodarone-induced pulmonary toxicity; however, these changes also are present in approximately 50% of all patients on amiodarone therapy. Use these cells as markers of therapy but not as evidence of toxicity. A diagnosis of amiodarone-induced interstitial/alveolar pneumonitis should lead, at a minimum, to dose reduction, or, preferably, to withdrawal of the amiodarone to establish reversibility, especially if other acceptable antiarrhythmic therapies are available. Where these measures have been instituted, a reduction in symptoms of amiodarone-induced pulmonary toxicity was usually noted within the first week, and a clinical improvement was greatest in the first 2 to 3 weeks. Chest x-ray changes usually resolve within 2 to 4 months. According to some experts, steroids may prove beneficial. Prednisone in doses of 40 to 60 mg/day or equivalent doses of other steroids have been given and tapered over the course of several weeks depending upon the condition of the patient. In some cases, rechallenge with amiodarone at a lower dose has not resulted in return of toxicity. Recent reports suggest that the use of lower loading and maintenance doses of amiodarone are associated with a decreased incidence of amiodarone-induced pulmonary toxicity.

If a diagnosis of amiodarone-induced interstitial/alveolar pneumonitis is made, institute steroid therapy, and, preferably, discontinue amiodarone or, at a minimum, reduce dosage. Some cases of amiodarone-induced interstitial/alveolar pneumonitis may resolve following a reduction in amiodarone dosage in conjunction with the administration of steroids. In some patients, rechallenge at a lower dose has not resulted in return of interstitial/alveolar pneumonitis; however, in some patients (perhaps because of severe alveolar damage), the pulmonary lesions have not been reversible.

➤*Cardiac effects:*

Proarrhythmia – Amiodarone, like other antiarrhythmics, can cause serious exacerbation of the presenting arrhythmia, a risk that may be enhanced by the presence of concomitant antiarrhythmics. Exacerbation has been reported in approximately 2% to 5% in most series and has included new ventricular fibrillation, incessant ventricular tachycardia, increased resistance to cardioversion, and polymorphic ventricular tachycardia associated with QTc prolongation (torsades de pointes). In addition, amiodarone has caused symptomatic bradycardia or sinus arrest with suppression of escape foci in 2% to 4% of patients.

See Drug Interactions for more information.

The need to coadminister amiodarone with any other drug known to prolong the QTc interval must be based on a careful assessment of the potential risks and benefits of doing so for each patient.

➤*Hepatic effects:* Elevations of hepatic enzyme levels are seen frequently in patients exposed to amiodarone and in most cases are asymptomatic. If the increase exceeds 3 times normal or doubles in a patient with an elevated baseline, consider discontinuation of amiodarone or dosage reduction. In a few cases in which biopsy has been done, the histology has resembled that of alcoholic hepatitis or cirrhosis. Hepatic failure has been a rare cause of death in patients treated with amiodarone.

➤*Ophthalmologic effects:* Cases of optic neuropathy and/or optic neuritis, usually resulting in visual impairment, have been reported in patients treated with amiodarone. In some cases, visual impairment has progressed to permanent blindness. Optic neuropathy and/or neuritis may occur at any time following initiation of therapy. A causal relationship to the drug has not been clearly established. If symptoms of visual impairment appear, such as changes in visual acuity and decreases in peripheral vision, prompt ophthalmic examination is recommended. Appearance of optic neuropathy and/or neuritis calls for reevaluation of amiodarone therapy. The risks and complications of antiarrhythmic therapy with amiodarone must be weighed against its benefits in patients whose lives are threatened by cardiac arrhythmias. Regular ophthalmic examination, including fundoscopy and slit-lamp examination, is recommended during administration of amiodarone.

Corneal microdeposits appear in the majority of adults treated with amiodarone. They are usually discernible only by slit-lamp examination, but give rise to symptoms such as visual halos or blurred vision in as many as 10% of patients. Corneal microdeposits are reversible upon reduction of dose or termination of treatment. Asymptomatic microdeposits alone are not a reason to reduce dose or discontinue treatment.

➤*CNS effects:* Chronic administration of oral amiodarone in rare instances may lead to the development of peripheral neuropathy that may resolve when amiodarone is discontinued, but this resolution has been slow and incomplete.

➤*Thyroid abnormalities:* Amiodarone inhibits peripheral conversion of thyroxine (T_4) to triiodothyronine (T_3) and may cause increased thyroxine levels, decreased T_3 levels, and increased levels of inactive reverse T_3 (rT_3) in clinically euthyroid patients. It is also a potential source of large amounts of inorganic iodine. Amiodarone contains iodine 37.3% by weight; each 200 mg tablet contains iodide 75 mg, which releases approximately 6 mg of iodide during the metabolism of the drug. Because of its release of inorganic iodine, or perhaps for other reasons, amiodarone can cause either hypothyroidism or hyperthyroidism. Monitor thyroid function prior to treatment and periodically thereafter, particularly in elderly patients, and in any patient with a history of thyroid nodules, goiter, or other thyroid dysfunction. Because of the slow elimination of amiodarone and its metabolites, high plasma iodide levels, altered thyroid function, and abnormal thyroid function tests may persist for several weeks or even months following amiodarone tablets withdrawal.

A careful assessment of the potential risks and benefits of administering amiodarone must be made in patients with thyroid dysfunction because of the possibility of arrhythmia breakthrough or exacerbation of arrhythmia in these patients.

Hypothyroidism – Hypothyroidism has been reported in 2% to 4% of patients in most series, but in 8% to 10% in some series. This condition may be identified by relevant clinical symptoms and particularly by elevated serum thyroid-stimulating hormone (TSH) levels. In some clinically hypothyroid amiodarone-treated patients, free thyroxine index values may be normal. Hypothyroidism is best managed by amiodarone dose reduction and/or thyroid hormone supplement. However, therapy must be individualized, and it may be necessary to discontinue amiodarone in some patients.

Hyperthyroidism – Hyperthyroidism occurs in approximately 2% of patients receiving amiodarone, but the incidence may be higher among patients with prior inadequate dietary iodine intake. Amiodarone-induced hyperthyroidism usually poses a greater hazard to the patient than hypothyroidism because of the possibility of thyrotoxicosis and/or arrhythmia breakthrough or aggravation, all of which may result in death. There have been reports of death associated with amiodarone-induced thyrotoxicosis. If any new signs of arrhythmia appear, consider the possibility of hyperthyroidism.

Hyperthyroidism is best identified by relevant clinical symptoms and signs, accompanied usually by abnormally elevated levels of serum T_3 radioimmunoassay, and further elevations of serum T_4, and a subnormal serum TSH level (using a sufficiently sensitive TSH assay). The finding of a flat TSH response to a thyroid-releasing hormone is confirmatory of hyperthyroidism and may be sought in equivocal cases. Since arrhythmia breakthroughs may accompany amiodarone-induced hyperthyroidism, aggressive medical treatment is indicated, including, if possible, dose reduction or withdrawal of amiodarone.

The institution of antithyroid drugs, beta-adrenergic blockers, and/or temporary corticosteroid therapy may be necessary. The action of antithyroid drugs may be especially delayed in amiodarone-induced thyrotoxicosis because of substantial quantities of preformed thyroid hormones stored in the gland. Radioactive iodine therapy is contraindicated because of the low radioiodine uptake associated with amiodarone-induced hyperthyroidism. Amiodarone-induced hyperthyroidism may be followed by a transient period of hypothyroidism.

When aggressive treatment of amiodarone-induced thyrotoxicosis has failed or amiodarone cannot be discontinued because it is the only drug effective against the resistant arrhythmia, surgical management may be an option. Experience with thyroidectomy as a treatment for amiodarone-induced thyrotoxicosis is limited and this form of therapy could induce thyroid storm. Therefore, surgical and anesthetic management require careful planning.

There have been postmarketing reports of thyroid nodules/thyroid cancer in patients treated with amiodarone. In some instances, hyperthyroidism was also present.

Thyrotoxicosis – Amiodarone-induced hyperthyroidism may result in thyrotoxicosis and/or the possibility of arrhythmia breakthrough or aggra-

AMIODARONE HYDROCHLORIDE — ORAL

vation. There have been reports of death associated with amiodarone-induced thyrotoxicosis. If any new signs of arrhythmia appear, consider the possibility of hyperthyroidism.

➤*Surgery:*

Adult respiratory distress syndrome – Postoperatively, occurrences of adult respiratory distress syndrome have been reported in patients receiving amiodarone therapy who have undergone either cardiac or noncardiac surgery. Although patients usually respond well to vigorous respiratory therapy, in rare instances the outcome has been fatal. Until further studies have been performed, it is recommended that fraction of inspired oxygen (FiO_2) and the determinants of oxygen delivery to the tissues (eg, arterial oxygen saturation [SaO_2], alveolar oxygen partial pressure [PaO_2]) be closely monitored in patients on amiodarone.

Corneal refractive laser surgery – Advise patients that most manufacturers of corneal refractive laser surgery devices contraindicate that procedure in patients taking amiodarone.

Hypotension post-bypass – Rare occurrences of hypotension upon discontinuation of cardiopulmonary bypass during open-heart surgery in patients receiving amiodarone have been reported. The relationship of this event to amiodarone therapy is unknown.

Volatile anesthetic agents – Close perioperative monitoring is recommended in patients undergoing general anesthetic who are on amiodarone therapy, as they may be more sensitive to the myocardial depressant and conduction effects of halogenated inhalational anesthetics.

➤*Electrolyte disturbances:* Because antiarrhythmic drugs may be ineffective or may be arrhythmogenic in patients with hypokalemia, correct any potassium or magnesium deficiency before instituting amiodarone therapy. Use caution when coadministering amiodarone with drugs that may induce hypokalemia and/or hypomagnesemia.

➤*Photosensitivity:* Amiodarone has induced photosensitization in approximately 10% of patients; some protection may be afforded by the use of sun-barrier creams or protective clothing. During long-term treatment, a blue-gray discoloration of the exposed skin may occur. The risk may be increased in patients of fair complexion or those with excessive sun exposure, and may be related to cumulative dose and duration of therapy.

➤*Pregnancy: Category D.* Amiodarone can cause fetal harm when administered to a pregnant woman. Although amiodarone use during pregnancy is uncommon, there have been a small number of published reports of congenital goiter/hypothyroidism and hyperthyroidism. If amiodarone is administered during pregnancy, or if the patient becomes pregnant while taking amiodarone, apprise the patient of the potential hazard to the fetus.

In general, use amiodarone during pregnancy only if the potential benefit to the mother justifies the unknown risk to the fetus.

➤*Lactation:* Amiodarone and one of its major metabolites, desethylamiodarone, are excreted in human milk, suggesting that breast-feeding could expose the breast-feeding infant to a significant dose of the drug. Breast-feeding offspring of lactating rats administered amiodarone have been shown to be less viable and have reduced body-weight gains. Therefore, when amiodarone therapy is indicated, advise the mother to discontinue breast-feeding.

➤*Children:* The safety and efficacy of amiodarone in children have not been established.

➤*Elderly:* In general, dose selection for an elderly patient should be cautious, usually starting at the low end of the dosing range, reflecting the greater frequency of decreased hepatic, renal, or cardiac function, and of concomitant disease or other drug therapy.

Per the Beers list, amiodarone is associated with QT interval problems, risk of provoking torsades de pointes, and lack of efficacy in older adults.

➤*Lab test abnormalities:* Elevations in liver enzymes (AST and ALT) can occur. Monitor liver enzymes in patients on relatively high maintenance doses on a regular basis. Consider reducing the maintenance dose of amiodarone or discontinuing therapy in the case of persistent significant elevations in the liver enzymes or hepatomegaly. Amiodarone alters the results of thyroid function tests, causing an increase in serum T_4 and serum reverse T_3, and a decline in serum T_3 levels. Despite these biochemical changes, most patients remain clinically euthyroid.

➤*Monitoring:* Perform baseline chest x-rays and pulmonary function tests, including diffusion capacity before therapy initiation. Repeat a history, physical exam, and chest x-ray every 3 to 6 months.

Monitor thyroid function at baseline and periodically during therapy, particularly in elderly patients and in any patient with a history of thyroid nodules, goiter, or other thyroid dysfunction.

Perform regular ophthalmic examinations, including a fundoscopy and slit-lamp examination, during administration of amiodarone.

Monitor liver enzymes on a regular basis.

Closely monitor FiO_2 and the determinants of oxygen delivery to the tissues (eg, SaO_2, PaO_2) in postoperative patients on amiodarone, in whom occurrences of adverse reactions have been reported.

Close perioperative monitoring is recommended in patients undergoing general anesthetic who are on amiodarone therapy, as they may be more sensitive to the myocardial depressant and conduction effects of halogenated inhalational anesthetics.

Close monitoring is indicated during the loading phase, particularly until the risk of recurrent ventricular tachycardia or ventricular fibrillation has abated.

Drug Interactions

➤*QT prolongation:* An additive effect of amiodarone with other drugs that prolong the QT interval cannot be excluded. The following drugs may prolong the QT interval and increase the risk of life-threatening cardiac arrhythmias, including torsade de pointes: Antiarrhythmic agents (eg, bretylium, disopyramide, dofetilide, procainamide, quinidine, and sotalol), arsenic trioxide, chlorpromazine, cisapride, dolasetron, droperidol, mefloquine, mesoridazine, moxifloxacin, pentamidine, pimozide, tacrolimus, thioridazine, and ziprasidone. For a more complete list of drugs that may prolong the QT interval, see the appendix, Drug-Induced Prolongation of the QT Interval and Torsade de Pointes.

Amiodarone Oral Drug Interactions

Precipitant drug	Object drug[a]		Description
Azole antifungals (eg, itraconazole)	Amiodarone	↑	The risk of life-threatening cardiac arrhythmias, including torsades de pointes, may be increased.
Cholestyramine	Amiodarone	↓	Increased enterohepatic elimination of amiodarone and reduced serum levels and half-life may occur.
Cimetidine	Amiodarone	↑	Increased serum amiodarone levels may occur.
Fentanyl	Amiodarone	↑	May cause hypotension, bradycardia, decreased cardiac output, and sinus arrest.
Fluoroquinolones (eg, sparfloxacin)	Amiodarone	↑	The risk of life-threatening cardiac arrhythmias, including torsades de pointes, may be increased.
Hydantoins (eg, phenytoin)	Amiodarone	↑	Chronic use (more than 2 weeks) of amiodarone impairs metabolism of phenytoin. Increased hydantoin concentrations with symptoms of toxicity may occur. Also, amiodarone serum levels may be decreased.
Amiodarone	Hydantoins (eg, phenytoin)	↑	
Loratadine	Amiodarone	↑	QT-interval prolongation and torsades de pointes have been reported with coadministration.
Macrolide antibiotics (eg, azithromycin, telithromycin)	Amiodarone	↑	The risk of life-threatening cardiac arrhythmias, including torsades de pointes, may be increased. Avoid coadministration of telithromycin and amiodarone.
Protease inhibitors (ie, atazanavir, indinavir, nelfinavir, ritonavir)	Amiodarone	↑	Increases in amiodarone concentrations may occur, increasing the risk of amiodarone toxicity. Ritonavir and nelfinavir are contraindicated in patients receiving amiodarone. Monitor amiodarone plasma levels and for toxicity.
Rifamycins (eg, rifampin)	Amiodarone	↓	Serum concentrations of amiodarone and its active metabolite may be decreased, reducing its pharmacologic effect.
St. John's wort	Amiodarone	↓	St. John's wort induces CYP3A4, possibly reducing amiodarone levels.
Trazodone	Amiodarone	↑	QT-interval prolongation and torsades de pointes have been reported with coadministration.
Amiodarone	Antiarrhythmics (eg, disopyramide, flecainide, procainamide, quinidine)	↑	Amiodarone may increase serum concentrations of these antiarrhythmics. Reduce dose of antiarrhythmic with coadministration.
Amiodarone	Anticoagulants (eg, warfarin)	↑	Potentiation of anticoagulant response is almost always seen in patients receiving amiodarone and can result in serious or fatal bleeding. A 30% to 50% anticoagulant dose reduction is typically required. Onset is 3 to 4 days and may persist for months after amiodarone discontinuation. Closely monitor prothrombin time and international normalized ratio.

AMIODARONE HYDROCHLORIDE — ORAL

Amiodarone Oral Drug Interactions

Precipitant drug	Object drug[a]		Description
Amiodarone	Beta-blockers (eg, propranolol)	⬆	Effects of beta-blockers eliminated by hepatic metabolism may be increased. Because amiodarone has weak beta-blocking activity, concomitant use can increase risk of AV block, hypotension, bradycardia, and sinus arrest.
Amiodarone	Calcium channel blockers (eg, diltiazem, verapamil)	⬆	Use amiodarone with caution with calcium channel blockers because of the possible potentiation of bradycardia, sinus arrest, and AV block.
Amiodarone	Cardiac glycosides (eg, digitoxin, digoxin)	⬆	Amiodarone taken concomitantly with digoxin increases the serum digoxin concentrations by 70% after 1 day. Reduce the dose of digitalis by 50% or discontinue.
Amiodarone	Cisapride	⬆	Risk of life-threatening cardiac arrhythmias, including torsades de pointes, may be increased because of possible additive prolongation of the QT interval.
Amiodarone	Clopidogrel	⬇	Coadministration may result in ineffective inhibition of platelet aggregation.
Amiodarone	Cyclosporine	⬆	Concomitant use has produced persistently elevated plasma cyclosporine levels, resulting in elevated creatinine despite reduction in dose of cyclosporine.
Amiodarone	Dextromethorphan	⬆	Chronic use (more than 2 weeks) of amiodarone administration impairs metabolism of dextromethorphan.
Amiodarone	HMG-CoA reductase inhibitors (eg, simvastatin)	⬆	Simvastatin in combination with amiodarone has been associated with reports of myopathy/rhabdomyolysis.
Amiodarone	Lidocaine	⬆	Sinus bradycardia has been reported with oral amiodarone in combination with lidocaine for local anesthesia. Seizure associated with increased lidocaine concentrations has been reported with coadministration of IV amiodarone.
Amiodarone	Methotrexate	⬆	Chronic use (more than 2 weeks) of amiodarone impairs metabolism of methotrexate. Methotrexate toxicity may be increased.
Amiodarone	Ranolazine	⬆	The risk of life-threatening cardiac arrhythmias, including torsades de pointes, may be increased.
Amiodarone	Thioridazine	⬆	The risk of life-threatening cardiac arrhythmias, including torsades de pointes, may be increased.
Amiodarone	Vardenafil	⬆	The risk of life-threatening cardiac arrhythmias, including torsades de pointes, may be increased.
Amiodarone	Ziprasidone	⬆	The risk of life-threatening cardiac arrhythmias, including torsades de pointes, may be increased.

[a] ⬆ = object drug increased; ⬇ = object drug decreased.

➤*Drug/Lab test interactions:* Amiodarone alters the results of thyroid function tests, causing an increase in serum T_4 and serum reverse T_3 levels, and a decline in serum T_3 levels. Despite these biochemical changes, most patients remain clinically euthyroid.

➤*Drug/Food interactions:* After a high-fat meal and an overnight fast, the AUC and C_{max} increased by 2.3 and 3.8 times, respectively, in the presence of food. Food also increased the rate of absorption of amiodarone, decreasing the time to T_{max} by 37%. The AUC and C_{max} metabolite desethylamiodarone increased by 55% and 32%, respectively, in the presence of food. Because of the food effect on absorption, administer amiodarone consistently with regard to meals.

Grapefruit juice inhibits metabolism of oral amiodarone in the intestinal mucosa, resulting in increased amiodarone AUC by 50% and C_{max} by 84%, and decreased desethylamiodarone to unquantifiable concentrations.

Adverse Reactions

Adverse reactions have been very common in virtually all series of patients treated with amiodarone for ventricular arrhythmias with relatively large doses of drug (400 mg/day and more), occurring in approximately three-fourths of all patients and causing discontinuation in 7% to 18%. The most serious reactions are exacerbation of arrhythmia, pulmonary toxicity, and rare serious liver injury, but other adverse reactions constitute important problems. They are often reversible with dose reduction or cessation of amiodarone treatment. Most of the adverse reactions appear to become more frequent with continued treatment beyond 6 months, although rates appear to remain relatively constant beyond 1 year. The time and dose relationships of adverse reactions are under continued study.

In surveys of almost 5,000 patients treated in open US studies and in published reports of treatment with amiodarone, the adverse reactions most frequently requiring discontinuation of drug included CHF, elevation of liver enzymes, paroxysmal ventricular tachycardia, and pulmonary infiltrates or fibrosis. Other symptoms causing discontinuations less often included bluish skin discoloration, hyperthyroidism, hypothyroidism, solar dermatitis, and visual disturbances.

➤*Cardiovascular:* Cardiovascular adverse reactions, other than exacerbation of the arrhythmias, include the uncommon occurrence of CHF (3%) and bradycardia. Bradycardia usually responds to dosage reduction but may require a pacemaker for control. CHF rarely requires drug discontinuation. Cardiac conduction abnormalities occur infrequently and are reversible upon discontinuation of drug.

Cardiac arrhythmias, CHF, sinoatrial node dysfunction (1% to 3%); cardiac conduction abnormalities, hypotension (less than 1%).

➤*CNS:* Neurologic problems are extremely common, occurring in 20% to 40% of patients and including malaise and fatigue, peripheral neuropathy, poor coordination and gait, and tremor and involuntary movements; they are rarely a reason to stop therapy and may respond to dose reductions or discontinuation.

Abnormal gait/ataxia, dizziness, lack of coordination, malaise and fatigue, paresthesias, tremor/abnormal involuntary movements (4% to 9%); decreased libido, headache, insomnia, sleep disturbances (1% to 3%).

➤*Dermatologic:* Dermatologic adverse reactions occur in approximately 15% of patients, with photosensitivity being most common (approximately 10%). Sunscreen and protection from sun exposure may be helpful, and drug discontinuation is not usually necessary. Prolonged exposure to amiodarone occasionally results in a blue-gray pigmentation. This is slowly and occasionally incompletely reversible upon discontinuation of drug but is of cosmetic importance only.

Solar dermatitis/photosensitivity (4% to 9%); alopecia, blue skin discoloration, rash, spontaneous ecchymosis (less than 1%).

➤*Endocrine:* Hyperthyroidism, hypothyroidism (1% to 3%).

➤*GI:* GI complaints, most commonly anorexia, constipation, nausea, and vomiting, occur in approximately 25% of patients but rarely require discontinuation of drug. These commonly occur during high-dose administration (ie, loading dose) and usually respond to dose reduction or divided doses.

Nausea, vomiting (10% to 33%); anorexia, constipation (4% to 9%); abdominal pain (1% to 3%).

➤*Hepatic:* Abnormal liver function tests (4% to 9%); nonspecific hepatic disorders (1% to 3%).

➤*Ophthalmic:* Ophthalmic abnormalities, including optic neuropathy and/or optic neuritis, in some cases progressing to corneal degeneration, eye discomfort, lens opacities, macular degeneration, papilledema, permanent blindness, photosensitivity, and scotoma, have been reported.

Asymptomatic corneal microdeposits are present in virtually all adult patients who have been on the drug for more than 6 months. Some patients develop eye symptoms of dry eyes, halos, and photophobia. Vision is rarely affected and drug discontinuation is rarely needed.

Visual disturbances (4% to 9%).

➤*Respiratory:* Fibrosis, pulmonary inflammation (4% to 9%).

➤*Miscellaneous:* Abnormal salivation, abnormal taste and smell, coagulation abnormalities, edema, flushing (1% to 3%).

➤*Postmarketing:*

Cardiovascular – Hypotension (sometimes fatal), sinus arrest, vasculitis.

CNS – Confusional state, delirium, disorientation, hallucination, pseudotumor cerebri.

Dermatologic – Erythema multiforme, exfoliative dermatitis, pruritus, skin cancer, Stevens-Johnson syndrome, toxic epidermal necrolysis (sometimes fatal).

Endocrine – Thyroid cancer, thyroid nodules.

GU – Epididymitis, impotence.

Hematologic – Agranulocytosis, aplastic anemia, hemolytic anemia, neutropenia, pancytopenia, thrombocytopenia.

Hepatic – Cholestatic hepatitis, cirrhosis, hepatitis.

Musculoskeletal – Muscle weakness, myopathy, rhabdomyolysis.

Renal – Acute renal failure, renal function impairment, renal insufficiency.

Respiratory – Bronchiolitis obliterans organizing pneumonia (possibly fatal), bronchospasm, cough, dyspnea, hemoptysis, hypoxia, pleuritis, possi-

AMIODARONE HYDROCHLORIDE — ORAL

bly fatal respiratory disorders (including adult respiratory distress syndrome, arrest, distress, and failure), pulmonary infiltrates and/or masses, wheezing.

Miscellaneous – Anaphylactic/anaphylactoid reaction (sometimes fatal), angioedema, fever, granuloma, pancreatitis, syndrome of inappropriate antidiuretic hormone secretion.

Overdosage

➤*Symptoms:* There have been cases, some fatal, of amiodarone overdose.

➤*Treatment:* In addition to general supportive measures, monitor the patient's cardiac rhythm and blood pressure, and if bradycardia ensues, a beta-adrenergic agonist or a pacemaker may be used. Treat hypotension with inadequate tissue perfusion with positive inotropic and/or vasopressor agents. Neither amiodarone nor its metabolite is dialyzable.

Patient Information

Instruct patients to read the accompanying Medication Guide each time they refill their prescription.

Instruct patients to not drink grapefruit juice during treatment with amiodarone. Grapefruit juice affects how amiodarone is absorbed in the stomach.

Instruct patients to avoid exposing their skin to the sun or sun lamps. Amiodarone can cause a photosensitive reaction. Instruct patients to wear sunblock cream or protective clothing when out in the sun.

Advise women to avoid pregnancy while on amiodarone because it may harm the fetus.

Instruct women not to breast-feed while taking amiodarone because it may pass into their milk and can harm the baby.

AMIODARONE HYDROCHLORIDE — INJECTION

Refer to the general introductory discussion concerning Antiarrhythmic Agents.

Indications

➤*Ventricular arrhythmias:* For initiation of treatment and prophylaxis of frequently recurring ventricular fibrillation and hemodynamically unstable ventricular tachycardia in patients refractory to other therapy. Amiodarone injection also can be used to treat patients with ventricular tachycardia/ventricular fibrillation for whom oral amiodarone is indicated but who are unable to take oral medication. During or after treatment with amiodarone injection, patients may be transferred to oral amiodarone therapy.

Use amiodarone injection for acute treatment until the patient's ventricular arrhythmias are stabilized. Most patients will require this therapy for 48 to 96 hours, but amiodarone injection may be safely administered for longer periods if necessary.

➤*Off-label uses:*

Atrioventricular nodal reentry tachycardia – [4] = Insufficient documentation. Amiodarone is a second-line therapeutic option for the treatment of atrioventricular (AV) nodal reentry tachycardia only in select adults based on expert opinion. Because of serious safety risks and weak efficacy data, amiodarone should be used only when other treatment options are inappropriate.

Conversion of atrial fibrillation to sinus rhythm – [2] = Fair documentation. Amiodarone is highly lipophilic and has a long half-life, which results in delayed onset of therapeutic effect. Serious safety issues limit its use. Amiodarone can serve as an alternative to other agents for patients without underlying cardiac disease, and it may be an appropriate first-line agent in patients with structural heart disease or congestive heart failure for whom other drug choices would be contraindicated. Consensus guidelines support the use of intravenous (IV) amiodarone for cardioversion of atrial fibrillation in adults.

Supraventricular tachycardia – Amiodarone is an effective therapeutic option with a variety of potential uses in the management of supraventricular tachycardia (SVT); however, safety risks limit its therapeutic use. In many cases, amiodarone is reserved for use in patients who have failed other therapies or who have structural heart disease, including left ventricular dysfunction.

Supraventricular tachycardia (adults): [3] = Safety concerns.

Supraventricular tachycardia (infants/children/adolescents): [3] = Safety concerns.

Other possible off-label uses – For postoperative conversion of atrial fibrillation and atrial flutter and prevention of recurrence of symptomatic paroxysmal and persistent atrial fibrillation after cardioversion.

Administration and Dosage

➤*General dosing considerations:* Administer amiodarone injection concentrations more than 2 mg/mL via a central venous catheter (see Administration).

Administer amiodarone via polyvinyl chloride (PVC) tubing using an in-line filter (see Administration).

Amiodarone injection infusions exceeding 2 hours must be administered in glass or polyolefin bottles containing dextrose 5% in water (see Administration).

➤*Adults:*

Ventricular arrhythmias –

Loading dose: Approximately 1,000 mg over the first 24 hours of therapy, delivered by IV infusion as follows: rapid administration of 150 mg over first 10 minutes (15 mg/min), followed by 360 mg over the next 6 hours (1 mg/min), then 540 mg over the remaining 18 hours (0.5 mg/min).

The first 24-hour dose may be individualized for each patient; however, in controlled clinical trials, mean daily doses of more than 2,100 mg were associated with an increased risk of hypotension.

Maintenance dosage: After the first 24 hours, continue the maintenance infusion rate of 0.5 mg/min (720 mg per 24 hours) using a concentration of 1 to 6 mg/mL (1.8 mg/mL [*Nexterone*]) at a rate of 0.278 mL/min. The rate of the maintenance infusion may be increased to achieve effective arrhythmia suppression.

In the event of breakthrough episodes of ventricular fibrillation or hemodynamically unstable ventricular tachycardia, supplemental infusions of amiodarone 150 mg may be administered. Administer such infusions over 10 minutes to minimize the potential for hypotension.

Based on the experience from clinical studies of amiodarone, a maintenance infusion of 0.5 mg/min can be cautiously continued for 2 to 3 weeks regardless of the patient's age, renal function, or left ventricular function. There has been limited experience in patients receiving amiodarone injection for more than 3 weeks.

Dosage adjustment: Amiodarone shows considerable interindividual variation in response. Thus, although a starting dose adequate to suppress life-threatening arrhythmias is necessary, close monitoring with dose adjustment is essential.

Conversion: Patients whose arrhythmias have been suppressed by amiodarone injection may be switched to oral amiodarone. The optimal dose for changing from IV to oral administration of amiodarone will depend on the dose of amiodarone injection already administered, as well as the bioavailability of oral amiodarone.

The suggested doses of oral amiodarone to be initiated after varying durations of amiodarone injection administration are made on the basis of a comparable total body amount of amiodarone delivered by the IV and oral routes, based on 50% bioavailability of oral amiodarone.

Amiodarone Recommendations for Oral Dosage After IV Infusion

Duration of amiodarone IV infusion[a]	Initial daily dose of oral amiodarone
Less than 1 week	800 to 1,600 mg
1 to 3 week	600 to 800 mg
More than 3 week[b]	400 mg

[a] Assuming 720 mg/day infusion (0.5 mg/min).
[b] Amiodarone IV is not intended for maintenance treatment.

Off-label dosing –

Atrioventricular nodal reentry tachycardia: [4] = Insufficient documentation. According to national guidelines for atrial fibrillation, the recommended IV dose of amiodarone is 150 mg over 10 minutes, followed by a maintenance dose of 0.5 to 1 mg/min. For long-term oral management in adults, the following schedule is recommended: 800 mg daily for 1 week, followed by 600 mg daily for 1 week, followed by 400 mg daily for 4 to 6 weeks, followed by maintenance therapy with 200 mg/day.

The largest reported experience with amiodarone used 5 mg/kg IV for acute termination of AV nodal reentry tachycardia, followed by daily oral maintenance therapy with 200 to 400 mg. Another small study reported starting dosages of 600 to 1,200 mg/day for the first 5 to 7 days, followed by maintenance dosing with an average of 245 mg/day.

In a case report, oral maintenance was initiated at 1,200 mg/day for 1 week, followed by 800 mg/day for 1 week, 600 mg/day for 1 week, and 400 mg/day thereafter.

Conversion of atrial fibrillation to sinus rhythm: [2] = Fair documentation.

• *IV/Oral* – 5 to 7 mg/kg IV over 30 to 60 minutes, then 1.2 to 1.8 g/day as a continuous IV infusion or in divided oral doses until 10 g total, then 200 to 400 mg/day oral maintenance.

Supraventricular tachycardia (adults): [3] = Safety concerns.

• *Initial dosage* – 50 mg IV over 10 minutes, followed by 0.5 to 1 mg/min, then switched to oral maintenance dosing.

• *Maintenance dosage* – 800 mg daily orally for 1 week, followed by 600 mg daily for 1 week, followed by 400 mg daily for 4 to 6 weeks, followed by maintenance therapy with 200 mg/day.

➤*Children:*

Off-label dosing –

Cardiovascular conditions:

Amiodarone Injection Off-Label Dosing in Children

Indication	Recommended dosage
Life-threatening or drug-resistant refractory cardiac arrhythmias (eg, ventricular tachycardia, junctional ectopic tachycardia)	5 mg/kg IV given over 20 to 60 minutes, followed by 5 mcg/kg/min continuous infusion. Infusion may be increased up to a maximum dose of 15 mcg/kg/min or 20 mcg/kg per 24 hours. May also administer by intraosseous route. Consider converting to oral therapy within 24 to 48 hours.

AMIODARONE HYDROCHLORIDE — INJECTION

Amiodarone Injection Off-Label Dosing in Children	
Indication	**Recommended dosage**
Ventricular fibrillation/pulseless ventricular tachycardia	5 mg/kg by rapid IV push if no pulse or over 15 to 20 minutes if there is a pulse. Repeat up to 15 mg/kg (maximum dose of 300 mg). May also administer by intraosseous route.

Supraventricular tachycardia (infants/children/adolescents): [3] = Safety concerns.

- *Initial dosage* – 5 mg/kg given IV over 1 hour, followed by 5 mg/kg/day for 47 hours.
- *Maintenance dosage* – 10 to 20 mg/kg/day for 7 to 10 days, followed by 3 to 20 mg/kg/day.

➤*Monitoring:* When changing to oral amiodarone therapy, clinical monitoring is recommended, particularly for elderly patients.

➤*Preparation for administration:*

Rapid loading infusion – Add 3 mL of amiodarone (150 mg) to 100 mL of dextrose 5% in water to yield a concentration of 1.5 mg/mL.

Subsequent slow (6-hour) loading infusion – Add 18 mL of amiodarone (900 mg) to 500 mL of dextrose 5% in water to yield a concentration of 1.8 mg/mL.

➤*Administration:* The initial infusion rate should not exceed 30 mg/min.

The surface properties of solutions containing injectable amiodarone are altered such that the drop size may be reduced. This reduction may lead to underdosage of the patient by up to 30% if drop-counter infusion sets are used. Amiodarone injection must be delivered by a volumetric infusion pump.

Administer amiodarone injection, whenever possible, through a central venous catheter dedicated to that purpose. Use an in-line filter during administration.

IV amiodarone loading infusions at much higher concentrations and rates of infusion much faster than recommended have resulted in hepatocellular necrosis and acute renal failure leading to death.

Amiodarone concentrations more than 3 mg/mL in dextrose 5% in water have been associated with a high incidence of peripheral vein phlebitis; however, concentrations of 2.5 mg/mL or less appear to be less irritating. Therefore, for infusions longer than 1 hour, amiodarone injection concentrations should not exceed 2 mg/mL unless a central venous catheter is used.

Amiodarone premixed injection (*Nexterone*) is available in *Galaxy* containers as a single-use, ready to use, iso-osmotic solution in dextrose for IV administration. No further dilution is required. Amiodarone should not be combined with any product in the same IV line or premixed container. Protect from light until ready to use.

Because the premixed container is for single use only, any unused portion should be discarded.

Do not use plastic containers in series connections. Such use could result in air embolism due to residual air being drawn from the primary container before the administration of the fluid from the secondary container is complete.

Nexterone – For loading infusions, rapidly administer 150 mg over the first 10 minutes (15 mg/min). Directly infuse amiodarone premixed injection (150 mg per 100 mL; 1.5 mg/mL) at a rate of 10 mL/min, followed by slow infusion of 360 mg over the next 6 hours (1 mg/min). Directly infuse amiodarone premixed injection (360 mg per 200 mL; 1.8 mg/mL) at a rate of 0.556 mL/min.

For maintenance infusions, administer 540 mg over the remaining 18 hours (0.5 mg/min). Decrease the rate of the slow loading infusion to 0.5 mg/min. Directly infuse amiodarone premixed injection (360 mg per 200 mL; 1.8 mg/mL) at a rate of 0.278 mL/min.

➤*Admixture compatibility:* It is well known that amiodarone adsorbs to PVC tubing, and the clinical trial dose administration schedule was designed to account for this adsorption. All of the clinical trials were conducted using PVC tubing and its use is therefore recommended. The concentrations and rates of infusion previously provided reflect doses identified in these studies. It is important that the recommended infusion regimen be followed closely.

Amiodarone has been found to leach out plasticizers, including di-(2-ethylhexyl) phthalate (DEHP) from IV tubing (including PVC tubing). The degree of leaching increases when infusing amiodarone at higher concentrations and lower flow rates than provided in this section.

Amiodarone injection infusions exceeding 2 hours must be administered in glass or polyolefin bottles containing dextrose 5% in water. Use of evacuated glass containers for admixing amiodarone injection is not recommended, as incompatibility with a buffer in the container may cause precipitation.

Amiodarone Y-Site Injection Incompatibility			
Drug	**Vehicle**	**Amiodarone concentration**	**Comments**
Aminophylline	Dextrose 5% in water	4 mg/mL	Precipitate
Cefamandole nafate	Dextrose 5% in water	4 mg/mL	Precipitate
Cefazolin sodium	Dextrose 5% in water	4 mg/mL	Precipitate
Mezlocillin sodium	Dextrose 5% in water	4 mg/mL	Precipitate
Heparin sodium	Dextrose 5% in water		Precipitate
Sodium bicarbonate	Dextrose 5% in water	3 mg/mL	Precipitate

➤*Storage/Stability:* Store at room temperature, 20° to 25°C (68° to 77°F); excursions are permitted between 15° and 30°C (59° and 86°F). Protect from light and excessive heat. Use carton to protect contents from light until used.

Amiodarone does not need to be protected from light during administration.

Amiodarone Solution Stability			
Solution	**Concentration (mg/mL)**	**Container**	**Comments**
Dextrose 5% in water	1 to 6	PVC	Physically compatible, with amiodarone loss less than 10% at 2 hours at room temperature.
Dextrose 5% in water	1 to 6	Polyolefin, glass	Physically compatible, with no amiodarone loss at 24 hours at room temperature.

Actions

➤*Pharmacology:* Amiodarone is generally considered a class III antiarrhythmic drug, but it possesses electrophysiologic characteristics of all 4 Vaughan-Williams classes. Like class I drugs, amiodarone blocks sodium channels at rapid pacing frequencies, and, like class II drugs, it exerts a noncompetitive antisympathetic action. One of its main effects, with prolonged administration, is to lengthen the cardiac action potential, a class III effect. The negative chronotropic effect of amiodarone in nodal tissues is similar to the effect of class IV drugs. In addition to blocking sodium channels, amiodarone blocks myocardial potassium channels, which contributes to slowing of conduction and prolongation of refractoriness. The antisympathetic action and the block of calcium and potassium channels are responsible for the negative dromotropic effects on the sinus node and for the slowing of conduction and prolongation of refractoriness in the atrioventricular (AV) node. Its vasodilatory action can decrease cardiac workload and consequently myocardial oxygen consumption.

Administration of amiodarone prolongs intranodal conduction (atrial-His) and effective refractory period (ERP) of the atrioventricular node (AVN), but has little or no effect on sinus cycle length, effective refractory period of the right atrium and right ventricle, repolarization (QTc), intraventricular conduction (QRS), and infranodal conduction (His-ventricular). A comparison of the electrophysiologic effects of amiodarone IV and oral amiodarone is shown in the following table.

Effects of IV and Oral Amiodarone on Electrophysiologic Parameters[a]								
Formulation	**SCL**	**QRS**	**QTc**	**AH**	**HV**	**ERP RA**	**ERP RV**	**ERP AVN**
IV	↔[b]	↔	↔	↑	↔	↔	↔	↑
Oral	↑	↔	↑	↑	↔	↑	↑	↑

[a] SCL = sinus cycle length; AH = atrial-His; RA = right atrium; RV = right ventricle; HV = His-ventricular.
[b] No change.

At higher doses (more than 10 mg/kg) of amiodarone, prolongation of the ERP right ventricle and modest prolongation of the QRS have been seen. These differences between oral and IV administration suggest that the initial acute effects of amiodarone may be predominantly focused on the AVN, causing an intranodal conduction delay and increased nodal refractoriness caused by slow channel blockade (class IV activity) and noncompetitive adrenergic antagonism (class II activity).

Pharmacodynamics – Amiodarone has been reported to produce negative inotropic and vasodilatory effects in animals and humans. In clinical studies in patients with refractory ventricular fibrillation or hemodynamically unstable ventricular tachycardia, treatment-emergent, drug-related hypotension occurred in 288 of 1,836 (16%) patients treated with amiodarone. No correlations were seen between the baseline ejection fraction and the occurrence of clinically significant hypotension during infusion of amiodarone.

➤*Pharmacokinetics:*

Absorption/Distribution – Amiodarone exhibits complex disposition characteristics after IV administration. Peak serum concentrations after single 5 mg/kg 15-minute IV infusions in healthy subjects range between 5 and 41 mg/L. Peak concentrations after 10-minute infusions of amiodarone 150 mg in patients with ventricular fibrillation or hemodynamically

AMIODARONE HYDROCHLORIDE — INJECTION

unstable ventricular tachycardia range between 7 and 26 mg/L. Because of rapid distribution, serum concentrations decline to 10% of peak values within 30 to 45 minutes after the end of the infusion. In clinical trials, after 48 hours of continued infusions (125, 500, or 1,000 mg/day) plus supplemental (150 mg) infusions (for recurrent arrhythmias), amiodarone mean serum concentrations between 0.7 and 1.4 mg/L were observed (n = 260).

There is no established relationship between drug concentration and therapeutic response for short-term IV use. Steady-state amiodarone concentrations of 1 to 2.5 mg/L have been associated with antiarrhythmic effects and acceptable toxicity following chronic oral amiodarone therapy.

The systemic availability of oral amiodarone in healthy subjects ranges between 33% and 65%. In in vitro studies, the protein binding of amiodarone is more than 96%. Amiodarone and desethylamiodarone cross the placenta and both appear in breast milk.

Metabolism / Excretion – N-desethylamiodarone is the major active metabolite of amiodarone in humans. Desethylamiodarone serum concentrations of 0.05 mg/L or more are not usually seen until after several days of continuous infusion, but with prolonged therapy reach approximately the same concentration as amiodarone. The enzymes responsible for the N-deethylation are believed to be the CYP-450 3A (CYP3A) subfamily, principally CYP-3A4. This isozyme is present in both the liver and intestines. The highly variable systemic availability of oral amiodarone may be attributed potentially to large interindividual variability in CYP-3A4 activity.

Amiodarone is eliminated primarily by hepatic metabolism and biliary excretion and there is negligible excretion of amiodarone or desethylamiodarone in urine. Neither amiodarone or desethylamiodarone is dialyzable.

Desethylamiodarone clearance and volume involve an unknown biotransformation factor.

In clinical studies of 2 to 7 days, clearance of amiodarone after IV administration in patients with ventricular tachycardia and ventricular fibrillation ranged between 220 and 440 mL/h/kg.

The following table summarizes the mean ranges of pharmacokinetic parameters of amiodarone reported in single-dose IV (5 mg/kg over 15 minutes) studies of healthy subjects.

Pharmacokinetic Profile After Amiodarone Injection Administration[a]

Drug	Clearance (mL/h/kg)	V_c (L/kg)	V_{ss} (L/kg)	t½ (days)
Amiodarone	90 to 158	0.2	40 to 84	20 to 47
Desethylamiodarone	197 to 290	NA	68 to 168	≥ amiodarone t½

[a] V_c = central volume of distribution from IV studies; V_{ss} = steady-state volume of distribution from IV studies; NA = not available; t½ = elimination half-life.

Special populations –

Hepatic function impairment: After a single dose of amiodarone injection in cirrhotic patients, significantly lower maximal drug concentration (C_{max}) and average concentration values are seen for desethylamiodarone, but mean amiodarone levels are unchanged.

Elderly: Healthy subjects older than 65 years of age show lower clearances (approximately 100 mL/h/kg) than younger subjects (approximately 150 mL/h/kg) and an increase in t½ from approximately 20 to 47 days.

Severe left ventricular dysfunction: In patients with severe left ventricular dysfunction, the pharmacokinetics of amiodarone are not significantly altered but the terminal disposition t½ of desethylamiodarone is prolonged.

Contraindications

Hypersensitivity to any of the components of amiodarone injection; cardiogenic shock; marked sinus bradycardia; second- or third-degree AV block, unless a functioning pacemaker is available.

Warnings/Precautions

➤*Cardiac effects:*

Hypotension – Hypotension is the most common adverse reaction seen with amiodarone. In clinical trials, treatment-emergent, drug-related hypotension was reported as an adverse reaction in 288 of 1,836 (16%) patients treated with amiodarone. Clinically significant hypotension during infusions was seen most often in the first several hours of treatment and was not dose related, but appeared to be related to the rate of infusion. Hypotension necessitating alterations in amiodarone therapy was reported in 3% of patients, with permanent discontinuation required in less than 2% of patients.

Initially treat by slowing the infusion; additional standard therapy may be needed, including the following: vasopressor drugs, positive inotropic agents, and volume expansion. Monitor the initial rate of infusion closely; do not let it exceed that prescribed.

In some cases, hypotension may be refractory, resulting in fatal outcome.

Bradycardia / AV block – Drug-related bradycardia occurred in 90 of 1,836 (4.9%) patients in clinical trials while they were receiving amiodarone for life-threatening ventricular tachycardia/ventricular fibrillation; it was not dose related. Treat bradycardia by slowing the infusion rate or discontinuing amiodarone. In some patients, inserting a pacemaker is required. Despite such measures, bradycardia was progressive and terminal in one patient during controlled trials. Treat patients with a known predisposition to bradycardia or AV block with amiodarone in a setting where a temporary pacemaker is available.

Proarrhythmia – Like all antiarrhythmic agents, amiodarone may cause a worsening of existing arrhythmias or precipitate a new arrhythmia. Proarrhythmia, primarily torsades de pointes, has been associated with prolongation by amiodarone of the QTc interval to 500 milliseconds or more. Although QTc prolongation occurred frequently in patients receiving amiodarone, torsades de pointes or new-onset ventricular fibrillation occurred infrequently (less than 2%). Monitor patients for QTc prolongation during infusion with amiodarone injection. Reserve combination of amiodarone with other antiarrhythmic therapy that prolongs the QTc for patients with life-threatening ventricular arrhythmias who are incompletely responsive to a single agent.

Fluoroquinolones, macrolide antibiotics, and azoles are known to cause QTc prolongation. There have been reports of QTc prolongation, with or without torsades de pointes, in patients taking amiodarone when fluoroquinolones, macrolide antibiotics, or azoles were coadministered.

The need to coadminister amiodarone with any other drug known to prolong the QTc interval must be based on a careful assessment of the potential risks and benefits of doing so for each patient.

A careful assessment of the potential risks and benefits of administering amiodarone must be made in patients with thyroid dysfunction because of the possibility of arrhythmia breakthrough or exacerbation of arrhythmia (which may result in death) in these patients.

➤*Long-term use:* There has been limited experience in patients receiving amiodarone IV for more than 3 weeks. Pulmonary toxicity is a well-recognized complication of long-term amiodarone use.

➤*Hepatic effects:* Elevations of blood hepatic enzyme values ALT, AST, and gamma-glutamyl transferase are seen commonly in patients with immediately life-threatening ventricular tachycardia/ventricular fibrillation. Interpreting elevated AST activity can be difficult because the values may be elevated in patients who have had recent myocardial infarction, congestive heart failure, or multiple electrical defibrillations. Approximately 54% of patients receiving amiodarone in clinical studies had baseline liver enzyme elevations and 13% had clinically significant elevations. In 81% of patients with both baseline and on-therapy data available, the liver enzyme elevations either improved during therapy or remained at baseline levels. Baseline abnormalities in hepatic enzymes are not a contraindication to treatment.

Rare cases of fatal hepatocellular necrosis after treatment with amiodarone have been reported. Two patients, one 28 years of age and the other 60 years of age, were treated for atrial arrhythmias with an initial infusion of 1,500 mg over 5 hours, a rate much higher than recommended. Both patients developed hepatic and renal failure within 24 hours after the start of amiodarone treatment and died on day 14 and day 4, respectively. Because these episodes of hepatic necrosis may have been caused by the rapid rate of infusion with possible rate-related hypotension, closely monitor the initial rate of infusion and do not let it exceed that prescribed.

In patients with life-threatening arrhythmias, weigh the potential risk of hepatic injury against the potential benefit of amiodarone therapy, but carefully monitor patients receiving amiodarone for evidence of progressive hepatic injury. Give consideration to reducing the rate of administration or withdrawing amiodarone in such cases.

➤*Pulmonary effects:*

Pulmonary toxicity – There have been postmarketing reports of acute-onset (days to weeks) pulmonary injury in patients treated with amiodarone IV. Findings have included pulmonary infiltrates on bronchospasm, cough, dyspnea, fever, hemoptysis, hypoxia, wheezing, and x-ray. Some cases have progressed to respiratory failure and/or death.

Adult respiratory distress syndrome – Two percent of patients were reported to have adult respiratory distress syndrome during clinical studies involving 48 hours of therapy. Adult respiratory distress syndrome is a disorder characterized by bilateral, diffuse pulmonary infiltrates with pulmonary edema and varying degrees of respiratory function impairment. The clinical and radiographic picture can arise after a variety of lung injuries, such as those resulting from trauma, shock, prolonged cardiopulmonary resuscitation, and aspiration pneumonia, conditions present in many of the patients enrolled in the clinical studies. There have been postmarketing reports of adult respiratory distress syndrome in amiodarone IV patients. Amiodarone IV may play a role in causing or exacerbating pulmonary disorders in those patients.

Postoperatively, occurrences of adult respiratory distress syndrome have been reported in patients receiving oral amiodarone therapy who have undergone either cardiac or noncardiac surgery. Although patients usually respond well to vigorous respiratory therapy, in rare instances the outcome has been fatal. Until further studies have been performed, it is recommended that fraction of inspired oxygen (FiO_2) and the determinants of oxygen delivery to the tissues (eg, arterial oxygen saturation [SaO_2], alveolar oxygen partial pressure [PaO_2]) be closely monitored in patients taking amiodarone.

Pulmonary fibrosis – Only 1 of more than 1,000 patients treated with amiodarone IV in clinical studies developed pulmonary fibrosis. In that patient, the condition was diagnosed 3 months after treatment with amiodarone injection, during which time she received oral amiodarone. Pulmonary toxicity is a well-recognized complication of long-term amiodarone use.

➤*Surgery:* Close perioperative monitoring is recommended in patients undergoing general anesthesia who are on amiodarone therapy, as they may be more sensitive to the myocardial depressant and conduction effects of halogenated inhalational anesthetics.

➤*Electrolyte disturbances:* Patients with hypokalemia or hypomagnesemia should have the condition corrected whenever possible before being treated with amiodarone, as these disorders can exaggerate the degree of QTc prolongation and increase the potential for torsades de pointes. Give

AMIODARONE HYDROCHLORIDE — INJECTION

special attention to electrolyte and acid-base balance in patients experiencing severe or prolonged diarrhea or in patients receiving concomitant diuretics.

➤*Pregnancy: Category D.* Although oral amiodarone use during pregnancy is uncommon, there have been a small number of published reports of congenital goiter/hypothyroidism and hyperthyroidism. If amiodarone injection is administered during pregnancy, apprise the patient of the potential hazard to the fetus.

In a reproductive study in which amiodarone was given IV to rabbits at doses of 5, 10, or 25 mg/kg/day (approximately 0.1, 0.3, and 0.7 times the maximum recommended human dose [MRHD] on a body surface area basis), maternal deaths occurred in all groups, including controls. Embryotoxicity (as manifested by fewer full-term fetuses and increased resorptions with concomitantly lower litter weights) occurred at doses of 10 mg/kg or more.

In a teratology study in which amiodarone was administered by continuous IV infusion to rats at doses of 25, 50, or 100 mg/kg/day (approximately 0.4, 0.7, and 1.4 times the MRHD when compared on a body surface area basis), maternal toxicity (as evidenced by reduced weight gain and food consumption) and embryotoxicity (as evidenced by increased resorptions, decreased live litter size, reduced body weights, and retarded sternum and metacarpal ossification) were observed in the 100 mg/kg group.

Only use amiodarone during pregnancy if the potential benefit to the mother justifies the risk to the fetus.

➤*Lactation:* Amiodarone and one of its major metabolites, desethylamiodarone, are excreted in human milk, suggesting that breast-feeding could expose the breast-feeding infant to a significant dose of the drug. Breast-feeding offspring of lactating rats administered amiodarone have demonstrated reduced viability and reduced body weight gains. Weigh the risk of exposing the infant to amiodarone against the potential benefit of arrhythmia suppression in the mother. Advise the mother to discontinue breast-feeding.

➤*Children:* The safety and efficacy of amiodarone in children have not been established; therefore, its use in children is not recommended.

In a trial of 61 children (30 days to 15 years of age), hypotension (36%), bradycardia (20%), and AV block (15%) were common dose-related adverse reactions, and were severe or life-threatening in some cases. Injection-site reactions were seen in 5 of the 20 (25%) patients receiving amiodarone through a peripheral vein irrespective of dose regimen.

Benzyl alcohol – Amiodarone injection may contain the preservative benzyl alcohol. There have been reports of fatal "gasping syndrome" in neonates (children younger than 1 month of age) following administration of IV solutions containing the preservative benzyl alcohol. Symptoms include a striking onset of gasping respiration, hypotension, bradycardia, and cardiovascular collapse.

➤*Elderly:* In general, dose selection for an elderly patient should be cautious, usually starting at the low end of the dosing range, reflecting the greater frequency of decreased hepatic, renal, or cardiac function, and of concomitant disease or other drug therapy.

Per the Beers list, amiodarone is associated with QT interval problems, risk of provoking torsades de pointes, and lack of efficacy in older adults.

➤*Monitoring:* Monitor for hypotension, especially during the first few hours of infusion. Monitor for QTc prolongation during infusion with amiodarone. Close perioperative monitoring is recommended in patients undergoing general anesthesia who are on amiodarone therapy.

Monitor liver enzymes on a regular basis.

Closely monitor FiO_2 and the determinants of oxygen delivery to the tissues (eg, SaO_2, PaO_2) in patients taking amiodarone.

Drug Interactions

➤*QT prolongation:* An additive effect of amiodarone with other drugs that prolong the QT interval cannot be excluded. The following drugs may prolong the QT interval and increase the risk of life-threatening cardiac arrhythmias, including torsade de pointes: Antiarrhythmic agents (eg, bretylium, disopyramide, dofetilide, procainamide, quinidine, and sotalol), arsenic trioxide, chlorpromazine, cisapride, dolasetron, droperidol, mefloquine, mesoridazine, moxifloxacin, pentamidine, pimozide, tacrolimus, thioridazine, and ziprasidone. For a more complete list of drugs that may prolong the QT interval, see the appendix, Drug-Induced Prolongation of the QT Interval and Torsade de Pointes.

Amiodarone Injection Drug Interactions

Precipitant drug	Object drug[a]		Description
Azole antifungals (eg, itraconazole)	Amiodarone	↑	The risk of life-threatening cardiac arrhythmias, including torsades de pointes, may be increased.
Cholestyramine	Amiodarone	↓	Increased enterohepatic elimination of amiodarone and reduced serum levels and half-life may occur.
Cimetidine	Amiodarone	↑	Increased serum amiodarone levels may occur.
Fentanyl	Amiodarone	↑	Concomitant use may cause hypotension, bradycardia, decreased cardiac output, and sinus arrest.
Fluoroquinolones (eg, sparfloxacin)	Amiodarone	↑	The risk of life-threatening cardiac arrhythmias, including torsades de pointes, may be increased.
Hydantoins (eg, phenytoin)	Amiodarone	↓	Chronic use (more than 2 weeks) of oral amiodarone impairs metabolism of phenytoin. Increased hydantoin concentrations with symptoms of toxicity may occur. Also, amiodarone serum levels may be decreased.
Amiodarone	Hydantoins (eg, phenytoin)	↑	
Iohexol	Amiodarone	↑	The risk of life-threatening cardiac arrhythmias may be increased.
Macrolide antibiotics (eg, azithromycin, telithromycin)	Amiodarone	↑	The risk of life-threatening cardiac arrhythmias, including torsades de pointes, may be increased. Avoid coadministration of telithromycin with amiodarone.
Protease inhibitors (ie, atazanavir, indinavir, nelfinavir, ritonavir)	Amiodarone	↑	Increases in amiodarone concentrations may occur, increasing the risk of amiodarone toxicity. Ritonavir and nelfinavir are contraindicated in patients receiving amiodarone. Monitor amiodarone plasma levels and for amiodarone toxicity.
Rifamycins (eg, rifampin)	Amiodarone	↓	Serum concentrations of oral amiodarone and its active metabolite may be decreased, reducing its pharmacologic effect.
St. John's wort	Amiodarone	↓	St. John's wort induces CYP3A4, possibly reducing amiodarone levels.
Trazodone	Amiodarone	↑	QT prolongation and torsades de pointes have been reported with coadministration of oral amiodarone and trazodone.
Amiodarone	Antiarrhythmics (eg, disopyramide, flecainide, procainamide, quinidine)	↑	Amiodarone may increase serum concentrations of these antiarrhythmics. Monitor patients closely. Reduce dose of antiarrhythmic with coadministration.
Amiodarone	Anticoagulants (eg, warfarin)	↑	Potentiation of anticoagulant response is almost always seen in patients receiving amiodarone and can result in serious or fatal bleeding. A 30% to 50% anticoagulant dose reduction is typically required. Onset is 3 to 4 days and may persist for months after amiodarone discontinuation. Closely monitor prothrombin time.
Amiodarone	Beta-blockers (eg, propranolol)	↑	Effects of beta-blockers eliminated by hepatic metabolism may be increased. Because amiodarone has weak beta-blocking activity, concomitant use can increase the risk of AV block, hypotension, bradycardia, and sinus arrest.
Amiodarone	Calcium channel blockers (eg, diltiazem, verapamil)	↑	Use amiodarone with caution with calcium channel blockers because of the possible potential of bradycardia, sinus arrest, and AV block.
Amiodarone	Cardiac glycosides (eg, digoxin, digitoxin)	↑	Oral amiodarone taken concomitantly with digoxin increases the serum digoxin concentration by 70% after 1 day. Reduce dose of digitalis therapy by 50% or discontinue.
Amiodarone	Cisapride	↑	Risk of life-threatening cardiac arrhythmias, including torsades de pointes, may be increased because of possible additive prolongation of the QT interval.

AMIODARONE HYDROCHLORIDE — INJECTION

Amiodarone Injection Drug Interactions			
Precipitant drug	Object drug[a]		Description
Amiodarone	Cyclosporine	↑	Concomitant use with oral amiodarone has produced persistently elevated plasma cyclosporine levels, resulting in elevated creatinine despite reduction in dose of cyclosporine.
Amiodarone	Dextromethorphan	↑	Oral amiodarone impairs metabolism of dextromethorphan.
Amiodarone	HMG-CoA reductase inhibitors (eg, simvastatin)	↑	Simvastatin in combination with amiodarone has been associated with reports of myopathy/rhabdomyolysis.
Amiodarone	Lidocaine	↑	Sinus bradycardia has been reported with oral amiodarone in combination with lidocaine for local anesthesia. Seizure, associated with increased lidocaine concentrations, has been reported with coadministration of IV amiodarone.
Amiodarone	Methotrexate	↑	Chronic use (more than 2 weeks) of oral amiodarone impairs metabolism of methotrexate. Methotrexate toxicity may be increased.
Amiodarone	Ranolazine	↑	The risk of life-threatening cardiac arrhythmias, including torsades de pointes, may be increased.
Amiodarone	Thioridazine	↑	The risk of life-threatening cardiac arrhythmias, including torsades de pointes, may be increased.
Amiodarone	Vardenafil	↑	The risk of life-threatening cardiac arrhythmias, including torsades de pointes, may be increased.
Amiodarone	Ziprasidone	↑	The risk of life-threatening cardiac arrhythmias, including torsades de pointes, may be increased.

[a] ↑ = object drug increased; ↓ = object drug decreased.

➤*Drug/Food interactions:* Grapefruit juice inhibits metabolism of oral amiodarone in the intestinal mucosa, resulting in increased amiodarone area under the curve by 50% and C_{max} by 84%, and decreased desethylamiodarone to unquantifiable concentrations. Consider this information when changing from IV amiodarone to oral amiodarone.

Adverse Reactions

The most important treatment-emergent adverse reactions were hypotension, asystole/cardiac arrest/electromechanical dissociation (EMD), cardiogenic shock, congestive heart failure, bradycardia, liver function test abnormalities, ventricular tachycardia, and AV block. Overall, treatment was discontinued for approximately 9% of the patients because of adverse reactions. The most common adverse reactions leading to discontinuation of amiodarone injection therapy were hypotension (1.6%), asystole/cardiac arrest/EMD (1.2%), ventricular tachycardia (1.1%), and cardiogenic shock (1%).

Amiodarone IV Adverse Reactions (≥ 2%)			
Adverse reaction	Controlled studies (n = 814)	Open-label studies (n = 1,022)	Total (n = 1,836)
Cardiovascular			
Bradycardia	6%	4%	4.9%
Congestive heart failure	2.2%	2%	2.1%
Heart arrest	3.5%	2.5%	2.9%
Hypotension	20.2%	12%	15.6%
Ventricular tachycardia	1.8%	2.9%	2.4%
GI			
Liver function tests abnormal	4.2%	2.8%	3.4%
Nausea	3.5%	4.2%	3.9%
Miscellaneous			
Fever	2.9%	1.2%	2%

➤*Other adverse reactions (less than 2%):* Other treatment-emergent, possibly drug related adverse reactions reported in less than 2% of patients receiving amiodarone injection in controlled and uncontrolled studies included the following:

Cardiovascular – Atrial fibrillation, nodal arrhythmia, prolonged QT interval, sinus bradycardia, ventricular fibrillation.

GI – Diarrhea, vomiting.

Hepatic – Increased ALT, increased AST.

Respiratory – Lung edema, respiratory disorder.

Miscellaneous – Abnormal kidney function, shock, Stevens-Johnson syndrome, thrombocytopenia.

➤*Postmarketing:*

Cardiovascular – Hypotension (sometimes fatal), sinus arrest.

CNS – Confusional state, delirium, disorientation, hallucination, pseudotumor cerebri.

Dermatologic – Erythema multiforme, exfoliative dermatitis, toxic epidermal necrolysis (sometimes fatal).

Hematologic – Neutropenia, pancytopenia.

Local – Cellulitis, edema, erythema, necrosis, pain, phlebitis, pigment changes, skin sloughing, thrombophlebitis, venous thrombosis.

Respiratory – Bronchospasm, cough, dyspnea, hemoptysis, hypoxia, possibly fatal respiratory disorders (including arrest, distress, failureand adult respiratory distress syndrome), pulmonary infiltrates, wheezing.

Miscellaneous – Anaphylactic/anaphylactoid reaction (including shock), angioedema, fever, syndrome of inappropriate antidiuretic hormone secretion.

Overdosage

➤*Symptoms:* Effects of an inadvertent overdose of amiodarone injection include AV block, bradycardia, cardiogenic shock, hepatotoxicity, and hypotension.

There have been cases, some fatal, of amiodarone overdose.

➤*Treatment:* Treat hypotension and cardiogenic shock by slowing the infusion rate or with standard therapy: vasopressor drugs, positive inotropic agents, and volume expansion. Bradycardia and AV block may require temporary pacing. Closely monitor hepatic enzyme concentrations. Amiodarone is not dialyzable.

ADENOSINE

Rx	**Adenosine** (Various, eg, Bedford, Sagent)	**Injection, solution:** 3 mg/mL	Sodium chloride 9 mg/mL. Preservative free. In 2 and 4 mL single-dose vials.
Rx	**Adenocard** (Astellas Pharma US)		Sodium chloride 9 mg/mL. Preservative free. In 2 and 4 mL syringes.

ADENOSINE — INJECTION

Indications

➤*Paroxysmal supraventricular tachycardia:* Conversion to sinus rhythm of paroxysmal supraventricular tachycardia (PSVT), including that associated with accessory bypass tracts (Wolff-Parkinson-White syndrome). When clinically advisable, attempt appropriate vagal maneuvers (eg, Valsalva maneuver) prior to use.

➤*Off-label uses:* Adenosine has been used in the noninvasive assessment of patients with suspected coronary artery disease in conjunction with thallium-201 tomography; results are similar to assessment with intravenous (IV) dipyridamole.

Administration and Dosage

➤*Adults:*

Paroxysmal supraventricular tachycardia –

Maximum dose: 12 mg per dose.

Initial dosage: 6 mg given as a rapid IV bolus (administered over a 1- to 2-second period).

Repeat administration: If the first dose does not result in elimination of the supraventricular tachycardia (SVT) within 1 to 2 minutes, give 12 mg. Repeat the 12 mg dose a second time if required. Doses of more than 12 mg are not recommended.

➤*Children:*

Paroxysmal supraventricular tachycardia –

50 kg or more: See Adults for dosing.

Less than 50 kg:

• *Maximum dose* – 0.3 mg/kg single dose (up to 12 mg).

• *Initial dosage* – 0.05 to 0.1 mg/kg as a rapid IV bolus given centrally or peripherally.

• *Repeat administration* – If conversion of PSVT does not occur within 1 to 2 minutes, additional bolus injections can be administered at incrementally higher doses, increasing the amount given by 0.05 to 0.1 mg/kg. Con-

ADENOSINE — INJECTION

tinue this process until sinus rhythm is established or a maximum single dose of 0.3 mg/kg (up to 12 mg) is used.

➤*Administration:* Give as a rapid bolus by the peripheral IV route only (administered over a 1- to 2-second period) in adults and children weighing more than 50 kg. In children weighing less than 50 kg, give centrally or peripherally. To be certain the solution reaches the systemic circulation, administer directly into a vein or, if given into an IV line, as proximal as possible, and follow with a rapid saline flush.

➤*Storage/Stability:* Store at 15° to 30°C (59° to 86°F). Do not refrigerate because crystallization may occur. If this occurs, let crystals warm to room temperature. Discard unused portion.

Actions

➤*Pharmacology:* Adenosine is an endogenous nucleoside occurring in all cells of the body. Adenosine slows conduction time through the atrioventricular (AV) node, can interrupt the reentry pathways through the AV node, and can restore normal sinus rhythm in patients with PSVT, including PSVT associated with Wolff-Parkinson-White syndrome.

➤*Pharmacokinetics:*

Distribution – IV administered adenosine is rapidly cleared from the circulation via cellular uptake, primarily by erythrocytes and vascular endothelial cells. This process involves a specific transmembrane nucleoside carrier system that is reversible, nonconcentrative, and bidirectionally symmetrical.

Metabolism/Excretion – Intracellular adenosine is rapidly metabolized via phosphorylation to adenosine monophosphate by adenosine kinase or via deamination to inosine by adenosine deaminase in the cytosol. Because adenosine kinase has a lower Michaelis-Menten dissociation constant and maximum velocity than adenosine deaminase, deamination plays a significant role only when cytosolic adenosine saturates the phosphorylation pathway. Inosine formed by deamination of adenosine can leave the cell intact or can be degraded to hypoxanthine, xanthine, and, ultimately, uric acid. Adenosine monophosphate formed by phosphorylation of adenosine is incorporated into the high-energy phosphate pool. While extracellular adenosine is primarily cleared by cellular uptake with a half-life of less than 10 seconds in whole blood, excessive amounts may be deaminated by an ecto-form of adenosine deaminase.

Contraindications

Second- or third-degree AV block (except in patients with a functioning artificial pacemaker); sinus node disease, such as sick sinus syndrome or symptomatic bradycardia (except in patients with a functioning artificial pacemaker); known hypersensitivity to adenosine.

Warnings/Precautions

➤*Heart block:* Adenosine exerts its effect by decreasing conduction through the AV node and may produce a short-lasting first-, second,- or third-degree heart block. Institute appropriate therapy as needed. Do not give patients who develop high-level block on 1 dose of adenosine additional doses. Because of the very short half-life, these effects are generally self-limiting. Ensure that appropriate resuscitative measures are available.

Transient or prolonged episodes of asystole have been reported with fatal outcomes in some cases. Rarely, ventricular fibrillation has been reported following adenosine administration, including resuscitated and fatal events. In most instances, these cases were associated with the concomitant use of digoxin and, less frequently, with digoxin and verapamil. Although no causal relationship or drug-drug interaction has been established, use adenosine with caution in patients receiving digoxin or digoxin and verapamil in combination.

➤*Arrhythmias:* At the time of conversion to normal sinus rhythm, a variety of new rhythms may appear on the electrocardiogram (ECG). They generally last only a few seconds without intervention and may take the form of atrial premature contractions, premature ventricular contractions, sinus bradycardia, sinus tachycardia, skipped beats, and varying degrees of AV nodal block. Such findings were seen in 55% of patients.

➤*Bronchoconstriction:* Adenosine is a respiratory stimulant (probably through activation of carotid body chemoreceptors), and IV administration in humans has been shown to increase minute ventilation and to reduce arterial partial pressure of carbon dioxide, causing respiratory alkalosis.

Adenosine administered by inhalation has been reported to cause bronchoconstriction in asthmatic patients, presumably because of mast cell degranulation and histamine release. These effects have not been observed in healthy subjects. Adenosine has been administered to a limited number of patients with asthma, and mild to moderate exacerbation of their symptoms has been reported. Respiratory compromise has occurred using adenosine infusion in patients with obstructive pulmonary disease. Use adenosine with caution in patients with obstructive lung disease not associated with bronchoconstriction (eg, bronchitis, emphysema), and avoid use in patients with bronchoconstriction or bronchospasm (eg, asthma). Discontinue adenosine in any patient who develops severe respiratory difficulties.

➤*Pregnancy: Category C.* Animal reproduction studies have not been conducted with adenosine, nor have studies been performed in pregnant women. Because adenosine is a naturally occurring material widely dispersed throughout the body, no fetal effects would be anticipated. However, because it is not known whether the drug can cause fetal harm when administered to pregnant women, use during pregnancy only if clearly needed.

➤*Lactation:* Because adenosine is used only by IV injection in acute care situations, it is doubtful that any reports will be located describing the use of adenosine during human lactation. In addition, the serum half-life is so short that it is unlikely that any of the drug will pass into human breast-milk.

➤*Children:* No controlled studies have been conducted in children to establish the safety and efficacy of adenosine for the conversion of PSVT. However, IV adenosine has been used for the treatment of PSVT in neonates, infants, children, and adolescents.

➤*Elderly:* In general, use adenosine with caution in elderly patients because this population may have a diminished cardiac function, nodal dysfunction, concomitant diseases, or drug therapy that may alter hemodynamic function and produce severe bradycardia or AV block.

➤*Monitoring:* Monitor blood pressure and cardiac rhythm during and after administration. Monitor for transient asystole.

Drug Interactions

Adenosine Drug Interactions

Precipitant drug	Object drug[a]		Description
Carbamazepine	Adenosine	⬆	Carbamazepine may increase the degree of heart block produced by other agents. Because the primary effect of adenosine is to decrease conduction through the AV node, higher degrees of heart block may be produced in the presence of carbamazepine. Closely monitor cardiac function.
Cardioactive drugs (eg, ACE[b] inhibitors [eg, captopril], antiarrhythmic agents [eg, quinidine], beta-adrenergic blocking agents [eg, propanolol], calcium channel blocking agents [eg, verapamil], cardiac glycosides [eg, digoxin])	Adenosine	⬆	Use adenosine with caution in the presence of these agents because of potential additive or synergistic depressant effects on the sinoatrial and AV nodes. The use of adenosine with digoxin and verapamil may rarely be associated with ventricular fibrillation. Closely monitor cardiac function.
Adenosine	Cardioactive drugs (eg, ACE inhibitors [eg, captopril], antiarrhythmic agents [eg, quinidine], beta-adrenergic blocking agents [eg, propranolol], calcium channel blocking agents [eg, verapamil], cardiac glycosides [eg, digoxin])		
Dipyridamole	Adenosine	⬆	The effects of adenosine are potentiated. Thus, smaller doses of adenosine may be effective in the presence of dipyridamole.
Methylxanthines (eg, caffeine, theophylline)	Adenosine	⬇	The effects of adenosine are antagonized. In the presence of methylxanthines, larger doses of adenosine may be required or adenosine may be ineffective.

[a] ⬆ = object drug increased; ⬇ = object drug decreased.
[b] ACE = angiotensin-converting enzyme.

Adverse Reactions

➤*Cardiovascular:* Facial flushing (18%); chest pain, hypotension, palpitations (less than 1%).

➤*CNS:* Headache, light-headedness (2%); dizziness, numbness, tingling in arms (1%); apprehension (less than 1%).

➤*GI:* Nausea (3%); metallic taste, pressure in groin, tightness in throat (less than 1%).

➤*Musculoskeletal:* Heaviness in arms, neck/back pain (less than 1%).

➤*Respiratory:* Dyspnea (12%); hyperventilation (less than 1%).

➤*Miscellaneous:* Chest pressure (7%); blurred vision, burning sensation, head pressure, sweating (less than 1%).

ADENOSINE — INJECTION

➤*Postmarketing:*

Cardiovascular – Atrial fibrillation, bradycardia, prolonged asystole, torsades de pointes, transient increase in blood pressure, ventricular fibrillation, ventricular tachycardia.

CNS – Loss of consciousness and seizure activity, including generalized tonic-clonic seizures.

Respiratory – Bronchospasm.

Overdosage

➤*Symptoms:* The half-life of adenosine is less than 10 seconds. Adverse effects are generally rapidly self-limiting.

➤*Treatment:* Individualize treatment of prolonged adverse effects and direct toward the specific effect. Methylxanthines, such as caffeine and theophylline, are competitive antagonists of adenosine. Refer to General Management of Acute Overdosage.

Patient Information

Instruct patients to report the following symptoms to their health care provider: chest pressure, dizziness, facial flushing, headache, light-headedness, nausea, numbness, shortness of breath, or tingling in arms.

DOFETILIDE

Rx	Tikosyn (Pfizer)	Capsules: 125 mcg	(TKN 125 PFIZER). Light orange/white. In 14s, 60s, and UD 40s.
		250 mcg	(TKN 250 PFIZER). Peach. In 14s, 60s, and UD 40s.
		500 mcg	(TKN 500 PFIZER). Peach/white. In 14s, 60s, and UD 40s.

DOFETILIDE — ORAL

WARNING

To minimize the risk of induced arrhythmia, patients initiated or re-initiated on dofetilide should be placed for a minimum of 3 days in a facility that can provide calculations of creatinine clearance, continuous electrocardiographic monitoring, and cardiac resuscitation. For detailed instructions regarding dose selection, see Administration and Dosage. Dofetilide is available only to hospitals and prescribers who have received appropriate dofetilide dosing and treatment initiation education.

Indications

➤*Maintenance of normal sinus rhythm (delay in AF/AFl recurrence):* Maintenance of normal sinus rhythm (delay in time to recurrence of atrial fibrillation/atrial flutter [AF/AFl]) in patients with atrial fibrillation/atrial flutter of more than 1 week duration who have been converted to normal sinus rhythm. Because dofetilide can cause life-threatening ventricular arrhythmia, it should be reserved for patients in whom atrial fibrillation/atrial flutter is highly symptomatic.

➤*Conversion of atrial fibrillation/flutter:* Conversion of atrial fibrillation and atrial flutter to normal sinus rhythm.

➤*Off-label uses:* Ventricular arrhythmias (inconclusive data).

Administration and Dosage

➤*General dosing considerations:* Therapy with dofetilide must be initiated (and, if necessary, reinitiated) in a setting that provides continuous electrocardiographic (ECG) monitoring and in the presence of personnel trained in the management of serious ventricular arrhythmias. Patients should continue to be monitored in this way for a minimum of 3 days. Additionally, patients should not be discharged within 12 hours of electrical or pharmacological conversion to normal sinus rhythm.

The dose of dofetilide must be individualized according to calculated creatinine clearance (CrCl) and QTc (QT interval should be used if the heart rate is less than 60 bpm. There are no data on use of dofetilide when the heart rate is less than 50 bpm).

Patients with AF should be anticoagulated according to usual medical practice prior to electrical or pharmacological cardioversion. Anticoagulant therapy may be continued after cardioversion according to usual medical practice for the treatment of people with AF. Hypokalemia should be corrected before initiation of dofetilide therapy.

Patients to be discharged on dofetilide therapy from an inpatient setting as described must have an adequate supply of dofetilide at the patient's individualized dose to allow uninterrupted dosing until the patient receives the first outpatient supply.

Dofetilide is distributed only to those hospitals and other appropriate institutions confirmed to have received applicable dosing and treatment initiation education programs. Inpatient and subsequent outpatient discharge and refill prescriptions are filled only upon confirmation that the prescribing health care provider has received applicable dosing and treatment initiation education programs. For this purpose, a list for use by pharmacists is maintained containing hospitals and health care providers who have received one of the education programs.

➤*Adults:*

Conversion of atrial fibrillation/flutter –

Maximum dose: The maximum recommended dose in patients with a calculated CrCl more than 60 mL/min is 500 mcg twice daily; doses more than 500 mcg twice daily have been associated with an increased incidence of torsade de pointes.

Initial dosage: Prior to administration of the first dose, the QTc must be determined using an average of 5 to 10 beats. If the QTc is more than 440 msec (500 msec in patients with ventricular conduction abnormalities), dofetilide is contraindicated. If heart rate is less than 60 bpm, QT interval should be used. Patients with heart rates less than 50 bpm have not been studied.

Dofetilide Starting Dose Determination	
Calculated CrCl	Dofetilide dose
> 60 mL/min	500 mcg twice daily
40 to 60 mL/min	250 mcg twice daily
20 to < 40 mL/min	125 mcg twice daily
< 20 mL/min	Dofetilide is contraindicated in these patients.

Administer the adjusted dofetilide dose and begin continuous ECG monitoring.

Dosage adjustment: At 2 to 3 hours after administering the first dose of dofetilide, determine the QTc. If the QTc has increased by more than 15% compared with the baseline established in step 1 or if the QTc is more than 500 msec (550 msec in patients with ventricular conduction abnormalities), subsequent dosing should be adjusted.

Subsequent Dofetilide Dosing	
If starting dose based on CrCl is:	Then the adjusted dose (for QTc prolongation) is:
500 mcg twice daily	250 mcg twice daily
250 mcg twice daily	125 mcg twice daily
125 mcg twice daily	125 mcg once daily

At 2 to 3 hours after each subsequent dose of dofetilide, determine the QTc (for in-hospital doses 2 to 5). No further down titration of dofetilide based on QTc is recommended.

Alternative dosage: In clinical trials, the highest dose of 500 mcg twice daily of dofetilide as modified by the dosing algorithm led to greater effectiveness than lower doses of 125 or 250 mcg twice daily as modified by the dosing algorithm. The risk of torsade de pointes, however, is related to dose as well as to patient characteristics. Health care providers, in consultation with their patients, may choose doses lower than determined by the algorithm in some cases. It is critically important that if at any time this lower dose is increased, the patient needs to be rehospitalized for 3 days. Previous toleration of higher doses does not eliminate the need for rehospitalization.

Conversion: Before initiating therapy when switching to dofetilide from class I or other class III antiarrhythmic therapy, previous antiarrhythmic therapy should be withdrawn under careful monitoring for a minimum of 3 plasma half-lives. Because of the unpredictable pharmacokinetics of amiodarone, dofetilide should not be initiated following amiodarone therapy until amiodarone plasma levels are below 0.3 mcg/mL or until amiodarone has been withdrawn for at least 3 months.

Discontinuation of therapy: If at any time after the second dose of dofetilide is given the QTc is more than 500 msec (550 msec in patients with ventricular conduction abnormalities), dofetilide should be discontinued.

If dofetilide needs to be discontinued to allow dosing of other potentially interacting drug(s), a washout period of at least 2 days should be followed before starting the other drug(s).

Monitoring: Patients are to be continuously monitored by ECG for a minimum of 3 days, or for a minimum of 12 hours after electrical or pharmacological conversion to normal sinus rhythm, whichever is greater.

Renal function and QTc should be reevaluated every 3 months or as medically warranted. If QTc exceeds 500 msec (550 msec in patients with ventricular conduction abnormalities), dofetilide therapy should be discontinued and patients should be carefully monitored until QTc returns to baseline levels. If renal function deteriorates, adjust dose as described in Initial Dosage.

Maintenance of normal sinus rhythm (delay in atrial fibrillation/atrial flutter recurrence) – See Conversion of atrial fibrillation/flutter for dosing.

➤*Elderly:* Because elderly patients are more likely to have decreased renal function with a reduced CrCl, care must be taken in dose selection.

➤*Renal function impairment:* The overall systemic clearance of dofetilide is decreased and plasma concentration increased with decreasing CrCl. The dose of dofetilide must be adjusted based on CrCl.

➤*Hepatic function impairment:* No additional dose adjustment is required for patients with mild or moderate hepatic impairment. Patients

DOFETILIDE — ORAL

with severe hepatic impairment have not been studied. Dofetilide should be used with particular caution in these patients.

➤*Cardioversion:* If patients do not convert to normal sinus rhythm within 24 hours of initiation of dofetilide therapy, electrical conversion should be considered. Patients continuing on dofetilide after successful electrical cardioversion should continue to be monitored by ECG for 12 hours postcardioversion, or a minimum of 3 days after initiation of dofetilide therapy, whichever is greater.

➤*Administration:* A patient who misses a dose should not double the next dose. The next dose should be taken at the usual time.

➤*Storage / Stability:* Store at 15° to 30°C (59° to 86°F). Protect from moisture and humidity.

Actions

➤*Pharmacology:* Dofetilide shows Vaughan Williams Class III antiarrhythmic activity. The mechanism of action is blockade of the cardiac ion channel carrying the rapid component of the delayed rectifier potassium current, I_{Kr}. At concentrations covering several orders of magnitude, dofetilide blocks only I_{Kr} with no relevant block of the other repolarizing potassium currents (eg, I_{Ks}, I_{K1}). At clinically relevant concentrations, dofetilide has no effect on sodium channels (associated with Class I effect), adrenergic alpha receptors, or adrenergic beta receptors.

➤*Pharmacokinetics:*

Absorption / Distribution – The oral bioavailability of dofetilide is more than 90%, with maximal plasma concentrations occurring at about 2 to 3 hours in the fasted state. Oral bioavailability is unaffected by food or antacid. The terminal half life of dofetilide is approximately 10 hours; steady state plasma concentrations are attained within 2 to 3 days, with an accumulation index of 1.5 to 2. Plasma concentrations are dose proportional. Plasma protein binding of dofetilide is 60% to 70%, is independent of plasma concentration, and is unaffected by renal impairment. Volume of distribution is 3 L/kg.

Metabolism / Excretion – Approximately 80% of a single dose of dofetilide is excreted in urine, of which approximately 80% is excreted as unchanged dofetilide with the remaining 20% consisting of inactive or minimally active metabolites. Renal elimination involves both glomerular filtration and active tubular secretion (via the cation transport system, a process that can be inhibited by cimetidine, trimethoprim, prochlorperazine, megestrol and ketoconazole). In vitro studies with human liver microsomes show that dofetilide can be metabolized by CYP3A4, but it has a low affinity for this isoenzyme. Metabolites are formed by N-dealkylation and N-oxidation. There are no quantifiable metabolites circulating in plasma, but 5 metabolites have been identified in urine.

Special populations –

Renal function impairment: In volunteers with varying degrees of renal impairment and patients with arrhythmias, the clearance of dofetilide decreases with decreasing creatinine clearance. As a result, and as seen in clinical studies, the half-life of dofetilide is longer in patients with lower creatinine clearances. Because increase in QT interval and the risk of ventricular arrhythmias are directly related to plasma concentrations of dofetilide, dosage adjustment based on calculated creatinine clearance is critically important. Patients with severe renal impairment (creatinine clearance less than 20 mL/min) were not included in clinical or pharmacokinetic studies.

Contraindications

Congenital or acquired long QT syndromes. Dofetilide should not be used in patients with a baseline QT interval or QTc more than 440 msec (500 msec in patients with ventricular conduction abnormalities).

Severe renal impairment (calculated creatinine clearance less than 20 mL/min).

Concomitant use with verapamil or the cation transport system inhibitors cimetidine, trimethoprim (alone or in combination with sulfamethoxazole) or ketoconazole; other known inhibitors of the renal cation transport system such as prochlorperazine and megestrol should not be used in patients on dofetilide.

Hypersensitivity to the drug.

Warnings/Precautions

➤*Ventricular arrhythmia:* Dofetilide can cause serious ventricular arrhythmias, primarily torsade de pointes (TdP) type ventricular tachycardia, a polymorphic ventricular tachycardia associated with QT interval prolongation. QT interval prolongation is directly related to dofetilide plasma concentration. Factors such as reduced creatinine clearance or certain dofetilide drug interactions will increase dofetilide plasma concentration. The risk of TdP can be reduced by controlling the plasma concentration through adjustment of the initial dofetilide dose according to creatinine clearance and by monitoring the ECG for excessive increases in the QT interval.

Treatment with dofetilide must therefore be started only in patients placed for a minimum of 3 days in a facility that can provide electrocardiographic monitoring and in the presence of personnel trained in the management of serious ventricular arrhythmias. Calculation of the creatinine clearance for all patients must precede administration of the first dose of dofetilide. For detailed instructions regarding dose selection, see Administration and Dosage.

The risk of dofetilide-induced ventricular arrhythmia was assessed in 3 ways in clinical studies:

1.) by description of the QT interval and its relation to the dose and plasma concentration of dofetilide;
2.) by observing the frequency of TdP in dofetilide-treated patients according to dose;
3.) by observing the overall mortality rate in patients with atrial fibrillation and in patients with structural heart disease.

Relation of QT interval to dose – The QT interval increases linearly with increasing dofetilide dose.

Frequency of torsade de pointes –

Summary of Torsade de Pointes in Patients Randomized to Dofetilide by Dose; Patients with Supraventricular Arrhythmias

	Dofetilide dose				
	< 250 mcg twice daily (n = 217)	250 mcg twice daily (n = 388)	> 250 to 500 mcg twice daily (n = 703)	> 500 mcg twice daily (n = 38)	All doses (n = 1,346)
Torsade de pointes	0	1 (0.3%)	6 (0.9%)	4 (10.5%)	11 (0.8%)

Incidence of Torsade de Pointes before and after Introduction of Dofetilide Dosing According to Renal Function

Population	Total n/N %	Before n/N %	After n/N %
Supraventricular arrhythmias	11/1,346 (0.8%)	6/193 (3.1%)	5/1,153 (0.4%)
DIAMOND CHF	25/762 (3.3%)	7/148 (4.7%)	18/614 (2.9%)
DIAMOND MI	7/749 (0.9%)	3/101 (3%)	4/648 (0.6%)
DIAMOND AF	4/249 (1.6%)	0/43 (0%)	4/206 (1.9%)

The majority of the episodes of TdP occurred within the first 3 days of dofetilide therapy (10/11 events in the studies of patients with supraventricular arrhythmias; 19/25 and 4/7 events in DIAMOND CHF and DIAMOND MI, respectively; 2/4 events in the DIAMOND AF subpopulation).

Mortality – In a pooled survival analysis of patients in the supraventricular arrhythmia population (low prevalence of structural heart disease), deaths occurred in 0.9% (12/1346) of patients receiving dofetilide and 0.4% (3/677) in the placebo group. Adjusted for duration of therapy, primary diagnosis, age, gender, and prevalence of structural heart disease, the point estimate of the hazard ratio for the pooled studies (dofetilide/placebo) was 1.1 (95% CI: 0.3, 4.3). The DIAMOND CHF and MI trials examined mortality in patients with structural heart disease (ejection fraction less than or equal to 35%). In these large, double-blind studies, deaths occurred in 36% (541/1511) of dofetilide patients and 37% (560/1517) of placebo patients. In an analysis of 506 DIAMOND patients with atrial fibrillation/flutter at baseline, 1–year mortality on dofetilide was 31% vs 32% on placebo.

Because of the small number of events, an excess mortality due to dofetilide cannot be ruled out with confidence in the pooled survival analysis of placebo-controlled trials in patients with supraventricular arrhythmias. However, it is reassuring that in 2 large placebo-controlled mortality studies in patients with significant heart disease (DIAMOND CHF/MI), there were no more deaths in dofetilide-treated patients than in patients given placebo.

➤*Women:* Female patients constituted 32% of the patients in the placebo-controlled trials of dofetilide. As with other drugs that cause torsade de pointes, dofetilide was associated with a greater risk of torsade de pointes in female patients than in male patients. During the dofetilide clinical development program the risk of torsade de pointes in females was approximately 3 times the risk in males. Unlike torsade de pointes, the incidence of other ventricular arrhythmias was similar in female patients receiving dofetilide and patients receiving placebo. Although no study specifically investigated this risk, in post-hoc analyses, no increased mortality was observed in females on dofetilide compared with females on placebo.

➤*Cardiac conduction disturbances:* Animal and human studies have not shown any adverse effects of dofetilide on conduction velocity. No effect on AV nodal conduction following dofetilide treatment was noted in healthy volunteers and in patients with first-degree heart block. Patients with sick sinus syndrome or with second— or third-degree heart block were not included in the Phase 3 clinical trials unless a functioning pacemaker was present. Dofetilide has been used safely in conjunction with pacemakers (53 patients in DIAMOND studies, 136 in trials in patients with ventricular and supraventricular arrhythmias).

➤*Renal function impairment:* The overall systemic clearance of dofetilide is decreased and plasma concentration increased with decreasing creatinine clearance. The dose of dofetilide must be adjusted based on creatinine clearance. Patients undergoing dialysis were not included in clinical studies, and appropriate dosing recommendations for these patients are unknown. There is no information about the effectiveness of hemodialysis in removing dofetilide from plasma.

➤*Hepatic function impairment:* After adjustment for creatinine clearance, no additional dose adjustment is required for patients with mild or moderate hepatic impairment. Patients with severe hepatic impairment have not been studied. Dofetilide should be used with particular caution in these patients.

➤*Pregnancy: Category C.* Dofetilide has been shown to adversely affect in utero growth and survival of rats and mice when orally administered during organogenesis at doses of 2 or more mg/kg/day. Other than an increased inci-

DOFETILIDE — ORAL

dence of nonossified fifth metacarpal, and the occurrence of hydroureter and hydronephroses at doses as low as 1 mg/kg/day in the rat, structural anomalies associated with drug treatment were not observed in either species at doses below 2 mg/kg/day. The clearest drug-effect associations were for sternebral and vertebral anomalies in both species; cleft palate, adactyly, levocardia, dilation of cerebral ventricles, hydroureter, hydronephroses, and unossified metacarpal in the rat; and increased incidence of unossified calcaneum in the mouse. The "no observed adverse effect dose" in both species was 0.5 mg/kg/day. The mean dofetilide $AUCs_{(0\text{-}24h)}$ at this dose in the rat and mouse are estimated to be about equal to the maximum likely human AUC and about half the likely human AUC, respectively. There are no adequate and well controlled studies in pregnant women. Therefore, dofetilide should only be administered to pregnant women where the benefit to the patient justifies the potential risk to the fetus.

➤*Lactation:* There is no information on the presence of dofetilide in breast milk. Patients should be advised not to breast-feed an infant if they are taking dofetilide.

➤*Children:* The safety and effectiveness of dofetilide in children (younger than 18 years old) has not been established.

➤*Elderly:* Because elderly patients are more likely to have decreased renal function with a reduced creatinine clearance, care must be taken in dose selection.

Drug Interactions

Because there is a linear relationship between dofetilide plasma concentration and QTc, concomitant drugs that interfere with the metabolism or renal elimination of dofetilide may increase the risk of arrhythmia (torsade de pointes). Dofetilide is metabolized to a small degree by the CYP3A4 isoenzyme of the cytochrome P450 system and an inhibitor of this system could increase systemic dofetilide exposure. More important, dofetilide is eliminated by cationic renal secretion, and 3 inhibitors of this process have been shown to increase systemic dofetilide exposure. The magnitude of the effect on renal elimination by cimetidine, trimethoprim and ketoconazole (all contraindicated concomitant uses with dofetilide) suggests that all renal cation transport inhibitors should be contraindicated.

➤*QT prolongation:* An additive effect of dofetilide with other drugs that prolong the QT interval cannot be excluded. The following drugs may prolong the QT interval and increase the risk of life-threatening cardiac arrhythmias, including torsade de pointes: Antiarrhythmic agents (eg, amiodarone, bretylium, disopyramide, procainamide, quinidine, and sotalol), arsenic trioxide, chlorpromazine, cisapride, dolasetron, droperidol, mefloquine, mesoridazine, moxifloxacin, pentamidine, pimozide, tacrolimus, thioridazine, and ziprasidone. For a more complete list of drugs that may prolong the QT interval, see the appendix, Drug-Induced Prolongation of the QT Interval and Torsade de Pointes.

➤*Potential drug interactions:* Dofetilide is eliminated in the kidney by cationic secretion. Inhibitors of renal cationic secretion are contraindicated with dofetilide. In addition, drugs that are actively secreted via this route (eg, triamterene, metformin, amiloride) should be coadministered with care as they might increase dofetilide levels.

Dofetilide is metabolized to a small extent by the CYP3A4 isoenzyme of the cytochrome P450 system. Inhibitors of the CYP3A4 isoenzyme could increase systemic dofetilide exposure. Inhibitors of this isoenzyme (eg, macrolide antibiotics, azole antifungal agents, protease inhibitors, serotonin reuptake inhibitors, amiodarone, cannabinoids, diltiazem, grapefruit juice, nefazadone, norfloxacin, quinine, zafirlukast) should be cautiously coadministered with dofetilide as they can potentially increase dofetilide levels. Dofetilide is not an inhibitor of CYP3A4 nor of other cytochrome P450 isoenzymes (eg, CYP2C9, CYP2D6) and is not expected to increase levels of drugs metabolized by CYP3A4.

Dofetilide Drug Interactions			
Precipitant drug	Object drug[a]		Description
Amiloride Metformin Megestrol Prochlorperazine Triamterene	Dofetilide	⬆	Inhibitors of dofetilide elimination of renal cationic secretion are contraindicated. Use caution when coadministering drugs actively secreted via cationic secretion as they might increase dofetilide levels.
Antiarrhythmic agents (Class I or Class III)	Dofetilide	⬆	Withhold Class I or Class III antiarrhythmic agents for ≥ 3 plasma half-lives prior to dofetilide dosing.
Bepridil Certain oral macrolides Cisapride Phenothiazines Tricyclic antidepressants	Dofetilide	⬆	Administration of drugs that prolong the QT interval have not been studied in conjunction with dofetilide administration and are not recommended for coadministration.
Cimetidine	Dofetilide	⬆	Concomitant use of cimetidine is contraindicated. Cimetidine increased dofetilide plasma levels by 58%. Use omeprazole, ranitidine, or antacids as an alternative to cimetidine.
Digoxin	Dofetilide	⬌	A higher occurrence of torsades de pointes was associated in patients concomitantly administered digoxin with dofetilide.
Ketoconazole	Dofetilide	⬆	Concomitant use of ketoconazole is contraindicated. Ketoconazole increased dofetilide C_{max} and AUC by 53% and 41% in males and 97% and 69% in females, respectively.
Potassium-depleting diuretics	Dofetilide	⬆	Hypokalemia or hypomagnesemia may occur with administration of potassium-depleting diuretics, increasing the potential for torsades de pointes. Potassium levels should be within normal range prior to administration of dofetilide and maintained in the normal range during dofetilide administration.
Trimethoprim Trimethoprim/sulfamethoxazole	Dofetilide	⬆	Concomitant use of trimethoprim alone or in combination with sulfamethoxazole is contraindicated. Coadministration increased dofetilide AUC by 103% and C_{max} by 93%
Verapamil	Dofetilide	⬆	Concomitant use of verapamil is contraindicated. Dofetilide peak plasma concentrations increased by 42% when coadministered with verapamil, although overall exposure to dofetilide was not significantly increased. Concomitant administration was associated with a higher occurrence of torsades de pointes.

[a] ⬆ = Object drug increased. ⬌ = Undetermined clinical effect.

➤*Drug/Food interactions:* Grapefruit juice can potentially increase dofetilide levels.

Adverse Reactions

In studies of patients with supraventricular arrhythmias a total of 1,346 and 677 patients were exposed to dofetilide and placebo for 551 and 207 patient years, respectively. A total of 8.7% of patients in the dofetilide groups were discontinued from clinical trials due to adverse events compared to 8% in the placebo groups. The most frequent reason for discontinuation (greater than 1%) was ventricular tachycardia (2% on dofetilide vs 1.3% on placebo). The most frequent adverse events were headache, chest pain, and dizziness.

➤*Serious arrhythmias and conduction disturbances:* Torsade de pointes is the only arrhythmia that showed a dose-response relationship to dofetilide treatment. It did not occur in placebo-treated patients. The incidence of torsade de pointes in patients with supraventricular arrhythmias was 0.8% (11 of 1,346). The incidence of torsade de pointes in patients who were dosed according to the recommended dosing regimen was 0.8% (4 of 525).

Dofetilide vs. Placebo: Incidence of Serious Arrhythmias and Conduction Disturbances in Patients with Supraventricular Arrhythmias					
	Dofetilide dose				
Arrhythmia event	< 250 mcg twice daily (n = 217)	250 mcg twice daily (n = 388)	> 250 to 500 mcg twice daily (n = 703)	> 500 mcg twice daily (n = 38)	Placebo (n = 677)
Ventricular arrhythmias[a,b]	3.7%	2.6%	3.4%	15.8%	2.7%
Ventricular fibrillation	0%	0.3%	0.4%	2.6%	0.1%
Ventricular tachycardia[b]	3.7%	2.6%	3.3%	13.2%	2.5%
Torsade de pointes	0%	0.3%	0.9%	10.5%	0%
Various forms of block					
AV block	0.9%	1.5%	0.4%	0%	0.3%
Bundle branch block	0%	0.5%	0.1%	0%	0.1%
Heart block	0%	0.5%	0.1%	0%	0.1%

[a] Patients with more than 1 arrhythmia are counted only once in this category.
[b] Ventricular arrhythmias and ventricular tachycardia include all cases of torsade de pointes.

DOFETILIDE — ORAL

In the DIAMOND trials a total of 1511 patients were exposed to dofetilide for 1757 patient years. The incidence of torsade de pointes was 3.3% in CHF patients and 0.9% in patients with a recent MI.

Dofetilide vs. Placebo: Incidence of Serious Arrhythmias and Conduction Disturbances in Patients with AF at Entry to the DIAMOND Studies		
Arrhythmia	Dofetilide (n = 249)	Placebo (n = 257)
Ventricular arrhythmias[a,b]	14.5%	13.6%
Ventricular fibrillation	4.8%	3.1%
Ventricular tachycardia[b]	12.4%	11.3%
Torsade de pointes	1.6%	0%
Various forms of block		
AV block	0.8%	2.7%
(Left) bundle branch block	0%	0.4%
Heart block	1.2%	0.8%

[a] Patients with more than 1 arrhythmia are counted only once in this category.
[b] Ventricular arrhythmias and ventricular tachycardia include all cases of torsade de pointes.

➤*Other adverse reactions:*

Adverse Reactions with Dofetilide vs Placebo in Patients with Supraventricular Arrhythmias (> 2%)		
Adverse reactions	Dofetilide	Placebo
Headache	11%	9%
Chest pain	10%	7%
Dizziness	8%	6%
Respiratory tract infection	7%	5%
Dyspnea	6%	5%
Nausea	5%	4%
Flu syndrome	4%	2%
Insomnia	4%	3%
Accidental injury	3%	1%
Back pain	3%	2%
Procedure (medical/surgical/ health service)	3%	2%
Diarrhea	3%	2%
Rash	3%	2%
Abdominal pain	3%	2%

Adverse events reported at a rate more than 2% but no more frequently on dofetilide than on placebo were angina pectoris, anxiety, arthralgia, asthenia, atrial fibrillation, complications (application, injection, incision, insertion, or device), hypertension, pain, palpitation, peripheral edema, supraventricular tachycardia, sweating, urinary tract infection, and ventricular tachycardia.

The following adverse events have been reported with a frequency of less than or equal to 2% and numerically more frequently with dofetilide than placebo in patients with supraventricular arrhythmias: angioedema, bradycardia, cerebral ischemia, cerebrovascular accident, edema, facial paralysis, flaccid paralysis, heart arrest, increased cough, liver damage, migraine, myocardial infarct, paralysis, paresthesia, sudden death, and syncope.

The incidences of clinically significant laboratory test abnormalities in patients with supraventricular arrhythmias were similar for patients on dofetilide and those on placebo. No clinically relevant effects were noted in serum alkaline phosphatase, serum GGT, LDH, AST, ALT, total bilirubin, total protein, blood urea nitrogen, creatinine, serum electrolytes (calcium, chloride, glucose, magnesium, potassium, sodium) or creatine kinase. Similarly, no clinically relevant effects were observed in hematologic parameters.

In the DIAMOND population, adverse events other than those related to the postinfarctionand heart failure patient population were generally similar to those seen in the supraventricular arrhythmia groups.

Overdosage

➤*Symptoms:* Dofetilide overdose was rare in clinical studies; there were two reported cases of dofetilide overdose in the oral clinical program. One patient received very high multiples of the recommended dose (28 capsules), was treated with gastric aspiration 30 minutes later, and experienced no events. One patient inadvertently received two 500 mcg doses 1 hour apart and experienced ventricular fibrillation and cardiac arrest 2 hours after the second dose.

In the supraventricular arrhythmia population only 38 patients received doses greater than 500 mcg twice daily, all of whom received 750 mcg twice daily irrespective of creatinine clearance. In this very small patient population the incidence of torsade de pointes was 10.5% (4/38 patients), and the incidence of new ventricular fibrillation was 2.6% (1/38 patients).

➤*Treatment:* There is no known antidote to dofetilide; treatment of overdose should therefore be symptomatic and supportive. The most prominent manifestation of overdosage is likely to be excessive prolongation of the QT interval.

In cases of overdose cardiac monitoring should be initiated. Charcoal slurry may be given soon after overdosing but has been useful only when given within 15 minutes of dofetilide administration. Treatment of torsade de pointes or overdose may include administration of isoproterenol infusion, with or without cardiac pacing. Administration of intravenous magnesium sulfate may be effective in the management of torsade de pointes. Close medical monitoring and supervision should continue until the QT interval returns to normal levels.

Isoproterenol infusion into anesthetized dogs with cardiac pacing rapidly attenuates the dofetilide-induced prolongation of atrial and ventricular effective refractory periods in a dose-dependent manner. Magnesium sulfate, administered prophylactically either intravenously or orally in a dog model, was effective in the prevention of dofetilide-induced torsade de pointes ventricular tachycardia. Similarly, in man, intravenous magnesium sulfate may terminate torsade de pointes, irrespective of cause.

Patient Information

Prior to initiation of dofetilide therapy, the patient should be advised to read the patient package insert and reread it each time therapy is renewed in case the patient's status has changed. The patient should be fully instructed on the need for compliance with the recommended dosing of dofetilide and the potential for drug interactions, and the need for periodic monitoring of QTc and renal function to minimize the risk of serious abnormal rhythms.

➤*Medications and supplements:* Assessment of patients' medication history should include all over-the-counter, prescription and herbal/natural preparations with emphasis on preparations that may affect the pharmacokinetics of dofetilide such as cimetidine (see Contraindications), trimethoprim alone or in combination with sulfamethoxazole (see Contraindications), prochlorperazine (see Contraindications), megestrol (see Contraindications), ketoconazole (see Contraindications), other cardiovascular drugs (especially verapamil - see Contraindications), phenothiazines, and tricyclic antidepressants (see Warnings). If a patient is taking dofetilide and requires antiulcer therapy, omeprazole, ranitidine or antacids (aluminum and magnesium hydroxides) should be used as alternatives to cimetidine, as these agents have no effect on the pharmacokinetics of dofetilide. Patients should be instructed to notify their health care providers of any change in over-the-counter, prescription or supplement use. If a patient is hospitalized or is prescribed a new medication for any condition, the patient must inform the health care provider of ongoing dofetilide therapy. Patients should also check with their health care provider and/or pharmacist prior to taking a new over-the-counter preparation.

➤*Electrolyte imbalance:* If patients experience symptoms that may be associated with altered electrolyte balance, such as excessive or prolonged diarrhea, sweating, vomiting, loss of appetite, or thirst, these conditions should immediately be reported to their health care provider.

➤*Dosing schedule:* Patients should be instructed not to double the next dose if a dose is missed. The next dose should be taken at the usual time.

Indications

Calcium Channel Blocking Agents – Summary of Indications[a]

Indications ✓ = labeled X = off-label	Amlodipine	Diltiazem	Diltiazem SR	Diltiazem ER	Diltiazem IV[i]	Felodipine	Isradipine	Nicardipine	Nicardipine SR	Nicardipine IV	Nifedipine	Nifedipine ER	Nimodipine	Nisoldipine	Verapamil	Verapamil SR	Verapamil ER	Verapamil IV
Angina pectoris																		
Vasospastic	✓	✓		✓							✓	✓[b]			✓		✓[c]	
Chronic stable	✓	✓		✓				✓			✓	✓[b]			✓		✓[c]	
Unstable															✓		✓[c]	
Hypertension	✓		✓	✓		✓	✓	✓	✓	✓		✓		✓	✓	✓	✓	
Pediatric hypertension						X[d]	X[d]					X[d]						
Pediatric hypertension urgency or emergency							X[d]			X[d]								
Subarachnoid hemorrhage													✓					
Atrial fibrillation/flutter					✓													✓
Paroxysmal supraventricular tachycardia					✓										✓[d]			✓
Unlabeled uses																		
Anal fissures		X[f]									X[f]							
Anal sphincter pressure reduction (topical)		X[g]																
Cluster headaches															X[h]			
Hypertrophic cardiomyopathy															X[h]			
Idiopathic muscle cramps		X[f]																
Postherpetic neuralgia								X[g]										
Prevention of migraine (adults)													X[g]		X[f]			
Pulmonary hypertension	X[h]	X[h]				X[h]					X[h]							
Raynaud phenomenon	X[h]	X[h]				X[h]	X[h]				X[e]							
Preterm labor											X[h]							
Ureteral stones											X[g]							
Wound healing (topical)											X[g]							

[a] For more detailed information, see the information below and individual drug monographs.
[b] Except *Adalat CC*.
[c] *Covera-HS* only.
[d] For prophylaxis of repetitive paroxysmal supraventricular tachycardia.
[e] Good documentation.
[f] Fair documentation.
[g] Insufficient documentation.
[h] Not rated.
[i] IV = intravenous; SR = sustained release; ER = extended-release.

➤*Vasospastic (Prinzmetal or variant) angina (amlodipine, diltiazem immediate release and ER, nifedipine immediate release and ER [except Adalat CC], verapamil immediate release and ER [Covera-HS only]):* Treatment of spontaneous coronary artery spasm presenting as Prinzmetal variant angina (resting angina with ST segment elevation during attacks).

➤*Chronic stable (classic effort-associated) angina (amlodipine, diltiazem immediate release and ER, nicardipine immediate release, nifedipine immediate release and ER [except Adalat CC], verapamil immediate release and ER [Covera-HS only]):* For the treatment of chronic stable angina, alone or in combination with other antianginals.

➤*Unstable angina at rest:* **Verapamil** immediate release and ER (*Covera-HS* only).

➤*Hypertension:* **Amlodipine**, **clevidipine** IV, **diltiazem** SR and ER, **felodipine**, **isradipine**, **nicardipine** immediate release and ER, **nicardipine** IV, **nifedipine** ER, **nisoldipine**, and oral **verapamil**.

➤*Subarachnoid hemorrhage (nimodipine only):* For the improvement of neurological outcome by reducing the incidence and severity of ischemic deficits in patients with subarachnoid hemorrhage (SAH) from ruptured intracranial berry aneurysms regardless of their post-ictus neurological condition (ie, Hunt and Hess Grades I to V).

➤*Paroxysmal supraventricular tachycardias (diltiazem IV and verapamil IV):* Rapid conversion of paroxysmal supraventricular tachycardias (PSVT) to sinus rhythm.

➤*Prophylaxis of repetitive PSVT:* **Verapamil** immediate release.

➤*Atrial fibrillation/flutter (diltiazem IV and verapamil IV):* For temporary control of rapid ventricular rate in atrial fibrillation or atrial flutter.

➤*Off-label uses:* Refer to individual monographs for further information.

Anal fissures –
Diltiazem (topical): [2] = Fair documentation.
Nifedipine: [2] = Fair documentation.

Anal sphincter pressure reduction (topical) –
Diltiazem (topical): [4] = Insufficient documentation.

Idiopathic muscle cramps –
Diltiazem: [2] = Fair documentation.

Pediatric hypertension –
Felodipine: [1] = Good documentation.
Isradipine: [1] = Good documentation.
Nifedipine: [1] = Good documentation.

Pediatric hypertensive urgency or emergency –
Isradipine: [1] = Good documentation.
Nicardipine: [1] = Good documentation.

Postherpetic neuralgia –
Nicardipine: [4] = Insufficient documentation.

Prevention of migraine (adults) –
Diltiazem: [5] = Poor documentation.
Nicardipine: [5] = Poor documentation.
Nifedipine: [5] = Poor documentation.
Nimodipine: [4] = Insufficient documentation.
Verapamil: [2] = Fair documentation.

Prevention of migraine (children/adolescents) –
Nimodipine: [5] = Poor documentation.

Raynaud phenomenon –
Nifedipine: [1] = Good documentation.

Ureteral stones –
Nifedipine: [4] = Insufficient documentation.

Wound healing –
Nifedipine (topical): [4] = Insufficient documentation.

Other possible off-label uses –
Verapamil (oral): Prevention of cluster headaches; management of hypertrophic cardiomyopathy.

Actions

➤*Pharmacology:* In specialized automatic and conducting cells in the heart, calcium is involved in genesis of action potential. In contractile cells of the myocardium, it links excitation to contraction and controls energy storage and use. Systemic and coronary arteries are influenced by movement of calcium across cell membranes of vascular smooth muscle. Contractile processes of cardiac and vascular smooth muscle depend on movement of extracellular calcium ions into these cells through specific ion channels.

The calcium channel blockers (ie, slow channel blockers, calcium antagonists), share the ability to inhibit movement of calcium ions across the cell membrane. The effects on the cardiovascular system include depression of mechanical contraction of myocardial and smooth muscle and depression of both impulse formation (automaticity) and conduction velocity. Calcium channel blockers are classified by structure as follows: Diphenylalkylamines – **verapamil**; benzothiazepines – **diltiazem**; dihydropyridines – **amlodipine**, **clevidipine**, **felodipine**, **isradipine**, **nicardipine**, **nifedipine**, **nimodipine**, **nisoldipine**.

Although these agents are similar in that they all act on the slow (calcium) channel, they have different degrees of selectivity in their effects on vascular smooth muscle, myocardium, or specialized conduction and pacemaker tissues. The resulting clinical effects depend on the direct activity of the drug, reflex physiological responses (primarily beta-adrenergic response to vasodilation), and the patient's cardiovascular status. This heterogeneity of the calcium blockers, in part, determines their clinical application and the different side effects produced by each agent.

In animals, **nimodipine** had a greater effect on cerebral arteries than on other arteries, possibly because it is highly lipophilic. While studies show a favorable effect on severity of neurological deficits caused by cerebral vasospasm following SAH, there is no arteriographic evidence that the drug prevents or relieves spasm of these arteries. Therefore, the actual mechanism of action is unknown.

Hemodynamic – (See Pharmacokinetics table.) These agents dilate the coronary arteries and arterioles in normal and ischemic regions and inhibit coronary artery spasm. This increases myocardial oxygen delivery in patients with coronary artery spasm and vasospastic (Prinzmetal or variant) angina.

The drugs reduce arterial blood pressure at rest and with exercise by dilating peripheral arterioles and reducing total peripheral resistance (afterload) against which the heart works. This reduces myocardial energy consumption and oxygen requirements and probably accounts for the efficacy in chronic stable angina.

These agents exhibit a negative inotropic effect, but this is rare because of reflex responses to vasodilation. In patients with normal ventricular function, there may be a small increase in cardiac index without major effects on ejection fraction or left ventricular end diastolic pressure or volume (LVEDP or LVEDV).Usual **verapamil** IV doses may slightly increase left ventricular filling pressure. Acute worsening of heart failure may be seen when **verapamil** is used in moderate to severe cardiac dysfunction. In patients with impaired ventricular function, most acute studies have shown some increase in ejection fraction and reduction in left ventricular filling pressure. **Nicardipine** use in coronary artery disease and normal or moderately abnormal left ventricular function significantly increased ejection fraction and cardiac output with no significant change or a small decrease in LVEDP. Administration of a single dose of **nisoldipine** leads to decreased systemic vascular resistance and blood pressure with a transient increase in heart rate.

Electrophysiology – **Verapamil** slows atrioventricular (AV) conduction and prolongs the effective refractory period (ERP) within the AV node in a rate-related manner, thus reducing ventricular rate because of atrial flutter or atrial fibrillation. By interrupting re-entry at the AV node, verapamil can restore normal sinus rhythm in patients with PSVT, including Wolff-Parkinson-White syndrome. It can interfere with sinus node impulse generation and induce sinus arrest or sinoatrial block in patients with sick sinus syndrome. AV block can occur in patients without preexisting conduction defects. Verapamil decreases the frequency of episodes of PSVT. Verapamil may shorten the antegrade ERP of the accessory bypass tracts. It does not alter the normal atrial action potential or intraventricular conduction time, but it depresses amplitude, velocity of depolarization, and conduction in depressed atrial fibers.

Patients with supraventricular tachycardia convert to normal sinus rhythm within 10 minutes after verapamil IV (approximately 60% to 80%). About 70% of patients with atrial flutter or fibrillation with a fast ventricular rate respond with a decrease in heart rate of at least 20%. Conversion of atrial flutter or fibrillation to sinus rhythm is uncommon (about 10%) after verapamil and may reflect the spontaneous conversion rate. Slowing of the ventricular rate in patients with atrial fibrillation/flutter lasts 30 to 60 minutes after a single injection.

Because a small fraction (less than 1%) of patients treated with verapamil have life-threatening adverse responses, the initial use of verapamil injection should, if possible, be in a treatment setting with monitoring and resuscitation facilities, including direct current (DC)–cardioversion capability. As familiarity with the patient's response is gained, use in an office setting may be acceptable.

Diltiazem decreases sinuatrial (SA) and AV conduction in isolated tissues. Diltiazem IV in doses of 20 mg prolongs AH conduction time and AV node functional and effective refractory periods by approximately 20%. Diltiazem-associated prolongation of the AH interval is not more pronounced in patients with first-degree heart block. In patients with sick sinus syndrome, diltiazem significantly prolongs sinus cycle length (up to 50%).

➤*Pharmacokinetics:*

Calcium Channel Blocking Agents: Pharmacokinetics[a]

	Parameters	Amlodipine	Diltiazem	Felodipine	Isradipine	Nicardipine	Nifedipine	Nimodipine	Nisoldipine	Verapamil
Pharmacokinetics	Extent of absorption (oral) (%)	nd	nd	≈ 100	90-95	≈ 100	100	nd	nd	> 90
	Absolute bioavailability (oral) (%)	64-90	40	≈ 20	15-24	≈ 35	45-75 (IR) 84-89 (ER)	≈ 13	≈ 5	20-35 (IR)
	Vd	nd	≈ 305 L (IV)	10 L/kg	3 L/kg	8.3 L/kg (IV)	nd	nd	nd	nd
	T_{max} (h)	6-12	2-4 (IR) 10-14 (ER) 6-11 (SR)	2.5-5	1.5 (IR) 7-18 (CR)	0.5-2 (IR) 1-4 (ER)	0.5 (IR) 6 (ER)	1	6-12	1-2 (IR) ≈ 11 (ER) ≈ 7-9 (SR)
	Protein binding (%)	93	70-80	> 99	95	> 95	92-98	> 95	> 99	≈ 90
	Metabolism	Hepatic	Hepatic	Hepatic	Hepatic	Hepatic	Hepatic	Hepatic	Hepatic	Hepatic
	Major metabolites	90% converted to inactive	Desacetyl-diltiazem[b]	6 inactive	Mono acids and cyclic lactone[c]	nd	Inactive	Numerous, inactive	5 major urinary metabolites	Norverapamil[d]
	Half-life, elimination (h)	30-50	3-4.5 (IR) 4-9.5 (ER) 5-7 (SR) ≈ 3.4 (IV)	11-16	8	8.6	≈ 2 (IR) ≈ 7 (ER)	≈ 8-9[e]	7-12	2.8-7.4[f] 4.5-12[g] ≈ 12 (SR) 2-5 (IV)
	Clearance, systemic	nd	≈ 65 L/h (IV)	≈ 0.8 L/min	1.4 L/min	0.4 L/h•kg (IV)	nd	nd	nd	nd
	Excreted unchanged in urine (%)	10	2-4	±	0	< 1	< 0.1	< 1	trace	3-4
	Excreted in urine (%)	nd	nd	70	60-65	60 (oral) 49 (IV)	60-80	nd	60-80	≈ 70
	Excreted in feces (%)	nd	nd	10	25-30	35 (oral) 43 (IV)	15	nd	nd	≥ 16

Calcium Channel Blocking Agents: Pharmacokinetics[a]

	Parameters	Amlodipine	Diltiazem	Felodipine	Isradipine	Nicardipine	Nifedipine	Nimodipine	Nisoldipine	Verapamil
ECG Changes	Heart rate	±	0-↓	↑↑	↑	↑↑	0-↑		±	±
	QRS complex	0	nd	0	0	0	nd		0	nd
	PR interval	0	↑	0	0	0	nd		0	↑
	QT interval	0	nd	0	↑	↑	nd		0	nd
Hemodynamics	Myocardial contractility	0-↓	0-↓	0-↓	↓	0-↓	0-↓	na	0-↓	↓↓
	Cardiac output/index	↑	0-↑	nd	↑	↑↑	↑		nd	±
	Peripheral vascular resistance	↓↓	↓↓[h]	↓↓[h]	↓↓	↓↓↓	↓↓↓		↓↓	↓↓

[a] ↑↑↑ or ↓↓↓ = pronounced effect; ↑↑ or ↓↓ = moderate effect; ↑ or ↓ = slight effect; ± = negligible amount or effect; nd = no data; na = not applicable; Vd = volume of distribution; IR = immediate release; T_{max} = time to maximum concentration.

[b] 25% to 50% as potent a coronary vasodilator as diltiazem; plasma levels are 10% to 20% of the parent drug.

[c] Of 6 metabolites identified, accounting for > 75%.

[d] Major metabolite; cardiovascular activity is ≈ 20% that of verapamil.

[e] Earlier elimination rates are much more rapid, equivalent to a half-life of 1 to 2 hours.

[f] After single doses.

[g] After repetitive doses.

[h] Dose-related.

Contraindications

Hypersensitivity to the drug; in patients with known hypersensitivity to dihydropyridine calcium channel blockers (**nisoldipine**); sick sinus syndrome or second- or third-degree AV block except with a functioning pacemaker, hypotension less than 90 mmHg systolic (**diltiazem**, and **verapamil**); concomitant administration with strong cytochrome P450 (CYP-450) inducers (eg, rifampin) or cardiogenic shock (nifedipine).

➤*Clevidipine:* Known allergy to soybeans, soy products, eggs or egg products; defective lipid metabolism (eg, pathologic hyperlipemia, lipoid nephrosis, or acute pancreatitis if accompanied by hyperlipidemia; severe aortic stenosis.

➤*Diltiazem:* Acute myocardial infarction (MI) and pulmonary congestion documented by x-ray on admission.

Injectable –

- Sick sinus syndrome except in the presence of a functioning ventricular pacemaker.
- Second- or third-degree AV block except in the presence of a functioning ventricular pacemaker.
- Severe hypotension or cardiogenic shock.
- IV diltiazem and IV beta-blockers should not be administered together or in close proximity (within a few hours).
- Atrial fibrillation or atrial flutter associated with an accessory bypass tract such as in Wolff-Parkinson-White syndrome or short PR syndrome.
- Initial use of injectable forms of diltiazem should be, if possible, in a setting where monitoring and resuscitation capabilities, including DC cardioversion/defibrillation, are present. Once familiarity of the patient's response is established, use in an office setting may be acceptable.
- Ventricular tachycardia.
- In newborns, because of the presence of benzyl alcohol (*Cardizem Lyo-Ject* syringe only).

➤*Nicardipine:* Advanced aortic stenosis.

➤*Verapamil:* Severe left ventricular dysfunction; cardiogenic shock and severe congestive heart failure (CHF), unless secondary to a supraventricular tachycardia amenable to verapamil therapy, and in patients with atrial flutter or atrial fibrillation and an accessory bypass tract.

Verapamil IV –

- Severe hypotension or cardiogenic shock.
- Second- or third-degree AV block (except in patients with a functioning artificial ventricular pacemaker).
- Sick sinus syndrome (except in patients with a functioning artificial ventricular pacemaker).
- Severe CHF (unless secondary to a supraventricular tachycardia amenable to verapamil therapy).
- IV beta-adrenergic blocking agents. IV verapamil and IV beta-adrenergic blocking drugs should not be administered in close proximity to each other (within a few hours) because both may have a depressant effect on myocardial contractility and AV conduction (see Drug Interactions).
- Patients with atrial flutter or atrial fibrillation and an accessory bypass tract (eg, Wolff-Parkinson-White, Lown-Ganong-Levine syndromes) are at risk to develop ventricular tachyarrhythmia, including ventricular fibrillation if verapamil is administered. Therefore, the use of verapamil in these patients is contraindicated.
- Ventricular tachycardia. Patients with wide-complex ventricular tachycardia (QRS greater than or equal to 0.12 sec) can result in marked hemodynamic deterioration and ventricular fibrillation.
- Known hypersensitivity.

Warnings/Precautions

➤*Hypotension:* Hypotension, usually modest and well tolerated, occasionally may occur during initial titration or with dosage increases, and may be more common in patients taking concomitant beta-blockers. Hypotensive episodes may be caused by excess vasodilation induced by **nifedipine** or by direct cardiopressor effects of **verapamil** and **diltiazem**. Nifedipine has the greatest effect on vascular smooth muscle; therefore, incidence of adverse reactions resulting from vasodilation (eg, headache, flushing) is greater. **Clevidipine** may produce systemic hypotension and reflex tachycardia. Because **amlodipine**-induced hypotension is gradual in onset, acute hypotension rarely has been reported. Nonetheless, exercise caution when administering amlodipine as with any other peripheral vasodilator, particularly in patients with severe aortic stenosis.

Systolic pressure less than 90 mmHg or diastolic pressure less than 60 mmHg was seen in 5% to 10% of patients with supraventricular tachycardia and in about 10% of the patients with atrial flutter/fibrillation who were given IV **verapamil**.

Carefully monitor blood pressure during initial administration and titration. Closely observe patients already taking antihypertensives.

➤*Congestive heart failure:* CHF has developed rarely, usually in patients receiving a beta-blocker, after beginning **nifedipine**. Patients with tight aortic stenosis may be at greater risk, as the unloading effect would be of less benefit to these patients because of their fixed impedance to flow across the aortic valve.

Isradipine and nicardipine – Exercise caution when using isradipine and nicardipine in CHF, particularly in combination with a beta-blocker.

Nisoldipine – Exercise caution when using nisoldipine in patients with heart failure or compromised ventricular function, particularly in combination with a beta-blocker.

Verapamil – Verapamil has a negative inotropic effect that is usually compensated by its afterload reduction (decreased systemic vascular resistance) properties without a net impairment of ventricular performance. In clinical studies with oral **verapamil**, 1.8% developed CHF or pulmonary edema. Avoid verapamil in patients with severe left ventricular dysfunction (ie, ejection fraction less than 30%) or moderate to severe symptoms of cardiac failure and in patients with any degree of ventricular dysfunction if they are receiving a beta-adrenergic blocker. Control patients with milder ventricular dysfunction, if possible, with digitalis or diuretics before verapamil treatment.

Use **diltiazem**, **nisoldipine**, **felodipine**, and **amlodipine** with caution in CHF patients.

➤*Cardiac conduction:* **Verapamil** IV slows AV nodal conduction and SA nodes; it rarely produces second- or third-degree AV block, bradycardia, and in extreme cases, asystole. This is more likely to occur in patients with sick sinus syndrome (which is more common in older patients). Asystole in patients other than those with sick sinus syndrome is usually of short duration (a few seconds or less), with spontaneous return to AV nodal or normal sinus rhythm.

Oral **verapamil** may lead to first-degree AV block and transient bradycardia, sometimes accompanied by nodal escape rhythms. PR-interval prolongation is correlated with verapamil plasma concentrations especially during the early titration phase of therapy. Higher degrees of AV block are infrequent (0.8%). Marked first-degree block or progressive development to second- or third-degree AV block requires dose reduction or discontinuation of verapamil and institution of appropriate therapy, depending on the clinical situation.

Patients with atrial flutter/fibrillation and an accessory AV pathway may develop increased antegrade conduction, producing a very rapid ventricular response or ventricular fibrillation after receiving IV verapamil (or digitalis). Although a risk of this occurring with oral verapamil has not been established, such patients receiving oral verapamil may be at risk and its use in these patients is contraindicated (see Contraindications). Treatment is usually DC cardioversion.

Diltiazem prolongs AV node refractory periods without significantly prolonging sinus node recovery time, except in sick sinus syndrome. This may rarely result in abnormally slow heart rates (particularly in sick sinus syndrome) or second- or third-degree AV block. Concomitant use with beta-adrenergic blockers or digitalis may be additive on cardiac conduction. A patient with Prinzmetal angina developed periods of asystole (2 to 5 seconds) after 60 mg diltiazem. If high-degree AV block occurs in sinus rhythm, discontinue diltiazem IV and institute appropriate supportive measures.

➤*Negative inotropy:* Dihydropyridine calcium channel blockers can produce negative inotropic effects and exacerbate heart failure. Monitor heart failure patients carefully.

➤*Premature ventricular contractions:* During conversion or marked reduction in ventricular rate, benign complexes of unusual appearance (sometimes resembling premature ventricular contractions [PVCs]) may occur after **verapamil** IV. Similar complexes of no clinical significance occur during spontaneous conversion of supraventricular tachycardia after DC cardioversion and other therapy. These complexes appear to have no clinical significance.

➤*Hypertrophic cardiomyopathy:* Serious adverse effects were seen in 120 patients with hypertrophic cardiomyopathy (most refractory or intolerant to propranolol) who received oral **verapamil** at doses up to 720 mg/day. Three patients died with pulmonary edema; all had severe left ventricular outflow obstruction and a history of left ventricular dysfunction. Eight had pulmonary edema or severe hypotension; most had abnormally high (greater than 20 mmHg) pulmonary wedge pressure and a marked left ventricular outflow obstruction. Coadministration of quinidine preceded the severe hypotension in 3 of the 8 patients (2 of whom developed pulmonary edema). Sinus bradycardia occurred in 11%, second-degree AV block in 4% and sinus arrest in 2%. Most adverse effects responded to dose reduction; discontinuation of verapamil was rare.

➤*Antiplatelet effects:* Calcium channel blockers, alone and with aspirin, have caused inhibition of platelet function. Episodes of bruising, petechiae, and bleeding have occurred.

Nifedipine – Decreases platelet aggregation in vitro. Limited clinical studies have demonstrated a moderate but statistically significant decrease in platelet aggregation and increase in bleeding time in some patients. This is thought to be a function of inhibition of calcium transport across the platelet membrane.

➤*Withdrawal syndrome:* Abrupt withdrawal of calcium channel blockers may cause increased frequency and duration of chest pain. The rebound angina is probably the result of the increased flow of calcium into cells causing coronary arteries to spasm. Gradually taper the dose under medical supervision. Results of other studies do not support the occurrence of a withdrawal syndrome; however, caution is still warranted when discontinuing these agents.

➤*Rebound hypertension:* Patients who receive prolonged **clevidipine** infusions and are not transitioned to other antihypertensive therapies should be monitored for the possibility of rebound hypertension for at least 8 hours after the infusion is stopped.

➤*Beta-blocker withdrawal:* Patients recently withdrawn from beta-blockers may develop a withdrawal syndrome with increased angina, probably related to increased sensitivity to catecholamines. Initiation of **nifedipine** will not prevent this occurrence and might exacerbate it by provoking reflex catecholamine release. Taper beta-blockers rather than stopping them abruptly before beginning nifedipine.

Nicardipine – Gradually reduce beta-blocker dose over 8 to 10 days with coadministration.

➤*Lipid intake:* **Clevidipine** contains approximately 0.2 g of lipid per mL (2 kcal). Lipid intake restrictions may be necessary for patients with significant disorders of lipid metabolism. For these patients, a reduction in the quantity of concurrently administered lipids may be necessary to compensate for the amount of lipid infused as part of the clevidipine formulation.

➤*Hepatic function impairment:* Patients with hepatic impairment (liver cirrhosis) have a longer disposition half-life and higher bioavailability of **nifedipine** than healthy volunteers. Protein binding may be greatly reduced in patients with renal or hepatic impairment.

Because **verapamil** is highly metabolized by the liver, it should be administered cautiously to patients with impaired hepatic function. Severe liver dysfunction prolongs the elimination half-life of verapamil to about 14 to 16 hours; therefore, administer approximately 30% of the dose given to patients with normal liver function to these patients. Carefully monitor for abnormal prolongation of the PR interval or other signs of excessive pharmacologic effects.

Bioavailability of nifedipine is increased in hepatic cirrhosis. With **nifedipine** IV, half-life and volume of distribution are increased and plasma protein binding is decreased. Carefully monitor for abnormal prolongation of the PR interval and other signs of excessive pharmacologic effects.

Because **amlodipine**, **diltiazem**, **nicardipine**, **felodipine**, **nisoldipine**, and **nimodipine** are extensively metabolized by the liver, use with caution in impaired hepatic function or reduced hepatic blood flow. In severe liver disease, elevated nicardipine blood levels (4-fold increase in area under the curve [AUC]) and prolonged half-life (19 hours) occurred; patients on nimodipine had an approximately doubled maximum drug concentration. Consider decreasing the dose of calcium channel blockers and monitor drug response (ie, blood pressure, PR interval) in cirrhosis patients.

➤*Renal function impairment:* The pharmacokinetics of **diltiazem** in patients with impaired renal function are similar to the pharmacokinetic profile of patients with normal renal function. However, caution is still advised. About 70% of a dose of **verapamil** is excreted as metabolites in the urine. Administer verapamil cautiously to patients with impaired renal function. Carefully monitor these patients for abnormal prolongation of the PR interval or other signs of overdosage (see Overdosage). Effects of single IV doses should not increase, although duration may be prolonged.

Nicardipine – Mean plasma concentrations, AUC, and maximum concentration were approximately 2-fold higher in patients with mild renal impairment. Doses must be adjusted.

Nifedipine – Although nifedipine has been used safely in patients with renal dysfunction and has exerted a beneficial effect in certain cases, rare, reversible elevations in serum urea nitrogen (BUN) and serum creatinine have occurred in patients with preexisting chronic renal insufficiency. The relationship to therapy is uncertain in most cases but probable in some.

➤*Increased angina:* About 7% of patients developed increased frequency, duration or severity of angina on starting **nicardipine** or at the time of dosage increases. Rarely, patients, particularly those who have severe obstructive coronary artery disease have developed increased frequency, duration, or severity of angina or acute MI on starting **nifedipine** or at the time of dosage increase. The mechanism of these effects have not been established.

➤*Increased intracranial pressure:* **Verapamil** IV has increased intracranial pressure in patients with supratentorial tumors at the time of anesthesia induction. Use with caution and perform appropriate monitoring.

➤*Duchenne muscular dystrophy:* **Verapamil** may decrease neuromuscular transmission in patients with Duchenne muscular dystrophy, prolong recovery from the neuromuscular blocking agent vecuronium, and cause a worsening of myasthenia gravis. It may be necessary to decrease dosage of verapamil when administering it to patients with attenuated neuromuscular transmission. Verapamil IV can precipitate respiratory muscle failure in these patients; therefore, use with caution.

➤*GI narrowing:* As with other nondeformable dosage forms, use caution when administering *Covera HS* in patients with preexisting severe GI narrowing.

➤*Acute hepatic injury:* In rare instances, symptoms consistent with acute hepatic injury, as well as significant elevations in enzymes such as alkaline phosphatase, creatine phosphokinase (CPK), lactate dehydrogenase (LDH), AST, and ALT have occurred with oral **diltiazem** and **nifedipine**. The potential for acute hepatic injury exists following administration of IV diltiazem. These were reversible on drug discontinuation. Drug relationship was uncertain in most cases, but probable in some. These laboratory abnormalities rarely have been associated with clinical symptoms; however, cholestasis with or without jaundice has occurred with nifedipine. Rare instances of allergic hepatitis also occurred with nifedipine.

Elevations of transaminases with and without concomitant elevations in alkaline phosphatase and bilirubin have occurred with **verapamil**. Elevations sometimes have been transient and may disappear with continued verapamil treatment. Several cases of hepatocellular injury related to verapamil have been proven by rechallenge; half of these cases had clinical symptoms (malaise, fever, or right upper quadrant pain) in addition to elevations of AST, ALT, and alkaline phosphatase. Periodically monitor liver function in patients treated with verapamil.

Isolated cases of elevated LDH, alkaline phosphatase, and ALT levels have occurred rarely with **nimodipine**.

➤*Edema:* Mild to moderate peripheral edema, typically associated with arterial vasodilation and not caused by left ventricular dysfunction, occurs in 10% to about 30% of patients receiving **nifedipine**. It occurs primarily in the lower extremities and usually responds to diuretic therapy. With patients whose angina is complicated by CHF, differentiate this peripheral edema from the effects of increasing left ventricular dysfunction.

Peripheral edema, generally mild and not associated with generalized fluid retention, may occur with **felodipine** within 2 to 3 weeks of therapy initiation. The incidence is both age- and dose-dependent, with frequency ranging from about 10% in patients under 50 years of age taking 5 mg/day to about 30% in patients over 60 years of age taking 20 mg/day.

➤*Pregnancy: Category C.* Teratogenic and embryotoxic effects have been demonstrated in small animals, usually at doses higher than the usual human dosage. There are no well-controlled studies in pregnant women. Use during pregnancy only when clearly needed and when potential benefits outweigh potential hazards to the fetus.

Amlodipine – Significantly decreased litter size (by about 50%) and significantly increased the number of intrauterine deaths (about 5-fold) in rats administered 10 mg/kg amlodipine for 14 days before mating and throughout mating and gestation. Gestation period and duration of labor is also prolonged.

Clevidipine – In animal studies, clevidipine caused increases in maternal and fetal mortality and length of gestation. There was decreased fetal survival when pregnant rats and rabbits were treated with clevidipine during organogenesis at doses 0.7 times the maximum recommended human dose (MRHD) in rats and 2 times the MRHD in rabbits.

Diltiazem – Doses given at 4 to 10 times the human dose resulted in embryo and fetal death and skeletal abnormalities; incidence of stillbirths was increased at 20 or more times the human dose.

Felodipine – In rabbits, doses 0.8 to 8 times the maximum dosage resulted in digital anomalies (dose-related) in the fetuses, and a prolongation of parturition with difficult labor and increased frequency of fetal and early postnatal deaths occurred in rats. Significant enlargement of the mammary glands also occurred in pregnant rabbits.

Isradipine – There was a significant reduction in maternal weight gain in rats with a dose 150 times the MRHD. Decrements in maternal body weight gain and increased fetal resorptions occurred in rabbits following doses 2.5, 7.5, and 25 times the MRHD. Also, reduced maternal body weight gain during late pregnancy in rats was associated with reduced birth weights and decreased peri- and postnatal pup survival.

Nicardipine – Nicardipine was embryocidal in animals at 150 mg/kg/day but not at 50 mg/kg/day 25 times the maximum human dose. However, dystocia, reduced birth weights, reduced neonatal survival, and reduced neonatal weight gain occurred at 50 times the human dose.

Nifedipine – Nifedipine administration was associated with a variety of embryotoxic, placentotoxic, and fetotoxic effects, including stunted fetuses (rats, mice, rabbits), rib deformities (mice), cleft palate (mice), small placentas, and underdeveloped chorionic villi (monkeys), embryonic and fetal deaths (rats, mice, rabbits), and prolonged pregnancy/decreased neonatal survival (rats; not evaluated on other species). On a mg/kg basis, all of the doses associated with teratogenic, embryotoxic, or fetotoxic effects in animals were higher (3.5 to 42 times) than the MRHD of 120 mg/day. The doses associated with placentotoxic effect in monkeys were equivalent to or lower than the MRHD on a mg/m^2 basis.

Nimodipine – In animals, nimodipine has resulted in malformations and stunted fetuses at dosages of 1 and 10 mg/kg/day but not at 3 mg/kg/day in 1 study. Dosages of 30 to 100 mg/kg/day resulted in stunted fetuses, stillbirths, and higher incidences of skeletal variation.

Nisoldipine – Nisoldipine was fetotoxic but not teratogenic in rats and rabbits at doses resulting in maternal toxicity (reduced maternal body weight gain). In pregnant rats, increased fetal resorption (postimplantation loss) was observed at 100 mg/kg/day and decreased fetal weight was observed at both 30 and 100 mg/kg/day. These doses are, respectively, about 5 and 16 times the MRHD when compared on a mg/m^2 basis. In pregnant rabbits, decreased fetal and placental weights were observed at a dosage of 30 mg/kg/day, about 10 times the MRHD when compared on a mg/m^2 basis. In a study in which pregnant monkeys (both treated and control) had high rates of abortion and mortality, the only surviving fetus from a group exposed to a maternal dosage of nisoldipine 100 mg/kg/day (about 30 times the MRHD when compared on a mg/m^2 basis) presented with forelimb and vertebral abnormalities not previously seen in control monkeys of the same strain.

Verapamil, oral – Oral verapamil in rats with doses 1.5 and 6 times the human dose was embryocidal and retarded fetal growth and development, probably due to reduced weight gains in dams. Verapamil crosses the placenta and can be detected in umbilical vein blood at delivery.

➤*Lactation:* **Verapamil**, **diltiazem**, **nicardipine** (minimal), and **nifedipine** are excreted in breast milk. One report suggests that diltiazem concentrations in breast milk may approximate serum levels. Significant concentrations of **nimodipine** appear in maternal milk of rats. It is not known if nimodipine, **clevidipine**, **isradipine**, **amlodipine**, **nisoldipine**, or **felodipine** are excreted in breast milk. Discontinue nursing while taking amlodipine, diltiazem, nicardipine, verapamil, or nimodipine. If using felodipine, isradipine, nifedipine, or nisoldipine, decide whether to discontinue nursing or discontinue the drug, taking into account the importance of the drug to the mother.

➤*Children:* Safety and efficacy of oral **verapamil**, **diltiazem**, **felodipine**, **amlodipine**, **nicardipine** (oral and IV), **nifedipine**, **nisoldipine**, **isradipine**, and IV **clevidipine** have not been established. Use of *Procardia* in the pediatric population is not recommended.

Controlled studies of IV **verapamil** have not been conducted in pediatric patients, but uncontrolled experience indicates that results of treatment are similar to those in adults. Patients under 6 months of age may not respond to IV verapamil; this resistance may be related to a developmental difference of AV node responsiveness. However, in rare instances, severe hemodynamic side effects, some of them fatal, have occurred following IV verapamil administration in neonates and infants. Therefore, use caution when administering verapamil to this group of pediatric patients. The most commonly used single doses in patients up to 12 months of age have ranged from 0.1 to 0.2 mg/kg of body weight, while in patients 1 to 15 years of age, the most commonly used single doses ranged from 0.1 to 0.3 mg/kg of body weight. Most of the patients received the lower dose of 0.1 mg/kg once, but in some cases, the dose was repeated once or twice every 10 to 30 minutes.

➤*Elderly:* Make dose selection for an elderly patient with caution, usually starting at the low end of the dosing range, reflecting the greater frequency of decreased hepatic, renal, or cardiac function and of concomitant disease or other drug therapy.

Per the Beers list, short acting **nifedipine** has the potential for hypotension and constipation. Short acting nifedipine is also considered a high risk medication for the elderly according to the Centers of Medicare and Medicaid Services.

Drug Interactions

➤*Cytochrome P450:* CYP3A4 has a major role in the metabolism of all the calcium channel blockers. Inducers and inhibitors of CYP3A4 can affect the metabolism of the dihydropyridines as well as **verapamil** and **diltiazem**. In general, diltiazem and verapamil inhibit other CYP3A4 substrates (eg, midazolam, carbamazepine), whereas the dihydropyridines do not.

Calcium Channel Blocker Drug Interactions

Precipitant drug	Object drug[a]		Description
Amiodarone	Calcium channel blockers–Diltiazem	↑	Coadministration may result in cardiotoxicity with bradycardia and decreased cardiac output. Monitor closely.
Azole antifungals	Calcium channel blockers–Nisoldipine	↑	Serum nisoldipine concentrations may be elevated. If coadministration cannot be avoided, observe clinical response, monitor cardiovascular status, and adjust nisoldipine dose accordingly.
Azole antifungals–Itraconazole	Calcium channel blockers–Felodipine, isradipine, nifedipine	↑	Serum concentrations of the calcium channel blocker may be increased. Observe clinical response, monitor cardiovascular status, and adjust calcium channel blocker dose accordingly.
Barbiturates (eg, phenobarbital)	Calcium channel blockers–Felodipine, nifedipine, verapamil	↓	Pharmacologic effects of the calcium channel blocker may be decreased.
Beta-blockers (eg, metoprolol)	Calcium channel blockers	↑	Coadministration may cause additive or synergistic effects. Do not administer IV verapamil an IV beta-blockers within a few hours of each other because both may have a depressant effect on myocardial contractility and AV conduction. Diltiazem, isradipine, nicardipine, nifedipine, and verapamil may inhibit the metabolism of certain beta-blockers. Monitor cardiac function and adjust dosages as needed.
Calcium channel blockers–Diltiazem, isradipine, nicardipine, nifedipine, verapamil	Beta-blockers (eg, metoprolol)		
Calcium salts	Calcium channel blockers–Verapamil	↓	Clinical effects and toxicities of verapamil may be reversed by calcium.
Carbamazepine, Oxcarbazepine	Calcium channel blockers–Felodipine	↓	Pharmacologic effects of felodipine may be decreased. Patients may require higher doses of felodipine.
Cisapride	Calcium channel blockers–Nifedipine	↑	Cisapride may increase nifedipine serum concentrations. Monitor closely and adjust dose of nifedipine as needed.
Clonidine	Calcium channel blockers–Verapamil	↑	Synergistic effects resulting in sinus bradycardia have been reported in association with coadministration of clonidine and verapamil. Monitor heart rate during concurrent use of verapamil and clonidine.
Calcium channel blockers–Verapamil	Clonidine		
Cyclosporine	Calcium channel blockers–Nifedipine, felodipine	↑	Pharmacologic and toxic effects of nifedipine or felodipine may be increased. Cyclosporine levels and toxicity may be increased when given concurrently with diltiazem, felodipine, nicardipine, or verapamil. However, verapamil may be nephroprotective when given before cyclosporine. Monitor cyclosporine levels and adjust the dose as needed.
Calcium channel blockers–Diltiazem, felodipine, nicardipine, verapamil	Cyclosporine		
Dantrolene	Calcium channel blockers–Verapamil	↑	Hyperkalemia and myocardial depression has been reported in a patient following coadministration of oral verapamil and IV dantrolene. Monitor serum potassium and cardiac function.
Calcium channel blockers–Verapamil	Dantrolene		

Calcium Channel Blocker Drug Interactions

Precipitant drug	Object drug[a]		Description
Dronedarone	Calcium channel blockers–Verapamil	↑	Plasma concentrations and pharmacologic effects of both agents may be increased. Verapamil may enhance the electrophysiologic effects of dronedarone. Initiate verapamil at low doses in patients receiving dronedarone. Monitor the ECG[b] and increase verapamil dosage if the ECG demonstrates tolerability.
Calcium channel blockers–Verapamil	Dronedarone		
Erythromycin	Calcium channel blockers–Felodipine		Coadministration may increase the effects of felodipine. Monitor cardiovascular status closely and adjust felodipine dose as needed.
H_2 antagonists–Cimetidine, ranitidine	Calcium channel blockers–Diltiazem, felodipine, isradipine, nicardipine, nifedipine, nimodipine, nisoldipine, verapamil	↑	Serum concentrations of the calcium channel blocker may be increased when given concurrently with cimetidine. Ranitidine also has been shown to affect diltiazem concentrations. Monitor cardiovascular status closely. Adjust dose as needed.
HMG-CoA reductase inhibitors (eg, atorvastatin, lovastatin)	Calcium channel blockers–Verapamil		Plasma concentrations of certain HMG-CoA reductase inhibitors may be elevated. Verapamil concentrations may also be elevated. If coadministration cannot be avoided, administer a conservative dose of the HMG-CoA reductase inhibitor. Monitor the clinical response and for adverse reactions to verapamil. Adjust the dose as needed.
Calcium channel blockers–Diltiazem, verapamil	HMG-CoA reductase inhibitors (eg, atorvastatin, lovastatin, simvastatin)		
Hydantoins (eg, phenytoin)	Calcium channel blockers–Felodipine, nisoldipine, verapamil	↓	The pharmacologic effects of the calcium channel blocker may be decreased. Monitor cardiovascular status closely. Adjust dose as needed.
Macrolide antibiotics (eg, clarithromycin, erythromycin, telithromycin)	Calcium channel blockers–Verapamil	↑	Erythromycin concentrations may be elevated, increasing the risk of cardiotoxicity. Verapamil concentrations may be elevated, increasing the pharmacologic effects and risk of toxicity. Monitor the clinical response of the patient and closely monitor cardiac function. Adjust treatment as needed.
Calcium channel blockers–Verapamil	Macrolide antibiotics (eg, erythromycin)		
Melatonin	Calcium channel blockers–Nifedipine	↓	Concurrent use may decrease the antihypertensive effects of nifedipine.
Nafcillin	Calcium channel blockers–Nifedipine	↓	Nafcillin administration results in a large reduction in the plasma concentration of nifedipine; loss of efficacy is likely to result. Nafcillin would be expected to reduce the plasma concentrations of other calcium channel blockers as well. Avoid coadministration.
Protease inhibitors (eg, amprenavir, indinavir, nelfinavir, ritonavir)	Calcium channel blocker Nicardipine	↑	Protease inhibitors may increase the antihypertensive and pharmacologic effects of nicardipine. Administer with caution.
Quinupristin/Dalfopristin	Calcium channel blockers–Nifedipine	↑	Concurrent use may increase the plasma concentration of nifedipine. The metabolism of other calcium channel blockers would likely be reduced by quinupristin/dalfopristin.
Rifampin	Calcium channel blockers–Diltiazem, isradipine, nicardipine, nifedipine, verapamil	↓	Coadministration may decrease the therapeutic effects of the calcium channel blocker. Monitor cardiovascular status closely. Adjust dose as needed.
St. John's Wort	Calcium channel blockers–Nifedipine, verapamil	↓	Coadministration may reduce the plasma concentration of nifedipine and verapamil. The metabolism of other calcium channel blockers would likely be increased by St. John's Wort as well.
Valproic acid	Calcium channel blockers–Nimodipine	↑	Valproic acid increases the AUC of nimodipine with no effect on the elimination half-life. Monitor closely.
Calcium channel blockers	Anesthetics	↑	Calcium channel blockers may potentiate the cardiac effects and vascular dilation associated with anesthetics. Severe hypotension has been reported during fentanyl anesthesia with concomitant use of a beta-blocker and a calcium channel blocker. Titrate doses carefully.
Calcium channel blockers–Verapamil	Antiarrhythmic agents–Disopyramide, flecainide	↑	Concomitant use of verapamil and flecainide may have additive effects. Until data on possible interactions between verapamil and disopyramide are obtained, the manufacturer recommends not administering disopyramide within 48 h before or 24 h after verapamil administration.
Calcium channel blockers–Verapamil	Antineoplastics–Doxorubicin, paclitaxel	↑	Verapamil appears to increase doxorubicin and paclitaxel serum concentrations.
Antineoplastics	Calcium channel blockers–Verapamil	↓	The absorption of verapamil can be reduced by the cyclophosphamide, oncovin, procarbazine, prednisone (COPP) and the vindesine, adriamycin, cisplatin (VAC) drug regimens.
Calcium channel blockers–Verapamil	Aspirin	↑	In a few reported cases, coadministration has led to increased bleeding times greater than observed with aspirin alone. Closely monitor bleeding times.
Calcium channel blockers–Diltiazem, verapamil	Benzodiazepines–Midazolam, triazolam	↑	Effects of certain benzodiazepines may be increased.
Calcium channel blockers–Diltiazem, verapamil	Buspirone	↑	Coadministration may increase the effects of buspirone. Monitor closely and adjust buspirone dose as needed.
Calcium channel blockers–Diltiazem, verapamil	Carbamazepine	↑	Serum carbamazepine concentrations may be increased. Monitor serum levels and adjust dosage as necessary.
Calcium channel blockers–Nifedipine	Calcium channel blockers–Diltiazem	↑	Diltiazem increases nifedipine plasma concentrations and nifedipine increases diltiazem plasma concentrations.
Calcium channel blockers–Diltiazem	Calcium channel blockers–Nifedipine		
Calcium channel blockers–Verapamil	Colchicine	↑	Colchicine plasma concentrations may be elevated, increasing the risk of toxicity. Use with caution and closely monitor for colchicine toxicity. The recommended colchicine dose for the treatment of gout flare in patients receiving verapamil is 1.2 mg for 1 dose. A 3-day lapse should occur before subsequent colchicine administration. The recommended maximum colchicine dose for treatment of familial Mediterranean fever in patients receiving verapamil is 1.2 mg daily.
Calcium channel blocker Nicardipine	Cyclosporine	↑	Increased cyclosporine blood or plasma concentrations may occur, possibly with renal toxicity. Monitor cyclosporine levels and reduce the dose accordingly.

Calcium Channel Blocker Drug Interactions			
Precipitant drug	Object drug[a]		Description
Calcium channel blockers–Diltiazem, nicardipine, nifedipine, verapamil	Digoxin	↑	Serum digoxin concentrations may be elevated, causing increased toxicity. Coadministration with diltiazem or nifedipine has produced conflicting reports. Monitor digoxin levels and adjust the dose as needed.
Calcium channel blockers–Verapamil	Dofetilide	↑	Concurrent use may increase dofetilide plasma concentration with increased risk of ventricular arrhythmias. Coadministration is contraindicated.
Calcium channel blockers–Verapamil	Eletriptan	↑	Eletriptan plasma concentrations may be elevated, increasing the pharmacologic effects and risk of adverse reactions.
Calcium channel blockers–Verapamil	Eplerenone	↑	Eplerenone plasma concentrations may be elevated, increasing the pharmacologic effects and risk of toxicity.
Calcium channel blockers–Verapamil	Ethanol	↑	Verapamil may cause increased and prolonged CNS effects of ethanol.
Calcium channel blockers–Verapamil	Everolimus	↑	Everolimus plasma concentrations may be elevated, increasing the pharmacologic effects and risk of toxicity. If coadministration cannot be avoided, closely monitor everolimus blood concentrations when verapamil is started or stopped. Adjust the everolimus dose as needed.
Calcium channel blockers–Nicardipine, verapamil	Fentanyl	↑	Fentanyl plasma concentrations may be elevated, increasing the pharmacologic effects and risk of toxicity. When coadministered, closely monitor patients for an extended period of time.
Calcium channel blockers–Isradipine	Lovastatin	↓	Plasma concentrations of lovastatin may be reduced, decreasing pharmacologic effect. Monitor clinical response and adjust therapy as needed.
Calcium channel blockers–Diltiazem, verapamil	Imipramine	↑	Coadministration increases imipramine serum concentrations.
Calcium channel blockers–Diltiazem, verapamil	Lithium	↑↓	Coadministration with verapamil has caused a reduction in lithium levels and toxicity. Coadministration with diltiazem has caused neurotoxicity.
Calcium channel blockers–Diltiazem	Methylprednisolone	↑	Pharmacologic and toxic effects of methylprednisolone may be increased.
Calcium channel blockers–Diltiazem	Moricizine	↑	Concurrent use may increase moricizine concentrations, while moricizine may decrease diltiazem concentrations.
Moricizine	Calcium channel blockers–Diltiazem	↓	
Calcium channel blockers–Verapamil	Nondepolarizing muscle relaxants	↑	Nondepolarizing muscle relaxant effects may be enhanced. Respiratory depression may be prolonged. Avoid concurrent use if possible.
Calcium channel blockers–Verapamil	Prazosin	↑	Concurrent use may increase serum prazosin concentrations and may increase the sensitivity to prazosin-induced postural hypotension.
Calcium channel blockers–Diltiazem, verapamil	Quinidine	↑	Coadministration may increase the therapeutic and adverse effects of quinidine. Use quinidine with verapamil only when no other alternative exists. Closely monitor quinidine serum levels and cardiac effects. In patients with hypertrophic cardiomyopathy, coadministration of verapamil and quinidine may cause clinically important hypotension; avoid concurrent use. Quinidine decreased the AUC of nisoldipine by 26% but not the peak concentration.
Quinidine	Calcium channel blockers–Nisoldipine	↓	
Calcium channel blockers–Nifedipine	Quinidine	↓	Serum levels and actions of quinidine may be decreased. Serum concentrations and actions of nifedipine may be increased.
Quinidine	Calcium channel blockers–Nifedipine	↑	
Calcium channel blockers–Verapamil	Ranolazine	↑	Ranolazine plasma concentrations may be elevated, increasing the pharmacologic effects and risk of toxicity. Limit the dose of ranolazine to 500 mg twice daily. Closely monitor for signs of ranolazine toxicity, including QT interval prolongation.
Calcium channel blockers–Verapamil	Risperidone	↑	Risperidone plasma concentrations may be elevated, increasing the pharmacologic effects and risk of toxicity.
Calcium channel blockers–Diltiazem	Sirolimus	↑	Coadministration may increase sirolimus plasma concentrations.
Calcium channel blockers–Diltiazem, nifedipine	Tacrolimus	↑	Tacrolimus levels may be elevated, increasing toxicity. Monitor serum levels and adjust dosage as needed.
Calcium channel blockers–Diltiazem, verapamil	Theophyllines	↑	Pharmacologic and toxic effects of theophyllines may be increased. Monitor serum levels and adjust dosage as needed.
Calcium channel blockers–Verapamil	Tolvaptan	↑	Tolvaptan plasma concentrations may be elevated, increasing the pharmacologic effects and risk of adverse reactions. Avoid coadministration.
Calcium channel blockers–Nifedipine	Vincristine	↑	Vincristine levels may be elevated, possibly increasing toxicity.

[a] ↑ = object drug increased. ↓ = object drug decreased. ↑↓ = object drug both increased and decreased.
[b] ECG = electrocardiogram.

➤*Drug/Food interactions:* Grapefruit juice may increase the serum concentrations of **felodipine**, **nicardipine**, **nifedipine**, **nisoldipine**, **verapamil**, and possibly **amlodipine**.

Diltiazem – Administration of certain diltiazem ER products with a high-fat breakfast increased AUC and maximum drug concentration (C_{max}).

Felodipine – When administered with either a high fat or carbohydrate diet, felodipine C_{max} is increased by approximately 60%; AUC is unchanged. Coadministration with grapefruit juice resulted in more than a 2-fold increase in the AUC and C_{max} but no prolongation in the half-life of felodipine.

Isradipine – Administration with food significantly increases isradipine's time to peak by about an hour but has no effect on the AUC. Food has been shown to decrease the extent of bioavailability of isradipine controlled release by up to 25%.

Nicardipine – When nicardipine was administered 1 or 3 hours after a high-fat meal, the mean C_{max} and AUC were lower (20% to 30%) than when given to fasting subjects. When nicardipine ER was administered with a high-fat breakfast, mean C_{max} was 45% lower, AUC was 25% lower, and trough levels were 75% higher than when given in the fasting state.

Nifedipine – When *Adalat CC* was given immediately after a high-fat meal in healthy volunteers, there was an average increase of 60% in the C_{max}, a prolongation in the T_{max}, but no significant change in the AUC. Coadministration of nifedipine with grapefruit juice resulted in up to a 2-fold increase in AUC and C_{max}. Avoid coadministration.

Nimodipine – Nimodipine administration following a standard breakfast resulted in a 68% lower C_{max} and 38% lower bioavailability relative to dosing under fasted conditions.

Nisoldipine – Food with a high-fat content had a pronounced effect on the release of nisoldipine from the coat-core formulation and resulted in a significant increase in C_{max} by up to 300%. However, total exposure was decreased about 25%, presumably because more of the drug was released proximally. Avoid concomitant intake of a high-fat meal with nisoldipine ER.

Do not administer nisoldipine with grapefruit juice, as this has been shown to result in a mean increase in C_{max} of about 3-fold (ranging up to 7-fold) and AUC of almost 2-fold (ranging up to 5-fold).

Verapamil – Administration of verapamil SR with food produced decreased AUC but a narrower peak-to-trough ratio.

Adverse Reactions

Calcium Channel Blocker Adverse Reactions (%)[a]

	Adverse Reactions	Amlodipine	Diltiazem Oral (IV)[b]	Felodipine	Isradipine[b]	Nicardipine Oral (IV)[b]	Nifedipine[b]	Nimodipine	Nisoldipine	Verapamil Oral (IV)[b]
Cardiovascular	Angina/Angina pectoris		< 2	0.5-1.5		†	≤ 1			≤ 1
	Angina increased					5.6[c]	≤ 1			
	Arrhythmia	≤ 1	< 2 (1[d])	0.5-1.5			≤ 1			
	Arrhythmia, ventricular		< 1				< 0.5			
	Atrial fibrillation	≤ 1	1.4		≤ 1		< 1		≤ 1	
	AV block (1°, 2°, or 3°)		≤ 7.6 (< 1)			(†)			≤ 1	0.8-1.7
	Bradycardia	≤ 1	≤ 6 (< 1)				< 1	≤ 1		1.4 (1.2)
	Chest pain	≤ 1	< 1	0.5-1.5	≤ 2.7	(0.7)	≤ 3		2	≤ 1
	CHF		< 2 (< 1)					< 1		1.8
	Edema	1.8-14.6[e]	≤ 6 (< 1)		3.5-35.9[c]	0.6-1	10-30[c]	≤ 1.2[c]		1.7-3
	ECG abnormalities		≤ 4.1			0.6 (1.4)		≤ 1.4		2
	Facial edema			0.5-1.5			≤ 1			
	Hypertension		< 1			(0.7)		< 1	≤ 1	1.7
	Hypotension	≤ 1	< 2	0.5-1.5	≤ 1	† (5.6)	< 1	≤ 8.1[c]	≤ 1	0.7-2.5
	Hypotension, postural	≤ 1	< 1			≤ 0.9 (1.4)	< 1		≤ 1	0.4
	Hypotension, symptomatic		(3.2)							(1.5)
	MI		< 1	0.5-1.5	≤ 1				≤ 1	≤ 1
	Palpitations	0.7-4.5[c]	≤ 2	0.4-2.5	1-5.1[c]	2.8-4.1	≤ 7	< 1	3	≤ 1
	Peripheral edema		2-15 (4.3)	2-17.4		(†)	7-29[c]		7-29[c]	3.7
	Sinus bradycardia		< 1							
	Supraventricular tachycardia					(0.7)			≤ 1	
	Syncope	≤ 1	< 2 (< 1)	0.5-1.5	≤ 1	0.8 (0.7)	≤ 1		≤ 1	≤ 1
	Tachycardia	≤ 1	< 2	0.5-1.5	≤ 3.4	0.8-3.4 (3.5)	≤ 1	≤ 1.4		
	Vasculitis	≤ 1								≤ 1
	Vasodilation		≤ 3			4.7 (0.7)			4	
	Ventricular extrasystoles	≤ 0.1	≤ 2			† (1.4)			≤ 1	
	Ventricular tachycardia	≤ 1	(< 1)			† (0.7)				
CNS	Abnormal dreams	≤ 1	< 2			0.4			≤ 1	
	Amnesia	≤ 0.1	< 2						≤ 1	
	Anxiety/Anxiety disorders	≤ 1		0.5-1.5		†	≤ 1		≤ 1	
	Asthenia	1-2	≤ 4 (< 1)	2.2-3.9		0.9-5.8 (0.7)	≤ 4			2
	Ataxia	≤ 0.1					≤ 1		≤ 1	
	Confusion					† (†)	< 1		≤ 1	≤ 1
	Depression	≤ 1	< 2	0.5-1.5	≤ 1	†	≤ 1	≤ 1.4	≤ 1	(†)
	Dizziness/Lightheadedness	≤ 3.4[c]	≤ 10 (< 1)	2.7-3.7	3.4-8	1.6-6.9 (1.4)	4-27	< 1	3-10[c]	3-4.7 (1.2)
	Drowsiness				≤ 1					
	Equilibrium disturbances						≤ 2			≤ 1
	Fatigue/Lethargy	4.5[c]			≤ 8.5[c]		4-5.9			1.7-4.5
	Headache	7.3	≤ 12 (< 1)	10.6-14.7	10.3-22	6.2-8.2 (14.6)	10-23	≤ 4.1[c]	22	2.2-12.1 (1.2)
	Hypesthesia	≤ 1				(0.7)	≤ 1		≤ 1	
	Insomnia	≤ 1	< 2	0.5-1.5	≤ 1	0.6	≤ 3		≤ 1	≤ 1
	Malaise	≤ 1	< 1			0.6	≤ 1		≤ 1	
	Migraine	≤ 0.1					≤ 1		≤ 1	
	Nervousness	≤ 1	≤ 2	0.5-1.5	≤ 1	0.6	≤ 7		≤ 1	
	Paresthesia	≤ 1	< 2 (< 1)	1.2-1.6	≤ 1	1 (0.7)	≤ 3		≤ 1	≤ 1
	Shakiness/Jitteriness						≤ 2			≤ 1
	Sleep disturbances						≤ 2			1.4
	Somnolence	1.3-1.6[e]	< 2	0.5-1.5		1.1-1.4	≤ 3		≤ 1	≤ 1
	Tremor	≤ 1	< 2			0.6	≤ 8		≤ 1	
	Vertigo	≤ 1	< 1			†	≤ 3		≤ 1	(†)
	Weakness				≤ 1.2		10-12			

Calcium Channel Blocker Adverse Reactions (%)[a]

	Adverse Reactions	Amlodipine	Diltiazem Oral (IV)[b]	Felodipine	Isradipine[b]	Nicardipine Oral (IV)[b]	Nifedipine[b]	Nimodipine	Nisoldipine	Verapamil Oral (IV)[b]
Dermatologic	Acne							≤ 1.4	≤ 1	
	Dermatitis	≤ 0.1	≤ 1				≤ 2			
	Erythema multiforme	≤ 1	< 1							≤ 1
	Hair loss	≤ 0.1	†				≤ 1		≤ 1	≤ 1
	Injection site reactions		(3.9)			(1.4)				
	Leukocytoclastic vasculitis		†	0.5						
	Pruritus	1-2	< 2 (< 1)		≤ 1		< 3	< 1	≤ 1	
	Rash	1-2	≤ 2	0.2-2	≤ 2.6	0.4-1.2	≤ 3	≤ 2.4	≤ 2	≤ 2.4
	Rash maculopapular	≤ 1							≤ 1	
	Stevens-Johnson syndrome		†				< 0.5			≤ 1
	Urticaria	≤ 0.1	< 1	0.5-1.5	≤ 1		≤ 2		≤ 1	≤ 1 (†)
GI	Abdominal discomfort	1.6	1	0.5-1.5	≤ 5.1	(0.7)	< 3			(0.6)
	Abdominal distention		≤ 2		1.2					
	Acid regurgitation			0.5-1.5						
	Anorexia	≤ 1	< 2						≤ 1	
	Appetite increase	≤ 0.1							≤ 1	
	Constipation	≤ 1	≤ 3.6 (< 1)	0.3-1.5	≤ 3.8	0.6	≤ 3.3			3.9-11.7
	Diarrhea	≤ 1	≤ 2	0.5-1.5	≤ 3.4		< 3	≤ 4.2	≤ 1	≤ 2.4
	Dry mouth	≤ 1	< 2 (< 1)	0.5-1.5	≤ 1	0.4-1.4	< 3		≤ 1	≤ 1
	Dysgeusia	≤ 0.1	< 2				≤ 1		≤ 1	
	Dysphagia	≤ 1							≤ 1	
	Dyspepsia	1-2	≤ 6	0.5-3.9		0.8-1.5 (†)	< 3		≤ 1	2.5-2.7
	Flatulence	≤ 1	< 1	0.5-1.5			< 3		≤ 1	
	Gastritis	≤ 0.1							≤ 1	
	GI distress									≤ 1
	GI hemorrhage		< 1				< 1	< 1	≤ 1	
	Gingival hyperplasia	≤ 1	†	< 0.5			≤ 1		≤ 1	≤ 1
	Nausea	2.9[c]	≤ 2.2 (< 1)	1-1.7	1-5.1	1.9-2.2 (4.9)	2-11	0.6-1.4	2	1.7-2.7 (0.9)
	Thirst	≤ 1	< 2							
	Vomiting	≤ 1	≤ 2 (< 1)	0.5-1.5	≤ 1.3	0.4-0.6 (4.9)	≤ 1	< 1		
GU	Decreased libido			0.5-1.5	≤ 1		≤ 1		≤ 1	
	Dysuria	≤ 0.1		0.5-1.5			≤ 1		≤ 1	
	Gynecomastia		< 2	0.5-1.5			< 0.5		≤ 1	
	Hematuria					(0.7)	≤ 1		≤ 1	
	Impotence		≤ 2	0.5-1.5	≤ 1	†	≤ 3		≤ 1	≤ 1
	Nocturia	≤ 1	< 2		≤ 1	0.4	≤ 1		≤ 1	
	Polyuria	≤ 1	< 2	0.5-1.5		(1.4)	< 3			
	Sexual difficulties	≤ 2	< 2				≤ 2			
	Urinary frequency	≤ 1		0.5-1.5	1.3-3.4	≤ 0.6 (†)	≤ 3		≤ 1	≤ 1
Hematologic	Anemia			0.5-1.5			< 0.5	< 1	≤ 1	
	Ecchymosis								≤ 1	≤ 1
	Leukopenia	≤ 1	†		≤ 1		< 0.5		≤ 1	
	Petechiae		< 2						≤ 1	
	Purpura	≤ 1	< 1				≤ 1			≤ 1
	Thrombocytopenia	≤ 1	†			(†)	< 0.5	< 1		
Musculoskeletal	Arthralgia	≤ 1	1.4	0.5-1.5		†	< 3		≤ 1	≤ 1
	Arthritis						≤ 1		≤ 1	
	Back pain	≤ 1	1.7-2.9	0.5-1.5			≤ 1			
	Hypertonia	≤ 0.1	< 1			(†)	≤ 1		≤ 1	
	Leg cramps				≤ 1		≤ 3			
	Leg pain			0.5-1.5			≤ 3			
	Muscle cramps	1-2	< 2	0.5-1.5			≤ 8	≤ 1.4		≤ 1
	Myalgia	≤ 1	≤ 2.3	0.5-1.5		1	≤ 1		≤ 1	1.1
	Neck pain		< 1			(†)	< 1			
	Rigors	≤ 1					≤ 1			

Calcium Channel Blocker Adverse Reactions (%)[a]

	Adverse Reactions	Amlodipine	Diltiazem Oral (IV)[b]	Felodipine	Isradipine[b]	Nicardipine Oral (IV)[b]	Nifedipine[b]	Nimodipine	Nisoldipine	Verapamil Oral (IV)[b]
Respiratory	Bronchitis		≤ 4	0.5-1.5						
	Cough	≤ 0.1		0.8-1.7	≤ 1		≤ 6			
	Cough increased		1-3				< 1		≤ 1	
	Dyspnea	1-2	≤ 6 (< 1)	0.5-1.5	≤ 3.4	0.6 (0.7)	≤ 6	≤ 1.2	≤ 1	1.4
	Epistaxis	≤ 1	< 2	0.5-1.5			≤ 3		≤ 1	
	Nasal congestion		< 2				≤ 6			
	Pharyngitis		1.4-6	0.5-1.5			< 1		≤ 5	3
	Respiratory disorder		< 1			(†)	≤ 1			
	Respiratory infection			0.5-1.5			≤ 1			
	Rhinitis	≤ 0.1	≤ 9.6			†			≤ 1	2.7
	Sinusitis		2	0.5-1.5		†	≤ 1		≤ 3	3
	Upper respiratory infection			0.7-3.9			≤ 1			5.4
	Wheezing						6	< 1		
Special senses	Abnormal vision	≤ 1				†	≤ 1		≤ 1	
	Amblyopia		(< 1)				< 1		≤ 1	
	Blurred vision		< 1			†	≤ 2			≤ 1
	Conjunctivitis	≤ 1				(†)			≤ 1	
	Tinnitus	≤ 1	< 2			† (†)	≤ 1		≤ 1	≤ 1
Miscellaneous	Accidental injury		≤ 1.3							1.5
	Angioedema	≤ 1		0.5-1.5			≤ 0.5			
	Chills						≤ 2		≤ 1	
	Fever		< 1			(†)	≤ 2		≤ 1	
	Flu-like illness/syndrome/ symptoms		≤ 2.3	0.5-1.5					≤ 1	3.7
	Flushing	0.7-4.5[e]	≤ 3 (1.7)	3.9-6.9	1.2-5.1[c]	5.6-9.7	≤ 25	≤ 2.1		0.6-0.8
	Gout		1-2				≤ 1		≤ 1	
	Hot flashes					†	≤ 1			
	Hyperglycemia	≤ 1	< 2							
	Infection		≤ 6			†				12.1
	Pain	≤ 1	≤ 6			0.6	< 3			
	Sore throat					†	6			
	Sweating		< 1 (< 1)			(1.4)	≤ 2	< 1	≤ 1	≤ 1
	Sweating increased	≤ 1				0.6	≤ 1			(†)
	Weight gain	≤ 1	< 2				≤ 1		≤ 1	
	Weight loss						< 1		≤ 1	

[a] Data are pooled from separate studies and are not necessarily comparable.
[b] Includes data for SR/ER form.
[c] Dose-related.
[d] Functional rhythm or isorhythmic dissociation.
[e] Dose-related and higher in females.
† Occurs, no incidence reported.

In addition to the adverse effects listed in the table, the following have been reported:

➤*Amlodipine:* Peripheral ischemia, peripheral neuropathy, rash erythematous, pancreatitis, micturition disorder, postural dizziness, depersonalization, allergic reaction, hot flushes, arthrosis, diplopia, eye pain (less than or equal to 1%); cardiac failure, pulse irregularity, skin discoloration/dryness, twitching, cold/clammy skin, apathy, agitation, loose stools, parosmia, muscle weakness, abnormal visual accommodation, xerophthalmia (less than or equal to 0.1%).

➤*Clevidipine:* Atrial fibrillation (21%); acute renal failure (9%); headache (6.3%); nausea (4.8%); vomiting (3.2%); MI, cardiac arrest, syncope, dyspnea (less than 1%).

➤*Diltiazem:* Asymptomatic hypotension (4.3%); bundle branch block, hallucination, personality change, photosensitivity, gait abnormalities, crystalluria, osteoarticular pain, neck rigidity, hyperuricemia, albuminuria (less than 2%); arthrosis (1%); eye irritation, pallor, phlebitis, tooth disorder, eructation, skin hypertrophy (nevus), cystitis, kidney calculus, dysmenorrhea, pyelonephritis, urinary tract infection, eye hemorrhage, ophthalmitis, otitis media, sinus pause, sinus node dysfunction, ventricular fibrillation, kidney failure, respiratory distress, contact dermatitis, stomach ulcers, colitis, neuropathy, myocardial ischemia, vaginitis, prostate disease, bursitis, bone pain, lymphadenopathy, ear pain, bigeminal extrasystole, asystole, atrial flutter (less than 1%).

➤*Felodipine:* Sneezing (less than or equal to 1.6%); rhinorrhea (0.2% to 1.6%); premature beats, irritability, erythema, urinary urgency, visual disturbances, influenza, arm/foot/hip/knee pain, contusion (0.5% to 1.5%); warm sensation (less than or equal to 1.5%).

➤*Isradipine:* Foot cramps, shortness of breath, ventricular fibrillation, numbness, tingling, transient ischemic attack, stroke, hyperhidrosis, visual disturbance, throat discomfort (less than or equal to 1%).

➤*Nicardipine:* Pedal edema (5.9% to 8%); hemopericardium, hypokalemia, intracranial hemorrhage, injection-site pain (0.7%); ST segment depression, inverted T wave, deep-vein thrombophlebitis, hypophosphatemia, ear disorder, allergic reaction, peripheral vascular disorder, hyperkinesia, atypical chest pain (rare).

➤*Nifedipine:* Giddiness (27%); heat sensation (4% to 25%); muscle tremor (8%); heartburn (11%); mood changes (less than or equal to 7%); transient hypotension (5%); abdominal cramps, joint stiffness; muscle inflammation, chest congestion (less than or equal to 2%); periorbital edema, eructation, GI reflux, melena, abnormal lacrimation, breast pain (less than or equal to 1%); cellulitis, pelvic pain, cardiac arrest, extrasystole, phlebitis, cutaneous angiectases, esophagitis, lymphadenopathy, rales, diplopia, kidney calculus, breast engorgement (less than 1%); erythromelalgia, allergenic hepatitis, arthritis with ANA (+), transient blindness, exfoliative dermatitis, toxic epidermal necrolysis, paranoia, psychiatric disturbances (less than 0.5%). Very rarely, therapy was associated with an increase in anginal pain, possibly caused by associated hypotension. Transient unilateral loss of vision also occurred.

In a subgroup of approximately 250 patients with a diagnosis of CHF as well as angina pectoris (about 10% of the total patient population), dizziness or lightheadedness, peripheral edema, headache, or flushing each occurred in 1 in 8 patients. Hypotension occurred in about 1 in 20 patients. Syncope occurred in approximately 1 patient in 250. MI or symptoms of CHF each occurred in about 1 patient in 15. Atrial or ventricular dysrhythmias each occurred in approximately 1 patient in 150.

➤*Nimodipine:* GI symptoms (less than or equal to 2.4%); rebound vasospasm, jaundice, hyponatremia, disseminated intravascular coagulation, deep-vein thrombosis, neurological deterioration, phenytoin toxicity, decreased platelet count, hepatitis, hematoma (less than 1%).

➤*Nisoldipine:* Cellulitis, cerebrovascular accident, jugular venous distension, systolic ejection murmur, venous insufficiency, colitis, glossitis, hepatomegaly, melena, mouth ulceration, diabetes mellitus, thyroiditis, hypokalemia, increased serum creatine kinase, increased nonprotein nitrogen, myasthenia, myositis, blepharitis, ear pain, glaucoma, itchy eyes, keratoconjunctivitis, otitis media, retinal detachment, watery eyes, temporary unilateral loss of vision, vitreous floater, increased BUN and serum creatinine, vaginal hemorrhage, vaginitis, tenosynovitis, abnormal thinking, cerebral ischemia, end inspiratory wheeze and fine rales, laryngitis, pleural effusion, dry skin, herpes simplex, herpes zoster, pustular rash, skin discoloration, skin ulcer, fungal dermatitis, exfoliative dermatitis, T wave abnormalities on ECG (flattening, inversion, nonspecific changes), asthma (less than or equal to 1%); chest tightness (rare).

➤*Verapamil:* Allergy aggravated (less than or equal to 2%); ankle edema (1.4%); pulmonary edema (1.8%); severe tachycardia (1%); atrioventricular dissociation, claudication, cerebrovascular accident, psychotic symptoms, exanthema, hyperkeratosis, macules, galactorrhea/hyperprolactinemia, spotty menstruation, bruising (less than or equal to 1%); broncho/laryngeal spasm, itch (rare); rotary nystagmus, sleepiness, muscle fatigue, seizures during injection (occasional); respiratory failure (low frequency).

In clinical trials related to the control of ventricular response in digitalized patients who had atrial fibrillation or flutter, ventricular rates below 50 at rest occurred in 15% of patients and asymptomatic hypotension occurred in 5% of patients.

Reversible (upon discontinuation of verapamil) nonobstructive paralytic ileus has been reported infrequently in association with the use of verapamil.

➤*Lab test abnormalities:* Rare, usually transient, but occasionally significant elevations of enzymes such as alkaline phosphatase, CPK, LDH, AST, and ALT have occurred with **diltiazem** and **nifedipine** (see Precautions). **Felodipine** patients experienced an ALT increase of 0.5% to 1.5%. Positive direct Coombs test with or without hemolytic anemia has occurred with **nifedipine**. Abnormal liver function test (1.2%), isolated cases of decreased platelet counts (0.3%), and elevated nonfasting serum glucose, LDH (0.4%), alkaline phosphatase (0.2%), and ALT (0.2%) have occurred rarely with **nimodipine**. Abnormal liver function tests have occurred with **nisoldipine**, elevated liver function tests have occurred with **isradipine**, elevated liver enzymes occurred with **verapamil** (1.4%), and abnormal liver chemistries were reported with **nicardipine**.

➤*Postmarketing experience:*

Amlodipine – Jaundice and hepatic enzyme elevations (mostly consistent with cholestasis or hepatitis), in some cases severe enough to require hospitalization, have been reported in association with use of amlodipine.

Diltiazem – Infrequently reported postmarketing events include the following: Allergic reactions; alopecia; asystole; angioedema; erythema multiforme; Stevens-Johnson syndrome; toxic epidermal necrolysis; extrapyramidal symptoms; gingival hyperplasia; hemolytic anemia; increased bleeding time; leukopenia; purpura; retinopathy; thrombocytopenia; generalized rash; leukocytoclastic vasculitis; exfoliative dermatitis.

Nifedipine – There have been rare reports of the following: Toxic epidermal necrolysis; exfoliative dermatitis; Stevens-Johnson syndrome; and photosensitivity reactions.

Nisoldipine – Systemic hypersensitivity reaction has been reported very rarely, which may include 1 or more of the following: Angioedema, shortness of breath, tachycardia, chest tightness, hypotension, rash.

Overdosage

➤*Symptoms:* Symptoms of overdosage include marked and prolonged hypotension and bradycardia, both of which may result in decreased cardiac output. Junctional rhythms and second- or third-degree AV block may be seen. Death has occurred. Toxic **diltiazem** blood levels in man are not known, but there have been 29 reports of diltiazem overdose in doses ranging from less than 1 to 10.8 g. Sixteen of these reports involved multiple drug ingestion.

Ingestion of 900 mg of **nifedipine** immediate release and 4800 mg **nifedipine** ER in 2 patients resulted in dizziness, palpitations, flushing, nervousness, loss of consciousness, nausea, vomiting, generalized edema, and profound hypotension. One patient had sinus bradycardia and varying degrees of AV block. Both patients recovered. Significant hyperglycemia was seen initially in the nifedipine immediate release patient, but plasma glucose levels rapidly normalized without further treatment.

One patient ingested 250 mg **amlodipine** and was asymptomatic. Another patient ingested 120 mg, underwent gastric lavage, and remained normotensive. A third patient took 105 mg and had hypotension (90/50 mmHg), which normalized following plasma expansion. A 19-month-old ingested 30 mg (2 mg/kg) and had no evidence of hypotension but had a heart rate of 180 bpm.

Ingestion of **nicardipine** 600 mg immediate-release and nicardipine ER 2,160 mg produced symptoms of marked hypotension, bradycardia, palpitations, flushing, drowsiness, confusion, and slurred speech.

➤*Treatment:* If the patient is seen shortly after oral ingestion, employ lavage, activated charcoal, and cathartics. Treatment is supportive. Refer to General Management of Acute Overdosage. Beta-adrenergic agonists and IV calcium have been used effectively. Treat cardiac failure with inotropic agents (isoproterenol, dopamine, or dobutamine) and diuretics. In patients with hypertrophic cardiomyopathy, use alpha-adrenergic agents (phenylephrine HCl or metaraminol bitartrate) to maintain blood pressure; avoid isoproterenol and norepinephrine. Monitor cardiac and respiratory function; elevate the extremities. Because these agents are highly protein bound, dialysis is not likely to help. Verapamil cannot be removed by hemodialysis.

Calcium Channel Blocker Overdosage: Suggested Treatment of Acute Cardiovascular Adverse Reactions[a]

Adverse reactions	Proven effective treatment[b]	Supportive treatment
Symptomatic hypotension requiring treatment	Dopamine Calcium chloride Isoproterenol HCl Metaraminol bitartrate Norepinephrine bitartrate	IV fluids Trendelenburg position
Bradycardia, AV block, asystole	Atropine Calcium chloride Cardiac pacing Isoproterenol HCl Norepinephrine bitartrate	IV fluids
Rapid ventricular rate (caused by antegrade conduction in flutter/fibrillation with Wolff-Parkinson-White or Lown-Ganong-Levine syndromes)	DC cardioversion Lidocaine Procainamide	IV fluids

[a] Actual treatment and dosage should depend on the severity of the clinical situation and the judgment and experience of the treating health care provider.
[b] Drug therapy is administered IV.

Patient Information

Notify health care provider if any of the following occurs: irregular heart beat, shortness of breath, swelling of the hands and feet, pronounced dizziness, constipation, nausea, or hypotension.

➤*Diltiazem (Dilacor XR)*: Swallow whole; do not open, crush, or chew.

➤*Felodipine:* Swallow whole; do not crush or chew.

Mild gingival hyperplasia has occurred; good dental hygiene decreases its incidence and severity.

➤*Isradipine:* Swallow controlled-release tablets whole. Do not chew, divide, or crush. The empty tablet shell is eliminated in the stool.

➤*Nifedipine ER:* Swallow whole; do not chew, divide, or crush. Take *Adalat CC* on an empty stomach. An empty tablet may appear in the stool; this is no cause for concern.

➤*Nisoldipine:* Nisoldipine is an extended-release tablet; swallow whole. Do not chew, divide, or crush the tablet. Do not administer with a high-fat meal. Grapefruit juice, which has been shown to increase significantly the bioavailability of nisoldipine and other dihydropyridine-type calcium channel blockers, should not be taken with nisoldipine.

➤*Verapamil ER / SR:* Do not crush or chew the contents of the pellet-filled capsule. When the sprinkle method of administration is prescribed, explain to patients the details of proper technique. Swallow *Covera-HS* tablets whole; do not break, crush, or chew. The patient should not be concerned if they occasionally observe this outer shell in their stool as it passes from the body.

NISOLDIPINE

Rx	**Sular** (Sciele Pharma)	**Tablets, extended-release; oral:** 8.5 mg	Lactose, polyethylene glycol. (SCI 500). Oyster. Film-coated. In 100s.
Rx	**Sular** (Sciele Pharma)	**Tablets, extended-release; oral:** 17 mg	Lactose, polyethylene glycol, tartrazine. (SCI 501). Yellow cream. Film-coated. In 100s.
Rx	**Nisoldipine** (Mylan)	**Tablets, extended-release; oral:** 20	Polydextrose. (M N 22). Beige, round. Film-coated. In 100s and 500s.
Rx	**Sular** (Sciele Pharma)	**Tablets, extended-release; oral:** 25.5 mg	Lactose, polyethylene glycol. (SCI 502). Mustard. Elliptic. Film-coated. In 100s.
Rx	**Nisoldipine** (Mylan)	**Tablets, extended-release; oral:** 30 mg	Polydextrose. (M N 23). Orange, round. Film-coated. In 100s and 500s.
Rx	**Sular** (Sciele Pharma)	**Tablets, extended-release; oral:** 34 mg	Lactose, polyethylene glycol. (SCI 503). Burnt orange. Elliptic. Film-coated. In 100s.
Rx	**Nisoldipine** (Mylan)	**Tablets, extended-release; oral:** 40 mg	Polydextrose. (M N 24). Yellow, round, film-coated. In 100s and 500s.

NISOLDIPINE — ORAL

For complete and comparative prescribing information, refer to the Calcium Channel Blockers group monograph.

Indications

➤*Hypertension:* Treatment of hypertension. It may be used alone or in combination with other antihypertensive agents.

Administration and Dosage

➤*General dosing considerations:* The dosage of nisoldipine must be adjusted to each patient's needs.

➤*Adults:*

Hypertension –

Maximum dose: Dosages beyond 34 mg once daily are not recommended.

Initial dosage: 17 mg orally once daily, then increased by 8.5 mg per week or longer intervals to attain adequate control of blood pressure.

Maintenance dosage: 17 to 34 mg once daily. Blood pressure response increases over the 8.5 to 34 mg daily dose range, but adverse reaction rates also increase.

Concomitant therapy: Nisoldipine has been used safely with diuretics, angiotensin-converting enzyme (ACE) inhibitors, and beta-blocking agents.

➤*Elderly:* Patients older than 65 years of age are expected to develop higher plasma concentrations of nisoldipine. Their blood pressure should be monitored closely during any dosage adjustment. A starting dose not exceeding 8.5 mg daily is recommended in these patient groups.

➤*Hepatic function impairment:* Initial dose should not exceed 8.5 mg daily.

➤*Administration:* Nisoldipine should be taken on an empty stomach (1 hour before or 2 hours after a meal).

Administration with a high-fat meal can lead to excessive peak drug concentration and should be avoided.

Grapefruit products should be avoided before and after dosing.

Nisoldipine is an extended-release dosage form; tablets should be swallowed whole, not bitten, divided, or crushed.

➤*Storage/Stability:* Store at 20° to 25°C (68° to 77°F); excursions are permitted to 15° to 30°C (59° to 86°F). Protect from light and moisture. Dispense in tight, light-resistant containers.

NIFEDIPINE

Rx	**Nifedipine** (Mylan)	**Tablets, extended-release; oral:** 30 mg	In 100s and 300s.
Rx	**Adalat CC** (Schering)		Lactose. (30 ADALAT CC). Pink, round. Film-coated. In 100s, 1,000s, and UD 100s.
Rx	**Afeditab CR** (Watson)		(ELN 30). Brick red. In 100s.
Rx	**Nifediac CC** (Teva)		(B 30). Mustard yellow. Film coated. In 100s, 300s, and 1000s.
Rx	**Nifedical XL** (Teva)		Lactose. (B 30). Reddish brown. Film-coated. In 100s and 300s.
Rx	**Procardia XL** (Pfizer)		(PROCARDIA XL 30). Rose pink. Film-coated. In 100s, 300s, 5000s, and UD 100s.
Rx	**Nifedipine** (Mylan)	**Tablets, extended-release; oral:** 60 mg	In 100s and 300s.
Rx	**Adalat CC** (Schering)		Lactose. (60 ADALAT CC). Salmon, round. Film-coated. In 100s, 1,000s, and UD 100s.
Rx	**Afeditab CR** (Watson)		(ELN 60). Brick red. In 100s.
Rx	**Nifediac CC** (Teva)		Lactose. (B 60). Mustard yellow. Film coated. In 100s, 300s, and 1000s.
Rx	**Nifedical XL** (Teva)		Lactose. (B 60). Reddish brown. Film-coated. In 100s and 300s.
Rx	**Procardia XL** (Pfizer)		(PROCARDIA XL 60). Rose pink. Film-coated. In 100s, 300s, 5000s, and UD 100s.
Rx	**Nifedipine** (Mylan)	**Tablets, extended-release; oral:** 90 mg	In 100s.
Rx	**Adalat CC** (Schering)		Lactose. (90 ADALAT CC). Dark red, round. Film-coated. In 100s and UD 100s.
Rx	**Nifediac CC** (Teva)		Lactose. (B 90). Yellow. Film coated. In 100s.
Rx	**Procardia XL** (Pfizer)		(PROCARDIA XL 90). Rose pink. Film-coated. In 100s and UD 100s.
Rx	**Nifedipine** (Various, eg, Purepac)	**Capsules; oral:** 10 mg	May be liquid-filled. In 100s and 300s.
Rx	**Procardia** (Pfizer)		Liquid-filled. Saccharin. (PROCARDIA PFIZER 260). Orange. In 100s and 300s.
Rx	**Nifedipine** (Various, eg, Major, Purepac)	**Capsules; oral:** 20 mg	May be liquid-filled. In 100s and 300s.
Rx	**Procardia** (Pfizer)		Liquid-filled. (PROCARDIA 20 PFIZER 261). Orange. In 100s.

NIFEDIPINE — ORAL

For complete and comparative prescribing information, refer to the Calcium Channel Blockers class monograph.

Indications

➤*Chronic stable angina (except Adalat CC, Afeditab CR, Nifediac CC):* Classic effort-associated angina without vasospasm in patients who remain symptomatic despite adequate doses of beta-blockers or organic nitrates or who cannot tolerate those agents.

➤*Hypertension (extended-release only):* For the treatment of hypertension. May be used alone or in combination with other antihypertensive agents.

➤*Vasospastic angina (except Adalat CC, Afeditab CR, Nifediac CC):* For the management of vasospastic angina confirmed by any of the following criteria: 1) classical pattern of angina at rest accompanied by ST segment elevation; 2) angina or coronary artery spasm provoked by ergonovine; or 3) angiographically demonstrated coronary artery spasm. In patients who have had angiography, the presence of significant fixed obstructive disease is not incompatible with the diagnosis of vasospastic angina, provided that the above criteria are satisfied. Also may be used when clinical presentation suggests a vasospastic component, but where vasospasm has not been confirmed (eg, where pain has a variable threshold on exertion, or in unstable angina where electrocardiographic findings are compatible with intermittent vasospasm, or when angina is refractory to nitrates or adequate doses of beta-blockers).

➤*Off-label uses:*

Anal fissures – [2] = Fair documentation. Initial data suggest nifedipine may be useful in the treatment of anal fissures for some patients.

Pediatric hypertension – [1] = Good documentation. Nifedipine is among the therapeutic options for pediatric hypertension identified by the National High Blood Pressure Education Program based on case series and expert opinion.

Prevention of migraine (adults) – [5] = Poor documentation. Data from several trials evaluating nifedipine for the prevention of migraine headaches in adults are conflicting, but generally do not support consistent efficacy. In addition, nifedipine was poorly tolerated; several patients discontinued therapy because of adverse effects. American Academy of Neurology practice guidelines consider nifedipine to be no better than placebo for the prevention of migraine. Nifedipine should not be used routinely for migraine prevention.

Raynaud phenomenon – [1] = Good documentation. Several controlled trials have reported efficacy of nifedipine in the treatment of Raynaud phenomenon.

Ureteral stones – [4] = Insufficient documentation. Nifedipine, alone or in combination with steroids, may have some benefit as adjunctive therapy in the management of ureteral stones. There are conflicting reports regarding its efficacy in comparison with other agents (eg, tamsulosin); thus, its place in therapy has not been established. In the meta-analysis performed for the guidelines statement, more patients (9%) receiving nifedipine passed stones compared with controls, a difference that was not statistically significant and showed only marginal benefit.

Wound healing – [4] = Insufficient documentation. Although limited data suggest that topical nifedipine may have some benefit in the promotion of wound healing, there is insufficient evidence to establish valid recommendations. A commercial topical preparation of this product is not currently available in the United States.

Administration and Dosage

➤*General dosing considerations:* Individualize dosage. Excessive doses can result in hypotension.

NIFEDIPINE — ORAL

➤*Adults:*

Angina –

Procardia:

• *Usual dosage* – 10 to 20 mg 3 times/day. Some patients, especially those with coronary artery spasm, respond only to higher doses, more frequent administration, or both. In such patients, 20 to 30 mg 3 or 4 times/day may be effective. Dosages above 120 mg/day are rarely necessary.

• *Maximum dose* – 180 mg/day; dosages above 120 mg/day are rarely necessary.

• *Initial dosage* – 10 mg 3 times/day; swallow whole.

• *Dosage titration* – Titrate throughout 7 to 14 days to assess response to each dose level; monitor blood pressure before proceeding to higher doses. If symptoms warrant, titrate more rapidly, but assess frequently based on physical activity level, attack frequency, and sublingual nitroglycerin consumption. Increase dosage from 10 to 20 mg 3 times/day, and then 30 mg 3 times/day throughout 3 days.

In hospitalized patients under close observation, the dose may be increased in 10 mg increments throughout 4- to 6-hour periods as required to control pain and arrhythmias caused by ischemia. A single dose should rarely exceed 30 mg.

• *Concomitant therapy* – Sublingual nitroglycerin may be taken as required for the control of acute manifestations of angina, particularly during nifedipine titration. Coadministration of nifedipine with beta-blockers or long-acting nitrates is usually well tolerated, but there have been occasional reports suggesting that the combination, especially with beta-blockers, may increase the likelihood of congestive heart failure, severe hypotension or exacerbation of angina.

Nifedical XL, Procardia XL:

• *Usual dosage* – 30 or 60 mg once daily.

• *Maximum dose* – 120 mg/day.

• *Dosage titration* – Titrate over 7 to 14 days. Titration may proceed more rapidly if the patient is frequently assessed. Titration to doses above 120 mg is not recommended.

• *Concomitant therapy* – Sublingual nitroglycerin may be taken as required for the control of acute manifestations of angina, particularly during nifedipine titration. Coadministration of nifedipine with beta-blockers or long-acting nitrates is usually well tolerated, but there have been occasional reports suggesting that the combination, especially with beta-blockers, may increase the likelihood of congestive heart failure, severe hypotension or exacerbation of angina.

• *Conversion* – Angina patients maintained on the nifedipine capsule formulation may be switched to the extended-release tablet at the nearest equivalent total daily dose. Experience with doses greater than 90 mg in angina is limited; therefore, use with caution and only when clinically warranted.

Hypertension (Adalat CC, Afeditab CR, Nifediac CC) –

Usual dosage: 30 to 60 mg once daily.

Maximum dose: 90 mg/day.

Initial dosage: 30 mg once daily.

Dosage titration: In general, titrate over 7 to 14 days. Base upward titration on therapeutic efficacy and safety. Titration to dosages above 90 mg/day is not recommended.

Off-label dosing –

Anal fissures: [2] = Fair documentation.

• *Topical* – Nifedipine 0.2% gel or ointment every 12 hours for 3 to 6 weeks.

• *Sublingual* – Nifedipine 20 mg.

Raynaud phenomenon: [1] = Good documentation. 5 to 20 mg given 3 times daily or 20 mg given in a slow-release formulation twice daily.

Ureteral stones: [4] = Insufficient documentation. Nifedipine administered with oral steroids (eg, methylprednisolone or deflazacort with misoprostol) as an immediate-release oral product (20 mg daily) or sustained-release preparation (30 mg daily) for up to 20 to 45 days or until stone expulsion.

Wound healing: [4] = Insufficient documentation. 1 mL of nifedipine 2% or 8% gel applied twice daily.

➤*Hepatic function impairment:* Careful monitoring and dose reduction may be necessary; consider initiating therapy with the lowest dose available.

➤*Therapeutic drug monitoring:* Because nifedipine decreases peripheral vascular resistance, monitor blood pressure during the initial administration and titration of nifedipine.

➤*Discontinuation of therapy:* No "rebound effect" has been observed upon discontinuation of nifedipine. However, if discontinuation of nifedipine is necessary, sound clinical practice suggests the dosage be decreased gradually with close health care provider supervision.

➤*Administration:* Avoid coadministration of nifedipine with grapefruit juice.

Tablet – Swallow whole; do not bite or divide tablet.

Adalat CC, Afeditab CR, and *Nifediac CC* should be taken on an empty stomach.

➤*Storage/Stability:*

Capsules – Store at 15° to 25°C (59° to 77°F). Protect from light, moisture, and humidity. Prevent freezing; capsules may be liquid-filled. Replace cap tightly after each opening.

Tablets – Store below 30°C (86°F). Protect from moisture and humidity.

NICARDIPINE HYDROCHLORIDE

Rx	**Nicardipine Hydrochloride** (Various, eg, Amneal, Mylan)	**Capsules; oral:** 20 mg	In 90s, 100s, and 500s.
Rx	**Nicardipine Hydrochloride** (Various, eg, Amneal, Mylan)	**Capsules; oral:** 30 mg	In 90s, 100s, and 500s.
Rx	**Cardene SR** (PDL Biopharma)	**Capsules, extended-release; oral:** 30 mg	Lactose. (CARDENE SR 30 mg/PDL Biopharma). Opaque, pink. In 60s and 200s.
		45 mg	Lactose. (CARDENE SR 45 mg/PDL Biopharma). Opaque, powder blue. In 60s and 200s.
		60 mg	Lactose. (CARDENE SR 60 mg/PDL Biopharma). Opaque, lt. blue/white. In 60s.
Rx	**Cardene I.V.** (EKR Therapeutics)	**Injection, solution:** 0.1 mg/mL	In 200 mL premixed, single-use *Galaxy* container in dextrose 4.8% or sodium chloride 0.86%.
		0.2 mg/mL	In 200 mL premixed, single-use *Galaxy* container in dextrose 5% or sodium chloride 0.83%.
Rx	**Nicardipine Hydrochloride** (Various, eg, Sandoz)	**Injection, solution, concentrate:** 2.5 mg/mL	In 10 mL single-use vials.
Rx	**Cardene I.V.** (EKR Therapeutics)		In 10 mL ampules.

NICARDIPINE HYDROCHLORIDE — ORAL

For complete and comparative prescribing information, refer to the Calcium Channel Blockers class monograph.

Indications

➤*Angina (immediate-release only):* For the management of patients with chronic stable angina (effort-associated angina).

➤*Hypertension:* For the treatment of hypertension. Nicardipine may be used alone or in combination with other antihypertensive drugs.

➤*Off-label uses:*

Postherpetic neuralgia – [4] = Insufficient documentation. The results from the trial evaluating the efficacy of nicardipine in patients with ophthalmic postherpetic neuralgia are favorable. American Academy of Neurology clinical practice guidelines state that the efficacy of nicardipine for the treatment of postherpetic neuralgia is unproven (level U, single class IV study). Until additional data are available defining the optimum dose and patent population, avoid routine use.

Prevention of migraine (adults) – [5] = Poor documentation. Nicardipine has been studied for the prevention of migraine headaches in adult patients, with limited data supporting its use for this indication. American Academy of Neurology clinical practice guidelines state that nicardipine is no more effective than placebo for the prevention of migraines.

Administration and Dosage

➤*Adults:*

Angina –

Immediate release:

• *Initial dosage* – 20 mg 3 times daily.

• *Maintenance dosage* – 20 to 40 mg 3 times daily.

• *Dosage adjustment* – Allow at least 3 days before increasing the dose to ensure achievement of steady-state plasma drug concentrations.

Hypertension –

Extended-release:

• *Initial dosage* – 30 mg 2 times daily.

• *Maintenance dosage* – 30 to 60 mg 2 times daily.

• *Conversion* – The total daily dose of immediate-release nicardipine may not be a useful guide in judging the effective dose of extended-release (ER) nicardipine. Patients currently receiving immediate-release nicardipine may be titrated with nicardipine ER starting at their current total daily dose of immediate-release nicardipine and then reexamined to assess the adequacy of blood pressure control.

Immediate release: See Angina for dosing.

NICARDIPINE HYDROCHLORIDE — ORAL

Off-label dosing –

Postherpetic neuralgia: [4] = Insufficient documentation. 40 mg daily for 2 weeks.

➤*Renal function impairment:* Careful dose titration beginning with 30 mg 2 times daily (ER) or 20 mg 3 times daily (immediate-release) is advised.

➤*Hepatic function impairment:* A suggested starting dosage of 20 mg twice daily (immediate release) is advised with individual titration.

➤*Administration:* Do not chew, crush, or open ER capsules. Avoid grapefruit juice during administration.

➤*Storage / Stability:* Store at 15° to 30°C (59° to 86°F). Protect from light.

NICARDIPINE HYDROCHLORIDE — INJECTION

For complete and comparative prescribing information, refer to the Calcium Channel Blockers class monograph.

Indications

➤*Hypertension:* For the short-term treatment of hypertension when oral therapy is not feasible or desirable.

➤*Off-label uses:*

Pediatric hypertensive urgency or emergency – [1] = Good documentation. Nicardipine is among the therapeutic options for pediatric hypertensive urgency or emergency identified by the National High Blood Pressure Education Program as most useful.

Postherpetic neuralgia – [4] = Insufficient documentation. The results from the one trial evaluating the efficacy of nicardipine in patients with ophthalmic postherpetic neuralgia are favorable. American Academy of Neurology clinical practice guidelines state that the efficacy of nicardipine for the treatment of postherpetic neuralgia is unproven (level U, single class IV study). Until additional data are available defining the optimum dose and patient population, avoid routine use.

Administration and Dosage

➤*Adults:*

Hypertension –

Maximum dose:

- *Premixed injection (0.1 mg / mL)* – 150 mL/h (15 mg/h).
- *Premixed injection (0.2 mg / mL)* – 75 mL/h (15 mg/h).
- *Vials / Ampules* – 150 mL/h (15 mg/h).

Initial dosage:

- *Premixed injection (0.1 mg / mL)* – 50 mL/h (5 mg/h) intravenous (IV) infusion.
- *Premixed injection (0.2 mg / mL)* – 25 mL/h (5 mg/h) IV infusion.
- *Vials / Ampules* – 50 mL/h (5 mg/h) IV infusion.

Dosage titration:

- *Premixed injection (0.1 mg / mL)* – If desired blood pressure reduction is not achieved at initial dosage, the infusion rate may be increased by 25 mL/h (2.5 mg/h) every 5 minutes (for rapid titration) to 15 minutes (for gradual titration), up to a maximum of 150 mL/h, until desired blood pressure reduction is achieved. Following achievement of the blood pressure goal utilizing rapid titration, decrease the infusion rate to 30 mL/h (3 mg/h).
- *Premixed injection (0.2 mg / mL)* – If desired blood pressure reduction is not achieved at initial dosage, the infusion rate may be increased by 12.5 mL/h (2.5 mg/h) every 5 minutes (for rapid titration) to 15 minutes (for gradual titration), up to a maximum of 75 mL/h, until desired blood pressure reduction is achieved. Following achievement of the blood pressure goal utilizing rapid titration, decrease the infusion rate to 15 mL/h (3 mg/h).
- *Vials / Ampules* – See Premixed Injection (0.1 mg/mL) for dosing.

Maintenance dosage: Adjust the rate of infusion as needed to maintain desired response.

Dosage adjustment:

- *Hypotension or tachycardia* – In case of hypotension or tachycardia, the infusion should be discontinued. When blood pressure has stabilized, infusion of nicardipine may be restarted at low doses and adjusted to maintain desired blood pressure.

  Premixed injection (0.1 mg / mL): 30 to 50 mL/h (3 to 5 mg/h).
  Premixed injection (0.2 mg / mL): 15 to 25 mL/h (3 to 5 mg/h).
  Vials / Ampules: 30 to 50 mL/h (3 to 5 mg/h).

Conversion:

- *Injection to oral therapy* – When switching to oral nicardipine, administer the first oral dose 1 hour prior to discontinuation of the infusion. If treatment includes transfer to an oral antihypertensive agent other than oral nicardipine, therapy should generally be initiated upon discontinuation of nicardipine infusion.
- *Oral therapy to injection –*

Nicardipine Oral and IV Equivalence

Oral nicardipine dosage	Equivalent IV infusion rate
20 mg every 8 h	0.5 mg/h
30 mg every 8 h	1.2 mg/h
40 mg every 8 h	2.2 mg/h

Off-label dosing –

Postherpetic neuralgia: [4] = Insufficient documentation. 40 mg daily for 2 weeks.

➤*Children:*

Off-label dosing –

Pediatric hypertensive urgency or emergency: [1] = Good documentation.

- *1 to 17 years of age* – IV infusion 1 to 3 mcg/kg/min. The goal is to reduce blood pressure by up to 25% over the first 8 hours from presentation, and then gradually normalize pressure over 26 to 48 hours.

The following are additional off-label dosing recommendations for the treatment of pediatric hypertensive urgency, emergency, or severe hypertension.

Nicardipine Injection Dosage in Children

Age	Initial dosage	Maintenance dosage	Dosage titration	Maximum dosage
Preterm neonates	0.5 mcg/kg/min	0.5 to 2 mcg/kg/min; has been used for up to 36 to 43 days	Titrate every 15 to 30 min until desired blood pressure is achieved	Initial: 10 mcg/kg/min Maintenance: 6 mcg/kg/min
Term neonates and infants	0.5 to 1 mcg/kg/min; 5 mcg/kg/min was used in 1 patient	1.5 to 3 mcg/kg/min	Titrate every 15 to 30 min until desired blood pressure is achieved	Initial: 10 mcg/kg/min Maintenance: 6 mcg/kg/min
1 to 17 years of age	1 to 5 mcg/kg/min; 10 mcg/kg/min has been used	2 to 3 (range, 1 to 6) mcg/kg/min	Titrate every 15 to 30 min until desired blood pressure is achieved	Initial: 10 mcg/kg/min Maintenance: 6 mcg/kg/min

➤*Renal function impairment:* Titrate slowly when treating patients with renal impairment.

➤*Hepatic function impairment:* Use with caution and titrate slowly in patients with impaired hepatic function or reduced hepatic blood flow. The use of a lower dosage should be considered; monitor closely.

➤*Special risk patients:* Use with caution and titrate slowly in patients with heart failure or significant left ventricular dysfunction.

➤*Preparation for administration:*

Premixed injection – Suspend container from eyelet support, remove protector from outlet port at bottom of container, and attach administration set. Refer to complete directions accompanying set.

No further dilution is required.

Vials / Ampules – Further dilution is required before infusion.

Each vial or ampule (25 mg) should be diluted with 240 mL of a compatible IV diluent, resulting in 250 mL of a solution at a concentration of 0.1 mg/mL. Nicardipine is normally light yellow in color.

➤*Administration:* Administer by slow continuous infusion at a concentration of 0.1 or 0.2 mg/mL. Administer by a central line or through a large peripheral vein. The infusion site should be changed every 12 hours if administered via peripheral vein.

Premixed injection – Do not use plastic container in series connections. Such use could result in air embolism because of residual air being drawn from the primary container before the administration of the fluid from the secondary container is complete.

➤*Admixture compatibility:*

Compatibility –

Vials / Ampules: Nicardipine has been found to be compatible and stable in glass or polyvinyl chloride containers for 24 hours at controlled room temperature with dextrose 5% injection, dextrose 5% and sodium chloride 0.45% injection, dextrose 5% and sodium chloride 0.9% injection, dextrose 5% with potassium 40 mEq, sodium chloride 0.45% injection, and sodium chloride 0.9% injection.

Incompatibility –

Premixed injection: Nicardipine should not be combined with any product in the same IV line or premixed container. Do not add supplementary medication to the bag.

Vials / Ampules: Nicardipine is not compatible with sodium bicarbonate 5% injection or Ringer's lactate injection.

➤*Storage / Stability:* Store at 20° to 25°C (68° to 77°F). The diluted solution is stable for 24 hours at room temperature. Because the premixed container is for single use, discard any unused portion. Protect from freezing. Freezing does not adversely affect the product in the vials or ampules, but avoid exposure to elevated temperatures. Avoid excessive heat. Protect from light until ready to use; store vials in carton until ready to use.

ISRADIPINE

Rx	**DynaCirc CR** (GlaxoSmithKline)	**Tablets, controlled-release; oral:** 5 mg	(DynaCirc CR 5). Lt. pink. Film-coated. In 30s and 100s.
		10 mg	(DynaCirc CR 10). Beige. Film-coated. In 30s and 100s.
Rx	**Isradipine** (Various, eg, Actavis Totowa)	**Capsules; oral:** 2.5 mg	May contain lactose. In 60s, 100s, and 500s.
Rx	**Isradipine** (Various, eg, Actavis Totowa)	**Capsules; oral:** 5 mg	May contain lactose. In 60s, 100s, and 500s.

[a] May contain benzyl alcohol and parabens.

ISRADIPINE — ORAL

For complete and comparative prescribing information, refer to the Calcium Channel Blockers group monograph.

Indications

➤*Hypertension:* Management of hypertension. It may be used alone or concurrently with thiazide-type diuretics.

➤*Off-label uses:*

Pediatric hypertension – [1] = Good documentation. Isradipine is among the therapeutic options for pediatric hypertension identified by the National High Blood Pressure Education Program (NHBEP) based on published case series and expert opinion.

Pediatric hypertensive urgency or emergency – [1] = Good documentation. Isradipine is among the therapeutic options for pediatric hypertensive urgency or emergency identified by the NHBPEP as occasionally useful.

Administration and Dosage

➤*Adults:*

Hypertension –

Capsules:

• *Maximum dose* – 20 mg/day.

• *Initial dosage* – 2.5 mg twice per day alone or in combination with a thiazide diuretic. An antihypertensive response usually occurs within 2 to 3 hours. Maximal response may require 2 to 4 weeks.

• *Dosage titration* – If a satisfactory reduction in blood pressure does not occur after this period, the dose may be adjusted in increments of 5 mg/day at 2- to 4-week intervals up to a maximum of 20 mg/day. Most patients, however, show no additional response to doses above 10 mg/day, and adverse effects are increased in frequency above 10 mg/day.

Controlled-release tablets:

• *Maximum dose* – 20 mg/day.

• *Initial dosage* – 5 mg once daily as monotherapy or in combination with a thiazide diuretic. An antihypertensive response usually occurs within 2 hours, with the peak antihypertensive response occurring 8 to 10 hours postdose; blood pressure reduction is maintained for at least 24 hours following drug administration.

• *Dosage titration* – If necessary, the dose may be adjusted in increments of 5 mg at 2- to 4-week intervals up to a maximum dose of 20 mg/day. Adverse effects are increased in frequency above 10 mg/day.

➤*Children:*

Off-label dosing –

Pediatric hypertension: [1] = Good documentation.

• *1 to 17 years of age* –

Maximum dose: 0.8 mg/kg/day (not to exceed 20 mg/day).

Initial dosage: 0.15 to 0.2 mg/kg orally every day in 3 to 4 divided doses (immediate-release) or in 1 to 2 doses (sustained-release).

Pediatric hypertensive urgency or emergency: [1] = Good documentation.

• *1 to 17 years of age* –

Usual dosage: 0.05 to 0.1 mg/kg orally per dose.

➤*Elderly:* The bioavailability of isradipine (increased AUC) is increased in elderly patients (older than 65 years of age). Ordinarily, the starting dose should still be 2.5 mg twice per day (capsules) and 5 mg once daily (controlled-release tablets) in these patients.

➤*Renal function impairment:* The bioavailability of isradipine (increased AUC) is increased in patients with renal impairment. Ordinarily, the starting dose should still be 2.5 mg twice per day (capsules) and 5 mg once daily (controlled-release tablets) in these patients.

➤*Hepatic function impairment:* The bioavailability of isradipine (increased AUC) is increased in patients with hepatic impairment. Ordinarily, the starting dose should still be 2.5 mg twice per day (capsules) and 5 mg once daily (controlled-release tablets) in these patients.

➤*Administration:* Isradipine controlled-release tablets should be swallowed whole and should not be bitten or divided.

➤*Storage/Stability:* Store below 30°C (86°F) in a tight container, protected from moisture, humidity, and light.

NIMODIPINE

Rx	**Nimodipine** (Various, eg, Barr, Caraco)	**Capsules, liquid-filled; oral:** 30 mg	In UD 30s and 100s.

NIMODIPINE — ORAL

For complete and comparative prescribing information, refer to the Calcium Channel Blockers group monograph.

WARNING

Do not administer nimodipine intravenously (IV) or by other parenteral routes. Deaths and serious, life-threatening adverse reactions have occurred when the contents of nimodipine capsules have been injected parenterally.

Indications

➤*Subarachnoid hemorrhage (SAH):* For the improvement of neurological outcome by reducing the incidence and severity of ischemic deficits in patients with SAH from ruptured intracranial berry aneurysms regardless of their postictus neurological condition (ie, Hunt and Hess grades I to V).

➤*Off-label uses:*

Prevention of migraine (adults) – [4] = Insufficient documentation. Results from several small, controlled trials evaluating the use of nimodipine for the prevention of migraine headaches in adults have been favorable. American Academy of Neurology practice guidelines state that while scientific evidence supports the use of nimodipine for migraine prevention, the evidence is not optimal. (See Administration and Dosage.)

Prevention of migraine (children/adolescents) – [5] = Poor documentation. Current practice guidelines state that nimodipine is not effective for the prevention of migraine headache in pediatric patients and that its use is not recommended.

Administration and Dosage

➤*Maximum dose:*

Adults – There is no well-established maximum dose for the approved indication according to the prescribing information.

➤*Adults:*

Subarachnoid hemorrhage – 60 mg (two 30 mg capsules) every 4 hours for 21 consecutive days, preferably not less than 1 hour before or 2 hours after meals. Oral nimodipine therapy should commence within 96 hours of the SAH.

Off-label dosing –

Prevention of migraine (adults): [4] = Insufficient documentation. 120 mg/day, given in 3 to 4 divided doses.

➤*Hepatic function impairment:* Patients with hepatic cirrhosis have substantially reduced clearance and approximately doubled maximal drug concentration (C_{max}). Dosage should be reduced to 30 mg every 4 hours, with close monitoring of blood pressure and heart rate.

➤*Administration:* Take no less than 1 hour before or 2 hours after meals.

Do not administer nimodipine IV or by other parenteral routes. If nimodipine is inadvertently administered IV, clinically significant hypotension may require cardiovascular support with pressor agents. Specific treatments for calcium channel blocker overdose should also be given promptly.

If the capsule cannot be swallowed (eg, at the time of surgery, or if the patient is unconscious) a hole should be made in both ends of the capsule with an 18-gauge needle, and the contents of the capsule extracted into a syringe. To help minimize administration errors, it is recommended that the syringe be labeled "Not for IV Use." The contents should then be emptied into the patient's in situ nasogastric tube and washed down the tube with 30 mL of normal saline (0.9%).

➤*Storage/Stability:* Store in the manufacturer's original foil package at 25°C (77°F); excursions are permitted to 15° to 30°C (59° to 86°F). Protect from light and freezing.

FELODIPINE

Rx	**Felodipine** (Mutual)	**Tablets, extended release:** 2.5 mg	(MP 771). Lt. green, film-coated. In 30s, 90s, 100s, 250s, 500s, and 1000s.
Rx	**Felodipine** (Mutual)	**Tablets, extended release:** 5 mg	(MP 772). Lt. orange, film-coated. In 30s, 90s, 100s, 250s, 500s, and 1000s.
Rx	**Felodipine** (Mutual)	**Tablets, extended release:** 10 mg	(MP 773). Brown, film-coated. In 30s, 90s, 100s, 250s, 500s, and 1000s.

FELODIPINE — ORAL

For complete and comparative prescribing information, refer to the Calcium Channel Blockers group monograph.

Indications

➤*Hypertension:* For the treatment of hypertension. Felodipine may be used alone or concomitantly with other antihypertensive agents.

➤*Off-label uses:*

Pediatric hypertension – [1] = Good documentation. Felodipine is among the therapeutic options for pediatric hypertension identified by the National High Blood Pressure Education Program based on randomized, controlled trials and expert opinion.

Administration and Dosage

➤*Adults:*

Hypertension –

Usual dosage: 2.5 to 10 mg once daily. In clinical trials, doses more than 10 mg daily increased blood pressure (BP) response, but a large increase in the rate of peripheral edema and other vasodilatory adverse events were reported.

Initial dosage: 5 mg once daily.

Dosage adjustment: Depending on the patient's response, the dosage can be decreased to 2.5 mg or increased to 10 mg once daily. These adjustments generally should occur at intervals of not less than 2 weeks.

➤*Children:*

Off-label dosing –

Pediatric hypertension: [1] = Good documentation.

- *1 to 17 years of age –*

  Maximum dose: 10 mg/day.

  Initial dosage: 2.5 mg orally daily.

➤*Elderly:* Patients older than 65 years of age are likely to develop higher plasma felodipine concentrations. In general, dose selection for an elderly patient should be cautious, usually starting at the low end of the dosing range (2.5 mg daily). Closely monitor BP during dosage adjustment.

➤*Hepatic function impairment:* Patients with impaired liver function may have elevated plasma drug concentrations and may respond to lower doses; closely monitor BP during dosage adjustment of felodipine.

➤*Administration:* Felodipine should be taken without food or with a light meal. Tablets should be swallowed whole and not crushed or chewed.

➤*Storage/Stability:* Store below 30°C (86°F). Keep container tightly closed. Protect from light.

AMLODIPINE

Rx	**Amlodipine Besylate** (Various, eg, Dr. Reddy's, Teva, Zydus, UDL)	**Tablets; oral:** 2.5 mg	In 90s, 100s, 300s, 500s, and UD 100s.
Rx	**Norvasc** (Pfizer)		(NORVASC 2.5). White, diamond shape. In 90s and 100s.
Rx	**Amlodipine Besylate** (Various, eg, Dr. Reddy's, Teva, Zydus, UDL)	**Tablets; oral:** 5 mg	In 90s, 100s, 300s, 500s, 1,000s, 2,500s, and UD 100s and 300s.
Rx	**Norvasc** (Pfizer)		(NORVASC 5). White, elongated octagon. In 90s, 100s, 300s, and UD 100s.
Rx	**Amlodipine Besylate** (Various, eg, Dr. Reddy's, Teva, Zydus, UDL)	**Tablets; oral:** 10 mg	In 90s, 100s, 300s, 500s, 1,000s, and UD 100s.
Rx	**Norvasc** (Pfizer)		(NORVASC 10). White. In 90s, 100s, and UD 100s.

AMLODIPINE BESYLATE — ORAL

For complete and comparative prescribing information, refer to the Calcium Channel Blockers group monograph.

Indications

➤*Hypertension:* For the treatment of hypertension. It may be used alone or in combination with other antihypertensive agents.

➤*Chronic stable angina:* For the treatment of chronic stable angina. Amlodipine may be used alone or in combination with other antianginal agents.

➤*Vasospastic angina (Prinzmetal's or variant angina):* For the treatment of confirmed or suspected vasospastic angina. Amlodipine may be used as monotherapy or in combination with other antianginal drugs.

Administration and Dosage

➤*Maximum dose:* 10 mg once daily, but it may differ depending on indication.

➤*Adults:*

Chronic stable or vasospastic angina – 5 to 10 mg daily. Most patients will require 10 mg for adequate effect.

Hypertension –

Maximum dose: 10 mg once daily.

Initial dosage: 5 mg once daily.

Dosage titration: In general, titration should proceed over 7 to 14 days so that the physician can fully assess the patient's response to each dose level. Titration may proceed more rapidly; however, if clinically warranted, provided the patient is assessed frequently.

Concomitant therapy: A dose of 2.5 mg once daily may be used when adding amlodipine to other antihypertensive therapy.

➤*Elderly:*

Chronic stable or vasospastic angina – 5 mg daily.

Hypertension – Elderly patients may be started on 2.5 mg once daily.

➤*Hepatic function impairment:*

Chronic stable or vasospastic angina – 5 mg daily.

Hypertension – Patients with hepatic function impairment may be started on 2.5 mg once daily.

➤*Debilitated patients:* See Elderly for dosing.

➤*Storage/Stability:* Store bottles at controlled room temperature, 15° to 30°C (59° to 86°F) and dispense in tight, light-resistant containers.

DILTIAZEM HYDROCHLORIDE

Rx	**Diltiazem HCl** (Various, eg, Mylan, Teva)	**Tablets; oral:** 30 mg	May contain lactose or methylparaben. In 100s, 500s, and 1,000s.
Rx	**Cardizem** (Biovail)		Lactose, methylparaben. (MARION 1771). Green. In 100s, 500s and UD 100s.
Rx	**Diltiazem HCl** (Various, eg, Mylan, Teva, Watson)	**Tablets; oral:** 60 mg	May contain lactose or methylparaben. In 100s, 500s, and 1,000s.
Rx	**Cardizem** (Biovail)		Lactose, methylparaben. (MARION 17 72). Yellow, scored. In 100s, 500s, and UD 100s.
Rx	**Diltiazem HCl** (Various, eg, Mylan, Teva, Watson)	**Tablets; oral:** 90 mg	May contain lactose or methylparaben. In 100s, 500s, and 1,000s.
Rx	**Cardizem** (Biovail)		Lactose, methylparaben. (CARDIZEM 90 mg). Green, scored. In 100s and UD 100s.
Rx	**Diltiazem HCl** (Various, eg, Mylan, Teva, Watson)	**Tablets; oral:** 120 mg	May contain lactose or methylparaben. In 100s, 500s, and 1,000s.
Rx	**Cardizem** (Biovail)		Lactose, methylparaben. (CARDIZEM 120 mg). Yellow, scored. In 100s and UD 100s.

DILTIAZEM HYDROCHLORIDE

Rx	**Cardizem LA** (Abbott)	**Tablets, extended-release; oral:** 120 mg	Sucrose. (B 120 mg). White, capsule shape. In 7s, 30s, 90s, and 1,000s.
Rx	**Matzim LA** (Watson Pharma)		Lactose, sucrose. (120 690). White, capsule shape. In 30s, 90s, and 1,000s.
Rx	**Cardizem LA** (Abbott)	**Tablets, extended-release; oral:** 180 mg	Sucrose. (B 180 mg). White, capsule shape. In 7s, 30s, 90s, and 1,000s.
Rx	**Matzim LA** (Watson Pharma)		Lactose, sucrose. (180 691). White, capsule shape. In 30s, 90s, and 1,000s.
Rx	**Cardizem LA** (Abbott)	**Tablets, extended-release; oral:** 240 mg	Sucrose. (B 240 mg). White, capsule shape. In 7s, 30s, 90s, and 1,000s.
Rx	**Matzim LA** (Watson Pharma)		Lactose, sucrose. (240 692). White, capsule shape. In 30s, 90s, and 1,000s.
Rx	**Cardizem LA** (Abbott)	**Tablets, extended-release; oral:** 300 mg	Sucrose. (B 300 mg). White, capsule shape. In 7s, 30s, 90s, and 1,000s.
Rx	**Matzim LA** (Watson Pharma)		Lactose, sucrose. (300 693). White, capsule shape. In 30s, 90s, and 1,000s.
Rx	**Cardizem LA** (Abbott)	**Tablets, extended-release; oral:** 360 mg	Sucrose. (B 360 mg). White, capsule shape. In 7s, 30s, 90s, and 1,000s.
Rx	**Matzim LA** (Watson Pharma)		Lactose, sucrose. (360 694). White, capsule shape. In 30s, 90s, and 1,000s.
Rx	**Cardizem LA** (Abbott)	**Tablets, extended-release; oral:** 420 mg	Sucrose. (B 420 mg). White, capsule shape. In 7s, 30s, 90s, and 1,000s.
Rx	**Matzim LA** (Watson Pharma)		Lactose, sucrose. (420 695). White, capsule shape. In 30s, 90s, and 1,000s.
Rx	**Diltiazem HCl Extended Release** (Various, eg, Mylan, Teva)	**Capsules, extended-release; oral:**[a] 60 mg	May contain sucrose or sugar spheres. In 100s.
Rx	**Diltiazem HCl Extended Release** (Various, eg, Mylan, Teva)	**Capsules, extended-release; oral:**[a] 90 mg	May contain sucrose or sugar spheres. In 100s.
Rx	**Diltiazem HCl Extended Release** (Various, eg, Mylan, Purepac, Teva)	**Capsules, extended-release; oral:**[a] 120 mg	May contain sucrose or sugar spheres. In 30s, 90s, 100s, 500s, and 1,000s.
Rx	**Cardizem CD** (Biovail)		Sucrose. (cardizem CD 120 mg). Lt. turquoise blue. In 30s, 90s, and UD 100s.
Rx	**Cartia XT** (Andrx Pharmaceuticals)		Sucrose. (Andrx 597 120 mg). White/Orange. In 30s, 90s, 500s, and 1,000s.
Rx	**Dilt-CD** (Apotex USA)		Sucrose. (APO 007). White. In 30s, 90s, and 500s.
Rx	**Dilt-XR** (Apotex USA)		(APO 014). Orange opaque/white. In 100s.
Rx	**Diltia XT** (Andrx Pharmaceuticals)		Lactose. (Andrx 548 120 mg). White. In 100s, 500s, and 1,000s.
Rx	**Diltzac** (Apotex)		(APO 120). Blue violet. In 30s, 90s, 100s, 500s, and 1,000s.
Rx	**Taztia XT** (Andrx Pharmaceuticals)		(ANDRX 696 120 mg). Pink. In 30s and 90s.
Rx	**Tiazac** (Forest)		Sucrose. (Tiazac 120). Lavender. In 7s, 30s, 90s, and 1,000s.
Rx	**Diltiazem HCl Extended Release** (Various, eg, Purepac, Teva)	**Capsules, extended-release; oral:**[a] 180 mg	May contain sucrose or sugar spheres. In 30s, 90s, 100s, 500s, and 1,000s.
Rx	**Cardizem CD** (Biovail)		Sucrose. (cardizem CD 180 mg). Lt. turquoise blue/Blue. In 30s, 90s, and UD 100s.
Rx	**Cartia XT** (Andrx Pharmaceuticals)		Sucrose. (Andrx 598 180 mg). Yellow/Orange. In 30s, 90s, 500s, and 1,000s.
Rx	**Dilt-CD** (Apotex USA)		Sucrose. (APO 008). Lt. blue. In 30s, 90s, and 500s.
Rx	**Dilt-XR** (Apotex USA)		(APO 015). Bright orange opaque/white. In 100s.
Rx	**Diltia XT** (Andrx Pharmaceuticals)		Lactose. (Andrx 549 180 mg). Gray/White. In 100s, 500s, and 1,000s.
Rx	**Diltzac** (Apotex)		(APO 180). White and blue green. In 30s, 90s, 100s, and 500s.
Rx	**Taztia XT** (Andrx Pharmaceuticals)		(ANDRX 697 180 mg). Lt. blue/Buff. In 30s and 90s.
Rx	**Tiazac** (Forest)		Sucrose. (Tiazac 180). White/Blue-green. In 7s, 30s, 90s, and 1,000s.
Rx	**Diltiazem HCl Extended Release** (Various, eg, Purepac, Teva)	**Capsules, extended-release; oral:**[a] 240 mg	May contain sucrose or sugar spheres. In 30s, 90s, 100s, 500s, and 1,000s.
Rx	**Cardizem CD** (Biovail)		Sucrose. (cardizem CD 240 mg). Blue. In 30s, 90s, and UD 100s.
Rx	**Cartia XT** (Andrx Pharmaceuticals)		Sucrose. (Andrx 599 240 mg). Lt. brown/Orange. In 30s, 90s, 500s, and 1,000s.
Rx	**Dilacor XR** (Watson)		(A Dilacor XR 240 mg). Lt. blue/Flesh. In 100s and 500s.
Rx	**Dilt-CD** (Apotex USA)		Sucrose. (APO 009). Lt. blue. In 30s, 90s, and 500s.
Rx	**Dilt-XR** (Apotex USA)		(APO 016). Brown opaque/white. In 100s.
Rx	**Diltia XT** (Andrx Pharmaceuticals)		Lactose. (Andrx 550 240 mg). Gray. In 100s, 500s, and 1,000s.
Rx	**Diltzac** (Apotex)		(APO 240). Blue violet and blue green. In 30s, 90s, 100s, and 500s.
Rx	**Taztia XT** (Andrx Pharmaceuticals)		(ANDRX 698 240 mg). Pink/Lt. blue. In 30s and 90s.
Rx	**Tiazac** (Forest)		Sucrose. (Tiazac 240). Blue-green/Lavender. In 7s, 30s, 90s, and 1,000s.

DILTIAZEM HYDROCHLORIDE

Rx	**Diltiazem HCl Extended Release** (Various, eg, Purepac, Teva)	**Capsules, extended-release; oral:**[a] 300 mg	May contain sucrose or sugar spheres. In 30s, 90s, 500s, and 1,000s.
Rx	**Cardizem CD** (Biovail)		Sucrose. (cardizem CD 300 mg). Lt. gray/Blue. In 30s, 90s, and UD 100s.
Rx	**Cartia XT** (Andrx Pharmaceuticals)		Sucrose. (Andrx 600 300 mg). Orange. In 30s, 90s, 500s, and 1,000s.
Rx	**Dilt-CD** (Apotex USA)		Sucrose. (APO 010). Lt. gray. In 30s, 90s, and 500s.
Rx	**Diltzac** (Apotex)		(APO 300). Blue violet and white. In 30s, 90s, 100s, and 500s.
Rx	**Taztia XT** (Andrx Pharmaceuticals)		(ANDRX 699 300 mg). Pink/Buff. In 30s and 90s.
Rx	**Tiazac** (Forest)		Sucrose. (Tiazac 300). White/Lavender. In 7s, 30s, 90s, and 1,000s.
Rx	**Diltiazem HCl** (Various, eg, Inwood)	**Capsules, extended-release; oral:**[a] 360 mg	In 90s.
Rx	**Cardizem CD** (Biovail)		Sucrose. (cardizem CD 360 mg). Lt. blue/White. In 90s.
Rx	**Diltzac** (Apotex)		(APO 360). Blue green. In 30s, 90s, 100s, and 500s.
Rx	**Taztia XT** (Andrx Pharmaceuticals)		(ANDRX 700 360 mg). Lt. blue. In 30s and 90s.
Rx	**Tiazac** (Forest)		Sucrose. (Tiazac 360). Blue-green. In 7s, 30s, 90s, and 1,000s.
Rx	**Diltiazem Hydrochloride** (Various, eg, Inwood)	**Capsules, extended-release; oral:**[a] 420 mg	May contain sucrose. In 30s, 90s, and 1,000s.
Rx	**Tiazac** (Forest)		Sucrose. (Tiazac 420). White. In 7s, 30s, 90s, and 1,000s.
Rx	**Diltiazem HCl** (Various, eg, Bedford, Bertek)	**Injection:** 5 mg/mL	In 5, 10, and 25 mL vials.
Rx	**Cardizem** (Biovail)		In 5 and 10 mL single-use vials.
Rx	**Cardizem** (Biovail)	**Powder for injection:** 25 mg	Single-use containers. Carton of 6 *Lyo-Ject* syringes with diluent.

[a] Note: The terms "extended-release" and "sustained-release" sometimes are used interchangeably.

DILTIAZEM HYDROCHLORIDE — ORAL

For complete and comparative prescribing information, refer to the Calcium Channel Blockers group monograph.

Indications

➤*Extended-release capsules and tablets:* For the treatment of hypertension. It may be used alone or in combination with other antihypertensive medications.

➤*Extended-release capsules and immediate-release tablets:* For the management of chronic stable angina and angina due to coronary artery spasm.

➤*Extended-release tablets:* For the management of chronic stable angina.

➤*Off-label uses:*

Anal fissures – [2] = Fair documentation. Topical diltiazem gel appears to be an effective therapy for the treatment of anal fissures and is associated with fewer adverse reactions than topical nitroglycerin.

Anal sphincter pressure reduction (topical) – [4] = Insufficient documentation. Topical diltiazem gel has been studied in 1 small trial as a single dose in several concentrations and compared with oral diltiazem and topical bethanecol. In a small number of volunteers, the maximum reduction of sphincter pressure was achieved with a 2% topical formulation and concentrations above this strength did not offer additional reductions. Single-dose topical application was more effective than single- or multiple-dose oral ingestion and was without adverse reactions.

Idiopathic muscle cramps – [2] = Fair documentation. Evidence-based pharmacologic treatments for idiopathic muscle cramps are limited. Although quinine derivatives are likely effective for the condition, the American Academy of Neurology recommended that they be considered only in cases in which cramps are disabling, no other agents provide relief, and adverse effects can be carefully monitored. Diltiazem was considered possibly effective; however, further research is needed to establish the appropriate therapy for idiopathic muscle cramps that offers an acceptable balance of efficacy and safety.

Prevention of migraine (adults) – [5] = Poor documentation. Diltiazem has been studied for the prevention of migraine headaches in adults in a single, small, open-label study. American Academy of Neurology practice guidelines state that diltiazem does not have any significant effect on prophylaxis of migraine, a consensus that was reached in the absence of relevant scientific evidence.

Hypertension – Diltiazem has been used in children for hypertension. (See also Administration and Dosage.)

Administration and Dosage

➤*Adults:*

Angina –

Extended-release capsules:
- *Maximum dose* – 480 mg once daily.
- *Initial dosage* – 120 to 180 mg once daily.
- *Dosage titration* – When necessary, titration may be carried out over a 7 to 14 day period.

Extended-release tablets:
- *Initial dosage* – 180 mg once daily.
- *Dosage titration* – Increase at intervals of 7 to 14 days if adequate response is not obtained.
- *Maintenance dosage* – Doses above 360 mg appear to confer no additional benefit.

Immediate-release tablets:
- *Usual dosage* – 180 to 360 mg/day divided 3 to 4 times a day.
- *Initial dosage* – 30 mg 4 times daily, before meals and at bedtime.
- *Dosage titration* – Increase gradually at 1 to 2 day intervals until optimum response is obtained.

Hypertension –

Usual dosage:
- *Extended-release capsules* – 120 to 480 mg once daily.
- *Extended-release tablets* – 120 to 540 mg once daily.

Maximum dose:
- *Extended-release capsules* – 480 mg once daily.
- *Extended-release tablets* – 540 mg once daily.

Initial dosage: 180 to 240 mg once daily when used as monotherapy.

Dosage titration: Maximum antihypertensive effect is usually observed by 14 days of chronic therapy; therefore, schedule dosage adjustments accordingly.

Concomitant therapy –

Antihypertensives: Diltiazem has an additive antihypertensive effect when used with other antihypertensive agents. Therefore, the dosage of diltiazem or the concomitant antihypertensives may need to be adjusted when adding one to the other.

Conversion – Patients controlled on diltiazem alone or in combination with other medications may be switched to diltiazem extended-release capsules or tablets at the nearest equivalent total daily dose. Higher doses of extended-release diltiazem may be needed in some patients. Closely monitor patients. Subsequent titration to higher or lower doses may be necessary and should be initiated as clinically warranted.

Off-label dosing –

Anal fissures: [2] = Fair documentation. Topical diltiazem 2% gel, ointment, or cream applied twice daily for 6 to 12 weeks. Three-times-daily administration also has been reported.

Anal sphincter pressure reduction (topical): [4] = Insufficient documentation. Topical diltiazem 0.1%, 0.5%, 1%, 2%, 5%, and 10% gels applied once.

Idiopathic muscle cramps: [2] = Fair documentation. 30 mg orally once daily. The optimal duration of therapy is not known.

➤*Children:*

Off-label dosing –

Hypertension:
- *Adolescents* –
  Immediate-release: 30 to 120 mg 3 to 4 times daily; usual range 180 to 360 mg/day.
  Extended-release: 120 to 300 mg/day divided 1 to 2 times daily depending on extended-release product selected. 540 mg/day.
- *Children* –
  Usual dosage: 1.5 to 2 mg/kg/day divided 3 to 4 times daily.
  Maximum dose: 3.5 mg/kg/day or 6 mg/kg/day up to 360 mg/day.

➤*Administration:*

Extended-release tablets – Intended for once-daily administration. The tablets should be swallowed whole and not chewed or crushed.

Tiazac extended-release capsules – May administer by carefully opening the capsule and sprinkling the capsule contents on a spoonful of applesauce. Immediately swallow the applesauce without chewing and follow with a glass of cool water to ensure complete swallowing of the capsule contents. The applesauce should not be hot, and it should be soft enough to be swallowed without chewing. Use any capsule contents/applesauce mixture immediately and do not store for future use. Subdividing the contents of the extended-release capsule is not recommended.

➤*Storage/Stability:* Store at 25°C (77°F); excursions permitted to 15° to 30°C (59° to 86°F).

DILTIAZEM HYDROCHLORIDE — INJECTION

For complete and comparative prescribing information, refer to the Calcium Channel Blockers group monograph.

Indications

➤*Atrial fibrillation or atrial flutter:* Temporary control of rapid ventricular rate in atrial fibrillation or atrial flutter. It should not be used in patients with atrial fibrillation or atrial flutter associated with an accessory bypass tract such as in Wolff-Parkinson-White (WPW) syndrome or short PR syndrome.

➤*Paroxysmal supraventricular tachycardia:* Rapid conversion of paroxysmal supraventricular tachycardias (PSVTs) to sinus rhythm. This includes AV nodal reentrant tachycardias and reciprocating tachycardias associated with an extranodal accessory pathway such as the WPW syndrome or short PR syndrome. Unless otherwise contraindicated, appropriate vagal maneuvers should be attempted prior to administration of diltiazem single-use solution for injection or diltiazem single-use syringe.

The use of diltiazem single-use syringe, diltiazem single-use solution, or diltiazem powder for reconstitution should be undertaken with caution when the patient is compromised hemodynamically or is taking other drugs that decrease any or all of the following: Peripheral resistance, myocardial filling, myocardial contractility, or electrical impulse propagation in the myocardium.

Administration and Dosage

➤*General dosing considerations:* Patients with low body weights should be dosed on a mg/kg basis.

➤*Adults:*

Atrial fibrillation / flutter –

Initial dosage: 0.25 mg/kg actual body weight as a bolus administered over 2 minutes (20 mg is a reasonable dose for the average patient). If response is inadequate after 15 minutes, administer a second bolus dose of 0.35 mg/kg actual body weight over 2 minutes (25 mg is a reasonable dose for the average patient). Subsequent IV bolus doses should be individualized.

Maintenance dosage: For continued reduction of heart rate (up to 24 hours) immediately following the bolus dose, administer an IV infusion. The initial infusion rate is 10 mg/h. Some patients may maintain response to an initial infusion rate of 5 mg/h. The infusion rate may be increased in 5 mg/h increments up to 15 mg/h as needed. Infusion duration exceeding 24 hours and infusion rates exceeding 15 mg/h are not recommended.

Alternative dosage: Some patients may respond to an initial bolus dose of 0.15 mg/kg, although duration of action may be shorter. Experience with this dose is limited.

Conversion: Transition to other antiarrhythmic agents following administration of diltiazem is generally safe. However, reference should be made to the respective agent manufacturer's package insert for information relative to dosage and administration.

Paroxysmal supraventricular tachycardia – See Atrial Fibrillation/ Flutter for dosing.

➤*Preparation for administration:* For continuous IV infusion, aseptically transfer the appropriate quantity of diltiazem to the desired volume of Normal Saline, D5W, or D5W/0.45% NaCl. Mix thoroughly.

Dilution of Diltiazem Injection or *Cardizem Lyo-Ject*				
Diluent volume (mL)	Quantity of diltiazem injection or *Cardizem Lyo-Ject* to add	Final concentration (mg/mL)	Administration dose[a] (mg/h)	Infusion rate (mL/h)
100	125 mg (25 mL)	1	10	10
			15	15
250	250 mg (50 mL)	0.83	10	12
			15	18

Dilution of Diltiazem Injection or *Cardizem Lyo-Ject*				
Diluent volume (mL)	Quantity of diltiazem injection or *Cardizem Lyo-Ject* to add	Final concentration (mg/mL)	Administration dose[a] (mg/h)	Infusion rate (mL/h)
500	250 mg (50 mL)	0.45	10	22
			15	33

[a] 5 mg/h may be appropriate for some patients.

➤*Admixture compatibility:*

Compatibility – Diltiazem up to 1 mg/mL was found to be physically compatible and chemically stable in the following parenteral solutions for at least 24 hours when stored in glass (diltiazem single-use solution for injection/diltiazem single-use syringe only) or polyvinylchloride (PVC) bags at controlled room temperature 15° to 30°C (59° to 86°F) or under refrigeration 2° to 8°C (36° to 46°F).

1.) Dextrose (5%) injection
2.) Sodium chloride (0.9%) injection
3.) Dextrose (5%) and sodium chloride (0.45%) injection

Diltiazem single-use syringe was found to be compatible with insulin (regular, 100 units/mL).

Diltiazem powder for reconstitution at a concentration of 1 mg/mL diluted in normal saline was infused in the same IV line and was found to be compatible with the following drugs: aminophylline, ampicillin sodium, ampicillin sodium/sulbactam sodium, cefamandole, hydrocortisone sodium succinate, regular insulin (100 units/mL), methylprednisolone sodium succinate, mezlocillin sodium, nafcillin sodium, and sodium bicarbonate.

Incompatibility – Because of potential physical incompatibilities, it is recommended that diltiazem not be mixed with any other drugs in the same container. If possible, it is recommended that diltiazem single-use solution for injection, diltiazem single-use syringe, or diltiazem powder for reconstitution not be co-infused in the same IV line.

Physical incompatibilities were observed when diltiazem single-use solution for injection or diltiazem single-use syringe was infused in the same IV line with the following drugs: Acetazolamide, acyclovir, aminophylline, ampicillin, ampicillin sodium/sulbactam sodium, cefamandole, cefoperazone, diazepam, furosemide, hydrocortisone sodium succinate, insulin, (regular: 100 units/mL), methylprednisolone sodium succinate, mezlocillin, nafcillin, phenytoin, rifampin, and sodium bicarbonate.

Physical incompatibilities (precipitate formation or cloudiness) were observed when diltiazem powder for reconstitution at a concentration of 1 mg/mL diluted in normal saline was infused in the same IV line with the following drugs: Acetazolamide, acyclovir, cefoperazone sodium, diazepam, furosemide, phenytoin, and rifampin.

➤*Storage / Stability:*

Diltiazem single-use solution for injection – Store product under refrigeration 2° to 8°C (36° to 46°F). Do not freeze. May be stored at room temperature for up to 1 month. Destroy after 1 month at room temperature. Keep diluted diltiazem single-use solution for injection refrigerated until use. Discard unused portion.

Diltiazem single-use syringe – Store at 15° to 30°C (59° to 86°F). Do not freeze. Reconstituted material is stable for 24 hours at room temperature. Discard unused portion.

Diltiazem powder for reconstitution – Store at 15° to 30°C (59° to 86°F). Do not freeze. Reconstituted material is stable for 24 hours at room temperature.

VERAPAMIL HYDROCHLORIDE

Rx	**Verapamil Hydrochloride** (Watson)	**Tablets; oral:** 40 mg	May contain lactose, polyethylene glycol. In 100s.
Rx	**Verapamil Hydrochloride** (Various, eg, Major, Mylan, Watson)	**Tablets; oral:** 80 mg	May contain lactose, polyethylene glycol. In 100s, 500s, and 1,000s.
Rx	**Calan** (Pfizer)		Lactose, polyethylene glycol. (CALAN 80). Peach, oval, scored. Film-coated. In 100s.
Rx	**Verapamil Hydrochloride** (Various, eg, Major, Mylan, Watson)	**Tablets; oral:** 120 mg	May contain lactose, polyethylene glycol. In 100s, 500s, and 1,000s.
Rx	**Calan** (Pfizer)		Lactose, polyethylene glycol. (CALAN 120). Brown, oval, scored. Film-coated. In 100s.
Rx	**Verapamil Hydrochloride Extended-Release** (Various, eg, Mylan, Teva)	**Tablets, extended-release; oral**[a]: 120 mg	In 30s, 100s, and UD 100s.
Rx	**Calan SR** (Pfizer)		Polyethylene glycol. (CALAN SR 120). Lt. violet, oval. Film-coated. In 100s.
Rx	**Isoptin SR** (Ranbaxy)		Polyethylene glycol. (p SC). Lt. violet, oval. Film-coated. In 100s.

VERAPAMIL HYDROCHLORIDE

Rx	**Verapamil Hydrochloride Extended-Release** (Various, eg, Mylan, Teva)	**Tablets, extended-release; oral**[a]: 180 mg	In 30s, 100s, 300s, 500s, and UD 100s.
Rx	**Calan SR** (Pfizer)		Polyethylene glycol. (CALAN SR 180). Lt. pink, oval, scored. Film-coated. In 100s.
Rx	**Covera-HS**[b] (Pfizer)		BHT, polyethylene glycol. (COVERA-HS 2011). Lavender, round. Film-coated. In 100s and UD 100s.
Rx	**Isoptin SR** (Ranbaxy)		Polyethylene glycol. (pp SK). Lt. pink, oval, scored. Film-coated. In 100s.
Rx	**Verapamil Hydrochloride Extended-Release** (Various, eg, Mylan, Teva)	**Tablets, extended-release; oral**[a]: 240 mg	In 30s, 90s, 100s, 300s, 500s, and UD 100s.
Rx	**Calan SR** (Pfizer)		Polyethylene glycol. (CALAN SR 240). Lt. green, capsule shape, scored. Film-coated. In 100s, 500s, and UD 100s.
Rx	**Covera-HS**[b] (Pfizer)		BHT, polyethylene glycol. (COVERA-HS 2021). Pale yellow, round. Film-coated. In 100s and UD 100s.
Rx	**Isoptin SR** (Ranbaxy)		Polyethylene glycol. (pp ST). Lt. green, capsule shape, scored. Film-coated. In 100s and 500s.
Rx	**Verapamil Hydrochloride** (Various, eg, Kremers Urban, Mylan)	**Capsules, extended-release; oral**[a]: 100 mg	May contain maltodextrin, polyethylene glycol, sugar. In 100s and 500s.
Rx	**Verelan PM**[b] (Schwarz Pharma)		Pellet-filled. Sugar. (SCHWARZ 4085/100 mg). White/Amethyst. In 100s.
Rx	**Verapamil Hydrochloride Extended-Release** (Various, eg, Mylan, UDL, Watson)	**Capsules, extended-release; oral**[a]: 120 mg	May be pellet-filled. May contain maltodextrin, polyethylene glycol, sugar. In 30s, 100s, 500s, and UD 100s.
Rx	**Verelan**[b] (Schwarz Pharma)		Pellet-filled. Sugar, parabens. (SCHWARZ 2490 VERELAN 120 mg). Yellow. In 100s.
Rx	**Verapamil Hydrochloride Extended-Release** (Various, eg, Mylan, Watson)	**Capsules, extended-release; oral**[a]: 180 mg	May be pellet-filled. May contain maltodextrin, polyethylene glycol, sugar. In 30s, 100s, and 500s.
Rx	**Verelan**[b] (Schwarz Pharma)		Pellet-filled. Sugar, parabens. (SCHWARZ 2489 VERELAN 180 mg). Lt. gray/yellow. In 100s.
Rx	**Verapamil Hydrochloride** (Various, eg, Kremers Urban, Mylan)	**Capsules, extended-release; oral**[a]: 200 mg	May contain maltodextrin, polyethylene glycol, sugar. In 100s and 500s.
Rx	**Verelan PM**[b] (Schwarz Pharma)		Pellet-filled. Sugar. (SCHWARZ 4086 200 mg). Amethyst. In 100s.
Rx	**Verapamil Hydrochloride Extended-Release** (Various, eg, Mylan, Watson)	**Capsules, extended-release; oral**[a]: 240 mg	May be pellet-filled. May contain maltodextrin, polyethylene glycol, sugar. In 30s, 100s, and 500s.
Rx	**Verelan**[b] (Schwarz Pharma)		Pellet-filled. Sugar, parabens. (SCHWARZ 2491 VERELAN 240 mg). Dk. blue/yellow. In 100s.
Rx	**Verapamil Hydrochloride** (Various, eg, Kremers Urban, Mylan)	**Capsules, extended-release; oral**[a]: 300 mg	May contain maltodextrin, polyethylene glycol, sugar. In 100s and 500s.
Rx	**Verelan PM**[b] (Schwarz Pharma)		Pellet-filled. Sugar. (SCHWARZ 4087 300 mg). Lavender/Amethyst. In 100s.
Rx	**Verapamil Hydrochloride Extended-Release** (Watson)	**Capsules, extended-release; oral**[a]: 360 mg	May be pellet-filled. In 100s.
Rx	**Verelan**[b] (Schwarz Pharma)		Pellet-filled. Sugar, parabens. (SCHWARZ 2495 VERELAN 360 mg). Lavender/Yellow. In 100s.
Rx	**Verapamil Hydrochloride** (Various, eg, Hospira)	**Injection, solution:** 2.5 mg/mL	May contain sodium chloride. In 2 mL amps and 2 and 4 mL vials. Also in 4 mL *Ansyr* syringe.

[a] The terms "extended-release" and "sustained-release" sometimes are used interchangeably.

[b] 24-hour formulation.

VERAPAMIL HYDROCHLORIDE — ORAL

For complete and comparative prescribing information, refer to the Calcium Channel Blockers class monograph.

Indications

➤*Angina:*

Immediate-release tablets – For the treatment of angina at rest, including vasospastic (Prinzmetal variant) angina and unstable (crescendo, preinfarction) angina. Also for the treatment of chronic stable angina (classic effort-associated angina).

Covera-HS – For the management of angina.

➤*Arrhythmias (immediate-release tablets only):* With digitalis to control ventricular rate at rest and during stress in chronic atrial flutter and/or fibrillation. May also be used for prophylaxis of repetitive paroxysmal supraventricular tachycardia (PSVT).

➤*Hypertension:* For the management of essential hypertension.

➤*Off-label uses:*

Prevention of migraine (adults) – 2 = Fair documentation. Results from trials evaluating verapamil for the prevention of migraine headache in adults have shown favorable results. American Academy of Neurology practice guidelines state that, while the scientific evidence is not optimal, some patients do show a clinically significant benefit from verapamil treatment. (See Administration and Dosage.)

Other possible off-label uses – Prevention of cluster headaches; management of hypertrophic cardiomyopathy.

Administration and Dosage

➤*General dosing considerations:* Individualize dose by titration.

Because the half-life of verapamil increases during chronic dosing, maximum response may be delayed.

➤*Adults:*

Angina –

Covera-HS:

• *Usual dosage* – 180 to 540 mg given once daily at bedtime.

• *Initial dosage* – 180 mg/day at bedtime.

• *Dosage adjustment* – If an adequate response is not obtained with 180 mg, the dose may be titrated upward in the following manner: 240 mg each evening; 360 mg each evening (2 × 180 mg); 480 mg each evening (2 × 240 mg).

Immediate-release tablet:

• *Usual dosage* – 80 to 120 mg 3 times/day. However, 40 mg 3 times/day may be warranted in patients who have increased response to verapamil (eg, decreased hepatic function, elderly patients).

• *Maximum dose* – The usefulness and safety of dosage exceeding 480 mg/day have not been established; therefore, this daily dosage should not be exceeded.

• *Dosage adjustment* – Base on safety and therapeutic efficacy; evaluate approximately 8 hours after dosing. Dosage may be increased daily (eg, unstable angina) or weekly until optimum clinical response is obtained.

VERAPAMIL HYDROCHLORIDE — ORAL

Arrhythmias –

Immediate-release tablet:

• *Usual dosage* – Dosage range in digitalized patients with chronic atrial fibrillation is 240 to 320 mg/day in divided doses 3 or 4 times/day. Dosage range for prophylaxis of PSVT (nondigitalized patients) is 240 to 480 mg/day in divided doses 3 or 4 times/day. Maximum effects will be apparent during the first 48 hours of therapy.

• *Maximum dose* – The usefulness and safety of dosage exceeding 480 mg/day have not been established; therefore, this daily dosage should not be exceeded.

Hypertension –

Calan SR, Isoptin SR:

• *Initial dosage* – 180 mg given in the morning. Lower initial dosages of 120 mg/day may be warranted in patients who may have an increased response to verapamil (eg, elderly patients, patients of small stature).

• *Dosage adjustment* – Base on therapeutic efficacy and safety; evaluate weekly and approximately 24 hours after the previous dose. The antihypertensive effects are evident within the first week of therapy. If adequate response is not obtained with 180 mg, the dosage may be titrated upward in the following manner: 240 mg each morning; 180 mg each morning plus 180 mg each evening, or 240 mg each morning plus 120 mg each evening; 240 mg every 12 hours.

• *Conversion* – When switching from immediate-release tablets to extended-release (ER) tablets, the total daily dose in milligrams may remain the same.

Covera-HS: See Angina for dosing.

Verelan:

• *Usual dosage* – 240 mg once daily in the morning.

• *Initial dosage* – Initial dosages of 120 mg/day may be warranted in patients who may have an increased response to verapamil (eg, elderly patients, patients of small stature).

• *Dosage adjustment* – Base on therapeutic efficacy and safety; evaluate approximately 24 hours after dosing. The antihypertensive effects are evident within the first week of therapy. If adequate response is not obtained with verapamil 120 mg, the dose may be titrated upward in the following manner: 180 mg in the morning; 240 mg in the morning; 360 mg in the morning; 480 mg in the morning.

• *Conversion* – When switching from immediate-release verapamil to ER capsules, the total daily dose in milligrams may remain the same.

Verelan PM:

• *Usual dosage* – 200 mg/day at bedtime.

• *Initial dosage* – Initial dosages of 100 mg/day may be warranted in patients who have an increased response to verapamil (eg, impaired renal or hepatic function, elderly patients, patients of small stature).

• *Dosage adjustment* – Base on safety and therapeutic efficacy; evaluate approximately 24 hours after dosing. Antihypertensive effects are evident within the first week of therapy. If an adequate response is not obtained with 200 mg, the dose may be titrated upward in the following manner: 300 mg each evening; 400 mg each evening (2 × 200 mg).

Immediate-release tablet:

• *Maximum dose* – The usefulness and safety of dosage exceeding 480 mg/day have not been established; therefore, this daily dosage should not be exceeded.

• *Initial dosage* – Initial monotherapy dosage is 80 mg 3 times/day (240 mg/day). Consider beginning titration at 40 mg 3 times/day in patients who might respond to lower doses (eg, elderly patients, patients of small stature).

• *Maintenance dosage* – Daily dosages of 360 and 480 mg have been used, but there is no evidence that dosages beyond 360 mg provide added effect.

• *Dosage adjustment* – Antihypertensive effects are evident within the first week of therapy. Base upward titration on therapeutic efficacy, assessed at the end of the dosing interval.

Off-label dosing –

Prevention of migraine (adults): [2] = Fair documentation. Verapamil dosages ranged from 160 to 320 mg daily, given in 3 to 4 divided doses.

➤*Elderly:* In general, lower initial doses of verapamil may be warranted in elderly patients.

➤*Renal function impairment:* Administer verapamil cautiously to patients with renal impairment.

➤*Hepatic function impairment:* Administer verapamil cautiously to patients with hepatic impairment. Administer approximately 30% of the dose given to patients with healthy liver function to patients with severe liver dysfunction.

➤*Monitoring:*

Extended release – When administered at bedtime, office evaluation of blood pressure during morning and early afternoon hours is essentially a measure of peak effect. The usual evaluation of trough effect, which sometimes might be needed to evaluate the appropriateness of any given dose, would be just prior to bedtime.

➤*Administration:*

Extended release –

Capsules: Administer once daily. Swallow the capsules whole or sprinkle onto applesauce; do not crush or chew the capsules.

May administer pellet-filled capsules by carefully opening the capsule and sprinkling the pellets on a spoonful of applesauce. Swallow the applesauce immediately without chewing and follow with a glass of cool water to ensure complete swallowing of the pellets. The applesauce used should not be hot, and it should be soft enough to be swallowed without chewing. Use any pellet/applesauce mixture immediately and do not store for future use. Subdividing the contents of the capsule is not recommended.

Administer *Verelan PM* at bedtime.

Tablets:

• *Calan SR, Isoptin SR* – Administer with food. Tablets may be divided in half.

• *Covera-HS* – Swallow tablets whole; do not chew, break, or crush the tablets.

➤*Storage / Stability:*

Capsules – Store at 20° to 25°C (68° to 77°F). Avoid excessive heat. Brief digressions above 25°C (77°F), while not detrimental, should be avoided. Protect from moisture.

Tablets – Store at 15° to 25°C (59° to 77°F). Protect from light and moisture. *Covera-HS*: Store at 20° to 25°C (68° to 77°F).

VERAPAMIL HYDROCHLORIDE — INJECTION

For complete and comparative prescribing information, refer to the Calcium Channel Blockers class monograph.

Indications

➤*Atrial flutter or fibrillation:* Temporary control of rapid ventricular rate in atrial flutter and/or atrial fibrillation, except when the atrial flutter or atrial fibrillation are associated with accessory bypass tracts (Wolff-Parkinson-White and Lown-Ganong-Levine syndromes).

➤*Supraventricular tachycardias:* Rapid conversion to sinus rhythm of paroxysmal supraventricular tachycardias, including those associated with accessory bypass tracts (Wolff-Parkinson-White and Lown-Ganong-Levine syndromes). When clinically advisable, attempt appropriate vagal maneuvers (eg, Valsalva maneuver) prior to verapamil administration.

Administration and Dosage

➤*Adults:*

Atrial flutter / fibrillation –

Initial dosage: 5 to 10 mg (0.075 to 0.15 mg/kg body weight) given as an intravenous (IV) bolus over at least 2 minutes.

Repeat dosage: 10 mg (0.15 mg/kg body weight) 30 minutes after the first dose if the initial response is not adequate. An optimal interval for subsequent IV doses has not been determined and should be individualized for each patient.

Supraventricular tachycardias – See Atrial flutter/fibrillation for dosing.

➤*Children:*

Atrial flutter / fibrillation –

1 to 15 years of age:

• *Maximum dose* – 5 mg (initial dosage) or 10 mg (repeat dosage) as a single dose.

• *Initial dosage* – 0.1 to 0.3 mg/kg body weight (usual single-dose range, 2 to 5 mg) as an IV bolus over at least 2 minutes. Do not exceed 5 mg.

• *Repeat dosage* – Repeat initial dose 30 minutes after the first dose if the initial response is not adequate. An optimal interval for subsequent IV doses has not been determined and should be individualized for each patient. Do not exceed 10 mg as a single dose.

0 to 1 year of age:

• *Initial dosage* – 0.1 to 0.2 mg/kg body weight (usual single-dose range, 0.75 to 2 mg) as an IV bolus over at least 2 minutes under continuous ECG monitoring.

• *Repeat dosage* – Repeat initial dose 30 minutes after the first dose if the initial response is not adequate (under continuous ECG monitoring). An optimal interval for subsequent IV doses has not been determined and should be individualized for each patient.

Supraventricular tachycardias – See Atrial flutter/fibrillation for dosing.

➤*Elderly:* Administer the dose over at least 3 minutes to minimize the risk of untoward drug effects.

➤*Administration:* For IV use only. Give as a slow IV injection over at least a 2-minute time period under continuous ECG and blood pressure monitoring.

➤*Admixture compatibility:* For stability reasons, this product is not recommended for dilution with sodium lactate injection in polyvinyl chloride bags. Verapamil is physically compatible and chemically stable for at least 24 hours at 25°C (77°F) protected from light in most common large-volume parenteral solutions. Avoid admixing verapamil injection with albumin, amphotericin B, hydralazine, and trimethoprim with sulfamethoxazole. Verapamil injection will precipitate in any solution with a pH above 6.

➤*Storage / Stability:* Store at 20° to 25°C (68° to 77°F). Protect from light by retaining in package until ready to use.

Discard any unused amount of the solution immediately following withdrawal of any portion of contents.

CLEVIDIPINE BUTYRATE

Rx	Cleviprex (The Medicines Company[a])	Injection, emulsion: 0.5 mg/mL	In 50 and 100 mL single-use vials.[b]

[a] The Medicine Company; 8 Campus Drive; Parsippany, NJ 07054; (973)656-1616; http://www.themedicinecompany.com.

[b] Contains soybean oil 200 mg/mL, glycerin 22.5 mg/mL, and purified egg yolk phospholipids 12 mg/mL.

CLEVIDIPINE BUTYRATE — INJECTION

For complete and comparative prescribing information, refer to the Calcium Channel Blockersgroup monograph.

Indications

➤*Hypertension:* For the reduction of blood pressure when oral therapy is not feasible or not desirable.

Administration and Dosage

➤*General dosing considerations:*

Rebound hypertension – Patients who receive prolonged clevidipine infusions and are not transitioned to other antihypertensive therapies should be monitored for the possibility of rebound hypertension for at least 8 hours after the infusion is stopped. These patients may need follow-up adjustments in blood pressure control.

➤*Adults:*

Hypertension –

Maximum dose: 32 mg/h or 1,000 mL (average of 21 mg/h) per 24-hour period.

Initial dosage: 1 to 2 mg/h by IV infusion.

Dosage titration: The dose may be doubled at short (90-second) intervals initially. As the blood pressure approaches the goal, the increase in doses should be less than doubling and the time between dose adjustments should be lengthened to every 5 to 10 minutes. An approximately 1 to 2 mg/h increase will generally produce an additional 2 to 4 mm Hg decrease in systolic pressure. Titrate drug to achieve the desired blood pressure reduction.

Maintenance dosage: 4 to 6 mg/h. Patients with severe hypertension may require doses of up to 32 mg/h, but there is limited experience at this dose rate.

Conversion: To convert to oral therapy, discontinue clevidipine or titrate downward while appropriate oral therapy is established. When an oral antihypertensive agent is being instituted, consider the lag time of onset of the oral agent's effect. Continue blood pressure monitoring until the desired effect is achieved.

➤*Renal function impairment:* 1 to 2 mg/h as an initial infusion rate is appropriate in patients with moderate to severe renal impairment.

➤*Hepatic function impairment:* 1 to 2 mg/h as an initial infusion rate is appropriate in patients with abnormal hepatic function (1 or more of the following: elevated serum bilirubin, AST, and ALT).

➤*Preparation for administration:* Clevidipine is a single-use parenteral product that contains phospholipids and can support microbial growth. Do not use if contamination is suspected. Once the stopper is punctured, use within 4 hours and discard any unused portion, including that which is currently being infused.

Invert vial gently several times before use to ensure uniformity of the emulsion prior to administration. Clevidipine should not be diluted.

➤*Administration:* For IV use. Administer clevidipine by a central or peripheral IV line using an infusion device allowing calibrated infusion rates. Commercially available standard plastic cannulae may be used to administer the infusion.

Dosing conversion from mg/h to mL/h –

Clevidipine Dose Conversion From mg/h to mL/h	
Dose (mg/h)	Dose (mL/h)
1	2
2	4
4	8
6	12
8	16
10	20
12	24
14	28
16	32
18	36
20	40
22	44
24	48
26	52
28	56
30	60
32	64

➤*Admixture compatibility:*

Incompatibility – Clevidipine should not be administered in the same line as other medications.

Compatibility – Clevidipine should not be diluted, but it can be administered with the following: water for injection, sodium chloride 0.9% injection, dextrose 5% injection, dextrose 5% in sodium chloride 0.9% injection, dextrose 5% in Ringer's lactate injection, Ringer's lactate injection, 10% amino acid.

➤*Storage/Stability:* Store at 2° to 8°C (36° to 46°F). Do not freeze. Vials in cartons may be transferred to 25°C (77°F) for a period not to exceed 2 months. Upon transfer to room temperature, mark vials in cartons when removed from the refrigerator. It must be used or discarded 2 months after this date or the labeled expiration date (whichever date comes first). Do not return to refrigerated storage after beginning room temperature storage. Discard any unused product, including product being infused, within 4 hours of stopper puncture.

Leave vials in cartons until use. Clevidipine is photosensitive and storage in cartons protects against photodegradation. Protection from light during administration is not required.

VASODILATORS

Nitrates

Indications

➤*Amyl nitrite:* For the rapid relief of angina pectoris. The effect of amyl nitrite appears within 30 seconds and lasts for approximately 3 to 5 minutes.

➤*Isosorbide dinitrate:*

Tablets, extended-release (ER) tablets, and sustained-release (SR) capsules – For the prevention of angina pectoris caused by coronary artery disease (CAD). The onset of action of immediate- and controlled-release oral isosorbide dinitrate is not sufficiently rapid for these products to be useful in aborting an acute anginal episode.

Sublingual tablets – For the prevention and treatment of angina pectoris caused by CAD. However, because the onset of action of sublingual isosorbide dinitrate is significantly slower than that of sublingual nitroglycerin, sublingual isosorbide dinitrate is not the drug of first choice for abortion of an acute anginal episode.

➤*Isosorbide mononitrate:*

Tablets, ER tablets – For the treatment (*Monoket* only) and prevention of angina pectoris caused by CAD. The onset of action of immediate- and controlled-release oral isosorbide mononitrate is not sufficiently rapid for these products to be useful in aborting an acute anginal episode.

➤*Nitroglycerin:*

Lingual spray, sublingual tablets – For the acute relief of an attack or prophylaxis of angina pectoris caused by CAD.

ER capsules, ointment, transdermal patch – For the prevention of angina pectoris caused by CAD. The onset of action of transdermal and oral nitroglycerin is not sufficiently rapid for this product to be useful in aborting an acute anginalattack.

Intravenous (IV) – For the treatment of perioperative hypertension; for control of congestive heart failure (CHF) in the setting of acute myocardial infarction (MI); for the treatment of angina pectoris in patients who have not responded to sublingual nitroglycerin and beta-blockers; for induction of intraoperative hypotension.

➤*Off-label uses:* Refer to individual monographs for further information.

Anal fissures (adults) –

Nitroglycerin (transdermal): [4] = Insufficient documentation.

Anal fissures (children) –

Nitroglycerin (topical): [2] = Fair documentation.

Extravasation treatment –

Nitroglycerin (topical): [4] = Insufficient documentation.

Prevention of variceal bleeding –

Isosorbide mononitrate: [1] = Good documentation.

Raynaud phenomenon –

Nitroglycerin (topical): [4] = Insufficient documentation.

Nitroglycerin (transdermal): [4] = Insufficient documentation.

Variant angina pectoris –

Nitroglycerin (sublingual): [1] = Good documentation.

Variceal bleeding –

Nitroglycerin (IV): [1] = Good documentation.

Other possible off-label uses –

Isosorbide dinitrate, oral: Used with hydralazine to increase survival among black patients with advanced heart failure; for the treatment of acute angle-closure glaucoma in emergency situations, not intended for long-term management; achalasia.

Nitroglycerin, IV: For the management of acute MI; treatment of hypertensive emergencies; used in combination with vasopressin to treat variceal bleeding; cocaine-induced acute coronary syndrome; management of Prinzmetal angina that occurs in patients without coronary heart disease.

Nitroglycerin, sublingual: For the management of acute MI.

Nitroglycerin, topical: For the management of acute MI; erectile dysfunction; management of Prinzmetal angina that occurs in patients without coronary heart disease.

Nitroglycerin, transdermal: For the management of an acute myocardial infarction; erectile dysfunction; management of Prinzmetal angina that occurs in patients without coronary heart disease.

Actions

➤*Pharmacology:* The principal pharmacological action of nitrates is relaxation of the vascular smooth muscle and consequent dilation of peripheral arteries and especially the veins. Dilation of the veins promotes peripheral pooling of blood and decreases venous return to the heart, thereby reducing left ventricular end-diastolic pressure and pulmonary capillary wedge pressure (preload). Arteriolar relaxation reduces systemic vascular resistance, systolic arterial pressure, and mean arterial pressure (afterload). Dilation of the coronary arteries also occurs. The relative importance of preload reduction, afterload reduction, and coronary dilation remains undefined.

Therapeutic doses of **nitroglycerin** may reduce systolic, diastolic, and mean arterial blood pressure. Effective coronary perfusion pressure is usually maintained but can be compromised if blood pressure falls excessively or increased heart rate decreases diastolic filling time. Heart rate is usually slightly increased, presumably because of a compensatory response to the fall in blood pressure. Cardiac index may be increased, decreased, or unchanged. Myocardial oxygen consumption or demand (as measured by the pressure-rate product, tension-time index, and stroke-work index) is decreased and a more favorable supply-demand ratio can be achieved. Patients with elevated left ventricular filling pressures and increased systemic vascular resistance in association with a depressed cardiac index are likely to experience an improvement in cardiac index. In contrast, when filling pressures and cardiac index are normal, cardiac index may be slightly reduced following nitroglycerin administration.

Nitroglycerin forms free radical nitric oxide (NO), which activates guanylate cyclase, resulting in an increase of guanosine 3'5' monophosphate (cyclic GMP) in smooth muscle and other tissues. These events lead to dephosphorylation of myosin light chains, which regulate the contractile state in smooth muscle and result in vasodilation.

Amyl nitrite causes a nonspecific relaxation of smooth muscle with the most prominent actions occurring in vascular smooth muscle. This effect on vascular smooth muscle results in coronary vasodilation and decreased systemic vascular resistance and left ventricular preload and afterload. Myocardial ischemia is relieved in patients with angina pectoris, with an abatement of chest pain and possibly other related symptoms.

➤*Pharmacokinetics:*

Amyl nitrite –

Absorption: Amyl nitrite vapors are absorbed rapidly through the pulmonary alveoli, manifesting therapeutic effect within 1 minute after inhalation.

Metabolism: The drug is metabolized rapidly, probably by hydrolytic denitration.

Elimination: Approximately one third of inhaled amyl nitrite is excreted in the urine.

Isosorbide dinitrate –

Absorption: Absorption of isosorbide dinitrate after oral dosing is nearly complete but bioavailability is highly variable (10% to 90%). Maximum serum levels are reached approximately 1 hour after ingestion. The average bioavailability of isosorbide dinitrate is approximately 25%; most studies have observed progressive increases in bioavailability during chronic therapy.

Distribution: The volume of distribution of isosorbide dinitrate is 2 to 4 L/kg, and this volume is cleared at a rate of 2 to 4 L/min; therefore, half-life in serum is approximately 1 hour.

Metabolism: Isosorbide dinitrate has extensive first-pass metabolism in the liver. Clearance is affected primarily by denitration to the 2-mononitrate (15% to 25%) and the 5-mononitrate (75% to 85%). Both metabolites have biological activity, especially the 5-mononitrate. The 5-mononitrate is cleared from the serum by denitration to isosorbide, glucuronidation to the 5-mononitrate glucuronide, and denitration/hydration to sorbitol. The 2-mononitrate has been less well studied, but it appears to participate in the same metabolic pathways.

Elimination: Isosorbide dinitrate has an overall elimination half-life of approximately 5 hours.

Isosorbide mononitrate –

Absorption: After oral administration of isosorbide mononitrate, T_{max} is achieved in 30 to 60 minutes, with an absolute bioavailability of approximately 100%.

Distribution: The volume of distribution of isosorbide mononitrate is approximately 0.6 L/kg; less than 5% is bound to plasma protein and distributed into blood cells and saliva.

Metabolism: Isosorbide mononitrate is primarily metabolized by the liver but is not subject to first-pass metabolism. It is cleared from the serum by denitration to isosorbide, glucuronidation to the mononitrate, and denitration/hydration to sorbitol. None of the metabolites are vasoactive.

Elimination: The overall elimination half-life is approximately 5 hours; 96% of the dose is excreted in the urine within 5 days and 1% eliminated in the feces. Renal clearance accounts for about 4% of total body clearance. The rate of clearance is the same in healthy young adults, in patients with various degrees of renal, hepatic, or cardiac dysfunction, and in the elderly.

Isosorbide Mononitrate Pharmacokinetic Parameters

Parameter	Single-dose studies		Multiple-dose studies	
	Isosorbide mononitrate 60 mg	Isosorbide mononitrate ER tablets 60 mg	Isosorbide mononitrate ER tablets 60 mg	Isosorbide mononitrate ER tablets 120 mg
C_{max} (ng/mL)	1,242 to 1,534	424 to 541	557 to 572	1,151 to 1,180
T_{max} (h)	0.6 to 0.7	3.1 to 4.5	2.9 to 4.2	3.1 to 3.2
AUC (ng•h/mL)	8,189 to 8,313	5,990 to 7,452	6,625 to 7,555	14,241 to 16,800
t½ (h)	4.8 to 5.1	6.3 to 6.6	6.2 to 6.3	6.2 to 6.4
Cl/F (mL/min)	120 to 122	151 to 187	132 to 151	119 to 140

Food effects: See Drug Interactions for more information. Isosorbide mononitrate is significantly removed from the blood during hemodialysis; however, an additional dose to compensate for drug lost is not necessary. In patients undergoing continuous ambulatory peritoneal dialysis, blood levels are similar to patients not on dialysis.

Nitroglycerin lingual spray –

Absorption: In a pharmacokinetic study when a single dose of nitroglycerin 0.8 mg lingual spray was administered to healthy volunteers (n = 24), the mean C_{max} and T_{max} were 1,041 pg/mL•min and 7.5 minutes, respectively. Additionally, in these subjects the mean AUC was 12,769 pg/mL•min.

Nitroglycerin sublingual –

Absorption: Nitroglycerin is rapidly absorbed following sublingual administration. Mean peak plasma concentrations occur at a mean time of approximately 6 to 7 minutes postdose. Maximal drug concentration (C_{max}) and area under the curve (AUC) increase dose proportionally following nitroglycerin 0.3 to 0.6 mg sublingual tablets. The absolute bioavailability is approximately 40% but tends to be variable because of factors influencing drug absorption, such as sublingual hydration and mucosal metabolism.

Mean peak 1,2- and 1,3-dinitroglycerin plasma concentrations occur at approximately 15 minutes postdose.

Mean Nitroglycerin (SD) Values

Parameter	2 × 0.3 mg *Nitrostat* tablets	1 × 0.6 mg *Nitrostat* tablets
C_{max} (ng/mL)	2.3 (1.7)	2.1 (1.5)
T_{max} (min)	6.4 (2.5)	7.2 (3.2)
$AUC_{(0-\infty)}$ (min)	14.9 (8.2)	14.9 (11.4)
t½ (min)	2.8 (1.1)	2.6 (0.6)

Distribution: At plasma concentrations between 50 and 500 ng/mL, the binding of nitroglycerin to plasma proteins is approximately 60%, while that of 1,2-dinitroglycerin and 1,3-dinitroglycerin is 60% and 30%, respectively.

Metabolism: Nitroglycerin is rapidly metabolized to dinitrates and mononitrates. A liver reductase enzyme is of primary importance in the metabolism of nitroglycerin to glycerol dinitrate and mononitrate metabolites and ultimately to glycerol and organic nitrate. Known sites of extrahepatic metabolism include red blood cells and vascular walls. The 1,2- and 1,3-dinitroglycerin metabolites have been reported to possess approximately 2% and 10% of the pharmacological activity of nitroglycerin. Glycerol mononitrate metabolites of nitroglycerin are biologically inactive.

Elimination: Nitroglycerin plasma concentrations decrease rapidly with a mean elimination half-life of 2 to 3 minutes (range, 1.5 to 7.5 minutes). Clearance (13.6 L/min) greatly exceeds hepatic blood flow. Metabolism is the primary route of drug elimination. The elimination half-life of 1,2- and 1,3-dinitroglycerin is 36 and 32 minutes, respectively.

Nitroglycerin ER –

Absorption: The maximum achievable daily duration of antianginal effect from nitroglycerin ER capsules is approximately 12 hours. Controlled trials of multiple-dose oral nitroglycerin have shown statistically significant antianginal efficacy 2.5 to 4 hours after a dose when oral nitroglycerin had been administered 4 times a day for 2 weeks or 3 times a day for 1 week.

Distribution: The volume of distribution of nitroglycerin is approximately 3 L/kg.

Metabolism: The first products in the metabolism of nitroglycerin are inorganic nitrate and the 1,2- and 1,3-dinitroglycerols. The dinitrates are less effective vasodilators than nitroglycerin, but they are longer lived in the serum and their net contribution to the overall effect of chronic nitroglycerin regimens is not known. The dinitrates are further metabolized to (nonvasoactive) mononitrates and, ultimately, to glycerol and carbon dioxide. Known sites of extrahepatic metabolism include red blood cells and vascular walls.

Elimination: Nitroglycerin is cleared at extremely rapid rates, with a resulting serum half-life of approximately 3 minutes. The observed clearance rates (close to 1 L/kg/min) greatly exceed hepatic blood flow.

Nitroglycerin transdermal, ointment –

Absorption: In healthy volunteers, steady-state plasma concentrations of nitroglycerin are reached in approximately 2 hours after application of the patch and are maintained for the duration of wearing the system (observations have been limited to 24 hours). The onset of action of transdermal nitroglycerin is not sufficiently rapid for it to be useful in aborting an acute anginal episode. It is reasonable to believe that the rate of nitroglycerin absorption from patches may vary with the site of application, but this relationship has not been adequately studied. Nitroglycerin levels rise to steady state within about 1 hour after nitroglycerin ointment application.

Distribution: The volume of distribution of nitroglycerin is approximately 3 L/kg.

Metabolism: The first products in the metabolism of nitroglycerin are inorganic nitrate and the 1,2- and 1,3-dinitroglycerols. The dinitrates are less effective vasodilators than nitroglycerin, but they are longer lived in the serum and their net contribution to the overall effect of chronic nitroglycerin regimens is not known. The dinitrates are further metabolized to (nonvasoactive) mononitrates and, ultimately, to glycerol and carbon dioxide. Known sites of extrahepatic metabolism include red blood cells and vascular walls.

Elimination: Nitroglycerin is cleared at extremely rapid rates, with a resulting serum half-life of approximately 3 minutes. The observed clearance rates (close to 1 L/kg/min) greatly exceed hepatic blood flow. Upon removal of the nitroglycerin transdermal patch, the plasma concentration declines, with a half-life of approximately 1 hour. After removal of ointment, levels wane with a half-life of approximately half an hour.

Nitroglycerin IV –

Absorption: The pharmacokinetic results from clinical trials with the IV formulation are consistent with results from other trials with other formulations of nitroglycerin and other nitrates.

Distribution: The volume of distribution of nitroglycerin is approximately 3 L/kg.

Metabolism: The first products in the metabolism of nitroglycerin are inorganic nitrate and the 1,2- and 1,3-dinitroglycerols. The dinitrates are less effective vasodilators than nitroglycerin, but they are longer lived in the serum and their net contribution to the overall effect of chronic nitroglycerin regimens is not known. The dinitrates are further metabolized to (nonvasoactive) mononitrates and, ultimately, to glycerol and carbon dioxide. Known sites of extrahepatic metabolism include red blood cells and vascular walls.

Elimination: Continuous IV nitroglycerin lost almost all of its hemodynamic effect after 48 hours. Nitroglycerin is cleared at extremely rapid rates, with a resulting serum half-life of approximately 3 minutes. The observed clearance rates (close to 1 L/kg/min) greatly exceed hepatic blood flow.

Contraindications

➤*Amyl nitrite:* Patients with glaucoma, recent head trauma, cerebral hemorrhage, and pregnancy.

➤*Isosorbide dinitrate:* Allergic reactions to isosorbide dinitrate or any of its ingredients.

➤*Isosorbide mononitrate:* Hypersensitivity or idiosyncratic reactions to other nitrates or nitrites.

➤*Nitroglycerin:* Allergic reactions to organic nitrates.

Patients who are using certain drugs for erectile dysfunction (eg, sildenafil citrate), because these drugs have been shown to potentiate the hypotensive effects of organic nitrates (sublingual tablets, lingual spray, transdermal).

Allergy to the adhesives used in the transdermal patches (transdermal).

Patients with early MI, severe anemia, increased intracranial pressure, known hypersensitivity to nitroglycerin (sublingual tablets).

Patients with pericardial tamponade, restrictive cardiomyopathy, constrictive pericarditis, solutions containing dextrose in patients with known allergy to corn or corn products (IV).

Warnings/Precautions

➤*Phosphodiesterase inhibitors:* See Drug Interactions for more information.

➤*Acute MI and/or CHF:* The benefits of nitrates (other than **nitroglycerin in dextrose**) in patients with acute MI or CHF have not been established. If electing to use these products, use careful clinical and hemodynamic monitoring to avoid the hazards of hypotension and tachycardia. Because the effects of **isosorbide mononitrate** and **isosorbide dinitrate** are so difficult to terminate rapidly, these products are not recommended in these settings.

➤*Arcing:* Do not discharge a cardioverter/defibrillator through a paddle electrode that overlies a **nitroglycerin transdermal** system patch. The arcing that may be seen in this situation is harmless in itself, but it may be associated with local current concentration that can cause damage to the paddles and burns to the patient.

➤*Polyvinyl chloride (PVC) tubing:* Because of the problem of nitroglycerin absorption by PVC tubing, use nitroglycerin IV with the least absorptive infusion tubing (ie, non-PVC tubing) available.

➤*IV filters:* Some in-line IV filters also absorb **nitroglycerin**; avoid these filters.

➤*Hemolysis/Pseudoagglutination:* Do not administer solutions containing dextrose without electrolytes through the same administration set as blood because this may result in pseudoagglutination or hemolysis.

➤*Electrolyte concentrations:* The IV administration of solutions may cause fluid overloading, resulting in dilution of serum electrolyte concentrations, overhydration, and congested states of pulmonary edema. The risk of dilutional states is inversely proportional to the electrolyte concentration in the injections. The risk of solute overload causing congested states with peripheral and pulmonary edema is directly proportional to the electrolyte concentration of the injections.

➤*Postural hypotension:* Transient episodes of dizziness, weakness, syncope, or other signs of cerebral ischemia caused by postural hypotension may develop following inhalation of **amyl nitrite**, particularly if the patient is standing immobile. This effect may be more frequent in patients who also have consumed alcohol. To hasten recovery, use measures that facilitate venous return (eg, head-low posture, deep breathing, movement of extremities).

➤*Flammability:* **Amyl nitrite** is very flammable. Do not use where it would become ignited.

➤*Angina:* Nitrate therapy may aggravate angina caused by hypertrophic cardiomyopathy.

➤*Tolerance:* Use only the smallest dose required for effective relief of the acute anginal attack. Excessive use of **sublingual nitroglycerin** may lead to the development of tolerance. In industrial workers who have had long-term exposure to unknown (presumably high) doses of organic nitrates, tolerance clearly occurs. As tolerance to other forms of nitroglycerin develops, the effects of sublingual nitroglycerin on exercise tolerance, although still observable, is blunted.

Tolerance to **amyl nitrite** may develop with repeated use of the drug for prolonged periods of time. Tolerance may be minimized by beginning with the smallest effective dose and alternating the drug with another coronary vasodilator.

➤*Severe hypotension:* Severe hypotension, particularly with upright posture, may occur with small doses of nitrates; therefore, use these drugs with caution in patients who may be volume depleted or who are already hypotensive. Hypotension induced by **nitroglycerin** may be accompanied by paradoxical bradycardia and increased angina pectoris.

➤*Withdrawal:* Chest pain, acute MI, and even sudden death have occurred during temporary withdrawal of nitrates from industrial workers who have had long-term exposure to unknown doses of organic nitrates, demonstrating the existence of true physical dependence.

➤*Nitrate-free interval:* Several clinical trials of nitroglycerin in patients with angina pectoris have evaluated regimens that incorporated a 10- to 12-hour nitrate-free interval. In some of these trials, an increase in the frequency of anginal attacks during the nitrate-free interval was observed in a small number of patients. In one trial, patients had decreased exercise tolerance at the end of the nitrate-free interval. Hemodynamic rebound has been observed rarely; on the other hand, few studies were designed that rebound, if it had occurred, would have been detected. The importance of these findings to the routine clinical use of nitrates is unknown.

➤*Fluid load:* Lower concentrations of **nitroglycerin IV** and **nitroglycerin in dextrose injection** increase the potential precision of dosing, but these concentrations increase the total fluid volume that must be delivered to patients. Total fluid load may be a dominant consideration in patients with compromised function of the heart, liver, and/or kidneys.

➤*Nitroglycerin infusions:* Administer nitroglycerin IV and nitroglycerin in dextrose infusions only via an infusion pump that can maintain a constant infusion rate. Intracoronary injection of nitroglycerin IV and nitroglycerin in dextrose infusions has not been studied.

➤*Diabetes mellitus:* Use solutions containing dextrose with caution in patients with known subclinical or overt diabetes mellitus.

➤*Methemoglobinemia:* See Overdose for more information.

➤*Discontinuation:* Discontinue **sublingual nitroglycerin** if blurring of vision or drying of the mouth occurs. Excessive dosages of nitroglycerin may produce severe headaches.

➤*Drug abuse and dependence:* Volatile nitrites, including **amyl nitrite**, are abused for sexual stimulation, with headache as a common side effect. Tolerance to nitrites can develop; conditions and duration have not been established.

➤*Pregnancy: Category C* – **nitroglycerin** (per manufacturers' prescribing information), **isosorbide dinitrate**, **isosorbide mononitrate** [ie, *ISMO*], **amyl nitrite**. *Category B* – **isosorbide mononitrate ER** (ie, *Imdur*), isosorbide mononitrate (ie, *Monoket*), nitroglycerin (per Briggs' *Drugs in Pregnancy and Lactation*).

Amyl nitrite can cause fetal harm to the fetus when it is administered to a pregnant woman because it significantly reduces systemic blood pressure and blood flow on the maternal side of the placenta.

There are no adequate and well-controlled studies in pregnant women with nitroglycerin. It is not known whether nitroglycerin can cause fetal harm when administered to a pregnant woman or can affect reproductive capacity. Give nitroglycerin to a pregnant woman only if clearly needed.

At oral doses 35 and 150 times the maximum recommended human daily dose, isosorbide dinitrate has been shown to cause a dose-related increase in embryotoxicity (increase in mummified pups) in rabbits.

➤*Lactation:* It is not known whether nitrates are excreted in human milk. Because many drugs are excreted in human milk, exercise caution when administering nitrates to a breast-feeding woman.

➤*Children:* Safety and efficacy in children have not been established.

➤*Elderly:* Clinical experience for organic nitrates reported in the literature identified a potential for severe hypotension and increased sensitivity to nitrates in the elderly. Nitrate therapy may aggravate the angina caused by hypertrophic cardiomyopathy, particularly in the elderly.

Elderly patients may have reduced baroreceptor function and may develop severe orthostatic hypotension when vasodilators are used. Use **isosorbide mononitrate ER** tablets with caution in elderly patients who may be volume depleted, on multiple medications, or who are already hypotensive. Hypotension induced by isosorbide mononitrate may be accompanied by paradoxical bradycardia and increased angina pectoris.

Use caution in dose selection for an elderly patient, usually starting at the low end of the dosing range, reflecting the greater frequency of decreased hepatic, renal, or cardiac function, and of concomitant disease or other drug therapy.

Drug Interactions

Nitrate Drug Interactions

Precipitant drug	Object drug[a]		Description
Alcohol	Nitrates	↑	Severe hypotension and cardiovascular collapse may occur.
Aspirin	Nitrates	↑	The vasodilatory and hemodynamic effects of nitrates may be enhanced by coadministration of aspirin.
Phosphodiesterase inhibitors (eg, sildenafil, tadalafil, vardenafil)	Nitrates	↑	Phosphodiesterase inhibitors have been shown to potentiate the hypotensive effects of organic nitrates. Concomitant use is contraindicated.
Vasodilators	Nitrates	↑	Additive hypotension may occur.
Nitrates	Antihypertensives Beta-blockers Calcium channel blockers	↑	Possible additive hypotension may occur. Marked orthostatic hypotension may occur with coadministration with calcium channel blockers. Dose adjustments of either class may be necessary.
Nitrates	Nondepolarizing muscle relaxants (eg, pancuronium)	↑	Nitrates may potentiate the actions of pancuronium, possibly resulting in profound and severe respiratory depression.
Nitrates	Phenothiazines	↑	Possible additive hypotension may occur. Dose adjustment of either class of agent may be necessary.
Nitrates, IV	Heparin	↓	Nitroglycerin IV reduces the anticoagulant effect of heparin; monitor aPTT in patients receiving these drugs concomitantly and adjust heparin dose as needed.
Nitrates, long-acting	Nitrates, sublingual	↓	A decrease in therapeutic effect of sublingual nitroglycerin may result from use of long-acting nitrates.
Nitrates, oral	Dihydroergotamine	↑	Oral administration of nitroglycerin markedly decreases the first-pass metabolism of dihydroergotamine and subsequently increases its oral bioavailability. Ergotamine is known to precipitate angina pectoris. Therefore, patients receiving sublingual nitroglycerin should avoid ergotamine and related drugs or be monitored for symptoms of ergotism if this is not possible.
Nitroglycerin	Alteplase	↓	Nitroglycerin administration decreases the thrombolytic effect of alteplase. Avoid concurrent use.

[a] ↑ = object drug increased; ↓ = object drug decreased.

➤*Drug/Lab test interactions:* Nitrates and nitrites may interfere with the *Zlatkis-Zak* color reaction causing falsely low readings in serum cholesterol determinations.

Because of the propylene glycol content of **nitroglycerin IV**, serum triglyceride assays that rely on glycerol oxidase may give falsely elevated results in patients receiving this medication.

➤*Drug/Food interactions:* Concomitant food intake may decrease the rate (increase in T_{max}) but not the extent (AUC) of absorption of **isosorbide mononitrate**.

Adverse Reactions

➤*Amyl nitrite:* Mild transitory headache, dizziness, and flushing of the face are common with the use of amyl nitrite. The following adverse reactions may occur in susceptible patients: cold sweat, hypotension, involuntary passing of urine and feces, nausea, pallor, restlessness, syncope, tachycardia, vomiting, weakness. Excessively high doses of amyl nitrite administered chronically may cause methemoglobinemia.

➤*Isosorbide mononitrate tablets:*

Cardiovascular – Cardiovascular disorder, chest pain (1% or more); acute MI, angina pectoris, apoplexy, arrhythmias, atrial fibrillation, bradycardia, edema, hypertension, hypotension, pallor, palpitations, postural hypotension, premature ventricular contractions, supraventricular tachycardia, syncope, tachycardia (less than 1%).

CNS – Dizziness, emotional lability, fatigue, headache (1% or more); agitation, anxiety, confusion, depression, hypesthesia, hypokinesia, impaired concentration, insomnia, nervousness, nightmares, restlessness, tremor, vertigo (less than 1%).

Dermatologic – Pruritus, rash (1% or more); sweating (less than 1%).

GI – Abdominal pain, diarrhea, nausea, vomiting (1% or more); anorexia, decreased weight, dry mouth, dyspepsia, tenesmus, thirst, tooth disorder (less than 1%).

GU – Dysuria, impotence, prostatic disorder, urinary frequency (less than 1%).

Musculoskeletal – Arthralgia, muscle cramps (less than 1%).

Respiratory – Increased cough, upper respiratory tract infection (1% or more); asthma, dyspnea, sinusitis (less than 1%).

Miscellaneous – Allergic reaction, flushing, pain (1% or more); amblyopia, asthenia, back pain, bitter taste, blurred vision, cold sweat, diplopia, increased appetite, malaise, neck pain, neck stiffness, paresthesia, rigors, susurrus aurium (less than 1%).

➤*Isosorbide mononitrate ER tablets:*

Cardiovascular – Angina pectoris aggravated, arrhythmia, arrhythmia atrial, atrial fibrillation, bradycardia, bundle branch block, cardiac failure, extrasystole, heart murmur, heart sound abnormal, hypertension, hypotension, MI, palpitation, Q-wave abnormality, tachycardia, ventricular tachycardia (5% or less); syncope (postmarketing).

CNS – Dizziness, headache (more than 5%); anxiety, concentration impaired, confusion, decreased libido, depression, dizziness, fatigue, headache, hypesthesia, insomnia, migraine, nervousness, neuritis, paroniria, paresis, paresthesia, somnolence, tremor, vertigo (5% or less).

Dermatologic – Acne, hair texture abnormal, increased sweating, pruritus, rash, skin nodule (5% or less).

GI – Abdominal pain, constipation, diarrhea, dry mouth, dyspepsia, flatulence, gastric ulcer, gastritis, glossitis, hemorrhagic gastric ulcer, hemorrhoids, loose stools, melena, nausea, vomiting (5% or less).

GU – Atrophic vaginitis, breast pain, impotence, polyuria, renal calculus, urinary tract infection (5% or less).

Hematologic – Hypochromic anemia, purpura, thrombocytopenia (5% or less).

Hepatic – ALT increase, AST increase (5% or less).

Metabolic/Nutritional – Edema, hyperuricemia, hypokalemia (5% or less).

Musculoskeletal – Arthralgia, frozen shoulder, muscle weakness, musculoskeletal pain, myalgia, myositis, tendon disorder, torticollis (5% or less).

Respiratory – Bronchitis, bronchospasm, coughing, dyspnea, increased sputum, nasal congestion, pharyngitis, pneumonia, pulmonary infiltration, rales, rhinitis, sinusitis (5% or less).

Special senses – Conjunctivitis, earache, photophobia, tinnitus, tympanic membrane perforation, vision abnormal (5% or less).

Miscellaneous – Asthenia, back pain, bacterial infection, chest pain, fever, flu-like symptoms, flushing, hot flushes, intermittent claudication, leg ulcer, malaise, moniliasis, ptosis, rigors, varicose vein, viral infection (5% or less).

➤*Nitroglycerin lingual spray:* Adverse reactions to oral nitroglycerin dosage forms, particularly headache and hypotension, are generally dose-related. In clinical trials at various doses of nitroglycerin, the following adverse reactions have been observed: headache which may be severe and persistent, is the most commonly reported side effect of nitroglycerin with an incidence of about 50% in some studies. Cutaneous vasodilation with flushing may occur. Transient episodes of dizziness and weakness as well as other signs of cerebral ischemia associated with postural hypotension may occasionally develop. Occasionally, an individual may exhibit marked sensitivity to the hypotensive effects of nitrates and severe responses (collapse, nausea, pallor, perspiration, restlessness, vomiting, and weakness) may occur even with therapeutic doses. Drug rash and/or exfoliative dermatitis have been reported in patients receiving nitrate therapy. Nausea and vomiting are uncommon.

More than 2% – Dizziness, headache, paresthesia.

2% or less – Abdominal pain, asthenia, dyspnea, peripheral edema, pharyngitis, rhinitis, vasodilation.

➤*Nitroglycerin sublingual:* Headache which may be severe and persistent may occur immediately after use. Dizziness, palpitation, vertigo, weakness, and other manifestations of postural hypotension may develop occasionally, particularly in erect, immobile patients. Marked sensitivity to the hypotensive effects of nitrates (manifested by collapse, diaphoresis, nausea, pallor, vomiting, and weakness) may occur at therapeutic doses. Syncope caused by nitrate vasodilation has been reported. Drug rash, exfoliative dermatitis, and flushing have been reported in patients receiving nitrate therapy.

➤*Nitroglycerin ointment, transdermal, IV, ER capsules, and isosorbide dinitrate:* Adverse reactions to nitroglycerin and isosorbide dinitrate are generally dose related, and almost all of these reactions are the result of the activity of these drugs as vasodilators. Headache, which may be severe, is the most commonly reported side effect. Headache may be recurrent with each daily dose, especially at higher doses. Transient episodes of lightheadedness, occasionally related to blood pressure changes, also may occur. Hypotension occurs infrequently, but in some patients it may be severe enough to warrant discontinuation of therapy. Syncope, crescendo angina, and rebound hypertension have been reported but are uncommon.

Allergic reactions to nitroglycerin are also uncommon, and the great majority of those reported have been cases of contact dermatitis or fixed drug eruptions in patients receiving nitroglycerin ointment or patch. There have been a few reports of anaphylactoid reactions; these reactions can probably occur in patients receiving nitroglycerin by any route.

Application-site irritation may occur with transdermal nitroglycerin but is rarely severe. The most frequent adverse reactions with transdermal nitroglycerin were as follows: headache (63%); light-headedness (6%); hypotension and/or syncope (4%); increased angina (2%).

Overdosage

➤*Symptoms:* The ill effects of nitrate overdose are generally the result of the capacity of nitrates to induce vasodilation, venous pooling, reduced cardiac output, and hypotension. These hemodynamic changes may have protean manifestations, including increased intracranial pressure, with any or all of the following; persistent throbbing headache, confusion, and moderate fever; vertigo; palpitations; visual disturbances; nausea and vomiting (possibly with colic and even bloody diarrhea); syncope (especially in the upright posture); air hunger and dyspnea, later followed by reduced ventilatory effort; diaphoresis, with the skin either flushed or cold or clammy; heart block and bradycardia; paralysis; coma; seizures; and death.

Inhaled doses of 5 to 10 drops of **amyl nitrite** may cause violent flushing of the face, accompanied by a feeling of imminent bursting of the head and very excessive heart action. The inhalation of larger amounts may produce a feeling of suffocation and muscular weakness. Symptoms comparable to shock may be produced (eg, incontinence, nausea, pallor, restlessness, sweating, syncope, vomiting, weakness) attributable to pooling of blood in the postarteriolar vessels and failure of the venous blood to return to the heart.

Methemoglobinemia – Methemoglobinemia has been reported in patients receiving other organic nitrates. Certainly, nitrate ions liberated during metabolism of nitrates can oxidize hemoglobin into methemoglobin. However, even in patients totally without cytochrome b_5 reductase activity and assuming that the nitrate moiety of the nitrate is quantitatively applied to oxidation of hemoglobin, approximately 2 mg/kg of **isosorbide mononitrate** or 1 mg/kg of **nitroglycerin** or **isosorbide dinitrate** should be required before any of these patients manifests clinically significant (10% or more) methemoglobinemia. In patients with normal reductase function, significant production of methemoglobin should require larger doses of the nitrate. In one study in which 36 patients received 2 to 4 weeks of continuous nitroglycerin therapy at 3.1 to 4.4 mg/h, the average methemoglobin level measured was 0.2%; this was comparable with that observed in parallel patients who received placebo.

Notwithstanding these observations, there are case reports of significant methemoglobinemia in association with moderate overdoses of organic nitrates. None of the affected patients were thought to be unusually susceptible.

➤*Treatment:* Dialysis is known to be ineffective in removing **isosorbide mononitrate** from the body. No specific antagonist to the vasodilator effects of nitrates is known, and no intervention has been subject to controlled study as a therapy of nitrate overdose. Because the hypotension associated with nitrate overdose is the result of venodilation and arterial hypovolemia, direct prudent therapy in this situation toward an increase in central fluid volume. Passive elevation of the patient's legs may be sufficient, but IV infusion of normal saline or similar fluid also may be necessary.

In patients with renal disease or CHF, therapy resulting in central volume expansion may be hazardous. Treatment of nitrate overdose in these patients may be subtle and difficult and invasive monitoring may be required.

Measures that facilitate venous return, such as head-low posture, deep breathing, and movement of extremities, may be used. The use of epinephrine aggravates the shock-like reaction. Inject methylene blue for treatment of severe methemoglobinemia with dyspnea. For treating cyanide poisoning, methylene blue is contraindicated where nitrites cause iatrogenic methemoglobinemia.

Patient Information

Instruct patients to carefully follow the prescribed schedule of dosing.

Instruct patients to take oral nitrates on an empty stomach with a glass of water.

Daily headaches sometimes accompany treatment with nitrates. In patients who get these headaches, the headaches are a marker of the activity of the drug. Instruct patients to resist the temptation to avoid headaches by altering the schedule of their treatment with nitrates because loss of headache is likely to be associated with simultaneous loss of antianginal efficacy.

Treatment with nitrates may be associated with light-headedness on standing, especially just after rising from a recumbent or seated position. This effect may be more frequent in patients who have also consumed alcohol. Aspirin or acetaminophen often successfully relieves nitrate-induced headaches with no deleterious effect on antianginal efficacy.

Instruct patients not to take nitrate products with certain drugs taken for erectile dysfunction (phosphodiesterase inhibitors) because of the risk of dangerously lowering their blood pressure.

Inform patients that the antianginal efficacy of **isosorbide mononitrate** or **isosorbide dinitrate** is strongly related to its dosing regimen and to carefully follow the prescribed schedule of dosing. For most patients taking isosorbide mononitrate ER tablets, this can be accomplished by taking the dose on arising. For most patients taking isosorbide mononitrate IR tablets, this can be accomplished by taking the first dose on awakening and the second dose 7 hours later.

Keep tablets and capsules in original container. Keep container closed tightly.

➤*Brand interchange:* Instruct patients not to change from one brand of this drug to another without consulting their pharmacist or health care provider. Products manufactured by different companies may not be equally effective.

➤*Amyl nitrite inhalant:* Instruct patients to use when lying down only. Amyl nitrite is highly flammable; advise patients not to use where it might be ignited. Advise patients to use amyl nitrite in a well-ventilated room.

➤*ER tablets, capsules:* Instruct patients to swallow whole and not chew. Not for sublingual use.

➤*Lingual spray:* Instruct patients to spray onto or under tongue. Instruct patients not to inhale spray.

➤*Sublingual tablets:* Instruct patients to dissolve tablet under tongue and not swallow. A lack of burning or stinging sensation does not indicate a loss of potency. Advise patients to use when seated and to take at the first sign of an anginal attack before severe pain develops. If angina is not relieved in 5 minutes, instruct patients to dissolve a second tablet under the tongue. If pain is not relieved within another 5 minutes, instruct patients to dissolve a third tablet. If pain continues or intensifies, advise patients to notify their health care provider immediately or report to the nearest emergency room.

Instruct patients to keep **nitroglycerin** in original glass container, tightly capped, and to discard the cotton once the bottle is opened.

➤*Transdermal patches:* Patient instructions are available with products. Advise patients that there is enough residual **nitroglycerin** in discarded patches that they are a potential hazard to children and pets. Instruct patients to use caution when discarding.

➤*Ointment:* Patient instructions are available with products. Instruct patients to spread a thin layer on skin using applicator or dose-measuring papers. Instruct patients not to use fingers and to not rub or massage. Instruct patients to keep tube tightly closed.

AMYL NITRITE

Rx	**Amyl Nitrite** (Various)	**Inhalant:** 0.3 mL	Covered glass capsules. In 12s.

AMYL NITRITE — INHALATIONAL

For complete prescribing information, refer to the Nitrates class monograph.

Indications

➤*Angina pectoris:* For the rapid relief of angina pectoris. The effect of amyl nitrite appears within 30 seconds and lasts for approximately 3 to 5 minutes.

Administration and Dosage

➤*Adults:*

Angina pectoris – Two to 6 inhalations of the vapors from the capsule are usually sufficient to promptly produce therapeutic effects. If necessary, the dose may be repeated in 3 to 5 minutes.

➤*Administration:* With the patient in recumbent or seated position, a capsule of amyl nitrite is held away from the face, crushed between the fingers, and held under the patient's nose. Caution is recommended to avoid inhalation of the drug when it is administered by someone other than the patient.

➤*Storage/Stability:* Store in a cool place, 2° to 8°C (36° to 46°F). Contents are flammable; protect from light.

ISOSORBIDE DINITRATE

Rx	**Isosorbide Dinitrate** (Various, eg, IVAX Pharm, Major, Par, Sandoz, West-Ward)	**Tablets; oral:** 5 mg	In 100s, 500s, 1,000s, and UD 100s.
Rx	**Isordil Titradose** (Wyeth)		Lactose. (WYETH 4152). Pink, scored. In 100s and 1,000s.
Rx	**Isosorbide Dinitrate** (Various, eg, IVAX Pharm, Major, Par, Sandoz, UDL, West-Ward)	**Tablets; oral:** 10 mg	In 100s, 500s, 1,000s and UD 100s.
Rx	**Isordil Titradose** (Wyeth)		Lactose. (WYETH 4153). White, scored. In 100s and 1,000s.
Rx	**Isosorbide Dinitrate** (Various, eg, IVAX Pharm, Major, Par, Sandoz, UDL, West-Ward)	**Tablets; oral:** 20 mg	In 100s, 1,000s, and UD 100s.
Rx	**Isordil Titradose** (Wyeth)		Lactose. (WYETH 4154). Green, scored. In 100s and 500s.
Rx	**Isosorbide Dinitrate** (Various, eg, Imiren, Par)	**Tablets; oral:** 30 mg	In 100s, 500s, 1,000s, and UD 100s.
Rx	**Isordil Titradose** (Wyeth)		Lactose. (WYETH 4159). Blue, scored. In 100s.
Rx	**Isordil Titradose** (Wyeth)	**Tablets; oral:** 40 mg	Lactose. (WYETH 4192). Lt. green, scored. In 100s.
Rx	**Isosorbide Dinitrate** (Corepharma)	**Tablets, extended-release; oral:** 40 mg	Lactose. In 100s.
Rx	**Isochron** (Forest)		Lactose. (IL/3613). Peach colored, scored. In 100s.
Rx	**Isosorbide Dinitrate** (Various, eg, Qualitest, West-Ward)	**Tablets, sublingual; oral:** 2.5 mg	May contain lactose. In 100s, 1,000s, and UD 100s.
Rx	**Isosorbide Dinitrate** (Various, eg, Qualitest, West-Ward)	**Tablets, sublingual; oral:** 5 mg	May contain lactose. In 100s, 1,000s, and UD 100s.
Rx	**Dilatrate-SR** (Schwarz Pharma)	**Capsules, sustained-release; oral:** 40 mg	Lactose, sucrose. (Schwarz 0920). Pink, opaque. In 100s.

ISOSORBIDE DINITRATE — ORAL

For complete and comparative prescribing information, refer to the Nitrates group monograph.

Indications

➤*Angina pectoris:* For the treatment (sublingual tablets only) and prevention of angina pectoris caused by coronary artery disease. The onset of action of oral isosorbide dinitrate is not sufficiently rapid for this product to be useful in aborting an acute anginal episode.

➤*Off-label uses:* Used with hydralazine to increase survival among black patients with advanced heart failure; for the treatment of acute angle-closure glaucoma in emergency situations, not intended for long-term management; achalasia.

Administration and Dosage

➤*General dosing considerations:* Tolerance to these agents may develop. Consider administering the short-acting preparations 2 or 3 times daily (last dose no later than 7 pm) and the sustained-release preparations once daily or twice daily at 8 am and 2 pm.

Every dosing regimen for isosorbide dinitrate must provide a daily dose-free interval to minimize the development of tolerance; one of the daily dose-free intervals must be longer than 14 hours.

➤*Adults:*

Angina pectoris –

Capsules, sustained-release:
- *Initial dosage* – 40 mg.
- *Maintenance dosage* – 40 to 80 mg every 8 to 12 hours.

Tablets:
- *Initial dosage* – 5 to 20 mg 2 or 3 times daily.
- *Maintenance dosage* – 10 to 40 mg 2 or 3 times daily is recommended.

Tablets, extended-release: See Capsules, sustained-release.

Tablets, sublingual:
- *Initial dosage* – 2.5 to 5 mg.
- *Dosage titration* – Titrate upward until angina is relieved or side effects limit the dose.
- *Prophylactic dosage* – 1 sublingual tablet (2.5 to 5 mg) approximately 15 minutes before the anticipated activity likely to cause angina is expected to begin. Isosorbide dinitrate sublingual tablets may be used to abort an acute anginal episode, but its use is recommended only in patients who fail to respond to sublingual nitroglycerin.

➤*Administration:*

Sublingual tablets – Do not crush or chew sublingual tablets.

Tablets, extended-release and capsules, sustained-release – Do not crush or chew these preparations.

➤*Storage/Stability:*

Capsules, sustained-release – Store at 15° to 30°C (59° to 86°F) in a dry place.

Tablets – Store at approximately 25°C (77°). Protect from light. Keep bottles tightly closed. Dispense in a light-resistant, tight container.

Tablets, extended-release – Store at 25°C (77°); excursions permitted to 15° to 30°C (59° to 86°F). Dispense in well-closed container.

Tablets, sublingual – Store at 15° to 30°C (59° to 86°F). Protect from light and moisture. Dispense in a tight, light-resistant container.

ISOSORBIDE MONONITRATE

Rx	**Isosorbide Mononitrate** (Various, eg, Kremers Urban, Purepac, Schwarz Pharma)	**Tablets:** 10 mg	May contain lactose. In 100s.
Rx	**Monoket** (Schwarz Pharma)		Lactose. (10 SCHWARZ 610). White, scored. In 100s.
Rx	**ISMO** (Reddy Pharmaceuticals)	**Tablets:** 20 mg	Lactose. (ISMO 20). Orange, scored. Film coated. In 100s and UD 100s.
Rx	**Isosorbide Mononitrate** (Various, eg, Kremers Urban, Purepac, Schwarz Pharma, Teva)		May contain lactose. In 100s and 500s.
Rx	**Monoket** (Schwarz Pharma)		Lactose. (20 SCHWARZ 620). White, scored. In 100s, 180s, and UD 100s.
Rx	**Isosorbide Mononitrate** (Various, eg, Ethex, Kremers Urban)	**Tablets, extended-release:** 30 mg	May contain lactose. In 100s and 1,000s.
Rx	**Imdur** (Key Pharmaceuticals)		(IMDUR 30). Rose colored, scored. In 100s and UD 100s.
Rx	**Isosorbide Mononitrate** (Various, eg, Ethex, Kremers Urban)	**Tablets, extended-release:** 60 mg	May contain lactose. In 100s and 1,000s.
Rx	**Imdur** (Key Pharmaceuticals)		(IMDUR 60). Yellow, scored. In 100s and UD 100s.
Rx	**Isosorbide Mononitrate** (Various, eg, Ethex, Kremers Urban)	**Tablets, extended-release:** 120 mg	May contain lactose. In 100s and 1,000s.
Rx	**Imdur** (Key Pharmaceuticals)		(IMDUR 120). White. In 100s and UD 100s.

ISOSORBIDE MONONITRATE — ORAL

For complete and comparative prescribing information, refer to the Nitrates group monograph.

Indications

➤*Angina pectoris:* For the treatment (*Monoket* only) and prevention of angina pectoris caused by coronary artery disease. The onset of action of oral isosorbide mononitrate is not sufficiently rapid for this product to be useful in aborting an acute angina episode.

➤*Off-label uses:*

Prevention of variceal bleeding – [1] = Good documentation. Because of its ability to enhance the effect of a nonselective beta-blocker, isosorbide mononitrate has been shown to decrease the variceal rebleeding rate when administered as adjunctive therapy. Four recent controlled trials compared combination pharmacological treatment with procedural intervention of endoscopic ligation. Although results were conflicting, a meta-analysis of the trials concluded that survival rates were similar among groups; thus, combination therapy with a nonselective beta-blocker and isosorbide mononitrate is a reasonable treatment option for prevention of variceal rebleeding.

Administration and Dosage

➤*Adults:*

Immediate release –

Angina pectoris:

• *Usual dose* – 20 mg twice daily, with the 2 doses given 7 hours apart.

• *Initial dosage* – A starting dose of 5 mg (one-half tablet of the 10 mg dosing strength) may be appropriate for people of particularly small stature, but should be increased to at least 10 mg by the second or third day of therapy. The suggested regimen is to give the first dose upon awakening and the second dose 7 hours later. The asymmetric (2 doses, 7 hours apart) dosing regimen provides a daily nitrate-free interval to minimize the development of tolerance.

Extended release –

Angina pectoris:

• *Initial dosage* – 30 mg (given as a single 30 mg tablet or one-half of a 60 mg tablet) or 60 mg (given as a single tablet) once daily.

• *Dosage titration* – After several days, the dosage may be increased to 120 mg (given as a single 120 mg tablet or as two 60 mg tablets) once daily. Rarely, 240 mg may be required.

Off-label dosing –

Prevention of variceal bleeding: [1] = Good documentation. Used as adjunctive therapy with a beta-blocker (eg, nadolol, propranolol) in oral doses, titrated up to a maximum of 40 mg twice daily.

➤*Administration:*

Extended release – The suggested regimen is to give the daily dose in the morning upon arising. Do not crush or chew extended-release tablets, and swallow them together with half a glassful of fluid.

➤*Storage/Stability:*

Immediate release – Store at 15° to 30°C (59° to 86°F). Keep tightly closed.

Extended release – Store at 25°C (77°F); excursions are permitted to 15° to 30°C (59° to 86°F). Protect from excessive moisture.

NITROGLYCERIN, INTRAVENOUS

Rx	**Nitroglycerin** (Various, eg, American Regent)	**Solution for injection**[a]: 5 mg/mL	In 5 and 10 mL single-dose vials.
Rx	**Nitroglycerin in 5% Dextrose** (Various, eg, Abbott, Baxter)	**Injection**: 100 mcg/mL	In 250 and 500 mL glass containers.
		200 mcg/mL	In 250 and 500 mL glass containers.
		400 mcg/mL	In 250 and 500 mL glass containers.

[a] Requires dilution.

NITROGLYCERIN — INJECTION

For complete and comparative prescribing information, refer to the Nitrates class monograph.

Indications

➤*Angina pectoris:* For the treatment of angina pectoris in patients who have not responded to sublingual nitroglycerin and beta-blockers.

➤*Congestive heart failure (CHF):* For control of CHF in the setting of acute myocardial infarction (MI).

➤*Intraoperative hypotension:* For induction of intraoperative hypotension.

➤*Perioperative hypertension:* For the treatment of perioperative hypertension.

➤*Off-label uses:*

Variceal bleeding – [1] = Good documentation. Nitroglycerin is recommended to always be coadministered with vasopressin when vasopressin is used for the treatment of active variceal bleeding. It is important to note that vasopressin is not the first-line treatment recommended in published guidelines. Primary pharmacological options include somatostatin or its analogs octreotide and vapreotide, as well as terlipressin. (See Administration and Dosage.)

Other possible off-label uses – For the management of an acute MI; cocaine-induced acute coronary syndrome; sympathomimetic-induced cardiopulmonary toxicities (eg, tachycardia); management of Prinzmetal angina that occurs in patients without coronary heart disease.

According to the American Heart Association's advanced cardiac life support (ACLS) guidelines, nitroglycerin injection is the initial treatment of choice for suspected ischemic-type pain or discomfort in patients with acute coronary syndromes. ACLS guidelines also recommend nitroglycerin for the management of hypertensive emergencies (especially if related to volume overload), congestive heart failure, and pulmonary congestion in patients with ST-elevation myocardial infarction associated with left ventricular failure. (See Off-label dosing.)

Administration and Dosage

➤*General dosing considerations:* Because of variations in the responsiveness of individual patients to the drug, carefully titrate each patient to the desired level of hemodynamic function. Continuously monitor physiologic parameters (eg, blood pressure, heart rate) and other measurements (eg, pulmonary capillary wedge presure [PCWP]) to achieve correct dose. Maintain adequate systemic blood and coronary perfusion pressures.

Dosage is affected by the type of container and administration set used.

Administration of nitroglycerin infusion for more than 24 hours without interruption produces tolerance.

➤*Adults:*

Angina pectoris –

Initial dosage:

• *Polyvinyl chloride (PVC) administration sets* – 25 mcg/min.

• *Nonabsorbing infusion set* – 5 mcg/min delivered through an infusion pump capable of exact and constant delivery of the drug.

Dosage titration: Adjust subsequent titration to the clinical situation, with dose increments becoming more cautious as partial response is seen. Initial titration should be in 5 mcg/min increments, with increases every 3 to 5 minutes until some response is noted. If no response occurs at 20 mcg/min, increments of 10 and even 20 mcg/min can be used. Once a partial blood pressure response is observed, reduce the dose and lengthen the interval between increments.

Some patients with normal or low left ventricular filling pressure or PCWP (eg, angina patients without other complications) may be hypersensitive to the effects of nitroglycerin and may respond fully to doses as small as 5 mcg/min. The nitroglycerin concentration should not exceed 400 mcg/mL.

Congestive heart failure – See angina pectoris for dosing.

Intraoperative hypotension – See angina pectoris for dosing.

Perioperative hypertension – See angina pectoris for dosing.

Off-label dosing –

ACLS guidelines:

• *Initial dosage* – 10 to 20 mcg/min as a continuous IV infusion. (See also Preparation for administration.)

• *Dosage titration* – Increase by 5 to 10 mcg/min every 5 to 10 minutes until the desired hemodynamic or clinical response occurs. Doses of 30 to 40 mcg/min primarily produce venodilation, while high doses (150 mcg/min and above) produce arteriolar dilatation.

Variceal bleeding: [1] = Good documentation. IV infusion started at 40 mcg/min, titrated to a maximum of 400 mcg/min to maintain systolic blood pressure greater than 90 mm Hg.

➤*Preparation for administration:* Nitroglycerin is a concentrated potent drug that must be diluted prior to its infusion. Invert the glass parenteral bottle several times to assure uniform dilution of the nitroglycerin.

Transfer the contents of 1 nitroglycerin vial (containing nitroglycerin 25 or 50 mg) into a 500 mL glass bottle of either dextrose 5% or sodium chloride 0.9%. This yields a final concentration of 50 mcg/mL or 100 mcg/mL. Diluting nitroglycerin 5 mg into 100 mL will also yield a final concentration of 50 mcg/mL. The nitroglycerin concentration should not exceed 400 mcg/mL. It is important to consider the fluid requirements of the patient as well as the expected duration of infusion in selecting the appropriate dilution of nitroglycerin injection.

Nitroglycerin Dilution

Milliliters of nitroglycerin injection		Final concentration		
		100 mcg/mL	200 mcg/mL	400 mcg/mL
Volume	mg	up to	up to	up to
5 mL	25 mg	250 mL	125 mL	
10 mL	50 mg	500 mL	250 mL	125 mL

NITROGLYCERIN — INJECTION

Nitroglycerin Dilution				
Milliliters of nitroglycerin injection		Final concentration		
		100 mcg/mL	200 mcg/mL	400 mcg/mL
Volume	mg	up to	up to	up to
20 mL	100 mg	1,000 mL	500 mL	250 mL
40 mL	200 mg	—	1,000 mL	500 mL

ACLS guidelines – Dilute 50 or 100 mg in 250 mL of dextrose 5% in water or sodium chloride 0.9%.

➤*Administration:* Use only with glass IV bottles and administration set provided. Total amount of nitroglycerin (20% to 60%) in the final diluted solution for infusion could be adsorbed by PVC tubing of IV administration sets in general use. Greater adsorption occurs with low flow rates, high concentrations, and long tubing. Although the rate of loss is highest during early administration (when flow rates are lowest), the loss is neither constant nor self-limiting; consequently, no simple calculation or correction can convert theoretical infusion rate (based on concentration of solution) to actual delivery rate. Manufacturers have developed non-PVC infusion tubing in which nitroglycerin loss is less than 5%. Use IV sets provided by manufacturers or use similar infusion sets.

Dosing instructions must be followed with care. When nitroglycerin IV administration set/nitroglycerin set with volumetric infusion pump is used, the calculated dose will be delivered to the patient because the loss of nitroglycerin seen with standard PVC tubing will be avoided. Relatively nonabsorptive IV administration sets are available. If IV nitroglycerin is administered through nonabsorptive tubing, doses based upon published reports will generally be too high. Some in-line IV filters also absorb nitroglycerin; avoid these filters.

Change in nitroglycerin concentration – If the concentration is adjusted, it is imperative to flush or replace the infusion set before a new concentration is used. If the set was not flushed or replaced, it could take minutes to hours, depending upon the flow rate and the dead space of the set, for the new concentration to reach the patient.

Flow rates –

Nitroglycerin for injection:

Nitroglycerin for Injection Flow Rate (microdrops/min = mL/h)			
Dose (mcg/min)	Solution concentration (mcg/mL)		
	100	200	400
5	3	—	—
10	6	3	—
15	9	—	—
20	12	6	3
30	18	9	—
40	24	12	6
60	36	18	9
80	48	24	12
120	72	36	18
160	96	48	24
240	—	72	36
320	—	96	48
480	—	—	72
640	—	—	96

Premixed nitroglycerin with dextrose:

Premixed Nitroglycerin with Dextrose Necessary Flow Rates (mL/h)[a]			
Desired dose (mcg/min)	Solution concentration (mcg/mL)		
	100	200	400
5	3	1.5	0.8
10	6	3	1.5
15	9	4.5	2.3
20	12	6	3
30	18	9	4.5
40	24	12	6
50	30	15	7.5
60	36	18	9
80	48	24	12
100	60	30	15
120	72	36	18
140	84	42	21
160	96	48	24
180	108	54	27
200	120	60	30
240	144	72	36
280	168	84	42
320	192	96	48
500	300	150	75

[a] With a set that produces 60 drops/mL, 1 mL/h = 1 drop/min.

➤*Admixture compatibility:* Nitroglycerin for injection and nitroglycerin in dextrose 5% should not be mixed with other drugs. Do not administer solutions containing dextrose without electrolytes through the same administration set as blood, as this may result in pseudoagglutination or hemolysis.

➤*Storage/Stability:*

Nitroglycerin for injection – Store at controlled room temperature 15° to 30°C (59° to 86°F). Discard unused portion. Protect from freezing and light.

Premixed nitroglycerin with dextrose – Store at room temperature (25°C); however, brief exposure up to 40°C does not adversely affect the product. Avoid excessive heat and protect from freezing.

NITROGLYCERIN ORAL

Rx	**Nitroglycerin** (Various, eg, Glenmark, Konec, Pliva)	**Tablets; sublingual:** 0.3 mg (1/200 grain)	May contain lactose. In 100s.
Rx	**Nitrostat** (Parke-Davis)		Lactose. (N 3). White. In 100s.
Rx	**Nitroglycerin** (Various, eg, Glenmark, Konec, Pliva)	**Tablets; sublingual:** 0.4 mg (1/150 grain)	May contain lactose. In 25s and 100s.
Rx	**Nitrostat** (Parke-Davis)		Lactose. (N 4). White. In 25s and 100s.
Rx	**Nitroglycerin** (Various, eg, Glenmark, Konec, Pliva)	**Tablets; sublingual:** 0.6 mg (1/100 grain)	May contain lactose. In 100s.
Rx	**Nitrostat** (Parke-Davis)		Lactose. (N 6). White. In 100s.
Rx	**Nitroglycerin** (Various, eg, Dixon-Shane, Goldline, Major, Moore, URL, Vitarine)	**Capsules, extended-release; oral:** 2.5 mg	In 60s, 100s, and UD 60s and 100s.
Rx	**Nitro-Time** (Time-Cap Labs)		Lactose, sucrose. (TCL-1221). Pink/clear. In 60s, 90s, and 100s.
Rx	**Nitroglycerin** (Various, eg, Dixon-Shane , Goldline, Major, Moore, URL, Vitarine)	**Capsules, extended-release; oral:** 6.5 mg	In 60s, 100s, and UD 100s.
Rx	**Nitro-Time** (Time-Cap Labs)		Lactose, sucrose. (TCL-1222). Blue/yellow. In 60s, 90s, and 100s.
Rx	**Nitroglycerin** (Various, eg, Dixon-Shane, Major, Moore, URL, Vitarine)	**Capsules, extended-release; oral:** 9 mg	In 30s, 60s, 100s, and UD 100s.
Rx	**Nitro-Time** (Time-Cap Labs)		Lactose, sucrose. (TCL-1223). Green/yellow. In 60s, 90s, and 100s.
Rx	**Nitrolingual** (Sciele Pharma)	**Aerosol spray; lingual:** 0.4 mg/metered spray	Alcohol 20%, peppermint oil. In 4.9 and 12 g (60 and 200 metered doses).
Rx	**NitroMist** (Akrimax Pharmaceuticals)		In 8.5 g (230 metered doses).

NITROGLYCERIN — ORAL

For complete and comparative prescribing information, refer to the Nitrates group monograph.

Indications

➤*Angina pectoris:* For acute relief of an attack (sublingual tablets, lingual spray only) or prophylaxis of angina pectoris caused by coronary artery disease.

The onset of action of nitroglycerin extended-release capsules is not sufficiently rapid for this product to be useful in aborting an acute anginal episode.

➤*Off-label uses:*

Variant angina pectoris – [1] = Good documentation. American College of Cardiology/American Heart Association (ACC/AHA) guidelines support the use of nitroglycerin as first-line therapy for variant (Prinzmetal) angina in patients without obstructive coronary artery lesions.

Other possible off-label uses –

Nitroglycerin sublingual: For the management of an acute myocardial infarction (MI).

Administration and Dosage

➤*Adults:*

Angina pectoris –

Spray:

• *Usual dosage* – 1 or 2 metered dose sprays onto or under the tongue. A spray may be repeated approximately every 5 minutes as needed. If chest pain persists, prompt medical attention is recommended. May be used prophylactically 5 to 10 minutes prior to engaging in activities that might precipitate an acute attack.

• *Maximum dose* – 3 metered doses per 15-minute period.

Capsules:

• *Initial dosage* – 2.5 to 6.5 mg 3 or 4 times daily.

• *Dosage titration* – Titrate upward to an effective dose until side effects limit the dose. Upward dose titration in these increments 2 to 4 times daily over a period of days or weeks can be attempted. In studies, doses as high as 26 mg given 4 times daily have been effective.

• *Maintenance dosage* – Give the smallest effective dose 2 to 4 times daily.

Sublingual tablets:

• *Usual dosage* – Dissolve 1 tablet under tongue or in buccal pouch at first sign of an acute anginal attack. Dose may be repeated approximately every 5 minutes until relief is obtained. If pain continues, prompt medical attention is recommended. May be used prophylactically 5 to 10 minutes prior to engaging in activities that might precipitate an acute attack.

• *Maximum dose* – 3 tablets per 15-minute period.

➤*Preparation for administration:*

Spray – Each metered spray of nitroglycerin delivers 48 mg of solution, which contains nitroglycerin 400 mcg after an initial priming of 1 spray. It will remain adequately primed for 6 weeks. If the product is not used within 6 weeks, it can be adequately reprimed with 1 spray. There are 60 or 200 metered sprays per bottle. However, the total number of available doses is dependent on the number of sprays per use (1 or 2 sprays) and the frequency of repriming.

➤*Administration:*

Spray – During application, the patient should rest, ideally in the sitting position. Do not shake container. The container should be held vertically with the valve head up and the spray orifice as close to the mouth as possible. The dose should preferably be sprayed onto the tongue by pressing the button firmly; the mouth should be closed immediately after each dose. Do not inhale spray. The medication should not be expectorated or the mouth rinsed for 5 to 10 minutes following administration. Instruct patients to familiarize themselves with the position of the spray orifice, which can be identified by the finger rest on top of the valve, in order to facilitate orientation for administration at night.

Capsules – Capsules must be swallowed; they are not to be chewed or used sublingually.

Sublingual tablets – Dissolve tablet under tongue or in buccal pouch (between cheek and gum). Do not swallow tablet. The patient should rest during administration, preferably in the sitting position.

➤*Storage/Stability:* Store at 25°C (77°F); excursions are permitted between 15° and 30°C (59° and 86°F). Protect sublingual tablets from moisture.

NITROGLYCERIN TOPICAL

Rx	**Nitroglycerin** (Various, eg, DHS)	**Ointment:** 2%	In 30 and 60 g tubes.
Rx	**Nitro-Bid** (Savage)		Lactose. In a lanolin-white petrolatum base. In 30 and 60 g tubes and UD 1 g.

NITROGLYCERIN — TRANSDERMAL OINTMENT

For complete and comparative prescribing information, refer to the Nitrates group monograph.

Indications

➤*Angina pectoris:* For the prevention of angina pectoris caused by coronary artery disease. The onset of action of nitroglycerin ointment is not sufficiently rapid for this product to be useful in aborting an acute anginal attack.

➤*Off-label uses:*

Anal fissures (children) – [2] = Fair documentation. In the majority of trials in children, topical nitroglycerin ointment has been effective for the treatment of anal fissures. (See Administration and Dosage.)

Extravasation treatment – [4] = Insufficient documentation. Data regarding the use of topical nitroglycerin for the reversal of peripheral ischemia caused by extravasation injuries are limited to isolated case reports only. However, in this small number of patients, topically applied nitroglycerin was effective in reversing peripheral ischemia caused by dopamine extravasation or parenteral extravasation. Improvement in pallor and ischemia were evident within minutes to hours after application. (See Administration and Dosage.)

Raynaud phenomenon (topical) – [4] = Insufficient documentation. Evidence from a limited number of controlled studies suggests that topical nitroglycerin may be of benefit for the treatment of Raynaud phenomenon. (See Administration and Dosage.)

Other possible off-label uses – Used topically in the treatment of anal fissures in children.

For the management of an acute myocardial infarction (MI);treatment of erectile dysfunction; management of Prinzmetal angina that occurs in patients without coronary heart disease.

Administration and Dosage

➤*Adults:*

Angina pectoris –

Usual dosage: Apply 2 daily ½ inch (7.5 mg) doses, 1 applied on rising in the morning and 1 applied 6 hours later.

Dosage titration: The dose can be doubled and even doubled again in patients tolerating this dose but failing to respond to it.

Off-label dosing –

Extravasation treatment: [4] = Insufficient documentation. 4 mm/kg or a 1-inch strip applied to affected areas.

Raynaud phenomenon: [4] = Insufficient documentation. Administered as ointment (2% or 1%) for 6 weeks (1% ointment).

➤*Children:*

Off-label dosing –

Anal fissures (children): [2] = Fair documentation. Nitroglycerin 0.2% ointment applied to the affected area twice daily for 6 to 8 weeks.

➤*Administration:* Each tube of ointment is supplied with a pad of ruled, impermeable paper applicators. To apply the ointment using 1 of the applicators, place the applicator on a flat surface, printed side down. Squeeze the necessary amount of ointment from the tube onto the applicator, place the applicator (ointment side down) on the desired area of the skin, and tape the applicator into place.

➤*Storage/Stability:* Store at 15° to 30°C (59° to 86°F). Close tightly immediately after use.

Nitrates

NITROGLYCERIN TRANSDERMAL

Rx	**Nitroglycerin Transdermal** (Mylan)	**Transdermal patch**: 0.1 mg/h	4 cm^2 surface area. In 30s.
Rx	**Minitran** (3M)	**Transdermal patch**: 0.1 mg/h (9 mg total nitroglycerin)	3.3 cm^2 surface area. In 30s.
Rx	**Nitro-Dur** (Key Pharmaceuticals)	**Transdermal patch**: 0.1 mg/h (20 mg total nitroglycerin)	5 cm^2 surface area. In 30s and UD 30s.
Rx	**Nitroglycerin Transdermal** (Various, eg, Hercon Labs, Major, Mylan)	**Transdermal patch**: 0.2 mg/h (16 to 62.5 mg[a] total nitroglycerin)	6 to 10 cm^2 surface area.[a] In 30s.
Rx	**Minitran** (3M)	**Transdermal patch**: 0.2 mg/h (18 mg total nitroglycerin)	6.7 cm^2 surface area. In 30s.
Rx	**Nitrek** (Bertek)	**Transdermal patch**: 0.2 mg/h (22.4 mg total nitroglycerin)	8 cm^2 surface area. In 30s.
Rx	**Nitro-Dur** (Key Pharmaceuticals)	**Transdermal patch**: 0.2 mg/h (40 mg total nitroglycerin)	10 cm^2 surface area. In 30s and UD 30s.
Rx	**Nitro-Dur** (Key Pharmaceuticals)	**Transdermal patch**: 0.3 mg/h (60 mg total nitroglycerin)	15 cm^2 surface area. In 30s and UD 30s.
Rx	**Nitroglycerin Transdermal** (Various, eg, Hercon Labs, Major, Mylan)	**Transdermal patch**: 0.4 mg/h (32 to 125 mg[a] total nitroglycerin)	13 to 20 cm^2 surface area.[a] In 30s.
Rx	**Minitran** (3M)	**Transdermal patch**: 0.4 mg/h (36 mg total nitroglycerin)	13.3 cm^2 surface area. In 30s.
Rx	**Nitrek** (Bertek)	**Transdermal patch**: 0.4 mg/h (44.8 mg total nitroglycerin)	16 cm^2 surface area. In 30s.
Rx	**Nitro-Dur** (Key Pharmaceuticals)	**Transdermal patch**: 0.4 mg/h (80 mg total nitroglycerin)	20 cm^2 surface area. In 30s and UD 30s.
Rx	**Nitroglycerin Transdermal** (Various, eg, Hercon Labs, Major, Mylan)	**Transdermal patch**: 0.6 mg/h (75 to 187.5 mg[a] total nitroglycerin)	20 to 30 cm^2 surface area.[a] In 30s.
Rx	**Minitran** (3M)	**Transdermal patch**: 0.6 mg/h (54 mg total nitroglycerin)	20 cm^2 surface area. In 30s.
Rx	**Nitrek** (Bertek)	**Transdermal patch**: 0.6 mg/h (67.2 mg total nitroglycerin)	24 cm^2 surface area. In 30s.
Rx	**Nitro-Dur** (Key Pharmaceuticals)	**Transdermal patch**: 0.6 mg/h (120 mg total nitroglycerin)	30 cm^2 surface area. In 30s and UD 30s.
Rx	**Nitro-Dur** (Key Pharmaceuticals)	**Transdermal patch**: 0.8 mg/h (160 mg total nitroglycerin)	40 cm^2 surface area. In 30s and UD 30s.

[a] Various systems have the same release rates but variable surface areas and nitroglycerin contents.

NITROGLYCERIN — TRANSDERMAL PATCH

For complete and comparative prescribing information, refer to the Nitrates group monograph.

Indications

➤*Angina pectoris:* For the prevention of angina pectoris caused by coronary artery disease. The onset of action of transdermal nitroglycerin is not sufficiently rapid for this product to be useful in aborting an acute anginal attack.

➤*Off-label uses:*

Anal fissures – [4] = Insufficient documentation. Information regarding the use of transdermal nitroglycerin in the management of chronic anal fissures is limited but suggests that it may produce healing rates similar to those of topical nitroglycerin ointment. A transdermal patch applied daily may be more convenient than multiple daily applications of nitroglycerin ointment and promote greater compliance. Larger controlled trials are needed to determine this drug's place in therapy.

Extravasation treatment – [4] = Insufficient documentation. Data regarding the use of topical nitroglycerin for the reversal of peripheral ischemia caused by extravasation injuries are limited to isolated case reports only. However, in this small number of patients, topically applied nitroglycerin was effective in reversing peripheral ischemia caused by dopamine extravasation or parenteral extravasation. Improvement in pallor and ischemia was evident within minutes to hours after application.

Raynaud phenomenon (transdermal) – [4] = Insufficient documentation. Evidence from a controlled study suggests that nitroglycerin patches may be of benefit for the treatment of Raynaud phenomenon.

Other possible off-label uses – For the management of an acute myocardial infarction (MI); erectile dysfunction; management of Prinzmetal angina that occurs in patients without coronary heart disease.

Administration and Dosage

➤*General dosing considerations:* Although the minimum nitrate-free interval has not been defined, data show that a nitrate-free interval of 10 to 12 hours is sufficient. Thus, an appropriate dosing schedule would include a daily patch-on period of 12 to 14 hours and a patch-off period of 10 to 12 hours. Tolerance is a major factor limiting efficacy when the system is used continuously for more than 12 hours each day.

➤*Adults:*

Angina pectoris –

Usual dosage: Doses between 0.4 and 0.8 mg/h have shown continued effectiveness for 10 to 12 hours daily for at least 1 month of intermittent administration.

Initial dosage: 0.2 to 0.4 mg/h for 12 to 14 hours daily.

Dosage titration: Titrate dose to response.

Off-label dosing –

Anal fissures: [4] = Insufficient documentation. Transdermal patch (10 mg per 24 hours) applied daily below the umbilicus at the flanks of the abdomen.

Raynaud phenomenon (transdermal): [4] = Insufficient documentation. Administered as a daily patch (0.2 mg/h) for 1 week.

➤*Children:*

Off-label dosing –

Extravasation treatment: [4] = Insufficient documentation. In a newborn infant, a 25 mg patch (delivering 5 mg per 24 hours) was applied to the affected area on the dorsum of the foot for 1 hour.

➤*Administration:* Apply once daily to a skin site free of hair and not subject to excessive movement. Do not apply to distal parts of extremities such as below the knee or elbow. The chest is the preferred site. Avoid areas with cuts or irritations. Do not apply the patch immediately after showering or bathing; it is best to wait until the skin is completely dry. Apply immediately upon removal from package. After applying the patch, wash hands to remove any drug. Once the patch is securely on, contact with water (eg, bathing, swimming, showering) will not affect the patch. In the unlikely event that a patch falls off, discard it and put a new one on a different skin site.

➤*Storage/Stability:* Store at controlled room temperature 15° to 30°C (59° to 86°F). Avoid extremes of temperature and/or humidity. Do not refrigerate. Do not store outside of the protective package. Apply immediately upon removal from package.

Peripheral Vasodilators

ISOXSUPRINE HYDROCHLORIDE

Rx	**Isoxsuprine HCl** (Various)	**Tablets**: 10 mg	In 60s, 100s, 500s, 1000s and UD 100s.
Rx	**Vasodilan** (Mead Johnson)		(10 MJ 543). In 100s, 1000s and UD 1000s.
Rx	**Voxsuprine** (Major)		In 100s, 250s, 1000s and UD 100s.
Rx	**Isoxsuprine HCl** (Various)	**Tablets**: 20 mg	In 60s, 100s, 500s, 1000s and UD 100s.
Rx	**Vasodilan** (Mead Johnson)		(20 MJ 544). In 100s and 1000s.
Rx	**Voxsuprine** (Major)		In 100s, 250s, 1000s and UD 100s.

ISOXSUPRINE HYDROCHLORIDE — ORAL

For complete prescribing information, refer to the Antihypertensives Treatment Guidelines in the Appendix.

Indications

➤*"Possibly effective":* For relief of symptoms associated with cerebral vascular insufficiency; peripheral vascular disease of arteriosclerosis obliterans, thromboangiitis obliterans (Buerger disease) and Raynaud disease.

➤*Off-label uses:* Isoxsuprine has been used in the treatment of dysmenorrhea and threatened premature labor, but efficacy has not been established.

Administration and Dosage

➤*Adults:*

Peripheral vascular disease of arteriosclerosis obliterans, thromboangiitis obliterans (Buerger disease), and Raynaud disease – 10 to 20 mg 3 or 4 times daily.

ISOXSUPRINE HYDROCHLORIDE — ORAL

Relief of symptoms associated with cerebral vascular insufficiency – 10 to 20 mg 3 or 4 times daily.

Actions

➤*Pharmacology:* Isoxsuprine is a vasodilator that acts primarily on blood vessels within skeletal muscle. In healthy subjects, resting blood flow in skeletal muscle is increased; cutaneous blood flow is usually not affected. Isoxsuprine is an alpha-adrenoreceptor antagonist with beta-adrenoreceptor stimulating properties; however, vasodilation is not blocked by propranolol. Isoxsuprine may act directly on vascular smooth muscle. The drug also causes cardiac stimulation (increased contractility, heart rate and cardiac output) and uterine relaxation. At high doses, it lowers blood viscosity and inhibits platelet aggregation.

Contraindications

Immediately postpartum; in the presence of arterial bleeding.

Warnings/Precautions

➤*Rash:* If rash appears, discontinue use. A causal relationship is not established.

➤*Pregnancy: Category C.* There are no reports of isoxsuprine causing congenital defects. Hypotension, hypocalcemia, hypoglycemia, ileus, tachycardia, and death have occurred when cord serum levels are more than 10 ng/mL. Pulmonary edema has been reported in mothers treated with beta-stimulants. Isoxsuprine is neither approved nor recommended for the treatment of premature labor.

➤*Lactation:* There are no data regarding the use of isoxsuprine in breast-feeding women.

➤*Elderly:* Per the Beers list, isoxsuprine has a lack of efficacy in the elderly population. Isoxsuprine is also considered a high risk medication for the elderly according to the centers of Medicare and Medicaid Services.

Adverse Reactions

➤*Cardiovascular:* Hypotension; tachycardia; chest pain.

➤*GI:* Nausea; vomiting; abdominal distress.

➤*Miscellaneous:* Dizziness; weakness; severe rash.

Patient Information

May cause palpitations or skin rash. Notify physician if these symptoms become particularly bothersome.

If dizziness (orthostatic hypotension) occurs, avoid sudden changes in posture.

PAPAVERINE HYDROCHLORIDE

Rx	Papaverine HCl (Various, eg, Eon, Qualitest, Time-Cap Labs)	Capsules, extended release: 150 mg	In 100s, 500s, and 1000s.
Rx	Papaverine HCl (Various)	Injection: 30 mg/mL	In 2 mL vials and 10 mL multiple-dose vials.

PAPAVERINE HYDROCHLORIDE — ORAL

For more information, refer to the Antihypertensives Treatment Guidelines in the Appendix.

Indications

➤*Ischemia:* For relief of cerebral and peripheral ischemia associated with arterial spasm and myocardial ischemia complicated by arrhythmias.

Administration and Dosage

➤*Adults:*

Ischemia – One capsule every 12 hours. In difficult cases, administration may be increased to 1 capsule every 8 hours or 2 capsules every 12 hours.

➤*Storage/Stability:* Store at controlled room temperature between 15° and 30°C (59° and 86°F). Dispense in tight, light resistant containers.

Warnings/Precautions

➤*Pregnancy: Category C.* No teratogenic effects were observed in rats when papaverine was administered subcutaneously as a single agent. It is not known whether papaverine can cause fetal harm when administered to a pregnant woman or can affect reproduction capacity. Give papaverine to a pregnant woman only if clearly needed.

➤*Lactation:* It is not known whether this drug is excreted in human milk. Because many drugs are excreted in human milk, exercise caution when papaverine is administered to a breast-feeding woman.

PAPAVERINE HYDROCHLORIDE — INJECTION

For more information, refer to the Antihypertensives Treatment Guidelines in the Appendix.

Indications

➤*Spasm of smooth muscle:* Papaverine is recommended in various conditions accompanied by spasm of smooth muscle, such as vascular spasm associated with acute MI (coronary occlusion), angina pectoris, peripheral and pulmonary embolism, peripheral vascular disease in which there is a vasospastic element, or certain cerebral angiospastic states; and visceral spasm, as in ureteral, biliary, or gastrointestinal colic.

Administration and Dosage

➤*Maximum dose:*

Adults – There is no well-established maximum dose for the approved indication according to the prescribing information.

➤*Adults:*

Various conditions accompanied by spasm of smooth muscle – For a list of conditions, refer to Indications.

Usual dosage: 1 to 4 mL IM or IV repeated every 3 hours as indicated.
Cardiac extrasystoles: 2 doses may be given 10 minutes apart.

➤*Administration:* Papaverine may be administered intravenously or intramuscularly. The intravenous route is recommended when an immediate effect is desired, but the drug must be injected slowly over the course of 1 or 2 minutes to avoid uncomfortable or alarming side effects.

➤*Admixture compatibility:*

Incompatibility – Papaverine injection should not be added to Ringer's lactate injection, because precipitation would result.

➤*Storage/Stability:* Store at controlled room temperature between 15° and 30°C (59° and 86°F). Protect from light. Retain in carton until time of use.

Actions

➤*Pharmacology:* The most characteristic effect of papaverine is relaxation of the tonus of all smooth muscle, especially when it has been spasmodically contracted. Papaverine apparently acts directly on the muscle itself. This relaxation is noted in the vascular system and bronchial musculature and in the gastrointestinal, biliary, and urinary tracts.

The main actions of papaverine are exerted on cardiac and smooth muscle. Papaverine relaxes various smooth muscles, especially those of larger arteries; this relaxation may be prominent if spasm exists. The antispasmodic effect is a direct one and unrelated to muscle innervation, and the muscle still responds to drugs and other stimuli causing contraction. Papaverine has minimal actions on the CNS, although very large doses tend to produce some sedation and sleepiness in some patients. In certain circumstances, mild respiratory stimulation can be observed, but this is therapeutically inconsequential. Papaverine stimulates respiration by acting on carotid and aortic body chemoreceptors.

Papaverine relaxes the smooth musculature of the larger blood vessels, including the coronary, cerebral, peripheral, and pulmonary arteries. This action is particularly evident when such vessels are in spasm, induced reflexly or by drugs, and it provides the basis for the clinical use of papaverine in peripheral or pulmonary arterial embolism.

Experimentally in dogs, the alkaloid has been shown to cause fairly marked and long-lasting coronary vasodilatation and an increase in coronary blood flow. However, it also appears to have a direct inotropic effect and, when increased mechanical activity coincides with decreased systemic pressure, increases in coronary blood flow may not be sufficient to prevent brief periods of hypoxic myocardial depression.

➤*Pharmacokinetics:*

Absorption – Papaverine is effective by all routes of administration. A considerable fraction of the drug localizes in fat depots and in the liver, with the remainder being distributed throughout the body.

Distribution – About 90% of the drug is bound to plasma protein. Although estimates of its biologic half-life vary widely, reasonably constant plasma levels can be maintained with oral administration at 6-hour intervals.

Metabolism – It is metabolized in the liver.

Excretion – The drug is excreted in the urine in an inactive form.

Contraindications

IV injection of papaverine is contraindicated in the presence of complete atrioventricular heart block. When conduction is depressed, the drug may produce transient ectopic rhythms of ventricular origin, either premature beats or paroxysmal tachycardia.

Papaverine is not indicated for the treatment of impotence by intracorporeal injection. The intracorporeal injection of papaverine has been reported to have resulted in persistent priapism requiring medical and surgical intervention.

Warnings/Precautions

➤*Cardiac:* Large doses can depress AV and intraventricular conduction and thereby produce serious arrhythmias. When conduction is depressed, it may produce transient ectopy of ventricular origin, either premature beats or paroxysmal tachycardia.

PAPAVERINE HYDROCHLORIDE — INJECTION

➤*Hepatic effects:* Chronic hepatitis, as evidenced by an increase in serum bilirubin and serum glutamic transaminase, has been reported in 3 cases following long-term papaverine therapy. One patient had jaundice, and another had abnormal liver function on biopsy.

The medication should be discontinued if hepatic hypersensitivity with GI symptoms, jaundice, or eosinophilia becomes evident or if liver function test values become altered.

➤*Special risk:* Use with caution in patients with glaucoma.

➤*Drug abuse and dependence:* Drug dependence resulting from the abuse of many of the selective depressants, including papaverine, has been reported.

➤*Pregnancy:* Category C. No teratogenic effects were observed in rats when papaverine was administered subcutaneously as a single agent. It is not known whether papaverine can cause fetal harm when administered to a pregnant woman or can affect reproduction capacity.

➤*Lactation:* It is not known whether this drug is excreted in human milk. Because many drugs are excreted in human milk, exercise caution when papaverine is administered to a breast-feeding woman.

➤*Children:* Safety and efficacy for use in children have not been established.

Drug Interactions

➤*QT prolongation:* An additive effect of papaverine with other drugs that prolong the QT interval cannot be excluded. The following drugs may prolong the QT interval and increase the risk of life-threatening cardiac arrhythmias, including torsades de pointes: Antiarrhythmic agents (eg, amiodarone, bretylium, disopyramide, dofetilide, procainamide, quinidine, and sotalol), arsenic trioxide, chlorpromazine, cisapride, dolasetron, droperidol, mefloquine, mesoridazine, moxifloxacin, pentamidine, pimozide, tacrolimus, thioridazine, and ziprasidone. For a more complete list of drugs that may prolong the QT interval, see the appendix, Drug-Induced Prolongation of the QT Interval and Torsades de Pointes.

➤*Levodopa:* Loss of control of Parkinson disease may occur following the introduction of papaverine. Although the mechanism is unknown, papaverine may block dopamine receptors in the striatum.

Adverse Reactions

The following adverse reactions have been reported: general discomfort, nausea, abdominal discomfort, anorexia, constipation or diarrhea, skin rash, malaise, vertigo, headache, intensive flushing of the face, perspiration, increase in the depth of respiration, increase in heart rate, a slight rise in blood pressure, and excessive sedation.

Hepatitis, probably related to an immune mechanism, has been reported infrequently. Rarely, this has progressed to cirrhosis.

Overdosage

➤*Symptoms:* The symptoms of toxicity from papaverine often result from vasomotor instability and include nausea, vomiting, weakness, central nervous system depression, nystagmus, diplopia, diaphoresis, flushing, dizziness, and sinus tachycardia. In large overdoses, papaverine is a potent inhibitor of cellular respiration and a weak calcium antagonist. Following an oral overdose of 15 g, metabolic acidosis with hyperventilation, hyperglycemia, and hypokalemia have been reported. No information on toxic serum concentrations is available.

➤*Treatment:* To obtain up-to-date information about the treatment of overdose, a good resource is your certified regional poison control center. In managing overdosage, consider the possibility of multiple drug overdoses, interaction among drugs, and unusual drug kinetics in your patient.

Protect the patient's airway and support ventilation and perfusion. Meticulously monitor vital signs, blood gases, blood chemistry values, and other variables.

If convulsions occur, consider diazepam, phenytoin, or phenobarbital. If the seizures are refractory, general anesthesia with thiopental or halothane and paralysis with a neuromuscular blocking agent may be necessary.

For hypotension, consider intravenous fluids, elevation of the legs, and an inotropic vasopressor, such as dopamine or norepinephrine (levarterenol). Theoretically, calcium gluconate may be helpful in treating some of the toxic cardiovascular effects of papaverine; monitor the ECG and plasma calcium concentrations.

Forced diuresis, peritoneal dialysis, hemodialysis, or charcoal hemoperfusion have not been established as beneficial for an overdose of papaverine.

HYDRALAZINE HYDROCHLORIDE

Rx	**Hydralazine** (Various, eg, Goldline, Schein)	**Tablets:** 10 mg	In 100s, 1000s and UD 100s.
Rx	**Apresoline** (Novartis)		Lactose. Yellow. In 100s and 1200s.
Rx	**Hydralazine** (Various, eg, Goldline)	**Tablets:** 25 mg	In 100s, 1000s and UD 100s.
Rx	**Apresoline** (Novartis)		Blue. In 100s and 1000s.
Rx	**Hydralazine** (Various, eg, Goldline)	**Tablets:** 50 mg	In 100s, 1000s and UD 100s.
Rx	**Apresoline** (Novartis)		Lactose. Light blue. In 100s and 1000s.
Rx	**Hydralazine** (Various, eg, Goldline)	**Tablets:** 100 mg	In 100s and 1000s.
Rx	**Apresoline** (Novartis)		Tartrazine. Peach. In 100s.
Rx	**Hydralazine** (Solopak)	**Injection:** 20 mg per mL	In 1 mL vials.

HYDRALAZINE HYDROCHLORIDE — ORAL

For more information, refer to the Antihypertensives Treatment Guidelines in the Appendix.

Indications

➤*Hypertension:* Essential hypertension, alone or as an adjunct.

➤*Off-label uses:* Hydralazine in doses up to 800 mg 3 times daily has been effective in reducing afterload in the treatment of congestive heart failure (CHF) and severe aortic insufficiency and after valve replacement.

Administration and Dosage

➤*General dosing considerations:* In a few resistant patients, up to 300 mg of hydralazine daily may be required. In such cases, a lower dosage of hydralazine combined with a thiazide or reserpine or a beta-blocker may be considered. However, when combining therapy, individual titration is essential to ensure the lowest possible therapeutic dose of each drug.

The incidence of toxic reactions, particularly the LE cell syndrome, is high in the group of patients receiving large doses of hydralazine.

➤*Adults:*

Essential hypertension –

Initial dosage: 10 mg 4 times daily for the first 2 to 4 days, 25 mg 4 times daily for the balance of the first week.

Dosage titration: 50 mg 4 times daily from the second week on.

Maintenance dosage: Adjust dosage to the lowest effective levels.

➤*Children:*

Essential hypertension –

1 year of age and older:

- *Maximum dose* – 7.5 mg/kg/day in 4 divided doses or 200 mg/day.
- *Initial dosage* – 0.75 mg/kg/day in 4 divided doses.
- *Dosage titration* – Increase gradually over 3 to 4 weeks, to a maximum of 7.5 mg/kg/day in 4 divided doses or 200 mg/day.

Off-label dosing –

Essential hypertension:

- *Less than 1 year of age –*

Maximum dose: 25 mg/dose; 5 mg/kg/day or 200 mg/day.

Initial dosage: 0.75 to 1 mg/kg/day in 2 to 4 divided doses.

Dosage titration: Increase gradually over 3 to 4 weeks, to a maximum of 5 mg/kg/day or 200 mg/day.

➤*Administration:* Administer with food to enhance absorption.

➤*Storage/Stability:* Do not store above 30°C (86°F).

Actions

➤*Pharmacology:* Although the precise mechanism of action of hydralazine is not fully understood, the major effects are on the cardiovascular system. Hydralazine apparently lowers blood pressure by exerting a peripheral, vasodilating effect through a direct relaxation of vascular smooth muscle. Hydralazine, by altering cellular calcium metabolism, interferes with the calcium movements within the vascular smooth muscle that are responsible for initiating or maintaining the contractile state.

The peripheral, vasodilating effect of hydralazine results in decreased arterial blood pressure (diastolic more than systolic); decreased peripheral vascular resistance; and an increased heart rate, stroke volume, and cardiac output. The preferential dilatation of arterioles, as compared to veins, minimizes postural hypotension and promotes the increase in cardiac output. Hydralazine usually increases renin activity in plasma, presumably as a result of increased secretion of renin by the renal juxtaglomerular cells in response to reflex sympathetic discharge. This increase in renin activity leads to the production of angiotensin II, which then causes stimulation of aldosterone and consequent sodium reabsorption. Hydralazine also maintains or increases renal and cerebral blood flow.

➤*Pharmacokinetics:*

Absorption/Distribution – Hydralazine is rapidly absorbed after oral administration, and peak plasma levels are reached at 1 to 2 hours. Plasma levels of apparent hydralazine decline with a half-life of 3 to 7 hours. Binding to human plasma protein is 87%. Plasma levels of hydralazine vary

HYDRALAZINE HYDROCHLORIDE — ORAL

widely among individuals. Hydralazine is subject to polymorphic acetylation; slow acetylators generally have higher plasma levels of hydralazine and require lower doses to maintain control of blood pressure.

Metabolism/Excretion – Hydralazine undergoes extensive hepatic metabolism; it is excreted mainly in the form of metabolites in the urine.

Contraindications

Hypersensitivity to hydralazine; coronary artery disease; mitral valvular rheumatic heart disease.

Warnings/Precautions

➤*Systemic erythematosus-like symptoms:* In a few patients, hydralazine may produce a clinical picture simulating systemic lupus erythematosus, including glomerulonephritis. In such patients, hydralazine should be discontinued unless the benefit-to-risk determination requires continued antihypertensive therapy with this drug. Symptoms and signs usually regress when the drug is discontinued, but residua have been detected many years later. Long-term treatment with steroids may be necessary.

➤*Peripheral neuritis:* Peripheral neuritis, evidenced by paresthesia, numbness, and tingling, has been observed. Published evidence suggests an antipyridoxine effect, and that pyridoxine should be added to the regimen if symptoms develop.

➤*Cardiovascular effects:* Myocardial stimulation produced by hydralazine hydrochloride can cause anginal attacks and ECG changes of myocardial ischemia. The drug has been implicated in the production of myocardial infarction (MI). It must, therefore, be used with caution in patients with suspected coronary artery disease.

The "hyperdynamic" circulation caused by hydralazine hydrochloride may accentuate specific cardiovascular inadequacies. For example, hydralazine hydrochloride may increase pulmonary artery pressure in patients with mitral valvular disease. The drug may reduce the pressor responses to epinephrine. Postural hypotension may result from hydralazine hydrochloride but is less common than with ganglionic-blocking agents. It should be used with caution in patients with cerebral vascular accidents.

➤*Renal effects:* In hypertensive patients with healthy kidneys who are treated with hydralazine hydrochloride, there is evidence of increased renal blood flow and a maintenance of glomerular filtration rate. In some instances where control values were below normal, improved renal function has been noted after administration of hydralazine hydrochloride. However, as with any antihypertensive agent, hydralazine hydrochloride should be used with caution in patients with advanced renal damage.

➤*Tartrazine sensitivity:* Some of these products may contain FD&C Yellow No. 5 (tartrazine), which may cause allergic-type reactions (including bronchial asthma) in certain susceptible individuals. Although the overall incidence of FD&C Yellow No. 5 (tartrazine) sensitivity in the general population is low, it is frequently seen in patients who are also hypersensitive to aspirin.

➤*Pregnancy: Category C.* Hydralazine is considered a second-line agent for the management of hypertension during pregnancy.

Animal studies indicate that hydralazine is teratogenic in mice at 20 to 30 times the maximum daily human dose of 200 to 300 mg and possibly in rabbits at 10 to 15 times the maximum daily human dose, but that it is nonteratogenic in rats. Teratogenic effects observed were cleft palate and malformations of facial and cranial bones.

There are no adequate and well-controlled studies in pregnant women. Although clinical experience does not include any positive evidence of adverse effects on the human fetus, hydralazine should be used during pregnancy only if the expected benefit justifies the potential risk to the fetus.

➤*Lactation:* Hydralazine has been shown to be excreted in breast milk. Because many drugs are excreted in human milk, caution should be exercised when hydralazine is administered to a breast-feeding woman.

➤*Children:* Safety and efficacy in pediatric patients have not been established in controlled clinical trials; although, there is experience with the use of hydralazine in these patients. The usual recommended oral starting dosage is 0.75 mg/kg of body weight daily in 4 divided doses. Dosage may be increased gradually over the next 3 to 4 weeks to a maximum of 7.5 mg/kg or 200 mg daily.

➤*Monitoring:* Complete blood counts and antinuclear antibody titer determinations are indicated before and periodically during prolonged therapy with hydralazine, even though the patient is asymptomatic. These studies are also indicated if the patient develops arthralgia, fever, chest pain, continued malaise, or other unexplained signs or symptoms.

A positive antinuclear antibody titer requires that the physician carefully weigh the implications of the test results against the benefits to be derived from antihypertensive therapy with hydralazine.

Drug Interactions

Hydralazine Drug Interactions

Precipitant drug	Object drug[a]		Description
Beta blockers Metoprolol Propranolol	Hydralazine	↑	Serum levels of either drug may be increased by concurrent use.
Hydralazine	Beta blockers Metoprolol Propranolol	↑	
Indomethacin	Hydralazine	↓	The pharmacologic effects of hydralazine may be decreased.

[a] ↑ = Object drug increased. ↓ = Object drug decreased.

MAO inhibitors should be used with caution in patients receiving hydralazine.

When other potent parenteral antihypertensive drugs, such as diazoxide, are used in combination with hydralazine, patients should be continuously observed for several hours for any excessive fall in blood pressure. Profound hypotensive episodes may occur when diazoxide injection and hydralazine hydrochloride are used concomitantly.

➤*Drug/Food interactions:* Administration of hydralazine with food results in higher plasma levels.

Adverse Reactions

Adverse reactions with hydralazine hydrochloride are usually reversible when dosage is reduced. However, in some cases it may be necessary to discontinue the drug.

The following adverse reactions have been observed, but there has not been enough systematic collection of data to support an estimate of their frequency.

➤*Common:*

Miscellaneous – Headache, anorexia, nausea, vomiting, diarrhea, palpitations, tachycardia, angina pectoris.

➤*Less frequent:*

Cardiovascular – Hypotension, paradoxical pressor response, edema.

CNS – Peripheral neuritis, evidenced by paresthesia, numbness, and tingling; dizziness; tremors; muscle cramps; psychotic reactions characterized by depression, disorientation, or anxiety.

GI – Constipation and paralytic ileus.

GU – Difficulty in urination.

Hematologic – Blood dyscrasias, consisting of reduction in hemoglobin and red cell count; leukopenia; agranulocytosis; purpura; lymphadenopathy; splenomegaly.

Hypersensitivity – Rash, urticaria, pruritus, fever, chills, arthralgia, eosinophilia, and, rarely, hepatitis.

Respiratory – Dyspnea.

Miscellaneous – Nasal congestion, flushing, lacrimation, conjunctivitis.

Overdosage

➤*Highest known dose survived:* Adults, 10 g orally.

➤*Symptoms:* Signs and symptoms of overdosage include hypotension, tachycardia, headache, and generalized skin flushing.

Complications can include myocardial ischemia and subsequent MI, cardiac arrhythmia, and profound shock.

➤*Treatment:* There is no specific antidote.

The gastric contents should be evacuated, taking adequate precautions against aspiration and for protection of the airway. An activated charcoal slurry may be instilled if conditions permit. These manipulations may have to be omitted or carried out after cardiovascular status has been stabilized, since they might precipitate cardiac arrhythmias or increase the depth of shock.

Support of the cardiovascular system is of primary importance. Shock should be treated with plasma expanders. If possible, vasopressors should not be given, but if a vasopressor is required, care should be taken not to precipitate or aggravate cardiac arrhythmia. Tachycardia responds to beta blockers. Digitalization may be necessary, and renal function should be monitored and supported as required.

No experience has been reported with extracorporeal or peritoneal dialysis.

Patient Information

Patients should be informed of possible side effects and advised to take the medication regularly and continuously as directed.

HYDRALAZINE HYDROCHLORIDE — INJECTION

For more information, refer to the Antihypertensives Treatment Guidelines in the Appendix.

Indications

➤*Severe hypertension:* Severe essential hypertension when the drug cannot be given orally or when there is an urgent need to lower blood pressure.

➤*Off-label uses:* Hydralazine in doses up to 800 mg 3 times daily has been effective in reducing afterload in the treatment of congestive heart failure (CHF), severe aortic insufficiency and after valve replacement.

Administration and Dosage

➤*General dosing considerations:* Hydralazine injection should be used only when the drug cannot be given orally.

HYDRALAZINE HYDROCHLORIDE — INJECTION

Blood pressure should be checked frequently. It may begin to fall within a few minutes after injection, with the average maximal decrease occurring in 10 to 80 minutes.

In cases where there has been increased intracranial pressure, lowering the blood pressure may increase cerebral ischemia.

Most patients can be transferred to hydralazine oral within 24 to 48 hours.

➤*Adults:*

Severe essential hypertension – 20 to 40 mg IM or IV repeated as necessary.

➤*Children:*

Severe essential hypertension – 1.7 to 3.5 mg/kg/day IM or IV divided into 4 to 6 doses.

Off-label dosing –

Hypertensive crisis:

- *1 to 17 years of age* –
  - *Usual dosage:* 1.7 to 3.5 mg/kg/day IM or IV divided into 4 to 6 doses.
  - *Maximum dose:* 20 mg/dose IM or IV. 2 mg/kg every 3 to 6 hours; cumulative daily dose not to exceed 9 mg/kg.
  - *Initial dosage:* 0.1 to 0.2 mg/kg/dose IM or IV every 4 to 6 hours as needed.
  - *Alternative dosage:* 0.2 to 0.6 mg/kg/dose IM or IV; dose every 4 hours for IV bolus administration.
- *3 months to 1 year* –
  - *Maximum dose:* 2 mg/kg IV every 6 hours.
  - *Initial dosage:* 0.1 to 0.5 mg/kg/dose IV every 6 to 8 hours.
  - *Dosage titration:* Dosage should be titrated for blood pressure control.

Congestive heart failure:

- *3 months to 1 year* –
  - *Maximum dose:* 2 mg/kg IV every 6 hours.
  - *Initial dosage:* 0.1 to 0.5 mg/kg/dose IV every 6 to 8 hours.
  - *Dosage titration:* Dosage should be titrated for blood pressure control.

➤*Renal function impairment:* Certain patients (especially those with marked renal damage) may require a lower dose.

➤*Preparation for administration:* Hydralazine may discolor upon contact with metal; discolored solutions should be discarded. Use immediately after the vial is opened.

➤*Administration:* When there is urgent need, therapy in the hospitalized patient may be initiated IM or as a rapid IV bolus injection directly into the vein.

➤*Admixture compatibility:* Hydralazine should not be added to infusion solutions.

To screen for specific compatibilities, see *Trissel's IV-Chek*.

➤*Storage/Stability:* Store between 15° and 30°C (59° and 86°F).

Actions

➤*Pharmacology:* Although the precise mechanism of action of hydralazine is not fully understood, the major effects are on the cardiovascular system. Hydralazine apparently lowers blood pressure by exerting a peripheral vasodilating effect through a direct relaxation of vascular smooth muscle. Hydralazine, by altering cellular calcium metabolism, interferes with the calcium movements within the vascular smooth muscle that are responsible for initiating or maintaining the contractile state.

The peripheral vasodilating effect of hydralazine results in decreased arterial blood pressure (diastolic more than systolic); decreased peripheral vascular resistance; and an increased heart rate, stroke volume, and cardiac output. The preferential dilatation of arterioles, as compared to veins, minimizes postural hypotension and promotes the increase in cardiac output. Hydralazine usually increases renin activity in plasma, presumably as a result of increased secretion of renin by the renal juxtaglomerular cells in response to reflex sympathetic discharge. This increase in renin activity leads to the production of angiotensin II, which then causes stimulation of aldosterone and consequent sodium reabsorption. Hydralazine also maintains or increases renal and cerebral blood flow.

The average maximal decrease in blood pressure usually occurs 10 to 80 minutes after administration of hydralazine injection. No other pharmacokinetic data on hydralazine injection are available.

Contraindications

Hypersensitivity to hydralazine; coronary artery disease; mitral valvular rheumatic heart disease.

Warnings/Precautions

➤*Systemic lupus erythematosus-like symptoms:* In a few patients hydralazine may produce a clinical picture simulating systemic lupus erythematosus including glomerulonephritis. In such patients hydralazine should be discontinued unless the benefit-to-risk determination requires continued antihypertensive therapy with this drug. Symptoms and signs usually regress when the drug is discontinued but residua have been detected many years later. Long-term treatment with steroids may be necessary.

➤*Cardiovascular changes:* Myocardial stimulation produced by hydralazine can cause anginal attacks and ECG changes of myocardial ischemia. The drug has been implicated in the production of myocardial infarction. It must, therefore, be used with caution in patients with suspected coronary artery disease.

The "hyperdynamic" circulation caused by hydralazine may accentuate specific cardiovascular inadequacies. For example, hydralazine may increase pulmonary artery pressure in patients with mitral valvular disease. The drug may reduce the pressor responses to epinephrine. Postural hypotension may result from hydralazine but is less common than with ganglionic blocking agents. It should be used with caution in patients with cerebral vascular accidents.

➤*Renal effects:* In hypertensive patients with normal kidneys who are treated with hydralazine, there is evidence of increased renal blood flow and a maintenance of glomerular filtration rate. In some instances where control values were below normal, improved renal function has been noted after administration of hydralazine. However, as with any antihypertensive agent, hydralazine should be used with caution in patients with advanced renal damage.

Peripheral neuritis – Peripheral neuritis, evidenced by paresthesia, numbness, and tingling, has been observed. Published evidence suggests an antipyridoxine effect, and that pyridoxine should be added to the regimen if symptoms develop.

➤*Pregnancy: Category C.* Hydralazine injection is a recommended agent for the emergency treatment of hypertension during pregnancy.

Teratogenic – Animal studies indicate that hydralazine is teratogenic in mice at 20 to 30 times the maximum daily human dose of 200 to 300 mg and possibly in rabbits at 10 to 15 times the maximum daily human dose, but that it is nonteratogenic in rats. Teratogenic effects observed were cleft palate and malformations of facial and cranial bones.

There are no adequate and well-controlled studies in pregnant women. Although clinical experience does not include any positive evidence of adverse effects on the human fetus, hydralazine should be used during pregnancy only if the expected benefit justifies the potential risk to the fetus.

➤*Lactation:* It is not known whether this drug is excreted in human milk. Because many drugs are excreted in human milk, caution should be exercised when hydralazine injection is administered to a breast-feeding woman.

➤*Children:* Safety and efficacy in pediatric patients have not been established in controlled clinical trials, although there is experience with the use of hydralazine hydrochloride in children. The usual recommended parenteral dosage, administered intramuscularly or intravenously, is 1.7 to 3.5 mg/kg of body weight daily, divided into 4 to 6 doses.

➤*Monitoring:* Complete blood counts and antinuclear antibody titer determinations are indicated before and periodically during prolonged therapy with hydralazine even though the patient is asymptomatic. These studies are also indicated if the patient develops arthralgia, fever, chest pain, continued malaise, or other unexplained signs or symptoms.

A positive antinuclear antibody titer requires that the physician carefully weigh the implications of the test results against the benefits to be derived from antihypertensive therapy with hydralazine hydrochloride.

Blood dyscrasias, consisting of reduction in hemoglobin and red cell count, leukopenia, agranulocytosis, and purpura, have been reported. If such abnormalities develop, therapy should be discontinued.

Drug Interactions

Hydralazine Drug Interactions

Precipitant drug	Object drug[a]		Description
Beta-blockers Metoprolol Propranolol	Hydralazine	↑	Serum levels of either drug may be increased by concurrent use.
Hydralazine	Beta-blockers Metoprolol Propranolol	↑	
Indomethacin	Hydralazine	↓	The pharmacologic effects of hydralazine may be decreased.

[a] ↑ = Object drug increased. ↓ = Object drug decreased.

MAO inhibitors should be used with caution in patients receiving hydralazine.

When other potent parenteral antihypertensive drugs, such as diazoxide, are used in combination with hydralazine, patients should be continuously observed for several hours for any excessive fall in blood pressure. Profound hypotensive episodes may occur when diazoxide injection and hydralazine injection are used concomitantly.

Adverse Reactions

Adverse reactions with hydralazine hydrochloride are usually reversible when dosage is reduced. However, in some cases it may be necessary to discontinue the drug.

The following adverse reactions have been observed, but there has not been enough systematic collection of data to support an estimate of their frequency.

➤*Common:*

Miscellaneous – Headache, anorexia, nausea, vomiting, diarrhea, palpitations, tachycardia, angina pectoris.

➤*Less frequent:*

Cardiovascular – Hypotension, paradoxical pressor response, edema.

CNS – Peripheral neuritis, evidenced by paresthesia, numbness, and tingling; dizziness; tremors; muscle cramps; psychotic reactions characterized by depression, disorientation, or anxiety.

HYDRALAZINE HYDROCHLORIDE — INJECTION

GI – Constipation, paralytic ileus.

GU – Difficulty in urination.

Hematologic – Blood dyscrasias, consisting of reduction in hemoglobin and red cell count, leukopenia, agranulocytosis, purpura; lymphadenopathy; splenomegaly.

Hypersensitivity – Rash, urticaria, pruritus, fever, chills, arthralgia, eosinophilia, and, rarely, hepatitis.

Respiratory – Dyspnea.

Miscellaneous – Nasal congestion, flushing, lacrimation, conjunctivitis.

Overdosage

➤*Highest known dose survived:* Adults, 10 g orally.

➤*Symptoms:* Signs and symptoms of overdosage include hypotension, tachycardia, headache, and generalized skin flushing.

Complications can include myocardial ischemia and subsequent myocardial infarction, cardiac arrhythmia, and profound shock.

➤*Treatment:* There is no specific antidote.

Support of the cardiovascular system is of primary importance. Shock should be treated with plasma expanders. If possible, vasopressors should not be given, but if a vasopressor is required, care should be taken not to precipitate or aggravate cardiac arrhythmia. Tachycardia responds to beta blockers. Digitalization may be necessary, and renal function should be monitored and supported as required.

No experience has been reported with extracorporeal or peritoneal dialysis.

MINOXIDIL

Rx	**Minoxidil** (Various, eg, PAR, Southwood, URL, Watson)	**Tablets:** 2.5 mg	In 100s, 500s, and 1000s.
Rx	**Minoxidil** (Various, eg, Major, PAR, Southwood, URL, Watson)	**Tablets:** 10 mg	In 100s, 500s and 1000s.

MINOXIDIL — ORAL

For complete prescribing information, refer to the Antihypertensives Treatment Guidelines in the Appendix.

WARNING

Minoxidil may produce serious adverse effects. It can cause pericardial effusion, occasionally progressing to tamponade, and it can exacerbate angina pectoris. Reserve for hypertensive patients who do not respond adequately to maximum therapeutic doses of a diuretic and 2 other antihypertensive agents.

In experimental animals, minoxidil caused several kinds of myocardial lesions and other adverse cardiac effects.

Administer under close supervision, usually concomitantly with a beta -adrenergic blocking agent, to prevent tachycardia and increased myocardial workload. Usually, it must be given with a diuretic, frequently one acting in the ascending limb of the loop of Henle to prevent serious fluid accumulation. When first administering minoxidil, hospitalize and monitor patients with malignant hypertension and those already receiving guanethidine to avoid too rapid or large orthostatic decreases in blood pressure.

Indications

➤*Severe hypertension:* Severe hypertension that is symptomatic or associated with target organ damage, and is not manageable with maximum therapeutic doses of a diuretic plus 2 other antihypertensives. Use in milder degrees of hypertension is not recommended because the benefit-risk ratio in such patients has not been defined.

➤*Alopecia androgenetica (topical only):* Topical minoxidil is used for the treatment of male pattern baldness (alopecia androgenetica) of the vertex of the scalp (see Minoxidil Topical Solution monograph in the Dermatological Agents chapter). Use of the tablets, in any formulation, to promote hair growth is not an approved use. Effects of extemporaneous formulations and dosages have not been shown to be safe and effective.

Administration and Dosage

➤*Adults:*

Severe hypertension –

Usual dosage: 10 to 40 mg orally daily.

Maximum dose: 100 mg/day.

Initial dosage: 5 mg/day as a single dose.

Dosage titration: Daily dosage can be increased to 10, 20, then 40 mg in single or divided doses if required. Must be carefully titrated and adjusted at 3-day or more intervals because full response to a given dose is not attained until then. If more rapid management is required, adjustments can be made every 6 hours with careful monitoring.

Dosage adjustment: The magnitude of within-day fluctuation of arterial pressure during therapy is directly proportional to the extent of pressure reduction. If supine diastolic pressure has been reduced less than 30 mm Hg, administer the drug only once a day; if reduced more than 30 mm Hg, divide the daily dosage into 2 equal parts.

Concomitant therapy:

• *Diuretics* – Use minoxidil with a diuretic in patients relying on renal function for maintaining salt and water balance. Diuretics have been used at the following dosages when starting minoxidil therapy: hydrochlorothiazide (50 mg twice daily) or other thiazides at equally effective doses; chlorthalidone (50 to 100 mg/day); furosemide (40 mg twice daily). If excessive salt and water retention results in a weight gain of more than 2.3 kg (5 lb), change diuretic therapy to furosemide. In furosemide-treated patients, increase dosage in accordance with their needs.

• *Beta-blockers/Other sympathetic nervous system suppressants* – When beginning therapy, the β-blocker dosage should be equal to propranolol 80 to 160 mg/day in divided doses. If β-blockers are contraindicated, use methyldopa 250 to 750 mg twice daily; give for at least 24 hours before starting minoxidil due to delay in onset. Clonidine may also be used to prevent tachycardia induced by minoxidil; usual dosage is 0.1 to 0.2 mg twice daily.

Sympathetic nervous system suppressants may not completely prevent a heart rate increase but usually prevent tachycardia. Typically, patients receiving a β-blocker prior to minoxidil have bradycardia; expect an increase in heart rate toward normal when minoxidil is added. Simultaneous treatment with minoxidil and a β-blocker or other sympathetic nervous system suppressant causes little change in heart rate because their opposing cardiac effects usually nullify each other.

➤*Children:*

Severe hypertension –

12 years of age and older: See Adults for dosing for children 12 years of age and older.

Younger than 12 years of age:

• *Usual dosage* – 0.25 to 1 mg/kg orally daily.
• *Maximum dose* – 50 mg/day.
• *Initial dosage* – 0.2 mg/kg orally as a single daily dose.
• *Dosage titration* – See Adults for Dosage titration.

Experience in children is limited, particularly in infants; monitor closely. Titrate carefully for optimal effects.

• *Dosage adjustment* – See Adults for Dosage adjustment.
• *Concomitant therapy* – See Adults for Concomitant therapy.

➤*Storage/Stability:* Store minoxidil at 15° to 30°C (59° to 86°F).

Actions

➤*Pharmacology:* Minoxidil is a direct-acting peripheral vasodilator. It does not interfere with vasomotor reflexes; therefore, it does not produce orthostatic hypotension. The drug does not affect CNS function.

Because it causes peripheral vasodilation, minoxidil elicits a reduction of peripheral arteriolar resistance. This action, with the associated fall in blood pressure, triggers sympathetic, vagal inhibitory, and renal homeostatic mechanisms, including an increase in renin secretion, which leads to increased cardiac rate and output, and salt and water retention. These adverse effects can usually be minimized by coadministration of a diuretic and a beta-adrenergic-blocking agent or other sympathetic nervous system suppressant.

Antihypertensive effects – Minoxidil reduces elevated systolic and diastolic blood pressure by decreasing peripheral vascular resistance. The blood pressure response to minoxidil is dose-related and proportional to the extent of hypertension. In humans, forearm and renal vascular resistance decline; forearm blood flow increases while renal blood flow and glomerular filtration rate (GFR) are preserved.

When used in severely hypertensive patients resistant to other therapy, frequently with an accompanying diuretic and β-adrenergic blocker, minoxidil decreased the blood pressure and reversed encephalopathy and retinopathy. The drug reduced supine diastolic blood pressure by 20 mm Hg, or by 90 mm Hg or less in approximately 75% of the patients studied.

➤*Pharmacokinetics:*

Absorption/Distribution – Minoxidil is not protein bound and is at least 90% absorbed from the GI tract. Plasma levels of the parent drug reach a maximum within the first hour and decline rapidly thereafter.

Onset/Duration: The extent and time course of blood pressure reduction by minoxidil do not correspond closely to its plasma concentration. After an effective single oral dose, blood pressure usually starts to decline within 30 minutes, reaches a minimum between 2 and 3 hours and recovers at a linear rate of about 30% per day. The total duration of effect is approximately 75 hours.

When minoxidil is administered chronically once or twice a day, the time required to achieve maximum effect on blood pressure is inversely related to the size of the dose. Thus, maximum effect is achieved on 10 mg/day within 7 days, on 20 mg/day within 5 days, and on 40 mg/day within 3 days.

Metabolism/Excretion – Predominantly by conjugation with glucuronic acid, 90% is metabolized. Metabolites exert much less pharmacologic effect than minoxidil itself; all are excreted principally in the urine. Renal clearance corresponds to the GFR. Minoxidil and its metabolites are hemodialyzable. Average plasma half-life is 4.2 hours.

Contraindications

Hypersensitivity to any component of the product; pheochromocytoma (because the drug may stimulate secretion of catecholamines from the tumor through its antihypertensive action).

MINOXIDIL — ORAL

Warnings/Precautions

➤*Mild hypertension:* Because of potential for serious adverse effects, use in milder degrees of hypertension is not recommended; benefit-risk ratio in such patients is not defined.

➤*Cardiac lesions:*

Animal toxicology – Minoxidil has produced cardiac lesions in animals in general, including grossly visible hemorrhagic lesions of the atrium, epicardium, endocardium, and walls of small arteries and arterioles; necrosis of papillary muscles and subendocardial areas of left ventricle. Cardiac hypertrophy and dilation occurred but was partly reversed by diuretics in monkeys, suggesting increased heart weight may be related to fluid overload. In a 1-year dog study, serosanguinous pericardial fluid was noted.

Human toxicology – Autopsies of 150 patients who died from various causes who had also received minoxidil did not reveal right atrial or other hemorrhagic pathology of the kind seen in dogs. Instances of necrotic areas in papillary muscles were seen, but occurred in the presence of known pre-existing ischemic heart disease and did not appear different from or more common than lesions in patients never exposed to minoxidil.

➤*ECG changes:* Rarely, a large negative amplitude of the T wave may encroach upon the ST segment, but the ST segment is not independently altered. These changes usually disappear with continuance of treatment and revert to the pretreatment state if therapy is discontinued. No symptoms, alterations in blood cell counts or plasma enzyme concentrations, or signs of myocardial damage have been noted. Long-term treatment of patients manifesting such changes has provided no evidence of deteriorating cardiac function. At present, the changes appear to be nonspecific and without identifiable clinical significance.

➤*Fluid and electrolyte balance:* Monitor fluid and electrolyte balance and body weight. Give with a diuretic to prevent fluid retention and possible CHF; a loop diuretic is usually required. If used without a diuretic, retention of several hundred mEq salt and corresponding volumes of water can occur in a few days, leading to increased plasma and interstitial fluid volume and local or generalized edema. Diuretics alone or with restricted salt intake usually minimize fluid retention, but reversible edema developed in approximately 10% of nondialysis patients so treated. Ascites has also occurred. Diuretic effectiveness is limited by impaired renal function. Condition of patients with pre-existing CHF occasionally deteriorates due to fluid retention, but because of the fall in blood pressure (afterload reduction), more than twice as many improve than worsen.

Refractory fluid retention rarely requires discontinuation of minoxidil. Under close medical supervision, it may be possible to resolve refractory salt retention by discontinuing the drug for 1 or 2 days, and then resuming treatment in conjunction with vigorous diuretic therapy.

➤*Tachycardia/Angina:* Minoxidil increases heart rate; this can be prevented by coadministration of a β-adrenergic blocking drug or other sympathetic nervous system suppressants (eg, clonidine, methyldopa). The ability of β-adrenergic blocking agents to minimize papillary muscle lesions in animals is further reason for such concomitant use.

In addition, angina may worsen or appear for the first time during treatment, probably because of the increased oxygen demands associated with increased heart rate and cardiac output. This can usually be prevented by sympathetic blockade or β-adrenergic blocking drugs.

➤*Pericardial effusion:* Occasionally with tamponade, it has occurred in about 3% of treated patients not on dialysis, especially those with inadequate or compromised renal function. Many cases were associated with connective tissue disease, the uremic syndrome, CHF, or fluid retention, but were instances in which these potential causes of effusion were not present. Observe patients closely for signs of pericardial disorder. Perform echocardiographic studies if suspicion arises. More vigorous diuretic therapy, dialysis, pericardiocentesis, or surgery may be required. If the effusion persists, consider drug withdrawal.

➤*Hazard of rapid control of blood pressure:* Too rapid control of very severe blood pressure elevation can precipitate syncope, cerebrovascular accidents, MI, and ischemia of special sense organs with resulting decrease or loss of vision or hearing. Patients with compromised circulation or cryoglobulinemia may also suffer ischemic episodes of affected organs. Although such events have not been unequivocally associated with minoxidil use, experience is limited.

Hospitalize any patient with malignant hypertension during initial treatment to assure that blood pressure is not falling more rapidly than intended.

➤*Hemodilution:* Hematocrit, hemoglobin, and erythrocyte count usually fall about 7% initially and then recover to pretreatment levels.

➤*Myocardial infarction:* Minoxidil has not been used in patients who have had an MI within the preceding month. A reduction in arterial pressure with the drug might further limit blood flow to the myocardium, although this might be compensated by decreased oxygen demand because of lower blood pressure.

➤*Hypertrichosis:* Elongation, thickening, and enhanced pigmentation of fine body hair develops within 3- to 6-weeks after starting therapy in approximately 80% of patients. It is usually first noticed on the temples, between the eyebrows, between the hairline and the eyebrows, or in the sideburn area of the upper lateral cheek, later extending to the back, arms, legs, and scalp. Upon discontinuation of the drug, new hair growth stops, but 1- to 6-months may be required for restoration to pretreatment appearance.

No endocrine abnormalities have been found to explain the abnormal hair growth; thus, it is hypertrichosis without virilism. Inform patients (especially children and women) about this effect before therapy.

➤*Hypersensitivity reactions:* Manifested as a skin rash, hypersensitivity reactions occur in fewer than 1% of patients and rare reports of bullous eruptions and Stevens-Johnson syndrome. Deciding whether the drug should be discontinued depends on treatment alternatives.

➤*Renal function impairment:* Renal failure or dialysis patients may require smaller doses; closely supervise to prevent precipitation of cardiac failure or exacerbation of renal failure.

➤*Pregnancy: Category C.* Minoxidil reduced conception rate and increased fetal absorption in small animals when administered at 5 times the human dose. There are no adequate and well-controlled studies in pregnant women. Use only when clearly needed and when potential benefits outweigh potential hazards to the fetus.

➤*Lactation:* Safety for use in the breast-feeding mother has not been established. Minoxidil is excreted in breast milk; do not breast-feed while taking minoxidil.

➤*Children:* Use in children is limited, particularly in infants. The recommendations under Administration and Dosage are only a rough guide; careful titration is essential.

➤*Elderly:* Clinical studies did not include sufficient numbers of subjects 65 years of age and older to determine whether they respond differently from younger subjects. Other reported clinical experience has not identified differences in responses between elderly and younger patients. In general, dose selection for an elderly patient should be cautious, usually starting at the low end of the dosing range, reflecting the greater frequency of decreased hepatic, renal, or cardiac function, and of concomitant disease or other drug therapy.

➤*Monitoring:* Monitor initially and periodically thereafter body weight, blood pressure, fluid, and electrolyte balance; signs and symptoms of pericardial effusion; ECG changes; CBC; alkaline phosphatase; renal function tests.

Repeat tests that are abnormal at initiation of minoxidil therapy (eg, urinalysis, renal function tests, ECG, chest x-ray, echocardiogram) to ascertain whether improvement or deterioration is occurring under therapy. Initially, perform such tests frequently, at 1- to 3-month intervals, and as stabilization occurs, at 6- to 12-month intervals.

Drug Interactions

➤*Guanethidine:* Although minoxidil does not cause orthostatic hypotension, use in patients on guanethidine can result in profound orthostatic effects. If possible, discontinue guanethidine well before minoxidil is instituted. If this is not possible, start minoxidil in the hospital and institutionalize the patient until severity of effects are no longer present or the patient has learned to avoid activities that provoke them.

Adverse Reactions

➤*Cardiovascular:* Pericardial effusion and occasionally with tamponade (3%). Changes in direction and magnitude of T waves occur (approximately 60%).

➤*GI:* Nausea; vomiting.

➤*Hematologic:* Initially, hematocrit, hemoglobin, and erythrocyte count usually fall about 7% and then recover to pretreatment levels. Thrombocytopenia and leukopenia (WBC fewer than 3,000/mm^3) have been reported rarely.

➤*Hypersensitivity:* Rashes including bullous eruptions (rare) and Stevens-Johnson syndrome. (See Warnings/Precautions.)

➤*Lab test abnormalities:* Alkaline phosphatase increased varyingly without other evidence of liver or bone abnormality. Serum creatinine increased an average of 6% and BUN slightly more but later declined to pretreatment levels.

➤*Miscellaneous:* Temporary edema (7%); breast tenderness (fewer than 1%).

Hypertrichosis – Elongation, thickening, and enhanced pigmentation of fine body hair develops within 3 to 6 weeks of starting therapy in approximately 80% of patients.

Overdosage

➤*Symptoms:* Exaggerated hypotension is likely in association with residual sympathetic nervous system blockade from previous therapy (guanethidine-like effects or alpha-adrenergic blockade), which prevents compensatory maintenance of blood pressure.

➤*Treatment:* Administer normal saline IV to maintain blood pressure and facilitate urine formation. Avoid sympathomimetics (eg, norepinephrine, epinephrine) with excessive cardiac stimulating action. Phenylephrine, angiotensin II, vasopressin, and dopamine reverse hypotension due to minoxidil, but use only in underperfusion of a vital organ.

Radioimmunoassay can determine plasma concentration. However, due to blood level variations, it is difficult to establish a warning level. At 100 mg/day, peak blood levels of 1,641 and 2,441 ng/mL were seen in two patients. Regard an increase greater than 2,000 ng/mL as overdosage unless the patient has taken no more than the maximum dose.

Patient Information

Patient package insert is available with product.

Peripheral Vasodilators

MINOXIDIL — ORAL

Minoxidil is usually taken with at least 2 other antihypertensive medications. Take all medications as prescribed; do not discontinue any except on advice of physician.

Enhanced growth and darkening of fine body hair (approximately 80% of patients) may occur; however, do not stop medication without consulting physician.

Notify physician immediately if any of the following occur: Heart rate increase of 20 bpm or more over normal; rapid weight gain of more than 5 pounds (2.3 kg); unusual swelling of extremities, face, or abdomen; breathing difficulty, especially when lying down; new or aggravated angina symptoms (chest, arm, or shoulder pain); severe indigestion; dizziness, lightheadedness, or fainting.

Nausea or vomiting may occur.

EPOPROSTENOL (PGI_2; PGX; Prostacyclin)

Rx	**Epoprostenol Sodium** (Various, eg, Teva, Sicor)	**Injection, powder for solution:** 0.5 mg	As epoprostenol sodium. May contain mannitol, sodium chloride. In 10 mL.
Rx	**Flolan** (GlaxoSmithKline)		As epoprostenol sodium. Mannitol 50 mg, sodium chloride. In 17 mL.
Rx	**Epoprostenol Sodium** (Various, eg, Teva, Sicor)	**Injection, powder for solution:** 1.5 mg	As epoprostenol sodium. May contain mannitol, sodium chloride. In 10 mL.
Rx	**Flolan** (GlaxoSmithKline)		As epoprostenol sodium. Mannitol 50 mg, sodium chloride. In 17 mL.
Rx	**Veletri** (Actelion)		As epoprostenol sodium. Mannitol 50 mg. In 10 mL.

EPOPROSTENOL SODIUM — INJECTION

For more information, refer to the Antihypertensives Treatment Guidelines in the Appendix.

Indications

➤*Pulmonary hypertension:* For the long-term intravenous treatment of primary pulmonary hypertension and pulmonary hypertension associated with the scleroderma spectrum of disease in New York Heart Association (NYHA) class III and class IV patients who do not respond adequately to conventional therapy.

Administration and Dosage

➤*Adults:*

Pulmonary hypertension –

Initial dosage: 2 ng/kg/min intravenously (IV). If the initial infusion rate is not tolerated, identify a lower dose that is tolerated by the patient.

Dosage titration: Increase in increments of 2 ng/kg/min every 15 minutes or longer until dose-limiting pharmacologic effects are elicited or until a tolerance limit to the drug is established and further increases in the infusion rate are not clinically warranted. If dose-limiting pharmacologic effects occur, then decrease the infusion rate to an appropriate long-term infusion rate whereby the pharmacologic effects of epoprostenol are tolerated.

Dosage adjustment: Base changes in the long-term infusion rate on persistence, recurrence, or worsening of the patient's symptoms of pulmonary hypertension and the occurrence of adverse reactions due to excessive doses of epoprostenol. In general, expect increases in dose from the initial chronic dose.

Consider increments in dose if symptoms of pulmonary hypertension persist or recur after improving. Increase the infusion by 1 to 2 ng/kg/min increments at intervals sufficient to allow assessment of clinical response; these intervals should be at least 15 minutes. In clinical trials, incremental increases in dose occurred at intervals of 24 to 48 hours or longer.

During long-term infusion, the occurrence of dose-limiting pharmacological events may necessitate a decrease in infusion rate, but the adverse reactions may occasionally resolve without dosage adjustment. Make dosage decreases gradually in 2 ng/kg/min decrements every 15 minutes or longer until the dose-limiting effects resolve.

Except in life-threatening situations (eg, unconsciousness, collapse), adjust infusion rates of epoprostenol only under the direction of a health care provider.

Tapering: In patients receiving lung transplants, doses of epoprostenol were tapered after the initiation of cardiopulmonary bypass.

Discontinuation of therapy: Avoid abrupt withdrawal of epoprostenol or sudden large reductions in infusion rates.

Monitoring: Following establishment of a new long-term infusion rate, observe the patient, and monitor standing and supine blood pressure and heart rate for several hours to ensure that the new dose is tolerated.

➤*Preparation for administration:* Select a concentration for the solution of epoprostenol that is compatible with the infusion pump being used with respect to minimum and maximum flow rates, reservoir capacity, and the infusion pump criteria listed.

Flolan – When administered long-term, prepare epoprostenol in a drug delivery reservoir appropriate for the infusion pump with a total reservoir volume of at least 100 mL. Prepare epoprostenol using 2 vials of sterile diluent for epoprostenol for use during a 24-hour period.

Veletri – When administered long-term, prepare epoprostenol in a drug delivery reservoir appropriate for the infusion pump for up to a 24-hour period.

Epoprostenol Reconstitution and Dilution Instructions

To make 100 mL of solution with final concentration (ng/mL) of:	Directions
3,000 ng/mL	Dissolve contents of one 0.5 mg (*Flolan* only) vial with 5 mL of sterile diluent for epoprostenol. Withdraw 3 mL and add to sufficient sterile diluent for epoprostenol to make a total of 100 mL.

Epoprostenol Reconstitution and Dilution Instructions

To make 100 mL of solution with final concentration (ng/mL) of:	Directions
5,000 ng/mL	Dissolve contents of one 0.5 mg (*Flolan* only) vial with 5 mL of sterile diluent for epoprostenol. Withdraw entire vial contents and add sufficient sterile diluent for epoprostenol to make a total of 100 mL.
10,000 ng/mL	Dissolve contents of two 0.5 mg (*Flolan* only) vials each with 5 mL of sterile diluent for epoprostenol. Withdraw entire vial contents and add sufficient sterile diluent for epoprostenol to make a total of 100 mL.
15,000 ng/mL[a]	Dissolve contents of one 1.5 mg (*Veletri* only) vial with 5 mL of sterile diluent for epoprostenol or sodium chloride 0.9% injection. Withdraw entire vial contents and add sufficient sterile diluent for epoprostenol to make a total of 100 mL.
30,000 ng/mL[a]	Dissolve contents of two 1.5 mg (*Veletri* only) vials each with 5 mL of sterile water for injection or sodium chloride 0.9% injection. Withdraw entire vial contents and add to a sufficient volume of the identical diluent to make a total of 100 mL.

[a] Higher concentrations may be required for patients who receive epoprostenol long-term.

Generally, 3,000 ng/mL and 10,000 ng/mL are satisfactory concentrations to deliver between 2 to 16 ng/kg/min in adults. Concentrations higher than 15,000 ng/mL may be required for patients who receive epoprostenol long-term.

The reconstitution and dilution instructions provide infusion delivery rates for doses up to 16 ng/kg/min based upon patient weight, drug delivery rate, and concentration of the solution of epoprostenol to be used. These instructions may be used to select the most appropriate concentration of epoprostenol that will result in an infusion rate between the minimum and maximum flow rates of the infusion pump, and which will allow the desired duration of infusion from a given reservoir volume. Higher infusion rates, and, therefore, more concentrated solutions may be necessary with long-term administration of epoprostenol.

Infusion Rates for Epoprostenol (*Flolan*) at a Concentration of 3,000 ng/mL

Patient weight (kg)	Dose or drug delivery rate (ng/kg/min)							
	2	4	6	8	10	12	14	16
	Infusion delivery rate (mL/h)							
10	—	—	1.2	1.6	2	2.4	2.8	3.2
20	—	1.6	2.4	3.2	4	4.8	5.6	6.4
30	1.2	2.4	3.6	4.8	6	7.2	8.4	9.6
40	1.6	3.2	4.8	6.4	8	9.6	11.2	12.8
50	2	4	6	8	10	12	14	16
60	2.4	4.8	7.2	9.6	12	14.4	16.8	19.2
70	2.8	5.6	8.4	11.2	14	16.8	19.6	22.4
80	3.2	6.4	9.6	12.8	16	19.2	22.4	25.6
90	3.6	7.2	10.8	14.4	18	21.6	25.2	28.8
100	4	8	12	16	20	24	28	32

EPOPROSTENOL SODIUM — INJECTION

Infusion Rates for Epoprostenol (*Flolan*) at a Concentration of 5,000 ng/mL

Patient weight (kg)	Dose or drug delivery rate (ng/kg/min)							
	2	4	6	8	10	12	14	16
	Infusion delivery rate (mL/h)							
10	—	—	—	1	1.2	1.4	1.7	1.9
20	—	1	1.4	1.9	2.4	2.9	3.4	3.8
30	—	1.4	2.2	2.9	3.6	4.3	5	5.8
40	1	1.9	2.9	3.8	4.8	5.8	6.7	7.7
50	1.2	2.4	3.6	4.8	6	7.2	8.4	9.6
60	1.4	2.9	4.3	5.8	7.2	8.6	10.1	11.5
70	1.7	3.4	5	6.7	8.4	10.1	11.8	13.4
80	1.9	3.8	5.8	7.7	9.6	11.5	13.4	15.4
90	2.2	4.3	6.5	8.6	10.8	13	15.1	17.3
100	2.4	4.8	7.2	9.6	12	14.4	16.8	19.2

Infusion Rates for Epoprostenol (*Flolan*) at a Concentration of 10,000 ng/mL

Patient weight (kg)	Dose or drug delivery rate (ng/kg/min)						
	4	6	8	10	12	14	16
	Infusion delivery rate (mL/h)						
20	—	—	1	1.2	1.4	1.7	1.9
30	—	1.1	1.4	1.8	2.2	2.5	2.9
40	1	1.4	1.9	2.4	2.9	3.4	3.8
50	1.2	1.8	2.4	3	3.6	4.2	4.8
60	1.4	2.2	2.9	3.6	4.3	5	5.8
70	1.7	2.5	3.4	4.2	5	5.9	6.7
80	1.9	2.9	3.8	4.8	5.8	6.7	7.7
90	2.2	3.2	4.3	5.4	6.5	7.6	8.6
100	2.4	3.6	4.8	6	7.2	8.4	9.6

Infusion Rates for Epoprostenol at a Concentration of 15,000 ng/mL

Patient weight (kg)	Dose or drug delivery rate (ng/kg/min)						
	4	6	8	10	12	14	16
	Infusion delivery rate (mL/h)						
20	—	—	—	—	1	1.1	1.3
30	—	—	1	1.2	1.4	1.7	1.9
40	—	1	1.3	1.6	1.9	2.2	2.6
50	—	1.2	1.6	2	2.4	2.8	3.2
60	1	1.4	1.9	2.4	2.9	3.4	3.8
70	1.1	1.7	2.2	2.8	3.4	3.9	4.5
80	1.3	1.9	2.6	3.2	3.8	4.5	5.1
90	1.4	2.2	2.9	3.6	4.3	5	5.8
100	1.6	2.4	3.2	4	4.8	5.6	6.4

Infusion Rates for Epoprostenol (*Veletri* only) at a Concentration of 30,000 ng/mL

Patient weight (kg)	Dose or drug delivery rate (ng/kg/min)					
	6	8	10	12	14	16
30	—	—	—	—	—	1
40	—	—	—	1	1.1	1.3
50	—	—	1	1.2	1.4	1.6
60	—	1	1.2	1.4	1.7	1.9
70	—	1.1	1.4	1.7	2	2.2
80	1	1.3	1.6	1.9	2.2	2.6
90	1.1	1.4	1.8	2.2	2.5	2.9
100	1.2	1.6	2	2.4	2.8	3.2

➤*Administration:* Epoprostenol, once prepared as directed, is administered by continuous IV infusion via a central venous catheter using an ambulatory infusion pump. During initiation of treatment, epoprostenol may be administered peripherally.

The ambulatory infusion pump used to administer epoprostenol should:

- Be small and lightweight.
- Be able to adjust infusion rates in 2 ng/kg/min increments.
- Have occlusion, end of infusion, and low battery alarms.
- Be accurate to ±6% of the programmed rate.
- Be positive pressure-driven (continuous or pulsatile) with intervals between pulses not exceeding 3 minutes at infusion rates used to deliver epoprostenol.

The reservoir should be made of polyvinyl chloride, polypropylene, or glass.

To avoid potential interruptions in drug delivery, the patient should have access to a backup infusion pump and IV infusion sets. A multilumen catheter should be considered if other IV therapies are routinely administered.

To facilitate extended use at ambient temperatures exceeding 25°C (77°F), a cold pouch with frozen gel packs was used in clinical trials. Any cold pouch used must be capable of maintaining the temperature of reconstituted epoprostenol between 2° and 8°C (35.6° and 46.4°F) for 12 hours.

During use, a single reservoir of reconstituted solution of epoprostenol can be administered at room temperature for a total duration of 8 hours, or it can be used with a cold pouch and administered up to 24 hours with the use of 2 frozen 6 oz gel packs in a cold pouch. When stored or in use, reconstituted epoprostenol must be insulated from temperatures greater than 25°C (77°F) and less than 0°C (32°F), and must not be exposed to direct sunlight.

➤*Admixture compatibility:* Epoprostenol is stable only when reconstituted with sterile diluent for epoprostenol or sodium chloride 0.9% injection (*Veletri*). Epoprostenol must not be reconstituted or mixed with any other parenteral medications or solutions prior to or during administration.

➤*Storage/Stability:* Store unopened vials of epoprostenol and sterile diluent at 15° to 25°C (59° to 77°F) and protected from light in the carton. Do not freeze.

Reconstituted solutions must be protected from light and must be refrigerated at 2° to 8°C (36° to 46°F) if not used immediately. Do not freeze reconstituted solutions. Discard any reconstituted solution that has been frozen. Discard any reconstituted solution if it has been refrigerated for more than 48 hours.

When administered at room temperature (15° to 25°C [59° to 77°F]), reconstituted solutions may be used for no longer than 8 hours. This 48-hour period allows the patient to reconstitute a 2-day supply (200 mL) of epoprostenol. Each 100 mL daily supply may be divided into 3 equal portions. Two of the portions are stored refrigerated at 2° to 8°C (36° to 46°F) until they are used.

Prior to infusion with the use of a cold pouch, solutions may be stored refrigerated at 2° to 8°C (36° to 46°F) for up to 24 hours. When a cold pouch is employed during the infusion, reconstituted solutions of epoprostenol may be used for no longer than 24 hours. Change the gel packs every 12 hours. Reconstituted solutions may be kept at 2° to 8°C (36° to 46°F), either in refrigerated storage or in a cold pouch or a combination of the two, for no more than 48 hours.

Veletri – Store the vials of *Veletri* at 20° to 25°C (68° to 77°F). Protect from light. Unopened vials of *Veletri* are stable until the date indicated on the package when stored at 20° to 25°C (68° to 77°F) and protected from light in the carton.

Prior to use, *Veletri* solutions reconstituted with 5 mL diluent must be protected from light and can be refrigerated at 2° to 8°C (36° to 46°F) for as long as 5 days or held at up to 25°C (77°F) for up to 48 hours prior to use. Do not freeze reconstituted solutions of *Veletri*. Discard any reconstituted solution that has been frozen. Discard any reconstituted solution if it has been refrigerated for more than 5 days, or if held at room temperature for more than 48 hours.

When the patient is then ready for the administration at room temperature, the dosing solutions may be prepared from the 5 mL solution as directed, by dilution with the same appropriate diluent to the needed concentration. This fully diluted solution can then be administered at room temperature for periods up to 24 hours. (If lower concentrations are chosen, the pump reservoirs should be changed every 12 hours when administered at room temperature.) Do not expose this solution to direct sunlight.

Actions

➤*Pharmacology:* Epoprostenol has 2 major pharmacological actions: Direct vasodilation of pulmonary and systemic arterial vascular beds, and inhibition of platelet aggregation. In animals, the vasodilatory effects reduce right and left ventricular afterload and increase cardiac output and stroke volume. The effect of epoprostenol on heart rate in animals varies with dose. At low doses, there is vagally mediated bradycardia, but at higher doses, epoprostenol causes reflex tachycardia in response to direct vasodilation and hypotension. No major effects on cardiac conduction have been observed. Additional pharmacologic effects of epoprostenol in animals include bronchodilation, inhibition of gastric acid secretion, and decreased gastric emptying.

➤*Pharmacokinetics:* Epoprostenol is rapidly hydrolyzed at neutral pH in blood and is also subject to enzymatic degradation. Animal studies using tritium-labelled epoprostenol have indicated a high clearance (93 mL/min/kg), small volume of distribution (357 mL/kg), and a short half-life (2.7 minutes). During infusions in animals, steady-state plasma concentrations of tritium-labelled epoprostenol were reached within 15 minutes and were proportional to infusion rates.

No available chemical assay is sufficiently sensitive and specific to assess the in vivo human pharmacokinetics of epoprostenol. The in vitro half-life of epoprostenol in human blood at 37°C (98.6°F), and pH 7.4 is approximately 6 minutes; the in vivo half-life of epoprostenol in humans is therefore expected to be no greater than 6 minutes. The in vitro pharmacologic half-life of epoprostenol in human plasma, based on inhibition of platelet aggregation, was similar for males (n = 954) and females (n = 1,024).

Tritium-labelled epoprostenol has been administered to humans in order to identify the metabolic products of epoprostenol. Epoprostenol is metabolized

EPOPROSTENOL SODIUM — INJECTION

to 2 primary metabolites: 6-keto-PGF$_{1\alpha}$ (formed by spontaneous degradation) and 6,15-diketo-13,14-dihydro-PGF$_{1\alpha}$ (enzymatically formed), both of which have pharmacological activity orders of magnitude less than epoprostenol in animal test systems. The recovery of radioactivity in urine and feces over a 1-week period was 82% and 4% of the administered dose, respectively. Fourteen additional minor metabolites have been isolated from urine, indicating that epoprostenol is extensively metabolized in humans.

Contraindications

A large study evaluating the effect of epoprostenol on survival in NYHA class III and IV patients with congestive heart failure (CHF) due to severe left ventricular systolic dysfunction was terminated after an interim analysis of 471 patients revealed a higher mortality in patients receiving epoprostenol plus conventional therapy than in those receiving conventional therapy alone. The long-term use of epoprostenol in patients with CHF due to severe left ventricular systolic dysfunction is therefore contraindicated.

Some patients with pulmonary hypertension have developed pulmonary edema during dose initiation, which may be associated with pulmonary veno-occlusive disease. Do not use epoprostenol long-term in patients who develop pulmonary edema during dose initiation.

Epoprostenol is also contraindicated in patients with known hypersensitivity to the drug or to structurally related compounds.

Warnings/Precautions

➤*Abrupt withdrawal:* Abrupt withdrawal (including interruptions in drug delivery) or sudden large reductions in dosage of epoprostenol may result in symptoms associated with rebound pulmonary hypertension, including dyspnea, dizziness, and asthenia. In clinical trials, one Class III PPH patient's death was judged attributable to the interruption of epoprostenol. Avoid abrupt withdrawal.

➤*Sepsis:* During long-term follow-up in the clinical trial of PPH, sepsis was reported at least once in 14% of patients and occurred at a rate of 0.32 infections/patient per year in patients treated with epoprostenol. This rate was higher than reported in patients using chronic indwelling central venous catheters to administer parenteral nutrition, but lower than reported in oncology patients using these catheters.

➤*Experienced clinicians:* Epoprostenol should be used only by clinicians experienced in the diagnosis and treatment of pulmonary hypertension. The diagnosis of PPH or PH/SSD should be carefully established.

Epoprostenol is a potent pulmonary and systemic vasodilator. Dose initiation with epoprostenol must be performed in a setting with adequate personnel and equipment for physiologic monitoring and emergency care. Dose initiation in controlled PPH clinical trials was performed during right heart catheterization. In uncontrolled PPH and controlled PH/SSD clinical trials, dose initiation was performed without cardiac catheterization. Carefully weigh the risk of cardiac catheterization in patients with pulmonary hypertension should be carefully weighed against the potential benefits. During dose initiation, asymptomatic increases in pulmonary artery pressure coincident with increases in cardiac output occurred rarely. In such cases, consider dose reduction, but such an increase does not imply that chronic treatment is contraindicated.

➤*Permanent IV catheter:* During chronic use, epoprostenol is delivered continuously on an ambulatory basis through a permanent indwelling central venous catheter. Unless contraindicated, administer anticoagulant therapy to PPH and PH/SSD patients receiving epoprostenol to reduce the risk of pulmonary thromboembolism or systemic embolism through a patent foramen ovale. In order to reduce the risk of infection, aseptic technique must be used in the reconstitution and administration of epoprostenol as well as in routine catheter care. Because epoprostenol is metabolized rapidly, even brief interruptions in the delivery of epoprostenol may result in symptoms associated with rebound pulmonary hypertension including dyspnea, dizziness, and asthenia. Base the decision to initiate therapy with epoprostenol upon the understanding that there is a high likelihood that IV therapy with epoprostenol will be needed for prolonged periods, possibly years, and carefully consider the patient's ability to accept and care for a permanent IV catheter and infusion pump.

➤*Pregnancy: Category B.* There are no adequate and well-controlled studies in pregnant women. Because animal reproduction studies are not always predictive of human response, use during pregnancy only if clearly needed.

➤*Lactation:* It is not known whether this drug is excreted in human milk. Because many drugs are excreted in human milk, exercise caution when epoprostenol is administered to a breast-feeding woman.

➤*Children:* Safety and efficacy in children have not been established.

➤*Elderly:* Clinical studies of epoprostenol in pulmonary hypertension did not include sufficient numbers of subjects aged 65 and over to determine whether they respond differently from younger patients. Other reported clinical experience has not identified differences in responses between the elderly and younger patients. In general, dose selection for an elderly patient should be cautious, usually starting at the low end of the dosing range, reflecting the greater frequency of decreased hepatic, renal, or cardiac function and of concomitant disease or other drug therapy.

➤*Monitoring:* Based on clinical trials, the acute hemodynamic response to epoprostenol did not correlate well with improvement in exercise tolerance or survival during chronic use of epoprostenol. Adjust dosage of epoprostenol during chronic use at the first sign of recurrence or worsening of symptoms attributable to pulmonary hypertension or the occurrence of adverse events associated with epoprostenol. Following dosage adjustments, closely monitor standing and supine blood pressure and heart rate for several hours.

Drug Interactions

Epoprostenol Drug Interactions			
Precipitant drug	Object drug[a]		Description
Epoprostenol	Diuretics Vasodilators	↑	Coadministration could cause additional reductions in blood pressure.
Epoprostenol	Antiplatelet agents Anticoagulants	↑	Coadministration can increase the risk of bleeding, although this did not occur in clinical trials.

[a] ↑ = object drug increased.

In a pharmacokinetic substudy in patients with congestive heart failure receiving furosemide or digoxin in whom therapy with epoprostenol was initiated, apparent oral clearance values for furosemide (n = 23) and digoxin (n = 30) were decreased by 13% and 15%, respectively, on the second day of therapy and had returned to baseline values by day 87. The change in furosemide clearance value is not likely to be clinically significant. However, patients on digoxin may show elevations of digoxin concentrations after initiation of therapy with epoprostenol, which may be clinically significant in patients prone to digoxin toxicity.

Adverse Reactions

➤*Adverse reactions during dose initiation and escalation:* During early clinical trials, epoprostenol was increased in 2 ng/kg/min increments until the patients developed symptomatic intolerance. The most common adverse events and the adverse events that limited further increases in dose were generally related to the major pharmacologic effect of epoprostenol, vasodilation. The most common dose-limiting adverse events (occurring in greater than or equal to 1% of patients) were nausea, vomiting, headache, hypotension, and flushing, but also include chest pain, anxiety, dizziness, bradycardia, dyspnea, abdominal pain, musculoskeletal pain, and tachycardia.

Epoprostenol Adverse Reactions During Dose Initiation and Escalation (≥ 1%)	
Adverse reactions	Epoprostenol (n = 391)
Abdominal pain	5%
Anxiety, nervousness, agitation	11%
Back pain	2%
Bradycardia	5%
Chest pain	11%
Dizziness	8%
Dyspnea	2%
Dyspepsia	1%
Flushing	58%
Headache	49%
Hypesthesia/Paresthesia	1%
Hypotension	16%
Musculoskeletal pain	3%
Nausea/Vomiting	32%
Sweating	1%
Tachycardia	1%

➤*Adverse reactions during chronic administration:* Interpretation of adverse events is complicated by the clinical features of PPH and PH/SSD, which are similar to some of the pharmacologic effects of epoprostenol (eg, dizziness, syncope). Adverse events probably related to the underlying disease include dyspnea, fatigue, chest pain, edema, hypoxia, right ventricular failure, and pallor. Several adverse events, on the other hand, can clearly be attributed to epoprostenol. These include headache, jaw pain, flushing, diarrhea, nausea and vomiting, flu-like symptoms, and anxiety/nervousness.

➤*Adverse reactions during chronic administration for PPH:* In an effort to separate the adverse effects of the drug from the adverse effects of the underlying disease, the table below lists adverse events that occurred at a rate at least 10% different in the 2 groups in controlled trials for PPH.

Adverse Reactions Regardless of Attribution Occurring in Patients with PPH with ≥ 10% Difference between Epoprostenol and Conventional Therapy Alone		
Adverse reaction	Epoprostenol (n = 52)	Conventional therapy (n = 54)
Occurrence more common with epoprostenol		
Cardiovascular		
Flushing	42%	2%
Tachycardia	35%	24%
CNS		
Anxiety/nervousness/tremor	21%	9%
Dizziness	83%	70%
Headache	83%	33%
Hypesthesia, hyperesthesia, paresthesia	12%	2%

EPOPROSTENOL SODIUM — INJECTION

Adverse Reactions Regardless of Attribution Occurring in Patients with PPH with ≥ 10% Difference between Epoprostenol and Conventional Therapy Alone		
Adverse reaction	Epoprostenol (n = 52)	Conventional therapy (n = 54)
GI		
Diarrhea	37%	6%
Nausea/vomiting	67%	48%
Musculoskeletal		
Jaw pain	54%	0%
Myalgia	44%	31%
Nonspecific musculoskeletal pain	35%	15%
Miscellaneous		
Chills/fever/sepsis/flu-like symptoms	25%	11%
Occurrence more common with conventional therapy		
Cardiovascular		
Heart failure	31%	52%
Shock	0%	13%
Syncope	13%	24%
Respiratory		
Hypoxia	25%	37%

Thrombocytopenia has been reported during uncontrolled clinical trials in patients receiving epoprostenol.

The following table lists additional adverse events reported in PPH patients receiving epoprostenol plus conventional therapy or conventional therapy alone during controlled clinical trials.

Adverse Reactions Regardless of Attribution Occurring in Patients with PPH with < 10% Difference Between Epoprostenol and Conventional Therapy Alone		
Adverse reaction	Epoprostenol (n = 52)	Conventional therapy (n = 54)
Cardiovascular		
Angina pectoris	19%	20%
Arrhythmia	27%	20%
Bradycardia	15%	9%
Cerebrovascular accident	4%	0%
Cyanosis	31%	39%
Hemorrhage	19%	11%
Hypotension	27%	31%
Myocardial ischemia	2%	6%
Pallor	21%	30%
Palpitation	63%	61%
Supraventricular tachycardia	8%	0%
CNS		
Confusion	6%	11%
Convulsion	4%	0%
Depression	37%	44%
Insomnia	4%	4%
Dermatologic		
Pruritus	4%	0%
Rash	10%	13%
Sweating	15%	20%
GI		
Abdominal pain	27%	31%
Anorexia	25%	30%
Ascites	12%	17%
Constipation	6%	2%
Metabolic		
Edema	60%	63%
Hypokalemia	6%	4%
Weight gain	6%	4%
Weight reduction	27%	24%
Musculoskeletal		
Arthralgia	6%	0%
Bone pain	0%	4%
Chest pain	67%	65%
Respiratory		
Cough increase	38%	46%
Dyspnea	90%	85%
Epistaxis	4%	2%
Pleural effusion	4%	2%
Special senses		
Amblyopia	8%	4%
Vision abnormality	4%	0%
Miscellaneous		
Asthenia	87%	81%

➤*Adverse events during chronic administration for PH/SSD:* In an effort to separate the adverse reactions of the drug from the adverse effects of the underlying disease, the table below lists adverse events that occurred at a rate at least 10% different in the 2 groups in controlled trial for patients with PH/SSD.

Adverse Reactions Regardless of Attribution Occurring in Patients with PH/SSD with ≥ 10% Difference between Epoprostenol and Conventional Therapy Alone		
Adverse reaction	Epoprostenol (n = 56)	Conventional therapy (n = 55)
Occurrence more common with epoprostenol		
Cardiovascular		
Flushing	23%	0%
Hypotension	13%	0%
CNS		
Headache	46%	5%
Dermatologic		
Eczema/rash/urticaria	25%	4%
Skin ulcer	39%	24%
GI		
Anorexia	66%	47%
Diarrhea	50%	5%
Nausea/vomiting	41%	16%
Musculoskeletal		
Jaw pain	75%	0%
Pain/neck pain/arthralgia	84%	65%
Occurrence more common with conventional therapy		
Cardiovascular		
Cyanosis	54%	80%
Pallor	32%	53%
Syncope	7%	20%
CNS		
Dizziness	59%	76%
GI		
Ascites	23%	33%
Esophageal reflux/gastritis	61%	73%
Metabolic		
Weight decrease	45%	56%
Respiratory		
Hypoxia	55%	65%

The following table lists additional adverse reactions reported in PH/SSD patients receiving epoprostenol plus conventional therapy or conventional therapy alone during controlled clinical trials.

Adverse Events Regardless of Attribution Occurring in Patients with PH/SSD with < 10% Difference Between Epoprostenol and Conventional Therapy Alone		
Adverse reaction[a]	Epoprostenol (n = 56)	Conventional therapy (n = 55)
Cardiovascular		
Heart failure/heart failure right	11%	13%
Myocardial infarction	4%	0%
Palpitation	63%	71%
Shock	5%	5%
Tachycardia	43%	42%
Vascular disorder	95%	89%
Vascular disorder peripheral	96%	100%
CNS		
Anxiety/hyperkinesia/nervousness/tremor	7%	5%
Depression/depression psychotic	13%	4%
Hyperesthesia/hypesthesia/paresthesia	5%	0%
Insomnia	9%	0%
Somnolence	4%	2%
Dermatologic		
Collagen disease	82%	84%
Pruritus	4%	2%
Sweat	41%	36%
GI		
Abdominal enlargement	4%	0%
Abdominal pain	14%	7%
Constipation	4%	2%
Flatulence	5%	4%
Hematologic/Lymphatic		
Thrombocytopenia	4%	0%
GU		
Hematuria	5%	0%
Urinary tract infection	7%	0%

EPOPROSTENOL SODIUM — INJECTION

Adverse Events Regardless of Attribution Occurring in Patients with PH/SSD with < 10% Difference Between Epoprostenol and Conventional Therapy Alone		
Adverse reaction[a]	Epoprostenol (n = 56)	Conventional therapy (n = 55)
Metabolic		
Edema/edema peripheral/edema genital	79%	87%
Hypercalcemia	48%	51%
Hyperkalemia	4%	0%
Thirst	0%	4%
Musculoskeletal		
Arthritis	52%	45%
Back pain	13%	5%
Chest pain	52%	45%
Leg cramps	5%	7%
Respiratory		
Cough increase	82%	82%
Dyspnea	100%	100%
Epistaxis	9%	7%
Pharyngitis	5%	2%
Pleural effusion	7%	0%
Pneumonia	5%	0%
Pneumothorax	4%	0%
Pulmonary edema	4%	2%
Respiratory disorder	7%	4%
Sinusitis	4%	4%
Miscellaneous		
Asthenia	100%	98%
Chills/fever/sepsis/flu-like symptoms	13%	11%
Hemorrhage/hemorrhage injection site/ hemorrhage rectal	11%	2%
Infection/rhinitis	21%	20%

[a] Adverse events which occurred in at least 2 patients in either treatment group.

Although the relationship to epoprostenol administration has not been established, pulmonary embolism has been reported in several patients taking epoprostenol, and there have been reports of hepatic failure.

➤*Adverse events attributable to the drug delivery system:* Chronic infusions of epoprostenol are delivered using a small, portable infusion pump through an indwelling central venous catheter. During controlled PPH trials of up to 12 weeks duration, up to 21% of patients reported a local infection and up to 13% of patients reported pain at the injection site. During a controlled PH/SSD trial of 12 weeks' duration, 14% of patients reported a local infection and 9% of patients reported pain at the injection site. During long-term follow-up in the clinical trial of PPH, sepsis was reported at least once in 14% of patients and occurred at a rate of 0.32 infections per patient per year in patients treated with epoprostenol. This rate was higher than reported in patients using chronic indwelling central venous catheters to administer parenteral nutrition, but lower than reported in oncology patients using these catheters. Malfunctions in the delivery system resulting in an inadvertent bolus of or a reduction in epoprostenol were associated with symptoms related to excess or insufficient epoprostenol, respectively (see Adverse events during chronic administration).

➤*Postmarketing:* In addition to adverse reactions reported from clinical trials, the following events have been identified during postapproval use of epoprostenol. Because they are reported voluntarily from a population of unknown size, estimates of frequency cannot be made. These events have been chosen for inclusion due to a combination of their seriousness, frequency of reporting, or potential causal connection to epoprostenol injection.

Endocrine – Hyperthyroidism.

Hematologic / Lymphatic – Anemia, hypersplenism, pancytopenia, splenomegaly.

Overdosage

➤*Symptoms:* Signs and symptoms of excessive doses of epoprostenol during clinical trials are the expected dose-limiting pharmacologic effects of epoprostenol, including flushing, headache, hypotension, tachycardia, nausea, vomiting, and diarrhea. Treatment will ordinarily require dose reduction of epoprostenol.

➤*Treatment:* One patient with secondary pulmonary hypertension accidentally received 50 mL of an unspecified concentration of epoprostenol. The patient vomited and became unconscious with an initially unrecordable blood pressure. Epoprostenol was discontinued and the patient regained consciousness within seconds. In clinical practice, fatal occurrences of hypoxemia, hypotension, and respiratory arrest have been reported following overdosage of epoprostenol.

Single IV doses of epoprostenol at 10 and 50 mg/kg (2,703 and 27,027 times the recommended acute phase human dose based on body surface area) were lethal to mice and rats, respectively. Symptoms of acute toxicity were hypoactivity, ataxia, loss of righting reflex, and deep slow breathing, and hypothermia.

Patient Information

Patients receiving epoprostenol sodium should receive the following information: Epoprostenol sodium must be reconstituted only with sterile diluent for epoprostenol sodium. Epoprostenol sodium is infused continuously through a permanent indwelling central venous catheter via a small, portable infusion pump. Thus, therapy with epoprostenol sodium requires commitment by the patient to drug reconstitution, drug administration, and care of the permanent central venous catheter. Sterile technique must be adhered to in preparing the drug and in the care of the catheter, and even brief interruptions in the delivery of epoprostenol sodium may result in rapid symptomatic deterioration. A patient's decision to receive epoprostenol sodium should be based upon the understanding that there is a high likelihood that therapy with epoprostenol sodium will be needed for prolonged periods, possibly years. The patient's ability to accept and care for a permanent intravenous catheter and infusion pump should also be carefully considered.

TREPROSTINIL

Rx	**Remodulin** (United Therapeutics)	**Injection, solution:** 1 mg/mL	As treprostinil sodium. Sodium chloride 5.3 mg/mL. In 20 mL multiuse vials.
		2.5 mg/mL	As treprostinil sodium. Sodium chloride 5.3 mg/mL. In 20 mL multiuse vials.
		5 mg/mL	As treprostinil sodium. Sodium chloride 5.3 mg/mL. In 20 mL multiuse vials.
		10 mg/mL	As treprostinil sodium. Sodium chloride 4 mg/mL. In 20 mL multiuse vials.
Rx	**Tyvaso** (United Therapeutics)	**Solution; inhalation:** 0.6 mg/mL	In 2.9 mL ampules.

TREPROSTINIL SODIUM — INJECTION

Indications

➤*Pulmonary arterial hypertension:* For the treatment of pulmonary arterial hypertension (PAH) in patients with New York Heart Association (NYHA) class II to IV symptoms to diminish symptoms associated with exercise.

➤*Transition from epoprostenol:* To diminish the rate of clinical deterioration in patients requiring transition from epoprostenol.

Administration and Dosage

➤*General dosing considerations:* Treprostinil can be administered as supplied or diluted for intravenous (IV) infusion with sterile water for injection, sodium chloride 0.9% injection, or epoprostenol sterile diluent for injection prior to administration.

The goal of chronic dosage adjustments is to establish a dose at which PAH symptoms are improved, while minimizing excessive pharmacologic effects of treprostinil (eg, anxiety, emesis, headache, infusion-site pain or reaction, nausea, restlessness).

The transition of epoprostenol to treprostinil should take place in a hospital with constant observation of response (eg, signs and symptoms of disease progression, walk distance).

Avoid abrupt cessation of therapy. See Discontinuation of Therapy.

➤*Adults:*

Pulmonary arterial hypertension –

Initial dosage: The infusion rate is initiated at 1.25 ng/kg/min. If this initial dose cannot be tolerated because of systemic effects, the infusion rate should be reduced to 0.625 ng/kg/min.

Dosage adjustment: The infusion rate should be increased in increments of no more than 1.25 ng/kg/min per week for the first 4 weeks and then no more than 2.5 ng/kg/min per week for the remaining duration of infusion, depending on clinical response. Dosage adjustments may be undertaken more often if tolerated. There is little experience with doses greater than 40 ng/kg/min. Restarting a treprostinil infusion within a few hours after an interruption can be done using the same dose rate. Interruptions for longer periods may require the dose of treprostinil to be retitrated.

Discontinuation of therapy: Abrupt cessation of infusion should be avoided. Abrupt withdrawal or sudden large reductions in dosage of treprostinil may result in worsening of PAH symptoms and should be avoided.

Transition from epoprostenol to treprostinil: Treprostinil should be initiated at a recommended dose of 10% of the current epoprostenol dose and then escalated as the epoprostenol dose is decreased.

Patients are individually titrated to a dose that allows transition from epoprostenol therapy to treprostinil while balancing prostacylin-limiting adverse reactions. Increases in the patient's symptoms of PAH should first be treated with increases in the dose of treprostinil. Adverse reactions normally associated with prostacylin and prostacylin analogs are to be first treated by decreasing the dose of epoprostenol.

TREPROSTINIL SODIUM — INJECTION

Epoprostenol to Treprostinil Transition: Recommended Dose Changes		
Step	Treprostinil dose	Epoprostenol dose
1	10% starting epoprostenol dose	Unchanged
2	30% starting epoprostenol dose	80% starting epoprostenol dose
3	50% starting epoprostenol dose	60% starting epoprostenol dose
4	70% starting epoprostenol dose	40% starting epoprostenol dose
5	90% starting epoprostenol dose	20% starting epoprostenol dose
6	110% starting epoprostenol dose	5% starting epoprostenol dose
7	110% starting epoprostenol dose + additional 5% to 10% increments as needed	0%

➤*Children:* Safety and efficacy in children have not been established. In general, use caution with dose selection.

➤*Elderly:* Dose selection for an elderly patient should be cautious.

➤*Renal function impairment:* Use with caution.

➤*Hepatic function impairment:* In patients with mild or moderate hepatic impairment, the initial dose of treprostinil should be decreased to 0.625 ng/kg/min ideal body weight and should be increased cautiously. Treprostinil has not been studied in patients with severe hepatic impairment.

➤*Administration:* Treprostinil is for subcutaneous or IV use only. Treprostinil is administered by continuous infusion. Treprostinil is preferably infused subcutaneously but can be administered by a central IV line if the subcutaneous route is not tolerated because of severe site pain or reaction. To avoid potential interruptions in drug delivery, the patient must have immediate access to a backup infusion pump and subcutaneous infusion sets.

Subcutaneous infusion – Treprostinil is administered subcutaneously by continuous infusion, via a self-inserted subcutaneous catheter, using an infusion pump designed for subcutaneous drug delivery.

For subcutaneous infusion, treprostinil is delivered without further dilution at a calculated subcutaneous infusion rate (mL/h) based on a patient's dose (ng/kg/min), weight (kg), and the vial strength (mg/mL) of treprostinil being used. The subcutaneous infusion rate is calculated using the following formula:

$$\text{Subcutaneous infusion rate (mL/h)} = \frac{\text{dose (ng/kg/min)} \times \text{weight (kg)} \times 0.00006}{\text{treprostinil vial strength (mg/mL)}}$$

In the above formula, conversion factor of 0.00006 = 60 min/h × 0.000001 mg/ng.

Intravenous infusion – Treprostinil must be diluted with either sterile water for injection, sodium chloride 0.9% injection, or epoprostenol sterile diluent for injection and is administered IV by continuous infusion via a surgically placed, indwelling, central venous catheter, using an infusion pump designed for IV drug delivery. If clinically necessary, a temporary peripheral IV cannula, preferably placed in a large vein, may be used for short-term administration of treprostinil. Use of a peripheral IV infusion for more than a few hours may be associated with an increased risk of thrombophlebitis. To avoid potential interruptions in drug delivery, the patient must have immediate access to a backup infusion pump and infusion sets.

When using an appropriate infusion pump and reservoir, a predetermined IV infusion rate should first be selected to allow for a desired infusion period length of up to 48 hours between system changeovers. Typical IV infusion system reservoirs have volumes of 50 or 100 mL. With this selected IV infusion rate (mL/h) and the patient's dose (ng/kg/min) and weight (kg), the diluted IV treprostinil concentration (mg/mL) can be calculated using the following formula:

Step 1:

$$\text{Diluted IV treprostinil concentration (mg/mL)} = \frac{\text{dose (ng/kg/min)} \times \text{weight (kg)} \times 0.00006}{\text{IV infusion rate (mL/h)}}$$

The amount of treprostinil needed to make the required diluted IV treprostinil concentration for the given reservoir size can then be calculated using the following formula:

Step 2:

$$\text{Amount of treprostinil (mL)} = \frac{\text{diluted IV treprostinil concentration (mg/mL)}}{\text{treprostinil vial strength (mg/mL)}} \times \text{total volume of diluted treprostinil in reservoir (mL)}$$

The calculated amount of treprostinil is then added to the reservoir along with the sufficient volume of diluent (sterile water for injection, sodium chloride 0.9% injection, or epoprostenol sterile diluent for injection) to achieve the desired total volume in the reservoir.

➤*Storage/Stability:* Unopened vials of treprostinil are stable until the date indicated when stored at 15° to 25°C (59° to 77°F). Store at 25°C (77°F); excursions are permitted to 15° to 30°C (59° to 86°F).

During use, a single reservoir (syringe) of undiluted treprostinil can be administered up to 72 hours at 37°C (98.6°F). Diluted treprostinil can be administered up to 48 hours at 37°C (98.6°F) when diluted to concentrations as low as 0.004 mg/mL in sterile water for injection, or sodium chloride 0.9% injection, or epoprostenol sterile diluent for injection. A single vial of treprostinil should be used for no more than 30 days after the initial introduction into the vial.

Actions

➤*Pharmacology:* The major pharmacologic actions of treprostinil are direct vasodilation of pulmonary and systemic arterial vascular beds and inhibition of platelet aggregation.

➤*Pharmacokinetics:*

Absorption – Treprostinil is relatively rapidly and completely absorbed after subcutaneous infusion, with an absolute bioavailability approximating 100%. Steady-state concentrations occurred in approximately 10 hours. Concentrations in patients treated with an average dose of 9.3 ng/kg/min were approximately 2 mcg/L.

The pharmacokinetics of continuous subcutaneous treprostinil are linear over the dose range of 1.25 to 125 ng/kg/min (corresponding to plasma concentrations of about 15 to 18,250 pg/mL) and can be described by a 2-compartment model.

Subcutaneous and IV administration of treprostinil demonstrated bioequivalence at steady state at a dose of 10 ng/kg/min.

Distribution – The volume of distribution of the drug in the central compartment is approximately 14 L per 70 kg ideal body weight. Treprostinil at in vitro concentrations ranging from 330 to 10,000 mcg/L was 91% bound to human plasma protein.

Metabolism – Treprostinil is substantially metabolized by the liver, but the precise enzymes responsible are unknown. Five metabolites have been described (HU1 through HU5). The biological activity and metabolic fate of these metabolites are unknown. The chemical structure of HU1 is unknown. HU5 is the glucuronide conjugate of treprostinil. The other metabolites are formed by oxidation of the 3-hydroxyoctyl side chain (HU2) and subsequent additional oxidation (HU3) or dehydration (HU4). Based on the results of in vitro human hepatic cytochrome P450 studies, treprostinil does not inhibit CYP1A2, 2C9, 2C19, 2D6, 2E1, or 3A. Whether treprostinil induces these enzymes has not been studied.

Excretion – The elimination of treprostinil is biphasic, with a terminal half-life of approximately 4 hours. Approximately 79% of an administered dose is excreted in the urine as unchanged drug (4%) and as the identified metabolites (64%). Approximately 13% of a dose is excreted in the feces. Systemic clearance is approximately 30 L/h for a 70 kg ideal body weight person.

Special populations –

Hepatic function impairment: In patients with portopulmonary hypertension and mild (n = 4) or moderate (n = 5) hepatic impairment, treprostinil at a subcutaneous dose of 10 ng/kg/min for 150 minutes had a maximal drug concentration that was increased 2- and 4-fold, respectively, and an area under the curve ($AUC_{0-\infty}$) that was increased 3- and 5-fold, respectively, compared with healthy subjects. Clearance in patients with hepatic impairment was reduced up to 80% compared with healthy adults.

See Administration and Dosage for more information.

Contraindications

None known.

Warnings/Precautions

➤*Intravenous administration adverse reactions:* Chronic IV infusions of treprostinil are delivered using an indwelling central venous catheter. This route is associated with the risk of bloodstream infections and sepsis, which may be fatal.

In an open-label study of IV treprostinil (n = 47), there were 7 catheter-related line infections during approximately 35 patient-years, or about 1 bloodstream infection event per 5 years of use. A Centers for Disease Control and Prevention survey of 7 sites that used IV treprostinil for the treatment of PAH found approximately 1 bloodstream infection (defined as any positive blood culture) event per 3 years of use.

➤*Administration:* Treprostinil should be used only by health care providers experienced in the diagnosis and treatment of PAH.

Treprostinil is a potent pulmonary and systemic vasodilator. Initiation of treprostinil must be performed in a setting with adequate personnel and equipment for physiological monitoring and emergency care. Therapy with treprostinil may be used for prolonged periods; carefully consider the patient's ability to administer injections and care for an infusion system.

➤*Dosage adjustments/withdrawal:* See Administration and Dosage for more information.

See Administration and Dosage for more information.

➤*Renal/Hepatic function impairment:* Use caution in patients with hepatic or renal impairment. See also Pharmacokinetics.

➤*Pregnancy: Category B*. Use treprostinil during pregnancy only if clearly needed.

In pregnant rabbits, effects of continuous, subcutaneous infusions of treprostinil during organogenesis were limited to an increased incidence of fetal skeletal variations (bilateral full rib or right rudimentary rib on lumbar 1) associated with maternal toxicity (reduction in body weight and food consumption) at an infusion rate of 150 ng/kg/min (about 41 times the starting human rate of infusion, on a ng/m^2 basis, and 5 times the average rate used in clinical trials).

➤*Lactation:* It is not known whether treprostinil is excreted in human milk or absorbed systemically after ingestion. Because many drugs are excreted in human milk, exercise caution when treprostinil is administered to a breast-feeding woman.

TREPROSTINIL SODIUM — INJECTION

➤*Children:* Safety and efficacy in children have not been established. In general, use caution in dose selection.

➤*Elderly:* In general, dose selection for an elderly patient should be cautious, reflecting the greater frequency of decreased hepatic, renal, or cardiac function, and of concomitant disease or other drug therapy.

Drug Interactions

➤*Anticoagulants:* Because treprostinil inhibits platelet aggregation, there is a potential for increased risk of bleeding, particularly among patients maintained on anticoagulants.

➤*Antihypertensive agents, diuretics, or vasodilators:* Reduction in blood pressure caused by treprostinil may be exacerbated by drugs that, by themselves, alter blood pressure, such as antihypertensive agents, diuretics, or vasodilators.

Adverse Reactions

➤*Subcutaneous infusion:* Patients receiving treprostinil as a subcutaneous infusion reported a wide range of adverse reactions, many potentially related to the underlying disease (eg, chest pain, dyspnea, fatigue, pallor, right ventricular heart failure). During clinical trials with subcutaneous infusion of treprostinil, infusion-site pain and reaction were the most common adverse reactions among those treated with treprostinil. Infusion-site reaction was defined as any local adverse reaction other than pain or bleeding/bruising at the infusion site and included symptoms such as erythema, induration, or rash. Infusion-site reactions were sometimes severe and led to discontinuation of treatment.

Treprostinil Subcutaneous Infusion-Site Adverse Reactions

	Reaction		Pain	
Adverse reactions	Treprostinil	Placebo	Treprostinil	Placebo
Severe	38%	1%	39%	2%
Requiring narcotics[a]	NA[b]	NA[b]	32%	1%
Leading to discontinuation	3%	0%	7%	0%

[a] Based on prescriptions for narcotics, not actual use.
[b] NA = not applicable; medications used to treat infusion-site pain were not distinguished from those used to treat site reactions.

Chronic subcutaneous administration –

Treprostinil (Subcutaneous) Adverse Reactions in Patients With PAH[a] (≥ 3%)

Adverse reactions	Treprostinil (n = 236)	Placebo (n = 233)
CNS		
Dizziness	9%	8%
Headache	27%	23%
Dermatologic		
Pruritus	8%	6%
Rash	14%	11%
GI		
Diarrhea	25%	16%
Nausea	22%	18%
Miscellaneous		
Edema	9%	3%
Hypotension	4%	2%
Infusion-site pain	85%	27%
Infusion-site reaction	83%	27%
Jaw pain	13%	5%
Vasodilation	11%	5%

[a] PAH = pulmonary arterial hypertension.

➤*Drug-delivery system adverse reactions:* In controlled studies of treprostinil administered subcutaneously, there were no reports of infection related to the drug-delivery system. There were 187 infusion system complications reported in 28% of patients (23% treprostinil, 33% placebo); 173 (93%) were pump related and 14 (7%) related to the infusion set. Eight of these patients (4 treprostinil, 4 placebo) reported nonserious adverse reactions resulting from infusion system complications. Adverse reactions resulting from problems with the delivery systems were typically related to either symptoms of excess treprostinil (eg, nausea) or return of PAH symptoms (eg, dyspnea). These reactions were generally resolved by correcting the delivery system pump or infusion set problem (eg, replacing the syringe or battery, reprogramming the pump, straightening a crimped infusion line). Adverse reactions resulting from problems with the delivery system did not lead to clinical instability or rapid deterioration. In addition to these adverse reactions due to the drug delivery system during subcutaneous administration, the following adverse reactions may be attributable to the IV mode of infusion including arm swelling, hematoma, pain, and paresthesias.

➤*Subcutaneous or IV infusion adverse reactions:* Other adverse reactions included diarrhea, edema, jaw pain, nausea, and vasodilation. These are generally considered to be related to the pharmacologic effects of treprostinil, whether administered subcutaneously or IV.

➤*Postmarketing:*

Cardiovascular – Thrombophlebitis associated with peripheral IV infusion.

Dermatologic – Cellulitis and generalized rashes, sometimes macular and papular in nature.

Hematologic – Thrombocytopenia.

Musculoskeletal – Bone pain.

Overdosage

➤*Symptoms:* Signs and symptoms of overdose with treprostinil during clinical trials are extensions of its dose-limiting pharmacologic effects and include diarrhea, flushing, headache, hypotension, nausea, and vomiting. In controlled clinical trials, 7 patients received some level of overdose; in open-label follow-on treatment, 7 additional patients received an overdose. These occurrences resulted from accidental bolus administration of treprostinil, errors in pump programmed rate of administration, and prescription of an incorrect dose. In only 2 cases did excess delivery of treprostinil produce a reaction of substantial hemodynamic concern (eg, hypotension, near-syncope).

One child was accidentally administered treprostinil 7.5 mg via a central venous catheter. Symptoms included flushing, headache, hypotension, nausea, seizure-like activity with loss of consciousness lasting several minutes, and vomiting. The patient subsequently recovered.

➤*Treatment:* Most reactions were self-limiting and resolved with reduction or withholding of treprostinil.

Patient Information

Treprostinil is infused continuously through a subcutaneous or surgically placed, indwelling, central venous catheter, via an infusion pump. Therapy with treprostinil will be needed for prolonged periods, possibly years. Carefully consider the patient's ability to accept and care for a catheter and to use an infusion pump.

Advise patients that to reduce the risk of infection aseptic technique must be used in the preparation and administration of treprostinil.

Inform patients that subsequent disease management may require the initiation of an alternative IV prostacyclin therapy, epoprostenol.

TREPROSTINIL — INHALATION

Indications

➤*Pulmonary arterial hypertension:* To increase walk distance in patients with World Health Organization (WHO) group I pulmonary arterial hypertension and New York Heart Association (NYHA) class III symptoms. The effects diminish over the minimum recommended dosing interval of 4 hours; treatment timing can be adjusted for planned activities.

Administration and Dosage

➤*Adults:*

Pulmonary arterial hypertension –

Maximum dose: 9 breaths per treatment session, 4 times daily.

Initial dosage: Therapy should begin with 3 breaths of treprostinil (18 mcg of treprostinil) per treatment session, 4 times daily. If 3 breaths are not tolerated, reduce to 1 or 2 breaths and subsequently increase to 3 breaths, as tolerated.

Dosage titration: Dosage should be increased by an additional 3 breaths at approximately 1- to 2-week intervals, if tolerated, until the target dose of 9 breaths (54 mcg of treprostinil) is reached per treatment session, 4 times daily. If adverse effects preclude titration to target dose, treprostinil should be continued at the highest tolerated dose.

Maintenance dosage: 9 breaths (54 mcg of treprostinil) per treatment session, 4 times daily.

If a scheduled treatment session is missed or interrupted, therapy should be resumed as soon as possible at the usual dose.

➤*Preparation for administration:* Treprostinil is intended for oral inhalation using the treprostinil inhalation system, which consists of the *Optineb*-ir model ON-100/7 (an ultrasonic, pulsed-delivery device) and its accessories. Treprostinil must be used only with the treprostinil inhalation system. Patients should follow the instructions for use for operation of the treprostinil inhalation system and for daily cleaning of the device components after the last treatment session of the day. To avoid potential interruptions in drug delivery because of equipment malfunction, patients should have access to a back-up *Optineb*-ir device.

➤*Administration:* One ampule of treprostinil contains a sufficient volume of medication for all 4 treatment sessions in a single day. Prior to the first treatment session, the patient should twist the top off a single treprostinil ampule and squeeze the entire contents into the medicine cup. Between each of the 4 daily treatment sessions, the device should be capped and stored upright with the remaining medication inside. At the end of each day, the medicine cup and any remaining medication must be discarded. The device must be cleaned each day according to the instructions for use.

Treprostinil is dosed in 4 separate, equally spaced treatment sessions per day, during waking hours. The treatment sessions should be approximately 4 hours apart.

TREPROSTINIL — INHALATION

Avoid skin or eye contact with treprostinil solution. Treprostinil solution should not be orally ingested.

➤*Admixture compatibility:* Do not mix treprostinil with other medications in the *Optineb*-ir device. Compatibility of treprostinil with other medications has not been studied.

➤*Storage/Stability:* The ampules should be stored at 25°C (77°F), with excursions permitted between 15° and 30°C (59° and 86°F). After opening the foil pouch, treprostinil should be used within 7 days. Treprostinil is light-sensitive; store unopened ampules in foil pouch. After a treprostinil ampule is opened and transferred to the medicine cup, the solution should remain in the device for no more than 24 hours. Discard any remaining solution at the end of the day.

Actions

➤*Pharmacology:* Treprostinil is a prostacyclin analogue. The major pharmacologic actions of treprostinil are direct vasodilation of pulmonary and systemic arterial vascular beds and inhibition of platelet aggregation.

Pharmacodynamics – In a clinical trial of 240 healthy volunteers, single doses of treprostinil 54 mcg (the target maintenance dose per session) and 84 mcg (supratherapeutic inhalation dose) prolonged the corrected QTc interval by approximately 10 ms. The QTc effect dissipated rapidly as the concentration of treprostinil decreased.

➤*Pharmacokinetics:*

Absorption/Distribution – In a 3-period crossover study, the bioavailability of 2 single doses of treprostinil (18 and 36 mcg) was compared with that of intravenous treprostinil in 18 healthy volunteers. Mean estimates of the 8 absolute systemic bioavailability of treprostinil after inhalation were approximately 64% (18 mcg) and 72% (36 mcg).

Treprostinil plasma exposure data were obtained from 2 studies at the target maintenance dose of 54 mcg. The mean C_{max} at the target dose was 0.91 and 1.32 ng/mL, with corresponding mean time to reach maximum concentration of 0.25 and 0.12 h, respectively. The mean AUC for the 54 mcg dose was 0.81 and 0.97 h•ng/mL, respectively.

Following parenteral infusion, the apparent steady state volume of distribution at steady state of treprostinil is approximately 14 L per 70 kg ideal body weight.

In vitro treprostinil is 91% bound to human plasma proteins over the 330 to 10,000 mcg/L concentration range.

Metabolism/Excretion – Of subcutaneously administered treprostinil, only 4% is excreted unchanged in urine. Treprostinil is substantially metabolized by the liver, primarily by CYP2C8. Metabolites are excreted in urine (79%) and feces (13%) over 10 days. Five apparently inactive metabolites were detected in the urine, each accounting for 10% to 15% of the dose administered. Four of the metabolites are products of oxidation of the 3-hydroxyloctyl side chain and 1 is a glucuroconjugated derivative (treprostinil glucuronide).

The elimination of treprostinil (following subcutaneous administration of treprostinil) is biphasic, with a terminal elimination half-life of approximately 4 hours using a 2-compartment model.

Special populations –

Renal function impairment: No studies have been performed in patients with renal insufficiency; therefore, because treprostinil and its metabolites are excreted mainly through the urinary route, there is the potential for an increase in both parent drug and its metabolites and an increase in systemic exposure.

Hepatic function impairment: Plasma clearance of treprostinil, delivered subcutaneously, was reduced up to 80% in subjects presenting with mild to moderate hepatic insufficiency. Treprostinil has not been studied in patients with severe hepatic insufficiency.

Contraindications

None known.

Warnings/Precautions

➤*Pulmonary disease/infections:* The safety and efficacy of treprostinil have not been established in patients with significant underlying lung disease (eg, asthma or chronic obstructive pulmonary disease). Carefully monitor patients with acute pulmonary infections to detect any worsening of lung disease and loss of drug effect.

➤*Hypotension:* Treprostinil is a pulmonary and systemic vasodilator. In patients with low systemic arterial pressure, treatment with treprostinil may produce symptomatic hypotension.

➤*Bleeding:* Because treprostinil inhibits platelet aggregation, there may be an increased risk of bleeding, particularly among patients receiving anticoagulant therapy.

➤*Renal function impairment:* Titrate slowly in patients with renal insufficiency because such patients will likely be exposed to greater systemic concentrations relative to patients with healthy renal function.

See Actions for more information.

➤*Hepatic function impairment:* Titrate slowly in patients with hepatic insufficiency, because such patients will likely be exposed to greater systemic concentrations relative to patients with healthy renal function.

See Actions for more information.

➤*Pregnancy:* Category B. There are no adequate and well-controlled studies with treprostinil in pregnant women. Animal reproduction studies have not been conducted with treprostinil administered by the inhalation route. However, studies in pregnant rabbits using continuous subcutaneous infusions of treprostinil at infusion rates higher than the recommended human subcutaneous infusion rate resulted in an increased incidence of fetal skeletal variations associated with maternal toxicity.

It is not known if treprostinil crosses the human placenta. The molecular weight (about 412) is low enough that passage to the fetus should be expected.

Animal reproduction studies are not always predictive of human response; treprostinil should be used during pregnancy only if clearly needed.

In pregnant rats, continuous subcutaneous infusions of treprostinil during organogenesis and late gestational development, at rates as high as treprostinil 900 ng/kg/min (about 117 times the recommended starting human subcutaneous infusion rate and about 16 times the average rate achieved in clinical trials, on a ng/m² basis), resulted in no evidence of harm to the fetus. In pregnant rabbits, effects of continuous subcutaneous infusions of treprostinil during organogenesis were limited to an increased incidence of fetal skeletal variations (bilateral full rib or right rudimentary rib on lumbar vertebra 1) associated with maternal toxicity (reduction in body weight and food consumption) at an infusion rate of treprostinil 150 ng/kg/min (about 41 times the starting human subcutaneous infusion rate and 5 times the average rate achieved in clinical trials, on a ng/m² basis).

➤*Lactation:* It is not known whether treprostinil is excreted in human milk.

The molecular weight (about 412) and method of administration (continuous subcutaneous infusion) suggest that the drug will be excreted into breast milk. Because many drugs are excreted in human milk, exercise caution when treprostinil is administered to breast-feeding women.

➤*Children:* Safety and effectiveness in children have not been established. Clinical studies of treprostinil did not include patients younger than 18 years of age to determine whether they respond differently from older patients.

➤*Elderly:* Dose selection for an elderly patient should be cautious, reflecting the greater frequency of hepatic, renal, or cardiac dysfunction, and of concomitant diseases or other drug therapy.

➤*Monitoring:* Carefully monitor patients with acute pulmonary infections to detect any worsening of lung disease and loss of drug effect.

Drug Interactions

Treprostinil Drug Interactions

Precipitant drug	Object drug[a]		Description
Antihypertensive agents (eg, ACE-[b] inhibitors [eg, captopril])	Treprostinil	⬆	Risk of symptomatic hypotension may be increased. Coadminister with caution. Monitor blood pressure. If an interaction is suspected, dosage adjustments or supportive treatment may be needed.
Treprostinil	Antihypertensive agents (eg, ACE inhibitors [eg, captopril])		
CYP2C8 inducers (eg, rifampin)	Treprostinil	⬇	Studies using an oral formulation of treprostinil indicate that treprostinil exposure may be decreased, decreasing the efficacy. Monitor the response of the patient and adjust the treprostinil treatment timing based on planned activity.
CYP2C8 inhibitors (eg, gemfibrozil)	Treprostinil	⬇	Studies using an oral formulation of treprostinil indicate that treprostinil exposure may be increased, increasing the pharmacologic effects and risk of adverse reactions. Monitor the response of the patient, and adjust the treprostinil treatment timing based on planned activity.
Diuretics (eg, chlorothiazide)	Treprostinil	⬆	Risk of symptomatic hypotension may be increased. Coadminister with caution. Monitor blood pressure. If an interaction is suspected, dosage adjustments or supportive treatment may be needed.
Treprostinil	Diuretics (eg, chlorothiazide)		
Vasodilators (eg, epoprostenol, hydralazine)	Treprostinil	⬆	Risk of symptomatic hypotension may be increased. Coadminister with caution. Monitor blood pressure. If an interaction is suspected, dosage adjustments or supportive treatment may be needed.
Treprostinil	Vasodilators (eg, epoprostenol, hydralazine)		

TREPROSTINIL — INHALATION

Treprostinil Drug Interactions

Precipitant drug	Object drug[a]		Description
Treprostinil	Anticoagulants (eg, heparin, warfarin)	↑	Treprostinil does not affect the pharmacokinetics or pharmacodynamics of warfarin. However, treprostinil inhibits platelet aggregation, which may increase the risk of bleeding, especially in patients maintained on anticoagulants. Use with caution in patients receiving anticoagulants. Monitor anticoagulant parameters and adjust the dose as needed.

[a] ↑ = object drug increased; ↓ = object drug decreased.
[b] ACE = angiotensin-converting enzyme.

Adverse Reactions

➤*Common adverse reactions:* In a 12-week, placebo-controlled study (TRIUMPH I) of 235 patients with pulmonary arterial hypertension (WHO group I and nearly all NYHA functional class III), the most commonly reported adverse reactions on treprostinil included cough and throat irritation; flushing; GI effects; headache; muscle, jaw, or bone pain; and syncope.

Treprostinil Adverse Reactions (≥ 4%)[a]

Adverse reaction	Treprostinil (n = 115)	Placebo (n = 120)
CNS		
Flushing	15%	< 1%
Headache	41%	23%
Respiratory		
Cough	54%	29%
Throat irritation/ pharyngolaryngeal pain	25%	14%
Miscellaneous		
Nausea	19%	11%
Syncope	6%	< 1%

[a] More than 3% greater than placebo.

➤*Respiratory:* Adverse reactions in the treated group during the double-blind and open-label phase reflecting irritation to the respiratory tract included cough, epistaxis, hemoptysis, pharyngeal pain, throat irritation, and wheezing.

➤*Serious adverse reactions:* Serious adverse events during the open-label portion of the study included pneumonia in 8 subjects. There were 3 serious episodes of hemoptysis (1 fatal) noted during the open-label experience.

Overdosage

➤*Symptoms:* Diarrhea, flushing, headache, hypotension, nausea, vomiting.

➤*Treatment:* Provide general supportive care until the symptoms of overdose have resolved.

Patient Information

Properly train patients in the administration process for treprostinil, including dosing, and *Optineb*-ir device setup, operation, cleaning, and maintenance, according to the instructions for use.

To avoid potential interruptions in drug delivery because of equipment malfunction, ensure that patients have access to a back-up *Optineb*-ir device.

In the event that a scheduled treatment session is missed or interrupted, resume therapy as soon as possible.

Advise patients to avoid skin or eye contact with treprostinil. If treprostinil comes in contact with the skin or eyes, instruct patients to rinse immediately with water.

PERIPHERAL VASODILATOR COMBINATIONS

Rx	**Lipo-Nicin/100 mg** (ICN Pharm)	**Tablets:** 100 mg niacin, 75 mg niacinamide, 150 mg vitamin C, 25 mg B_1, 2 mg B_2 and 10 mg B_6. *Dose: 1 tablet daily.*	Blue. In 100s.
Rx	**Lipo-Nicin/300 mg** (ICN Pharm)	**Capsules, timed release:** 300 mg niacin, 150 mg vitamin C, 25 mg B_1, 2 mg B_2 and 10 mg B_6. *Dose: 1 capsule daily.*	Clear. In 100s.

PERIPHERAL VASODILATOR COMBINATIONS

In these combinations: *NIACIN* (see Vitamins monograph) is used for its vasodilating action.

Human B-Type Natriuretic Peptide

NESIRITIDE

Rx	**Natrecor** (Scios)	**Powder for injection, lyophilized:** 1.5 mg	Mannitol. In single-use vials.

NESIRITIDE — INJECTION

Indications

➤*Congestive heart failure:* For the intravenous treatment of patients with acutely decompensated congestive heart failure who have dyspnea at rest or with minimal activity. In this population, the use of nesiritide reduced pulmonary capillary wedge pressure and improved dyspnea.

Administration and Dosage

➤*General dosing considerations:* Blood pressure should be monitored closely during nesiritide administration.

If hypotension occurs during the administration of nesiritide, the dose should be reduced or discontinued and other measures to support blood pressure should be started (IV fluids, changes in body position). In the vasodilation in the management of acute congestive heart failure (VMAC) trial, when symptomatic hypotension occurred, nesiritide was discontinued and subsequently could be restarted at a dose that was reduced by 30% (with no bolus administration) once the patient was stabilized. Because hypotension caused by nesiritide may be prolonged (up to hours), a period of observation may be necessary before restarting the drug.

➤*Adults:*

Congestive heart failure –

Usual dosage: An IV bolus of 2 mcg/kg followed by a continuous infusion at a dose of 0.01 mcg/kg/min. Nesiritide should not be initiated at a dose that is above the recommended dose.

Dosage adjustment: The dose-limiting side effect of nesiritide is hypotension. In the VMAC trial there was limited experience with increasing the dose of nesiritide above the recommended dose of a 2 mcg/kg bolus followed by an infusion of 0.01 mcg/kg/min. (23 patients, all of whom had central hemodynamic monitoring). In those patients, the infusion dose of nesiritide was increased by 0.005 mcg/kg/min (preceded by a bolus of 1 mcg/kg), no more frequently than every 3 hours up to a maximum dose of 0.03 mcg/kg/min. Nesiritide should not be titrated at frequent intervals as is done with other IV agents that have a shorter half-life.

➤*Preparation for administration:* Prime the IV tubing with an infusion of 25 mL prior to connecting to the patient's vascular access port and prior to administering the bolus or starting the infusion.

1.) Reconstitute one 1.5 mg vial of nesiritide by adding 5 mL of diluent removed from a pre-filled 250 mL plastic IV bag containing the diluent of choice. The following preservative-free diluents are recommended for reconstitution: dextrose 5% injection; sodium chloride 0.9% injection; dextrose 5% and sodium chloride 0.45% injection, or dextrose 5% and sodium chloride 0.2% injection.
2.) Do not shake the vial. Rock the vial gently so that all surfaces, including the stopper, are in contact with the diluent to ensure complete reconstitution. Use only a clear, essentially colorless solution.
3.) Withdraw the entire contents of the reconstituted nesiritide vial and add to the 250 mL plastic IV bag. This will yield a solution with a concentration of nesiritide of approximately 6 mcg/mL. The IV bag should be inverted several times to ensure complete mixing of the solution.

See Storage and Stability for storage instructions.

➤*Administration:* Nesiritide is for intravenous (IV) use only. Give as an IV bolus dose followed by a continuous infusion.

There is limited experience with administering nesiritide for longer than 48 hours.

Bolus followed by infusion – After preparation of the infusion bag, withdraw the bolus volume (see data below) from the nesiritide infusion bag, and administer it over approximately 60 seconds through an IV port in the tubing. Immediately following the administration of the bolus, infuse nesiritide at a flow rate of 0.1 mL/kg/h. This will deliver a nesiritide infusion dose of 0.01 mcg/kg/min.

To calculate the appropriate bolus volume and infusion flow rate to deliver a 0.01 mcg/kg/min dose, use the following formulas (or refer to the following dosing data).

NESIRITIDE — INJECTION

Bolus volume:

Bolus volume (mL) = 0.33 × Patient weight (kg)

Infusion flow rate:

Infusion flow rate (mL/h) = 0.1 × Patient weight (kg)

Nesiritide Weight-Adjusted Bolus Volume and Infusion Flow Rate (2 mcg/kg Bolus Followed by a 0.01 mcg/kg/min Dose)		
Patient weight (kg)	Volume of bolus (mL)	Rate of infusion (mL/h)
60	20	6
70	23.3	7
80	26.7	8
90	30	9
100	33.3	10
110	36.7	11

➤*Admixture compatibility:*

Compatibility – See Preparation for administration.

Incompatibility – Nesiritide is physically or chemically incompatible with injectable formulations of heparin, insulin, ethacrynate sodium, bumetamide, enalaprilat, hydralazine, and furosemide. These drugs should not be coadministered as infusions with nesiritide through the same IV catheter.

The preservative sodium metabisulfite is incompatible with nesiritide. Injectable drugs that contain sodium metabisulfite should not be administered in the same infusion line as nesiritide.

The catheter must be flushed between administration of nesiritide and incompatible drugs.

Nesiritide binds to heparin and therefore could bind to the heparin lining of a heparin-coated catheter, decreasing the amount of nesiritide delivered to the patient for some period of time. Therefore, nesiritide must not be administered through a central heparin-coated catheter. Concomitant administration of a heparin infusion through a separate catheter is acceptable.

➤*Storage/Stability:* Store nesiritide at controlled room temperature (20° to 25°C; 68° to 77°F); excursions permitted to 15° to 30°C (59° to 86°F; see USP controlled room temperature), or refrigerated (2° to 8°C; 36° to 46°F). Keep in carton until time of use.

Reconstituted vials of nesiritide may be left at controlled room temperature (20° to 25°C; 68° to 77°F) as per United States Pharmacopeia (USP) or may be refrigerated (2° to 8°C; 36° to 46°F) for up to 24 hours.

Actions

➤*Pharmacology:* Human BNP binds to the particulate guanylate cyclase receptor of vascular smooth muscle and endothelial cells, leading to increased intracellular concentrations of guanosine 3'5'-cyclic monophosphate (cGMP) and smooth muscle cell relaxation. Cyclic GMP serves as a second messenger to dilate veins and arteries. Nesiritide has been shown to relax isolated human arterial and venous tissue preparations that were precontracted with either endothelin-1 or the alpha-adrenergic agonist, phenylephrine.

In human studies, nesiritide produced dose-dependent reductions in pulmonary capillary wedge pressure (PCWP) and systemic arterial pressure in patients with heart failure.

➤*Pharmacokinetics:*

Absorption – The recommended dosing regimen of nesiritide is a 2 mcg/kg IV bolus followed by an intravenous infusion dose of 0.01 mcg/kg/min. With this dosing regimen, 60% of the 3-hour effect on PCWP reduction is achieved within 15 minutes after the bolus, reaching 95% of the 3-hour effect within 1 hour. Approximately 70% of the 3-hour effect on SBP reduction is reached within 15 minutes. The pharmacodynamic (PD) half-life of the onset and offset of the hemodynamic effect of nesiritide is longer than what the PK half-life of 18 minutes would predict. For example, in patients who developed symptomatic hypotension in the VMAC trial, half of the recovery of SBP toward the baseline value after discontinuation or reduction of the dose of nesiritide was observed in about 60 minutes. When higher doses of nesiritide were infused, the duration of hypotension was sometimes several hours.

Distribution – In patients with congestive heart failure (CHF), nesiritide administered intravenously by infusion or bolus exhibits biphasic disposition from the plasma.

In these patients, the mean volume of distribution of the central compartment (Vc) of nesiritide was estimated to be 0.073 L/kg, the mean steady-state volume of distribution (V_{ss}) was 0.19 L/kg, and the mean clearance (CL) was approximately 9.2 mL/min/kg. At steady state, plasma BNP levels increase from baseline endogenous levels by approximately 3- to 6-fold with nesiritide infusion doses ranging from 0.01 to 0.03 mcg/kg/min.

Excretion – The mean terminal elimination half-life ($t_{1/2}$) of nesiritide is approximately 18 minutes and was associated with approximately ⅔ of the area-under-the-curve (AUC). The mean initial elimination phase was estimated to be approximately 2 minutes.

Human BNP is cleared from the circulation via the following 3 independent mechanisms, in order of decreasing importance:

1.) Binding to cell surface clearance receptors with subsequent cellular internalization and lysosomal proteolysis.
2.) Proteolytic cleavage of the peptide by endopeptidases, such as neutral endopeptidase, which are present on the vascular lumenal surface.
3.) Renal filtration.

Contraindications

Hypersensitivity to any components of the product. Nesiritide should not be used as primary therapy for patients with cardiogenic shock or in patients with a systolic blood pressure less than 90 mm Hg.

Warnings/Precautions

➤*Low cardiac filling pressures:* Administration of nesiritide should be avoided in patients suspected of having, or known to have, low cardiac filling pressures.

➤*Cardiovascular:* Nesiritide may cause hypotension. In the VMAC trial, in patients given the recommended dose (2 mcg/kg bolus followed by a 0.01 mcg/kg/min infusion) or the adjustable dose, the incidence of symptomatic hypotension in the first 24 hours was similar for nesiritide (4%) and IV nitroglycerin (5%). When hypotension occurred, however, the duration of symptomatic hypotension was longer with nesiritide (mean duration was 2.2 hours) than with nitroglycerin (mean duration was 0.7 hours). In earlier trials, when nesiritide was initiated at doses greater than the 2 mcg/kg bolus followed by a 0.01 mcg/kg/min infusion (ie, 0.015 and 0.030 mcg/kg/min preceded by a small bolus), there were more hypotensive episodes and these episodes were of greater intensity and duration. They were also more often symptomatic or more likely to require medical intervention. Nesiritide should be administered only in settings where blood pressure can be monitored closely, and the dose of nesiritide should be reduced or the drug discontinued in patients who develop hypotension. The rate of symptomatic hypotension may be increased in patients with a blood pressure less than 100 mmHg at baseline, and nesiritide should be used cautiously in these patients. The potential for hypotension may be increased by combining nesiritide with other drugs that may cause hypotension. For example, in the VMAC trial in patients treated with either nesiritide or nitroglycerin therapy, the frequency of symptomatic hypotension in patients who received an oral ACE inhibitor was 6%, compared with a frequency of symptomatic hypotension of 1% in patients who did not receive an oral ACE inhibitor.

➤*Renal effects:* Nesiritide may affect renal function in susceptible individuals. In patients with severe heart failure whose renal function may depend on the activity of the renin-angiotensin-aldosterone system, treatment with nesiritide may be associated with azotemia. When nesiritide was initiated at doses more than 0.01 mcg/kg/min (0.015 and 0.030 mcg/kg/min), there was an increased rate of elevated serum creatinine over baseline compared with standard therapies, although the rate of acute renal failure and need for dialysis was not increased. In the 30-day follow-up period in the VMAC trial, 5 patients in the nitroglycerin group (2%) and 9 patients in the nesiritide group (3%) required first-time dialysis.

➤*Hypersensitivity reactions:* Parenteral administration of protein pharmaceuticals or *E. coli*-derived products should be attended by appropriate precautions in case of an allergic or untoward reaction. No serious allergic or anaphylactic reactions have been reported with nesiritide.

➤*Special risk:* Nesiritide is not recommended for patients for whom vasodilating agents are not appropriate, such as patients with significant valvular stenosis, restrictive or obstructive cardiomyopathy, constrictive pericarditis, pericardial tamponade, or other conditions in which cardiac output is dependent upon venous return, or for patients suspected to have low cardiac filling pressures.

➤*Pregnancy: Category C.* Animal reproductive studies have not been conducted with nesiritide. It is also not known whether nesiritide can cause fetal harm when administered to pregnant women or can affect reproductive capacity. Nesiritide should be used during pregnancy only if the potential benefit justifies any possible risk to the fetus.

➤*Lactation:* It is not known whether this drug is excreted in human milk. Therefore, caution should be exercised when nesiritide is administered to a breast-feeding woman.

➤*Children:* The safety and efficacy of nesiritide in children have not been established.

Drug Interactions

None known.

Adverse Reactions

Adverse reactions that occurred with at least a 3% frequency during the first 24 hours of nesiritide infusion are shown in the following table.

Human B-Type Natriuretic Peptide

NESIRITIDE — INJECTION

Nesiritide Adverse Reactions (≥ 3%)

Adverse reaction	VMAC Trial: Nitroglycerin (n = 216)	VMAC Trial: Nesiritide Recommended dose (n = 273)	Other Long Infusion Trials: Control[a] (n = 256)	Other Long Infusion Trials: Nesiritide mcg/kg/min 0.015 (n = 253)	Other Long Infusion Trials: Nesiritide mcg/kg/min 0.03 (n = 246)
Cardiovascular					
Hypotension	25 (12%)	31 (11%)	20 (8%)	56 (22%)	87 (35%)
Symptomatic hypotension	10 (5%)	12 (4%)	8 (3%)	28 (11%)	42 (17%)
Asymptomatic hypotension	17 (8%)	23 (8%)	13 (5%)	31 (12%)	49 (20%)
Ventricular tachycardia (VT)	11 (5%)	9 (3%)	25 (10%)	25 (10%)	10 (4%)
Non-sustained VT	11 (5%)	9 (3%)	23 (9%)	24 (9%)	9 (4%)
Ventricular extrasystoles	2 (1%)	7 (3%)	15 (6%)	10 (4%)	9 (4%)
Angina pectoris	5 (2%)	5 (2%)	6 (2%)	14 (6%)	6 (2%)
Bradycardia	1 (< 1%)	3 (1%)	1 (< 1%)	8 (3%)	13 (5%)
CNS					
Insomnia	9 (4%)	6 (2%)	7 (3%)	15 (6%)	15 (6%)
Dizziness	4 (2%)	7 (3%)	7 (3%)	16 (6%)	12 (5%)
Anxiety	6 (3%)	8 (3%)	2 (1%)	8 (3%)	4 (2%)
GI					
Nausea	13 (6%)	10 (4%)	12 (5%)	24 (9%)	33 (13%)
Vomiting	4 (2%)	4 (1%)	2 (1%)	6 (2%)	10 (4%)
Miscellaneous					
Headache	44 (20%)	21 (8%)	23 (9%)	23 (9%)	17 (7%)
Abdominal pain	11 (5%)	4 (1%)	10 (4%)	6 (2%)	8 (3%)
Back pain	7 (3%)	10 (4%)	4 (2%)	5 (2%)	3 (1%)

[a] Includes dobutamine, milrinone, nitroglycerin, placebo, dopamine, nitroprusside, or amrinone.

➤*Other adverse reactions that occurred in at least 1%:* Adverse reactions that are not listed in the above table that occurred in at least 1% of patients who received any of the above nesiritide doses included:

Miscellaneous – Tachycardia, atrial fibrillation, AV node conduction abnormalities, catheter pain, fever, injection site reaction, confusion, paresthesia, somnolence, tremor, increased cough, hemoptysis, apnea, increased creatinine, sweating, pruritus, rash, leg cramps, amblyopia, anemia. All reported events (at least 1%) are included except those already listed, those too general to be informative, and those not reasonably associated with the use of the drug because they were associated with the condition being treated or are very common in the treated population.

➤*Placebo and active-controlled clinical trials:*

Cardiovascular – In placebo and active-controlled clinical trials, nesiritide has not been associated with an increase in atrial or ventricular tachyarrhythmias. In placebo-controlled trials, the incidence of VT in both nesiritide and placebo patients was 2%. In the PRECEDENT (prospective randomized evaluation of cardiac ectopy with dobutamine or nesiritide therapy) trial, the effects of nesiritide (n = 163) and dobutamine (n = 83) on the provocation or aggravation of existing ventricular arrhythmias in patients with decompensated CHF was compared using Holter monitoring. Treatment with nesiritide (0.015 and 0.03 mcg/kg/min without an initial bolus) for 24 hours did not aggravate preexisting VT or the frequency of premature ventricular beats, compared to a baseline 24-hour holter tape.

➤*Effect on mortality:* In the VMAC trial, the mortality rates at 6 months in the patients receiving nesiritide and nitroglycerin were 25.1% (95% confidence interval, 20.0% to 30.5%) and 20.8% (95% confidence interval, 15.5% to 26.5%), respectively. In all controlled trials combined, the mortality rates for nesiritide and active control (including nitroglycerin, dobutamine, nitroprusside, milrinone, amrinone, and dopamine) patients were 21.5% and 21.7%, respectively.

➤*Lab test abnormalities:* In the PRECEDENT trial, the incidence of elevations in serum creatinine to more than 0.5 mg/dL above baseline through day 14 was higher in the nesiritide 0.015 mcg/kg/min group (17%) and the nesiritide 0.03 mcg/kg/min group (19%) than with standard therapy (11%). In the VMAC trial, through day 30, the incidence of elevations in creatinine to more than 0.5 mg/dL above baseline was 28% and 21% in the nesiritide (2 mcg/kg bolus followed by 0.01 mcg/kg/min) and nitroglycerin groups, respectively.

Overdosage

No data are available with respect to overdosage in humans. The expected reaction would be excessive hypotension, which should be treated with drug discontinuation or reduction and appropriate measures.

Endothelin Receptor Antagonist

BOSENTAN

Rx	**Tracleer** (Actelion)	**Tablets; oral:** 62.5 mg	(62,5). Orange and white, round. Film-coated. In 60s.
		125 mg	(125). Orange and white, oval. Film-coated. In 60s.

BOSENTAN — ORAL

WARNING

Distribution program – Because of the risk of liver injury and birth defects, bosentan is available only through a special restricted distribution program called the *Tracleer* Access Program (TAP), by calling 1-866-228-3546. Only prescribers and pharmacies registered with TAP may prescribe and distribute bosentan. In addition, bosentan may be dispensed only to patients who are enrolled in and meet all conditions of TAP.

Liver injury – In clinical studies, bosentan caused at least a 3-fold upper limit of normal (ULN) elevation of liver aminotransferases (ALT and AST) in approximately 11% of patients, accompanied by elevated bilirubin in a small number of cases. Because these changes are a marker for potential serious liver injury, serum aminotransferase levels must be measured prior to initiation of treatment and then monthly. In the postmarketing period, in the setting of close monitoring, rare cases of unexplained hepatic cirrhosis were reported after prolonged (more than 12 months) therapy with bosentan in patients with multiple comorbidities and drug therapies. There have also been reports of liver failure. The contribution of bosentan in these cases could not be excluded.

WARNING (cont.)

In at least 1 case, the initial presentation of liver injury (after more than 20 months of treatment) included pronounced elevations in aminotransferases and bilirubin levels accompanied by nonspecific symptoms, all of which resolved slowly over time after discontinuation of bosentan. This case reinforces the importance of strict adherence to the monthly monitoring schedule for the duration of treatment and the treatment algorithm, which includes stopping bosentan if a rise of aminotransferase accompanied by signs or symptoms of liver dysfunction occurs.

Elevations in aminotransferases require close attention. Avoid using bosentan in patients with elevated aminotransferases (greater than 3 times the ULN) at baseline because monitoring liver injury may be more difficult. Stop treatment if liver aminotransferase elevations are accompanied by clinical symptoms of liver injury (eg, abdominal pain, fever, jaundice, nausea, unusual lethargy or fatigue, vomiting) or increases in bilirubin greater than or equal to 2 times the ULN. There is no experience with the reintroduction of bosentan in these circumstances.

BOSENTAN — ORAL

WARNING (cont.)

Pregnancy – Bosentan is likely to cause major birth defects if used by pregnant women based on animal data. Pregnancy must be excluded before the start of treatment with bosentan. Throughout treatment and for 1 month after stopping bosentan, women of childbearing potential must use 2 reliable methods of contraception unless the patient has a tubal sterilization or Copper T 380A intrauterine device (IUD) or levonorgestrel 20 mcg/day intrauterine system (IUS) inserted, in which case no other contraception is needed. Hormonal contraceptives, including oral, injectable, transdermal, and implantable contraceptives, should not be used as the sole means of contraception because these may not be effective in patients receiving bosentan. Obtain monthly pregnancy tests.

Indications

➤*Pulmonary arterial hypertension:* For the treatment of pulmonary arterial hypertension (World Health Organization [WHO] group 1), to improve exercise ability and decrease the rate of clinical worsening.

➤*Off-label uses:*

Prevention of digital ulcers in systemic sclerosis – [3] = Safety concerns. Based on the limited patient population for which data are available, bosentan may be effective for patients with digital ulcers caused by systemic sclerosis. Bosentan has been found to decrease the number of new ulcers, but has not been found to improve healing of existing ulcers. Enrollment of patients into the TAP is required because bosentan cannot be dispensed through traditional retail pharmacies. To enroll a patient in this program, the prescriber is asked to sign a statement, "I certify that I am prescribing *Tracleer* (bosentan) for this patient for a medically appropriate use in the treatment of pulmonary arterial hypertension, as described in the *Tracleer* full prescribing information. I have reviewed the liver and pregnancy warning with the patient and commit to undertaking appropriate blood testing for monitoring liver function in this patient and testing for pregnancy (if the patient is a female of childbearing potential)."

Prevention of Raynaud phenomenon – [3] = Safety concerns. Initial data from a limited number of trials suggest bosentan may be of symptomatic benefit in patients with Raynaud phenomenon. However, conflicting data regarding efficacy in objective measures require further study in larger, controlled trials before this agent can be recommended for routine use.

Administration and Dosage

➤*General dosing considerations:* See the Warning box for more information.

Liver aminotransferase levels must be measured prior to initiation of treatment and then monthly. If elevated aminotransferase levels are seen, changes in monitoring and treatment must be initiated.

➤*Adults:*

Pulmonary arterial hypertension –

Initial dosage: 62.5 mg twice daily for 4 weeks. In patients with a body weight of less than 40 kg, the recommended initial dosage is 62.5 mg twice daily.

Maintenance dosage: 125 mg twice daily. In patients with a body weight of less than 40 kg, the recommended maintenance dosage is 62.5 mg twice daily.

Dosage adjustment: Discontinue treatment if liver aminotransferase elevations are accompanied by clinical symptoms of liver injury (eg, abdominal pain, fever, jaundice, nausea, unusual lethargy or fatigue, vomiting) or increases in bilirubin of 2 times the ULN or more. There is no experience with the reintroduction of bosentan in these circumstances.

Bosentan Dosage Adjustment For Aminotransferase Elevations > 3 × ULN

ALT/AST levels	Treatment and monitoring recommendations
> 3 and ≤ 5 × ULN	Confirm by another aminotransferase test. If confirmed, reduce the dosage to 62.5 mg twice daily or interrupt treatment and monitor aminotransferase levels at least every 2 weeks. If the aminotransferase levels return to pretreatment values, continue or reintroduce[a] the treatment as appropriate.
> 5 and ≤ 8 × ULN	Confirm by another aminotransferase test. If confirmed, stop treatment and monitor aminotransferase levels at least every 2 weeks. Once the aminotransferase levels return to pretreatment values, consider reintroduction[a] of the treatment.
> 8 × ULN	Treatment should be stopped and reintroduction of bosentan should not be considered. There is no experience with the reintroduction of bosentan in these circumstances.

[a] If bosentan is reintroduced it should be at the starting dose; aminotransferase levels should be checked within 3 days and thereafter at least every 2 weeks.

Off-label dosing –

Prevention of digital ulcers in systemic sclerosis: [3] = Safety concerns. 62.5 mg orally twice daily, increased to 125 mg twice daily.

Prevention of Raynaud phenomenon: [3] = Safety concerns. Initial dosage was 62.5 mg orally twice daily for 1 month and then increased to 125 mg twice daily for up to 1 year.

➤*Hepatic function impairment:*

Moderate to severe hepatic impairment – Bosentan should generally be avoided in patients with moderate or severe hepatic impairment.

➤*Concomitant therapy:* Discontinue use of bosentan at least 36 hours prior to initiation of ritonavir. After at least 10 days following the initiation of ritonavir, resume bosentan at 62.5 mg once daily or every other day based on individual tolerability. In patients who have been receiving ritonavir for at least 10 days, start bosentan at 62.5 mg once daily or every other day based on individual tolerability.

➤*Discontinuation of therapy:* There is limited experience with abrupt discontinuation of bosentan. No evidence for acute rebound has been observed. To avoid the potential for clinical deterioration, gradual dosage reduction (62.5 mg twice daily for 3 to 7 days) should be considered.

➤*Administration:* Administer in the morning and evening, with or without food.

➤*Storage/Stability:* Store at 20° to 25°C (68° to 77°F). Excursions are permitted between 15° and 30°C (59° and 86°F).

Actions

➤*Pharmacology:* Endothelin-1 (ET-1) is a neurohormone, the effects of which are mediated by binding to ET_A and ET_B receptors in the endothelium and vascular smooth muscle. ET-1 concentrations are elevated in plasma and lung tissue of patients with pulmonary arterial hypertension, suggesting a pathogenic role for ET-1 in this disease. Bosentan is a specific and competitive antagonist at endothelin receptor types ET_A and ET_B. Bosentan has a slightly higher affinity for ET_A receptors than for ET_B receptors. The clinical impact of dual endothelin blockage is unknown.

➤*Pharmacokinetics:*

Absorption/Distribution – After oral administration, maximum concentrations (C_{max}) of bosentan are attained within 3 to 5 hours in healthy adult subjects. The exposure to bosentan after intravenous (IV) and oral administration is approximately 2-fold higher in adult patients with pulmonary arterial hypertension than in healthy adult subjects. Steady state is reached within 3 to 5 days.

The absolute bioavailability of bosentan in healthy volunteers is approximately 50% and is unaffected by food. The volume of distribution is approximately 18 L. Bosentan is highly bound (more than 98%) to plasma proteins, mainly albumin. Bosentan does not penetrate into erythrocytes.

Metabolism/Excretion – Bosentan has 3 metabolites, one of which is pharmacologically active and may contribute 10% to 20% of the effect of bosentan. Bosentan is an inducer of cytochrome P-450 (CYP)–2C9 and 3A4 and possibly also of CYP2C19. Total clearance after a single IV dose is approximately 4 L/h in patients with pulmonary arterial hypertension. Upon multiple oral dosing, plasma concentrations decrease gradually to 50% to 65% of those seen after single-dose administration, probably the effect of autoinduction of the metabolizing liver enzymes. Bosentan is eliminated by biliary excretion following metabolism in the liver. Less than 3% of an administered oral dose is recovered in urine.

The terminal elimination half-life is approximately 5 hours in healthy adult subjects.

Special populations –

Renal function impairment: In patients with severe renal impairment (creatinine clearance, 15 to 30 mL/min), plasma concentrations of bosentan were essentially unchanged and plasma concentrations of the 3 metabolites were increased approximately 2-fold compared with subjects with healthy renal function. These differences do not appear to be clinically important.

Hepatic function impairment: In vitro and in vivo evidence showing extensive hepatic metabolism of bosentan suggests that hepatic impairment would significantly increase exposure (C_{max} and area under the curve [AUC]) of bosentan. In a study comparing 8 patients with mild hepatic impairment (as indicated by the Child-Pugh method) with 8 controls, the single- and multiple-dose pharmacokinetics of bosentan were not altered in patients with mild hepatic impairment. The influence of moderate or severe hepatic impairment on the pharmacokinetics of bosentan has not been evaluated. There are no specific data to guide dosing in hepatically impaired patients; exercise caution in patients with mildly impaired liver function. Generally, avoid using bosentan in patients with moderate or severe liver abnormalities and/or elevated aminotransferases greater than 3 times the ULN.

Contraindications

In women who are or may become pregnant (see also Warning Box and Warnings/Precautions); concomitant use with cyclosporine A or glyburide; hypersensitivity to bosentan or any component of the product.

Warnings/Precautions

➤*Hepatotoxicity:* Elevations in ALT or AST by more than 3 times the ULN were observed in 11% of bosentan-treated patients (n = 658) compared with 2% of placebo-treated patients (n = 280). Three-fold increases were seen in 12% of 95 pulmonary arterial hypertension patients taking 125 mg twice daily and 14% of 70 pulmonary arterial hypertension patients taking 250 mg twice daily. Eight-fold increases were seen in 2% of pulmonary arterial hypertension patients taking 125 mg twice daily and 7% of pulmonary

BOSENTAN — ORAL

arterial hypertension patients taking 250 mg twice daily. Bilirubin increases to at least 3 times the ULN were associated with aminotransferase increases in 0.3% of patients treated with bosentan.

The combination of hepatocellular injury (increases in aminotransferases of greater than 3 times the ULN) and increases in total bilirubin (at least 3 times the ULN) is a marker for potential serious liver injury.

Elevations of AST and/or ALT associated with bosentan are dose dependent, occur both early and late in treatment, usually progress slowly, are typically asymptomatic, and, to date, have been reversible after treatment interruption or cessation. These aminotransferase elevations may reverse spontaneously while continuing treatment with bosentan.

Liver aminotransferase levels must be measured prior to initiation of treatment and then monthly. If elevated aminotransferase levels are seen, initiate changes in monitoring and treatment.

See the Warning box for more information.

➤*Fluid retention:* Peripheral edema is a known clinical consequence of pulmonary arterial hypertension and worsening pulmonary arterial hypertension and is also a known effect of other endothelin receptor antagonists. In pulmonary arterial hypertension clinical trials with bosentan, combined adverse events of fluid retention or edema were reported in 1.7% (placebo-corrected) of patients.

In addition, there have been numerous postmarketing reports of fluid retention in patients with pulmonary hypertension occurring within weeks after starting bosentan. Patients required intervention with a diuretic, fluid management, or hospitalization for decompensating heart failure.

If clinically significant fluid retention develops, with or without associated weight gain, undertake further evaluation to determine the cause, such as bosentan or underlying heart failure, and the possible need for treatment or discontinuation of bosentan therapy.

➤*Decreased sperm counts:* An open-label, single-arm, multicenter, safety study evaluated the effect on testicular function of bosentan 62.5 mg twice daily for 4 weeks, followed by 125 mg twice daily for 5 months. Twenty-five men with WHO functional class III and IV pulmonary arterial hypertension and normal baseline sperm count were enrolled. Twenty-three completed the study and 2 discontinued because of adverse reactions not related to testicular function. There was a decline in sperm count of at least 50% in 25% of the patients after 3 to 6 months of treatment with bosentan. Sperm count remained within the normal range in all 22 patients with data after 6 months and no changes in sperm morphology, sperm motility, or hormone levels were observed. One patient developed marked oligospermia at 3 months and the sperm count remained low with 2 follow-up measurements over the subsequent 6 weeks. Bosentan was discontinued, and, after 2 months, the sperm count had returned to baseline levels. Based on these findings and preclinical data from endothelin receptor antagonists, it cannot be excluded that endothelin receptor antagonists, such as bosentan, have an adverse effect on spermatogenesis.

➤*Hematologic effects:* Treatment with bosentan caused a dose-related decrease in hemoglobin and hematocrit. Monitor hemoglobin levels after 1 and 3 months of treatment and then every 3 months.

If a marked decrease in hemoglobin concentration occurs, undertake further evaluation to determine the cause and need for specific treatment.

The overall mean decrease in hemoglobin concentration for bosentan-treated patients was 0.9 g/dL (change to end of treatment). Most of this decrease of hemoglobin concentration was detected during the first few weeks of bosentan treatment and hemoglobin levels stabilized by 4 to 12 weeks of bosentan treatment. In placebo-controlled studies of all uses of bosentan, marked decreases in hemoglobin (greater than 15% decrease from baseline resulting in values less than 11 g/dL) were observed in 6% of bosentan-treated patients and 3% of placebo-treated patients. In patients with pulmonary arterial hypertension treated with dosages of 125 and 250 mg twice daily, marked decreases in hemoglobin occurred in 3% compared with 1% in placebo-treated patients.

A decrease in hemoglobin concentration by at least 1 g/dL was observed in 57% of bosentan-treated patients, compared with 29% of placebo-treated patients. In 80% of those patients whose hemoglobin decreased by at least 1 g/dL, the decrease occurred during the first 6 weeks of bosentan treatment.

During the course of treatment, the hemoglobin concentration remained within normal limits in 68% of bosentan-treated patients compared with 76% of placebo patients. The explanation for the change in hemoglobin is not known, but it does not appear to be hemorrhage or hemolysis.

➤*Pulmonary veno-occlusive disease:* If signs of pulmonary edema occur when bosentan is administered, consider the possibility of associated pulmonary veno-occlusive disease and discontinue bosentan.

➤*Distribution program:* See the Warning box for more information.

➤*Hypersensitivity reactions:* Bosentan is contraindicated in patients who are hypersensitive to bosentan or any component of the product. Observed reactions include rash and angioedema.

➤*Hepatic function impairment:* Avoid using bosentan in patients with moderate to severe liver impairment. In addition, generally avoid using bosentan in patients with elevated aminotransferases (greater than 3 times the ULN) because monitoring liver injury in these patients may be more difficult.

➤*Pregnancy: Category X.* Use of bosentan is contraindicated in women who are or may become pregnant. While there are no adequate and well controlled studies in pregnant women, animal studies show that bosentan is likely to cause major birth defects when administered during pregnancy. Bosentan caused teratogenic effects in animals, including malformations of the head, mouth, face, and large blood vessels. If this drug is used during pregnancy or if a patient becomes pregnant while taking this drug, apprise the patient of the potential hazard to the fetus.

Bosentan was teratogenic in rats given oral doses 2 times the maximum recommended human dose (MRHD) (on a mg/m^2 basis). In an embryofetal toxicity study in rats, bosentan showed dose-dependent teratogenic effects, including malformations of the head, mouth, face, and large blood vessels. Bosentan administration increased stillbirths and pup mortality at oral doses 2 (60 mg/kg/day) and 10 (300 mg/kg/day) times the MRHD (on a mg/m^2 basis). Although birth defects were not observed in rabbits given oral dosages of up to 1,500 mg/kg/day, plasma concentrations of bosentan in rabbits were lower than those reached in the rat. The similarity of malformations induced by bosentan and those observed in ET-1 knockout mice and in animals treated with other endothelin receptor antagonists indicates that teratogenicity is a class effect of these drugs.

Women of childbearing potential should have a negative pregnancy test before starting treatment with bosentan. Do not dispense a prescription for bosentan without documenting a negative urine or serum pregnancy test performed during the first 5 days of a normal menstrual period and at least 11 days after the last unprotected act of sexual intercourse. Obtain follow-up urine or serum pregnancy tests monthly in women of childbearing potential taking bosentan. Advise the patient to contact her health care provider immediately for pregnancy testing if onset of menses is delayed or pregnancy is suspected. If the pregnancy test is positive, the health care provider and patient must discuss the risks to her, the pregnancy, and the fetus.

Drug interaction studies show that bosentan reduces serum levels of the estrogen and progestin in oral contraceptives. Based on these findings, hormonal contraceptives (including oral, injectable, transdermal, and implantable contraceptives) may be less effective for preventing pregnancy in patients using bosentan and should not be used as a patient's only contraceptive method. Women of childbearing potential using bosentan must use 2 reliable forms of contraception unless she has a tubal sterilization or has a Copper T 380A IUD or levonorgestrel 20 mcg/day IUS. In these cases, no additional contraception is needed. Contraception should be continued until 1 month after completing bosentan therapy. Women of childbearing potential using bosentan should seek contraception counseling from a gynecologist or other expert as needed.

➤*Lactation:* It is not known whether bosentan is excreted into human milk. The molecular weight (approximately 570) is low enough that excretion into breast milk should be expected. Because many drugs are excreted in human milk, and because of the potential for serious adverse reactions in breast-feeding infants from bosentan, make a decision to discontinue breast-feeding or the drug, taking into account the importance of the drug to the mother.

➤*Children:* Safety and efficacy in children have not been established.

➤*Elderly:* Exercise caution in dose selection for elderly patients given the greater frequency of decreased hepatic, renal, or cardiac function, and of concomitant disease or other drug therapy in this age group.

➤*Monitoring:* Obtain monthly follow-up urine or serum pregnancy tests in women of childbearing potential taking bosentan.

Liver aminotransferase levels must be measured prior to initiation of treatment and then monthly. If elevated aminotransferase levels are seen, changes in monitoring and treatment must be initiated.

Monitor hemoglobin levels after 1 and 3 months of treatment and then every 3 months.

Drug Interactions

Bosentan Drug Interactions

Precipitant drug	Object drug[a]		Description
Clarithromycin	Bosentan	⬆	The risk of bosentan hepatotoxicity may be increased. Close clinical and laboratory monitoring is warranted. If an interaction is suspected, stop 1 or both drugs.
Cyclosporine A	Bosentan	⬆⬇	Coadministration increased bosentan trough concentrations ≈ 30-fold and steady-state concentrations 3- to 4-fold. Cyclosporine A plasma concentrations decreased ≈ 50%. Coadministration is contraindicated.
Bosentan	Cyclosporine A		
Glyburide	Bosentan	⬇	Glyburide plasma concentrations were decreased ≈ 40% when administered with bosentan, whereas the plasma concentrations of bosentan were also decreased ≈ 30%. Coadministration is contraindicated because an increased risk of elevated liver enzymes was observed in patients receiving concomitant therapy with glyburide.
Bosentan	Glyburide		

BOSENTAN — ORAL

Bosentan Drug Interactions			
Precipitant drug	Object drug[a]		Description
Ketoconazole	Bosentan	↑	Coadministration increased bosentan plasma concentrations ≈ 2-fold. No dosage adjustment is necessary, but consider increased effects of bosentan. Additional monitoring is warranted.
PDE5[b] inhibitors (eg, sildenafil)	Bosentan	↑↓	Coadministration may elevate bosentan plasma concentrations, increasing the pharmacologic effects and risk of toxicity. PDE5 inhibitor concentrations may be reduced, decreasing the pharmacologic effects. Coadminister these agents with caution. Closely monitor the clinical response and for adverse reactions. Adjust therapy as needed.
Bosentan	PDE5 inhibitors (eg, sildenafil)		
Rifampin	Bosentan	↑↓	Coadministration may increase bosentan trough concentrations after the first concomitant dose and decrease bosentan trough concentrations at steady state. Measure liver function weekly for the first 4 weeks of concurrent use before reverting to normal monitoring.
Ritonavir-containing regimens	Bosentan	↑	Coadministration may increase bosentan trough concentrations. In patients receiving ritonavir for at least 10 days, start bosentan at 62.5 mg once daily or every other day based on tolerability. In patients receiving bosentan, stop bosentan at least 36 hours before starting ritonavir. At least 10 days after starting ritonavir, resume bosentan at 62.5 mg once daily or every other day based on tolerability.
Tacrolimus	Bosentan	↑	Although not studied in humans, coadministration resulted in markedly increased plasma concentrations of bosentan in animals. Use with caution.
Bosentan	Hormonal contraceptives (including oral, transdermal, injectable, and implantable)	↓	There is a possibility of contraceptive failure when bosentan is coadministered. Women should not rely on hormonal contraception alone when taking bosentan. Because animal studies indicate that bosentan can cause teratogenic effects, females of child bearing potential must use 2 reliable methods of contraception during treatment and for 1 month after stopping bosentan.
Bosentan	Statins (eg, atorvastatin, lovastatin, simvastatin)	↓	The plasma concentrations of simvastatin and its metabolite decreased ≈ 50% when coadministered with bosentan. Bosentan is also expected to reduce plasma concentrations of other statins metabolized by CYP3A4 (ie, atorvastatin, lovastatin). Monitor cholesterol levels and adjust statin dose accordingly.
Bosentan	Warfarin	↓	Coadministration decreased the plasma concentrations of S-warfarin and R-warfarin 29% and 38%, respectively. Clinically relevant changes in INR[b] or warfarin dose were not seen in patients with pulmonary arterial hypertension during clinical trials. Because warfarin has a narrow therapeutic index, monitor coagulation parameters and adjust the warfarin dose as needed.

[a] ↑ = object drug increased; ↓ = object drug decreased; ↑↓= object drug increased and then decreased.
[b] PDE5 = phosphodiesterase type 5; INR = international normalized ratio.

Adverse Reactions

➤*Discontinuation:* Treatment discontinuation because of adverse reactions other than those related to pulmonary hypertension during the clinical trials in patients with pulmonary arterial hypertension were more frequent with bosentan (6%) than with placebo (3%). In this database, the only cause of discontinuations more than 1% and occurring more often with bosentan was abnormal liver function.

➤*Adverse reactions (at least 3%):*

Bosentan Adverse Reactions[a] (≥ 3%)		
Adverse reactions	Bosentan 125 or 250 mg twice daily (n = 258)	Placebo (n = 172)
Cardiovascular		
Flushing	4%	3%
Hypotension	4%	2%
Palpitations	4%	2%
Syncope	5%	4%
Respiratory		
Respiratory tract infection	22%	17%
Sinusitis	4%	2%
Miscellaneous		
Anemia	3%	—
Arthralgia	4%	2%
Chest pain	5%	5%
Edema	11%	9%
Headache	15%	14%
Liver function test abnormal	4%	2%

[a] Only adverse reactions with onset from start of treatment to 1 calendar day after end of treatment are included. Combined data from study 351, BREATHE-1, and EARLY.

➤*Postmarketing:*

Dermatologic – Rash.

Hematologic/Lymphatic – Anemia requiring transfusion, leukopenia, neutropenia, thrombocytopenia.

Hepatic – Jaundice, liver failure, unexplained hepatic cirrhosis

Hypersensitivity – There have been several postmarketing reports of angioneurotic edema associated with the use of bosentan. The onset of the reported cases occurred within a range of 8 hours to 21 days after starting therapy. Some patients were treated with an antihistamine and signs of angioedema resolved without discontinuing bosentan.

Overdosage

➤*Symptoms:* The most common adverse reaction was headache of mild to moderate intensity. In the cyclosporine A interaction study, in which dosages of 500 and 1,000 mg twice daily of bosentan were given concomitantly with cyclosporine A, trough plasma concentrations of bosentan increased 30-fold, resulting in severe headache, nausea, and vomiting, but no serious adverse reactions. Mild decreases in blood pressure and increases in heart rate were observed.

In the postmarketing period, there was 1 reported overdose of 10,000 mg of bosentan taken by an adolescent boy. He had symptoms of nausea, vomiting, hypotension, dizziness, sweating, and blurred vision. He recovered within 24 hours with blood pressure support.

➤*Treatment:* Bosentan is unlikely to be effectively removed by dialysis because of the high molecular weight and extensive plasma protein binding.

Patient Information

Discuss with patients the importance of monthly monitoring of serum aminotransferases.

Advise patients that bosentan is likely to cause birth defects based on animal studies. Only initiate bosentan treatment in women of childbearing

BOSENTAN — ORAL

potential following a negative pregnancy test. Women of childbearing potential must have monthly pregnancy tests and need to use 2 different forms of contraceptive methods. Advise females of childbearing potential that they must have monthly pregnancy tests and need to use 2 different forms of contraception while taking bonsentan and for 1 month after discontinuing bonsentan. Tell women who have tubal ligation or a Copper T 380A IUD or levonorgestrol 20 IUS that they can use those contraceptive methods alone. Instruct women to immediately contact their health care provider if they suspect they may be pregnant and advise them to seek contraceptive advice from a gynecologist or similar expert as needed.

Discuss with patients possible drug interactions with bosentan and which medications should not be taken with bosentan. Discuss with patients the importance of disclosing all concomitant or new medications.

Instruct patients to immediately report any of the following symptoms to a health care provider: nausea, vomiting, fever, abdominal pain, jaundice, unusual lethargy, fatigue.

AMBRISENTAN

Rx	**Letairis** (Gilead Sciences)	**Tablets; oral:** 5 mg	Lactose. (5 GSI). Pale pink, square. Film-coated. In UD 30s.
		10 mg	Lactose. (10 GSI). Deep pink, oval. Film-coated. In UD 30s.

AMBRISENTAN — ORAL

WARNING

Pregnancy – Ambrisentan is contraindicated during pregnancy. Ambrisentan is very likely to produce serious birth defects if used by pregnant women. This effect has been seen consistently when it is administered to animals; therefore, pregnancy must be excluded before the initiation of treatment with ambrisentan and prevented during treatment and for 1 month after stopping treatment by the use of at least 2 acceptable methods of contraception, unless the patient has had a tubal sterilization or chooses to use a Copper T 380A intrauterine device (IUD) or levonorgestrel 20 mcg/day intrauterine system (IUS), in which case no other contraception is needed. Obtain monthly pregnancy tests.

Dispensing program – Because of the risks of birth defects, ambrisentan is available only through a special restricted distribution program called the *Letairis* Education and Access Program (LEAP) by calling 1-866-664-5327. Only prescribers and pharmacies registered with LEAP may prescribe and distribute ambrisentan. In addition, ambrisentan may be dispensed only to patients who are enrolled in and meet all conditions of LEAP.

Indications

➤*Pulmonary arterial hypertension:* For the treatment of pulmonary arterial hypertension (World Health Organization [WHO] group 1) to improve exercise ability and delay clinical worsening.

Studies establishing effectiveness included predominately patients with WHO functional class II to III symptoms and etiologies of idiopathic or heritable pulmonary arterial hypertension (64%) or pulmonary arterial hypertension associated with connective tissue diseases (32%).

Administration and Dosage

➤*General dosing considerations:* See the Warning box for more information.

Because of the risk of birth defects, ambrisentan may be prescribed only through LEAP by calling 1-866-664-LEAP (5327) or logging on to http://www.letairis.com.

➤*Adults:*

Pulmonary arterial hypertension –

Initial dosage: 5 mg once daily.

Dosage adjustment: May increase dosage to 10 mg once daily if 5 mg is tolerated.

➤*Hepatic function impairment:* Not recommended in patients with moderate or severe hepatic impairment.

➤*Administration:* Tablets may be administered with or without food. Tablets should not be split, crushed, or chewed.

➤*Storage/Stability:* Store at 25°C (77°F); excursions are permitted between 15° and 30°C (59° and 86°F). Store in original packaging.

Actions

➤*Pharmacology:* Ambrisentan is an endothelin receptor antagonist that is selective for the endothelin type A (ET_A) receptor. Endothelin-1 (ET-1) is a potent autocrine and paracrine peptide. Two receptor subtypes, ET_A and ET_B, mediate the effects of ET-1 in the vascular smooth muscle and endothelium. The primary actions of ET_A are vasoconstriction and cell proliferation, while the predominant actions of ET_B are vasodilation, antiproliferation, and ET-1 clearance.

In patients with pulmonary arterial hypertension, plasma ET-1 concentrations are increased as much as 10-fold and correlate with increased mean right atrial pressure and disease severity. ET-1 and ET-1–messenger RNA concentrations are increased as much as 9-fold in the lung tissue of patients with pulmonary arterial hypertension, primarily in the endothelium of pulmonary arteries. These findings suggest that ET-1 may play a critical role in the pathogenesis and progression of pulmonary arterial hypertension.

➤*Pharmacokinetics:*

Absorption/Distribution – The pharmacokinetics of ambrisentan (S-ambrisentan) in healthy subjects are dose proportional. The absolute bioavailability of ambrisentan is not known. Ambrisentan is rapidly absorbed, with peak concentrations occurring approximately 2 hours after oral administration in healthy subjects and patients with pulmonary arterial hypertension. Ambrisentan is highly bound to plasma proteins (99%).

Metabolism – Studies with human liver tissue indicate that ambrisentan is metabolized by cytochrome P450 (CYP) 3A, CYP2C19, and uridine 5′-diphosphate glucuronosyltransferases (UGTs) 1A9S, 2B7S, and 1A3S. In plasma, the area under the curve (AUC) of 4-hydroxymethyl ambrisentan accounts for approximately 4% relative to parent ambrisentan AUC. The in vivo inversion of S-ambrisentan to R-ambrisentan is negligible.

Excretion – The elimination of ambrisentan is predominantly by nonrenal pathways, but the relative contributions of metabolism and biliary elimination have not been well characterized. Based on in vitro data, interactions with strong inhibitors of P-glycoprotein, organic anion transport protein (OATP), CYP3A4, CYP2C19, and UGTs are possible. The mean oral clearance of ambrisentan is 38 mL/min and 19 mL/min in healthy subjects and in patients with pulmonary arterial hypertension, respectively. Although ambrisentan has a 15-hour terminal half-life, the mean trough concentration of ambrisentan at steady state is about 15% of the mean peak concentration, and the accumulation factor is about 1.2 after long-term daily dosing, indicating that the effective half-life of ambrisentan is approximately 9 hours.

Special populations –

Hepatic function impairment: The influence of preexisting hepatic impairment on the pharmacokinetics of ambrisentan has not been evaluated. Because there is in vitro and in vivo evidence of significant metabolic and biliary contribution to the elimination of ambrisentan, hepatic impairment would be expected to have significant effects on the pharmacokinetics of ambrisentan.

Contraindications

Women who are or may become pregnant.

Warnings/Precautions

➤*Hepatic effects:* See the Warning box for more information.

Liver function tests were closely monitored in all clinical studies with ambrisentan. For all ambrisentan-treated patients (n = 483), the 12-week incidence of aminotransferases of more than 3 times the ULN was 0.8% and of more than 8 times the ULN was 0.2%. For placebo-treated patients, the 12-week incidence of aminotransferases of more than 3 times the ULN was 2.3% and of more than 8 times the ULN was 0%. The 1-year rate of aminotransferase elevations of more than 3 times the ULN with ambrisentan was 2.8% and of more than 8 times the ULN was 0.5%. One case of aminotransferase elevations of more than 3 times the ULN has been accompanied by bilirubin elevations of more than 2 times the ULN.

Measure liver chemistries prior to initiation of ambrisentan and at least every month thereafter. If there are aminotransferase elevations of more than 3 times the ULN or 5 times the ULN or less, remeasure them. If the confirmed level is more than 3 times the ULN or 5 times the ULN or less, reduce the daily dose or interrupt treatment and continue to monitor every 2 weeks until the levels are less than 3 times the ULN. If there are aminotransferase elevations of more than 5 times the ULN or 8 times the ULN or less, discontinue ambrisentan and monitor until the levels are less than 3 times the ULN. Ambrisentan can then be reinitiated with more frequent measurements of aminotransferase levels. If there are aminotransferase elevations of more than 8 times the ULN, stop treatment and do not reinitiate.

Ambrisentan is not recommended in patients with elevated aminotransferases (more than 3 times the ULN) at baseline because monitoring liver injury may be more difficult. If aminotransferase elevations are accompanied by clinical symptoms of liver injury (such as anorexia, fatigue, fever, itching, jaundice, malaise, nausea, right upper quadrant abdominal discomfort, or vomiting) or increases in bilirubin of more than 2 times the ULN, stop ambrisentan treatment. There is no experience with the reintroduction of ambrisentan in these circumstances.

➤*Hematologic effects:* Decreases in hemoglobin concentration and hematocrit have followed administration of other endothelin receptor antagonists and were observed in clinical studies with ambrisentan. These decreases were observed within the first few weeks of treatment with ambrisentan and stabilized thereafter. The mean decrease in hemoglobin from baseline to end of treatment for those patients receiving ambrisentan in the 12-week, placebo-controlled studies was 0.8 g/dL.

Marked decreases in hemoglobin (more than 15% decrease from baseline resulting in a value below the lower limit of normal) were observed in 7% of all patients receiving ambrisentan (and 10% of patients receiving 10 mg) compared with 4% of patients receiving placebo. The cause of the decrease in hemoglobin is unknown, but it does not appear to result from hemorrhage or hemolysis.

Monitor hemoglobin prior to initiation of ambrisentan, at 1 month, and periodically thereafter. Initiation of ambrisentan therapy is not recommended for patients with clinically significant anemia. If a clinically significant

AMBRISENTAN — ORAL

decrease in hemoglobin is observed and other causes have been excluded, consider discontinuing ambrisentan.

➤*Fluid retention:* Peripheral edema is a known class effect of endothelin receptor antagonists and is also a clinical consequence of pulmonary arterial hypertension and worsening pulmonary arterial hypertension. In the placebo-controlled studies, there was an increased incidence of peripheral edema in patients treated with doses of ambrisentan 5 or 10 mg compared with placebo. Most edema was mild to moderate in severity, and it occurred with greater frequency and severity in elderly patients.

In addition, there have been postmarketing reports of fluid retention occurring within weeks after starting ambrisentan in patients with pulmonary hypertension. Patients required intervention with a diuretic, fluid management, or, in some cases, hospitalization for decompensating heart failure.

If clinically significant fluid retention develops, with or without associated weight gain, undertake further evaluation to determine the cause, such as ambrisentan or underlying heart failure, and the possible need for specific treatment or discontinuation of ambrisentan therapy.

➤*Decreased sperm counts:* In a 6-month study of another endothelin receptor antagonist, bosentan, 25 men with WHO functional class III and IV pulmonary arterial hypertension and normal baseline sperm count were evaluated for effects on testicular function. There was a decline in sperm count of at least 50% in 25% of the patients after 3 or 6 months of treatment with bosentan. One patient developed marked oligospermia at 3 months and the sperm count remained low with 2 follow-up measurements over the subsequent 6 weeks. Bosentan was discontinued and after 2 months, the sperm count had returned to baseline levels. In 22 patients who completed 6 months of treatment, sperm count remained within the normal range and no changes in sperm morphology, sperm motility, or hormone levels were observed. Based on these findings and preclinical data from endothelin receptor antagonists, it cannot be excluded that endothelin receptor antagonists such as ambrisentan have an adverse effect on spermatogenesis.

➤*Pulmonary venoocclusive disease:* If patients develop acute pulmonary edema during initiation of therapy with vasodilating agents such as ambrisentan, the possibility of pulmonary venoocclusive disease should be considered, and if confirmed, ambrisentan should be discontinued.

➤*Prescribing and distribution program:* See the Warning box for more information.

To enroll in LEAP, prescribers must complete the LEAP prescriber enrollment and agreement form indicating agreement to the following (see LEAP prescriber enrollment and agreement form for full prescriber agreement):

- Read the prescribing information and Medication Guide for ambrisentan.
- Enroll all patients in LEAP and reenroll patients after the first 12 months of treatment and annually thereafter.
- Review the ambrisentan Medication Guide and patient education brochure(s) with every patient.
- Educate patients on the risks of ambrisentan, including the risks of hepatotoxicity and teratogenicity.
- Educate and counsel women of childbearing potential to use highly reliable contraception during ambrisentan treatment and for 1 month after stopping treatment. If the patient has had a tubal sterilization or chooses to use a Copper T 380 IUD or levonorgestrel 20 mcg/day IUS for pregnancy prevention, no additional contraception is needed. Women who do not choose 1 of these methods should always use 2 acceptable forms of contraception: 1 hormone method and 1 barrier method, or 2 barrier methods where 1 method is the male condom. Acceptable hormone methods include: progesterone injectables, progesterone implants, combination oral contraceptives, transdermal patch, and vaginal ring. Acceptable barrier methods include: diaphragm (with spermicide), cervical cap (with spermicide), and the male condom. Partner's vasectomy must be used along with a hormone method or barrier method.
- Order and review liver function tests (including aminotransferases and bilirubin) prior to initiation of ambrisentan treatment and monthly during treatment.
- For women of childbearing potential, order and review a pregnancy test prior to initiation of ambrisentan treatment and monthly during treatment.
- Counsel patients who fail to comply with the program requirements.
- Notify LEAP of any adverse reactions, including liver injury, or if any patient becomes pregnant during ambrisentan treatment.

➤*Hepatic function impairment:* Ambrisentan is not recommended in patients with moderate or severe hepatic impairment. There is no information on the use of ambrisentan in patients with mild preexisting impaired liver function; however, exposure to ambrisentan may be increased in these patients.

➤*Pregnancy:* Category X. Ambrisentan may cause fetal harm when administered to a pregnant woman. If this drug is used during pregnancy, or if the patient becomes pregnant while taking this drug, apprise the patient of the potential hazard to a fetus. Ambrisentan was teratogenic at oral dosages of 15 mg/kg/day or more in rats and 7 mg/kg/day or more in rabbits; it was not studied at lower doses. In both species, there were abnormalities of the lower jaw and hard and soft palate, malformation of the heart and great vessels, and failure of formation of the thymus and thyroid. Teratogenicity is a class effect of endothelin receptor antagonists. There are no data on the use of ambrisentan in pregnant women.

See the Warning box for more information.

➤*Lactation:* It is not known whether ambrisentan is excreted in human milk. Breast-feeding while receiving ambrisentan is not recommended. A preclinical study in rats has shown decreased survival of newborn pups (mid and high doses) and effects on testicle size and fertility of pups (high dose) following maternal treatment with ambrisentan from late gestation through weaning. Doses tested were 17, 51, and 170 times (low, mid, and high dose, respectively) the maximum oral human dose of 10 mg on a mg/m^2 basis.

➤*Children:* Safety and efficacy of ambrisentan in children have not been established.

➤*Elderly:* Elderly patients (65 years of age and older) showed less improvement in walk distances with ambrisentan than younger patients, but the results of such subgroup analyses must be interpreted cautiously. Peripheral edema was more common in elderly patients than in younger patients.

➤*Monitoring:* Measure hemoglobin prior to initiation of ambrisentan, at 1 month post initiation, and periodically thereafter.

Monitor liver function tests (including aminotransferases and bilirubin) prior to initiation of ambrisentan treatment and monthly during treatment.

For women of childbearing potential, order and review a pregnancy test prior to initiation of ambrisentan treatment and monthly during treatment.

Drug Interactions

Ambrisentan Drug Interactions

Precipitant drug	Object drug[a]		Description
Cyclosporine	Ambrisentan	⬆	Cyclosporine may cause increased concentrations of ambrisentan. Use with caution. Limit the dosage of ambrisentan to 5 mg daily when coadministered with cyclosporine.
Inducers of P-glycoprotein, CYPs, and UGTs (eg, rifampin)	Ambrisentan	⟷	In healthy volunteers, coadministration of ambrisentan with rifampin was associated with a transient 2-fold increase in ambrisentan AUC; however, by day 7, rifampin had no clinically important effect on ambrisentan AUC or C_{max}. Use with caution.

[a] ⬆ = object drug increased; ⟷ = undetermined clinical effect.

Adverse Reactions

Ambrisentan Adverse Reactions (> 3%)[a]: ARIES-1 and ARIES-2

Adverse reactions	Ambrisentan (n = 261)	Ambrisentan Placebo-adjusted	Placebo (n = 132)
GI			
Abdominal pain	3%	2%	1%
Constipation	4%	2%	2%
Respiratory			
Dyspnea	4%	1%	3%
Nasal congestion	6%	4%	2%
Nasopharyngitis	3%	2%	1%
Sinusitis	3%	3%	0%
Miscellaneous			
Flushing	4%	3%	1%
Headache	15%	1%	14%
Palpitations	5%	3%	2%
Peripheral edema	17%	6%	11%

[a] This table includes all adverse reactions of > 3% incidence in the combined ambrisentan treatment group and more frequent than in the placebo group, with a difference of > 1% between the ambrisentan and placebo groups.

Most adverse drug reactions were mild to moderate, and only nasal congestion was dose dependent. Fewer patients receiving ambrisentan had adverse reactions related to liver function tests compared with placebo.

➤*Peripheral edema:* Few notable differences in the incidence of adverse drug reactions were observed for patients by age or sex. Peripheral edema was similar in younger patients (younger than 65 years of age) receiving ambrisentan (14%) or placebo (13%) and was greater in elderly patients (65 years of age and older) receiving ambrisentan (29%) compared with placebo (4%). The results of such subgroup analyses must be interpreted cautiously.

➤*Serious adverse reactions:* The incidence of patients with serious adverse reactions other than those related to pulmonary hypertension during the clinical trials in patients with pulmonary arterial hypertension was similar for placebo (7%) and for ambrisentan (5%).

Overdosage

➤*Symptoms:* In healthy volunteers, single doses of 50 and 100 mg (5 to 10 times the maximum recommended dose) were associated with headache,

Endothelin Receptor Antagonist

AMBRISENTAN — ORAL

flushing, dizziness, nausea, and nasal congestion. Massive overdosage could potentially result in hypotension that may require intervention.

Patient Information

Advise patients that ambrisentan may cause fetal harm. Only initiate ambrisentan treatment in women of childbearing potential following a negative pregnancy test.

Inform women of childbearing potential of the importance of monthly pregnancy tests and the need to use highly reliable contraception during ambrisentan treatment and for 1 month after stopping treatment. If the patient has had a tubal sterilization or chooses to use a Copper T 380A IUD or levonorgestrel 20 mcg/day IUS for pregnancy prevention, no additional contraception is needed. Women who do not choose 1 of these methods should always use 2 acceptable forms of contraception: 1 hormone method and 1 barrier method, or 2 barrier methods where 1 method is the male condom. Acceptable hormone methods include: progesterone injectables, progesterone implants, combination oral contraceptives, transdermal patch, and vaginal ring. Acceptable barrier methods include: diaphragm (with spermicide), cervical cap (with spermicide), and the male condom. Partner's vasectomy must be used along with a hormone method or a barrier method.

Instruct patients to immediately contact their health care provider if they suspect they may be pregnant.

Advise patients of the importance of monthly liver function testing, and instruct them to immediately report any symptoms of potential liver injury (such as anorexia, nausea, vomiting, fever, malaise, fatigue, right upper quadrant abdominal discomfort, jaundice, dark urine, or itching) to their health care provider.

Advise patients of the importance of hemoglobin testing.

Advise patients not to split, crush, or chew tablets.

Prostacyclin Analog

ILOPROST

Rx	**Ventavis** (Actelion Pharm)	**Solution; inhalation:** 10 mcg/mL	Preservative free. Ethanol 0.81 mg. In 1 mL single-dose ampules.
		20 mcg/mL	Preservative free. Ethanol 1.62 mg. In 1 mL single-dose ampules.

ILOPROST — INHALATION

Indications

➤*Pulmonary arterial hypertension:* For the treatment of pulmonary arterial hypertension (World Health Organization [WHO] group I) in patients with New York Heart Association (NYHA) class III or IV symptoms.

➤*Off-label uses:* Intravenous (IV) administration of iloprost for the treatment of severe Raynaud phenomenon associated with systemic sclerosis.

Administration and Dosage

➤*General dosing considerations:* Iloprost is intended to be inhaled using either of 2 pulmonary drug delivery devices: the *I-neb AAD* (Adaptive Aerosol Delivery) or *Prodose AAD* system.

Iloprost Delivered Doses		
Nebulizer	10 mcg/mL	20 mcg/mL
I-neb AAD	2.5 or 5 mcg from 1 ampule	5 mcg from 1 ampule
Prodose AAD	2.5 or 5 mcg from 2 ampules	Not applicable

The 20 mcg/mL concentration is intended for patients who are maintained at the 5 mcg dose and who have repeatedly experienced extended treatment times that could result in incomplete dosing. Transitioning patients to the 20 mcg/mL concentration using the *I-neb AAD* system will decrease treatment times to help maintain patient compliance.

To avoid potential interruptions in drug delivery caused by equipment malfunctions, the patient should have easy access to a backup *I-neb AAD* or *Prodose AAD* system.

If patients deteriorate while on this treatment, consider alternative treatments. Several patients whose status deteriorated while on iloprost were successfully switched to IV epoprostenol.

➤*Adults:*

Pulmonary arterial hypertension –

Maximum dose: 45 mcg (5 mcg 9 times per day).

Initial dosage: The first inhaled dose should be 2.5 mcg (as delivered at the mouthpiece). If this dose is well tolerated, increase dosing to 5 mcg and maintain that dose; otherwise, maintain the dose at 2.5 mcg. Take iloprost 6 to 9 times/day (no more than every 2 hours) during waking hours, according to individual need and tolerability.

Maintenance dosage: 2.5 to 5 mcg per dose, 6 to 9 times per day.

➤*Preparation for administration:* Iloprost ampules may be opened with an ampule breaker or with a rubber pad. With one hand, hold the bottom of the ampule with the blue dot facing away from the body. With the other hand, wrap the included rubber pad around the entire ampule. Using thumbs, break open the neck of the ampule by snapping the top toward the body and then carefully dispose of the top of the ampule into a sharps bin.

When using an ampule breaker, align the blue dot on the iloprost ampule with the dot on the ampule breaker, if available, and then insert the top of the ampule into the ampule breaker. Gently break open the neck of the ampule by levering away from the dot on the iloprost ampule to snap off the ampule lid. Carefully dispose of the top of the ampule into a sharps bin.

After opening the ampules, use the small tube (pipette) to transfer the entire contents of the ampule into the medication chamber of the *I-neb AAD* or *Prodose AAD* system. If using the *Prodose AAD* system, two 10 mcg/mL ampules need to be added to the medication chamber. Safely dispose of the open ampule and pipette, out of the reach of children and as instructed by a health care provider. Follow the instructions provided by the drug manufacturer for administration of the iloprost dose and maintenance of the *I-neb AAD* or *Prodose AAD* system.

➤*Administration:* For each inhalation session, transfer the entire contents of each opened ampule of iloprost into either the *I-neb AAD* or *Prodose AAD* system medication chamber immediately before use. After each inhalation session, discard any solution remaining in the medication chamber. Use of the remaining solution will result in unpredictable dosing. Follow the manufacturer's instructions for cleaning the *I-neb AAD* or *Prodose AAD* system components after each dose administration.

Administer iloprost 6 to 9 times per day (no more than every 2 hours) during waking hours.

➤*Admixture compatibility:* Direct mixing of iloprost with other medications in the *I-neb AAD* or *Prodose AAD* system has not been evaluated.

➤*Storage / Stability:* Store at 20° to 25°C (68° to 77°F); excursions are permitted to 15° to 30°C (59° to 86°F).

Actions

➤*Pharmacology:* Iloprost is a synthetic analog of prostacyclin PGI_2. Iloprost dilates systemic and pulmonary arterial vascular beds. It also affects platelet aggregation; however, the relevance of this effect to the treatment of pulmonary hypertension is unknown. The 2 diastereoisomers of iloprost differ in their potency in dilating blood vessels, with the 4S isomer substantially more potent than the 4R isomer.

➤*Pharmacokinetics:* In pharmacokinetic studies in animals, there was no evidence of interconversion of the 2 diastereoisomers of iloprost. In human pharmacokinetic studies, the 2 diastereoisomers were not individually assayed.

Absorption – Iloprost administered IV has linear pharmacokinetics over the dosage range of 1 to 3 ng/kg/min.

The absolute bioavailability of inhaled iloprost has not been determined. Following inhalation of iloprost (5 mcg), patients with pulmonary hypertension have iloprost peak serum levels of approximately 150 pg/mL. Iloprost was generally not detectable in the plasma 30 minutes to 1 hour after inhalation.

Distribution – Following IV infusion, the apparent steady-state volume of distribution was 0.7 to 0.8 L/kg in healthy subjects. Iloprost is approximately 60% protein bound, mainly to albumin, and this ratio is concentration independent in the range of 30 to 3,000 pg/mL.

Metabolism / Excretion – Clearance in healthy subjects was approximately 20 mL/min/kg. Iloprost is metabolized principally via beta-oxidation of the carboxyl side chain. The main metabolite is tetranor-iloprost, which is found in the urine in free and conjugated form.

In vitro studies reveal that cytochrome P-450–dependent metabolism plays only a minor role in the biotransformation of iloprost. A mass-balance study using IV and oral [^{3}H]-iloprost in healthy subjects (n = 8) showed that recovery of total radioactivity more than 14 hours postdose was 81%, with 68% and 12% recoveries in urine and feces, respectively.

The half-life of iloprost is 20 to 30 minutes.

Special populations –

Renal function impairment: Inhaled iloprost has not been evaluated in subjects with impaired renal function. In a study with IV infusion of iloprost in patients with end-stage renal failure requiring intermittent dialysis treatment (n = 7), the mean area under the plasma concentration-time curve ($AUC_{0\text{-}4h}$) was 230 pg•h/mL compared with 54 pg•h/mL in patients with renal failure (n = 8) not requiring intermittent dialysis and 48 pg•h/mL in healthy patients. The half-life was similar in both groups.

Hepatic function impairment: Inhaled iloprost has not been evaluated in subjects with impaired hepatic function. In an IV iloprost study in patients with liver cirrhosis, the mean clearance in Child-Pugh class B subjects (n = 5) was approximately 10 mL/min/kg (half that of healthy patients). Following oral administration, the mean $AUC_{0\text{-}8h}$ in Child-Pugh class B patients (n = 3) was 1,725 pg•h/mL compared with 117 pg•h/mL in healthy subjects (n = 4) receiving the same oral iloprost dose. In Child-Pugh class A subjects (n = 5), the mean $AUC_{0\text{-}8h}$ was 639 pg•h/mL. Although exposure increased with hepatic impairment, there was no effect on half-life.

ILOPROST — INHALATION

Contraindications

None known.

Warnings/Precautions

➤*Administration:* See Administration and Dosage for more information.

➤*Syncope:* Because of the risk of syncope, monitor vital signs while initiating iloprost. In patients with low systemic blood pressure, take care to avoid further hypotension. Do not initiate iloprost in patients with systolic blood pressure less than 85 mm Hg. Be alert to the presence of concomitant conditions or drugs that might increase the risk of syncope. Syncope can also occur in association with pulmonary arterial hypertension, particularly in association with physical exertion. The occurrence of exertional syncope may reflect a therapeutic gap or insufficient efficacy; consider the need to adjust dose or change therapy.

➤*Pulmonary edema:* If signs of pulmonary edema occur when inhaled iloprost is administered in patients with pulmonary hypertension, stop the treatment immediately. This may be a sign of pulmonary venous hypotension.

➤*Contact with iloprost solution:* Do not allow iloprost solution to come into contact with the skin or eyes; avoid oral ingestion of iloprost solution.

➤*Renal function impairment:* Dose adjustment is not required in patients not on dialysis. Use caution in treating patients on dialysis.

➤*Hepatic function impairment:* Because iloprost elimination is reduced in patients with impaired liver function, exercise caution during iloprost therapy in patients with at least Child-Pugh class B hepatic impairment.

➤*Pregnancy: Category C.* In developmental toxicity studies in pregnant Han-Wistar rats, continuous IV administration of iloprost at a dosage of 0.01 mg/kg/day (serum levels not available) led to shortened digits of the thoracic extremity in fetuses and pups. In comparable studies in pregnant Sprague-Dawley rats that received iloprost clathrate (13% iloprost by weight) orally at dosages of up to 50 mg/kg/day (maximum plasma concentration [C_{max}] of 90 ng/mL), in pregnant rabbits at IV dosages of up to 0.5 mg/kg/day (C_{max} of 86 ng/mL), and in pregnant monkeys at dosages of up to 0.04 mg/kg/day (serum levels of 1 ng/mL), no such digital anomalies or other gross-structural abnormalities were observed in the fetuses/pups. However, in gravid Sprague-Dawley rats, iloprost clathrate (13% iloprost) significantly increased the number of nonviable fetuses at a maternally toxic oral dosage of 250 mg/kg/day and in Han-Wistar rats was found to be embryolethal in 15 of 44 litters at an IV dosage of 1 mg/kg/day. There are no adequate and well-controlled studies in pregnant women. Use during pregnancy only if the potential benefit justifies the potential risk to the fetus.

➤*Lactation:* It is not known whether iloprost is excreted in human milk. In studies with Han-Wistar rats, higher mortality was observed in pups of lactating dams receiving iloprost IV at 1 mg/kg/day. In Sprague-Dawley rats, higher mortality was also observed in nursing pups at a maternally toxic oral dosage of 250 mg/kg/day of iloprost clathrate (13% iloprost by weight). It is not known whether this drug is excreted in human milk. Because many drugs are excreted in human milk and because of the potential for serious adverse reactions in breast-feeding infants from iloprost, decide whether to discontinue breast-feeding or the drug, taking into account the importance of the drug to the mother.

➤*Children:* Safety and efficacy in children have not been established.

➤*Monitoring:* Because of the risk of syncope, monitor vital signs while initiating iloprost. Do not initiate iloprost in patients with systolic blood pressure less than 85 mm Hg.

Drug Interactions

➤*Vasodilators/antihypertensive agents:* Iloprost has the potential to increase the hypotensive effect of vasodilators and antihypertensive agents.

Adverse Reactions

Safety data on iloprost were obtained from 215 patients with pulmonary arterial hypertension receiving iloprost in two 12-week clinical trials and 2 long-term extensions. Patients received inhaled iloprost for periods ranging from 1 day to more than 3 years. The mean number of weeks of exposure was 15 weeks. Forty patients completed 12 months of open-label treatment with iloprost.

The following table shows adverse reactions reported by at least 4 iloprost patients and reported at least 3% more frequently for iloprost patients than placebo patients in the 12-week, placebo-controlled study.

Iloprost Adverse Reactions

Adverse reaction	Iloprost (n = 101)	Placebo (n = 102)	Placebo subtracted
Cardiovascular			
Hypotension	11%	6%	5%
Palpitations	7%	4%	3%
Syncope	8%	5%	3%
Vasodilation (flushing)	27%	9%	18%
CNS			
Headache	30%	20%	10%
Insomnia	8%	2%	6%
GI			
Nausea	13%	8%	5%
Vomiting	7%	2%	5%
Lab test abnormalities			
Abnormal lab test	7%	3%	4%
Increased alkaline phosphatase	6%	1%	5%
Increased gamma-glutamyltransferase (GGT)	6%	3%	3%
Respiratory			
Hemoptysis	5%	2%	3%
Increased cough	39%	26%	13%
Pneumonia	4%	1%	3%
Miscellaneous			
Back pain	7%	3%	4%
Flu syndrome	14%	10%	4%
Muscle cramps	6%	3%	3%
Tongue pain	4%	0%	4%
Trismus	12%	3%	9%

Serious adverse reactions reported with the use of inhaled iloprost and not shown in the previous table include chest pain, congestive heart failure, dyspnea, kidney failure, peripheral edema, and supraventricular tachycardia.

In a small clinical trial (the STEP trial), safety trends in patients receiving concomitant bosentan and iloprost were consistent with those observed in the larger experience of the phase 3 study in patients receiving only iloprost.

➤*Adverse reactions with higher doses:* In a study in healthy volunteers (n = 160), inhaled doses of iloprost solution were given every 2 hours, beginning with 5 mcg and increasing up to 20 mcg for a total of 6 dose inhalations (total cumulative dose of 70 mcg) or up to the highest dose tolerated in a subgroup of 40 volunteers. There were 13 subjects (32%) who failed to reach the highest scheduled dose (20 mcg). Five were unable to increase the dose because of mild to moderate transient chest pain/discomfort/tightness, usually accompanied by headache, nausea, and dizziness. The remaining 8 subjects discontinued for other reasons.

Overdosage

➤*Symptoms:* In clinical trials of iloprost, no case of overdose was reported. Signs and symptoms to be anticipated are extensions of the dose-limiting pharmacological effects, including diarrhea, flushing, headache, hypotension, nausea, and vomiting.

➤*Treatment:* A specific antidote is not known. Interruption of the inhalation session, monitoring, and symptomatic measures are recommended.

Patient Information

Advise patients receiving iloprost to use the drug only as prescribed with either of 2 pulmonary drug delivery devices, the *I-neb AAD* or *Prodose AAD* system following the manufacturer's instructions. Train patients in proper administration techniques, including dosing frequency, ampule dispensing, *I-neb AAD* or *Prodose AAD* system operation, and equipment cleaning.

Advise patients that they may have a fall in blood pressure with iloprost, so they may become dizzy or even faint. Instruct patients to stand up slowly when they get out of a chair or bed. If fainting gets worse, advise patients to consult their health care provider about dose adjustment.

Advise patients to inhale iloprost at intervals of not less than 2 hours and that the acute benefits of iloprost may not last 2 hours.

Advise patients to avoid oral ingestion or skin contact of iloprost solution.

Advise patients that the most common adverse reactions with iloprost include flushing, increased cough, hypotension, headache, nausea, spasms of the jaw muscles that cause trouble opening the mouth, and syncope.

Advise patients not to put any other medicines in the *I-neb AAD* or *Prodose AAD* system while using iloprost.

ISOSORBIDE DINITRATE and HYDRALAZINE HYDROCHLORIDE

Rx	BiDil (NitroMed[a])	Tablets: 20 mg isosorbide dinitrate/ 37.5 mg hydralazine hydrochloride	Lactose. (N 20). Orange, scored. Film-coated. In 180s.

[a] NitroMed, Inc., 15 Ingram Boulevard, Lavergne, TN 37086; (781) 266-4186.

ISOSORBIDE DINITRATE and HYDRALAZINE HYDROCHLORIDE — ORAL

For additional prescribing information, refer to the Nitratesclass monograph and the Hydralazine individual monograph.

Indications

➤*Heart failure:* For the treatment of heart failure as an adjunct to standard therapy in self-identified black patients to improve survival, to prolong time to hospitalization for heart failure, and to improve patient-reported functional status. There is little experience in patients with the New York Heart Association class IV heart failure.

Administration and Dosage

➤*Adults:*

Heart failure –

Usual dosage: One tablet 3 times a day.

Maximum dose: May be titrated to a maximum tolerated dose not to exceed 2 tablets 3 times a day.

Initial dosage: One tablet 3 times a day.

Dosage titration: Although titration can be rapid (3 to 5 days), some patients may experience adverse effects and may take longer to reach their maximum tolerated dose. The dosage may be decreased to as little as one-half tablet 3 times a day if intolerable adverse effects occur. Efforts should be made to titrate up as soon as adverse effects subside.

➤*Children:* Safety and effectiveness in children have not been established.

➤*Storage / Stability:* Store at 25°C (77°F), excursions are permitted to 15° to 30°C (59° to 86°F).

Warnings/Precautions

➤*Pregnancy: Category C.* The molecular weight (about 236) of isosorbide dinitrate is low enough that passage to the fetus should be expected. Hydralazine readily crosses the placenta to the fetus. Serum concentrations in the fetus are equal to or greater than those in the mother. Hydralazine was associated with significantly more maternal hypotension, placental abruption, cesarean sections, and oliguria, with more adverse effects on fetal heart rate and with lower Apgar scores. There are no studies using isosorbide dinitrate in pregnant women. Therefore, isosorbide dinitrate should be used with caution during pregnancy only if the potential benefit justifies the potential risk to the fetus.

➤*Lactation:* Hydralazine is excreted into breast milk. The molecular weight (about 236) of isosorbide dinitrate is low enough that excretion into breast milk should be expected. Exercise caution when isosorbide dinitrate/hydralazine is administered to a breast-feeding woman.

ANTIADRENERGICS/SYMPATHOLYTICS

Beta-Adrenergic Blocking Agents (Beta Blockers)

WARNING

Atenolol, metoprolol, nadolol, propranolol, timolol – There have been reports of exacerbation of angina and, in some cases, myocardial infarction and ventricular arrythmias, following abrupt discontinuance of beta-adrenergic blocking agents therapy. Therefore, when discontinuance of beta-adrenergic blocking agents is planned, gradually reduce the dosage over at least a few weeks, and caution the patient against interruption or cessation of therapy without a physician's advice. If beta-adrenergic blocking agents therapy is interrupted and exacerbation of angina occurs or acute coronary insufficiency develops, it is usually advisable to promptly reinstitute beta-adrenergic blocking agents therapy and take other measures appropriate for the management of angina pectoris. Because coronary artery disease may be unrecognized, it may be prudent to follow the above advice in patients who are given beta-adrenergic blocking agents for other indications.

Sotalol – To minimize the risk of induced arrhythmia, place patients initiated or reinitiated on sotalol or sotalol AF for a minimum of 3 days (on their maintenance dose) in a facility that can provide cardiac resuscitation, continuous electrocardiographic monitoring, and calculations of creatinine clearance. For detailed instructions regarding dose selection and special cautions for people with renal impairment, see Administration and Dosage.

Do not substitute sotalol for sotalol AF because of significant differences in labeling (eg, patient package insert, dosing administration, safety administration).

Indications

➤*Hypertension (all except esmolol and sotalol):* Used alone as initial drug choice or in combination with other drugs, particularly a thiazide diuretic. Not indicated for treatment of hypertensive emergencies.

➤*Angina pectoris (nadolol, propranolol, atenolol, metoprolol):* Long-term management.

➤*Hypertrophic subaortic stenosis (propranolol):* Useful in managing exertional or other stress-induced angina, palpitations, and syncope. Improves exercise performance. Efficacy appears to be caused by reduction of elevated outflow pressure gradient that is exacerbated by beta receptor stimulation. Clinical improvement may be temporary.

➤*Cardiac arrhythmias (acebutolol, esmolol, propranolol, sotalol):* Use acebutolol for ventricular premature beats only. Use sotalol for documented life-threatening ventricular arrhythmias, such as sustained ventricular tachycardia.

Supraventricular arrhythmias (propranolol) – Paroxysmal atrial tachycardias, particularly those arrhythmias induced by catecholamines or digitalis or associated with the Wolff-Parkinson-White syndrome); persistent sinus tachycardia that is noncompensatory and impairs the well-being of the patient.

Tachycardias and arrhythmias caused by thyrotoxicosis when they cause distress or increased hazard and when immediate effect is necessary as adjunctive, short-term (2 to 4 weeks) therapy. May be used with, but not in place of, specific therapy.

Persistent atrial extrasystoles that impair the well-being of the patient and do not respond to conventional measures. Atrial flutter and fibrillation when ventricular rate cannot be controlled by digitalis alone, or when digitalis is contraindicated.

Supraventricular tachycardia (esmolol) – Rapid control of ventricular rate in patients with atrial fibrillation or atrial flutter in perioperative, postoperative, or other emergent circumstances in which short-term control of ventricular rate with a short-acting agent is desirable.

Sinus tachycardia (esmolol) – Noncompensatory sinus tachycardia in which the rapid heart rate requires intervention. Esmolol is not intended for use in chronic settings where transfer to another agent is anticipated.

Intraoperative and postoperative tachycardia and hypertension (esmolol) – Treatment of tachycardia and hypertension that may occur during induction and tracheal intubation, during surgery, on emergence from anesthesia, and in the postoperative period, when in the physician's judgment such specific intervention is indicated.

Ventricular tachycardias (propranolol) – In ventricular tachycardias, with the exception of those induced by catecholamines or digitalis, propranolol is not the drug of first choice. In critical situations when cardioversion techniques or other drugs are not indicated or are ineffective, propranolol may be considered.

Persistent premature ventricular extrasystoles that impair the well-being of the patient and do not respond to conventional measures.

Tachyarrhythmias of digitalis intoxication (propranolol) – If it is persistent following discontinuation of digitalis and correction of electrolyte abnormalities, tachyarrhythmias are usually reversible with oral propranolol. Severe bradycardia may occur. Reserve IV propranolol for life-threatening arrhythmias. Temporary maintenance with oral therapy may be indicated.

Resistant tachyarrhythmias caused by excessive catecholamine action during anesthesia (propranolol) – All general inhalation anesthetics produce some degree of myocardial depression; therefore, use propranolol with extreme caution.

Maintenance of normal sinus rhythm (sotalol) – In patients with highly symptomatic atrial fibrillation/atrial flutter (AFIB/AFL) who are currently in sinus rhythm (*Betapace AF* only).

➤*MI (propranolol, timolol):* Indicated in clinically stable patients who have survived the acute phase of an MI to reduce cardiovascular mortality and risk of reinfarction. Initiate treatment within 1 to 4 weeks after infarction.

Metoprolol and atenolol – Both are also indicated in the treatment of hemodynamically stable patients with definite or suspected acute MI. Treatment can be initiated as soon as the patient's clinical condition allows or within 3 to 10 days of the acute event.

➤*Congestive heart failure (metoprolol):* Treatment of stable, symptomatic (NYHA Class II or III) heart failure of ischemic, hypertensive, or cardiomyopathic origin (*Toprol-XL* 25 mg only). Studied in patients already receiving ACE inhibitors, diuretics, and, in the majority of cases, digitalis. In this population, *Toprol-XL* decreased the rate of mortality plus hospitalization, largely through a reduction in cardiovascular mortality and hospitalizations for heart failure.

➤*Pheochromocytoma (propranolol):* After primary treatment with an alpha-adrenergic blocking agent has been instituted, propranolol may be useful as adjunctive therapy if the control of tachycardia becomes necessary before or during surgery.

With inoperable or metastatic pheochromocytoma, propranolol may be useful as an adjunct to the management of symptoms caused by excessive beta receptor stimulation.

➤*Migraine (propranolol, timolol):* For the prophylaxis of common migraine headache.

➤*Essential tremor (propranolol):* For the management of familial or hereditary essential tremor consisting of involuntary, rhythmic, and oscillatory movements. Propranolol causes a reduction in the tremor amplitude but not in the tremor frequency. It is not indicated for the treatment of tremor associated with Parkinsonism.

➤*Off-label uses:* Refer to individual monographs for further information.

Fibromyalgia –
Pindolol: [4] = Insufficient documentation.

Pediatric hypertension –
Atenolol: [3] = Safety concerns.
Metoprolol: [3] = Safety concerns.

Pediatric hypertensive urgency or emergency –
Esmolol: [1] = Good documentation.

Prevention of migraine (adults) –
Atenolol: [2] = Fair documentation.
Metoprolol: [2] = Fair documentation.
Nadolol: [1] = Good documentation.
Pindolol: [5] = Poor documentation.

Prevention of migraine (children/adolescents) –
Propranolol: [4] = Insufficient documentation.

Prevention of supraventricular arrhythmia –
Atenolol: [4] = Insufficient documentation.

Prevention of variceal bleeding –
Atenolol: [5] = Poor documentation.

Smoking cessation –
Propranolol: [5] = Poor documentation.

Thyrotoxicosis –
Acebutolol: [4] = Insufficient documentation.

Traumatic brain injury –
Pindolol: [2] = Fair documentation.
Propranolol: [2] = Fair documentation.

Ventricular tachycardia –
Acebutolol: [1] = Good documentation.

Other possible off-label uses – The agents listed have been evaluated for use in the following conditions:

Akathisia (antipsychotic-induced): Propranolol (30 to 120 mg/day), metoprolol (50 to 400 mg/day).

Atrial fibrillation (rapid heart rate control): Metoprolol (2.5 to 5 mg IV bolus over 2 minutes, up to 3 doses).

Atrial fibrillation (maintenance heart rate control): Metoprolol (25 to 100 mg twice daily).

Angina (stable): Acebutolol, bisoprolol.

Angina (unstable): Atenolol (5 mg over 5 minutes IV, up to 3 doses; 25 to 100 mg/day orally), esmolol (500 mcg/kg bolus and infusion of 10 to 200 mcg/kg/minute), metoprolol (5 mg over 5 minutes IV, up to 3 doses; 25 to 100 mg twice daily orally).

Congestive heart failure (stable): Immediate-release metoprolol (initial dose of 12.5 mg twice daily, increase to up to 50 mg twice daily), bisoprolol (initial dose of 2.5 mg daily, increase to up to 10 mg daily).

Generalized anxiety disorder: Propranolol (initial dose of 10 mg twice daily; maximum daily dose is 360 mg).

Hypertensive crises: Esmolol (loading dose of 500 mcg/kg over 1 minute, followed by infusion at 25 to 50 mcg/kg/min, which may be increased by 25 mcg/kg/min every 10 to 20 minutes until the desired response is obtained; maximum dose is 300 mcg/kg/min).

Hyperthyroidism adjunctive therapy: Propranolol and nadolol may provide symptomatic improvement until euthyroid state is achieved.

Parkinsonian tremor: Propranolol SR (initial dose of 60 mg in the morning; may be increased up to 160 mg/day); nadolol.

Prevention of variceal bleeding caused by portal hypertension: Propranolol (initial dose of 40 mg twice daily; average maintenance dose is 160 mg/day), nadolol (80 mg/day), atenolol, timolol, metoprolol.

Supraventricular arrhythmias: Atenolol 50 mg/day, started 72 hours before coronary artery bypass operations, appears effective in reducing the incidence of supraventricular arrhythmias.

Beta-Adrenergic Blocking Agents – Summary of Indications[a]

Indications ✓ = labeled x = unlabeled	Acebutolol	Atenolol	Betaxolol	Bisoprolol	Esmolol	Metoprolol[b]	Nadolol	Nebivolol	Penbutolol	Pindolol	Propranolol	Sotalol	Timolol
Hypertension	✓	✓	✓	✓		✓	✓	✓	✓	✓	✓		✓
Pediatric hypertensive urgency or emergency					x[g]	x[i]							
Angina pectoris		✓				✓	✓				✓		
Cardiac arrhythmias													
Supraventricular arrhythmias/tachycardias		x[j]			✓						✓		
Sinus tachycardia					✓								
Intraoperative and postoperative tachycardia and hypertension					✓								
Ventricular arrhythmias/tachycardias	x[g]										✓	✓[c]	
Premature ventricular contractions (PVCs)	✓										✓		
Digitalis-induced tachyarrhythmias											✓		
Resistant tachyarrhythmias (during anesthesia)											✓		
Atrial ectopy						x[k]							
Maintenance of normal sinus rhythm												✓	
MI		✓				✓					✓		✓
CHF (stable)[d]				x[k]		✓[e]							
Pheochromocytoma											✓		
Migraine prevention(adults)		x[h]				x[h]	x[g]				✓		✓
Migraine prevention (children/adolescents)											x[j]		
Hypertrophic subaortic stenosis											✓		
Parkinsonian tremors							x[k]				x[f]		
Akathisia, antipsychotic-induced						x[k]					x[k]		
Variceal bleeding in portal hypertension						x[k]	x[k]				x[k]		x[k]
Atrial fibrillation													
Rapid heart rate control						x[k]							
Maintenance heart rate control						x[k]							
Generalized anxiety disorder											x[k]		
Angina													
Stable	x[k]			x[k]									
Unstable		x[k]			x[k]	x[k]							

Beta-Adrenergic Blocking Agents (Beta Blockers)

Beta-Adrenergic Blocking Agents – Summary of Indications[a]

Indications ✓= labeled x = unlabeled	Acebutolol	Atenolol	Betaxolol	Bisoprolol	Esmolol	Metoprolol[b]	Nadolol	Nebivolol	Penbutolol	Pindolol	Propranolol[b]	Sotalol	Timolol
Fibromyalgia										x[i]			
Thyrotoxicosis	x[i]												

[a] For more detailed information, see preceding Indications and individual monographs.
[b] Includes long-acting formulation.
[c] Not *Betapace AF*.
[d] See Precautions or Warnings.
[e] *Toprol-XL* 25 mg only.
[f] Sustained-release only.
[g] Good documentation.
[h] Fair documentation.
[i] Safety concerns.
[j] Insufficient documentation.
[k] Not rated.

Actions

➤*Pharmacology:*

Pharmacologic/Pharmacokinetic Properties of Beta-Adrenergic Blocking Agents

Drug (0 – none; + – low; ++ – moderate; +++ – high)	Adrenergic-receptor blocking activity	Membrane stabilizing activity	Intrinsic sympathomimetic activity	Lipid solubility	Extent of absorption (%)	Absolute oral bioavailability (%)	Half-life (hrs)	Protein binding (%)	Metabolism/Excretion
Acebutolol	β_1[a]	+[b]	+	Low	90	20-60	3-4	26	Hepatic; renal excretion 30% to 40%; nonrenal excretion 50% to 60% (bile; intestinal wall)
Atenolol	β_1[a]	0	0	Low	50	50-60	6-7	6-16	≈ 50% excreted unchanged in feces
Betaxolol	β_1[a]	+	0	Low	≈ 100	89	14-22	≈ 50	Hepatic; > 80% recovered in urine, 15% unchanged
Bisoprolol	β_1[a]	0	0	Low	≥ 90	80	9-12	≈ 30	≈ 50% excreted unchanged in urine, remainder as inactive metabolites; < 2% excreted in feces.
Esmolol	β_1[a]	0	0	Low	na[c]	na[c]	0.15	55	Rapid metabolism by esterases in cytosol of red blood cells
Metoprolol	β_1[a]	0[b]	0	Moderate	≈ 100	40-50	3-7	12	Hepatic; renal excretion,
Metoprolol, long-acting						77[d]			
Nadolol	β_1 β_2	0	0	Low	30	30-50	20-24	30	Urine, unchanged
Nebivolol	β_1[a]	0	0	High	nd[f]	nd[f]	12 (extensive metabolizers) 19 (poor metabolizers)	98	38% excreted in urine and 44% in feces (extensive metabolizers); 67% in urine and 13% in feces (poor metabolizers)
Penbutolol	β_1 β_2	0	+	High	≈ 100	≈ 100	≈ 5	80-98	Hepatic (conjugation, oxidation); renal excretion of metabolites (17% as conjugate)
Pindolol	β_1 β_2	0	+++	Low	> 95	≈ 100	3-4[e]	40	Urinary excretion of metabolites (60% to 65%) and unchanged drug (35% to 40%)
Propranolol	β_1 β_2	++	0	High	< 90	30	3-5	90	Hepatic; < 1% excreted unchanged in urine
Propranolol, long-acting						9-18	8-11		
Sotalol	β_1 β_2	0	0	Low	nd[f]	90-100	12	0	Not metabolized; excreted unchanged in urine
Timolol	β_1 β_2	0	0	Low to moderate	90	75	4	< 10	Hepatic; urinary excretion of metabolites and unchanged drug

[a] Inhibits β_2 receptors (bronchial and vascular) at higher doses.
[b] Detectable only at doses much greater than required for beta blockade.
[c] Not applicable (available IV only).
[d] Average bioavailability; not absolute.
[e] In elderly hypertensive patients with normal renal function, t½ variable: 7 to 15 hours.
[f] No data.

Beta-adrenergic receptor blocking agents compete with beta-adrenergic agonists for available beta receptor sites. Propranolol, nadolol, timolol, penbutolol, sotalol, and pindolol inhibit both the β_1 receptors (located chiefly in myocardium, kidney, and eye) and β_2 receptors (located chiefly in adipose tissue, pancreas, liver, and smooth and skeletal muscle), inhibiting the chronotropic, inotropic, and vasodilator responses to β-adrenergic stimulation. Metoprolol, acebutolol, bisoprolol, nebivolol, esmolol, betaxolol, and atenolol are cardioselective and preferentially inhibit β_1 receptors.

Propranolol and, to a lesser extent, acebutolol and betaxolol, exert a quinidine-like (anesthetic) membrane action (membrane stabilizing activity; MSA), which affects cardiac action potential. Pindolol, penbutolol, and acebutolol have intrinsic sympathomimetic activity (ISA) in therapeutic dosage ranges. ISA or partial agonist activity is mediated directly at adrenergic receptor sites and may be blocked by other β antagonists. ISA is manifested by a smaller reduction in resting cardiac output and resting heart rate (4 to 8 beats per minute [BPM]) than is seen with drugs lacking ISA; clinical significance has not been evaluated and there is no evidence that exercise cardiac output is less affected by pindolol.

➤*Pharmacokinetics:*

Absorption – Systemic bioavailability following oral administration of metoprolol, acebutolol, timolol, and propranolol is low because of significant first-pass hepatic metabolism. Pindolol and sotalol have no significant first-pass effect; first-pass metabolism of bisoprolol is ≈ 20%. Ingestion with food enhances the bioavailability of propranolol and metoprolol, and reduces the absorption of sotalol; this effect is not noted with nadolol, nebivolol, pindolol, bisoprolol, or betaxolol.

Distribution – There is no simple correlation between dose or plasma level and therapeutic effect; the dose-sensitivity range observed in clinical practice is wide because sympathetic tone varies widely among individuals. There is no reliable test to estimate sympathetic tone or to determine whether total β-blockade has been achieved; proper dosage requires titration. There appear to be significant correlations between acebutolol plasma levels and both the reduction in resting heart rate and the percent of β-blockade of exercise-induced tachycardia.

Metoprolol and propranolol readily enter the CNS. Because of their high water solubility, sotalol, acebutolol, nadolol, and atenolol do not pass the blood-brain barrier; these drugs may have a lower incidence of CNS side effects.

Contraindications

Sinus bradycardia; greater than first-degree heart block; cardiogenic shock; CHF unless secondary to a tachyarrhythmia treatable with beta-blockers; overt cardiac failure; hypersensitivity to beta-blocking agents.

➤*Acebutolol:* Persistently severe bradycardia.

➤*Propranolol, nadolol, timolol, penbutolol, sotalol, and pindolol:* Bronchial asthma, including severe chronic obstructive pulmonary disease.

➤*Metoprolol:* Treatment of MI in patients with a heart rate less than 45 BPM; significant heart block greater than first-degree (PR interval greater than or equal to 0.24 sec); systolic blood pressure less than 100 mm Hg; moderate to severe cardiac failure.

➤*Nebivolol:* Severe bradycardia, sick sinus syndrome (unless a permanent pacemaker is in place), severe hepatic impairment (Child-Pugh greater than class B).

➤*Sotalol:* Congenital or acquired long QT syndromes.

Warnings/Precautions

➤*Mortality:* The National Heart Lung and Blood Institute conducted the Cardiac Arrhythmia Suppression Trial (CAST-I), a long-term, multicenter, randomized, double-blind study in patients with asymptomatic non-life-threatening ventricular ectopy who had an MI > 6 days but < 2 years previously. An excessive mortality or nonfatal cardiac arrest was seen in patients treated with encainide or flecainide (56/730) compared with that seen in patients assigned to matched placebo-treated groups (22/725), and a similar excess has been seen with moricizine. The average duration of treatment with encainide or flecainide in this study was 10 months.

CAST-II originally was designed as a blinded, randomized trial divided into a 14-day exposure phase to evaluate the risk of initiating treatment with moricizine after MI, and a long-term phase to evaluate survival after MI. The study was stopped early because the first 14-day period of treatment with moricizine after MI was associated with excess mortality, as compared with no treatment or placebo. As with the antiarrhythmic agents used in CAST-I, the use of moricizine to reduce mortality after MI is not only ineffective, but also harmful.

The applicability of these results to other populations (eg, those without recent MI) and to other than Class I antiarrhythmic agents is uncertain. **Sotalol** is devoid of Class I effects, and in a large controlled trial in patients with a recent MI who did not necessarily have ventricular arrhythmias, sotalol did not produce increased mortality at doses up to 320 mg/day. Conversely, in the large postinfarction study using a nontitrated initial dose of 320 mg once daily and in a second small randomized trial in high-risk postinfarction patients treated with high doses (320 mg twice daily), there have been suggestions of an excess of early sudden deaths.

➤*Proarrhythmia:* Like other antiarrhythmic agents, sotalol can provoke new or worsened ventricular arrhythmias in some patients, including sustained ventricular tachycardia or ventricular fibrillation, with potentially fatal consequences. Because of its effect on cardiac repolarization (QTc interval prolongation), torsades de pointes (a polymorphic ventricular tachycardia with prolongation of the QT interval and a shifting electrical axis) is the most common form of proarrhythmia associated with sotalol, occurring in about 4% of high-risk (history of sustained ventricular tachycardia/ventricular fibrillation [VT/VF]) patients. The risk of torsades de pointes progressively increases with prolongation of the QT interval and is worsened also by reduction in heart rate and reduction in serum potassium.

Overall, 4.3% of patients experienced a new or worsened ventricular arrhythmia. Of this 4.3%, there was new or worsened sustained ventricular tachycardia in approximately 1% of patients and torsades de pointes in 2.4%. Additionally, in approximately 1% of patients, deaths were considered possibly drug-related and may have been associated with proarrhythmic events. In patients with a history of sustained ventricular tachycardia, the incidence of torsades de pointes was 4% and worsened VT approximately 1%; in patients with other, less serious, ventricular and supraventricular arrhythmias, the incidence of torsades de pointes was 1% and 1.4%, respectively. Torsade de pointes arrhythmias were dose related.

In addition to dose and presence of sustained VT, other risk factors for torsades de pointes were gender (females had a higher incidence), excessive prolongation of the QTc interval, and history of cardiomegaly or CHF. Patients with sustained ventricular tachycardia and a history of CHF appear to have the highest risk for serious proarrhythmia (7%). Of the patients experiencing torsades de pointes, ≈ ⅔ spontaneously reverted to their baseline rhythm. The others were either converted electrically (D/C cardioversion or overdrive pacing) or treated with other drugs. Although **sotalol** therapy was discontinued in most patients experiencing torsades de pointes, 17% were continued on a lower dose. Nonetheless, use with particular caution if the QTc is > 500 msec on-therapy and give serious consideration to reducing the dose or discontinuing therapy when the QTc exceeds 550 msec. However, because of the multiple risk factors associated with torsades de pointes, exercise caution regardless of the QTc interval.

Proarrhythmic events must be anticipated not only on initiating sotalol therapy, but with every upward dose adjustment. Proarrhythmic events most often occur within 7 days of initiating therapy or of an increase in dose; 75% of serious proarrhythmias (torsades de pointes and worsened VT) occurred within 7 days of initiating therapy, while 60% of such events occurred within 3 days of initiation or a dosage change. Initiating therapy at 80 mg twice daily with gradual upward dose titration and appropriate evaluations for efficacy and safety prior to dose escalation, should reduce the risk of proarrhythmia. Avoiding excessive accumulation of sotalol in patients with diminished renal function, by appropriate dose reduction, should also reduce the risk of proarrhythmia.

➤*Cardiac failure:* Sympathetic stimulation is a vital component supporting circulatory function in CHF, and beta-blockade carries the potential hazard of further depressing myocardial contractility and precipitating more severe failure. Administer cautiously in hypertensive patients who have CHF controlled by digitalis and diuretics. Beta-blockers do not abolish the inotropic action of digitalis on heart muscle. Digitalis and beta-blockers slow AV conduction. If cardiac failure persists, withdraw beta-blocker therapy. Although cardiac failure rarely occurs in properly selected patients, advise patients to consult a physician at the first sign or symptom of impending CHF or unexplained respiratory symptoms.

In patients without a history of cardiac failure, continued myocardial depression can lead to cardiac failure. At the first sign or symptom of impending cardiac failure, fully digitalize patients or treat with diuretics and closely observe the response. If cardiac failure continues, withdraw therapy (gradually, if possible).

Studies suggest that in certain patients with CHF, beta blockers may result in symptomatic and hemodynamic improvements. β_1 selective agents are the drugs of choice; start with a low dose and titrate upward. They should not be used as routine therapy nor for acute heart failure. In these studies, most patients had idiopathic dilated cardiomyopathy. Further study is needed to identify patients most likely to benefit from therapy as well as the appropriate drug.

➤*Wolff-Parkinson-White syndrome:* In several cases, the tachycardia was replaced by a severe bradycardia requiring a demand pacemaker after **propranolol** administration with as little as 5 mg.

➤*Abrupt withdrawal:* The occurrence of a β-blocker withdrawal syndrome is controversial. However, hypersensitivity to catecholamines has been observed in patients withdrawn from β-blocker therapy. Exacerbation of angina, MI, ventricular arrhythmias, and death have occurred after abrupt discontinuation of therapy. When discontinuing chronically administered β-blocking agents, particularly in patients with ischemic heart disease, reduce dosage gradually over 1 to 2 weeks and carefully monitor the patient. If therapy with an alternative β-adrenergic blocker is desired, the patient may be transferred directly to comparable doses of another agent without interrupting β-blocking therapy. If angina markedly worsens or acute coronary insufficiency develops, reinstitute administration promptly, at least temporarily, and employ other measures to manage unstable angina.

Because coronary artery disease may be unrecognized, do not discontinue therapy abruptly, even in patients treated only for hypertension, as abrupt withdrawal may result in transient symptoms (eg, tremulousness, sweating, palpitations, headache, malaise).

It has been suggested that β-adrenergic blockers may be discontinued abruptly during acute MI if indicated because the withdrawal phenomenon is not a major clinical problem in these patients.

➤*Peripheral vascular disease:* Treatment with β-antagonists reduces cardiac output and can precipitate or aggravate the symptoms of arterial insufficiency in patients with peripheral or mesenteric vascular disease. Exercise caution with such patients and observe closely for evidence of progression of arterial obstruction.

➤*Nonallergic bronchospasm (eg, chronic bronchitis, emphysema):* In general, do not administer β-blockers to patients with bronchospastic diseases. Administer **nadolol**, **timolol**, **penbutolol**, **propranolol**, **sotalol**, and **pindolol** with caution, because they may block bronchodilation produced by endogenous or exogenous catecholamine stimulation of β_2 receptors.

Because of their relative β_1 selectivity, low doses of **metoprolol**, **nebivolol**, **acebutolol**, **betaxolol**, **bisoprolol**, and **atenolol** may be used with caution in patients with bronchospastic disease who do not respond to, or cannot tolerate, other antihypertensive treatment. Because β_1 selectivity is not absolute, use the lowest possible dose of a β_2-stimulating agent. It may be advisable initially to administer in smaller divided doses, instead of larger doses twice daily, to avoid the higher plasma levels associated with the longer dosing interval. **Esmolol** may also be used with caution in patients with asthma if an IV agent is required.

Because it is unknown to what extent β_2-stimulating agents may exacerbate myocardial ischemia and the extent of infarction, β-blockers should not be used prophylactically. If bronchospasm not related to CHF occurs, discontinue β-blockers. A theophylline derivative or a β_2 agonist may be administered cautiously, depending on the clinical condition of the patient. Both theophylline derivatives and β_2 agonists may produce serious cardiac arrhythmias.

➤*Bradycardia:*

Metoprolol – Metoprolol produces a decrease in sinus heart rate in most patients; this decrease is greatest among patients with high initial heart rates and least among patients with low initial heart rates. Acute MI (particularly inferior infarction) may, in itself, produce significant lowering of the sinus rate. If the sinus rate decreases to < 40 BPM, particularly if associated with lowered cardiac output, give IV atropine (0.25 to 0.5 mg). If treatment with atropine is not successful, discontinue metoprolol and consider cautious administration of isoproterenol or installation of a cardiac pacemaker.

➤*Pheochromocytoma:* It is hazardous to use **propranolol** or **atenolol** unless α-adrenergic blocking drugs are already in use, because this would predispose to serious blood pressure elevation. Blocking only the peripheral dilator (β) action of epinephrine leaves its constrictor (α) action unopposed. In the event of hemorrhage or shock, there is a disadvantage in having both β and α blockade; the combination prevents the increase in heart rate and peripheral vasoconstriction needed to maintain blood pressure.

➤*Sinus bradycardia (heart rate < 50 bpm):* This occurred in 13% of patients receiving **sotalol** in clinical trials, and led to discontinuation in about 3%. Bradycardia itself increases risk of torsades de pointes. Sinus pause, sinus arrest, and sinus node dysfunction occur in less than 1% of patients. Incidence of 2nd- or 3rd- degree AV block is approximately 1%.

➤*Electrolyte disturbances:* Do not use **sotalol** in patients with hypokalemia or hypomagnesemia prior to correction of imbalance, as these conditions can exaggerate the degree of QT prolongation and increase the potential for torsades de pointes. Give special attention to electrolyte and acid-base balance in patients experiencing severe or prolonged diarrhea or patients receiving concomitant diuretic drugs.

➤*Hypotension:* If hypotension (systolic blood pressure ≤ 90 mmHg) occurs, discontinue drug and carefully assess patient's hemodynamic status and extent of myocardial damage. Invasive monitoring of central venous, pulmonary capillary wedge, and arterial pressures may be required. Institute fluids, positive inotropic agents, balloon counterpulsation or other appropriate therapy. If hypotension is associated with sinus bradycardia or AV block, direct treatment at reversing these.

In clinical trials, 20% to 50% of patients treated with **esmolol** have had hypotension, generally defined as systolic pressure < 90 mmHg or diastolic pressure < 50 mmHg. About 12% of the patients have been symptomatic (mainly diaphoresis or dizziness). Hypotension can occur at any dose, but is dose-related; therefore, doses > 200 mcg/kg/min are not recommended. Closely monitor patients, especially if pretreatment blood pressure is low. Decrease of dose or termination of infusion reverses hypotension, usually within 30 minutes.

➤*Anaphylaxis:* Anaphylaxis has occurred and may include symptoms such as profound hypotension, bradycardia with or without AV nodal block, severe sustained bronchospasm, hives, and angioedema. Deaths have occurred. Refer to Management of Acute Hypersensitivity Reactions. However, patients have been resistant to conventional therapy, especially epinephrine. Aggressive therapy may be required.

➤*Anesthesia and major surgery:* Necessity, or desirability, of withdrawing β-blockers prior to major surgery is controversial. β-blockade impairs the heart's ability to respond to β-adrenergically mediated reflex stimuli. While this might help prevent arrhythmic response, risk of excessive myocardial depression during general anesthesia may be enhanced, and difficulty restarting and maintaining heart beat has occurred. If β-blockers are withdrawn, allow several days between the last dose and anesthesia. If treatment is continued, take particular care when using anesthetics that depress the myocardium, such as ether, cyclopropane and trichlorethylene; use the lowest possible β-blocker doses. Others may recommend withdrawal of β-blockers well before surgery takes place.

In the event of emergency surgery, effects of β-blockers can be reversed by β-receptor agonists (eg, isoproterenol, dopamine, dobutamine, norepinephrine).

➤*AV block:* **Metoprolol** slows AV conduction and may produce significant first (PR interval greater than or equal to 0.26 sec), second, or third-degree heart block. Acute MI also produces heart block.

If heart block occurs, discontinue metoprolol and give IV atropine (0.25 to 0.5 mg). If treatment with atropine is not successful, consider cautious administration of isoproterenol or installation of a cardiac pacemaker.

➤*Sick sinus syndrome:* Use **sotalol** only with extreme caution in patients with sick sinus syndrome associated with symptomatic arrhythmias because it may cause sinus bradycardia, sinus pauses, or sinus arrest.

➤*Concomitant use of calcium channel blockers (atenolol):* Bradycardia and heart block can occur and the left ventricular end diastolic pressure can rise when beta-blockers are administered with verapamil or diltiazem. Patients with preexisting conduction abnormalities or left ventricular dysfunction are particularly susceptible.

➤*Recent acute MI (sotalol):* Sotalol can be used safely and effectively in the long-term treatment of life-threatening ventricular arrhythmias following an MI. However, experience in the use of sotalol to treat cardiac arrhythmias in the early phase of recovery from acute MI is limited and at least at high initial doses is not reassuring. In the first 2 weeks post-MI, caution is advised and careful dose titration is especially important, particularly in patients with markedly impaired ventricular function.

➤*Intraoperative and postoperative tachycardia and hypertension:* Do not use esmolol as the treatment for hypertension in patients in whom the increased blood pressure is primarily caused by the vasoconstriction associated with hypothermia.

➤*Diabetes/Hypoglycemia:* β-adrenergic blockade may blunt premonitory signs and symptoms (eg, pulse rate, tachycardia, blood pressure changes) of acute hypoglycemia, but other manifestations such as dizziness and sweating may not be significantly affected. Hypoglycemic attacks may be accompanied by a precipitous elevation of blood pressure in patients on **propranolol**. Nonselective β-blockers may potentiate insulin-induced hypoglycemia. This is less likely with cardioselective agents. **Atenolol** does not potentiate insulin-induced hypoglycemia and, unlike nonselective β-blockers, does not delay recovery of blood glucose to normal levels.

Use with caution in diabetic patients, especially those with labile diabetes. β blockade reduces the release of insulin in response to hyperglycemia; it may be necessary to adjust the dose of antidiabetic drugs.

Propranolol therapy, particularly in infants and children, diabetic or not, has been associated with hypoglycemia, especially during fasting as in preparation for surgery. Hypoglycemia also has been found after this type of drug therapy and prolonged physical exertion and has occurred in renal insufficiency, both during dialysis and sporadically, in patients on propranolol.

➤*Thyrotoxicosis:* β-adrenergic blockers may mask clinical signs (eg, tachycardia) of developing or continuing hyperthyroidism. Abrupt withdrawal may exacerbate symptoms of hyperthyroidism, including thyroid storm; therefore, monitor closely and withdraw the drug slowly.

Propranolol may change thyroid-function tests, increasing T_4 and reverse T_3, and decreasing T_3.

➤*Serum lipid concentrations:* Although study results conflict, β-blockers may alter serum lipids including an increase in the concentration of total triglycerides, total cholesterol and LDL and VLDL cholesterol, and a decrease in the concentration of HDL cholesterol; however, this finding is not clinically significant. Other studies suggest **pindolol** does not significantly alter serum lipid concentrations and **acebutolol** actually lowers total and LDL cholesterol levels; **bisoprolol** did not significantly alter total cholesterol and triglycerides. Further studies are needed.

➤*Muscle weakness:* Beta-blockade has potentiated muscle weakness consistent with certain myasthenic symptoms (eg, diplopia, ptosis, generalized weakness). **Timolol** rarely increased muscle weakness in some patients with myasthenia gravis or myasthenic symptoms.

➤*Renal/Hepatic function impairment:* Use with caution. **Timolol**'s half-life is essentially unchanged in moderate renal insufficiency; however, marked hypotensive responses have been seen in patients with marked renal impairment undergoing dialysis. Dosage reduction may be necessary in impaired renal or hepatic function.

Because **nadolol**, **sotalol**, and **atenolol** are eliminated primarily by the kidney, half-life increases in renal failure; dosage adjustments are necessary.**Bisoprolol**'s half-life is increased in patients with creatinine clearance less than 40 mL/min and in cirrhosis; adjust dosage. Although **acebutolol** is excreted through the GI tract, the active metabolite, diacetolol, is eliminated primarily by the kidney; reduce daily acebutolol dose. Administer **esmolol** with caution in impaired renal function because its acid metabolite is primarily excreted unchanged by the kidney. Elimination half-life of the acid metabolite was prolonged 10-fold and plasma level was considerably elevated in end-stage renal disease. Poor renal function has only minor effects on **pindolol** clearance, but poor hepatic function may cause pindolol blood levels to increase substantially. Expect **penbutolol** conjugate accumulation upon multiple dosing in renal insufficiency. **Metoprolol**'s systemic availability and half-life in renal failure do not differ significantly from those in normal subjects; dosage reduction is usually not needed. **Betaxolol** is primarily metabolized in the liver to metabolites that are inactive and then excreted by the kidneys; clearance is somewhat reduced in patients with renal failure but little changed in patients with hepatic disease. Reduce dosage in patients with severe renal impairment and those on dialysis; dosage reductions have not routinely been necessary in hepatic insufficiency.

Nebivolol clearance was reduced by 53% in patients with severe renal function impairment (CrCl less than 30 mL/min). Adjust the dose of nebivolol in patients with severe renal impairment. In patients with moderate hepatic impairment (Child-Pugh class B), reduce the starting dose. Nebivolol is contraindicated in patients with severe hepatic impairment.

➤*Pregnancy: Category D* (**atenolol**; bisoprolol [if used in the second or third trimesters per Briggs' *Drugs in Pregnancy and Lactation*]). Atenolol can cause fetal harm when administered to a pregnant woman. Atenolol crosses the placental barrier and appears in cord blood. Administration of atenolol, starting in the second trimester of pregnancy, has been associated with the birth of infants that are small for gestational age. No studies have been performed on the use of atenolol in the first trimester and the possibility of fetal injury cannot be excluded.

Category C (**betaxolol**, **esmolol**, **metoprolol**, **nadolol**, **nebivolol**, **timolol**, **propranolol**, **penbutolol**, **bisoprolol**). Embryotoxic effects have been demonstrated in animals at doses 5 to 600 times higher than the maximum recommended doses in humans.

Category B (**acebutolol**, **pindolol**, **sotalol**). Acebutolol and its major metabolite, diacetolol, cross the placenta. Neonates of mothers who received acebutolol during pregnancy have reduced birth weight and decreased blood pressure and heart rate. Sotalol crosses the placenta and is found in amniotic fluid; subnormal birth weight has occurred.

Safety for use during pregnancy has not been established. Use only when clearly needed and when the potential benefits outweigh the potential hazards to the fetus.

Although cases of teratogenicity in humans have not been reported, problems have occurred during delivery. These include the following: Neonatal bradycardia, hypoglycemia and apnea, low Apgar scores, maternal and fetal bradycardia, hypothermia, oliguria, poor peripheral perfusion, and small birth weight infants (caused by chronic therapy). Some of the effects on the neonate may last up to 72 hours postpartum.

➤*Lactation:* **Propranolol**, **pindolol**, **timolol**, **sotalol**, **betaxolol**, and **nadolol** are excreted in breast milk. **Acebutolol** and diacetolol (its major metabolite) appear in breast milk with a milk:plasma ratio of 7.1 and 12.2, respectively. **Metoprolol** is excreted in breast milk in very small quantities; an infant consuming 1 L of breast milk would receive a dose of < 1 mg of the drug. **Atenolol** is excreted in breast milk at a ratio of 1.5 to 6.8. In one patient, the peak atenolol milk:plasma ratio was 3.6 and the estimated infant dose (maternal dose, 100 mg/day) was 0.13 mg/feeding (75 mL). Another infant developed cyanosis and 2 incidences of bradycardia following maternal atenolol ingestion (100 mg/day). Small amounts of **bisoprolol** (< 2% of the dose) are detected in the breast milk of rats; it is not known if it is excreted in human breast milk. Betaxolol is excreted in sufficient amounts to have pharmacological effects in the infant. It is not known if **penbutolol**, **nebivolol**, or **esmolol** are excreted in breast milk. Nursing should not be undertaken by mothers receiving these drugs.

➤*Children:* Safety and efficacy for use in children have not been established.

IV administration of **propranolol** is not recommended in children; however, oral propranolol has been used (see Administration and Dosage).

Drug Interactions

Beta-Blocker Drug Interactions

Precipitant drug	Object drug[a]		Description
Aluminum salts Barbiturates Calcium salts Cholestyramine Colestipol Penicillins (ampicillin) Rifampin	β-blockers	↓	The bioavailability and plasma levels of certain β-blockers may be decreased by these agents, possibly resulting in a decreased pharmacologic effect.
Calcium channel blockers	β-blockers	↑	Pharmacologic effects of β-blockers as well as nifedipine and verapamil may be synergistic or additive. Diltiazem and nicardipine may decrease the metabolism of certain beta blockers, thus increasing the pharmacologic effects.
Catecholamine-depleting agents (ie, guanethidine, reserpine)	Nebivolol	↑	Closely monitor concomitant use of catecholamine-depleting agents and nebivolol because coadministration may produce excessive reduction in sympathetic activity.
Cimetidine	β-blockers Metoprolol Propranolol	↑	Pharmacokinetic parameters of β-blockers metabolized by cytochrome P450 may be altered by cimetidine; pharmacodynamic effects may be increased.
Contraceptives, oral	β-blockers	↑	Bioavailability and plasma levels of certain β-blockers may be increased.
Digitalis glycosides	Nebivolol	↑	Both digitalis glycosides and nebivolol slow atrioventricular conduction and decrease heart rate. Concomitant use can increase the risk of bradycardia. Monitor cardiac function and heart rate. If an interaction is suspected, adjust treatment as needed.
Nebivolol	Digitalis glycosides		
Diphenhydramine	β-blockers	↑	Diphenhydramine may increase plasma concentrations and cardiovascular effects of certain β-blockers through inhibition of CYP2D6-mediated metabolism.
Flecainide	β-blockers	↑	The bioavailability of either agent may be increased, possibly increasing the pharmacologic effects.
β-blockers	Flecainide		
Haloperidol	β-blockers Propranolol	↑	Pharmacologic effects (hypotensive episodes) of both drugs may be increased.
β-blockers Propranolol	Haloperidol		
Hydralazine	β-blockers Metoprolol Propranolol	↑	Serum levels and, hence, pharmacologic effects of β-blockers and hydralazine may be enhanced.
β-blockers Metoprolol Propranolol	Hydralazine		
Hydroxychloroquine	β-blockers	↑	Plasma concentrations and cardiovascular effects of certain β-blockers may be increased because hydroxychloroquine inhibits the CYP2D6-mediated β-blocker metabolism.
Loop diuretics	β-blockers Propranolol	↑	Propranolol plasma levels and cardiovascular effects may be enhanced. Atenolol was not affected.
MAO inhibitors	β-blockers Metoprolol Nadolol	↑	Bradycardia may develop during concurrent use.

Beta-Blocker Drug Interactions

Precipitant drug	Object drug[a]		Description
Mibefradil	Nebivolol	↑	Coadministration may result in additive effects, increasing the risk of cardiovascular toxicity, including lowering of heart rate and suppression of sinoarterial node activity. Avoid coadministration, especially in patients with lowered heart rates and/or sick sinus syndrome.
Nebivolol	Mibefradil		
NSAIDs Salicylates Sulfinpyrazone	β-blockers	↓	NSAIDs, salicylates, and sulfinpyrazone may inhibit the synthesis of prostaglandins involved in the antihypertensive activity of β-blockers.
Phenothiazines	β-blockers Propranolol	↑	Propranolol bioavailability and plasma levels and phenothiazine plasma levels may be increased, possibly resulting in increased effects.
β-blockers Propranolol	Phenothiazines		
Propafenone	β-blockers Metoprolol Propranolol	↑	Plasma levels of β-blockers metabolized by the liver may be increased.
Quinidine	β-blockers	↑	Plasma β-blocker levels may be increased in "extensive metabolizers," possibly resulting in increased effects.
Quinolones Ciprofloxacin	β-blockers	↑	Bioavailability of β-blockers metabolized by cytochrome P450 may be increased.
SSRIs	β-blockers Metoprolol Propranolol	↑	Certain SSRIs may inhibit the metabolism (CYP2D6) of certain β-blockers, leading to excessive β-blockade.
Thioamines	β-blockers Metoprolol Propranolol	↑	The pharmacokinetics of the β-blockers may be altered, increasing the pharmacologic effects.
Thyroid hormones	β-blockers Metoprolol Propranolol	↓	The actions of certain β-blockers may be impaired when the hypothyroid patient is converted to the euthyroid state.
β-blockers Propranolol	Anticoagulants	↑	Propranolol may increase the anticoagulant effect of warfarin.
β-blockers Metoprolol Propranolol	Benzodiazepines	↑	Effects of certain benzodiazepines may be increased by lipophilic β-blockers. Atenolol does not interact.
β-blockers	Clonidine	↑	Life-threatening and fatal increases in blood pressure have occurred after discontinuation of clonidine in patients receiving a β-blocker or after simultaneous withdrawal.
β-blockers	Disopyramide	↔	Difficult to predict; disopyramide clearance may be decreased; adverse effects may occur (eg, sinus bradycardia, hypotension) or there may be no occurrence of synergistic or additive negative inotropic effects.
β-blockers	Epinephrine	↑	Nonselective β-blockade allows alpha receptor effects of epinephrine to predominate. Increasing vascular resistance leads to initial hypertensive episode followed by bradycardia.
β-blockers	Ergot alkaloids	↑	Peripheral ischemia manifested by cold extremities, possible peripheral gangrene may develop due to ergot alkaloid-mediated vasoconstriction and β-blocker-mediated blockade of peripheral β_2 receptors, allowing for unopposed ergot action.
β-blockers Propranolol	Gabapentin	↑	Gabapentin adverse reactions may be increased.

Beta-Blocker Drug Interactions

Precipitant drug	Object drug[a]		Description
β-blockers	Lidocaine	↑	Increased lidocaine levels may occur, resulting in toxicity.
β-blockers	Nondepolarizing muscle relaxants	↔	β-blockers may potentiate, counteract, delay, or have no effect on the actions of the nondepolarizing muscle relaxants.
β-blockers	Prazosin	↑	Concurrent administration may increase the postural hypotension produced by prazosin.
β-blockers	Sulfonylureas	↓	Hypoglycemic effects of sulfonylureas may be attenuated.
β-blockers Nonselective	Theophylline	↔	Reduced elimination of theophylline may occur. Pharmacologic antagonism can also be expected, thus reducing the effects of one or both agents. Cardioselective agents may be preferred.

[a] ↑ = Object drug increased. ↓ = Object drug decreased. ↔ = Undetermined clinical effect.

➤*Drug/Lab test interactions:* These agents may produce hypoglycemia and interfere with **glucose** or **insulin** tolerance tests. **Propranolol** and **betaxolol** may interfere with the glaucoma screening test because of a reduction in intraocular pressure.

➤*Drug/Food interactions:* Food enhances the bioavailability of **metoprolol** and **propranolol**; food does not enhance the bioavailability of **nadolol, bisoprolol**, or **pindolol**. The rate of **penbutolol** absorption is slowed by the presence of food; however, extent of absorption is not appreciably affected. **Sotalol** absorption is reduced ≈ 20% by a standard meal.

Adverse Reactions

Most adverse effects are mild and transient and rarely require withdrawal of therapy.

➤*Cardiovascular:* Bradycardia; torsades de pointes and other serious new ventricular arrhythmias (see Warnings/Precautions); cardiovascular disorder; automatic implantable cardioverter/defibrillator (AICD) discharge; development of mitral regurgitation; cardiac reinfarction; total cardiac arrest; nonfatal cardiac arrest; cardiogenic shock; development of ventricular septal defect; chest pain; hypertension; hypotension (including asymptomatic and orthostatic); peripheral ischemia; flushing; worsening of angina and arterial insufficiency; shortness of breath; peripheral vascular insufficiency (cold extremities, paresthesia of hands); arterial insufficiency; claudication (including intermittent); heart failure; CHF; sinoatrial block; cerebral vascular accident; edema; pulmonary edema; vasodilation; presyncope and syncope; tachycardia (including ventricular); palpitations; conduction disturbances; first-, second- and third-degree heart block; intensification of AV block; abnormal ECG; bundle branch block plus major axis deviation; supraventricular tachycardia (including atrial fibrillation and flutter); angina pectoris; AV block; MI; thrombosis; cerebrovascular disorder; leg cramps; thrombophlebitis; disturbance rhythm atrial; disturbance rhythm subjective; diaphoresis; proarrhythmia; peripheral vascular disorder.

➤*CNS:* Dizziness; vertigo; tiredness/fatigue; headache; mental depression (lassitude, weakness); peripheral neuropathy; paralysis; paresthesias; hypesthesia; hyperesthesia; lethargy; anxiety; nervousness; diminished concentration/memory; somnolence; restlessness; insomnia; sleep disturbances; nightmares; bizarre or many dreams; sedation; change in behavior; altered consciousness; mood change; slightly clouded sensorium; incoordination; reversible mental depression progressing to catatonia; hallucinations; an acute reversible syndrome characterized by disorientation of time and place, short-term memory loss, emotional lability, decreased performance on neuropsychometrics, slurred speech, tinnitus and lightheadedness; increase in signs and symptoms of myasthenia gravis; ataxia; neuralgia; neuropathy; numbness; stupor; abnormal thinking; amnesia; impaired concentration; confusion; seizures; local weakness; stroke.

It has been suggested that the more lipophilic the β-blocker, the higher the CNS penetration and subsequent incidence of adverse CNS effects. These effects may improve or disappear when a less lipophilic agent is substituted.

➤*Dermatologic:* Rash; pruritus; skin irritation; increased pigmentation; sweating/hyperhidrosis; alopecia (including reversible); dry skin; psoriasis (often reversible); acne; eczema; flushing; exfoliative dermatitis; peripheral skin necrosis; psoriasiform rash or exacerbation of psoriasis; erythematous rash; hypertrichosis; skin disorders; erythema, skin discoloration; burning at infusion site; thrombophlebitis; local skin necrosis; cutaneous vasculitis.

➤*Endocrine:* Hyperglycemia; hypoglycemia; unstable diabetes.

➤*GI:* Gastric/epigastric pain; flatulence; gastritis; constipation; nausea; diarrhea; colon problem; dry mouth; vomiting; heartburn; appetite disorder; anorexia; bloating; abdominal discomfort/pain; mesenteric arterial thrombosis; ischemic colitis; retroperitoneal fibrosis; hepatomegaly; dyspepsia; taste distortion; elevated liver enzymes (see Lab Test Abnormalities); elevated bilirubin; acute hepatitis with jaundice; GI disorder; increased appetite; mouth ulceration; rectal disorders; dysphagia; abnormal taste; taste loss; abdominal distension; taste perversion; digestive tract disorders; indigestion.

➤*GU:* Sexual dysfunction; impotence or decreased libido; dysuria; nocturia; pollakiuria; urinary retention or frequency; urinary tract infection; cystitis; renal colic; GU disorder; renal failure; cystitis; micturition disorder; oliguria; proteinuria; abnormal renal function; renal pain; menstrual disorders; prostatitis.

➤*Hematologic:* Agranulocytosis; nonthrombocytopenic or thrombocytopenic purpura; bleeding; thrombocytopenia; eosinophilia; leukopenia; pulmonary emboli; hyperlipidemia; anemia; leukocytosis; lymphadenopathy; purpura.

➤*Hypersensitivity:* Pharyngitis; photosensitivity reaction; erythematous rash; fever combined with aching and sore throat; laryngospasm; respiratory distress; angioedema; anaphylaxis (see Warnings/Precautions).

➤*Lab test abnormalities:* **Propranolol** may elevate blood urea levels in patients with severe heart disease. **Propranolol** and **metoprolol** may cause elevated serum transaminase, alkaline phosphatase, and LDH. **Timolol** may produce slight increases in BUN, serum potassium, and serum uric acid, and slight decreases in hemoglobin and hematocrit and HDL cholesterol; however, these alterations are not progressive and are not associated with clinical manifestations. Increases in liver function tests have been reported.

Minor persistent elevations in AST and ALT have occurred in 7% of patients treated with **pindolol**, but progressive elevations were not observed and liver injury has not been reported. Alkaline phosphatase, LDH, and uric acid are also elevated on rare occasions. The significance of this is unknown. Elevations of AST and ALT of 1 to 2 times normal have occurred with **bisoprolol** (3.9% to 6.2%). Small increases in uric acid, creatinine, BUN, serum potassium, glucose, and phosphorus, and decreases in WBC and platelets have also occurred, although they were generally not of clinical importance. Liver abnormalities (increased AST and ALT) have occurred in a small number of patients receiving **acebutolol**.

Nebivolol was associated with an increase in serum urea nitrogen (BUN), uric acid, and triglycerides, and a decrease in high-density lipoprotein cholesterol and platelet count.

The development of antinuclear antibodies (ANA) has been associated with β-blocker therapy. Symptoms of arthralgia and myalgias were infrequent and reversed upon drug discontinuation.

➤*Musculoskeletal:* Joint pain; arthralgia; muscle cramps/pain; back/neck pain; arthritis; twitching/tremor; localized pain; extremity pain; myalgia; pain; shoulder pain; joint disorder; arthropathy; tendonitis; chest pain; muscle cramps.

➤*Ophthalmic:* Eye irritation/discomfort; visual disturbances; dry/burning eyes; blurred vision; conjunctivitis; ocular pain/pressure; abnormal lacrimation; ptosis; eye disorder; abnormal vision; blepharitis; ocular hemorrhage; iritis; cataract; scotoma; diplopia.

➤*Respiratory:* Bronchospasm; dyspnea; cough; bronchial obstruction; rales; wheeziness; nasal stuffiness; pharyngitis; rhonchi; laryngospasm with respiratory distress; asthma; rhinitis; sinusitis; pulmonary problem; upper respiratory tract problem; cold symptoms; flu symptoms; bronchitis; lung disorder; cough; epistaxis; pneumonia; tracheobronchitis.

➤*Miscellaneous:* Facial swelling; weight gain; weight loss; peripheral edema; decreased exercise tolerance; lupus syndrome and lupus-like reactions; Peyronie's disease; Raynaud's phenomenon; speech disorder; rigors; earache; gout; asthenia; malaise; infection; fever; death; tinnitus; injury; salivation; sweating; allergy; breast pain; breast fibroadenosis; labyrinth disorders; deafness; acidosis; diabetes; hypercholesterolemia; hyperglycemia; hyperkalemia; hyperlipemia; hyperuricemia; hypokalemia; thirst; cold sensation; systemic lupus erythematosus (rarely); speech disorder; midscapular pain; pemphigoid rash; hypertensive reaction in patients with pheochromocytoma.

Overdosage

➤*Symptoms:* Bradycardia, hypotension, low-output cardiac failure, and cardiogenic shock are the most common effects of beta-blocker intoxication.

Cardiovascular – Asystole; tachycardia (partial agonists); prolonged QT interval (sotalol); prolonged QRS complex (membrane-stabilizing agents); ventricular dysrhythmias (membrane-stabilizing agents, sotalol); hypotension; hypertension (partial agonists); bradycardia; AV block.

CNS – Seizures; coma; depressed level of consciousness.

GI – Mesenteric ischemia; esophageal spasms.

Metabolic – Hyperkalemia; hypoglycemia.

Respiratory – Apnea; cyanosis; respiratory depression; bronchospasm.

Miscellaneous – Renal failure.

➤*Treatment:* Perform evaluation of the "ABCs" (airway, breathing, and circulation) as well as rapid assessment of serum glucose levels with correction of hypoglycemia using IV glucagon. Early ventilatory control is essential in addition to chest radiography, serum electrolytes, and arterial blood gases. Administer activated charcoal to all patients and perform gastric lavage in patients who present within 1 to 2 hours after ingestion. In patients who ingest sustained-release preparations, consider whole-bowel irrigation with polyethylene glycol solution. Treat seizures with initial administration of benzodiazepines. Use barbiturates if benzodiazepines are ineffective. **Atenolol**, **acebutolol**, **sotalol**, and **nadolol** are the only beta-blockers that can successfully be removed by hemodialysis. Although rare, bronchospasm should be treated with β-agonists. Parenteral epinephrine may be required in severe cases. See Management of Acute Overdosage.

Other treatments for cardiovascular complications include the following:

1.) *Catecholamine agents:* Epinephrine had the greatest effect of all agents. High-dose isoproterenol and dopamine also have been used for β-blocker toxicity.
2.) *Phosphodiesterase inhibitors:* A positive inotropic effect without an increase in myocardial oxygen demand has been shown in the canine model using amrinone. Milrinone, aminophylline, and theophylline also have been employed for β-blocker toxicity.
3.) *Atropine:* Atropine is the least effective agent in the treatment of β-blocker toxicity, although it is the most frequently used. The lack of effect of a 1 mg dose of atropine may be diagnostic for β-blocker poisoning.
4.) *Pacing:* External cardiac pacing or transvenous pacing is often attempted to treat β-blocker-induced bradycardia; however, it may be ineffective. Overdrive pacing may be necessary in cases of torsades de pointes associated with sotalol intoxification.
5.) *Intra-aortic balloon pump:* If other measures fail, insertion of an intra-aortic balloon pump may restore perfusion.

Patient Information

Do not discontinue medication abruptly, except on advice of physician. Sudden cessation of therapy may precipitate or exacerbate angina.

Consult pharmacist or physician before using other products that may contain α-adrenergic stimulants (eg, nasal decongestants, *otc* cold preparations).

Notify physician if symptoms of CHF occur (eg, difficult breathing, especially on exertion or when lying down; night cough; swelling of the extremities).

Notify physician if any of the following occur: Slow pulse rate, dizziness, lightheadedness, confusion or depression, skin rash, fever, sore throat, unusual bleeding or bruising.

May produce drowsiness, dizziness, lightheadedness, blurred vision; patient should observe caution while driving or performing other tasks requiring alertness, coordination, or physical dexterity.

➤*Diabetics:* These agents may mask signs of hypoglycemia or alter blood glucose levels.

➤*Propranolol and metoprolol:* Food may enhance bioavailability; take at the same time each day.

➤*Nadolol, nebivolol, pindolol, acebutolol, atenolol, bisoprolol, betaxolol, and penbutolol:* May be taken without regard to meals.

➤*Sotalol:* Food may reduce absorption. Take on an empty stomach.

ATENOLOL

Rx	**Atenolol** (Various, eg, Caraco, Teva)	**Tablets; oral:** 25 mg	In 30s, 60s, 90s, 100s, and 1,000s.
Rx	**Tenormin** (AstraZeneca)		(T 107). White. In 100s.
Rx	**Atenolol** (Various, eg, Caraco, Teva)	**Tablets; oral:** 50 mg	In 30s, 60s, 90s, 100s, and 1,000s.
Rx	**Tenormin** (AstraZeneca)		(Tenormin 105). Round. White, scored. In 100s.
Rx	**Atenolol** (Various, eg, Caraco, Teva)	**Tablets; oral:** 100 mg	In 30s, 60s, 90s, 100s, 500s, and 1,000s.
Rx	**Tenormin** (AstraZeneca)		(Tenormin 101). White. In 100s.

ATENOLOL — ORAL

For complete and comparative prescribing information, refer to the Beta-Adrenergic Blocking Agents class monograph.

WARNING

Advise patients with coronary artery disease who are being treated with atenolol against abrupt discontinuation of therapy. Severe exacerbation of angina and the occurrence of myocardial infarction (MI) and ventricular arrhythmias have been reported in patients with angina following the abrupt discontinuation of therapy with beta-blockers. The last 2 complications may occur with or without preceding exacerbation of the angina pectoris. As with other beta-blockers, when discontinuation of atenolol is planned, observe the patient carefully and advise the patient to limit physical activity to a minimum. If the angina worsens or acute coronary insufficiency develops, it is recommended that atenolol be promptly reinstituted, at least temporarily. Because coronary artery disease is common and may be unrecognized, it may be prudent not to discontinue atenolol therapy abruptly, even in patients treated only for hypertension.

Indications

➤*Acute myocardial infarction:* For the management of hemodynamically stable patients with definite or suspected acute MI to reduce cardiovascular mortality. Treatment can be initiated as soon as the patient's clinical condition allows. In general, there is no basis for treating patients like those who were excluded from the International Study of Infarct Survival (ISIS-1) trial (blood pressure less than 100 mm Hg systolic, heart rate less than 50 bpm) or who have other reasons to avoid beta-blockade. Some subgroups (eg, elderly patients with systolic blood pressure below 120 mm Hg) seem less likely to benefit.

➤*Angina pectoris caused by coronary atherosclerosis:* For the long-term management of patients with angina pectoris.

➤*Hypertension:* For the management of hypertension. Atenolol may be used alone or concomitantly with other antihypertensive agents, particularly with a thiazide-type diuretic.

➤*Off-label uses:*

Pediatric hypertension – [3] = Safety concerns. Atenolol is among the therapeutic options for pediatric hypertension identified by the National High Blood Pressure Education Program, based on published case series in children.

Prevention of migraine (adults) – [2] = Fair documentation. Three controlled trials suggest that atenolol is as effective as propranolol and better than placebo in preventing migraine headache. American Academy of Neurology practice guidelines consider atenolol to be efficacious, despite the lack of optimal scientific evidence.

Prevention of supraventricular arrhythmia – [4] = Insufficient documentation. Data suggest that atenolol is effective as prophylaxis for supraventricular arrhythmias after cardiac surgery, but results are mixed. Atenolol has not been shown to be more effective than any other drug that has been evaluated for prophylaxis of this condition, and both sotalol and carvedilol have been reported to be more effective than atenolol. Combination therapy with digoxin was more effective than either drug alone compared with placebo in one study, but atenolol monotherapy in that study was no more effective than placebo. More studies are needed to determine the most appropriate patients for atenolol therapy.

Prevention of variceal bleeding – [5] = Poor documentation. Because of evidence-based guidelines indicating less effectiveness in the prevention of variceal hemorrhage with selective beta-blockers compared with nonselective beta-blockers, atenolol is not recommended for use in cirrhotic patients with nonbleeding varices.

Unstable angina – [1] = Good documentation. Current guidelines recommend using beta-blocker therapy in unstable angina (UA)/non–ST-segment elevation myocardial infarction (NSTEMI) within 24 hours if no contraindications exist. However, recommendations do not specify any particular beta-blocking agent for optimal treatment of unstable angina. Thus, clinicians must use practical experience to determine proper therapy in managing patients with unstable angina. Additionally, oral beta-blockers are recommended for secondary prevention of UA/NSTEMI in patients with heart failure or left ventricle systolic dysfunction.

Administration and Dosage

➤*General dosing considerations:* In patients with definite or suspected acute MI, treatment with atenolol intravenous (IV) injection should be initiated as soon as possible after the patient's arrival at the hospital and after eligibility is established. Atenolol is an additional treatment to standard coronary care unit therapy. Treatment with beta-blockers that are effective in the postinfarction setting may be continued for 1 to 3 years if there are no contraindications.

If bradycardia or hypotension requiring treatment or any other untoward effects occur, atenolol should be discontinued.

Twenty-four-hour control of angina pectoris with once-daily dosing is achieved by giving doses larger than necessary to achieve an immediate maximum effect. The maximum early effect on exercise tolerance occurs with doses of 50 to 100 mg, but at these doses, the effect at 24 hours is attenuated, averaging approximately 50% to 75% of that observed with 200 mg once daily.

➤*Adults:*

Acute myocardial infarction –

Initial dosage: Note: The atenolol IV formulation has been discontinued in the United States. 5 mg IV over 5 minutes, followed by 5 mg IV 10 minutes later. In patients who tolerate the full IV dose (10 mg), 50 mg orally should be initiated 10 minutes after the last IV dose, followed by another 50 mg oral dose 12 hours later.

Maintenance dosage: 100 mg daily or 50 mg twice daily for a further 6 to 9 days or until discharge from the hospital occurs.

Angina pectoris –

Initial dosage: 50 mg daily.

Dosage adjustment: If an optimal response is not achieved within 1 week, the dosage should be increased to 100 mg daily.

Alternative dosage: Some patients may require 200 mg daily for optimal effect.

Discontinuation of therapy: If withdrawal of atenolol is planned, gradually decrease dosage and observe and advise the patient to limit his/her physical activity to a minimum.

Hypertension –

Initial dosage: 50 mg daily, either alone or added to diuretic therapy. The full effect of this dose will usually be seen within 1 to 2 weeks.

Dosage adjustment: If an optimal response is not achieved, the dosage should be increased to 100 mg daily. Increasing the dosage beyond 100 mg daily is unlikely to produce any further benefit.

Concomitant therapy: Atenolol may be used alone or with other antihypertensive agents, including thiazide-type diuretics, hydralazine, prazosin, and alpha-methyldopa.

ATENOLOL — ORAL

Off-label dosing –

Prevention of migraine (adults): [2] = Fair documentation. 100 mg daily for 6 to 12 weeks.

Prevention of supraventricular arrhythmia: [4] = Insufficient documentation. 50 mg daily beginning up to 3 days before surgery until 7 days postsurgery. In 1 study, atenolol 5 mg IV was used before oral atenolol 50 mg daily was begun.

➤*Children:*

Off-label dosing –

Pediatric hypertension: [3] = Safety concerns.

• *1 to 17 years of age –*

Maximum dose: 2 mg/kg/day, up to 100 mg/day.

Initial dosage: 0.5 to 1 mg/kg/day, given once daily or divided for twice-daily administration.

Unstable angina: [1] = Good documentation. Current guidelines address the use of oral beta-blocker therapy in patients with unstable angina; however, specific agents and dosages are not outlined. As maintenance therapy, oral atenolol 50 to 200 mg/day is suggested.

➤*Elderly:* Initial dosage is 25 mg daily.

➤*Renal function impairment:* Atenolol is excreted by the kidneys; dosage should be adjusted in cases of severe renal impairment. No significant accumulation of atenolol occurs until creatinine clearance (CrCl) falls below 35 mL/min per 1.73 m^2.

Atenolol Dosage Adjustment in Renal Impairment

CrCl (mL/min per 1.73 m^2)	Atenolol elimination half-life (h)	Maximum dosage
15 to 35	16 to 27	50 mg daily
< 15	> 27	25 mg daily

Hemodialysis – Patients on hemodialysis should be given 25 or 50 mg after each dialysis; this should be done under hospital supervision, as marked falls in blood pressure can occur.

➤*Monitoring:* Assessment of efficacy should include measurement of blood pressure just prior to the next dose ("trough" blood pressure).

➤*Storage/Stability:* Store at 20° to 25°C (68° to 77°F).

ESMOLOL HYDROCHLORIDE

Rx	**Esmolol** (Baxter)	**Injection, solution:** 10 mg/mL	Preservative free. In 10 mL vials.
Rx	**Brevibloc** (Baxter)		Preservative free. Sodium chloride. In ready-to-use 10 mL vials and 250 mL premixed bags.
Rx	**Brevibloc Double Strength** (Baxter)	**Injection, solution:** 20 mg/mL	Preservative free. Sodium chloride. In ready-to-use 5 mL vials and 100 mL premixed bags.

[a] With 25% propylene glycol.

ESMOLOL HYDROCHLORIDE — INJECTION

For complete and comparative prescribing information, refer to the Beta-Adrenergic Blocking Agents group monograph.

Indications

➤*Supraventricular tachycardia:* For the rapid control of ventricular rate in patients with atrial fibrillation or atrial flutter in perioperative, postoperative, or other emergent circumstances where short-term control of ventricular rate with a short-acting agent is desirable. Esmolol hydrochloride is also indicated in noncompensatory sinus tachycardia where, in the physician's judgment, the rapid heart rate requires specific intervention. Esmolol hydrochloride is not intended for use in chronic settings where transfer to another agent is anticipated.

➤*Intraoperative and postoperative tachycardia or hypertension:* For the treatment of tachycardia and hypertension that occur during induction and tracheal intubation, during surgery, on emergence from anesthesia, and in the postoperative period, when in the physician's judgment such specific intervention is considered indicated.

Use of esmolol hydrochloride to prevent such events is not recommended.

➤*Off-label uses:*

Pediatric hypertensive urgency or emergency – [1] = Good documentation. Esmolol is among the therapeutic options for pediatric hypertensive urgency or emergency identified by the National High Blood Pressure Education Program as most useful.

Other possible off-label uses – For unstable angina, 2 to 24 mg/min as a continuous infusion.

Administration and Dosage

➤*General dosing considerations:* Dosage needs to be titrated, using ventricular rate as the guide for treatment of supraventricular tachycardia.

Higher dosages (250 to 300 mcg/kg/min) may be required for adequate control of blood pressure than those required for the treatment of atrial fibrillation, flutter and sinus tachycardia. One-third of the postoperative hypertensive patients required these higher doses.

➤*Adults:*

Supraventricular tachycardia –

Usual dosage: The following table summarizes the above and assumes that 3 loading doses (the maximum recommended) are infused over 1 minute and incremental maintenance doses are required after each loading dose. There should be no 4th loading dose, but the maintenance dose may be increased by 1 more increment.

Esmolol Loading And Maintenance Dose

Elapsed time (min)	Loading dose (over 1 min) mcg/kg/min	Maintenance dose (over 4 min) mcg/kg/min
0 to 1	500 mcg/kg/min	
1 to 5		50 mcg/kg/min
5 to 6	500 mcg/kg/min	
6 to 10		100 mcg/kg/min
10 to 11	500 mcg/kg/min	
11 to 15		150 mcg/kg/min
15 to 16	—	
16 to 20		200 mcg/kg/min[a]
> 20		Maintenance dose titrated to heart rate or other clinical end point.

[a] As the desired heart rate or end point is approached, the loading infusion may be omitted and the maintenance infusion titrated to 300 mcg/kg/min or downward as appropriate. Maintenance dosages above 200 mcg/kg/min have not been shown to have significantly increased benefits. The interval between titration steps may be increased.

Responses to esmolol hydrochloride usually (over 95%) occur within the range of 50 to 200 mcg/kg/min. The average effective dosage is approximately 100 mcg/kg/min, although dosages as low as 25 mcg/kg/min have been adequate in some patients. Dosage of esmolol hydrochloride in supraventricular tachycardia must be individualized by titration in which each step consists of a loading dosage followed by a maintenance dosage. This specific dosage regimen has not been studied intraoperatively and, because of the time required for titration, may not be optimal for intraoperative use.

Maximum dose: 200 mcg/kg/min.

Loading dose: 500 mcg/kg infused over a minute duration followed by a maintenance infusion of 50 mcg/kg/min for the next 4 minutes is recommended. This should give a rough guide with respect to the responsiveness of ventricular rate.

Maintenance dosage: After the 4 minutes of initial maintenance infusion (total treatment duration, 5 minutes), depending upon the desired ventricular response, the maintenance infusion may be continued at 50 mcg/kg/min or increased step-wise (eg, 100 mcg/kg/min, 150 mcg/kg/min, to a maximum of 200 mcg/kg/min) with each step being maintained for 4 or more minutes.

Alternative dosage: If more rapid slowing of ventricular response is imperative, the 500 mcg/kg loading dose infused over a 1-minute period may be repeated, followed by a maintenance infusion of 100 mcg/kg/min for 4 minutes. Then, depending upon ventricular rate, another (and final) loading dose of 500 mcg/kg/min infused over a 1-minute period may be administered followed by a maintenance infusion of 150 mcg/kg/min. If needed, after 4 minutes of the 150 mcg/kg/min maintenance infusion, the maintenance infusion may be increased to a maximum of 200 mcg/kg/min.

Duration of therapy: The use of infusions of esmolol hydrochloride up to 24 hours has been well documented; in addition, limited data from 24 to 48 hours (n = 48) indicate that esmolol hydrochloride is well tolerated up to 48 hours.

Conversion: After achieving an adequate control of the heart rate and a stable clinical status in patients with supraventricular tachycardia, transition to alternative antiarrhythmic agents, such as propranolol, digoxin, or verapamil, may be accomplished. A recommended guideline for such a transition is given below but the health care provider should carefully consider the labeling instructions for the alternative agent selected.

Guidelines for Transitioning to Alternate Agents from Esmolol

Alternative agent	Dosage
Propranolol hydrochloride	10 to 20 mg every 4 to 6 hours
Digoxin	0.125 to 0.5 mg every 6 hours (oral or IV[a])
Verapamil	80 mg every 6 hours

[a] IV = intravenous.

ESMOLOL HYDROCHLORIDE — INJECTION

The dosage of esmolol hydrochloride should be reduced as follows:

1.) Thirty minutes following the first dose of the alternative agent, reduce the infusion rate of esmolol hydrochloride by one-half.
2.) Following the second dose of the alternative agent, monitor the patient's response and, if satisfactory control is maintained for the first hour, discontinue esmolol hydrochloride.

Intraoperative tachycardia and hypertension – In the intraoperative and postoperative settings, it is not always advisable to slowly titrate the dose of esmolol hydrochloride to a therapeutic effect. Therefore, 2 dosing options are presented: Immediate control dosing and a gradual control when the physician has time to titrate.

Immediate control:

• *Usual dosage* – For intraoperative treatment of tachycardia or hypertension, give an 80 mg (approximately 1 mg/kg) bolus dose over 30 seconds followed by a 150 mcg/kg/min infusion, if necessary.

• *Dosage adjustment* – Adjust the infusion rate as required up to 300 mcg/kg/min to maintain desired heart rate or blood pressure.

Postoperative tachycardia and hypertension – In the intraoperative and postoperative settings it is not always advisable to slowly titrate the dose of esmolol hydrochloride to a therapeutic effect. Therefore, 2 dosing options are presented: Immediate control dosing and a gradual control when the physician has time to titrate.

Gradual control:

• *Usual dosage* – For postoperative tachycardia and hypertension, the dosing schedule is the same as that used in supraventricular tachycardia. (See Supraventricular tachycardia).

• *Loading dose* – To initiate treatment, administer a loading dosage infusion of 500 mcg/kg/min of esmolol hydrochloride for 1 minute followed by a 4 minute maintenance infusion of 50 mcg/kg/min. If an adequate therapeutic effect is not observed within 5 minutes, repeat the same loading dosage and follow with a maintenance infusion increased to 100 mcg/kg/min.

Off-label dosing –

Unstable angina: 2 to 24 mg/min as a continuous infusion.

➤*Children:*

Off-label dosing –

Acute, severe hypertension:

• *1 to 17 years of age* –

Initial dosage: Following the loading dose, initiate 25 to 100 mcg/kg/min IV infusion.

Loading dose: 100 to 500 mcg/kg IV over 1 minute.

Dosage titration: Titrate to individual response. Readminister loading dose or increase maintenance dose by 25 to 50 mcg/kg/min every 5 to 10 minutes as needed to achieve the desired response.

Maintenance dosage: 50 to 500 mcg/kg/min; dosages as high as 1000 mcg/kg/min have been administered.

• *Younger than 1 year of age* –

Maximum dose: 200 mcg/kg/min.

Initial dosage: 50 mcg/kg/min by continuous IV infusion.

Dosage titration: Titrate to desired blood pressure, increasing by 25 to 50 mcg/kg/min every 5 minutes. Rarely titrate above 300 mcg/kg/min because of adverse effects.

Pediatric hypertensive urgency or emergency: [1] = Good documentation. IV infusion of 100 to 500 mcg/kg/min. A constant infusion is preferred because esmolol is very short acting. The goal is to reduce blood pressure by up to 25% over the first 8 hours from presentation and then gradually normalize pressure over 26 to 48 hours.

Supraventricular tachycardia:

• *1 to 17 years of age* – See Children: Acute, Severe Hypertension.

• *Younger than 1 year of age* –

Initial dosage: 100 mcg/kg/min by continuous IV infusion.

Dosage titration: Titrate for control of ventricular rate, increasing by 50 to 100 mcg/kg/min every 5 minutes.

➤*Discontinuation of therapy:* In the event of an adverse reaction, the dosage of esmolol hydrochloride may be reduced or discontinued. If a local infusion site reaction develops, an alternate infusion site should be used and caution should be taken to prevent extravasation. The use of butterfly needles should be avoided.

Abrupt cessation of esmolol hydrochloride in patients has not been reported to produce the withdrawal effects which may occur with abrupt withdrawal of beta blockers following chronic use in coronary artery disease (CAD) patients. However, caution should still be used in abruptly discontinuing infusions of esmolol hydrochloride in CAD patients.

➤*Storage/Stability:* Store at 25°C (77°F). Excursions permitted to 15° to 30°C (59° to 86°F). Protect from freezing. Avoid excessive heat.

BETAXOLOL HYDROCHLORIDE

Rx	**Betaxolol Hydrochloride** (KVK Tech)	**Tablets; oral:** 10 mg	Lactose, PEG. (K 13). White, round, scored. Film-coated. In 100s.
Rx	**Kerlone** (Sanofi)		Lactose. (KERLONE 10). White, scored. Film-coated. In 100s.
Rx	**Betaxolol Hydrochloride** (KVK Tech)	**Tablets; oral:** 20 mg	Lactose, PEG. (K 14). White, round. Film-coated. In 100s.
Rx	**Kerlone** (Sanofi)		Lactose. (KERLONE 20 β). White. Film-coated. In 100s.

BETAXOLOL HYDROCHLORIDE — ORAL

For complete and comparative prescribing information, refer to the Beta-Adrenergic Blocking Agents group monograph.

Indications

➤*Hypertension:* Management of hypertension. It may be used alone or concomitantly with other antihypertensive agents, particularly thiazide diuretics.

Administration and Dosage

➤*Adults:*

Hypertension –

Initial dosage: 10 mg once daily either alone or added to diuretic therapy.

Dosage titration: The full antihypertensive effect is usually seen within 7 to 14 days. If the desired response is not achieved, the dose can be doubled after 7 to 14 days. Increasing the dose beyond 20 mg has not been shown to produce a statistically significant additional antihypertensive effect, but the 40 mg dose has been studied and is well tolerated. An increased effect (reduction) on heart rate should be anticipated with increasing dosage.

Concomitant therapy: If monotherapy with betaxolol does not produce the desired response, the addition of a diuretic agent or other antihypertensive should be considered.

Nifedipine, chlorthalidone, and hydrochlorothiazide have been coadministered with betaxolol and have not altered its pharmacokinetics. Calcium antagonists may be used in combination with beta-adrenergic blocking agents when heart function is normal, but should be avoided in patients with impaired cardiac function. Catecholamine-depleting drugs may have an additive effect when given with beta-blocking agents. Use with caution.

➤*Elderly:* Consideration should be given to reducing the starting dose to 5 mg in elderly patients. These patients are especially prone to beta-blocker–induced bradycardia, which appears to be dose related and sometimes responds to reductions in dose.

➤*Renal function impairment:* In patients with renal impairment, clearance of betaxolol declines with decreasing renal function.

Maximum dose – 20 mg/day.

Initial dosage – In patients with severe renal impairment and those undergoing dialysis, the initial dose of betaxolol is 5 mg once daily.

Dose titration – If the desired response is not achieved, dosage may be increased by 5 mg/day increments every 2 weeks to a maximum dose of 20 mg/day.

➤*Hepatic function impairment:* Patients with hepatic disease do not have significantly altered clearance. Dosage adjustments are not routinely needed.

➤*Discontinuation of therapy:* If withdrawal of betaxolol therapy is planned, it should be achieved gradually over a period of about 2 weeks. Patients should be carefully observed and advised to limit physical activity to a minimum.

➤*Storage/Stability:* Store between 15° and 25°C (59° and 77°F).

PENBUTOLOL SULFATE

Rx	**Levatol** (Schwarz Pharma)	**Tablets; oral:** 20 mg	(RC22). Yellow, scored, capsule shape. In 100s.

PENBUTOLOL — ORAL

For complete and comparative prescribing information, refer to the Beta-Adrenergic Blocking Agents group monograph.

Indications

➤*Arterial hypertension:* Penbutolol is indicated in the treatment of mild to moderate arterial hypertension. It may be used alone or in combination with other antihypertensive agents, especially thiazide-type diuretics.

Administration and Dosage

➤*Adults:*

Arterial hypertension –

Usual dosage: 20 mg given once daily used alone or in combination with other antihypertensive agents, such as thiazide-type diuretics. Doses of 40 and 80 mg have been well-tolerated but have not been shown to give a greater antihypertensive effect. The full effect of a 20 or 40 mg dose is seen by the end of 2 weeks. A dose of 10 mg also lowers blood pressure, but the full effect is not seen for 4 to 6 weeks.

➤*Storage/Stability:* Store at controlled room temperature 15° to 30°C (59° to 86°F). Keep tightly closed and protect from light.

NEBIVOLOL

Rx	**Bystolic** (Forest Pharmaceuticals)	**Tablets; oral:** 2.5 mg	As nebivolol hydrochloride. Lactose. (FL 2½). Lt. blue, triangular. In 30s, 100s, and UD 100s.
		5 mg	As nebivolol hydrochloride. Lactose. (FL 5). Beige, triangular. In 30s, 100s, and UD 100s.
		10 mg	As nebivolol hydrochloride. Lactose. (FL 10). Pinkish purple, triangular. In 30s, 100s, and UD 100s.
		20 mg	As nebivolol hydrochloride. Lactose. (FL 20). Lt. blue, triangular. In 30s, 100s, and UD 100s.

For complete and comparative prescribing information, refer to the Beta-Adrenergic Blocking Agents class monograph.

NEBIVOLOL HYDROCHLORIDE — ORAL

Indications

➤*Hypertension:* For the treatment of hypertension; may be used alone or in combination with other antihypertensive agents.

Administration and Dosage

➤*General dosing considerations:* The dose of nebivolol should be individualized to the needs of the patient.

May be used alone or in combination with other antihypertensive agents.

➤*Adults:*

Hypertension –

Usual dosage: 5 mg once daily with or without food.

Dosage titration: For patients requiring further reduction in blood pressure, increase dose at 2-week intervals, up to 40 mg. A more frequent dosing regimen is unlikely to be beneficial.

Discontinuation of therapy: As with other beta-blockers, when discontinuation of nebivolol is planned, carefully observe patients and advise them to minimize physical activity. Taper nebivolol over 1 to 2 weeks when possible. If the angina worsens or acute coronary insufficiency develops, it is recommended that nebivolol be reinstituted promptly, at least temporarily.

➤*Renal function impairment:* In patients with severe renal impairment (creatinine clearance [CrCl] less than 30 mL/min), the recommended initial dosage is 2.5 mg once daily; upward titration should be performed slowly if needed. Nebivolol has not been studied in patients receiving dialysis.

➤*Hepatic function impairment:* In patients with moderate hepatic impairment, the recommended initial dosage is 2.5 mg once daily; upward titration should be performed slowly, if needed. Nebivolol has not been studied in patients with severe hepatic impairment and, therefore, is not recommended in that population.

➤*Storage/Stability:* Store at 20° to 25°C (68° to 77°F). Dispense in a tight, light-resistant container.

CARTEOLOL HYDROCHLORIDE

Rx	**Cartrol** (Abbott)	**Tablets:** 2.5 mg	Lactose. Gray. In 100s.
		5 mg	Lactose. White. In 100s.

CARTEOLOL HYDROCHLORIDE — ORAL

For complete and comparative prescribing information, refer to the Beta-Adrenergic Blocking Agents group monograph.

Indications

➤*Hypertension:* Carteolol hydrochloride is indicated in the management of hypertension. It may be used alone or in combination with other antihypertensive agents, especially thiazide diuretics. Preliminary data indicate that carteolol does not have a favorable effect on arrhythmias.

Administration and Dosage

➤*Adults:*

Hypertension –

Usual dosage: The usual maintenance dose of carteolol is 2.5 or 5 mg once daily.

Initial dosage: 2.5 mg given as a single daily oral dose either alone or added to diuretic therapy.

Dosage titration: If an adequate response is not achieved, the dose can be gradually increased to 5 and 10 mg as single daily doses. Increasing the dose above 10 mg/day is unlikely to produce further substantial benefits and, in fact, may decrease the response.

➤*Renal function impairment:* Carteolol is excreted principally by the kidneys. When administering carteolol to patients with renal impairment, the dosage regimen should be adjusted individually by the health care provider. Guidelines for dose interval adjustment based upon creatinine clearance (CrCl) (mL/h) are as follows:

- For CrCl more than 60 mL/h, the dosage interval is every 24 hours.
- For CrCl 20 to 60 mL/h, the dosage interval is every 48 hours.
- For CrCl less than 20 mL/h, the dosage interval is every 72 hours.

➤*Storage/Stability:* Store at 15° to 30°C (59° to 86°F).

BISOPROLOL FUMARATE

Rx	**Bisoprolol Fumarate** (Eon)	**Tablets:** 5 mg	In 30s and 100s.
Rx	**Zebeta** (Barr)		(B1 LL). Pink, scored, heart shape, biconvex. Film-coated. In 30s.
Rx	**Bisoprolol Fumarate** (Eon)	10 mg	In 30s and 100s.
Rx	**Zebeta** (Barr)		(B3 LL). White, heart shape, biconvex. Film-coated. In 30s.

BISOPROLOL FUMARATE — ORAL

For complete and comparative prescribing information, refer to the Beta-Adrenergic Blocking Agents group monograph.

Indications

➤*Hypertension:* Used alone or in combination with other antihypertensive agents.

Administration and Dosage

➤*General dosing considerations:* Individualize dosage.

➤*Adults:*

Hypertension –

Initial dosage: 5 mg once daily. In some patients, 2.5 mg may be appropriate.

Dosage titration: If the antihypertensive effect of 5 mg is inadequate, the dose may be increased to 10 mg and then, if necessary, to 20 mg once daily.

➤*Elderly:* Dose adjustment is not necessary unless there is also significant renal or hepatic dysfunction.

➤*Renal function impairment:* In patients with renal dysfunction (creatinine clearance less than 40 mL/min), use an initial daily dose of 2.5 mg and use caution in dose titration. Because limited data suggest that bisoprolol is not dialyzable, drug replacement is not necessary in patients undergoing hemodialysis.

➤*Hepatic function impairment:* In patients with hepatic impairment (hepatitis or cirrhosis), use an initial daily dose of 2.5 mg and use caution in dose titration.

➤*Administration:* May be given without regard to meals.

➤*Storage/Stability:* Store at 20° to 25°C (68° to 77°F), protected from moisture.

PINDOLOL

Rx	**Pindolol** (Various, eg, Mutual, Mylan, URL, Watson)	**Tablets**: 5 mg	In 100s, 500s, and 1000s.
Rx	**Visken** (Novartis)		(Visken 5 V). White, heart shape. In 100s.
Rx	**Pindolol** (Various, eg, Mutual, Mylan, URL, Watson)	**Tablets**: 10 mg	In 100s, 500s, and 1000s.
Rx	**Visken** (Novartis)		(Visken 10 V). White, heart shape. In 100s.

PINDOLOL — ORAL

For complete and comparative prescribing information, refer to the Beta-Adrenergic Blocking Agents group monograph.

Indications

➤*Hypertension:* Pindolol tablets are indicated in the management of hypertension. They may be used alone or concomitantly with other antihypertensive agents, particularly with a thiazide-type diuretic.

➤*Off-label uses:*

Fibromyalgia – [4] = Insufficient documentation. Preliminary data from a limited number of patients (fewer than 20) indicate that pindolol may be effective for the treatment of fibromyalgia.

Prevention of migraine (adults) – [5] = Poor documentation. Pindolol failed to show efficacy over placebo in 2 controlled trials. American Academy of Neurology practice guidelines consider pindolol to be no more effective than placebo for the prevention of migraines.

Traumatic brain injury – [2] = Fair documentation. Beta-blockers are recommended by the Neurobehavioral Guidelines Working Group at the guideline level, making them a second-tier recommendation after standard-level recommendations. Among the beta-blockers, pindolol has the most support from published studies. Although the preponderance of evidence supports the use of beta-blockers in the management of aggression after traumatic brain injury (TBI), case reports have documented lack of response to various beta-blockers, and some patients in the studies with pindolol did not benefit from therapy. Thus, monitor patients receiving pindolol for neurobehavioral sequelae of TBI for adequate response.

Administration and Dosage

➤*Adults:*

Hypertension –

Maximum dose: 60 mg/day.

Initial dosage: 5 mg twice daily alone or in combination with other antihypertensive agents. An antihypertensive response usually occurs within the first week of treatment. Maximal response, however, may take as long as or occasionally longer than 2 weeks.

Dosage adjustment: If a satisfactory reduction in blood pressure does not occur within 3 to 4 weeks, the dose may be adjusted in increments of 10 mg/day at these intervals up to a maximum of 60 mg/day.

Off-label dosing

Fibromyalgia: [4] = Insufficient documentation. Initial dosage of 2.5 mg 3 times daily for 2 weeks. Maintenance dosage of 10 to 15 mg daily in divided doses for up to 12 weeks.

Traumatic brain injury: [2] = Fair documentation. 10 mg per day orally, increased in increments of 10 mg per day at 3- to 4-day intervals. In 1 study, optimal response was observed at dosages of 40 to 60 mg per day. The maximum recommended dosage is 100 mg per day. Pindolol has been studied in patients with TBI over 10 weeks; however, the optimal duration of therapy has not been established, and long-term administration may be required to maintain symptom control.

➤*Children:* Safety and effectiveness in children have not been established.

➤*Renal function impairment:* Should be used with caution in patients with impaired renal function.

➤*Hepatic function impairment:* Should be used with caution in patients with impaired hepatic function.

➤*Storage/Stability:* Store at controlled room temperature, 15° to 30°C (59° to 86°F). Protect from light. Dispense in a tight, light-resistant container using a child-resistant closure.

METOPROLOL

Rx	**Metoprolol Tartrate** (Various, eg, Caraco, Mylan)	**Tablets; oral**: 25 mg	In 30s, 90s, 100s, and 1000s.
Rx	**Metoprolol Tartrate** (Various, eg, Mylan, Qualitest, Teva, URL, Watson)	**Tablets; oral**: 50 mg	In 100s and 1000s.
Rx	**Lopressor** (Novartis)		Lactose. (GEIGY 51 51). Pink, scored, capsule shape, biconvex. In 100s, 1000s, and UD 100s.
Rx	**Metoprolol Tartrate** (Various, eg, Mylan, Qualitest, Teva, URL, Watson)	**Tablets; oral**: 100 mg	In 100s and 1000s.
Rx	**Lopressor** (Novartis)		Lactose. (GEIGY 71 71). Light blue, scored, capsule shape, biconvex. In 100s and 1000s.
Rx	**Metoprolol Succinate** (Various, eg, Par, Sandoz)	**Tablets, extended-release; oral**: 25 mg	23.75 mg metoprolol succinate equivalent to 25 mg metoprolol tartrate. Film-coated. In 100s and 1,000s.
Rx	**Toprol XL** (AstraZeneca)		(AB). White, scored, oval, biconvex. Film-coated. In 100s.
Rx	**Metoprolol Succinate** (Various, eg, Ethex, Par)	**Tablets, extended-release; oral**: 50 mg	47.5 mg metoprolol succinate equivalent to 50 mg metoprolol tartrate. Film-coated. In 100s.
Rx	**Toprol XL** (AstraZeneca)		(A mo). White, scored, biconvex. Film-coated. In 100s.

METOPROLOL

Rx	**Metoprolol Succinate** (Various, eg, Ethex, Par)	**Tablets, extended-release; oral:** 100 mg	95 mg metoprolol succinate equivalent to 100 mg metoprolol tartrate. May contain maltodextrin, polydextrose. Film-coated. In 100s 1,000s, and UD 100s.
Rx	**Toprol XL** (AstraZeneca)		(A ms). White, scored, biconvex. Film-coated. In 100s.
Rx	**Metoprolol Succinate** (Various, eg, Ethex, Par)	**Tablets, extended-release; oral:** 200 mg	190 mg metoprolol succinate equivalent to 200 mg metoprolol tartrate. May contain maltodextrin, polydextrose. Film-coated. In 100s, 1,000s, and UD 100s.
Rx	**Toprol XL** (AstraZeneca)		(A my). White, scored, oval, biconvex. Film-coated. In 100s.
Rx	**Metoprolol Tartrate** (Hospira)	**Injection:** 1 mg/mL	In amps and *Carpuject* sterile cartridge units with Luer-Lock.
Rx	**Lopressor** (Novartis)		In 5 mL amps.

METOPROLOL TARTRATE – ORAL

For complete and comparative prescribing information, refer to the Beta-Adrenergic Blocking Agents group monograph.

WARNING

Ischemic heart disease – Following abrupt cessation of therapy with certain beta-blocking agents, exacerbations of angina pectoris and, in some cases, myocardial infarction have occurred. When discontinuing chronically administered metoprolol tartrate, particularly in patients with ischemic heart disease, gradually reduce the dosage over a period of 1 to 2 weeks and carefully monitor the patient. If angina markedly worsens or acute coronary insufficiency develops, reinstate metoprolol tartrate administration promptly, at least temporarily, and take other measures appropriate for the management of unstable angina. Warn patients against interruption or discontinuation of therapy without the physician's advice. Because coronary artery disease is common and may be unrecognized, it may be prudent not to discontinue metoprolol tartrate therapy abruptly, even in patients treated only for hypertension.

Bronchospastic diseases – Patients with bronchospastic diseases should, in general, not receive beta blockers, including metoprolol tartrate. Because of its relative $beta_1$ selectivity, however, metoprolol tartrate may be used with caution in patients with bronchospastic disease who do not respond to or cannot tolerate, other antihypertensive treatment. Since beta selectivity is not absolute, a $beta_2$-stimulating agent should be administered concomitantly, and the lowest possible dose of metoprolol tartrate should be used. In these circumstances it would be prudent initially to administer metoprolol tartrate in smaller doses 3 times daily, instead of larger doses 2 times daily, to avoid the higher plasma levels associated with the longer dosing interval.

Major surgery – The necessity or desirability of withdrawing beta-blocking therapy, including metoprolol tartrate, prior to major surgery is controversial; the impaired ability of the heart to respond to reflex adrenergic stimuli may augment the risks of general anesthesia and surgical procedures.

Metoprolol tartrate, like other beta blockers, is a competitive inhibitor of beta-receptor agonists, and its effects can be reversed by administration of such agents (eg, dobutamine or isoproterenol). However, such patients may be subject to protracted severe hypotension. Difficulty in restarting and maintaining the heart beat has also been reported with beta blockers.

Diabetes and hypoglycemia – Metoprolol tartrate should be used with caution in diabetic patients if a beta-blocking agent is required. Beta blockers may mask tachycardia occurring with hypoglycemia, but other manifestations, such as dizziness and sweating may not be significantly affected.

Pheochromocytoma – In patients known to have, or suspected of having, a pheochromocytoma, metoprolol tartrate is contraindicated. If metoprolol tartrate is required, it should be given in combination with an alpha blocker, and only after the alpha blocker has been initiated. Administration of beta blockers alone in the setting of pheochromocytoma has been associated with a pardoxical increase in blood pressure due to the attenuation of beta-mediated vasodilatation in skeletal muscle.

Thyrotoxicosis – Beta-adrenergic blockade may mask certain clinical signs (eg, tachycardia) of hyperthyroidism. Patients suspected of developing thyrotoxicosis should be managed carefully to avoid abrupt withdrawal of beta blockade, which might precipitate a thyroid storm.

Indications

➤*Hypertension:* For the treatment of hypertension. May be used alone or in combination with other antihypertensive agents.

➤*Angina pectoris:* Long-term treatment of angina pectoris.

➤*Myocardial infarction:* Treatment of hemodynamically stable patients with definite or suspected acute myocardial infarction to reduce cardiovascular mortality. Treatment with intravenous metoprolol tartrate can be initiated as soon as the patient's clinical condition allows. Alternatively, treatment can begin within 3 to 10 days of the acute event.

➤*Off-label uses:*

Pediatric hypertension – [3] = Safety concerns. Metoprolol is among the therapeutic options for pediatric hypertension identified by the National High Blood Pressure Education Program, based on published case series.

Prevention of migraine (adults) – [2] = Fair documentation. Controlled trials comparing metoprolol with placebo, propanolol, or other agents for the prophylaxis of migraine have shown it to be an effective agent. American Academy of Neurology practice guidelines state that metoprolol is an efficacious treatment option that has limited strength of evidence.

Administration and Dosage

➤*General dosing considerations:* The dosage of metoprolol should be individualized.

While once-daily dosing is effective and can maintain a reduction in blood pressure throughout the day, lower doses (especially 100 mg) may not maintain a full effect at the end of the 24-hour period, and larger or more frequent daily doses may be required. This can be evaluated by measuring blood pressure near the end of the dosing interval to determine whether satisfactory control is being maintained throughout the day. Beta-1 selectivity diminishes as the dose of metoprolol is increased.

➤*Adults:*

Angina pectoris –

Usual dosage: 100 to 400 mg/day taken with or immediately following meals; dosages above 400 mg/day have not been studied.

Initial dosage: 100 mg daily, given in 2 divided doses.

Dosage titration: The dosage may be gradually increased at weekly intervals until optimum clinical response has been obtained or there is pronounced slowing of the heart rate.

Discontinuation of therapy: If treatment is to be discontinued, the dosage should be reduced gradually over a period of 1 to 2 weeks.

Hypertension –

Usual dosage: 100 to 450 mg/day taken with or immediately following meals; dosages above 450 mg/day have not been studied.

Initial dosage: 100 mg daily in single or divided doses, whether used alone or added to a diuretic.

Dosage titration: The dosage may be increased at weekly (or longer) intervals until optimum blood pressure reduction is achieved. In general, the maximum effect of any given dosage level will be apparent after 1 week of therapy.

Myocardial infarction –

Early treatment: During the early phase of definite or suspected acute myocardial infarction, treatment with metoprolol can be initiated as soon as possible after the patient's arrival in the hospital. Such treatment should be initiated in a coronary care or similar unit immediately after the patient's hemodynamic condition has stabilized. During the intravenous administration of metoprolol, blood pressure, heart rate, and electrocardiogram should be carefully monitored.

- *Initial dosage* – 3 bolus injections of 5 mg of metoprolol each; given at approximately 2-minute intervals.
- *Maintenance dosage* –

Patients who tolerate the full intravenous dose (15 mg): Start metoprolol tablets, 50 mg every 6 hours, 15 minutes after the last intravenous dose and continue for 48 hours. Thereafter, patients should receive a maintenance dosage of 100 mg twice daily.

Patients unable to tolerate the full intravenous dose: Start metoprolol tablets either 25 mg or 50 mg every 6 hours (depending on the degree of intolerance) 15 minutes after the last intravenous dose or as soon as the clinical condition allows. In patients with severe intolerance, treatment with metoprolol should be discontinued.

Late treatment: Patients with contraindications to treatment during the early phase of suspected or definite myocardial infarction, patients who appear not to tolerate the full early treatment, and patients in whom the health care provider wishes to delay therapy for any other reason should be started on metoprolol tablets, 100 mg twice daily, as soon as their clinical condition allows. Therapy should be continued for at least 3 months. Although the efficacy of metoprolol beyond 3 months has not been conclusively established, data from studies with other beta blockers suggest that treatment should be continued for 1 to 3 years.

Off-label dosing –

Prevention of migraine (adults): [2] = Fair documentation. 100 to 200 mg daily.

➤*Storage/Stability:* Store between 15° to 30°C (59° to 86°F). Protect from moisture. Dispense in tight, light-resistant container.

METOPROLOL SUCCINATE — ORAL

For complete and comparative prescribing information, refer to the Beta-Adrenergic Blocking Agents group monograph.

WARNING

Ischemic heart disease – Following abrupt cessation of therapy with certain beta-blocking agents, exacerbations of angina pectoris and, in some cases, myocardial infarction have occurred. When discontinuing chronically administered metoprolol, particularly in patients with ischemic heart disease, gradually reduce the dosage over a period of 1 to 2 weeks and carefully monitor the patient. If angina markedly worsens or acute coronary insufficiency develops, reinstate metoprolol administration promptly, at least temporarily, and take other measures appropriate for the management of unstable angina. Warn patients against interruption or discontinuation of therapy without the physician's advice. Because coronary artery disease is common and may be unrecognized, it may be prudent not to discontinue metoprolol therapy abruptly, even in patients treated only for hypertension.

Indications

➤*Hypertension:* Treatment of hypertension. They may be used alone or in combination with other antihypertensive agents.

➤*Angina pectoris:* Long-term treatment of angina pectoris.

➤*Heart failure:* Treatment of stable, symptomatic (NYHA class II or III) heart failure of ischemic, hypertensive, or cardiomyopathic origin. It was studied in patients already receiving ACE inhibitors, diuretics, and, in the majority of cases, digitalis. In this population, metoprolol succinate extended-release tablets decreased the rate of mortality plus hospitalization, largely through a reduction in cardiovascular mortality and hospitalizations for heart failure.

➤*Off-label uses:*

Prevention of migraine (adults) – [2] = Fair documentation. Controlled trials comparing metoprolol with placebo, propanolol, or other agents for the prophylaxis of migraine have shown it to be an effective agent. American Academy of Neurology practice guidelines state that metoprolol is an efficacious treatment option that has limited strength of evidence.

Administration and Dosage

➤*General dosing considerations:* An extended-release tablet intended for once-daily administration. When switching from immediate-release metoprolol tablet to metoprolol extended-release, the same total daily dose of metoprolol should be used.

As with immediate-release metoprolol, dosages of extended-release metoprolol should be individualized and titration may be needed in some patients.

➤*Adults:*

Angina pectoris –

Usual dosage: 100 mg daily in a single dose; dosages above 400 mg/day have not been studied.

Dosage titration: The dosage may be gradually increased at weekly intervals until optimum clinical response has been obtained or there is a pronounced slowing of the heart rate.

Discontinuation of therapy: If treatment is to be discontinued, the dosage should be reduced gradually over a period of 1 to 2 weeks.

Heart failure – Dosage must be individualized and closely monitored during up-titration. Prior to initiation of extended-release metoprolol, the dosing of diuretics, ACE inhibitors, and digitalis (if used) should be stabilized.

Initial dosage: 25 mg once daily for 2 weeks in patients with NYHA class II heart failure; 12.5 mg once daily in patients with more severe heart failure.

Dosage titration: The dose should then be doubled every 2 weeks to the highest dosage level tolerated by the patient or up to 200 mg of extended-release metoprolol. Initial difficulty with titration should not preclude later attempts to introduce extended-release metoprolol. If heart failure patients experience symptomatic bradycardia, the dose of extended-release metoprolol should be reduced.

Worsening heart failure: If transient worsening of heart failure occurs, it may be treated with increased doses of diuretics, and it may also be necessary to lower the dose of extended-release metoprolol or temporarily discontinue it. The dose of extended-release metoprolol should not be increased until symptoms of worsening heart failure have been stabilized.

Hypertension –

Initial dosage: 25 to 100 mg daily in a single dose, whether used alone or added to a diuretic; dosages above 400 mg/day have not been studied.

Dosage titration: The dosage may be increased at weekly (or longer) intervals until optimum blood pressure reduction is achieved. In general, the maximum effect of any given dosage level will be apparent after 1 week of therapy.

Off-label dosing –

Prevention of migraine (adults): [2] = Fair documentation. 100 to 200 mg daily.

➤*Administration:* Metoprolol extended-release tablets are scored and can be divided; however, the whole or half tablet should be swallowed whole and not chewed or crushed.

➤*Storage/Stability:* Store at 25°C (77°F). Excursions permitted to 15° to 30°C (59° to 86°F).

METOPROLOL TARTRATE — INJECTION

For complete and comparative prescribing information, refer to the Beta-Adrenergic Blocking Agents group monograph.

WARNING

Ischemic heart disease – Following abrupt cessation of therapy with certain beta-blocking agents, exacerbations of angina pectoris and, in some cases, myocardial infarction have occurred. When discontinuing chronically administered metoprolol, particularly in patients with ischemic heart disease, gradually reduce the dosage over a period of 1 to 2 weeks and carefully monitor the patient. If angina markedly worsens or acute coronary insufficiency develops, reinstate metoprolol administration promptly, at least temporarily, and take other measures appropriate for the management of unstable angina. Warn patients against interruption or discontinuation of therapy without the physician's advice. Because coronary artery disease is common and may be unrecognized, it may be prudent not to discontinue metoprolol therapy abruptly, even in patients treated only for hypertension.

Indications

➤*Myocardial infarction:* Treatment of hemodynamically stable patients with definite or suspected acute myocardial infarction to reduce cardiovascular mortality. Treatment with intravenous metoprolol tartrate can be initiated as soon as the patient's clinical condition allows. Alternatively, treatment can begin within 3 to 10 days of the acute event.

Administration and Dosage

➤*Adults:*

Myocardial infarction –

Early treatment: During the early phase of definite or suspected acute myocardial infarction, treatment with metoprolol can be initiated as soon as possible after the patient's arrival in the hospital. Such treatment should be initiated in a coronary care or similar unit immediately after the patient's hemodynamic condition has stabilized. During the intravenous administration of metoprolol, blood pressure, heart rate, and electrocardiogram should be carefully monitored.

- *Initial dosage –* See also Off-label dosing recommendations from the American Heart Association.

3 bolus injections of 5 mg of metoprolol each; given at approximately 2-minute intervals.

- *Maintenance dosage –*

  Patients who tolerate the full intravenous dose (15 mg): See also Off-label dosing recommendations from the American Heart Association.

  Start metoprolol tablets, 50 mg every 6 hours, 15 minutes after the last intravenous dose and continue for 48 hours. Thereafter, patients should receive a maintenance dosage of 100 mg twice daily.

  Patients unable to tolerate the full intravenous dose: Start metoprolol tablets either 25 mg or 50 mg every 6 hours (depending on the degree of intolerance) 15 minutes after the last intravenous dose or as soon as the clinical condition allows. In patients with severe intolerance, treatment with metoprolol should be discontinued.

Late treatment: Patients with contraindications to treatment during the early phase of suspected or definite myocardial infarction, patients who appear not to tolerate the full early treatment, and patients in whom the health care provider wishes to delay therapy for any other reason should be started on metoprolol tablets, 100 mg twice daily, as soon as their clinical condition allows. Therapy should be continued for at least 3 months. Although the efficacy of metoprolol beyond 3 months has not been conclusively established, data from studies with other beta blockers suggest that treatment should be continued for 1 to 3 years.

Off-label dosing –

Acute coronary syndrome (ST-elevation MI, non-ST-elevation MI, and unstable angina): 5 mg by slow IV push at 5 minute intervals to a total of 15 mg.

Atrial fibrillation: 2.5 to 5 mg IV bolus over 2 minutes, repeat every 5 minutes, up to 3 doses.

➤*Storage/Stability:* Do not store above 30°C (86°F). Protect from light.

TIMOLOL MALEATE

Rx	**Timolol Maleate** (Various, eg, Mylan)	**Tablets:** 5 mg	In 100s.
Rx	**Blocadren** (Merck)		(MSD 59 BLOCADREN). Light blue. In 100s.
Rx	**Timolol Maleate** (Various, eg, Mylan)	**Tablets:** 10 mg	In 100s.
Rx	**Timolol Maleate** (Various, eg, Mylan)	**Tablets:** 20 mg	In 100s.
Rx	**Blocadren** (Merck)		(MSD 437 BLOCADREN). Light blue, scored, capsule shape. In 100s.

TIMOLOL MALEATE — ORAL

For complete and comparative prescribing information, refer to the Beta-Adrenergic Blocking Agents group monograph.

WARNING

Exacerbation of ischemic heart disease following abrupt withdrawal – Hypersensitivity to catecholamines has been observed in patients withdrawn from beta-blocker therapy; exacerbation of angina and, in some cases, myocardial infarction have occurred after abrupt discontinuation of such therapy. When discontinuing chronically administered timolol, particularly in patients with ischemic heart disease, gradually reduce the dosage over a period of one to two weeks and carefully monitor the patient. If angina markedly worsens or acute coronary insufficiency develops, reinstitute timolol administration promptly, at least temporarily, and take other measures appropriate for the management of unstable angina. Warn patients against interruption of discontinuation of therapy without the physician's advice. Because coronary artery disease is common and may be unrecognized, it may be prudent not to discontinue timolol therapy abruptly, even in patients treated only for hypertension.

Indications

➤*Hypertension:* Treatment of hypertension. It may be used alone or in combination with other antihypertensive agents, especially thiazide-type diuretics.

➤*Myocardial infarction:* In patients who have survived the acute phase of myocardial infarction, and are clinically stable, to reduce cardiovascular mortality and the risk of reinfarction.

➤*Migraine:* Prophylaxis of migraine headache.

Administration and Dosage

➤*Adults:*

Hypertension –

Usual dosage: 20 to 40 mg/day divided into 2 doses.

Maximum dose: 60 mg/day divided into 2 doses.

Initial dosage: 10 mg twice a day, whether used alone or added to diuretic therapy.

Dosage adjustment: Dosage may be increased or decreased depending on heart rate and blood pressure response. Increases in dosage to a maximum of 60 mg/day divided into 2 doses may be necessary. There should be an interval of at least 7 days between increases in dosages.

Concomitant therapy: May be used with a thiazide diuretic or with other antihypertensive agents. Patients should be observed carefully during initiation of such concomitant therapy.

Migraine –

Usual dosage: 10 mg daily to 30 mg daily given in divided doses.

Maximum dose: 30 mg daily, given in divided doses.

Initial dosage: 10 mg twice a day.

Maintenance dosage: During maintenance therapy, the 20 mg daily dosage may be administered as a single dose.

Dosage adjustment: Total daily dosage may be increased to a maximum of 30 mg, given in divided doses, or decreased to 10 mg once per day, depending on clinical response and tolerability.

Discontinuation of therapy: If a satisfactory response is not obtained after 6 to 8 weeks use of the maximum daily dosage, therapy with timolol should be discontinued.

Myocardial infarction –

Usual dosage: The recommended dosage for long-term prophylactic use in patients who have survived the acute phase of a myocardial infarction is 10 mg given twice daily.

➤*Renal function impairment:* Because timolol is excreted mainly by the kidneys, dosage reductions may be necessary when renal insufficiency is present.

Marked hypotensive responses have been seen in patients with marked renal impairment undergoing dialysis after 20 mg doses. Dosing in such patients should be especially cautious.

➤*Hepatic function impairment:* Because timolol is partially metabolized in the liver, dosage reductions may be necessary when hepatic insufficiency is present.

➤*Storage/Stability:* Store at 15° to 30°C (59° to 86°F). Protect from light.

SOTALOL HYDROCHLORIDE

Rx	**Sotalol Hydrochloride** (Various, eg, Eon, Global, Par)	**Tablets; oral:** 80 mg	Lactose. In 100s, 500s, and 1,000s.
Rx	**Betapace** (Bayer)		Lactose. (Betapace 80 mg). Lt. blue, capsule shape, scored. In 100s and UD 100s.
Rx	**Sotalol Hydrochloride** (Various, eg, Eon, Global, Par)	**Tablets; oral:** 120 mg	Lactose. In 100s, 500s, and 1,000s.
Rx	**Betapace** (Bayer)		Lactose. (Betapace 120 mg). Lt. blue, capsule shape, scored. In 100s and UD 100s.
Rx	**Sotalol Hydrochloride** (Various, eg, Global, Par, Teva)	**Tablets; oral:** 160 mg	Lactose. In 100s, 500s, and 1,000s.
Rx	**Betapace** (Bayer)		Lactose. (Betapace 160 mg). Lt. blue, capsule shape, scored. In 100s and UD 100s.
Rx	**Sotalol Hydrochloride** (Various, eg, Eon, Par)	**Tablets; oral:** 240 mg	Lactose. In 100s, 500s, and 1,000s.
Rx	**Betapace** (Bayer)		Lactose. (Betapace 240 mg). Lt. blue, capsule shape, scored. In 100s and UD 100s.
Rx	**Sotalol Hydrochloride AF** (Apotex USA)	**Tablets; oral:** 80 mg	(APO AF 80). White to off-white, capsule shape, scored. In 100s.
Rx	**Betapace AF** (Bayer)		Lactose. White, capsule shape, scored. In UD 60s and 100s.
Rx	**Sotalol Hydrochloride AF** (Apotex USA)	**Tablets; oral:** 120 mg	(APO AF 120). White to off-white, capsule shape, scored. In 100s.
Rx	**Betapace AF** (Bayer)		Lactose. White, capsule shape, scored. In UD 60s and 100s.
Rx	**Sotalol Hydrochloride AF** (Apotex USA)	**Tablets; oral:** 160 mg	(APO AF 160). White to off-white, capsule shape, scored. In 100s.
Rx	**Betapace AF** (Bayer)		Lactose. White, scored, capsule shape. In UD 60s and 100s.
Rx	**Sotalol Hydrochloride** (Academic Pharmaceutical)	**Injection, solution, concentrate:** 15 mg/mL	In 10 mL vials.

SOTALOL HYDROCHLORIDE — ORAL

For complete prescribing information, refer to the Beta-Adrenergic Blocking Agents group monograph.

WARNING

To minimize the risk of induced arrhythmia, place patients initiated or reinitiated on sotalol AF or sotalol for a minimum of 3 days (on their maintenance dose) in a facility that can provide cardiac resuscitation, continuous electrocardiographic (ECG) monitoring, and calculations of creatinine clearance. Calculate creatinine clearance prior to dosing. Do not substitute sotalol for sotalol AF because of significant differences in labeling (ie, patient package insert, dosing administration, safety information).

Indications

➤*Betapace*: Oral *Betapace* (sotalol) is indicated for the treatment of documented ventricular arrhythmias, such as sustained ventricular tachycardia, that in the judgment of the physician are life-threatening. Because of the proarrhythmic effects of sotalol, including a 1.5% to 2% rate of torsade de pointes or new ventricular tachycardia (VT)/ventricular fibrillation (VF) in patients with either nonsustained ventricular tachycardia (NSVT) or supraventricular arrhythmias, its use in patients with less severe arrhythmias, even if the patients are symptomatic, is generally not recommended. Treatment of patients with asymptomatic ventricular premature contractions should be avoided.

Initiation of sotalol treatment or increasing doses, as with other antiarrhythmic agents used to treat life-threatening arrhythmias, should be carried out in the hospital. The response to treatment should then be evaluated by a suitable method (eg, PES or Holter monitoring) prior to continuing the patient on chronic therapy. Various approaches have been used to determine the response to antiarrhythmic therapy, including sotalol.

In the Electrophysiologic Study Versus Electrocardiographic Monitoring Trial (ESVEM) trial, response by Holter monitoring was tentatively defined as 100% suppression of ventricular tachycardia, 90% suppression of nonsustained VT, 80% suppression of paired ventricular premature contractions (VPCs), and 75% suppression of total VPCs in patients who had at least 10 VPCs/hour at baseline; this tentative response was confirmed if VT lasting 5 or more beats was not observed during treadmill exercise testing using a standard Bruce protocol. The programmed electrical stimulation (PES) protocol utilized a maximum of 3 extra stimuli at 3 pacing cycle lengths and 2 right ventricular pacing sites. Response by PES was defined as prevention of induction of the following:

1.) Monomorphic VT lasting over 15 seconds.
2.) Nonsustained polymorphic VT containing more than 15 beats of monomorphic VT in patients with a history of monomorphic VT.
3.) Polymorphic VT or VF greater than 15 beats in patients with VF or a history of aborted sudden death without monomorphic VT.
4.) Two episodes of polymorphic VT or VF of greater than 15 beats in a patient presenting with monomorphic VT. Sustained VT or NSVT producing hypotension during the final treadmill test was considered a drug failure.

In a multicenter, open-label, long-term study of sotalol in patients with life-threatening ventricular arrhythmias that had proven refractory to other antiarrhythmic medications, response by Holter monitoring was defined as in ESVEM. Response by PES was defined as noninducibility of sustained VT by at least double extrastimuli delivered at a pacing cycle length of 400 msec. Overall survival and arrhythmia recurrence rates in this study were similar to those seen in ESVEM, although there was no comparative group to allow a definitive assessment of outcome.

Antiarrhythmic drugs have not been shown to enhance survival in patients with ventricular arrhythmias.

➤*Betapace AF*: *Betapace AF* is indicated for the maintenance of normal sinus rhythm [delay in time to recurrence of atrial fibrillation/atrial flutter (AFIB/AFL)] in patients with symptomatic AFIB/AFL who are currently in sinus rhythm. Because *Betapace AF* can cause life-threatening ventricular arrhythmias, it should be reserved for patients in whom AFIB/AFL is highly symptomatic. Patients with paroxysmal AFIB whose AFIB/AFL that is easily reversed (by Valsalva maneuver, for example) should usually not be given *Betapace AF*.

In general, antiarrhythmic therapy for AFIB/AFL aims to prolong the time in normal sinus rhythm. Recurrence is expected in some patients.

Sotalol is also indicated for the treatment of documented life-threatening ventricular arrhythmias and is marketed under the trade name *Betapace* (sotalol HCl). *Betapace*, however, must not be substituted for *Betapace AF* because of significant differences in labeling (see entire monograph).

➤*Off-label uses:* For the treatment of refractory ventricular and supraventricular tachyarrhythmias in children. (See Administration and Dosage.)

Administration and Dosage

➤*General dosing considerations:* As with other antiarrhythmic agents, sotalol should be initiated and doses increased in a hospital with facilities for cardiac rhythm monitoring and assessment. Sotalol should be administered only after appropriate clinical assessment, and the dosage of sotalol must be individualized for each patient on the basis of therapeutic response and tolerance. Patients should continue to be monitored in this way for a minimum of 3 days on the maintenance dose. In addition, patients should not be discharged within 12 hours of electrical or pharmacological conversion to normal sinus rhythm.

Proarrhythmic reactions can occur not only at initiation of therapy, but also with each upward dosage adjustment.

The dose of *Betapace AF* must be individualized according to calculated creatinine clearance (CrCl).

Patients with atrial fibrillation should be anticoagulated according to usual medical practice. Hypokalemia should be corrected before initiation of *Betapace AF* therapy.

➤*Adults:*

Betapace –

Ventricular arrhythmias:

• *Usual dosage* – 160 to 320 mg/day, given in 2 or 3 divided doses. Some patients with life-threatening refractory ventricular arrhythmias may require doses as high as 480 to 640 mg/day.

• *Initial dosage* – 80 mg twice daily.

• *Dosage adjustment* – Dosage of sotalol should be adjusted gradually, allowing 3 days between dosing increments in order to attain steady-state plasma concentrations, and to allow monitoring of QT intervals. Graded dose adjustment will help prevent the usage of doses that are higher than necessary to control the arrhythmia.

Doses may be increased, if necessary, after appropriate evaluation to 240 or 320 mg/day (120 to 160 mg twice daily). Some patients with life-threatening refractory ventricular arrhythmias may require doses as high as 480 to 640 mg/day; however, these doses should only be prescribed when the potential benefit outweighs the increased risk of adverse reactions, in particular proarrhythmia.

Betapace AF –

Maintenance of normal sinus rhythm:

• *Maximum dose* – 160 mg twice daily.

• *Initial dosage* – 80 mg; frequency determined by CrCl.

Step 1: Prior to administration of the first dose, the QT interval must be determined using an average of 5 beats. If the baseline QT is greater than 450 msec (JT greater than or equal to 330 msec if QRS over 100 msec), use is contraindicated.

Step 2: Prior to the administration of the first dose, the patient's CrCl should be calculated.

Step 3:

CrCl greater than 60 mL/min – 80 mg twice daily.

CrCl 40 to 60 mL/min – 80 mg once daily.

CrCl less than 40 mL/min – Contraindicated.

Step 4: Administer the appropriate daily dose and begin continuous ECG monitoring with QT interval measurements 2 to 4 hours after each dose.

Step 5: If the 80 mg dose level is tolerated and the QT interval remains less than 500 msec after at least 3 days (after 5 or 6 doses if patient receives once-daily dosing), the patient can be discharged. Alternatively, during hospitalization, the dose can be increased to 120 mg twice daily and the patient followed for 3 days on this dose (followed for 5 or 6 doses if patient receives once-daily doses).

• *Dosage titration* – If the 80 mg dose level does not reduce the frequency of relapses of AFIB/AFL and is tolerated without excessive QT interval prolongation (ie, greater than or equal to 520 msec), the dose level may be increased to 120 mg (twice daily or once daily, depending upon the CrCl). As proarrhythmic reactions can occur not only at initiation of therapy, but also with each upward dosage adjustment, steps 2 through 5 used during initiation should be followed when increasing the dose level.

If the 120 mg dose does not reduce the frequency of early relapse of AFIB/AFL and is tolerated without excessive QT interval prolongation (greater than or equal to 520 msec), an increase to 160 mg (twice daily or once daily, depending upon the CrCl), can be considered. Steps 2 through 5 used during the initiation of therapy should be used again to introduce such an increase.

• *Maintenance dosage* – Renal function and QT should be reevaluated regularly if medically warranted. If QT is 520 msec or greater (JT 430 msec or greater if QRS is greater than 100 msec), the dose should be reduced and patients should be carefully monitored until QT returns to less than 520 msec. If the QT interval is greater than or equal to 520 msec while on the lowest maintenance dose level (80 mg), the drug should be discontinued. If renal function deteriorates, reduce the daily dose in half by administering the drug once daily (see step 3, Initial dosage).

• *Conversion* – Patients with a history of symptomatic AFIB/AFL who are currently receiving *Betapace* for the maintenance of normal sinus should be transferred to *Betapace AF* because of the significant differences in labeling (ie, patient package insert, dosing administration, and safety information).

➤*Children:* Use with particular caution in children if the QTc is greater than 500 msec on therapy and serious consideration should be given to reducing the dose or discontinuing therapy when QTc exceeds 550 msec.

Betapace –

Approximately 2 years of age and older: Doses normalized for body surface area are appropriate for both initial and incremental dosing. Since the class III potency in children is not very different from that in adults, reaching plasma concentrations that occur within the adult dose range is an appropriate guide.

• *Maximum dose* – 60 mg/m^2 3 times a day.

• *Initial dosage* – 30 mg/m^2 3 times a day (90 mg/m^2 total daily dose).

• *Dosage titration* – Subsequent titration to a maximum of 60 mg/m^2 can occur. Titration should be guided by clinical response, heart rate, and QTc, with increased dosing being preferably carried out in-hospital. At least 36 hours should be allowed between dose increments to attain steady-state plasma concentrations of sotalol in patients.

Approximately 2 years of age or younger: The dosage for children 2 years of age and older should be reduced by a factor that depends heavily upon age,

SOTALOL HYDROCHLORIDE — ORAL

with age plotted on a logarithmic scale in months. For a child aged 20 months, the dosing suggested for children aged 2 years or older should be multiplied by approximately 0.97; the initial starting dose would be $(30 \times 0.97) = 29.1 \text{ mg/m}^2$, administered 3 times daily. For a child aged 1 month, the starting dose should be multiplied by 0.68; the initial starting dose would be $(30 \times 0.68) = 20 \text{ mg/m}^2$, administered 3 times daily. For a child aged about 1 week, the initial starting dose should be multiplied by 0.3; the starting dose would be $(30 \times 0.3) = 9 \text{ mg/m}^2$. Similar calculations should be made for with decreasing age (below about 2 years), time to steady state will also increase. Thus, in neonates the time to steady-state may be as long as a week or longer.

Off-label dosing –

Refractory ventricular/supraventricular tachyarrhythmias:

- *Maximum dose* – 4 mg/kg every 12 hours.
- *Initial dosage* – 1 mg/kg every 12 hours.
- *Dosage titration* – Increase gradually every 3 to 5 days as needed until rhythm is stable.

➤*Renal function impairment:*

Adults –

Betapace:

Dose escalations in renal impairment should be done after administration of at least 5 to 6 doses at appropriate intervals.

Sotalol Oral Dosing Intervals in Renal Function Impairment

CrCl	Dosing[a] interval
> 60 mL/min	12 hours
30 to 59 mL/min	24 hours
10 to 29 mL/min	36 to 48 hours
< 10 mL/min	Dose should be individualized.

[a] The initial dose of 80 mg and subsequent doses should be administered at these intervals.

Betapace AF: In patients with CrCl greater than 60 mL/min, sotalol is administered twice daily, while in those with CrCl between 40 and 60 mL/min, the dose is administered once daily. In patients with CrCl less than 40 mL/min, use is contraindicated.

Children – The use of sotalol in children with renal impairment has not been investigated. Sotalol elimination is predominantly via the kidney in the unchanged form. Use of sotalol in any age group with decreased renal function should be at lower doses or at increased intervals between doses. Monitoring of heart rate and QTc is more important and it will take much longer to reach steady state with any dose and/or frequency of administration.

➤*Concomitant therapy:* Before starting sotalol, previous antiarrhythmic therapy should generally be withdrawn under careful monitoring for a minimum of 2 to 3 plasma half-lives if the patient's clinical condition permits. Treatment has been initiated in some patients receiving IV lidocaine without ill effect. After discontinuation of amiodarone, sotalol should not be initiated until the QT interval is normalized.

➤*Preparation for administration:*

Betapace suspension – Sotalol 5 mg/mL can be compounded using simple syrup containing sodium benzoate 0.1% (syrup, NF) as follows: Measure 120 mL of simple syrup. Transfer the syrup to a 6-ounce amber plastic (polyethylene terephthalate [PET]) prescription bottle. Note: An oversized bottle is used to allow for a headspace, so that there will be more effective mixing during shaking of the bottle. Add 5 sotalol 120 mg tablets to the bottle. These tablets are added intact; it is not necessary to crush the tablets. Note: The addition of the tablets can also be done first. The tablets can also be crushed if preferred. If the tablets are crushed, care should be taken to transfer the entire quantity of tablet powder into the bottle containing the syrup. Shake the bottle to wet the entire surface of the tablets. If the tablets have been crushed, shake the bottle until the end point is achieved. Allow the tablets to hydrate for approximately 2 hours. After at least 2 hours have elapsed, shake the bottle intermittently over the course of at least another 2 hours until the tablets are completely disintegrated. Note: The tablets can be allowed to hydrate overnight to simplify the disintegration process. The end point is achieved when a dispersion of fine particles in the syrup is obtained. This compounding procedure results in a solution containing 5 mg/mL of sotalol HCl. The fine solid particles are the water-insoluble inactive ingredients of the tablets. This extemporaneously prepared oral solution of sotalol (with suspended inactive particles) must be shaken well prior to administration. This is to ensure that the amount of inactive solid particles per dose remains constant throughout the duration of use.

➤*Administration:* Because of the long terminal elimination half-life of sotalol, dosing on more than a twice-daily regimen is usually not necessary. A patient who misses a dose should not double the next dose. The next dose should be taken at the usual time.

➤*Storage/Stability:* Store at 15° to 30°C (59° to 86°F). Stability studies indicate that the suspension is stable when stored at 15° to 30°C (59° to 86°F) and ambient humidity for 3 months.

SOTALOL HYDROCHLORIDE — INJECTION

For complete and comparative prescribing information, refer to the Beta-Adrenergic Blocking Agents class monograph.

WARNING

Life-threatening proarrhythmia – To minimize the risk of induced arrhythmia, patients initiated or reinitiated on intravenous (IV) sotalol, and patients who are converted from IV to oral administration should be hospitalized in a facility that can provide cardiac resuscitation, continuous electrocardiographic (ECG) monitoring, and calculations of creatinine clearance (CrCl).

Sotalol can cause life-threatening ventricular tachycardia associated with QT interval prolongation. Do not initiate sotalol therapy if the baseline QTc is longer than 450 msec. If the QT interval prolongs to 500 msec or longer, the dose must be reduced, the duration of the infusion prolonged, or the drug discontinued. Adjust the dosing interval based on CrCl.

Indications

➤*Symptomatic atrial fibrillation/atrial flutter:* For the maintenance of normal sinus rhythm (delay in time to recurrence of atrial fibrillation/atrial flutter [AFib/AFL]) in patients with symptomatic AFib/AFL who are currently in sinus rhythm. Reserve sotalol for patients in whom AFib/AFL is highly symptomatic because sotalol can cause life-threatening ventricular arrhythmias. Patients with paroxysmal AFib whose AFib/AFL is easily reversed (eg, by Valsalva maneuver) usually should not be given sotalol. In general, antiarrhythmic therapy for AFib/AFL aims to prolong the time in normal sinus rhythm. Recurrence is expected in some patients.

Patients with atrial fibrillation should be anticoagulated according to usual medical practice.

➤*Ventricular arrhythmia:* For the treatment of documented life-threatening ventricular arrhythmias. Because of the proarrhythmic effects of sotalol, including a 1.5% to 2% rate of torsades de pointes or new ventricular tachycardia (VT)/ventricular fibrillation (VF) in patients with either nonsustained VT or supraventricular arrhythmias, its use in patients with less severe arrhythmias, even if the patients are symptomatic, is generally not recommended. Avoid treatment of patients with asymptomatic ventricular premature contractions. In life-threatening ventricular arrhythmias, evaluate the response to treatment by a suitable method (eg, programmed electrical stimulation, Holter monitoring) at steady-state blood levels of the drug prior to continuing the patient on long-term therapy. Antiarrhythmic drugs may not enhance survival in patients with ventricular arrhythmias.

IV sotalol can be substituted for oral sotalol in patients who are unable to take sotalol orally.

Administration and Dosage

➤*General dosing considerations:* To minimize the risk of induced arrhythmia, patients initiated or reinitiated on sotalol should be hospitalized for at least 3 days, or until steady-state drug levels are achieved, in a facility that can provide cardiac resuscitation and continuous ECG monitoring. Initiate sotalol IV therapy in the presence of personnel trained in the management of serious ventricular arrhythmias.

Perform a baseline ECG to determine the QT interval, and measure and normalize serum potassium and magnesium levels before initiating therapy with sotalol injection. If the baseline QT is longer than 450 msec (JT longer than 330 msec if QRS over 100 msec), sotalol is not recommended. Start sotalol therapy only if the baseline QT interval is less than 450 msec. During initiation and titration, monitor the QT interval after the completion of each infusion. If the QT interval prolongs to 500 msec or longer, reduce the dose, decrease the infusion rate, or discontinue the drug.

Measure serum creatinine and calculate an estimated CrCl in order to establish the appropriate dosing interval for sotalol.

Do not abruptly withdrawal sotalol, if possible (see Discontinuation of Therapy).

Dosing interval is based on CrCl (see Renal Function Impairment).

➤*Adults:*

Symptomatic atrial fibrillation/atrial flutter –

Usual dosage: 112.5 mg IV once or twice daily based on CrCl.

Initial dosage: 75 mg once or twice daily based on CrCl. Monitor ECG for excessive increase in QTc.

Dosage titration: If the dose of sotalol 75 mg IV does not reduce the frequency of relapses of symptomatic AFib/AFL and is tolerated without excessive (to longer than 500 msec) QTc prolongation, increase the dosage to 112.5 mg once or twice daily, depending on CrCl. Continue to monitor QTc during dose escalations.

If the dose of 112.5 mg does not reduce the frequency of early relapse of arrythmia at steady state and is tolerated without excessive QTc prolongation (longer than 520 msec), increase the dosage to 150 mg IV once or twice daily based on CrCl.

The 75 mg dose can be titrated upward to 112.5 or 150 mg after at least 3 days.

Ventricular arrhythmia –

Usual dosage: 75 to 150 mg IV once or twice daily based on CrCl. Dosages as high as 225 to 300 mg IV once or twice daily have been used in patients with refractory life-threatening arrhythmias.

Initial dosage: 75 once or twice daily based on CrCl. Monitor ECG for excessive increase in QTc.

Dosage titration: If the 75 mg dose of IV sotalol does not reduce the frequency of relapses of life-threatening ventricular arrhythmias and is tolerated without excessive (to longer than 500 msec) QTc prolongation, increase

SOTALOL HYDROCHLORIDE — INJECTION

the dosage to 112.5 mg once or twice daily, depending on CrCl. Continue to monitor QTc during dose escalations.

The 75 mg dose can be titrated upward to 112.5 or 150 mg after at least 3 days.

Dosage adjustment: The dosage may be increased in increments of 75 mg/day every 3 days.

➤*Children:* IV sotalol has not been studied in children. As in adults, the following precautionary measures should be considered when initiating sotalol treatment in children: initiation of treatment in the hospital after appropriate clinical assessment, individualized regimen as appropriate, gradual increase of doses if required, careful assessment of therapeutic response and tolerability, and frequent monitoring of the QTc interval and heart rate. Doses normalized for body surface area are appropriate for both initial and incremental dosing. Because the class III potency in children is not very different from that in adults, reaching plasma concentrations that occur within the adult dose range is an appropriate guide. In all children, individualization of dosage is required. As in adults, sotalol should be used with particular caution in children if the QTc is longer than 500 msec on therapy, and serious consideration should be given to reducing the dose or discontinuing therapy when QTc exceeds 550 msec.

2 years of age and older –

Maximum dose: 60 mg/m^2 3 times a day.

Initial dosage: 30 mg/m^2 three times a day (90 mg/m^2 total daily dose) is approximately equivalent to the initial 160 mg total oral daily dose for adults.

Dosage titration: Subsequent titration to a maximum of 60 mg/m^2 (approximately equivalent to the 360 mg total daily dose for adults) should be guided by clinical response, heart rate, and QTc, with increased dosing being carried out in-hospital. At least 36 hours should be allowed between dose increments to attain steady-state plasma concentrations of sotalol in patients with age-adjusted healthy renal function.

2 years of age and younger – The previously stated pediatric dosage should be reduced by a factor that depends heavily upon age, determined by plotting the child's age on the manufacturer-provided logarithmic scale.

For a child 20 months of age, the dosing suggested for children 2 years of age and older with healthy renal function should be multiplied by approximately 0.97; the initial starting dose would be (30×0.97) = 29.1 mg/m^2 administered orally 3 times daily. For a child 1 month of age, the starting dose should be multiplied by 0.68; the initial starting dose would be (30×0.68) = 20 mg/m^2, administered orally 3 times daily. For a child 1 week of age, the initial starting oral dose should be multiplied by 0.3; the starting dose would be (30×0.3) = 9 mg/m^2. Similar calculations should be made for increased doses as titration proceeds. Because the half-life of sotalol decreases with decreasing age (younger than approximately 2 years of age), time to steady state will also increase. Thus, in neonates, the time to steady state may be as long as a week or longer.

➤*Renal function impairment:*

Adults –

CrCl greater than 60 mL/min: Administer sotalol twice daily in patients with CrCl greater than 60 mL/min.

CrCl between 40 and 60 mL/min: Administer sotalol once daily in patients with CrCl between 40 and 60 mL/min.

CrCl less than 40 mL/min: Not recommended in patients with CrCl less than 40 mL/min.

Children – The use of oral sotalol in children with renal impairment has not been investigated. Use of sotalol in any age group with decreased renal function should be at lower doses or at increased intervals between doses. Monitoring of heart rate and QTc is most important. It will take much longer to reach steady state with any dose and/or frequency of administration in these children.

➤*Conversion from oral to IV:*

Conversion From Oral to IV Sotalol

Oral dose	IV dose
80 mg	75 mg (sotalol 5 mL injection)
120 mg	112.5 mg (sotalol 7.5 mL injection)
160 mg	150 mg (sotalol 10 mL injection)

➤*Discontinuation of therapy:* When discontinuing sotalol administered long-term, particularly in patients with ischemic heart disease, carefully monitor the patient and consider the temporary use of an alternative beta-blocker if appropriate. If possible, the dosage of sotalol should be gradually reduced over a period of 1 to 2 weeks. If angina or acute coronary insufficiency develops, institute appropriate therapy promptly. Because coronary artery disease (CAD) is common and may be unrecognized in patients receiving sotalol, abrupt discontinuation in patients with arrhythmias may unmask coronary insufficiency.

➤*Preparation for administration:* IV sotalol must be diluted for infusion. Appropriate diluents are saline, dextrose 5% in water, or Ringer's lactate. Usually prepare in a volume of 100 to 250 mL. Use a volumetric infusion pump to infuse IV sotalol at a constant rate. The following table compensates for dead space in the infusion set.

Sotalol Infusion Preparation

Target dose	Sotalol injection	Diluent	Volume prepared	Volume to infuse
75 mg	6 mL	114 mL	120 mL	100 mL
112.5 mg	9 mL	111 mL		100 mL
150 mg	12 mL	108 mL		100 mL
75 mg	6 mL	294 mL	300 mL	250 mL
112.5 mg	9 mL	291 mL		250 mL
150 mg	12 mL	288 mL		250 mL

➤*Administration:* Infuse dose over 5 hours once or twice daily based on CrCl.

➤*Admixture compatibility:* Appropriate diluents are saline, dextrose 5% in water, or Ringer's lactate.

➤*Storage/Stability:* Store at 25°C (77°F); excursions are permitted to 15° to 30°C (59° to 86°F). Protect from freezing and light.

ACEBUTOLOL HYDROCHLORIDE

Rx	**Acebutolol HCl** (Various, eg, Mylan, Watson)	**Capsules:** 200 mg	In 100s and 1000s.
Rx	**Sectral** (Reddy Pharmaceuticals)		(Wyeth 4177 Sectral 200). Purple/orange. In 100s and *Redipak* 100s.
Rx	**Acebutolol HCl** (Various, eg, Mylan, Watson)	**Capsules:** 400 mg	In 100s and 1000s.
Rx	**Sectral** (Reddy Pharmaceuticals)		(Wyeth 4179 Sectral 400). Brown/orange. In 100s.

ACEBUTOLOL HYDROCHLORIDE — ORAL

For complete and comparative prescribing information, refer to the Beta-Adrenergic Blocking Agents group monograph.

Indications

➤*Hypertension:* Management of hypertension in adults. It may be used alone or in combination with other antihypertensive agents, especially thiazide-type diuretics.

➤*Ventricular arrhythmias:* Management of ventricular premature beats; it reduces the total number of premature beats, as well as the number of paired and multiform ventricular ectopic beats, and R-on-T beats.

➤*Off-label uses:*

Essential tremor – [5] = Poor documentation. Evidence-based guidelines recommend propranolol and primidone as first-line agents for the treatment of essential tremor. Current guidelines do not provide specific information about acebutolol. Because of a lack of evidence, additional research is needed to determine if acebutolol has a place in the treatment of essential tremor.

Thyrotoxicosis – [4] = Insufficient documentation. Initial research indicates that acebutolol may decrease thyroid hormone levels as well as thyroglobulin levels. Acebutolol has been shown to have symptomatic improvement in patients with hyperthyroidism. However, additional research is needed.

Ventricular tachycardia – [1] = Good documentation. Initial data from limited trials indicate that acebutolol reduces ventricular ectopic beats and may be beneficial in patients with ventricular tachycardia. American Heart Association guidelines also recommend the use of beta-blockers as first-line therapy for the treatment of ventricular tachycardia.

Administration and Dosage

➤*Adults:*

Hypertension –

Usual dosage: An optimal response is usually achieved with dosages of 400 to 800 mg/day; however, some patients have been maintained on as little as 200 mg/day.

Initial dosage: The initial dosage of acebutolol in uncomplicated, mild to moderate hypertension is 400 mg. This can be given as a single daily dose, but in occasional patients, twice-daily dosing may be required for adequate 24-hour blood pressure control.

Dosage titration: Patients with more severe hypertension or who have demonstrated inadequate control may respond to a total of 1,200 mg daily (administered twice daily). Beta-1 selectivity diminishes as dosage is increased.

Concomitant therapy: Patients with more severe hypertension or who have demonstrated inadequate control may respond to the addition of a second antihypertensive agent.

Ventricular arrhythmia –

Usual dosage: 600 to 1,200 mg/day.

Initial dosage: The usual initial dose of acebutolol is 400 mg daily given as 200 mg twice daily.

Dosage titration: Dosage should be increased gradually until an optimal clinical response is obtained, generally at 600 to 1,200 mg/day.

Discontinuation of therapy: If treatment is to be discontinued, the dosage should be reduced gradually over a period of approximately 2 weeks.

ACEBUTOLOL HYDROCHLORIDE — ORAL

Off-label dosing –

Thyrotoxicosis: [4] = Insufficient documentation. 200 mg 2 to 3 times daily for 7 to 10 days.

Ventricular tachycardia: [1] = Good documentation. 200 to 400 mg 3 times daily.

➤*Elderly:* Elderly patients have an approximately 2-fold increase in bioavailability and may require lower maintenance doses. Doses greater than 800 mg/day should be avoided in elderly patients.

➤*Renal function impairment:* The daily dose of acebutolol should be reduced by 50% when creatinine clearance (CrCl) is less than 50 mL/min and by 75% when CrCl is less than 25 mL/min.

➤*Hepatic function impairment:* Acebutolol should be used cautiously in patients with impaired hepatic function.

➤*Storage/Stability:* Store at approximately 25°C (77°F). Keep tightly closed. Protect from light.

NADOLOL

Rx	**Nadolol** (Various, eg, Apothecon, Mylan, UDL)	**Tablets:** 20 mg	In 100s and UD 100s.
Rx	**Corgard** (Monarch)		(CORGARD 20 BL 232). Scored. In 100s and *Unimatic* 100s.
Rx	**Nadolol** (Various, eg, Apothecon, Mylan, UDL, Zenith)	**Tablets:** 40 mg	In 100s, 1000s, and UD 100s.
Rx	**Nadolol** (Various, eg, Apothecon, Mylan, UDL, Zenith)	**Tablets:** 80 mg	In 30s, 100s, 500s, 1000s, and UD 100s.
Rx	**Nadolol** (Various, eg, Apothecon, Zenith)	**Tablets:** 120 mg	In 100s, 500s, and 1000s.
Rx	**Corgard** (Monarch)		(CORGARD 120 MG BL 208). Scored. In 100s and 1000s.
Rx	**Nadolol** (Various, eg, Apothecon, Zenith)	**Tablets:** 160 mg	In 100s, 500s, and 1000s.
Rx	**Corgard** (Monarch)		(246). Scored. In 100s.

NADOLOL — ORAL

For complete and comparative prescribing information, refer to the Beta-Adrenergic Blocking Agents group monograph.

WARNING

Exacerbation of ischemic heart disease following abrupt withdrawal –

Hypersensitivity to catecholamines has been observed in patients withdrawn from beta-blocker therapy; exacerbation of angina and, in some cases, myocardial infarction have occurred after abrupt discontinuation of such therapy. When discontinuing chronically administered nadolol, particularly in patients with ischemic heart disease, gradually reduce the dosage over a period of one to two weeks and carefully monitor the patient. If angina markedly worsens or acute coronary insufficiency develops, reinstitute nadolol administration promptly, at least temporarily, and take other measures appropriate for the management of unstable angina. Warn patients against interruption or discontinuation of therapy without the physician's advice. Because coronary artery disease is common and may be unrecognized, it may be prudent not to discontinue nadolol therapy abruptly, even in patients treated only for hypertension.

Indications

➤*Angina pectoris:* Nadolol is indicated for the long-term management of patients with angina pectoris.

➤*Hypertension:* Nadolol is indicated in the management of hypertension; it may be used alone or in combination with other antihypertensive agents, especially thiazide diuretics.

➤*Off-label uses:*

Prevention of migraine (adults) – [1] = Good documentation. Nadolol was studied for migraine prophylaxisin the 1980s in both placebo- and drug-controlled trials with favorable results. American Academy of Neurology practice guidelines consider nadolol to be efficacious, despite the lack of optimal scientific evidence.

Administration and Dosage

➤*General dosing considerations:* Dosage must be individualized.

➤*Adults:*

Angina pectoris –

Usual dosage: 40 or 80 mg administered once daily.

Initial dosage: 40 mg once daily.

Dosage titration: Dosage may be gradually increased in 40 to 80 mg increments at 3- to 7-day intervals until optimum clinical response is obtained, or there is pronounced slowing of the heart rate. Doses may be titrated up to 160 or 240 mg administered once daily if needed.

Hypertension –

Usual dosage: 40 to 80 mg administered once daily.

Initial dosage: 40 mg once daily, whether it is used alone or in addition to diuretic therapy.

Dosage titration: Dosage may be gradually increased in increments of 40 to 80 mg until optimum blood pressure reduction is achieved. Doses of up to 240 or 320 mg administered once daily may be needed.

Off-label dosing –

Prevention of migraine (adults): [1] = Good documentation. 80 to 240 mg daily for 2 to 18 months.

➤*Renal function impairment:* Absorbed nadolol is excreted principally by the kidneys and, although nonrenal elimination does occur, dosage adjustments are necessary in patients with renal impairment. The following dose intervals are recommended.

Nadolol Dosage Intervals in Renal Impairment

CrCl[a] (mL/min/1.73 m²)	Dosage interval (hours)
> 50	24
31 to 50	24 to 36
10 to 30	24 to 48
< 10	40 to 60

[a] CrCl = creatinine clearance.

➤*Discontinuation of therapy:* If treatment is to be discontinued, reduce the dosage gradually over a period of 1 to 2 weeks.

➤*Administration:* Nadolol may be administered without regard to meals.

➤*Storage/Stability:* Store at 15° to 30°C (59° to 86°F). Protect from light. Dispense in a tight, light-resistant container using a child-resistant closure.

PROPRANOLOL HYDROCHLORIDE

Rx	**Propranolol Hydrochloride** (Various, eg, Heritage, Major, Mylan, Watson)	**Tablets; oral:** 10 mg	May contain lactose. In 30s, 100s, and 1,000s.
Rx	**Propranolol Hydrochloride** (Various, eg, Heritage, Major, Mylan, Watson)	**Tablets; oral:** 20 mg	May contain lactose. In 30s, 100s, and 1,000s.
Rx	**Propranolol Hydrochloride** (Various, eg, Heritage, Major, Mylan, Watson)	**Tablets; oral:** 40 mg	May contain lactose. In 30s, 100s, and 1,000s.
Rx	**Propranolol Hydrochloride** (Various, eg, Heritage, Major)	**Tablets; oral:** 60 mg	May contain lactose. In 30s, 100s, and 1,000s.
Rx	**Propranolol Hydrochloride** (Various, eg, Heritage, Major, Mylan, Watson)	**Tablets; oral:** 80 mg	May contain lactose. In 30s, 100s, and 1,000s.
Rx	**Propranolol Hydrochloride** (Various, eg, Mylan, Par)	**Capsules, extended-release; oral:** 60 mg	In 100s, 500s, and 1,000s.
Rx	**Inderal LA** (Akrimax)		(INDERAL LA 60). White/Light blue. In 100s.
Rx	**Propranolol Hydrochloride** (Various, eg, Mylan, Par)	**Capsules, extended-release; oral:** 80 mg	In 100s, 500s, and 1,000s.
Rx	**Inderal LA** (Akrimax)		(INDERAL LA 80). Light blue. In 100s.
Rx	**InnoPran XL** (GlaxoSmithKline)		Contains sustained-release beads. Sugar spheres. (80 InnoPran XL). Gray/White. In 30s and 100s.

PROPRANOLOL HYDROCHLORIDE

Rx	**Propranolol Hydrochloride** (Various, eg, Mylan, Par)	**Capsules, extended-release; oral:** 120 mg	In 100s, 500s, and 1,000s.
Rx	**Inderal LA** (Akrimax)		(INDERAL LA 120). Light blue/Dark blue. In 100s.
Rx	**InnoPran XL** (GlaxoSmithKline)		Contains sustained-release beads. Sugar spheres. (120 InnoPran XL). Gray/Off-white. In 30s and 100s.
Rx	**Propranolol Hydrochloride** (Various, eg, Mylan, Par)	**Capsules, extended-release; oral:** 160 mg	In 100s, 500s, and 1,000s.
Rx	**Inderal LA** (Akrimax)		(INDERAL LA 160). Dark blue. In 100s.
Rx sf	**Propranolol Hydrochloride** (Roxane)	**Solution; oral:** 4 mg/mL (20 mg per 5 mL)	Alcohol 0.6%, parabens, saccharin, sorbitol, disodium edetate. Dye free. Strawberry-mint flavor. In 500 mL.
		8 mg/mL (40 mg per 5 mL)	Alcohol 0.6%, parabens, saccharin, sorbitol, disodium edetate. Dye free. Strawberry-mint flavor. In 500 mL.
Rx	**Propranolol Hydrochloride** (Various, eg, Bedford, Sandoz, Westward)	**Injection, solution:** 1 mg/mL	In 1 mL vials.

PROPRANOLOL HYDROCHLORIDE — ORAL

WARNING

Angina pectoris – There have been reports of exacerbation of angina and, in some cases, myocardial infarction (MI), following abrupt discontinuance of propranolol therapy. Therefore, when discontinuance of propranolol is planned, the dosage should be gradually reduced over at least a few weeks, and the patient should be cautioned against interruption or cessation of therapy without a health care provider's advice. If propranolol therapy is interrupted and exacerbation of angina occurs, it is usually advisable to reinstitute propranolol therapy and take other measures appropriate for the management of angina pectoris. Because coronary artery disease may be unrecognized, it may be prudent to follow the above advice in patients considered at risk of having occult atherosclerotic heart disease who are given propranolol for other indications.

Indications

Propranolol is approved for use in adults for the following indications:

➤*Angina pectoris due to coronary atherosclerosis (excluding InnoPran XL)*: To decrease angina frequency and increase exercise tolerance in patients with angina pectoris.

➤*Atrial fibrillation (excluding extended-release products):* To control ventricular rate in patients with atrial fibrillation and a rapid ventricular response.

➤*Essential tremor (excluding extended-release products):* Management of familial or hereditary essential tremor. Familial or essential tremor consists of involuntary, rhythmic, oscillatory movements, usually limited to the upper limbs. It is absent at rest but occurs when the limb is held in a fixed posture or position against gravity and during active movement. Propranolol causes a reduction in the tremor amplitude but not in the tremor frequency. Propranolol is not indicated for the treatment of tremor associated with parkinsonism.

➤*Hypertension:* Management of hypertension. It may be used alone or in combination with other antihypertensive agents, particularly a thiazide diuretic. Propranolol is not indicated in the management of hypertensive emergencies.

➤*Hypertrophic subaortic stenosis (excluding InnoPran XL)*: Propranolol improves New York Heart Association (NYHA) functional class in symptomatic patients with hypertrophic subaortic stenosis.

➤*Migraine prevention(excluding InnoPran XL)*: Prophylaxis of common migraine headache. The efficacy of propranolol in the treatment of a migraine attack that has started has not been established and propranolol is not indicated for such use.

➤*Myocardial infarction (excluding extended-release products):* To reduce cardiovascular mortality in patients who have survived the acute phase of MI and are clinically stable.

➤*Pheochromocytoma (excluding extended-release products):* As an adjunct to alpha-adrenergic blockade to control blood pressure and reduce symptoms of catecholamine-secreting tumors.

➤*Off-label uses:*

Migraine prevention(children / adolescents) – [4] = Insufficient documentation. Published data on the use of propranolol for the prevention of migraine headaches in children are limited by small population size and conflicting results. Consideration for use must also take into account the safety concerns, which may limit propranolol's use in this patient population.

Smoking cessation – [5] = Poor documentation. In the only study conducted to date of propranolol treatment for smoking cessation, no benefit from therapy was detected. Guidelines from the Public Health Service specifically note the lack of beneficial effect of propranolol in smoking cessation. Rational use cannot be established because of this evidence of lack of efficacy coupled with the availability of better-established Food and Drug Administration–approved pharmacotherapy options.

Traumatic brain injury – [2] = Fair documentation. Beta-blockers are recommend by the Neurobehavioral Guidelines Working Group at the guideline level, making them a second-tier recommendation after standard-level recommendations. Among the beta-blockers, propranolol and pindolol are supported by published results. Although the preponderance of evidence supports the use of beta-blockers in the management of aggression after traumatic brain injury (TBI), case reports have documented a lack of response to various beta-blockers. Thus, monitor patients receiving propranolol for neurobehavioral sequelae of TBI for adequate response to therapy.

Administration and Dosage

➤*General dosing considerations:* Dosage must be individualized.

When discontinuing propranolol, the dosage should be gradually reduced over at least a few weeks. See Discontinuation of Therapy.

➤*Adults:*

Immediate-release tablets and oral solution –

Angina pectoris because of coronary atherosclerosis:

• *Usual dosage* – 80 to 320 mg daily administered twice a day, 3 times a day, or 4 times a day has been shown to increase exercise tolerance to reduce ischemic change in the electrocardiogram (ECG).

• *Discontinuation of therapy* – If treatment is to be discontinued, reduce dosage gradually over a period of several weeks.

Atrial fibrillation: 10 to 30 mg 3 or 4 times daily before meals and at bedtime.

Essential tremor:

• *Initial dosage* – 40 mg twice daily.

• *Maintenance dosage* – Optimum reduction of essential tremor is usually achieved with a dosage of 120 mg/day. Occasionally, it may be necessary to administer 240 to 320 mg/day.

Hypertension:

• *Initial dosage* – 40 mg twice daily, whether used alone or added to a diuretic.

• *Dosage titration* – Dosage may be increased gradually until adequate blood pressure control is achieved. The time needed for full hypertensive response to a given dosage is variable and may range from a few days to several weeks.

• *Maintenance dosage* – 120 to 240 mg/day. In some instances, a dose of 640 mg may be required.

• *Alternative dosage* – While twice-daily dosing is effective and can maintain a reduction in blood pressure throughout the day, some patients, especially when lower doses are used, may experience a modest rise in blood pressure toward the end of the 12-hour dosing interval. This can be evaluated by measuring blood pressure near the end of the dosing interval to determine whether satisfactory control is being maintained throughout the day. If control is not adequate, a larger dose, or dosing 3 times daily, may achieve better control.

Hypertrophic subaortic stenosis: 20 to 40 mg 3 or 4 times daily before meals and at bedtime.

Migraine prevention:

• *Initial dosage* – 80 mg daily in divided doses.

• *Dosage titration* – The dosage may be increased gradually to achieve optimal migraine prophylaxis.

• *Maintenance dosage* – 160 to 240 mg/day.

• *Discontinuation of therapy* – If a satisfactory response is not obtained within 4 to 6 weeks after reaching the maximum dose, propranolol therapy should be discontinued. It may be advisable to withdraw the drug gradually over a period of several weeks.

Myocardial infarction:

• *Initial dosage* – 40 mg 3 times/day was the initial dosage in the Beta-Blocker Heart Attack Trial (BHAT).

• *Dosage titration* – After 1 month, titrate to 60 to 80 mg 3 times daily, as tolerated.

• *Maintenance dosage* – 180 to 240 mg/day in divided doses.

The effectiveness and safety of daily dosages greater than 240 mg for prevention of cardiac mortality have not been established. However, higher dosages may be needed to effectively treat coexisting diseases such as angina or hypertension.

Pheochromocytoma:

• *Management of inoperable tumor* – 30 mg/day in divided doses, concomitantly with an alpha-adrenergic blocking agent.

• *Preoperatively* – 60 mg/day in divided doses for 3 days prior to surgery, concomitantly with an alpha-adrenergic blocking agent.

Extended-release capsules (excluding InnoPran XL) –

Angina pectoris because of coronary atherosclerosis:

• *Initial dosage* – 80 mg once daily.

• *Dosage titration* – Dosage should be gradually increased at 3- to 7-day intervals until optimal response is obtained.

PROPRANOLOL HYDROCHLORIDE — ORAL

• *Maintenance dosage* – Although individual patients may respond at any dosage level, the average optimal dosage appears to be 160 mg once daily. In angina pectoris, the value and safety of dosages exceeding 320 mg/day have not been established.

• *Discontinuation of therapy* – If treatment is to be discontinued, reduce dosage gradually over a period of a few weeks.

Hypertension:

• *Initial dosage* – 80 mg once daily, whether used alone or added to a diuretic.

• *Dosage titration* – The dosage may be increased to 120 mg once daily or higher until adequate blood pressure control is achieved. The time needed for full hypertensive response to a given dosage is variable and may range from a few days to several weeks.

• *Maintenance dosage* – Usual maintenance dosage is 120 to 160 mg once daily. In some instances, a dose of 640 mg may be required.

Hypertrophic subaortic stenosis: 80 to 160 mg once daily.

Migraine prevention:

• *Initial dosage* – 80 mg once daily.

• *Dosage titration* – The dosage may be increased gradually to achieve optimal migraine prophylaxis.

• *Maintenance dosage* – 160 to 240 mg once daily.

• *Discontinuation of therapy* – If a satisfactory response is not obtained within 4 to 6 weeks after reaching the maximal dose, therapy should be discontinued. It may be advisable to withdraw the drug gradually over a period of several weeks depending on the patient's age, comorbidity, and dose of propranolol sustained-release.

Extended-release capsules (InnoPran XL only) –

Hypertension:

• *Initial dosage* – 80 mg once daily at bedtime (approximately 10 PM).

• *Dosage titration* – Titration may be needed to a dose of 120 mg. The time needed for full antihypertensive response is variable but is usually achieved within 2 to 3 weeks.

Off-label dosing –

Traumatic brain injury: [2] = Fair documentation. 60 mg per day orally, increased in increments of 60 mg per day every third day until agitation ceases, adverse reactions occur, or the maximum recommended dosage of 520 mg/day is reached. Propranolol use has been studied in patients with TBI for longer than 14 weeks; however, the optimal duration of therapy has not been established, and long-term administration may be required to maintain symptom control.

➤*Children:*

Off-label dosing –

Migraine prevention (children/adolescents): [4] = Insufficient documentation. Propranolol oral doses varied widely; fixed dosages were 60 to 120 mg daily, and weight-based dosages were 1 to 3 mg/kg/day.

Arrhythmias:

• *Infants and children* –
  - *Maximum dose:* 60 mg/day or 16 mg/kg/day.
  - *Initial dosage:* 0.5 to 1 mg/kg/day given in divided doses every 6 to 8 hours.
  - *Dosage titration:* Increase dosage every 3 to 5 days as needed.
  - *Maintenance dosage:* 2 to 5 mg/kg/day given in divided doses every 6 to 8 hours.

• *Neonates* –
  - *Maximum dose:* 3.5 mg/kg every 6 hours.
  - *Initial dosage:* 0.25 mg/kg every 6 hours.

Hypertension:

• *Children* –
  - *Maximum dose:* 4 to 8 mg/kg/day up to 640 mg/day.
  - *Initial dosage:* 0.5 to 2 mg/kg/day given in divided doses every 6 to 12 hours.
  - *Dosage titration:* Increase dosage every 3 to 5 days as needed.
  - *Maintenance dosage:* 2 to 4 mg/kg/day given in divided doses every 6 to 8 hours.

• *Neonates* –
  - *Maximum dose:* 3.5 mg/kg every 6 hours.
  - *Initial dosage:* 0.25 mg/kg every 6 hours.

Infundibular spasm ("tet spell"):

• *Children* –
  - *Usual dosage:* 4 to 8 mg/kg/day given in divided doses every 6 hours as needed.
  - *Initial dosage:* 2 to 4 mg/kg/day given in divided doses every 6 hours as needed.

• *Neonates* –
  - *Maximum dose:* 3.5 mg/kg every 6 hours.
  - *Initial dosage:* 0.25 mg/kg every 6 hours.

Thyrotoxicosis:

• *Adolescents* – 10 to 40 mg every 6 hours.

• *Children* – 2.5 to 10 mg 2 or 3 times/day. In severe cases, dosage may be increased to 4 to 6 mg/kg/day.

• *Neonates* –
  - *Maximum dose:* 3.5 mg/kg every 6 hours.
  - *Initial dosage:* 0.25 mg/kg every 6 hours (1 to 2 mg/kg/day).

➤*Conversion:* If patients are switched from propranolol immediate-release tablets to propranolol extended-release (ER) capsules, care should be taken to ensure that the desired therapeutic effect is maintained. Propranolol ER capsules should not be considered a simple mg-for-mg substitute for conventional propranolol. Propranolol ER capsules have different kinetics and produce lower blood levels. Retitration may be necessary, especially to maintain effectiveness at the end of the 24-hour dosing interval.

➤*Discontinuation of therapy:* There have been reports of exacerbation of angina and, in some cases, MI, following abrupt discontinuance of propranolol therapy. Therefore, when discontinuance of propranolol is planned, the dosage should be gradually reduced over at least a few weeks, and the patient should be cautioned against interruption or cessation of therapy without a health care provider's advice. If propranolol therapy is interrupted and exacerbation of angina occurs, it is usually advisable to reinstitute propranolol therapy and take other measures appropriate for the management of angina pectoris.

➤*Administration:* *InnoPran XL* should be administered once daily at bedtime (approximately 10 PM) and should be taken consistently either on an empty stomach or with food.

➤*Storage/Stability:* Store at 20° to 25°C (68° to 77°F); excursions are permitted to 15° to 30°C (59° to 86°F). Dispense in a tight, light-resistant container. Protect the ER capsules from light, moisture, freezing, and excessive heat.

PROPRANOLOL HYDROCHLORIDE — INJECTION

For complete and comparative prescribing information, refer to the Beta-Adrenergic Blocking Agents class monograph.

WARNING

Angina pectoris – There have been reports of exacerbation of angina and, in some cases, myocardial infarction (MI), following abrupt discontinuance of propranolol therapy. Therefore, when discontinuance of propranolol is planned, gradually reduce the dosage over at least a few weeks, and caution the patient against interruption or cessation of therapy without a health care provider's advice. If propranolol therapy is interrupted and exacerbation of angina occurs, it is usually advisable to reinstitute propranolol therapy and take other measures appropriate for the management of angina pectoris. Because coronary artery disease may be unrecognized, it may be prudent to follow the above advice in patients considered at risk of having occult atherosclerotic heart disease who are given propranolol for other indications.

Indications

Intravenous (IV) administration is usually reserved for life-threatening arrhythmias or those occurring under anesthesia.

➤*Supraventricular arrhythmias:* For the short-term treatment of supraventricular tachycardia, including Wolff-Parkinson-White syndrome and thyrotoxicosis, to decrease ventricular rate. Use in patients with atrial flutter or atrial fibrillation should be reserved for arrhythmias unresponsive to standard therapy or when more prolonged control is required. Reversion to normal sinus rhythm has occasionally been observed, predominantly in patients with sinus or atrial tachycardia.

➤*Ventricular tachycardias:* With the exception of those induced by catecholamines or digitalis, propranolol is not the drug of first choice. In critical situations when cardioversion techniques or other drugs are not indicated or are not effective, propranolol may be considered. If, after consideration of the risks involved, propranolol is used, it should be given IV in low dosage and very slowly, as the failing heart requires some sympathetic drive for maintenance of myocardial tone. Some patients may respond with complete reversion to normal sinus rhythm, but reduction in ventricular rate is more likely. Ventricular arrhythmias do not respond to propranolol as predictably as do the supraventricular arrhythmias.

IV propranolol is indicated for the treatment of persistent premature ventricular extrasystoles that impair the well-being of the patient and do not respond to conventional measures.

➤*Tachyarrhythmias of digitalis intoxication:* To control ventricular rate in life-threatening digitalis-induced arrhythmias. Severe bradycardia may occur.

➤*Resistant tachyarrhythmias caused by excessive catecholamine action during anesthesia:* To abolish tachyarrhythmias caused by excessive catecholamine action during anesthesia when other measures fail. These arrhythmias may arise because of release of endogenous catecholamines or administration of catecholamines. All general inhalation anesthetics produce some degree of myocardial depression. Therefore, when propranolol is used to treat arrhythmias during anesthesia, it should be used with extreme caution, usually with constant monitoring of the electrocardiogram (ECG) and central venous pressure.

➤*Off-label uses:* Infundibular spasm ("tet spell"), thyrotoxicosis, arrhythmias, and hypertensive emergencies in children.

Administration and Dosage

➤*General dosing considerations:* Reserve IV use for life-threatening arrhythmias or those occurring under anesthesia.

When discontinuing propranolol, the dosage should be gradually reduced over at least a few weeks. (See Discontinuation of Therapy.)

Propranolol is not indicated for the treatment of hypertensive emergencies.

PROPRANOLOL HYDROCHLORIDE — INJECTION

➤*Adults:*

Cardiac arrhythmias –

Usual dosage: 1 to 3 mg IV under careful monitoring (eg, central venous pressure, ECG). The rate of administration should not exceed 1 mg/min to avoid lowering blood pressure and causing cardiac standstill. Allow sufficient time for the drug to reach the site of action, even when slow circulation is present. If necessary, give a second dose after 2 minutes. Thereafter, additional propranolol should not be given in less than 4 hours.

Duration of therapy: Additional propranolol should not be given after the desired alteration in rate or rhythm is achieved. Transfer to oral therapy as soon as possible.

➤*Children:*

Off-label dosing –

Arrhythmias:

• *Infants and children –*

Usual dosage: 0.01 to 0.25 mg/kg administered IV over 10 minutes. Do not exceed 1 mg/min. Repeat every 6 to 8 hours as needed.

Maximum dose:

Infants: 1 mg/dose.

Children: 3 mg/dose.

• *Neonates –*

Maximum dose: 0.15 mg/kg/dose.

Initial dosage: 0.01 mg/kg administered IV every 6 hours over 10 minutes.

Dosage adjustment: Dosage may be increased up to a maximum of 0.15 mg/kg administered every 6 hours.

Hypertensive emergencies: Labetalol is a more preferred agent; however, if propranolol is used, then the dosage is 0.01 to 0.05 mg/kg administered IV over 1 hour.

Infundibular spasm ("tet spell"):

• *Infants and children –*

Usual dosage: 0.01 to 0.25 mg/kg administered IV over 10 minutes. If needed, may repeat this dose once in 15 minutes.

Maximum dose: 1 mg (maximum initial dose).

• *Neonates –*

Maximum dose: 0.15 mg/kg/dose.

Initial dosage: 0.01 mg/kg administered IV every 6 hours over 10 minutes.

Dosage adjustment: Dosage may be increased up to a maximum of 0.15 mg/kg administered every 6 hours.

Thyrotoxicosis:

• *Adolescents* – 1 to 3 mg/kg administered IV over 10 minutes. May repeat dose in 4 to 6 hours.

• *Neonates –*

Maximum dose: 0.15 mg/kg/dose.

Initial dosage: 0.01 mg/kg administered IV every 6 hours over 10 minutes.

Dosage adjustment: Dosage may be increased up to a maximum of 0.15 mg/kg administered every 6 hours.

➤*Hepatic function impairment:* Consideration should be given to lowering the dose of IV-administered propranolol in patients with hepatic insufficiency.

➤*Discontinuation of therapy:* There have been reports of exacerbation of angina and, in some cases, MI, following abrupt discontinuance of propranolol therapy. Therefore, when discontinuance of propranolol is planned, gradually reduce the dosage over at least a few weeks, and caution the patient against interruption or cessation of therapy without a health care provider's advice. If propranolol therapy is interrupted and exacerbation of angina occurs, it is usually advisable to reinstitute propranolol therapy and take other measures appropriate for the management of angina pectoris.

➤*Administration:* The rate of IV administration should not exceed 1 mg/min.

➤*Storage/Stability:* Store at approximately 25°C (77°F). Protect from light, freezing, and excessive heat. Discard unused portion. Retain in carton until time of use.

LABETALOL HYDROCHLORIDE

Rx	**Labetalol hydrochloride** (Various, eg, Apothecon, Eon, Ivax, Mutual, UDL, URL, Watson)	**Tablets:** 100 mg	In 30s, 100s, 250s, 500s, and 1000s.
Rx	**Trandate** (Faro Pharmaceuticals, Inc.)		(Trandate 100). Lt. orange, scored. Film-coated. In 100s, 500s, and UD 100s.
Rx	**Labetalol HCl** (Various, eg, Apothecon, Eon, Ivax, Mutual, UDL, URL, Watson)	**Tablets:** 200 mg	In 30s, 100s, 250s, 500s, and 1000s.
Rx	**Trandate** (Faro Pharmaceuticals, Inc.)		(Trandate 200). White, scored. Film-coated. In 100s, 500s, and UD 100s.
Rx	**Labetalol HCl** (Various, eg, Apothecon, Eon, Ivax, Mutual, Teva, URL, Watson)	**Tablets:** 300 mg	In 30s, 100s, 250s, 500s, and 1000s.
Rx	**Trandate** (Faro Pharmaceuticals, Inc.)		(Trandate 300). Peach, scored. Film-coated. In 100s, 500s, and UD 100s.
Rx	**Labetalol HCl** (Various, eg, Apothecon, Bedford Labs)	**Injection:** 5 mg/mL[1]	Dextrose, EDTA, parabens. In 20 and 40 mL multidose vials.

[1] With 0.1 mg EDTA and 0.8 mg methylparaben and 0.1 mg propylparaben.

LABETALOL HYDROCHLORIDE — ORAL

Indications

➤*Hypertension:* Management of hypertension. Labetalol tablets may be used alone or in combination with other antihypertensive agents, especially thiazide and loop diuretics.

➤*Off-label uses:*

Pediatric hypertension – [1] = Good documentation. Guidelines for the management of pediatric hypertension generally recommend the same drug classes that are indicated for management of adult hypertension. Particular consideration should be given to medications for which published pediatric experience is available, including appropriate dosing ranges. Similar to adults, prescribers should assess for concomitant disease states that would present a compelling indication for use of a particular drug. Other patient-specific factors, such as concomitant asthma, heart failure, or diabetes, may limit selection. Labetalol is among the therapeutic options for pediatric hypertension identified by the National High Blood Pressure Education Program based on case series and expert opinion.

Pediatric hypertensive urgency or emergency – [1] = Good documentation. Guidelines for the management of pediatric hypertension generally recommend the same drug classes that are indicated for management of adult hypertension. Particular consideration should be given to medications for which published pediatric experience is available, including appropriate dosing ranges. Labetalol is among the therapeutic options for pediatric hypertensive urgency or emergency identified by the NHBPEP as most useful.

Other possible off-label uses – Labetalol has effectively lowered blood pressure and relieved symptoms in patients with pheochromocytoma; higher IV doses may be required. However, paradoxical hypertensive responses have occurred; therefore, use caution when administering labetalol. Labetalol has been used to treat clonidine withdrawal hypertension.

Administration and Dosage

➤*General dosing considerations:* Labetalol tablets may be used alone or in combination with other antihypertensive agents, especially thiazide and loop diuretics.

Patients with severe hypertension may require from 1,200 to 2,400 mg/day, with or without thiazide diuretics. If side effects (principally nausea or dizziness) occur with these doses administered twice daily, the same total daily dose administered 3 times daily may improve tolerability and facilitate further titration. Titration increments should not exceed 200 mg twice daily.

➤*Adults:*

Hypertension –

Inpatient: Subsequent oral dosing with labetalol hydrochloride tablets should begin when it has been established that the supine diastolic blood pressure has begun to rise.

• *Usual dose* – 200 mg, followed in 6 to 12 hours by an additional dose of 200 or 400 mg, depending on the blood pressure response. (see Dosage titration.)

• *Dosage titration* – Titration increments should not exceed 200 mg twice daily.

Inpatient Labetalol Oral Titration Instructions

Regimen	Daily dose[a]
200 mg twice a day	400 mg
400 mg twice a day	800 mg
800 mg twice a day	1,600 mg
1,200 mg twice a day	2,400 mg

[a] If needed, the total daily dose may be given in 3 divided doses.

While in the hospital, the dosage of labetalol hydrochloride tablets may be increased at 1-day intervals to achieve the desired blood pressure reduction.

LABETALOL HYDROCHLORIDE — ORAL

Outpatient:

• *Usual dose* – 200 and 400 mg twice daily; dosage must be individualized.

• *Initial dosage* – 100 mg twice daily.

• *Dosage titration* – After 2 or 3 days, using standing blood pressure as an indicator, dosage may be titrated in increments of 100 mg twice a day every 2 or 3 days.

• *Concomitant therapy* – When a diuretic is added, an additive antihypertensive effect can be expected. In some cases this may necessitate a labetalol dosage adjustment. As with most antihypertensive drugs, optimal dosages of labetalol tablets are usually lower in patients also receiving a diuretic.

When transferring patients from other antihypertensive drugs, labetalol tablets should be introduced as recommended and the dosage of the existing therapy progressively decreased.

➤*Children:*

Off-label dosing –

Pediatric hypertension: [1] = Good documentation. Initial dosage is 1 to 3 mg/kg/day orally, divided for twice-daily administration. The maximum recommended dose is 10 to 12 mg/kg/day up to 1,200 mg/day.

Therapy should be initiated using the lowest recommended dose and increased until the target blood pressure is reached, the highest recommended dose is reached, or the child experiences adverse effects. A second drug from a different class may be added for patients who reach the maximum recommended dose or experience adverse effects. In some patients, a step-down may be attempted after an extended course of good blood pressure control. In these cases, the dose is reduced gradually, with the goal of complete discontinuation. Step-down dosing may be particularly appropriate for children with uncomplicated primary hypertension who successfully implement new lifestyle modifications, such as losing weight.

Pediatric hypertensive urgency or emergency: [1] = Good documentation. IV bolus 0.2 to 1 mg/kg per dose up to a maximum of 40 mg per dose; IV infusion 0.25 to 3 mg/kg/h. The goal is to reduce blood pressure by up to 25% over the first 8 hours from presentation and then gradually normalize pressure over 26 to 48 hours.

➤*Elderly:*

Hypertension –

Usual dosage: The majority of elderly patients will require between 100 and 200 mg twice a day.

Initial dosage: 100 mg twice daily.

Dosage titration: Titrate upwards in increments of 100 mg twice a day as required for control of blood pressure.

➤*Storage / Stability:* Labetalol tablets should be stored between 2° and 30°C (36° and 86°F). Labetalol tablets in the unit dose boxes should be protected from excessive moisture.

Actions

➤*Pharmacology:* Labetalol combines both selective, competitive, alpha-1-adrenergic blocking and nonselective, competitive, beta-adrenergic blocking activity in a single substance. In man, the ratios of alpha- to beta-blockade have been estimated to be approximately 1:3 and 1:7 following oral and IV administration, respectively. Beta-2-agonist activity has been demonstrated in animals with minimal beta-1-agonist (ISA) activity detected. In animals, at doses greater than those required for alpha- or beta-adrenergic blockage, a membrane-stabilizing effect has been demonstrated.

➤*Pharmacokinetics:*

Absorption – Labetalol is completely absorbed from the GI tract with peak plasma levels occurring 1 to 2 hours after oral administration. The relative bioavailability of labetalol tablets compared to an oral solution is 100%. The absolute bioavailability (fraction of drug reaching systemic circulation) of labetalol when compared to an IV infusion is 25%; this is due to extensive "first-pass" metabolism. Despite "first-pass" metabolism, there is a linear relationship between oral doses of 100 to 3000 mg and peak plasma levels. The absolute bioavailability of labetalol is increased when administered with food.

The plasma half-life of labetalol following oral administration is about 6 to 8 hours. Steady-state plasma levels of labetalol during repetitive dosing are reached by about the third day of dosing. In patients with decreased hepatic or renal function, the elimination half-life of labetalol is not altered; however, the relative bioavailability in hepatically impaired patients is increased due to decreased "first-pass" metabolism.

Metabolism / Excretion – The metabolism of labetalol is mainly through conjugation to glucuronide metabolites. These metabolites are present in plasma and are excreted in the urine and, via the bile, into the feces. Approximately 55% to 60% of a dose appears in the urine as conjugates or unchanged labetalol within the first 24 hours of dosing.

Labetalol has been shown to cross the placental barrier in humans. Only negligible amounts of the drug crossed the blood-brain barrier in animal studies. Labetalol is approximately 50% protein bound. Neither hemodialysis nor peritoneal dialysis removes a significant amount of labetalol from the general circulation (less than 1%).

Elderly patients: Some pharmacokinetic studies indicate that the elimination of labetalol is reduced in elderly patients. Therefore, although elderly patients may initiate therapy at the currently recommended dosage of 100 mg twice a day, elderly patients will generally require lower maintenance dosages than nonelderly patients.

Contraindications

Bronchial asthma, overt cardiac failure, greater-than-first-degree heart block, cardiogenic shock, severe bradycardia, other conditions associated with severe and prolonged hypotension, and hypersensitivity to any component of the product.

Beta-blockers, even those with apparent cardioselectivity, should not be used in patients with a history of obstructive airway disease, including asthma.

Warnings/Precautions

➤*Hepatic injury:* Severe hepatocellular injury, confirmed by rechallenge in at least 1 case, occurs rarely with labetalol therapy. The hepatic injury is usually reversible, but hepatic necrosis and death have been reported. Injury has occurred after both short- and long-term treatment and may be slowly progressive despite minimal symptomatology. Similar hepatic events have been reported with a related research compound, dilevalol, including 2 deaths. Dilevalol is 1 of the 4 isomers of labetalol. Thus, for patients taking labetalol, periodic determination of suitable hepatic laboratory tests would be appropriate. Appropriate laboratory testing should be done at the first symptom/sign of liver dysfunction (eg, pruritus, dark urine, persistent anorexia, jaundice, right upper quadrant tenderness, or unexplained "flu-like" symptoms). If the patient has laboratory evidence of liver injury or jaundice, labetalol should be stopped and not restarted.

➤*Cardiac failure:* Sympathetic stimulation is a vital component supporting circulatory function in congestive heart failure. Beta blockade carries a potential hazard of further depressing myocardial contractility and precipitating more severe failure. Although beta-blockers should be avoided in overt congestive heart failure, if necessary, labetalol can be used with caution in patients with a history of heart failure who are well compensated. Congestive heart failure has been observed in patients receiving labetalol. Labetalol HCl does not abolish the inotropic action of digitalis on heart muscle.

➤*In patients without a history of cardiac failure:* In patients with latent cardiac insufficiency, continued depression of the myocardium with beta-blocking agents over a period of time can, in some cases, lead to cardiac failure. At the first sign or symptom of impending cardiac failure, patients should be fully digitalized or be given a diuretic, and the response should be observed closely. If cardiac failure continues despite adequate digitalization and diuretic, therapy with labetalol tablets should be withdrawn (gradually, if possible).

➤*Exacerbation of ischemic heart disease following abrupt withdrawal:* Angina pectoris has not been reported upon labetalol discontinuation. However, hypersensitivity to catecholamines has been observed in patients withdrawn from beta blocker therapy; exacerbation of angina and, in some cases, myocardial infarction have occurred after abrupt discontinuation of such therapy. When discontinuing chronically administered labetalol tablets, particularly in patients with ischemic heart disease, the dosage should be gradually reduced over a period of 1 to 2 weeks and the patient should be carefully monitored. If angina markedly worsens or acute coronary insufficiency develops, therapy with labetalol tablets should be reinstituted promptly, at least temporarily, and other measures appropriate for the management of unstable angina should be taken. Patients should be warned against interruption or discontinuation of therapy without the physician's advice. Because coronary artery disease is common and may be unrecognized, it may be prudent not to discontinue therapy with labetalol tablets abruptly in patients being treated for hypertension.

➤*Nonallergic bronchospasm (eg, chronic bronchitis and emphysema):* Patients with bronchospastic disease should, in general, not receive beta blockers. Labetalol tablets may be used with caution, however, in patients who do not respond to, or cannot tolerate, other antihypertensive agents. It is prudent, if labetalol tablets are used, to use the smallest effective dose, so that inhibition of endogenous or exogenous beta agonists is minimized.

➤*Pheochromocytoma:* Labetalol has been shown to be effective in lowering blood pressure and relieving symptoms in patients with pheochromocytoma. However, paradoxical hypertensive responses have been reported in a few patients with this tumor; therefore, use caution when administering labetalol to patients with pheochromocytoma.

➤*Diabetes mellitus and hypoglycemia:* Beta-adrenergic blockade may prevent the appearance of premonitory signs and symptoms (eg, tachycardia) of acute hypoglycemia. This is especially important with labile diabetics. Beta-blockade also reduces the release of insulin in response to hyperglycemia; it may therefore be necessary to adjust the dose of antidiabetic drugs.

➤*Major surgery:* The necessity or desirability of withdrawing beta-blocking therapy before major surgery is controversial. Protracted severe hypotension and difficulty in restarting or maintaining a heartbeat have been reported with beta blockers. The effect of labetalol's alpha-adrenergic activity has not been evaluated in this setting.

➤*Hepatic function impairment:* Labetalol tablets should be used with caution in patients with impaired hepatic function since metabolism of the drug may be diminished.

➤*Pregnancy: Category C.* Labetalol is a recommended agent for the management of hypertension during pregnancy. It has a long history of safety, although it has been associated with fetal growth restriction in some studies.

Teratogenic – Teratogenic studies were performed with labetalol in rats and rabbits at oral doses up to approximately 6 and 4 times the maximum

LABETALOL HYDROCHLORIDE — ORAL

recommended human dose (MRHD), respectively. No reproducible evidence of fetal malformations was observed. Increased fetal resorptions were seen in both species at doses approximating the MRHD. A teratology study performed with labetalol in rabbits at IV doses up to 1.7 times the MRHD revealed no evidence of drug-related harm to the fetus. There are no adequate and well-controlled studies in pregnant women. Labetalol should be used during pregnancy only if the potential benefit justifies the potential risk to the fetus.

Nonteratogenic – Hypotension, bradycardia, hypoglycemia, and respiratory depression have been reported in infants of mothers who were treated with labetalol for hypertension during pregnancy. Oral administration of labetalol to rats during late gestation through weaning at doses of 2 to 4 times the MRHD caused a decrease in neonatal survival.

Labor and delivery – Labetalol given to pregnant women with hypertension did not appear to affect the usual course of labor and delivery.

➤*Lactation:* Small amounts of labetalol (approximately 0.004% of the maternal dose) are excreted in human milk. Caution should be exercised when labetalol tablets are administered to a breast-feeding woman.

➤*Children:* Safety and efficacy in children have not been established.

➤*Elderly:* As in the general population, some elderly patients (60 years of age and older) have experienced orthostatic hypotension, dizziness, or lightheadedness during treatment with labetalol. Because elderly patients are generally more likely than younger patients to experience orthostatic symptoms, they should be cautioned about the possibility of such side effects during treatment with labetalol.

➤*Monitoring:* As with any new drug given over prolonged periods, laboratory parameters should be observed over regular intervals. In patients with concomitant illnesses, such as impaired renal function, appropriate tests should be done to monitor these conditions.

Drug Interactions

➤*Tricyclic antidepressants:* In 1 survey, 2.3% of patients taking labetalol in combination with tricyclic antidepressants experienced tremor, as compared to 0.7% reported to occur with labetalol alone. The contribution of each of the treatments to this adverse reaction is unknown, but the possibility of a drug interaction cannot be excluded.

➤*Beta-agonists:* Drugs possessing beta-blocking properties can blunt the bronchodilator effect of beta-receptor agonist drugs in patients with bronchospasm; therefore, doses greater than the normal antiasthmatic dose of beta agonist bronchodilator drugs may be required.

➤*Cimetidine:* Cimetidine has been shown to increase the bioavailability of labetalol. Since this could be explained either by enhanced absorption or by an alteration of hepatic metabolism of labetalol, special care should be used in establishing the dose required for blood pressure control in such patients.

➤*Halothane:* Synergism has been shown between halothane anesthesia and intravenously administered labetalol. During controlled hypotensive anesthesia using labetalol in association with halothane, high concentrations (3% or above) of halothane should not be used because the degree of hypotension will be increased and because of the possibility of a large reduction in cardiac output and an increase in central venous pressure. The anesthesiologist should be informed when a patient is receiving labetalol.

➤*Nitroglycerin:* Labetalol blunts the reflex tachycardia produced by nitroglycerin without preventing its hypotensive effect. If labetalol is used with nitroglycerin in patients with angina pectoris, additional antihypertensive effects may occur.

➤*Calcium channel blockers:* Care should be taken if labetalol is used concomitantly with calcium antagonists of the verapamil type.

➤*Risk of anaphylactic reaction:* While taking beta-blockers, patients with a history of severe anaphylactic reaction to a variety of allergens may be more reactive to repeated challenge, either accidental, diagnostic, or therapeutic. Such patients may be unresponsive to the usual doses of epinephrine used to treat allergic reaction.

➤*Drug/Lab test interactions:* The presence of labetalol metabolites in the urine may result in falsely elevated levels of urinary catecholamines, metanephrine, normetanephrine, and vanillylmandelic acid when measured by fluorimetric or photometric methods. In screening patients suspected of having a pheochromocytoma and being treated with labetalol, a specific method, such as a high performance liquid chromatographic assay with solid phase extraction (eg, *J Chromatogr* 385:241,1987) should be employed in determining levels of catecholamines.

Labetalol has also been reported to produce a false-positive test for amphetamine when screening urine for the presence of drugs using the commercially available assay methods *Toxi-Lab A* (thin-layer chromatographic assay) and *Emit-d.a.u.* (radioenzymatic assay). When patients being treated with labetalol have a positive urine test for amphetamine using these techniques, confirmation should be made by using more specific methods, such as a gas chromatographic-mass spectrometer technique.

Adverse Reactions

Most adverse effects are mild and transient and occur early in the course of treatment. In controlled clinical trials of 3 to 4 months' duration, discontinuation of labetalol tablets due to 1 or more adverse effects was required in 7% of all patients. In these same trials, other agents with solely beta-blocking activity used in the control groups led to discontinuation in 8% to 10% of patients, and a centrally acting alpha agonist led to discontinuation in 30% of patients.

The incidence rates of adverse reactions listed in the following table were derived from multicenter, controlled clinical trials comparing labetalol, placebo, metoprolol, and propranolol over treatment periods of 3 and 4 months. Where the frequency of adverse effects for labetalol and placebo is similar, causal relationship is uncertain. The rates are based on adverse reactions considered probably drug related by the investigator. If all reports are considered, the rates are somewhat higher (eg, dizziness, 20%; nausea, 14%; fatigue, 11%), but the overall conclusions are unchanged.

Labetalol vs Propranolol and Metoprolol Adverse Reactions

Adverse reactions	Labetalol (n = 227)	Placebo (n = 98)	Propranolol (n = 84)	Metoprolol (n = 49)
Autonomic nervous system				
Nasal stuffiness	3%	0%	0%	0%
Ejaculation failure	2%	0%	0%	0%
Impotence	1%	0%	1%	3%
Increased sweating	< 1%	0%	0%	0%
Cardiovascular				
Edema	1%	0%	0%	0%
Postural hypotension	1%	0%	0%	0%
Bradycardia	0%	0%	5%	12%
CNS				
Dizziness	11%	3%	4%	4%
Paresthesia	< 1%	0%	0%	0%
Drowsiness	< 1%	2%	2%	2%
Dermatologic				
Rash	1%	0%	0%	0%
GI				
Nausea	6%	1%	1%	2%
Vomiting	< 1%	0%	0%	0%
Dyspepsia	3%	1%	1%	0%
Abdominal pain	0%	0%	1%	2%
Diarrhea	< 1%	0%	2%	0%
Taste distortion	1%	0%	0%	0%
Respiratory				
Dyspnea	2%	0%	1%	2%
Special senses				
Vertigo	2%	1%	0%	0%
Vision abnormality	1%	0%	0%	0%
Miscellaneous				
Fatigue	5%	0%	12%	12%
Asthenia	1%	1%	1%	0%
Headache	2%	1%	1%	2%

The adverse effects were reported spontaneously and are representative of the incidence of adverse effects that may be observed in a properly selected hypertensive patient population, ie, a group excluding patients with bronchospastic disease, overt congestive heart failure, or other contraindications to beta blocker therapy.

Clinical trials also included studies utilizing daily doses up to 2400 mg in more severely hypertensive patients. Certain of the side effects increased with increasing dose, as shown in the following table that depicts the entire US therapeutic trials data base for adverse reactions that are clearly or possibly dose related.

Labetalol Adverse Reactions by Dose

	Daily dose								
Adverse reactions	200 mg (n = 522)	300 mg (n = 181)	400 mg (n = 606)	600 mg (n = 608)	800 mg (n = 503)	900 mg (n = 117)	1,200 mg (n = 411)	1,600 mg (n = 242)	2,400 mg (n = 175)
Dizziness	2%	3%	3%	3%	5%	1%	9%	13%	16%
Fatigue	2%	1%	4%	4%	5%	3%	7%	6%	10%
Nausea	< 1%	0%	1%	2%	4%	0%	7%	11%	19%
Vomiting	0%	0%	< 1%	< 1%	< 1%	0%	1%	2%	3%
Dyspepsia	1%	0%	2%	1%	1%	0%	2%	2%	4%
Paresthesia	2%	0%	2%	2%	1%	1%	2%	5%	5%
Nasal stuffiness	1%	1%	2%	2%	2%	2%	4%	5%	6%

LABETALOL HYDROCHLORIDE — ORAL

Labetalol Adverse Reactions by Dose									
	Daily dose								
Adverse reactions	200 mg (n = 522)	300 mg (n = 181)	400 mg (n = 606)	600 mg (n = 608)	800 mg (n = 503)	900 mg (n = 117)	1,200 mg (n = 411)	1,600 mg (n = 242)	2,400 mg (n = 175)
Ejaculation failure	0%	2%	1%	2%	3%	0%	4%	3%	5%
Impotence	1%	1%	1%	1%	2%	4%	3%	4%	3%
Edema	1%	0%	1%	1%	1%	0%	1%	2%	2%

In addition, a number of other less common adverse events have been reported.

➤*Cardiovascular:* Hypotension, and rarely, syncope, bradycardia, heart block.

➤*CNS:* Paresthesia, most frequently described as scalp tingling. In most cases, it was mild and transient and usually occurred at the beginning of treatment.

➤*Dermatologic:* Rashes of various types, such as generalized maculopapular, lichenoid, urticarial, bullous lichen planus, psoriasiform, and facial erythema; Peyronie's disease; reversible alopecia.

➤*GU:* Difficulty in micturition, including acute urinary bladder retention.

➤*Hepatic:* Hepatic necrosis, hepatitis, cholestatic jaundice, elevated liver function tests.

➤*Hypersensitivity:* Rare reports of hypersensitivity (eg, rash, urticaria, pruritus, angioedema, dyspnea) and anaphylactoid reactions.

➤*Immunologic:* Antimitochondrial antibodies.

➤*Musculoskeletal:* Muscle cramps, toxic myopathy.

➤*Ophthalmic:* Dry eyes.

➤*Respiratory:* Bronchospasm.

➤*Miscellaneous:* Fever. Systemic lupus erythematosus, positive antinuclear factor.

➤*Lab test abnormalities:* There have been reversible increases of serum transaminases in 4% of patients treated with labetalol and tested and, more rarely, reversible increases in blood urea.

Overdosage

➤*Symptoms:* Overdosage with labetalol causes excessive hypotension that is posture sensitive and, sometimes, excessive bradycardia. Patients should be placed supine and their legs raised if necessary to improve the blood supply to the brain. If overdosage with labetalol follows oral ingestion, gastric lavage or pharmacologically induced emesis (using syrup of ipecac) may be useful for removal of the drug shortly after ingestion. The following additional measures should be employed if necessary.

➤*Treatment:*

Excessive bradycardia – Administer atropine or epinephrine.

Cardiac failure – Administer a digitalis glycoside and a diuretic. Dopamine or dobutamine may also be useful.

Hypotension – Administer vasopressors (eg, norepinephrine). There is pharmacologic evidence that norepinephrine may be the drug of choice.

Bronchospasm – Administer epinephrine or an aerosolized beta-2-agonist.

Seizures – Administer diazepam. In severe beta-blocker overdose resulting in hypotension or bradycardia, glucagon has been shown to be effective when administered in large doses (5 to 10 mg rapidly over 30 seconds, followed by continuous infusion of 5 mg per hour that can be reduced as the patient improves).

Neither hemodialysis nor peritoneal dialysis removes a significant amount of labetalol from the general circulation (less than 1%).

Patient Information

As with all drugs with beta-blocking activity, certain advice to patients being treated with labetalol is warranted. This information is intended to aid in the safe and effective use of this medication. It is not a disclosure of all possible adverse or intended effects. While no incident of the abrupt withdrawal phenomenon (exacerbation of angina pectoris) has been reported with labetalol, dosing with labetalol tablets should not be interrupted or discontinued without a physician's advice. Patients being treated with labetalol tablets should consult a physician at any signs or symptoms of impending cardiac failure or hepatic dysfunction. Also, mild transient scalp tingling may occur, usually when treatment with labetalol tablets is initiated.

LABETALOL HYDROCHLORIDE — INJECTION

Indications

➤*Severe hypertension:* For control of blood pressure in severe hypertension.

Administration and Dosage

➤*General dosing considerations:* Labetalol injection is intended for IV use in hospitalized patients. Dosage must be individualized depending upon the severity of hypertension and the response of the patient during dosing.

Patients should always be kept in a supine position during the period of IV drug administration. A substantial fall in blood pressure on standing should be expected in these patients. The patient's ability to tolerate an upright position should be established before permitting any ambulation, such as using toilet facilities.

➤*Adults:*

Severe hypertension –

Repeated IV injection:

• *Initial dosage* – Labetalol 20 mg (which corresponds to 0.25 mg/kg for an 80 kg patient) by slow IV injection over a 2-minute period.

• *Maintenance dosage* – Additional injections of 40 mg or 80 mg can be given at 10-minute intervals until a desired supine blood pressure is achieved or a total of labetalol 300 mg has been injected. The maximum effect usually occurs within 5 minutes of each injection.

Slow continuous infusion: 50 to 200 mg; A total dose of up to 300 mg may be required in some patients at a rate of 2 mg/min. The rate of infusion of the diluted solution may be adjusted according to the blood pressure response, at the discretion of the health care provider.

➤*Children:*

Off-label dosing –

Severe hypertension:

• *1 to 17 years of age* –

Intermittent infusion: Start at lowest dose and titrate to desired effect. 0.2 to 1 mg/kg IV over a 2 minute period every 10 minutes as needed. The maximum hypotensive effect usually occurs within 5 to 15 minutes.1 2 3 40 mg/dose.

Continuous infusion: 0.25 to 3 mg/kg/hour.

➤*Monitoring:* Immediately before each injection and at 5 and 10 minutes after injection, supine blood pressure should be measured to evaluate response.

The blood pressure should be monitored during and after completion of the infusion or IV injections. Rapid or excessive falls in either systolic or diastolic blood pressure during IV treatment should be avoided. In patients with excessive systolic hypertension, the decrease in systolic pressure should be used as an indicator of effectiveness in addition to the response of the diastolic pressure.

➤*Preparation for administration:* Labetalol injection is prepared for IV continuous infusion by diluting the contents with commonly used IV fluids (see Admixture compatibility). Examples of methods of preparing the infusion solution are as follows:

The contents of either two 20 mL vials (40 mL), or one 40 mL vial, are added to 160 mL of a commonly used IV fluid, such that the resultant 200 mL of solution contains 200 mg of labetalol , 1 mg/mL. The diluted solution should be administered at a rate of 2 mL/min to deliver 2 mg/min.

Alternatively, the contents of either two 20 mL vials (40 mL), or one 40 mL vial, of labetalol injection are added to 250 mL of a commonly used IV fluid. The resultant solution will contain 200 mg of labetalol, approximately 2 mg per 3 mL. The diluted solution should be administered at a rate of 3 mL/min to deliver approximately 2 mg/min.

➤*Admixture compatibility:* Labetalol injection was tested for compatibility with commonly used IV fluids at final concentrations of 1.25 to 3.75 mg labetalol per mL of mixture. Labetalol injection was found to be compatible with and stable (for 24 hours refrigerated or at room temperature) in mixtures with the following solutions: Ringer's injection; Ringer's lactated injection; dextrose 5% and Ringer's injection; Ringer's lactated 5% and dextrose 5% injection; dextrose 5% injection; sodium chloride 0.9% injection; dextrose 5% and sodium chloride 0.2% injection; dextrose 2.5% and sodium chloride 0.45% injection; dextrose 5% and sodium chloride 0.9% injection; dextrose 5% and sodium chloride 0.33% injection.

Labetalol injection was not compatible with sodium bicarbonate 5% injection. Care should be taken when administering alkaline drugs, including furosemide, in combination with labetalol. Compatibility should be ensured prior to administering these drugs together.

➤*Storage/Stability:* Store between 2° and 30°C (36° and 86°F). Protect from freezing and light.

Actions

➤*Pharmacology:* Labetalol combines both selective, competitive alpha-1-adrenergic-blocking and nonselective, competitive beta-adrenergic-blocking activity in a single substance. In man, the ratios of alpha- to beta-blockade have been estimated to be approximately 1:3 and 1:7 following oral and IV administration, respectively. Beta-2-agonist activity has been demonstrated in animals with minimal beta-1-agonist (ISA) activity detected. In animals, at doses greater than those required for alpha- or beta-adrenergic blockade, a membrane-stabilizing effect has been demonstrated.

LABETALOL HYDROCHLORIDE — INJECTION

➤*Pharmacokinetics:*

Distribution – Labetalol has been shown to cross the placental barrier in humans. Only negligible amounts of the drug crossed the blood-brain barrier in animal studies. Labetalol is approximately 50% protein bound. Neither hemodialysis nor peritoneal dialysis removes a significant amount of labetalol from the general circulation (less than 1%).

Metabolism/Excretion – Following IV infusion, the elimination half-life is about 5.5 hours, and the total body clearance is approximately 33 mL/min/kg. The plasma half-life of labetalol following oral administration is about 6 to 8 hours. In patients with decreased hepatic or renal function, the elimination half-life of labetalol is not altered; however, the relative bioavailability in hepatically impaired patients is increased due to decreased "first-pass" metabolism.

The metabolism of labetalol is mainly through conjugation to glucuronide metabolites. These metabolites are present in plasma and are excreted in the urine and, via the bile, into the feces. Approximately 55% to 60% of a dose appears in the urine as conjugates or unchanged labetalol within the first 24 hours of dosing.

Contraindications

Bronchial asthma, overt cardiac failure, greater than first-degree heart block, cardiogenic shock, severe bradycardia, other conditions associated with severe and prolonged hypotension, hypersensitivity to any component of the product.

Beta-blockers, even those with apparent cardioselectivity, should not be used in patients with a history of obstructive airway disease, including asthma.

Warnings/Precautions

➤*Cardiac failure:* Sympathetic stimulation is a vital component supporting circulatory function in congestive heart failure. Beta blockade carries a potential hazard of further depressing myocardial contractility and precipitating more severe failure. Although beta blockers should be avoided in overt congestive heart failure, if necessary, labetalol can be used with caution in patients with a history of heart failure who are well compensated. Congestive heart failure has been observed in patients receiving labetalol. Labetalol does not abolish the inotropic action of digitalis on heart muscle.

Patients without histories of cardiac failure – In patients with latent cardiac insufficiency, continued depression of the myocardium with beta-blocking agents over a period of time can lead, in some cases, to cardiac failure. At the first sign or symptom of impending cardiac failure, patients should be fully digitalized or be given a diuretic, and the response observed closely. If cardiac failure continues, despite adequate digitalization and diuretic, labetalol therapy should be withdrawn (gradually if possible).

➤*Ischemic heart disease:* Angina pectoris has not been reported upon labetalol discontinuation. However, following abrupt cessation of therapy with some beta-blocking agents in patients with coronary artery disease, exacerbations of angina pectoris and, in some cases, myocardial infarction have been reported. Therefore, such patients should be cautioned against interruption of therapy without the physician's advice. Even in the absence of overt angina pectoris, when discontinuation of labetalol is planned, the patient should be carefully observed and should be advised to limit physical activity. If angina markedly worsens or acute coronary insufficiency develops, labetalol administration should be reinstituted promptly, at least temporarily, and other measures appropriate for the management of unstable angina should be taken.

➤*Nonallergic bronchospasm (eg, chronic bronchitis, emphysema):* Since labetalol injection at the usual IV therapeutic doses has not been studied in patients with nonallergic bronchospastic disease, it should not be used in such patients.

➤*Pheochromocytoma:* IV labetalol has been shown to be effective in lowering the blood pressure and relieving symptoms in patients with pheochromocytoma; higher than usual doses may be required. However, paradoxical hypertensive responses have been reported in a few patients with this tumor; therefore, use caution when administering labetalol to patients with pheochromocytoma.

➤*Diabetes mellitus and hypoglycemia:* Beta-adrenergic blockade may prevent the appearance of premonitory signs and symptoms (eg, tachycardia) of acute hypoglycemia. This is especially important with labile diabetics. Beta blockade also reduces the release of insulin in response to hyperglycemia; it may therefore be necessary to adjust the dose of antidiabetic drugs.

➤*Major surgery:* The necessity or desirability of withdrawing beta-blocking therapy prior to major surgery is controversial. Protracted severe hypotension and difficulty in restarting or maintaining a heartbeat have been reported with beta-blockers. The effect of labetalol's alpha-adrenergic activity has not been evaluated in this setting.

Several deaths have occurred when labetalol injection was used during surgery (including when used in cases to control bleeding).

➤*Rapid decreases of blood pressure:* Caution must be observed when reducing severely elevated blood pressure. Although such findings have not been reported with IV labetalol, a number of adverse reactions, including cerebral infarction, optic nerve infarction, angina, and ischemic changes in the electrocardiogram, have been reported with other agents when severely elevated blood pressure was reduced over time courses of several hours to as long as 1 or 2 days. The desired blood pressure lowering should therefore be achieved over as long a period of time as is compatible with the patient's status.

➤*Hepatic effects:* Severe hepatocellular injury, confirmed by rechallenge in at least 1 case, occurs rarely with labetalol therapy. The hepatic injury is usually reversible, but hepatic necrosis and death have been reported. Injury has occurred after both short- and long-term treatment and may be slowly progressive despite minimal symptomatology. Similar hepatic events have been reported with a related compound, dilevalol HCl, including 2 deaths. Dilevalol hydrochloride is 1 of the 4 isomers of labetalol hydrochloride. Thus, for patients taking labetalol, periodic determination of suitable hepatic laboratory tests would be appropriate. Laboratory testing should also be done at the very first symptom or sign of liver dysfunction (eg, pruritus, dark urine, persistent anorexia, jaundice, right upper quadrant tenderness, unexplained "flu-like" symptoms). If the patient has jaundice or laboratory evidence of liver injury, labetalol should be stopped and not restarted.

➤*Following coronary artery bypass surgery:* In 1 uncontrolled study, patients with low cardiac indices and elevated systemic vascular resistance following IV labetalol experienced significant declines in cardiac output with little change in systemic vascular resistance. One of these patients developed hypotension following labetalol HCl treatment. Therefore, use of labetalol should be avoided in such patients.

➤*High-dose labetalol:* Administration of up to 3 g/day as an infusion for up to 2 to 3 days has been anecdotally reported; several patients experienced hypotension or bradycardia.

➤*Hypotension:* Symptomatic postural hypotension (incidence, 58%) is likely to occur if patients are tilted or allowed to assume the upright position within 3 hours of receiving labetalol injection. Therefore, the patient's ability to tolerate an upright position should be established before permitting any ambulation.

➤*Hypersensitivity reactions:* While taking beta-blockers, patients with histories of severe anaphylactic reactions to a variety of allergens may be more reactive to repeated challenge, either accidental, diagnostic, or therapeutic. Such patients may be unresponsive to the usual doses of epinephrine used to treat allergic reactions.

➤*Hepatic function impairment:* Use labetalol injection with caution in patients with impaired hepatic function since metabolism of the drug may be diminished.

➤*Pregnancy: Category C.* Labetalol injection is a recommended agent for the emergency treatment of hypertension during pregnancy. Labetalol has a long history of safety, although it has been associated with fetal growth restriction in some studies.

Teratogenic – Teratogenic studies have been performed with labetalol in rats and rabbits at oral doses up to approximately 6 and 4 times the maximum recommended human dose (MRHD), respectively. No reproducible evidence of fetal malformations was observed. Increased fetal resorptions were seen in both species at doses approximating the MRHD. A teratology study performed with labetalol in rabbits at IV doses up to 1.7 times the MRHD revealed no evidence of drug-related harm to the fetus. There are no adequate and well-controlled studies in pregnant women. Labetalol should be used during pregnancy only if the potential benefit justifies the potential risk to the fetus.

Nonteratogenic – Hypotension, bradycardia, hypoglycemia, and respiratory depression have been reported in infants of mothers who were treated with labetalol for hypertension during pregnancy. Oral administration of labetalol to rats during late gestation through weaning at doses of 2 to 4 times the MRHD caused a decrease in neonatal survival.

Labor and delivery – Labetalol given to pregnant women with hypertension did not appear to affect the usual course of labor and delivery.

➤*Lactation:* Small amounts of labetalol (approximately 0.004% of the maternal dose) are excreted in human milk. Caution should be exercised when labetalol injection is administered to a breast-feeding woman.

➤*Children:* Safety and efficacy in pediatric patients have not been established.

➤*Monitoring:* Routine laboratory tests are ordinarily not required before or after IV labetalol. In patients with concomitant illnesses, such as impaired renal function, appropriate tests should be done to monitor these conditions.

Drug Interactions

➤*Other antihypertensive agents:* Because labetalol injection may be administered to patients already being treated with other medications, including other antihypertensive agents, careful monitoring of these patients is necessary to detect and treat promptly any undesired effect from concomitant administration.

➤*Tricyclic antidepressants:* In 1 survey, 2.3% of patients taking labetalol orally in combination with tricyclic antidepressants experienced tremor compared with 0.7% reported to occur with labetalol alone. The contribution of each of the treatments to this adverse reaction is unknown but the possibility of a drug interaction cannot be excluded.

➤*Beta-agonist bronchodilators:* Drugs possessing beta-blocking properties can blunt the bronchodilator effect of beta-receptor agonist drugs in patients with bronchospasm; therefore, doses greater than the normal anti-asthmatic dose of beta-agonist bronchodilator drugs may be required.

➤*Halothane:* Synergism has been shown between halothane anesthesia and IV labetalol. During controlled hypotensive anesthesia using labetalol in association with halothane, high concentrations (3% or above) of halothane should not be used because the degree of hypotension will be increased and because of the possibility of a large reduction in cardiac out-

LABETALOL HYDROCHLORIDE — INJECTION

put and an increase in central venous pressure. The anesthesiologist should be informed when a patient is receiving labetalol.

➤*Nitroglycerin:* Labetalol blunts the reflex tachycardia produced by nitroglycerin without preventing its hypotensive effect. If labetalol hydrochloride is used with nitroglycerin in patients with angina pectoris, additional antihypertensive effects may occur.

➤*Calcium-channel blockers:* Care should be taken if labetalol is used concomitantly with calcium antagonists of the verapamil type.

➤*Furosemide:* When drug products that are alkaline, such as furosemide, have been administered in combination with labetalol, a white precipitate has been noted. Therefore, these drugs should not be administered in the same infusion line.

➤*Drug/Lab test interactions:* The presence of labetalol metabolites in the urine may result in falsely elevated levels of urinary catecholamines, metanephrine, normetanephrine, and vanillylmandelic acid (VMA) when measured by fluorimetric or photometric methods. In screening patients suspected of having a pheochromocytoma and being treated with labetalol, a specific method, such as a high-performance liquid chromatographic assay with solid phase extraction should be employed in determining levels of catecholamines.

Labetalol has also been reported to produce a false-positive test for amphetamine when screening urine for the presence of drugs using the commercially available assay methods *Toxi-Lab A* (thin-layer chromatographic assay) and *Emit-d.a.u.* (radioenzymatic assay). When patients being treated with labetalol have a positive urine test for amphetamine using these techniques, confirmation should be made by using more specific methods, such as a gas chromatographic-mass spectrometer technique.

Adverse Reactions

Labetalol injection is usually well tolerated. Most adverse reactions have been mild and transient, and in controlled trials involving 92 patients did not require labetalol withdrawal. Symptomatic postural hypotension (incidence, 58%) is likely to occur if patients are tilted or allowed to assume the upright position within 3 hours of receiving labetalol hydrochloride injection. Moderate hypotension occurred in 1 of 100 patients while supine. Increased sweating was noted in 1 of 100 patients, and flushing occurred in 1 of 100 patients.

The following also were reported with labetalol HCl injection with the incidence per 100 patients noted:

➤*Cardiovascular:* Ventricular arrhythmia in 1.

➤*CNS:* Dizziness in 9; tingling of the scalp/skin in 7; hypesthesia (numbness) and vertigo, 1 each.

➤*Dermatologic:* Pruritus in 1.

➤*GI:* Nausea in 13; vomiting in 4; dyspepsia and taste distortion, 1 each.

➤*Metabolic:* Transient increases in blood urea nitrogen and serum creatinine levels occurred in 8 of 100 patients; these were associated with drops in blood pressure, generally patients with prior renal insufficiency.

➤*Psychiatric:* Somnolence/yawning in 3.

➤*Respiratory:* Wheezing in 1.

Overdosage

➤*Treatment:* Overdosage with labetalol hydrochloride injection causes excessive hypotension that is posture-sensitive, and sometimes, excessive bradycardia. Patients should be placed supine and their legs raised if necessary to improve the blood supply to the brain. If overdosage with labetalol follows oral ingestion, gastric lavage or pharmacologically induced emesis (using syrup of ipecac) may be useful for removal of the drug shortly after ingestion. The following additional measures should be employed if necessary:

Excessive bradycardia – Administer atropine or epinephrine.

Cardiac failure – Administer a digitalis glycoside and a diuretic. Dopamine or dobutamine may also be useful.

Hypotension – Administer vasopressors (eg, norepinephrine). There is pharmacological evidence that norepinephrine may be the drug of choice.

Bronchospasm – Administer epinephrine or an aerosolized beta-2 agonist.

Seizures – Administer diazepam.

Other – In severe beta-blocker overdose resulting in hypotension or bradycardia, glucagon has been shown to be effective when administered in large doses (5 to 10 mg rapidly over 30 seconds, followed by continuous infusion of 5 mg/hr that can be reduced as the patient improves).

Neither hemodialysis nor peritoneal dialysis removes a significant amount of labetalol from the general circulation (less than 1%).

Patient Information

The following information is intended to aid in the safe and effective use of this medication. It is not a disclosure of all possible adverse or intended effects. During and immediately following (for up to 3 hours) labetalol injection, the patient should remain supine. Subsequently, the patient should be advised on how to proceed gradually to become ambulatory, and should be observed at the time of first ambulation.

When the patient is started on labetalol hydrochloride tablets, following adequate control of blood pressure with labetalol injection, appropriate directions for titration of dosage should be provided.

As with all drugs with beta-blocking activity, certain advice to patients being treated with labetalol is warranted: While no incident of the abrupt withdrawal phenomenon (exacerbation of angina pectoris) has been reported with labetalol, dosing with labetalol tablets should not be interrupted or discontinued without a physician's advice. Patients being treated with labetalol tablets should consult a physician at any signs or symptoms of impending cardiac failure or hepatic dysfunction. Also, transient scalp tingling may occur, usually when treatment with labetalol tablets is initiated.

CARVEDILOL

Rx	**Carvedilol** (Various, eg, Apotex, Caraco, Dr. Reddy's Laboratories, Inc, Zydus Pharmaceuticals)	**Tablets; oral:** 3.125 mg	May contain mannitol, lactose, and sucrose. Film-coated. In 28s, 30s, 100s, 500s, 1000s, UD 100s, and blister pack 100s.
Rx	**Coreg** (GlaxoSmithKline)		Lactose, sucrose. (39 SB). White, oval. Film-coated. In 100s.
Rx	**Carvedilol** (Various, eg, Apotex, Caraco, Dr. Reddy's Laboratories, Inc, Zydus Pharmaceuticals)	**Tablets; oral:** 6.25 mg	May contain mannitol, lactose, and sucrose. Film-coated. In 28s, 30s, 100s, 500s, 1,000s, UD 100s, and blister pack 100s.
	Coreg (GlaxoSmithKline)		Lactose, sucrose. (4140 SB). White, oval. Film-coated. In 100s.
Rx	**Carvedilol** (Various, eg, Apotex, Caraco, Dr. Reddy's Laboratories, Inc, Zydus Pharmaceuticals)	**Tablets; oral:** 12.5 mg	May contain mannitol, lactose, and sucrose. Film-coated. In 28s, 30s, 100s, 500s, 1,000s, UD 100s, and blister pack 100s.
Rx	**Coreg** (GlaxoSmithKline)		Lactose, sucrose. (4141 SB). White, oval. Film-coated. In 100s.
Rx	**Carvedilol** (Various, eg, Apotex, Caraco, Dr. Reddy's Laboratories, Inc, Zydus Pharmaceuticals)	**Tablets; oral:** 25 mg	May contain mannitol, lactose, and sucrose. Film-coated. In 28s, 30s, 100s, 500s, 1,000s, UD 100s, and blister pack 100s.
Rx	**Coreg** (GlaxoSmithKline)		Lactose, sucrose. (4142 SB). White, oval. Film-coated. In 100s.
Rx	**Coreg CR** (GlaxoSmithKline)	**Capsules, extended-release; oral**[a]: 10 mg (as phosphate)	(GSK Coreg CR 10 mg). White/green. In 30s and 90s.
		20 mg (as phosphate)	(GSK Coreg CR 20 mg). White/yellow. In 30s and 90s.
		40 mg (as phosphate)	(GSK Coreg CR 40 mg). Yellow/green. In 30s and 90s.
		80 mg (as phosphate)	(GSK Coreg CR 80 mg). White. In 30s and 90s.

[a] Contains immediate- and controlled-release microparticles.

CARVEDILOL — ORAL

Indications

➤*Congestive heart failure (CHF):* Treatment of mild to severe heart failure of ischemic or cardiomyopathic origin, usually in addition to diuretics, angiotensin-converting enzyme (ACE) inhibitors, and digitalis, to increase survival and to reduce the risk of hospitalization.

➤*Hypertension:* Management of essential hypertension. It can be used alone or in combination with other antihypertensive agents, especially thiazide-type diuretics.

➤*Left ventricular dysfunction following myocardial infarction (MI)* : To reduce cardiovascular mortality in clinically stable patients who have survived the acute phase of a MI and have a left ventricular ejection fraction of 40% or less (with or without symptomatic heart failure).

➤*Off-label uses:*

Chronic stable angina – [1] = Good documentation. Beta-blockers are recommended (class IB evidence) by American College of Cardiology/American Heart Association (ACC/AHA) guidelines as initial therapy, in the absence of contraindications, to prevent MI and death caused by chronic stable angina in patients with prior MI. In patients without prior MI, beta-blockers, as a class, are recommended for use in chronic stable angina as class IIC evidence. Individual beta-blockers are not specified within guidelines.

Hiccups (singultus) – [4] = Insufficient documentation. The available data, while favorable, are limited to a single case report.

Idiopathic cardiomyopathy – In general, beta-blockers should be used with caution, but it appears that carvedilol has an advantage over other beta-blockers because it does not block beta-1 adrenergic activity. Therefore, it can decrease heart rate, increase contractility, improve myocardial blood flow reserves, and decrease sympathetic activity that could damage heart tissue. Studies in small populations have demonstrated potential benefit in acute hemodynamic effects in patients with idiopathic dilated cardiomyopathy. However, large studies are needed to confirm these results and show improvements in the survivability of these patients. Currently, patients with idiopathic dilated cardiomyopathy show only a 33% to 66% 5-year survival rate.

Idiopathic cardiomyopathy (adults): [2] = Fair documentation.

Idiopathic cardiomyopathy (children/adolescents): [4] = Insufficient documentation.

Administration and Dosage

➤*General dosing considerations:* Dosage must be individualized and closely monitored during up-titration.

Patients should be advised that initiation of treatment and, to a lesser extent, dosage increases may be associated with transient symptoms of dizziness or light-headedness and syncope (rarely) within the first hour after dosing. Thus, during these periods patients should avoid situations such as driving or hazardous tasks, where symptoms could result in injury. In addition, carvedilol should be taken with food to slow the rate of absorption.

Episodes of dizziness or fluid retention during initiation of carvedilol generally can be managed without discontinuation of treatment and do not preclude subsequent successful titration of, or a favorable response to, carvedilol.

➤*Adults:*

Congestive heart failure – Prior to initiation of carvedilol, it is recommended that fluid retention be minimized.

Maximum dose: 50 mg twice daily has been administered to patients with mild to moderate heart failure weighing more than 85 kg (187 lbs).

Initial dosage: 3.125 mg twice daily for 2 weeks.

Dosage titration: Patients who tolerate a dosage of 3.125 mg twice daily may have their dosage increased to 6.25, 12.5, and 25 mg twice daily over successive intervals of at least 2 weeks. Patients should be maintained on lower doses if higher doses are not tolerated.

The dose of carvedilol should not be increased until symptoms of worsening heart failure or vasodilation have been stabilized.

The dose of carvedilol should be reduced if patients experience bradycardia (heart rate less than 55 beats/min).

Concomitant therapy: Vasodilatory symptoms often do not require treatment, but it may be useful to separate the time of dosing of carvedilol from that of the ACE inhibitor or to reduce temporarily the dose of the ACE inhibitor.

Fluid retention (with or without transient worsening heart failure symptoms) should be treated by an increase in the dose of diuretics.

Hypertension – Carvedilol should be taken with food to slow the rate of absorption and reduce the incidence of orthostatic effects.

Maximum dose: 50 mg daily.

Initial dosage: 6.25 mg twice daily.

Dosage adjustment: If initial dose is tolerated, using standing systolic pressure measured about 1 hour after dosing as a guide, the dose should be maintained for 7 to 14 days and then increased to 12.5 mg twice daily if needed (based on trough blood pressure), again using standing systolic pressure 1 hour after dosing as a guide for tolerance. This dose should be maintained for 7 to 14 days and can then be adjusted upward to 25 mg twice daily if tolerated and needed. The full antihypertensive effect of carvedilol is seen within 7 to 14 days.

Concomitant therapy: Addition of a diuretic to carvedilol, or carvedilol to a diuretic, can be expected to produce additive effects and exaggerate the orthostatic component of carvedilol action.

Left ventricular dysfunction following myocardial infarction – Treatment may be started as inpatient or outpatient treatment and should be started after the patient is hemodynamically stable and fluid retention has been minimized.

Initial dosage: 6.25 mg twice daily.

Dosage titration: Increase after 3 to 10 days, based on tolerability, to 12.5 mg twice daily, then again to the target dose of 25 mg twice daily.

Alternative dosage: Lower starting dose may be used (3.125 mg twice daily) and/or the rate of up-titration may be slowed if clinically indicated (eg, because of low blood pressure or heart rate, fluid retention). Patients should be maintained on lower doses if higher doses are not tolerated. The recommended dosing regimen need not be altered in patients who received treatment with an intravenous (IV) or oral beta-blocker during the acute phase of the MI.

Off-label dosing –

Chronic stable angina: [1] = Good documentation. 12.5, 25, or 50 mg orally twice daily for 2 to 12 weeks.

Hiccups (singultus): [4] = Insufficient documentation. Initial oral doses were 3.125 mg administered 4 times daily and doubled to 6.25 mg administered 4 times daily on day 2 for several months.

Idiopathic cardiomyopathy (adults): [2] = Fair documentation. 2.5 mg/day orally initially and increase as tolerated; dosages of up to 75 mg/day have been studied, and therapy has been continued for at least 6 to 8 months.

➤*Hepatic function impairment:* Carvedilol should not be given to patients with severe hepatic function impairment.

➤*Storage/Stability:* Store below 30°C (86°F). Protect from moisture. Dispense in a tight, light-resistant container.

Actions

➤*Pharmacology:* Carvedilol is a racemic mixture in which nonselective beta-adrenoreceptor blocking activity is present in the S(−) enantiomer and alpha-adrenergic blocking activity is present in both R(+) and S(−) enantiomers at equal potency. Carvedilol has no intrinsic sympathomimetic activity.

Pharmacodynamics –

CHF: The basis for the beneficial effects of carvedilol in CHF is not established.

Two placebo-controlled studies compared the acute hemodynamic effects of carvedilol with baseline measurements in 59 and 49 patients with New York Heart Association (NYHA) class II-IV heart failure receiving diuretics, ACE inhibitors, and digitalis. There were significant reductions in systemic blood pressure, pulmonary artery pressure, pulmonary capillary wedge pressure, and heart rate. Initial effects on cardiac output, stroke volume index, and systemic vascular resistance were small and variable.

These studies measured hemodynamic effects again at 12 to 14 weeks. Carvedilol significantly reduced systemic blood pressure, pulmonary artery pressure, right atrial pressure, systemic vascular resistance, and heart rate, while stroke volume index was increased.

Among 839 patients with NYHA class II-III heart failure treated for 26 to 52 weeks in 4 US placebo-controlled trials, the average left ventricular ejection fraction, measured by radionuclide ventriculography, increased by 9 ejection fraction units (%) in carvedilol patients and by 2 ejection fraction units in placebo patients at a target dose of 25 to 50 mg twice daily. The effects of carvedilol on ejection fraction were related to dose. Doses of 6.25 mg twice daily, 12.5 mg twice daily, and 25 mg twice daily were associated with placebo-corrected increases in ejection fraction of 5 ejection fraction units, 6 ejection fraction units, and 8 ejection fraction units, respectively; each of these effects were nominally statistically significant.

Left ventricular dysfunction following MI: The basis for the beneficial effects of carvedilol in patients with left ventricular dysfunction following an acute MI is not established.

Hypertension: The mechanism by which beta-blockade produces an antihypertensive effect has not been established.

Beta-adrenoreceptor blocking activity has been demonstrated in animal and human studies showing that carvedilol reduces cardiac output in healthy subjects, reduces exercise- and/or isoproterenol-induced tachycardia, and reduces reflex orthostatic tachycardia. Significant beta-adrenoreceptor blocking effect is usually seen within 1 hour of drug administration.

Alpha-1-adrenoreceptor blocking activity has been demonstrated in human and animal studies, showing that carvedilol attenuates the pressor effects of phenylephrine, causes vasodilation, and reduces peripheral vascular resistance. These effects contribute to the reduction of blood pressure and usually are seen within 30 minutes of drug administration.

Because of the alpha-1-receptor blocking activity of carvedilol, blood pressure is lowered more in the standing than in the supine position, and symptoms of postural hypotension (1.8%), including rare instances of syncope, can occur.

Following oral administration, when postural hypotension has occurred, it has been transient and is uncommon when carvedilol is administered with food at the recommended starting dose and titration increments are closely followed.

In hypertensive patients with healthy renal function, therapeutic doses of carvedilol decreased renal vascular resistance with no change in glomerular filtration rate or renal plasma flow. Changes in excretion of sodium, potassium, uric acid, and phosphorus in hypertensive patients with healthy renal function were similar after carvedilol and placebo.

CARVEDILOL — ORAL

Carvedilol has little effect on plasma catecholamines, plasma aldosterone, or electrolyte levels, but it significantly reduces plasma renin activity when given for at least 4 weeks. It also increases levels of atrial natriuretic peptide.

➤*Pharmacokinetics:*

Absorption/Distribution – Carvedilol is rapidly and extensively absorbed following oral administration, with absolute bioavailability of approximately 25% to 35% due to a significant degree of first-pass metabolism. Following oral administration, the apparent mean terminal elimination half-life of carvedilol generally ranges from 7 to 10 hours. Plasma concentrations achieved are proportional to the oral dose administered. When administered with food, the rate of absorption is slowed, as evidenced by a delay in the time to reach peak plasma levels (C_{max}), with no significant difference in extent of bioavailability. Taking carvedilol with food should minimize the risk of orthostatic hypotension.

Carvedilol is more than 98% bound to plasma proteins, primarily with albumin. The plasma-protein binding is independent of concentration over the therapeutic range. Carvedilol is a basic lipophilic compound with a steady-state volume of distribution of approximately 115 L, indicating substantial distribution into extravascular tissues. Plasma clearance ranges from 500 to 700 mL/min.

Metabolism/Excretion – Carvedilol is extensively metabolized. Following oral administration of radiolabeled carvedilol to healthy volunteers, carvedilol accounted for only about 7% of the total radioactivity in plasma as measured by area under the curve (AUC). Less than 2% of the dose was excreted unchanged in the urine. Carvedilol is metabolized primarily by aromatic ring oxidation and glucuronidation. The oxidative metabolites are further metabolized by conjugation via glucuronidation and sulfation. The metabolites of carvedilol are excreted primarily via the bile into the feces. Demethylation and hydroxylation at the phenol ring produce 3 active metabolites with β-receptor blocking activity. Based on preclinical studies, the 4′-hydroxyphenyl metabolite is approximately 13 times more potent than carvedilol for β-blockade.

Compared with carvedilol, the 3 active metabolites exhibit weak vasodilating activity. Plasma concentrations of the active metabolites are about one tenth of those observed for carvedilol and have pharmacokinetics similar to the parent.

Carvedilol undergoes stereoselective first-pass metabolism with plasma levels of R(+)-carvedilol approximately 2 to 3 times higher than S(−)-carvedilol following oral administration in healthy subjects. The mean apparent terminal elimination half-lives for R(+)-carvedilol range from 5 to 9 hours compared with 7 to 11 hours for the S(−)-enantiomer.

The primary P-450 enzymes responsible for the metabolism of both R(+) and S(−)-carvedilol in human liver microsomes were CYP2D6 and CYP2C9 and, to a lesser extent, CYP3A4, 2C19, 1A2, and 2E1. CYP2D6 is thought to be the major enzyme in the 4′- and 5′-hydroxylation of carvedilol, with a potential contribution from 3A4. CYP2C9 is thought to be of primary importance in the O-methylation pathway of S(−)-carvedilol.

Carvedilol is subject to the effects of genetic polymorphism, with poor metabolizers of debrisoquin (a marker for CYP-450 2D6) exhibiting 2- to 3-fold higher plasma concentrations of R(+)-carvedilol compared with extensive metabolizers. In contrast, plasma levels of S(−)-carvedilol are increased only about 20% to 25% in poor metabolizers, indicating this enantiomer is metabolized to a lesser extent by CYP-450 2D6 than R(+)-carvedilol. The pharmacokinetics of carvedilol do not appear to be different in poor metabolizers of S-mephenytoin (patients deficient in CYP-450 2C19).

Special populations –

Renal function impairment: Although carvedilol is metabolized primarily by the liver, plasma concentrations of carvedilol have been reported to be increased in patients with renal function impairment. Based on mean AUC data, approximately 40% to 50% higher plasma concentrations of carvedilol were observed in hypertensive patients with moderate to severe renal function impairment compared with a control group of hypertensive patients with healthy renal function. However, the ranges of AUC values were similar for both groups. Changes in mean C_{max} levels were less pronounced, approximately 12% to 26% higher in patients with renal function impairment.

Consistent with its high degree of plasma protein binding, carvedilol does not appear to be cleared significantly by hemodialysis.

Hepatic function impairment: Compared with healthy subjects, patients with cirrhotic liver disease exhibit significantly higher concentrations of carvedilol (approximately 4- to 7-fold) following single-dose therapy.

Elderly: Plasma levels of carvedilol average about 50% higher in elderly subjects compared with younger subjects.

CHF: Steady-state plasma concentrations of carvedilol and its enantiomers increased proportionally over the 6.25 to 50 mg dose range in patients with CHF. Compared with healthy subjects, CHF patients had increased mean AUC and C_{max} values for carvedilol and its enantiomers, with up to 50% to 100% higher values observed in 6 patients with NYHA class IV heart failure.

Contraindications

Bronchial asthma (2 cases of death from status asthmaticus have been reported in patients receiving single doses of carvedilol) or related bronchospastic conditions, second- or third-degree atrioventricular (AV) block, sick sinus syndrome or severe bradycardia (unless a permanent pacemaker is in place), cardiogenic shock or decompensated heart failure requiring the use of IV inotropic therapy (such patients should first be weaned from IV therapy before initiating carvedilol), clinically manifest hepatic function impairment, hypersensitivity to any component of the drug.

Warnings/Precautions

➤*Cessation of therapy:* Advise patients with coronary artery disease who are being treated with carvedilol against abrupt discontinuation of therapy. Severe exacerbation of angina and the occurrence of MI and ventricular arrhythmias have been reported in angina patients following the abrupt discontinuation of therapy with beta-blockers. The last 2 complications may occur with or without preceding exacerbation of the angina pectoris. As with other beta-blockers, when discontinuation of carvedilol is planned, carefully observe patients and advise them to limit physical activity to a minimum. Discontinue carvedilol over 1 to 2 weeks whenever possible. If the angina worsens or acute coronary insufficiency develops, it is recommended that carvedilol be promptly reinstituted, at least temporarily. Because coronary artery disease is common and may be unrecognized, it may be prudent not to discontinue carvedilol therapy abruptly even in patients treated only for hypertension or heart failure.

➤*Hypotension and postural hypotension:* In clinical trials of primarily mild to moderate heart failure, hypotension and postural hypotension occurred in 9.7% and syncope in 3.4% of patients receiving carvedilol compared with 3.6% and 2.5% of placebo patients, respectively. The risk for these events was highest during the first 30 days of dosing, corresponding to the up-titration period, and was a cause for discontinuation of therapy in 0.7% of carvedilol patients, compared with 0.4% of placebo patients. In a long-term, placebo-controlled trial in severe heart failure (COPERNICUS), hypotension and postural hypotension occurred in 15.1% and syncope in 2.9% of heart failure patients receiving carvedilol, compared with 8.7% and 2.3% of placebo patients, respectively. These events were a cause for discontinuation of therapy in 1.1% of carvedilol patients, compared with 0.8% of placebo patients.

Postural hypotension occurred in 1.8% and syncope in 0.1% of hypertensive patients, primarily following the initial dose or at the time of dose increase and was a cause for discontinuation of therapy in 1% of patients.

In the CAPRICORN study of survivors of an acute MI, hypotension or postural hypotension occurred in 20.2% of patients receiving carvedilol, compared with 12.6% of placebo patients. Syncope was reported in 3.9% and 1.9% of patients, respectively. These events were a cause for discontinuation of therapy in 2.5% of patients receiving carvedilol, compared with 0.2% of placebo patients.

➤*Peripheral vascular disease:* Beta-blockers can precipitate or aggravate symptoms of arterial insufficiency in patients with peripheral vascular disease. Exercise caution in such individuals.

➤*Anesthesia and major surgery:* If carvedilol treatment is to be continued perioperatively, take particular care when anesthetic agents that depress myocardial function, such as ether, cyclopropane, and trichloroethylene, are used.

➤*Diabetes and hypoglycemia:* In general, beta-blockers may mask some of the manifestations of hypoglycemia, particularly tachycardia. Nonselective beta-blockers may potentiate insulin-induced hypoglycemia and delay recovery of serum glucose levels. Caution patients subject to spontaneous hypoglycemia, or diabetic patients receiving insulin or oral hypoglycemic agents, about these possibilities. In CHF patients, there is a risk of worsening hyperglycemia.

➤*Effects on glycemic control in patients with type 2 diabetes:* In CHF patients with diabetes, carvedilol therapy may lead to worsening hyperglycemia, which responds to intensification of hypoglycemic therapy. It is recommended that blood glucose be monitored when carvedilol dosing is initiated, adjusted, or discontinued. Studies designed to examine the effects of carvedilol on glycemic control in patients with diabetes and heart failure have not been conducted.

In a study designed to examine the effects of carvedilol on glycemic control in a population with mild to moderate hypertension and well-controlled type 2 diabetes mellitus, carvedilol had no adverse effect on glycemic control based on glycosylated hemoglobin (HbA_{1c}) measurements.

➤*Thyrotoxicosis:* Beta-adrenergic blockade may mask clinical signs of hyperthyroidism, such as tachycardia. Abrupt withdrawal of beta-blockade may be followed by an exacerbation of the symptoms of hyperthyroidism or may precipitate thyroid storm.

➤*Pheochromocytoma:* In patients with pheochromocytoma, initiate an alpha-blocking agent prior to the use of any beta-blocking agent. Although carvedilol has both alpha- and beta-blocking pharmacologic activities, there has been no experience with its use in this condition. Therefore, take caution in the administration of carvedilol to patients suspected of having pheochromocytoma.

➤*Worsening cardiac failure:* Worsening cardiac failure or fluid retention may occur during up-titration of carvedilol. If such symptoms occur, increase diuretics and do not advance the carvedilol dose until clinical stability resumes. Occasionally it is necessary to lower the carvedilol dose or temporarily discontinue it. Such episodes do not preclude subsequent successful titration of, or favorable response to, carvedilol. In a placebo-controlled trial of patients with severe heart failure, worsening heart failure during the first 3 months was reported to a similar degree with carvedilol and with placebo. When treatment was maintained beyond 3 months, worsening heart failure was reported less frequently in patients treated with carvedilol than with placebo. Worsening heart failure observed during long-term therapy is more likely to be related to the patient's underlying disease than to treatment with carvedilol.

➤*Prinzmetal variant angina:* Agents with nonselective beta-blocking activity may provoke chest pain in patients with Prinzmetal variant angina. There has been no clinical experience with carvedilol in these patients,

CARVEDILOL — ORAL

although the alpha-blocking activity may prevent such symptoms. However, take caution in the administration of carvedilol to patients suspected of having Prinzmetal variant angina.

➤*Cardiovascular effects:* In clinical trials, carvedilol caused bradycardia in about 2% of hypertensive patients, 9% of CHF patients, and 6.5% of MI patients with left ventricular dysfunction. If pulse rate drops below 55 beats/min, reduce the dosage.

To decrease the likelihood of syncope or excessive hypotension, initiate treatment with 3.125 mg twice daily for CHF patients and 6.25 mg twice daily for hypertensive patients and survivors of an acute MI with left ventricular dysfunction. Increase dosage slowly, according to dosage recommendations, and advise patients to take the drug with food. During initiation of therapy, caution patients to avoid situations such as driving or hazardous tasks where injury could result if syncope occurs.

➤*Nonallergic bronchospasm (eg, chronic bronchitis, emphysema):* Patients with bronchospastic disease should, in general, not receive beta-blockers. However, carvedilol may be used with caution in patients who do not respond to, or cannot tolerate, other antihypertensive agents. It is prudent, if carvedilol is used, to use the smallest effective dose so that inhibition of endogenous or exogenous beta-agonists is minimized.

In clinical trials of patients with CHF, patients with bronchospastic disease were enrolled if they did not require oral or inhaled medication to treat their bronchospastic disease. In such patients, it is recommended that carvedilol be used with caution. Follow the dosing recommendations closely and lower the dose if any evidence of bronchospasm is observed during up-titration.

➤*Hypersensitivity reactions:* While taking beta-blockers, patients with a history of severe anaphylactic reaction to a variety of allergens may be more reactive to repeated challenge, either accidental, diagnostic, or therapeutic. Such patients may be unresponsive to the usual doses of epinephrine used to treat allergic reaction.

➤*Renal function impairment:* Rarely, use of carvedilol in patients with CHF has resulted in deterioration of renal function. Patients at risk appear to be those with low blood pressure (systolic blood pressure less than 100 mm Hg), ischemic heart disease and diffuse vascular disease, and/or underlying renal function impairment. Renal function has returned to baseline when carvedilol was stopped. In patients with these risk factors, it is recommended that renal function be monitored during up-titration of carvedilol and that the drug be discontinued or dosage reduced if worsening of renal function occurs.

➤*Pregnancy: Category C.*

Teratogenic – Studies performed in pregnant rats and rabbits given carvedilol revealed increased postimplantation loss in rats at doses of 300 mg/kg/day (50 times the MRHD as mg/m^2) and in rabbits at doses of 75 mg/kg/day (25 times the MRHD as mg/m^2). In the rats, there was also a decrease in fetal body weight at the maternally toxic dose of 300 mg/kg/day (50 times the MRHD as mg/m^2), which was accompanied by an elevation in the frequency of fetuses with delayed skeletal development (missing or stunted 13th rib). In rats, the no-observed-effect level for developmental toxicity was 60 mg/kg/day (10 times the MRHD as mg/m^2); in rabbits it was 15 mg/kg/day (5 times the MRHD as mg/m^2). There are no adequate and well-controlled studies in pregnant women. Use carvedilol during pregnancy only if the potential benefit justifies the potential risk to the fetus.

➤*Lactation:* It is not known whether this drug is excreted in human milk. Studies in rats have shown that carvedilol or its metabolites (as well as other beta-blockers) cross the placental barrier and are excreted in breast milk. There was increased mortality at 1 week postpartum in neonates from rats treated with 60 mg/kg/day (10 times the MRHD as mg/m^2) and above during the last trimester through day 22 of lactation. Because many drugs are excreted in human milk and because of the potential for serious adverse reactions in breast-feeding infants from beta-blockers, especially bradycardia, decide whether to discontinue breast-feeding or the drug, taking into account the importance of the drug to the mother. The effects of other alpha- and beta-blocking agents have included perinatal and neonatal distress.

➤*Children:* Safety and efficacy in patients younger than 18 years of age have not been established.

➤*Elderly:* With the exception of dizziness in hypertensive patients (incidence 8.8% in the elderly patients vs 6% in younger patients), no overall differences in the safety or efficacy were observed between the older subjects and younger subjects in each of these populations. Similarly, other reported clinical experience has not identified differences in responses between elderly subjects and younger subjects, but greater sensitivity of some older individuals cannot be ruled out.

➤*Monitoring:* Regular monitoring of blood glucose is recommended in patients taking insulin or oral hypoglycemics. Monitor renal function during up-titration, discontinuation, or dosage reduction in patients at risk for renal function deterioration. Monitor for worsening of heart failure or fluid retention.

Drug Interactions

Carvedilol Drug Interactions

Precipitant drug	Object drug[a]		Description
Cimetidine	Carvedilol	↑	Cimetidine increased carvedilol AUC by ≈ 30% but caused no change in C_{max}.
CYP-450 2D6 inhibitors (eg, propafenone, quinidine)	Carvedilol	↑	CYP-450 2D6 inhibitors may increase blood levels of the R(+) enantiomer of carvedilol.
Diphenhydramine	Carvedilol	↑	Diphenhydramine may inhibit carvedilol metabolism, resulting in increased plasma concentrations and cardiovascular effects of carvedilol.
Hydroxychloroquine	Carvedilol	↑	Hydroxychloroquine may inhibit metabolism of carvedilol, resulting in increased plasma concentrations and cardiovascular effects. Monitor patients when hydroxychloroquine is started or stopped.
Rifampin	Carvedilol	↓	Rifampin reduced AUC and C_{max} of carvedilol by ≈ 70%.
Salicylates	Carvedilol	↓	The blood pressure–lowering effect of carvedilol may be attenuated by salicylates. In addition, the beneficial effects of carvedilol on left ventricular ejection fraction in patients with chronic heart failure may be attenuated. Monitor blood pressure during concomitant administration.
SSRIs[b] (eg, fluoxetine, paroxetine)	Carvedilol	↑	Certain SSRIs may inhibit metabolism of carvedilol; possible excessive beta blockade (bradycardia) may occur. Monitor cardiac function during coadministration.
Carvedilol	Antidiabetic agents (ie, insulin, oral hypoglycemics)	↑	Carvedilol may enhance the glucose-reducing effect of insulin or oral hypoglycemics. Regular blood glucose monitoring is recommended in the patients.
Carvedilol	Calcium channel blockers (eg, diltiazem, verapamil)	↑	Isolated cases of conduction disturbances (rarely with hemodynamic compromise) have been observed when carvedilol is coadministered with diltiazem. If carvedilol is to be administered orally with calcium channel blockers of the verapamil or diltiazem type, monitor electrocardiogram and blood pressure.
Carvedilol	Catecholamine-depleting agents (eg, monoamine oxidase inhibitors, reserpine)	↑	Closely observe patients taking agents with beta-blocking properties and a drug that can deplete catecholamines for signs of hypotension or severe bradycardia.
Carvedilol	Clonidine	↑	Coadministration of clonidine with carvedilol may potentiate blood pressure and heart rate–lowering effects. When stopping both carvedilol and clonidine, discontinue carvedilol first. Clonidine therapy can then be discontinued several days later by gradually decreasing the dosage.
Carvedilol	Cyclosporine	↑	Coadministration of carvedilol and cyclosporine may cause an increase in mean trough cyclosporine concentrations. Monitor cyclosporine concentrations closely after carvedilol initiation.
Carvedilol	Digoxin	↑	Digoxin concentrations are increased by approximately 15% during concurrent use. Monitor digoxin level when initiating, adjusting, or discontinuing carvedilol.

[a] ↑ = object drug increased; ↓ = object drug decreased.
[b] SSRIs = selective serotonin reuptake inhibitors.

CARVEDILOL — ORAL

➤*Drug/Food interactions:* When administered with food, the rate of absorption is slowed, as evidenced by a delay in the time to reach peak plasma levels (C_{max}), with no significant difference in extent of bioavailability. Taking carvedilol with food should minimize the risk of orthostatic hypotension.

Adverse Reactions

➤*CHF:* In placebo-controlled clinical trials, the only cause of discontinuation greater than 1%, and occurring more often with carvedilol, was dizziness (1.3% with carvedilol, 0.6% with placebo in the COPERNICUS trial).

Carvedilol Adverse Reactions in Heart Failure Trials (> 3%)

Adverse reactions	Mild to moderate heart failure		Severe heart failure	
	Carvedilol (n = 765)	Placebo (n = 437)	Carvedilol (n = 1,156)	Placebo (n = 1,133)
Cardiovascular				
Angina pectoris	2%	3%	6%	4%
Bradycardia	9%	1%	10%	3%
Hypotension	9%	3%	14%	8%
Syncope	3%	3%	8%	5%
CNS				
Asthenia	7%	7%	11%	9%
Dizziness	32%	19%	24%	17%
Fatigue	24%	22%	-	-
Headache	8%	7%	5%	3%
GI				
Diarrhea	12%	6%	5%	3%
Nausea	9%	5%	4%	3%
Vomiting	6%	4%	1%	2%
Metabolic				
BUN[a] increased	6%	5%	-	-
Hypercholesterolemia	4%	3%	1%	1%
Hyperglycemia	12%	8%	5%	3%
Nonprotein nitrogen increased	6%	5%	-	-
Peripheral edema	2%	1%	7%	6%
Weight increase	10%	7%	12%	11%
Musculoskeletal				
Arthralgia	6%	5%	1%	1%
Respiratory				
Increased cough	8%	9%	5%	4%
Rales	4%	4%	4%	2%
Special senses				
Abnormal vision	5%	2%	-	-
Miscellaneous				
Dependent edema	4%	2%	-	-
Digoxin level increased	5%	4%	2%	1%
Generalized edema	5%	3%	6%	5%

[a] BUN = serum urea nitrogen.

Cardiac failure and dyspnea were also reported in these studies, but the rates were equal or greater in patients who received placebo.

➤*Other adverse reactions (more than 1% to 3%):* The following adverse reactions were reported with a frequency of more than 1% to 3% and more frequently with carvedilol in either the US placebo-controlled trials in patients with mild to moderate heart failure or in patients with severe heart failure in the COPERNICUS trial.

Cardiovascular – Aggravated angina pectoris, AV block, fluid overload, hypertension, palpitation, postural hypotension.

CNS – Hypesthesia, malaise, paresthesia, somnolence, vertigo.

GI – Melena, periodontitis.

GU – Impotence.

Hematologic – Prothrombin decreased, purpura, thrombocytopenia.

Hepatic – ALT increased, AST increased.

Metabolic/Nutritional – Diabetes mellitus, glycosuria, hyperkalemia, hyperuricemia, hypervolemia, hypoglycemia, hyponatremia, increased alkaline phosphatase, increased creatinine, increased gamma-glutamyl transferase, weight loss.

Musculoskeletal – Muscle cramps.

Renal – Albuminuria, hematuria, renal function impairment.

Special senses – Blurred vision.

Miscellaneous – Allergy, fever, hypovolemia, leg edema.

➤*Left ventricular dysfunction following MI:* The most common adverse reactions reported with carvedilol in the CAPRICORN trial were consistent with the profile of the drug in the US heart failure trials and the COPERNICUS trial. The only additional adverse reactions reported in CAPRICORN in greater than 3% of the patients and more commonly with carvedilol were anemia, dyspnea, and lung edema. The following adverse reactions were reported with a frequency of greater than 1% but less than or equal to 3% and more frequently with carvedilol: arthritis, cerebrovascular accident, depression, flu syndrome, GI pain, gout, hypotonia, and peripheral vascular disorder. The overall rates of discontinuations due to adverse reactions were similar in both groups of patients. In this database, the only cause of discontinuation greater than 1% and occurring more often with carvedilol was hypotension (1.5% with carvedilol, 0.2% with placebo).

➤*Hypertension:* Although there was no overall difference in discontinuation rates, discontinuations were more common in the carvedilol group for postural hypotension (1% vs 0%). The overall incidence of adverse reactions in US placebo-controlled trials was found to increase with increasing doses of carvedilol. For individual adverse reactions, this could only be distinguished for dizziness, which increased in frequency from 2% to 5% as the total daily dose increased from 6.25 to 50 mg.

Carvedilol Adverse Reactions in Hypertension Trials[a] (≥ 1%)

Adverse reactions	Carvedilol (n = 1,142)	Placebo (n = 462)
Cardiovascular		
Bradycardia	2%	-
Peripheral edema	1%	-
Postural hypotension	2%	-
CNS		
Dizziness	6%	5%
Insomnia	2%	1%
GI		
Diarrhea	2%	1%
Hematologic		
Thrombocytopenia	1%	-
Metabolic		
Hypertriglyceridemia	1%	-

[a] Shown are reactions with rates greater than 1% rounded to nearest integer. Dyspnea and fatigue were also reported in these studies, but the rates were equal or greater in patients who received placebo.

➤*Other adverse reactions (more than 0.1% to 1%):*

Cardiovascular – Peripheral ischemia, tachycardia.

CNS – Abnormal thinking, aggravated depression, emotional lability, hypokinesia, impaired concentration, nervousness, paroniria, sleep disorder.

Dermatologic – Erythematous rash, maculopapular rash, photosensitivity reaction, pruritus, psoriasiform rash.

GU – Decreased libido (men), increased micturition frequency.

Hematologic/Lymphatic – Anemia, bilirubinemia, leukopenia.

Hepatic – Increased hepatic enzymes (0.2% of hypertension patients and 0.4% of CHF patients were discontinued from therapy because of increases in hepatic enzymes).

Metabolic/Nutritional – Hypertriglyceridemia, hypokalemia.

Respiratory – Asthma.

Special senses – Tinnitus.

Miscellaneous – Dry mouth, increased sweating. The following reactions were reported in less than or equal to 0.1% of patients and are potentially important: alopecia, amnesia, anaphylactoid reaction, atypical lymphocytes, bronchospasm, bundle branch block, cerebrovascular disorder, complete AV block, convulsions, decreased hearing, decreased high-density lipoprotein (HDL), exfoliative dermatitis, GI hemorrhage, increased BUN, migraine, myocardial ischemia, neuralgia, pancytopenia, paresis, pulmonary edema, and respiratory alkalosis.

➤*Lab test abnormalities:* Reversible elevations in serum transaminases (ALT or AST) have been observed during treatment with carvedilol. Rates of transaminase elevations (2 to 3 times the upper limit of normal) observed during controlled clinical trials have generally been similar between patients treated with carvedilol and those treated with placebo. However, transaminase elevations, confirmed by rechallenge, have been observed with carvedilol. In a long-term, placebo-controlled trial in severe heart failure, patients treated with carvedilol had lower values for hepatic transaminases than patients treated with placebo, possibly because carvedilol-induced improvements in cardiac function led to less hepatic congestion and/or improved hepatic blood flow.

➤*Postmarketing:* Reports of aplastic anemia and severe skin reactions (eg, erythema multiforme, Stevens-Johnson syndrome, toxic epidermal necrolysis) have been rare and were received only when carvedilol was coadministered with other medications associated with such reactions. Urinary incontinence in women (which resolved upon discontinuation of the medication) and interstitial pneumonitis have been reported rarely.

CARVEDILOL — ORAL

Overdosage

➤*Symptoms:* Overdosage may cause bradycardia, cardiac arrest, cardiac insufficiency, cardiogenic shock, and severe hypotension. Bronchospasms, generalized seizures, lapses of consciousness, respiratory problems, and vomiting may also occur.

Cases of overdosage with carvedilol alone or in combination with other drugs have been reported. Quantities ingested in some cases exceeded 1,000 mg. Symptoms experienced included low blood pressure and heart rate. Standard supportive treatment was provided and individuals recovered.

➤*Treatment:* Place the patient in a supine position and, where necessary, keep under observation and treat under intensive-care conditions. Gastric lavage may be used shortly after ingestion. The following agents may be administered

For excessive bradycardia – Atropine 2 mg IV.

To support cardiovascular function – Glucagon 5 to 10 mg IV rapidly over 30 seconds, followed by a continuous infusion of 5 mg/h; sympathomimetics (eg, epinephrine, dobutamine, isoprenaline) at doses according to body weight and effect.

If peripheral vasodilation dominates, it may be necessary to administer epinephrine or norepinephrine with continuous monitoring of circulatory conditions. For therapy-resistant bradycardia, perform pacemaker therapy. For bronchospasm, give beta-sympathomimetics (as aerosol or IV) or aminophylline IV. In the event of seizures, slow IV injection of diazepam or clonazepam is recommended.

In the event of severe intoxication where there are symptoms of shock, treatment with antidotes must be continued for a sufficiently long period of time consistent with the 7- to 10-hour half-life of carvedilol.

Patient Information

Advise patients taking carvedilol not to interrupt or discontinue use of carvedilol without a health care provider's advice.

Advise CHF patients to consult their health care provider if they experience signs or symptoms of worsening heart failure, such as weight gain or increasing shortness of breath. They may experience a drop in blood pressure when standing, resulting in dizziness and, rarely, fainting. Patients should sit or lie down when these symptoms of lowered blood pressure occur.

If patients experience dizziness or fatigue, they should avoid driving or performing hazardous tasks.

Advise patients to consult a health care provider if they experience dizziness or faintness; their dosage may need to be adjusted.

Advise patients to take carvedilol with food.

Advise diabetic patients to report any changes in blood sugar levels to their health care provider.

Contact lens wearers may experience decreased lacrimation.

CARVEDILOL PHOSPHATE — ORAL

Indications

➤*Heart failure:* For the treatment of mild to severe heart failure of ischemic or cardiomyopathic origin, usually in addition to diuretics, angiotensin-converting enzyme (ACE) inhibitors, and digitalis, to increase survival, and also to reduce the risk of hospitalization.

➤*Hypertension:* For the treatment of essential hypertension. It can be used alone or in combination with other antihypertensive agents, especially thiazide-type diuretics.

➤*Left ventricular dysfunction following myocardial infarction (MI):* To reduce cardiovascular (CV) mortality in clinically stable patients who have survived the acute phase of an MI and have a left ventricular ejection fraction of 40% or less (with or without symptomatic heart failure).

➤*Off-label uses:* Immediate-release (IR) carvedilol has been shown to be beneficial in the treatment of chronic stable angina and as adjunctive treatment in unstable angina.

Administration and Dosage

➤*General dosing considerations:* Carvedilol phosphate is an extended-release (ER) capsule intended for once-daily administration.

Dosage must be individualized and closely monitored by a health care provider during up-titration.

Patients should be advised that initiation of treatment and, to a lesser extent, dosage increases may be associated with transient symptoms of dizziness or light-headedness (and rarely syncope) within the first hour after dosing. Thus, during these periods, patients should avoid situations such as driving or hazardous tasks in which symptoms could result in injury.

Episodes of dizziness or fluid retention during initiation of carvedilol can generally be managed without discontinuation of treatment and do not preclude subsequent successful titration of or favorable response to carvedilol.

➤*Adults:*

Heart failure – Prior to initiation of carvedilol, it is recommended that fluid retention be minimized.

Initial dosage: 10 mg once daily for 2 weeks.

Dosage titration: Patients who tolerate a dosage of 10 mg once daily may have their dose increased to 20, 40, and 80 mg over successive intervals of at least 2 weeks. Patients should be maintained on lower doses if higher doses are not tolerated.

The dose of carvedilol should not be increased until symptoms of worsening heart failure or vasodilation have been stabilized.

The dose of carvedilol should be reduced if patients experience bradycardia (heart rate of less than 55 bpm).

Concomitant therapy: Vasodilatory symptoms often do not require treatment, but it may be useful to separate the time of dosing of carvedilol from that of the ACE inhibitor or to reduce temporarily the dose of the ACE inhibitor.

Fluid retention (with or without transient worsening heart failure symptoms) should be treated by an increase in the dose of diuretics.

Hypertension –

Maximum dose: Total daily dose should not exceed 80 mg.

Initial dosage: 20 mg once daily.

Dosage titration: If this dosage is tolerated, using standing systolic pressure measured approximately 1 hour after dosing as a guide, the dosage should be maintained for 7 to 14 days, then increased to 40 mg once daily if needed, based on trough blood pressure, again using standing systolic pressure 1 hour after dosing as a guide for tolerance. This dosage should also be maintained for 7 to 14 days, and then it can be adjusted upward to 80 mg once daily, if tolerated and needed. Although not specifically studied, it is anticipated that the full antihypertensive effect of carvedilol would be seen within 7 to 14 days, as had been demonstrated with carvedilol immediate release.

Concomitant therapy: Addition of a diuretic to carvedilol or carvedilol to a diuretic can be expected to produce additive effects and exaggerate the orthostatic component of carvedilol action.

Left ventricular dysfunction following myocardial infarction – Treatment with carvedilol may be started as an in- or outpatient and should be started after the patient is hemodynamically stable and fluid retention has been minimized.

Initial dosage: 20 mg once daily.

Dosage titration: Increase after 3 to 10 days, based on tolerability, to 40 mg once daily, then again to the target dosage of 80 mg once daily.

Alternative dosage: A lower starting dose (10 mg once daily) may be used and/or the rate of up-titration may be slowed if clinically indicated (eg, low blood pressure or heart rate, fluid retention). Patients should be maintained on lower doses if higher doses are not tolerated. The recommended dosing regimen need not be altered in patients who received treatment with an intravenous (IV) or oral beta-blocker during the acute phase of the MI.

➤*Elderly:* Greater sensitivity of some older individuals cannot be ruled out.

➤*Renal function impairment:* It is recommended that renal function be monitored during up-titration of carvedilol ER and the drug discontinued or dosage reduced if worsening of renal function occurs.

➤*Hepatic function impairment:* Carvedilol should not be given to patients with severe hepatic function impairment.

➤*Conversion:* Patients controlled with carvedilol immediate-release tablets alone or in combination with other medications may be switched to carvedilol ER capsules based on the total daily doses shown in the following table. Subsequent titration to higher or lower doses may be necessary as clinically warranted.

Carvedilol Dosing Conversion	
Daily dosage of carvedilol immediate release tablets	Daily dosage of carvedilol ER capsules
6.25 mg (3.125 mg twice daily)	10 mg once daily
12.5 mg (6.25 mg twice daily)	20 mg once daily
25 mg (12.5 mg twice daily)	40 mg once daily
50 mg (25 mg twice daily)	80 mg once daily

➤*Administration:* Carvedilol should be taken once daily in the morning with food. It should be swallowed as a whole capsule. Carvedilol and/or its contents should not be crushed, chewed, or taken in divided doses.

The administration of carvedilol with alcohol, including prescription and over-the-counter medications that contain ethanol, should be separated by at least 2 hours.

The capsules may be carefully opened and the beads sprinkled over a spoonful of applesauce. The applesauce should not be warm because it could affect the modified-release properties of this formulation. The mixture of drug and applesauce should be consumed immediately in its entirety. The drug and applesauce mixture should not be stored for future use. Absorption of the beads sprinkled on other foods has not been tested.

➤*Storage/Stability:* Store at 25°C (77°F); excursions are permitted to 15° to 30°C (59° to 86°F).

Actions

➤*Pharmacology:* Carvedilol is a racemic mixture in which nonselective beta-adrenoreceptor blocking activity is present in the S(−) enantiomer and $alpha_1$-adrenergic blocking activity is present in both R(+) and S(−) enantiomers at equal potency. Carvedilol has no intrinsic sympathomimetic activity.

Pharmacodynamics –

Hypertension: Beta-adrenoreceptor blocking activity has been demonstrated in animal and human studies showing that carvedilol (1) reduces cardiac output in healthy subjects, (2) reduces exercise- and/or

CARVEDILOL PHOSPHATE — ORAL

isoproterenol-induced tachycardia, and (3) reduces reflex orthostatic tachycardia. Significant beta-adrenoreceptor blocking effect is usually seen within 1 hour of drug administration.

$Alpha_1$-adrenoreceptor blocking activity has been demonstrated in human and animal studies, showing that carvedilol (1) attenuates the pressor effects of phenylephrine, (2) causes vasodilation, and (3) reduces peripheral vascular resistance. These effects contribute to the reduction of blood pressure and usually are seen within 30 minutes of drug administration.

Carvedilol has little effect on plasma catecholamines, plasma aldosterone, or electrolyte levels, but it does significantly reduce plasma renin activity when given for at least 4 weeks. It also increases levels of atrial natriuretic peptide.

➤*Pharmacokinetics:*

Absorption – Carvedilol is rapidly and extensively absorbed following oral administration of carvedilol IR tablets, with an absolute bioavailability of approximately 25% to 35% due to a significant degree of first-pass metabolism. Carvedilol ER capsules have approximately 85% of the bioavailability of carvedilol IR tablets. For corresponding dosages, the exposure (area under the curve [AUC], peak concentration [C_{max}], trough concentration) of carvedilol as carvedilol ER capsules is equivalent to those of carvedilol IR tablets when both are administered with food. The absorption of carvedilol from carvedilol ER capsules is slower and more prolonged compared with the carvedilol IR tablet with C_{max} achieved approximately 5 hours after administration. Plasma concentrations of carvedilol increase in a dose-proportional manner over the dosage range of carvedilol ER 10 to 80 mg. Within-subject and between-subject variability for AUC and C_{max} is similar for carvedilol ER and carvedilol IR.

Effect of food: Administration of carvedilol ER with a high-fat meal resulted in increases (approximately 20%) in AUC and C_{max} compared with carvedilol administered with a standard meal. Decreases in AUC (27%) and C_{max} (43%) were observed when carvedilol ER was administered in the fasted state compared with administration after a standard meal. Instruct patients to take carvedilol ER with food. In a study with adult subjects, sprinkling the contents of the carvedilol ER capsule on applesauce did not appear to have a significant effect on AUC compared with administration of the intact capsule following a standard meal but did result in a decrease in C_{max} (18%).

Distribution – Carvedilol is more than 98% bound to plasma proteins, primarily with albumin. The plasma-protein binding is independent of concentration over the therapeutic range. Carvedilol is a basic lipophilic compound with a steady-state volume of distribution of approximately 115 L, indicating substantial distribution into extravascular tissues.

Metabolism/Excretion – Carvedilol is extensively metabolized. Following oral administration of radiolabelled carvedilol to healthy volunteers, carvedilol accounted for only about 7% of the total radioactivity in plasma as measured by AUC. Less than 2% of the dose was excreted unchanged in the urine. Carvedilol is metabolized primarily by aromatic ring oxidation and glucuronidation. The oxidative metabolites are further metabolized by conjugation via glucuronidation and sulfation. The metabolites of carvedilol are excreted primarily via the bile into the feces. Demethylation and hydroxylation at the phenol ring produce 3 active metabolites with beta-receptor blocking activity. Based on preclinical studies, the 4'-hydroxyphenyl metabolite is approximately 13 times more potent than carvedilol for beta-blockade.

Compared with carvedilol, the 3 active metabolites exhibit weak vasodilating activity. Plasma concentrations of the active metabolites are about one tenth of those observed for carvedilol and have pharmacokinetics similar to the parent.

Carvedilol undergoes stereoselective first-pass metabolism with plasma levels of R(+)-carvedilol approximately 2 to 3 times higher than S(−)-carvedilol following oral administration of carvedilol in healthy subjects. Apparent clearance is 90 and 213 L/h for R(+)- and S(−)-carvedilol, respectively.

The primary P-450 enzymes responsible for the metabolism of both R(+)- and S(−)-carvedilol in human liver microsomes were CYP2D6 and CYP2C9 and, to a lesser extent, CYP3A4, 2C19, 1A2, and 2E1. CYP2D6 is thought to be the major enzyme in the 4'- and 5'-hydroxylation of carvedilol, with a potential contribution from 3A4. CYP2C9 is thought to be of primary importance in the O-methylation pathway of S(−)-carvedilol.

Carvedilol is subject to the effects of genetic polymorphism with poor metabolizers of debrisoquin (a marker for CYP-450 2D6) exhibiting 2- to 3-fold higher plasma concentrations of R(+)-carvedilol compared with extensive metabolizers. In contrast, plasma levels of S(−)-carvedilol are increased only about 20% to 25% in poor metabolizers, indicating this enantiomer is metabolized to a lesser extent by CYP-450 2D6 than R(+)-carvedilol. The pharmacokinetics of carvedilol do not appear to be different in poor metabolizers of S-mephenytoin (patients deficient in CYP-450 2C19).

Special populations –

Renal function impairment: No studies have been performed with carvedilol ER in patients with renal function impairment. Although carvedilol is metabolized primarily by the liver, plasma concentrations of carvedilol have been reported to be increased in patients with renal function impairment after dosing with carvedilol IR. Based on mean AUC data, approximately 40% to 50% higher plasma concentrations of carvedilol were observed in hypertensive patients with moderate to severe renal function impairment compared with a control group of hypertensive patients with healthy renal function. However, the ranges of AUC values were similar for both groups. Changes in mean peak plasma levels were less pronounced, approximately 12% to 26% higher in patients with renal function impairment. Consistent with its high degree of plasma protein binding, carvedilol does not appear to be cleared significantly by hemodialysis.

Hepatic function impairment: No studies have been performed with carvedilol ER in patients with hepatic function impairment. Compared with healthy subjects, patients with cirrhotic liver disease exhibit significantly higher concentrations of carvedilol (approximately 4- to 7-fold) following single-dose therapy with carvedilol IR.

Elderly: Plasma levels of carvedilol average about 50% higher in the elderly compared with younger subjects after administration of carvedilol IR.

Heart failure: Following administration of carvedilol IR tablets, steady-state plasma concentrations of carvedilol and its enantiomers increased proportionally over the dose range in patients with heart failure. Compared with healthy subjects, heart failure patients had increased mean AUC and C_{max} values for carvedilol and its enantiomers, with up to 50% to 100% higher values observed in 6 patients with New York Heart Association (NYHA) class IV heart failure. The mean apparent terminal elimination half-life for carvedilol was similar to that observed in healthy subjects.

Contraindications

Bronchial asthma (2 cases of death from status asthmaticus have been reported in patients receiving single doses of carvedilol IR) or bronchospastic conditions; second- or third-degree atrioventricular (AV) block, sick sinus syndrome, or severe bradycardia (unless a permanent pacemaker is in place); cardiogenic shock or decompensated heart failure requiring the use of IV inotropic therapy (such patients should first be weaned from IV therapy before initiation of carvedilol ER); clinically manifest hepatic function impairment; hypersensitivity to any component of the drug.

Warnings/Precautions

➤*Anesthesia and major surgery:* If treatment with carvedilol ER is to be continued perioperatively, take particular care when anesthetic agents that depress MI, such as ether, cyclopropane, and trichloroethylene, are used.

➤*Cessation of therapy:* Advise patients with coronary artery disease who are being treated with carvedilol ER against abrupt discontinuation of therapy. Severe exacerbation of angina and the occurrence of MI and ventricular arrhythmias have been reported in angina patients following the abrupt discontinuation of therapy with beta-blockers. The last 2 complications may occur with or without preceding exacerbation of the angina pectoris. As with other beta-blockers, when discontinuation of carvedilol ER is planned, carefully observe the patients and advise them to limit physical activity to a minimum. Discontinue carvedilol ER over 1 to 2 weeks whenever possible. If the angina worsens or acute coronary insufficiency develops, it is recommended that carvedilol ER be promptly reinstituted, at least temporarily. Because coronary artery disease is common and may be unrecognized, it may be prudent not to discontinue carvedilol ER therapy abruptly even in patients treated only for hypertension or heart failure.

➤*Diabetes and hypoglycemia:* In general, beta-blockers may mask some of the manifestations of hypoglycemia, particularly tachycardia. Nonselective beta-blockers may potentiate insulin-induced hypoglycemia and delay recovery of serum glucose levels. Caution patients subject to spontaneous hypoglycemia or diabetic patients receiving insulin or oral hypoglycemic agents about these possibilities. In heart failure patients, there is a risk of worsening hyperglycemia.

➤*Peripheral vascular disease:* Beta-blockers can precipitate or aggravate symptoms of arterial insufficiency in patients with peripheral vascular disease. Exercise caution in such individuals.

➤*Thyrotoxicosis:* Beta-adrenergic blockade may mask clinical signs of hyperthyroidism, such as tachycardia. Abrupt withdrawal of beta-blockade may be followed by an exacerbation of the symptoms of hyperthyroidism or may precipitate thyroid storm.

➤*General:* In clinical trials of carvedilol in patients with hypertension (338 subjects) and in patients with left ventricular dysfunction following an MI or heart failure (187 subjects), the profile of adverse reactions observed with carvedilol phosphate was generally similar to that observed with the administration of carvedilol IR. Therefore, the information included within this section is based on data from controlled clinical trials with carvedilol ER as well as carvedilol IR.

➤*Cardiovascular effects:* In clinical trials with carvedilol IR, bradycardia was reported in about 2% of hypertensive patients, 9% of heart failure patients, and 6.5% of MI patients with left ventricular dysfunction. Bradycardia was reported in 0.5% of patients receiving carvedilol ER in a study of heart failure patients and MI patients with left ventricular dysfunction. There were no reports of bradycardia in the clinical trial of carvedilol ER in hypertension. However, if pulse rate drops below 55 beats/minute, reduce the dosage of carvedilol ER.

To decrease the likelihood of syncope or excessive hypotension, initiate treatment with carvedilol ER with 10 mg once daily for heart failure patients and at 20 mg once daily for hypertensive patients and survivors of an acute MI with left ventricular dysfunction. Then increase dosage slowly, according to recommendations in the Dosage and administration section, and instruct the patient to take the drug with food. During initiation of therapy, caution the patient to avoid situations such as driving or hazardous tasks, in which injury could result should syncope occur.

➤*Worsening heart failure/fluid retention:* Worsening heart failure or fluid retention may occur during up-titration of carvedilol. If such symptoms occur, increase diuretics and do not advance the dose of carvedilol ER until clinical stability resumes. Occasionally, it is necessary to lower the dose of carvedilol ER or temporarily discontinue it. Such episodes do not preclude subsequent successful titration of or a favorable response to carvedilol ER. In a placebo-controlled trial of patients with severe heart failure, worsening heart failure during the first 3 months was reported to a similar degree with

CARVEDILOL PHOSPHATE — ORAL

carvedilol IR and with placebo. When treatment was maintained beyond 3 months, worsening heart failure was reported less frequently in patients treated with carvedilol than with placebo. Worsening heart failure observed during long-term therapy is more likely to be related to the patient's underlying disease than to treatment with carvedilol.

➤*Pheochromocytoma:* In patients with pheochromocytoma, initiate an alpha-blocking agent prior to the use of any beta-blocking agent. Although carvedilol has both alpha- and beta-blocking pharmacologic activities, there has been no experience with its use in this condition. Therefore, use caution in the administration of carvedilol to patients suspected of having pheochromocytoma.

➤*Prinzmetal variant angina:* Agents with nonselective beta-blocking activity may provoke chest pain in patients with Prinzmetal variant angina. There has been no clinical experience with carvedilol in these patients, although the alpha-blocking activity may prevent such symptoms. However, use caution in the administration of carvedilol to patients suspected of having Prinzmetal variant angina.

➤*Effects on glycemic control in type 2 diabetic patients:* In heart failure patients with diabetes, carvedilol therapy may lead to worsening hyperglycemia, which responds to intensification of hypoglycemic therapy. It is recommended that blood glucose be monitored when dosing with carvedilol is initiated, adjusted, or discontinued. Studies designed to examine the effects of carvedilol on glycemic control in patients with diabetes and heart failure have not been conducted.

➤*Nonallergic bronchospasm (eg, chronic bronchitis, emphysema):* Patients with bronchospastic disease should, in general, not receive beta-blockers. Carvedilol ER may be used with caution, however, in patients who do not respond to or cannot tolerate other antihypertensive agents. If carvedilol ER is used, it is prudent to use the smallest effective dose, so that inhibition of endogenous or exogenous beta-agonists is minimized. In clinical trials of patients with heart failure, patients with bronchospastic disease were enrolled if they did not require oral or inhaled medication to treat their bronchospastic disease. In such patients, it is recommended that carvedilol ER be used with caution. Follow the dosing recommendations closely and lower the dose if any evidence of bronchospasm is observed during up-titration.

➤*Hypersensitivity reactions:* While taking beta-blockers, patients with a history of severe anaphylactic reaction to a variety of allergens may be more reactive to repeated challenge, either accidental, diagnostic, or therapeutic. Such patients may be unresponsive to the usual doses of epinephrine used to treat allergic reaction.

➤*Renal function impairment:* Rarely, use of carvedilol in patients with heart failure has resulted in deterioration of renal function. Patients at risk appear to be those with low blood pressure (systolic blood pressure less than 100 mm Hg), ischemic heart disease and diffuse vascular disease, and/or underlying renal function impairment. Renal function has returned to baseline when carvedilol was stopped. In patients with these risk factors, it is recommended that renal function be monitored during up-titration of carvedilol ER and the drug discontinued or dosage reduced if worsening of renal function occurs.

➤*Pregnancy: Category C.*

Teratogenic – Studies performed in pregnant rats and rabbits given carvedilol revealed increased postimplantation loss in rats at doses of 300 mg/kg/day (50 times the MRHD as mg/m^2) and in rabbits at doses of 75 mg/kg/day (25 times the MRHD as mg/m^2). In the rats, there was also a decrease in fetal body weight at the maternally toxic dose of 300 mg/kg/day (50 times the MRHD as mg/m^2) that was accompanied by an elevation in the frequency of fetuses with delayed skeletal development (missing or stunted thirteenth rib). In rats, the no-observed-effect level for developmental toxicity was 60 mg/kg/day (10 times the MRHD as mg/m^2); in rabbits it was 15 mg/kg/day (5 times the MRHD as mg/m^2). There are no adequate and well-controlled studies in pregnant women. Use carvedilol ER during pregnancy only if the potential benefit justifies the potential risk to the fetus.

➤*Lactation:* It is not known whether this drug is excreted in human milk. Studies in rats have shown that carvedilol and/or its metabolites (as well as other beta-blockers) cross the placental barrier and are excreted in breast milk. There was increased mortality at 1 week postpartum in neonates from rats treated with 60 mg/kg/day (10 times the MRHD as mg/m^2) and above during the last trimester through day 22 of lactation. Because many drugs are excreted in human milk and because of the potential for serious adverse reactions in breast-feeding infants from beta-blockers, especially bradycardia, decide whether to discontinue breast-feeding or the drug, taking into account the importance of the drug to the mother. The effects of other alpha- and beta-blocking agents have included perinatal and neonatal distress.

➤*Children:* Safety and efficacy of carvedilol in patients younger than 18 years of age have not been established.

Drug Interactions

Carvedilol Drug Interactions[a]

Precipitant drug	Object drug[b]		Description
Alcohol	Carvedilol ER	↑	Alcohol may affect the modified release properties of carvedilol ER. Separate the administration of carvedilol ER and alcohol by at least 2 hours.
Catecholamine-depleting agents (eg, MAOIs, reserpine)	Carvedilol ER	↑	Closely observe patients taking agents with beta-blocking properties and a drug that can deplete catecholamines for signs of hypotension or severe bradycardia.
Carvedilol phosphate	Catecholamine-depleting agents (eg, MAO inhibitors, reserpine)		
Cimetidine	Carvedilol ER	↑	Cimetidine increased carvedilol AUC by approximately 30% but caused no change in C_{max}.
Clonidine	Carvedilol ER	↑	Coadministration of clonidine with agents with beta-blocking properties may potentiate BP- and heart-rate–lowering effects. When concomitant treatment with agents with beta-blocking properties and clonidine is to be terminated, discontinue the beta-blocking agent first. Clonidine therapy can then be discontinued several days later by gradually decreasing the dosage.
Carvedilol ER	Clonidine		
Diphenhydramine	Carvedilol ER	↑	Diphenhydramine may inhibit carvedilol metabolism, resulting in increased plasma concentrations and cardiovascular effects of carvedilol.
Hydroxychloroquine	Carvedilol ER	↑	Hydroxychloroquine may inhibit the metabolism of carvedilol, resulting in increased plasma concentrations and cardiovascular effects. Monitor patients when hydroxychloroquine is started or stopped.
Rifampin	Carvedilol ER	↓	Rifampin reduced AUC and C_{max} of carvedilol by approximately 70%.
Salicylates	Carvedilol ER	↓	The blood-pressure effects of carvedilol ER may be attenuated by salicylates. In addition, the beneficial effects of carvedilol ER on left ventricular ejection fraction in patients with chronic heart failure may be attenuated.
SSRIs (ie, fluoxetine, paroxetine)	Carvedilol ER	↑	Certain SSRIs may inhibit metabolism of some beta-blockers; possible excessive beta blockade (bradycardia) may occur. Monitor cardiac function during coadministration.
Carvedilol ER	Antidiabetic agents	↑	Agents with beta-blocking properties may enhance the blood sugar–reducing effect of insulin and oral hypoglycemics. In patients taking insulin or oral hypoglycemics, regular monitoring of blood glucose is recommended.
Carvedilol ER	Calcium channel blockers (eg, diltiazem, verapamil)	↑	Isolated cases of conduction disturbance (rarely with hemodynamic compromise) have been observed when carvedilol is coadministered with diltiazem. As with other agents with beta-blocking properties, if carvedilol ER is to be administered orally with calcium channel blockers of the verapamil or diltiazem type, it is recommended that ECG and BP be monitored.
Carvedilol ER	Cyclosporine	↑	Coadministration of carvedilol and cyclosporine may cause an increase in mean trough cyclosporine concentrations. Monitor cyclosporine concentrations closely after carvedilol ER initiation and adjust the cyclosporine dose as appropriate.

CARVEDILOL PHOSPHATE — ORAL

Carvedilol Drug Interactions[a]			
Precipitant drug	Object drug[b]		Description
Carvedilol ER	Digoxin	⬆	Digoxin concentrations are increased by approximately 15% during concurrent use. Therefore, increased monitoring of digoxin is recommended when initiating, adjusting, or discontinuing carvedilol ER.
Carvedilol ER	Disopyramide	⬆	Clearance of disopyramide may be decreased by beta-blockers, resulting in increased adverse reactions (eg, sinus bradycardia, hypotension). Monitor patients closely during coadministration.

[a] ⬆ = object drug increased; ⬇ = object drug decreased.
[b] MAOIs = monoamine oxidase inhibitors; BP = blood pressure; SSRI = selective serotonin reuptake inhibitors; ECG = electrocardiogram.

Adverse Reactions

Carvedilol has been evaluated for safety in patients with heart failure (mild, moderate, and severe), in patients with left ventricular dysfunction following MI, and in hypertensive patients. The observed adverse reaction profile was consistent with the pharmacology of the drug and the health status of the patients in the clinical trials. Adverse reactions reported for each of these patient populations reflecting the use of either carvedilol ER or carvedilol IR are provided in the following sections. Excluded are adverse reactions considered too general to be informative and those not reasonably associated with the use of the drug because they were associated with the condition being treated or are very common in the treated population. Rates of adverse reactions were generally similar across demographic subsets (men and women, elderly and nonelderly, blacks and nonblacks). Carvedilol ER has been evaluated for safety in a 4-week (2 weeks of carvedilol IR and 2 weeks of carvedilol ER) clinical study (N = 187) that included 157 patients with stable, mild, moderate, or severe chronic heart failure and 30 patients with left ventricular dysfunction following acute MI. The profile of adverse reactions observed with carvedilol ER in this small, short-term study was generally similar to that observed with carvedilol IR. Differences in safety would not be expected based on the similarity in plasma levels for carvedilol ER and carvedilol IR.

➤*Heart failure:* The following information describes the safety experience in heart failure with carvedilol IR.

Carvedilol IR Adverse Reactions in Heart Failure Trials (> 3%)[a]				
	Mild to moderate heart failure		Severe heart failure	
Adverse reaction	Carvedilol (n = 765)	Placebo (n = 437)	Carvedilol (n = 1,156)	Placebo (n = 1,133)
Cardiovascular				
Angina pectoris	2%	3%	6%	4%
Bradycardia	9%	1%	10%	3%
Hypotension	9%	3%	14%	8%
Syncope	3%	3%	8%	5%
CNS				
Dizziness	32%	19%	24%	17%
Headache	8%	7%	5%	3%
GI				
Diarrhea	12%	6%	5%	3%
Nausea	9%	5%	4%	3%
Vomiting	6%	4%	1%	2%
Metabolic				
BUN increased	6%	5%		
Edema peripheral	2%	1%	7%	6%
Hypercholesterolemia	4%	3%	1%	1%
Hyperglycemia	12%	8%	5%	3%
NPN increased	6%	5%		
Weight increase	10%	7%	12%	11%
Musculoskeletal				
Arthralgia	6%	5%	1%	1%
Respiratory				
Cough increased	8%	9%	5%	4%
Rales	4%	4%	4%	2%
Special senses				
Vision abnormal	5%	2%		
Miscellaneous				
Asthenia	7%	7%	11%	9%
Digoxin level increased	5%	4%	2%	1%
Edema dependent	4%	2%		
Edema generalized	5%	3%	6%	5%
Fatigue	24%	22%		

[a] BUN = Serum urea nitrogen; NPN = nonprotein nitrogen.

➤*Incidence more than 1% to 3%:*

Cardiovascular – Aggravated angina pectoris, AV block, fluid overload, hypertension, palpitation, postural hypotension.

CNS – Hypesthesia, paresthesia, somnolence, vertigo.

GI – Melena, periodontitis.

GU – Albuminuria, hematuria, impotence, renal function impairment.

Hematologic – Prothrombin decreased, purpura, thrombocytopenia.

Hepatic – ALT increased, AST increased.

Metabolic/Nutritional – Creatinine increased, diabetes mellitus, gamma-glutamyl transferase increased, glycosuria, hyperkalemia, hyperuricemia, hypervolemia, hypoglycemia, hyponatremia, increased alkaline phosphatase, weight loss.

Musculoskeletal – Muscle cramps.

Special senses – Blurred vision.

Miscellaneous – Allergy, fever, hypovolemia, leg edema, malaise.

➤*Left ventricular dysfunction following MI:* The following information describes the safety experience in left ventricular dysfunction following acute MI with carvedilol IR.

Carvedilol has been evaluated for safety in survivors of an acute MI with left ventricular dysfunction in the CAPRICORN trial, which involved 969 patients who received carvedilol and 980 who received placebo. Approximately 75% of the patients received carvedilol for at least 6 months and 53% received carvedilol for at least 12 months. Patients were treated for an average of 12.9 and 12.8 months with carvedilol and placebo, respectively.

The most common adverse reactions reported with carvedilol in the CAPRICORN trial were consistent with the profile of the drug in the US heart failure trials and the COPERNICUS trial. The only additional adverse reactions reported in CAPRICORN in more than 3% of the patients and more commonly on carvedilol were anemia, dyspnea, and lung edema. The following adverse reactions were reported with a frequency of more than 1% but no more than 3% and more frequently with carvedilol: arthritis, cerebrovascular accident, depression, flu syndrome, GI pain, gout, hypotonia, and peripheral vascular disorder. The overall rates of discontinuations due to adverse reactions were similar in both groups of patients. In this database, the only cause of discontinuation of more than 1% and occurring more often on carvedilol was hypotension (1.5% on carvedilol, 0.2% on placebo).

➤*Hypertension:* Carvedilol ER was evaluated for safety in an 8-week, double-blind trial in 337 subjects with essential hypertension. The profile of adverse reactions observed with carvedilol ER was generally similar to that observed with carvedilol IR. The overall rates of discontinuations due to adverse reactions were similar between carvedilol ER and placebo.

Carvedilol ER Adverse Reactions in Patients with Hypertension (≥ 1%)		
Adverse reactions	Placebo (n = 84)	Carvedilol ER (n = 253)
CNS		
Dizziness	1%	2%
Insomnia	0%	1%
Paresthesia	0%	1%
GI		
Diarrhea	0%	1%
Nausea	0%	2%
Metabolic		
Edema peripheral	1%	2%
Respiratory		
Nasal congestion	0%	1%
Nasopharyngitis	0%	4%
Sinus congestion	0%	1%

The following information describes the safety experience in hypertension with carvedilol IR.

Carvedilol has been evaluated for safety in hypertension in more than 2,193 patients in US clinical trials and in 2,976 patients in international clinical trials. Approximately 36% of the total treated population received carvedilol for at least 6 months. In general, carvedilol was well tolerated at doses up to 50 mg daily. Most adverse reactions reported during carvedilol therapy were of mild to moderate severity. In US controlled clinical trials directly compar-

CARVEDILOL PHOSPHATE — ORAL

ing carvedilol monotherapy in doses up to 50 mg (n = 1,142) with placebo (n = 462), 4.9% of carvedilol patients discontinued for adverse reactions versus 5.2% of placebo patients. Although there was no overall difference in discontinuation rates, discontinuations were more common in the carvedilol group for postural hypotension (1% vs 0%). The overall incidence of adverse reactions in US placebo-controlled trials was found to increase with an increasing dose of carvedilol. For individual adverse reactions, this could only be distinguished for dizziness, which increased in frequency from 2% to 5% as total daily dose increased from 6.25 to 50 mg as single or divided doses.

The following table shows adverse reactions in US placebo-controlled clinical trials for hypertension that occurred with an incidence of more than 1% regardless of causality and that were more frequent in drug-treated patients than placebo-treated patients.

Carvedilol IR Adverse Reactions in Patients with Hypertension (≥ 1%)[a]

Adverse reactions	Placebo (n = 462)	Carvedilol (n = 1,142)
Cardiovascular		
Bradycardia		2%
Postural hypotension		2%
CNS		
Dizziness	5%	6%
Insomnia	1%	2%
GI		
Diarrhea	1%	2%
Hematologic		
Thrombocytopenia		1%
Metabolic		
Hypertriglyceridemia		1%
Peripheral edema		1%

[a] Shown are reactions with rate >1% to nearest integer.

Dyspnea and fatigue were also reported in these studies, but the rates were equal or greater in patients who received placebo.

➤*Incidence more than 0.1% to 1%:* The following adverse reactions not previously described were reported as possibly or probably related to carvedilol in worldwide open or controlled trials with carvedilol in patients with hypertension or heart failure.

Cardiovascular – Peripheral ischemia, tachycardia.

CNS – Abnormal thinking, aggravated depression, emotional lability, hypokinesia, impaired concentration, nervousness, paroniria, sleep disorder.

Dermatologic – Photosensitivity reaction, pruritus, rash erythematous, rash maculopapular, rash psoriasiform.

GI – Bilirubinemia, dry mouth, increased hepatic enzymes (0.2% of hypertension patients and 0.4% of heart failure patients were discontinued from therapy because of increases in hepatic enzymes).

GU – Male: decreased libido, micturition frequency increased.

Hematologic – Anemia, leukopenia.

Metabolic/Nutritional – Hypertriglyceridemia, hypokalemia.

Respiratory – Asthma.

Special senses – Tinnitus.

Miscellaneous – Sweating increased. The following reactions were reported in 0.1% or less of patients and are potentially important: alopecia, amnesia, anaphylactoid reaction, atypical lymphocytes, bronchospasm, bundle branch block, cerebrovascular disorder, complete AV block, convulsions, decreased high-density lipoprotein, decreased hearing, exfoliative dermatitis, GI hemorrhage, increased BUN, migraine, myocardial ischemia, neuralgia, pancytopenia, paresis, pulmonary edema, respiratory alkalosis.

➤*Lab test abnormalities:* Reversible elevations in serum transaminases (ALT or AST) have been observed during treatment with carvedilol. Rates of transaminase elevations (2 to 3 times the upper limit of normal) observed during controlled clinical trials have generally been similar between patients treated with carvedilol and those treated with placebo. However, transaminase elevations, confirmed by rechallenge, have been observed with carvedilol. In a long-term, placebo-controlled trial in severe heart failure, patients treated with carvedilol had lower values for hepatic transaminases than patients treated with placebo, possibly because carvedilol-induced improvements in cardiac function led to less hepatic congestion and/or improved hepatic blood flow.

➤*Postmarketing:* Reports of aplastic anemia and severe skin reactions (eg, erythema multiforme, Stevens-Johnson syndrome, toxic epidermal necrolysis) have been rare and received only when carvedilol was coadministered with other medications associated with such reactions. Urinary incontinence in women (which resolved upon discontinuation of the medication) and interstitial pneumonitis have been reported rarely.

Overdosage

➤*Symptoms:* The acute oral median lethal doses in male and female mice and male and female rats are more than 8,000 mg/kg. Overdosage may cause severe hypotension, bradycardia, cardiac insufficiency, cardiogenic shock, and cardiac arrest. Respiratory problems, bronchospasms, vomiting, lapses of consciousness, and generalized seizures may also occur.

➤*Treatment:* Place the patient in a supine position and, when necessary, keep under observation and treat under intensive-care conditions. Gastric lavage may be used shortly after ingestion. The following agents may be administered: for excessive bradycardia: atropine, 2 mg IV. To support CV function: glucagon 5 to 10 mg IV rapidly over 30 seconds, followed by a continuous infusion of 5 mg/hour; sympathomimetics (eg, dobutamine, epinephrine, isoproterenol, norepinephrine) at doses according to body weight and effect. If peripheral vasodilation dominates, it may be necessary to administer epinephrine or norepinephrine with continuous monitoring of circulatory conditions. For therapy-resistant bradycardia, perform pacemaker therapy. For bronchospasm, give beta-sympathomimetics (as aerosol or IV) or aminophylline IV. In the event of seizures, slow IV injection of diazepam or clonazepam is recommended.

There is no experience of overdosage with carvedilol ER. Cases of overdosage with carvedilol alone or in combination with other drugs have been reported. Quantities ingested in some cases exceeded 1,000 mg. Symptoms experienced included low blood pressure and heart rate. Standard supportive treatment was provided and individuals recovered.

Note – In the event of severe intoxication in which there are symptoms of shock, treatment with antidotes must be continued for a sufficiently long period of time consistent with the 7- to 10-hour half-life of carvedilol.

Patient Information

Advise patients taking carvedilol of the following:

- They should not interrupt or discontinue using carvedilol ER without a health care provider's advice.
- Heart failure patients should consult their doctor if they experience signs or symptoms of worsening heart failure, such as weight gain or increasing shortness of breath.
- They may experience a drop in blood pressure when standing, resulting in dizziness and, rarely, fainting. Patients should sit or lie down when these symptoms of lowered blood pressure occur.
- If patients experience dizziness or fatigue, they should avoid driving or hazardous tasks.
- They should consult a health care provider if they experience dizziness or faintness, in case the dosage should be adjusted.
- They should not crush or chew carvedilol ER capsules.
- They should take carvedilol ER with food.
- They should separate the administration of carvedilol ER from alcohol consumption (including prescription and nonprescription medications that contain ethanol) by at least 2 hours.
- Diabetic patients should report any changes in blood sugar levels to their health care provider.
- Contact lens wearers may experience decreased lacrimation.

Antiadrenergic Agents — Centrally Acting

METHYLDOPA AND METHYLDOPATE HYDROCHLORIDE

Rx	**Methyldopa** (Various, eg, Ivax, Mylan, Teva, UDL)	**Tablets; oral:** 250 mg	May contain edetate disodium, polyethylene glycol. In 100s, 500s, 1,000s, and UD 100s.
Rx	**Methyldopa** (Various, eg, Ivax, Mylan, Teva, UDL)	**Tablets; oral:** 500 mg	May contain edetate disodium, polyethylene glycol, polysorbate 80. In 100s, 500s, and UD 100s.
Rx	**Methyldopate Hydrochloride** (American Regent)	**Injection, solution:** 50 mg/mL	May contain sulfites,[a] edetate disodium, parabens. In 5 mL single-dose vials.

[a] Refer to individual product package insert for sulfite content.

METHYLDOPA — ORAL

Indications

➤*Hypertension:* For the treatment of hypertension.

➤*Off-label uses:* Hypertension in pregnancy.

Administration and Dosage

➤*Adults:*

Hypertension –

Maximum dose: 3 g/day.

Initial dosage: 250 mg 2 or 3 times/day in the first 48 hours.

Maintenance dosage: 500 mg to 2 g/day in 2 to 4 doses. Once an effective dosage range is attained, a smooth blood pressure response occurs in most patients in 12 to 24 hours.

Dosage adjustment: Adjust dosage at intervals of not less than 2 days until an adequate response is achieved. To minimize sedation, increase dosage in the evening. By adjusting dosage, morning hypotension may be prevented without sacrificing control of afternoon blood pressure.

➤*Children:*

Hypertension –

Maximum dose: 65 mg/kg or 3 g/day, whichever is less.

Initial dosage: 10 mg/kg/day in 2 to 4 doses. The daily dosage is then increased or decreased until an adequate response is achieved.

➤*Elderly:* Syncope in older patients may be related to increased sensitivity and advanced arteriosclerotic vascular disease. This may be avoided with lower doses.

➤*Renal function impairment:* Methyldopa is largely excreted by the kidneys; patients with impaired renal function may respond to smaller doses.

➤*Concomitant therapy:* A thiazide may be added at anytime during methyldopa therapy and is recommended if therapy was not started with a thiazide or if effective control of blood pressure cannot be maintained on methyldopa 2 g/day.

When methyldopa is given with antihypertensives other than thiazides, limit the initial dosage to 500 mg/day in divided doses. The dosage of the concomitant antihypertensive may need to be adjusted; when added to a thiazide, the dosage of thiazide does not need to be changed.

➤*Tolerance:* Tolerance may occur, usually between the second and third month of therapy. Adding a diuretic or increasing the dosage of methyldopa frequently restores blood pressure control.

➤*Discontinuation of therapy:* Methyldopa has a relatively short duration of action; therefore, withdrawal is followed by return of hypertension, usually within 48 hours. This is not complicated by an overshoot of blood pressure.

➤*Storage/Stability:* Store at 20° to 25°C (68° to 77°F). Dispense in a well-closed container.

Actions

➤*Pharmacology:* Methyldopa is an aromatic-amino-acid decarboxylase inhibitor in animals and humans. The mechanism of action of methyldopa has not been conclusively demonstrated but is probably because of the drug's metabolism to alpha-methylnorepinephrine, which lowers arterial pressure by the stimulation of central inhibitory alpha-adrenergic receptors, false neurotransmission, and/or reduction of plasma renin activity. Methyldopa causes a net reduction in tissue concentrations of serotonin, dopamine, norepinephrine, and epinephrine.

Only methyldopa, the L-isomer of alpha-methyldopa, has the ability to inhibit dopa decarboxylase and to deplete animal tissues of norepinephrine. In humans, the antihypertensive activity appears to be due solely to the L-isomer. About twice the dose of the racemate (DL-alpha-methyldopa) is required for equal antihypertensive effect.

Pharmacodynamics –

Normal or elevated plasma renin activity may decrease in the course of methyldopa therapy.

Methyldopa reduces standing and supine blood pressure. It usually produces highly effective lowering of supine pressure with infrequent symptomatic postural hypotension. Exercise hypotension and diurnal blood pressure variations rarely occur.

The maximum decrease in blood pressure occurs 4 to 6 hours after oral dosage. Once an effective dosage level is attained, a smooth blood pressure response occurs in most patients in 12 to 24 hours. After withdrawal, blood pressure usually returns to pretreatment levels within 24 to 48 hours.

➤*Pharmacokinetics:*

Absorption/Distribution – Methyldopa crosses the placental barrier, appears in cord blood, and appears in breast milk.

Metabolism/Excretion – Methyldopa is extensively metabolized. The known urinary metabolites include the following: alpha-methyldopa mono-O-sulfate; 3-0-methyl-alpha-methyldopa; 3,4,-dihydroxyphenylacetone; alpha-methyldopamine; 3-0-methyl-alpha-methyldopamine and their conjugates.

Approximately 70% of the drug that is absorbed is excreted in the urine as methyldopa and its mono-O-sulfate conjugate. The renal clearance is about 130 mL/min in healthy subjects and is diminished in renal insufficiency. The plasma half-life of methyldopa is 105 minutes. After oral doses, excretion is essentially complete in 36 hours.

Contraindications

Active hepatic disease, such as acute hepatitis or active cirrhosis; if previous methyldopa therapy has been associated with liver disorders; coadministration with monoamine oxidase inhibitors (MAOIs); hypersensitivity to any component of these formulations.

Warnings/Precautions

➤*Positive Coombs test/Hemolytic anemia:* It is important to recognize that a positive Coombs test, hemolytic anemia, and liver disorders may occur with methyldopa therapy. The rare occurrences of hemolytic anemia or liver disorders could lead to potentially fatal complications unless properly recognized and managed.

With prolonged therapy, 10% to 20% of patients develop a positive direct Coombs test, usually between 6 and 12 months of starting therapy. The lowest incidence reported was at a dosage of 1 g/day or less. This is rarely associated with hemolytic anemia, which could lead to potentially fatal complications, and is difficult to predict. Prior existence or development of a positive direct Coombs test is not a contraindication to methyldopa, but if it develops during therapy, determine whether hemolytic anemia exists and whether the positive Coombs test may be a problem. For example, in addition to a positive direct Coombs test, there is less often a positive indirect Coombs test that may interfere with cross-matching of blood.

Before treatment is started, it is desirable to do a blood cell count (hematocrit, hemoglobin, or red cell count) for a baseline or to establish whether there is anemia. Perform periodic blood cell counts to detect hemolytic anemia. A direct Coombs test may be useful before therapy and at 6 and 12 months later. If Coombs-positive hemolytic anemia occurs, discontinue methyldopa; anemia usually remits promptly. If not, corticosteroids may be given; consider other causes. If hemolytic anemia is related to methyldopa, do not reinstitute.

When methyldopa produces a positive Coombs test alone or with hemolytic anemia, the red cell is usually coated with gamma globulin of the immunoglobulin G (IgG) (gamma G) class only. The positive Coombs test may not revert to normal until weeks to months after methyldopa is stopped.

➤*Blood transfusions:* Should the need for transfusion arise in a patient receiving methyldopa, perform a direct and indirect Coombs test. In the absence of hemolytic anemia, usually only the direct Coombs test will be positive. A positive direct Coombs test alone will not interfere with typing or cross-matching. If the indirect Coombs test is also positive, problems may arise in the major cross-match, and the assistance of a hematologist or transfusion expert will be needed.

➤*Hepatic effects:* Fever has occasionally occurred within the first 3 weeks of therapy, sometimes associated with eosinophilia or abnormalities in 1 or more liver function tests (eg, alkaline phosphatase, AST, ALT, bilirubin, prothrombin time). Jaundice with or without fever may occur, usually within the first 2 to 3 months of therapy. In some patients, the findings are consistent with cholestasis. In others, the findings are consistent with hepatitis and hepatocellular injury. Fatal hepatic necrosis has rarely been reported. These hepatic changes may represent hypersensitivity reactions. Periodic determinations of hepatic function should be assessed, particularly during the first 6 to 12 weeks of therapy or whenever an unexplained fever occurs. If fever, abnormalities in liver function tests, or jaundice appear, discontinue therapy; temperature and abnormalities in liver function revert to normal when the drug is discontinued. Do not reinstitute methyldopa in such patients.

➤*Hematologic effects:* Rarely, a reversible reduction of the white blood cell count (WBC) with a primary effect on granulocytes has been seen but promptly returns to normal upon drug discontinuation. Rare cases of granulocytopenia have been reported. WBC returned to normal after drug discontinuation. Reversible thrombocytopenia occurs rarely.

➤*Edema/Weight gain:* Some patients taking methyldopa experience clinical edema or weight gain, which may be controlled by the use of a diuretic. Do not continue methyldopa if edema progresses or signs of heart failure appear.

➤*Choreoathetotic movements:* Involuntary choreoathetotic movements have been observed rarely in patients with severe bilateral cerebrovascular disease. Should these occur, discontinue methyldopa therapy.

➤*Renal function impairment:* This drug is known to be substantially excreted by the kidney, and the risk of toxic reactions to this drug may be greater in patients with impaired renal function. Hypertension has recurred occasionally after dialysis in patients given methyldopa because the drug is removed by this procedure.

➤*Hepatic function impairment:* Use with caution in patients with previous liver disease or dysfunction.

➤*Pregnancy: Category B.* Methyldopa is considered a first-line agent for the management of hypertension during pregnancy.

Reproduction studies performed with methyldopa at oral doses up to 1,000 mg/kg in mice, 200 mg/kg in rabbits, and 100 mg/kg in rats revealed no evidence of harm to the fetus. These doses are 16.6, 3.3, and 1.7 times, respectively, the maximum daily human dose when compared on the basis of body weight; 1.4, 1.1, and 0.2 times, respectively, when compared on the basis of body surface area; calculations assume a patient weight of 50 kg. However, there are no adequate and well-controlled studies in pregnant women in the first trimester of pregnancy. Because animal reproduction studies are not always predictive of human response, use methyldopa during pregnancy only if clearly needed.

METHYLDOPA — ORAL

Published reports of methyldopa use during all trimesters indicate that if this drug is used during pregnancy, the possibility of fetal harm appears remote. In 5 studies, 3 of which were controlled, involving 332 pregnant hypertensive women, treatment with methyldopa was associated with an improved fetal outcome. The majority of these women were in the third trimester when methyldopa therapy was begun.

In 1 study, women who had begun methyldopa treatment between weeks 16 and 20 of pregnancy gave birth to infants whose average head circumference was reduced by a small amount (34.2 ± 1.7 cm vs 34.6 ± 1.3 cm [mean ± 1 standard deviation]). Long-term follow up of 97.5% of the children born to methyldopa-treated pregnant women (including those who began treatment between weeks 16 and 20) failed to uncover any significant adverse effect in the children. At 4 years of age, the developmental delay commonly seen in children born to hypertensive mothers was less evident in those whose mothers were treated with methyldopa during pregnancy than those whose mothers were untreated. The children of the treated group scored consistently higher than the children of the untreated group on 5 major indices of intellectual and motor development. At 7.5 years of age, developmental scores and intelligence indices showed no significant differences in children of treated or untreated hypertensive women.

➤*Lactation:* Methyldopa appears in breast milk. Therefore, exercise caution when methyldopa is given to a breast-feeding woman. After 750 to 2,000 mg/day, milk levels of free and conjugated methyldopa ranged from 0.1 to 0.9 mcg/mL. The American Academy of Pediatrics considers methyldopa to be compatible with breast-feeding.

➤*Children:* There are no well-established clinical trials in children. Information on dosing in pediatric patients is supported by evidence from published literature regarding the treatment of hypertension in pediatric patients. See Administration and Dosage.

➤*Elderly:* Because elderly patients are more likely to have decreased renal function, care should be taken in dose selection and it may be useful to monitor renal function.

See Administration and Dosage for more information.

Per the Beers list, methyldopa may cause bradycardia and exacerbate depression in elderly patients.

➤*Monitoring:* Before treatment is started, it is desirable to do a blood cell count (hematocrit, hemoglobin, or red cell count) for a baseline or to establish whether there is anemia. Perform periodic blood cell counts to detect hemolytic anemia. A direct Coombs test may be useful before therapy and at 6 and 12 months later. Perform periodic determinations of hepatic function, particularly during the first 6 to 12 weeks of therapy or when an unexplained fever occurs.

Drug Interactions

Methyldopa Drug Interactions

Precipitant drug	Object drug[a]		Description
Beta-blockers, nonselective (eg, propranolol)	Methyldopa	↑	Coadministration of nonselective beta-blockers and methyldopa would rarely cause a hypertensive crisis. Closely monitor for acute increases in blood pressure. If an acute increase occurs, discontinuation of the beta-blocker and treatment with an alpha-adrenergic blocking agent (eg, phentolamine) may be needed.
Ferrous sulfate or gluconate	Methyldopa	↓	A decrease in the bioavailability of methyldopa when it is ingested with ferrous sulfate or ferrous gluconate has been demonstrated. Coadministration is not recommended.
Levodopa	Methyldopa	↑	Blood pressure–lowering effects of methyldopa may be potentiated by levodopa. Central effects of levodopa in Parkinson disease may be potentiated by methyldopa. Monitor blood pressure and for signs of toxicity. If either occurs, adjust the dose of either drug as needed.
Methyldopa	Levodopa		
Tizanidine	Methyldopa	↑	Additive hypotensive effects may occur. If coadministration cannot be avoided, closely monitor blood pressure and adjust treatment as needed.
Methyldopa	Tizanidine		
Methyldopa	Anesthetics	↑	Reduced doses of anesthetics may be required. Hypotension during anesthesia can be controlled by vasopressors because adrenergic receptors remain sensitive.
Methyldopa	Antihypertensives	↑	When methyldopa is used with other hypotensive agents, the hypotensive effect may be potentiated. Closely monitor the patient to detect adverse reactions or manifestations of idiosyncratic reactions.
Methyldopa	Haloperidol	↑	Methyldopa may potentiate the antipsychotic effects of haloperidol or the combination may produce psychosis. If adverse mental symptoms occur, discontinue one or both drugs.
Methyldopa	Lithium	↑	Lithium toxicity characterized by GI symptoms, polyuria, muscle weakness, lethargy, and tremor has been reported following methyldopa coadministration. Closely monitor the patient for signs and symptoms of lithium toxicity and adjust the lithium dose as needed.
Methyldopa	MAOIs (eg, phenelzine)	↑	Metabolites of methyldopa stimulate release of endogenous catecholamines that are usually metabolized by MAOIs, thereby leading to excessive sympathetic stimulation. Coadministration is contraindicated.
Methyldopa	Phenothiazines	↑	Serious elevations in blood pressure may occur. Closely monitor blood pressure. If hypertension occurs, discontinue one or both drugs.
Methyldopa	Sympathomimetics (eg, norepinephrine)	↑	Methyldopa may potentiate the pressor effects of sympathomimetics and lead to hypertension. Monitor blood pressure. If hypertension occurs, discontinuation of the sympathomimetic agent or treatment with an alpha-adrenergic blocking agent (eg, phentolamine) may be needed.

[a] ↑ = object drug increased; ↓ = object drug decreased.

➤*Drug/Lab test interactions:* Methyldopa may interfere with tests for the following: Urinary uric acid by phosphotungstate method; serum creatinine by alkaline picrate method; AST by colorimetric methods. Interference with spectrophotometric methods for AST analysis is not reported.

Because methyldopa causes fluorescence in urine samples at the same wavelengths as catecholamines, falsely high levels of urinary catecholamines may occur and will interfere with the diagnosis of pheochromocytoma. Methyldopa does not interfere with measurement of vanillylmandelic acid (VMA) by methods converting VMA to vanillin.

Adverse Reactions

➤*Cardiovascular:* Aggravation of angina pectoris, bradycardia, congestive heart failure, edema, weight gain, orthostatic hypotension (decrease daily dosage), prolonged carotid sinus hypersensitivity.

➤*CNS:* Bell palsy; decreased mental acuity; dizziness; headache, asthenia, or weakness (may be early, transient symptoms); involuntary choreoathetotic movements; light-headedness; paresthesias; parkinsonism; psychic disturbances, including nightmares and reversible mild psychoses or depression; sedation, usually transient, may occur during initial therapy or whenever the dose is increased; symptoms of cerebrovascular insufficiency.

➤*Dermatologic:* Rash, toxic epidermal necrolysis.

➤*Endocrine:* Breast enlargement, gynecomastia, hyperprolactinemia, lactation.

➤*GI:* Colitis, constipation, diarrhea, distention, dry mouth, flatus, nausea, pancreatitis, sialoadenitis, sore or "black" tongue, vomiting.

➤*GU:* Amenorrhea, decreased libido, impotence.

➤*Hematologic:* Bone marrow depression; eosinophilia; granulocytopenia; hemolytic anemia; leukopenia; positive Coombs test; positive tests for antinuclear antibody, lupus erythematosus cells, and rheumatoid factor; thrombocytopenia.

➤*Hepatic:* Liver disorders including abnormal liver function tests, hepatitis, jaundice.

➤*Hypersensitivity:* Drug-related fever, lupus-like syndrome, myocarditis, pericarditis, vasculitis.

➤*Musculoskeletal:* Arthralgia with or without joint swelling, myalgia.

➤*Miscellaneous:* Nasal stuffiness, rise in serum urea nitrogen.

Overdosage

➤*Symptoms:* Acute overdosage may produce acute hypotension with other responses, attributable to brain and GI malfunction (excessive sedation, weakness, bradycardia, dizziness, light-headness, constipation, distention, flatus, diarrhea, nausea, vomiting).

➤*Treatment:* In the event of overdosage, employ symptomatic and supportive measures. When overdosage is recent, gastric lavage may reduce absorption. When overdosage has been earlier, infusions may be helpful to promote

METHYLDOPA — ORAL

urinary excretion. Otherwise, management includes special attention to cardiac rate and output, blood volume, electrolyte imbalance, paralytic ileus, urinary function, and cerebral activity. Refer to General Management of Acute Overdosage. Sympathomimetic drugs (eg, norepinephrine, epinephrine, metaraminol bitartrate) may be indicated. Methyldopa is dialyzable.

Patient Information

Caution patient not to stop taking drug abruptly.

Instruct patient to report the following symptoms to their health care provider: fever, flu-like symptoms, jaundice, muscle aches.

Advise patient that drowsiness may occur and to use caution while driving and performing other activities requiring mental alertness.

METHYLDOPATE HYDROCHLORIDE — INJECTION

Indications

➤*Hypertension:* For the treatment of hypertension, when parenteral medication is indicated. The treatment of hypertensive crises may be initiated with methyldopate injection.

Administration and Dosage

➤*General dosing considerations:* Methyldopate when given intravenously (IV) in effective doses, causes a decline in blood pressure that may begin 4 to 6 hours and last 10 to 16 hours after injection.

➤*Adults:*

Hypertension –

Usual dosage: 250 to 500 mg IV every 6 hours as required.

Maximum dose: 1 g every 6 hours.

Conversion: When control has been obtained, substitute oral therapy starting with the same parenteral dosage schedule.

➤*Children:*

Hypertension –

Usual dosage: 20 to 40 mg/kg/day IV in divided doses every 6 hours.

Maximum dose: 65 mg/kg or 3 g daily, whichever is less.

Conversion: When blood pressure control has been obtained, substitute oral therapy starting with the same parenteral dosage schedule.

➤*Elderly:* Syncope in older patients may be related to increased sensitivity and advanced arteriosclerotic vascular disease. This may be avoided with lower doses.

➤*Renal function impairment:* Methyldopa is largely excreted by the kidneys and patients with impaired renal function may respond to smaller doses.

➤*Concomitant therapy:* A thiazide may be added at any time during methyldopa therapy and is recommended if therapy has not been started with a thiazide or if effective control of blood pressure cannot be maintained with methyldopa 2 g daily.

➤*Tolerance:* Occasionally tolerance may occur, usually between the second and third month of therapy. Adding a diuretic or increasing the dosage of methyldopa frequently will restore effective blood pressure control.

➤*Discontinuation of therapy:* Because methyldopate has a relatively short duration of action, withdrawal is followed by return of hypertension usually within 48 hours. This is not complicated by an overshoot of blood pressure.

➤*Preparation for administration:* Add the desired dose of methyldopate to 100 mL of dextrose 5% injection. Alternatively, the desired dose may be given in dextrose 5% in water in a concentration of 100 mg per 10 mL.

➤*Administration:* Give by slow IV infusion over a period of 30 to 60 minutes.

➤*Storage/Stability:* Store at 20° to 25°C (68° to 77°F); excursions permitted to 15° to 30°C (59° to 86°F).

Actions

➤*Pharmacology:* Methyldopate, an antihypertensive agent, is an aromatic-amino-acid decarboxylase inhibitor in animals and humans. Although the mechanism of action has yet to be conclusively demonstrated, the antihypertensive effect of methyldopa is probably due to its metabolism to alpha-methyl-norepinephine, which then lowers arterial pressure by stimulation of central inhibitory alpha-adrenergic receptors, false neurotransmission, and/or reduction of plasma renin activity. Methyldopa has been shown to cause a net reduction in the tissue concentration of serotonin, dopamine, norepinephrine, and epinephrine.

Only methyldopa, the L-isomer of alpha-methyldopa, has the ability to inhibit dopa decarboxylase and to deplete animal tissues of norepinephrine. In humans, the antihypertensive activity appears to be due solely to the L-isomer. About twice the dose of the racemate (DL-alpha-methyldopa) is required for equal antihypertensive effect.

Methyldopate is the ethyl ester of methyldopa and possesses the same pharmacologic attributes.

Pharmacodynamics –

Normal or elevated plasma renin activity may decrease in the course of methyldopa therapy.

Methyldopa reduces supine and standing blood pressure. It usually produces highly effective lowering of the supine pressure with infrequent symptomatic postural hypotension. Exercise hypotension and diurnal blood pressure variations rarely occur.

Following IV administration of methyldopate a decrease in blood pressure may occur in 4 to 6 hours and last 10 to 16 hours.

➤*Pharmacokinetics:*

Absorption/Distribution – Methyldopa crosses the placental barrier, appears in cord blood, and appears in breast milk.

Metabolism/Excretion – Methyldopa is extensively metabolized. The known urinary metabolites are alpha-methyldopa mono-O-sulfate; 3-0-methyl-alpha-methyldopa; 3,4-dihydroxyphenylacetone; alpha-methyldopamine; 3-0-methyl-alpha-methyldopamine and their conjugates.

Approximately 49% of the dose of methyldopate is excreted in the urine as methyldopa and its mono-O-sulfate. The renal clearance of methyldopa following methyldopate is about 156 mL/min in healthy subjects and is diminished in renal insufficiency. Following methyldopate injection, the plasma half-life of methyldopa is 90 to 127 minutes. Approximately 17% of a dose of methyldopate given to healthy subjects appears in plasma as free methyldopa.

Contraindications

Active hepatic disease, such as acute hepatitis and active cirrhosis; liver disorders associated with previous methyldopa therapy; hypersensitivity to any component of this product, including sulfites; therapy with monoamine oxidase inhibitors (MAOIs).

Warnings/Precautions

➤*Positive Coombs test/Hemolytic anemia:* It is important to recognize that a positive Coombs test, hemolytic anemia, and liver disorders may occur with methyldopa therapy. The rare occurrences of hemolytic anemia or liver disorders could lead to potentially fatal complications unless properly recognized and managed.

With prolonged methyldopa therapy, 10% to 20% of patients develop a positive direct Coombs test, which usually occurs between 6 and 12 months of starting methyldopa therapy. The lowest incidence is at a daily dosage of 1 g or less. On rare occasions, this may be associated with hemolytic anemia, which could lead to potentially fatal complications. It cannot be predicted which patients with a positive direct Coombs test may develop hemolytic anemia.

Prior existence or development of a positive direct Coombs test is not in itself a contraindication to use methyldopa. If a positive Coombs test develops during methyldopa therapy, determine whether hemolytic anemia exists and whether the positive Coombs test may be a problem. For example, in addition to a positive direct Coombs test, there is less often a positive indirect Coombs test, which may interfere with cross-matching of blood.

Before treatment is started, perform a blood cell count (hematocrit, hemoglobin, or red cell count) for a baseline or to establish whether there is anemia. Periodic blood cell counts should be done during therapy to detect hemolytic anemia. It may be useful to do a direct Coombs test before therapy and at 6 and 12 months after the start of therapy.

If Coombs-positive hemolytic anemia occurs, the cause may be methyldopa, and the drug should be discontinued. Usually the anemia remits promptly. If not, corticosteroids may be given and other causes of anemia should be considered. If the hemolytic anemia is related to methyldopa, the drug should not be reinstituted.

When methyldopa causes Coombs positivity alone or with hemolytic anemia, the red cell is usually coated with gamma globulin of the immunoglobulin G (IgG) (gamma G) class only. The positive Coombs test may not revert to normal until weeks to months after methyldopa is stopped.

➤*Blood transfusions:* Should the need for transfusion arise in a patient receiving methyldopa, perform a direct and indirect Coombs test. In the absence of hemolytic anemia, usually only the direct Coombs test will be positive. A positive direct Coombs test alone will not interfere with typing or cross-matching. If the indirect Coombs test is also positive, problems may arise in the major cross-match and the assistance of a hematologist or transfusion expert will be needed.

➤*Hepatic effects:* Occasionally, fever has occurred within the first 3 weeks of methyldopa therapy, associated in some cases with eosinophilia or abnormalities in 1 or more liver function tests, such as serum alkaline phosphatase, serum transaminases (ALT, AST), bilirubin, and prothrombin time. Jaundice, with or without fever, may occur with onset usually within the first 2 to 3 months of therapy. In some patients, the findings are consistent with those of cholestasis. In others, the findings are consistent with hepatitis and hepatocellular injury.

Rarely, fatal hepatic necrosis has been reported after the use of methyldopa. These hepatic changes may represent hypersensitivity reactions. Periodic determination of hepatic function should be assessed particularly during the first 6 to 12 weeks of therapy or whenever an unexplained fever occurs. If fever, abnormalities in liver function tests, or jaundice appear, stop therapy with methyldopa. If caused by methyldopa, the temperature and abnormalities in liver function characteristically have reverted to normal when the drug was discontinued. Do not reinstitute methyldopa in such patients.

➤*Hematologic effects:* Rarely, a reversible reduction of the white blood cell count (WBC) with a primary effect on the granulocytes has been seen. The granulocyte count returned promptly to normal on discontinuance of the

METHYLDOPATE HYDROCHLORIDE — INJECTION

drug. Rare cases of granulocytopenia have been reported. In each instance, upon stopping the drug, the WBC count returned to normal. Reversible thrombocytopenia has occurred rarely.

➤*Edema/Weight gain:* Some patients taking methyldopa experience clinical edema or weight gain, which may be controlled by use of a diuretic. Do not continue methyldopa if edema progresses or signs of heart failure appear.

➤*Paradoxical pressor responses:* A paradoxical pressor response has been reported with IV administration of methyldopate.

➤*Choreoathetotic movements:* Rarely, involuntary choreoathetotic movements have been observed during therapy with methyldopa in patients with severe bilateral cerebrovascular disease. Should these movements occur, stop therapy.

➤*Sulfite sensitivity:* Some products may contain sodium bisulfite, a sulfite that may cause allergic-type reactions, including anaphylactic symptoms and life-threatening or less severe asthmatic episodes in certain susceptible people. The overall prevalence of sulfite sensitivity in the general population is unknown and probably low. Sulfite sensitivity is seen more frequently in asthmatic than in nonasthmatic people.

➤*Renal function impairment:* See Administration and Dosage for more information. Hypertension has recurred occasionally after dialysis in patients given methyldopa because the drug is removed by this procedure.

➤*Hepatic function impairment:* Use methyldopa with caution in patients with a history of previous liver disease or dysfunction.

➤*Pregnancy: Category C.* Animal reproduction studies have not been conducted with methyldopate. It is also not known whether methyldopate can affect reproduction capacity or can cause fetal harm when given to a pregnant woman. Give methyldopate to a pregnant woman only if clearly needed.

Methydopa has been used frequently during pregnancy for the treatment of hypertension.

➤*Lactation:* Methyldopa appears in breast milk. Therefore, exercise caution when methyldopa is given to a breast-feeding woman.

The American Academy of Pediatrics classifies methyldopa as compatible with breast-feeding.

➤*Children:* There are no well-controlled clinical trials in children. Information on dosing in children is supported by evidence from published literature regarding the treatment of hypertension in children.

➤*Elderly:* See Administration and Dosage for more information.

Per the Beers list, methyldopa may cause bradycardia and exacerbate depression in elderly patients.

➤*Monitoring:* Before treatment is started, perform a blood cell count (hematocrit, hemoglobin, or red cell count) for a baseline or to establish whether there is anemia. Periodic blood cell counts should be done during therapy to detect hemolytic anemia. It may be useful to do a direct Coombs test before therapy and at 6 and 12 months after the start of therapy. Periodic determinations of hepatic function should be done particularly during the first 6 to 12 weeks of therapy or whenever an unexplained fever occurs.

Drug Interactions

Methyldopate Drug Interactions

Precipitant drug	Object drug[a]		Description
Beta-blockers, nonselective (eg, propranolol)	Methyldopate	↑	Coadministration of nonselective beta-blockers and methyldopa would rarely cause a hypertensive crisis. Closely monitor for acute increases in blood pressure. If an acute increase occurs, discontinuation of the beta-blocker and treatment with an alpha-adrenergic blocking agent (eg, phentolamine) may be needed.
Levodopa	Methyldopate	↑	Blood pressure–lowering effects of methyldopa may be potentiated by levodopa. Central effects of levodopa in Parkinson disease may be potentiated by methyldopa. Monitor blood pressure and for signs of toxicity. If either occurs, adjust the dose of either drug as needed.
Methyldopate	Levodapa		
Tizanidine	Methyldopate	↑	Additive hypotensive effects may occur. If coadministration cannot be avoided, closely monitor blood pressure and adjust treatment as needed.
Methyldopate	Tizanidine		

Methyldopate Drug Interactions

Precipitant drug	Object drug[a]		Description
Methyldopate	Anesthetics	↑	Reduced doses of anesthetics may be required. Hypotension during anesthesia can be controlled by vasopressors because adrenergic receptors remain sensitive.
Methyldopate	Antihypertensives	↑	When methyldopa is used with other hypotensive agents, the hypotensive effect may be potentiated. Closely monitor the patient to detect adverse reactions or manifestations of idiosyncratic reactions.
Methyldopate	Haloperidol	↑	Methyldopa may potentiate the antipsychotic effects of haloperidol or the combination may produce psychosis. If adverse mental symptoms occur, discontinue one or both drugs.
Methyldopate	Lithium	↑	Lithium toxicity characterized by GI symptoms, polyuria, muscle weakness, lethargy, and tremor has been reported following methyldopa coadministration. Closely monitor the patient for signs and symptoms of lithium toxicity, and adjust the lithium dose as needed.
Methyldopate	MAOIs (eg, phenelzine)	↑	Metabolites of methyldopa stimulate the release of endogenous catecholamines that are usually metabolized by MAOIs, thereby leading to excessive sympathetic stimulation. Coadministration is contraindicated.
Methyldopate	Phenothiazines	↑	Serious elevations in blood pressure may occur. Closely monitor blood pressure. If hypertension occurs, discontinue one or both drugs.
Methyldopate	Sympathomimetics (eg, norepinephrine)	↑	Methyldopa may potentiate the pressor effects of sympathomimetics and lead to hypertension. Monitor blood pressure. If hypertension occurs, discontinuation of the sympathomimetic agent or treatment with an alpha-adrenergic blocking agent (eg, phentolamine) may be needed.

[a] ↑ = object drug increased.

➤*Drug/Lab test interactions:* Methyldopa may interfere with tests for the following: urinary uric acid by the phosphotungstate method, serum creatinine by the alkaline picrate method, and AST by colorimetric methods. Interference with spectrophotometric methods for AST analysis has not been reported.

Because methyldopa causes fluorescence in urine samples at the same wavelengths as catecholamines, falsely high levels of urinary catecholamines may occur and will interfere with the diagnosis of pheochromocytoma. Methyldopa does not interfere with measurement of vanillylmandelic acid (VMA) by methods converting VMA to vanillin.

Adverse Reactions

Significant adverse effects due to methyldopa have been infrequent; this agent is usually well tolerated.

The following adverse reactions have been reported.

➤*Cardiovascular:* Aggravation of angina pectoris, bradycardia, congestive heart failure, edema and weight gain, prolonged carotid sinus hypersensitivity, paradoxical pressor response with IV use, orthostatic hypotension (decrease daily dosage).

➤*CNS:* Sedation, usually transient, may occur during the initial period of therapy or whenever the dose is increased. Headache, asthenia, or weakness may be noted as early and transient symptoms.

Asthenia or weakness, Bell palsy, choreoathetotic movements, decreased mental acuity, dizziness, headache, light-headedness, paresthesias, Parkinsonism, psychic disturbances including nightmares and reversible mild psychosis or depression, sedation, symptoms of cerebrovascular insufficiency.

➤*Dermatologic:* Rash, toxic epidermal necrolysis.

➤*Endocrine:* Breast enlargement, gynecomastia, hyperprolactinemia, lactation.

METHYLDOPATE HYDROCHLORIDE — INJECTION

➤*GI:* Colitis, constipation, diarrhea, distension, dryness of mouth, flatus, nausea, pancreatitis, sialadenitis, sore or "black" tongue, vomiting.

➤*GU:* Amenorrhea, decreased libido, impotence.

➤*Hematologic:* Bone marrow depression, granulocytopenia, hemolytic anemia, leukopenia, lupus erythematosus cells, positive Coombs tests, positive tests for antinuclear antibody, rheumatoid factor, thrombocytopenia.

➤*Hepatic:* Liver disorders including abnormal liver function tests, hepatitis, jaundice.

➤*Hypersensitivity:* Drug-related fever, eosinophilia, lupus-like syndrome, myocarditis, pericarditis, vasculitis.

➤*Musculoskeletal:* Arthralgia, with or without joint swelling, myalgia.

➤*Miscellaneous:* Nasal stuffiness, rise in serum urea nitrogen.

Overdosage

➤*Symptoms:* Acute overdosage may produce acute hypotension with other responses attributable to brain and GI malfunction (excessive sedation, weakness, bradycardia, dizziness, lightheadedness, constipation, distension, flatus, diarrhea, nausea, vomiting).

➤*Treatment:* In the event of overdosage, employ symptomatic and supportive measures. Management includes special attention to cardiac rate and output, blood volume, electrolyte balance, paralytic ileus, urinary function, and cerebral activity.

Sympathomimetic drugs (eg, norepinephrine, epinephrine, metaraminol bitartrate) may be indicated.

CLONIDINE HYDROCHLORIDE

Rx	**Clonidine** (Various, eg, Actavis, Mylan, UDL)	**Tablets; oral:** 0.1 mg	May contain lactose. In 30s, 100s, 500s, 1,000s, UD 25s, and UD 100s.
Rx	**Catapres** (Boehringer Ingelheim)		Equiv. to clonidine base 0.087 mg. Lactose. (BI-6). Tan. In 100s.
Rx	**Clonidine** (Various, eg, Actavis, Mylan, UDL)	**Tablets; oral:** 0.2 mg	May contain lactose. In 30s, 100s, 500s, 1,000s, UD 25s, UD 100s, and UD 300s.
Rx	**Catapres** (Boehringer Ingelheim)		Lactose. (BI-7). Orange. In 100s.
Rx	**Clonidine** (Various, eg, Actavis, Mylan, UDL)	**Tablets; oral:** 0.3 mg	May contain lactose. In 30s, 100s, 500s, 1,000s, and UD 100s.
Rx	**Catapres** (Boehringer Ingelheim)		Lactose. (BI-11). Peach. In 100s.
Rx	**Jenloga** (UPM)	**Tablets, modified-release; oral:** 0.1 mg	Equiv. to clonidine base 0.087 mg. Lactose. (651). White, round. In 60s and 180s.
Rx	**Kapvay** (Shionogi Pharma)	**Tablets, extended-release; oral:** 0.1 mg	Equiv. to clonidine base 0.087 mg. Lactose. (651). White, round. In 60s and 180s.
		0.2 mg	Equiv. to clonidine base 0.174 mg. Lactose. (652). White, oval. In 60s and 180s.
Rx	**Nexiclon XR** (Nextwave Pharmaceuticals)	**Suspension, extended-release; oral:** 0.09 mg/mL	Corn syrup, glycerin, parabens, polysorbate 80, sucrose. In 118 mL.

CLONIDINE HYDROCHLORIDE — ORAL

For complete prescribing information, refer to the Antihypertensives Treatment Guidelines in the Appendix.

Indications

➤*Attention deficit hyperactivity disorder (extended release only):* For the treatment of attention deficit hyperactivity disorder (ADHD) in children as monotherapy and as adjunctive therapy to stimulant medications.

➤*Hypertension (immediate release and modified release only):* Treatment of hypertension.

➤*Off-label uses:*

Alcohol withdrawal syndrome – [4] = Insufficient documentation. Initial data comparing clonidine with chlordiazepoxide suggest that clonidine may have a role in alcohol withdrawal syndrome; however, subsequent trials may have diminished the role of clonidine in the disorder because of better efficacy and fewer adverse reactions with other agents, such as short-acting benzodiazepines. Larger, well-designed controlled studies are needed to show evidence that clonidine is effective and safe for alcohol withdrawal syndrome.

Attention deficit hyperactivity disorder (immediate-release) – [1] = Good documentation. None of the alpha-2 adrenergic agonists are indicated for psychiatric indications, nor are they considered first-line treatment for ADHD. However, in an official American Academy of Child and Adolescent Psychiatry (AACAP) statement, clonidine as monotherapy was suggested as a useful alternative in modulating mood and activity level in children with ADHD, particularly those with sleep difficulties who are nonresponsive to stimulants, or in children with tic disorders in whom stimulants may cause tic exacerbations. Despite widespread use, the addition of clonidine to existing stimulant therapy should be carefully considered because several safety issues have been recognized and there is limited published information from controlled trials regarding efficacy of these combinations.

Diabetic diarrhea – [4] = Insufficient documentation. Initial data from a limited number of trials suggest that clonidine may be beneficial for the treatment of diabetic diarrhea.

Growth hormone stimulation test – [1] = Good documentation. Current guidelines support the use of clonidine to assess growth hormone (GH) secretion in potential GH-deficient patients. Trials have demonstrated the efficacy of clonidine, and it remains an effective tool for the diagnosis of GH deficiency in adults and children.

Hot flashes – [2] = Fair documentation. In controlled trials of a limited number of postmenopausal women, clonidine demonstrated variable results, significantly reducing the frequency, duration, and severity of hot flashes with transdermal therapy (0.1 mg patch every 7 days) or higher oral clonidine dosages (0.1 to 0.4 mg twice daily) compared with placebo, but demonstrated no benefit with lower oral dosages (50 mcg twice daily).

Hyperhidrosis – [4] = Insufficient documentation. Clonidine may provide some benefit in the management of hyperhidrosis based on data from a few case reports, although the small number of patients studied makes it difficult to accurately state the true effect of clonidine on excessive sweating. Larger, controlled trials are needed to provide a better evaluation of clonidine's place in the treatment of hyperhidrosis.

Methadone withdrawal – [1] = Good documentation. Methadone is the only Food and Drug Administration–approved medication used in the treatment of opiate withdrawal. Clonidine has been used effectively to alleviate some withdrawal symptoms during the termination of methadone maintenance treatment after patients have reached a methadone dosage of 40 mg/day or less.

Opiate withdrawal – [1] = Good documentation. Methadone and buprenorphine are widely used μ-receptor agonists for the treatment of opiate dependence and withdrawal. Clonidine, an alpha-2 adrenergic receptor agonist, has been proven safe and effective to decrease catecholamine-induced symptoms associated with opiate withdrawal, and, according to American Psychological Association guidelines, its use with or without naltrexone is an option for patients with opiate withdrawal.

Postherpetic neuralgia – [2] = Fair documentation. Although guidelines do not list clonidine as a preferred treatment for postherpetic neuralgia, published data indicate patients received benefit from oral doses of clonidine 0.2 mg or repetitive paravertebral block injections of combination bupivacaine and clonidine. All patients had failed other treatment options but found pain relief with clonidine treatment. Reports showed a high tolerability and significant effect on pain with clonidine treatment.

Prevention of migraine (adults) – [5] = Poor documentation. Although early results using clonidine for prophylaxis of migrainewere positive, several controlled trials demonstrated little to no efficacy. A review written in 1990 considered the use of clonidine for migraine prophylaxisto be obsolete. American Academy of Neurology practice guidelines state that clonidine is no more effective than placebo for the prevention of migraine.

Prevention of migraine (children/adolescents) – [5] = Poor documentation. In studies (published in 1977 and 1982) evaluating clonidine use for the prevention of migraine headaches in children, it was no more effective than placebo; it has not been studied further. Current practice guidelines state that clonidine is not effective for the prevention of migraine in children and its use is not recommended.

Restless legs syndrome – [4] = Insufficient documentation. Limited data suggest that clonidine may be beneficial in treating restless legs syndrome (RLS) in patients refractory to other medications or with RLS of an idiopathic nature. Guidelines are conflicting relative to effectiveness; clonidine is probably effective for relieving symptoms with short-term use in primary RLS. Larger, controlled trials are needed to confirm these findings and establish an adequate dosing regimen.

Smoking cessation – [1] = Good documentation. Because of its adverse effect profile and its potential to cause rebound withdrawal symptoms upon discontinuation, clonidine is recommended as a second-line agent when nicotine replacement, bupropion sustained-release, or varenicline have been ineffective or are contraindicated. Clonidine may be targeted to those who will benefit from its sedative effects, such as those who experience high levels of anxiety when they quit smoking.

Tourette syndrome (adults) – [4] = Insufficient documentation. Although results are conflicting, there is evidence that clonidine may improve motor tics in patients with Tourette syndrome.

Tourette syndrome (children/adolescents) – [4] = Insufficient documentation. Although results are conflicting, there is evidence that clonidine may improve motor tics in patients with Tourette syndrome.

CLONIDINE HYDROCHLORIDE — ORAL

Ulcerative colitis – [2] = Fair documentation. Mesalamine, administered orally or rectally, is considered first-line therapy for ulcerative colitis. Corticosteroids and intravenous (IV) cyclosporine can be used for severe acute ulcerative colitis, but they are not appropriate as maintenance therapy. Azathioprine and mercaptopurine have been effective as maintenance therapy but are associated with severe adverse reactions. Immunosuppressives may require up to 6 months of treatment to see improvements. Based on data from controlled trials in fewer than 100 patients, clonidine may provide some benefit in the management of ulcerative colitis. Larger, controlled trials would provide a better evaluation of clonidine's place in treating ulcerative colitis.

Other possible off-label uses –

Atrial fibrillation: 75 mcg oral single dose or twice daily, alone or with digoxin.

Constitutional growth delay in children: 37.5 to 150 mcg/m^2/day.

Gilles de la Tourette syndrome: 150 to 200 mcg/day.

Hypertensive "urgencies" (diastolic more than 120 mm Hg): Initially 100 to 200 mcg, followed by 50 to 100 mcg/h to a maximum of 800 mcg.

Opiate detoxification: 15 to 16 mcg/kg/day.

Pheochromocytoma diagnosis (overnight clonidine suppression test): 300 mcg.

Psychosis in schizophrenic patients: 900 mcg/day or less.

Unlabeled route of administration: Sublingual clonidine, using a dosage of 200 to 400 mcg/day, may be effective in hypertensive patients unable to take oral medication. Onset occurs within 30 to 60 minutes and blood pressure appears to be maintained on a twice-daily regimen.

Administration and Dosage

➤*Adults:*

Hypertension –

Usual dosage: 0.2 to 0.6 mg/day given in divided doses (tablets); 0.17 mg (2 mL) to 0.52 mg (6 mL) once daily.

Maximum dose: 2.4 mg/day (immediate release); 0.52 mg (6 mL)/day.

Dosages of modified-release clonidine higher than 0.6 mg/day (0.3 mg twice daily) were not evaluated in clinical trials and are not recommended. Doses of clonidine suspension higher than 0.52 mg (6 mL) per day were not evaluated and are not recommended.

Initial dosage: 0.1 mg twice daily (immediate release), 0.1 mg at bedtime (modified release), or 0.17 mg (2 mL) once daily (suspension).

Dosage adjustment: Increments of 0.1 mg/day (0.09 mg [1 mL] for suspension) may be made at weekly intervals if necessary until the desired response is achieved.

Off-label dosing –

Alcohol withdrawal syndrome: [4] = Insufficient documentation. Clonidine in oral doses of up to 0.3 mg initially, decreased as alcohol withdrawal symptoms subside.

Diabetic diarrhea: [4] = Insufficient documentation. 0.1 mg every 12 hours titrated to 0.5 or 0.6 mg every 12 hours over the following 3 days followed by maintenance dosing for up to 24 months has been studied. In one study, 0.3 mg was administered 1.5 or 4.5 hours before diarrhea was induced by intragastric infusion of balanced electrolyte solutions.

Growth hormone stimulation test: [1] = Good documentation. 200 mcg or 0.15 mg/m^2 orally.

Hot flashes: [2] = Fair documentation. 0.05 to 0.4 mg twice daily.

Hyperhidrosis: [4] = Insufficient documentation. Dosages of 0.3 to 0.6 mg/day orally for several months and 3.5 mg/day orally for several weeks have been studied.

Methadone withdrawal: [1] = Good documentation. Clonidine dosages of 0.2 mg 3 to 4 times daily are usually sufficient to suppress withdrawal symptoms; however, initial dosing and dose titration should be specialized to the patient's individual needs. Within 2 to 3 weeks, clonidine can typically be discontinued.

Opiate withdrawal: [1] = Good documentation.

• *Clonidine monotherapy* – Clonidine 0.1 mg 3 times daily titrated to withdrawal symptoms.

• *Clonidine adjunctive therapy with naltrexone* – Titrate both medications to specific patient needs.

Postherpetic neuralgia: [2] = Fair documentation. 0.2 mg orally.

Restless legs syndrome: [4] = Insufficient documentation. Titrate oral doses of clonidine according to patient symptoms. Clonidine doses of 0.1 to 0.9 mg have shown improvement in RLS when used before bedtime. In guidelines, the recommended oral clonidine dose is 0.5 mg administered 2 hours before onset of symptoms for 2 to 3 weeks.

Smoking cessation: [1] = Good documentation. 0.15 to 0.75 mg/day orally for 3 to 10 weeks. Initial dosing should start up to 3 days prior to the quit date and is typically 0.1 mg orally twice daily, increasing by 0.1 mg weekly if needed.

Tourette syndrome (adults): [4] = Insufficient documentation. 0.0025 to 0.015 mg/kg/day for 6 weeks to 3 months.

Ulcerative colitis: [2] = Fair documentation. 0.3 mg orally 3 times per day for 6 weeks has been studied.

➤*Children:*

Hypertension –

Immediate release:

• *Children 12 years of age and older* –

Usual dosage: 0.2 to 0.6 mg/day given in divided doses.

Maximum dose: 2.4 mg/day.

Initial dosage: 0.1 mg tablet twice daily (morning and bedtime).

Dosage adjustment: Increments of 0.1 mg/day may be made at weekly intervals, if necessary, until the desired response is achieved.

Attention deficit hyperactivity disorder –

Extended release:

• *Children 6 years of age and older* –

Maximum dose: 0.4 mg/day.

Initial dosage: 0.1 mg at bedtime.

Dosage adjustment: Adjust in increments of 0.1 mg/day at weekly intervals until the desired response is achieved.

Clonidine ER[a] Dosing		
Total daily dose	Morning dose	Bedtime dose
0.1 mg/day	—	0.1 mg
0.2 mg/day	0.1 mg	0.1 mg
0.3 mg/day	0.1 mg	0.2 mg
0.4 mg/day	0.2 mg	0.2 mg

[a] ER = extended release.

Duration of therapy: The effectiveness of clonidine ER for longer-term use (more than 5 weeks) has not been systematically evaluated in controlled trials. Therefore, the health care provider electing to use clonidine ER for extended periods should periodically reevaluate the long-term usefulness of the drug for the individual patient.

Concomitant therapy: When clonidine ER is being added to a psychostimulant, the dose of the psychostimulant can be adjusted depending on the patient's response to clonidine ER.

Off-label dosing –

Attention deficit hyperactivity disorder (immediate-release tablets): [1] = Good documentation. Initial oral dosages of 0.05 mg daily with increases of 0.05 mg every 3 to 7 days to a maximum dosage of 0.3 to 0.4 mg daily. Mean daily doses in reviewed studies have ranged from 0.19 to 0.245 mg daily. Daily doses have typically been administered 3 or 4 times daily. Practice parameters published by the AACAP have suggested that clonidine be initiated at a dose of 0.05 mg at bedtime to maximize efficacy and minimize initial sedation. Dose titration should be performed over several weeks to 0.15 to 0.3 mg daily in 3 or 4 divided doses.

Hypertension:

• *Maximum dose* – 25 mcg/kg/day up to 0.9 mg/day.

• *Initial dosage* – 5 to 10 mcg/kg/day divided every 8 to 12 hours.

• *Dosage adjustment* – If needed, increase to 5 to 25 mcg/kg/day in 4 divided doses at 5- to 7-day intervals.

Growth hormone stimulation test: [1] = Good documentation. 200 mcg or 0.15 mg/m^2 orally.

Tourette syndrome (children/adolescents): [4] = Insufficient documentation. 0.0025 to 0.015 mg/kg/day for 6 weeks to 3 months.

➤*Elderly:* Elderly patients may benefit from a lower initial dose.

➤*Renal function impairment:* Adjust dosage according to the degree of impairment and uptitrate slowly. Monitor patients carefully to prevent excessive blood pressure lowering or bradycardia.

➤*Bioequivalence:* While modified-release clonidine is dosed twice daily (the same as the immediate-release formulation), it is not to be used interchangeably with the immediate-release formulation. Substitution may necessitate further dose adjustment based on tolerability or blood pressure response.

Clonidine ER is dosed twice a day (the same as the immediate-release formulation), but it is not to be used interchangeably with the immediate-release formulation.

Because of the lack of controlled clinical trial data and differing pharmacokinetic profiles, substitution of clonidine ER for other clonidine products on a mg-per-mg basis is not recommended.

➤*Discontinuation of therapy:* Reduce the dose gradually over 2 to 4 days to avoid withdrawal symptomatology.

If therapy is to be discontinued in patients receiving a beta-blocker and clonidine concurrently, the beta-blocker should be withdrawn several days before the gradual discontinuation of clonidine.

Extended release – When discontinuing clonidine ER, the total daily dose should be tapered in decrements of no more than 0.1 mg every 3 to 7 days.

➤*Administration:* Dosages above 0.1 mg/day should be divided and taken in the morning and at bedtime. Taking the larger portion of the oral daily dose at bedtime may minimize transient adjustment effects of dry mouth and drowsiness.

Extended release – Swallow ER tablet whole and never crush, cut, or chew. Clonidine ER may be taken with or without food. Doses should be taken twice a day, with an equal or higher split dosage given at bedtime.

➤*Storage/Stability:* Store immediate-release tablets at 25°C (77°F). Excursions are permitted between 15° and 30°C (59° and 86°F). Store modified-release and ER tablets between 20° and 25°C (68° and 77°F).

Actions

➤*Pharmacology:* Clonidine is a centrally acting alpha-2 adrenergic agonist that stimulates alpha-adrenoreceptors in the brain stem. This action results in reduced sympathetic outflow from the CNS and decreased in peripheral resistance, renal vascular resistance, heart rate, and blood pressure.

CLONIDINE HYDROCHLORIDE — ORAL

Other studies in patients taking immediate-release clonidine have provided evidence of a reduction in plasma renin activity and in the excretion of aldosterone and catecholamines. The exact relationship of these pharmacologic actions to the antihypertensive effect of clonidine has not been fully elucidated.

Clonidine acutely stimulates GH release in both children and adults, but does not produce a chronic elevation of GH with long-term use.

Clonidine is not a CNS stimulant. The mechanism of action of clonidine in ADHD is not known.

Pharmacodynamics – Clonidine acts relatively rapidly. The patient's blood pressure declines within 30 to 60 minutes after an immediate-release oral dose, and the maximum decrease occurs within 2 to 4 hours. Renal blood flow and glomerular filtration rate remain essentially unchanged. Normal postural reflexes are intact; therefore, orthostatic symptoms are mild and infrequent.

Acute studies with clonidine in humans have demonstrated a moderate reduction (15% to 20%) of cardiac output in the supine position, with no change in the peripheral resistance. At a 45° tilt, there is a smaller reduction in cardiac output and a decrease of peripheral resistance. During long-term therapy, cardiac output tends to return to control values, while peripheral resistance remains decreased. Slowing of the pulse rate has been observed in most patients given clonidine, but the drug does not alter normal hemodynamic response to exercise.

Tolerance to the antihypertensive effect may develop in some patients, necessitating a reevaluation of therapy.

➤*Pharmacokinetics:*

Absorption – The plasma level of clonidine immediate release peaks in approximately 3 to 5 hours.

Following oral administration of modified-release clonidine, peak clonidine levels are reached in 4 to 7 hours.

The peak-to-trough ratio (maximal/minimal plasma concentrations) of clonidine following repeat dosing with modified-release clonidine ranges from 1.4 to 1.5. The plasma concentrations of clonidine increased proportionately with increase in dose over 0.1 to 0.6 mg twice daily.

After administration of clonidine ER, maximum clonidine concentrations were approximately 50% of the immediate-release clonidine maximum concentrations and occurred approximately 5 hours later relative to immediate-release clonidine. Total systemic bioavailability following clonidine ER was approximately 89% of that following immediate-release clonidine.

Clonidine Pharmacokinetic Parameters in Adults[a]

	Immediate-release clonidine fasted (n = 15)		Clonidine ER fed (n = 15)		Clonidine ER fasted (n = 14)	
Parameter	Mean	SD	Mean	SD	Mean	SD
C_{max} (pg/mL)	443	59.6	235	34.7	258	33.3
AUC_{inf} (h•pg/mL)	7313	1812	6505	1728	6729	1650
T_{max} (h)	2.07	0.5	6.8	3.61	6.5	1.23
t½ (h)	12.57	3.11	12.67	3.76	12.65	3.56

[a] SD = standard deviation; C_{max} = maximum plasma concentration; AUC = area under the curve; T_{max} = time to C_{max}; t½ = half-life.

Bioequivalence: Immediate-release and clonidine ER have different pharmacokinetic characteristics; dose substitution on a mg-for-mg basis will result in differences in exposure. A comparison across studies suggests that the C_{max} is 50% lower for clonidine ER compared with immediate-release clonidine.

Effect of food: The absorption of clonidine from modified-release clonidine is not affected by food.

Food had no effect on plasma concentrations, bioavailability, or elimination half-life of clonidine ER.

Metabolism/Excretion – The plasma half-life of immediate-release clonidine ranges from 12 to 16 hours. The plasma half-life of modified-release clonidine averages 13 hours. The elimination half-life of clonidine ER was similar to that of immediate-release clonidine. Following oral administration, about 40% to 60% of the absorbed immediate-release dose is recovered in the urine as unchanged drug in 24 hours. About 50% of the absorbed dose is metabolized in the liver.

Special populations –

Renal function impairment: The half-life of immediate-release clonidine increases up to 41 hours in patients with severe renal impairment.

Children: Plasma clonidine (0.1 and 0.2 mg twice daily) concentrations in children and adolescents with ADHD are greater than those of adults, with hypertension with children and adolescents receiving higher doses on a mg/kg basis. Body weight–normalized clearance (CL/F) in children and adolescents was higher than CL/F observed in adults with hypertension. Clonidine concentrations in plasma increased with increases in dose over the dosage range of 0.2 to 0.4 mg/day. Clonidine CL/F was independent of dose administered over the 0.2 to 0.4 mg/day dosage range. Clonidine CL/F appeared to decrease slightly with increases in age over the range of 6 to 17 years, and females had a 23% lower CL/F than males. The incidence of "sedation-like" adverse reactions (somnolence and fatigue) appeared to be independent of clonidine dose or concentration within the studied dose range in the titration study. Results from the add-on study showed that clonidine CL/F was 11% higher in patients who were receiving methylphenidate and 44% lower in those receiving amphetamine compared with subjects not on adjunctive therapy.

Contraindications

Known hypersensitivity (eg, rash, angioedema) to clonidine.

Warnings/Precautions

➤*Withdrawal:* Instruct patients not to discontinue therapy without consulting their health care provider. In adults with hypertension, sudden cessation of immediate-release clonidine treatment has, in some cases, resulted in symptoms such as agitation, headache, nervousness, and tremor accompanied or followed by a rapid rise in blood pressure and elevated plasma catecholamine concentrations. In adults with hypertension, sudden cessation of modified-release clonidine treatment in the 0.2 to 0.6 mg/day range resulted in reports of anxiety, brief lightheadedness, flushing, headache, nausea, tachycardia, tightness in the chest, or warm feeling. Rebound hypertension, as assessed by ambulatory blood pressure monitoring, was not noted. The likelihood of such reactions to discontinuation of clonidine therapy appears to be greater after administration of higher doses or continuation of concomitant beta-blocker treatment; therefore, special caution is advised in these situations. Rare instances of hypertensive encephalopathy, cerebrovascular accidents, and death have been reported after clonidine withdrawal. When discontinuing therapy with clonidine, reduce the dose gradually over 2 to 4 days to avoid withdrawal symptomatology.

No studies evaluating abrupt discontinuation of clonidine ER in children with ADHD have been conducted. In children and adolescents with ADHD, gradually reduce the dose of clonidine ER in decrements of no more than 0.1 mg every 3 to 7 days. Instruct patients not to discontinue clonidine ER therapy without consulting their health care provider because of the potential risk of withdrawal effects.

An excessive rise in blood pressure following discontinuation of clonidine therapy can be reversed by administration of oral clonidine or IV phentolamine. If therapy is to be discontinued in patients receiving a beta-blocker and clonidine concurrently, withdraw the beta-blocker several days before the gradual discontinuation of clonidine.

➤*Cardiovascular effects:* Treatment with clonidine ER can cause dose-related decreases in blood pressure and heart rate. See Adverse Reactions for more information.

Measure heart rate and blood pressure prior to initiation of therapy, following dose increases, and periodically while the patient is on therapy. Use clonidine ER with caution in patients with a history of hypotension, heart block, bradycardia, or cardiovascular disease because it can decrease blood pressure and heart rate. Use caution in treating patients who have a history of syncope or may have a condition that predisposes them to syncope, such as hypotension, orthostatic hypotension, bradycardia, or dehydration. Use clonidine ER with caution in patients treated concomitantly with antihypertensives or other drugs that can reduce blood pressure or heart rate, or increase the risk of syncope.

➤*Perioperative use:* Continue administration of clonidine to within 4 hours of surgery and resume as soon as possible thereafter. Monitor blood pressure carefully during surgery and ensure that additional measures to control blood pressure are available if required.

➤*CNS effects:* Somnolence and sedation were commonly reported adverse reactions in clinical studies of clonidine ER. In patients who completed 5 weeks of therapy in a controlled, fixed-dose pediatric monotherapy study, 31% of patients treated with 0.4 mg/day and 38% treated with 0.2 mg/day versus 7% of placebo-treated patients reported somnolence as an adverse reaction. In patients who completed 5 weeks of therapy in a controlled, flexible-dose pediatric adjunctive to stimulants study, 19% of patients treated with clonidine ER plus stimulant versus 8% treated with placebo plus stimulant reported somnolence. Before using clonidine ER with other centrally active depressants (eg, phenothiazines, barbiturates, benzodiazepines), consider the potential for additive sedative effects. Caution patients against operating heavy equipment or driving until they know how they respond to treatment with clonidine ER.

➤*Ophthalmic effects:* In view of the retinal degeneration seen in rats, eye examinations were performed during clinical trials in 908 patients before and periodically after the start of clonidine therapy for hypertension. In 353 of these 908 patients, the eye examinations were carried out over periods of 24 months or longer. Except for some dryness of the eyes, no drug-related abnormal ophthalmological findings were recorded and, according to specialized tests such as electroretinography and macular dazzle, retinal function was unchanged.

➤*Adult use in attention deficit hyperactivity disorder:* Clonidine ER has not been studied in adult patients with ADHD.

➤*Hypersensitivity reactions:* In patients who have developed localized contact sensitization to transdermal clonidine, continuation of transdermal clonidine or substitution of oral clonidine therapy may be associated with the development of a generalized skin rash.

In patients who develop an allergic reaction to transdermal clonidine, substitution of oral clonidine may also elicit an allergic reaction, including generalized rash, urticaria, or angioedema.

➤*Renal function impairment:* See Administration and Dosage for more information.

➤*Special risk:* Uptitrate clonidine slowly and use with caution in patients with severe coronary insufficiency, conduction disturbances, recent myocardial infarction, cerebrovascular disease, or chronic renal failure.

CLONIDINE HYDROCHLORIDE — ORAL

➤*Hazardous tasks:* Advise patients who engage in potentially hazardous activities, such as operating machinery or driving, of a possible sedative effect of clonidine. Also inform patients that this sedative effect may be increased by concomitant use of alcohol, barbiturates, or other sedating drugs.

➤*Pregnancy:* *Category C.* No adequate, well-controlled studies have been conducted in pregnant women. Because animal reproduction studies are not always predictive of human response, use this drug during pregnancy only if it is clearly needed.

Teratogenic – In rats, doses as low as one-third the oral maximum recommended human dosage (MRHD) (15 mcg/kg/day; human equivalent dosage [HED], 2.4 mcg/kg/day; 1/15 the MRHD on a mg/m² basis) of clonidine were associated with increased resorptions in a study in which dams were treated continuously from 2 months prior to mating and throughout gestation. Increased resorptions were not associated with treatment at the same time or at higher dose levels (up to 3 times the oral MRHD [up to 150 mcg/kg/day [HED, 24 mcg/kg/day]) when the dams were treated on gestation days 6 to 15. Increases in resorption were observed at much higher dose levels (40 times the oral MRHD on a mg/kg basis [HED, 80 mcg/kg/day] for rats; 4 to 8 times the MRHD on a mg/m² basis [HED, 40 mcg/kg/day] for mice) in mice and rats treated on gestation days 1 to 14 (lowest dose employed in the study was 500 mcg/kg).

A study was conducted in which young rats were treated orally with clonidine hydrochloride from 21 days of age to adulthood at doses of up to 300 mcg/kg/day, which is approximately 3 times the MRHD of 0.4 mg/day on a mg/m² basis. A slight delay in onset of preputial separation was seen in males treated with the highest dose (no-effect dose of 100 mcg/kg/day, which is approximately equal to the MRHD), but there were no drug effects on fertility or other measures of sexual or neurobehavioral development.

➤*Lactation:* Because clonidine is excreted in human milk, exercise caution when clonidine is administered to a breast-feeding woman. Clonidine modified-release tablets should generally not be administered to a breast-feeding woman.

➤*Children:* Safety and efficacy of the immediate-release tablets in children younger than 12 years of age or the modified-release tablets in children younger than 18 years of age have not been established. Clonidine ER has not been studied in children with ADHD younger than 6 years of age.

Because children commonly have GI illnesses that lead to vomiting, they may be particularly susceptible to hypertensive episodes resulting from an abrupt inability to take medication.

➤*Elderly:* Per the Beers list, clonidine has the potential for orthostatic hypotension and CNS adverse effects in elderly patients. (See also Administration and Dosage for more information.)

➤*Monitoring:* Monitor patients with renal impairment carefully to prevent excessive blood pressure lowering or bradycardia.

Measure heart rate and blood pressure prior to initiation of therapy, following dose increases, and periodically while on therapy.

Drug Interactions

Clonidine Oral Drug Interactions

Precipitant drug	Object drug[a]		Description
Beta-adrenergic blocking agents (eg, atenolol)	Clonidine	↑↓	Attenuation or reversal of antihypertensive effect and potentially life-threatening increases in blood pressure may occur. Because of a potential for additive effects, such as bradycardia and AV[b] block, caution is warranted in patients receiving clonidine concomitantly with agents known to affect sinus node function or AV nodal conduction (eg, beta-blockers). If clonidine therapy is discontinued in patients receiving a beta-blocker, withdraw the beta-blocker several days before gradual discontinuation of clonidine. Monitor heart rate.
Clonidine	Beta-adrenergic blocking agents (eg, atenolol)		
Calcium channel blockers (eg, verapamil)	Clonidine	↑	Because of a potential for additive effects, such as bradycardia and AV block, caution is warranted in patients receiving clonidine concomitantly with agents known to affect sinus node function or AV nodal conduction (eg, calcium channel blockers). Sinus bradycardia resulting in hospitalization and pacemaker insertion has been associated with concurrent use of clonidine and diltiazem or verapamil. Monitor heart rate and blood pressure. Adjust the dose of either agent as needed.
Clonidine	Calcium channel blockers (eg, verapamil)		
Digitalis	Clonidine	↑	Because of a potential for additive effects, such as bradycardia and AV block, caution is warranted in patients receiving clonidine concomitantly with agents known to affect sinus node function or AV nodal conduction (eg, digitalis). Monitor heart rate.
Clonidine	Digitalis		
Mirtazapine	Clonidine	↓	The pharmacologic effects of clonidine may be decreased by mirtazapine. Closely monitor blood pressure when mirtazapine is started or stopped. If an interaction is suspected, adjust the clonidine dose as needed.
Prazosin	Clonidine	↓	The antihypertensive effectiveness of clonidine may be decreased. Monitor blood pressure when prazosin is started or stopped. Adjust the clonidine dose as needed.
Tizanidine	Clonidine	↑	Possible additive hypotensive effects may occur when clonidine and tizanidine are coadministered. Avoid coadministration. If both drugs must be given, closely monitor for signs of hypotension during dose increases.
Clonidine	Tizanidine		
Tricyclic antidepressants (eg, amitriptyline)	Clonidine	↓	Tricyclic antidepressants may block antihypertensive effects of clonidine and potentially life-threatening elevations in blood pressure may occur. The hypotensive effect of clonidine may be reduced, necessitating an increase in the clonidine dose.
Clonidine	CNS depressants (eg, alcohol, barbiturates)	↑	Clonidine may potentiate the CNS depressant effects of sedating drugs. Monitor the response of the patient and adjust the CNS depressant dose as needed. Advise patients of the increased sedative effect.
Clonidine	Cyclosporine	↑	The pharmacologic and toxic effects of cyclosporine may be increased by clonidine. Monitor cyclosporine concentrations and observe the clinical response of the patient. If an interaction is suspected, decrease the cyclosporine dose or stop clonidine.

[a] ↑ = object drug increased; ↓ = object drug decreased; ↑↓ = object drug both increased and decreased; ↔ = undetermined clinical effect.
[b] AV = atrioventricular; CV = cardiovascular.

➤*Amitriptyline:* Amitriptyline in combination with clonidine enhances the manifestation of corneal lesions in rats.

Adverse Reactions

➤*Immediate-release tablets:*

Most frequent adverse reactions – Most adverse reactions are mild and tend to diminish with continued therapy. The most frequent adverse reactions (which appear to be dose related) are dry mouth (40%), drowsiness (33%), dizziness (16%), and constipation and sedation (10%).

Cardiovascular – Bradycardia; congestive heart failure; electrocardiographic abnormalities (ie, sinus node arrest, functional bradycardia, high-degree AV block, arrhythmias); orthostatic symptoms; palpitations; Raynaud phenomenon; sinus bradycardia and AV block, both with and without the use of concomitant digitalis; syncope; tachycardia.

CNS – Agitation, anxiety, delirium, delusional perception, fatigue, headache, insomnia, malaise, mental depression, nervousness, other behavioral changes, paresthesia, restlessness, sleep disorder, visual and auditory hallucinations, vivid dreams or nightmares.

Dermatologic – Alopecia, angioneurotic edema, hives, pruritus, rash, urticaria.

GI – Abdominal pain; anorexia; hepatitis; mild transient abnormalities in liver function tests; nausea; parotitis; pseudo-obstruction, including colonic pseudo-obstruction; salivary gland pain; vomiting.

GU – Decreased sexual activity, difficulty in micturition, erectile dysfunction, loss of libido, nocturia, urinary retention.

CLONIDINE HYDROCHLORIDE — ORAL

Metabolic – Gynecomastia, transient elevation of blood glucose or serum creatine phosphokinase, weight gain.

Musculoskeletal – Leg cramps, muscle or joint pain.

Special senses – Accommodation disorder, blurred vision, burning of the eyes, decreased lacrimation, dryness of the eyes, dryness of the nasal mucosa.

Miscellaneous – Fever, increased sensitivity to alcohol, pallor, thrombocytopenia, weakly positive Coombs' test, weakness, withdrawal syndrome.

➤*Modified-release tablets:* The incidence of adverse reactions progressively increased with higher doses and was notably less in the 0.2 mg/day treatment group compared with the 0.4 and 0.6 mg/day treatment groups. The majority of adverse reactions were mild. Adverse reactions of moderate severity occurred in 6 patients and included 2 reports of insomnia and 2 reports of dry mouth. One patient in the 0.4 mg/day group experienced symptomatic sinus bradycardia 2 weeks after initiating the study drug. This reaction was the only severe adverse reaction, the only serious adverse reaction, and the only adverse reaction that led to discontinuation of the study drug. Because the number of subjects is small and the duration of exposure is short, no inferences regarding differences in adverse reactions between modified-release clonidine and other clonidine formulations is warranted.

Clonidine Modified-Release Tablet Adverse Reactions

	Clonidine modified-release tablet			
Adverse reactions	0.2 mg/day (n = 12)	0.4 mg/day (n = 15)	0.6 mg/day (n = 15)	Total (N = 42)
At least 1 adverse reaction reported	42%	67%	80%	64%
CNS				
Dizziness	0%	20%	13%	12%
Fatigue	17%	27%	27%	24%
Headache	8%	7%	13%	10%
Insomnia	0%	0%	13%	5%
Somnolence	0%	7%	7%	5%
GI				
Dry mouth	0%	53%	53%	38%
Nausea	8%	7%	7%	7%

➤*Extended-release tablets:*

Common adverse reactions (≥ 5%) – Most common adverse reactions, reported during the treatment period were constipation, dry mouth, ear pain, emotional disorder, fatigue, increased body temperature, insomnia, irritability, nasal congestion, nightmares, somnolence, throat pain, and upper respiratory tract infection. The most common adverse reactions that were reported during the taper phase were upper abdominal pain and GI virus.

Discontinuation – Of patients receiving clonidine ER, 13% discontinued from the pediatric monotherapy study because of adverse reactions, compared with 1% in the placebo group. The most common adverse reactions leading to discontinuation in clonidine ER monotherapy–treated patients were somnolence/sedation (5%) and fatigue (4%). Less common adverse reactions leading to discontinuation (occurring in approximately 1% of patients) included formication, increased heart rate, prolonged QT, rash, and vomiting. In the pediatric adjunctive treatment to stimulants study, 1 patient discontinued from clonidine the ER plus stimulant group because of bradyphrenia.

Fixed-dose monotherapy –

Clonidine ER Fixed-Dose Monotherapy Adverse Reactions (≥ 2%)

Adverse reactions	Clonidine ER 0.4 mg/day (n = 78)	Clonidine ER 0.2 mg/day (n = 76)	Placebo (n = 76)
CNS			
Abnormal sleep-related event	1%	3%	0%
Aggression	1%	3%	1%
Dizziness	3%	7%	5%
Emotional disorder	5%	4%	1%
Fatigue[a]	13%	16%	1%
Headache	19%	29%	18%
Insomnia	6%	4%	1%
Irritability	6%	9%	3%
Nightmare	9%	3%	0%
Sleep terror	0%	3%	0%
Somnolence[b]	31%	38%	5%
Tremor	3%	1%	0%
GI			
Constipation	6%	1%	0%
Diarrhea	1%	4%	3%
Dry mouth	5%	0%	1%
GI viral	0%	7%	4%
Nausea	8%	5%	4%
Thirst	3%	1%	0%
Upper abdominal pain	13%	20%	17%
GU			
Enuresis	4%	0%	0%
Pollakiuria	0%	3%	0%
Respiratory			
Asthma	1%	3%	1%
Lower respiratory tract infection	0%	3%	1%
Upper respiratory tract infection	6%	11%	4%
Special senses			
Ear pain	0%	5%	1%
Epistaxis	0%	3%	0%
Nasal congestion	5%	3%	1%
Nasopharyngitis	3%	3%	1%
Tearfulness	3%	1%	0%
Throat pain	6%	8%	3%
Miscellaneous			
Body temperature increased	1%	5%	3%
Bradycardia	4%	0%	0%
Influenza-like illness	3%	1%	1%

[a] Fatigue includes the terms "fatigue" and "lethargy."
[b] Somnolence includes the terms "somnolence" and "sedation."

Clonidine ER Fixed-Dose Monotherapy – Taper Period[a] Adverse Reactions (≥ 2%)

Adverse reactions	Clonidine ER 0.4 mg/day (n = 78)	Clonidine ER 0.2 mg/day (n = 76)	Placebo (n = 76)
CNS			
Headache	2%	5%	3%
Somnolence	3%	2%	0%
GI			
Abdominal pain upper	6%	0%	3%
GI viral	5%	0%	0%
Miscellaneous			
Heart rate increased	3%	0%	0%
Otitis media acute	0%	3%	0%

[a] Taper period: 0.2 mg dose, week 8; 0.4 mg dose, weeks 6 to 8; placebo dose, weeks 6 to 8.

Flexible-dose as adjunctive therapy to psychostimulants –

Flexible-Dose Clonidine ER[a] Adjunctive to Stimulant Therapy Trial – Treatment Period (Study 2)

Adverse reactions	Clonidine ER + stimulant therapy (n = 102)	Placebo + stimulant therapy (n = 96)
CNS		
Anxiety	2%	0%
Dizziness	4%	2%
Fatigue[b]	16%	4%
Insomnia	4%	2%
Somnolence[c]	19%	8%
GI		
Abdominal pain	2%	1%
Abdominal pain upper	12%	7%
Decreased appetite	5%	4%
Special senses		
Epistaxis	3%	0%
Nasal congestion	6%	5%
Rhinorrhea	3%	0%
Throat pain	6%	3%

CLONIDINE HYDROCHLORIDE — ORAL

Flexible-Dose Clonidine ER[a] Adjunctive to Stimulant Therapy Trial – Treatment Period (Study 2)

Adverse reactions	Clonidine ER + stimulant therapy (n = 102)	Placebo + stimulant therapy (n = 96)
Miscellaneous		
Body temperature increased	4%	2%
Pain in extremity	2%	0%

[a] Clonidine ER was initiated at 0.1 mg/day and titrated up to 0.4 mg/day over a 3-week period.
[b] Fatigue includes the terms "fatigue" and "lethargy."
[c] Somnolence includes the terms "somnolence" and "sedation."

Flexible-Dose Clonidine ER Adjunctive to Stimulant Therapy Trial – Taper Period[a] Adverse Reactions (≥ 2%)

Adverse reactions	Clonidine ER + stimulant therapy (n = 102)	Placebo + stimulant therapy (n = 96)
CNS		
Headache	3%	1%
Irritability	3%	2%
Special senses		
Nasal congestion	4%	2%
Throat pain	3%	1%
Miscellaneous		
Gastroenteritis viral	2%	0%
Rash	2%	0%

[a] Taper period: weeks 6 to 8.

Cardiovascular – In patients who completed 5 weeks of treatment in a controlled, fixed-dose monotherapy study in children, the maximum placebo-subtracted mean change in systolic blood pressure during the treatment period was −4 mm Hg on clonidine ER 0.2 mg/day and −8.8 mm Hg on clonidine ER 0.4 mg/day. The maximum placebo-subtracted mean change in diastolic blood pressure was −4 mm Hg on clonidine ER 0.2 mg/day and −7.3 mm Hg on clonidine ER 0.4 mg/day. The maximum placebo-subtracted mean change in heart rate was −4 beats per minute (bpm) on clonidine ER 0.2 mg/day and −7.7 bpm on clonidine ER 0.4 mg/day.

During the taper period of the fixed-dose monotherapy study, the maximum placebo-subtracted mean change in systolic blood pressure was +3.4 mm Hg on clonidine ER 0.2 mg/day and −5.6 mm Hg on clonidine ER 0.4 mg/day. The maximum placebo-subtracted mean change in diastolic blood pressure was +3.3 mm Hg on clonidine ER 0.2 mg/day and −5.4 mm Hg on clonidine ER 0.4 mg/day. The maximum placebo-subtracted mean change in heart rate was −0.6 bpm on clonidine ER 0.2 mg/day and −3 bpm on clonidine ER 0.4 mg/day.

Overdosage

➤*Symptoms:* Hypertension may develop early and may be followed by hypotension, bradycardia, respiratory depression, hypothermia, drowsiness, decreased or absent reflexes, weakness, irritability, or miosis. The frequency of CNS depression may be higher in children than adults. Large overdoses may result in reversible cardiac conduction defects or dysrhythmias, apnea, coma, and seizures. Signs and symptoms of overdose generally occur within 30 minutes to 2 hours after exposure. As little as 0.1 mg of clonidine has produced signs of toxicity in children.

The largest overdose reported to date involved a 28-year-old man who ingested 100 mg of clonidine powder. This patient developed hypertension followed by hypotension, bradycardia, apnea, hallucinations, semicoma, and premature ventricular contractions. The patient fully recovered after intensive treatment. Plasma clonidine levels were 60 ng/mL after 1 hour, 190 ng/mL after 1.5 hours, 370 ng/mL after 2 hours, and 120 ng/mL after 5.5 and 6.5 hours.

➤*Treatment:* There is no specific antidote for clonidine overdosage. Gastric lavage may be indicated following recent and/or large ingestions. Administration of activated charcoal and/or a cathartic may be beneficial. Supportive care may include atropine for bradycardia, IV fluids or vasopressor agents for hypotension, and vasodilators for hypertension. Naloxone may be a useful adjunct for the management of clonidine-induced respiratory depression, hypotension, and/or coma; monitor blood pressure because the administration of naloxone has occasionally resulted in paradoxical hypertension. Tolazoline administration has yielded inconsistent results and is not recommended as first-line therapy. Dialysis is not likely to significantly enhance the elimination of clonidine.

Patient Information

Caution patients against interruption of clonidine therapy without their health care provider's advice.

Advise patients to avoid becoming dehydrated or overheated.

Advise patients to avoid use with alcohol.

Caution patients who wear contact lenses that treatment with clonidine tablets may cause dryness of the eyes.

Advise patients who engage in potentially hazardous activities, such as operating machinery or driving, of a possible sedative effect of clonidine. Also inform them that this sedative effect may be increased by concomitant use of alcohol, barbiturates, or other sedating drugs.

Advise patients not to discontinue clonidine ER abruptly. In order to minimize potential withdrawal effects, when discontinuing clonidine ER therapy, instruct patients to decrease their total daily dose of in decrements of no more than 0.1 mg every 3 to 7 days.

Advise patients who have developed an allergic reaction from clonidine transdermal system that substitution of oral clonidine may also elicit an allergic reaction (including generalized rash, urticaria, or angioedema).

Instruct patients that if the total daily dose of clonidine does not allow equal doses to be given in the morning and at bedtime, to take the higher of the 2 doses at bedtime.

Clonidine ER must be swallowed whole and never crushed, cut, or chewed.

Advise patients to consult their health care provider if they are breastfeeding, pregnant, or thinking of becoming pregnant while taking clonidine.

Inform patients that they may take clonidine ER with or without food.

Advise patients that if they miss a dose of clonidine ER, to skip the missed dose and take the next dose as scheduled. Do not take more than the prescribed total daily amount of clonidine ER in any 24-hour period.

CLONIDINE HYDROCHLORIDE

	Product/Distributor	Release Rate (mg/24 h)	Surface Area (cm^2)	Total Clonidine Content (mg)	How Supplied
Rx	**Clonidine** (Par Pharmaceutical)	0.1	10.8	3.67	In 4s.
Rx	**Catapres-TTS-1** (Boehringer Ingelheim)	0.1	3.5	2.5	Mineral oil. In 12s.
Rx	**Clonidine** (Par Pharmaceutical)	0.2	21.6	7.34	In 4s.
Rx	**Catapres-TTS-2** (Boehringer Ingelheim)	0.2	7	5	Mineral oil. In 12s.
Rx	**Clonidine** (Par Pharmaceutical)	0.3	32.4	11.02	In 4s.
Rx	**Catapres-TTS-3** (Boehringer Ingelheim)	0.3	10.5	7.5	Mineral oil. In 4s.

CLONIDINE — TRANSDERMAL

Indications

Treatment of hypertension. It may be employed alone or concomitantly with other antihypertensive agents.

➤*Off-label uses:*

Attention deficit hyperactivity disorder (children/adolescents) – [1] = Good documentation. None of the alpha-2 adrenergic agonists are indicated for psychiatric indications, nor are they considered first-line treatment for ADHD. However, in an official American Academy of Child and Adolescent Psychiatry (AACAP) statement, clonidine as monotherapy was suggested as a useful alternative in modulating mood and activity level in children with ADHD, particularly those with sleep difficulties who are nonresponsive to stimulants, or in children with tic disorders (where stimulants may cause tic exacerbations). Despite widespread use, the addition of clonidine to existing stimulant therapy should be carefully considered because several safety issues have been recognized and there is limited published information from controlled trials regarding efficacy of these combinations.

Hot flashes – [2] = Fair documentation. In controlled trials of a limited number of postmenopausal women, clonidine demonstrated variable results, significantly reducing the frequency, duration, and severity of hot flashes with transdermal therapy (0.1 mg patch every 7 days) or higher oral clonidine dosages (0.1 to 0.4 mg twice daily) when compared with placebo, but demonstrated no benefit with lower oral dosages (50 mcg twice daily).

Hyperhidrosis – [4] = Insufficient documentation. Clonidine may provide some benefit in the management of hyperhidrosis based on data from a few case reports, although the small number of patients studied makes it difficult to accurately state the true effect of clonidine on excessive sweating. Larger, controlled trials are needed to provide a better evaluation of clonidine's place in the treatment of hyperhidrosis.

Postherpetic neuralgia (transdermal) – [5] = Poor documentation. Published data assessing the efficacy of topical clonidine in patients with postherpetic neuralgia (PHN) are limited, but show some benefit. American Academy of Neurology clinical practice guidelines do not address the efficacy of topical clonidine for PHN.

CLONIDINE — TRANSDERMAL

Prevention of migraine (adults) – [5] = Poor documentation. Although early results using clonidine for migraine prophylaxis were positive, several controlled trials demonstrated little to no efficacy. A review written in 1990 considered the use of clonidine for migraine prophylaxisto be obsolete. American Academy of Neurology practice guidelines state that clonidine is no more effective than placebo for the prevention of migraine.

Prevention of migraine (children/adolescents) – [5] = Poor documentation. In studies (published in 1977 and 1982) evaluating clonidine use for the prevention of migraine headaches in pediatric patients, it was no more effective than placebo. It has not been studied further. Current practice guidelines state that clonidine is not effective for the prevention of migraine in pediatric patients and its use is not recommended.

Smoking cessation – [1] = Good documentation. Because of its adverse reaction profile and its potential to cause rebound withdrawal symptoms upon discontinuation, clonidine is recommended as a second-line agent when nicotine replacement, bupropion sustained release, or varenicline have been ineffective or are contraindicated. Clonidine may be targeted to those who will benefit from its sedative effects, such as those who experience high levels of anxiety when they quit smoking.

Ulcerative colitis – [2] = Fair documentation. Mesalamine, administered orally or rectally, is considered first-line therapy for ulcerative colitis. Corticosteroids and intravenous (IV) cyclosporine can be used for severe acute ulcerative colitis, but they are not appropriate as maintenance therapy. Azathioprine and mercaptopurine have been effective as maintenance therapy, but are associated with severe adverse effects. Immunosuppressives may require up to 6 months of treatment to see improvements. Based on data from controlled trials in fewer than 100 patients, clonidine may provide some benefit in the management of ulcerative colitis. Larger, controlled trials would provide a better evaluation of clonidine's place in treating ulcerative colitis.

Other possible off-label uses –

Cyclosporine-associated nephrotoxicity: 100 to 200 mcg/day transdermal.

Diabetic diarrhea: 100 to 600 mcg every 12 hours or 300 mcg per 24-hour patch (1 to 2 patches/week).

Administration and Dosage

➤*General dosing considerations:* Clonidine transdermal dosage should be titrated according to individual therapeutic requirements.

➤*Adults:*

Hypertension –

Initial dosage: Clonidine 0.1 mg transdermal system.

Dosage adjustment: If after 1 or 2 weeks the desired reduction in blood pressure is not achieved, increase the dosage by adding another clonidine 0.1 mg transdermal system or changing to a larger system. An increase in dosage more than 2 clonidine 0.3 mg transdermal systems is usually not associated with additional efficacy.

Conversion: When substituting clonidine transdermal for oral clonidine or for other antihypertensive drugs, health care provider should be aware that the antihypertensive effect of clonidine transdermal may not commence until 2 to 3 days after initial application. Therefore, gradual reduction of prior drug dosage is advised. Some or all previous antihypertensive treatment may have to be continued, particularly in patients with more severe forms of hypertension.

Off-label dosing –

Hot flashes: [2] = Fair documentation. 0.1 mg patch every 7 days.

Hyperhidrosis: [4] = Insufficient documentation. 0.2 mg/day via transdermal patch for 14 days has been studied.

Smoking cessation: [1] = Good documentation. 0.1 to 0.2 mg/day transdermally for 3 to 10 weeks. Initial dosing should start up to 3 days prior to the quit date and is typically 0.1 mg/day applied transdermally each week, increasing by 0.1 mg weekly if needed.

Ulcerative colitis: [2] = Fair documentation. Dosages of 15 mg/wk via transdermal patch for up to 8 weeks have been studied.

➤*Children:*

Children 12 years of age and older – See Adults.

Off-label dosing –

Attention deficit hyperactivity disorder: One study transferred 8 patients who had favorable results with oral clonidine to equivalent daily doses of transdermal clonidine. In 3 children, slightly higher clonidine dosing (0.3 mg/day vs 0.2 mg/day) was required to maintain similar clinical response. An AACAP practice statement has suggested that patients may be transferred to equivalent daily doses of transdermal therapy after oral therapy has been established. Onset of action may not be evident for several weeks.

➤*Renal function impairment:* Adjust dosage according to the degree of impairment and carefully monitor patients. Because only a minimal amount of clonidine is removed during routine hemodialysis, there is no need to give supplemental clonidine following dialysis.

➤*Discontinuation of therapy:* Patients should be instructed not to discontinue therapy without consulting their health care provider. Reduce the dose gradually over 2 to 4 days to avoid withdrawal symptomatology.

If therapy is to be discontinued in patients receiving a beta-blocker and clonidine concurrently, the beta-blocker should be withdrawn several days before the gradual discontinuation of clonidine.

➤*Administration:* Apply transdermal clonidine once every 7 days to a hairless area of intact skin on the upper outer arm or chest. Each new application of clonidine transdermal should be on a different skin site from the previous location. If the system loosens during 7-day wearing, apply adhesive overlay directly over the system to ensure good adhesion. There have been rare reports of the need for patch changes prior to 7 days to maintain blood pressure control.

➤*Storage/Stability:* Store below 30°C (86°F).

Actions

➤*Pharmacology:* Clonidine stimulates alpha-adrenoreceptors in the brain stem. This action results in reduced sympathetic outflow from the central nervous system and in decreases in peripheral resistance, renal vascular resistance, heart rate, and blood pressure. Renal blood flow and glomerular filtration rate remain essentially unchanged. Normal postural reflexes are intact; therefore, orthostatic symptoms are mild and infrequent.

Acute studies with clonidine hydrochloride in humans have demonstrated a moderate reduction (15% to 20%) of cardiac output in the supine position with no change in the peripheral resistance; at a 45° tilt there is a smaller reduction in cardiac output and a decrease of peripheral resistance.

During long-term therapy, cardiac output tends to return to control values, while peripheral resistance remains decreased. Slowing of the pulse rate has been observed in most patients given clonidine, but the drug does not alter normal hemodynamic responses to exercise.

Tolerance to the antihypertensive effect may develop in some patients, necessitating a reevaluation of therapy.

Other studies in patients have provided evidence of a reduction in plasma resin activity and in the excretion of aldosterone and catecholamines. The exact relationship of these pharmacologic actions to the antihypertensive effect of clonidine has not been fully elucidated.

Clonidine acutely stimulates the release of growth hormone in children as well as adults but does not produce a chronic elevation of growth hormone with long-term use.

➤*Pharmacokinetics:* The plasma half-life of clonidine is 12.7 ± 7 hours. Following oral administration, about 40% to 60% of the absorbed dose is recovered in the urine as unchanged drug within 24 hours. The remainder of the absorbed dose is metabolized in the liver.

Contraindications

Hypersensitivity to clonidine or any component of the therapeutic system.

Warnings/Precautions

➤*Withdrawal:* Patients should be instructed not to discontinue therapy without consulting their physician. Sudden cessation of clonidine treatment has, in some cases, resulted in symptoms such as nervousness, agitation, headache, and confusion accompanied or followed by a rapid rise in blood pressure and elevated catecholamine concentrations in the plasma. The likelihood of such reactions to discontinuation of clonidine therapy appears to be greater after administration of higher doses or continuation of concomitant beta blocker treatment and special caution is therefore advised in these situations. Rare instances of hypertensive encephalopathy, cerebrovascular accidents and death have been reported after clonidine withdrawal. When discontinuing clonidine transdermal therapy, the physician should reduce the dose gradually over 2 to 4 days to avoid withdrawal symptomatology.

An excessive rise in blood pressure following discontinuation of clonidine transdermal therapy can be reversed by administration of oral clonidine hydrochloride or by intravenous phentolamine. If therapy is to be discontinued in patients receiving a beta blocker and clonidine concurrently, the beta blocker should be withdrawn several days before the gradual discontinuation of clonidine transdermal.

➤*Skin rash:* In patients who have developed localized contact sensitization to clonidine transdermal, continuation of clonidine transdermal or substitution of oral clonidine hydrochloride therapy may be associated with development of a generalized skin rash.

In patients who develop an allergic reaction to clonidine transdermal, substitution of oral clonidine hydrochloride may also elicit an allergic reaction (including generalized rash, urticaria, or angioedema).

➤*Perioperative use:* Clonidine transdermal therapy should not be interrupted during the surgical period. Blood pressure should be carefully monitored during surgery and additional measures to control blood pressure should be available if required. Physicians considering starting clonidine transdermal therapy during the perioperative period must be aware that therapeutic plasma clonidine levels are not achieved until 2 to 3 days after initial application of clonidine transdermal (see Administration and Dosage).

➤*Defibrillation or cardioversion:* The transdermal clonidine systems should be removed before attempting defibrillation or cardioversion because of the potential for altered electrical conductivity which may increase the risk of arcing, a phenomenon associated with the use of defibrillators.

➤*Ophthalmologic effects:* In several studies with oral clonidine hydrochloride, a dose-dependent increase in the incidence and severity of spontaneous retinal degeneration was seen in albino rats treated for 6 months or longer. Tissue distribution studies in dogs and monkeys showed a concentration of clonidine in the choroid.

In view of the retinal degeneration seen in rats, eye examinations were performed during clinical trials in 908 patients before, and periodically after, the start of clonidine therapy. In 353 of these 908 patients, the eye examinations were carried out over periods of 24 months or longer. Except for some dryness of the eyes, no drug-related abnormal ophthalmological findings were recorded and, according to specialized tests such as electroretinography and macular dazzle, retinal function was unchanged.

CLONIDINE — TRANSDERMAL

In combination with amitriptyline, clonidine hydrochloride administration led to the development of corneal lesions in rats within 5 days.

➤*Special risk:* Clonidine transdermal should be used with caution in patients with severe coronary insufficiency, conduction disturbances, recent MI, cerebrovascular disease, or chronic renal failure.

In rare instances, loss of blood pressure control has been reported in patients using clonidine transdermal according to the instructions for use.

➤*Pregnancy: Category C.*

Teratogenic – In rats, doses as low as ⅓ the oral MRDHD (1/15 the MRDHD on a mg/m² basis) of clonidine were associated with increased resorptions in a study in which dams were treated continuously from 2 months prior to mating. Increased resorptions were not associated with treatment at the same or at higher dose levels (up to 3 times the oral MRDHD) when the dams were treated on gestation days 6 to 15. Increases in resorption were observed at much higher dose levels (40 times the oral MRDHD on a mg/kg basis; 4 to 8 times the MRDHD on a mg/m² basis) in mice and rats treated on gestation days 1 to 14 (lowest dose employed in the study was 500 mcg/kg).

No adequate well-controlled studies have been conducted in pregnant women. Because animal reproduction studies are not always predictive of human response, this drug should be used during pregnancy only if clearly needed.

➤*Lactation:* As clonidine is excreted in human milk, caution should be exercised when clonidine transdermal is administered to a breast-feeding woman.

➤*Children:* Safety and effectiveness in pediatric patients below the age of 12 have not been established (see Withdrawal).

➤*Elderly:* Per the Beers list, clonidine has the potential for orthostatic hypotension and CNS adverse effects.

Drug Interactions

Clonidine Transdermal Drug Interactions

Precipitant drug	Object drug[a]		Description
Beta-adrenergic blocking agents (eg, atenolol)	Clonidine	↑↓	Attenuation or reversal of antihypertensive effect and potentially life-threatening increases in blood pressure may occur. Because of a potential for additive effects, such as bradycardia and AV[b] block, caution is warranted in patients receiving clonidine concomitantly with agents known to affect sinus node function or AV nodal conduction (eg, beta-blockers). If clonidine therapy is discontinued in patients receiving a beta-blocker, withdraw the beta-blocker several days before gradual discontinuation of clonidine. Monitor heart rate.
Clonidine	Beta-adrenergic blocking agents (eg, atenolol)		
Calcium channel blockers (eg, verapamil)	Clonidine	↑	Because of a potential for additive effects such as bradycardia and AV block, caution is warranted in patients receiving clonidine concomitantly with agents known to affect sinus node function or AV nodal conduction (eg, calcium channel blockers). Sinus bradycardia resulting in hospitalization and pacemaker insertion has been associated with concurrent use of clonidine and diltiazem or verapamil. Monitor heart rate and blood pressure. Adjust the dose of either agent as needed.
Clonidine	Calcium channel blockers (eg, verapamil)		
Digitalis	Clonidine	↑	Use with caution because of a potential for additive effects such as bradycardia and AV block. Monitor heart rate in patients receiving clonidine concomitantly with agents known to affect sinus node function or AV nodal conduction such as digitalis. Adjust the dose of either agent as needed.
Clonidine	Digitalis		
Prazosin	Clonidine	↓	The antihypertensive effectiveness of clonidine may be decreased. Monitor blood pressure when prazosin is started or stopped. Adjust the clonidine dose as needed.
Tizanidine	Clonidine	↑	Possible additive hypotensive effects may occur when clonidine and tizanidine are coadministered. Avoid coadministration. If both drugs must be given, closely monitor for signs of hypotension during dose increases.
Clonidine	Tizanidine		
Tricyclic antidepressants (eg, amitriptyline)	Clonidine	↓	Tricyclic antidepressants may block antihypertensive effects of clonidine and potentially life-threatening elevations in blood pressure may occur. The hypotensive effect of clonidine may be reduced, necessitating an increase in the clonidine dose.
Clonidine	CNS depressants (eg, alcohol, barbiturates)	↑	Clonidine may potentiate the CNS depressant effects of sedating drugs. Monitor the response of the patient and adjust the CNS depressant dose as needed. Advise patients of the increased sedative effect.
Clonidine	Cyclosporine	↑	The pharmacologic and toxic effects of cyclosporine may be increased by clonidine. Monitor cyclosporine concentrations and observe the clinical response of the patient. If an interaction is suspected, decrease the cyclosporine dose or stop clonidine.

[a] ↑ = object drug increased; ↓ = object drug decreased; ↑↓ = object drug both increased and decreased; ↔ = undetermined clinical effect.
[b] AV = atrioventricular; CV = cardiovascular.

➤*Amitriptyline:* Amitriptyline, in combination with clonidine enhances the manifestation of corneal lesions in rats.

Adverse Reactions

➤*Clinical trials:* Most systemic adverse effects during clonidine transdermal therapy have been mild and have tended to diminish with continued therapy. In a 3-month multiclinic trial of clonidine transdermal in 101 hypertensive patients, the systemic adverse reactions were: dry mouth (25 patients) and drowsiness (12), fatigue (6), headache (5), lethargy and sedation (3 each), insomnia, dizziness, impotence/sexual dysfunction, dry throat (2 each) and constipation, nausea, change in taste and nervousness (1 each).

In the above mentioned 3-month controlled clinical trial, as well as other uncontrolled clinical trials, the most frequent adverse reactions were dermatological and are described below.

In the 3-month trial, 51 of the 101 patients had localized skin reactions such as erythema (26 patients) and/or pruritus, particularly after using an adhesive overlay throughout the 7-day dosage interval. Allergic contact sensitization to clonidine transdermal was observed in 5 patients. Other skin reactions were localized vesiculation (7 patients), hyperpigmentation (5), edema (3), excoriation (3), burning (3), papulas (1), throbbing (1), blanching (1), and a generalized macular rash (1).

In additional clinical experience, contact dermatitis resulting in treatment discontinuation was observed in 128 of 673 patients (about 19 in 100) after a mean duration of treatment of 37 weeks. The incidence of contact dermatitis was about 34 in 100 among white women, about 18 in 100 in white men, about 14 in 100 in black women, and ≈ 8 in 100 in black men. Analysis of skin reaction data showed that the risk of having to discontinue clonidine transdermal treatment because of contact dermatitis was greatest between treatment weeks 6 and 26, although sensitivity may develop either earlier or later in treatment.

In a large-scale clinical acceptability and safety study by 451 physicians in a total of 3539 patients, other allergic reactions were recorded for which a causal relationship to clonidine transdermal was not established; maculopapular rash (10 cases); urticaria (2 cases); and angioedema of the face (2 cases), which also affected the tongue in one of the patients.

➤*Postmarketing:* Other adverse effects reported since the drug has been marketed are listed below by body system. In this setting, an incidence or causal relationship cannot always be accurately determined. However, none of the events listed below occurred in a frequency more than 0.5%.

Cardiovascular – Congestive heart failure; cerebrovascular accident; electrocardiographic abnormalities (i.e., bradycardia, sick sinus syndrome disturbances and arrhythmias); chest pain; orthostatic symptoms; syncope, increases in blood pressure; sinus bradycardia and atrioventricular block with and without the use of concomitant digitalis; Raynaud's phenomenon; tachycardia; bradycardia; and palpitations.

Dermatologic – Angioneurotic edema; localized or generalized rash; hives; urticaria; contact dermatitis; pruritus; alopecia; and localized hypo- or hyperpigmentation.

GI – Anorexia and vomiting.

GU – Difficult micturition; loss of libido; and decreased sexual activity.

CLONIDINE — TRANSDERMAL

Metabolic – Gynecomastia or breast enlargement and weight gain.

Musculoskeletal – Muscle or joint pain; and leg cramps.

Ophthalmic – Blurred vision; burning of the eyes and dryness of the eyes.

Psychiatric – Delirium; mental depression; visual and auditory hallucinations; localized numbness; vivid dreams or nightmares; restlessness; anxiety; agitation; irritability; other behavioral changes; and drowsiness.

Miscellaneous – Fever; malaise; weakness; and pallor; and withdrawal syndrome.

Overdosage

➤*Symptoms:* Hypertension may develop early and may be followed by hypotension, bradycardia, respiratory depression, hypothermia, drowsiness, decreased or absent reflexes, weakness, irritability and miosis. The frequency of CNS depression may be higher in children than adults. Large overdoses may result in reversible cardiac conduction defects or arrhythmias, apnea, coma and seizures. Signs and symptoms of overdose generally occur within 30 minutes to 2 hours after exposure. As little as 0.1 mg of clonidine has produced signs of toxicity in children.

If symptoms of poisoning occur following dermal exposure, remove all clonidine transdermal systems. After their removal, the plasma clonidine levels will persist for about 8 hours, then decline slowly over a period of several days. Rare cases of clonidine transdermal poisoning due to accidental or deliberate mouthing or ingestion of the patch have been reported, many of them involving children.

The largest overdose reported to date, involved a 28-year-old male who ingested 100 mg of clonidine hydrochloride powder. This patient developed hypertension followed by hypotension, bradycardia, apnea, hallucinations, semicoma, and premature ventricular contractions. The patient fully recovered after intensive treatment. Plasma clonidine levels were 60 ng/mL after 1 hour, 190 ng/mL after 1.5 hours, 370 ng/mL after 2 hours, and 120 ng/mL after 5.5 and 6.5 hours. In mice and rats, the oral LD_{50} of clonidine is 206 and 465 mg/kg, respectively.

➤*Treatment:* There is no specific antidote for clonidine overdosage. Ipecac syrup-induced vomiting and gastric lavage would not be expected to remove significant amounts of clonidine following dermal exposure. If the patch is ingested, whole bowel irrigation may be considered and the administration of activated charcoal or cathartic may be beneficial. Supportive care may include atropine sulfate for bradycardia, intravenous fluids or vasopressor agents for hypotension and vasodilators for hypertension. Naloxone may be a useful adjunct for the management of clonidine-induced respiratory depression, hypotension and/or coma; blood pressure should be monitored since the administration of naloxone has occasionally resulted in paradoxical hypertension. Totazoline administration has yielded inconsistent results and is not recommended as first-line therapy. Dialysis is not likely to significantly enhance the elimination of clonidine.

Patient Information

Patients should be cautioned against interruption of clonidine transdermal therapy without their physician's advice.

Patients who engage in potentially hazardous activities, such as operating machinery or driving, should be advised of a possible sedative effect of clonidine. They should also be informed that this sedative effect may be increased by concomitant use of alcohol, barbiturates, or other sedating drugs.

Patients should be instructed to consult their physicians promptly about the possible need to remove the patch if they observe moderate to severe localized erythema or vesicle formation at the site of application or generalized skin rash.

If a patient experiences isolated, mild localized skin irritation before completing 7 days of use, the system may be removed and replaced with a new system applied to a fresh skin site.

If the system should begin to loosen from the skin after application, the patient should be instructed to place the adhesive overlay directly over the system to ensure adhesion during its 7-day use.

Used clonidine transdermal patches contain a substantial amount of their initial drug content which may be harmful to infants and children if accidentally applied or ingested. Therefore, patients should be cautioned to keep both used and unused clonidine transdermal patches out of the reach of children. After use, clonidine transdermal should be folded in half with the adhesive sides together and discarded away from children's reach.

Instructions for use, storage and disposal of the system are provided in each box of clonidine transdermal.

GUANFACINE

Rx	**Guanfacine Hydrochloride** (Various, eg, Amneal Pharmaceuticals, Watson Pharma)	**Tablets; oral:** 1 mg	As guanfacine hydrochloride. May contain lactose. In 100s and 500s.
Rx	**Tenex** (Promius Pharma)		As guanfacine hydrochloride. Lactose. (1 RP Tenex). Light pink, diamond shape. In 100s and 500s.
Rx	**Guanfacine Hydrochloride** (Various, eg, Amneal Pharmaceuticals, Watson Pharma)	**Tablets; oral:** 2 mg	As guanfacine hydrochloride. May contain lactose. In 100s and 500s.
Rx	**Tenex** (Promius Pharma)		As guanfacine hydrochloride. Lactose. (2 RP Tenex). Yellow, diamond shape. In 100s.
Rx	**Intuniv** (Shire)	**Tablets, extended-release; oral:** 1 mg	As guanfacine hydrochloride. Lactose. (503/1mg). White, round. In 100s.
		2 mg	As guanfacine hydrochloride. Lactose. (503/2mg). White, capsule shape. In 100s.
		3 mg	As guanfacine hydrochloride. Lactose. (503/3mg). Green, round. In 100s.
		4 mg	As guanfacine hydrochloride. Lactose. (503/4mg). Green, capsule shape. In 100s.

GUANFACINE HYDROCHLORIDE — ORAL

Indications

➤*Attention deficit hyperactivity disorder (extended-release only):* For the treatment of attention deficit hyperactivity disorder (ADHD) as monotherapy and as adjunctive therapy to stimulant medications.

➤*Hypertension (excluding extended-release):* Management of hypertension. Guanfacine may be given alone or in combination with other antihypertensive agents, especially thiazide-type diuretics.

➤*Off-label uses:*

Tourette syndrome (children/adolescents) – [2] = Fair documentation. Although most trials evaluating the use of guanfacine in the treatment of Tourette syndrome showed benefit, 1 double-blind, controlled trial showed no benefit. This could have been attributed to a lower dose and shorter treatment period. Some trials have shown a significant improvement. (See Administration and Dosage.)

Other possible off-label uses – Guanfacine (0.03 to 1.5 mg/day) may be beneficial in ameliorating withdrawal symptoms when discontinuing heroin usage.

In a small study, guanfacine (1 mg/day for 12 weeks) significantly reduced the frequency of migraine headache and reduced nausea and vomiting.

Administration and Dosage

➤*General dosing considerations:* The frequency of rebound hypertension is low but can occur 2 to 4 days after withdrawal of the drug. In most cases, blood pressure returns to pretreatment levels slowly (within 2 to 4 days), without ill effects.

Do not substitute guanfacine extended-release (ER) for guanfacine immediate-release tablets on a mg-per-mg basis because of differing pharmacokinetic profiles.

➤*Adults:*

Hypertension (excluding guanfacine extended-release) –

Initial dosage: 1 mg daily given at bedtime, alone or in combination with another antihypertensive drug.

Dosage adjustment: If after 3 to 4 weeks of therapy, 1 mg does not give a satisfactory result, a dose of 2 mg may be given; although, most of the effect of guanfacine is seen at 1 mg. Higher daily doses have been used, but adverse reactions increase significantly with dosages above 3 mg/day.

➤*Children:*

Attention deficit hyperactivity disorder (extended-release only) –

6 to 17 years of age:

- *Initial dosage* – 1 mg/day.
- *Dosage titration* – Adjust in increments of no more than 1 mg/wk for both monotherapy and adjunctive therapy to a psychostimulant.
- *Maintenance dosage* – 1 to 4 mg once daily, depending on clinical response and tolerability for both monotherapy and adjunctive therapy to a psychostimulant.
- *Alternative dosage* – 0.05 to 0.08 mg/kg once daily showed clinically relevant improvements in monotherapy trials. Efficacy increased with increasing weight-adjusted dose (mg/kg). If well tolerated, dosages of up to 0.12 mg/kg once daily may provide additional benefit. Dosages of more than 4 mg/day have not been studied.

  In the adjunctive trial, the majority of subjects reached optimal dosages in the 0.05 to 0.12 mg/kg/day range.
- *Conversion* – If switching from immediate-release guanfacine, discontinue that treatment, and titrate with guanfacine ER 1 mg/day.
- *Discontinuation of therapy* – The dose should generally be tapered in decrements of no more than 1 mg every 3 to 7 days.

GUANFACINE HYDROCHLORIDE — ORAL

• *Missed dose* – When reinitiating patients on guanfacine ER to the previous maintenance dose after 2 or more missed consecutive doses, health care providers should consider titration based on patient tolerability.

Off-label dosing –

Tourette syndrome (children/adolescents): [2] = Fair documentation.

➤*Renal function impairment:*

Immediate-release – When prescribing for patients with renal impairment, the low end of the dosing range should be used. Patients on dialysis also can be given usual doses of guanfacine because the drug is poorly dialyzed.

Extended-release – It may be necessary to adjust the dose in patients with significant renal impairment.

➤*Hepatic function impairment:*

Extended-release – It may be necessary to adjust the dose in patients with significant hepatic impairment.

➤*Administration:* Administer guanfacine immediate-release at bedtime to minimize somnolence.

Guanfacine ER should be dosed once daily. Tablets should not be crushed, chewed, or broken before swallowing because this will increase the rate of guanfacine release. Do not administer with high fat meal because of increased exposure.

➤*Storage/Stability:* Store guanfacine immediate-release at 20° to 25°C (68° to 77°F). Dispense in tight, light-resistant container. Store guanfacine ER tablets at 25°C (77°F); excursions are permitted to 15° to 30°C (59° to 86°F).

Actions

➤*Pharmacology:*

ADHD – Guanfacine is a selective alpha-2A adrenergic receptor agonist. Guanfacine is not a CNS stimulant. The mechanism of action of guanfacine in ADHD is unknown.

Hypertension – Guanfacine is an orally active antihypertensive agent whose principal mechanism of action appears to be stimulation of central alpha-2 adrenergic receptors. By stimulating these receptors, guanfacine reduces sympathetic nerve impulses from the vasomotor center to the heart and blood vessels. This results in a decrease in peripheral vascular resistance and a reduction in heart rate.

➤*Pharmacokinetics:*

Absorption/Distribution –

Immediate-release: The drug is approximately 70% bound to plasma proteins, independent of drug concentration.

Relative to an intravenous (IV) dose of 3 mg, the absolute oral bioavailability of guanfacine is about 80%. Peak plasma concentrations occur from 1 to 4 hours with an average of 2.6 hours after single oral doses or at steady state.

The area under the curve (AUC) increases linearly with the dose.

The whole body volume of distribution is high (a mean of 6.3 L/kg), which suggests a high distribution of drug to the tissues.

Extended-release: After oral administration of guanfacine ER, the time to peak plasma concentration is approximately 5 hours in children and adolescents with ADHD. Following administration of guanfacine ER in single doses of 1, 2, 3, and 4 mg to adults, maximal drug concentration (C_{max}) and $AUC_{0-\infty}$ of guanfacine were proportional to dose.

A comparison across studies suggests that the C_{max} is 60% lower and $AUC_{0-\infty}$ 43% lower, respectively, for guanfacine ER compared with guanfacine immediate-release. Therefore, the relative bioavailability of guanfacine ER to guanfacine immediate-release is 58%.

Guanfacine Pharmacokinetic Parameters in Adults[a]

Parameter	Guanfacine ER 1 mg once daily (n = 52)	Guanfacine immediate-release 1 mg once daily (n = 12)
C_{max} (ng•mL)	1 ± 0.3	2.5 ± 0.6
$AUC_{0-\infty}$ (ng•h/mL)	32 ± 9	56 ± 15
T_{max} (h)	6 (4 to 8)	3 (1.5 to 4)
Half-life (h)	18 ± 4	16 ± 3

[a] Values are mean ± standard deviation (SD), except for time to reach maximum concentration (T_{max}), which is median (range).

• *Effect of food* – The pharmacokinetics were affected by intake of food when a single dose of guanfacine ER 4 mg was administered with a high-fat breakfast. The mean exposure increased (C_{max} approximately 75% and AUC approximately 40%) compared with dosing in a fasted state.

Metabolism/Excretion –

Immediate-release: In patients with healthy renal function, the average elimination half-life is approximately 17 hours (range, 10 to 30 hours). Younger patients tend to have shorter elimination half-lives (13 to 14 hours), while older patients tend to have half-lives at the upper end of the range. Steady-state blood levels were attained within 4 days in most subjects.

In patients with healthy renal function, guanfacine and its metabolites are excreted primarily in the urine. Approximately 50% (40% to 75%) of the dose is eliminated in the urine as unchanged drug; the remainder is eliminated mostly as conjugates of metabolites produced by oxidative metabolism of the aromatic ring.

The guanfacine-to-creatinine clearance ratio is greater than 1, which would suggest that tubular secretion of drug occurs.

Extended-release: In vitro studies with human liver microsomes and recombinant CYPs demonstrated that guanfacine was primarily metabolized by CYP3A4. Guanfacine is a substrate of CYP3A4/5 and exposure is affected by CYP3A4/5 inducers/inhibitors.

Special populations –

Renal function impairment:

• *Immediate-release* – The clearance of guanfacine in patients with varying degrees of renal insufficiency is reduced, but plasma levels of drug are only slightly increased compared with patients with healthy renal function. When prescribing for patients with renal impairment, use the low end of the dosing range. Patients on dialysis also can be given usual doses of guanfacine as the drug is poorly dialyzed.

Children: Exposure to guanfacine was higher in children (6 to 12 years of age) compared with adolescents (13 to 17 years of age) and adults. After oral administration of multiple doses of guanfacine ER 4 mg, the C_{max} was 10 ng/mL compared with 7 ng/mL and the AUC was 162 ng•h/mL compared with 116 ng•h/mL in children (6 to 12 years of age) and adolescents (13 to 17 years of age), respectively. These differences are probably attributable to the lower body weight of children compared with adolescents and adults.

Contraindications

Hypersensitivity to guanfacine or any components of the product(s).

Warnings/Precautions

➤*Cardiovascular effects:* Treatment of ADHD with guanfacine ER can cause decreases in blood pressure and heart rate. In the pediatric, short-term (8 to 9 weeks), controlled trials, the maximum mean changes from baseline in systolic blood pressure, diastolic blood pressure, and pulse were −5 mm Hg, −3 mm Hg, and −6 beats/min, respectively, for all dose groups combined (generally 1 week after reaching target dosages of 1, 2, 3, or 4 mg/day). These changes were dose dependent. Decreases in blood pressure and heart rate were usually modest and asymptomatic; however, hypotension and bradycardia can occur. Hypotension was reported as an adverse event for 6% of the guanfacine ER group and 4% of the placebo group. Orthostatic hypotension was reported for 1% of the guanfacine ER group and none in the placebo group. In long-term, open-label studies (mean exposure of approximately 10 months), maximum decreases in systolic and diastolic blood pressure occurred in the first month of therapy. Decreases were less pronounced over time. Syncope occurred in 1% of pediatric subjects in the clinical program. The majority of these cases occurred in the long-term, open-label studies.

Measure heart rate and blood pressure prior to initiation of therapy, following dose increases, and periodically while on therapy. Use guanfacine ER with caution in patients with a history of hypotension, heart block, bradycardia, or cardiovascular disease, because it can decrease blood pressure and heart rate. Use caution in treating patients who have a history of syncope or may have a condition that predisposes them to syncope, such as hypotension, orthostatic hypotension, bradycardia, or dehydration. Use guanfacine ER with caution in patients treated concomitantly with antihypertensives or other drugs that can reduce blood pressure or heart rate or increase the risk of syncope. Advise patients to avoid becoming dehydrated or overheated.

➤*Sedation:* Guanfacine, like other orally active central alpha-2 adrenergic agonists, causes sedation or drowsiness, especially when beginning therapy. These symptoms are dose related. When guanfacine is used with other centrally active depressants (eg, barbiturates, benzodiazepines, phenothiazines), consider the potential for additive sedative effects. Advise patients to avoid use with alcohol.

➤*Rebound:* Abrupt cessation of therapy with orally active central alpha-2 adrenergic agonists may be associated with increases (from depressed on-therapy levels) in plasma and urinary catecholamines, symptoms of "nervousness and anxiety," and, less commonly, increases in blood pressure to levels significantly higher than those prior to therapy.

➤*Renal function impairment:* In adult patients with impaired renal function, the cumulative urinary excretion of guanfacine and the renal clearance diminished as renal function decreased. In patients on hemodialysis, the dialysis clearance was about 15% of the total clearance. The low dialysis clearance suggests that the hepatic elimination (metabolism) increases as renal function decreases. It may be necessary to adjust the dose in patients with significant renal function impairment.

➤*Hepatic function impairment:* Guanfacine in adults is cleared by the liver and the kidney, and approximately 50% of the clearance of guanfacine is hepatic. It may be necessary to adjust the dose in patients with significant hepatic function impairment.

➤*Special risk:* Like other antihypertensive agents, use guanfacine immediate-release with caution in patients with severe coronary insufficiency, recent myocardial infarction, cerebrovascular disease, or chronic renal or hepatic failure.

➤*Hazardous tasks:* Advise patients who receive guanfacine to exercise caution when operating dangerous machinery or driving motor vehicles until it is determined that they do not become drowsy or dizzy from the medication.

➤*Pregnancy:* Category B. Higher doses (100 and 200 times the MRHD in rabbits and rats, respectively) were associated with reduced fetal survival and maternal toxicity. Rat experiments have shown that guanfacine crosses the placenta.

GUANFACINE HYDROCHLORIDE — ORAL

However, there are no adequate and well-controlled studies in pregnant women. Because animal reproduction studies are not always predictive of human response, use this drug during pregnancy only if clearly needed.

Labor and delivery – Guanfacine immediate-release is not recommended in the treatment of acute hypertension associated with toxemia of pregnancy. There is no information available on the effects of guanfacine on the course of labor and delivery.

➤*Lactation:* It is not known whether guanfacine is excreted in human milk. Experiments with rats have shown that guanfacine is excreted in milk. The molecular weight (about 247 for the free base) is low enough that excretion into human milk should be expected. Because many drugs are excreted in human milk, exercise caution when guanfacine is administered to a breast-feeding woman.

➤*Children:*

Immediate-release – Safety and efficacy of guanfacine immediate-release in children younger than 12 years of age have not been demonstrated; use in this age group is not recommended.

There have been spontaneous postmarketing reports of mania and aggressive behavioral changes in children with ADHD receiving guanfacine immediate-release. The reported cases were from a single center. All patients had medical or family risk factors for bipolar disorder. All patients recovered upon discontinuation of guanfacine immediate-release.

Extended-release – The safety and efficacy of guanfacine extended-release in children younger than 6 years of age have not been established. For children and adolescents 6 years of age and older, efficacy past 9 weeks and safety past 2 years of treatment have not been established.

➤*Elderly:* In general, dose selection of guanfacine immediate-release for an elderly patient should be cautious, usually starting at the low end of the dosing range, reflecting the greater frequency of decreased hepatic, renal, or cardiac function, and of concomitant disease or other drug therapy.

➤*Monitoring:* When treating ADHD with guanfacine ER, measure heart rate and blood pressure prior to initiation of therapy, following dose increases, and periodically while on therapy.

Drug Interactions

➤*CYP-450 system:* Because guanfacine is metabolized mainly by the CYP3A enzyme systems, substances known to inhibit these enzymes may decrease metabolism or increase bioavailability of guanfacine, as indicated by increased plasma concentrations. Drugs known to induce these enzyme systems may result in an increased metabolism of guanfacine or decreased bioavailability, as indicated by decreased plasma concentrations. Monitoring of plasma concentrations and appropriate dosage adjustments are essential when such drugs are used concomitantly.

Guanfacine Drug Interactions

Precipitant drug	Object drug[a]		Description
Alpha-2 adrenergic agonists (eg, tizanidine)	Guanfacine	↑	Additive hypotension effects may occur. Avoid coadministration. If concurrent use cannot be avoided, closely monitor for signs of hypotension.
Guanfacine	Alpha-2 adrenergic agonists (eg, tizanidine)		
Antihypertensive agents or other drugs that can reduce blood pressure, decrease heart rate, or increase risk of syncope	Guanfacine	↑	Pharmacodynamic effects may be additive (eg, hypotension, syncope).
Guanfacine	Antihypertensive agents or other drugs that can reduce blood pressure, decrease heart rate, or increase risk of syncope		
CNS depressants (eg, alcohol, antipsychotics, benzodiazepines [eg, diazepam], sedative/ hypnotics [eg, phenobarbital])	Guanfacine	↑	Pharmacodynamic effects may be additive (eg, sedation, somnolence). Avoid coadministration.
Guanfacine	CNS depressants (eg, alcohol, antipsychotics [eg, chlorpromazine], benzodiazepines [eg, diazepam], sedative/ hypnotics [eg, phenobarbital], tricyclic antidepressants [eg, amitriptyline])		
CYP3A4 inducers (eg, phenobarbital, phenytoin, rifampin)	Guanfacine	↓	Guanfacine plasma concentrations may be reduced, decreasing the efficacy. Monitor the response of the patient. Consider increasing the guanfacine dose within the recommended dose range. Coadministration of rifampin reduced guanfacine exposure 70%.
CYP3A4/5 strong inhibitors (eg, ketoconazole)	Guanfacine	↑	Guanfacine plasma concentrations may be elevated, increasing the pharmacologic effects and risk of adverse reactions. Coadministration of ketoconazole increased guanfacine exposure 3-fold. Monitor the response of the patient and adjust the guanfacine dose as needed.
Tricyclic antidepressants (eg, amitriptyline)	Guanfacine	↓	The antihypertensive effect of guanfacine may be decreased. Carefully monitor blood pressure during coadministration and when stopping tricyclic antidepressants. Adjust the guanfacine dose as needed.
Valproic acid	Guanfacine	↑	Valproic acid plasma concentrations may be elevated. Consider monitoring valproic acid concentrations and observing the patient for additive CNS effects (eg, sedation). Adjust the valproic acid dose as needed.
Guanfacine	Valproic acid		

[a] ↑ = object drug increased; ↓ = object drug decreased.

➤*Drug/Food interactions:* Taking guanfacine with high-fat meals increases drug exposure compared with dosing in a fasted state. Do not administer guanfacine with high-fat meals.

Adverse Reactions

➤*Immediate-release:* The following adverse reactions noted with guanfacine are similar to those of other drugs of the central alpha-2 adrenoreceptor agonist class: constipation, dizziness, dry mouth, impotence, sedation (somnolence), and weakness (asthenia). While the reactions are common, most are mild and tend to disappear on continued dosing.

Skin rash with exfoliation has been reported in a few cases; although clear cause-and-effect relationships to guanfacine could not be established, if a rash occurs, discontinue guanfacine and appropriately monitor the patient.

Guanfacine Dose-Response Monotherapy Study

Adverse reactions	0.5 mg (n = 60)	1 mg (n = 61)	2 mg (n = 60)	3 mg (n = 59)	Placebo (n = 59)
CNS					
Asthenia	2%	3%	7%	3%	0%
Dizziness	12%	2%	8%	15%	8%
Fatigue	2%	5%	8%	10%	2%
Headache	13%	7%	5%	3%	8%
Somnolence	5%	10%	13%	39%	8%

GUANFACINE HYDROCHLORIDE — ORAL

Guanfacine Dose-Response Monotherapy Study					
Adverse reactions	0.5 mg (n = 60)	1 mg (n = 61)	2 mg (n = 60)	3 mg (n = 59)	Placebo (n = 59)
GI					
Constipation	2%	0%	5%	15%	0%
Dry mouth	10%	10%	42%	54%	0%
Miscellaneous					
Impotence	0%	0%	7%	3%	0%

Discontinuation of therapy –

Guanfacine Monotherapy Dropout Rates Due to Adverse Reactions by Dosage Group					
	0.5 mg	1 mg	2 mg	3 mg	Placebo
Percent dropouts	2%	5%	13%	32%	0%

The most common reasons for dropouts among patients who received guanfacine were constipation, dizziness, dry mouth, fatigue, somnolence, and weakness.

Combination therapy with chlorthalidone –

Guanfacine/Chlorthalidone Dose-Response Study					
Adverse reactions	0.5 mg (n = 72)	1 mg (n = 72)	2 mg (n = 72)	3 mg (n = 72)	Placebo (n = 73)
CNS					
Asthenia	3%	0%	2%	10%	0%
Dizziness	1%	4%	8%	4%	2%
Fatigue	3%	3%	6%	4%	3%
Headache	3%	4%	1%	2%	4%
Somnolence	4%	0%	1%	14%	1%
GI					
Constipation	0%	0%	1%	1%	0%
Dry mouth	5%	8%	11%	28%	7%
Miscellaneous					
Impotence	0%	0%	1%	4%	1%

In a second 12-week, placebo-controlled, combination therapy study in which the dose could be adjusted upward to 3 mg/day in 1 mg increments at 3-week intervals (ie, a setting more similar to ordinary clinical use), the most commonly recorded reactions were dry mouth (47%), constipation (16%), fatigue (12%), somnolence (10%), asthenia (6%), dizziness (6%), headache (4%), and insomnia (4%).

Discontinuation of therapy:

Guanfacine/Chlorthalidone Dropout Rates Due to Adverse Reactions by Guanfacine Dosage Group					
	0.5 mg	1 mg	2 mg	3 mg	Placebo
Percent dropouts	4.2%	3.2%	6.9%	8.3%	6.9%

Reasons for dropouts among patients who received guanfacine were conjunctivitis, constipation, dermatitis, dizziness, dry mouth, headache, impotence, insomnia, paresthesia, somnolence, syncope, urinary incontinence, and weakness.

Reasons for dropouts in the second trial among patients who received guanfacine were confusion, constipation, depression, dizziness, dry mouth, impotence, palpitations, and somnolence.

Comparison with clonidine –

Guanfacine vs Clonidine Adverse Reactions		
Adverse reactions	Guanfacine (n = 279)	Clonidine (n = 278)
CNS		
Dizziness	11%	8%
Fatigue	9%	8%
Headache	4%	4%
Insomnia	4%	3%
Somnolence	21%	35%
GI		
Constipation	10%	5%
Dry mouth	30%	37%

Combination therapy with a diuretic – Adverse reactions occurring in 3% or less of patients in the 3 controlled trials of guanfacine with a diuretic were the following:

Cardiovascular: Bradycardia, palpitations, substernal pain.

CNS: Amnesia, confusion, depression, insomnia, libido decrease, malaise, paresthesia, paresis.

Dermatologic: Dermatitis, pruritus, purpura, sweating.

GI: Abdominal pain, diarrhea, dyspepsia, dysphagia, nausea.

GU: Testicular disorder, urinary incontinence.

Musculoskeletal: Leg cramps, hypokinesia.

Ophthalmic: Conjunctivitis, iritis, vision disturbance.

Respiratory: Dyspnea, rhinitis.

Special senses: Taste perversion, tinnitus.

Adverse reactions in an open-label trial of 1 year –

Guanfacine Adverse Reactions		
Adverse reactions	Incidence of adverse reactions at any time during the study (n = 580)	Incidence of adverse reactions at end of 1 year (n = 580)
CNS		
Dizziness	15%	1%
Drowsiness	33%	6%
Headache	4%	0.2%
Insomnia	5%	0%
Weakness	5%	1%
GI		
Constipation	14%	3%
Dry mouth	60%	15%

Discontinuation of therapy: There were 52 (8.9%) dropouts caused by adverse effects in this 1-year trial. The causes were as follows: constipation (n = 7), depression (n = 1), dry mouth (n = 20), headache (n = 1), insomnia (n = 1), nausea (n = 3), orthostatic hypotension (n = 2), nightmares (n = 1), rash (n = 1), somnolence (n = 3), and weakness (n = 12).

➤*Extended-release:*

Discontinuation of therapy – Twelve percent of patients taking guanfacine ER discontinued from the clinical studies because of adverse reactions compared with 4% in the placebo group. The most common adverse reactions leading to discontinuation of guanfacine ER-treated patients from the studies were fatigue (2%) and somnolence/sedation (6%). Less common adverse reactions leading to discontinuation (occurring in approximately 1% of patients) included dizziness, headache, and hypotension/decreased blood pressure.

Eighteen percent of patients receiving guanfacine ER discontinued from long-term studies because of adverse reactions. The most frequent adverse reactions leading to discontinuation (2% or more) were depression (2%), fatigue (2%), increased weight (2%), somnolence (3%), and syncopal events (2%). Other adverse reactions leading to discontinuation in the long-term studies (occurring in approximately 1% of patients) included headache, hypotension/decreased blood pressure, lethargy, and sedation.

Dose-related adverse reactions – Adverse reactions that were dose-related included abdominal pain, constipation, dizziness, dry mouth, hypotension/decreased blood pressure, sedation, and somnolence.

Common adverse reactions –

Guanfacine ER Adverse Reactions in Short-Term Studies 1 and 2 (≥ 2%)		
Adverse reactions	All doses of guanfacine ER (n = 513)	Placebo (n = 149)
CNS		
Dizziness	6%	4%
Fatigue	14%	3%
Headache	24%	19%
Irritability	6%	4%
Lethargy	6%	3%
Somnolence[a]	38%	12%
GI		
Abdominal pain (upper)	10%	7%
Constipation	3%	1%
Dry mouth	4%	1%
Nausea	6%	2%
Miscellaneous		
Decreased appetite	5%	3%
Hypotension/Decreased blood pressure	6%	4%

[a] The somnolence term includes hypersomnia, sedation, and somnolence.

GUANFACINE HYDROCHLORIDE — ORAL

Guanfacine ER Adverse Reactions During Long-Term Follow-Up Studies (≥ 5%)	
Adverse reactions	All doses of guanfacine ER (n = 446)
CNS	
Dizziness	7%
Fatigue	15%
Headache	26%
Irritability	6%
Somnolence[a]	45%
GI	
Abdominal pain (upper)	11%
Nausea	7%
Vomiting	9%
Miscellaneous	
Hypotension/Decreased blood pressure	10%
Weight increased	7%

[a] The somnolence term includes somnolence, sedation, and hypersomnia.

Other short-term treatment adverse reactions (less than 2%) –
Cardiovascular: Atrioventricular block, bradycardia, increased blood pressure, orthostatic hypotension, sinus arrhythmia.
CNS: Asthenia, postural dizziness.
GU: Enuresis, increased urinary frequency.
Hepatic: Increased ALT.
Miscellaneous: Asthma, chest pain, dyspepsia, increased weight, pallor.

In addition, the following less common (less than 2%) psychiatric disorders occurred in more than 1 patient receiving guanfacine ER and were more common than in the placebo group. The relationship to guanfacine ER could not be determined because these events may also occur as symptoms in pediatric patients with ADHD: agitation, anxiety, depression, emotional lability, interrupted sleep, nightmares.

Long-term treatment adverse reactions: Adverse reactions that occurred in less than 5% of patients but 2% or more in open-label, long-term studies that are considered possibly related to guanfacine ER include constipation, decreased appetite, diarrhea, dry mouth, hypertension/increased blood pressure, insomnia, lethargy, stomach discomfort, and syncopal events.

Serious adverse reactions – In long-term, open-label studies, serious adverse reactions occurring in more than 1 patient were convulsion (0.4%) and syncope (2%).

Effects on height, weight, and body mass index – Patients taking guanfacine ER demonstrated similar growth compared with normative data. Patients taking guanfacine ER had a mean increase in weight of 1 kg (2 lb) compared with those receiving placebo over a comparative treatment period. Patients receiving guanfacine ER for at least 12 months in open-label studies gained an average of 8 kg (17 lb) in weight and 8 cm (3 in) in height. The height, weight, and body mass index percentile remained stable in patients at 12 months in the long-term studies compared with when they began receiving guanfacine ER.

➤*Effects on heart rate and QT interval:* The effect of 2 dose levels of immediate-release guanfacine (4 and 8 mg) on the QT interval was evaluated in a double-blind, randomized, placebo- and active-controlled, crossover study in healthy adults.

A dose-dependent decrease in heart rate was observed during the first 12 hours, at time of maximal concentrations. The mean change in heart rate was −13 beats/min at 4 mg and −22 beats/min at 8 mg.

An apparent increase in mean QTc was observed for both doses. However, guanfacine does not appear to interfere with cardiac repolarization of the form associated with proarrhythmic drugs. This finding has no known clinical relevance.

➤*Postmarketing (immediate-release):* An open-label postmarketing study involving 21,718 patients was conducted to assess the safety of guanfacine immediate-release 1 mg/day given at bedtime for 28 days. Guanfacine was administered with or without other antihypertensive agents. Adverse reactions reported in the postmarketing study at an incidence of more than 1% included dizziness, dry mouth, fatigue, headache, nausea, and somnolence. The most commonly reported adverse reactions in this study were the same as those observed in controlled clinical trials.

Less frequent, possibly guanfacine immediate-release–related reactions observed in the postmarketing study or reported spontaneously include the following:

Cardiovascular – Bradycardia, palpitations, syncope, tachycardia.

CNS – Agitation, anxiety, asthenia, confusion, depression, insomnia, malaise, nervousness, paresthesias, tremor, vertigo.

Dermatologic – Alopecia, dermatitis, exfoliative dermatitis, pruritus, rash.

GI – Abdominal pain, constipation, diarrhea, dyspepsia.

GU – Impotence, nocturia, urinary frequency.

Hepatic – Abnormal liver function tests.

Musculoskeletal – Arthralgia, leg cramps, leg pain, myalgia.

Miscellaneous – Alterations in taste, blurred vision, chest pain, dyspnea, edema.

Rare, serious disorders – Rare, serious disorders with no definitive cause and effect relationship to guanfacine have been reported spontaneously or in the postmarketing study. These events include acute renal failure, cardiac fibrillation, cerebrovascular accident, congestive heart failure, heart block, and myocardial infarction.

Overdosage

➤*Symptoms:*

Immediate-release – Bradycardia, drowsiness, hypotension, and lethargy have been observed following overdose with guanfacine. Similar symptoms have been described in voluntary reports to the American Association of Poison Control Center's National Poison Data System. Miosis of the pupils may be noted on examination. No fatal overdoses of guanfacine have been reported in published literature.

A 25-year-old woman intentionally ingested 60 mg. She presented with severe drowsiness and bradycardia of 45 beats/min. Gastric lavage was performed and an infusion of isoproterenol (0.8 mg in 12 hours) was administered. She recovered quickly and without sequelae.

A 28-year-old woman who ingested 30 to 40 mg developed only lethargy, was treated with activated charcoal and a cathartic, was monitored for 24 hours, and was discharged in good health.

A 2-year-old male weighing 12 kg, who ingested up to 4 mg of guanfacine, developed lethargy. Gastric lavage (followed by activated charcoal and sorbitol slurry via nasogastric tube) removed some tablet fragments within 2 hours after ingestion, and vital signs were normal. During 24-hour observation in the intensive care unit, systolic pressure was 58 and heart rate 70 at 16 hours postingestion. No intervention was required, and the child was discharged fully recovered the next day.

Extended-release – Two cases of accidental overdose of guanfacine ER were reported in clinical trials in pediatric ADHD patients. These reports included adverse reactions of bradycardia and sedation in one patient and dizziness and somnolence in the other patient.

➤*Treatment:* Consult a certified poison control center for up to date guidance and advice. Gastric lavage may be indicated if performed soon after ingestion. Activated charcoal may be useful in limiting absorption. Guanfacine is not dialyzable in clinically significant amounts (2.4%).

Management of guanfacine overdose should include monitoring for and the treatment of bradycardia, hypotension, lethargy, and respiratory depression. Observe patients who develop lethargy for the development of more serious toxicity, including coma, bradycardia, and hypotension for up to 24 hours, because of the possibility of delayed onset hypotension.

Patient Information

Instruct patients to swallow guanfacine ER whole with water, milk, or other liquid. Tablets should not be crushed, chewed, or broken prior to administration because this may increase the rate of release of the active drug.

Instruct patients not to take guanfacine ER with a high-fat meal, because this can raise blood levels of guanfacine ER.

Instruct the parent or caregiver to supervise the child or adolescent taking guanfacine ER and to keep the bottle of tablets out of the reach of children.

Instruct patients on how to properly taper the medication, if the health care provider decides to discontinue treatment.

Advise patients that sedation can occur, particularly early in treatment or with dose increases. Caution against operating heavy equipment or driving until they know how they respond to treatment with guanfacine. Headache and abdominal pain can also occur. If any of these symptoms persist, or other symptoms occur, advise the patient to discuss the symptoms with the health care provider.

Advise patients to avoid becoming dehydrated or overheated, and to avoid use with alcohol.

Inform patients that guanfacine immediate-release and guanfacine ER contain the same active ingredient (guanfacine) and that the 2 should not be used in combination.

GUANABENZ ACETATE

Rx	**Guanabenz Acetate** (Various, eg, Ivax, Watson)	**Tablets:** 4 mg	In 100s and 500s.
Rx	**Wytensin** (Wyeth-Ayerst)		(Wyeth 73/W4). Orange. In 100s, 500s and Redipak 100s.
Rx	**Guanabenz Acetate** (Various, eg, Ivax, Watson)	8 mg	In 100s and 500s.
Rx	**Wytensin** (Wyeth-Ayerst)		(Wyeth 74/W8). Gray, scored. In 100s.

GUANABENZ ACETATE — ORAL

Indications

➤*Hypertension:* Treatment of hypertension. It may be employed alone or in combination with a thiazide diuretic.

Administration and Dosage

➤*General dosing considerations:* Dosage with guanabenz acetate tablets should be individualized.

➤*Adults:*

Hypertension –

Maximum dose: 32 mg twice daily, but doses as high as this are rarely needed.

Initial dosage: A starting dose of 4 mg orally twice per day is recommended, whether guanabenz is used alone or with a thiazide diuretic.

Dosage adjustment: Dosage may be increased in increments of 4 to 8 mg/day every 1 to 2 weeks, depending on the patient's response.

➤*Storage/Stability:* Store at 20° to 25°C (68° to 77°F).

Actions

➤*Pharmacology:* Guanabenz acetate is an orally active central alpha-2-adrenergic agonist. Its antihypertensive action appears to be mediated via stimulation of central alpha adrenergic receptors, resulting in a decrease of sympathetic outflow from the brain at the bulbar level to the peripheral circulatory system.

➤*Pharmacokinetics:* In human studies, approximately 75% of an orally administered dose of guanabenz acetate is absorbed and metabolized with less than 1% of unchanged drug recovered from the urine. Peak plasma concentrations of unchanged drug occur between 2 and 5 hours after a single oral dose. The average half-life for guanabenz is approximately 6 hours. The site or sites of metabolism of guanabenz have not been determined. The effect of meals on the absorption of guanabenz acetate tablets has not been studied.

Contraindications

Sensitivity to the drug.

Warnings/Precautions

➤*Sedation:* Guanabenz causes sedation or drowsiness in a large fraction of patients. When guanabenz is used with centrally-active depressants, such as phenothiazines, barbiturates, and benzodiazepines, the potential for additive sedative effects should be considered.

➤*Vascular insufficiency:* Guanabenz, like other antihypertensive agents, should be used with caution in patients with severe coronary insufficiency, recent MI, cerebrovascular disease, or severe hepatic or renal failure.

➤*Rebound:* Sudden cessation of therapy with central alpha agonists like guanabenz may rarely result in "overshoot" hypertension and more commonly produces an increase in serum catecholamines and subjective symptomatology.

➤*Renal function impairment:* The disposition of orally administered guanabenz acetate is altered modestly in patients with renal impairment. Guanabenz half-life is prolonged and clearance decreased, more so in patients on hemodialysis. The clinical significance of these findings is unknown.

➤*Hazardous tasks:* Patients who receive guanabenz should be advised to exercise caution when operating dangerous machinery or driving motor vehicles until it is determined that they do not become drowsy or dizzy from the medication (see Patient Information).

➤*Pregnancy: Category C.*

Teratogenic – Guanabenz acetate may have adverse effects on the fetus when administered to pregnant women. A teratology study in mice has indicated a possible increase in skeletal abnormalities when guanabenz acetate is given orally at doses of 3 to 6 times the maximum recommended human dose of 1 mg/kg. These abnormalities, principally costal and vertebral, were not noted in similar studies in rats and rabbits. However, increased fetal loss has been observed after oral guanabenz acetate administration to pregnant rats (14 mg/kg) and rabbits (20 mg/kg). Reproductive studies of guanabenz in rats have shown slightly decreased live-birth indices, decreased fetal survival rate, and decreased pup body weight at oral doses of 6.4 and 9.6 mg/kg. There are no adequate, well-controlled studies in pregnant women. Guanabenz should be used during pregnancy only if the potential benefit justifies the potential risk to the fetus.

➤*Lactation:* Because no information is available on the excretion of guanabenz in human milk, it should not be administered to breast-feeding mothers.

➤*Children:* The safety and efficacy of guanabenz acetate in children younger than 12 years of age have not been demonstrated. Therefore, its use in this age group cannot be recommended at this time.

➤*Monitoring:* Careful monitoring of blood pressure during guanabenz dose titration is suggested in patients with coexisting hypertension, coexisting chronic hepatic dysfunction, or renal impairment.

Drug Interactions

Guanabenz has not been demonstrated to cause any drug interactions when administered with other drugs, such as digitalis, diuretics, analgesics, anxiolytics, and anti-inflammatory or anti-infective agents, in clinical trials. However, the potential for increased sedation when guanabenz is administered concomitantly with CNS-depressant drugs should be noted.

Adverse Reactions

The following table shows the incidence of adverse effects, occurring in 5% or more of patients in a study comparing guanabenz acetate to placebo, at a starting dose of 8 mg twice daily.

Most Common Guanabenz Adverse Reactions

Adverse reactions	Placebo (n = 102)	Guanabenz acetate (n = 109)
Dizziness	7%	17%
Drowsiness or sedation	12%	39%
Dry mouth	7%	28%
Headache	6%	5%
Weakness	7%	10%

In other controlled clinical trials at the starting dose of 16 mg/day in 476 patients, the incidence of dry mouth was slightly higher (38%) and that of dizziness was slightly lower (12%), but the incidence of the most frequent adverse effects was similar to the placebo-controlled trial.

Although these side effects were not serious, they led to discontinuation of treatment approximately 15% of the time. In more recent studies using an initial dose of 8 mg/day in 274 patients, the incidence of drowsiness or sedation was lower, approximately 20%.

Other adverse effects were reported during clinical trials with guanabenz but are not clearly distinguishable from placebo effects and occurred with a frequency of less than or equal to 3%:

➤*Cardiovascular:* Chest pain, edema, arrhythmias, palpitations.

In very rare instances atrioventricular dysfunction, up to and including complete AV block, has been caused by guanabenz.

➤*CNS:* Anxiety, ataxia; depression; sleep disturbances.

➤*GI:* Nausea; epigastric pain; diarrhea; vomiting; constipation; abdominal discomfort.

➤*GU:* Urinary frequency; disturbances of sexual function (decreased libido; impotence).

➤*Dermatologic:* Rash; pruritus.

➤*Musculoskeletal:* Aches in extremities; muscle aches.

➤*Respiratory:* Dyspnea.

➤*Special senses:* Blurring of vision; nasal congestion.

➤*Miscellaneous:* Gynecomastia; taste disorders.

Overdosage

➤*Symptoms:* Accidental ingestion of guanabenz caused hypotension, somnolence, lethargy, irritability, miosis, and bradycardia in 2 children aged 1 and 3 years. Gastric lavage and administration of pressor substances, fluids, atropine, ipecac and oral activated charcoal resulted in complete and uneventful recovery within 12 hours in both patients.

➤*Treatment:* Because experience with accidental overdosage is limited, the suggested treatment is mainly supportive while the drug is being eliminated from the body and until the patient is no longer symptomatic. Vital signs and fluid balance should be carefully monitored. An adequate airway should be maintained and, if indicated, assisted respiration instituted. There is no data available on the dialyzability of guanabenz.

Patient Information

Patients who receive guanabenz should be advised to exercise caution when operating dangerous machinery or driving motor vehicles until it is determined that they do not become drowsy or dizzy from the medication. Patients should be warned that their tolerance for alcohol and other CNS depressants may be diminished. Patients should be advised not to discontinue therapy abruptly.

RESERPINE

Rx	**Reserpine** (Various, eg, Eon, Moore)	**Tablets:** 0.1 mg	In 100s, 1000s and 5000s.
Rx	**Reserpine** (Various, eg, Eon, Moore, URL)	**Tablets:** 0.25 mg	In 100s, 1000s and 5000s.

RESERPINE — ORAL

Indications

➤*Hypertension:* Mild essential hypertension.

Adjunctive therapy with other antihypertensive agents in more severe forms of hypertension.

➤*Psychotic states:* Relief of symptoms in agitated psychotic states (eg, schizophrenia), primarily in those individuals unable to tolerate phenothiazine derivatives or in those who also require antihypertensive medication.

Administration and Dosage

➤*Adults:*

Hypertension –

Initial dosage: In the average patient not receiving other antihypertensive agents, the usual initial dosage is 0.5 mg daily for 1 or 2 weeks.

Maintenance dosage: Reduce to 0.1 to 0.25 mg daily.

Use higher dosages cautiously because occurrence of serious mental depression and other adverse reactions may increase considerably.

Psychiatric disorders –

Initial dosage: 0.5 mg daily, but may range from 0.1 to 1 mg.

Dosage adjustment: Adjust dosage upward or downward according to the patient's response.

➤*Children:* The manufacturer does not recommend the use of reserpine in children.

Maximum dose – 250 mcg/day (0.25 mg/day).

Initial dose – 20 mcg/kg/day.

➤*Elderly:* See Warnings/Precautions for more information.

➤*Renal function impairment:* Exercise caution when treating hypertensive patients with renal insufficiency, because they adjust poorly to lowered blood pressure levels.

➤*Storage/Stability:* Store between 59° and 86°F (15° and 30 °C). Store away from heat, moisture, and light.

Actions

➤*Pharmacology:* Reserpine depletes stores of catecholamine and 5-hydroxytryptamine in many organs, including the brain and adrenal medulla. Most of its pharmacological effects have been attributed to this action. Depletion is slower and less complete in the adrenal medulla than in other tissues. The depression of sympathetic nerve function results in a decreased heart rate and a lowering of arterial blood pressure. The sedative and tranquilizing properties of reserpine are thought to be related to depletion of catecholamine and 5-hydroxytryptamine from the brain.

➤*Pharmacokinetics:* Reserpine is characterized by slow onset of action and sustained effects. Both cardiovascular and CNS effects may persist for a period of time following withdrawal of the drug.

Mean maximum plasma levels of 1.54 ng/mL were attained after a median of 3.5 hours in six healthy subjects receiving a single oral 1 mg dose. Bioavailability was ≈ 50% of that of a corresponding IV dose. Plasma levels of reserpine after IV administration declined with a mean half-life of 33 hours. Reserpine is extensively bound (96%) to plasma proteins. No definitive studies on the metabolism of reserpine have been made.

Contraindications

Hypersensitivity; mental depression or history of mental depression (especially with suicidal tendencies); active peptic ulcer; ulcerative colitis; patients receiving electroconvulsive therapy.

Warnings/Precautions

➤*Depression:* Exercise extreme caution in treating patients with a history of mental depression. Reserpine may cause mental depression. Recognition of depression may be difficult, because this condition may often be disguised by somatic complaints (masked depression). Discontinue the drug at first signs of depression (eg, despondency, early morning insomnia, loss of appetite, impotence or self-deprecation). Drug-induced depression may persist for several months after drug withdrawal and may be severe enough to result in suicide.

➤*Ulcers:* Since reserpine increases GI motility and secretion, use cautiously in patients with a history of peptic ulcer, ulcerative colitis or gallstones (biliary colic may be precipitated).

➤*Cardiovascular effects:* Preoperative withdrawal of reserpine does not assure that circulatory instability will not occur. It is important that the anesthesiologist be aware of the patient's drug intake and consider this in the overall management, since hypotension has occurred in patients receiving reserpine. Anticholinergic or adrenergic drugs (eg, metaraminol, norepinephrine) have been employed to treat adverse vagocirculatory effects.

➤*Renal function impairment:* Exercise caution when treating hypertensive patients with renal insufficiency, since they adjust poorly to lowered blood pressure levels.

➤*Pregnancy: Category C.* There are no adequate and well controlled studies of reserpine in pregnant women. Reserpine crosses the placental barrier. Increased respiratory tract secretions, nasal congestion, cyanosis and anorexia may occur in neonates of reserpine-treated mothers. Use during pregnancy only if the potential benefit justifies the potential risk to the fetus.

➤*Lactation:* Reserpine is excreted in breast milk. Increased respiratory tract secretions, nasal congestion, cyanosis and anorexia may occur in breastfed infants. Because of the potential for adverse reactions in nursing infants and the potential for tumorigenicity, decide whether to discontinue nursing or to discontinue the drug, taking into account the importance of the drug to the mother.

➤*Children:* Safety and efficacy have not been established by means of controlled clinical trials, although there is experience with the use of reserpine in children. Because of adverse effects such as emotional depression and lability, sedation and stuffy nose, reserpine is not usually recommended as a Step-2 drug in the treatment of hypertension in children.

➤*Elderly:* See Administration and Dosage for more information.

Drug Interactions

Reserpine Drug Interactions

Precipitant drug	Object drug[a]		Description
MAO inhibitors	Reserpine	↔	Avoid MAO inhibitors or use with extreme caution.
Tricyclic antidepressants	Reserpine	↓	Concurrent use may decrease the antihypertensive effect of reserpine.
Reserpine	Digitalis glycosides Quinidine	↑	Use reserpine cautiously with digitalis and quinidine, since cardiac arrhythmias have occurred.
Reserpine	Sympathomimetics, direct-acting	↑	Closely monitor concurrent use of reserpine and direct- or indirect-acting sympathomimetics. The action of direct-acting amines (eg, epinephrine, isoproterenol, phenylephrine, metaraminol) may be prolonged when given to patients taking reserpine. The action of indirect-acting amines (eg, ephedrine, tyramine, amphetamines) is inhibited.
	Sympathomimetics, indirect-acting	↓	

[a] ↑ = Object drug increased. ↓ = Object drug decreased. ↔ = Undetermined clinical effect.

Adverse Reactions

The following adverse reactions are listed in decreasing order of severity, not frequency.

➤*Cardiovascular:* Arrhythmias (particularly when used concurrently with digitalis or quinidine); syncope; angina-like symptoms; bradycardia; edema.

➤*CNS:* Parkinsonian syndrome and other extrapyramidal tract symptoms (rare); dizziness; headache; paradoxical anxiety; depression; nervousness; nightmares; dull sensorium; drowsiness.

➤*GI:* Vomiting; diarrhea; nausea; anorexia; dryness of mouth; hypersecretion.

➤*GU:* Pseudolactation; impotence; dysuria; gynecomastia; decreased libido; breast engorgement.

➤*Respiratory:* Dyspnea; epistaxis; nasal congestion.

➤*Special senses:* Deafness; optic atrophy; glaucoma; uveitis; conjunctival injection.

➤*Miscellaneous:* Hypersensitivity reactions: Purpura, rash, pruritus; weight gain; muscular aches.

Overdosage

➤*Symptoms:* No deaths due to acute poisoning with reserpine have been reported.

Highest known doses survived – Children, 1,000 mg (age and sex not specified), young children, 200 mg (20-month-old boy). The clinical picture of acute poisoning is characterized chiefly by signs and symptoms due to the reflex parasympathomimetic effect of reserpine.

Impairment of consciousness may occur and may range from drowsiness to coma, depending on the severity of overdosage. Flushing of the skin, conjunctival injection and pupillary constriction are to be expected. Hypotension, hypothermia, central respiratory depression and bradycardia may develop in cases of severe overdosage. Increased salivary secretion, gastric secretion and diarrhea also may occur.

➤*Treatment:* There is no specific antidote. Evacuate stomach contents, taking adequate precautions against aspiration and for protection of the airway. Activated charcoal slurry should be instilled.

RESERPINE — ORAL

Treat the effects of reserpine overdosage symptomatically. If hypotension is severe enough to require treatment with a vasopressor, use one having a direct action upon vascular smooth muscle (eg, phenylephrine, norepinephrine, metaraminol). Since reserpine is long-acting, observe the patient carefully for at least 72 hours, and administer treatment as required.

Patient Information

Inform patients of possible side effects and advise them to take the medication regularly and continuously as directed.

ALPHA-1 ADRENERGIC BLOCKERS

Indications

➤*Hypertension (doxazosin immediate release, prazosin, and terazosin only):* For the treatment of hypertension, alone or in combination with other antihypertensive agents.

➤*Benign prostatic hyperplasia:*

Terazosin – Treatment of symptomatic benign prostatic hyperplasia (BPH).

Doxazosin – Treatment of urinary outflow obstruction and obstructive symptoms (hesitation, intermittency, dribbling, weak urinary stream, incomplete emptying of the bladder) and irritative symptoms (nocturia, daytime frequency, urgency, burning) associated with BPH.

Alfuzosin / silodosin / tamsulosin – Treatment of the signs and symptoms of BPH.

➤*Off-label uses:* Refer to individual monographs for further information.

Benign prostatic hyperplasia –

Prazosin: [5] = Poor documentation.

Pediatric hypertension –

Doxazosin: [1] = Good documentation.

Prazosin: [1] = Good documentation.

Terazosin: [1] = Good documentation.

Raynaud phenomenon –

Prazosin: [2] = Fair documentation.

Ureteral stones – In the meta-analysis performed for the guidelines statement, significantly more patients (29%) receiving alpha-blocker therapy passed stones compared with controls. The guidelines state that alpha-blockers are the preferred agents for medical expulsive therapy to facilitate the passage of stones or stone fragments.

Doxazosin: [1] = Good documentation.

Tamsulosin: [1] = Good documentation.

Terazosin: [1] = Good documentation.

Other possible off-label uses –

Terazosin: Symptomatic treatment of chronic abacterial prostatitis.

Actions

➤*Pharmacology:* **Alfuzosin** and **silodosin** exhibit selectivity for alpha-1 adrenergic receptors in the lower urinary tract. **Alfuzosin** and **silodosin** are not intended for use as antihypertensive drugs.

Doxazosin, **prazosin**, and **terazosin** selectively block alpha-1 adrenergic receptors. This blockade causes a reduction in systemic vascular resistance, thus causing an antihypertensive effect. The degree of smooth muscle tone in the prostate and bladder neck is mediated by the alpha-1 adrenergic receptor, which is present in high density in the prostatic stroma, prostatic capsule, and bladder neck. Blockade of the alpha-1 adrenergic receptor decreases urethral resistance and may relieve the obstruction and improve urine flow and BPH symptoms.

Doxazosin causes maximum reductions in blood pressure 2 to 6 hours after dosing, which is associated with a small increase in standing heart rate. Doxazosin has a greater effect on blood pressure and heart rate in the standing position.

Prazosin lowers blood pressure in the supine and standing positions. This effect is most pronounced on the diastolic blood pressure. The antihypertensive action usually is not accompanied by a reflex tachycardia.

Tamsulosin selectively inhibits the alpha-1A-adrenergic receptor. Approximately 70% of the alpha-1 adrenergic receptors in human prostate are of the alpha-1A subtype. Tamsulosin is not intended for use as an antihypertensive drug.

Terazosin decreases blood pressure gradually within 15 minutes following oral administration. Terazosin treatment in normotensive men with BPH did not result in a clinically significant blood pressure-lowering effect.

➤*Pharmacokinetics:*

Pharmacokinetics of Alpha-1 Adrenergic Blockers

Parameter	Alfuzosin	Doxazosin	Prazosin	Silodosin	Tamsulosin	Terazosin
Oral bioavailability	49% (fed state)	≈ 65%	nd	32%	> 90% (fasting state)	nd
T_{max}	8 h (fed state)	≈ 2 to 3 h	≈ 3 h	Approximately 2.6 h	4 to 5 h (fasting state) 6 to 7 h (fed state)	≈ 1 h
Protein binding	82% to 90%	≈ 98%	High	97%	94% to 99%[a]	90% to 94%
Metabolism	Extensively metabolized by the liver, mainly by oxidation, o-demethylation, and N-dealkylation.	First-pass metabolism; extensively metabolized by the liver, mainly by O-demethylation or hydroxylation	Extensively metabolized, primarily by demethylation and conjugation	Extensive metabolism through glucuronidation, alcohol, and aldehyde dehydrogenase, and CYP3A4 pathways.	CYP450	nd
Half-life, elimination	10 h	≈ 22 h	2 to 3 h	Approximately 13.3 h	9 to 15 h	≈ 12 h
Excretion	Urine (24%) Feces (69%)	Urine (≈ 9%) Feces (≈ 63%)[d]	Bile and feces	Urine (33.5%) Feces (54.9%)	Urine (76%) Feces (21%)	Urine (≈ 40%)[b] Feces (≈ 60%)[c]

* nd = no data.
[a] Primarily bound to alpha-1 acid glycoprotein.
[b] Approximately 10% of an oral dose is excreted as parent drug in the urine.
[c] Approximately 20% of an oral dose is excreted as parent drug in the feces.
[d] 4.8% of the dose is excreted as unchanged drug in the feces and a trace amount is excreted in the urine as unchanged drug.

Absorption – Enterohepatic recycling of **doxazosin** is suggested by secondary peaking of plasma concentrations. Plasma elimination of doxazosin is biphasic. After morning dosing of doxazosin, the AUC was 11% less than after evening dosing and the time to peak concentration after evening dosing occurred significantly later than after morning dosing (5.6 vs 3.5 hours).

Distribution – The mean steady-state apparent volume of distribution of **tamsulosin** after IV administration was 16 L, which is suggestive of distribution into extracellular fluids in the body. Tamsulosin is widely distributed to most tissues. The volume of distribution following **alfuzosin** IV administration was 3.2 L/kg. **Silodosin** has an apparent volume of distribution of 49.5 L.

Metabolism – **Terazosin** undergoes minimal hepatic first-pass metabolism and nearly all the circulating dose is in the form of the parent drug. The cytochrome P450 enzymes that primarily catalyze the Phase I metabolism of tamsulosin have not been conclusively identified. The metabolites of tamsulosin undergo extensive conjugation to glucuronide or sulfate prior to renal excretion.

ALPHA-1 ADRENERGIC BLOCKERS

Special populations –

Renal function impairment: Relative to subjects with healthy renal function, the **alfuzosin** mean C_{max} and AUC values were increased by approximately 50% in patients with mild, moderate, or severe renal impairment.

In a study with 6 subjects with moderate renal impairment, the total **silodosin** (bound and unbound) AUC, C_{max}, and elimination half-life were 3.2-, 3.1-, and 2-fold higher, respectively, compared with 7 subjects with healthy renal function. The unbound silodosin AUC and C_{max} were 2- and 1.5- fold higher, respectively, in subjects with moderate renal impairment compared with the healthy controls.

Hepatic function impairment: Administration of a single dose of doxazosin 2 mg to patients with cirrhosis (Child-Pugh Class A) showed a 40% increase in exposure to **doxazosin**. In patients with moderate or severe hepatic insufficiency (Child-Pugh categories B and C), the **alfuzosin** plasma apparent clearance (CL/F) was reduced to approximately one-third to one-fourth that observed in healthy subjects. This reduction in clearance results in 3- to 4-fold higher plasma concentrations of alfuzosin in these patients compared with healthy subjects. Therefore, alfuzosin hydrochloride extended release is contraindicated in patients with moderate to severe hepatic impairment.

Elderly: In patients 70 years of age and older taking **terazosin**, plasma clearance decreased by 31.7%, compared with younger patients. For **tamsulosin**, a 40% higher AUC in those 55 to 75 years of age was seen compared with younger subjects. For **silodosin**, the AUC and elimination half-life were approximately 15% and 20%, respectively, greater in elderly (mean age, 69 years) patients. For **alfuzosin**, trough level concentrations in patients older than 75 years of age were approximately 35% greater than in those younger than 65 years of age.

Contraindications

Hypersensitivity to quinazolines (eg, **doxazosin**, **prazosin**, **tamsulosin**, **terazosin**) or to any components of the products.

➤*Alfuzosin:* Moderate or severe hepatic insufficiency (Child-Pugh categories B and C); coadministration with potent CYP3A4 inhibitors (eg, ketoconazole, itraconazole, ritonavir).

➤*Silodosin:* Severe renal impairment (CrCl less than 30 mL/min); severe hepatic impairment (Child-Pugh score of 10 or more); coadministration with strong CYP3A4 inhibitors (eg, ketoconazole, clarithromycin, itraconazole, ritonavir).

Warnings/Precautions

➤*"First-dose" effect and orthostatic hypotension:* **Alfuzosin, doxazosin, prazosin, silodosin, tamsulosin,** and **terazosin**, like other α-adrenergic blocking agents, can cause marked hypotension (especially postural hypotension) and syncope with sudden loss of consciousness with the first few doses. Anticipate a similar effect if therapy is interrupted for more than a few doses, if dosage is increased rapidly, or if another antihypertensive drug is introduced. Syncope is due to an excessive postural hypotensive effect, although the syncopal episode has occasionally been preceded by severe supraventricular tachycardia with heart rates of 120 to 160 beats per minute.

The "first-dose" phenomenon may be minimized by limiting the initial dose to 1 mg of **terazosin** or **prazosin** (given at bedtime) or **doxazosin**. Slowly increase dosage of these drugs. Add additional antihypertensives with caution. Caution patients to avoid situations where injury could result should syncope occur during initiation of therapy. Hypotension may develop in patients also receiving a β-adrenergic blocker.

If syncope occurs, place patient in recumbent position and treat supportively. More common than loss of consciousness are dizziness and lightheadedness.

Syncopal episodes have usually occurred within 30 to 90 minutes of the initial dose of **prazosin**; the incidence is approximately 1% with an initial dose of 2 mg or greater. Syncope occurred in about 1% of **terazosin** patients and was not necessarily associated with early doses. There is evidence that the orthostatic effect of terazosin is greater, even in chronic use, shortly after dosing. Syncope occurred in 0.7% of **doxazosin** patients with dose titration every 1 to 2 weeks; none of these events were reported at the starting dose of 1 mg and 1.2% occurred at 16 mg/day. Other symptoms of lowered blood pressure (eg, dizziness, lightheadedness palpitations) are more common, occurring in approximately 28% of terazosin patients and up to 23% of doxazosin patients (approximately 2% of doxazosin patients discontinued therapy).

➤*Patients with congenital or acquired QT prolongation:* In a study of QT effect in 45 healthy men, the QT effect appeared less with **alfuzosin** 10 mg than with 40 mg. This observation should be considered in clinical decisions to prescribe alfuzosin for patients with a known history of QT prolongation or patients who are taking medications known to prolong QT.

➤*Priapism:* Rarely (probably less frequently than once in every several thousand patients), alpha-$_1$ antagonists have been associated with priapism (painful penile erection, sustained for hours and unrelieved by sexual intercourse or masturbation). Because this condition can lead to permanent impotence if not promptly treated, patients must be advised about the seriousness of the condition.

➤*Coronary insufficiency:* If symptoms of angina pectoris should newly appear or worsen, **alfuzosin** should be discontinued.

➤*Hemodilution:* Small but statistically significant decreases in hematocrit, hemoglobin, white blood cells, total protein, and albumin were observed in controlled clinical trials with **terazosin**. These laboratory findings suggest the possibility of hemodilution.

➤*Leukopenia/Neutropenia:* In hypertensive patients receiving **doxazosin**, mean WBC and neutrophil counts were decreased by 2.4% and 1%, respectively, compared with placebo, a phenomenon seen with other alpha blocking drugs. In BPH patients, the incidence of clinically significant WBC abnormalities was 0.4%. No patients became symptomatic as a result of the low counts. WBCs and neutrophil counts returned to normal after drug discontinuation.

➤*Intraoperative floppy iris syndrome:* Intraoperative floppy iris syndrome has been observed during cataract surgery in some patients on alpha-1 blockers or previously treated with alpha-1 blockers. This variant of small pupil syndrome is characterized by the combination of a flaccid iris that billows in response to intraoperative irrigation currents; progressive intraoperative miosis despite preoperative dilation with standard mydriatic drugs; and potential prolapse of the iris toward the phacoemulsification incisions.

➤*Weight gain:* There was a tendency for patients to gain weight during **terazosin** therapy. In placebo-controlled monotherapy trials, male and female patients receiving terazosin gained a mean of 0.8 and 1 kg, respectively, compared with losses of 0.1 and 0.5 kg, respectively, in the placebo group. Patients receiving **doxazosin** gained a mean of 0.6 kg compared with a mean loss of 0.1 kg for placebo patients.

➤*Cholesterol:* During controlled clinical studies, patients receiving **terazosin** monotherapy had a small but statistically significant decrease (3%) in total cholesterol and the combined LDL and VLDL fractions. No significant changes were observed in HDL fraction and triglycerides. In clinical trials involving normocholesterolemic patients, **doxazosin** reduced total serum cholesterol by 2% to 3% and LDL by 4%, and increased HDL to total cholesterol ratio by 4%. The clinical significance is unknown.

➤*Cardiotoxicity:* An increased incidence of myocardial necrosis or fibrosis occurred in rats and mice following 6 to 18 months of **doxazosin** 40 to 80 mg/kg/day. There is no evidence that similar lesions occur in humans.

➤*Prostatic cancer:* Carcinoma of the prostate and BPH cause many of the same symptoms and frequently co-exist. Therefore, examine patients thought to have BPH prior to starting **terazosin** therapy to rule out prostate carcinoma.

➤*Renal function impairment:* Exercise caution when **alfuzosin** is administered in patients with severe renal insufficiency. Reduce **silodosin** dose in patients with moderate renal impairment; exercise caution and monitor for adverse reactions. Silodosin is contraindicated in patients with severe renal impairment.

➤*Hepatic function impairment:* Administer **doxazosin** with caution to patients with evidence of impaired hepatic function or to patients receiving drugs known to influence hepatic metabolism. **Silodosin** is contraindicated in patients with severe hepatic impairment. **Alfuzosin** should not be given to patients with moderate or severe hepatic insufficiency.

➤*Hazardous tasks:* Caution patients about driving, operating machinery, or performing hazardous tasks when initiating therapy with an alpha-1 adrenergic blocker.

➤*Pregnancy: Category C* (**prazosin, terazosin, doxazosin**). *Category B* (**alfuzosin, silodosin, tamsulosin**). A **doxazosin** dosage of 82 mg/kg/day in rabbits was associated with reduced fetal survival. In rats, maternal doxazosin doses 8 times the human AUC exposure (12 mg/day) delayed postnatal development. **Terazosin** doses 280 times the maximum recommended human dose in rats resulted in fetal resorptions; increased fetal resorptions, decreased fetal weight, and increased number of supernumerary ribs occurred with doses 60 times the maximum recommended human dose. Significantly more rat pups died in the group dosed with terazosin (more than 75 times the maximum recommended human dose) vs controls.

An embryo/fetal study in rabbits showed decreased maternal body weight at 200 mg/kg/day (approximately 13 to 25 times the exposure of the MRHD of **silodosin** via AUC).

Gestation was slightly prolonged in rats with a maternal dose of **alfuzosin** greater than 5 mg/kg/day (oral gavage), which corresponds to systemic exposure levels (based on AUC of unbound drug) 12 times higher than human exposure levels, but there were no difficulties with parturition.

There are no adequate and well-controlled studies in pregnant women. Safety for use during pregnancy has not been established. Use only when clearly needed and when the potential benefits outweigh the potential hazards to the fetus. **Tamsulosin** is not indicated for use in women.

➤*Lactation:* **Doxazosin** accumulates in breast milk of lactating rats following a single 1 mg/kg dose with a maximum concentration about 20 times greater than the maternal plasma concentration. It is not known whether **terazosin** or **tamsulosin** are excreted in breast milk. **Tamsulosin** and **alfuzosin** are not indicated for use in women. **Prazosin** is excreted in small amounts in breast milk. Exercise caution when administering these drugs to a nursing woman.

No effects on physical or behavioral development of offspring were observed when rats were treated during pregnancy and lactation with **silodosin** up to 300 mg/kg/day.

➤*Children:* Safety and efficacy for use in children have not been established.

➤*Elderly:* Per the Beers list, there is the potential for hypotension, dry mouth, and urinary problems with **doxazosin** use in the elderly.

ALPHA-1 ADRENERGIC BLOCKERS

Drug Interactions

Alpha-1 Antiadrenergic Blocker Drug Interactions			
Precipitant drug	Object drug[a]		Description
Alcohol	Alpha-1 adrenergic blockers	↑	Coadministration may cause increased risk of hypotension. Advise patients to avoid alcohol.
Beta blockers	Alpha-1 adrenergic blockers Alfuzosin Prazosin	↑	Beta-blockers may enhance the acute postural hypotensive reaction following the first dose of prazosin. Coadministration of atenolol with alfuzosin increased alfuzosin C_{max} and AUC values by 28% and 21%, respectively. Alfuzosin increased atenolol C_{max} and AUC values by 26% and 14%, respectively. In this study, the combination of alfuzosin with atenolol caused significant reductions in mean blood pressure and in mean heart rate. Terazosin and doxazosin have been combined with beta blockers with no adverse reaction.
Alpha-1 adrenergic blockers Alfuzosin	Beta-blockers		
Cimetidine	Alpha-1 adrenergic blockers Alfuzosin Tamsulosin	↑	Cimetidine decreased the clearance of tamsulosin 26% and increased the AUC 44%. Use with caution. Repeated administration of cimetidine 1 g/day increased both alfuzosin C_{max} and AUC by 20%.
CYP 3A4 inhibitors (eg, clarithromycin, itraconazole, ketoconazole, ritonavir)	Alpha-1 adrenergic blockers Alfuzosin Silodosin	↑	May increase plasma levels. Concomitant use of strong CYP3A4 inhibitors is contraindicated.
CYP 3A4 inhibitors (moderate) (eg, diltiazem, erythromycin, verapamil)	Alpha-1 adrenergic blockers Alfuzosin Silodosin	↑	May increase plasma levels. Exercise caution and monitor patients for adverse reactions.
Indomethacin	Alpha-1 adrenergic blockers Prazosin	↓	The antihypertensive action of prazosin may be decreased. No interaction occurred in patients receiving doxazosin, terazosin, and NSAIDs.
Phosphodiesterase type 5 inhibitors (eg, sildenafil, tadalafil)	Alpha-1 adrenergic blockers Silodosin	↑	There was an increased incidence of orthostatic adverse reactions when these agents were used together.
Alpha-1 adrenergic blockers Silodosin	Phosphodiesterase type 5 inhibitors (eg, sildenafil, tadalafil)		
P-gp inhibitors (eg, cyclosporine)	Alpha-1 adrenergic blockers Silodosin	↑	May increase plasma levels. Concomitant use with strong P-gp inhibitors is not recommended.
Verapamil	Alpha-1 adrenergic blockers Prazosin Terazosin	↑	Verapamil appears to increase serum prazosin levels and may increase the sensitivity to prazosin-induced postural hypotension. Verapamil increased terazosin AUC 24%, C_{max} 25%, and C_{min} 32% and decreased T_{max} 0.5 h.
Alpha$_1$-adrenergic blockers Prazosin	Clonidine	↓	The antihypertensive effect of clonidine may be decreased.

[a] ↑ = object drug increased; ↓ = object drug decreased.

➤*Drug/Lab test interactions:* In a study of 5 patients given **prazosin** 12 to 24 mg/day for 10 to 14 days, there was an average increase of 42% in the urinary metabolite of norepinephrine and an average increase in urinary vanillylmandelic acid (VMA) of 17%. Therefore, false-positive results may occur in screening tests for pheochromocytoma in patients who are being treated with **prazosin**. If an elevated VMA is found, discontinue prazosin and retest the patient after 1 month.

Doxazosin and **terazosin** do not affect plasma concentrations of prostate specific antigen (PSA) in patients treated for up to 3 years (doxazosin), 2 years (terazosin), or 1 year (**tamsulosin**).

➤*Drug/Food interactions:* Administration of **terazosin** capsules immediately after meals delayed T_{max} by about 40 minutes. For **tamsulosin**, the T_{max} is reached by 4 to 5 hours under fasting conditions and by 6 to 7 hours after administration with food. Taking tamsulosin under fasted conditions results in a 30% increase in AUC and 40% to 70% increase in C_{max} compared with fed conditions. The effect of a moderate-fat, moderate-calorie meal was variable and decreased **silodosin** C_{max} by approximately 18% to 43% and AUC by 4% to 49%. **Alfuzosin** extent of absorption is 50% lower under fasting conditions; therefore, take immediately following a meal.

Adverse Reactions

Alpha-1 Adrenergic Blocker Adverse Reactions (%)[a]									
	Hypertension				BPH				
Adverse Reaction	Doxazosin	Prazosin	Terazosin	Alfuzosin	Doxazosin	Silodosin	Tamsulosin 0.4 mg	Tamsulosin 0.8 mg	Terazosin
Cardiovascular									
Palpitations	2%	5.3%	4.3%		1.2%		-		0.9%
Postural hypotension/ hypotension	0.3% to 1%	1% to 4%	1.3%	0.4 %	0.3% to 1.7%	2.6%	0.2%	0.4%	0.6% to 3.9%
Tachycardia	0.3%	< 1%	1.9%		0.9%		-	-	-
Arrhythmia	1%	-	≥ 1%		-		-	-	-
Chest pain	2%	-	≥ 1%		1.2%		4%	4.1%	-
Vasodilation	-	-	≥ 1%		-		-	-	-
Syncope	0.5% to 1%	1% to 4%	-	0.2%	0.5%		0.2%	0.4%	0.6%
Peripheral ischemia	0.3%	-	-		-		-	-	-
Angina pectoris	< 0.5%	-	-		0.6%		-	-	-
CNS									
Depression	1%	1% to 4%	0.3%		-		-	-	-
Dizziness	19%	10.3%	19.3%	5.7%	15.6%[b]	3.2%	14.9%	17.1%	9.1%
Decreased libido/ sexual dysfunction	2%	-	0.6%		0.8%		1%	2%	-
Nervousness	2%	1% to 4%	2.3%		-		-	-	-
Paresthesia	1%	< 1%	2.9%		-		-	-	-
Somnolence	5%	-	5.4%		3%		3%	4.3%	3.6%
Anxiety	-	-	≥ 1%		1.1%		-	-	-
Insomnia	1%	-	≥ 1%		1.2%	1% to 2%	2.4%	1.4%	-
Asthenia	1% to 12%	≈ 7%	11.3%[c]		-	1% to 2%	7.8%	8.5%	7.4%[c]
Fatigue	-	-	-	2.7%	8%		-	-	-
Drowsiness	-	7.6%	-		-		-	-	-
Ataxia	1%	-	-		-		-	-	-

ALPHA-1 ADRENERGIC BLOCKERS

Alpha-1 Adrenergic Blocker Adverse Reactions (%)[a]									
	Hypertension			BPH					
Adverse Reaction	Doxazosin	Prazosin	Terazosin	Alfuzosin	Doxazosin	Silodosin	Tamsulosin 0.4 mg	Tamsulosin 0.8 mg	Terazosin
Hypertonia	1%	-	-		-		-	-	-
Hallucinations	-	< 1%	-		-		-	-	-
Kinetic disorders	1%	-	-		-		-	-	-
Dermatologic									
Pruritus	1%	< 1%	≥ 1%		-		-	-	-
Rash	1%	1% to 4%	≥ 1%	1% to 2%	-		-	-	-
Sweating	0.5% to 1%	-	≥ 1%		1.1%		-	-	-
Alopecia/Lichen planus	< 0.5%	< 1%	-		-		-	-	-
GI									
Nausea	3%	4.9%	4.4%	1% to 2%	1.5%		2.6%	3.9%	1.7%
Vomiting	≤ 2%	1% to 4%	≥ 1%		1.4%		-	-	-
Dry mouth	-	1% to 4%	≥ 1%		-		-	-	-
Diarrhea	2%	1% to 4%	≥ 1%		2.3%	2.6%	6.2%	4.3%	-
Constipation	1%	1% to 4%	≥ 1%	1% to 2%	-		-	-	-
Abdominal discomfort/pain	0%	< 1%	≥ 1%	1% to 2%	2.4%	1% to 2%	-	-	-
Flatulence	1%	-	≥ 1%		-		-	-	-
Liver function abnormalities	-	< 1%	-		-		-	-	-
Pancreatitis	-	< 1%	-		-		-	-	-
Tooth disorder	-	-	-		-		1.2%	2%	-
Dyspepsia	1%	-	≥ 1%	1% to 2%	1.7%		-	-	-
GU									
Impotence	-	< 1%	1.2%	1% to 2%	1.1%		-	-	1.6%
Urinary frequency	0%	1% to 4%	≥ 1%		-		-	-	-
Urinary tract infection	-	-	≥ 1%		1.4%		-	-	1.3%
Incontinence	1%	< 1%	≥ 1%[4]		-		-	-	-
Polyuria	2%	-	-		-		-	-	-
Priapism	-	< 1%	-		-		-	-	-
Abnormal ejaculation	-	-	-		-	28.1%[e]	8.4%	18.1%	-
Dysuria	-	-	-		0.5%		-	-	-
Musculoskeletal									
Shoulder/Neck/Back/ Extremity pain	-	-	1% to 3.5%		-		7%	8.3%	-
Arthritis, joint disorder/muscle pain, gout, cramps	1%	-	≥ 1%		-		-	-	-
Arthralgia	1%	< 1%	≥ 1%		-		-	-	-
Myalgia	1%	-	≥ 1%		-		-	-	-
Muscle weakness	1%	-	-		-		-	-	-
Respiratory									
Dyspnea	1%	1% to 4%	3.1%		2.6%		-	-	1.7%
Nasal congestion	-	1% to 4%	5.9%		-	2.1%	-	-	1.9%
Sinusitis	< 0.5%	-	2.6%	1% to 2%	-	1% to 2%	2.2%	3.7%	-
Bronchitis/Cold symptoms/ bronchospasm	< 0.5%	-	≥ 1%	1% to 2%	-		-	-	-
Epistaxis	1%	1% to 4%	≥ 1%		-		-	-	-
Flu symptoms	< 0.5%	-	≥ 1%		1.1%		-	-	2.4%
Increased cough	< 0.5%	-	≥ 1%		-		3.4%	4.5%	-
Pharyngitis/Rhinitis	< 0.5%/3%	-	≥ 1%	1% to 2%	< 0.5%	2.4%	5.8%/13.1%	5.1%/17.9%	1.9%
Special senses									
Blurred vision/ amblyopia	-	1% to 4%	1.6%		-		-	-	1.3%
Abnormal vision	2%	-	≥ 1%		1.4%		-	-	0.6%
Conjunctivitis, reddened sclera/eye pain	1%	1% to 4%	≥ 1%		-		-	-	-
Tinnitus	1%	< 1%	≥ 1%		-		-	-	-
Vertigo	2%	1% to 4%	-		-		0.6%	1%	1.4%
Amblyopia	-	-	-		-		0.2%	2%	1.3%
Miscellaneous									
Headache	14%	7.8%	16.2%	1% to 2%	9.9%	2.4%	19.3%	21.1%	4.9%
Edema	4%	1% to 4%	0.9%		2.7%		-	-	-
Peripheral edema	-	-	5.5%		-		-	-	0.9%
Weight gain	0.5 to 1%	-	0.5%		-		-	-	0.5%
Facial edema	1%	-	≥ 1%		-		-	-	-
Fever	< 0.5%	< 1%	≥ 1%		-		-	-	-
Flushing	1%	-	-		-		-	-	-
Diaphoresis	-	< 1%	-		-		-	-	-
Positive ANA titer	-	< 1%	-		-		-	-	-
Infection	< 0.5%	-	-		-		9%	10.8%	-

ALPHA-1 ADRENERGIC BLOCKERS

Alpha-1 Adrenergic Blocker Adverse Reactions (%)[a]

	Hypertension			BPH					
Adverse Reaction	Doxazosin	Prazosin	Terazosin	Alfuzosin	Doxazosin	Silodosin	Tamsulosin 0.4 mg	Tamsulosin 0.8 mg	Terazosin
Pain	2%	-	-	1% to 2%	2%		-	-	
Lack of energy	-	6.9%	-		-		-	-	
Weakness	-	6.5%	-		-		-	-	
Fatigue/Malaise	12%	-	-	2.7%	-		-	-	
Gout	-	-	≥ 1%		-		-	-	

[a] Data are pooled from separate studies and are not necessarily comparable.
[b] Includes vertigo.
[c] Includes weakness, tiredness, lassitude, and fatigue.
[d] Primarily reported in postmenopausal women.
[e] Reported as retrograde ejaculation.

➤*Doxazosin (hypertension):*

Cardiovascular – MI, cerebrovascular accident (fewer than 0.5%).

CNS – Hypesthesia, agitation (0.5% to 1%); paresis, tremor, twitching, confusion, migraine, impaired concentration, paroniria, amnesia, emotional lability, abnormal thinking, depersonalization (fewer than 0.5%).

Dermatologic – Dry skin, eczema (fewer than 0.5%).

GI – Increased appetite, anorexia, fecal incontinence, gastroenteritis (fewer than 0.5%).

GU – Breast pain, renal calculus (fewer than 0.5%).

Hematologic – Lymphadenopathy, purpura (fewer than 0.5%).

Metabolic/Nutritional – Thirst, gout, hypokalemia (fewer than 0.5%).

Special senses – Parosmia, earache, taste perversion, photophobia, abnormal lacrimation (fewer than 0.5%).

Miscellaneous – Pallor, hot flushes, fever/rigors, decreased weight (fewer than 0.5%).

➤*Postmarketing:*

Cardiovascular –

Prazosin: Angina pectoris, bradycardia, hypotension.
Alfuzosin: Tachycardia.

CNS –

Prazosin: Flushing, insomnia.

GU –

Doxazosin: Priapism, gynecomastia, hematuria, micturition disorder, micturition frequency, nocturia.
Alfuzosin: Priapism.

Hematologic –

Doxazosin: Leukopenia, thrombocytopenia.

Hepatic –

Doxazosin: Hepatitis, hepatitis cholestatic.
Silodosin: Impaired hepatic function associated with increased transaminase values, jaundice.

Miscellaneous –

Alfuzosin: Chest pain, rash.
Doxazosin: Allergic reaction, urticaria, bronchospasm aggravated, vomiting, hypesthesia, bradycardia.
Prazosin: Allergic reaction, asthenia, malaise, pain, gynecomastia, urticaria, vasculitis, eye pain.
Silodosin: Purpura, toxic skin eruption.
Tamsulosin: Allergic-type reactions (eg, skin rash, pruritus, angioedema of the tongue, lips, and face, urticaria) have been reported with positive rechallenge in some cases; priapism (rare); palpitations, constipation, vomiting (infrequent).
Terazosin: Allergic reactions, including anaphylaxis; priapism; thrombocytopenia; atrial fibrillation.

Overdosage

➤*Symptoms:* **Silodosin** was evaluated at dosages of up to 48 mg/day in healthy men. The dose-limiting adverse reaction was postural hypotension.

Accidental ingestion of at least 50 mg **prazosin** in a 2-year-old child produced profound drowsiness and depressed reflexes. No decrease in blood pressure was noted. Recovery was uneventful.

Several cases of **doxazosin** overdose have been reported (doses ranging from 1 to 40 mg in children and 60 to 70 mg in adults). All children made full recoveries. One adult developed hypotension that responded to fluid therapy. The other adult (with chronic renal failure, epilepsy, and depression) died; death was attributed to a grand mal seizure resulting from hypotension. The most likely manifestation of overdosage would be hypotension.

One patient reported an overdose of thirty 0.4 mg **tamsulosin** capsules. Following the ingestion of the capsules, the patient reported a severe headache.

➤*Treatment:* Restore blood pressure and normalize heart rate by keeping the patient supine. Treat shock with volume expanders. If necessary, use vasopressors and monitor and support renal function. These drugs are highly protein bound; dialysis may not be of benefit. Refer to General Management of Acute Overdosage.

Patient Information

Inform patients of the possibility of syncopal and orthostatic symptoms, especially at the initiation of therapy. Avoid driving or hazardous tasks for 12 to 24 hours after the first dose, after a dosage increase, and after interruption of therapy when treatment is resumed. Use caution when rising from a sitting or lying position. If dizziness or palpitations are bothersome, contact the physician for possible dose adjustment. These effects also may occur if patients drink alcohol, stand for long periods of time, or exercise, or if the weather is hot.

Drowsiness or somnolence may occur. Use caution when driving or operating heavy machinery.

Advise patients about the possibility of priapism as a result of treatment with alpha-$_1$ antagonists. Let patients know that this adverse event is very rare. If they experience priapism, advise them to bring it to immediate medical attention because, if not treated promptly, it can lead to permanent erectile dysfunction (impotence).

Advise patients not to crush, chew, or open **tamsulosin** capsules.

Inform patients to take alfuzosin with food and not to crush or chew the extended-release tablets.

Instruct the patient to tell their ophthalmologist about the use of silodosin before cataract surgery or other procedures involving the eyes, even if the patient is no longer taking silodosin.

SILODOSIN

Rx	**Rapaflo** (Watson Pharma)	**Capsules; oral:** 4 mg	(WATSON 151 4 mg). White/Opaque. In 30s and 90s.
		8 mg	(WATSON 152 8 mg). White/Opaque. In 30s, 90s, and 1,000s.

SILODOSIN — ORAL

For complete and comparative prescribing information, refer to the Alpha-1-Adrenergic Blockers class monograph.

Indications

➤*Benign prostatic hyperplasia:* For the treatment of the signs and symptoms of benign prostatic hyperplasia (BPH).

Administration and Dosage

➤*Adults:*

Benign prostatic hyperplasia – 8 mg once daily with a meal.

➤*Renal function impairment:* Silodosin is contraindicated in patients with severe renal impairment (creatinine clearance [CrCl] less than 30 mL/min). In patients with moderate renal impairment (CrCl 30 to 50 mL/min), the dosage should be reduced to 4 mg once daily taken with a meal. No dosage adjustment is needed in patients with mild renal impairment (CrCl 50 to 80 mL/min).

➤*Hepatic function impairment:* Silodosin has not been studied in patients with severe hepatic impairment (Child-Pugh score of 10 or greater) and is therefore contraindicated in these patients. No dosage adjustment is needed in patients with mild or moderate hepatic impairment.

➤*Administration:* Take with a meal.

➤*Storage/Stability:* Store at 25°C (77°F); excursions are permitted between 15° and 30°C (59° and 86°F). Protect from light and moisture.

PRAZOSIN HYDROCHLORIDE

Rx	**Prazosin HCl** (Various, eg, Ivax)	**Capsules:** 1 mg (as base)	In 100s, 250s, 500s, and 1000s.
Rx	**Minipress** (Pfizer)		(431). White. In 250s.
Rx	**Prazosin HCl** (Various, eg, Ivax)	**Capsules:** 2 mg (as base)	In 100s, 250s, 500s, and 1000s.
Rx	**Minipress** (Pfizer)		(437). Pink/white. In 250s.
Rx	**Prazosin HCl** (Various, eg, Ivax)	**Capsules:** 5 mg (as base)	In 100s, 250s, and 500s.
Rx	**Minipress** (Pfizer)		(438). Blue/white. In 250s.

PRAZOSIN HYDROCHLORIDE — ORAL

For complete and comparative prescribing information, refer to the Alpha-1-Adrenergic Blockers group monograph.

Indications

➤*Hypertension:* Treatment of hypertension. It can be used alone or in combination with other antihypertensive drugs such as diuretics or beta-adrenergic-blocking agents.

➤*Off-label uses:*

Benign prostatic hyperplasia – [5] = Poor documentation. The use of prazosin therapy for the management of benign prostatic hyperplasia (BPH) cannot be recommended at this time based on limited data and the availability of other effective agents in this class. American Urological Association guidelines on the management of BPH state that data are insufficient to support a recommendation for the use of prazosin as treatment of lower urinary tract symptoms secondary to BPH.

Pediatric hypertension – [1] = Good documentation. Prazosin is among the therapeutic options for pediatric hypertension identified by the National High Blood Pressure Education Program, based on expert opinions.

Raynaud phenomenon – [2] = Fair documentation. Initial data from controlled studies are conflicting; however, prazosin may have a beneficial role in the treatment of Raynaud phenomenon.

Administration and Dosage

➤*Adults:*

Hypertension –

Initial dosage: 1 mg 2 or 3 times per day.

Syncopal episodes usually have occurred within 30 to 90 minutes of the initial dose of the drug; occasionally, they have been reported in association with rapid dosage increases or the introduction of another antihypertensive drug into the regimen of a patient taking high doses of prazosin. The incidence of syncopal episodes is approximately 1% in patients given an initial dose of 2 mg or greater. Clinical trials conducted during the investigational phase of this drug suggest that syncopal episodes can be minimized by limiting the initial dose of the drug to 1 mg by subsequently increasing the dosage slowly and by introducing any additional antihypertensive drugs into the patient's regimen with caution.

Maintenance dosage: Dosage may be slowly increased to a total daily dose of 20 mg given in divided doses. The therapeutic dosages most commonly employed have ranged from 6 to 15 mg daily given in divided doses. Doses higher than 20 mg usually do not increase efficacy; however, a few patients may benefit from further increases, up to a daily dose of 40 mg given in divided doses. After initial titration, some patients can be maintained adequately on a twice-daily dosage regimen.

Concomitant therapy: When adding a diuretic or other antihypertensive agent, the dose of prazosin hydrochloride should be reduced to 1 or 2 mg 3 times per day and retitration then carried out.

Off-label dosing –

Raynaud phenomenon: [2] = Fair documentation. 1 mg 3 times daily orally.

➤*Children:*

Off-label dosing –

Pediatric hypertension: [1] = Good documentation.

- *1 to 17 years of age* –
  - *Maximum dose:* 0.5 mg/kg orally divided 3 times daily.
  - *Initial dosage:* 0.05 to 0.1 mg/kg orally divided 3 times daily.
  - *Dosage titration:* Dosage should be titrated to the needs of the individual patient.
  - *Concomitant therapy:* Coadministration with other antihypertensives may be necessary if blood pressure goals are not attained or if adverse effects are experienced. The use of combination products cannot generally be recommended.

➤*Storage/Stability:* Store at controlled room temperature, 15° to 30°C (59° to 86°F). Protect from moisture and light. Dispense in a tight, light-resistant container using a child-resistant closure.

TERAZOSIN HYDROCHLORIDE

Rx	**Terazosin HCl** (Geneva)	**Tablets:** 1 mg (as base)	In 100s and 1000s.
		2 mg (as base)	In 100s and 1000s.
		5 mg (as base)	In 100s and 1000s.
		10 mg (as base)	In 100s and 1000s.
Rx	**Terazosin HCl** (Various, eg, Apotex USA, Geneva, Teva)	**Capsules:** 1 mg (as base)	May contain lactose. In 100s and 500s.
Rx	**Hytrin** (Abbott)		Parabens. (HH). Grey. In 100s and UD 100s.
Rx	**Terazosin HCl** (Various, eg, Apotex USA, Geneva, Teva)	**Capsules:** 2 mg (as base)	May contain lactose. In 100s and 500s.
Rx	**Hytrin** (Abbott)		Parabens. (HY). Yellow. In 100s and UD 100s.
Rx	**Terazosin HCl** (Various, eg, Apotex USA, Geneva, Teva)	**Capsules:** 5 mg (as base)	May contain lactose. In 100s and 500s.
Rx	**Hytrin** (Abbott)		Parabens. (HK). Red. In 100s and UD 100s.
Rx	**Terazosin HCl** (Various, eg, Apotex USA, Geneva, Teva)	**Capsules:** 10 mg (as base)	May contain lactose. In 100s and 500s.
Rx	**Hytrin** (Abbott)		Parabens. (HN). Blue. In 100s. and UD 100s

TERAZOSIN HYDROCHLORIDE — ORAL

For complete and comparative prescribing information, refer to the Alpha-1-Adrenergic Blockers group monograph.

Indications

➤*Benign prostatic hyperplasia (BPH):* Treatment of symptomatic benign prostatic hyperplasia (BPH). There is a rapid response, with approximately 70% of patients experiencing an increase in urinary flow and improvement in symptoms of BPH when treated with terazosin. The long-term effects of terazosin on the incidence of surgery, acute urinary obstruction, or other complications of BPH are yet to be determined.

➤*Hypertension:* Treatment of hypertension. It can be used alone or in combination with other antihypertensive agents such as diuretics or beta-adrenergic-blocking agents.

➤*Off-label uses:*

Pediatric hypertension – [1] = Good documentation. Terazosin is among the therapeutic options for pediatric hypertension identified by the National High Blood Pressure Education Program, based on expert opinion.

Ureteral stones – [1] = Good documentation. In limited trials, terazosin was as effective as doxazosin or tamsulosin in the management of ureteral stones. In the meta-analysis performed for the guidelines statement, significantly more patients (29%) receiving alpha-blocker therapy passed stones compared with controls. The guidelines panel states that alpha-blockers are the preferred agents for medical expulsive therapy to facilitate the passage of stones or stone fragments.

Administration and Dosage

➤*General dosing considerations:* If terazosin administration is discontinued for several days, therapy should be reinstituted using the initial dosing regimen.

Postural hypotension and syncope are highly associated with the first dose, the first 7 days of therapy, immediately following dosage increases, and restarting therapy when interrupted for several days. Rapid dosage increases are also associated with postural hypotension and syncope. There is evidence that the orthostatic effect of terazosin is greater, even in chronic use, shortly after dosing.

TERAZOSIN HYDROCHLORIDE — ORAL

➤*Adults:*

Benign prostatic hyperplasia (BPH) –

Usual dosage: Doses of 10 mg once daily are generally required for clinical response. Treatment with 10 mg for a minimum of 4 to 6 weeks may be required to assess whether a beneficial response has been achieved.

Initial dosage: 1 mg once daily at bedtime. This dose should not be exceeded as an initial dose. Patients should be closely monitored during initial administration in order to minimize the risk of severe hypotensive response.

Dosage titration: The dose should be increased in a stepwise fashion to 2 mg, 5 mg, or 10 mg once daily to achieve the desired improvement of symptoms or flow rates. Some patients may not achieve a clinical response despite appropriate titration.

Although some patients responded at a 20 mg daily dose, there were an insufficient number of patients studied to draw definitive conclusions about this dose. There are insufficient data to support the use of higher doses for those patients who show inadequate or no response to 20 mg daily.

Concomitant therapy: When using terazosin and other antihypertensive agents concomitantly (especially the calcium channel blocker verapamil), dosage reduction and retitration of either agent may be necessary to avoid the possibility of developing significant hypotension.

Hypertension –

Usual dosage: 1 to 5 mg administered once a day; however, some patients may benefit from doses as high as 20 mg/day. Doses over 20 mg do not appear to provide further blood pressure effect and doses over 40 mg have not been studied.

Initial dosage: 1 mg once a day at bedtime. This initial dosing regimen should be strictly observed to minimize the potential for severe hypotensive effects.

Dosage titration: The dose may be slowly increased to achieve the desired blood pressure response.

Dosage adjustment: The dose interval (12 or 24 hours) should be adjusted according to the patient's individual blood pressure response. Blood pressure should be monitored at 2 to 3 hours after dosing and at the end of the dosing interval to ensure maximum and minimum responses are similar. If response is substantially diminished at the end of the dosing interval of a once daily regimen, an increased dose or use of a twice daily regimen can be considered.

Off-label dosing –

Ureteral stones: [1] = Good documentation.

• *Usual dose* – Used as adjunctive therapy in dosages of 2 to 5 mg daily for up to 1 month or until expulsion.

➤*Children:*

Off-label dosing –

Pediatric hypertension: [1] = Good documentation.

• *Children 1 to 17 years of age* – Initial dosage is 1 mg/day orally once daily. The maximum recommended dosage is 20 mg/day.

➤*Administration:* In clinical trials for hypertension, the dose was given in the morning with the exception of the initial dose.

➤*Storage/Stability:* Store at 15° to 30°C (59° to 86°F). Protect from light and moisture.

DOXAZOSIN MESYLATE

Rx	**Doxazosin Mesylate** (Various, eg, Ethex, Ivax, Mylan, Teva)	**Tablets**: 1 mg (as base)	May contain lactose. In 100s, 500s, 1,000s, and UD 100s.
Rx	**Cardura** (Pfizer)		Lactose. (Cardura 1 mg). White. In 100s and UD 100s.
Rx	**Doxazosin Mesylate** (Various, eg, Ethex, Ivax, Mylan, Teva)	**Tablets**: 2 mg (as base)	May contain lactose. In 100s, 500s, 1,000s, and UD 100s.
Rx	**Cardura** (Pfizer)		Lactose. (Cardura 2 mg). Yellow. In 100s and UD 100s.
Rx	**Doxazosin Mesylate** (Various, eg, Ethex, Ivax, Mylan, Teva)	**Tablets**: 4 mg (as base)	May contain lactose. In 100s, 500s, 1,000s, and UD 100s.
Rx	**Cardura** (Pfizer)		Lactose. (Cardura 4 mg). Orange. In 100s and UD 100s.
Rx	**Doxazosin Mesylate** (Various, eg, Ethex, Ivax, Mylan, Teva)	**Tablets**: 8 mg (as base)	May contain lactose. In 100s, 500s, 1,000s, and UD 100s.
Rx	**Cardura** (Pfizer)		Lactose. (Cardura 8 mg). Green. In 100s and UD 100s.
Rx	**Cardura XL** (Pfizer)	**Tablets, extended-release**: 4 mg (as base)	(CXL 4). In 30s.
		8 mg (as base)	(CXL 8). In 30s.

DOXAZOSIN MESYLATE — ORAL

For complete and comparative prescribing information, refer to the Alpha-1-Adrenergic Blockers group monograph.

Indications

➤*Benign prostatic hyperplasia:* Treatment of both the urinary outflow obstruction and obstructive and irritative symptoms associated with benign prostatic hyperplasia (BPH): obstructive symptoms (hesitation, intermittency, dribbling, weak urinary stream, incomplete emptying of the bladder), and irritative symptoms (nocturia, daytime frequency, urgency, burning). Doxazosin mesylate may be used in all BPH patients whether hypertensive or normotensive. In patients with hypertension and BPH, both conditions were effectively treated with doxazosin mesylate monotherapy. Doxazosin mesylate provides rapid improvement in symptoms and urinary flow rate in 66% to 71% of patients. Sustained improvements with doxazosin mesylate were seen in patients treated for up to 14 weeks in double-blind studies and up to 2 years in open-label studies.

➤*Hypertension (not extended-release):* Treatment of hypertension. Doxazosin mesylate may be used alone or in combination with diuretics, beta-adrenergic blocking agents, calcium channel blockers or angiotensin-converting enzyme inhibitors.

➤*Off-label uses:*

Pediatric hypertension – [1] = Good documentation. Doxazosin is among the therapeutic options for pediatric hypertension identified by the National High Blood Pressure Education Program, based on expert opinion.

Ureteral stones – [1] = Good documentation. In limited trials, doxazosin was as effective as terazosin or tamsulosin in the management of ureteral stones and may be more effective in promoting expulsion of larger stones (5 to 10 mm) than smaller ones (smaller than 5 mm). Larger, controlled trials are needed to identify which types of stones may be most responsive to this therapy. In the meta-analysis performed for the guidelines statement, significantly more patients (29%) receiving alpha-blocker therapy passed stones compared with controls. The guidelines state that alpha-blockers are the preferred agents for medical expulsive therapy to facilitate the passage of stones or stone fragments.

Administration and Dosage

➤*General dosing considerations:* The starting dose is intended to minimize the frequency of postural hypotension and first-dose syncope associated with doxazosin. Postural effects are most likely to occur between 2 and 6 hours postdose. Therefore, blood pressure measurements should be taken during this time period after the first dose and with each increase in dose. If doxazosin administration is discontinued for several days, therapy should be restarted using the initial dosing regimen.

➤*Adults:*

Benign prostatic hyperplasia –

Extended-release tablets:

• *Maximum dose* – 8 mg once daily.

• *Initial dosage* – 4 mg once daily with breakfast.

• *Dosage titration* – Dose may be increased to 8 mg at 3- to 4-week intervals.

• *Conversion* – If switching from immediate- to extended-release tablets, therapy should be initiated with the lowest dose (4 mg once daily). Prior to starting therapy with extended-release tablets, the final evening dose of immediate-release tables should not be taken.

Immediate-release tablets:

• *Maximum dose* – 8 mg once daily.

• *Initial dosage* – 1 mg once daily in the morning or evening.

• *Dosage titration* – Dosage may be increased to 2 mg and to 4 and 8 mg once daily at 1- to 2-week intervals thereafter. Blood pressure should be evaluated routinely in these patients.

Hypertension –

Immediate-release tablets:

• *Maximum dose* – 16 mg once daily.

• *Initial dosage* – 1 mg once daily.

• *Dosage titration* – Depending on the individual patient's standing blood pressure response (based on measurements taken at 2 to 6 hours postdose and 24 hours postdose), dosage may then be increased to 2 mg and, if necessary, to 4, 8, and 16 mg thereafter to achieve the desired reduction in blood pressure. Increases in dose beyond 4 mg increase the likelihood of excessive postural effects, including syncope, postural dizziness/vertigo, and postural hypotension. At a titrated dose of 16 mg once daily, the frequency of postural effects is about 12% compared with 3% for placebo.

Off-label dosing –

Ureteral stones: [1] = Good documentation. As adjunctive therapy in dosages of 4 mg daily for up to 1 month or time of expulsion.

➤*Children:*

Off-label dosing –

Pediatric hypertension: [1] = Good documentation. Initial dosage is 1 mg/day orally once daily. The maximum recommended dosage is 4 mg/day.

DOXAZOSIN MESYLATE — ORAL

➤*Hepatic function impairment:* Doxazosin mesylate should be administered with caution to patients with evidence of impaired hepatic function.

➤*Administration:*

Extended-release tablets – Tablets should be swallowed whole, and they must not be chewed, divided, cut, or crushed.

➤*Storage/Stability:* Store at 15° to 30°C (59° to 86°F).

TAMSULOSIN HYDROCHLORIDE

Rx	**Tamsulosin** (Various, eg, Global Pharmaceuticals, Wockhardt)	**Capsules; oral:** 0.4 mg	May contain sugar spheres. In 30s, 100s, 500s, 1,000s, and UD 16s and 30s.
Rx	**Flomax** (Boehringer Ingelheim)		(Flomax 0.4 mg BI 58). Olive green/orange. In 100s and 1,000s.

TAMSULOSIN HYDROCHLORIDE — ORAL

For complete and comparative prescribing information, refer to the Alpha-1-Adrenergic Blockers group monograph.

Indications

➤*Benign prostatic hyperplasia (BPH):* Treatment of the signs and symptoms of benign prostatic hyperplasia (BPH). Tamsulosin capsules are not indicated for the treatment of hypertension.

➤*Off-label uses:*

Ureteral stones – [1] = Good documentation. Initial data suggest that tamsulosin may have some benefit as adjunctive therapy in the management of ureteral stones. In a study comparing the efficacy of tamsulosin with doxazosin and terazosin, all 3 alpha-blockers produced similar rates of efficacy as measured by expulsion rates, time to expulsion, and lower analgesia use. In the meta-analysis performed for the guidelines statement, significantly more patients (29%) receiving alpha-blocker therapy passed stones compared with controls. The guidelines panel states that alpha-blockers are the preferred agents for medical expulsive therapy to facilitate the passage of stones or stone fragments. (See Administration and Dosage.)

Administration and Dosage

➤*Adults:*

Benign prostatic hyperplasia –

Usual dosage: 0.4 mg once daily 30 minutes following the same meal each day.

Alternative dosage: For patients who fail to respond to the 0.4 mg dose after 2 to 4 weeks, the dose of tamsulosin can be increased to 0.8 mg once daily.

Discontinuation of therapy: If tamsulosin capsules administration is discontinued or interrupted for several days at either the 0.4 mg or 0.8 mg dose, therapy should be started again with the 0.4 mg once daily dose.

Off-label dosing –

Ureteral stones: [1] = Good documentation. Used as adjunctive therapy in dosages of 0.4 mg daily for up to 6 weeks or until expulsion.

➤*Renal function impairment:* Patients with renal impairment do not require an adjustment in dosing.

➤*Hepatic function impairment:* Patients with moderate hepatic dysfunction do not require an adjustment in dosage.

➤*Storage/Stability:* Store at 20° to 25°C (68° to 77°F).

ALFUZOSIN HYDROCHLORIDE

Rx	**Uroxatral** (Sanofi-Syntholabo)	**Tablets, extended-release; oral:** 10 mg	Hydrogenated castor oil, mannitol. (X10). Round, white, yellow. In 30s, 100s, and UD 100s.

ALFUZOSIN HYDROCHLORIDE — ORAL

For complete and comparative prescribing information, refer to the Alpha-1-Adrenergic Blockers class monograph.

Indications

➤*Benign prostatic hyperplasia:* Treatment of the signs and symptoms of benign prostatic hyperplasia (BPH).

Administration and Dosage

➤*Adults:*

Benign prostatic hyperplasia – 10 mg daily to be taken immediately after the same meal each day.

➤*Children:* Alfuzosin is not indicated for use in children.

➤*Elderly:* No overall differences in safety or effectiveness were observed between these subjects and younger subjects.

➤*Renal function impairment:* Caution should be exercised when alfuzosin is administered in patients with severe renal insufficiency.

➤*Hepatic function impairment:* Alfuzosin is contraindicated in patients with moderate to severe hepatic impairment.

➤*Administration:* The tablets should not be chewed or crushed.

➤*Storage/Stability:* Store at 25°C (77°F); excursions permitted between 15° and 30°C (59° and 86°F). Protect from light and moisture.

RENIN ANGIOTENSIN SYSTEM ANTAGONISTS

Angiotensin-Converting Enzyme Inhibitors

WARNING

Pregnancy – When used in pregnancy during the second and third trimesters, angiotensin-converting enzyme (ACE) inhibitors can cause injury to and even death in the developing fetus. When pregnancy is detected, discontinue the ACE inhibitor as soon as possible. Refer to the general discussion of these products in the Antihypertensives Introduction.

Indications

➤*General information:* Refer to individual monographs for specific indications.

ACE Inhibitor Indications

Indications ✓ = FDA approved X = Unlabeled	Benazepril	Captopril	Enalapril	Enalaprilat	Fosinopril	Lisinopril	Moexipril	Perindopril	Quinapril	Ramipril	Trandolapril
Diabetic nephropathy		✓	X[a]							X[a]	
Heart failure	X[b]	✓	✓		✓	✓			✓	✓[c]	✓[c]
Hypertension	✓	✓	✓	✓	✓	✓	✓	✓	✓	✓	✓
Pediatric hypertension		X[d]							X[d]		
Hypertensive emergencies/ urgencies		X[a]		X[d]							
Improve survival post-MI[e]						✓					
Left ventricular dysfunction, post-MI		✓									✓
Left ventricular dysfunction, asymptomatic			✓								
Nondiabetic nephropathy	X[b]									X[a]	
Prevention of migraine (adults)						X[f]					
Prevention of recurrent stroke	X[g]										
Raynaud phenomenon		X[g]									
Reduce risk of MI, stroke, and death from cardiovascular causes										✓	

ACE Inhibitor Indications											
Indications ✔ = FDA approved X = Unlabeled	Benazepril	Captopril	Enalapril	Enalaprilat	Fosinopril	Lisinopril	Moexipril	Perindopril	Quinapril	Ramipril	Trandolapril
Reduce risk of nonfatal MI or cardiovascular mortality								✔			

[a] Not rated.
[b] Good documentation.
[c] Following MI.
[d] Safety concerns.
[e] MI = myocardial infarction.
[f] Insufficient documentation.
[g] Fair documentation.

➤*Hypertension:* The ACE inhibitors are effective alone and in combination with other antihypertensives, especially thiazide-type diuretics. Blood pressure-lowering effects of ACE inhibitors and thiazides are approximately additive.

Per the Joint National Committee Seventh Report (JNC 7) guidelines, use thiazide-type diuretics as initial therapy for most patients with hypertension, either alone or in combination with 1 or the other classes (eg, ACE inhibitors).

➤*Heart failure:* **Captopril**, **enalapril**, **fosinopril**, **lisinopril**, and **quinapril** are indicated in the treatment of (congestive) heart failure, usually in combination with diuretics and/or digitalis. **Ramipril** and **trandolapril** are indicated in stable patients who are symptomatic from congestive heart failure (CHF) within the first few days after sustaining acute MI.

➤*Left ventricular dysfunction:* **Enalapril** is indicated to treat clinically stable asymptomatic patients with left ventricular dysfunction (ejection fraction 35% or less). It has been shown to decrease the rate of developing overt heart failure and decrease the incidence of hospitalization for heart failure.

Captopril is indicated to improve survival following MI in clinically stable patients with left ventricular dysfunction manifested as an ejection fraction of 40% or less and to reduce the incidence of overt heart failure and subsequent hospitalizations for CHF in these patients.

Trandolapril is indicated in stable patients who have evidence of left ventricular systolic dysfunction (identified by wall motion abnormalities).

➤*Myocardial infarction:* **Lisinopril** is indicated in the treatment of hemodynamically stable patients within 24 hours of acute MI to improve survival.

➤*Reduction in risk of myocardial infarction, stroke, and death from cardiovascular causes:* **Ramipril** is indicated in patients 55 years or older who are at high risk of developing a major cardiovascular event because of a history of coronary artery disease, stroke, peripheral vascular disease, or diabetes that is accompanied by at least 1 other cardiovascular risk factor (eg, hypertension, elevated total cholesterol levels, low HDL levels, cigarette smoking, documented microalbuminuria), to reduce the risk of MI, stroke, or death from cardiovascular causes.

➤*Diabetic nephropathy:* **Captopril** is indicated for the treatment of diabetic nephropathy (proteinuria over 500 mg/day) in patients with type 1 insulin-dependent diabetes mellitus and retinopathy. Captopril decreases the rate of progression of renal insufficiency and development of serious adverse clinical outcomes (death or need for renal transplantation or dialysis).

➤*Off-label uses:* Refer to individual monographs for further information.

Heart failure –
Benazepril: [1] = Good documentation.

Nephropathy (nondiabetic) –
Benazepril: [1] = Good documentation.

Pediatric hypertension –
Captopril: [3] = Safety concerns.
Quinapril: [3] = Safety concerns.

Pediatric hypertensive urgency or emergency –
Enalaprilat: [3] = Safety concerns.

Prevention of migraine (adults) –
Lisinopril: [4] = Insufficient documentation.

Prevention of recurrent stroke –
Benazepril: [2] = Fair documentation.

Raynaud phenomenon –
Captopril: [2] = Fair documentation.
Enalapril: [5] = Poor documentation.

Other possible off-label uses –

Bartter syndrome: ACE inhibitors may be of benefit in the management of Bartter syndrome.

Diabetic nephropathy: Other ACE inhibitors (eg, **enalapril**, **ramipril**) have been shown to be effective in the treatment of diabetic nephropathy in normotensive patients.

Hypertensive emergencies/urgencies: **Enalaprilat** (1.25 mg intravenously (IV) over 5 minutes every 6 hours; titrate by 1.25 mg increments up to a maximum dose of 5 mg) may be useful in the management of hypertensive emergencies. **Captopril** (25 to 50 mg at 1- or 2-hour intervals) may be useful for hypertensive urgencies.

JNC 7 guidelines: Per JNC 7 guidelines, ACE inhibitors have been shown in clinical trials to be beneficial in the following: heart failure, post-MI, high coronary disease risk, diabetes, chronic kidney disease, and recurrent stroke prevention.

Nondiabetic nephropathy: **Ramipril**has been shown to have favorable effects on the progression of nondiabetic nephropathy.

Renovascular hypertension: ACE inhibitors have shown effectiveness in the treatment of renovascular hypertension.

Sclerodermal renal crisis: Prompt treatment of sclerodermal renal crisis with ACE inhibitors may reverse acute renal failure.

Stroke prevention: **Perindopril**, alone and in combination with a diuretic, has been shown to reduce the risk of stroke among hypertensive and nonhypertensive individuals with a history of stroke or transient ischemic attack.

Actions

➤*Pharmacology:* The ACE inhibitors appear to act primarily through suppression of the renin-angiotensin-aldosterone system. Based on chemical structure, they can be classified into 3 groups: Sulfhydryl-containing (**captopril**); dicarbocyl-containing (**enalapril**, **lisinopril**, **benazepril**, **quinapril**, **moexipril**, **perindopril**, **trandolapril**, **ramipril**); and phosphorus-containing (**fosinopril**).

Synthesized by the kidneys, renin is released into the circulation where it acts on angiotensinogen to produce angiotensin I, a relatively inactive decapeptide. Angiotensin I is then converted by the ACE to angiotensin II, a potent endogenous vasoconstrictor that also stimulates aldosterone secretion from the adrenal cortex, contributing to sodium and fluid retention. ACE inhibitors prevent the conversion of angiotensin I to angiotensin II by inhibiting ACE; they do not alter pressor responses to other agents.

Inhibiting ACE results in decreased plasma angiotensin II and increased plasma renin activity (PRA), the latter resulting from loss of negative feedback on renin release caused by reduction in angiotensin II. This leads to decreased aldosterone secretion, resulting in small increases in serum potassium along with sodium and fluid loss.

Increased prostaglandin synthesis also may play a role in the antihypertensive action of ACE inhibitor. ACE is identical to bradykininase (kininase II); thus, ACE inhibitors can increase bradykinin levels. Because bradykinin stimulates prostaglandin biosynthesis, these peptides may contribute to the pharmacological effects of ACE inhibitors.

The ACE inhibitors produce a reduction of peripheral arterial resistance in hypertensive patients, an increase in cardiac output, and little or no change in heart rate. Renal blood flow increases, but glomerular filtration rate (GFR) is usually unchanged.

Blood pressure reduction may be progressive. To achieve maximal effects, several weeks of therapy may be required. Blood pressure–lowering effects of ACE inhibitors and thiazide-type diuretics are additive, but **captopril** and beta-blockers have a less than additive effect. Standing and supine blood pressures are lowered to about the same extent. Orthostatic effects and tachycardia are infrequent but may occur in volume- or salt-depleted patients. Abrupt withdrawal is not associated with a rapid increase in blood pressure.

The ACE inhibitors are antihypertensive, even in low-renin hypertensive patients. They are antihypertensive in all races studied, but black hypertensive patients (usually low-renin hypertensive patients) show a smaller average response to monotherapy than nonblacks.

Some ACE inhibitors have demonstrated a beneficial effect on the severity of heart failure and an improvement in maximal exercise tolerance in patients with heart failure. In these patients, ACE inhibitors significantly decrease peripheral (systemic vascular) resistance, blood pressure (afterload), pulmonary capillary wedge pressure (preload), and pulmonary vascular resistance, and increase cardiac output and exercise tolerance time. These effects occur after the first dose and persist for the duration of therapy.

➤*Pharmacokinetics:*

Absorption/Distribution – The presence of food in the GI tract reduces the absorption of **captopril** by about 30% to 40%. Food intake also reduces **moexipril** maximum drug concentration (C_{max}) 70% to 80% and area under the curve (AUC) 40% to 50%. Therefore, take **captopril** and **moexipril** 1 hour before meals (see Drug Interactions).

Animal studies indicate that **benazepril** (and metabolites), **enalapril**, **lisinopril**, **captopril**, and **perindopril** cross the blood-brain barrier poorly, if at all. **Enalaprilat**, **fosinopril**/fosinoprilat, and **quinapril** do not cross the blood-brain barrier.

Metabolism/Excretion – With the exception of **captopril** and **lisinopril**, most of the ACE inhibitors are prodrugs that are rapidly converted to their active metabolites following oral administration.

The effective half-lives for accumulation are as follows: 10 to 11 hours for **benazeprilat**, 11 hours for **enalaprilat**, 11.5 hours for **fosinoprilat**, 12 hours for **lisinopril**, 12 hours for **moexiprilat**, and 3 hours for **quinaprilat**.

Special populations –

Renal function impairment:

• *Benazepril –* In patients with creatinine clearance (CrCl) 30 mL/min or less, peak benazeprilat levels and the initial (alpha phase) half-life increase, and the time to steady state may be delayed. In patients with renal failure, biliary clearance may compensate to an extent.

• *Captopril* – Excretion rates are reduced and retention of captopril occurs in patients with impaired renal function. **Captopril** can be removed by hemodialysis.

• *Enalapril/Enalaprilat* – With GFR of 30 mL/min or less, peak and trough enalapril levels increase, time to reach C_{max} (T_{max}) increases, and time to steady state may be delayed. Enalaprilat is dialyzable at the rate of 62 mL/min.

• *Fosinopril* – In patients with end-stage renal disease (CrCl less than 10 mL/min), the total body clearance of fosinoprilat is approximately one-half of that in patients with healthy renal function. **Fosinopril** is not well dialyzed.

• *Lisinopril* – Impaired renal function (GFR less than 30 mL/min) decreases **lisinopril** elimination, increases peak and trough levels, increases T_{max}, and time to attain steady state is prolonged. **Lisinopril** can be removed by hemodialysis.

• *Moexipril* – The effective elimination half-life and AUC of **moexipril** and moexiprilat are increased with decreasing renal function. At CrCl in the range of 10 to 40 mL/min, the half-life of moexiprilat is increased by a factor of 3 to 4.

• *Perindopril* – Perindoprilat AUC increases with decreasing renal function. At CrCl of 30 to 80 mL/min, AUC is about double that of 100 mL/min. When CrCl drops below 30 mL/min, AUC increases more markedly. **Perindopril** dialysis clearance ranges from 40 to 80 mL/min and perindoprilat dialysis clearance ranges from 40 to 90 mL/min.

• *Quinapril* – The half-life of quinaprilat increases as CrCl decreases. There is a linear correlation between plasma quinaprilat clearance and CrCl. Chronic hemodialysis or continuous ambulatory peritoneal dialysis has little or no effect on the elimination of quinapril and quinaprilat.

• *Ramipril* – In patients with CrCl less than 40 mL/min, peak levels of ramiprilat are approximately doubled, and trough levels may be as much as 5 times higher. In multiple dose regimens, the ramiprilat AUC is 3 to 4 times as large as it is in patients with normal renal function.

• *Trandolapril* – The plasma concentrations of **trandolapril** and trandolaprilat are approximately 2-fold greater and renal clearance is reduced by about 85% in patients with CrCl below 30 mL/min and in patients on hemodialysis.

Hepatic function impairment:

• *Fosinopril* – In patients with hepatic insufficiency (alcoholic or biliary cirrhosis), the rate of hydrolysis of **fosinopril** may be slowed. The apparent total body clearance of fosinoprilat is approximately one-half of that in patients with normal hepatic function.

• *Moexipril* – In patients with mild to moderate cirrhosis given single 15 mg doses, the C_{max} of moexipril was increased by about 50% and the AUC increased by about 120%, while the C_{max} for moexiprilat was decreased by about 50% and the AUC increased by about 300%.

• *Perindopril* – The bioavailability of perindoprilat is increased, and plasma concentrations were about 50% higher than those with healthy liver function.

• *Quinapril* – Quinaprilat concentrations are reduced in patients with alcoholic cirrhosis because of impaired deesterification of **quinapril**.

• *Ramipril* – The metabolism of **ramipril** to ramiprilat appears to be slowed, and plasma **ramipril** levels are increased about 3-fold.

• *Trandolapril* – Following oral administration in patients with mild to moderate alcoholic cirrhosis, plasma concentrations of **trandolapril** and trandolaprilat were, respectively, 9- and 2-fold greater than in healthy subjects, but inhibition of ACE activity was not affected.

Elderly:

• *Lisinopril* – Older patients have (approximately doubled) higher blood levels and AUC than younger patients.

• *Moexipril* – The AUC and C_{max} of moexipril is about 30% greater than in younger subjects.

• *Perindopril* – Plasma concentrations of **perindopril** and perindoprilat in patients older than 70 years are approximately twice those observed in younger patients.

• *Quinapril* – Elimination of quinaprilat may be reduced in patients 65 years and older.

• *Ramipril* – Peak ramiprilat levels and AUC are higher in older patients.

• *Trandolapril* – The plasma concentration of **trandolapril** is increased in elderly hypertensive patients, but the plasma concentration of trandolaprilat and inhibition of ACE activity are similar in elderly and young hypertensive patients.

Heart failure:

• *Fosinopril* – The effective half-life of fosinoprilat was 14 hours.

• *Perindopril* – Perindoprilat clearance is reduced in CHF patients, resulting in 40% higher-dose interval AUC.

• *Quinapril* – Elimination of quinaprilat may be reduced in patients with heart failure.

Pharmacokinetics of the Active Moieties of ACE Inhibitors

ACE inhibitor	Onset (h)	Peak effect (h)	Duration (h)	Bioavailability (%)	T_{max} (h)	Protein binding	Effect of food on absorption	Active metabolite	Elimination half-life (h)	Routes of elimination
Benazepril	1	2-4	24	≥ 37	0.5-1 (1-4)[a,b]	≈ 96.7% (≈ 95.3%)[a]	slows absorption	benazeprilat		renal (20%)[a] bile (11%-12%)[a]
Captopril	≤ 0.5	1-1.5	6-10 (dose-related)	≥ 75	1	≈ 25%-30%	absorption reduced by ≈ 30%-40%		< 2	renal (> 95%)
Enalapril	1	4-6	≥ 24	≈ 60	1 (3-4)[a]		none	enalaprilat		renal feces
Enalaprilat	0.25	1-4	≈ 6	NA[c]			NA			renal (> 90%)
Fosinopril	1	2-6	24	≈ 36	3	99.4%[a]	slows absorption	fosinoprilat	≈ 12[a]	renal (≈ 50%) feces (≈ 50%)
Lisinopril	1	6	24	≈ 25	7	none	none			renal (100%)
Moexipril	≈ 1	3-6	24	≈ 13	≈ 1.5[a]	≈ 50%[a]	markedly reduced	moexiprilat	2-9[a]	renal (13%) feces (53%)
Perindopril				≈ 75	≈ 1 (3-7)[a]	≈ 60% (10%-20%)[a]	reduces bioavailability of metabolite	perindoprilat	≈ 0.8-1 (3-10)[a]	renal
Quinapril	≤ 1	2-4	24	≥ 60	1 (≈ 2)[a]	≈ 97%	moderately reduced	quinaprilat	≈ 2[a]	renal
Ramipril	1-2	3-6	24	≥ 50-60	1 (2-4)[a]	≈ 73% (≈ 56%)[a]	slows absorption	ramiprilat	9-18[a]	renal (60%) feces (40%)
Trandolapril		4-8	24	≈ 10 (70)[a]	1 (4-10)[a]	≈ 80%	slows absorption	trandolaprilat	≈ 6 (10)[a]	renal (≈ 33%) feces (≈ 66%)

[a] Active metabolite.
[b] 1 to 2 hours in fasting state and 2 to 4 hours in nonfasting state.
[c] NA = not available.

Contraindications

Hypersensitivity to these products and in patients with a history of angioedema related to previous treatment with an ACE inhibitor; in patients with hereditary or idiopathic angioedema (**enalapril, enalaprilat, lisinopril, perindopril**).

Warnings/Precautions

➤*Hematologic effects:* Neutropenia (less than 1,000/mm³) with myeloid hypoplasia resulted from use of **captopril**. About half of the neutropenic patients developed systemic or oral cavity infections or other features of agranulocytosis. The risk of neutropenia is dependent on the patient's clinical status. In hypertension with healthy renal function (serum creatinine less than 1.6 mg/dL, no collagen vascular disease [eg, systemic lupus erythematosus, scleroderma]), neutropenia occurred in 1 patient in more than 8,600 exposed. In patients with some degree of renal failure (serum creatinine at least 1.6 mg/dL) but no collagen vascular disease, the risk of neutropenia was about 1 in 500. Daily doses of **captopril** were relatively high. Concomitant **allopurinol** and **captopril** have been associated with neutropenia. In collagen vascular diseases and impaired renal function, neutropenia has occurred in 3.7% of patients. In heart failure, the same risk factors for neutropenia appear present; about half of cases had serum creatinine at least 1.6 mg/dL, and more than 75% also were on **procainamide**.

Neutropenia usually has been detected within 3 months after **captopril** initiation. Bone marrow examinations consistently showed myeloid hypoplasia, frequently accompanied by erythroid hypoplasia and decreased numbers of megakaryocytes (eg, hypoplastic bone marrow, pancytopenia); anemia and thrombocytopenia were sometimes seen. In general, neutrophils returned to normal about 2 weeks after **captopril** was discontinued; serious infections were limited to clinically complex patients. About 13% of neutropenia cases were fatal, but almost all were in patients with serious illness having collagen vascular disease, renal failure, heart failure, immunosuppressant therapy, or a combination of these factors. Discontinuation of captopril and other drugs has generally led to prompt return of the normal WBC count; upon confirmation of neutropenia, withdraw the drug and closely observe the patient.

Neutropenia/leukopenia/agranulocytosis has occurred rarely with **enalapril** or **lisinopril** and in 1 patient on **quinapril**; a causal relationship cannot be excluded. Data are insufficient to show that **moexipril**, **perindopril**, **ramipril**, **benazepril**, **trandolapril**, or **fosinopril** do not cause agranulocytosis at similar rates. Periodically monitor white blood cell (WBC) counts.

➤*Anaphylactoid and possibly related reactions:* Presumably because ACE inhibitors affect the metabolism of eicosanoids and polypeptides, including endogenous bradykinin, patients receiving ACE inhibitors may be subject to a variety of adverse reactions, some of them serious.

Angioedema – Angioedema has occurred in patients treated with ACE inhibitors. It may occur at any time during treatment with **enalapril** (0.2%); **captopril**, **lisinopril**, **perindopril**, **quinapril** (0.1%); **trandolapril** (0.13%); **benazepril** (about 0.5%); **moexipril** (less than 0.5%); **ramipril** (0.3%); or **fosinopril** (0.2% to 1%). Angioedema of the face, extremities, lips, mucous membranes, tongue, glottis, or larynx has occurred. In instances where swelling has been confined to the face and lips, the condition has generally resolved without treatment, although antihistamines have been useful in relieving symptoms. Angioedema associated with laryngeal edema may be fatal. If laryngeal stridor or angioedema of the face, tongue, larynx, or glottis occurs and appears likely to cause airway obstruction, discontinue treatment and institute appropriate therapy (eg, epinephrine solution 1:1000 subcutaneous) immediately. Use with extreme caution in patients with hereditary angioedema (caused by a deficiency of C1 esterase inhibitor). Intestinal angioedema has been reported in patients treated with ACE inhibitors. These patients presented with abdominal pain (with or without nausea or vomiting); in some cases there was no history of facial angioedema and C1 esterase levels were normal. The angioedema was diagnosed by procedures including abdominal CT scan or ultrasound, or at surgery, and symptoms resolved after stopping the ACE inhibitor. Include intestinal angioedema in the differential diagnosis of patients on ACE inhibitors presenting with abdominal pain. Symptoms resolved after stopping ACE inhibitors. Patients with a history of angioedema unrelated to ACE inhibitor therapy may be at increased risk of angioedema while receiving an ACE inhibitor. Black patients receiving ACE inhibitor monotherapy have been reported to have a higher incidence of angioedema compared with nonblacks.

Anaphylactoid reactions during desensitization – Two patients undergoing desensitizing treatment with Hymenoptera venom while receiving ACE inhibitors sustained life-threatening anaphylactoid reactions. In the same patients, these reactions were avoided when ACE inhibitors were temporarily withheld, but they reappeared upon inadvertent rechallenge.

Anaphylactoid reactions during membrane exposure – Anaphylactoid reactions have been reported in patients dialyzed with high-flux membranes and treated concomitantly with an ACE inhibitor. In such patients, immediately stop dialysis and initiate aggressive therapy for anaphylactoid reactions. Symptoms have not been relieved by antihistamines in these situations. Consider a different type of dialysis membrane or a different class of medication. Anaphylactoid reactions also have occurred in patients undergoing low-density lipoprotein apheresis with dextran sulfate absorption.

➤*Proteinuria:* Total urinary proteins of more than 1 g/day were seen in about 0.7% of **captopril** patients. About 90% of affected patients showed evidence of prior renal disease or received relatively high dosages of **captopril** (more than 150 mg/day) or both. Nephrotic syndrome occurred in approximately one-fifth of these cases. In most cases, proteinuria cleared within 6 months, regardless of whether **captopril** was continued; creatinine and serum urea nitrogen (BUN) were seldom altered.

➤*Hypotension:*

First-dose effect – ACE inhibitors may cause a profound fall in blood pressure following the first dose. Excessive hypotension is rare in uncomplicated hypertensive patients, but is possible with ACE inhibitor use in severely salt/volume-depleted people, such as those treated vigorously with diuretics or patients on dialysis. Patients at risk of excessive hypotension, sometimes associated with oliguria and/or progressive azotemia, and rarely with acute renal failure and/or death, include those with the following conditions or characteristics: heart failure, hyponatremia, high-dose diuretic therapy, recent intensive diuresis or increase in diuretic dose, renal dialysis, or severe volume and/or salt depletion. Correct volume and/or salt depletion before initiating treatment. Excessive perspiration, dehydration, vomiting, and/or diarrhea may also lead to an excessive fall in blood pressure because of reduction in fluid volume.

Minimize the possibility of hypotension either by discontinuing the diuretic or by increasing salt intake about 1 week prior to initiating ACE inhibitors, or initiate with small doses. Alternatively, provide medical supervision for at least 2 hours after the initial dose and until blood pressure has stabilized for at least an additional hour.

A transient hypotensive response is not a contraindication for further doses of these agents, which usually can be given without difficulty once the blood pressure has stabilized. If excessive hypotension occurs, place patient in supine position and, if necessary, give normal saline IV. A dose reduction or discontinuation of the ACE inhibitor or concomitant diuretic may be necessary.

Heart failure – In heart failure where the blood pressure was either normal or low, transient decreases in mean blood pressure more than 20% occurred in about half of patients taking **captopril**. Transient hypotension may occur after the first several doses. This effect is usually well tolerated, and it is asymptomatic or produces brief, mild light-headedness. It rarely has been associated with arrhythmia or conduction defects. Start therapy under close medical supervision. Follow patients closely for the first 2 weeks and whenever the dose of ACE inhibitor or diuretic is increased. Also follow patients with ischemic heart, aortic stenosis, or cerebrovascular disease in whom an excessive fall in blood pressure could result in MI or cerebrovascular accident.

Hypotension is not a reason to discontinue the ACE inhibitor. Some decrease in systemic blood pressure is common and desirable in heart failure. The magnitude of the decrease is greatest early in treatment, stabilizes within 1 to 2 weeks, and generally returns to pretreatment levels without a decrease in efficacy within 2 months.

Acute myocardial infarction – In a study, patients with an acute MI had a higher incidence of persistent hypotension (systolic blood pressure less than 90 mm Hg for more than 1 hour) when treated with **lisinopril**. Treatment must not be initiated in acute MI patients at risk of further serious hemodynamic deterioration after treatment with a vasodilator (eg, systolic blood pressure of 100 mm Hg or lower) or cardiogenic shock.

➤*Hepatic failure:* Rarely ACE inhibitors have been associated with a syndrome that starts with cholestatic jaundice and progresses to fulminant hepatic necrosis and (sometimes) death. The mechanism of this syndrome is not understood. Patients receiving ACE inhibitors who develop jaundice or marked elevations of hepatic enzymes should discontinue the ACE inhibitor and receive appropriate medical follow-up.

➤*Hyperkalemia:* Elevated serum potassium (at least 0.5 mEq/L greater than the upper limit of normal) was observed in **perindopril**, in 0.4% of hypertensive patients given **trandolapril**; about 1% of hypertensive patients given **benazepril**, **enalapril**, **ramipril**, or **moexipril**; about 2% of patients receiving **lisinopril** or **quinapril**, about 2.6% of hypertensive patients given **fosinopril**, and about 4.8% of CHF patients given **lisinopril**. In most cases, these were resolved despite continued therapy. Hyperkalemia was a cause of therapy discontinuation in 0.28% of hypertensive patients on **enalapril**, about 0.1% with **lisinopril** and **fosinopril**, less than 0.1% with **quinapril**, no patients on **ramipril** and **trandolapril**, 2% of type 1 diabetics with proteinuria receiving **captopril**, 0.6% of heart failure patients on **lisinopril**, and 0.1% of MI patients on **lisinopril**. Risk factors of development of hyperkalemia may include renal insufficiency, diabetes mellitus, and concomitant use of agents that increase serum potassium (eg, potassium-sparing diuretics, potassium supplements, and/or potassium-containing salt substitutes).

➤*Valvular stenosis:* Theoretically, patients with aortic stenosis might be at risk of decreased coronary perfusion when treated with vasodilators, because they do not develop as much afterload reduction as others. Use with caution in patients with obstruction in the outflow tract of the left ventricle (eg, aortic stenosis, hypertrophic cardiomyopathy).

➤*Surgery/Anesthesia:* In patients undergoing major surgery or during anesthesia with agents that produce hypotension, ACE inhibitors will block angiotensin II formation secondary to compensatory renin release. Hypotension can be corrected by volume expansion.

➤*Cough:* Chronic cough has occurred with the use of all ACE inhibitors, presumably caused by the inhibition of the degradation of endogenous bradykinin. Characteristically, the cough is nonproductive, persistent, and resolves within 1 to 7 days (but can take as long as 2 weeks) after therapy discontinuation. Consider ACE inhibitor–induced cough as part of the differential diagnosis of cough.

The cough appears to have a higher incidence in women. The incidence of cough, although still reported as 0.5% to 3% by some manufacturers, appears to range from 5% to 25% and has been reported to be as high as 39%, resulting in discontinuation rates as high as 15%. The use of sulindac, diclofenac, indomethacin, nifedipine, cromolyn, or nebulized bupivacaine may be effective in managing cough; although, this is only based on a small number of patients. Further study is needed.

➤*Renal function impairment:* Some hypertensive patients with unilateral or bilateral renal artery stenosis have developed increases in BUN and serum creatinine after reduction of blood pressure (20% of patients with **enalapril**). Monitor renal function in such patients during the first few weeks of therapy. Dosage reduction and/or discontinuation of the ACE inhibitor and/or diuretic may be required. For some patients, it may not be possible to normalize blood pressure and maintain adequate renal perfusion.

About 20% of heart failure patients develop stable elevations of BUN and serum creatinine more than 20% above normal or baseline with long-term **captopril**. Less than 5% of patients, generally those with severe preexisting renal disease, require treatment discontinuation; subsequent improvement probably relies on the severity of underlying renal disease.

In patients with severe CHF whose renal function may depend on the activity of the renin-angiotensin-aldosterone system, treatment with ACE inhibitors may be associated with oliguria and/or progressive azotemia and, rarely, with acute renal failure and/or death.

Some hypertensive or heart failure patients with no apparent preexisting renal vascular disease have developed increases in BUN and serum creatinine; these are usually minor and transient, especially when the ACE inhibitor was given with a diuretic. This is more likely to occur in patients with preexisting renal impairment. Dosage adjustment and/or discontinuation of the diuretic and/or ACE inhibitor may be required. However, captopril has shown renal protective effects in hypertensive patients with some renal dysfunction.

Impaired renal function decreases **lisinopril** elimination, which is excreted principally through the kidneys, but this decrease becomes clinically important only when the GFR is less than 30 mL/min. The elimination half-life of quinaprilat increases as creatinine clearance decreases. Dosage adjustment may be necessary for **quinapril**, **benazepril**, **ramipril**, **captopril**, **trandolapril**, **moexipril**, **enalapril**, **perindopril**, and **lisinopril**. Impaired renal function decreases total clearance of fosinoprilat and approximately doubles the AUC. However, in general, no dosing adjustment is needed (see Pharmacokinetics).

➤*Hepatic function impairment:* Patients with impaired liver function could develop markedly elevated plasma levels of unchanged **fosinopril**, **moexipril**, or **ramipril**. No formal pharmacokinetic studies with **ramipril** have been done in hypertensive patients with impaired liver function. In patients with alcoholic or biliary cirrhosis, the rate, but not extent, of **fosinopril** hydrolysis was reduced; the total body clearance of fosinoprilat was decreased and AUC approximately doubled. Quinaprilat concentrations are reduced in patients with alcoholic cirrhosis caused by impaired deesterification of **quinapril**. Consider lower **trandolapril** doses in patients with mild to moderate alcoholic cirrhosis; plasma concentrations of **trandolapril** and trandolaprilat were increased. Perindoprilat plasma concentrations may be elevated.

➤*Photosensitivity:* Photosensitization may occur; therefore, caution patients to take protective measures (ie, sunscreens, protective clothing) against exposure to ultraviolet light or sunlight until tolerance is determined.

➤*Pregnancy: Category C* (first trimester), except **perindopril**; *Category D* (**perindopril** and second and third trimesters for all others). ACE inhibitors can cause fetal and neonatal morbidity and death when administered to pregnant women. Several dozen cases have been reported in the world literature. When pregnancy is detected, discontinue ACE inhibitors as soon as possible.

The use of ACE inhibitors during the second and third trimesters of pregnancy has been associated with fetal and neonatal injury, including hypotension, neonatal skull hypoplasia, anuria, reversible or irreversible renal failure, and death. Oligohydramnios also has occurred, presumably resulting from decreased fetal renal function; oligohydramnios in this setting has been associated with fetal limb contractures, craniofacial deformation, and hypoplastic lung development. Prematurity, intrauterine growth retardation, and patent ductus arteriosus also have been reported, although it is not clear whether these occurrences were caused by the ACE inhibitor exposure.

These adverse effects do not appear to have resulted from intrauterine ACE inhibitor exposure that has been limited to the first trimester. Inform mothers whose embryos and fetuses are exposed to ACE inhibitors only during the first trimester. Nonetheless, when patients become pregnant, make every effort to discontinue the use of the ACE inhibitor as soon as possible.

Rarely (probably less often than 1 in every 1000 pregnancies), no alternative to ACE inhibitors will be found. In these rare cases, apprise the mother of the potential hazards to the fetus, and perform serial ultrasound examinations to assess the intra-amniotic environment.

If oligohydramnios is observed, discontinue the ACE inhibitor unless it is considered lifesaving for the mother. Contraction stress testing, a nonstress test, or biophysical profiling may be appropriate, depending on the week of pregnancy. However, patients and health care providers should be aware that oligohydramnios may not appear until after the fetus has sustained irreversible injury.

Closely observe infants with histories of in utero exposure to ACE inhibitors for hypotension, oliguria, and hyperkalemia. If oliguria occurs, direct attention toward support of blood pressure and renal perfusion. Exchange transfusion or dialysis may be required as a means of reversing hypotension or substituting for disordered renal function. Some of these agents may be removed from neonatal circulation by exchange transfusion or dialysis (see Overdosage); however, limited experience has not shown that such removal is central to the treatment of these infants.

➤*Lactation:* Several ACE inhibitors have been detected in breast milk. Do not administer **trandolapril**, **captopril**, **fosinopril**, **enalapril**, **quinapril**, or **ramipril** to breast-feeding mothers. It is not known whether **lisinopril**, **moexipril**, or **perindopril** are excreted in breast milk. Because of the potential for serious adverse effects, exercise caution when these drugs are administered to breast-feeding women. Decide whether to discontinue breast-feeding or discontinue the drug, taking into account the importance of the drug to the mother.

Minimal amounts of unchanged **benazepril** and of benazeprilat are excreted in the breast milk of breast-feeding women treated with benazepril. A newborn child ingesting entirely breast milk would receive less than 0.1% of the mg/kg maternal dose of **benazepril** and benazeprilat.

➤*Children:* Treatment with **benazepril** is not recommended in pediatric patients younger than 6 years. Safety and efficacy have not been established. However, there is limited experience with the use of **captopril** in children. Dosage, on a weight basis, was comparable to or less than that used in adults. Infants, especially newborns, may be more susceptible to the adverse hemodynamic effects of captopril. Excessive, prolonged, and unpredictable decreases in blood pressure and associated complications, including oliguria and seizures, have occurred. Use **captopril** in children only when other measures for controlling blood pressure have not been effective.

Antihypertensive effects of **enalapril** have been established in hypertensive pediatric patients 1 month to 16 years of age and with **lisinopril** in patients 6 to 16 years of age. **Enalapril**, **benazepril**, and **lisinopril** are not recommended in neonates and in pediatric patients with GFR less than 30 mL/min/1.73 m^2, because no data is available.

Safety and efficacy of **perindopril** has not been established in children.

➤*Elderly:* Elderly patients may have higher blood levels and AUC of **lisinopril**, ramiprilat, **perindopril**, quinaprilat, and moexiprilat. This may relate to decreased renal function rather than to age itself. No overall differences in effectiveness or safety were observed between elderly patients receiving **trandolapril**, **fosinopril**, or **benazepril**; however, greater sensitivity of some older individuals cannot be ruled out.

➤*Monitoring:* Patients with impaired renal function should have WBC and differential counts monitored prior to starting treatment and at approximately 2-week intervals for about 3 months, then periodically. Consider periodic monitoring of WBCs in patients with collagen vascular disease and renal disease. Periodically monitor patients' serum potassium. Monitor elderly patients for dizziness because of the potential for falls.

Drug Interactions

ACE Inhibitor Drug Interactions

Precipitant drug	Object drug[a]		Description
Aldosterone blockers (eg, eplerenone)	ACE inhibitors	⬆	The risk of serious hyperkalemia may be increased, resulting in cardiac arrhythmias or arrest. Periodic monitoring of serum potassium level is recommended until the effect of the aldosterone blocker is established. Dose reduction of the aldosterone blocker may be necessary to decrease potassium levels.
ACE inhibitors	Aldosterone blockers (eg, eplerenone)		
Aliskiren	ACE inhibitors	⬆	The risk of hyperkalemia may be increased. Use with caution. Closely monitor potassium concentrations.
ACE inhibitors	Aliskiren		
Angiotensin II receptor antagonists (eg, telmisartan)	ACE inhibitors	⬆	Coadministration may be associated with an increased risk of renal dysfunction. Coadministration is not recommended.
ACE inhibitors	Angiotensin II receptor antagonists (eg, telmisartan)		
Antacids (eg, aluminum and magnesium hydroxide, simethicone)	ACE inhibitors	⬇	Bioavailability of ACE inhibitors may be decreased. May be more likely with **captopril** and **fosinopril**. Separate the administration times by 1 to 2 hours if an interaction is suspected.
Capsaicin	ACE inhibitors	⬆	Capsaicin may cause or exacerbate coughing associated with ACE inhibitor treatment and vice versa.
Cyclosporine	ACE inhibitors Perindopril	⬆	The risk of hyperkalemia may be increased. Frequent monitoring of serum potassium is warranted.
ACE inhibitors Perindopril	Cyclosporine		
Diuretics	ACE inhibitors	⬆	Possible excessive reduction in blood pressure, especially in those patients with intravascular volume depletion, can occur. Consider discontinuing the diuretic or increasing salt intake prior to initiation of treatment with an ACE inhibitor. If this is not possible, consider reduction of initial ACE inhibitor dose.
Everolimus	ACE inhibitors Perindopril	⬆	The risk of angioedema may be increased. If an interaction is suspected, stop one or both drugs.
Heparin	ACE inhibitors Perindopril	⬆	The risk of hyperkalemia may be increased. Frequent monitoring of serum potassium is warranted.
ACE inhibitors Perindopril	Heparin		
Iron salts	ACE inhibitors Captopril	⬇	Oral iron preparations may reduce captopril blood levels. Separate administration by at least 2 hours.
NSAIDs[b] (eg, indomethacin)	ACE inhibitors Perindopril	⬆⬇	This combination reduced hypotensive effects of ACE inhibitors. More prominent in low-renin or volume-dependent hypertensive patients; concomitant use may further deteriorate renal function. Monitor blood pressure and renal function. In addition, the risk of hyperkalemia may be increased. Frequently monitor serum potassium.
ACE inhibitors Perindopril	NSAIDs (eg, indomethacin)		

Angiotensin-Converting Enzyme Inhibitors

ACE Inhibitor Drug Interactions			
Precipitant drug	Object drug[a]		Description
Rifampin	ACE inhibitors Enalapril	↓	Pharmacologic effects of enalapril may be decreased.
Salicylates (eg, aspirin)	ACE inhibitors	↓	The hypotensive and vasodilator effects of benazepril may be reduced. Consider increasing the dosage of ACE inhibitor or stopping the salicylate if blood pressure control or renal function deteriorates. A decease in the salicylate dose may avoid the interaction.
Trimethoprim	ACE inhibitors	↑	The risk of serious hyperkalemia may be increased, resulting in cardiac arrhythmias or arrest. Closely monitor serum potassium level and the clinical response of the patient. If an interaction, occurs, discontinuation of one or both drugs may be necessary.
ACE inhibitors	Trimethoprim		
ACE inhibitors Captopril	Allopurinol	↑	A higher risk of hypersensitivity reaction is possible when these drugs are given concurrently.
ACE inhibitors	Diuretics (eg, loop diuretics)	↓	The effect of loop diuretics may be decreased, and inhibition of angiotensin II production by ACE inhibitors is possible.
ACE inhibitors	Gold salts (eg, sodium aurothiomalate)	↑	The risk of nitritoid reactions (eg, facial flushing, hypotension, nausea, vomiting) may be increased. Carefully monitor patients for signs and symptoms of nitritoid. If an interaction occurs, one of the agents may need to be discontinued.
ACE inhibitors	Lithium	↑	Increased serum lithium levels and symptoms of toxicity may occur; monitor lithium levels frequently.
ACE inhibitors	Hypoglycemic agents/insulin	↑	Rarely, hypoglycemia has been reported during concomitant therapy. Monitor symptoms of hypoglycemia during initiation of therapy.
ACE inhibitors	Potassium preparations/ Potassium-sparing diuretics	↑	Coadministration may result in elevated serum potassium concentrations. Use with caution; monitor potassium levels and renal function frequently.
ACE inhibitors Perindopril	Sulfonylureas (eg, glyburide)	↑	The risk of hypoglycemia may be increased. Close clinical and laboratory monitoring are warranted.
ACE inhibitors Quinapril	Tetracycline	↓	Tetracycline absorption was reduced 28% to 37%, possibly caused by the high magnesium content of quinapril tablets.

[a] ↑ = object drug increased; ↓ = object drug decreased; ↑↓ = object drug both increased and decreased.
[b] NSAIDs = nonsteroidal anti-inflammatory drugs.

➤*Drug/Lab test interactions:* **Captopril** may cause a false-positive urine test for acetone.

Fosinopril may cause a false-low measurement of serum digoxin levels with the *Digi-Tab RIA Kit for Digoxin*. Other kits, such as the *Coat-A-Count RIA Kit*, may be used.

➤*Drug/Food interactions:* Food significantly reduces the absorption of **captopril** 30% to 40%. Administer **captopril** 1 hour before meals. Food intake reduces the C_{max} and AUC of **moexipril** about 70% and 40%, respectively, after a low-fat breakfast and 80% and 50%, respectively, after a high-fat breakfast; take **moexipril** in the fasting state and administer 1 hour before meals. Food reduces the biotransformation of **perindopril** to the active metabolite perindoprilat by approximately 43%, resulting in a reduction in the plasma ACE inhibition curve of approximately 20%. The rate and extent of **quinapril** absorption are diminished moderately (about 25% to 30%) when administered during a high-fat meal. The rate, but not extent, of **ramipril**, **fosinopril**, and **trandolapril** absorption is reduced by food. Food does not reduce the GI absorption of **benazepril**, **enalapril**, and **lisinopril**.

Adverse Reactions

Adverse Reactions Shared by the ACE inhibitors[a] (%)										
✓ = Reported; no incidence given. Adverse reactions	Benazepril	Captopril	Enalapril/ Enalaprilat	Fosinopril	Lisinopril	Moexipril	Perindopril	Quinapril	Ramipril	Trandolapril
Cardiovascular										
Angina pectoris	< 1	0.2-0.3	1.5	0.2-1		< 1		< 0.5	< 1-3	
Bradycardia			0.5-1	0.4-1	0.3-1				< 1	0.3-4.7
Cardiac arrest		✓[b]	0.5-1	✓	0.3-1		✓[b]		< 1	
Cerebrovascular accident		✓[b]	0.5-1	0.2-1	0.3-1	< 1		< 0.5	< 1	
Chest pain		1	2.1	0.2-2.2	3.4	> 1		2.4	< 1	0.3-1
Hypotension[c]	0.3	✓	0.9-6.7	0.2-4.4	1.2-9.7	0.51	0.3	2.9	0.5-11	0.3-11
MI		0.2-0.3	0.5- 1.2	0.2-1	0.3-1	< 1		< 0.5	< 1	
Orthostatic hypotension/effects	0.4	✓[b]	1.2-2.2	≤ 1.2-1.9	0.3- 1.2	0.51	0.8	< 0.5	2	
Palpitations	< 1	1	0.5-1	0.2-1	0.3-1	< 1		0.5-1	< 1	0.3-1
Peripheral edema	< 1				0.3-1	> 1				
Rhythm disturbances		✓[b]	0.5-1	≤ 0.2-1.4		< 1		< 0.5		
Tachycardia		1	0.5-1	0.4-1	0.3-1			0.5-1	< 1	
CNS										
Anxiety	< 1					< 1			< 1	0.3-1
Ataxia		✓[b]	0.5-1		0.3-1					
Confusion		✓[b]	0.5-1	0.2-1	0.3-1					
Depression		✓[b]	0.5-1	0.4-1				0.5-1	< 1	
Dizziness	3.6		0.5-7.9	1.6-11.9	5.4-11.8	4.3		3.9-7.7	1.9-4	1.3-23
Fatigue	2.4		0.5-3	≥ 1	2.5	2.4		2.6	2	
Headache	6.2		1.8-5.2	≥ 1	4.4-5.7	> 1		1.7		
Insomnia/Sleep disturbances	< 1		0.5-1	0.2-1	0.3-1	< 1		0.5-1	< 1	0.3-1
Malaise					0.3-1	< 1		0.5-1	< 1	
Nervousness	< 1	✓[b]	0.5-1		0.3-1	< 1		0.5-1	< 1	

Adverse Reactions Shared by the ACE inhibitors[a] (%)

✓ = Reported; no incidence given.

Adverse reactions	Benazepril	Captopril	Enalapril/ Enalaprilat	Fosinopril	Lisinopril	Moexipril	Perindopril	Quinapril	Ramipril	Trandolapril
Paresthesias	< 1		0.5-1	0.2-1	0.3-1			0.5-1	< 1	0.3-1
Peripheral edema	< 1					> 1				
Somnolence/Drowsiness	1.6	✓[b]	0.5-1	0.2-1	0.3-1	< 1		0.5-1	< 1	0.3-1
Vertigo			1.6	0.2-1	0.2			0.5-1	< 1-2	0.3-1
Dermatologic										
Alopecia	< 1		0.5-1		0.3-1	< 1		0.5-1		
Diaphoresis/Sweating	< 1		0.5-1	0.2-1	0.3-1	< 1		0.5-1	< 1	
Erythema multiforme		✓[b]	0.5-1						< 1	
Exfoliative dermatitis		✓[b]	0.5-1	✓			✓[b]	< 0.5		
Flushing	< 1	0.2-0.5	0.5-1	0.2-1	0.3-1	1.6				0.3-1
Pemphigus/Pemphigoid	< 1	✓	0.5-1		0.3-1		✓[b]	0.5-1		0.3-1
Photosensitivity	< 1	✓	0.5-1	0.2-1	0.3-1	< 1		< 0.5	< 1	
Pruritus	< 1	2	0.5-1	0.2-1		< 1		0.5-1	< 1	0.3-1
Rash	< 1	4-7	0.5-1.4	0.2-1	0.01-1.7	1.6	✓[b]	1.4	< 1	0.3-1
Stevens-Johnson syndrome	< 1	✓[b]	0.5-1		rare				< 1	
Toxic epidermal necrolysis			0.5-1		rare				< 1	
Urticaria			0.5-1	0.2-1	0.3-1	< 1		< 1	< 1	
GI										
Abdominal pain			1.6	0.2-1	2.2	< 1		1	< 1	0.3-1
Anorexia			0.5-1						< 1	
Constipation	< 1		0.5-1	0.2-1	0.3-1	< 1		0.5-1	< 1	0.3-1
Diarrhea			1.4-2.1	> 1	2.7-3.7	3.1		1.7	≤ 1	0.3-1
Dry mouth			0.5-1	0.2-1	0.3-1	< 1		0.5-1	< 1	
Dysgeusia		2-4								
Dyspepsia		✓[b]	0.5-1		0.3-1	> 1		< 0.5	< 1	0.3-6.4
Hepatitis		✓[b]	0.5-1	0.2-1	0.3-1	< 1		< 0.5	< 1	
Nausea	1.3		1.3-1.4	1.2-2.2	2	> 1		2.4	2	
Pancreatitis	< 1	✓[b]	0.5-1	0.2-1	0.3-1	< 1	✓[b]	< 0.5	< 1	0.3-1
Vomiting	< 1		1.3	1.2-2.2	0.3-1.1	< 1		2.4	2	0.3-1
GU										
Decreased libido	< 1			0.2-1	0.4					0.3-1
Impotence	< 1	✓[b]	0.5-1		1			0.5-1	< 1	0.3-1
Oliguria		0.1-0.2	0.5-1		0.3-1	< 1				
UTI[f]	< 1		1.3		0.3-1			0.5-1		
Musculoskeletal										
Arthralgia	< 1	✓	✓	0.2-1	0.3-1	< 1	✓[b]	0.5-1	< 1	
Arthritis	< 1		✓	✓	0.3-1		✓[b]		< 1	
Muscle cramps			0.5-1	0.2-1	0.5					0.3-1
Myalgia	< 1	✓[b]	✓	0.2-1	0.3-1	1.3	✓[b]		< 1	4.7
Respiratory										
Asthma	< 1	✓	0.5-1		0.3-1					
Bronchitis	< 1		1.3		0.3-1					
Bronchospasm	< 1	✓[b]	0.5-1	0.2-1	0.3-1	< 1				
Cough[d]	1.2	0.5-2	1.3-2.2	2.2-9.7	0.5-3.5	6.1	✓	2-4.3	8	1.9-35
Dyspnea	< 1		1.3	≥ 1	0.3-1	< 1			< 1	0.3-1
Pharyngitis				0.2-1	0.3-1	1.8		0.5-1		
Rhinitis		✓[b]		0.2-1	0.3-1	> 1				
Sinusitis	< 1			0.2-1	0.3-1	> 1				
Upper respiratory tract infection			0.5-1	2.2	1.5-2.1	> 1			✓	0.3-1
Miscellaneous										
Anemia[e]	✓	≤ 0.2		✓	0.3-1	< 1	✓[b]	< 0.5	< 1	
Angioedema[c]	0.5	0.1	✓	0.2-1	0.1	< 1	0.1	0.1	0.3	0.13
Asthenia	< 1	✓[b]	1.1-1.6		1.3				2	3.3
Blurred vision		✓[b]	0.5-1		0.3-1					
Eosinophilia		✓	✓	✓	0.3-1		✓[b]		< 1	
Fever		✓	0.5-1	0.4-1	0.3-1		✓[b]		< 1	

Adverse Reactions Shared by the ACE inhibitors[a] (%)										
✓ = Reported; no incidence given. Adverse reactions	Benazepril	Captopril	Enalapril/ Enalaprilat	Fosinopril	Lisinopril	Moexipril	Perindopril	Quinapril	Ramipril	Trandolapril
Syncope	0.1	✓[b]	0.5-2.2	0.2-1	0.3-1.8	0.51		0.5-1	< 1-2	5.9
Tinnitus			0.5-1	0.2-1	0.3-1	< 1			< 1	
Vasculitis		✓	✓		0.3-1		✓[b]		< 1	

[a] Data are pooled from separate studies and are not necessarily comparable. Data included for both hypertension and heart failure indications.
[b] Postmarketing.
[c] See Warnings or Precautions.
[d] See Precautions. Although still reported at 0.5% to 3% by some manufacturers, the incidence appears to range from 5% to 25% and has been reported to be as high as 39%.
[e] Including aplastic and hemolytic.
[f] UTI = urinary tract infection.

➤*Cardiovascular:*

Benazepril – Postural dizziness (1.5%); postural hypotension (0.4%); electrocardiogram changes (rare).

Captopril – Raynaud syndrome, CHF (0.2% to 0.3%).

Enalapril – Pulmonary embolism and infarction, pulmonary edema, atrial fibrillation, Raynaud phenomenon (0.5 to 1%).

Fosinopril – Hypertensive crisis, claudication, hypertension, conduction disorder, cerebral infarction, sudden death, cardiorespiratory arrest, shock, transient ischemic attacks (0.2% to 1%).

Lisinopril – Ventricular/atrial tachycardia; pulmonary embolism, premature ventricular contractions, pulmonary infarction, paroxysmal nocturnal dyspnea, decreased blood pressure, chest discomfort, atrial fibrillation, arrhythmias, transient ischemic attack (0.3 to 1%); postinfarction angina (0.3%).

Quinapril – Vasodilation (0.5% to 1%); heart failure, hypertensive crisis, cardiogenic shock (less than 0.5%).

Ramipril – CHF, arrhythmia, transient ischemic attack (less than 1%).

Trandolapril – Stroke (3.3%); cardiogenic shock (3.8%); first-degree AV block (0.3% to 1%).

➤*CNS:*

Enalapril – Peripheral neuropathy, dream abnormality, dysesthesia (0.5% to 1%).

Fosinopril – Memory disturbance, tremor, mood change, numbness, behavior change (0.2% to 1%).

Lisinopril – Stroke, memory impairment, tremor, irritability, hypersomnia, peripheral neuropathy, spasm (0.3% to 1%).

Moexipril – Mood changes (less than 1%).

Ramipril – Amnesia, convulsions, hearing loss, neuralgia, neuropathy, tremor, vision disturbances (less than 1%); angioneurotic edema (0.3%).

➤*Dermatologic:*

Benazepril – Dermatitis (less than 1%).

Captopril – Rash, often with pruritus and sometimes with fever, arthralgia, and eosinophilia occurred in 4 to 7 of 100 patients, usually during the first 4 weeks of therapy. It is usually maculopapular and rarely urticarial. The rash is usually mild and disappears within a few days of dosage reduction, short-term treatment with an antihistaminic agent, and/or discontinuing therapy; remission may occur even if captopril is continued. Between 7% and 10% of patients with rash have shown an eosinophilia and/or positive antinuclear antibody (ANA) titers. Pallor (0.2% to 0.5%).

Enalapril – Herpes zoster (0.5% to 1%).

Lisinopril – Erythema, herpes zoster, skin lesions, skin infections (0.3% to 1%).

Quinapril – Dermatopolymyositis (less than 0.5%).

Ramipril – Purpura, onycholysis (less than 1%).

➤*GI:*

Benazepril – Gastritis, melena (less than 1%).

Captopril – Weight loss may be associated with taste loss; taste impairment is reversible and usually self-limited (2 to 3 months) even with continuous administration (2% to 4%).

Enalapril – Hepatic failure, stomatitis, ileus, taste alterations, melena, glossitis (0.5% to 1%).

Fosinopril – Dysphagia, abdominal distention, flatulence, heartburn, appetite/weight change, hepatomegaly (0.2% to 1%); hepatic failure, jaundice (hepatocellular or cholestatic).

Lisinopril – Flatulence, gastritis, heartburn, GI cramps, weight loss/gain, taste disturbances, hepatocellular/cholestatic jaundice (0.3% to 1%).

Moexipril – Appetite/weight change, taste alterations (less than 1%).

Quinapril – GI hemorrhage (less than 0.5%); flatulence, dry throat (0.5% to 1%).

Ramipril – Abdominal pain occurs sometimes with enzyme changes suggesting pancreatitis; dysphagia, gastroenteritis, increased salivation, taste disturbance (less than 1%).

Trandolapril – Gastritis (4.2%); abdominal distention (0.3% to 1%).

➤*Hematologic:* Small decreases in hemoglobin and/or hematocrit have been attributed to many ACE inhibitors but are rarely of clinical importance unless another cause of anemia coexists.

Benazepril – Thrombocytopenia, hemolytic anemia, leukopenia (less than 1%).

Captopril – Neutropenia/agranulocytosis). Cases of anemia, thrombocytopenia, and pancytopenia have been reported.

Enalapril – Neutropenia, thrombocytopenia, bone marrow suppression (0.5% to 1%); hemolytic anemia, including cases of hemolysis in patients with glucose-6-phosphate dehydrogenase (G6PD) deficiency, has been reported.

Fosinopril – Lymphadenopathy (0.2% to 1%); neutropenia, leukopenia.

Lisinopril – Rare cases of bone marrow depression, hemolytic anemia, leukopenia/neutropenia, thrombocytopenia.

Perindopril – Leukopenia (including neutropenia) (0.1%).

Quinapril – Hemolytic anemia, agranulocytosis, thrombocytopenia (less than 0.5%).

Ramipril – Pancytopenia, hemolytic anemia, thrombocytopenia (less than 1%); leukopenia (rare).

Trandolapril – Decreased leukocytes, decreased neutrophils, low lymphocytes, thrombocytopenia (0.3% to 1%).

➤*Lab test abnormalities:* Hyperkalemia; hyponatremia, elevated liver transaminases and serum bilirubin.

Benazepril – Elevations in uric acid and blood glucose.

Captopril – Elevation of alkaline phosphatase.

Fosinopril – Elevations of lactate dehydrogenase and alkaline phosphatase.

Moexipril – Elevations of uric acid (rare).

Perindopril – Elevations in ALT (1.6%) and AST (0.5%).

Ramipril – Elevations of uric acid and blood glucose (rare).

Trandolapril – Elevated serum uric acid (15%).

➤*Renal:* Elevation, usually transient and minor, in serum creatinine and BUN.

Benazepril – Proteinuria (rare; see Warnings).

Captopril – Proteinuria (1%; see Warnings); renal insufficiency, renal failure, nephrotic syndrome, polyuria, urinary frequency (0.1% to 0.2%).

Enalapril – Renal failure, renal dysfunction (0.5% to 1%).

Fosinopril – Renal insufficiency, urinary frequency, abnormal urination, kidney pain (0.2% to 1%).

Lisinopril – Renal dysfunction (2%); acute renal failure, anuria, uremia, progressive azotemia, pyelonephritis, dysuria (0.3% to 1%).

Moexipril – Urinary frequency (more than 1%); renal insufficiency (less than 1%).

Quinapril – Acute renal failure, worsening renal failure (less than 0.5%).

Ramipril – Abnormal kidney function (1%); proteinuria (rare).

➤*Respiratory:* Eosinophilic pneumonitis has been attributed to many ACE inhibitors.

Enalapril – Rhinorrhea, sore throat, hoarseness, pulmonary infiltrates (0.5% to 1%).

Fosinopril – Pleuritic chest pain, tracheobronchitis, abnormal breathing, sinus abnormalities (0.4% to 1%); laryngitis/hoarseness, epistaxis (0.2% to 1%); a symptom-complex of cough, bronchospasm, and eosinophilia has been observed in 2 patients.

Lisinopril – Common cold (1.1%); nasal congestion (0.4%); influenza (0.3%); malignant lung neoplasms, hemoptysis, pulmonary infiltrates, pleural effusion, wheezing, orthopnea, painful respiration, epistaxis, laryngitis, rhinorrhea, pneumonia, pharyngeal pain (0.3% to 1%).

Trandolapril – Epistaxis, throat inflammation (0.3% to 1%).

➤*Miscellaneous:* Anaphylactoid reactions have occurred (see Warnings).

A symptom complex has occurred and may include the following: Positive ANA, elevated erythrocyte sedimentation rate, arthralgia, arthritis, myalgia/myositis, fever, interstitial nephritis, vasculitis, rash, eosinophilia, serositis, leukocytosis, photosensitivity, other dermatologic manifestations.

Benazepril – Hypertonia, infection (less than 1%).

Enalapril – Anosmia, conjunctivitis, dry eyes, tearing, flank pain, gynecomastia, myositis, serositis (0.5% to 1%).

Fosinopril – Musculoskeletal pain (0.2% to 3.3%); weakness (1.4%); edema, vision/taste disturbance, eye irritation, sexual dysfunction, hyperhidrosis, fall, gout, influenza, cold sensation, pain, swelling/weakness of extremities, abnormal vocalization, abnormal urination, kidney pain, weight gain, muscle ache (0.2% to 1%).

Lisinopril – Neck/hip/leg/knee/arm/joint/shoulder/low back pain, gout, lumbago, fluid overload, dehydration, diabetes mellitus, chills, virus infection, pain, pelvic/flank pain, edema, facial edema, visual loss, diplopia, photophobia, breast pain (0.3% to 1%).

Moexipril – Flu syndrome (3.1%); pain, urinary frequency (more than 1%).

Perindopril – Back pain (5.8%).

Quinapril – Back pain (0.5% to 1.2%); amblyopia, viral infections, edema (0.5% to 1%); agranulocytosis (less than 0.5%).

Ramipril – Flu syndrome, edema, epistaxis, weight gain, hypoglycemia (less than 1%).

Trandolapril – Hypocalcemia (4.7%); intermittent claudication (3.8%); edema, extremity pain, gout (0.3% to 1%).

Postmarketing –

Benazepril: Agranulocytosis, anaphylactoid reactions, hyperkalemia, neutropenia, small bowel angioedema.

Captopril: Anaphylactoid reactions; gynecomastia; cerebrovascular insufficiency; bullous pemphigus; glossitis; jaundice; hepatitis, including rare cases of necrosis; cholestasis; symptomatic hyponatremia; myasthenia; eosinophilic pneumonitis.

Perindopril: Acute renal failure, eosinophilic pneumonitis, falls, hepatic failure, hyponatremia, jaundice (hepatocellular or cholestatic), nephritis, neutropenia/agranulocytosis, pancytopenia, psoriasis, thrombocytopenia.

Overdosage

➤*Symptoms:* Hypotension is most common. Systolic blood pressures of 95 and 80 mm Hg have occurred following **lisinopril** and **captopril** overdoses, respectively. One reported case of **perindopril** overdose developed hypothermia and circulatory arrest, then died following ingestion of up to 180 mg.

➤*Treatment:* Treatment includes usual supportive measures. Refer to General Management of Acute Overdosage. The primary concern is correction of hypotension. Volume expansion with an IV infusion of normal saline is the treatment of choice to restore blood pressure.

Captopril, **enalaprilat**, trandolaprilat, **lisinopril**, and **perindopril** may be removed by hemodialysis. There are inadequate data concerning the efficacy of removing **captopril** by hemodialysis in neonates and children. Enalaprilat has been removed from neonatal circulation by peritoneal dialysis. **Benazepril** is only slightly dialyzable, but dialysis might be considered in overdosed patients with severely impaired renal function. It is not known if **ramipril**, **moexipril**, or ramiprilat are removed by hemodialysis. Hemodialysis and peritoneal dialysis have little effect on the elimination of fosinoprilat, **quinapril**, and quinaprilat. Use caution with concurrent use of ACE inhibitors and polyacrylonitrile dialyzers because of the possibility of severe, sudden, and sometimes fatal reactions. Stop the dialysis immediately and begin measures to treat anaphylactoid reactions.

Patient Information

Apprise female patients of childbearing age about the consequences of second and third trimester exposure to ACE inhibitors and that these consequences do not appear to have resulted from intrauterine ACE inhibitor exposure limited to the first trimester. Ask these patients to report pregnancies to their health care providers as soon as possible.

Take **captopril** and **moexipril** 1 hour before meals.

Stop taking the drug and notify health care provider if any of the following occurs: sore throat, fever, swelling of hands or feet, irregular heartbeat, chest pains, signs of angioedema (eg, swelling of face, eyes, lips, tongue, difficulty swallowing or breathing, hoarseness).

Excessive perspiration, dehydration, vomiting, and diarrhea may lead to a fall in blood pressure.

May cause dizziness, fainting, or lightheadedness, especially during the first days of therapy; avoid sudden changes in posture. If actual syncope occurs, discontinue drug until health care provider has been contacted. Heart failure patients should avoid rapid increases in physical activity.

May cause rash or impaired taste perception. Notify health care provider if these persist.

Do not use potassium supplements or salt substitutes containing potassium without consulting a health care provider.

A persistent dry cough may occur and usually does not subside unless the medication is stopped. If this effect becomes bothersome, consult a health care provider.

Advise patients planning to undergo any surgery and/or anesthesia to inform their health care provider that they are taking an ACE inhibitor that has a long duration of action.

Tell patients to promptly report any indication of infection (eg, sore throat, fever) that could be a sign of neutropenia.

Tell patients to immediately report signs or symptoms suggestive of angioedema (eg, swelling of the face, extremities, eyes, lips, or tongue; hoarseness or difficulty swallowing or breathing), and stop taking the drug until a health care provider has been consulted.

BENAZEPRIL HYDROCHLORIDE

Rx	**Benazepril Hydrochloride** (Various, eg, Ivax, Teva)	**Tablets; oral:** 5 mg	In 30s, 100s, 500s, and 1,000s.
Rx	**Lotensin** (Novartis)		Lactose, castor oil. (LOTENSIN 5). Light yellow. In 100s.
Rx	**Benazepril Hydrochloride** (Various, eg, Ivax, Teva)	**Tablets; oral:** 10 mg	In 30s, 100s, 500s, and 1,000s.
Rx	**Lotensin** (Novartis)		Lactose, castor oil. (LOTENSIN 10). Dark yellow. In 100s.
Rx	**Benazepril Hydrochloride** (Various, eg, Ivax, Teva)	**Tablets; oral:** 20 mg	In 30s, 100s, 500s, and 1,000s.
Rx	**Lotensin** (Novartis)		Lactose, castor oil. (LOTENSIN 20). Pink. In 100s.
Rx	**Benazepril Hydrochloride** (Various, eg, Ivax, Teva)	**Tablets; oral:** 40 mg	In 30s, 100s, 500s, and 1,000s.
Rx	**Lotensin** (Novartis)		Lactose. (LOTENSIN 40). Dark rose. In 100s.

BENAZEPRIL HYDROCHLORIDE — ORAL

For complete and comparative prescribing information, refer to the Angiotensin-Converting Enzyme Inhibitors class monograph.

WARNING

Use during pregnancy – When used during pregnancy, angiotensin-converting enzyme (ACE) inhibitors can cause injury and even death to the developing fetus. When pregnancy is detected, discontinue benazepril as soon as possible.

Indications

➤*Hypertension:* For the treatment of hypertension. It may be used alone or in combination with thiazide diuretics.

➤*Off-label uses:*

Heart failure – [1] = Good documentation. ACE inhibitors have an established role for the treatment of congestive heart failure. There is no reason to suspect that benazepril would act any differently than other ACE inhibitors that have documented symptom relief and long-term benefit. However, only one randomized, controlled trial with benazepril has demonstrated improvement in symptoms of heart failure and in exercise tolerance. Further research is needed. It is important to use other appropriate medications along with the ACE inhibitor to control heart failure.

Nephropathy(nondiabetic) – [1] = Good documentation. Data and consensus guidelines support the use of benazepril for nondiabetic nephropathy. The Kidney Disease Outcomes Quality Initiative guidelines recommend using ACE inhibitors and angiotensin receptor blockers at moderate to high doses for patients with chronic kidney disease to help control blood pressure and reduce proteinuria. Guidelines for HIV-induced nephropathy recommend the addition of ACE inhibitors, angiotensin receptor blockers, and/or prednisone in patients with HIV-associated nephropathy if highly active antiretroviral therapy alone does not improve kidney function. ACE inhibitors and angiotensin receptor blockers are also the drugs of choice for hypertension in this patient population.

Prevention of recurrent stroke – [2] = Fair documentation. In general, antihypertensives have clearly demonstrated that when blood pressure can be reduced, there will be reduction in recurrent strokes. There is evidence that some ACE inhibitors reduce the recurrence of strokes in patients with and without hypertension. There is no reason to suspect that benazepril would differ from other ACE inhibitors in preventing recurrence of stroke, but no studies have addressed this issue directly. It would appear that, for ACE inhibitors to be optimally effective, they should be used in conjunction with a diuretic to maximize the reduction in blood pressure.

Other possible off-label uses – Nondiabetic neuropathy; per Joint National Committee on the Prevention, Detection, Evaluation, and Treat-

BENAZEPRIL HYDROCHLORIDE — ORAL

ment of High Blood Pressure (JNC) guidelines, ACE inhibitors have been shown in clinical trials to be beneficial in postmyocardial infarction, high coronary disease risk, diabetes, and chronic kidney disease.

Administration and Dosage

➤*Adults:*

Hypertension –

Initial dosage:

• *Patients taking a diuretic* – 5 mg once daily to avoid excessive hypotension.

• *Patients not taking a diuretic* – 10 mg once daily.

Maintenance dosage: 20 to 40 mg/day administered as a single dose or 2 equally divided doses. A dose of 80 mg gives an increased response, but experience with this dose is limited. Total daily doses greater than 80 mg have not been evaluated.

Dosage adjustment: Base dosage adjustment on measurement of peak (2 to 6 hours after dosing) and trough responses.

Concomitant therapy: Coadministration of benazepril with potassium supplements, potassium salt substitutes, or potassium-sparing diuretics can lead to increases of serum potassium.

If blood pressure is not controlled with benazepril alone, a diuretic can be added.

In patients who are currently being treated with a diuretic, symptomatic hypotension occasionally can occur following the initial dose of benazepril. To reduce the likelihood of hypotension, if possible, discontinue the diuretic 2 to 3 days prior to beginning therapy with benazepril. Then, if blood pressure is not controlled with benazepril alone, resume diuretic therapy.

Off-label dosing –

Heart failure: [1] = Good documentation. 10 mg/day orally initially and increased at monthly intervals, with a maintenance dosage generally between 20 and 40 mg/day. Evaluate for potential hypotension within 2 weeks of any change in dose.

Nephropathy (nondiabetic): [1] = Good documentation. 10 to 20 mg daily has been studied for up to 3 years. Less common doses are as low as 1.25 to 5 mg daily.

Prevention of recurrent stroke: [2] = Fair documentation. 10 mg/day orally in combination with a diuretic and increased at monthly intervals, with a maintenance dosage generally between 20 and 40 mg/day. Evaluate for potential hypotension within 2 weeks of any change in benazepril dose.

➤*Children:*

Hypertension –

6 years of age and older:

• *Usual dosage* – Dosages between 0.1 and 0.6 mg/kg once daily have been studied, and doses greater than 0.1 mg/kg were shown to reduce blood pressure.

• *Maximum dose* – Doses higher than 0.6 mg/kg (or in excess of 40 mg daily) have not been studied in children.

• *Initial dosage* – 0.2 mg/kg once per day as monotherapy.

• *Alternative dosage* – For children who cannot swallow tablets or for whom the calculated dosage (mg/kg) does not correspond to the available tablet strengths for benazepril, follow the suspension preparation instructions to administer benazepril as a suspension. See Preparation for Administration.

➤*Renal function impairment:*

Adults –

Maximum dose: 40 mg/day.

Initial dosage: 5 mg once daily for patients with a creatinine clearance (CrCl) of less than 30 mL/min per 1.73 m^2 (serum creatinine greater than 3 mg/dL).

Dosage titration: Dosage may be titrated upward until blood pressure is controlled or to a maximum total daily dose of 40 mg.

Children – Treatment with benazepril is not advised for children with a glomerular filtration rate (GFR) of less than 30 mL because there are insufficient data available to support a dosing recommendation in this group.

➤*Preparation for administration:*

Preparation of suspension (for 150 mL of a 2 mg/mL suspension) – Add 75 mL of *Ora-Plus* oral suspending vehicle to an amber polyethylene terephthalate (PET) bottle containing 15 benazepril 20 mg tablets and shake for at least 2 minutes. Allow the suspension to stand for a minimum of 1 hour. After the standing time, shake the suspension for a minimum of 1 additional minute. Add 75 mL of *Ora-Sweet* oral syrup vehicle to the bottle and shake the suspension to disperse the ingredients.

➤*Administration:* The divided regimen was more effective in controlling trough (predosing) blood pressure than the same dose given as a once-daily regimen. If a once-daily regimen does not give adequate trough response, consider an increase in dosage or divided administration. Shake the suspension before each use.

➤*Storage/Stability:* Do not store the tablets above 30°C (86°F). Protect the tablets from moisture.

Refrigerate the suspension at 2° to 8°C (36° to 46°F); it can be stored for up to 30 days in the PET bottle with a child-resistant screw-cap closure.

CAPTOPRIL

Rx	**Captopril** (Various, eg, Geneva, Mylan, Teva, UDL, Watson, West-Ward)	**Tablets; oral:** 12.5 mg	In 100s, 500s, 1000s, 5000s, UD 100s, and blister 600s.
Rx	**Capoten** (Par)		Lactose. White, oval. In 100s and UD 100s.
Rx	**Captopril** (Various, eg, Geneva, Mylan, Teva, UDL, Watson, West-Ward)	**Tablets; oral:** 25 mg	In 100s, 500s, 1000s, 5000s, UD 100s, and blister 600s.
Rx	**Capoten** (Par)		Lactose. White, rounded square, quadrisected. In 100s, 1000s, and UD 100s.
Rx	**Captopril** (Various, eg, Geneva, Mylan, Teva, UDL, Watson, West-Ward)	**Tablets; oral:** 50 mg	In 100s, 500s, 1000s, 5000s, UD 100s, and blister 600s.
Rx	**Capoten** (Par)		Lactose. White, oval. In 100s, 1000s, and UD 100s.
Rx	**Captopril** (Various, eg, Geneva, Mylan, Teva, UDL, Watson, West-Ward)	**Tablets; oral:** 100 mg	In 100s, 500s,1000s, UD 100s, and blister 600s.
Rx	**Capoten** (Par)		Lactose. White, oval. In 100s.

CAPTOPRIL — ORAL

For complete and comparative prescribing information, refer to the Angiotensin-Converting Enzyme Inhibitors group monograph.

WARNING

Pregnancy – When used in pregnancy during the second and third trimesters, angiotensin-converting enzyme (ACE) inhibitors can cause injury and even death to the developing fetus. When pregnancy is detected, captopril should be discontinued as soon as possible.

Indications

➤*Hypertension:* Captopril is indicated for the treatment of hypertension.

Captopril tablets may be used as initial therapy for patients with normal renal function, in whom the risk is relatively low. In patients with impaired renal function, particularly those with collagen vascular disease, captopril should be reserved for hypertensive patients who have either developed unacceptable side effects on other drugs, or have failed to respond satisfactorily to drug combinations.

Captopril is effective alone and in combination with other antihypertensive agents, especially thiazide diuretics. The blood pressure-lowering effects of captopril and thiazides are approximately additive.

➤*Heart failure:* Captopril is indicated in the treatment of congestive heart failure usually in combination with diuretics and digitalis. The beneficial effect of captopril in heart failure does not require the presence of digitalis; however, most controlled clinical trial experience with captopril has been in patients receiving digitalis, as well as diuretic treatment.

➤*Left ventricular dysfunction after myocardial infarction:* Captopril is indicated to improve survival in clinically stable patients with myocardial infarction following left ventricular dysfunction manifested as an ejection fraction less than 40% and to reduce the incidence of overt heart failure and subsequent hospitalizations for congestive heart failure in these patients.

In considering use of captopril, it should be noted that in controlled clinical trials, ACE inhibitors have an effect on blood pressure that is less in black patients than in nonblack patients.

➤*Off-label uses:*

Pediatric hypertension – [3] = Safety concerns. Captopril is among the therapeutic options for pediatric hypertension identified by the National High Blood Pressure Education Program, based on published case series and randomized, controlled trials.

Raynaud phenomenon – [2] = Fair documentation. Initial data from limited trials indicate that captopril may be beneficial for the treatment of Raynaud phenomenon. Greater benefit may be seen with captopril in patients with Raynaud phenomenon who do not have systemic sclerosis. Dose reductions or discontinuation of therapy may be necessary to alleviate adverse effects.

Administration and Dosage

➤*General dosing considerations:* Initiation of therapy requires consideration of recent antihypertensive drug treatment, the extent of blood pres-

CAPTOPRIL — ORAL

sure elevation, salt restriction, and other clinical circumstances. If possible, discontinue the patient's previous antihypertensive drug regimen for 1 week before starting captopril.

Concomitant sodium restriction may be beneficial when captopril is used alone.

When necessitated by the patient's clinical condition, the daily dose of captopril may be increased every 24 hours or less under continuous medical supervision until a satisfactory blood pressure response is obtained or the maximum dose of captopril is reached. In this regimen, addition of a more potent diuretic (eg, furosemide) may also be indicated.

➤*Adults:*

Hypertension –

Usual dosage: 25 to 150 mg 2 or 3 times daily.
Maximum dose: 450 mg daily.
Initial dosage: 25 mg 2 or 3 times daily.
Dosage adjustment: If satisfactory reduction of blood pressure has not been achieved after 1 or 2 weeks, the dose may be increased to 50 mg 2 or 3 times daily. If further blood pressure reduction is required, the dose of captopril may be increased to 100 mg 2 or 3 times daily and then, if necessary, to 150 mg 2 or 3 times daily (while continuing the diuretic).
Concomitant therapy: If the blood pressure has not been satisfactorily controlled after 1 to 2 weeks at 50 mg 3 times daily (and the patient is not already receiving a diuretic), a modest dose of a thiazide-type diuretic (eg, hydrochlorothiazide, 25 mg daily), should be added. The diuretic dose may be increased at 1- to 2-week intervals until its highest usual antihypertensive dose is reached.
Severe hypertension: For patients with severe hypertension (eg, accelerated or malignant hypertension), when temporary discontinuation of current antihypertensive therapy is not practical or desirable, or when prompt titration to more normotensive blood pressure levels is indicated, diuretic should be continued but other current antihypertensive medication stopped and captopril dosage promptly initiated at 25 mg 2 or 3 times daily, under close medical supervision.

Heart failure –

Usual dosage: 50 or 100 mg 3 times daily.
Maximum dose: 450 mg daily.
Initial dosage: 25 mg 3 times daily. In patients with either normal or low blood pressure, who have been vigorously treated with diuretics and who may be hyponatremic and/or hypovolemic, a starting dose of 6.25 or 12.5 mg 3 times daily may minimize the magnitude or duration of the hypotensive effect; for these patients, titration to the usual daily dosage can then occur within the next several days.
Dosage adjustment: After a dose of 50 mg 3 times daily is reached, further increases in dosage should be delayed, where possible, for at least 2 weeks to determine if a satisfactory response occurs.
Concomitant therapy: Captopril should generally be used in conjunction with a diuretic and digitalis.

Left ventricular dysfunction after myocardial infarction –

Initial dosage: After a single dose of 6.25 mg, initiate at 12.5 mg 3 times daily. Therapy may be initiated as early as 3 days following a myocardial infarction.
Maintenance dosage: 50 mg 3 times daily.
Dosage adjustment: Increase to 25 mg 3 times daily during the next several days and to a target dose of 50 mg 3 times daily over the next several weeks as tolerated.
Single dose: 6.25 mg.
Concomitant therapy: May be used in patients treated with other postmyocardial infarction therapies (eg, thrombolytics, aspirin, beta-blockers).

Off-label dosing –

Raynaud phenomenon: [2] = Fair documentation. 12.5 mg twice daily (initial) titrated gradually up to 25 mg 3 times daily.

➤*Children:*

Off-label dosing –

Pediatric hypertension: [3] = Safety concerns.
- *1 to 17 years of age –*
  Maximum dose: 6 mg/kg/day.
  Initial dosage: 0.3 to 0.5 mg/kg 3 times per day. Captopril may be compounded into a suspension to facilitate pediatric use.

Hypertension: The following are additional off-label dosing recommendations for the treatment of pediatric hypertension.
- *Older than 6 months of age –*
  Maximum dose: 6 mg/kg/day, up to 450 mg/day.
  Initial dosage: 0.3 to 0.5 mg/kg 2 to 3 times daily.
  Dosage titration: Titrate as needed.
- *30 days to younger than 6 months of age –*
  Maximum dose: 6 mg/kg/day.
  Initial dosage: 0.01 to 0.5 mg/kg 2 to 3 times daily.
  Dosage titration: Titrate as needed.
- *29 days of age and younger* – 0.01 to 0.05 mg/kg every 8 to 12 hours.

➤*Renal function impairment:* For patients with significant renal impairment, initial daily dosage of captopril should be reduced, and smaller increments utilized for titration, which should be quite slow (1- to 2-week intervals). After the desired therapeutic effect has been achieved, the dose should be slowly back-titrated to determine the minimal effective dose. When concomitant diuretic therapy is required, a loop diuretic (eg, furosemide), rather than a thiazide diuretic, is preferred in patients with severe renal impairment.

➤*Administration:* Take 1 hour before or 2 hours after meals.

➤*Storage/Stability:* Store at 15° to 30°C (59° to 86°F). Protect from moisture.

ENALAPRIL MALEATE

Rx	**Enalapril Maleate** (Various, eg, Geneva, Mylan, Teva, Watson)	**Tablets:** 2.5 mg	In 100s and 1000s.
Rx	**Vasotec** (Biovail)		Lactose. (VASOTEC MSD 14). Yellow, barrel-shape, scored. In 100s, 1000s, 10,000s, unit-of-use 90s, and UD 100s.
Rx	**Enalapril Maleate** (Various, eg, Geneva, Mylan, Teva, Watson)	**Tablets:** 5 mg	In 100s and 1000s.
Rx	**Vasotec** (Biovail)		Lactose. (MSD 712 VASOTEC). White, barrel-shape, scored. In 100s, 1000s,10,000s, unit-of-use 90s, and UD 100s.
Rx	**Enalapril Maleate** (Various, eg, Geneva, Mylan, Teva, Watson)	**Tablets:** 10 mg	In 100s and 1000s.
Rx	**Vasotec** (Biovail)		Lactose. (MSD 713 VASOTEC). Salmon, barrel-shape. In 100s, 1000s, 10,000s, unit-of-use 90s, and UD 100s.
Rx	**Enalapril Maleate** (Various, eg, Geneva, Mylan, Teva, Watson)	**Tablets:** 20 mg	In 100s and 1000s.
Rx	**Vasotec** (Biovail)		Lactose. (MSD 714 VASOTEC). Peach, barrel-shape. In 100s, 1000s, 10,000s, unit-of-use 90s, and UD 100s.
Rx	**Enalaprilat** (Various, eg, Hospira, Bedford	**Injection:** 1.25 mg enalaprilat/mL	In 1 and 2 mL vials.

ENALAPRIL MALEATE — ORAL

For complete and comparative prescribing information, refer to the Angiotensin-Converting Enzyme Inhibitors group monograph.

WARNING

Use in pregnancy – When used in pregnancy during the second and third trimesters, ACE inhibitors can cause injury and even death to the developing fetus. When pregnancy is detected, enalapril maleate should be discontinued as soon as possible.

Indications

➤*Hypertension:* Enalapril maleate is indicated for the treatment of hypertension.

Enalapril maleate is effective alone or in combination with other antihypertensive agents, especially thiazide-type diuretics. The blood pressure-lowering effects of enalapril maleate and thiazides are approximately additive.

➤*Heart failure:* Enalapril maleate is indicated for the treatment of symptomatic congestive heart failure, usually in combination with diuretics and digitalis. In these patients enalapril maleate improves symptoms, increases survival, and decreases the frequency of hospitalization.

➤*Asymptomatic left ventricular dysfunction:* In clinically stable asymptomatic patients with left ventricular dysfunction (ejection fraction less than or equal to 35%), enalapril maleate decreases the rate of development of overt heart failure and decreases the incidence of hospitalization for heart failure.

➤*Off-label uses:*

Raynaud phenomenon – [5] = Poor documentation. Data from 2 small, controlled crossover trials indicate that enalapril is not effective in the management of Raynaud phenomenon. These trials were limited by small populations and limited duration of treatment. Until further data demonstrate beneficial results, this drug should not be used in the management of Raynaud phenomenon.

ENALAPRIL MALEATE — ORAL

Administration and Dosage

➤*Adults:*

Asymptomatic left ventricular dysfunction –
Initial dosage: 2.5 mg twice daily.
Dosage titration: Titrate as tolerated to the targeted daily dose of 20 mg (in divided doses).

Heart failure –
Usual dosage: Range is 2.5 to 20 mg given twice a day.
Maximum dose: 40 mg in divided doses.
Initial dosage: 2.5 mg.
Dosage titration: Titrate dose upward, as tolerated, over a period of a few days or weeks up to 40 mg, administered in 2 divided doses.
Concomitant therapy: Enalapril is indicated for the treatment of symptomatic heart failure, usually in combination with diuretics and digitalis.
If possible, reduce the dose of any concomitant diuretic that may diminish the likelihood of hypotension. The appearance of hypotension after the initial dose of enalapril does not preclude subsequent careful dose titration with the drug, following effective management of the hypotension.
Monitoring: After the initial dose of enalapril, the patient should be observed under medical supervision for at least 2 hours and until blood pressure has stabilized for at least an additional hour.

Hypertension –
Usual dosage: 10 to 40 mg/day as a single dose or 2 divided doses.
In some patients treated once daily, the antihypertensive effect may diminish toward the end of the dosing interval. In such patients, an increase in dosage or twice-daily administration should be considered.
Initial dosage: 5 mg once a day.
In patients who are currently being treated with a diuretic, symptomatic hypotension occasionally may occur following the initial dose of enalapril. If possible, discontinue the diuretic for 2 to 3 days before beginning therapy with enalapril to reduce the likelihood of hypotension. If the patient's blood pressure is not controlled with enalapril alone, diuretic therapy may be resumed. If the diuretic cannot be discontinued, use an initial dose of 2.5 mg under medical supervision for at least 2 hours and until blood pressure has stabilized for at least an additional hour.
Concomitant therapy: If blood pressure is not controlled with enalapril alone, a diuretic may be added.
Coadministration of enalapril with potassium supplements, potassium salt substitutes, or potassium-sparing diuretics may lead to increases of serum potassium. Risk factors for the development of hyperkalemia include renal insufficiency, diabetes mellitus, and the concomitant use of potassium-sparing diuretics, potassium supplements, or potassium-containing salt substitutes, which should be used cautiously, if at all, with enalapril.
Patients at risk for excessive hypotension, sometimes associated with oliguria or progressive azotemia, and rarely with acute renal failure or death, include those with the following conditions or characteristics: heart failure, hyponatremia, high dose diuretic therapy, recent intensive diuresis or increase in diuretic dose, renal dialysis, or severe volume or salt depletion of any etiology. It may be advisable to eliminate the diuretic (except in patients with heart failure), reduce the diuretic dose, or increase salt intake cautiously before initiating therapy with enalapril in patients at risk for excessive hypotension who are able to tolerate such adjustments. In patients at risk for excessive hypotension, start therapy under very close medical supervision and follow such patients closely for the first 2 weeks of treatment and whenever the dose of enalapril or diuretic is increased. Similar considerations may apply to patients with ischemic heart or cerebrovascular disease, in whom an excessive fall in blood pressure could result in a myocardial infarction or cerebrovascular accident.

➤*Children:* Enalapril is not recommended in neonates or in pediatric patients with glomerular filtration rate less than 30 mL/min per 1.73 m^2, as no data are available.

2 months to 16 years of age –
Hypertension:
• *Initial dosage* – 0.08 mg/kg (up to 5 mg) once daily.

Off-label dosing –
Hypertension:
• *Adolescents –*
Maximum dose: 40 mg/day divided once or twice daily.
Initial dosage: 2.5 to 5 mg/day.
• *Infants and children –*
Usual dosage: 0.1 mg/kg/day up to 5 mg/day divided once to twice daily.
Maximum dose: 0.6 mg/kg/day up to 40 mg/day.
Dosage titration: Increase as needed over 14 days.

➤*Renal function impairment:*

Enalapril Dosage Adjustments in Hypertensive Patients With Renal Function Impairment

Renal status	Creatinine clearance mL/min	Initial dose mg/day
Normal renal function	> 80 mL/min	5 mg
Mild impairment	≤ 80 to 30 mL/min	5 mg
Moderate to severe impairment	≤ 30 mL/min	2.5 mg
Dialysis patients[a]	—	2.5 mg on dialysis day[b]

[a] Anaphylactoid reactions have been reported in patients dialyzed with high-flux membranes and treated concomitantly with an ACE inhibitor. Anaphylactoid reactions have also been reported in patients undergoing low-density lipoprotein apheresis with dextran sulfate absorption.
[b] Dosage on nondialysis days should be adjusted depending on the blood pressure response.

➤*Heart failure and renal impairment or hyponatremia:* In patients with heart failure who have hyponatremia (serum sodium less than 130 mEq/L) or with serum creatinine greater than 1.6 mg/dL.

Maximum dose – 40 mg daily.

Initial dosage – 2.5 mg daily under close medical supervision (see Heart Failure).

Dosage titration – Increase to 2.5 mg twice daily, then 5 mg twice daily, and higher as needed, usually at intervals of 4 days or more if, at the time of dosage adjustment, there is not excessive hypotension or significant deterioration of renal function.

➤*Preparation for administration:*

Preparation of suspension (for 200 mL of a 1 mg/mL suspension) – Add 50 mL of *Bicitra* (sodium citrate dihydrate, citric acid, monohydrate, and sodium ion) to a polyethylene terephthalate (PET) bottle containing ten 20 mg tablets of enalapril and shake for at least 2 minutes. Let concentrate stand for 60 minutes. Following the 60-minute hold time, shake the concentrate for an additional minute. Add 150 mL of *Ora Sweet SF* (sugar-free syrup vehicle) to the concentrate in the PET bottle and shake the suspension to disperse the ingredients.

➤*Storage/Stability:* Store at 15° to 30°C (59° to 86°F). Avoid transient temperatures above 50°C (122°F). Protect from moisture.

The suspension should be refrigerated at 2° to 8°C (36° to 46°F) and can be stored for up to 30 days. Shake the suspension before each use.

ENALAPRILAT — INJECTION

For complete and comparative prescribing information, refer to the Angiotensin-Converting Enzyme Inhibitors group monograph.

WARNING

Use in pregnancy – When used in pregnancy during the second and third trimesters, angiotensin-converting enzyme (ACE) inhibitors can cause injury and even death to the developing fetus. When pregnancy is detected, discontinue enalaprilat as soon as possible.

Indications

➤*Hypertension:* Enalaprilat is indicated for the treatment of hypertension when oral therapy is not practical.

➤*Off-label uses:*

Pediatric hypertensive urgency or emergency – [3] = Safety concerns. Enalaprilat is among the therapeutic options for pediatric hypertensive urgency or emergency identified by the National High Blood Pressure Education Program as occasionally useful.

Administration and Dosage

➤*General dosing considerations:* A clinical response is usually seen within 15 minutes. Peak effects after the first dose may not occur for up to 4 hours after dosing, although most of the effect is usually apparent within the first hour. The peak effects of the second and subsequent doses may exceed those of the first.

➤*Adults:*

Hypertension –
Usual dosage: 1.25 mg IV every 6 hours over a 5-minute period.
Maintenance dosage: No dosage regimen for enalaprilat has been clearly demonstrated to be more effective in treating hypertension than 1.25 mg IV every 6 hours. However, in controlled clinical studies in hypertension, doses as high as 5 mg IV every 6 hours were well tolerated for up to 36 hours. There has been inadequate experience with dosages greater than 20 mg/day.
Conversion: The dosage for patients being converted to enalaprilat from oral therapy for hypertension with enalapril maleate is 1.25 mg IV every 6 hours. For conversion from IV to oral therapy, the recommended initial dose of enalapril maleate is 5 mg once a day, with subsequent dosage adjustments as necessary.

Hypertensive patients at risk of excessive hypotension – Patients at risk include those with the following concurrent conditions or characteristics: heart failure, hyponatremia, high dose diuretic therapy, recent intensive diuresis or increase in diuretic dose, renal dialysis, or severe volume or salt depletion of any etiology. Single doses of enalaprilat as low as 0.2 mg have produced excessive hypotension in normotensive patients with these diagnoses. Because of the potential for an extreme hypotensive response in these patients, therapy should be started under very close medical supervision.
Concomitant therapy: Enalaprilat may be administered with diuretic therapy.
• *Initial dosage* – 0.625 mg IV over a period of no less than 5 minutes and preferably longer (up to 1 hour).

ENALAPRILAT — INJECTION

• *Maintenance dosage* – If there is an inadequate clinical response after 1 hour, the 0.625 mg IV dose may be repeated. Additional doses of 1.25 mg IV may be administered at 6-hour intervals.

• *Conversion* – For conversion from IV to oral therapy, the recommended initial dosage of enalapril maleate for patients who have responded to 0.625 mg of enalaprilat every 6 hours is 2.5 mg once a day, with subsequent dosage adjustment as necessary.

➤*Renal function impairment:* The usual dosage of enalaprilat 1.25 mg every 6 hours is recommended for patients with a creatinine clearance greater than 30 mL/min (serum creatinine of up to approximately 3 mg/dL). For patients with creatinine clearance 30 mL/min or less (serum creatinine to 3 mg/dL), the initial dose is 0.625 mg.

For dialysis patients, see the information on patients at risk of excessive hypotension.

If there is an inadequate clinical response after 1 hour, the 0.625 mg dose may be repeated. Additional doses of 1.25 mg may be administered at 6-hour intervals.

Conversion – For conversion from IV to oral therapy, the recommended initial dosage is enalapril maleate 5 mg once a day for patients with creatinine clearance greater than 30 mL/min and 2.5 mg once daily for patients with creatinine clearance 30 mL/min or less. Dosage should then be adjusted according to blood pressure response.

➤*Monitoring:* Closely follow patients whenever the dose of enalaprilat is adjusted or the diuretic is increased.

➤*Duration of therapy:* In studies of patients with hypertension, enalaprilat has not been administered for periods longer than 48 hours. In other studies, patients have received enalaprilat for as long as 7 days.

➤*Preparation for administration:* May be diluted with up to 50 mL of a compatible diluent. For neonates, mix 1 mL (1.25 mg) in 49 mL dextrose 5% in water or normal saline for a 0.025 mg/mL concentration.

➤*Administration:* Administer as a slow IV infusion over 5 minutes. It may be administered as provided or after dilution.

➤*Admixture compatibility:* Enalaprilat as supplied and mixed with the following IV diluents has been found to maintain full activity for 24 hours at room temperature:

1.) 5% dextrose injection
2.) 0.9% sodium chloride injection
3.) 0.9% sodium chloride injection in 5% dextrose
4.) 5% dextrose in Ringer's lactate injection
5.) McGaw Isolyte E

➤*Storage/Stability:* Store at 25°C (77°F); excursions permitted to 15° to 30°C (59° to 86°F).

FOSINOPRIL SODIUM

Rx	**Fosinopril Sodium** (Teva)	**Tablets:** 10 mg	Isopropyl alcohol, lactose. (9 3 72 22). White to off-white, rectangular, scored. In 90s and 1000s.
Rx	**Monopril** (Bristol-Myers Squibb)		Lactose. (BMS MONOPRIL 10). White to off-white, biconvex flat-end, diamond shape, scored. In 90s and 1000s.
Rx	**Fosinopril Sodium** (Teva)	**Tablets:** 20 mg	Isopropyl alcohol, lactose. (93 7223). White to off-white, capsule shape, scored. In 90s and 1000s.
Rx	**Monopril** (Bristol-Myers Squibb)		Lactose. (BMS MONOPRIL 20). White to off-white, oval. In 90s, 1000s, and UD 100s.
Rx	**Fosinopril Sodium** (Teva)	**Tablets:** 40 mg	Isopropyl alcohol, lactose. (93 7224). White to off-white, round, scored. In 90s and 1000s.
Rx	**Monopril** (Bristol-Myers Squibb)		Lactose. (BMS MONOPRIL 40). White to off-white, biconvex hexagonal. In 90s.

FOSINOPRIL SODIUM — ORAL

For complete prescribing information, refer to the Angiotensin-Converting Enzyme Inhibitors group monograph.

WARNING

Use in pregnancy – When used in pregnancy during the second and third trimesters, angiotensin-converting enzyme (ACE) inhibitors can cause injury and even death to the developing fetus. When pregnancy is detected, discontinue fosinopril as soon as possible.

Indications

➤*Hypertension:* Fosinopril is indicated for the treatment of hypertension. It may be used alone or in combination with thiazide diuretics.

➤*Heart failure:* Fosinopril is indicated in the management of heart failure as adjunctive therapy when added to conventional therapy, including diuretics with or without digitalis.

Administration and Dosage

➤*Adults:*

Heart failure –

Usual dosage: 20 to 40 mg orally once daily.

Maximum dose: 40 mg once daily.

Initial dosage: 10 mg once daily. Following the initial dose of fosinopril, the patient should be observed under medical supervision for at least 2 hours for the presence of hypotension or orthostasis and, if present, until blood pressure stabilizes. An initial dose of 5 mg is preferred in heart failure patients with moderate to severe renal failure or those who have been vigorously diuresed.

Dosage titration: Dosage should be increased over a several week period to a dose that is maximal and tolerated but not exceeding 40 mg once daily.

The appearance of hypotension, orthostasis, or azotemia early in dose titration should not preclude further careful dose titration. Consider reducing the dose of concomitant diuretic.

Concomitant therapy: Digitalis is not required for fosinopril to manifest improvements in exercise tolerance and symptoms. Most placebo-controlled clinical trial experience has been with both digitalis and diuretics present as background therapy.

Hypertension –

Usual dosage: 20 to 40 mg orally once daily, but some patients appear to have a further response to 80 mg. In some patients treated with once daily dosing, the antihypertensive effect may diminish toward the end of the dosing interval. If trough response is inadequate, consider dividing the daily dose.

Initial dosage: 10 mg once a day, both as monotherapy and when the drug is added to a diuretic. Dosage should then be adjusted according to blood pressure response at peak (2 to 6 hours) and trough (about 24 hours after dosing) blood levels.

Concomitant therapy: If blood pressure is not adequately controlled with fosinopril alone, a diuretic may be added.

In patients who are currently being treated with a diuretic, symptomatic hypotension occasionally can occur following the initial dose of fosinopril. To reduce the likelihood of hypotension, discontinue the diuretic, if possible, 2 to 3 days prior to beginning therapy with fosinopril. Then, if blood pressure is not controlled with fosinopril alone, resume diuretic therapy. If diuretic therapy cannot be discontinued, use an initial dose of fosinopril 10 mg with careful medical supervision for several hours and until blood pressure has stabilized.

➤*Children:*

Hypertension –

Weight greater than 50 kg:

• *Maximum dose* – 40 mg/day.
• *Initial dosage* – 5 to 10 mg/day orally.

➤*Storage/Stability:* Store at 25°C (77°F); excursions are permitted between 15° and 30°C (59° and 86°F). Protect from moisture by keeping bottle tightly closed.

LISINOPRIL

Rx	**Lisinopril** (Various, eg, Aurobindo Pharma, Eon, Mylan, Sandoz, Watson)	**Tablets; oral:** 2.5 mg	In 30, 100s, 500s, 1,000s, and UD 100s.
Rx	**Zestril** (AstraZeneca)		Mannitol. (ZESTRIL 2½ 135). White. In 100s.
Rx	**Lisinopril** (Various, eg, Aurobindo Pharma, Eon, Ivax, Par, Watson, West-Ward)	**Tablets; oral:** 5 mg	In 30s, 100s, 500s, 1,000s, UD 100s and UD 300s.
Rx	**Zestril** (AstraZeneca)		Mannitol. (ZESTRIL 130). Pink, capsule shape, bisected. In 100s.

LISINOPRIL

Rx	**Lisinopril** (Various, eg, Aurobindo Pharma, Ivax, Mylan, Ranbaxy, West-Ward)	**Tablets; oral:** 10 mg	In 30s, 100s, 500s, 1,000s, UD 25s, UD 100s, and UD 300s.
Rx	**Prinivil** (Merck)		Mannitol. (MSD 106). Light yellow, oval shape. In unit-of-use 90s.
Rx	**Zestril** (AstraZeneca)		Mannitol. (ZESTRIL 10 131). Pink. In 100s.
Rx	**Lisinopril** (Various, eg, Aurobindo Pharma, Eon, Ivax, Par, Sandoz, UDL Labs)	**Tablets; oral:** 20 mg	In 30s, 100s, and 1,000s.
Rx	**Prinivil** (Merck)		Mannitol. (MSD 207). Peach, oval shape. In unit-of-use 90s.
Rx	**Zestril** (AstraZeneca)		Mannitol. (ZESTRIL 20 132). Red. In 100s.
Rx	**Lisinopril** (Various, eg, Aurobindo Pharma, Eon, Ivax , Par, Sandoz)	**Tablets; oral:** 30 mg	In 30s, 100s, 500s, and 1,000s.
Rx	**Zestril** (AstraZeneca)		Mannitol. (ZESTRIL 30 133). Red. In 100s.
Rx	**Lisinopril** (Various, eg, Aurobindo Pharma, Ivax, Par, Sandoz, UDL Labs)	**Tablets; oral:** 40 mg	In 30s, 100s, 500s, 1,000s, UD 25s, and UD 100s.
Rx	**Zestril** (AstraZeneca)		Mannitol. (ZESTRIL 40 134). Yellow. In 100s.

LISINOPRIL — ORAL

For complete and comparative prescribing information, refer to the Angiotensin-Converting Enzyme Inhibitors group monograph.

WARNING

Use in pregnancy – When used in pregnancy during the second and third trimesters, angiotensin-converting enzyme (ACE) inhibitors can cause injury and even death to the developing fetus. When pregnancy is detected, discontinue lisinopril as soon as possible.

Indications

➤*Acute myocardial infarction (MI):* For the treatment of hemodynamically stable patients within 24 hours of acute MI, to improve survival. Patients should receive, as appropriate, the standard recommended treatments, such as thrombolytics, aspirin, and beta-blockers.

➤*Heart failure:* As adjunctive therapy in the management of heart failure in patients who are not responding adequately to diuretics and digitalis.

➤*Hypertension:* For the treatment of hypertension. Lisinopril may be used alone as initial therapy or concomitantly with other classes of antihypertensive agents.

➤*Off-label uses:*

Prevention of migraine (adults) – [4] = Insufficient documentation. Evidence from a limited number of controlled and noncontrolled studies evaluating the use of lisinopril in the prevention of migraine headache suggests that there may be some benefit.

Administration and Dosage

➤*Adults:*

Acute MI –

Hemodynamically stable:

• *Usual dosage* – 10 mg once daily.

• *Initial dosage* – 5 mg within 24 hours of the onset of symptoms of acute MI, followed by 5 mg after 24 hours and 10 mg after 48 hours.

• *Duration of therapy* – 6 weeks.

• *Concomitant therapy* – Patients should receive, as appropriate, the standard recommended treatments, such as thrombolytics, aspirin, and beta-blockers.

Systolic blood pressure 120 mm Hg or less when treatment is started or during the first 3 days after the infarct:

• *Initial dosage* – 2.5 mg.

• *Maintenance dosage* – 5 mg may be given, with temporary reductions to 2.5 mg if needed. If prolonged hypotension occurs (systolic blood pressure less than 90 mm Hg for more than 1 hour), lisinopril should be withdrawn.

Heart failure –

Usual dosage: 5 to 20 mg/day (*Prinivil*) and 5 to 40 mg/day (*Zestril*) as a single daily dose.

Initial dosage: 5 mg once a day with diuretics and digitalis. In patients with heart failure who have hyponatremia (serum sodium less than 130 mEq/L) or moderate to severe renal function impairment (creatinine clearance [CrCl] 30 mL/min or less or serum creatinine more than 3 mg/dL), initiate lisinopril at a dose of 2.5 mg once a day under close medical supervision.

Dosage adjustment: The dose of *Zestril* can be increased by increments of no more than 10 mg at intervals of no less than 2 weeks to the highest tolerated dose, up to a maximum of 40 mg daily. Dose adjustment should be based on the clinical response of individual patients.

Concomitant therapy: The concomitant diuretic dose should be reduced, if possible, to help minimize hypovolemia, which may contribute to hypotension.

Hypertension –

Usual dosage: 20 to 40 mg/day as a single daily dose. Dosage should be adjusted according to the patient's blood pressure response.

Initial dosage: 10 mg once a day.

Dosage adjustment: The antihypertensive effect may diminish toward the end of the dosing interval, regardless of the administered dose, but most commonly with a dose of 10 mg/day. This can be evaluated by measuring blood pressure just prior to dosing to determine whether satisfactory control is being maintained for 24 hours. If it is not, an increase in dose should be considered. Doses of up to 80 mg have been used but do not appear to have a greater effect.

Concomitant therapy: If blood pressure is not controlled with lisinopril alone, a low dose of a diuretic may be added. Hydrochlorothiazide 12.5 mg has been shown to provide an additive effect. After the addition of a diuretic, it may be possible to reduce the dose of lisinopril.

In hypertensive patients who are currently being treated with a diuretic, symptomatic hypotension may occur occasionally following the initial dose of lisinopril. The diuretic should be discontinued, if possible, for 2 to 3 days before beginning therapy with lisinopril to reduce the likelihood of hypotension. The dosage of lisinopril should be adjusted according to blood pressure response. If the patient's blood pressure is not controlled with lisinopril alone, diuretic therapy may be resumed as previously described.

If the diuretic cannot be discontinued, an initial dose of 5 mg should be used under medical supervision for at least 2 hours and until blood pressure has stabilized for at least an additional hour.

Coadministration of lisinopril with potassium supplements, potassium salt substitutes, or potassium-sparing diuretics may lead to increases of serum potassium.

Off-label dosing –

Prevention of migraine (adults): [4] = Insufficient documentation. 5 to 20 mg/day orally for up to 11 weeks; lisinopril was administered in an open-label trial for up to 3 years.

➤*Children:*

Hypertension –

6 years of age and older:

• *Usual dosage* – 0.07 mg/kg once daily (up to 5 mg total). Adjust according to blood pressure response.

• *Maximum dose* – 5 mg per dose initially; 40 mg/day.

• *Dosage titration* – Titrate dose up to 0.61 mg/kg/day or 40 mg/day.

➤*Renal function impairment:*

Adults –

Heart failure:

• *CrCl 30 mL/min or less or serum creatine more than 3 mg/dL* – Initiate dose at 2.5 mg once a day under close medical supervision.

Hypertension:

• *CrCl 10 mL/min to 30 mL/min or serum creatine 3 mg/dL or more* – 5 mg/day.

• *CrCl less than 10 mL/min (dialysis patients)* – 2.5 mg/day. Dosage or dosing interval should be adjusted, depending on patient's blood pressure response, to a maximum of 40 mg/day.

Children – Not recommended in children with a glomerular filtration rate of 30 mL/min per 1.73 min^2 or less.

➤*Monitoring:* Evaluation of patients with hypertension, heart failure, or MI should always include assessment of renal function.

➤*Preparation for administration:*

Preparation of suspension (for 200 mL of a 1 mg/mL suspension) – Add 10 mL of purified water to a polyethylene terephthalate bottle (PET) containing 10 lisinopril 20 mg tablets and shake for at least 1 minute. Add *Bicitra* diluent 30 mL and *Ora-Sweet SF* 160 mL to the concentrate in the PET bottle and gently shake for several seconds to disperse the ingredients. Shake the suspension before each use.

➤*Storage/Stability:*

Tablets – Store at 15° to 30°C (59° to 86°F), and protect from moisture, freezing, and excessive heat.

Suspension – Store at or below 25°C (77°F); lisinopril can be stored for up to 4 weeks. Protect from moisture. Dispense in a tight container.

MOEXIPRIL HYDROCHLORIDE

Rx	**Moexipril Hydrochloride** (Various, eg, Kremers Urban, Paddock)	**Tablets:** 7.5 mg	Lactose. Scored. Film-coated. In unit of use 90s, 100s, and 500s.
Rx	**Univasc** (Schwarz Pharma)		Lactose. (707 SP 7.5). Pink, scored. Film-coated. In 100s and unit-of-use 90s.
Rx	**Moexipril Hydrochloride** (Various, eg, Kremers Urban, Paddock)	**Tablets:** 15 mg	Lactose. Scored. Film-coated. In unit of use 90s, 100s, and 500s.
Rx	**Univasc** (Schwarz Pharma)		Lactose. (715 SP 15). Salmon, scored. Film-coated. In 100s and unit-of-use 90s.

MOEXIPRIL HYDROCHLORIDE — ORAL

For complete and comparative prescribing information, refer to the Angiotensin-Converting Enzyme Inhibitors group monograph.

Indications

➤*Hypertension:* Moexipril hydrochloride is indicated for treatment of patients with hypertension. It may be used alone or in combination with thiazide diuretics.

Administration and Dosage

➤*Adults:*

Hypertension –

Usual dosage: 7.5 to 30 mg daily, administered in 1 or 2 divided doses, 1 hour before meals. For patients who are currently being treated with a diuretic that cannot be discontinued, an initial dose of 3.75 mg of moexipril should be used. (See Concomitant therapy.)

Initial dosage: 7.5 mg, 1 hour prior to meals, once daily.

Dosage adjustment: Dosage should be adjusted according to blood pressure response. The antihypertensive effect of moexipril may diminish towards the end of the dosing interval. Measure blood pressure prior to dosing to determine whether satisfactory blood pressure control is obtained. If control is not adequate, increase dose or divide the dosing interval.

Concomitant therapy: In patients who are currently being treated with a diuretic, symptomatic hypotension may occasionally occur following the initial dose of moexipril. The diuretic should, if possible, be discontinued for 2 to 3 days before therapy with moexipril is begun, to reduce the likelihood of hypotension. If the patient's blood pressure is not controlled with moexipril alone, diuretic therapy may then be reinstituted. If diuretic therapy cannot be discontinued, an initial dose of 3.75 mg of moexipril should be used with medical supervision until blood pressure has stabilized.

➤*Renal function impairment:* For patients with a creatinine clearance less than or equal to 40 mL/min/1.73 m^2, an initial dose of 3.75 mg once daily should be given cautiously. Doses may be titrated upward to a maximum daily dose of 15 mg.

➤*Administration:* Administer in 1 or 2 divided doses 1 hour before meals.

➤*Storage/Stability:* Store, tightly closed, at controlled room temperature. Protect from excessive moisture. If product package is subdivided, dispense in tight containers.

PERINDOPRIL ERBUMINE

Rx	**Perindopril Erbumine** (Roxane)	**Tablets; oral:** 2 mg	May contain lactose. In 30s and 100s.
Rx	**Aceon** (Solvay)		Lactose. (ACN 2 SLV SLV). White, oblong, scored. In 100s.
Rx	**Perindopril Erbumine** (Roxane)	**Tablets; oral:** 4 mg	May contain lactose. In 30s, 100s, and 500s.
Rx	**Aceon** (Solvay)		Lactose. (ACN 4 SLV SLV). Pink, oblong, scored. In 100s.
Rx	**Perindopril Erbumine** (Roxane)	**Tablets; oral:** 8 mg	May contain lactose. In 30s, 100s, and 500s.
Rx	**Aceon** (Solvay)		Lactose. (ACN 8 SLV SLV). Salmon, oblong, scored. In 100s.

PERINDOPRIL ERBUMINE — ORAL

For complete and comparative prescribing information, refer to the Angiotensin-Converting Enzyme (ACE) Inhibitors class monograph.

WARNING

Pregnancy – Avoid use in pregnancy. When pregnancy is detected, discontinue perindopril as soon as possible. Drugs that act on the renin-angiotensin system can cause injury or death of the developing fetus.

Indications

➤*Hypertension:* For the treatment of patients with essential hypertension. Perindopril may be used alone or with other classes of antihypertensives, especially thiazide diuretics.

➤*Stable coronary artery disease:* Perindopril is indicated in patients with stable coronary artery disease (CAD) to reduce the risk of cardiovascular mortality or nonfatal myocardial infarction (MI). Perindopril can be used with conventional treatment for management of CAD, such as antiplatelet, antihypertensive, or lipid-lowering therapy.

Administration and Dosage

➤*Adults:*

Hypertension (uncomplicated) –

Maximum dose: 16 mg/day.

Initial dosage: 4 mg once a day.

Dosage titration: The dosage may be titrated upward as needed or a maximum of 16 mg/day.

Maintenance dosage: 4 to 8 mg administered as a single daily dose or in 2 divided doses.

Concomitant therapy: In patients currently being treated with a diuretic, symptomatic hypotension occasionally can occur following the initial dose of perindopril. Consider reducing the dose of diuretic prior to starting perindopril.

Stable coronary artery disease –

Initial dosage: 4 mg once daily for 2 weeks, and then increased as tolerated.

Maintenance dosage: 8 mg once daily.

➤*Elderly:*

Hypertension –

Older than 65 years of age:

- *Usual dose –* 4 mg daily in 1 or 2 divided doses.

Experience with perindopril is limited in elderly patients at doses exceeding 8 mg. Doses greater than 8 mg should be administered with careful blood pressure monitoring and dose titration.

Stable coronary artery disease –

70 years of age and older:

- *Initial dosage –* 2 mg once daily in the first week, followed by 4 mg once daily in the second week.
- *Maintenance dosage –* 8 mg once daily, if tolerated.

➤*Renal function impairment:*

Creatinine clearance greater than 30 mL/min – Initial dosage should be 2 mg/day and dosage should not exceed 8 mg/day.

Creatinine clearance less than 30 mL/min – Not recommended.

➤*Storage/Stability:* Store at controlled room temperature (20° to 25°C [68° to 77°F]). Protect from moisture.

QUINAPRIL HYDROCHLORIDE

Rx	**Quinapril Hydrochloride** (Various, eg, Greenstone, Mylan, Par, Teva)	**Tablets:** 5 mg	May contain lactose. In 90s and 500s.
Rx	**Accupril** (Pfizer)		Lactose. (PD 527 5). Brown, elliptical, scored. Film-coated. In 90s and UD 100s.
Rx	**Quinapril Hydrochloride** (Various, eg, Greenstone, Mylan, Par, Teva)	**Tablets:** 10 mg	May contain lactose. In 90s and 500s.
Rx	**Accupril** (Pfizer)		Lactose. (PD 530 10). Brown, triangular. Film-coated. In 90s and UD 100s.
Rx	**Quinapril Hydrochloride** (Various, eg, Greenstone, Mylan, Par, Teva)	**Tablets:** 20 mg	May contain lactose. In 90s and 500s.
	Accupril (Pfizer)		Lactose. (PD 532 20). Brown. Film-coated. In 90s and UD 100s.
Rx	**Quinapril Hydrochloride** (Various, eg, Greenstone, Mylan, Par, Teva)	**Tablets:** 40 mg	May contain lactose. In 90s and 500s.
Rx	**Accupril** (Pfizer)		Lactose. (PD 535 40). Brown, elliptical. Film-coated. In 90s.

QUINAPRIL HYDROCHLORIDE — ORAL

For complete and comparative prescribing information, refer to the Angiotensin-Converting Enzyme Inhibitors group monograph.

WARNING

Use in pregnancy – When used in pregnancy during the second and third trimesters, ACE inhibitors can cause injury and even death to the developing fetus. When pregnancy is detected, quinapril should be discontinued as soon as possible.

Indications

➤*Hypertension:* Quinapril is indicated for the treatment of hypertension. It may be used alone or in combination with thiazide diuretics.

➤*Heart failure:* Quinapril is indicated in the management of heart failure as adjunctive therapy when added to conventional therapy including diuretics or digitalis. In using quinapril, consideration should be given to the fact that another angiotensin-converting enzyme (ACE) inhibitor, captopril, has caused agranulocytosis, particularly in patients with renal impairment or collagen vascular disease. Available data are insufficient to show that quinapril does not have a similar risk.

➤*Off-label uses:*

Pediatric hypertension – [3] = Safety concerns. Quinapril is among the therapeutic options for pediatric hypertension identified by National High Blood Pressure Education Program, based on randomized, controlled trials and expert opinion. All ACE inhibitors, including quinapril, are contraindicated in pregnancy. Females of childbearing age should use reliable contraception if quinapril is selected for management of pediatric hypertension.

Administration and Dosage

➤*Adults:*

Heart failure –

Usual dosage: 20 to 40 mg daily in 2 equally divided doses.

Initial dosage: 5 mg twice daily.

Dosage titration: Titrate patients at weekly intervals until an effective dose is reached or undesirable hypotension, orthostatis, or azotemia prohibit reaching this dose. The appearance of hypotension, orthostasis, or azotemia early in dose titration should not preclude further careful dose titration.

Concomitant therapy: Consider reducing the dose of concomitant diuretics.

Monitoring: Following the initial dose of quinapril, observe the patient under medical supervision for at least 2 hours for the presence of hypotension or orthostatis and, if present, until blood pressure stabilizes.

Hypertension –

Usual dosage: 20, 40, or 80 mg as a single dose or in 2 equally divided doses.

Initial dosage: 10 or 20 mg once daily in patients not on diuretics.

Dosage adjustment: Adjust dosage at intervals of at least 2 weeks according to blood pressure response measured at peak (2 to 6 hours after dosing) and trough (predosing).

Concomitant therapy: If blood pressure is not adequately controlled with quinapril monotherapy, a diuretic may be added.

In patients who are currently being treated with a diuretic, symptomatic hypotension occasionally can occur following the initial dose of quinapril. To reduce the likelihood of hypotension, the diuretic should, if possible, be discontinued 2 to 3 days prior to beginning therapy with quinapril. Then, if blood pressure is not controlled with quinapril alone, resume diuretic therapy.

If the diuretic cannot be discontinued, use an initial dose of 5 mg with careful medical supervision for several hours and until blood pressure has stabilized.

The dosage should subsequently be titrated to the optimal response.

➤*Elderly:* The recommended initial dosage of quinapril for hypertension is 10 mg given once daily, followed by titration to the optimal response.

➤*Renal function impairment:*

Heart failure –

Initial dosage:

- *CrCl greater than 30 mL/min* – 5 mg daily.
- *CrCl 10 to 30 mL/min* – 2.5 mg daily.

Dosage titration: If the initial dose is well tolerated, administer the following day as a twice-daily regimen. In the absence of excessive hypotension or significant deterioration of renal function, the dose may be increased at weekly intervals based on clinical and hemodynamic response.

Hypertension –

Initial dosage:

- *CrCl greater than 60 mL/min* – 10 mg.
- *CrCl 30 to 60 mL/min* – 5 mg.
- *CrCl 10 to 30 mL/min* – 2.5 mg.

Dosage adjustment: See Adults for information.

➤*Administration:* In some patients treated once daily, the antihypertensive effect may diminish toward the end of the dosing interval. In such patients, an increase in dosage or twice-daily administration may be warranted.

➤*Storage/Stability:* Store at 15° to 30°C (59° to 86°F). Protect from light.

RAMIPRIL

Rx	**Ramipril** (Various. eg, Cobalt, Actavis Elizabeth)	**Capsules; oral:** 1.25 mg	In 30s, 100s, and 500s.
Rx	**Altace** (Monarch)		Gelatin. Yellow. In 100s and UD 100s.
Rx	**Ramipril** (Various. eg, Cobalt, Actavis Elizabeth)	**Capsules; oral:** 2.5 mg	In 30s, 100s, 500s, and 1,000s.
Rx	**Altace** (Monarch)		Gelatin. Orange. In 100s, 500s, 1000s, UD 100s, and bulk pack 5000s.
Rx	**Ramipril** (Various. eg, Cobalt, Actavis Elizabeth)	**Capsules; oral:** 5 mg	In 30s, 100s, 500s, and 1,000s.
Rx	**Altace** (Monarch)		Gelatin. Red. In 100s, 500s, 1000s, UD 100s, and bulk pack 5000s.
Rx	**Ramipril** (Various. eg, Cobalt, Actavis Elizabeth)	**Capsules; oral:** 10 mg	In 30s, 100s, 500s, and 1,000s.
Rx	**Altace** (Monarch)		Gelatin. Blue. In 100s, 500s, and 1000s.
Rx	**Ramipril** (Actavis Elizabeth)	**Tablets; oral:** 1.25 mg	(P 2694). White. In 100s and 500s.
Rx	**Ramipril** (Actavis Elizabeth)	**Tablets; oral:** 2.5 mg	(R 2695). Yellow. In 100s, 500s, and 1,000s.
Rx	**Ramipril** (Actavis Elizabeth)	**Tablets; oral:** 5 mg	In 100s.
Rx	**Ramipril** (Actavis Elizabeth)	**Tablets; oral:** 10 mg	In 100s.

RAMIPRIL — ORAL

For complete and comparative prescribing information, refer to the Angiotensin-Converting Enzyme Inhibitors group monograph.

WARNING

Use in pregnancy – When used in pregnancy during the second and third trimesters, angiotensin-converting enzyme (ACE) inhibitors can cause injury and even death to the developing fetus. When pregnancy is detected, ramipril should be discontinued as soon as possible.

Indications

➤*Reduction in risk of myocardial infarction, stroke, and death from cardiovascular causes:* Ramipril is indicated in patients 55 years or older at high risks of developing major cardiovascular events because of a history of coronary artery disease, stroke, peripheral vascular disease, or diabetes that is accompanied by at least 1 other cardiovascular risk factor (eg, hypertension, elevated total cholesterol levels, low HDL levels, cigarette smoking, documented microalbuminuria) to reduce the risk of myocardial infarction, stroke, or death from cardiovascular causes. Ramipril can be used in addition to other needed treatments (such as antihypertensive, antiplatelet or lipid-lowering therapy).

➤*Hypertension:* Ramipril is indicated for the treatment of hypertension. It may be used alone or in combination with thiazide diuretics. In using ramipril, consideration should be given to the fact that another ACE inhibitor, captopril, has caused agranulocytosis, particularly in patients with renal impairment or collagen-vascular disease. Available data are insufficient to show that ramipril does not have a similar risk.

➤*Heart failure postmyocardial infarction:* Ramipril is indicated in stable patients who have demonstrated clinical signs of congestive heart failure within the first few days after sustaining acute myocardial infarction (MI). Administration of ramipril to such patients has been shown to decrease the risk of death (principally cardiovascular death) and to decrease the risks of failure-related hospitalization and progression to severe/resistant heart failure.

Administration and Dosage

➤*General dosing considerations:* Decreases in blood pressure associated with any dose of ramipril depend, in part, on the presence or absence of volume depletion (eg, past and current diuretic use) or the presence or absence of renal artery stenosis. If such circumstances are suspected to be present, the initial starting dose should be 1.25 mg once daily.

➤*Adults:*

RAMIPRIL — ORAL

Heart failure postmyocardial infarction –

Initial dosage: 2.5 mg twice daily (5 mg/day). A patient who becomes hypotensive at this dose may be switched to 1.25 mg twice daily.

Dosage titration: Titrate all patients (as tolerated) toward a target dose of 5 mg twice daily, with dose increases about 3 weeks apart. The appearance of hypotension after the initial dose of ramipril does not preclude subsequent careful dose titration with the drug, following effective management of the hypotension.

Concomitant therapy: To reduce the likelihood of hypotension, the diuretic should, if possible, be discontinued 2 to 3 days prior to beginning therapy with ramipril. Then, if blood pressure is not controlled with ramipril alone, diuretic therapy should be resumed.

If the diuretic cannot be discontinued, an initial dose of ramipril 1.25 mg should be used to avoid excess hypotension.

Coadministration of ramipril with potassium supplements, potassium salt substitutes, or potassium-sparing diuretics can lead to increases of serum potassium.

Monitoring: After the initial dose of ramipril, observe the patient under medical supervision for 2 hours or more and until blood pressure has stabilized for at least an additional hour.

Hypertension –

Usual dosage: 2.5 to 20 mg/day administered as a single dose or in 2 equally divided doses.

Initial dosage: 2.5 mg once a day for patients not receiving a diuretic.

Dosage adjustment: Adjust according to the blood pressure response.

Concomitant therapy: If blood pressure is not controlled with ramipril alone, a diuretic can be added.

Reduction in risk of myocardial infarction, stroke, and death from cardiovascular causes –

Initial dosage: 2.5 mg once daily for 1 week, 5 mg once daily for the next 3 weeks.

Dosage titration: Increase as tolerated to a maintenance dose of 10 mg once daily.

Maintenance dosage: 10 mg once daily. If the patient is hypertensive or recently postmyocardial infarction, it can also be given as a divided dose.

➤*Renal function impairment:* In patients with creatinine clearance less than 40 mL/min per 1.73 m^2 (serum creatinine approximately greater than 2.5 mg/dL), expect doses only 25% of those normally used to induce full therapeutic levels.

Heart failure postmyocardial infarction –

Maximum dose: 2.5 mg twice daily.

Initial dosage: 1.25 mg once daily.

Dosage adjustment: Increase to 1.25 mg twice daily and up to a maximum dose of 2.5 mg twice daily, depending upon clinical response and tolerability.

Hypertension –

Maximum dose: 5 mg daily.

Initial dosage: 1.25 mg once daily.

Dosage adjustment: Titrate upward until blood pressure is controlled or to a maximum total daily dose of 5 mg.

➤*Administration:* The ramipril capsule is usually swallowed whole.

In some patients treated once daily, the antihypertensive effect may diminish toward the end of the dosing interval. In such patients, an increase in dosage or twice-daily administration should be considered.

The ramipril capsule can also be opened and the contents sprinkled on a small amount (approximately 4 oz) of applesauce or mixed in 4 oz (120 mL) of water or apple juice. To be sure that ramipril is not lost when such a mixture is used, consume the mixture in its entirety.

➤*Storage/Stability:* Store at 15° to 30°C (59° to 86°F).

Ramipril/apple sauce or water or apple juice mixture – Can be stored for up to 24 hours at room temperature or up to 48 hours under refrigeration.

TRANDOLAPRIL

Rx	**Trandolapril** (Various, eg, Aurobindo, Cobalt, Lupin, Teva)	**Tablets; oral:** 1 mg	May contain lactose. In 100s.
Rx	**Mavik** (Abbott)		Lactose. (FT). Salmon, scored. In 100s and UD 100s.
Rx	**Trandolapril** (Various, eg, Aurobindo, Cobalt, Lupin, Teva)	**Tablets; oral:** 2 mg	May contain lactose. In 100s.
Rx	**Mavik** (Abbott)		Lactose. (FX). Yellow. In 100s and UD 100s.
Rx	**Trandolapril** (Various, eg, Aurobindo, Cobalt, Lupin, Teva)	**Tablets; oral:** 4 mg	May contain lactose. In 100s.
Rx	**Mavik** (Abbott)		Lactose. (FZ). Rose. In 100s and UD 100s.

TRANDOLAPRIL — ORAL

For complete and comparative prescribing information, refer to the Angiotensin-Converting Enzyme Inhibitors group monograph.

WARNING

Use in pregnancy – When used in pregnancy during the second and third trimesters, ACE inhibitors can cause injury and even death to the developing fetus. When pregnancy is detected, trandolapril should be discontinued as soon as possible. See Warnings, Pregnancy.

Indications

➤*Hypertension:* Trandolapril is indicated for the treatment of hypertension. It may be used alone or in combination with other antihypertensive medication such as hydrochlorothiazide.

➤*Heart failure post-myocardial infarction or left-ventricular dysfunction post-myocardial infarction:* Trandolapril is indicated in stable patients who have evidence of left-ventricular systolic dysfunction (identified by wall motion abnormalities) or who are symptomatic from congestive heart failure within the first few days after sustaining acute myocardial infarction. Administration of trandolapril to white patients has been shown to decrease the risk of death (principally cardiovascular death) and to decrease the risk of heart failure-related hospitalization.

Administration and Dosage

➤*General dosing considerations:* In patients who are currently being treated with a diuretic, symptomatic hypotension occasionally can occur following the initial dose of trandolapril.

Coadministration of trandolapril with potassium supplements, potassium salt substitutes, or potassium-sparing diuretics can lead to increases of serum potassium.

➤*Adults:*

Heart failure post myocardial infarction –

Initial dosage: 1 mg once daily.

Dosage titration: All patients should be titrated (as tolerated) toward a target dose of 4 mg once daily. If a 4 mg dose is not tolerated, patients can continue therapy with the greatest tolerated dose.

Hypertension –

Usual dosage: Most patients have required dosages of 2 to 4 mg once daily. There is little clinical experience with doses greater than 8 mg.

Initial dosage: For patients not receiving a diureticm, 1 mg once daily in nonblack patients and 2 mg in black patients.

Dosage adjustment: Dosage should be adjusted according to the blood pressure response. Generally, dosage adjustments should be made at intervals of at least 1 week.

Patients inadequately treated with once-daily dosing at 4 mg may be treated with twice-daily dosing.

Concomitant therapy: If blood pressure is not adequately controlled with trandolapril monotherapy, a diuretic may be added.

In patients who are currently being treated with a diuretic, symptomatic hypotension occasionally can occur following the initial dose of trandolapril. To reduce the likelihood of hypotension, the diuretic should, if possible, be discontinued 2 to 3 days prior to beginning therapy with trandolapril. Then, if blood pressure is not controlled with trandolapril alone, diuretic therapy should be resumed. If the diuretic cannot be discontinued, an initial dose of trandolapril 0.5 mg should be used with careful medical supervision for several hours until blood pressure has stabilized. The dosage should subsequently be titrated to the optimal response.

Coadministration of trandolapril with potassium supplements, potassium salt substitutes, or potassium-sparing diuretics can lead to increases of serum potassium.

Left-ventricular dysfunction post myocardial infarction – See Heart Failure Post Myocardial Infarction for dosing information.

➤*Elderly:* Greater sensitivity of some older individual patients cannot be ruled out.

➤*Renal function impairment:* For patients with a creatinine clearance of less than 30 mL/min, the recommended starting dose is 0.5 mg daily. Subsequently, patients should have their dosage titrated to the optimal response.

➤*Hepatic function impairment:* For patients with hepatic cirrhosis, the recommended starting dose is 0.5 mg daily. Subsequently, patients should have their dosage titrated to the optimal response.

➤*Storage/Stability:* Store at 20° to 25°C (68° to 77°F).

WARNING

When used in pregnancy during the second and third trimesters, drugs that act directly on the renin-angiotensin system can cause injury and even death to the developing fetus. When pregnancy is detected, discontinue angiotensin II receptor antagonists (AIIRAs) as soon as possible.

Indications

Angiotensin Receptor Blockers Products

Generic name	Candesartan	Eprosartan	Irbesartan	Losartan	Olmesartan	Telmisartan	Valsartan
Trade name	*Atacand*	*Teveten*	*Avapro*	*Cozaar*	*Benicar*	*Micardis*	*Diovan*
Dosage forms and strengths	Tablets: 4, 8, 16, 32 mg	Tablets: 400, 600 mg	Tablets: 75, 150, 300 mg	Tablets: 25, 50, 100 mg	Tablets: 5, 20, 40 mg	Tablets: 20, 40, 80 mg	Tablets: 40, 80, 160, 320 mg
Combination products[a]	Candesartan + hydrochlorothiazide (*Atacand HCT*) 16/12.5, 32/12.5, 32/25 mg	Eprosartan + hydrochlorothiazide (*Teveten HCT*) 600/12.5, 600/25 mg	Irbesartan + hydrochlorothiazide (*Avalide*) 150/12.5, 300/12.5, 300/25 mg	Losartan + hydrochlorothiazide (*Hyzaar*) 50/12.5, 100/12.5, 100/25 mg	Olmesartan + hydrochlorothiazide (*Benicar HCT*) 20/12.5, 40/12.5, 40/25 mg	Telmisartan + hydrochlorothiazide (*Micardis HCTZ*) 40/12.5, 80/12.5, 80/25 mg	Valsartan + hydrochlorothiazide (*Diovan HCT*) 80/12.5, 160/12.5, 160/25, 320/12.5, 320/25 mg
Hypertension							
Initial dosage[b]	16 mg once daily	600 mg once daily	150 mg once daily	50 mg once daily	20 mg once daily	40 mg once daily	80 to 160 mg once daily
Maintenance dosage	8 to 32 mg once daily	400 to 800 mg/day divided once or twice daily	150 to 300 mg once daily	25 to 100 mg/day divided once or twice daily	20 to 40 mg once daily	20 to 80 mg once daily	80 to 320 mg once daily
Heart failure							
Approval status	FDA[c] approved			Off-label			FDA approved
ACC/AHA[c] Initial dosage	4 to 8 mg once daily			25 to 50 mg once daily			20 to 40 mg twice daily
ACC/AHA Maximum dosage	32 mg once daily			50 to 100 mg once daily			160 mg twice daily

[a] Combination products are approved for hypertension only.
[b] Initial dosage in normovolemic patients: Refer to individual drug monograph for initial dosage in hypovolemic patients.
[c] FDA = Food and Drug Administration; ACC/AHA = American College of Cardiology/American Heart Association.

➤*Hypertension:* For the treatment of hypertension, alone or in combination with other antihypertensive agents.

➤*Nephropathy in type 2 diabetics (losartan and irbesartan):* For the treatment of diabetic nephropathy with an elevated serum creatinine and proteinuria (urinary albumin to creatinine ratio 300 mg/g or more with losartan; greater than 300 mg/day with irbesartan) in patients with type 2 diabetes and a history of hypertension. In this population, losartan and irbesartan reduced the rate of progression of nephropathy as measured by the occurrence of doubling of serum creatinine or end-stage renal disease (need for dialysis or renal transplantation).

➤*Heart failure (valsartan):* For the treatment of heart failure (NYHA class II to IV) in patients who are intolerant of angiotensin-converting enzyme inhibitors (ACEIs).

➤*Hypertension with left ventricular hypertrophy (losartan):* To reduce the risk of stroke in patients with hypertension and left ventricular hypertrophy, but there is evidence that this benefit does not apply to black patients.

➤*Off-label uses:* Refer to individual monographs for further information.

Prevention of migraine (adults) –

Candesartan: [4] = Insufficient documentation.
Olmesartan: [4] = Insufficient documentation.

Actions

➤*Pharmacology:* **Candesartan**, **eprosartan**, **irbesartan**, **losartan**, **olmesartan**, **telmisartan**, and **valsartan** are angiotensin II receptor (type AT_1) antagonists. Angiotensin II (formed from angiotensin I in a reaction catalyzed by angiotensin-converting enzyme [ACE; kininase II]) is a potent vasoconstrictor, the primary vasoactive hormone of the renin-angiotensin system, and an important component in the pathophysiology of hypertension. Its effects are vasoconstriction, stimulation of synthesis and release of aldosterone, cardiac stimulation, and renal reabsorption of sodium. AIIRAs block the vasoconstrictor and aldosterone-secreting effects of angiotensin II by selectively blocking the binding of angiotensin II to the AT_1 receptor in many tissues (eg, vascular smooth muscle, adrenal gland). There is also an AT_2 receptor in many tissues, but it is not known to be associated with cardiovascular homeostasis. AIIRAs have much greater affinity (greater than 10,000-fold, candesartan; 1000 times greater, eprosartan; greater than 8,500-fold, irbesartan; approximately 1,000-fold, losartan; greater than 12,500-fold, olmesartan; greater than 3,000-fold, telmisartan; approximately 20,000-fold, valsartan) for the AT_1 than for the AT_2 receptor and do not exhibit any agonist activity. In vitro binding studies indicate that losartan is a reversible, competitive inhibitor of the AT_1 receptor. The active metabolite is 10 to 40 times more potent by weight than losartan and appears to be a reversible, noncompetitive inhibitor of the AT_1 receptor. The primary metabolite of valsartan is essentially inactive with an affinity for the AT_1 receptor approximately 1⁄200 of valsartan itself.

AIIRAs do not inhibit ACE (kininase II, the enzyme that converts angiotensin I to angiotensin II and degrades bradykinin), nor do they bind to or block other hormone receptors or ion channels known to be important in cardiovascular regulation.

AIIRAs inhibit the pressor effect of angiotensin II (as well as angiotensin I) infusions. Removal of the negative feedback of angiotensin II causes a 2- to 3-fold rise in plasma renin activity and a consequent rise in angiotensin II plasma concentration in hypertensive patients. The resulting increased plasma renin activity and angiotensin II circulating levels are insufficient to alter the effects of AIIRAs on blood pressure. AIIRAs do not affect the response to bradykinin, whereas ACE inhibitors do increase the response. AIIRAs have very little effect on serum potassium. There was a small uricosuric effect with losartan leading to a minimal decrease in serum uric acid (mean decrease less than 0.4 mg/dL) during chronic oral administration.

➤*Pharmacokinetics:*

Angiotensin II Antagonist Pharmacokinetics

Parameters	Candesartan	Eprosartan	Irbesartan	Losartan (metabolite)[a]	Olmesartan	Telmisartan	Valsartan
Bioavailability	≈ 15%	≈ 13%	60% to 80%	≈ 33%	≈ 26%	42%/58% (40 mg/160 mg)	≈ 25%
Food effect (AUC/C_{max})	no effect	↓< 25%	no effect	↓10%/↓14%	no effect	↓6%/↓20% (40 mg AUC/160 mg AUC)	↓40%/↓50%
Plasma bound	> 99%	≈ 98%	90%	98.7% (99.8%)	99%	> 99.5%	95%
T_{max}	3 to 4 h	1 to 2 h	1.5 to 2 h	1 h (3 to 4 h)	1 to 2 h	0.5 to 1 h	2 to 4 h
Volume of distribution	0.13 L/kg	308 L	53 to 93 L	≈ 34 L (≈ 12 L)	≈ 17L	≈ 500 L	17 L[b]
Converted to metabolites	minor	minor	< 20%	≈ 14%	none	≈ 11%	≈ 20%

Angiotensin II Antagonist Pharmacokinetics

Parameters	Candesartan	Eprosartan	Irbesartan	Losartan (metabolite)[a]	Olmesartan	Telmisartan	Valsartan
Metabolism	O-deethylation	glucuronidation	CYP2C9	CYP2C9; CYP3A4	none	conjugation	unknown
Terminal half-life	≈ 9 hr	5 to 9 h	11 to 15 h	≈ 2 h (6 to 9 h)	≈ 13 h	≈ 24 h	≈ 6 h[b]
Total plasma clearance	0.37 mL/min/kg	≈ 130 mL/min[b]	157 to 176 mL/min	≈ 600 mL/min (≈ 50 mL/min)	1.3 L/h	> 800 mL/min	≈ 2 L/h[b]
Renal clearance	0.19 mL/min/kg	≈30 to 40 mL/min	3 to 3.5 mL/min	≈ 75 mL/min (≈ 25 mL/min)	0.6 L/h	nd[c]	≈ 0.62 L/h[b]
Recovered in the urine	≈ 33%	≈ 7%	≈ 20%	≈ 45/≈ 35% (IV/oral)	35% to 50%	0.91%/ 0.49% (IV/oral)	≈ 13%
Recovered in the feces	≈ 67%	≈ 90%	≈ 80%	≈ 50/≈ 60% (IV/oral)	50% to 65%	> 97%	≈ 83%

[a] Active.
[b] IV dosing.
[c] nd = no data AIIRAs do not accumulate in plasma upon repeated once-daily dosing.

Losartan undergoes substantial first-pass metabolism and is converted to an active carboxylic acid metabolite (14% of dose) that is responsible for most of the angiotensin II receptor antagonism. Cytochrome P-450 2C9 and 3A4 isozymes are involved in losartan's biotransformation.

The enzyme(s) responsible for **valsartan** metabolism have not been identified but do seem to be cytochrome P-450 isozymes.

In vitro studies of **irbesartan** oxidation by cytochrome P-450 isoenzymes indicated irbesartan was oxidized primarily by 2C9; metabolism by 3A4 was negligible. Irbesartan was neither metabolized by, nor did it substantially induce or inhibit, isoenzymes commonly associated with drug metabolism (1A1, 1A2, 2A6, 2B6, 2D6, 2E1). There was no induction or inhibition of 3A4.

Telmisartan is metabolized by conjugation to form a pharmacologically inactive acylglucuronide; the glucuronide of the parent compound is the only metabolite that has been identified in human plasma and urine. After a single dose, the glucuronide represents approximately 11% of the measured radioactivity in plasma. The cytochrome P450 isoenzymes are not involved in the metabolism of telmisartan.

Candesartan is rapidly and completely bioactivated by ester hydrolysis during absorption from the GI tract to candesartan, a selective AT_1 subtype angiotensin II receptor antagonist. Candesartan is mainly excreted unchanged in urine and feces (via bile). It undergoes minor hepatic metabolism by O-deethylation to an inactive metabolite. Candesartan and its inactive metabolite do not accumulate in serum upon repeated once-daily dosing.

Olmesartan shows linear pharmacokinetics following single oral doses of up to 320 mg and multiple oral doses of up to 80 mg. Steady-state levels are achieved within 3 to 5 days, and no accumulation in plasma occurs with once-daily dosing. Following the rapid and complete conversion of olmesartan medoxomil to olmesartan during absorption, there is virtually no further metabolism of olmesartan. Olmesartan crossed the blood-brain barrier poorly, if at all. It passed across the placental barrier in rats and was distributed to the fetus. It was distributed to milk at low levels in rats.

Absolute bioavailability following a single 300 mg oral dose of **eprosartan** is approximately 13%. Eprosartan plasma concentrations peak at 1 to 2 hours after an oral dose in the fasted state. Plasma concentrations of eprosartan increase in a slightly less than dose-proportional manner over the 100 to 800 mg dose range. The terminal elimination half-life following oral administration is typically 5 to 9 hours.

Contraindications

Hypersensitivity to any component of these products.

Warnings/Precautions

➤*Hypotension/volume- or salt-depleted patients:* In patients who are intravascularly volume depleted (eg, those treated with diuretics), symptomatic hypotension may occur. Correct these conditions prior to administration or start treatment under close medical supervision with a reduced dose.

If hypotension occurs, place the patient in the supine position and, if necessary, give an IV infusion of normal saline. A transient hypotensive response is not a contraindication to further treatment, which usually can be continued once the blood pressure has stabilized.

➤*Race:* **Losartan** and **olmesartan** were effective in reducing blood pressure regardless of race, although the effect was somewhat less in black patients (usually a low-renin population).In healthy black subjects, **irbesartan** AUC values were approximately 25% greater than in white subjects; there were no differences in C_{max} values.

➤*Gender:* Plasma concentrations of **telmisartan** are generally 2 to 3 times higher in women than in men. However, in clinical trials, no significant increases in blood pressure response or in the incidence of orthostatic hypotension were found in women. No dosage adjustment is necessary.

➤*Cough:* In trials where **valsartan** was compared with an ACE inhibitor with or without placebo, the incidence of dry cough was significantly greater in the ACE inhibitor group (7.9%) than in the groups who received valsartan (2.6%) or placebo (1.5%). In patients who had dry cough when previously receiving ACE inhibitors, the incidences of cough in patients who received AIIRAs, hydrochlorothiazide, or lisinopril were approximately 20%, approximately 19%, and 69%, respectively.

There was no significant difference in the incidence of cough between **losartan**, **olmesartan**, **eprosartan**, or **telmisartan** and placebo. **Irbesartan** use was not associated with an increased incidence of dry cough, as is typically associated with ACE inhibitor use.

➤*Potassium supplements:* Tell patients receiving **losartan** not to use potassium supplements or salt substitutes containing potassium without consulting the prescribing physician.

➤*Renal function impairment:* As a consequence of inhibiting the renin-angiotensin-aldosterone system, changes in renal function may be anticipated in susceptible individuals. In patients whose renal function may depend on the activity of the renin-angiotensin-aldosterone system (eg, patients with severe CHF), treatment with ACE inhibitors and angiotensin receptor antagonists has been associated with oliguria or progressive azotemia and rarely, with acute renal failure or death. In studies of ACE inhibitors in patients with unilateral or bilateral renal artery stenosis, increases in serum creatinine or BUN have been reported. AIIRAs would be expected to behave similarly. In some patients, these effects were reversible upon discontinuation of therapy. No dosage adjustment is necessary for patients with renal impairment unless they are volume-depleted.

Losartan – Plasma concentrations of losartan are not altered in patients with Ccr above 30 mL/min. In patients with lower Ccr, AUCs are about 50% greater and they are doubled in hemodialysis patients. Plasma concentrations of the active metabolite are not significantly altered in patients with renal impairment or in hemodialysis patients.

Valsartan – There is no apparent correlation between renal function (measured by Ccr) and exposure (measured by AUC) to valsartan in patients with different degrees of renal impairment. Consequently, dose adjustment is not required in patients with mild to moderate renal dysfunction. No studies have been performed in patients with severe impairment of renal function (Ccr less than 10 mL/min).Valsartan is not removed from plasma by hemodialysis. In the case of severe renal disease, exercise care with valsartan dosing.

In a 4-day trial of valsartan in 12 patients with unilateral renal artery stenosis, no significant increases in serum creatinine or BUN were observed. There has been no long-term use of valsartan in patients with unilateral or bilateral renal artery stenosis, but anticipate an effect similar to that seen with ACE inhibitors.

Irbesartan – The pharmacokinetics of irbesartan are not altered in patients with renal impairment or in patients on hemodialysis. Irbesartan is not removed by hemodialysis.

Candesartan – In hypertensive patients with renal insufficiency, serum concentrations of candesartan were elevated. After repeated dosing, the AUC and C_{max} were approximately doubled in patients with severe renal impairment (Ccr less than 30 mL/min/1.73 m^2) compared with patients with normal kidney function. The pharmacokinetics of candesartan in hypertensive patients undergoing hemodialysis are similar to those in hypertensive patients with severe renal impairment. Candesartan cannot be removed by hemodialysis. No initial dosage adjustment is necessary in patients with renal insufficiency.

Telmisartan – Renal excretion does not contribute to telmisartan clearance. Based on modest experience in patients with mild-to-moderate renal impairment (Ccr of 30 to 80 mL/min, mean clearance approximately 50 mL/min), no dosage adjustment is necessary in patients with decreased renal function. Telmisartan is not removed from blood by hemofiltration.

Eprosartan – Following administration of 600 mg once daily, there was an almost 2-fold increase in AUC and a 50% and 30% increase in C_{max} in moderate and severe renal impairment. The unbound eprosartan fractions increased by 35% and 59% in patients with moderate and severe renal impairment. No initial dosing adjustment is generally necessary in patients with moderate and severe renal impairment, with maximum dose not exceeding 600 mg daily. Eprosartan was poorly removed by hemodialysis (CL_{HD} less than 1 L/h).

Olmesartan – Patients with renal insufficiency have elevated serum concentrations of olmesartan compared with subjects with healthy renal function. After repeated dosing, the AUC was approximately tripled in patients with severe renal impairment (CrCl less than 20 mL/min). No initial dosage adjustment is recommended for patients with moderate to marked renal impairment (CrCl less than 40 mL/min).

➤*Hepatic function impairment:*

Candesartan – No differences in the pharmacokinetics were observed in patients with mild to moderate chronic liver disease. No initial dosage adjustment is necessary in patients with mild hepatic disease.

Irbesartan – The pharmacokinetics of irbesartan following repeated oral administration were not significantly affected in patients with mild to moderate cirrhosis of the liver. No dosage adjustment is necessary in patients with hepatic insufficiency.

Losartan – Following administration in patients with mild to moderate alcoholic cirrhosis of the liver, plasma concentrations of losartan and its active metabolite were, respectively, 5 times and about 1.7 times those in young male volunteers. Compared with healthy subjects, the total plasma clearance in patients with hepatic insufficiency was about 50% lower and the oral bioavailability was about 2 times higher. A lower starting dose is recommended for patients with a history of hepatic impairment.

Based on pharmacokinetic data that demonstrate significantly increased plasma concentrations of losartan in cirrhotic patients, consider a lower dose for patients with impaired hepatic function.

Olmesartan – Increases in $AUC_{0-\infty}$ and C_{max} were observed in patients with moderate hepatic impairment compared with those in matched controls, with an increase in AUC of about 60%.

Telmisartan – As the majority of telmisartan is eliminated by biliary excretion, patients with biliary obstructive disorders or hepatic insufficiency can be expected to have reduced clearance. Use telmisartan with caution in these patients. In patients with hepatic insufficiency, plasma concentrations of telmisartan are increased, and absolute bioavailability approaches 100%.

Valsartan – On average, patients with mild to moderate chronic liver disease have twice the exposure (measured by AUC values) to valsartan of healthy volunteers (matched by age, sex, and weight). In general, no dosage adjustment is needed in patients with mild to moderate liver disease. However, exercise care in this patient population.

As the majority of valsartan is eliminated in the bile, patients with mild to moderate hepatic impairment, including patients with biliary obstructive disorders, showed lower valsartan clearance (higher AUCs). Exercise care in administering valsartan to these patients.

Eprosartan – Eprosartan AUC (but not C_{max}) values increased, on average, by approximately 40% in men with decreased hepatic function compared with healthy men after a single 100 mg oral dose of eprosartan. The extent of eprosartan plasma protein binding was not influenced by hepatic dysfunction. No dosage adjustment is necessary for patients with hepatic impairment.

➤*Pregnancy: Category C* (first trimester); *Category D* (second and third trimesters).

Fetal / Neonatal morbidity / mortality – Drugs that act directly on the renin-angiotensin system can cause fetal and neonatal morbidity and death when administered to pregnant women. Several dozen cases have been reported in patients who were taking ACE inhibitors. When pregnancy is detected, discontinue AIIRAs as soon as possible.

The use of drugs that act directly on the renin-angiotensin system during the second and third trimesters of pregnancy has been associated with fetal and neonatal injury, including hypotension, neonatal skull hypoplasia, anuria, reversible or irreversible renal failure, and death. Oligohydramnios has also been reported, presumably resulting from decreased fetal renal function; oligohydramnios, in this setting, has been associated with fetal limb contractures, craniofacial deformation, and hypoplastic lung development. Prematurity, intrauterine growth retardation, and patent ductus arteriosus have also occurred, although it is not clear whether these occurrences were caused by exposure to the drug. These adverse effects do not appear to have resulted from intrauterine drug exposure in the first trimester.

Inform mothers whose embryos and fetuses are exposed to an AIIRA only during the first trimester. Nonetheless, when patients become pregnant, physicians should have the patient discontinue the use of AIIRAs as soon as possible.

Rarely (probably less often than once in every 1000 pregnancies), no alternative to an AIIRA will be found. In these rare cases, apprise the mother of the potential hazards to her fetus, and perform serial ultrasound examinations to assess the intra-amniotic environment.

If oligohydramnios is observed, discontinue the drug unless it is considered lifesaving for the mother. Contraction stress testing (CST), a non-stress test (NST), or biophysical profiling (BPP) may be appropriate, depending on the week of pregnancy. However, patients and physicians should be aware that oligohydramnios may not appear until after the fetus has sustained irreversible injury.

Closely observe infants with histories of in utero exposure to an AIIRA for hypotension, oliguria, and hyperkalemia. If oliguria occurs, direct attention toward support of blood pressure and renal perfusion. Exchange transfusion or dialysis may be required as means of reversing hypotension or substituting for disordered renal function.

Candesartan – Oral doses of 10 mg/kg/day or greater of candesartan administered to pregnant rats during late gestation and continued through lactation were associated with reduced survival and an increased incidence of hydronephrosis in the offspring. The 10 mg/kg/day dose in rats is approximately 2.8 times the maximum recommended human dose (MRHD) of 32 mg on a mg/m^2 basis (comparison assumes human body weight of 50 kg). Candesartan given to pregnant rabbits at an oral dose of 3 mg/kg/day (approximately 1.7 times the MRHD on a mg/m^2 basis) caused maternal toxicity (decreased body weight and death) but, in surviving dams, had no adverse effects on fetal survival, fetal weight, or external, visceral, or skeletal development. No maternal toxicity or adverse effects on fetal development were observed when oral doses up to 1000 mg/kg/day of candesartan (approximately 138 times the MRHD on a mg/m^2 basis) were administered to pregnant mice.

Eprosartan – Eprosartan has been shown to produce maternal and fetal toxicities (maternal and fetal mortality, low maternal body weight and food consumption, resorptions, abortions, and litter loss) in pregnant rabbits given oral doses as low as 10 mg/kg/day of eprosartan. No maternal or fetal adverse effects were observed at 3 mg/kg/day; this oral dose yielded a systemic exposure (AUC) to unbound eprosartan 0.8 times that achieved in humans given 400 mg twice daily. No adverse effects on in utero or postnatal development and maturation of offspring were observed when eprosartan was administered to pregnant rats at oral doses up to 1000 mg/kg/day of eprosartan (the 1000 mg/kg/day dose in nonpregnant rats yielded systemic exposure to unbound eprosartan approximately 0.6 times the exposure achieved in humans given 400 mg twice daily).

Irbesartan – When pregnant rats were dosed with irbesartan from day 0 to day 20 of gestation (oral doses of 50, 180, and 650 mg/kg/day), increased incidences of renal pelvic cavitation, hydroureter, or absence of renal papilla were observed in fetuses at doses of at least 50 mg/kg/day (approximately equivalent to the MRHD, 300 mg/day, on a body surface area basis). Subcutaneous edema was observed in fetuses at doses of at least 180 mg/kg/day (about 4 times the MRHD on a body surface area basis). As these abnormalities were not observed in rats in which irbesartan exposure (oral doses of 50, 150, and 450 mg/kg/day) was limited to gestation days 6 to 15, they appear to reflect late gestational effects of the drug. In pregnant rabbits, oral doses of 30 mg/kg/day of irbesartan were associated with maternal mortality and abortion. Surviving females receiving this dose (about 1.5 times the MRHD on a body surface area basis) had a slight increase in early resorptions and a corresponding decrease in live fetuses. Irbesartan was found to cross the placental barrier in rats and rabbits.

Radioactivity was present in the rat and rabbit fetus during late gestation and in rat milk following oral doses of radiolabeled irbesartan.

Losartan – Losartan has been shown to produce adverse effects in rat fetuses and neonates, including decreased body weight, delayed physical and behavioral development, mortality, and renal toxicity. With the exception of neonatal weight gain (which was affected at doses as low as 10 mg/kg/day), doses associated with these effects exceeded 25 mg/kg/day (approximately 3 times the MRHD of 100 mg on a mg/m^2 basis). These findings are attributed to drug exposure in late gestation and during lactation. Significant levels of losartan and its active metabolite were shown to be present in rat fetal plasma during late gestation and in rat milk.

Olmesartan – In rats, significant decreases in pup birth weight and weight gain were observed at doses of 1.6 mg/kg/day or more, and delays in developmental milestones (delayed separation of ear auricula, eruption of lower incisors, appearance of abdominal hair, descent of testes, and separation of eyelids) and dose-dependent increases in the incidence of dilation of the renal pelvis were observed at doses of 8 mg/kg/day or more.

Telmisartan – In rabbits, embryolethality associated with maternal toxicity (reduced body weight gain and food consumption) was observed at 45 mg/kg/day of telmisartan (about 6.4 times the MRHD of 80 mg on a mg/m^2 basis). In rats, maternally toxic (reduction in body weight gain and food consumption) telmisartan doses of 15 mg/kg/day (about 1.9 times the MRHD on a mg/m^2 basis), administered during late gestation and lactation, were observed to produce adverse effects in neonates, including reduced viability, low birth weight, delayed maturation, and decreased weight gain. Telmisartan has been shown to be present in rat fetuses during late gestation and in rat milk. The no-observed-effect doses for developmental toxicity in rats and rabbits, 5 and 15 mg/kg/day, respectively, are about 0.64 and 3.7 times, on a mg/m^2 basis, the MRHD of telmisartan (80 mg/day).

➤*Lactation:* AIIRAs were present in rat milk. It is not known if AIIRAs are excreted in human breast milk. Because of the potential for adverse effects on the nursing infant, decide whether to discontinue nursing or discontinue the drug, taking into account the importance of the drug to the mother.

➤*Children:* Safety and efficacy have not been established. Safety and efficacy have been established for treatment of hypertension in children 6 to 16 years of age (**olmesartan**).

➤*Elderly:* No dosage adjustment is necessary when initiating AIIRAs in the elderly. No overall differences in effectiveness or safety of **candesartan**, **irbesartan**, **losartan**, **olmesartan**, **eprosartan**, or **telmisartan** were observed between elderly patients and younger patients, but greater sensitivity of some older individuals cannot be ruled out.

Based on the pooled data from randomized trials, the decrease in diastolic blood pressure and systolic blood pressure with eprosartan was slightly less in patients 65 years of age and older compared with younger patients. Adverse experiences were similar in younger and older patients.

➤*Lab test abnormalities:*

Liver function tests – Occasional elevations (more than 150% in **valsartan**-treated patients) of liver enzymes or serum bilirubin have occurred.Three patients (less than 0.1%) treated with valsartan discontinued treatment for elevated liver chemistries.Minor elevations of ALT, AST, and alkaline phosphatase occurred for comparable percentages of patients taking **eprosartan** or placebo in controlled clinical trials.

Creatinine/Blood urea nitrogen (BUN) – Minor increases in BUN or serum creatinine were observed infrequently with **candesartan**, in less than 0.1% of patients with essential hypertension treated with **losartan** alone, in 0.8% of patients taking **valsartan**, less than 0.7% with **irbesartan**, and 0.6% and 1.3%, respectively, of patients taking **eprosartan**. At least a 0.5 mg/dL rise in creatinine was observed in 0.4% of **telmisartan** patients compared with 0.3% of placebo patients.

Hemoglobin and hematocrit – A greater than 2 g/dL decrease in hemoglobin was observed in 0.8% of **telmisartan** patients compared with 0.3% of placebo patients. No patients discontinued therapy because of anemia.

Small decreases in hemoglobin and hematocrit occurred frequently in patients treated with **losartan** alone but were rarely of clinical importance.

Decreases of more than 20% in hemoglobin and hematocrit were observed in 0.4% and 0.8%, respectively, of **valsartan** patients, vs 0.1% and 0.1% with placebo. One valsartan patient discontinued treatment for microcytic anemia. Neutropenia was observed in 1.9% of patients treated with valsartan and 0.8% of patients treated with placebo.

Mean decreases in hemoglobin of 0.2 g/dL were observed in 0.2% of patients receiving **irbesartan**. Neutropenia (less than 1000 cells/mm^3) occurred at similar frequencies (0.3%).

Small decreases in hemoglobin and hematocrit (mean decreases of approximately 0.2 g/dL and 0.5 volume percent, respectively) were observed in patients treated with **candesartan** alone but were rarely of clinical importance. Anemia, leukopenia, and thrombocytopenia were associated with withdrawal of 1 patient each from clinical trials.

A greater than 20% decrease in hemoglobin was observed in 0.1% of patients taking **eprosartan**. Leukopenia (WBC count of up to 3 × 10^3/mm^3) occurred in 0.3% of patients taking eprosartan and in 0.3% of patients given placebo in controlled clinical trials. Neutropenia (neutrophil count of up to 1.5 × 10^3/mm^3) occurred in 1.3% of patients taking eprosartan and in 1.4% of patients given placebo in controlled clinical trials. Thrombocytopenia (platelet count of up to 100 × 10^9/L) occurred in 0.3% of patients taking eprosartan (1 patient) and in no patient given placebo in controlled clinical trials. Four patients receiving eprosartan in clinical trials were withdrawn for thrombocytopenia.

Small decreases in hemoglobin and hematocrit (mean decreases of approximately 0.3 g/dL and 0.3 volume percent, respectively) were observed with **olmesartan**.

Serum potassium – Increases of more than 20% in serum potassium were observed in 4.4% of **valsartan**-treated patients vs 2.9% of placebo-treated patients.

A small increase (mean increase of 0.1 mEq/L) was observed in patients treated with **candesartan** alone but was rarely of clinical importance. One patient from a CHF trial was withdrawn for hyperkalemia (serum potassium, 7.5 mEq/L). This patient was also receiving spironolactone.

A potassium value of at least 5.6 mmol/L occurred in 0.9% of patients taking **eprosartan** and 0.3% of patients given placebo in controlled clinical trials. One patient was withdrawn from clinical trials for hyperkalemia and 3 for hypokalemia.

Hyperuricemia – Hyperuricemia was rarely found (0.6% with **candesartan** vs 0.5% with placebo).

Drug Interactions

Angiotensin II Receptor Antagonist Drug Interactions

Precipitant drug	Object drug[a]		Description
Cimetidine	Losartan	↑	Coadministration led to an increase of ≈ 18% in AUC of losartan but did not affect the pharmacokinetics of its active metabolite.
Fluconazole	Losartan	↑	Fluconazole may inhibit the metabolism of losartan (CYP2C9), causing increased antihypertensive and adverse effects. Fluconazole did not affect the pharmacokinetics of eprosartan.
Indomethacin	Losartan	↓	The hypotensive effect of losartan may be reduced.
Phenobarbital	Losartan	↓	Coadministration led to a reduction of ≈ 20% in the AUC of losartan and its active metabolite.
Rifamycins	Losartan	↓	Rifamycins may increase the metabolism of losartan, thereby decreasing antihypertensive effects.
Telmisartan	Digoxin	↑	Median increases in digoxin peak plasma concentration (49%) and in trough concentration (20%) were seen with coadministration.
Telmisartan	Warfarin	↔	Telmisartan administered for 10 days slightly decreased the mean warfarin trough plasma concentration; this decrease did not result in a change in the International Normalized Ratio.

[a] ↑ = Object drug increased. ↓ = Object drug decreased. ↔ = Undetermined clinical effect.

➤*CYP450:* In vitro studies show significant inhibition of the formation of the active metabolite of **losartan** by inhibitors of cytochrome P450 3A4 (eg, ketoconazole, troleandomycin) or P450 2C9 (sulfaphenazole). The pharmacodynamic consequences of concomitant use of losartan and these inhibitors have not been examined.

In vitro studies show significant inhibition of the formation of oxidized **irbesartan** metabolites with the known cytochrome CYP2C9 substrates/inhibitors, tolbutamide, and nifedipine. However, clinical consequences were negligible.

➤*Potassium:* As with other drugs that block angiotensin II or its effects, concomitant use of potassium-sparing diuretics (eg, spironolactone, triamterene, amiloride), potassium supplements, or salt substitutes containing potassium may lead to increases in serum potassium.

➤*Drug/Food interactions:* A meal has only minor effects on **losartan** AUC or on the AUC of the metabolite (about 10% decrease). Food decreases **valsartan**'s C_{max} by 50% and its AUC by 40%. Food slightly reduces the bioavailability of **telmisartan**, with an AUC reduction of about 6% with the 40 mg tablet and about 20% after a 160 mg dose. Food does not affect the bioavailability of **irbesartan**, **olmesartan**, or **candesartan**. Administering **eprosartan** with food delays absorption and causes variable changes (less than 25%) in C_{max} and AUC values that do not appear clinically important.

Adverse Reactions

In general, treatment with AIIRAs is well tolerated. In controlled clinical trials, discontinuation of therapy because of adverse reactions was required in 2.3% of patients treated with **losartan** or **valsartan**, 2.4% with **olmesartan** and **candesartan**, 2.8% with **telmisartan**, 3.3% with **irbesartan** , and 4% with **eprosartan** vs 3.7%, 2%, 2.7%, 3.4%, 6.1%, 4.5%, and 6.5%, respectively, given placebo.

Angiotensin II Receptor Antagonist Adverse Reactions (%)[a]

Adverse reaction	Candesartan (n = 2350)	Eprosartan (n = 1202)	Irbesartan (n = 1965)	Losartan (n = 1075)	Olmesartan (n = 3278)	Telmisartan (n = 1455)	Valsartan (n = 2316)
CNS							
Dizziness	4	≥ 1	≥ 1	3.5	3	1	> 1
Insomnia	-	< 1	-	1.4	> 0.5	> 0.3	> 0.2
Headache	≥ 1	≥ 1	≥ 1	≥ 1	> 1	1	> 1
Fatigue	> 1	2	4	-	> 0.5	1	2
Anxiety/Nervousness	≥ 0.5	< 1	≥ 1	< 1	-	> 0.3	> 0.2
Depression	≥ 0.5	1	< 1	< 1	-	> 0.3	-
GI							
Diarrhea	> 1	≥ 1	3	2.4	> 1	3	> 1
Dyspepsia/Heartburn	≥ 0.5	≥ 1	2	1.3	> 0.5	1	> 0.2
Nausea/Vomiting	> 1	< 1	≥ 1	≥ 1	-	1	> 1
Abdominal pain	> 1	2	≥ 1	≥ 1	> 0.5	1	2

Angiotensin II Receptor Antagonists

Angiotensin II Receptor Antagonist Adverse Reactions (%)[a]							
Adverse reaction	Candesartan (n = 2350)	Eprosartan (n = 1202)	Irbesartan (n = 1965)	Losartan (n = 1075)	Olmesartan (n = 3278)	Telmisartan (n = 1455)	Valsartan (n = 2316)
Musculoskeletal							
Arthralgia	> 1	2	-	< 1	> 0.5	> 0.3	> 1
Pain[b]	3	< 1	≥ 1	1 to 1.8	> 1	1 to 3	> 0.2
Muscle cramp	-	-	-	1.1		-	> 0.2
Myalgia	≥ 0.5	≥ 1	-	1	> 0.5	1	> 0.2
Trauma	-	-	2	-	-	-	-
Respiratory							
Upper respiratory tract infection	6	8	9	7.9	> 1	7	> 1
Cough[c]	> 1	4	2.8	3.4	-	1	> 1
Nasal congestion	-	-	-	2		-	-
Sinus disorder	-	-	≥ 1	1.5		-	-
Sinusitis	> 1	≥ 1	-	1	> 1	3	> 1
Pharyngitis	2	4	≥ 1	≥ 1	> 1	1	> 1
Rhinitis	2	4	≥ 1	< 1	> 1	> 0.3	> 1
Influenza/Influenza-like symptoms	-	< 1	≥ 1	< 1	> 1	1	-
Bronchitis	> 1	≥ 1	-	< 1	> 1	> 0.3	-
Miscellaneous							
Viral infection	-	2	-	-		-	3
Edema	-	≥ 1	≥ 1	≥ 1	-	-	> 1
Chest pain	> 1	≥ 1	≥ 1	≥ 1	> 0.5	1	
Rash	≥ 0.5	< 1	≥ 1	< 1	> 0.5	> 0.3	> 0.2
Tachycardia	≥ 0.5	< 1	≥ 1	< 1	> 0.5	> 0.3	-
Urinary tract infection	-	4	≥ 1	< 1	> 0.5	1	
Peripheral edema	> 1		-		> 0.5	1	
Albuminuria	> 1	< 1	-	-	-		
Hypertension	-	-	-			1	
Hypertriglyceridemia	≥ 0.5	1	-		> 1	-	
Creatine phosphokinase increased	≥ 0.5	< 1	-	-	> 1	-	
Hyperglycemia	≥ 0.5	< 1	-	-	> 1	-	
Hematuria	≥ 0.5	< 1	-	-	> 1	-	
Inflicted injury	-	2	-	-	> 1	-	

[a] Data are pooled from separate studies and are not necessarily comparable.
[b] This includes back and leg pain.
[c] See Warnings.

➤*Candesartan:*

Cardiovascular – Palpitation (at least 0.5%).

CNS – Paresthesia, vertigo, somnolence (at least 0.5%).

Metabolic/Nutritional – Hyperuricemia (at least 0.5%).

Miscellaneous – Asthenia, fever, epistaxis, dyspnea, sweating increased, gastroenteritis (at least 0.5%).

Other reported events observed less frequently included angina pectoris, MI, and angioedema.

Adverse reactions occurred at about the same rates in men and women, older and younger patients, and black and nonblack patients.

Postmarketing experience: Abnormal hepatic function, hepatitis, neutropenia, leukopenia, agranulocytosis, pruritus, urticaria.

➤*Eprosartan:*

Cardiovascular – Angina pectoris, bradycardia, abnormal ECG, specific abnormal ECG, extrasystoles, atrial fibrillation, hypotension (including orthostatic hypotension), palpitations (less than 1%).

CNS – Ataxia, migraine, neuritis, nervousness, paresthesia, somnolence, tremor, vertigo (less than 1%).

Dermatologic – Eczema, furunculosis, pruritus, maculopapular rash, increased sweating (less than 1%).

GI – Anorexia, constipation, dry mouth, esophagitis, flatulence, gastritis, gastroenteritis, gingivitis, periodontitis, toothache (less than 1%).

GU – Cystitis, micturition frequency, polyuria, renal calculus, urinary incontinence (less than 1%).

Hematologic – Anemia, purpura (less than 1%).

Hepatic – Increased ALT and AST (less than 1%).

Metabolic/Nutritional – Diabetes mellitus, glycosuria, gout, hypercholesterolemia, hyperkalemia, hypokalemia, hyponatremia (less than 1%).

Musculoskeletal – Arthritis, aggravated arthritis, arthrosis, skeletal pain, tendinitis (less than 1%).

Respiratory – Asthma, epistaxis (less than 1%).

Special senses – Conjunctivitis, abnormal vision, xerophthalmia, tinnitus (less than 1%).

Miscellaneous – Alcohol intolerance, asthenia, substernal chest pain, peripheral edema, fever, hot flushes, malaise, rigors, herpes simplex, otitis externa, otitis media, leg cramps, peripheral ischemia (less than 1%).

Facial edema was reported in 5 patients receiving eprosartan. Angioedema has been reported with other AIIRAs.

➤*Irbesartan:*

Cardiovascular – Flushing, hypertension, cardiac murmur, MI, angina pectoris, arrhythmic/conduction disorder, cardiorespiratory arrest, heart failure, hypertensive crisis (less than 1%).

CNS – Sleep disturbance, numbness, somnolence, emotional disturbance, paresthesia, tremor, transient ischemic attack, cerebrovascular accident (less than 1%).

Dermatologic – Pruritus, dermatitis, ecchymosis, face erythema, urticaria (less than 1%).

Endocrine – Sexual dysfunction, libido change, gout (less than 1%).

GI – Constipation, oral lesion, gastroenteritis, flatulence, abdominal distention (less than 1%).

GU – Abnormal urination, prostate disorder (less than 1%).

Musculoskeletal – Extremity swelling, muscle cramp, arthritis, muscle ache, musculoskeletal chest pain, joint stiffness, bursitis, muscle weakness (less than 1%).

Respiratory – Epistaxis, tracheobronchitis, congestion, pulmonary congestion, dyspnea, wheezing (less than 1%).

Special senses – Vision disturbance, hearing abnormality, ear infection, ear pain, conjunctivitis, other eye disturbance, eyelid abnormality, ear abnormality (less than 1%).

Miscellaneous – Fever, chills, facial edema, upper extremity edema (less than 1%).

The incidence of hypotension or orthostatic hypotension was low in irbesartan-treated patients (0.4%), unrelated to dosage, and similar to the incidence among placebo-treated patients (0.2%). Dizziness, syncope, and vertigo were reported with equal or less frequency in patients receiving irbesartan compared with placebo.

Postmarketing: Urticaria, angioedema (involving swelling of the face, lips, pharynx, or tongue), increased liver function tests, jaundice. Hyperkalemia has been reported rarely.

➤*Losartan:*

Cardiovascular – Angina pectoris, second degree AV block, CVA, hypotension, MI, arrhythmias including atrial fibrillation, palpitation, sinus bradycardia, ventricular tachycardia, ventricular fibrillation (less than 1%).

CNS – Anxiety disorder, ataxia, confusion, dream abnormality, hypesthesia, decreased libido, memory impairment, migraine, paresthesia, peripheral neuropathy, panic disorder, sleep disorder, somnolence, tremor, vertigo (less than 1%).

Dermatologic – Alopecia, dermatitis, dry skin, ecchymosis, erythema, flushing, photosensitivity, pruritus, sweating, urticaria (less than 1%).

GI – Anorexia, constipation, dental pain, dry mouth, flatulence, gastritis (less than 1%).

GU – Impotence, nocturia, urinary frequency (less than 1%).

Musculoskeletal – Arm pain, hip pain, joint swelling, knee pain, shoulder pain, stiffness, arthritis, fibromyalgia, muscle weakness (less than 1%).

Respiratory – Dyspnea, pharyngeal discomfort, epistaxis, respiratory congestion (less than 1%).

Special senses – Blurred vision, burning/stinging in the eye, conjunctivitis, taste perversion, tinnitus, decrease in visual acuity (less than 1%).

Miscellaneous – Asthenia/fatigue (at least 1%); facial edema, fever, orthostatic effects, syncope, anemia, gout (less than 1%).

A patient with known hypersensitivity to aspirin and penicillin, when treated with losartan, was withdrawn from the study because of swelling of the lips and eyelids and facial rash, reported as angioedema, which returned to normal 5 days after therapy was discontinued.

Superficial peeling of palms and hemolysis was reported in 1 subject.

Postmarketing experience: Hepatitis (rare); dry cough (including positive rechallenges), hyperkalemia, hyponatremia. Angioedema, including swelling of the larynx and glottis, causing airway obstruction or swelling of the face, lips, pharynx, or tongue has been reported rarely in patients treated with losartan; some of these patients previously experienced angioedema with other drugs including ACE inhibitors. Vasculitis, including Henoch-Schönlein purpura, has been reported. Anaphylactic reactions have been reported.

➤*Olmesartan:*

GI – Gastroenteritis, nausea (greater than 0.5%).

Metabolic/Nutritional – Hypercholesterolemia, hyperlipemia, hyperuricemia (greater than 0.5%).

Musculoskeletal – Arthritis, skeletal pain (greater than 0.5%).

Miscellaneous – Pain, vertigo (greater than 0.5%).

Facial edema was reported in 5 patients receiving olmesartan. Angioedema has been reported with other AIIRAs.

➤*Telmisartan:*

Cardiovascular – Palpitation, dependent edema, angina pectoris, leg edema, abnormal ECG (more than 0.3%).

CNS – Somnolence, migraine, vertigo, paresthesia, involuntary muscle contractions, hypesthesia (greater than 0.3%).

Dermatologic – Dermatitis, eczema, pruritus (greater than 0.3%).

GI – Flatulence, constipation, gastritis, vomiting, dry mouth, hemorrhoids, gastroenteritis, enteritis, gastroesophageal reflux, toothache, nonspecific GI disorders (greater than 0.3%).

GU – Micturition frequency, cystitis (greater than 0.3%).

Metabolic – Gout, hypercholesterolemia, diabetes mellitus (greater than 0.3%).

Musculoskeletal – Arthritis, leg cramps (greater than 0.3%).

Respiratory – Asthma, dyspnea, epistaxis (greater than 0.3%).

Special senses – Abnormal vision, conjunctivitis, tinnitus, earache (greater than 0.3%).

Miscellaneous – Impotence, increased sweating, flushing, allergy, fever, leg pain, malaise, infection, fungal infection, abscess, otitis media, cerebrovascular disorder (greater than 0.3%).

A single case of angioedema was reported (among a total of 3,781 patients treated with telmisartan).

➤*Valsartan:*

CNS – Paresthesia, somnolence (greater than 0.2%).

GU – Constipation, dry mouth, flatulence (greater than 0.2%).

Miscellaneous – Allergic reaction, asthenia, palpitations, dyspnea, vertigo, impotence, pruritus (greater than 0.2%).

Other reported events seen less frequently in clinical trials included chest pain, syncope, anorexia, vomiting, and angioedema.

Dose-related orthostatic effects were seen in less than 1% of patients. An increase in the incidence of dizziness was observed in patients treated with 320 mg valsartan (8%) compared with 10 to 160 mg (2% to 4%).

Postmarketing experience: Hepatitis (very rare), elevated liver enzymes, angioedema (rare), impaired renal function, hyperkalemia, alopecia.

Overdosage

Limited data are available. The most likely manifestation of overdosage with an AIIRA would be hypotension, dizziness, and tachycardia; bradycardia could occur from parasympathetic (vagal) stimulation. If symptomatic hypotension should occur, institute supportive treatment. Refer to General Management of Acute Overdosage. AIIRAs cannot be removed by hemodialysis.

Patient Information

Tell patients of childbearing age about the consequences of second- and third-trimester exposure to drugs that act on the renin-angiotensin system, and tell them that these consequences do not appear to have resulted from intrauterine drug exposure that has been limited to the first trimester. Ask these patients to report pregnancies to their physicians as soon as possible.

AZILSARTAN MEDOXOMIL

Rx	**Edarbi** (Takeda)	**Tablets; oral:** 40 mg	Equiv. to azilsartan kamedoxomil 42.68 mg. Mannitol. (ASL 40). White, round. In 30s and 90s.
		80 mg	Equiv. to azilsartan kamedoxomil 85.36 mg. Mannitol. (ASL 80). White, round. In 30s and 90s.

AZILSARTAN MEDOXOMIL — ORAL

WARNING

Avoid use in pregnancy. When pregnancy is detected, discontinue azilsartan as soon as possible. Drugs that act directly on the renin-angiotensin system can cause injury and death to the developing fetus.

Indications

➤*Hypertension:* For the treatment of hypertension alone or in combination with other antihypertensive agents.

Administration and Dosage

➤*Adults:*

Hypertension –

Usual dosage: 80 mg once daily.

Concomitant therapy:

• *Antihypertensives* – If blood pressure is not controlled with azilsartan alone, additional blood pressure reduction can be achieved by taking azilsartan with other antihypertensive agents.

• *Diuretics* – Consider a starting dose of azilsartan 40 mg for patients who are treated with high doses of diuretics.

➤*Storage/Stability:* Store at 25°C (77°F); excursions are permitted to 15° to 30°C (59° to 86°F). Protect from moisture and light. Do not repackage; dispense and store in original container.

LOSARTAN POTASSIUM

Rx	**Losartan Potassium** (ZyGenerics)	**Tablets; oral:** 25 mg	May contain lactose, PEG, 2.12 mg potassium. In 30s, 90s, 100s, 1,000s, 5,000s and 10,000s.
Rx	**Cozaar** (Merck)		Lactose, 2.12 mg potassium. (MRK 951). Lt. green, teardrop shape. Film-coated. In 1000s, unit-of-use 90s and 100s, and UD 100s.
Rx	**Losartan Potassium** (ZyGenerics)	**Tablets; oral:** 50 mg	May contain lactose, PEG, 4.24 mg potassium. In 30s, 90s, 100s, 1,000s, and 10,000s.
Rx	**Cozaar** (Merck)		Lactose, 4.24 mg potassium. (MRK 952 COZAAR). Green, teardrop shape. Film-coated. In 1000s, unit-of-use 30s, 90s, and 100s, and UD 100s.
Rx	**Losartan Potassium** (ZyGenerics)	**Tablets; oral:** 100 mg	May contain lactose, PEG, 8.48 mg potassium. In 30s, 90s, 100s, 1,000s, and 5,000s.
Rx	**Cozaar** (Merck)		Lactose, 8.48 mg potassium. (960 MRK). Dk. green, teardrop shape. Film-coated. In 1000s, unit-of-use 30s, 90s, and 100s, and UD 100s.

LOSARTAN POTASSIUM — ORAL

For complete and comparative prescribing information, refer to the Angiotensin II Receptor Antagonists group monograph.

WARNING

When used in pregnancy during the second and third trimesters, drugs that act directly on the remin-angiotensin system can cause injury and even death to the developing fetus. When pregnancy is detected, losartan should be discontinued as soon as possible.

Indications

➤*Hypertension:* Losartan is indicated for the treatment of hypertension. It may be used alone or in combination with other antihypertensive agents, including diuretics.

➤*Hypertensive patients with left ventricular hypertrophy:* Losartan is indicated to reduce the risk of stroke in patients with hypertension and left ventricular hypertrophy, but there is evidence that this benefit does not apply to black patients. In the Losartan Intervention For End point reduction (LIFE) in hypertension study, black patients treated with atenolol were at lower risk of experiencing the primary composite end point compared with black patients treated with losartan. In the subgroup of black patients (n = 533; 6% of the LIFE study patients), there were 29 primary end points among 263 patients on atenolol (11%, 26 per 1,000 patient-years) and 46 primary end points among 270 patients (17%, 42 per 1,000 patient-years) on losartan. This finding could not be explained on the basis of differences in the populations other than race or on any imbalances between treatment groups. In addition, blood pressure reductions in both treatment groups were consistent between black and nonblack patients. Given the difficulty in interpreting subset differences in large trials, it cannot be known whether the observed difference is the result of chance. However, the LIFE study provides no evidence that the benefits of losartan potassium on reducing the risk of cardiovascular events in hypertensive patients with left ventricular hypertrophy apply to black patients.

➤*Nephropathy in patients with type 2 diabetes:* Losartan is indicated for the treatment of diabetic nephropathy with an elevated serum creatinine and proteinuria (urinary albumin to creatinine ratio greater than or equal to 300 mg/g) in patients with type 2 diabetes and a history of hypertension. In this population, losartan reduces the rate of progression of nephropathy as measured by the occurrence of doubling of serum creatinine or end-stage renal disease (need for dialysis or renal transplantation).

Administration and Dosage

➤*General dosing considerations:* Dosing must be individualized.

In patients who are intravascularly volume-depleted (eg, those treated with diuretics), symptomatic hypotension may occur after initiation of therapy with losartan. Correct these conditions prior to administration of losartan potassium, or a lower starting dose should be used.

If the antihypertensive effect measured at trough using once-a-day dosing is inadequate, a twice-a-day regimen at the same total daily dose or an increase in dose may give a more satisfactory response. The effect of losartan is substantially present within 1 week, but in some studies, the maximal effect occurred in 3 to 6 weeks.

➤*Adults:*

Hypertension –

Usual dosage: 25 to 100 mg total dose given once or twice daily.

Initial dosage: 50 mg once daily. In patients with possible depletion of intravascular volume (eg, patients treated with diuretics), the initial dose is 25 mg once daily.

Concomitant therapy: Losartan may be administered with other antihypertensive agents. If blood pressure is not controlled by losartan alone, a low dose of a diuretic may be added. Hydrochlorothiazide has been shown to have an additive effect. Addition of a low dose of hydrochlorothiazide (12.5 mg) to losartan 50 mg once daily resulted in placebo-adjusted blood pressure reductions of 15.5 per 9.2 mm Hg.

Hypertension with left ventricular hypertrophy –

Usual dosage: Hydrochlorothiazide 12.5 mg daily should be added, or the dose of losartan should be increased to 100 mg once daily followed by an increase in hydrochlorothiazide to 25 mg once daily based on blood pressure response.

Initial dosage: 50 mg once daily.

Nephropathy in patients with type 2 diabetes mellitus –

Usual dosage: The dose should be increased to 100 mg once daily based on blood pressure response.

Initial dosage: 50 mg once daily.

Concomitant therapy: Losartan may be administered with insulin and other commonly used hypoglycemic agents (eg, sulfonylureas, glitazones, glucosidase inhibitors).

➤*Children:*

Hypertension –

6 years of age and older:

• *Usual dosage* – 0.7 mg/kg once daily (up to 50 mg total) administered as a tablet or suspension. Dosage should be adjusted according to blood pressure response.

• *Maximum dose* – Doses higher than 1.4 mg/kg/day (or in excess of 100 mg) have not been studied in children.

➤*Renal function impairment:*

Children – Losartan is not recommended in pediatric patients with glomerular filtration rates of less than 30 mL/min per 1.73 m^2.

➤*Hepatic function impairment:* 25 mg once daily as usual starting dosage. A lower starting dose is recommended for patients with a history of hepatic impairment.

➤*Preparation for administration:*

Preparation of suspension (for 200 mL of a 2.5 mg/mL suspension) – Add 10 mL of purified water to an 8 ounce (240 mL) amber polyethylene terephthalate (PET) bottle containing ten 50 mg losartan tablets. Immediately shake for at least 2 minutes. Let the concentrate stand for 1 hour and then shake for 1 minute to disperse the tablet contents. Separately, prepare a 50/50 volumetric mixture of *Ora-Plus* and *Ora-Sweet SF*. Add 190 mL of the 50/50 *Ora-Plus/Ora-Sweet SF* mixture to the tablet and water slurry in the PET bottle and shake for 1 minute to disperse the ingredients. The suspension should be refrigerated at 2° to 8°C (36° to 46°F) and can be stored for up to 4 weeks. Shake the suspension prior to each use, and return it promptly to the refrigerator.

➤*Administration:* Losartan may be administered with or without food.

➤*Storage/Stability:*

Tablets – Store at 25°C (77°F); excursions are permitted to 15° to 30°C (59° to 86°F). Keep container tightly closed. Protect from light.

Suspension – Refrigerate at 2° to 8°C (36° to 46°F). May be stored for up to 4 weeks.

VALSARTAN

Rx	**Diovan** (Novartis)	**Tablets; oral:** 40 mg	Polyethylene glycol 8000. (NVR DO). Yellow, ovaloid shape. Scored. In 30s and UD 100s.
		80 mg	Polyethylene glycol 8000. (NVR DV). Pale red, almond shape. In 90s and UD 100s.
		160 mg	Polyethylene glycol 8000. (NVR DX). Gray-orange, almond shape. In 90s and UD 100s.
		320 mg	Polyethylene glycol 8000. (NVR DXL). Dark grayish violet, almond shape. In 90s.

VALSARTAN — ORAL

For complete and comparative prescribing information, refer to the Angiotensin II Receptor Antagonists group monograph.

WARNING

Use in pregnancy – When used in pregnancy, drugs that act directly on the renin-angiotensin system can cause injury and even death to the developing fetus. When pregnancy is detected, discontinue valsartan as soon as possible (see Warnings/Precautions).

Indications

➤*Heart failure:* For the treatment of heart failure (New York Heart Association [NYHA] class II to IV).

➤*Hypertension:* For the treatment of hypertension for adults and children 6 to 16 years of age. It may be used alone or in combination with other antihypertensive agents.

➤*Post–myocardial infarction (MI):* To reduce cardiovascular mortality in clinically stable patients with left ventricular failure or left ventricular dysfunction following MI.

Administration and Dosage

➤*Adults:*

Heart failure –

Maximum dose: 320 mg/day in divided doses.

Initial dosage: 40 mg twice daily.

Dosage titration: Up titration to 80 and 160 mg twice daily should be done to the highest dose, as tolerated by the patient.

Concomitant therapy: Consideration should be given to reducing the dose of concomitant diuretics.

Hypertension –

Usual dosage: Range of 80 to 320 mg once daily.

Maximum dose: 320 mg daily.

Initial dosage: 80 or 160 mg once daily when used as monotherapy in patients who are not volume-depleted. Patients requiring greater reductions may be started at a higher dose.

Dosage adjustment: The antihypertensive effect is substantially present within 2 weeks and maximal reduction is generally attained after 4 weeks. If additional antihypertensive effect is required over the starting dose range,

VALSARTAN — ORAL

the dose may be increased to a maximum of 320 mg/day, or a diuretic may be added. The addition of a diuretic has a greater effect than dose increases above 80 mg.

Concomitant therapy: Valsartan may be administered with other antihypertensive agents.

Postmyocardial infarction –

Initial dosage: 20 mg twice daily initiated as early as 12 hours after an MI.

Dosage titration: Patients may be up-titrated within 7 days to 40 mg twice daily, with subsequent titrations to a target maintenance dosage of 160 mg twice daily, as tolerated by the patient. If symptomatic hypotension or renal function impairment occur, consideration should be given to a dosage reduction.

Concomitant therapy: Valsartan may be given with other standard post-MI treatments, including thrombolytics, aspirin, beta-blockers, and statins.

➤*Children:* Valsartan is not recommended for treatment of children of any age with a glomerular filtration rate of less than 30 mL/min per 1.73 m^2.

6 to 16 years of age –

Hypertension:

- *Initial dosage* – 1.3 mg/kg once daily (up to 40 mg total).
- *Dosage adjustment* – Adjust dosage according to blood pressure response. Dosages higher than 2.7 mg/kg (up to 160 mg) once daily have not been studied in children 6 to 16 years of age.

➤*Elderly:* No initial dosage adjustment is required for elderly patients.

➤*Renal function impairment:* No initial dosage adjustment is required for patients with mild or moderate renal function impairment. Exercise care with dosing of valsartan in patients with severe renal function impairment.

➤*Hepatic function impairment:* No initial dosage adjustment is required for patients with mild or moderate hepatic function impairment. Exercise care with dosing of valsartan in patients with hepatic function impairment.

➤*Preparation for administration:*

Preparation of suspension (for 160 mL of a 4 mg/mL suspension) – Add 80 mL of *Ora-Plus* oral suspending vehicle to an amber glass bottle containing 8 valsartan 80 mg tablets and shake for a minimum of 2 minutes. Allow the suspension to stand for a minimum of 1 hour. After the standing time, shake the suspension for a minimum of 1 additional minute. Add 80 mL of *Ora-Sweet SF* oral sweetening vehicle to the bottle and shake the suspension for at least 10 seconds to disperse the ingredients. Shake the bottle well (for at least 10 seconds) prior to dispensing the suspension.

➤*Administration:* May be administered with or without food.

For children who cannot swallow tablets, or children for whom the calculated dosage (mg/kg) does not correspond to the available tablet strengths of valsartan, the use of a suspension is recommended (see Preparation of suspension). When the suspension is replaced by a tablet, the dose of valsartan may have to be increased. The exposure to valsartan with the suspension is 1.6 times more than with the tablet.

➤*Storage/Stability:* Store at 25°C (77°F); excursions are permitted to 15° to 30°C (59° to 86°F). Protect from moisture.

The suspension is homogeneous and can be stored for either up to 30 days at room temperature (below 30°C [below 86°F]) or up to 75 days at refrigerated conditions (2° to 8°C [35° to 46°F]) in the glass bottle with a child-resistant screw-cap closure.

IRBESARTAN

Rx	**Avapro** (Bristol-Myers Squibb Sanofi-Synthelabo Partnership)	**Tablets:** 75 mg	Lactose. (2771). White to off-white, oval. In 30s and 90s.
		150 mg	Lactose. (2772). White to off-white, oval. In 30s, 90s, 500s, and UD 100s.
		300 mg	Lactose. (2773). White to off-white, oval. In 30s, 90s, and 500s.

IRBESARTAN — ORAL

For complete and comparative prescribing information, refer to the Angiotensin II Receptor Antagonists group monograph.

WARNING

When used in pregnancy during the second and third trimesters, drugs that act directly on the renin-angiotensin system can cause injury and even death to the developing fetus. When pregnancy is detected, irbesartan should be discontinued as soon as possible.

Indications

➤*Hypertension:* Irbesartan is indicated for the treatment of hypertension; it may be used alone or in combination with other antihypertensive agents.

➤*Nephropathy in type 2 diabetic patients:* Irbesartan is indicated for the treatment of diabetic nephropathy with an elevated serum creatinine and proteinuria (greater than 300 mg/day) in patients with type 2 diabetes and hypertension. In this population, irbesartan reduces the rate of progression of nephropathy as measured by the occurrence of doubling of serum creatinine or end-stage renal disease (need for dialysis or renal transplantation).

Administration and Dosage

➤*Adults:*

Hypertension –

Usual dosage: 150 mg once daily. Patients requiring further reduction in blood pressure should be titrated to 300 mg once daily.

Maximum dose: 300 mg once daily.

Dosage titration: Patients not adequately treated by the maximum dose of 300 mg once daily are unlikely to derive additional benefit from a higher dose or twice-daily dosing.

Concomitant therapy: A low dose of a diuretic may be added if blood pressure is not controlled by irbesartan alone. Hydrochlorothiazide has been shown to have an additive effect. In controlled trials, the addition of irbesartan to hydrochlorothiazide doses of 6.25, 12.5, or 25 mg produced further dose-related reductions in blood pressure similar to those achieved with the same monotherapy dose of irbesartan.

Nephropathy in type 2 diabetes – 300 mg once daily. There are no data on the clinical effects of lower doses of irbesartan on diabetic nephropathy.

➤*Children:*

Off-label dosing –

Hypertension:

- *13 years of age and older* –
  Usual dosage: 150 to 300 mg/day.
  Initial dosage: 150 mg once daily.
- *6 to 12 years of age* –
  Usual dosage: 75 to 150 mg/day orally.
  Initial dosage: 75 mg once daily.

➤*Volume- and salt-depleted patients:* Volume depletion should be corrected prior to administration of antihypertensive therapy, or a low starting dose of irbesartan should be used. Closely monitor the patient. A lower initial dose of irbesartan 75 mg is recommended in patients with depletion of intravascular volume or salt (eg, patients treated vigorously with diuretics or on hemodialysis).

➤*Storage/Stability:* Store between 15° and 30°C (59° and 86°F).

CANDESARTAN CILEXETIL

Rx	**Atacand** (AstraZeneca)	**Tablets:** 4 mg	Lactose. (ACF 004). White to off-white. In unit-of-use 30s.
		8 mg	Lactose. (ACG 008). Lt. pink. In unit-of-use 30s.
		16 mg	Lactose. (ACH 016). Pink. In unit-of-use 30s and 90s and UD 100s.
		32 mg	Lactose. (ACL 032). Pink. In unit-of-use 30s and 90s and UD 100s.

CANDESARTAN CILEXETIL — ORAL

For complete and comparative prescribing information, refer to the Angiotensin II Receptor Antagonists group monograph.

WARNING

Use in pregnancy – When used in pregnancy during the second and third trimesters, drugs that act directly on the renin-angiotensin system can cause injury and even death to the developing fetus. When pregnancy is detected, discontinue candesartan as soon as possible. Drugs that act directly on the renin-angiotensin system can cause fetal and neonatal morbidity and death when administered to pregnant women.

Indications

➤*Hypertension:* Candesartan is indicated for the treatment of hypertension. It may be used alone or in combination with other antihypertensive agents.

➤*Heart failure:* Candesartan is indicated for the treatment of heart failure (New York Heart Association [NYHA] class II to IV and ejection fraction up to 40%) to reduce the risk of death from cardiovascular causes and reduce hospitalizations for heart failure.

➤*Off-label uses:*

Prevention of migraine (adults) – [4] = Insufficient documentation. Use of candesartan as preventive therapy for migraine is limited to one randomized, placebo-controlled, double-blind, crossover trial and several case reports. Larger controlled trials are needed to establish the role of this agent in migraine prophylaxis.

Administration and Dosage

➤*General dosing considerations:* Dosage must be individualized. Blood pressure response is dose related over the range of 2 to 32 mg.

Most of the antihypertensive effect is present within 2 weeks, and maximal blood pressure reduction is generally obtained within 4 to 6 weeks of treatment with candesartan.

➤*Adults:*

Heart failure –

Initial dosage: The recommended initial dosage is 4 mg once daily.

Dosage titration: Double the dose at approximately 2-week intervals, as tolerated by the patient.

Maintenance dosage: The target dosage is 32 mg once daily.

Hypertension –

Usual dosage: Total daily doses ranging from 8 to 32 mg. Larger doses do not appear to have a greater effect, and there is relatively little experience with such doses.

Initial dosage: The usual recommended starting dosage is 16 mg once daily when it is used as monotherapy in patients who are not volume depleted.

Concomitant therapy: If blood pressure is not controlled by candesartan alone, a diuretic may be added. Candesartan may be administered with other antihypertensive agents.

Off-label dosing –

Prevention of migraine (adults): [4] = Insufficient documentation. 8 to 16 mg/day for up to 12 weeks.

➤*Elderly:* No initial dosage adjustment is necessary for elderly patients.

➤*Renal function impairment:* No initial dosage adjustment is necessary for patients with mildly impaired renal function.

➤*Hepatic function impairment:* No initial dosage adjustment is necessary for patients with mildly impaired hepatic function. In patients with moderate hepatic impairment, consider initiating candesartan at a lower dose.

➤*Volume-depleted patients:* For patients with possible depletion of intravascular volume (eg, patients treated with diuretics, particularly those with impaired renal function), initiate candesartan under close medical supervision and consider administering a lower dose.

➤*Administration:* Candesartan may be administered with or without food. Candesartan can be administered once or twice daily.

➤*Storage/Stability:* Store at 25°C (77°F); excursions are permitted to 15° to 30°C (59° to 86°F).

TELMISARTAN

Rx	**Micardis** (Boehringer Ingelheim)	**Tablets; oral:** 20 mg	Sorbitol. (50H). White to off-white, round. In UD 30s.
		40 mg	Sorbitol. (51H). White to off-white, oblong. In UD 30s.
		80 mg	Sorbitol. (52H). White to off-white, oblong. In UD 30s.

TELMISARTAN — ORAL

For complete and comparative prescribing information, refer to the Angiotensin II Receptor Antagonists class monograph.

WARNING

Use in pregnancy – When used in pregnancy, drugs that act directly on the renin-angiotensin system can cause injury and even death to the developing fetus. When pregnancy is detected, discontinue telmisartan as soon as possible.

Indications

➤*Cardiovascular risk reduction:* For reduction of the risk of myocardial infarction (MI), stroke, or death from cardiovascular causes in patients 55 years of age and older at high risk of developing major cardiovascular events who are unable to take angiotensin-converting enzyme (ACE) inhibitors.

➤*Hypertension:* For the treatment of hypertension. It may be used alone or in combination with other antihypertensive agents.

➤*General information:* Use of telmisartan with an ACE inhibitor is not recommended.

Administration and Dosage

➤*Adults:*

Cardiovascular risk reduction – 80 mg once a day.

Hypertension –

Usual dosage: 20 to 80 mg daily.

Initial dosage: 40 mg once daily.

Concomitant therapy: May be administered with other antihypertensive agents. When additional blood pressure reduction beyond that achieved with 80 mg is required, a diuretic may be added.

➤*Hepatic function impairment:* Initiate at low doses and titrate slowly in patients with biliary obstructive disorders or hepatic insufficiency.

➤*Volume depletion:* Correct the condition of patients with depletion of intravascular volume or initiate therapy under close supervision or with a reduced dose.

➤*Administration:* May be administered with or without food.

➤*Storage/Stability:* Store at 25°C (77°F); excursions are permitted to between 15° and 30°C (59° and 86°F). Tablets should not be removed from blisters until immediately before administration.

EPROSARTAN MESYLATE

Rx	**Teveten** (Abbott)	**Tablets; oral:** 400 mg	Lactose, PEG. (SOLVAY 5044). Pink, oval shape. Film-coated. In 100s.
		600 mg	Lactose, PEG. (SOLVAY 5046). White, capsule shape. Film-coated. In 100s.

EPROSARTAN MESYLATE — ORAL

For complete and comparative prescribing information, refer to the Angiotensin II Receptor Antagonists group monograph.

WARNING

Use in pregnancy – When used in pregnancy during the second and third trimesters, drugs that act directly on the renin-angiotensin system can cause injury and even death to the developing fetus. When pregnancy is detected, eprosartan mesylate tablets should be discontinued as soon as possible (see Warnings, Fetal/Neonatal morbidity and mortality).

Indications

➤*Hypertension:* Eprosartan mesylate tablets are indicated for the treatment of hypertension. It may be used alone or in combination with other antihypertensives such as diuretics and calcium channel blockers.

Administration and Dosage

➤*Adults:*

Hypertension –

Usual dosage: Administered once or twice daily with total daily doses ranging from 400 to 800 mg. There is limited experience with doses beyond 800 mg/day.

Initial dosage: 600 mg once daily when used as monotherapy in patients who are not volume depleted.

Dosage titration: If the antihypertensive effect measured at trough using once-daily dosing is inadequate, a twice-a-day regimen at the same total daily dose or an increase in dose may give a more satisfactory response. Achievement of maximum blood pressure reduction in most patients may take 2 to 3 weeks.

Angiotensin II Receptor Antagonists

EPROSARTAN MESYLATE — ORAL

Concomitant therapy: Eprosartan may be used in combination with other antihypertensive agents, such as thiazide diuretics or calcium channel blockers, if additional blood pressure-lowering effect is required.

➤*Elderly:* No initial dosing adjustment is generally necessary for elderly patients.

➤*Renal function impairment:* No initial dosing adjustment is generally necessary with renal impairment. In patients with moderate and severe renal impairment, the maximum dose should not exceed 600 mg daily.

➤*Hepatic function impairment:* No initial dosing adjustment is generally necessary for hepatically impaired patients.

➤*Discontinuation of therapy:* Discontinuation of treatment with eprosartan does not lead to a rapid rebound increase in blood pressure.

➤*Administration:* Eprosartan mesylate tablets may be taken with or without food once or twice daily.

➤*Storage/Stability:* Store at 20° to 25°C (68° to 77°F).

OLMESARTAN MEDOXOMIL

Rx	Benicar (Daiichi Sankyo)	Tablets; oral: 5 mg	Lactose. (Sankyo C12). Yellow, round. Film-coated. In 30s.
		20 mg	Lactose. (Sankyo C14). White, round. Film-coated. In 30s, 90s, and UD 100s.
		40 mg	Lactose. (Sankyo C15). White, oval. Film-coated. In 30s, 90s, and UD 100s.

OLMESARTAN MEDOXOMIL — ORAL

For complete and comparative prescribing information, refer to the Angiotensin II Receptor Antagonists class monograph.

WARNING

When pregnancy is detected, discontinue olmesartan as soon as possible. Drugs that act directly on the renin-angiotensin system can cause injury and even death to the developing fetus.

Indications

➤*Hypertension:* For the treatment of hypertension.

➤*Off-label uses:*

Prevention of migraine (adults) – [4] = Insufficient documentation. Although there are limited noncontrolled data regarding the use of olmesartan for the prevention of migraines, it may be useful in patients with migraines and hypertension. Larger, controlled trials are needed to establish the role of this agent in migraine prophylaxis.

Administration and Dosage

➤*General dosing considerations:* For children who cannot swallow tablets, the same dose can be given using an extemporaneous suspension. Follow the suspension preparation instructions to administer olmesartan as a suspension. (See Preparation for administration.)

➤*Adults:*

Hypertension –

Initial dosage: 20 mg once daily when used as monotherapy in patients who are not volume contracted.

Dosage adjustment: After 2 weeks of therapy, the dose may be increased to 40 mg.

Concomitant therapy: If blood pressure is not controlled by olmesartan alone, a diuretic may be added. Olmesartan may be administered with other antihypertensive agents.

Off-label dosing –

Prevention of migraine (adults): [4] = Insufficient documentation. 10 to 40 mg daily for 3 months up to 1 year.

➤*Children:*

Hypertension –

6 to 16 years of age:

- *20 to less than 35 kg –*
  Maximum dose: 20 mg once daily.
  Initial dosage: 10 mg once daily.
  Dosage adjustment: After 2 weeks of therapy, the dosage may be increased to a maximum of 20 mg once daily.
- *35 kg or more –*
  Maximum dose: 40 mg once daily.
  Initial dosage: 20 mg once daily.
  Dosage adjustment: After 2 weeks of therapy, the dosage may be increased to a maximum of 40 mg once daily.

➤*Intravascular volume depletion:* For patients with possible depletion of intravascular volume (eg, patients treated with diuretics, particularly those with impaired renal function), initiate olmesartan under close medical supervision, and consider giving a lower starting dose.

➤*Preparation for administration:*

Preparation of suspension (2 mg/mL) – Add 50 mL of purified water to an amber polyethylene terephthalate bottle containing 20 olmesartan 20 mg tablets and allow to stand for a minimum of 5 minutes. Shake the container for at least 1 minute and allow the suspension to stand for at least 1 minute. Repeat 1-minute shaking and 1-minute standing 4 additional times. Add 100 mL of *Ora-Sweet* and 50 mL of *Ora-Plus* to the suspension and shake well for at least 1 minute.

➤*Administration:* Olmesartan may be administered with or without food. Shake the prepared suspension well before each use.

➤*Storage/Stability:* Store at 20° to 25°C (68° to 77°F). The extemporaneously prepared suspension should be refrigerated at 2° to 8°C (36° to 46°F) and can be stored for up to 4 weeks.

Direct Renin Inhibitors

ALISKIREN

Rx	Tekturna (Novartis)	Tablets; oral: 150 mg	As aliskiren hemifumarate. (NVR IL). Lt. pink, round. Film-coated. In 30s, 90s, and UD 100s.
		300 mg	As aliskiren hemifumarate. (NVR IU). Lt. red, oval. Film-coated. In 30s, 90s, and UD 100s.

ALISKIREN HEMIFUMARATE — ORAL

WARNING

Use in pregnancy – Drugs that act directly on the renin-angiotensin system can cause injury and even death to the developing fetus. When pregnancy is detected, discontinue aliskiren as soon as possible.

Indications

➤*Hypertension:* For the treatment of hypertension. It may be used alone or in combination with other antihypertensive agents.

Administration and Dosage

➤*General dosing considerations:* Patients should establish a routine pattern for taking aliskiren with regard to meals. High-fat meals decrease absorption substantially.

➤*Adults:*

Hypertension –

Initial dosage: 150 mg once daily.

Dosage titration: In patients whose blood pressure is not adequately controlled, the daily dose may be increased to 300 mg. Doses higher than 300 mg did not attain an increased blood pressure response, but increased the rate of diarrhea. The antihypertensive effect of a given dose is substantially attained (85% to 90%) by 2 weeks.

Concomitant therapy: Aliskiren may be administered with other antihypertensive agents. Most exposure to date is with diuretics and an angiotensin receptor blocker (valsartan); the drugs together have a greater effect at their maximum recommended doses than either drug alone. It is not known whether additive effects are present when aliskiren is used with angiotensin-converting enzyme (ACE) inhibitors or beta-blockers.

➤*Storage/Stability:* Store at 25°C (77°F); excursions are permitted to 15° to 30°C (59° to 86°F). Protect from moisture.

Actions

➤*Pharmacology:* Renin is secreted by the kidney in response to decreases in blood volume and renal perfusion. Renin cleaves angiotensinogen to form the inactive decapeptide angiotensin I (Ang I). Ang I is converted to the active octapeptide angiotensin II (Ang II) by ACE and non-ACE pathways. Ang II is a powerful vasoconstrictor that leads to the release of catecholamines from the adrenal medulla and prejunctional nerve endings. It also promotes aldosterone secretion and sodium reabsorption. Together, these effects increase blood pressure. Ang II also inhibits renin release, thus providing a negative feedback to the system. This cycle, from renin through angiotensin to aldosterone and its associated negative feedback loop, is known as the renin-angiotensin-aldosterone system (RAAS). Aliskiren is a direct renin inhibitor, decreasing plasma renin activity (PRA) and inhibiting the conversion of angiotensinogen to Ang I. Whether aliskiren affects other RAAS components (ie, ACE or non-ACE pathways) is not known.

All agents that inhibit the RAAS, including renin inhibitors, suppress the negative feedback loop, leading to a compensatory rise in plasma renin concentration. When this rise occurs during treatment with ACE inhibitors and

ALISKIREN HEMIFUMARATE — ORAL

angiotensin receptor blockers, the result is increased levels of PRA. However, during treatment with aliskiren, the effect of increased renin levels is blocked so that PRA, Ang I, and Ang II are all reduced whether aliskiren is used as monotherapy or in combination with other antihypertensive agents.

➤*Pharmacokinetics:*

Absorption/Distribution – Aliskiren is a poorly absorbed (bioavailability about 2.5%) drug with an approximate accumulation half-life of 24 hours. Steady-state blood levels are reached in about 7 to 8 days. Following oral administration, peak plasma concentrations of aliskiren are reached within 1 to 3 hours.

Food effects: When taken with a high-fat meal, mean area under the curve (AUC) and maximum drug concentration (C_{max}) of aliskiren are decreased 71% and 85%, respectively. In clinical trials, aliskiren was administered without requiring a fixed relation to administration of meals.

Metabolism/Excretion – Approximately one-fourth of the absorbed dose appears in the urine as parent drug. How much of the absorbed dose that is metabolized is unknown. Based on in vitro studies, the major enzyme responsible for aliskiren metabolism appears to be CYP3A4.

Contraindications

None well documented.

Warnings/Precautions

➤*Fetal/Neonatal morbidity and mortality:* Drugs that act directly on the renin-angiotensin system can cause fetal and neonatal morbidity and death when administered to pregnant women. If this drug is used during pregnancy, or if the patient becomes pregnant while taking this drug, apprise the patient of the potential hazard to the fetus. In several dozen published cases, ACE inhibitor use during the second and third trimesters of pregnancy was associated with fetal and neonatal injury, including hypotension, neonatal skull hypoplasia, anuria, reversible or irreversible renal failure, and death. In addition, first trimester use of ACE inhibitors has been associated with birth defects in retrospective data.

➤*Head and neck angioedema:* Angioedema of the face, extremities, lips, tongue, glottis, and/or larynx has been reported in patients treated with aliskiren and has necessitated hospitalization and intubation. This may occur at any time during treatment and has occurred in patients with and without a history of angioedema with ACE inhibitors or angiotensin receptor antagonists. If angioedema involves the throat, tongue, glottis, or larynx, or if the patient has a history of upper respiratory surgery, airway obstruction may occur and be fatal. Patients who experience these effects, even without respiratory distress, require prolonged observation because treatment with antihistamines and corticosteroids may not be sufficient to prevent respiratory involvement. Prompt administration of subcutaneous epinephrine solution 1:1,000 (0.3 to 0.5 mL) and measures to ensure a patient airway may be necessary. Discontinue aliskiren immediately in patients who develop angioedema, and do not readminister.

➤*Hypotension:* An excessive fall in blood pressure was rarely seen (0.1%) in patients with uncomplicated hypertension treated with aliskiren alone in controlled trials and in less than 1% during combination therapy with other antihypertensive agents. In patients with an activated renin-angiotensin system, such as volume- or salt-depleted patients (ie, those receiving high doses of diuretics), symptomatic hypotension could occur after initiation of treatment with aliskiren. Correct this condition prior to administration of aliskiren or start the treatment under close medical supervision.

If an excessive fall in blood pressure occurs, place the patient in the supine position and, if necessary, give an intravenous infusion of normal saline. A transient hypotensive response is not a contraindication to further treatment, which usually can be continued without difficulty once the blood pressure has stabilized.

➤*Hyperkalemia:* Increases in serum potassium of more than 5.5 mEq/L were infrequent with aliskiren alone (0.9% compared with 0.6% with placebo). However, when used in combination with an ACE inhibitor in a diabetic population, increases in serum potassium were more frequent (5.5%). Routine monitoring of electrolytes and renal function is indicated in this population.

➤*Renal artery stenosis:* No data are available on the use of aliskiren in patients with unilateral or bilateral renal artery stenosis or stenosis of the artery to a solitary kidney.

➤*Renal function impairment:* Patients with greater than moderate renal impairment (creatinine 1.7 mg/dL for women and 2 mg/dL for men and/or estimated glomerular filtration rate less than 30 mL/min), a history of dialysis, nephrotic syndrome, or renovascular hypertension were excluded from hypertension clinical trials of aliskiren. Consider periodic determinations of serum electrolytes to detect possible electrolyte imbalances, particularly in patients with severe renal impairment.

➤*Pregnancy: Category C* (first trimester); *Category D* (second and third trimesters).

There is no clinical experience with the use of aliskiren in pregnant women.

Fetal/Neonatal morbidity and mortality – Drugs that act directly on the renin-angiotensin system can cause fetal and neonatal morbidity and death when administered to pregnant women. Several dozen cases have been reported in the world literature in patients who were taking ACE inhibitors. Discontinue aliskiren as soon as possible when pregnancy is detected.

The use of drugs that act directly on the renin-angiotensin system during the second and third trimesters of pregnancy has been associated with fetal and neonatal injury, including hypotension, neonatal skull hypoplasia, anuria, reversible or irreversible renal failure, and death. Oligohydramnios also has been reported, presumably resulting from decreased fetal renal function; oligohydramnios in this setting has been associated with fetal limb contractures, craniofacial deformation, and hypoplastic lung development. Prematurity, intrauterine growth retardation, and patent ductus arteriosus also have been reported, although it is not clear whether these occurrences were caused by exposure to the drug.

In addition, first trimester use of ACE inhibitors, a specific class of drugs acting on the renin-angiotensin system, has been associated with a potential risk of birth defects in retrospective data. Health care providers that prescribe drugs acting directly on the renin-angiotensin system should counsel women of childbearing potential about the potential risks of these agents during pregnancy. Rarely (probably less than 1 in every 1,000 pregnancies), no alternative to a drug acting on the renin-angiotensin system will be found. In these rare cases, apprise mothers of the potential hazards to their fetuses and perform serial ultrasound examinations to assess the intra-amniotic environment.

If oligohydramnios is observed, discontinue aliskiren unless it is considered lifesaving for the mother. Contraction stress testing, a nonstress test, or biophysical profiling may be appropriate, depending upon the week of pregnancy. However, patients and health care providers should be aware that oligohydramnios may not appear until after the fetus has sustained irreversible injury.

Closely observe infants with histories of in utero exposure to a renin inhibitor for hypotension, oliguria, and hyperkalemia. If oliguria occurs, direct attention toward support of blood pressure and renal perfusion. Exchange transfusion or dialysis may be required as means of reversing hypotension and/or substituting for disordered renal function.

Fetal birth weight was adversely affected in rabbits at 50 mg/kg/day (3.2 times the maximum recommended human dose (MRHD) on a mg/m^2 basis). Aliskiren was present in the placenta, amniotic fluid, and fetuses of pregnant rabbits.

➤*Lactation:* It is not known whether aliskiren is excreted in human milk. Aliskiren was secreted in the milk of lactating rats. Because of the high molecular weight and low oral absorption (3%) of aliskiren, breast-feeding infants would not be likely to absorb enough to receive a therapeutic dose. Because of the potential for adverse reactions in the breast-feeding infant, decide whether to discontinue breast-feeding or the drug, taking into account the importance of the drug to the mother.

➤*Children:* Safety and efficacy in children have not been established.

➤*Monitoring:* Aliskiren, when used in combination with an ACE inhibitor in a diabetic population, caused increases in serum potassium. Routine monitoring of electrolytes and renal function is indicated in this population.

Consider periodic determinations of serum electrolytes to detect possible electrolyte imbalances, particularly in patients with severe renal impairment.

Drug Interactions

Aliskiren Drug Interactions

Precipitant drug	Object drug[a]		Description
Irbesartan	Aliskiren	↓	Multiple dose administration may result in reduced aliskiren AUC, decreasing the pharmacologic effect. Use with caution and monitor blood pressure. Adjust the aliskiren dose as needed.
Potent P-glycoprotein inhibitors (eg, atorvastatin, cyclosporine, ketoconazole)	Aliskiren	↑	Aliskiren plasma concentrations may be elevated, increasing the pharmacologic effects and risk of adverse reactions. Monitor the clinical response of the patient and adjust the aliskiren dose as needed. Coadministration of aliskiren and cyclosporine is not recommended.
Thiazide diuretics (eg, hydrochlorothiazide)	Aliskiren	↑	Additive increases in serum uric acid levels may occur. Use with caution, especially in patients at risk for hyperuricemia.
Aliskiren	Thiazide diuretics (eg, hydrochlorothiazide)		
Aliskiren	ACE inhibitors (eg, captopril)	↑	Increased risk of elevated serum potassium occurred in diabetic patients. Routinely monitor electrolytes and renal function when these agents are coadministered, especially in diabetic patients.

ALISKIREN HEMIFUMARATE — ORAL

Aliskiren Drug Interactions			
Precipitant drug	Object drug[a]		Description
Aliskiren	Drugs that increase potassium levels, potassium-sparing diuretics (eg, spironolactone), potassium supplements, salt substitutes containing potassium	↑	Increased serum potassium may occur. Use with caution. Monitor electrolytes.
Aliskiren	Furosemide	↓	The furosemide AUC and C_{max} may be reduced, decreasing the efficacy. Monitor the diuretic response and adjust the furosemide dose as needed.

[a] ↑ = object drug increased; ↓ = object drug decreased.

➤*Drug/Food interactions:* High-fat meals substantially reduce aliskiren absorption (ie, AUC and C_{max} 71% and 85%, respectively). Patients should establish a routine pattern for taking aliskiren with regard to meals.

Adverse Reactions

➤*Discontinuation of therapy:* Aliskiren has been evaluated for safety in more than 6,460 patients, including more than 1,740 treated for longer than 6 months and more than 1,250 treated for longer than 1 year. In placebo-controlled clinical trials, discontinuation of therapy because of a clinical adverse reaction, including uncontrolled hypertension, occurred in 2.2% of patients treated with aliskiren versus 3.5% of patients given placebo.

➤*Angioedema:* Two cases of angioedema with respiratory symptoms were reported with aliskiren use in the clinical studies. Two other cases of periorbital edema without respiratory symptoms were reported as possible angioedema and resulted in discontinuation. The rate of these angioedema cases in the completed studies was 0.06%.

In addition, 26 other cases of edema involving the face, hands, or whole body were reported with aliskiren use, including 4 leading to discontinuation.

However, in the placebo-controlled studies, the incidence of edema involving the face, hands, or whole body was 0.4% with aliskiren compared with 0.5% with placebo. In a long-term, active-control study with aliskiren and hydrochlorothiazide arms, the incidence of edema involving the face, hands, or whole body was 0.4% in both treatment arms.

➤*Cough:* Aliskiren was associated with a slight increase in cough in the placebo-controlled studies (1.1% for any aliskiren use vs 0.6% for placebo). In active-controlled trials with ACE inhibitor (lisinopril, ramipril) arms, the rates of cough for the aliskiren arms were about one-third to one-half the rates in the ACE inhibitor arms.

➤*GI:* Aliskiren produces dose-related GI adverse reactions. Diarrhea was reported by 2.3% of patients at 300 mg compared with 1.2% in placebo patients. In women and elderly (65 years of age and older) patients, increases in diarrhea rates were evident starting at a dosage of 150 mg daily, with rates for these subgroups at 150 mg comparable with those seen at 300 mg for men or younger patients (all rates about 2% to 2.3%). Other GI symptoms included abdominal pain, dyspepsia, and gastroesophageal reflux, although increased rates for abdominal pain and dyspepsia were distinguished from placebo only at 600 mg daily. Diarrhea and other GI symptoms were typically mild and rarely led to discontinuation.

➤*Seizures:* Single episodes of tonic-clonic seizures with loss of consciousness were reported in 2 patients treated with aliskiren in the clinical trials. One of these patients had predisposing causes for seizures and had a negative electroencephalogram (EEG) and cerebral imaging following the seizures (for the other patient, EEG and imaging results were not reported). Aliskiren was discontinued, and there was no rechallenge.

➤*Other adverse reactions:* Other adverse reactions with increased rates for aliskiren compared with placebo included rash (1% vs 0.3%), elevated uric acid (0.4% vs 0.1%), gout (0.2% vs 0.1%), and renal stones (0.2% vs 0%).

The following adverse reactions occurred in placebo-controlled clinical trials at an incidence of more than 1% of patients treated with aliskiren but also occurred at about the same or greater incidence in patients receiving placebo: back pain, cough, dizziness, fatigue, headache, nasopharyngitis, and upper respiratory tract infection.

➤*Lab test abnormalities:*

Blood urea nitrogen, creatinine – Minor increases in blood urea nitrogen or serum creatinine were observed in less than 7% of patients with essential hypertension treated with aliskiren alone versus 6% for placebo.

Creatine kinase – Increases in creatine kinase of more than 300% were recorded in about 1% of aliskiren monotherapy patients versus 0.5% of placebo patients. Five cases of creatine kinase increases, 3 leading to discontinuation and 1 diagnosed as subclinical rhabdomyolysis and another as myositis, were reported as adverse reactions with aliskiren use in the clinical trials. No cases were associated with renal function impairment.

Hemoglobin and hematocrit – Small decreases in hemoglobin and hematocrit (mean decreases of approximately 0.08 g/dL and 0.16 volume percent, respectively, for all aliskiren monotherapy) were observed. The decreases were dose-related and were 0.24 g/dL and 0.79 volume percent for 600 mg daily. This effect is also seen with other agents acting on the renin-angiotensin system, such as angiotensin inhibitors and angiotensin receptor blockers, and may be mediated by reduction of Ang II, which stimulates erythropoietin production via the AT1 receptor. These decreases, which led to slight increases in rates of anemia, were observed with aliskiren compared with placebo (0.1% for any aliskiren use, 0.3% for aliskiren 600 mg daily, versus 0% for placebo). No patients discontinued therapy because of anemia.

Serum potassium – Increases in serum potassium greater than 5.5 mEq/L were infrequent in patients with essential hypertension treated with aliskiren alone (0.9% compared with 0.6% with placebo). However, when used in combination with an ACE inhibitor in a diabetic population, increases in serum potassium were more frequent (5.5%); routine monitoring of electrolytes and renal function is indicated in this population.

Serum uric acid – Aliskiren monotherapy produced small median increases in serum uric acid levels (about 6 mcmol/L), while hydrochlorothiazide produced larger increases (approximately 30 mcmol/L). The combination of aliskiren with hydrochlorothiazide appears to be additive (approximately a 40 mcmol/L increase). The increases in uric acid appear to lead to slight increases in the following uric acid–related adverse reactions: elevated uric acid (0.4% vs 0.1%), gout (0.2% vs 0.1%), and renal stones (0.2% vs 0%).

Overdosage

➤*Symptoms:* Limited data are available related to overdosage in humans. The most likely manifestation of overdosage would be hypotension.

➤*Treatment:* If symptomatic hypotension occurs, initiate supportive treatment.

Patient Information

Advise women of childbearing age about the consequences of second- and third-trimester exposure to drugs that act on the renin-angiotensin system. Discuss other treatment options with women planning to become pregnant. Ask these patients to report pregnancy to their health care provider as soon as possible.

Advise patients that angioedema, including laryngeal edema, may occur at any time during treatment with aliskiren. Instruct patients to immediately report any signs or symptoms suggesting angioedema (swelling of face, extremities, eyes, lips, tongue, difficulty in swallowing or breathing) and not to take any more of the drug until they have consulted with the prescribing health care provider.

Caution patients receiving aliskiren that light-headedness can occur, especially during the first days of therapy, and that it should be reported to the prescribing health care provider. Tell patients that if syncope occurs to discontinue aliskiren until the health care provider has been consulted.

Caution all patients that inadequate fluid intake, excessive perspiration, diarrhea, or vomiting can lead to an excessive fall in blood pressure, with the same consequences of light-headedness and possible syncope.

Tell patients receiving aliskiren not to use potassium supplements or salt substitutes containing potassium without consulting the prescribing health care provider.

Patients should establish a routine pattern for taking aliskiren with regard to meals. High-fat meals decrease absorption substantially.

EPLERENONE

Rx	**Eplerenone** (Apotex)	**Tablets; oral:** 25 mg	(EP 25 APO). Yellow, round. Film-coated. In 30s, 90s, 500s, 1,000s, and blister 100s.
Rx	**Inspra** (Pfizer)		Lactose. (Pfizer NSR/25). Yellow, diamond shape. Film-coated. In 30s, 90s, and unit doses.
Rx	**Eplerenone** (Apotex)	**Tablets; oral:** 50 mg	(EP 50 APO). Yellow, round. Film-coated. In 30s, 90s, 1,000s, and blister 100s.
Rx	**Inspra** (Pfizer)		Lactose. (Pfizer NSR/50). Yellow, diamond shape. Film-coated. In 30s and 90s.

EPLERENONE — ORAL

Indications

➤*Congestive heart failure (CHF) post-myocardial infarction (MI):* Eplerenone is indicated to improve survival of stable patients with left ventricular systolic dysfunction (ejection fraction less than or equal to 40%) and clinical evidence of CHF after an acute MI.

➤*Hypertension:* Eplerenone is indicated for the treatment of hypertension. Eplerenone may be used alone or in combination with other antihypertensive agents.

➤*Off-label uses:* Possible therapy used alone or in combination with an angiotensin-converting enzyme (ACE) inhibitor for reducing left ventricular hypertrophy (LVH); as adjunctive therapy to reduce microalbuminuria in diabetic hypertensive patients.

Administration and Dosage

➤*General dosing considerations:* Measure serum potassium before initiating eplerenone therapy, within the first week and at 1 month after the start of treatment or dosage adjustment.

➤*Adults:*

Congestive heart failure post-myocardial infarction –

Usual dosage: The recommended dosage of eplerenone is 50 mg once daily.

Initial dosage: 25 mg once daily.

Dosage titration: Titrate to the target dosage of 50 mg once daily, preferably within 4 weeks as tolerated by the patient.

Dosage adjustment: Adjust the dosage based on the serum potassium level and as shown in the table.

Eplerenone Dosage Adjustment in Congestive Heart Failure

Serum potassium (mEq/L)	Action	Dosage adjustment
< 5	Increase	25 mg every other day to 25 mg daily; 25 mg daily to 50 mg daily
5 to 5.4	Maintain	No adjustment
5.5 to 5.9	Decrease	50 mg to 25 mg daily; 25 mg daily to 25 mg every other day; 25 mg every other day to withhold
≥ 6	Withhold	

Rechallenge: Following withholding eplerenone because of serum potassium greater than or equal to 6 mEq/L, eplerenone can be restarted at a dosage of 25 mg every other day when serum potassium levels have fallen below 5.5 mEq/L.

Monitoring: Measure serum potassium before initiating eplerenone therapy, within the first week and at 1 month after the start of treatment or dosage adjustment. Assess serum potassium periodically thereafter.

Factors such as patient characteristics and serum potassium levels may indicate that additional monitoring is appropriate. In the eplerenone post-acute myocardial infarction heart failure efficacy and survival study (EPHESUS), the majority of hyperkalemia was observed within the first 3 months after randomization.

Hypertension –

Maximum dose: Higher dosages of eplerenone are not recommended either because they have no greater effect on blood pressure than 100 mg or because they are associated with an increased risk of hyperkalemia.

Initial dosage: 50 mg administered once daily.

Dosage titration: The full therapeutic effect of eplerenone is apparent within 4 weeks. For patients with an inadequate blood pressure response to 50 mg once daily, increase the dosage of eplerenone to 50 mg twice daily.

Concomitant therapy: For patients receiving weak CYP3A4 inhibitors, such as erythromycin, saquinavir, verapamil, and fluconazole, reduce the starting dosage to 25 mg once daily.

Use eplerenone alone or in combination with other antihypertensive agents.

➤*Elderly:* No adjustment of the starting dose is recommended for elderly patients.

➤*Renal function impairment:* Eplerenone is contraindicated in patients with serum potassium greater than 5.5 mEq/L at initiation and/or creatinine clearance less than or equal to 30 mL/min.

➤*Hepatic function impairment:* No adjustment of the starting dose is recommended for patients with mild to moderate hepatic impairment.

The use of eplerenone in patients with severe hepatic impairment has not been evaluated.

➤*Administration:* Administer eplerenone with or without food.

➤*Storage/Stability:* Store at 25°C (77°F); excursions are permitted to 15° to 30°C (59° to 86°F).

Actions

➤*Pharmacology:* Eplerenone binds to the mineralocorticoid receptor and blocks the binding of aldosterone, a component of the renin-angiotensin-aldosterone-system (RAAS). Aldosterone synthesis, which occurs primarily in the adrenal gland, is modulated by multiple factors, including angiotensin II and non-RAAS mediators such as corticotropin and potassium. Aldosterone binds to mineralocorticoid receptors in both epithelial (eg, kidney) and nonepithelial (eg, heart, blood vessels, brain) tissues and increases blood pressure through induction of sodium reabsorption and possibly other mechanisms.

Eplerenone has been shown to produce sustained increases in plasma renin and serum aldosterone, consistent with inhibition of the negative regulatory feedback of aldosterone on renin secretion. The resulting increased plasma renin activity and aldosterone circulating levels do not overcome the effect of eplerenone.

Eplerenone selectively binds to recombinant human mineralocorticoid receptors compared with its binding to recombinant human glucocorticoid, progesterone, and androgen receptors.

➤*Pharmacokinetics:*

Absorption – Absorption is not affected by food.

Mean peak plasma concentrations of eplerenone are reached approximately 1.5 hours following oral administration. The absolute bioavailability of eplerenone is unknown. Both peak plasma levels (C_{max}) and area under the curve (AUC) are dose proportional over doses of 25 to 100 mg and less than proportional at doses above 100 mg.

Distribution – The plasma protein binding of eplerenone is about 50% and is primarily bound to alpha-1 acid glycoproteins. The apparent volume of distribution at steady state ranged from 43 to 90 L. Eplerenone does not preferentially bind to red blood cells. Inhibitors of CYP3A4 (eg, ketoconazole, saquinavir) increase blood levels of eplerenone.

Metabolism – Eplerenone metabolism is primarily mediated via CYP3A4. No active metabolites of eplerenone have been identified in human plasma. Eplerenone is cleared predominantly by cytochrome P-450 (CYP) 3A4 metabolism, with an elimination half-life of 4 to 6 hours. Steady state is reached within 2 days.

Excretion – Less than 5% of an eplerenone dose is recovered as unchanged drug in the urine and feces. Following a single oral dose of radiolabeled drug, approximately 32% of the dose was excreted in the feces and approximately 67% was excreted in the urine. The elimination half-life of eplerenone is approximately 4 to 6 hours. The apparent plasma clearance is approximately 10 L/h.

Special populations –

Renal function impairment: The pharmacokinetics of eplerenone were evaluated in patients with varying degrees of renal impairment and in patients undergoing hemodialysis. Compared with control subjects, steady-state AUC and C_{max} were increased by 38% and 24%, respectively, in patients with severe renal function impairment and were decreased by 26% and 3%, respectively, in patients undergoing hemodialysis. No correlation was observed between plasma clearance of eplerenone and creatinine clearance. Eplerenone is not removed by hemodialysis.

Hepatic function impairment: The pharmacokinetics of eplerenone 400 mg have been investigated in patients with moderate (Child-Pugh class B) hepatic function impairment and compared with healthy subjects. Steady-state C_{max} and AUC of eplerenone were increased by 3.6% and 42%, respectively.

Elderly: The pharmacokinetics of eplerenone at a dosage of 100 mg once daily have been investigated in the elderly (65 years of age and older).

At steady state, elderly subjects had increases in C_{max} (22%) and AUC (45%) compared with younger subjects (18 to 45 years of age).

Gender: The pharmacokinetics of eplerenone at a dosage of 100 mg once daily have been investigated in men and women.

The pharmacokinetics of eplerenone did not differ significantly between men and women.

Race: The pharmacokinetics of eplerenone at a dosage of 100 mg once daily have been investigated in black patients.

At steady state, C_{max} was 19% lower and AUC was 26% lower in black patients.

Heart failure: The pharmacokinetics of eplerenone 50 mg were evaluated in 8 patients with heart failure (New York Heart Association [NYHA] classification II-IV), and 8 matched (gender, age, weight) healthy controls. Compared with the controls, steady state AUC and C_{max} in patients with stable heart failure were 38% and 30% higher, respectively.

Contraindications

Eplerenone is contraindicated in all patients with the following:

1.) Serum potassium greater than 5.5 mEq/L at initiation.
2.) Creatinine clearance less than or equal to 30 mL/min.
3.) Concomitant use with the following potent CYP3A4 inhibitors: clarithromycin, itraconazole, ketoconazole, nefazodone, nelfinavir, ritonavir, and troleandomycin. Do not use eplerenone with other drugs noted to be potent CYP3A4 inhibitors.

➤*Hypertension:* Eplerenone is also contraindicated for the treatment of hypertension in patients with the following:

1.) Type 2 diabetes with microalbuminuria.
2.) Serum creatinine greater than 2 mg/dL in men or greater than 1.8 mg/dL in women.
3.) Creatinine clearance less than 50 mL/min.
4.) Concomitant use of potassium supplements or potassium-sparing diuretics (amiloride, spironolactone, or triamterene).

EPLERENONE — ORAL

Warnings/Precautions

➤*Hyperkalemia:* The principal risk of eplerenone is hyperkalemia. Hyperkalemia can cause serious, sometimes fatal, arrhythmias. Patients who develop hyperkalemia (greater than 5.5 mEq/L) may still benefit from eplerenone with proper dose adjustment. Minimize hyperkalemia by patient selection, avoidance of certain concomitant treatments, and periodic monitoring until the effect of eplerenone has been established. Dose reduction of eplerenone has been shown to decrease potassium levels.

➤*Diabetes:* Treat diabetic patients with CHF post-MI, including those with proteinuria, with caution. The subset of patients in EPHESUS with both diabetes and proteinuria on the baseline urinalysis had increased rates of hyperkalemia.

➤*Renal function impairment:* Eplerenone is contraindicated in patients with serum potassium greater than 5.5 mEq/L at initiation and/or creatinine clearance less than or equal to 30 mL/min.

Treat patients with CHF post-MI who have serum creatinine levels greater than 2 mg/dL (men) or greater than 1.8 mg/dL (women) or creatinine clearance less than or equal to 50 mL/min with caution. The rates of hyperkalemia increased with declining renal function.

➤*Pregnancy:* Category B. There are no adequate and well-controlled studies in pregnant women. Use eplerenone during pregnancy only if the potential benefit justifies the potential risk to the fetus.

Teratogenic – Embryo-fetal development studies were conducted with dosages up to 1,000 mg/kg/day in rats and 300 mg/kg/day in rabbits (exposures up to 32 and 31 times the human AUC for the 100 mg/day therapeutic dosage, respectively). No teratogenic effects were seen in rats or rabbits, although decreased body weight in maternal rabbits and increased rabbit fetal resorptions and postimplantation loss were observed at the highest administered dosage. Because animal reproduction studies are not always predictive of human response, use eplerenone during pregnancy only if clearly needed.

➤*Lactation:* The concentration of eplerenone in human breast milk after oral administration is unknown. However preclinical data show that eplerenone and/or metabolites are present in rat breast milk (0.85:1 [milk:plasma] AUC ratio) obtained after a single oral dose. Peak concentrations in plasma and milk were obtained from 0.5 to 1 hour after dosing. Rat pups exposed by this route developed normally. Because many drugs are excreted in human milk and because of the unknown potential for adverse reactions on the breast-feeding infant, make a decision whether to discontinue breast-feeding or discontinue the drug, taking into account the importance of the drug to the mother.

➤*Children:* The safety and efficacy of eplerenone have not been established in children.

➤*Elderly:*

Data from CHF post-MI trials – Of the total number of patients in EPHESUS, 3,340 (50%) were 65 years of age and older, while 1,326 (20%) were 75 years of age and older. Patients older than 75 years of age did not appear to benefit from the use of eplerenone. No differences in the overall incidence of adverse reactions were observed between elderly and younger patients. However, due to age-related decreases in creatinine clearance, the incidence of laboratory-documented hyperkalemia was increased in patients 65 years of age and older.

Data from hypertension trials – Of the total number of subjects in clinical hypertension studies of eplerenone, 1,123 (23%) were 65 years of age and older, while 212 (4%) were 75 years of age and older. No overall differences in safety or efficacy were observed between elderly subjects and younger subjects.

Drug Interactions

➤*Inhibitors of CYP450 3A4:* Eplerenone metabolism is predominantly mediated via CYP3A4. A pharmacokinetic study evaluating the administration of a single dose of eplerenone 100 mg with ketoconazole 200 mg twice daily, a potent inhibitor of the CYP3A4 pathway, showed a 1.7-fold increase in C_{max} of eplerenone and a 5.4-fold increase in AUC of eplerenone. Do not use eplerenone with drugs described as strong inhibitors of CYP3A4 in their labeling.

➤*Administration with other CYP3A4 inhibitors:* Administration of eplerenone with other CYP3A4 inhibitors (eg, erythromycin 500 mg twice daily, verapamil 240 mg daily, saquinavir 1,200 mg 3 times daily, fluconazole 200 mg daily) resulted in increases in C_{max} of eplerenone ranging from 1.4- to 1.6-fold and AUC from 2- to 2.9-fold.

➤*Angiotensin-converting enzyme (ACE) inhibitors and angiotensin II receptor antagonists:*

Data from CHF post-MI studies – In EPHESUS, 3,020 (91%) patients receiving eplerenone 25 to 50 mg also received ACE inhibitors or angiotensin II receptor antagonists. Rates of patients with maximum potassium levels greater than 5.5 mEq/L were similar regardless of the use of ACE inhibitors or angiotensin II receptor antagonists.

Data from hypertension studies – In clinical studies of patients with hypertension, the addition of eplerenone 50 to 100 mg to ACE inhibitors and angiotensin II receptor antagonists increased mean serum potassium slightly (about 0.09 to 0.13 mEq/L). In a study in diabetics with microalbuminuria eplerenone 200 mg combined with the ACE inhibitor enalapril 10 mg increased the frequency of hyperkalemia (serum potassium greater than 5.5 mEq/L) from 17% on enalapril alone to 38%.

➤*Lithium:* A drug interaction study of eplerenone with lithium has not been conducted. Lithium toxicity has been reported in patients receiving lithium concomitantly with diuretics and ACE inhibitors. Monitor serum lithium levels frequently if eplerenone is coadministered with lithium.

➤*Nonsteroidal anti-inflammatory drugs (NSAIDs):* A drug interaction study of eplerenone with an NSAID has not been conducted. The administration of other potassium-sparing antihypertensives with NSAIDs has been shown to reduce the antihypertensive effect in some patients and result in severe hyperkalemia in patients with impaired renal function. Therefore, when eplerenone and NSAIDs are used concomitantly, observe patients to determine whether the desired effect on blood pressure is obtained.

Eplerenone Drug Interactions

Precipitant drug	Object drug[a]		Description
ACE inhibitors Angiotensin II antagonists	Eplerenone	⬆	Increased risk of hyperkalemia with coadministration.
CYP3A4 inhibitors	Eplerenone	⬆	Coadministration of potent inhibitors (eg, ketoconazole) resulted in increased exposure of about 5-fold; less potent inhibitors yielded about a 2-fold increase (see Administration and Dosage and Contraindications).
NSAIDs	Eplerenone	⬆⬇	Coadministration of NSAIDs with other potassium-sparing antihypertensives may cause decreased antihypertensive effect and results in severe hyperkalemia in patients with impaired renal function.
St. John's wort	Eplerenone	⬇	Approximately 30% decrease in eplerenone AUC.
Eplerenone	Lithium	⬆	Coadministration of lithium with diuretics and ACE inhibitors may lead to lithium toxicity; frequently monitor serum lithium levels if coadministered with eplerenone.

[a] ⬆ = object drug increased; ⬇ = object drug decreased.

➤*Drug/Food interactions:* Coadministration with grapefruit juice produced a small increase (about 25%) in exposure.

Adverse Reactions

➤*Data from CHF post-MI trials:* In EPHESUS, safety was evaluated in 3,307 patients treated with eplerenone and 3,301 placebo-treated patients. The overall incidence of adverse reactions reported with eplerenone (78.9%) was similar to placebo (79.5%). Adverse reactions occurred at a similar rate regardless of age, gender, or race. Patients discontinued treatment due to an adverse reaction at similar rates in either treatment group (4.4% eplerenone vs 4.3% placebo).

Adverse reactions that occurred more frequently in patients treated with eplerenone than placebo were hyperkalemia (3.4% vs 2%) and increased creatinine (2.4% vs 1.5%). Discontinuations due to hyperkalemia or abnormal renal function were less than 1% in both groups. Hypokalemia occurred less frequently in patients treated with eplerenone (0.6% vs 1.6%).

The rates of sex hormone-related adverse reactions are shown in the following table.

Rates of Sex Hormone-Related Adverse Reactions in EPHESUS

	Rates in men			Rates in women
	Gynecomastia	Mastodynia	Either	Abnormal vaginal bleeding
Eplerenone	0.4%	0.1%	0.5%	0.4%
Placebo	0.5%	0.1%	0.6%	0.4%

➤*Data from hypertension trials:* Eplerenone has been evaluated for safety in 3,091 patients treated for hypertension. A total of 690 patients were treated for over 6 months, and 106 patients were treated for over 1 year.

In placebo-controlled studies, the overall rates of adverse reactions were 47% with eplerenone and 45% with placebo. Adverse reactions occurred at a similar rate regardless of age, gender, or race. Therapy was discontinued due to an adverse reaction in 3% of patients treated with eplerenone and 3% of patients given placebo. The most common reasons for discontinuation of eplerenone were headache, dizziness, angina pectoris/MI, and increased gamma-glutamyl-transferase (GGT). The adverse reactions that were reported at a rate of at least 1% of patients and at a higher rate in patients treated with eplerenone in daily doses of 25 to 400 mg versus placebo are shown in the following table.

Adverse Reactions Hypertension Studies with Eplerenone (25 to 400 mg) (≥ 1%)

Adverse reactions	Eplerenone (n = 945)	Placebo (n = 372)
CNS		
Dizziness	3%	2%
GI		
Abdominal pain	1%	0%

EPLERENONE — ORAL

Adverse Reactions Hypertension Studies with Eplerenone (25 to 400 mg) (≥ 1%)		
Adverse reactions	Eplerenone (n = 945)	Placebo (n = 372)
Diarrhea	2%	1%
GU		
Albuminuria	1%	0%
Metabolic		
Hypercholesterolemia	1%	0%
Hypertriglyceridemia	1%	0%
Respiratory		
Coughing	2%	1%
Miscellaneous		
Fatigue	2%	1%
Influenza-like symptoms	2%	1%

Note – Adverse reactions that are too general to be informative or are very common in the treated population are excluded.

Gynecomastia and abnormal vaginal bleeding were reported with eplerenone but not with placebo. The rates of these sex hormone-related adverse reactions are shown in the following table. The rates increased slightly with increasing duration of therapy. In females, abnormal vaginal bleeding was also reported in 0.8% of patients on antihypertensive medications (other than spironolactone) in active-control arms of the studies with eplerenone.

Rates of Sex Hormone-Related Adverse Reactions with Eplerenone in Hypertension Clinical Studies				
	Rates in men			Rates in women
	Gynecomastia	Mastodynia	Either	Abnormal vaginal bleeding
All controlled studies	0.5%	0.8%	1%	0.6%
Controlled studies lasting ≥ 6 months	0.7%	1.3%	1.6%	0.8%
Open-label, long-term study	1%	0.3%	1%	2.1%

➤*Clinical laboratory test findings:*

Data from CHF post-MI trials –

Creatinine: Increases of more than 0.5 mg/dL were reported for 6.5% of patients administered eplerenone and for 4.9% of placebo-treated patients.

Potassium: In EPHESUS, the frequency of patients with changes in potassium (less than 3.5 mEq/L or greater than 5.5 mEq/L or greater than or equal to 6 mEq/L) receiving eplerenone compared with placebo are displayed in the following table.

Hypokalemia (< 3.5 mEq/L) or Hyperkalemia (> 5.5 or ≥ 6 mEq/L) in EPHESUS		
Potassium (mEq/L)	Eplerenone (n = 3,251)	Placebo (n = 3,237)
< 3.5	273 (8.4%)	424 (13.1%)
> 5.5	508 (15.6%)	363 (11.2%)
≥ 6	180 (5.5%)	126 (3.9%)

The following table shows the rates of hyperkalemia in EPHESUS as assessed by baseline renal function (creatinine clearance).

Rates of Hyperkalemia (> 5.5 mEq/L) in EPHESUS by Baseline Creatinine Clearance[a]		
Baseline creatinine clearance (mL/min)	Eplerenone	Placebo
≤ 30	31.5%	22.6%
31 to 50	24.1%	12.7%
51 to 70	16.9%	13.1%
> 70	10.8%	8.7%

[a] Estimated using the Cockroft-Gault formula.

The following table shows the rates of hyperkalemia in EPHESUS as assessed by 2 baseline characteristics: presence/absence of proteinuria from baseline urinalysis and presence/absence of diabetes.

Rates of Hyperkalemia (> 5.5 mEq/L) in Ephesus by Proteinuria and History of Diabetes[a]		
	Eplerenone	Placebo
Proteinuria, no diabetes	16%	11%
Diabetes, no proteinuria	18%	13%
Proteinuria and diabetes	26%	16%

[a] Diabetes assessed as positive medical history at baseline; proteinuria assessed by positive dipstick urinalysis at baseline.

Data from hypertension trials –

Potassium: In placebo-controlled fixed-dose studies, the mean increases in serum potassium were dose related and are shown in the following table along with the frequencies of values greater than 5.5 mEq/L.

Changes in Serum Potassium in the Placebo-Controlled, Fixed-Dose Eplerenone Hypertension Studies			
Daily dosage	n	Mean change (mEq/L)	% > 5.5 mEq/L
Placebo	194	0	1
25	97	0.08	0
50	245	0.14	0
100	193	0.09	1
200	139	0.19	1
400	104	0.36	8.7

Patients with both type 2 diabetes and microalbuminuria are at increased risk of developing persistent hyperkalemia. In a study in such patients taking eplerenone 200 mg, the frequencies of maximum serum potassium levels greater than 5.5 mEq/L were 33% with eplerenone given alone and 38% when eplerenone was given with enalapril.

Rates of hyperkalemia increased with decreasing renal function. In all studies serum potassium elevations greater than 5.5 mEq/L were observed in 10.4% of patients treated with eplerenone with baseline calculated creatinine clearance less than 70 mL/min, 5.6% of patients with baseline creatinine clearance of 70 to 100 mL/min, and 2.6% of patients with baseline creatinine clearance of greater than 100 mL/min.

Sodium: Serum sodium decreased in a dose-related manner. Mean decreases ranged from 0.7 mEq/L at 50 mg daily to 1.7 meq/L at 400 mg daily. Decreases in sodium (less than 135 mEq/L) were reported for 2.3% of patients administered eplerenone and 0.6% of placebo-treated patients.

Triglycerides – Serum triglycerides increased in a dose-related manner. Mean increases ranged from 7.1 mg/dL at 50 mg daily to 26.6 mg/dL at 400 mg daily. Increases in triglycerides (above 252 mg/dL) were reported for 15% of patients administered eplerenone and 12% of placebo-treated patients.

Cholesterol – Serum cholesterol increased in a dose-related manner. Mean changes ranged from a decrease of 0.4 mg/dL at 50 mg daily to an increase of 11.6 mg/dL at 400 mg daily. Increases in serum cholesterol values greater than 200 mg/dL were reported for 0.3% of patients administered eplerenone and 0% of placebo-treated patients.

Liver function tests – Serum ALT and GGT increased in a dose-related manner. Mean increases ranged from 0.8 units/L at 50 mg daily to 4.8 units/L at 400 mg daily for ALT and 3.1 units/L at 50 mg daily to 11.3 units/L at 400 mg daily for GGT. Increases in ALT levels greater than 120 units/L (3 times the upper limit of normal [ULN]) were reported for 15 of 2,259 patients administered eplerenone and 1 of 351 placebo-treated patients. Increases in ALT levels greater than 200 units/L (5 times the ULN) were reported for 5 of 2,259 of patients administered eplerenone and 1 of 351 placebo-treated patients. Increases of ALT greater than 120 units/L and bilirubin greater than 1.2 mg/dL were reported in 1 of 2,259 patients administered eplerenone and 0 of 351 placebo-treated patients. Hepatic failure was not reported in patients receiving eplerenone.

Serum urea nitrogen/creatinine – Serum creatinine increased in a dose-related manner. Mean increases ranged from 0.01 mg/dL at 50 mg daily to 0.03 mg/dL at 400 mg daily. Increases in serum urea nitrogen to greater than 30 mg/dL and serum creatinine to greater than 2 mg/dL were reported for 0.5% and 0.2%, respectively, of patients administered eplerenone and 0% of placebo-treated patients.

Uric acid – Increases in uric acid to greater than 9 mg/dL were reported in 0.3% of patients administered eplerenone and 0% of placebo-treated patients.

Overdosage

No cases of human overdosage with eplerenone have been reported. Lethality was not observed in mice, rats, or dogs after single oral doses that provided C_{max} exposures at least 25 times higher than in humans receiving eplerenone 100 mg/day. Dogs showed emesis, salivation, and tremors at a C_{max} 41 times the human therapeutic C_{max}, progressing to sedation and convulsions at higher exposures.

The most likely manifestation of human overdosage would be anticipated to be hypotension or hyperkalemia. Eplerenone cannot be removed by hemodialysis. Eplerenone has been shown to bind extensively to charcoal. If symptomatic hypotension occurs, institute supportive treatment. If hyperkalemia develops, initiate standard treatment.

Patient Information

Inform patients receiving eplerenone not to use potassium supplements, salt substitutes containing potassium, or contraindicated drugs without consulting their doctors.

ANTIHYPERTENSIVE COMBINATIONS

Content given per capsule or tablet.

	Product and Distributor	Diuretic	Other Content	How Supplied
Rx	**Nadolol and Bendroflumethiazide Tablets** (IMPAX Laboratories)	5 mg bendroflumethiazide	40 mg nadolol	Lactose, mannitol. (G 531). Scored. In 100s and 500s.
Rx	**Corzide Tablets 40/5** (King Pharma)			Lactose. (CORZIDE 40/5 BL 283). In 100s.
Rx	**Nadolol and Bendroflumethiazide Tablets** (IMPAX Laboratories)	5 mg bendroflumethiazide	80 mg nadolol	Lactose, mannitol. (G 532). Scored. In 100s and 500s.
Rx	**Corzide Tablets 80/5** (King Pharma)			Lactose. (CORZIDE 80/5 BL 284). In 100s.
Rx	**Rauwolfia/Bendroflumethiazide Tablets** (Various)	4 mg bendroflumethiazide	50 mg powdered *Rauwolfia serpentina*	In 100s.
Rx	**Atenolol/Chlorthalidone Tablets** (Various, eg, Zenith-Goldline)	25 mg chlorthalidone	50 mg atenolol	In 50s, 100s, 250s, 500s, and 1000s.
Rx	**Tenoretic 50 Tablets** (AstraZeneca)			(ICI 115). White, scored. In 100s.
Rx	**Atenolol/Chlorthalidone Tablets** (Various, eg, Zenith-Goldline)	25 mg chlorthalidone	100 mg atenolol	In 50s, 100s, 250s, 500s, and 1000s.
Rx	**Tenoretic 100 Tablets** (AstraZeneca)			(ICI 117). White, scored. In 100s.
Rx	**Clorpres Tablets** (Mylan)	15 mg chlorthalidone	0.1 mg clonidine HCl	(M1). Yellow, scored. In 100s.
		15 mg chlorthalidone	0.2 mg clonidine HCl	(M27). Yellow, scored. In 100s.
		15 mg chlorthalidone	0.3 mg clonidine HCl	(M72). Yellow, scored. In 100s.
Rx	**Tekturna HCT** (Novartis Consumer Health)	12.5 mg hydrochlorothiazide	150 mg aliskiren	Lactose. (NVR LCI). White, oval. Film-coated. In 30s, 90s, and blister 100s.
		25 mg hydrochlorothiazide	150 mg aliskiren	Lactose. (NVR CLL). Pale yellow, oval. Film-coated. In 30s, 90s, and blister 100s.
		12.5 mg hydrochlorothiazide	300 mg aliskiren	Lactose. (NVR CVI). Violet/white, oval. Film-coated. In 30s, 90s, and blister 100s.
		25 mg hydrochlorothiazide	300 mg aliskiren	Lactose. (NVR CVV). Light yellow, oval. Film-coated. In 30s, 90s, and blister 100s.
Rx	**Benazepril HCl/Hydrochlorothiazide** (Sandoz)	6.25 mg hydrochlorothiazide	5 mg benazepril	Lactose. (GG 364). White. In 100s.
Rx	**Lotensin HCT Tablets** (Novartis)			Lactose. (Lotensin HCT 57). White, oblong, scored. In 100s.
Rx	**Benazepril HCl/Hydrochlorothiazide** (Sandoz)	12.5 mg hydrochlorothiazide	10 mg benazepril	Lactose. (GG 365). Light pink. In 100s.
Rx	**Lotensin HCT Tablets** (Novartis)			Lactose. (Lotensin HCT 72). Lt. pink, oblong, scored. In 100s.
Rx	**Benazepril HCl/Hydrochlorothiazide** (Sandoz)	12.5 mg hydrochlorothiazide	20 mg benazepril	Lactose. (GG 366). Grayish-violet. In 100s.
Rx	**Lotensin HCT Tablets** (Novartis)			Lactose. (Lotensin HCT 74). Grayish-violet, oblong, scored. In 100s.
Rx	**Benazepril HCl/Hydrochlorothiazide** (Sandoz)	25 mg hydrochlorothiazide	20 mg benazepril	Lactose. (GG 367). Red. In 100s.
Rx	**Lotensin HCT Tablets** (Novartis)			Lactose. (Lotensin HCT 75). Red, oblong, scored. In 100s.
Rx	**Benazepril HCl/Hydrochlorothiazide** (Sandoz)	6.25 mg hydrochlorothiazide	5 mg benazepril	Lactose. (GG 364). White. In 100s.
Rx	**Lotensin HCT Tablets** (Novartis)			Lactose. (Lotensin HCT 57). White, oblong, scored. In 100s.
Rx	**Benazepril HCl/Hydrochlorothiazide** (Sandoz)	12.5 mg hydrochlorothiazide	10 mg benazepril	Lactose. (GG 365). Light pink. In 100s.
Rx	**Lotensin HCT Tablets** (Novartis)			Lactose. (Lotensin HCT 72). Lt. pink, oblong, scored. In 100s.
Rx	**Benazepril HCl/Hydrochlorothiazide** (Sandoz)	12.5 mg hydrochlorothiazide	20 mg benazepril	Lactose. (GG 366). Grayish-violet. In 100s.
Rx	**Lotensin HCT Tablets** (Novartis)			Lactose. (Lotensin HCT 74). Grayish-violet, oblong, scored. In 100s.
Rx	**Benazepril HCl/Hydrochlorothiazide** (Sandoz)	25 mg hydrochlorothiazide	20 mg benazepril	Lactose. (GG 367). Red. In 100s.
Rx	**Lotensin HCT Tablets** (Novartis)			Lactose. (Lotensin HCT 75). Red, oblong, scored. In 100s.
Rx	**Bisoprolol Fumarate/Hydrochlorothiazide Tablets** (Various, eg, Mylan, Purepac, Ivax)	6.25 mg hydrochlorothiazide	2.5 mg bisoprolol fumarate	In 100s, 500s, and 1000s.
Rx	**Ziac Tablets** (Teva)			(LL B 12). In 30s and 100s.
Rx	**Bisoprolol Fumarate/Hydrochlorothiazide Tablets** (Various, eg, Mylan, Purepac, Ivax)	6.25 mg hydrochlorothiazide	5 mg bisoprolol fumarate	In 100s, 500s, and 1000s.
Rx	**Ziac Tablets** (Teva)			(LL B 13). In 30s and 100s.
Rx	**Bisoprolol Fumarate/Hydrochlorothiazide Tablets** (Various, eg, Mylan, Purepac, Ivax)	6.25 mg hydrochlorothiazide	10 mg bisoprolol fumarate	In 30s, 100s, 500s, and 1000s.
Rx	**Ziac Tablets** (Teva)			(LL B 14). In 30s.

ANTIHYPERTENSIVE COMBINATIONS

	Product and Distributor	Diuretic	Other Content	How Supplied
Rx	**Bisoprolol Fumarate/Hydrochlorothiazide Tablets** (Various, eg, Mylan, Purepac, Ivax)	6.25 mg hydrochlorothiazide	2.5 mg bisoprolol fumarate	In 100s, 500s, and 1000s.
Rx	**Ziac Tablets** (Teva)			(LL B 12). In 30s and 100s.
Rx	**Bisoprolol Fumarate/Hydrochlorothiazide Tablets** (Various, eg, Mylan, Purepac, Ivax)	6.25 mg hydrochlorothiazide	5 mg bisoprolol fumarate	In 100s, 500s, and 1000s.
Rx	**Ziac Tablets** (Teva)			(LL B 13). In 30s and 100s.
Rx	**Bisoprolol Fumarate/Hydrochlorothiazide Tablets** (Various, eg, Mylan, Purepac, Ivax)	6.25 mg hydrochlorothiazide	10 mg bisoprolol fumarate	In 30s, 100s, 500s, and 1000s.
Rx	**Ziac Tablets** (Teva)			(LL B 14). In 30s.
Rx	**Atacand HCT** (AstraZeneca)	12.5 mg hydrochlorothiazide	16 mg candesartan cilexetil	Lactose. (ACS 162). Peach, oval. In UD 100s and unit-of-use 90s.
		12.5 mg hydrochlorothiazide	32 mg candesartan cilexetil	Lactose. (ACJ 322). Yellow, oval. In UD 100s, and unit-of-use 90s.
		25 mg hydrochlorothiazide	32 mg candesartan	Lactose. (ACD). Pink, oval, scored. In unit-of-use 90s.
Rx	**Captopril and Hydrochlorothiazide Tablets** (Teva)	15 mg hydrochlorothiazide	25 mg captopril	In 100s and 1000s.
Rx	**Capozide 25/15 Tablets** (Par)			(CAPOZIDE 25/15). White and orange mottled, square, scored. In 100s.
Rx	**Captopril and Hydrochlorothiazide Tablets** (Teva)	15 mg hydrochlorothiazide	50 mg captopril	In 100s and 1000s.
Rx	**Capozide 50/15 Tablets** (Par)			(CAPOZIDE 50/15). White and orange mottled, oval, scored. In 100s.
Rx	**Captopril and Hydrochlorothiazide Tablets** (Teva)	25 mg hydrochlorothiazide	25 mg captopril	In 100s and 1000s.
Rx	**Capozide 25/25 Tablets** (Par)			(CAPOZIDE 25/25). Peach, square, scored. In 100s.
Rx	**Captopril and Hydrochlorothiazide Tablets** (Teva)	25 mg hydrochlorothiazide	50 mg captopril	In 100s and 1000s.
Rx	**Capozide 50/25 Tablets** (Par)			(CAPOZIDE 50/25). Peach, oval. In 100s.
Rx	**Enalapril Maleate/Hydrochlorothiazide Tablets** (Eon)	12.5 mg hydrochlorothiazide	5 mg enalapril maleate	Lactose. (E 151). Green. In 100s and 1000s.
Rx	**Vaseretic Tablets** (Valeant)			Lactose. (MSD 173). Green, squared capsule shape. In 100s.
Rx	**Enalapril Maleate/Hydrochlorothiazide Tablets** (Eon)	25 mg hydrochlorothiazide	10 mg enalapril maleate	Lactose. (E 172). Salmon. In 100s and 1000s.
Rx	**Vaseretic Tablets** (Valeant)			Lactose. (Vaseretic MSD 720). Rust, squared capsule shape. In 100s.
Rx	**Teveten HCT** (Abbott)	12.5 mg hydrochlorothiazide	600 mg eprosartan	Lactose. (SOLVAY 5147). Butterscotch, capsule shape. Film-coated. In 100s.
Rx	**Fosinopril Sodium/Hydrochlorothiazide Tablets** (Ranbaxy)	12.5 mg hydrochlorothiazide	10 mg fosinopril sodium	Lactose. (RC 3). White to off-white. In 30s, 100s, and 1,000s.
Rx	**Monopril-HCT Tablets** (Bristol-Myers Squibb)			Lactose. (1492). Peach. In 100s.
Rx	**Fosinopril Sodium/Hydrochlorothiazide Tablets** (Ranbaxy)	12.5 mg hydrochlorothiazide	20 mg fosinopril sodium	Lactose. (RC 4). White to off-white. In 30s, 100s, and 1,000s.
Rx	**Monopril-HCT Tablets** (Bristol-Myers Squibb)			Lactose. (1493). Peach. In 100s.
Rx	**Hydrochlorothiazide/Hydralazine Caps** (Various, eg, Moore, Zenith-Goldline)	25 mg hydrochlorothiazide	25 mg hydralazine HCl	In 100s, 500s and 1000s.
Rx	**Hydrochlorothiazide/Hydralazine Caps** (Various, eg, Moore, Zenith-Goldline)	50 mg hydrochlorothiazide	50 mg hydralazine HCl	In 100s, 500s and 1000s.
Rx	**Avalide Tablets** (Bristol-Myers Squibb)	12.5 mg hydrochlorothiazide	150 mg irbesartan	Lactose. (2775). Peach, oval. In 30s and 90s.
		12.5 mg hydrochlorothiazide	300 mg irbesartan	Lactose. (2776). Peach, oval. In 30s and 90s.
		25 mg hydrochlorothiazide	300 mg irbesartan	Lactose. (2788). Pink, oval. Film-coated. In 30s and 90s.
Rx	**Lisinopril/Hydrochlorothiazide Tablets** (Various, eg, Ivax, Sandoz)	12.5 mg hydrochlorothiazide	10 mg lisinopril	In 100s, 500s, 1000s, and UD 100s.
Rx	**Prinzide Tablets** (Merck)			Mannitol. (145). Blue, hexagonal. In unit-of-use 100s.
Rx	**Zestoretic Tablets** (AstraZeneca)			Mannitol. (Zestoretic 141). Peach, round. In 100s.
Rx	**Lisinopril/Hydrochlorothiazide Tablets** (Various, eg, Ivax, Sandoz)	12.5 mg hydrochlorothiazide	20 mg lisinopril	In 100s, 500s, 1000s, and UD 100s.
Rx	**Prinzide Tablets** (Merck)			Mannitol. (MSD 140). Yellow, hexagonal, scored. In unit-of-use 100s.
Rx	**Zestoretic Tablets** (AstraZeneca)			Mannitol. (142 Zestoretic). White, round. In 100s.

ANTIHYPERTENSIVE COMBINATIONS

	Product and Distributor	Diuretic	Other Content	How Supplied
Rx	**Lisinopril/Hydrochlorothiazide Tablets** (Various, eg, Ivax, Sandoz)	25 mg hydrochlorothiazide	20 mg lisinopril	In 100s, 500s, 1000s, and UD 100s.
Rx	**Prinzide Tablets** (Merck)			Mannitol. (MSD 142 Prinzide). Peach, round. In unit-of-use 30s and 100s.
Rx	**Zestoretic Tablets** (AstraZeneca)			Mannitol. (145 Zestoretic). Peach, round. In 100s.
Rx	**Losartan Potassium/Hydrochlorothiazide Tablets** (ZyGenerics)	12.5 mg hydrochlorothiazide	50 mg losartan potassium	May contain lactose, PEG, 4.24 mg potassium. In 30s, 90s, 1,000s, and 5,000s.
Rx	**Hyzaar Tablets** (Merck)			4.24 mg potassium, lactose. (MRK 717 HYZAAR). Yellow, teardrop shape. In 30s, 90s, 1,000s, 5,000s, and UD 100s.
Rx	**Losartan Potassium/Hydrochlorothiazide Tablets** (Various, eg, Roxane, Teva)	12.5 mg hydrochlorothiazide	100 mg losartan potassium	May contain lactose, PEG, 8.48 mg potassium. In 30s, 90s, 500s, and 1,000s.
Rx	**Hyzaar Tablets** (Merck)			8.48 mg potassium, lactose. (745). White, oval. In 30s, 90s, 1,000s, 5,000s, and UD 100s.
Rx	**Losartan Potassium/Hydrochlorothiazide Tablets** (ZyGenerics)	25 mg hydrochlorothiazide	100 mg losartan potassium	May contain lactose, PEG, 8.48 mg potassium. In 30s, 90s, 1,000s, and 4,000s.
	Hyzaar Tablets (Merck)			8.48 mg potassium, lactose. (MRK 747 HYZAAR). Lt. yellow, teardrop shape. In 30s, 90s, 1000s, 4000s, and UD 100s.
Rx	**Methyldopa/Hydrochlorothiazide Tablets** (Various, eg, Mylan, Zenith-Goldline)	15 mg hydrochlorothiazide	250 mg methyldopa	In 100s, 500s, 1000s and UD 100s.
Rx	**Methyldopa/Hydrochlorothiazide Tablets** (Various, eg, Goldline, Mylan)	25 mg hydrochlorothiazide	250 mg methyldopa	In 100s, 500s, 1000s and UD 100s.
Rx	**Methyldopa/Hydrochlorothiazide Tablets** (Various)	30 mg hydrochlorothiazide	500 mg methyldopa	In 100s, 250s and 500s.
Rx	**Methyldopa/Hydrochlorothiazide Tablets** (Various)	50 mg hydrochlorothiazide	500 mg methyldopa	In 100s, 250s, and 500s.
Rx	**Metoprolol Tartrate/Hydrochlorothiazide Tablets** (Mylan)	25 mg hydrochlorothiazide	50 mg metoprolol tartrate	Lactose. (M 424). Peach, scored. In 100s and 500s.
Rx	**Lopressor HCT 50/25 Tablets** (Novartis)			Lactose, sucrose. (GEIGY 35 35). White-mottled blue, capsule shape, scored. In 100s.
Rx	**Metoprolol Tartrate/Hydrochlorothiazide Tablets** (Mylan)	25 mg hydrochlorothiazide	100 mg metoprolol tartrate	Lactose. (M 434). Peach, oval, scored. In 100s and 500s.
Rx	**Lopressor HCT 100/25 Tablets** (Novartis)			Lactose, sucrose. (GEIGY 53 53). White-mottled pink, capsule shape, scored. In 100s.
Rx	**Metoprolol Tartrate/Hydrochlorothiazide Tablets** (Mylan)	50 mg hydrochlorothiazide	100 mg metoprolol tartrate	Lactose. (M 445). Peach, capsule shape, scored. In 100s and 500s.
Rx	**Lopressor HCT 100/50 Tablets** (Novartis)			Lactose, sucrose. (GEIGY 73 73). White-mottled yellow, capsule shape, scored. In 100s.
Rx	**Moexipril Hydrochloride/Hydrochlorothiazide Tablets** (Teva)	12.5 mg hydrochlorothiazide	7.5 mg moexipril hydrochloride	Tartrazine. (9 3 5213). Yellow, capsule shape, scored. Film-coated. In 100s.
Rx	**Uniretic Tablets** (Schwarz Pharma)			Lactose. (712 S P). Yellow, oval, scored. Film-coated. In 100s.
Rx	**Moexipril Hydrochloride/Hydrochlorothiazide Tablets** (Teva)	12.5 mg hydrochlorothiazide	15 mg moexipril HCl	(9 3 5214). White, capsule shape, scored. Film-coated. In 100s.
Rx	**Uniretic Tablets** (Schwarz Pharma)			Lactose. (720 S P). White, oval, scored. Film-coated. In 100s.
Rx	**Moexipril Hydrochloride/Hydrochlorothiazide Tablets** (Teva)	25 mg hydrochlorothiazide	15 mg moexipril HCl	Tartrazine. (9 3 5215). Yellow, capsule shape, scored. Film-coated. In 100s.
Rx	**Uniretic Tablets** (Schwarz Pharma)			Lactose. (725 S P). Yellow, oval, scored. Film-coated. In 100s.
Rx	**Benicar HCT** (Sankyo Pharma)	12.5 mg hydrochlorothiazide	20 mg olmesartan medoxomil	Lactose. (Sankyo C22). Red-yellow, round. Film-coated. In 30s, 90s, 1000s, and UD 100s.
		12.5 mg hydrochlorothiazide	40 mg olmesartan medoxomil	Lactose. (Sankyo C23). Red-yellow, oval. Film-coated. In 30s, 90s, 1000s, and UD 100s.
		25 mg hydrochlorothiazide	40 mg olmesartan medoxomil	Lactose. (Sankyo C25). Pink, oval. Film-coated. In 30s, 90s, 1000s, and UD 100s.
Rx	**Propranolol/Hydrochlorothiazide Tablets** (Various, eg, Mylan)	25 mg hydrochlorothiazide	40 mg propranolol hydrochloride	In 100s.
Rx	**Propranolol/Hydrochlorothiazide Tablets** (Various, eg, Mylan)	25 mg hydrochlorothiazide	80 mg propranolol hydrochloride	In 100s and 1000s.
Rx	**Quinapril Hydrochloride/Hydrochlorothiazide Tablets** (Greenstone)	12.5 mg hydrochlorothiazide	10 mg quinapril hydrochloride	Lactose. (G 222). Pink, elliptical, scored. Film-coated. In 90s.
Rx	**Accuretic** (Parke-Davis)			Lactose. (PD 222). Pink, elliptical, scored. Film-coated. In 30s.
Rx	**Accuretic Tablets** (Amide)			(A238). Peach, oval. Film-coated. In 30s, 100s, and 500s.

ANTIHYPERTENSIVE COMBINATIONS

	Product and Distributor	Diuretic	Other Content	How Supplied
Rx	**Quinapril Hydrochloride/Hydrochlorothiazide Tablets** (Greenstone)	12.5 mg hydrochlorothiazide	20 mg quinapril hydrochloride	Lactose. (G 220). Pink, triangular, scored. Film-coated. In 90s.
Rx	**Accuretic** (Parke-Davis)			Lactose. (PD 220). Pink, triangular, scored. Film-coated. In 30s.
Rx	**Quinaretic Tablets** (Amide)			(A239). Peach, triangular. Film-coated. In 30s, 100s, and 500s.
Rx	**Quinapril Hydrochloride/Hydrochlorothiazide Tablets** (Greenstone)	25 mg hydrochlorothiazide	20 mg quinapril HCl	Lactose. (G 223). Pink. Film-coated. In 90s.
Rx	**Accuretic** (Parke-Davis)			Lactose. (PD 223). Pink, scored. Film-coated. In 30s.
Rx	**Quinaretic Tablets** (Amide)			(A240). Peach. Film-coated. In 30s, 100s, and 500s.
Rx	**Micardis HCT Tablets** (Boehringer Ingelheim)	12.5 mg hydrochlorothiazide	40 mg telmisartan	Sorbitol, lactose. (H4). Bilayered (red and white, possibly with red specks), oblong. In blister pack 30s.
		12.5 mg hydrochlorothiazide	80 mg telmisartan	Sorbitol, lactose. (H8). Bilayered (red and white, possibly with red specks), oblong. In blister pack 30s.
		25 mg hydrochlorothiazide	80 mg telmisartan	Sorbitol, lactose. (H9). Bilayered (yellow and white, possibly with yellow specks), oblong. In blister pack 30s.
Rx	**Maxzide-25 Tablets** (Mylan)	25 mg hydrochlorothiazide	37.5 mg triamterene	(B M9 MAXZIDE). Green, bow-tie shape, scored. In 100s.
Rx	**Maxzide Tablets** (Mylan)	50 mg hydrochlorothiazide	75 mg triamterene	(B M8 MAXZIDE). Yellow, bow-tie shape, scored. In 100s and 500s.
Rx	**Diovan HCT Tablets** (Novartis)	12.5 mg hydrochlorothiazide	80 mg valsartan	(CG HGH). Lt. orange, ovaloid. In 90s and UD 100s.
		12.5 mg hydrochlorothiazide	160 mg valsartan	(CG HHH). Dk. red, ovaloid. In 90s and UD 100s.
		12.5 mg hydrochlorothiazide	320 mg valsartan	(NVR HIL). Pink, ovaloid. In 90s and UD 100s.
		25 mg hydrochlorothiazide	160 mg valsartan	(NVR HXH). Brown orange, ovaloid. In 90s and UD 100s.
		25 mg hydrochlorothiazide	320 mg valsartan	(NVR CTI). Yellow, ovaloid. In 90s and UD 100s.
Rx	**Exforge HCT Tablets** (Novartis)	12.5 mg hydrochlorothiazide	5 mg amlodipine, 160 mg valsartan	(NVR VCL). White, ovaloid. Film-coated. In 30s and 90s.
		12.5 mg hydrochlorothiazide	10 mg amlodipine, 160 mg valsartan	(NVR VDL). Pale yellow, ovaloid. Film-coated. In 30s and 90s.
		25 mg hydrochlorothiazide	5 mg amlodipine, 160 mg valsartan	(NVR VEL). Yellow, ovaloid. Film-coated, In 30s and 90s.
		25 mg hydrochlorothiazide	10 mg amlodipine, 160 mg valsartan	(NVR VHL). Brown-yellow, ovaloid. Film-coated. In 30s and 90s.
		25 mg hydrochlorothiazide	10 mg amlodipine, 320 mg valsartan	(NyVR VFL). Brown-yellow, ovaloid. Film-coated. In 30s and 90s.
Rx	**Tekamlo** (Novartis)		5 mg amlodipine besylate, 150 mg aliskiren	As aliskiren hemifumarate. PEG. (T2 NVR). Lt. yellow, ovaloid. Film-coated. In 30s, 90s, and UD 100s.
			10 mg amlodipine besylate, 150 mg aliskiren	As aliskiren hemifumarate. PEG. (T7 NVR). Yellow, ovaloid. Film-coated. In 30s, 90s, and UD 100s.
			5 mg amlodipine besylate, 300 mg aliskiren	As aliskiren hemifumarate. PEG. (T11 NVR). Dark yellow, ovaloid. Film-coated. In 30s, 90s, and UD 100s.
			10 mg amlodipine besylate, 300 mg aliskiren	As aliskiren hemifumarate. PEG. (T12 NVR). Brown/yellow, ovaloid. Film-coated. In 30s, 90s, and UD 100s.
Rx	**Valturna** (Novartis)		150 mg aliskiren, 160 mg valsartan	(NVR HDU). Lt. red, ovaloid. Film-coated. In 30s, 90s, and UD 100s.
			300 mg aliskiren, 320 mg valsartan	(NVR SNB). Lt. brown, ovaloid. Film-coated. In 30s, 90s, and UD 100s.
Rx	**Amlodipine Besylate/Benazepril Hydrochloride** (Various, eg, Sandoz, Teva)		2.5 mg amlodipine, 10 mg benazepril hydrochloride	May contain lactose. In 100s.
Rx	**Lotrel Capsules** (Novartis)			(LOTREL 2255). White/gold bands. In 100s.
Rx	**Amlodipine Besylate/Benazepril Hydrochloride** (Various, eg, Sandoz, Teva)		5 mg amlodipine, 10 mg benazepril hydrochloride	May contain lactose. In 100s.
Rx	**Lotrel Capsules** (Novartis)			(LOTREL 2260). Lt. brown/white bands. In 100s.
Rx	**Amlodipine Besylate/Benazepril Hydrochloride** (Various, eg, Sandoz, Teva)		5 mg amlodipine, 20 mg benazepril hydrochloride	May contain lactose. In 100s.
Rx	**Lotrel Capsules** (Novartis)			(LOTREL 2265). Pink/white bands. In 100s.
Rx	**Amlodipine Besylate/Benazepril Hydrochloride Capsules** (Various, eg, Par, Sandoz)		5 mg amlodipine, 40 mg benazepril HCl	May contain lactose. In 100s and 500s.
Rx	**Lotrel Capsules** (Novartis)			Lactose. (Lotrel 0384). Light blue w/ 2 white bands. In 100s.

ANTIHYPERTENSIVE COMBINATIONS

	Product and Distributor	Diuretic	Other Content	How Supplied
Rx	**Amlodipine Besylate/Benazepril Hydrochloride** (Various, eg, Sandoz, Teva)		10 mg amlodipine, 20 mg benazepril hydrochloride	May contain lactose. In 100s.
Rx	**Lotrel Capsules** (Novartis)			Lactose. (Lotrel 0364). Purple. In 100s.
Rx	**Amlodipine Besylate/Benazepril Hydrochloride Capsules** (Various, eg, Par, Sandoz)		10 mg amlodipine, 40 mg benazepril HCl	May contain lactose. In 100s and 500s.
Rx	**Lotrel Capsules** (Novartis)			Lactose. (Lotrel 0379). Dark blue w/ 2 white bands. In 100s.
Rx	**Exforge Tablets** (Novartis)		5 mg amlodipine besylate, 160 mg valsartan	(NVR ECE). Dark yellow, oval. Film coated. In 30s, 90s, and UD 100s.
			5 mg amlodipine besylate, 320 mg valsartan	(NVR CSF). Dark yellow, oval. Film coated. In 30s, 90s, and UD 100s.
			10 mg amlodipine besylate, 160 mg valsartan	(NVR UIC). Light yellow, oval. Film coated. In 30s, 90s, and UD 100s.
			10 mg amlodipine besylate, 320 mg valsartan	(NVR LUF). Dark yellow, oval. Film coated. In 30s, 90s, and UD 100s.
Rx	**Azor Tablets** (Daiichi Sankyo)		5 mg amlodipine besylate, 20 mg olmesartan medoxomil	(C73). White. In 30s, 90s, 1,000s, and UD 100s.
			10 mg amlodipine besylate, 20 mg olmesartan medoxomil	(C74). Grayish orange. In 30s, 90s, 100s, 1,000s, and UD 100s.
			5 mg amlodipine besylate, 40 mg olmesartan medoxomil	(C75). Cream. In 30s, 90s, 1,000s, and UD 100s.
			10 mg amlodipine besylate, 40 mg olmesartan medoxomil	(C77). Brownish red. In 30s, 90s, 1,000s, and UD 100s.
Rx	**Lexxel Extended-Release Tablets** (AstraZeneca)		5 mg enalapril maleate, 5 mg felodipine	Lactose. (LEXXEL 1, 5-5). White. Film-coated. In unit-of-use 30s and 100s.
Rx	**Trandolapril/Verapamil** (Glenmark Pharmaceuticals)		1 mg trandolapril/240 mg verapamil hydrochloride	Extended release. Lactose. (294). White to pinkish-white, oval. Film-coated. In 100s.
Rx	**Tarka Tablets** (Abbott)			Lactose. (241). White, oval. Film-coated. In 100s.
Rx	**Trandolapril/Verapamil** (Glenmark Pharmaceuticals)		2 mg trandolapril/180 mg verapamil hydrochloride	Extended release. Lactose. (295). Pink, oval. Film-coated. In 100s.
Rx	**Tarka Tablets** (Abbott)			Lactose. (182). Pink, oval. Film-coated. In 100s.
Rx	**Trandolapril/Verapamil** (Glenmark Pharmaceuticals)		2 mg trandolapril/240 mg verapamil hydrochloride	Extended release. Lactose. (296). Cream, oval. Film-coated. In 100s.
Rx	**Tarka Tablets** (Abbott)			Lactose. (242). Gold, oval. Film-coated. In 100s.
Rx	**Trandolapril/Verapamil** (Glenmark Pharmaceuticals)		4 mg trandolapril/240 mg verapamil hydrochloride	Extended release. Lactose. (G38). Brown, oval. Film-coated. In 100s.
Rx	**Tarka Tablets** (Abbott)			Lactose. (244). Reddish-brown, oval. Film-coated. In 100s.
Rx	**Twynsta Tablets** (Boehringer Ingelheim)		5 mg amlodipine besylate/40 mg telmisartan	Sorbitol. (A1). White-off-white/blue, oval. In blister pack 30s and 90s.
			10 mg amlodipine besylate/40 mg telmisartan	Sorbitol. (A2). White-off-white/blue, oval. In blister pack 30s and 90s.
			5 mg amlodipine besylate/80 mg telmisartan	Sorbitol. (A3). White-off-white/blue, oval. In blister pack 30s and 90s.
			10 mg amlodipine besylate/80 mg telmisartan	Sorbitol. (A4). White-off-white/blue, oval. In blister pack 30s and 90s.

AMLODIPINE/OLMESARTAN MEDOXOMIL

Rx	**Azor** (Daiichi Sankyo)	**Tablets; oral:** amlodipine 5 mg/olmesartan medoxomil 20 mg	(C73). White. In 30s, 90s, 1,000s, and UD 100s.
		amlodipine 5 mg/olmesartan medoxomil 40 mg	(C74). Grayish orange. In 30s, 90s, 1,000s, and UD 100s.
		amlodipine 10 mg/olmesartan medoxomil 20 mg	(C75). Cream. In 30s, 90s, 1,000s, and UD 100s.
		amlodipine 10 mg/olmesartan medoxomil 40 mg	(C77). Brownish red. In 30s, 90s, 1,000s, and UD 100s.

AMLODIPINE/OLMESARTAN MEDOXOMIL

The following is an abbreviated monograph. For complete prescribing information, refer to the Amlodipine and Olmesartan Medoxomil individual monographs.

WARNING

When pregnancy is detected, discontinue amlodipine/olmesartan as soon as possible. When used in pregnancy during the second and third trimesters, drugs that act directly on the renin-angiotensin system can cause injury and even death to the developing fetus

Indications

Treatment of hypertension.

Administration and Dosage

➤*General dosing considerations:* Max antihypertensive effects are attained within 2 wk after a dose change. Dose may be increased after 2 wk.

Amlodipine/olmesartan combination may be substituted for individually titrated components.

➤*Adults:*

Hypertension –

Maximum dose: 10 mg amlodipine, 40 mg olmesartan.

Initial dosage: 5 mg/20 mg once daily.

Dosage titration: Increase after 1 to 2 weeks to a max of 10 mg/40 mg once daily.

Concomitant therapy: May be administered with other antihypertensive agents.

Replacement therapy: When substituting for individual components, the dose of one or both of the components can be increased if blood pressure control has not been satisfactory.

Add-on therapy: Amlodipine/olmesartan may be used to provide additional blood pressure lowering for patients not adequately controlled with amlodipine (or another dihydropyridine calcium channel blocker) alone or with olmesartan (or another angiotensin receptor blocker).

➤*Children:* Safety and efficacy not established.

➤*Elderly:* Initial therapy with amlodipine/olmesartan is not recommended in patients 75 years of age and older.

➤*Hepatic function impairment:* Initial therapy with amlodipine/olmesartan is not recommended.

➤*Administration:* May be taken with or without food.

➤*Storage/Stability:* Store at 59° to 86°F; protect from moisture.

Actions

➤*Pharmacology:*

Amlodipine – Causes peripheral artery vasodilation by inhibiting the transmembrane influx of calcium ions into vascular smooth muscle.

Olmesartan – Blocks vasoconstrictor effects of angiotensin II by selectively blocking its binding to the AT_1 receptor in vascular smooth muscle.

Contraindications

None well documented.

Warnings/Precautions

➤*Angina or MI:* Increased frequency, duration, or severity of angina or acute MI may occur.

➤*Congestive heart failure:* Use with caution in patients with history of congestive heart failure.

➤*Hypotension:*

Amlodipine – Acute hypotension may occur.

Olmesartan – Symptomatic hypotension may occur after initiation of treatment, especially in patients with an activated renin-angiotensin system (eg, volume- and/or salt-depleted patients)

➤*Renal function impairment:* In patients whose renal function may depend on activity of the renin-angiotensin-aldosterone system (eg, patients with severe CHF), olmesartan treatment may be associated with oliguria and progressive azotemia, which may rarely result in acute renal failure and death.

➤*Hepatic function impairment:* Use with caution. Initial therapy with amlodipine/olmesartan is not recommended in patients with hepatic impairment.

➤*Pregnancy: Category C* (first trimester); *Category D* (second and third trimesters). Drugs that act directly on the renin-angiotensin system can cause fetal and neonatal morbidity and death when administered to pregnant women. There have been several dozen cases reported in the world literature of patients who were taking angiotensin converting enzyme inhibitors. During the second and third trimesters of pregnancy, these drugs have been associated with fetal injury that includes hypotension, neonatal skull hypoplasia anuria, reversible or irreversible renal failure and death. Oligohydramnios has also been reported, presumably resulting from decreased fetal renal function; oligohydramnios in this setting has been associated with fetal limb contractures, craniofacial deformation, and hypoplastic lung development. Prematurity, intrauterine growth retardation, and patent ductus arteriosus have also been reported, although it is not clear whether these occurrences were due to exposure to the drug. When pregnancy is detected, discontinue amlodipine/olmesartan as soon as possible.

➤*Lactation:* It is not known whether the amlodipine or olmesartan components of amlodipine/olmesartan are excreted in human milk, but olmesartan is secreted at low concentrations in the milk of lactating rats. Because of the potential for adverse effects on the nursing infant, a decision should be made whether to discontinue nursing or discontinue the drug, taking into account the importance of the drug to the mother.

➤*Children:* Safety and efficacy not established.

➤*Elderly:* Use with caution, usually starting at the low end of the dosage range, because of the greater frequency of decreased hepatic, renal, or cardiac function, and of concomitant diseases or other drug therapy. Initial therapy with amlodipine/olmesartan is not recommended in patients 75 years of age and older.

➤*Monitoring:* Monitor blood pressure at regular intervals during therapy.

Drug Interactions

➤*Conivaptan, diltiazem, potassium-sparing diuretics, protease inhibitors (eg, ritonavir):* Amlodipine plasma concentrations may be elevated, increasing the pharmacologic effects and adverse reactions. Coadministration of olmesartan and potassium-sparing diuretics may cause elevated serum potassium concentrations.

Adverse Reactions

➤*Cardiovascular:*

Amlodipine – Palpitation (5%).

➤*CNS:*

Amlodipine – Dizziness (3%); somnolence (2%).

Olmesartan – Dizziness (3%); asthenia (postmarketing).

➤*Dermatologic:*

Amlodipine – Flushing (3%).

Olmesartan – Alopecia, pruritus, urticaria (postmarketing).

➤*GI:*

Olmesartan – Vomiting (postmarketing).

➤*GU:*

Olmesartan – Acute renal failure (postmarketing).

➤*Hepatic:*

Amlodipine – Hepatic enzyme elevations, jaundice (postmarketing).

➤*Musculoskeletal:*

Olmesartan – Rhabdomyolysis (postmarketing).

➤*Miscellaneous:*

Amlodipine – Edema (11%).

Olmesartan – Angioedema (postmarketing).

Overdosage

➤*Symptoms:*

Amlodipine – Excessive peripheral vasodilation with marked hypotension and possibly reflex tachycardia is expected to occur.

Olmesartan – Hypotension, tachycardia, and bradycardia (from parasympathetic stimulation) are expected to occur.

Patient Information

Inform female patients of childbearing age to report pregnancy to health care provider as soon as possible.

IRBESARTAN/HYDROCHLOROTHIAZIDE

	Product and Distributor	Diuretic	Other Content	How Supplied
Rx	**Avalide** (Bristol-Myers Squibb)	12.5 mg hydrochlorothiazide	150 mg irbesartan	Lactose. (2775). Peach, oval. In 30s and 90s.
		12.5 mg hydrochlorothiazide	300 mg irbesartan	Lactose. (2776). Peach, oval. In 30s and 90s.
		25 mg hydrochlorothiazide	300 mg irbesartan	Lactose. (2788). Pink, oval. Film-coated. In 30s and 90s.

IRBESARTAN/HYDROCHLOROTHIAZIDE

The following is an abbreviated monograph. For complete prescribing information, refer to the Hydrochlorothiazide and Irbesartan individual monographs.

WARNING

Can cause injury and death to developing fetus when used during second and third trimester of pregnancy.

Indications

➤*Hypertension:* Treatment of hypertension.

Administration and Dosage

➤*Maximum dose:* Irbesartan 300 mg/hydrochlorothiazide 25 mg once daily.

➤*General dosing considerations:* May be administered with other antihypertensives.

Maximum antihypertensive effects are attained within 2 to 4 weeks after a change in dose.

Not recommended as initial therapy in patients with intravascular volume depletion.

➤*Adults:*

Hypertension –

Maximum dose: Irbesartan 300 mg/hydrochlorothiazide 25 mg once daily.

Initial dosage: Irbesartan 150 mg/hydrochlorothiazide 12.5 mg once daily.

Dosage titration: Increase after 1 to 2 weeks of therapy to a maximum of irbesartan 300 mg/hydrochlorothiazide 25 mg once daily.

Conversion: May be substituted for the titrated components.

➤*Renal function impairment:*

CrCl 30 mL/min or less – Use is not recommended.

➤*Administration:* Take with or without food.

➤*Storage/Stability:* Store between 59° and 86°F.

Actions

➤*Pharmacology:*

Irbesartan – Antagonizes the effect of angiotensin II (vasoconstriction and aldosterone secretion) by blocking the angiotensin II (AT_1 receptor) in vascular smooth muscle and the adrenal gland, producing decreased BP.

Hydrochlorothiazide – Increases chloride, sodium, and water excretion by interfering with transport of sodium ions across renal tubular epithelium.

Contraindications

Anuria; hypersensitivity to sulfonamide-derivatives or any component of the product.

Warnings/Precautions

➤*Diabetes:* May require adjustments of insulin or oral hypoglycemic agents. Hyperglycemia may occur with thiazide diuretics.

➤*Fluid/Electrolyte imbalance:* Hyponatremia, hypochloremic alkalosis, hypokalemia, and/or hypomagnesemia may occur.

➤*Hyperuricemia:* Hyperuricemia or frank gout may be precipitated.

➤*Lipid disturbances:* Increases in cholesterol and triglyceride levels may occur.

➤*Post-sympathectomy:* Antihypertensive effects the drugs may be enhanced.

➤*Systemic lupus erythematosus:* Activation or exacerbation may occur.

➤*Volume or salt depletion:* Symptomatic hypotension may occur after initiation of treatment in patients with an activated renin-angiotensin system (eg, volume- or salt-depleted patients).

➤*Hypersensitivity reactions:* May occur in patients with or without a history of allergy or bronchial asthma.

➤*Renal function impairment:* Decreases in renal function may occur in patients whose renal function is dependent on the renin-angiotensin system; oliguria and/or progressive azotemia and rarely with acute renal failure and/or death may occur. Patients with renal artery stenosis may experience increases in serum creatinine or BUN. In addition, hydrochlorothiazide may precipitate azotemia and cumulative effects of the drug may develop in patients with impaired renal function. Not recommended in patients with severe renal disease.

➤*Hepatic function impairment:* Use with caution in patients with impaired hepatic function or progressive liver disease.

➤*Pregnancy: Category D.* Drugs that act directly on the renin-angiotensin system can cause fetal and neonatal morbidity, including hypotension, neonatal skull hypoplasia, anuria, reversible or irreversible renal failure, and death when administered to pregnant women during the second and third trimesters. Oligohydramnios has also been reported, and has been associated with fetal limb contractures, craniofacial deformation, and hypoplastic lung development. Prematurity, intrauterine growth retardation, and patent ductus arteriosus have also been reported, although it is not clear whether these occurrences were due to exposure to the drug. Mothers whose embryos and fetuses are exposed to an angiotensin II receptor antagonist only during the first trimester should be so informed. Nonetheless, when patients become pregnant, physicians should have the patient discontinue the use of irbesartan as soon as possible.

➤*Lactation:* It is not known whether this drug is excreted in human milk, but irbesartan or some metabolite of irbesartan is secreted at low concentration in the milk of lactating rats. Thiazides appear in human milk. Because of the potential for adverse effects on the breast-feeding infant, a decision should be made whether to discontinue breast-feeding or discontinue the drug, taking into account the importance of the drug to the mother.

➤*Children:* Safety and efficacy not established.

➤*Monitoring:* Perform periodic determinations of serum and urine electrolytes to detect possible electrolyte imbalance.

Drug Interactions

➤*Alcohol, barbiturates, narcotics:* Potentiation of orthostatic hypotension may occur.

➤*Antidiabetic agents (oral agents and insulin):* Dosage adjustments of the antidiabetic agent may be needed.

➤*Antihypertensive agents:* Effects may be additive or potentiated.

➤*Cholestyramine, colestipol:* Hydrochlorothiazide absorption may be reduced up to 85%.

➤*Corticosteroids:* Increased risk of electrolyte depletion (eg, hypokalemia).

➤*Lithium:* Increased risk of lithium toxicity caused by reduced clearance. Do not coadminister.

➤*Nondepolarizing skeletal muscle relaxants (eg, tubocurarine):* Effect of muscle relaxant may be enhanced.

➤*NSAIDs (eg, ibuprofen):* The antihypertensive effect of hydrochlorothiazide may be reduced.

➤*Pressor amines (eg, norepinephrine):* Effect of pressor amine may be reduced.

➤*Drug/Lab test interactions:* Hydrochlorothiazide may decrease serum protein-bound iodine levels without signs of thyroid disturbance; may cause diagnostic interference of serum electrolyte levels, blood and urine glucose levels, serum bilirubin levels, and serum uric acid levels; may cause intermittent and slight elevations in serum calcium without known disorders of calcium metabolism.

Adverse Reactions

➤*CNS:* Dizziness (8%); fatigue (7%); orthostatic dizziness (1%).

➤*GI:* Nausea, vomiting (3%); abdominal pain, dyspepsia/heartburn (2%).

➤*Hepatic:* Hepatitis, jaundice (postmarketing).

➤*Lab test abnormalities:* Increased BUN (2%); increased serum creatinine (1%); elevations of liver function tests and/or bilirubin; hyperkalemia (postmarketing).

➤*Miscellaneous:* Musculoskeletal pain (7%); edema, influenza (3%); abnormal urination (2%); chest pain (2%); allergy, tachycardia (1%); angioedema involving swelling of face, lips, pharynx, and/or tongue, urticaria (postmarketing).

Overdosage

➤*Symptoms:* Bradycardia, dehydration, electrolyte depletion (ie, hypochloremia, hypokalemia, hyponatremia), hypotension, tachycardia.

Patient Information

Explain name, dose, action, and potential side effects of drug. Advise patient to take every day as prescribed, without regard to meals. Advise patient to try to take at the same time each day.

Inform patient that drug controls, but not does cure, hypertension and to continue taking drug as prescribed even when blood pressure is not elevated. Caution patient not to change the dose or stop taking unless advised to do so by health care provider.

Caution patient to avoid sudden position changes to prevent orthostatic hypotension.

Instruct patient to lie or sit down if they experience dizziness or lightheadedness when standing.

Caution patient that inadequate fluid intake, excessive perspiration, diarrhea, or vomiting can lead to excessive fall in blood pressure resulting in lightheadedness or fainting.

IRBESARTAN/HYDROCHLOROTHIAZIDE

Instruct diabetic patient to monitor blood glucose more frequently when drug is started or dose is changed and to inform health care provider of significant changes in readings.

Caution patient to avoid unnecessary exposure to UV light (eg, sunlight, tanning booths) and to use sunscreen and wear protective clothing when exposed to UV light to avoid photosensitivity reaction.

Emphasize to hypertensive patient importance of other modalities on blood pressure: weight control, regular exercise, smoking cessation, and moderate intake of alcohol and salt.

Instruct women to notify health care provider if they become pregnant, plan on becoming pregnant, or are breastfeeding.

Instruct patient to stop taking drug and immediately report any of the following symptoms to health care provider: fainting or swelling of the face, lips, eyelids or tongue.

Caution patient to not take any prescription or OTC medications, salt substitutes, or dietary supplements unless advised to do so by health care provider.

METOPROLOL TARTRATE/HYDROCHLOROTHIAZIDE

	Product and Distributor	Diuretic	Other Content	How Supplied
Rx	**Metoprolol Tartrate/Hydrochlorothiazide Tablets** (Mylan)	25 mg hydrochlorothiazide	50 mg metoprolol tartrate	Lactose. (M 424). Peach, scored. In 100s and 500s.
Rx	**Lopressor HCT 50/25 Tablets** (Novartis)			Lactose, sucrose. (GEIGY 35 35). White-mottled blue, capsule shape, scored. In 100s.
Rx	**Metoprolol Tartrate/Hydrochlorothiazide Tablets** (Mylan)	25 mg hydrochlorothiazide	100 mg metoprolol tartrate	Lactose. (M 434). Peach, oval, scored. In 100s and 500s.
Rx	**Lopressor HCT 100/25 Tablets** (Novartis)			Lactose, sucrose. (GEIGY 53 53). White-mottled pink, capsule shape, scored. In 100s.
Rx	**Metoprolol Tartrate/Hydrochlorothiazide Tablets** (Mylan)	50 mg hydrochlorothiazide	100 mg metoprolol tartrate	Lactose. (M 445). Peach, capsule shape, scored. In 100s and 500s.
Rx	**Lopressor HCT 100/50 Tablets** (Novartis)			Lactose, sucrose. (GEIGY 73 73). White-mottled yellow, capsule shape, scored. In 100s.

METOPROLOL TARTRATE/HYDROCHLOROTHIAZIDE

The following is an abbreviated monograph. For complete prescribing information, refer to the Hydrochlorothiazide and Metoprolol individual monographs.

WARNING

Ischemic heart disease – Following abrupt cessation of therapy with certain beta-blocking agents, exacerbations of angina pectoris and, in some cases, myocardial infarction have occurred. Even in the absence of overt angina pectoris, when discontinuing therapy, metoprolol should not be withdrawn abruptly, and patients should be cautioned against interruption of therapy without the physician's advice.

Indications

➤*Hypertension:* For the management of hypertension.

Administration and Dosage

➤*General dosing considerations:* Dosage should be determined by individual titration.

Dosing regimens that exceed hydrochlorothiazide 50 mg/day are not recommended.

➤*Adults:*

Hypertension –

Usual dosage: Hydrochlorothiazide is usually given at a dose of 12.5 to 50 mg/day. The usual initial dose of metoprolol is 100 mg/day in single or divided doses. Metoprolol is effective in the dose range of 100 to 450 mg/day.

Dosage titration: Increase gradually until optimum blood pressure control is achieved.

Dosage adjustment: In general, once-daily dosing is effective and can maintain a reduction in blood pressure throughout the day; however, lower doses of metoprolol, especially 100 mg, may not maintain full effect at end of 24-h period and larger or more frequent doses may be required.

Concomitant therapy: Another antihypertensive agent may be added gradually, beginning with 50% of the usual recommended starting dose to avoid an excessive fall in blood pressure.

➤*Storage/Stability:* Store at 25°C (77°F); excursions permitted between 15° and 30°C (59° to 86°F). Protect from moisture.

Actions

➤*Pharmacology:*

Metoprolol – Blocks beta receptors, primarily affecting the CV system (decreases heart rate, contractility, and blood pressure) and lungs (promotes bronchospasm).

Hydrochlorothiazide – Enhances excretion of sodium, chloride, and water by interfering with transport of sodium ions across renal tubular epithelium.

Contraindications

Sinus bradycardia; heart block greater than first degree; cardiogenic shock; overt cardiac failure; sick-sinus syndrome; severe peripheral arterial circulatory disorder; anuria; hypersensitivity to any component of the product, beta-blockers, or sulfonamide-derivatives.

Warnings/Precautions

➤*Cardiac failure:* Use with caution in patients controlled by digitalis and diuretics.

➤*Ischemic heart disease:* May occur following abrupt discontinuation of metoprolol.

➤*Bronchospastic disease:* Patients with bronchospastic disease should, in general, not receive beta blockers. Use with caution; administer in smaller divided doses.

➤*Major surgery:* The necessity or desirability of withdrawing beta-blocking therapy prior to major surgery is controversial; the impaired ability of the heart to respond to reflex adrenergic stimuli may augment the risks of general anesthesia and surgical procedures.

➤*Diabetes and hypoglycemia:* Metoprolol may mask tachycardia associated with hypoglycemia. Latent diabetes may become manifest with hydrochlorothiazide therapy.

➤*Pheochromocytoma:* Administration of beta blockers alone in the setting of pheochromocytoma has been associated with a paradoxical increase in blood pressure due to the attenuation of beta-mediated vasodilatation in skeletal muscle.

➤*Thyrotoxicosis:* Metoprolol may mask clinical signs of developing or continuing hyperthyroidism. Abrupt withdrawal of metoprolol may exacerbate symptoms of hyperthyroidism, including thyroid storm.

➤*Lupus erythematosus:* Exacerbation or activation may occur.

➤*Electrolyte and fluid balance:* All patients receiving diuretic therapy should be observed for evidence of fluid or electrolyte imbalance: Namely, hyponatremia, hypochloremic alkalosis, and hypokalemia.

➤*Hyperuricemia:* Hyperuricemia or frank gout may be precipitated.

➤*Postsympathectomy patients:* Hydrochlorothiazide may enhance antihypertensive effects.

➤*Hypersensitivity reactions:* May occur in patients with or without history of allergy or bronchial asthma; cross-sensitivity with sulfonamides may occur.

➤*Renal function impairment:* Use with caution in patients with severe renal disease; hydrochlorothiazide may precipitate azotemia.

➤*Hepatic function impairment:* Use with caution. Minor alterations of fluid and electrolyte imbalance may precipitate hepatic coma.

➤*Pregnancy: Category C.*

➤*Lactation:* Hydrochlorothiazide and metoprolol are excreted in breast milk.

➤*Children:* Safety and effectiveness in children have not been established.

➤*Elderly:* Use with caution, usually starting at low end of dosage range because of greater frequency of decreased hepatic, renal, or cardiac function, and of concomitant diseases or other drug therapy.

➤*Monitoring:* Periodic determination of serum electrolytes to detect possible electrolyte imbalance should be done at appropriate intervals.

Drug Interactions

➤*Barbiturates:* Metoprolol bioavailability may be decreased.

➤*Bile acid sequestrants (eg, cholestyramine):* May reduce hydrochlorothiazide absorption; give at least 2 hours before the sequestrant.

➤*Catecholamine-depleting drugs (eg, reserpine):* May have additive effect when given with metoprolol.

➤*Clonidine:* May enhance or reverse antihypertensive effect. Potentially life-threatening situations may occur, especially on abrupt withdrawal of clonidine.

➤*Diazoxide:* May increase the risk of hyperglycemia.

➤*Digitalis glycosides:* Diuretic-induced hypokalemia and hypomagnesemia may precipitate digitalis-induced arrhythmias.

METOPROLOL TARTRATE/HYDROCHLOROTHIAZIDE

➤*General anesthetics:* Metoprolol cardiodepressant effects may be increased.

➤*Hydralazine:* Serum levels of hydralazine and metoprolol may increase.

➤*Insulin, sulfonylureas:* Hypoglycemic effect may be decreased. May need higher doses of sulfonylurea or insulin.

➤*Lidocaine:* Lidocaine levels may increase, leading to toxicity.

➤*Lithium:* Renal excretion of lithium may be decreased.

➤*Loop diuretics:* Synergistic effects may result in profound diuresis and serious electrolyte abnormalities.

➤*NSAIDs:* Some agents may impair antihypertensive effect.

➤*Potent inhibitors of CYP2D6 (eg, antiarrhythmic agents [eg, propafenone, quinidine], antifungal agents [eg, terbinafine], antihistamines [eg, diphenhydramine], antimalarial agents [eg, hydroxychloroquine], antipsychotic agents [eg, thioridazine], antiulcer agents [eg, cimetidine], antiviral agents [eg, ritonavir], bupropion, fluoxetine, paroxetine):* May elevate metoprolol plasma levels, increasing the risk of adverse reactions.

➤*Prazosin:* Orthostatic hypotension may be increased.

➤*Rifampin:* Effects of metoprolol may be decreased.

➤*Verapamil:* Effects of verapamil or metoprolol may be increased.

➤*Drug/Lab test interactions:* Antinuclear antibodies may develop but are usually reversible on discontinuation. Serum protein-bound iodine levels may be reduced without signs of thyroid disturbance. May cause diagnostic interference of serum electrolyte levels, blood and urine glucose levels, serum bilirubin levels, and serum uric acid levels.

Adverse Reactions

➤*Cardiovascular:* Bradycardia (about 6%); shortness of breath (3%); decreased exercise tolerance (about 1%); congestive heart failure, intensification of AV block.

➤*CNS:* Dizziness, drowsiness, fatigue, headache, lethargy, somnolence, tiredness, vertigo (about 10%); depression (5%); nightmares (about 1%).

➤*Dermatologic:* Purpura, sweating (1%); Stevens-Johnson syndrome.

➤*GI:* Diarrhea (5%); constipation, digestive disorder, dry mouth, flatulence, gastric pain, heartburn, nausea, vomiting (about 1%).

➤*GU:* Impotence (1%).

➤*Hematologic/Lymphatic:* Agranulocytosis, aplastic anemia, leukopenia, nonthrombocytopenic purpura, thrombocytopenia, thrombocytopenic purpura.

➤*Hepatic:* Elevated alkaline phosphatase, elevated lactate dehydrogenase and transaminase, hepatic function impairment, hepatitis, jaundice (postmarketing).

➤*Metabolic/Nutritional:* Hypokalemia (less than 10%); anorexia, edema, gout (1%).

➤*Musculoskeletal:* Muscle pain (1%).

➤*Respiratory:* Dyspnea (about 1%).

➤*Special senses:* Blurred vision, earache, tinnitus (1%).

➤*Miscellaneous:* Flu syndrome (about 10%); gangrene, hypersensitivity including fever with aching and sore throat, laryngospasm and respiratory distress, necrotizing angiitis.

Overdosage

➤*Symptoms:* Alkalosis, anuria, bradycardia, bronchospasm, cardiac failure, confusion, cramps of the calf muscles, dizziness, fatigue, hypochloremia, hypokalemia, hyponatremia, hypotension, impairment of consciousness, increased serum urea nitrogen, nausea, oliguria, paresthesia, polyuria, shock, tachycardia, thirst, vomiting, weakness.

Patient Information

Instruct patients that if a dose is missed, to take only the next scheduled dose without doubling the dose.

Advise patient to take this medication regularly and continuously, as directed.

Advise patient to avoid operating machinery and driving, or engaging in other tasks requiring alertness until the response to therapy has been determined.

Advise patients to contact health care provider if any difficulty breathing occurs.

Instruct patients to inform health care provider before any type of surgery that metoprolol is being taken.

OLMESARTAN/HYDROCHLOROTHIAZIDE

Rx	**Benicar HCT** (Daiichi Sankyo)	**Tablets; oral:** olmesartan medoxomil 20 mg/hydrochlorothiazide 12.5 mg	Lactose. (Sankyo C22), Red-yellow, round. Film-coated. In 30s, 90s, 1,000s, and UD 100s.
		olmesartan medoxomil 40 mg/ hydrochlorothiazide 12.5 mg	Lactose. (Sankyo C23), Red-yellow, oval. Film-coated. In 30s, 90s, 1,000s, and UD 100s.
		olmesartan medoxomil 40 mg/ hydrochlorothiazide 25 mg	Lactose. (Sankyo C25), Pink, oval. Film-coated. In 30s, 90s, 1,000s, and UD 100s.

OLMESARTAN/HYDROCHLOROTHIAZIDE

The following is an abbreviated monograph. For complete prescribing information, refer to the Olmesartan Medoxomil and Hydrochlorothiazide individual monographs or the Angiotensin II Receptor Antagonists class monograph.

WARNING

When pregnancy is detected, discontinue olmesartan/hydrochlorothiazide as soon as possible. Drugs that act directly on the renin-angiotensin system can cause injury and even death to the developing fetus.

Indications

➤*Hypertension:* For the treatment of hypertension.

Administration and Dosage

➤*Adults:*

Hypertension –

Usual dosage: 1 tablet once daily.

Initial dosage: Titrate the dose based on individual response to each component as monotherapy.

• *Olmesartan* – The usual starting dosage of olmesartan is 20 mg once daily as monotherapy. If further reduction of blood pressure is needed after 2 wk of therapy, the dose may be increased to 40 mg. If blood pressure is not controlled by olmesartan alone, hydrochlorothiazide may be added, starting with 12.5 mg and then titrating to 25 mg once daily.

• *Hydrochlorothiazide* – If a patient is taking hydrochlorothiazide, olmesartan may be added, starting with 20 mg once daily and titrating to 40 mg. Consider reducing larger doses of hydrochlorothiazide to 12.5 mg before adding olmesartan.

Dosage titration: Depending on the blood pressure response, the dose may be titrated at intervals of 2 to 4 weeks.

Concomitant therapy: May be given with other antihypertensive agents.

➤*Renal function impairment:* Not recommended in severe renal impairment.

➤*Administration:* May be given with or without food.

➤*Storage/Stability:* Store between 20° and 25°C (68° and 77°F).

Actions

➤*Pharmacology:*

Olmesartan – Blocks the vasoconstrictor effects of angiotensin II by selectively blocking the binding of angiotensin II to the AT_1 receptor in vascular smooth muscle. Its action is, therefore, independent of the pathways for angiotensin II synthesis.

Hydrochlorothiazide – Increases chloride, sodium, and water excretion by interfering with transport of sodium ions across renal tubular epithelium.

Contraindications

Anuria; hypersensitivity to sulfonamide-derivatives or any component of the product.

Warnings/Precautions

➤*Hyperglycemia:* Hyperglycemia may occur; latent diabetes mellitus may become manifest.

➤*Hyperuricemia:* Hyperuricemia or frank gout may be precipitated.

➤*Lipid disorders:* Increases in cholesterol and triglyceride levels may occur.

➤*Systemic lupus erythematosus:* Activation or exacerbation may occur.

➤*Volume or salt depletion:* Symptomatic hypotension may occur after initiation of treatment in patients with an activated renin-angiotensin system (eg, volume- or salt-depleted patients).

➤*Hypersensitivity reactions:* May occur in patients with or without a history of allergy or bronchial asthma.

➤*Renal function impairment:* Not recommended in patients with severe renal function impairment; cumulative effects may develop in patients with impaired renal function.

➤*Hepatic function impairment:* Use with caution in patients with impaired hepatic function or progressive liver disease.

➤*Pregnancy:* *Category C* (first trimester) and *Category D* (second and third trimesters). Can cause injury and death to fetus if used during second or

OLMESARTAN/HYDROCHLOROTHIAZIDE

third trimester. There is no clinical experience with the use of olmesartan-hydrochlorothiazide in pregnant women. Drugs that act directly on the renin-angiotensin system can cause fetal and neonatal morbidity, including hypotension, neonatal skull hypoplasia, anuria, reversible or irreversible renal failure, and death when administered to pregnant women during the second and third trimesters. Oligohydramnios has also been reported, and has been associated with fetal limb contractures, craniofacial deformation, and hypoplastic lung development. Prematurity, intrauterine growth retardation, and patent ductus arteriosus have also been reported, although it is not clear whether these occurrences were due to exposure to the drug. Mothers whose embryos and fetuses are exposed to an angiotensin II receptor antagonist only during the first trimester should be so informed. Nonetheless, when patients become pregnant, physicians should have the patient discontinue the use of irbesartan as soon as possible.

➤*Lactation:* It is not known whether olmesartan is excreted in human milk, but olmesartan is secreted at low concentration in the milk of lactating rats. Thiazides appear in human milk. Because of the potential for adverse effects on the breast-feeding infant, a decision should be made whether to discontinue breast-feeding or discontinue the drug, taking into account the importance of the drug to the mother.

➤*Children:* Safety and efficacy not established.

➤*Elderly:* Use with caution, usually starting at the low end of the dosage range, because of the greater frequency of decreased hepatic, renal, or cardiac function, and concomitant diseases or other drug therapy.

➤*Monitoring:* Perform periodic determinations of serum electrolytes to detect possible electrolyte imbalance.

Drug Interactions

➤*Alcohol, barbiturates, narcotics:* Potentiation of orthostatic hypotension may occur.

➤*Antidiabetic agents (oral agents and insulin):* Dosage adjustments of the antidiabetic agent may be needed.

➤*Antihypertensive agents:* Effects may be additive or potentiated.

➤*Cholestyramine, colestipol:* Hydrochlorothiazide absorption may be reduced up to 85%.

➤*Corticosteroids:* Increased risk of electrolyte depletion (eg, hypokalemia).

➤*Lithium:* Increased risk of lithium toxicity caused by reduced clearance. Do not coadminister.

➤*Nondepolarizing skeletal muscle relaxants (eg, tubocurarine):* Effect of muscle relaxant may be enhanced.

➤*NSAIDs (eg, ibuprofen):* The antihypertensive effect of hydrochlorothiazide may be reduced.

➤*Pressor amines (eg, norepinephrine):* Effect of pressor amine may be reduced.

➤*Drug/Lab test interactions:* Hydrochlorothiazide may decrease serum protein-bound iodine levels without signs of thyroid disturbance; may cause diagnostic interference of serum electrolyte levels, blood and urine glucose levels, serum bilirubin levels, and serum uric acid levels; may cause intermittent and slight elevations in serum calcium without known disorders of calcium metabolism.

Adverse Reactions

➤*CNS:* Dizziness (9%); vertigo (greater than 1%); asthenia (postmarketing).

➤*Dermatologic:* Rash (greater than 1%); alopecia, pruritus, urticaria (postmarketing).

➤*GI:* Nausea (3%); abdominal pain, diarrhea, dyspepsia, gastroenteritis (greater than 1%); vomiting (postmarketing).

➤*GU:* Hematuria (greater than 1%); acute renal failure, increased blood creatinine levels (postmarketing).

➤*Hepatic:* Increased AST, ALT, and glucose tolerance test (greater than 1%).

➤*Lab test abnormalities:* Increased serum urea nitrogen and serum creatinine (1%).

➤*Metabolic/Nutritional:* Hyperuricemia (4%); increased creatine phosphokinase, hyperglycemia, hyperlipidemia (greater than 1%).

➤*Musculoskeletal:* Arthralgia, arthritis, back pain, myalgia (greater than 1%); rhabdomyolysis (postmarketing).

➤*Respiratory:* Upper respiratory tract infection (7%); coughing (greater than 1%).

➤*Miscellaneous:* Chest pain, peripheral edema (greater than 1%); angioedema (postmarketing).

Overdosage

➤*Symptoms:* Bradycardia, dehydration, electrolyte depletion (ie, hypochloremia, hypokalemia, hyponatremia), hypotension, tachycardia.

➤*Treatment:* If symptomatic hypotension occurs, initiate supportive treatment. The dialyzability of olmesartan is unknown.

Patient Information

Inform female patients of childbearing age to report pregnancy to health care provider as soon as possible.

Caution patients to inform health care provider if light-headedness occurs. If syncope occurs, the drug should be stopped until the health care provider is contacted.

Instruct patient to take exactly as prescribed and not to change the dose or discontinue therapy unless advised by health care provider.

TELMISARTAN/AMLODIPINE

Rx	Twynsta (Boehringer Ingelheim)	**Tablets; oral:** telmisartan 40 mg/amlodipine 5 mg	Sorbitol. (A1), White-off white/blue, oval. In blister pack 30s and 90s.
		telmisartan 40 mg/amlodipine 10 mg	Sorbitol. (A2), White-off white/blue, oval. In blister pack 30s and 90s.
		telmisartan 80 mg/amlodipine 5 mg	Sorbitol. (A3), White-off white/blue, oval. In blister pack 30s and 90s.
		telmisartan 80 mg/amlodipine 10 mg	Sorbitol. (A4), White-off white/blue, oval. In blister pack 30s and 90s.

TELMISARTAN/AMLODIPINE

The following is an abbreviated monograph. For complete prescribing information, refer to the Telmisartan and Amlodipine individual monographs.

WARNING

When used in pregnancy, drugs that act directly on the rennin-angiotensin system can cause injury and even death to the developing fetus. When pregnancy is detected, discontinue therapy as soon as possible.

Indications

➤*Hypertension:* Treatment of hypertension.

Administration and Dosage

➤*General dosing considerations:* Dosage must be individualized.

Most of the antihypertensive effect is apparent within 2 weeks and maximal reduction is generally attained after 4 weeks.

Correct imbalances of intravascular volume or salt depletion before initiating therapy with telmisartan/amlodipine.

➤*Adults:*

Hypertension –

Usual dosage: 1 tablet (telmisartan 20 to 80 mg/amlodipine 2.5 to 10 mg) by mouth per day.

Maximum dose: Telmisartan 80 mg/amlodipine 10 mg once daily.

Initial dosage: Telmisartan 40 mg/amlodipine 5 mg once daily. Patients requiring larger blood pressure reductions may be started on telmisartan 80 mg/amlodipine 5 mg.

Dosage titration: Dosage may be increased after at least 2 weeks.

Replacement therapy: Patients receiving amlodipine and telmisartan from separate tablets may instead receive telmisartan/amlodipine tablets containing the same component doses once daily.

Add-on therapy in patients not adequately controlled on monotherapy: Switch patients who experience dose-limiting adverse reactions (eg, edema) on amlodipine 10 mg to telmisartan 40 mg/amlodipine 5 mg once daily.

➤*Elderly:* Initiate amlodipine therapy at 2.5 mg once daily. Titrate slowly in patients 75 years of age and older. Not recommended as initial therapy in patients 75 years of age and older.

➤*Renal function impairment:* No initial dosage adjustment is required for patients with mild or moderate renal impairment. Titrate slowly in patients with severe renal impairment.

➤*Hepatic function impairment:* Initiate amlodipine therapy at 2.5 mg once daily. Titrate slowly. Not recommended as initial therapy in patients with hepatic impairment.

➤*Administration:* May be taken with or without food.

➤*Storage/Stability:* Store at 25°C (77°F); excursions permitted between 15° and 30°C (59° and 86°F). Protect from moisture and light. Do not remove from blisters until immediately before administration.

Actions

➤*Pharmacology:*

Amlodipine – Inhibits movement of calcium ions across cell membranes in systemic and coronary vascular smooth muscle.

Telmisartan – Antagonizes the effect of angiotensin II (vasoconstriction and aldosterone secretion) by blocking the angiotensin II receptor (AT_1 receptor) in vascular smooth muscle and the adrenal gland, producing decreased blood pressure.

Contraindications

None well documented.

TELMISARTAN/AMLODIPINE

Warnings/Precautions

➤*Cardiovascular effects:* Increased frequency, duration, or severity of angina or acute MI may occur. Use with caution in patients with heart failure or severe aortic stenosis.

➤*Hyperkalemia:* May occur in patients on angiotensin II receptor blockers, especially in patients with advanced renal impairment, heart failure, on renal replacement therapy, or those on potassium supplements, potassium-sparing diuretics, potassium-containing salt substitutes, or other drugs that increase potassium levels.

➤*Hypotension / Volume-depleted patients:* Symptomatic hypotension may occur after initiation of telmisartan in patients who are intravascularly volume-depleted (eg, those treated with diuretics). Correct these conditions prior to administration of telmisartan or start treatment under close medical supervision.

➤*Renal function impairment:* In patients whose renal function may depend on the activity of the renin-angiotensin-aldosterone system (eg, patients with severe CHF or renal dysfunction), telmisartan treatment may be associated with oliguria and/or progressive azotemia, which may rarely result in acute renal failure and death.

➤*Hepatic function impairment:* Use with caution; not recommended as initial therapy in patients with hepatic impairment.

➤*Pregnancy: Category C* (first trimester); *Category D* (second and third trimester). Drugs that act directly on the renin-angiotensin system can cause fetal and neonatal morbidity and death when administered to pregnant women. Several dozen cases have been reported in the world literature in patients who were taking angiotensin-converting enzyme inhibitors. When pregnancy is detected, discontinue the medication as soon as possible.

➤*Lactation:* Undetermined. Because the molecular weight (515 for telmisartan) and (about 567 for the amlodipine besylate salt) is low enough, excretion into human breast milk should be expected. The effects of this exposure on a nursing infant are unknown.

➤*Children:* Safety and efficacy not established.

➤*Elderly:* Reduced initial dosage of amlodipine is required in patients 75 years of age and older. Use as initial therapy is not recommended in these patients.

➤*Monitoring:* Monitor blood pressure at regular intervals during therapy. Assess renal function in heart failure and post-MI patients. Periodically monitor serum electrolytes to detect possible electrolyte imbalances. Closely monitor patients with heart failure.

Drug Interactions

➤*Azole antifungals (eg, itraconazole, ketoconazole), conivaptan, diltiazem, protease inhibitors (eg, ritonavir):* Amlodipine plasma concentrations may be elevated, increasing the pharmacologic effects and adverse reactions.

➤*Clopidogrel:* Platelet inhibition may be reduced by coadministration with amlodipine.

➤*Cyclosporine:* Plasma levels and pharmacologic effects may be increased by amlodipine.

➤*Digoxin:* Telmisartan may increase plasma levels of digoxin, increasing toxicity. Monitor digoxin levels when initiating, adjusting, or discontinuing telmisartan.

➤*Lithium:* Plasma concentrations may be elevated by telmisartan, increasing the pharmacologic and toxic effects of lithium. Monitor lithium serum levels.

➤*Potassium-sparing diuretics (eg, spironolactone), potassium supplements:* Coadministration with telmisartan may cause elevated potassium concentrations and, in heart failure patients, increased serum creatinine. Amlodipine plasma concentrations may be elevated.

➤*Ramipril:* Increases ramipril exposure and possibly increases incidence of renal impairment; coadministration of telmisartan and ramipril is not recommended.

➤*Drug / Lab test interactions:* None well documented.

Adverse Reactions

➤*Cardiovascular:* Orthostatic hypotension (6%); atrial fibrillation, BP increased, bradycardia, CHF, MI, syncope (postmarketing).

➤*CNS:* Dizziness (3%); headache (1%).

➤*GI:* Diarrhea (3%).

➤*GU:* Erectile dysfunction, renal impairment including acute renal failure, urinary tract infection (postmarketing).

➤*Hematologic:* Anemia, eosinophilia, thrombocytopenia (postmarketing).

➤*Metabolic:* Peripheral edema (5%).

➤*Respiratory:* Upper respiratory tract infection (7%); sinusitis (3%); pharyngitis (1%).

➤*Miscellaneous:* Back pain (3%).

Overdosage

➤*Symptoms:* Bradycardia, dizziness, hypotension, peripheral vasodilation, tachycardia.

Patient Information

Advise patient to take once daily as prescribed without regard to meals, but to take with food if GI upset occurs.

Inform patient that drug controls, but does not cure, hypertension and to continue taking drug as prescribed even when blood pressure is not elevated.

Instruct patient to avoid the use of supplements or salt substitutes containing potassium without first consulting health care provider.

Advise patient to monitor and record blood pressure and pulse at home and to inform health care provider if abnormal measurements are noted.

Caution patient to avoid sudden position changes to prevent orthostatic hypotension.

Inform women of childbearing age to report pregnancy to health care provider as soon as possible.

Advise women not to breast-feed while taking this medication.

AGENTS FOR PHEOCHROMOCYTOMA

PHENTOLAMINE MESYLATE

Rx	**Phentolamine Mesylate** (Bedford Laboratories)	**Injection, lyophilized powder for solution:** 5 mg	Mannitol. In 2 mL vials.
Rx	**OraVerse** (Novalar Pharmaceuticals)	**Injection; solution:** 0.4 mg per 1.7 mL	Preservative free. D-mannitol, edetate disodium. In dental cartridge.

PHENTOLAMINE MESYLATE — INJECTION

Indications

➤*Dermal necrosis from norepinephrine extravasation:* For the prevention or treatment of dermal necrosis and sloughing following intravenous (IV) administration or extravasation of norepinephrine.

➤*Hypertensive episodes in patients with pheochromocytoma (excluding OraVerse):* For the prevention or control of hypertensive episodes that may occur in patients with pheochromocytoma as a result of stress or manipulation during preoperative preparation and surgical excision.

➤*Pheochromocytoma diagnosis (excluding OraVerse):* For the diagnosis of pheochromocytoma by the phentolamine blocking test.

➤*Reversal of soft-tissue anesthesia (OraVerse only):* Reversal of the soft-tissue anesthesia (ie, anesthesia of the lip and tongue) and the associated functional deficits resulting from intraoral submucosal injection of a local anesthetic containing a vasoconstrictor.

Phentolamine is not recommended for use in children younger than 6 years of age or who weigh less than 15 kg (33 lbs).

➤*Off-label uses:* Phentolamine has been used to treat hypertensive crises secondary to monoamine oxidase inhibitor/sympathomimetic amine interactions and rebound hypertension on withdrawal of clonidine, propranolol, or other antihypertensives. It has also been used in combination with papaverine as an intracavernous injection for impotence.

Administration and Dosage

➤*General dosing considerations:* The recommended dose of *OraVerse* is based on the number of cartridges of local anesthetic with vasoconstrictor administered.

OraVerse should be administered following the dental procedure using the same location(s) and technique(s) (infiltration or block injection) employed for the administration of the local anesthetic.

The diagnosis of pheochromocytoma (phentolamine blocking test) is not to be performed on a patient who is normotensive.

For the diagnosis of pheochromocytoma (phentolamine blocking test), the patient should be kept at rest in a supine position throughout the test, preferably in a quiet, darkened room.

➤*Adults:*

Dermal necrosis from norepinephrine extravasation (excluding OraVerse) –

Prevention: Phentolamine 10 mg is added to each liter of solution containing norepinephrine. The pressor effect of norepinephrine is not affected.

Treatment: Phentolamine 5 to 10 mg in 10 mL of saline is injected into the area of extravasation within 12 hours.

Hypertensive episodes in patients with pheochromocytoma (excluding OraVerse) –

Preoperative: 5 mg IV or intramuscularly (IM) 1 or 2 hours before surgery and repeated if necessary.

PHENTOLAMINE MESYLATE — INJECTION

Surgery: 5 mg IV during surgery to help prevent or control paroxysms of hypertension, tachycardia, respiratory depression, convulsions, or other effects of epinephrine intoxication.

Postoperatively, norepinephrine may be given to control the hypotension that commonly follows complete removal of a pheochromocytoma.

Pheochromocytoma diagnosis (phentolamine blocking test [excluding OraVerse]) – The test is most reliable in detecting pheochromocytoma in patients with sustained hypertension and least reliable in those with paroxysmal hypertension. False-positive tests may occur in patients with hypertension without pheochromocytoma.

Usual dosage: 5 mg IV or IM.

Concomitant therapy: Sedatives, analgesics, and all other medications except those that might be deemed essential (ie, digitalis, insulin) are withheld for at least 24 hours, and preferably 48 to 72 hours, prior to the test. Antihypertensive drugs are withheld until blood pressure returns to the untreated, hypertensive level.

Interpretation of phentolamine blocking test: A positive response after IV administration, suggestive of pheochromocytoma, is indicated when the blood pressure is reduced more than 35 mm Hg systolic and 25 mm Hg diastolic. A typical positive response is a reduction in pressure of 60 mm Hg systolic and 25 mm Hg diastolic. Usually, maximal effect is evident within 2 minutes after injection. A return to preinjection pressure commonly occurs within 15 to 30 minutes but may occur more rapidly.

A positive response after IM administration is indicated when the blood pressure is reduced 35 mm Hg systolic and 25 mm Hg diastolic, or more, within 20 minutes following injection.

If blood pressure decreases to a dangerous level, the patient should be treated as outlined in Overdosage.

A positive response should always be confirmed by other diagnostic procedures, preferably by measurement of urinary catecholamines or their metabolites.

A negative response is indicated when the blood pressure is elevated, unchanged, or reduced less than 35 mm Hg systolic and 25 mm Hg diastolic after injection of phentolamine. A negative response to this test does not exclude the diagnosis of pheochromocytoma, especially in patients with paroxysmal hypertension in whom the incidence of false-negative responses is high.

Reversal of soft-tissue anesthesia (OraVerse only) –

Phentolamine Recommended Dosage

Amount of local anesthetic administered	Dose of phentolamine (mg)	Dose of phentolamine (cartridge)
½ cartridge	0.2 mg	½ cartridge
1 cartridge	0.4 mg	1 cartridge
2 cartridges	0.8 mg	2 cartridges

➤*Children:*

Hypertensive episodes in patients with pheochromocytoma (excluding OraVerse) –

Preoperative: 1 mg IV or IM 1 or 2 hours before surgery and repeated if necessary.

Surgery: 1 mg IV during surgery to help prevent or control paroxysms of hypertension, tachycardia, respiratory depression, convulsions, or other effects of epinephrine intoxication.

Postoperatively, norepinephrine may be given to control the hypotension that commonly follows complete removal of a pheochromocytoma.

Pheochromocytoma diagnosis (excluding OraVerse) – 1 mg IV or 3 mg IM.

Reversal of soft-tissue anesthesia (OraVerse only) –

More than 30 kg and 6 years of age and older:

• *Usual dosage* – See Adults for dosing.

• *Maximum dose* – A dose of more than 0.4 mg (1 cartridge) has not been studied in children younger than 12 years of age.

15 to 30 kg and 6 years of age and older:

• *Maximum dose* – ½ cartridge (0.2 mg).

➤*Preparation for administration:*

Diagnosis of pheochromocytoma – For IV or IM administration, dissolve 5 mg in 1 mL of sterile water for injection.

➤*Administration:* May be administered IV (excluding *OraVerse*), IM (excluding *OraVerse*), or by submucosal oral injection (*OraVerse* only).

Diagnosis of pheochromocytoma (phentolamine blocking test) – The syringe needle is inserted into the vein, and injection is delayed until pressor response to venipuncture has subsided. Phentolamine is injected rapidly.

Blood pressure is recorded immediately after IV administration, at 30-second intervals for the first 3 minutes, and at 60-second intervals for the next 7 minutes.

Blood pressure is recorded every 5 minutes for 30 to 45 minutes following IM administration.

➤*Storage/Stability:* Store at controlled room temperature, 15° to 30°C (59° to 86°F).

The reconstituted solution should be used upon preparation and should not be stored.

OraVerse – Store at controlled room temperature, 20° to 25°C (68° to 77°F), with brief excursions permitted between 15° and 30°C (59° and 86°F). Protect from direct heat and light. Do not allow to freeze.

Actions

➤*Pharmacology:* Phentolamine produces an alpha-adrenergic block of relatively short duration, resulting in vasodilatation when applied to vascular smooth muscle. It also has direct, but less marked, positive inotropic and chronotropic effects on cardiac muscle and vasodilator effects on vascular smooth muscle.

The mechanism by which *OraVerse* accelerates reversal of soft-tissue anesthesia and the associated functional deficits is not fully understood.

➤*Pharmacokinetics:*

Absorption – Following *OraVerse* administration, phentolamine is 100% available from the submucosal injection site, and peak concentrations are achieved 10 to 20 minutes after injection. Phentolamine systemic exposure increased linearly after 0.8 mg compared with 0.4 mg of phentolamine intraoral submucosal injection.

Metabolism/Excretion – Phentolamine has a half-life in the blood of 19 minutes following IV administration. The terminal elimination half-life of *OraVerse* in the blood was approximately 2 to 3 hours. Approximately 13% of a single IV dose appears in the urine as unchanged drug.

Special populations –

Children: Following *OraVerse* administration, the phentolamine maximal drug concentration (C_{max}) was higher (approximately 3.5-fold) in children who weighed between 15 and 30 kg (33 and 66 lbs) than in children who weighed more than 30 kg. However, phentolamine AUC was similar between the 2 groups. It is recommended that in children weighing 15 to 30 kg, the maximum dose of phentolamine be limited to ½ cartridge (0.2 mg).

The pharmacokinetics of phentolamine in adults and children who weighed more than 30 kg (66 lbs) are similar after intraoral submucosal injection.

Phentolamine has not been studied in children younger than 3 years of age or weighing less than 15 kg (33 lbs). The pharmacokinetics of phentolamine after administration of more than 1 cartridge (0.4 mg) have not been studied in children.

Contraindications

Myocardial infarction (MI), history of MI, coronary insufficiency, angina, or other evidence suggestive of coronary artery disease; hypersensitivity to phentolamine or related compounds.

➤*OraVerse*: None known.

Warnings/Precautions

➤*Cardiovascular events:* MI, cerebrovascular spasm, and cerebrovascular occlusion have been reported to occur following the administration of phentolamine, usually in association with marked hypotensive episodes producing shock-like states.

Tachycardia and cardiac arrhythmias may occur with the use of phentolamine or other alpha-adrenergic blocking agents. When possible, administration of cardiac glycosides should be deferred until cardiac rhythm returns to normal.

➤*Diagnosis of pheochromocytoma:* For screening tests in patients with hypertension, the generally available urinary assay of catecholamines or other biochemical assays have largely replaced the phentolamine and other pharmacological tests for reasons of accuracy and safety. None of the chemical or pharmacological tests is infallible in the diagnosis of pheochromocytoma. The phentolamine blocking test is not the procedure of choice and should be reserved for cases in which additional confirmatory evidence is necessary and the relative risks involved in conducting the test have been considered.

➤*Pregnancy: Category C.* There are no adequate and well-controlled studies in pregnant women. Phentolamine has been used for the short-term management of severe hypertension caused by pheochromocytoma, including those cases occurring during surgery to deliver the fetus or to resect the tumor. No adverse effects on the fetus or newborn attributable to phentolamine from this use have been reported, but fetal hypoxia is a potential complication. Use phentolamine during pregnancy only if the potential benefit justifies the potential risk to the fetus.

Teratogenic – Administration of phentolamine to pregnant rats and mice at oral doses 24 to 30 times the usual daily human dose (based on a 60 kg human) resulted in slightly decreased growth and slight skeletal immaturity of the fetuses. Immaturity was manifested by increased incidence of incomplete or unossified calcanei and phalangeal nuclei of the hind limb and of incompletely ossified sternebrae. At oral doses at least 60 times the usual daily human dose (based on a 60 kg human), a slightly lower rate of implantation was found in rats.

Phentolamine did not affect embryonic or fetal development in rabbits at oral doses 20 times the usual daily human dose (based on a 60 kg human). No teratogenic or embryotoxic effects were observed in the rat, mouse, or rabbit studies.

➤*Lactation:* It is not known whether this drug is excreted in human milk. Because many drugs are excreted in human milk and because of the potential for serious adverse reactions in breast-feeding infants from phentolamine, decide whether to discontinue breast-feeding or the drug, taking into account the importance of the drug to the mother. Weigh the unknown risks of limited infant exposure to phentolamine through breast milk following a single maternal dose against the known benefits of breast-feeding.

➤*Children:* In clinical studies, children between 3 and 17 years of age received *OraVerse*. The safety and effectiveness of *OraVerse* have been established in children 6 to 17 years of age. Effectiveness in children younger than 6 years of age has not been established. Use of *OraVerse* in patients between 6 and 17 years of age is supported by evidence from adequate and well-controlled studies of *OraVerse* in adults, with additional adequate and

PHENTOLAMINE MESYLATE — INJECTION

well-controlled studies of *OraVerse* in children 12 to 17 years of age (studies 1 [mandibular procedures] and 2 [maxillary procedures]) and 6 to 11 years of age (study 3 [mandibular and maxillary procedures]). The safety, but not the efficacy, of *OraVerse* has been evaluated in children younger than 6 years of age. Dosages in children may need to be limited based on body weight.

➤*Elderly:* Of the total number of patients in clinical studies of *OraVerse*, 55 were 65 years of age and older, while 21 were 75 years of age and older. No overall differences in safety or effectiveness were observed between these patients and younger patients, and other reported clinical experience has not identified differences in responses between elderly and younger patients, but greater sensitivity of some older individuals cannot be ruled out.

Drug Interactions

None known.

Adverse Reactions

➤*OraVerse*: In clinical trials, the most common adverse reaction with phentolamine that was greater than the control group was injection-site pain.

Dental patients were administered a dose of phentolamine 0.2, 0.4, or 0.8 mg. The majority of adverse reactions were mild and resolved within 48 hours. There were no serious adverse reactions and no discontinuations because of adverse reactions.

Phentolamine Adverse Reactions (≥ 3%)

Adverse reaction	Phentolamine 0.2 mg (n = 83)	0.4 mg (n = 284)	0.8 mg (n = 51)	Total (n = 418)	Control Total (n = 359)
Patients with adverse reactions	18%	29%	39%	28%	27%
Cardiovascular					
Bradycardia	0%	2%	4%	2%	0.3%
Tachycardia	0%	6%	4%	5%	6%
Miscellaneous					
Headache	0%	4%	6%	3%	4%
Injection-site pain	6%	5%	4%	5%	4%
Postprocedural pain	4%	6%	10%	6%	6%

Oral pain – Results from the pain assessments in studies 1 and 2, involving mandibular and maxillary procedures, respectively, indicated that the majority of dental patients in the phentolamine and control groups experienced no or mild oral pain, with less than 10% of patients in each group reporting moderate oral pain, with a similar distribution between the phentolamine and control groups. No patient experienced severe pain in theses studies.

Less common adverse reactions (less than 3%) – Adverse reactions reported by less than 3% but at least 2 dental patients receiving phentolamine and occurring at a greater incidence than those receiving control included diarrhea, facial swelling, increased blood pressure/hypertension, injection-site reactions, jaw pain, oral pain, paresthesia, pruritus, tenderness, upper abdominal pain, and vomiting. The majority of these adverse reactions were mild and resolved within 48 hours. The few reports of paresthesia were mild and transient and resolved during the same time period.

➤*Postmarketing:*

Cardiovascular – Acute and prolonged hypotensive episodes, cardiac arrhythmias, flushing, orthostatic hypotension, tachycardia.

CNS – Dizziness, weakness.

GI – Diarrhea, nausea, vomiting.

Miscellaneous – Nasal stuffiness.

Overdosage

➤*Symptoms:* Overdosage with phentolamine is characterized chiefly by cardiovascular disturbances, such as arrhythmias, tachycardia, hypotension, and possibly shock. In addition, the following might occur: excitation, headache, sweating, pupillary contraction, visual disturbances; nausea, vomiting, diarrhea; hypoglycemia.

No deaths because of acute poisoning with phentolamine have been reported. Oral median lethal dose (LD_{50}) in mice is 1,000 mg/kg; in rats, it is 1,250 mg/kg.

➤*Treatment:* There is no specific antidote.

Treat a decrease in blood pressure to dangerous levels or other evidence of shock-like conditions vigorously and promptly. Keep the patient's legs raised and administer a plasma expander. If necessary, include IV infusion or norepinephrine, titrated to maintain blood pressure at the normotensive level, and all available supportive measures. Do not use epinephrine because it may cause a paradoxical reduction in blood pressure.

Patient Information

Instruct patients to avoid sudden position changes to prevent orthostatic hypotension.

Instruct patients to notify their health care provider if chest pain develops during infusion.

Advise patients to report the following symptoms to their health care provider: dizziness, fainting spells, or weakness.

PHENOXYBENZAMINE HYDROCHLORIDE

Rx	**Dibenzyline** (Wellspring)	**Capsules:** 10 mg	(SKF E33). Red. In 100s

PHENOXYBENZAMINE HYDROCHLORIDE— ORAL

Indications

➤*Pheochromocytoma:* Pheochromocytoma, to control episodes of hypertension and sweating. If tachycardia is excessive, it may be necessary to use a beta-blocking agent concomitantly.

➤*Off-label uses:*

Benign prostatic hyperplasia – [5] = Poor documentation. The use of phenoxybenzamine for the management of benign prostatic hyperplasia (BPH) cannot be recommended at this time based on limited published data, its adverse effect profile, and the availability of other effective agents approved for this indication. American Urological Association guidelines on the management of BPH state that data are insufficient to support a recommendation for the use of phenoxybenzamine as treatment of lower urinary tract symptoms secondary to BPH.

Administration and Dosage

➤*General dosing considerations:* The dosage should be adjusted to fit the needs of each patient. Small initial doses should be slowly increased until the desired effect is obtained or the side effects from blockade become troublesome. After each increase, the patient should be observed on that level before instituting another increase. The dosage should be carried to a point where symptomatic relief or objective improvements are obtained, but not so high that the adverse effects from blockade become troublesome.

➤*Adults:*

Pheochromocytoma –

Initial dosage: 10 mg twice a day.

Dosage titration: Dosage should be increased every other day, usually to 20 to 40 mg 2 or 3 times a day, until an optimal dosage is obtained, as judged by blood pressure control.

Off-label dosing –

➤*Storage / Stability:* Store between 15° and 30°C (59° and 86°F).

Actions

➤*Pharmacology:* Phenoxybenzamine hydrochloride is a long-acting, adrenergic, alpha-receptor blocking agent which can produce and maintain chemical sympathectomy by oral administration. It increases blood flow to the skin, mucosa and abdominal viscera, and lowers both supine and erect blood pressures. It has no effect on the parasympathetic system.

➤*Pharmacokinetics:*

Absorption / Distribution – Twenty percent to 30% of orally administered phenoxybenzamine appears to be absorbed in the active form.

The half-life of orally administered phenoxybenzamine hydrochloride is not known; however, the half-life of IV administered drug is ≈ 24 hours. Demonstrable effects with IV administration persist for at least 3 to 4 days, and the effects of daily administration are cumulative for nearly a week.

Contraindications

Conditions where a fall in blood pressure may be undesirable.

Warnings/Precautions

➤*Hypotension:* Phenoxybenzamine-induced alpha-adrenergic blockade leaves beta-adrenergic receptors unopposed. Compounds that stimulate both types of receptors may therefore produce an exaggerated hypotensive response and tachycardia.

➤*Special risk:* Administer with caution in patients with marked cerebral or coronary arteriosclerosis or renal damage. Adrenergic-blocking effect may aggravate symptoms of respiratory infections.

➤*Pregnancy: Category C.*

Teratogenic – Adequate reproductive studies have not been performed with phenoxybenzamine hydrochloride. It is also not known whether phenoxybenzamine hydrochloride can cause fetal harm when administered to a pregnant woman. Phenoxybenzamine should be given to a pregnant woman only if clearly needed.

➤*Lactation:* It is not known whether this drug is excreted in human milk. Because many drugs are excreted in human milk, and because of the potential for serious adverse reactions from phenoxybenzamine hydrochloride, a decision should be made whether to discontinue breast-feeding or the drug, taking into account the importance of the drug to the mother.

➤*Children:* Safety and efficacy in children have not been established.

Drug Interactions

Phenoxybenzamine hydrochloride may interact with compounds that stimulate both alpha- and beta-adrenergic receptors (ie, epinephrine) to produce an exaggerated hypotensive response and tachycardia.

PHENOXYBENZAMINE HYDROCHLORIDE— ORAL

Phenoxybenzamine blocks hyperthermia production by levarterenol and blocks hypothermia production by reserpine.

Adverse Reactions

The following adverse reactions have been observed, but there are insufficient data to support an estimate of their frequency.

➤*CNS:*

Autonomic nervous system – Postural hypotension, tachycardia, inhibition of ejaculation, nasal congestion, miosis.

➤*Miscellaneous:* GI irritation, drowsiness, fatigue.

These so-called side effects are actually evidence of adrenergic blockade and vary according to the degree of blockade.

Overdosage

➤*Symptoms:* These are largely the result of block of the sympathetic nervous system and of the circulating epinephrine. They may include the following: postural hypotension resulting in dizziness or fainting; tachycardia, particularly postural; vomiting; lethargy; shock.

➤*Treatment:* When symptoms and signs of overdosage exist, discontinue the drug. Treatment of circulatory failure, if present, is a prime consideration. In cases of mild overdosage, recumbent position with legs elevated usually restores cerebral circulation. In the more severe cases, the usual measures to combat shock should be instituted. Usual pressor agents are not effective. Epinephrine is contraindicated because it stimulates both alpha and beta receptors; since alpha receptors are blocked, the net effect of epinephrine administration is vasodilation and a further drop in blood pressure (epinephrine reversal).

The patient may have to be kept flat for 24 hours or more in the case of overdose, as the effect of the drug is prolonged. Leg bandages and an abdominal binder may shorten the period of disability.

IV infusion of levarterenol bitartrate may be used to combat severe hypotensive reactions, because it stimulates alpha receptors primarily. Although phenoxybenzamine hydrochloride is an alpha-adrenergic blocking agent, a sufficient dose of levarterenol bitartrate will overcome this effect.

The oral LD_{50} for phenoxybenzamine is approximately 2,000 mg/kg in rats and approximately 500 mg/kg in guinea pigs.

METYROSINE

Rx	**Demser** (Aton Pharma)	**Capsules; oral:** 250 mg	(MSD 690 DEMSER). Two-tone blue. In 100s.

METYROSINE — ORAL

Indications

➤*Pheochromocytoma:* Metyrosine is indicated in the treatment of patients with pheochromocytoma for:

1.) Preoperative preparation of patients for surgery.
2.) Management of patients when surgery is contraindicated.
3.) Chronic treatment of patients with malignant pheochromocytoma.

Administration and Dosage

➤*Adults:*

Pheochromocytoma –

Usual dosage: 2 and 3 g/day in divided doses.

Maximum dose: 4 g/day in divided doses.

Initial dosage: 250 mg orally 4 times daily.

Dosage titration: The dose may be increased by 250 to 500 mg every day to a maximum of 4 g/day in divided doses. Optimally effective dosages usually are between 2 and 3 g/day, and the dose should be titrated by monitoring clinical symptoms and catecholamine excretion. In patients who are hypertensive, dosage should be titrated to achieve normalization of blood pressure and control of clinical symptoms. In patients who are usually normotensive, dosage should be titrated to the amount that will reduce urinary metanephrines and/or vanillylmandelic acid by 50% or more.

Duration of therapy: When used for preoperative preparation, the optimally effective dosage of metyrosine should be given for at least 5 to 7 days.

Concomitant therapy: If patients are not adequately controlled by the use of metyrosine, an alpha-adrenergic blocking agent (phenoxybenzamine) should be added.

➤*Children:*

Pheochromocytoma – See Adults for dosing for children 12 years of age and older.

Actions

➤*Pharmacology:* Metyrosine inhibits tyrosine hydroxylase, which catalyzes the first transformation in catecholamine biosynthesis (ie, the conversion of tyrosine to dihydroxyphenylalanine [DOPA]). Because the first step is also the rate-limiting step, blockade of tyrosine hydroxylase activity results in decreased endogenous levels of catecholamines, usually measured as decreased urinary excretion of catecholamines and their metabolites.

In patients with pheochromocytoma, who produce excessive amounts of norepinephrine and epinephrine, administration of 1 to 4 g of metyrosine per day has reduced catecholamine biosynthesis from approximately 35% to 80% as measured by the total excretion of catecholamines and their metabolites (metanephrine and vanillylmandelic acid). The maximum biochemical effect usually occurs within 2 to 3 days, and the urinary concentration of catecholamines and their metabolites usually returns to pretreatment levels within 3 to 4 days after metyrosine is discontinued. In some patients the total excretion of catecholamines and catecholamine metabolites may be lowered to normal or near normal levels (less than 10 mg per 24 hours). In most patients the duration of treatment has been 2 to 8 weeks, but several patients have received metyrosine for periods of 1 to 10 years.

Most patients with pheochromocytoma treated with metyrosine experience decreased frequency and severity of hypertensive attacks with their associated headache, nausea, sweating, and tachycardia. In patients who respond, blood pressure decreases progressively during the first 2 days of therapy with metyrosine; after withdrawal, blood pressure usually increases gradually to pretreatment values within 2 to 3 days.

➤*Pharmacokinetics:* Metyrosine is well absorbed from the GI tract. From 53% to 88% (mean 69%) was recovered in the urine as unchanged drug following maintenance oral doses of 600 to 4,000 mg per 24 hours in patients with pheochromocytoma or essential hypertension. Less than 1% of the dose was recovered as catechol metabolites. These metabolites are probably not present in sufficient amounts to contribute to the biochemical effects of metyrosine. The quantities excreted, however, are sufficient to interfere with accurate determination of urinary catecholamines determined by routine techniques.

Plasma half-life of metyrosine determined over an 8-hour period after single oral doses was 3 to 3.7 hours in 3 patients.

Contraindications

Known hypersensitivity to this compound.

Warnings/Precautions

➤*Maintain fluid volume during and after surgery:* When metyrosine is used preoperatively, alone or especially in combination with alpha-adrenergic blocking drugs, adequate intravascular volume must be maintained intraoperatively (especially after tumor removal) and postoperatively to avoid hypotension and decreased perfusion of vital organs resulting from vasodilatation and expanded volume capacity. Following tumor removal, large volumes of plasma may be needed to maintain blood pressure and central venous pressure within the normal range.

In addition, life-threatening arrhythmias may occur during anesthesia and surgery, and may require treatment with a beta-blocker or lidocaine. During surgery, patients should have continuous monitoring of blood pressure and electrocardiogram.

➤*Intraoperative effects:* While the preoperative use of metyrosine in patients with pheochromocytoma is thought to decrease intraoperative problems with blood pressure control, metyrosine does not eliminate the danger of hypertensive crises or arrhythmias during manipulation of the tumor, and the alpha-adrenergic blocking drug, phentolamine, may be needed.

➤*Interaction with alcohol:* Metyrosine may add to the sedative effects of alcohol and other CNS depressants (eg, hypnotics, sedatives, tranquilizers).

➤*Long-term use:* The total human experience with the drug is quite limited and few patients have been studied long-term. Chronic animal studies have not been carried out. Therefore, suitable laboratory tests should be carried out periodically in patients requiring prolonged use of metyrosine and caution should be observed in patients with impaired hepatic or renal function.

➤*Metyrosine crystalluria:* Crystalluria and urolithiasis have been found in dogs treated with metyrosine at doses similar to those used in humans, and crystalluria has also been observed in a few patients. To minimize the risk of crystalluria, patients should be urged to maintain water intake sufficient to achieve a daily urine volume of more than 2,000 mL, particularly when doses more than 2 g/day are given. Routine examination of the urine should be carried out. Metyrosine will crystallize as needles or rods. If metyrosine crystalluria occurs, fluid intake should be increased further. If crystalluria persists, the dosage should be reduced or the drug discontinued.

➤*Hazardous tasks:* When receiving metyrosine, patients should be warned about engaging in activities requiring mental alertness and motor coordination, such as driving a motor vehicle or operating machinery. metyrosine may have additive sedative effects with alcohol and other CNS depressants (eg, hypnotics, sedatives, tranquilizers).

➤*Pregnancy: Category C.* Animal reproduction studies have not been conducted with metyrosine. It is also not known whether metyrosine can cause fetal harm when administered to a pregnant woman or can affect reproduction capacity. Metyrosine should be given to a pregnant woman only if clearly needed.

➤*Lactation:* It is not known whether metyrosine is excreted in human milk. Because many drugs are excreted in human milk, caution should be exercised when metyrosine is administered to a nursing woman.

➤*Children:* Safety and efficacy in children younger than 12 years of age have not been established.

Drug Interactions

Caution should be observed in administering metyrosine to patients receiving phenothiazines or haloperidol because the extrapyramidal effects of these drugs can be expected to be potentiated by inhibition of catecholamine synthesis.

Concurrent use of metyrosine with alcohol or other CNS depressants can increase their sedative effects.

METYROSINE — ORAL

➤*Drug/Lab test interactions:* Spurious increases in urinary catecholamines may be observed in patients receiving metyrosine due to the presence of metabolites of the drug.

Adverse Reactions

➤*CNS:*

Sedation – The most common adverse reaction to metyrosine is moderate to severe sedation, which has been observed in almost all patients. It occurs at both low and high dosages. Sedative effects begin within the first 24 hours of therapy, are maximal after 2 to 3 days, and tend to wane during the next few days. Sedation usually is not obvious after 1 week unless the dosage is increased, but at dosages more than 2,000 mg/day some degree of sedation or fatigue may persist.

In most patients who experience sedation, temporary changes in sleep pattern occur following withdrawal of the drug. Changes consist of insomnia that may last for 2 or 3 days and feelings of increased alertness and ambition. Even patients who do not experience sedation while on metyrosine may report symptoms of psychic stimulation when the drug is discontinued.

Extrapyramidal signs – Extrapyramidal signs such as drooling, speech difficulty, and tremor have been reported in approximately 10% of patients. These occasionally have been accompanied by trismus and frank parkinsonism.

Anxiety and psychic disturbances – Anxiety and psychic disturbances such as depression, hallucinations, disorientation, and confusion may occur. These effects seem to be dose dependent and may disappear with reduction of dosage.

➤*GI:* Diarrhea occurs in approximately 10% of patients and may be severe. Antidiarrheal agents may be required if continuation of metyrosine is necessary.

➤*Miscellaneous:* Infrequently, slight swelling of the breast, galactorrhea, nasal stuffiness, decreased salivation, dry mouth, headache, nausea, vomiting, abdominal pain, and impotence or failure of ejaculation may occur. Crystalluria and transient dysuria and hematuria have been observed in a few patients. Hematologic disorders (including eosinophilia, anemia, thrombocytopenia, and thrombocytosis), increased AST levels, peripheral edema, and hypersensitivity reactions such as urticaria and pharyngeal edema have been reported rarely.

Overdosage

➤*Symptoms:* Signs of metyrosine overdosage include those central nervous system effects observed in some patients even at low dosages.

At doses exceeding 2,000 mg/day, some degree of sedation or feeling of fatigue may persist. Doses of 2,000 to 4,000 mg/day can result in anxiety or agitated depression, neuromuscular effects (including fine tremor of the hands, gross tremor of the trunk, tightening of the jaw with trismus), diarrhea, and decreased salivation with dry mouth.

➤*Treatment:* Reduction of drug dose or cessation of treatment results in the disappearance of these symptoms.

The acute toxicity of metyrosine was 442 mg/kg and 752 mg/kg in the female mouse and rat respectively.

Patient Information

Patients should be advised to maintain a liberal fluid intake.

When receiving metyrosine, patients should be warned about engaging in activities requiring mental alertness and motor coordination, such as driving a motor vehicle or operating machinery. metyrosine may have additive sedative effects with alcohol and other CNS depressants (eg, hypnotics, sedatives, tranquilizers).

AGENTS FOR HYPERTENSIVE EMERGENCIES

NITROPRUSSIDE SODIUM

Rx	**Sodium Nitroprusside** (Various)	**Powder for Injection**: 50 mg per vial	In single dose 5 mL vials.
Rx	**Nitropress** (Hospira)		In single dose 2 mL Fliptop Vials.

NITROPRUSSIDE SODIUM — INJECTION

WARNING

After reconstitution, nitroprusside is not suitable for direct injection. The reconstituted solution must be further diluted in dextrose 5% injection before infusion.

Nitroprusside can cause precipitous decreases in blood pressure. In patients not properly monitored, these decreases can lead to irreversible ischemic injuries or death. Use only when available equipment and personnel allow blood pressure to be continuously monitored.

Except when used briefly or at low (less than 2 mcg/kg/min) infusion rates, nitroprusside injection gives rise to important quantities of cyanide ion, which can reach toxic, potentially lethal levels. The usual dose rate is 0.5 to 10 mcg/kg/min, but infusion at the maximum dose rates should never last more than 10 minutes. If blood pressure has not been adequately controlled after 10 minutes of infusion at the maximum rate, terminate administration immediately.

Although acid-base balance and venous oxygen concentration should be monitored and may indicate cyanide toxicity, these laboratory tests provide imperfect guidance.

Indications

➤*Hypertensive crises:* Immediate reduction of blood pressure of patients in hypertensive crises. Administer concomitant longer-acting antihypertensive medication so that the duration of treatment with nitroprusside can be minimized.

➤*Bleeding reduction during surgery:* Production of controlled hypotension in order to reduce bleeding during surgery.

➤*Acute congestive heart failure (CHF):* For use in acute congestive heart failure.

➤*Off-label uses:* Myocardial infarction with coadministration of dopamine; left ventricular failure with coadministration of oxygen, morphine and a loop diuretic.

Administration and Dosage

➤*Maximum dose:* 10 mcg/kg/min IV for the approved indications according to the prescribing information.

➤*General dosing considerations:* While the average effective rate is about 3 mcg/kg/min, some patients will become dangerously hypotensive at this rate. Therefore, start at a very low rate with gradual upward titration.

Do not infuse through ordinary IV apparatus regulated only by gravity and mechanical clamps. (See Administration.)

The blood pressure must be continuously monitored. (See Monitoring.)

When more than 500 mcg/kg of nitroprusside is administered faster than 2 mcg/kg/min, cyanide is generated faster than the unaided patient can eliminate it.

Rare patients receiving more than 10 mg/kg of nitroprusside will develop methemoglobinemia; other patients, especially those with impaired renal function, will predictably develop thiocyanate toxicity after prolonged, rapid infusions. Test patients for these toxicities.

➤*Adults:*

Acute congestive heart failure –

Usual dosage: 3 mcg/kg/min IV. Some patients require much lower doses, especially if other hypotensive agents are used.

Maximum dose: 10 mcg/kg/min IV.

Initial dosage: 0.3 mcg/kg/min IV. Titrate upward gradually every few minutes until desired effect is achieved or the maximum dose is reached.

Dosage titration: Titrate by increasing the infusion rate until measured cardiac output is no longer increasing, systemic blood pressure cannot be further reduced without compromising the perfusion of vital organs, or the maximum recommended infusion rate has been reached, whichever comes earliest.

Bleeding reduction during surgery –

Usual dosage: 3 mcg/kg/min IV. Some patients require much lower doses, especially if other hypotensive agents are used.

Maximum dose: 10 mcg/kg/min IV.

Initial dosage: 0.3 mcg/kg/min IV. Titrate upward gradually every few minutes until desired effect is achieved or the maximum dose is reached.

Hypertensive crises –

Usual dosage: 3 mcg/kg/min IV. Some patients require much lower doses, especially if other hypotensive agents are used.

Maximum dose: 10 mcg/kg/min IV.

Initial dosage: 0.3 mcg/kg/min IV. Titrate upward gradually every few minutes until desired effect is achieved or the maximum dose is reached.

➤*Children:*

Acute congestive heart failure –

Usual dosage: 3 mcg/kg/min IV. Some patients require much lower doses, especially if other hypotensive agents are used.

Maximum dose: 10 mcg/kg/min IV.

Initial dosage: 0.3 mcg/kg/min IV. Titrate upward gradually every few minutes until desired effect is achieved or the maximum dose is reached.

Dosage titration: Titrate by increasing the infusion rate until measured cardiac output is no longer increasing, systemic blood pressure cannot be further reduced without compromising the perfusion of vital organs, or the maximum recommended infusion rate has been reached, whichever comes earliest.

Bleeding reduction during surgery –

Usual dosage: 3 mcg/kg/min IV. Some patients require much lower doses, especially if other hypotensive agents are used.

Maximum dose: 10 mcg/kg/min IV.

Initial dosage: 0.3 mcg/kg/min IV. Titrate upward gradually every few minutes until desired effect is achieved or the maximum dose is reached.

Off-label dosing –

Hypertensive crises:

- *3 months of age and older* –

  Usual dosage: 3 mcg/kg/min IV. Some patients require much lower doses, especially if other hypotensive agents are used.

  Maximum dose: 10 mcg/kg/min IV.

  Initial dosage: 0.3 mcg/kg/min IV. Titrate upward gradually every few minutes until desired effect is achieved or the maximum dose is reached.

  Alternative dosage: 0.53 to 10 mcg/kg/min IV.

NITROPRUSSIDE SODIUM — INJECTION

Tapering: Tapering may be required to avoid rebound hypertension.

• *Younger than 3 months of age –*

Maximum dose: 10 mcg/kg/min IV for 10 minutes or less.

Initial dosage: 0.25 to 0.5 mcg/kg/min IV.

Maintenance dosage: Typically less than 2 mcg/kg/min IV.

Refractory heart failure:

• *Younger than 3 months of age –*

Maximum dose: 10 mcg/kg/min IV for 10 minutes or less.

Initial dosage: 0.25 to 0.5 mcg/kg/min IV.

Maintenance dosage: Typically less than 2 mcg/kg/min IV.

➤*Elderly:* Use special caution because elderly patients may be more sensitive to the hypotensive effects of the drug.

➤*Hepatic function impairment:* Because cyanide is metabolized by hepatic enzymes, it may accumulate in patients with severe liver impairment. Therefore, use with caution in patients with hepatic insufficiency.

➤*Therapeutic drug monitoring:* Because nitroprusside can induce essentially unlimited blood pressure reduction, the blood pressure of a patient receiving this drug must be continuously monitored, using either a continually reinflated sphygmomanometer or, preferably, an intra-arterial pressure sensor.

➤*Preparation for administration:* Dissolve the contents of a 50 mg vial in 2 to 3 mL of dextrose in water or sterile water for injection. Depending on the desired concentration, the initially reconstituted solution containing 50 mg must be further diluted in 250 to 1,000 mL of dextrose 5% injection.

Nitroprusside can be inactivated by reactions with trace contaminants. Products of these reactions are often blue, green, or red, and much brighter than the faint brownish color of unreacted nitroprusside. Do not use discolored solutions, or solutions with particulate matter visible.

➤*Administration:* Because nitroprusside's hypotensive effect is very rapid in onset and in dissipation, small variations in infusion rate can lead to wide, undesirable variations in blood pressure. Do not infuse through an ordinary IV apparatus regulated only by gravity and mechanical clamps. Use only an infusion pump, preferably a volumetric pump.

Some infusion rates are so slow or so rapid as to be impractical, and these practicalities must be considered when the concentration to be used is selected. Note that when the concentration used in a given patient is changed, the tubing is still filled with a solution at the previous concentration.

Infusion Rates to Achieve Initial (0.3 mcg/kg/min) and Maximal (10 mcg/kg/min) Dosing of Nitroprusside

Patient weight		Nitroprusside concentration					
		200 mcg/mL		100 mcg/mL		50 mcg/mL	
		Infusion rate (mL/h)		Infusion rate (mL/h)		Infusion rate (mL/h)	
kg	lbs	Initial	Maximal	Initial	Maximal	Initial	Maximal
10	22	1	30	2	60	4	120
20	44	2	60	4	120	7	240
30	66	3	90	5	180	11	360
40	88	4	120	7	240	14	480
50	110	5	150	9	300	18	600
60	132	5	180	11	360	22	720
70	154	6	210	13	420	25	840
80	176	7	240	14	480	29	960
90	198	8	270	16	540	32	1,080
100	220	9	300	18	600	36	1,200

➤*Admixture compatibility:* Esmolol and nitroprusside are compatible.

To screen for specific compatibilities, see Trissel's *IV-Chek*.

➤*Storage/Stability:* Store at 15° to 30°C (59° to 86°F). If properly protected from light, the freshly reconstituted and diluted solution is stable for 24 hours. Protect the diluted solution from light by promptly wrapping with the supplied opaque sleeve, aluminum foil, or other opaque material. It is not necessary to cover the infusion drip chamber or the tubing.

Actions

➤*Pharmacology:* Nitroprusside is a potent IV antihypertensive agent. The principal pharmacological action of nitroprusside is relaxation of vascular smooth muscle and consequent dilation of peripheral arteries and veins. Other smooth muscle (eg, uterus, duodenum) is not affected. Nitroprusside is more active on veins than on arteries, but this selectivity is much less marked than that of nitroglycerin. Dilation of the veins promotes peripheral pooling of blood and decreases venous return to the heart, thereby reducing left ventricular end-diastolic pressure and pulmonary capillary wedge pressure (preload). Arteriolar relaxation reduces systemic vascular resistance, systolic arterial pressure and mean arterial pressure (afterload). Dilation of the coronary arteries also occurs.

In association with the decrease in blood pressure, nitroprusside administered IV to hypertensive and normotensive patients produces slight increases in heart rate and a variable effect on cardiac output. In hypertensive patients, moderate doses induce renal vasodilation roughly proportional to the decrease in systemic blood pressure, so there is no appreciable change in renal blood flow or glomerular filtration rate.

In normotensive subjects, acute reduction of mean arterial pressure to 60 to 75 mm Hg by infusion of nitroprusside caused a significant increase in renin activity. In the same study, 10 renovascular-hypertensive patients given nitroprusside had significant increases in renin release from the involved kidney at mean arterial pressures of 90 to 137 mm Hg.

The hypotensive effect of nitroprusside is seen within 1 to 2 minutes after the start of an adequate infusion, and it dissipates almost as rapidly after an infusion is discontinued. The effect is augmented by ganglionic blocking agents and inhaled anesthetics.

➤*Pharmacokinetics:*

Absorption/Distribution – Infused nitroprusside is rapidly distributed to a volume that is approximately coextensive with the extracellular space. The drug is cleared from this volume by intraerythrocytic reaction with hemoglobin (HgB), and nitroprusside's resulting circulatory half-life is about 2 minutes.

Metabolism/Excretion – The products of the nitroprusside/HgB reaction are cyanmethemoglobin (cyanmetHgB) and cyanide ion (CN^-). Safe use of nitroprusside injection must be guided by knowledge of the further metabolism of these products. The essential features of nitroprusside metabolism are: One molecule of nitroprusside is metabolized by combination with HgB to produce one molecule of cyanmethemoglobin and four CN^- ions; methemoglobin, obtained from HgB, can sequester cyanide as cyanmethemoglobin; thiosulfate reacts with cyanide to produce thiocyanate (SCN^-); thiocyanate is eliminated in the urine; cyanide, not otherwise removed, binds to cytochromes; cyanide is much more toxic than methemoglobin or thiocyanate.

When the Fe^{+++} of cytochromes is bound to cyanide, the cytochromes are unable to participate in oxidative metabolism. In this situation, cells may be able to provide for their energy needs by utilizing anaerobic pathways, but they thereby generate an increasing body burden of lactic acid. Other cells may be unable to utilize these alternate pathways, and they may die hypoxic deaths.

When CN^- is infused or generated within the bloodstream, essentially all of it is bound to methemoglobin until intraerythrocytic methemoglobin has been saturated. At healthy steady state, most people have < 1% of their HgB in the form of methemoglobin. Nitroprusside metabolism can lead to methemoglobin formation (a) through dissociation of cyanmethemeglobin formed in the original reaction of nitroprusside with HgB and (b) by direct oxidation of HgB by the released nitroso group. Relatively large quantities of nitroprusside, however, are required to produce significant methemoglobinemia.

When thiosulfate is supplied only by normal physiologic mechanisms, conversion of CN^- to SCN^- generally proceeds at about 1 mcg/kg/min. This rate of CN^- clearance corresponds to steady-state processing of a nitroprusside infusion of slightly more than 2 mcg/kg/min. CN^- accumulates when nitroprusside infusions exceed this rate.

In patients with normal renal function, clearance of SCN^- is primarily renal, with a half-life of about 3 days. In renal failure, the half-life can be doubled or tripled.

Contraindications

Treatment of compensatory hypertension, where the primary hemodynamic lesion is aortic coarctation or arteriovenous shunting; to produce hypotension during surgery in patients with known inadequate cerebral circulation or in moribund patients (A.S.A. Class 5E) coming to emergency surgery; patients with congenital (Leber's) optic atrophy or with tobacco amblyopia (these rare conditions are probably associated with defective or absent rhodanese and patients with unusually high cyanide/thiocyanate ratios); acute CHF associated with reduced peripheral vascular resistance such as high-output heart failure that may be seen in endotoxic sepsis.

Warnings/Precautions

➤*Excessive hypotension:* Small transient excesses in the infusion rate of nitroprusside can result in excessive hypotension, sometimes to levels so low as to compromise the perfusion of vital organs. These hemodynamic changes may lead to a variety of associated symptoms. Nitroprusside-induced hypotension will be self-limited within 1 to 10 minutes after discontinuation of the infusion; during these few minutes, it may be helpful to put the patient into a head-down (Trendelenburg) position to maximize venous return. If

NITROPRUSSIDE SODIUM — INJECTION

hypotension persists more than a few minutes after discontinuation of the infusion, nitroprusside is not the cause, and the true cause must be sought.

➤*Cyanide toxicity:* Nitroprusside infusions at rates more than 2 mcg/kg/min generate CN^- faster than the body can normally dispose of it. (When sodium thiosulfate is given, the body's capacity for CN^- elimination is greatly increased.) Methemoglobin normally present in the body can buffer a certain amount of CN^-, but the capacity of this system is exhausted by the CN^- produced from nitroprusside 500 mcg/kg. This amount of nitroprusside is administered in less than 1 hour when the drug is administered at 10 mcg/kg/min (the maximum recommended rate). Thereafter, the toxic effects of CN^- may be rapid, serious and even lethal.

The true rates of clinically important cyanide toxicity cannot be assessed from spontaneous reports or published data. Most patients reported to have experienced such toxicity have received relatively prolonged infusions, and the only patients whose deaths have been unequivocally attributed to nitroprusside-induced cyanide toxicity have been patients who had received nitroprusside infusions at rates much greater than those now recommended (30 to 120 mcg/kg/min). Elevated cyanide levels, metabolic acidosis and marked clinical deterioration, however, have occasionally been reported in patients who received infusions at recommended rates for only a few hours and even, in one case, for only 35 minutes. In some of these cases, infusion of sodium thiosulfate caused dramatic clinical improvement, supporting the diagnosis of cyanide toxicity.

Cyanide toxicity may manifest itself as venous hyperoxemia with bright red venous blood, as cells become unable to extract the oxygen delivered to them; metabolic (lactic) acidosis; air hunger; confusion; death. Cyanide toxicity due to causes other than nitroprusside has been associated with angina pectoris and myocardial infarction, ataxia, seizures and stroke, and other diffuse ischemic damage.

➤*Hypertensive patients:* Hypertensive patients and patients concomitantly receiving other antihypertensive medications may be more sensitive to the effects of nitroprusside.

➤*Methemoglobinemia:* Nitroprusside infusions can cause sequestration of hemoglobin as methemoglobin. The back-conversion process is normally rapid, and clinically significant methemoglobinemia (more than 10%) is only seen rarely. Even patients congenitally incapable of back-converting methemoglobin should demonstrate 10% methemoglobinemia only after they have received about 10 mg/kg nitroprusside; a patient receiving nitroprusside at the maximum recommended rate (10 mcg/kg/min) would take more than 16 hours to reach this total accumulated dose.

Methemoglobin levels can be measured by most clinical laboratories. Suspect the diagnosis in patients who have received more than 10 mg/kg of nitroprusside and who exhibit signs of impaired oxygen delivery despite adequate cardiac output and adequate arterial pO_2. Classically, methemoglobinemic blood is described as chocolate brown, without color change on exposure to air.

When methemoglobinemia is diagnosed, the treatment of choice is 1 to 2 mg/kg of methylene blue, administered IV over several minutes. In patients likely to have substantial amounts of cyanide bound to methemoglobin as cyanmethemoglobin, treatment of methemoglobinemia with methylene blue must be undertaken with extreme caution.

➤*Thiocyanate toxicity:* Most of the cyanide produced during metabolism of nitroprusside is eliminated in the form of thiocyanate. When cyanide elimination is accelerated by the coinfusion of thiosulfate, thiocyanate production is increased. Thiocyanate is mildly neurotoxic (eg, tinnitus, miosis, hyperreflexia) at serum levels of 1 mmol/L (60 mg/L). Thiocyanate toxicity is life-threatening when levels are 3 or 4 times higher (200 mg/L).

The steady-state thiocyanate level after prolonged infusions of nitroprusside is increased with increased infusion rate, and the half-time of accumulation is 3 to 4 days. To keep the steady-state thiocyanate level < 1 mmol/L, a prolonged infusion should not be more rapid than 3 mcg/kg/min; in anuric patients, the corresponding limit is just 1 mcg/kg/min. When prolonged infusions are more rapid than these, measure thiocyanate levels daily.

Physiologic maneuvers (eg, those that alter the pH of the urine) are not known to increase the elimination of thiocyanate. Thiocyanate clearance rates during dialysis, on the other hand, can approach the blood flow rate of the dialyzer.

Thiocyanate interferes with iodine uptake by the thyroid.

➤*Intracranial pressure:* Like other vasodilators, nitroprusside can cause increases in intracranial pressure. In patients whose intracranial pressure is already elevated, use only with extreme caution.

➤*Anesthesia:* When nitroprusside (or any other vasodilator) is used for controlled hypotension during anesthesia, the patient's capacity to compensate for anemia and hypovolemia may be diminished. If possible, correct preexisting anemia and hypovolemia prior to use.

Hypotensive anesthetic techniques may also cause abnormalities of the pulmonary ventilation/perfusion ratio. Patients intolerant of these abnormalities may require a higher fraction of inspired oxygen.

Exercise extreme caution in patients who are especially poor surgical risks (A.S.A. Classes 4 and 4E).

➤*Hepatic function impairment:* Because cyanide is metabolized by hepatic enzymes, it may accumulate in patients with severe liver impairment. Therefore, use with caution in patients with hepatic insufficiency.

➤*Pregnancy: Category C.* Nitroprusside injection is an alternative agent for the emergency treatment of hypertension during pregnancy. However, there is a risk for cyanide toxicity if used in high doses and/or for extended periods of time. See also Warnings/Precautions.

In 3 studies in pregnant ewes, nitroprusside crossed the placental barrier. Fetal cyanide levels were dose-related to maternal levels of nitroprusside. The metabolic transformation of nitroprusside given to pregnant ewes led to fatal levels of cyanide in the fetuses. The infusion of 25 mcg/kg/min nitroprusside for 1 hour in pregnant ewes resulted in the death of all fetuses. There are no adequate or well controlled studies in pregnant women. It is not known whether nitroprusside can cause fetal harm when administered to a pregnant woman or can affect reproductive capacity. Give to a pregnant woman only if clearly needed.

The effects of administering sodium thiosulfate in pregnancy, either by itself or as a co-infusion with sodium nitroprusside, are completely unknown.

➤*Lactation:* It is not known whether nitroprusside and its metabolites are excreted in breast milk. Because of the potential for serious adverse reactions in nursing infants, decide whether to discontinue breast-feeding or the drug, taking into account the importance of the drug to the mother.

➤*Children:* See Administration and Dosage.

➤*Elderly:* Use special caution because elderly patients may be more sensitive to the hypotensive effects of the drug.

➤*Monitoring:* The cyanide-level assay is technically difficult, and cyanide levels in body fluids other than packed red blood cells are difficult to interpret. Cyanide toxicity will lead to lactic acidosis and venous hyperoxemia, but these findings may not be present until more than 1 hour after the cyanide capacity of the body's red-cell mass has been exhausted.

Adverse Reactions

➤*Cardiovascular:* Bradycardia; ECG changes; tachycardia.

➤*Hematologic:* Decreased platelet aggregation; methemoglobinemia.

➤*Miscellaneous:* Thiocyanate toxicity; flushing; venous streaking; irritation at the infusion site; rash; hypothyroidism; ileus; increased intracranial pressure).

Rapid blood pressure reduction – Abdominal pain, apprehension, diaphoresis, dizziness, headache, muscle twitching, nausea, palpitations, restlessness, retching and retrosternal discomfort have been noted when the blood pressure was reduced too rapidly. Symptoms quickly disappeared when the infusion was slowed or discontinued, and they did not reappear with a continued (or resumed) slower infusion.

Overdosage

➤*Symptoms:* Toxicity has occurred at doses well below the recommended maximum infusion rate of 10 mcg/kg/min. Overdosage of nitroprusside can be manifested as excessive hypotension, cyanide toxicity or as thiocyanate toxicity.

The acute IV mean lethal doses (LD_{50}) of nitroprusside in rabbits, dogs, mice and rats are 2.8, 5, 8.4 and 11.2 mg/kg, respectively.

➤*Treatment:* Measure cyanide levels and blood gases for venous hyperoxemia or acidosis. Acidosis may not appear until more than 1 hour after the appearance of dangerous cyanide levels; do not wait for laboratory tests. Reasonable suspicion of cyanide toxicity is adequate grounds for initiation of treatment.

Treatment of cyanide toxicity consists of: Discontinuing the administration of nitroprusside; providing a buffer for cyanide by using sodium nitrite to convert as much HgB into methemoglobin as the patient can safely tolerate; and then infusing sodium thiosulfate in sufficient quantity to convert the cyanide into thiocyanate.

The medications for treatment are contained in commercially available cyanide antidote kits. Alternatively, discrete stocks of medications can be used. Hemodialysis is ineffective in removal of cyanide, but it will eliminate most thiocyanate.

Antidote kits – Cyanide antidote kits contain both amyl nitrite and sodium nitrite for induction of methemoglobinemia. The amyl nitrite is supplied in the form of inhalant ampules, for use where IV administration of sodium nitrite may be delayed. In a patient who already has a patent IV line, use of amyl nitrite confers no benefit that is not provided by infusion of sodium nitrite.

Nitrite-thiosulfate regimen – Sodium nitrite is available in a 3% solution; inject 4 to 6 mg/kg (about 0.2 mL/kg) over 2 to 4 minutes. This dose converts about 10% of the patient's HgB into methemoglobin; this level of methemoglobinemia is not associated with any important hazard of its own. The nitrite infusion may cause transient vasodilation and hypotension, and this hypotension must, if it occurs, be routinely managed.

Immediately after infusion of the sodium nitrite, infuse sodium thiosulfate. This agent is available in 10% and 25% solutions, and the recommended dose is 150 to 200 mg/kg; a typical adult dose is 50 mL of the 25% solution. Thiosulfate treatment of an acutely cyanide-toxic patient will raise thiocyanate levels, but not to a dangerous degree.

The nitrite-thiosulfate regimen may be repeated, at half the original doses, after 2 hours.

Hydroxocobalamin – No concrete guidelines have been developed for hydroxocobalamin.

Prophylactically during surgery: Doses of 25 mg/h for 4 hours.

Treatment: A dose of 4 to 5 g of hydroxocobalamin alone, or a combination of 8 g of sodium thiosulfate and 4 g of hydroxocobalamin.

FENOLDOPAM MESYLATE

Rx	**Corlopam** (Hospira)	**Injection, concentrate:** 10 mg/mL	In 1 and 2 mL single-dose ampules.[a]
Rx	**Fenoldopam Mesylate** (Baxter)	**Injection:** 10 mg/mL	In 1 and 2 mL single-dose ampules.[b]

[a] With 1 mg sodium metabisulfite.

[b] With sodium metabisulfite.

FENOLDOPAM — INJECTION

Indications

➤*Severe hypertension:*

Adults – For the in-hospital, short-term (up to 48 hours) management of severe hypertension when rapid, but quickly reversible, emergency reduction of blood pressure is clinically indicated, including malignant hypertension with deteriorating end-organ function. Transition to oral therapy with another agent can begin at any time after blood pressure is stable during fenoldopam infusion.

Children – For the in-hospital, short-term (up to 4 hours) reduction in blood pressure.

➤*Off-label uses:*

Prevention of contrast media nephrotoxicity – [5] = Poor documentation. Although initial data regards the use of fenoldopam as a preventive agent for radiocontrast-induced nephrotoxicity, more recent information from controlled trials suggests that this drug with hydration is no better than hydration alone or with N-acetylcysteine. Based on this new data, this drug is not recommended for the prevention of radiocontrast nephropathy in cardiovascular interventions.

Administration and Dosage

➤*General dosing considerations:* Fenoldopam should be administered by continuous intravenous (IV) infusion.

The fenoldopam injection ampule concentrate must be diluted in sodium chloride 0.9% injection or dextrose 5% injection. (See Preparation for Administration.)

➤*Adults:*

Severe hypertension –

Usual dosage: The drug dose rate must be individualized according to body weight and according to the desired rapidity and extent of pharmacodynamic effect. The following table provides the calculated infusion volume in mL/h for a range of doses and body weights. The infusion should be administered using a calibrated mechanical infusion pump that can accurately and reliably deliver the desired infusion rate.

Fenoldopam Infusion Rates (mL/h) for Adults (> 40 kg)

Body weight (kg)	Infusion rate										
	0.025 (mcg/kg/ min)	0.05 (mcg/kg/ min)	0.1 (mcg/kg/ min)	0.2 (mcg/kg/ min)	0.3 (mcg/kg/ min)	0.5 (mcg/kg/ min)	0.8 (mcg/kg/ min)	1 (mcg/kg/ min)	1.2 (mcg/kg/ min)	1.4 (mcg/kg/ min)	1.6 (mcg/kg/ min)
	Infusion rates (mL/h) of 40 mcg/mL solution										
40	1.5	3	6	12	18	30	48	60	72	84	96
50	1.9	3.8	7.5	15	22.5	37.5	60	75	90	105	120
60	2.3	4.5	9	18	27	45	72	90	108	126	144
70	2.6	5.3	10.5	21	31.5	52.5	84	105	126	147	168
80	3	6	12	24	36	60	96	120	144	158	192
90	3.4	6.8	13.5	27	40.5	67.5	108	135	162	189	216
100	3.8	7.5	15	30	45	75	120	150	180	210	240
110	4.1	8.3	16.5	33	49.5	82.5	132	165	198	231	264
120	4.5	9	18	36	54	90	144	180	216	252	288
130	4.9	9.8	19.5	39	58.5	97.5	156	195	234	273	312
140	5.3	10.5	21	42	63	105	168	210	252	294	336
150	5.6	11.3	22.5	45	67.5	112.5	180	225	270	315	360

Initial dosage: An initial fenoldopam dose that produces the desired magnitude and rate of blood pressure reduction in a given clinical situation may be chosen from the following table.

Doses less than 0.1 mcg/kg/min have very modest effects and appear only marginally useful in this population. In general, as the initial dosage increases, there is a greater and more rapid blood pressure reduction. However, lower initial dosages (0.03 to 0.1 mcg/kg/min) titrated slowly have been associated with less reflex tachycardia than higher initial dosages (at least 0.3 mcg/kg/min). In clinical trials, dosages from 0.01 to 1.6 mcg/kg/min have been studied. Most of the effect of a given infusion rate is attained in 15 minutes.

Pharmacodynamic Effects of Fenoldopam in Adult Hypertensive Emergency Patients

Time point and pharmacodynamic parameters	Drug dosage (mcg/kg/min) 0.01 (n = 25)	0.03 (n = 24)	0.1 (n = 22)	0.3 (n = 23)
Preinfusion baseline				
Systolic blood pressure — mean ± standard error (SE)	210 ± 21	208 ± 26	205 ± 24	211 ± 17
Diastolic blood pressure — mean ± SE	136 ± 16	135 ± 11	133 ± 14	136 ± 15
Heart rate — mean ± SE	87 ± 20	84 ± 14	81 ± 19	80 ± 14
15 minutes of infusion[a]				
Systolic blood pressure	−5 ± 4	−7 ± 4	−16 ± 4	−19 ± 4
Diastolic blood pressure	−5 ± 3	−8 ± 3	−12 ± 2	−21 ± 2
Heart rate	−2 ± 3	+1 ± 1	+2 ± 1	+11 ± 2
30 minutes of infusion[a]				
Systolic blood pressure	−6 ± 4	−11 ± 4	−21 ± 3	−16 ± 4
Diastolic blood pressure	−10 ± 3	−12 ± 3	−17 ± 3	−20 ± 2
Heart rate	−2 ± 3	−1 ± 1	+3 ± 2	+12 ± 3
1 hour of infusion[a]				
Systolic blood pressure	−5 ± 3	−9 ± 4	−19 ± 4	−22 ± 4
Diastolic blood pressure	−8 ± 3	−13 ± 3	−18 ± 2	−23 ± 2
Heart rate	−1 ± 3	0 ± 2	+3 ± 2	+11 ± 3

Pharmacodynamic Effects of Fenoldopam in Adult Hypertensive Emergency Patients

Time point and pharmacodynamic parameters	Drug dosage (mcg/kg/min) 0.01 (n = 25)	0.03 (n = 24)	0.1 (n = 22)	0.3 (n = 23)
4 hours of infusion[a]				
Systolic blood pressure	−14 ± 4	−20 ± 5	−23 ± 4	−37 ± 4
Diastolic blood pressure	−12 ± 3	−18 ± 3	−21 ± 3	−29 ± 3
Heart rate	−2 ± 4	0 ± 2	+4 ± 2	+11 ± 2

[a] Mean change from baseline ± SE.

➤*Children:*

Severe hypertension –

Usual dosage: The following table provides the calculated infusion volume in mL/h for a range of drug doses and body weights. The infusion should be administered using a calibrated mechanical infusion pump that can accurately and reliably deliver the desired infusion rate. Because low flow rates (eg, less than 0.5 mL/h) may not be practical and because of volume overload, it may be necessary to increase the concentration of fenoldopam in the infused solutions.

Fenoldopam Infusion Rates for Children Between 5 and 70 kg

Body weight (kg)	Infusion rate				
	0.2 mcg/kg/ min	0.5 mcg/kg/ min	0.8 mcg/kg/ min	1 mcg/kg/ min	1.2 mcg/kg/ min
	Infusion rates (mL/h) of 60 mcg/mL solution				
5	1	2.5	4	5	6
10	2	5	8	10	12
20	4	10	16	20	24
30	6	15	24	30	36
40	8	20	32	40	48
50	10	25	40	50	60
60	12	30	48	60	72

FENOLDOPAM — INJECTION

Fenoldopam Infusion Rates for Children Between 5 and 70 kg					
	Infusion rate				
Body weight (kg)	0.2 mcg/kg/min	0.5 mcg/kg/min	0.8 mcg/kg/min	1 mcg/kg/min	1.2 mcg/kg/min
70	14	35	56	70	84

Initial dosage: 0.2 mcg/kg/min. Effect on mean arterial pressure (MAP) evident within 5 minutes. At a constant infusion rate, the effect was maximal after 20 to 25 minutes. An initial fenoldopam dose that produces the desired magnitude and rate of blood pressure reduction in a given clinical situation may be chosen from the following table.

Pharmacodynamic Effects of Fenoldopam in Children Baseline Mean and Mean Change ± SE					
	Drug Dosage (mcg/kg/min)				
	Placebo (n = 16)	0.05 (n = 15[a])	0.2 (n = 16)	0.8 (n = 15)	3.2 (n = 15)
Preinfusion baseline					
MAP	81 ± 4	77 ± 5	75 ± 4	88 ± 6	74 ± 4
Systolic blood pressure	108 ± 5	103 ± 6	104 ± 6	117 ± 7	98 ± 4
Diastolic blood pressure	62 ± 4	61 ± 4	57 ± 3	69 ± 6	56 ± 3
Heart rate	106 ± 8	110 ± 7	119 ± 7	125 ± 6	122 ± 6
Change at 5 minutes of infusion					
MAP	4 ± 2	3 ± 3	−2 ± 2	−3 ± 3	−6 ± 3
Systolic blood pressure	5 ± 3	3 ± 3	−2 ± 3	−5 ± 3	−8 ± 3
Diastolic blood pressure	4 ± 2	6 ± 2	−1 ± 2	−2 ± 2	−4 ± 2
Heart rate	2 ± 3	−2 ± 3	−1 ± 3	4 ± 3	−2 ± 3
Change at 30 minutes of infusion (LOCF[b])					
MAP	0 ± 3	−1 ± 3	−2 ± 3	−10 ± 3	−10 ± 3
Systolic blood pressure	−3 ± 4	0 ± 4	−3± 4	−12 ± 4	−10 ± 4
Diastolic blood pressure	0 ± 3	1 ± 3	−2 ± 3	−8 ± 3	−6 ± 3
Heart rate	−6 ± 4	−4 ± 4	5 ± 4	7 ± 4	14 ± 4

[a] For MAP, n = 14; otherwise, n = 15.
[b] Dropouts were accounted for using the Last Observation Carried Forward (LOCF) method of analysis.

Dosage titration: Increased dosages of up to 0.3 to 0.5 mcg/kg/min every 20 to 30 minutes were generally well tolerated. Tachycardia without further decrease in MAP occurred at dosages greater than 0.8 mcg/kg/min.

Discontinuation of therapy: Upon discontinuation of the fenoldopam infusion after an average of 4 hours of therapy, blood pressure and heart rate returned to near baseline within 30 minutes.

Off-label dosing –

Acute, severe hypertension:

- *Usual dose* – 0.2 to 0.8 mcg/kg/min by IV infusion.

➤*Monitoring:*

Adults – In clinical trials, fenoldopam treatment was safely performed without the need for intra-arterial blood pressure monitoring; blood pressure and heart rate were monitored at frequent intervals, typically every 15 minutes. Frequent blood pressure monitoring is recommended.

Children – Monitoring of blood pressure should be continuous, usually by way of an intra-arterial line. Heart rate should also be continuously monitored.

➤*Preparation for administration:* Contents of ampules must be diluted before infusion. Each ampule is for single use only.

Dilution – The fenoldopam injection ampule concentrate must be diluted in sodium chloride 0.9% injection or dextrose 5% injection using the following dilution schedule:

Adults:

Dilution of Fenoldopam for Adults		
mL of concentrate (mg of drug)	Added to	Final concentration
4 mL (40 mg)	1,000 mL	40 mcg/mL
2 mL (20 mg)	500 mL	40 mcg/mL
1 mL (10 mg)	250 mL	40 mcg/mL

Children:

Dilution of Fenoldopam for Children		
mL of concentrate (mg of drug)	Added to	Final concentration
3 mL (30 mg)	500 mL	60 mcg/mL
1.5 mL (15 mg)	250 mL	60 mcg/mL
0.6 mL (6 mg)	100 mL	60 mcg/mL

➤*Administration:*

Adults – Fenoldopam should be administered by continuous IV infusion. A bolus dose should not be used. Hypotension and rapid decreases of blood pressure should be avoided. The initial dose should be titrated upward or downward, no more frequently than every 15 minutes (and less frequently as goal pressure is approached) to achieve the desired therapeutic effect. The recommended increments for titration are 0.05 to 0.1 mcg/kg/min.

Use of a calibrated, mechanical infusion pump is recommended for proper control of infusion rate during fenoldopam infusion.

The fenoldopam infusion can be abruptly discontinued or gradually tapered prior to discontinuation. Oral antihypertensive agents can be added during fenoldopam infusion or following its discontinuation. Patients in controlled clinical trials have received IV fenoldopam for as long as 48 hours.

Children – Fenoldopam should be administered IV by a continuous infusion pump appropriate for the delivery of low infusion rates.

➤*Storage/Stability:* Store at 2° to 30°C (36° to 86°F). The diluted solution is stable under normal ambient light and temperature conditions for at least 24 hours. Diluted solution that is not used within 24 hours of preparation should be discarded.

Actions

➤*Pharmacology:* Fenoldopam is a rapidly acting vasodilator. It is an agonist for D_1-like dopamine receptors and binds with moderate affinity to α_2-adrenoceptors. It has no significant affinity for D_2-like receptors, alpha-1 and beta adrenoceptors, 5-HT_1 and 5-HT_2 receptors, or muscarinic receptors. Fenoldopam is a racemic mixture with the R-isomer responsible for the biological activity. The R-isomer has approximately 250-fold higher affinity for D_1-like receptors than does the S-isomer. In nonclinical studies, fenoldopam had no agonist effect on presynaptic D_2-like dopamine receptors, or alpha- or beta-adrenoceptors, nor did it affect angiotensin-converting enzyme (ACE) activity. Fenoldopam may increase norepinephrine plasma concentration.

In animals, fenoldopam has vasodilating effects in coronary, renal, mesenteric, and peripheral arteries. All vascular beds, however, do not respond uniformly to fenoldopam. Vasodilating effects have been demonstrated in renal efferent and afferent arterioles.

➤*Pharmacokinetics:*

Absorption/Distribution –

Adults: Fenoldopam administered as a constant infusion at dosages of 0.01 to 1.6 mcg/kg/min produced steady-state plasma concentrations that were proportional to infusion rates. Steady-state concentrations are attained in about 20 minutes (4 half-lives). The steady-state plasma concentrations of fenoldopam, at comparable infusion rates, were similar in normotensive patients and in patients with mild-to-moderate hypertension or hypertensive emergencies. In radiolabeled studies in rats, no more than 0.005% of fenoldopam crossed the blood-brain barrier.

Metabolism/Excretion – Radiolabeled studies show that about 90% of infused fenoldopam is eliminated in urine, 10% in feces. Elimination is largely by conjugation, without participation of cytochrome P-450 enzymes. The principal routes of conjugation are methylation, glucuronidation, and sulfation. Only 4% of the administered dose is excreted unchanged. Animal data indicate that the metabolites are inactive. The elimination half-life was about 5 minutes in mild to moderate hypertensive patients, with little difference between the R (active) and S isomers.

Contraindications

None known.

Warnings/Precautions

➤*Intraocular pressure:* In a clinical study of 12 patients with open-angle glaucoma or ocular hypertension (mean baseline intraocular pressure was 29.2 mm Hg with a range of 22 to 33 mm Hg), infusion of fenoldopam at escalating doses ranging from 0.05 to 0.5 mcg/kg/min over a 3.5-hour period caused a dose-dependent increase in intraocular pressure (IOP). At the peak effect, the IOP was raised by a mean of 6.5 mm Hg (range −2 to +8.5 mm Hg, corrected for placebo effect). Upon discontinuation of the fenoldopam infusion, the IOP returned to baseline values within 2 hours. Undertake fenoldopam administration to patients with glaucoma or intraocular hypertension with caution.

➤*Tachycardia:* Fenoldopam causes a dose-related tachycardia, particularly with infusion rates above 0.1 mcg/kg/min. Tachycardia in adults diminishes over time but remains substantial at higher doses. Tachycardia in children persists for at least 4 hours at dosages greater than 0.8 mcg/kg/min.

➤*Hypotension:* Fenoldopam may occasionally produce symptomatic hypotension, and close monitoring of blood pressure during administration is essential. It is particularly important to avoid systemic hypotension when administering the drug to patients who have sustained an acute cerebral infarction or hemorrhage. In children, fenoldopam was only administered to patients with an indwelling intra-arterial line.

➤*Hypokalemia:* Decreases in serum potassium occasionally to values below 3 mEq/L were observed after less than 6 hours of fenoldopam infusion. It is not clear if the hypokalemia reflects a pressure natriuresis with enhanced potassium-sodium exchange or a direct drug effect. During clinical trials, electrolytes were monitored at intervals of 6 hours. Hypokalemia was treated with either oral or IV potassium supplementation. Patient management should include appropriate attention to serum electrolytes.

➤*Sulfite sensitivity:* Contains sodium metabisulfite, a sulfite that may cause allergic-type reactions including anaphylactic symptoms and life-threatening or less severe asthmatic episodes in certain susceptible people. The overall prevalence of sulfite sensitivity in the general population is unknown and probably low. Sulfite sensitivity is seen more frequently in asthmatic than in nonasthmatic people.

➤*Pregnancy: Category B.* Oral reproduction studies have been performed in rats and rabbits at dosages of 12.5 to 200 mg/kg/day and 6.25 to 25 mg/kg/day, respectively. Studies have revealed maternal toxicity at the highest doses tested but no evidence of impaired fertility or harm to the fetus due to fenoldo-

FENOLDOPAM — INJECTION

pam. However, there are no adequate and well-controlled studies in pregnant women. Since animal reproduction studies are not always predictive of human response, use fenoldopam in pregnancy only if clearly needed.

➤*Lactation:* Fenoldopam is excreted in milk in rats. It is not known whether this drug is excreted in human milk. Because many drugs are excreted in human milk, exercise caution when fenoldopam is administered to a breast-feeding woman.

➤*Children:* Antihypertensive effects of fenoldopam have been studied in children younger than 1 month of age (at least 2 kg or full term) to 12 years of age requiring blood pressure reduction.

Clinical studies of fenoldopam did not include subjects 12 to 16 years of age to determine if they respond differently from younger subjects or adults. The pharmacokinetics of fenoldopam are independent of age when corrected for body weight. Consider the patient's clinical condition and concomitant drug therapy when making a dose selection for patients 12 to 16 years of age.

➤*Elderly:* Clinical studies of fenoldopam did not include sufficient numbers of subjects 65 years of age and older to determine whether they respond differently from younger subjects. Other reported clinical experience has not identified differences in responses between the elderly and younger patients. In general, dose selection for an elderly patient should be cautious, usually starting at the low end of the dosing range, reflecting the greater frequency of decreased hepatic, renal, or cardiac function, and of concomitant disease or other drug therapy.

➤*Monitoring:* Monitor blood pressure and heart rate at frequent intervals, typically every 15 minutes to avoid hypotension and rapid decreases of blood pressure. In children, continuously monitor blood pressure by way of an intra-arterial line. Monitor electrolytes every 6 hours.

Drug Interactions

➤*Drug interactions with beta-blockers:* Avoid concomitant use of fenoldopam with beta-blockers. If the drugs are used together, exercise caution because unexpected hypotension could result from beta-blocker inhibition of the sympathetic reflex response to fenoldopam.

Adverse Reactions

➤*Adults:* Fenoldopam causes a dose-related fall in blood pressure and increase in heart rate. In controlled clinical studies of severe hypertension in patients with end-organ damage, 3% (4/137) of patients withdrew because of excessive falls in blood pressure. Increased heart rate could, in theory, lead to ischemic cardiac events or worsened heart failure, although these events have not been observed. The most common events reported as associated with fenoldopam use are headache, cutaneous dilation (flushing), nausea, and hypotension, each reported in greater than 5% of patients.

➤*Cardiovascular:*

Tachycardia – See Warnings/Precautions for more information.

Hypotension – See Warnings/Precautions for more information.

➤*Adverse reactions in hypertensive adult patients:* Adverse reactions occurring more than once in any dosing group (once if potentially important or plausibly drug related) in the fixed-dose constant-infusion studies are presented in the following table by infusion-rate group. There was no clear dose relationship, except possibly for headache, nausea, and flushing.

Fenoldopam Adverse Reactions[a] in Adults						
	Fenoldopam dosage (mcg/kg/min)					
Adverse reaction	Placebo (n = 7)	0.01 (n = 26)	0.03 to 0.04 (n = 31)	0.1 (n = 28)	0.3 to 0.4 (n = 29)	0.6 to 0.8 (n = 11)
Cardiovascular						
ST-T abnormalities (primarily T-wave inversion)	0	2	4	0	1	0
Flushing	0	0	0	0	1	3
Hypotension[b]	0	0	0	2	0	2
Postural hypotension	0	2	0	0	0	0
Tachycardia[b]	0	0	0	0	0	2
CNS						
Headache	1	5	4	7	8	6
Nervousness/Anxiety	0	0	1	0	0	2
Insomnia	0	2	0	0	0	0
Dizziness	0	1	1	2	2	0
GI						
Nausea	0	3	0	3	5	4
Vomiting	0	2	0	2	1	2
Abdominal pain/fullness	0	2	0	0	2	1
Constipation	0	0	0	0	0	2
Diarrhea	0	0	0	0	2	0
Metabolic/Nutritional						
Increased creatinine[b]	0	0	2	0	0	0
Hypokalemia[b]	0	2	2	0	1	0
Miscellaneous						
Back pain	0	1	0	1	2	2
Injection site reaction	0	1	3	0	3	2
Nasal congestion	0	0	0	0	0	2
Sweating	0	0	0	1	1	2
Urinary tract infection	0	2	0	1	0	0

[a] Includes events reported by 2 or more patients receiving fenoldopam treatment across all dose groups.

[b] Investigator defined; no protocol definition.

➤*Additional adverse reactions (0.5% to 5%):*

Cardiovascular – Angina pectoris, bradycardia, extrasystoles, heart failure, ischemic heart disease, myocardial infarction, palpitations.

Hematologic/Lymphatic – Bleeding, leukocytosis.

Metabolic – Elevated lactate dehydrogenase, elevated serum glucose, elevated serum urea nitrogen (BUN), elevated transaminase.

Respiratory – Dyspnea, upper respiratory tract disorder.

Miscellaneous – Limb cramp, nonspecific chest pain, oliguria, pyrexia.

Children – In children, the most common adverse reactions reported during short-term administration in controlled trials (30 minutes) were hypotension and tachycardia. However, because of the short exposure, there is limited experience with defining adverse reactions in children. The long-term effects of fenoldopam on growth and development have not been studied.

Overdosage

➤*Symptoms:* Intentional fenoldopam overdosage has not been reported. The most likely reaction would be excessive hypotension.

➤*Treatment:* Treat excessive hypotension with drug discontinuation and appropriate supportive measures.

Patient Information

This product contains sulfite, which can cause allergic reactions in certain individuals (eg, asthma patients).

Before taking this medicine, tell your health care provider if you have glaucoma or increased pressure in the eye, or if you are taking beta-blockers.

ANTIHYPERLIPIDEMIC AGENTS

Lowering cholesterol levels can arrest or reverse in all vascular beds and can significantly decrease the morbidity and mortality associated with atherosclerosis. Each 10% reduction in cholesterol levels is associated with an approximate 20% to 30% reduction in the incidence of coronary heart disease. Hyperlipidemia, particularly elevated serum cholesterol and low-density lipoprotein (LDL) levels, is a risk factor in the development of atherosclerotic cardiovascular disease.

Individually assess potential benefits and risks of therapy. The cornerstone of treatment in primary hyperlipidemia is diet restriction and weight reduction. Limit or eliminate alcohol intake. Use drug therapy in conjunction with diet and after maximal efforts to control serum lipids by diet alone prove unsatisfactory, when tolerance to or compliance with diet is poor, or when hyperlipidemia is severe and risk of complications is high. Treat contributory diseases such as hypothyroidism or diabetes mellitus.

Elevated blood cholesterol levels are a major cause of coronary artery disease. Lowering these levels (specifically, LDL cholesterol) will reduce the risk of heart attacks caused by coronary heart disease (CHD).

➤*Risk factors:* Positive risk factors for CHD (other than high LDL) include: age (men 45 years of age and older; women 55 years of age and older or women who go through premature menopause without estrogen replacement therapy); family history of premature CHD; smoking; hypertension (greater than 140/90 mmHg); low HDL cholesterol (less than 35 mg/dL); obesity (greater than 30% overweight); and diabetes mellitus. Physical inactivity is not listed but should also be considered.

➤*Negative:* Negative risk factors include: High HDL cholesterol (greater than or equal to 60 mg/dL); subtract one risk factor if the patient's HDL is at this level.

All Americans (except children younger than 2 years old) should adopt a diet that reduces total dietary fat, decreases intake of saturated fat, increases intake of polyunsaturated fat, and reduces daily cholesterol intake to less than or equal to 250 to 300 mg.

The following treatments guidelines are provided by the National Cholesterol Education Program Expert Panel on Detection, Evaluation and Treatment of High Blood Cholesterol in Adults 20 years of age and older.

Classification of Total and HDL-Cholesterol Levels (Adults ≥ 20 years of Age)

Level (mg/dL) (mmol/L)	Classification
< 200 (5.2)	desirable
200 to 239 (5.2 to 6.2)	borderline high
≥ 240 (6.2)	high
HDL < 35 (0.9)	low

1.) Total blood cholesterol less than 200 mg/dL: HDL greater than or equal to 35 mg/dL, repeat total cholesterol and HDL measurements within 5 years or with physical exam; provide education on general population eating pattern, physical activity, and risk factor education. HDL less than 35 mg/dL, do lipoprotein analysis; base further action on LDL levels.
2.) Total blood cholesterol 200 to 239 mg/dL: HDL greater than or equal to 35 mg/dL and less than 2 risk factors, provide information on dietary modification, physical activity, and risk factor reduction; reevaluate in 1 to 2 years, repeat total and HDL cholesterol measurements, and reinforce nutrition and physical activity education. HDL less than 35 mg/dL or greater than or equal to 2 risk factors, analyze lipoprotein; base further action on LDL levels.
3.) Total blood cholesterol greater than or equal to 240 mg/dL: Analyze lipoprotein; base further action on LDL levels.

Classification of LDL-Cholesterol Levels

Level (mg/dL) (mmol/L)	Classification
< 130 (3.4)	desirable
130 to 159 (3.4 to 4.1)	borderline high
≥ 160 (4.1)	high

1.) LDL greater than or equal to 160 mg/dL without CHD and with less than 2 risk factors: Dietary treatment.
2.) LDL greater than or equal to 130 mg/dL without CHD and with greater than or equal to 2 risk factors: Dietary treatment.
3.) LDL greater than or equal to 190 mg/dL without CHD and with less than 2 other risk factors, or LDL greater than or equal to 160 mg/dL without CHD and with greater than or equal to 2 other risk factors: Drug treatment.

➤*Hyperlipidemias:* Elevation of serum cholesterol, triglycerides, or both is characteristic of hyperlipidemias. Differentiation of the specific biochemical abnormality requires identification of specific lipoprotein fractions in the serum. Lipoproteins transport serum lipids and are identified by their density and electrophoretic mobility. Chylomicrons are the largest and least dense of the lipoproteins, followed in order of increasing density and decreasing size by very low density lipoproteins (VLDL or pre-β), intermediate low density lipoproteins (ILDL or broad-β), low density lipoproteins (LDL or β) and high density lipoproteins (HDL or α). Triglycerides are transported primarily by chylomicrons and VLDL; the predominant cholesterol transporting lipoprotein is LDL.

Elevations and treatment associated with each type of hyperlipidemia follow:

Hyperlipidemias and Their Treatment[a]

Hyperlipidemia type	I	IIa	IIb	III	IV	V
Lipids						
Cholesterol	N-⇧	↑	↑	N-↑	N-⇧	N-↑
Triglycerides	↑	N	↑	N-↑	↑	↑
Lipoproteins						
Chylomicrons	↑	N	N	N	N	↑
VLDL (pre-β)	N-⇧	N-↓	↑	N-⇧	↑	↑
ILDL (broad-β)[b]				↑		
LDL (β)	↓	↑	↑	↑	N-⇩	↓
HDL (α)	↓	N	N	N	N-⇩	↓
Treatment	Diet	Diet HMG-CoA reductase inhibitors Bile acid sequestrants Nicotinic acid	Diet HMG-CoA reductase inhibitors Bile acid sequestrants[c] Gemfibrozil[d] Nicotinic acid	Diet Nicotinic acid Gemfibrozil	Diet Gemfibrozil Nicotinic acid Fenofibrate	Diet Gemfibrozil Nicotinic acid[e] Fenofibrate

[a] N = normal ↑ = increase ↓ = decrease ⇧ = slight increase ⇩ = slight decrease
[b] An abnormal lipoprotein.
[c] Particularly useful if hypercholesterolemia predominates.
[d] In patients with inadequate response to weight loss, bile acid sequestrants, nicotinic acid.
[e] Norethindrone acetate (women) and oxandrolone (men) are effective, but use is not FDA-approved.

The following table summarizes the effects of the various antihyperlipidemic drugs on serum lipids and lipoproteins:

Antihyperlipidemic Drug Effects[a]

	Lipids		Lipoproteins		
Drug	Cholesterol	Triglycerides	VLDL (pre-β)	LDL (β)	HDL
Atorvastatin	↓	↓	↓	↓	↑
Cerivastatin	↓	↓	↓	↓	↑
Cholestyramine	↓	→↑	→↑	↓	→↑
Colestipol	↓	→↑	↑	↓	→↑
Fenofibrate	↓	↓	↓	↑	↑
Fluvastatin	↓	↓	↓	↓	↑
Gemfibrozil	↓	↓	↓	→↓	↑
Lovastatin	↓	↓	↓	↓	↑
Nicotinic acid	↓	↓	↓	↓	↑
Pravastatin	↓	↓	↓	↓	↑
Simvastatin	↓	↓	↓	↓	↑

[a] ↓ = decrease ↑ = increase → = unchanged

➤*General considerations:*
1.) Define the type of hyperlipoproteinemia, and establish baseline serum cholesterol and triglyceride levels.
2.) Institute a trial of diet, weight reduction and physical activity, which are extremely important elements of therapy for high blood cholesterol. Remind patients to restrict their dietary intake of cholesterol and saturated fats and to adhere to prescribed dietary regimens. Drug therapy does not reduce the importance of adhering to diet.
3.) Carefully monitor the patient during treatment, including serum cholesterol and triglyceride levels.
4.) Consider failure of cholesterol level to fall or a significant rise in triglyceride level as indications to discontinue medication.

➤*Dietary treatment:* Reducing elevated cholesterol levels and maintaining adequate nutrition is the aim of dietary therapy. Step I and Step II diets are specifically designed to progressively reduce saturated fatty acids and cholesterol intake and promote weight loss in overweight individuals by eliminating excess total calories and increasing physical activity.

Step I – Total fat intake less than or equal to 30% of calories; saturated fatty acid intake less than 8% to 10% of calories; cholesterol intake less than 300 mg/day. Measure serum total cholesterol and adherence to diet at 4 to 6 weeks and at 3 months. If cholesterol and LDL level goals are met, monitor quarterly the first year and twice a year thereafter. If response is insufficient, proceed to Step II.

Step II – Saturated fatty acid intake less than 7% of calories; cholesterol intake less than 200 mg/day. Measure serum total cholesterol and adherence to diet at 4 to 6 weeks and at 3 months. Begin long-term monitoring if goal has been met. Consider drug therapy if goal has not been attained. Carry out intensive diet therapy and counseling for greater than or equal to 6 months before starting drug therapy. Continue dietary treatment during drug treatment.

➤*Drug treatment:* **Cholestyramine** and **colestipol** are used to lower cholesterol. HMG-CoA reductase inhibitors, **gemfibrozil**, **nicotinic acid**, and **fenofibrate** are used to lower both cholesterol and triglycerides. Gemfibrozil and fenofibrate lower serum triglycerides much more effectively than cholesterol levels. When both cholesterol and triglycerides are elevated, treatment of the hypertriglyceridemia should take precedence. When hypercholesterolemia is treated first, an exacerbation of the hypertriglyceridemia may occur. Serum cholesterol often falls to normal levels without specific therapy following treatment of the hypertriglyceridemia.

First choice – Drugs of first choice include HMG-CoA reductase inhibitors, gemfibrozil or nicotinic acid. Measure LDL-cholesterol levels at 4 to 6 weeks and at 3 months. The target LDL level for treatment is less than or equal to 130 mg/dL. If the response is adequate, monitor every 4 months; if inadequate, switch to another agent or use a combination of 2 drugs. Refer patients who fail to respond to combination therapy to a lipid disorder specialist.

Estrogen – Estrogen replacement therapy can be considered in postmenopausal women with high serum cholesterol because estrogens have been shown to reduce total and LDL- and raise HDL-cholesterol levels.

Combination therapy – Because drug therapy of different hyperlipoproteinemias involves different mechanisms and pharmacologic actions, consider a combined drug regimen in stubborn cases. However, experience with combination therapy is limited. The coadministration of a bile acid sequestrant with either nicotinic acid or an HMG-CoA reductase inhibitor can lower LDL-cholesterol levels by greater than or equal to 40% to 50%. Use HMG-CoA reductase inhibitors and gemfibrozil concomitantly with caution because of the risks of myopathy, rhabdomyolysis and acute renal failure.

Bile Acid Sequestrants

Refer to general discussions on these agents in Antihyperlipidemic Agents Introduction.

Indications

➤*Hyperlipidemia:* Adjunctive therapy to diet for the reduction of elevated serum cholesterol in patients with primary hypercholesterolemia (elevated low-density lipoprotein [LDL]) who do not respond adequately to diet.

These agents may lower LDL cholesterol in patients who also have hypertriglyceridemia, but they are not indicated where hypertriglyceridemia is the abnormality of most concern.

Bile acid sequestrants may raise serum triglyceride levels and are not recommended as monotherapy in patients with triglyceride levels higher than 400 mg/dL or in patients with familial dysbetalipoproteinemia. They may be used as monotherapy in patients with triglyceride levels less than 200 mg/dL. Per the National Cholesterol Education Program (NCEP) Third Report, bile acid sequestrants should be considered as LDL-lowering therapy in patients with moderately elevated LDL cholesterol; women who are considering pregnancy and have elevated LDL cholesterol; patients who need only modest reductions in their LDL cholesterol level to reach their target goal; and for use as combination therapy with an HMG-CoA reductase inhibitor in patients with very high LDL cholesterol levels.

➤*Pruritus (cholestyramine only):* Relief of pruritus associated with partial biliary obstruction. Cholestyramine has been shown to have a variable effect on serum cholesterol in these patients.

➤*Off-label uses:* Refer to individual monographs for further information.

Cholestatic pruritus (adults) –

Colesevelam: [5] = Poor documentation.

Diarrhea –

Cholestyramine: [2] = Fair documentation.

Hyperoxaluria –

Cholestyramine: [4] = Insufficient documentation.

Other possible off-label uses –

Cholestyramine: Postvagotomy diarrhea.

Colestipol: Relief of pruritus associated with partial biliary obstruction (including primary biliary cirrhosis and various other forms of bile stasis).

Cholestyramine and colestipol: Binds to the toxin produced by *Clostridium difficile* in patients with *C. difficile*–associated diarrhea.; bile salt-mediated diarrhea; adjunctive treatment for hyperthyroidism; digitalis toxicity (see Cardiac Glycosides monograph); hyperoxaluria.

Administration and Dosage

Mix dry granules with liquid. Swallow tablets whole.

Cholesterol reduction should occur during the first month of therapy. Continue therapy to sustain cholesterol reduction. If adequate reduction is not attained, discontinue therapy.

➤*Concomitant therapy:* Evidence suggests that the cholesterol-lowering effects of these agents and an HMG-CoA reductase inhibitor are additive. Additive effects on LDL cholesterol also are seen with combined cholestyramine and nicotinic acid therapy.

Actions

➤*Pharmacology:* Cholesterol is the major, and probably sole, precursor of bile acids. During normal digestion, bile acids are secreted via the bile from the liver and gallbladder into the intestines to emulsify the fat and lipid materials in food, thus facilitating absorption. A major portion of the bile acids secreted is reabsorbed from the intestines and returned via the portal circulation to the liver, which completes the enterohepatic cycle.

Bile-acid-sequestering resins bind bile acids in the intestine to form an insoluble complex that is excreted in the feces. This results in a partial removal of bile acids from the enterohepatic circulation, preventing their absorption. Because these agents are anion-exchange resins, the chloride anions of the resin are replaced by other anions. These agents are hydrophilic but insoluble in water. They remain unchanged in the GI tract and are not absorbed.

The increased fecal loss of bile acids leads to an increased oxidation of cholesterol to bile acids. This results in an increased number of LDL receptors, increased hepatic uptake of LDL, decreased beta lipoprotein or LDL serum levels, and decreased serum cholesterol levels. Although bile-acid-sequestering resins produce an increase in the hepatic synthesis of cholesterol, serum cholesterol levels fall. Plasma cholesterol levels fall secondary to an increased rate of clearance of cholesterol-rich lipoproteins from the plasma. Serum triglyceride levels may increase or remain unchanged in treated patients.

The decline in serum cholesterol is usually evident within 1 month. When the resins are discontinued, serum cholesterol levels usually return to baseline within 1 month. Determine serum cholesterol levels periodically.

In patients with partial biliary obstruction, reduction of serum bile acid levels by **cholestyramine** reduces bile acid deposits in the dermal tissues with a resultant decrease in pruritus.

➤*Pharmacokinetics:*

Absorption – Bile acid sequestrants are hydrophilic but virtually water insoluble (99.75%), not hydrolyzed by digestive enzymes, and not absorbed.

Excretion – After administration of 1.9 g of **colesevelam** twice per day for 28 days, an average of 0.05% of a single dose was excreted in the urine. For **colestipol**, administration of 20 g per day for 60 days, less than 0.17% of a single dose was excreted in the urine.

Contraindications

Hypersensitivity to bile acid sequestering resins or any components of the products; complete biliary obstruction (cholestyramine only); bowel obstruction (colesevelam only).

Warnings/Precautions

➤*Phenylketonurics:* Some products may contain phenylalanine. See individual monographs.

➤*Powder / Granules:* Avoid accidental inhalation or esophageal distress; do not take dry. Mix with fluids before ingesting.

➤*Calcified material:* Calcified material has been observed in the biliary tree and the gall bladder; however, this may be due to liver disease and not drug-related. One patient experienced biliary colic on each of 3 occasions on which he took **cholestyramine**. Another patient, diagnosed with an acute abdominal symptom complex, showed a "pasty mass" in the transverse colon on x-ray.

➤*Diet:* Before instituting therapy, vigorously attempt to control serum cholesterol with an appropriate dietary regimen and weight reduction.

➤*Thyroid function:* While there have been no reports of hypothyroidism induced in individuals with normal thyroid function, the theoretical possibility exists, particularly in patients with limited thyroid reserve.

➤*Contributing diseases:* Prior to initiating therapy, investigate and treat diseases contributing to increased blood cholesterol (eg, alcoholism, diabetes mellitus, dysproteinemias, hypothyroidism, nephrotic syndrome, obstructive liver disease, other drug therapy).

➤*Malabsorption:* Because they sequester bile acids, these resins may interfere with normal fat absorption and digestion and may prevent absorption of fat-soluble vitamins such as A, D, K, and folic acid.

Chronic use may increase bleeding tendencies due to hypoprothrombinemia associated with vitamin K deficiency. This usually responds promptly to parenteral vitamin K_1; prevent recurrences by giving oral vitamin K_1.

➤*Reduced folate:* Reduction of serum or red cell folate has been reported over long-term administration of **cholestyramine**. Consider supplementation with folic acid.

➤*Hyperchloremic acidosis:* Prolonged use of chloride anion-exchange resins may cause hyperchloremic acidosis, especially for younger and smaller patients in which relative dosage may be higher.

➤*GI disorders:* The safety and efficacy of colesevelam in patients with dysphagia, swallowing disorders, severe GI motility disorders, or major GI tract surgery have not be established. Use with caution.

➤*Constipation:* These agents may produce or severely worsen preexisting constipation. Fecal impaction may occur and hemorrhoids may be aggravated. Avoid constipation in patients with symptomatic coronary artery disease. Most instances of constipation are mild, transient, and controlled with standard treatment. Some patients require decreased dosage or discontinuation of therapy.

Gradually increase the dosage to minimize the risk of developing fecal impaction. Encourage increased fluid intake and inclusion of additional dietary fiber to alleviate constipation; a stool softener may be added if needed.

Colestipol tablets – In patients with preexisting constipation, the starting dosage should be 2 g once or twice daily.

Colestipol and cholestyramine oral suspension – In patients with preexisting constipation, the starting dosage is 1 packet or 1 scoop once daily for 5 to 7 days, increasing to twice daily with monitoring of constipation and of serum lipoproteins, at least twice, 4 to 6 weeks apart.

➤*Pregnancy:* *Category B* – **colesevelam**; **cholestyramine** and **colestipol** per Briggs' *Drugs in Pregnancy and Lactation*. *Category C* – **cholesty-**

ramineand **colestipol** per manufacturer's prescribing information. These agents are not absorbed systemically, and are not expected to cause fetal harm when administered during pregnancy in recommended doses. There are no adequate and well-controlled studies in pregnant women, and the known interference with fat-soluble vitamin absorption may be detrimental even with supplementation. No adverse fetal effects were observed when **cholestyramine** was used for the treatment of cholestasis of pregnancy. Weigh the potential benefits against the risks.

➤*Lactation:* Exercise caution when administering to a breast-feeding woman. The possible lack of proper vitamin absorption may have an effect on breast-feeding infants.

➤*Children:*

Cholestyramine – Dosage schedules have not been established. Standard texts list a usual pediatric dosage of anhydrous cholestyramine resin 240 mg/kg/day in 2 to 3 divided doses, normally not to exceed 8 g/day with dose titration based on response and tolerance. In calculating pediatric dosages, anhydrous cholestyramine resin 80 mg is contained in 110 mg of *Prevalite*; anhydrous cholestyramine 44.4 mg is contained in 100 mg of *Questran*; and anhydrous cholestyramine 62.7 mg is contained in 100 mg of *Questran Light*. The effects of long-term administration and efficacy in maintaining lowered cholesterol levels are unknown.

Colestipol and colesevelam – Safety and efficacy have not been established.

➤*Monitoring:* Determine serum cholesterol levels at baseline, then frequently during the first few months of therapy and periodically thereafter. Periodically measure serum triglyceride levels to detect significant changes.

Drug Interactions

Bile Acid Sequestrant (BAS) Drug Interactions

Precipitant drug	Object drug[a]		Description
BAS	Anticoagulants	⬇	Cholestyramine may decrease anticoagulant effect; separate the administration of these agents.
BAS	Mycophenolate	⬇	≈ 40% decrease in the area under the curve (AUC) by cholestyramine.
BAS	Thyroid hormones	⬇	Possible loss of efficacy of thyroid and potential hypothyroidism with concurrent cholestyramine. Separate administration by 6 h.
BAS	Verapamil, sustained-release	⬇	Colesevelam decreased the maximum plasma concentration (C_{max}) and AUC of sustained-release verapamil by approximately 31% and 11%, respectively.
BAS	Vitamins A, D, E, K, folic acid	⬇	Malabsorption may occur during administration of bile acid sequestrants (see Precautions).

[a] ⬇ = Object drug decreased.

For cholestyramine and colestipol, binding in the GI tract may delay or reduce the absorption of concomitant oral medication. Take other drugs at least 1 hour before or 4 to 6 hours after these agents. Discontinuation of a resin could pose a hazard if a potentially toxic, significantly bound drug has been titrated to a maintenance level while on the resin.

Cholestyramine and Colestipol Drug Interactions (Decreased Serum Levels or GI Absorption)

Corticosteroids	HMG-CoA reductase inhibitors	Phosphate supplements
Digitalis glycosides	Hydrocortisone	Propranolol
Doxepin	Imipramine	Tetracyclines
Estrogens/progestins	NSAIDs	Thiazide diuretics
Furosemide	Penicillin G	Ursodiol
Gemfibrozil	Phenobarbital	Valproic acid
Glipizide		

Adverse Reactions

➤*Colesevelam:*

Colesevelam Adverse Reactions (> 2%)

Adverse reaction	Placebo (n = 258)	Colesevelam only (n = 807)
CNS		
Asthenia	2	4
Headache	8	6
GI		
Abdominal pain	5	5
Constipation	7	11
Diarrhea	7	5
Dyspepsia	3	8
Flatulence	14	12
Nausea	4	4
Musculoskeletal		
Back pain	6	3
Myalgia	0	2
Respiratory		
Cough increased	2	2
Pharyngitis	2	3
Rhinitis	3	3
Sinusitis	4	2
Miscellaneous		
Accidental injury	3	4
Flu syndrome	3	3
Infection	13	10
Pain	7	5

➤*Cholestyramine/colestipol:*

Cardiovascular – Chest pain, angina, tachycardia (colestipol); syncope (cholestyramine).

CNS – Dizziness, fatigue, headache (eg, migraine, sinus).

Cholestyramine: Anxiety, drowsiness, femoral nerve pain, paresthesia, tinnitus, vertigo.

Colestipol: Insomnia, light-headedness, weakness.

GI –

Cholestyramine/Colestipol: Abdominal discomfort/pain/cramping, aggravated or bleeding hemorrhoids, anorexia, blood in the stool, constipation, diarrhea, intestinal gas (bloating and flatulence), nausea, vomiting.

Colestipol: Heartburn, indigestion, loose stools; cholecystitis, cholelithiasis, peptic ulceration. (rare).

Cholestyramine: Bleeding from known duodenal ulcer, diverticulitis, dyspepsia, dysphagia, eructation, hiccups, pancreatitis, rectal pain, steatorrhea, sour taste, ulcer attack; rare reports of intestinal obstruction, including 2 deaths, in pediatric patients. Occasional calcified material has been observed in the biliary tree, including calcification of the gallbladder; however, this may be a manifestation of liver disease and not drug related (see Warnings). One patient experienced biliary colic on 3 occasions; one patient was diagnosed with acute abdominal symptom complex and was found to have a "pasty mass" in the transverse colon on x-ray.

Hematologic – Anemia, ecchymosis, increased prothrombin time (cholestyramine).

Hypersensitivity –

Cholestyramine: Asthma, shortness of breath, urticaria, wheezing.

Colestipol: Rash; dermatitis, urticaria (rare).

Musculoskeletal – Aches and pains in the extremities, arthritis, backache, muscle/joint pains.

Renal – Burnt odor to urine, diuresis, dysuria, hematuria (cholestyramine).

Miscellaneous –

Colestipol: Shortness of breath, swelling of hands or feet.

Cholestyramine: Bleeding tendencies due to hypoprothrombinemia (vitamin K deficiency); edema; dental bleeding; dental caries; erosion of tooth enamel; hyperchloremic acidosis in children (see Precautions); rash and irritation of the skin, tongue, and perianal area; increased libido; osteoporosis; swollen glands; tooth discoloration; uveitis; vitamin A (1 case of night blindness) and D deficiencies; weight loss/gain.

Lab test abnormalities –

Colestipol: Transient, modest elevations of AST, ALT, and alkaline phosphatase.

Cholestyramine: Liver function abnormalities.

Overdosage

The main potential harm is GI tract obstruction. Location and degree of obstruction and status of gut motility determine treatment. Overdosage has been reported in a patient taking 150% of the maximum recommended daily dose of **cholestyramine** for several weeks; no ill effects were reported.

Patient Information

Instruct patients not to take the powder in dry form but to mix with beverages, highly fluid soups, cereals, or pulpy fruits (see Administration and Dosage in individual monographs).

Instruct patients to swallow **colestipol** tablets whole 1 at a time and not to cut, crush, or chew.

Medication may interfere with absorption of concomitant drugs. Advise patients to take other drugs 1 hour before or 4 to 6 hours after **cholestyramine**, **colestipol**, or **colesevelam** (see Drug Interactions).

Constipation, flatulence, nausea, and heartburn may occur and may disappear with continued therapy. Advise patients to notify health care provider if these effects become bothersome or if unusual bleeding (eg, from the gums or rectum) occurs.

Sipping or holding the resin suspension in the mouth for prolonged periods may lead to changes in the surface of the teeth, resulting in discoloration, erosion of enamel, or decay; instruct patients to maintain good oral hygiene.

Instruct patient to inform health care provider if pregnant, planning to become pregnant, or breastfeeding.

CHOLESTYRAMINE

Rx	**Cholestyramine** (Various, eg, Eon, Novopharm)	**Powder for oral suspension:** anhydrous cholestyramine resin 4 g per 9 g powder	May contain sucrose, sorbitol. In 9 g packets (42s and 60s) and 378 g cans.
Rx	**Questran** (Par)		Sucrose. In 9 g packets (60s) and 378 g cans.
Rx	**Cholestyramine (Light)** (Various, eg, Eon, Novopharm)	**Powder for oral suspension:** anhydrous cholestyramine resin 4 g per 5.7 g powder	May contain aspartame. In 5 and 5.7 g packets (60s) and 210, 231, and 239 g cans.
Rx	**Prevalite** (Upsher Smith)	**Powder for oral suspension:** anhydrous cholestyramine resin 4 g per 5.5 g powder	Aspartame, phenylalanine 14.1 mg per 5.5 g. Orange flavor. In 5.5 g packets (42s and 60s) and 231 g cans (42 doses).
Rx	**Questran Light** (Par)	**Powder for oral suspension:** anhydrous cholestyramine resin 4 g per 6.4 g powder	Maltodextrin, aspartame, phenylalanine 28.1 mg per 6.4 g. Orange vanilla flavor. In 6.4 g packets (60s) and 268 g cans.

CHOLESTYRAMINE — ORAL

For complete and comparative prescribing information, refer to the Bile Acid Sequestrants group monograph.

Indications

➤*Hyperlipidemia:* Adjunctive therapy to diet for reduction of elevated serum cholesterol in patients with primary hypercholesterolemia (elevated low-density lipoprotein [LDL] cholesterol) who do not respond adequately to diet. May be useful to lower LDL cholesterol in patients who also have hypertriglyceridemia, but it is not indicated where hypertriglyceridemia is the abnormality of most concern.

➤*Pruritus:* Relief of pruritus associated with partial biliary obstruction.

➤*Off-label uses:*

Diarrhea – [2] = Fair documentation. The data available from small studies suggest that cholestyramine may have some benefits as an adjunctive therapy in the management of bile acid malabsorption diarrhea. Because of the drug's limited adverse event profile, it may be a viable option in patients refractory to other therapy.

Hyperoxaluria – [4] = Insufficient documentation. Studies performed in the 1970s suggest that cholestyramine is an effective treatment for hyperoxaluria in symptomatic patients who have a history of ileal resection. However, more recent studies have shown insignificant changes in oxalate excretion after cholestyramine administration.

Other possible off-label uses – Binds to the toxin produced by *Clostridium difficile* in patients with *C. difficile*–associated diarrhea; digitalis toxicity (see Cardiac Glycosides monograph); adjunctive treatment for hyperthyroidism.

For the treatment of diarrhea associated with excess fecal bile acids or pseudomembranous colitis and pruritus associated with elevated bile acids in children.

Administration and Dosage

➤*Adults:*

Hyperlipidemia – 4 g (1 packet or 1 full scoop) 1 to 2 times daily. Individualize dosage.

Maintenance dosage: 2 to 4 packets or full scoops daily (anhydrous cholestyramine resin 8 to 16 g) divided into 2 doses. Increase dose gradually.

Dosage adjustment: In patients with preexisting constipation, the starting dosage should be 1 packet or 1 scoop once daily for 5 to 7 days, increasing to twice daily, with monitoring of constipation and serum lipoproteins at least twice, 4 to 6 weeks apart.

Alternative dosage: Although the recommended dosing schedule is twice daily, cholestyramine may be administered in 1 to 6 doses/day.

Concomitant therapy: Because cholestyramine resin may bind other drugs given concurrently, it is recommended that patients take other drugs at least 1 hour before or 4 to 6 hours after (or at as large an interval as possible) cholestyramine to avoid impeding their absorption.

Monitoring: Periodic assessment of lipid/lipoprotein levels at intervals of at least 4 weeks.

Off-label dosing –

Diarrhea: [2] = Fair documentation. Used as adjunctive therapy in doses of up to 4 g four times per day for 2 weeks.

Hyperoxaluria: [4] = Insufficient documentation. 4 g administered 4 times daily. Dosages of 2 and 8 g 4 times daily have also been studied with no significant difference in effect noted.

➤*Children:*

Hyperlipidemia –

Usual dosage: Although an optimal dosage schedule has not been established, the usual dose is 240 mg/kg/day of anhydrous cholestyramine resin in 2 to 3 divided doses.

Maximum dose: 8 g/day.

Dosage titration: Base dosage titration on response and tolerance.

Duration of therapy: The effects of long-term drug administration and the effect in maintaining lowered cholesterol levels in children are unknown.

Off-label dosing –

Diarrhea associated with excess fecal bile acids or pseudomembranous colitis:

- *Usual dose* – 240 mg/kg/day in 3 divided doses.
- *Maximum dose* – 8 g/day.

Pruritus associated with elevated bile acids:

- *Usual dose* – 240 mg/kg/day in 3 divided doses.
- *Maximum dose* – 8 g/day.

➤*Preparation for administration:* Mix the contents of 1 powder packet or 1 level scoopful with 60 to 180 mL (2 to 6 fl oz) of water or noncarbonated beverage. Stir to a uniform consistency and drink. Do not take in dry form. Always mix with water or other fluids, highly fluid soups, or pulpy fruits, such as applesauce or crushed pineapple.

➤*Administration:* Recommended administration time is at mealtime; this may be modified to avoid interference with absorption of concomitant medications.

➤*Storage/Stability:* Store at 15° to 30°C (59° to 86°F).

COLESEVELAM HYDROCHLORIDE

Rx	**Welchol** (Daiichi Sankyo)	**Tablets; oral:** 625 mg	(Sankyo C01). Off-white, oval. Film-coated. In 180s.
		Powder for suspension; oral: 1.875 g	Aspartame, phenylalanine 24 mg. Citrus flavored. In single-dose packets.
		Powder for suspension; oral: 3.75 g	Aspartame, phenylalanine 48 mg. Citrus flavored. In single-dose packets.

COLESEVELAM HYDROCHLORIDE — ORAL

For complete and comparative prescribing information, refer to the Bile Acid Sequestrants group monograph.

Indications

➤*Primary hyperlipidemia:* Adjunctive therapy to diet and exercise and used alone or in combination with a 3-hydroxy-3-methylglutaryl coenzyme A (HMG-CoA) reductase inhibitor to reduce elevated low-density lipoprotein-cholesterol (LDL-C) in adults with primary hyperlipidemia (Fredrickson type IIa).

Colesevelam is indicated as monotherapy or in combination with a statin to reduce LDL-C levels in boys and postmenarchal girls, 10 to 17 years of age, with heterozygous familial hypercholesterolemia if after an adequate trial of diet therapy the following findings are present: LDL-C remains at least 190 mg/dL, or LDL-C remains at least 160 mg/dL and there is a positive family history of premature cardiovascular disease or 2 or more other cardiovascular disease risk factors are present in the pediatric patient.

Use lipid-altering agents in addition to a diet restricted in saturated fat and cholesterol when response to diet and nonpharmacological interventions alone has been inadequate. Colesevelam has not been studied in Fredrickson type I, III, IV, and V dyslipidemias.

Colesevelam has not been studied in children younger than 10 years of age or in premenarchal girls.

➤*Type 2 diabetes mellitus:* As an adjunct to diet and exercise to improve glycemic control in adults with type 2 diabetes mellitus.

➤*Off-label uses:*

Cholestatic pruritus (adults) – [5] = Poor documentation. Current evidence from controlled trials in a limited number of patients indicates that colesevelam is not superior to placebo in the management of cholestatic pruritus. The Association for the Study of Liver Diseases practice guideline for the management of primary biliary cirrhosis recommends cholestyramine as the first-line drug for the treatment of pruritus associated with liver disease. In patients who are intolerant of or who fail therapy with cholestyramine, rifampin is recommended as a second-line agent.

COLESEVELAM HYDROCHLORIDE — ORAL

Administration and Dosage

➤*General dosing considerations:* After initiation of colesevelam, lipid levels should be analyzed within 4 to 6 weeks.

➤*Adults:*

Primary hyperlipidemia –

Usual dosage: 6 tablets once daily or 3 tablets twice daily whether used as monotherapy or in combination with a statin or 3.75 g powder once daily or 1.875 g powder twice daily.

Concomitant therapy: Colesevelam can be dosed at the same time as a statin, or the 2 drugs can be dosed apart.

Type 2 diabetes mellitus – 6 tablets once daily or 3 tablets twice daily or 3.75 g powder once daily or 1.875 g powder twice daily.

Off-label dosing –

➤*Children:*

Primary hypercholesterolemia –

10 to 17 years of age:

• *Usual dosage –* 3.75 g powder once daily or 1.875 g powder twice daily taken with meals.

Because of the tablet size, colesevelam tablets are not recommended for use in children.

➤*Elderly:* Greater sensitivity of some older patients cannot be ruled out.

➤*Renal function impairment:* No overall differences in safety or effectiveness were observed between patients with creatinine clearance (CrCl) of less than 50 mL/min (n = 53) and those with a CrCl of 50 mL/min or more (n = 1,075).

➤*Preparation for administration:* To prepare oral suspension, the entire contents of 1 packet should be emptied into a glass or cup. Add ½ or 1 cup (4 to 8 oz) of water. Advise patient to stir well and drink.

➤*Administration:* Colesevelam tablets should be taken with a meal and liquid. Colesevelam for oral suspension should be taken with meals. To avoid esophageal distress, colesevelam for oral suspension should not be taken in its dry form.

➤*Storage/Stability:* Store tablets and powder for oral suspension at 25°C (77°F); excursions are permitted to 15° to 30°C (59° to 86°F). Brief exposure of tablets to 40°C (104°F) does not adversely affect the product. Protect tablets and powder from moisture.

COLESTIPOL HYDROCHLORIDE

Rx	**Colestipol Hydrochloride** (Various, eg, Global, Greenstone)	**Tablets; oral:** 1 g	In 120s and 500s.
Rx	**Colestid** (Pharmacia)		(U). Yellow, elliptical. In 120s and 500s.
Rx	**Colestipol Hydrochloride**	**Granules for oral suspension; oral:** 5 g per packet/scoop	In 5 g packets (30s and 90s) and 500 g bottles.
Rx	**Colestid** (Pharmacia)	**Granules for oral suspension; oral:** colestipol hydrochloride 5 g per 7.5 g granules	Unflavored: In 300 and 500 g bottles and 5 g packets (30s and 90s). Flavored: Aspartame, mannitol. Orange flavor. In 450 g bottles (60 doses) and 7.5 g packets (60s).

COLESTIPOL HYDROCHLORIDE — ORAL

For complete and comparative prescribing information, refer to the Bile Acid Sequestrants group monograph.

Indications

➤*Hyperlipidemia:* Adjunctive therapy to diet for the reduction of elevated serum total and low-density lipoprotein (LDL) cholesterol in patients with primary hypercholesterolemia (elevated LDL cholesterol) who do not respond adequately to diet.

Generally, colestipol has no clinically significant effect on serum triglycerides, but with its use, triglyceride levels may be raised in some patients.

➤*Off-label uses:*

Pruritus with primary biliary obstruction – [4] = Insufficient documentation. No primary studies have been published investigating the use of colestipol for treatment of pruritus associated with primary biliary cirrhosis. Current guidelines recommend the use of cholestyramine as first-line therapy, and review literature has stated that colestipol is an alternative treatment option for those patients who do not tolerate the adverse reactions of cholestyramine. This recommendation is based on empirical knowledge that cholestyramine is highly effective for this indication and is in the same classification as colestipol. Therefore, it would be sensible for patients to attempt colestipol as treatment for pruritus related to primary biliary obstruction before trying other medical alternatives.

Other possible off-label uses – Treatment of digitalis toxicity (see Cardiac Glycosides monograph); hyperoxaluria; diarrhea due to bile acids; adjunctive treatment for hyperthyroidism; binds to the toxin produced by *Clostridium difficile* in patients with *C. difficile*–associated diarrhea.

Administration and Dosage

➤*General dosing considerations:* Patients should take other drugs at least 1 hour before or 4 hours after colestipol to minimize possible interference with its absorption.

➤*Adults:*

Hyperlipidemia –

Granules:

• *Usual dosage –* 5 to 30 g/day (1 to 6 packets or level scoopfuls) given once daily or in divided doses.

• *Initial dosage –* 5 g once or twice daily.

• *Dosage titration –* Daily increment of 5 g at 1- or 2-month intervals.

Tablets:

• *Usual dosage –* 2 to 16 g/day given once or in divided doses.

• *Initial dosage –* 2 g once or twice daily.

• *Dosage titration –* Increases of 2 g, once or twice daily, should occur at 1- or 2-month intervals. Periodically assess lipid/lipoprotein levels.

• *Concomitant therapy –* If the desired effect is not obtained at the recommended dose, consider combined therapy or alternate treatment.

Off-label dosing –

Pruritus with primary biliary obstruction: [4] = Insufficient documentation. Colestipol 5 to 30 g/day has typically been used. Initiate at 5 g orally once or twice daily with increases of 5 g/day every 1 to 2 months. Maximum dosage was 30 g/day divided into 2 to 4 doses.

➤*Constipation:*

Granules – In patients with pre-existing constipation, the starting dosage should be 1 packet or 1 scoop once daily for 5 to 7 days, increasing to twice daily with monitoring of constipation and serum lipoproteins, at least twice, 4 to 6 weeks apart.

Tablets – In patients with pre-existing constipation, the starting dosage should be 2 g once or twice per day.

➤*Administration:*

Granules – Mix in liquids, soups, cereals, or pulpy fruits (eg, crushed pineapple, pears, peaches). Do not take dry. Add the prescribed amount to a glassful (90 mL or more) of liquid; stir until completely mixed. A heavy or pulpy juice may minimize complaints about consistency. Colestipol will not dissolve. It may also be mixed with carbonated beverages slowly stirred in a large glass; however, this mixture may be associated with GI complaints. Rinse glass with a small amount of additional beverage to ensure that all of the medication is taken.

Tablets – Swallow tablets whole, 1 at a time; do not cut, chew, or crush. The tablets may be taken with plenty of water or other appropriate fluids.

➤*Storage/Stability:* Store at 20° to 25°C (68° to 77°F).

HMG-CoA Reductase Inhibitors (Statins)

Refer to the general discussion of these products in the Antihyperlipidemic Agents Introduction.

Indications

HMG-CoA Reductase Inhibitors – Summary of Indications[a]

Indication	Atorvastatin	Fluvastatin	Lovastatin	Pitavastatin	Pravastatin	Rosuvastatin	Simvastatin
Food and Drug Administration–approved indications							
Primary prevention of CV disease in patients with multiple risk factors for CHD, diabetes, peripheral vascular disease, history of stroke, or other cerebrovascular disease to:							
Reduce angina risk	✓		✓				
Reduce MI risk	✓				✓		✓
Reduce stroke risk	✓						✓
Reduce risk for revascularization procedures	✓		✓		✓		✓
Reduce risk of CV mortality					✓		✓
Secondary prevention of CV events in patients with clinically evident CHD to:							
Reduce risk of MI	✓				✓		✓
Reduce risk of stroke	✓				✓		✓
Reduce risk for revascularization procedures	✓	✓			✓		✓
Reduce risk of hospitalization for CHF	✓						
Reduce angina risk	✓						
Slow progression of coronary atherosclerosis		✓	✓		✓	✓	
Reduce risk of total mortality by reducing coronary death					✓		✓
Hypercholesterolemia							
Primary hypercholesterolemia (heterozygous familial and nonfamilial)	✓	✓	✓	✓	✓	✓	✓
Adolescents with heterozygous familial hypercholesterolemia	✓	✓	✓		✓		✓
Homozygous familial hypercholesterolemia	✓					✓	✓
Mixed dyslipidemia (Fredrickson types IIa and IIb)	✓	✓	✓	✓	✓	✓	✓
Hypertriglyceridemia (Fredrickson type IV)	✓				✓	✓	✓
Primary dysbetalipoproteinemia (Fredrickson type III)	✓				✓	✓	✓

[a] HMG-CoA = 3-hydroxy-3-methylglutaryl coenzyme A; CV = cardiovascular; CHD = coronary heart disease; MI = myocardial infarction; CHF = congestive heart failure.

➤*General information:* Use HMG-CoA reductase inhibitors in addition to a diet restricted in saturated fat and cholesterol when diet and other nonpharmacological therapies alone have produced inadequate response.

Before initiating treatment with HMG-CoA reductase inhibitors, exclude secondary causes of hypercholesterolemia (eg, poorly controlled diabetes mellitus, hypothyroidism, nephrotic syndrome, dysproteinemias, obstructive liver disease, other drug therapy, alcoholism). Perform a lipid profile to measure total cholesterol (total-C), low-density lipoprotein cholesterol (LDL-C), high-density lipoprotein cholesterol (HDL-C), and triglycerides (TGs). Estimate LDL-C in patients with TG less than 400 mg/dL (less than 4.5 mmol/L) using the following equation: LDL-C = total-C − (⅕ TG + HDL-C). Determine LDL-C by ultracentrifugation for patients with TG greater than 400 mg/dL because this equation is less accurate.

➤*Off-label uses:* Refer to individual monographs for further information.

Juvenile rheumatoid arthritis –

Atorvastatin: [4] = Insufficient documentation.

Multiple sclerosis –

Simvastatin: [5] = Poor documentation.

Rheumatoid arthritis –

Atorvastatin: [4] = Insufficient documentation.

Actions

➤*Pharmacology:* These agents, also referred to as the statins, competitively inhibit HMG-CoA reductase, the enzyme that catalyzes the conversion of HMG-CoA to mevalonate. This conversion is an early rate-limiting step in cholesterol biosynthesis. By inhibiting this enzyme, statins markedly reduce plasma concentrations of LDL and total-C and to a lesser extent apolipoprotein B (Apo-B) and TGs, and increase levels of HDL-C. The mechanism of the LDL-lowering effect may involve both reduction of very low density lipoprotein synthesis and induction of the LDL receptor, leading to reduced production and/or increased uptake and catabolism of LDL (by increasing the number of hepatic LDL receptors on the cell surface). **Lovastatin** and **simvastatin** are inactive lactone prodrugs that are rapidly hydrolyzed to their active beta-hydroxyacid forms. The other statins are administered in their active forms.

These agents are highly effective in reducing total-C and LDL in heterozygous familial and nonfamilial forms of hypercholesterolemia and mixed hyperlipidemia. A marked response was seen within 1 to 2 weeks, and the maximum therapeutic response occurred within 4 to 6 weeks. The response was maintained during therapy. Reductions in LDL are dose dependent and log linear; therefore, LDL levels decreased by 6% with each doubling of the statin dose. In patients with TG levels higher than 200 mg/dL, TGs decrease in direct proportion to LDL decreases. In patients with very high TG levels, the LDL decreases are less than observed in patients with low TG levels.

In studies of some agents, single daily doses given in the evening were more effective than in the morning, perhaps because cholesterol is synthesized mainly at night. However, **atorvastatin** and its metabolites have long half-lives and thus administration in the morning is equally effective.

The rank order for statins, based on LDL-C–lowering potencies, is as follows: **rosuvastatin > atorvastatin > simvastatin > pravastatin = lovastatin > fluvastatin**.

➤*Pharmacokinetics:*

HMG-CoA Reductase Inhibitor Pharmacokinetics[a]

	Atorvastatin	Fluvastatin	Lovastatin	Pitavastatin	Pravastatin	Rosuvastatin	Simvastatin
Pharmacology							
Lipophilicity	Lipophilic	Hydrophilic	Lipophilic	Lipophilic	Hydrophilic	Hydrophilic	Lipophilic
Pharmacokinetics							
Prodrug	No	No	Yes	No	No	No	Yes
Bioavailability	≈ 14%; first-pass metabolism (CYP3A4)	24%; saturable first-pass metabolism (CYP2C9); mean relative bioavailability is ≈ 29% for ER compared with IR	< 5%; extensive first-pass metabolism (CYP3A4); bioavailability for ER was 190% compared with IR	51%	34% absorbed; absolute bioavailability 17%; extensive first-pass metabolism	≈ 20%	< 5%; extensive first-pass metabolism (CYP3A4)
Time to peak	1 to 2 h	< 1 h (IR); 3 h (ER)	2 to 4 h	1 h	1 to 1.5 h	3 to 5 h	1.3 to 2.4 h

HMG-CoA Reductase Inhibitor Pharmacokinetics[a]

	Atorvastatin	Fluvastatin	Lovastatin	Pitavastatin	Pravastatin	Rosuvastatin	Simvastatin
Effect of food	Decreased rate and extent of absorption 25% and 9%, respectively; not clinically significant	Decreased rate, but not extent, of absorption (IR); Delayed T_{max} (6 h) and increased bioavailability by ≈ 50% (ER)	Decreased bioavailability (ER)	Decreased rate by 43%, but does not significantly reduce extent	Decreased bioavailability; not clinically significant	Decreased rate 20%, but not extent of absorption	
Protein binding	≥ 98%	98%	> 95%	> 99%	≈ 50%	88%	≈ 95%
Half-life	14 h[b]	< 3 h (IR); ≈ 9 (ER)	3 to 4 h (IR)	12 h	77 h[c]	≈ 19 h	
Metabolic enzymes	Extensive CYP3A4	Extensive CYP2C9, CYP3A4	Extensive CYP3A4	Marginal CYP2C9	Extensive sulfation	Minor CYP2C9	Extensive CYP3A4
Active metabolites	Yes	No	Yes	Yes	No	No	Yes
Excretion	Biliary; < 2% (urine)	≈ 5% (urine); ≈ 90% (feces)	10% (urine); 83% (feces)	15% (urine); 79% (feces)	≈ 20% (urine); 70% (feces)	90% (feces)	13% (urine); 60% (feces)
Effects of renal/hepatic impairment	Plasma levels not affected by renal disease; markedly increased with chronic alcoholic liver disease; C_{max} and AUC are 4-fold greater and 16-fold greater in patients with Child-Pugh score A disease and Child-Pugh score B disease, respectively.	Potential drug accumulation with hepatic insufficiency.	Increased plasma concentration with severe renal disease.	Plasma concentrations are increased in mild to moderate hepatic impairment; rate and extent of absorption are increased 60% and 79%, respectively, in patients with moderate renal impairment.	Potential drug accumulation with renal or hepatic insufficiency; mean AUC varied 18-fold in cirrhotic patients, and peak values varied 47-fold.	Increased plasma concentrations with severe renal impairment and hepatic disease.	Higher systemic exposure may occur in hepatic and severe renal insufficiency.

[a] IR = immediate-release; C_{max} = maximal drug concentration; T_{max} = time to maximal drug concentration; AUC = area under the curve.
[b] For unmetabolized **atorvastatin** only. The half-life of inhibitory activity for HMG-CoA reductase is 20 to 30 hours because of the contribution of active metabolites.
[c] Parent plus metabolites.

Contraindications

Hypersensitivity to any component of these products; active liver disease or unexplained persistent elevations of hepatic transaminases; pregnancy, lactation (see Warnings/Precautions); coadministration with cyclosporine (**pitavastatin** only).

Warnings/Precautions

➤*Skeletal muscle effects:* Cases of rhabdomyolysis with acute renal failure secondary to myoglobinuria have been reported with statins, and rare fatalities have occurred. Myopathy (ie, muscle pain, tenderness, or weakness with creatine phosphokinase [CPK] values above 10 times the upper limit of normal [ULN]) and uncomplicated myalgia have also been reported with drugs in this class. The risk of myopathy is increased by high levels of HMG-CoA reductase inhibitory activity in plasma. Factors that may predispose patients to myopathy with HMG-CoA reductase inhibitors include advanced age (65 years of age and older), inadequately treated or uncontrolled hypothyroidism, and renal insufficiency. The risk of myopathy/rhabdomyolysis is dose related and also increases when statins are given concomitantly with other drugs that inhibit their metabolism (eg, cyclosporine, erythromycin, azole antifungals) or other drugs that can cause myopathy when given alone (eg, fibrates, lipid-lowering doses of niacin). Generally avoid concomitant use of these agents with statins. If combination use is being considered, carefully weigh the benefit against the potential risks of these combinations, and carefully monitor patients for any signs or symptoms of muscle pain, tenderness, or weakness, particularly during the initial months of therapy and during any periods of upward dosage titration of either drug. Consider periodic CPK determinations in such situations; however, there is no assurance that such monitoring will prevent the occurrence of severe myopathy. For dosage adjustments, refer to the individual monographs. See also Drug Interactions.

Consider myopathy in any patient with diffuse myalgias, muscle tenderness or weakness, and/or marked CPK elevation. Advise patients to promptly report muscle pain, tenderness, or weakness, particularly with malaise or fever. Discontinue the drug if markedly elevated CPK levels occur or if myopathy is diagnosed or suspected. For **lovastatin** and **simvastatin**, most cases of muscle symptoms and CPK increases resolved when treatment was promptly discontinued.

Consider temporarily withholding or discontinuing drug therapy in any patient with an acute, serious condition suggestive of a myopathy or with a risk factor predisposing them to the development of renal failure secondary to rhabdomyolysis, including the following: severe acute infection; sepsis; hypotension; major surgery; trauma; severe metabolic, endocrine, or electrolyte disorders; uncontrolled seizures. Temporarily stop statin therapy a few days prior to elective major surgery and when any major medical or surgical condition supervenes.

➤*Hepatic effects:* Statins have been associated with biochemical abnormalities of liver function. Elevations in hepatic transaminases were dose dependent. Marked persistent increases (greater than 3 times the ULN occurring on 2 or more occasions) in serum transaminases have occurred. The incidence of these abnormalities with **lovastatin** was 0.1%, 0.9%, and 1.5% for 20, 40, and 80 mg, respectively. However, in postmarketing experience with **lovastatin**, symptomatic liver disease has been reported rarely at all dosages. The incidence of these abnormalities with **rosuvastatin** was 1.1%. The incidence of these abnormalities with **fluvastatin** was 0.2%, 1.5%, and 2.7% with 20, 40, and 80 mg, respectively. The incidence of these abnormalities with **pravastatin** was 1.2% or less. The incidence of these abnormalities with **simvastatin** was approximately 1%. The incidence of these abnormalities with **atorvastatin** was 0.2%, 0.2%, 0.6%, and 2.3% for 10, 20, 40, and 80 mg, respectively. The incidence of these abnormalities with **pitavastatin** was 0.5% for 4 mg. When the drug was interrupted or discontinued or the drug dosage was reduced, transaminase levels usually fell slowly to pretreatment levels.

Liver enzyme changes generally occur in the first 3 months of treatment with **atorvastatin** or **fluvastatin**, and within 3 to 12 months of starting **lovastatin** or **simvastatin**. Consider a second liver function evaluation to confirm the finding in patients who develop increased transaminases. Monitor patients who develop increased transaminase levels until the abnormalities resolve. If an increase in ALT or AST greater than 3 times the ULN persists, reduce dose or withdraw therapy. According to National Cholesterol Education Program (NCEP) guidelines, if a statin has been discontinued because of elevated transaminase levels, rechallenge or selection of another statin often does not produce a reoccurrence of elevated transaminases.

➤*Endocrine effects:* Statins interfere with cholesterol synthesis and lower circulating cholesterol levels and, as such, might theoretically blunt adrenal or gonadal steroid hormone production. Small declines in total testosterone with no commensurate elevation in luteinizing hormone have been noted with the use of **fluvastatin**. **Pravastatin** showed inconsistent results with regard to possible effects on basal steroid hormone levels; **atorvastatin**, **lovastatin**, **rosuvastatin**, and **simvastatin** did not reduce basal plasma cortisol concentration or basal plasma testosterone concentration or impair adrenal reserve. Appropriately evaluate patients who display clinical evidence of endocrine dysfunction. Exercise caution when administering HMG-

CoA reductase inhibitors with drugs that affect steroid levels or activity, such as ketoconazole, spironolactone, and cimetidine.

➤*CNS/Ophthalmologic effects:* CNS vascular lesions characterized by perivascular hemorrhage, edema, mononuclear cell infiltration of perivascular spaces and other similar CNS vascular lesions have been observed in animals with drugs in this class.

Other effects seen in animals include optic nerve degeneration (Wallerian degeneration of retinogeniculate fibers); brain hemorrhage; optic nerve vacuolation; tonic-clonic convulsion; edema, hemorrhage, and partial necrosis in the interstitium of the choroid plexus; corneal opacity; cataracts; retinal dysplasia; retinal loss; decreased activity; ataxia; loss of righting reflex; ptosis; prominent bilateral posterior Y suture lines in the ocular lens; vestibulocochlear Wallerian-like degeneration; retinal ganglion cell chromatolysis; perivascular fibrin deposits; necrosis of small vessels; and periaxonal vacuolation.

There was a high prevalence of baseline leticular opacities in the patient population included in the early clinical trials with **lovastatin**. During these trials, new opacities appeared in both the **lovastatin** and placebo groups. There was no clinically significant change in visual acuity in the patients who had new opacities reported, nor was any patient, including those with opacities noted at baseline, discontinued from therapy because of a decrease in visual acuity.

➤*Homozygous familial hypercholesterolemia:* HMG-CoA reductase inhibitors are reported to be less effective in patients with rare homozygous familial hypercholesterolemia, possibly because these patients have few functional LDL receptors.

➤*Hypersensitivity reactions:* An apparent hypersensitivity syndrome has occurred rarely with drugs in this class. See also Adverse Reactions. Refer to Management of Acute Hypersensitivity Reactions.

➤*Renal function impairment:* A single 20 mg dose of **pravastatin** was given to patients with varying degrees of renal impairment. Although no effect on the pharmacokinetics of **pravastatin** or its 3 alpha-hydroxy-isomeric metabolite was observed, a small increase in mean AUC values and half-life was seen for the inactive hydroxylation metabolite. Closely monitor patients with renal impairment. Higher systemic exposure of **simvastatin** may occur in severe renal insufficiency. Plasma concentrations of total inhibitors after a single dose of **lovastatin** were approximately 2-fold higher in patients with severe renal insufficiency. Plasma concentrations of **rosuvastatin** increased to a clinically significant extent (approximately 3-fold) in patients with severe renal impairment. In patients with moderate renal impairment (glomerular filtration rate [GFR] 30 to less than 60 mL/min per 1.73 m^2) and end-stage renal disease receiving hemodialysis, **pitavastatin** $AUC_{0-\infty}$ is 79% and 86% higher than those of healthy patients, respectively, while C_{max} is 60% and 40% higher, respectively. Dosage adjustment is required.

➤*Hepatic function impairment:* Use with caution in patients who consume substantial quantities of alcohol, who have a history of liver disease, or who have signs suggestive of liver disease (eg, unexplained aminotransferase elevations, jaundice). Active liver disease or unexplained persistent transaminase elevations are contraindications for the use of HMG-CoA reductase inhibitors.

➤*Pregnancy: Category X.* Contraindicated during pregnancy. Congenital anomalies and/or skeletal malformations have occurred in animals. There have been reports of infants with malformations following in utero exposure to HMG-CoA reductase inhibitors. There has been 1 report of severe congenital bony deformity, tracheo-esophageal fistula, and anal atresia (vertebral defects, anal atresia, tracheoesophageal fistula with esophageal atresia, and radial and renal anomalies [VATER] association) in a baby born to a woman who took **lovastatin** with dextroamphetamine during the first trimester of pregnancy. In a review of about 100 prospectively followed pregnancies in women exposed to **simvastatin** or **lovastatin**, the incidences of congenital anomalies, spontaneous abortions, and fetal deaths/stillbirths did not exceed the rate expected in the general population. However, this study was only able to exclude a 3- to 4-fold increased risk of congenital anomalies over the background incidence. In 89% of the prospectively followed pregnancies, drug treatment was initiated prior to pregnancy and was discontinued at some point in the first trimester when pregnancy was identified.

Cholesterol and cholesterol derivatives are needed for healthy fetal development. Because HMG-CoA reductase inhibitors can decrease synthesis of cholesterol and possibly other biologically active substances derived from cholesterol, they may cause fetal harm when given to pregnant women. Give to women of childbearing age only if they are highly unlikely to conceive and have been informed of potential hazards. Women of childbearing potential who require treatment with a HMG-CoA reductase inhibitor should be advised to use effective contraception. If a patient becomes pregnant while on the drug, immediately discontinue the drug and apprise her of the potential hazard to the fetus. Discontinuing lipid-lowering drugs during pregnancy should have little impact on the outcome of long-term therapy of primary hypercholesterolemia.

It is unknown if **atorvastatin** (or its active metabolites) or **rosuvastatin** cross the placenta in humans. **Atorvastatin** is unlikely to cross the placenta because of its relatively high molecular weight and extensive protein binding. **Rosuvastatin's** low metabolism and prolonged elimination half-life suggest that it may cross the placenta.

Evidence suggests that **pravastatin** may have a lower risk of developmental toxicity because of its hydrophilic properties.

➤*Lactation:* **Atorvastatin** and **rosuvastatin** are excreted in the milk of rats and are likely to be excreted in breast milk; it is not known whether **lovastatin**, **pitavastatin**, or **simvastatin** are excreted in breast milk;a small amount of **pravastatin** is excreted in breast milk; **fluvastatin** is present in breast milk in a 2:1 ratio (milk:plasma). Because of the potential for serious adverse reactions in breast-feeding infants, caution women taking these drugs not to breast-feed their infants.

➤*Children:* Safety and efficacy have not been established for **atorvastatin**, **simvastatin**, and **lovastatin** immediate-release in prepubertal patients and patients younger than 10 years of age. Safety and efficacy have not been established in patients younger than 8 years of age for **pravastatin**. Safety and efficacy of **lovastatin ER**, **pitavastatin**, and **rosuvastatin** have not been established in children.

➤*Elderly:* Elderly patients are at higher risk of myopathy; use HMG-CoA reductase inhibitors with caution in elderly patients.

Pharmacokinetic studies with **lovastatin** and **simvastatin** showed the mean plasma level of HMG-CoA reductase inhibitory activity to be approximately 45% higher in elderly patients (70 to 78 years of age). Plasma concentrations are higher for **atorvastatin** (approximately 30% for AUC), **pitavastatin** (approximately 30% for AUC), and **pravastatin** (approximately 25% to 50% for AUC) compared with healthy young patients.

Elderly patients (65 years of age and older) demonstrated a greater treatment response to LDL-C, total-C, and LDL/HDL ratio than patients younger than 65 years of age with **fluvastatin**.

➤*Monitoring:*

HMG-CoA Reductase Inhibitors – Recommended Monitoring

	Atorvastatin	Fluvastatin	Lovastatin	Pitavastatin	Pravastatin	Rosuvastatin	Simvastatin
Efficacy							
Lipids	2 to 4 weeks after initiation or dosage titration	4 weeks after initiation and periodically thereafter	Periodically	4 weeks after initiation or dosage titration	4 weeks after initiation or dosage titration	2 to 4 weeks after initiation or dosage titration	4 weeks after initiation and periodically thereafter
Toxicity							
Liver function tests	Before initiation, at 12 weeks after initiation and any dose increase, and semiannually thereafter	Before initiation and at 12 weeks after initiation and any dose increase	Before initiation in patients with a history of liver disease, or when clinically indicated; in all patients prior to use of 40 mg/day dosage; and when clinically indicated	Before initiation, at 12 weeks following the initiation of therapy and any elevation of dose, and periodically (eg, semiannually) thereafter	Before initiation and when clinically indicated	Before initiation, at 12 weeks after initiation and any dose increase, and semiannually thereafter	Before initiation and when clinically indicated; for dosages of 80 mg/day, patients should receive an additional test prior to titration, 3 months after titration, and semiannually for the first year

Pay special attention to patients who develop elevated serum transaminase levels. If transaminase levels progress, particularly if they rise to 3 times the ULN and are persistent, discontinue the drug. Monitor patients who develop increased transaminase levels with a second liver function evaluation to confirm the finding and follow them thereafter with frequent liver function tests until the abnormality(ies) return to normal. If an increase in AST or ALT of 3 times the ULN or greater persists, withdrawal of **simvastatin**, **lovastatin**, **pitavastatin**, **pravastatin**, or **fluvastatin** therapy is recommended, or a reduction of dose or withdrawal of **atorvastatin**, **pitavastatin**, or **rosuvastatin** is recommended.

Periodic creatine kinase (CK) determinations may be considered in patients starting therapy with **simvastatin** or **lovastatin** or patients whose dose is being increased, but there is no assurance that such monitoring will prevent myopathy.

Because HMG-CoA reductase inhibitors may increase CPK and transaminase levels, consider this in the differential diagnosis of chest pain in patients treated with these agents.

Closely monitor patients with renal impairment receiving **pravastatin** or **simvastatin**.

Drug Interactions

➤*CYP-450 system:* **Atorvastatin**, **lovastatin**, and **simvastatin** are primarily metabolized by CYP3A4; they may interact with CYP3A4 inhibitors (eg, itraconazole, erythromycin, protease inhibitors [eg, ritonavir, saquinavir], nefazodone, cyclosporine), thereby increasing the risk of myopathy and rhabdomyolysis by reducing the elimination of the HMG-CoA reductase inhibitors.

Fluvastatin is primarily metabolized by CYP2C9; it may interact with CYP2C9 inhibitors. **Fluvastatin** is also metabolized by CYP2C8 and CYP3A4 to a much less extent. In vivo drug interaction studies with CYP3A4 inhibitors/substrates resulted in minimal changes in **fluvastatin** pharmacokinetics.

Pitavastatin is marginally metabolized by CYP2C9 and, to a lesser extent, by CYP2C8.

HMG-CoA Reductase Inhibitors Drug Interactions

Precipitant drug	Object drug[a]		Description
Amiodarone	HMG-CoA reductase inhibitors Atorvastatin Lovastatin Simvastatin	↑	Amiodarone may inhibit the metabolism (CYP3A4) of certain HMG-CoA reductase inhibitors, increasing the risk of toxicity (eg, myopathy). If coadministration cannot be avoided, use the lowest possible HMG-CoA reductase inhibitor dose.
Antacids	HMG-CoA reductase inhibitors Rosuvastatin Atorvastatin	↓	Coadministration with aluminum hydroxide/magnesium hydroxide suspension decreased **atorvastatin** levels by approximately 35%; LDL-C reduction was not altered. Coadministration of **rosuvastatin** and an aluminum/magnesium combination antacid decreased **rosuvastatin** levels by 54%. Administer antacids at least 2 hours after **rosuvastatin**.
Azole antifungals (eg, fluconazole, itraconazole, ketoconazole)	HMG-CoA reductase inhibitors	↑	Azole antifungal agents may inhibit the metabolism of HMG-CoA reductase inhibitors, increasing the risk of toxicity (eg, myopathy). Itraconazole is contraindicated with HMG-CoA reductase inhibitors metabolized by CYP3A4. If coadministration of other agents cannot be avoided, consider suspending the dose of the HMG-CoA reductase inhibitor during the course of therapy. **Pravastatin** and **rosuvastatin** levels are affected the least.
Bile acid sequestrants (eg, cholestyramine, colestipol)	HMG-CoA reductase inhibitors Atorvastatin Pravastatin Fluvastatin	↓	The HMG-CoA reductase inhibitor may adsorb to the bile acid sequestrant, reducing the GI absorption of the HMG-CoA reductase inhibitor. Administer **pravastatin** 1 hour before or 4 hours after bile acid sequestrants. Administer **fluvastatin** at least 2 hours after a bile acid sequestrant. Plasma levels of **atorvastatin** decreased approximately 25% with coadministration with colestipol; however, LDL-C reduction was greater when **atorvastatin** and colestipol were coadministered than when either drug was given alone.
Bosentan	HMG-CoA reductase inhibitors Atorvastatin Lovastatin Simvastatin	↓	Bosentan may induce the metabolism (CYP3A4) of certain HMG-CoA reductase inhibitors, decreasing the therapeutic effect. Monitor closely and adjust dosage as needed.
Carbamazepine	HMG-CoA reductase inhibitors Atorvastatin Lovastatin Simvastatin	↓	Carbamazepine may induce the metabolism (CYP3A4) of certain HMG-CoA reductase inhibitors, decreasing the therapeutic effect. Monitor closely and adjust dosage as needed.
Cilostazole	HMG-CoA reductase inhibitors Atorvastatin Lovastatin Simvastatin	↑	Cilostazole may inhibit the metabolism (CYP3A4) of certain HMG-CoA reductase inhibitors, increasing the risk of toxicity (eg, myopathy). Monitor closely and adjust dosage as needed.
Cisapride[b]	HMG-CoA reductase inhibitors Simvastatin	↑↓	Coadministration may decrease **simvastatin** levels, and cisapride levels may be elevated.
HMG-CoA reductase inhibitors Simvastatin	Cisapride[b]		
Colchicine	HMG-CoA reductase inhibitors	↑	Coadministration may increase the risk of myopathy or rhabdomyolysis. If coadministration cannot be avoided, then use with caution and closely monitor CK.
HMG-CoA reductase inhibitors	Colchicine		
Cyclosporine	HMG-CoA reductase inhibitors	↑	Coadministration may increase HMG-CoA reductase inhibitor plasma levels and increase the risk of myopathy or rhabdomyolysis. If coadministration cannot be avoided, consider decreasing HMG-CoA reductase inhibitor dose and monitor closely. **Lovastatin** ER should not be coadministered with cyclosporine; however, reduced dosage of immediate-release **lovastatin** may be considered. Coadministration with **pitavastatin** is contraindicated.
Danazol	HMG-CoA reductase inhibitors Lovastatin Simvastatin	↑	Coadministration may cause myopathy or rhabdomyolysis. If coadministration cannot be avoided, consider decreasing the HMG-CoA reductase inhibitor dose and monitor closely.
Diltiazem	HMG-CoA reductase inhibitors Atorvastatin Lovastatin Simvastatin	↑	Diltiazem may inhibit the metabolism (CYP3A4) of certain HMG-CoA reductase inhibitors, increasing the risk of toxicity (eg, myopathy).
Fibric acid derivatives (ie, fenofibrate, gemfibrozil)	HMG-CoA reductase inhibitors	↑	Severe myopathy or rhabdomyolysis may occur. Avoid concurrent use if possible. If used, consider a reduced dosage of the HMG-CoA reductase inhibitor.
HMG-CoA reductase inhibitors	Fibric acid derivatives (ie, fenofibrate, gemfibrozil)		
Glyburide	HMG-CoA reductase inhibitors Fluvastatin	↑	Coadministration increased glyburide C_{max}, AUC, and half-life approximately 50%, 69%, and 121%, respectively. Coadministration also led to an increase in **fluvastatin** C_{max} and AUC by 44% and 51%, respectively. Monitor patients.
HMG-CoA reductase inhibitors Fluvastatin	Glyburide		

HMG-CoA Reductase Inhibitors Drug Interactions

Precipitant drug	Object drug[a]		Description
Histamine H_2 antagonists (ie, cimetidine, ranitidine)	HMG-CoA reductase inhibitors Fluvastatin	↑	Coadministration of **fluvastatin** with cimetidine and ranitidine resulted in a significant increase in **fluvastatin** C_{max} and AUC by 44% and 51%, respectively. Monitor patients.
Hydantoins (eg, phenytoin)	HMG-CoA reductase inhibitors Atorvastatin Fluvastatin Simvastatin	↑↓	Coadministration may result in decreased plasma levels of certain HMG-CoA reductase inhibitors, producing a decrease in therapeutic effect. Coadministration of **fluvastatin** and phenytoin increased the levels of both drugs.
HMG-CoA reductase inhibitors Fluvastatin	Hydantoins (eg, phenytoin)		
Imatinib	HMG-CoA reductase inhibitors Atorvastatin Lovastatin Simvastatin	↑	Imatinib may inhibit the metabolism (CYP3A4) of certain HMG-CoA reductase inhibitors, increasing the risk of toxicity (eg, myopathy).
Isradipine	HMG-CoA reductase inhibitors Lovastatin	↓	Isradipine may increase clearance of lovastatin and its metabolites by increasing hepatic blood flow. Monitor the clinical response and adjust the lovastatin dosage as necessary.
Macrolides Clarithromycin Erythromycin	HMG-CoA reductase inhibitors	↑	Certain macrolides may inhibit the metabolism of HMG-CoA reductase inhibitors metabolized by CYP3A4. Coadministration increases the risk of severe myopathy or rhabdomyolysis. If coadministration is unavoidable, suspend therapy with an HMG-CoA reductase inhibitor during the course of macrolide therapy. Do not exceed a dosage of **pitavastatin** 1 mg once daily during coadministration.
Nefazodone	HMG-CoA reductase inhibitors	↑	Nefazodone may inhibit the metabolism (CYP3A4) of certain HMG-CoA reductase inhibitors, increasing the risk of toxicity (eg, myopathy). Avoid use if possible.
Niacin (nicotinic acid)	HMG-CoA reductase inhibitors	↑	Coadministration of HMG-CoA reductase inhibitors with niacin (dosages of at least 1 g/day) increases the risk of severe myopathy or rhabdomyolysis. If coadministration cannot be avoided, use the lowest possible HMG-CoA reductase inhibitor dose.
HMG-CoA reductase inhibitors	Niacin (nicotinic acid)		
NNRTIs[c] (eg, delavirdine, efavirenz, nevirapine)	HMG-CoA reductase inhibitors Atorvastatin Lovastatin Pravastatin Simvastatin	↑↓	Delavirdine may inhibit the metabolism (CYP3A4) of certain HMG-CoA reductase inhibitors, increasing the risk of toxicity (eg, myopathy). However, efavirenz and nevirapine may induce CYP3A4 and reduce HMG-CoA reductase inhibitor levels.
Omeprazole	HMG-CoA reductase inhibitors Fluvastatin	↑	Coadministration of **fluvastatin** with omeprazole resulted in a significant increase in **fluvastatin** C_{max} (50%) and AUC (24% to 33%), with an 18% to 23% decrease in plasma clearance.
Propranolol	HMG-CoA reductase inhibitors Simvastatin	↔	Coadministration resulted in a significant decrease in **simvastatin** C_{max}, but no change in AUC. No dosage adjustment is needed.
Protease inhibitors (eg, nelfinavir, ritonavir)	HMG-CoA reductase inhibitors	↑↓	Concomitant use may result in elevated plasma levels of certain HMG-CoA reductase inhibitors, increasing the risk of toxicity (eg, myopathy). Darunavir or nelfinavir is contraindicated in patients taking **lovastatin** or **simvastatin**; avoid coadministration with ritonavir or atazanavir. However, concomitant use of a protease inhibitor with **pravastatin** may decrease **pravastatin** plasma levels, possibly decreasing efficacy. Avoid use if possible.
Quinine	HMG-CoA reductase inhibitors Atorvastatin	↑	Quinine may inhibit the metabolism (CYP3A4) of **atorvastatin**, increasing the risk of toxicity (eg, myopathy).
Rifamycins (eg, rifampin)	HMG-CoA reductase inhibitors Atorvastatin Fluvastatin Pitavastatin Pravastatin	↑↓	Coadministration may reduce levels of certain HMG-CoA reductase inhibitors. However, **pravastatin** and **pitavastatin** levels may be increased in some patients. Do not exceed a dosage of **pitavastatin** 2 mg once daily during coadministration.
St. John's wort	HMG-CoA reductase inhibitors Atorvastatin Lovastatin Simvastatin	↓	St. John's wort may induce the metabolism (CYP3A4) of certain HMG-CoA reductase inhibitors, decreasing therapeutic effect.
Telithromycin	HMG-CoA reductase inhibitors Atorvastatin Lovastatin Simvastatin	↑	Telithromycin may inhibit the metabolism (CYP3A4) of certain HMG-CoA reductase inhibitors, increasing the risk of toxicity (eg, myopathy).
Verapamil	HMG-CoA reductase inhibitors Atorvastatin Lovastatin Simvastatin	↑	Verapamil may inhibit the metabolism (CYP3A4) of certain HMG-CoA reductase inhibitors, increasing the risk of toxicity (eg, myopathy). If coadministration cannot be avoided, consider decreasing the HMG-CoA reductase inhibitor dose and monitor closely. **Atorvastatin** may also increase the levels of verapamil.
HMG-CoA reductase inhibitors Atorvastatin	Verapamil		

HMG-CoA Reductase Inhibitors Drug Interactions			
Precipitant drug	Object drug[a]		Description
HMG-CoA reductase inhibitors Atorvastatin	Benzodiazepines (ie, midazolam)	↑	**Atorvastatin** may decrease the oxidative metabolism (CYP3A4) of certain benzodiazepines. The effects of the benzodiazepines may be increased and prolonged.
HMG-CoA reductase inhibitors Atorvastatin Fluvastatin Lovastatin Simvastatin	Clopidogrel	↓	Data for this interaction are conflicting. Certain HMG-CoA reductase inhibitors may interfere with clopidogrel platelet inhibition. One case of rhabdomyolysis has been reported. No special precautions are needed based on available data.
HMG-CoA reductase inhibitors Atorvastatin Rosuvastatin	Contraceptives, hormonal	↑	Coadministration with **atorvastatin** increased the AUC for norethindrone and ethinyl estradiol by approximately 30% and 20%, respectively. Coadministration with **rosuvastatin** increased the AUC for norgestrel and ethinyl estradiol by approximately 34% and 26%, respectively.
HMG-CoA reductase inhibitors Fluvastatin	Diclofenac	↑	Coadministration increased the mean diclofenac C_{max} and AUC by 60% and 25%, respectively.
HMG-CoA reductase inhibitors Atorvastatin Fluvastatin Rosuvastatin Simvastatin	Digoxin	↑	Coadministration may increase digoxin plasma concentrations. Monitor digoxin levels and adjust the dosage as needed.
HMG-CoA reductase inhibitors Fluvastatin Lovastatin Pitavastatin Rosuvastatin Simvastatin	Warfarin	↑	The anticoagulant effect of warfarin may increase. Bleeding also has been reported in a few patients. Monitor anticoagulation parameters when starting, stopping, or adjusting the HMG-CoA reductase inhibitor dosage.

[a] ↑ = object drug increased; ↓ = object drug decreased; ↔ = undetermined clinical effect; ↑↓ = object drug both increased and decreased.

[b] Available from the manufacturer on a limited-access protocol.

[c] NNRTIs = nonnucleoside reverse transcriptase inhibitors.

➤*Drug/Food interactions:* Under fasting conditions, **lovastatin** (immediate-release) levels are approximately two-thirds of those found when given immediately after meals; **lovastatin** (immediate-release) should be taken with meals. When **lovastatin** (ER) was given after a meal, plasma concentrations were approximately 0.5 to 0.6 times those found when **lovastatin** (ER) was administered in a fasting state.

Pitavastatin administration with a high-fat meal (50% fat content) decreased C_{max} by 43%. AUC is not significantly reduced. C_{max} and AUC of **pitavastatin** did not differ following evening or morning administration. Give **pitavastatin** any time of day with or without food.

Fibers such as oat bran and pectin may decrease GI absorption of HMG-CoA reductase inhibitors. If coadministration cannot be avoided, separate the administration times by as much as possible.

Grapefruit juice – Coadministration with large quantities of grapefruit juice (at least 1 quart daily) may result in increased plasma levels of **lovastatin**, **simvastatin**, or **atorvastatin**, increasing the risk of myopathy. Avoid concurrent use.

Adverse Reactions

➤*Adults:*

Discontinuation – In placebo-controlled trials, 5.6% of **rosuvastatin**-treated patients, 4.6% of lovastatin-treated patients, 3.9% of **fluvastatin** (ER)-treated patients and **pitavastatin**-treated patients, less than 2% of **atorvastatin**-treated patients, 1.7% of **pravastatin**-treated patients, 1.4% of **simvastatin**-treated patients, and 1% of **fluvastatin** (immediate-release)-treated patients discontinued treatment because of adverse reactions.

HMG-CoA Reductase Inhibitor Adverse Reactions[a]							
Adverse reaction	Atorvastatin	Fluvastatin[b]	Lovastatin[b]	Pitavastatin	Pravastatin[c]	Rosuvastatin	Simvastatin
Cardiovascular							
Angina pectoris	< 2%	—	—	—	3.1%	—	—
Atrial fibrillation	—	—	—	—	—	—	5.7%
Hypertension	< 2%	—	—	—	—	—	—
CNS							
Asthenia	≤ 3.8%	—	1.2% to 3%	—	PM[d]	2.7%	✓[d]
Depression	< 2%	✓	—	—	1%	—	PM[d]
Dizziness	≥ 2%	✓	0.5% to 2%	—	1% to 2.2%	4%	PM[d]
Headache	2.5% to 16.7%	4.7% to 8.9%	2.1% to 7%	✓	1.7% to 1.9%	5.5% to 6.4%	7.4%
Insomnia	≥ 2%	0.8% to 2.7%	0.5% to 1%	—	< 1%	—	4%
Paresthesia	< 2%	✓	0.5% to 1%	—	< 1%	—	PM[d]
Vertigo	—	✓	✓	—	< 1%	—	4.5%
Dermatologic							
Alopecia	< 2%	✓	0.5% to 1%	—	< 1%	—	PM[d]
Eczema	< 2%	—	—	—	—	—	4.5%
Pruritus	< 2%	✓	0.5% to 1%	—	< 1%	✓[d]	PM[d]
Rash	1.1% to 3.9%	—	0.8% to 1.3%	—	1.3% to 2.1%	✓[d]	✓[d]
GI							
Abdominal pain/cramps	≤ 3.8%	3.7% to 4.9%	2% to 2.5%	—	2% to 2.4%	2.4%	7.3%
Acid regurgitation	—	—	0.5% to 1%	—	—	—	—
Constipation	≤ 2.5%	—	2% to 3.5%	3.6%	1.2% to 2.4%	2.4%	6.6%
Diarrhea	≤ 5.3%	3.3% to 4.9%	2.2% to 3%	2.6%	2%	—	✓[d]
Dry mouth	< 2%	—	0.5% to 1%	—	—	—	—
Dysgeusia	< 2%	—	0.8%	—	—	—	—
Dyspepsia	1.3% to 2.8%	3.5% to 7.9%	1% to 1.6%	—	3.5%	—	✓[d]
Flatulence	1.1% to 2.8%	1.4% to 2.6%	3.7% to 4.5%	—	1.2% to 2.7%	—	✓[d]
Gastroenteritis/Gastritis	< 2%	—	—	—	—	≥ 2%	4.9%
Heartburn	—	—	1.6%	—	2%	—	—
Nausea	≥ 2%	2.5% to 3.2%	1.9% to 2.5%	—	1.6% to 2.9%	3.4%	5.4%
Tooth disorder	—	—	—	—	—	—	—
Vomiting	< 2%	✓	0.5% to 1%	—	1.6% to 2.9%	—	PM[d]
GU							
Albuminuria	≥ 2%	—	—	—	—	—	—
Hematuria	≥ 2%	—	—	—	—	✓[d]	—

HMG-CoA Reductase Inhibitors (Statins)

HMG-CoA Reductase Inhibitor Adverse Reactions[a]

Adverse reaction	Atorvastatin	Fluvastatin[b]	Lovastatin[b]	Pitavastatin	Pravastatin[c]	Rosuvastatin	Simvastatin
Urinary abnormality	—	—	—	—	0.7% to 1%	—	—
Urinary tract infection	≥ 2%	1.6% to 2.7%	2% to 3%		—	—	3.2%
Lab test abnormalities							
ALT > 3 × ULN	0.2% to 2.3%	0.2% to 4.9%	1.9%	—	≤ 1.2%	2.2%	≈1%
Elevated CPK	< 2%	✓[d]	✓[d]		✓[d]	2.6%	✓[d]
Musculoskeletal							
Arthralgia	≤ 5.1%	✓	0.5% to 5%	✓	PM[d]	10.1%	PM[d]
Arthritis	≥ 2%	1.3% to 2.1%	—	—	✓[d]	PM[d]	
Arthropathy	—	3.2%	—	—	—	—	
Back pain	≤ 3.8%	—	5%	3.9%	—	—	
Leg pain	< 2%	—	0.5% to 1%		—	—	
Localized pain			0.5% to 1%		1.4%		
Muscle cramps/pain	—	✓	0.6% to 1.1%		2% to 6%	12.7%	PM[d]
Myalgia	≤ 5.6%	3.8% to 5%	1.8% to 3%	3.1%	0.6% to 1.4%	2.8%	3.7%
Myopathy	✓[d]	✓[d]	✓[d]	—	PM[d]	✓[d]	0.02% to 0.53%
Rhabdomyolysis	PM[d]	✓[d]	✓[d]	—	PM[d]	✓[d]	✓[d]
Shoulder pain	—	—	0.5% to 1%	—	—	—	—
Ophthalmic							
Blurred vision	—	—	0.9% to 1.2%	—	—	—	—
Eye irritation	—	—	0.5% to 1%	—	—	—	—
Visual disturbance	—	—	—	—	1.6%	—	—
Respiratory							
Bronchitis	≥ 2%	1.8% to 2.6%	—	—	—	—	6.6%
Cough					0.1% to 1%		
Dyspnea	< 2%	—			1.6%	—	—
Pharyngitis	≤ 2.5%	—			—	—	—
Rhinitis	≥ 2%	—	—	—	0.1%	—	—
Sinusitis	≤ 6.4%	2.6% to 3.5%	4% to 6%	—	—	—	2.3%
Upper respiratory tract infection	—	—	—	—	1.3%	—	9%
Miscellaneous							
Accidental trauma	≤ 4.2%	4.2% to 5.1%	4% to 6%	—	—	—	—
Allergy/Hypersensitivity	≤ 2.8%	1% to 2.3%		✓	< 1%	✓[d]	PM[d]
Chest pain	≥ 2%	—	0.5% to 1%	—	0.1% to 2.6%	—	—
Diabetes mellitus	—					—	4.2%
Edema/Swelling	< 2%	—		—	—	—	2.7%
Fatigue	PM[d]	1.6% to 2.7%		—	1.9% to 3.4%	—	—
Flu syndrome	≤ 3.2%	5.1% to 7.1%	5%			—	—
Infection	2.8% to 10.3%		11% to 16%	—		—	—
Pain	—	—	3% to 5%	—	1.4%	≥ 2%	—
Peripheral edema	≥ 2%	—	—	—		≥ 2%	—

[a] All reactions. Data are pooled from separate studies and are not necessarily comparable.
[b] Immediate-release and ER combined.
[c] Includes short-term and long-term studies.
[d] ✓ = reported, no evidence given; PM = postmarketing

The following are additional adverse reactions reported for HMG-CoA reductase inhibitors.

Cardiovascular –

Atorvastatin: Arrhythmia, palpitation, phlebitis, postural hypotension, syncope, vasodilation (less than 2%).

CNS –

Atorvastatin: Abnormal dreams, amnesia, emotional lability, facial paralysis, hyperkinesia, hypertonia, hypesthesia, incoordination, libido decreased, migraine, peripheral neuropathy, somnolence, torticollis (less than 2%).

Fluvastatin and lovastatin: Anxiety, dysfunction of certain cranial nerves (including alteration of taste, facial paresis, and impairment of extraocular movement), memory loss, peripheral nerve palsy, peripheral neuropathy, psychic disturbances, tremor.

Pravastatin: Memory impairment, neuropathy (including peripheral neuropathy), tremor (less than 1%).

Dermatologic –

Atorvastatin: Acne, contact dermatitis, dry skin, seborrhea, skin ulcer, sweating, urticaria (less than 2%).

Fluvastatin and lovastatin: Photosensitivity reaction (less than 2%). A variety of skin changes (eg, changes to hair/nails, discoloration, dryness of skin/mucous membranes, nodules) have been reported.

Pravastatin: Dermatitis, skin dryness, scalp hair abnormality, urticaria (less than 1%).

GI –

Atorvastatin: Anorexia, biliary pain, cheilitis, cholestatic jaundice, colitis, duodenal ulcer, dysphagia, enteritis, eructation, esophagitis, glossitis, gum hemorrhage, hepatitis, increased appetite, liver function tests abnormal, melena, mouth ulceration, pancreatitis, rectal hemorrhage, stomach ulcer, stomatitis, tenesmus, ulcerative stomatitis (less than 2%).

Fluvastatin and lovastatin: Anorexia, cholestatic jaundice, cirrhosis, fatty change in liver, hepatic necrosis, hepatitis (including chronic active hepatitis), hepatoma, pancreatitis.

Pravastatin: Decreased appetite (less than 1%).

Rosuvastatin: Pancreatitis.

GU –

Atorvastatin: Abnormal ejaculation, breast enlargement, cystitis, dysuria, epididymitis, fibrocystic breast, impotence, kidney calculus, metrorrhagia, nephritis, nocturia, urinary frequency, urinary incontinence, urinary retention, urinary urgency, uterine hemorrhage, vaginal hemorrhage (less than 2%).

Fluvastatin and lovastatin: Erectile dysfunction, gynecomastia, loss of libido.

Pravastatin: Libido change, sexual dysfunction (less than 1%).

Hematologic/Lymphatic –

Atorvastatin: Anemia, ecchymosis, lymphadenopathy, petechia, thrombocytopenia (less than 2%).

Hypersensitivity – An apparent hypersensitivity syndrome has been reported rarely that has included 1 or more of the following features: anaphylaxis, angioedema, arthralgia, arthritis, asthenia, chills, dermatomyositis, dyspnea, eosinophilia, erythema multiforme (including Stevens-Johnson syndrome), erythrocyte sedimentation rate increase, fever, flushing, hemolytic anemia, leukopenia, lupus erythematosus-like syndrome, malaise, photosensitivity, polymyalgia rheumatica, positive antinuclear antibody (ANA), purpura, thrombocytopenia, toxic epidermal necrolysis, urticaria, vasculitis.

Lab test abnormalities –

Fluvastatin and lovastatin: Anemia, leukopenia, thrombocytopenia; bilirubin, elevated alkaline phosphatase, gamma-glutamyl transpeptidase (GGT), and transaminases; thyroid function abnormalities. Large increases in CK have sometimes been reported.

Pitavastatin: Elevated alkaline phosphatase, bilirubin, and glucose.

Pravastatin: Increases in serum transaminase (ALT, AST). Transient, asymptomatic eosinophilia has been reported. Eosinophil counts usually returned to normal despite continued therapy. In 2 controlled trials, 4 of 464 patients taking pravastatin 80 mg had a single elevation of CK greater than 10 times the ULN compared with none of the 115 patients taking pravastatin 40 mg.

Rosuvastatin: Dipstick-positive proteinuria; elevated transaminases, glucose, gamma-glutamyl transpeptidase, alkaline phosphatase, and bilirubin; thyroid function abnormalities.

Simvastatin: Marked persistent increases in hepatic transaminases; alkaline phosphatase and gamma-glutamyl transpeptidase. Approximately 5% of patients had elevations of CK levels of 3 or more times the normal value on 1 or more occasions. This was attributable to the noncardiac function of CK.

Metabolic/Nutritional –

Atorvastatin: Gout, hyperglycemia, hypoglycemia, weight gain (less than 2%).

Musculoskeletal –

Atorvastatin: Bursitis, leg cramps, myasthenia, myositis, tendinous contracture, tenosynovitis (less than 2%).

Pravastatin: Muscle weakness (less than 1%).

Simvastatin: Myopathy/rhabdomyolysis (less than 0.1%).

Respiratory –
Atorvastatin: Asthma, epistaxis, pneumonia (less than 2%).

Special senses –
Fluvastatin and lovastatin: Ophthalmoplegia, progression of cataracts (lens opacities).
Atorvastatin: Amblyopia, deafness, dry eyes, eye hemorrhage, glaucoma, parosmia, refraction disorder, taste loss, taste perversion, tinnitus (less than 2%).
Pravastatin: Lens opacity (less than 1%).

Miscellaneous –
Atorvastatin: Face edema, fever, malaise, neck rigidity, photosensitivity (less than 2%).
Pitavastatin: Pain in extremity (23%); influenza and nasopharyngitis.
Pravastatin: Edema head/neck, fever, flushing, taste disturbance (less than 1%).

Postmarketing –
Atorvastatin: Anaphylaxis, angioneurotic edema, bullous rashes (including erythema multiforme, Stevens-Johnson syndrome, and toxic epidermal necrolysis), hepatic failure, tendon rupture.
Pravastatin: Anaphylaxis, angioedema, chills, cholestatic jaundice, cirrhosis, dermatomyositis, dysfunction of certain cranial nerves (including alteration of taste, facial paresis, and impairment of extraocular movement), erythema multiforme (including Stevens-Johnson syndrome), erythrocyte sedimentation rate increase, fatty change in liver, fulminant hepatic necrosis, gynecomastia, hemolytic anemia, hepatitis (including chronic active hepatitis), hepatoma, liver function test abnormalities, lupus erythematosus-like syndrome, malaise, pancreatitis, peripheral nerve palsy, photosensitivity, polymyalgia rheumatica, positive ANA, purpura, skin changes (eg, changes to hair/nails, discoloration, dryness of mucous membranes, nodules), thyroid function abnormalities, toxic epidermal necrolysis, vasculitis.
Rosuvastatin: Hepatic failure, hepatitis, jaundice, memory loss.
Simvastatin: Anemia, hepatic failure, hepatitis/jaundice, memory impairment, pancreatitis, peripheral neuropathy, pruritus, rhabdomyolysis, a variety of skin changes (eg, changes to hair/nails, discoloration, dryness of mucous membranes, nodule).

➤*Children:* In children receiving **atorvastatin**, **lovastatin**, or **pravastatin**, the safety and tolerability were generally similar to that of placebo. The most common adverse reactions in children receiving **fluvastatin** were influenza and infections. The most common adverse reactions in children receiving **simvastatin** were upper respiratory tract infections, headache, abdominal pain, and nausea.

Overdosage

➤*Treatment:* Treat symptomatically and institute supportive measures as required. Refer to General Management of Acute Overdosage.

Patient Information

Advise patients of the risk of myopathy. Advise patients to promptly report unexplained muscle pain, tenderness, or weakness, especially if accompanied by fever or malaise.

Some HMG-CoA reductase inhibitors may cause photosensitivity (sensitivity to sunlight). Avoid prolonged exposure to the sun and other ultraviolet light. Advise patients to use sunscreen and wear protective clothing until tolerance is determined.

If the patient becomes pregnant, discontinue the drug immediately to avoid harmful effects in the developing fetus. Advise women of childbearing potential who require treatment with a HMG-CoA reductase inhibitor to use effective contraception.

Caution women taking these drugs not to breast-feed their infants.

Advise patients to follow dietary and exercise recommendations.

Take **lovastatin** with meals; **fluvastatin**, **pravastatin**, **simvastatin**, **atorvastatin**, **pitavastatin**, and **rosuvastatin** may be taken without regard to meals.

Coadministration with large quantities of grapefruit juice (at least 1 quart daily) may result in increased plasma levels of **lovastatin**, **simvastatin**, or **atorvastatin**, increasing the risk of myopathy. Avoid concurrent use.

Advise patients to swallow lovastatin ER tablets whole; do not chew, crush, or cut.

When patients are taking **rosuvastatin** with an aluminum and magnesium hydroxide combination antacid, advise them to take the antacid at least 2 hours after **rosuvastatin** administration.

LOVASTATIN (Mevinolin)

Rx	**Lovastatin** (Various, eg, Eon, Mylan, Purepac, Teva)	**Tablets; oral:** 10 mg	May contain lactose. In 30s, 60s, 100s, 500s, and 1000s.
Rx	**Lovastatin** (Various, eg, Eon, Mylan, Purepac, Teva)	**Tablets; oral:** 20 mg	May contain lactose. In 30s, 60s, 90s, 100s, 500s, and 1000s.
Rx	**Mevacor** (Merck)		Lactose. (MSD 731 MEVACOR). Lt. blue, octagonal. In 1000s, 10,000s, unit-of-use 60s and 90s, and UD 100s.
Rx	**Lovastatin** (Various, eg, Eon, Mylan, Purepac, Teva)	**Tablets; oral:** 40 mg	May contain lactose. In 30s, 60s, 90s, 100s, 500s, and 1000s.
Rx	**Mevacor** (Merck)		Lactose. (MSD 732 MEVACOR). Green, octagonal. In 1000s, 10,000s, and unit-of-use 60s and 90s.
Rx	**Altoprev** (Sciele)	**Tablets, extended-release; oral:** 10 mg	Sugar, lactose. (10). Dk. orange. In 30s.
		20 mg	Sugar, lactose. (20). Orange. In 30s.
		40 mg	Sugar, lactose. (40). Peach. In 30s.
		60 mg	Sugar, lactose. (60). Lt. peach. In 30s.

LOVASTATIN — ORAL

For complete and comparative prescribing information, refer to the HMG-CoA Reductase Inhibitors group monograph.

Indications

➤*General information:* Therapy with lovastatin should be a component of multiple-risk factor intervention in those individuals with dyslipidemia at risk for atherosclerotic vascular disease. Lovastatin should be used in addition to a diet restricted in saturated fat and cholesterol as part of a treatment strategy to lower total cholesterol (total-C) and low-density lipoprotein cholesterol (LDL-C) to target levels when the response to diet and other nonpharmacological measures alone has been inadequate to reduce risk.

➤*Primary prevention of coronary heart disease (CHD):* In individuals without symptomatic cardiovascular disease, average to moderately elevated total-C and LDL-C, and below average high-density lipoprotein cholesterol (HDL-C), lovastatin is indicated to reduce the risk of the following: Myocardial infarction (MI); unstable angina; coronary revascularization procedures.

➤*Coronary heart disease:* Lovastatin is indicated to slow the progression of coronary atherosclerosis in patients with coronary heart disease as part of a treatment strategy to lower total-C and LDL-C to target levels.

➤*Hypercholesterolemia:* Therapy with lipid-altering agents should be a component of multiple-risk factor intervention in those individuals at significantly increased risk for atherosclerotic vascular disease due to hypercholesterolemia. Lovastatin is indicated as an adjunct to diet for the reduction of elevated total-C and LDL-C levels in patients with primary hypercholesterolemia (types IIa and IIb), when the response to diet restricted in saturated fat and cholesterol and to other nonpharmacological measures alone has been inadequate.

Extended-release tablets – Lovastatin is indicated as an adjunct to diet for the reduction of elevated total-C, LDL-C, Apo B, and TG, and to increase HDL-C in patients with primary hypercholesterolemia (heterozygous familial and non-familial) and mixed dyslipidemia (Fredrickson types IIa and IIb, see information below) when the response to diet restricted in saturated fat and cholesterol and to other nonpharmacological measures alone has been inadequate.

➤*Off-label uses:*
Extended-interval dosing (alternate-day dosing) – [4] = Insufficient documentation. Two small trials suggest that alternate-day dosing with lovastatin may be comparable with daily dosing in maintaining similar reductions in total cholesterol and LDL-C concentrations. The authors of these studies suggest that annual cost-savings may benefit patients without loss of efficacy. Compliance with an alternate-day regimen appears to be acceptable (98%). (See Administration and Dosage.)

Administration and Dosage

➤*General dosing considerations:* The patient should be placed on a standard cholesterol-lowering diet before receiving lovastatin and should continue on this diet during treatment with lovastatin.

Doses should be individualized according to the recommended goal of therapy.

➤*Adults:*
Immediate-release –
Hypercholesterolemia:
- *Usual dosage –* 10 to 80 mg/day in single or 2 divided doses.
- *Maximum dose –* 80 mg/day.
- *Initial dosage –* 20 mg once a day given with the evening meal. Patients requiring reductions in LDL-C of 20% or more to achieve their goal should

LOVASTATIN — ORAL

be started on 20 mg/day of lovastatin. A starting dose of 10 mg may be considered for patients requiring smaller reductions.

• *Dosage adjustment* – Adjustments should be made at intervals of 4 weeks or more.

• *Concomitant therapy* – Lovastatin is effective alone or when used concomitantly with bile-acid sequestrants. If lovastatin is used in combination with gemfibrozil, other fibrates, or lipid-lowering doses (greater than or equal to 1 g/day) of niacin, the dose of lovastatin should not exceed 20 mg/day.

Dosage in patients taking cyclosporine: In patients taking cyclosporine concomitantly with lovastatin immediate release, therapy should begin with 10 mg of lovastatin and should not exceed 20 mg/day.

Dosage in patients taking amiodarone or verapamil: In patients taking amiodarone or verapamil concomitantly with lovastatin immediate release, the dose should not exceed 40 mg/day.

Extended-release –

Hypercholesterolemia:

• *Usual dosage* – 10 to 60 mg/day, in single doses.

• *Initial dosage* – 20, 40, or 60 mg once daily given in the evening at bedtime. A starting dose of 10 mg may be considered for patients requiring smaller reductions.

• *Dosage adjustment* – Adjustments should be made at intervals of 4 weeks or more.

• *Concomitant therapy* – Use of lovastatin extended-release tablets with fibrates or niacin should generally be avoided. However, if lovastatin extended-release tablets are used in combination with fibrates or niacin, the dose of lovastatin extended-release should generally not exceed 20 mg.

Dosage in patients taking cyclosporine: In patients taking cyclosporine concomitantly with lovastatin extended-release, therapy should begin with 10 mg of lovastatin and should not exceed 20 mg/day.

Dosage in patients taking amiodarone or verapamil: In patients taking amiodarone or verapamil concomitantly with lovastatin extended-release, the dose should not exceed 40 mg/day.

Off-label dosing –

Extended-interval dosing (alternate-day dosing): [4] = Insufficient documentation. 20 mg every other day.

➤*Children:*

Heterozygous familial hypercholesterolemia –

10 to 17 years and older:

• *Usual dose* – 10 to 40 mg/day.

• *Maximum dose* – 40 mg/day.

• *Initial dosage* – Patients requiring reductions in LDL-C of 20% or more to achieve their goal should be started on 20 mg/day of lovastatin. A starting dose of 10 mg may be considered for patients requiring smaller reductions.

• *Dosage adjustment* – Adjustments should be made at intervals of 4 weeks or more.

➤*Renal function impairment:* In patients with severe renal insufficiency (CrCl less than 30 mL/min), dosage increases above 20 mg/day should be carefully considered and, if deemed necessary, implemented cautiously.

➤*Hepatic function impairment:* The drug should be used with caution in patients who consume substantial quantities of alcohol or have a history of liver disease. Active liver disease or unexplained transaminase elevations are contraindications to the use of lovastatin.

As with other lipid-lowering agents, moderate (less than 3 times the upper limit of normal) elevations of serum transaminases have been reported following therapy with lovastatin. These changes appeared soon after initiation of therapy with lovastatin, were often transient, were not accompanied by any symptoms and interruption of treatment was not required.

➤*Monitoring:* Cholesterol levels should be monitored periodically and consideration should be given to reducing the dosage of lovastatin if cholesterol levels fall significantly below the targeted range.

It is recommended that liver function tests be performed before the initiation of treatment, at 6 and 12 weeks after initiation of therapy or elevation in dose, and periodically thereafter (eg, semiannually). Patients who develop increased transaminase levels should be monitored with a second liver function evaluation to confirm the finding and be followed thereafter with frequent liver function tests until the abnormality(ies) returns to normal. Should an increase in AST or ALT of 3 times the upper limit of normal or greater persist, withdrawal of therapy with lovastatin is recommended.

➤*Administration:* Lovastatin immediate-release tablets should be given with meals. The extended-release tablets should be swallowed whole and not crushed, chewed, or cut.

➤*Storage/Stability:*

Immediate-release tablets – Store between 5° to 30°C (41° to 86°F). Lovastatin tablets must be protected from light and stored in a well-closed, light-resistant container.

Extended-release tablets – Store at 20° to 25°C (68° to 77°F). Avoid excessive heat and humidity.

SIMVASTATIN

Rx	**Simvastatin** (Various, eg, Aurobindo, Ranbaxy, Sandoz, Teva)	**Tablets; oral:** 5 mg	May contain lactose. Film-coated. In 30s, 60s, 90s, 100s, 500s, 1,000s, and UD 100s.
Rx	**Zocor** (Merck)		Lactose. (MSD 726 ZOCOR 5). Buff, oval. Film-coated. In unit-of-use 30s and 90s.
Rx	**Simvastatin** (Various, eg, Aurobindo, Sandoz, Teva, UDL Laboratories)	**Tablets; oral:** 10 mg	May contain lactose. Film-coated. In 30s, 60s, 90s, 500s, 1,000s, 10,000s, and UD 100s.
Rx	**Zocor** (Merck)		Lactose. (MSD 735). Peach, oval. Film-coated. In 1,000s and unit-of-use 30s and 90s.
Rx	**Simvastatin** (Various, eg, Aurobindo, Sandoz, Teva, UDL Laboratories)	**Tablets; oral:** 20 mg	May contain lactose. Film-coated. In 30s, 60s, 90s, 500s, 1,000s, 10,000, and UD 100s.
Rx	**Zocor** (Merck)		Lactose. (MSD 740). Tan, oval. Film-coated. In 1,000s and unit-of-use 30s and 90s.
Rx	**Simvastatin** (Various, eg, Aurobindo, McKesson, Sandoz, Teva, UDL Laboratories)	**Tablets; oral:** 40 mg	May contain lactose. Film-coated. In 30s, 60s, 90s, 500s, 1,000s, 5,000s, and UD 100s.
Rx	**Zocor** (Merck)		Lactose. (MSD 749). Brick red, oval. Film-coated. In 1,000s and unit-of-use 30s and 90s.
Rx	**Simvastatin** (Various, eg, Aurobindo, Dr. Reddy's, Ranbaxy, Sandoz, Teva)	**Tablets; oral:** 80 mg	May contain lactose. Film-coated. In 30s, 60s, 90s, 500s, and 1,000s.
Rx	**Zocor** (Merck)		Lactose. (543 80). Brick red, capsule shape. Film-coated. In 1,000s, unit-of-use 30s and 90s, and UD 100s.
Rx	**Simvastatin** (Synthon Pharmaceuticals)	**Tablets, disintegrating; oral:** 10 mg	Sucralose. (S10 ODT). Mint menthol. Yellow. In 30s and 90s.
		20 mg	Sucralose. (S20 ODT). Mint menthol. Peach. In 30s and 90s.
		40 mg	Sucralose. (S40 ODT). Mint menthol. Pink. In 30s and 90s.
		80 mg	Sucralose. (S80 ODT). Mint menthol. In 30s and 90s.

SIMVASTATIN — ORAL

For complete and comparative prescribing information, refer to the HMG-CoA Reductase Inhibitors class monograph.

Indications

➤*General information:* Therapy with lipid-altering agents should be only one component of multiple risk factor intervention in individuals at significantly increased risk for atherosclerotic vascular disease due to hypercholesterolemia. Drug therapy is indicated as an adjunct to diet when the response to a diet restricted in saturated fat and cholesterol and other nonpharmacologic measures alone has been inadequate. In patients with coronary heart disease or at high risk of coronary heart disease, simvastatin can be started simultaneously with diet.

➤*Heterozygous familial hypercholesterolemia in adolescents (10 to 17 years of age):* As an adjunct to diet to reduce total cholesterol (total-C), low-density lipoprotein cholesterol (LDL-C), and apolipoprotein B (apo B) levels in adolescent boys and girls (10 to 17 years of age) who are at least 1 year postmenarche with heterozygous familial hypercholesterolemia, if, after an adequate trial of diet therapy, the following findings are present: LDL cholesterol remains 190 mg/dL or higher, or LDL cholesterol remains 160 mg/dL or higher and there is a positive family history of premature cardiovascular disease or 2 or more other cardiovascular disease risk factors present in the adolescent patient.

SIMVASTATIN — ORAL

➤*Hyperlipidemia:* To reduce elevated total-C, LDL-C, apo B, and triglyceride (TG) levels, and increase high-density lipoprotein cholesterol (HDL-C) in patients with primary hyperlipidemia (Fredrickson type IIa, heterozygous familial and nonfamilial) and mixed dyslipidemia (Frederickson type IIb); for the treatment of patients with hypertriglyceridemia (Fredrickson type IV hyperlipidemia); reduce elevated TG and very low density lipoprotein C (VLDL-C) in patients with primary dysbetalipoproteinemia (Fredrickson type III hyperlipidemia); to reduce total-C and LDL-C in patients with homozygous familial hypercholesterolemia as an adjunct to other lipid-lowering treatments (eg, LDL apheresis) or if such treatments are unavailable.

➤*Prevention of coronary events:* In patients at high risk of coronary events because of existing coronary heart disease, diabetes, peripheral vessel disease, or history of stroke or other cerebrovascular disease, simvastatin is indicated to reduce the risk of total mortality by reducing coronary heart disease deaths, reduce the risk of nonfatal myocardial infarction (MI) and stroke, and reduce the need for coronary and noncoronary revascularization procedures.

➤*Off-label uses:*

Extended-interval dosing (alternate-day, twice-weekly dosing) – [4] = Insufficient documentation. Initial small trials suggest that twice-weekly or alternate-day simvastatin dosing with or without fenofibrate may be comparable with daily dosing in maintaining similar reductions in total-C and LDL-C concentrations. These studies suggest that patients on an alternate-day regimen may see annual cost savings without loss of clinical efficacy. Compliance with these regimens was comparable with that observed with daily therapy. (See Administration and Dosage.)

Multiple sclerosis – [5] = Poor documentation. Preliminary data suggest that simvastatin administration could inhibit inflammatory processes in multiple sclerosis (MS) associated with neurological disability. However, the clinical significance of these effects has yet to be determined.

Administration and Dosage

➤*General dosing considerations:* Place the patient on a standard cholesterol-lowering diet. In patients with coronary heart disease or who are at high risk of coronary heart disease, simvastatin can be started simultaneously with diet.

Use simvastatin as an adjunct to other lipid-lowering treatments (eg, LDL apheresis) in patients with homozygous familial hypercholesterolemia or if such treatments are unavailable.

➤*Adults:*

Hyperlipidemia –

Usual dosage: 5 to 80 mg daily.

Initial dosage: 20 to 40 mg once a day in the evening. For patients at high risk for a CHD event caused by existing CHD, diabetes, peripheral vascular disease, history of stroke, or other cerebrovascular disease, the recommended starting dosage is 40 mg/day.

Homozygous familial hypercholesterolemia: 40 mg once a day in the evening or 80 mg/day in three divided doses of two 20 mg doses and one evening dose of 40 mg.

Prevention of coronary events –

Usual dosage: 5 to 80 mg daily.

Initial dosage: 20 to 40 mg once a day in the evening. For patients at high risk for a CHD event caused by existing CHD, diabetes, peripheral vessel disease, history of stroke, or other cerebrovascular disease, the recommended starting dosage is 40 mg/day.

Off-label dosing –

Extended-interval dosing (alternate-day, twice-weekly dosing): [4] = Insufficient documentation.

• *Alternate-day dosing* – In 1 study, simvastatin 10 mg and fenofibrate 250 mg were administered every other day for 6 months. In a small study of male outpatients who had already achieved NCEP goals for LDL-C, the daily simvastatin dose was doubled and administered every other day.

• *Twice-weekly dosing* – In a small outpatient study, patients receiving simvastatin 10 mg daily were converted to 40 mg twice weekly for 12 weeks. Patients receiving simvastatin 20 mg daily were converted to 80 mg twice weekly for 12 weeks. Twice-weekly dosing was administered on Mondays and Thursdays. For both groups, the weekly dose was approximately 14% larger with the twice-weekly dosing.

➤*Children:*

Heterozygous familial hypercholesterolemia –

10 to 17 years of age:

• *Usual dosage* – 10 to 40 mg daily.
• *Maximum dose* – 40 mg daily.
• *Initial dosage* – 10 mg once a day in the evening.
• *Dosage adjustment* – Make adjustments at intervals of 4 weeks or more.

➤*Renal function impairment:* Caution should be exercised when simvastatin is administered to patients with severe renal impairment. Start patients with severe renal impairment at 5 mg daily and monitor closely.

➤*Hepatic function impairment:* Use the drug with caution in patients who consume substantial quantities of alcohol and/or have a history of liver disease.

➤*Chinese patients:* Because of an increased risk for myopathy, caution should be used when treating Chinese patients with simvastatin coadministered with lipid-modifying doses (at least 1 g/day of niacin) of niacin-containing products. Because the risk for myopathy is dose-related, Chinese patients should not receive simvastatin 80 mg coadministered with lipid-modifying doses of niacin-containing products. The cause of the increased risk of myopathy is not known. It is also unknown if the risk for myopathy with coadministration of simvastatin with lipid-modifying doses of niacin-containing products observed in Chinese patients applies to other Asian patients.

➤*Concomitant amiodarone or verapamil therapy:* Do not exceed 20 mg daily of simvastatin.

➤*Concomitant cyclosporine or danazol therapy:* Begin therapy with simvastatin 5 mg daily and do not exceed 10 mg daily.

➤*Concomitant gemfibrozil therapy:* Do not exceed 10 mg daily of simvastatin.

➤*Patients taking diltiazem:* The dosage of simvastatin should not exceed 40 mg/day.

➤*Administration:*

Orally disintegrating tablets – Place the orally disintegrating tablet on the tongue where it will dissolve and then be swallowed with saliva. If necessary, follow with water.

➤*Storage/Stability:* Store tablets between 5° and 30°C (41° and 86°F). Store orally disintegrating tablets at 20° to 25°C (68° to 77°F); excursions are permitted to 15° to 30°C (59° to 86°F).

PRAVASTATIN SODIUM

Rx	**Pravastatin Sodium** (Various, eg, Par, Sandoz, Teva)	**Tablets**: 10 mg	Lactose. In 30s, 90s, 100s, 500s, and 1,000s.
Rx	**Pravachol** (Bristol-Myers Squibb)		Lactose. (P PRAVACHOL 10). Pink to peach, rectangular. In 90s.
Rx	**Pravastatin Sodium** (Various, eg, Par, Sandoz, Teva, UDL)	**Tablets**: 20 mg	May contain lactose. In 30s, 90s, 100s, 500s, and 1,000s.
Rx	**Pravachol** (Bristol-Myers Squibb)		Lactose. (P PRAVACHOL 20). Yellow, rectangular. In 90s, 1,000s, and UD 100s.
Rx	**Pravastatin Sodium** (Various, eg, Par, Sandoz, Teva)	**Tablets**: 40 mg	Lactose. In 30s, 90s, 100s, 500s, and 1,000s.
Rx	**Pravachol** (Bristol-Myers Squibb)		Lactose, FD&C Blue No 1. (P PRAVACHOL 40). Green, rectangular. In 90s and UD 100s.
Rx	**Pravastatin Sodium** (Various, eg, Ranbaxy, Watson)	**Tablets**: 80 mg	Lactose. In 90s, 100s, 500s, and 1,000s.
Rx	**Pravachol** (Bristol-Myers Squibb)		Lactose. (BMS 80). Yellow, oval. In 90s, 500s, and UD 100s.

PRAVASTATIN SODIUM — ORAL

For complete and comparative prescribing information, refer to the HMG-CoA Reductase Inhibitors group monograph.

Indications

➤*General information:* Consider pravastatin therapy in patients at increased risk for atherosclerosis-related clinical events as a function of cholesterol level, the presence or absence of coronary heart disease, and other risk factors.

➤*Primary prevention of coronary events:* In hypercholesterolemic patients without clinically evident coronary heart disease (CHD), pravastatin is indicated to reduce the risk of the following: cardiovascular mortality with no increase in death from noncardiovascular causes, myocardial infarction (MI), and undergoing myocardial revascularization procedures.

➤*Secondary prevention of cardiovascular events:* In patients with clinically evident CHD, pravastatin is indicated to slow the progression of coronary atherosclerosis and reduce the risk of the following: MI, stroke and stroke/transient ischemic attack (TIA), total mortality by reducing coronary death, and undergoing myocardial revascularization procedures.

➤*Hyperlipidemia:* An adjunct to diet to reduce elevated total cholesterol (total-C), low-density lipoprotein cholesterol (LDL-C), apolipoprotein B (apo

PRAVASTATIN SODIUM — ORAL

B), and triglyceride levels, and to increase high-density lipoprotein cholesterol (HDL-C) in patients with primary hypercholesterolemia and mixed dyslipidemia (Fredrickson type IIa and IIb).

As adjunctive therapy to diet for the treatment of patients with elevated serum triglyceride levels (Fredrickson type IV).

For the treatment of patients with primary dysbetalipoproteinemia (Fredrickson type III) who do not respond adequately to diet.

➤*Children (8 years of age and older) with heterozygous familial hypercholesterolemia (HeFH):* As an adjunct to diet and lifestyle modification for treatment of HeFH in children and adolescent patients 8 years of age and older if, after an adequate trial of diet, the following findings are present: LDL-C remains at 190 mg/dL or more; or LDL-C remains at 160 mg/dL or more and there is a positive family history of premature cardiovascular disease (CVD) or 2 or more other CVD risk factors are present in the patient.

➤*The National Cholesterol Education Program's (NCEP) Treatment Guidelines:*

NCEP Treatment Guidelines

Risk category	LDL goal (mg/dL)	LDL levels at which to initiate therapeutic lifestyle changes (mg/dL)	LDL level at which to consider drug therapy (mg/dL)
CHD[a] or CHD risk equivalents (10-year risk > 20%)	< 100	≥ 100	≥ 130 (100 to 129: drug optional)[b]
+2 risk factors (10-year risk ≤ 20%)	< 130	≥ 130	10-year risk 10% to 20%: ≥ 130
			10-year risk < 10%: ≥ 160
0 to 1 risk factor[c]	< 160	≥ 160	≥ 190 (160 to 189: LDL-lowering drug optional)

[a] CHD = coronary heart disease.

[b] Some authorities recommend the use of LDL-lowering drugs in this category if an LDL-C level of < 100 mg/dL cannot be achieved by therapeutic lifestyle changes. Others prefer use of drugs that primarily modify triglycerides and HDL-C (eg, nicotinic acid or fibrate). Clinical judgement also may call for deferring drug therapy in this subcategory.

[c] Almost all people with 0 to 1 risk factor have 10-year risk < 10%; thus, 10-year risk assessment in people with 0 to 1 risk factor is not necessary.

After the LDL-C goal has been achieved, if the triglyceride level is still 200 mg/dL or more, non–HDL-C (total-C minus HDL-C) becomes a secondary target of therapy. Non–HDL-C goals are set 30 mg/dL higher than LDL-C goals for each risk category.

At the time of hospitalization for an acute coronary event, consider initiating drug therapy at discharge if the LDL-C is 130 mg/dL or more.

Because the goal of treatment is to lower LDL-C, the NCEP recommends that LDL-C levels be used to initiate and assess treatment response. Use the total-C to monitor therapy only if the LDL-C levels are not available.

As with other lipid-lowering therapy, pravastatin is not indicated when hypercholesterolemia is caused by hyperalphalipoproteinemia (elevated HDL-C).

The NCEP classification of cholesterol levels in children with a familial history of hypercholesterolemia or premature CVD is summarized in the following table.

NCEP Classification for Children

Category	Total-C (mg/dL)	LDL-C (mg/dL)
Acceptable	< 170	< 110
Borderline	170 to 199	110 to 129
High	≥ 200	≥ 130

Administration and Dosage

➤*General dosing considerations:* Place the patient on a standard cholesterol-lowering diet before starting pravastatin and continue on this diet during treatment.

Pravastatin can be administered as a single dose at any time of the day, with or without food. Because the maximal effect of a given dose is seen within 4 weeks, perform periodic lipid determinations at this time and adjust dosage according to the patient's response to therapy and established treatment guidelines.

➤*Adults:*

Hyperlipidemia –

Usual dosage: 40 mg once daily.

Dosage adjustment: If a daily dose of 40 mg does not achieve desired cholesterol levels, 80 mg once daily is recommended.

➤*Children:*

Hyperlipidemia – Reevaluate children and adolescents treated with pravastatin in adulthood and make appropriate changes to their cholesterol-lowering regimen to achieve adult goals for LDL-C.

14 to 18 years of age:

• *Usual dosage* – 40 mg once daily. Doses greater than 40 mg have not been studied in this patient population.

8 to 13 years of age, inclusive:

• *Usual dosage* – 20 mg once daily. Doses greater than 20 mg have not been studied in this patient population.

➤*Renal function impairment:* In patients with a history of significant renal function impairment, a starting dosage of 10 mg daily is recommended.

➤*Hepatic function impairment:* In patients with a history of significant hepatic function impairment, a starting dosage of 10 mg daily is recommended.

➤*Concomitant immunosuppressants:* In patients taking immunosuppressive drugs such as cyclosporine concomitantly with pravastatin, begin therapy with pravastatin 10 mg once daily at bedtime and titrate to higher doses with caution. Most patients treated with this combination received a maximum dose of pravastatin 20 mg/day.

➤*Concomitant lipid-lowering therapy:* The lipid-lowering effects of pravastatin on total and LDL-C are enhanced when combined with a bile acid-binding resin. When administering a bile acid-binding resin (eg, cholestyramine, colestipol) and pravastatin, give pravastatin 1 hour or more before or at least 4 hours following the resin.

➤*Storage/Stability:* Store at 25°C (77°F); excursions are permitted to 15° to 30°C (59° to 86°F). Protect from light and moisture.

ROSUVASTATIN CALCIUM

Rx	**Crestor** (AstraZeneca)	**Tablets**; **oral:** 5 mg	Lactose. (CRESTOR 5). Yellow, round. Film-coated. In 90s.
		10 mg	Lactose. (CRESTOR 10). Pink, round. Film-coated. In 90s and UD 100s.
		20 mg	Lactose. (CRESTOR 20). Pink, round. Film-coated. In 90s and UD 100s.
		40 mg	Lactose. (CRESTOR 40). Pink, oval. Film-coated. In 30s.

ROSUVASTATIN CALCIUM — ORAL

For complete and comparative prescribing information, refer to the HMG-CoA Reductase Inhibitors class monograph.

Indications

➤*Atherosclerosis:* As adjunctive therapy to diet to slow the progression of atherosclerosis in adult patients as part of a treatment strategy to lower total cholesterol and low-density lipoprotein cholesterol (LDL-C) to target levels.

➤*Heterozygous familial hypercholesterolemia in children:* As an adjunct to diet to reduce total cholesterol, LDL-C, and apolipoprotein B (apo B) levels in adolescent boys and girls who are at least 1 year postmenarche and are 10 to 17 years of age with heterozygous familial hypercholesteremia if after an adequate trial of diet therapy the following findings are present: LDL-C more than 190 mg/dL or more than 160 mg/dL and there is a positive family history of premature cardiovascular (CV) disease or 2 or more other CV disease risk factors.

➤*Homozygous familial hypercholesterolemia:* To reduce LDL-C, total cholesterol, and apo B in adult patients with homozygous familial hypercholesterolemia as an adjunct to other lipid-lowering treatments (eg, LDL apheresis) or alone if such treatments are unavailable.

➤*Hyperlipidemia and mixed dyslipidemia:* As adjunctive therapy to diet to reduce elevated total cholesterol, LDL-C, apo B, non–high-density lipoprotein cholesterol (HDL-C), and triglyceride levels, and to increase HDL-C in patients with primary hyperlipidemia or mixed dyslipidemia.

➤*Hypertriglyceridemia:* As an adjunct to diet for the treatment of adult patients with hypertriglyceridemia.

➤*Primary dysbetalipoproteinemia (type III hyperlipoproteinemia):* As an adjunct to diet for the treatment of patients with primary dysbetalipoproteinemia (type III hyperlipoproteinemia).

➤*Primary prevention of cardiovascular disease:* To reduce the risk of stroke, reduce the risk of myocardial infarction, and reduce the risk of arterial revascularization procedures in individuals without clinically evident coronary heart disease, but with an increased risk of CV disease based on age of 50 years and older in men and 60 years and older in women, high-sensitivity C-reactive protein of at least 2 mg/L, and the presence of at least 1 additional CV disease risk factor such as hypertension, low HDL-C, smoking, or a family history of premature coronary heart disease.

ROSUVASTATIN CALCIUM — ORAL

Administration and Dosage

➤*General dosing considerations:* Lipid-altering agents should be used in addition to a diet restricted in saturated fat and cholesterol when response to diet and nonpharmacologic interventions alone has been inadequate. When initiating rosuvastatin therapy or switching from another HMG-CoA reductase inhibitor therapy, the appropriate rosuvastatin starting dose should be utilized first, and only then titrated according to the patient's response and individualized goal of therapy.

The 40 mg dose of rosuvastatin should be used only for those patients who have not achieved their LDL-C goal utilizing the 20 mg dose.

➤*Adults:*

Atherosclerosis –

Usual dosage: 5 to 40 mg orally once daily.

Initial dosage: 10 to 20 mg once daily.

Dosage titration: After initiation or upon titration of rosuvastatin, lipid levels should be analyzed within 2 to 4 weeks and the dosage adjusted accordingly.

Homozygous familial hypercholesterolemia –

Usual dosage: 5 to 40 mg orally once daily.

Initial dosage: 20 mg once daily. Response to therapy should be estimated from preapheresis LDL-C levels.

Hyperlipidemia and mixed dyslipidemia – See Atherosclerosis for dosing.

Hypertriglyceridemia – See Atherosclerosis for dosing.

Primary dysbetalipoproteinemia (type III hyperlipoproteinemia) – See Atherosclerosis for dosing.

Primary prevention of cardiovascular disease –

Usual dosage: 5 to 40 mg orally once daily.

Initial dosage: 10 to 20 mg once daily.

➤*Children:*

Heterozygous familial hypercholesteremia –

10 to 17 years of age:

• *Usual dose* – 5 to 20 mg/day.

• *Maximum dose* – 20 mg/day (doses greater than 20 mg have not been studied in this patient population).

• *Dosage adjustment* – Doses should be individualized according to the recommended goal of therapy. Adjustments should be made at intervals of 4 weeks or more.

➤*Renal function impairment:* For patients with severe renal impairment (creatinine clearance [CrCl] less than 30 mL/min per 1.73 m^2) not on hemodialysis, dosing of rosuvastatin should be started at 5 mg once daily and not exceed 10 mg once daily.

➤*Hepatic function impairment:* Use with caution in patients who consume substantial quantities of alcohol or have a history of liver disease. Active liver disease or unexplained persistent transaminase elevations are contraindications to the use of rosuvastatin.

➤*Asian patients:* Consider initiation of rosuvastatin therapy with 5 mg once daily for Asian patients.

➤*Concomitant therapy:*

Cyclosporine – In patients taking cyclosporine, therapy should be limited to 5 mg once daily.

Lipid-lowering therapy – The risk of skeletal muscle effects may be enhanced when used in combination with niacin or fenofibrate; a reduction in rosuvastatin dosage should be considered in this setting. Combination therapy with gemfibrozil should be avoided because of an increase in rosuvastatin exposure with concomitant use. If rosuvastatin is used in combination with gemfibrozil, the dosage of rosuvastatin should be limited to 10 mg once daily.

Lopinavir/Ritonavir or atazanavir/ritonavir – In patients taking a combination of lopinavir and ritonavir or atazanavir and ritonavir, the dosage of rosuvastatin should be limited to 10 mg once daily.

➤*Administration:* Administer as a single dose at any time of the day, with or without food.

➤*Storage/Stability:* Store at 20° to 25°C (68° to 77°F). Protect from moisture.

FLUVASTATIN

Rx	**Lescol XL** (Novartis)	**Tablets, extended-release; oral:** 80 mg	As fluvastatin sodium. (Lescol XL 80). Yellow. Film-coated. In 30s and 100s.
Rx	**Lescol** (Novartis)	**Capsules; oral:** 20 mg	As fluvastatin sodium. May contain benzyl alcohol, parabens, EDTA. (20 LESCOL). Brown/Lt. brown. In 30s and 100s.
		40 mg	As fluvastatin sodium. May contain benzyl alcohol, parabens, EDTA. (40 LESCOL). Brown/Gold. In 30s and 100s.

FLUVASTATIN SODIUM — ORAL

For complete and comparative prescribing information, refer to the HMG-CoA Reductase Inhibitors group monograph.

Indications

➤*Atherosclerosis:* To slow the progression of coronary atherosclerosis in patients with coronary heart disease as part of a treatment strategy to lower total cholesterol (total-C) and low-density lipoprotein cholesterol (LDL-C) to target levels.

➤*Heterozygous familial hypercholesterolemia in children:* As an adjunct to diet to reduce total-C, LDL-C, and apolipoprotein B (apoB) levels in adolescent boys and girls (who are at least 1 year postmenarche) 10 to 16 years of age with heterozygous familial hypercholesterolemia whose response to dietary restriction has not been adequate and for whom the following findings are present: LDL-C remains at 190 mg/dL or more; or LDL-C remains at 160 mg/dL or more and there is a positive family history of premature cardiovascular disease or 2 or more other cardiovascular disease risk factors are present.

➤*Hypercholesterolemia (heterozygous familial and nonfamilial) and mixed dyslipidemia:* To reduce elevated total-C, LDL-C, triglycerides (TG), and apoB levels, and to increase high-density lipoprotein cholesterol (HDL-C) in patients with primary hypercholesterolemia and mixed dyslipidemia (Fredrickson types IIa and IIb) whose response to dietary restriction of saturated fat and cholesterol and other nonpharmacological measures has not been adequate.

➤*Secondary prevention of coronary events:* To reduce the risk of undergoing coronary revascularization procedures in patients with coronary heart disease.

➤*Off-label uses:*

Extended-interval dosing (alternate-day dosing) – [4] = Insufficient documentation. One small nonblinded crossover trial suggests that alternate-day dosing with fluvastatin may be comparable to daily dosing in maintaining similar reductions in total cholesterol and LDL concentrations.

Administration and Dosage

➤*General dosing considerations:* The patient should be placed on a standard cholesterol-lowering diet before receiving fluvastatin and should continue on this diet during treatment with fluvastatin.

➤*Adults:*

Atherosclerosis –

Usual dosage: 20 to 80 mg/day.

Initial dosage:

• *Patients requiring LDL-C reduction to a goal of at least 25%* – 40 mg as 1 capsule in the evening, 80 mg as 1 extended-release tablet administered as a single dose at any time of the day, or 80 mg in divided doses of the 40 mg capsule given twice daily.

• *Patients requiring LDL-C reduction to a goal of less than 25%* – 20 mg daily.

Dosage adjustment: Because the maximal reductions in LDL-C of a given dose are seen within 4 weeks, periodic lipid determinations should be performed and dosage adjustment made according to the patient's response to therapy and established treatment guidelines. The therapeutic effect of fluvastatin is maintained with prolonged administration.

Hypercholesterolemia (heterozygous familial and nonfamilial) – See Atherosclerosis.

Mixed dyslipidemia – See Atherosclerosis.

Secondary prevention of coronary events – See Atherosclerosis.

Off-label dosing –

Extended-interval dosing (alternate-day dosing) (off-label): [4] = Insufficient documentation. 40 mg every other night.

➤*Children:*

Heterozygous familial hypercholesterolemia –

9 to 16 years of age:

• *Initial dosage* – 20 mg daily.

• *Dosage adjustment* – Dosage adjustments, up to a maximum daily dose, administered either as fluvastatin 40 mg capsules twice daily or 1 fluvastatin 80 mg extended-release tablet once daily, should be made at 6-week intervals. Doses should be individualized according to the goal of therapy.

➤*Concomitant therapy:* Lipid-lowering effects on total-C and LDL-C are additive when immediate-release fluvastatin is combined with a bile-acidbinding resin or niacin. When administering a bile-acid resin (eg, cholestyramine) and fluvastatin, fluvastatin should be administered at bedtime, at least 2 hours following the resin to avoid a significant interaction caused by drug binding to resin.

➤*Administration:* Fluvastatin may be taken without regard to meals because there are no apparent differences in the lipid-lowering effects of fluvastatin administered with the evening meal or 4 hours after the evening meal.

FLUVASTATIN SODIUM — ORAL

Do not break, crush, or chew fluvastatin tablets, or open capsules prior to administration.

Administer capsule in the evening or in divided doses twice a day.

Administer extended-release tablet as a single dose at any time of the day.

➤*Storage/Stability:* Store at 25°C (77°F); excursions are permitted between 15° and 30°C (59° and 86°F). Dispense in a tight container. Protect from light.

ATORVASTATIN

Rx	**Lipitor** (Pfizer)	**Tablets; oral:** 10 mg	Lactose. (PD 155 10). White, elliptical. Film-coated. In 90s, 5,000s, and UD 100s.
		20 mg	Lactose. (PD 156 20). White, elliptical. Film-coated. In 90s, 5,000s, and UD 100s.
		40 mg	Lactose. (PD 157 40). White, elliptical. Film-coated. In 90s and 500s.
		80 mg	Lactose. (PD 158 80). White, elliptical. Film-coated. In 90s and 500s.

ATORVASTATIN — ORAL

For complete and comparative prescribing information, refer to the HMG-CoA Reductase Inhibitors group monograph.

Indications

➤*Clinically evident coronary heart disease (CHD):* To reduce the risk of nonfatal myocardial infarction (MI), fatal and nonfatal stroke, revascularization procedures, hospitalization for CHF, and angina in patients with clinically evident CHD.

➤*Dysbetalipoproteinemia:* For the treatment of patients with primary dysbetalipoproteinemia (Fredrickson type III) who do not respond adequately to diet.

➤*Heterozygous familial and nonfamilial hypercholesterolemia and mixed dyslipidemia:* As an adjunct to diet to reduce elevated total cholesterol (total-C), low-density lipoprotein cholesterol (LDL-C), apolipoprotein B (apo B), and triglyceride levels, and to increase high-density lipoprotein cholesterol (HDL-C) in patients with primary hypercholesterolemia (heterozygous familial and nonfamilial) and mixed dyslipidemia (Fredrickson type IIa and IIb).

➤*Heterozygous familial hypercholesterolemia (FH) in children 10 to 17 years of age:* As an adjunct to diet to reduce total-C, LDL-C, and apo B levels in boys and postmenarchal girls 10 to 17 years of age with heterozygous FH if after an adequate trial of diet therapy the following findings are present: LDL-C remains 190 mg/dL or higher, or LDL-C remains 160 mg/dL or higher, and there is a positive family history of premature cardiovascular disease (CVD) or 2 or more other CVD risk factors are present in the child.

➤*Homozygous FH:* To reduce total-C and LDL-C in patients with homozygous FH as an adjunct to other lipid-lowering treatments (eg, LDL apheresis) or if such treatments are unavailable.

➤*Hypertriglyceridemia:* As an adjunct to diet for the treatment of patients with elevated serum triglyceride levels (Fredrickson type IV).

➤*Prevention of CVD:* In adult patients without clinically evident CHD but with multiple risk factors for CHD, such as age, smoking, hypertension, low HDL-C, or a family history of early CHD, atorvastatin is indicated to reduce the risk of MI and stroke and the risk for revascularization procedures and angina.

In patients with type 2 diabetes and without clinically evident CHD but with multiple risk factors for CHD, such as retinopathy, albuminuria, smoking, or hypertension, atorvastatin is indicated to reduce the risk of MI and stroke.

➤*National Cholesterol Education Program (NCEP) guidelines:* Therapy with lipid-altering agents should be a component of multiple risk factor intervention in individuals at increased risk for atherosclerotic vascular disease caused by hypercholesterolemia. Use lipid-altering agents, in addition to a diet restricted in saturated fat and cholesterol, only when the response to diet and other nonpharmacological measures has been inadequate (see the following NCEP guidelines).

NCEP Treatment Guidelines: LDL-C Goals and Cutpoints for Therapeutic Lifestyle Changes and Drug Therapy in Different Risk Categories

Risk category	LDL-C goal (mg/dL)	LDL level at which to initiate therapeutic lifestyle changes (mg/dL)	LDL level at which to consider drug therapy (mg/dL)
CHD or CHD risk equivalents (10-year risk > 20%)	< 100	≥ 100	≥ 130 (100 to 129: drug optional)[a]
≥ 2 risk factors (10-year risk ≤ 20%)	< 130	≥ 130	10-year risk 10% to 20%: ≥ 130
			10-year risk < 10%: ≥ 160
0 to 1 risk factor[b]	< 160	≥ 160	≥ 190 (160 to 189: LDL-lowering drug optional)

[a] Some authorities recommend use of LDL-lowering drugs in this category if an LDL-C level < 100 mg/dL cannot be achieved by therapeutic lifestyle changes. Others prefer use of drugs that primarily modify triglycerides and HDL-C (eg, fibrate, nicotinic acid). Clinical judgment also may call for deferring drug therapy in this subcategory.
[b] Almost all people with 0 to 1 risk factor have a 10-year risk

After the LDL-C goal has been achieved, if the triglyceride level is still 200 mg/dL or higher, non–HDL-C (total-C minus HDL-C) becomes a secondary target of therapy. Non–HDL-C goals are set 30 mg/dL higher than LDL-C goals for each risk category.

NCEP classification for children – The NCEP classification of cholesterol levels in children with a familial history of hypercholesterolemia or premature CVD is summarized in the following table:

NCEP Classification of Cholesterol Levels in Children

Category	Total-C (mg/dL)	LDL-C (mg/dL)
Acceptable	< 170	< 110
Borderline	170 to 199	110 to 129
High	≥ 200	≥ 130

➤*Off-label uses:*

Extended-interval dosing (alternate-day, weekly dosing) – [4] = Insufficient documentation. One small, open-label trial in approximately 20 patients comparing weekly versus daily dosing suggested there were significant differences between the 2 groups for LDL cholesterol and total cholesterol levels, although both regimens produced significant reductions when compared with pretherapy levels.

Two small trials enrolling approximately 50 patients with alternate-day atorvastatin dosing suggest this regimen may be comparable with daily dosing in maintaining similar reductions in total cholesterol and LDL concentrations. (See Administration and Dosage.)

Juvenile rheumatoid arthritis – [4] = Insufficient documentation. There is little information on the therapeutic benefit of this agent in children with arthritis. More information is needed before this drug can be recommended for this use in children. (See Administration and Dosage.)

Rheumatoid arthritis – [4] = Insufficient documentation. Initial results suggest that atorvastatin may affect markers for cardiac disease as well as some parameters for clinical inflammatory changes in patients with rheumatoid arthritis (RA) (eg, swollen joint count, disease activity score). However, larger, controlled trials with stricter controls for disease-state assessment and adjunctive therapy are needed before this therapy is established as effective. (See Administration and Dosage.)

Administration and Dosage

➤*Adults:*

Heterozygous familial and nonfamilial hypercholesterolemia and mixed dyslipidemia (Fredrickson type IIa and IIb) –

Initial dosage: 10 or 20 mg once daily. Patients who require a large reduction in LDL-C (more than 45%) may be started at 40 mg once daily.

Maintenance dosage: 10 to 80 mg once daily.

Dosage adjustment: After initiation and/or upon titration of atorvastatin, lipid levels should be analyzed within 2 to 4 weeks and dosage adjusted accordingly.

Homozygous familial hypercholesterolemia –

Initial dosage: 10 to 80 mg daily.

Concomitant therapy: Atorvastatin should be used as an adjunct to other lipid-lowering treatments (eg, LDL apheresis) in these patients or if such treatments are unavailable.

Off-label dosing –

Extended-interval dosing (alternate-day, weekly dosing): [4] = Insufficient documentation. 20 mg weekly or 10 to 20 mg every other day.

Rheumatoid arthritis: [4] = Insufficient documentation.

- *Adults* – 20 mg for 3 months or 40 mg daily for 6 months.

➤*Children:*

Heterozygous familial hypercholesterolemia in children 10 to 17 years of age –

Maximum dose: 20 mg/day (doses of more than 20 mg have not been studied in this patient population).

Initial dosage: 10 mg daily.

Dosage adjustment: Adjustments should be made at intervals of 4 weeks or more.

Off-label dosing –

Juvenile rheumatoid arthritis: [4] = Insufficient documentation.

HMG-CoA Reductase Inhibitors (Statins)

ATORVASTATIN — ORAL

- *Children* – 10 to 30 mg daily (1.5 mg/kg/day) (duration unspecified).

➤*Concomitant lipid-lowering therapy:* Atorvastatin may be used in combination with a bile acid-binding resin for additive effect. The combination of 3-hydroxy-3-methylglutaryl coenzyme A (HMG-CoA) reductase inhibitors and fibrates (eg, gemfibrozil) should generally be avoided.

➤*Therapeutic drug monitoring:* Because the goal of treatment is to lower LDL-C, the NCEP recommends that LDL-C levels be used to initiate and assess treatment response. Total-C should be used to monitor therapy only if LDL-C levels are not available.

➤*Administration:* Atorvastatin can be administered as a single dose at any time of the day, with or without food.

➤*Storage/Stability:* Store at controlled room temperature, 20° to 25°C (68° to 77°F).

PITAVASTATIN

Rx	**Livalo** (Lilly)	Tablets; oral: 1 mg	Equiv. to pitavastatin calcium 1.045 mg. Lactose. (KC 1). White, round. Film-coated. In 90s.
		2 mg	Equiv. to pitavastatin calcium 2.09 mg. Lactose. KC 2). White, round. Film-coated. In 90s.
		4 mg	Equiv. to pitavastatin calcium 4.18 mg. Lactose. KC 4). White, round. Film-coated. In 90s.

PITAVASTATIN CALCIUM — ORAL

Indications

➤*Primary hyperlipidemia and mixed dyslipidemia:* As an adjunctive therapy to diet to reduce elevated total cholesterol (TC), low-density lipoprotein cholesterol (LDL-C), apolipoprotein B (Apo B), and triglycerides (TG), and to increase high-density lipoprotein cholesterol (HDL-C) in adult patients with primary hyperlipidemia or mixed dyslipidemia.

Administration and Dosage

➤*Adults:*

Primary hyperlipidemia and mixed dyslipidemia –

Maximum dose: 4 mg once daily.

Initial dosage: 2 mg orally once daily at any time of the day with or without food.

Maintenance dosage: 1 to 4 mg orally once daily.

Dosage adjustment: After initiation or upon titration of pitavastatin, lipid levels should be analyzed after 4 weeks and the dosage adjusted accordingly.

➤*Renal function impairment:*

Moderate renal impairment – Patients with moderate renal impairment (GFR 30 to less than 60 mL/min per 1.73 m^2) should receive a starting dosage of pitavastatin 1 mg once daily and a maximum dose of 2 mg once daily.

Severe renal impairment – Pitavastatin should not be used in patients with severe renal impairment (GFR less than 30 mL/min per 1.73 m^2) not yet on hemodialysis.

Hemodialysis – Patients with end-stage renal disease (ESRD) receiving hemodialysis should receive a starting dosage of 1 mg once daily and a maximum dose of 2 mg once daily.

➤*Hepatic function impairment:* Pitavastatin is contraindicated in patients with active liver disease.

➤*Concomitant medications:*

Erythromycin – 1 mg once daily should not be exceeded in patients taking erythromycin.

Rifampin – 2 mg once daily should not be exceeded in patients taking rifampin.

➤*Administration:* Pitavastatin should be taken orally once daily at any time of the day with or without food.

➤*Storage/Stability:* Store at room temperature, between 15° and 30°C (59° and 86°F). Protect from light.

Fibric Acid Derivatives

GEMFIBROZIL

Rx	**Gemfibrozil** (Various, eg, Mylan, UDL, Warner Chilcott)	Tablets: 600 mg	In 60s, 500s, blister pack 25s, and UD 100s.
Rx	**Lopid** (Parke-Davis)		(LOPID P-D 737). Parabens. White, scored, elliptical. Film-coated. In 60s, 500s, and UD 100s.

GEMFIBROZIL — ORAL

Refer to the general discussion of these products in the Antihyperlipidemic Agents Introduction.

Indications

➤*Hypertriglyceridemia:* Gemfibrozil is indicated as adjunctive therapy to diet for treatment of adult patients with very high elevations of serum triglyceride levels (type IV and type V hyperlipidemia) who present a risk of pancreatitis and who do not respond adequately to a determined dietary effort to control them. Patients who present such risk typically have serum triglycerides over 2,000 mg/dL and have elevations of very low-density lipoproteins (VLDL) cholesterol and fasting chylomicrons (type V hyperlipidemia). Subjects who consistently have total serum or plasma triglycerides less than 1,000 mg/dL are unlikely to present a risk of pancreatitis. Gemfibrozil therapy may be considered for those subjects with triglyceride elevations between 1,000 and 2,000 mg/dL who have a history of pancreatitis or of recurrent abdominal pain typical of pancreatitis. It is recognized that some type IV patients with triglycerides less than 1,000 mg/dL may, through dietary or alcoholic indiscretion, convert to a type V pattern with massive triglyceride elevations accompanying fasting chylomicronemia, but the influence of gemfibrozil therapy on the risk of pancreatitis in such situations has not been adequately studied. Drug therapy is not indicated for patients with type I hyperlipoproteinemia, who have elevations of chylomicrons and plasma triglycerides, but who have normal levels of VLDL. Inspection of plasma refrigerated for 14 hours is helpful in distinguishing types I, IV, and V hyperlipoproteinemia.

➤*Prevention of cardiovascular disease:* Gemfibrozil is indicated as adjunctive therapy to diet for reducing the risk of developing coronary heart disease only in type IIb patients without history of or symptoms of existing coronary heart disease who have had an inadequate response to weight loss, dietary therapy, exercise, and other pharmacologic agents (such as bile acid sequestrants and nicotinic acid, known to reduce low-density lipoprotein [LDL] and raise high-density lipoprotein [HDL] cholesterol) and who have the following triad of lipid abnormalities: Low HDL cholesterol levels in addition to elevated LDL cholesterol and elevated triglycerides. The National Cholesterol Education Program has defined a serum HDL cholesterol value that is consistently less than 35 mg/dL as constituting an independent risk factor for coronary heart disease. Patients with significantly elevated triglycerides should be closely observed when treated with gemfibrozil. In some patients with high triglyceride levels, treatment with gemfibrozil is associated with a significant increase in LDL cholesterol. Because of potential toxicity such as malignancy, gallbladder disease, abdominal pain leading to appendectomy, and other abdominal surgeries, an increased incidence in noncoronary mortality, and the 44% relative increase during the trial period in age-adjusted all-cause mortality seen with the chemically and pharmacologically related drug, clofibrate, the potential benefit of gemfibrozil in treating type IIa patients with elevations of LDL cholesterol only is not likely to outweigh the risks. Gemfibrozil is also not indicated for the treatment of patients with low HDL cholesterol as their only lipid abnormality.

➤*General information:* The initial treatment for dyslipidemia is dietary therapy specific for the type of lipoprotein abnormality. Excess body weight and excess alcohol intake may be important factors in hypertriglyceridemia and should be managed prior to any drug therapy. Physical exercise can be an important ancillary measure, and has been associated with rises in HDL cholesterol. Diseases contributory to hyperlipidemia, such as hypothyroidism or diabetes mellitus, should be looked for and adequately treated. Estrogen therapy is sometimes associated with massive rises in plasma triglycerides, especially in subjects with familial hypertriglyceridemia. In such cases, discontinuation of estrogen therapy may obviate the need for specific drug therapy of hypertriglyceridemia. The use of drugs should be considered only when reasonable attempts have been made to obtain satisfactory results with nondrug methods. If the decision is made to use drugs, the patient should be instructed that this does not reduce the importance of adhering to diet.

Administration and Dosage

➤*Adults:*

Usual dosage – 1,200 mg administered in 2 divided doses 30 minutes before the morning and evening meals.

➤*Renal function impairment:* Contraindicated in patients with severe renal impairment. Use with caution in patients with mild to moderate renal impairment.

➤*Hepatic function impairment:* Contraindicated in patients with hepatic impairment.

GEMFIBROZIL — ORAL

➤*Monitoring:*

Initial therapy – Laboratory studies should be done to ascertain that the lipid levels are consistently abnormal. Before instituting gemfibrozil therapy, every attempt should be made to control serum lipids with appropriate diet, exercise, and weight loss in obese patients, and to control any medical problems such as diabetes mellitus and hypothyroidism that are contributing to the lipid abnormalities.

Continued therapy – Periodic determination of serum lipids should be obtained, and the drug withdrawn if lipid response is inadequate after 3 months of therapy.

Actions

➤*Pharmacology:* The mechanism of action of gemfibrozil has not been definitely established. In man, gemfibrozil has been shown to inhibit peripheral lipolysis and to decrease the hepatic extraction of free fatty acids, thus reducing hepatic triglyceride production. Gemfibrozil inhibits synthesis and increases clearance of VLDL carrier apolipoprotein B, leading to a decrease in VLDL production.

➤*Pharmacokinetics:*

Absorption/Distribution – Gemfibrozil is well absorbed from the GI tract after oral administration. Peak plasma levels occur in 1 to 2 hours with a plasma half-life of 1.5 hours following multiple doses. Gemfibrozil is completely absorbed after oral administration of gemfibrozil tablets, reaching peak plasma concentrations 1 to 2 hours after dosing. Gemfibrozil pharmacokinetics are affected by the timing of meals relative to time of dosing. In 1 study, both the rate and extent of absorption of the drug were significantly increased when administered 0.5 hour before meals. Average AUC was reduced by 14% to 44% when gemfibrozil was administered after meals compared to 0.5 hour before meals. In a subsequent study, rate of absorption of gemfibrozil was maximum when administered 0.5 hour before meals with the C_{max} 50% to 60% greater than when given either with meals or fasting. In this study, there were no significant effects on AUC of timing of dose relative to meals.

Gemfibrozil is highly bound to plasma proteins and there is potential for displacement interactions with other drugs such as with HMG-CoA-reductase inhibitors and anticoagulants.

Metabolism – Gemfibrozil mainly undergoes oxidation of a ring methyl group to successively form a hydroxymethyl and a carboxyl metabolite.

Excretion – Approximately 70% of the administered human dose is excreted in the urine, mostly as the glucuronide conjugate, with less than 2% excreted as unchanged gemfibrozil. Six percent (6%) of the dose is accounted for in the feces.

Contraindications

Hepatic or severe renal dysfunction, including primary biliary cirrhosis; preexisting gallbladder disease; hypersensitivity to gemfibrozil; concurrent use with repaglinide.

Warnings/Precautions

➤*Gallstones:* A gallstone prevalence substudy of 450 Helsinki Heart Study participants showed a trend toward a greater prevalence of gallstones during the study within the gemfibrozil treatment group (7.5% vs 4.9% for the placebo group, a 55% excess for the gemfibrozil group). A trend toward a greater incidence of gallbladder surgery was observed for the gemfibrozil group (17 vs 11 subjects, a 54% excess). This result did not differ statistically from the increased incidence of cholecystectomy observed in the WHO study in the group treated with clofibrate. Both clofibrate and gemfibrozil may increase cholesterol excretion into the bile leading to cholelithiasis. If cholelithiasis is suspected, gallbladder studies are indicated. Gemfibrozil therapy should be discontinued if gallstones are found.

➤*General information:* Because a reduction of mortality from coronary heart disease has not been demonstrated and because liver and interstitial cell testicular tumors were increased in rats, gemfibrozil should be administered only to those patients described in Indications. If a significant serum lipid response is not obtained, gemfibrozil should be discontinued.

➤*Concomitant anticoagulants:* Caution should be exercised when anticoagulants are given in conjunction with gemfibrozil. The dosage of the anticoagulant should be reduced to maintain the prothrombin time at the desired level to prevent bleeding complications. Frequent prothrombin determinations are advisable until it has been definitely determined that the prothrombin level has stabilized.

➤*Skeletal muscle effects:* Concomitant therapy with gemfibrozil and an HMG-CoA reductase inhibitor is associated with an increased risk of skeletal muscle toxicity manifested as rhabdomyolysis, markedly elevated creatine kinase (CPK) levels and myoglobinuria, leading in a high proportion of cases to acute renal failure and death. Because of an observed marked increased risk of myopathy and rhabdomyolysis, the specific combination of gemfibrozil and cerivastatin is absolutely contraindicated. In patients who have had an unsatisfactory lipid response to either drug alone, the benefit of combined therapy with gemfibrozil and HMG-CoA reductase inhibitors other than cerivastatin does not outweigh the risks of severe myopathy, rhabdomyolysis, and acute renal failure. The use of fibrates alone, including gemfibrozil, may occasionally be associated with myositis. Patients receiving gemfibrozil and complaining of muscle pain, tenderness, or weakness should have prompt medical evaluation for myositis, including serum creatine kinase level determination. If myositis is suspected or diagnosed, gemfibrozil therapy should be withdrawn.

➤*Cataracts:* Subcapsular bilateral cataracts occurred in 10% and unilateral in 6.3% of male rats treated with gemfibrozil at 10 times the human dose.

➤*Renal function impairment:* There have been reports of worsening renal insufficiency upon the addition of gemfibrozil therapy in individuals with baseline plasma creatinine greater than 2 mg/dL. In such patients, the use of alternative therapy should be considered against the risks and benefits of a lower dose of gemfibrozil.

➤*Hepatic function impairment:* Abnormal liver function tests have been observed occasionally during gemfibrozil administration, including elevations of AST, ALT, LDH, bilirubin, and alkaline phosphatase. These are usually reversible when gemfibrozil is discontinued. Therefore, periodic liver function studies are recommended and gemfibrozil therapy should be terminated if abnormalities persist.

➤*Pregnancy: Category C.* Gemfibrozil has been shown to produce adverse effects in rats and rabbits at doses between 0.5 and 3 times the human dose (based on surface area). There are no adequate and well-controlled studies in pregnant women. Gemfibrozil should be used during pregnancy only if the potential benefit justifies the potential risk to the fetus. Administration of gemfibrozil to female rats at 2 times the human dose (based on surface area) before and throughout gestation caused a dose-related decrease in conception rate and, at the high dose, an increase in stillborns and a slight reduction in pup weight during lactation. There were also dose-related increased skeletal variations. Anophthalmia occurred, but rarely.

Administration of 0.6 and 2 times the human dose (based on surface area) of gemfibrozil to female rats from gestation day 15 through weaning caused dose-related decreases in birth weight and suppressions of pup growth during lactation.

Administration of 1 and 3 times the human dose (based on surface area) of gemfibrozil to female rabbits during organogenesis caused a dose-related decrease in litter size and, at the high dose, an increased incidence of parietal bone variations.

➤*Lactation:* It is not known whether this drug is excreted in human milk. Because many drugs are excreted in human milk and because of the potential for tumorigenicity shown for gemfibrozil in animal studies, a decision should be made whether to discontinue nursing or to discontinue the drug, taking into account the importance of the drug to the mother.

➤*Children:* Safety and efficacy in children have not been established.

➤*Lab test abnormalities:* Mild hemoglobin, hematocrit, and white blood cell decreases have been observed in occasional patients following initiation of gemfibrozil therapy. However, these levels stabilize during long-term administration. Rarely, severe anemia, leukopenia, thrombocytopenia, and bone marrow hypoplasia have been reported. Therefore, periodic blood counts are recommended during the first 12 months of gemfibrozil administration.

➤*Monitoring:*

Initial therapy – Laboratory studies should be done to ascertain that the lipid levels are consistently abnormal. Before instituting gemfibrozil therapy, every attempt should be made to control serum lipids with appropriate diet, exercise, weight loss in obese patients, and control of any medical problems such as diabetes mellitus and hypothyroidism that are contributing to the lipid abnormalities.

Continued therapy – Periodic determination of serum lipids should be obtained, and the drug withdrawn if lipid response is inadequate after 3 months of therapy.

Hepatic function – Abnormal liver function tests have been observed occasionally during gemfibrozil administration, including elevations of AST, ALT, LDH, bilirubin, and alkaline phosphatase. These are usually reversible when gemfibrozil is discontinued. Periodic liver function studies are recommended and gemfibrozil therapy should be terminated if abnormalities persist.

Drug Interactions

Gemfibrozil Drug Interactions

Precipitant drug	Object drug[a]		Description
Colestipol	Gemfibrozil	⬇	The gemfibrozil pharmacologic effect may be decreased. Separate the administration times by at least 2 hours.
Gemfibrozil	Anticoagulants (eg, warfarin)	⬆	Gemfibrozil may enhance the pharmacologic effects of these agents. If this combination cannot be avoided, observe for signs of bleeding and monitor prothrombin time. Adjust the anticoagulant dose as needed.
Gemfibrozil	Bexarotene	⬆	Bexarotene plasma concentrations may be elevated, increasing the pharmacologic effects and risk of adverse reactions. Monitor the clinical response and for adverse reactions. Adjust the bexarotene dose as needed.

GEMFIBROZIL — ORAL

Gemfibrozil Drug Interactions			
Precipitant drug	Object drug[a]		Description
Gemfibrozil	Cyclosporine	⬇	The pharmacologic effect of cyclosporine may be decreased. Monitor whole blood cyclosporine concentrations. Adjust the dose of cyclosporine as indicated and observe the patient for signs of toxicity or rejection when gemfibrozil therapy is stopped or started.
Gemfibrozil	HMG-CoA reductase inhibitors (eg, lovastatin)	⬆	Rhabdomyolysis has been associated with the administration of HMG-CoA reductase inhibitors and gemfibrozil. If combined use cannot be avoided, frequently monitor for symptoms and signs of rhabdomyolysis and myopathy. If myositis is suspected or diagnosed, discontinue gemfibrozil treatment.
Gemfibrozil	Loperamide	⬆	Loperamide plasma concentrations may be elevated, increasing the risk of adverse reactions (eg, respiratory depression). Monitor for loperamide adverse reactions and adjust treatment as needed.
Gemfibrozil	Montelukast	⬆	The montelukast plasma concentrations may be elevated, increasing the pharmacologic effects and risk of adverse reactions. Monitor the clinical response when gemfibrozil is started or stopped. Adjust the montelukast dose as needed.
Gemfibrozil	Repaglinide	⬆	The repaglinide plasma concentrations may be greatly increased and prolonged, increasing the risk of severe and protracted hypoglycemia. Coadministration is contraindicated.
Gemfibrozil	Sulfonylureas (eg, glyburide)	⬆	Increased hypoglycemic effects may occur. Monitor blood glucose levels when gemfibrozil is started or stopped. Adjust the sulfonylurea dose accordingly.
Gemfibrozil	Thiazolidinediones (eg, pioglitazone)	⬆	The risk of hypoglycemia and other adverse reactions (eg, peripheral edema) may be increased. Monitor blood glucose concentrations and for adverse reactions when gemfibrozil is started or stopped. Adjust the thiazolidinedione dose accordingly.
Gemfibrozil	Tiagabine	⬆	The tiagabine plasma concentrations may be elevated, increasing the pharmacologic effects and risk of toxicity (eg, confusion, lightheadedness). Monitor the clinical response and adjust the tiagabine dose as needed.

[a] ⬆ = object drug increased; ⬇ = object drug decreased.

Adverse Reactions

In the double-blind, controlled phase of the primary prevention component of the Helsinki Heart Study, 2046 patients received gemfibrozil for up to 5 years. In that study, the following adverse reactions were statistically more frequent in subjects in the gemfibrozil group:

Gemfibrozil Adverse Reactions		
Adverse reaction	Gemfibrozil (n = 2046)	Placebo (n = 2035)
GI reactions	34.2%	23.8%
Dyspepsia	19.6%	11.9%
Abdominal pain	9.8%	5.6%
Acute appendicitis (histologically confirmed in most cases)	1.2%	0.6%
Atrial fibrillation	0.7%	0.1%
Adverse reactions reported by > 1% of subjects, but without a significant difference between groups		
Diarrhea	7.2%	6.5%
Fatigue	3.8%	3.5%
Nausea/vomiting	2.5%	2.1%
Eczema	1.9%	1.2%
Rash	1.7%	1.3%
Vertigo	1.5%	1.3%
Constipation	1.4%	1.3%
Headache	1.2%	1.1%

➤*Gallbladder surgery:* Gallbladder surgery was performed in 0.9% of gemfibrozil and 0.5% of placebo subjects in the primary prevention component, a 64% excess, which is not statistically different from the excess of gallbladder surgery observed in the clofibrate compared to the placebo group of the WHO study. Gallbladder surgery was also performed more frequently in the gemfibrozil group compared to placebo (1.9% vs 0.3%, $P = 0.07$) in the secondary prevention component. A statistically significant increase in appendectomy in the gemfibrozil group was seen also in the secondary prevention component (6 on gemfibrozil vs 0 on placebo, $P = 0.014$).

Nervous system and special senses adverse reactions were more common in the gemfibrozil group. These included hypesthesia, paresthesias, and taste perversion. Other adverse reactions that were more common among gemfibrozil treatment group subjects but where a causal relationship was not established include cataracts, peripheral vascular disease, and intracerebral hemorrhage.

From other studies it seems probable that gemfibrozil is causally related to the occurrence of musculoskeletal symptoms, and to abnormal liver function tests and hematologic changes.

Reports of viral and bacterial infections (eg, common cold, cough, urinary tract infections) were more common in gemfibrozil treated patients in other controlled clinical trials of 805 patients. Additional adverse reactions that have been reported for gemfibrozil are listed below by system. These are categorized according to whether a causal relationship to treatment with gemfibrozil is probable or not established.

➤*Adverse events in which a causal relationship to treatment with gemfibrozil is probable:*

CNS – Dizziness; somnolence; paresthesia; peripheral neuritis; decreased libido; depression; headache.

Dermatologic – Exfoliative dermatitis; rash; dermatitis; pruritus.

GI – Cholestatic jaundice.

GU – Impotence.

Hematologic – Anemia; leukopenia; bone marrow hypoplasia; eosinophilia.

Hypersensitivity – Angioedema; laryngeal edema; urticaria.

Lab test abnormalities – Increased creatine phosphokinase; increased bilirubin; increased liver transaminases (AST, ALT); increased alkaline phosphatase.

Musculoskeletal – Myopathy; myasthenia; myalgia; painful extremities; arthralgia; synovitis; rhabdomyolysis (see Warnings).

Ophthalmic – Blurred vision.

➤*Adverse events in which a causal relationship to treatment with gemfibrozil has not been established:*

Cardiovascular – Extrasystoles.

CNS – Confusion; convulsions; syncope.

Dermatologic – Alopecia; photosensitivity.

GI – Pancreatitis; hepatoma; colitis.

GU – Decreased male fertility; renal dysfunction.

Hematologic – Thrombocytopenia.

Hypersensitivity – Anaphylaxis; Lupus-like syndrome; vasculitis.

Lab test abnormalities – Positive antinuclear antibody.

Ophthalmic – Retinal edema.

Miscellaneous – Weight loss.

Overdosage

➤*Symptoms:* There have been reported cases of overdosage with gemfibrozil. In one case, a 7-year-old child recovered after ingesting up to 9 g of gemfibrozil. Symptoms reported with overdosage were abdominal cramps, abnormal liver function tests, diarrhea, increased CPK, joint and muscle pain, nausea and vomiting.

➤*Treatment:* Symptomatic supportive measures should be taken if an overdose occurs.

FENOFIBRATE

Rx	**Fibricor** (Mutual Pharmaceutical)	**Tablets; oral:** 35 mg	(AR 787). White, round. In 30s, 60s, 90s, 100s, 250s, 500s, and 1,000s.
Rx	**Fenoglide** (Shore Therapeutics)	**Tablets; oral:** 40 mg	Lactose, PEG. (FLO). White to off-white, oval. In 90s.
Rx	**Tricor** (Abbott)	**Tablets; oral:** 48 mg	Lactose, sucrose. (FI). Yellow. In 90s.
Rx	**Triglide** (Sciele Pharma)	**Tablets; oral:** 50 mg	Lactose. (FH 50). Off-white. In 90s.
Rx	**Fenofibrate** (Various, eg, Ranbaxy, Teva)	**Tablets; oral:** 54 mg	In 10s, 90s, 500s, and 1,000s.
Rx	**Lofibra** (Gate)		Lactose. (93 7330). Yellow. Film coated. In 90s.
Rx	**Fibricor** (Mutual Pharmaceutical)	**Tablets; oral:** 105 mg	(AR 788). White, oval. In 30s, 60s, 90s, 100s, 250s, 500s, and 1,000s.
Rx	**Fenofibrate** (Various, eg, Par Pharm, Ranbaxy)	**Tablets; oral:** 107 mg	In 10s, 90s, and 1,000s.
Rx	**Fenoglide** (Shore Therapeutics)	**Tablets; oral:** 120 mg	Lactose, PEG. (FHI). White to off-white, oval. In 90s.
Rx	**Tricor** (Abbott)	**Tablets; oral:** 145 mg	Lactose, sucrose. (FO). White. In 90s.
Rx	**Fenofibrate** (Global Pharmaceutical)	**Tablets; oral:** 160 mg	Polydextrose. (G 352). White, film-coated, capsule shaped. In 90s, 100s, 500s, and 1,000s.
Rx	**Lofibra** (Gate)		Lactose. (93 7331). White to off-white, oval. Film coated. In 90s.
Rx	**Triglide** (Sciele Pharma)		Lactose. (FH 160). Off-white. In 90s.
Rx	**Antara** (Reliant)	**Capsules; oral:** 43 mg (micronized fenofibrate)	Sugar spheres. (43 ANTARA). Lt. green/white to off-white. In 30s and 100s.
Rx	**Lipofen** (Kowa Pharm)	**Capsules; oral:** 50 mg	(50 G 246). In 90s.
Rx	**Fenofibrate** (Various, eg, Global Pharm)	**Capsules; oral:** 67 mg (micronized fenofibrate)	In 100s.
Rx	**Lofibra** (Gate)		Lactose. (Lofibra 67 mg Gate 322). Opaque pink. In 100s.
Rx	**Antara** (Reliant)	**Capsules; oral:** 130 mg (micronized fenofibrate)	Sugar spheres. (130 ANTARA). Dk. green/white. In 30s and 100s.
Rx	**Fenofibrate** (Various, eg, Global Pharm)	**Capsules; oral:** 134 mg (micronized fenofibrate)	In 100s.
Rx	**Lofibra** (Gate)		Lactose. (Lofibra 134 mg Gate 323). Opaque lt. blue. In 100s.
Rx	**Lipofen** (Kowa Pharm)	**Capsules; oral:** 150 mg	(150 G 248). In 90s.
Rx	**Fenofibrate** (Various, eg, Global Pharm)	**Capsules; oral:** 200 mg (micronized fenofibrate)	In 100s.
Rx	**Lofibra** (Gate)		Lactose. (Lofibra 200 mg Gate 324). Opaque orange. In 100s.
Rx	**Trilipix** (Abbott Laboratories)	**Capsules, delayed-release; oral:** 45 mg	As fenofibric acid. (A 45). Reddish brown/yellow. In 90s.
		135 mg	As fenofibric acid. (A 135). Blue/yellow. In 90s.

FENOFIBRATE — ORAL

Refer to the general discussion of these agents in the Antihyperlipidemic Agents introduction.

Indications

➤*Hypercholesterolemia:* Adjunctive therapy to diet for the reduction of low-density lipoprotein-cholesterol (LDL-C), total cholesterol (total-C), triglycerides, and apolipoprotein B (apo B), and to increase high-density lipoprotein-cholesterol (HDL-C) in adult patients with primary hypercholesterolemia or mixed dyslipidemia (Fredrickson types IIa and IIb). Use lipid-altering agents in addition to a diet restricted in saturated fat and cholesterol when response to diet and nonpharmacological interventions alone has been inadequate.

➤*Hypertriglyceridemia:* Adjunctive therapy to diet for treatment of adult patients with hypertriglyceridemia (Fredrickson types IV and V hyperlipidemia).

Improving glycemic control in diabetic patients showing fasting chylomicronemia will usually reduce fasting triglycerides and eliminate chylomicronemia, thereby obviating the need for pharmacologic intervention.

➤*Combination therapy with statins for mixed dyslipidemia (fenofibric acid):* As an adjunct to diet in combination with a statin to reduce triglycerides and increase HDL-C in patients with mixed dyslipidemia and coronary heart disease (CHD) or a CHD risk equivalent who are on optimal statin therapy to achieve their LDL-C goal.

CHD risk equivalents comprise:

- other clinical forms of atherosclerotic disease (eg, abdominal aortic aneurysm, peripheral arterial disease, symptomatic carotid artery disease),
- diabetes,
- multiple risk factors that confer a 10-year risk for CHD greater than 20%.

No incremental benefit of fenofibric acid on cardiovascular morbidity and mortality over and above that demonstrated for statin monotherapy has been established. Fenofibrate at a dose equivalent to fenofibric acid 135 mg was not shown to reduce CHD morbidity and mortality in a large, randomized controlled trial of patients with type 2 diabetes mellitus.

➤*Off-label uses:*

Hyperuricemia – [2] = Fair documentation. Data from some studies suggest that fenofibrate reduces uric acid levels in patients with gout and hyperuricemia in other disease states. This drug may be useful as adjunctive therapy in patients who continue to have acute gout attacks during allopurinal therapy. (See Administration and Dosage.)

Other possible off-label uses –

Hypertriglyceridemia associated with HIV lipodystrophy: Treatment of hypertriglyceridemia associated with HIV lipodystrophy.

Administration and Dosage

➤*General dosing considerations:* Patients should be placed on an appropriate lipid-lowering diet before receiving fenofibrate and should continue on this diet during treatment.

➤*Adults:*

Fenofibrate dosing recommendations –

Fenofibrate Dosing Recommendations

Dosing regimen	*Antara*	*Lipofen*[a]	*Lofibra* tablets[a]	*Lofibra* capsules[a]	*Tricor*	*Triglide*
Hypertriglyceridemia						
Maximum dosage	130 mg/day	150 mg/day	160 mg/day	200 mg/day	145 mg/day	160 mg/day
Initial dosage	43 to 130 mg/day	50 to 150 mg/day	54 to 160 mg/day	67 to 200 mg/day	48 to 145 mg/day	50 to 160 mg/day
Mixed hyperlipidemia, initial dosage	130 mg/day	150 mg/day	160 mg/day	200 mg/day	145 mg/day	160 mg/day
Primary hypercholesterolemia, initial dosage	130 mg/day	150 mg/day	160 mg/day	200 mg/day	145 mg/day	160 mg/day

[a] Taken with meals.

FENOFIBRATE — ORAL

Dosage adjustment: Individualize dosage according to patient response and adjust if necessary following repeat lipid determinations at 4- to 8-week intervals. Monitor lipid levels periodically and consider reducing the dose of fenofibrate if lipid levels fall significantly below the targeted range.

Discontinuation of therapy: Withdraw therapy in patients who do not have an adequate response after 2 months of treatment with the maximum recommended dose.

Off-label dosing –

Hyperuricemia: [2] = Fair documentation. 200 mg/day (micronized formulation) for up to 12 months. Other regimens have included 100 mg 3 times/day for 6 weeks.

➤*Elderly:* Fenofibric acid is known to be substantially excreted by the kidney, and the risk of adverse reactions to this drug may be greater in patients with renal function impairment. Because elderly patients are more likely to have decreased renal function, take care in dose selection.

Fenofibrate Initial Dosing Recommendations for Elderly Patients					
Antara	Lipofen[a]	Lofibra tablets[a]	Lofibra capsules[a]	Tricor	Triglide
43 mg/day	50 mg/day	54 mg/day	67 mg/day	48 mg/day	50 mg/day

[a] Taken with meals.

➤*Renal function impairment:* See the dosing table. Increase dosage only after evaluation of the effects on renal function and lipid levels. Minimize the dosage of fenofibrate in patients with severe renal function impairment; no modification of dosage is required in patients with moderate renal function impairment.

Fenofibrate Initial Dosing Recommendations for Renal Function Impairment					
Antara	Lipofen[a]	Lofibra tablets[a]	Lofibra capsules[a]	Tricor	Triglide
43 mg/day	50 mg/day	54 mg/day	67 mg/day	48 mg/day	50 mg/day

[a] Taken with meals.

➤*Hepatic function impairment:* No pharmacokinetic studies have been conducted in patients with hepatic function impairment.

➤*Monitoring:* Obtain periodic determination of serum lipids during initial therapy in order to establish the lowest effective dose of fenofibrate. Withdraw therapy in patients who do not have an adequate response after 2 months of treatment with the maximum recommended dose. Perform liver function tests regularly, including serum ALT, for the duration of therapy with fenofibrate; discontinue therapy if enzyme levels persist above 3 times the normal limit. Periodic blood cell counts also are recommended during the first 12 months of fenofibrate administration.

➤*Administration:* Give *Lofibra* capsules and tablets and *Lipofen* capsules with meals to optimize the bioavailability of the medication. The other fenofibrate formulations (*Antara, Tricor, Triglide*) can be given without regard to meals.

➤*Storage/Stability:* Store at 20° to 25°C (68° to 77°F); excursions are permitted to 15° to 30°C (59° to 86°F). Dispense in a tightly closed container. Keep out of the reach of children. Protect from moisture and light.

Actions

➤*Pharmacology:* Fenofibric acid, the active metabolite of fenofibrate, produces reductions in total-C, LDL-C, apo B, total triglycerides, and triglyceride-rich lipoprotein in treated patients. In addition, treatment with fenofibrate results in increases in HDL and apoproteins apo AI and apo AII.

Through the activation of the peroxisome proliferator–activated receptor alpha (PPARα), fenofibrate increases lipolysis and elimination of triglyceride-rich particles from plasma by activating lipoprotein lipase and reducing production of apoprotein C III (an inhibitor of lipoprotein lipase activity). The resulting fall in triglycerides produces an alteration in the size and composition of LDL from small, dense particles (which are thought to be atherogenic because of their susceptibility to oxidation) to large, buoyant particles. These larger particles have a greater affinity for cholesterol receptors and are catabolized rapidly.

Activation of PPARα also induces an increase in the synthesis of apo, AI, AII, and HDL-C.

Fenofibrate also reduces serum uric acid levels in hyperuricemic and healthy individuals by increasing the urinary excretion of uric acid.

➤*Pharmacokinetics:*

Absorption/Distribution – Fenofibrate is well absorbed from the GI tract. The 2 different formulations of fenofibrate, micronized and nonmicronized, demonstrate bioequivalence.

Plasma concentrations of fenofibric acid after administration of 3 *Tricor* 48 mg tablets or one *Tricor* 145 mg tablet are equivalent under fed conditions to one 200 mg micronized capsule.

Peak plasma levels of fenofibric acid occur within 3 to 8 hours (depending on product) after administration, and steady-state plasma levels are achieved within 5 to 7 days of dosing. Accumulation following multiple doses does not occur. Serum protein binding is approximately 99%.

Plasma concentrations of fenofibric acid after administration of *Lofibra* 54 mg and 160 mg tablets are equivalent under fed conditions to 67 mg and 200 mg micronized capsules, respectively.

Food effect:

• *Fenofibrate tablets* – The extent of absorption is comparable (*Tricor, Triglide*) or increased by approximately 35% (*Lofibra*) under fed as compared with fasting conditions. Food increases the rate of absorption by approximately 55% (*Triglide*).

Micronized fenofibrate capsules: The absorption of micronized fenofibrate is increased by 26% to 35% (depending on product) under fed as compared with fasted conditions.

Metabolism – Fenofibrate is rapidly hydrolyzed by esterases to the active metabolite, fenofibric acid; no unchanged fenofibrate is detected in plasma. Fenofibric acid is primarily conjugated with glucuronic acid and then excreted in urine. A small amount of fenofibric acid is reduced at the carbonyl moiety to a benzhydrol metabolite, which is, in turn, conjugated with glucuronic acid and excreted in urine.

In vivo metabolism data indicate that neither fenofibrate nor fenofibric acid undergo oxidative metabolism (eg, CYP-450) to a significant extent.

Excretion – Fenofibrate is eliminated with a half-life of 16 to 23 hours, allowing once-daily administration. It is mainly excreted in urine in the form of metabolites, primarily fenofibric acid and fenofibric acid glucuronide; about 60% of the dose appears in urine and 25% in feces.

Special populations –

Renal function impairment: In a study in patients with severe renal function impairment (creatinine clearance [Ccr] less than 50 mL/min), the rate of clearance of fenofibric acid was greatly reduced, and the compound accumulated during chronic dosage. However, in patients with moderate renal function impairment (Ccr of 50 to 90 mL/min), the oral clearance and the oral volume of distribution of fenofibric acid are increased compared with healthy adults (2.1 L/h and 95 L versus 1.1 L/h and 30 L, respectively). Therefore, minimize the dosage of fenofibrate in patients with severe renal function impairment; no modification of dosage is required in patients with moderate renal function impairment.

Contraindications

Hepatic dysfunction, including primary biliary cirrhosis, and unexplained, persistent liver function abnormality; severe renal dysfunction; preexisting gallbladder disease; hypersensitivity to fenofibrate.

Warnings/Precautions

➤*Cholelithiasis:* Fenofibrate, like clofibrate and gemfibrozil, may increase cholesterol excretion into the bile, leading to cholelithiasis. If cholelithiasis is suspected, gallbladder studies are indicated. Discontinue fenofibrate therapy if gallstones are found.

➤*Hepatic effects:* Fenofibrate is associated with increases in serum transaminase (AST or ALT). Increases to more than 3 times the upper limit of normal (ULN) occurred in 5.3% of patients taking fenofibrate versus 1.1% of patients treated with placebo.

See Warnings/Precautions for more information.

➤*Hematologic changes:* Mild to moderate hemoglobin, hematocrit, and white blood cell decreases have been observed in patients following initiation of fenofibrate therapy. However, these levels stabilize during long-term administration. Extremely rare spontaneous reports of thrombocytopenia and agranulocytosis have been received during postmarketing surveillance outside of the United States. Periodic blood counts are recommended during the first 12 months of fenofibrate administration.

➤*Initial therapy:* Ascertain that lipid levels are consistently abnormal before instituting fenofibrate therapy. Make every attempt to control serum lipids with appropriate diet, exercise, weight loss in obese patients, and control of any medical problems (eg, diabetes mellitus, hypothyroidism) that are contributing to the lipid abnormalities. If possible, discontinue or change medications known to exacerbate hypertriglyceridemia (eg, beta-blockers, thiazides, estrogens) prior to consideration of triglyceride-lowering drug therapy.

➤*Pancreatitis:* Pancreatitis has been reported in patients taking fenofibrate, gemfibrozil, and clofibrate. This occurrence may represent a failure of efficacy in patients with severe hypertriglyceridemia, a direct drug effect, or a secondary phenomenon mediated through biliary tract stone or sludge formation with obstruction of the common bile duct.

➤*Skeletal muscle effects:* The use of fibrates alone, including fenofibrate, may occasionally be associated with myopathy. Treatment with drugs of the fibrate class has been associated on rare occasions with rhabdomyolysis, usually in patients with renal function impairment. Consider myopathy in any patient with diffuse myalgias, muscle tenderness or weakness, and/or marked elevations of creatine phosphokinase (CPK) levels.

Assess CPK levels in patients reporting muscle pain, tenderness, or weakness, and discontinue therapy if markedly elevated CPK levels occur or myopathy is diagnosed.

➤*Hypersensitivity reactions:* Acute hypersensitivity reactions, including severe skin rashes requiring patient hospitalization and treatment with steroids, have occurred very rarely during treatment with fenofibrate, including rare spontaneous reports of Stevens-Johnson syndrome and toxic epidermal necrolysis. Urticaria was seen in 1.1% versus 0% and rash in 1.4% versus 0.8% of fenofibrate and placebo patients, respectively, in controlled trials.

➤*Renal function impairment:* In patients with Ccr less than 50 mL/min, the rate of clearance of fenofibric acid was greatly reduced, and it accumulated during chronic dosage. In patients with Ccr 50 to 90 mL/min, the oral clearance and the oral volume of distribution of fenofibric acid are increased, compared with healthy adults (2.1 L/h and 95 L versus 1.1 L/h and 30 L, respectively). Therefore, minimize the dosage in patients who have Ccr less than 50 mL/min.

FENOFIBRATE — ORAL

➤*Pregnancy: Category C.* Fenofibrate is embryocidal and teratogenic in rats when given in doses 7 to 10 times the MRHD and embryocidal in rabbits when given at 9 times the MRHD. There are no adequate and well-controlled studies in pregnant women. Use during pregnancy only if the potential benefit justifies the potential risk to the fetus.

Administration of 9 times the MRHD of fenofibrate to female rats before and throughout gestation caused 100% of dams to delay delivery and resulted in a 60% increase in postimplantation loss, a decrease in litter size, a decrease in birth weight, a 40% survival of pups at birth, a 4% survival of pups as neonates, and a 0% survival of pups to weaning, and an increase in spina bifida.

Administration of 10 times the MRHD to female rats on days 6 to 15 of gestation caused an increase in gross, visceral, and skeletal findings in fetuses (domed head/hunched shoulders/rounded body/abnormal chest, kyphosis, stunted fetuses, elongated sternal ribs, malformed sternebrae, extra foramen in palatine, misshapen vertebrae, supernumerary ribs).

Administration of 7 times the MRHD to female rats from day 15 of gestation through weaning caused a delay in delivery, a 40% decrease in live births, a 75% decrease in neonatal survival, and decreases in pup weight at birth, as well as on days 4 and 21 postpartum.

Administration of 9 and 18 times the MRHD to female rabbits caused abortions in 10% of dams at 9 times and 25% of dams at 18 times the MRHD, and death in 7% of fetuses at 18 times the MRHD.

➤*Lactation:* Do not use fenofibrate in breast-feeding mothers. Because of the potential for tumorigenicity seen in animal studies, decide whether to discontinue breast-feeding or the drug.

➤*Children:* Safety and efficacy in children have not been established.

➤*Elderly:* Fenofibric acid is known to be substantially excreted by the kidney, and the risk of adverse reactions to this drug may be greater in patients with renal function impairment. Because elderly patients are more likely to have decreased renal function, take care in dose selection.

➤*Monitoring:* Obtain periodic determination of serum lipids during initial therapy in order to establish the lowest effective dose of fenofibrate. Withdraw therapy in patients who do not have an adequate response after 2 months of treatment with the maximum recommended dose. Perform liver function tests regularly, including serum ALT, for the duration of therapy with fenofibrate; discontinue therapy if enzyme levels persist above 3 times the normal limit. Periodic blood cell counts also are recommended during the first 12 months of fenofibrate administration.

Drug Interactions

Fenofibrate Drug Interactions

Precipitant drug	Object drug[a]		Description
Bile acid sequestrants	Fenofibrate	⬇	Because bile acid sequestrants may bind other drugs given concurrently, advise patients to take fenofibrate at least 1 hour before or 4 to 6 hours after a bile acid–binding resin to avoid impeding its absorption.
Fenofibrate	Anticoagulants, oral	⬆	Potentiation of coumarin-type anticoagulants has been observed with prolongation of the prothrombin time (PT)/international normalized ratio (INR). Frequent PT/INR determinations and anticoagulant dosage reduction are advisable.
Fenofibrate	Cyclosporine	⬆	Coadministration may lead to increased risk of nephrotoxicity. Carefully consider the benefits and risks of using fenofibrate with immunosuppressants and other potentially nephrotoxic agents, and employ the lowest effective dose.
Fenofibrate	HMG-CoA reductase inhibitors	⬆	The combined use of fenofibrate and HMG-CoA reductase inhibitors has been associated with rhabdomyolysis, markedly elevated creatine kinase levels, and myoglobinuria, leading in a high proportion of cases to acute renal failure. Avoid this drug combination unless the benefit of further alterations in lipid levels is likely to outweigh the increased risk of this drug combination.

[a] ⬆ = object drug increased; ⬇ = object drug decreased.

➤*Drug/Food interactions:* Administration of fenofibrate with food has little effect (*Tricor*) or increases absorption by 26% to 35% (*Antara, Lofibra*). Food has no effect on the extent of absorption (*Triglide*) but increases the rate of absorption by approximately 55%.

Adverse Reactions

Adverse reactions led to discontinuation of treatment in 5% of patients treated with fenofibrate and in 3% treated with placebo. Increases in liver function tests were the most frequent events causing discontinuation (1.6%) of fenofibrate treatment.

Adverse reactions reported by 2% or more of patients treated with fenofibrate during the double-blind, placebo-controlled trials, regardless of causality, are listed in the following table.

Fenofibrate Adverse Reactions (%)

Adverse reaction	Fenofibrate[a] (n = 439)	Placebo (n = 365)
GI		
Abdominal pain	4.6%	4.4%
Constipation	2.1%	1.4%
Diarrhea	2.3%	4.1%
Nausea	2.3%	1.9%
Lab test abnormalities		
ALT increased	3%	1.6%
AST increased	3.4%[b]	0.5%
CPK increased	3%	1.4%
Liver function tests abnormal	7.5%[b]	1.4%
Respiratory		
Respiratory disorder	6.2%	5.5%
Rhinitis	2.3%	1.1%
Miscellaneous		
Asthenia	2.1%	3%
Back pain	3.4%	2.5%
Flu syndrome	2.1%	2.7%
Headache	3.2%	2.7%

[a] Dose equivalent to micronized fenofibrate 200 mg.
[b] Significantly different from placebo.

The following are additional adverse reactions reported by at least 3 patients in placebo-controlled trials or reported in other controlled or open trials, regardless of causality.

➤*Cardiovascular:* Abnormal electrocardiogram, angina pectoris, arrhythmia, atrial fibrillation, cardiovascular disorder, coronary artery disorder, extrasystoles, hypertension, hypotension, myocardial infarction, palpitation, peripheral vascular disorder, phlebitis, tachycardia, varicose vein, vascular disorder, vasodilation, ventricular extrasystoles.

➤*CNS:* Anxiety, decreased libido, depression, dizziness, dry mouth, hypertonia, insomnia, migraine, nervousness, neuralgia, paresthesia, somnolence, vertigo.

➤*Dermatologic:* Acne, alopecia, contact dermatitis, eczema, fungal dermatitis, herpes simplex, herpes zoster, maculopapular rash, nail disorder, pruritus, rash, skin disorder, skin ulcer, sweating, urticaria.

➤*GI:* Anorexia, cholecystitis, cholelithiasis, colitis, diarrhea, duodenal ulcer, dyspepsia, eructation, esophagitis, flatulence, gastritis, gastroenteritis, GI disorder, increased appetite, liver fatty deposit, nausea, nausea/vomiting, peptic ulcer, rectal disorder, rectal hemorrhage, tooth disorder, vomiting.

➤*GU:* Abnormal kidney function, cystitis, dysuria, gynecomastia, prostatic disorder, unintended pregnancy, urinary frequency, urolithiasis, vaginal moniliasis.

➤*Hematologic/Lymphatic:* Anemia, ecchymosis, eosinophilia, leukopenia, lymphadenopathy, thrombocytopenia.

➤*Lab test abnormalities:* Creatinine increased, increased gamma glutamyl transpeptidase.

➤*Metabolic/Nutritional:* Edema, gout, hyperuricemia, hypoglycemia, peripheral edema, weight gain, weight loss.

➤*Musculoskeletal:* Arthralgia, arthritis, arthrosis, bursitis, joint disorder, leg cramps, myalgia, myasthenia, myositis, tenosynovitis.

➤*Respiratory:* Allergic pulmonary alveolitis, asthma, bronchitis, dyspnea, increased cough, laryngitis, pharyngitis, pneumonia, sinusitis.

➤*Special senses:* Abnormal vision, amblyopia, cataract specified, conjunctivitis, ear pain, eye disorder, otitis media, refraction disorder.

➤*Miscellaneous:* Accidental injury, allergic reaction, chest pain, cyst, diabetes mellitus, fever, hernia, infection, malaise, pain (unspecified), photosensitivity reaction.

Overdosage

➤*Treatment:* If indicated, use gastric lavage to achieve elimination of unabsorbed drug; observe usual precautions to maintain the airway. Because fenofibrate is highly bound to plasma proteins, do not consider hemodialysis.

Patient Information

Advise patients to promptly report unexplained muscle pain, tenderness, or weakness, particularly if accompanied by malaise or fever.

NIACIN (Nicotinic acid)

For complete prescribing information, refer to the Niacin monograph in the Nutrients and Nutritional Agents chapter.

EZETIMIBE

Rx	**Zetia** (Merck/Schering-Plough)	**Tablets:** 10 mg	Lactose. (414). Capsule shape. In 30s, 90s, 500s, and UD 100s.

EZETIMIBE — ORAL

Indications

➤*Homozygous familial hypercholesterolemia:* In combination with atorvastatin or simvastatin for the reduction of elevated total-C and LDL-C levels in patients with homozygous familial hypercholesterolemia as an adjunct to other lipid-lowering treatments (eg, LDL apheresis) or if such treatments are unavailable.

➤*Homozygous sitosterolemia:* As adjunctive therapy to diet for the reduction of elevated sitosterol and campesterol levels in patients with homozygous familial sitosterolemia.

➤*Mixed hyperlipidemia:*

Combination therapy with fenofibrate – In combination with fenofibrate as adjunctive therapy to diet for the reduction of total-C, LDL-C, apo B, and non–high-density lipoprotein cholesterol (non–HDL-C) in patients with mixed hyperlipidemia.

➤*Primary hypercholesterolemia:*

Combination therapy with beta-hydroxy-beta-methylglutaryl-CoA (HMG-CoA) reductase inhibitors – In combination with an HMG-CoA reductase inhibitor as adjunctive therapy to diet for the reduction of elevated total-C, LDL-C, and apo B in patients with primary (heterozygous familial and nonfamilial) hypercholesterolemia.

Monotherapy – As adjunctive therapy to diet for the reduction of elevated total cholesterol (total-C), low-density lipoprotein cholesterol (LDL-C), and apolipoprotein B (apo B) in patients with primary (heterozygous familial and nonfamilial) hypercholesterolemia.

Administration and Dosage

➤*General dosing considerations:* The patient should be placed on a standard cholesterol-lowering diet before receiving ezetimibe and should continue on this diet during treatment with ezetimibe.

➤*Adults:*

Usual dosage – 10 mg once daily with or without food.

➤*Children:*

10 years of age and older – See Adults for dosing.

➤*Hepatic function impairment:* Because of the unknown effects of the increased exposure to ezetimibe in patients with moderate or severe hepatic function impairment, ezetimibe is not recommended in these patients.

➤*Administration:*

Coadministration with bile acid sequestrants – Dosing of ezetimibe should occur at least 2 hours before or at least 4 hours after administration of a bile acid sequestrant.

➤*Storage/Stability:* Store at 25°C (77°F); excursions are permitted to 15° to 30°C (59° to 86°F). Protect from moisture.

Actions

➤*Pharmacology:* Ezetimibe reduces total-C, LDL-C, apo B, and triglycerides, and increases HDL-C in patients with hypercholesterolemia. Administration of ezetimibe with an HMG-CoA reductase inhibitor is effective in improving serum total-C, LDL-C, apo B, triglycerides, and HDL-C beyond either treatment alone. Administration of ezetimibe with fenofibrate is effective in improving serum total-C, LDL-C, apo B, and non–HDL-C in patients with mixed hyperlipemia as compared with either treatment alone. The effects of ezetimibe given either alone or in addition to an HMG-CoA reductase inhibitor on cardiovascular morbidity and mortality have not been established.

Ezetimibe has a mechanism of action that differs from those of other classes of cholesterol-reducing compounds (HMG-CoA reductase inhibitors, bile acid sequestrants [resin], fibric acid derivatives, and plant stanols).

Ezetimibe does not inhibit cholesterol synthesis in the liver, or increase bile acid excretion. Instead, ezetimibe localizes and appears to act at the brush border of the small intestine and inhibits the absorption of cholesterol, leading to a decrease in the delivery of intestinal cholesterol to the liver. This causes a reduction of hepatic cholesterol stores and an increase in clearance of cholesterol from the blood; this distinct mechanism is complementary to that of HMG-CoA reductase inhibitors and of fenofibrate.

➤*Pharmacokinetics:*

Absorption – After oral administration, ezetimibe is absorbed and extensively conjugated to a pharmacologically active phenolic glucuronide (ezetimibe-glucuronide). After a single dose of ezetimibe 10 mg to fasted adults, mean ezetimibe peak plasma concentrations (C_{max}) of 3.4 to 5.5 ng/mL were attained within 4 to 12 hours time to peak plasma concentration ($_{max}$]). Ezetimibe-glucuronide mean C_{max} values of 45 to 71 ng/mL were achieved between 1 and 2 hours (T_{max}). There was no substantial deviation from dose proportionality between 5 and 20 mg. The absolute bioavailability of ezetimibe cannot be determined because the compound is virtually insoluble in aqueous media suitable for injection. Ezetimibe has variable bioavailability; the coefficient of variation, based on intersubject variability, was 35% to 60% for area under the curve (AUC) values.

Food effects: Coadministration with food (high- or non-fat meals) had no effect on the extent of absorption of ezetimibe when administered as ezetimibe 10 mg tablets. The C_{max} value of ezetimibe was increased 38% with consumption of high-fat meals. Ezetimibe can be administered with or without food.

Distribution – Ezetimibe and ezetimibe-glucuronide are highly bound (greater than 90%) to human plasma proteins.

Metabolism/Excretion – Ezetimibe is primarily metabolized in the small intestine and liver via glucuronide conjugation (a phase 2 reaction) with subsequent biliary and renal excretion. Minimal oxidative metabolism (a phase 1 reaction) has been observed in all species evaluated.

In humans, ezetimibe is rapidly metabolized to ezetimibe-glucuronide. Ezetimibe and ezetimibe-glucuronide are the major drug-derived compounds detected in plasma, constituting approximately 10% to 20% and 80% to 90% of the total drug in plasma, respectively. Both ezetimibe and ezetimibe-glucuronide are slowly eliminated from plasma with a half-life of approximately 22 hours for both ezetimibe and ezetimibe-glucuronide. Plasma concentration-time profiles exhibit multiple peaks, suggesting enterohepatic recycling.

Following oral administration of ^{14}C-ezetimibe (20 mg) to human subjects, total ezetimibe (ezetimibe + ezetimibe-glucuronide) accounted for approximately 93% of the total radioactivity in plasma. After 48 hours, there were no detectable levels of radioactivity in the plasma.

Approximately 78% and 11% of the administered radioactivity were recovered in the feces and urine, respectively, over a 10-day collection period. Ezetimibe was the major component in feces and accounted for 69% of the administered dose, while ezetimibe-glucuronide was the major component in urine and accounted for 9% of the administered dose.

Special populations –

Renal function impairment: After a single 10 mg dose of ezetimibe in patients with severe renal disease (n = 8; mean creatinine clearance [Ccr] less than or equal to 30 mL/min/1.73 m^2), the mean AUC values for total ezetimibe, ezetimibe-glucuronide, and ezetimibe were increased approximately 1.5-fold, compared with healthy subjects (n = 9).

Hepatic function impairment: After a single dose of ezetimibe 10 mg, the AUC for total ezetimibe was increased approximately 1.7-fold in patients with mild hepatic function impairment (Child-Pugh score 5 to 6), compared with healthy subjects. The mean AUC values for total ezetimibe and ezetimibe were increased approximately 3- to 4-fold and 5- to 6-fold, respectively, in patients with moderate (Child-Pugh score 7 to 9) or severe hepatic impairment (Child-Pugh score 10 to 15). In a 14-day, multiple-dose study (10 mg daily) in patients with moderate hepatic function impairment, the mean AUC values for total ezetimibe and ezetimibe were increased approximately 4-fold on day 1 and 14 compared with healthy subjects. Because of the unknown effects of the increased exposure to ezetimibe in patients with moderate or severe hepatic function impairment, ezetimibe is not recommended in these patients.

Elderly: In a multiple-dose study with ezetimibe 10 mg given once daily for 10 days, plasma concentrations for total ezetimibe were about 2-fold higher in older (at least 65 years of age) healthy subjects compared with younger subjects.

Gender: In a multiple-dose study with ezetimibe 10 mg given once daily for 10 days, plasma concentrations for total ezetimibe were slightly higher (less than 20%) in women than in men.

Contraindications

Hypersensitivity to any component of this medication.

The combination of ezetimibe with an HMG-CoA reductase inhibitor is contraindicated in patients with active liver disease or unexplained persistent elevations in serum transaminases.

All HMG-CoA reductase inhibitors are contraindicated in pregnant and breast-feeding women. When ezetimibe is administered with an HMG-CoA reductase inhibitor to a woman of childbearing potential, refer to the pregnancy category and product labeling for the HMG-CoA reductase inhibitor.

Warnings/Precautions

➤*Hepatic effects:* In controlled clinical monotherapy studies, the incidence of consecutive elevations (at least 3 times the ULN) in serum transaminases was similar between ezetimibe (0.5%) and placebo (0.3%).

➤*Hyperlipidemia, secondary causes:* Prior to initiating therapy with ezetimibe, exclude or, if appropriate, treat secondary causes for dyslipidemia (ie, diabetes, hypothyroidism, obstructive liver disease, chronic renal failure, drugs that increase LDL-C and decrease HDL-C [progestins, anabolic steroids, and corticosteroids]). Perform a lipid profile to measure total-C, LDL-C, HDL-C, and triglycerides. For triglyceride levels greater than 400 mg/dL (greater than 4.5 mmol/L), determine LDL-C concentrations by ultracentrifugation.

➤*Skeletal muscle:* In clinical trials, there was no excess of myopathy or rhabdomyolysis associated with ezetimibe compared with the relevant control arm (placebo or HMG-CoA reductase inhibitor alone). However, myopathy and rhabdomyolysis are known adverse reactions to HMG-CoA reductase inhibitors and other lipid-lowering drugs. In clinical trials, the

EZETIMIBE — ORAL

incidence of creatine phosphokinase (CPK) greater than 10 times the ULN was 0.2% for ezetimibe versus 0.1% for placebo, and 0.1% for ezetimibe coadministered with an HMG-CoA reductase inhibitor versus 0.4% for HMG-CoA reductase inhibitors alone.

In postmarketing experience with ezetimibe, cases of myopathy and rhabdomyolysis have been reported regardless of causality. Most patients who developed rhabdomyolysis were taking an HMG-CoA reductase inhibitor prior to initiating ezetimibe. However, rhabdomyolysis has been reported very rarely with ezetimibe monotherapy and very rarely with the addition of ezetimibe to agents known to be associated with increased risk of rhabdomyolysis, such as fibrates. Advise all patients starting therapy with ezetimibe of the risk of myopathy and tell them to promptly report any unexplained muscle pain, tenderness, or weakness. Immediately discontinue ezetimibe and any HMG-CoA reductase inhibitor or fibrate that the patient is taking concomitantly if myopathy is diagnosed or suspected. The presence of these symptoms and a CPK level greater than 10 times the ULN indicates myopathy.

➤*Hepatic function impairment:* Because of the unknown effects of the increased exposure to ezetimibe in patients with moderate or severe hepatic function impairment, ezetimibe is not recommended in these patients.

➤*Pregnancy: Category C.* There are no adequate and well-controlled studies of ezetimibe in pregnant women. Use ezetimibe during pregnancy only if the potential benefit justifies the risk to the fetus.

In oral (gavage) embryo-fetal development studies of ezetimibe conducted in rats and rabbits during organogenesis, there was no evidence of embryolethal effects at the dosages tested (250, 500, 1,000 mg/kg/day). In rats, increased incidences of common fetal skeletal findings (extra pair of thoracic ribs, unossified cervical vertebral centra, shortened ribs) were observed at 1,000 mg/kg/day (approximately 10 times the human exposure at 10 mg daily based on $AUC_{0\text{-}24h}$ for total ezetimibe). In rabbits treated with ezetimibe, an increased incidence of extra thoracic ribs was observed at 1,000 mg/kg/day (150 times the human exposure at 10 mg daily based on $AUC_{0\text{-}24h}$ for total ezetimibe). Ezetimibe crossed the placenta when pregnant rats and rabbits were given multiple oral doses.

Multiple-dose studies of ezetimibe given in combination with HMG-CoA reductase inhibitors (statins) in rats and rabbits during organogenesis resulted in higher ezetimibe and statin exposures. Reproductive findings occur at lower doses in combination therapy compared with monotherapy.

All HMG-CoA reductase inhibitors are contraindicated in pregnant and breast-feeding women. When ezetimibe is administered with an HMG-CoA reductase inhibitor to a woman of childbearing potential, refer to the pregnancy category and package labeling for the HMG-CoA reductase inhibitor.

➤*Lactation:* In rat studies, exposure to total ezetimibe in nursing pups was up to half of that observed in maternal plasma. It is not known whether ezetimibe is excreted into human breast milk; therefore, do not use ezetimibe in breast-feeding mothers unless the potential benefit justifies the potential risk to the infant.

➤*Children:* The pharmacokinetics of ezetimibe in adolescents (10 to 18 years of age) have been shown to be similar to those in adults. Treatment experience with ezetimibe in children is limited to 4 patients (9 to 17 years of age) in the sitosterolemia study and 5 patients (11 to 17 years of age) in the homozygous familial hypercholesterolemia study. Treatment with ezetimibe in children (younger than 10 years of age) is not recommended.

➤*Monitoring:* Prior to initiating therapy with ezetimibe, exclude secondary causes for dyslipidemia. Obtain a lipid panel before therapy and periodically thereafter. At the time of hospitalization for an acute coronary event, take lipid measurements on admission or within 24 hours. These values can guide the initiation of LDL-lowering therapy before or at discharge.

When ezetimibe is coadministered with an HMG-CoA reductase inhibitor, perform liver function tests at initiation of therapy and according to the recommendations of the HMG-CoA reductase inhibitor.

Drug Interactions

Ezetimibe Drug Interactions

Precipitant drug	Object drug[a]		Description
Antacids	Ezetimibe	↓	Administration of an aluminum- and magnesium-containing antacid decreased the C_{max} of ezetimibe 30% but had no significant effect on the AUC.
Cholestyramine	Ezetimibe	↓	Coadministration decreased the mean AUC of ezetimibe ≈ 55%. The incremental LDL-C reduction caused by adding ezetimibe to cholestyramine may be reduced.
Cyclosporine	Ezetimibe	↑	Coadministration increased the AUC and C_{max} of total ezetimibe 3.4- and 3.9-fold, respectively, in 8 post–renal transplant patients with healthy to mildly impaired renal function. In another study with healthy patients, ezetimibe increased cyclosporine AUC by 15%. Monitor closely.
Ezetimibe	Cyclosporine		
Fibric acid derivatives Fenofibrate Gemfibrozil	Ezetimibe	↑	Coadministration of ezetimibe with fenofibrate or gemfibrozil increased the total ezetimibe concentration 1.5- and 1.7-fold, respectively. Because fibrates may increase cholesterol excretion into the bile, leading to cholelithiasis, and ezetimibe was shown in animal studies to increase cholesterol in the gallbladder bile, concomitant use is not recommended until use in patients is studied.

[a] ↑ = Object drug increased. ↓ = Object drug decreased.

➤*Drug/Food interactions:* The C_{max} value of ezetimibe was increased 38% with consumption of high-fat meals. Ezetimibe may be administered with or without food.

Adverse Reactions

➤*Monotherapy:* Adverse reactions reported in at least 2% of patients treated with ezetimibe and at an incidence greater than placebo in placebo-controlled studies of ezetimibe, regardless of causality assessment, are shown in the following table.

Ezetimibe Adverse Reactions (≥ 2%)[a]

Adverse reaction	Placebo (n = 795)	Ezetimibe 10 mg (n = 1,691)
GI		
Abdominal pain	2.8%	3%
Diarrhea	3%	3.7%
Musculoskeletal		
Arthralgia	3.4%	3.8%
Back pain	3.9%	4.1%
Respiratory		
Coughing	2.1%	2.3%
Pharyngitis	2.1%	2.3%
Sinusitis	2.8%	3.6%
Miscellaneous		
Fatigue	1.8%	2.2%
Viral infection	1.8%	2.2%

[a] Includes patients who received placebo or ezetimibe alone.

The frequency of less common adverse reactions was comparable between ezetimibe and placebo.

➤*Combination with an HMG-CoA reductase inhibitor:* Ezetimibe has been evaluated for safety in combination studies in more than 2,000 patients.

In general, adverse reactions were similar between ezetimibe administered with HMG-CoA reductase inhibitors and HMG-CoA reductase inhibitors alone. However, the frequency of increased transaminases was slightly higher in patients receiving ezetimibe administered with HMG-CoA reductase inhibitors than in patients treated with HMG-CoA reductase inhibitors alone.

Clinical adverse reactions reported in at least 2% of patients and at an incidence greater than placebo in 4 placebo-controlled trials in which ezetimibe was administered alone or initiated concurrently with various HMG-CoA reductase inhibitors, regardless of causality assessment, are shown in the following table.

Ezetimibe Adverse Reactions (≥ 2%)[a]

Adverse reaction	Placebo (n = 259)	Ezetimibe 10 mg (n = 262)	All statins[b](%) (n = 936)	Ezetimibe + all statins[b] (n = 925)
CNS				
Dizziness	1.2%	2.7%	1.4%	1.8%
Fatigue	1.9%	1.9%	1.4%	2.8%
Headache	5.4%	8%	7.3%	6.3%
GI				
Abdominal pain	2.3%	2.7%	3.1%	3.5%
Diarrhea	1.5%	3.4%	2.9%	2.8%
Musculoskeletal				
Arthralgia	2.3%	3.8%	4.3%	3.4%
Back pain	3.5%	3.4%	3.7%	4.3%

EZETIMIBE — ORAL

Ezetimibe Adverse Reactions (≥ 2%)[a]				
Adverse reaction	Placebo (n = 259)	Ezetimibe 10 mg (n = 262)	All statins[b](%) (n = 936)	Ezetimibe + all statins[b] (n = 925)
Myalgia	4.6%	5%	4.1%	4.5%
Respiratory				
Pharyngitis	1.9%	3.1%	2.5%	2.3%
Sinusitis	1.9%	4.6%	3.6%	3.5%
Upper respiratory tract infection	10.8%	13%	13.6%	11.8%
Miscellaneous				
Chest pain	1.2%	3.4%	2%	1.8%

[a] Includes 4 placebo-controlled combination studies in which ezetimibe was initiated concurrently with an HMG-CoA reductase inhibitor.
[b] All statins = all doses of all HMG-CoA reductase inhibitors.

➤*Combination with fenofibrate:* In a clinical study involving 625 patients treated for up to 12 weeks and 576 patients treated for up to an additional 48 weeks, coadministration of ezetimibe and fenofibrate was well tolerated. This study was not designed to compare treatment groups for infrequent reactions. Incidence rate (95% confidence interval) for clinically important elevations (greater than 3 times the ULN, consecutive) in serum transaminases were 4.5% (1.9, 8.8) and 2.7% (1.2, 5.4) for fenofibrate monotherapy and ezetimibe coadministered with fenofibrate, respectively, adjusted for treatment exposure. Corresponding incidence rates for cholecystectomy were 0.6% (0, 3.1) and 1.7% (0.6, 4) for fenofibrate monotherapy and ezetimibe coadministered with fenofibrate, respectively. The numbers of patients exposed to coadministration therapy as well as fenofibrate and ezetimibe monotherapy were inadequate to assess gallbladder disease risk. There were no CPK elevations greater than 10 times the ULN in any of the treatment groups.

➤*Postmarketing:* The following adverse reactions have been reported in postmarketing experience, regardless of causality assessment.

GI – Nausea, pancreatitis.

Hepatic – Cholecystitis, cholelithiasis, elevations in liver transaminases, hepatitis, thrombocytopenia.

Hypersensitivity – Hypersensitivity reactions, including anaphylaxis, angioedema, rash, and urticaria.

Lab test abnormalities – Elevated CPK.

Musculoskeletal – Arthralgia, myalgia, myopathy/rhabdomyolysis (very rare).

Overdosage

In clinical studies, administration of ezetimibe 50 mg/day to 15 healthy subjects for up to 14 days, or 40 mg/day to 18 patients with primary hypercholesterolemia for up to 56 days, was generally well tolerated.

➤*Treatment:* A few cases of overdosage with ezetimibe have been reported; most have not been associated with adverse reactions. Reported adverse reactions have not been serious. In the event of an overdose, employ symptomatic and supportive measures.

ANTIHYPERLIPIDEMIC COMBINATION PRODUCTS

AMLODIPINE BESYLATE/ATORVASTATIN CALCIUM

Rx	**Caduet** (Pfizer)	**Tablets:** 2.5 mg amlodipine besylate/10 mg atorvastatin calcium (as base)	Calcium carbonate. (Pfizer CDT 251). White. Film coated. In 30s.
		2.5 mg amlodipine besylate/20 mg atorvastatin calcium (as base)	Calcium carbonate. (Pfizer CDT 252). White. Film coated. In 30s.
		2.5 mg amlodipine besylate/40 mg atorvastatin calcium (as base)	Calcium carbonate. (Pfizer CDT 254). White. Film coated. In 30s.
		5 mg amlodipine besylate/10 mg atorvastatin calcium (as base)	Calcium carbonate. (Pfizer CDT 051). White. Film coated. In 30s.
		5 mg amlodipine besylate/20 mg atorvastatin calcium (as base)	Calcium carbonate. (Pfizer CDT 052). White. Film coated. In 30s.
		5 mg amlodipine besylate/40 mg atorvastatin calcium (as base)	Calcium carbonate. (Pfizer CDT 054). White. Film coated. In 30s.
		5 mg amlodipine besylate/80 mg atorvastatin calcium (as base)	Calcium carbonate. (Pfizer CDT 058). White. Film coated. In 30s.
		10 mg amlodipine besylate/10 mg atorvastatin calcium (as base)	Calcium carbonate. (Pfizer CDT 101). Blue. Film coated. In 30s.
		10 mg amlodipine besylate/20 mg atorvastatin calcium (as base)	Calcium carbonate. (Pfizer CDT 102). Blue. Film coated. In 30s.
		10 mg amlodipine besylate/40 mg atorvastatin calcium (as base)	Calcium carbonate. (Pfizer CDT 104). Blue. Film coated. In 30s.
		10 mg amlodipine besylate/80 mg atorvastatin calcium (as base)	Calcium carbonate. (Pfizer CDT 108). Blue. Film coated. In 30s.

AMLODIPINE BESYLATE/ATORVASTATIN CALCIUM — ORAL

For additional prescribing information, refer to the individual monographs for Amlodipine and Atorvastatin Calcium.

Indications

➤*Amlodipine:* For the treatment of hypertension, chronic stable angina, and confirmed or suspected vasospastic angina (Prinzmetal or Variant angina).

➤*Atorvastatin:* As an adjunct to diet to reduce elevated total-cholesterol (C), LDL-C, apo B, and triglyceride (TG) levels and to increase HDL-C in patients with primary hypercholesterolemia (heterozygous familial and nonfamilial) and mixed dyslipidemia (Fredrickson types IIa and IIb); as an adjunct to diet for the treatment of patients with elevated serum TG levels (Fredrickson type IV); for the treatment of patients with primary dysbetalipoproteinemia (Fredrickson type III); to reduce total-C and LDL-C in patients with homozygous familial hypercholesterolemia as an adjunct to other lipid-lowering treatments (eg, LDL apheresis) or if such treatments are unavailable; to reduce total-C, LDL-C, and apo B levels in boys and postmenarchal girls (10 to 17 years of age with heterozygous familial hypercholesterolemia).

Administration and Dosage

➤*Maximum dose:*

Adults – Amlodipine 10 mg/day, atorvastatin 80 mg/day according to the prescribing information.

➤*General dosing considerations:* Amlodipine/atorvastatin may be substituted for its individually titrated components.

Individualize dosage. Lipid-altering agents should be used in addition to a diet restricted in saturated fat and cholesterol, only when the response to diet and other nonpharmacological measures has been inadequate.

➤*Adults:*

As initial therapy for one indication and continuation of treatment of the other – The recommended starting dose of amlodipine/atorvastatin should be selected based on the continuation of the component being used and the recommended starting dose of the added monotherapy.

As continuation of treatment for both components – Amlodipine/atorvastatin may be substituted for its individually titrated components. Patients may be given the equivalent dose of amlodipine/atorvastatin or a dose of amlodipine/atorvastatin with increased amounts of amlodipine, atorvastatin, or both for additional antianginal effects, blood pressure lowering, or lipid-lowering effect.

Concomitant therapy – Atorvastatin may be used in combination with a bile acid-binding resin for additive effect. The combination of HMG-CoA reductase inhibitors and fibrates generally should be avoided.

➤*Elderly:* Elderly patients have decreased clearance of amlodipine with a resulting increase in AUC of approximately 40% to 60%, and a lower initial dose may be required.

Clinical data suggest a greater degree of LDL-lowering at any atorvastatin dose in the elderly patient population compared with younger adults.

➤*Renal function impairment:* No dosage adjustment is needed for patients with renal impairment.

➤*Hepatic function impairment:* Patients with hepatic function impairment have decreased clearance of amlodipine, with a resulting increase in AUC of approximately 40% to 60%; a lower initial dose may be required.

In patients with chronic alcoholic liver disease, plasma concentrations of atorvastatin are markedly increased. Atorvastatin is contraindicated in patients with active liver disease or unexplained persistent elevations of serum transaminases.

➤*Storage/Stability:* Store at 25°C (77°F); excursions permitted to 15° to 30°C (59° to 86°F).

Warnings/Precautions

➤*Pregnancy: Category X.* Safety in pregnant women has not been established. Amlodipine/Atorvastatin should be administered to women of childbearing potential only when such patients are highly unlikely to conceive and have been informed of the potential hazards. If the woman becomes pregnant while taking this medication, it should be discontinued and the patient advised again as to the potential hazards to the fetus.

The molecular weight of amlodipine (approximately 567 for the besylate salt) is low enough that excretion to the fetus should be expected. The high

AMLODIPINE BESYLATE/ATORVASTATIN CALCIUM — ORAL

molecular weight of atorvastatin (approximately 1,161 for the nonhydrated form) and extensive protein binding suggest that transfer across the placenta will be inhibited.

Rare reports of congenital anomalies have been received following intrauterine exposure to HMG-CoA reductase inhibitors. There has been one report of severe congenital boney deformity, tracheo-esophageal fistula, and anal atresia (VATER association) in a baby born to a woman who took lovastatin with dextroamphetamine during the first trimester of pregnancy.

➤*Lactation:* It is not known whether amlodipine is excreted in human milk. Breast-feeding rat pups taking atorvastatin had plasma and liver drug levels of 50% and 40%, respectively, of that in their mother's milk. Because of the potential for adverse reactions in breast-feeding infants, women should not breast-feed. The molecular weight of amlodipine suggests that excretion into breast milk should be expected. The high molecular weight of atorvastatin suggests that excretion into milk would be inhibited. However, atorvastatin is excreted into the milk of lactating rats, so excretion into human milk should be expected.

NIACIN/LOVASTATIN

Rx	**Advicor** (Abbott)	**Tablets, extended-release; oral** Niacin extended-release 500 mg/lovastatin 20 mg	(KOS 502). Lt. yellow, capsule shape. In 90s.
		Niacin extended-release 1,000 mg/lovastatin 20 mg	(KOS 1002). Dk. pink/lt. purple, capsule shape. In 90s.
		Niacin extended-release 1,000 mg/lovastatin 40 mg	(KOS 1004). Reddish brown, capsule shape. In 90s.

NIACIN/LOVASTATIN — ORAL

For complete and comparative prescribing information, refer to the HMG-CoA Reductase Inhibitors group monograph and the Niacin (B_3; Nicotinic Acid) monograph. Refer to the general discussion of these products in the Antihyperlipidemic Agents Introduction.

Indications

➤*Primary hypercholesterolemia/mixed dyslipidemia:* For the treatment of primary hypercholesterolemia (heterozygous familial and nonfamilial) and mixed dyslipidemia (Frederickson Types IIa and IIb) in the following: Patients treated with lovastatin who require further TG-lowering or HDL-raising who may benefit from having niacin added to their regimen; patients treated with niacin who require further LDL-lowering who may benefit from having lovastatin added to their regimen.

Administration and Dosage

➤*General dosing considerations:* A relative bioavailability study indicated that niacin extended-release/lovastatin tablet strengths (ie, two tablets of 500 mg/20 mg and one tablet of 1,000 mg/40 mg) are not interchangeable.

Flushing of the skin may be reduced in frequency or severity by pretreatment with aspirin (taken up to approximately 30 minutes prior to niacin extended-release/lovastatin tablets) or other nonsteroidal anti-inflammatory drugs. Flushing, pruritus, and GI distress also are greatly reduced by slowly increasing the dose of niacin and avoiding administration on an empty stomach.

➤*Adults:*

Hypercholesterolemia –

Maximum dose: Doses of niacin extended-release/lovastatin more than 2,000 mg/40 mg daily are not recommended.

Initial dosage: 500 mg/20 mg tablet once daily at bedtime.

Dosage titration: Niacin extended-release tablets must be titrated and the dose should not be increased by more than 500 mg every 4 weeks up to a maximum dose of 2,000 mg/day to reduce the incidence and severity of side effects.

Conversion: Patients already receiving a stable dose of niacin extended-release tablets may be switched directly to a niacin-equivalent dose of niacin extended-release/lovastatin tablets. Patients previously receiving niacin products other than niacin extended-release tablets should be started on niacin extended-release tablets with the recommended niacin extended-release tablets titration schedule, and the dose should subsequently be individualized.

Patients already receiving a stable dose of lovastatin may receive concomitant dosage titration with niacin extended-release tablets, and switch to niacin extended-release/lovastatin tablets once a stable dose of niacin extended-release tablets has been reached.

Mixed dyslipidemia – See Hypercholesterolemia.

➤*Renal function impairment:* In patients with severe renal insufficiency (CrCl less than 30 mL/min), dosage increases more than 20 mg/day should be carefully considered, and if deemed necessary, implemented cautiously. Use with caution in patients with renal dysfunction.

➤*Hepatic function impairment:* Use is contraindicated in patients with significant or unexplained hepatic dysfunction.

➤*Discontinuation of therapy:* If niacin extended-release/lovastatin therapy is discontinued for an extended period (more than 7 days), reinstitution of therapy should begin with the lowest dose of niacin extended-release/lovastatin.

➤*Administration:* Niacin extended-release/lovastatin tablets should be taken at bedtime with a low-fat snack, and the dose should be individualized according to patient response.

Niacin extended-release/lovastatin tablets should be taken whole and not broken, chewed, or crushed before swallowing.

➤*Storage/Stability:* Store at room temperature (20° to 25°C; 68° to 77°F).

Warnings/Precautions

➤*Pregnancy: Category X.* Niacin extended-release/lovastatin tablets should be administered to women of childbearing potential only when such patients are highly unlikely to conceive and have been informed of the potential hazard. Safety in pregnant women has not been established, and there is no apparent benefit to therapy with niacin extended-release/lovastatin tablets during pregnancy. Treatment should be immediately discontinued as soon as pregnancy is recognized.

Rare reports of congenital anomalies have been received following intrauterine exposure to HMG-CoA reductase inhibitors. In a review of approximately 100 prospectively followed pregnancies in women exposed to lovastatin or another structurally related HMG-CoA reductase inhibitor, the incidences of congenital anomalies, spontaneous abortions, and fetal deaths/stillbirths did not exceed what would be expected in the general population. The number of cases is adequate only to exclude a 3-to 4-fold increase in congenital anomalies over the background incidence. In 89% of the prospectively followed pregnancies, drug treatment was initiated prior to pregnancy and was discontinued at some point in the first trimester when pregnancy was identified.

Lovastatin has been shown to produce skeletal malformations at plasma levels 40 times the human exposure (for mouse fetus) and 80 times the human exposure (for rat fetus) based on mg/m_2 surface area (doses were 800 mg/kg/day).

➤*Lactation:* Because of the potential for serious adverse reactions in breast-feeding infants from lipid-altering doses of niacin and lovastatin, niacin extended-release/lovastatin tablets should not be taken while a woman is breast-feeding.

Niacin has been reported to be excreted in human milk. It is not known whether lovastatin is excreted in human milk. A small amount of another drug in this class is excreted in human breast milk.

EZETIMIBE/SIMVASTATIN

Rx	**Vytorin** (Merck/Schering-Plough)	**Tablets; oral:** ezetimibe 10 mg/simvastatin 10 mg	Lactose. (311). White to off-white, capsule shape. In 30s, 90s, 1,000s, 10,000s, and UD 100s.
		ezetimibe 10 mg/simvastatin 20 mg	Lactose. (312). White to off-white, capsule shape. In 30s, 90s, 1,000s, 10,000s, and UD 100s.
		ezetimibe 10 mg/simvastatin 40 mg	Lactose. (313). White to off-white, capsule shape. In 30s, 90s, 500s, 5,000s, and UD 50s.
		ezetimibe 10 mg/simvastatin 80 mg	Lactose. (315). White to off-white, capsule shape. In 30s, 90s, 500s, 2,500s, and UD 50s.

EZETIMIBE/SIMVASTATIN — ORAL

Indications

➤*Homozygous familial hypercholesterolemia:* For reducing elevated total cholesterol (total-C) and low-density lipoprotein cholesterol (LDL-C) in patients with homozygous familial hypercholesterolemia, as an adjunct to other lipid-lowering treatments (eg, LDL apheresis), or if such treatments are unavailable.

National Cholesterol Education Program (NCEP) Adult Treatment Panel (ATP) III guidelines – Therapy with lipid-altering agents should be a component of multiple risk-factor intervention in individuals at increased risk for atherosclerotic vascular disease due to hypercholesterolemia. Use lipid-altering agents in addition to an appropriate diet (including restriction of saturated fat and cholesterol) and when the response to diet and other nonpharmacological measures has been inadequate.

EZETIMIBE/SIMVASTATIN — ORAL

➤*Primary hyperlipidemia:* For the reduction of elevated total-C, LDL-C, apolipoprotein B (apo B), triglycerides, and non–high-density lipoprotein cholesterol (HDL-C), and to increase HDL-C in patients with primary (heterozygous familial and nonfamilial) hyperlipidemia or mixed hyperlipidemia.

No incremental benefit of ezetimibe/simvastatin on cardiovascular morbidity and mortality over and above that demonstrated for simvastatin has been established. Ezetimibe/simvastatin has not been studied in Fredrickson type I, III, IV, and V dyslipidemias.

Administration and Dosage

➤*General dosing considerations:* Place the patient on a standard cholesterol-lowering diet before the patient receives ezetimibe/simvastatin. Continue this diet during treatment with ezetimibe/simvastatin. Individualize the dosage according to the baseline LDL-C level, the recommended goal of therapy, and the patient's response.

➤*Adults:*

Homozygous familial hypercholesterolemia – Dosage is ezetimibe 10 mg/simvastatin 40 mg daily or ezetimibe 10 mg/simvastatin 80 mg daily in the evening. Use ezetimibe/simvastatin as an adjunct to other lipid-lowering treatments (eg, LDL apheresis) in these patients or if such treatments are unavailable.

Primary hypercholesterolemia –

Usual dosage: Ezetimibe 10 mg/simvastatin 10 mg daily to ezetimibe 10 mg/simvastatin 80 mg daily.

Initial dosage: Ezetimibe 10 mg/simvastatin 20 mg daily. Consider initiation of therapy with ezetimibe 10 mg/simvastatin 10 mg daily for patients requiring less aggressive LDL-C reductions. Start patients who require a larger reduction in LDL-C (greater than 55%) at ezetimibe 10 mg/simvastatin 40 mg daily.

Dosage adjustment: After initiation or titration of ezetimibe/simvastatin, lipid levels may be analyzed after 2 or more weeks and dosage adjusted.

➤*Renal function impairment:* No dosage adjustment is necessary in patients with mild or moderate renal function impairment.

For patients with severe renal function impairment, do not start ezetimibe/simvastatin unless the patient has already tolerated treatment with simvastatin at a dose of 5 mg or higher. Exercise caution when ezetimibe/simvastatin is administered to these patients and monitor them closely.

➤*Hepatic function impairment:* No dosage adjustment is necessary in patients with mild hepatic function impairment.

Use is not recommended in patients with moderate or severe hepatic function impairment.

➤*Chinese patients taking lipid-modifying doses (niacin 1 g/day or more) of niacin-containing products:* Because of an increased risk for myopathy, caution should be used when treating Chinese patients with ezetimibe/simvastatin coadministered with lipid-modifying doses (niacin 1 g/day or more) of niacin-containing products. Because the risk for myopathy is dose-related, Chinese patients should not receive ezetimibe 10 mg/simvastatin 80 mg coadministered with lipid-modifying doses of niacin-containing products. The cause of the increased risk of myopathy is not known. It is also unknown if the risk for myopathy with coadministration of simvastatin and lipid-modifying doses of niacin-containing products observed in Chinese patients applies to other Asian patients.

➤*Concomitant amiodarone or verapamil:* In patients taking amiodarone or verapamil concomitantly with ezetimibe/simvastatin, do not exceed ezetimibe 10 mg/simvastatin 20 mg daily.

➤*Concomitant bile acid sequestrants:* Give ezetimibe/simvastatin either 2 hours or more before or 4 hours or more after administration of a bile acid sequestrant.

➤*Concomitant cyclosporine or danazol:* Exercise caution when initiating ezetimibe/simvastatin in the setting of cyclosporine. In patients taking cyclosporine or danazol, do not start ezetimibe/simvastatin unless the patient has already tolerated treatment with simvastatin at a dose of 5 mg or higher. Do not exceed ezetimibe 10 mg/simvastatin 10 mg daily.

➤*Concomitant diltiazem:* Do not exceed ezetimibe 10 mg/simvastatin 40 mg daily.

➤*Concomitant lipid-lowering therapy:* The safety and efficacy of ezetimibe administered with fibrates have not been established. Therefore, the combination of ezetimibe/simvastatin and fibrates should be avoided.

There is an increased risk of myopathy when simvastatin is used concomitantly with fibrates (especially gemfibrozil). Therefore, although not recommended, if ezetimibe/simvastatin is used in combination with gemfibrozil, the dose should not exceed ezetimibe 10 mg/simvastatin 10 mg daily.

➤*Administration:* Ezetimibe/simvastatin should be taken as a single daily dose in the evening with or without food.

➤*Storage/Stability:* Store at 20° to 25°C (68° to 77°F). Keep the container tightly closed. Store in the original container until time of use. When the product container is subdivided, repackage it into a tightly closed, light-resistant container. The entire contents must be repackaged immediately upon opening.

NIACIN/SIMVASTATIN

Rx	**Simcor** (Abbott)	**Tablets, extended-release; oral:** niacin extended-release 500 mg/simvastatin 20 mg	Lactose, PEG. (A 500-20). Blue. In 90s.
		niacin extended-release 500 mg/simvastatin 40 mg	Lactose, PEG. (A 500-40). Dark blue. In 90s.
		niacin extended-release 750 mg/simvastatin 20 mg	Lactose, PEG. (A 750-20). Blue. In 90s.
		niacin extended-release 1,000 mg/simvastatin 20 mg	Lactose, PEG. (A 1000-20). Blue. In 90s.
		niacin extended-release 1,000 mg/simvastatin 40 mg	Lactose, PEG. (A 1000-40). Dark blue. In 90s.

NIACIN/SIMVASTATIN — ORAL

Indications

➤*Hypercholesterolemia:* For the reduction of total cholesterol, low-density lipoprotein cholesterol (LDL-C), apolipoprotein B (apo B), non–high-density liproprotein cholesterol (HDL-C), or triglycerides, or to increase HDL-C in patients with primary hypercholesterolemia and mixed dyslipidemia when treatment with simvastatin monotherapy or niacin extended-release (ER) monotherapy is considered inadequate.

➤*Hypertriglyceridemia:* For the reduction of triglycerides in patients with hypertriglyceridemia when treatment with simvastatin monotherapy or niacin ER monotherapy is considered inadequate.

Administration and Dosage

➤*General dosing considerations:* Because of the increased risk of hepatotoxicity with other modified-release (sustained-release or time-release) niacin preparations or immediate-release (crystalline) niacin, niacin ER/simvastatin should only be substituted for equivalent doses of niacin ER (*Niaspan*).

➤*Adults:*

Hypercholesterolemia –

Maximum dose: The efficacy and safety of doses of niacin ER/simvastatin of more than 2,000 mg/40 mg daily have not been studied and, therefore, are not recommended.

Initial dosage:

• *Niacin ER naive* – 500 mg/20 mg tablet daily at bedtime, for patients not taking niacin ER and patients taking niacin products other than niacin ER.

• *Patients currently taking simvastatin* – Patients already taking simvastatin 20 to 40 mg who need additional management of their lipid levels may be started on a niacin ER/simvastatin dosage of 500 mg/40 mg once daily at bedtime.

Maintenance dosage: 1,000 mg/20 mg to 2,000 mg/40 mg (two 1,000 mg/20 mg tablets) once daily, depending on patient tolerability and lipid levels.

Dosage adjustment: The dose of niacin ER should not be increased by more than 500 mg daily every 4 weeks.

Recommended Niacin ER Initial Titration Schedule

Week(s)	Daily dose of niacin ER
1 to 4	500 mg
5 to 8	1,000 mg
[a]	1,500 mg
[a]	2,000 mg

[a] After week 8, titrate to patient response and tolerance. If response to 1,000 mg daily is inadequate, increase dose to 1,500 mg daily; may subsequently increase dose to 2,000 mg daily. Daily dose should not be increased more than 500 mg in a 4-week period, and doses higher than 2,000 mg daily are not recommended.

Interruption of therapy: If niacin/simvastatin therapy is discontinued for an extended period of time (more than 7 days), retitration as tolerated is recommended.

Pretreatment: Flushing may be reduced in frequency or severity by pretreatment with aspirin up to the recommended dose of 325 mg (approximately 30 minutes prior to niacin/simvastatin dose). Flushing, pruritus, and GI distress are also reduced by gradually increasing the dose of niacin and avoiding administration on an empty stomach. Concomitant alcohol, hot drinks, or spicy foods may increase the adverse reactions of flushing and pruritus and should be avoided around the time of niacin/simvastatin ingestion.

Hypertriglyceridemia – See Hypercholesterolemia.

➤*Renal function impairment:* For patients with severe renal function impairment, do not start niacin/simvastatin unless the patient has already tolerated treatment with simvastatin at a dose of 10 mg or higher.

NIACIN/SIMVASTATIN — ORAL

➤*Administration:* Niacin/simvastatin tablets should be taken whole and not broken, crushed, or chewed before swallowing. They should be taken as a single daily dose at bedtime, with a low-fat snack.

➤*Storage/Stability:* Store at 20° to 25°C (68° to 77°F).

VASOPRESSORS USED IN SHOCK

➤*Shock:* Shock is a state of inadequate tissue perfusion. It can be caused by, or cause, a decreased supply of, or an increased demand for, oxygen and nutrients. The imbalance between supply and demand interferes with normal cellular function. Widespread cellular dysfunction can result in death. Inadequate tissue perfusion can occur even if cardiac output, peripheral resistance, and other factors that determine blood pressure (eg, blood volume) are normal or elevated. Therefore, hypotension need not be present for the patient to be in shock.

Shock produces various physiologic responses. Some, such as lactic acidosis, occur as a direct result of tissue hypoperfusion. Others, such as catecholamine release, also serve to compensate for the absolute or relative reduction in tissue perfusion. The systemic responses to shock can be beneficial in the early stages and classically consist of an increase in circulating catecholamines, vasodilation, and increased vascular permeability. These early responses produce a "hyperdynamic" state, which may be referred to as "warm" shock, so named because blood flow to the skin and extremities is still maintained. If left uncorrected, however, these responses become counterproductive and contribute to the relentless progression of the shock state. Profound vascular decompensation occurs, which is associated with a further loss of blood flow to the vital organs, skin, and extremities. Thus, more advanced shock is "cold" shock.

➤*Clinical manifestations:* Clinical manifestations of shock are variable and nonspecific. In addition, underlying or concurrent disease states, drug therapy, and patient age may alter the response to hypoperfusion. Signs and symptoms of shock include:

Skin – Pallor, cyanosis, cold and clammy, sweating.

CNS – Agitation, confusion, disorientation, coma.

Cardiovascular – Tachycardia, arrhythmias, wide pulse pressure, gallop rhythm, hypotension.

Pulmonary – Tachypnea, pulmonary edema.

Renal – Oliguria (< 0.5 mL/kg/hr).

Metabolic – Acidosis, hypoglycemia or hyperglycemia.

➤*Causes:* The causes of shock are varied. Despite the etiology, advanced shock tends to follow a common clinical course. However, identifying the underlying cause may assist in the selection of general supportive therapy and is essential for selecting specific therapy.

➤*Types of shock:*

Hypovolemic shock – Hypovolemic shock occurs when intravascular volume is reduced by > 15% to 25%. The volume loss can be absolute (eg, hemorrhage, fluid loss due to burns, diarrhea or vomiting, excess diuresis, diabetes) or relative (eg, sequestration of body fluids, capillary leak).

Cardiogenic shock – Cardiogenic shock occurs when the heart is unable to deliver an adequate cardiac output to maintain vital organ perfusion. This can be caused by an acute MI, sustained ventricular arrhythmias, severe cardiomyopathy, or CHF.

Septic shock – Septic shock occurs as a result of circulatory insufficiency associated with overwhelming infection.

Obstructive shock – Obstructive shock occurs when obstruction of blood flow results in inadequate tissue perfusion. Massive pulmonary embolism, pericardial tamponade, restrictive pericarditis, and severe cardiac valve dysfunction can reduce blood flow enough to produce shock.

Neurogenic shock – An uncommon form of shock that occurs as a result of blockade of neurohumoral outflow. The neurohumoral blockade may be induced by pharmacologic agents (eg, spinal anesthesia) or by direct injury to the spinal cord.

Other causes of shock – Other causes include anaphylaxis, hypoglycemia, hypothyroidism and hypoadrenalism (ie, Addison disease).

➤*Management:* Management of shock is aimed at providing basic life support (eg, airway, breathing, circulation) while attempting to correct the underlying cause. Antibiotics, inotropes, hormones (eg, insulin, thyroid) and other agents may be used to treat the underlying disease states in the shock patient. However, initial pharmacologic interventions are primarily aimed at supporting the circulation.

Blood pressure is a function of the peripheral vascular resistance and the cardiac output. Cardiac output is determined by the heart rate and stroke volume. The stroke volume is a function of the contractile state of the heart and the volume of blood in the ventricle available to be pumped out (ie, preload). Manipulation of any of these parameters can produce a change in blood pressure.

Fluids – Relative or absolute volume depletion occurs in most shock states, especially in the early or "warm" phase in which vasodilation is prominent. Adequate volume repletion is necessary to maintain cardiac output, urine flow, and the integrity of the microcirculation. Attempts to support the circulation with vasopressors or inotropes will be unsuccessful if the intravascular volume is depleted.

The choice of fluids is probably irrelevant in the early stages. Although whole blood might be preferred for the patient with hemorrhagic shock, the delay in availability of blood products often negates any advantage. There is no clear superiority of crystalloids or colloids in emergency fluid resuscitation. Hydroxyethyl starch and the dextrans are also suitable plasma volume expanders.

Vasopressors – Sympathomimetic agents are used in shock to treat hypoperfusion in normovolemic patients and in patients unresponsive to whole blood or plasma volume expanders. These agents increase myocardial contractility, constrict capacitance vessels, and dilate resistance vessels. In cardiogenic shock or advanced shock from other causes associated with a low cardiac output, they may be combined with vasodilators (eg, nitroprusside, nitroglycerin) to maintain blood pressure while the vasodilator improves myocardial performance. Nitroprusside is used to reduce preload and afterload and improve cardiac output. Nitroglycerin directly relaxes the venous vasculature and decreases preload.

Pharmacology – Sympathomimetic agents produce α-adrenergic stimulation (vasoconstriction), β_1-adrenergic stimulation (increase myocardial contractility, heart rate, automaticity, and AV conduction), and β_2-adrenergic activity (peripheral vasodilation). Dopamine also causes vasodilation of the renal and mesenteric, cerebral and coronary beds by dopaminergic receptor activation. Adrenergic agents are useful in improving hemodynamic status by improving myocardial contractility and increasing heart rate, which results in increased cardiac output. Peripheral resistance is increased by vasoconstriction. Increased cardiac output and increased peripheral resistance increase blood pressure. The relative activity and predominance of these actions result in a number of hemodynamic responses which may affect coronary perfusion, renal perfusion, cardiac output, total peripheral resistance and blood pressure. These actions are summarized in the Sites of Action/Hemodynamic Response table. The actual response of an individual patient will depend largely on clinical status at time of administration.

Other drugs – A number of other drug classes have been used as supportive therapy in shock patients. However, with the exception of vasodilator treatment of cardiogenic shock, none of these treatments appear superior to vasopressor therapy. These drugs include: Opiate antagonists, prostaglandin inhibitors, corticosteroids, and thyrotropin-releasing hormone.

Monitoring – The monitoring of shock patients and their response to drugs requires special vigilance. Monitor heart rate, blood pressure, and ECG continuously. Record urine output and fluid intake frequently. Due to rapid and life-threatening changes that can occur in the hemodynamically unstable patient, optimal drug selection, dose titration, and management is probably best achieved with the use of invasive hemodynamic monitoring. Monitoring of central venous pressures via a central venous catheter will provide an estimation of the patient's fluid status by approximating the diastolic pressure of the right ventricle. When warranted, additional hemodynamic data can be obtained through the use of a pulmonary artery catheter (ie, Swan-Ganz). Changes in the pulmonary artery wedge pressure (a measure of left ventricular end diastolic volume), cardiac output, and peripheral vascular resistance can be monitored and therapy adjusted accordingly.

Administration – Administration should only be via the IV route using a large-bore, free-flowing IV in the antecubital vein or a central vein because of unpredictable absorption. Small IVs in the extremities are both unreliable and unsafe for vasopressor administration. Frequent monitoring of the IV sites for extravasation injury is essential when vasopressor agents are being used.

Prolonged, high-dose therapy – Prolonged, high-dose therapy can produce cyanosis and tissue necrosis of distal extremities. The principle of using the lowest dose that produces an adequate response for the shortest period of time is very important when using these agents.

Plasma volume depletion – Prolonged use of vasopressors may result in plasma volume depletion; this should be corrected by appropriate fluid and electrolyte replacement therapy. If plasma volumes are not corrected, hypotension may recur when these drugs are discontinued. Blood pressure may be maintained at the risk of severe peripheral vasoconstriction with diminution in blood flow and tissue perfusion.

Acidosis – Acidosis lessens the response to vasopressors; therefore, correct acidosis if it exists or develops during the course of vasopressor therapy.

Avoid continuous IV therapy – Acute tolerance develops during continuous IV administration. High concentration/low volume (250 mL) vasopressor solutions administered with the aid of an infusion control device allows for maximum dosing flexibility since fluids and drugs can be regulated independently, and the development of tolerance is minimized.

Effects of Vasopressors Used in Shock

+++ pronounced effect
++ *moderate effect*
\+ *slight effect*
0 *no effect*
↑ *increase*
↓ *decrease*

		Sites of Action: Heart		Sites of Action: Blood Vessels		Hemodynamic Response			
		Contractility (Inotropic)	SA Node Rate (Chronotropic)	Vasoconstriction	Vasodilatation	Renal Perfusion	Cardiac Output	Total Peripheral Resistance	Blood Pressure
		β1	β1	α	β2				
Inotropic	Isoproterenol	+++	+++	0	+++	↑[a] or ↓[b]	↑	↓	↑[c]↓[d]
	Dobutamine	+++	0 to +[e]	0 to +[e]	+	0	↑	↓	↑
	Dopamine	+++	+ to ++[e]	+ to +++[e]	0 to +[f]	↑[e]	↑	↓[e] or ↑	0 to ↑
Mixed	Epinephrine	+++	+++	+++[e]	++[e]	↓	↑	↓	↑[c]↓[d]
	Norepinephrine	++	++[g]	+++	0	↓	0 or ↓	↑	↑
	Ephedrine	++	++	+	0 to +	↓	↑	↑ or ↓	↑
	Mephentermine	+	+	+	++	↑ or ↓	↑	0 to ↑	↑
	Metaraminol	+	+	++	0	↓	↓	↑	↑
Pressors	Methoxamine	0	0[g]	+++	0	↓	0 or ↓	↑	↑
	Phenylephrine	0	0[g]	+++	0	↓	↓	↑	↑

[a] Cardiogenic or septicemic shock.
[b] Normotensive patient.
[c] Systolic effect.
[d] Diastolic effect.
[e] Effects are dose dependent.
[f] Dilates renal and splanchnic beds via dopaminergic effect at doses
[g] Decreased heart rate may result from reflex mechanisms.

Common Dilutions and Infusion Rates for Selected Drugs Used in Shock

Drug	Usual Dilution for IV Infusion	Infusion Rate
Isoproterenol	2 mg (10 mL) in 500 mL D5W (4 mcg/mL) or 1 mg (5 mL) in 250 mL D5W	5 mcg/min
Dobutamine	250 mg in 250 to 500 mL NS or D5W (500 to 1000 mcg/mL)	2.5 to 15 mcg/kg/min
Dopamine	200 to 800 mg in 250 to 500 mL NS or D5W (400 to 3200 mcg/mL)	Low dose – 2.5 to 10 mcg/kg/min High dose – 20 to 50 mcg/kg/min
Norepinephrine	4 mg in 250 mL of D5W (16 mcg/mL)	Initial: 8 to 12 mcg/min Maintenance: 2 to 4 mcg/min

ISOPROTERENOL HYDROCHLORIDE

Rx	**Isoproterenol** (Various, eg, Abbott)	**Injection, solution:** 1:5,000 (0.2 mg/mL)[a]	In 5 and 10 mL vials.
Rx	**Isuprel** (Hospira)		In 1 and 5 mL ampules.

[a] With sodium metabisulfite.

ISOPROTERENOL HYDROCHLORIDE — INJECTION

Refer to the general discussion of these products in the Vasopressors Used in Shock class monograph.

Indications

➤*Heart block:* For mild or transient episodes of heart block that do not require electric shock or pacemaker therapy.

➤*Heart block and Adams-Stokes attacks:* For serious episodes of heart block and Adams-Stokes attacks (except when caused by ventricular tachycardia or fibrillation).

➤*Cardiac arrest:* In cardiac arrest until electric shock or pacemaker therapy, the treatments of choice, is available.

➤*Bronchospasm:* For bronchospasm occurring during anesthesia.

➤*Treatment of hypovolemic and septic shock, low cardiac output (hypoperfusion) states, CHF, cardiogenic shock:* As an adjunct to fluid and electrolyte replacement therapy and the use of other drugs and procedures in the treatment of these conditions.

Administration and Dosage

➤*General dosing considerations:* Isoproterenol should generally be started at the lowest recommended dose and the rate of administration gradually increased if necessary while carefully monitoring the patient.

The usual route of administration is by IV infusion or bolus IV injection. In dire emergencies, the drug may be administered by intracardiac injection. If time is not of the utmost importance, initial therapy by intramuscular or subcutaneous injection is preferred.

➤*Adults:*

Bronchospasm occurring during anesthesia –

Recommended Isoproterenol Dosage for Adults With Bronchospasm Occurring During Anesthesia

Route of administration	Preparation of dilution	Initial dose	Subsequent dose
Bolus IV injection	Dilute 1 mL (0.2 mg) of 1:5,000 solution to 10 mL with sodium chloride injection or 5% dextrose injection	0.01 to 0.02 mg (0.5 to 1 mL of diluted solution) 0.01 to 0.02 mg (0.5 to 1 mL)	The initial dose may be repeated when necessary.

Adams-Stokes attacks, cardiac arrest, or heart block –

Recommended Isoproterenol Dosage for Adults With Heart Block, Adams-Stokes Attacks, and Cardiac Arrest

Route of administration	Preparation of dilution	Initial dose	Subsequent dose range[a]
Bolus IV injection	Dilute 1 mL (0.2 mg) of 1:5,000 solution to 10 mL with sodium chloride injection or 5% dextrose injection	0.02 to 0.06 mg (1 to 3 mL of diluted solution) 0.02 to 0.06 mg (1 to 3 mL)	0.01 to 0.2 mg (0.5 to 10 mL of diluted solution)

ISOPROTERENOL HYDROCHLORIDE — INJECTION

Recommended Isoproterenol Dosage for Adults With Heart Block, Adams-Stokes Attacks, and Cardiac Arrest			
Route of administration	Preparation of dilution	Initial dose	Subsequent dose range[a]
IV infusion	Dilute 10 mL (2 mg) of 1:5,000 solution in 500 mL of 5% dextrose injection	5 mcg/min (1.25 mL of diluted solution per minute)	
Intramuscular	Use solution 1:5,000 undiluted	0.2 mg (1 mL)	0.02 to 1 mg (0.1 to 5 mL)
Subcutaneous	Use solution 1:5,000 undiluted	0.2 mg (1 mL)	0.15 to 0.2 mg (0.75 to 1 mL)
Intracardiac[b]	Use solution 1:5,000 undiluted	0.02 mg (0.1 mL)	

[a] Subsequent dosage and method of administration depend on the ventricular rate and the rapidity with which the cardiac pacemaker can take over when the drug is gradually withdrawn.
[b] This route of administration may be used in dire emergencies.

Hypoperfusion states or shock –

Recommended Isoproterenol Dosage for Adults With Shock and Hypoperfusion States		
Route of administration	Preparation of dilution[a]	Infusion rate[b]
IV infusion	Dilute 5 mL (1 mg) of 1:5,000 solution in 500 mL of 5% dextrose injection	0.5 to 5 mcg/min (0.25 to 2.5 mL of diluted solution)

[a] Concentrations up to 10 times greater have been used when limitation of volume is essential.
[b] Rates over 30 mcg per minute have been used in advanced stages of shock. The rate of infusion should be adjusted on the basis of heart rate, central venous pressure, systemic blood pressure, and urine flow. If the heart rate exceeds 110 beats per minute, it may be advisable to decrease or temporarily discontinue the infusion.

➤*Children:*

Off-label dosing – There are no well-controlled studies in children to establish appropriate dosing; however, the American Heart Association recommends the following:

Adams-Stokes attacks:
- *IV infusion –*
  Usual dosage: 0.1 to 1 mcg/kg/min.
  Initial dosage: 0.1 mcg/kg/min.

Cardiac arrest:
- *IV infusion –*
  Usual dosage: 0.2 to 1 mcg/kg/min.
  Initial dosage: 0.1 mcg/kg/min.

Heart block:
- *IV infusion –*
  Usual dosage: 0.3 to 1 mcg/kg/min.
  Initial dosage: 0.1 mcg/kg/min.

➤*Preparation for administration:* See the previous tables within adult dosing for diluting instructions for each indication.

➤*Storage/Stability:* Store at 15° to 30°C (59° to 86°F). Protect from light. Retain in carton until time of use. Do not use the injection if its color is pinkish or darker than slightly yellow or if it contains a precipitate.

Actions

➤*Pharmacology:* Isoproterenol is a potent nonselective beta-adrenergic agonist with very low affinity for alpha-adrenergic receptors. IV infusion of isoproterenol in man lowers peripheral vascular resistance, primarily in skeletal muscle but also in renal and mesenteric vascular beds. Diastolic pressure falls. Renal blood flow is decreased in normotensive subjects but is increased markedly in shock. Systolic blood pressure may remain unchanged or rise although mean arterial pressure typically falls. Cardiac output is increased because of the positive inotropic and chronotropic effects of the drug in the face of diminished peripheral vascular resistance. The cardiac effects of isoproterenol may lead to palpitations, sinus tachycardia, and more serious arrhythmias; large doses of isoproterenol may cause myocardial necrosis in animals.

➤*Pharmacokinetics:* Isoproterenol is readily absorbed when given parenterally or as an aerosol. It is metabolized primarily in the liver and other tissues by catechol-O-methyl transferase (COMT). Isoproterenol is a relatively poor substrate for monoamine oxidase (MAO) and is not taken up by sympathetic neurons to the same extent as are epinephrine and norepinephrine. The duration of action of isoproterenol may therefore be longer than that of epinephrine, but is still brief.

Contraindications

Tachyarrhythmias; tachycardia or heart block caused by digitalis intoxication; ventricular arrhythmias which require inotropic therapy; and angina pectoris.

Warnings/Precautions

➤*Use following an MI:* Isoproterenol, by increasing myocardial oxygen requirements while decreasing effective coronary perfusion, may have a deleterious effect on the injured or failing heart. Most experts discourage its use as the initial agent in treating cardiogenic shock following myocardial infarction. However, when a low arterial pressure has been elevated by other means, isoproterenol hydrochloride injection may produce beneficial hemodynamic and metabolic effects.

➤*Cardiac effects:* In a few patients, presumably with organic disease of the AV node and its branches, isoproterenol hydrochloride injection has paradoxically been reported to worsen heart block or to precipitate Adams-Stokes attacks during normal sinus rhythm or transient heart block.

There are case reports of occasional fatal cardiac dysrhythmia and myocardial necrosis at autopsy as a result of intravenous isoproterenol. ECG changes and serum CPK-MB level elevation consistent with transient myocardial ischemia and abnormal echocardiographic findings suggestive of myocardial dysfunction have been documented with the use of intravenous isoproterenol hydrochloride infusion for the treatment of severe asthma exacerbations in children. Care should be taken to ensure that oxygen is always administered during isoproterenol infusions in patients with asthma. Heart rate, blood pressure, arrhythmias and evidence of myocardial ischemia by ECG should be monitored. Arterial blood gases should also be monitored carefully and PaO_2 maintained above 60 torr. Where ECG suggests myocardial ischemia, cardiac enzymes including cardiac-specific CPK-MB isoenzyme levels should be determined.

➤*Lowest recommended dose:* Isoproterenol should generally be started at the lowest recommended dose. This may be gradually increased, if necessary, while carefully monitoring the patient. Doses sufficient to increase the heart rate to more than 130 beats per minute may increase the likelihood of inducing ventricular arrhythmias. Such increases in heart rate will also tend to increase cardiac work and oxygen requirements which may adversely affect the failing heart or the heart with a significant degree of arteriosclerosis.

➤*Special populations:* Particular caution is necessary in administering isoproterenol to patients with coronary artery disease, coronary insufficiency, diabetes, hyperthyroidism, and sensitivity to sympathomimetic amines.

➤*Volume expanders:* Adequate filling of the intravascular compartment by suitable volume expanders of primary importance in most cases of shock, and should precede the administration of vasoactive drugs. In patients with normal cardiac function, determination of central venous pressure is a reliable guide during volume replacement. If evidence of hypoperfusion persists after adequate volume replacement, isoproterenol hydrochloride injection may be given.

➤*Sulfite sensitivity:* Contains sodium metabisulfite, a sulfite that may cause allergic-type reactions including anaphylactic symptoms and life-threatening or less severe asthmatic episodes in certain susceptible people. The overall prevalence of sulfite sensitivity in the general population is unknown and probably low. Sulfite sensitivity is seen more frequently in asthmatic than in nonasthmatic people.

➤*Pregnancy: Category C.* Animal reproduction studies have not been conducted with isoproterenol. It is also not known whether isoproterenol can cause fetal harm when administered to a pregnant woman or can affect reproduction capacity. Isoproterenol should be given to a pregnant woman only if clearly needed.

➤*Lactation:* It is not known whether this drug is excreted in human milk. Because many drugs are excreted in human milk, caution should be exercised when isoproterenol is administered to a nursing woman.

➤*Children:* The safety and effectiveness of isoproterenol in children have not been established.

➤*Monitoring:* In addition to the routine monitoring of systemic blood pressure, heart rate, urine flow, and the electrocardiograph, the response to therapy should also be monitored by frequent determination of the central venous pressure and blood gases. Patients in shock should be closely observed during isoproterenol hydrochloride injection administration. If the heart rate exceeds 110 beats per minute, it may be advisable to decrease the infusion rate or temporarily discontinue the infusion. Determinations of cardiac output and circulation time may also be helpful. Appropriate measures should be taken to ensure adequate ventilation. Careful attention should be paid to acid-base balance and to the correction of electrolyte disturbances. In cases of shock associated with bacteremia, suitable antimicrobial therapy is, of course, imperative.

Suggested minimal precautions while infusing isoproterenol hydrochloride continuously include careful monitoring of blood pressure and pulse, ECG monitoring of heart rate, arrhythmias, and evidence of myocardial ischemia, and where ECG evidence suggests myocardial ischemia, daily determination of cardiac enzymes including the more specific CPK-MB isoenzyme, monitoring arterial pH and blood gases carefully and maintaining PaO_2 above 60 torr by administration of supplemental oxygen.

Drug Interactions

➤*QT prolongation:* An additive effect of isoproterenol with other drugs that prolong the QT interval cannot be excluded. The following drugs may

ISOPROTERENOL HYDROCHLORIDE — INJECTION

prolong the QT interval and increase the risk of life-threatening cardiac arrhythmias, including torsades de pointes: Antiarrhythmic agents (eg, amiodarone, bretylium, disopyramide, dofetilide, procainamide, quinidine, and sotalol), arsenic trioxide, chlorpromazine, cisapride, dolasetron, droperidol, mefloquine, mesoridazine, moxifloxacin, pentamidine, pimozide, tacrolimus, thioridazine, and ziprasidone. For a more complete list of drugs that may prolong the QT interval, see the appendix, Drug-Induced Prolongation of the QT Interval and Torsades de Pointes.

Isoproterenol Drug Interactions

Precipitant drug	Object drug [a]		Description
Bretylium	Isoproterenol	↑	Bretylium potentiates the action of vasopressors on adrenergic receptors, possibly resulting in arrhythmias.
Guanethidine	Isoproterenol	↑	Guanethidine may increase the pressor response of the direct-acting vasopressors, possibly resulting in severe hypertension.
Halogenated hydrocarbon anesthetics	Isoproterenol	↑	Halogenated hydrocarbon anesthetics may sensitize the myocardium to the effects of catecholamines. Use of vasopressors may lead to serious arrhythmias; use with caution.
Oxytocic drugs	Isoproterenol	↑	In obstetrics, if vasopressor drugs are used either to correct hypotension or added to the local anesthetic solution, some oxytocic drugs may cause severe persistent hypertension.
Tricyclic antidepressants	Isoproterenol	↑	The pressor response of the direct-acting vasopressors may be potentiated by these agents; use with caution.

[a] ↑ = Object drug increased.

➤*Epinephrine:* Isoproterenol and epinephrine should not be administered simultaneously because both drugs are direct cardiac stimulants and their combined effects may induce serious arrhythmias. The drugs may, however, be administered alternately provided a proper interval has elapsed between doses.

➤*Inhalation anesthetics:* Isoproterenol should be used with caution, if at all, when potent inhalational anesthetics such as halothane are employed because of potential to sensitize the myocardium to effects of sympathomimetic amines.

➤*IV methylxanthines and IV steroids:* Cautions should be maintained when using continuous IV isoproterenol infusions in conjunction with intravenous methyl xanthines (aminophylline, theophylline) and intravenous corticosteroids. The use of isoproterenol with aminophylline and corticosteroids may be additive in cardiotoxic properties and can lead to myocardial necrosis and death. Severe cardiac symptoms of sympathetic overactivation (ie, hypertension, tachycardia, arrhythmias, seizures, myocardial ischemia, and fatal myocardial necrosis) have been reported.

Adverse Reactions

The following reactions to isoproterenol have been reported:

➤*Cardiovascular:* Tachycardia, palpitations, angina, Adams-Stokes attacks, pulmonary edema, hypertension, hypotension, ventricular arrhythmias, tachyarrhythmias. In a few patients, presumably with organic disease of the AV node and its branches, isoproterenol hydrochloride injection has been reported to precipitate Adams-Stokes seizures during normal sinus rhythm or transient heart block.

➤*CNS:* Nervousness, headache, dizziness.

➤*Miscellaneous:* Flushing of the skin, sweating, mild tremors, weakness.

The following reactions to isoproterenol have been reported in healthy adult controls undergoing upright tilt testing:

Isoproterenol Adverse Reactions in Upright Tilt Testing

Symptoms	Patients (n = 15)	Control group I (n = 13)	Control group II (n = 9)
Warmth	87%	93%	78%
Diaphoresis	87%	77%	56%
Dizziness	80%	77%	56%
Pallor	40%	69%	78%
Visual blurring[a]	33%	77%	56%
Nausea	40%	39%	22%
Shakiness	20%	8%	22%
Weakness	27%	15%	0%
Headache	33%	8%	0%
Dyspnea	29%	15%	0%

[a] $P = 0.03$ (difference between patients vs controls).

Overdosage

The acute toxicity of isoproterenol in animals is much less than that of epinephrine. Excessive doses in animals or man can cause a striking drop in blood pressure, and repeated large doses in animals may result in cardiac enlargement and focal myocarditis.

Cardiotoxicity is quite common with use of intravenous isoproterenol infusions. Cardiotoxicity is characterized by ventricular tachyarrhythmias frequently culminating in ventricular fibrillation and sudden death and is associated histologically with well-defined areas of myocardial necrosis.

Cardiotoxicity is highly associated with elevation of CPK-MB isoenzyme levels and ECG abnormalities which should be looked for. There is reason to suspect that there may be a subgroup of patients with asthma who are at increased risk when receiving both beta-adrenergic agonists and methyl xanthines. Risk factors for cardiotoxicity with isoproterenol infusions during treatment of severe asthma include the presence of hypercapnia (Pco_2 greater than 50 mmHg), acidosis (pH less than 7.3) and/or concomitant use of other medications such as corticosteroids or particularly aminophylline and methyl xanthines which may potentiate the cardiotoxic effects of isoproterenol.

In case of accidental overdosage as evidenced mainly by tachycardia or other arrhythmias, palpitations, angina, hypotension, or hypertension, reduce rate of administration or discontinue isoproterenol injection until patient's condition stabilizes. Blood pressure, pulse, respiration, and EKG should be monitored.

It is not known whether isoproterenol is dialyzable.

The oral LD_{50} of isoproterenol in mice is 3,850 mg/kg ± 1,190 mg/kg of pure drug in solution.

DOBUTAMINE

Rx	**Dobutamine** (Various, eg, Bedford, Hospira)	**Injection, solution, concentrate**: 12.5 mg/mL	As dobutamine hydrochloride. May contain sulfites. In 20 and 40 mL single-use vials and 100 mL pharmacy bulk packages.
Rx	**Dobutamine Hydrochloride in 5% Dextrose Injection** (Various, eg, Hospira)	**Injection, solution**: 250 mg per 250 mL (1 mg/mL)	May contain sulfites. In 250 mL single-use containers.
		500 mg per 500 mL (1 mg/mL)	In 500 mL single-use containers.
		500 mg per 250 mL (2 mg/mL)	In 250 mL single-use containers.
		1,000 mg per 250 mL (4 mg/mL)	In 250 mL single-use containers.

DOBUTAMINE HYDROCHLORIDE — INJECTION

Refer to the general discussion of these products in the Vasopressors Used in Shock class monograph.

Indications

➤*Cardiac decompensation:* Dobutamine is indicated when parenteral therapy is necessary for inotropic support in the short-term treatment of adults with cardiac decompensation caused by depressed contractility resulting from organic heart disease or from cardiac surgical procedures. Experience with intravenous (IV) dobutamine in controlled trials does not extend beyond 48 hours of repeated boluses and/or continuous infusions.

Administration and Dosage

➤*General dosing considerations:* According to the American Heart Association guidelines, it is recommended to optimize treatment with dobutamine based on hemodynamic end points rather than a specific dose.

➤*Adults:*

Cardiac decompensation –

Maximum dose: 40 mcg/kg/min.

Initial dosage: 0.5 to 1 mcg/kg/min as a continuous IV infusion.

Dosage titration: Titrate every few minutes guided by the patient response, including systemic blood pressure, urine flow, frequency of ectopic

DOBUTAMINE HYDROCHLORIDE — INJECTION

activity, heart rate, and, whenever possible, measurements of cardiac output, central venous pressure, and/or pulmonary capillary wedge pressure.

Maintenance dosage: 2 to 20 mcg/kg/min as a continuous infusion. On rare occasions, up to 40 mcg/kg/min has been required.

Duration of therapy: Adjust duration of therapy according to patient response, as determined by heart rate, presence of ectopic activity, blood pressure, urine flow, and, whenever possible, measurements of central venous or pulmonary wedge pressure and cardiac output.

➤*Children:* Dobutamine in dextrose 5% injection may be inappropriate for the dosage requirements for children weighing less than 30 kg. Other dosage forms may be more appropriate.

Cardiac decompensation – Refer to Adults for dosing.

Off-label dosing –

Cardiac output maintenance:

• *Usual dose* – According to the American Heart Association's pediatric advanced life support guidelines, the dosage ranges from 2 to 20 mcg/kg/min administered either IV or intraosseously. Titrate infusion to desired effect.

• *Maximum dose* – 40 mcg/kg/min.

➤*Elderly:* Start at the low end of the dosage range. Elderly patients have a significantly decreased response to dobutamine.

➤*Preparation for administration:*

Conventional vials – At the time of administration, dobutamine must be further diluted in an IV container. Dilute 20 mL of dobutamine in at least 50 mL of diluent and dilute 40 mL of dobutamine in at least 100 mL of diluent. Use one of the following IV solutions as a diluent for the conventional vials: dextrose 5% injection, dextrose 5% and sodium chloride 0.45% injection, dextrose 5% and sodium chloride 0.9% injection, dextrose 10% injection, *Isolyte M* with dextrose 5% injection, Ringer's lactate injection, dextrose 5% in Ringer's lactate injection, *Normosol-M* in dextrose 5% in water, mannitol 20% in water for injection, sodium chloride 0.9% injection, or sodium lactate injection. IV solutions should be used within 24 hours.

Children – The following formula for preparation of the infusion has been suggested:

$$6 \times \frac{\text{desired dose (mcg/kg/min)}}{\text{desired rate (mL/h)}} \times \text{wt (kg)} = \frac{\text{mg drug}}{\text{100 mL fluid}}$$

➤*Administration:* Administer by IV infusion. Not for IV bolus. A calibrated electronic infusion device is recommended for controlling the rate of flow in mL per hour or drops per minute.

Concentrations of up to 5,000 mcg/mL have been administered (250 mg per 50 mL). Determine the final volume administered by the fluid requirements of the patient.

Infusion Rates of Various Dilutions of Dobutamine

Desired delivery rate (mcg/kg/min)	Infusion rate (mL/kg/min)		
	250 mcg/mL[a]	500 mcg/mL[b]	1,000 mcg/mL[c]
2.5	0.01	0.005	0.0025
5	0.02	0.01	0.005
7.5	0.03	0.015	0.0075
10	0.04	0.02	0.01
12.5	0.05	0.025	0.0125
15	0.06	0.03	0.015

[a] 250 mcg/mL of diluent.
[b] 500 mcg/mL or 250 mg per 500 mL of diluent.
[c] 1,000 mcg/mL or 250 mg per 250 mL of diluent.

➤*Admixture compatibility:*

Compatibility – Use one of the following IV solutions as a diluent for the conventional vials: dextrose 5% injection, dextrose 5% and sodium chloride 0.45% injection, dextrose 5% and sodium chloride 0.9% injection, dextrose 10% injection, *Isolyte M* with dextrose 5% injection, Ringer's lactate injection, dextrose 5% in Ringer's lactate injection, *Normosol-M* in dextrose 5% in water, mannitol 20% in water for injection, sodium chloride 0.9% injection, or sodium lactate injection.

Incompatibility – Do not add dobutamine to sodium bicarbonate 5% injection or to any other strongly alkaline solution because dobutamine is inactivated in alkaline solution. Because of potential physical incompatibilities, it is recommended that dobutamine not be mixed with other drugs in the same solution. Dobutamine should not be used in conjunction with other agents or diluents containing both sodium bisulfite and ethanol.

Solutions containing dextrose should not be administered through the same administration set as blood, as this may result in pseudoagglutination or hemolysis.

➤*Storage/Stability:* Store at 15° to 30°C (59° to 86°F). Avoid excessive heat. Protect from freezing. Use IV solutions within 24 hours.

Dobutamine in dextrose 5% injection solutions may exhibit a pink color that, if present, will increase with time. This color change is caused by a slight oxidation of the drug, but there is no significant loss of potency. Do not administer unless solution is clear and container is undamaged. Discard unused portion.

Actions

➤*Pharmacology:* Dobutamine, a synthetic catecholamine, is a direct-acting inotropic agent whose primary activity results from stimulation of the beta receptors of the heart while producing comparatively mild chronotropic, hypertensive, arrhythmogenic, and vasodilative effects. It does not cause the release of endogenous norepinephrine, as does dopamine. In animal studies, dobutamine produces less increase in heart rate and less decrease in peripheral vascular resistance for a given inotropic effect than does isoproterenol.

In patients with depressed cardiac function, dobutamine and isoproterenol increase the cardiac output to a similar degree. In the case of dobutamine, this increase is usually not accompanied by marked increases in heart rate (although tachycardia is occasionally observed), and the cardiac stroke volume is usually increased. In contrast, isoproterenol increases the cardiac index primarily by increasing the heart rate while stroke volume changes little or declines.

The effective infusion rate of dobutamine varies widely from patient to patient, and titration is always necessary. At least in pediatric patients, dobutamine-induced increases in cardiac output and systemic pressure are generally seen in any given patient at lower infusion rates than those that cause substantial tachycardia.

➤*Pharmacokinetics:*

Absorption/Distribution – The onset of action of dobutamine is within 1 to 2 minutes; however, as much as 10 minutes may be required to obtain the peak effect of a particular infusion rate.

Metabolism/Excretion – The plasma half-life of dobutamine in humans is 2 minutes. The principal routes of metabolism are methylation of the catechol and conjugation. In human urine, the major excretion products are the conjugates of dobutamine and 3-O-methyl dobutamine. The 3-O-methyl derivative of dobutamine is inactive.

Contraindications

Idiopathic hypertrophic subaortic stenosis; hypersensitivity to dobutamine.

Do not administer dextrose solutions without electrolytes simultaneously with blood through the same infusion set because of the possibility that pseudoagglutination of red cells may occur.

Warnings/Precautions

➤*Cardiovascular effects:*

Increase in heart rate or blood pressure – Dobutamine may cause a marked increase in heart rate or blood pressure, especially systolic pressure. Approximately 10% of adult patients in clinical studies have had rate increases of 30 beats/min or more, and approximately 7.5% have had a 50 mm Hg or higher increase in systolic pressure. Usually, reduction of dosage promptly reverses these effects. Because dobutamine facilitates atrioventricular conduction, patients with atrial fibrillation are at risk of developing rapid ventricular response. In patients who have atrial fibrillation with rapid ventricular response, use a digitalis preparation prior to institution of therapy with dobutamine. Patients with preexisting hypertension appear to face an increased risk of developing an exaggerated pressor response.

Ectopic activity – Dobutamine may precipitate or exacerbate ventricular ectopic activity, but it rarely has caused ventricular tachycardia.

Use following acute myocardial infarction – Clinical experience with dobutamine following myocardial infarction has been insufficient to establish the safety of the drug for this use. There is concern that any agent that increases contractile force and heart rate may increase the size of an infarction by intensifying ischemia, but it is not known whether dobutamine does this.

➤*Hypovolemia:* Correct hypovolemia with suitable volume expanders before treatment with dobutamine is instituted.

➤*Bolus administration:* Avoid bolus administration of the drug. Clinical evaluation and periodic laboratory determinations are necessary to monitor changes in fluid balance, electrolyte concentrations, and acid-base balance during prolonged parenteral therapy or whenever the condition of the patient warrants such evaluation.

➤*Fluid overload:* The IV administration of solutions may cause fluid and/or solute overloading, resulting in dilution of serum electrolyte concentrations, overhydration, congested states, or pulmonary edema.

➤*Hypokalemia:* Excess administration of potassium-free solutions may result in significant hypokalemia.

Dobutamine, like other beta-2 agonists, can produce a mild reduction in serum potassium concentration, rarely to hypokalemic levels. Accordingly, consider monitoring serum potassium.

➤*Hypersensitivity reactions:* Reactions suggestive of hypersensitivity associated with administration of dobutamine, including skin rash, fever, eosinophilia, and bronchospasm, have been reported occasionally.

➤*Sulfite sensitivity:* Dobutamine products may contain sodium metabisulfite, a sulfite that may cause allergic-type reactions, including anaphylactic symptoms and life-threatening or less severe asthmatic episodes, in certain susceptible people. The overall prevalence of sulfite sensitivity in the general population is unknown and probably low. Sulfite sensitivity is seen more frequently in asthmatic than in nonasthmatic persons.

➤*Special risk:* Use dobutamine and dextrose 5% with caution in patients with known subclinical or overt diabetes mellitus.

➤*Pregnancy:* *Category B.* There are no adequate and well-controlled studies in pregnant women. Passage of dobutamine to the fetus is expected

DOBUTAMINE HYDROCHLORIDE — INJECTION

because of the drug's relativity low molecular weight. Use this drug during pregnancy only if clearly needed.

➤*Lactation:* It is not known whether this drug is excreted in human milk. However, any dobutamine in milk is unlikely to affect an infant because of the drug's poor oral bioavailability and short half-life. Exercise caution when dobutamine is administered to a breast-feeding woman. If a mother requires dobutamine treatment, discontinue breast-feeding for the duration of the treatment.

➤*Children:* Dobutamine has been shown to increase cardiac output and systemic pressure in pediatric patients of every age group. In premature neonates, however, dobutamine is less effective than dopamine in raising systemic blood pressure without causing undue tachycardia, and dobutamine has not been shown to provide any added benefit when given to infants already receiving optimal infusions of dopamine.

➤*Elderly:* Other reported clinical experience suggests that the incidence of significant hypotension is a function of both dose and age; older individuals having a greater incidence of hypotension. According to the American Heart Association guidelines, elderly patients have a significantly reduced response to dobutamine.

In general, cautiously select dosage for an elderly patient, usually starting at the low end of the dosing range, reflecting the greater frequency of decreased hepatic, renal, or cardiac function, and of concomitant disease or drug therapy.

➤*Monitoring:* During the administration of dobutamine, as with any adrenergic agent, continuously monitor electrocardiogram and blood pressure. In addition, monitor pulmonary wedge pressure and cardiac output whenever possible to aid in the safe and effective infusion of dobutamine. Also consider monitoring serum potassium. Clinical evaluation and periodic laboratory determinations are necessary to monitor changes in fluid balance, electrolyte concentrations, and acid-base balance during prolonged parenteral therapy or whenever the condition of the patient warrants such evaluation.

Drug Interactions

Dobutamine Drug Interactions

Precipitant drug	Object drug[a]		Description
Beta-blocking agents (eg, metoprolol, propranolol)	Dobutamine	⬇	Animal studies indicate that dobutamine may be ineffective in patients who have recently received a beta-blocking drug. In such a case, the peripheral vascular resistance may increase. Monitor the clinical response of the patient.
Cimetidine	Dobutamine	⬆	Pharmacologic effects of dobutamine may be increased. Monitor blood pressure. If an interaction is suspected, decrease the dosage of dobutamine.
COMT[b] inhibitors (eg, entacapone, tolcapone)	Dobutamine	⬆	Coadministration of dobutamine and COMT inhibitors may result in inhibition of the pathway responsible for normal catecholamine metabolism. Excessive sympathetic stimulation may result. Use with caution and monitor closely.
Desflurane	Dobutamine	⬆	Death associated with cardiac ischemia has been reported. This drug interaction has not been proven; however, because of its severity, consider the possibility of this drug interaction. Closely monitor for clinical response of the patient.
Guanethidine[c]	Dobutamine	⬆	Guanethidine may increase the pressor response of the direct-acting vasopressors, possibly resulting in severe hypertension. Also, the hypotensive action of guanethidine may be reversed.
Dobutamine	Guanethidine	⬇	
Linezolid	Dobutamine	⬆	Pharmacologic effects of dobutamine may be increased by linezolid. Headache, hyperpyrexia, and hypertension may occur. Coadministration is not recommended without careful monitoring for increases in blood pressure. If coadministration is considered necessary, reduce the initial dose of dobutamine and titrate to desired effect. If severe hypertension occurs, give phentolamine or other alpha-adrenergic blocker.
Methyldopa	Dobutamine	⬆	Coadministration may result in an increased pressor response, possibly resulting in hypertension. Monitor blood pressure closely. If an interaction is suspected, be prepared to discontinue dobutamine or administer phentolamine.
Nitroprusside	Dobutamine	⬆	Preliminary studies indicate that the concomitant use of dobutamine and nitroprusside results in a higher cardiac output and, usually, a lower pulmonary wedge pressure than when either drug is used alone.
Dobutamine	Nitroprusside		
Oxytocic drugs (eg, ergonovine, oxytocin)	Dobutamine	⬆	Coadministration may result in hypertension. The incidence of hypertension decreases when dobutamine is not used prior to administration of the oxytocic drug.
Reserpine	Dobutamine	⬆	Reserpine may potentiate the pressor response of dobutamine, resulting in hypertension. If these agents must be used together, monitor blood pressure and adjust dobutamine dose as needed.
Tricyclic antidepressants (eg, amitriptyline)	Dobutamine	⬆	The pressor response of dobutamine may be potentiated by these agents; use with caution. Closely monitor patients for dysrhythmias and hypertension. Adjust the dobutamine dose as needed.

[a] ⬆ = object drug increased; ⬇ = object drug decreased.
[b] COMT = catechol-o-methyltransferase.
[c] No longer marketed in the United States.

Adverse Reactions

➤*Cardiovascular:*

Increased heart rate, blood pressure, and ventricular ectopic activity – A 10 to 20 mm Hg increase in systolic blood pressure and an increase in heart rate of 5 to 15 beats/min have been noted in most patients (see Warnings/Precautions regarding exaggerated chronotropic and pressor effects). Approximately 5% of patients have had increased premature ventricular beats during infusions. These effects are dose related.

Hypotension – Precipitous decreases in blood pressure have occasionally been described in association with dobutamine therapy. Decreasing the dose or discontinuing the infusion typically results in rapid return of blood pressure to baseline values. In rare cases, however, intervention may be required and reversibility may not be immediate.

Other – Anginal pain, palpitations (1% to 3%).

➤*Local:* Phlebitis has occasionally been reported. Local inflammatory changes have been described following inadvertent infiltration. Isolated cases of cutaneous necrosis (destruction of skin tissue) have been reported.

➤*Miscellaneous:* Nausea, headache, nonspecific chest pain, shortness of breath (1% to 3%). Isolated cases of thrombocytopenia have been reported.

➤*Lab test abnormalities:* Mild reduction in serum potassium concentration, rarely to hypokalemic levels.

Overdosage

➤*Symptoms:* Overdoses of dobutamine have been reported rarely. The following is provided to serve as a guide if such an overdose is encountered.

Toxicity from dobutamine is usually caused by excessive cardiac beta-receptor stimulation. The duration of action of dobutamine is generally short (half-life, 2 minutes) because it is rapidly metabolized by COMT. The symptoms of tox-

DOBUTAMINE HYDROCHLORIDE — INJECTION

icity may include anorexia, nausea, vomiting, tremor, anxiety, palpitations, headache, shortness of breath, and anginal and nonspecific chest pain. The positive inotropic and chronotropic effects of dobutamine on the myocardium may cause hypertension, tachyarrhythmias, myocardial ischemia, and ventricular fibrillation. Hypotension may result from vasodilation.

➤*Treatment:* To obtain up-to-date information about the treatment of overdose, contact a certified regional poison control center at 1-800-222-1222. In managing overdosage, consider the possibility of multiple-drug overdoses, interaction among drugs, and unusual drug kinetics in your patient.

The initial actions to be taken in a dobutamine overdose are discontinuing administration, establishing an airway, and ensuring oxygenation and ventilation. Promptly initiate resuscitative measures. Severe ventricular tachyarrhythmias may be successfully treated with propranolol or lidocaine. Hypertension usually responds to a reduction in dose or discontinuation of therapy.

Protect the patient's airway and support ventilation and perfusion. If needed, meticulously monitor and maintain, within acceptable limits, the patient's vital signs, blood gases, and serum electrolytes.

If the product is ingested, unpredictable absorption may occur from the mouth and the GI tract. Absorption of drugs from the GI tract may be decreased by giving activated charcoal, which, in many cases, is more effective than emesis or lavage; consider charcoal instead of or in addition to gastric emptying. Repeated doses of charcoal over time may hasten elimination of some drugs that have been absorbed. Safeguard the patient's airway when employing gastric emptying or charcoal.

Forced diuresis, peritoneal dialysis, hemodialysis, or charcoal hemoperfusion have not been established as beneficial for an overdose of dobutamine.

Patient Information

Some of these products contain sulfites, which cause allergic reactions in some individuals.

DOPAMINE

Rx	**Dopamine Hydrochloride** (Various, eg, American Regent, Hospira)	**Injection, solution, concentrate**: 40 mg/mL	May contain sodium metabisulfite. In 5 and 10 mL vials.
		80 mg/mL	May contain sodium metabisulfite. In 5 and 10 mL vials.
		160 mg/mL	May contain sodium metabisulfite. In 5 mL vials.
Rx	**Dopamine Hydrochloride in Dextrose 5% Injection** (Various, eg, Baxter, B. Braun McGaw, Hospira)	**Injection, solution**: 200 mg per 250 mL (0.8 mg/mL)	May contain sulfites. In 250 mL premixed single-use containers.
		400 mg per 500 mL (0.8 mg/mL)	May contain sulfites. In 500 mL premixed single-use containers.
		400 mg per 250 mL (1.6 mg/mL)	May contain sulfites. In 250 mL premixed single-use containers.
		800 mg per 500 mL (1.6 mg/mL)	May contain sulfites. In 500 mL premixed single-use containers.
		800 mg per 250 mL (3.2 mg/mL)	May contain sulfites. In 250 mL premixed single-use containers.

DOPAMINE HYDROCHLORIDE — INJECTION

Refer to the general discussion of these products in the Vasopressors Used in Shock class monograph.

WARNING

Antidote for peripheral ischemia – To prevent sloughing and necrosis in ischemic areas, the area should be infiltrated as soon as possible with 10 to 15 mL of sodium chloride 0.9% injection containing phentolamine 5 to 10 mg, an adrenergic blocking agent. Pediatric dosage of phentolamine should be 0.1 to 0.2 mg/kg up to a maximum of 10 mg per dose. A syringe with a fine hypodermic needle should be used, and the solution liberally infiltrated throughout the ischemic area. Sympathetic blockade with phentolamine causes immediate and conspicuous local hyperemic changes if the area is infiltrated within 12 hours. Therefore, phentolamine should be given as soon as possible after the extravasation is noted.

Indications

➤*Hypotension:* Hypotension due to inadequate cardiac output can be managed by administration of low to moderate doses of dopamine, which have little effect on systemic vascular resistance (SVR). At high therapeutic doses, the alpha-adrenergic activity of dopamine becomes more prominent and, thus, may correct hypotension because of diminished SVR. As in the case of other circulatory decompensation states, prognosis is better in patients whose blood pressure and urine flow have not undergone profound deterioration. Therefore, administer dopamine as soon as a definite trend toward decreased systolic and diastolic pressure becomes evident.

➤*Low cardiac output:* Increased cardiac output is related to the direct inotropic effect of dopamine on the myocardium. Increased cardiac output at low or moderate doses appears to be related to a favorable prognosis. Increase in cardiac output has been associated with either static or decreased SVR. Static or decreased SVR associated with low or moderate increments in cardiac output is believed to be a reflection of differential effects on specific vascular beds with increased resistance in peripheral beds (eg, femoral) and concomitant decreases in mesenteric and renal vascular beds. Redistribution of blood flow parallels these changes so that an increase in cardiac output is accompanied by an increase in mesenteric and renal blood flow. In many instances, the renal fraction of the total cardiac output has been found to increase. The increase in cardiac output produced by dopamine is not associated with substantial decreases in systemic vascular resistance as may occur with isoproterenol.

➤*Poor perfusion of vital organs:* Urine flow appears to be one of the better diagnostic signs by which adequacy of vital organ perfusion can be monitored. Nevertheless, observe the patient for signs of reversal of mental confusion or comatose condition. Loss of pallor, increase in toe temperature, and/or adequacy of nail bed capillary filling may also be used as indices of adequate dosage. Clinical studies have shown that when dopamine is administered before urine flow has diminished to levels approximating 0.3 mL/min, prognosis is more favorable. Nevertheless, in a number of oliguric or anuric patients, administration of dopamine has resulted in an increase in urine flow, which, in some cases, reached normal levels. Dopamine may also increase urine flow in patients whose output is within normal limits and, thus, may be of value in reducing the degree of preexisting fluid accumulation. It should be noted that at doses above those optimal for the individual patient, urine flow may decrease, necessitating reduction of dosage. Coadministration of dopamine and diuretic agents may produce an additive or potentiating effect.

➤*Shock:* For the correction of hemodynamic imbalances present in the shock syndrome due to myocardial infarctions, trauma, endotoxic septicemia, open heart surgery, renal failure, and chronic cardiac decompensation as in refractory congestive failure.

➤*Off-label uses:*

Other possible off-label uses – Chronic obstructive pulmonary disease (COPD) (4 mcg/kg/min); congestive heart failure (CHF) (2 to 5 mcg/kg/min); respiratory distress syndrome (RDS) in infants (starting at 5 mcg/kg/min).

Calcium channel blocker overdosage, beta-blocker overdosage, and drug-induced hypovolemic shock.

Administration and Dosage

➤*General dosing considerations:* Dopamine is a potent drug. Dopamine in conventional vials must be diluted before administration.

When appropriate, increase blood volume with whole blood or plasma until central venous pressure is 10 to 15 cm H_2O or pulmonary wedge pressure is 14 to 18 mm Hg.

Treatment of all patients requires constant evaluation of therapy in terms of blood volume, augmentation of cardiac contractility, urine flow, cardiac output, blood pressure, and distribution of peripheral perfusion.

For information on tapering dopamine dosage, see the Discontinuation of Therapy section.

Dosage of dopamine should be adjusted according to the patient's response, with particular attention to diminution of established urine flow rate, increasing tachycardia, or development of new dysrhythmias as indices for decreasing or temporarily suspending the dosage.

As with all potent intravenously (IV) administered drugs, care should be taken to control the rate of administration so as to avoid inadvertent administration of a bolus of drug.

Each patient must be individually titrated to the desired hemodynamic and/or renal response with dopamine. In titrating to the desired increase in systolic blood pressure, the optimum dosage rate for renal response may be exceeded, thus necessitating a reduction in rate after the hemodynamic condition is stabilized.

If a disproportionate rise in diastolic pressure (ie, a marked decrease in pulse pressure) is observed in patients receiving dopamine, the infusion rate should be decreased and the patient observed carefully for further evidence of predominant vasoconstrictor activity, unless such an effect is desired.

➤*Adults:*

Hypotension –

Usual dosage: More than 50% of patients have been satisfactorily maintained on doses of less than 20 mcg/kg/min.

Initial dosage: Begin infusion with 2 to 5 mcg/kg/min in patients who are likely to respond to modest increments of heart force and renal perfusion.

In more severely ill patients, begin with 5 mcg/kg/min.

Dosage titration: In more severely ill patients, increase the dose gradually, using 5 to 10 mcg/kg/min increments, up to 20 to 50 mcg/kg/min as needed.

DOPAMINE HYDROCHLORIDE — INJECTION

If doses in excess of 50 mcg/kg/min are required, check urine output frequently. Should urinary flow begin to decrease in the absence of hypotension, reduction of dopamine dosage should be considered.

Concomitant therapy: Patients who have been treated with monoamine oxidase inhibitors (MAOIs) within 2 to 3 weeks prior to the administration of dopamine should receive initial doses of dopamine not greater than one-tenth of the usual dose.

Low cardiac output –

Usual dosage: More than 50% of patients have been satisfactorily maintained on doses of less than 20 mcg/kg/min.

Initial dosage: Begin infusion with 2 to 5 mcg/kg/min in patients who are likely to respond to modest increments of heart force and renal perfusion.

In more severely ill patients, begin with 5 mcg/kg/min.

Dosage titration: In more severely ill patients, increase the dose gradually, using 5 to 10 mcg/kg/min increments, up to 20 to 50 mcg/kg/min as needed. If doses in excess of 50 mcg/kg/min are required, check urine output frequently. Should urinary flow begin to decrease in the absence of hypotension, reduction of dopamine dosage should be considered.

Concomitant therapy: Patients who have been treated with MAOIs within 2 to 3 weeks prior to the administration of dopamine should receive initial doses of dopamine not greater than one-tenth of the usual dose.

Poor perfusion of vital organs –

Usual dosage: More than 50% of patients have been satisfactorily maintained on doses of less than 20 mcg/kg/min.

Initial dosage: Begin infusion with 2 to 5 mcg/kg/min in patients who are likely to respond to modest increments of heart force and renal perfusion.

In more severely ill patients, begin with 5 mcg/kg/min.

Dosage titration: In more severely ill patients, increase the dose gradually, using 5 to 10 mcg/kg/min increments, up to 20 to 50 mcg/kg/min as needed. If doses in excess of 50 mcg/kg/min are required, check urine output frequently. Should urinary flow begin to decrease in the absence of hypotension, reduction of dopamine dosage should be considered.

Concomitant therapy: Patients who have been treated with MAOIs within 2 to 3 weeks prior to the administration of dopamine should receive initial doses of dopamine not greater than one-tenth of the usual dose.

Shock –

Usual dosage: More than 50% of patients have been satisfactorily maintained on doses of less than 20 mcg/kg/min.

Initial dosage: Begin infusion with 2 to 5 mcg/kg/min in patients who are likely to respond to modest increments of heart force and renal perfusion.

In more severely ill patients, begin with 5 mcg/kg/min.

Dosage titration: In more severely ill patients, increase the dose gradually, using 5 to 10 mcg/kg/min increments, up to 20 to 50 mcg/kg/min as needed. If doses in excess of 50 mcg/kg/min are required, check urine output frequently. Should urinary flow begin to decrease in the absence of hypotension, reduction of dopamine dosage should be considered.

Concomitant therapy: Patients who have been treated with MAOIs within 2 to 3 weeks prior to the administration of dopamine should receive initial doses of dopamine not greater than one-tenth of the usual dose.

➤*Children:* Most reports in children describe dosing that is similar (on a mcg/kg/min basis) to that used in adults. There are scattered reports of infusion rates in neonates up to 125 mcg/kg/min.

Refer to the previous Adults section for more information.

Off-label dosing –

Cardiac output maintenance: According to the American Heart Association's pediatric advanced life support (PALS) guidelines, the dosage ranges from 2 to 20 mcg/kg/min administered either IV or IO (intraosseous). Infusion rates greater than 20 mcg/kg/min may result in excessive vasoconstriction.

Dosages higher than 5 mcg/kg/min produce stimulation of cardiac beta-adrenergic receptors; however, this effect may be reduced in infants and those patients with chronic congestive heart failure.

➤*Elderly:* Start at the low end of the dosage range.

Refer to the previous Adults section for more information.

➤*Discontinuation of therapy:* When discontinuing the infusion, it may be necessary to gradually decrease the dose of dopamine while expanding blood volume with IV fluids, because sudden cessation may result in marked hypotension.

➤*Preparation for administration:* Do not administer if solution is darker than slightly yellow or discolored in any other way. Do not administer unless solution is clear and container is undamaged. Discard unused portion.

Conventional vials – Transfer contents of 1 or more vials by aseptic technique to either 250 or 500 mL of a sterile IV solution (see the Admixture compatibility section).

Parenteral drug products should be inspected visually for particulate matter and discoloration prior to administration, whenever solution and container permit.

➤*Administration:* Dopamine in conventional vials must be diluted before administration.

Dopamine is administered IV through a suitable IV catheter or needle. An IV drip chamber or other suitable metering device is essential for controlling the rate of flow in drops/min. Dopamine should be infused into a large vein whenever possible to prevent the infiltration of perivascular tissue adjacent to the infusion site. Extravasation may cause necrosis and sloughing of the surrounding tissue. Large veins of the antecubital fossa are preferred to veins of the dorsum of the hand or ankle. Less suitable infusion sites should be used only when larger veins are unavailable and the patient's condition requires immediate attention. Administration into an umbilical artery catheter is not recommended. There should be a switch to a more suitable site as soon as possible and the infusion site in use should be continuously monitored for free flow.

➤*Extravasation:* Infuse dopamine into a large vein whenever possible to prevent the possibility of extravasation into tissue adjacent to the infusion site. Extravasation may cause necrosis and sloughing of surrounding tissue. Large veins of the actecubital fossa are preferred to veins in the dorsum of the hand or ankle. Administration into an umbilical arterial catheter is not recommended. Only use less suitable infusion sites when larger veins are unavailable and if the patient's condition requires immediate attention. Switch to more suitable sites as rapidly as possible. Continuously monitor the infusion site for free flow.

If signs or symptoms of extravasation occur, stop the infusion immediately. If possible, withdraw 3 to 5 mL of blood to remove some of the drug. Remove the infusion needle. Delineate the infiltrated area on the patient's skin with a felt-tip marker. Cleanse the area with povidone-iodine and inject phentolamine 5 to 10 mg (reconstituted with 10 mL sodium chloride 0.9% injection) as soon as possible under the skin using a 25-gauge needle. Insert the needle at a 15 degree angle, bevel up, so that a raised area appears. Change the needle after each injection if using multiple injections. (For children, the maximum dose is phentolamine 0.1 to 0.2 mg/kg or 5 mg). Phentolamine may not be effective if more than 12 hours has elapsed since injury. Application of warm compresses to the area for 15 minutes every 6 hours for 48 hours may be useful. Elevate for 48 hours above heart level using a sling or stockinette dressing with an observation window cut in the dressing. Avoid pressure or friction. Do not rub area. Observe for signs of increased erythema, pain, or skin necrosis. If increased symptoms occur, consult a plastic surgeon. Ensure that no medication is given distally to extravasation site. After 48 hours, encourage the patient to use the extremity normally to promote full range of motion.

➤*Admixture compatibility:*

Compatibility – Dopamine is compatible with the following IV solutions: sodium chloride injection; dextrose 5% injection; dextrose 5% and sodium chloride 0.9% injection; dextrose 5% in sodium chloride 0.45% solution; dextrose 5% in lactated Ringer's solution; sodium lactate (⅙ molar) injection; lactated Ringer's injection.

Dopamine has been found to be stable for a minimum of 24 hours after dilution in the sterile IV solutions previously listed. However, as with all IV admixtures, dilution should be made just prior to administration.

Incompatibility – Do not add dopamine injection to sodium bicarbonate or other alkaline IV solutions, since the drug is inactivated in alkaline solution.

Avoid contact with alkalis (including sodium bicarbonate), oxidizing agents, or iron salts.

Mixing of dopamine with alteplase in the same container should be avoided as visible particulate matter has been observed.

It is recommended that dopamine not be added to amphotericin B solutions because amphotericin B is physically unstable in dopamine-containing solutions.

Dextrose solutions without electrolytes should not be administered simultaneously with blood through the same infusion set because of the possibility that pseudoagglutination of red cells may occur.

➤*Storage/Stability:* Store vials at controlled room temperature, 15° to 30°C (59° to 86°F), and premixed single-use containers at 20° to 25°C (68° to 77°F). Brief exposure of premixed single-use containers of up to 40°C (104°F) does not adversely affect the product.

Exposure of pharmaceutical products to heat should be minimized. Avoid excessive heat. Protect from freezing.

Avoid contact with alkalies (including sodium bicarbonate), oxidizing agents, or iron salts. Dopamine has been found to be stable for a minimum of 24 hours after dilution in the sterile IV solutions previously listed. However, as with all IV admixtures, dilution should be made just prior to administration.

Actions

➤*Pharmacology:* Dopamine is a natural catecholamine formed by the decarboxylation of 3,4-dihydroxyphenylalanine (DOPA). It is a precursor to norepinephrine in noradrenergic nerves and is also a neurotransmitter in certain areas of the CNS, especially in the nigrostriatal tract, and in a few peripheral sympathetic nerves.

Dopamine produces positive chronotropic and inotropic effects on the myocardium, resulting in increased heart rate and cardiac contractility. This is accomplished directly by exerting an agonist action on beta-adrenoceptors and indirectly by causing release of norepinephrine from storage sites in sympathetic nerve endings.

➤*Pharmacokinetics:*

Absorption/Distribution – Dopamine's onset of action occurs within 5 minutes of IV administration, and with dopamine's plasma half-life of about 2 minutes, the duration of action is less than 10 minutes. If MAOIs are present, however, the duration may increase to 1 hour. The drug is widely distributed in the body but does not cross the blood-brain barrier to a significant extent.

Metabolism/Excretion – Dopamine is metabolized in the liver, kidney, and plasma by MAO and catechol-O-methyltransferase to the inactive compounds homovanillic acid (HVA) and 3,4-dihydroxyphenylacetic acid. About 25% of the dose is taken up into specialized neurosecretory vesicles (the adrenergic nerve terminals), where it is hydroxylated to form norepinephrine. It has been reported that about 80% of the drug is excreted in the

DOPAMINE HYDROCHLORIDE — INJECTION

urine within 24 hours, primarily as HVA and its sulfate and glucuronide conjugates and as 3,4-dihydroxyphenylacetic acid. A very small portion is excreted unchanged.

Special populations –

Children: The reported clearance rate of dopamine in critically ill infants and children has ranged from 46 to 168 mL/kg/min, with the higher values seen in the younger patients. The apparent volume of distribution in neonates is reported as 0.6 to 4 L/kg, leading to an elimination half-life of 5 to 11 minutes.

Contraindications

Pheochromocytoma; uncorrected tachyarrhythmias; ventricular fibrillation. Solutions containing dextrose may be contraindicated in patients with known allergy to corn or corn products.

Warnings/Precautions

➤*Discontinuation of therapy:* When discontinuing the infusion, it may be necessary to gradually decrease the dose of dopamine while expanding blood volume with IV fluids, since sudden cessation may result in marked hypotension.

➤*Cardiovascular effects:*

Ventricular arrhythmias – If an increased number of ectopic beats are observed, reduce the dose if possible.

Decreased pulse pressure – If a disproportionate rise in the diastolic pressure (ie, a marked decrease in the pulse pressure) is observed in patients receiving dopamine, decrease the infusion rate and the carefully observe the patient for further evidence of predominant vasoconstrictor activity, unless such an effect is desired.

Hypotension – At lower infusion rates, if hypotension occurs, rapidly increase the infusion rate until adequate blood pressure is obtained. If hypotension persists, discontinue dopamine and administer a more potent vasoconstrictor agent, such as norepinephrine.

➤*Fluid overload:* The IV administration of solutions can cause fluid and/or solute overloading, resulting in dilution of serum electrolyte concentrations, overhydration, congested states, or pulmonary edema.

➤*Hypokalemia:* Excess administration of potassium-free solutions may result in significant hypokalemia.

➤*Pump device:* Control of the rate of infusion is essential to avoid inadvertent administration of a bolus of the drug. If administration is controlled by a pumping device, care must be taken to discontinue pumping action before the container runs dry or air embolism may result.

➤*Hypovolemia:* Prior to treatment with dopamine, ensure that hypovolemia is fully corrected, if possible, with either whole blood or plasma as indicated. Monitoring of central venous pressure or left ventricular filling pressure may be helpful in detecting and treating hypovolemia.

➤*Hypoxia, hypercapnia, acidosis:* These conditions, which may also reduce the effectiveness and/or increase the incidence of adverse reactions of dopamine, must be identified and corrected prior to, or concurrently with, administration of dopamine.

➤*Occlusive vascular disease:* Closely monitor patients with a history of occlusive vascular disease (eg, atherosclerosis, arterial embolism, Raynaud disease, cold injury [eg, frostbite], diabetic endarteritis, Buerger disease) for any changes in color or temperature of the skin in the extremities. If a change in skin color or temperature occurs and is thought to be the result of compromised circulation to the extremities, weigh the benefits of continued dopamine infusion against the risk of possible necrosis. This condition may be reversed by either decreasing the rate or discontinuing the infusion.

➤*Extravasation:* See Administration and Dosage for more information.

➤*Sulfite sensitivity:* Some of these products contain sodium metabisulfite or sodium bisulfite; these sulfites may cause allergic-type reactions, including anaphylactic symptoms, and life-threatening or less severe asthmatic episodes in certain susceptible people. The overall prevalence of sulfite sensitivity in the general population is unknown and is probably low. Sulfite sensitivity is seen more frequently in asthmatic than in nonasthmatic people.

➤*Special risk:* Use solutions containing dextrose with caution in patients with known subclinical or overt diabetes mellitus.

➤*Pregnancy: Category C.* There are no adequate and well-controlled studies in pregnant women, and it is not known if dopamine crosses the placental barrier. Dopamine has been used in women with severe toxemia to prevent renal failure in oliguric or anuric eclamptic women, women with severe preeclampsia and oliguria, and women with hypotension undergoing cesarean section. No adverse reactions attributed to dopamine were noted in the fetuses or newborns in these studies. Use dopamine during pregnancy only if the potential benefit justifies the potential risk to the fetus.

Teratogenic – Teratogenicity studies in rats and rabbits at dopamine dosages of up to 6 mg/kg/day IV during organogenesis produced no detectable teratogenic or embryotoxic effects, although maternal toxicity consisting of mortalities, decreased body weight gain, and pharmacotoxic signs were observed in rats. In a published study, dopamine administered at 10 mg/kg subcutaneously for 30 days markedly prolonged metestrus and increased mean pituitary and ovary weights in female rats. Similar administration to pregnant rats throughout gestation or for 5 days starting on gestation day 10 or 15 resulted in decreased body weight gains, increased mortalities, and slight increases in cataract formation among the offspring.

Labor and delivery – In obstetrics, if vasopressor drugs are used to correct hypotension or are added to a local anesthetic solution, the interaction with some oxytocic drugs may cause severe hypertension.

➤*Lactation:* It is not known whether this drug is excreted in human milk. Because many drugs are excreted in human milk, exercise caution when dopamine is administered to a breast-feeding mother. However, according to Briggs' *Drugs in Pregnancy and Lactation*, dopamine is considered to be probably compatible with breast-feeding, although there are no human data.

➤*Children:* Safety and effectiveness in children have not been established. Dopamine has been used in a limited number of children, but such use has been inadequate to fully define proper dosage and limitations for use. Peripheral gangrene has been reported in neonates and children.

Dopamine infusions have been used in patients of every age from birth onwards. There are scattered reports of infusion rates in neonates of up to 125 mcg/kg/min, but most reports in children describe dosing that is similar (on a mcg/kg/min basis) to that used in adults. Except for vasoconstrictive effects caused by inadvertent infusion of dopamine into the umbilical artery, adverse reactions unique to the pediatric population have not been identified, nor have adverse reactions identified in adults been found to be more common in children.

➤*Elderly:* In general, dose selection for an elderly patient should be cautious, usually starting at the low end of the dosing range, reflecting the frequency of decreased hepatic, renal, or cardiac function, and of concomitant disease or other drug therapy.

➤*Lab test abnormalities:* Infusion of dopamine suppresses pituitary secretion of thyroid-stimulating hormone, growth hormone, and prolactin.

➤*Monitoring:* Close monitoring of urine flow, cardiac output, pulmonary wedge pressure, and blood pressure during dopamine infusion is necessary, as in the case of any adrenergic agent. Continuously monitor the infusion site for free flow.

Closely monitor patients with a history of occlusive vascular disease (eg, atherosclerosis, arterial embolism, Raynaud disease, cold injury [eg, frostbite], diabetic endarteritis, Buerger disease) for any changes in color or temperature of the skin in the extremities (see previous section "Occlusive vascular disease").

Monitoring of central venous pressure or left ventricular filling pressure may be helpful in detecting and treating hypovolemia.

Drug Interactions

Dopamine Drug Interactions

Precipitant drug	Object drug[a]		Description
Alpha-blocking agents	Dopamine	⬇	The peripheral vasoconstriction caused by high doses of dopamine are antagonized by alpha-blocking agents. Dopamine-induced renal and mesenteric vasodilation are not antagonized.
Beta-blocking agents (eg, metoprolol, propranolol)	Dopamine	⬇	Cardiac effects of dopamine are antagonized by beta-blocking agents.
Cyclopropane Halogenated hydrocarbon anesthetics (eg, desflurane)	Dopamine	⬆	Halogenated hydrocarbon anesthetics may sensitize the myocardium to the effects of catecholamines. Use of vasopressors may lead to serious arrhythmias; use with extreme caution. Death associated with cardiac ischemia has been reported in patients receiving desflurane with dopamine or dobutamine. This drug interaction has not been proven; however, because of its severity, consider the possibility of this drug interaction.
Diuretics (eg, furosemide)	Dopamine	⬆	Concurrent use of low-dose dopamine and diuretics may cause additive or potentiating effect on urine flow.
Dopamine	Diuretics (eg, furosemide)		
Guanethidine[b]	Dopamine	⬆	Guanethidine may increase the pressor response of the direct-acting vasopressors, possibly resulting in severe hypertension. Also, the hypotensive action of guanethidine may be reversed.
Dopamine	Guanethidine[b]	⬇	
Haloperidol	Dopamine	⬇	Haloperidol can suppress the dopaminergic renal and mesenteric vasodilation induced with low-dose dopamine.

DOPAMINE HYDROCHLORIDE — INJECTION

Dopamine Drug Interactions

Precipitant drug	Object drug[a]		Description
Hydantoins (eg, phenytoin)	Dopamine	↓	The administration of phenytoin during a dopamine infusion may result in profound hypotension and possibly cardiac arrest. Use phenytoin with extreme caution in patients receiving a dopamine infusion. Consider an alternative anticonvulsant.
Methyldopa	Dopamine	↑	Coadministration may result in an increased pressor response, possibly resulting in hypertension. Monitor blood pressure closely.
MAOIs (eg, phenelzine)	Dopamine	↑	Dopamine is metabolized by MAOIs, and inhibition of this enzyme prolongs and potentiates the effect of dopamine. This may result in hypertensive crisis. Avoid coadministration. Patients who have been treated with MAOIs within 2 to 3 weeks prior to dopamine should receive no more than one-tenth of the usual initial dosage. If given inadvertently and hypertension occurs, administer phentolamine.
Oxytocic drugs (eg, oxytocin, ergonovine)	Dopamine	↑	Coadministration may result in hypertension.
Phenothiazines (eg, prochlorperazine)	Dopamine	↓	Phenothiazines can suppress the dopaminergic renal and mesenteric vasodilation induced with low-dose dopamine.
Reserpine	Dopamine	↑	Reserpine may potentiate the pressor response of dopamine, resulting in hypertension. If these agents must be used together, monitor blood pressure.
Tricyclic antidepressants (eg, amitriptyline)	Dopamine	↑	The pressor response of dopamine may be potentiated by these agents; use with caution.

[a] ↑ = object drug increased; ↓ = object drug decreased.
[b] No longer marketed in the United States.

Adverse Reactions

For more information on cardiovascular effects (eg, pulse pressure, blood pressure), sulfite hypersensitivity, and allergic reactions, refer to the Warnings/Precautions section.

The following adverse reactions have been observed, but there are not enough data to support an estimate of their frequency.

➤*Cardiovascular:* Anginal pain; bradycardia; cardiac conduction abnormalities; ectopic beats; hypertension; hypotension; palpitation; tachycardia; vasoconstriction; ventricular arrhythmia (at very high doses); widened QRS complex.

➤*CNS:* Anxiety, headache.

➤*GI:* Nausea, vomiting.

➤*Miscellaneous:* Azotemia, dyspnea, piloerection. Gangrene of the extremities has occurred when moderate to high doses were administered for prolonged periods or in patients with occlusive vascular disease receiving low doses of dopamine. A few cases of peripheral cyanosis have been reported.

Reactions that may occur because of the solution or the technique of administration include febrile response, infection at the injection site, venous thrombosis or phlebitis extending from the injection site, extravasation, and hypervolemia. If an adverse reaction does occur, discontinue the infusion, evaluate the patient, institute appropriate therapeutic countermeasures, and save the remainder of the fluid for examination, if deemed necessary.

Overdosage

➤*Treatment:* In case of accidental overdosage, as evidenced by excessive blood pressure elevation, reduce rate of administration or temporarily discontinue dopamine until the patient's condition stabilizes. Since the duration of action of dopamine is quite short, no additional remedial measures are usually necessary. If these measures fail to stabilize the patient's condition, consider use of the short-acting alpha-adrenergic blocking agent, phentolamine.

Patient Information

Some of these products contain sulfites, which can cause allergic reactions in some individuals.

EPINEPHRINE (Adrenaline)

otc	**Epinephrine Mist** (Various, eg, Alpharma, Major)	**Aerosol; inhalation:** 0.22 mg/spray	May contain alcohol. In 15 mL.
otc	**Primatene Mist** (Armstrong)		With 34% alcohol, CFC[a] 12 and 114. Sulfite-free. In 15 mL with mouthpiece or 15 mL refills.
otc	**S2** (Nephron)	**Solution; inhalation:** 1.125%	Equiv. to racepinephrine hydrochloride 2.25%. With edetate disodium. In 0.5 mL single-use vials.
Rx	**Adrenalin Chloride** (JHP Pharmaceuticals)	**Solution; intranasal:** 1:1,000 (1 mg/mL)	As hydrochloride. With chlorobutanol and sodium bisulfite. In 30 mL.
Rx	**Epinephrine** (Various, eg, Amphastar, Hospira)	**Injection, solution:** 1:10,000 (0.1 mg/mL)	As hydrochloride. May contain sulfites. In 10 mL prefilled syringe and vials.
Rx	**EpiPen Jr** (Dey)	**Injection, solution:** 1:2,000 (0.15 mg per 0.3 mL)	With sodium metabisulfite. Latex-free. In 0.3 mL single-dose auto-injectors.[b]
Rx	**Epinephrine** (Greenstone)	**Injection, solution:** 1:1,000 (0.15 mg per 0.15 mL)	May contain chlorobutanol and sodium bisulfite. In single-dose injectors.
Rx	**Twinject** (Sciele)		With chlorobutanol and sodium bisulfite. Latex-free. In dual-dose auto-injectors.
Rx	**Epinephrine** (Various, eg, Adamis Labs, Greenstone)	**Injection, solution:** 1:1,000 (0.3 mg per 0.3 mL)	May contain chlorobutanol, sodium bisulfite, sodium metabisulfite. In prefilled single dose syringes.
Rx	**EpiPen** (Dey)		With sodium bisulfite. Latex-free. In 0.3 mL single-dose auto-injectors.[b]
Rx	**Twinject** (Sciele)		With chlorobutanol and sodium bisulfite. Latex-free. In dual-dose auto-injectors.
Rx	**Epinephrine** (Various, eg, American Regent, Amphastar,[c] Hospira)	**Injection, solution:** 1:1,000 (1 mg/mL)	As hydrochloride. May contain sulfites. In 1 mL amps and 30 mL vials.
Rx	**Adrenalin Chloride** (JHP Pharmaceuticals)		As hydrochloride. In 1 mL (with sodium bisulfite) and 30 mL (with chlorobutanol and sodium bisulfite) vials.

[a] CFC = chlorofluorocarbon.
[b] Single-dose auto-injectors contain a total of epinephrine 2 mL injection solution.
[c] Product is preservative free, sulfite free.

EPINEPHRINE — INHALATION

Refer to the general discussion of these products in the Vasopressors Used in Shock group monograph. See also Bronchodilators in the Respiratory Agents chapter and Agents for Glaucoma in the Ophthalmic and Otic Agents chapter.

Indications

➤*Bronchial asthma (Rx and OTC):* For temporary relief of shortness of breath, tightness of chest, and wheezing due to bronchial asthma. The inhalation of epinephrine solution 1:100 eases breathing for asthma patients by reducing spasms of bronchial muscles.

Administration and Dosage

➤*Adults:*

Bronchial asthma –

Rx: Treatment should be started at the first symptoms. 1 to 3 inhalations not more often than every 3 hours.

OTC: Start with 1 inhalation, then wait at least 1 minute. If not relieved, use once more. Do not use again for at least 3 hours. Each inhalation delivers epinephrine 0.22 mg.

➤*Children:*

Bronchial asthma – The use of this product by children and adolescents should be supervised by an adult.

4 years of age and older: See Adults for dosing.

➤*Administration:*

Rx – Epinephrine solution 1:100 should be applied with a glass or plastic nebulizer capable of delivering a very fine spray, and which will work with a very small amount of solution.

Approximately 10 drops (not more) of epinephrine solution 1:100 are placed in the reservoir of the nebulizer, the nozzle of which is placed just inside the partially opened mouth. As the bulb is squeezed once or twice, the patient inhales deeply, drawing the vaporized solution into the lungs. Rinsing the mouth with water immediately after using epinephrine solution 1:100 will help prevent the sensation of dryness of mouth and throat, which may otherwise follow.

➤*Storage/Stability:* Do not use the inhalation solution if it is pinkish or darker than slightly yellow or if it contains a precipitate.

Rx – Store between 15° and 25°C (59° and 77°F). Protect from light and freezing.

When the nebulizer contains any liquid and is not in use, it should be stoppered and kept in an upright position. Because of oxidation, epinephrine solution 1:100 will turn pink to brown when exposed to air. Light, heat, alkalies, and certain metals (eg, copper, iron, zinc) will also promote deterioration. A discolored inhalation solution or one containing a precipitate should not be used.

OTC – Store at room temperature 15° and 30°C (59° and 86°F).

Contents under pressure. Do not puncture or throw container into incinerator. Using or storing near open flame or heating above 49°C (120°F) may cause bursting.

Warnings/Precautions

➤*Proper diagnosis:* Do not use this product unless a diagnosis of asthma has been made by a physician.

➤*Hypodermic injection:* Epinephrine solution 1:100 is supplied for use by oral (not nasal) inhalation only. Because of the relatively high concentration, epinephrine solution 1:100 is not suitable for hypodermic injection.

➤*Symptomatic relief:* Do not continue to use this product, but seek medical assistance immediately, if symptoms are not relieved within 20 minutes or become worse.

➤*Excessive use:* Do not use this product more frequently or at higher doses than recommended unless directed by a physician. Excessive use may cause nervousness and rapid heart beat and possibly, adverse effects on the heart.

➤*Special risk:* Do not use this product if you have heart disease, high blood pressure, thyroid disease, or difficulty in urination due to enlargement of the prostate gland unless directed by a physician.

Do not use this product if you have ever been hospitalized for asthma or if you are taking any prescription drug for asthma unless directed by a physician.

➤*Pregnancy: Category C* (per Briggs' *Drugs in Pregnancy and Lactation*) Epinephrine readily crosses the placenta. As with any drug, if you are pregnant, seek the advice of a health professional before using this product.

➤*Lactation:* Epinephrine is excreted in breast milk. As with any drug, if you are breast-feeding a baby, seek the advice of a health professional before using this product.

➤*Children:* Keep this and all drugs out of the reach of children. In case of accidental overdose, seek professional assistance or contact a poison control center immediately.

Drug Interactions

Epinephrine Inhalation Drug Interactions

Precipitant drug	Object drug [a]		Description
Alpha-adrenergic blockers (eg, phentolamine)	Epinephrine	↓	The vasoconstricting and hypertensive effects are antagonized by alpha-adrenergic blocking drugs.
Beta-adrenergic blockers, nonspecific	Epinephrine	↑	Coadministration allows alpha-receptor effects of epinephrine to predominate, causing hypertension and reflex bradycardia.
Cardiac glycosides	Epinephrine	↑	Cardiac glycosides may sensitize the myocardium to the actions of sympathomimetics.
Chlorpromazine	Epinephrine	↓	Chlorpromazine may reverse the pressor effects of epinephrine.
Diuretic drugs	Epinephrine	↓	Diuretic agents may decrease vascular response to pressor drugs such as epinephrine.
Furazolidone	Epinephrine	↑	Furazolidone may increase the pressor sensitivity to epinephrine, possibly resulting in hypertension. Avoid coadministration if possible.
Halogenated hydrocarbon anesthetics, cyclopropane	Epinephrine	↑	Halogenated hydrocarbon anesthetics and cyclopropane may sensitize the myocardium to the effects of epinephrine and may lead to serious arrhythmias; use with extreme caution.
Levothyroxine Antihistamines (eg, chlorpheniramine, tripelennamine, diphenhydramine)	Epinephrine	↑	The pressor response of the direct-acting vasopressors may be potentiated by these agents; use with caution.
Monoamine oxidase inhibitors (MAOIs)	Epinephrine	↑	Although coadministration of an MAOI with an indirect- or mixed-acting sympathomimetic may cause severe headache, hypertension, high fever, and hypertensive crisis, direct-acting sympathomimetics (eg, epinephrine) appear to interact minimally.
Methyldopa	Epinephrine	↑	Coadministration may result in increased pressor response, possibly resulting in hypertension.
Oxytocic drugs	Epinephrine	↑	Coadministration may result in hypertension.
Reserpine	Epinephrine	↑	Reserpine may potentiate the pressor response of epinephrine, resulting in hypertension.
Sympathomimetic drugs (eg, isoproterenol)	Epinephrine	↑	Do not coadminister epinephrine with other sympathomimetic drugs because of possible additive effects and increased toxicity. Combined effects may induce serious cardiac arrhythmias. They may be administered alternately when the preceding effect of other such drugs has subsided.
Tricyclic antidepressants	Epinephrine	↑	The pressor response of the direct-acting vasopressors may be potentiated by these agents; use with caution.
Epinephrine	Guanethidine	↓	Epinephrine may antagonize the effects of guanethidine, resulting in decreased antihypertensive effect and requiring increased dosage of guanethidine.

[a] ↑ = Object drug increased. ↓ = Object drug decreased.

Do not use this product if you are presently taking a prescription drug for high blood pressure or depression without first consulting your physician.

➤*MAOIs:* Do not use this product if you are now taking a prescription monoamine oxidase inhibitor (MAOI) (certain drugs for depression, psychiatric, emotional conditions, or Parkinsons disease), or for weeks after stop-

EPINEPHRINE — INHALATION

ping MAOI drug. If you are uncertain whether your prescription drug contains an MAOI, consult a health professional before taking this product.

Patient Information

➤*OTC:*

Directions for use of mouthpiece – The mouthpiece, which is enclosed in the *Primatene Mist* 15 mL (not the refill size), should be used for inhalation only with *Primatene Mist*.

Take plastic cap off mouthpiece. (For refills, use mouthpiece from previous purchase.)

Care of mouthpiece: The *Primatene Mist* mouthpiece should be washed once a day with hot, soapy water, rinsed thoroughly, and dried with a clean, lint-free cloth.

If the unit becomes clogged and fails to spray, please write and send the clogged unit to: Whitehall-Robins Healthcare, PO Box 26609, Richmond, VA 23261-6609.

EPINEPHRINE — INJECTION

Refer to the general discussion of these products in the Vasopressors Used in Shock group monograph. See also Bronchodilators in the Respiratory Agents chapter and Agents for Glaucoma in the Ophthalmic and Otic Agents chapter.

Indications

➤*1:1,000 (1 mg/mL solution):* Epinephrine 1:1,000 is used to relieve respiratory distress due to bronchospasm, to provide rapid relief of hypersensitivity reactions to drugs and other allergens, and to prolong the action of anesthetics used in local and regional anesthesia. Its cardiac effects may be of use in restoring cardiac rhythm in cardiac arrest due to various causes, but it is not used in cardiac failure or in hemorrhagic, traumatic, or cardiogenic shock.

Epinephrine is used as a hemostatic agent. It is also used in treating mucosal congestion of hay fever, rhinitis, and acute sinusitis; to relieve bronchial asthmatic paroxysms; in syncope because of complete heart block or carotid sinus hypersensitivity; for symptomatic relief of serum sickness, urticaria, or angioneurotic edema; for resuscitation in cardiac arrest following anesthetic accidents; in simple (open-angle) glaucoma; for relaxation of uterine musculature and to inhibit uterine contractions.

➤*1:10,000 (0.1 mg/mL solution):* Epinephrine 1:10,000 injection is indicated for intravenous (IV) injection in the treatment of acute hypersensitivity (anaphylactoid reactions to drugs, animal serums, and other allergens) and in acute asthmatic attacks to relieve bronchospasm not controlled by inhalation or subcutaneous administration of other solutions of the drug.

Epinephrine is used in the treatment and prophylaxis of cardiac arrest in the absence of ventricular fibrillation and attacks of transitory atrioventricular (AV) heart block with syncopal seizures (Stokes-Adams syndrome), but it is not used in cardiac failure or in hemorrhagic, traumatic, or cardiogenic shock. It may also be used to stimulate the heart in syncope due to complete heart block or carotid sinus sensitivity and is used for resuscitation in cardiac arrest following anesthetic accidents.

In acute attacks of ventricular standstill, physical measures should be applied first. When external cardiac compression and attempts to restore the circulation by electrical defibrillation or use of a pacemaker fail, intracardiac puncture and intramyocardial injection of epinephrine may be effective. Note: Intracardiac injection is no longer recommended in Advanced Cardiac Life Support (ACLS) guidelines.

➤*Auto-injectors:* Epinephrine by auto-injector is indicated in the emergency treatment of allergic reactions (type 1) such as anaphylaxis to insect stings or bites, foods, drugs, diagnostic testing substances (eg, radiocontrast media), and other allergens, as well as idiopathic or exercise-induced anaphylaxis. The epinephrine auto-injectors are intended for immediate self-administration by patients who are determined to be at increased risk for anaphylaxis, including those with a history of an anaphylactic reaction. Such reactions may occur within minutes after exposure and consist of flushing, apprehension, syncope, tachycardia, thready or unobtainable pulse associated with a fall in blood pressure, convulsions, vomiting, diarrhea and abdominal cramps, involuntary voiding, wheezing, dyspnea caused by laryngeal spasm, pruritus, rashes, urticaria, or angioedema. The epinephrine auto-injectors are designed as emergency supportive therapy only and are not replacements or substitutes for immediate medical or hospital care.

➤*Off-label uses:* Endoscopic injection therapy with epinephrine or a mixture of epinephrine and saline has been shown to be a safe and effective hemostatic option in the management of acute lower GI bleeding.

Epinephrine is also effective for the treatment of tricyclic antidepressant (and other sodium channel blockers) overdosage, calcium channel blocker overdosage, and beta-blocker overdosage.

In patients with symptomatic bradycardia or hypotension who have failed to respond to atropine and transcutaneous pacing, or if transcutaneous pacing is not available (eg, in the out-of-hospital setting), epinephrine may be used.

Administration and Dosage

➤*General dosing considerations:*

Warning – Medication errors (some resulting in death) have occurred because of inadvertent administration of the 1:1,000 (1 mg/mL) concentration instead of 1:10,000 (0.1 mg/mL). The 1:1,000 (1 mg/mL) solution must be diluted before administering IV.

The following dosing information is according to the prescribing information. See also Off-Label Dosing for recommendations from the American Heart Association.

➤*Adults:*

Anaphylaxis – See also Off-Label Dosing for recommendations from the American Heart Association.

1:1,000 (1 mg/mL) solution: 0.2 to 1 mg (mL) subcutaneously or intramuscularly (IM). Start with a small dose and increase if required. Repeat every 10 to 15 minutes as needed.

1:10,000 (0.1 mg/mL) solution: 0.1 to 0.25 mg (1 to 2.5 mL) administered slowly IV. May repeat every 5 to 15 minutes as needed.

Epinephrine auto-injectors: 0.3 mg IM or subcutaneously into the anterolateral aspect of the thigh, through clothing if necessary. Repeat injection with an additional epinephrine auto-injector as necessary. (See also Administration.)

Asthma – See also Off-Label Dosing for recommendations from the American Heart Association.

1:1,000 (1 mg/mL) solution: 0.2 to 1 mg (mL) subcutaneously. Start with a small dose and increase if required. May also be given IM, but the subcutaneous route is preferred.

1:10,000 (0.1 mg/mL) solution: 0.1 to 0.25 mg (1 to 2.5 mL) injected slowly IV.

Cardiac stimulation – See also Off-Label Dosing for recommendations from the American Heart Association.

1:1,000 (1 mg/mL) solution: The effect of IV administration of 1:10,000 (0.1 mg/mL) may only last a few minutes, so the IV dose may be followed with 0.3 mg (0.3 mL) of 1:1,000 (1 mg/mL) solution administered subcutaneously.

A previous dosing recommendation for cardiac resuscitation was 0.5 mg (mL) diluted to 10 mL with sodium chloride injection and administered IV or intracardially to restore myocardial contractility. External cardiac massage should follow intracardial administration to permit the drug to enter coronary circulation. The drug should be used secondarily to unsuccessful attempts with physical or electromechanical methods. Note: Intracardiac injection is no longer recommended in ACLS guidelines.

Intracardiac injection should only be administered by personnel well trained in the technique, if there has not been sufficient time to establish an IV route.

1:10,000 (0.1 mg/mL) solution: 0.1 to 1 mg (1 to 10 mL) of 1:10,000 (0.1 mg/mL) solution, repeated every 5 minutes, if necessary. Epinephrine is administered by IV injection and/or, in cardiac arrest, by intracardiac injection into the left ventricular chamber. Intracardiac injection should only be administered by personnel well trained in the technique, if there has not been sufficient time to establish an IV route. Note: Intracardiac injection is no longer recommended in ACLS guidelines.

Intraspinal use – Usual dose is 0.2 to 0.4 mL (0.2 to 0.4 mg) of 1:1,000 (1 mg/mL) solution added to anesthetic spinal fluid mixture. Epinephrine 1:100,000 (0.01 mg/mL) to 1:20,000 (0.05 mg/mL) is the usual concentration employed for use with local anesthetics. Intraspinal injection should only be administered by a trained specialist.

Ophthalmologic use – For producing conjunctival decongestion, controlling hemorrhage, producing mydriasis, and reducing intraocular pressure, use a concentration of 1:10,000 (0.1 mg/mL) to 1:1,000 (1 mg/mL).

Off-label dosing – The following dosages are according to the American Heart Association guidelines for cardiopulmonary resuscitation and emergency cardiovascular care.

Anaphylaxis: 0.3 to 0.5 mg IM every 15 to 20 minutes as needed. The 1:1,000 (1 mg/mL) concentration is recommended.

If the anaphylaxis is severe with life-threatening symptoms, administer epinephrine 0.1 mg by slow IV injection over 5 minutes. A 1:10,000 (0.1 mg/mL) concentration is recommended. If frequent epinephrine injections are anticipated, a continuous IV infusion (1 to 4 mcg/min) may be used.

For anaphylactic reaction progressing to cardiac arrest, use high-dose epinephrine in a sequence such as 1 to 3 mg IV over 3 minutes followed by 3 to 5 mg IV over 3 minutes, and then 4 to 10 mcg/min infusion.

Asthma: For acute severe asthma, the recommend dosage is 0.01 mg/kg divided into 3 doses of approximately 0.3 mg administered subcutaneously at 20-minute intervals. The 1:1,000 (1 mg/mL) concentration is recommended.

Asystole/Pulseless electrical activity: 1 mg IV push or intraosseous push every 3 to 5 minutes until return of spontaneous circulation.

Epinephrine may also be given via endotracheal tube at a dose of 2 to 2.5 mg. Dilute the endotracheal tube dose in 5 to 10 mL of sterile water or 50% isotonic chloride solution.

Symptomatic bradycardia or hypotension: As a second-line treatment for symptomatic bradycardia or hypotension, the initial dosage is 1 mcg/min IV infusion titrated to desired hemodynamic response, which is typically achieved at a dose of 2 to 10 mcg/min.

Ventricular fibrillation/pulseless ventricular tachycardia: The dosage for adult cardiac arrest is 1 mg IV push or intraosseous push every 3 to 5 minutes until return of spontaneous circulation.

Epinephrine may also be given via endotracheal tube at a dose of 2 to 2.5 mg. Dilute the dose in 5 to 10 mL of sterile water or 50% isotonic chloride solution.

➤*Children:*

Anaphylaxis –

1:1,000 (1 mg/mL) solution:

- *Usual dosage* – 0.01 mg/kg (or 0.3 mg/m^2) up to a maximum of 0.5 mg administered subcutaneously. Repeat every 15 minutes for 2 doses, then every 4 hours as needed.
- *Maximum dose* – 0.5 mg/dose.

EPINEPHRINE — INJECTION

1:10,000 (0.1 mg/mL) solution: 0.3 mg (3 mL) of 1:10,000 (0.1 mg/mL) solution administered slowly IV, repeated every 15 minutes for 3 or 4 doses, if necessary.

Epinephrine auto-injectors: Dosage based on patient body weight: 15 to 29 kg, 0.15 mg IM; 30 kg or more, 0.3 mg IM. Repeat injections as necessary. (See also Administration.)

Asthma –

Children:

• *Usual dosage* – 0.01 mg/kg (or 0.3 mg/m^2) of 1:1,000 (1 mg/mL) solution to a maximum of 0.5 mg subcutaneously, repeated every 4 hours as needed.

• *Maximum dose* – 0.5 mg/dose.

Infants: 0.05 mg subcutaneously is an adequate initial dose, and this may be repeated at 20- to 30-minute intervals in the management of asthma attacks.

Neonates: 0.01 mg/kg of 1:1,000 (1 mg/mL) solution subcutaneously.

Cardiac stimulation – See also Off-Label Dosing for recommendations from the American Heart Association.

1:10,000 (0.1 mg/mL) solution: 0.005 to 0.01 mg/kg (0.05 to 0.1 mL) of 1:10,000 (0.1 mg/mL) solution by IV injection and/or in cardiac arrest, by intracardiac injection into the left ventricular chamber, repeated every 5 minutes, if necessary.

Off-label dosing –

Asystole/Pulseless electrical activity:

• *Children –*

Usual dosage: 0.01 mg/kg (0.1 mL/kg) of 1:10,000 (0.1 mg/mL) solution administered by IV push or intraosseous push every 3 to 5 minutes until return of spontaneous circulation.

Higher epinephrine doses may be used in exceptional circumstances (eg, beta-blocker overdosage). Routine use of high-dose epinephrine (0.2 mg/kg) has not been shown to improve survival benefit, and it may actually be harmful (particularly in asphyxia).

Maximum dose: 1 mg IV push or intraosseous push; 10 mg endotracheal tube.

Alternative dosage: If epinephrine is given via endotracheal tube, the dose is 0.1 mg/kg (0.1 mL/kg) of 1:1,000 (1 mg/mL) solution. Follow each endotracheal tube dose with at least 5 mL of 50% isotonic chloride solution.

• *Neonates –*

Usual dosage: 0.01 to 0.03 mg/kg/dose given by IV push every 3 to 5 minutes as needed. Higher doses are not recommended. Use the 1:10,000 (0.1 mg/mL) concentration.

Alternative dosage: While IV access is being obtained, consider administering up to 0.1 mg/kg through the endotracheal tube. Low-dose epinephrine via endotracheal tube is not effective. Follow the endotracheal tube dose with at least 5 mL of 50% isotonic chloride solution. Use the 1:10,000 (0.1 mg/mL) concentration.

Maintenance of cardiac output: Because of great interpatient variability, the infusion should be titrated to the desired effect. Low dosages (less than 0.3 mcg/kg/min) usually result in beta-adrenergic action (potent inotropy and decreased systemic vascular resistance). Higher dosages (more than 0.3 mcg/kg/min) produce alpha-adrenergic vasoconstriction.

Symptomatic bradycardia:

• *Children –*

Usual dosage: 0.01 mg/kg (0.1 mL/kg) of 1:10,000 (0.1 mg/mL) solution administered by IV push or intraosseous push every 3 to 5 minutes until return of spontaneous circulation.

Maximum dose: 1 mg IV push or intraosseous push; 10 mg endotracheal tube.

Alternative dosage: If epinephrine is given via endotracheal tube, the dose is 0.1 mg/kg (0.1 mL/kg) of 1:1,000 (1 mg/mL) solution. May repeat every 3 to 5 minutes. Follow each endotracheal tube dose with at least 5 mL of 50% isotonic chloride solution.

• *Neonates –*

Usual dosage: 0.01 to 0.03 mg/kg/dose given by IV push every 3 to 5 minutes as needed. Higher doses are not recommended. Use the 1:10,000 (0.1 mg/mL) concentration.

Alternative dosage: While IV access is being obtained, consider administering up to 0.1 mg/kg through the endotracheal tube. Low-dose epinephrine via endotracheal tube is not effective. Follow the endotracheal tube dose with at least 5 mL of 50% isotonic chloride solution. Use the 1:10,000 (0.1 mg/mL) concentration.

Ventricular fibrillation/pulseless ventricular tachycardia:

• *Children –*

Usual dosage: 0.01 mg/kg (0.1 mL/kg) of 1:10,000 (0.1 mg/mL) solution administered by IV push or intraosseous push every 3 to 5 minutes until return of spontaneous circulation.

Maximum dose: 1 mg IV push or intraosseous push; 10 mg endotracheal tube.

Alternative dosage: If epinephrine is given via endotracheal tube, the dose is 0.1 mg/kg (0.1 mL/kg) of 1:1,000 (1 mg/mL) solution. Follow each endotracheal tube dose with at least 5 mL of 50% isotonic chloride solution.

• *Neonates –*

Usual dosage: 0.01 to 0.03 mg/kg/dose given by IV push every 3 to 5 minutes as needed. Higher doses are not recommended. Use the 1:10,000 (0.1 mg/mL) concentration.

Alternative dosage: While IV access is being obtained, consider administering up to 0.1 mg/kg through the endotracheal tube. Low-dose epinephrine via endotracheal tube is not effective. Follow the endotracheal tube dose with at least 5 mL of 50% isotonic chloride solution. Use the 1:10,000 (0.1 mg/mL) concentration.

➤*Elderly:* Use with caution.

➤*Extravasation:* Tissue necrosis may develop if extravasation occurs. To treat extravasation, initial therapy may consist of applying warm compresses, submersion into warm water, and/or topical application of nitroglycerin paste. Consultation with a hand specialist is also recommended.

If the noninvasive therapies are inadequate, consider infiltrating phentolamine within 12 hours of extravasation. For adults, infiltrate 5 to 10 mg (diluted in 10 mL of 50% isotonic chloride solution) into the site of extravasation. (Do not exceed 0.1 to 0.2 mg/kg or 5 mg total.) For children, infiltrate phentolamine 0.1 to 0.2 mg/kg (diluted in 10 mL of 50% isotonic chloride solution) into the area of extravasation. If phentolamine is effective, then hyperemia should return within 1 hour.

A combination of phentolamine/lidocaine has also been used for treatment of epinephrine-induced ischemia of the hands and digits. For adults, dilute phentolamine 1.5 mg in 1 mL solution plus 1 mL of lidocaine 2%. For children, dilute phentolamine 0.015 to 0.02 mg/kg in 0.5 mL solution plus 0.5 mg/kg of lidocaine 2%. Inject subcutaneously into the area proximal to the site of extravasation; observe for return of hyperemia.

➤*Preparation for administration:* Do not remove ampules from carton until ready to use. Do not use the injection if its color is pinkish or darker than slightly yellow or if it contains a precipitate. Do not administer unless solution is clear and container is intact. Discard unused portion.

➤*Administration:* Subcutaneous administration results in slower absorption and delayed attainment of maximal plasma levels. If given IM, injection into the buttocks should be avoided.

1:1,000 (1 mg/mL) solution – May be administered subcutaneously, IM, and, when diluted, it may be administered intracardially or IV. Administer intraspinally by adding to anesthetic spinal fluid mixture. Note: Intracardiac injection is no longer recommended in ACLS guidelines.

For bronchial asthma and certain allergic manifestations (eg, angioedema, urticaria, serum sickness, anaphylactic shock), use epinephrine subcutaneously. According to ACLS guidelines, IM injection is the preferred route of administration for patients with anaphylaxis with signs of systemic reaction. See also Off-Label Dosing for recommendations from the American Heart Association.

1:10,000 (0.1 mg/mL) solution – Epinephrine 1:10,000 (1 mg/mL) injection is administered by IV injection or, in cardiac arrest, by intracardiac injection into the left ventricular chamber or via endotracheal tube directly into the bronchial tree. Note: Intracardiac injection is no longer recommended in ACLS guidelines. See also Adults Off-Label Dosing for recommendations from the American Heart Association.

Auto-injectors – Do not inject IV. Only inject into the anterolateral aspect of the thigh. Do not inject into the buttock because this may not provide effective treatment of anaphylaxis. More than 2 sequential doses should only be administered under direct medical supervision. The epinephrine auto-injectors are designed as emergency supportive therapy only and are not replacements or substitutes for immediate medical or hospital care.

Before using, check to make sure the solution in the auto-injector is not discolored. Replace the auto-injector if the solution is discolored or contains a precipitate. Avoid possible inadvertent intravascular administration.

Epinephrine auto-injectors, which provide a dose of 0.15 mg, may be more appropriate for patients weighing less than 30 kg. However, the prescribing health care provider has the option of prescribing more or less than 0.15 mg, based on careful assessment of each individual patient and recognizing the life-threatening nature of the reactions for which this drug is being prescribed. Consider using other forms of injectable epinephrine if doses lower than 0.15 mg are felt to be necessary.

Twinject is capable of delivering 2 doses of either 0.15 mg or 0.3 mg each. The first dose is available for auto-injection by the patient, and the second dose is available for manual injection by the patient following a partial disassembly of *Twinject*.

➤*Storage/Stability:* Store at controlled room temperature, 15° to 30°C (59° to 86°F). Protect from light and store in light-resistant containers. Do not freeze.

Vial and contents must be discarded 30 days after initial use.

Epinephrine deteriorates rapidly on exposure to air or light, turning pink from oxidation to adrenochrome and brown from the formation of melanin. Solutions that show evidence of discoloration should be replaced. Do not use if the injection is pinkish or darker than slightly yellow or it contains a precipitate.

Epinephrine is readily destroyed by alkalies and oxidizing agents. In the latter category are oxygen, chlorine, bromine, iodine, permanganates, chromates, nitrites, and salts of easily reducible metals, especially iron.

Actions

➤*Pharmacology:* Epinephrine is a sympathomimetic drug. It activates an adrenergic receptive mechanism on effector cells and imitates all actions of the sympathetic nervous system except those on the arteries of the face and sweat glands. The actions of epinephrine resemble the effects of stimulation of adrenergic nerves. To a variable degree it acts on both alpha and beta receptor sites of sympathetic effector cells, and is the most potent alpha receptor activator. Its most prominent actions are on the beta receptors of the heart, vascular and other smooth muscle. When given by rapid IV injection, it produces a rapid rise in blood pressure, mainly systolic, by:

1.) direct stimulation of cardiac muscle which increases the strength of ventricular contraction

EPINEPHRINE — INJECTION

2.) increasing the heart rate
3.) constriction of the arterioles in the skin, mucosa, and splanchnic areas of the circulation

When given by slow IV injection, epinephrine usually produces only a moderate rise in systolic and a fall in diastolic pressure. Although some increases in pulse pressure occurs, there is usually no great elevation in mean blood pressure. Accordingly, the compensatory reflex mechanisms that come into play with a pronounced increase in blood pressure do not antagonize the direct cardiac actions of epinephrine as much as with catecholamines that have a predominant action on alpha receptors.

Total peripheral resistance decreases by action of epinephrine on beta receptors of the skeletal muscle vasculature and blood flow is thereby enhanced. Usually, this vasodilator effect of the drug on the circulation predominates so that the modest rise in systolic pressure that follows slow injection or absorption is mainly the result of direct cardiac stimulation and increase in cardiac output. In some instances, peripheral resistance is not altered or may even rise owing to a greater ratio of alpha to beta activity in different vascular areas.

Epinephrine relaxes the smooth muscles of the bronchi and iris and is a physiologic antagonist of histamine. The drug also produces an increase in blood sugar and glycogenolysis in the liver.

➤*Pharmacokinetics:*

Absorption / Distribution – IV injection produces an immediate and intensified response. Following IV injection, epinephrine disappears rapidly from the bloodstream.

Metabolism / Excretion – The large portion of injection doses is excreted in the urine as inactivated compounds. The remainder is excreted in the urine as unchanged or conjugated compounds.

The drug becomes fixed in the tissues and is rapidly inactivated chiefly by enzymatic transformation in the liver and other tissues to metanephrine or normetanephrine, either of which is subsequently conjugated and excreted in the urine in the form of sulfates and glucuronides. Either sequence results in the formation of 3-methoxy-4-hydroxy-mandelic acid (vanillylmandelic acid: VMA), which also is detectable in the urine.

Contraindications

Hypersensitivity to sympathomimetic amines; narrow-angle glaucoma; shock (nonanaphylactic); during general anesthesia with halogenated hydrocarbons or cyclopropane; organic brain damage. Epinephrine is also contraindicated with local anesthesia of certain areas (eg, fingers, toes) because of the danger of vasoconstriction producing sloughing of tissue; in labor because it may delay the second stage; in cardiac dilatation and coronary insufficiency.

Except as diluted for admixture with local anesthetics to reduce absorption and prolong action, epinephrine should not ordinarily be used in those cases where vasopressor drugs may be contraindicated (eg, in thyrotoxicosis, diabetes, in obstetrics when maternal blood pressure is in excess of 130/80 and in hypertension and other cardiovascular disorders).

There are no absolute contraindications to the use of epinephrine in a life-threatening situation.

Warnings/Precautions

➤*Extravasation:* Tissue necrosis may develop if extravasation occurs. (See also Administration and Dosage.)

Accidental injection into the digits, hands, or feet may result in loss of blood flow to the affected area and should be avoided. If there is an accidental injection into these areas, advise the patient to go immediately to the nearest emergency room for treatment. Epinephrine auto-injectors should only be injected into the anterolateral aspect of the thigh. (See also Administration and Dosage.)

➤*Cardiovascular effects:* Inadvertently induced high arterial blood pressure may result in angina pectoris (especially when coronary insufficiency is present) or aortic rupture.

Epinephrine may induce potentially serious cardiac arrhythmias in patients not suffering from heart disease, patients with organic heart disease, or patients who are receiving drugs that sensitize the myocardium. With epinephrine 1:10,000 (0.1 mg/mL), a paradoxical but transient lowering of blood pressure, bradycardia, and apnea may occur immediately after injection.

Although epinephrine can produce ventricular fibrillation, its actions in restoring electrical activity in asystole and in enhancing defibrillation are well documented. However, use it with caution in patients with ventricular fibrillation.

In patients with prefibrillatory rhythm, IV epinephrine must be used with extreme caution because of its excitatory action on the heart. Since the myocardium is sensitized to the drug by many anesthetic agents, epinephrine may convert asystole to ventricular fibrillation if used in the treatment of anesthetic cardiac accidents.

➤*Cerebrovascular effects:* Overdosage or inadvertent IV injection may cause cerebrovascular hemorrhage resulting from the sharp rise in blood pressure.

➤*Pulmonary edema:* Fatalities may result from pulmonary edema because of the peripheral constriction and cardiac stimulation produced.

➤*Hypovolemia:* Use is not a substitute for the replacement of blood, plasma, fluids, and electrolytes, which should be restored promptly when loss has occurred.

➤*Sulfite sensitivity:* Epinephrine is the preferred treatment for serious allergic or other emergency situations, even though some of these products may contain sodium metabisulfite, a sulfite that may in other products cause allergic-type reactions, including anaphylactic symptoms or life-threatening or less severe asthmatic episodes in certain susceptible persons. The alternatives to using epinephrine in a life-threatening situation may not be satisfactory. The presence of a sulfite in this product should not deter administration of the drug for treatment of serious allergic or other emergency situations.

➤*Renal function impairment:* Parenterally administered epinephrine initially may produce constriction of renal blood vessels and decrease urine formation.

➤*Special risk:* Use epinephrine cautiously in patients with hyperthyroidism, hypertension, diabetes, bronchial asthma and emphysema with degenerative heart disease, and psychoneurotic illness. All vasopressors should be used cautiously in patients taking MAO inhibitors.

Administer with extreme caution to patients who have cardiovascular disease.

Epinephrine auto-injectors – Some patients may be at greater risk of developing adverse reactions after epinephrine administration. These include the following: hyperthyroid persons, persons with cardiovascular disease, hypertension, or diabetes, elderly patients, pregnant women and pediatric patients under 30 kg (66 lbs) body weight using *EpiPen* and pediatric patients under 15 kg (33 lbs) body weight using *EpiPen Jr*.

Despite these concerns, epinephrine is essential for the treatment of anaphylaxis. Therefore, patients with these conditions or any other person who might be in a position to administer epinephrine auto-injectors to patients experiencing anaphylaxis should be carefully instructed in regard to the circumstances under which this lifesaving medication should be used.

➤*Pregnancy: Category C.* Epinephrine readily crosses the placenta but human teratogenicity has not been suspected. A mother was given epinephrine IV as treatment for severe hypotension secondary to an allergic reaction, and her 28-week-old fetus developed intrauterine anoxic insult. Epinephrine may have contributed to this effect on the fetus. The fetus, delivered at 34 weeks' gestation, had evidence of intracranial hemorrhage at birth and died 4 days later. Based on epinephrine's pharmacologic action, it may theoretically decrease uterine blood flow. If a pressor agent is required for maternal hypotension, consider using ephedrine.

Epinephrine has been shown to be teratogenic in small animals when given in doses about 25 times the human dose. Epinephrine has been shown to have developmental effects when administered subcutaneously in rabbits at a dose of 1.2 mg/kg daily for 2 to 3 days (approximately 30 times the maximum recommended daily subcutaneous or IM dose on a mg/m^2 basis), in mice at a subcutaneous dose of 1 mg/kg daily for 10 days (approximately 7 times the maximum daily subcutaneous or IM dose on a mg/m^2 basis), and in hamsters at a subcutaneous dose of 0.5 mg/kg daily for 4 days (approximately 5 times the maximum daily subcutaneous or IM dose on a mg/m^2 basis). These effects were not seen in mice at a subcutaneous dose of 0.5 mg/kg daily for 10 days (approximately 3 times the maximum recommended daily subcutaneous or IM dose on a mg/m^2 basis). There are no adequate and well-controlled studies in pregnant women. It is also not known whether epinephrine can cause fetal harm when administered to a pregnant woman or can affect reproduction capacity. Give epinephrine to a pregnant woman only if clearly needed and if anticipated benefits outweigh possible hazards.

Labor and delivery – Parenteral administration of epinephrine if used to support blood pressure during low or other spinal anesthesia for delivery can cause acceleration of fetal heart rate and should not be used in obstetrics when maternal blood pressure exceeds 130/80.

➤*Lactation:* Epinephrine is likely to be excreted in breast milk. However, it is destroyed in the infant's GI tract and therefore it is unlikely that any would be absorbed (unless the infant is in the early neonatal period or premature). Decide whether to discontinue breast-feeding or the drug, taking into account the importance of the drug to the mother.

➤*Children:* Epinephrine may be given safely to pediatric patients at a dosage appropriate to body weight. Syncope has occurred following the administration of epinephrine to asthmatic children.

➤*Elderly:* Administer with caution to elderly patients.

Drug Interactions

Epinephrine Injection Drug Interactions

Precipitant drug	Object drug[a]		Description
Alpha-adrenergic blockers (eg, phentolamine), nitrites	Epinephrine	⬇	The vasoconstricting and pressor effects of epinephrine are antagonized by alpha-adrenergic blocking drugs and nitrites.
Antihistamines (eg, chlorpheniramine, diphenhydramine)	Epinephrine	⬆	The pressor response of the direct-acting vasopressors may be potentiated by these agents; use with caution.
Beta-adrenergic blockers, nonspecific (eg, propranolol)	Epinephrine	⬆	Coadministration allows alpha-receptor effects of epinephrine to predominate, causing hypertension and reflex bradycardia.
Cardiac glycosides (eg, digoxin)	Epinephrine	⬆	Cardiac glycosides may sensitize the myocardium to the actions of sympathomimetics.

EPINEPHRINE — INJECTION

Epinephrine Injection Drug Interactions

Precipitant drug	Object drug[a]		Description
Chlorpromazine	Epinephrine	⬇	Chlorpromazine may reverse the pressor effects of epinephrine.
COMT[b] inhibitors (ie, entacapone, tolcapone)	Epinephrine	⬆	Coadministration may result in inhibition of the pathway responsible for normal catecholamine metabolism. Excessive sympathetic stimulation may result.
Diuretic agents	Epinephrine	⬇	Diuretic agents may decrease vascular response to pressor drugs such as epinephrine.
Furazolidone[c]	Epinephrine	⬆	Furazolidone may increase the pressor sensitivity to epinephrine, possibly resulting in headache, hyperpyrexia, and hypertension (possibly hypertensive crisis and intracranial hemorrhage). Avoid coadministration if possible.
Halogenated hydrocarbon anesthetics (eg, halothane), cyclopropane	Epinephrine	⬆	Halogenated hydrocarbon anesthetics and cyclopropane may sensitize the myocardium to the arrhythmic action of epinephrine and may lead to serious arrhythmias; coadministration is contraindicated.
Levothyroxine	Epinephrine	⬆	The pressor response of the direct-acting vasopressors may be potentiated by levothyroxine; use with caution.
Linezolid	Epinephrine	⬆	Linezolid may increase the pharmacologic effects of sympathomimetics, possibly resulting in headache, hyperpyrexia, and hypertension. Careful monitoring for increases in blood pressure is needed if used concurrently. Adjust the epinephrine dosage as needed. This interaction is most commonly seen with indirect- and mixed-acting sympathomimetics; direct-acting sympathomimetics (eg, epinephrine) appear to interact minimally.
Methyldopa	Epinephrine	⬆	Coadministration may result in increased pressor response, possibly resulting in hypertension.
MAOIs	Epinephrine	⬆	Use with caution.
Oxytocic drugs	Epinephrine	⬆	Coadministration may result in hypertension.
Rauwolfia alkaloids (ie, reserpine)	Epinephrine	⬆	Reserpine may potentiate the pressor response of epinephrine, resulting in hypertension.
Sympathomimetic drugs (eg, isoproterenol)	Epinephrine	⬆	Do not coadminister epinephrine with other sympathomimetic drugs because of possible additive effects and increased toxicity. Combined effects may induce serious cardiac arrhythmias. They may be administered alternately when the preceding effect of other such drugs has subsided.
Tricyclic antidepressants (eg, amitriptyline, imipramine)	Epinephrine	⬆	The pressor response of the direct-acting vasopressors may be potentiated by these agents; use with caution.
Epinephrine	Bromocriptine	⬆	Epinephrine may increase the risk of bromocriptine toxicity. If concurrent use cannot be avoided, then closely monitor the patient.
Epinephrine	Guanethidine[c]	⬇	Epinephrine may antagonize the effects of guanethidine, resulting in decreased antihypertensive effect and requiring increased dosage of guanethidine.

[a] ⬆ = object drug increased; ⬇ = object drug decreased.
[b] COMT = Catechol-O-methyltransferase.
[c] This drug is no longer marketed in the United States.

➤*Digitalis glycosides and diuretic agents:* Use of epinephrine with excessive doses of digitalis, mercurial diuretics, quinidine, or other drugs that sensitize the heart to arrhythmias is not recommended. Anginal pain may be induced when coronary insufficiency is present.

➤*Drug/Lab test interactions:*
Noninteraction – Sodium chloride added to render the solution isotonic for injection of the active ingredient is present in amounts insufficient to affect serum electrolyte balance of sodium (Na^+) and chloride (Cl^-) ions.

Adverse Reactions

➤*Cardiovascular:* Anginal pain in patients with angina pectoris or coronary artery disease; cardiac arrhythmias; excessive rise in blood pressure (which has caused cerebral hemorrhage); palpitations (transient).

Arrhythmias, including fatal ventricular fibrillation, have been reported in patients with underlying cardiac disease or certain drugs.

➤*CNS:* Apprehensiveness; dizziness; restlessness; cerebral hemorrhage; hemiplegia; subarachnoid hemorrhage; transient symptoms of anxiety, fear, headache; tremor; weakness.

➤*Dermatologic:* Pallor, sweating.

➤*GI:* Nausea, vomiting.

➤*Local:* Repeated local injections can result in necrosis at sites of injection from vascular constriction.

Accidental injection into the digits, hands, or feet may result in loss of blood flow to the affected area. Other symptoms may include increased heart rate, local reactions, including injection-site pallor, coldness, and hypoesthesia or injury at the injection site resulting in bruising, bleeding, discoloration, erythema, or skeletal injury. (See also Administration and Dosage.)

➤*Miscellaneous:* Respiratory difficulty. "Epinephrine-fastness" can occur with prolonged use.

Overdosage

➤*Symptoms:* Erroneous administration of large doses of epinephrine may lead to precordial distress, vomiting, headache, and dyspnea, as well as unusually elevated blood pressure.

Overdosage of epinephrine may cause cerebral hemorrhage resulting from a sharp rise in blood pressure. Pulmonary edema may develop because of peripheral vascular constriction together with cardiac stimulation. Transient bradycardia followed by tachycardia may also develop, and these may be accompanied by potentially fatal cardiac arrhythmias. Premature ventricular contractions may appear within 1 minute after injection and may be followed by multifocal ventricular fibrillation (prefibrillation rhythm). Subsidence of the ventricular effects may be followed by atrial tachycardia and occasionally by atrioventricular block.

Overdosage sometimes results in extreme pallor and coldness of the skin, metabolic acidosis, and kidney failure.

➤*Treatment:* Epinephrine is rapidly inactivated in the body and treatment following overdosage with epinephrine is primarily supportive.

Most toxic effects of overdosage can be counteracted by injection of an alpha-adrenergic blocker and a beta-adrenergic blocker. In the event of a sharp rise in blood pressure, rapid-acting vasodilators, such as the nitrites, or alpha-adrenergic-blocking agents can be given to counteract the marked pressor effect of large doses of epinephrine.

Treatment of pulmonary edema consists of a rapidly acting alpha-adrenergic blocking agent and/or respiratory support.

Treatment of arrhythmias consists of administration of a beta-blocking drug (eg, propranolol).

Patient Information

Epinephrine may produce symptoms and signs that include an increase in heart rate, the sensation of a more forceful heartbeat, palpitations, sweating, nausea and vomiting, difficulty breathing, pallor, dizziness, weakness or shakiness, headache, apprehension, nervousness, or anxiety. These symptoms and signs usually subside rapidly, especially with rest, quiet, and recumbency. Patients with hypertension or hyperthyroidism may develop more severe or persistent effects, and patients with coronary artery disease could experience angina. Patients with diabetes may develop increased blood glucose levels following epinephrine administration. Patients with Parkinson disease may notice a temporary worsening of symptoms.

Epinephrine is essential for the treatment of anaphylaxis. Carefully instruct patients about the circumstances under which this lifesaving medication should be used.

A health care provider who prescribes epinephrine auto-injectors should take appropriate steps to ensure that the patient (or parent) understands the indications and use of these devices thoroughly. The health care provider should review with the patient, or any other person who might be in a position to administer epinephrine auto-injectors to a patient experiencing anaphylaxis, in detail, the patient instructions and operation of the *EpiPen* or *EpiPen Jr* auto-injector.

In case of accidental injection, advise the patient to immediately go to the emergency room for treatment. Because epinephrine is a strong vasoconstrictor when injected into the digits, hands, or feet, direct treatment at vasodilation if there is such an inadvertent administration to these areas. (See also Administration and Dosage.)

EPINEPHRINE — TOPICAL

Refer to the general discussion of these products in the Vasopressors Used in Shock class monograph. See also Bronchodilators in the Respiratory Agents chapter and Agents for Glaucoma in the Ophthalmic and Otic Agents chapter.

Indications

➤*Nasal decongestant:* For use as a nasal decongestant.

Administration and Dosage

➤*Maximum dose:* There is no well-established maximum dose for the approved indication according to the prescribing information.

➤*Adults:*

Nasal decongestant – Apply locally as drops or spray or with a sterile swab, as required. See product labeling for dilution instructions.

➤*Children:*

Nasal decongestant –

6 years of age and older: See Adults for dosing.

➤*Storage/Stability:* Store between 15° and 25°C (59° and 77°F). Protect from light and freezing. Do not use solution if it is pinkish or darker than slightly yellow or if it contains a precipitate.

Warnings/Precautions

➤*Pregnancy:* *Category C.* Epinephrine readily crosses the placenta. Epinephrine is teratogenic in some animal species, but human teratogenicity has not been suspected.

➤*Lactation:* Although likely to be secreted in milk, epinephrine is rapidly destroyed in the GI tract. It is unlikely that any would be absorbed by the infant unless it is in the early neonatal period or premature.

NOREPINEPHRINE BITARTRATE (Levarterenol; Noradrenaline)

Rx	**Norepinephrine Bitartrate** (Abbott)	**Injection:** 1 mg (as base) per mL	In 4 mL amps.[a]
Rx	**Levophed** (Hospira)		In 4 mL amps.[b]

[a] Contains sodium metabisulfite 0.46 mg and sodium chloride 8.2 mg.

[b] Contains ≤ metabisulfite 2 mg.

NOREPINEPHRINE BITARTRATE — INJECTION

Refer to the general discussion of these products in the Vasopressors Used in Shock class monograph.

WARNING

Antidote for extravasation ischemia – To prevent sloughing and necrosis in areas in which extravasation has taken place, the area should be infiltrated as soon as possible with 10 to 15 mL of saline solution containing from 5 to 10 mg of phentolamine, an adrenergic blocking agent. A syringe with a fine hypodermic needle should be used, with the solution being infiltrated liberally throughout the area, which is easily identified by its cold, hard, and pallid appearance. Sympathetic blockade with phentolamine causes immediate and conspicuous local hyperemic changes if the area is infiltrated within 12 hours. Therefore, phentolamine should be given as soon as possible after the extravasation is noted.

Indications

➤*Blood pressure control in acute hypotensive states:* For blood pressure control in certain acute hypotensive states (eg, pheochromocytomectomy, sympathectomy, poliomyelitis, spinal anesthesia, MI, septicemia, blood transfusion, and drug reactions).

➤*Cardiac arrest:* As an adjunct in the treatment of cardiac arrest and profound hypotension.

➤*Off-label uses:* For the management of calcium channel blocker overdosage, beta-blocker overdosage, tricyclic antidepressant overdosage, and drug-induced distributive shock.

Administration and Dosage

➤*General dosing considerations:* Always correct blood volume depletion as fully as possible before any vasopressor is administered. When, as an emergency measure, intra-aortic pressures must be maintained to prevent cerebral or coronary artery ischemia, norepinephrine can be administered before and concurrently with blood volume replacement.

Record the blood pressure every 2 minutes from the time administration is started until the desired blood pressure is obtained, then every 5 minutes if administration is to be continued. The rate of flow must be watched constantly; never leave the patient unattended while receiving norepinephrine. Headache may be a symptom of hypertension due to overdosage.

Avoid abrupt withdrawal of infusions. (See Discontinuation of Therapy.)

Administer using an IV drip chamber. (See Administration.)

➤*Adults:*

Off-label dosing –

Severe hypotension: According to the American Heart Association's ACLS guidelines, norepinephrine may be used as second-line therapy for severe hypotension. The initial dosage is 0.5 to 1 mcg/min (as base) and then titrated to desired effect. (See also Preparation for Administration.)

➤*Children:*

Off-label dosing –

Blood pressure control in acute hypotensive states:

- *Maximum dose* – 1 to 2 mcg/kg/min.
- *Initial dosage* – 0.05 to 0.1 mcg/kg/min titrated to desired effect.
- *Cardiac output maintenance* – According to the American Heart Association's pediatric advanced life support guidelines, the dosage ranges from 0.1 to 2 mcg/kg/min. Titrate infusion to desired effect.

➤*Duration of therapy:* Continue therapy until adequate blood pressure and tissue perfusion are maintained without therapy.

➤*Discontinuation of therapy:* Reduce infusions of norepinephrine gradually, avoiding abrupt withdrawal.

➤*Preparation for administration:* Dilute norepinephrine in dextrose 5% or dextrose 5% and sodium chloride. Administration in saline solution alone is not recommended.

Add a 4 mL ampul (4 mg) of norepinephrine bitartrate to 1,000 mL of a dextrose 5%–containing solution. Each mL of this dilution contains 4 mcg of norepinephrine bitartrate base.

According to the ACLS guidelines, add norepinephrine 4 mg (norepinephrine bitartrate 8 mg) to 250 mL of dextrose 5% in water or dextrose 5% in normal saline (but not in normal saline alone). This results in a concentration of norepinephrine 16 mcg/mL (norepinephrine bitartrate 32 mcg/mL).

The degree of dilution depends on clinical fluid volume requirements. If large volumes of fluid (dextrose) are needed at a flow rate that would involve an excessive dose of the pressor agent per unit of time, use a solution more dilute than 4 mcg/mL. On the other hand, when large volumes of fluid are clinically undesirable, a concentration more than 4 mcg/mL may be necessary.

Do not use the solution if its color is pinkish or darker than slightly yellow, or if it contains a precipitate.

➤*Administration:* Give this solution by IV infusion in a large vein. Insert a plastic IV catheter through a suitable bore needle well advanced centrally into the vein and securely fixed with adhesive tape, avoiding, if possible, a catheter tie-in technique, as this promotes stasis. An IV drip chamber or other suitable metering device is essential to permit an accurate estimation of the rate of flow in drops per minute.

Norepinephrine infusions should not be administered into the leg veins in elderly patients.

➤*Extravasation:* The infusion site should be checked frequently for free flow. Care should be taken to avoid extravasation of norepinephrine bitartrate injection into the tissues, as local necrosis might ensue due to the vasoconstrictive action of the drug. Blanching along the course of the infused vein, sometimes without obvious extravasation, has been attributed to vasa vasorum constriction with increased permeability of the vein wall, permitting some leakage.

This also may progress on rare occasions to superficial slough, particularly during infusion into leg veins in elderly patients or in those with obliterative vascular disease. Hence, if blanching occurs, consideration should be given to the advisability of changing the infusion site at intervals to allow the effects of local vasoconstriction to subside.

If signs or symptoms of extravasation occur, stop the infusion immediately. If possible, withdraw 3 to 5 mL of blood to remove some of the drug. Remove the infusion needle. Delineate the infiltrated area on the patient's skin with a felt-tip marker. Cleanse the area with povidone-iodine and inject phentolamine 5 to 10 mg (reconstituted with 10 mL sodium chloride 0.9% injection) as soon as possible under the skin using a 25-gauge needle. Insert the needle at a 15 degree angle, bevel up, so that a raised area appears. Change the needle after each injection if using multiple injections. (For children, the maximum dose is phentolamine 0.1 to 0.2 mg/kg or 5 mg). Phentolamine may not be effective if more than 12 hours has elapsed since injury. Application of warm compresses to the area for 15 minutes every 6 hours for 48 hours may be useful. Elevate for 48 hours above heart level using a sling or stockinette dressing with an observation window cut in the dressing. Avoid pressure or friction. Do not rub area. Observe for signs of increased erythema, pain, or skin necrosis. If increased symptoms occur, consult a plastic surgeon. Ensure that no medication is given distally to extravasation site. After 48 hours, encourage the patient to use the extremity normally to promote full range of motion.

➤*Admixture compatibility:* Avoid contact with iron salts, alkalis, or oxidizing agents.

Administer whole blood or plasma separately (ie, by use of a Y-tube and individual containers if given simultaneously).

To screen for specific compatibilities, see *Trissel's IV-Chek*.

➤*Storage/Stability:* Store at 25°C (77°F); excursions are permitted to 15° to 30°C (59° to 86°F). Protect from light.

NOREPINEPHRINE BITARTRATE — INJECTION

Actions

➤*Pharmacology:* Norepinephrine bitartrate functions as a peripheral vasoconstrictor (alpha-adrenergic action) and as an inotropic stimulator of the heart and dilator of coronary arteries (beta-adrenergic action).

Contraindications

➤*Emergency use only:* Norepinephrine bitartrate should not be given to patients who are hypotensive from blood volume deficits except as an emergency measure to maintain coronary and cerebral artery perfusion until blood volume replacement therapy can be completed. If norepinephrine bitartrate is continuously administered to maintain blood pressure in the absence of blood volume replacement, the following may occur: Severe peripheral and visceral vasoconstriction, decreased renal perfusion and urine output, poor systemic blood flow despite "normal" blood pressure, tissue hypoxia, and lactate acidosis.

➤*Mesenteric or peripheral vascular thrombosis:* Norepinephrine bitartrate should also not be given to patients with mesenteric or peripheral vascular thrombosis (because of the risk of increasing ischemia and extending the area of infarction) unless, in the opinion of the attending physician, the administration of norepinephrine bitartrate is necessary as a lifesaving procedure.

Cardiac arrhythmias may result from the use of norepinephrine bitartrate injection in patients with profound hypoxia or hypercarbia.

Cyclopropane and halothane anesthetics increase cardiac autonomic irritability and therefore seem to sensitize the myocardium to the action of IV administered epinephrine or norepinephrine. Hence, the use of norepinephrine bitartrate injection during cyclopropane and halothane anesthesia is generally considered contraindicated because of the risk of producing ventricular tachycardia or fibrillation.

Warnings/Precautions

➤*Concomitant therapy:* See Drug Interactions for more information.

➤*Site of infusion:* Whenever possible, infusions of norepinephrine bitartrate injection should be given into a large vein, particularly an antecubital vein because, when administered into this vein, the risk of necrosis of the overlying skin from prolonged vasoconstriction is apparently very slight. Some authors have indicated that the femoral vein is also an acceptable route of administration. A catheter tie-in technique should be avoided, if possible, since the obstruction to blood flow around the tubing may cause stasis and increased local concentration of the drug. Occlusive vascular diseases (eg, atherosclerosis, arteriosclerosis, diabetic endarteritis, Buerger's disease) are more likely to occur in the lower than in the upper extremity. Therefore, one should avoid the veins of the leg in elderly patients or in those suffering from such disorders. Gangrene has been reported in a lower extremity when infusions of norepinephrine bitartrate injection were given in an ankle vein.

➤*Extravasation:* See Administration and Dosage for more information.

➤*Sulfite sensitivity:* Norepinephrine bitartrate injection contains sodium metabisulfite, a sulfite that may cause allergic-type reactions including anaphylactic symptoms and life-threatening or less severe asthmatic episodes in certain susceptible people. The overall prevalence of sulfite sensitivity in the general population is unknown. Sulfite sensitivity is seen more frequently in asthmatic than in nonasthmatic people.

➤*Pregnancy: Category C.* Animal reproduction studies have not been conducted with norepinephrine bitartrate. It is also not known whether norepinephrine bitartrate can cause fetal harm when administered to a pregnant woman or can affect reproduction capacity. Norepinephrine bitartrate should be given to a pregnant woman only if clearly needed.

➤*Lactation:* It is not known whether this drug is excreted in human milk. Because many drugs are excreted in human milk, caution should be exercised when norepinephrine bitartrate is administered to a breast-feeding woman.

➤*Children:* Safety and effectiveness in pediatric patients have not been established.

➤*Elderly:* Clinical studies of norepinephrine bitartrate did not include sufficient numbers of patients aged 65 and over to determine whether they respond differently from younger subjects. Other reported clinical experience has not identified differences in responses between the elderly and younger patients. In general, dose selection for an elderly patient should be cautious, usually starting at the low end of the dosing range, reflecting the greater frequency of decreased hepatic, renal, or cardiac function, and of concomitant disease or other drug therapy.

Norepinephrine bitartrate injection infusions should not be administered into the veins in the leg in elderly patients.

➤*Monitoring:* Because of the potency of norepinephrine bitartrate and because of varying response to pressor substances, the possibility always exists that dangerously high blood pressure may be produced with overdoses of this pressor agent. It is desirable, therefore, to record the blood pressure every 2 minutes from the time administration is started until the desired blood pressure is obtained, then every 5 minutes if administration is to be continued.

The rate of flow must be watched constantly, and the patient should never be left unattended while receiving norepinephrine bitartrate injection. Headache may be a symptom of hypertension due to overdosage.

Drug Interactions

➤*Cyclopropane and halothane anesthetics:* Cyclopropane and halothane anesthetics increase cardiac autonomic irritability and therefore seem to sensitize the myocardium to the action of IV administered epinephrine or norepinephrine. Hence, the use of norepinephrine bitartrate injection during cyclopropane and halothane anesthesia is generally considered contraindicated because of the risk of producing ventricular tachycardia or fibrillation. The same type of cardiac arrhythmias may result from the use of norepinephrine bitartrate injection in patients with profound hypoxia or hypercarbia.

➤*MAO inhibitors (MAOIs):* Norepinephrine bitartrate injection should be used with extreme caution in patients receiving monoamine oxidase inhibitors (MAOI) or antidepressants of the triptyline or imipramine types, because severe, prolonged hypertension may result.

Adverse Reactions

➤*Cardiovascular:* Bradycardia, probably as a reflex result of a rise in blood pressure, arrhythmias.

➤*CNS:* Anxiety, transient headache.

➤*Dermatologic:* Extravasation necrosis at injection site.

➤*Respiratory:* Respiratory difficulty.

➤*Miscellaneous:* Ischemic injury due to potent vasoconstrictor action and tissue hypoxia.

➤*Prolonged administration or overdosage:* Prolonged administration of any potent vasopressor may result in plasma volume depletion which should be continuously corrected by appropriate fluid and electrolyte replacement therapy. If plasma volumes are not corrected, hypotension may recur when norepinephrine bitartrate injection is discontinued, or blood pressure may be maintained at the risk of severe peripheral and visceral vasoconstriction (eg, decreased renal perfusion) with diminution in blood flow and tissue perfusion with subsequent tissue hypoxia and lactic acidosis and possible ischemic injury. Gangrene of extremities has been rarely reported.

Hypersensitivity – Overdoses or conventional doses in hypersensitive persons (eg, hyperthyroid patients) cause severe hypertension with violent headache, photophobia, stabbing retrosternal pain, pallor, intense sweating, and vomiting.

Overdosage

Overdosage with norepinephrine bitartrate may result in headache, severe hypertension, reflex bradycardia, marked increase in peripheral resistance, and decreased cardiac output. In case of accidental overdosage, as evidenced by excessive blood pressure elevation, discontinue norepinephrine bitartrate injection until the condition of the patient stabilizes.

EPHEDRINE

otc	**Ephedrine Sulfate** (West-Ward)	**Capsules:** 25 mg	In 100s.
Rx	**Ephedrine Sulfate** (Various, eg, UDL)	**Injection:** 50 mg/mL	In 1 mL single-dose vials
Rx	**Ephedrine Sulfate** (Hospira)		Preservative free. In 1 mL single-dose amps.

EPHEDRINE SULFATE — ORAL

Refer to the general discussion of these products in the Vasopressors Used in Shock group monograph and the Sympathomimetic Bronchodilator group monographRespiratory Agents in the chapter.

Indications

➤*Asthma:* Oral ephedrine is indicated for temporary relief of shortness of breath, tightness of chest, wheezing, and for easing breathing in bronchial asthma.

Administration and Dosage

➤*Adults:*

Asthma –

Usual dosage: 12.5 to 25 mg every 4 hours.

Maximum dose: Not to exceed 150 mg in 24 hours.

➤*Children:*

12 years of age and older – See Adults for dosing.

EPHEDRINE SULFATE — INJECTION

Refer to the general discussion of these products in the Vasopressors Used in Shock group monographand the Sympathomimetic Bronchodilator group monograph in the Respiratory Agents chapter.

Indications

➤*Allergic disorders:* Treatment of allergic disorders, such as bronchial asthma. The drug has long been used as a pressor agent, particularly during spinal anesthesia when hypotension frequently occurs. In Stokes-Adams syndrome with complete heart block, ephedrine has a value similar to that of epinephrine. It is indicated as a CNS stimulant in narcolepsy and depressive states. It is also used in myasthenia gravis.

Administration and Dosage

➤*Adults:*

Allergic disorders – The usual parenteral dose is 25 to 50 mg, given subcutaneously or intramuscularly (IM). Intravenously, 5 to 25 mg may be administered slowly, repeated in 5 to 10 minutes, if necessary.

➤*Children:*

Allergic disorders – The usual subcutaneous or IM dose is 0.5 mg/kg of body weight or 16.7 mg/m^2 of body surface every 4 to 6 hours.

➤*Storage/Stability:* Store at 15° to 25°C (59° to 77°F). Protect from light.

Actions

➤*Pharmacology:* Ephedrine sulfate is a potent sympathomimetic that stimulates both α and β receptors and has clinical uses related to both actions. Its peripheral actions, which it owes in part to the release of norepinephrine, simulate responses that are obtained when adrenergic nerves are stimulated. These include an increase in blood pressure, stimulation of heart muscle, constriction of arterioles, relaxation of the smooth muscle of the bronchi and gastrointestinal tract, and dilation of the pupils. In the bladder, relaxation of the detrusor muscle is not prominent, but the tone of the trigone and vesicle sphincter is increased.

Ephedrine sulfate also has a potent effect on the CNS. It stimulates the cerebral cortex and subcortical centers, which accounts for its use in narcolepsy.

The cardiovascular responses reported in man include moderate tachycardia, unchanged or augmented stroke volume, enhanced cardiac output, variable alterations in peripheral resistance and usually a rise in blood pressure. The action of ephedrine is more prominent on the heart than on the blood vessels. Ephedrine sulfate increases the flow of coronary, cerebral and muscle blood.

In patients with myasthenia gravis, administration of ephedrine sulfate injection, USP produces a real but modest increase in motor power. The exact mechanism by which ephedrine sulfate affects skeletal muscle contractions is unknown.

Contraindications

Allergic reactions to ephedrine sulfate are rare. The hypersensitivity, if known, is a specific contraindication. Patients hypersensitive to other sympathomimetics may also be hypersensitive to ephedrine sulfate.

Warnings/Precautions

➤*Special risk:* Special care should be used when administering ephedrine sulfate injection to patients with heart disease, angina pectoris, diabetes, hyperthyroidism, prostatic hypertrophy or hypertension and to patients receiving digitalis. Prolonged use may produce a syndrome resembling an anxiety state. Tolerance to ephedrine sulfate may develop, but temporary discontinuance to the drug restores its original effectiveness.

➤*Drug abuse and dependence:* Prolonged abuse of ephedrine sulfate injection can lead to symptoms of paranoid schizophrenia. When this occurs, patients exhibit such physical signs as tachycardia, poor nutrition and hygiene, fever, cold sweat and dilated pupils.

Some measure of tolerance may develop with prolonged or excessive use but addiction does not occur. Temporary cessation of medication and subsequent readministration restores its effectiveness.

➤*Pregnancy: Category C.* Animal reproduction studies have not been conducted with ephedrine sulfate injection, USP. Also, it is not known whether the drug can cause fetal harm when administered to a pregnant woman or can affect reproduction capacity. Ephedrine sulfate injection, USP should be given to a pregnant woman only if clearly indicated.

It is not known what effect ephedrine sulfate injection, USP may have on the newborn or on the child's later growth and development when the drug is administered to the mother just before or during labor.

➤*Lactation:* Ephedrine sulfate is excreted in breast milk. Use by breastfeeding mothers is not recommended because of the higher than usual risks for infants.

Drug Interactions

➤*General anesthetics and digitalis glycosides:* Concurrent use of ephedrine sulfate with general anesthetics, especially cyclopropane or halogenated hydrocarbons or digitalis glycosides may cause cardiac arrhythmias, since these medications may sensitize the myocardium to the effects of ephedrine sulfate.

➤*Guanethidine, bethanidine, debrisoquin:* Therapeutic doses of ephedrine sulfate can inhibit the hypotensive effect of guanethidine, bethanidine, and debrisoquin by displacing the adrenergic blockers from their site of action in the sympathetic neurons. The effect in man is seen as a relative or a complete blockade of the antihypertensive drug by a sudden rise in blood pressure. Concomitant use of ephedrine sulfate injection, USP and oxytocics may cause severe hypotension.

➤*MAOIs:* Monoamine oxidase inhibitors may potentiate the pressor effect of ephedrine sulfate, possibly resulting in a hypertensive crisis. Ephedrine sulfate injection should not be administered during or within 14 days following the administration of MAO inhibitors.

Adverse Reactions

With large doses of ephedrine sulfate most patients will experience nervousness, insomnia, vertigo, headache, tachycardia, palpitation and sweating. Some patients have nausea, vomiting and anorexia. Vesical sphincter spasm may occur and result in difficult and painful urination. Urinary retention may develop in males with prostatism.

Precordial pain and cardiac arrhythmias may occur following administration of ephedrine sulfate injection.

Overdosage

➤*Symptoms:* The principal manifestation of ephedrine sulfate poisoning is convulsions. In acute poisoning the following signs and symptoms may occur: nausea, vomiting, chills, cyanosis, irritability, nervousness, fever, suicidal behavior, tachycardia, dilated pupils, blurred vision, opisthotonos, spasms, convulsions, pulmonary edema, gasping respirations, coma and respiratory failure. Initially, the patient may have hypertension, followed later by hypotension accompanied by anuria.

➤*Treatment:* If respirations are shallow or cyanosis is present, artificial respiration should be administered. Vasopressors are contraindicated. In cardiovascular collapse blood pressure should be maintained.

Antidote – For hypertension, 5 mg phentolamine mesylate diluted in saline may be administered slowly intravenously, or 100 mg may be given orally. Convulsions may be controlled by diazepam or paraldehyde. Cool applications and dexamethasone 1 mg/kg, administered slowly intravenously, may control pyrexia.

PHENYLEPHRINE HYDROCHLORIDE

Rx	**Phenylephrine Hydrochloride** (Various, eg, American Regent)	**Injection:** 1% (10 mg/mL)	In 1 and 5 mL vials.
Rx	**Neo-Synephrine** (Hospira)		In 1 mL *Uni-Nest* amps.[a]

[a] With sodium bisulfite.

PHENYLEPHRINE HYDROCHLORIDE — INJECTION

Refer to the general discussion of these products in the Vasopressors Used in Shock group monograph.

WARNING

Physicians should completely familiarize themselves with the complete contents of this monograph before prescribing phenylephrine injection.

Indications

➤*Blood pressure maintenance:* Maintenance of an adequate level of blood pressure during spinal and inhalation anesthesia and for the treatment of vascular failure in shock, shock-like states and drug-induced hypotension or hypersensitivity. It is also employed to overcome paroxysmal supraventricular tachycardia, to prolong spinal anesthesia, and as a vasoconstrictor in regional analgesia.

➤*Off-label uses:*

Other possible off-label uses – For the management of drug-induced distributive shock.

Administration and Dosage

➤*General dosing considerations:* Phenylephrine injection is generally injected subcutaneously, IM, slowly IV, or in dilute solution as a continuous IV infusion. In patients with paroxysmal supraventricular tachycardia and, if indicated, in case of emergency, phenylephrine injection is administered directly IV. The dose should be adjusted according to the pressor response.

➤*Adults:*

Mild or moderate hypotension –

Subcutaneously or IM:

- *Usual dosage* – 2 to 5 mg, with a range of 1 to 10 mg. Injections should not be repeated more often than every 10 to 15 minutes.
- *Initial dosage* – Should not exceed 5 mg.

PHENYLEPHRINE HYDROCHLORIDE — INJECTION

IV:

• *Usual dosage* – 0.2 mg with a range of 0.1 to 0.5 mg. Injections should not be repeated more often than every 10 to 15 minutes.

• *Initial dosage* – Should not exceed 0.5 mg.

Paroxysmal supraventricular tachycardia – Rapid IV injection (within 20 to 30 seconds) is recommended.

Initial dosage: Should not exceed 0.5 mg.

Dosage adjustment: Subsequent doses, which are determined by the initial blood pressure response, should not exceed the preceding dose by more than 0.1 to 0.2 mg and should never exceed 1 mg.

Prolongation of spinal anesthesia – The addition of 2 to 5 mg of phenylephrine to the anesthetic solution increases the duration of motor block by as much as approximately 50% without any increase in the incidence of complications, such as nausea, vomiting, or blood pressure disturbances.

Severe hypotension and shock (including drug-related hypotension) – Blood-volume depletion should always be corrected as fully as possible before any vasopressor is administered. When, as an emergency measure, intraaortic pressures must be maintained to prevent cerebral or coronary artery ischemia, phenylephrine can be administered before and concurrently with blood-volume replacement.

Hypotension and occasionally severe shock may result from overdosage or idiosyncrasy following the administration of certain drugs, especially adrenergic- and ganglionic-blocking agents, rauwolfia and veratrum alkaloids, and phenothiazine tranquilizers. Patients who receive a phenothiazine derivative as preoperative medication are especially susceptible to these reactions. As an adjunct in the management of such episodes, phenylephrine injection is a suitable agent for restoring blood pressure.

Higher initial and maintenance doses of phenylephrine are required in patients with persistent or untreated severe hypotension or shock. Hypotension produced by powerful peripheral adrenergic-blocking agents, chlorpromazine, or pheochromocytomectomy may also require more intensive therapy.

Continuous infusion: Add 10 mg of the drug (1 mL of 1% solution) to 500 mL of dextrose injection or sodium chloride injection (providing a 1:50,000 solution). To raise the blood pressure rapidly, start the infusion at about 100 mcg to 180 mcg/min (based on 20 drops/mL, this would be 100 to 180 drops/min). When the blood pressure is stabilized (at a low normal level for the individual), a maintenance rate of 40 to 60 mcg/min usually suffices (based on 20 drops/mL, this would be 40 to 60 drops/min). If the drop size of the infusion system varies from the 20 drops/mL, the dose must be adjusted accordingly.

If a prompt initial pressor response is not obtained, additional increments of phenylephrine (10 mg or more) can be added to the infusion bottle. The rate of flow is then adjusted until the desired blood-pressure level is obtained. In some cases, a more potent vasopressor, such as norepinephrine bitartrate, may be required. Hypertension should be avoided. The blood pressure should be checked frequently. Headache or bradycardia may indicate hypertension. Arrhythmias are rare.

Spinal anesthesia-hypotension – Routine parenteral use of phenylephrine has been recommended for the prophylaxis and treatment of hypotension during spinal anesthesia. It is recommended to be administered subcutaneously or IM 3 or 4 minutes before injection of the spinal anesthetic

Usual dosage: The total requirement for high anesthetic levels is usually 3 mg, and for lower levels, 2 mg.

Initial dosage: For hypotensive emergencies during spinal anesthesia, phenylephrine may be injected IV, using an initial dose of 0.2 mg.

Dosage adjustment: Any subsequent dose should not exceed the previous dose by more than 0.1 to 0.2 mg, and no more than 0.5 mg should be administered in a single dose.

Vasoconstrictor for regional analgesia – Concentrations about 10 times those employed when epinephrine is used as a vasoconstrictor are recommended. The optimum strength is 1:20,000 (made by adding 1 mg of phenylephrine to every 20 mL of local anesthetic solution). Some pressor responses can be expected when 2 mg or more are injected.

➤*Children:*

Spinal anesthesia-hypotension – To combat hypotension during spinal anesthesia in children, a dose of 0.5 to 1 mg per 25 pounds body weight administered subcutaneously or IM is recommended.

➤*Elderly:* Use with extreme caution in the elderly.

➤*Preparation for administration:* Parenteral drug products should be inspected visually for particulate matter and discoloration prior to administration, whenever solution and container permit.

Phenylephrine Injection Dosage Calculations

Dose required	Use phenylephrine injection 1%
10 mg	1 mL
5 mg	0.5 mL
1 mg	0.1 mL

For convenience in intermittent IV administration, dilute 1 mL phenylephrine injection 1% with 9 mL of sterile water for injection to yield 0.1% phenylephrine injection.

Phenylephrine Injection Dilution

Dose required	Use diluted phenylephrine injection 0.1%
0.1 mg	0.1 mL
0.2 mg	0.2 mL
0.5 mg	0.5 mL

➤*Extravasation:* Tissue necrosis may develop if extravasation occurs. To treat extravasation, consider infiltrating phentolamine 5 to 10 mg (diluted in 10 to 15 mL normal saline) into the site extravasation.

➤*Storage/Stability:* Store at controlled room temperature 15° to 30°C (59° to 86°F). Protect from light. Keep covered in carton until time of use. For single use only. Discard unused portion.

Actions

➤*Pharmacology:* Phenylephrine is a powerful postsynaptic, alpha-receptor stimulant with little effect on the beta receptors of the heart. In therapeutic doses, it produces little if any stimulation of either the spinal cord or cerebrum. A singular advantage of this drug is the fact that repeated injections produce comparable effects.

Contraindications

Severe hypertension or ventricular tachycardia; hypersensitivity to phenylephrine or to any of the components.

Warnings/Precautions

➤*Extravasation:* See Administration and Dosage for more information.

➤*Sulfite sensitivity:* Some of these products contain sodium metabisulfite, a sulfite that may cause allergic-type reactions including anaphylactic symptoms and life-threatening or less severe asthmatic episodes in certain susceptible people. The overall prevalence of sulfite sensitivity in the general population is unknown and probably low. Sulfite sensitivity is seen more frequently in asthmatic than in nonasthmatic people.

➤*Special risk:* Use only with extreme caution in elderly patients or in patients with hyperthyroidism, bradycardia, partial heart block, myocardial disease or severe arteriosclerosis.

➤*Pregnancy:* Category C.

Teratogenic – Animal reproduction studies have not been conducted with phenylephrine. It is also not known whether phenylephrine can cause fetal harm when administered to a pregnant woman or can affect reproduction capacity. Phenylephrine should be given to a pregnant woman only if clearly needed.

Labor and delivery – If vasopressor drugs are either used to correct hypotension or added to the local anesthetic solution, the obstetrician should be cautioned that some oxytocic drugs may cause severe persistent hypertension and that even a rupture of a cerebral blood vessel may occur during the postpartum period (see Warnings).

➤*Lactation:* It is not known whether this drug is excreted in human milk. Because many drugs are excreted in human milk, caution should be exercised when phenylephrine is administered to a breast-feeding woman.

➤*Children:* To combat hypotension during spinal anesthesia in children, a dose of 0.5 to 1 mg per 25 pounds of body weight, administered subcutaneously, or IM, is recommended.

Drug Interactions

➤*Vasopressors:* Vasopressors, particularly metaraminol, may cause serious cardiac arrhythmias during halothane anesthesia and therefore should be used only with great caution or not at all.

➤*Oxytoxic drugs:* If used in conjunction with oxytocic drugs, the pressor effect of sympathomimetic pressor amines is potentiated. The pressor effect of sympathomimetic pressor amines is markedly potentiated in patients receiving monamine oxidase inhibitors (MAOIs). Therefore, when initiating pressor therapy in these patients, the initial dose should be small and used with due caution. The pressor response of adrenergic agents may also be potentiated by tricyclic antidepressants. The obstetrician should be warned that some oxytocic drugs may cause severe persistent hypertension and that even a rupture of a cerebral blood vessel may occur during the postpartum period.

➤*MAO inhibitors:* The pressor effect of sympathomimetic pressor amines is markedly potentiated in patients receiving monoamine oxidase inhibitors (MAOI). Therefore, when initiating pressor therapy in these patients, the initial dose should be small and used with due caution. The pressor response of adrenergic agents may also be potentiated by tricyclic antidepressants.

Adverse Reactions

Headache, reflex bradycardia, excitability, restlessness and rarely arrhythmias.

Overdosage

The oral LD_{50} in the rat is 350 mg/kg, in the mouse 120 mg/kg.

➤*Symptoms:* Overdosage may induce ventricular extrasystoles and short paroxysms of ventricular tachycardia, a sensation of fullness in the head and tingling of the extremities.

➤*Treatment:* Should an excessive elevation of blood pressure occur, it may be immediately relieved by an alpha-adrenergic-blocking agent (eg, phentolamine).

MIDODRINE HYDROCHLORIDE

Rx	**Midodrine Hydrochloride** (Global)	**Tablets:** 2.5 mg	(G 421). White. In 100s, 500s, and 1,000s.
Rx	**ProAmatine** (Shire)		(RPC 2.5 003). White, scored. In 100s.
Rx	**Midodrine Hydrochloride** (Global)	**Tablets:** 5 mg	(G 422). Lt. orange. In 100s, 500s, and 1,000s.
Rx	**ProAmatine** (Shire)		(RPC 5 004). Orange, scored. In 100s.
Rx	**ProAmatine** (Shire)	**Tablets:** 10 mg	(RPC 10 007). Blue, scored. In 100s.

MIDODRINE HYDROCHLORIDE — ORAL

WARNING

Because midodrine can cause marked elevation of supine blood pressure, it should be used in patients whose lives are considerably impaired despite standard clinical care. The indication for use of midodrine in the treatment of symptomatic orthostatic hypotension is based primarily on a change in a surrogate marker of effectiveness, an increase in systolic blood pressure measured 1 minute after standing, a surrogate marker considered likely to correspond to a clinical benefit. At present, however, clinical benefits of midodrine, principally improved ability to carry out activities of daily living, have not been verified.

Indications

➤*Orthostatic hypotension:* Treatment of symptomatic orthostatic hypotension. Because midodrine can cause marked elevation of supine blood pressure (BP greater than 200 mmHg systolic), it should be used in patients whose lives are considerably impaired despite standard clinical care, including nonpharmacologic treatment (such as support stockings), fluid expansion, and lifestyle alterations. The indication is based on midodrine's effect on increases in 1-minute standing systolic blood pressure, a surrogate marker considered likely to correspond to a clinical benefit. At present however, clinical benefits of midodrine principally improved ability to perform life activities have not been established. Further clinical trials are underway to verify and describe the clinical benefits of midodrine.

After initiation of treatment, midodrine should be continued only for patients who report significant symptomatic improvement.

➤*Off-label uses:* Management of urinary incontinence (2.5 to 5 mg 2 to 3 times a day).

Administration and Dosage

➤*General dosing considerations:* The supine and standing blood pressure should be monitored regularly, and the administration of midodrine should be stopped if supine blood pressure increases excessively.

➤*Adults:*

Orthostatic hypotension –

Usual dosage: 10 mg 3 times daily during daytime hours when the patient needs to be upright.

Alternative dosage: Single doses as high as 20 mg have been given to patients, but severe and persistent systolic supine hypertension occurs at a high rate (approximately 45%) at this dose.

Total daily doses greater than 30 mg have been tolerated by some patients, but their safety and usefulness have not been studied systematically or established.

Discontinuation of therapy: Because of the risk of supine hypertension, midodrine should be continued only in patients who appear to attain symptomatic improvement during initial treatment.

Administration of midodrine should be stopped if supine blood pressure increases excessively.

➤*Renal function impairment:* Because desglymidodrine is excreted renally, dosing in patients with abnormal renal function should be cautious; it is recommended that treatment of these patients be initiated using 2.5 mg doses.

➤*Administration:* A suggested dosing schedule of approximately 4-hour intervals is as follows: shortly before, or upon arising in the morning, midday, and late afternoon (not later than 6 pm). Doses may be given in 3-hour intervals, if required, to control symptoms, but not more frequently.

In order to reduce the potential for supine hypertension during sleep, midodrine should not be given after the evening meal or less than 4 hours before bedtime.

➤*Storage/Stability:* Store at 25°C (77°F). Excursions permitted to 15° to 30°C (59° to 86°F).

Actions

➤*Pharmacology:* Midodrine forms an active metabolite, desglymidodrine, that is an alpha-1 agonist, and exerts its actions via activation of the alpha-adrenergic receptors of the arteriolar and venous vasculature, producing an increase in vascular tone and elevation of blood pressure. Desglymidodrine does not stimulate cardiac beta-adrenergic receptors. Desglymidodrine diffuses poorly across the blood-brain barrier, and is therefore not associated with effects on the central nervous system.

➤*Pharmacokinetics:*

Absorption/Distribution – Midodrine is a prodrug (ie, the therapeutic effect of orally administered midodrine is due to the major metabolite desglymidodrine) formed by deglycination of midodrine. After oral administration, midodrine is rapidly absorbed. The plasma levels of the prodrug peak after about half an hour, and decline with a half-life of approximately 25 minutes, while the metabolite reaches peak blood concentrations about 1 to 2 hours after a dose of midodrine and has a half-life of about 3 to 4 hours. The absolute bioavailability of midodrine (measured as desglymidodrine) is 93%. The bioavailability of desglymidodrine is not affected by food. Approximately the same amount of desglymidodrine is formed after intravenous and oral administration of midodrine. Neither midodrine nor desglymidodrine is bound to plasma proteins to any significant extent.

Metabolism – Thorough metabolic studies have not been conducted, but it appears that deglycination of midodrine to deglymidodrine takes place in many tissues, and both compounds are metabolized in part by the liver. Neither midodrine nor desglymidodrine is a substrate for monoamine oxidase.

Excretion – Renal elimination of midodrine is insignificant. The renal clearance of desglymidodrine is of the order of 385 mL/min, most, about 80%, by active renal secretion. The actual mechanism of active secretion has not been studied, but it is possible that it occurs by the base-secreting pathway responsible for the secretion of several other drugs that are bases.

Contraindications

Severe organic heart disease, acute renal disease, urinary retention, pheochromocytoma, thyrotoxicosis, persistent and excessive supine hypertension.

Warnings/Precautions

➤*Supine hypertension:* The most potentially serious adverse reaction associated with midodrine therapy is marked elevation of supine arterial blood pressure (supine hypertension). Systolic pressure of about 200 mmHg were seen overall in about 13.4% of patients given 10 mg of midodrine. Systolic elevations of this degree were most likely to be observed in patients with relatively elevated pretreatment systolic blood pressures (mean, 170 mmHg). There is no experience in patients with initial supine systolic pressure above 180 mmHg, as those patients were excluded from the clinical trials. Use of midodrine in such patients is not recommended. Sitting blood pressures were also elevated by midodrine therapy. It is essential to monitor supine and sitting blood pressures in patients maintained on midodrine.

➤*Potential for supine and sitting hypertension:* The potential for supine and sitting hypertension should be evaluated at the beginning of midodrine therapy. Supine hypertension can often be controlled by preventing the patient from becoming fully supine (ie, sleeping with the head of the bed elevated). The patient should be cautioned to report symptoms of supine hypertension immediately. Symptoms may include cardiac awareness, pounding in the ears, headache, blurred vision, etc. The patient should be advised to discontinue the medication immediately if supine hypertension persists.

➤*Slight slowing of the heart rate:* A slight slowing of the heart rate may occur after administration of midodrine, primarily due to vagal reflex. Caution should be exercised when midodrine is used concomitantly with cardiac glycosides (eg, digitalis), psychopharmacologic agents, beta blockers or other agents that directly or indirectly reduce heart rate. Patients who experience any signs or symptoms suggesting bradycardia (pulse slowing, increased dizziness, syncope, cardiac awareness) should be advised to discontinue midodrine and should be reevaluated.

➤*Renal function impairment:* Midodrine use has not been studied in patients with renal impairment. Because desglymidodrine is eliminated via the kidneys, and higher blood levels would be expected in such patients, midodrine should be used with caution in patients with renal impairment, with a starting dose of 2.5 mg. Renal function should be assessed prior to initial use of midodrine.

➤*Hepatic function impairment:* Midodrine use has not been studied in patients with hepatic impairment. Midodrine should be used with caution in patients with hepatic impairment, as the liver has a role in the metabolism of midodrine.

➤*Special risk:*

Patients with urinary retention problems – Use cautiously in patients with urinary retention problems, as desglymidodrine acts on the alpha-adrenergic receptors of the bladder neck.

Orthostatic hypotensive patients – Use with caution in orthostatic hypotensive patients who are also diabetic, as well as those with a history of visual problems who are also taking fludrocortisone acetate, which is known to cause an increase in intraocular pressure and glaucoma.

➤*Pregnancy:* *Category C.* Midodrine increased the rate of embryo resorption, reduced fetal body weight in rats and rabbits, and decreased fetal survival in rabbits when given in doses 13 (rat) and 7 (rabbit) times the maximum human dose based on body surface area (mg/m^2). There are no adequate and well-controlled studies in pregnant women. Midodrine should be used during pregnancy only if the potential benefit justifies the potential risk to the fetus. No teratogenic effects have been observed in studies in rats and rabbits.

➤*Lactation:* It is not known whether this drug is excreted in human milk. Because many drugs are excreted in human milk, caution should be exercised when midodrine is administered to a breast-feeding woman.

MIDODRINE HYDROCHLORIDE — ORAL

➤*Children:* Safety and efficacy in pediatric patients have not been established.

➤*Monitoring:* Blood pressure should be monitored carefully when midodrine is used concomitantly with other agents that cause vasoconstriction (eg, phenylephrine, ephedrine, dihydroergotamine, phenylpropanolamine, pseudoephedrine).

Because desglymidodrine is eliminated by the kidneys and the liver has a role in its metabolism, evaluation of the patient should include assessment of renal and hepatic function prior to initiating therapy and subsequently, as appropriate.

Drug Interactions

Midodrine Drug Interactions

Precipitant drug	Object drug[a]		Description
Alpha-adrenergic blocking agent (eg, prazosin, terazosin, doxazosin)	Midodrine	↓	Alpha-adrenergic antagonist agents can antagonize the effects of midodrine.
Metformin, H_2 antagonists, procainamide, triamterene, flecainide, quinidine	Midodrine	↔	There may be a potential for interactions with these drugs.
Phenylephrine, pseudoephedrine, ephedrine, dihydroergotamine	Midodrine	↑	The use of drugs that stimulate alpha-adrenergic agonists may enhance or potentiate the pressor effects of midodrine.
Midodrine	Cardiac glycosides, psychopharmacologics, beta-blockers	↑	When coadministered with midodrine, cardiac glycosides, psychopharmacologic agents, or beta-blockers may enhance or precipitate bradycardia, A-V block, or arrhythmia (see Precautions).
Midodrine	Steroid therapy (eg, fludrocortisone)	↑	Concomitant use may increase the risk of supine hypertension. Reduce the dose of fludrocortisone or decrease the salt intake prior to initiation of treatment with midodrine. Fludrocortisone also causes an increase in intraocular pressure and glaucoma (see Precautions).

[a] ↑ = object drug increased; ↓ = object drug decreased; ↔ = undetermined clinical effect.

Adverse Reactions

Most frequent adverse reactions – Supine and sitting hypertension; paresthesia and pruritus, mainly of the scalp; goosebumps; chills; urinary urge; urinary retention and urinary frequency.

The frequency of these reactions in a 3-week placebo-controlled trial is shown in the following table:

Midodrine Adverse Reactions

Adverse reaction	Placebo (n = 88)		Midodrine (n = 82)	
	Number of reports	Percent of patients	Number of reports	Percent of patients
Total number of reports	22		77	
Paresthesia[a]	4	4.5%	15	18.3%
Piloerection	0	0%	11	13.4%
Dysuria[b]	0	0%	11	13.4%
Pruritus[c]	2	2.3%	10	12.2%
Supine hypertension[d]	0	0%	6	7.3%
Chills	0	0%	4	4.9%
Pain[e]	0	0%	4	4.9%
Rash	1	1.1%	2	2.4%

[a] Includes hyperesthesia and scalp paresthesia.
[b] Includes dysuria (1), increased urinary frequency (2), impaired urination (1), urinary retention (5), urinary urgency (2).
[c] Includes scalp pruritus.
[d] Includes patients who experienced an increase in supine hypertension.
[e] Includes abdominal pain and pain increase.

Less frequent adverse reactions – Headache; feeling of pressure/fullness in the head; vasodilation/flushing face; confusion/thinking abnormality; dry mouth; nervousness/anxiety, and rash.

Other adverse reactions (rare) – Visual field defect; dizziness; skin hyperesthesia; insomnia; somnolence; erythema multiforme; canker sore; dry skin; dysuria; impaired urination; asthenia; backache; pyrosis; nausea; gastrointestinal distress; flatulence, and leg cramps.

Most potentially serious adverse reaction – Supine hypertension. The feelings of paresthesia, pruritus, piloerection and chills are pilomotor reactions associated with the action of midodrine on the alpha-adrenergic receptors of the hair follicles. Feelings of urinary urgency, retention, and frequency are associated with the action of midodrine on the alpha-receptors of the bladder neck.

Overdosage

➤*Symptoms:* Symptoms of overdose could include hypertension, piloerection (goosebumps), a sensation of coldness and urinary retention. There are 2 reported cases of overdosage with midodrine, both in young males. One patient ingested midodrine drops, 250 mg, experienced systolic blood pressure greater than 200 mmHg, was treated with an IV injection of 20 mg of phentolamine, and was discharged the same night without any complaints. The other patient ingested 205 mg of midodrine (41 [5 mg] tablets), and was found lethargic and unable to talk, unresponsive to voice but responsive to painful stimuli, hypertensive and bradycardic. Gastric lavage was performed, and the patient recovered fully by the next day without sequelae.

The single doses that would be associated with symptoms of overdosage or would be potentially life-threatening are unknown. The oral LD_{50} is approximately 30 to 50 mg/kg in rats, 675 mg/kg in mice, and 125 to 160 mg/kg in dogs.

➤*Treatment:* Desglymidodrine is dialyzable.

Recommended general treatment, based on the pharmacology of the drug, includes induced emesis and administration of alpha-sympatholytic drugs (eg, phentolamine).

Patient Information

Patients should be told that certain agents in over-the-counter products, such as cold remedies and diet aids, can elevate blood pressure, and therefore, should be used cautiously with midodrine, as they may enhance or potentiate the pressor effects of midodrine. These agents include phenylephrine, pseudoephedrine, ephedrine, and phenylpropanolamine. Patients should also be made aware of the possibility of supine hypertension. They should be told to avoid taking their dose if they are to be supine for any length of time (ie, they should take their last daily dose of midodrine 3 to 4 hours before bedtime to minimize nighttime supine hypertension).

POTASSIUM REMOVING RESINS

SODIUM POLYSTYRENE SULFONATE

Rx	**SPS** (Carolina Medical Products)	**Suspension; oral or rectal:** 15 g per 60 mL	Alcohol 0.3%, parabens, propylene glycol, saccharin, sodium 1.5 g (65 mEq) per 60 mL, sorbitol 20 g per 60 mL. Cherry flavor. In 120, 473, and UD 60 mL.
Rx	**Kionex** (Paddock Laboratories)		Alcohol 0.2%, parabens, propylene glycol, saccharin, sodium 1.5 g (65 mEq) per 60 mL, sorbitol 19.3 g per 60 mL. Raspberry flavor. In 480 and UD 60 mL.
Rx	**Kayexalate** (Sanofi-Aventis)	**Powder for suspension; oral or rectal:** Finely ground sodium polystyrene sulfonate	Sodium ≈ 100 mg (4.1 mEq)/g. In 453.6 g.
Rx	**Kionex** (Paddock Laboratories)		Sodium ≈ 100 mg (4.1 mEq)/g. In 454 g.
Rx	**Sodium Polystyrene Sulfonate** (Various, eg, Carolina Medical, Harvard Drug, Major)		In 454 g.

SODIUM POLYSTYRENE SULFONATE — ORAL

Indications

➤*Hyperkalemia:* For the treatment of hyperkalemia.

Administration and Dosage

➤*General dosing considerations:* The intensity and duration of therapy depend upon the severity and resistance of hyperkalemia.

Each 60 mL of sodium polystyrene sulfonate suspension contains sodium 1,500 mg (65 mEq).

One gram of sodium polystyrene sulfonate powder contains sodium 100 mg (4.1 mEq); 1 level teaspoon of sodium polystyrene sulfonate powder contains approximately 3.5 g of sodium polystyrene sulfonate and sodium 15 mEq. A heaping teaspoon may contain as much as 10 to 12 g of sodium polystyrene sulfonate.

Because the in vivo efficiency of sodium potassium exchange resins is approximately 33%, approximately one-third of the resin's actual sodium content is being delivered to the body.

Coadministration with sorbitol is not recommended. (See also Warnings/Precautions.)

Rectal administration produces less effective results.

➤*Adults:*

Hyperkalemia –

Powder for suspension: 15 to 60 g/day, administered as a suspension. This is best provided by administering sodium polystyrene sulfonate 15 g (approximately 4 level teaspoons) 1 to 4 times daily. (See also Preparation for Administration.)

Suspension: 15 (60 mL) to 60 g (240 mL)/day. This is best provided by administering 15 g (60 mL) 1 to 4 times daily.

➤*Children:* In smaller children and infants, lower doses should be employed by using as a guide a rate of potassium 1 mEq/g of resin as the basis of calculation.

Off-label dosing –

Hyperkalemia: 1 g/kg every 6 hours.

➤*Elderly:* See Warnings/Precautions for more information.

➤*Renal function impairment:* See Warnings/Precautions for more information.

➤*Duration of therapy:* Because intracellular potassium deficiency is not always reflected by serum potassium levels, the level at which treatment with sodium polystyrene sulfonate should be discontinued must be determined individually for each patient. Important aids in making this determination are the patient's clinical condition and electrocardiogram (ECG).

➤*Preparation for administration:* Each dose of the powder should be given as a suspension in a small quantity of water or, for greater palatability, in syrup. The amount of fluid usually ranges from 20 to 100 mL, depending on the dose, or may be simply determined by allowing 3 to 4 mL/g of resin.

Shake suspension well before using.

➤*Administration:* Follow full aspiration precautions when administering sodium polystyrene sulfonate, such as placing and maintaining the patient in an upright position while the resin is being administered.

The suspension may be introduced into the stomach through a plastic tube and, if desired, given with a diet appropriate for a patient with renal failure.

➤*Storage/Stability:* Store at 20° to 25°C (68° to 77°F); excursions are permitted to 15° to 30°C (59° to 86°F).

Sodium polystyrene sulfonate should not be heated; doing so may alter the exchange properties of the resin.

Powder – The suspension should be freshly prepared from powder and not stored for longer than 24 hours.

Suspension – Dispense in a tight container. If repackaging into other containers, store in refrigerator and use within 14 days of packaging.

Actions

➤*Pharmacology:* Sodium polystyrene sulfonate is a cation-exchange resin. As the sodium polystyrene sulfonate resin passes along the intestine or is retained in the colon after administration by enema, the sodium ions are partially released and are replaced by potassium ions. This action occurs mostly in the large intestine, which excretes potassium ions to a greater degree than does the small intestine. The efficiency of this process is limited and unpredictably variable. It commonly approximates the order of 33%, but the range is so large that definitive indices of electrolyte balance must be clearly monitored.

Contraindications

Hypokalemia; hypersensitivity to polystyrene sulfonate resins; obstructive bowel disease; oral administration in neonates; rectal administration in neonates (suspension only); neonates with reduced gut motility (postoperatively or drug induced) (powder only); any postoperative patient until normal bowel function resumes (suspension only).

Warnings/Precautions

➤*Alternative therapy in severe hyperkalemia:* Because the effective lowering of serum potassium with sodium polystyrene sulfonate may take hours to days, treatment with this drug alone may be insufficient to rapidly correct severe hyperkalemia associated with states of rapid tissue breakdown (eg, burns and renal failure) or hyperkalemia so marked as to constitute a medical emergency. Therefore, always consider other definitive measures, including dialysis, which may be imperative.

➤*Hypokalemia:* Serious potassium deficiency can occur from sodium polystyrene sulfonate therapy. The effect must be carefully controlled by frequent serum potassium determinations within each 24-hour period. Because intracellular potassium deficiency is not always reflected by serum potassium levels, the level at which to discontinue treatment with sodium polystyrene sulfonate must be determined individually for each patient. Important aids in making this determination are the patient's clinical condition and electrocardiogram. Early clinical signs of severe hypokalemia include a pattern of irritable confusion and delayed thought processes. Electrocardiographically, severe hypokalemia is often associated with a lengthened QT interval, widening, flattening, or inversion of the T wave, and prominent U waves. Also, cardiac arrhythmias may occur, such as premature atrial, nodal, and ventricular contractions, and supraventricular and ventricular tachycardias. The toxic effects of digitalis are likely to be exaggerated. Marked hypokalemia can also be manifested by severe muscle weakness, at times extending into frank paralysis.

➤*Electrolyte disturbances:* Like all cation-exchange resins, sodium polystyrene sulfonate is not totally selective (for potassium) in its actions, and small amounts of other cations, such as magnesium and calcium, can also be lost during treatment. Accordingly, monitor patients receiving sodium polystyrene sulfonate for all applicable electrolyte disturbances.

➤*Systemic alkalosis:* Systemic alkalosis has been reported after cation-exchange resins were administered orally in combination with nonabsorbable cation-donating antacids and laxatives, such as magnesium hydroxide and aluminum carbonate. Do not administer magnesium hydroxide with sodium polystyrene sulfonate. One case of grand mal seizure has been reported in a patient with chronic hypocalcemia of renal failure who was given sodium polystyrene sulfonate with magnesium hydroxide as a laxative. (See Drug Interactions for more information.)

➤*Intestinal necrosis:* Cases of intestinal necrosis, which may be fatal, and other serious GI adverse reactions (bleeding, ischemic colitis, perforation) have been reported in association with sodium polystyrene sulfonate use. The majority of these cases reported the concomitant use of sorbitol. Risk factors for GI adverse events were present in many of the cases, including prematurity, history of intestinal disease or surgery, hypovolemia, and renal insufficiency and failure. Coadministration of sorbitol is not recommended.

➤*Sodium:* Caution is advised when sodium polystyrene sulfonate is administered to patients who cannot tolerate even a small increase in sodium loads (ie, severe congestive heart failure, severe hypertension, or marked edema). In such instances, compensatory restriction of sodium intake from other sources may be indicated.

➤*Patients undergoing surgery:* Do not administer sodium polystyrene sulfonate to patients following surgery until normal bowel function resumes.

➤*Constipation:* If clinically significant constipation occurs, discontinue treatment with sodium polystyrene sulfonate until normal bowel motion is resumed. Do not use magnesium-containing laxatives or sorbitol.

➤*Aspiration:* Position the patient carefully when ingesting the resin in order to avoid aspiration, which may lead to bronchopulmonary complications.

➤*Renal function impairment:* Caution is advised when sodium polystyrene sulfonate is administered to patients with end-stage diabetic renal disease.

➤*Pregnancy: Category C.* Animal reproduction studies have not been conducted with sodium polystyrene sulfonate. It is also not known whether sodium polystyrene sulfonate can cause fetal harm when administered to a pregnant woman or can affect reproduction capacity. Give sodium polystyrene sulfonate to a pregnant woman only if clearly needed.

➤*Lactation:* It is not known whether this drug is excreted in human milk. Because many drugs are excreted in human milk, exercise caution when sodium polystyrene sulfonate is administered to a breast-feeding woman.

➤*Children:* The effectiveness of sodium polystyrene sulfonate in children has not been established. Oral administration of sodium polystyrene sulfonate is contraindicated in neonates and especially in premature infants.

Due to the risk of digestive hemorrhage or intestinal necrosis, observe particular care in premature infants or low birth weight infants.

➤*Elderly:* Large doses in elderly individuals may cause fecal impaction.

➤*Monitoring:* Frequently monitor serum potassium levels. Regularly monitor other electrolytes (eg, magnesium, calcium, sodium). Monitor ECG in select patients.

SODIUM POLYSTYRENE SULFONATE — ORAL

Drug Interactions

Sodium Polystyrene Sulfonate Drug Interactions

Precipitant drug	Object drug[a]		Description
Antacids	Sodium polystyrene sulfonate	↑↓	The simultaneous oral administration of sodium polystyrene sulfonate with nonabsorbable cation-donating antacids and laxatives may reduce the resin's potassium exchange capability. Systemic alkalosis has been reported after cation-exchange resins were administered orally in combination with nonabsorbable cation-donating antacids and laxatives, such as magnesium hydroxide and aluminum carbonate. One case of grand mal seizure has been reported in a patient with chronic hypocalcemia of renal failure who was given sodium polystyrene sulfonate with magnesium hydroxide as a laxative. Intestinal obstruction due to concretions of aluminum hydroxide when used in combination with sodium polystyrene sulfonate has been reported. If these agents are used concurrently, separate the administration times by at least several hours. Magnesium hydroxide should not be administered with sodium polystyrene sulfonate.
Digoxin	Sodium polystyrene sulfonate	↑	The toxic effects of digitalis on the heart, especially various ventricular arrhythmias and atrioventricular nodal dissociation, are likely to be exaggerated by hypokalemia, even in the face of serum digoxin concentrations in the "normal range." Close clinical and laboratory monitoring are warranted.
Sorbitol	Sodium polystyrene sulfonate	↑	Concomitant use of sorbitol with sodium polystyrene sulfonate has been implicated in cases of intestinal necrosis, which may be fatal. Concurrent use is not recommended.
Sodium polystyrene sulfonate	Lithium	↓	Lithium absorption may be reduced, decreasing the pharmacologic effect. Close clinical and laboratory monitoring is warranted. If an interaction is suspected, adjust lithium therapy as needed.
Sodium polystyrene sulfonate	Thyroid hormones (eg, levothyroxine)	↓	Thyroxine absorption may be reduced, decreasing the pharmacologic effect. Closely monitor thyroid function and adjust thyroid hormone treatment as needed.

[a] ↑ = object drug increased; ↓ = object drug decreased; ↑↓ = object drug both increased and decreased.

Adverse Reactions

➤*GI:* Sodium polystyrene sulfonate may cause some degree of gastric irritation. Anorexia, nausea, vomiting, and constipation may occur, especially if high doses are given. Diarrhea occasionally develops. Large doses in elderly individuals may cause fecal impaction. Rare instances of intestinal necrosis have been reported. Intestinal obstruction due to concretions of aluminum hydroxide, when used in combination with sodium polystyrene sulfonate, has been reported.

➤*Metabolic:* Hypokalemia, hypocalcemia, and significant sodium retention (and their related clinical manifestations) may occur. Cases of hypomagnesemia have been reported.

➤*Postmarketing:*

GI – Fecal impaction following rectal administration, particularly in children; GI concretions (bezoars) following oral administration; ischemic colitis or GI tract ulceration or necrosis, which could lead to intestinal perforation. Intestinal necrosis has been reported with concomitant use of sorbitol.

Respiratory – Rare cases of acute bronchitis and/or bronchopneumonia associated with inhalation of particles of polystyrene sulfonate.

Overdosage

➤*Symptoms:* Overdosage may result in electrolyte disturbances, including hypokalemia, hypocalcemia, and hypomagnesemia. Biochemical disturbances resulting from overdosage may give rise to clinical signs and symptoms of hypokalemia, including irritability, confusion, delayed thought processes, muscle weakness, hyporeflexia (which may progress to frank paralysis), and/or apnea. Hypocalcemic tetany may occur. ECG changes may be consistent with hypokalemia or hypercalcemia; cardiac arrhythmias may occur.

➤*Treatment:* Take appropriate measures to correct serum electrolytes (potassium, calcium, magnesium); remove the resin from the alimentary tract by appropriate use of laxatives or enemas.

Patient Information

Instruct patients to shake suspension well before taking this medicine. Inform patients not to take this medicine with magnesium hydroxide or sorbitol. Advise patients to report any of the following symptoms to their health care provider: anorexia, nausea, vomiting; changes in bowel function; confusion, trouble thinking; severe muscle weakness; palpitations.

SODIUM POLYSTYRENE SULFONATE — RECTAL

Indications

➤*Hyperkalemia:* For the treatment of hyperkalemia.

Administration and Dosage

➤*General dosing considerations:* The intensity and duration of therapy depend upon the severity and resistance of hyperkalemia.

Each 60 mL of sodium polystyrene sulfonate suspension contains sodium 1,500 mg (65 mEq).

One gram of sodium polystyrene sulfonate powder contains sodium 100 mg (4.1 mEq); 1 level teaspoon of sodium polystyrene sulfonate powder contains approximately 3.5 g of sodium polystyrene sulfonate and sodium 15 mEq. A heaping teaspoon may contain as much as 10 to 12 g of sodium polystyrene sulfonate.

Because the in vivo efficiency of sodium potassium exchange resins is approximately 33%, about one-third of the resin's actual sodium content is being delivered to the body.

Coadministration with sorbitol is not recommended. (See also Warnings/Precautions.)

Compared with oral administration of sodium polystyrene sulfonate, rectal administration produces less effective results.

➤*Adults:*

Hyperkalemia – 30 g (120 mL) to 50 g (200 mL) every 6 hours as a retention enema. When using sodium polystyrene sulfonate powder, each dose is administered as a warm emulsion (at body temperature) in 100 mL of aqueous vehicle. The emulsion should be agitated gently during administration. The enema should be retained as long as possible and followed by a cleansing enema. (See also Administration.)

➤*Children:* In smaller children and infants, lower doses should be employed by using as a guide a rate of 1 mEq of potassium per gram of resin as the basis of calculation.

Off-label dosing –

Hyperkalemia: 1 g/kg every 2 to 6 hours.

➤*Elderly:* See Warnings/Precautions for more information.

➤*Renal function impairment:* See Warnings/Precautions for more information.

➤*Duration of therapy:* Because intracellular potassium deficiency is not always reflected by serum potassium levels, the level at which treatment with sodium polystyrene sulfonate should be discontinued must be determined individually for each patient. Important aids in making this determination are the patient's clinical condition and electrocardiogram (ECG).

➤*Preparation for administration:* Shake suspension well before using.

➤*Administration:* After an initial cleansing enema, a soft, large-size (French 28) rubber tube is inserted into the rectum for a distance of 20 cm, with the tip well into the sigmoid colon and taped in place. When using the premixed suspension, the suspension is introduced at body temperature by gravity. When using the powder, the resin is suspended in the appropriate amount of aqueous vehicle at body temperature and introduced by gravity,

SODIUM POLYSTYRENE SULFONATE — RECTAL

while the particles are kept in suspension by stirring. The suspension is flushed with 50 or 100 mL of fluid, following which the tube is clamped and left in place. If back leakage occurs, the hips are elevated on pillows or a knee-chest position is taken temporarily. A somewhat thicker suspension may be used, but care should be taken that no paste is formed because the latter has a greatly reduced exchange surface and will be particularly ineffective if deposited in the rectal ampulla. The suspension is kept in the sigmoid colon for several hours, if possible. Then the colon is irrigated with a sodium-free cleansing enema at body temperature in order to remove the resin. Two quarts of flushing solution may be necessary. The returns are drained constantly through a Y tube connection. While the use of sorbitol is not recommended, particular attention should be paid to this cleansing enema if sorbitol has been used. Sorbitol is present in the vehicle of the premixed suspension.

➤*Storage / Stability:* Store at 20° to 25°C (68° to 77°F); excursions are permitted to 15° to 30°C (59° to 86°F).

Sodium polystyrene sulfonate should not be heated; doing so may alter the exchange properties of the resin.

Powder – The suspension should be freshly prepared from powder and not stored longer than 24 hours.

Suspension – Dispense in a tight container. If repackaging into other containers, store in refrigerator and use within 14 days of packaging.

Actions

➤*Pharmacology:* Sodium polystyrene sulfonate is a cation-exchange resin. As the sodium polystyrene sulfonate resin passes along the intestine or is retained in the colon after administration by enema, the sodium ions are partially released and are replaced by potassium ions. This action occurs mostly in the large intestine, which excretes potassium ions to a greater degree than does the small intestine. The efficiency of this process is limited and unpredictably variable. It commonly approximates the order of 33%, but the range is so large that definitive indices of electrolyte balance must be clearly monitored.

Contraindications

Hypokalemia; hypersensitivity to polystyrene sulfonate resins; obstructive bowel disease; oral administration in neonates; rectal administration in neonates (suspension only); neonates with reduced gut motility (postoperatively or drug induced) (powder only); any postoperative patient until normal bowel function resumes (suspension only).

Warnings/Precautions

➤*Alternative therapy in severe hyperkalemia:* Because the effective lowering of serum potassium with sodium polystyrene sulfonate may take hours to days, treatment with this drug alone may be insufficient to rapidly correct severe hyperkalemia associated with states of rapid tissue breakdown (eg, burns and renal failure) or hyperkalemia so marked as to constitute a medical emergency. Therefore, always consider other definitive measures, including dialysis, which may be imperative.

➤*Hypokalemia:* Serious potassium deficiency can occur from sodium polystyrene sulfonate therapy. The effect must be carefully controlled by frequent serum potassium determinations within each 24-hour period. Because intracellular potassium deficiency is not always reflected by serum potassium levels, determine the level at which to discontinue treatment with sodium polystyrene sulfonate individually for each patient. Important aids in making this determination are the patient's clinical condition and electrocardiogram. Early clinical signs of severe hypokalemia include a pattern of irritable confusion and delayed thought processes. Electrocardiographically, severe hypokalemia is often associated with a lengthened QT interval, widening, flattening, or inversion of the T wave, and prominent U waves. Also, cardiac arrhythmias may occur, such as premature atrial, nodal, and ventricular contractions, and supraventricular and ventricular tachycardias. The toxic effects of digitalis are likely to be exaggerated. Marked hypokalemia can also be manifested by severe muscle weakness, at times extending into frank paralysis.

➤*Electrolyte disturbances:* Like all cation-exchange resins, sodium polystyrene sulfonate is not totally selective (for potassium) in its actions, and small amounts of other cations, such as magnesium and calcium, can also be lost during treatment. Accordingly, monitor patients receiving sodium polystyrene sulfonate for all applicable electrolyte disturbances.

➤*Systemic alkalosis:* Systemic alkalosis has been reported after cation-exchange resins were administered orally in combination with nonabsorbable cation-donating antacids and laxatives, such as magnesium hydroxide and aluminum carbonate. Do not administer magnesium hydroxide with sodium polystyrene sulfonate. One case of grand mal seizure has been reported in a patient with chronic hypocalcemia of renal failure who was given sodium polystyrene sulfonate with magnesium hydroxide as a laxative.

➤*Intestinal necrosis:* Cases of intestinal necrosis, which may be fatal, and other serious GI adverse reactions (bleeding, ischemic colitis, perforation) have been reported in association with sodium polystyrene sulfonate use. The majority of these cases reported the concomitant use of sorbitol. Risk factors for GI adverse events were present in many of the cases, including prematurity, history of intestinal disease or surgery, hypovolemia, and renal insufficiency and failure. Coadministration of sorbitol is not recommended.

➤*Sodium:* Caution is advised when sodium polystyrene sulfonate is administered to patients who cannot tolerate even a small increase in sodium loads (ie, severe congestive heart failure, severe hypertension, or marked edema). In such instances, compensatory restriction of sodium intake from other sources may be indicated.

➤*Patients undergoing surgery:* Do not administer sodium polystyrene sulfonate to patients following surgery until normal bowel function resumes.

➤*Constipation:* If clinically significant constipation occurs, discontinue treatment with sodium polystyrene sulfonate until normal bowel motion is resumed. Do not use magnesium-containing laxatives or sorbitol.

➤*Cleansing enema:* Take precautions to ensure the use of adequate volumes of sodium-free cleansing enemas after rectal administration.

➤*Renal function impairment:* Caution is advised when sodium polystyrene sulfonate is administered to patients with end-stage diabetic renal disease.

➤*Pregnancy:* *Category C.* Animal reproduction studies have not been conducted with sodium polystyrene sulfonate. It is also not known whether sodium polystyrene sulfonate can cause fetal harm when administered to a pregnant woman or can affect reproduction capacity. Give sodium polystyrene sulfonate to a pregnant woman only if clearly needed.

➤*Lactation:* It is not known whether this drug is excreted in human milk. Because many drugs are excreted in human milk, exercise caution when sodium polystyrene sulfonate is administered to a breast-feeding woman.

➤*Children:* The effectiveness of sodium polystyrene sulfonate in children has not been established. Rectal administration of the premixed suspension is contraindicated in neonates. The powder for suspension is contraindicated in neonates with reduced gut motility. In both children and neonates, observe particular care with rectal administration, as excessive dosage or inadequate dilution could result in impaction of the resin. Take precautions to ensure the use of adequate volumes of sodium-free cleansing enemas after rectal administration.

Due to the risk of digestive hemorrhage or intestinal necrosis, observe particular care in premature infants or low birth weight infants.

➤*Elderly:* Large doses in elderly individuals may cause fecal impaction.

➤*Monitoring:* Frequently monitor serum potassium levels. Regularly monitor other electrolytes (eg, magnesium, calcium, sodium). Monitor ECG in select patients.

Drug Interactions

Sodium Polystyrene Sulfonate Drug Interactions

Precipitant drug	Object drug[a]		Description
Digoxin	Sodium polystyrene sulfonate	↑	The toxic effects of digitalis on the heart, especially various ventricular arrhythmias and atrioventricular nodal dissociation, are likely to be exaggerated by hypokalemia, even in the face of serum digoxin concentrations in the "normal range." Close clinical and laboratory monitoring are warranted.
Sorbitol	Sodium polystyrene sulfonate	↑	Concomitant use of sorbitol with sodium polystyrene sulfonate has been implicated in cases of intestinal necrosis, which may be fatal. Concurrent use is not recommended.

[a] ↑ = object drug increased.

Adverse Reactions

➤*GI:* Sodium polystyrene sulfonate may cause some degree of gastric irritation. Anorexia, nausea, vomiting, and constipation may occur, especially if high doses are given. Diarrhea occasionally develops. Large doses in elderly individuals may cause fecal impaction. Rare instances of intestinal necrosis have been reported. Intestinal obstruction due to concretions of aluminum hydroxide, when used in combination with sodium polystyrene sulfonate, has been reported.

➤*Metabolic:* Hypokalemia, hypocalcemia, and significant sodium retention (and their related clinical manifestations) may occur. Cases of hypomagnesemia have been reported.

➤*Postmarketing:*

GI – Fecal impaction following rectal administration, particularly in children; GI concretions (bezoars) following oral administration; ischemic colitis or GI tract ulceration or necrosis, which could lead to intestinal perforation. Intestinal necrosis has been reported with concomitant use of sorbitol.

Respiratory – Rare cases of acute bronchitis and/or bronchopneumonia associated with inhalation of particles of polystyrene sulfonate.

Overdosage

➤*Symptoms:* Overdosage may result in electrolyte disturbances, including hypokalemia, hypocalcemia, and hypomagnesemia. Biochemical disturbances resulting from overdosage may give rise to clinical signs and symptoms of hypokalemia, including irritability, confusion, delayed thought processes, muscle weakness, hyporeflexia (which may progress to frank paralysis) and/or apnea. Hypocalcemic tetany may occur. ECG changes may be consistent with hypokalemia or hypercalcemia; cardiac arrhythmias may occur.

➤*Treatment:* Take appropriate measures to correct serum electrolytes (potassium, calcium, magnesium); remove the resin from the alimentary tract by appropriate use of laxatives or enemas.

SODIUM POLYSTYRENE SULFONATE — RECTAL

Patient Information

Instruct patients to shake suspension well before taking this medicine. Inform patients not to take this medicine with magnesium hydroxide or sorbitol. Advise patients to report any of the following symptoms to their health care provider: anorexia, nausea, vomiting; changes in bowel function; confusion, trouble thinking; severe muscle weakness; palpitations.

CARDIOPLEGIC SOLUTIONS

CARDIOPLEGIC SOLUTION

Rx	**Plegisol** (Hospira)	**Solution:** 17.6 mg calcium chloride dihydrate, 325.3 mg magnesium chloride hexahydrate, 119.3 mg potassium chloride and 643 mg sodium chloride per 100 mL (approx. 260 mOsm/L)	In single-dose 1000 mL flexible plastic container.

CARDIOPLEGIC SOLUTION — INJECTION

Indications

➤*Open heart surgery:* With ischemia and hypothermia, induces cardiac arrest during open heart surgery.

Administration and Dosage

➤*General dosing considerations:* The volumes of solution instilled into the aortic root may vary depending on the duration or type of open heart surgical procedure.

➤*Adults:*

Open heart surgery –

Initial dosage: The initial rate of infusion may be 300 mL/m²/min (about 540 mL/min in a 1.8 meter, 70 kg adult with 1.8 square meters of surface area) given for 2 to 4 minutes.

If myocardial electromechanical activity persists or recurs, the solution may be reinfused at a rate of 300 mL/m²/min for 2 minutes. Repeat every 20 to 30 minutes or sooner if myocardial temperature rises above 15° to 20°C or returning cardiac activity is observed.

Concomitant therapy: Concurrent external cooling (regional hypothermia of the pericardium) may be accomplished by instilling a refrigerated (4°C) physiologic solution such as *Normosol-R* (balanced electrolyte replacement solution) or Ringer's Injection into the chest cavity.

The regional hypothermia solution around the heart also may be replenished continuously or periodically in order to maintain adequate hypothermia. Suction may be used to remove warmed infusates. An implanted thermistor probe may be used to monitor myocardial temperature.

➤*Preparation for administration:* The solution contains no preservatives and is intended only for a single operative procedure. After adjusting pH with sodium bicarbonate, extemporaneous alternative buffering is not recommended. Discard the unused portion.

Add 10 mL (840 mg) of 8.4% sodium bicarbonate injection (10 mEq each of sodium and bicarbonate) to each 1000 mL of the cardioplegic solution just prior to administration to adjust pH to approximately 7.8 when measured at room temperature. Use of any other Sodium Bicarbonate Injection may not achieve this pH due to the varying pH's of Sodium Bicarbonate Injections. Cool the buffered solution with added sodium bicarbonate to 4°C prior to administration and use within 24 hours of mixing.

➤*Administration:* Following institution of cardiopulmonary bypass at perfusate temperatures of 28° to 30°C, (82° to 86°F) and cross-clamping of the ascending aorta, administer the buffered solution by rapid infusion into the aortic root.

➤*Admixture compatibility:* Additives may be incompatible. Consult with pharmacist, if possible. When introducing additives, use aseptic technique, mix thoroughly and do not store.

➤*Storage / Stability:* Store at 25°C (77°F); however, brief exposure up to 40°C (104°F) does not adversely affect the product. Protect from freezing and extreme heat.

Actions

➤*Pharmacology:* Cardioplegic solution with added sodium bicarbonate, when cooled and instilled into the coronary artery vasculature, causes prompt arrest of cardiac electromechanical activity, combats intracellular ion losses and buffers ischemic acidosis. When used with hypothermia and ischemia, the action may be characterized as cold ischemic potassium-induced cardioplegia. This provides a quiet, relaxed heart and bloodless field of operation. The component electrolytes and their physiologic effects are listed below:

➤*Pharmacokinetics:*

Calcium (Ca^{++}) ion – Maintains integrity of cell membrane to ensure against calcium paradox during reperfusion.

Magnesium (Mg^{++}) ion – May help stabilize the myocardial membrane by inhibiting a myosin phosphorylase, which protects adenosine triphosphate (ATP) reserves for postischemic activity. The protective effects of magnesium and potassium are additive.

Potassium (K^{++}) ion – Causes prompt cessation of mechanical myocardial contractile activity. The immediacy of the arrest thus preserves energy supplies for postischemic contractile activity in diastole.

Chloride (Cl^-) and sodium (Na^+) ions – Sodium is essential to maintain ionic integrity of myocardial tissue. Chloride ions maintain the electroneutrality of the solution and have no specific role in the production of cardiac arrest.

Bicarbonate (HCO_{3^-}) anion – Acts as a buffer to render the solution slightly alkaline and compensate for the metabolic acidosis that accompanies ischemia.

Contraindications

Do not administer without the addition of 8.4% Sodium Bicarbonate Injection.

Not for IV injection; only for instillation into cardiac vasculature.

Warnings/Precautions

➤*Intended use:* Only those trained to perform open heart surgery should use this solution. It is intended only for use during cardiopulmonary bypass when the coronary circulation is isolated from the systemic circulation.

➤*Right heart venting:* Right heart venting is recommended. If large volumes of cardioplegic solution are infused and allowed to return to the heart lung machine without any venting from the right heart, plasma magnesium and potassium levels may rise. Development of severe hypotension and metabolic acidosis while on bypass has occurred when large volumes (8 to 10 L) of solution are instilled and allowed to enter the pump and then the systemic circulation.

➤*Do not administer:* Do not administer unless solution is clear and container is undamaged.

➤*Pregnancy: Category C.* Safety for use during pregnancy has not been established. Use only when clearly needed and when the potential benefits outweigh the potential hazards to the fetus.

➤*Lactation:* There are no data regarding the use of cardioplegic solution in breast-feeding patients.

➤*Monitoring:* Monitor myocardial temperature during surgery to maintain hypothermia.

Continuous ECG monitoring of myocardial activity during the procedure is essential.

Appropriate equipment to defibrillate the heart following cardioplegia and inotropic agents during postoperative recovery should be readily available.

Adverse Reactions

Potential hazards of open heart surgery include myocardial infarction, ECG abnormalities and arrhythmias, including ventricular fibrillation. Spontaneous recovery may be delayed or absent when circulation is restored. Defibrillation by electric shock may be required to restore normal cardiac function.

Overdosage

Overzealous instillation may result in unnecessary dilatation of the myocardial vasculature and leakage into the perivascular myocardium, possibly causing tissue edema.

ALPROSTADIL (Prostaglandin E_1; PGE_1)

Rx	**Prostin VR Pediatric** (Upjohn)	**Injection:** 500 mcg/mL[a]	In 1 mL amps.

[a] In 1 mL dehydrated alcohol.

ALPROSTADIL — INJECTION

WARNING

Apnea is experienced by about 10% to 12% of neonates with congenital heart defects treated with alprostadil pediatric sterile solution. Apnea is most often seen in neonates weighing less than 2 kg at birth and usually appears during the first hour of drug infusion. Therefore, monitor respiratory status throughout treatment, and use alprostadil pediatric injection where ventilatory assistance is immediately available.

Indications

➤*Patent ductus arteriosus:* For palliative, not definitive, therapy to temporarily maintain the patency of the ductus arteriosus until corrective or palliative surgery can be performed in neonates who have congenital heart defects and who depend upon the patent ductus for survival. Such congenital heart defects include pulmonary atresia, pulmonary stenosis, tricuspid atresia, tetralogy of Fallot, interruption of the aortic arch, coarctation of the aorta, or transposition of the great vessels, with or without other defects.

➤*Off-label uses:*

Raynaud phenomenon – [2] = Fair documentation. Initial data suggest alprostadil is effective for the treatment of Raynaud phenomenon, decreasing both subjective and objective measures of the disease. Alprostadil appears to be well tolerated with only minor adverse effects. (See Administration and Dosage.)

Administration and Dosage

➤*Children:*

Patent ductus arteriosus –

Initial dosage: Begin infusion with 0.05 to 0.1 mcg alprostadil per kg of body weight per minute.

Dosage adjustment: After a therapeutic response is achieved (increased pO_2 in infants with restricted pulmonary blood flow or increased systemic blood pressure and blood pH in infants with restricted systemic blood flow), reduce the infusion rate to provide the lowest possible dosage that maintains the response. This may be accomplished by reducing the dosage from 0.1 to 0.05 to 0.025 to 0.01 mcg/kg of body weight per minute. If response to 0.05 mcg/kg of body weight per minute is inadequate, dosage can be increased up to 0.4 mcg/kg of body weight per minute; although, in general, higher infusion rates do not produce greater effects.

Off-label dosing –

Raynaud phenomenon: [2] = Fair documentation. IV doses have ranged from a loading dose for 5 days followed by 2 maintenance doses once every 30 days at a dosage of 20 mcg/h over 3 hours. Alternative dosages include 60 mcg daily infused over 3 hours for 6 days or 40 mcg at a rate of 3 to 5 ng/kg/min given twice daily. The treatment duration was a minimum of 7 days repeated every 3 to 4 weeks.

➤*Preparation for administration:* To prepare infusion solutions, dilute 1 mL of alprostadil pediatric sterile solution with sodium chloride injection or dextrose injection.

When using a volumetric infusion chamber, the appropriate amount of IV infusion solution should be added to the chamber first. The undiluted alprostadil pediatric sterile solution should then be added to the IV infusion solution, avoiding direct contact of the undiluted solution with the walls of the volumetric infusion chamber.

Dilute to volumes appropriate for the pump delivery system available. Prepare fresh infusion solutions every 24 hours. Discard any solution more than 24 hours old.

Sample Dilutions and Infusion Rates to Provide an Alprostadil Dosage of 0.1 mcg/kg of Body Weight per Minute

Add 1 ampule (500 mcg) alprostadil to:	Approximate concentration of resulting solution (mcg/mL)	Infusion rate (mL/min/kg of body weight)
250 mL	2	0.05
100 mL	5	0.02
50 mL	10	0.01
25 mL	20	0.005

Example – To provide 0.1 mcg/kg of body weight per minute to an infant weighing 2.8 kg using a solution of 1 ampule alprostadil pediatric injection in 100 mL of saline or dextrose: Infusion rate = 0.02 mL/min/kg × 2.8 kg = 0.056 mL/min or 3.36 mL/h.

➤*Administration:* The preferred route of administration for alprostadil pediatric sterile solution is continuous intravenous (IV) infusion into a large vein. Alternatively, alprostadil pediatric injection may be administered through an umbilical artery catheter placed at the ductal opening. Increases in blood pO_2 (torr) have been the same in neonates who received the drug by either route of administration.

Alprostadil pediatric sterile solution must be diluted before it is administered.

➤*Admixture compatibility:* Dilute with sodium chloride injection or dextrose injection.

Undiluted alprostadil pediatric sterile solution may interact with the plastic sidewalls of volumetric infusion chambers, causing a change in the appearance of the chamber and creating a hazy solution. Should this occur, the solution and the volumetric infusion chamber should be replaced.

➤*Storage/Stability:* Store alprostadil at 2° to 8°C (36° to 46°F).

Actions

➤*Pharmacology:* Alprostadil (prostaglandin E_1) is one of a family of naturally occurring acidic lipids with various pharmacologic effects. Vasodilation, inhibition of platelet aggregation, and stimulation of intestinal and uterine smooth muscle are among the most notable of these effects. IV doses of 1 to 10 mcg of alprostadil per kg of body weight lower the blood pressure in mammals by decreasing peripheral resistance. Reflex increases in cardiac output and rate accompany the reduction in blood pressure.

Smooth muscle of the ductus arteriosus is especially sensitive to alprostadil, and strips of lamb ductus markedly relax in the presence of the drug. In addition, administration of alprostadil reopened the closing ductus of newborn rats, rabbits, and lambs. These observations led to the investigation of alprostadil in infants who had congenital defects which restricted the pulmonary or systemic blood flow and who depended on a patent ductus arteriosus for adequate blood oxygenation and lower body perfusion.

In infants with restricted pulmonary blood flow, about 50% responded to alprostadil infusion with at least a 10 torr increase in blood pO_2 (mean increase about 14 torr and mean increase in oxygen saturation about 23%). In general, patients who responded best had low pretreatment blood pO_2 and were 4 days old or less.

In infants with restricted systemic blood flow, alprostadil often increased pH in those having acidosis, increased systemic blood pressure, and decreased the ratio of pulmonary artery pressure to aortic pressure.

➤*Pharmacokinetics:*

Metabolism/Excretion – Alprostadil must be infused continuously because it is very rapidly metabolized. As much as 80% of the circulating alprostadil may be metabolized in 1 pass through the lungs, primarily by β- and ω- oxidation. The metabolites are excreted primarily by the kidney, and excretion is essentially complete within 24 hours after administration. No unchanged alprostadil has been found in the urine, and there is no evidence of tissue retention of alprostadil or its metabolites.

Contraindications

None.

Warnings/Precautions

➤*Apnea:* Apnea is experienced by about 10% to 12% of neonates with congenital heart defects treated with alprostadil pediatric sterile solution. Apnea is most often seen in neonates weighing less than 2 kg at birth and usually appears during the first hour of drug infusion. Therefore, monitor respiratory status throughout treatment, and use alprostadil pediatric injection where ventilatory assistance is immediately available.

➤*Gastric outlet obstruction:* The administration of alprostadil pediatric injection to neonates may result in gastric outlet obstruction secondary to antral hyperplasia. This effect appears to be related to duration of therapy and cumulative dose of the drug. Closely monitor neonates receiving alprostadil pediatric injection at recommended doses for more than 120 hours for evidence of antral hyperplasia and gastric outlet obstruction.

➤*Duration of infusion:* Infuse alprostadil pediatric injection for the shortest time and at the lowest dose that will produce the desired effects. Weigh the risks of long-term infusion of alprostadil pediatric injection against the possible benefits that critically ill infants may derive from its administration.

➤*Skeletal effects:* Cortical proliferation of the long bones, first observed in dogs, has also been observed in infants during long-term infusions of alprostadil. The cortical proliferation in infants regressed after withdrawal of the drug.

➤*Causes of death unrelated to ductus arteriosus:* In infants treated with alprostadil pediatric injection at the usual doses for 10 hours to 12 days, and who died of causes unrelated to ductus structural weakness, tissue sections of the ductus and pulmonary arteries have shown intimal lacerations, a decrease in medial muscularity and disruption of the medial and internal elastic lamina. Localized and aneurysmal dilatations and vessel wall edema also were seen compared to a series of pathological specimens from infants not treated with alprostadil pediatric injection. The incidence of such structural alterations has not been defined.

➤*Hematologic effects:* Because alprostadil inhibits platelet aggregation, use alprostadil pediatric injection cautiously in neonates with bleeding tendencies.

➤*Respiratory distress syndrome:* Do not use alprostadil pediatric injection in neonates with respiratory distress syndrome. A differential diagnosis should be made between respiratory distress syndrome (hyaline membrane disease) and cyanotic heart disease (restricted pulmonary blood flow). If full diagnostic facilities are not immediately available, cyanosis (pO_2 less than

ALPROSTADIL — INJECTION

40 torr) and restricted pulmonary blood flow apparent on an x-ray are appropriate indicators of congenital heart defects.

➤*Pregnancy: Category: Undetermined.* Alprostadil is not indicated for use in adults.

➤*Lactation:* Alprostadil is not indicated for use in adults.

➤*Monitoring:* In all neonates, monitor arterial pressure intermittently by umbilical artery catheter, auscultation, or with a Doppler transducer. Should arterial pressure fall significantly, decrease the rate of infusion immediately.

In infants with restricted pulmonary blood flow, measure efficacy of alprostadil pediatric injection by monitoring improvement in blood oxygenation. In infants with restricted systemic blood flow, measure efficacy by monitoring improvement of systemic blood pressure and blood pH.

Drug Interactions

None known.

Adverse Reactions

➤*Cardiovascular:* The most common cardiovascular adverse reactions reported have been flushing in about 10% of patients (more common after intra-arterial dosing), bradycardia in about 7%, hypotension in about 4%, tachycardia in about 3%, cardiac arrest in about 1%, and edema in about 1%. The following reactions have been reported in less than 1% of the patients: congestive heart failure, hyperemia, second degree heart block, shock, spasm of the right ventricle infundibulum, supraventricular tachycardia, and ventricular fibrillation.

➤*CNS:* Apnea has been reported in about 12% of the neonates treated. Other common adverse reactions reported have been fever in about 14% of the patients treated and seizures in about 4%. The following reactions have been reported in less than 1% of the patients: Cerebral bleeding, hyperextension of the neck, hyperirritability, hypothermia, jittering, lethargy, and stiffness.

➤*GI:* The most common GI adverse reaction reported has been diarrhea in about 2% of the patients. The following reactions have been reported in less than 1% of the patients: gastric regurgitation and hyperbilirubinemia.

➤*GU:* Anuria and hematuria have been reported in less than 1% of the patients.

➤*Hematologic:* The most common hematologic event reported has been disseminated intravascular coagulation in about 1% of the patients. The following events have been reported in less than 1% of the patients: anemia, bleeding, and thrombocytopenia.

➤*Musculoskeletal:* Cortical proliferation of the long bones has been reported.

➤*Respiratory:* The following reactions have been reported in less than 1% of the patients: Bradypnea, bronchial wheezing, hypercapnia, respiratory depression, respiratory distress, and tachypnea.

➤*Miscellaneous:* Sepsis has been reported in about 2% of the patients. Peritonitis has been reported in less than 1% of the patients. Hypokalemia has been reported in about 1%, and hypoglycemia and hyperkalemia have been reported in less than 1% of the patients.

Overdosage

➤*Symptoms:* Apnea, bradycardia, pyrexia, hypotension, and flushing may be signs of drug overdosage.

➤*Treatment:* If apnea or bradycardia occurs, discontinue the infusion, and provide appropriate medical treatment. Use caution in restarting the infusion. If pyrexia or hypotension occurs, reduce the infusion rate until these symptoms subside. Flushing is usually a result of incorrect intraarterial catheter placement, and the catheter should be repositioned.

IBUPROFEN LYSINE

Rx	**Neoprofen** (Ovation)	**Solution for injection**: ibuprofen lysine 17.1 mg/mL (equivalent to 10 mg/mL (±) -ibuprofen)	Preservative free. In single-use vials.

IBUPROFEN LYSINE — INJECTION

Indications

➤*Patent ductus arteriosus (PDA):* To close a clinically significant PDA in premature infants weighing between 500 and 1,500 g who are no more than 32 weeks of gestational age when usual medical management (eg, diuretics, fluid restriction, respiratory support) is ineffective. The clinical trial was conducted among infants with asymptomatic PDA. However, the consequences beyond 8 weeks after treatment have not been evaluated; therefore, reserve treatment for infants with clear evidence of a clinically significant PDA.

Administration and Dosage

➤*General dosing considerations:* If anuria or marked oliguria (urinary output less than 0.6 mL/kg/h) is evident at the scheduled time of the second or third dose, no additional dosage should be given until laboratory studies indicate that renal function has returned to normal.

Because ibuprofen lysine is potentially irritating to tissues, it should be administered carefully to avoid extravasation. (See Administration.)

➤*Children:*

Patent ductus arteriosus –

Initial dosage: 10 mg/kg IV, followed by 2 doses of 5 mg/kg each, after 24 and 48 hours. A course of therapy is 3 doses administered IV (administration via an umbilical arterial line has not been evaluated). All doses should be based on birth weight.

If the ductus arteriosus closes or is significantly reduced in size after completion of the first course of ibuprofen lysine, no further doses are necessary. If during continued medical management the ductus arteriosus fails to close or reopens, then a second course of ibuprofen, alternative pharmacological therapy, or surgery may be necessary.

Duration of therapy: There are no long-term evaluations of the infants treated with ibuprofen at durations of more than the 36 weeks of postconceptual age observation period.

➤*Preparation for administration:* For administration, ibuprofen lysine should be diluted to an appropriate volume with dextrose or saline.

➤*Administration:* For intravenous (IV) administration only.

Ibuprofen lysine should be prepared for infusion and administered within 30 minutes of preparation and infused continuously over a period of 15 minutes. The drug should be administered via the IV port that is nearest the insertion site. After the first withdrawal from the vial, any solution remaining must be discarded because ibuprofen lysine contains no preservative.

Because ibuprofen lysine is potentially irritating to tissues, it should be administered carefully to avoid extravasation.

➤*Admixture compatibility:* Ibuprofen lysine should not be simultaneously administered in the same IV line with total parenteral nutrition (TPN). If necessary, TPN should be interrupted for a 15-minute period prior to and after drug administration. Line patency should be maintained by using dextrose or saline.

➤*Storage/Stability:* Store at 20° to 25°C (68° to 77°F); excursions are permitted to 15° to 30°C (59° to 86°F). Protect from light. Store vials in carton until contents have been used.

Actions

➤*Pharmacology:* The mechanism of action through which ibuprofen causes closure of a PDA in neonates is not known. In adults, ibuprofen is an inhibitor of prostaglandin synthesis.

➤*Pharmacokinetics:*

Absorption/Distribution – The population volume of distribution value of racemic ibuprofen for premature infants at birth was 320 mL/kg.

Metabolism/Excretion – The metabolism and excretion of ibuprofen in premature infants have not been studied. In adults, renal elimination of unchanged ibuprofen accounts for only 10% to 15% of the dose. The excretion of ibuprofen and metabolites occurs rapidly in both urine and feces. Approximately 80% of the dose administered orally is recovered in urine as hydroxyl and carboxyl metabolites as a mixture of conjugated and unconjugated forms. Ibuprofen is eliminated primarily by metabolism in the liver where CYP2C9 mediates the 2- and 3-hydroxylations of R- and S-ibuprofen. Ibuprofen and its metabolites are further conjugated to acyl glucuronides.

The population average clearance value of racemic ibuprofen for premature infants at birth was 3 mL/kg/h. Clearance increased rapidly with postnatal age (an average increase of approximately 0.5 mL/kg/h/day). Interindividual variability in clearance and volume of distribution were 55% and 14%, respectively. In general, the half-life in infants is more than 10 times longer than in adults. In neonates, renal function and the enzymes associated with drug metabolism are underdeveloped at birth and substantially increase in the days after birth.

Contraindications

Preterm infants with proven or suspected infection that is untreated; preterm infants with congenital heart disease in whom patency of the PDA is necessary for satisfactory pulmonary or systemic blood flow (eg, pulmonary atresia, severe coarctation of the aorta, severe tetralogy of Fallot); preterm infants who are bleeding, especially those with active intracranial hemorrhage or GI bleeding; preterm infants with thrombocytopenia; preterm infants with coagulation defects; preterm infants who have or who are suspected of having necrotizing enterocolitis; preterm infants with significant renal function impairment.

Warnings/Precautions

➤*Bleeding:* Ibuprofen lysine, like other NSAIDs, can inhibit platelet aggregation. Observe preterm infants for signs of bleeding. Ibuprofen has been shown to prolong bleeding time (but within the normal range) in healthy adult subjects. This effect may be exaggerated in patients with underlying hemostatic defects.

➤*Extravasation:* Carefully administer ibuprofen lysine to avoid extravascular injection or leakage because the solution may irritate tissue.

IBUPROFEN LYSINE — INJECTION

➤*Long-term use:* There are no long-term evaluations of the infants treated with ibuprofen at durations of more than the 36 weeks of postconceptual age observation period. Ibuprofen's effects on neurodevelopmental outcome and growth as well as disease processes associated with prematurity (such as retinopathy of prematurity and chronic lung disease) have not been assessed.

➤*Special risk:* Ibuprofen lysine may alter the usual signs of infection. Be continually alert and use the drug with extra care in the presence of controlled infection and in infants at risk of infection.

Ibuprofen has been shown to displace bilirubin from albumin-binding sites; therefore, use the drug with caution in patients with elevated total bilirubin.

➤*Pregnancy:* Category B. Category D. if used in the third trimester or near delivery (per Briggs' *Drugs in Pregnancy and Lactation*). Ibuprofen lysine is not indicated for use in pregnant women.

➤*Lactation:* Ibuprofen lysine is not recommended for use in breast-feeding women.

Drug Interactions

None known.

Adverse Reactions

Ibuprofen Lysine Adverse Reactions[a]

Adverse reactions	Ibuprofen lysine	Placebo
Dermatologic		
Skin lesion/irritation	16%	6%
GI		
GI disorders (non-necrotizing enterocolitis)	22%	18%
GU		
Urinary tract infection	9%	4%
Urine output reduced	3%	1%
Hematologic		
Anemia	32%	25%
IVH[b], all grades	29%	24%
IVH, grades 1/2	15%	13%
IVH, grades 3/4	15%	10%
Other bleeding	6%	13%
Total bleeding[c]	32%	29%
Lab test abnormalities		
Blood urea increased	7%	4%
Blood urea increased with hematuria	1%	1%
Metabolic/Nutritional		
Hypernatremia	7%	4%
Hypocalcemia	12%	9%
Hypoglycemia	12%	6%
Renal		
Blood creatinine increased	3%	1%
Renal failure	1%	3%
Renal insufficiency, impairment	6%	4%
Total renal events[c]	21%	15%
Respiratory		
Apnea	28%	26%
Atelectasis	4%	1%
Respiratory failure	10%	4%
Respiratory tract infection	19%	13%
Miscellaneous		
Adrenal insufficiency	7%	1%
Edema	4%	0%
Sepsis	43%	37%

[a] Within 30 days of therapy, with a reaction rate greater on ibuprofen lysine than on placebo, and greater than 2 reactions on ibuprofen lysine.
[b] IVH = intraventricular hemorrhage.
[c] A given subject may have experienced more than 1 specific reaction within these adverse reaction categories. Only the most severe grade of IVH counted for a given subject.

➤*Renal:* Compared with placebo, there was a small decrease in urinary output in the ibuprofen group on days 2 through 6 of life, with a compensatory increase in urine output on day 9. In other studies, adverse reactions classified as renal insufficiency, including elevated creatinine, elevated serum urea nitrogen, oliguria, or renal failure, were reported in ibuprofen-treated infants.

➤*Additional adverse reactions:*
Cardiovascular – Cardiac failure, hypotension, tachycardia.
CNS – Convulsions.
GI – Abdominal distension, gastritis, gastroesophageal reflux, ileus.
GU – Inguinal hernia.
Hepatic – Cholestasis, jaundice.
Lab test abnormalities – Various laboratory abnormalities, including hyperglycemia, neutropenia, and thrombocytopenia.
Local – Injection site reactions.
Miscellaneous – Feeding problems, various infections.

Overdosage

➤*Symptoms:* The following signs and symptoms have occurred in individuals (not necessarily in premature infants) following an overdose of oral ibuprofen: breathing difficulties, coma, drowsiness, irregular heartbeat, kidney failure, low blood pressure, seizures, and vomiting.

➤*Treatment:* There are no specific measures to treat acute overdosage with ibuprofen lysine. Follow the patient for several days because GI ulceration and hemorrhage may occur.

INDOMETHACIN

Rx	**Indomethacin** (Various, eg, APP Pharmaceutical, Bedford Labs)	**Injection, lyophilized powder for solution:** 1 mg	As indomethacin sodium. In single-dose vials.
Rx	**Indocin I.V.** (Lundbeck)		As indomethacin sodium. In single-dose vials.

INDOMETHACIN SODIUM – INJECTION

For information on oral indomethacin, see Nonsteroidal Anti-inflammatory Agents.

Indications

➤*Patent ductus arteriosus:* To close a hemodynamically significant patent ductus arteriosus in premature infants weighing between 500 and 1,750 g when after 48 hours usual medical management (eg, fluid restriction, diuretics, digitalis, respiratory support) is ineffective. Clear-cut clinical evidence of a hemodynamically significant patent ductus arteriosus should be present, such as respiratory distress, a continuous murmur, a hyperactive precordium, cardiomegaly, and pulmonary plethora on chest x-ray.

➤*Off-label uses:* Indomethacin IV has been used prophylactically to reduce the incidence of symptomatic patent ductus arteriosus in premature infants with a high probability of developing this condition; a single dose of 0.2 mg/kg 24 hours after birth has been used. However, no study has shown a significant decrease in neonatal morbidity.

Administration and Dosage

➤*General dosing considerations:* Dosage recommendations for closure of the ductus arteriosus depends on the age of the infant at the time of therapy.

➤*Children:*
Patent ductus arteriosus –
Usual dosage: A course of therapy is defined as 3 IV doses of indomethacin sodium trihydrate IV given at 12- to 24-hour intervals, with careful attention to urinary output. If anuria or marked oliguria (urinary output less than 0.6 mL/kg/h) is evident at the scheduled time of the second or third dose of indomethacin sodium trihydrate IV, no additional doses should be given until laboratory studies indicate that renal function has returned to normal.

Dosage according to age at first dose is as follows:

Indomethacin Sodium Trihydrate Dosage According to Age at First Dose

Age at 1st dose	Dosage (mg/kg)		
Less than 48 hours	1st (0.2)	2nd (0.1)	3rd (0.1)
2 to 7 days	0.2	0.2	0.2
Over 7 days	0.2	0.25	0.25

If the ductus arteriosus closes or is significantly reduced in size after an interval of 48 hours or more from completion of the first course of indomethacin sodium trihydrate IV, no further doses are necessary. If the ductus arteriosus reopens, a second course of 1 to 3 doses may be given, each dose separated by a 12- to 24-hour interval as described above.

INDOMETHACIN SODIUM — INJECTION

If the neonate remains unresponsive to therapy with indomethacin sodium trihydrate IV after 2 courses, surgery may be necessary for closure of the ductus arteriosus. If severe adverse reactions occur, stop the drug.

Discontinuation of therapy: If clinical signs and symptoms consistent with liver disease develop in the neonate, or if systemic manifestations occur, indomethacin sodium trihydrate IV should be discontinued.

➤*Preparation for administration:* The solution should be prepared only with 1 to 2 mL of preservative-free sterile sodium chloride 0.9% injection or preservative-free sterile water for injection. Benzyl alcohol as a preservative has been associated with toxicity in neonates. Therefore, all diluents should be preservative free.

If 1 mL of diluent is used, the concentration of indomethacin in the solution will equal approximately 0.1 mg per 0.1 mL; if 2 mL of diluent are used, the concentration of the solution will equal approximately 0.05 mg per 0.1 mL.

Further dilution with IV infusion solutions is not recommended.

Any unused portion of the solution should be discarded because there is no preservative contained in the vial. A fresh solution should be prepared just prior to each administration.

➤*Administration:* For IV administration only.

While the optimal rate of injection has not been established, published literature suggests an infusion rate over 20 to 30 minutes.

The drug should be administered carefully to avoid extravascular injection or leakage as the solution may be irritating to tissue.

➤*Admixture compatibility:* Indomethacin sodium trihydrate IV is not buffered, and reconstitution with solutions at pH values less than 6 may result in precipitation of the insoluble indomethacin free acid moiety.

➤*Storage/Stability:* Store below 30°C (86°F). Protect from light. Store container in carton until contents have been used.

Actions

➤*Pharmacology:* Although the exact mechanism of action through which indomethacin causes closure of a patent ductus arteriosus is not known, it is believed to be through inhibition of prostaglandin synthesis. Indomethacin has been shown to be a potent inhibitor of prostaglandin synthesis, both in vitro and in vivo. In human newborns with certain congenital heart malformations, PGE 1 dilates the ductus arteriosus. In fetal and newborn lambs, E type prostaglandins have also been shown to maintain the patency of the ductus, and as in human newborns, indomethacin causes its constriction.

Studies in healthy young animals and in premature infants with patent ductus arteriosus indicated that, after the first dose of IV indomethacin, there was a transient reduction in cerebral blood flow velocity and cerebral blood flow. Similar decreases in mesenteric blood flow and velocity have been observed. The clinical significance of these effects has not been established.

➤*Pharmacokinetics:*

Absorption/Distribution – The disposition of indomethacin following IV administration (0.2 mg/kg) in preterm neonates with patent ductus arteriosus has not been extensively evaluated. Even though the plasma half-life of indomethacin was variable among premature infants, it was shown to vary inversely with postnatal age and weight. In one study, of 28 neonates who could be evaluated, the plasma half-life in those less than 7 days old averaged 20 hours (range: 3 to 60 hours, n = 18). In neonates over 7 days, the mean plasma half-life of indomethacin was 12 hours (range: 4 to 38 hours, n = 10). Grouping the neonates by weight, mean plasma half-life in those weighing less than 1000 g was 21 hours (range: 9 to 60 hours, n = 10); in those neonates weighing greater than 1000 g, the mean plasma half-life was 15 hours (range: 3 to 52 hours, n = 18).

In adults, approximately 99% of indomethacin is bound to protein in plasma over the expected range of therapeutic plasma concentrations. The percent bound in neonates has not been studied. In controlled trials in premature infants, however, no evidence of bilirubin displacement has been observed as evidenced by increased incidence of bilirubin encephalopathy (kernicterus). Indomethacin has been found to cross the blood-brain barrier and the placenta.

Metabolism/Excretion – Following IV administration in adults, indomethacin is eliminated via renal excretion, metabolism, and biliary excretion. Indomethacin undergoes appreciable enterohepatic circulation. The mean plasma half-life of indomethacin is 4.5 hours. In the absence of enterohepatic circulation, it is 90 minutes.

Contraindications

Contraindicated in neonates with proven or suspected infection that is untreated; neonates who are bleeding, especially those with active intracranial hemorrhage or GI bleeding; neonates with thrombocytopenia; neonates with coagulation defects; neonates with or who are suspected of having necrotizing enterocolitis; neonates with significant impairment of renal function; neonates with congenital heart disease in whom patency of the ductus arteriosus is necessary for satisfactory pulmonary or systemic blood flow (eg, pulmonary atresia, severe tetralogy of Fallot, severe coarctation of the aorta).

Warnings/Precautions

➤*GI effects:* In the collaborative study, major GI bleeding was no more common in those neonates receiving indomethacin than in those neonates on placebo. However, minor GI bleeding (ie, chemical detection of blood in the stool) was more commonly noted in those neonates treated with indomethacin. Severe GI effects have been reported in adults with various arthritic disorders treated chronically with oral indomethacin (for further information, see monograph for indomethacin sodium trihydrate capsules).

➤*CNS effects:* Prematurity per se, is associated with an increased incidence of spontaneous intraventricular hemorrhage. Because indomethacin may inhibit platelet aggregation, the potential for intraventricular bleeding may be increased. However, in the large multicenter study of indomethacin sodium trihydrate IV, the incidence of intraventricular hemorrhage in neonates treated with indomethacin sodium trihydrate IV was not significantly higher than in the control neonates.

➤*Renal effects:* Indomethacin sodium trihydrate IV may cause significant reduction in urine output (greater than or equal to 50%) with concomitant elevations of blood urea nitrogen and creatinine, and reductions in glomerular filtration rate and creatinine clearance. These effects in most neonates are transient, disappearing with cessation of therapy with indomethacin sodium trihydrate IV. However, because adequate renal function can depend upon renal prostaglandin synthesis, indomethacin sodium trihydrate IV may precipitate renal insufficiency, including acute renal failure, especially in neonates with other conditions that may adversely affect renal function (eg, extracellular volume depletion from any cause, congestive heart failure, sepsis, concomitant use of any nephrotoxic drug, hepatic dysfunction). When significant suppression of urine volume occurs after a dose of indomethacin sodium trihydrate IV, no additional dose should be given until the urine output returns to normal levels.

Because renal function may be reduced by indomethacin sodium trihydrate IV, consideration should be given to reduction in dosage of those medications that rely on adequate renal function for their elimination.

➤*Hepatic effects:* Severe hepatic reactions have been reported in adults treated chronically with oral indomethacin for arthritic disorders (for further information, see monograph for indomethacin sodium trihydrate capsules). If clinical signs and symptoms consistent with liver disease develop in the neonate, or if systemic manifestations occur, indomethacin sodium trihydrate IV should be discontinued.

➤*Infection:* Indomethacin sodium trihydrate may mask the usual signs and symptoms of infection. Therefore, the physician must be continually on the alert for this and should use the drug with extra care in the presence of existing controlled infection.

➤*Platelet aggregation:* Indomethacin sodium trihydrate IV may inhibit platelet aggregation. In one small study, platelet aggregation was grossly abnormal after indomethacin therapy (given orally to premature infants to close the ductus arteriosus). Platelet aggregation returned to normal by the tenth day. Premature infants should be observed for signs of bleeding.

➤*Pregnancy:* *Category C* (per manufacturer prescribing information). *Category B* (Briggs' *Drugs in Pregnancy and Lactation*); *Category D* if used for longer than 48 hours or after 34 weeks. This drug is not indicated for use in adults.

In rats and mice, oral indomethacin 4 mg/kg/day given during the last 3 days of gestation caused a decrease in maternal weight gain and some maternal and fetal deaths. An increased incidence of neuronal necrosis in the diencephalon in the live-born fetuses was observed. At 2 mg/kg/day, no increase in neuronal necrosis was observed as compared to the control groups. Administration of 0.5 or 4 mg/kg/day during the first 3 days of life did not cause an increase in neuronal necrosis at either dose level.

Pregnant rats, given 2 mg/kg/day and 4 mg/kg/day during the last trimester of gestation, delivered offspring whose pulmonary blood vessels were both reduced in number and excessively muscularized. These findings are similar to those observed in the syndrome of persistent pulmonary hypertension of the neonate.

➤*Lactation:* This drug is not indicated for use in adults. AAP lists indomethacin as compatible with breast-feeding.

➤*Elderly:* Per the Beers list, of all available NSAIDs, indomethacin produces the most CNS adverse reactions.

➤*Monitoring:* Indomethacin sodium trihydrate IV in preterm infants may suppress water excretion to a greater extent than sodium excretion. When this occurs, a significant reduction in serum sodium values (ie, hyponatremia) may result. Neonates should have serum electrolyte determinations done during therapy with indomethacin sodium trihydrate IV. Renal function and serum electrolytes should be monitored. Since renal function may be reduced by indomethacin sodium trihydrate IV, consideration should be given to reduction in dosage of those medications that rely on adequate renal function for their elimination. If anuria or marked oliguria (urinary output less than 0.6 mL/kg/h) is evident at the scheduled time of the second or third dose of indomethacin sodium trihydrate IV, no additional doses should be given until laboratory studies indicate that renal function has returned to normal.

Drug Interactions

➤*Digitalis:* Because the half-life of digitalis (given frequently to preterm infants with patent ductus arteriosus and associated cardiac failure) may be prolonged when given concomitantly with indomethacin, the neonate should be observed closely; frequent ECGs and serum digitalis levels may be required to prevent or detect digitalis toxicity early.

➤*Aminoglycosides :* In one study of premature infants treated with indomethacin sodium trihydrate IV and also receiving either gentamicin or amikacin, both peak and trough levels of these aminoglycosides were significantly elevated.

➤*Furosemide:* Therapy with indomethacin may blunt the natriuretic effect of furosemide. This response has been attributed to inhibition of prostaglandin synthesis by nonsteroidal anti-inflammatory drugs. In a

INDOMETHACIN SODIUM — INJECTION

study of 19 premature infants with patent ductus arteriosus treated with either indomethacin sodium trihydrate IV alone or a combination of indomethacin sodium trihydrate IV and furosemide, results showed that neonates receiving both indomethacin sodium trihydrate IV and furosemide had significantly higher urinary output, higher levels of sodium and chloride excretion, and higher glomerular filtration rates than did those receiving indomethacin sodium trihydrate IV alone. In this study, the data suggested that therapy with furosemide helped to maintain renal function in the premature infant when indomethacin sodium trihydrate IV was added to the treatment of patent ductus arteriosus.

Adverse Reactions

In a double-blind, placebo-controlled trial of 405 premature infants weighing less than or equal to 1750 g with evidence of large ductal shunting, in those neonates treated with indomethacin (n = 206), there was a statistically significantly greater incidence of bleeding problems, including gross or microscopic bleeding into the GI tract, oozing from the skin after needle stick, pulmonary hemorrhage, and disseminated intravascular coagulopathy. There was no statistically significant difference between treatment groups with reference to intracranial hemorrhage.

The neonates treated with indomethacin sodium trihydrate also has a significantly higher incidence of transient oliguria and elevations of serum creatinine (greater than or equal to 1.8 mg/dL) than did the neonates treated with placebo.

The incidences of retrolental fibroplasia (grades 3 and 4) and pneumothorax in neonates treated with indomethacin sodium trihydrate IV were not greater than in placebo controls and were statistically significantly lower than in surgically treated neonates.

The following additional adverse reactions in neonates have been reported from the collaborative study, anecdotal case reports, from other studies using rectal, oral, or IV indomethacin for treatment of patent ductus arteriosus or in marketed use. The rates are calculated from a database that contains experience of 849 indomethacin-treated neonates reported in the medical literature, regardless of the route of administration. One-year follow-up is available on 175 neonates and shows no long-term sequelae that could be attributed to indomethacin. In controlled clinical studies, only electrolyte imbalance and renal dysfunction (of the reactions listed below) occurred statistically significantly more frequently after indomethacin sodium trihydrate IV than after placebo. Reactions marked with a single asterisk (*) occurred in 3% to 9% of indomethacin-treated neonates; those marked with a double asterisk (**) occurred in 3% to 9% of both indomethacin- and placebo-treated neonates. Unmarked reactions occurred in less than 3% of neonates.

➤*Cardiovascular:* Intracranial bleeding**; pulmonary hypertension.

➤*GI:* GI bleeding*; vomiting; abdominal distention; transient ileus; localized perforation(s) of the small and/or large intestines.

➤*Hematologic:* Decreased platelet aggregation.

Indomethacin sodium trihydrate IV may inhibit platelet aggregation. In one small study, platelet aggregation was grossly abnormal after indomethacin therapy (given orally to premature infants to close the ductus arteriosus). Platelet aggregation returned to normal by the tenth day. Premature infants should be observed for signs of bleeding.

➤*Metabolic:* Hyponatremia*; elevated serum potassium*; reduction in blood sugar, including hypoglycemia, increased weight gain (fluid retention).

➤*Renal:* Renal dysfunction in 41% of neonates, including greater than or equal to 1 of the following: Reduced urinary output; reduced urine sodium, chloride, or potassium, urine osmolality, free water clearance, or glomerular filtration rate; elevated serum creatinine or BUN; uremia.

➤*Additional adverse reactions:* The following adverse reactions have been reported in neonates treated with indomethacin, however, a causal relationship to therapy with indomethacin IV has not been established.

Cardiovascular – Bradycardia.

GI – Necrotizing enterocolitis.

Hematologic – Disseminated intravascular coagulation.

Ophthalmic – Retrolental fibroplasia**.

Metabolic – Acidosis/alkalosis.

Respiratory – Apnea; exacerbation of preexisting pulmonary infection.

Patient Information

Because renal function may be reduced by indomethacin sodium trihydrate IV, consideration should be given to reduction in dosage of those medications that rely on adequate renal function for their elimination.

SCLEROSING AGENTS

Indications

➤*Varicose veins:* Treatment of small, uncomplicated varicose veins of the lower extremities.

Sclerosing agents may be useful as a supplement to venous ligation to obliterate residual varicosed veins or in patients who have conditions which increase the risk of surgery. Ineffective sclerotherapy may decrease the potential success of later surgery.

➤*Morrhuate sodium:* This has been used for the treatment of internal hemorrhoids; there is no substantial evidence for this indication.

➤*Off-label uses:* Sclerosing agents have been used to treat esophageal varices, introduced via a flexible fiberoptic esophagoscope.

Actions

➤*Pharmacology:* These agents are mild sclerosing drugs used in the treatment of varicose veins. They produce their effect by irritation and inflammation of the venous intimal endothelium and formation of a thrombus. This blood clot occludes the injected vein and fibrous tissue develops, resulting in the obliteration of the vein.

Morrhuate sodium is a mixture of the sodium salts of the saturated and unsaturated fatty acids of cod liver oil.

Contraindications

Hypersensitivity to any component of these drugs; acute superficial thrombophlebitis; underlying arterial disease; varicosities caused by abdominal and pelvic tumors; uncontrolled diabetes mellitus; sepsis; blood dyscrasia; thyrotoxicosis; tuberculosis; neoplasms; asthma; acute respiratory or skin diseases; any condition which causes the patient to be bedridden; extensive injection treatment in patients who are severely debilitated or senile; an unusual local reaction at the injection site or any systemic reaction; persistent occlusion of deep veins.

Delay treatment if there is any acute local or systemic reaction, including infected ulcers.

Do not use if there is significant valvular or deep venous incompetence.

Warnings/Precautions

➤*Hypersensitivity reactions:* Anaphylactoid and allergic reactions have occurred. Anaphylactoid reactions may occur within a few minutes after the injection and are most likely to occur when therapy is reinstituted after several weeks. Refer to Management of Acute Hypersensitivity Reactions.

➤*Deep vein thrombosis:* Do not undertake sclerotherapy for the treatment of varicosities unless valvular competency and deep vein patency and competency are determined. Perform the Trendelenburg test, Perthes' test and angiography. Because of the danger of extension of thrombosis into the deep veins, perform a thorough preinjection evaluation for valvular competence and slowly inject a small amount (not more than 2 mL) of the preparation into the varicosity. Necrosis may result from direct injection of sclerosing agents.

➤*Initial treatment:* Initially treat most patients with symptomatic primary varicosed veins with compression stockings. If this treatment is inadequate, surgery may be required.

➤*Administration:* For IV use only. Inadvertent intra-arterial injection may result in severe ischemic damage.

➤*Pregnancy:* Safety for use during pregnancy has not been established. Use only when clearly needed and when the potential benefits outweigh the potential hazards to the fetus.

Adverse Reactions

➤*CNS:* Drowsiness and headache may occur rarely with morrhuate.

➤*Hypersensitivity:* Dizziness; weakness; vascular collapse; asthma; respiratory depression; GI disturbances (ie, nausea and vomiting); urticaria (rare).

➤*Local:* Burning; cramping sensations; urticaria; tissue sloughing and necrosis may occur with extravasation (morrhuate).

➤*Respiratory:* Pulmonary embolism has occurred.

➤*Miscellaneous:* Postoperative sloughing can occur.

ETHANOLAMINE OLEATE

Rx	Ethamolin (Questcor)	Injection: 5%	In 2 mL amps.[a]

[a] With 2% benzyl alcohol.

ETHANOLAMINE OLEATE — INJECTION

Refer to the general discussion of these products in the Sclerosing Agents group monograph.

Indications

➤*Esophageal varices:* Ethanolamine oleate injection is indicated for the treatment of patients with esophageal varices that have recently bled, to prevent rebleeding.

Ethanolamine oleate is not indicated for the treatment of patients with esophageal varices that have not bled. There is no evidence that treatment of this population decreases the likelihood of bleeding.

Administration and Dosage

➤*Adults:*

Esophageal varices –

Usual dosage: 1.5 to 5 mL IV per varix. To obliterate the varix, injections may be made at the time of the acute bleeding episode and then after 1 week, 6 weeks, 3 months, and 6 months as indicated.

Maximum dose: The maximum dose per treatment session should not exceed 20 mL.

➤*Hepatic function impairment:* Patients with significant liver dysfunction (Child class C) or concomitant cardiopulmonary disease should usually receive less than the recommended maximum dose.

➤*Administration:* Submucosal injections are not recommended because they are reportedly more likely to result in ulceration at the injection site.

➤*Storage/Stability:* Store at controlled room temperature, 15° to 30°C (59° to 86°F). Protect from light.

Actions

➤*Pharmacology:* When injected IV, ethanolamine oleate injection acts primarily by irritation of the intimal endothelium of the vein and produces a sterile dose-related inflammatory response. This results in fibrosis and possible occlusion of the vein. Ethanolamine oleate injection also rapidly diffuses through the venous wall and produces a dose-related extravascular inflammatory reaction.

The oleic acid component of the ethanolamine oleate injection is responsible for the inflammatory response, and may also activate coagulation in vivo by release of tissue factor and activation of Hageman factor. The ethanolamine component, however, may inhibit fibrin clot formation by chelating calcium, so that a procoagulant action of ethanolamine oleate has not been demonstrated.

After injection, ethanolamine oleate disappears from the injection site within 5 minutes via the portal vein. When volumes larger than 20 mL are injected, some ethanolamine oleate also flows into the azygos vein through the periesophageal vein. In human autopsy studies it was found that within 4 days after injection there is neutrophil infiltration of the esophageal wall and hemorrhage within 6 days. Granulation tissue is first seen at 10 days, red thrombi obliterating the varices by 20 days, and sclerosis of the varices by 2.5 months. The time course of these findings suggests that sclerosis of esophageal varices will be a delayed rather than an immediate effect of the drug.

The minimum lethal dose of ethanolamine oleate injection administered IV to rabbits is 130 mg/kg.

In dogs, ethanolamine oleate injected into the right atrium at a dose of 1 mL/kg over 1 minute has been shown to increase extravascular lung water. The maximum recommended human dose is 20 mL, or 0.4 mL/kg for a 50 kg person. The concentration of ethanolamine oleate reaching the lung in human treatment will be less than in the dog studies, but pleural effusions, pulmonary edema, pulmonary infiltration and pneumonitis have been reported in clinical trials, and minimizing the total per session dose, especially in patients with concomitant cardiopulmonary disease, is recommended.

Contraindications

Known hypersensitivity to ethanolamine, oleic acid, or ethanolamine oleate.

Warnings/Precautions

➤*Varicosities of the leg:* The practice of injecting varicosities of the leg with ethanolamine oleate injection is not supported by adequately controlled clinical trials. Therefore, such use is not recommended.

➤*Severe injection necrosis:* The physician should bear in mind that severe injection necrosis may result from direct injection of sclerosing agents, especially if excessive volumes are used. At least 1 fatal case of extensive esophageal necrosis and death has been reported. The drug should be administered by physicians who are familiar with an acceptable injection technique.

➤*Child class C:* Patients in Child class C are more likely to develop esophageal ulceration than those in classes A and B. Complications of ulceration, necrosis, and delayed esophageal perforation appear to occur more frequently when ethanolamine oleate injection is injected submucosally. This route is not recommended.

➤*Cardiorespiratory disease:* In patients with concomitant cardiorespiratory disease, careful monitoring and minimization of the total dose per session is recommended.

➤*Hypersensitivity reactions:* Fatal anaphylactic shock was reported following injection of a larger than normal volume of ethanolamine oleate injection into a man who had a known allergic disposition. Although there are only 3 known reports of anaphylaxis, the possibility of an anaphylactic reaction should be kept in mind, and the physician should be prepared to treat it appropriately. In extreme emergencies, 0.25 mL of a 1:1000 IV solution of epinephrine (0.25 mg) should be used and allergic reactions should be controlled with antihistamines.

➤*Renal function impairment:* Acute renal failure with spontaneous recovery followed injection of 15 to 20 mL of ethanolamine oleate injection into 2 women.

➤*Pregnancy: Category C.*

Ethanolamine oleate injection should be used in pregnant women only when clearly needed.

Teratogenic – Animal reproduction studies have not been conducted with ethanolamine oleate injection. It is also not known whether ethanolamine oleate injection can cause fetal harm when administered to a pregnant woman or can affect reproduction capacity. Ethanolamine oleate injection should be given to a pregnant woman only if clearly needed.

➤*Lactation:* It is not known whether this drug is excreted in human milk. Because many drugs are excreted in human milk, caution should be exercised when ethanolamine oleate injection is administered to a nursing woman.

➤*Children:* Safety and efficacy in pediatric patients have not been established.

➤*Elderly:* Fatal aspiration pneumonia has occurred in elderly patients undergoing esophageal variceal sclerotherapy with ethanolamine oleate injection. This adverse event appears to be procedure related rather than drug related, but as aspiration of blood or stomach contents is not uncommon in patients with bleeding esophageal varices, special precautions should be taken to prevent its occurrence, especially in the elderly and critically ill subjects.

Adverse Reactions

The reported frequency of complications/adverse events per injection session was 13%. The most common complications were pleural effusion/infiltration (2.1%), esophageal ulcer (2.1%), pyrexia (1.8%), retrosternal pain (1.6%), esophageal stricture (1.3%), and pneumonia (1.2%).

➤*Local:* Other adverse local esophageal reactions have also been reported at rates of 0.1% to 0.4%, including esophagitis, tearing of the esophagus, sloughing of the mucosa overlying the injected varix, ulceration, stricture, necrosis, periesophageal abscess and perforation. These complications appear to be dependent upon the dose and the patient's clinical state.

➤*Miscellaneous:* Bacteremia has been observed in patients following injection of esophageal varices with ethanolamine oleate. Pyrexia and retrosternal pain are not infrequently observed during the postinjection period. Fatal aspiration pneumonia has occurred in patients with esophageal varices who underwent ethanolamine oleate injection sclerotherapy. Anaphylactic shock and acute renal failure with spontaneous recovery have occurred. A case of disseminated intravascular coagulation has been reported.

Spinal cord paralysis due to occlusion of the anterior spinal artery has been reported in 1 child 8 hours after ethanolamine oleate sclerotherapy.

Overdosage

➤*Symptoms:* Overdosage of ethanolamine oleate injection can result in severe intramural necrosis of the esophagus. Complications resulting from such overdosage have resulted in death.

SODIUM TETRADECYL SULFATE

Rx	**Sotradecol** (AngioDynamics[a])	**Injection, solution:** 10 mg/mL	Benzyl alcohol 0.02 mL. In 2 mL vials.
		30 mg/mL	Benzyl alcohol 0.02 mL. In 2 mL vials.

[a] AngioDynamics, Inc., 603 Queensbury Ave., Queensbury, NY 12804; 518-798-1215; 800-772-6446; http://www.angiodynamics.com.

SODIUM TETRADECYL SULFATE — INJECTION

Indications

➤*Varicose veins:* Sodium tetradecyl sulfate is indicated in the treatment of small uncomplicated varicose veins of the lower extremities that show simple dilation with competent valves. Consider the benefit-to-risk ratio in selected patients who are at great surgical risks.

➤*Off-label uses:* Bleeding esophageal varices.

Administration and Dosage

➤*General dosing considerations:* The strength of solution required depends on the size and degree of varicosity.

➤*Adults:*

Varicose veins –

Usual dosage: In general, the 1% solution will be found most useful with the 3% solution preferred for larger varicosities. Keep the dose small, using 0.5 to 2 mL (preferably 1 mL maximum) for each injection, and do not exceed the maximum 10 mL single treatment.

Maximum dose: 10 mL single treatment.

➤*Children:* Safety and efficacy in children have not been established.

➤*Administration:* Sodium tetradecyl sulfate injection is for intravenous (IV) use only.

Visually inspect parenteral drug products for particulate matter and discoloration prior to administration. Do not use if precipitated or discolored.

➤*Admixture compatibility:* Do not include heparin in the same syringe as sodium tetradecyl sulfate because they are incompatible.

➤*Storage/Stability:* Store at 20° to 25°C (68° to 77°F).

Actions

➤*Pharmacology:* Sodium tetradecyl sulfate is a sclerosing agent. IV injection causes intima inflammation and thrombus formation. This usually occludes the injected vein. Subsequent formation of fibrous tissue results in partial or complete vein obliteration that may or may not be permanent.

Contraindications

Sodium tetradecyl sulfate is contraindicated in previous hypersensitivity reactions to the drug; in acute superficial thrombophlebitis; valvular or deep vein incompetence; huge superficial veins with wide open communications to deeper veins; phlebitis migrans; acute cellulitis; allergic conditions; acute infections; varicosities caused by abdominal and pelvic tumors (unless the tumor has been removed); bedridden patients; uncontrolled systemic diseases, such as diabetes, toxic hyperthyroidism, tuberculosis, asthma, neoplasm, sepsis, blood dyscrasias, and acute respiratory or skin diseases.

Warnings/Precautions

➤*Administration:* Sodium tetradecyl sulfate should be administered only by a health care provider familiar with venous anatomy, the diagnosis and treatment of conditions affecting the venous system, and proper injection technique. Severe adverse local reactions, including tissue necrosis, may occur following extravasation; therefore, extreme care in IV needle placement and use of the minimal effective volume at each injection site are important.

➤*Deep vein thrombosis/pulmonary embolism:* Because of the danger of thrombosis extension into the deep venous system, carry out thorough preinjection evaluation for valvular competency and slowly inject a small amount (not over 2 mL) of the preparation into the varicosity. Deep venous patency must be determined by angiography or noninvasive testing, such as duplex ultrasound. Venous sclerotherapy should not be undertaken if tests, such as Trendelenberg, Perthes, and angiography, show significant valvular or deep venous incompetence.

The development of deep vein thrombosis and pulmonary embolism have been reported following sclerotherapy treatment of superficial varicosities. Patients should have posttreatment follow-up of sufficient duration to assess for the development of deep vein thrombosis. Embolism may occur as long as 4 weeks after injection of sodium tetradecyl sulfate. Adequate posttreatment compression may decrease the incidence of deep vein thrombosis.

➤*Arterial disease:* Exercise extreme caution in the presence of underlying arterial disease, such as marked peripheral arteriosclerosis or thromboangiitis obliterans (Buerger disease).

➤*Benzyl alcohol:* Benzyl alcohol, contained in this product as a preservative, has been associated with an increased incidence of neurological and other complications in premature infants that are sometimes fatal.

➤*Hypersensitivity reactions:* Emergency resuscitation equipment should be immediately available. Allergic reactions, including fatal anaphylaxis, have been reported. As a precaution against anaphylactic shock, it is recommended that sodium tetradecyl sulfate 0.5 mL be injected into a varicosity, followed by observation of the patient for several hours before administration of a second or larger dose. Keep the possibility of an anaphylactic reaction in mind, and be prepared to treat it appropriately.

➤*Pregnancy: Category C.* Animal reproduction studies have not been conducted with sodium tetradecyl sulfate. It also is not known whether sodium tetradecyl sulfate can cause fetal harm when administered to a pregnant woman or can affect reproduction capacity. Administer sodium tetradecyl sulfate to a pregnant woman only if clearly needed and the benefits outweigh the risks.

➤*Lactation:* It is not known whether this drug is excreted in human milk. Because many drugs are excreted in human milk, exercise caution when sodium tetradecyl sulfate is administered to a breastfeeding woman.

➤*Children:* Safety and efficacy in children have not been established.

Drug Interactions

➤*Antiovulatory drugs:* No well-controlled studies have been performed in patients taking antiovulatory agents (eg, oral contraceptives). Use judgment and evaluate any patient taking antiovulatory drugs prior to initiating treatment with sodium tetradecyl sulfate.

Adverse Reactions

➤*Hypersensitivity:* Allergic reactions, such as hives, asthma, hay fever, and anaphylactic shock, have been reported. Mild systemic reactions that have been reported include headache, nausea, and vomiting.

At least 6 deaths have been reported with the use of sodium tetradecyl sulfate. Four cases of anaphylactic shock leading to death have been reported in patients who received sodium tetradecyl sulfate. One of these 4 patients reported a history of asthma, a contraindication to the administration of sodium tetradecyl sulfate.

➤*Local:* Local reactions consisting of pain, urticaria, or ulceration may occur at the site of injection. A permanent discoloration may remain along the path of the sclerosed vein segment. Sloughing and necrosis of tissue may occur following extravasation of the drug.

➤*Miscellaneous:* One death has been reported in a patient who received sodium tetradecyl sulfate and who had been receiving an antiovulatory agent. Another death (fatal pulmonary embolism) has been reported in a 36-year-old woman treated with sodium tetradecyl acetate and who was not taking oral contraceptives.

Overdosage

The IV LD_{50} of sodium tetradecyl sulfate in mice was reported to be 90 ± 5 mg/kg.

In rats, the acute IV LD_{50} of sodium tetradecyl sulfate was estimated to be between 72 and 108 mg/kg.

Purified sodium tetradecyl sulfate was found to have an LD_{50} of 2 g/kg when administered orally by stomach tube as a 25% aqueous solution to rats. In rats given 0.15 g/kg in drinking water for 30 days, no appreciable toxicity was seen, although some growth inhibition was discernible.

MORRHUATE SODIUM

Rx	**Morrhuate Sodium** (Various, eg, American Regent)	**Injection; solution:** 50 mg/mL	May contain 2% benzyl alcohol. In 30 mL multiple-use vials.
Rx	**Scleromate** (Glenwood)		In 30 mL multiple-use vials.

MORRHUATE SODIUM — INJECTION

Indications

➤*Varicose veins:* For the obliteration of primary varicosed veins that consist of simple dilation with competent valves.

Administration and Dosage

➤*General dosing considerations:* Dosage of morrhuate sodium depends on the size and degree of varicosity.

➤*Adults:*

Varicose veins –

Usual dosage:

- *Small or medium veins* – 50 to 100 mg (1 to 2 mL of the 5% injection).
- *Large veins* – 150 to 250 mg (3 to 5 mL of the injection).

Test dose: To determine possible sensitivity to the drug, some clinicians recommend injection of 0.25 to 1 mL of morrhuate sodium 5% injection into a varicosity 24 hours before administration of a large dose.

Duration of therapy: The drug may be given as multiple injections at one time or in single doses. Therapy may be repeated at 5 to 7 day intervals, according to the patient's response.

➤*Post-injection:* Following injection of morrhuate sodium, the vein promptly becomes hard and swollen for 2 to 4 inches, depending on the size and response of the vein. After 24 hours, the vein is hard and slightly tender to the touch (with little or no periphlebitis). The skin around the injection becomes light-bronze; this color usually disappears shortly. An aching sensation and feeling of stiffness usually occur and last approximately 48 hours.

➤*Preparation for administration:* When small veins are injected, the injection solution is cold, or if solid matter has separated in the solution, the vial should be warmed by immersing in hot water. The solution should become clear on warming; only a clear solution should be used. The injection should not be used if the solid matter does not dissolve completely on warming. Because the solution froths easily, a large bore needle should be used to fill the syringe; however, a small bore needle should be used for the injection.

➤*Administration:* Morrhuate sodium is administered only by intravenous injection. Care must be taken to avoid extravasation. Specialized references should be consulted for specific procedures and techniques of administration.

➤*Storage/Stability:* Store below 40°C (104°F), preferably between 15° and 30°C (59° and 86°F).

MISCELLANEOUS ANTIANGINAL AGENTS

RANOLAZINE

Rx	**Ranexa** (Gilead Sciences)	**Tablets, extended-release; oral:** 500 mg	PEG. (CVT 500). Lt. orange, oblong. Film-coated. In 60s and 500s.
		1,000 mg	Lactose, PEG. (CVT 1000). Pale yellow, oblong. Film-coated. In 60s and 500s.

RANOLAZINE — ORAL

Indications

➤*Chronic angina:* For the treatment of chronic angina.

Ranolazine may be used with beta-blockers, nitrates, calcium channel blockers, antiplatelet therapy, lipid-lowering therapy, angiotensin-converting enzyme (ACE) inhibitors, and angiotensin-receptor blockers.

Administration and Dosage

➤*Adults:*

Chronic angina –

Initial dosage: Initiate dosage at 500 mg twice daily and increase to 1,000 mg twice daily as needed, based on clinical symptoms. If a dose of ranolazine is missed, the prescribed dosage should be taken at the next scheduled time. The next dose should not be doubled.

Concomitant therapy: Dosage adjustments may be needed when ranolazine is taken in combination with certain other drugs. Limit the maximum dosage of ranolazine to 500 mg twice daily in patients on diltiazem, verapamil, and other moderate CYP3A inhibitors. Down-titrate ranolazine based on clinical response in patients concomitantly treated with P-glycoprotein inhibitors, such as cyclosporine.

➤*Administration:* Ranolazine may be taken with or without meals. Ranolazine should be swallowed whole and not crushed, broken, or chewed.

➤*Storage/Stability:* Store at 25°C (77°F); excursions are permitted between 15° and 30°C (59° and 86°F).

Actions

➤*Pharmacology:* Ranolazine has antianginal and anti-ischemic effects that do not depend upon reductions in heart rate or blood pressure. The mechanism of action of ranolazine's antianginal effects has not been determined. It does not affect the rate-pressure product, a measure of myocardial work, at maximal exercise. Ranolazine at therapeutic levels can inhibit the cardiac late sodium current (I_{Na}). However, the relationship of this inhibition to angina symptoms is uncertain.

The QT prolongation effect of ranolazine on the surface electrocardiogram (ECG) is the result of inhibition of I_{Kr}, which prolongs the ventricular action potential.

➤*Pharmacokinetics:*

Absorption/Distribution – Ranolazine is extensively metabolized in the gut and liver, and its absorption is highly variable. For example, at a dosage of 1,000 mg twice daily, the mean steady-state maximum effective plasma concentration (C_{max}) was 2,600 ng/mL; 95% confidence interval values were between 400 and 6,100 ng/mL. The pharmacokinetics of the (+) R- and (−) S-enantiomers of ranolazine are similar in healthy volunteers. Steady state is generally achieved within 3 days of twice-daily dosing with ranolazine. At steady state over the dosage range 500 to 1,000 mg twice daily, C_{max} and area under the curve $(AUC)_{0-\tau}$ increase slightly more than proportionally to dose, 2.2- and 2.4-fold, respectively. With twice-daily dosing, the peak-to-trough ratio of the ranolazine plasma concentration is 0.3 to 0.6.

After oral administration of ranolazine, peak plasma concentrations of ranolazine are reached between 2 and 5 hours. After oral administration of ^{14}C-ranolazine as a solution, 73% of the dose is systemically available as ranolazine or metabolites. The bioavailability of ranolazine from ranolazine tablets relative to that from a solution of ranolazine is 76%. Because ranolazine is a substrate of P-gp, inhibitors of P-gp may increase the absorption of ranolazine. Over the concentration range of 0.25 to 10 mcg/mL, ranolazine is approximately 62% bound to human plasma proteins.

Food effect: Food (high-fat breakfast) has no important effect on the C_{max} and AUC of ranolazine. Therefore, ranolazine may be taken without regard to meals.

Metabolism/Excretion – The apparent terminal half-life of ranolazine is 7 hours. Following a single oral dose of ranolazine solution, approximately 75% of the dose is excreted in urine and 25% in feces. Ranolazine is metabolized rapidly and extensively in the liver and intestine; less than 5% is excreted unchanged in urine and feces. The pharmacologic activity of the metabolites has not been well characterized. After dosing to steady state with 500 to 1,500 mg twice daily, the 4 most abundant metabolites in plasma have AUC values ranging from about 5% to 33% that of ranolazine, and display apparent half-lives ranging from 6 to 22 hours. Ranolazine is metabolized mainly by CYP3A and to a lesser extent by CYP2D6.

Special populations –

Renal function impairment: See Warnings/Precautions for more information.

Hepatic function impairment: See Warnings/Precautions for more information.

Contraindications

Patients taking strong inhibitors of CYP3A, patients taking inducers of CYP3A, and those with clinically significant hepatic impairment.

Warnings/Precautions

➤*QT prolongation:* Ranolazine blocks I_{Kr} and prolongs the QTc interval in a dose-related manner. Clinical experience in an acute coronary syndrome population did not show an increased risk of proarrhythmia or sudden death. However, there is little experience with high doses (more than 1,000 mg twice daily) or exposure, other QT-prolonging drugs, or potassium channel variants resulting in a long QT interval.

Dose- and plasma concentration–related increases in the QTc interval, reductions in T-wave amplitude, and, in some cases, notched T-waves, have been observed in patients treated with ranolazine. These effects are believed to be caused by ranolazine and not by its metabolites. The relationship between the change in QTc and ranolazine plasma concentrations is linear with a slope of about 2.6 msec per 1,000 ng/mL, through exposures corresponding to doses several-fold higher than the maximum recommended dosage of 1,000 mg twice daily. The variable blood levels attained after a given dose of ranolazine give a wide range of effects on QTc. At T_{max} following repeat dosing at 1,000 mg twice daily, the mean change in QTc is about 6 msec, but in the 5% of the population with the highest plasma concentrations, the prolongation of QTc is at least 15 msec. In subjects with mild or moderate hepatic impairment, the relationship between plasma level of ranolazine and QTc is much steeper.

➤*Tumor promotion:* A published study reported that ranolazine promoted tumor formation and progression to malignancy when given to transgenic adenomatous polyposis coli (APC) (min/+) mice at a dosage of 30 mg/kg twice daily. The clinical significance of this finding is unclear.

RANOLAZINE — ORAL

➤*Use in patients with heart failure:* Heart failure (NYHA class I to IV) had no significant effect on ranolazine pharmacokinetics. Ranolazine had minimal effects on heart rate and blood pressure in patients with angina and heart failure NYHA class I to IV. No dose adjustment of ranolazine is required in patients with heart failure.

➤*Use in patients with diabetes mellitus:* A population pharmacokinetic evaluation of data from angina patients and healthy subjects showed no effect of diabetes on ranolazine pharmacokinetics. No dose adjustment is required in patients with diabetes.

Ranolazine produces small reductions in hemoglobin A_{1c} (HbA_{1c}) in patients with diabetes, the clinical significance of which is unknown. Ranolazine should not be considered a treatment for diabetes.

➤*Renal function impairment:* In patients with varying degrees of renal impairment, ranolazine plasma levels increased up to 50%. The pharmacokinetics of ranolazine have not been assessed in patients on dialysis.

➤*Hepatic function impairment:* Ranolazine is contraindicated in patients with clinically significant hepatic impairment. Plasma concentrations of ranolazine were increased by 30% in patients with mild (Child-Pugh class A) and by 60% in patients with moderate (Child-Pugh class B) hepatic impairment. This was not enough to account for the 3-fold increase in QT prolongation seen in patients with mild to severe hepatic impairment.

➤*Pregnancy:* *Category C.* There are no adequate and well-controlled studies in pregnant women. Use ranolazine during pregnancy only when the potential benefit to the patient justifies the potential risk to the fetus.

In animal studies, ranolazine at exposures 1.5 (rabbit) to 2 (rat) times the usual human exposure caused maternal toxicity and misshapen sternebrae, and reduced ossification in offspring. These doses in rats and rabbits were associated with an increased maternal mortality rate.

➤*Lactation:* It is not known whether ranolazine is excreted in human milk. Because many drugs are excreted in human milk and because of the potential for serious adverse reactions from ranolazine in breast-feeding infants, decide whether to discontinue breast-feeding or ranolazine, taking into account the importance of the drug to the mother.

➤*Children:* Safety and efficacy in children have not been established.

➤*Elderly:* Of the chronic angina patients treated with ranolazine in controlled studies, 496 (48%) were 65 years of age and older, and 114 (11%) were 75 years of age and older. No overall differences in efficacy were observed between older and younger patients. There were no differences in safety for patients 65 years of age and older compared with younger patients, but patients 75 years of age and older taking ranolazine, compared with placebo, had a higher incidence of adverse reactions, serious adverse reactions, and drug discontinuations because of adverse reactions. In general, use caution when selecting dosage for an elderly patient, usually starting at the low end of the dosing range, reflecting the greater frequency of decreased cardiac, hepatic, or renal function, and of concomitant disease or other drug therapy.

➤*Lab test abnormalities:* Ranolazine produces small reductions in HbA_{1c}. Ranolazine is not a treatment for diabetes.

Ranolazine produces elevations of serum creatinine by 0.1 mg/dL, regardless of previous renal function. The elevation has a rapid onset, shows no signs of progression during long-term therapy, is reversible after discontinuation of ranolazine, and is not accompanied by changes in serum urea nitrogen. In healthy volunteers, ranolazine 1,000 mg twice daily had no effect upon the glomerular filtration rate. The elevated creatinine levels are likely because of a blockage of creatinine's tubular secretion by ranolazine or one of its metabolites.

➤*Monitoring:* Obtain baseline and follow-up ECGs to evaluate effects on QT interval. Monitor HbA_{1c} regularly during therapy.

Drug Interactions

➤*Cytochrome P450 system:* Because ranolazine is metabolized mainly by the CYP3A, do not use ranolazine with potent CYP3A inhibitors (ketoconazole, clarithromycin). Substrates known to inhibit CYP3A and CYP2D6 may decrease metabolism or increase bioavailability of ranolazine, as indicated by decreased whole blood or plasma concentrations. Drugs known to induce these enzyme systems may result in an increased metabolism of ranolazine or decreased bioavailability, as indicated by decreased whole blood or plasma concentrations. Monitoring of blood concentrations and appropriate dosage adjustments are essential when such drugs are used concomitantly.

➤*P-glycoprotein:* Ranolazine is a substrate for P-glycoprotein. Drugs that affect P-glycoprotein may alter the pharmacokinetics of ranolazine. Also, ranolazine may alter the pharmacokinetics of drugs that are substrates for P-glycoprotein.

➤*QT prolongation:* An additive effect of ranolazine with other drugs that prolong the QT interval cannot be excluded. The following drugs may prolong the QT interval and increase the risk of life-threatening cardiac arrhythmias, including torsades de pointes: antiarrhythmic agents (eg, amiodarone, bretylium, disopyramide, dofetilide, procainamide, quinidine, sotalol), arsenic trioxide, chlorpromazine, cisapride, dolasetron, droperidol, mefloquine, mesoridazine, moxifloxacin, pentamidine, pimozide, tacrolimus, thioridazine, and ziprasidone. For a more complete list of drugs that may prolong the QT interval, see the appendix Drug Induced Prolongation of the QT Interval and Torsades de Pointes.

Ranolazine Drug Interactions

Precipitant drug	Object drug[a]		Description
Aprepitant	Ranolazine	↑	Concomitant use may increase ranolazine plasma levels and QTc prolongation. Adjust the dose of ranolazine. Limit the ranolazine dosage to 500 mg twice daily in patients receiving aprepitant.
Azole antifungals (eg, itraconazole, ketoconazole)	Ranolazine	↑	Ketoconazole increases average steady-state plasma concentrations of ranolazine 3.2-fold. Concomitant use is contraindicated.
Carbamazepine	Ranolazine	↓	Carbamazepine may increase clearance of ranolazine, decreasing plasma concentration. Concomitant use is contraindicated.
Clarithromycin	Ranolazine	↑	Concomitant use may increase ranolazine plasma levels and QTc prolongation. Concomitant use is contraindicated.
Cyclosporine	Ranolazine	↑	Cyclosporine may increase the absorption of ranolazine. Downtitrate the dose of ranolazine based on clinical response.
Diltiazem	Ranolazine	↑	Diltiazem causes dose-dependent mean increases in average ranolazine steady-state concentrations of about 2-fold. Adjust the dose of ranolazine. Limit the maximum dosage of ranolazine to 500 mg twice daily in patients taking diltiazem.
Fluconazole	Ranolazine	↑	Fluconazole may increase ranolazine concentrations, increasing the risk of adverse reactions, including dose-related QTc prolongation. Limit the dosage of ranolazine to 500 mg twice daily in patients taking fluconazole.
Macrolide antibiotics (eg, erythromycin)	Ranolazine	↑	Concomitant use may increase ranolazine plasma levels and QTc prolongation. Adjust the dose of ranolazine. Limit the ranolazine dosage to 500 mg twice daily in patients receiving erythromycin.
Nefazodone	Ranolazine	↑	Concomitant use may increase ranolazine plasma levels and QTc prolongation. Concomitant use is contraindicated.
Paroxetine	Ranolazine	↑	Paroxetine increases average steady-state plasma concentrations of ranolazine 1.2-fold. However, no ranolazine dosage adjustment is needed.
Phenobarbital	Ranolazine	↓	Phenobarbital may increase clearance of ranolazine, decreasing plasma concentration. Coadministration is contraindicated.
Phenytoin	Ranolazine	↓	Phenytoin may increase clearance of ranolazine, decreasing plasma concentration. Coadministration is contraindicated.
Protease inhibitors (eg, indinavir, nelfinavir, ritonavir, saquinavir)	Ranolazine	↑	Concomitant use may increase ranolazine plasma levels and QTc prolongation. Concomitant use is contraindicated.
Rifamycins (eg, rifampin)	Ranolazine	↓	Rifampin decreases the plasma concentration of ranolazine by 95%. Coadministration is contraindicated.
St. John's wort	Ranolazine	↓	St. John's wort may increase the clearance of ranolazine, decreasing plasma concentration. Coadministration is contraindicated.

RANOLAZINE — ORAL

Ranolazine Drug Interactions			
Precipitant drug	Object drug[a]		Description
Verapamil	Ranolazine	↑	Verapamil increases ranolazine steady-state plasma concentrations about 2-fold. Adjust the dose of ranolazine.
Ranolazine	Antipsychotics	↑	Plasma concentrations of antipsychotic agents may be elevated, increasing the pharmacologic effects and risk of adverse reactions. A lower dose of the antipsychotic may be needed during concurrent use of ranolazine.
Ranolazine	Digoxin	↑	Coadministration of ranolazine and digoxin results in a 1.5-fold elevation of digoxin plasma concentrations. May need to reduce digoxin dose.
Ranolazine	Metoprolol	↑	Ranolazine 750 mg twice daily increased plasma concentrations of a single dose of immediate-release metoprolol 100 mg by 1.8-fold. A lower metoprolol dose may be needed during concurrent use of ranolazine.
Ranolazine	Simvastatin	↑	Coadministration of ranolazine and simvastatin results in about a 2-fold increase in plasma concentrations of simvastatin and its active metabolites. However, no simvastatin dosage adjustment is needed.
Ranolazine	Tricyclic antidepressants (eg, amitriptyline)	↑	Tricyclic antidepressant plasma concentrations may be elevated, increasing the pharmacologic effects and risk of adverse reactions. A lower dose of tricyclic antidepressant may be needed during concurrent use of ranolazine.

[a] ↑ = object drug increased; ↓ = object drug decreased.

➤*Drug/Food interactions:*

Grapefruit – Concomitant use may increase ranolazine plasma levels and QTc prolongation. Adjust the dose of ranolazine with coadministration. Limit the ranolazine dose to 500 mg twice daily in patients receiving grapefruit juice or grapefruit-containing products.

Adverse Reactions

In controlled clinical trials of angina patients, the most frequently reported treatment-emergent adverse reactions (more than 4%), occurring more often with ranolazine than placebo, were dizziness (6.2%), headache (5.5%), constipation (4.5%), and nausea (4.4%). Dizziness may be dose related. In open-label, long-term treatment studies, a similar adverse reaction profile was observed in patients treated with ranolazine.

At recommended doses, about 6% of patients discontinued treatment with ranolazine because of an adverse reaction in controlled studies in patients with angina compared with about 3% on placebo. The most common adverse reactions that led to discontinuation more frequently on ranolazine than placebo were dizziness (1.3% vs 0.1%) and nausea (1% vs 0%), asthenia, constipation, and headache (each about 0.5% vs 0%). Dosages above 1,000 mg twice daily are poorly tolerated.

➤*Adverse reactions occurring among all ranolazine-treated patients with chronic angina:* The following additional adverse reactions occurred at an incidence of more than 0.5% to less than 2% in patients treated with ranolazine, and were more frequent than the incidence observed in placebo-treated patients.

Cardiovascular – Bradycardia, hypotension, orthostatic hypotension, palpitations.

GI – Abdominal pain, dry mouth, vomiting.

Special senses – Tinnitus, vertigo.

Miscellaneous – Dyspnea, peripheral edema.

➤*Less common adverse reactions:* Other rarer (0.5% or less) but potentially medically important adverse reactions observed more frequently with ranolazine than placebo treatment in all controlled studies included: angioedema, blurred vision, confusional state, eosinophilia, hematuria, hypesthesia, leukopenia, pancytopenia, paresthesia, pulmonary fibrosis, renal failure, thrombocytopenia, and tremor.

A large clinical trial in acute coronary syndrome patients was unsuccessful in demonstrating a benefit for ranolazine, but there was no apparent proarrhythmic effect in these high-risk patients.

Overdosage

➤*Symptoms:* High oral doses of ranolazine produce dose-related increases in dizziness, nausea, and vomiting. High intravenous exposure also produces diplopia, paresthesia, confusion, and syncope.

➤*Treatment:* Since ranolazine is about 62% bound to plasma proteins, hemodialysis is unlikely to be effective in clearing ranolazine. In addition to general supportive measures, continuous ECG monitoring may be warranted in the event of overdose.

PHENAZOPYRIDINE HYDROCHLORIDE (Phenylazo Diamino Pyridine HCl)

otc	**Azo-Standard** (Alcon)	**Tablets; oral:** 95 mg	(W). In 30s.
otc	**Prodium** (Breckenridge)		In 12s and 30s.
Rx	**Phenazopyridine Hydrochloride** (Various, eg, Moore, Parmed, URL)	**Tablets; oral:** 100 mg	In 100s, 1,000s, and UD 100s.
otc	**Baridium** (Pfeiffer)		In 32s.
Rx	**Geridium** (Goldline)		Burgundy. Sugar coated. In 100s and 1,000s.
Rx	**Pyridium** (Warner Chilcott)		Sucrose, lactose. (WC 180). Maroon. In 100s, 1,000s, and UD 100s.
Rx	**Urogesic** (Edwards)		In 100s.
Rx	**UTI Relief** (Consumers Choice Systems)	**Tablets; oral:** 97.2 mg	In 12s.
Rx	**Phenazopyridine Hydrochloride** (Various, eg, Moore, Parmed, URL)	**Tablets; oral:** 200 mg	In 100s, 1,000s, and UD 100s.
Rx	**Geridium** (Goldline)		Burgundy. Sugar coated. In 100s.
Rx	**Pyridium** (Warner Chilcott)		Sucrose, lactose. (P-D 181). Maroon. In 100s, 1,000s, and UD 100s.

PHENAZOPYRIDINE HYDROCHLORIDE — ORAL

Urinary analgesics in combination with urinary anti-infectives are listed in the Anti-Infectives chapter.

Indications

➤*Dysuria, symptomatic relief:* Phenazopyridine HCl is indicated for the symptomatic relief of pain, burning, urgency, frequency, and other discomforts arising from irritation of the lower urinary tract mucosa caused by infection, trauma, surgery, endoscopic procedures, or the passage of sounds or catheters. The use of phenazopyridine HCl for relief of symptoms should not delay definitive diagnosis and treatment of causative conditions. Because it provides only symptomatic relief, prompt appropriate treatment of the cause of pain must be instituted and phenazopyridine HCl should be discontinued when symptoms are controlled.

The analgesic action may reduce or eliminate the need for systemic analgesics or narcotics. It is, however, compatible with antibacterial therapy and can help to relieve pain and discomfort during the interval before antibacterial therapy controls the infection. Treatment of a urinary tract infection with phenazopyridine HCl should not exceed 2 days because there is a lack of evidence that the combined administration of phenazopyridine HCl and an antibacterial provides greater benefit than administration of the antibacterial alone after 2 days.

Administration and Dosage

➤*Adults:*

Irritation of lower urinary tract mucosa – 100 to 200 mg 3 times/day.

➤*Children:*

Irritation of lower urinary tract mucosa –

Children over 12 years of age: 100 to 200 mg 3 times/day.

Off-label dosing –

Irritation of lower urinary tract mucosa:

- *6 to 12 years of age* – 12 mg/kg/day divided into 3 oral doses for 2 days.

➤*Renal function impairment:* Contraindicated in patients with renal insufficiency. A yellowish tinge of the skin or sclera may indicate accumulation due to impaired renal excretion and the need to discontinue therapy.

➤*Duration of therapy:* When used concomitantly with an antibacterial agent for the treatment of a urinary tract infection, administration should not exceed 2 days.

➤*Administration:* Administer after meals.

➤*Storage/Stability:* Store at 15° to 30°C (59° to 86°F). Protect from light and moisture.

Actions

➤*Pharmacology:* Phenazopyridine HCl is excreted in the urine where it exerts a topical analgesic effect on the mucosa of the urinary tract. This action helps to relieve pain, burning, urgency, and frequency. The precise mechanism of action is not known. Phenazopyridine is compatible with antibacterial therapy and can help relieve pain and discomfort before antibacterial therapy controls the infection.

➤*Pharmacokinetics:*

Excretion – The pharmacokinetic properties of phenazopyridine HCl have not been determined. Phenazopyridine HCl is rapidly excreted by the kidneys, with as much as 65% of an oral dose being excreted unchanged in the urine.

Contraindications

Phenazopyridine HCl should not be used in patients who have previously exhibited hypersensitivity to it. The use of phenazopyridine HCl is contraindicated in patients with renal insufficiency.

Warnings/Precautions

➤*Skin/sclera discoloration:* A yellowish tinge of the skin or sclera may indicate accumulation due to impaired renal excretion and the need to discontinue therapy. The decline in renal function associated with advanced age should be kept in mind.

➤*Duration of therapy:* Treatment of a urinary tract infection (UTI) with phenazopyridine should not exceed 2 days because there is a lack of evidence that the combined administration of phenazopyridine and an antibacterial provides greater benefit than administration of the antibacterial alone after 2 days.

➤*Urine discoloration:* Patients should be informed that phenazopyridine HCl produces a reddish-orange discoloration of the urine and may stain fabric. This is not abnormal and represents no cause for alarm.

➤*Contact lenses:* Staining of contact lenses has been reported.

➤*Renal function impairment:* The use of phenazopyridine HCl is contraindicated in patients with renal insufficiency.

➤*Pregnancy: Category B.* Reproduction studies have been performed in rats at doses up to 50 mg/kg/day and have revealed no evidence of impaired fertility or harm to the fetus due to phenazopyridine HCl. There are, however, no adequate and well controlled studies in pregnant women. Because animal reproduction studies are not always predictive of human response, this drug should be used during pregnancy only if clearly needed.

➤*Lactation:* No information is available on the appearance of phenazopyridine HCl, or its metabolites in human milk.

➤*Children:* Do not give to children younger than 12 years of age unless directed by physician.

➤*Elderly:* A yellowish tinge of the skin or sclera may indicate accumulation due to impaired renal excretion and the need to discontinue therapy. The decline in renal function associated with advanced age should be kept in mind.

➤*Lab test abnormalities:* Due to its properties as an azo dye, phenazopyridine HCl may interfere with urinalysis based on spectrometry or color reactions.

Adverse Reactions

Headache; rash; pruritus; occasional gastrointestinal disturbance. An anaphylactoid-like reaction has been described. Methemoglobinemia, hemolytic anemia, renal and hepatic toxicity have been described, usually at overdosage levels.

Staining of contact lenses has been reported.

Overdosage

➤*Symptoms:* Exceeding the recommended dose in patients with good renal function or administering the usual dose to patients with impaired renal function (common in elderly patients) may lead to increased serum levels and toxic reactions. Methemoglobinemia generally follows a massive, acute overdose. Oxidative Heinz body hemolytic anemia may also occur, and "bite cells" (degmacytes) may be present in a chronic overdosage situation. Red blood cell G-6-PD deficiency may predispose to hemolysis. Renal and hepatic impairment and occasional failure, usually due to hypersensitivity, may also occur.

➤*Treatment:* Methylene blue, 1 to 2 mg/kg/body weight intravenously or ascorbic acid 100 to 200 mg, given orally should cause prompt reduction of the methemoglobinemia and disappearance of the cyanosis which is an aid in diagnosis.

Patient Information

Phenazopyridine HCl may cause GI upset; take after meals.

Phenazopyridine HCl produces an orange to red color in the urine and may stain fabric. This is not abnormal and represents no cause for alarm. Staining of contact lenses has also occurred.

Do not use long term to treat undiagnosed urinary tract pain. This drug treats painful symptoms but not the source or cause of the pain.

PENTOSAN POLYSULFATE SODIUM

Rx	**Elmiron** (Janssen)	**Capsule; oral:** 100 mg	(BNP7600). White. In 100s.

PENTOSAN POLYSULFATE SODIUM — ORAL

Indications

➤*Relief of bladder pain/discomfort:* For the relief of bladder pain or discomfort associated with interstitial cystitis.

Administration and Dosage

➤*Adults:*

Interstitial cystitis –

Usual dosage: 100 mg 3 times daily.

Duration of therapy: Patients should be reassessed after 3 months. If improvement has not occurred and if limiting adverse reactions are not present, pentosan may be continued for another 3 months.

➤*Children:*

Interstitial cystitis –

16 years of age and older: See Adults for dosing.

➤*Administration:* Administer with water at least 1 hour before meals or 2 hours after meals.

➤*Storage/Stability:* Store at 15° to 30°C (59° to 86°F).

Actions

➤*Pharmacology:* Pentosan polysulfate sodium is a low molecular weight heparin-like compound. It has anticoagulant and fibrinolytic effects. The mechanism of action of pentosan polysulfate sodium in interstitial cystitis is not known.

Pharmacodynamics – The mechanism by which pentosan polysulfate sodium achieves its effects in patients is unknown. In preliminary clinical models, pentosan polysulfate sodium adhered to the bladder wall mucosal membrane. The drug may act as a buffer to control cell permeability preventing irritating solutes in the urine from reaching the cells.

➤*Pharmacokinetics:*

Absorption – In preliminary clinical studies with different doses of radiolabeled pentosan polysulfate sodium, absorption was ≈ 3% of the administered dose (n = 3).

Food effects: The effect of food on absorption of pentosan polysulfate sodium is not known. In clinical trials, pentosan polysulfate sodium was administered with water 1 hour before or 2 hours after meals.

Distribution – Preclinical studies with parenterally administered radiolabeled pentosan polysulfate sodium showed distribution to the uroepithelium of the genitourinary tract with lesser amounts found in the liver, spleen, lung, skin, periosteum, and bone marrow. Erythrocyte penetration is low in animals.

Metabolism – Preliminary literature studies of metabolism in 5 healthy volunteers with radiolabeled drug suggest that 68% of the dose, at about 1 hour after IV administration, undergoes partial desulfation in the liver and spleen. In another study of 3 healthy volunteers, partial depolymerization occurs in the kidney. Both the desulfation and depolymerization can be saturated with continued dosing.

Excretion – In preliminary clinical studies in 8 healthy male volunteers, the elimination half-life of pentosan polysulfate sodium had a mean value at 24 hours after IV injection of 40 mg.

The elimination half-life in urine following orally administered radiolabeled pentosan polysulfate sodium was determined to be 4.8 hours for the unchanged drug.

In preliminary human studies in 3 healthy male volunteers, after single doses of radiolabeled drug, urinary excretion averaged 3.5% of the administered dose. After multiple doses of pentosan polysulfate sodium, urine excretion of radioactivity averaged 11% of the administered dose.

Further analyses of the urinary fraction obtained after repeated dosing showed that about 3% of the dose may be unchanged pentosan polysulfate sodium.

Special populations –

Renal function impairment: Dose adjustments were not studied in patients with renal function impairment.

Hepatic function impairment: Dose adjustments were not studied in patients with hepatic function impairment.

Elderly: Dose adjustments were not studied in elderly patients.

Contraindications

Hypersensitivity to the drug, structurally related compounds, or excipients.

Warnings/Precautions

➤*Bleeding risks:* Pentosan polysulfate sodium is a weak anticoagulant (1/15 the activity of heparin). Bleeding complications of ecchymosis, epistaxis, and gum hemorrhage have been reported (see Adverse Reactions). Patients undergoing invasive procedures or having signs/symptoms of underlying coagulopathy or other increased risk of bleeding (due to other therapies such as coumarin anticoagulants, heparin, t-PA, streptokinase, or high dose aspirin) should be evaluated for hemorrhage. Patients with diseases such as aneurysms, thrombocytopenia, hemophilia, gastrointestinal ulcerations, polyps, or diverticula should be carefully evaluated before starting pentosan polysulfate sodium.

➤*Delayed immunoallergic thrombocytopenia:* A similar product that was given subcutaneously, sublingually, or intramuscularly (and not initially metabolized by the liver) is associated with delayed immunoallergic thrombocytopenia with symptoms of thrombosis and hemorrhage. Caution should be exercised when using pentosan polysulfate sodium in patients who have a history of heparin induced thrombocytopenia.

➤*Alopecia:* Alopecia is associated with pentosan polysulfate sodium and with heparin products. In clinical trials of pentosan polysulfate sodium, alopecia could begin within the first 4 weeks of treatment. Ninety-seven percent (97%) of the cases of alopecia reported were alopecia areata, limited to a single area on the scalp.

➤*Hepatic function impairment:* Pentosan polysulfate sodium is desulfated by both the liver and the spleen. The extent to which hepatic insufficiency or splenic disorders may increase the bioavailability of the parent or active metabolites of pentosan polysulfate sodium is not known. Caution should be exercised when using pentosan polysulfate sodium in these patients.

Mildly (< 2.5 × normal) elevated transaminase, alkaline phosphatase, gamma-glutamyl transpeptidase, and lactic dehydrogenase occurred in 1.2% of patients. The increases usually appeared 3 to 12 months after the start of pentosan polysulfate sodium therapy, and were not associated with jaundice or other clinical signs or symptoms. These abnormalities are usually transient, may remain essentially unchanged, or may rarely progress with continued use. Increases in PTT and PT (< 1% for both) or thrombocytopenia (0.2%) were noted.

➤*Pregnancy: Category B.* Reproduction studies have been performed in mice and rats with intravenous daily doses of 15 mg/kg, and in rabbits with 7.5 mg/kg. These doses are 0.42 and 0.14 times the daily oral human doses of pentosan polysulfate sodium when normalized to body surface area. These studies did not reveal evidence of impaired fertility or harm to the fetus from pentosan polysulfate sodium. Direct in vitro bathing of cultured mouse embryos with pentosan polysulfate sodium (PPS) at a concentration of 1 mg/mL may cause reversible limb bud abnormalities. Adequate and well controlled studies have not been performed in pregnant women. Because animal studies are not always predictive of human response, this drug should be used in pregnancy only if clearly needed.

➤*Lactation:* It is not known whether this drug is excreted in human milk. Because many drugs are excreted in human milk, caution should be exercised when pentosan polysulfate sodium is administered to a nursing woman.

➤*Children:* Safety and effectiveness in pediatric patients below the age of 16 years have not been established.

➤*Lab test abnormalities:* Pentosan polysulfate sodium did not affect prothrombin time (PT) or partial thromboplastin time (PTT) up to 1200 mg per day in 24 healthy male subjects treated for 8 days. Pentosan polysulfate sodium also inhibits the generation of factor Xa in human plasma and inhibits thrombin-induced platelet aggregation in human platelet rich plasma ex vivo. (See Warnings for additional information.)

Drug Interactions

Not studied.

Adverse Reactions

Pentosan polysulfate sodium was evaluated in clinical trials in a total of 2,627 patients (2,343 women, 262 men, 22 unknown) with a mean age of 47 [range 18 to 88 with 581 (22%) over 60 years of age]. Of the 2,627 patients, 128 patients were in a 3-month trial, and the remaining 2,499 patients were in a long term unblinded trial.

Deaths occurred in 6/2,627 (0.2%) patients who received the drug over a period of 3 to 75 months. The deaths appear to be related to other concurrent illnesses or procedures, except in one patient for whom the cause was not known.

Serious adverse events occurred in 33/2,627 (1.3%) patients. Two patients had severe abdominal pain or diarrhea and dehydration that required hospitalization. Because there was not a control group of patients with interstitial cystitis who were concurrently evaluated, it is difficult to determine which events are associated with pentosan polysulfate sodium and which events are associated with concurrent illness, medicine, or other factors.

Adverse Reactions in Placebo-Controlled Clinical Trials of Pentosan Polysulfate Sodium 100 mg 3 Times a Day for 3 Months

Body system/adverse reaction		Pentosan polysulfate sodium (n = 128)	Placebo (n = 130)
CNS	Overall number of patients*	3	5
	Insomnia	1	0
	Headache	1	3
	Severe emotional lability/depression	2	1
	Nystagmus/dizziness	1	1
	Hyperkinesia	1	1

PENTOSAN POLYSULFATE SODIUM — ORAL

Adverse Reactions in Placebo-Controlled Clinical Trials of Pentosan Polysulfate Sodium 100 mg 3 Times a Day for 3 Months

Body system	Adverse reaction	Pentosan polysulfate sodium (n = 128)	Placebo (n = 130)
GI	Overall number of patients*	7	7
	Nausea	3	3
	Diarrhea	3	6
	Dyspepsia	1	0
	Jaundice	0	1
	Vomiting	0	2
Dermatologic/allergic	Overall number of patients*	2	4
	Rash	0	2
	Pruritus	0	2
	Lacrimation	1	1
	Rhinitis	1	1
	Increased sweating	1	0
Miscellaneous	Overall number of patients*	1	3
	Amenorrhea	0	1
	Arthralgia	0	1
	Vaginitis	1	1
Total reactions		17	27
Total number of patient reporting adverse reactions		13	19

* Within a body system, the individual reactions do not sum to equal overall number of patients because a patient may have more than one reaction.

The adverse events described below were reported in an unblinded clinical trial of 2,499 interstitial cystitis patients treated with pentosan polysulfate sodium. Of the original 2,499 patients, 1,192 (48%) received pentosan polysulfate sodium for 3 months; 892 (36%) received pentosan polysulfate sodium for 6 months; and 598 (24%) received pentosan polysulfate sodium for one year, 355 (14%) received pentosan polysulfate sodium for 2 years, and 145 (6%) for 4 years.

➤*Frequency (1 to 4%):*

Miscellaneous – Alopecia (4%), diarrhea (4%), nausea (4%), headache (3%), rash (3%), dyspepsia (2%), abdominal pain (2%), liver function abnormalities (1%), dizziness (1%).

➤*Frequency (≤1%):* The adverse events described below were reported in an unblinded clinical trial of 2,499 interstitial cystitis patients treated with pentosan polysulfate sodium. Of the original 2,499 patients, 1,192 (48%) received pentosan polysulfate sodium for 3 months; 892 (36%) received pentosan polysulfate sodium for 6 months; and 598 (24%) received pentosan polysulfate sodium for one year, 355 (14%) received pentosan polysulfate sodium for 2 years, and 145 (6%) for 4 years.

Dermatologic – Pruritus, urticaria.

GI – Vomiting, mouth ulcer, colitis, esophagitis, gastritis, flatulence, constipation, anorexia, gum hemorrhage.

Hematologic – Anemia, ecchymosis, increased prothrombin time, increased partial thromboplastin time, leukopenia, thrombocytopenia.

Hypersensitivity – Allergic reaction, photosensitivity.

Respiratory – Pharyngitis, rhinitis, epistaxis, dyspnea.

Special senses – Conjunctivitis, tinnitus, optic neuritis, amblyopia, retinal hemorrhage.

Overdosage

Overdose has not been reported. Based upon the pharmacodynamics of the drug, toxicity is likely to be reflected as anticoagulation, bleeding, thrombocytopenia, liver function abnormalities, and gastric distress. (See Pharmacokinetics, Warnings, and Precautions.) In the event of acute overdosage, the patient should be given gastric lavage if possible, carefully observed and given symptomatic and supportive treatment.

Patient Information

Patients should take the drug as prescribed, in the dosage prescribed, and no more frequently than prescribed. Patients should be reminded that pentosan polysulfate sodium has a weak anticoagulant effect. This effect may increase bleeding times.

DIMETHYL SULFOXIDE (DMSO)

Rx	**Dimethyl Sulfoxide** (Bioniche)	**Solution:** 50% aqueous solution	In 50 mL.
Rx	**Rimso-50** (Research Industries)		In 50 mL.

DIMETHYL SULFOXIDE — INTRAVESICAL

Indications

➤*Interstitial cystitis, symptomatic relief:* For the symptomatic relief of patients with interstitial cystitis. Dimethyl sulfoxide has not been approved as being safe and effective for any other indication. There is no clinical evidence of effectiveness of dimethyl sulfoxide in the treatment of bacterial infections of the urinary tract.

Administration and Dosage

➤*Adults:*

Interstitial cystitis –

Usual dosage: 50 mL instilled directly into the bladder and allowed to remain for 15 minutes. The medication is expelled by spontaneous voiding.

Duration of therapy: Repeat every 2 weeks until maximum symptomatic relief is obtained. Thereafter, time intervals between therapy may be increased appropriately.

Concomitant therapy: Administration of oral analgesic medication or suppositories containing belladonna and opium prior to the instillation of dimethyl sulfoxide can reduce bladder spasm.

➤*Administration:* For intravesical use. Dimethyl sulfoxide should not be given IM or IV. Instillation of dimethyl sulfoxide directly into the bladder may be accomplished by catheter or aseptic syringe. Application of an analgesic lubricant gel such as lidocaine jelly to the urethra is suggested prior to insertion of the catheter to avoid spasm. In patients with severe interstitial cystitis with very sensitive bladders, the initial treatment, and possibly the second and third (depending on patient response) should be done under anesthesia. (Saddle block has been suggested.)

➤*Storage/Stability:* Store at 59° to 86°F (15° to 30°C). Do not autoclave. Protect from strong light.

Actions

➤*Pharmacology:* Dimethyl sulfoxide is metabolized in man by oxidation to dimethyl sulfone or by reduction to dimethyl sulfide. Dimethyl sulfoxide and dimethyl sulfone are excreted in the urine and feces. Dimethyl sulfide is eliminated through the breath and skin and is responsible for the characteristic odor from patients on dimethyl sulfoxide medication. Dimethyl sulfone can persist in serum for longer than two weeks after a single intravesical instillation. No residual accumulation of dimethyl sulfoxide has occurred in man or lower animals who have received treatment for protracted periods of time. Following topical application, dimethyl sulfoxide is absorbed and generally distributed in the tissues and body fluids.

Contraindications

None known.

Warnings/Precautions

➤*Ophthalmic effects:* Changes in the refractive index and lens opacities have been seen in monkeys, dogs and rabbits given high doses of dimethyl sulfoxide chronically. Since lens changes were noted in animals, full eye evaluations, including slit lamp examinations, are recommended prior to and periodically during treatment.

➤*Intravesical instillation:* Intravesical instillation of dimethyl sulfoxide may be harmful to patients with urinary tract malignancy because of dimethyl sulfoxide-induced vasodilation.

➤*Drug interactions:* Some data indicate that dimethyl sulfoxide potentiates other concomitantly administered medications.

➤*Hypersensitivity reactions:* Dimethyl sulfoxide can initiate the liberation of histamine and there has been occasional hypersensitivity reaction with topical administration of dimethyl sulfoxide. This hypersensitivity has been reported in one patient receiving intravesical dimethyl sulfoxide. The physician should be cognizant of this possibility in prescribing dimethyl sulfoxide. If anaphylactoid symptoms develop, appropriate therapy should be instituted.

➤*Drug abuse and dependence:* None known.

➤*Pregnancy: Category C.* Dimethyl sulfoxide caused teratogenic responses in hamsters, rats and mice when administered intraperitoneally at high doses (2.5-12 g/kg). Oral or topical doses of dimethyl sulfoxide did not cause problems of reproduction in rats, mice and hamsters. Topical doses (5 g/kg first two days, then 2.5 g/kg - last eight days) produced terata in rabbits, but in another study, topical doses of 1.1 gm/kg days 3 through 16 of gestation failed to produce any abnormalities. There are no adequate and well controlled studies in pregnant women. Dimethyl sulfoxide should be used during pregnancy only if the potential benefit justifies the potential risk to the fetus.

➤*Lactation:* It is not known whether this drug is excreted in human milk. Because many drugs are excreted in human milk, caution should be exercised when dimethyl sulfoxide is administered to a nursing woman.

➤*Children:* Safety and effectiveness in children have not been established.

DIMETHYL SULFOXIDE — INTRAVESICAL

➤*Monitoring:* Approximately every six months, patients receiving dimethyl sulfoxide should have a biochemical screening, particularly liver and renal function tests and complete blood count.

Adverse Reactions

A garlic-like taste may be noted by the patient within a few minutes after instillation of dimethyl sulfoxide. This taste may last several hours and because of the presence of metabolites, an odor on the breath and skin may remain for 72 hours.

Transient chemical cystitis has been noted following instillation of dimethyl sulfoxide.

The patient may experience moderately severe discomfort on administration. Usually this becomes less prominent with repeated administration.

Overdosage

The oral LD_{50} of dimethyl sulfoxide in the dog is greater than 10 g/kg. It is improbable that this dosage level could be obtained with intravesical instillation of dimethyl sulfoxide in the patient.

In case of accidental oral ingestion, specific measures should be taken to induce emesis. Additional measures which may be considered are gastric lavage, activated charcoal and forced diuresis.

Patient Information

Dimethyl sulfoxide is a sterile solution of 50% dimethyl sulfoxide (DMSO) and 50% water that has been approved by the U.S. Food and Drug Administration for use in the symptomatic relief of patients with interstitial cystitis.

Dimethyl sulfoxide will be instilled in the bladder on an inpatient or outpatient basis, which will be determined by your physician.

Some data indicate that dimethyl sulfoxide could change the effectiveness of any medication(s) that you may be presently receiving. Be sure to mention the name and dosage of all medications you are taking to your physician before a dimethyl sulfoxide instillation.

A garlic-like taste may be noted by the patient within a few minutes after instillation of dimethyl sulfoxide. This taste may last several hours. An odor on the breath and skin may be present and remain for up to 72 hours.

Some patients may experience discomfort on administration of the drug. Usually this becomes less prominent with repeated administration.

If you are pregnant or nursing, ask your physician about the advisability of using dimethyl sulfoxide.

Some eye changes have been observed in animals treated with DMSO in large doses for prolonged periods. Therefore your doctor may want you to have eye evaluations, including slit lamp examinations prior to and periodically during treatment.

PHENAZOPYRIDINE/BUTABARBITAL/HYOSCYAMINE

Rx	**Phenazopyridine Plus** (Breckenridge)	**Tablets; oral:** phenazopyridine hydrochloride 150 mg, hyoscyamine hydrobromide 0.3 mg, butabarbital 15 mg	(B-251). Dark brown. In 30s.
Rx	**PhenazoForte Plus** (Creekwood)		Lactose, mineral oil, PEG. (C 070). Maroon. Film-coated. In 30s.

PHENAZOPYRIDINE/BUTABARBITAL/HYOSCYAMINE — ORAL

For complete prescribing information, refer to the Phenazopyridine Hydrochloride individual monograph, the Gastrointestinal Anticholinergic/Antispasmodic class monograph, and the Barbiturates class monograph.

Indications

➤*Dysuria, symptomatic relief:* For the symptomatic relief of pain, burning, frequency, urgency, and dysuria, particularly when accompanied by the detrusor muscle spasm and apprehension. These symptoms may arise from infection, trauma, surgery, endoscopic procedures, or the passage of sounds or catheters.

Therapy does not interfere with antibacterial therapy and can help relieve symptoms of pain and discomfort before definitive treatment is effective. The use for symptomatic relief should not delay definitive diagnosis and treatment. Treatment of a urinary tract infection with this product should not exceed 2 days because there is a lack of evidence that the combined administration of phenazopyridine hydrochloride and an antibacterial provides greater benefit than administration of the antibacterial alone after 2 days.

In the absence of infection, this product may be the only medication required.

Administration and Dosage

➤*Adults:*

Irritation of lower urinary tract mucosa – One tablet 4 times a day. When used concomitantly with an antibacterial agent for the treatment of a urinary tract infection, administration should not exceed 2 days.

➤*Administration:* Take after meals and at bedtime.

➤*Storage/Stability:* Store at 25°C (77°F); excursions permitted to 15° to 30°C (59° to 86°F).

CELLULOSE SODIUM PHOSPHATE

CELLULOSE SODIUM PHOSPHATE

Rx	**Calcibind** (Mission)	**Powder:** Inorganic phosphate content 31% to 36% and sodium content ≈ 11%	In 300 g bulk powder.

CELLULOSE SODIUM PHOSPHATE — ORAL

Indications

➤*Absorptive hypercalciuria Type I:* Cellulose sodium phosphate (CSP) is indicated only for absorptive hypercalciuria Type I with recurrent calcium oxalate or calcium phosphate nephrolithiasis. Appropriate use of CSP substantially reduces the incidence of new stone formation in these patients. Causes of hypercalciuria other than hyperabsorption cannot be expected to respond to CSP. Treatment with CSP is not needed for absorptive hypercalciuria Type II because dietary calcium restriction provides adequate treatment. In patients without hyperabsorption of calcium, CSP would be expected to cause excessive parathyroid hormone secretion and possible hyperparathyroid bone disease.

Absorptive hypercalciuria Type I is characterized by

1.) recurrent passage or formation of calcium oxalate and/or calcium phosphate renal stones,
2.) no evidence of bone disease,
3.) normal serum calcium and phosphorus,
4.) increased intestinal calcium absorption,
5.) hypercalciuria,
6.) normal urinary calcium during fasting,
7.) normal parathyroid function,
8.) lack of renal "leak" or excessive skeletal mobilization of calculi. Minimal diagnostic tests include serum calcium and phosphorus, parathyroid hormone (PTH) level obtained before breakfast, 24-hour urinary calcium on a diet restricted in calcium and sodium, and a fasting urinary excretion of calcium.

The diagnosis of absorptive hypercalciuria Type I can be made if there is: a) recurrent calcium nephrolithiasis without clinical evidence of bone disease, b) normal serum calcium and phosphorus (borderline values should be repeated), c) 24-hour urinary calcium greater than 200 mg/day on a diet of 400 mg calcium and 100 mEq sodium/day, d) normal serum immunoreactive PTH, and e) normal fasting urinary calcium. A definite diagnosis requires, in addition, evidence of high intestinal calcium absorption (eg, urinary calcium greater than 0.2 mg/mg creatinine after oral load of 1 g calcium.)

Administration and Dosage

➤*General dosing considerations:* The amount of dietary calcium bound depends upon actual mixing of cellulose sodium phosphate with a meal. Consequently, cellulose sodium phosphate should be taken with a meal; the amount of dietary calcium bound by cellulose sodium phosphate is considerably reduced when cellulose sodium phosphate is administered more than 1 hour after a meal. Both the initial and maintenance doses of cellulose sodium phosphate are based on measurements of 24-hour urinary calcium excretion.

➤*Adults:*

Absorptive hypercalciuria Type I –

Initial dosage: 15 g/day (5 g with each meal) in patients with urinary calcium greater than 300 mg/day (on moderate calcium-restricted diet, ie, avoidance of dairy products). Patients with controlled urinary calcium on moderate calcium-restricted diet of less than 300 mg/day (but greater than 200 mg/day) should begin on 10 g/day (5 g with supper, 2.5 g each with remaining meal).

Dosage adjustment: When urinary calcium declines to less than 150 mg/day, the dosage should be reduced to 10 g/day (5 g with supper, 2.5 g each with remaining meal).

Concomitant therapy: Fluid intake should be encouraged to achieve a minimum urine output of 2 L/day. The dose of oral magnesium gluconate supplements depends upon the dose of cellulose sodium phosphate. Those receiving 15 g of cellulose sodium phosphate/day should take 1.5 g of magnesium gluconate before breakfast and again at bedtime (separately from cellulose sodium phosphate). Those taking 10 g of cellulose sodium phosphate/day should take 1 g of magnesium gluconate twice a day.

Dietary restrictions: A moderate calcium intake is recommended, by avoidance of dairy products. A moderate dietary oxalate restriction should be imposed by discouraging ingestion of spinach (and similar dark greens), rhubarb, chocolate, and brewed tea. Vitamin C supplementation should be denied because of its potential metabolism to oxalate. A high sodium intake should be discouraged by advising avoidance of salty foods and salt shakers, in an attempt to achieve an intake of less than 150 mEq/day.

➤*Administration:* It is recommended that each dose of cellulose sodium phosphate (in the powder form) be suspended in a glass of water, soft drink

CELLULOSE SODIUM PHOSPHATE — ORAL

or fruit juice, and ingested within 30 minutes of the meal. It should not be given with magnesium. To avoid binding of magnesium by cellulose sodium phosphate, supplemental magnesium should be given at least 1 hour before or after a dose of cellulose sodium phosphate.

➤*Storage/Stability:* Store at 2° to 8°C (36° to 46°F).

Actions

➤*Pharmacology:* CSP alters urinary composition of calcium, magnesium, phosphate and oxalate by affecting their absorption in the intestinal tract. When it is given orally with meals, CSP binds dietary and secreted calcium, and reduces urinary calcium by approximately 50 mg/5 g of CSP. It also binds dietary Mg and lowers urinary Mg. Oral magnesium supplementation given separately from CSP partly overcomes this effect.

CSP administration increases urinary phosphorus (P) and oxalate. The usual rise in urinary P of 150 to 250 mg/15 g CSP largely reflects the hydrolysis of 7% to 30% of CSP in the intestinal tract and absorption of released P. An increase in urinary oxalate occurs. Since CSP binds divalent cations, the cations are not available to complex oxalate and thereby limit its absorption. The rise in urinary oxalate may be largely prevented by moderate dietary oxalate restriction and the use of a modest dose of CSP (10 to 15 g/day).

The marked reduction in urinary calcium with only slightly increased urinary phosphorus and oxalate leads to a reduction in urinary saturation and propensity for spontaneous nucleation of calcium oxalate and calcium phosphate (brushite).

CSP does not apparently alter the metabolism of trace metals, since it does not significantly change the serum concentration of copper, zinc or iron.

Contraindications

CSP is contraindicated in

1.) primary or secondary hyperparathyroidism, including renal hypercalciuria (renal calcium leak),
2.) hypomagnesemic states (serum magnesium less than 1.5 mg/dL),
3.) bone disease (osteoporosis, osteomalacia, osteitis),
4.) hypocalcemic states (eg, hypoparathyroidism, intestinal malabsorption),
5.) normal or low intestinal absorption and renal excretion of calcium,
6.) enteric hyperoxaluria. It should not be used in patients with high fasting urinary calcium or hypophosphatemia, unless a high skeletal mobilization of calcium can be excluded.

Warnings/Precautions

➤*Congestive heart failure/ascites:* In patients with congestive heart failure or ascites, sodium contained in CSP (35 to 48 mEq exchangeable sodium/15 g CSP) may represent a hazard.

➤*Hyperparathyroidism:* By inhibiting intestinal calcium absorption, CSP may stimulate parathyroid function leading to hyperparathyroid hormone levels. CSP treatment has been shown to maintain parathyroid function within normal limits, if it is used only in patients with absorptive hypercalciuria Type I (increased intestinal calcium restricted diet), at a dosage just sufficient to restore normal calcium absorption but not sufficient to cause subnormal absorption.

➤*Long-term use:* The following additional complications may potentially develop during long-term use of CSP: Hyperoxaluria and hypomagnesiuria, which would negate the beneficial effect of hypocalciuria on new stone formation; magnesium depletion; depletion of trace metals (copper, zinc, iron). All of these effects may be minimized by restricting the use of CSP to absorptive hypercalciuria Type I only, and by taking precautionary measures (see Administration and Dosage) and by monitoring serum calcium, magnesium, copper, zinc, iron, parathyroid hormone, and complete blood count every 3 to 6 months.

➤*Dietary restriction:* A moderate calcium intake is recommended, by avoidance of dairy products. A moderate dietary oxalate restriction should be imposed by discouraging ingestion of spinach (and similar dark greens), rhubarb, chocolate and brewed tea. Vitamin C supplementation should be denied because of its potential metabolism to oxalate. A high sodium intake should be discouraged by advising avoidance of "salty" foods and salt shakers, in an attempt to achieve an intake of less than 150 mEq/day.

➤*Fluid intake:* Fluid intake should be encouraged to achieve a minimum urine output of 2 L/day.

➤*Inadequate response:* If there is an inadequate hypocalciuric response to CSP treatment (a reduction in urinary calcium of less than 30 mg/5 g of CSP), while patients are maintained on moderate calcium and sodium restriction, the treatment may be considered ineffective and should be stopped.

➤*Discontinuation of therapy:* Cessation of treatment should be considered if urinary oxalate exceeds 55 mg/day on moderate dietary oxalate restriction.

➤*Pregnancy: Category C.* Animal reproduction studies have not been conducted with CSP. It is also not known whether CSP can cause fetal harm when administered to a pregnant woman or can affect reproduction capacity. However, because of the increased requirement of dietary calcium in pregnant women, CSP should be given to pregnant women only if clearly needed.

➤*Lactation:* There is no information regarding the use of cellulose sodium phosphate in breast-feeding women.

➤*Children:* Because of the increased requirement for dietary calcium in growing children, the use of CSP in children less than 16 years of age is not recommended.

➤*Monitoring:* Borderline values for parathyroid hormone and calcium should be repeated promptly. Serum PTH should be obtained at least once between the first 2 weeks to 3 months of treatment and the treatment should be adjusted or stopped if a rise in serum PTH above normal appears.

Adverse Reactions

Some patients may have gastrointestinal complaints manifested by poor taste of the drug, loose bowel movements, diarrhea or dyspepsia.

IMPOTENCE AGENTS

ALPROSTADIL (Prostaglandin E_1; PGE_1)

Rx	**Caverject** (Pharmacia & Upjohn)	**Injection, aqueous**: 10 mcg/mL	In 1 mL ampules and kit.[a]
		20 mcg/mL	In 1 mL ampules and kit.[a]
		40 mcg/2 mL	In 2 mL ampules and kit.[a]
Rx	**Caverject** (Pharmacia & Upjohn)	**Powder for injection, lyophilized**: 5 mcg/mL (after reconstitution)	With 8.4 mg benzyl alcohol and lactose. In vials with diluent syringes.
		10 mcg/mL (after reconstitution)	With 8.4 mg benzyl alcohol and lactose. In vials and vials with diluent syringes.
		20 mcg/mL (after reconstitution)	With 8.4 mg benzyl alcohol and lactose. In vials and vials with diluent syringes.
		40 mcg/mL (after reconstitution)	With 8.4 mg benzyl alcohol and lactose. In vials with diluent syringes.
Rx	**Caverject Impulse** (Pharmacia & Upjohn)	**Powder for injection, lyophilized**: 10 mcg/0.5 mL (after reconstitution)[b]	With 4.45 mg benzyl alcohol and lactose. In blister tray.[c]
		20 mcg/0.5 mL (after reconstitution)[d]	With 4.45 mg benzyl alcohol and lactose. In blister tray.[c]
Rx	**Edex** (Schwarz Pharma)	**Powder for injection, lyophilized**: 5 mcg/mL (after reconstitution)	Lactose. In single-dose vials and kit.[e]
		10 mcg/mL (after reconstitution)	Lactose. In single-dose vials and kit.[e]
		20 mcg/mL (after reconstitution)	Lactose. In single-dose vials and kit.[e]
		40 mcg/mL (after reconstitution)	Lactose. In single-dose vials and kit.[e]
Rx	**Muse** (Vivus)	**Pellet**: 125 mcg	In individual foil pouches.
		250 mcg	In individual foil pouches.
		500 mcg	In individual foil pouches.
		1000 mcg	In individual foil pouches.

[a] Kit contains 2 mL *Luer-lock* syringe, 2 one-half inch needles (one 27-gauge and one 30-gauge), alcohol swab.
[b] Amounts can be delivered in increments of 10 mcg/0.5 mL, 2.5 mcg/0.125 mL, 5 mcg/0.25 mL, or 7.5 mcg/0.375 mL.
[c] Blister tray contains 1 dual chamber syringe system, 1 needle, 2 alcohol swabs.
[d] Amounts can be delivered in increments of 20 mcg/0.5 mL, 5 mcg/0.125 mL, 10 mcg/0.25 mL, or 15 mcg/0.375 mL.
[e] Kit contains prefilled syringe (with 1.2 mL of 0.9% sodium chloride), plunger rod, 2 one-half inch needles (one 27-gauge and one 30-gauge), 2 alcohol swabs, tape.

ALPROSTADIL — INTRACAVERNOSAL

For information on the use of alprostadil for patent ductus arteriosus, refer to the specific monograph in the Cardiovasculars chapter.

Indications

➤*Erectile dysfunction:* For the treatment of erectile dysfunction due to neurogenic, vasculogenic, psychogenic, or mixed etiology.

May be a useful adjunct to other diagnostic tests in the diagnosis of erectile dysfunction.

Administration and Dosage

➤*General dosing considerations:* Advise the patient not to exceed the optimum dose, which was determined in the health care provider's office. In general, always use the lowest possible effective dose.

The first injections must be done at the health care provider's office by medically trained personnel. Self-injection therapy by the patient can be started only after the patient is properly instructed and well trained in the self-injection technique. The health care provider should make a careful assessment of the patient's skills and competence with this procedure.

➤*Adults:*

Adjunct to the diagnosis of erectile dysfunction – Use a single dose of alprostadil that induces an erection with firm rigidity.

Erectile dysfunction of vasculogenic, psychogenic, or mixed etiology –

Usual dosage:

• *Caverject formulations* – In clinical studies, patients were treated with alprostadil sterile powder in doses ranging from 0.2 to 140 mcg; however, because 99% of patients received doses of 60 mcg or less, doses of greater than 60 mcg are not recommended.

• *Edex* – 1 to 40 mcg. Give the injection over a 5- to 10-second interval.

Maximum dose: 60 mcg/dose (*Caverject* formulations).

Initial dosage: 2.5 mcg.

Dosage titration: If there is a partial response, the dose may be increased by 2.5 mcg to a dose of 5 mcg and then in increments of 5 to 10 mcg, depending on erectile response, until the dose that produces an erection suitable for intercourse and not exceeding a duration of 1 hour. If the duration of erection is longer than 1 hour, reduce the dose. If there is no response to the initial 2.5 mcg dose, the second dose may be increased to 7.5 mcg, followed by increments of 5 to 10 mcg. The patient must stay in the health care providers office until complete detumescence occurs. If there is no response, then the next higher dose may be given within 1 hour. If there is a response, then there should be at least a 1-day interval before the next dose is given.

Maintenance dosage: Use the lowest effective dose at home. Initiate self-injection therapy for use at home at the dose that was determined in the health care provider's office; however, make dose adjustment, if required (up to 57% of patients in 1 clinical study), only after consultation with the health care provider. Adjust the dose in accordance with the titration guidelines. The recommended frequency of injection is no more than 3 times weekly, with at least 24 hours between each dose.

Exercise careful and continuous follow-up of the patient while in the self-injection program. This is especially true for the initial self-injections because adjustments in the dose of alprostadil may be needed. While on self-injection treatment, it is recommended that the patient visit the prescribing health care provider's office every 3 months. At that time, assess the efficacy and safety of the therapy and the dose of alprostadil, if needed.

Erectile dysfunction of pure neurogenic etiology (spinal cord injury) –

Usual dosage: See Erectile Dysfunction of Vasculogenic, Psychogenic, or Mixed Etiology.

Maximum dose: 60 mcg/dose (*Caverject* formulations).

Initial dosage: 1.25 mcg.

Dosage titration: The dose may be increased by 1.25 mcg to a dose of 2.5 mcg, followed by an increment of 2.5 mcg to a dose of 5 mcg, and then in 5 mcg increments until the dose that produces an erection suitable for intercourse and not exceeding a duration of 1 hour. The patient must stay in the health care provider's office until complete detumescence occurs. If there is no response, then the next higher dose may be given within 1 hour. If there is a response, then there should be at least a 1-day interval before the next dose is given.

Maintenance dosage: See Maintenance dosage under Erectile Dysfunction of Vasculogenic, Psychogenic, or Mixed Etiology.

➤*Elderly:* Always use the lowest possible effective dose.

➤*Preparation for administration:*

Aqueous solution – To prepare a dose for administration, remove the ampule from the foil wrapping. Allow the ampule contents to warm to room temperature. The ampule should not be cool to the touch. Do not immerse in water. Do not microwave. Shake the ampule vigorously for at least 30 seconds. Next, hold the shorter tab closest to the neck of the ampule and shake it downward with a quick snap to clear any solution from the neck. Holding the ampule by the edges, twist the top of the ampule and lift upward to remove it. Make sure the open end of the ampule does not touch your hands or any other surface. After opening the ampule, immediately transfer the solution to a syringe and use promptly.

Sterile powder – Bacteriostatic water for injection or sterile water, both preserved with benzyl alcohol 0.945% w/v, must be used as the diluent for reconstitution. After reconstitution with 1 mL of diluent, the volume of the resulting solution is 1.13 mL. One mL of this solution will contain 5.4, 10.5, 20.5, or 41.1 mcg of alprostadil, depending on vial strength. The deliverable amount of alprostadil is 5, 10, 20, or 40 mcg/mL because approximately 0.4 mcg for the 5 mcg strength, 0.5 mcg for the 10 and 20 mcg strengths, and 1.1 mcg for the 40 mcg strength is lost because of adsorption to the vial and syringe.

Caverject dual-chamber system – When reconstituted and used as directed, the deliverable amount for the 10 mcg strength is 10 mcg per 0.5 mL or an increment of 10 mcg per 0.5 mL, 2.5 mcg per 0.125 mL, 5 mcg per 0.25 mL, or 7.5 mcg per 0.375 mL of alprostadil, and the deliverable amount for the 20 mcg strength is 20 mcg per 0.5 mL or an increment of 20 mcg per 0.5 mL, 5 mcg per 0.125 mL, 10 mcg per 0.25 mL, or 15 mcg per 0.375 mL of alprostadil.

Edex dual-chamber cartridge – The *Edex* injection device is used to reconstitute the single-dose, dual-chamber cartridge. The plunger is used to force the sterile sodium chloride 0.9% (1.075 mL) in 1 chamber into the chamber containing alprostadil. After reconstitution, the *Edex* injection device is used to administer the intracavernosal injection of alprostadil. When the cartridge is placed into the *Edex* injection device and reconstituted, the deliverable amount of alprostadil in each mL is 10, 20, or 40 mcg, respectively.

Prepare the *Edex* solution immediately before use. The *Edex* cartridge contains a solid layer or lyophilized cake of dry white powder approximately ⅜ inch in thickness for the cartridge. A normal cake may appear cracked or crumbled. If the cartridge is damaged, the cake may shrink in size. Do not use the cartridge if it appears damaged or the cake is substantially reduced in size.

➤*Administration:* The intracavernosal injection must be done under sterile conditions. The injection site is usually along the dorsolateral aspect of the proximal third of the penis. Avoid visible veins. Alternate the side of the penis that is injected and the injection site; cleanse the injection site with an alcohol swab.

Aqueous solution and sterile powder – A ½-inch, 27- to 30-gauge needle is generally recommended. Determine the most suitable size needle for the patient, and instruct the patient on the appropriate size to use for self-injection.

Caverject dual-chamber system – Uses a superfine (29-gauge) needle.

➤*Admixture compatibility:* Do not add any drugs or solutions to the *Edex* solution.

➤*Storage/Stability:* All formulations of alprostadil are intended for single use only and should be discarded after use. Instruct the user in the proper disposal of the injection materials (eg, device, syringes, needles, ampoule, reconstituted vial). Instruct the patient to discard any needles that become bent during the reconstitution or self-injection procedure because these needles may break.

Aqueous solution – Store alprostadil injection frozen at 20° to 10°C (4° to 14°F) until dispensed. After dispensing, store in a freezer at 20° to 10°C (4° to 14°F) for up to 3 months. During this 3-month period, alprostadil injection may be moved to and kept in a refrigerator at 2° to 8°C (36° to 46°F) for up to 7 days. Once refrigerated, use within 7 days or discard; do not refreeze. Once removed from the foil wrapping, use the solution in the ampule immediately after allowing it to warm to room temperature or discard it. Use open ampules of alprostadil injection immediately.

Sterile powder – Store at 2° to 8°C (36° to 46°F) until dispensed. After dispensing, store at or below 25°C (77°F) for 3 months or until expiration date, whichever occurs first. Use the reconstituted solution within 24 hours when stored at or below 25°C (77°F) and do not refrigerate or freeze.

Caverject dual-chamber system – Store the unreconstituted product at 25°C (77°F); excursions are permitted to 15° to 30°C (59° to 86°F). Use the reconstituted solution within 24 hours when stored at or below 25°C (77°F). Following a single use, properly discard the injection device and any remaining solution.

Edex cartridge – Store at 25°C (77°F); excursions are permitted between 15° and 30°C (59° to 86°F). Do not store the reconstituted *Edex* solution. The reusable *Edex* injection device is for use only with the cartridges and needles included in the Edex cartridge packs.

Actions

➤*Pharmacology:* Alprostadil (PGE_1) is 1 of the prostaglandins, a family of naturally occurring acidic lipids with various pharmacological effects. Endogenous PGE_1 is derived from dihomo-gamma-linolenic acid, a fatty acid found within the phospholipids of cellular membranes. As an endogenous substance, PGE_1 exerts its biological effects either directly or indirectly by regulating and modifying the synthesis and effects of other hormones and mediators.

Alprostadil is a smooth muscle relaxant. Precontracted isolated preparations of the human corpus cavernosum, corpus spongiosum, and cavernous artery are relaxed by alprostadil. Alprostadil has been shown to bind to specific receptors in human penile tissue. Two types of receptors that differ in their PGE_1-binding affinity have been identified. The binding of alprostadil to its receptors is accompanied by an increase in intracellular cAMP levels. Human cavernous smooth muscle cells respond to alprostadil by releasing intracellular calcium into the surrounding medium. Smooth muscle relaxation is associated with a reduction of cytoplasmic free calcium concentration. Alprostadil also attenuates presynaptic norepinephrine release in the corpus cavernosum, which is essential for the maintenance of a flaccid and nonerect penis.

Alprostadil has a wide variety of pharmacological actions; vasodilation and inhibition of platelet aggregation are among the most notable of these effects. In most animal species tested, alprostadil relaxed retractor penis and corpus cavernosum urethrae in vitro. Alprostadil also relaxed isolated preparations of human corpus cavernosum and spongiosum, as well as cavernous arterial segments contracted by either norepinephrine or $PGF_{2\alpha}$ in vitro. In pigtail monkeys (*Macaca nemestrina*), alprostadil increased cavernous arterial blood flow in vivo. The degree and duration of cavernous smooth muscle relaxation in this animal model was dose dependent.

ALPROSTADIL — INTRACAVERNOSAL

Alprostadil induces erection by relaxation of trabecular smooth muscle and by dilation of cavernosal arteries. This leads to expansion of lacunar spaces and entrapment of blood by compressing the venules against the tunica albuginea, a process referred to as the corporal veno-occlusive mechanism.

➤*Pharmacokinetics:*

Absorption – For the treatment of erectile dysfunction, alprostadil is administered by injection into the corpora cavernosa. The absolute bioavailability of alprostadil estimated from systemic exposure was about 98% as compared to the same dose given by a short-term IV infusion.

Edex: After intracavernosal injection of 20 mcg of *Edex* in 24 patients with erectile dysfunction, mean systemic plasma concentrations of PGE_1 increased from baseline of 0.8 ± 0.6 pg/mL to a peak (C_{max}) of 16.8 ± 18.9 pg/mL (corrected for baseline) within 2 to 5 minutes and dropped to endogenous plasma levels within 2 hours (see the following table). The absolute bioavailability of alprostadil estimated from systemic exposure was about 98% as compared to the same dose given by a short-term IV infusion.

Distribution – After intracavernosal injection of 20 mcg of alprostadil in 24 patients with erectile dysfunction, mean systemic plasma concentrations of PGE_1 increased from baseline of 0.8 ± 0.6 pg/mL to a peak (C_{max}) of 16.8 ± 18.9 pg/mL (corrected for baseline) within 2 to 5 minutes and dropped to endogenous plasma levels within 2 hours.

Plasma levels of PGE_1 were measured using a radioimmunoassay method. PGE_1 is bound in plasma primarily to albumin (81% bound) and, to a lesser extent, α-globulin IV-4 fraction (55% bound). No significant binding to erythrocytes or white blood cells was observed.

Edex: The volume of distribution for PGE_1 was not estimated. Approximately 93% of PGE_1 found in plasma is protein bound.

After reconstitution, PGE_1 immediately dissociates from the alpha-cyclodextrin inclusion; the in vivo disposition of both components occurs independently after administration.

After intracavernosal administration in monkeys, radiolabeled α-cyclodextrin was rapidly distributed from the injection site, with less than 0.1% of the dose remaining in the penis 1 hour after administration. There was no evidence of tissue retention of radiolabeled α-cyclodextrin in monkeys.

Metabolism – PGE_1 is metabolized in the corpus cavernosum after intracavernosal administration. PGE_1 entering the systemic circulation is rapidly and extensively metabolized in the lungs with a first-pass pulmonary elimination of 60% to 90% of PGE_1. Enzymatic oxidation of the C15-hydroxy group followed by reduction of the C13, 14-double bond produces the primary metabolites, 15-keto-PGE_1, 15-keto-PGE_0, and PGE_0. 15-keto-PGE_1 has only been detected in vitro in homogenized lung preparations, whereas 15-keto-PEG_0 and PGE_0 have been measured in plasma. Unlike the 15-keto metabolites, which are less pharmacologically active than the parent compound, PGE_0 is similar in potency to PGE_1 in vitro using isolated animal organs.

After intracavernosal injection of 20 mcg of alprostadil to 24 patients with erectile dysfunction, mean systemic plasma 15-keto-PGE_0 levels increased within 7 minutes from endogenous levels of 12.9 ± 11.8 pg/mL to a C_{max} of 421 ± 337 pg/mL (corrected for baseline), followed by a decrease to baseline levels in several hours. Mean systemic plasma PGE_0 levels increased within 20 minutes from endogenous levels of 0.6 ± 0.5 pg/mL to a C_{max} of 3.9 ± 2.3 pg/mL (corrected for baseline), followed by a decrease to baseline levels in several hours.

Excretion – After further degradation of PGE_1 by beta and omega oxidation, the main metabolites are excreted primarily in urine (88%) and feces (12%) over 72 hours, and total excretion is essentially complete (92%) within 24 hours after administration. No unchanged PGE_1 has been found in the urine, and there is no evidence of tissue retention of PGE_1 and its metabolites. After intracavernosal injection of 20 mcg of alprostadil in patients with erectile dysfunction, the terminal half-lives ($t_{1/2}$) of 15-keto-PGE_0 and PGE_0 were calculated to be 40.9 ± 16.5 minutes and 63.2 ± 31.1 minutes, respectively. The terminal half-life of PGE_1 in healthy volunteers was calculated to be around 9 to 11 minutes, which is consistent with that reported in the literature (8 minutes).

Mean total body clearance of PGE_1 in patients with erectile dysfunction was calculated to be around 115 L/min after an IV infusion of 20 mcg alprostadil. The above value exceed cardiac output, indicating extensive and rapid elimination of PGE_1 in the lungs or blood.

Edex: After IV infusion of radiolabeled α-cyclodextrin to healthy volunteers, the radiolabeled components were rapidly eliminated within 24 hours, urine accounting for 81% to 83% of radioactivity and feces for 0.1%. There was no evidence of significant accumulation of radiolabeled α-cyclodextrin in the body even after 7 days of repeated IV injection.

Special populations –

Renal function impairment: In a study in symptomatic subjects with end-stage renal disease undergoing hemodialysis and age/weight/sex-matched healthy volunteers, 120 mcg of alprostadil was administered by IV infusion over 2 hours. The mean C_{max} value of PGE_1 in renally impaired patients was 37% lower as compared to that in healthy volunteers, whereas mean C_{max} values of 15-keto-PGE_0 and PGE_0 in these patients increased 104% and 145% respectively as compared to those in healthy volunteers. The terminal half-lives of PGE_1, PGE_0, and 15-keto-PGE_0 and plasma albumin levels were similar in these patients vs healthy volunteers. The mechanism responsible for the observed discrepancies between renally impaired subjects and healthy volunteers is not known.

Hepatic function impairment: In a study in symptomatic subjects with impaired hepatic function and age/weight/sex-matched healthy volunteers, 120 mcg of alprostadil was administered by IV infusion over 2 hours. The mean C_{max} value of PGE_1 in hepatically impaired patients was 96% higher than in healthy volunteers. Mean C_{max} values of both 15-keto-PGE_0 and PGE_0 increased 65% as compared to those in healthy volunteers. Due to the fact that PGE_1 is primarily metabolized in the lung, the observed differences between hepatically impaired subjects and healthy volunteers were not anticipated; the mechanism responsible for the observed discrepancies is not known.

Pulmonary disease: The pulmonary extraction of alprostadil following intravascular administration was reduced by 15% (66 ± 3.2% vs 78 ± 2.4%) in patients with ARDS compared with a control group of patients with normal respiratory function who were undergoing cardiopulmonary bypass surgery. Pulmonary clearance was found to vary as a function of cardiac output and pulmonary intrinsic clearance in a group of 14 patients with ARDS or at risk of developing ARDS following trauma or sepsis. In this study, the extraction efficiency of alprostadil ranged from subnormal (11%) to normal (90%), with an overall mean of 67%.

Contraindications

Hypersensitivities to the drug or other prostaglandins; patients who have conditions that might predispose them to priapism, such as sickle cell anemia or trait, multiple myeloma, or leukemia; patients with anatomical deformations of the penis, such as angulation, cavernosal fibrosis, or Peyronie's disease; patients with penile implants; men for whom sexual activity is inadvisable or contraindicated.

Alprostadil is intended for use in adult men only. Alprostadil is not indicated for use in women, children, or newborns.

Warnings/Precautions

➤*Priapism and prolonged erection:* Prolonged erection, defined as erection lasting greater than 4 to less than or equal to 6 hours in duration, occurred in 4% of 1,861 patients treated up to 18 months in studies of alprostadil sterile powder. The incidence of priapism (erections lasting greater than 6 hours in duration) was 0.4% with the same length of use. Pharmacologic intervention or aspiration of blood from the corpora cavernosum was performed in 2 of the 7 patients with priapism. To minimize the chances of prolonged erection or priapism, titrate alprostadil injection slowly to the lowest effective dose. Instruct the patient to immediately report to his prescribing physician, or, if unavailable, to seek immediate medical assistance for any erection that persists longer than 4 hours. If priapism is not treated immediately, penile tissue damage and permanent loss of potency may result. Treat priapism according to established medical practice.

Edex – Prolonged erections greater than 4 hours in duration occurred in 4% of all patients treated up to 24 months. The incidence of priapism (erections greater than 6 hours in duration) was less than 1% with long-term use for up to 24 months. In the majority of cases, spontaneous detumescence occurred. Pharmacologic intervention or aspiration of blood from the corpora was necessary in 1.6% of 311 patients with prolonged erections/priapism.

➤*Penile fibrosis:* The overall incidence of penile fibrosis, including Peyronie's disease, reported in clinical studies with alprostadil was 3%. In 1 self-injection clinical study where duration of use was up to 18 months, the incidence of fibrosis was 7.8%.

➤*Hypotension:* Intracavernosal injections of alprostadil can lead to increased peripheral blood levels of PGE_1 and its metabolites, especially in those patients with significant corpora cavernosa venous leakage. Increased peripheral blood levels of PGE_1 and its metabolites may lead to hypotension or dizziness.

➤*Anticoagulants:* See Drug Interactions for more information.

➤*Other medical causes:* Diagnose and treat underlying treatable medical causes of erectile dysfunction prior to initiation of therapy with alprostadil.

➤*Vasoactive agents:* The safety and efficacy of combinations of alprostadil and other vasoactive agents have not been systematically studied. Therefore, the use of such combinations is not recommended.

➤*Bleeding disorder:* After injection of the alprostadil solution, compression of the injection site for 5 minutes, or until bleeding stops, is necessary. Patients on anticoagulants, such as warfarin or heparin, may have increased propensity for bleeding after intracavernosal injection.

➤*Caverject dual-chamber system:* Alprostadil dual-chamber system is designed for one use only. Following a single use, properly discard the injection device and any remaining solution.

Alprostadil dual-chamber system uses a superfine (29-gauge) needle. As with all superfine needles, the possibility of needle breakage exists. Careful instruction in proper handling and injection techniques may minimize the potential for needle breakage.

➤*Pregnancy: Category C* (urogenital suppository). Alprostadil is not indicated for use in women. Alprostadil has been shown to be embryotoxic (decreased fetal weight). When administered as a subcutaneous bolus to pregnant rats at doses as low as 500 mcg/kg/day. Doses of 2,000 mcg/kg/day resulted in increased resorptions, reduced numbers of live fetuses, increased incidences of visceral and skeletal variations (primarily left umbilical artery and generalized reduction in ossification of the entire skeleton) and gross visceral and skeletal malformations (primarily edema, hydrocephaly, anophthalmia/microphthalmia, and skeletal anomalies). The latter dose produced maternal toxicity (ataxia, lethargy, diarrhea, and retarded body weight gain). When administered by continuous intravenous infusion, evidence of embryotoxicity (decreased fetal weight gain and increased incidence of hydroureter) was observed at 2,000 mcg/kg/day, a dose that was also associated with a decrease in maternal weight gain. Intravaginal administration of up to 4,000 mcg/day of alprostadil to pregnant rabbits (1,100 mcg/kg/day or about 12.5 times the maximum recommended daily dose adjusted for body surface area) resulted in no evidence of harm to the fetus.

➤*Lactation:* Alprostadil is not indicated for use in women.

➤*Children:* Alprostadil is not indicated for use in pediatric patients.

ALPROSTADIL — INTRACAVERNOSAL

➤*Elderly:* Of the approximately 1,065 patients who entered the in-office dose-titration period in clinical studies, 25% were 65 and older. In clinical studies, geriatric patients required, on average, higher minimally effective doses and had higher rates of lack of effect (optimum dose not determined). Overall differences in safety were not observed between these geriatric patients and younger patients. Dose and titrate geriatric patients according to the same recommendations as younger patients, and always use the lowest possible effective dose.

This drug is known to be substantially excreted by the kidney, and the risk of toxic reactions to this drug may be greater in patients with impaired renal function. Because elderly patients are more likely to have decreased renal function, take care in dose selection, and it may be useful to monitor renal function.

➤*Monitoring:* Regular follow-up of patients, with careful examination of the penis at the start of therapy and at regular intervals (eg, 3 months), is strongly recommended to detect signs of penile fibrosis. Discontinue treatment with alprostadil in patients who develop penile angulation, cavernosal fibrosis, or Peyronie's disease. Treatment can be resumed if the penile abnormality subsides.

Drug Interactions

Alprostadil Drug Interactions

Precipitant drug	Object drug[a]		Description
Alprostadil	Anticoagulants	↑	Patients on anticoagulants (eg, warfarin, heparin) may have increased propensity for bleeding after intracavernosal injection. Coadministration with heparin resulted in a 140% and 120% increase in PTT and TT, respectively. Use caution with coadministration.
Alprostadil	Vasoactive agents	↔	The safety and efficacy of combinations of alprostadil and other vasoactive agents have not been systematically studied. Therefore, the use of such combinations is not recommended.

[a] ↑ = object drug increased; ↔ = undetermined clinical effect.

Adverse Reactions

➤*Local adverse reactions:* The following local adverse reaction information was derived from controlled and uncontrolled studies, including an uncontrolled 18-month safety study.

Local Adverse Reactions Reported by ≥ 1% of Patients Treated with Alprostadil Injection for up to 18 Months[a]

Event	Alprostadil injection (n = 1,861)
Injection site ecchymosis	2%
Injection site hematoma	3%
Penis disorder[b]	3%
Penile edema	1%
Penile fibrosis[c]	3%
Penile pain	37%
Penile rash	1%
Prolonged erection	4%

[a] Except for penile pain (2%), no significant local adverse reactions were reported by 294 patients who received 1 to 3 injections of placebo.
[b] Includes numbness, yeast infection, irritation, sensitivity, phimosis, pruritus, erythema, venous leak, penile skin tear, strange feeling of penis, discoloration of penile head, itch at tip of penis.
[c] The overall incidence of penile fibrosis, including Peyronie's disease, reported in clinical studies with alprostadil was 3%. In 1 self-injection clinical study where duration of use was up to 18 months, the incidence of fibrosis was 7.8%. Regular follow-up of patients, with careful examination of the penis, is strongly recommended to detect signs of penile fibrosis. Treatment with alprostadil should be discontinued in patients who develop penile angulation, cavernosal fibrosis, or Peyronie's disease.

➤*Penile pain:* Penile pain after intracavernosal administration of alprostadil was reported at least once by 37% of patients in clinical studies of up to 18 months in duration. In the majority of the cases, penile pain was rated mild or moderate in intensity. Three percent (3%) of patients discontinued treatment because of penile pain. The frequency of penile pain was 2% in 294 patients who received 1 to 3 injections of placebo.

➤*Prolonged erection/priapism:* In clinical trials, prolonged erection was defined as an erection that lasted for 4 to 6 hours; priapism was defined as erection that lasted 6 hours or longer. The frequency of prolonged erection after intracavernosal administration of alprostadil was 4%, while the frequency of priapism was 0.4%. In the majority of cases, spontaneous detumescence occurred.

See Warnings/Precautions for more information.

➤*Hematoma/ecchymosis:* The frequency of hematoma and ecchymosis was 3% and 2%, respectively. In most cases, hematoma/ecchymosis was judged to be a complication of a faulty injection technique. Accordingly, proper instruction of the patient in self-injection is of importance to minimize the potential of hematoma/ecchymosis.

The following local adverse reactions were reported by less than 1% of patients after injection of alprostadil: Balanitis; injection site hemorrhage; injection site inflammation; injection site itching; injection site swelling; injection site edema; urethral bleeding; penile warmth; numbness; yeast infection; irritation; sensitivity; phimosis; pruritus; erythema; venous leak; painful erection; and abnormal ejaculation.

➤*Systemic adverse events:* The following systemic adverse event information was derived from controlled and uncontrolled studies, including an uncontrolled 18-month safety study.

Alprostadil Adverse Reactions (≥ 1%)[a]

Adverse reaction	Alprostadil (n = 1,861)
Cardiovascular	
Hypertension	2%
CNS	
Dizziness	1%
Headache	2%
GU	
Prostatic disorder[b]	2%
Musculoskeletal	
Back pain	1%
Respiratory	
Cough	1%
Flu syndrome	2%
Nasal congestion	1%
Sinusitis	2%
Upper respiratory tract infection	4%
Miscellaneous	
Localized pain[c]	2%
Trauma[d]	2%

[a] No significant adverse events were reported by 294 patients who received 1 to 3 injections of placebo.
[b] Prostatitis, pain, hypertrophy, enlargement.
[c] Pain in various anatomical structures other than injection site.
[d] Injuries, fractures, abrasions, lacerations, dislocations.

The following systemic events, which were reported for less than 1% of patients in clinical studies, were judged by investigators to be possibly related to use of alprostadil: Testicular pain, scrotal disorder, scrotal edema, hematuria, testicular disorder, impaired urination, urinary frequency, urinary urgency, pelvic pain, hypotension, vasodilation, peripheral vascular disorder, supraventricular extrasystoles, vasovagal reactions, hypesthesia, nongeneralized weakness, diaphoresis, rash, nonapplication site pruritus, skin neoplasm, nausea, dry mouth, increased serum creatinine, leg cramps, and mydriasis.

Hemodynamic changes, manifested as decreases in blood pressure and increases in pulse rate, were observed during clinical studies, principally at doses above 20 mcg and above 30 mcg of alprostadil, respectively, and appeared to be dose-dependent. However, these changes were usually clinically unimportant; only 3 patients discontinued the treatment because of symptomatic hypotension.

➤*Needle breakage:* During postmarketing surveillance, needle breakage requiring surgical extraction has been reported with the administration of alprostadil sterile powder. Careful instruction in proper patient handling and injection techniques may minimize the potential of needle breakage.

➤*Caverject dual-chamber system vs sterile powder:* The safety of alprostadil dual-chamber system was evaluated in a study that compared the formulation of alprostadil for injection contained in the alprostadil dual-chamber system with the formulation contained in alprostadil sterile powder. The doses used by the 87 patients in this crossover study were the same for both formulations. The number and type of events reported for alprostadil dual-chamber system were consistent between formulations in this study and in other controlled and uncontrolled studies with alprostadil sterile powder.

➤*Edex dual-chamber cartridge: Edex*, administered by intracavernosal injection in doses ranging from 1 to 40 mcg per injection for periods up to 24 months, has been evaluated in clinical trials for safety in over 1,065 patients with erectile dysfunction. Discontinuation of therapy due to a side effect in clinical trials was required in approximately 9% of patients treated with *Edex*, and less than 1% of patients treated with placebo.

Local – The following local adverse reactions were reported in studies including 1,065 patients treated with *Edex* for up to 2 years.

Penile pain: With use of up to 24 months, penile pain was reported at least once by 29% of patients during injection, 35% of patients during erection, and 30% of patients after erection. On a per injection basis, 15% of injections were associated with penile pain. Penile pain was judged by patients to be mild in intensity for 80% of painful injections, moderate in intensity for 16% of painful injections, and severe in intensity for 4% of painful injections. The frequency of penile pain reports decreased over time; 41% of the patients experienced pain during the first 2 months and 3% of the patients experienced pain during months 21 to 24. In placebo-controlled studies, penile pain was reported by 31% of patients after *Edex* and by 9% of patients after placebo injection.

Prolonged erection/priapism: Prolonged erections greater than 4 hours in duration occurred in 4% of all patients treated up to 24 months. In placebo-controlled studies, 3% of patients treated with *Edex* and less than 1% of patients treated with placebo reported prolonged erections greater than 4 hours. The incidence of priapism (erections greater than 6 hours in duration) was less than 1% with long-term use for up to 24 months. In the majority of cases, spontaneous detumescence occurred. A higher incidence of

ALPROSTADIL — INTRACAVERNOSAL

prolonged erections was found in younger patients (less than 40 years), nondiabetic patients, and patients treated with psychogenic etiology of erectile dysfunction.

Hematoma/ecchymosis: In patients treated with *Edex* for up to 24 months, local bleeding, hematoma, and ecchymosis were observed in 15%, 5%, and 4% of patients, respectively. In placebo-controlled studies, the frequency of local bleeding was 6% with injection of *Edex* and 3% with injection of placebo. In most cases, these reactions were attributed to faulty injection technique.

Alprostadil Local Adverse Reactions (≥ 1%)[a]

Local reaction	*Edex* (n = 1,065) n (%)
Penile pain after erection	317 (30%)
Penile pain during injection	305 (29%)
Penile pain during erection	368 (35%)
Penile pain (other)[b]	116 (11%)
Prolonged erection	
> 4 to ≤ 6 hours	44 (4%)
> 6 hours	6 (< 1%)
Bleeding	158 (15%)
Cavernous body fibrosis	20 (2%)
Ecchymosis	44 (4%)
Erythema	17 (2%)
Faulty injection technique[c]	59 (6%)
Hematoma	56 (5%)
Penile angulation	72 (7%)
Penis disorder	28 (3%)
Penile fibrosis	52 (5%)
Peyronie's disease	11 (1%)

[a] Protocol numbers KU-620-001, KU-620-002, KU-620-003, F-8653.
[b] Penile pain reported without an association to injection site or erection, such as pain in penis and scrotum, pain in glans penis, and burning penile pain.
[c] Examples include injection into glans penis, urethra, or subcutaneously.

Hemodynamic changes – Hemodynamic changes, manifested as increases or decreases in blood pressure and pulse rate, were observed during clinical studies but did not appear to be dose dependent. Four patients (less than 1%) reported clinical symptoms of hypotension such as dizziness or syncope.

***Edex* Adverse Reactions (≥ 1%)**

Adverse reaction	*Edex* (n = 1,065)
Cardiovascular	
Abnormal ECG	12 (1%)
Hypertension	17 (2%)
Myocardial infarction	13 (1%)
Dermatologic	
Skin disorder	14 (1%)
GU	
Inguinal hernia	11 (1%)
Prostate disorder	15 (1%)
Testicular pain	13 (1%)
Metabolic/nutritional	
Hypercholesterolemia	12 (1%)
Hyperglycemia	12 (1%)
Hypertriglyceridemia	17 (2%)
Musculoskeletal	
Back pain	23 (2%)
Leg pain	13 (1%)
Respiratory	
Sinusitis	14 (1%)
Upper respiratory tract infection	58 (5%)
Special senses	
Abnormal vision	11 (1%)
Miscellaneous	
Headache	20 (2%)
Infection	18 (2%)
Influenza-like symptoms	35 (3%)
Pain	16 (2%)

Overdosage

➤*Edex:* Limited data are available in regard to *Edex* overdose in humans. Systemic reactions are uncommon with intracavernosal injection of *Edex*. Hypotension occurred in less than 1% of patients treated with *Edex*.

A single dose rising tolerance study in healthy volunteers indicated that single IV doses of alprostadil from 1 to 120 mcg were well tolerated. Beginning with a 40 mcg bolus IV dose, the frequency of drug-related systemic adverse events increased in a dose-dependent manner, characterized mainly by facial flushing.

➤*Symptoms:* The primary symptom of an overdose is a prolonged erection or priapism.

➤*Treatment:* Because of the potential for tissue hypoxia and possible necrosis, it is strongly recommended to treat an erection lasting more than 6 hours. The patient is strongly encouraged to go to the nearest emergency room if his personal physician is not available.

Overdosage was not observed in clinical trials with alprostadil. If intracavernous overdose of alprostadil occurs, the patient should be under medical supervision until any systemic effects have resolved or until penile detumescence has occurred. Symptomatic treatment of any systemic symptoms would be appropriate.

Patient Information

To ensure safe and effective use of alprostadil, thoroughly instruct and train the patient in the self-injection technique before he begins intracavernosal treatment with alprostadil at home. Establish the desirable dose in the physician's office.

Instruct the patient not to reuse or to share needles, syringes, or cartridges. As with all prescription medicines, the patient should not allow anyone else to use his medicine.

The dose of alprostadil that is established in the physician's office should not be changed by the patient without consulting the physician. The patient may expect an erection to occur within 5 to 20 minutes. A standard treatment goal is to produce an erection lasting no longer than 1 hour. Generally, do not use alprostadil more than 3 times per week, with at least 24 hours between each use.

Patients should be aware of possible side effects of therapy with alprostadil; the most frequently occurring is penile pain after injection, usually mild to moderate in severity. A potentially serious adverse reaction with intracavernosal therapy is priapism. Accordingly, instruct the patient to contact the physician's office immediately or, if unavailable, to seek immediate medical assistance if an erection persists for longer than 4 hours.

The patient should report any penile pain that was not present before or that increased in intensity, as well as the occurrence of nodules or hard tissue in the penis to his physician as soon as possible. As with any intravenous injection, an infection is a possibility. Instruct patients to report to the physician any penile redness, swelling, tenderness, or curvature of the erect penis. The patient must visit the physician's office for regular checkups for assessment of the therapeutic benefit and safety of treatment with alprostadil.

Individuals who are sexually active should be counseled about the protective measures that are necessary to guard against the spread of sexually transmitted diseases, including the human immunodeficiency virus (HIV). Use of intracavernosal alprostadil offers no protection from the transmission of sexually transmitted or bloodborne diseases. The injection of alprostadil can induce a small amount of bleeding at the site of injection. In patients infected with bloodborne diseases, this could increase the risk of transmission of bloodborne diseases between partners.

➤*Aqueous solution:* Instruct the patient to transfer the solution from the pharmacy to his home freezer or refrigerator as soon as possible. Brief (2 hours or less) exposure to conditions as warm as 25°C (77°F) will not harm the product.

Discard any ampule containing sterile solution with precipitates or discoloration. The ampule is designed for 1 use only and should be discarded after withdrawal of proper volume of the solution. Properly discard needles after use; do not reuse or share with other persons. Patient instructions for administration are included in each package of alprostadil.

➤*Caverject sterile powder:* Carefully follow the instructions for preparation of the solution of alprostadil sterile powder for intracavernosal injection. Discard vials with precipitates or discoloration. The reconstituted vial is designed for 1 use only and should be discarded after withdrawal of proper volume of the solution. Do not shake the content of the reconstituted vial. Properly discard the needle after use; do not reuse or share with other persons. Patient instructions for administration are included in each package of alprostadil sterile powder.

➤*Caverject dual-chamber system:* Discard any reconstituted solution with precipitates or discoloration. The alprostadil dual-chamber syringe system is designed for 1 use only and should be discarded after use. Properly discard the device and the needle after use.

➤*Edex dual-chamber cartridge:* Carefully follow the instructions for the preparation of the *Edex* solution. The reconstituted solution may initially appear cloudy due to small air bubbles. Do not use the solution if it remains cloudy, contains precipitates, or is discolored. Gently mix the reconstituted solution. Do not shake it. A patient information pamphlet is included in each package of *Edex* kits and cartridges.

Use *Edex* immediately after reconstitution. The patient should follow the instructions in the patient information pamphlet to limit the possibility of bacterial contamination. The reconstituted cartridge is designed for 1 use only and should be discarded after use.

The *Edex* cartridge contains a solid layer or lyophilized of dry white powder approximately 3/16" in thickness for the vial and 3/8" in thickness for the cartridge. A normal cake may appear cracked or crumbled. If the vial or cartridge is damaged, the cake may shrink in size. Do not use the vial or cartridge if they appear damaged or if the cake is substantially reduced in size.

If the dosage prescribed is less than 1 mL of *Edex* solution, excess solution will be expelled through the needle as the plunger is pushed and the upper rim of the top stopper reaches the correct volume mark for the prescribed dose. Properly discard the needle after use; do not reuse or share with other persons.

The dose of *Edex* that is established in the physician's office should not be changed by the patient without consulting the physician. The patient may expect an erection to occur within 5 to 20 minutes. A standard treatment

ALPROSTADIL — INTRACAVERNOSAL

goal is to produce an erection lasting no longer than 1 hour. Do not use *Edex* more than 3 times per week, with at least 24 hours between each use.

➤*Note:* Use of intracavernosal alprostadil offers no protection from the transmission of sexually transmitted diseases. Counsel individuals who use alprostadil about the protective measures that are necessary to guard against the spread of sexually transmitted diseases, including the human immunodeficiency virus (HIV).

The injection of alprostadil can induce a small amount of bleeding at the site of injection. In patients infected with bloodborne diseases, this could increase the risk of transmission of bloodborne diseases between partners.

ALPROSTADIL — UROGENITAL

For information on the use of alprostadil for patent ductus arteriosus, refer to the specific monograph in the Cardiovasculars chapter.

Indications

➤*Erectile dysfunction:* For the treatment of erectile dysfunction. Studies that established benefit demonstrated improvements in success rates for sexual intercourse compared with similarly administered placebo.

Administration and Dosage

➤*General dosing considerations:* The onset of effect is within 5 to 10 minutes after administration. The duration of effect is approximately 30 to 60 minutes. However, the actual duration will vary from patient to patient.

➤*Adults:*

Erectile dysfunction –

Maximum dose: 2 systems per 24-hour period.

Initial dosage: Lower doses (125 or 250 mcg) are recommended.

Dosage adjustment: If necessary, the dose should be increased (or decreased) on separate occasions in a step-wise manner until the patient achieves an erection that is sufficient for sexual intercourse.

Dose titration should be undertaken under the supervision of a health care provider to test a patient's responsiveness to alprostadil, to demonstrate proper administration technique (see detailed instructions for alprostadil administration in patient package insert), and to monitor for evidence of hypotension.

➤*Administration:* Alprostadil should be administered as needed to achieve an erection. Each patient should be instructed by a medical professional on proper technique for administering alprostadil prior to self-administration.

➤*Storage / Stability:* Store unopened foil pouches in a refrigerator at 2° to 8°C (36° to 46°F). Do not expose to temperatures above 30°C (86°F). May be kept at room temperature (below 30°C or 86°F) for up to 14 days prior to use. Each alprostadil urethral suppository is for single use only and should be properly discarded after use.

Actions

➤*Pharmacology:* Prostaglandin E1 is a naturally occurring acidic lipid that is synthesized from fatty acid precursors by most mammalian tissues and has a variety of pharmacologic effects. Human seminal fluid is a rich source of prostaglandins, including PGE_1 and PGE_2, and the total concentration of prostaglandins in ejaculate has been estimated to be approximately 100 to 200 mcg/mL. In vitro, alprostadil (PGE_1) has been shown to cause dose-dependent smooth muscle relaxation in isolated corpus cavernosum and corpus spongiosum preparations. Additionally, vasodilation has been demonstrated in isolated cavernosal artery segments that were precontracted with either norepinephrine or prostaglandin $F_2\alpha$. When alprostadil was injected into the corpus cavernosum of pigtail monkeys in vivo, dose-dependent increases in cavernosal artery blood flow were observed.

In human studies using Doppler duplex ultrasonography, intraurethral administration of 500 mcg of alprostadil resulted in an increase in cavernosal artery diameter and a 5- to 10-fold increase in peak systolic flow velocities. These results suggest that intraurethral alprostadil is absorbed from the urethra, transported throughout the erectile bodies by communicating vessels between the corpus spongiosum and corpora cavernosa, and able to induce vasodilation of the targeted vascular beds.

The vasodilatory effects of alprostadil on the cavernosal arteries and the trabecular smooth muscle of the corpora cavernosa result in rapid arterial inflow and expansion of the lacunar spaces within the corpora. As the expanded corporal sinusoids are compressed against the tunica albuginea, venous outflow through subtunical vessels is impeded and penile rigidity develops. This process is referred to as the corporal veno-occlusive mechanism.

The most notable systemic effects of alprostadil are vasodilation, inhibition of platelet aggregation, and stimulation of intestinal and uterine smooth muscle. Intravenous doses of 1 to 10 mcg/kg of body weight lower blood pressure in mammals by decreasing peripheral resistance. Reflex increases in cardiac output and heart rate may accompany these effects.

➤*Pharmacokinetics:*

Absorption – About 80% of alprostadil administered by alprostadil urethral suppository is absorbed within 10 minutes and is rapidly cleared from the systemic circulation by the lungs, leaving barely detectable systemic blood levels.

Alprostadil urethral suppository is designed to deliver alprostadil directly to the urethral lining for transfer via the corpus spongiosum to the corpora cavernosa. Intraurethral administration of alprostadil urethral suppository is preceded by urination, and the residual urine disperses the medicated pellet, permitting alprostadil to be absorbed by the urethral mucosa. The transurethral absorption of alprostadil after alprostadil urethral suppository administration is biphasic. Initial absorption is rapid, with approximately 80% of an administered dose absorbed within 10 minutes. The mean time to the maximum plasma PGE_1 concentration after a 1000 mcg intraurethral dose of alprostadil urethral suppository is approximately 16 minutes.

In 10 healthy human volunteers, endogenous PGE_1 levels in the ejaculate averaged 31 mcg (range 0 to 161 mcg). In these same volunteers, an average of 123 mcg of additional PGE_1 (range 30 to 369 mcg) was present in the ejaculate obtained 10 minutes after the highest dose (1000 mcg) of alprostadil urethral suppository. The mean total endogenous PGE content (PGE_1, PGE_2, 19-OH-PGE_1, and 19-OH-PGE_2) of the ejaculate in these subjects was 444 mcg (range 0 to 1423 mcg).

Distribution – Following alprostadil urethral suppository administration, alprostadil is absorbed from the urethral mucosa into the corpus spongiosum. A portion of the administered dose is transported to the corpora cavernosa through collateral vessels, while the remainder passes into the pelvic venous circulation through veins draining the corpus spongiosum. The half-life of alprostadil in humans is short, varying between 30 seconds and 10 minutes, depending on the body compartment in which it is measured and the physiological status of the subject. Nearly all of the alprostadil entering the central venous circulation is removed in a single pass through the lungs; thus peripheral venous plasma levels of PGE_1 are low or undetectable (less than 2 pg/mL) after alprostadil urethral suppository administration. The mean maximum plasma PGE_1 concentration following intraurethral administration of the highest dose of alprostadil urethral suppository (1000 mcg) was barely detectable (11.4 pg/mL). In a study of 14 subjects, the plasma PGE_1 level was shown to be undetachable within 60 minutes of alprostadil urethral suppository administration in most subjects.

Metabolism – Alprostadil is rapidly metabolized locally by enzymatic oxidation of the 15-hydroxyl group to 15-keto-PGE_1. The enzyme catalyzing this process has been isolated from many tissues in the lower genito-urinary tract including the urethra, prostate, and corpus cavernosum. 15-keto-PGE_1 retains little (1% to 2%) of the biological activity of PGE_1. 15-keto-PGE_1 is rapidly reduced at the C_{13}-C_{14} position to form the most abundant metabolite in plasma, 13,14-dihydro,15-keto PGE_1 (DHK-PGE_1), which is biologically inactive. The majority of DHK-PGE_1 is further metabolized to smaller prostaglandin remnants that are cleared primarily by the kidney and liver. Between 60% and 90% of PGE_1 has been shown to be metabolized after 1 pass through the pulmonary capillary beds.

Excretion – After intravenous administration of tritium-labeled alprostadil in man, labeled drug disappears rapidly from the blood in the first 10 minutes, and by 1 hour radioactivity in the blood reaches a low level. The metabolites of alprostadil are excreted primarily by the kidney, with approximately 90% of an administered intravenous dose excreted in the urine within 24 hours of dosing. The remainder is excreted in the feces. There is no evidence of tissue retention of alprostadil or its metabolites following intravenous administration.

Special populations –

Pulmonary disease: The near-complete pulmonary first-pass metabolism of PGE_1 is the primary factor influencing the systemic pharmacokinetics of alprostadil urethral suppository and is a reason that peripheral venous plasma levels of PGE_1 are low or undetectable (less than 2 pg/mL) following alprostadil urethral suppository administration.

Patients with pulmonary disease therefore may have a reduced capacity to clear the drug. In patients with the adult respiratory distress syndrome (ARDS), pulmonary extraction of intravascularly administered alprostadil was reduced by approximately 15% compared to a control group of patients with normal respiratory function (66 ± 3.2% vs 78 ± 2.4%).

Contraindications

Hypersensitivity to alprostadil; in patients with urethral stricture, balanitis (inflammation/infection of the glans of the penis), severe hypospadias and curvature, and in patients with acute or chronic urethritis; in patients who are prone to venous thrombosis or who have a hyperviscosity syndrome and are therefore at increased risk of priapism (rigid erection lasting 6 or more hours). Alprostadil urethral suppository should not be used in men for whom sexual activity is inadvisable (see General Precautions) or for sexual intercourse with a pregnant woman unless the couple uses a condom barrier.

Warnings/Precautions

➤*Hypotension / Syncope:* Because of the potential for symptomatic hypotension and syncope, which occurred in 3% and 0.4%, respectively, of patients during in-clinic dosing, alprostadil urethral suppository titration should be carried out under medical supervision. During post-marketing surveillance syncope occurring within one hour of administration has been reported. Patients should be cautioned to avoid activities, such as driving or hazardous tasks, where injury could result if hypotension or syncope were to occur after alprostadil urethral suppository administration.

➤*Medical history / physical exam:* A complete medical history and physical examination should be undertaken to exclude reversible causes of erectile dysfunction prior to the initiation of alprostadil urethral suppository therapy. In addition, underlying disorders that might preclude the use of alprostadil urethral suppository (see Contraindications) should be sought.

➤*Cardiovascular effects:* During in-clinic dosing, patients should be monitored for symptoms of hypotension, and the lowest effective dose of alprostadil urethral suppository should be prescribed.

➤*Hematologic effects:* Patients administering alprostadil urethral suppository improperly may be at risk of urethral abrasion resulting in minor bleeding or spotting. Patients on anticoagulant therapy or with bleeding dis-

ALPROSTADIL — UROGENITAL

orders may be at higher risk of bleeding. Patients on anticoagulant therapy have been safely treated with alprostadil urethral suppository; however, the risk/benefit ratio in these patients should be considered prior to prescribing alprostadil urethral suppository.

➤*Resumption of sexual activity:* Sexual intercourse is considered a vigorous physical activity, and it increases heart rate as well as cardiac work. Physicians may want to examine the cardiac fitness of patients prior to treating erectile dysfunction.

➤*Priapism and prolonged erection:* In clinical trials of alprostadil urethral suppository, priapism (rigid erection lasting more than 6 hours) and prolonged erection (rigid erection between 4 and 6 hours) were reported infrequently (less than 0.1% and 0.3% of patients, respectively). Nevertheless, these events are a potential risk of pharmacologic therapy and can cause penile injury. Physicians should lower the dose or consider discontinuing alprostadil urethral suppository treatment in any patient who develops priapism or prolonged erection.

➤*Pregnancy: Category C.* Alprostadil has been shown to be embryo toxic (decreased fetal weight) when administered as a subcutaneous bolus to pregnant rats at doses as low as 500 mcg/kg/day. Doses of 2000 mcg/kg/day resulted in increased resorptions, reduced numbers of live fetuses, increased incidences of visceral and skeletal variations (primarily left umbilical artery and generalized reduction in ossification of the entire skeleton) and gross visceral and skeletal malformations (primarily edema, hydrocephaly, anophthalmia/microphthalmia, and skeletal anomalies). The latter dose produced maternal toxicity (ataxia, lethargy, diarrhea, and retarded body weight gain). When administered by continuous intravenous infusion, evidence of embryotoxicity (decreased fetal weight gain and increased incidence of hydroureter) was observed at 2000 mcg/kg/day, a dose that was also associated with a decrease in maternal weight gain. Intravaginal administration of up to 4000 mcg/day of alprostadil to pregnant rabbits (1100 mcg/kg/day or about 12.5 times the maximum recommended daily dose adjusted for body surface area) resulted in no evidence of harm to the fetus.

➤*Children:* Not indicated for use in newborns or children.

Drug Interactions

Because there are low or undetectable (less than 2 pg/mL) amounts of alprostadil found in the peripheral venous circulation following alprostadil urethral suppository administration, systemic drug-drug interactions with alprostadil urethral suppository are unlikely. The presence of medications in the circulation that attenuate erectile function, however, may influence the response to alprostadil urethral suppository.

Adverse Reactions

➤*In-clinic titration:* In the 2 largest double-blind, parallel, placebo-controlled trials, 1511 patients received alprostadil urethral suppository at least 1 time in the clinic setting. The most frequently reported drug-related side effects during in-clinic titration included pain in the penis (36%), urethra (13%), or testes (5%). These discomforts were most commonly reported as mild and transient, but about 7% of patients withdrew at this stage because of adverse events. Urethral bleeding/spotting and other minor abrasions to the urethra were reported in approximately 3% of patients. Symptomatic lowering of blood pressure (hypotension) occurred in 3% of patients. Dizziness was reported in 4% of patients. Syncope (fainting) was reported by 0.4% of patients.

➤*Home treatment:* Nine hundred ninety-six patients (66% of those who began titration) were studied during the home treatment portion of 2 phase III placebo-controlled studies. Fewer than 2% of patients discontinued from these studies primarily because of adverse events. The following information summarizes the frequency of adverse events reported by patients using alprostadil urethral suppository or placebo.

Alprostadil Urogenital Adverse Reactions (≥ 2%)

Adverse reaction	Alprostadil urethral suppository (n = 486)	Placebo (n = 511)
GU		
Penile pain	32%	3%
Urethral burning	12%	4%
Minor urethral bleeding/spotting	5%	1%
Testicular pain	5%	1%
CNS		
Dizziness	2%	< 1%
Miscellaneous		
Flu symptoms	4%	2%
Headache	3%	2%
Pain	3%	1%
Accidental injury	3%	2%
Back pain	2%	1%
Pelvic pain	2%	< 1%
Respiratory		
Rhinitis	2%	< 1%
Infection	3%	2%

➤*Female partner adverse events:* The most common drug-related adverse event reported by female partners during placebo-controlled clinical studies was vaginal burning/itching, reported by 5.8% of partners of patients on active vs 0.8% of partners of patients on placebo. It is unknown whether this adverse event experienced by female partners was a result of the medication or a result of resuming sexual intercourse, which occurred much more frequently in partners of patients on active medication.

Overdosage

Overdosage has not been reported with alprostadil urethral suppository. Overdosage with alprostadil urethral suppository may result in hypotension, persistent penile pain, and possibly priapism (rigid erection lasting greater than or equal to 6 hours). Priapism can result in permanent worsening of erectile function. Patients suspected of overdosage who develop these symptoms should be kept under medical supervision until systemic or local symptoms have resolved.

Patient Information

Patients should be informed that alprostadil urethral suppository offers no protection from the transmission of sexually transmitted diseases. Patients and partners who use alprostadil urethral suppository need to be counseled about the protective measures that are necessary to guard against the spread of sexually transmitted agents, including the human immunodeficiency virus (HIV).

Although unreported in clinical trials, there is the possibility that an overdosage of alprostadil urethral suppository can cause priapism, a painful erection of the penis sustained for hours and unrelieved by sexual intercourse or masturbation. This condition is serious and, if untreated, it can lead to permanent inability to have an erection. Patients who experience a prolonged erection should seek prompt medical attention.

Patients should be instructed how to administer alprostadil urethral suppository. A patient package insert must be given to each patient at the initiation of alprostadil urethral suppository therapy.

➤*Information for partners:* Partners of patients using alprostadil urethral suppository should be informed that alprostadil urethral suppository offers no protection from the transmission of sexually transmitted diseases. Patients and partners who use alprostadil urethral suppository should be counseled about the protective measures that are necessary to guard against the spread of sexually transmitted agents, including the human immunodeficiency virus (HIV). Human semen contains PGE_1, but additional amounts may be present from alprostadil urethral suppository administration (see Pharmacokinetics). Partners who have experienced an extended period of sexual abstinence should be encouraged to seek advice from a healthcare professional prior to resuming sexual intercourse. The use of a water-based lubricant may facilitate vaginal penetration.

It is recommended that couples using alprostadil urethral suppository employ adequate contraception if the female partner is of childbearing potential. There is no information on the effects on early pregnancy of PGE_1 at the levels received by female partners. Alprostadil urethral suppository has no contraceptive properties. Alprostadil urethral suppository should not be used if the female partner is pregnant, unless the couple uses a condom barrier.

YOHIMBINE HYDROCHLORIDE

Rx	**Yohimbine HCl** (Various, eg, Eon)	**Tablets:** 5.4 mg	May contain lactose. In 100s, 500s, and 1000s.
Rx	**Aphrodyne** (Star)		(APHRODYNE). Aqua, scored. In 100s and 1000s.
Rx	**Yocon** (Glenwood)		In 100s and 1000s.

YOHIMBINE HYDROCHLORIDE — ORAL

Indications

Yohimbine has no FDA sanctioned indications.

➤*Off-label uses:* Sympatholytic and mydriatic. It may have activity as an aphrodisiac.

Impotence – Impotence has been successfully treated with yohimbine in male patients with vascular or diabetic origins and psychogenic origins (18 mg/day).

Orthostatic hypotension – Orthostatic hypotension may be favorably affected by yohimbine.

Administration and Dosage

➤*Adults:*

Off-label dosing –

Male erectile impotence:

- *Usual dose* – 1 tablet (5.4 mg) 3 times per day.
- *Dosage adjustment* – If adverse effects occur, reduce to one-half tablet 3 times per day, followed by gradual increases to 1 tablet 3 times per day.

➤*Children:* Do not use in children.

➤*Elderly:* Not for use in elderly patients.

YOHIMBINE HYDROCHLORIDE — ORAL

➤*Renal function impairment:* Contraindicated in renal disease.

➤*Special risk patients:* Not for use in psychiatric or cardiorenal patients with a history of gastric or duodenal ulcer; generally, not for use in women.

➤*Storage/Stability:* Store at controlled room temperature 15° to 30°C (59° to 86°F).

Actions

➤*Pharmacology:* Yohimbine, an indolalkylamine alkaloid, has chemical similarity to reserpine. It is the principal alkaloid of the bark of the *Corynanthe yohimbi* tree and also is found in *Rauwolfia serpentina* (L) Benth.

Yohimbine blocks presynaptic α_2-adrenergic receptors. Its peripheral autonomic nervous system effect is to increase parasympathetic (cholinergic) and decrease sympathetic (adrenergic) activity. In male sexual performance, erection is linked to cholinergic activity and α_2-adrenergic blockade, which theoretically results in increased penile blood inflow, decreased outflow, or both. Yohimbine exerts a stimulating action on mood and may increase anxiety. Such actions appear to require high doses. Yohimbine has a mild antidiuretic action, probably via stimulation of hypothalmic centers and release of posterior pituitary hormone.

Its action on peripheral blood vessels resembles that of reserpine, though it is weaker and of shorter duration. The drug reportedly exerts no significant influence on cardiac stimulation.

➤*Pharmacokinetics:*

Absorption/Distribution – Oral absorption appears to be extremely rapid, with a mean T_{max} of less than 1 hour. The low bioavailability of approximately 30% is thought to be caused by first-pass metabolism rather than poor absorption. The mean distribution half-life is less than 30 minutes, and the mean apparent volume of distribution ranged from 24.6 to 226 L. Approximately 82% of yohimbine is bound to plasma proteins.

Metabolism/Excretion – Yohimbine undergoes extensive first-pass metabolism that results in poor but highly variable bioavailability. It also undergoes extensive biotransformation in the liver and extrahepatic sites, and at least 2 hydroxylated metabolites have been identified. After single-dose administration, the terminal half-life of yohimbine is 0.25 to 2.5 hours. The active metabolite (11-hydroxy-yohimbine) has a longer elimination half-life of 6 hours. Less than 1% of the yohimbine dose is recovered in the urine as unchanged drug.

Contraindications

Renal disease; hypersensitivity to any component.

Warnings/Precautions

➤*Special risk patients:* Not for use in geriatric, psychiatric, or cardiorenal patients with a history of gastric or duodenal ulcer. Generally, not for use in females.

➤*Pregnancy: Category: Undetermined.* This drug is not proposed for use in females. Do not use during pregnancy.

➤*Lactation:* This drug is not proposed for use in females.

➤*Children:* Do not use in children.

Drug Interactions

➤*Antidepressants:* Do not use with yohimbine.

Adverse Reactions

Yohimbine readily penetrates the CNS and produces a complex pattern of responses in lower doses than those required to produce peripheral α-adrenergic blockade. These include antidiuresis and central excitation including elevated blood pressure and heart rate, increased motor activity, nervousness, irritability, and tremor. Dizziness, nausea, headache, and skin flushing have been reported.

Overdosage

Yohimbine may be toxic if ingested in high doses. The drug causes severe hypotension, abdominal distress, and weakness. Larger doses may cause CNS stimulation and paralysis.

Phosphodiesterase Type 5 Inhibitors

Indications

➤*Erectile dysfunction (except Adcirca and Revatio):* For the treatment of erectile dysfunction.

➤*Pulmonary arterial hypertension (Revatio and Adcirca only):* For the treatment of pulmonary arterial hypertension (PAH) (World Health Organization [WHO] Group I) to improve exercise ability. Also indicated to delay clinical worsening (*Revatio* only).

➤*Off-label uses:* The use of **sildenafil** in women with sexual dysfunction has been evaluated in small clinical trials. The results are mixed, with many studies unable to demonstrate efficacy.

Actions

➤*Pharmacology:* **Sildenafil**, **tadalafil**, and **vardenafil** are selective inhibitors of phosphodiesterase type 5 (PDE5). The physiologic mechanism of penile erection involves release of nitric oxide (NO) in the corpus cavernosum during sexual stimulation. NO activates the enzyme guanylate cyclase, resulting in increased synthesis of cyclic guanosine monophosphate (cGMP) in the smooth muscle cells of the corpus cavernosum. The cGMP, in turn, triggers smooth muscle relaxation, allowing increased blood flow into the penis, resulting in erection. Sildenafil, tadalafil, and vardenafil enhance the effects of NO by inhibiting PDE5 that is responsible for the degradation of cGMP in the smooth muscle cells of the corpus cavernosum. Because sexual stimulation is required to initiate the local release of NO, the inhibition of PDE5 by sildenafil, tadalafil, or vardenafil has no effect in the absence of sexual stimulation.

PDE5 also is found in lower concentrations in other tissues, including platelets, vascular and visceral smooth muscle, and skeletal muscle. In these tissues, inhibition of PDE5 may be the basis for the enhanced platelet antiaggregatory activity of NO, inhibition of platelet thrombus formation, and peripheral arterial-venous dilation.

Sildenafil and tadalafil – Sildenafil and tadalafil are also inhibitors of cGMP PDE5 in the smooth muscle of the pulmonary vasculature, where PDE5 is responsible for degradation of cGMP. Sildenafil and tadalafil, therefore, increase cGMP within pulmonary vascular smooth muscle cells, resulting in relaxation. In patients with pulmonary hypertension, this can lead to vasodilation of the pulmonary vascular bed, and, to a lesser degree, vasodilation in the systemic circulation.

Sildenafil is more potent on PDE5 than on other known phosphodiesterases (more than 10-fold for PDE6, more than 80-fold for PDE1, more than 700-fold for PDE2, PDE3, PDE4, PDE7, PDE8, PDE9, PDE10, and PDE11). The approximate 4,000-fold selectivity for PDE5 versus PDE3 is important because PDE3 is involved in the control of cardiac contractility. Sildenafil is only about 10-fold as potent for PDE5 compared with PDE6, an enzyme found in the retina. This lower selectivity is thought to be the basis for abnormalities related to color vision observed with higher doses or plasma levels.

Tadalafil – Tadalafil is more potent on PDE5 than on other phosphodiesterases. Studies have shown that tadalafil is more than 10,000-fold more potent for PDE5 than for PDE1, PDE2, PDE4, and PDE7 enzymes, which are found in the heart, brain, blood vessels, liver, leukocytes, skeletal muscle, and other organs. Tadalafil is more than 10,000-fold more potent for PDE5 than for PDE3, an enzyme found in the heart and blood vessels. Additionally, tadalafil is 700-fold more potent for PDE5 than for PDE6, which is found in the retina and is responsible for phototransduction. Tadalafil is more than 9,000-fold more potent for PDE5 than for PDE8, PDE9, PDE10. Tadalafil is 14-fold more potent for PDE5 than for PDE11A1 and 40-fold more potent for PDE5 than for PDE11A4. PDE11 is an enzyme found in human prostate, testes, skeletal muscle, and other tissues. Tadalafil inhibits human recombinant PDE11A1 activity at concentrations within the therapeutic range. The physiological role and clinical consequence of PDE11 inhibition in humans have not been defined.

Vardenafil – The inhibitory effect of vardenafil is more selective on PDE5 than for other known phosphodiesterases (more than 15-fold relative to PDE6, more than 130-fold relative to PDE1, more than 300-fold relative to PDE11, and more than 1,000-fold relative to PDE2, PDE3, PDE4, PDE7, PDE8, PDE9, and PDE10).

Effects on blood pressure (BP) –

Sildenafil: Single oral doses of sildenafil 100 mg produced a mean maximum decrease of 8/5 mm Hg in healthy volunteers. The decrease in BP was most notable approximately 1 to 2 hours after dosing and was not different than placebo at 8 hours. Similar effects on BP were noted with sildenafil 25, 50, and 100 mg. Larger effects were recorded among patients receiving concomitant nitrates.

Vardenafil: In a clinical pharmacology study of patients with erectile dysfunction, single doses of vardenafil 20 mg caused a mean maximum decrease in supine BP of 7 mm Hg systolic and 8 mm Hg diastolic (compared with placebo), accompanied by a mean maximum increase in heart rate of 4 beats/minute. The maximum decrease in BP occurred between 1 and 4 hours after dosing. Following multiple dosing for 31 days, similar BP responses were observed on day 31 as on day 1.

➤*Pharmacokinetics:*

Absorption/Distribution –

Phosphodiesterase Type 5 Inhibitor Pharmacokinetics

Parameters	Sildenafil	Tadalafil	Vardenafil
Bioavailability	≈ 40%	Not determined	≈ 15%
T_{max}	0.5 to 2 h (median, 1 h)[a]	0.5 to 6 h (median, 2 h) (ED) 2 to 8 h (median, 4 h) (PAH)[b]	0.5 to 2 h (median, 1 h)[c]
Effect of food (high-fat meal)	C_{max} reduced 29% T_{max} increased 1 h	No effect	C_{max} reduced 18% to 50%
Onset of action	≈ 30 min (ED)	≈ 30 min (ED)	≈ 20 min[d]
Maximum effect	no data	no data	45 to 90 min[d]
Duration of action	≥ 4 h (ED)	36 h (ED)	< 5 h
Volume of distribution[e]	105 L	≈ 63 L (ED) ≈ 77 L (PAH)	208 L
Protein binding[f]	≈ 96%	94%	≈ 95%
Metabolism	CYP3A4 (major) CYP2C9 (minor)	CYP3A4	CYP3A4 (major) CYP3A5, CYP2C isoforms (minor)
Active metabolite	Yes[g]	No	Yes[h]

Phosphodiesterase Type 5 Inhibitor Pharmacokinetics			
Parameters	Sildenafil	Tadalafil	Vardenafil
Terminal half-life	≈ 4 h	17.5 h (ED) 35 h (PAH)	4 to 5 h
Excretion	Feces (≈ 80%) Urine (≈ 13%)	Feces (≈ 61%) Urine (≈ 36%)	Feces (≈ 91% to 95%) Urine (≈ 2% to 6%)
Clearance	no data	2.5 L/h (ED) 1.6 L/h (PAH)	56 L/h

[a] Oral dosing in the fasted state.
[b] Single oral dose.
[c] Single oral dose of 20 mg; fasted state.
[d] Based on animal studies.
[e] At steady state.
[f] For parent drug and major circulating metabolite.
[g] Accounts for approximately 20% of sildenafil's pharmacologic activity.
[h] Accounts for approximately 7% of vardenafil's pharmacologic activity.

Sildenafil and **vardenafil** are rapidly absorbed. The pharmacokinetics of sildenafil and vardenafil are dose-proportional over the recommended dose range. Protein binding for both drugs is independent of total drug concentrations.

Based on measurements of sildenafil in semen of healthy volunteers 90 minutes after dosing, less than 0.001% of the administered dose may appear in the semen of patients. Following a single vardenafil 20 mg oral dose in healthy volunteers, a mean of 0.00018% of the administered dose was obtained in semen 90 minutes after dosing. Less than 0.0005% of the administered **tadalafil** dose appeared in the semen of healthy subjects.

Sildenafil injection: A 10 mg dose of sildenafil injection can be expected to provide the pharmacological effect of sildenafil and its metabolite equivalent to that of a 20 mg oral dose.

Metabolism/Excretion – **Sildenafil**, **tadalafil**, and **vardenafil** are cleared predominantly by the CYP3A4 (major route), 3A5 (minor route; vardenafil), and CYP2C9 (minor route; sildenafil and vardenafil) hepatic microsomal isoenzymes. Sildenafil is converted into an active metabolite by N-desmethylation and is further metabolized. This metabolite has a PDE selectivity profile similar to sildenafil and an in vitro potency for PDE5 approximately 50% of the parent drug. Plasma concentrations of this metabolite are approximately 40% of those seen for sildenafil, so that the metabolite accounts for approximately 20% of sildenafil's pharmacologic effects. However, in patients with PAH, the ratio of the metabolite to sildenafil is higher. Both sildenafil and the metabolite have terminal half-lives of approximately 4 hours. The major circulating metabolite of vardenafil, M1, results from desethylation at the piperazine moiety of vardenafil. M1 is subject to further metabolism. The plasma concentration of M1 is approximately 26% that of the parent compound. M1 accounts for approximately 7% of total pharmacologic activity. Tadalafil is predominantly metabolized by CYP3A4 to a catechol metabolite. The catechol metabolite undergoes extensive methylation and glucuronidation to form the methylcatechol and methylcatechol glucuronide conjugate, respectively. The major circulating metabolite is the methylcatechol glucuronide. In vitro data suggests that metabolites are not expected to be pharmacologically active at observed metabolite concentrations.

Special populations –

Renal function impairment: In volunteers with severe renal impairment (creatinine clearance [CrCl] 30 mL/min or less), **sildenafil** clearance was reduced, resulting in approximately double the area under the curve (AUC) and C_{max}, compared with age-matched volunteers with no renal impairment. In the moderate (CrCl 30 to 50 mL/min) or severe (CrCl less than 30 mL/min) renal impairment groups, the AUC of **vardenafil** was 20% to 30% higher compared with that observed in a control group with normal (CrCl greater than 80 mL/min) renal function. In studies using single-dose **tadalafil** (5 to 10 mg), tadalafil AUC doubled in subjects with mild (CrCl 51 to 80 mL/min) or moderate (CrCl 31 to 50 mL/min) renal insufficiency. In subjects with end-stage renal disease on hemodialysis, there was a 2-fold increase in C_{max} and 2.7- to 4.1-fold increase in AUC following single-dose administration of tadalafil 10 or 20 mg.

Hepatic function impairment: In volunteers with mild to moderate hepatic cirrhosis (Child-Pugh class A and B), **sildenafil** clearance was reduced, resulting in increases in AUC (84%) and C_{max} (47%), compared with age-matched volunteers with no hepatic impairment. In volunteers with mild hepatic impairment (Child-Pugh class A), the C_{max} and AUC following a **vardenafil** 10 mg dose were increased by 22% and 17%, respectively, compared with healthy control subjects. In volunteers with moderate hepatic impairment (Child-Pugh class B), the C_{max} and AUC following a vardenafil 10 mg dose were increased by 130% and 160%, respectively, compared with healthy control subjects.

Elderly: Healthy elderly volunteers (65 years of age and older) had a reduced clearance of **sildenafil**, resulting in an 84% higher plasma concentration, with free plasma concentrations approximately 45% greater than those seen in healthy younger volunteers (18 to 45 years of age). In a study of healthy elderly (65 years of age and older) and younger (18 to 45 years of age) men, mean C_{max} and AUC of **vardenafil** were 34% and 52% higher, respectively, in elderly men. Healthy elderly men (65 years of age and older) had a lower oral clearance of **tadalafil**, resulting in a 25% higher AUC with no effect on C_{max} relative to that observed in healthy subjects 19 to 45 years of age.

Pulmonary hypertension: In patients with pulmonary hypertension, the average steady-state concentrations of a **sildenafil** dose were 20% to 50% higher when compared with those of healthy volunteers. There was also a doubling of C_{min} levels compared with healthy volunteers. Also, in patients with PAH, not receiving bosentan, the average tadalafil exposure at steady-state after 40 mg dose was 26% higher when compared with healthy volunteers. These findings suggest a lower clearance and/or a higher oral bioavailability of sildenafil and tadalafil in patients with pulmonary hypertension compared with healthy volunteers.

Contraindications

Hypersensitivity to any component of the tablet; administration with nitrates (either regularly and/or intermittently) and NO donors because of the potentiation of hypotension (see Drug Interactions).

Warnings/Precautions

➤*Priapism and prolonged erection:* Prolonged erections lasting longer than 4 hours and priapism (painful erections longer than 6 hours in duration) have been reported infrequently for this class of compounds. In the event of an erection that persists longer than 4 hours, whether painful or not, advise the patient to seek immediate medical assistance. If priapism is not treated immediately, penile tissue damage and permanent loss of potency may result.

Use with caution in patients who have conditions that might predispose them to priapism (eg, sickle cell anemia, multiple myeloma, leukemia) or in patients with anatomical deformation of the penis (eg, angulation, cavernosal fibrosis, Peyronie disease).

➤*Cardiovascular effects:* There is a potential for cardiac risk associated with sexual activity. Treatments for erectile dysfunction, including these agents, generally should not be used in men for whom sexual activity is inadvisable because of their underlying cardiovascular status. Consider the cardiovascular status of patients to determine whether patients with underlying cardiovascular disease could be adversely affected by vasodilatory effects (eg, transient decreases in BP) of these drugs, especially in combination with sexual activity.

Patients with the following underlying conditions can be particularly sensitive to the actions of vasodilators, including **sildenafil**, **tadalafil**, and **vardenafil**: those with left ventricular outflow obstruction (eg, aortic stenosis, idiopathic hypertrophic subaortic stenosis) and those with severely impaired autonomic control of BP.

There are no controlled clinical data on the safety or efficacy of sildenafil in patients who have suffered a myocardial infarction (MI), stroke, or life-threatening arrhythmia within the last 6 months; patients with resting hypotension (BP lower than 90/50 mm Hg) or hypertension (BP higher than 170/110 mm Hg); patients with cardiac failure (*Viagra* only) or coronary artery disease causing unstable angina; patients with retinitis pigmentosa; or patients on bosentan therapy (*Revatio* only). Use caution when prescribing sildenafil in these groups. Use of vardenafil is not recommended in the patients listed above and in severe hepatic impairment (Child-Pugh class C) and end-stage renal disease requiring dialysis.

The following groups of patients with cardiovascular disease were not included in clinical safety and efficacy trials for tadalafil, and, therefore, the use of tadalafil is not recommended in these groups until further information is available:

- Patients with an MI within the previous 90 days
- patients with unstable angina or angina occurring during sexual intercourse
- patients with New York Heart Association class 2 or greater heart failure in the last 6 months
- patients with uncontrolled arrhythmias, hypotension (BP lower than 90/50 mm Hg), or uncontrolled hypertension (BP higher than 170/100 mm Hg)
- patients with a stroke within the previous 6 months
- patients with clinically significant aortic and mitral valve disease; pericardial constriction; restrictive or congestive cardiomyopathy; significant left ventricular dysfunction; life-threatening arrhythmias; symptomatic coronary artery disease.

Sildenafil/Tadalafil – Serious cardiovascular, cerebrovascular, and vascular events, including MI, sudden cardiac death, ventricular arrhythmia, cerebrovascular hemorrhage, transient ischemic attack, hypertension, subarachnoid and intracerebral hemorrhages, and pulmonary hemorrhage have been reported postmarketing in temporal association with sildenafil or tadalafil. Most of these patients had preexisting cardiovascular risk factors. Many of these events were reported to occur during or shortly after sexual activity, and a few were reported to occur shortly after the use of sildenafil or tadalafil without sexual activity. Others were reported to have occurred hours to days after sildenafil or tadalafil use and sexual activity. It is not possible to determine whether these events are directly related to sildenafil or tadalafil, to sexual activity, to the patient's underlying cardiovascular disease, to a combination of these factors, or to other factors.

Pulmonary vasodilators may worsen the cardiovascular status of patients with pulmonary veno-occlusive disease. Since there are not data on the administration of *Adcirca* or *Revatio* to patients with veno-occlusive disease, administration to such patients is not recommended. Should signs of pulmonary edema occur when *Adcirca* or *Revatio* is administered, the possibility of associated pulmonary veno-occlusive disease should be considered.

Tadalafil – The effect of a single dose of tadalafil 100 mg on the QT interval was evaluated at the time of peak tadalafil concentration in a randomized, double-blind, placebo- and active (IV ibutilide)-controlled crossover study in 90 healthy men 18 to 53 years of age. The mean change in QTc (Fridericia QT correction) for tadalafil, relative to placebo, was 3.5 msec. The mean change in QTc (individual QT correction) for tadalafil, relative to placebo, was 2.8 msec. In this study, the mean increase in heart rate associated with a tadalafil 100 mg dose compared with placebo was 3.1 beats/minute.

Vardenafil –

Congenital or acquired QT prolongation: In a study of the effects of vardenafil on QT interval in 59 healthy men, therapeutic (10 mg) and supratherapeutic (80 mg) doses of vardenafil and the active control moxifloxacin (400 mg) produced similar increases in QTc interval. Consider this observation in clinical decisions when prescribing vardenafil. Patients with congenital QT prolongation and those taking class IA (eg, quinidine, procainamide) or class III (eg, amiodarone, sotalol) antiarrhythmic medications should avoid using vardenafil.

➤*Erectile dysfunction:* Undertake thorough medical history and physical examination to diagnose erectile dysfunction, determine potential underlying causes, and identify appropriate treatment.

The safety and efficacy of combinations of **sildenafil**, **tadalafil**, or **vardenafil** with other treatments for erectile dysfunction have not been studied. Therefore, the use of such combinations is not recommended.

➤*Deformation of penis:* Use these agents with caution in patients with anatomical deformation of the penis (eg, angulation, cavernosal fibrosis, Peyronie disease) or in patients who have conditions that may predispose them to priapism (eg, sickle cell anemia, multiple myeloma, leukemia).

➤*Hematologic effects:* **Sildenafil**, **tadalafil**, or **vardenafil** have no effect on bleeding time when taken alone or with aspirin. In vitro studies with human platelets indicate that sildenafil potentiates the antiaggregatory effect of sodium nitroprusside (a NO donor). In rabbits, the combination of heparin and sildenafil had an additive effect on bleeding time, but this interaction has not been studied in humans. There is no safety information on the administration of sildenafil, tadalafil, or vardenafil to patients with bleeding disorders or active peptic ulceration.

The incidence of epistaxis was higher in patients with PAH secondary to connective tissue disease (sildenafil 13%, placebo 0%) than in primary pulmonary hypertension patients (sildenafil 3%, placebo 2%). The incidence of epistaxis was also higher in sildenafil-treated patients with concomitant oral vitamin K antagonists (9% vs 2% in those not treated with concomitant vitamin K antagonists).

➤*Visual disturbances:* Single oral doses of PDE inhibitors have demonstrated transient, dose-related impairment of color discrimination (blue/green), with peak effects near the time of peak plasma levels. The findings were most evident 1 hour after administration, diminishing but still present 6 hours after administration. This finding is consistent with the inhibition of PDE6, which is involved in phototransduction in the retina. An evaluation of visual function of **sildenafil** up to 200 mg and **tadalafil** 40 mg revealed no effects on visual acuity, intraocular pressure, or pupillometry. In a single-dose study of 25 healthy men, **vardenafil** 40 mg, twice the maximum daily recommended dose, did not alter visual acuity, intraocular pressure, or fundoscopic and slit-lamp findings.

➤*Non-arteritic anterior ischemic optic neuropathy:* Advise patients to seek immediate medical attention in the event of sudden vision loss in one or both eyes. This may be a sign of non-arteritic anterior ischemic optic neuropathy (NAION), a cause of decreased vision, including permanent vision loss that has been reported rarely postmarketing in temporal association with the use of all PDE5 inhibitors. It is not possible to determine if these events are related directly to the use of PDE5 inhibitors or other factors. The risk may be increased in individuals who have already experienced NAION in one eye.

➤*Hearing impairment:* Sudden decrease or loss of hearing, sometimes accompanied by dizziness and tinnitus, has been reported in temporal association to the intake of PDE5 inhibitors. It is not possible to determine whether these events are related directly to the use of PDE5 inhibitors or to other factors.

➤*Retinitis pigmentosa:* A minority of patients with retinitis pigmentosa have genetic disorders of retinal phosphodiesterases. There is no safety information on the administration of **sildenafil**, **tadalafil**, or **vardenafil** to patients with known hereditary degenerative retinal disorders, including retinitis pigmentosa. Therefore, use is not recommended.

➤*Renal function impairment:* In volunteers with severe renal impairment (CrCl 30 mL/min or less), **sildenafil** clearance was reduced, resulting in approximately double the AUC and C_{max}. For erectile dysfunction, consider an initial sildenafil 25 mg dose in these patients; for PAH, no dosage dysfunction is required. There are no clinical data on the safety or efficacy of **vardenafil** in patients with end-stage renal disease requiring dialysis, and, therefore, its use is not recommended.

For erectile dysfunction, limit **tadalafil** to 5 mg not more than once every 72 hours in patients with severe renal insufficiency or end-stage renal disease on hemodialysis. The starting dose in patients with a moderate degree of renal insufficiency should be 5 mg not more than once daily, and the maximum dose should be limited to 10 mg not more than once every 48 hours. No dose adjustment is required in patients with mild renal insufficiency. For PAH, start tadalafil at 20 mg once daily in patients with mild or moderate renal impairment; increase the dose to 40 mg once daily based on individual tolerability. In patients with severe renal impairment, avoid use of tadalafil because of increased exposure (AUC), limited clinical experience, and the lack of ability to influence clearance by dialysis.

In patients with moderate (CrCl 30 to 50 mL/min) to severe (CrCl less than 30 mL/min) renal impairment, the AUC of vardenafil was 20% to 30% higher compared with that observed in a control group with normal renal function (CrCl more than 80 mL/min). No dosage adjustment for vardenafil is required.

➤*Hepatic function impairment:* In volunteers with hepatic cirrhosis, **sildenafil** clearance was reduced, resulting in increases in AUC (84%) and C_{max} (47%). Consider an initial sildenafil 25 mg dose for erectile dysfunction in these patients; no dosage adjustment is required for PAH. In patients with mild or moderate hepatic impairment, do not exceed a **tadalafil** 10 mg dose for as-needed dosing for erectile dysfunction; consider a starting dose of 20 mg once daily in these patients when treating PAH. Because of insufficient information in patients with severe hepatic impairment, use of tadalafil in these patients is not recommended. In volunteers with mild hepatic impairment (Child-Pugh class A), the C_{max} and AUC following a **vardenafil** 10 mg dose were increased by 22% and 17%, respectively, compared with healthy control subjects. In volunteers with moderate hepatic impairment (Child-Pugh class B), the C_{max} and AUC following a vardenafil 10 mg dose were increased by 130% and 160%, respectively, compared with healthy control subjects. Consequently, a starting dose of 5 mg is recommended for patients with moderate hepatic impairment, and the maximum dose should not exceed 10 mg. Vardenafil has not been evaluated in patients with severe (Child-Pugh class C) hepatic impairment and its use is not recommended in these patients.

➤*Pregnancy: Category B.* The agents for erectile dysfunction are not indicated for use in women. There are no adequate and well-controlled studies of these agents in pregnant women. **Tadalafil** and/or its metabolites cross the placenta, resulting in fetal exposure in rats. In a rat prenatal and postnatal development study at doses of tadalafil 60, 200, and 1,000 mg/kg, there was a reduction in postnatal survival of pups. Retarded physical development of pups in the absence of maternal effects was observed following maternal exposure to **vardenafil** 1 and 8 mg/kg, possibly because of vasodilation and/or secretion of the drug into milk. The number of living pups born to rats exposed pre- and postnatally was reduced at 60 mg/kg/day.

➤*Lactation:* The agents for erectile dysfunction are not indicated for use in women. **Tadalafil** and/or its metabolites were secreted into the milk of lactating rats at concentrations approximately 2.4-fold greater than found in the plasma. **Vardenafil** was secreted into the milk of lactating rats at concentrations approximately 10-fold greater than found in plasma. Following a single oral dose of 3 mg/kg, 3.3% of the administered dose was excreted into the milk within 24 hours. It is not known if the drugs are excreted in human breast milk.

➤*Children:* These agents for erectile dysfunction are not indicated for use in newborns or children.

Safety and efficacy of **sildenafil** or **tadalafil** in pediatric pulmonary hypertension patients have not been established.

➤*Elderly:* Healthy elderly volunteers (65 years of age and older) had reduced **sildenafil** clearance reulsting in an 84% higher plasma concentration, with free plasma concentrations approximately 45% greater than those in healthy younger volunteers 18 to 45 years of age. Consider an initial sildenafil 25 mg dose in these patients for erectile dysfunction. Healthy male elderly subjects (65 years of age and older) had a lower oral clearance of **tadalafil**, resulting in a 25% higher AUC with no effect on C_{max} relative to that observed in healthy subjects 19 to 45 years of age. In a study of healthy elderly (65 years of age and older) and younger (18 to 45 years of age) men, mean C_{max} and AUC of **vardenafil** were 34% and 52% higher, respectively, in elderly men. Consequently, consider a lower starting dose of vardenafil (5 mg) in patients 65 years of age and older.

Drug Interactions

➤*CYP450 system:* PDE5 inhibitors are metabolized principally by the cytochrome P-450 (CYP) isoforms 3A4 (major route), 3A5 (major route; **vardenafil**), and 2C9 (minor route; **sildenafil**, vardenafil). Therefore, inhibitors of these isoenzymes may increase PDE5 inhibitor concentrations and inducers of these isoenzymes (eg, carbamazepine, phenytoin, phenobarbital) may decrease PDE5 inhibitor concentrations. See Administration and Dosage sections of the individual monographs for dosing recommendations.

➤*Alpha-blockers:* Caution is advised when PDE5 inhibitors are coadministered with alpha-blockers. PDE5 inhibitors and alpha-adrenergic blocking agents are both vasodilators with BP-lowering effects. When vasodilators are used in combination, an additive effect on BP may be anticipated. In some patients, concomitant use of these 2 drug classes can lower BP significantly, leading to symptomatic hypotension (eg, fainting). Give consideration to the following:

- Patients should be stable on alpha-blocker therapy prior to initiating a PDE5 inhibitor. Patients who demonstrate hemodynamic instability on alpha-blocker therapy alone are at increased risk of symptomatic hypotension with concomitant use of PDE5 inhibitors.
- In those patients who are stable on alpha-blocker therapy, initiate PDE5 inhibitors at the lowest recommended starting dose.
- In those patients already taking an optimized dose of a PDE5 inhibitor, initiate alpha-blocker therapy at the lowest dose. Stepwise increases in alpha-blocker dose may be associated with further lowering of BP in patients taking a PDE5 inhibitor.
- Safety of combined use of PDE5 inhibitors and alpha-blockers may be affected by other variables, including intravascular volume depletion and other antihypertensive drugs.

PDE5 Inhibitor Drug Interactions

Precipitant drug	Object drug[a]		Description
Alcohol	PDE5 inhibitors	↑	Alcohol and PDE5 inhibitors are mild systemic vasodilators. Substantial consumption of alcohol in combination with a PDE5 inhibitor may produce decreases in BP, postural dizziness, and orthostatic hypotension.
Alpha-blockers (eg, doxazosin, terazosin)	PDE5 inhibitors	↑	Coadministration of a PDE5 inhibitor with an alpha-blocker may cause BP to be significantly lowered. Dose modifications may be required (see Administration and Dosage).
PDE5 inhibitors	Alpha-blockers (eg, doxazosin, terazosin)		
Amlodipine	PDE5 inhibitors Sildenafil Tadalafil	↑	Coadministration of sildenafil and amlodipine produced an additional mean reduction in BP of 8/7 mm Hg. Amlodipine administered with tadalafil reduced mean supine systolic/diastolic BP by 3/2 mm Hg.
PDE5 inhibitors Sildenafil Tadalafil	Amlodipine		
Angiotensin II receptor blockers	PDE5 inhibitors Tadalafil	↑	Coadministration of tadalafil and an angiotensin II receptor blocker produced a mean reduction in supine BP of 8/4 mm Hg.
PDE5 inhibitors Tadalafil	Angiotensin II receptor blockers		
Antacids	PDE5 inhibitors Tadalafil	↓	Simultaneous administration of tadalafil with an antacid (magnesium hydroxide/aluminum hydroxide) reduced the rate of tadalafil absorption without altering the AUC.
Azole antifungals (eg, ketoconazole, itraconazole)	PDE5 inhibitors	↑	Ketoconazole and itraconazole are CYP3A4 inhibitors and therefore would reduce the PDE5 inhibitor clearance. Coadministration of vardenafil with ketoconazole produced a 10-fold increase in vardenafil AUC and a 4-fold increase in C_{max}. Dose adjustments are recommended (see Administration and Dosage).
Beta-blockers, (nonspecific)	PDE5 inhibitors Sildenafil	↑	The AUC of sildenafil's active metabolite, N-desmethyl sildenafil, was increased 102% by nonspecific beta-blockers. This effect is not expected to be of clinical consequence.
Bosentan	PDE5 inhibitors Sildenafil	↓	Coadministration of bosentan and sildenafil resulted in a decrease in sildenafil AUC by 63% and C_{max} by 55%. Sildenafil (at steady state) increased bosentan AUC by 50% and C_{max} by 42%.
PDE5 inhibitors Sildenafil	Bosentan	↑	
Cimetidine	PDE5 inhibitors Sildenafil	↑	Coadministration yielded a 56% increase in sildenafil plasma concentrations.
Ciprofloxacin	PDE5 inhibitors Sildenafil	↑	Coadministration may increase sildenafil plasma levels, increasing the risk of adverse reactions. Consider a lower starting dose of sildenafil in patients taking ciprofloxacin. Monitor for adverse reactions. If an interaction is suspected, discontinue one or both drugs.
Delavirdine	PDE5 inhibitors Sildenafil	↑	Use with caution. Coadministration may substantially increase sildenafil plasma levels. Consider a maximum dose of sildenafil 25 mg in a 48-hour period for treatment of ED in patients taking delavirdine.

PDE5 Inhibitor Drug Interactions

Precipitant drug	Object drug[a]		Description
Diuretics	PDE5 inhibitors Sildenafil Tadalafil	↑	The AUC of sildenafil's active metabolite, N-desmethyl sildenafil, was increased 62% by loop diuretics and potassium-sparing diuretics. This effect is not expected to be of clinical consequence. Coadministration of tadalafil with a thiazide diuretic caused a decrease in BP.
Enalapril	PDE5 inhibitors Tadalafil	↑	Coadministration of tadalafil and enalapril produced a mean reduction in supine BP of 4/1 mm Hg.
PDE5 inhibitors Tadalafil	Enalapril		
Macrolides (eg, erythromycin)	PDE5 inhibitors	↑	Coadministration of sildenafil and erythromycin (CYP3A4 inhibitor) resulted in a 182% increase in sildenafil systemic exposure. Erythromycin produced a 4-fold increase in vardenafil AUC and a 3-fold increase in C_{max}. Also consider interactions with clarithromycin and troleandomycin.
Metoprolol	PDE5 inhibitors Tadalafil	↑	Coadministration of tadalafil and metoprolol produced a mean reduction in supine BP of 5/3 mm Hg.
PDE5 inhibitors Tadalafil	Metoprolol		
Nifedipine	PDE5 inhibitors Vardenafil	↑	Coadministration of vardenafil and nifedipine produced an additional mean reduction in supine BP of 6/5 mm Hg.
PDE5 inhibitors Vardenafil	Nifedipine		
Nitrates (eg, isosorbide dinitrate, nitroglycerin)	PDE5 inhibitors	↑	Concomitant use is contraindicated. PDE5 inhibitors potentiate the vasodilatory effect of circulating nitric oxide, resulting in a significant and potentially fatal drop in BP.
PDE5 inhibitors	Nitrates (eg, isosorbide dinitrate, nitroglycerin)		
Protease inhibitors (eg, ritonavir, indinavir, saquinavir)	PDE5 inhibitors	↑	When coadministered with a protease inhibitor, the PDE5 inhibitor plasma concentrations may be substantially elevated, resulting in severe and potentially fatal hypotension. Dose modifications are recommended (see Administration and Dosage). Concomitant use of vardenafil with ritonavir or indinavir may lead to a decrease in the protease inhibitor plasma concentration.
PDE5 inhibitors Vardenafil	Protease inhibitors (ie, ritonavir, indinavir)	↓	
Rifampin	PDE5 inhibitors Sildenafil Tadalafil	↓	Rifampin and other CYP3A4 inducers increase sildenafil and tadalafil clearance.
Serotonin reuptake inhibitors (eg, fluvoxamine)	PDE5 inhibitors Sildenafil	↑	Sildenafil plasma concentrations may be elevated, increasing the risk of adverse reactions. Use with caution. Consider reducing the sildenafil starting dose.
Tacrolimus	PDE5 inhibitors Sildenafil	↑	Sildenafil plasma concentrations may be elevated, increasing risk of side effects.
PDE5 inhibitors Sildenafil	Anticoagulants (vitamin K-dependent)	↑	In pulmonary arterial hypertension patients, the concomitant use of vitamin K antagonists and sildenafil resulted in a greater incidence of bleeding (primarily epistaxis).

[a] ↑ = Object drug increased. ↓ = Object drug decreased.

➤*Drug/Food interactions:* Although specific interactions have not been studied, grapefruit juice (CYP3A4 inhibitor) would likely increase PDE5 inhibitor exposure. When taken with a high-fat meal, the rate of **sildenafil** absorption is reduced, with a mean delay in T_{max} of 60 minutes and a mean reduction in C_{max} of 29%. High-fat meals caused a reduction in **vardenafil** C_{max} by 18% to 50%.

Adverse Reactions

➤*Erectile dysfunction:*

Phosphodiesterase Type 5 Inhibitors Adverse Reactions (%)[a]					
	Sildenafil	Vardenafil	Tadalafil		
			5 mg	10 mg	20 mg
Adverse reaction	(n = 734)[b]	(n = 2,203)[c]	(N = 151)	(N = 394)	(N = 635)
CNS					
Dizziness	2%	2%	—	—	—
Headache	16%	15%	11%	11%	15%
GI					
Diarrhea	3%	< 2%	—	—	—
Dyspepsia	7%	4%	4%	8%	10%
Nausea	—	2%	—	—	—
Respiratory					
Nasal congestion	4%	—	2%	3%	3%
Rhinitis	—	9%	—	—	—
Sinusitis	< 2%	3%	—	—	—
Miscellaneous					
Abnormal vision[d]	3%	< 2%	—	—	—
Accidental injury	< 2%	3%	—	—	—
Back pain	> 2%[e]	2%	3%	5%	6%
Flu syndrome	> 2%[e]	3%			
Flushing[f]	10%	11%	2%	3%	3%
Increased creatine kinase	—	2%	—	—	—
Limb pain	—	—	1%	3%	3%
Myalgia	< 2%	< 2%	1%	4%	3%
Rash	2%	< 2%	—	—	—
Urinary tract infection	3%	—	—	—	—

[a] Data are pooled from separate studies and are not necessarily comparable.
[b] As needed flexible-dose studies.
[c] Fixed and flexible-dose studies. Flexible-dose studies started all patients at vardenafil 10 mg and allowed a decrease in dose to 5 mg or increase in dose to 20 mg based on side effects and efficacy.
[d] Mild and transient, predominantly color tinge to vision but also increased sensitivity to light or blurred vision. Only 1 patient discontinued because of abnormal vision.
[e] Incidence is equally common with placebo.
[f] The term flushing includes facial flushing and flushing.

In fixed-dose studies, dyspepsia (17%) and abnormal vision (11%) were more common at the **sildenafil** 100 mg dose than at lower doses.

Placebo-controlled trials suggested a dose effect in the incidence of some adverse reactions (headache, flushing, dyspepsia, nausea, rhinitis) over the **vardenafil** 5, 10, and 20 mg doses.

The following adverse reactions were reported in less than 2% of patients.

Cardiovascular – Angina pectoris, chest pain, hypotension, palpitation, postural hypotension, syncope, tachycardia, abnormal electrocardiogram, AV block, cardiac arrest, cardiomyopathy, cerebral thrombosis, heart failure, myocardial ischemia, hypertension, MI, stroke, sudden cardiac death, ventricular arrhythmia.

Many of these events reported were either during or shortly after sexual activity, and few were reported without sexual activity. It is not possible to determine if these events are related to the use of PDE5 Inhibitors, to sexual activity, to the patient's underlying cardiovascular disease, to a combination of these factors, or to other factors not stated.

CNS – Hypesthesia, insomnia, paresthesia, somnolence, vertigo, abnormal dreams, ataxia, depression, hypertonia, migraine, neuralgia, neuropathy, reflexes decreased, tremor, dizziness.

Dermatologic – Pruritus, sweating, contact dermatitis, exfoliative dermatitis, herpes simplex, photosensitivity reaction, skin ulcer, urticaria, rash.

GI – Abnormal liver function tests, dry mouth, dysphagia, esophagitis, gastritis, vomiting, abdominal pain, colitis, gastroenteritis, gingivitis, glossitis, rectal hemorrhage, stomatitis, diarrhea, gamma-glutamyl transpeptidase (GGTP) increased, gastroesophageal reflux, loose stools, nausea, upper abdominal pain.

GU – Abnormal ejaculation, anorgasmia, breast enlargement, cystitis, genital edema, nocturia, urinary frequency, urinary incontinence, erection increased, spontaneous penile erection, priapism (including prolonged or painful erections).

Hematologic – Anemia, leukopenia.

Metabolic/Nutritional – Edema, gout, hyperglycemia, hypernatremia, hyperuricemia, hypoglycemia reaction, peripheral edema, thirst, unstable diabetes.

Musculoskeletal –

Sildenafil: Arthritis, arthrosis, bone pain, myasthenia, synovitis, tendon rupture, tenosynovitis, arthralgia, neck pain.

Tadalafil: In tadalafil clinical pharmacology trials, back pain or myalgia generally occurred 12 to 24 hours after dosing and typically resolved within 48 hours. The back pain/myalgia associated with tadalafil treatment was characterized by diffuse bilateral lower lumbar, gluteal, thigh, or thoracolumbar muscular discomfort and was exacerbated by recumbancy. In general, pain was reported as mild or moderate in severity and resolved without medical treatment, but severe back pain was reported infrequently (less than 5% of all reports). When medical treatment was necessary, acetaminophen or nonsteroidal anti-inflammatory drugs were generally effective; however, in a small percentage of subjects who required treatment, a mild narcotic (eg, codeine) was used. Overall, approximately 0.5% of all tadalafil-treated subjects discontinued treatment as a consequence of back pain/myalgia. Diagnostic testing, including measures for inflammation, muscle injury, or renal damage revealed no evidence of medically significant underlying pathology.

Respiratory – Dyspnea, pharyngitis, asthma, bronchitis, cough increased, laryngitis, sputum increased, epistaxis.

Special senses – Conjunctivitis, eye pain, cataract, deafness, dry eyes, ear pain, eye hemorrhage, mydriasis, photophobia, tinnitus, blurred vision, conjunctival hyperemia, eyelid swelling, lacrimation increased, changes in color vision, chromatopsia, dim vision, glaucoma, watery eyes.

Miscellaneous – Asthenia, face edema, pain, accidental fall, allergic reaction, chills, shock, anaphylactic reaction (including laryngeal edema).

Postmarketing – Nonarteritic anterior ischemic optic neuropathy (NAION), a cause of decreased vision including permanent loss of vision, has been reported rarely postmarketing in temporal association with the use of PDE5 inhibitors. Most, but not all, of these patients had underlying anatomic or vascular risk factors for developing NAION, including but not necessarily limited to: low cup or disc ratio ("crowded disc"), age older than 50 years, diabetes, hypertension, coronary artery disease, hyperlipidemia, and smoking. It is not possible to determine whether these events are related directly to the use of PDE5 inhibitors, to the patient's underlying vascular risk factors or anatomical defects, to a combination of these factors, or to other factors.

Sildenafil: Anxiety, diplopia, epistaxis, hematuria, increased intraocular pressure, ocular burning, ocular redness or bloodshot appearance, ocular swelling/pressure, paramacular edema, priapism, prolonged erection, retinal vascular disease or bleeding, seizure, temporary vision loss/decreased vision, vitreous detachment/traction.

Tadalafil: Hypersensitivity reactions including exfoliative dermatitis, Stevens-Johnson syndrome, urticaria; priapism; retinal vein occlusion; visual field defects (see also Warnings/Precautions).

Vardenafil: Visual disturbances, including vision loss (temporary or permanent), such as visual field defect, retinal vein occlusion, and reduced visual acuity, also have been reported rarely in postmarketing experience. It is not possible to determine whether these reactions are related directly to the use of vardenafil.

➤*Pulmonary arterial hypertension:*

Sildenafil Adverse Reactions in Pulmonary Arterial Hypertension Clinical Trial (≥ 3%)		
Adverse reaction	Sildenafil 20 mg 3 times daily (n = 69)	Tadalafil 40 mg (n = 79)
CNS		42%
Headache	46%	
Insomnia	7%	
GI		
Diarrhea, not otherwise specified	9%	
Dyspepsia	13%	10%
Gastritis not otherwise specified	3%	
Nausea		11%
Respiratory		
Dyspnea exacerbated	7%	
Nasopharyngitis		13%
Respiratory tract infection (upper and lower)		13%
Rhinitis not otherwise specified	4%	
Sinusitis	3%	9%
Miscellaneous		
Back pain		10%
Epistaxis	9%	
Erythema	6%	
Flushing	10%	13%
Myalgia	7%	14%
Pain in extremity		11%
Paresthesia	3%	
Pyrexia	6%	

At doses higher than the recommended 20 mg 3 times daily dose, there was a greater incidence of some adverse reactions including diarrhea, flushing, myalgia, and visual disturbances. Visual disturbances were identified as mild and transient, and were predominantly color-tinge to vision but also included increased sensitivity to light or blurred vision.

In the pivotal study, the incidence of retinal hemorrhage at the recommended sildenafil 20 mg 3 times daily dose was 1.4% versus 0% placebo and for all sildenafil doses studied was 1.9% versus 0% placebo. The incidence of eye hemorrhage at both the recommended dose and at all doses studied was 1.4% for sildenafil versus 1.4% for placebo. The patients experiencing these events had risk factors for hemorrhage including concurrent anticoagulant therapy.

Overdosage

➤*Symptoms:* In studies with healthy volunteers of single **sildenafil** doses up to 800 mg, adverse reactions were similar to those seen at lower doses, but incidence rates were increased. The maximum dose of **vardenafil** for which human data are available is a single 120 mg dose administered to 8 healthy men. The majority of these subjects experienced reversible back pain/myalgia and/or abnormal vision. Single **tadalafil** doses up to 500 mg have been given to healthy subjects, and multiple daily doses up to 100 mg have been given to patients. Adverse reactions were similar to those seen at lower doses.

➤*Treatment:* In cases of overdose, adopt standard supportive measures as required. Refer to General Management of Acute Overdosage. Renal dialysis is not expected to accelerate clearance as these drugs are highly bound to plasma proteins and are not significantly eliminated in urine.

Patient Information

Discuss with patients the contraindication of these agents with concurrent organic nitrates. Concomitant use with nitrates could cause BP to suddenly drop to an unsafe level, resulting in dizziness, syncope, or even heart attack or stroke.

Discuss with patients the potential for **tadalafil** to augment the BP-lowering effect of alpha-blockers and antihypertensive medications.

Discuss with patients the potential cardiac risk of sexual activity in patients with preexisting cardiovascular risk factors. Advise patients who experience symptoms (eg, angina pectoris, dizziness, nausea) upon initiation of sexual activity to refrain from further activity and discuss the episode with their physician.

Advise patients to stop use of all PDE5 inhibitors and to seek medical attention in the event of a sudden loss of vision in 1 or both eyes. Such an event may be a sign of NAION, a cause of decreased vision, including permanent loss of vision that has been reported rarely postmarketing in temporal association with the use of all PDE5 inhibitors. It is not possible to determine whether these events are related directly to the use of PDE5 inhibitors or other factors. Also discuss with patients the increased risk of NAION in individuals who have already experienced NAION in 1 eye, including whether such individuals could be adversely affected by use of vasodilators such as PDE5 inhibitors.

These agents offer no protection against sexually transmitted diseases. Consider counseling patients about the protective measures necessary to guard against sexually transmitted diseases, including HIV.

Advise patients that these agents have no effect in the absence of sexual stimulation. Sexual stimulation is required for an erection to occur after taking these agents.

Warn patients to seek immediate medical attention if erections last for longer than 4 hours.

Advise patients to contact the prescribing physician if new medications that may interact with these agents are prescribed by another health care provider.

Inform patients that substantial consumption of alcohol (eg, 5 units or greater) in combination with a PDE5 inhibitor can increase the potential for orthostatic signs and symptoms, including increase in heart rate, decrease in standing BP, dizziness, and headache.

Advise patients not to take other PDE5 inhibitors.

Advise patients to seek medical attention in the event of sudden decrease or loss of hearing. These events may be accompanied by tinnitus and dizziness.

SILDENAFIL CITRATE

Rx	**Revatio** (Pfizer)	**Tablets; oral:** 20 mg	Lactose. (RVT20). White, round. Film-coated. In 90s.
Rx	**Viagra** (Pfizer)	**Tablets; oral:** 25 mg	Lactose. (VGR25 PFIZER). Blue, rounded-diamond shape. Film-coated. In 30s.
		50 mg	Lactose. (VGR50 PFIZER). Blue, rounded-diamond shape. Film-coated. In 30s and 100s.
		100 mg	Lactose. (VGR100 PFIZER). Blue, rounded-diamond shape. Film-coated. In 30s and 100s.
Rx	**Revatio** (Pfizer)	**Injection, solution:** 10 mg per 12.5 mL	Dextrose 50.5 mg/mL. In 12.5 mL single-use vials.

SILDENAFIL CITRATE — ORAL

For complete and comparative prescribing information, refer to the Phosphodiesterase Type 5 Inhibitors class monograph.

Indications

➤*Erectile dysfunction (Viagra only):* For the treatment of erectile dysfunction (ED).

➤*Pulmonary arterial hypertension (Revatio only):* For the treatment of pulmonary arterial hypertension (World Health Organization [WHO] group 1) to improve exercise ability and delay clinical worsening.

➤*Off-label uses:*

Achalasia/Esophageal motility disorders – [4] = Insufficient documentation. Initial trials in healthy subjects indicate that sildenafil affects lower esophageal sphincter pressure and amplitude, suggestive of beneficial activity for patients with certain types of esophageal motility disorders. To date, the limited data available regarding the use of sildenafil in the treatment of achalasia and other esophageal motility disorders also suggest beneficial results. However, before sildenafil can be recommended for this indication, larger controlled trials evaluating efficacy and safety are needed. (See Administration and Dosage.)

Anal fissures – [4] = Insufficient documentation. Topical sildenafil cream appears to reduce maximum resting anal pressure in patients with anal fissures and is associated with fewer adverse reactions than topical nitroglycerin. Larger controlled trials, particularly those with comparative nitroglycerin data, may be useful in determining the utility of this drug in promoting healing of anal fissures. (See Administration and Dosage.)

Antidepressant/Antipsychotic-induced sexual dysfunction – [2] = Fair documentation. Most of the published information suggests that sildenafil may be effective in antidepressant/antipsychotic-induced sexual dysfunction, although a mechanism of action for this use has not been established. It is unclear if these benefits would remain with long-term therapy or if potential drug interactions may limit usefulness in antidepressant-induced sexual dysfunction. (See Administration and Dosage.)

Pulmonary hypertension in children – [4] = Insufficient documentation. There are limited data available regarding the use of sildenafil in the management of pulmonary hypertension associated with disease progress or induced via nitric oxide withdrawal. Before this product can be recommended for this indication, larger controlled trials that evaluate efficacy, optimal dosing, and safety are needed. (See Administration and Dosage.)

Raynaud phenomenon – [4] = Insufficient documentation. Data from limited studies and cases in a small number of patients (approximately 11) suggest that sildenafil may have some benefit in reducing the severity and frequency of Raynaud phenomenon attacks. Because sildenafil is associated with several potentially serious drug interactions, the use of safer conventional treatments may be recommended as first-line therapy. (See Administration and Dosage.)

Sexual dysfunction in women – [4] = Insufficient documentation. It is not clear why initial data suggest that sildenafil may be effective in antidepressant-induced sexual dysfunction because a mechanism of action for this use has not been established. Preliminary data from a very small controlled trial (fewer than 20 patients) also suggest that this agent may have beneficial effects in women with sexual dysfunction related to spinal cord injury. Effects in pre- and postmenopausal women have been variable. Results from these trials suggest that sildenafil may be useful in some women. However, it is unclear if these benefits would remain with long-term therapy or if potential drug interactions may limit usefulness in antidepressant-induced sexual dysfunction. (See Administration and Dosage.)

Administration and Dosage

➤*Adults:*

Erectile dysfunction (Viagra only) –

Usual dosage: 50 mg taken, as needed, approximately 1 hour before sexual activity. However, it may be taken anywhere from 4 to 0.5 hours before sexual activity.

Maximum dose: 100 mg once per day. The maximum recommended dosing frequency is once per day.

Dosage adjustment: May be increased to a maximum recommended dose of 100 mg or decreased to 25 mg, based on efficacy and toleration.

Concomitant therapy:

• *Nitrates* – Sildenafil was shown to potentiate the hypotensive effects of nitrates; its administration in patients who use nitric oxide donors or nitrates in any form is therefore contraindicated.

• *Ritonavir* – Ritonavir greatly increased the systemic level of sildenafil in a study of healthy, non–HIV-infected volunteers (11-fold increase in area under the curve [AUC]). Based on these pharmacokinetic data, it is recommended not to exceed a maximum single dose of sildenafil 25 mg in a 48-hour period in patients taking ritonavir.

• *Alpha-blockers* – When sildenafil is coadministered with an alpha-blocker, patients should be on stable alpha-blocker therapy prior to initiating treatment and should be initiated on sildenafil at the lowest dose.

• *CYP3A4 inhibitors* – Coadministration of potent CYP3A4 inhibitors (eg, erythromycin, itraconazole, ketoconazole, saquinavir) with sildenafil substantially increases serum concentrations of sildenafil. Consider a sildenafil starting dose of 25 mg.

Pulmonary arterial hypertension (Revatio only) –

Usual dosage: 20 mg 3 times daily, taken approximately 4 to 6 hours apart with or without food.

Maximum dose: 20 mg 3 times daily.

Concomitant therapy:

• *Nitrates* – Sildenafil was shown to potentiate the hypotensive effects of nitrates; its administration in patients who use nitric oxide donors or nitrates in any form is, therefore, contraindicated.

SILDENAFIL CITRATE — ORAL

• *Alpha-blockers* – Use caution when coadministering with alpha-blockers because of additive blood pressure–lowering effects.

• *CYP3A4 inhibitors* – Coadministration of potent CYP3A4 inhibitors (eg, ritonavir) with sildenafil substantially increases serum concentrations of sildenafil. Concomitant use is not recommended.

Off-label dosing –

Achalasia/Esophageal motility disorders: [4] = Insufficient documentation. Sildenafil 50 mg dissolved in 10 mL of water and infused via esophageal gastric probe or administered orally as 50 mg. One study used 0.8 mg/kg dissolved in distilled water.

Anal fissures: [4] = Insufficient documentation. 10% cream, 0.75 mL (75 mg), applied topically.

Antidepressant/Antipsychotic-induced sexual dysfunction: [2] = Fair documentation. 50 to 100 mg at least 1 hour and not more than 2 hours prior to sexual intercourse.

Raynaud phenomenon: [4] = Insufficient documentation. 50 mg nightly. Higher doses have been used in patients with pulmonary hypertension (50 mg 4 times per day) who also have Raynaud phenomenon.

Sexual dysfunction in women: [4] = Insufficient documentation. 25, 50, or 100 mg at least 1 hour and not more than 2 hours prior to sexual intercourse. Duration of therapy not specified in most reports, although some controlled trials allowed as-needed use for 6 to 12 weeks.

➤*Children:*

Off-label dosing –

Pulmonary hypertension in children: [4] = Insufficient documentation.

• *Children* – 2 mg/kg 4 times daily orally every 4 hours (based on 1 case report).

• *Neonates* – 1 to 1.1 mg administered via nasogastric tube during nitric oxide withdrawal attempts (based on 3 case reports).

• *Additional recommendations* – The following are additional off-label dosing recommendations for the treatment of pulmonary hypertension.

Children: 0.25 to 0.5 mg/kg/dose orally every 4 to 8 hours. Increase to 1 mg/kg/dose every 4 to 8 hours if needed and tolerated.

Neonates: 0.3 to 1 mg/kg/dose orally every 6 to 12 hours. 3 mg/kg single oral doses have been used to facilitate weaning from inhaled nitric oxide in select patients.

➤*Elderly:*

Viagra – Consider lowering the starting dose to 25 mg.

➤*Renal function impairment:*

Viagra – Consider lowering the starting dose to 25 mg in patients with severe renal impairment (CrCl less than 30 mL/min).

➤*Hepatic function impairment:*

Viagra – Consider lowering the starting dose to 25 mg.

➤*Administration: Revatio* can be taken with or without food.

➤*Storage/Stability:* Store at 25°C (77°F); excursions are permitted between 15° and 30°C (59° and 86°F).

SILDENAFIL CITRATE — INJECTION

For complete and comparative prescribing information, refer to the Phosphodiesterase Type 5 Inhibitors class monograph.

Indications

➤*Pulmonary arterial hypertension:* For the treatment of pulmonary arterial hypertension (World Health Organization [WHO] group I) to improve exercise ability and delay clinical worsening.

Administration and Dosage

➤*General dosing considerations:* Sildenafil injection is for the continued treatment of patients with pulmonary arterial hypertension who are currently prescribed oral sildenafil and who are temporarily unable to take oral medication.

A dose of sildenafil 10 mg injection is predicted to provide pharmacological effect of sildenafil and its N-desmethyl metabolite equivalent to that of a 20 mg oral dose.

➤*Adults:*

Pulmonary arterial hypertension –

Usual dosage: 10 mg (corresponding to 12.5 mL) administered as an intravenous (IV) bolus injection 3 times a day.

The dose of sildenafil does not need to be adjusted for body weight.

Concomitant therapy:

• *Nitrates* – Sildenafil was shown to potentiate the hypotensive effects of nitrates; its administration in patients who use nitric oxide donors or nitrates in any form is, therefore, contraindicated.

• *Alpha-blockers* – Use caution when coadministering with alpha-blockers because of additive blood pressure–lowering effects.

• *CYP3A4 inhibitors* – Coadministration of potent CYP3A4 inhibitors (eg, ritonavir) with sildenafil substantially increases serum concentrations of sildenafil. Concomitant use is not recommended.

➤*Storage/Stability:* Store at 25°C (77°F); excursions are permitted between 15° and 30°C (59° and 86°F).

TADALAFIL

Rx	**Cialis** (Eli Lilly)	**Tablets; oral:** 2.5 mg	Lactose. (C 2½). Yellow, almond shape. Film-coated. In blisters of 2 × 15.
		5 mg	Lactose. (C 5). Yellow, almond shape. Film-coated. In 10s and blisters of 2 × 15.
		10 mg	Lactose. (C 10). Yellow, almond shape. Film-coated. In 30s.
		20 mg	Lactose. (C 20). Yellow, almond shape. Film-coated. In 30s.
Rx	**Adcirca** (Eli Lilly)	**Tablets; oral:** 20 mg	Lactose. (4467). Orange, almond shape. Film-coated. In 60s.

TADALAFIL — ORAL

For complete and comparative prescribing information, refer to the Phosphodiesterase Type 5 Inhibitors class monograph.

Indications

➤*Erectile dysfunction (Cialis only):* For the treatment of erectile dysfunction.

➤*Pulmonary arterial hypertension (Adcirca only):* For the treatment of pulmonary arterial hypertension (PAH) (World Health Organization group 1) to improve exercise ability.

➤*Off-label uses:*

Raynaud phenomenon – [4] = Insufficient documentation. Data from 1 case report suggest that tadalafil may have some benefit in the reduction of the severity and frequency of Raynaud phenomenon attacks. Because tadalafil is associated with several potentially serious drug interactions, the use of safer conventional treatment may be recommended as first-line therapy.

Administration and Dosage

➤*General dosing considerations:* Dosage adjustment required for patients with renal insufficiency. (See Renal Function Impairment.)

Dosage adjustment required for patients with hepatic insufficiency. (See Hepatic Function Impairment.)

➤*Adults:*

Erectile dysfunction –

As-needed use:

• *Initial dosage* – 10 mg taken prior to anticipated sexual activity.

• *Dosage adjustment* – Increase to 20 mg or decrease to 5 mg based on individual efficacy and tolerability. The maximum recommended dosing frequency is once per day in most patients.

• *Concomitant therapy –*

Alpha-blockers: Patients should be stable on alpha-blocker therapy prior to initiating tadalafil treatment, and tadalafil should be initiated at the lowest recommended dose.

CYP3A4 inhibitors: The maximum recommended dose of tadalafil is 10 mg, not to exceed once every 72 hours.

Nitrates: Concomitant use is contraindicated. In a life-threatening situation, at least 48 hours should elapse after the last dose of tadalafil before nitrate administration is considered.

Once-daily use:

• *Initial dosage* – 2.5 mg taken at approximately the same time every day without regard to timing of sexual activity.

• *Dosage adjustment* – May be increased to 5 mg based on individual efficacy and tolerability.

• *Concomitant therapy –*

Alpha-blockers: Patients should be stable on alpha-blocker therapy prior to initiating tadalafil treatment, and tadalafil should be initiated at the lowest recommended dose.

CYP3A4 inhibitors: The once-daily dose should not exceed 2.5 mg.

Nitrates: Concomitant use is contraindicated. In a life-threatening situation, at least 48 hours should elapse after the last dose of tadalafil before nitrate administration is considered.

Pulmonary arterial hypertension –

Usual dosage: 40 mg (two 20 mg tablets) taken once daily.

Concomitant therapy: In patients receiving ritonavir for at least 1 week, start tadalafil at 20 mg once daily. Increase to 40 mg once daily based on individual tolerability. Avoid use of tadalafil during the initiation of ritonavir. Stop tadalafil at least 24 hours prior to starting ritonavir. After at least 1 week following the initiation of ritonavir, resume tadalafil 20 mg once daily. Increase to 40 mg once daily based on individual tolerability.

Off-label dosing –

Raynaud phenomenon: [4] = Insufficient documentation. 10 mg/day.

TADALAFIL — ORAL

➤*Renal function impairment:*

Erectile dysfunction –

As-needed use:

• *Moderate renal insufficiency (CrCl 31 to 50 mL/min)* – A starting dose of 5 mg not more than once daily is recommended, and the maximum dose should be limited to 10 mg not more than once every 48 hours.

• *Severe renal insufficiency (CrCl less than 30 mL/min and on hemodialysis)* – The maximum recommended dosage is 5 mg once every 72 hours.

Once-daily use:

• *Severe renal insufficiency (creatinine clearance [CrCl] less than 30 mL/min and on hemodialysis)* – Once-daily use is not recommended.

Pulmonary arterial hypertension –

Mild to moderate renal insufficiency (CrCl 31 to 80 mL/min): Start dosing at 20 mg once daily. Increase to 40 mg once daily based on individual tolerability.

Severe renal insufficiency (CrCl less than 30 mL/min and on hemodialysis): Avoid use because of increased tadalafil exposure (area under the curve [AUC]), limited clinical experience, and the lack of ability to influence clearance by dialysis.

➤*Hepatic function impairment:*

Erectile dysfunction –

As-needed use:

• *Mild or moderate hepatic impairment (Child-Pugh class A or B)* – The dosage should not exceed 10 mg once daily.

• *Severe hepatic impairment (Child-Pugh class C)* – Not recommended.

Once-daily use:

• *Mild or moderate hepatic insufficiency (Child-Pugh class A or B)* – Caution is advised.

• *Severe hepatic insufficiency (Child-Pugh class C)* – Use is not recommended.

Pulmonary arterial hypertension –

Mild or moderate hepatic impairment (Child-Pugh class A or B): Consider a starting dosage of 20 mg once per day.

Severe hepatic cirrhosis (Child-Pugh class C): Avoid use.

➤*Administration:* May be taken without regard to food.

➤*Storage/Stability:* Store at 25°C (77°F); excursions are permitted between 15° and 30°C (59° and 86°F).

VARDENAFIL HYDROCHLORIDE

Rx	**Levitra** (Schering-Plough)	**Tablets:** 2.5 mg	(BAYER 2.5). Orange, round. Film-coated. In 30s.
		5 mg	(BAYER 5). Orange, round. Film-coated. In 30s.
		10 mg	(BAYER 10). Orange, round. Film-coated. In 30s.
		20 mg	(BAYER 20). Orange, round. Film-coated. In 30s.
Rx	**Staxyn** (Schering-Plough)	**Tablets, disintegrating; oral:** 10 mg	Equiv. to vardenafil hydrochloride 11.85 mg. Phenylalanine 1.01 mg, aspartame, mannitol, sorbitol. White, round. In UD 4s and 40s.

VARDENAFIL HYDROCHLORIDE — ORAL

For complete prescribing information, refer to the Phosphodiesterase Type 5 Inhibitors class monograph.

Indications

➤*Erectile dysfunction:* For the treatment of erectile dysfunction.

➤*Off-label uses:*

Raynaud phenomenon (film-coated tablets only) –

[3] = Safety concerns. Data from 1 open-label trial suggest vardenafil film-coated tablets may have some benefit in reducing the severity and frequency of Raynaud phenomenon attacks. (See Administration and Dosage.)

Administration and Dosage

➤*Adults:*

Erectile dysfunction –

Usual dosage: 10 mg, taken approximately 60 minutes before sexual activity.

Maximum dose:

• *Film-coated tablets* – 20 mg/dose once daily.

• *Orally disintegrating tablets* – 10 mg/day according to the prescribing information.

Dosage adjustment:

• *Film-coated tablets* – The dose may be increased to a maximum recommended dose of 20 mg or decreased to 5 mg based on efficacy and adverse reactions.

Off-label dosing –

Raynaud phenomenon (film-coated tablets only): [3] = Safety concerns. 10 mg twice daily for 2 weeks.

➤*Elderly:*

Film-coated tablets – A starting dose of 5 mg should be considered in patients 65 years of age and older.

➤*Hepatic function impairment:*

Film-coated tablets – Vardenafil clearance is reduced in patients with moderate hepatic impairment (Child-Pugh class B), and a starting dose of vardenafil 5 mg is recommended. The maximum dose in patients with moderate hepatic impairment should not exceed 10 mg.

Orally disintegrating tablets – Do not use in patients with moderate (Child-Pugh B) or severe (Child-Pugh C) hepatic impairment.

➤*Concomitant therapy with alpha-blockers:*

Film-coated tablets – Caution is advised when vardenafil is used concomitantly with alpha-blockers because of the potential for an additive effect on blood pressure. In some patients, concomitant use of these 2 drugs can lower blood pressure significantly, leading to symptomatic hypotension (eg, fainting). Concomitant treatment should be initiated only if the patient is stable on alpha-blocker therapy. In those patients who are stable on alpha-blocker therapy, vardenafil should be initiated at a dose of 5 mg (2.5 mg when used concomitantly with certain CYP3A4 inhibitors.)

Orally disintegrating tablets – In those patients who are stable on alpha-blocker therapy, phosphodiesterase type 5 (PDE5) inhibitors should be initiated at the lowest recommended starting dose. In patients taking alpha-blockers, do not initiate vardenafil therapy. Lower doses of vardenafil film-coated tablets should be used as initial therapy in these patients. Patients taking alpha-blockers who have previously used vardenafil film-coated tablets may change to orally disintegrated tablets at the advice of their health care provider.

➤*Concomitant therapy with CYP3A4 inhibitors:*

Film-coated tablets – The dosage of vardenafil may require adjustment in patients receiving certain CYP3A4 inhibitors (eg, erythromycin, indinavir, itraconazole, ketoconazole, ritonavir). For ritonavir, a single dose of vardenafil 2.5 mg should not be exceeded in a 72-hour period. For indinavir, ketoconazole 400 mg daily, and itraconazole 400 mg daily, a single dose of vardenafil 2.5 mg should not be exceeded in a 24-hour period. For ketoconazole 200 mg daily, itraconazole 200 mg daily, and erythromycin, a single dose of vardenafil 5 mg should not be exceeded in a 24-hour period.

Orally disintegrating tablets – Do not use with potent or moderate CYP3A4 inhibitors, such as ketoconazole, itraconazole, ritonavir, indinavir, saquinavir, atazanavir, clarithromycin, and erythromycin.

➤*Concomitant therapy with nitrates:*

Orally disintegrating tablets – Concomitant use with nitrates in any form is contraindicated.

➤*Administration:* May be taken with or without food. Administer orally, as needed, approximately 60 minutes before sexual activity.

Orally disintegrating tablets – Should be placed on the tongue where it will disintegrate. Should be taken without liquid, immediately upon removal from the blister.

➤*Storage/Stability:* Store at 25°C (77°F); excursions are permitted to 15° to 30°C (59° to 86°F).

ACETOHYDROXAMIC ACID

Rx	**Lithostat** (Mission)	**Tablets:** 250 mg	(Mission MPC 500). White. In unit-of-use 100s.

ACETOHYDROXAMIC ACID — ORAL

Indications

➤*Chronic urea-splitting urinary infection:* Adjunctive therapy in patients with chronic urea-splitting urinary infection. Acetohydroxamic acid is intended to decrease urinary ammonia and alkalinity, but it should not be used in lieu of curative surgical treatment (for patients with stones) or antimicrobial treatment. Long-term treatment with acetohydroxamic acid may be warranted to maintain urease inhibition as long as urea-splitting infection is present. Experience with acetohydroxamic acid does not go beyond 7 years. A patient monograph should be distributed to each patient who receives acetohydroxamic acid.

Administration and Dosage

➤*Adults:*

Chronic urea-splitting urinary infection –

Usual dosage: 1 tablet 3 to 4 times a day in a total daily dose of 10 to 15 mg/kg/day.

Maximum dose: 1.5 g/day.

Initial dosage: 12 mg/kg/day, administered at 6- to 8-hour intervals.

➤*Children:*

Chronic urea-splitting urinary infection –

Initial dosage: 10 mg/kg/day taken in 2 or 3 divided doses.

Dosage adjustment: Titration of the dose to higher or lower levels may be required to obtain an optimum therapeutic effect or to reduce the risk of adverse effects.

➤*Renal function impairment:* Contraindicated in patients with advanced renal insufficiency (ie, serum creatinine greater than 2.5 mg/dL or creatinine clearance less than 20 mL/min). Patients whose serum creatinine is greater than 1.8 mg/dL should take no more than 1 g/day; such patients should be dosed at 12-hour intervals. Further reductions in dosage to prevent the accumulation of toxic concentrations in the blood may also be desirable. Insufficient data exists to accurately characterize the optimum dose or dose interval in patients with moderate degrees of renal insufficiency.

➤*Administration:* Should be administered orally on an empty stomach.

➤*Storage / Stability:* Store in a dry place at 15° to 30°C (59° to 86°F).

Actions

➤*Pharmacology:* Acetohydroxamic acid reversibly inhibits the bacterial enzyme urease, thereby inhibiting the hydrolysis of urea and production of ammonia in urine infected with urea-splitting organisms. The reduced ammonia levels and decreased pH enhance the effectiveness of antimicrobial agents and allow an increased cure rate of these infections.

Acetohydroxamic acid has been evaluated clinically in patients with urea-splitting urinary infections, often accompanied by struvite stone disease, that were recalcitrant to other forms of medical and surgical management. In these clinical trials, acetohydroxamic acid reduced the pathologically elevated urinary ammonia and pH levels that result from the hydrolysis of urea by the enzyme, urease.

Acetohydroxamic acid does not acidify urine directly nor does it have a direct antibacterial effect. The usefulness of reducing ammonia levels and decreasing urinary pH is suggested by single (not yet replicated) clinical trials in which urease inhibition allowed successful antibiotic treatment of urea-splitting *Proteus* infections after surgical removal of struvite stones in patients not cured by 3 months of antibacterial treatment alone, and reduced the rate of stone growth in patients who were not candidates for surgical removal of stones.

➤*Pharmacokinetics:*

Absorption / Distribution – Acetohydroxamic acid is well absorbed from the gastrointestinal tract after oral administration; peak blood levels occur from 0.25 to 1 hour after dosing. The compound is distributed throughout body water, and there is no known binding to any tissue. Acetohydroxamic acid chelates with dietary iron within the gut. This reaction may interfere with absorption of acetohydroxamic acid and with iron. Concomitant hypochromic anemia should be treated with intramuscular iron.

Metabolism / Excretion – In rodents, the metabolic fate of acetohydroxamic acid is well known; 55% is excreted unchanged in urine, 25% is excreted as acetamide or acetate and 7% is excreted by the lungs as carbon dioxide. Less than 1% is excreted in the feces. Approximately 5% of the administered dose is unaccounted for. In rodents, acetohydroxamic acid shows a dose-related change in pharmacokinetics; with increasing dose, there is an increase in the half-life and an increase in the percent of the administered dose recovered in urine as unchanged acetohydroxamic acid.

Pharmacokinetics in man are generally similar to rodents including the dose-related increase in half-life, but they are not as well characterized as in the rodent. Thirty-six to sixty-five percent (36% to 65%) of the oral dosage is excreted unchanged in the urine. It is unaltered acetohydroxamic acid in the urine that provides the therapeutic effect, but the precise concentration of acetohydroxamic acid in urine that is necessary to inhibit urease is incompletely delineated. Therapeutic benefit may be obtained from concentrations as low as 8 mcg/mL; higher concentrations (ie, 30 mcg/mL) are expected to provide more complete inhibition of urease. The plasma half-life of acetohydroxamic acid is approximately 5 to 10 hours in subjects with normal renal function and is prolonged in patients with reduced renal function.

Contraindications

Patients whose physical state and disease are amenable to definitive surgery and appropriate antimicrobial agents; patients whose urine is infected by nonurease-producing organisms; patients whose urinary infections can be controlled by culture-specific oral antimicrobial agents; patients whose renal function is poor (ie, serum creatinine greater than 2.5 mg/dL or creatinine clearance less than 20 mL/min); female patients who do not evidence a satisfactory method of contraception; patients who are pregnant (see Warnings/Precautions).

Warnings/Precautions

➤*Coombs negative hemolytic anemia:* A Coombs negative hemolytic anemia has occurred in patients receiving acetohydroxamic acid. Gastrointestinal upset characterized by nausea, vomiting, anorexia, and generalized malaise has accompanied the most severe forms of hemolytic anemia. Approximately 15% of patients receiving acetohydroxamic acid have had only laboratory findings of an anemia. However, most patients developed a mild reticulocytosis. The untoward reactions have reverted to normal following cessation of treatment. A complete blood count, including a reticulocyte count, is recommended after 2 weeks of treatment. If the reticulocyte count exceeds 6%, a reduced dosage should be entertained. A CBC and reticulocyte count are recommended at 3-month intervals for the duration of treatment.

➤*Hematologic effects:* Bone marrow depression (leukopenia, anemia, and thrombocytopenia) has occurred in experimental animals receiving large doses of acetohydroxamic acid, but has not been seen in man to date. Acetohydroxamic acid is a known inhibitor of DNA synthesis and also chelates metals, notably iron. Its bone marrow suppressant effect is probably related to its ability to inhibit DNA synthesis, but anemia could also be related to depletion of iron stores. To date, the only clinical effect noted has been hemolysis, with a decrease in the circulating red blood cells, hemoglobin and hematocrit. Abnormalities in platelet or white blood cell count have not been noted. However, clinical monitoring of the platelet and white cell count is recommended.

➤*Renal function impairment:* Since acetohydroxamic acid is eliminated primarily by the kidneys, patients with significantly impaired renal function should be closely monitored, and a reduction of daily dose may be needed to avoid excessive drug accumulation (see Administration and Dosage).

➤*Hepatic function impairment:* Abnormalities of liver function have not been reported to date. However, a chloro-benzene derivative of acetohydroxamic acid caused significant liver dysfunction in an unrelated study. Therefore, close monitoring of liver function is recommended (see Carcinogenesis for discussion of possible hepatic carcinogenesis).

➤*Pregnancy: Category X.* Acetohydroxamic acid may cause fetal harm when administered to a pregnant woman. Acetohydroxamic acid was teratogenic (retarded or clubbed rear leg at 750 mg/kg and above and exencephaly and encephalocele at 1500 mg/kg) when given intraperitoneally to rats. Acetohydroxamic acid is contraindicated in women who are or may become pregnant. If this drug is used during pregnancy, or if the patient becomes pregnant while taking this drug, the patient should be informed of the potential hazard to the fetus.

➤*Lactation:* It is not known whether acetohydroxamic acid is secreted in human milk. Because many drugs are excreted in human milk, and because of the potential for serious adverse reactions in nursing infants from acetohydroxamic acid, a decision should be made whether to discontinue nursing or the drug, taking into account the significance of the drug to the mother's well-being.

➤*Children:* Children with chronic, recalcitrant, urea-splitting urinary infection may benefit from treatment with acetohydroxamic acid. However, detailed studies involving dosage and dose intervals in children have not been established. Children have tolerated a dose of 10 mg/kg/day, taken in 2 or 3 divided doses, satisfactorily for periods up to 1 year. Close monitoring of such patients is mandatory.

Drug Interactions

AHA Drug Interactions

Precipitant drug	Object drug[a]		Description
Alcoholic beverages	AHA	↑	Alcoholic beverages taken with AHA have caused rash
AHA	Heavy metals	↓	AHA chelates heavy metals, notably iron. The absorption of iron and AHA from the intestinal lumen may be reduced when both drugs are taken concomitantly. When iron is indicated, administer IM.

[a] ↑ = Object drug increased. ↓ = Object drug decreased.

Acetohydroxamic acid has been used concomitantly with insulin, oral and parenteral antibiotics, and progestational agents. No clinically significant interactions have been noted, but until wider clinical experience is obtained, acetohydroxamic acid should be used with caution in patients receiving other therapeutic agents.

ACETOHYDROXAMIC ACID — ORAL

➤*Drug/Food interactions:* Acetohydroxamic acid taken in association with alcoholic beverages has resulted in a rash (see Adverse Reactions).

Adverse Reactions

Experience with acetohydroxamic acid is limited. About 150 patients have been treated, most for periods of more than a year.

Adverse reactions have occurred in up to 30% of the patients receiving acetohydroxamic acid. In some instances the reactions were symptomatic; in others only changes in laboratory parameters were noted. Adverse reactions seem to be more prevalent in patients with preexisting thrombophlebitis or phlebothrombosis or in patients with advanced degrees of renal insufficiency. The risk of adverse reactions is highest during the first year of treatment. Chronic treatment does not seem to increase the risk nor the severity of adverse reactions.

The following reactions have been reported:

➤*Cardiovascular:* Superficial phlebitis involving the lower extremities has occurred in several patients on acetohydroxamic acid during the early (phase II) clinical trials. Several of the affected patients had had phlebitic episodes prior to treatment. One patient developed deep vein thrombosis of the lower extremities. The patient with phlebothrombosis had an associated traumatic injury to the groin. It is unclear whether the phlebitis was related to or exacerbated by treatment with acetohydroxamic acid. No patient in the 3 year controlled (phase III) clinical trial developed phlebitis. In all instances these vascular abnormalities returned to normal following appropriate medical therapy. Embolic phenomena have been reported in 3 patients taking acetohydroxamic acid in the phase II trial. The phlebitis and emboli resolved following discontinuation of acetohydroxamic acid and implementation of appropriate medical therapy. Several patients have resumed treatment with acetohydroxamic acid without ill effect. Palpitations have also been reported in patients taking acetohydroxamic acid.

➤*CNS:* Mild headaches are commonly reported (about 30%) during the first 48 hours of treatment. These headaches are mild, responsive to oral salicylate-type analgesics, and usually disappear spontaneously. The headaches have not been associated with vertigo, tinnitus, or visual or auditory abnormalities. Tremulousness and nervousness have also been reported.

➤*Dermatologic:* A nonpruritic, macular skin rash has occurred in the upper extremities and on the face of several patients taking acetohydroxamic acid on a long-term basis, usually when acetohydroxamic acid has been taken concomitantly with alcoholic beverages, but in a few patients in the absence of alcohol consumption. The rash commonly appears 30 to 45 minutes after ingestion of alcoholic beverages; it characteristically disappears spontaneously in 30 to 60 minutes. The rash may be associated with a general sensation of warmth. In some patients the rash is sufficiently severe to warrant discontinuation of treatment, but most patients have continued treatment, avoiding alcohol or using smaller quantities of it. Alopecia has also been reported in patients taking acetohydroxamic acid.

➤*GI:* Gastrointestinal symptoms, nausea, vomiting, anorexia, and malaise have occurred in 20% to 25% of patients. In most patients the symptoms were mild, transitory, and did not result in interruption of treatment. Approximately 3% of patients developed a hemolytic anemia of sufficient magnitude to warrant interruption in treatment; several of these patients also had symptoms of gastrointestinal upset.

➤*Hematologic:* Approximately 15% of patients have had laboratory findings characteristic of a hemolytic anemia. A mild reticulocytosis (5% to 6%) without anemia, is even more prevalent. The laboratory findings are occasionally accompanied by systemic symptoms such as malaise, lethargy and fatigue, and gastrointestinal symptoms. Symptoms and laboratory findings have invariably improved following cessation of treatment with acetohydroxamic acid. The hematological abnormalities are more prevalent in patients with advanced renal failure.

➤*Psychiatric:* Depression, anxiety, nervousness, and tremulousness have been observed in approximately 20% of patients taking acetohydroxamic acid. In most patients the symptoms were mild and transitory, but in about 6% of patients the symptoms were sufficiently distressing to warrant interruption or discontinuation of treatment.

➤*Respiratory:* No symptoms have been reported. Radiographic evidence of small pulmonary emboli has been seen in three patients with phlebitis in their lower legs.

Overdosage

➤*Symptoms:* Acute deliberate overdosage in man has not occurred, but would be expected to induce the following symptoms: Anorexia, malaise, lethargy, diminished sense of well-being, tremulousness, anxiety, nausea and vomiting. Laboratory findings are likely to include an elevated reticulocyte count and a severe hemolytic reaction requiring hospitalization, symptomatic treatment, and possibly blood transfusions. Concomitant reduction in platelets or white blood cells should be anticipated.

Milder overdosages resulting in hemolysis have occurred in an occasional patient with reduced renal function after several weeks or months of continuous treatment.

The acute LD_{50} of acetohydroxamic acid in animals (rats) is 4.8 g/kg.

➤*Treatment:* Recommended treatment for an overdosage reaction consists of cessation of treatment, close monitoring of hematologic status, symptomatic treatment, and blood transfusions as required by the clinical circumstances. The drug is probably dialyzable, but this property has not been tested clinically.

Patient Information

Advise patients that the daily dosage of acetohydroxamic acid is important to the proper treatment of their condition. Advise patients to report any unusual side effects to their health care provider.

GENITOURINARY IRRIGANTS

NEOMYCIN/POLYMYXIN B SULFATE IRRIGATION

Rx	**Neomycin/Polymyxin B Sulfates** (Watson)	**Solution, intravesical:** 40 mg neomycin and 200,000 units polymyxin B sulfate per mL	As neomycin sulfate. In 1 ml amps (10s and 50s).
Rx	**Neosporin G.U. Irrigant** (GlaxoWellcome)		As neomycin sulfate. In 1 ml amps (10s and 50s) and 20 ml multidose vials.[a]

[a] With methylparaben.

NEOMYCIN/POLYMYXIN B SULFATE — IRRIGATION

Indications

➤*Urinary bladder irrigant:* Continuous irrigant or rinse for short-term use (up to 10 days) in the urinary bladder of abacteriuric patients to help prevent bacteriuria and gram-negative rod bacteremia associated with the use of indwelling catheters.

Administration and Dosage

➤*Adults:*

Urinary bladder irrigant – 1 mL a day for up to 10 days.

➤*Preparation for administration:* Add 1 mL irrigant to 1 L isotonic saline solution.

➤*Administration:* Not for injection. Connect the container to the inflow lumen of the 3-way catheter. Connect the outflow lumen via a sterile disposable plastic tube to a disposable plastic collection bag. Stringent procedures, such as taping the inflow and outflow junction at the catheter, should be observed when necessary to ensure the junctional integrity of the system. Adjust flow rate to 1 L/24 hours. If the patient's urine output exceeds 2 L/day, increase flow rate to 2 L/24 hours. The rinse of the bladder must be continuous. Do not interrupt the inflow or rinse solution for more than a few minutes.

➤*Storage/Stability:* Store at 2° to 8°C (26° to 36°F). Store prepared solution at 4°C and use within 48 hours following preparation to reduce the risk of contamination with resistant microorganisms.

Actions

➤*Pharmacology:* Polymyxin B sulfate is bactericidal to most gram-negative bacilli, particularly against *Pseudomonas* infections. Neomycin sulfate is bactericidal against a wide range of gram-negative organisms including *Proteus vulgaris* and gram-positive organisms. When used topically, these drugs are rarely irritating.

Contraindications

Hypersensitivity to any component.

Warnings/Precautions

➤*Recent UT surgery:* Safety and efficacy have not been established for use in patients with recent lower urinary tract surgery.

➤*Neomycin toxicity:* Neomycin is nephrotoxic and ototoxic, particularly when given parenterally in higher than recommended doses. Cases of nephrotoxicity or ototoxicity have been reported following its topical use for extensive burns and wound irrigation. Although the possibility of these reactions is remote with use of the minimal amount in bladder irrigations, such reactions may occur if irrigations are continued beyond the recommended maximum of 10 days; observe caution.

➤*Superinfection:* Use of antibiotics (especially prolonged or repeated therapy) may result in bacterial or fungal overgrowth of nonsusceptible organisms. Such overgrowth may lead to a secondary infection. Appropriate measures should be taken if superinfection occurs.

➤*Pregnancy: Category C* (neomycin); *Category B* (polymyxin B) per Briggs' *Drugs in Pregnancy and Lactation.*

➤*Lactation:* It is unknown if continuous irrigation of the urinary bladder in breast-feeding women would affect the breast-feeding infant.

Adverse Reactions

The prevalence of neomycin hypersensitivity has increased; however, topical application to mucous membranes rarely results in local or systemic reactions.

CITRIC ACID/GLUCONO-DELTA-LACTONE/MAGNESIUM CARBONATE IRRIGANT (Hemiacidrin)

Rx	**Renacidin** (Guardian)	**Solution:** 6.602 g citric acid (anhydrous), 0.198 g glucono-delta-lactone, 3.177 g magnesium carbonate and 0.023 g benzoic acid/100 mL	In 500 mL.

CITRIC ACID/GLUCONO-DELTA-LACTONE/MAGNESIUM CARBONATE (Hemiacidrin) — IRRIGATION

Indications

➤*Solution:* Local irrigation for dissolution of renal calculi composed of apatite (a calcium carbonate-phosphate compound) or struvite (magnesium ammonium phosphates) in patients who are not candidates for surgical removal of the calculi.

As adjunctive therapy to dissolve residual apatite or struvite calculi and fragments after surgery or to achieve partial dissolution of renal calculi to facilitate surgical removal.

For dissolution of bladder calculi of the struvite or apatite variety by local intermittent irrigation through a urethral catheter or cystostomy catheter as an alternative or adjunct to surgical procedures.

For use as an intermittent irrigating solution to prevent or minimize encrustations of indwelling urinary tract catheters.

➤*Off-label uses:* Hemiacidrin has been used as a renal pelvis irrigation, with meticulous attention to intrapelvic pressure and urosepsis.

Administration and Dosage

➤*Maximum dose:* There are no well-established maximum doses for the approved indications according to the prescribing information.

➤*General dosing considerations:*

Bladder calculi – In the presence of bladder spasm and associated high pressure reflux, all precautions required for irrigation of the renal pelvis must be observed.

Renal calculi – It is essential that patients be free from urinary tract infections prior to initiating chemolytic therapy. (See Warning/Precautions.)

➤*Adults:*

Bladder calculi –

Usual dosage: Following appropriate studies to evaluate possible vesicoureteral reflux, 30 mL is instilled through a urinary catheter into the bladder and the catheter is clamped for 30 to 60 minutes. The clamp is then released and the bladder is drained. This is repeated 4 to 6 times a day.

Alternative dosage: A continuous drip through a 3-way Foley catheter is an alternative means of dissolving bladder stones.

Indwelling urinary tract catheter encrustation – Instill 30 mL of the solution through the catheter and then clamping the catheter for 10 minutes, after which the clamp is removed to allow drainage of the bladder. This process is repeated 3 times a day.

Renal calculi – Irrigation of the renal pelvis is begun with sterile saline only after a sterile urine has been demonstrated. The saline is infused at a rate of 60 mL/hr initially, and the rate is increased until pain or an elevated pressure (25 cm H_2O) appears, or until a maximum flow rate of 120 mL/hr is achieved. If no leakage or flank pain occurs, start irrigation with hemiacidrin with a flow rate equal to maximum rate achieved with the saline solution. Place a clamp on the inflow tube and instruct patients and nursing personnel to stop the irrigating solution whenever pain develops. If stones fail to change size after several days of adequate irrigation, discontinue the procedure. Upon demonstration of complete dissolution of the calculus, the inflow tube is clamped and left in place for a few days to ensure that no obstruction exists, after which time the nephrostomy tube is removed.

➤*Administration:*

Bladder calculi – Instill 30 mL through a urinary catheter into the bladder, and the catheter is clamped for 30 to 60 minutes. The clamp is then released and the bladder is drained.

Indwelling urinary tract catheter encrustation – Instill 30 mL through the catheter and then clamping the catheter for 10 minutes, after which the clamp is removed to allow drainage of the bladder.

Renal calculi – A nephrostomy tube is placed at surgery or percutaneously to permit lavage of the calculi. A single catheter may be sufficient if the calculus is not obstructing the ureter or ureteropelvic junction. In patients with an obstructed ureter, a retrograde catheter can be placed through the ureter to the renal pelvis via a cystoscope. This second catheter is used to irrigate the calculus while the percutaneous nephrostomy tube is used for drainage. Pressure measurements are made under fluoroscopy to assure that 2 to 3 mL/min can be infused without causing pain, pyelovenous or pyelotubular backflow or manometric evidence of elevated pressure within the collecting system.

For postoperative patients, irrigation should not be started before the fourth or fifth postoperative day. Irrigation of the renal pelvis is begun with sterile saline only after a sterile urine has been demonstrated. The saline is infused at a rate of 60 mL/hr initially, and the rate is increased until pain or an elevated pressure (25 cm H_2O) appears, or until a maximum flow rate of 120 mL/hr is achieved. Inspect the site of insertion for leakage. If leakage occurs, the irrigation is discontinued temporarily to allow for complete healing around the nephrostomy tube.

If no leakage or flank pain occurs, start irrigation with hemiacidrin with a flow rate equal to maximum rate achieved with the saline solution. Place a clamp on the inflow tube and instruct patients and nursing personnel to stop the irrigating solution whenever pain develops. Nursing personnel who are responsible for performing the irrigation must be instructed concerning location of the nephrostomy tube(s) and direction of flow of irrigating solution to ensure against misconnection of inflowing and egress tubes. Perform nephrostomograms periodically to assure proper placement of catheter tip and to assess efficacy. If stones fail to change size after several days of adequate irrigation, discontinue the procedure.

Upon demonstration of complete dissolution of the calculus, the inflow tube is clamped and left in place for a few days to ensure that no obstruction exists, after which time the nephrostomy tube is removed.

➤*Storage/Stability:* Store solution at 15° to 30°C (59° to 86°F). Avoid excessive heat or cold (keep from freezing). Brief exposure to temperatures of up to 40°C (104°F) or temperatures down to 5°C (41°F) does not adversely affect the product.

Actions

➤*Pharmacology:* The action of hemiacidrin on susceptible apatite calculi results from an exchange of magnesium from the irrigating solution for the insoluble calcium contained in the stone matrix or calcification. The magnesium salts thereby formed are soluble in the gluconocitrate irrigating solution resulting in the dissolution of the calculus. Struvite calculi are composed mainly of magnesium ammonium phosphates which are solubilized by hemiacidrin due to its acidic pH.

Hemiacidrin is not effective for dissolution of calcium oxalate, uric acid or cysteine stones.

Contraindications

Urinary tract infections (see Warnings); presence of demonstrable urinary tract extravasation.

Warnings/Precautions

➤*Urinary tract infection:* Stop the drug immediately if patient develops fever, urinary tract infection, signs and symptoms consistent with urinary tract infection, persistent flank pain, or if hypermagnesemia or elevated serum creatinine develops.

Urea-splitting bacteria reside within struvite and apatite stones which therefore serve as a source of infection. Dissolution therapy with hemiacidrin in the presence of an infected urinary tract may lead to sepsis and death. Obtain urine specimens for culture prior to initiating chemolytic therapy of the renal pelvis. Institute appropriate antibiotic therapy to treat any infection detected. A sterile urine must be present prior to initiating therapy. An infected stone can serve as a continual source for infection; therefore, continue antibiotic therapy throughout the course of dissolution therapy.

➤*Severe hypermagnesemia:* Severe hypermagnesemia has occurred. Use caution when irrigating the renal pelvis of patients with impaired renal function. Observe patients for early signs and symptoms of hypermagnesemia including nausea, lethargy, confusion and hypotension. Severe hypermagnesemia may result in hyporeflexia, dyspnea, apnea, coma, cardiac arrest and subsequent death. Monitor serum magnesium levels and evaluate deep tendon reflexes. Treatment of hypermagnesemia should include discontinuation of hemiacidrin followed by therapy with IV calcium gluconate, fluids and diuresis in severe cases.

➤*Not indicated:* Not indicated for dissolution of calcium oxalate, uric acid or cysteine calculi.

➤*Vesicoureteral reflux:* Vesicoureteral reflux frequently occurs in patients with indwelling urethral or cystostomy catheters. Cystogram prior to initiation of hemiacidrin is essential for such patients. If reflux is demonstrated, all precautions recommended for renal pelvis irrigation must be taken.

➤*Catheter care:* Hospitalization is prolonged for days to weeks when chemolytic therapy is used in lieu of, or following, surgery. Reserve this therapy for selected patients. Care must be taken during chemolysis of renal calculi with hemiacidrin to maintain the patency of the irrigating catheter. Calculus fragments and debris may obstruct the outflow catheter. Continued irrigation under those circumstances leads to increased intrapelvic pressure with a danger of tissue damage or absorption of the irrigating solution. Catheter outflow blockage may be prevented by flushing the catheter with saline and repositioning of the catheter. Frequent monitoring of the system should be performed by a nurse, an aide or any person with sufficient skills to be able to detect any problems with the patency of the catheter. At the first sign of obstruction, discontinue the irrigation and disconnect the system.

➤*Intrapelvic pressures:* Intrapelvic pressures must be maintained at or below 25 cm of water. The preferred method of pressure control is the insertion of an open Y connection pop-off valve into the infusion line allowing immediate decompression if pressure exceeds 25 cm of water. An alternative method has been proposed to direct or stop the flow of the irrigating solution to prevent increased intrapelvic pressure: Placement of a pinch clamp on the inflow line which can be used by the patient or nurse to stop the irrigation at the first sign of flank pain. However, extreme caution must be taken when relying on cooperation of the patient. Patients may not be sufficiently alert to detect signs and symptoms of outflow obstruction. This is especially true in elderly patients, sedated patients or those with severe neurological dysfunction with varying degrees of sensory loss or motor paralysis.

➤*Monitoring:* Throughout the course of therapy, monitor patients to ensure safety. Obtain serum creatinine phosphate and magnesium every few days. Collect urine specimens for culture and antibacterial sensitivity every 3 days or less and at the first sign of fever. Stop the irrigation if any culture exhibits growth and initiate appropriate antibacterial therapy. The irrigation may be started again after a course of antibacterial therapy upon demonstration of a sterile urine. Struvite calculi frequently contain bacteria within the stone; therefore, continue antibacterial therapy throughout the

CITRIC ACID/GLUCONO-DELTA-LACTONE/ MAGNESIUM CARBONATE (Hemiacidrin) — IRRIGATION

course of dissolution therapy. Hypermagnesemia or an elevated serum creatinine level are indications to halt the irrigation until they return to preirrigation levels. Evidence of severe urothelial edema on X-ray is also an indication for temporarily halting the irrigation until the complication resolves.

➤*Pregnancy: Category C.* It is not known whether hemiacidrin can cause fetal harm when administered to a pregnant woman or can affect reproduction capacity. Give to a pregnant woman only if clearly needed.

➤*Lactation:* Magnesium is known to be excreted into breast milk. However, it is not known whether hemiacidrin is excreted in breast milk. Exercise caution when hemiacidrin is administered to a nursing woman.

Drug Interactions

➤*Magnesium-containing medications:* Concurrent use may contribute to production of hypermagnesemia and is not recommended.

Adverse Reactions

The most common adverse reaction in selected case series is transient flank pain which occurs in most patients. Additional reactions include: Urothelial ulceration or edema (13%); fever (20% but up to 40% in some case series); urinary tract infection, back pain, dysuria, transient hematuria, nausea, hypermagnesemia, hyperphosphatemia, elevated serum creatinine, candidiasis, bladder irritability (1% to 10%); septicemia, ileus, vomiting, thrombophlebitis (less than 1%). Death from sepsis has occurred.

Hexitol Irrigants

Indications

➤*Urologic irrigation:* In transurethral prostatic resection or other transurethral surgical procedures.

Administration and Dosage

Do not use unless solution is clear and seal unbroken. Use as required for irrigation.

➤*Storage/Stability:* Promptly use the contents of opened containers; discard unused portions of the solution. Do not warm above 66°C (150°F). Protect from freezing and avoid storage at temperatures above 40°C (104°F).

Actions

➤*Pharmacology:* Hexitol irrigants are nonelectrolytic and nonhemolytic urologic irrigation solutions. The amount of solution absorbed intravascularly during transurethral prostatic surgery is variable and depends primarily on the extent and duration of the surgery. Mannitol is confined to the extracellular space, only slightly metabolized, rapidly excreted in the urine and is, therefore, an effective osmotic diuretic. The sorbitol-containing products will be metabolized to carbon dioxide (70%) and dextrose (30%) or excreted by the kidneys.

Contraindications

Anuria; injection.

Warnings/Precautions

➤*Special risk:* Use caution in significant cardiopulmonary or renal dysfunction (see Precautions).

➤*Systemic effects:* Irrigating fluids used during transurethral prostatectomy may enter the systemic circulation in relatively large volumes. Therefore, the irrigation solution must be considered as a systemic drug. The osmotic diuresis it may produce can significantly alter cardiopulmonary and renal dynamics.

➤*Diabetes mellitus:* Hyperglycemia from metabolism of sorbitol may occur in patients with diabetes mellitus.

➤*Sorbitol solution:* Use with caution in patients unable to metabolize sorbitol rapidly enough to avoid the development of hyperosmolar states.

➤*Cardiovascular effects:* Carefully evaluate cardiovascular status of the patient, particularly one with cardiac disease, before and during transurethral prostatic resection when mannitol irrigant is used. The quantity of fluid absorbed into systemic circulation may cause expansion of extracellular fluid, leading to fulminating CHF.

➤*Fluid and electrolyte balance:* Systemic absorption of the solutions may cause a shift of sodium-free intracellular fluid into the extracellular compartment, lowering serum sodium concentration and aggravating any preexisting hyponatremia.

A significant diuresis resulting from the irrigating solution may obscure and intensify inadequate hydration or hypovolemia. Excessive loss of water and electrolytes may lead to hypernatremia.

Adverse Reactions

Since significant systemic absorption occurs, the potential for systemic effects must be considered. The following effects have been noted from intravenous infusion:

➤*Cardiovascular:* Pulmonary congestion; hypotension; tachycardia; angina-like pains; thrombophlebitis.

➤*Electrolyte disturbance:* Acidosis; electrolyte loss; marked diuresis; urinary retention; edema; dry mouth; thirst; dehydration.

➤*Miscellaneous:* Blurred vision; convulsions; nausea; vomiting; rhinitis; chills; vertigo; backache; urticaria; diarrhea.

Additional reactions associated with sorbitol solution include slight increases in postoperative serum glucose and inhibition of intestinal absorption of vitamin B_{12}.

MANNITOL

For complete prescribing information, refer to the Mannitol monograph in the Osmotic Diuretics section.

SORBITOL IRRIGATION

Rx	**Sorbitol** (B. Braun Medical)	**Solution:** 3.3% (183 mOsm/L)	In 2,000 mL.
Rx	**Sorbitol** (Travenol)	**Solution:** 3% (165 mOsm/L)	In 1,500 and 3,000 mL.

SORBITOL — IRRIGATION

For complete and comparative prescribing information, refer to the Hexitol Irrigants group monograph.

MANNITOL/SORBITOL

Rx	**Sorbitol-Mannitol** (Hospira)	**Solution:** 0.54 g mannitol and 2.7 g sorbitol/100 mL (178 mOsm/L)	In 1,500 and 3,000 mL.

MANNITOL/SORBITOL — IRRIGATION

For complete and comparative prescribing information, refer to the Hexitol Irrigants group monograph.

GENITOURINARY IRRIGANTS

ACETIC ACID IRRIGATION

Rx	**Acetic Acid Irrigation** (Various, eg, Hospira)	**Solution:** 0.25%	In 250, 500 and 1,000 mL.

ACETIC ACID — IRRIGATION

Indications

➤*Bladder irrigation:* For bladder irrigation.

Administration and Dosage

Acetic acid 0.25% irrigation may be administered by gravity drip via an administration set connected to an indwelling catheter designed for continuous or intermittent 2-way flow. A disposable dispensing set should be used. A bulb or piston syringe may be used for periodic irrigation of an indwelling catheter.

For continuous or intermittent irrigation, the rate of administration will correspond roughly to the rate of urine flow and should be adjusted to maintain a urinary effluent pH of 4.5 to 5. Nitrazine or other pH paper may be used to monitor pH, preferably at least 4 times daily. Drip rate should be adjusted as necessary to maintain desired pH; increasing flow rate reduces pH value and vice versa. With continuous or intermittent irrigation, each patient will require a volume of approximately 500 to 1,500 mL per 24 hours.

For periodic irrigation of an indwelling catheter to maintain patency, about 50 mL is required for each irrigation and may be administered using a bulb or piston syringe for injection and aspiration as often as desired.

Parenteral drug products should be inspected visually for particulate matter and discoloration prior to administration, whenever solution and container permit.

➤*Storage/Stability:* Exposure of pharmaceutical products to heat should be minimized. Avoid excessive heat. Protect from freezing. Store at 20° to 25°C (68° to 77°F).

ACETIC ACID — IRRIGATION

Warnings/Precautions

➤*Pregnancy: Category C.* Animal reproduction studies have not been conducted with acetic acid irrigation. It is also not known whether acetic acid irrigation can cause fetal harm when administered to a pregnant woman or can affect reproduction capacity. Acetic acid irrigation should be given to a pregnant woman only if clearly needed.

➤*Lactation:* Caution should be exercised when acetic acid irrigation is administered to a breast-feeding woman.

GLYCINE (AMINOACETIC ACID)

Rx	**Glycine for Irrigation** (Various, eg, Hospira)	**Solution:** 1.5%	In 1500, 2000, 3000, 4000 and 5000 mL.

GLYCINE — IRRIGATION

Indications

➤*Urologic irrigation:* Glycine irrigation 1.5% is indicated for use as irrigating fluid during transurethral prostatic resection and other transurethral surgical procedures.

Administration and Dosage

➤*Adults:*

Irrigant for transurethral surgical procedures – The total volume of solution used for irrigation is solely at the discretion of the surgeon.

➤*Renal function impairment:* Do not use in patients with anuria.

➤*Administration:* For urologic irrigation only. Not for injection by usual parenteral routes. Glycine should be administered only by transurethral instillation with appropriate urologic instrumentation. Aseptic technique is essential with the use of sterile solutions for irrigation.

A disposable irrigation set should be used. The administration set should be attached promptly. A fresh container of appropriate size should be used for the start-up of each cycle or repeat procedure. Height of container(s) above the operating table in excess of 60 cm (approximately 2 ft) has been reported to increase intravascular absorption of the irrigating fluid.

➤*Admixture compatibility:* Additives may be incompatible. When introducing additives, use aseptic technique, mix thoroughly and do not store.

➤*Storage/Stability:* Store at 25°C (77°F). Avoid excessive heat. Protect from freezing. Do not heat container above 66°C (150°F). Unused portions should be discarded.

SODIUM CHLORIDE IRRIGATION

Rx	**Sodium Chloride for Irrigation** (Various, eg, Abbott, Kendall McGaw)	**Solution (Isotonic):** 0.9%	In 150, 250, 500, 1000, 1500, 2000 and 4000 mL.
Rx	**Sodium Chloride for Irrigation** (Various, eg, Abbott)	**Solution (Hypotonic):** 0.45%	In 500, 1000 and 1500 mL.

STERILE WATER IRRIGATION

Rx	**Sterile Water for Irrigation** (Various, eg, Abbott)	In 250, 500, 1,000, 2,000 and 4,000 mL.

STERILE WATER — IRRIGATION

Indications

➤*Irrigation:* For use as an irrigating solution.

CYSTINE-DEPLETING AGENTS

CYSTEAMINE BITARTRATE

Refer to the Cysteamine bitartrate monograph in the Endocrine Metabolic Agents chapter for full prescribing information.

TIOPRONIN

Rx	**Thiola** (Mission)	**Tablets:** 100 mg	(Mission SS 121). White. Sugar coated. In 100s.

TIOPRONIN — ORAL

Indications

➤*Kidney stones:* For the prevention of cystine (kidney) stone formation in patients with severe homozygous cystinuria with urinary cystine greater than 500 mg/day, who are resistant to treatment with conservative measures of high fluid intake, alkali and diet modification, or who have adverse reactions to d-penicillamine.

Administration and Dosage

➤*General dosing considerations:* A conservative treatment program should be attempted first. (See Conservative treatment program.)

The dose should not be arbitrary but should be based on that amount required to reduce urinary cystine concentration to below its solubility limit (generally less than 250 mg/L). The extent of the decline in cystine excretion is generally dependent on the tiopronin dosage. Urinary cystine should be measured at 1 month after tiopronin treatment and every 3 months thereafter.

➤*Adults:*

Kidney stones –

Initial dosage: 800 mg 3 times/day.

Dosage adjustment: Dosage should be readjusted depending on the urinary cystine value. In a multiclinic trial, average dose was approximately 1,000 mg/day. However, some patients require a smaller dose.

Conversion: Tiopronin may also be substituted for d-penicillamine in patients who have developed toxicity to the latter drug. In these patients, tiopronin might be started at a lower dosage. The conservative treatment program should be continued.

➤*Children:*

Kidney stones –

9 years of age and older:

- *Initial dosage* – 15 mg/kg/day.
- *Dosage adjustment* – Dosage should be readjusted depending on the urinary cystine value.

➤*Conservative treatment program:* At least 3 L of fluid (ten 10 oz glassfuls) should be provided, including 2 glasses with each meal and at bedtime. The patients should be expected to awake at night to urinate; they should drink 2 more glasses of fluids before returning to bed. Additional fluids should be consumed if there is excessive sweating or intestinal fluid loss. A minimum urine output of 2 L/day on a consistent basis should be sought. A modest amount of alkali should be provided in order to maintain urinary pH at a high normal range (6.5 to 7). Potassium alkali is advantageous over sodium alkali because they do not cause hypercalciuria and are less likely to cause the complication of calcium stones. Excessive alkali therapy is not advisable. When urinary pH increases above 7 with alkali therapy, the complication of calcium phosphate nephrolithiasis may ensue because of the enhanced urinary supersaturation of hydroxyapatite in an alkaline environment.

In patients who continue to form cystine stones on the conservative program, tiopronin may be added to the treatment program.

➤*Administration:* Administer at least 1 hour before or 2 hours after meals.

➤*Storage/Stability:* Store at 25°C (77°F); excursions are permitted to 15° to 30°C (59° to 86°F).

Actions

➤*Pharmacology:* Tiopronin is an active reducing agent which undergoes thiol-disulfide exchange with cystine to form a mixed disulfide of Thiola-cysteine.

From this reaction, a water-soluble mixed disulfide is formed and the amount of sparingly soluble cystine is reduced.

➤*Pharmacokinetics:* When tiopronin is given orally, up to 48% of dose appears in urine during the first 4 hours and up to 78% by 72 hours. Thus, in patients with cystinuria, sufficient amount of tiopronin or its active metabolites could appear in urine to react with cystine, lowering cystine excretion.

The decrement in urinary cystine produced by tiopronin is generally proportional to the dose. A reduction in urinary cystine of 250 to 350 mg/day at a tiopronin dosage of 1 g/day, and a decline of approximately 500 mg/day at a dosage of 2 g/day, might be expected. Tiopronin causes a sustained reduction in cystine excretion without apparent loss of effectiveness. Tiopronin has a rapid onset and offset of action, showing a fall in cystine excretion on the first day of administration and a rise on the first day of drug withdrawal.

TIOPRONIN — ORAL

Contraindications

The use of tiopronin during pregnancy is contraindicated, except in those with severe cystinuria where the anticipated benefit of inhibited stone formation clearly outweighs possible hazards of treatment (see Warnings).

Tiopronin should not be begun again in patients with a history of developing agranulocytosis, aplastic anemia or thrombocytopenia on this medication.

Mothers maintained on tiopronin treatment should not nurse their infants.

Warnings/Precautions

➤*Hematologic effects:* Leukopenia of the granulocytic series may develop without eosinophilia. Thrombocytopenia may be immunologic in origin or occur on an idiosyncratic basis. The reduction in peripheral blood white count to less than 3500/mm^3 or in platelet count to below 100,000 mm^3 mandates cessation of therapy. Patients should be instructed to report promptly the occurrence of any symptom or sign of these hematological abnormalities, such as fever, sore throat, chills, bleeding or easy bruisability.

Despite apparent lower toxicity of tiopronin, tiopronin may potentially cause all the serious adverse reactions reported for d-penicillamine. Thus, although no death has been reported to result directly from tiopronin treatment, a fatal outcome from tiopronin is possible, as has been reported with d-penicillamine therapy from such complications as aplastic anemia, agranulocytosis, thrombocytopenia, Goodpasture's syndrome or myasthenia gravis.

➤*Proteinuria:* Proteinuria, sometimes sufficiently severe to cause nephrotic syndrome, may develop from membranous glomerulopathy. A close observation of affected patients is mandatory.

➤*Complications:* The following complications, though rare, have been reported during d-penicillamine therapy and could occur during tiopronin treatment. When there are abnormal urinary findings associated with hemoptysis and pulmonary infiltrates suggestive of Goodpasture's syndrome, tiopronin treatment should be stopped. Appearance of myasthenic syndrome or myasthenia gravis requires cessation of treatment. When pemphigus-type reactions develop, tiopronin therapy should be stopped. Steroid treatment may be necessary.

➤*Complications:* Patients should be advised of the potential development of complications and to report promptly the occurrence of any symptom or sign of them.

➤*Pregnancy: Category C.* D-penicillamine has been shown to cause skeletal defects and cleft palates in the fetus when given to pregnant rats at 10 times the dose recommended for human use. A similar teratogenicity might be expected for tiopronin although no such findings could be related to the drug in studies in mice and rats at doses up to 10 times the highest recommended human dose. There are no adequate and well-controlled studies in pregnant women. Tiopronin should be used during pregnancy only if the potential benefit justifies potential risk to the fetus.

➤*Lactation:* Because tiopronin may be excreted in milk and because of the potential serious adverse reactions of nursing infants from tiopronin, mothers taking tiopronin should not nurse their infants.

➤*Children:* Safety and effectiveness below the age of 9 years have not been established.

➤*Monitoring:* To help monitor potential complications, the following tests are recommended: peripheral blood counts, direct platelet count, hemoglobin, serum albumin, liver function tests, 24-hour urinary protein and routine urinalysis at 3– to 6–month intervals during treatment. In order to assess effect on stone disease, urinary cystine analysis should be monitored frequently during the first 6 months when the optimum dose schedule is being determined, and at 6-month intervals thereafter. Abdominal roentogenogram (KUB) is advised on a yearly basis to monitor the size and appearance/disappearance of stone(s).

Adverse Reactions

Some patients may develop drug fever, usually during the first month of therapy. Tiopronin treatment should be discontinued until the fever subsides. It may be reinstated at a small dose, with a gradual increase in dosage until the desired level is achieved.

A generalized rash (erythematous, maculopapular or morbilliform) accompanied by pruritus may develop during the first few months of treatment. It may be controlled by antihistamine therapy, typically recedes when tiopronin treatment is discontinued, and seldom recurs when tiopronin treatment is restarted at a lower dosage. Less commonly, rash may appear late in the course of treatment (of more than 6 months). Located usually in the trunk, the late rash is associated with intense pruritus, recedes slowly after discontinuing treatment, and usually recurs upon resumption of treatment.

A drug reaction simulating lupus erythematous, manifested by fever, arthralgia and lymphadenopathy may develop. It may be associated with a positive antinuclear antibody test, but not necessarily with nephropathy. It may require discontinuance of tiopronin treatment.

A reduction in taste perception may develop. It is believed to be the result of chelation of trace metals by tiopronin. Hypogeusia is often self-limiting.

Unlike during d-penicillamine therapy, vitamin B_6 deficiency is uncommonly associated with tiopronin treatment.

Some patients may complain of wrinkling and friability of skin. This complication usually occurs after long-term treatment, and is believed to result from the effect of tiopronin on collagen.

A multiclinic trial involving 66 cystinuric patients in the United States indicated that tiopronin is associated with fewer or less severe adverse reactions than d-penicillamine. Among those who had to stop taking d-penicillamine due to toxicity, 64.7% could take tiopronin. In those without history of d-penicillamine treatment, only 5.9% developed reactions of sufficient severity to require tiopronin withdrawal. A review of available literature supports the findings from this trial.

Despite this apparent reduced toxicity to tiopronin relative to d-penicillamine, tiopronin treatment may potentially be associated with all the adverse reactions reported with d-penicillamine. They include:

➤*CNS:* Myasthenic syndrome in about 1 in 50 patients.

➤*Dermatologic:* Pharyngitis, oral ulcers, rash, ecchymosis, pruritus, urticaria, warts, skin wrinkling, pemphigus, elastosis perforans serpiginosa in about 1 in 6 patients.

➤*GI:* Nausea, emesis, diarrhea or soft stools, anorexia, abdominal pain, bloating or flatus in about 1 in 6 patients.

➤*Hematologic:* Increased bleeding, anemia, leukopenia, thrombocytopenia, eosinophilia in about 1 in 25 patients.

➤*Hepatic:* Jaundice and abnormal liver function tests have been reported during tiopronin therapy for non-cystinuric conditions. A direct cause and effect relationship, based upon these foreign reports, has not been established. Although such complications were not encountered in the small multi-center trials in the United States, patients should be carefully monitored and if any abnormalities are noted, the drug should be discontinued and the patient treated by appropriate measures.

➤*Hypersensitivity:* Laryngeal edema, dyspnea, respiratory distress, fever, chills, arthralgia, weakness, fatigue, myalgia, adenopathy in about 1 in 25 patients.

➤*Pulmonary:* Bronchiolitis, hemoptysis, pulmonary infiltrates, dyspnea in about 1 in 50 patients.

➤*Renal:* Proteinuria, nephrotic syndrome, hematuria in about 1 in 20 patients.

➤*Special senses:* Impairment in taste and smell in about 1 in 25 patients.

These reactions are more likely to develop during tiopronin therapy among patients who had previously shown toxicity to d-penicillamine.

In patients who had previously manifested adverse reactions to d-penicillamine, adverse reactions to tiopronin are more likely to occur than in patients who took tiopronin for the first time. A close supervision with a careful monitoring of potential side effects is mandatory during tiopronin treatment. Patients should be told to report promptly any symptoms suggesting toxicity. The treatment with tiopronin should be stopped if severe toxicity develops.

PENICILLAMINE

Rx	**Cuprimine** (Aton Pharma)	**Capsules; oral:** 250 mg	Lactose. (MSD 602). Ivory. In 100s.
Rx	**Depen** (Wallace)	**Tablets, titratable; oral:** 250 mg	Lactose, EDTA. (37-4401). Oval, scored. In 100s.

PENICILLAMINE — ORAL

WARNING

Physicians planning to use penicillamine should thoroughly familiarize themselves with its toxicity, special dosage considerations, and therapeutic benefits. Penicillamine should never be used casually. Each patient should remain constantly under the close supervision of the physician. Patients should be warned to report promptly any symptoms suggesting toxicity.

Indications

➤*Rheumatoid arthritis:* For the treatment of patients with severe, active rheumatoid arthritis who have failed to respond to an adequate trial of conventional therapy.

Because penicillamine can cause severe adverse reactions, restrict its use in rheumatoid arthritis to patients who have severe, active disease and who have failed to respond to an adequate trial of conventional therapy. Even then, carefully consider the benefit-to-risk ratio. Use other measures, such as rest, physiotherapy, salicylates, and corticosteroids, when indicated, in conjunction with penicillamine.

Administration and Dosage

➤*General dosing considerations:* Because penicillamine increases the requirement for pyridoxine, patients may require a daily supplement of pyridoxine.

➤*Adults:*

Cystinuria –

Usual dosage: 2 g/day; range, 1 to 4 g/day.
Initial dosage: 250 mg/day and increase gradually.
Maintenance dosage: Must be individualized to an amount that limits cystine excretion to 100 to 200 mg/day in those with no history of stones, and below 100 mg/day in those who have had stone formation and/or pain.

PENICILLAMINE — ORAL

Alternative dosage: If 4 equal doses are not feasible, give the larger portion at bedtime. If adverse reactions necessitate a reduction in dosage, it is important to retain the bedtime dose.

Concomitant therapy: It is recommended that penicillamine be used along with conventional therapy. In addition to taking penicillamine, patients should drink copiously. It is especially important to drink about a pint of fluid at bedtime and another pint once during the night when urine is more concentrated and more acidic than during the day. The greater the fluid intake, the lower the required dosage of penicillamine.

Rheumatoid arthritis –

Maximum dose: 1.5 g daily.

Initial dosage: 125 or 250 mg once daily.

Dosage titration: Increase at 1- to 3-month intervals, by 125 or 250 mg/day, as patient response and tolerance indicate. If there is no improvement and there are no signs of potentially serious toxicity after 2 to 3 months of treatment with doses of 500 to 750 mg/day, increases of 250 mg/day at 2- to 3-month intervals may be continued until a satisfactory remission occurs or signs of toxicity develop. In those patients who do respond, but who evidence incomplete suppression of their disease after the first 6 to 9 months of treatment, the daily dosage may be increased by 125 or 250 mg/day at 3-month intervals.

Maintenance dosage: 500 to 700 mg/day. If a satisfactory remission of symptoms is achieved, continue the dose associated with the remission. Changes in maintenance dosage levels may not be reflected clinically or in the erythrocyte sedimentation rate for 2 to 3 months after each dosage adjustment.

Rechallenge: When treatment with penicillamine has been interrupted because of adverse reactions or other reasons, reintroduce the drug cautiously by starting with a lower dosage and increasing slowly.

Duration of therapy: The optimum duration of therapy has not been determined. If the patient has been in remission for 6 months or more, a gradual, stepwise dosage reduction in decrements of 125 or 250 mg/day at approximately 3-month intervals may be attempted.

Concomitant therapy: Do not use penicillamine in patients who are receiving gold therapy, antimalarial or cytotoxic drugs, oxyphenbutazone, or phenylbutazone. Other measures, such as salicylates, other nonsteroidal anti-inflammatory drugs, or systemic corticosteroids, may be continued when penicillamine is initiated. After improvement commences, analgesic and anti-inflammatory drugs may be slowly discontinued as symptoms permit. Steroid withdrawal must be done gradually, and many months of treatment with penicillamine may be required before steroids can be completely eliminated.

Discontinuation of therapy: If there is no discernible improvement after 3 to 4 months of treatment with 1,000 to 1,500 mg/day, it may be assumed the patient will not respond and penicillamine should be discontinued.

Management of exacerbations: Patients may experience an exacerbation of disease activity following an initial good response. These may be self-limited and can subside within 12 weeks. They are usually controlled by the addition of nonsteroidal anti-inflammatory drugs, and only if the patient has demonstrated a true "escape" phenomenon (as evidenced by failure of the flare to subside within this time period) should an increase in the maintenance dose ordinarily be considered.

Wilson disease – Optimal dosage can be determined by measurement of urinary copper excretion and the determination of free copper in the serum. The urine must be collected in copper-free glassware, and should be quantitatively analyzed for copper before and soon after initiation of therapy with penicillamine. Determination of 24–hour urinary copper excretion is of greatest value in the first week of therapy. In the absence of drug reactions, continue a dose between 0.75 and 1.5 g that results in an initial 24-hour cupriuresis of over 2 mg for about 3 months.

Maximum dose: It is seldom necessary to exceed a dosage of 2 g/day.

Alternative dosage: In patients who cannot tolerate as much as 1 g/day initially, initiate with 250 mg/day, and increase gradually.

Monitoring: The most reliable method of monitoring maintenance treatment is the determination of free copper in the serum. This equals the difference between quantitatively determined total copper and ceruloplasmin-copper. Adequately treated patients will usually have less than 10 mcg free copper/dL of serum.

➤*Children:*

Cystinuria – 30 mg/kg/day divided into 4 doses. Titrate doses so that urinary cystine excretion is maintained at less than 100 to 200 mg/day.

Off-label dosing –

Arsenic poisoning:

- *Usual dose* – 25 mg/kg every 6 hours for 5 days.
- *Maximum dose* – 1 g/day.

Juvenile rheumatoid arthritis: 5 mg/kg once daily (or 2.5 mg/kg twice daily) for 2 months followed by 10 mg/kg once daily (or 5 mg/kg twice daily) for 4 months.

- *Concomitant therapy* – Pyridoxine 25 to 50 mg/day.

Lead poisoning (third-line therapy):

- *Usual dose* – 30 to 40 mg/kg/day (or 600 to 750 mg/m^2/day) divided 3 to 4 times a day.
- *Maximum dose* – 1.5 g/day.
- *Duration of therapy* – 1 to 6 months.

Wilson disease:

- *Usual dose* – 20 mg/kg/day divided 2 to 4 times a day. Urinary copper excretion should be titrated to greater than 1 mg/day.
- *Maximum dose* – 1 g/day.
- *Concomitant therapy* – Pyridoxine 25 to 50 mg/day.

➤*Administration:* Give on an empty stomach, at least 1 hour before meals or 2 hours after meals, and at least 1 hour apart from any other drug, food, or milk.

Dosages up to 500 mg/day can be given as a single daily dose. Administer dosages in excess of 500 mg/day in divided doses.

➤*Storage/Stability:* Store at 59° to 86°F. Protect from moisture.

Actions

➤*Pharmacology:* Penicillamine is a chelating agent recommended for the removal of excess copper in patients with Wilson's disease. From in vitro studies which indicate that 1 atom of copper combines with 2 molecules of penicillamine, it would appear that 1 g of penicillamine should be followed by the excretion of about 200 mg of copper; however, the actual amount excreted is about 1% of this.

Penicillamine also reduces excess cystine excretion in cystinuria. This is done, at least in part, by disulfide interchange between penicillamine and cystine, resulting in formation of penicillamine-cysteine disulfide, a substance that is much more soluble than cystine and is excreted readily.

Penicillamine interferes with the formation of cross-links between tropocollagen molecules and cleaves them when newly formed.

The mechanism of action of penicillamine in rheumatoid arthritis is unknown although it appears to suppress disease activity. Unlike cytotoxic immunosuppressants, penicillamine markedly lowers IgM rheumatoid factor but produces no significant depression in absolute levels of serum immunoglobulins. Also unlike cytotoxic immunosuppressants which act on both, penicillamine in vitro depresses T-cell activity but not B-cell activity.

In vitro, penicillamine dissociates macroglobulins (rheumatoid factor) although the relationship of the activity to its effect in rheumatoid arthritis is not known.

In rheumatoid arthritis, the onset of therapeutic response to penicillamine may not be seen for 2 or 3 months. In those patients who respond, however, the first evidence of suppression of symptoms such as pain, tenderness, and swelling is generally apparent within 3 months. The optimum duration of therapy has not been determined. If remissions occur, they may last from months to years, but usually require continued treatment.

In all patients receiving penicillamine, it is important that penicillamine be given on an empty stomach, at least 1 hour before meals or 2 hours after meals, and at least 1 hour apart from any other drug, food, or milk. This permits maximum absorption and reduces the likelihood of inactivation by metal binding in the gastrointestinal tract.

➤*Pharmacokinetics:*

Absorption – Penicillamine is absorbed rapidly but incompletely (40% to 70%) from the gastrointestinal tract, with wide interindividual variations. Food, antacids, and iron reduce absorption of the drug. The peak plasma concentration of penicillamine occurs 1 to 3 hours after ingestion; it is approximately 1 to 2 mg/L after an oral dose of 250 mg. The drug appears in the plasma as free penicillamine, penicillamine disulfide, and cysteine-penicillamine disulfide. When prolonged treatment is stopped, there is a slow elimination phase lasting 4 to 6 days.

More than 80% of plasma penicillamine is bound to proteins. The drug also binds to erythrocytes and macrophages.

Metabolism/Excretion – A small fraction of the dose is metabolized in the liver to s-methyl-D-penicillamine. Drug excretion is primarily renal, mainly as disulfides.

Contraindications

Except for the treatment of Wilson's disease or certain cases of cystinuria, use of penicillamine during pregnancy is contraindicated.

Although breast milk studies have not been reported in animals or humans, mothers on therapy with penicillamine should not nurse their infants.

Patients with a history of penicillamine-related aplastic anemia or agranulocytosis should not be restarted on penicillamine.

Because of its potential for causing renal damage, penicillamine should not be administered to rheumatoid arthritis patients with a history or other evidence of renal insufficiency.

Warnings/Precautions

➤*Fatalities:* The use of penicillamine has been associated with fatalities due to certain diseases such as aplastic anemia, agranulocytosis, thrombocytopenia, Goodpasture's syndrome, and myasthenia gravis.

➤*Hematologic effects:* Leukopenia and thrombocytopenia have been reported to occur in up to 5% of patients during penicillamine therapy. Leukopenia is of the granulocytic series and may or may not be associated with an increase in eosinophils. A confirmed reduction in WBC below 3,500/mm^3 mandates discontinuance of penicillamine therapy. Thrombocytopenia may be on an idiosyncratic basis, with decreased or absent megakaryocytes in the marrow, when it is part of an aplastic anemia. In other cases the thrombocytopenia is presumably on an immune basis since the number of megakaryocytes in the marrow has been reported to be normal or sometimes increased. The development of a platelet count below 100,000/mm^3, even in the absence of clinical bleeding, requires at least temporary cessation of penicillamine therapy. A progressive fall in either platelet count or WBC in 3 successive determinations, even though values are still within the normal range, likewise requires at least temporary cessation.

➤*Goodpasture's syndrome:* Goodpasture's syndrome has occurred rarely. The development of abnormal urinary findings associated with hemoptysis and pulmonary infiltrates on x-ray requires immediate cessation of penicillamine.

➤*Obliterative bronchiolitis:* Obliterative bronchiolitis has been reported rarely. Caution the patient to report immediately pulmonary symptoms such as exertional dyspnea, unexplained cough or wheezing. Pulmonary function studies should be considered at that time.

PENICILLAMINE — ORAL

➤*CNS effects:* Onset of new neurologic symptoms has been reported with penicillamine. Occasionally, neurologic symptoms become worse during initiation of therapy with penicillamine. Myasthenic syndrome sometimes progressing to myasthenia gravis has been reported. Ptosis and diplopia, with weakness of the extraocular muscles, are often early signs of myasthenia. In the majority of cases, symptoms of myasthenia have receded after withdrawal of penicillamine.

➤*Pemphigus vulgaris:* Most of the various forms of pemphigus have occurred during treatment with penicillamine. Pemphigus vulgaris and pemphigus foliaceus are reported most frequently, usually as a late complication of therapy. The seborrhea-like characteristics of pemphigus foliaceus may obscure an early diagnosis. When pemphigus is suspected, discontinue penicillamine. Treatment has consisted of high doses of corticosteroids alone or, in some cases, concomitantly with an immunosuppressant. Treatment may be required for only a few weeks or months, but may need to be continued for more than a year.

➤*Administration:* Once instituted for Wilson's disease or cystinuria, treatment with penicillamine should, as a rule, be continued on a daily basis. Interruptions for even a few days have been followed by sensitivity reactions after reinstitution of therapy.

➤*Drug fever:* Some patients may experience drug fever, a marked febrile response to penicillamine, usually in the second to third week following initiation of therapy. Drug fever may sometimes be accompanied by a macular cutaneous eruption.

In the case of drug fever in patients with Wilson's disease or cystinuria, temporarily discontinue penicillamine until the reaction subsides. Then reinstitute penicillamine with a small dose that is gradually increased until the desired dosage is attained. Systemic steroid therapy may be necessary, and is usually helpful, in such patients in whom drug fever and rash develop several times.

In the case of drug fever in rheumatoid arthritis patients, because other treatments are available, discontinue penicillamine and try another therapeutic alternative. Experience indicates that the febrile reaction will recur in a very high percentage of patients upon readministration of penicillamine.

➤*Antibody development:* Certain patients will develop a positive antinuclear antibody (ANA) test and some of these may show a lupus erythematosus-like syndrome similar to drug-induced lupus associated with other drugs. The lupus erythematosus-like syndrome is not associated with hypocomplementemia and may be present without nephropathy. The development of a positive ANA test does not mandate discontinuance of the drug; however, be alert to the possibility that a lupus erythematosus-like syndrome may develop in the future.

➤*Oral ulcerations:* Some patients may develop oral ulcerations which in some cases have the appearance of aphthous stomatitis. The stomatitis usually recurs on rechallenge but often clears on a lower dosage. Although rare, cheilosis, glossitis and gingivostomatitis have also been reported. These oral lesions are frequently dose-related and may preclude further increase in penicillamine dosage or require discontinuation of the drug.

➤*Hypogeusia:* Hypogeusia (a blunting or diminution in taste perception) has occurred in some patients. This may last 2 to 3 months or more and may develop into a total loss of taste; however, it is usually self-limited despite continued penicillamine treatment. Such taste impairment is rare in patients with Wilson's disease.

➤*Concomitant medications:* See Drug Interactions for more information.

➤*Cross-sensitivity:* Patients who are allergic to penicillin may theoretically have cross-sensitivity to penicillamine. The possibility of reactions from contamination of penicillamine by trace amounts of penicillin has been eliminated now that penicillamine is being produced synthetically rather than as a degradation product of penicillin.

➤*Vitamin supplementation:* Give patients with Wilson's disease or cystinuria 25 mg/day pyridoxine during therapy, since penicillamine increases the requirement for this vitamin. Patients also may receive benefit from a multivitamin preparation, although there is no evidence that deficiency of any vitamin other than pyridoxine is associated with penicillamine. In Wilson's disease, multivitamin preparations must be copper-free.

Rheumatoid arthritis patients whose nutrition is impaired should also be given a daily supplement of pyridoxine. Do not give mineral supplements because they may block the response to penicillamine.

Iron deficiency may develop, especially in pediatric patients and in menstruating women. In Wilson's disease, this may be a result of adding the effects of the low copper diet, which is probably also low in iron, and the penicillamine to the effects of blood loss or growth. In cystinuria, a low methionine diet may contribute to iron deficiency, since it is necessarily low in protein. If necessary, iron may be given in short courses, but a period of 2 hours should elapse between administration of penicillamine and iron, since oral iron has been shown to reduce the effects of penicillamine.

➤*Collagen and elastin effects:* Penicillamine causes an increase in the amount of soluble collagen. In the rat this results in inhibition of normal healing and also a decrease in tensile strength of intact skin. In man this may be the cause of increased skin friability at sites especially subject to pressure or trauma, such as shoulders, elbows, knees, toes, and buttocks. Extravasations of blood may occur and may appear as purpuric areas, with external bleeding if the skin is broken, or as vesicles containing dark blood. Neither type is progressive. There is no apparent association with bleeding elsewhere in the body and no associated coagulation defect has been found. Therapy with penicillamine may be continued in the presence of these lesions. They may not recur if dosage is reduced. Other reported effects probably due to the action of penicillamine on collagen are excessive wrinkling of the skin and development of small, white papules at venipuncture and surgical sites.

The effects of penicillamine on collagen and elastin make it advisable to consider a reduction in dosage to 250 mg/day, when surgery is contemplated. Delay reinstitution of full therapy until wound healing is complete.

➤*Hypersensitivity reactions:* Observe the skin and mucous membranes for allergic reactions. Early and late rashes have occurred. Early rash occurs during the first few months of treatment and is more common. It is usually a generalized pruritic, erythematous, maculopapular, or morbilliform rash and resembles the allergic rash seen with other drugs. Early rash usually disappears within days after stopping penicillamine and seldom recurs when the drug is restarted at a lower dosage. Pruritus and early rash may often be controlled by the concomitant administration of antihistamines. Less commonly, a late rash may be seen, usually after 6 months or more of treatment, and requires discontinuation of penicillamine. It is usually on the trunk, is accompanied by intense pruritus, and is usually unresponsive to topical corticosteroid therapy. Late rash may take weeks to disappear after penicillamine is stopped and usually recurs if the drug is restarted.

The appearance of a drug eruption accompanied by fever, arthralgia, lymphadenopathy, or other allergic manifestations usually requires discontinuation of penicillamine.

➤*Renal function impairment:* Proteinuria and/or hematuria may develop during therapy and may be warning signs of membranous glomerulopathy which can progress to a nephrotic syndrome. Close observation of these patients is essential. In some patients the proteinuria disappears with continued therapy; in others, penicillamine must be discontinued. When a patient develops proteinuria or hematuria, the physician must ascertain whether it is a sign of drug-induced glomerulopathy or is unrelated to penicillamine.

Rheumatoid arthritis patients who develop moderate degrees of proteinuria may be continued cautiously on penicillamine therapy, provided that quantitative 24-hour urinary protein determinations are obtained at intervals of 1 to 2 weeks. Do not increase the penicillamine dosage under these circumstances. Proteinuria which exceeds 1 g per 24 hours, or proteinuria which is progressively increasing, requires either discontinuance of the drug or a reduction in the dosage. In some patients, proteinuria has been reported to clear following reduction in dosage.

In rheumatoid arthritis patients, penicillamine should be discontinued if unexplained gross hematuria or persistent microscopic hematuria develops.

In patients with Wilson's disease or cystinuria, the risks of continued penicillamine therapy in patients manifesting potentially serious urinary abnormalities must be weighed against the expected therapeutic benefits.

Up to 1 year or more may be required for any urinary abnormalities to disappear after penicillamine has been discontinued.

➤*Pregnancy:* Category D (per Briggs' *Drugs in Pregnancy and Lactation*). Penicillamine has been shown to be teratogenic in rats when given in doses 6 times higher than the highest dose recommended for human use. Skeletal defects, cleft palates and fetal toxicity (resorptions) have been reported.

There are no controlled studies on the use of penicillamine in pregnant women. Although normal outcomes have been reported, characteristic congenital cutis laxa and associated birth defects have been reported in infants born of mothers who received therapy with penicillamine during pregnancy. Use penicillamine in women of childbearing potential only when the expected benefits outweigh the possible hazards. Apprise women on therapy with penicillamine who are of childbearing potential of this risk. Advise them to report promptly any missed menstrual periods or other indications of possible pregnancy, and to follow closely for early recognition of pregnancy.

See Contraindications for more information.

Wilson's disease – Reported experience shows that continued treatment with penicillamine throughout pregnancy protects the mother against relapse of the Wilson's disease, and that discontinuation of penicillamine has deleterious effects on the mother.

If penicillamine is administered during pregnancy to patients with Wilson's disease, it is recommended that the daily dosage be limited to 750 mg. If cesarean section is planned, reduce the daily dose to 250 mg, but not lower, for the last 6 weeks of pregnancy and postoperatively until wound healing is complete.

Cystinuria – If possible, do not give penicillamine during pregnancy to women with cystinuria. There are reports of women with cystinuria on therapy with penicillamine who gave birth to infants with generalized connective tissue defects who died following abdominal surgery. If stones continue to form in these patients, the benefits of therapy to the mother must be evaluated against the risk to the fetus.

Rheumatoid arthritis – Do not administer penicillamine to rheumatoid arthritis patients who are pregnant, and discontinue the drug promptly in patients in whom pregnancy is suspected or diagnosed.

There is a report that a woman with rheumatoid arthritis treated with less than 1 g a day of penicillamine during pregnancy gave birth (cesarean delivery) to an infant with growth retardation, flattened face with broad nasal bridge, low set ears, short neck with loose skin folds, and unusually lax body skin.

➤*Lactation:* Although breast milk studies have not been reported in animals or humans, mothers on therapy with penicillamine should not nurse their infants.

➤*Children:* The efficacy of penicillamine in juvenile rheumatoid arthritis has not been established.

PENICILLAMINE — ORAL

➤*Monitoring:* Because of the potential for serious hematological and renal adverse reactions to occur at any time, routine urinalysis, white and differential blood cell count, hemoglobin determination, and direct platelet count must be done twice weekly, together with monitoring of the patient's skin, lymph nodes and body temperature, during the first month of therapy, every 2 weeks for the next 5 months, and monthly thereafter. Patients should be instructed to report promptly the development of signs and symptoms of granulocytopenia and/or thrombocytopenia such as fever, sore throat, chills, bruising, or bleeding. The above laboratory studies should then be promptly repeated.

When penicillamine is used in cystinuria, an annual x-ray for renal stones is advised. Cystine stones form rapidly, sometimes in 6 months.

Because of rare reports of intrahepatic cholestasis and toxic hepatitis, liver function tests are recommended every 6 months for the duration of therapy. In Wilson's disease, these are recommended every 3 months, at least during the first year of treatment.

Drug Interactions

Penicillamine Drug Interactions

Precipitant drug	Object drug[a]		Description
Penicillamine	Digoxin	↓	Digoxin serum levels may be reduced, possibly decreasing its pharmacological effects. The digoxin dose may need to be increased.
Penicillamine	Gold therapy, antimalarial or cytotoxic drugs, oxyphenbutazone or pheylbutazone	↑	Do not use these drugs in patients who are concurrently receiving penicillamine. These drugs are associated with similar serious hematologic and renal reactions.
Penicillamine	Gold salts	↑	Patients who have had **gold salt** therapy discontinued due to a major toxic reaction may be at greater risk of serious adverse reactions with penicillamine, but not necessarily of the same type. However, this is controversial.
Antacids	Penicillamine	↓	The absorption of penicillamine is decreased by 66% with coadministration of antacids.
Iron salts	Penicillamine	↓	The absorption of penicillamine is decreased by 35% with coadministration of iron salts.

[a] ↑ = Object drug increased. ↓ = Object drug decreased.

➤*Drug/Food interactions:* The absorption of penicillamine is decreased by 52% when taken with food.

Adverse Reactions

Penicillamine is a drug with a high incidence of untoward reactions, some of which are potentially fatal. Therefore, it is mandatory that patients receiving penicillamine therapy remain under close medical supervision throughout the period of drug administration.

Reported incidences (%) for the most commonly occurring adverse reactions in rheumatoid arthritis patients are noted, based on 17 representative clinical trials reported in the literature (1,270 patients).

➤*Allergic:* Generalized pruritus, early and late rashes (5%), pemphigus, and drug eruptions which may be accompanied by fever, arthralgia, or lymphadenopathy have occurred. Some patients may show a lupus erythematosus-like syndrome similar to drug-induced lupus produced by other pharmacological agents.

Urticaria and exfoliative dermatitis have occurred.

Thyroiditis has been reported; hypoglycemia in association with anti-insulin antibodies has been reported. These reactions are extremely rare.

Some patients may develop a migratory polyarthralgia, often with objective synovitis.

➤*CNS:* Tinnitus, optic neuritis and peripheral sensory and motor neuropathies (including polyradiculoneuropathy [ie, Guillain-Barré syndrome]) have been reported. Muscular weakness may or may not occur with the peripheral neuropathies. Visual and psychic disturbances; mental disorders; and agitation and anxiety have been reported.

➤*GI:* Anorexia, epigastric pain, nausea, vomiting, or occasional diarrhea may occur (17%).

Isolated cases of reactivated peptic ulcer have occurred, as have hepatic dysfunction including hepatic failure, and pancreatitis. Intrahepatic cholestasis and toxic hepatitis have been reported rarely. There have been a few reports of increased serum alkaline phosphatase, lactic dehydrogenase, and positive cephalin flocculation and thymol turbidity tests.

Some patients may report a blunting, diminution, or total loss of taste perception (12%); or may develop oral ulcerations. Although rare, cheilosis, glossitis, and gingivostomatitis have been reported.

Gastrointestinal side effects are usually reversible following cessation of therapy.

➤*Hematologic:* Penicillamine can cause bone marrow depression. Leukopenia (2%) and thrombocytopenia (4%) have occurred. Fatalities have been reported as a result of thrombocytopenia, agranulocytosis, aplastic anemia, and sideroblastic anemia.

Thrombotic thrombocytopenic purpura, hemolytic anemia, red cell aplasia, monocytosis, leukocytosis, eosinophilia, and thrombocytosis have also been reported.

➤*Renal:* Patients on penicillamine therapy may develop proteinuria (6%) and/or hematuria which, in some, may progress to the development of the nephrotic syndrome as a result of an immune complex membranous glomerulopathy. Renal failure has been reported.

➤*Miscellaneous:*

Neuromuscular – Myasthenia gravis; dystonia. Adverse reactions that have been reported rarely include thrombophlebitis; hyperpyrexia; falling hair or alopecia; lichen planus; polymyositis; dermatomyositis; mammary hyperplasia; elastosis perforans serpiginosa; toxic epidermal necrolysis; anetoderma (cutaneous macular atrophy); and Goodpasture's syndrome, a severe and ultimately fatal glomerulonephritis associated with intra-alveolar hemorrhage. Vasculitis, including fatal renal vasculitis, has also been reported. Allergic alveolitis, obliterative bronchiolitis, interstitial pneumonitis and pulmonary fibrosis have been reported in patients with severe rheumatoid arthritis, some of whom were receiving penicillamine. Bronchial asthma also has been reported.

Increased skin friability, excessive wrinkling of skin, and development of small white papules at venipuncture and surgical sites have been reported; yellow nail syndrome.

The chelating action of the drug may cause increased excretion of other heavy metals such as zinc, mercury and lead.

There have been reports associating penicillamine with leukemia. However, circumstances involved in these reports are such that a cause and effect relationship to the drug has not been established.

URINARY ALKALINIZERS

SODIUM BICARBONATE

For complete prescribing information, refer to the oral sodium bicarbonate monograph in the systemic alkalinizers section of the nutritionals chapter or the parenteral sodium bicarbonate monograph in the IV nutritionals section. Also see the Antacids group monograph.

POTASSIUM CITRATE

Rx	**Potassium Citrate** (Rising)	**Tablets, extended-release; oral:** 5 mEq	In 100s.
Rx	**Urocit-K** (Mission)		(MPC 600). Tan/yellowish, ball shape. In 100s.
Rx	**Potassium Citrate** (Rising)	**Tablets, extended-release; oral:** 10 mEq	In 100s.
Rx	**Urocit-K** (Mission)		(MISSION MPC 610). Tan/yellowish, elliptical. In 100s.
Rx	**Potassium Citrate** (Rising)	**Tablets, extended-release; oral:** 15 mEq	(M 15). Elliptical shape. Tan/yellowish. In 100s.
Rx	**Urocit-K** (Mission)		(M 15). Tan/yellowish, rectangular. In 100s.

POTASSIUM CITRATE — ORAL

For complete prescribing information on citrate and citric acid, see monograph in the Nutrients and Nutritionals chapter.

Indications

➤*Kidney stones:* For the management of renal tubular acidosis (RTA) with calcium stones, hypocitraturic calcium oxalate nephrolithiasis of any etiology, and uric acid lithiasis with or without calcium stones.

Administration and Dosage

➤*Adults:*

Hypocitraturia –

Maximum dose: Dosages greater than 100 mEq/day have not been studied and should be avoided.

Initial dosage:

• *Mild to moderate (urinary citrate greater than 150 mg/day)* – 30 mEq/day in divided dosage (10 mEq 3 times/day).

• *Severe (urinary citrate of less than 150 mg/day)* – 60 mEq/day in divided dosage (20 mEq 3 times/day or 15 mEq 4 times/day).

POTASSIUM CITRATE — ORAL

Dosage adjustment: Twenty four-hour urinary citrate and/or urinary pH measurements should be used to determine the adequacy of the initial dosage and to evaluate the effectiveness of any dosage change.

Concomitant therapy: Treatment with potassium should be added to a regimen that limits salt intake (avoidance of foods with high salt content and of added salt at the table) and encourages high fluid intake (urine volume should be at least 2 L/day).

➤*Renal function impairment:* Contraindicated in patients with renal insufficiency (glomerular filtration rate of less than 0.7 mL/kg/min).

➤*Monitoring:* Urinary citrate and/or pH should be measured every 4 months.

➤*Administration:* Administer with meals or within 30 minutes after meals or bedtime snack.

➤*Storage/Stability:* Store in a cool, dry place.

POTASSIUM CITRATE COMBINATIONS

Rx	**Citrolith** (Beach Pharm.)	**Tablets; oral:** 50 mg potassium citrate and 950 mg sodium citrate	(Beach 1136). In 100s & 500s.

POTASSIUM CITRATE COMBINATIONS — ORAL

For complete prescribing information on citrate and citric acid, see monograph in the Nutrients and Nutritionals chapter.

Administration and Dosage

➤*Adults:*

Urinary alkalinizer – 1 to 4 tablets after meals and at bedtime.

➤*Administration:* Take with a full glass of water (8 ounces) after meals and at bedtime. Drink more water or juice after taking this medication unless otherwise directed by your doctor. Do not lie down for 30 minutes after taking this medication.

➤*Storage/Stability:* Store between 68° and 77°F away from heat, light, and moisture.

Warnings/Precautions

➤*Pregnancy: Category A* (potassium citrate) (per Briggs' *Drugs in Pregnancy and Lactation*). Citric acid is widely distributed in nature and is a key ingredient in intermediary metabolism. In addition, potassium is a natural constituent of human tissues and fluids. The primary risk appears to be from hyperkalemia, as this product could produce this in patients who have a condition predisposing them to high blood potassium levels. Because high levels are detrimental to maternal and embryo/fetal cardiac function, closely monitor maternal serum potassium levels.

➤*Lactation:* Because potassium freely passes into and out of milk, the use of potassium citrate by a lactating woman with normal plasma potassium levels would have no adverse effect on a breast-feeding infant. However, if the woman has hyperkalemia, this could result in higher milk potassium concentrations. In this case, observe breast-feeding infants for GI complaints commonly observed in adults with oral potassium, and monitor plasma potassium concentrations.

SODIUM CITRATE/CITRIC ACID SOLUTION (Shohl's Solution, Modified)

Rx sf	**Sodium Citrate/Citric Acid** (Pharmaceutical Associates)	**Solution:** 500 mg sodium citrate/334 mg citric acid per 5 ml (1 mEq sodium equiv. to 1 mEq bicarbonate/ml)	In 473 mL.
Rx sf	**Bicitra** (Alza Corp.)		Grape flavored. In 120 and 473 ml and UD 15 and 30 ml.
Rx	**Oracit** (Carolina Medical Products)	**Solution:** 490 mg sodium citrate/640 mg citric acid per 5 ml (1 mEq sodium equiv. to 1 mEq bicarbonate/ml)	In 500 ml and UD 15 and 30 ml.

SODIUM CITRATE/CITRIC ACID SOLUTION — ORAL

Administration and Dosage

➤*Adults:*

Systemic alkalinization – 10 to 30 mL diluted in 30 to 90 mL water, after meals and at bedtime.

Neutralizing buffer – 15 mL diluted in 15 mL water, as a single dose.

➤*Children:*

Systemic alkalinization –

2 years of age and older: 5 to 15 mL diluted in 30 to 90 mL water, after meals and at bedtime.

➤*Renal function impairment:* Contraindicated in patients with impaired renal function with oliguria, azotemia, or anuria.

➤*Administration:* Dilute each dose with 1 to 3 oz of cold water and take after meals if possible to prevent laxative effect. Additional water may follow the dose if desired.

➤*Storage/Stability:* Store at 59° to 86°F. Protect from freezing, excessive heat, and moisture.

URINARY ACIDIFIERS

ASCORBIC ACID

For information on the use of ascorbic acid as a urinary acidifier, see the vitamin C monograph in the Nutritional Agents chapter.

Acid Phosphates

Indications

➤*Elevated urinary pH:* To acidify the urine and lower urinary calcium concentration.; increase the antibacterial activity of methenamine; reduce odor and rash caused by ammoniacal urine.

Contraindications

Renal insufficiency (less than 30% of normal), infected magnesium ammonium phosphate stones, hyperphosphatemia and hyperkalemia. Also use with caution if potassium regulation is desired. Use sodium acid phosphate cautiously in patients on sodium restriction.

Warnings/Precautions

➤*Concurrent potassium supplementation:* Consider potassium content of these products. Decrease supplemental potassium dosage to avoid hyperkalemia.

➤*Special risk:* Cardiac disease (particularly digitalized patients), Addison's disease, acute dehydration, severe renal insufficiency or chronic renal disease, extensive tissue breakdown (such as severe burns), myotonia congenita, cardiac failure, cirrhosis of the liver or severe hepatic disease, peripheral and pulmonary edema, hypernatremia, hypertension, toxemia of pregnancy, hypoparathyroidism, acute pancreatitis and rickets.

➤*Pregnancy: Category C.* Safe use during pregnancy is not established. Use only when clearly needed and when potential benefits outweigh potential hazards to the fetus.

➤*Lactation:* Safety for use in the nursing mother has not been established. It is not known whether this drug is excreted in breast milk. Exercise caution when administering to a nursing woman.

➤*Lab test abnormalities:* Carefully monitor renal function and serum electrolytes (calcium, phosphorus, potassium) at periodic intervals during phosphate therapy if required. High serum phosphate levels increase incidence of extraskeletal calcification.

Drug Interactions

Acid Phosphate Drug Interactions

Precipitant drug	Object drug[a]		Description
Acid phosphates	Salicylates	↑	Acidified urine reduces excretion of salicylates and may lead to salicylate toxicity.
Antacids	Acid phosphates	↓	Antacids containing magnesium, calcium or aluminum in conjunction with phosphate preparations may bind the phosphate and prevent absorption.
Antihypertensives; Corticosteroids	Acid phosphates	↑	Antihypertensives, especially diazoxide, guanethidine, hydralazine, methyldopa or rauwolfia alkaloids; or corticosteroids, especially mineralocorticoids or corticotropin; used concurrently with sodium phosphate may result in hypernatremia.

Acid Phosphate Drug Interactions			
Precipitant drug	Object drug[a]		Description
Potassium-containing medications	Acid phosphates	↑	Potassium-containing medications or potassium-sparing diuretics may cause hyperkalemia when used concurrently with potassium salts. Perform periodic serum potassium level determinations.

[a] ↑ = Object drug increased. ↓ = Object drug decreased.

Adverse Reactions

Mild laxation may occur; it usually subsides with dosage reduction. If it persists, discontinue use. Abdominal discomfort, diarrhea, nausea and vomiting may occur.

Less frequent – Fast or irregular heartbeat, dizziness, headache, mental confusion, seizures, weakness or heaviness of legs, unusual tiredness, muscle cramps, numbness, tingling, pain or weakness in hands or feet, numbness or tingling around lips, shortness of breath or troubled breathing, swelling of feet or legs, unusual weight gain, low urine output, thirst, bone and joint pain.

Patient Information

Notify physician if abdominal pain, nausea or vomiting occurs.

Warn patients with kidney stones of the possibility of passing old stones when phosphate therapy is started.

Advise patients to avoid antacids containing aluminum, calcium or magnesium which may prevent phosphate absorption.

To assure against GI injury associated with oral ingestion of concentrated potassium salt preparations, instruct patients to dissolve tablets completely in an appropriate amount of water before taking.

POTASSIUM ACID PHOSPHATE

Rx	**K-Phos Original** (Beach)	**Tablets:** 500 mg (contains 3.7 mEq potassium)	Sodium free. (Beach 1111). White, scored. In 100s and 500s.

POTASSIUM ACID PHOSPHATE — ORAL

For complete prescribing information, refer to the Acid Phosphates group monograph.

Indications

➤*Elevated urinary pH:* For use in patients with elevated urinary pH. Potassium acid phosphate helps keep calcium soluble and reduces odor and rash caused by ammoniacal urine. Also, by acidifying the urine, it increases the antibacterial activity of methenamine mandelate and methenamine hippurate.

Administration and Dosage

➤*Adults:*

Elevated urinary pH – Two tablets dissolved in 6 to 8 oz of water 4 times daily with meals and at bedtime.

➤*Renal function impairment:* Contraindicated in patients with severely impaired renal function (less than 30% of normal).

➤*Administration:* For best results, let the tablets soak in water for 2 to 5 minutes, or more if necessary, and stir. If any tablet particles remain undissolved, they may be crushed and stirred vigorously to speed dissolution.

➤*Storage/Stability:* Store at 20° to 25°C (68° to 77°F).

POTASSIUM ACID PHOSPHATE AND SODIUM ACID PHOSPHATE

Rx	**K-Phos Neutral** (Beach)	**Tablets; oral:** 852 mg dibasic sodium phosphate anhydrous, 155 mg monobasic potassium phosphate and 130 mg monobasic sodium phosphate monohydrate (contains 1.1 mEq potassium and 13.0 mEq sodium)	(Beach 1125). White, film coated. In 100s and 500s.
Rx	**Phospha 250 Neutral** (Rising Pharmaceuticals)	**Tablets; oral:** 852 mg dibasic sodium phosphate, 155 mg monobasic potassium phosphate and 130 mg monobasic sodium phosphate monohydrate (contains 1.1 mEq potassium and 13 mEq sodium), and 250 mg phosphorus	(CPC 2369). White, capsule shape. Film-coated. In 100s.
Rx	**K-Phos M.F.** (Beach)	**Tablets; oral:** 155 mg potassium acid phosphate and 350 mg sodium acid phosphate (contains 1.1 mEq potassium and 2.9 mEq sodium)	(Beach 1135). White, scored. In 100s and 500s.
Rx	**K-Phos No. 2** (Beach)	**Tablets; oral:** 305 mg potassium acid phosphate and 700 mg sodium acid phosphate (contains 2.3 mEq potassium and 5.8 mEq sodium)	(Beach 1134). Brown. In 100s and 500s.

POTASSIUM ACID PHOSPHATE AND SODIUM ACID PHOSPHATE — ORAL

For complete and comparative prescribing information, refer to the Acid Phosphates class monograph.

Indications

➤*Urinary phosphate excretion:* Increases urinary phosphate and pyrophosphate.

Administration and Dosage

➤*Adults:*

Urinary phosphate excretion –

Usual dosage: 1 to 2 tablets 4 times daily. When the urine is difficult to acidify, administer 1 tablet every 2 hours.

Maximum dose: 8 tablets in 24 hours.

➤*Administration:* Tablets should be taken with a full glass of water.

Warnings/Precautions

➤*Pregnancy: Category C.* Animal reproduction studies have not been conducted. It is also not known whether these products can cause fetal harm when administered to a pregnant woman or can affect reproductive capacity. This product should be given to a pregnant woman only if clearly needed.

➤*Lactation:* It is not known whether these drugs are excreted in human milk. Because many drugs are excreted in human milk, caution should be exercised when these products are administered to a breast-feeding woman.

ANTICHOLINERGICS

FLAVOXATE HYDROCHLORIDE

Rx	**Flavoxate** (Global)	**Tablets:** 100 mg	(G 181). Off-white. Film-coated. In 100s.
Rx	**Urispas** (Ortho-McNeil)		Castor oil. (URISPAS SKF). White. Film-coated. In UD 100s.

FLAVOXATE HYDROCHLORIDE — ORAL

Indications

➤*Urinary tract symptoms:* For symptomatic relief of dysuria, urgency, nocturia, suprapubic pain, frequency and incontinence as may occur in cystitis, prostatitis, urethritis, urethrocystitis/urethrotrigonitis. Flavoxate hydrochloride is not indicated for definitive treatment, but is compatible with drugs used for the treatment of urinary tract infections.

Administration and Dosage

➤*Adults:*

Urinary tract symptoms – 100 to 200 mg 3 or 4 times a day. With improvement of symptoms, the dose may be reduced.

➤*Children:*

Urinary tract symptoms – See Adults for dosing for children 12 years of age and older.

➤*Storage/Stability:* Store between 15° and 30°C (59° and 86°F).

Actions

➤*Pharmacology:* Flavoxate hydrochloride counteracts smooth muscle spasm of the urinary tract and exerts its effect directly on the muscle.

➤*Pharmacokinetics:* In a single study of 11 healthy male subjects, the time to onset of action was 55 minutes. The peak effect was observed at 112 minutes.

FLAVOXATE HYDROCHLORIDE — ORAL

Fifty-seven percent of the flavoxate HCl was excreted in the urine within 24 hours.

Contraindications

Pyloric or duodenal obstruction, obstructive intestinal lesions or ileus, achalasia, GI hemorrhage and obstructive uropathies of the lower urinary tract.

Warnings/Precautions

➤*Glaucoma:* Give cautiously to patients with suspected glaucoma.

➤*Hazardous tasks:* Patients should be informed that if drowsiness and blurred vision occur, they should not operate a motor vehicle or machinery or participate in activities where alertness is required.

➤*Pregnancy: Category B.* Reproduction studies have been performed in rats and rabbits at doses up to 34 times the human dose and revealed no evidence of impaired fertility or harm to the fetus due to flavoxate HCl. There are, however, no well-controlled studies in pregnant women. Because animal reproduction studies are not always predictive of human response, this drug should be used during pregnancy only if clearly needed.

➤*Lactation:* It is not known whether this drug is excreted in human milk. Because many drugs are excreted in human milk, caution should be exercised when flavoxate HCl is administered to a nursing woman.

➤*Children:* Safety and efficacy in children younger than 12 years of age have not been established.

Adverse Reactions

➤*Allergic:* Urticaria and other dermatoses, eosinophilia and hyperpyrexia.

➤*Cardiovascular:* Tachycardia and palpitation.

➤*CNS:* Vertigo, headache, mental confusion, especially in the elderly, drowsiness, nervousness.

➤*GI:* Nausea, vomiting, dry mouth.

➤*Hematologic:* Leukopenia (1 case which was reversible upon discontinuation of the drug).

➤*Ophthalmic:* Increased ocular tension, blurred vision, disturbance in eye accommodation.

➤*Renal:* Dysuria.

Overdosage

The oral LD_{50} for flavoxate HCl in rats is 4273 mg/kg. The oral LD_{50} for flavoxate HCl in mice is 1837 mg/kg.

➤*Treatment:* It is not known whether flavoxate HCI is dialyzable.

Patient Information

Patients should be informed that if drowsiness and blurred vision occur, they should not operate a motor vehicle or machinery or participate in activities where alertness is required.

OXYBUTYNIN CHLORIDE

Rx	**Oxybutynin Chloride** (Various, eg, Pliva, Sidmak, UDL)	**Tablets; oral:** 5 mg	In 100s, 500s, 1,000s, blister pack 25s, and UD 100s.
Rx	**Oxybutynin Chloride** (Various, eg, Mylan, UDL)	**Tablets, extended-release; oral:** 5 mg	In 100s and 500s.
Rx	**Ditropan XL** (Janssen)		Lactose. (5 XL). Pale yellow. In 100s.
Rx	**Oxybutynin Chloride** (Various, eg, Mylan, UDL)	**Tablets, extended-release; oral:** 10 mg	In 100s and 500s.
Rx	**Ditropan XL** (Janssen)		Lactose. (10 XL). Pink. In 100s.
Rx	**Oxybutynin Chloride** (Various, eg, Mylan, Teva)	**Tablets, extended-release; oral:** 15 mg	May contain lactose. In 100s.
Rx	**Ditropan XL** (Janssen)		Lactose. (15 XL). Gray. In 100s.
Rx	**Oxybutynin Chloride** (Various, eg, Cypress, Morton Grove)	**Syrup; oral:** 5 mg per 5 mL	In 473 mL.
Rx	**Oxytrol** (Watson)	**Transdermal system; topical:** oxybutynin 36 mg delivering oxybutynin 3.9 mg/day.	(OXYTROL). 39 cm^2 system. In patient calendar boxes of 8 systems.
Rx	**Gelnique** (Watson)	**Gel; topical:** 10%	Alcohol. In 1 g sachets. Carton of 30s.

OXYBUTYNIN CHLORIDE — ORAL

Indications

➤*Tablets and syrup:* For the relief of symptoms of bladder instability associated with voiding in patients with uninhibited neurogenic or reflex neurogenic bladder (ie, urgency, frequency, urinary leakage, urge incontinence, dysuria).

➤*Extended-release tablets:* For the treatment of overactive bladder with symptoms of urge urinary incontinence, urgency, and frequency.

Oxybutynin chloride is also indicated in the treatment of pediatric patients aged 6 years and older with symptoms of detrusor overactivity associated with a neurological condition (eg, spina bifida).

➤*Off-label uses:*

Hyperhidrosis – [4] = Insufficient documentation. There is limited information regarding the use of oxybutynin in the management of hyperhidrosis. Data regarding the use of oxybutynin in the treatment of hyperhidrosis are limited to 1 open-label trial and a case report, a total of 15 patients. In an open-label trial, the majority of patients (approximately 78%) with hyperhidrosis responded to oxybutynin therapy. (See Administration and Dosage.)

Administration and Dosage

➤*Maximum dose:*

Adults –

Extended-release tablets: 30 mg/day according to the prescribing information.

Syrup and tablets: 5 mg 4 times daily according to the prescribing information.

Children older than 5 years of age –

Extended-release tablets: 20 mg/day according to the prescribing information.

Syrup and tablets: 5 mg 3 times daily according to the prescribing information.

➤*Adults:*

Bladder instability –

Syrup and tablets:

- *Usual dosage* – 5 mg (1 tsp of the 5 mg/5 mL syrup) 2 to 3 times daily.
- *Maximum dose* – 5 mg 4 times daily.

Overactive bladder –

Extended-release tablets:

- *Usual dosage* – 5 mg once daily.
- *Maximum dose* – 30 mg/day.
- *Dosage adjustment* – May be adjusted in 5 mg increments at approximately weekly intervals to achieve a balance of efficacy and tolerability (up to a maximum of 30 mg/day).

Off-label dosing –

Hyperhidrosis: [4] = Insufficient documentation. 2.5 mg 3 times daily or 5 mg twice daily for 4 weeks.

➤*Children:*

Detrusor overactivity associated with a neurological condition –

Extended-release tablets:

- *6 years of age and older* –

  Usual dosage: 5 mg once daily.

  Maximum dose: 20 mg/day.

  Dosage adjustment: Dosage may be adjusted in 5 mg increments to achieve a balance of efficacy and tolerability (up to a maximum of 20 mg/day).

Syrup and tablets:

- *Older than 5 years of age* –

  Usual dosage: 5 mg (1 tsp of the 5 mg/5 mL syrup) 2 times a day.

  Maximum dose: 5 mg 3 times daily.

Off-label dosing –

Children younger than 5 years of age:

- *Usual dose* – 0.2 mg/kg/dose 2 to 4 times per day.
- *Maximum dose* – 15 mg in 24 hours.

➤*Elderly:*

Tablets and syrup – For frail elderly patients, a lower initial starting dose of 2.5 mg given 2 or 3 times a day has been recommended because of a prolongation of the elimination half-life from 2 to 3 hours to 5 hours.

➤*Administration:* Extended-release tablets must be swallowed whole with the aid of liquids, and must not be chewed, divided, or crushed. May be administered with or without food.

➤*Storage/Stability:*

Tablets and syrup – Store at controlled room temperature, 15° to 30°C (59° to 86°F). Dispense in tight, light-resistant container.

Extended-release tablets – Store at 25°C (77°F); excursions permitted to 15° to 30°C (59° to 86°F). Protect from moisture and humidity.

OXYBUTYNIN CHLORIDE — ORAL

Actions

➤*Pharmacology:* Oxybutynin chloride exerts a direct antispasmodic effect on smooth muscle and inhibits the muscarinic action of acetylcholine on smooth muscle. Oxybutynin chloride exhibits only one-fifth of the anticholinergic activity of atropine on the rabbit detrusor muscle, but 4 to 10 times the antispasmodic activity. No blocking effects occur at skeletal neuromuscular junctions or autonomic ganglia (antinicotinic effects).

Oxybutynin chloride relaxes bladder smooth muscle. In patients with conditions characterized by involuntary bladder contractions, cystometric studies have demonstrated that oxybutynin increases bladder (vesical) capacity, diminishes the frequency of uninhibited contractions of the detrusor muscle, and delays the initial desire to void. Oxybutynin thus decreases urgency and the frequency of both incontinent episodes and voluntary urination.

Antimuscarinic activity resides predominately in the R-isomer. A metabolite, desethyloxybutynin, has pharmacological activity similar to that of oxybutynin in in vitro studies.

➤*Pharmacokinetics:*

Absorption –

Tablets and syrup: Following oral administration, oxybutynin is rapidly absorbed achieving C_{max} within an hour, following which plasma concentration decreases with an effective half-life of approximately 2 to 3 hours. The absolute bioavailability of oxybutynin is reported to be about 6% (range 1.6% to 10.9%) for both the tablet and syrup. Wide interindividual variation in pharmacokinetic parameters is evident following oral administration of oxybutynin.

The mean pharmacokinetic parameters for R- and S-oxybutynin are summarized below. The plasma concentration-time profiles for R- and S-oxybutynin are similar in shape.

Mean (SD) R- and S-Oxybutynin Pharmacokinetic Parameters Following 3 Doses of 5 mg Oxybutynin Every 8 Hours (n = 23)

Parameters (units)	R-oxybutynin	S-oxybutynin
C_{max} (ng/mL)	3.6 (2.2)	7.8 (4.1)
t_{max} (hr)	0.89 (0.34)	0.65 (0.32)
AUC_t (ng•hr/mL)	22.6 (11.3)	35 (17.3)
AUC_{inf} (ng•hr/mL)	24.3 (12.3)	37.3 (18.7)

Oxybutynin chloride steady-state pharmacokinetics was also studied in 23 pediatric patients with detrusor overactivity associated with a neurological condition (eg, spina bifida). These pediatric patients were on oxybutynin chloride tablets (n = 11) with total daily dose ranging from 7.5 mg to 15 mg (0.22 to 0.53 mg/kg) or oxybutynin chloride syrup (n = 12) with total daily dose ranging from 5 mg to 22.5 mg (0.26 to 0.75 mg/kg). Overall, most patients (86.9%) were taking a total daily oxybutynin chloride dose between 10 mg and 15 mg. Sparse sampling technique was used to obtain serum samples. When all available data are normalized to an equivalent of 5 mg twice daily oxybutynin chloride, the mean pharmacokinetic parameters derived for R- and S-oxybutynin and R- and S-desethyloxybutynin are summarized below for tablet and syrup. The plasma-time concentration profile for R- and S-oxybutynin are similar in shape.

Mean ± SD R- and S-Oxybutynin and R- and S-Desethyloxybutynin Pharmacokinetic Parameters in Children 5 to 15 Years of Age After 7.5 to 15 mg Total Daily Dose of Oxybutynin Tablets (n = 11)[a]

Parameters (units)	R-oxybutynin	S-oxybutynin	R-desethyloxybutynin	S-desethyloxybutynin
C_{max}[b] (ng/mL)	6.1 ± 3.2	10.1 ± 7.5	55.4 ± 17.9	28.2 ± 10
t_{max} (hr)	1	1	2	2
AUC[c] (ng•hr/mL)	19.8 ± 7.4	28.4 ± 12.7	238.8 ± 77.6	119.5 ± 50.7

[a] All available data normalized to an equivalent of oxybutynin chloride tablets 5 mg 2 times a day or 3 times a day at steady rates.
[b] Reflects C_{max} for pooled data.
[c] $AUC_{0\text{-end of dosing interval}}$.

Mean ± SD R- and S-Oxybutynin and R- and S-Desethyloxybutynin Pharmacokinetic Parameters in Children 5 to 15 Years of Age After 5 to 22.5 mg Total Daily Dose of Oxybutynin Syrup (n = 12)[a]

Parameters (units)	R-oxybutynin	S-oxybutynin	R-desethyloxybutynin	S-desethyloxybutynin
C_{max}[b] (ng/mL)	5.7 ± 6.2	7.3 ± 7.3	54.2 ± 34	27.8 ± 20.7
t_{max} (hr)	1	1	1	1
AUC[c] (ng•hr/mL)	16.3 ± 17.1	20.2 ± 20.8	209.1 ± 174.2	99.1 ± 87.5

[a] All available data normalized to an equivalent of oxybutynin chloride syrup 5 mg 2 times a day or 3 times a day at steady rates.
[b] Reflects C_{max} for pooled data.
[c] $AUC_{0\text{-end of dosing interval}}$.

Extended-release tablets: Following the first dose of oxybutynin chloride extended-release tablets, oxybutynin plasma concentrations rise for 4 to 6 hours; thereafter steady concentrations are maintained for up to 24 hours, minimizing fluctuations between peak and trough concentrations associated with oxybutynin.

The relative bioavailabilities of R- and S-oxybutynin from oxybutynin chloride extended-release tablets are 156% and 187%, respectively, compared with oxybutynin. The mean pharmacokinetic parameters for R- and S-oxybutynin are summarized below. The plasma concentration-time profiles for R- and S-oxybutynin are similar in shape.

Pharmacokinetic parameters of oxybutynin and desethyloxybutynin (C_{max} and AUC) following administration of 5 to 20 mg of oxybutynin chloride extended-release tablets are dose proportional.

Mean (SD) R- and S-Oxybutynin Pharmacokinetic Parameters After a Single Dose of Oxybutynin 10 mg Extended-Release Tablets (n = 43)

Parameters (units)	R-oxybutynin	S-oxybutynin
C_{max} (ng/mL)	1 (0.6)	1.8 (1)
t_{max} (hr)	12.7 (5.4)	11.8 (5.3)
$t_{1/2}$ (hr)	13.2 (6.2)	12.4 (6.1)
$AUC_{(0\text{-}48)}$ (ng•hr/mL)	18.4 (10.3)	34.2 (16.9)
AUC_{inf} (ng•hr/mL)	21.3 (12.2)	39.5 (21.2)

Steady-state oxybutynin plasma concentrations are achieved by day 3 of repeated oxybutynin chloride extended-release tablet dosing, with no observed drug accumulation or change in oxybutynin and desethyloxybutynin pharmacokinetic parameters.

Oxybutynin chloride steady-state pharmacokinetics was studied in 19 children aged 5 to 15 years with detrusor overactivity associated with a neurological condition (eg, spina bifida). The children were on oxybutynin chloride total daily dose ranging from 5 to 20 mg (0.1 to 0.77 mg/kg). Sparse sampling technique was used to obtain serum samples. When all available data are normalized to an equivalent of 5 mg per day oxybutynin chloride, the mean pharmacokinetic parameters derived for R- and S-oxybutynin and R- and S-desethyloxybutynin are summarized below. The plasma-time concentration profiles for R- and S-oxybutynin are similar in shape.

Mean ± SD R- and S-Oxybutynin and R- and S-Desethyloxybutynin Pharmacokinetic Parameters in Children 5 to 15 Years of Age After Once–Daily 5 to 20 mg Oxybutynin Extended-Release Tablets (n = 19)[a]

Parameters (units)	R-oxybutynin	S-oxybutynin	R-desethyloxybutynin	S-desethyloxybutynin
C_{max} (ng/mL)	0.7 ± 0.4	1.3 ± 0.8	7.8 ± 3.7	4.2 ± 2.3
t_{max} (hr)	5	5	5	5
AUC (ng•hr/mL)	12.8 ± 7	23.7 ± 14.4	125.1 ± 66.7	73.6 ± 47.7

[a] All available data normalized to an equivalent of oxybutynin chloride extended-release tablets 5 mg once daily.

Mean steady state (±SD) R-oxybutynin plasma concentrations following administration of 5 to 20 mg oxybutynin chloride once daily in children aged 5 to 15. Plot represents all available data normalized to an equivalent of oxybutynin chloride 5 mg once daily.

• *Food effects –*

Tablets and syrup: Data in the literature suggests that oxybutynin chloride solution coadministered with food resulted in a slight delay in absorption and an increase in its bioavailability by 25% (n = 18).

Extended-release tablets: The rate and extent of absorption and metabolism of oxybutynin chloride are similar under fed and fasted conditions.

Distribution – Plasma concentrations of oxybutynin decline biexponentially following IV or oral administration. The volume of distribution is 193 L after IV administration of 5 mg oxybutynin chloride.

Metabolism – Oxybutynin chloride is metabolized primarily by the cytochrome P450 enzyme systems, particularly CYP3A4 found mostly in the liver and gut wall. Its metabolic products include phenylcyclohexyl-glycolic acid, which is pharmacologically inactive, and desethyloxybutynin, which is pharmacologically active.

Extended-release tablets: Following oxybutynin chloride extended-release tablet administration, plasma concentrations of R- and S-desethyloxybutynin are 73% and 92%, respectively, of concentrations observed with oxybutynin.

Excretion – Oxybutynin chloride is extensively metabolized by the liver, with less than 0.1% of the administered dose excreted unchanged in the urine. Also, less than 0.1% of the administered dose is excreted as the metabolite desethyloxybutynin.

Contraindications

Urinary retention, gastric retention and other severe decreased GI motility conditions, uncontrolled narrow-angle glaucoma and in patients who are at risk for these conditions; hypersensitivity to the drug substance or other components of the product.

Warnings/Precautions

➤*Urinary retention:* Oxybutynin chloride should be administered with caution to patients with clinically significant bladder outflow obstruction because of the risk of urinary retention. Oxybutynin chloride is contraindicated in patients with urinary retention and in patients who are at risk for urinary retention.

➤*Gastrointestinal disorders:* Oxybutynin chloride should be administered with caution to patients with gastrointestinal obstructive disorders because of the risk of gastric retention. Oxybutynin chloride is contraindicated in patients with gastric retention and other severe decreased gastrointestinal motility conditions and in patients at risk for these conditions.

Oxybutynin chloride like other anticholinergic drugs, may decrease gastrointestinal motility and should be used with caution in patients with conditions such as ulcerative colitis, and intestinal atony.

Oxybutynin chloride should be used with caution in patients who have gastroesophageal reflux or who are concurrently taking drugs (such as bisphosphonates) that can cause or exacerbate esophagitis.

OXYBUTYNIN CHLORIDE — ORAL

Extended-release tablets – As with any other nondeformable material, caution should be used when administering oxybutynin chloride extended-release tablets to patients with preexisting severe gastrointestinal narrowing (pathologic or iatrogenic). There have been rare reports of obstructive symptoms in patients with known strictures in association with the ingestion of other drugs in nondeformable controlled-release formulations.

➤*Renal function impairment:*

Extended-release tablets – Oxybutynin chloride extended-release tablets should be used with caution in patients with renal impairment. There is no experience with the use of oxybutynin chloride extended-release tablets in patients with renal insufficiency.

➤*Hepatic function impairment:*

Extended-release tablets – There is no experience with the use of oxybutynin chloride extended-release tablets in patients with hepatic insufficiency. Oxybutynin chloride extended-release tablets should be used with caution in patients with hepatic impairment.

➤*Special risk:*

Tablets and syrup – Oxybutynin chloride should be used with caution in the frail elderly, in patients with hepatic or renal impairment, and in patients with myasthenia gravis. Oxybutynin chloride may aggravate the symptoms of hyperthyroidism, coronary heart disease, congestive heart failure, cardiac arrhythmias, hiatal hernia, tachycardia, hypertension, myasthenia gravis, and prostatic hypertrophy. Administration of oxybutynin chloride to patients with ulcerative colitis may suppress intestinal motility to the point of producing a paralytic ileus and precipitate or aggravate toxic megacolon, a serious complication of the disease.

Extended-release tablets – Oxybutynin chloride should be used with caution in patients with hepatic or renal impairment and in patients with myasthenia gravis due to the risk of symptom aggravation.

➤*Pregnancy: Category B.* The safety of oxybutynin chloride administration to women who are or who may become pregnant has not been established. Therefore, oxybutynin chloride should not be given to pregnant women unless, in the judgment of the physician, the probable clinical benefits outweigh the possible hazards.

➤*Lactation:* It is not known whether oxybutynin chloride is excreted in human milk. Because many drugs are excreted in human milk, caution should be exercised when oxybutynin chloride is administered to a nursing woman.

➤*Children:*

Tablets and syrup – The safety and efficacy of oxybutynin chloride administration have been demonstrated for children 5 years of age or older. However, as there is insufficient clinical data for children younger than 5 years of age, oxybutynin chloride is not recommended for this age group.

Extended-release tablets – The safety and efficacy of oxybutynin chloride were studied in 60 children in a 24-week, open-label trial. Patients were aged 6 to 15 years, all had symptoms of detrusor overactivity in association with a neurological condition (eg, spina bifida), all used clean intermittent catheterization, and all were current users of oxybutynin chloride. Study results demonstrated that administration of oxybutynin chloride 5 to 20 mg/day was associated with an increase from baseline in mean urine volume per catheterization from 108 mL to 136 mL, an increase from baseline in mean urine volume after morning awakening from 148 mL to 189 mL, and an increase from baseline in the mean percentage of catheterizations without a leaking episode from 34% to 51%.

Urodynamic results were consistent with clinical results. Administration of oxybutynin chloride resulted in an increase from baseline in mean maximum cystometric capacity from 185 mL to 254 mL, a decrease from baseline in mean detrusor pressure at maximum cystometric capacity from 44 cm H_2O to 33 cm H_2O, and a reduction in the percentage of patients demonstrating uninhibited detrusor contractions (of at least 15 cm H_2O) from 60% to 28%.

Oxybutynin chloride is not recommended in pediatric patients who can not swallow the tablet whole without chewing, dividing, or crushing, or in children under the age of 6 years.

➤*Elderly:*

Tablets and syrup – Clinical studies of oxybutynin chloride did not include sufficient numbers of subjects 65 years of age and older to determine whether they respond differently from younger patients. Other reported clinical experience has not identified differences in responses between healthy elderly and younger patients; however, a lower initial starting dose of 2.5 mg given 2 or 3 times a day has been recommended for the frail elderly due to a prolongation of the elimination half-life from 2 to 3 hours to 5 hours. In general, dose selection for an elderly patient should be cautious, usually starting at the low end of the dosing range, reflecting the greater frequency of decreased hepatic, renal or cardiac function, and of concomitant disease or other drug therapy.

Per the Beers list, most muscle relaxants and antispasmodic drugs are poorly tolerated by elderly patients, because these cause anticholinergic adverse effects, sedation, and weakness. Additionally, their effectiveness at doses tolerated by elderly patients is questionable.

Drug Interactions

Oxybutynin Drug Interactions

Precipitant drug	Object drug[a]		Description
Oxybutynin	Anticholinergic agents	↑	Concomitant use may increase the frequency and/or severity of anticholinergic-like effects. Anticholinergic agents may potentially alter the absorption of some concomitantly administered drugs because of anticholinergic effects on GI motility.
Anticholinergic agents	Oxybutynin		
Oxybutynin	Beta blockers Atenolol	↑	The bioavailability of atenolol may be increased. If an increase in beta blockade is suspected, tailoring the beta blocker dose downward may be necessary.
Oxybutynin	Digoxin	↑	Serum levels of digoxin administered as slow-dissolution oral tablets may be increased and actions enhanced. Serum level monitoring may assist in tailoring dosage. Problems may be avoided with use of digoxin elixir or capsules.
Oxybutynin	Haloperidol	↔	Effects are variable. Use oxybutynin only when clearly needed. Routinely monitor these patients; discontinue anticholinergic or tailor haloperidol if necessary.
Oxybutynin	Phenothiazines	↓	Pharmacologic/therapeutic actions of phenothiazines may be decreased by anticholinergics. Tailor the phenothiazine dose as needed.
Amantadine	Oxybutynin	↑	Anticholinergic side effects may be increased. Decrease the dose of oxybutynin during coadministration. Monitor patient response and adjust the dose accordingly.

[a] ↑ = object drug increased; ↓ = object drug decreased; ↔ = undetermined clinical effect.

➤*Tablets and syrup:* Mean oxybutynin chloride plasma concentrations were approximately 3- to 4-fold higher when oxybutynin chloride was administered with ketoconazole, a potent CYP3A4 inhibitor.

➤*Extended-release tablets:* Mean oxybutynin chloride plasma concentrations were approximately 2-fold higher when oxybutynin was administered with ketoconazole, a potent CYP3A4 inhibitor.

Other inhibitors of the cytochrome P450 3A4 enzyme system, such as antimycotic agents (eg, itraconazole and miconazole) or macrolide antibiotics (eg, erythromycin and clarithromycin), may alter oxybutynin mean pharmacokinetic parameters (ie, C_{max} and AUC). The clinical relevance of such potential interactions is not known. Caution should be used when such drugs are coadministered.

Adverse Reactions

➤*Tablets and syrup:* The safety and efficacy of oxybutynin chloride was evaluated in a total of 199 patients in 3 clinical trials comparing oxybutynin chloride with oxybutynin chloride extended-release (see below). These participants were treated with oxybutynin chloride 5 to 20 mg/day for up to 6 weeks. The table below shows the incidence of adverse events judged by investigator to be at least possibly related to treatment and reported by at least 5% of patients.

Oxybutynin Oral Adverse Reactions (> 5%)

Adverse reaction	Oxybutynin chloride (5 to 20 mg/day) (n = 199)
General	
Abdominal pain	6.5%
Headache	6%
GI	
Dry mouth	71.4%
Constipation	12.6%
Nausea	10.1%
Dyspepsia	7%
Diarrhea	5%
CNS	
Dizziness	15.6%
Somnolence	12.6%
Special senses	
Blurred vision	9%

OXYBUTYNIN CHLORIDE — ORAL

Oxybutynin Oral Adverse Reactions (> 5%)	
Adverse reaction	Oxybutynin chloride (5 to 20 mg/day) (n = 199)
GU	
Impaired urination	10.6%
Increased post void residuals	5%
Urinary tract infection	5%

The most common adverse events reported by patients receiving oxybutynin chloride 5 to 20 mg/day were the expected side effects of anticholinergic agents. The incidence of dry mouth was dose-related.

In addition, the following adverse events were reported by 2% to less than 5% of patients using oxybutynin chloride (5 to 20 mg/day) in all studies.

Cardiovascular – Palpitation.

CNS – Insomnia, nervousness, confusion.

Dermatologic – Dry skin.

Metabolic/Nutritional – Peripheral edema.

Special senses – Dry eyes, taste perversion.

Miscellaneous – Asthenia, dry nasal and sinus mucous membranes.

Other adverse events that have been reported include tachycardia, hallucinations, cycloplegia, mydriasis, impotence, suppression of lactation, vasodilatation, rash, decreased gastrointestinal motility, flatulence, urinary retention, convulsions, and decreased sweating.

➤*Symptoms associated with the use of other anticholinergic drugs:* Following administration of oxybutynin chloride, the symptoms that can be associated with the use of other anticholinergic drugs may occur:

Cardiovascular – Palpitations, tachycardia, vasodilatation.

CNS – Asthenia, dizziness, drowsiness, hallucinations, insomnia, restlessness.

Dermatologic – Decreased sweating, rash.

GI – Constipation, decreased gastrointestinal motility, dry mouth, nausea.

GU – Urinary hesitance and retention.

Ophthalmic – Amblyopia, cycloplegia, decreased lacrimation, mydriasis.

Miscellaneous – Impotence, suppression of lactation.

➤*Extended-release tablets:* The safety and efficacy of oxybutynin chloride extended-release tablets was evaluated in a total of 580 participants who received oxybutynin chloride extended-release tablets in clinical trials (429 patients, 151 healthy volunteers). These participants were treated with 5 to 30 mg/day for up to 4.5 months. Safety information is provided for 429 patients from 3 controlled clinical studies and one open label study. The adverse reactions are reported regardless of causality.

Oxybutynin Extended-Release Oral Adverse Reactions (≥ 5%)	
Adverse reaction	Oxybutynin chloride 5 to 30 mg/day (n = 429)
Miscellaneous	
Headache	9.8%
Asthenia	6.8%
Pain	6.8%
GI	
Dry mouth	60.8%
Constipation	13.1%
Diarrhea	9.1%
Nausea	8.9%
Dyspepsia	6.8%
CNS	
Somnolence	11.9%
Dizziness	6.3%
Respiratory	
Rhinitis	5.6%
Special senses	
Blurred vision	7.7%
Dry eyes	6.1%
GU	
Urinary tract infection	5.1%

The most common adverse reactions reported by patients receiving 5 to 30 mg/day oxybutynin chloride extended-release tablets were the expected side effects of anticholinergic agents. The incidence of dry mouth was dose-related.

The discontinuation rate for all adverse reactions was 6.8%. The most frequent adverse reaction causing early discontinuation of study medication was nausea (1.9%), while discontinuation due to dry mouth was 1.2%.

➤*Adverse reactions were reported by 2% to less than 5% of patients using oxybutynin chloride extended-release tablets (5 to 30 mg/day):*

Cardiovascular – Hypertension, palpitation, vasodilatation.

CNS – Insomnia, nervousness, confusion.

Dermatologic – Dry skin, rash.

GI – Flatulence, gastroesophageal reflux.

GU – Impaired urination (hesitancy), increased post void residual volume, urinary retention, cystitis.

Musculoskeletal – Arthritis.

Respiratory – Upper respiratory tract infection, cough, sinusitis, bronchitis, pharyngitis.

Miscellaneous – Abdominal pain, dry nasal and sinus mucous membranes, accidental injury, back pain, flu syndrome.

Other adverse reactions have been reported with oxybutynin chloride: Tachycardia, hallucinations, cycloplegia, mydriasis, impotence, and suppression of lactation.

Additional rare adverse events reported from worldwide postmarketing experience with oxybutynin chloride include peripheral edema, cardiac arrhythmia, tachycardia, hallucinations, convulsions, and impotence.

Additional adverse events reported with some other oxybutynin chloride formulations include cycloplegia, mydriasis, and suppression of lactation.

Overdosage

➤*Tablets and syrup:*

Symptoms – Overdosage with oxybutynin chloride has been associated with anticholinergic effects including central nervous system excitation (eg, restlessness, tremor, irritability, convulsions, delirium, hallucinations), flushing, fever, dehydration, cardiac arrhythmia, vomiting, and urinary retention. Other symptoms may include hypotension or hypertension, respiratory failure, paralysis, and coma.

Ingestion of 100 mg oxybutynin chloride in association with alcohol has been reported in a 13-year-old boy who experienced memory loss, and a 34 year old woman who developed stupor, followed by disorientation and agitation on awakening, dilated pupils, dry skin, cardiac arrhythmia, and retention of urine. Both patients fully recovered with symptomatic treatment.

Treatment – Treatment should be symptomatic and supportive. Activated charcoal may be administered as well as a cathartic.

➤*Extended-release tablets:* The continuous release of oxybutynin from oxybutynin chloride extended-release tablets should be considered in the treatment of overdosage. Patients should be monitored for at least 24 hours. Treatment should be symptomatic and supportive. Activated charcoal as well as a cathartic may be administered.

Overdosage with oxybutynin chloride has been associated with anticholinergic effects including CNS excitation, flushing, fever, dehydration, cardiac arrhythmia, vomiting, and urinary retention.

Ingestion of 100 mg oxybutynin chloride in association with alcohol has been reported in a 13-year-old boy who experienced memory loss, and a 34-year-old woman who developed stupor, followed by disorientation and agitation on awakening, dilated pupils, dry skin, cardiac arrhythmia, and retention of urine. Both patients fully recovered with symptomatic treatment.

Patient Information

Patients should be informed that heat prostration (fever and heat stroke due to decreased sweating) can occur when anticholinergics such as oxybutynin chloride are administered in the presence of high environmental temperature.

Because anticholinergic agents such as oxybutynin chloride may produce drowsiness (somnolence) or blurred vision, patients should be advised to exercise caution.

Patients should be informed that alcohol may enhance the drowsiness caused by anticholinergic agents such as oxybutynin chloride.

Patients should be informed that oxybutynin chloride extended-release tablets should be swallowed whole with the aid of liquids. Patients should not chew, divide, or crush tablets. The medication is contained within a nonabsorbable shell designed to release the drug at a controlled rate. The tablet shell is eliminated from the body; patients should not be concerned if they occasionally notice in their stool something that looks like a tablet.

OXYBUTYNIN — TRANSDERMAL PATCH

Indications

➤*Overactive bladder:* For the treatment of overactive bladder with symptoms of urge urinary incontinence, urgency, and frequency.

Administration and Dosage

➤*Adults:*

Overactive bladder – One 3.9 mg/day system applied twice weekly (every 3 to 4 days).

➤*Elderly:* No overall differences in safety or effectiveness were observed between elderly and younger patients.

➤*Administration:* Apply immediately after removal from the protective pouch. Apply to dry, intact skin on the abdomen, hip, or buttock. The waistline area should be avoided. A new application site should be selected with each new system to avoid reapplication to the same site within 7 days.

The patch should not be exposed to sunlight. Therefore, it should be worn underneath clothing.

OXYBUTYNIN — TRANSDERMAL PATCH

➤*Storage/Stability:* Store at 25°C (77°F); excursions are permitted to 15° to 30°C (59° to 86°F). Protect from moisture and humidity. Discard used transdermal system in household trash in a manner that prevents accidental application or ingestion by children, pets, or others. Do not store outside the sealed pouch.

Actions

➤*Pharmacology:* The free base form of oxybutynin is pharmacologically equivalent to oxybutynin hydrochloride. Oxybutynin acts as a competitive antagonist of acetylcholine at postganglionic muscarinic receptors, resulting in relaxation of bladder smooth muscle. In patients with conditions characterized by involuntary detrusor contractions, cystometric studies have demonstrated that oxybutynin increases maximum urinary bladder capacity and increases the volume to first detrusor contraction. Oxybutynin thus decreases urinary urgency and the frequency of both incontinence episodes and voluntary urination.

Oxybutynin is a racemic (50:50) mixture of R- and S-isomers. Antimuscarinic activity resides predominantly in the R-isomer. The active metabolite, N-desethyloxybutynin, has pharmacological activity on the human detrusor muscle that is similar to that of oxybutynin in in vitro studies.

➤*Pharmacokinetics:*

Absorption – Oxybutynin is transported across intact skin and into the systemic circulation by passive diffusion across the stratum corneum. The average daily dose of oxybutynin absorbed from the 39 cm^2 oxybutynin transdermal system is 3.9 mg. The average (SD) nominal dose, 0.1 (0.02) mg oxybutynin per cm^2 surface area, was obtained from analysis of residual oxybutynin content of systems worn over a continuous 4-day period during 303 separate occasions in 76 healthy volunteers. Following application of the first oxybutynin transdermal system 3.9 mg/day system, oxybutynin plasma concentration increases for approximately 24 to 48 hours, reaching average maximum concentrations of 3 to 4 ng/mL. Thereafter, steady concentrations are maintained for up to 96 hours. Absorption of oxybutynin is bioequivalent when oxybutynin transdermal system is applied to the abdomen, buttocks, or hip. Average plasma concentrations were measured during a randomized, crossover study of the 3 recommended application sites in 24 healthy men and women.

Steady-state conditions are reached during the second oxybutynin transdermal system application. Average steady-state plasma concentrations were 3.1 ng/mL for oxybutynin and 3.8 ng/mL for N-desethyloxybutynin. The following information provides a summary of pharmacokinetic parameters of oxybutynin in healthy volunteers after single and multiple applications of oxybutynin transdermal system (see the following figure).

Mean (SD) Oxybutynin Pharmacokinetic Parameters from Single and Multiple Studies in Healthy Men and Women Volunteers after Abdominal Application of Oxybutynin Chloride Transdermal System

Dosing	C_{max} (ng/mL)	T_{max}[a] (h)	C_{avg} (ng/mL)	AUC (ng/mL×h)
Single	3	48		245[b]
	3.4	36		279[b]
Multiple	6.6	10	4.2	408[c]
	4.2	28	3.1	259[d]

[a] T_{max} given as median.
[b] AUC_{inf}.
[c] AUC_{0-96}.
[d] AUC_{0-84}.

Distribution – Oxybutynin is widely distributed in body tissues following systemic absorption. The volume of distribution was estimated to be 193 L after IV administration of oxybutynin chloride 5 mg.

Metabolism – Oxybutynin is metabolized primarily by the cytochrome P450 enzyme systems, particularly CYP3A4, found mostly in the liver and gut wall. Metabolites include phenylcyclohexylglycolic acid, which is pharmacologically inactive, and N-desethyloxybutynin, which is pharmacologically active.

After oral administration of oxybutynin, presystemic first-pass metabolism results in an oral bioavailability of approximately 6% and higher plasma concentration of the N-desethyl metabolite compared with oxybutynin. The plasma concentration AUC ratio of N-desethyl metabolite to parent compound following a single oral dose of oxybutynin chloride 5 mg was 11.9:1.

Transdermal administration of oxybutynin bypasses the first-pass gastrointestinal and hepatic metabolism, reducing the formation of the N-desethyl metabolite. Only small amounts of CYP3A4 are found in skin, limiting presystemic metabolism during transdermal absorption. The resulting plasma concentration AUC ratio of N-desethyl metabolite to parent compound following multiple oxybutynin transdermal applications was 1.3:1.

Excretion – Oxybutynin is extensively metabolized by the liver, with less than 0.1% of the administered dose excreted unchanged in the urine. Also, less than 0.1% of the administered dose is excreted as the metabolite N-desethyloxybutynin.

Following intravenous administration, the elimination half-life of oxybutynin is approximately 2 hours. Following removal of oxybutynin transdermal system, plasma concentrations of oxybutynin and N-desethyloxybutynin decline with an apparent half-life of approximately 7 to 8 hours.

Special populations –

Race: Japanese volunteers demonstrated a somewhat lower metabolism of oxybutynin to N-desethyloxybutynin compared with white volunteers.

Contraindications

Urinary retention, gastric retention, or uncontrolled narrow-angle glaucoma and in patients who are at risk for these conditions; hypersensitivity to oxybutynin or other components of these product.

Warnings/Precautions

➤*Urinary retention:* Oxybutynin transdermal system should be administered with caution to patients with clinically significant bladder outflow obstruction because of the risk of urinary retention. Oxybutynin is contraindicated in patients with urinary retention.

➤*GI disorders:* Administer oxybutynin transdermal system with caution to patients with GI obstructive disorders because of the risk of gastric retention. Oxybutynin is contraindicated in patients with gastric retention.

Oxybutynin, like other anticholinergic drugs, may decrease GI motility. Use with caution in patients with conditions such as ulcerative colitis, intestinal atony, and myasthenia gravis. Use oxybutynin with caution in patients who have gastroesophageal reflux or who are concurrently taking drugs (such as bisphosphonates) that can cause or exacerbate esophagitis.

➤*Renal/Hepatic function impairment:* Use with caution in patients with hepatic or renal impairment.

➤*Pregnancy:* Category B.

Teratogenic – The safety of oxybutynin transdermal system administration to women who are or who may become pregnant has not been established. Therefore, oxybutynin transdermal system should not be given to pregnant women unless, in the judgment of the health care provider, the probable clinical benefits outweigh the possible hazards.

➤*Lactation:* It is not known whether oxybutynin is excreted in human milk. Because many drugs are excreted in human milk, exercise caution when oxybutynin transdermal system is administered to a breast-feeding woman.

➤*Children:* Safety and effectiveness have not been established.

➤*Elderly:* No overall differences in safety or effectiveness were observed between these subjects and younger subjects

Of the total number of patients in the clinical studies of oxybutynin transdermal system, 49% were 65 and over. Other reported clinical experience has not identified differences in response between elderly and younger patients, but greater sensitivity of some older individuals cannot be ruled out.

Drug Interactions

Oxybutynin Drug Interactions

Precipitant drug	Object drug[a]		Description
Oxybutynin	Anticholinergic agents	↑	Concomitant use may increase the frequency and/or severity of anticholinergic-like effects. Anticholinergic agents may potentially alter the absorption of some concomitantly administered drugs because of anticholinergic effects on GI motility.
Anticholinergic agents	Oxybutynin		
Oxybutynin	Beta blockers Atenolol	↑	The bioavailability of atenolol may be increased. If an increase in beta blockade is suspected, tailoring the beta blocker dose downward may be necessary.
Oxybutynin	Digoxin	↑	Serum levels of digoxin administered as slow-dissolution oral tablets may be increased and actions enhanced. Serum level monitoring may assist in tailoring dosage. Problems may be avoided with use of digoxin elixir or capsules.
Oxybutynin	Haloperidol	↔	Effects are variable. Use oxybutynin only when clearly needed. Routinely monitor these patients; discontinue anticholinergic or tailor haloperidol if necessary.
Oxybutynin	Phenothiazines	↓	Pharmacologic/therapeutic actions of phenothiazines may be decreased by anticholinergics. Tailor the phenothiazine dose as needed.
Amantadine	Oxybutynin	↑	Anticholinergic side effects may be increased. Decrease the dose of oxybutynin during coadministration. Monitor patient response and adjust the dose accordingly.

[a] ↑ = Object drug increased. ↓ = Object drug decreased.
↔ = Undetermined clinical effect.

OXYBUTYNIN — TRANSDERMAL PATCH

Adverse Reactions

Oxybutynin Transdermal System Adverse Reactions (≥ 2%) (Study 1)		
Adverse reaction[a]	Placebo (n = 132)	Oxybutynin transdermal system (3.9 mg/day) (n = 125)
Application-site pruritus	6.1%	16.8%
Dry mouth	8.3%	9.6%
Application-site erythema	2.3%	5.6%
Application-site vesicles	0%	3.2%
Diarrhea	2.3%	3.2%
Dysuria	0%	2.4%

[a] Includes adverse reactions judged by the investigator as possibly, probably, or definitely treatment-related.

Oxybutynin Transdermal System Adverse Reactions (≥ 2%) (Study 2)		
Adverse reaction[a]	Placebo (n = 117)	Oxybutynin transdermal system (3.9 mg/day) (n = 121)
Application-site pruritus	4.3%	14%
Application-site erythema	1.7%	8.3%
Dry mouth	1.7%	4.1%
Constipation	0%	3.3%
Application-site rash	0.9%	3.3%
Application-site macules	0%	2.5%
Abnormal vision	0%	2.5%

[a] Includes adverse reactions judged by the investigator as possibly, probably, or definitely treatment-related.

Other adverse reactions reported by greater than 1% of oxybutynin transdermal system-treated patients, and judged by the investigator to be possibly, probably, or definitely related to treatment include: Abdominal pain, nausea, flatulence, fatigue, somnolence, headache, flushing, rash, application site burning, and back pain.

Most treatment-related adverse reactions were described as mild or moderate in intensity. Severe application site reactions were reported by 6.4% of oxybutynin transdermal system-treated patients in study 1 and by 5% of oxybutynin transdermal system-treated patients in study 2.

Treatment-related adverse reactions that resulted in discontinuation were reported by 11.2% of oxybutynin transdermal system-treated patients in study 1 and 10.7% of oxybutynin transdermal system-treated patients in study 2. Most of these were secondary to application site reaction. In the 2 pivotal studies, no patient discontinued oxybutynin transdermal system treatment due to dry mouth.

In the open-label extension, the most common treatment-related adverse reactions were: Application site pruritus, application site erythema, and dry mouth.

➤*Postmarketing:* The following has been reported in association with oxybutynin chloride transdermal system use in clinical practice: dizziness. Because spontaneously reported events are from worldwide postmarketing experiences, the frequency of events an the role of oxybutynin chloride transdermal system in their causation cannot be ruled out.

Overdosage

Plasma concentration of oxybutynin declines within 1 to 2 hours after removal of transdermal system(s). Patients should be monitored until symptoms resolve.

➤*Symptoms:* Overdosage with oxybutynin has been associated with anticholinergic effects including CNS excitation, flushing, fever, dehydration, cardiac arrhythmia, vomiting, and urinary retention. Ingestion of 100 mg oral oxybutynin chloride in association with alcohol has been reported in a 13-year-old boy who experienced memory loss, and in a 34-year-old woman who developed stupor, followed by disorientation and agitation on awakening, dilated pupils, dry skin, cardiac arrhythmia, and retention of urine.

➤*Treatment:* Both patients recovered fully with symptomatic treatment.

OXYBUTYNIN CHLORIDE — TRANSDERMAL GEL

Indications

➤*Overactive bladder:* For the treatment of overactive bladder with symptoms of urge urinary incontinence, urgency, and frequency.

Administration and Dosage

➤*Adults:*

Overactive bladder – Apply 1 g (1 sachet) once daily to dry, intact skin on the abdomen, upper arms/shoulders, or thighs.

➤*Administration:* The contents of 1 sachet should be applied once daily to dry intact skin on the abdomen, upper arms/shoulders, or thighs. Application sites should be rotated. Oxybutynin gel should not be applied to the same site on consecutive days.

Oxybutynin gel is for topical application only and should not be ingested. Apply immediately after the sachets are opened and contents expelled.

➤*Storage/Stability:* Store at 25°C (77°F); excursions are permitted to 15° to 30°C (59° to 86°F). Protect from moisture and humidity. Discard used sachets in household trash in a manner that prevents accidental application or ingestion by children, pets, or others.

Actions

➤*Pharmacology:* Oxybutynin is an antispasmodic, antimuscarinic agent and acts as a competitive antagonist of acetylcholine at postganglionic muscarinic receptors, resulting in relaxation of bladder smooth muscle. In patients with conditions characterized by involuntary detrusor contractions, cystometric studies have demonstrated that oxybutynin increases maximum urinary bladder capacity and the volume to first detrusor contraction.

Oxybutynin is a racemic (50:50) mixture of R- and S-isomers. Antimuscarinic activity resides predominantly in the R-isomer. The active metabolite N-desethyloxybutynin has pharmacological activity on the human detrusor muscle that is similar to that of oxybutynin in in vitro studies.

➤*Pharmacokinetics:*

Absorption – Oxybutynin is transported across intact skin and into the systemic circulation by passive diffusion across the stratum corneum. Steady-state concentrations are achieved within 7 days of continuous dosing. Absorption of oxybutynin is similar when oxybutynin gel is applied to the abdomen, upper arm/shoulders, or thighs.

Average steady-state plasma oxybutynin concentrations were 4.7, 5.2, and 5.5 ng/mL for the abdomen, upper arm/shoulder, and thigh application sites, respectively.

Mean (SD) Steady-State Pharmacokinetic Parameters for Oxybutynin Following Oxybutynin Gel Application to the Abdomen, Upper Arm/Shoulder, and Thigh (N = 39)[a]			
Application site	AUC_{0-24} (ng•h/mL)	C_{max} (ng/mL)	C_{avg} (ng/mL)
Abdomen	112.7 (58)	6.8 (3.93)	4.7 (2.39)
Upper arm/shoulder	133.8 (81.58)	8.3 (5.97)	5.5 (3.37)
Thigh	125.1 (84.67)	7 (4.95)	5.2 (3.5)

[a] SD = standard deviation; AUC_{0-24} = area under the curve; C_{max} = maximum drug concentration; C_{avg} = average steady-state plasma concentration.

Person-to-person transference: The potential for dermal transfer of oxybutynin from a treated person to an untreated person was evaluated in a single-dose study in which subjects dosed with oxybutynin gel engaged in vigorous contact with an untreated partner for 15 minutes, either with (n = 14 couples) or without (n = 12 couples) clothing covering the application area. The untreated partners not protected by clothing demonstrated detectable plasma concentrations of oxybutynin (mean C_{max}, 0.94 ng/mL). Two of the 14 untreated subjects participating in the clothing-to-skin contact regimen had measurable oxybutynin plasma concentrations (C_{max}, 0.1 ng/mL or less) during the 48 hours following contact with treated subjects; oxybutynin was not detectable with the remaining 12 untreated subjects.

Use of sunscreen: The effect of sunscreen on the absorption of oxybutynin when applied 30 minutes before or 30 minutes after oxybutynin application was evaluated in a single-dose, randomized, crossover study (N = 16). Concomitant application of sunscreen, either before or after oxybutynin application, had no effect on the systemic exposure of oxybutynin.

Showering: The effect of showering on the absorption of oxybutynin was evaluated in a randomized, steady-state, crossover study under conditions of no shower or showering 1, 2, or 6 hours after oxybutynin application (N = 20). The results of the study indicate that showering after an hour does not affect the overall systemic exposure to oxybutynin.

Distribution – Oxybutynin is widely distributed in body tissues following systemic absorption. The volume of distribution was estimated to be 193 L after intravenous (IV) administration of oxybutynin 5 mg.

Metabolism – Oxybutynin is metabolized primarily by the cytochrome P450 (CYP-450) enzyme systems, particularly CYP3A4, found mostly in the liver and gut wall. Metabolites include phenylcyclohexylglycolic acid, which is pharmacologically inactive, and N-desethyloxybutynin, which is pharmacologically active.

Transdermal administration of oxybutynin bypasses the first-pass GI and hepatic metabolism, reducing the formation of the N-desethyloxybutynin metabolite. Only small amounts of CYP3A4 are found in skin, limiting presystemic metabolism during transdermal absorption. The resulting plasma concentration AUC ratio of N-desethyloxybutynin metabolite to parent compound following multiple oxybutynin transdermal applications was 1:1.

Excretion – Following IV administration, the elimination half-life of oxybutynin is approximately 2 hours. After the final steady-state dose of oxybutynin gel, oxybutynin and N-desethyloxybutynin demonstrated biphasic elimination, with plasma concentrations beginning to decrease 24 hours after dosing. Elimination was more rapid between 24 and 48 hours after dosing, during which time plasma concentrations of oxybutynin and N-desethyloxybutynin declined by approximately one-half. This rapid elimi-

OXYBUTYNIN CHLORIDE — TRANSDERMAL GEL

nation phase was followed by a more prolonged terminal elimination phase. The apparent elimination half-lives, including the terminal elimination phase, were 64 and 82 hours for oxybutynin and N-desethyloxybutynin, respectively.

Oxybutynin is extensively metabolized by the liver, with less than 0.1% of the administered dose excreted unchanged in the urine. Also, less than 0.1% of the administered dose is excreted as the metabolite N-desethyloxybutynin.

Contraindications

Urinary retention, gastric retention, or uncontrolled narrow-angle glaucoma; known hypersensitivity to oxybutynin, including skin hypersensitivity.

Warnings/Precautions

➤*Urinary retention:* Administer oxybutynin gel with caution to patients with clinically significant bladder outflow obstruction because of the risk of urinary retention.

➤*GI disorders:* Administer oxybutynin gel with caution to patients with GI obstructive disorders because of the risk of gastric retention. Oxybutynin is contraindicated in patients with gastric retention.

Oxybutynin, like other anticholinergic drugs, may decrease GI motility. Use with caution in patients with conditions such as ulcerative colitis or intestinal atony. Use oxybutynin with caution in patients who have gastroesophageal reflux and/or who are concurrently taking drugs (such as bisphosphonates) that can cause or exacerbate esophagitis.

➤*Skin transference:* Transfer of oxybutynin to another person can occur when vigorous skin-to-skin contact is made with the application site. To minimize the potential transfer of oxybutynin from oxybutynin-treated skin to another person, instruct patients to cover the application site with clothing after the gel has dried if direct skin-to-skin contact at the application site is anticipated. Advise patients to wash their hands immediately after application of oxybutynin.

➤*Flammable gel:* Oxybutynin is an alcohol-based gel and is therefore flammable. Instruct patients to avoid open fire or smoking until gel has dried.

➤*Myasthenia gravis:* Administer oxybutynin with caution in patients with myasthenia gravis, a disease characterized by decreased cholinergic activity at the neuromuscular junction.

➤*Hypersensitivity reactions:* In a controlled clinical trial of skin sensitization, 1 of 200 (0.5%) patients demonstrated skin hypersensitivity to oxybutynin gel. Discontinue drug treatment in patients who develop skin hypersensitivity to oxybutynin.

➤*Pregnancy: Category B.* There are no adequate and well-controlled studies of topical or oral oxybutynin use in pregnant women. The safety of oxybutynin gel administration to women who are or who may become pregnant has not been established. Therefore, oxybutynin gel should not be given to pregnant women unless, in the judgment of the health care provider, the probable clinical benefits outweigh the possible hazards.

➤*Lactation:* It is not known whether oxybutynin is excreted in human milk. Because many drugs are excreted in human milk, exercise caution when oxybutynin gel is administered to a breast-feeding woman.

➤*Children:* Safety and effectiveness have not been established.

➤*Elderly:* No overall differences in safety or effectiveness were observed between elderly and younger patients.

Of the 496 patients exposed to oxybutynin in the randomized, double-blind, placebo-controlled, 12-week study and the 14-week safety extension study, 188 (38%) patients were 65 years of age and older.

Drug Interactions

Oxybutynin Gel Drug Interactions

Precipitant drug	Object drug[a]		Description
Anticholinergic agents	Oxybutynin	↑	Concomitant use may increase the frequency and/or severity of anticholinergic-like effects (eg, dry mouth, constipation, blurred vision). Anticholinergic agents may potentially alter the absorption of some coadministered drugs because of anticholinergic effects on GI motility.
Oxybutynin	Anticholinergic agents		
Oxybutynin	Beta-blockers Atenolol	↑	The bioavailability of atenolol may be increased. If an increase in beta blockade is suspected, tailoring the beta-blocker dose downward may be necessary.
Oxybutynin	Digoxin	↑	Serum levels of digoxin administered as slow-dissolution oral tablets may be increased and actions enhanced. Serum level monitoring may assist in tailoring dosage. Interaction may be avoided with use of digoxin elixir or tablets.
Oxybutynin	Haloperidol	↔	Effects are variable. Worsening of schizophrenic symptoms, decreased serum concentrations of haloperidol, and development of tardive dyskinesia were reported during coadministration. Use oxybutynin only when clearly needed. Routinely monitor these patients; discontinue the anticholinergic or tailor haloperidol if necessary.
Oxybutynin	Phenothiazines	↓	Pharmacologic/therapeutic actions of phenothiazines may be decreased by anticholinergics. Tailor the phenothiazine dose as needed.
Oxybutynin	Potassium preparations	↑	Anticholinergic agents may stop or delay passage of potassium tablets through the GI tract. Coadministration is not recommended.
Amantadine	Oxybutynin	↑	Anticholinergic adverse effects may be increased. Decrease the dose of oxybutynin during coadministration. Monitor patient response and adjust the dose accordingly.

[a] ↑ = object drug increased; ↓ = object drug decreased; ↔ = undetermined clinical effect.

Adverse Reactions

Because clinical trials are conducted under widely varying conditions, adverse reaction rates observed in the clinical trials of a drug cannot be directly compared with rates in the clinical trial of another drug and may not reflect the rates observed in practice.

The safety of oxybutynin was evaluated in 789 patients (389 randomized to oxybutynin 1 g and 400 randomized to placebo) during a randomized, placebo-controlled, double-blind, 12-week clinical efficacy and safety study. A subset of these 789 patients (n = 216) participated in the 14-week, open-label safety extension that followed the placebo-controlled study. Of 216 patients in the safety extension, 107 were randomized to placebo gel during the double-blind, placebo-controlled, 12-week study. In the combined double-blind, placebo-controlled study and the open-label safety extension, 496 patients were exposed to at least 1 dose of oxybutynin. A total of 431 patients received at least 12 weeks of oxybutynin treatment and 85 patients received 26 weeks of oxybutynin treatment. The study population primarily consisted of white women (approximately 90%) with an average age of 59 years who had overactive bladder with urge urinary incontinence.

The following table lists adverse reactions, regardless of causality, that were reported in the randomized, double-blind, placebo-controlled, 12-week study at an incidence greater than placebo and in more than 2% of patients treated with oxybutynin.

Oxybutynin Gel Adverse Reactions

Adverse reactions	Placebo (n = 400)	Oxybutynin 1 g gel (n = 389)
CNS		
Dizziness	1%	2.8%
Fatigue	1%	2.1%
GI		
Dry mouth	2.8%	7.5%
Gastroenteritis viral	1.8%	2.1%
Respiratory		
Nasopharyngitis	2.3%	2.8%
Upper respiratory tract infection	5%	5.4%
Miscellaneous		
Application-site reactions[a]	1%	5.4%
Urinary tract infection	4.3%	6.9%

[a] Includes application-site pruritus, dermatitis, papules, anesthesia, erythema, irritation, and pain.

➤*Most common adverse reactions:* The most common adverse reactions, defined as adverse reactions judged by the investigator to be reasonably associated with the use of study drug, that were reported in 1% or more of oxybutynin-treated patients were dry mouth (6.9%), application-site reactions (5.4%), headache (1.5%), dizziness (1.5%), constipation (1.3%), and pruritus (1.3%). Application-site pruritus (2.1%) and application-site dermatitis (1.8%) were the most commonly reported application-site reactions. A majority of treatment-related adverse reactions were described as mild or moderate in intensity, except for 2 patients reporting severe headache.

No serious adverse reactions were judged by the investigator to be treatment-related during the randomized, double-blind, placebo-controlled,

OXYBUTYNIN CHLORIDE — TRANSDERMAL GEL

12-week study. The most common adverse reaction leading to drug discontinuation was application-site reaction (0.8% with oxybutynin vs 0.3% with placebo).

The most common adverse reactions reported during the 14-week, open-label extension study were application-site reactions (6%) and dry mouth (1.9%). The most common reason for premature discontinuation was application-site reactions (9 [4.2%] patients). Two of these 9 patients experienced application-site reactions of severe intensity (dermatitis, erythema, and urticaria).

Overdosage

➤*Symptoms:* Overdosage with oxybutynin has been associated with anticholinergic effects, including CNS excitation, flushing, fever, dehydration, cardiac arrhythmia, vomiting, and urinary retention. Ingestion of oral oxybutynin 100 mg in association with alcohol has been reported in a boy 13 years of age who experienced memory loss, and in a woman 34 years of age who developed stupor, followed by disorientation and agitation upon awakening, dilated pupils, dry skin, cardiac arrhythmia, and retention of urine. If overexposure occurs, monitor patients until symptoms resolve.

➤*Treatment:* Plasma concentrations of oxybutynin begin to decline 24 hours after oxybutynin gel application. Both patients recovered fully with symptomatic treatment.

Patient Information

Oxybutynin gel is for topical application only and should not be ingested. Advise patients not to apply oxybutynin gel to recently shaved skin surfaces. Also advise patients to wash their hands immediately after product application. Advise patients not to subject application sites to showering or water immersion for 1 hour after product application. Advise patients to cover application sites with clothing if close skin-to-skin contact at the application site is anticipated.

Alcohol-based gels are flammable. Avoid open fire or smoking until the gel has dried.

➤*Important anticholinergic adverse reactions:* Inform patients that anticholinergic (antimuscarinic) agents, such as oxybutynin gel, may produce clinically significant adverse reactions related to anticholinergic pharmacological activity, including constipation, urinary retention, and blurred vision. Heat prostration (because of decreased sweating) can occur when anticholinergics such as oxybutynin gel are used in a hot environment. Because anticholinergic (antimuscarinic) agents, such as oxybutynin gel, may produce dizziness or blurred vision, advise patients to exercise caution in decisions to engage in potentially dangerous activities until oxybutynin gel effects have been determined.

Inform patients that alcohol may enhance the drowsiness caused by anticholinergic (antimuscarinic) agents such as oxybutynin gel.

TOLTERODINE TARTRATE

Rx	**Detrol** (Pfizer)	**Tablets:** 1 mg	(TO). White. Film-coated. In 60s, 500s, and UD 140s.
		2 mg	(DT). White. Film-coated. In 60s, 500s, and UD 140s.
Rx	**Detrol LA** (Pfizer)	**Capsules, extended-release:** 2 mg	Sucrose. (2). Blue-green. In 30s, 90s, 500s, and UD blister 100s.
		4 mg	Sucrose. (4). Blue. In 30s, 90s, 500s, and UD blister 100s.

TOLTERODINE TARTRATE — ORAL

Indications

➤*Overactive bladder:* For the treatment of patients with an overactive bladder with symptoms of urge urinary incontinence, urgency, and frequency.

Administration and Dosage

➤*Adults:*

Overactive bladder –

Extended-release capsules:

• *Usual dosage* – 4 mg/day taken once daily.

• *Dosage adjustment* – Lower the dose to 2 mg daily based on individual response and tolerability; however, limited efficacy data is available for 2 mg extended-release capsules.

Immediate-release tablets:

• *Usual dosage* – 2 mg twice daily.

• *Dosage adjustment* – Lower the dose to 1 mg twice daily based on individual response and tolerability.

➤*Renal function impairment:* For patients with significantly reduced renal function, the recommended dose is 2 mg daily for extended-release capsules or 1 mg twice daily for immediate-release tablets.

➤*Hepatic function impairment:* For patients with significantly reduced hepatic function, the recommended dose is 2 mg daily for extended-release capsules or 1 mg twice daily for immediate-release tablets.

➤*Concomitant therapy:* For patients currently taking potent inhibitors of CYP3A4, the recommended dose is 2 mg daily for extended-release capsules or 1 mg twice daily for immediate-release tablets.

➤*Administration:* Extended-release capsules should be taken once daily with liquids and swallowed whole.

➤*Storage/Stability:* Store at controlled room temperature, 25°C (77°F); excursions are permitted to 15° to 30°C (59° to 86°F). Protect extended-release capsules from light.

Actions

➤*Pharmacology:* Tolterodine is a competitive muscarinic receptor antagonist. Both urinary bladder contraction and salivation are mediated via cholinergic muscarinic receptors.

After oral administration, tolterodine is metabolized in the liver, resulting in the formation of the 5-hydroxymethyl derivative, a major pharmacologically active metabolite. The 5-hydroxymethyl metabolite, which exhibits an antimuscarinic activity similar to that of tolterodine, contributes significantly to the therapeutic effect. Both tolterodine and the 5-hydroxymethyl metabolite exhibit a high specificity for muscarinic receptors, since both show negligible activity or affinity for other neurotransmitter receptors and other potential cellular targets, such as calcium channels.

Tolterodine has a pronounced effect on bladder function. Effects on urodynamic parameters before and 1 and 5 hours after a single 6.4 mg dose of immediate-release tolterodine were determined in healthy volunteers. The main effects of tolterodine at 1 and 5 hours were an increase in residual urine, reflecting an incomplete emptying of the bladder, and a decrease in detrusor pressure. These findings are consistent with antimuscarinic action on the lower urinary tract.

➤*Pharmacokinetics:*

Absorption –

Immediate-release tablets: In a study of ^{14}C-tolterodine in healthy volunteers who received a 5 mg oral dose, at least 77% of the radiolabeled dose was absorbed. Immediate-release tolterodine is rapidly absorbed, and maximum serum concentrations (C_{max}) typically occur within 1 to 2 hours after dose administration. C_{max} and area under the concentration-time curve (AUC) determined after dosage of immediate-release tolterodine are dose proportional over the range of 1 to 4 mg.

• *Effect of food* – Food intake increases the bioavailability of tolterodine (average increase 53%), but does not affect the levels of the 5-hydroxymethyl metabolite in extensive metabolizers. This change is not expected to be a safety concern, and adjustment of dose is not needed.

Extended-release capsules: In a study with ^{14}C-tolterodine solution in healthy volunteers who received a 5 mg oral dose, at least 77% of the radiolabeled dose was absorbed. C_{max} and area under the concentration-time curve (AUC) determined after dosage of immediate-release tolterodine are dose proportional over the range of 1 to 4 mg. Based on the sum of unbound serum concentrations of tolterodine and the 5-hydroxymethyl metabolite ("active moiety"), the AUC of 4 mg/day extended-release tolterodine is equivalent to 4 mg (2 mg twice daily) immediate-release tolterodine. C_{max} and C_{min} levels of extended-release tolterodine are about 75% and 150% of immediate-release tolterodine, respectively. Maximum serum concentrations of extended-release tolterodine are observed 2 to 6 hours after dose administration.

Distribution – Tolterodine is highly bound to plasma proteins, primarily α_1-acid glycoprotein. Unbound concentrations of tolterodine average 3.7% ± 0.13% over the concentration range achieved in clinical studies. The 5-hydroxymethyl metabolite is not extensively protein bound, with unbound fraction concentrations averaging 36% ± 4%. The blood-to-serum ratio of tolterodine and the 5-hydroxymethyl metabolite averages 0.6 and 0.8, respectively, indicating that these compounds do not distribute extensively into erythrocytes. The volume of distribution of tolterodine following administration of a 1.28 mg IV dose is 113 ± 26.7 L.

Metabolism – Tolterodine is extensively metabolized by the liver following oral dosing. The primary metabolic route involves the oxidation of the 5-methyl group and is mediated by the cytochrome P450 2D6 (CYP2D6) and leads to the formation of a pharmacologically active 5-hydroxymethyl metabolite. Further metabolism leads to formation of the 5-carboxylic acid and N-dealkylated 5-carboxylic acid metabolites, which account for 51% ± 14% and 29% ± 6.3% of the metabolites recovered in the urine, respectively.

Variability in metabolism: A subset (about 7%) of the white population is devoid of CYP2D6, the enzyme responsible for the formation of the 5-hydroxymethyl metabolite of tolterodine. The identified pathway of metabolism for these individuals ("poor metabolizers") is dealkylation via cytochrome P450 3A4 (CYP3A4) to N-dealkylated tolterodine. The remainder of the population is referred to as "extensive metabolizers." Pharmacokinetic studies revealed that tolterodine is metabolized at a slower rate in poor metabolizers than in extensive metabolizers; this results in significantly higher serum concentrations of tolterodine and in negligible concentrations of the 5-hydroxymethyl metabolite.

• *Immediate-release tablets* – Because of differences in the protein-binding characteristics of tolterodine and the 5-hydroxymethyl metabolite, the sum of unbound serum concentrations of tolterodine and the 5-hydroxymethyl metabolite is similar in extensive and poor metabolizers at steady state. Since tolterodine and the 5-hydroxymethyl metabolite have similar antimuscarinic effects, the net activity of tolterodine immediate-release tablets is expected to be similar in extensive and poor metabolizers.

Excretion – Following administration of a 5 mg oral dose of ^{14}C-tolterodine to healthy volunteers, 77% of radioactivity was recovered in urine and 17% was recovered in feces in 7 days. Less than 1% (less than 2.5% in poor metabolizers) of the dose was recovered as intact tolterodine, and 5% to 14% (less than 1% in poor metabolizers) was recovered as the active 5-hydroxymethyl metabolite.

TOLTERODINE TARTRATE — ORAL

Immediate-release tablets: Most of the radioactivity was recovered within the first 24 hours, which is consistent with the apparent half-life of tolterodine: 1.9 to 3.7 hours in pharmacokinetic studies.

A summary of mean (± standard deviation) pharmacokinetic parameters of immediate-release tolterodine and the 5-hydroxymethyl metabolite in extensive and poor metabolizers is provided in the following tables. These data were obtained following single and multiple doses of 4 mg tolterodine administered twice daily to 16 healthy male volunteers (8 extensive metabolizers, 8 poor metabolizers).

Summary of Mean (± SD) Pharmacokinetic Parameters of Tolterodine and Its Active Metabolite (5-hydroxymethyl Metabolite) in Healthy Volunteers[a]

Phenotype (CYP2D6)	Tolterodine					5-hydroxymethyl metabolite			
	t_{max} (hr)	C_{max}[b] (mcg/L)	C_{avg}[b] (mcg/L)	t½ (hr)	CL/F (L/hr)	t_{max} (hr)	C_{max}[b] (mcg/L)	C_{avg}[b] (mcg/L)	t½ (hr)
Single dose									
EM	1.6 ± 1.5	1.6 ± 1.2	0.5 ± 0.35	2 ± 0.7	534 ± 697	1.8 ± 1.4	1.8 ± 0.7	0.62 ± 0.26	3.1 ± 0.7
PM	1.4 ± 0.5	10 ± 4.9	8.3 ± 4.3	6.5 ± 1.6	17 ± 7.3	NA	NA	NA	NA
Multiple dose									
EM	1.2 ± 0.5	2.6 ± 2.8	0.58 ± 0.54	2.2 ± 0.4	415 ± 377	1.2 ± 0.5	2.4 ± 1.3	0.92 ± 0.46	2.9 ± 0.4
PM	1.9 ± 1	19 ± 7.5	12 ± 5.1	9.6 ± 1.5	11 ± 4.2	NA	NA	NA	NA

[a] C_{max} = Maximum plasma concentration; t_{max} = time of occurrence of C_{max}; C_{avg} = Average plasma concentration; t½ = Terminal elimination half-life; CL/F = Apparent oral clearance; EM = Extensive metabolizers; PM = Poor metabolizers.
[b] Parameter was dose-normalized from 4 mg to 2 mg.

Extended-release capsules: A summary of mean (± standard deviation) pharmacokinetic parameters of extended-release tolterodine and the 5-hydroxymethyl metabolite in extensive and poor metabolizers is provided in the table below. These data were obtained following single and multiple doses of extended-release tolterodine administered daily to 17 healthy male volunteers (13 extensive metabolizers, 4 poor metabolizers).

Summary of Mean (± SD) Pharmacokinetic Parameters of Extended-Release Tolterodine and Its Active Metabolite (5-hydroxymethyl Metabolite) in Healthy Volunteers[a]

	Tolterodine				5-hydroxymethyl metabolite			
	t_{max}[b] (hr)	C_{max} (mcg/L)	C_{avg} (mcg/L)	t½ (hr)	t_{max}[b] (hr)	C_{max} (mcg/L)	C_{avg} (mcg/L)	t½ (hr)
Single dose 4 mg[c]								
EM	4 (2 to 6)	1.3 (0.8)	0.8 (0.57)	8.4 (3.2)	4 (3 to 6)	1.6 (0.5)	1 (0.32)	8.8 (5.9)
Multiple dose 4 mg								
EM	4 (2 to 6)	3.4 (4.9)	1.7 (2.8)	6.9 (3.5)	4 (2 to 6)	2.7 (0.9)	1.4 (0.6)	9.9 (4)
PM	4 (3 to 6)	19 (16)	13 (11)	18 (16)	NA	NA	NA	NA

[a] C_{max} = Maximum plasma concentration; t_{max} = Time of occurrence of C_{max}; C_{avg} = Average plasma concentration; t½ = Terminal elimination half-life; CL/F = Apparent oral clearance.
[b] Data presented as median (range).
[c] Parameter dose-normalized from 8 to 4 mg for the single-dose data.

Special populations –

Renal function impairment:

• *Immediate-release tablets* – Renal impairment can significantly alter the disposition of immediate-release tolterodine and its metabolites. In a study conducted in patients with creatinine clearance between 10 and 30 mL/min, immediate-release tolterodine and the 5-hydroxymethyl metabolite levels were approximately 2 to 3 fold higher in patients with renal impairment than in healthy volunteers. Exposure levels of other metabolites of tolterodine (eg, tolterodine acid, N-dealkylated tolterodine acid, N-dealkylated tolterodine, and N-dealkylated hydroxylated tolterodine) were significantly higher (10- to 30-fold) in renally impaired patients as compared with the healthy volunteers. The recommended dosage for patients with significantly reduced renal function is 1 mg tolterodine twice daily.

• *Extended-release capsules* – Renal impairment can significantly alter the disposition of immediate-release tolterodine and its metabolites. In a study conducted in patients with creatinine clearance between 10 and 30 mL/min, immediate-release tolterodine and the 5-hydroxymethyl metabolite levels were approximately 2- to 3-fold higher in patients with renal impairment than in healthy volunteers. Exposure levels of other metabolites of tolterodine (eg, tolterodine acid, N-dealkylated tolterodine acid, N-dealkylated tolterodine and N-dealkylated hydroxy tolterodine) were significantly higher (10- to 30-fold) in renally impaired patients as compared to the healthy volunteers. The recommended dose for patients with significantly reduced renal function is 2 mg/day tolterodine.

Hepatic function impairment: Liver impairment can significantly alter the disposition of immediate-release tolterodine. In a study conducted in cirrhotic patients, the elimination half-life of immediate-release tolterodine was longer in cirrhotic patients (mean, 7.8 hours) than in healthy, younger and elderly volunteers (mean, 2 to 4 hours). The clearance of orally administered tolterodine was substantially lower in cirrhotic patients (1 ± 1.7 L/hr/kg) than in healthy volunteers (5.7 ± 3.8 L/hr/kg). The recommended dose for patients with significantly reduced hepatic function is 1 mg immediate-release tolterodine twice daily or 2 mg/day extended-release tolterodine.

Children:

• *Extended-release capsules* – The pharmacokinetics of tolterodine extended-release capsules have been evaluated in pediatric patients ranging in age from 11 to 15 years. The dose-plasma concentration relationship was linear over the range of doses assessed. Parent/metabolite ratios differed according to CYP2D6 metabolizer status: Extensive metabolizers had low serum concentrations of tolterodine and high concentrations of the active 5-hydroxymethyl metabolite, while poor metabolizers had high concentrations of tolterodine and negligible active metabolite concentrations.

Contraindications

Urinary retention, gastric retention, or uncontrolled narrow-angle glaucoma; hypersensitivity to the drug or its ingredients.

Warnings/Precautions

➤*Risk of urinary retention and gastric retention:* Administer tolterodine with caution to patients with clinically significant bladder outflow obstruction because of the risk of urinary retention and to patients with GI obstructive disorders, such as pyloric stenosis, because of the risk of gastric retention.

➤*Controlled narrow-angle glaucoma:* Use tolterodine with caution in patients being treated for narrow-angle glaucoma.

➤*Renal/Hepatic function impairment:*

Immediate-release tablets – For patients with significantly reduced hepatic function or renal function, the recommended dose of tolterodine is 1 mg twice daily.

Extended-release capsules – For patients with significantly reduced hepatic function or renal function, the recommended dose is 2 mg/day extended-release tolterodine.

➤*Pregnancy:* *Category C.* When given at doses of 30 to 40 mg/kg/day, tolterodine has been shown to be embryolethal and reduce fetal weight, and increase the incidence of fetal abnormalities (cleft palate, digital abnormalities, intra-abdominal hemorrhage, and various skeletal abnormalities, primarily reduced ossification) in mice. At these doses, the AUC values were about 20- to 25-fold higher than in humans. Rabbits treated subcutaneously at a dose of 0.8 mg/kg/day achieved an AUC of 100 mcg•hr/L, which is about 3-fold higher than that resulting from the human dose. This dose did not result in any embryotoxicity or teratogenicity. There are no studies of tolterodine in pregnant women. Therefore, only use tolterodine during pregnancy if the potential benefit for the mother justifies the potential risk for the fetus.

➤*Lactation:* Tolterodine is excreted into the milk in mice. Offspring of female mice treated with tolterodine 20 mg/kg/day during the lactation period had slightly reduced body-weight gain. The offspring regained the weight during the maturation phase. It is not known whether tolterodine is excreted in human milk; therefore, do not administer tolterodine during nursing. Decide whether to discontinue nursing or to discontinue tolterodine in nursing mothers.

➤*Children:* Safety and efficacy have not been established.

Extended-release capsules – A total of 710 pediatric patients (486 on extended-release tolterodine, 224 on placebo) 5 to 10 years of age with urinary frequency and urge incontinence were studied in two phase 3 randomized, placebo-controlled, double-blind, 12-week studies. The percentage of patients with urinary tract infections was higher in patients treated with extended-release tolterodine (6.6%) compared with patients who received placebo (4.5%). Aggressive, abnormal, and hyperactive behavior and attention disorders occurred in 2.9% of children treated with extended-release tolterodine compared with 0.9% of children treated with placebo.

Drug Interactions

➤*CYP3A4 inhibitors:* Ketoconazole, an inhibitor of the drug metabolizing enzyme CYP3A4, significantly increased plasma concentrations of tolterodine when coadministered to subjects who were poor metabolizers. For patients receiving ketoconazole or other potent CYP3A4 inhibitors such as other azole antifungals (eg, itraconazole, miconazole) or macrolide antibiotics (eg, erythromycin, clarithromycin), or cyclosporine or vinblastine, the recommended dose is 1 mg twice daily of immediate-release tolterodine or 2 mg/day extended-release tolterodine.

➤*Fluoxetine:* Fluoxetine is a selective serotonin reuptake inhibitor (SSRI) and a potent inhibitor of cytochrome P450 2D6 activity. In a study to assess the effect of fluoxetine on the pharmacokinetics of immediate-release tolterodine and its metabolites, it was observed that fluoxetine significantly inhibited the metabolism of immediate-release tolterodine in extensive metabolizers, resulting in a 4.8-fold increase in tolterodine AUC. There was a 52% decrease in C_{max} and a 20% decrease in AUC of the 5-hydroxymethyl metabolite. Fluoxetine thus alters the pharmacokinetics in patients who would otherwise be extensive metabolizers of immediate-release tolterodine to resemble the pharmacokinetic profile in poor metabolizers. The sums of unbound serum concentrations of immediate-release tolterodine and the 5-hydroxymethyl metabolite are only 25% higher during the interaction. No dose adjustment is required when tolterodine and fluoxetine are coadministered.

Adverse Reactions

➤*Immediate-release tablets:* The phase 2 and 3 clinical trial program for tolterodine included 3,071 patients who were treated with tolterodine (n = 2,133) or placebo (n = 938). The patients were treated with 1, 2, 4, or

TOLTERODINE TARTRATE — ORAL

8 mg/day for up to 12 months. No differences in the safety profile of tolterodine were identified based on age, gender, race, or metabolism.

The data described below reflect exposure to 2 mg tolterodine twice daily in 986 patients and to placebo in 683 patients exposed for 12 weeks in 5 phase 3, controlled clinical studies. Because clinical trials are conducted under widely varying conditions, adverse reaction rates observed in the clinical trials of a drug cannot be directly compared with rates in the clinical trials of another drug and may not reflect the rates observed in practice. The adverse reaction information from clinical trials does, however, provide a basis for identifying the adverse reactions that appear to be related to drug use and approximating rates.

Sixty-six percent (66%) of patients receiving 2 mg tolterodine twice daily reported adverse reactions versus 56% of placebo patients. The most common adverse reactions reported by patients receiving tolterodine were dry mouth, headache, constipation, vertigo/dizziness, and abdominal pain. Dry mouth, constipation, abnormal vision (accommodation abnormalities), urinary retention, and xerophthalmia are expected side effects of antimuscarinic agents.

Dry mouth was the most frequently reported adverse reaction for patients treated with 2 mg tolterodine twice daily in the phase 3 clinical studies, occurring in 34.8% of patients treated with tolterodine and 9.8% of placebo-treated patients. One percent (1%) of patients treated with tolterodine discontinued treatment due to dry mouth.

The frequency of discontinuation due to adverse reactions was highest during the first 4 weeks of treatment. Seven percent (7%) of patients treated with tolterodine 2 mg twice daily discontinued treatment due to adverse reactions verses 6% of placebo patients. The most common adverse reactions leading to discontinuation were dizziness and headache.

Three percent (3%) of patients treated with 2 mg tolterodine twice daily reported a serious adverse reaction versus 4% of placebo patients. Significant ECG changes in QT and QTc have not been demonstrated in clinical-study patients treated with tolterodine 2 mg twice daily. The table below lists the adverse reactions reported in 1% or more of the patients treated with 2 mg tolterodine twice daily in the 12-week studies. The adverse reactions are reported regardless of causality.

Tolterodine Adverse Reactions[a] (> 1%)

Adverse reaction	% Tolterodine (n = 986)	% Placebo (n = 683)
Autonomic nervous		
Accommodation abnormal	2	1
Dry mouth	35	10
CNS		
Somnolence	3	2
Vertigo/dizziness	5	3
Dermatologic		
Dry skin	1	0
GI		
Abdominal pain	5	3
Constipation	7	4
Diarrhea	4	3
Dyspepsia	4	1
GU		
Dysuria	2	1
Metabolic/Nutritional		
Weight gain	1	0
Musculoskeletal		
Arthralgia	2	1
Special senses		
Xerophthalmia	3	2
Miscellaneous		
Chest pain	2	1
Fatigue	4	3
Headache	7	5
Infection	1	0
Influenza-like symptoms	3	2

[a] In nearest integer.

➤*Extended-release capsules:* The phase 2 and 3 clinical trial program for tolterodine extended-release capsules included 1,073 patients who were treated with tolterodine extended-release capsules (n = 537) or placebo (n = 536). The patients were treated with 2, 4, 6, or 8 mg/day for up to 15 months. Because clinical trials are conducted under widely varying conditions, adverse reaction rates observed in the clinical trials of a drug cannot be directly compared with rates in the clinical trials of another drug and may not reflect the rates observed in practice. The adverse reaction information from clinical trials does, however, provide a basis for identifying the adverse reactions that appear to be related to drug use and for approximating rates. The data described below reflect exposure to 4 mg extended-release tolterodine capsules once daily every morning in 505 patients and to placebo in 507 patients exposed for 12 weeks in the phase 3, controlled clinical study.

Adverse reactions were reported in 52% (n = 263) of patients receiving tolterodine extended-release capsules and in 49% (n = 247) of patients receiving placebo. The most common adverse reactions reported by patients receiving tolterodine extended-release capsules were dry mouth, headache, constipation, and abdominal pain. Dry mouth was the most frequently reported adverse reaction for patients treated with tolterodine extended-release capsules, occurring in 23.4% of patients treated with tolterodine extended-release capsules and 7.7% of placebo-treated patients. Dry mouth, constipation, abnormal vision (accommodation abnormalities), urinary retention, and dry eyes are expected side effects of antimuscarinic agents. A serious adverse reaction was reported by 1.4% (n = 7) of patients receiving tolterodine extended-release capsules and by 3.6% (n = 18) of patients receiving placebo.

The frequency of discontinuation due to adverse reactions was highest during the first 4 weeks of treatment. Similar percentages of patients treated with tolterodine extended-release capsules or placebo discontinued treatment due to adverse reactions. Treatment was discontinued due to adverse reactions and dry mouth was reported as an adverse reaction in 2.4% (n = 12) of patients treated with tolterodine extended-release capsules and in 1.2% (n = 6) of patients treated with placebo.

The table below lists the adverse reactions reported in greater than or equal to 1% of patients treated with 4 mg tolterodine extended-release capsules once daily in the 12-week study. The adverse reactions were reported regardless of causality.

Tolterodine Adverse Reactions[a] (≥ 1%)

Adverse reaction	% Tolterodine extended-release capsules (n = 505)	% Placebo (n = 507)
Autonomic nervous system		
Dry mouth	23	8
CNS		
Anxiety	1	0
Dizziness	2	1
Somnolence	3	2
GI		
Abdominal pain	4	2
Constipation	6	4
Dyspepsia	3	1
GU		
Dysuria	1	0
Respiratory		
Sinusitis	2	1
Special senses		
Abnormal vision	1	0
Xerophthalmia	3	2
Miscellaneous		
Fatigue	2	1
Headache	6	4

[a] In nearest integer.

➤*Postmarketing:* The following events have been reported in association with tolterodine use in clinical practice: Anaphylactoid reactions, including angioedema; tachycardia; palpitations; peripheral edema; and hallucinations. Because these spontaneously reported reactions are from the worldwide postmarketing experience, the frequency of reactions and the role of tolterodine in their causation cannot be reliably determined.

Overdosage

A 27-month-old child who ingested 5 to 7 immediate-release tablets of 2 mg tolterodine was treated with a suspension of activated charcoal and was hospitalized overnight with symptoms of dry mouth. The child fully recovered.

➤*Treatment:* Overdosage with tolterodine immediate-release tablets or extended-release capsules can potentially result in severe central anticholinergic effects and should be treated accordingly.

ECG monitoring is recommended in the event of overdosage. In dogs, changes in the QT interval (slight prolongation of 10% to 20%) were observed at a suprapharmacologic dose of 4.5 mg/kg, which is about 68 times higher than the recommended human dose. In clinical trials of healthy volunteers and patients, QT interval prolongation was not observed with immediate-release tolterodine at doses up to 4 mg twice daily of tolterodine (higher doses were not evaluated).

Patient Information

Inform patients that antimuscarinic agents such as tolterodine may produce blurred vision, dizziness, or drowsiness.

TROSPIUM CHLORIDE

Rx	**Trospium Chloride** (Paddock Laboratories)	**Tablets; oral:** 20 mg	Lactose. (PAD 145). White, round. Film-coated. In 60s.
Rx	**Sanctura** (Odyssey, Indevus)		Lactose, sucrose. Brownish yellow, biconvex. Glossy-coated. In 60s, 500s, and blister 14s.
Rx	**Sanctura XR** (Allergan)	**Capsules, extended-release; oral:** 60 mg	Sugar spheres. (SAN 60). White/orange. In 30s.

TROSPIUM CHLORIDE — ORAL

Indications

➤*Overactive bladder:* For the treatment of overactive bladder with symptoms of urge urinary incontinence, urgency, and urinary frequency.

Administration and Dosage

➤*Adults:*

Overactive bladder –

Extended-release capsules: 60 mg daily in the morning.

Immediate-release tablets: 20 mg twice daily.

➤*Elderly:* In patients 75 years of age or older, dosage may be titrated down to 20 mg once daily based upon tolerability.

➤*Renal function impairment:*

Extended-release capsules – Not recommended for use in patients with severe renal impairment (creatinine clearance [CrCl] less than 30 mL/minute).

Immediate-release tablets – For patients with severe renal impairment (CrCl less than 30 mL/min), the recommended dosage is 20 mg once daily at bedtime.

➤*Administration:* Dose at least 1 hour before meals or on an empty stomach.

➤*Storage/Stability:* Store at 20° to 25°C (68° to 77°F). Excursions are permitted at 15° to 30°C (59° to 86°F).

Actions

➤*Pharmacology:* Trospium is an antispasmodic, antimuscarinic agent.

Trospium antagonizes the effect of acetylcholine on muscarinic receptors in cholinergically innervated organs. Its parasympatholytic action reduces the tonus of smooth muscle in the bladder. Receptor assays showed that trospium has negligible affinity for nicotinic receptors as compared with muscarinic receptors at concentrations obtained from therapeutic doses.

Pharmacodynamics – Placebo-controlled studies employing urodynamic variables were conducted in patients with conditions characterized by involuntary detrusor contractions. The results demonstrate that trospium increases maximum cystometric bladder capacity and volume at first detrusor contraction.

➤*Pharmacokinetics:* A summary of mean (± standard deviation) pharmacokinetic parameters for a single 20 mg trospium dose is provided in the following table.

Mean (± SD) Pharmacokinetic Parameter Estimates for a Single 20 mg Trospium Dose in Healthy Volunteers

C_{max} (ng/mL)	$AUC_{0-\infty}$ (ng/mL•hr)	T_{max} (hr)	t½ (hr)
3.5 ± 4	36.4 ± 21.8	5.3 ± 1.2	18.3 ± 3.2

Absorption – After oral administration, less than 10% of the dose is absorbed. Mean absolute bioavailability of a 20 mg dose is 9.6% (range, 4% to 16.1%). Peak plasma concentrations (C_{max}) occur between 5 to 6 hours post-dose. Mean C_{max} increases greater than dose-proportionally; a 3-fold and 4-fold increase in C_{max} was observed for dose increases from 20 to 40 mg and from 20 to 60 mg, respectively. AUC exhibits dose linearity for single doses up to 60 mg. Trospium exhibits diurnal variability in exposure with a decrease in C_{max} and AUC of up to 59% and 33%, respectively, for evening relative to morning doses.

Effect of food: Administration with a high fat meal resulted in reduced absorption, with AUC and C_{max} values 70% to 80% lower than those obtained when trospium was administered while fasting. Therefore, it is recommended that trospium should be taken at least 1 hour prior to meals or on an empty stomach.

Distribution – Protein binding ranged from 50% to 85% when therapeutic concentration levels (0.5 to 50 ng/mL) were incubated with human serum in vitro.

The ^{3}H-trospium ratio of plasma to whole blood was 1.6:1. This ratio indicates that the majority of ^{3}H-trospium is distributed in plasma. The apparent volume of distribution for a 20 mg oral dose is 395 (± 140) L.

Metabolism – The metabolic pathway of trospium in humans has not been fully defined. Of the 10% of the dose absorbed, metabolites account for approximately 40% of the excreted dose following oral administration. The major metabolic pathway is hypothesized as ester hydrolysis with subsequent conjugation of benzylic acid to form azoniaspironortropanol with glucuronic acid. Cytochrome P450 is not expected to contribute significantly to the elimination of trospium. In vitro data from human liver microsomes investigating the inhibitory effect of trospium on seven cytochrome P450 isoenzyme substrates (CYP1A2, 2A6, 2C9, 2C19, 2D6, 2E1, and 3A4) suggest a lack of inhibition at clinically relevant concentrations of trospium.

Excretion – The plasma half-life for trospium following oral administration is approximately 20 hours. After administration of oral ^{14}C-trospium chloride, the majority of the dose (85.2%) was recovered in feces and a smaller amount (5.8% of the dose) was recovered in urine; 60% of the radioactivity excreted in urine was unchanged trospium.

The mean renal clearance for trospium (29.07 L/hr) is 4-fold higher than average glomerular filtration rate, indicating that active tubular secretion is a major route of elimination for trospium. There may be competition for elimination with other compounds that are also renally eliminated. Carefully monitor patients receiving such drugs.

Special populations –

Renal function impairment: Severe renal impairment significantly altered the disposition of trospium. A 4.5-fold and 2-fold increase in mean $AUC_{0-\infty}$ and C_{max}, respectively, and the appearance of an additional elimination phase with a long half-life (approximately 33 hours) was detected in patients with severe renal insufficiency (Ccr less than 30 mL/min) compared with healthy, nearly age-matched subjects. The different pharmacokinetic behavior of trospium in patients with severe renal insufficiency necessitates adjustment of dosage frequency. The pharmacokinetics of trospium have not been studied in people with moderate or mild renal impairment (Ccr ranging from 30 to 80 mL/min).

Hepatic function impairment: There is no information regarding the effect of severe hepatic impairment on exposure to trospium. Maximum trospium concentration (C_{max}) increased 12% and 63% in subjects with mild and moderate hepatic impairment, respectively, compared with healthy subjects. Mean area under the plasma concentration-time curve (AUC) was similar. Use caution when administering trospium to patients with moderate and severe hepatic dysfunction. Use caution when administering trospium in patients with moderate or severe hepatic dysfunction.

Elderly: Age did not appear to significantly affect the pharmacokinetics of trospium; however, increased anticholinergic side effects unrelated to drug exposure were observed in patients 75 years of age or older.

Gender: Studies comparing the pharmacokinetics in different genders had conflicting results. When a single 40 mg trospium dose was administered to 16 elderly subjects, exposure was 45% lower in elderly women compared to elderly men. When 20 mg trospium was dosed twice daily for 4 days to 6 elderly men and 6 elderly women (60 to 75 years), AUC and C_{max} were 26% and 68% higher, respectively, in women without hormone replacement therapy than in men.

Contraindications

Urinary retention, gastric retention, or uncontrolled narrow-angle glaucoma and in patients who are at risk for these conditions; hypersensitivity to the drug or its ingredients.

Warnings/Precautions

➤*Risk of urinary retention:* Administer trospium with caution to patients with clinically significant bladder outflow obstruction because of the risk of urinary retention.

➤*Decreased GI motility:* Administer trospium with caution to patients with GI obstructive disorders because of the risk of gastric retention. Trospium, like other anticholinergic drugs, may decrease GI motility; use with caution in patients with conditions such as ulcerative colitis, intestinal atony, and myasthenia gravis.

➤*Controlled narrow-angle glaucoma:* In patients being treated for narrow-angle glaucoma, use trospium only if the potential benefits outweigh the risks, and, in that circumstance, only with careful monitoring.

➤*Renal function impairment:* See Administration and Dosage for more information.

➤*Hepatic function impairment:* Use caution when administering trospium in patients with moderate or severe hepatic dysfunction.

➤*Pregnancy: Category C.* Trospium has been shown to cause maternal toxicity in rats and a decrease in fetal survival in rats administered approximately 10 times the expected clinical exposure (AUC). The no effect levels for maternal and fetal toxicity were approximately equivalent to the expected clinical exposure in rats, and about 5 to 6 times the expected clinical exposure in rabbits. No malformations or developmental delays were observed. There are no adequate and well-controlled studies in pregnant women. Use trospium during pregnancy only if the potential benefit justifies the potential risk to the fetus.

➤*Lactation:* Trospium (2 mg/kg orally and 50 mcg/kg IV) was excreted, to a limited extent (less than 1%), into the milk of lactating rats. The activity observed in the milk was primarily from the parent compound. It is not known whether this drug is excreted in human milk. Because many drugs are excreted in human milk, exercise caution when trospium is administered to a nursing woman. Use trospium during lactation only if the potential benefit justifies the potential risk to the child.

➤*Children:* Safety and efficacy have not been established.

➤*Elderly:* Of the 591 patients with overactive bladder who received treatment with trospium in the 2 US, placebo-controlled, efficacy and safety studies, 249 patients (42%) were 65 years of age and older. Eighty-eight trospium-treated patients (15%) were 75 years of age and older.

In these 2 studies, the incidence of commonly reported anticholinergic adverse events in patients treated with trospium (including dry mouth, constipation, dyspepsia, urinary tract infection, and urinary retention) was higher in patients 75 years of age and older as compared with younger

TROSPIUM CHLORIDE — ORAL

patients. This effect may be related to an enhanced sensitivity to anticholinergic agents in this patient population. Therefore, based upon tolerability, the dose frequency of trospium may be reduced to 20 mg once daily in patients 75 years of age and older.

Drug Interactions

The concomitant use of trospium with other anticholinergic agents that produce dry mouth, constipation, and other anticholinergic pharmacological effects may increase the frequency and/or severity of such effects. Anticholinergic agents may potentially alter the absorption of some concomitantly administered drugs due to anticholinergic effects on GI motility.

➤*Drugs eliminated by active tubular secretion:* Although studies to assess drug-drug interactions with trospium have not been conducted, trospium has the potential for pharmacokinetic interactions with other drugs that are eliminated by active tubular secretion (eg, digoxin, procainamide, pancuronium, morphine, vancomycin, metformin, tenofovir). Coadministration of trospium with drugs that are eliminated by active renal tubular secretion may increase the serum concentration of trospium and/or the coadministered drug due to competition for this elimination pathway. Carefully monitor patients receiving such drugs.

Adverse Reactions

The 2 most common adverse events reported by patients receiving 20 mg trospium twice daily were dry mouth and constipation. The single most frequently reported adverse event for trospium, dry mouth, occurred in 20.1% of trospium treated patients and 5.8% of patients receiving placebo. In the 2 phase 3 US studies, dry mouth led to discontinuation in 1.9% of patients treated with 20 mg trospium twice daily. For the patients who reported dry mouth, most had their first occurrence of the event within the first month of treatment.

Trospium Adverse Reactions (≥ 1%)

Adverse reaction	Placebo (n = 590)	Trospium 20 mg twice daily (n = 591)
CNS		
Headache	12 (2%)	25 (4.2%)
GI		
Abdominal pain upper	7 (1.2%)	9 (1.5%)
Constipation	27 (4.6%)	57 (9.6%)
Constipation aggravated	5 (0.8%)	8 (1.4%)
Dry mouth	34 (5.8%)	119 (20.1%)
Dyspepsia	2 (0.3%)	7 (1.2%)
Flatulence	5 (0.8%)	7 (1.2%)
GU		
Urinary retention	2 (0.3%)	7 (1.2%)
Ophthalmic		
Dry eyes (not otherwise specified)	2 (0.3%)	7 (1.2%)
Miscellaneous		
Fatigue	8 (1.4%)	11 (1.9%)

Other adverse events from the phase 3, US, placebo-controlled trials judged possibly related to treatment with trospium by the investigator, occurring in greater than or equal to 0.5% of trospium-treated patients, and more common with trospium than placebo are tachycardia (not otherwise specified), vision blurred, abdominal distension, vomiting (not otherwise specified), dysgeusia, dry throat, and dry skin.

During controlled clinical studies, 1 event of angioneurotic edema was reported.

➤*Postmarketing:* Additional spontaneous adverse events, regardless of relationship to drug, reported from marketing experience with trospium include the following: anaphylactic reaction, chest pain, gastritis, hallucinations and delirium, "hypertensive crisis," palpitations, rhabdomyolysis, Stevens-Johnson syndrome, supraventricular tachycardia, syncope, vision abnormal.

Overdosage

➤*Symptoms:* Overdosage with trospium may result in severe anticholinergic effects.

A baby 7 months of age experienced tachycardia and mydriasis after administration of a single dose of trospium 10 mg given by a sibling. The baby's weight was reported as 5 kg. Following admission into the hospital and about 1 hour after ingestion of the trospium, medicinal charcoal was administered for detoxification. While hospitalized, the baby experienced mydriasis and tachycardia up to 230 bpm. Therapeutic intervention was not deemed necessary. The baby was discharged as completely recovered the following day.

➤*Treatment:* Treatment should be provided according to symptoms and supportive care. In the event of overdosage, ECG monitoring is recommended.

Patient Information

Inform patients that anticholinergic agents, such as trospium, may produce clinically significant adverse reactions related to anticholinergic pharmacological activity. For example, heat prostration (fever and heat stroke due to decreased sweating) can occur when anticholinergics such as trospium are used in a hot environment. Because anticholinergics such as trospium may also produce dizziness or blurred vision, advise patients to exercise caution. Inform patients that alcohol may enhance the drowsiness caused by anticholinergic agents.

Take trospium 1 hour prior to meals or on an empty stomach. If a dose is skipped, advise patients to take the next dose 1 hour prior to their next meal.

SOLIFENACIN SUCCINATE

Rx	Vesicare (Astellas)	Tablets; oral: 5 mg	Lactose, PEG 8000. (VESIcare 150). Lt. yellow, round. Film-coated. In 30s, 90s, and UD 100s.
		10 mg	Lactose, PEG 8000. (VESIcare 151). Lt. pink, round. Film-coated. In 30s, 90s, and UD 100s.

SOLIFENACIN SUCCINATE — ORAL

Indications

➤*Overactive bladder:* For the treatment of overactive bladder with symptoms of urge urinary incontinence, urgency, and urinary frequency.

Administration and Dosage

➤*Adults:*

Overactive bladder –

Initial dosage: 5 mg once daily.

Dosage titration: If the 5 mg dose is well tolerated, the dose may be increased to 10 mg once daily.

Concomitant therapy: When administered with therapeutic doses of ketoconazole or other potent cytochrome P450 enzyme 3A4 (CYP3A4) inhibitors, a daily dose greater than 5 mg is not recommended.

➤*Renal function impairment:* A daily dose greater than 5 mg is not recommended for patients with severe renal impairment (creatinine clearance [CrCl] less than 30 mL/min).

➤*Hepatic function impairment:*

Moderate hepatic impairment (Child-Pugh B) – A daily dose greater than 5 mg is not recommended.

Severe hepatic impairment (Child-Pugh C) – Use is not recommended.

➤*Administration:* Take with liquids and swallow whole. Administer with or without food.

➤*Storage/Stability:* Store at 25°C (77°F); excursions are permitted between 15° and 30°C (59° and 86°F).

Actions

➤*Pharmacology:* Solifenacin is a competitive muscarinic receptor antagonist. Muscarinic receptors play an important role in several major cholinergically mediated functions, including contractions of urinary bladder smooth muscle and stimulation of salivary secretion.

Pharmacodynamics –

Cardiac electrophysiology: The median difference from baseline in heart rate associated with solifenacin 10 and 30 mg compared with placebo was −2 and 0 beats/min, respectively. Because a significant period effect on QTc was observed, the QTc effects were analyzed utilizing the parallel placebo-control arm rather than the prespecified intrapatient analysis.

Solifenacin QTc Changes in msec (90% CI) From Baseline at T_{max} (Relative to Placebo)[a]

Drug/Dose	Fridericia method (using mean difference)
Solifenacin 10 mg	2 (−3 to 6)
Solifenacin 30 mg	8 (4 to 13)

[a] CI = confidence interval; T_{max} = time to peak plasma levels; results displayed are those derived from the parallel-design portion of the study and represent the comparison of group 1 to time-matched placebo effects in group 2.

Moxifloxacin was included as a positive control in this study and, given the length of the study, its effect on the QT interval was evaluated in 3 different sessions. The placebo-subtracted mean changes (90% CI) in QTcF for moxifloxacin in the 3 sessions were 11 (7 to 14), 12 (8 to 17), and 16 (12 to 21), respectively.

The QT interval–prolonging effect appeared greater for the 30 mg dose compared with the dose of solifenacin 10 mg. Although the effect of the highest solifenacin dose (3 times the maximum therapeutic dose) studied did not appear as large as that of the positive control moxifloxacin at its therapeutic dose, the confidence intervals overlapped. This study was not designed to draw direct statistical conclusions between the drugs or the dose levels.

SOLIFENACIN SUCCINATE — ORAL

➤*Pharmacokinetics:*

Absorption – After oral administration of solifenacin to healthy volunteers, peak plasma levels (C_{max}) of solifenacin are reached within 3 to 8 hours of administration, and, at steady state, ranged from 32.3 to 62.9 ng/mL for the solifenacin 5 and 10 mg tablets, respectively. The absolute bioavailability of solifenacin is approximately 90%, and plasma concentrations of solifenacin are proportional to the dose administered.

Distribution – Solifenacin is approximately 98% (in vivo) bound to human plasma proteins, principally to alpha-1-acid glycoprotein. Solifenacin is highly distributed to non-CNS tissues, having a mean steady-state volume of distribution of 600 L.

Metabolism – Solifenacin is metabolized extensively in the liver. The primary pathway for elimination is by way of CYP3A4; however, alternate metabolic pathways exist. The primary metabolic routes of solifenacin are through N-oxidation of the quinuclidin ring and 4R-hydroxylation of the tetrahydroisoquinoline ring. One pharmacologically active metabolite (4R-hydroxy solifenacin) occurring at low concentrations and unlikely to contribute significantly to clinical activity, and 3 pharmacologically inactive metabolites (N-glucuronide and the N-oxide and 4R-hydroxy-N-oxide of solifenacin) have been found in human plasma after oral dosing.

Excretion – Following the administration of ^{14}C-solifenacin 10 mg to healthy volunteers, 69.2% of the radioactivity was recovered in the urine and 22.5% in the feces over 26 days. Less than 15% (as mean value) of the dose was recovered in the urine as intact solifenacin. The major metabolites identified in urine were N-oxide of solifenacin, 4R-hydroxy solifenacin, and 4R-hydroxy-N-oxide of solifenacin; the major metabolite identified in feces was 4R-hydroxy solifenacin. The elimination half-life of solifenacin following long-term dosing is approximately 45 to 68 hours.

Special populations –

Renal function impairment: Use solifenacin with caution in patients with renal impairment. There is a 2.1-fold increase in area under the curve (AUC) and a 1.6-fold increase in half-life of solifenacin in patients with severe renal impairment.

See Administration and Dosage for more information.

Hepatic function impairment: Use solifenacin with caution in patients with reduced hepatic function. There is a 2-fold increase in the half-life and a 35% increase in AUC of solifenacin in patients with moderate hepatic impairment.

See Administration and Dosage for more information.

Elderly: Multiple-dose studies of solifenacin in elderly volunteers (65 to 80 years of age) showed that C_{max}, AUC, and half-life values were 20% to 25% higher compared with younger volunteers (18 to 55 years of age).

Contraindications

Gastric retention, hypersensitivity to the drug substance or other components of the product, uncontrolled narrow-angle glaucoma, and urinary retention.

Warnings/Precautions

➤*Bladder outflow obstruction:* As with other anticholinergic drugs, administer solifenacin with caution to patients with clinically significant bladder outflow obstruction because of the risk of urinary retention.

➤*GI motility:* As with other anticholinergics, use solifenacin with caution in patients with decreased GI motility.

➤*Glaucoma:* Use solifenacin with caution in patients being treated for narrow-angle glaucoma. Solifenacin is contraindicated in patients with uncontrolled narrow-angle glaucoma.

➤*QT prolongation:* In a study of the effect of solifenacin on the QT interval in 76 healthy women, the QT-prolonging effect appeared less with solifenacin 10 mg than with 30 mg (3 times the maximum recommended dose), and the effect of solifenacin 30 mg did not appear as large as that of the positive-control moxifloxacin at its therapeutic dose. Consider this observation in clinical decisions to prescribe solifenacin for patients with a history of QT prolongation or patients who are taking medications known to prolong the QT interval.

➤*Hypersensitivity reactions:* Angioedema of the face, lips, tongue, and/or larynx have been reported with solifenacin. In some cases, angioedema occurred after the first dose. Angioedema associated with upper airway swelling may be life-threatening. If involvement of the hypopharynx, larynx, or tongue occurs, promptly discontinue solifenacin and promptly provide appropriate therapy and/or measures necessary to ensure a patent airway.

➤*Renal function impairment:* Use solifenacin with caution in patients with reduced renal function.

See Administration and Dosage for more information.

➤*Hepatic function impairment:* Use solifenacin with caution in patients with reduced hepatic function.

See Administration and Dosage for more information.

➤*Pregnancy:* *Category C.* Reproduction studies have been performed in mice, rats, and rabbits. After oral administration of ^{14}C-solifenacin to pregnant mice, drug-related material was shown to cross the placental barrier. No embryotoxicity or teratogenicity was observed in mice treated with 30 mg/kg/day (1.2 times exposure at the maximum recommended human dose [MRHD]). Administration of solifenacin to pregnant mice at doses of 100 mg/kg and greater (3.6 times exposure at the MRHD) during the major period of organ development resulted in reduced fetal body weights. Administration of 250 mg/kg (7.9 times exposure at the MRHD) to pregnant mice resulted in an increased incidence of cleft palate. In utero and lactational exposures to maternal dosages of solifenacin 100 mg/kg/day and greater (3.6 times exposure at the MRHD) resulted in reduced peripartum and postnatal survival, reductions in body weight gain, and delayed physical development (eye opening and vaginal patency). An increase in the percentage of male offspring was also observed in litters from offspring exposed to maternal dosages of 250 mg/kg/day. No embryotoxic effects were observed in rats at up to 50 mg/kg/day (less than 1 times exposure at the MRHD) or in rabbits at up to 50 mg/kg/day (1.8 times exposure at the MRHD).

There are no adequate and well-controlled studies in pregnant women. Because animal reproduction studies are not always predictive of human response, use solifenacin during pregnancy only if the potential benefit justifies the potential risk to the fetus.

➤*Lactation:* After oral administration of ^{14}C-solifenacin to lactating mice, radioactivity was detected in maternal milk. There were no adverse observations in mice treated with 30 mg/kg/day (1.2 times exposure at the MRHD). Pups of female mice treated with 100 mg/kg/day (3.6 times exposure at the MRHD) or greater revealed delays in the onset of reflex and physical development, postpartum pup mortality, or reduced body weights during the lactation period.

It is not known whether solifenacin is excreted in human milk. The molecular weight (approximately 363 for the free base) and prolonged plasma elimination half-life suggest that the drug and/or its metabolites will be excreted into breast milk. The effects of solifenacin exposure on a breast-feeding infant are unknown, but the risk of toxicity probably is low.

Because many drugs are excreted in human milk, do not administer solifenacin during breast-feeding. Decide whether to discontinue breast-feeding or solifenacin in breast-feeding mothers.

➤*Children:* Safety and efficacy have not been established.

➤*Monitoring:* Monitor for improvement in symptoms of overactive bladder, including incontinence, urinary urgency, and frequency.

Drug Interactions

Solifenacin Drug Interactions

Precipitant drug	Object drug[a]		Description
Potent CYP3A4 inhibitors (eg, atazanavir, clarithromycin, indinavir, itraconazole, ketoconazole, nefazodone, nelfinavir, ritonavir, saquinavir, telithromycin, voriconazole)	Solifenacin	⬆	Solifenacin plasma concentrations may be elevated, increasing the pharmacologic effects and risk of adverse reactions. Following the administration of solifenacin 10 mg in the presence of ketoconazole 400 mg, a potent inhibitor of CYP3A4, the mean C_{max} and AUC of solifenacin increased 1.5- and 2.7-fold, respectively. Therefore, it is recommended not to exceed a 5 mg daily dose of solifenacin when administered with a therapeutic dose of ketoconazole or other potent CYP3A4 inhibitors.
Strong CYP3A4 inducers (eg, rifampin)	Solifenacin	⬇	Solifenacin plasma concentrations may be reduced, decreasing the pharmacologic effect.
Solifenacin	Potassium preparations (eg, potassium chloride)	⬇	Passage of solid doseforms of potassium chloride through the GI tract may be delayed or arrested because of slowing of GI motility by solifenacin. Coadministration of solid dosage forms of potassium chloride and solifenacin is contraindicated. Potassium chloride liquid may be a suitable alternative.

[a] ⬆ = object drug increased; ⬇ = object drug decreased.

Adverse Reactions

➤*Most common adverse reactions:* Expected adverse effects of antimuscarinic agents are dry mouth, constipation, blurred vision (accommodation abnormalities), urinary retention, and dry eyes. The most common adverse reactions reported in patients treated with solifenacin were dry mouth and constipation, and the incidence of these side effects was higher in the 10 mg compared with the 5 mg dose group.

➤*Serious adverse reactions:* In the four 12-week, double-blind clinical trials, there were 3 intestinal serious adverse events in patients, all treated with solifenacin 10 mg (1 fecal impaction, 1 colonic obstruction, and 1 intestinal obstruction). The overall rate of serious adverse reactions in the double-blind trials was 2%. Angioneurotic edema was reported in 1 patient taking solifenacin 5 mg.

➤*Discontinuation of therapy:* The most frequent reason for discontinuation because of an adverse reaction was dry mouth (1.5%).

SOLIFENACIN SUCCINATE — ORAL

➤*Adverse reactions (1% or more):*

Solifenacin Adverse Reactions (≥ 1%)			
Adverse reactions	Solifenacin 5 mg (n = 578)	Solifenacin 10 mg (n = 1,233)	Placebo (n = 1,216)
Number of patients with treatment-emergent adverse reactions	265	773	634
CNS			
Depression, NOS[a]	1.2%	0.8%	0.8%
Dizziness	1.9%	1.8%	1.8%
Fatigue	1%	2.1%	1.1%
GI			
Abdominal pain, upper	1.9%	1.2%	1%
Constipation	5.4%	13.4%	2.9%
Dry mouth	10.9%	27.6%	4.2%
Dyspepsia	1.4%	3.9%	1%
Nausea	1.7%	3.3%	2%
Vomiting, NOS	0.2%	1.1%	0.9%
GU			
Urinary retention	0	1.4%	0.6%
Urinary tract infection, NOS	2.8%	4.8%	2.8%
Respiratory			
Cough	0.2%	1.1%	0.2%
Pharyngitis, NOS	0.3%	1.1%	1%
Special senses			
Dry eyes, NOS	0.3%	1.6%	0.6%
Vision blurred	3.8%	4.8%	1.8%
Miscellaneous			
Edema, lower limb	0.3%	1.1%	0.7%
Hypertension	1.4%	0.5%	0.6%
Influenza	2.2%	0.9%	1.3%

[a] NOS = not otherwise specified.

➤*Postmarketing:*

Cardiovascular – QT prolongation, torsades de pointes.

CNS – Confusion, hallucinations, headache.

Hypersensitivity – Hypersensitivity reactions, including angioedema with airway obstruction, pruritus, rash, and urticaria.

Miscellaneous – Peripheral edema.

Overdosage

➤*Symptoms:*

Short-term – Overdosage with solifenacin can potentially result in severe anticholinergic effects; treat accordingly. The highest dose ingested in an accidental overdose of solifenacin was 280 mg in a 5-hour period. This case was associated with mental status changes. Some cases reported a decrease in the level of consciousness.

Long-term – Intolerable anticholinergic side effects (fixed and dilated pupils, blurred vision, failure of heel-to-toe exam, tremors, and dry skin) occurred on day 3 in healthy volunteers taking 50 mg daily (5 times the maximum recommended therapeutic dose) and resolved within 7 days following discontinuation of drug.

➤*Treatment:* In the event of overdose with solifenacin, treat with gastric lavage and appropriate supportive measures. ECG monitoring is also recommended.

Patient Information

Advise patients to swallow tablets whole with liquid and not to crush, chew, or break tablets.

Inform patients that antimuscarinic agents such as solifenacin have been associated with constipation and blurred vision. Advise patients to contact their health care provider if they experience severe abdominal pain or become constipated for 3 or more days. Because solifenacin may cause blurred vision, advise patients to exercise caution in decisions to engage in potentially dangerous activities until the drug's effect on the patient's vision has been determined.

Inform patients that solifenacin may produce angioedema, which could result in life-threatening airway obstruction. Advise patients to promptly discontinue solifenacin therapy and seek immediate attention if they experience edema of the tongue or laryngopharynx, or difficulty breathing.

Advise patients that heat prostration (caused by decreased sweating) can occur when anticholinergic drugs, such as solifenacin, are used in a hot environment.

DARIFENACIN HYDROBROMIDE

Rx	**Enablex** (Novartis)	**Tablets, extended-release**: 7.5 mg	Lactose. (DF 7.5). White. In 30s, 90s, and UD 100s.
		15 mg	Lactose. (DF 15). Lt. peach. In 30s, 90s, and UD 100s.

DARIFENACIN HYDROBROMIDE — ORAL

Indications

➤*Overactive bladder:* For the treatment of overactive bladder with symptoms of urge urinary incontinence, urgency, and frequency.

Administration and Dosage

➤*Adults:*

Overactive bladder –

Initial dosage: 7.5 mg once daily.

Dosage titration: The dose may be increased to 15 mg once daily as early as 2 weeks after starting therapy.

Concomitant therapy: When coadministered with potent CYP3A4 inhibitors (eg, ketoconazole, itraconazole, ritonavir, nelfinavir, clarithromycin, nefazodone), the daily dose should not exceed 7.5 mg.

➤*Hepatic function impairment:* For patients with moderate hepatic impairment, the daily dose of darifenacin should not exceed 7.5 mg. Darifenacin is not recommended for use in patients with severe hepatic impairment.

➤*Administration:* Administer with liquid. Swallow whole; do not chew, divide, or crush. May be taken with or without food.

➤*Storage/Stability:* Store at 25°C (77°F); excursions permitted to 15° to 30°C (59° to 86°F). Protect from light.

Actions

➤*Pharmacology:* Darifenacin is a competitive muscarinic receptor antagonist. Muscarinic receptors play an important role in several major cholinergically mediated functions, including contractions of the urinary bladder smooth muscle and stimulation of salivary secretion.

In vitro studies using human recombinant muscarinic receptor subtypes show that darifenacin has greater affinity for the M_3 receptor than for the other known muscarinic receptors (9- and 12-fold greater affinity for M_3 compared with M_1 and M_5, respectively, and 59-fold greater affinity for M_3 compared with both M_2 and M_4). M_3 receptors are involved in contraction of human bladder and GI smooth muscle, saliva production, and iris sphincter function. Adverse drug effects, such as dry mouth, constipation, and abnormal vision, may be mediated through effects on M_3 receptors in these organs.

Pharmacodynamics – In 3 cystometric studies performed in patients with involuntary detrusor contractions, increased bladder capacity was demonstrated by an increased volume threshold for unstable contractions and diminished frequency of unstable detrusor contractions after darifenacin extended-release tablet treatment. These findings are consistent with an antimuscarinic action on the urinary bladder.

➤*Pharmacokinetics:*

Absorption – The mean oral bioavailability of darifenacin in EMs at steady state is estimated to be 15% and 19% for 7.5 and 15 mg tablets, respectively.

After oral administration of darifenacin to healthy volunteers, peak plasma concentrations of darifenacin are reached approximately 7 hours after multiple dosing; steady state plasma concentrations are achieved by the sixth day of dosing.

Mean (SD) Steady State Pharmacokinetic Parameters From Darifenacin 7.5 mg and 15 mg Extended-Release Tablets Based On Pooled Data By Predicted CYP2D6 Phenotype										
	Darifenacin 7.5 mg (N = 68 EM, 5 PM)					Darifenacin 15 mg (N = 102 EM, 17 PM)				
	AUC_{24} (ng•h/mL)	C_{max} (ng/mL)	C_{avg} (ng/mL)	T_{max} (h)	t½ (h)	AUC_{24} (ng•h/mL)	C_{max} (ng/mL)	C_{avg} (ng/mL)	T_{max} (h)	t½ (h)
EM	29.24 (15.47)	2.01 (1.04)	1.22 (0.64)	6.49 (4.19)	12.43 (5.64)[a]	88.9 (67.87)	5.76 (4.24)	3.7 (2.83)	7.61 (5.06)	12.05 (12.37)[b]
PM	67.56 (13.13)	4.27 (0.98)	2.81 (0.55)	5.2 (1.79)	19.95[c]	157.71 (77.08)	9.99 (5.09)	6.58 (3.22)	6.71 (3.58)	7.4[d]

[a] N = 25
[b] N = 8
[c] N = 2
[d] N = 1

Distribution – Darifenacin is approximately 98% bound to plasma proteins (primarily to alpha-1-acid glycoprotein). The steady-state volume of distribution (Vss) is estimated to be 163 L.

Metabolism – Darifenacin is extensively metabolized by the liver following oral dosing.

DARIFENACIN HYDROBROMIDE — ORAL

Metabolism is mediated by cytochrome P450 enzymes CYP2D6 and CYP3A4. The 3 main metabolic routes are as follows

1.) monohydroxylation in the dihydrobenzofuran ring
2.) dihydrobenzofuran ring opening
3.) N-dealkylation of the pyrrolidine nitrogen

The initial products of the hydroxylation and N-dealkylation pathways are the major circulating metabolites, but they are unlikely to contribute significantly to the overall clinical effect of darifenacin.

A subset of individuals (approximately 7% white and 2% black) are PMs of CYP2D6 metabolized drugs. Individuals with normal CYP2D6 activity are referred to as EMs. The metabolism of darifenacin in PMs will be principally mediated via CYP3A4. The darifenacin ratios (PM:EM) for C_{max} and area under the curve (AUC) following darifenacin 15 mg once-daily at steady state were 1.9 and 1.7, respectively.

Excretion – Following administration of an oral dose of ^{14}C-darifenacin solution to healthy volunteers, approximately 60% of the radioactivity was recovered in the urine and 40% in the feces. Only a small percentage of the excreted dose was unchanged darifenacin (3%). Estimated darifenacin clearance is 40 L/h for EMs and 32 L/h for PMs. The elimination half-life of darifenacin following chronic dosing is approximately 13 to 19 hours.

Special populations –

Hepatic function impairment: The daily dose of darifenacin should not exceed 7.5 mg once daily for patients with moderate hepatic impairment (Child-Pugh B). No dose adjustment is recommended for patients with mild hepatic impairment (Child-Pugh A).

Darifenacin pharmacokinetics were investigated in subjects with mild (Child-Pugh A) or moderate (Child-Pugh B) impairment of hepatic function given darifenacin 15 mg once daily to steady state. Mild hepatic impairment had no effect on the pharmacokinetics of darifenacin. However, protein binding of darifenacin was affected by moderate hepatic impairment. After adjusting for plasma protein binding, unbound darifenacin exposure was estimated to be 4.7-fold higher in subjects with moderate hepatic impairment than subjects with normal hepatic function. Subjects with severe hepatic impairment (Child-Pugh C) have not been studied; therefore, darifenacin is not recommended for use in these patients.

Elderly: No dose adjustment is recommended for the elderly. A population pharmacokinetic analysis of patient data indicated a trend for clearance of darifenacin to decrease with age (6% per decade relative to a median age of 44). Following administration of darifenacin 15 mg once daily, darifenacin exposure at steady state was approximately 12% to 19% higher in volunteers between 45 and 65 years of age compared with younger volunteers aged 18 to 44 years of age.

Gender: No dose adjustment is recommended based on gender. Pharmacokinetic parameters were calculated for 22 male and 25 female healthy volunteers. Darifenacin C_{max} and AUC at steady state were approximately 57% to 79% and 61% to 73% higher in females than in males, respectively.

Contraindications

Urinary retention, gastric retention, or uncontrolled narrow-angle glaucoma and in patients who are at risk for these conditions; hypersensitivity to the drug or its ingredients.

Warnings/Precautions

➤*Controlled narrow-angle glaucoma:* Use darifenacin with caution in patients being treated for narrow-angle glaucoma and only where the potential benefits outweigh the risks.

➤*Decreased GI motility:* Administer darifenacin with caution to patients with GI obstructive disorders because of the risk of gastric retention. Darifenacin, like other anticholinergic drugs, may decrease GI motility; use with caution in patients with conditions such as severe constipation, ulcerative colitis, and myasthenia gravis.

➤*Risk of urinary retention:* Administer darifenacin extended-release tablets with caution to patients with clinically significant bladder outflow obstruction because of the risk of urinary retention.

➤*Hepatic function impairment:* See Administration and Dosage for more information.

➤*Pregnancy:* Category C. Darifenacin was not teratogenic in rats and rabbits at doses up to 50 and 30 mg/kg/day, respectively. At the dose of 50 mg/kg in rats, there was a delay in the ossification of the sacral and caudal vertebrae that was not observed at 10 mg/kg (approximately 13 times the AUC of free plasma concentration at MRHD). Exposure in this study at 50 mg/kg corresponds to approximately 59 times the AUC of free plasma concentration at MRHD. Dystocia was observed in dams at 10 mg/kg/day (17 times the AUC of free plasma concentration at MRHD). Slight developmental delays were observed in pups at this dose. At 3 mg/kg/day (5 times the AUC of free plasma concentration at MRHD), there were no effects on dams or pups. At the dose of 30 mg/kg in rabbits, darifenacin was shown to increase post-implantation loss but not at 10 mg/kg (9 times the AUC of free plasma concentration at MRHD). Exposure to unbound drug at 30 mg/kg in this study corresponds to approximately 28 times the AUC at MRHD. In rabbits, dilated ureter and/or kidney pelvis was observed in offspring at 30 mg/kg/day and one case was observed at 10 mg/kg/day along with urinary bladder dilation consistent with pharmacological action of darifenacin. No effect was observed at 3 mg/kg/day (2.8 times the AUC of free plasma concentration at MRHD). There are no studies of darifenacin in pregnant women. Because animal reproduction studies are not always predictive of human response, use darifenacin during pregnancy only if the benefit to the mother outweighs the potential risk to the fetus.

➤*Lactation:* Darifenacin is excreted into the milk of rats. It is not known whether darifenacin is excreted into human milk. Use caution before administering darifenacin to a breast-feeding woman.

➤*Children:* The safety and efficacy of darifenacin in pediatric patients have not been established.

Drug Interactions

Darifenacin Drug Interactions

Precipitant Drug	Object Drug[a]		Description
Moderate CYP3A4 inhibitors (eg, diltiazem, erythromycin, fluconazole, verapamil)	Darifenacin	⬆	Darifenacin levels may be increased; no dosing adjustments are recommended.
Potent CYP3A4 inhibitors (eg, clarithromycin, itraconazole, ketoconazole, nefazodone, protease inhibitors [eg, nelfinavir, ritonavir])	Darifenacin	⬆	Darifenacin levels may be increased; darifenacin should not exceed 7.5 mg when coadministered with potent CYP3A4 inhibitors.
Darifenacin	Anticholinergic drugs	⬆	Additive anticholinergic adverse effects may occur.
Darifenacin	CYP2D6 substrates (eg, flecainide, thioridazine, tricyclic antidepressants [eg, desipramine, imipramine])	⬆	Use caution when darifenacin is used with drugs metabolized by CYP2D6 and that have a narrow therapeutic window. The mean C_{max} and AUC of imipramine were increased 57% and 70%, respectively, in the presence of steady state darifenacin 30 mg once daily; active metabolite of imipramine, desipramine increased 3.6-fold.
Darifenacin	Digoxin	⬆	Darifenacin 30 mg daily coadministered with digoxin 0.25 mg at steady state resulted in 16% increase in digoxin; monitor digoxin.

[a] ⬆ = Object drug increased.

Adverse Reactions

During the clinical development of darifenacin extended-release tablets, a total of 7,363 patients and volunteers were treated with doses of darifenacin from 3.75 to 75 mg once daily.

The safety of darifenacin was evaluated in phase II and III controlled clinical trials in a total of 8,830 patients, 6,001 of whom were treated with darifenacin. Of this total, 1,069 patients participated in three 12-week, phase III, fixed-dose efficacy and safety studies. Of this total, 337 and 334 patients received darifenacin 7.5 and 15 mg daily, respectively. In all long-term trials combined, 1,216 and 672 patients received treatment with darifenacin for at least 24 and 52 weeks, respectively.

In all placebo-controlled trials combined, the incidence of serious adverse reactions for 7.5 mg, 15 mg, and placebo was similar.

In all fixed-dose phase III studies combined, 3.3% of patients treated with darifenacin discontinued because of all adverse reactions versus 2.6% in placebo. Dry mouth leading to study discontinuation occurred in 0%, 0.9%, and 0% of patients treated with darifenacin 7.5 mg daily, darifenacin 15 mg daily, and placebo respectively. Constipation leading to study discontinuation occurred in 0.6%, 1.2%, and 0.3% of patients treated with darifenacin 7.5 mg daily, darifenacin 15 mg daily, and placebo, respectively.

The table below lists the adverse reactions reported (regardless of causality) in 2% or more of patients treated with 7.5 or 15 mg darifenacin extended-release tablets and greater than placebo in the 3 fixed-dose, placebo-controlled phase III studies (studies 1, 2, and 3). Adverse reactions were reported by 54% and 66% of patients receiving 7.5 and 15 mg once daily darifenacin extended-release tablets, respectively, and by 49% of patients receiving placebo. In these studies, the most frequently reported adverse reactions were dry mouth and constipation. The majority of adverse reactions in darifenacin-treated subjects were mild or moderate in severity and most occurred during the first 2 weeks of treatment.

Darifenacin Adverse Reactions[a] (≥ 2%) (Studies 1, 2, and 3)

Adverse reaction	Percentage of Subjects With Adverse Reaction (%)		
	Darifenacin 7.5 mg (N = 337)	Darifenacin 15 mg (N = 334)	Placebo (N = 388)
CNS			
Dizziness	0.9	2.1	1.3
GI			
Abdominal pain	2.4	3.9	0.5
Constipation	14.8	21.3	6.2
Diarrhea	2.1	0.9	1.8

DARIFENACIN HYDROBROMIDE — ORAL

Darifenacin Adverse Reactions[a] (≥ 2%) (Studies 1, 2, and 3)			
	Percentage of Subjects With Adverse Reaction (%)		
Adverse reaction	Darifenacin 7.5 mg (N = 337)	Darifenacin 15 mg (N = 334)	Placebo (N = 388)
Dry mouth	20.2	35.3	8.2
Dyspepsia	2.7	8.4	2.6
Nausea	2.7	1.5	1.5
GU			
Urinary tract infection	4.7	4.5	2.6
Ophthalmic			
Dry eyes	1.5	2.1	0.5
Miscellaneous			
Asthenia	1.5	2.7	1.3

[a] Regardless of causality.

Other adverse reactions reported, regardless of causality, by at least 1% of darifenacin patients in either the 7.5 or 15 mg once-daily darifenacin dose groups in these fixed-dose, placebo-controlled phase III studies include the following: abnormal vision, accidental injury, arthralgia, back pain, bronchitis, dry skin, flu syndrome, hypertension, pain, peripheral edema, pharyngitis, pruritus, rash, rhinitis, sinusitis, urinary tract disorder, vaginitis, vomiting, and weight gain.

Study 4 was a 12-week, placebo-controlled, dose-titration regimen study in which darifenacin was administered in accordance with dosing recommendations. All patients initially received placebo or darifenacin 7.5 mg daily, and after 2 weeks, patients and physicians were allowed to adjust upward to darifenacin 15 mg if needed. In this study, the most commonly reported adverse reactions also were constipation and dry mouth. The incidence of discontinuation because of all adverse reactions was 3.1% and 6.7% for placebo and for darifenacin, respectively.

Darifenacin Adverse Reactions[a] (> 3%) (Study 4)		
Adverse reaction	Darifenacin 7.5 mg per 15 mg (N = 268)	Placebo (N = 127)
CNS		
Headache	18 (6.7%)	7 (5.5%)
GI		
Constipation	56 (20.9%)	10 (7.9%)
Dry mouth	50 (18.7%)	11 (8.7%)
Dyspepsia	12 (4.5%)	2 (1.6%)
Nausea	11 (4.1%)	2 (1.6%)
GU		
Urinary tract infection	10 (3.7%)	4 (3.1%)
Miscellaneous		
Accidental injury	8 (3%)	3 (2.4%)
Flu syndrome	8 (3%)	3 (2.4%)

[a] Regardless of causality.

➤*GI:* Constipation was reported as a serious adverse reaction in 6 patients in the darifenacin phase I to III clinical trials, including 1 patient with benign prostatic hypertrophy (BPH), one overactive bladder (OAB) patient taking darifenacin 30 mg daily, and only one OAB patient taking the recommended doses. The latter patient was hospitalized for investigation with colonoscopy after reporting 9 months of chronic constipation that was reported as being moderate in severity.

➤*GU:* Acute urinary retention (AUR) requiring treatment was reported in a total of 16 patients in the darifenacin phase I to III clinical trials. Of these 16 cases, 7 were reported as serious adverse reactions, including 1 patient with detrusor hyperreflexia secondary to a stroke, 1 patient with BPH, 1 patient with irritable bowel syndrome (IBS), and 4 OAB patients taking darifenacin 30 mg daily. Of the remaining 9 cases, none were reported as serious adverse reactions. Three occurred in OAB patients taking the recommended doses, and 2 of these required bladder catheterization for 1 to 2 days.

Overdosage

➤*Symptoms:* Overdosage with antimuscarinic agents, including darifenacin extended-release tablets can result in severe antimuscarinic effects.

➤*Treatment:* Treatment should be symptomatic and supportive. In the event of overdosage, ECG monitoring is recommended. Darifenacin has been administered in clinical trials at doses up to 75 mg (5 times the maximum therapeutic dose) and signs of overdose were limited to abnormal vision.

Patient Information

Inform patients that anticholinergic agents, such as darifenacin, may produce clinically significant adverse events related to anticholinergic pharmacological activity including constipation, urinary retention, and blurred vision. Heat prostration (caused by decreased sweating) can occur when anticholinergics such as darifenacin are used in a hot environment.

Because anticholinergics, such as darifenacin, may produce dizziness or blurred vision, advise patients to exercise caution in decisions to engage in potentially dangerous activities until the drug's effects have been determined.

Advise patients to read the patient information leaflet before starting therapy with darifenacin.

Instruct patients that darifenacin may be taken with or without food. Darifenacin should be taken once daily with liquid.

Advise patients to swallow darifenacin tablets whole and not to chew, crush, or divide the tablets.

Inform patients that dry mouth may occur.

FESOTERODINE FUMARATE

Rx	**Toviaz** (Pfizer)	**Tablets, extended-release; oral:** 4 mg	Lactose, PEG, polyvinyl alcohol. (FS). Light blue, oval. Film-coated. In 30s, 90s, and UD 100s.
		8 mg	Lactose, PEG, polyvinyl alcohol. (FT). Blue, oval. Film-coated. In 30s, 90s, and UD 100s.

FESOTERODINE FUMARATE — ORAL

Indications

➤*Overactive bladder:* For the treatment of overactive bladder with symptoms of urge urinary incontinence, urgency, and frequency.

Administration and Dosage

➤*Adults:*

Overactive bladder –

Usual dosage: 8 mg once daily based upon individual response and tolerability.

Initial dosage: 4 mg once daily.

Concomitant therapy: The daily dose should not exceed 4 mg in patients taking potent CYP3A4 inhibitors (eg, clarithromycin, itraconazole, ketaconazole).

➤*Renal function impairment:* Doses of fesoterodine more than 4 mg are not recommended in patients with severe renal insufficiency.

➤*Hepatic function impairment:* Fesoterodine is not recommended for use in patients with severe hepatic function impairment.

➤*Administration:* Fesoterodine tablets should be taken with liquid and swallowed whole; do not chew, divide, or crush the tablets. May be administered with or without food.

➤*Storage/Stability:* Store at 20° to 25°C (68° to 77°F); excursions are permitted between 15° and 30°C (59° and 86°F). Protect from moisture.

Actions

➤*Pharmacology:* Fesoterodine is a competitive muscarinic receptor antagonist. After oral administration, fesoterodine is rapidly and extensively hydrolyzed by nonspecific esterases to its active metabolite, 5-hydroxymethyl tolterodine, which is responsible for the antimuscarinic activity of fesoterodine.

Muscarinic receptors play a role in contractions of urinary bladder smooth muscle and stimulation of salivary secretion. Inhibition of these receptors in the bladder is presumed to be the mechanism by which fesoterodine produces its effects.

➤*Pharmacokinetics:*

Absorption – After oral administration, fesoterodine is well absorbed. Because of rapid and extensive hydrolysis by nonspecific esterases to its active metabolite, fesoterodine cannot be detected in plasma. Bioavailability of the active metabolite is 52%. After single- or multiple-dose oral administration of fesoterodine 4 to 28 mg, plasma concentrations of the active metabolite are proportional to the dose. Maximum plasma levels are reached after approximately 5 hours. No accumulation occurs after multiple-dose administration.

A summary of pharmacokinetic parameters for the active metabolite after a single dose of fesoterodine 4 and 8 mg in extensive and poor metabolizers of CYP2D6 is provided in the following table.

Fesoterodine Summary of Mean CV[a] Pharmacokinetic Parameters for Fesoterodine 4 and 8 mg in Extensive and Poor CYP2D6 Metabolizers				
	Fesoterodine 4 mg		Fesoterodine 8 mg	
	EM[a] (n = 16)	PM[a] (n = 8)	EM[a] (n = 16)	PM[a] (n = 8)
C_{max}[b] (ng/mL)	1.89 (43%)	3.45 (54%)	3.98 (28%)	6.90 (39%)
$AUC_{0\text{-}tz}$[b] (ng•h/mL)	21.2 (38%)	40.5 (31%)	45.3 (32%)	88.7 (36%)

FESOTERODINE FUMARATE — ORAL

Fesoterodine Summary of Mean CV[a] Pharmacokinetic Parameters for Fesoterodine 4 and 8 mg in Extensive and Poor CYP2D6 Metabolizers				
	Fesoterodine 4 mg		Fesoterodine 8 mg	
	EM[a] (n = 16)	PM[a] (n = 8)	EM[a] (n = 16)	PM[a] (n = 8)
T_{max}[b] (h)[c]	5 (2 to 6)	5 (5 to 6)	5 (3 to 6)	5 (5 to 6)
t½ (h)	7.31 (27%)	7.31 (30%)	8.59 (41%)	7.66 (21%)

[a] EM = CYP2D6 extensive metabolizer, PM = CYP2D6 poor metabolizer, CV = coefficient of variation
[b] C_{max} = maximum plasma concentrations; AUC_{0-tz} = area under the concentration time curve from zero up to the last measurable plasma concentration; t_{max} = time to reach C_{max}; t½= terminal half-life.
[c] Data presented as median (range).

Distribution – Plasma protein binding of the active metabolite is low (approximately 50%) and is primarily bound to albumin and alpha-1 acid glycoprotein. The mean steady-state volume of distribution following intravenous (IV) infusion of the active metabolite is 169 L.

Metabolism – After oral administration, fesoterodine is rapidly and extensively hydrolyzed to its active metabolite. The active metabolite is further metabolized in the liver to its carboxy, carboxy-N-desisopropyl, and N-desisopropyl metabolites via 2 major pathways involving CYP2D6 and CYP3A4. None of these metabolites contribute significantly to the antimuscarinic activity of fesoterodine.

A subset of individuals (approximately 7% white and 2% black) are poor metabolizers for CYP2D6. The remainder of the population is referred to as extensive metabolizers. C_{max} and AUC of the active metabolite are increased 1.7- and 2-fold, respectively, in CYP2D6 poor metabolizers as compared to extensive metabolizers.

Excretion – Hepatic metabolism and renal excretion contribute significantly to the elimination of the active metabolite. After oral administration of fesoterodine, approximately 70% of the administered dose was recovered in urine as the active metabolite (16%), carboxy metabolite (34%), carboxy-N-desisopropyl metabolite (18%), or N-desisopropyl metabolite (1%), and a smaller amount (7%) was recovered in feces.

The t½ of the active metabolite is approximately 4 hours following an IV administration. The apparent t½ following oral administration is approximately 7 hours.

Special populations –

Renal function impairment: In patients with mild or moderate renal function impairment (CrCl ranging from 30 to 80 mL/min), C_{max} and AUC of the active metabolite are increased up to 1.5- and 1.8-fold, respectively, as compared with healthy subjects. In patients with severe renal function impairment (CrCl less than 30 mL/min), C_{max} and AUC are increased 2- and 2.3-fold, respectively.

In patients with mild or moderate renal function impairment, no dose adjustment is recommended. Doses of fesoterodine of more than 4 mg are not recommended in patients with severe renal function impairment.

Hepatic function impairment: In patients with moderate (Child-Pugh class B) hepatic function impairment, C_{max} and AUC of the active metabolite are increased 1.4- and 2.1-fold, respectively, as compared with healthy subjects.

No dose adjustment is recommended in patients with mild or moderate hepatic function impairment. Subjects with severe hepatic function impairment (Child-Pugh class C) have not been studied; therefore, fesoterodine is not recommended for use in these patients.

Contraindications

Urinary retention; gastric retention; uncontrolled narrow-angle glaucoma; known hypersensitivity to the drug or its ingredients.

Warnings/Precautions

➤*Bladder outlet obstruction:* Administer fesoterodine with caution to patients with clinically significant bladder outlet obstruction because of the risk of urinary retention.

➤*GI motility:* Use fesoterodine, like other antimuscarinic drugs, with caution in patients with decreased GI motility, such as those with severe constipation.

➤*Controlled narrow-angle glaucoma:* Use fesoterodine with caution in patients being treated for narrow-angle glaucoma and only when the potential benefits outweigh the risks.

➤*Myasthenia gravis:* Use fesoterodine with caution in patients with myasthenia gravis, a disease characterized by decreased cholinergic activity at the neuromuscular junction.

➤*Renal function impairment:* There are no dosing adjustments for patients with mild or moderate renal insufficiency. Doses of fesoterodine of more than 4 mg are not recommended in patients with severe renal insufficiency.

➤*Hepatic function impairment:* There are no dosing adjustments for patients with mild or moderate hepatic function impairment. Fesoterodine has not been studied in patients with severe hepatic function impairment and, therefore, is not recommended for use in this patient population.

➤*Pregnancy:* *Category C.* In mice treated orally with 75 mg/kg/day (6 to 27 times the expected exposure at the maximum recommended human dose [MRHD] based on AUC and greater than 77 times the expected C_{max}), increased resorptions and decreased live fetuses were observed. One fetus with cleft palate was observed at each dosage (15, 45, and 75 mg/kg/day), at an incidence within the background historical range. In rabbits treated orally with 27 mg/kg/day (3- to 11-fold by AUC and 19- to 62-fold by C_{max}), incompletely ossified sternebrae (retardation of bone development) were observed in fetuses. In rabbits treated by subcutaneous administration with 4.5 mg/kg/day (9- to 11-fold by AUC and 43- to 53-fold by C_{max}), maternal toxicity and incompletely ossified sternebrae were observed in fetuses (at an incidence within the background historical range). At 1.5 mg/kg/day subcutaneously (3-fold by AUC and 11- to 13-fold by C_{max}), decreased maternal food consumption in the absence of any fetal effects was observed. Oral administration of fesoterodine 30 mg/kg/day to mice in a pre- and postnatal development study resulted in decreased body weight of the dams and delayed ear opening of the pups. No effects were noted on mating and reproduction of the F_1 dams or on the F_2 offspring.

There are no adequate or well-controlled studies using fesoterodine in pregnant women. Therefore, use fesoterodine during pregnancy only if the potential benefit outweighs the potential risk to the fetus.

➤*Lactation:* It is not known whether fesoterodine is excreted in human milk. The molecular weight of the active metabolite 5-HT (about 342), its low plasma protein binding (about 50%), and its long terminal half-life (about 6 to 9 hours with a range of about 4 to 20 hours) suggest that it will be excreted into breast milk. Do not administer during breast-feeding unless the potential benefit outweighs the potential risk to the neonate.

➤*Children:* The safety and effectiveness of fesoterodine in children have not been established.

➤*Elderly:* The incidence of antimuscarinic adverse reactions, including constipation, dizziness (at 8 mg only), dry mouth, dyspepsia, increase in residual urine, and urinary tract infection, was higher in patients 75 years of age and older as compared with younger patients.

Drug Interactions

Fesoterodine Drug Interactions			
Precipitant drug	Object drug[a]		Description
CYP3A4 inducers (eg, rifampin)	Fesoterodine	⬇	Coadministration decreased fesoterodine C_{max} and AUC by approximately 70% and 75%, respectively. No dosing adjustments are recommended in the presence of CYP3A4 inducers.
CYP3A4 inhibitors (eg, clarithromycin, erythromycin, itraconazole, ketoconazole)	Fesoterodine	⬆	Coadministration of potent CYP3A4 inhibitors with fesoterodine may increase the C_{max} and AUC of the active metabolite of fesoterodine. Doses of fesoterodine of more than 4 mg are not recommended in patients taking potent CYP3A4 inhibitors.
Fesoterodine	Anticholinergic agents	⬆	Concomitant use may increase the frequency and/or severity of anticholinergic-like effects (eg, constipation, dry mouth, urinary retention). Anticholinergic agents may potentially alter the absorption of some coadministered drugs because of anticholinergic effects on GI motility.
Anticholinergic agents	Fesoterodine		

[a] ⬆ = object drug increased; ⬇ = object drug decreased.

Adverse Reactions

➤*Serious adverse reactions:* In phase 2 and 3, placebo-controlled trials combined, the incidences of serious adverse reactions in patients receiving placebo, fesoterodine 4 mg, and fesoterodine 8 mg were 1.9%, 3.5%, and 2.9%, respectively. All serious adverse reactions were judged to be not related or unlikely to be related to study medication by the investigator, except for 4 patients receiving fesoterodine who reported 1 serious adverse reaction each: angina, chest pain, gastroenteritis, and QT prolongation on ECG.

➤*Most common adverse reactions:* The most commonly reported adverse reactions in patients treated with fesoterodine was dry mouth. The incidence of dry mouth was higher in those taking 8 mg/day (35%) and in those taking 4 mg/day (19%), as compared to placebo (7%). Dry mouth led to discontinuation in 0.4%, 0.4%, and 0.8% of patients receiving placebo, fesoterodine 4 mg, and fesoterodine 8 mg, respectively. For those patients who reported dry mouth, most had their first occurrence of the event within the first month of treatment.

The second most commonly reported adverse event was constipation. The incidence of constipation was 2% in those taking placebo, 4% in those taking 4 mg/day, and 6% in those taking 8 mg.

➤*Adverse reactions (at least 1%):* Adverse reactions, regardless of causality, were reported in the combined phase 3, randomized, placebo-controlled trials at an incidence greater than placebo and in 1% or more of patients treated with fesoterodine 4 or 8 mg once daily for up to 12 weeks.

Fesoterodine Adverse Reactions (≥1%)			
Adverse reactions	Placebo (n = 554)	Fesoterodine 4 mg/day (n = 554)	Fesoterodine 8 mg/day (n = 566)
GI			
Abdominal pain upper	0.5%	1.1%	0.5%
Constipation	2%	4.2%	6%

FESOTERODINE FUMARATE — ORAL

Fesoterodine Adverse Reactions (≥1%)			
Adverse reactions	Placebo (n = 554)	Fesoterodine 4 mg/day (n = 554)	Fesoterodine 8 mg/day (n = 566)
Dry mouth	7%	18.8%	34.6%
Dyspepsia	0.5%	1.6%	2.3%
Nausea	1.3%	0.7%	1.9%
GU			
Dysuria	0.7%	1.3%	1.6%
Urinary retention	0.2%	1.1%	1.4%
Urinary tract infection	3.1%	3.2%	4.2%
Lab test abnormalities			
ALT[a] increase	0.9%	0.5%	1.2%
GGT[a] increased	0.4%	0.4%	1.2%
Respiratory			
Cough	0.5%	1.6%	0.9%
Dry throat	0.4%	0.9%	2.3%
Upper respiratory tract infection	2.2%	2.5%	1.8%
Miscellaneous			
Back pain	0.4%	2.0%	0.9%
Dry eyes	0%	1.4%	3.7%
Edema peripheral	0.7%	0.7%	1.2%
Insomnia	0.5%	1.3%	0.4%
Rash	0.5%	0.7%	1.1%

[a] GGT = gamma glutamyltransferase.

➤*Long-term use adverse reactions:* Patients also received fesoterodine for up to 3 years in open-label extension phases of one phase 2 and two phase 3 controlled trials. In all open-label trials combined, 857, 701, 529, and 105 patients received fesoterodine for at least 6 months, 1 year, 2 years, and 3 years, respectively. The adverse reactions observed during long-term, open-label studies were similar to those observed in the 12-week, placebo-controlled studies, and included abdominal pain, constipation, dry eyes, dry mouth, and dyspepsia. Similar to the controlled studies, most adverse reactions of dry mouth and constipation were mild to moderate in intensity. Serious adverse reactions, judged to be at least possibly related to study medication by the investigator, and reported more than once during the open-label treatment period of up to 3 years, included urinary retention and diverticulitis (3 cases each); constipation, irritable bowel syndrome, and electrocardiogram QTc interval prolongation (2 cases each).

Overdosage

➤*Symptoms:* Overdosage with fesoterodine can result in severe anticholinergic effects.

➤*Treatment:* Treatment should be symptomatic and supportive. In the event of overdosage, ECG monitoring is recommended.

Patient Information

Inform patients that fesoterodine, like other antimuscarinic agents, may produce clinically significant adverse reactions related to antimuscarinic pharmacological activity, including constipation and urinary retention.

Fesoterodine, like other antimuscarinics, may be associated with blurred vision; therefore, advise patients to exercise caution until the drug effects on the patient have been determined.

Heat prostration (because of decreased sweating) can occur when fesoterodine, like other antimuscarinic drugs, is used in a hot environment.

Inform patients that alcohol may enhance the drowsiness caused by fesoterodine, like other anticholinergic agents.

Advise patients to read the patient information before starting therapy with fesoterodine.

URINARY CHOLINERGICS

BETHANECHOL CHLORIDE

Rx	**Bethanechol Chloride** (Various, eg, Goldline, Ivax, Qualitest, UDL)	**Tablets; oral:** 5 mg	In 100s, 1000s, and UD 100s.
Rx	**Urecholine** (Barr/Duramed)		Lactose. (OP 697). Scored. In 100s.
Rx	**Bethanechol Chloride** (Various, eg, Goldline, Ivax, Qualitest, UDL)	**Tablets; oral:** 10 mg	In 100s, 250s, 1000s, and UD 100s.
Rx	**Urecholine** (Barr/Duramed)		Lactose. (OP 703). Scored. In 100s.
Rx	**Bethanechol Chloride** (Various, eg, Goldline, Ivax, Qualitest, UDL)	**Tablets; oral:** 25 mg	In 100s, 250s, 1000s, and UD 100s.
Rx	**Urecholine** (Barr/Duramed)		Lactose. (OP 704). Yellow, scored. In 100s.
Rx	**Bethanechol Chloride** (Various, eg, Goldline, Ivax, Qualitest, UDL)	**Tablets; oral:** 50 mg	In 100s, 500s, 1000s, and UD 100s.
Rx	**Urecholine** (Barr/Duramed)		Lactose. (OP 700). Yellow, scored. In 100s.

BETHANECHOL CHLORIDE — ORAL

Indications

➤*Urinary retention:* For the treatment of acute postoperative and postpartum nonobstructive (functional) urinary retention and for neurogenic atony of the urinary bladder with retention.

➤*Off-label uses:*

Gastroesophageal reflux disease – [2] = Fair documentation. American College of Gastroenterology guidelines for the management of gastroesophageal reflux disease (GERD) state that bethanechol may be used in select patients as adjunctive therapy with other acid-suppressing agents. Despite scattered trials supporting the use of bethanechol for the treatment of GERD, it has not been widely accepted because of inconsistent efficacy reports and a substantial adverse effect profile.

Gastroesophageal reflux disease (children) – [5] = Poor documentation. Practice guidelines for the management of GERD in infants and children state that there is insufficient evidence to support the use of prokinetic agents, with the exception of cisapride. However, cisapride is a less practical option based on the availability of more effective therapies.

Administration and Dosage

➤*General dosing considerations:* The effects of the drug sometimes appear within 30 minutes and usually within 60 to 90 minutes. The drug's effects persist for about 1 hour.

The effects of the drug can be abolished promptly by atropine.

➤*Adults:*

Urinary retention –

Usual dosage: 10 to 50 mg 3 or 4 times a day.

Maximum dose: 50 mg single dose.

Initial dosage: The minimum effective dose is determined by giving 5 or 10 mg initially and repeating the same amount at hourly intervals until satisfactory response occurs or until a maximum of 50 mg has been given.

Off-label dosing –

Gastroesophageal reflux disease: [2] = Fair documentation. 25 mg orally 4 times a day.

➤*Administration:* Give the drug when the stomach is empty. If taken soon after eating, nausea and vomiting may occur.

➤*Storage/Stability:* Store at 20° to 25°C (68° to 77°F).

Actions

➤*Pharmacology:* Bethanechol chloride acts principally by producing the effects of stimulation of the parasympathetic nervous system. It increases the tone of the detrusor urinae muscle, usually producing a contraction sufficiently strong to initiate micturition and empty the bladder. It stimulates gastric motility, increases gastric tone, and often restores impaired rhythmic peristalsis.

Stimulation of the parasympathetic nervous system releases acetylcholine at the nerve endings. When spontaneous stimulation is reduced and therapeutic intervention is required, acetylcholine can be given, but it is rapidly hydrolyzed by cholinesterase, and its effects are transient. Bethanechol chloride is not destroyed by cholinesterase and its effects are more prolonged than those of acetylcholine.

Effects on the GI and urinary tracts sometimes appear within 30 minutes after oral administration of bethanechol chloride, but more often 60 to 90 minutes are required to reach maximum effectiveness. Following oral administration, the usual duration of action of bethanechol is 1 hour, although large doses (300 to 400 mg) have been reported to produce effects for up to 6 hours. SC injection produces a more intense action on bladder muscle than does oral administration of the drug.

Because of the selective action of bethanechol, nicotinic symptoms of cholinergic stimulation are usually absent or minimal when orally or subcutaneously administered in therapeutic doses, while muscarinic effects are prominent. Muscarinic effects usually occur within 5 to 15 minutes after SC injection, reach a maximum in 15 to 30 minutes, and disappear within 2 hours. Doses that stimulate micturition and defecation and increase peristalsis do not ordinarily stimulate ganglia or voluntary muscles. Therapeutic test doses in healthy human subjects have little effect on heart rate, blood pressure, or peripheral circulation.

➤*Pharmacokinetics:* Bethanechol chloride does not cross the blood-brain barrier because of its charged quaternary amine moiety. The metabolic fate and mode of excretion of the drug have not been elucidated.

BETHANECHOL CHLORIDE — ORAL

Contraindications

Hypersensitivity to bethanechol chloride, hyperthyroidism, peptic ulcer, latent or active bronchial asthma, pronounced bradycardia or hypotension, vasomotor instability, coronary artery disease, epilepsy, and parkinsonism.

Bethanechol chloride should not be employed when the strength or integrity of the GI or bladder wall is in question, or in the presence of mechanical obstruction; when increased muscular activity of the GI tract or urinary bladder might prove harmful, as following recent urinary bladder surgery, GI resection and anastomosis, or when there is possible GI obstruction; in bladder neck obstruction, spastic GI disturbances, acute inflammatory lesions of the GI tract, or peritonitis; or in marked vagotonia.

Warnings/Precautions

➤*Reflex infection:* In urinary retention, if the sphincter fails to relax as bethanechol chloride contracts the bladder, urine may be forced up the ureter into the kidney pelvis. If there is bacteriuria, this may cause reflux infection.

➤*Tartrazine sensitivity:* Some of these products contain tartrazine, which may cause allergic-type reactions (including bronchial asthma) in susceptible individuals. Although the incidence of sensitivity is low, it is frequently seen in patients who also have aspirin hypersensitivity.

➤*Pregnancy: Category C.* Animal reproduction studies have not been conducted with bethanechol chloride. It is also not known whether bethanechol chloride can cause fetal harm when administered to a pregnant woman or can affect reproduction capacity. Bethanechol chloride should be given to a pregnant woman only if clearly needed.

➤*Lactation:* It is not known whether this drug is excreted in human milk. Because many drugs are excreted in human milk and because of the potential for serious adverse reactions from bethanechol chloride in nursing infants, a decision should be made whether to discontinue nursing or to discontinue the drug, taking into account the importance of the drug to the mother.

➤*Children:* Safety and efficacy in children have not been established.

Drug Interactions

Bethanechol Drug Interactions			
Precipitant drug	Object drug[a]		Description
Cholinergic drugs	Bethanechol	↑	Additive effects may occur, particularly with cholinesterase inhibitors.
Ganglionic blocking compounds	Bethanechol	↑	A critical fall in blood pressure may occur that is usually preceded by severe abdominal symptoms.
Quinidine Procainamide	Bethanechol	↓	Quinidine or procainamide may antagonize cholinergic effects of bethanechol.

[a] ↑ = object drug increased; ↓ = object drug decreased.

Adverse Reactions

➤*Cardiovascular:* A fall in blood pressure with reflex tachycardia; vasomotor response.

➤*CNS:* Headache.

➤*Dermatologic:* Flushing producing a feeling of warmth; sensation of heat about the face; sweating.

➤*GI:* Abdominal cramps or discomfort; colicky pain; nausea and belching; diarrhea; borborygmi (rumbling/gurgling of stomach); salivation.

➤*Renal:* Urinary urgency.

➤*Respiratory:* Bronchial constriction; asthmatic attacks.

➤*Special senses:* Lacrimation; miosis.

➤*Miscellaneous:* Malaise.

➤*Casual relationship unknown :*
CNS – Seizures.

Overdosage

➤*Symptoms:* Early signs of overdosage are abdominal discomfort, salivation, flushing of the skin (hot feeling), sweating, nausea, and vomiting.

The oral LD_{50} of bethanechol chloride is 1510 mg/kg in the mouse.

➤*Treatment:* Atropine sulfate is a specific antidote. The recommended dose for adults is 0.6 mg. Repeat doses can be given every 2 hours, according to clinical response. The recommended dosage in infants and children up to 12 years of age is 0.01 mg/kg (to a maximum single dose of 0.4 mg) repeated every 2 hours as needed until the desired effect is obtained, or adverse effects of atropine preclude further usage. SC injection of atropine is preferred except in emergencies when the IV route may be employed.

Patient Information

Bethanechol chloride tablets should preferably be taken 1 hour before or 2 hours after meals to avoid nausea or vomiting. If taken soon after eating, nausea and vomiting may occur.

Dizziness, lightheadedness or fainting may occur, especially when getting up from a lying or sitting position.

May cause abdominal discomfort, salivation, sweating, or flushing; notify physician if these effects are pronounced.

NEOSTIGMINE METHYLSULFATE

Refer to the Neostigmine methylsulfate monograph in the CNS chapter for full prescribing information.

PHOSPHATE BINDERS

LANTHANUM

Rx	**Fosrenol** (Shire)	**Tablets, chewable:** 500 mg	As lanthanum carbonate. (S405 500). White to off-white, round. In 90s.
		750 mg	As lanthanum carbonate. (S405 750). White to off-white, round. In 90s.
		1,000 mg	As lanthanum carbonate. (S405 1000). White to off-white, round. In 90s.

LANTHANUM CARBONATE — ORAL

Indications

➤*Phosphate reduction:* To reduce serum phosphate in patients with end-stage renal disease (ESRD).

Administration and Dosage

➤*Adults:*

Phosphate reduction –

Initial dosage: The recommended initial total daily dose of lanthanum is 1,500 mg.

Dosage titration: Doses were generally titrated in increments of 750 mg/day. Titrate the dose every 2 to 3 weeks until an acceptable serum phosphate level is reached. Monitor serum phosphate levels as needed during dose titration and on a regular basis thereafter.

Maintenance dosage: In clinical studies of ESRD patients, lanthanum doses of up to 3,750 mg were evaluated. Most patients required a total daily dose between 1,500 and 3,000 mg to reduce plasma phosphate levels to less than 6 mg/dL.

➤*Administration:* Chew tablets completely before swallowing. To aid in chewing, tablets may be crushed. Do not swallow intact tablets. Divide the total daily dose of lanthanum and take with meals.

➤*Storage/Stability:* Store at 25°C (77°F); excursions are permitted to 15° to 30°C (59° to 86°F). Protect from moisture.

Actions

➤*Pharmacology:* Patients with ESRD can develop hyperphosphatemia that may be associated with secondary hyperparathyroidism and elevated calcium phosphate product. Elevated calcium phosphate product increases the risk of ectopic calcification. Treatment of hyperphosphatemia usually includes all of the following: reduction in dietary intake of phosphate, removal of phosphate by dialysis, and inhibition of intestinal phosphate absorption with phosphate binders.

Pharmacodynamics – Lanthanum dissociates in the acid environment of the upper GI tract to release lanthanum ions that bind dietary phosphate released from food during digestion. Lanthanum inhibits absorption of phosphate by forming highly insoluble lanthanum phosphate complexes, consequently reducing serum phosphate and calcium phosphate product.

➤*Pharmacokinetics:*

Absorption/Distribution – Following single-dose or multiple-dose oral administration of lanthanum to healthy subjects, the concentration of lanthanum in plasma was very low (bioavailability less than 0.002%). Following oral administration in ESRD patients, the mean lanthanum C_{max} was 1 ng/mL. During long-term administration (52 weeks) in ESRD patients, the mean lanthanum concentration in plasma was approximately 0.6 ng/mL. There was minimal increase in plasma lanthanum concentrations with increasing doses within the therapeutic dose range. The effect of food on the bioavailability of lanthanum has not been evaluated, but the timing of food intake relative to lanthanum administration (during and 30 minutes after food intake) has a negligible effect on the systemic level of lanthanum.

In vitro, lanthanum is highly bound (more than 99%) to human plasma proteins, including human serum albumin, α1-acid glycoprotein, and transferrin. Binding to erythrocytes in vivo is negligible in rats.

In 105 bone biopsies from patients treated with lanthanum for up to 4.5 years, rising levels of lanthanum were noted over time. Estimates of elimination half-life from bone ranged from 2 to 3.6 years. Steady-state bone concentrations were not reached during the period studied.

Metabolism/Excretion – Lanthanum is not metabolized and is not a substrate of CYP450. In vitro metabolic inhibition studies showed that lanthanum at concentrations of 10 and 40 mcg/mL does not have relevant

LANTHANUM CARBONATE — ORAL

inhibitory effects on any of the CYP450 isoenzymes tested (1A2, 2C9/10, 2C19, 2D6, and 3A4/5). Lanthanum was cleared from plasma following discontinuation of therapy with an elimination half-life of 53 hours.

No information is available regarding the mass balance of lanthanum in humans after oral administration. In rats and dogs, the mean recovery of lanthanum after an oral dose was approximately 99% and 94%, respectively, and was essentially all from feces. Biliary excretion is the predominant route of elimination for circulating lanthanum in rats. In healthy volunteers administered intravenous (IV) lanthanum as the soluble chloride salt (120 mcg), renal clearance was less than 2% of total plasma clearance. Quantifiable amounts of lanthanum were not measured in the dialysate of treated ESRD patients.

Contraindications

None known.

Warnings/Precautions

➤*Long-term effects:* There were no differences in the rates of fracture or mortality in patients treated with lanthanum compared with alternative therapy for up to 3 years. The duration of treatment exposure and time of observation in the clinical program are too short to conclude that lanthanum does not affect the risk of fracture or mortality beyond 3 years.

➤*Special risk:* Patients with acute peptic ulcer, ulcerative colitis, Crohn disease, or bowel obstruction were not included in lanthanum clinical studies. Use this drug with caution in patients with these conditions.

➤*Pregnancy: Category C.* No adequate and well-controlled studies have been conducted in pregnant women. The effect of lanthanum on the absorption of vitamins and other nutrients has not been studied in pregnant women. Lanthanum is not recommended for use during pregnancy.

In pregnant rabbits, oral administration of lanthanum at 1,500 mg/kg/day (5 times the MRHD) was associated with a reduction in maternal body weight gain and food consumption, increased postimplantation loss, reduced fetal weights, and delayed fetal ossification. Lanthanum administered to rats from implantation through lactation at 2,000 mg/kg/day (3.4 times the MRHD) caused delayed eye opening, reduction in body weight gain, and delayed sexual development (preputial separation and vaginal opening) of the offspring.

➤*Lactation:* It is not known whether lanthanum is excreted in human milk. Because many drugs are excreted in human milk, exercise caution when lanthanum is administered to a nursing woman.

➤*Children:* While growth abnormalities were not identified in long-term animal studies, lanthanum was deposited into developing bone, including growth plate. The consequences of such deposition in developing bone in pediatric patients are unknown. Therefore, the use of lanthanum in this population is not recommended.

Drug Interactions

An in vitro study showed no evidence that lanthanum forms insoluble complexes with warfarin, digoxin, furosemide, phenytoin, metoprolol, and enalapril in simulated gastric fluid. However, it is recommended that compounds known to interact with antacids not be taken within 2 hours of dosing with lanthanum.

Adverse Reactions

The most common adverse reactions for lanthanum were GI events, such as nausea and vomiting, and they generally abated over time with continued dosing.

Lanthanum Adverse Reactions

Adverse reaction	Lanthanum (N = 180)	Placebo (N = 95)
GI		
Abdominal pain	5%	0%
Nausea	11%	5%
Vomiting	9%	4%
Miscellaneous		
Dialysis graft occlusion	8%	1%

The safety of lanthanum was studied in 2 long-term clinical trials that included 1,215 patients treated with lanthanum and 943 patients with alternative therapy. Fourteen percent of patients in these comparative, open-label studies discontinued therapy in the lanthanum-treated group because of adverse reactions. GI adverse reactions, such as nausea, diarrhea, and vomiting, were the most common type of event leading to discontinuation.

The most common adverse reactions (5% or more in either treatment group) in both the long-term (2 year), open-label, active-controlled study of lanthanum vs alternative therapy (study A) and the 6-month, comparative study of lanthanum vs calcium carbonate (study B) are shown in the following table. Study A events have been adjusted for mean exposure differences between treatment groups (with a mean exposure of 0.9 years on lanthanum and 1.3 years on alternative therapy). The adjustment for mean exposure was achieved by multiplying the observed adverse reaction rates in the alternative therapy group by 0.71.

Lanthanum Adverse Reactions (≥ 5%)

Adverse reaction	Study A: Lanthanum (N = 682)	Study A: Alternative therapy adjusted rates (N = 676)	Study B: Lanthanum (N = 533)	Study B: Calcium carbonate (N = 267)
Cardiovascular				
Hypotension	16%	17%	8%	9%
CNS				
Headache	21%	20%	5%	6%
GI				
Abdominal pain	17%	17%	5%	3%
Constipation	14%	13%	6%	7%
Diarrhea	23%	22%	13%	10%
Nausea	36%	28%	16%	13%
Vomiting	26%	21%	18%	11%
Metabolic				
Hypercalcemia	4%	8%	0%	20%
Respiratory				
Bronchitis	5%	6%	5%	6%
Rhinitis	5%	7%	7%	6%
Miscellaneous				
Dialysis graft complication	26%	25%	3%	5%
Dialysis graft occlusion	21%	20%	4%	6%

Overdosage

There is no experience with lanthanum overdosage. Lanthanum was not acutely toxic in animals by the oral route. No deaths and no adverse effects occurred in mice, rats, or dogs after single oral doses of 2,000 mg/kg. In clinical trials, daily lanthanum doses up to 4,718 mg were well tolerated in healthy adults when administered with food, with the exception of GI symptoms. Given the topical activity of lanthanum in the gut, and the excretion in feces of the majority of the dose, supportive therapy is recommended for overdosage.

Patient Information

Instruct patients to take lanthanum tablets with or immediately after meals. Tablets should be chewed completely before swallowing; intact tablets should not be swallowed.

SEVELAMER

Rx	**Renagel** (Genzyme)	**Tablets; oral:** 400 mg	As sevelamer hydrochloride. (RENAGEL 400). Oval. Film-coated. In 360s.
		800 mg	As sevelamer hydrochloride. (RENAGEL 800). Oval. Film-coated. In 180s.
Rx	**Renvela** (Genzyme)	**Tablets; oral:** 800 mg	As sevelamer carbonate. (RENVELA 800). White, oval. Film-coated. In 30s and 270s.
		Powder for suspension; oral: 0.8 g per packet	As sevelamer carbonate. Sucralose. Citrus cream flavor. In 90s.
		2.4 g per packet	As sevelamer carbonate. Sucralose. Citrus cream flavor. In 90s.

SEVELAMER HYDROCHLORIDE — ORAL

Indications

➤*Hyperphosphatemia:* For the control of serum phosphorus in patients with chronic kidney disease on dialysis.

➤*Off-label uses:* Treatment of hyperuricemia in patients undergoing hemodialysis.

Administration and Dosage

➤*Adults:*

Hyperphosphatemia –

Usual dosage: 3 sevelamer 800 mg tablets per meal.

Maximum dose: 13 g daily.

SEVELAMER HYDROCHLORIDE — ORAL

Initial dosage:

• *Patients not taking a phosphate binder* –

Sevelamer Starting Dose for Dialysis Patients Not Taking a Phosphate Binder		
Serum phosphorus	Sevelamer 800 mg	Sevelamer 400 mg
> 5.5 and < 7.5 mg/dL	1 tablet 3 times daily with meals	2 tablets 3 times daily with meals
≥ 7.5 and < 9 mg/dL	2 tablets 3 times daily with meals	3 tablets 3 times daily with meals
≥ 9 mg/dL	2 tablets 3 times daily with meals	4 tablets 3 times daily with meals

• *Patients switching from calcium acetate* –

Sevelamer Starting Dose for Dialysis Patients Switching From Calcium Acetate to Sevelamer		
Calcium acetate 667 mg (tablets per meal)	Sevelamer 800 mg (tablets per meal)	Sevelamer 400 mg (tablets per meal)
1 tablet	1 tablet	2 tablets
2 tablets	2 tablets	3 tablets
3 tablets	3 tablets	5 tablets

Dosage titration: Adjust dosage based on serum phosphorus concentration, with a goal of lowering serum phosphorus to 5.5 mg/dL or less. The dosage may be increased or decreased by 1 tablet per meal at 2-week intervals as necessary.

Sevelamer Dose Titration Guideline	
Serum phosphorus	Sevelamer dosage
> 5.5 mg/dL	Increase by 1 tablet per meal at 2-week intervals
3.5 to 5.5 mg/dL	Maintain current dosage
< 3.5 mg/dL	Decrease by 1 tablet per meal

➤*Elderly:* Dose selection for an elderly patient should be cautious, usually starting at the low end of the dosing range.

➤*Concomitant medication:* When administering any other oral drug for which alteration in blood levels could have a clinically significant effect on safety or efficacy, administer the drug at least 1 hour before or 3 hours after sevelamer, or consider monitoring blood levels of the drug.

➤*Administration:* Administer sevelamer 3 times a day with meals.

➤*Storage/Stability:* Store at 25°C (77°F); excursions are permitted between 15° and 30°C (59° and 86°F). Protect from moisture.

Actions

➤*Pharmacology:* Sevelamer is a nonabsorbed binding crosslinked polymer. It contains multiple amines separated by 1 carbon from the polymer backbone. These amines exist in a protonated form in the intestine and interact with phosphate molecules through ionic and hydrogen bonding. By binding phosphate in the dietary tract and decreasing absorption, sevelamer lowers the phosphate concentration in the serum.

Sevelamer taken with meals has been shown to decrease serum phosphorus concentrations in patients with chronic kidney disease who are on dialysis.

➤*Pharmacokinetics:*

Absorption – A mass balance study using ^{14}C-sevelamer in 16 healthy men and women volunteers showed that sevelamer is not systemically absorbed.

Contraindications

Hypophosphatemia; bowel obstruction.

Warnings/Precautions

➤*GI disorders:* The safety of sevelamer in patients with dysphagia, swallowing disorders, severe GI motility disorders (including severe constipation), or major GI tract surgery have not been established. Exercise caution when sevelamer is used in patients with these GI disorders.

➤*Vitamin deficiencies:* In preclinical studies in rats and dogs, sevelamer reduced vitamin D, E, and K (coagulation parameters) and folic acid levels at doses of 6 to 10 times the recommended human dose. In short-term clinical trials, there was no evidence of reduction in serum levels of vitamins, with the exception of a 1-year clinical trial in which sevelamer treatment was associated with reduction of 25-hydroxyvitamin D (healthy range, 10 to 55 ng/mL) from 39 ± 22 ng/mL to 34 ± 22 ng/mL ($P < 0.01$). Most (approximately 75%) patients in sevelamer clinical trials received vitamin supplements, which is typical of patients on dialysis.

➤*Pregnancy: Category C.* In pregnant rats given dietary doses of sevelamer 0.5, 1.5, and 4.5 g/kg/day during organogenesis, reduced or irregular ossification of fetal bones, probably because of a reduced absorption of fat-soluble vitamin D, occurred in the mid- and high-dosage groups (human equivalent doses less than the maximum clinical trial dose of 13 g). In pregnant rabbits given oral dosages of 100, 500, and 1,000 mg/kg/day of sevelamer by gavage during organogenesis, an increase of early resorptions occurred in the high-dose group (human equivalent dose twice the maximum clinical trial dose).

The effect of sevelamer on the absorption of vitamins and other nutrients has not been studied in pregnant women. Requirements for vitamins and other nutrients are increased in pregnancy. Supplementation with higher oral doses of vitamins, especially fat-soluble vitamins (except vitamin A), might be required, or consider intravenous (IV) vitamins.

➤*Lactation:* Sevelamer is not absorbed into the systemic circulation, but it may cause vitamin deficiencies in the mother by preventing intestinal vitamin absorption, especially of fat-soluble vitamins. Because vitamins are excreted into breast milk, thereby further reducing maternal vitamin concentrations, women who are taking sevelamer might need to take higher oral doses of vitamins, especially fat-soluble vitamins (except vitamin A), or consider IV vitamin administration.

➤*Children:* The safety and efficacy have not been established.

➤*Elderly:* In general, dose selection for an elderly patient should be cautious, usually starting at the low end of the dosing range.

➤*Monitoring:* Monitor serum calcium, phosphorus, bicarbonate, and chloride levels.

Closely monitor patients on peritoneal dialysis to ensure the reliable use of appropriate aseptic technique with the prompt recognition and management of any signs and symptoms associated with peritonitis.

Drug Interactions

Sevelamer Drug Interactions			
Precipitant drug	Object drug[a]		Description
Sevelamer	Ciprofloxacin	⬇	Administration of a single dose of sevelamer 2.8 g reduced the bioavailability of ciprofloxacin approximately 50%. If coadministration cannot be avoided, separate the administration times by at least 4 hours.
Sevelamer	Mycophenolate	⬇	Sevelamer may reduce mycophenolic acid plasma concentrations, decreasing the efficacy. Administer sevelamer 2 hours after mycophenolate mofetil.
Sevelamer	Thyroid hormones (eg, levothyroxine)	⬇	The efficacy of thyroid hormones may be decreased with coadministration of sevelamer, resulting in hypothyroidism. Separate the administration times by at least 4 hours. Monitor thyroid-stimulating hormone levels and patients for signs of hypothyroidism.

[a] ⬇ = object drug decreased.

➤*Drug/Lab test interactions:* None well documented.

Adverse Reactions

➤*Adverse reactions (more than 5%):*

GI – Vomiting (22%), nausea (20%), diarrhea (19%), dyspepsia (16%), abdominal pain (9%), constipation (8%), flatulence (8%).

➤*Discontinuation:* A total of 27 patients treated with sevelamer and 10 patients treated with comparator withdrew from the study because of adverse reactions.

Based on studies of 8 to 52 weeks' duration, the most common reason for withdrawal from sevelamer was GI adverse reactions (3% to 16%).

➤*Dialysis patients:* In 143 patients on peritoneal dialysis studied for 12 weeks, most adverse reactions were similar to adverse reactions observed in hemodialysis patients. The most frequently occurring treatment-emergent serious adverse reaction was peritonitis (8 reactions in 8 [8%] patients in the sevelamer group and 2 reactions in 2 [4%] patients on active control). Thirteen (14%) in the sevelamer group and 9 (20%) patients in the active control group discontinued, mostly because of GI adverse reactions. Closely monitor patients on peritoneal dialysis to ensure the reliable use of appropriate aseptic technique with the prompt recognition and management of any signs and symptoms associated with peritonitis.

➤*Postmarketing:*

Dermatologic – Pruritus, rash.

GI – Abdominal pain; fecal impaction; uncommon cases of ileus, intestinal obstruction, and intestinal perforation. Give appropriate medical management to patients who develop constipation or have worsening of existing constipation to avoid severe complications.

Patient Information

Inform patients to take sevelamer with meals and adhere to their prescribed diets.

Give instructions on concomitant medications that should be dosed apart from sevelamer.

Advise patients that sevelamer may cause constipation that, if left untreated, may lead to severe complications. Advise patients to report new onset of constipation or worsening of existing constipation promptly to their health care provider.

SEVELAMER CARBONATE — ORAL

Indications

➤*Hyperphosphatemia:* For the control of serum phosphorus in patients with chronic kidney disease on dialysis.

Administration and Dosage

➤*Adults:*

Hyperphosphatemia –

Usual dosage: 7.2 g daily.

Maximum dose: 14 g daily.

Initial dosage:

• *Patients not taking a phosphate binder –*

Sevelamer Starting Dose for Dialysis Patients Not Taking a Phosphate Binder		
Serum phosphorus	Sevelamer 800 mg tablet	Sevelamer powder
> 5.5 and < 7.5 mg/dL	1 tablet 3 times daily with meals	0.8 g 3 times daily with meals
≥ 7.5 mg/dL	2 tablets 3 times daily with meals	1.6 g 3 times daily with meals

• *Patients switching from sevelamer hydrochloride* – Use the same dosage in grams. Further titration to the desired phosphate levels may be necessary.

• *Patients switching between sevelamer carbonate tablets and powder* – Use the same dosage in grams. Further titration may be necessary to achieve desired phosphorus levels.

• *Patients switching from calcium acetate –*

Sevelamer Starting Dose for Dialysis Patients Switching From Calcium Acetate to Sevelamer		
Calcium acetate 667 mg (tablets per meal)	Sevelamer 800 mg (tablets per meal)	Sevelamer powder
1 tablet	1 tablet	0.8 g
2 tablets	2 tablets	1.6 g
3 tablets	3 tablets	2.4 g

Dosage titration: Titrate the sevelamer dosage by 0.8 g 3 times daily with meals at 2-week intervals as necessary, with the goal of controlling serum phosphorus within the target range.

➤*Elderly:* Dose selection for an elderly patient should be cautious, usually starting at the low end of the dosing range.

➤*Concomitant medication:* When administering any other oral drug for which alteration in blood levels could have a clinically significant effect on its safety or efficacy, administer the drug at least 1 hour before or 3 hours after sevelamer, or consider monitoring blood levels of the drug.

➤*Preparation for administration:*

Powder – The entire contents of each 0.8 g packet should be placed in a cup and mixed thoroughly with 30 mL of water; the entire contents of each 2.4 g packet should be placed in a cup and mixed thoroughly with 60 mL of water. Multiple packets may be mixed together with the appropriate amount of water. Patients should be instructed to stir the mixture vigorously (it does not dissolve).

➤*Administration:* Administer 3 times a day with meals.

Sevelamer powder preparation should be used within 30 minutes of mixing or resuspended right before drinking.

➤*Storage/Stability:* Store at 25°C (77°F); excursions are permitted to 15° to 30°C (59° to 86°F). Protect from moisture.

Actions

➤*Pharmacology:* Sevelamer is a nonabsorbed, phosphate-binding, crosslinked polymer, free of metal and calcium. It contains multiple amines separated by 1 carbon from the polymer backbone. These amines exist in a protonated form in the intestine and interact with phosphate molecules through ionic and hydrogen bonding. By binding phosphate in the dietary tract and decreasing absorption, sevelamer lowers the phosphate concentration in the serum.

➤*Pharmacokinetics:*

Absorption – A mass balance study using ^{14}C-sevelamer hydrochloride in 16 healthy men and women showed that sevelamer hydrochloride is not systemically absorbed.

Contraindications

Bowel obstruction.

Warnings/Precautions

➤*GI disorders:* The safety of sevelamer has not been established in patients with dysphagia, swallowing disorders, severe GI motility disorders (including severe constipation), or major GI tract surgery. Uncommon cases of bowel obstruction and perforation have been reported.

➤*Vitamin deficiencies:* In preclinical studies in rats and dogs, sevelamer hydrochloride, which contains the same active moiety as sevelamer carbonate, reduced vitamins D, E, and K (coagulation parameters) and folic acid levels at doses of 6 to 10 times the recommended human dose. In short-term clinical trials, there was no evidence of reduction in serum levels of vitamins. However, in a 1-year clinical trial, 25-hydroxyvitamin D (normal range, 10 to 55 ng/mL) fell from 39 ± 22 ng/mL to 34 ± 22 ng/mL ($P < 0.01$) with sevelamer hydrochloride treatment. Most patients (approximately 75%) in sevelamer hydrochloride clinical trials received vitamin supplements, which is typical of patients on dialysis.

➤*Pregnancy: Category C.* In pregnant rats given dietary dosages of 0.5, 1.5, or 4.5 g/kg/day of sevelamer hydrochloride during organogenesis, reduced or irregular ossification of fetal bones, probably because of a reduced absorption of fat-soluble vitamin D, occurred in mid- and high-dose groups (human equivalent doses approximately equal to and 3.4 times the maximum clinical trial dose of 13 g). In pregnant rabbits given oral dosages of 100, 500, or 1,000 mg/kg/day of sevelamer hydrochloride by gavage during organogenesis, an increase of early resorptions occurred in the high-dose group (human equivalent dose twice the maximum clinical trial dose).

There are no adequate and well-controlled studies in pregnant women. The effect of sevelamer hydrochloride on the absorption of vitamins and other nutrients has not been studied in pregnant women. Requirements for vitamins and other nutrients are increased in pregnancy. Supplementation with higher oral doses of vitamins, especially fat-soluble vitamins (except vitamin A), might be required, or consider intravenous (IV) vitamins. Use sevelamer during pregnancy only if the potential benefit justifies the potential risk to the fetus.

➤*Lactation:* Sevelamer is not absorbed into the systemic circulation, but it may cause vitamin deficiencies in the mother by preventing intestinal vitamin absorption, especially of fat-soluble vitamins. Because vitamins are excreted into breast milk, thereby further reducing maternal vitamin concentrations, women who are taking sevelamer might need to take higher oral doses of vitamins, especially fat-soluble vitamins (except vitamin A), or consider IV vitamin administration.

➤*Children:* The safety and efficacy have not been established.

➤*Elderly:* In general, use caution when selecting a dose for an older patient, usually starting at the low end of the dosing range.

➤*Monitoring:* Monitor serum calcium, phosphorus, bicarbonate, and chloride levels.

Closely monitor patients on peritoneal dialysis to ensure the reliable use of appropriate aseptic technique with the prompt recognition and management of any signs and symptoms associated with peritonitis.

Drug Interactions

Sevelamer Drug Interactions			
Precipitant drug	Object drug[a]		Description
Sevelamer	Ciprofloxacin	⬇	Administration of a single dose of sevelamer 2.8 g reduced the bioavailability of ciprofloxacin approximately 50%. If coadministration cannot be avoided, separate the administration times by at least 4 hours.
Sevelamer	Mycophenolate	⬇	Sevelamer may reduce mycophenolic acid plasma concentrations, decreasing the efficacy. Administer sevelamer 2 hours after mycophenolate mofetil.
Sevelamer	Thyroid hormones (eg, levothyroxine)	⬇	The efficacy of thyroid hormones may be decreased with coadministration of sevelamer, resulting in hypothyroidism. Separate the administration times by at least 4 hours. Monitor thyroid-stimulating hormone levels and patients for signs of hypothyroidism.

[a] ⬇ = object drug decreased.

➤*Drug/Lab test interactions:* None well documented.

Adverse Reactions

➤*Sevelamer hydrochloride:*

GI – Vomiting (22%), nausea (20%), diarrhea (19%), dyspepsia (16%), abdominal pain (9%), constipation (8%), flatulence (8%).

Discontinuation – A total of 27 patients treated with sevelamer and 10 patients treated with the comparator withdrew from the study because of adverse reactions.

Based on studies of 8 to 52 weeks' duration, the most common reason for withdrawal from sevelamer hydrochloride was GI adverse reactions (3% to 16%).

Dialysis patients – In 143 patients on peritoneal dialysis studied for 12 weeks using sevelamer hydrochloride, most adverse reactions were similar to adverse reactions observed in patients on hemodialysis. The most frequently occurring serious treatment-emergent adverse reaction was peritonitis (8 reactions in 8 [8%] patients in the sevelamer group and 2 reactions in 2 [4%] patients on active control). Thirteen (14%) patients in the sevelamer group and 9 (20%) patients in the active control group discontinued, mostly because of GI adverse reactions. Closely monitor patients on peritoneal dialysis to ensure the reliable use of appropriate aseptic technique with the prompt recognition and management of any signs and symptoms associated with peritonitis.

SEVELAMER CARBONATE — ORAL

➤*Postmarketing:*

Dermatologic – Pruritus, rash.

GI – Abdominal pain; fecal impaction; uncommon cases of ileus, intestinal obstruction, and intestinal perforation. Give appropriate medical management to patients who develop constipation or have worsening of existing constipation to avoid severe complications.

Patient Information

Inform patients to take sevelamer with meals and adhere to their prescribed diets.

Give instructions on concomitant medications that should be dosed apart from sevelamer.

Advise patients that sevelamer may cause constipation that, if left untreated, may lead to severe complications. Caution patients to report new onset of constipation or worsening of existing constipation promptly to their health care provider.

For sevelamer powder, instruct the patient on preparation of the powder in water.

VAGINAL PREPARATIONS

Vaginal Antifungal Agents

Indications

➤*Candidiasis:* Local treatment of vulvovaginal candidiasis (eg, moniliasis, vaginal yeast infection).

Actions

➤*Pharmacology:* Treatment of vaginal candidiasis (moniliasis) is complicated by a high recurrence rate because of the ubiquitous nature of *Candida albicans* and non-albicans species of *Candida*. Predisposing factors include diabetes, antibiotics, pregnancy, corticosteroids, oral contraceptives containing 75 to 150 mcg of estrogen, intrauterine devices, and decreased host immunity (eg, HIV).

Agents approved for local treatment of vulvovaginal candidiasis include **nystatin** (a polyene antibiotic), the imidazoles (**butoconazole**, **clotrimazole**, **miconazole**, **tioconazole**), and **terconazole** (a triazole derivative).

Nystatin and imidazoles – Nystatin and imidazoles bind to sterols in the cell membrane of the fungus with a resultant change in membrane permeability allowing leakage of intracellular components.

Terconazole – Terconazole's exact pharmacologic mode of action is uncertain. It may exert antifungal activity by disruption of normal fungal cell membrane permeability.

➤*Pharmacokinetics:*

Butoconazole – Approximately 1.7% is absorbed after vaginal administration. Peak plasma levels (13.6 to 18.6 ng/mL) of the drug and its metabolites were attained between 12 and 24 hours.

Terconazole – Following daily intravaginal administration of 0.8% terconazole 40 mg (0.8% cream × 5 g) for 7 days to healthy humans, plasma concentrations were low and gradually rose to a daily peak (mean of 5.9 ng/mL) at 6.6 hours. Following oral (30 mg) administration of terconazole, the harmonic half-life of elimination from the blood for the parent terconazole was 6.9 hours (range, 4 to 11.3). Terconazole is extensively metabolized. In vitro, terconazole is highly protein bound (94.9%) and the degree of binding is independent of the drug concentration.

Nystatin – Nystatin is not absorbed from intact skin or mucous membranes.

➤*Microbiology:* **Miconazole** is active against susceptible strains of *Trichophyton* spp., *Epidermophyton* spp., *Candida albicans*, and *Microsporium* spp. **Clotrimazole**, **tioconazole**, **nystatin**, **terconazole**, and **butoconazole** are active against *Candida* spp. (*Candida albicans*). Other pathogens commonly associated with vulvovaginitis (*Trichomonas* and *Gardnerella vaginalis*) do not respond to these antifungal agents.

Contraindications

Hypersensitivity to specific drug or component of the product.

Warnings/Precautions

➤*Diagnosis:* It is important that vaginal infections be differentiated, as bacterial vaginosis, trichomoniasis, and vulvovaginal candidiasis may produce common symptoms. The diagnosis of vulvovaginitis (*Trichomonas vaginalis* and *Haemophilus vaginalis*) may be confirmed prior to therapy by KOH smears or cultures. This does not apply to *otc* use of these agents, which requires self-diagnosis by the patient.

➤*OTC products:*

Other conditions – If abdominal pain, fever, or offensive-smelling vaginal discharge is present, do not use these products. If there is no improvement within 3 to 7 days, stop using these products. Consult a doctor, a condition more serious than a yeast infection may be present.

Vaginal itch/discomfort – Patients should consult a physician before using these products if it is their first experience with vaginal itch and discomfort.

Recurrent infections – For patients with frequently recurrent candidal vaginitis, it is important to consider factors that predispose to infection. The discontinuation of oral contraceptives decreases the frequency of yeast vaginitis for many women. Eliminating nylon and tight-fitting garments can also be helpful. Many diabetic patients with poor glycemic control have recurring yeast vaginitis. Patients with recurrent yeast vaginitis should be tested for HIV.

➤*For vaginal use only:* Do not use creams in mouth or eyes.

➤*Irritation:* If irritation, sensitization, fever, chills, or flu-like symptoms occur, discontinue use.

➤*Chronic or recurrent candidiasis:* Chronic or recurrent candidiasis may be a symptom of unrecognized diabetes mellitus or a damaged immune system (including HIV infection). A persistently resistant infection may actually be caused by reinfection; evaluate sources of reinfection.

➤*Refractory patients:* If there is lack of response, repeat microbiological studies to confirm diagnosis and rule out other pathogens before reinstituting antifungal therapy.

➤*Pregnancy:* *Category A* – **nystatin**; *Category B* – **clotrimazole**, **nystatin** (Briggs GG, et al. *Drugs in Pregnancy and Lactation* 5th ed.); *Category C* – **butoconazole**, **terconazole**, **miconazole**. During pregnancy, use of a vaginal applicator may be contraindicated; manual insertion of vaginal tablets may be preferred. Use only on advice of physician.

Because small amounts of these drugs may be absorbed from the vagina, use during the first trimester only when essential. Use of **butoconazole** during the second and third trimesters has been approved. Possible exposure of the fetus through direct transfer of **terconazole** from an irritated vagina to the fetus by diffusion across amniotic membranes may occur.

➤*Lactation:* Because nystatin is poorly absorbed, if at all, serum and milk levels would not occur with **nystatin**. It is not known whether the other drugs are excreted in breast milk. Safety for use during lactation has not been established. Exercise caution or temporarily discontinue nursing during administration.

Terconazole – Because of the potential for adverse reactions in nursing infants from terconazole, decide whether to discontinue nursing or to discontinue the drug, taking into account the importance of the drug to the mother.

➤*Children:* Safety and efficacy have not been established with **butoconazole**, **terconazole**, **nystatin**, and **miconazole** (*Monistat Dual-Pak* only). Safety and efficacy have not been established in children younger than 12 years of age with **clotrimazole**, **tioconazole**, and **miconazole**.

Drug Interactions

➤*Miconazole:* Concomitant use of warfarin and miconazole intravaginal cream or suppository may cause an increase in PT, INR, and bleeding. Monitor appropriately.

Adverse Reactions

Irritation; sensitization; vulvovaginal burning.

Clotrimazole – Skin irritation with symptoms of redness, itching, burning, blistering, peeling, urticaria, or skin fissures.

Miconazole – Burning, irritation, pruritus, discharge, edema, and pain have occurred at the administration site. Other adverse reactions include GI cramping, nausea, and headache. Genital erythema, vaginal tenderness, dysuria, allergic reaction, dry mouth, flatulence, perianal burning, pelvic cramping, rash, urticaria, skin irritation, periorbital edema, and conjunctival pruritus occurred in less than 1% of patients in trials.

Butoconazole – Vulvar/vaginal burning, itching, soreness and swelling, pelvic or abdominal pain or cramping, or a combination of 2 or more of these symptoms.

Terconazole – Headache (21% to 26%); dysmenorrhea (6%); pain of the female genitalia (5%); body pain (2.1%); abdominal pain (3.4%); fever (1% to 1.7%); chills (0.4%); vulvovaginal burning (5.2%); itching (2.3%); irritation (3.1%). Most frequent reason for discontinuing therapy was vulvovaginal itching (0.6% to 0.7%).

Photosensitivity reactions may occur following repeated dermal application under conditions of filtered artificial ultraviolet light.

Tioconazole – Vaginal swelling or redness; difficult or burning urination; headache; abdominal pain/cramping; upper respiratory tract infection.

Patient Information

Patient instructions are enclosed with product. Patients should carefully read *otc* product labeling.

Open applicator just prior to administration to prevent contamination. Clean reusable applicators after use with mild soap solution and rinse thoroughly with water.

Insert high into the vagina (except during pregnancy).

Complete full course of therapy. Use continuously, even during menstrual period.

Notify physician if burning or irritation, skin rash, or hives occur.

Refrain from sexual intercourse.

Use sanitary napkin or minipad to prevent staining of clothing. Do not use a tampon.

The base used in some of these formulations may interact with (weaken) certain latex products such as condoms, diaphragms, or vaginal spermicides. Concurrent use (within 72 hours) is not recommended. The effect is temporary and occurs only during treatment.

Vaginal Antifungal Agents

CLOTRIMAZOLE

otc	**Clotrimazole** (Various, eg, Taro)	**Suppositories; vaginal:** 200 mg	In 3s with applicator.
otc	**Gyne-Lotrimin 3** (Schering-Plough)		In 3s with applicator.
otc	**Clotrimazole** (Various, eg, Taro)	**Cream; vaginal:** 2%	In 21 g tube with 3 disposable applicators.
otc	**Gyne-Lotrimin 3** (Schering-Plough)		Benzyl alcohol. In 21 g tube with 3 disposable applicators.
otc	**Clotrimazole** (Various, eg, Alpharma, Major, Warrick)	**Cream; vaginal:** 1%	In 15, 30, and 45 g with applicator(s).
otc	**Mycelex-7** (Ortho McNeil)		Benzyl alcohol, cetostearyl alcohol. In 45 g with 1 applicator or 45 g with 7 disposable applicators.
otc	**Gyne-Lotrimin 7** (Schering-Plough)		In 45 g with 1 applicator, 45 g with 7 applicators, or 45 g with 7 prefilled applicators.
otc	**Mycelex-7 Combination Pack** (Ortho McNeil)	**Suppositories; vaginal:** 100 mg	Lactose, povidone. In 7s with applicator.
		Cream; vaginal: 1%	Benzyl alcohol, cetostearyl alcohol. Polysorbate 80. In 7 g tubes.
otc	**Clotrimazole Combination Pack** (Various, eg, Taro)	**Suppositories; vaginal:** 200 mg	In 3s with applicator.
		Cream; vaginal: 1%	In tubes.
otc	**Gyne-Lotrimin 3 Combination Pack** (Schering-Plough)	**Suppositories; vaginal:** 200 mg	Lactose. In 3s with applicator.
		Cream; vaginal: 1%	Benzyl alcohol, cetyl stearyl alcohol. In 7 g tubes.

CLOTRIMAZOLE — VAGINAL

Refer to the general discussion of these products in the Vaginal Antifungal agents group monograph. For information on oral and topical clotrimazole, refer to individual monographs.

Indications

➤*Vaginal yeast infections:* For the treatment of vaginal yeast (candidiasis) infections and for the relief of external vulvar itching and irritation associated with vaginal yeast infections.

Administration and Dosage

➤*General dosing considerations:* If there is no improvement within 3 to 7 days, stop using these products and consult a physician.

➤*Adults:*

Candidiasis –

Cream: Insert 1 applicatorful per day, preferably at bedtime, for 7 consecutive days with the 1% cream and 3 days with the 2% cream.

Suppositories: 1 suppository once daily, preferably at bedtime for 7 consecutive days with the 100 mg and 3 consecutive days with the 200 mg suppository.

➤*Children:*

Candidiasis –

12 years of age and older: See Adults for dosing.

➤*Concomitant therapy:* For relief of external vulvar itching, squeeze a small amount of clotrimazole cream onto your finger and gently spread the cream onto the irritated area of the vulva. Use once or twice a day for up to 7 days as needed to relieve external vulvar itching. The cream should not be used for vulvar itching due to causes other than a yeast infection.

➤*Administration:* For vaginal or external vulvar use only. Do not use in the eyes or mouth.

➤*Storage/Stability:* Store at 15° to 30°C (59° to 86°F). Avoid excessive heat above 30°C (86°F). Avoid freezing.

MICONAZOLE NITRATE

otc	**Monistat-7** (Personal Products)	**Suppository; vaginal:** 100 mg	In 7s with applicator.
otc	**Miconazole 7** (Rugby)		Hydrogenated vegetable oil base. In 7s with applicator.
Rx	**Miconazole** (Actavis Mid Atlantic)	**Suppository; vaginal:** 200 mg	Hydrogenated vegetable oil base. In 3s with applicator.
otc	**Monistat** (Personal Products)	**Cream; topical:** 2%	In 9 g tubes.
otc	**Miconazole Nitrate** (Various, eg, Alpharma, E. Fougera, G & W Labs, Major, Taro)	**Cream; vaginal:** 2%	In 15, 30, and 45 g with applicator(s).
otc	**Monistat 7** (Personal Products)		In 35 and 45 g tubes with 1 applicator or 7 *Ultraslim* disposable applicators, or in 7 prefilled applicators with 5 g cream.
otc	**Monistat 3** (Personal Products)		In 3 prefilled applicators.
Rx	**Monistat 1 Combination Pack** (Personal Products)	**Suppository; vaginal:** 1200 mg	Glycerin, mineral oil, petrolatum. In 1s with applicator.
		Cream; topical: 2%	Steryl and cetyl alcohol. In 9 g tubes.
otc	**Monistat 3 Combination Pack** (Personal Products)	**Suppository; vaginal:** 200 mg	In 3s with 1 reusable applicator or 3 disposable applicators.
		Cream; topical: 2%	In tubes.
otc	**Vagistat-3 Combination Pack** (Novartis Consumer Health)	**Suppository; vaginal:** 200 mg	Hydrogenated vegetable oil. In 3s with 3 disposable applicators.
		Cream; topical: 2%	Mineral oil. In 9 g tube.
otc	**Monistat 7 Combination Pack** (Personal Products)	**Suppository; vaginal:** 100 mg	In 7s with 1 applicator.
		Cream; topical: 2%	In tubes.

MICONAZOLE NITRATE — VAGINAL

Refer to the general discussion of these products in the Vaginal Antifungal Agents class monograph. For information on topical miconazole, refer to the monograph in the Dermatologicals chapter.

Indications

➤*Suppositories:* For the treatment of vulvovaginal candidiasis (moniliasis).

➤*Cream:* For the relief of external vulvar itching and irritation associated with a yeast infection.

Administration and Dosage

➤*General dosing considerations:* Repeat course if necessary, after ruling out other pathogens.

➤*Adults:*

Candidiasis –

Cream: 1 applicatorful intravaginally at bedtime for 3 days (4%) or 7 days (2%).

Suppositories: 1 vaginal suppository at bedtime for 1 day (1,200 mg), 3 consecutive days (200 mg), or 7 consecutive days (100 mg).

➤*Children:*

Candidiasis –

12 years of age and older: See Adults for dosing.

➤*Concomitant therapy:* Apply topical cram to affected areas twice daily (morning and evening) for up to 7 days or as needed for external symptoms.

➤*Administration:* Administer intravaginally at bedtime.

➤*Storage/Stability:* Store at 15° to 30°C (59° to 86°F).

MICONAZOLE NITRATE — VAGINAL

Warnings/Precautions

➤*Pregnancy: Category C.* Small amounts of miconazole are absorbed from the vagina. Use in pregnant patients with vulvovaginal candidiasis (moniliasis) has not been associated with an increase in congenital malformations. Per Briggs' *Drugs in Pregnancy and Lactation*, miconazole applied topically is compatible for use in pregnant women.

➤*Lactation:* Because miconazole has poor oral bioavailability, it is unlikely to adversely affect the breast-fed infant, including topical application to the nipples. Remove any excess cream or ointment from the nipples before breast-feeding.

TIOCONAZOLE

otc	**Vagistat-1** (Novartis Consumer Health)	**Ointment; vaginal**: 6.5%	White petrolatum. In 300 mg prefilled, single-dose applicator.
otc	**Monistat 1** (Personal Products)		In 4.6 g prefilled, single-dose applicator.

TIOCONAZOLE — VAGINAL

Refer to the general discussion of these products in the Vaginal Antifungal Agents group monograph.

Indications

➤*Candidiasis:* For the treatment of recurrent vaginal yeast infections (candidiasis).

Administration and Dosage

➤*Adults:*

Candidiasis – 1 applicatorful at bedtime as a single dose.

➤*Children:*

Candidiasis –

12 years of age and older: 1 applicatorful at bedtime as a single dose.

➤*Administration:* Open the foil packet just before use. Remove blue cap. Insert entire contents of applicator into the vagina, preferably at bedtime, even during a menstrual period.

➤*Storage / Stability:* Store at 15° to 30°C (59° to 86°F). Dispose of applicator after use.

NYSTATIN

Rx	**Nystatin** (Various, eg, Goldline)	**Vaginal tablets**: 100,000 units	In 15s and 30s with applicator(s).

NYSTATIN — VAGINAL

Refer to the general discussion of these products in the Vaginal Antifungal Agents class monograph. For information on oral nystatin suspension and troches for oral candidiasis, oral nystatin tablets for intestinal candidiasis, and topical nystatin, refer to the individual monographs.

Indications

➤*Yeast infections:* For the treatment of vulvovaginal candidiasis (moniliasis).

➤*Off-label uses:*

Oral administration – [4] = Insufficient documentation. Although oral administration of vaginal nystatin dosage forms is acknowledged in a variety of tertiary references, the paucity of supporting study data precludes routine recommendations for use. Solid vaginal dosage forms might be appropriate in cases in which oral pastilles or troches are unavailable and the patient has difficulty retaining nystatin suspension in the mouth for the required time.

Administration and Dosage

➤*General dosing considerations:* Symptomatic relief may occur in a few days; continue the full course of treatment.

➤*Adults:*

Yeast infection – The usual dosage is 1 tablet inserted high in the vagina by means of the applicator daily for 2 weeks.

Off-label dosing –

Oral administration: [4] = Insufficient documentation. One 100,000 unit vaginal tablet or suppository dissolved slowly in the mouth 3 to 5 times daily for at least 7 to 14 days for up to 3 months.

➤*Storage / Stability:* Store at 15° to 30°C (59° to 86°F).

TERCONAZOLE

Rx	**Terconazole** (Various, eg, Taro, Watson)	**Cream; vaginal**: 0.4%	Alcohols. In 45 g tubes.
Rx	**Terazol 7** (Ortho-McNeil)		Cetyl alcohol, stearyl alcohol. In 45 g tube with 1 measured-dose applicator.
Rx	**Terconazole** (Various, eg, Taro, Watson)	**Cream; vaginal**: 0.8%	Alcohols. In 20 g tubes.
Rx	**Terazol 3** (Ortho-McNeil)		In 20 g tube with measured-dose applicator.
Rx	**Zazole** (PharmaDerm)		Alcohols. In 20 g tube with measured-dose applicator.
Rx	**Terconazole** (Perrigo)	**Suppositories; vaginal**: 80 mg	Coconut oil/palm kernel oil. White to off-white, elliptically shaped. In 2.5 g. In 3s with applicator.
Rx	**Terazol 3** (Ortho-McNeil)		Coconut oil/palm kernel oil. White to off-white, eliptically shaped. In 2.5 g. In 3s.

TERCONAZOLE — VAGINAL

Refer to the general discussion of these products in the Vaginal Antifungal Agents group monograph.

Indications

➤*Candidiasis:* For the local treatment of vulvovaginal candidiasis (moniliasis). As terconazole is effective only for vulvovaginitis caused by the genus *Candida*, the diagnosis should be confirmed by KOH smears or cultures.

Administration and Dosage

➤*Adults:*

Candidiasis – 1 applicatorful (5 g) or 1 vaginal suppository once daily at bedtime for 3 consecutive days (7 days for the 0.4% cream). Before prescribing another course of therapy, the diagnosis should be reconfirmed by smears or cultures and other pathogens commonly associated with vulvovaginitis ruled out.

➤*Administration:* Administer intravaginally at bedtime.

The base contained in the suppository formulation may interact with certain rubber or latex products, such as those used in vaginal contraceptive diaphragms; therefore, concurrent use is not recommended.

➤*Storage / Stability:* Store at 15° to 30°C (59° to 86°F).

BUTOCONAZOLE NITRATE

Rx	**Gynazole•1** (Ther-Rx)	**Cream; vaginal**: 2%	EDTA, parabens, mineral oil. In 5 g prefilled, single-dose applicator (1s).
otc	**Mycelex-3** (Ortho McNeil)		Cetyl and stearyl alcohol, parabens, mineral oil. In 3 prefilled, single-dose applicators, or in 20 g with 3 disposable applicators.

BUTOCONAZOLE NITRATE — VAGINAL

Refer to the general discussion of these products in the Vaginal Antifungal Agents group monograph.

Indications

➤*Candidiasis:* For the local treatment of vulvovaginal candidiasis (infections caused by *Candida*). The diagnosis may be confirmed by KOH smears or cultures.

Vaginal Antifungal Agents

BUTOCONAZOLE NITRATE — VAGINAL

Administration and Dosage

➤*Adults:*

Candidiasis –

Rx formulation: 1 applicatorful (approximately 5 g) intravaginally as a single dose.

OTC formulation: Insert 1 applicator full of cream into the vagina for 3 consecutive days, preferably at bedtime.

➤*Children:*

OTC formulation –

12 years of age and older: See Adults for dosing.

Younger than 12 years of age: Do not use.

➤*Administration:* One applicatorful intravaginally. Dispose of applicator after use.

➤*Storage / Stability:* Store at 25°C (77°F); excursions permitted to 15° to 30°C (59° to 86°F). Avoid heat above 30°C (86°F), and avoid freezng.

Miscellaneous Anti-infectives

SULFANILAMIDE

Rx	**AVC** (Pharmelle)	**Cream:** 15%	Methylparaben. In 120 g tube with applicator.

SULFANILAMIDE — VAGINAL

Indications

➤*Vulvovaginitis caused by Candida albicans:* For the treatment of vulvovaginitis caused by *Candida albicans*.

Administration and Dosage

➤*Adults:*

Vulvovaginitis caused by Candida albicans –

Usual dosage: One applicatorful (about 6 g) or 1 suppository once or twice daily.

Duration of therapy: Improvements in symptoms should occur within a few days, but treatment should be continued for a period of 30 days.

➤*Administration:* For intravaginal use. Douching with a suitable solution before insertion may be recommended for hygienic purposes.

➤*Storage / Stability:*

Cream – Store at room temperature, below 30°C (86°F). Protect from cold. Products darken with age. Potency is maintained throughout labeled shelf life when stored as directed.

Suppositories – Store at room temperature, below 30°C (86°F). Protect from excessive cold and moisture.

Actions

➤*Pharmacology:* Sulfanilamide has been a useful ingredient of vaginal formulations for about 4 decades. It blocks certain metabolic processes essential for the growth of susceptible bacteria. In sulfanilamide, the sulfanilamide is in a specially compounded base buffered to the pH (about 4.3) of the healthy vagina to encourage the presence of the normally occurring Döderlein's bacilli of the vagina.

The use of sulfanilamide for the treatment of vulvovaginitis caused by *Candida albicans* is supported by 3 clinical investigations. The 3 studies that show sulfanilamide to be significantly more effective ($p \leq 0.01$) than placebo are as follows:

In study I, the ratio of effectiveness was 71% for sulfanilamide vs 49% for placebo with 30 days of treatment.

In study II, the percentages were 48% vs 24%, respectively, with 15 days of treatment.

In study III, the percentages were 66% vs 33%, respectively, with 30 days of treatment.

Contraindications

Sulfanilamide should not be used in patients known to be sensitive to this product or to the sulfonamides.

Warnings/Precautions

➤*Goiter production:* Goiter production, diuresis, and hypoglycemia have reportedly occurred rarely in patients receiving oral sulfonamides. Cross-sensitivity may exist with these agents. Rats appear to be especially susceptible to the goitrogenic effects of sulfonamides, and long-term administration has reportedly produced thyroid malignancies in this species.

➤*Use with caution:* Vaginal applicators or inserters should be used with caution after the seventh month of pregnancy.

➤*Hypersensitivity reactions:* Deaths associated with administration of oral sulfonamides have reportedly occurred from hypersensitivity reactions, agranulocytosis, aplastic anemia, and other blood dyscrasias.

➤*Drug abuse and dependence:* Tolerance, abuse, or dependence with sulfanilamide has not been reported.

➤*Pregnancy: Category C.*

Teratogenic – Animal reproductive studies have been conducted with sulfonamides, including sulfanilamide (see below). It is not known whether sulfanilamide can cause fetal harm when administered to a pregnant woman or can affect reproductive capacity. Sulfanilamide should be given to a pregnant woman only if clearly needed.

Sulfonamides, including sulfanilamide, readily pass through the placenta and reach fetal circulation. The concentration in the fetus is from 5090% of that in the maternal blood and if high enough, can cause toxic effects. The safe use of sulfonamides, including sulfanilamide, in pregnancy has not been established. The teratogenic potential of most sulfonamides has not been thoroughly investigated in either animals or humans. However, a significant increase in the incidence of cleft palate and other bony abnormalities of offspring has been observed with certain sulfonamides of the short-, intermediate-, and long-acting types (including sulfanilamide) when given to pregnant rats and mice at high oral doses (7 to 25 times the human therapeutic oral dose).

➤*Lactation:* Sulfanilamide should be avoided in nursing mothers because absorbed sulfonamides will appear in maternal milk, and have caused kernicterus in the newborn. Because of the potential for serious adverse reactions in nursing infants from sulfonamides, a decision should be made whether to discontinue nursing or to discontinue the drug.

➤*Children:* Safety and efficacy of sulfanilamide in pediatric patients have not been established.

➤*Monitoring:* Because sulfonamides are absorbed from the vaginal mucosa, the usual precautions for oral sulfonamides apply. Patients should be observed for skin rash or evidence of systemic toxicity, and if these develop, the medications should be discontinued.

Drug Interactions

Drug interactions have not been documented with sulfanilamide.

Adverse Reactions

Local sensitivity reactions such as increased discomfort or a burning sensation have occasionally been reported following the use of topical sulfonamides. With the use of sulfanilamide cream, sensitivity reactions (only local) were reported for 0.2% of the investigational patients.

Treatment should be discontinued if either local or systemic manifestations of sulfonamide toxicity or sensitivity occur.

Overdosage

➤*Symptoms:* There have been no reports of accidental overdosage with sulfanilamide. The acute oral LD_{50} of sulfanilamide is 3700 to 4200 mg/kg in mice.

The minimum human lethal dose of sulfanilamide has not been established.

➤*Treatment:* It is not known if sulfanilamide is dialyzable.

Patient Information

The doctor should advise the patient that in the event unusual local itching and burning occur, or other unusual symptoms develop, medication should be discontinued and not restarted without further consultation.

CLINDAMYCIN PHOSPHATE

Rx	**Clindamycin Phosphate** (Greenstone)	**Cream:** 2%	Benzyl alcohol, cetostearyl alcohol, mineral oil. In 40 g tube with 7 disposable applicators.
Rx	**Cleocin** (Pfizer)		Benzyl alcohol, cetostearyl alcohol, mineral oil. In 40 g tube with 7 disposable applicators.
Rx	**Clindesse** (KV Pharma)		EDTA, mineral oil, parabens. In carton of 1 single-dose prefilled disposable applicator.
Rx	**Cleocin** (Pfizer)	**Suppositories:** 100 mg (as base)	In cartons of 3 with applicator.

CLINDAMYCIN PHOSPHATE — INTRAVAGINAL

Indications

➤*Bacterial vaginosis:* For the treatment of bacterial vaginosis (formerly referred to as *Haemophilus* vaginitis, *Gardnerella* vaginitis, nonspecific vaginitis, *Corynebacterium* vaginitis, or anaerobic vaginosis) in nonpregnant women.

Cleocin cream only – Clindamycin cream can be used to treat pregnant women during the second and third trimester.

Administration and Dosage

➤*General dosing considerations:* These products contain an oleaginous base that may weaken latex or rubber products such as condoms or vaginal contraceptive diaphragms. Therefore, the use of such barrier contraceptives is not recommended concurrently or for 72 hours (5 days for *Clindesse*) following treatment. During this time period, condoms may not be reliable for preventing pregnancy or for protecting against transmission of HIV and other sexually transmitted diseases.

➤*Adults:*

Bacterial vaginosis –

Cleocin cream: One applicatorful (5 g containing approximately clindamycin 100 mg) intravaginally, preferably at bedtime, for 3 or 7 consecutive days in nonpregnant women and for 7 consecutive days in pregnant women.

Clindesse cream: One applicatorful (5 g containing approximately clindamycin 100 mg) administered once intravaginally at anytime of the day.

Suppositories: One suppository (clindamycin 100 mg per 2.5 g suppository) intravaginally per day, preferably at bedtime, for 3 consecutive days.

➤*Administration:* For vaginal use only.

➤*Storage/Stability:*

Cream – Store at controlled room temperature, 20° to 25°C (68° to 77°F). Protect from freezing.

Suppositories – Store at 25°C (77°F); excursions are permitted to 15° to 30°C (59° to 86°F). Avoid heat over 30°C (86°F) and high humidity.

Actions

➤*Pharmacology:* Clindamycin is a water soluble ester of the semi-synthetic antibiotic produced by a 7(S)-chloro-substitution of the 7(R)-hydroxyl group of the parent antibiotic lincomycin. Clindamycin inhibits bacterial protein synthesis at the level of the bacterial ribosome. The antibiotic binds preferentially to the 50S ribosomal subunit and affects the process of peptide chain initiation. Although clindamycin is inactive in vitro, rapid in vivo hydrolysis converts this compound to the antibacterially active clindamycin.

➤*Pharmacokinetics:*

Cream – Following a once-daily intravaginal dose of 100 mg clindamycin vaginal cream administered to 6 healthy female volunteers for 7 days, approximately 5% of the administered dose was absorbed systemically. The peak serum clindamycin concentration averaged 18 and 25 ng/mL on day 1 and day 7, respectively. These peak concentrations were attained approximately 10 hours postdosing.

Following a once-daily intravaginal dose of 100 mg clindamycin vaginal cream administered for 7 consecutive days to 5 women with bacterial vaginosis, absorption was slower and less variable than that observed in healthy females. Approximately 5% of the dose was absorbed systemically. The peak serum clindamycin concentration averaged 13 and 16 ng/mL on day 1 and day 7, respectively. These peak concentrations were attained approximately 14 hours postdosing.

There was little or no systemic accumulation of clindamycin after repeated vaginal dosing of clindamycin vaginal cream. The systemic half life was 1.5 to 2.6 hours.

Suppositories – Systemic absorption of clindamycin was estimated following an intravaginal dose of 1 clindamycin suppository (equivalent to 100 mg clindamycin) administered once daily to 11 healthy female volunteers for 3 days. Approximately 30% of the administered dose was absorbed systemically on day 3 of dosing based on AUC. The mean AUC following day 3 of the suppository dosing was 3.2 mcg•h/mL. The C_{max} observed on day 3 of the suppository dosing averaged 0.27 mcg/mL and was observed approximately 5 hours after dosing. The mean apparent elimination half life after the suppository dosing was 11 hours and is considered to be limited by the absorption rate.

➤*Microbiology:* Clindamycin is active in vitro against most strains of the following organisms that have been reported to be associated with bacterial vaginosis: *Bacteroides* spp., *Gardnerella vaginalis*; *Mobiluncus* spp.; *Mycoplasma hominis*; *Peptostreptococcus* spp.

Contraindications

Hypersensitivity to clindamycin, lincomycin, or any components of the products; regional enteritis; ulcerative colitis; "antibiotic-associated" colitis.

Warnings/Precautions

➤*Pseudomembranous colitis:* Pseudomembranous colitis has been reported with nearly all antibacterial agents, including clindamycin, and may range in severity from mild to life-threatening. Orally and parenterally administered clindamycin has been associated with severe colitis that may end fatally. Diarrhea, bloody diarrhea, and colitis (including pseudomembranous colitis) have been reported with the use of orally and parenterally administered clindamycin as well as with topical (dermal) formulations of clindamycin. Therefore, it is important to consider this diagnosis in patients who present with diarrhea subsequent to the administration of clindamycin, even when administered by the vaginal route, because approximately 5% (cream) and 30% (suppository) of the clindamycin dose is systemically absorbed from the vagina.

Treatment with antibacterial agents alters the normal flora of the colon and may permit overgrowth of clostridia. Studies indicate that a toxin produced by *Clostridium difficile* is a primary cause of "antibiotic-associated" colitis.

After the diagnosis of pseudomembranous colitis has been established, initiate therapeutic measures. Mild cases of pseudomembranous colitis usually respond to discontinuation of the drug alone. In moderate to severe cases, give consideration to management with fluids and electrolytes, protein supplementation, and treatment with an antibacterial drug clinically effective against *C. difficile* colitis.

Onset of pseudomembranous colitis symptoms may occur during or after antimicrobial treatment.

➤*Mineral oil/oleaginous base:* The cream contains mineral oil and the suppositories contain an oleaginous base, both which can weaken latex or rubber products such as condoms or vaginal contraceptive diaphragms. Use of such products within 72 hours (*Cleocin*) or 5 days (*Clindesse*) following treatment with clindamycin is not recommended.

➤*Diagnosis:* A clinical diagnosis of bacterial vaginosis is usually defined by the presence of a homogeneous vaginal discharge that has a pH of greater than 4.5, emits a "fishy" amine odor when mixed with a 10% KOH solution, and contains clue cells on microscopic examination. Gram's stain results consistent with a diagnosis of bacterial vaginosis include markedly reduced or absent *Lactobacillus* morphology, predominance of *Gardnerella* morphotype, and absent or few white blood cells.

Rule out other pathogens commonly associated with vulvovaginitis (eg, *Trichomonas vaginalis*, *Chlamydia trachomatis*, *Neisseria gonorrhoeae*, *Candida albicans*, and herpes simplex virus).

➤*For intravaginal use only:* Avoid contact with the eyes. Clindamycin contains ingredients that will cause burning and irritation of the eye. In the event of accidental contact, rinse the eye with copious amounts of cool tap water.

➤*Overgrowth of nonsusceptible organisms:* The use of clindamycin may result in the overgrowth of nonsusceptible organisms, particularly yeasts, in the vagina. In studies using clindamycin suppositories, treatment-related moniliasis was reported in 2.7% of women patients and vaginitis in 3.6%. In women who received clindamycin cream treatment for 3 days, *C. albicans* was reported in 8.8% and vaginitis in 9% of patients; in the 7-day treatment, *C. albicans* was detected in 10.5% and vaginitis in 10.7% of patients.

➤*Pregnancy: Category B.* Clindamycin cream has been studied in pregnant women during the second trimester. In women treated for 7 days, abnormal labor was reported in 1.1% of patients who received clindamycin cream compared with 0.5% of patients who received placebo. There are no adequate and well-controlled studies in pregnant women during the first trimester of pregnancy treated with clindamycin cream; there are no adequate and well-controlled studies in pregnant women treated with clindamycin suppositories. Use during pregnancy only if clearly needed.

➤*Lactation:* It is not known if clindamycin is excreted in breast milk following the use of vaginally administered clindamycin. However, clindamycin has been detected in breast milk after oral or parenteral administration. Because of the potential for serious adverse reactions in nursing infants, decide whether to discontinue nursing or discontinue the drug, taking into account the importance of the drug to the mother.

➤*Children:* Safety and efficacy in children have not been established.

Drug Interactions

➤*Neuromuscular blocking agents:* Clindamycin has been shown to have neuromuscular blocking properties that may enhance the action of other neuromuscular blocking agents; use with caution in patients receiving such agents.

Adverse Reactions

➤*Cream:*

Nonpregnant women – In clinical trials involving nonpregnant women, 1.8% of 600 patients who received treatment with clindamycin cream for 3 days and 2.7% of 1325 patients who received treatment for 7 days discontinued therapy because of drug-related adverse events. Medical events judged to be related, probably related, possibly related, or of unknown relationship to vaginally administered clindamycin cream were reported for 20.7% of the patients receiving treatment for 3 days and 21.3% of the patients receiving treatment for 7 days.

Clindamycin Cream Adverse Reactions (≥ 1%)

Adverse reaction	Clindamycin cream 3 day (n = 600)	Clindamycin cream 7 day (n = 1325)
GU		
Trichomonal vaginitis	0	1.3
Vaginal moniliasis	7.7	10.4
Vulvovaginal disorder	3.2	5.3
Vulvovaginitis	6	4.4

CLINDAMYCIN PHOSPHATE — INTRAVAGINAL

Clindamycin Cream Adverse Reactions (≥ 1%)		
	Clindamycin cream	
Adverse reaction	3 day (n = 600)	7 day (n = 1325)
Miscellaneous		
Moniliasis (body)	1.3	0.2

Other adverse events (less than 1%):
- *CNS* – Dizziness, headache, vertigo.
- *Dermatologic* – Erythema, maculopapular rash, moniliasis, pruritus (nonapplication site), rash, urticaria.
- *GI* – Abdominal cramps, constipation, diarrhea, dyspepsia, flatulence, generalized abdominal pain, GI disorder, localized abdominal pain, nausea, vomiting.
- *GU* – Endometriosis, menstrual disorder, metrorrhagia, urinary tract infection, vaginal discharge, vaginal pain, vaginitis/vaginal infection.
- *Respiratory* – Epistaxis.
- *Miscellaneous* – Allergic reaction, bacterial infection, fungal infection, halitosis, hyperthyroidism, inflammatory swelling, taste perversion.

Pregnant women – In a clinical trial involving pregnant women during the second trimester, 1.7% of 180 patients who received treatment for 7 days discontinued therapy because of drug-related adverse events. Medical events judged to be related, probably related, possibly related, or of unknown relationship to vaginally administered clindamycin cream were reported for 22.8% of pregnant patients.

Clindamycin Cream Adverse Reactions (≥ 1%)		
	Clindamycin cream	Placebo
Adverse reaction	7 day (n = 180)	7 day (n = 184)
GU		
Abnormal labor	1.1	0.5
Vaginal moniliasis	13.3	7.1
Vulvovaginal disorder	6.7	7.1
Miscellaneous		
Fungal infection	1.7	
Pruritus, nonapplication site	1.1	0

Other adverse events (less than 1%):
- *Dermatologic* – Erythema, pruritus (topical application site).
- *GU* – Dysuria, metrorrhagia, trichomonal vaginitis, vaginal pain.
- *Miscellaneous* – Upper respiratory infection.

➤*Suppositories:* In clinical trials involving nonpregnant women, 3 of 589 (0.5%) patients who received treatment with clindamycin suppositories discontinued therapy because of drug-related adverse events. Adverse events judged to have a reasonable possibility of having been caused by clindamycin suppositories were reported for 10.5% of patients. Events reported by 1% or more of patients receiving clindamycin suppositories were as follows:

GU – Vulvovaginal disorder (3.4%), vaginal pain (1.9%), vaginal moniliasis (1.5%).

Miscellaneous – Fungal infection (1%).

Other adverse events (less than 1%) –
Dermatologic: Application-site pain, application-site pruritus, nonapplication-site pruritus, rash.
GI: Abdominal cramps, diarrhea, localized abdominal pain, nausea, vomiting.
GU: Dysuria, menstrual disorder, pyelonephritis, vaginal discharge, vaginitis/vaginal infection.
Miscellaneous: Fever, flank pain, generalized pain, headache, localized edema, moniliasis.

➤*Other clindamycin formulations:* Clindamycin vaginal cream and suppositories afford minimal peak serum levels and systemic exposure of clindamycin compared with 100 mg oral clindamycin dosing. Although these lower levels of exposure are less likely to produce the common reactions seen with oral clindamycin, the possibility of these and other reactions cannot be excluded presently. Refer to the Clindamycin and Lincomycin monographs in the Anti-Infectives chapter.

Overdosage

Vaginally applied cream or suppositories could be absorbed in sufficient amounts to produce systemic effects.

Patient Information

Instruct patients not to engage in vaginal intercourse or use other vaginal products (eg, tampons, douches) during treatment with this product.

Advise patients that the cream contains mineral oil and the suppositories contain an oleaginous base, both which can weaken latex or rubber products such as condoms or vaginal contraceptive diaphragms. Use of such products within 72 hours following treatment with clindamycin is not recommended.

METRONIDAZOLE

Rx	**Metronidazole Gel** (Prasco)	**Gel; vaginal:** 0.75%	EDTA, parabens. In 70 g tubes with 5 applicators.
Rx	**MetroGel-Vaginal** (Graceway Pharmaceuticals)		EDTA, parabens. In 70 g tube with 5 applicators.
Rx	**Vandazole** (Upsher-Smith Laboratories, Inc.)	**Gel; topical:** 0.75%	EDTA, parabens. In 70 g tube with 5 applicators.

METRONIDAZOLE — VAGINAL

Metronidazole is also available for topical and systemic use. For further information, refer to the individual monographs in the Anti-infectives chapter and the Dermatological Agents chapter.

Indications

➤*Bacterial vaginosis:* For the treatment of bacterial vaginosis (formerly referred to as *Haemophilus* vaginitis, *Gardnerella* vaginitis, nonspecific vaginitis, *Corynebacterium* vaginitis, or anaerobic vaginosis).

Administration and Dosage

➤*General dosing considerations:* Medicine is to be used intravaginally only.

Do not to engage in vaginal intercourse during treatment with this product.

Caution patients about drinking alcohol while being treated with metronidazole vaginal gel.

➤*Adults:*

Bacterial vaginosis – 1 applicatorful (approximately 5 g containing metronidazole 37.5 mg) intravaginally once or twice daily for 5 days. For once-a-day dosing, administer at bedtime.

➤*Children:*

Off-label dosing –
Adolescents (13 to 17 years of age):
- *Bacterial vaginosis* – 1 applicatorful (5 g) intravaginally twice daily for 5 days.

➤*Storage/Stability:* Store at 15° to 30°C (59° to 86°F). Protect from freezing.

Actions

➤*Pharmacology:* Metronidazole, a member of the imidazole class, is classified therapeutically as an antiprotozoal and antibacterial agent. The intracellular target of action of metronidazole on anaerobes are largely unknown. The 5-nitro group of metronidazole is reduced by metabolically active anaerobes, and studies have demonstrated that the reduced form of the drug interacts with bacterial DNA. However, it is not clear whether interaction with DNA alone is an important component in the bactericidal action of metronidazole.

➤*Pharmacokinetics:* A single intravaginal 5 g dose of metronidazole vaginal gel (equivalent to 37.5 mg metronidazole) to 12 healthy subjects resulted in a mean maximum serum metronidazole concentration of 237 ng/mL (range, 152 to 368 ng/mL). This is approximately 2% of the mean maximum serum metronidazole concentration reported in the same subjects administered a single oral 500 mg dose of metronidazole (mean C_{max} = 12,785 ng/mL; range, 10,013 to 17,400 ng/mL). These peak concentrations were obtained 6 to 12 hours after dosing with metronidazole vaginal gel and 1 to 3 hours after dosing with oral metronidazole.

The extent of exposure (AUC) of metronidazole, when administered as a single intravaginal 5 g dose was approximately 4% of the AUC of a single oral 500 mg dose (4977 ng•h/mL and approximately 125,000 ng•h/mL, respectively). When administered vaginally, absorption was approximately half that of an equivalent oral dose.

Patients with bacterial vaginosis – Single and multiple 5 g doses of metronidazole vaginal gel to 4 patients with bacterial vaginosis resulted in a mean maximum serum metronidazole concentration of 214 ng/mL on day 1 and 294 ng/mL on day 5. Steady-state metronidazole serum concentrations following oral dosages of 400 to 500 mg twice daily have been reported to range from 6000 to 20,000 ng/mL.

➤*Microbiology:* Metronidazole is active in vitro against most strains of the following organisms that have been reported to be associated with bacterial vaginosis: *Bacteroides* sp.; *Gardnerella vaginalis*; *Mobiluncus* sp.; *Peptostreptococcus* sp.

Contraindications

Hypersensitivity to metronidazole, parabens, or other ingredients of the formulation or other nitroimidazole derivatives.

Warnings/Precautions

➤*Convulsive seizures and peripheral neuropathy:* Convulsive seizures and peripheral neuropathy, the latter characterized mainly by numb-

METRONIDAZOLE — VAGINAL

ness or paresthesia of an extremity, have been reported in patients treated with oral or IV metronidazole. The appearance of abnormal neurologic signs demands the prompt discontinuation of metronidazole vaginal gel therapy. Administer with caution to patients with CNS diseases.

➤*Psychotic reactions:* Psychotic reactions have been reported in alcoholic patients who were using oral metronidazole and disulfiram concurrently. Do not administer metronidazole vaginal gel to patients who have taken disulfiram within the last 2 weeks.

➤*Diagnosis:* A clinical diagnosis of bacterial vaginosis is usually defined by the presence of a homogeneous vaginal discharge that has a pH of greater than 4.5, emits a "fishy" amine odor when mixed with a 10% KOH solution, and contains clue cells on microscopic examination. Gram's stain results consistent with a diagnosis of bacterial vaginosis include markedly reduced or absent *Lactobacillus* morphology, predominance of *Gardnerella* morphotype, and absent or few white blood cells.

Rule out other pathogens commonly associated with vulvovaginitis (eg, *Trichomonas vaginalis*, *Chlamydia trachomatis*, *Neisseria gonorrheae*, *Candida albicans*, herpes simplex virus).

➤*Vaginal candidiasis:* Known or previously unrecognized vaginal candidiasis may present more prominent symptoms during metronidazole vaginal gel therapy; approximately 6% to 10% of patients developed symptomatic *Candida* vaginitis during or immediately after therapy.

➤*For intravaginal use only:* Avoid contact with the eyes. Metronidazole vaginal gel contains ingredients that may cause burning and irritation of the eye. In the event of accidental contact with the eye, rinse with copious amounts of cool tap water.

➤*Hepatic function impairment:* Patients with severe hepatic disease metabolize metronidazole slowly. This results in the accumulation of metronidazole and its metabolites in the plasma. Accordingly, administer metronidazole vaginal gel cautiously in these patients.

➤*Pregnancy: Category B.* Metronidazole crosses the placental barrier and rapidly enters the fetal circulation. There are no adequate and well-controlled studies in pregnant women. Use during pregnancy only if clearly needed.

➤*Lactation:* Specific studies of metronidazole levels in breast milk following intravaginally administered metronidazole have not been performed. However, metronidazole is secreted in breast milk in concentrations similar to those found in plasma following oral administration. Decide whether to discontinue nursing or to discontinue the drug, taking into account the importance of the drug to the mother.

➤*Children:* Safety and efficacy in children have not been established.

Drug Interactions

Metronidazole Vaginal Gel Interactions

Precipitant drug	Object drug[a]		Description
Cimetidine	Metronidazole	↑	Use of cimetidine with oral metronidazole may prolong the half-life and decrease plasma clearance of metronidazole. Consider this possibility with the vaginal gel.
Metronidazole	Anticoagulants	↑	Oral metronidazole may potentiate the anticoagulant effect of warfarin, resulting in a prolongation of prothrombin time. Consider this possibility with the vaginal gel.
Metronidazole	Disulfiram	↑	Concurrent use may result in acute psychosis or a confusional state. Do not administer vaginal gel to patients who have taken disulfiram within the last 2 weeks.
Metronidazole	Ethanol	↑	Disulfiram-like reaction to alcohol has occurred with oral metronidazole. Consider the possibility of such a reaction with the vaginal gel.
Metronidazole	Lithium	↑	In patients stabilized on relatively high doses of lithium, short-term oral metronidazole therapy has been associated with elevation of serum lithium levels and, in a few cases, signs of lithium toxicity. Consider this possibility with the vaginal gel.

[a] ↑ = object drug increased.

➤*Drug/Lab test interactions:* Metronidazole may interfere with certain types of determinations of serum chemistry values, such as AST, ALT, LDH, triglycerides, and glucose hexokinase; values of zero may be observed.

Adverse Reactions

In a randomized, single-blind clinical trial of 505 nonpregnant women who received metronidazole vaginal gel once or twice/day, 2 patients (1 from each regimen) discontinued therapy early because of drug-related adverse events. One patient discontinued the drug because of moderate abdominal cramping and loose stools, while the other patient discontinued the drug because of mild vaginal burning. These symptoms resolved after discontinuation of the drug.

Medical events judged to be related, probably related, or possibly related to administration of metronidazole vaginal gel once or twice/day were reported for 39% (195/505) of patients.

➤*CNS:* Headache (5%); dizziness (2%); depression, fatigue (less than 1%).

➤*Dermatologic:* Generalized itching or rash (less than 1%).

➤*GI:* GI discomfort (7%); nausea and/or vomiting (4%); unusual taste (2%); decreased appetite, diarrhea/loose stools (1%); abdominal bloating/gas, dry mouth, thirst (less than 1%).

➤*GU:* Vaginal discharge (12%); symptomatic *Candida* cervicitis/vaginitis (10%); vulva/vaginal irritative symptoms (9%); pelvic discomfort (3%); darkened urine (less than 1%).

➤*Miscellaneous:* Unspecified cramping (1%).

➤*Other metronidazole formulations:* Other effects that have been reported in association with the use of topical (dermal) formulations of metronidazole include skin irritation, transient skin erythema, and mild skin dryness and burning (2% or less).

Metronidazole vaginal gel affords minimal peak serum levels and systemic exposure of metronidazole compared with 500 mg oral dosing. Although these lower levels of exposure are less likely to produce the common reactions seen with oral metronidazole, the possibility of these and other reactions cannot be excluded. Refer to the Metronidazole Oral monograph in the Anti-Infectives chapter.

Overdosage

Vaginally applied metronidazole gel could be absorbed in sufficient amounts to produce systemic effects (see Warnings/Precautions).

Patient Information

Caution patients about drinking alcohol while being treated with metronidazole vaginal gel. While blood levels are significantly lower than with usual doses of oral metronidazole, a possible interaction with alcohol cannot be excluded.

Instruct patients not to engage in vaginal intercourse during treatment with this product.

Advise patients that this medicine is to be used intravaginally only.

MISCELLANEOUS VAGINAL PREPARATIONS

otc	**Lubrin** (Kenwood/Bradley)	**Inserts; vaginal**: Caprylic/capric triglyceride, glycerin *Indication*: Prolonged lubrication for sexual intercourse. *Dosage*: 1 intravaginally 5 to 30 minutes before intercourse. Allow 5 to 10 minutes for insert to dissolve.	In 5s and 12s.
otc	**Astroglide** (BioFilm)	**Gel; vaginal**: Glycerin, propylene glycol, parabens *Indication*: Vaginal lubricant. *Dosage*: Apply externally or internally.	In 66.5 ml bottle and 5 ml travel packets.
otc	**Lubricating Jelly** (Taro)	**Jelly; vaginal**: Glycerin, propylene glycol *Indication*: Provides additional vaginal moisture. *Dosage*: Apply as needed.	In 60 and 125 g.

MISCELLANEOUS VAGINAL PREPARATIONS

otc	**K-Y** (Johnson & Johnson)	**Jelly; vaginal:** Glycerin, hydroxyethyl cellulose, methylparaben *Indication*: Vaginal lubricant *Dosage*: Apply as needed.	Sterile or regular. In 12, 60 and 120 g.
otc	**Surgel** (Ulmer)	**Gel; vaginal:** Propylene glycol, glycerin *Indication*: Vaginal lubricant.	In 120 and 240 ml and 1 gal.
Rx	**Fem pH** (Pharmics)	**Vaginal jelly; vaginal:** 0.9% glacial acetic acid, 0.025% oxyquinoline sulfate, glycerin, lactic acid, PEG 4500 *Indication*: Adjunctive therapy when restoration and maintenance of vaginal acidity is desirable *Dosage*: 1 applicatorful administered intravaginally morning and evening.	In 50 g with applicator.
otc	**Trimo-San** (Cooper Surgical[a])	**Jelly; vaginal:** 0.025% oxyquinoline sulfate, 0.7% sodium borate, 0.1% sodium lauryl sulfate, glycerin, methylparaben *Indication*: Controls odor-causing bacteria. Helps maintain normal vaginal pH 4. *Dosage*: ½ applicator 2 or 3 times per week.	In 120 g with applicator.
Rx	**Amino-Cerv** (Cooper Surgical)	**Cream; vaginal:** 8.34% urea, 0.5% sodium propionate, 0.83% methionine, 0.35% cystine, 0.83% inositol *Indications*: Treatment of mild cervicitis and postpartum cervicitis/cervical tears, postconization and for postsurgical procedures. *Dosage*: See manufacturer's information.	Water miscible base. In 82.5 g with applicator. Buffered to pH 5.5 in water-miscible creme base.
otc	**Yeast X** (Fleet)	**Suppositories; vaginal:** Pulsatilla 28× *Indication*: Relieves vaginal irritation, itching and burning. *Dosage*: One suppository daily as needed.	In 12s with applicator.
otc	**Norforms** (Fleet)	**Suppositories; vaginal:** PEG-18, PEG-32, PEG-20 stearate, methylparaben *Indication*: Feminine deodorant. *Dosage*: One suppository daily as needed.	In 12s and 24s with applicator.
otc	**Moist Again** (Lake Consumer)	**Gel; vaginal:** Aloe vera, EDTA, methylparaben, glycerin *Indication*: Vaginal lubricant. *Dosage*: Apply as needed.	In 70.8 g.
otc	**H-R Lubricating Jelly** (Carter-Wallace)	**Jelly; vaginal:** Hydroxypropyl, methylcellulose, parabens *Indication*: Vaginal lubricant. *Dosage*: Apply as needed.	In 150 g.
otc	**Acid Jelly** (Hope Pharmaceuticals)	**Jelly; vaginal:** 0.025% oxyquinoline sulfate, 0.7% ricinoleic acid, 0.921% glacial acetic acid, 5% glycerin, propylparaben *Indication*: As adjunctive therapy in those cases where restoration and maintenance of vaginal acidity is desirable. *Dosage*: 1 applicatorful, morning and evening.	In 85 g with applicator.
otc	**Surgilube** (Savage)	**Jelly; vaginal:** Chlorhexidine gluconate *Indication*: May be used where a sterile, water soluble, nonstaining lubrication jelly is indicated. *Dosage*: Apply as needed.	In 5 g and 120.49 g.
otc	**Vagi-Gard Maximum Strength** (Lake)	**Cream; vaginal:** 20% benzocaine, 3% resorcinol, methylparaben, sodium sulfite, EDTA, mineral oil *Indication*: Relieves external vaginal irritation, itching and burning. *Dosage*: Apply externally 3 to 4 times/day.	In 45 g.
otc	**Vagi-Gard Advanced Sensitive Formula** (Lake)	**Cream; vaginal:** 5% benzocaine, 2% resorcinol, methylparaben, sodium sulfite, EDTA, mineral oil *Indication*: Relieves external vaginal irritation, itching and burning. *Dosage*: Apply externally 3 to 4 times/day.	In 45 g.
otc	**UTI Feminine Hygiene Pack** (Consumers Choice Systems)	**Kit:** *Indication*: For temporary relief of minor irritations and burning. *Dosage*: Apply to the affected area ≤ 3 to 4 times daily.	
		Wipes; vaginal: Polysorbate 20, EDTA, methylparaben.	In 20s.
		Cream; vaginal: Oat beta glucan, aloe. Cetyl alcohol, cetearyl alcohol, EDTA, parabens.	In 15 g.
otc	**Massengill Feminine Cleansing Wash** (SmithKline Beecham)	**Liquid; vaginal:** Sodium laureth sulfate, sodium oleth sulfate, magnesium oleth sulfate, PEG-120 methyl glucose dioleate, parabens *Indication*: Vaginal cleansing. *Dosage*: Apply externally.	In 240 ml.
otc	**Vagisil** (Combe)	**Powder; vaginal:** Cornstarch, aloe, mineral oil, magnesium stearate, silica, benzethonium chloride, fragrance *Indication*: Absorbs moisture. *Dosage*: Apply externally.	In 198 and 312 g.
otc	**Maxilube** (Mission)	**Jelly; vaginal:** Water, silicone oil, glycerin, carbomer 934, triethanolamine, sodium lauryl sulfate, parabens *Indication*: Vaginal lubricant.	In 90 and 150 g.

[a] Cooper Surgical, 95 Corporate Drive, Trumbull, CT, 06611; 1-(800) 243-2974; fax 1-(800) 262-0105.

DIURETICS

Thiazides and Related Diuretics

Indications

➤*Edema:* Adjunctive therapy in edema associated with congestive heart failure (CHF), hepatic cirrhosis, and corticosteroid and estrogen therapy. Useful in edema caused by renal dysfunction (eg, nephrotic syndrome, acute glomerulonephritis, chronic renal failure).

Indapamide – Indapamide alone is indicated for edema associated with CHF.

Metolazone, rapidly acting (Mykrox) – Metolazone, rapidly acting (*Mykrox*) has not been evaluated for the treatment of CHF or fluid retention caused by renal or hepatic disease, and the correct dosage for these conditions and other edematous states has not been established. Because a safe and effective diuretic dose has not been established, do not use *Mykrox* when diuresis is desired.

➤*Hypertension:* As the sole therapeutic agent or to enhance other antihypertensive drugs in more severe forms of hypertension.

➤*Off-label uses:*

Pediatric hypertension –

Chlorthalidone: [1] = Good documentation.

Other possible off-label uses –

Calcium nephrolithiasis: Thiazide diuretics have been used alone and in combination with amiloride or allopurinol to prevent formation and recurrence of calcium nephrolithiasis in hypercalciuric and normal calciuric patients. Thiazides correct hypercalciuria, reduce urinary saturation, enhance inhibitor activity against spontaneous nucleation of calcium oxalate and brushite, and restore normal parathyroid function and intestinal calcium absorption. Doses of hydrochlorothiazide 50 or 100 mg daily, trichloromethiazide 4 mg/day, chlorthalidone 50 mg/day, and indapamide 2.5 mg/day have been used.

Osteoporosis: Thiazide diuretics may be useful in reducing the incidence of osteoporosis in postmenopausal women, alone or in combination with calcium or estrogen. Further studies are necessary to confirm this use.

Although data conflict, use of thiazides in older patients may be associated with a reduced risk of hip fracture.

Diabetes insipidus: Thiazide diuretics reduce urine volume by 30% to 50%. They constitute the mainstay of therapy for nephrogenic diabetes insipidus.

Administration and Dosage

➤*Edema:* Intermittent therapy may be advantageous. With administration every other day, or on a 3- to 5-day per week schedule, electrolyte imbalance is less likely.

➤*Hypertension:* Reduce dosage of other agents as soon as thiazides are added to the regimen to prevent excessive hypotension. As blood pressure falls, a further reduction in dosage may be necessary.

➤*Renal function impairment:* If the patient has a creatinine clearance (Ccr) less than 40 to 50 mL/min, a glomerular filtration rate (GFR) less than 25 mL/min or is not responsive to thiazides, a loop diuretic may be more effective. **Metolazone** is the only thiazide-like diuretic that may produce diuresis in patients with GFR less than 20 mL/min. Indapamide may also be effective in patients with renal function impairment.

➤*Coadministration:* Concurrent metolazone and furosemide (and probably other loop diuretics) have been used in the management of patients refractory to furosemide or other diuretics administered alone because of their synergistic effect on diuresis (see Drug Interactions). Metolazone 2.5 to 10 mg is added to the therapy, and the dose is doubled every 24 hours until the desired response is achieved. Decrease the furosemide dose if synergism occurs with the first dose of metolazone. Hydrochlorothiazide 50 mg may be used and may be safer because of its shorter action. This effect also has been noted with other thiazides in combination with other loop diuretics.

Actions

➤*Pharmacology:* Thiazide diuretics increase the urinary excretion of sodium and chloride in approximately equivalent amounts. They inhibit reabsorption of sodium and chloride in the cortical thick ascending limb of the loop of Henle and the early distal tubules. Many of these compounds possess some degree of carbonic anhydrase inhibition activity (metolazone has no activity) because of the sulfonamide moiety; however, this is unlikely to be encountered clinically. Other common actions include increased potassium and bicarbonate excretion, decreased calcium excretion, and uric acid retention. At maximal therapeutic dosages all thiazides are approximately equal in diuretic efficacy, but metolazone may be more effective in patients with impaired renal function. Metolazone (a quinazoline derivative), chlorthalidone (a phthalimidine derivative), and indapamide (an indoline) are included here because of their structural and pharmacological similarities to the thiazides.

The exact antihypertensive mechanism of the thiazides is unknown, although sodium depletion appears to be of primary importance. During initial therapy, cardiac output decreases and extracellular volume diminishes. With chronic therapy, cardiac output normalizes, peripheral vascular resistance falls, and there is a persistent small reduction in extracellular volume.

In hypertensive patients, daily doses of indapamide have no appreciable cardiac inotropic or chronotropic effect, and little or no effect on GFR or renal plasma flow. The drug decreases peripheral resistance, with little or no effect on cardiac output, rate or rhythm. Indapamide had an antihypertensive effect in patients with varying degrees of renal impairment, although in general, diuretic effects declined as renal function decreased.

➤*Pharmacokinetics:* The antihypertensive action requires several days to produce effects. Administration for up to 2 to 4 weeks is usually required for optimal therapeutic effect. The duration of the antihypertensive effect of the thiazides is sufficiently long to adequately control blood pressure with a single daily dose. Despite extensive use of diuretics, pharmacokinetic data are limited. It is important to emphasize the lack of relationship between plasma levels and diuretic effect.

Pharmacokinetics of Thiazides and Related Diuretics

Diuretic	Onset (h)	Peak (h)	Duration (h)	Equivalent dose (mg)	Percent absorbed	Half-life (h)
Bendroflumethiazide	2	4	16 to 12	5	≈ 100	3 to 3.9
Chlorothiazide	2[a]	4[a]	16 to 12	500	10 to 21[b]	0.75 to 2
Chlorthalidone	2 to 3	2 to 6	24 to 72	50	64[b]	40
Hydrochlorothiazide	2	4 to 6	16 to 12	50	65 to 75	5.6 to 14.8
Indapamide	1 to 2	within 2	up to 36	2.5	93	≈ 14
Methyclothiazide	2	6	24	5	nd[c]	nd[c]
Metolazone[d]	1	2	12 to 24	5	65	nd[c]
Trichlormethiazide	2	6	24	2	nd[c]	2.3 to 7.3

[a] Following IV use, onset of action is 15 minutes; peak occurs in 30 minutes.
[b] Bioavailability may be dose-dependent.
[c] nd = No data.
[d] *Mykrox*: Peak plasma concentrations reached in 2 to 4 h, t½ approximately 14 h.

Contraindications

Anuria; renal decompensation; hypersensitivity to thiazides or related diuretics or sulfonamide-derived drugs; hepatic coma or precoma (**metolazone**).

Warnings/Precautions

➤*Parenteral use:* Use IV **chlorothiazide** only when patients are unable to take oral medication or in an emergency. In infants and children, IV use is not recommended.

Avoid simultaneous administration of chlorothiazide with whole blood or its derivatives.

➤*Lupus erythematosus:* Lupus erythematosus exacerbation or activation has occurred.

➤*Fluid/electrolyte balance:* Serum and urine electrolyte determinations are particularly important in patients vomiting excessively or receiving parenteral fluids, in patients subject to electrolyte imbalance (including those with heart failure, kidney disease and cirrhosis), and in patients on a salt restricted diet. Warning signs of imbalance include the following: dry mouth, thirst, weakness, lethargy, drowsiness, restlessness, muscle pains or cramps, confusion, seizures, muscular fatigue, hypotension, oliguria, tachycardia, and GI disturbances.

Hypokalemia – Hypokalemia may develop (with consequent weakness, cramps, cardiac dysrhythmias) during concomitant corticosteroids, ACTH and especially with brisk diuresis, with severe liver disease or cirrhosis, vomiting or diarrhea, or after prolonged therapy. Inadequate oral electrolyte intake also contributes to hypokalemia. Hypokalemia may cause cardiac arrhythmias and sensitize or exaggerate the heart's response to toxic effects of digitalis (eg, increased ventricular irritability). Avoid or treat hypokalemia by using potassium-sparing diuretics, potassium supplements, or foods with high potassium content. Hypokalemia is a particular hazard in digitalized patients, or patients who have or have had a ventricular arrhythmia; dangerous or fatal arrhythmias may be precipitated. Hypokalemia is dose-related.

Hyponatremia/Hypochloremia – A chloride deficit is generally mild and usually does not require specific treatment, except in extraordinary circumstances (as in liver or renal disease). However, treatment of metabolic or hypochloremic alkalosis may require chloride replacement. Dilutional hyponatremia may occur in edematous patients in hot weather; appropriate therapy is water restriction, rather than salt administration, except in rare life-threatening instances. Thiazide-induced hyponatremia has been associated with death and neurologic damage in elderly patients. CNS manifestations include seizures, coma, and extensor-plantar response. Infrequently, severe hyponatremia accompanied by hypokalemia has occurred with recommended **indapamide** doses, primarily in elderly women.

Rarely, the rapid onset of severe hyponatremia or hypokalemia has occurred following initial doses of thiazide and non-thiazide diuretics. When symptoms consistent with electrolyte imbalance appear rapidly, discontinue the drug and initiate supportive measures immediately. Parenteral electrolytes may be required.

Hypomagnesemia – Thiazide diuretics have been shown to increase urinary excretion of magnesium, resulting in hypomagnesemia.

Hypercalcemia – Calcium excretion may be decreased by thiazide diuretics. Thiazides may cause a slight intermittent elevation of serum calcium in the absence of calcium metabolism disorders. Serum calcium levels return to normal upon discontinuation. Pathologic changes in the parathyroid glands with hypercalcemia and hypophosphatemia may occur in a few patients on prolonged thiazide therapy. Marked hypercalcemia may be evidence of hidden hyperparathyroidism. Common complications of hyperparathyroidism, such as renal lithiasis, bone resorption, and peptic ulceration, are not seen. Discontinue thiazides before performing parathyroid function tests.

➤*Glucose tolerance:* Hyperglycemia may occur with thiazide diuretics. Insulin or oral hypoglycemic agent dosage requirements in diabetic patients may be altered. Latent diabetes mellitus may become manifest during thiazide diuretic administration; diabetic complications may occur. Monitor serum glucose concentrations (see Drug Interactions). Administration time (ie, morning vs evening) may influence glucose tolerance; in a small study, blood glucose levels were higher when trichlormethiazide was taken in the evening.

➤*Hyperuricemia:* Hyperuricemia may occur or acute gout may be precipitated in certain patients receiving thiazides, even in those patients without a history of gouty attacks. Hyperuricemia with infrequent gouty attacks may occur in patients with a history of gout. Monitor serum uric acid concentrations periodically during treatment. One report suggests that it is not necessary to lower uric acid levels with pharmacologic measures in patients receiving thiazide diuretics who are without renal damage or history of gout. Serum uric acid increased by an average of 1 mg/dL in patients on **indapamide**.

➤*Post-sympathectomy:* Antihypertensive effects may be enhanced in the postsympathectomy patient.

➤*Lipids:* Use thiazides with caution in patients with moderate or high cholesterol concentrations and in patients with elevated triglyceride levels. Thiazides may cause increased concentrations of total serum cholesterol, total triglycerides, and low-density lipoproteins (LDL) (but not high-density lipoproteins [HDL]) in some patients, although these appear to return to pretreatment levels with long-term therapy. **Indapamide** does not appear to increase serum cholesterol.

➤*Hypersensitivity reactions:* Hypersensitivity reactions may occur in patients with or without a history of allergy or bronchial asthma; cross-sensitivity with sulfonamides may also occur. Have epinephrine 1:1,000 immediately available. Refer to Management of Acute Hypersensitivity Reactions.

➤*Tartrazine sensitivity:* Some of these products contain tartrazine (FD&C Yellow No. 5), which may cause allergic-type reactions (including bronchial asthma) in susceptible individuals. Although the incidence of sensitivity is low, it is frequently seen in patients who also have aspirin hypersensitivity. Specific products containing tartrazine are identified in the product listings.

➤*Renal function impairment:* Use with caution in severe renal disease because these agents may precipitate azotemia. Cumulative effects of the drug may develop in patients with impaired renal function. Monitor renal function periodically. If progressive renal impairment becomes evident, indicated by a rising nonprotein nitrogen (NPN) or BUN, consider withholding or discontinuing therapy. If the patient has a Ccr less than 40 to 50 mL/min, a GFR less than 25 mL/min or is not responsive to thiazides, a loop diuretic may be more effective. **Metolazone** is the only thiazide-like diuretic that may produce diuresis in patients with GFR less than 20 mL/min. Indapamide may also be useful in patients with impaired renal function.

➤*Hepatic function impairment:* Use with caution because minor alterations of fluid and electrolyte balance may precipitate hepatic coma.

➤*Photosensitivity:* Photosensitization may occur; therefore, caution patients to take protective measures (eg, sunscreens, protective clothing) against exposure to ultraviolet light and/or sunlight until tolerance is determined.

➤*Pregnancy: Category B* (**chlorothiazide**, **chlorthalidone**, **hydrochlorothiazide**, **indapamide**, **metolazone**); *Category C* (**bendroflumethiazide**, **methyclothiazide**, **trichlormethiazide**). Routine use during normal pregnancy is inappropriate. Diuretics decrease plasma volume and can decrease placental perfusion. Diuretics do not prevent development of toxemia, nor are they useful in the treatment of toxemia.

Thiazides are indicated in pregnancy when edema is due to pathologic causes, just as they are in the absence of pregnancy. Dependent edema in pregnancy, resulting from restriction of venous return by the gravid uterus, is not properly treated by the use of diuretics. In rare instances, hypervolemia during normal pregnancy results in edema that may cause extreme discomfort that is not relieved by rest; a short course of diuretics may provide relief.

Thiazides cross the placental barrier and appear in cord blood. Use only when clearly needed and when potential benefits outweigh the potential hazards to the fetus. These hazards include fetal or neonatal jaundice, thrombocytopenia, hemolytic anemia, electrolyte imbalances and hypoglycemia.

➤*Lactation:* Thiazides may appear in breast milk. **Chlorthalidone** has a low milk to plasma ratio of 0.05. Discontinue breast-feeding or the drug, taking into account the importance of the drug to the mother.

➤*Children:* **Bendroflumethiazide**, **chlorthalidone**, **hydrochlorothiazide**, **methyclothiazide**, **metolazone**, **trichlormethiazide** – Safety and efficacy have not been established. **Metolazone** is not recommended for use in children. In infants and children, IV use of **chlorothiazide** has been limited and is generally not recommended.

➤*Monitoring:* Perform initial and periodic determinations of serum electrolytes, BUN, uric acid, and glucose. Observe patients for clinical signs of fluid or electrolyte imbalance (eg, hyponatremia, hypochloremic alkalosis, hypokalemia, hypomagnesemia, changes in serum and urinary calcium).

Drug Interactions

Thiazides and Related Diuretic Drug Interactions

Precipitant drug	Object drug[a]		Description
Thiazides	Allopurinol	↑	Concurrent use may increase the incidence of hypersensitivity reactions to allopurinol.
Thiazides	Anesthetics	↑	Effects of these drugs may be potentiated by thiazide administration; dosage adjustments may be required. Monitor and correct fluid and electrolyte imbalance prior to surgery if feasible.
Thiazides	Anticoagulants	↓	Anticoagulant effects may be diminished.
Thiazides	Antigout agents	↓	Because thiazide diuretics may raise blood uric acid levels, dosage adjustment of antigout agents may be necessary.
Thiazides	Antineoplastics	↑	Thiazides may prolong antineoplastic-induced leukopenia.
Thiazides	Calcium salts	↑	Hypercalcemia resulting from renal tubular reabsorption or bone release of calcium may be amplified by exogenous calcium.
Thiazides	Diazoxide	↑	Hyperglycemia, often with symptoms and similar to frank diabetes, may occur.
Thiazides	Digitalis glycosides	↑	Diuretic-induced hypokalemia and hypomagnesemia may precipitate digitalis-induced arrhythmias.
Thiazides	Lithium	↑	Thiazides may induce lithium toxicity by decreasing its renal excretion. However, they have been used together for therapeutic reasons and can be coadministered safely with close lithium level monitoring.
Thiazides	Loop diuretics	↑	Both groups have synergistic effects that may result in profound diuresis and serious electrolyte abnormalities. Certain combinations have been used therapeutically in patients refractory to furosemide (see Administration and Dosage).
Thiazides	Methyldopa	↑	There have been rare occurrences of hemolytic anemia with concomitant use.
Thiazides	Nondepolarizing muscle relaxants	↑	Neuromuscular-blocking effects may be increased; respiratory depression may be prolonged.
Thiazides	Sulfonylureas insulin	↓	Thiazides increase fasting blood glucose and may decrease sulfonylurea hypoglycemia. Hyponatremia also may occur. The dosage may need to be adjusted.
Thiazides	Vitamin D	↑	The biological actions of vitamin D may be enhanced. Hypercalcemia could manifest.
Amphotericin B, Corticosteroids	Thiazides	↑	Electrolyte depletion may be intensified, particularly hypokalemia. Monitor potassium levels.
Anticholinergics	Thiazides	↑	Anticholinergics may substantially increase thiazide diuretic absorption.
Bile acid sequestrants (cholestyramine, colestipol)	Thiazides	↓	Bile acid sequestrants bind thiazides and reduce their absorption from the GI tract up to 85%. Thiazides should be given ≥ 2 hours before the resin.
Methenamines	Thiazides	↓	Possible decreased effectiveness of thiazides because of the alkalinization of urine.
NSAIDs	Thiazides	↓	Some NSAIDs (particularly indomethacin) may reduce the diuretic, natriuretic, and antihypertensive effects of thiazide diuretics. Observe closely to determine if the desired diuretic effects are obtained. Sulindac may enhance the diuretic effect.

[a] ↑ = Object drug increased. ↓ = Object drug decreased

➤*Drug/Lab test interactions:* Thiazides may decrease serum protein-bound iodine (PBI) levels without signs of thyroid disturbance. Thiazides also may cause diagnostic interference of serum electrolyte levels, blood and urine glucose levels (usually only in patients with a predisposition to glucose intolerance), serum bilirubin levels (by displacement from albumin binding), and serum uric acid levels. In uremic patients, serum magnesium levels may be increased. **Bendroflumethiazide** and **trichlormethiazide** may interfere with the **phenolsulfonphthalein test** because of decreased excretion. In the **phentolamine** and **tyramine tests**, bendroflumethiazide may produce false-negative and trichlormethiazide may produce false-positive results.

Adverse Reactions

Adverse Reactions of Thiazides and Related Diuretics

Adverse reaction	Bendroflumethiazide	Chlorothiazide	Chlorthalidone	Hydrochlorothiazide	Indapamide	Methyclothiazide	Metolazone	Trichlormethiazide
Cardiovascular								
Hypotension		✓						
Orthostatic hypotension	✓	✓		✓	< 5%	✓	< 2%[a]	✓
Palpitations					< 5%		< 2%[b]	✓
CNS								
Anxiety					≥ 5%		< 2%[c]	
Blurred vision (may be transient)	✓	✓		✓	< 5%	✓	✓[c]	
Depression					< 5%		< 2%[b]	✓
Dizziness/Lightheadedness	✓	✓	✓	✓	≥ 5%	✓	10%[b]	✓
Drowsiness					< 5%		✓[c]	✓
Fatigue/Lethargy/Malaise/Lassitude					≥ 5%		4%[b]	✓
Headache	✓	✓	✓	✓	≥ 5%	✓	9%[b]	✓
Nervousness					≥ 5%		< 2%[c]	✓
Paresthesias	✓	✓	✓	✓		✓	✓[c]	✓
Restlessness/Insomnia	✓	✓	✓	✓	< 5%	✓	✓[c]	✓
Vertigo	✓	✓	✓	✓	< 5%	✓	✓[c]	✓
Weakness	✓	✓	✓	✓	≥ 5%	✓	< 2%[b]	✓
Xanthopsia	✓	✓	✓	✓		✓		✓
Dermatologic								
Alopecia		✓[e]		✓				
Anaphylactic reactions	✓	✓		✓[d]		✓		
Erythema multiforme, Stevens-Johnson syndrome		✓[e]		✓		✓		
Exfoliative dermatitis/ toxic epidermal necrolysis	✓	✓[e]	✓	✓				
Fever	✓	✓		✓		✓		
Necrotizing angiitis, vasculitis, cutaneous vasculitis	✓	✓	✓	✓	< 5%	✓	✓[b]	✓
Photosensitivity/Photosensitivity dermatitis	✓	✓	✓	✓		✓	✓[c]	✓
Pruritus	✓				< 5%		< 2%[a]	
Purpura	✓	✓	✓	✓		✓	✓[c]	✓
Rash	✓	✓	✓	✓	< 5%	✓	< 2%[b]	✓
Urticaria	✓	✓	✓	✓		✓	✓[c]	✓
GI								
Abdominal pain/cramping/bloating	✓	✓	✓	✓	< 5%	✓	< 2%[b]	✓
Anorexia	✓	✓	✓	✓	< 5%	✓	✓[c]	✓
Constipation	✓	✓	✓	✓	< 5%	✓	< 2%[b]	✓
Diarrhea	✓	✓	✓	✓	< 5%	✓	< 2%[b]	✓
Dry mouth					< 5%		< 2%[a]	✓
Gastric irritation/epigastric distress	✓	✓	✓	✓	< 5%	✓		✓
Hepatitis	✓						✓[c]	
Jaundice (intrahepatic/cholestatic)	✓	✓	✓	✓		✓	✓[c]	✓
Nausea	✓	✓	✓	✓	< 5%	✓	< 2%[b]	✓
Pancreatitis	✓	✓	✓	✓		✓	✓[c]	✓
Sialadenitis	✓	✓		✓		✓		
Vomiting	✓	✓	✓	✓	< 5%	✓	< 2%[b]	✓
GU								
Impotence/Reduced libido	✓	✓	✓	✓	< 5%	✓	< 2%[b]	✓
Interstitial nephritis		✓		✓				
Nocturia					< 5%		< 2%[a]	
Renal failure/dysfunction		✓		✓				
Hematologic								
Agranulocytosis	✓	✓	✓	✓		✓	✓[c]	✓
Aplastic/Hypoplastic anemia	✓	✓	✓	✓		✓	✓[c]	✓
Hemolytic anemia	✓	✓		✓		✓		
Leukopenia	✓	✓	✓	✓		✓	✓[c]	✓
Thrombocytopenia	✓	✓	✓	✓		✓		✓
Metabolic								
Electrolyte imbalance		✓		✓		✓		
Glycosuria	✓	✓	✓	✓	< 5%	✓	✓[c]	✓
Hyperglycemia	✓	✓	✓	✓	< 5%	✓	✓[c]	✓
Hyperuricemia	✓	✓	✓	✓	< 5%	✓		✓
Miscellaneous								
Muscle cramp/spasm	✓	✓	✓	✓	≥ 5%	✓	6%[b]	✓
Respiratory distress (including pneumonitis/ pulmonary edema)	✓	✓		✓		✓		

[a] Rapidly acting doseform only.

[b] Percentage of occurrence refers to rapidly acting doseform; however, this adverse reaction also occurred with the slow-acting doseform.

[c] Slow-acting doseform only.

[d] Possibly with life-threatening anaphylactic shock.

[e] IV doseform.

Whenever adverse reactions are moderate or severe, reducing the thiazide dosage or withdrawing therapy will generally reverse the effect.

➤*Cardiovascular:*

Hydrochlorothiazide – Allergic myocarditis.

Indapamide – Premature ventricular contractions, irregular heartbeat (less than 5%).

Metolazone –

Rapidly acting: Chest pain, precordial pain (3%); cold extremities, edema (less than 2%).

Slow-acting: Venous thrombosis, chest pain, excessive volume depletion, hemoconcentration.

➤*CNS:*

Indapamide – Loss of energy, numbness of extremities, tension, irritability, agitation (greater than 5%); tingling of extremities (less than 5%).

Metolazone –

Slow-acting: Syncope, neuropathy.

Rapidly acting: Weird feeling, neuropathy (less than 2%).

➤*GI:* Cholecystitis (possible increased risk in patients with gallstones).

Metolazone –

Rapidly acting: Bitter taste (less than 2%).

➤*GU:*

Bendroflumethiazide – Allergic glomerulonephritis.

Chlorothiazide IV – Hematuria.

Indapamide – Frequent urination, polyuria (less than 5%).

➤*Dermatologic:*

Bendroflumethiazide – Ecchymosis.

Indapamide – Hives (less than 5%).

Metolazone –
Rapidly acting: Dry skin (less than 2%).

Trichlormethiazide – Lichenoid dermatitis.

➤*Musculoskeletal:*

Metolazone – Joint pain; back pain (rapidly acting; less than 2%); swelling (slow-acting).

➤*Respiratory:*

Indapamide – Rhinorrhea (less than 5%).

Metolazone –
Rapidly acting: Cough, epistaxis, sinus congestion, sore throat (less than 2%).

Trichlormethiazide – Dyspnea.

➤*Miscellaneous:* Neutropenia.

Bendroflumethiazide – Metabolic acidosis in diabetics.

Indapamide – Flushing, weight loss (less than 5%).

Methyclothiazide – Inappropriate antidiuretic hormone (ADH) secretion.

Metolazone –
Slow-acting: Chills, acute gouty attack.
Rapidly acting: Eye itching, tinnitus (less than 2%).

➤*Lab test abnormalities:* Hypercalcemia, hypokalemia, hyponatremia; hypomagnesemia, hypochloremia, hypochloremic alkalosis, hypophosphatemia, increase in BUN, elevation of creatinine, decreased serum PBI levels.

Clinical hypokalemia – Clinical hypokalemia occurred in 3% and 7% of patients given **indapamide** 2.5 and 5 mg, respectively.

Increases in plasma levels of total cholesterol, triglycerides, and LDL cholesterol have been associated with thiazide diuretics (see Warnings/Precautions).

Fluid/electrolyte imbalance – There are isolated reports of nonedematous individuals developing severe fluid and electrolyte derangements after only brief exposure to normal doses of thiazides. This condition usually is manifested as severe dilutional hyponatremia, hypokalemia and hypochloremia. It may be because of inappropriately increased ADH secretion and appears to be idiosyncratic. Potassium replacement is apparently the most important therapy along with removal of the offending drug.

Overdosage

➤*Symptoms:* Changes caused by plasma volume depletion (eg, orthostatic hypotension, dizziness, drowsiness, syncope, electrolyte abnormalities, hemoconcentration, hemodynamic changes); signs of potassium deficiency (eg, confusion, dizziness, muscular weakness, GI disturbances); nausea; vomiting. In severe instances, hypotension and depressed respiration may occur. Lethargy of varying degrees may progress to coma within a few hours, with minimal depression of respiration and cardiovascular function and without significant serum electrolyte changes or dehydration. GI irritation and hypermotility, temporary BUN elevation, CNS effects, cardiac abnormalities, and seizures also have been reported, especially in patients with compromised renal function.

➤*Treatment:* Perform gastric lavage or induce emesis; give activated charcoal. Prevent aspiration. Avoid cathartics because electrolyte and fluid loss may be enhanced. GI effects are usually of short duration, but may require symptomatic treatment. Monitor serum electrolyte levels and renal function. Maintain hydration, electrolyte balance, respiration and cardiovascular-renal function. Asymptomatic hyperuricemia usually responds to fluids, but if clinical gout is suspected, indomethacin may be started. Support respiration and cardiac circulation if hypotension and depressed respiration occur. Refer to General Management of Acute Overdosage. Dialysis is unlikely to be effective.

Patient Information

May cause GI upset; may be taken with food or milk.

Drug will initially increase urination, which should subside after a few weeks; advise patients to take early during the day or as directed.

Advise patients to notify health care provider if muscle pain, weakness or cramps, nausea, vomiting, restlessness, excessive thirst, tiredness, drowsiness, increased heart rate or pulse, diarrhea, or dizziness occurs.

May cause photosensitivity (sensitivity to sunlight). Advise patients to avoid prolonged exposure to the sun and other ultraviolet light. Instruct them to use sunscreens and wear protective clothing until tolerance is determined.

May increase blood sugar levels in patients with diabetes.

Patients should not drink alcohol or take other medications without health care provider's approval; this includes nonprescription medicines for appetite control, asthma, colds, cough, hay fever, or sinus.

Advise patients to not interrupt, discontinue, or adjust the dose even if feeling well and to follow health care provider's instructions regarding missed doses.

May cause gout attacks. Instruct patients to contact health care provider if significant sudden joint pain occurs.

CHLOROTHIAZIDE

Rx	**Chlorothiazide** (Various, eg, Mylan, UDL, West-Ward)	**Tablets; oral:** 250 mg	In 100s.
Rx	**Chlorothiazide** (Various, eg, Mylan, UDL, West-Ward)	**Tablets; oral:** 500 mg	In 100s.
Rx	**Diuril** (Salix)	**Suspension; oral:** 250 mg per 5 mL	Alcohol 0.5%, parabens, saccharin, sucrose. In 237 mL.
Rx	**Diuril** (Ovation)	**Injection, lyophilized, powder for solution:** 500 mg	As chlorothiazide sodium. Preservative free. In single-use vials.

CHLOROTHIAZIDE — ORAL

For complete and comparative prescribing information, refer to the Thiazides and Related Diuretics group monograph.

Indications

➤*Edema:* As adjunctive therapy in edema associated with congestive heart failure, corticosteroid and estrogen therapy, and hepatic cirrhosis. Chlorothiazide has also been found useful in edema due to various forms of renal function impairment, such as acute glomerulonephritis, chronic renal failure, and nephrotic syndrome.

➤*Hypertension:* For the management of hypertension, as the sole therapeutic agent or to enhance the effectiveness of other antihypertensive drugs in the more severe forms of hypertension.

➤*Off-label uses:* Calcium nephrolithiasis; osteoporosis; diabetes insipidus.

Administration and Dosage

➤*Adults:*

Edema –
Usual dosage: 0.5 to 1 g (10 to 20 mL) once or twice a day.
Alternative dosage: Many patients respond to intermittent therapy (ie, administration on alternate days or 3 to 5 days each week). With an intermittent schedule, excessive response and the resulting undesirable electrolyte imbalance are less likely to occur.

Hypertension –
Initial dosage: 0.5 or 1 g (10 to 20 mL) a day as a single or divided dose.
Dosage adjustment: The dosage is increased or decreased according to blood pressure response. Rarely, some patients may require up to 2 g (40 mL) a day in divided doses.

➤*Children:*

Edema –
6 months of age and older:
- *Usual dosage* – 10 to 20 mg/kg/day in single or 2 divided doses.
- *Maximum dose* –
  2 to 12 years of age: 1 g/day.
  2 years of age and younger: 375 mg/day (2.5 to 7.5 mL per day).

Younger than 6 months of age:
- *Usual dosage* – Doses of up to 30 mg/kg/day in 2 divided doses may be required.
- *Maximum dose* – 375 mg/day (2.5 to 7.5 mL per day).

Hypertension – See Edema dosing in children.

➤*Elderly:* Dose selection for elderly patients should be made with caution, usually starting at the low end of the dosing range, reflecting the greater frequency of decreased hepatic, renal, or cardiac function, and of concomitant disease or other drug therapy.

➤*Administration:* May be taken with food or milk.

➤*Storage/Stability:* Store tablets at 20° to 25°C (68° to 77°F). Store oral suspension at 15° to 30°C (59° to 86°F). Protect from freezing (−20°C [−4°F]).

CHLOROTHIAZIDE SODIUM — INJECTION

For complete and comparative prescribing information, refer to the Thiazides and Related Diuretics group monograph.

Indications

➤*Edema:* As adjunctive therapy in edema associated with congestive heart failure, corticosteroid and estrogen therapy, and hepatic cirrhosis. Chlorothiazide has also been found useful in edema caused by various forms of renal function impairment, such as acute glomerulonephritis, chronic renal failure, and nephrotic syndrome.

➤*Off-label uses:* Calcium nephrolithiasis; osteoporosis; diabetes insipidus.

Administration and Dosage

➤*Adults:*

Edema –

Usual dosage: 0.5 to 1 g once or twice a day.

Alternative dosage: Many patients with edema respond to intermittent therapy (ie, administration on alternate days or on 3 to 5 days each week). With an intermittent schedule, excessive response and the resulting undesirable electrolyte imbalance are less likely to occur.

Conversion: When medication can be taken orally, therapy with chlorothiazide tablets or oral suspension may be substituted for IV therapy, using the same dosage schedule as for the parenteral route.

➤*Elderly:* Dose selection for elderly patients should be made with caution, usually starting at the low end of the dosing range, reflecting the greater frequency of decreased hepatic, renal, or cardiac function, and of concomitant disease or other drug therapy.

➤*Renal function impairment:* Use with caution in severe renal disease.

➤*Preparation for administration:* Because IV chlorothiazide contains no preservative, a fresh solution should be prepared immediately prior to each administration. Add 18 mL of sterile water for injection to the vial to form an isotonic solution for IV injection; never add less than 18 mL. When reconstituted with 18 mL of sterile water for injection, the final concentration is 28 mg/mL.

➤*Administration:* May be given slowly by direct IV injection or IV infusion. Extravasation must be rigidly avoided. Do not give subcutaneously or intramuscularly.

➤*Admixture compatibility:* The solution is compatible with dextrose or sodium chloride solutions for IV infusion. Avoid simultaneous administration with whole blood or its derivatives.

➤*Storage/Stability:* Store between 2° and 25°C (36° and 77°F). The unused portion should be discarded.

CHLORTHALIDONE

Rx	**Thalitone** (Monarch)	**Tablets; oral:** 15 mg	Lactose. (M 024). White. Kidney shaped. In 100s.
Rx	**Chlorthalidone** (Various, eg, Geneva, Goldline)	**Tablets; oral:** 25 mg	In 100s, 1000s.
Rx	**Chlorthalidone** (Various, eg, Geneva, Goldline, Major, Schein)	**Tablets; oral:** 50 mg	In 100s, 250s, and 1000s.
Rx	**Chlorthalidone** (Various, eg, Goldline, Schein)	**Tablets; oral:** 100 mg	In 100s, 500s and 1000s.

CHLORTHALIDONE — ORAL

For complete and comparative prescribing information, refer to the Thiazides and Related Diuretics group monograph.

Indications

➤*Hypertension:* Management of hypertension either alone or in combination with other antihypertensive drugs.

➤*Edema:* Adjunctive therapy in edema associated with congestive heart failure, hepatic cirrhosis, and corticosteroid and estrogen therapy.

Chlorthalidone has also been found useful in edema due to various forms of renal dysfunction such as nephrotic syndrome, acute glomerulonephritis, and chronic renal failure.

➤*Off-label uses:*

Pediatric hypertension – [1] = Good documentation. Chlorthalidone is among the therapeutic options for pediatric hypertension identified by the National High Blood Pressure Education Program, based on expert opinion.

Administration and Dosage

➤*Adults:*

Edema –

Initial dosage: 50 to 100 mg daily or 100 mg on alternate days. Some patients may require 150 to 200 mg at these intervals or up to 200 mg daily.

Maintenance dosage: Maintenance doses may often be lower than initial doses and should be adjusted according to the individual patient. Effectiveness is well sustained during continued use.

Hypertension –

Initial dosage: 25 mg as single daily dose.

Dosage titration: If the response is insufficient after a suitable trial, the dosage may be increased to 50 mg. If additional control is required, increase to 100 mg once daily or a second antihypertensive drug may be added.

Maintenance dosage: Maintenance doses may often be lower than initial doses and should be adjusted according to the individual patient. Effectiveness is well sustained during continued use.

➤*Children:*

Off-label dosing –

Pediatric hypertension: [1] = Good documentation.

- *1 to 17 years of age –*
  Maximum dose: 2 mg/kg/day, up to 50 mg/day.
  Initial dosage: 0.3 mg/kg/day once daily.

➤*Administration:* A single dose given in the morning with food is recommended; divided doses are unnecessary.

➤*Storage/Stability:* Store at 20° to 25°C (68° to 77°F). Protect from light.

HYDROCHLOROTHIAZIDE

Rx	**Hydrochlorothiazide** (Various, eg, Actavis Elizabeth)	**Tablets; oral:** 12.5 mg	In 100s and 1,000s.
Rx	**Hydrochlorothiazide** (Various, eg, Major, Schein, Zenith)	**Tablets; oral:** 25 mg	In 30s, 100s, 500s, 1,000s, 5,000s, UD 32s and UD 100s.
Rx	**HydroDIURIL** (Merck)		Lactose. (MSD 42). Peach, scored. In 100s and 1,000s.
Rx	**Hydro-Par** (Parmed)		Peach, scored. In 1,000s.
Rx	**Hydrochlorothiazide** (Various, eg, Danbury, Schein, Zenith)	**Tablets; oral:** 50 mg	In 30s, 100s, 500s, 1,000s, 5,000s, and UD 100s.
Rx	**Ezide** (Econo Med)		In 100s and 1,000s.
Rx	**Hydro-Par** (Parmed)		In 1,000s and 5,000s.
Rx	**Hydrochlorothiazide** (Various, eg, Schein)	**Tablets; oral:** 100 mg	In 30s, 100s, 250s, 500s, 1,000s, and UD 100s.
Rx	**Hydrochlorothiazide** (Various, eg, Mylan, Watson)	**Capsules; oral:** 12.5 mg	In 100s and 500s.
Rx	**Microzide Capsules** (Watson)		Lactose. (Microzide 12.5). Light teal/teal. In 100s.

HYDROCHLOROTHIAZIDE — ORAL

For complete and comparative prescribing information, refer to the Thiazides and Related Diuretics class monograph.

Indications

➤*Edema:* Adjunctive therapy in edema associated with congestive heart failure, hepatic cirrhosis, and corticosteroid and estrogen therapy.

Hydrochlorothiazide has also been found useful in edema due to various forms of renal dysfunction, such as nephrotic syndrome, acute glomerulonephritis, and chronic renal failure.

➤*Hypertension:* Management of hypertension, either as the sole therapeutic agent or in combination with other antihypertensives. Unlike potassium-sparing combination diuretic products, hydrochlorothiazide may be used in those patients in whom the development of hyperkalemia cannot be risked, including patients taking angiotensin-converting enzyme (ACE) inhibitors.

Hydrochlorothiazide is indicated in the management of hypertension, either as the sole therapeutic agent or to enhance the effectiveness of other antihypertensive drugs in the more severe forms of hypertension.

Administration and Dosage

➤*Adults:*

Capsules –

Hypertension:

- *Usual dosage* – 12.5 mg daily given alone or in combination with other antihypertensives.
- *Maximum dose* – 50 mg daily.

HYDROCHLOROTHIAZIDE — ORAL

Tablets –
Edema:
• *Usual dosage* – 25 to 100 mg daily as a single or divided dose.
• *Alternative dosage* – Many patients respond to intermittent therapy (ie, administration on alternate days or on 3 to 5 days each week). With an intermittent schedule, excessive response and the resulting undesirable electrolyte imbalance are less likely to occur.
Hypertension:
• *Initial dosage* – 25 mg daily as a single dose.
• *Dosage adjustment* – The dosage may be increased to 50 mg daily, as a single or 2 divided doses. Doses above 50 mg are often associated with marked reductions in serum potassium. Patients usually do not require doses in excess of 50 mg daily when used concomitantly with other antihypertensive agents.

➤*Children:*
Tablets –
Diuresis:
• *6 months to 12 years of age –*
Usual dosage: 1 to 2 mg/kg per day in single or 2 divided doses.
Maximum dose: 100 mg/day for children 2 to 12 years of age; 37.5 mg/day for children 6 months to 2 years of age.
• *Younger than 6 months of age* – Doses up to 3 mg/kg per day in 2 divided doses may be required.
Hypertension: See Diuresis for dosing.

➤*Elderly:* A greater blood pressure reduction and an increase in adverse effects may be observed. Therefore, starting treatment with the lowest available dose (12.5 mg) is recommended. If further titration is required, 12.5 mg increments should be utilized.

➤*Storage / Stability:* Store at room temperature between 15° and 30°C (59° and 86°F). Keep container tightly closed. Protect from light, moisture, and freezing (−20°C [−4°F]).

METHYCLOTHIAZIDE

Rx	**Methyclothiazide** (Various, eg, Zenith)	**Tablets:** 2.5 mg	In 100s and 1000s.
Rx	**Methyclothiazide** (Various, eg, Geneva, Parmed, Zenith)	**Tablets:** 5 mg	In 1000s.
Rx	**Enduron** (Abbott)		(Enduron). Salmon. Square. In 100s, 1000s, 5000s and *Abbo-Pac* 100s.

METHYCLOTHIAZIDE — ORAL

For complete and comparative prescribing information, see Thiazides and Related Diuretics group monograph.

Indications

➤*Hypertension:* Management of hypertension, either as the sole therapeutic agent or to enhance the effect of other antihypertensive drugs in the more severe forms of hypertension.

➤*Edema:* Adjunctive therapy in edema associated with congestive heart failure, hepatic cirrhosis, and corticosteroid and estrogen therapy.

Methyclothiazide tablets have also been found useful in edema due to various forms of renal dysfunction such as the nephrotic syndrome, acute glomerulonephritis, and chronic renal failure.

Administration and Dosage

➤*Adults:*
Edema –
Usual dosage: 2.5 to 10 mg/day.
Maximum dose: 10 mg/day.

Hypertension –
Usual dosage: 2.5 to 5 mg/day. If control of blood pressure is not satisfactory after 8 to 12 weeks of therapy with 5 mg once daily, another antihypertensive drug should be added. Increasing the dosage of methyclothiazide will usually not result in further lowering of blood pressure.
Concomitant therapy:
When other antihypertensive agents are to be added to the regimen, this should be accomplished gradually. An enhanced response frequently follows its coadministration with deserpidine so that dosage of both drugs may be reduced. Ganglionic-blocking agents should be given at only half the usual dose because their effect is potentiated by pretreatment with methyclothiazide tablets.

➤*Renal function impairment:* Contraindicated in anuria. If progressive renal impairment becomes evident as indicated by a rising nonprotein nitrogen or blood urea nitrogen, a careful reappraisal of therapy is necessary with consideration given to withholding or discontinuing diuretic therapy.

➤*Administration:* Administer orally.

➤*Storage / Stability:* Store below 30°C (86°F).

INDAPAMIDE

Rx	**Indapamide** (Various, eg, Major, Mylan, Purepac, Teva, Watson, Zenith)	**Tablets; oral:** 1.25 mg	In 100s, 500s, and 1000s.
Rx	**Indapamide** (Mylan)	**Tablets; oral:** 2.5 mg	Lactose. (M 80). Film-coated. In 100s and 1,000s.

INDAPAMIDE — ORAL

For complete and comparative prescribing information, see Thiazides and Related Diuretics group monograph.

Indications

➤*Hypertension:* For the treatment of hypertension, alone or in combination with other antihypertensive drugs.

➤*Edema of congestive heart failure:* For the treatment of salt and fluid retention associated with congestive heart failure.

Administration and Dosage

➤*Adults:*
Edema of congestive heart failure –
Initial dosage: 2.5 mg once daily in the morning.
Dosage titration: If the response is not satisfactory after 1 week, the dose may be increased to 5 mg once daily.

Hypertension –
Initial dosage: 1.25 mg once daily dose in the morning.
Dosage titration: If the response is not satisfactory after 4 weeks, the dose may be increased to 2.5 mg once daily. If the response is not satisfactory after 4 weeks, the dose may be increased to 5 mg once daily, but adding another antihypertensive should be considered.
Concomitant therapy: If the antihypertensive response is insufficient, indapamide may be combined with other antihypertensive drugs, with careful monitoring of blood pressure. It is recommended that the usual dose of other agents be reduced by 50% during initial combination therapy. As the blood pressure response becomes evident, further dosage adjustments may be necessary.

➤*Renal function impairment:* Contraindicated in anuria. If progressive renal impairment is observed, withholding or discontinuing therapy should be considered.

➤*Administration:* May be taken with food or milk if GI upset occurs. Administer as morning dose to prevent nocturia.

➤*Storage / Stability:* Store at 15° to 30°C (59° to 86°F). Avoid excessive heat.

METOLAZONE

Rx	**Metolazone** (Various, eg, Eon, Mylan)	**Tablets; oral:** 2.5 mg	In 100s and 1000s.
Rx	**Zaroxolyn** (UCB Pharma)		(2 1/2 Zaroxolyn). Pink. In 100s, 1000s and UD 100s.
Rx	**Metolazone** (Various, eg, Eon)	**Tablets; oral:** 5 mg	In 100s.
Rx	**Zaroxolyn** (UCB Pharma)		(5 Zaroxolyn). Blue. In 100s, 1000s and UD 100s.
Rx	**Metolazone** (Various, eg, Eon)	**Tablets; oral:** 10 mg	In 100s.

METOLAZONE — ORAL

For complete and comparative prescribing information, refer to the Thiazides and Related Diuretics group monograph.

WARNING

Do not interchange – Do not interchange *Zaroxolyn* tablets and other formulations of metolazone that share its slow and incomplete bioavailability.

Indications

➤*Hypertension:* For the treatment of hypertension, alone or in combination with other antihypertensive drugs of a different class.

➤*Salt and water retention:* For the treatment of salt and water retention, including the following: edema accompanying congestive heart failure; edema accompanying renal diseases, including the nephrotic syndrome and states of diminished renal function.

➤*Off-label uses:* Osteoporosis; diabetes insipidus.

Administration and Dosage

➤*Adults:*

Edema –

Usual dosage: 5 to 20 mg once daily.

Dosage adjustment: When a desired therapeutic effect has been obtained, it may be advisable to reduce the dose if possible. Base a decision to change the daily dose on the results of thorough clinical and laboratory evaluations. For patients who tend to experience paroxysmal nocturnal dyspnea, it may be advisable to employ a larger dose to ensure prolongation of diuresis and saluresis for a full 24-hour period.

Concomitant therapy: If antihypertensive drugs or diuretics are given concurrently with metolazone, more careful dosage adjustment may be necessary.

Hypertension –

Usual dosage: 2.5 to 5 mg once daily.

➤*Renal function impairment:* Contraindicated in anuria. If azotemia and oliguria worsen during treatment of patients with severe renal disease, discontinue metolazone.

➤*Hepatic function impairment:* Contraindicated in hepatic coma or precoma.

➤*Administration:* Administer once daily in the morning.

➤*Storage/Stability:* Store at 20° to 25°C (68° to 77°F). Protect from light.

Loop Diuretics

WARNING

These agents are potent diuretics; excess amounts can lead to a profound diuresis with water and electrolyte depletion. Careful medical supervision is required and dosage must be individualized.

Indications

➤*Edema:* Edema associated with CHF, hepatic cirrhosis and renal disease, including the nephrotic syndrome. Particularly useful when greater diuretic potential is desired.

Parenteral administration is indicated when a rapid onset of diuresis is desired (eg, acute pulmonary edema), when GI absorption is impaired or when oral use is not practical for any reason. As soon as it is practical, replace with oral therapy.

➤*Hypertension (furosemide, oral; torsemide, oral):* Alone or in combination with other antihypertensive drugs. Hypertensive patients who are inadequately controlled with thiazides may not be adequately controlled with furosemide alone.

➤*Ethacrynic acid: Ascites:* Short-term management of ascites due to malignancy, idiopathic edema, and lymphedema.

Congenital heart disease, nephrotic syndrome – Short-term management of hospitalized pediatric patients, other than infants.

Pulmonary edema, acute – Adjunctive therapy.

➤*Off-label uses:* Refer to individual monographs for further information.

Pediatric hypertension –

Furosemide: [3] = Safety concerns.

Other possible off-label uses – Ethacrynic acid is being investigated for the treatment of glaucoma; a single injection into the eye may reduce intraocular pressure for a week or more. Further study is needed.

Bumetanide 1 mg may be beneficial in the treatment of adult nocturia; it is not effective in males with prostatic hypertrophy.

Administration and Dosage

Refer to the individual drug monograph for dosing information.

Actions

➤*Pharmacology:* Furosemide and ethacrynic acid inhibit primarily reabsorption of sodium and chloride, not only in proximal and distal tubules, but also the loop of Henle. High efficacy is largely due to unique site of action. Action on distal tubule is independent of any inhibitory effect on carbonic anhydrase or aldosterone.

In contrast, bumetanide is more chloruretic than natriuretic and may have an additional action in the proximal tubule; it does not appear to act on the distal tubule.

Torsemide acts from within the lumen of the thick ascending portion of the loop of Henle, where it inhibits the $Na^+/K^+/2Cl^-$-carrier system; effects in other segments of the nephron have not been demonstrated. Diuretic activity thus correlates better with the rate of drug excretion in urine than with the blood concentration. Torsemide increases the urinary excretion of sodium, chloride, and water, but does not significantly alter glomerular filtration rate, renal plasma flow or acid-base balance.

Because ethacrynic acid inhibits the reabsorption of filtered sodium to a much greater proportion than most other diuretics, it may be effective in many patients with significant degrees of renal insufficiency.

➤*Pharmacokinetics:* These agents are metabolized and excreted primarily through the urine. Protein binding of these agents exceeds 90%. Furosemide is metabolized approximately 30% to 40%, and its urinary excretion is 60% to 70%. Significantly more furosemide is excreted in urine after IV injection than after the tablet or oral solution. Recent evidence suggests that furosemide glucuronide is the only, or at least the major, biotransformation product of furosemide.

Oral administration of bumetanide revealed that 81% was excreted in urine, 45% of it as unchanged drug. Bumetanide increases potassium excretion in a dose-related fashion; it also decreases uric acid excretion and increases serum uric acid. Urinary and biliary metabolites are formed by oxidation of the N-butyl side chain. Biliary excretion of bumetanide amounted to only 2% of the administered dose.

Torsemide is cleared from the circulation by both hepatic metabolism (approximately 80% of total clearance) and excretion into the urine (approximately 20% of total clearance). The major metabolite in humans is the carboxylic acid derivative, which is biologically inactive. Two of the lesser metabolites possess some diuretic activity, but for practical purposes metabolism terminates the action of the drug. Most renal clearance occurs via active secretion of the drug by the proximal tubules into tubular urine. Simultaneous food intake delays the time to C_{max} by about 30 minutes, but overall bioavailability and diuretic activity are unchanged.

Pharmacokinetic Parameters of the Loop Diuretics

Diuretic	Bioavailability (%)	Half-life (min)	Onset of action (min)	Peak (min)	Duration (hr)	Dosage (mg)	Relative potency	Doses/day
Furosemide								
Oral	60-64[a]	≈ 120[b]	within 60	60-120[d]	6-8	20-80	1	1-2
IV or IM			within 5[c]	30	2	20-40	1	
Ethacrynic acid								
Oral	≈100	60	within 30	120	6-8	50-100	0.6-0.8	1-2
IV			within 5	15-30	2	50	0.6-0.8	1-2
Bumetanide								
Oral	72-96	60-90[e]	30-60	60-120	4-6	0.5-2	≈ 40	1
IV			within minutes	15-30	0.5-1	0.5-1	≈ 40	1-3
Torsemide								
Oral	≈ 80	210	within 60	60-120	6-8	5-20	2-4	1
IV			within 10	within 60	6-8	5-20	2-4	1

[a] Decreased in uremia and nephrosis.
[b] Prolonged in renal failure, uremia and in neonates.
[c] Somewhat delayed after IM administration.
[d] Decreased in CHF.
[e] Prolonged in renal disease.

Contraindications

Anuria; hypersensitivity to these compounds or to sulfonylureas; infants (ethacrynic acid); patients with hepatic coma or in states of severe electrolyte depletion until the condition is improved or corrected (bumetanide); patients who have experienced severe, watery diarrhea with previous use (ethacrynic acid).

Warnings/Precautions

➤*Dehydration:* Excessive diuresis may result in dehydration and reduction in blood volume with circulatory collapse and the possibility of vascular thrombosis and embolism, particularly in elderly patients.

➤*Hepatic cirrhosis and ascites:* In these patients, sudden alterations of electrolyte balance may precipitate hepatic encephalopathy and coma. Do not institute therapy until the basic condition is improved. Initiate therapy in the hospital with small doses and careful monitoring. Supplemental potassium chloride and, if required, an aldosterone antagonist help to prevent hypokalemia and metabolic alkalosis.

➤*Ototoxicity:* Tinnitus, reversible and irreversible hearing impairment, deafness and vertigo with a sense of fullness in the ears have been reported. Deafness is usually reversible and of short duration (1 to 24 hours); however, irreversible hearing impairment has occurred. Usually, ototoxicity is associated with rapid injection, with severe renal impairment, with doses several times the usual dose and with concurrent use with other ototoxic drugs.

➤*Systemic lupus erythematosus:* Systemic lupus erythematosus may be exacerbated or activated.

➤*Diarrhea:* In a few patients, ethacrynic acid has produced severe, watery diarrhea. If this occurs, discontinue the drug and do not readminister.

Because of the amount of sorbitol in the **furosemide** solution vehicle, the possibility of diarrhea, especially in children, exists when higher dosages are given.

➤*Thrombocytopenia:* Since there have been rare spontaneous reports of thrombocytopenia with **bumetanide**, observe regularly for possible occurrence.

➤*Cardiovascular effects:* Too vigorous a diuresis, as evidenced by rapid and excessive weight loss, may induce an acute hypotensive episode. In elderly cardiac patients, avoid rapid contraction of plasma volume and the resultant hemoconcentration to prevent thromboembolic episodes, such as cerebral vascular thromboses and pulmonary emboli.

➤*Electrolyte imbalance:* Electrolyte imbalance may occur, especially in patients receiving high doses with restricted salt intake. Perform periodic determinations of serum electrolytes. Observe patients for signs of fluid or electrolyte imbalance (eg, hyponatremia, hypochloremic alkalosis, hypokalemia, hypomagnesemia, hypocalcemia). Digitalis therapy may exaggerate metabolic effects of hypokalemia with reference to myocardial activity. Serum and urine electrolyte determinations are important in patients who are vomiting excessively, in patients who are receiving parenteral fluids, corticosteroids or ACTH, during brisk diuresis or when cirrhosis is present. Warning signs are dryness of mouth, thirst, anorexia, weakness, lethargy, drowsiness, restlessness, muscle pains or cramps, muscle fatigue, tetany (rarely), hypotension, oliguria, tachycardia, arrhythmia and GI disturbances (eg, nausea/vomiting).

Profound electrolyte and water loss may be avoided by weighing the patient periodically, adjusting dosage, initiating treatment with small doses and using the drugs intermittently. When excessive diuresis occurs, withdraw the drugs until homeostasis is restored. If excessive electrolyte loss occurs, reduce dosage or withdraw the drug temporarily.

Hypokalemia – Hypokalemia prevention requires particular attention to the following: Patients receiving digitalis and diuretics for CHF, hepatic cirrhosis and ascites; in aldosterone excess with normal renal function; potassium-losing nephropathy; certain diarrheal states; or where hypokalemia is an added risk to the patient (eg, history of ventricular arrhythmias).

Possible drug-related deaths occurred with **ethacrynic acid** in critically ill patients refractory to other diuretics. There are two categories: Patients with severe myocardial disease who received digitalis and developed acute hypokalemia with fatal arrhythmia; or patients with severely decompensated hepatic cirrhosis with ascites, with or without encephalopathy, who had electrolyte imbalances and died because of intensification of the electrolyte defect. Liberalization of salt intake and supplementary potassium are often necessary.

Hypomagnesemia – Loop diuretics increase the urinary excretion of magnesium.

Hypocalcemia – Serum calcium levels may be lowered (rare cases of tetany have occurred).

➤*Gastric hemorrhage:* **Ethacrynic acid** may increase the risk of gastric hemorrhage associated with corticosteroid treatment.

➤*Hyperuricemia:* Asymptomatic hyperuricemia can occur, and rarely, gout may be precipitated. Reversible elevations of BUN may be seen, usually in association with dehydration, particularly in patients with renal insufficiency. Serum creatinine may also be increased.

➤*Glucose:* Increases in blood glucose and alterations in glucose tolerance tests (fasting and 2 hour postprandial sugar) have been observed. Rare cases of precipitation of diabetes mellitus have occurred. Although these effects have not been reported with **bumetanide**, the possibility of an effect on glucose metabolism exists.

➤*Lipids:* Increases in LDL and total cholesterol and triglycerides with minor decreases in HDL cholesterol may occur.

➤*Hypersensitivity reactions:* Patients with known sulfonamide sensitivity may show allergic reactions to **furosemide**, **torsemide** or **bumetanide**. Bumetanide use following instances of allergic reactions to furosemide suggests a lack of cross-sensitivity. Refer to Management of Acute Hypersensitivity Reactions.

➤*Renal function impairment:* If increasing azotemia, oliguria or reversible increases in BUN or creatinine occur during treatment of severe progressive renal disease, discontinue therapy.

If high-dose parenteral **furosemide** therapy is used, controlled IV infusion is advisable. For adults, an infusion rate less than or equal to 4 mg/min has been used.

➤*Photosensitivity:* Photosensitization (photoallergy or phototoxicity) may occur; therefore, caution patients to take protective measures (ie, sunscreens, protective clothing) against exposure to sunlight or ultraviolet light (eg, tanning beds) until tolerance is determined.

➤*Pregnancy:* *Category B* (ethacrynic acid, torsemide); *Category C* (furosemide, bumetanide); *Category D* (bumetanide and ethacrynic acid if used in gestational hypertension per Briggs' *Drugs in Pregnancy and Lactation*). There are no adequate and well controlled studies in pregnant women. Use only when clearly needed and when the potential benefits outweigh the potential hazards to the fetus.

Furosemide – Furosemide caused unexplained maternal deaths and abortions in rabbits when 25 to 100 mg/kg (2 to 8 times the maximum recommended human dose) was administered. No pregnant rabbits survived a dose of 100 mg/kg. Data indicate that fetal lethality can precede maternal deaths. Studies in mice and rabbits showed an increased incidence of fetal hydronephrosis. Since furosemide may increase the incidence of patent ductus arteriosus in preterm infants with respiratory-distress syndrome (see Children), use caution when administering before delivery.

Bumetanide – Bumetanide appears to be nonteratogenic, but has a slight embryocidal effect in rats when given in doses of 3400 times the maximum human therapeutic dose and in rabbits at doses of 3.4 times the maximum human therapeutic dose. In rabbits, a decrease in litter size and an increase in resorption rate were noted at oral doses 3.4 to 10 times the maximum human therapeutic dose.

Torsemide – Fetal and maternal toxicity (decrease in average body weight, increase in fetal resorption and delayed fetal ossification) occurred in rabbits and rats.

➤*Lactation:* **Furosemide** appears in breast milk; such transfer of **ethacrynic acid**, **torsemide** and **bumetanide** is unknown. Because of the potential for adverse reactions in nursing infants, decide whether to discontinue nursing or to discontinue the drug, taking into account the importance of the drug to the mother.

➤*Children:* Safety and efficacy for use of **torsemide** in children, **bumetanide** in children younger than 18 years old, and **ethacrynic acid** in infants (oral) and children (IV) have not been established.

Furosemide – Furosemide stimulates renal synthesis of prostaglandin E_2 and may increase the incidence of patent ductus arteriosus when given in the first few weeks of life, to premature infants with respiratory-distress syndrome. Renal calcifications (from barely visible on x–ray to staghorn) have occurred in some severely premature infants treated with IV furosemide for edema due to patent ductus arteriosus and hyaline membrane disease. Concurrent use of chlorothiazide has reportedly decreased hypercalciuria and dissolved some calculi.

➤*Elderly:* Per the Beers list, **ethacrynic acid** has the potential for hypertension and fluid imbalances. Safer alternatives are available.

➤*Monitoring:* Observe for blood dyscrasias, liver or kidney damage or idiosyncratic reactions. Perform frequent serum electrolyte, calcium, glucose, uric acid, CO_2, creatinine and BUN determinations during the first few months of therapy and periodically thereafter (see Electrolyte imbalance and Laboratory test abnormalities).

Drug Interactions

Loop Diuretic Drug Interactions

Precipitant drug	Object drug[a]		Description
Loop diuretics	Aminoglycosides, certain cephalosporins	⬆	Auditory toxicity appears to be increased with concurrent use. Hearing loss of varying degrees may occur.
Loop diuretics	Anticoagulants	⬆	Anticoagulant activity may be enhanced.
Loop diuretics Furosemide	Beta blockers Propranolol	⬆	Plasma levels of propranolol may be increased.
Loop diuretics	Chloral hydrate	⬆	Although rare, transient diaphoresis, hot flashes, hypertension, tachycardia, weakness and nausea may occur with concurrent use.
Loop diuretics	Digitalis glycosides	⬆	Diuretic-induced electrolyte disturbances may predispose to digitalis-induced arrhythmias.
Loop diuretics	Lithium	⬆	Possible increased plasma lithium levels and toxicity.

Loop Diuretic Drug Interactions			
Precipitant drug	Object drug[a]		Description
Loop diuretics	Nondepolarizing muscle relaxants	↔	The actions of the muscle relaxants may be antagonized or potentiated, perhaps dependent on the loop diuretic dosage.
Loop diuretics	Sulfonylureas	↓	Loop diuretics may decrease glucose tolerance, resulting in hyperglycemia in patients previously well controlled on sulfonylureas.
Loop diuretics	Theophyllines	↔	The actions of theophyllines may be altered, enhanced or inhibited.
Loop diuretics Ethacrynic acid	Warfarin	↑	Warfarin may be displaced from plasma protein. Monitor coagulation parameters and adjust the warfarin dose as needed.
Charcoal	Loop diuretics Furosemide	↓	Charcoal can reduce the absorption of furosemide. Depending on the clinical situation, this will reduce its effectiveness or toxicity.
Cisplatin	Loop diuretics	↑	Additive ototoxicity may occur.
Clofibrate	Loop diuretics Furosemide	↑	An exaggerated diuretic response may occur.
Hydantoins Phenytoin	Loop diuretics Furosemide	↓	Hydantoins may reduce the diuretic effects of furosemide.
NSAIDs	Loop diuretics	↓	Effects of the loop diuretics may be decreased.
Probenecid	Loop diuretics	↓	The actions of the loop diuretics may be reduced.
Salicylates	Loop diuretics	↓	The diuretic response may be impaired in patients with cirrhosis and ascites.
Thiazide diuretics	Loop diuretics	↑	Both groups have synergistic effects that may result in profound diuresis and serious electrolyte abnormalities.

[a] ↑ = object drug increased; ↓ = object drug decreased; ↔ = undetermined clinical effect.

➤*Drug/Food interactions:* The bioavailability of **furosemide** is decreased and its degree of diuresis reduced when administered with food.

Adverse Reactions

➤*Furosemide:*

GI – Anorexia; nausea; vomiting; diarrhea; oral and gastric irritation; cramping; constipation; pancreatitis; jaundice; ischemic hepatitis.

CNS – Vertigo with a sense of fullness in the ears; headache; blurred vision; hearing loss; dizziness; paresthesia; xanthopsia; restlessness; fever.

Hematologic – Anemia; leukopenia; purpura; aplastic anemia; thrombocytopenia; agranulocytosis.

Dermatologic – Photosensitivity; urticaria; pruritus; necrotizing angiitis (vasculitis, cutaneous vasculitis); interstitial nephritis; exfoliative dermatitis; erythema multiforme; rash; occasionally, local irritation and pain with parenteral use.

Cardiovascular – Orthostatic hypotension; thrombophlebitis; chronic aortitis.

Miscellaneous Glycosuria; muscle spasm; weakness; urinary bladder spasm; hyperuricemia; hyperglycemia.

➤*Ethacrynic acid:*

GI – Anorexia; nausea; vomiting; diarrhea; pancreatitis (acute); jaundice; discomfort; pain; sudden watery, profuse diarrhea; GI bleeding; dysphagia.

Hematologic – Severe neutropenia has occurred in a few critically ill patients also receiving agents known to produce this effect. Rare instances of Henoch-Schoenlein purpura have occurred in patients with rheumatic heart disease. Thrombocytopenia; agranulocytosis.

Miscellaneous – Fever; chills; hematuria; apprehension; confusion; fatigue; malaise; acute gout; abnormal liver function tests in seriously ill patients on multiple drug therapy that included ethacrynic acid (rare); vertigo; headache; blurred vision; tinnitus; hearing loss (irreversible); rash; occasionally, local irritation and pain have occurred with parenteral use; hyperuricemia; hyperglycemia. Acute symptomatic hypoglycemia with convulsions occurred in two uremic patients who received doses above those recommended.

➤*Bumetanide:*

CNS – Asterixis; encephalopathy with preexisting liver disease; impaired hearing; ear discomfort; vertigo; headache; dizziness.

GI – Upset stomach; dry mouth; nausea; vomiting; diarrhea; pain.

GU – Premature ejaculation; difficulty maintaining erection; renal failure.

Musculoskeletal – Weakness; arthritic pain; pain; muscle cramps; fatigue.

Cardiovascular – Hypotension; ECG changes; chest pain.

Miscellaneous – Hives; pruritus; itching; dehydration; sweating; hyperventilation; nipple tenderness; rash; thrombocytopenia.

Lab test abnormalities – Diuresis rarely (less than or equal to 1%) accompanied by changes in LDH, total serum bilirubin, serum proteins, AST, ALT, alkaline phosphatase, cholesterol and creatinine clearance; deviations in hemoglobin, prothrombin time, hematocrit, WBC, platelet counts and differential counts; increases in urinary glucose and protein; hyperuricemia; hypochloremia; hypokalemia; azotemia; hyponatremia; increased serum creatinine; hyperglycemia; variations in phosphorus, CO_2 content, bicarbonate and calcium (see Warnings/Precautions).

➤*Torsemide:*

CNS – Headache (7.3%); dizziness (3.2%); asthenia (2%); insomnia (1.2%); nervousness (1.1%); syncope.

GI – Diarrhea (2%); constipation, nausea (1.8%); dyspepsia (1.6%); edema (1.1%); GI hemorrhage; rectal bleeding.

Cardiovascular – ECG abnormality (2%); sore throat (1.6%); chest pain (1.2%); atrial fibrillation; hypotension; ventricular tachycardia; shunt thrombosis.

Respiratory – Rhinitis (2.8%); cough increase (2%).

Musculoskeletal – arthralgia (1.8%); myalgia (1.6%).

Lab test abnormalities – Hyperglycemia; hyperuricemia; hypokalemia; hypovolemia.

Miscellaneous – Excessive urination (6.7%); rash.

Overdosage

➤*Symptoms:* Acute profound water loss, volume and electrolyte depletion, dehydration, reduction of blood volume, and circulatory collapse with a possibility of vascular thrombosis and embolism. Electrolyte depletion may be manifested by weakness, dizziness, mental confusion, anorexia, lethargy, vomiting and cramps.

➤*Treatment:* Replace fluid and electrolyte losses by careful monitoring of the urine and electrolyte output and serum electrolyte levels. Assure adequate drainage in urinary bladder outlet obstruction (such as prostatic hypertrophy). Hemodialysis does not accelerate furosemide or torsemide elimination. Perform gastric lavage. If required, give oxygen or artificial respiration. Treatment includes supportive measures. Refer to General Management of Acute Overdosage.

Patient Information

May cause GI upset; take with food or milk (see Drug Interactions). Torsemide may be given without regard to meals. Ethacrynic acid should be given after a meal.

Drug will increase urination; take early in the day.

Notify physician if muscle weakness, cramps, nausea or dizziness occurs.

Orthostatic hypotension may occur; get up slowly.

➤*Diabetes mellitus patients:* May increase blood glucose levels, affecting urine glucose tests.

➤*Photosensitivity:* Photosensitivity may occur in some patients. Caution patients to take protective measures (ie, sunscreens, protective clothing) against exposure to ultraviolet light or sunlight.

➤*Hypertensive patients:* Hypertensive patients should avoid medications that may increase blood pressure, including *otc* products for appetite suppression and cold symptoms.

FUROSEMIDE

Rx	**Furosemide** (Various, eg, Danbury, Geneva, Major, Mylan, Parmed, Roxane, Schein, Zenith)	**Tablets:** 20 mg	In 100s, 500s, 1000s and UD 100s.
Rx	**Lasix** (Aventis)		Lactose. (Lasix Hoechst). White. Oval. In 100s, 500s, 1000s and UD 100s.
Rx	**Furosemide** (Various, eg, Danbury, Geneva, Major, Mylan, Parmed, Roxane, Schein, Zenith)	**Tablets:** 40 mg	In 60s, 100s, 500s and 1000s and UD 100s.
Rx	**Lasix** (Aventis Pharm)		Lactose. (Lasix 40). White, scored. In 500s, 1000s, UD 100s and unit-of-use 100s.

FUROSEMIDE

Rx	**Furosemide** (Various, eg, Danbury, Geneva, Mylan, Parmed, Roxane, Schein)	**Tablets:** 80 mg	In 100s, 500s, 1000s and UD 100s.
Rx	**Lasix** (Aventis Pharm)		Lactose. (Lasix 80). White. In 50s, 500s and UD 100s.
Rx	**Furosemide** (Various, eg, Geneva, Roxane)	**Oral Solution:** 10 mg/ml	In 60 and 120 ml.
Rx	**Furosemide** (Roxane)	**Oral Solution:** 40 mg/5 ml	Pineapple/peach flavor. In 500 ml and UD 5 & 10 ml.
Rx	**Furosemide** (Various, eg, American Regent, Sanofi Winthrop)	**Injection:** 10 mg/ml	In 10 ml and 2, 4, and 10 ml single-dose vials.

FUROSEMIDE — ORAL

For complete and comparative prescribing information, refer to the Loop Diuretics group monograph.

WARNING

Furosemide is a potent diuretic which, if given in excessive amounts, can lead to a profound diuresis with water and electrolyte depletion. Therefore, careful medical supervision is required and dose and schedule must be adjusted to the individual patient's needs (see Administration and Dosage).

Indications

➤*Edema:* Furosemide is indicated in adult and pediatric patients for the treatment of edema associated with congestive heart failure, cirrhosis of the liver, and renal disease, including the nephrotic syndrome. Furosemide is particularly useful when an agent with greater diuretic potential is desired.

➤*Hypertension:* Oral furosemide may be used in adults for the treatment of hypertension alone or in combination with other antihypertensive agents. Hypertensive patients who cannot be adequately controlled with thiazides will probably also not be adequately controlled with furosemide alone.

➤*Off-label uses:*

Pediatric hypertension – [3] = Safety concerns. Furosemide is among the therapeutic options for pediatric hypertension identified by the National High Blood Pressure Educations Program, based on expert opinion.

Sublingual administration – [4] = Insufficient documentation. Initial data from one small pharmacokinetic/dynamic trial suggest that sublingual administration of furosemide may be a useful and effective alternative to oral administration, particularly in patients with decompensated heart failure when intestinal absorption may be diminished. Further studies are needed.

Administration and Dosage

➤*General dosing considerations:* When doses exceeding 80 mg/day are given for prolonged periods, careful clinical observations and laboratory monitoring are particularly advisable.

➤*Adults:*

Edema – Edema may be most efficiently and safely mobilized by dosing on 2 to 4 consecutive days each week.

Initial dosage: 20 to 80 mg given as a single dose. Ordinarily a prompt diuresis ensues. The same dose can be administered 6 to 8 hours later or the dose may be increased, if needed.

Dosage titration: The dose may be raised by 20 to 40 mg and given not sooner than 6 to 8 hours after the previous dose until the desired diuretic effect has been obtained. The dose may be carefully titrated up to 600 mg/day for patients with severe edema.

Maintenance dosage: The individually determined single dose should then be given once or twice daily.

Hypertension –

Initial dosage: 80 mg, usually divided into 40 mg twice a day. Doses should be adjusted according to response.

Concomitant therapy: If response is not satisfactory, add other antihypertensive agents. Changes in blood pressure must be carefully monitored when furosemide is used with other antihypertensive drugs, especially during initial therapy. To prevent excessive drop in blood pressure, the dosage of other agents should be reduced by at least 50 percent when furosemide is added to the regimen. As the blood pressure falls under the potentiating effect of furosemide, a further reduction in dosage or even discontinuation of other antihypertensive drugs may be necessary.

Off-label dosing –

Sublingual administration: [4] = Insufficient documentation. Single doses of 20 mg administered sublingually. Before administration, 180 mL of water was ingested. The tablet was placed under the tongue and held there for 5 minutes without swallowing.

➤*Children:*

Edema – For ease of administration, and to allow maximum flexibility in dosing, the use of oral solution is suggested.

Maximum dose: 6 mg/kg.

Initial dosage: 2 mg/kg body weight, given as a single dose.

Dosage titration: If the diuretic response is not satisfactory, dosage may be increased by 1 or 2 mg/kg not sooner than 6 to 8 hours after the previous dose (up to 6 mg/kg).

Maintenance dosage: The dose should be adjusted to the minimum effective level.

Off-label dosing –

Pediatric hypertension: [3] = Safety concerns. Initial dosage is 0.5 to 2 mg/kg per dose orally once or twice daily. The maximum recommended daily dose is 6 mg/kg.

➤*Storage / Stability:*

Oral solution – Store at controlled room temperature, 15° to 30°C (59° to 86°F). Dispense in original or light-resistant containers as defined in the USP with graduated dropper or graduated spoon (dropper graduated in 5 mg increments at 5, 10, 15, and 20 mg corresponding to 0.5, 1, 1.5, and 2 mL; dispensing spoon graduated in 20 mg increments at 20, 40, 60, and 80 mg corresponding to 2, 4, 6, and 8 mL). Discard opened bottle after 60 days. Protect from light.

Tablets – Store at controlled room temperature 15° to 30°C (59° to 86°F). Dispense in well-closed, light-resistant containers. Exposure to light might cause a slight discoloration. Discolored tablets should not be dispensed.

FUROSEMIDE — INJECTION

For complete and comparative prescribing information, refer to the Loop Diuretics group monograph.

Indications

➤*Edema:* For the treatment of edema associated with congestive heart failure, cirrhosis of the liver, and renal disease, including the nephrotic syndrome. Furosemide is particularly useful when an agent with greater diuretic potential is desired.

Furosemide is indicated as adjunctive therapy in acute pulmonary edema. The intravenous (IV) administration of furosemide is indicated when a rapid onset of diuresis is desired (eg, in acute pulmonary edema).

If GI absorption is impaired or oral medication is not practical for any reason, furosemide is indicated by the IV or intramuscular (IM) route. Parenteral use should be replaced with oral furosemide as soon as practical.

➤*Off-label uses:*

Dyspnea in cancer patients (nebulized furosemide) – [4] = Insufficient documentation. Preliminary data reveal inconsistent benefits with the administration of nebulized furosemide for the treatment of severe dyspnea in terminally ill cancer patients. It is difficult to determine if differences in effect were related to dosing regimens (single dose vs 4 times/day), the type and cause of dyspnea, or the dilution of the drug. Larger controlled trials are needed before this drug can be recommended on a routine basis. (See Administration and Dosage.)

Administration and Dosage

➤*Adults:*

Acute pulmonary edema –

Initial dosage: 40 mg injected slowly intravenously (IV) over 1 to 2 minutes.

Dosage titration: If a satisfactory response does not occur within 1 hour, the dose may be increased to 80 mg injected slowly IV over 1 to 2 minutes.

Concomitant therapy: If necessary, additional therapy (eg, digitalis, oxygen) may be administered.

Edema –

Initial dosage: 20 to 40 mg given as a single dose, injected intramuscularly (IM) or slowly IV over 1 to 2 minutes. Ordinarily a prompt diuresis ensues. If needed, another dose may be administered in the same manner 2 hours later or the dose may be increased.

Dosage titration: The dose may be raised by 20 mg and given not sooner than 2 hours after the previous dose until the desired diuretic effect has been obtained.

Maintenance dosage: The individually determined single dose should then be given once or twice daily.

Off-label dosing –

Dyspnea in cancer patients (nebulized furosemide): [4] = Insufficient documentation. 20 mg diluted in 2 to 3 mL of isotonic sodium chloride solution, administered via nebulizer for 10 to 15 minutes as a single dose or 4 times/day.

➤*Children:*

Edema – See also Off-label dosing.

Maximum dose: 6 mg/kg/dose; the dose for premature infants should not exceed 1 mg/kg/day.

Initial dosage: 1 mg/kg body weight slowly IV or IM and should be given under close medical supervision.

Dosage titration: If the diuretic response is not satisfactory, dosage may be increased by 1 mg/kg not sooner than 2 hours after the previous dose, until the desired diuretic effect has been obtained (up to 6 mg/kg).

Off-label dosing –

Edema:

• *Neonates* –

Usual dosage: 0.5 to 1 mg/kg given IV or IM every 8 to 24 hours.

FUROSEMIDE — INJECTION

Maximum dose: 2 mg/kg/dose.

• *Infants and children* – 0.5 to 2 mg/kg given IV or IM every 6 to 24 hours. When administered as a continuous IV infusion, suggested dosages have ranged from 0.05 to 0.4 mg/kg/hour, titrated to effect.

➤*Preparation for administration:* If the physician elects to use high dose parenteral therapy, add the furosemide to either Sodium Chloride Injection, Lactated Ringer's Injection, or Dextrose (5%) Injection after pH has been adjusted to above 5.5. (See also Administration.)

Do not use if solution is discolored.

➤*Administration:* IV dosing should be given slowly (over 1 to 2 minutes). High dose therapy should be administered as a controlled IV infusion at a rate not greater than 4 mg/min.

➤*Admixture compatibility:*

Compatibility – Furosemide is compatible with Sodium Chloride Injection, Lactated Ringer's Injection, or Dextrose (5%) Injection.

Incompatibility – Furosemide injection is a buffered alkaline solution with a pH of about 9 and drug may precipitate at pH values below 7. Care must be taken to ensure that the pH of the prepared infusion solution is in the weakly alkaline to neutral range. Acid solutions, including other parenteral medications (eg, labetalol, ciprofloxacin, amrinone, milrinone) must not be administered concurrently in the same infusion because they may cause precipitation of the furosemide. In addition, furosemide injection should not be added to a running IV line containing any of these acidic products.

➤*Storage/Stability:* Store at controlled room temperature 15° to 30°C (59° to 86°F). Protect from light.

BUMETANIDE

Rx	**Bumetanide** (Teva)	**Tablets; oral:** 0.5 mg	Lactose. (0.5 4232). Lt. green, scored. In 100s.
Rx	**Bumetanide** (Teva)	**Tablets; oral:** 1 mg	Lactose. (1 4233). Yellow, scored. In 100s and 1,000s.
Rx	**Bumetanide** (Teva)	**Tablets; oral:** 2 mg	Lactose. (2 4234). Peach, scored. In 100s and 1,000s.
Rx	**Bumetanide** (Various, eg, Bedford, Hoffman-LaRoche, Sanofi Winthrop)	**Injection:** 0.25 mg per ml	In 2 ml amps, 2, 4 and 10 ml vials and 4 ml fill in 5 ml vials.

BUMETANIDE — ORAL

For complete and comparative prescribing information, refer to the Loop Diuretics group monograph.

WARNING

Bumetanide is a potent diuretic which, if given in excessive amounts, can lead to a profound diuresis with water and electrolyte depletion. Therefore, careful medical supervision is required and dose and dosage schedule have to be adjusted to the individual patient's needs.

Indications

➤*Edema:* For the treatment of edema associated with congestive heart failure, hepatic and renal disease, including the nephrotic syndrome.

➤*Off-label uses:* Adult nocturia.

Administration and Dosage

➤*General dosing considerations:* Almost equal diuretic response occurs after oral and parenteral administration of bumetanide. Therefore, if impaired GI absorption is suspected or oral administration is not practical, bumetanide should be given by the IM or IV route.

Dosage should be individualized with careful monitoring of patient response.

Because cross-sensitivity with furosemide has rarely been observed, bumetanide can be substituted at approximately a 1:40 ratio of bumetanide to furosemide in patients allergic to furosemide.

Successful treatment with bumetanide following instances of allergic reactions to furosemide suggests a lack of cross-sensitivity.

➤*Adults:*

Edema –

Usual dosage: 0.5 to 2 mg daily given as a single dose.

Maximum dose: 10 mg daily.

Maintenance dosage: An intermittent dose schedule, whereby bumetanide is given on alternate days or for 3 to 4 days with rest periods of 1 to 2 days in between, is recommended as the safest and most effective method for the continued control of edema.

Dosage adjustment: If initial dose of bumetanide is not adequate, in view of its rapid onset and short duration of action, a second or third dose may be given at 4- to 5-hour intervals up to a maximum daily dose of 10 mg.

➤*Children:*

Off-label dosing –

Edema:

• *Infants and children older than 6 months of age* –

Usual dosage: 0.015 to 0.1 mg/kg per dose given daily or every other day.

Maximum dose: 10 mg daily.

• *Neonates and infants 6 months of age and younger* –

Usual dosage: 0.01 to 0.05 mg/kg per dose given daily or every other day. Maximal diuretic effect has been reported at 0.04 mg/kg per dose, with greater efficacy at lower dosages.

Caution: May displace bilirubin in critically ill neonates. Drug elimination has been reported to be slower in neonates with respiratory disorders.

➤*Elderly:* In general, dose selection for an elderly patient should be cautious, usually starting at the low end of the dosing range, reflecting the greater frequency of decreased hepatic, renal, or cardiac function, and of concomitant disease or other drug therapy. (See Adults for dosing.)

➤*Hepatic function impairment:* In patients with hepatic cirrhosis and ascites, sudden alterations of electrolyte balance may precipitate hepatic encephalopathy and coma. Treatment in such patients is best initiated in the hospital with small doses and careful monitoring of the patient's clinical status and electrolyte balance. Supplemental potassium and/or spironolactone may prevent hypokalemia and metabolic alkalosis in these patients.

In patients with hepatic failure, the dosage should be kept to a minimum and, if necessary, dosage increased very carefully.

➤*Storage/Stability:* Store between 15° and 30°C (59° and 86°F). Protect from light.

BUMETANIDE — INJECTION

For complete and comparative prescribing information, refer to the Loop Diuretics group monograph.

WARNING

Bumetanide is a potent diuretic which, if given in excessive amounts, can lead to a profound diuresis with water and electrolyte depletion. Therefore, careful medical supervision is required, and dose and dosage schedule have to be adjusted to the individual patient's needs (see Administration and Dosage).

Indications

➤*Edema:* For the treatment of edema associated with congestive heart failure, and hepatic and renal disease, including the nephrotic syndrome.

Administration and Dosage

➤*General dosing considerations:* If impaired GI absorption is suspected or oral administration is not practical, give bumetanide by the intramuscular (IM) or intravenous (IV) route.

Terminate parenteral treatment and institute oral treatment as soon as possible.

Individualize dosage, with careful monitoring of patient response.

Because cross-sensitivity with furosemide has rarely been observed, bumetanide can be substituted at approximately a 1:40 ratio of bumetanide to furosemide in patients allergic to furosemide.

Successful treatment with bumetanide following instances of allergic reactions to furosemide suggests a lack of cross-sensitivity.

➤*Adults:*

Edema –

Maximum dose: 10 mg daily.

Initial dosage: 0.5 to 1 mg IV or IM. If the response to an initial dose is deemed insufficient, a second or third dose may be given at intervals of 2 to 3 hours.

➤*Children:*

Off-label dosing –

Edema:

• *Infants and children older than 6 months of age* –

Usual dosage: 0.015 to 0.1 mg/kg per dose given daily or every other day IV or IM.

Maximum dose: 10 mg daily.

• *Neonates and infants 6 months of age and younger* –

Usual dosage: 0.01 to 0.05 mg/kg per dose IV or IM daily or every other day. Maximal diuretic effect has been reported at 0.04 mg/kg per dose, with greater efficacy at lower dosages.

Caution: May displace bilirubin in critically ill neonates. Drug elimination has been reported to be slower in neonates with respiratory disorders.

➤*Hepatic function impairment:* In patients with hepatic failure, the dosage should be kept to a minimum, and if necessary, dosage increased very carefully.

BUMETANIDE — INJECTION

➤*Administration:* Administer IV or IM. Give IV administration over a period of 1 to 2 minutes.

➤*Admixture compatibility:* The compatibility tests of bumetanide injection (0.25 mg/mL, 2 mL ampules) with dextrose 5% in water, sodium chloride 0.9%, and lactated Ringer's solution in both glass and plasticized polyvinyl chloride (*Viaflex*) containers have shown no significant absorption effect with either containers, nor a measurable loss of potency due to degradation of the drug.

➤*Storage/Stability:* Store at controlled room temperature 15° to 30°C (59° to 86°F).

Solutions should be freshly prepared and used within 24 hours.

ETHACRYNATE

Rx	**Edecrin** (Aton Pharma)	**Tablets; oral:** 25 mg	As ethacrynic acid. Lactose. (ATON 205/Edecrin). White, capsule shape, scored. In 100s.
Rx	**Sodium Edecrin** (Aton Pharma)	**Injection, powder for solution:** 50 mg	As ethacrynate sodium. Mannitol. In vials.

ETHACRYNIC ACID — ORAL

For complete and comparative prescribing information, refer to the Loop Diuretics class monograph.

WARNING

Ethacrynic acid is a potent diuretic that, if given in excessive amounts, may lead to profound diuresis with water and electrolyte depletion. Therefore, careful medical supervision is required, and dose and dose schedule must be adjusted to the individual patient's needs.

Indications

➤*Edema:* For the treatment of edema when an agent with greater diuretic potential than those commonly employed is required, including the following:
- Treatment of edema associated with congestive heart failure, cirrhosis of the liver, and renal disease, including the nephrotic syndrome.
- Short-term management of ascites caused by malignancy, idiopathic edema, and lymphedema.
- Short-term management of hospitalized children, other than infants, with congenital heart disease or the nephrotic syndrome.

Administration and Dosage

➤*General dosing considerations:* Salt liberalization usually prevents the development of hyponatremia and hypochloremia. During treatment with ethacrynic acid, salt may be liberalized to a greater extent than with other diuretics. Patients with cirrhosis, however, usually require at least moderate salt restriction with diuretic therapy.

➤*Adults:*

Edema –

Initial dosage: Onset of diuresis usually occurs at 50 to 100 mg. The smallest dose required to produce gradual weight loss (about 1 to 2 lbs/day) is recommended.
- *Day 1* – 50 mg once daily after a meal.
- *Day 2* – 50 mg twice daily after meals, if necessary.
- *Day 3* – 100 mg in the morning and 50 to 100 mg following the afternoon or evening meal, depending on the response to the morning dose.

Maintenance dosage: It is usually possible to reduce the dose and frequency of administration once dry weight has been achieved. After diuresis has been achieved, the minimally effective dosage (usually between 50 and 200 mg daily) may be given on a continuous or intermittent dosage schedule. A few patients may require initial and maintenance dosages as high as 200 mg twice daily. These higher dosages, which should be achieved gradually, are most often required in patients with severe, refractory edema.

Ethacrynic acid may be given intermittently after an effective diuresis is obtained with the initial dosage regimen. Dosing may be on an alternate-day schedule, or more prolonged periods of diuretic therapy may be interspersed with rest periods.

Dosage adjustment: Dose adjustments are usually in 25 to 50 mg increments to avoid derangement of water and electrolyte excretion. Small alterations in dose should effectively prevent a massive diuretic response.

➤*Children:*

Edema –

13 months and older:
- *Initial dosage* – 25 mg.
- *Dosage titration* – Careful stepwise increments in doses of 25 mg should be made to achieve effective maintenance.

12 months and younger: Use is contraindicated.

➤*Renal function impairment:* Contraindicated in patients with anuria. If increasing electrolyte imbalance, azotemia, and/or oliguria occur during treatment of severe, progressive renal disease, the diuretic should be discontinued.

➤*Concomitant therapy:*

Carbonic anhydrase inhibitors – Ethacrynic acid may potentiate the action of carbonic anhydrase inhibitors, with augmentation of natriuresis and kaliuresis. Therefore, when adding ethacrynic acid, the initial dose and changes in dose should be in 25 mg increments to avoid electrolyte depletion. Rarely, patients who failed to respond to ethacrynic acid have responded to older established agents.

Other diuretics – Ethacrynic acid has additive effects when used with other diuretics. For example, a patient who is on a maintenance dosage of an oral diuretic may require additional intermittent diuretic therapy, such as an organomercurial, for the maintenance of basal weight. The intermittent use of ethacrynic acid orally may eliminate the need for injections of organomercurials. Small doses of ethacrynic acid may be added to existing diuretic regimens to maintain basal weight.

Supplemental chloride – The chloruretic effect of this agent may give rise to retention of bicarbonate and a metabolic alkalosis. This may be corrected by giving chloride (ammonium chloride or arginine chloride). Ammonium chloride should not be given to patients with cirrhosis.

Supplemental potassium – While many patients do not require supplemental potassium, the use of potassium chloride or potassium-sparing agents, or both, during treatment with ethacrynic acid is advisable, especially in patients and in patients with cirrhosis or nephrosis and in patients receiving digitalis.

➤*Administration:* Administer after a meal.

➤*Storage/Stability:* Store at 25°C (77°F); excursions are permitted between 15° and 30°C (59° and 86°F).

ETHACRYNATE SODIUM — INJECTION

For complete and comparative prescribing information, refer to the Loop Diuretics class monograph.

WARNING

Ethacrynic acid is a potent diuretic that, if given in excessive amounts, may lead to profound diuresis with water and electrolyte depletion. Therefore, careful medical supervision is required, and dose and dose schedule must be adjusted to the individual patient's needs.

Indications

➤*Edema:* When a rapid onset of diuresis is desired (eg, in acute pulmonary edema) or when GI absorption is impaired or oral medication is not practicable.

Administration and Dosage

➤*Adults:*

Edema – 50 mg, or 0.5 to 1 mg/kg IV. Usually only 1 dose has been necessary; occasionally, a second dose at a new injection site may be required to avoid possible thrombophlebitis. A single IV dose not exceeding 100 mg has been used in critical situations.

➤*Children:* Contraindicated in infants.

Off-label dosing –

Children: 0.5 to 1 mg/kg IV. May repeat every 8 to 12 hours if needed.

➤*Renal function impairment:* Contraindicated in patients with anuria. If increasing electrolyte imbalance, azotemia, and/or oliguria occur during treatment of severe, progressive renal disease, the diuretic should be discontinued.

➤*Preparation for administration:* To reconstitute the dry material, add 50 mL of dextrose 5% injection or sodium chloride injection to the vial. Occasionally, some dextrose 5% injection solutions may have a low pH (below 5). The resulting solution with such a diluent may be hazy or opalescent. IV use of such a solution is not recommended.

➤*Administration:* The solution may be given slowly through the tubing of a running infusion or by direct IV injection over a period of several minutes. Ethacrynic acid should not be given subcutaneously or intramuscularly because of local pain and irritation. Use a new injection site to avoid possible thrombophlebitis for any additional doses.

➤*Admixture compatibility:* Do not mix the solution with whole blood or its derivatives.

➤*Storage/Stability:* Store at 25°C (77°F); excursions are permitted between 15° and 30°C (59° and 86°F). Discard unused reconstituted solution after 24 hours.

TORSEMIDE

Rx	**Torsemide** (Teva)	**Tablets; oral:** 5 mg	Lactose. In 100s.
Rx	**Demadex** (Meda Pharmaceuticals)		Lactose. (102 5). White, scored. Oval. In UD 100s.
Rx	**Torsemide** (Teva)	**Tablets; oral:** 10 mg	Lactose. In 100s.
Rx	**Demadex** (Meda Pharmaceuticals)		Lactose. (103 10). White, scored. Oval. In UD 100s.
Rx	**Torsemide** (Teva)	**Tablets; oral:** 20 mg	Lactose. In 100s.
Rx	**Demadex** (Meda Pharmaceuticals)		Lactose. (104 20). White, scored. Oval. In UD 100s.
Rx	**Torsemide** (Teva)	**Tablets; oral:** 100 mg	Lactose. In 100s.
Rx	**Demadex** (Meda Pharmaceuticals)		Lactose. (105 100). White, scored. Capsule shape. In UD 100s.

TORSEMIDE — ORAL

For complete and comparative prescribing information, refer to the Loop Diuretics group monograph.

Indications

➤*Edema:* For the treatment of edema associated with congestive heart failure, renal disease, or hepatic disease. Use of torsemide has been found to be effective for the treatment of edema associated with chronic renal failure. Chronic use of any diuretic in hepatic disease has not been studied in adequate and well-controlled trials.

➤*Hypertension:* For the treatment of hypertension alone or in combination with other antihypertensive agents.

Administration and Dosage

➤*General dosing considerations:* Because of the high bioavailability of torsemide, oral and IV doses are therapeutically equivalent, so patients may be switched to and from the IV form with no change in dose.

➤*Adults:*

Edema associated with chronic renal failure –

Initial dosage: 20 mg once daily.

Dosage titration: If the diuretic response is inadequate, the dose should be titrated upward by approximately doubling until the desired diuretic response is obtained.

Edema associated with congestive heart failure –

Initial dosage: 10 mg or 20 mg once daily.

Dosage titration: If the diuretic response is inadequate, the dose should be titrated upward by approximately doubling until the desired diuretic response is obtained.

Edema associated with hepatic cirrhosis –

Initial dosage: 5 or 10 mg once daily, administered together with an aldosterone antagonist or a potassium-sparing diuretic.

Dosage titration: If the diuretic response is inadequate, the dose should be titrated upward by approximately doubling until the desired diuretic response is obtained.

Hypertension –

Initial dosage: 5 mg once daily.

Dosage titration: If the 5 mg dose does not provide adequate reduction in blood pressure within 4 to 6 weeks, the dose may be increased to 10 mg once daily. If the response to 10 mg is insufficient, an additional antihypertensive agent should be added to the treatment regimen.

➤*Hepatic function impairment:* In patients with hepatic disease, diuresis with torsemide (or any other diuretic) is best initiated in the hospital. To prevent hypokalemia and metabolic alkalosis, an aldosterone antagonist or potassium-sparing drug should be used concomitantly with torsemide.

➤*Special risk patients:* In patients with decompensated congestive heart failure, a smaller fraction of any given dose is delivered to the intraluminal site of action because of reduced renal clearance, so at any given dose there is less natriuresis in patients with congestive heart failure than in healthy subjects.

➤*Administration:* Torsemide may be given at any time in relation to a meal, as convenient.

➤*Storage/Stability:* Store at 15° to 30°C (59° to 86°F).

TORSEMIDE — INJECTION

For complete and comparative prescribing information, refer to the Loop Diuretics group monograph.

Indications

➤*Edema:* For the treatment of edema associated with congestive heart failure, renal disease, or hepatic disease. Use of torsemide has been found to be effective for the treatment of edema associated with chronic renal failure. Chronic use of any diuretic in hepatic disease has not been studied in adequate and well-controlled trials. Torsemide is indicated for the treatment of hypertension alone or in combination with other antihypertensive agents.

Torsemide IV injection is indicated when a rapid onset of diuresis is desired or when oral administration is impractical.

Administration and Dosage

➤*General dosing considerations:* Because of the high bioavailability of torsemide, oral and IV doses are therapeutically equivalent, so patients may be switched to and from the IV form with no change in dose.

➤*Adults:*

Edema associated with chronic renal failure –

Initial dosage: 20 mg once daily.

Dosage titration: If the diuretic response is inadequate, the dose should be titrated upward by approximately doubling until the desired diuretic response is obtained.

Edema associated with congestive heart failure –

Initial dosage: 10 or 20 mg once daily.

Dosage titration: If the diuretic response is inadequate, the dose should be titrated upward by approximately doubling until the desired diuretic response is obtained.

Edema associated with hepatic cirrhosis –

Initial dosage: 5 or 10 mg once daily, administered together with an aldosterone antagonist or a potassium-sparing diuretic.

Dosage titration: If the diuretic response is inadequate, the dose should be titrated upward by approximately doubling until the desired diuretic response is obtained.

Hypertension –

Initial dosage: 5 mg once daily.

Dosage titration: If the 5 mg dose does not provide adequate reduction in blood pressure within 4 to 6 weeks, the dose may be increased to 10 mg once daily. If the response to 10 mg is insufficient, an additional antihypertensive agent should be added to the treatment regimen.

➤*Children:* Safety and efficacy in children have not been established.

➤*Administration:* Torsemide IV injection should be administered either slowly as a bolus over a period of 2 minutes or administered as a continuous infusion.

If torsemide is administered through an IV line, it is recommended that, as with other injections, the IV line be flushed with normal saline (sodium chloride injection) before and after administration. Torsemide injection is formulated above pH 8.3. Flushing the line is recommended to avoid the potential for incompatibilities caused by differences in pH, which could be indicated by color change, haziness, or the formation of a precipitate in the solution.

➤*Storage/Stability:* Store all dosage forms between 15° and 30°C (59° and 86°F). Do not freeze.

Stability – If torsemide is administered as a continuous infusion, stability has been demonstrated through 24 hours at room temperature in plastic containers for the following fluids and concentrations:

Torsemide Injection Stability[a]

Torsemide concentrations	Fluids
200 mg torsemide (10 mg/mL) added to:	250 mL dextrose 5% in water
	250 mL 0.9% sodium chloride
	500 mL 0.45% sodium chloride
50 mg torsemide (10 mg/mL) added to:	500 mL dextrose 5% in water
	500 mL 0.9% sodium chloride
	500 mL 0.45% sodium chloride

[a] Demonstrated stability through 24 hours at room temperature in plastic containers.

Potassium-Sparing Diuretics

Actions

➤*Pharmacology:* In the kidney, potassium is filtered at the glomerulus and then absorbed parallel to sodium throughout the proximal tubule and thick ascending limb of the loop of Henle, so that only minor amounts reach the distal convoluted tubule. As a result, potassium appearing in urine is secreted at the distal tubule and collecting duct. The potassium-sparing diuretics interfere with sodium reabsorption at the distal tubule, thus decreasing potassium secretion. They exert a weak diuretic and antihypertensive effect when used alone. Their major use is to enhance the action and counteract the kaliuretic effect of thiazide and loop diuretics.

Spironolactone – Spironolactone, a competitive inhibitor of aldosterone, binds to aldosterone receptors of the distal tubule and prevents the formation of a protein important in sodium transport. The dose of spironolactone required to produce an effect varies according to the amount of aldosterone present. It is effective in primary and secondary hyperaldosteronism. Spironolactone is effective in lowering systolic and diastolic blood pressure in both primary hyperaldosteronism and essential hypertension, although aldosterone secretion may be normal in benign essential hypertension. In addition, spironolactone interferes with testosterone synthesis and may increase peripheral conversion of testosterone to estradiol. This action may be responsible for endocrine abnormalities occasionally noted with therapy.

Amiloride/Triamterene – Amiloride and triamterene not only inhibit sodium reabsorption induced by aldosterone, but they also inhibit basal sodium reabsorption. They are not aldosterone antagonists, but act directly on the renal distal tubule, cortical collecting tubule and collecting duct. They induce a reversal of polarity of the transtubular electrical-potential difference and inhibit active transport of sodium and potassium. Amiloride may inhibit sodium, potassium-ATPase. Amiloride decreases the enhanced urinary excretion of magnesium that occurs when a thiazide or loop diuretic is used alone; it also decreases calcium excretion.

Potassium-Sparing Diuretics: Pharmacological and Pharmacokinetic Properties

Parameters	Amiloride	Spironolactone	Triamterene
Pharmacology			
Tubular site of action	Proximal = distal	Distal	Distal
Mechanism of action	Na^+, K^+–ATPase inhibition; Na^+/H^+ exchange mechanism inhibition (proximal tubule)	Aldosterone antagonism	Membrane effect
Action:			
Onset (hours)	2	24 to 48	2 to 4
Peak (hours)	6 to 10	48 to 72	6 to 8
Duration (hours)	24	48 to 72	12 to 16
Pharmacokinetics			
Bioavailability	15% to 25%	> 90%	30% to 70%
Protein binding	23%	≥ 98%[a]	50% to 67%
Half-life (hours)	6 to 9	20[b]	3
Active metabolites	none	canrenone	hydroxytriamterene sulfate
Peak plasma levels (hours)	3 to 4	canrenone: 2 to 4[c]	3
Excreted unchanged in urine	≈ 50%[d]	—[d]	≈ 21%
Daily dose (mg)	5 to 20	25 to 400	200 to 300

[a] Canrenone greater than 98%.
[b] 10 to 35 hours for canrenone.
[c] 40% excreted in stool within 72 hours.
[d] Metabolites primarily excreted in urine, but also in bile.

AMILORIDE HYDROCHLORIDE

Rx	**Midamor** (Merck)	**Tablets:** 5 mg	(MSD 92). Yellow. Diamond shape. In 100s.

AMILORIDE — ORAL

Refer to the general discussion of these agents in the Potassium-Sparing Diuretics introduction.

WARNING

Hyperkalemia – Like other potassium-conserving agents, amiloride may cause hyperkalemia (serum potassium levels greater than 5.5 mEq per liter) which, if uncorrected, is potentially fatal. Hyperkalemia occurs commonly (about 10%) when amiloride is used without a kaliuretic diuretic. This incidence is greater in patients with renal impairment, diabetes mellitus (with or without recognized renal insufficiency), and in the elderly. When amiloride is used concomitantly with a thiazide diuretic in patients without these complications, the risk of hyperkalemia is reduced to about 1% to 2%. It is thus essential to monitor serum potassium levels carefully in any patient receiving amiloride, particularly when it is first introduced, at the time of diuretic dosage adjustments, and during any illness that could affect renal function.

Indications

➤*Congestive heart failure/hypertension:* Adjunctive treatment with thiazide diuretics or other kaliuretic-diuretic agents in congestive heart failure or hypertension to:

1.) help restore normal serum potassium levels in patients who develop hypokalemia on the kaliuretic diuretic
2.) prevent development of hypokalemia in patients who would be exposed to particular risk if hypokalemia were to develop (eg, digitalized patients or patients with significant cardiac arrhythmias).

The use of potassium-conserving agents is often unnecessary in patients receiving diuretics for uncomplicated essential hypertension when such patients have a normal diet. Amiloride has little additive diuretic or antihypertensive effect when added to a thiazide diuretic.

➤*Off-label uses:*

Lithium-induced polyuria – [4] = Insufficient documentation. A limited number of studies have evaluated amiloride use in lithium-induced polyuria. Because amiloride is a potassium-sparing diuretic, potassium supplementation is unnecessary when amiloride is used in combination with thiazides to decrease sodium levels and urine output. Before amiloride is added to therapy, attempt reduction of the lithium dose and dosing frequency, along with potassium supplementation. Careful monitoring of electrolytes and serum lithium levels is required if amiloride therapy is implemented.

Pediatric hypertension – [3] = Safety concerns. Amiloride is among the therapeutic options for pediatric hypertension identified by the National High Blood Pressure Education Program, based on expert opinion.

Other possible off-label uses – Aerosolized amiloride (drug dissolved in saline 0.3% delivered by nebulizer) appears to slow the progression of pulmonary function reduction in adults with cystic fibrosis.

Administration and Dosage

➤*General dosing considerations:* Amiloride should rarely be used alone. It has weak (compared with thiazides) diuretic and antihypertensive effects. Used as single agents, potassium sparing diuretics, including amiloride, result in an increased risk of hyperkalemia (approximately 10% with amiloride). Amiloride should be used alone only when persistent hypokalemia has been documented and only with careful titration of the dose and close monitoring of serum electrolytes.

➤*Adults:*

Hypokalemia or prevention of hypokalemia –

Initial dosage:

- *Adjunctive therapy* – 5 mg daily should be added to the usual antihypertensive or diuretic dosage of a kaliuretic diuretic.
- *Monotherapy* – 5 mg daily.

Dosage titration: May increase to 10 mg/day, if necessary. More than two 5 mg tablets/day usually are not needed, and there is little controlled experience with such doses. If persistent hypokalemia is documented with 10 mg, the dose can be increased to 15 mg, then 20 mg, with careful monitoring of electrolytes.

Off-label dosing –

Lithium-induced polyuria: [4] = Insufficient documentation. 10 to 20 mg daily used alone or in combination with thiazide diuretics.

➤*Children:*

Off-label dosing –

Pediatric hypertension: [3] = Safety concerns.

- *1 to 17 years of age* –
  Usual dosage: 0.4 to 0.625 mg/kg/day as a single dose.
  Maximum dose: 20 mg/day.

➤*Renal function impairment:* Contraindicated in patients with anuria, acute or chronic renal insufficiency, and evidence of diabetic nephropathy.

➤*Congestive heart failure:* After an initial diuresis has been achieved, potassium loss may also decrease and the need for amiloride should be reevaluated. Dosage adjustment may be necessary. Maintenance therapy may be on an intermittent basis.

➤*Administration:* Amiloride should be administered with food.

➤*Storage/Stability:* Protect from moisture, freezing, and excessive heat.

AMILORIDE — ORAL

Actions

➤*Pharmacology:* In the kidney, potassium is filtered at the glomerulus and then absorbed parallel to sodium throughout the proximal tubule and thick ascending limb of the loop of Henle, so that only minor amounts reach the distal convoluted tubule. As a result, potassium appearing in urine is secreted at the distal tubule and collecting duct. The potassium-sparing diuretics interfere with sodium reabsorption at the distal tubule, thus decreasing potassium secretion.

Amiloride is a potassium-conserving (antikaliuretic) drug that possesses weak (compared with thiazide diuretics) natriuretic, diuretic, and antihypertensive activity. These effects have been partially additive to the effects of thiazide diuretics in some clinical studies. When administered with a thiazide or loop diuretic, amiloride has been shown to decrease the enhanced urinary excretion of magnesium which occurs when a thiazide or loop diuretic is used alone. Amiloride has potassium-conserving activity in patients receiving kaliuretic-diuretic agents.

Amiloride is not an aldosterone antagonist and its effects are seen even in the absence of aldosterone.

Amiloride exerts its potassium sparing effect through the inhibition of sodium reabsorption at the distal convoluted tubule, cortical collecting tubule and collecting duct; this decreases the net negative potential of the tubular lumen and reduces both potassium and hydrogen secretion and their subsequent excretion. This mechanism accounts in large part for the potassium sparing action of amiloride.

➤*Pharmacokinetics:*

Absorption / Distribution – Approximately 15% to 25% of a dose of amiloride is absorbed from the gastrointestinal tract following oral administration and amiloride is not highly protein bound (23%). Amiloride usually begins to act within 2 hours after an oral dose. Its effect on electrolyte excretion reaches a peak between 6 and 10 hours and lasts about 24 hours. Peak plasma levels are obtained in 3 to 4 hours and the plasma half-life varies from 6 to 9 hours. Effects on electrolytes increase with single doses of amiloride up to approximately 15 mg.

Metabolism / Excretion – Amiloride is not metabolized by the liver but is excreted unchanged by the kidneys. About 50 percent of a 20 mg dose of amiloride is excreted in the urine and 40% in the stool within 72 hours. Amiloride has little effect on glomerular filtration rate or renal blood flow. Because amiloride is not metabolized by the liver, drug accumulation is not anticipated in patients with hepatic dysfunction, but accumulation can occur if the hepatorenal syndrome develops.

Contraindications

➤*Hyperkalemia:* Amiloride should not be used in the presence of elevated serum potassium levels (greater than 5.5 mEq/L).

➤*Antikaliuretic therapy or potassium supplementation:* Amiloride should not be given to patients receiving other potassium-conserving agents, such as spironolactone or triamterene. Potassium supplementation in the form of medication, potassium-containing salt substitutes or a potassium-rich diet should not be used with amiloride except in severe and/or refractory cases of hypokalemia. Such concomitant therapy can be associated with rapid increases in serum potassium levels. If potassium supplementation is used, careful monitoring of the serum potassium level is necessary.

➤*Renal impairment:* Anuria, acute or chronic renal insufficiency, and evidence of diabetic nephropathy are contraindications to the use of amiloride. Patients with evidence of renal functional impairment (blood urea nitrogen [BUN] levels over 30 mg/100 mL or serum creatinine levels over 1.5 mg/100 mL) or diabetes mellitus should not receive the drug without careful, frequent and continuing monitoring of serum electrolytes, creatinine, and BUN levels. Potassium retention associated with the use of an antikaliuretic agent is accentuated in the presence of renal impairment and may result in the rapid development of hyperkalemia.

➤*Hypersensitivity:* Amiloride is contraindicated in patients who are hypersensitive to this product.

Warnings/Precautions

➤*Hyperkalemia:* The risk of hyperkalemia may be increased when potassium-conserving agents, including amiloride, are administered concomitantly with an angiotensin-converting enzyme inhibitor (see Drug Interactions). Warning signs or symptoms of hyperkalemia include paresthesias, muscular weakness, fatigue, flaccid paralysis of the extremities, bradycardia, shock, and ECG abnormalities. Monitoring of the serum potassium level is essential because mild hyperkalemia is not usually associated with an abnormal ECG.

When abnormal, the ECG in hyperkalemia is characterized primarily by tall, peaked T waves or elevations from previous tracings. There may also be lowering of the R wave and increased depth of the S wave, widening and even disappearance of the P wave, progressive widening of the QRS complex, prolongation of the PR interval, and ST depression.

➤*Diabetes mellitus:* In diabetic patients, hyperkalemia has been reported with the use of all potassium-conserving diuretics, including amiloride, even in patients without evidence of diabetic nephropathy. Therefore, amiloride should be avoided, if possible, in diabetic patients and, if it is used, serum electrolytes and renal function must be monitored frequently.

Amiloride should be discontinued at least 3 days before glucose tolerance testing.

➤*Metabolic or respiratory acidosis:* Antikaliuretic therapy should be instituted only with caution in severely ill patients in whom respiratory or metabolic acidosis may occur, such as patients with cardiopulmonary disease or poorly controlled diabetes. If amiloride is given to these patients, frequent monitoring of acid-base balance is necessary. Shifts in acid-base balance alter the ratio of extracellular/intracellular potassium, and the development of acidosis may be associated with rapid increases in serum potassium levels.

➤*Electrolyte imbalance and BUN increases:* Hyponatremia and hypochloremia may occur when amiloride is used with other diuretics and increases in BUN levels have been reported. These increases usually have accompanied vigorous fluid elimination, especially when diuretic therapy was used in seriously ill patients, such as those who had hepatic cirrhosis with ascites and metabolic alkalosis, or those with resistant edema. Therefore, when amiloride is given with other diuretics to such patients, careful monitoring of serum electrolytes and BUN levels is important.

➤*Hepatic function impairment:* In patients with pre-existing severe liver disease, hepatic encephalopathy manifested by tremors, confusion, and coma, and increased jaundice, have been reported in association with diuretics, including amiloride.

➤*Pregnancy: Category B.* Teratogenicity studies with amiloride in rabbits and mice given 20 and 25 times the maximum human dose, respectively, revealed no evidence of harm to the fetus, although studies showed that the drug crossed the placenta in modest amounts. Reproduction studies in rats at 20 times the expected maximum daily dose for humans showed no evidence of impaired fertility. At approximately 5 or more times the expected maximum daily dose for humans, some toxicity was seen in adult rats and rabbits and a decrease in rat pup growth and survival occurred. There are, however, no adequate and well-controlled studies in pregnant women. Because animal reproduction studies are not always predictive of human response, this drug should be used during pregnancy only if clearly needed.

➤*Lactation:* Studies in rats have shown that amiloride is excreted in milk in concentrations higher than those found in blood, but it is not known whether amiloride is excreted in human milk. Because many drugs are excreted in human milk and because of the potential for serious adverse reactions in nursing infants from amiloride, a decision should be made whether to discontinue nursing or to discontinue the drug, taking into account the importance of the drug to the mother.

➤*Children:* Safety and efficacy have not been established.

Drug Interactions

Amiloride Drug Interactions

Precipitant drug	Object drug[a]		Description
Amiloride	Digoxin	⬇	In six healthy subjects, amiloride increased the renal clearance and decreased the nonrenal clearance of digoxin. It also appeared to decrease the inotropic effect of digoxin.
Amiloride	Potassium preparations	⬆	Concurrent administration may result in severe hyperkalemia, possibly with cardiac arrhythmias or cardiac arrest. Avoid concomitant use.
ACE inhibitors	Amiloride	⬆	Use of ACE inhibitors may result in elevated serum potassium concentration. Concurrent use with amiloride may lead to significant hyperkalemia.
NSAIDs	Amiloride	⬇	NSAIDs may reduce the therapeutic effect of amiloride. Also, since indomethacin may be associated with increased potassium levels, consider this effect when amiloride is used concurrently.

[a] ⬆ = object drug increased; ⬇ = object drug decreased.

Lithium generally should not be given with diuretics because they reduce its renal clearance and add a high risk of lithium toxicity. However, amiloride may be given to reduce lithium-induced polyuria (see Unlabeled Uses). Read monographs for lithium preparations before use of such concomitant therapy.

Adverse Reactions

Amiloride is usually well tolerated and, except for hyperkalemia (serum potassium levels greater than 5.5 mEq/L, see Warnings/Precautions), significant adverse effects have been reported infrequently. Minor adverse reactions were reported relatively frequently (about 20%) but the relationship of many of the reports to amiloride is uncertain and the overall frequency was similar in hydrochlorothiazide treated groups. Nausea/anorexia, abdominal pain, flatulence, and mild skin rash have been reported and probably are related to amiloride. Other adverse experiences that have been reported with amiloride are generally those known to be associated with diuresis, or with the underlying disease being treated.

The incidence for column 1 was determined from clinical studies conducted in the United States (837 patients treated with amiloride). The adverse effects listed in column 2 include reports from the same clinical studies and voluntary reports since marketing. The probability of a causal relationship exists between amiloride and these adverse reactions, some of which have been reported only rarely.

AMILORIDE — ORAL

Amiloride Adverse Reactions	
Incidence > 1%	**Incidence ≤ 1%**
Miscellaneous	
Headache[a] Weakness Fatigability	Back pain Chest pain Neck/shoulder ache Pain, extremities
Cardiovascular	
None	Angina pectoris Orthostatic hypotension Arrhythmia Palpitation
GI	
Nausea/anorexia[a] Diarrhea[a] Vomiting[a] Abdominal pain Gas pain Appetite changes Constipation	Jaundice GI bleeding Abdominal fullness GI disturbance Thirst Heartburn Flatulence Dyspepsia
Metabolic	
Elevated serum potassium levels (> 5.5 mEq/L)[b]	None
Dermatologic	
None	Skin rash Itching Dryness of mouth Pruritus Alopecia
Musculoskeletal	
Muscle cramps	Joint pain Leg ache
CNS	
Dizziness Encephalopathy	Paresthesia Tremors Vertigo
Psychiatric	
None	Nervousness Mental confusion Insomnia Decreased libido Depression Somnolence
Respiratory	
Cough Dyspnea	Shortness of breath
Special senses	
None	Visual disturbances Nasal congestion Tinnitus Increased intraocular pressure
GU	
Impotence	Polyuria Dysuria Urinary frequency Bladder spasms Gynecomastia

[a] Reactions occurring in 3% to 8% of patients treated with amiloride. (Those reactions occurring in less than 3% of the patients are unmarked.)
[b] See Warnings/Precautions.

➤*Causal relationship unknown:* Other reactions have been reported but occurred under circumstances where a causal relationship could not be established. However, in these rarely reported events, that possibility cannot be excluded. Therefore, these observations are listed to serve as alerting information to physicians: activation of probable pre-existing peptic ulcer, aplastic anemia, neutropenia, abnormal liver function.

Overdosage

➤*Symptoms:* No data are available in regard to overdosage in humans.

It is not known whether the drug is dialyzable.

The most likely signs and symptoms to be expected with overdosage are dehydration and electrolyte imbalance. These can be treated by established procedures.

➤*Treatment:* Therapy with amiloride should be discontinued and the patient observed closely. There is no specific antidote. Emesis should be induced or gastric lavage performed. Treatment is symptomatic and supportive. If hyperkalemia occurs, active measures should be taken to reduce the serum potassium levels.

Patient Information

May cause GI upset; take with food.

Notify physician if any of the following occurs: Muscular weakness; fatigue; muscle cramps.

May cause dizziness, headache, or visual disturbances; observe caution while driving or performing other tasks requiring alertness, coordination or physical dexterity.

Avoid large quantities of potassium-rich food.

SPIRONOLACTONE

Rx	**Spironolactone** (Various, eg, Actavis Elizabeth, Mylan)	**Tablets; oral:** 25 mg	In 60s, 100s, 500s, and 1,000s.
Rx	**Aldactone** (Searle)		PEG. (Searle 1001 Aldactone 25). Lt. yellow, round. Film-coated. In 100s and 500s.
Rx	**Spironolactone** (Various, eg, Greenstone, Mylan)	**Tablets; oral:** 50 mg	In 30s, 60s, 100s, 500s, and 1,000s.
Rx	**Aldactone** (Searle)		PEG. (Searle 1041 Aldactone 50). Lt. orange, oval, scored. Film-coated. In 100s.
Rx	**Spironolactone** (Various, eg, Greenstone, Mylan)	**Tablets; oral:** 100 mg	In 100s and 500s.
Rx	**Aldactone** (Searle)		PEG. (Searle 1031 Aldactone 100). Peach, round, scored. Film-coated. In 100s.

SPIRONOLACTONE — ORAL

Refer to the general discussion of these agents in the Potassium-Sparing Diuretics introduction.

WARNING

Spironolactone has been shown to be a tumorigen in chronic toxicity studies in rats. Use spironolactone only in those conditions for which it is indicated. Avoid unnecessary use of this drug.

Indications

➤*Edematous conditions:*

Congestive heart failure – For the management of edema and sodium retention when the patient is only partially responsive to, or is intolerant of, other therapeutic measures; for patients with congestive heart failure taking digitalis when other therapies are considered inappropriate.

Cirrhosis of the liver accompanied by edema and/or ascites – For maintenance therapy together with bed rest and the restriction of fluid and sodium. Aldosterone levels may be exceptionally high in this condition.

Nephrotic syndrome – For nephrotic patients when treatment of the underlying disease, restriction of fluid and sodium intake, and the use of other diuretics do not provide an adequate response.

➤*Essential hypertension:* Usually in combination with other drugs, for patients who cannot be treated adequately with other agents or for whom other agents are considered inappropriate.

➤*Hypokalemia:* For the treatment of patients with hypokalemia when other measures are considered inappropriate or inadequate; for the prophylaxis of hypokalemia in patients taking digitalis when other measures are considered inadequate or inappropriate.

➤*Primary hyperaldosteronism:* Establishing the diagnosis of primary hyperaldosteronism by therapeutic trial; short-term preoperative treatment of patients with primary hyperaldosteronism; long-term maintenance therapy for patients with discrete aldosterone-producing adrenal adenomas who are judged to be poor operative risks or who decline surgery; and for long-term maintenance therapy for patients with bilateral micro- or macronodular adrenal hyperplasia (idiopathic hyperaldosteronism).

SPIRONOLACTONE — ORAL

➤*Severe heart failure (New York Heart Association [NYHA] class III to IV):* To increase survival and to reduce the need for hospitalization for heart failure when used in addition to standard therapy.

➤*Pregnancy:* The routine use of diuretics in an otherwise healthy woman is inappropriate and exposes mother and fetus to unnecessary hazard. Diuretics do not prevent development of toxemia of pregnancy, and there is no satisfactory evidence that they are useful in the treatment of developing toxemia.

Spironolactone is indicated in pregnancy when edema is caused by pathologic causes, just as it is in the absence of pregnancy. However, there are no adequate and well-controlled studies with spironolactone in pregnant women. Spironolactone has known endocrine effects in animals, including progestational and antiandrogenic effects. The antiandrogenic effects can result in apparent estrogenic side effects in humans, such as gynecomastia. Therefore, the use of spironolactone in pregnant women requires that the anticipated benefit be weighed against the possible hazards to the fetus. Dependent edema in pregnancy, resulting from restriction of venous return by the expanded uterus, is properly treated through elevation of the lower extremities and use of support hose; use of diuretics to lower intravascular volume in this case is unsupported and unnecessary. There is hypervolemia during normal pregnancy that is not harmful to either the fetus or the mother (in the absence of cardiovascular disease), but which is associated with edema, including generalized edema, in the majority of pregnant women. If this edema produces discomfort, increased recumbency will often provide relief. In rare instances, this edema may cause extreme discomfort that is not relieved by rest. In these cases, a short course of diuretics may provide relief and may be appropriate.

➤*Off-label uses:*

Hirsutism in women – [1] = Good documentation. Guidelines primarily based on expert consensus recommend the use of spironolactone in combination with an oral contraceptive for treatment of polycystic ovary syndrome (PCOS) hirsutism. Trials in patients with PCOS and idiopathic hirsutism have been small and not well defined but have demonstrated benefit. Meta-analyses have not been able to confirm results; therefore, further investigation is needed.

Male precocious puberty – [4] = Insufficient documentation. Initial data suggest that the combination of spironolactone and testolactone, along with the addition of deslorelin at the onset of central precocious puberty, may be effective in the treatment of boys with male precocious puberty. However, long-term trials and follow-up reports to current studies are necessary to determine the effects that the combination therapy has throughout the patients' adult lives. Larger controlled trials comparing different therapies (such as ketoconazole vs spironolactone plus testolactone) would also be beneficial in evaluating effectiveness. Testolactone and deslorelin are not available in the United States.

Pediatric hypertension – [3] = Safety concerns. Spironolactone is among the therapeutic options for pediatric hypertension identified by the National High Blood Pressure Education Program, based on expert opinion.

Other possible off-label uses – Studies have shown that the use of spironolactone (alone or in combination therapy) for the treatment of acne has produced a 50% to 70% improvement of acne. (See Administration and Dosage.)

Administration and Dosage

➤*Adults:*

Edema conditions –

Usual dosage: 25 to 200 mg daily.

Initial dosage: 100 mg daily in either single or divided doses. When given as the sole agent for diuresis, continue for at least 5 days at the initial dosage level, after which it may be adjusted to the optimal therapeutic or maintenance level administered in either single or divided daily doses.

Concomitant therapy: If, after 5 days, an adequate diuretic response has not occurred, a second diuretic that acts more proximally in the renal tubule may be added to the regimen. Because of the additive effect of spironolactone when coadministered with such diuretics, an enhanced diuresis usually begins on the first day of combined treatment; combined therapy is indicated when more rapid diuresis is desired. The dosage of spironolactone should remain unchanged when other diuretic therapy is added.

Essential hypertension –

Initial dosage: 50 to 100 mg daily in single or divided doses.

Dosage adjustment: Dosage should be adjusted according to the response of the patient.

Duration of therapy: Treatment should be continued for at least 2 weeks, because the maximum response may not occur before this time.

Concomitant therapy: May be given with diuretics that act more proximally in the renal tubule or with other antihypertensive agents.

Hypokalemia – 25 to 100 mg daily.

Primary hyperaldosteronism –

Usual dosage: 100 to 400 mg daily in preparation for surgery.

Maintenance dosage: For patients who are considered unsuitable for surgery, administer long-term maintenance therapy at the lowest effective dosage determined for the individual patient.

Diagnosis:

- *Long test* – 400 mg daily for 3 to 4 weeks. Correction of hypokalemia and of hypertension provides presumptive evidence for the diagnosis of primary hyperaldosteronism.
- *Short test* – 400 mg daily for 4 days. If serum potassium increases during spironolactone administration but drops when spironolactone is discontinued, a presumptive diagnosis of primary hyperaldosteronism should be considered.

Severe heart failure (NYHA class III to IV) –

Initial dosage: 25 mg once daily if the patient's serum potassium is 5 mEq/L or less and the patient's serum creatinine is 2.5 mg/dL or less.

Dosage adjustment: Patients who tolerate 25 mg once daily may have their dosage increased to 50 mg once daily as clinically indicated. Patients who do not tolerate the 25 mg once-daily dose may have their dosage reduced to 25 mg every other day.

Off-label dosing –

Acne: 50 to 200 mg/day.

Hirsutism in women: [1] = Good documentation. Used as monotherapy or in combination therapy at dosages ranging from 50 to 200 mg daily in 1 to 2 divided doses.

➤*Children:*

Off-label dosing –

Diagnosis of primary aldosteronism: 125 to 375 mg/m²/day orally divided 2 to 4 times daily.

Diuretic:

- *Older than 29 days* – 1 to 3.3 mg/kg/day orally divided up to 4 times daily.
- *29 days and younger* – 1 to 3 mg/kg/day orally divided up to twice daily.

Male precocious puberty: [4] = Insufficient documentation. 1.5 or 2 mg/kg/day in 2 divided doses in weeks 1 and 2, 3 or 4 mg/kg/day in weeks 3 and 4, and 5.7 mg/kg/day thereafter. In each trial, testolactone was given in combination with spironolactone, and in 1 study, deslorelin was added. In a case report, spironolactone monotherapy was given in 2 divided doses of 4 mg/kg/day for 6 months. Testolactone (discontinued in February 2008) and deslorelin are not available in the United States.

Pediatric hypertension: [3] = Safety concerns.

- *1 to 17 years of age* –

  Maximum dose: 3.3 mg/kg/day, up to 100 mg/day.

  Initial dosage: 1 mg/kg/day orally once daily or divided for twice-daily administration.

➤*Renal function impairment:* Contraindicated in patients with anuria, acute renal insufficiency, and/or significant impairment of renal excretory function.

➤*Storage/Stability:* Store below 25°C (77°F).

Actions

➤*Pharmacology:* Spironolactone is a specific pharmacologic antagonist of aldosterone, acting primarily through competitive binding of receptors at the aldosterone-dependent sodium-potassium exchange site in the distal convoluted renal tubule. Spironolactone causes increased amounts of sodium and water to be excreted, while potassium is retained. Spironolactone acts both as a diuretic and as an antihypertensive drug by this mechanism. It may be given alone or with other diuretic agents that act more proximally in the renal tubule.

Aldosterone antagonist activity – Increased levels of the mineralocorticoid, aldosterone, are present in primary and secondary hyperaldosteronism. Edematous states in which secondary aldosteronism is usually involved include congestive heart failure, hepatic cirrhosis, and the nephrotic syndrome. By competing with aldosterone for receptor sites, spironolactone provides effective therapy for the edema and ascites in those conditions. Spironolactone counteracts secondary aldosteronism induced by the volume depletion and associated sodium loss caused by active diuretic therapy.

Spironolactone is effective in lowering the systolic and diastolic blood pressure in patients with primary hyperaldosteronism. It is also effective in most cases of essential hypertension, despite the fact that aldosterone secretion may be within normal limits in benign essential hypertension.

Through its action in antagonizing the effect of aldosterone, spironolactone inhibits the exchange of sodium for potassium in the distal renal tubule and helps to prevent potassium loss.

➤*Pharmacokinetics:*

Absorption/Distribution –

Spironolactone Pharmacokinetic Data[a]

	Accumulation factor: AUC (0 to 24 h, day 15)/ AUC (0-24 h, day 1)	Mean peak serum concentration	Mean (SD) post–steady-state half-life
7-α-(thiomethyl) spirolactone (TMS)	1.25	391 ng/mL at 3.2 h	13.8 h (6.4) (terminal)
6-β-hydroxy-7-α-(thiomethyl) spirolactone (HTMS)	1.5	125 ng/mL at 5.1 h	15 h (4) (terminal)
Canrenone (C)	1.41	181 ng/mL at 4.3 h	16.5 h (6.3) (terminal)
Spironolactone	1.3	80 ng/mL at 2.6 h	Approximately 1.4 h (0.5) (β half-life)

[a] AUC = area under the curve; SD = standard deviation.

SPIRONOLACTONE — ORAL

Both spironolactone and its metabolites are more than 90% bound to plasma proteins.

Effect of food: See Drug Interactions for more information.

Metabolism/Excretion – Spironolactone is rapidly and extensively metabolized. Sulfur-containing products are the predominant metabolites and are thought to be primarily responsible, together with spironolactone, for the therapeutic effects of the drug.

The pharmacological activity of spironolactone metabolites in humans is not known. However, in the adrenalectomized rat, the antimineralocorticoid activities of the metabolites C, TMS, and HTMS, relative to spironolactone, were 1.1, 1.28, and 0.32, respectively. Relative to spironolactone, their binding affinities to the aldosterone receptors in rat kidney slices were 0.19, 0.86, and 0.06, respectively.

The metabolites are excreted primarily in the urine and secondarily in bile.

Contraindications

Anuria, acute renal insufficiency, significant impairment of renal excretory function, or hyperkalemia.

Warnings/Precautions

➤*Hyperkalemia:* Potassium supplementation, either in the form of medication or as a diet rich in potassium, should not ordinarily be given in association with spironolactone therapy. Excessive potassium intake may cause hyperkalemia in patients receiving spironolactone.

If hyperkalemia is suspected (warning signs include paresthesia, muscle weakness, fatigue, flaccid paralysis of the extremities, bradycardia and shock), obtain an electrocardiogram (ECG). However, it is important to monitor serum potassium levels because mild hyperkalemia may not be associated with ECG changes.

If hyperkalemia is present, discontinue spironolactone immediately. With severe hyperkalemia, the clinical situation dictates the procedures to be employed. These include the intravenous administration of calcium chloride solution, sodium bicarbonate solution, and/or the oral or parenteral administration of glucose with a rapid-acting insulin preparation. These are temporary measures to be repeated as required. Cationic exchange resins such as sodium polystyrene sulfonate may be orally or rectally administered. Persistent hyperkalemia may require dialysis.

Hyperkalemia may be fatal. It is critical to monitor and manage serum potassium in patients with severe heart failure receiving spironolactone. Avoid using other potassium-sparing diuretics. Avoid using oral potassium supplements in patients with serum potassium more than 3.5 mEq/L. RALES study excluded patients with a serum creatinine more than 2.5 mg/dL or a recent increase in serum creatinine more than 25%. The recommended monitoring for potassium and creatinine is 1 week after initiation or increase in dose of spironolactone, monthly for the first 3 months, then quarterly for a year, and then every 6 months. Discontinue or interrupt treatment for serum potassium more than 5 mEq/L or for serum creatinine more than 4 mg/dL.

➤*Fluid and electrolyte imbalance:* Serum and urine electrolyte determinations are particularly important when the patient is vomiting excessively or receiving parenteral fluids. Warning signs or symptoms of fluid and electrolyte imbalance, irrespective of cause, include dryness of the mouth, thirst, weakness, lethargy, drowsiness, restlessness, muscle pains or cramps, muscular fatigue, hypotension, oliguria, tachycardia, and GI disturbances such as nausea and vomiting. Hyperkalemia may occur in patients with impaired renal function or excessive potassium intake and can cause cardiac irregularities, which may be fatal. Consequently, no potassium supplement should ordinarily be given with spironolactone.

Periodically determine serum electrolytes to detect possible electrolyte imbalance at appropriate intervals, particularly in elderly patients and patients with significant renal or hepatic impairment.

➤*Hyperchloremic metabolic acidosis:* Reversible hyperchloremic metabolic acidosis, usually in association with hyperkalemia, has been reported to occur in some patients with decompensated hepatic cirrhosis, even in the presence of healthy renal function.

➤*Hyponatremia:* Dilutional hyponatremia, manifested by dryness of the mouth, thirst, lethargy, and drowsiness, and confirmed by a low serum sodium level, may be caused or aggravated, especially when spironolactone is administered in combination with other diuretics, and dilutional hyponatremia may occur in edematous patients in hot weather; appropriate therapy is water restriction rather than administration of sodium, except in rare instances when the hyponatremia is life-threatening.

➤*Gynecomastia:* Gynecomastia may develop in association with the use of spironolactone; health care providers should be alert to its possible onset. The development of gynecomastia appears to be related to both dosage level and duration of therapy and is normally reversible when spironolactone is discontinued. In rare instances, some breast enlargement may persist when spironolactone is discontinued.

➤*Renal effects:* Spironolactone therapy may cause a transient elevation of serum urea nitrogen (BUN), especially in patients with preexisting renal impairment. Spironolactone may cause mild acidosis.

➤*Hepatic function impairment:* Spironolactone should be used with caution in patients with impaired hepatic function because minor alterations of fluid and electrolyte balance may precipitate hepatic coma.

➤*Pregnancy: Category C. Category D* if used in gestational hypertension per Briggs' *Drugs in Pregnancy and Lactation*.

See Indications for more information.

Teratology studies with spironolactone have been carried out in mice and rabbits at dosages of up to 20 mg/kg/day. On a body surface area basis, this dose in the mouse is substantially below the maximum recommended human dose and, in the rabbit, approximates the maximum recommended human dose. No teratogenic or other embryotoxic effects were observed in mice, but the 20 mg/kg dose caused an increased rate of resorption and a lower number of live fetuses in rabbits. Because of its antiandrogenic activity and the requirement of testosterone for male morphogenesis, spironolactone may have the potential for adversely affecting sex differentiation of the male during embryogenesis. When administered to rats at 200 mg/kg/day between gestation days 13 and 21 (late embryogenesis and fetal development), feminization of male fetuses was observed. Offspring exposed during late pregnancy to 50 and 100 mg/kg/day dosages of spironolactone exhibited changes in the reproductive tract, including dose-dependent decreases in weights of the ventral prostate and seminal vesicle in males, ovaries and uteri that were enlarged in females, and other indications of endocrine dysfunction, that persisted into adulthood.

➤*Lactation:* Canrenone, a major (and active) metabolite of spironolactone, appears in human breast milk. Because spironolactone has been found to be tumorigenic in rats, decide whether to discontinue the drug, taking into account the importance of the drug to the mother. If the drug is deemed essential, institute an alternative method of infant feeding.

➤*Children:* Safety and effectiveness have not been established.

➤*Monitoring:* All patients receiving diuretic therapy should be observed for evidence of fluid or electrolyte imbalance (eg, hypomagnesemia, hyponatremia, hypochloremic alkalosis, hyperkalemia). Perform periodic determination of serum electrolytes at appropriate intervals, particularly in elderly patients and patients with significant renal or hepatic impairment.

Drug Interactions

Spironolactone Drug Interactions

Precipitant drug	Object drug[a]		Description
ACE inhibitors (eg, lisinopril), angiotensin II receptor antagonists (eg, losartan), eplerenone	Spironolactone	↑	Coadministration may lead to severe hyperkalemia. Use with caution. Use with eplerenone is contraindicated.
Spironolactone	ACE[b] inhibitors (eg, lisinopril), angiotensin II receptor antagonists (eg, losartan), eplerenone		
Alcohol, barbiturates, narcotics	Spironolactone	↑	Potentiation of orthostatic hypotension may occur.
Spironolactone	Alcohol, barbiturates, narcotics		
Corticosteroids, corticotropin (ACTH)	Spironolactone	↑	Intensified electrolyte depletion, particularly hypokalemia, may occur.
NSAIDs[b] (eg, diclofenac, indomethacin)	Spironolactone	↑↓	Effects of spironolactone may be decreased. Coadministration has also been associated with severe hyperkalemia.
Salicylates	Spironolactone	↓	The diuretic effect of spironolactone may be decreased by concurrent salicylate use.
Spironolactone	Anticoagulants (eg, warfarin)	↓	The hypoprothrombinemic effect of anticoagulants may be decreased.
Spironolactone	Digoxin	↑	Spironolactone has been shown to increase the half-life of digoxin and subsequent toxicity may occur. Monitor carefully during coadministration.
Spironolactone	Lithium	↑	Spironolactone may reduce lithium renal clearance and increase the risk of lithium toxicity.
Spironolactone	Mitotane	↓	Adrenolytic effects of mitotane may be blocked by spironolactone.
Spironolactone	Pressor amines (eg, norepinephrine)	↓	Spironolactone reduces the vascular responsiveness to norepinephrine. Exercise caution in the management of patients subjected to regional or general anesthesia while being treated with spironolactone.

SPIRONOLACTONE — ORAL

Spironolactone Drug Interactions

Precipitant drug	Object drug[a]		Description
Spironolactone	Potassium preparations, potassium-sparing diuretics (eg, triamterene)	↑	Coadministration may result in hyperkalemia, possibly with cardiac arrythmias or cardiac arrest. Avoid concurrent use.
Spironolactone	Skeletal muscle relaxants, nondepolarizing (eg, tubocurarine)	↑	Possible increased responsiveness to the muscle relaxant may result.

[a] ↑ = object drug increased; ↓ = object drug decreased; ↑↓ = object drug both increased and decreased.

[b] ACE = angiotensin-converting enzyme; NSAIDs = nonsteroidal anti-inflammatory drugs.

➤*Drug/Lab test interactions:* Several reports of possible interference with digoxin radioimmunoassays by spironolactone or its metabolites have appeared in the literature. Neither the extent nor the potential clinical significance of its interference (which may be assay-specific) has been fully established.

➤*Drug/Food interactions:* Food increased the bioavailability of unmetabolized spironolactone by almost 100%.

Adverse Reactions

➤*CNS:* Mental confusion, ataxia, headache, drowsiness, lethargy.

➤*Endocrine:* Gynecomastia, inability to achieve or maintain erection, irregular menses or amenorrhea, postmenopausal bleeding. The development of gynecomastia appears to be related to both dosage level and duration of therapy and is normally reversible when spironolactone is discontinued. In rare instances, some breast enlargement may persist when spironolactone is discontinued. Carcinoma of the breast has been reported in patients taking spironolactone, but a cause and effect relationship has not been established.

➤*GI:* Diarrhea and cramping, gastric bleeding, gastritis, nausea, ulceration, vomiting.

➤*Hepatic:* A very few cases of mixed cholestatic/hepatocellular toxicity, with 1 reported fatality, have been reported with spironolactone administration.

➤*Hypersensitivity:* Anaphylactic reactions, fever, maculopapular or erythematous cutaneous eruptions, urticaria, vasculitis.

➤*Miscellaneous:* Agranulocytosis, hyperkalemia, renal dysfunction (including renal failure).

Overdosage

➤*Symptoms:*

Animal toxicology – Acute overdosage of spironolactone may be manifested by drowsiness, mental confusion, maculopapular or erythematous rash, nausea, vomiting, dizziness, or diarrhea. Rarely, instances of hyponatremia, hyperkalemia, or hepatic coma may occur in patients with severe liver disease, but these are unlikely due to acute overdosage. Hyperkalemia may occur, especially in patients with impaired renal function.

➤*Treatment:* Evacuate the stomach by lavage. There is no specific antidote. Treatment is supportive to maintain hydration, electrolyte balance, and vital functions.

Patients who have renal impairment may develop spironolactone-induced hyperkalemia. In such cases, discontinue spironolactone immediately. With severe hyperkalemia, the clinical situation dictates the procedures to be employed. These include the intravenous administration of calcium chloride solution, sodium bicarbonate solution, and/or the oral or parenteral administration of glucose with a rapid-acting insulin preparation. These are temporary measures to be repeated as required. Cationic exchange resins such as sodium polystyrene sulfonate may be orally or rectally administered. Persistent hyperkalemia may require dialysis.

Patient Information

Advise patients who receive spironolactone to avoid potassium supplements and foods containing high levels of potassium, including salt substitutes.

Advise patients to notify health care provider if any of the following occurs: muscular weakness, fatigue, muscle cramps. May cause drowsiness, headache, or mental confusion. Instruct patients to observe caution while driving or performing other tasks requiring alertness.

TRIAMTERENE

Rx	Dyrenium (SmithKline Beecham)	Capsules: 50 mg	(Dyrenium 50). Red. In 100s and UD 100s.
		100 mg	(Dyrenium 100). Red. In 100s, 1000s and UD 100s.

TRIAMTERENE — ORAL

Refer to the general discussion of these agents in the Potassium-Sparing Diuretics introduction.

Indications

➤*Edema:* For the treatment of edema associated with congestive heart failure, cirrhosis of the liver and the nephrotic syndrome; also in steroid-induced edema, idiopathic edema and edema due to secondary hyperaldosteronism.

➤*Off-label uses:*

Pediatric hypertension – [3] = Safety concerns. Triamterene is among the therapeutic options for pediatric hypertension identified by the National High Blood Pressure Education Program, based on expert opinion.

Administration and Dosage

➤*General dosing considerations:* Triamterene may be used alone or with other diuretics either for its added diuretic effect or its potassium-sparing potential. It also promotes increased diuresis when patients prove resistant or only partially responsive to thiazides or other diuretics because of secondary hyperaldosteronism.

Dosage should be titrated to the needs of the individual patient.

➤*Adults:*

Edema –

Maximum dose: The total daily dosage should not exceed 300 mg/day.

Initial dosage: When used alone, the usual starting dose is 100 mg twice daily after meals.

Concomitant therapy: When combined with another diuretic or antihypertensive agent, the total daily dosage of each agent should usually be lowered initially and adjusted to the patient's needs.

When triamterene is added to other diuretic therapy or when patients are switched to triamterene from other diuretics, all potassium supplementation should be discontinued.

➤*Children:*

Off-label dosing –

Pediatric hypertension: [3] = Safety concerns.

- *1 to 17 years of age* –
  - *Maximum dose:* 3 to 4 mg/kg/day, up to 300 mg/day.
  - *Initial dosage:* 1 to 2 mg/kg/day orally, divided for twice-daily administration.

➤*Storage/Stability:* Store between 15° and 30°C (59° and 86°F). Protect from light.

Actions

➤*Pharmacology:* Triamterene has a unique mode of action; it inhibits the reabsorption of sodium ions in exchange for potassium and hydrogen ions at that segment of the distal tubule under the control of adrenal mineralocorticoids (especially aldosterone). This activity is not directly related to aldosterone secretion or antagonism; it is a result of a direct effect on the renal tubule.

The fraction of filtered sodium reaching this distal tubular exchange site is relatively small, and the amount that is exchanged depends on the level of mineralocorticoid activity. Thus, the degree of natriuresis and diuresis produced by inhibition of the exchange mechanism is necessarily limited. Increasing the amount of available sodium and the level of mineralocorticoid activity by the use of more proximally acting diuretics will increase the degree of diuresis and potassium conservation.

Triamterene occasionally causes increases in serum potassium, which can result in hyperkalemia. It does not produce alkalosis because it does not cause excessive excretion of titratable acid and ammonium.

Triamterene has been shown to cross the placental barrier and appear in the cord blood of animals.

➤*Pharmacokinetics:*

Absorption/Distribution – Onset of action is 2 to 4 hours after ingestion. In healthy volunteers the mean peak serum levels were 30 ng/mL at 3 hours. Triamterene is rapidly absorbed, with somewhat less than 50% of the oral dose reaching the urine. Most patients will respond to triamterene during the first day of treatment. Maximum therapeutic effect, however, may not be seen for several days.

Metabolism/Excretion – Triamterene is primarily metabolized to the sulfate conjugate of hydroxytriamterene. Both the plasma and urine levels of this metabolite greatly exceed triamterene levels. The average percent of drug recovered in the urine (0 to 48 hours) was 21%. Duration of diuresis depends on several factors, especially renal function, but it generally tapers off 7 to 9 hours after administration.

Contraindications

Anuria. Severe or progressive kidney disease or dysfunction with the possible exception of nephrosis. Severe hepatic disease. Hypersensitivity to the drug.

Triamterene should not be used in patients with preexisting elevated serum potassium, as is sometimes seen in patients with impaired renal function or azotemia, or in patients who develop hyperkalemia while on the drug. Patients should not be placed on dietary potassium supplements, potassium salts or potassium-containing salt substitutes in conjunction with triamterene.

TRIAMTERENE — ORAL

Triamterene should not be given to patients receiving other potassium-sparing agents such as spironolactone, amiloride hydrochloride or other formulations containing triamterene. Two deaths have been reported in patients receiving concomitant spironolactone and triamterene or formulations containing triamterene. Although dosage recommendations were exceeded in 1 case and in the other serum electrolytes were not properly monitored, these 2 drugs should not be given concomitantly.

Warnings/Precautions

➤*Hyperkalemia:* Abnormal elevation of serum potassium levels (≥ 5.5 mEq/L) can occur with all potassium-sparing agents, including triamterene. Hyperkalemia is more likely to occur in patients with renal impairment and diabetes (even without evidence of renal impairment), and in the elderly or severely ill. Since uncorrected hyperkalemia may be fatal, serum potassium levels must be monitored at frequent intervals especially in patients receiving triamterene, when dosages are changed or with any illness that may influence renal function.

If hyperkalemia is present or suspected, an electrocardiogram (ECG) should be obtained. If the ECG shows no widening of the QRS or arrhythmia in the presence of hyperkalemia, it is usually sufficient to discontinue triamterene and any potassium supplementation and substitute a thiazide alone. Sodium polystyrene sulfonate may be administered to enhance the excretion of excess potassium. The presence of a widened QRS complex or arrhythmia in association with hyperkalemia requires prompt additional therapy. For tachyarrhythmia, infuse 44 mEq of sodium bicarbonate or 10 mL of 10% calcium gluconate or calcium chloride over several minutes. For asystole, bradycardia or A-V block transvenous pacing is also recommended.

The effect of calcium and sodium bicarbonate is transient and repeated administration may be required. When indicated by the clinical situation, excess K+ may be removed by dialysis or oral or rectal administration of sodium polystyrene sulfonate. Infusion of glucose and insulin has also been used to treat hyperkalemia.

➤*Electrolyte imbalance:* Electrolyte imbalance often encountered in such diseases as congestive heart failure, renal disease or cirrhosis may be aggravated or caused independently by any effective diuretic agent including triamterene. The use of full doses of a diuretic when salt intake is restricted can result in a low-salt syndrome.

➤*Nitrogen retention:* Triamterene can cause mild nitrogen retention, which is reversible upon withdrawal of the drug and is seldom observed with intermittent (every-other-day) therapy.

➤*Metabolic acidosis:* Triamterene may cause a decreasing alkali reserve with the possibility of metabolic acidosis.

➤*Hematologic effects:* By the very nature of their illness, cirrhotics with splenomegaly sometimes have marked variations in their blood pictures. Since triamterene is a weak folic acid antagonist, it may contribute to the appearance of megaloblastosis in cases where folic acid stores have been depleted. Therefore, periodic blood studies in these patients are recommended. They should also be observed for exacerbations of underlying liver disease.

➤*Uric acid:* Triamterene has elevated uric acid, especially in persons predisposed to gouty arthritis.

➤*Renal stones:* Triamterene has been reported in renal stones in association with other calculus components. Triamterene should be used with caution in patients with histories of renal stones.

➤*Hypersensitivity reactions:* There have been isolated reports of hypersensitivity reactions; therefore, patients should be observed regularly for the possible occurrence of blood dyscrasias, liver damage or other idiosyncratic reactions.

➤*Special risk:* Triamterene tends to conserve potassium rather than to promote the excretion as do many diuretics and, occasionally, can cause increases in serum potassium which, in some instances, can result in hyperkalemia. In rare instances, hyperkalemia has been associated with cardiac irregularities.

➤*Pregnancy: Category C. Category D* if used in gestational hypertension per Briggs' *Drugs in Pregnancy and Lactation*.

The routine use of diuretics in an otherwise healthy woman is inappropriate and exposes mother and fetus to unnecessary hazard. Diuretics do not prevent development of toxemia of pregnancy, and there is no satisfactory evidence that they are useful in the treatment of developed toxemia.

Edema during pregnancy may arise from pathological causes or from the physiologic and mechanical consequences of pregnancy. Diuretics are indicated in pregnancy when edema is due to pathologic causes, just as they are in the absence of pregnancy (see Precautions). Dependent edema in pregnancy, resulting from restriction of venous return by the expanded uterus, is properly treated through elevation of the lower extremities and use of support hose; use of diuretics to lower intravascular volume in this case is illogical and unnecessary. There is hypervolemia during healthy pregnancy that is harmful to neither the fetus nor the mother (in the absence of cardiovascular disease), but that is associated with edema, including generalized edema, in the majority of pregnant women. If this edema produces discomfort, increased recumbency will often provide relief. In rare instances, this edema may cause extreme discomfort which is not relieved by rest. In these cases, a short course of diuretics may provide relief and may be appropriate.

Reproduction studies have been performed in rats at doses as high as 20 times the MRHD on the basis of body weight, and 6 times the MRHD on the basis of body surface area without evidence of harm to the fetus due to triamterene. Because animal reproduction studies are not always predictive of human response, this drug should be used during pregnancy only if clearly needed.

Triamterene has been shown to cross the placental barrier and appear in the cord blood. The use of triamterene in pregnant women requires that the anticipated benefits be weighed against possible hazards to the fetus. These possible hazards include adverse reactions that have occurred in the adult.

➤*Lactation:* Triamterene has not been studied in nursing mothers. Triamterene appears in animal milk and is likely present in human milk. If use of the drug product is deemed essential, the patient should stop nursing.

➤*Children:* Safety and effectiveness have not been established.

➤*Lab test abnormalities:* Hyperkalemia will rarely occur in patients with adequate urinary output, but it is a possibility if large doses are used for considerable periods of time. If hyperkalemia is observed, triamterene should be withdrawn. The healthy adult range of serum potassium is 3.5 to 5 mEq/L with 4.5 mEq often being used for a reference point. Potassium levels persistently above 6 mEq/L require careful observation and treatment. Normal potassium levels tend to be higher in neonates (7.7 mEq/L) than in adults.

Serum potassium levels do not necessarily indicate true body potassium concentration. A rise in plasma pH may cause a decrease in plasma potassium concentration and an increase in the intracellular potassium concentration. Because triamterene conserves potassium, it has been theorized that in patients who have received intensive therapy or been given the drug for prolonged periods, a rebound kaliuresis could occur upon abrupt withdrawal. In such patients, withdrawal of triamterene should be gradual.

➤*Monitoring:* Periodic BUN and serum potassium determinations should be made to check kidney function, especially in patients with suspected or confirmed renal insufficiency. It is particularly important to make serum potassium determinations in elderly or diabetic patients receiving the drug; these patients should be observed carefully for possible serum potassium increases.

Drug Interactions

Triamterene Drug Interactions

Precipitant drug	Object drug[a]		Description
Triamterene	Amantadine	↑	Amantadine plasma levels may increase and urinary excretion may decrease, possibly increasing the risk for developing adverse effects.
Triamterene	Potassium preparations	↑	Concurrent administration may result in severe hyperkalemia, possibly with cardiac arrhythmias or cardiac arrest. Avoid concomitant use.
ACE inhibitors	Triamterene	↑	Use of ACE inhibitors may elevate serum potassium. Concurrent use with triamterene may lead to significant hyperkalemia.
Cimetidine	Triamterene	↑	Cimetidine may increase the bioavailability and decrease the renal clearance and hydroxylation of triamterene.
Indomethacin	Triamterene	↑	Rapid progress into acute renal failure has occurred with concurrent use. Use this combination only when clearly needed.

[a] ↑ = object drug increased.

Caution should be used when lithium and diuretics are used concomitantly because diuretic-induced sodium loss may reduce the renal clearance of lithium and increase serum lithium levels with risk of lithium toxicity. Patients receiving such combined therapy should have serum lithium levels monitored closely and the lithium dosage adjusted if necessary.

The effects of the following drugs may be potentiated when given together with triamterene: Antihypertensive medication, other diuretics, preanesthetic and anesthetic agents, skeletal muscle relaxants (nondepolarizing).

Triamterene may raise blood glucose levels; for adult-onset diabetes, dosage adjustments of hypoglycemic agents may be necessary during and after therapy; concurrent use with chlorpropamide may increase the risk of severe hyponatremia.

➤*Drug/Lab test interactions:* Triamterene and quinidine have similar fluorescence spectra; thus, triamterene will interfere with the fluorescent measurement of quinidine.

Adverse Reactions

Adverse reactions are listed below. All adverse reactions occur rarely (that is, 1 in 1000, or less).

➤*CNS:* Weakness, fatigue, dizziness, headache, dry mouth.

➤*GI:* Jaundice or liver enzyme abnormalities, nausea and vomiting, diarrhea.

➤*Hematologic:* Thrombocytopenia, megaloblastic anemia.

➤*Hypersensitivity:* Anaphylaxis, rash, photosensitivity.

TRIAMTERENE — ORAL

➤*Metabolic:* Hyperkalemia, hypokalemia.

➤*Renal:* Azotemia, elevated BUN and creatinine, renal stones, acute interstitial nephritis (rare), acute renal failure (1 case of irreversible renal failure has been reported).

Overdosage

➤*Symptoms:* In the event of overdosage it can be theorized that electrolyte imbalance would be the major concern, with particular attention to possible hyperkalemia. Other symptoms that might be seen would be nausea and vomiting, other GI disturbances and weakness. It is conceivable that some hypotension could occur.

➤*Treatment:* Immediate evacuation of the stomach should be induced through emesis and gastric lavage. Careful evaluation of the electrolyte pattern and fluid balance should be made. There is no specific antidote.

Reversible acute renal failure following ingestion of 50 tablets of a product containing a combination of 50 mg triamterene and 25 mg hydrochlorothiazide has been reported. The oral LD_{50} in mice is 380 mg/kg. The amount of drug in a single dose ordinarily associated with symptoms of overdose or likely to be life-threatening is not known. Although triamterene is 67% protein-bound, there may be some benefit to dialysis in cases of overdosage.

Patient Information

To help avoid stomach upset, it is recommended that the drug be taken after meals. If a single daily dose is prescribed, it may be preferable to take it in the morning to minimize the effect of increased frequency of urination on nighttime sleep.

If a dose is missed, the patient should not take more than the prescribed dose at the next dosing interval.The fourth report on the diagnosis, evaluation, and treatment of high blood pressure in children and adolescents.

Indications

➤*Glaucoma:* For adjunctive treatment of chronic simple (open-angle) glaucoma and secondary glaucoma; preoperatively in acute angle-closure glaucoma when delay of surgery is desired to lower intraocular pressure (IOP).

➤*Acetazolamide:*

Tablets and extended-release capsules – For the prevention or amelioration of symptoms associated with acute mountain sickness in climbers attempting rapid ascent and in those who are susceptible to acute mountain sickness despite gradual ascent.

Tablets and injection only – For adjunctive treatment of edema due to chronic heart failure (CHF), drug-induced edema and centrencephalic epilepsy (petit mal, unlocalized seizures).

➤*Off-label uses:* Refer to individual monographs for further information.

Familial periodic paralysis –
Acetazolamide: [4] = Insufficient documentation.

Malignant glaucoma –
Acetazolamide: [4] = Insufficient documentation.

Prevention of cystine renal calculi (adjunctive therapy) –
Acetazolamide: [4] = Insufficient documentation.

Prevention of migraine (adults) –
Acetazolamide: [4] = Insufficient documentation.

Prevention of uric acid renal calculi (adjunctive therapy) –
Acetazolamide: [4] = Insufficient documentation.

Tardive dyskinesia –
Acetazolamide: [4] = Insufficient documentation.

Actions

➤*Pharmacology:* These agents are nonbacteriostatic sulfonamides that inhibit the enzyme carbonic anhydrase. This action reduces the rate of aqueous humor formation, resulting in decreased IOP. This action is independent of systemic acid-base balance.

By inhibiting hydrogen ion secretion by the renal tubule, these agents cause increased excretion of sodium, potassium, bicarbonate and water, thus producing an alkaline diuresis. Carbonic anhydrase inhibitors (CAIs) cause a decrease in renal blood flow and glomerular filtration rate. Redistribution of flow to the renal cortex occurs. These changes are mild and unrelated to diuretic activity.

Evidence seems to indicate that **acetazolamide** has utility as an adjuvant in the treatment of certain dysfunctions of the CNS (eg, epilepsy). Inhibition of carbonic anhydrase in this area appears to retard abnormal, paroxysmal, excessive discharge from CNS neurons.

➤*Pharmacokinetics:*

Pharmacokinetics of Carbonic Anhydrase Inhibitors

CAI	IOP Lowering Effects: Onset (h)	Peak effect (h)	Duration (h)	Relative inhibitor potency
Acetazolamide				
Tablets	1 to 1.5	1 to 4	8 to 12	1
Extended-release capsules	2	3 to 6	18 to 24	
Injection (IV)	2 min	15 min	4 to 5	
Methazolamide	2 to 4	6 to 8	10 to 18	–[a]

[a] Quantitative data not available; reported to be more active than acetazolamide.

Methazolamide – Peak plasma concentrations for the 25, 50 and 100 mg twice daily regimens were 2.5, 5.1 and 10.7 mcg/mL, respectively. Approximately 55% is bound to plasma proteins. The mean steady-state plasma elimination half-life is approximately 14 hours. At steady state approximately 25% of the dose is recovered unchanged in the urine. Renal clearance accounts for 20% to 25% of the total clearance of drug. After repeated dosing, methazolamide accumulates to steady-state concentrations in 7 days.

Contraindications

Hypersensitivity to these agents; depressed sodium and/or potassium serum levels; marked kidney and liver disease or dysfunction; suprarenal gland failure; hyperchloremic acidosis; adrenocortical insufficiency; cirrhosis (**acetazolamide, methazolamide**); long-term use in chronic noncongestive angle-closure glaucoma.

Warnings/Precautions

➤*Electrolyte imbalances:* Electrolyte imbalances, including hyponatremia, hypokalemia, and metabolic acidosis, may occur. Hypokalemia may develop when severe cirrhosis is present, during concomitant use of steroids or adrenocorticotropic hormone, and with interference with adequate oral electrolyte intake. Hypokalemia can sensitize or exaggerate the response of the heart to the toxic effects of digitalis (eg, increased ventricular irritability). Hypokalemia may be avoided or treated with potassium supplements or foods with high potassium content.

➤*Dose increases:* Increasing the dose of **acetazolamide** does not increase diuresis and may increase drowsiness or paresthesia; it often results in decreased diuresis. However, very large doses have been given with other diuretics to promote diuresis in complete refractory failure.

➤*Pulmonary conditions:* These drugs may precipitate or aggravate acidosis. Use with caution in patients with pulmonary obstruction or emphysema when alveolar ventilation may be impaired.

➤*Cross-sensitivity:* Cross-sensitivity between antibacterial sulfonamides and sulfonamide derivative diuretics, including **acetazolamide** and various thiazides, has been reported.

➤*Diabetes:* Both increase and decrease in blood glucose have occurred with **acetazolamide** administration.

➤*Hypersensitivity reactions:* Fatalities have occurred, although rarely, due to severe reactions to sulfonamides, including Stevens-Johnson syndrome, toxic epidermal necrolysis, fulminant hepatic necrosis, agranulocytosis, aplastic anemia, and other blood dyscrasias. If signs of hypersensitivity or other serious reactions occur, discontinue use of this drug.

➤*Renal function impairment:* Use **acetazolamide** with caution in patients with conditions that are associated with or predispose a patient to electrolyte and acid/base imbalances, such as impaired renal function.

➤*Hepatic function impairment:* Use of **methazolamide** in this condition may precipitate hepatic coma.

➤*Pregnancy: Category C.* Animal studies with some of these drugs have demonstrated teratogenicity (skeletal anomalies). Do not use during pregnancy, especially during the first trimester, unless the potential benefits outweigh the potential hazards.

➤*Lactation:* Safety for use in the nursing mother has not been established. It is not known whether all carbonic anhydrase inhibitors are excreted in breast milk. **Acetazolamide** appeared in breast milk of a patient taking 500 mg twice daily. However, the infant ingested only 0.06% of the dose, an amount unlikely to cause adverse reactions. The American Academy of Pediatrics classifies **acetazolamide** as compatible with breast-feeding.

➤*Children:* Safety and efficacy for use in children have not been established; safety and efficacy of **acetazolamide** extended-release capsules have not been established in children younger than 12 years of age.

➤*Elderly:* Metabolic acidosis, which can be severe, may occur in the elderly with reduced renal function.

➤*Monitoring:* Obtain baseline complete blood cell count and platelet counts before therapy and at regular intervals during therapy. Periodic monitoring of serum electrolytes is recommended.

Drug Interactions

CAI Drug Interactions

Precipitant drug	Object drug[a]		Description
Acetazolamide	Cyclosporine	⬆	Increased trough cyclosporine levels with possible nephrotoxicity and neurotoxicity may occur.
Acetazolamide	Primidone	⬇	Primidone serum and urine concentrations may be decreased.

CAI Drug Interactions

Precipitant drug	Object drug[a]		Description
CAIs	Salicylates	↑	Concurrent use may result in accumulation and toxicity of the CAI, including CNS depression and metabolic acidosis. Also, CAI-induced acidosis may allow increased CNS penetration by salicylates.
Salicylates	CAIs	↑	
Diflunisal	CAIs	↑	Concurrent use may result in a significant decrease in intraocular pressure; the effect may be less pronounced with methazolamide. Increased side effects may also occur.

[a] ↑ = object drug increased; ↓ = object drug decreased.

Adverse Reactions

Sulfonamide-type adverse reactions may occur (see Systemic Sulfonamides monograph in the Anti-Infectives chapter).

➤*CNS:* Ataxia, confusion, convulsions, depression, disorientation, dizziness, drowsiness, excitement, fatigue, headache, lassitude, malaise, nervousness, paresthesias of the extremities, tremor, weakness.

➤*GI:* Anorexia, constipation, diarrhea, loss of appetite, melena, nausea, taste alteration, vomiting.

➤*GU:* Crystalluria, glycosuria, hematuria, nephrolithiasis with long-term acetazolamide therapy, phosphaturia, polyuria, renal calculi, renal colic, renal failure, urinary frequency.

➤*Hematologic:* Agranulocytosis, aplastic anemia, bone marrow depression, hemolytic anemia, leukopenia, pancytopenia, thrombocytopenia, thrombocytopenic purpura.

➤*Hepatic:* Abnormal liver function, cholestatic jaundice, fulminant hepatic necrosis, hepatic insufficiency.

➤*Hypersensitivity:* Allergic skin reactions, including erythema multiforme, photosensitivity, Stevens-Johnson syndrome, toxic epidermal necrolysis, urticaria; anaphylaxis; pruritus; rash.

➤*Metabolic:* Metabolic acidosis, electrolyte imbalance (hypokalemia, hyponatremia), hyperglycemia, hypoglycemia.

➤*Special senses:* Hearing dysfunction, tinnitus, transient myopia.

➤*Miscellaneous:* Decreased/absent libido, electrolyte imbalance, fever, flaccid paralysis, flushing, growth retardation in children, hepatic insufficiency, impotence, pain at injection site, transient myopia, weight loss.

Overdosage

➤*Symptoms:* Symptoms of overdosage or toxicity may include anorexia, ataxia, development of an acidosis state, dizziness, drowsiness, electrolyte imbalances, nausea, paresthesias, tinnitus, tremor, and vomiting.

➤*Treatment:* In the event of overdosage, perform gastric lavage. The electrolyte disturbance most likely to be encountered from overdosage is hyperchloremic acidosis that may respond to bicarbonate administration. Potassium supplementation may be required. Observe carefully; give supportive treatment.

Patient Information

Advise patient that if GI upset occurs, to take with food.

Instruct patient to avoid prolonged exposure to sunlight or sunlamps; this medicine may cause photosensitivity.

This medicine may cause drowsiness; advise patients to observe caution while driving or performing other tasks requiring alertness, coordination, or physical dexterity.

Instruct patient to notify health care provider if sore throat, fever, unusual bleeding or bruising, tingling or tremors in the hands or feet, flank or loin pain, or skin rash occurs.

Inform patients with diabetes that both increases and decreases in blood glucose may occur.

ACETAZOLAMIDE

Rx	**Acetazolamide** (Various, eg, Taro)	**Tablets; oral:** 125 mg	May contain glycerin and/or lactose. In 100s.
Rx	**Acetazolamide** (Various, eg, Lannett, Taro)	**Tablets; oral:** 250 mg	May contain glycerin and/or lactose. In 100s, 500s, and 1,000s.
Rx	**Acetazolamide** (Various, eg, Barr Labs, ZyGenerics)	**Capsules, extended-release; oral:** 500 mg	In 100s and 1,000s.
Rx	**Diamox Sequels** (Barr)		(Diamox 754). Orange, opaque. In 100s.
Rx	**Acetazolamide** (Various, eg, Bedford Labs)	**Injection, lyophilized powder for solution:** 500 mg	As acetazolamide sodium. Preservative free. In vials.

ACETAZOLAMIDE — ORAL

For complete and comparative prescribing information, see Carbonic Anhydrase Inhibitors class monograph.

WARNING

Fatalities have occurred, although rarely, because of severe reactions to sulfonamides, including Stevens-Johnson syndrome, toxic epidermal necrolysis, fulminant hepatic necrosis, agranulocytosis, and aplastic anemia and other blood dyscrasias. Sensitizations may recur when a sulfonamide is readministered, irrespective of the route of administration. If signs of hypersensitivity or other serious reactions occur, discontinue use of this drug.

Caution is advised for patients receiving concomitant high-dose aspirin and acetazolamide because anorexia, tachypnea, lethargy, coma, and death have been reported.

Indications

➤*Acute mountain sickness:* For the prevention or amelioration of symptoms associated with acute mountain sickness in climbers attempting rapid ascent and in those who are very susceptible to acute mountain sickness, despite gradual ascent.

➤*Edema (tablets only):* For adjunctive treatment of edema because of congestive heart failure; drug-induced edema.

➤*Glaucoma:* For adjunctive treatment of chronic simple (open-angle) glaucoma, secondary glaucoma, and preoperatively in acute angle-closure glaucoma where delay of surgery is desired in order to lower intraocular pressure.

➤*Seizures (tablets only):* For adjunctive treatment of centrencephalic epilepsies (petit mal, unlocalized seizures).

➤*Off-label uses:*

Familial periodic paralysis – [4] = Insufficient documentation. Limited data from controlled trials and case reports suggest that acetazolamide may have some benefit in the treatment of hypokalemic and hyperkalemic periodic paralysis. Studies have shown that acetazolamide improves muscle strength in patients with hypokalemic periodic paralysis. In patients with hyperkalemic periodic paralysis, acetazolamide may decrease the steady-state potassium exchange rates and increase potassium uptake by other tissues, resulting in protection from hyperkalemic paralysis.

Malignant glaucoma – [4] = Insufficient documentation. Acetazolamide has been used only in combination therapy for the treatment of malignant glaucoma. In case reports, adjunctive therapy with acetazolamide showed no definite benefit in reducing intraocular pressure, and more invasive surgical measures were required. However, none of the cases followed the dosage recommendations of 250 mg 4 times per day. A review article reported that 5 days of treatment with a combination of carbonic anhydrase inhibitors, hyperosmotic agents, and mydriatic-cycloplegic drops is effective in treating half of malignant glaucoma cases. However, no trials or case reports supporting this claim could be identified.

Prevention of cystine renal calculi (adjunctive therapy) – [4] = Insufficient documentation. Case reports suggest that acetazolamide may have some benefits as adjunctive therapy in the management of alkalinizing the urine. However, these reports did not conclude that the use of acetazolamide was safe or effective at preventing cystine renal calculi formation.

Prevention of migraine (adults) – [4] = Insufficient documentation. Although poorly tolerated, data from a recent noncontrolled trial suggest acetazolamide may be effective for migraine prophylaxis in adults. However, an earlier controlled trial showed no benefit compared with placebo and was stopped early because of safety concerns. Additional data are needed to determine the optimal dosing regimen, the patient population that would most benefit from therapy, and the safety profile. Until these data are available, acetazolamide should not be routinely used for this indication.

Prevention of uric acid renal calculi (adjunctive therapy) – [4] = Insufficient documentation. Published case reports suggest that acetazolamide may have some benefits as adjunctive therapy in urine alkalinization. However, these reports did not conclude that the use of acetazolamide was safe or effective at preventing uric acid renal calculi from forming.

Tardive dyskinesia – [4] = Insufficient documentation. There is very little evidence on the use of acetazolamide in the treatment of tardive dyskinesia. One clinical trial demonstrated possible efficacy in reducing symptoms of tardive dyskinesia; however, additional controlled trials are needed to verify these results. Furthermore, thiamine is recommended with acetazolamide to prevent the formation of kidney stones. Also, because there was a complete relapse in every incident within a week of discontinuing this medication, it is thought that this medication is palliative therapy, not curative.

ACETAZOLAMIDE — ORAL

Administration and Dosage

➤*Adults:*

Acute congestive (closed-angle) glaucoma –

Extended-release capsules:

• *Usual dosage* – 500 mg 2 times a day.

• *Dosage adjustment* – It may be necessary to adjust the dose, but it has usually been found that a dose in excess of 1 g does not produce an increased effect. The dosage should be adjusted with careful individual attention both to symptomatology and intraocular tension. In all cases, continuous supervision by a health care provider is advisable.

• *Conversion* – In those unusual instances in which adequate control is not obtained by the twice-a-day administration of acetazolamide extended-release capsules, the desired control may be established by means of tablets or parenteral.

Tablets:

• *Usual dosage* – 250 mg every 4 hours, although some cases have responded to 250 mg twice daily on short-term therapy. In some acute cases, it may be more satisfactory to administer an initial dose of 500 mg followed by 125 or 250 mg every 4 hours, depending on the individual case.

• *Concomitant therapy* – A complementary effect has been noted when used in conjunction with miotics or mydriatics as the case demanded.

Acute mountain sickness –

Usual dosage: 500 to 1,000 mg daily in divided doses using tablets or extended-release capsules as appropriate. In circumstances of rapid ascent, such as in rescue or military operations, the higher dose level of 1,000 mg is recommended. It is preferable to initiate dosing 24 to 48 hours before ascent.

Duration of therapy: Continue for 48 hours while at high altitude, or longer as necessary to control symptoms.

Chronic simple (open-angle) glaucoma –

Extended-release capsules: See Acute Congestive (Closed-Angle) Glaucoma for dosing.

Tablets:

• *Usual dosage* – 250 mg to 1 g/day, usually in divided doses for amounts over 250 mg. It has usually been found that a dose in excess of 1 g per 24 hours does not produce an increased effect.

• *Dosage adjustment* – The dosage should be adjusted with careful individual attention both to symptomatology and ocular tension.

Congestive heart failure –

Tablets:

• *Initial dosage* – 250 to 375 mg once daily in the morning (5 mg/kg).

• *Dosage adjustment* – If, after an initial response, the patient fails to continue to lose edema fluid, do not increase the dose but allow for kidney recovery by skipping medication for a day. Acetazolamide yields best diuretic results when given on alternate days, or for 2 days alternating with a day of rest. Failures in therapy may be because of overdosage or too frequent dosage.

• *Concomitant therapy* – The use of acetazolamide does not eliminate the need for other therapy such as digitalis, bed rest, and salt restriction.

Drug-induced edema –

Tablets: 250 to 375 mg once a day for 1 or 2 days, alternating with a day of rest.

Secondary glaucoma –

Extended-release capsules: See Acute Congestive (Closed-Angle) Glaucoma.

Tablets: See Acute Congestive (Closed-Angle) Glaucoma for dosing.

Seizures –

Tablets:

• *Usual dosage* – 8 to 30 mg/kg in divided doses. Although some patients respond to a low dose, the optimum range appears to be from 375 to 1,000 mg daily. However, some investigators feel that daily doses in excess of 1 g do not produce any better results than a 1 g dose.

• *Concomitant therapy* – When given in combination with other anticonvulsants, it is suggested that the starting dosage should be 250 mg once daily in addition to the existing medications. This can be increased to levels as previously indicated.

Off-label dosing –

Familial periodic paralysis: [4] = Insufficient documentation. As monotherapy, the following dosage regimens have been studied: 120 mg twice daily, 250 mg/day, 125 mg 3 times daily, and 250 mg every 6 hours for up to 2 weeks.

Malignant glaucoma: [4] = Insufficient documentation. 250 mg orally 4 times daily as adjunctive therapy has been recommended, although lesser dosages have been used.

Prevention of cystine renal calculi (adjunctive therapy): [4] = Insufficient documentation. 250 to 500 mg at bedtime.

Prevention of migraine (adults): [4] = Insufficient documentation. 62.5 to 250 mg twice daily.

Prevention of uric acid renal calculi (adjunctive therapy): [4] = Insufficient documentation. 250 to 500 mg at bedtime.

Tardive dyskinesia: [4] = Insufficient documentation. 2 g daily in 3 divided doses, plus thiamine 1.5 g daily in 3 divided doses given concomitantly.

➤*Children:*

Extended-release capsules –

12 years of age and older:

• *Acute mountain sickness –*

Usual dosage: 500 to 1,000 mg daily, in divided doses as appropriate. In circumstances of rapid ascent, such as in rescue or military operations, the higher dose level of 1,000 mg is recommended. It is preferable to initiate dosing 24 to 48 hours before ascent.

Concomitant therapy: Continue for 48 hours while at high altitude, or longer as necessary to control symptoms.

• *Glaucoma –*

Usual dosage: 500 mg 2 times a day.

Dosage adjustment: It may be necessary to adjust the dose, but it has usually been found that a dose in excess of 1 g does not produce an increased effect. The dosage should be adjusted with careful individual attention both to symptomatology and intraocular tension. In all cases, continuous supervision by a health care provider is advisable.

➤*Elderly:*

Off-label dosing –

Tardive dyskinesia: [4] = Insufficient documentation. 1.5 g daily in 3 divided doses, plus thiamine 1.5 g daily in 3 divided doses given concomitantly.

➤*Administration:*

Extended-release capsules – Usually 1 capsule is administered in the morning and 1 capsule in the evening.

➤*Storage/Stability:* Store tablets and capsules at 20° to 25°C (68° to 77°F). Excursions for tablets are permitted to 15° to 30°C (59° to 86°F).

ACETAZOLAMIDE SODIUM — INJECTION

For complete and comparative prescribing information, see Carbonic Anhydrase Inhibitors class monograph.

Indications

➤*Edema:* For adjunctive treatment of edema caused by congestive heart failure; drug-induced edema.

➤*Glaucoma:* For the adjunctive treatment of chronic simple (open-angle) glaucoma, secondary glaucoma, and preoperatively in acute angle-closure glaucoma where delay of surgery is desired in order to lower intraocular pressure.

➤*Seizures:* For the adjunctive treatment of centrencephalic epilepsies (petit mal, unlocalized seizures).

➤*Off-label uses:*

Familial periodic paralysis – [4] = Insufficient documentation. Limited data from controlled trials and case reports suggest that acetazolamide may have some benefit in the treatment of hypokalemic and hyperkalemic periodic paralysis. Studies have shown that acetazolamide improves muscle strength in patients with hypokalemic periodic paralysis. In patients with hyperkalemic periodic paralysis, acetazolamide may decrease the steady-state potassium exchange rates and increase potassium uptake by other tissues, resulting in protection from hyperkalemic paralysis.

Prevention of migraine (adults): [4] = Insufficient documentation. Although poorly tolerated, data from a recent noncontrolled trial suggest acetazolamide may be effective for migraine prophylaxis in adults. However, an earlier controlled trial showed no benefit compared with placebo and was stopped early because of safety concerns. Additional data are needed to determine the optimal dosing regimen, the patient population that would most benefit from therapy, and the safety profile. Until these data are available, acetazolamide should not be routinely used for this indication.

Administration and Dosage

➤*Adults:*

Acute congestive (closed-angle) glaucoma –

Usual dosage: 250 mg intravenous (IV) every 4 hours, although some cases have responded to 250 mg IV twice daily on short-term therapy. In some acute cases, it may be more satisfactory to administer an initial dose of 500 mg followed by 125 or 250 mg every 4 hours, depending on the individual case.

Concomitant therapy: A complementary effect has been noted when used in conjunction with miotics or mydriatics, as the case demanded.

Congestive heart failure –

Initial dosage: 250 to 375 mg IV once daily in the morning (5 mg/kg).

Dosage adjustment: If the patient fails to continue to lose edema fluid after an initial response, do not increase the dose; allow for kidney recovery by skipping medication for a day. Acetazolamide yields best diuretic results when given on alternate days or for 2 days alternating with a day of rest. Failures in therapy may be caused by overdosage or too frequent dosage.

Concomitant therapy: The use of acetazolamide does not eliminate the need for other therapy, such as digitalis, bed rest, and salt restriction.

Drug-induced edema – 250 to 375 mg IV once a day for 1 or 2 days, alternating with a day of rest.

Chronic simple (open-angle) glaucoma –

Usual dosage: 250 mg to 1 g/day IV, usually in divided doses for amounts more than 250 mg. It has usually been found that a dosage in excess of 1 g/day does not produce an increased effect.

Dosage adjustment: The dosage should be adjusted with careful individual attention to symptomatology and ocular tension.

Secondary glaucoma – See Acute Congestive (Closed-Angle) Glaucoma for dosing.

ACETAZOLAMIDE SODIUM — INJECTION

Seizures –

Usual dosage: 8 to 30 mg/kg IV in divided doses. Although some patients respond to a low dose, the optimum range appears to be from 375 to 1,000 mg daily. However, some investigators feel that daily doses in excess of 1 g do not produce any better results than a 1 g dose.

Concomitant therapy: When given in combination with other anticonvulsants, it is suggested that the starting dosage should be 250 mg once daily in addition to the existing medications. This can be increased to levels as previously indicated.

Off-label dosing –

Familial periodic paralysis: [4] = Insufficient documentation. As monotherapy, the following dosage regimens have been studied: 120 mg twice daily, 250 mg/day, 125 mg 3 times daily, and 250 mg every 6 hours for up to 2 weeks.

Prevention of migraine (adults): [4] = Insufficient documentation. 62.5 to 250 mg twice daily.

➤*Preparation for administration:* Each vial should be reconstituted with at least 5 mL of sterile water for injection prior to use.

➤*Administration:* The direct IV route of administration is preferred. Intramuscular administration is not recommended.

➤*Storage/Stability:* Store at 15° to 30°C (59° to 86°F). Discard unused portion. Reconstituted solutions retain their physical and chemical properties for 3 days under refrigeration at 2° to 8°C (36° to 46°F), or 12 hours at room temperature, 15° to 30°C (59° to 86°F).

METHAZOLAMIDE

Rx	**Methazolamide** (Various, eg, Mikart)	**Tablets:** 25 mg	In 100s.
		50 mg	In 100s.

METHAZOLAMIDE — ORAL

For complete and comparative prescribing information, refer to the Carbonic Anhydrase Inhibitor group monograph.

Indications

➤*Glaucoma:* Methazolamide is indicated in the treatment of ocular conditions where lowering intraocular pressure is likely to be of therapeutic benefit, such as chronic open-angle glaucoma, secondary glaucoma, and preoperatively in acute angle-closure glaucoma where lowering the intraocular pressure is desired before surgery.

Administration and Dosage

➤*Adults:*

Glaucoma –

Usual dosage: 50 to 100 mg 2 to 3 times daily.

Concomitant therapy: May be used concomitantly with miotic and osmotic agents.

➤*Renal function impairment:* Contraindicated in cases of marked kidney disease or dysfunction.

➤*Hepatic function impairment:* Contraindicated in cases of marked liver disease or dysfunction.

➤*Storage/Stability:* Store at 15° to 30°C (59° to 86°F).

DIURETIC COMBINATIONS

Rx	**Amiloride/Hydrochlorothiazide** (Various, eg, Goldline, Warner Chilcott)	**Tablets:** 5 mg amiloride HCl and 50 mg hydrochlorothiazide	In 100s, 500s and 1000s.
Rx	**Moduretic** (Merck)		Lactose. (917). Peach, scored. Diamond shape. In 100s and UD 100s.
Rx	**Spironolactone/Hydrochlorothiazide** (Various, eg, Danbury, Goldline, Mylan)	**Tablets:** 25 mg spironolactone and 25 mg hydrochlorothiazide	In 100s, 250s, 500s and 1000s.
Rx	**Aldactazide** (Searle)		(Searle 1011 Aldactazide 25). Tan. Film coated. In 100s, 500s, 1000s and UD 100s.
Rx	**Aldactazide** (Searle)	**Tablets:** 50 mg spironolactone and 50 mg hydrochlorothiazide	(Searle 1021 Aldactazide 50). Tan, scored. In 100s and UD 100s.
Rx	**Triamterene/Hydrochlorothiazide** (Various, eg, Geneva)	**Tablets:** 37.5 mg triamterene and 25 mg hydrochlorothiazide	In 100s, 500s and 1000s.
Rx	**Maxzide-25MG** (Bertek)		(Maxzide LL M9). Lt. green, scored. Bow-tie shape. In 100s, UD 100s.
Rx	**Triamterene/Hydrochlorothiazide** (Duramed)	**Capsules:** 37.5 mg triamterene and 25 mg hydrochlorothiazide	Lactose. (DPI/488). White. In 1000s.
Rx	**Dyazide** (GlaxoSmithKline)		Lactose. (Dyazide). Red and white. In 1000s, unit-of-use 100s and UD 100s.
Rx	**Triamterene/Hydrochlorothiazide** (Various, eg, Geneva, Goldline, Zenith)	**Capsules:** 50 mg triamterene and 25 mg hydrochlorothiazide	In 100s and 1000s.
Rx	**Triamterene/Hydrochlorothiazide** (Various, eg, Barr, Danbury, Geneva, Goldline, Major, Schein, UDL, Warner Chilcott)	**Tablets:** 75 mg triamterene and 50 mg hydrochlorothiazide	In 100s, 250s, 500s, 1000s, and UD 100s.
Rx	**Maxzide** (Bertek)		(Maxzide LL M8). Lt. yellow, scored. Bow-tie shape. In 100s, 500s, UD 100s.

DIURETIC COMBINATIONS — ORAL

For complete information concerning the components of the combined diuretic products, consult the appropriate drug monographs in the Diuretics section.

Administration and Dosage

➤*General dosing considerations:* Dosage for each combination/strength varies. Refer to labeling for specific guidelines.

Fixed-dose combination drugs are not indicated for initial therapy of edema or hypertension, they require therapy titrated to the individual patient. If the fixed combination represents the determined dosage, its use may be more convenient in patient management.

The treatment of hypertension and edema is not static; reevaluate as conditions in each patient warrant.

➤*Adults:*

Edema –

Amiloride/Hydrochlorothiazide: 1 to 2 tablets daily with meals.

Triamterene/Hydrochlorothiazide:

- *37.5 mg/25 mg* – 1 or 2 tablets/capsules daily.
- *50 mg/25 mg* – 1 or 2 capsules twice daily after meals
- *75 mg/50 mg* – 1 tablet daily.

Spironolactone/Hydrochlorothiazide:

- *25 mg/25 mg* – 1 to 8 tablets daily.
- *50 mg/50 mg* – 1 to 4 tablets daily

Hypertension – See Edema for dosing.

➤*Renal function impairment:*

Amiloride/Hydrochlorothiazide – Contraindicated in patients with impaired renal function.

Spironolactone/Hydrochlorothiazide – Contraindicated in patients with anuria, acute renal insufficiency, and significant impairment of renal excretory function.

Triamterene/Hydrochlorothiazide – Contraindicated in patients with anuria and renal decompensation.

➤*Hepatic function impairment:*

Spironolactone/Hydrochlorothiazide – Contraindicated in patients with severe hepatic failure.

Triamterene/Hydrochlorothiazide – Contraindicated in patients with severe hepatic disease.

DIURETIC COMBINATIONS — ORAL

➤*Storage/Stability:* Store at 15° to 30°C (59° to 86°F). Protect from moisture, freezing, and excessive heat.

Actions

➤*Pharmacology:* The combination of a thiazide and a potassium-sparing diuretic provides additive diuretic activity and antihypertensive effects through different mechanisms of action and also minimizes the potassium depletion characteristics of thiazides.

Warnings/Precautions

➤*Triamterene/Hydrochlorothiazide:*

Bioavailability – Use caution when changing to another triamterene/hydrochlorothiazide combination product. Combination products are not equivalent.

➤*Pregnancy:* Category B (hydrochlorothiazide, amiloride). *Category C* (spironolactone, triamterene). *Category D* if used in gestational hypertension per Briggs' *Drugs in Pregnancy and Lactation*. Hydrochlorothiazide and triamterene cross the placental barrier and appear in the cord blood. Use only when clearly needed and when the potential benefits outweigh the potential hazards to the fetus.

➤*Lactation:* Thiazides and canrenone, a major and active metabolite of spironolactone, appear in human breast milk. It is unknown if triamterene or amiloride is present in human milk. Decide whether to discontinue breast-feeding or the drug, taking into account the importance of the drug to the mother.

Osmotic Diuretics

Actions

➤*Pharmacology:* Osmotic agents induce diuresis by elevating the osmolarity of the glomerular filtrate, thereby hindering the tubular reabsorption of water. Excretion of sodium and chloride is increased. These agents are freely filtered at the glomerulus; poorly reabsorbed by the renal tubule; not secreted by the tubule; relatively pharmacologically inert; usually resistant to metabolic alteration (except glycerin). Activity in the kidneys depends on the concentration of osmotically active particles in solution.

The main indication for osmotic diuretics (primarily mannitol) is prophylaxis of acute renal failure in conditions in which glomerular filtration is greatly reduced (ie, severe trauma, cardiovascular operations). By maintaining a flow of dilute urine, damage to the nephron by high concentrations of toxic solute does not occur. They are also employed to reduce intracranial pressure and elevated intraocular pressure. In the eyes, these agents act by creating an osmotic gradient between the plasma and ocular fluids.

Mannitol is the most widely used osmotic diuretic. The other agents include urea, glycerin and isosorbide. For specific approved indications, refer to individual drug monographs.

➤*Pharmacokinetics:* **Mannitol** is only slightly metabolized, while the rest is freely filtered by the glomeruli and excreted intact in urine. About 7% is reabsorbed by the renal tubules. Approximately 90% of an injected dose is recovered in urine after 24 hours. In severe renal insufficiency, the rate of mannitol excretion is greatly reduced; retained mannitol may increase extracellular tonicity, expand the extracellular fluid and induce an apparent hyponatremia with increased serum osmolality.

Osmotic Diuretics Pharmacokinetics

Diuretic	Route	Onset (min)	Peak (hrs)	Duration (hrs)	Half-life	Metabolized (%)	Ocular penetration	Distribution
Glycerin	PO	10-30	1-1.5	4-5	30-45 minutes	80	poor	E[a]
Isosorbide	PO	10-30	1-1.5	5-6	5-9.5 hrs	0	good	TBW[b]
Mannitol	IV	30-60	1	6-8	15-100 minutes	7-10	very poor	E[a]
Urea	IV	30-45	1	5-6	-		good	TBW[b]

[a] E = extracellular water

[b] TBW = total body water

MANNITOL

Rx	**Osmitrol** (Baxter)	**Injection:** 5%	In 1000 mL.
		10%	In 500 and 1000 mL.
		15%	In 500 mL.
		20%	In 250 and 500 mL.
Rx	**Mannitol** (Various, eg, Abbott, American Regent-,IMS, B. Braun McGaw, Pasadena)	**Injection:** 10%	In 1000 mL.
		Injection: 15%	In 150 and 500 mL.
		Injection: 20%	In 250 and 500 mL.
		Injection: 25%	In 50 mL vials and syringes.
Rx	**Mannitol** (B. Braun McGaw)	**Solution:** 5 g/100 mL in distilled water (275 mOsm/L)	In 2000 mL.

MANNITOL — INJECTION

Refer to the general discussion of these agents in the Osmotic Diuretics Introduction.

Indications

➤*Acute renal failure:* Promotion of diuresis, in the prevention or treatment of the oliguric phase of acute renal failure before irreversible renal failure becomes established.

➤*Intracranial pressure/cerebral edema:* For the reduction of intracranial pressure and treatment of cerebral edema by reducing brain mass.

➤*Elevated intraocular pressure:* Reduction of elevated intraocular pressure when the pressure cannot be lowered by other means.

➤*Urinary excretion of toxins:* Promotion of urinary excretion of toxins.

➤*Urologic irrigation:* Mannitol solution, 25% is indicated as an irrigation solution in transurethral prostatic resection or other transurethral surgical procedures.

Administration and Dosage

➤*General dosing considerations:* The adult dosage ranges from 50 to 200 g in a 24-hour period, but in most cases an adequate response will be achieved at a usual dosage of approximately 100 g/24 hours.

Lower mannitol concentrations and solutions containing sodium chloride are useful in preventing dehydration and electrolyte depletion.

➤*Adults:*

Adjunctive therapy for intoxications – 10% or 20% mannitol is indicated. The concentration will depend upon the fluid requirement and urinary output of the patient. Generally, a bolus dose of 20% mannitol is given, followed by a slower infusion of 10% mannitol (with electrolytes) to maintain urine output at the desired level.

Prevention of acute renal failure (oliguria) –

Usual dosage: When used during cardiovascular and other types of surgery, immediately postoperatively or following trauma, 50 to 100 g of mannitol as a 5% to 25% solution may be given. The concentration and amount will depend upon the fluid requirements of the patient. Following suspected or actual hemolytic transfusion reactions, 20 g of mannitol may be given IV over a 5-minute period to provoke diuresis. If diuresis does not occur, the 20 g dose may be repeated. If there is an adequate urine flow (30 to 50 mL/hr) then IV fluids containing not more than 50 to 75 mEq of sodium per liter should be given in sufficient volume to match the desired urine flow (100 mL/hr) until fluids can be taken orally.

Test dose: A test dose of mannitol should be given prior to instituting therapy for patients with marked oliguria or those believed to have inadequate renal function. Such test doses may be approximately 0.2 g/kg (about 75 mL of a 20% solution or 50 mL of a 25% solution) infused in a period of 3 to 5 minutes to produce a urine flow of at least 30 to 50 mL/hr. If urine flow does not increase within 2 or 3 hours, a second test dose may be given. If response is inadequate, the patient should be reevaluated.

Reduction of intracranial pressure – 25% mannitol is recommended. When used before or after surgery, a total dose of 1.5 to 2 g/kg can be given over a period of 30 to 60 minutes.

MANNITOL — INJECTION

Reduction of cerebral edema – 25% mannitol is recommended. When used before or after surgery, a total dose of 1.5 to 2 g/kg can be given over a period of 30 to 60 minutes.

Reduction of intraocular pressure – 25% mannitol is recommended. When used before or after surgery, a total dose of 1.5 to 2 g/kg can be given over a period of 30 to 60 minutes.

Treatment of oliguria – 50 to 100 g administered as a 15% to 25% solution.

Urinary excretion of toxic substances –

Usual dosage: 25% to 25% mannitol as an infusion as long as indicated if the level of urinary output remains high.

Concomitant therapy: The concentration will depend upon the fluid requirement and urinary output. IV water and electrolytes must be given to replace the loss of these substances in the urine, sweat and expired air.

Discontinuation of therapy: If benefits are not observed after 200 g of mannitol are given, discontinue it.

➤*Renal function impairment:* Contraindicated in well-established anuria. Use with caution in patients with significant renal dysfunction. A test dose should be utilized in patients with severe impairment of renal function. A second test dose may be tried if there is an inadequate response, but no more than 2 test doses should be attempted.

➤*Administration:* For IV use only using sterile equipment. The rate of administration is usually adjusted to maintain a urine flow of at least 30 to 50 mL/hr. An administration set with a filter should be used for IV infusions of solutions containing 20% or more of mannitol. Do not use plastic container in series connection. If administration is controlled by a pumping device, care must be taken to discontinue pumping action before the container runs dry or air embolism may result. It is recommended that IV administration apparatus be replaced at least once every 24 hours.

20% – Administer through a blood filter set to ensure against infusion of mannitol crystals. When a hypertonic solution is to be administered peripherally, it should be slowly infused through a small bore needle, placed well within the lumen of a large vein to minimize venous irritation. Carefully avoid infiltration.

25% – An administration set with a filter should be used.

Excel container – Tear overwrap down at notch and remove solution container. Check for minute leaks by squeezing solution container firmly. If leaks are found, discard solution as sterility may be impaired. Remove plastic protector from sterile set port at bottom of container. Attach administration set.

Vials with flip-tear top seals – If it is necessary to introduce filtered air into the vial, this must be done slowly and with caution. If the vial has been warmed, allow vial to cool to room temperature before use.

➤*Extravasation:* Extravasation may occur during administration of mannitol. If signs or symptoms of extravasation occur, stop the infusion immediately. If possible, withdraw 3 to 5 mL of blood to remove some of the drug. Remove the infusion needle. Delineate the infiltrated area on the patient's skin with a felt-tip marker. Hyaluronidase is an effective antidote for hyperosmolar drug infiltrations; administer promptly within the first few minutes to 1 hour after extravasation. Higher doses (150 units) have primarily been used in adults while lower doses (15 units) have been used in children. Administer hyaluronidase according to the following steps. Dilute hyaluronidase to desired concentration, depending on the dose and product used. (Note: Some products do not require dilution.) For example, if the total dose is 15 units, make 15 units/mL dilution. If the total dose is 150 units, make 150 units'mL dilution. Cleanse area with povidone-iodine. Inject hyaluronidase locally, subcutaneously or intradermally, using a 25-gauge needle or smaller. The dose is given as five 0.2 mL injections at the leading edge of the extravasation site. Change needle after each injection. Elevate for 48 hours above heart level using a sling or stockinette dressing with an observation window cut in the dressing. Avoid pressure or friction. Do not rub area. Observe for signs of increased erythema, pain, or skin necrosis. If increased symptoms occur, consult a plastic surgeon. Ensure that no medication is given distally to extravasation site. After 48 hours, encourage the patient to use the extremity normally to promote full range of motion.

➤*Admixture compatibility:* Do not admix with other drugs. A white flocculant mannitol precipitate may result from contact with PVC surfaces which act as nuclei for rapid rate crystallization of small crystals. This condition has also been reported to occur when mannitol has come in contact with other plastic and rough glass surfaces. Attempting to resolubilize the white flocculant precipitate with the aid of heat is not useful because crystallization may recur in a short period of time.

➤*Storage/Stability:* Store at 15° to 30°C (59° to 86°F). Avoid excessive heat. Protect from freezing. Solutions of mannitol may crystallize when exposed to low temperatures. Concentrations greater than 15% have a greater tendency to crystallization. If crystals are observed, the container should be warmed by appropriate means to not greater than 60°C (140°F), shaken, then cooled to body temperature before administering. If all crystals cannot be completely redissolved, the container must be rejected. Use of any other method to heat the vial may result in its explosion. 25% solution is preservative free; discard unused portion.

Actions

➤*Pharmacology:* Mannitol is an obligatory osmotic diuretic.

Mannitol occurs naturally in fruits and vegetables and is metabolically inert in humans.

➤*Pharmacokinetics:*

Absorption – Mannitol is poorly absorbed from the GI tract.

Metabolism/Excretion – After IV injection, mannitol is confined to the extracellular space, only slightly metabolized, and rapidly excreted by the kidneys. Approximately 80% of a typical dose appears in the urine within 3 hours. Mannitol is freely filtered by the glomeruli with less than 10% tubular reabsorption; it is not secreted by tubular cells. It induces diuresis by elevating the osmolarity of the glomerular filtrate and thereby hinders tubular reabsorption of water. Urinary output of water and excretion of sodium and chloride are enhanced.

Mannitol injection is free of electrolytes and is used in urology as a nonhemolytic irrigant. The amount of mannitol absorbed intravascularly during transurethral prostatic surgery is variable and depends primarily on the extent of the surgery. Such mannitol is excreted by the kidneys and produces osmotic diuresis.

Contraindications

Well-established anuria due to severe renal disease; severe pulmonary congestion or frank pulmonary edema; active intracranial bleeding except during craniotomy; severe dehydration; progressive renal damage or dysfunction after institution of mannitol therapy, including increasing oliguria and azotemia; progressive heart failure or pulmonary congestion after institution of mannitol therapy.

Warnings/Precautions

➤*Fluid and electrolyte imbalance:* Excessive loss of water and electrolytes may lead to serious imbalances. Serum sodium and potassium should be carefully monitored during mannitol therapy.

The diuresis after rapid infusion of mannitol may increase preexisting hemoconcentration. With continued use of mannitol, a loss of water in excess of electrolytes can cause hypernatremia.

Shift of sodium-free intracellular fluid into the extracellular compartment after mannitol infusion may lower serum sodium concentration and aggravate preexisting hyponatremia.

➤*Transurethral prostatectomy:* Irrigating solutions used in transurethral prostatectomy have been shown to enter the systemic circulation in relatively large volumes, exert a systemic effect and may significantly alter cardiopulmonary and renal dynamics.

➤*Cardiovascular:* The cardiovascular status of the patient should be carefully evaluated before mannitol is administered by rapid IV injection or before and during transurethral resection since expansion of the extracellular fluid may lead to fulminating congestive heart failure.

➤*Hypovolemia:* By sustaining diuresis, mannitol administration may obscure and intensify inadequate hydration or hypovolemia.

➤*Pseudoagglutination:* Electrolyte-free mannitol solutions should not be given conjointly with blood.

Unless it is essential, electrolyte-free mannitol solutions should not be combined with blood. When it is essential to give the combination, at least 20 mEq of sodium chloride should be added per L of mannitol solution to avoid agglomeration of erythrocytes. The contents of opened containers should be used promptly, and unused contents should be discarded.

➤*Crystallization (25% mannitol):* Crystals, if present in mannitol injection, 25% may be dissolved by placing the vial in a hot water bath maintained at 60° to 80°C (140° to 176°F), with occasional shaking. The resulting solution should be allowed to cool to body temperature before injection.

An administration set with a filter should be used for IV infusions of solutions containing 20% or more of mannitol.

A white flocculant mannitol precipitate may result from contact with PVC surfaces which act as nuclei for rapid rate crystallization of small crystals. This condition has also been reported to occur when mannitol has come in contact with other plastic and rough glass surfaces. Attempting to resolubilize the white flocculant precipitate with the aid of heat is not useful because crystallization may recur in a short period of time.

Solutions of mannitol may crystallize when exposed to low temperatures. Concentrations greater than 15% have a greater tendency to crystallization. If crystals are observed, the container should be warmed by appropriate means to not greater than 60°C (140°F), shaken, then cooled to body temperature before administering. If all crystals cannot be completely redissolved, the container must be rejected.

Note – Use of any other method to heat the vial may result in its explosion.

➤*Administration:* Do not use plastic container in series connection.

If administration is controlled by a pumping device, care must be taken to discontinue pumping action before the container runs dry or air embolism may result.

These solutions are intended for IV administration using sterile equipment. It is recommended that IV administration apparatus be replaced at least once every 24 hours.

➤*Extravasation:* See Administration and Dosage for more information.

➤*Renal function impairment:* A test dose should be utilized in patients with severe impairment of renal function. A second test dose may be tried if there is an inadequate response, but no more than 2 test doses should be attempted.

➤*Special risk:* Mannitol solution must be used with caution in patients with significantly cardiopulmonary or renal dysfunction.

Mannitol solutions should be used with care in patients with hypervolemia, renal insufficiency, urinary tract obstruction, or impending or frank cardiac decompensation.

MANNITOL — INJECTION

➤*Pregnancy:* Category B. This drug should be used during pregnancy only if clearly needed.

➤*Lactation:* It is not known whether this drug is excreted in human milk. Because many drugs are excreted in human milk, caution should be exercised when mannitol injection is administered to a nursing mother.

➤*Children:* Dosage requirements in children below 12 years of age have not been established.

➤*Monitoring:* Clinical evaluation and periodic laboratory determinations are necessary to monitor changes in fluid balance, electrolyte concentrations, and acid-base balance during parenteral therapy with mannitol solutions.

Excessive loss of water and electrolytes may lead to serious imbalances. Serum sodium and potassium should be carefully monitored during mannitol therapy.

Closely monitor the urine output and discontinue mannitol infusion promptly if output is low. Inadequate urine output results in accumulation of mannitol, expansion of extracellular fluid volume and could result in water intoxication or congestive heart failure. Renal function must be closely monitored during mannitol infusion.

Adverse Reactions

Reactions which may occur because of the solution or the technique of administration include febrile response, infection at the site of injection, venous thrombosis or phlebitis extending from the site of injection, extravasation and hypervolemia.

Isolated cases of adverse reactions, such as pulmonary congestion, fluid and electrolyte imbalance, acidosis, electrolyte loss, dryness of the mouth, thirst, marked diuresis, urinary retention, edema, headache, blurred vision, convulsions, nausea, vomiting, rhinitis, arm pain, skin necrosis, thrombophlebitis, chills, dizziness, urticaria, dehydration, hypotension, hypertension, tachycardia, fever, and angina-like chest pains have been reported during or following mannitol infusion.

Too rapid infusion of hypertonic solutions may cause local pain and venous irritation. Rate of administration should be adjusted according to tolerance. Use of the largest peripheral vein and a small bore needle is recommended.

If an adverse reaction does occur, discontinue the infusion, evaluate the patient, institute appropriate therapeutic countermeasures and save the remainder of the fluid for examination if deemed necessary.

➤*25% mannitol:* Reactions are infrequent and may include:

Cardiovascular – Pulmonary edema, edema, hypotension, hypertension, tachycardia, angina-like chest pain.

CNS – Headache, convulsions, dizziness.

Dermatologic – Skin necrosis, thrombophlebitis.

GI – Dryness of mouth, nausea, vomiting, diarrhea.

GU – Osmotic nephrosis, urinary retention.

Hypersensitivity – Urticaria.

Metabolic – Fluid and electrolyte imbalance, acidosis, dehydration.

Special senses – Blurred vision, rhinitis.

Miscellaneous – Thirst, arm pain, chills, fever.

Overdosage

➤*Symptoms:* Larger doses than recommended may result in increased electrolyte excretion, particularly sodium, chloride, and potassium. Sodium depletion can result in orthostatic tachycardia or hypotension and decreased central venous pressure. Chloride metabolism closely follows that of sodium. Potassium deficit can impair neuromuscular function and cause intestinal dilatation and ileus.

Mannitol may cause pulmonary edema or water intoxication if urine flow is inadequate.

➤*Treatment:* In the event of a fluid or solute overload during parenteral therapy, reevaluate the patient's condition, and institute appropriate corrective treatment.

UREA

Rx	**Ureaphil** (Abbott)	**Injection:** 40 g per 150 ml	In single-dose containers.

STERILE UREA — INJECTION

Refer to the general discussion of these agents in the Osmotic Diuretics Introduction.

Indications

➤*Intracranial / intraocular pressure reduction:* When administered as a 30% solution, this preparation is indicated for the reduction of intracranial pressure (in the control of cerebral edema) and of intraocular pressure.

➤*Off-label uses:* Intra-amniotic injection has been used to induce abortion.

Administration and Dosage

➤*General dosing considerations:* The amount to be administered is generally estimated on the basis of gram of urea per kg of body weight. Dosage also must take into account the clinical condition of the patient, especially the state of hydration, electrolyte balance and integrity of renal function.

➤*Adults:*

Reduction of increased intracranial pressure –
Usual dosage: 1 to 1.5 g (3.3 to 5 mL) per kg of body weight.
Maximum dose: 120 g/day.

Reduction of increased intraocular pressure –
Usual dosage: 1 to 1.5 g (3.3 to 5 mL) per kg of body weight.
Maximum dose: 120 g/day.

➤*Children:*

2 years of age and older –
Reduction of increased intracranial pressure:
- *Usual dosage* – 0.5 to 1.5 g per kg of body weight.
- *Maximum dose* – 120 g/day.

Reduction of increased intraocular pressure:
- *Usual dosage* – 0.5 to 1.5 g per kg of body weight.
- *Maximum dose* – 120 g/day.

Infants up to 2 years of age –
Reduction of increased intracranial pressure: As little as 0.1 g/kg may be adequate.
Reduction of increased intraocular pressure: As little as 0.1 g/kg may be adequate.

➤*Elderly:* Urea should not be infused in veins of the lower extremities of elderly patients because phlebitis and thrombosis of superficial and deep veins may occur.

➤*Renal function impairment:* Contraindicated in severely impaired renal function. Patients exhibiting a temporary reduction in urine volume are generally able to maintain a satisfactory elimination of urea. However, if diuresis does not follow the injection of urea to such patients within 6 to 12 hours, the drug should be withdrawn pending further evaluation of renal function.

➤*Hepatic function impairment:* Contraindicated in frank liver failure. If used in patients with some liver impairment, urea should be administered with great caution since there may be a significant rise in blood ammonia levels.

➤*Preparation for administration:* Urea should be freshly prepared in each case. Sterile urea is prepared by adding an appropriate volume of 5% or 10% dextrose injection. The desired diluent can be added directly to the urea container.

To prepare 135 mL of a 30% solution of sterile urea, the contents of one 40 g container are mixed with 105 mL of the diluent, or 2 such containers are mixed with 210 mL of diluent to prepare 270 mL of a 30% solution. Each mL of a 30% solution provides 300 mg of urea. The reconstituted solution should be clear.

➤*Administration:* Sterile urea is administered as a 30% solution by slow intravenous (IV) infusion. The rate of injection should not exceed 4 mL/min. Rapid IV administration of hypertonic solutions of urea may be associated with hemolysis as well as a direct effect on the cerebral vasomotor centers which may result in increased capillary bleeding. These effects usually can be avoided by not exceeding an infusion rate of 4 mL/min.

➤*Admixture compatibility:* Solutions of urea should not be administered through the same administration set through which blood is being infused.

➤*Storage / Stability:* Store at 15° to 30°C (59° to 86°F). Discard solution if not used within 24 hours after reconstitution.

Actions

➤*Pharmacology:* The reduction of intracranial edema and abnormally elevated cerebrospinal fluid pressure which occurs following intravenous administration of hypertonic urea solutions, depends upon osmotic pressure gradients between the blood, extracellular and intracellular fluid compartments. Thus, the primary mechanism of action appears to be physical. Hypertonic urea rapidly increases blood tonicity thus effecting a greater urea concentration gradient in the blood than in the extravascular fluid. This results in transudation of fluid from the tissues, including the brain and cerebrospinal fluid into the blood.

As the concentration of urea in the glomerular filtrate increases, reabsorption of a proportional amount of water is prevented. Such retardation of proximal tubular reabsorption increases the rate and volume of urine flow.

Contraindications

Severely impaired renal function; active intracranial bleeding; marked dehydration; frank liver failure.

Urea should not be infused in veins of the lower extremities of elderly patients because phlebitis and thrombosis of superficial and deep veins may occur.

Do not administer unless seal of urea container is intact and reconstituted solution is clear. Discard unused portion.

STERILE UREA — INJECTION

Warnings/Precautions

➤*Electrolyte imbalance:* Urea may cause depletion of electrolytes which can result in hyponatremia and hypokalemia. Early signs of such depletion may indicate the need for supplementation before serum levels are reduced.

➤*Extravasation:* Extreme care is essential to prevent accidental extravasation of the solution at the site of injection since this may cause local reactions ranging from mild irritation to tissue necrosis.

➤*Comatose patients:* An indwelling urethral catheter should be used in comatose patients receiving urea for injection to insure bladder emptying.

➤*Rapid IV administration:* Rapid intravenous (IV) administration of hypertonic solutions of urea may be associated with hemolysis as well as a direct effect on the cerebral vasomotor centers which may result in increased capillary bleeding. These effects usually can be avoided by not exceeding an infusion rate of 4 mL min. Solutions of urea should not be administered through the same administration set through which blood is being infused.

➤*Intracranial bleeding:* Although arterial oozing has been reported as a nuisance when intracranial surgery is performed on patients following treatment with urea, it has not been a significant problem. However, sterile urea should not be used in the presence of active intracranial bleeding unless such use is preliminary to prompt surgical intervention to control hemorrhage. It should be kept in mind that reduction of brain edema induced by urea may result in reactivation of intracranial bleeding.

➤*Blood loss:* As with other infused solutions, urea may temporarily maintain circulatory volume and blood pressure in spite of considerable blood loss. Consequently, when excessive blood loss occurs within a short period of time, blood replacement should be adequate and simultaneous with the infusion of urea.

➤*Hypothermia:* Hypothermia when used with urea infusion may increase the risk of venous thrombosis and hemoglobinuria.

➤*Renal function impairment:* In the presence of kidney disease, urea should be administered with caution. Mild elevation of blood urea nitrogen does not preclude its use or continued use, but frequent laboratory studies should be made to determine if kidney function is adequate to eliminate the infused urea as well as that produced endogenously.

Patients exhibiting a temporary reduction in urine volume are generally able to maintain a satisfactory elimination of urea. However, if diuresis does not follow the injection of urea to such patients within 6 to 12 hours, the drug should be withdrawn pending further evaluation of renal function.

➤*Hepatic function impairment:* If used in patients with some liver impairment, urea should be administered with great caution since there may be a significant rise in blood ammonia levels.

➤*Pregnancy: Category C.* Animal reproduction studies have not been conducted with sterile urea. It is also not known whether sterile urea can cause fetal harm when given to a pregnant woman or can affect reproduction capacity. Sterile urea should be given to a pregnant woman only if clearly needed.

➤*Lactation:* It is not known whether this drug is excreted in human milk. Because many drugs are excreted in human milk, caution should be exercised when sterile urea is administered to a nursing mother.

Adverse Reactions

Headaches (reported to be similar to those which occur in some patients following lumbar puncture), nausea and vomiting, occasionally syncope and disorientation have been known to occur following intravenous administration. Less often reported is a transient agitated confusional state. No serious reactions have been noted when solutions have been infused slowly provided renal function is not seriously impaired or there is no evidence of active intracranial bleeding. Chemical phlebitis and thrombosis near the site of injection have been reported infrequently.

Reactions which may occur because of the solution (reconstituted) or the technique of administration include febrile response, infection at the site of injection, venous thrombosis or phlebitis extending from the site of injection, extravasation and hypervolemia.

If an adverse reaction does occur, discontinue the infusion, evaluate the patient, institute appropriate therapeutic countermeasures and save the remainder of the fluid for examination if deemed necessary.

Overdosage

In the event of overdosage as reflected by unusually elevated blood urea nitrogen (BUN) levels, discontinue the drug, evaluate the patient and institute corrective measures as indicated. (See Warnings/Precautions and Administration and Dosage.)

NONPRESCRIPTION DIURETICS

otc	**Maximum Strength Aqua•Ban** (Thompson Medical)	**Tablets:** 50 mg pamabrom	Lactose. In 30s.

NONPRESCRIPTION DIURETICS — ORAL

Indications

➤*Premenstrual/menstrual symptoms:* For the relief of temporary water weight gain, bloating, swelling, or full feeling associated with the premenstrual and menstrual periods.

Administration and Dosage

➤*Adults:*

Premenstrual and menstrual discomfort –

Usual dosage: 1 tablet 4 times/day.

Maximum dose: 4 tablets per 24 hours.

➤*Children:* Not indicated for use in children.

➤*Storage/Stability:* Store at 15° to 30°C (59° to 86°F).

WARNING

Long-acting beta-2 agonists may increase the risk of asthma-related death. Data from a large placebo-controlled US study that compared the safety of salmeterol or placebo added to usual asthma therapy showed an increase in asthma-related deaths in patients receiving salmeterol. This finding is considered a class effect of long-acting beta-2 agonists. All long-acting beta-2 agonists are contraindicated in patients with asthma without the use of a long-term asthma control medication. Currently available data are inadequate to determine whether current use of inhaled corticosteroids or other long-term asthma control drugs mitigates the increased risk of asthma related-death from long-acting beta-2 adrenergic agonists.

Once asthma control is achieved and maintained, assess the patient at regular intervals and step down therapy (eg, discontinue long-acting beta-2 agonist) if possible without loss of asthma control and maintain the patient on a long-term asthma control medication, such as an inhaled corticosteroid. Do not use long-acting beta-2 agonists for patients whose asthma is adequately controlled on low- or medium-dose inhaled corticosteroids.

Children and adolescents – Available data from controlled clinical trials suggest that long-acting beta-2 agonists increase the risk of asthma-related hospitalization in children and adolescents. For children and adolescents with asthma who require addition of a long-acting beta-2 agonists to an inhaled corticosteroid, a fixed-dose combination product containing both an inhaled corticosteroid and a long-acting beta-2 agonist should ordinarily be used to ensure adherence with both drugs. In cases where use of a separate long-term asthma control medication (eg, inhaled corticosteroid) and a long-acting beta-2 agonists is clinically indicated, appropriate steps must be taken to ensure adherence with both treatment components. If adherence cannot be ensured, a fixed-dose combination product containing both an inhaled corticosteroid and a long-acting beta-2 agonist is recommended.

Indications

➤*Bronchodilation:* Relief of reversible bronchospasm associated with acute and chronic bronchial asthma, exercise-induced bronchospasm (EIB), and chronic obstructive pulmonary disease (COPD) (eg, chronic bronchitis, emphysema).

According to the National Asthma Education and Prevention Program's Expert Panel Report 3, short-acting beta-2 agonists (eg, albuterol, levalbuterol, pirbuterol) are recommended as drugs of choice for the treatment of acute asthma symptoms and exacerbations and also for the prevention of EIB. Long-acting beta-2 agonists (eg, salmeterol, formoterol) are recommended for use with inhaled corticosteroids for the long-term control of asthma symptoms. These long-acting agents are not recommended as monotherapy for long-term control of persistent asthma nor are they recommended for treatment of acute asthma symptoms or exacerbations.

Refer to individual monographs for indications of specific agents.

Sympathomimetic Bronchodilators[a]: Summary of FDA-Approved Indications

	Asthma/ bronchospasm (acute treatment)	Asthma/ bronchospasm (prevention)	COPD	Exercise-induced bronchospasm
Short-acting beta-2 agonists				
Albuterol	X	X		X
Levalbuterol	X	X		
Metaproterenol	X	X		
Pirbuterol	X	X		
Terbutaline	X	X	X	X
Long-acting beta-2 agonists				
Arformoterol			X	
Formoterol		X[b]	X	X[b]
Salmeterol		X	X	X

[a] For information on the use of ephedrine, epinephrine, and isoproterenol, see the monographs in the Vasopressors Used in Shock section in the Cardiovascular Agents chapter.
[b] Inhalation powder only.

➤*Off-label uses:* Refer to individual monographs for further information.

Hyperkalemia –
Albuterol (by nebulization): [1] = Good documentation.

Premature labor –
Terbutaline (injection): [1] = Good documentation.

Actions

➤*Pharmacology:* Sympathomimetic agents are used to produce bronchodilation. They relieve reversible bronchospasm by relaxing the smooth muscles of the bronchioles in conditions associated with asthma, bronchitis, emphysema, or bronchiectasis. Bronchodilation may additionally facilitate expectoration. Some agents are also used for other purposes. See monographs for Vasopressors Used in Shock, Nasal Decongestants, and Ophthalmic Decongestants.

The pharmacologic actions of these agents include: alpha-adrenergic stimulation (vasoconstriction, nasal decongestion, pressor effects); beta-1 adrenergic stimulation (increased myocardial contractility and conduction); and beta-2 adrenergic stimulation (bronchial dilation and vasodilation, enhancement of mucociliary clearance, and inhibition of cholinergic neurotransmission). Beta-adrenergic drugs stimulate adenyl cyclase, the enzyme that catalyzes the formation of cyclic-3′, 5′ adenosine monophosphate (cyclic AMP) from adenosine triphosphate (ATP). Cyclic AMP that is formed inhibits the release of mediators of immediate hypersensitivity from inflammatory cells, especially from mast cells and basophils. This increase of cyclic AMP leads to activation of protein kinase A, which inhibits the phosphorylation of myosin and lowers intracellular ionic calcium concentrations, resulting in relaxation.

Other adrenergic actions include alpha receptor–mediated contraction of GI and urinary sphincters; alpha and beta receptor–mediated lipolysis; alpha and beta receptor–mediated decrease in GI tone; and changes in renin secretion, uterine relaxation, hepatic glycogenolysis/gluconeogenesis, and pancreatic beta cell secretion.

The relative selectivity of action of sympathomimetic agents is the primary determinant of clinical usefulness; it can predict the most likely adverse effects. Beta-2 selective agents provide the greatest benefit with minimal adverse effects. Direct administration via inhalation provides prompt effects and minimizes systemic activity. These drugs also inhibit histamine release from mast cells, produce vasodilation, and increase ciliary motility. Isoproterenol is one of the most potent bronchodilators available.

Sympathomimetic Bronchodilators: Summary of Pharmacologic and Pharmacokinetic Properties

Sympathomimetic	Adrenergic receptor activity	β_2 potency[a]	Route	Onset (min)	Duration (h)
Albuterol[b]	$\beta_1 < \beta_2$	2	Oral	within 30	6 to 12
			Inhalation[c]	within 5	3 to 6
Arformoterol	$\beta_1 < \beta_2$	—	Inhalation	within 7	—
Ephedrine	α β_1 β_2	—	Oral	15 to 60	3 to 5
			Subcutaneous	> 20	≤ 1
			IM[d]	10 to 20	≤ 1
			IV[d]	immediate	—
Epinephrine	α β_1 β_2	—	Subcutaneous	5 to 10	4 to 6
			IM	—	1 to 4
			Inhalation[c]	1 to 5	1 to 3
Formoterol	$\beta_1 < \beta_2$	—	Inhalation	within 12	12
Isoproterenol	β_1 β_2	1	IV	immediate	< 1
			Inhalation[c]	2 to 5	1 to 3
Levalbuterol	$\beta_1 < \beta_2$	—	Inhalation	5 to 17	3 to 8
Metaproterenol[b]	$\beta_1 < \beta_2$	15	Oral	≈ 30	4
Pirbuterol[b]	$\beta_1 < \beta_2$	5	Inhalation	within 5	5
Salmeterol[b]	$\beta_1 < \beta_2$	0.5	Inhalation	5 to 45	12

Sympathomimetic Bronchodilators: Summary of Pharmacologic and Pharmacokinetic Properties					
Sympathomimetic	Adrenergic receptor activity	β_2 potency[a]	Route	Onset (min)	Duration (h)
Terbutaline[b]	$\beta_1 < \beta_2$	4	Oral	30	4 to 8
			Subcutaneous	5 to 15	1.5 to 4
			Inhalation	5 to 30	3 to 6

[a] Relative molar potency: 1 = most potent.
[b] These agents all have minor β_1 activity.
[c] May be administered via aerosol or bulb nebulizer or intermittent positive-pressure breathing (IPPB) administration.
[d] IM = intramuscular; IV = intravenous.

Contraindications

Hypersensitivity to any component (allergic reactions are rare); patients with asthma without use of a long-term asthma control medication (**arformoterol**, **formoterol**, **salmeterol**); cardiac arrhythmias associated with tachycardia (**metaproterenol**); angina, preexisting cardiac arrhythmias associated with tachycardia, known hypersensitivity to sympathomimetic amines, ventricular arrhythmias requiring inotropic therapy, tachycardia or heart block caused by digitalis intoxication (**isoproterenol**); patients with organic brain damage, local anesthesia of certain areas (eg, fingers, toes) because of the risk of tissue sloughing, labor, cardiac dilatation, coronary insufficiency, cerebral arteriosclerosis, organic heart disease (**epinephrine**); in those cases in which vasopressors may be contraindicated, narrow-angle glaucoma, nonanaphylactic shock during general anesthesia with halogenated hydrocarbons or cyclopropane (**epinephrine**, **ephedrine**).

Warnings/Precautions

➤*Asthma-related death:* Long-acting beta-2 agonists may increase the risk of asthma-related death. Data from a large placebo-controlled US study that compared the safety of salmeterol or placebo added to usual asthma therapy showed an increase in asthma-related deaths in patients receiving salmeterol. This finding is considered a class effect of long-acting beta-2 agonists. All long-acting beta-2 agonists are contraindicated in patients with asthma without the use of a long-term asthma control medication. Data are not available to determine whether the rate of death in patients with COPD is increased by long-acting beta-2 agonists. (See Black Box Warning for more information.)

Excessive use of inhalants – Deaths from excessive use of inhaled sympathomimetics have been reported; the exact cause is unknown, but cardiac arrest following an unexpected severe acute asthmatic crisis and subsequent hypoxia is suspected.

➤*Acute symptoms/deterioration of disease:* If the patient's short-acting, inhaled beta-2 agonist becomes less effective (eg, the patient needs more inhalations than usual), obtain medical evaluation immediately. Increasing its use in this situation is inappropriate.

Do not use long-acting beta-2 agonists (eg, **salmeterol**, **arformoterol**, **formoterol**) to treat acute asthma or COPD symptoms. Do not use **salmeterol**, **arformoterol**, or **formoterol** more frequently than twice daily (morning and evening) at the recommended dose. When prescribing long-acting beta-2 agonists, provide patients with a short-acting, inhaled beta-2 agonist (eg, albuterol) for treatment of symptoms that occur despite regular twice-daily (morning and evening) use of long-acting beta-2 agonists.

COPD and asthma may deteriorate acutely over a period of hours or chronically over several days. In this setting, increased use of inhaled, short-acting beta-2 agonists is a marker of destabilization of disease and requires immediate reevaluation of the patient. Consider alternative treatment regimens, especially inhaled or systemic corticosteroids. If the patient uses at least 4 inhalations/day of a short-acting beta-2 agonist on a regular basis, or if more than 1 canister (200 inhalations per canister) is used in an 8-week period, have the patient see their health care provider for reevaluation of treatment.

Close supervision is recommended in patients requiring more than 3 **isoproterenol** aerosolized treatments. Further therapy with the bronchodilator aerosol alone is inadvisable when 3 to 5 treatments within 6 to 12 hours produce minimal or no relief. Reduce **epinephrine** dose if bronchial irritation, nervousness, restlessness, or sleeplessness occurs. Do not continue to use epinephrine, but seek medical assistance immediately if symptoms are not relieved within 20 minutes or become worse.

Use with short-acting beta-2 agonists – When patients begin treatment with **salmeterol**, **arformoterol**, or **formoterol**, advise those who have been taking short-acting, inhaled beta-2 agonists on a regular daily basis to discontinue their regular daily dosing regimen, and clearly instruct them to use short-acting, inhaled beta-2 agonists only for symptomatic relief if they develop asthma symptoms while taking salmeterol.

➤*Paradoxical bronchospasm:* Occasionally patients have developed severe paradoxical airway resistance with repeated, excessive use of inhalation preparations; the cause is unknown. Discontinue the drug immediately and institute alternative therapy. It should be recognized that paradoxical bronchospasm, when associated with inhaled formulations, frequently occurs with the first use of a new canister.

➤*Combined therapy:* Concomitant use with other sympathomimetic agents is not recommended, as it may lead to deleterious cardiovascular effects. This does not preclude the judicious use of an adrenergic stimulant aerosol bronchodilator in patients receiving tablets. Do not give on a routine basis. If regular coadministration is required, consider alternative therapy.

Do not use 2 or more beta-adrenergic aerosol bronchodilators simultaneously because of the potential of additive effects.

Patients must be warned not to stop or reduce corticosteroid therapy without medical advice, even if they feel better when they are being treated with beta-2 agonists. These agents are not to be used as a substitute for oral or inhaled corticosteroids.

➤*Cardiovascular effects:* Use with caution in patients with cardiovascular disorders, including coronary insufficiency, ischemic heart disease, coronary artery disease, cardiac arrhythmias, congestive heart failure (CHF), and hypertension.

Beta-adrenergic agonists can produce significant cardiovascular effects measured by pulse rate, blood pressure, and/or electrocardiogram (ECG) changes (eg, flattening of T waves, prolongation of the QTc interval, ST-segment depression).

Isoproterenol doses sufficient to increase the heart rate more than 130 bpm may increase the likelihood of inducing ventricular arrhythmias.

These agents may cause toxic symptoms through idiosyncratic response or overdosage. If cardiac rate increases sharply, angina patients may experience anginal pain until the cardiac rate decreases.

Closely monitor patients receiving **epinephrine**. Inadvertently induced high arterial blood pressure may result in angina pectoris, aortic rupture, or cerebral hemorrhage. Cardiac arrhythmias develop in some individuals even after therapeutic doses. Epinephrine causes changes in the ECG, including a decrease in amplitude of the T wave, even in healthy people.

Ephedrine may cause hypertension, resulting in intracranial hemorrhage. It may induce anginal pain in patients with coronary insufficiency or ischemic heart disease.

Large doses of inhaled or oral **salmeterol** (12 to 20 times the recommended dose) have been associated with clinically significant prolongation of the QTc interval, which has the potential for producing ventricular arrhythmias.

Significant changes in systolic and diastolic blood pressure can occur in some patients after use of any beta-adrenergic aerosol bronchodilator.

➤*Diabetes:* Large doses of IV **albuterol** and IV **terbutaline** may aggravate preexisting diabetes mellitus and ketoacidosis. Relevance to the use of oral or inhaled albuterol and oral terbutaline is unknown. Diabetic patients receiving any of these agents may require an increase in dosage of insulin or oral hypoglycemic agents.

➤*CNS effects:* Sympathomimetics may produce CNS stimulation.

IV **albuterol** sulfate in animals has demonstrated that it crosses the blood-brain barrier and reaches brain concentrations of approximately 5% of the plasma concentrations.

Long-term use – Prolonged use of **ephedrine** may produce a syndrome resembling an anxiety state. Many patients develop nervousness, and a sedative may be needed. After prolonged use or overdosage, elevated serum lactic acid levels with severe metabolic acidosis have occurred, as have transient blood glucose elevations.

➤*Overdosage/IV injection:* Overdosage or inadvertent IV injection of conventional subcutaneous **epinephrine** doses may cause extremely elevated arterial pressure, which may result in cerebrovascular hemorrhage, particularly in elderly patients; severe peripheral constriction and cardiac stimulation resulting in pulmonary arterial hypertension and potentially fatal pulmonary edema; and ventricular hyperirritability, which may result in death from ventricular fibrillation. Epinephrine is rapidly inactivated in the body, and treatment is primarily supportive. If necessary, pressor effects may be counteracted by rapidly acting vasodilators or alpha-adrenergic blocking drugs. If prolonged hypotension follows such measures, it may be necessary to administer another pressor drug, such as norepinephrine. If an epinephrine overdose induces pulmonary edema that interferes with respiration, treatment consists of a rapidly acting alpha-adrenergic–blocking drug (eg, phentolamine) or intermittent positive-pressure respiration. Transient bradycardia followed by tachycardia may also result, and these may be accompanied by potentially fatal cardiac arrhythmias. Ventricular, premature contractions may appear within 1 minute after injection and may be followed by multifocal, ventricular tachycardia (prefibrillation rhythm). Subsidence of the ventricular effects may be followed by atrial tachycardia and occasionally by atrioventricular (AV) block. Treatment of arrhythmias consists of administration of a beta-adrenergic–blocking drug, such as propranolol. Overdosage sometimes also results in extreme pallor and coldness of skin, metabolic acidosis, and kidney failure. Take suitable corrective measures.

Administer **epinephrine** with great caution and in carefully circumscribed quantities in areas of the body served by end arteries or with otherwise limited blood supply (eg, fingers, toes, nose, ears, genitals) or if peripheral vascular disease is present to avoid vasoconstriction-induced tissue sloughing.

➤*Benzyl alcohol:* Benzyl alcohol, contained in some of these products as a preservative, has been associated with a fatal "gasping syndrome" in premature infants.

➤*Parkinson disease:* **Epinephrine** may temporarily increase rigidity and tremor.

➤*Hypersensitivity reactions:* Hypersensitivity (allergic) reactions can occur after administration of **albuterol**, **levalbuterol**, **metaproterenol**, **terbutaline**, **ephedrine**, **salmeterol**, **arformoterol**, **formoterol**, and possibly other bronchodilators, as demonstrated by cases of urticaria, angioedema, rash, and bronchospasm. See Management of Acute Hypersensitivity Reactions.

Formoterol inhalation powder contains lactose, which contains trace levels of milk proteins. Allergic reactions to products containing milk proteins may occur in patients with severe milk protein allergy.

➤*Sulfite sensitivity:* Some of these products contain sulfites that may cause allergic-type reactions, including anaphylactic symptoms and life-threatening or less severe asthmatic episodes in certain susceptible persons. The overall prevalence of sulfite sensitivity in the general population is unknown and possibly low. It is seen more frequently in asthmatic or atopic nonasthmatic persons.

➤*Special risk:* Administer with caution to patients with diabetes mellitus, hyperthyroidism, thyrotoxicosis, prostatic hypertrophy (**ephedrine**), or a history of seizures; patients who are unusually sensitive to sympathomimetic amines; elderly patients; psychoneurotic individuals; or patients with long-standing bronchial asthma and emphysema who have developed degenerative heart disease (**epinephrine**).

In patients with status asthmaticus and abnormal blood gas tensions, improvement in vital capacity and blood gas tensions may not accompany apparent relief of bronchospasm following isoproterenol. Facilities for administering oxygen and ventilatory assistance are necessary.

➤*Drug abuse and dependence:* Prolonged abuse of **ephedrine** can lead to symptoms of paranoid schizophrenia. Patients exhibit such signs as tachycardia, poor nutrition and hygiene, fever, cold sweat, and dilated pupils. Some measure of tolerance develops, but addiction does not occur. With all sympathomimetic aerosols, cardiac arrest and even death may be associated with abuse.

➤*Pregnancy: Category B* (**terbutaline**). *Category C* (**albuterol**, **arformoterol**, **ephedrine**, **epinephrine**, **formoterol**, **isoproterenol**, **levalbuterol**, **metaproterenol**, **salmeterol**, **pirbuterol**). Several of these agents are teratogenic and embryocidal in animal studies. There is no evidence that these class effects in animals are relevant to use in humans. There are no adequate and well-controlled studies in pregnant women. Use only when clearly needed and when potential benefits outweigh potential hazards to the fetus.

According to the 2004 Working Group Report on Managing Asthma During Pregnancy, albuterol is the preferred short-acting beta-2 agonist and is recommended in patients with intermittent asthma in need of a quick relief medication. Albuterol is also the recommended treatment for patients with intermittent asthma who experience exercise-induced bronchospasm. For treating moderate or severe persistent asthma, a long-acting beta-2 agonist with an inhaled corticosteroid is one of the preferred treatment options. Short-acting beta-2 agonists have not been shown to cause fetal injury, and it is expected that long-acting beta-2 agonists have a similar safety profile during pregnancy. Available observational data during pregnancy for salmeterol and formoterol is limited; salmeterol may be a preferred option as it has been available in the U.S. longer.

Labor and delivery – The 2004 Working Group Report on Managing Asthma During Pregnancy recommends that asthma medications be continued during labor and delivery. However, beta-2 agonists may inhibit uterine contractions. Adverse reactions include increased heart rate, transient hyperglycemia, hypokalemia, cardiac arrhythmias, pulmonary edema, cerebral and myocardial ischemia, and increased fetal heart rate and hypoglycemia in the neonate. Although these effects are unlikely with aerosol use, consider the potential for untoward effects.

Oral **albuterol** has the potential to delay preterm labor. There are no well-controlled studies that demonstrate that they stop preterm labor or prevent labor at term. Therefore, use cautiously in pregnant patients when given for relief of bronchospasm to avoid interference with uterine contractility. **Terbutaline** is not indicated for the management of preterm labor. Maternal death has occurred with terbutaline and other drugs in this class. (See Indications for information on the off-label use of terbutaline in preterm labor.)

Parenteral administration of **ephedrine** to maintain blood pressure during low or other spinal anesthesia for delivery can cause acceleration of fetal heart rate; do not use in obstetrics when maternal blood pressure exceeds 130/80 mm Hg.

➤*Lactation:* **Terbutaline**, **ephedrine**, and **epinephrine** are excreted in breast milk. It is not known whether other agents are excreted in breast milk. Decide whether to discontinue breast-feeding or the drug, taking into account the importance of the drug to the mother.

According to the 2004 Working Group Report on Managing Asthma During Pregnancy, beta-2 agonists are not contraindications to breast-feeding. It is recommended to manage asthma during breast-feeding the same as during pregnancy.

➤*Children:*

Inhalation – Safety and efficacy for use of **pirbuterol** in children 12 years of age and younger have not been established. **Salmeterol** and **albuterol** aerosol and inhalation powder in children younger than 4 years of age and **albuterol** solution for inhalation in children younger than 2 years of age have not been established. For **levalbuterol**, safety and efficacy in children younger than 6 years of age (inhalation solution) and in children younger than 4 years of age (inhalation aerosol) have not been established. Safety and efficacy of **arformoterol** in children have not been established. Safety and efficacy of **formoterol** inhalation powder in children younger than 5 years of age have not been established; formoterol inhalation solution is not indicated for use in children.

Injection – Parenteral **terbutaline** is not recommended for use in children younger than 12 years of age. Administer **epinephrine** with caution to infants and children. Syncope has occurred following administration to asthmatic children.

Oral – **Metaproterenol** is not recommended for use in children younger than 6 years of age. **Terbutaline** is not recommended for use in children younger than 12 years of age. Safety and efficacy have not been established for **albuterol** in children younger than 2 years of age (syrup) and younger than 6 years of age (tablets and extended-release tablets).

Benzyl alcohol – Benzyl alcohol, contained in some of these products as a preservative, has been associated with a fatal "gasping syndrome" in premature infants.

➤*Elderly:* Lower doses may be required because of increased sympathomimetic sensitivity. Observe special caution when using in elderly patients who have concomitant cardiovascular disease that could be adversely affected by this class of drug. Based on available data, no adjustment of **salmeterol** dosage in elderly patients is warranted.

➤*Lab test abnormalities:*

Hypokalemia – Decreases in serum potassium levels have occurred, possibly through intracellular shunting, which can produce adverse cardiovascular effects. The decrease is usually transient, not requiring supplementation.

➤*Monitoring:* Monitor patients for significant cardiovascular effects, such as pulse rate, blood pressure, and/or ECG changes (eg, flattening of T waves, prolongation of the QTc interval, ST-segment depression. Monitor patients for worsening of asthma or COPD. Consider periodic monitoring of potassium and glucose levels during therapy.

Drug Interactions

➤*QT prolongation:* An additive effect of certain sympathomimetics (eg, albuterol, formoterol, isoproterenol, salmeterol, terbutaline) with other drugs that prolong the QT interval cannot be excluded. The following drugs may prolong the QT interval and increase the risk of life-threatening cardiac arrhythmias, including torsades de pointes: antiarrhythmic agents (eg, amiodarone, bretylium, disopyramide, dofetilide, procainamide, quinidine, sotalol), arsenic trioxide, chlorpromazine, cisapride, dolasetron, droperidol, mefloquine, mesoridazine, moxifloxacin, pentamidine, pimozide, tacrolimus, thioridazine, and ziprasidone. For a more complete list of drugs that may prolong the QT interval, see the appendix Drug-Induced Prolongation of the QT Interval and Torsades de Pointes.

Most interactions listed apply to sympathomimetics when used as vasopressors; however, consider the interaction when using the bronchodilator sympathomimetics.

Sympathomimetic Bronchodilators Drug Interactions

Precipitant drug	Object drug[a]		Description
Alpha-adrenergic blockers (eg, phentolamine)	Sympathomimetics Ephedrine Epinephrine	⬇	Vasoconstricting and hypertensive effects are antagonized.
Antihistamines	Sympathomimetics Epinephrine	⬆	**Epinephrine** effects may be potentiated.
Beta-blockers, nonselective (eg, propranolol)	Sympathomimetics	⬆⬇	Concomitant use may inhibit cardiac, bronchodilating, and vasodilating effects. Severe bronchospasms may be produced in asthmatic patients taking beta-2 agonists. Consider cardioselective beta-blockers, and use with caution if there are no alternatives to beta-blocker therapy. With **epinephrine**, hypertension and reflex bradycardia may develop.
Cardiac glycosides (eg, digoxin)	Sympathomimetics Epinephrine Ephedrine Isoproterenol	⬆	The potential for the myocardium to be sensitized to the effects of sympathomimetic amines is increased. Arrhythmias may result with coadministration and may respond to beta-blockers. Digoxin serum levels may be decreased by **albuterol**.
Sympathomimetics Albuterol	Cardiac glycosides (ie, digoxin)	⬇	
COMT[b] inhibitors (ie, entacapone, tolcapone)	Sympathomimetics	⬆	Coadministration may result in inhibition of the pathway responsible for normal catecholamine metabolism. Excessive sympathetic stimulation may result.

Sympathomimetic Bronchodilators Drug Interactions			
Precipitant drug	Object drug[a]		Description
CYP3A4 strong inhibitors (eg, atazanavir, clarithromycin, indinavir, itraconazole, ketoconazole, nefazodone, nelfinavir, ritonavir, saquinavir, telithromycin)	Sympathomimetics Salmeterol	↑	**Salmeterol** plasma concentrations may be elevated. Coadministration of salmeterol and ketoconazole has been associated with more frequent increases in QTc interval. Concomitant use of salmeterol and strong CYP3A4 inhibitors is not recommended.
Diuretics	Sympathomimetics Ephedrine Epinephrine	↓	Vascular response to pressor drugs such as **epinephrine** may be decreased. ECG changes and/or hypokalemia associated with non–potassium-sparing diuretics may worsen with coadministration of certain sympathomimetics.
Sympathomimetics	Diuretics (eg, loop diuretics, thiazide diuretics)	↑	
Ergot alkaloids	Sympathomimetics Epinephrine Isoproterenol	↑↓	Coadministration of ergot alkaloids with **isoproterenol** may result in additive peripheral vasoconstriction. Pressor effects of **epinephrine** may be reversed.
Sympathomimetics Isoproterenol	Ergot alkaloids		
Erythromycin	Sympathomimetics Salmeterol	↑	Coadministration increased salmeterol C_{max} 40% and increased heart rate and QTc interval. Coadminister with caution.
Furazolidone[c]	Sympathomimetics	↑	The pressor sensitivity to mixed-acting sympathomimetics (eg, **ephedrine**) may be increased. Direct-acting agents (eg, **epinephrine**) are not affected.
General anesthetics (eg, cyclopropane, halothane)	Sympathomimetics Isoproterenol Epinephrine Ephedrine	↑	The potential for the myocardium to be sensitized to the effects of sympathomimetic amines is increased. Arrhythmias may result with coadministration and may respond to beta-blockers.
Guanethidine	Sympathomimetics		Guanethidine potentiates the effects of the direct-acting sympathomimetics (eg, **epinephrine**) and inhibits the effects of the mixed-acting agents (eg, **ephedrine**). Guanethidine hypotensive action may also be reversed, requiring increased guanethidine dosage.
	Direct	↑	
	Mixed	↓	
Sympathomimetics	Guanethidine	↓	
Levothyroxine	Sympathomimetics Epinephrine	↑	**Epinephrine** effects may be potentiated.
Linezolid	Sympathomimetics	↑	Pharmacologic effects of sympathomimetics may be increased by linezolid. Headache, hyperpyrexia, and hypertension may occur. Most direct-acting sympathomimetics (eg, **epinephrine, isoproterenol**) appear to have minimal or no interaction liability.
Methyldopa	Sympathomimetics	↑	Coadministration may result in an increased pressor response.
Monoamine oxidase inhibitors (MAOIs)	Sympathomimetics	↑	Coadministration of MAOIs and mixed-acting sympathomimetics (eg, **ephedrine**) may result in severe headache, hypertension, and hyperpyrexia, resulting in hypertensive crisis. MAOIs also potentiate the actions of beta-adrenergic agonists on the vascular system. Direct-acting agents (eg, **epinephrine**) interact minimally. Avoid coadministration with sympathomimetics or within 2 weeks.
Sympathomimetics	MAOIs		
Nitrites	Sympathomimetics Epinephrine	↓	Pressor effects of epinephrine may be reversed.
Oxytocic drugs (eg, ergonovine)	Sympathomimetics Epinephrine	↑	Coadministration may result in severe hypertension.
Phenothiazines (eg, chlorpromazine)	Sympathomimetics Epinephrine	↓	Pressor effects of epinephrine may be reversed.
Rauwolfia alkaloids (ie, reserpine)	Sympathomimetics		Reserpine potentiates the pressor response of the direct-acting sympathomimetics (eg, **epinephrine**), which may result in hypertension. The pressor response of the mixed-acting agents (eg, **ephedrine**) is decreased.
	Direct	↑	
	Mixed	↓	
Steroids	Sympathomimetics	↑	Concomitant treatment may potentiate any hypokalemic effect of the sympathomimetic.
Tricyclic antidepressants (TCAs) (eg, amitriptyline, imipramine)	Sympathomimetics		TCAs potentiate the pressor response of direct-acting sympathomimetics (eg, **epinephrine**); dysrhythmias have occurred. The pressor response of mixed-acting agents (eg, **ephedrine**) is decreased. TCAs also potentiate the actions of beta-adrenergic agonists on the vascular system. If coadministration cannot be avoided, coadminister with extreme caution.
	Direct	↑	
	Mixed	↓	
Xanthine derivatives (eg, aminophylline, theophylline)	Sympathomimetics	↑↓	Concomitant treatment may potentiate any hypokalemic effect of the sympathomimetic. Enhanced toxicity, particularly cardiotoxicity, has also been noted. Decreased theophylline levels may occur. **Ephedrine** may cause theophylline toxicity.
Sympathomimetics	Xanthine derivatives (ie, theophylline)		
Sympathomimetics	Bromocriptine	↑	Sympathomimetics (eg, epinephrine) may increase the risk of bromocriptine toxicity. If concurrent use cannot be avoided, closely monitor the patient.

[a] ↑ = object drug increased; ↓ = object drug decreased; ↑↓ = object drug both increased and decreased.
[b] COMT = catechol-O-methyltransferase.
[c] No longer marketed in the United States.

➤*Drug/Lab test interactions:* **Isoproterenol** causes false elevations of bilirubin as measured in vitro by a sequential multiple analyzer. Isoproterenol inhalation may result in enough absorption of the drug to produce elevated urinary **epinephrine** values. Although small with standard doses, the effect is likely to increase with larger doses.

Adverse Reactions

Adverse reactions	Albuterol	Arformoterol	Ephedrine	Epinephrine	Formoterol	Isoproterenol	Levalbuterol	Metaproterenol	Pirbuterol	Salmeterol	Terbutaline
Sympathomimetic Bronchodilators: Summary of Adverse Reactions[a]											
Cardiovascular											
Blood pressure changes/hypertension	1%			✔	✔	2% to 5%	< 2%	0.4%		4%	< 1%
Chest tightness/pain/discomfort, angina	< 1%	7%		≤ 2.6%	1.9% to 3.2%	✔	< 2%	0.2%	< 1.3%		1.3% to 1.5%
Palpitations	5%		✔	7.8% to 30%	✔[b]	< 5% to 22%		4%	1.3% to 1.7%	✔	≤ 23%
PVCs[c], arrhythmias, skipped beats			✔	✔	✔	< 1% to 3%			< 1%		≈ 4%
Tachycardia	7%		✔	≤ 2.6%	✔	2% to 12%	2.7% to 2.8%	6% to 17%	1.2% to 1.3%	✔	1.3% to 3%
CNS											
Dizziness/Vertigo	1.5% to 7%		✔	3.3% to 7.8%	1.6% to 2.4%	1.5% to 5%	1.4% to 2.7%	2.4%	0.6% to 1.2%	4%	1.3% to 10%
Drowsiness	< 1%			8.2% to 14%		< 5%		0.6%			< 5% to 11.7%
Headache	3% to 19%		✔	3.3% to 10%	✔	1.5% to 10%	7.6% to 11.9%	1.1% to 7%	1.3% to 2%	13% to 17%	7.8% to 10%
Hyperactivity/Hyperkinesia, excitement	2% to 20%					✔			< 1%		
Insomnia	1% to 2%			✔	1.5% to 2.4%	1.5%	< 2%	1.8%	< 1%		✔
Migraine	1% to 2%										
Restlessness	< 1%			✔							
Shakiness/Nervousness/Tension	4% to 20%		✔	8.5% to 31%	✔	< 15%	2.8% to 9.6%	4.8% to 20.2%	4.5% to 7%	✔	< 5% to 31%
Tremor	7% to 24%	< 2%		16% to 18%	1.9%	< 15%	≤ 6.8%	1.6% to 16.9%	1.3% to 6%	✔	< 5% to 38%
Weakness	1% to 2%			1.6% to 2.6%		✔		0.2%	< 1%		≤ 1.3%
GI											
Diarrhea		6%			4.9%		≤ 6%	1.2%	< 1.3%		
Dry mouth	< 3%				1.2% to 3.3%		< 2%	0.4%	< 1.3%		
Heartburn/GI distress/disorder	1%					≤ 5% to 10%	1.4% to 2.7%	3%		2%	< 10%
Nausea/Vomiting	2% to 10%		✔	1% to 11.5%	2.4% to 4.9%	< 15%	< 10.5%	0.8% to 3.6%	≤ 1.7%	3%	1.3% to 10%
Musculoskeletal											
Back pain	4%	6%			4.2%						
Muscle cramps	3%										
Musculoskeletal pain	5%										
Leg cramps		4%			1.7%		≤ 2.7%				
Respiratory											
Asthma/Bronchospasm	8% to 13%					≤ 18%	9% to 9.4%			3% to 4%	
Bronchitis/Upper respiratory tract infection	1% to 21%										
Cough	< 1% to 5%					1% to 5%	1.4% to 4.1%	0.2%	1.2%	5%	
Dyspnea		4%		≤ 2%	2.1%	≤ 1.5%					≤ 2%
Lung disorder	6%	2%									
Nasal/Sinus congestion	1% to 3%									4% to 9%	
Rhinitis	4% to 22%									4% to 5%	
Sinusitis		5%			2.7%					4%	

Sympathomimetic Bronchodilators: Summary of Adverse Reactions[a]											
Adverse reactions	Albuterol	Arformoterol	Ephedrine	Epinephrine	Formoterol	Isoproterenol	Levalbuterol	Metaproterenol	Pirbuterol	Salmeterol	Terbutaline
Throat dryness/ irritation, pharyngitis	1% to 14%				3.5%	3.1%	3% to 10.4%	0.4%	< 1%	≥ 3%	✓
Wheezing	1%					1.5%					✓
Miscellaneous											
Anorexia/ Appetite loss	1%		✓	✓					< 1%		
Flu syndrome	3%	3%								5%	
Flushing	< 1%3%			≤ 1.3%		✓			< 1%		≤ 2.4%
Pain		8%								1% to < 3%	
Peripheral edema		3%									
Rash		4%			1.1%					4%	
Sweating	< 1%		✓	✓		✓		0.2%			≤ 2.4%
Unusual/bad taste or taste/smell change	< 1%							0.8%	< 1%		✓
Viral infection	4% to 7%				17.2%						

[a] Data pooled for all routes of administration, all age groups, from separate studies, and are not necessarily comparable.
[b] ✓ = reported; no incidence given.
[c] PVCs = premature ventricular contractions.
[d] Reported terms coded to lung disorder were predominantly pulmonary or chest congestion.

Adverse reactions are generally transient, and no cumulative effects have been reported. It is usually not necessary to discontinue treatment; however, in selected cases temporarily reduce dosage. After the reaction has subsided, increase dosage in small increments to optimal dosage. In addition to the table, other adverse reactions are as follows:

➤*Albuterol:*

CNS – CNS stimulation, malaise (1.5%); aggressive behavior, emotional lability, fatigue, nightmares (1%); disturbed sleep, irritability, lightheadedness (less than 1%).

Respiratory – Epistaxis (1% to 3%); hoarseness (rare in adults; 2% in children 4 to 12 years of age).

Miscellaneous – Increased appetite, stomachache (3%); muscle cramps (1% to 3%); anorexia, conjunctivitis, dyspepsia, pallor, teeth discoloration (1%); dilated pupils, epigastric pain, micturition difficulty, muscle spasm, voice changes (less than 1%); angioedema, bronchospasm, oropharyngeal edema (rare with oral and inhaled albuterol), rash, urticaria. Rarely, erythema multiforme and Stevens-Johnson syndrome have been associated with the administration of albuterol sulfate syrup in children. There have been rare reports of GI obstruction in such patients in association with ingestion of products containing delivery systems similar to that contained in albuterol sulfate extended-release tablets.

➤*Arformoterol:*

Cardiovascular – Arteriosclerosis, atrial flutter, AV block, CHF, heart block, inverted T wave, myocardial infarct, QT interval prolonged, supraventricular tachycardia (less than 2%).

CNS – Agitation, cerebral infarct, circumoral paresthesia, hypokinesia, paralysis, somnolence (less than 2%).

Dermatologic – Dry skin, herpes simplex, herpes zoster, skin discoloration, skin hypertrophy (less than 2%).

GI – Constipation, gastritis, melena, oral moniliasis, periodontal abscess, rectal hemorrhage (less than 2%).

GU – Breast neoplasm, calcium crystalluria, cystitis, glycosuria, hematuria, kidney calculus, nocturia, prostate-specific antigen increase, pyuria, urinary tract disorder, urine abnormality (less than 2%).

Metabolic/Nutritional – Dehydration, edema, glucose tolerance decreased, gout, hyperglycemia, hyperlipemia, hypoglycemia, hypokalemia (less than 2%).

Musculoskeletal – Arthralgia, arthritis, bone disorder, rheumatoid arthritis, tendinous contracture (less than 2%).

Respiratory – Carcinoma of the lung, respiratory disorder, voice alteration (less than 2%).

Special senses – Abnormal vision, glaucoma (less than 2%).

Miscellaneous – Abscess, allergic reaction, digitalis intoxication, fever, hernia, neck rigidity, neoplasm, pelvic pain, retroperitoneal hemorrhage (less than 2%).

➤*Ephedrine:* Contact dermatitis after topical application, precordial pain. *Parenteral:* Cerebral hemorrhage; confusion, delirium, hallucinations; urinary retention in men with prostatism; vesical sphincter spasm from repeated injections resulting in difficult and painful urination.

➤*Epinephrine:* Anxiety, fear, pallor. *Parenteral:* Assaultive behavior; cerebral hemorrhage; direct vasoconstrictive effect on the renal circulation; disorientation; fatal ventricular fibrillation; hallucinations; hemiplegia; impairment of memory; induce or aggravate psychomotor agitation; local tissue necrosis from vascular constriction caused by repeated injections at the same site; occlusion of the central retinal artery, shock, and angina in coronary-artery disease; pain at injection site (1.6% to 2.6%); panic; schizophrenic-type thought disorders or paranoid delusions; subarachnoid and cerebral hemorrhage; suicidal or homicidal tendencies; syncope in children; temporary rigidity and tremor in patients with Parkinson disease; urticaria, wheal, and hemorrhage at injection site.

➤*Formoterol:*

Dermatologic – Pruritus (1.5%).

Musculoskeletal – Leg cramps, muscle cramps (1.7%).

Respiratory – Upper respiratory tract infection (7.4%); serious asthma exacerbations (some have been fatal) (0% to 6.4%); bronchitis (4.6%); nasopharyngitis (3.3%); chest infection (2.7%); tonsillitis (1.2%); dysphonia (1%).

Miscellaneous – Viral infection (17.2%); back pain (4.2%); fever (2.2%); anxiety, sputum increased (1.5%); angina, fatigue, hyperglycemia, hypokalemia, malaise, metabolic acidosis.

Postmarketing – Rare reports of anaphylactic reactions, including severe hypotension and angioedema, have been reported with formoterol inhalation powder.

➤*Isoproterenol:*

Cardiovascular – Adams-Stokes attacks, cardiac arrest, hypotension, precordial ache/distress. In a few patients, presumably with organic disease of the AV node and its branches, isoproterenol has precipitated Adams-Stokes seizures during normal sinus rhythm or transient heart block.

Respiratory – Bronchitis (5%); sputum increase (1.5%); coronary insufficiency, paradoxical airway resistance, pulmonary edema, rebound bronchospasm.

➤*Levalbuterol:*

Cardiovascular – ECG abnormal, ECG change, hypertension, hypotension, syncope (less than 2%).

CNS – Anxiety, migraine (0% to 2.7%); hypesthesia of the hand, paresthesia (less than 2%).

Dermatologic – Rash (0% to 7.5%); urticaria (0% to 3%); acne (less than 2%).

GI – Abdominal pain (0% to 1.5%); constipation, dry throat, dyspepsia, gastroenteritis (less than 2%).

Musculoskeletal – Myalgia (less than 2%).

Respiratory – Rhinitis (2.7% to 11.1%); bronchitis (2.6%); sinusitis (1.4% to 4.2%); turbinate edema (1.4% to 2.8%); epistaxis, lung disorder (less than 2%).

Miscellaneous – Viral infection (6.9% to 12.3%); fever (3% to 9.1%); flu syndrome (1.4% to 4.2%); accidental injury (0% to 9.2%); asthenia (3%); pain (1.4% to 4%); chest pain, chills, eye itch, lymphadenopathy (less than 3%); conjunctivitis, cyst, dysmenorrhea, ear pain, hematuria, herpes simplex, vaginal moniliasis (less than 2%).

Postmarketing – Angioedema, anaphylaxis, arrhythmias (including atrial fibrillation, supraventricular tachycardia, extrasystoles), asthma, chest pain, cough increased, dyspnea, nausea, nervousness, rash, tachycardia, tremor, urticaria.

➤*Metaproterenol:*

Dermatologic – Pruritus (0.4%); hives (0.2%).

Musculoskeletal – Pain, spasms (0.2%).

Miscellaneous – GI distress (3%); asthma exacerbation (2%); fatigue (1.4%); feverish, syncope (0.4%); blurred vision, chatty, chills, clonus noted on flexing foot, edema, facial and finger puffiness, flu symptoms, laryngeal changes, sensory disturbances (0.2%).

➤*Pirbuterol:*

CNS – Anxiety, confusion, depression, fatigue, syncope (less than 1%).

Dermatologic – Alopecia, bruising, edema, pruritus, rash (less than 1%).

GI – Abdominal pain/cramps, glossitis, stomatitis (less than 1%).

Miscellaneous – Hypotension, numbness in extremities, weight gain (less than 1%).

➤*Salmeterol:*

CNS – Anxiety, migraines, paresthesia, sinus headache, sleep disturbance (1% to 3%).

Dermatologic – Urticaria (3%); contact dermatitis, eczema (1% to 3%); photodermatitis (1% to 2%).

GI – Candidiasis mouth/throat, dyspeptic symptoms, hyposalivation, dental discomfort and pain, GI infections, oral mucosal abnormality (1% to less than 3%).

Musculoskeletal – Musculoskeletal pain (12%); muscle cramps and spasms (3%); arthralgia, articular rheumatism, muscle pain, bone and skeletal pain, musculoskeletal inflammation, muscle stiffness, pain in joint, tightness, rigidity (1% to less than 3%).

Respiratory – Tracheitis/bronchitis (7%); lower respiratory signs and symptoms (1% to less than 3%).

Musculoskeletal – Joint/back pain, muscle cramp/contraction, myalgia/myositis, muscular soreness (1% to 3%).

Special senses – Ear signs and symptoms (3% to 4%); conjunctivitis, keratitis (1% to less than 3%).

Miscellaneous – Localized aches and pains, pyrexia of unknown origin (1% to 3%); viral respiratory infection (5%), edema, hyperglycemia, swelling (1% to less than 3%).

Postmarketing – Arrhythmias (including atrial fibrillation, supraventricular tachycardia, extrasystoles); upper airway symptoms of laryngeal spasm, irritation, or swelling such as stridor or choking; oropharyngeal irritation; anaphylaxis; very rare anaphylactic reaction in patients with severe milk protein allergy; serious exacerbations of asthma, including some that have been fatal).

➤*Terbutaline:*

Miscellaneous – Central stimulation; ECG changes, such as sinus pause, atrial premature beats, AV block, ventricular premature beats, ST-T wave depression, T wave inversion, sinus bradycardia, and atrial escape beat with aberrant conduction; increased heart rate; muscle cramps; pain at injection site (0.5% to 2.6%); elevations in liver enzymes, hypersensitivity vasculitis, seizures (rare).

➤*Hyperglycemia:* **Isoproterenol** causes less hyperglycemia than **epinephrine**. Isoproterenol and epinephrine are equally effective in stimulating the release of free fatty acids and energy production.

Glycogenolysis in the liver is increased by **ephedrine**, but not as much as by **epinephrine**; usual doses of ephedrine are unlikely to produce hyperglycemia.

Overdosage

➤*Inhalation:*

Symptoms – Exaggeration of the effects listed under Adverse Reactions can occur (eg, seizures, hypokalemia, anginal pain, hyperglycemia, hypotension, hypertension, tachycardia with rates up to 200 beats/min, arrhythmias, nervousness, headache, tremor, muscle cramps, dry mouth, palpitation, nausea, dizziness, fatigue, malaise, insomnia). Metabolic acidosis may also occur. Clinically significant prolongation with QTc interval and cardiac arrest have been reported with use. Cardiac arrest and death may be associated with abuse.

Treatment – Discontinue medication with general supportive measures. Monitor blood pressure and ECG. The judicious use of a cardioselective beta-receptor blocker (ie, metoprolol, atenolol) is suggested, bearing in mind the danger of inducing an asthmatic attack. Dialysis is not appropriate.

➤*Systemic:*

Symptoms – Palpitations; tachycardia; transient arrhythmias; bradycardia; extrasystoles; heart block; angina; hyperglycemia and increased insulin levels, followed by rebound hypoglycemia; hypokalemia; hypo- or hypertension; significant drop in blood pressure caused by peripheral vasodilation; fever; chills; cold perspiration; blanching of the skin; nausea; vomiting; mydriasis. Central actions produce insomnia, anxiety, nervousness, drowsiness, muscle cramps, headache, sweating, and tremor. Delirium, convulsions, collapse, and coma may occur.

The principal manifestation of **ephedrine** sulfate poisoning is convulsions. The following signs and symptoms may also occur: Initially, the patient may have hypertension, followed later by hypotension accompanied by anuria. Nausea, vomiting, chills, cyanosis, irritability, nervousness, fever, suicidal behavior, tachycardia, dilated pupils, blurred vision, opisthotonos, spasms, convulsions, pulmonary edema, gasping respirations, coma, and respiratory failure.

Treatment – Discontinue medication or reduce dosage. Gastric lavage or charcoal may be useful following overdosage with oral agents. If pronounced, a beta-adrenergic blocker (propranolol) may be used, but consider the possibility of aggravation of airway obstruction; phentolamine may be used to block strong alpha-adrenergic actions. Treatment includes usual supportive measures. Monitor blood pressure, pulse respiration, and ECG. If respirations are shallow or cyanosis is present, administer artificial respiration. Vasopressors are contraindicated. In cardiovascular collapse, maintain blood pressure. For hypertension, phentolamine mesylate 5 mg diluted in saline may be administered slowly IV, or 100 mg may be given orally. Convulsions may be controlled by diazepam or paraldehyde. Cool applications and dexamethasone 1 mg/kg administered slowly IV may control pyrexia. Refer to General Management of Acute Overdosage.

Patient Information

Instruct patients not to exceed recommended dosage; excessive use may lead to adverse effects or loss of effectiveness. Do not stop or adjust the dose.

Advise patients not to change brands without consulting their health care provider or pharmacist.

Inform patients that long-acting beta-2 agonists increase the risk of asthma-related death. All long-acting beta-2 agonists should not be used in patients with asthma without use of a long-term asthma control medication.

Advise patients to notify their health care provider if treatment is less effective, symptoms worsen, or the need to use this product increases in frequency. Usual adverse events include palpitations, chest pain, rapid heart rate, and tremor or nervousness.

Inform patients that isoproterenol may cause the patient's saliva to turn pinkish red.

Long-acting beta-2 agonists are not meant to relieve acute asthmatic symptoms, which should be treated with an inhaled, short-acting bronchodilator. The bronchodilator action usually lasts for 12 or more hours; therefore, do not use more often than every 12 hours. While using long-acting beta-2 agonists, seek medical attention immediately if the short-acting bronchodilator treatment becomes less effective for symptom relief, if more inhalations than usual are needed, or if more than the maximum number of inhalations of short-acting bronchodilator treatment prescribed for a 24-hour period are needed.

Warn patients that adverse cardiovascular effects may occur (eg, palpitations, chest pain, rapid heart rate, tremor, nervousness).

Instruct patients that if palpitations, tachycardia, chest pain, muscle tremors, dizziness, headache, flushing, or difficult urination (ephedrine) occurs or if breathing difficulty persists to notify their health care provider.

ISOPROTERENOL HYDROCHLORIDE

For complete prescribing information, see the isoproterenolmonograph in the Vasopressors Used in Shock section.

EPHEDRINE SULFATE

For complete prescribing information refer to the Ephedrine monograph in the Vasopressors Used in Shock section.

EPINEPHRINE (Adrenaline)

For complete prescribing information, refer to the Epinephrine monograph in the Vasopressors Used in Shock section.

LEVALBUTEROL

Rx	**Xopenex** (Sepracor)	**Solution; inhalation:** 0.31 mg per 3 mL	As levalbuterol hydrochloride. Preservative free. Sulfuric acid. In UD 3 mL vials.
		0.63 mg per 3 mL	As levalbuterol hydrochloride. Preservative free. Sulfuric acid. In UD 3 mL vials.
		1.25 mg per 3 mL	As levalbuterol hydrochloride. Preservative free. Sulfuric acid. In UD 3 mL vials.
Rx	**Levabuterol** (Mylan)	**Solution, concentrate; inhalation:** 1.25 mg per 0.5 mL	As levalbuterol hydrochloride. Preservative free. Sulfuric acid. In UD 0.5 mL vials.
Rx	**Xopenex** (Sepracor)		As levalbuterol hydrochloride. Preservative free. In 0.5 mL UD vials.
Rx	**Xopenex HFA** (Sepracor)	**Aerosol; inhalation:** 45 mcg per actuation	As levalbuterol tartrate. Contains no CFCs. In 15 g (200 inhalations).

LEVALBUTEROL — INHALATION

For complete and comparative prescribing information, refer to the Sympathomimetic Bronchodilator group monograph.

Indications

➤*Bronchospasm:* For the treatment or prevention of bronchospasm in patients with reversible obstructive airway disease.

Administration and Dosage

➤*Maximum dose:*

Children 6 to 11 years of age –

Nebulization solution: 0.63 mg three times daily according to the prescribing information.

➤*Adults:*

Bronchospasm –

Xopenex:

• *Usual dosage* – 0.63 mg administered 3 times/day (every 6 to 8 hours) by nebulization.

• *Dosage titration* – Patients with severe asthma or who do not respond adequately to initial dose may benefit from a dosage of 1.25 mg 3 times/day. Closely monitor patients receiving the higher dose for adverse systemic effects and balance the risks of such effects against the potential for improved efficacy.

Xopenex HFA: 2 inhalations (90 mcg) repeated every 4 to 6 hours; in some patients, 1 inhalation every 4 hours may be sufficient. More frequent administrations or a larger number of inhalations is not routinely recommended.

Off-label dosing –

Asthma exacerbations: The following dosing is from the National Asthma Education and Prevention guidelines.

• *Inhalation aerosol (metered-dose inhaler)* – 4 to 8 inhalations every 20 minutes up to 4 hours, then every 1 to 4 hours as needed.

• *Inhalation solution (nebulizer)* – 1.25 to 2.5 mg every 20 minutes for 3 doses, then 1.25 to 5 mg every 1 to 4 hours as needed.

➤*Children:*

Bronchospasm –

Xopenex:

• *12 years of age and older –*

Usual dosage: 0.63 mg administered 3 times/day (every 6 to 8 hours) by nebulization.

Dosage titration: Patients with severe asthma or who do not respond adequately to initial dose may benefit from a dosage of 1.25 mg 3 times/day. Closely monitor patients receiving the higher dose for adverse systemic effects and balance the risks of such effects against the potential for improved efficacy.

• *6 to 11 years of age* – 0.31 mg administered 3 times/day by nebulization. Do not exceed routine dosing of 0.63 mg 3 times/day.

Xopenex HFA:

• *4 years of age and older* – 2 inhalations (90 mcg) repeated every 4 to 6 hours; in some patients, 1 inhalation every 4 hours may be sufficient. More frequent administrations or a larger number of inhalations is not routinely recommended.

Off-label dosing – The following dosing is from the National Asthma Education and Prevention guidelines.

Asthma (quick relief):

• *Inhalation solution (nebulizer)* – 5 to 11 years of age: 0.31 to 0.63 mg every 8 hours as needed.

4 years of age and younger: 0.31 to 1.25 mg (in 3 mL) every 4 to 6 hours as needed.

Asthma exacerbations:

• *Older than 12 years of age –*

Inhalation aerosol (metered-dose inhaler): 4 to 8 inhalations every 20 minutes up to 4 hours, then every 1 to 4 hours as needed.

Inhalation solution (nebulizer): 1.25 to 2.5 mg every 20 minutes for 3 doses, then 1.25 to 5 mg every 1 to 4 hours as needed.

• *12 years of age and younger –*

Inhalation aerosol (metered-dose inhaler): 4 to 8 inhalations every 20 minutes for 3 doses, then every 1 to 4 hours inhalation maneuver as needed. Use valved holding chamber; add mask in children younger than 4 years of age.

Inhalation solution (nebulizer): 0.075 mg/kg (minimum dose 1.25 mg) every 20 minutes for 3 doses, then 0.075 to 0.15 mg/kg up to 5 mg every 1 to 4 hours as needed.

➤*Elderly:* Dosage should be started at levalbuterol 0.63 mg inhalation solution. The dose may be increased as tolerated, in conjunction with frequent clinical and laboratory monitoring, to the maximum recommended daily dose.

➤*Preparation for administration:*

Xopenex – Dilute the concentrated solution (1.25 mg per 0.5 mL) with sterile normal saline before administration by nebulization.

Xopenex HFA – It is recommended to prime the inhaler before using for the first time and in cases in which the inhaler has not been used for more than 3 days by releasing 4 test sprays into the air, away from the face.

To maintain proper use of this product, it is critical that the actuator be washed and dried thoroughly at least once a week. The inhaler may cease to deliver medication if not properly cleaned and dried thoroughly. Keeping the plastic actuator clean is very important to prevent medication build-up and blockage. If the actuator becomes blocked with the drug, washing the actuator will remove the blockage.

➤*Administration:*

Xopenex – The safety and efficacy of levalbuterol inhalation solution have been established in clinical trials when administered using the *PARI LC Jet* and the *PARI LC Plus* nebulizers, and the *PARI Master Dura-Neb 2000* and *Dura-Neb 3000* compressors. The safety and efficacy of levalbuterol inhalation solution when administered using other nebulizer systems have not been established.

➤*Admixture compatibility:* Levalbuterol inhalation solution may be mixed with budesonide inhalant suspension.

➤*Storage/Stability:*

Xopenex – Store in the protective foil pouch between 20° and 25°C (68° and 77°F). Protect from light and excessive heat. Keep unopened vials in the foil pouch. Once the foil pouch is opened, use the vials within 2 weeks. If the individual vial is removed from the foil pouch and is not used immediately, protect from light and use within 1 week. Discard the vial if the solution is not colorless.

Xopenex HFA – Store between 20° and 25°C (68° and 77°F). Protect from freezing temperatures and direct sunlight. Store inhaler with the actuator (or mouthpiece) down. Do not puncture or incinerate. Exposure to temperatures above 49°C (120°F) may cause bursting.

SALMETEROL

Rx	**Serevent Diskus** (GlaxoSmithKline)	**Powder; inhalation:** 50 mcg	As salmeterol xinafoate. Lactose. In 60 blisters and institutional pack containing 28 blisters.

SALMETEROL XINAFOATE — INHALATION

For complete and comparative prescribing information, refer to the Sympathomimetics class monograph.

WARNING

Long-acting beta-2 adrenergic agonists, such as salmeterol, increase the risk of asthma-related death. Data from a large placebo-controlled US study that compared the safety of salmeterol or placebo added to usual asthma therapy showed an increase in asthma-related deaths in patients receiving salmeterol (13 deaths out of 13,176 patients treated for 28 weeks on salmeterol versus 3 deaths out of 13,179 patients on placebo). Currently available data are inadequate to determine whether concurrent use of inhaled corticosteroids or other long-term asthma control drugs mitigates the increased risk of asthma-related death from long-acting beta-2 adrenergic agonists.

Because of this risk, use of salmeterol for the treatment of asthma without a concomitant long-term asthma control medication, such as an inhaled corticosteroid, is contraindicated. Use salmeterol only as additional therapy for patients with asthma who are currently taking but are inadequately controlled on a long-term asthma control medication, such as an inhaled corticosteroid. Once asthma control is achieved and maintained, assess the patient at regular intervals and step down therapy (eg, discontinue salmeterol) if possible without loss of asthma control and maintain the patient on a long-term asthma control medication, such as an inhaled corticosteroid. Do not use salmeterol for patients whose asthma is adequately controlled on low- or medium-dose inhaled corticosteroids.

Children and adolescents – Available data from controlled clinical trials suggest that long-acting beta-2 adrenergic agonists increase the risk of asthma-related hospitalization in children and adolescents. For children and adolescents with asthma who require addition of a long-acting beta-2 adrenergic agonist to an inhaled corticosteroid, a fixed-dose combination product containing both an inhaled corticosteroid and a long-acting beta-2 adrenergic agonist should ordinarily be used to ensure adherence with both drugs. In cases where use of a separate long-term asthma control medication (eg, inhaled corticosteroid) and a long-acting beta-2 adrenergic agonist is clinically indicated, appropriate steps must be taken to ensure adherence with both treatment components. If adherence cannot be ensured, a fixed-dose combination product containing both an inhaled corticosteroid and a long-acting beta-2 adrenergic agonist is recommended.

Indications

➤*Asthma/Bronchospasm:* For the treatment of asthma and the prevention of bronchospasmonly as concomitant therapy with a long-term asthma control medication, such as an inhaled corticosteroid, in patients 4 years of age and older with reversible obstructive airway disease, including patients with symptoms of nocturnal asthma.

➤*Chronic obstructive pulmonary disease:* For the long-term, twice-daily (morning and evening) administration in the maintenance treatment of bronchospasm associated with chronic obstructive pulmonary disease (COPD) (including emphysema and chronic bronchitis).

➤*Prevention of exercise-induced bronchospasm:* For the prevention of exercise-induced bronchospasm (EIB) in patients 4 years of age and older. Use of salmeterol as a single agent for the prevention of EIB may be clinically indicated in patients who do not have persistent asthma. In patients with persistent asthma, use of salmeterol for the prevention of EIB may be clinically indicated, but the treatment of asthma should include a long-term asthma control medication, such as an inhaled corticosteroid.

Administration and Dosage

➤*General dosing considerations:* See the Warning box for more information.

Do not use in patients whose asthma can be managed by occasional use of inhaled, short-acting beta-2 agonists or whose asthma can be successfully managed by inhaled corticosteroids or other controller medications along with occasional use of inhaled, short-acting beta-2 agonists.

➤*Adults:*

Asthma/Bronchospasm –

Usual dosage: 1 inhalation (50 mcg) twice daily (morning and evening, approximately 12 hours apart).

Dosage adjustment: If a previously effective dosage regimen fails to provide the usual response, patients should seek medical advice immediately because this is often a sign of destabilization of asthma. Under these circumstances, reevaluate the therapeutic regimen.

Concomitant therapy: When initiating salmeterol in patients receiving oral or inhaled corticosteroids for treatment of asthma, patients should be continued on a suitable dose of corticosteroids to maintain clinical stability even if they feel better as a result of initiating salmeterol. Make any change in corticosteroid dosage only after clinical evaluation.

When prescribing salmeterol, also provide the patient with an inhaled, short-acting beta-2 agonist (eg, albuterol) for treatment of symptoms that occur acutely, despite regular twice-daily (morning and evening) use of salmeterol.

When beginning treatment with salmeterol, instruct patients who have been taking inhaled, short-acting beta-2 agonists on a regular basis (eg, 4 times a day) to discontinue the regular use of these drugs and to use them only for symptomatic relief of acute asthma or COPD symptoms.

Chronic obstructive pulmonary disease –

Usual dosage: 1 inhalation (50 mcg) twice daily (morning and evening, approximately 12 hours apart).

Maximum dose: 1 inhalation (50 mcg) twice daily.

Prevention of exercise-induced bronchospasm – 1 inhalation (50 mcg) at least 30 minutes before exercise. When used intermittently as needed for prevention of EIB, this protection may last up to 9 hours. Additional doses of salmeterol should not be used for 12 hours after the administration of this drug. Patients who are receiving salmeterol twice daily (morning and evening) should not use additional salmeterol for prevention of EIB.

➤*Children:*

Asthma/Bronchospasm –

4 years of age and older: See Adults.

• *Maximum dose –* 1 inhalation (50 mcg) twice daily.

Prevention of exercise-induced bronchospasm –

4 years of age and older: See Adults.

➤*Administration:* Only administer by the orally inhaled route. Instruct patient not to exhale into the inhalation device. Only activate and use the inhalation device in a level, horizontal position. Do not use a spacer.

➤*Storage/Stability:* Store at 20° to 25°C (68° to 77°F), in a dry place away from direct heat or sunlight. Discard 6 weeks after removal from the moisture-protective foil overwrap pouch or after all blisters have been used (when the dose indicator reads "0"), whichever comes first. The inhalation device is not reusable. Do not attempt to take the inhalation device apart.

ALBUTEROL (Salbutamol)

Rx	**Albuterol** (Various, eg, Mylan, UDL)	**Tablets; oral:** 2 mg	Equiv. to albuterol sulfate 2.4 mg. May contain lactose. In 100s, 500s, 600s, and UD 100s.
Rx	**Albuterol** (Various, eg, Mylan, UDL)	**Tablets; oral:** 4 mg	Equiv. to albuterol sulfate 4.8 mg. May contain lactose. In 100s, 500s, 600s, and UD 100s.
Rx	**Albuterol** (Mylan)	**Tablets, extended-release; oral:** 4 mg	Equiv. to albuterol sulfate 4.8 mg. May contain PEG, polydextrose. In 100s and 500s.
Rx	**VoSpire ER** (Dava)		Equiv. to albuterol sulfate 4.8 mg. Lactose, PEG. (V 4). Green, round. Film-coated. In 100s.
Rx	**Albuterol Sulfate** (Mylan)	**Tablets, extended-release; oral:** 8 mg	Equiv. to albuterol sulfate 9.6 mg. May contain PEG, polydextrose. (M 24). In 100s and 500s.
Rx	**VoSpire ER** (Dava)		Equiv. to albuterol sulfate 9.6 mg. Lactose, PEG. (V 8). White, round. Film-coated. In 100s.
Rx	**Albuterol** (Various, eg, Hi-Tech, Qualitest, Teva)	**Syrup; oral:** 2 mg per 5 mL	Equiv. to albuterol sulfate 2.4 mg. May contain sorbitol. In 473 mL.

ALBUTEROL (Salbutamol)

Rx	**Albuterol** (Various, eg, Barr)	**Aerosol; inhalation:** 90 mcg/actuation	Equiv. to albuterol sulfate 108 mcg. In 6.8 g (≥ 80 inhalations) and 17 g (≥ 200 inhalations).
Rx	**ProAir HFA** (Teva)		Equiv. to albuterol sulfate 108 mcg. In 8.5 g (200 inhalations).
Rx	**Proventil HFA** (Schering)		Equiv. to albuterol sulfate 108 mcg. In 6.7 g (200 inhalations).
Rx	**Ventolin HFA** (GlaxoSmithKline)		Equiv. to albuterol sulfate 108 mcg. In 18 g (200 inhalations) and 8 g (60 actuations).
Rx	**Albuterol** (Watson)	**Solution; inhalation:** 0.021% (0.63 mg per 3 mL)	Equiv. to albuterol sulfate 0.75 mg. Preservative free. In 3 mL UD vials.
Rx	**AccuNeb** (Dey)		Equiv. to albuterol sulfate 0.75 mg. Preservative free. In 3 mL UD vials.
Rx	**Albuterol** (Watson)	**Solution; inhalation:** 0.042% (1.25 mg per 3 mL)	Equiv. to albuterol sulfate 1.5 mg. Preservative free. In 3 mL UD vials.
Rx	**AccuNeb** (Dey)		Equiv. to albuterol sulfate 1.5 mg. Preservative free. In 3 mL UD vials.
Rx	**Albuterol** (Various, eg, Nephron)	**Solution; inhalation:** 0.083% (2.5 mg per 3 mL)	Equiv. to albuterol sulfate 1 mg. Preservative free. In 3 mL UD vials.
Rx	**Albuterol** (Various, eg, Nephron)	**Solution; inhalation:** 0.5% (5 mg/mL)	Equiv. to albuterol sulfate 3 mg. Preservative free. In 0.5 mL UD vials.

ALBUTEROL SULFATE — ORAL

For complete and comparative prescribing information, refer to the Sympathomimetic Bronchodilator class monograph.

Indications

➤*Bronchospasm:* For the relief of bronchospasm in patients with reversible obstructive airway disease.

Administration and Dosage

➤*General dosing considerations:* The following dosages are expressed in terms of albuterol base.

➤*Adults:*

Bronchospasm –

Extended-release tablets:

- *Usual dosage* – 8 mg every 12 hours. In some patients, 4 mg every 12 hours may be sufficient.
- *Maximum dose* – 32 mg/day.
- *Dosage adjustment* – The dosage may be cautiously increased stepwise.
- *Alternative dosage* – In unusual circumstances, such as adults of low body weight, it may be desirable to use a starting dosage of 4 mg every 12 hours and progress to 8 mg every 12 hours according to response.

Syrup and immediate-release tablets:

- *Maximum dose* – 32 mg/day.
- *Initial dosage* – 2 or 4 mg 3 or 4 times a day. An initial dosage of 2 mg 3 or 4 times a day is recommended in patients sensitive to beta-adrenergic stimulators.
- *Dosage adjustment* – The dosage should be cautiously increased stepwise. A dosage above 4 mg 4 times a day should be used only when the patient fails to respond.

➤*Children:*

Bronchospasm –

Extended-release tablets:

- *13 years of age and older –*
  Usual dosage: 8 mg every 12 hours. In some patients, 4 mg every 12 hours may be sufficient.
  Maximum dose: 32 mg/day.
  Dosage adjustment: The dosage may be cautiously increased stepwise.
  Alternative dosage: In unusual circumstances, it may be desirable to use a starting dosage of 4 mg every 12 hours and progress to 8 mg every 12 hours according to response.
- *6 to 12 years of age –*
  Usual dosage: 4 mg every 12 hours.
  Maximum dose: 24 mg/day.
  Dosage adjustment: The dosage may be cautiously increased stepwise.

Syrup:

- *15 years of age and older –*
  Maximum dose: 32 mg/day.
  Initial dosage: 2 or 4 mg 3 or 4 times a day. The initial dosage should be restricted to 2 mg 3 or 4 times a day in patients sensitive to beta-adrenergic stimulators.
  Dosage adjustment: The dosage should be cautiously increased stepwise. A dosage above 4 mg 4 times a day should be used only when the patient fails to respond.
- *6 to 14 years of age –*
  Maximum dose: 24 mg/day.
  Initial dosage: 2 mg 3 or 4 times a day.
  Dosage adjustment: The dosage may be cautiously increased stepwise.
- *2 to 5 years of age –*
  Maximum dose: 12 mg/day.
  Initial dosage: 0.1 mg/kg 3 times a day. This starting dose should not exceed 2 mg 3 times a day.
  Dosage adjustment: Increase stepwise to 0.2 mg/kg 3 times a day.
- *23 months of age and younger* – See Off-label Dosing.

Immediate-release tablets:

- *13 years of age and older –*
  Maximum dose: 32 mg/day.
  Initial dosage: 2 or 4 mg 3 or 4 times a day. An initial dosage of 2 mg 3 or 4 times a day is recommended in patients sensitive to beta-adrenergic stimulators.
  Dosage adjustment: The dosage should be cautiously increased stepwise. A dosage above 4 mg 4 times a day should be used only when the patient fails to respond.
- *6 to 12 years of age –*
  Maximum dose: 24 mg/day.
  Initial dosage: 2 mg 3 or 4 times a day.
  Dosage adjustment: The dosage may be cautiously increased stepwise.

Off-label dosing –

Bronchospasm:

- *Neonates* – 0.1 to 0.3 mg/kg every 6 to 8 hours.

➤*Elderly:*

Immediate-release tablets and syrup – An initial dosage of 2 mg 3 or 4 times a day is recommended. If adequate bronchodilation is not obtained, dosage may be increased gradually up to 8 mg 3 or 4 times a day.

➤*Conversion:* Patients currently maintained on immediate-release tablets or syrup can be switched to extended-release (ER) tablets. For example, the administration of one 4 mg ER tablet every 12 hours is comparable to one 2 mg tablet every 6 hours. Multiples of this regimen up to the maximum recommended daily dose also apply.

➤*Administration:* ER tablets must be swallowed whole with the aid of liquids. Do not chew or crush these tablets.

➤*Storage/Stability:* Store tablets at 20° to 25°C (68° to 77°F). Protect from light.

ALBUTEROL SULFATE — INHALATION

For complete and comparative prescribing information, refer to the Sympathomimetic Bronchodilator class monograph.

Indications

➤*Asthma/Bronchospasm:* For the treatment and prevention of bronchospasm in patients with reversible obstructive airway disease; for acute attacks of bronchospasm (inhalation solution 0.083% and 0.5%); and for prevention of exercise-induced bronchospasm.

➤*Off-label uses:*

Hyperkalemia – [1] = Good documentation. Evidence-based guidelines confirm the effectiveness of albuterol for treatment of moderate to severe hyperkalemia. Use of albuterol results in temporary correction of the serum potassium level; therefore, monitor patients and administer adjunctive treatments that promote potassium excretion from the body (eg, diuresis, kayexalate, dialysis) when appropriate. (See Administration and Dosage.)

ALBUTEROL SULFATE — INHALATION

Administration and Dosage

➤*General dosing considerations:* If a previously effective dosage regimen fails to provide the usual response, this may be a marker of destabilization of asthma and requires reevaluation of the patient and treatment regimen, giving special consideration to the possible need for anti-inflammatory treatment (eg, corticosteroids).

It is recommended to prime the inhaler before using for the first time, and in cases where the inhaler has not been used for more than 2 weeks, by releasing 4 test sprays into the air, away from the face (see Preparation for Administration).

➤*Adults:*

Asthma / Bronchospasm –

Aerosol:
- *Usual dosage* – 1 to 2 inhalations every 4 to 6 hours as needed.
- *Maximum dose* – 12 inhalations/24 hours.

Inhalation solution:
- *Usual dosage* – 1 vial (2.5 mg/vial) 3 to 4 times/day by nebulization over 5 to 15 minutes.
- *Maximum dose* – 4 vials (10 mg)/24 hours.

Prevention of exercise-induced bronchospasm –
Aerosol: 2 inhalations 15 to 30 minutes prior to exercise.

Off-label dosing – The following dosing is from the National Asthma Education and Prevention guidelines.

Asthma (quick relief):
- *Aerosol (metered-dose inhaler)* – 2 inhalations every 4 to 6 hours as needed.
- *Inhalation solution (nebulizer)* – 1.25 to 5 mg (in 3 mL of saline) every 4 to 6 hours as needed. Dose may be doubled in severe exacerbations.

Asthma exacerbations:
- *Older than 12 years of age –*
  Aerosol (metered-dose inhaler): 4 to 8 inhalations every 20 minutes up to 4 hours, then every 1 to 4 hours as needed.

Hyperkalemia: [1] = Good documentation. 10 to 20 mg administered via nebulization over 15 minutes, given in combination with other recommended therapy.

➤*Children:*

Asthma / Bronchospasm – (See also Off-Label Dosing for guideline dosing).

AccuNeb:
- *2 to 12 years of age –*
  Maximum dose: 4 vials (5 mg)/24 hours.
  Initial dosage: 1 vial (1.25 or 0.63 mg/vial) 3 or 4 times/day, as needed over 5 to 15 minutes. Patients 6 to 12 years of age with more severe asthma (baseline forced expiratory volume in 1 second [FEV_1] less than 60% predicted), weight more than 40 kg, or patients 11 to 12 years of age may achieve better initial response with the 1.25 mg dose.

Aerosol:
- *4 years of age and older.* – See Adults for dosing.

Inhalation solution:
- *13 years of age* – See Adults for dosing.
- *2 to 12 years of age –*
  Usual dosage:

➤*Weight less than 15 kg:* Use the 0.5% solution (2.5 mg/0.5 mL) 3 to 4 times/day by nebulization over 5 to 15 minutes.

➤*Weight 15 kg or more:* 1 vial (2.5 mg/3 mL) 3 to 4 times/day by nebulization over 5 to 15 minutes.
Maximum dose: 4 vials (10 mg)/24 h.

Prevention of exercise-induced bronchospasm –
Aerosol:
- *4 years of age and older* – 2 inhalations 15 to 30 minutes prior to exercise.

Off-label dosing – The following dosing is from the National Asthma Education and Prevention guidelines.

Asthma (quick relief):
- *Aerosol (metered-dose inhaler)* – 2 inhalations every 4 to 6 hours as needed.
- *Inhalation solution (nebulizer) –*
  1 year of age and older: 1.25 to 5 mg (in 3 mL of saline) every 4 to 8 hours as needed. Dose may be doubled in severe exacerbations.
  4 years of age and younger: 0.63 to 2.5 mg (in 3 mL of saline) every 4 to 6 hours as needed.

For children younger than 1 year of age, another reference suggests 0.05 to 0.15 mg/kg every 4 to 6 hours as needed.

Asthma exacerbations:
- *Older than 12 years of age –*
  Aerosol (metered-dose inhaler): 4 to 8 inhalations every 20 minutes up to 4 hours, then every 1 to 4 hours as needed.
  Inhalation solution (nebulizer): 2.5 to 5 mg every 20 minutes for 3 doses, then 2.5 to 10 mg every 1 to 4 hours as needed, or 10 to 15 mg/h continuously.
- *12 years of age and younger –*
  Aerosol (metered-dose inhaler): 4 to 8 inhalations every 20 minutes for 3 doses, then every 1 to 4 hours as needed. Use valved holding chamber; add mask in children younger than 4 years of age.
  Inhalation solution (nebulizer): 0.15 mg/kg (minimum dose 2.5 mg) every 20 minutes for 3 doses, then 0.15 to 0.3 mg/kg up to 10 mg every 1 to 4 hours as needed, or 0.5 mg/kg/h by continuous nebulization.

➤*Preparation for administration:*

Aerosol – Shake well before each spray. Prime the inhaler before using for the first time, when the inhaler has not been used for more than 2 weeks, or when the inhaler has been dropped. To prime, release 3 to 4 sprays into the air away from the face, shaking well before each spray.

Inhalation solution 0.083% or AccuNeb – Requires no dilution before administration; empty the entire contents of 1 sterile unit dose vial into nebulizer.

Inhalation solution 0.5% – Dilute 0.5 mL of 1 sterile unit dose vial to a total volume of 3 mL with sterile normal saline solution in nebulizer.

➤*Administration:* For oral inhalation only.

Inhalation solution – Administer via jet nebulizer connected to an air compressor with adequate air flow, equipped with a mouthpiece or suitable face mask. Adjust flow rate to deliver albuterol over 5 to 15 minutes.

AccuNeb: The safety and efficacy have been established using the *Pari LC Plus* nebulizer and *Pari PRONEB* compressor. The safety and efficacy when administering with other nebulizers has not been established.

➤*Admixture compatibility:* The drug compatibility (physical and chemical), clinical efficacy, and safety of albuterol when mixed with other drugs in a nebulizer has not been established.

To screen for specific compatibilities, see *Trissel's IV-Chek*

➤*Storage / Stability:*

Aerosol – Store between 15° and 25°C (59° and 77°F). Protect from freezing temperatures and prolonged exposure to sunlight. Store canister with mouthpiece down. For best results, the canister should be at room temperature before use. Contents under pressure; do not puncture or incinerate. Do not use or store near heat or open flame. Exposure to temperatures above 48.8°C (120°F) may cause bursting. Never throw container into fire or incinerator.

The actuator supplied with the aerosol should not be used with any other product canisters, and actuators from other products should not be used with the supplied canister. The correct amount of medication in each canister cannot be ensured after 200 actuations, even though the canister is not completely empty. The canister should be discarded when 200 actuations have been used or 12 months after removal from the moisture-protective foil pouch, whichever comes first.

To maintain proper use of the metered-dose inhaler, it is important that the actuator be washed with warm running water for 30 seconds and dried thoroughly at least once a week. The inhaler may cease to deliver medication if not properly cleaned and dried thoroughly. Keeping the plastic actuator clean is very important to prevent medication buildup and blockage. If the actuator becomes blocked with the drug, washing the actuator will remove the blockage.

Ventolin HFA: *Ventolin HFA* has a dose counter attached to the canister that starts at 204 or 64 and counts down each time a spray is released. When the counter reads 000, discard.

Inhalation solution – Store between 2° and 25°C (36° and 77°F). Protect from light and excessive heat. Store unit dose vials in protective foil pouch at all times. Once removed from the foil pouch, use with 1 week. Discard the vial if the solution is not colorless.

METAPROTERENOL SULFATE

Rx	**Metaproterenol Sulfate** (Various, eg, Par)	**Tablets**: 10 mg	In 100s and 1000s.
		20 mg	In 100s and 1000s.
Rx	**Metaproterenol Sulfate** (Silarx)	**Syrup**: 10 mg per 5 mL	Saccharin, sorbitol, EDTA. Black cherry flavor. In 473 mL.

[a] For use with an IPPB device.

METAPROTERENOL SULFATE — ORAL

For complete and comparative prescribing information, refer to the Sympathomimetic Bronchodilator group monograph.

Indications

➤*Asthma/Bronchospasm:* Bronchial asthma and for reversible bronchospasm which may occur in association with bronchitis and emphysema.

Administration and Dosage

➤*Adults:*

Bronchial asthma – 20 mg (10 mL) 3 or 4 times per day.

Reversible bronchospasm – 20 mg (10 mL) 3 or 4 times per day.

➤*Children:*

Older than 9 years of age or weight over 60 lbs – See Adults for dosing.

6 to 9 years of age or weight under 60 lbs –

Bronchial asthma: 10 mg (5 mL) 3 or 4 times per day.

Reversible bronchospasm: 10 mg (5 mL) 3 or 4 times per day.

Younger than 6 years of age – Clinical trial experience is limited. Of 40 children treated with metaproterenol syrup for at least 1 month, daily doses of approximately 1.3 to 2.6 mg/kg were well tolerated. Metaproterenol tablets are not recommended for use in children younger than 6 years.

➤*Storage/Stability:* Store between 15° and 30°C (59° and 86°F). Protect from light and moisture.

PIRBUTEROL ACETATE

Rx	**Maxair Autohaler** (Graceway)	**Inhalation aerosol:** Delivers 0.2 mg (as acetate)/actuation	In 2.8 g (80 inhalations) and 14 g (400 inhalations).

PIRBUTEROL ACETATE — INHALATION

For complete and comparative prescribing information, refer to the Sympathomimetic Bronchodilator group monograph.

Indications

➤*Asthma/Bronchospasm:* For the prevention and reversal of bronchospasm in patients 12 years of age and older with reversible bronchospasm including asthma. It may be used with or without concurrent theophylline and/or corticosteroid therapy.

Administration and Dosage

➤*Adults:*

Asthma/Bronchospasm –

Usual dosage: 2 inhalations (400 mcg) repeated every 4 to 6 hours. One inhalation (200 mcg) repeated every 4 to 6 hours may be sufficient for some patients.

Maximum dose: 12 inhalations/day.

➤*Children:*

Asthma/Bronchospasm –

12 years of age and older: See Adults for dosing.

➤*Elderly:* Lower doses may be required.

➤*Preparation for administration:* Shake well before using. It is recommended to "test spray" pirbuterol inhaler into the air before using for the first time and in cases in which the aerosol has not been used for a prolonged period of time.

➤*Administration:* Avoid spraying in eyes. Wait at least 1 to 2 minutes before administering the second inhalation.

➤*Storage/Stability:* Store between 15° and 30°C (59° and 86°F). Failure to use this product within this temperature range may result in improper dosing. For optimal results, the canister should be at room temperature before use. The contents are under pressure. Do not puncture. Do not use or store near heat or open flame. Exposure to temperature above 120°F may cause bursting. Never throw container into fire or incinerator. The light blue plastic actuator supplied should not be used with any other product canisters, and actuators from other product should not be used with pirbuterol acetate inhalation aerosol canister.

TERBUTALINE SULFATE

Rx	**Terbutaline Sulfate** (Global Pharmaceuticals)	**Tablets; oral:** 2.5 mg	Lactose. (G 2611). Off-white, oval. In 100s, 500s, and 1,000s.
		5 mg	Lactose. (G 2622). Off-white, round. In 100s, 500s, and 1,000s.
Rx	**Terbutaline Sulfate** (Various, eg, American Pharmaceutical Partners, Sicor)	**Injection:** 1 mg/mL	In 1 mL single-use vials.

TERBUTALINE SULFATE — ORAL

For complete and comparative prescribing information, refer to the Sympathomimetic Bronchodilator group monograph.

WARNING

Tocolysis – Oral terbutaline has not been approved and should not be used for acute or maintenance tocolysis. In particular, do not use terbutaline for maintenance tocolysis in the outpatient or home setting. Serious adverse reactions, including death, have been reported after administration of terbutaline to pregnant women. In mothers, these adverse reactions include increased heart rate, transient hyperglycemia, hypokalemia, cardiac arrhythmias, pulmonary edema, and myocardial ischemia. Increased fetal heart rate and neonatal hypoglycemia may occur as a result of maternal administration.

Indications

➤*Asthma/Bronchospasm:* For the prevention and reversal of bronchospasm in patients 12 years of age and older with asthma and reversible bronchospasm associated with bronchitis and emphysema.

➤*Off-label uses:*

Premature labor – [5] = Poor documentation. Several randomized, controlled trials involving tocolytic agents have been published; however, most are small and have limitations in study design. Oral terbutaline is contraindicated for the treatment or prevention of preterm labor because it has not been shown to be effective and has safety concerns.

Administration and Dosage

➤*Adults:*

Asthma/Bronchospasm –

Usual dosage: 5 mg 3 times daily at approximately 6-hour intervals while awake.

Maximum dose: 15 mg/day.

Dosage adjustment: If adverse effects are particularly disturbing, the dose may be reduced to 2.5 mg 3 times daily and still provide a clinically significant improvement in pulmonary function.

Off-label dosing –

➤*Children:*

Asthma/Bronchospasm –

12 to 15 years of age:

- *Usual dosage* – 2.5 mg 3 times daily.
- *Maximum dose* – 7.5 mg/day.

Off-label dosing –

Asthma/Bronchospasm:

- *12 years of age or younger* –

  Maximum dose: 5 mg/day or 0.15 mg/kg/dose every 8 hours.

  Initial dosage: 0.05 mg/kg/dose every 8 hours. May increase dose if needed.

➤*Storage/Stability:* Store at 15° to 30°C (59° to 86°F). Dispense in tightly closed, light-resistant container.

TERBUTALINE SULFATE — INJECTION

For complete and comparative prescribing information, refer to the Sympathomimetic Bronchodilator group monograph.

Indications

➤*Asthma/Bronchospasm:* Prevention and reversal of bronchospasm in patients 12 years of age and older with asthma and reversible bronchospasm associated with bronchitis and emphysema.

➤*Off-label uses:*

Premature labor – [3] = Safety concerns. Several randomized, controlled trials involving tocolytic agents have been published; however, most are small and have limitations in study design. Recent changes in product labeling (boxed warnings, contraindications) warn that injectable terbutaline should not be used in pregnant women for prevention or prolonged treatment (beyond 48 to 72 hours) of preterm labor in either the hospital or outpatient settings because of the potential for serious maternal heart problems and death. The statement also recognizes that there may be certain urgent obstetrical conditions for which the health care provider may decide that the

TERBUTALINE SULFATE — INJECTION

benefit of terbutaline injection for an individual patient in a hospital setting clearly outweighs the risk.

Administration and Dosage

➤*Adults:*

Asthma/Bronchospasm –

Usual dosage: 0.25 mg subcutaneously. If significant clinical improvement does not occur within 15 to 30 minutes, a second dose of 0.25 mg may be administered. If the patient then fails to respond within another 15 to 30 minutes, other therapeutic measures should be considered.

Maximum dose: Total dose within 4 hours should not exceed 0.5 mg.

Off-label dosing –

Premature labor: [3] = Safety concerns. The recommended starting dosage of terbutaline is 0.25 mg subcutaneously every 20 minutes to 3 hours. Dosing should be held if the pulse exceeds 120 beats per minute. In a recent survey of obstetricians, the majority of the respondents said they would continue tocolysis for a maximum of 48 hours.

➤*Children:*

Asthma/Bronchospasm –

13 years of age and older: See Adults for dosing.

Off-label dosing –

12 years of age or younger for asthma/bronchospasm:

- *Continuous infusion –*
  - *Loading dose:* 2 mcg/kg (given IV over 5 minutes) up to 10 mcg/kg (given IV over 30 minutes).
  - *Maintenance dosage:* Follow loading dose with IV infusion at a rate of 0.08 to 0.4 mcg/kg/min. Titrate in increments of 0.1 to 0.2 mcg/kg/min every 30 minutes depending on response. Doses as high as 5 to 10 mcg/kg/min have been used.
- *Subcutaneous –*
  - *Usual dosage:* 0.005 to 0.01 mg/kg/dose every 15 to 20 minutes as needed for 3 doses, then every 2 to 6 hours as needed.
  - *Maximum dose:* 0.4 mg/dose.

➤*Administration:* Subcutaneous injections should be made into the lateral deltoid area. Ampuls should be used only for subcutaneous administration and not IV infusion. Discard unused portion after single patient use.

➤*Storage/Stability:* Store at 15° to 30°C (59° to 86°F). Protect from light by storing ampuls in original carton until dispensed.

FORMOTEROL FUMARATE

Rx	**Foradil Aerolizer** (Schering)	**Powder contained in capsule;inhalation:** 12 mcg	Lactose. (CG FXF). In UD 12s and 60s with *Aerolizer* inhaler.
Rx	**Perforomist** (Dey)	**Solution; inhalation:** 10 mcg/mL	In 2 mL vials. In UD 60s.

FORMOTEROL FUMARATE — INHALATION

For complete and comparative prescribing information, refer to the Sympathomimetics class monograph.

WARNING

Asthma-related death – Long-acting beta-2 adrenergic agonists, such as formoterol, increase the risk of asthma-related death. Data from a large placebo-controlled US study that compared the safety of another long-acting beta-2 adrenergic agonist (salmeterol) or placebo added to usual asthma therapy showed an increase in asthma-related deaths in patients receiving salmeterol. This finding with salmeterol is considered a class effect of long-acting beta-2 adrenergic agonists, including formoterol. Currently available data are inadequate to determine whether concurrent use of inhaled corticosteroids or other long-term asthma control drugs mitigates the increased risk of asthma-related death from long-acting beta-2 adrenergic agonists.

Because of this risk, use of formoterol for the treatment of asthma without a concomitant long-term asthma control medication, such as an inhaled corticosteroid, is contraindicated. Use formoterol only as additional therapy for patients with asthma who are currently taking but are inadequately controlled on a long-term asthma control medication, such as an inhaled corticosteroid. Once asthma control is achieved and maintained, assess the patient at regular intervals and step down therapy (eg, discontinue formoterol) if possible without loss of asthma control, and maintain the patient on a long-term asthma control medication, such as an inhaled corticosteroid. Do not use formoterol for patients whose asthma is adequately controlled on low- or medium-dose inhaled corticosteroids.

Children and adolescent patients – Available data from controlled clinical trials suggest that long-acting beta-2 adrenergic agonists increase the risk of asthma-related hospitalization in children and adolescents. For children and adolescents with asthma who require the addition of a long-acting beta-2 adrenergic agonist to an inhaled corticosteroid, a fixed-dose combination product containing an inhaled corticosteroid and long-acting beta-2 adrenergic agonist should ordinarily be considered to ensure adherence with both drugs. In cases in which use of a separate long-term asthma control medication (eg, inhaled corticosteroid) and long-acting beta-2 adrenergic agonist is clinically indicated, appropriate steps must be taken to ensure adherence with both treatment components. If adherence cannot be ensured, a fixed-dose combination product containing an inhaled corticosteroid and long-acting beta-2 adrenergic agonist is recommended.

Indications

➤*Asthma/Bronchospasm (inhalation powder only):* For the treatment of asthma and in the prevention of bronchospasm only as concomitant therapy with a long-term asthma control medication, such as an inhaled corticosteroid, in adults and children 5 years of age and older with reversible obstructive airway disease, including patients with symptoms of nocturnal asthma.

➤*Chronic obstructive pulmonary disease:* For the long-term, twice-daily (morning and evening) administration in the maintenance treatment of bronchoconstriction in patients with chronic obstructive pulmonary disease (COPD), including chronic bronchitis and emphysema.

➤*Exercise-induced bronchospasm (inhalation powder only):* For the short-term prevention of exercise-induced bronchospasm (EIB) in adults and children 5 years of age and older when administered on an occasional, as-needed basis.

Administration and Dosage

➤*Adults:*

Asthma/Bronchospasm (inhalation powder only) –

Usual dosage: 12 mcg every 12 hours using the inhaler supplied. More frequent administration or administration of a larger number of inhalations is not recommended.

Maximum dose: 24 mcg total daily dose.

Concomitant therapy: If symptoms arise between doses, an inhaled, short-acting beta-2 agonist should be taken for immediate relief.

Chronic obstructive pulmonary disease –

Inhalation powder:

- *Usual dosage* – 12 mcg every 12 hours using the inhaler supplied.
- *Maximum dose* – 24 mcg/day.

Inhalation solution:

- *Usual dosage* – 20 mcg twice daily (morning and evening) by nebulization.
- *Maximum dose* – 40 mcg/day.

Exercise-induced bronchospasm (inhalation powder only) –

Usual dosage: 12 mcg using the inhaler supplied, administered at least 15 minutes before exercise on an occasional, as-needed basis. When used intermittently as needed for prevention, protection may last up to 12 hours. Additional doses should not be used for 12 hours after the administration of this drug.

➤*Children:*

Inhalation powder –

5 years of age and older:

- *Asthma/Bronchospasm* – See Adults for dosing.

➤*Administration:*

Inhalation powder – Administer only by the oral inhalation route and only using the inhaler supplied. The patient must not exhale into the device. Formoterol capsules should not be ingested (ie, swallowed) orally. Formoterol capsules should be used with the supplied inhaler only, and the inhaler should not be used with any other capsules.

To use the delivery system, a formoterol capsule is placed in the well of the inhaler supplied, and the capsule is pierced by pressing and releasing the buttons on the side of the device. The formoterol formulation is dispersed into the airstream when the patient inhales rapidly and deeply through the mouthpiece.

Inhalation solution – Administer by the orally inhaled route via a standard jet nebulizer connected to an air compressor. Dilution is not required prior to administration. The safety and efficacy of formoterol inhalation solution have been established in clinical trials when administered using the *Pari-LC Plus* nebulizer (with a facemask or mouthpiece) and the *Proneb Ultra* compressor.

➤*Storage/Stability:* Store in a refrigerator between 2° and 8°C (36° and 46°F) prior to dispensing to the patient.

Inhalation powder – After dispensing to the patient, store between 20° and 25°C (68° and 77°F). Protect from heat and moisture. Always store capsules in the blister and only remove from the blister immediately before use. Always discard the formoterol capsules and inhaler by the "use by" date and always use the new inhaler provided with each new prescription.

Inhalation solution – After dispensing to the patient, store between 2° and 25°C (36° and 77°F) for up to 3 months. Protect pouch from heat. Always store in the foil pouch and only remove immediately before use. Contents of any partially used container should be discarded. Discard the container and top after use.

Sympathomimetics

ARFORMOTEROL

Rx	**Brovana** (Sepracor)	**Solution; inhalation:** 7.5 mcg/mL	Equiv. to arformoterol tartrate 11 mcg. In 2 mL unit-dose vials.

ARFORMOTEROL TARTRATE — INHALATION

For complete and comparative prescribing information, refer to the Sympathomimetics class monograph.

WARNING

Asthma-related death – Long-acting beta-2 adrenergic agonists may increase the risk of asthma-related death. Data from a large placebo-controlled US study that compared the safety of another long-acting beta-2 adrenergic agonist (salmeterol) or placebo added to usual asthma therapy showed an increase in asthma-related deaths in patients receiving salmeterol. This finding with salmeterol is considered a class effect of long-acting beta-2 agonists, including arformoterol. The safety and efficacy of arformoterol in patients with asthma have not been established. All long-acting beta-2 agonists, including arformoterol, are contraindicated in patients with asthma without use of a long-term asthma control medication.

Indications

➤*Chronic obstructive pulmonary disease:* For the long-term, twice-daily (morning and evening) maintenance treatment of bronchoconstriction in patients with chronic obstructive pulmonary disease (COPD), including chronic bronchitis and emphysema.

Administration and Dosage

➤*General dosing considerations:* Do not use more often or at higher doses than recommended or with other long-acting beta agonists. Do not use to treat acute symptoms of COPD. If the recommended maintenance treatment regimen fails to provide the usual response, medical advice should be sought immediately because this is often a sign of destabilization of COPD. Under these circumstances, the therapeutic regimen should be reevaluated and additional therapeutic options should be considered.

➤*Adults:*

Chronic obstructive pulmonary disease –

Usual dosage: 15 mcg twice a day (morning and evening) by nebulization.

Maximum dose: 30 mcg/day.

Concomitant therapy: Discontinue use of inhaled, short-acting beta-2 agonists on a regular basis (eg, 4 times a day) and use them only for symptomatic relief of acute respiratory symptoms.

➤*Preparation for administration:* Dilution is not required. Discard any vial if the solution is not colorless.

➤*Administration:* For use by nebulization only. Arformoterol should not be swallowed. Administer by the inhaled route via a standard jet nebulizer connected to an air compressor. The safety and efficacy of arformoterol have been established in clinical trials when administered using the *Pari LC Plus* nebulizers and *Pari Dura-Neb 3000* compressors.

➤*Storage/Stability:* Store in the protective foil pouch at 2° to 8°C (36° to 46°F). Protect from light and excessive heat. After opening the pouch, unused vials should be returned to, and stored in, the pouch. Use an opened vial right away. Unopened foil pouches can also be stored at 20° to 25°C (68° to 77°F) for up to 6 weeks and discarded if not used after 6 weeks or if past the expiration date, whichever is sooner.

Xanthine Derivatives

Indications

➤*Asthma/reversible bronchospasm:* Symptomatic relief or prevention of bronchial asthma and reversible bronchospasm associated with chronic bronchitis and emphysema.

➤*Off-label uses:* Treatment of apnea and bradycardia of prematurity. Doses of 2 mg/kg/day have been used to maintain serum concentrations between 3 and 5 mcg/mL.

Theophylline 300 mg/day was effective in reducing essential tremor in one study of 20 patients.

Theophylline 10 mg/kg/day may significantly improve pulmonary function and dyspnea in patients with chronic obstructive pulmonary disease.

Administration and Dosage

➤*Parenteral administration:* See theophylline and dextrose and aminophylline.

Individualize dosage. Base dosage adjustments on clinical response and improvement in pulmonary function with careful monitoring of serum levels. If possible, monitor serum levels to maintain levels in the therapeutic range of 10 to 20 mcg/mL. Levels more than 20 mcg/mL may produce toxicity, and it may even occur with levels between 15 to 20 mcg/mL, particularly when factors known to reduce theophylline clearance are present (see Warnings/Precautions). Once stabilized on a dosage, serum levels tend to remain constant. Data are available that indicate that the serum theophylline concentrations required to produce maximum physiologic benefit may fluctuate with the degree of bronchospasm present and are variable.

Calculate dosages on the basis of lean body weight, since theophylline does not distribute into fatty tissue. Regardless of salt used, dosages should be equivalent based on anhydrous theophylline content.

➤*Individualize frequency of dosing:* With immediate-release products, dosing every 6 hours generally is required, especially in children; intervals up to 8 hours may be satisfactory in adults. Some children and adults requiring higher than average doses (those having rapid rates of clearance; eg, half-lives less than 6 hours) may be more effectively controlled during chronic therapy with sustained-release products. Determine dosage intervals to produce minimal fluctuations between peak and trough serum theophylline concentrations. Consider the absorption profile and the elimination rate. When converting from an immediate-release to a sustained-release product, the total daily dose should remain the same, and only the dosing interval adjusted.

➤*Acute symptoms requiring rapid theophyllinization in patients not receiving theophylline:* To achieve a rapid effect, an initial loading dose is required. Dosage recommendations are for theophylline anhydrous.

Dosage Guidelines for Rapid Theophyllinization[a]

Patient group	Oral loading	Maintenance
Children 1 to 9 years of age	5 mg/kg	4 mg/kg q 6 hr
Children 9 to 16 years of age and young adult smokers	5 mg/kg	3 mg/kg q 6 hr
Otherwise healthy non-smoking adults	5 mg/kg	3 mg/kg q 8 hr
Older patients, patients with cor pulmonale	5 mg/kg	2 mg/kg q 8 hr
Patients with CHF	5 mg/kg	1 to 2 mg/kg q 12 hr

[a] In patients not receiving theophylline.

➤*Infants (preterm to younger than 1 year):*

Theophylline Dosage Guidelines for Infants

Age	Initial maintenance dose
Premature infants	
≤ 24 days postnatal	1 mg/kg q 12 hr
> 24 days postnatal	1.5 mg/kg q 12 hr
Infants (6 to 52 weeks)	(× age in weeks] + 5) × kg = 24 hr dose in mg
≤ 26 weeks	Divide into q 8 hr dosing
26 to 52 weeks	Divide into q 6 hr dosing

Guide final dosage by serum concentration after a steady state has been achieved.

➤*Acute symptoms requiring rapid theophyllinization in patients receiving theophylline:* Each 0.5 mg/kg theophylline administered as a loading dose will increase the serum theophylline concentration by approximately 1 mcg/mL. Ideally, defer the loading dose if a serum theophylline concentration can be obtained rapidly.

If this is not possible, exercise clinical judgment. When there is sufficient respiratory distress to warrant a small risk, then 2.5 mg/kg of theophylline administered in rapidly absorbed form is likely to increase serum concentration by approximately 5 mcg/mL. If the patient is not experiencing theophylline toxicity, this is unlikely to result in dangerous adverse effects. Maintenance doses are in the Dosage Guidelines table.

➤*Chronic therapy:* Slow clinical titration is generally preferred.

Initial dose – 16 mg/kg/24 hours or 400 mg/24 hours, whichever is less, of anhydrous theophylline in divided doses at 6 or 8 hour intervals.

Increasing dose – The above dosage may be increased in approximately 25% increments at 3-day intervals so long as the drug is tolerated or until the maximum dose (indicated below) is reached.

➤*Maximum dose (where the serum concentration is not measured):* Do not attempt to maintain any dose that is not tolerated.

Maximum Daily Theophylline Dose Based on Age

Age	Maximum daily dose[a]
1 to 9 years	24 mg/kg/day
9 to 12 years	20 mg/kg/day
12 to 16 years	18 mg/kg/day
> 16 years	13 mg/kg/day

[a] Not to exceed listed dose or 900 mg, whichever is less.

Exercise caution in younger children who cannot complain of minor side effects. Older adults and those with cor pulmonale, CHF, or liver disease may have unusually low dosage requirements; they may experience toxicity at the maximal dosages recommended.

➤*Measurement of serum theophylline concentrations during chronic therapy:* Measurement of serum theophylline concentrations during chronic therapy is recommended. Obtain the serum sample at the time of peak absorption, 1 to 2 hours after administration for immediate-release products and 5 to 9 hours after the morning dose for most sustained-release formulations. The patient must not miss doses during the previous 48 hours, and dosing intervals must have been reasonably typical during that period of time. The table below provides guidance to dosage adjustments based on serum theophylline level determinations:

Dosage Adjustment After Serum Theophylline Measurement		
If serum theophylline is:		Directions
Too low	5 to 10 mcg/mL	Increase dose by ≈ 25% at 3-day intervals until either the desired clinical response or serum concentration is achieved.[a]
Within desired range	10 to 20 mcg/mL	Maintain dosage if tolerated. Recheck serum theophylline concentration at 6 to 12 month intervals.[b]
Too high	20 to 25 mcg/mL	Decrease doses by ≈ 10%. Recheck serum theophylline concentration after 3 days.[b]
	25 to 30 mcg/mL	Skip next dose and decrease subsequent doses by about 25%. Recheck serum theophylline after 3 days.
	> 30 mcg/mL	Skip next 2 doses and decrease subsequent doses by 50%. Recheck serum theophylline after 3 days.

[a] The total daily dose may need to be administered at more frequent intervals if asthma symptoms occur repeatedly at the end of a dosing interval.

[b] Finer adjustments in dosage may be needed for some patients.

➤*Timed-release capsules:* These dosage forms gradually release the active medication so that the total daily dosage may be administered in 1 to 3 doses divided by 8 to 24 hours, depending on the patient's pharmacokinetic profile, thus reducing the number of daily doses required. In the following timed-release capsule product listings, the manufacturer's recommended average dosing intervals are presented in parentheses. Nevertheless, frequency of dosing must be individualized based on the absorption profile of the drug and the rate of elimination of the drug from the patient. These products are not necessarily interchangeable. If patients are switched from one brand to another, closely monitor their theophylline serum levels; serum concentrations may vary greatly following brand interchange.

Actions

➤*Pharmacology:* The methylxanthines (theophylline, its soluble salts and derivatives) directly relax the smooth muscle of the bronchi and pulmonary blood vessels, stimulate the CNS, induce diuresis, increase gastric acid secretion, reduce lower esophageal sphincter pressure, and inhibit uterine contractions. Theophylline is also a central respiratory stimulant. Aminophylline has a potent effect on diaphragmatic contractility in healthy people and may then be capable of reducing fatigability and thereby improve contractility in patients with chronic obstructive airway disease. The exact mode of action is unclear.

For many years, the proposed main mechanism of action of the xanthines was inhibition of phosphodiesterase, which results in an increase in cyclic adenosine monophosphate (cAMP). However, this effect is negligible at therapeutic concentrations. Other effects that appear to occur at therapeutic concentrations and may collectively play a role in the mechanism of the xanthines include the following: Inhibition of extracellular adenosine (which causes bronchoconstriction), although it is unlikely that this is a main mechanism; stimulation of endogenous catecholamines, although this also does not appear to be a major mechanism; antagonism of prostaglandins PGE_2 and $PGF_{2}\alpha$; direct effect on mobilization of intracellular calcium resulting in smooth muscle relaxation; beta-adrenergic agonist activity on the airways. None of these mechanisms have been proven.

➤*Pharmacokinetics:*

Absorption – Theophylline is well absorbed from oral liquids and uncoated plain tablets; maximal plasma concentrations are reached in 2 hours. Rectal absorption from suppositories is slow and erratic, the oral route is generally preferred. Enteric coated tablets and some sustained release dosage forms may be unreliably absorbed. Food may alter bioavailability and absorption pattern of some sustained release preparations; close monitoring is advised (see Drug Interactions).

Distribution – Average volume of distribution is 0.45 L/kg (range, 0.3 to 0.7 L/kg). Theophylline does not distribute into fatty tissue, but readily crosses the placenta and is excreted into breast milk. Approximately 40% is bound to plasma protein. Therapeutic serum levels generally range from 10 to 20 mcg/mL. Although some bronchodilatory effect occurs at lower concentrations, stabilization of hyperreactive airways is most evident at levels more than 10 mcg/mL, and adverse effects are uncommon at levels less than 20 mcg/mL. Once a patient is stabilized, serum levels tend to remain constant with the same dosage.

Metabolism/Excretion – Xanthines are biotransformed in the liver (85% to 90%) to 1, 3–dimethyluric acid, 3–methylxanthine and 1–methyluric acid; 3–methylxanthine accumulates in concentrations approximately 25% of those of theophylline.

Excretion is by the kidneys; less than 15% of the drug is excreted unchanged. Elimination kinetics vary greatly. Plasma elimination half-life averages about 3 to 15 hours in adult nonsmokers, 4 to 5 hours in adult smokers (1 to 2 packs per day), 1 to 9 hours in children and 20 to 30 hours for premature neonates. In the neonate, theophylline is metabolized partially to caffeine. The premature neonate excretes about 50% unchanged theophylline and may accumulate the caffeine metabolite.

A prolonged half-life may occur in congestive heart failure, liver dysfunction, alcoholism, respiratory infections and patients receiving certain other drugs (see Drug Interactions). Total clearance appears relatively unaffected by renal failure.

Equivalent dose – Because of differing theophylline content, the various salts and derivatives are not equivalent on a weight basis. The table below indicates percentage of anhydrous theophylline and approximate equivalent dose of each compound. Product listings include anhydrous theophylline dosage equivalents.

Theophylline Content and Equivalent Dose of Various Theophylline Salts		
Theophylline salts	Theophylline %	Equivalent dose
Theophylline anhydrous	100	100 mg
Theophylline monohydrate	91	110 mg
Aminophylline anhydrous	86	116 mg
Aminophylline dihydrate	79	127 mg

Dyphylline – A chemical derivative of theophylline, it is not a theophylline salt as are the other agents. It is about one-tenth as potent as theophylline. Following oral administration, dyphylline is 68% to 82% bioavailable. Peak plasma concentrations are reached within 1 hour, and its half-life is 2 hours. The minimal effective therapeutic concentration is 12 mcg/mL. It is not metabolized to theophylline and 83% ± 5% is excreted unchanged in the urine.

Contraindications

Hypersensitivity to any xanthine; peptic ulcer; underlying seizure disorders (unless receiving appropriate anticonvulsant medication).

➤*Aminophylline:* Hypersensitivity to ethylenediamine.

➤*Aminophylline rectal suppositories:* Irritation or infection of rectum or lower colon.

Warnings/Precautions

➤*Status asthmaticus:* This is a medical emergency and is not rapidly responsive to usual doses of conventional bronchodilators. Optimal therapy frequently requires both parenteral medication and close monitoring, preferably in an intensive care setting. Oral theophylline products alone are not appropriate for status asthmaticus.

➤*Toxicity:* Excessive doses may cause severe toxicity; monitor serum levels to assure maximum benefit with minimum risk. Incidence of toxicity increases significantly at serum levels more than 20 mcg/mL (75% of patients with levels more than 25 mcg/mL). Serum levels more than 20 mcg/mL are rare after appropriate use of recommended doses. However, if theophylline plasma clearance is reduced for any reason (eg, hepatic impairment; patients older than 55 years of age, particularly males and those with chronic lung disease; cardiac failure; sustained high fever; infants younger than 1 year old), even conventional doses may result in increased serum levels and potential toxicity. Frequently, such patients have markedly prolonged levels following drug discontinuation.

Serious side effects such as ventricular arrhythmias, convulsions or even death may appear as the first sign of toxicity without any previous warning. Less serious signs of toxicity (eg, nausea, restlessness) may occur frequently when initiating therapy, but are usually transient; when such signs are persistent during maintenance therapy, they are often associated with serum concentrations greater than 20 mcg/mL. Serious toxicity is not reliably preceded by less severe side effects.

➤*Cardiac effects:* Theophylline may cause dysrhythmias or worsen preexisting arrhythmias. Any significant change in cardiac rate or rhythm warrants monitoring and further investigation. Many patients who require theophylline may exhibit tachycardia due to underlying disease; the relationship to elevated serum theophylline concentrations may not be appreciated. Ventricular arrhythmias respond to lidocaine.

➤*Use with caution:* Cardiac disease; hypoxemia; hepatic disease; hypertension; congestive heart failure (CHF); alcoholism; elderly (particularly males); and neonates.

➤*GI effects:* Use cautiously in peptic ulcer. Local irritation may occur; centrally mediated GI effects may occur with serum levels more than 20 mcg/mL. Reduced lower esophageal pressure may cause reflux, aspiration and worsening of airway obstruction.

➤*Alcohol:* The addition of alcohol in liquid formulations is not necessary for absorption and may be potentially harmful.

➤*Pregnancy: Category C.* It is not known whether theophylline can cause fetal harm when administered to a pregnant woman or can affect reproduction capacity. Give only if clearly needed. Theophylline has been found in cord serum and crosses the placenta; newborns may have therapeutic serum levels. Apnea has been associated with theophylline withdrawal in a neonate. Theophylline-related human congenital defects or malformations have not been reported.

➤*Lactation:* Theophylline distributes readily into breast milk with a milk:plasma ratio of 0.7 and may cause irritability or other signs of toxicity in nursing infants. Decide whether to discontinue nursing or to discontinue the drug, taking into account the importance of the drug to the mother.

➤*Children:* Sufficient numbers of infants younger than 1 year of age have not been studied in clinical trials to support use in this age group; however, there is evidence that the use of dosage recommendations for older infants and young children may result in the development of toxic serum levels. Carefully consider associated benefits and risks in this age group.

Drug Interactions

Agents that Decrease Theophylline Levels		
Aminoglutethimide	Rifampin	Carbamazepine[a]
Barbiturates	Smoking (cigarettes and marijuana)	Isoniazid[a]
Charcoal	Sulfinpyrazone	Loop diuretics[a]
Hydantoins[b]	Sympathomimetics (β-agonists)	
Ketoconazole	Thioamines[c]	

Agents that Increase Theophylline Levels		
Allopurinol	Disulfiram	Quinolones
Beta blockers (non-selective)	Ephedrine	Thiabendazole
Calcium channel blockers	Influenza virus vaccine	Thyroid hormones[d]
Cimetidine	Interferon	Carbamazepine[a]
Contraceptives, oral	Macrolides	Isoniazid[a]
Corticosteroids	Mexiletine	Loop diuretics[a]

[a] May increase or decrease theophylline levels.
[b] Decreased hydantoin levels may also occur.
[c] Increased theophylline clearance in hyperthyroid patients.
[d] Decreased theophylline clearance in hypothyroid patients.

➤*Benzodiazepines:* The sedative effects of benzodiazepines may be antagonized by theophyllines, although their pharmacokinetics do not appear to be altered. Coadministration may be beneficial in reversing sedation produced by benzodiazepines.

➤*Beta-agonists:* Acts synergistically with theophylline in vitro; an additive effect has also been demonstrated in vivo.

➤*Halothane:* Coadministration with theophylline has resulted in catecholamine-induced arrhythmias.

➤*Ketamine:* Coadministration with theophylline has resulted in extensor-type seizures.

➤*Lithium:* Plasma levels may be reduced by theophyllines.

➤*Nondepolarizing muscle relaxants:* A dose-dependent reversal of neuromuscular blockade by theophyllines may occur.

➤*Probenecid:* May increase the pharmacologic effects of dyphylline due to decreased dyphylline renal excretion.

➤*Propofol:* Theophyllines may antagonize the sedative effects of propofol.

➤*Ranitidine:* Case reports suggest that theophylline plasma levels may be increased by ranitidine, possibly increasing pharmacologic and toxic effects. However, several controlled studies indicate that an interaction does not occur. It appears that if this interaction occurs, it is rare.

➤*Tetracyclines:* The incidence of theophylline adverse reactions may possibly be enhanced by concurrent tetracyclines.

➤*Drug/Lab test interactions:* Currently available analytical methods for measuring serum theophylline levels are specific, and metabolites and other drugs generally do not affect the results. However, be aware of the specific laboratory method used and whether other factors will interfere with the assay for theophylline.

➤*Drug/Food interactions:* Theophylline elimination is increased (half-life shortened) by a low carbohydrate, high protein diet and charcoal broiled beef (due to a high polycyclic carbon content). Conversely, elimination is decreased (prolonged half-life) by a high carbohydrate low protein diet. Food may alter the bioavailability and absorption pattern of certain sustained release preparations. Some sustained release preparations may be subject to rapid release of their contents when taken with food, resulting in toxicity. It appears that consistent administration in the fasting state allows predictability of effects.

Adverse Reactions

Adverse reactions/toxicity are uncommon at serum theophylline levels less than 20 mcg/mL.

Levels more than 20 mcg/mL – 75% of patients experience adverse reactions (eg, nausea, vomiting, diarrhea, headache, insomnia, irritability).

Levels more than 35 mcg/mL – Hyperglycemia; hypotension; cardiac arrhythmias; tachycardia (more than 10 mcg/mL in premature newborns); seizures; brain damage; death.

➤*Cardiovascular:* Palpitations; tachycardia; extrasystoles; hypotension; circulatory failure; life-threatening ventricular arrhythmias.

➤*CNS:* Irritability; restlessness; headache; insomnia; reflex hyperexcitability; muscle twitching; convulsions.

➤*GI:* Nausea; vomiting; epigastric pain; hematemesis; diarrhea; rectal irritation or bleeding (aminophylline suppositories). Therapeutic doses of theophylline may induce gastroesophageal reflux during sleep or while recumbent, increasing the potential for aspiration which can aggravate bronchospasm.

➤*Renal:* Proteinuria; potentiation of diuresis.

➤*Respiratory:* Tachypnea; respiratory arrest.

➤*Miscellaneous:* Fever; flushing; hyperglycemia; inappropriate antidiuretic hormone syndrome; rash; alopecia. Ethylenediamine in aminophylline can cause sensitivity reactions, including exfoliative dermatitis and urticaria.

Overdosage

➤*Symptoms:* Anorexia; nausea; vomiting; nervousness; insomnia; agitation; irritability; headache; tachycardia; extrasystoles; tachypnea; fasciculation; tonic/clonic convulsions. Convulsions or ventricular arrhythmias may be the first signs of toxicity. Hyperamylasemia, simulating pancreatitis, has also been noted. Other symptoms of intoxication are listed under Adverse Reactions.

Serious adverse effects are rare at serum theophylline concentrations less than 20 mcg/mL. Between 20 and 40 mcg/mL, sinus tachycardia and cardiac arrhythmias occur. Above 40 mcg/mL, seizures and cardiorespiratory arrest can occur. However, convulsions and death have been reported at concentrations as low as 25 mcg/mL.

Acute overdosage appears to be better tolerated with the more serious reactions (eg, seizures) occurring with chronic overdosage (levels more than 40 mcg/mL), but rarely in the acute situation unless levels exceed 100 mcg/mL. Also, symptoms such as hypokalemia, hypercalcemia, hyperglycemia and decreased serum bicarbonate concentrations occur more frequently with acute overdosage.

Overdosage with sustained release preparations may cause a dramatic increase in serum theophylline concentrations much later (at least 12 hours) than the increases that occur with other preparations. Early treatment will help but not prevent these delayed elevated levels.

➤*Treatment:*

Treatment if seizure has not occurred – Induce vomiting, even if emesis has occurred spontaneously; ipecac syrup is preferred. However, do not induce emesis in patients with impaired consciousness. Take precautions against aspiration, especially in infants and children. If vomiting is unsuccessful or contraindicated, perform gastric lavage (of no value at least 1 hour post-ingestion). Administer a cathartic (particularly for sustained-release preparations; sorbitol may be useful) and activated charcoal. Prophylactic phenobarbital may increase the seizure threshold.

If seizure occurs – Establish an airway and administer oxygen. Administer IV diazepam 0.1 to 0.3 mg/kg, up to 10 mg. Monitor vital signs, maintain blood pressure and provide adequate hydration.

Post-seizure coma – Maintain airway and oxygenation. Perform intubation and lavage instead of inducing emesis. Introduce the cathartic and activated charcoal via a large bore gastric lavage tube. Provide full supportive care and adequate hydration while the drug is metabolized. If repeated oral activated charcoal is ineffective, charcoal hemoperfusion may be indicated.

Supportive care – Employ usual supportive measures. Refer to General Management of Acute Overdosage. Do not use stimulants (analeptic agents). Continuously monitor cardiac function. Verapamil has been used to treat atrial arrhythmias; lidocaine or procainamide may be used for ventricular arrhythmias. May need IV fluids to treat dehydration, acid-base imbalance and hypotension; the latter may also be treated with vasopressors. Apnea will require ventilatory support. Treat hyperpyrexia, especially in children, with tepid water sponge baths or a hypothermic blanket.

Monitor theophylline serum level until it falls below 20 mcg/mL because secondary rises of plasma theophylline may occur from redistribution, delayed absorption, etc.; this has been reported with sustained release products.

Dialysis – Charcoal hemoperfusion rapidly removes theophylline and may be indicated when the serum concentration is more than 60 mcg/mL, even in the absence of obvious toxicity. Forced diuresis, peritoneal dialysis and extracorporeal methods are inadequate. However, hemodialysis appears capable of removing approximately 36% to 40% of serum theophylline.

"Gastric dialysis": With oral activated charcoal, 20 to 40 g every 4 hours until serum level is less than 20 mcg/mL, may shorten half-life and speed removal, regardless of route. Mechanism may include enhancing drug concentration gradient into the GI lumen, a disruption of an enterohepatic recycling process or binding unabsorbed drug.

Patient Information

If GI upset occurs with liquid or non-sustained release forms, take with food.

Do NOT chew or crush enteric coated or sustained release tablets or capsules.

Take at the same time, with or without food, each day.

Notify physician if nausea, vomiting, insomnia, jitteriness, headache, rash, severe GI pain, restlessness, convulsions or irregular heartbeat occurs.

Avoid large amounts of caffeine-containing beverages, such as tea, coffee, cocoa and cola drinks or large amounts of chocolate; these products may increase side effects.

➤*Brand interchange:* Do not change from one brand to another without consulting your pharmacist or physician. Products manufactured by different companies may not be equally effective.

Individual doses are determined by response (decrease in symptoms). Blood levels must be checked regularly to avoid underdosing and overdosing. Do not change the dose of your medication without consulting your physician.

THEOPHYLLINE

Rx	**Theophylline** (Various, eg, Inwood, Ivax, Major, Pliva)	**Tablets, extended-release (12-hour); oral**[a]: 100 mg	In 100s.
Rx	**Theochron** (Forest)		(IL/3584). Scored. Convex. In 100s and 1,000s.
Rx	**Theophylline** (Various, eg, Inwood, Ivax, Major, Pliva)	**Tablets, extended-release (12-hour); oral**[a]: 200 mg	In 100s, 500s, and 1,000s.
Rx	**Theochron** (Forest)		(IL/3583). Oval, scored. Convex. In 100s, 500s, 1000s.
Rx	**Theophylline** (Various, eg, Inwood, Ivax, Major, Pliva)	**Tablets, extended-release (12-hour); oral**[a]: 300 mg	In 100s, 500s, and 1,000s.
Rx	**Theochron** (Forest)		(IL/3581). Scored. Capsule shape. In 100s, 500s, 1000s.
Rx	**Theophylline** (Various, eg, Inwood, Ivax, Major, Pliva)	**Tablets, extended-release (12-hour); oral**[a]: 450 mg	In 100s and 1,000s.
Rx	**Theochron** (Forest)		(IL3614/450). Off-white, capsule shape, scored. In 100s, 500s, and 1000s.
Rx	**Theophylline** (Inwood)	**Capsules, extended-release (12-hour); oral**[a]: 125 mg	May be pellet filled. In 100s.
Rx	**Theophylline** (Inwood)	**Capsules, extended-release (12-hour); oral**[a]: 200 mg	May be pellet filled. In 100s.
Rx	**Theo-24** (UCB Pharma)	**Capsules, extended-release (24-hour); oral**[a]: 100 mg	Pellet filled. Sucrose. (Theo-24 100 mg ucb 2832). Yellow-orange and clear. In 100s.
		200 mg	Pellet filled. Sucrose. (Theo-24 200 mg ucb 2842). Red-orange and clear. In 100s and 500s.
		300 mg	Pellet filled. Sucrose. (Theo-24 300 mg ucb 2852). Red and clear. In 100s and 500s.
		400 mg	Pellet filled. Sucrose. (Theo-24 400 mg ucb 2902). Pink and clear. In 100s.
Rx	**Elixophyllin** (Caraco)	**Elixir; oral**: 80 mg per 15 mL	Alcohol 20% per 15 mL. Saccharin, glycerin. Mixed fruit flavor. In 473, 946, and 3,785 mL.
Rx	**Theophylline** (Various, eg, Hospira)	**Injection; solution**: 0.8 mg/mL	In dextrose 5%. In 500 and 1,000 mL.
		1.6 mg/mL	In dextrose 5%. In 250 and 500 mL.
		2 mg/mL	In dextrose 5%. In 100 mL.
		3.2 mg/mL	In dextrose 5%. In 250 mL.
		4 mg/mL	In dextrose 5%. In 50 and 100 mL.

[a] Also may be given once every 24 hours. See Administration and Dosage.

THEOPHYLLINE — ORAL

For complete and comparative prescribing information, refer to the Xanthine Derivatives group monograph.

Indications

➤*Reversible airflow obstruction:* For the treatment of the symptoms and reversible airflow obstruction associated with chronic asthma and other chronic lung diseases (eg, emphysema, chronic bronchitis).

➤*Off-label uses:* Apnea in preterm infants.

Administration and Dosage

➤*General dosing considerations:* Theophylline distributes poorly into body fat; therefore, mg/kg dose should be calculated on the basis of ideal body weight.

Application of the general dosing recommendations to individual patients must take into account the unique clinical characteristics of each patient. In general, these recommendations should serve as the upper limit for dosage adjustments in order to decrease the risk of potentially serious adverse reactions associated with unexpected, large increases in serum theophylline concentration.

The steady-state peak serum theophylline concentration is a function of the dose, the dosing interval, and the rate of absorption and clearance in the individual patient. Because of marked individual differences in the rate of clearance, the dose required to achieve a peak serum concentration in the 10 to 20 mcg/mL range varies 4-fold among otherwise similar patients in the absence of factors known to alter theophylline clearance (eg, 400 to 1,600 mg/day in adults younger than 60 years of age and 10 to 36 mg/kg/day in children 1 to 9 years of age). For a given population, there is no single theophylline dose that will provide both safe and effective serum concentrations for all patients. Administration of the median dose required to achieve a therapeutic serum concentration in a given population may result in either subtherapeutic or potentially toxic serum concentrations in individual patients. For example, at a dose of 900 mg/day in adults younger than 60 years of age or 22 mg/kg/day in children 1 to 9 years of age, the steady-state peak serum concentration will be less than 10 mcg/mL in about 30% of patients, 10 to 20 mcg/mL in about 50% of patients, and 20 to 30 mcg/mL in about 20% of patients.

➤*Adults:*

Reversible airflow obstruction –

Loading dose: For acute bronchospasm, a single 5 mg/kg dose of theophylline in a patient who has not received any theophylline in the previous 24 hours will produce an average peak serum theophylline concentration of 10 mcg/mL (range, 5 to 15 mcg/mL).

If dosing with theophylline is to be continued beyond the loading dose, follow the guidelines in the following tables and monitor serum theophylline concentrations at 24-hour intervals to adjust final dosage.

If an inhaled or parenteral beta-agonist is not available, a loading dose of an oral immediate-release theophylline can be used as a temporary measure.

Maintenance dosage:

• *Patients without risk factors for impaired clearance –*

Theophylline Dosing Initiation and Titration for Adults Without Risk Factors for Impaired Clearance

Titration step	*Elixophyllin*	Theophylline extended-release capsules	Theophylline extended-release tablets, *Theochron*	*Theo-24, Uniphyl*
Starting dosage	300 mg/day, divided every 6 to 8 hours[b]	300 mg/day, divided every 8 to 12 hours[b]	300 mg/day, divided every 12 hours[b]	300 to 400 mg/day,[a] given once every 24 hours[b]

THEOPHYLLINE — ORAL

Theophylline Dosing Initiation and Titration for Adults Without Risk Factors for Impaired Clearance

After 3 days, if tolerated, increase dose to:	400 mg/day, divided every 6 to 8 hours[b]	400 mg/day, divided every 8 to 12 hours[b]	400 mg/day, divided every 12 hours[b]	400 to 600 mg/day,[a] given once every 24 hours[b]
After 3 more days, if tolerated and needed, increase dose to:	600 mg/day, divided every 6 to 8 hours[b]	600 mg/day, divided every 8 to 12 hours[b]	600 mg/day, divided every 12 hours[b]	As with all theophylline products, doses greater than 600 mg should be titrated according to blood level.

[a] If caffeine-like adverse reactions occur, consideration should be given to using a lower dose and titrating the dose more slowly.

[b] Patients with more rapid metabolism (clinically identified by higher-than-average dose requirements) should receive a smaller dose more frequently to prevent breakthrough symptoms resulting from low trough concentrations before the next dose. A reliably absorbed slow-release formulation will decrease fluctuations and permit longer dosing intervals.

• *Patients with risk factors for impaired clearance and patients not feasible to monitor serum theophylline concentrations* – Final dose should not exceed 400 mg/day.

Dosage adjustment: Transient caffeine-like adverse reactions and excessive serum concentrations in slow metabolizers can be avoided in most patients by starting with a sufficiently low dose and slowly increasing the dose, if judged to be clinically indicated, in small increments. Dose increases should only be made if the previous dosage is well tolerated and should be made at intervals of no less than 3 days to allow serum theophylline concentrations to reach the new steady state. Dosage adjustment should be guided by serum theophylline concentration measurement. Health care providers should instruct patients and care givers to discontinue any dosage that causes adverse reactions, to withhold the medication until these symptoms are gone, and to then resume therapy at a lower, previously tolerated dosage.

Dosage Adjustment Guided by Serum Theophylline Concentrations

Theophylline concentration	Theophylline dosage adjustment
< 9.9 mcg/mL	If symptoms are not controlled and current dosage is tolerated, increase dose about 25%. Recheck serum concentration after 3 days for further dosage adjustment.
10 to 14.9 mcg/mL	If symptoms are controlled and current dosage is tolerated, maintain dose and recheck serum concentration at 6- to 12-month intervals.[a] If symptoms are not controlled and current dosage is tolerated, consider adding additional medication(s) to treatment regimen.
15 to 19.9 mcg/mL	Consider 10% decrease in dose to provide greater margin of safety even if current dosage is tolerated.[a]
20 to 24.9 mcg/mL	Decrease dose by 25%, even if no adverse reactions are present. Recheck serum concentration after 3 days to guide further dosage adjustment.
25 to 30 mcg/mL	Skip next dose and decrease subsequent doses at least 25%, even if no adverse reactions are present. Recheck serum concentration after 3 days to guide further dosage adjustment. If symptomatic, consider whether overdose treatment is indicated.
> 30 mcg/mL	Treat overdose as indicated. If theophylline is subsequently resumed, decrease dose by at least 50%, and recheck serum concentration after 3 days to guide further dosage adjustment.

[a] Dose reduction and/or serum theophylline concentration measurement is indicated whenever adverse reactions are present, physiologic abnormalities that can reduce theophylline clearance occur (eg, sustained fever), or a drug that interacts with theophylline is added or discontinued.

➤***Children:*** See Adults for dosing for children 16 years of age and older.

Reversible airflow obstruction –

Loading dose: For acute bronchospasm, a single 5 mg/kg dose of theophylline in a patient who has not received any theophylline in the previous 24 hours will produce an average peak serum theophylline concentration of 10 mcg/mL (range, 5 to 15 mcg/mL). If dosing with theophylline is continued beyond the loading dose, follow the guidelines in the previous tables and monitor serum theophylline concentrations at 24-hour intervals to adjust final dosage.

Maintenance dosage:

• *Younger than 1 year of age (Elixophyllin)* –

Theophylline Dosing Initiation and Titration in Infants < 1 Year of Age[a]

Age	Initial dosage	Final dosage
Premature neonates		Adjusted to maintain a peak steady-state serum theophylline concentration of 5 to 10 mcg/mL in neonates and 10 to 15 mcg/mL in older infants. Because the time required to reach steady state is a function of theophylline half-life, up to 5 days may be required to achieve steady state in a premature neonate, while only 2 to 3 days may be required in an infant 6 months of age without other risk factors for impaired clearance in the absence of a loading dose. If a serum theophylline concentration is obtained before steady state is achieved, the maintenance dose should not be increased, even if the serum theophylline concentration is less than 10 mcg/mL.
< 24 days postnatal	1 mg/kg every 12 hours	
≥ 24 days postnatal	1.5 mg/kg every 12 hours	
Full-term infants and infants ≤ 52 weeks of age		
Up to 26 weeks of age	Divide dose[a] into 3 equal amounts, administered at 8-hour intervals	
26 weeks of age and older	Divide dose[a] into 4 equal amounts, administered at 6-hour intervals	

[a] Total daily dose (mg) = $[(0.2 \times \text{age in weeks}) + 5] / (\text{kg body weight})$.

THEOPHYLLINE — ORAL

• *1 to 15 years of age (weighing less than 45 kg) without risk factors for impaired clearance* –

Theophylline Dosing Initiation and Titration for Children < 45 kg Without Risk Factors for Impaired Clearance

Titration step	Children (1 to 15 years of age) *Elixophyllin*	Children (1 to 15 years of age) Theophylline extended-release capsules	Children (6 to 15 years of age) Theophylline extended-release tablets, *Theochron*	Children (12 to 15 years of age) *Theo-24, Uniphyl*
Starting dosage	12 to 14 mg/kg/day, up to a maximum of 300 mg/day divided every 4 to 6 hours[a]	12 to 14 mg/kg/day, up to a maximum of 300 mg/day divided every 8 to 12 hours[a]	12 to 14 mg/kg/day, up to a maximum of 300 mg/day divided every 12 hours[a]	12 to 14 mg/kg/day, up to a maximum of 300 mg/day given once every 24 hours[a]
After 3 days, if tolerated, increase dose to:	16 mg/kg/day up to a maximum of 400 mg/day, divided every 4 to 6 hours[a]	16 mg/kg/day up to a maximum of 400 mg/day, divided every 8 to 12 hours[a]	16 mg/kg/day up to a maximum of 400 mg/day, divided every 12 hours[a]	16 mg/kg/day up to a maximum of 400 mg/day, given once every 24 hours[a]
After 3 more days, if tolerated and needed, increase dose to:	20 mg/kg/day, up to a maximum of 600 mg/day, divided every 4 to 6 hours[a]	20 mg/kg/day, up to a maximum of 600 mg/day, divided every 8 to 12 hours[a]	20 mg/kg/day, up to a maximum of 600 mg/day, divided every 12 hours[a]	20 mg/kg/day, up to a maximum of 600 mg/day, given once every 24 hours[a]

[a] Patients with more rapid metabolism, clinically identified by higher-than-average dose requirements, should receive a smaller dose more frequently to prevent breakthrough symptoms resulting from low trough concentrations before the next dose. A reliably absorbed slow-release formulation will decrease fluctuations and permit longer dosing intervals.

• *1 to 15 years of age (weighing more than 45 kg) without risk factors for impaired clearance* –

Theophylline Dosing Initiation and Titration for Children > 45 kg Without Risk Factors for Impaired Clearance

Titration step	*Elixophyllin*	Theophylline extended- release capsules	Theophylline extended- release tablets, *Theochron*	Theo-24, *Uniphyl*
Starting dosage	300 mg/day, divided every 6 to 8 hours[b]	300 mg/day, divided every 8 to 12 hours[b]	300 mg/day, divided every 12 hours[b]	300 to 400 mg/day,[a] given once every 24 hours[b]
After 3 days, if tolerated, increase dose to:	400 mg/day divided every 6 to 8 hours[b]	400 mg/day divided every 8 to 12 hours[b]	400 mg/day divided every 12 hours[b]	400 to 600 mg/day[a] given once every 24 hours[b]
After 3 more days, if tolerated and needed, increase dose to:	600 mg/day divided every 6 to 8 hours[b]	600 mg/day divided every 8 to 12 hours[b]	600 mg/day divided every 12 hours[b]	As with all theophylline products, doses greater than 600 mg should be titrated according to blood level.

[a] If caffeine-like adverse reactions occur, consideration should be given to using a lower dose and titrating the dose more slowly.

[b] Patients with more rapid metabolism, clinically identified by higher-than-average dose requirements, should receive a smaller dose more frequently to prevent breakthrough symptoms resulting from low trough concentrations before the next dose. A reliably absorbed slow-release formulation will decrease fluctuations and permit longer dosing intervals.

• *Patients with risk factors for impaired clearance, and patients for whom it is not feasible to monitor serum theophylline concentrations* – Final theophylline dose should not exceed 16 mg/kg/day, up to a maximum of 400 mg/day.

Dosage adjustment: See Adults for more information.

Off-label dosing –

Neonatal apnea:

• *Loading dose* – 5 mg/kg as a single dose.

• *Maintenance dosage* – 3 to 6 mg/kg/day in divided doses given every 6 to 8 hours.

➤*Elderly:* The maximum daily dose of theophylline in patients older than 60 years of age ordinarily should not exceed 400 mg/day unless the patient continues to be symptomatic and the peak steady-state serum theophylline concentration is less than 10 mcg/mL. Prescribe theophylline doses more than 400 mg/day with caution in elderly patients.

➤*Hepatic function impairment:* Final dose should not exceed 400 mg/day.

➤*Once-daily dosing:* The slow absorption rate of theophylline 12-hour extended-release capsules and tablets may allow once-daily administration in adult nonsmokers with appropriate total body clearance and other patients with low dosage requirements. Once-daily dosing should be considered only after the patient has been gradually and satisfactorily treated to therapeutic levels with every-12-hour dosing. Once-daily dosing should be based on the dosing guidelines in the previous tables and should be initiated at the end of the last every-12-hour dosing interval. The trough concentration (C_{min}) obtained following conversion to once-daily dosing may be lower (especially in high clearance patients), and the peak concentration (C_{max}) may be higher (especially in low clearance patients) than that obtained with every-12-hour dosing. If symptoms recur, or signs of toxicity appear during the once-daily dosing interval, dosing on the every-12-hour basis should be reinstituted.

Patients who metabolize theophylline rapidly (eg, younger patients, smokers, some nonsmoking adults) and who have symptoms repeatedly at the end of a dosing interval will require either increased doses given once a day or, preferably, are likely to be better controlled by a schedule of twice-daily doing. Patients who require increased daily doses are more likely to experience relatively wide peak-trough differences and may be candidates for twice-daily dosing with theophylline extended-release capsules (12- and 24-hour) or extended-release tablets (12-hour).

It is essential that serum theophylline concentrations be monitored before and after transfer to once-daily dosing. Food and posture, along with changes associated with circadian rhythm, may influence the rate of absorption and/or clearance rates of theophylline from extended-release dosage forms administered at night. The exact relationship of these and other forms to nighttime serum concentrations and the clinical significance of such findings require additional study. Therefore, it is not recommended that theophylline extended-release capsules or tablets be administered at night when they are used as a once-a-day product.

➤*Therapeutic drug monitoring:* The therapeutic serum concentration range for theophylline is 10 to 20 mcg/mL. Serum theophylline concentration measurements are readily available and should be used to determine whether the dosage is appropriate. Specifically, the serum theophylline concentration should be measured as follows:

- When initiating therapy to guide final dosage adjustment after titration.
- Before making a dose increase to determine whether the serum concentration is subtherapeutic in a patient who continues to be symptomatic.
- Whenever signs or symptoms of theophylline toxicity are present.
- Whenever there is a new illness, worsening of a chronic illness, or a change in the patient's treatment regimen that may alter theophylline clearance (eg, fever greater than 38.8°C [102°F] sustained for at least 24 hours; hepatitis; adding a drug that inhibits theophylline metabolism [eg, cimetidine, erythromycin, tacrine]; stopping a coadministered drug that enhances theophylline metabolism [eg, carbamazepine, rifampin]).
- Careful attention to dose reduction and frequent monitoring of serum theophylline concentrations are required in patients who stop smoking in the third trimester of pregnancy, who have sepsis with multiple organ failure, and who have hypothyroidism.
- Monitor theophylline concentrations at 6-month intervals for rapidly growing children and at yearly intervals for all others.

➤*Administration:*

Theo-24 – Patients should be instructed to take this medicine each morning at approximately the same time and not to exceed the prescribed dose.

Recent studies suggest that dosing of extended-release theophylline products at night (after the evening meal) results in serum concentrations of theophylline that are not identical to those recorded during waking hours and may be characterized by early trough and delayed peak levels. This appears to occur whether the drug is given as an immediate-release, extended-release, or IV product. To avoid this phenomenon when 2 doses per

THEOPHYLLINE — ORAL

day are prescribed, it is recommended that the second dose be given 10 to 12 hours after the morning dose and before the evening meal.

Food and posture, along with changes associated with circadian rhythm, may influence the rate of absorption and/or clearance rates of theophylline from extended-release dosage forms administered at night. The exact relationship of these and other factors to nighttime serum concentrations and the clinical significance of such findings require additional study. Therefore, it is not recommended that *Theo-24* (when used as a once-a-day product) be administered at night.

Patients who require a relatively high dose of theophylline (ie, a dose of 900 mg or more or 13 mg/kg, whichever is less) should not take *Theo-24* less than 1 hour before a high-fat meal because this may result in a significant increase in peak serum level and the extent of absorption of theophylline, compared with administration in the fasted state.

12-hour extended-release capsules – Extended-release capsules may be administered by carefully opening the capsule and sprinkling the beaded contents on a spoonful of soft food such as applesauce or pudding; the soft food should be swallowed immediately without chewing and followed with a glass of cool water or juice to ensure complete swallowing of the beads. The food used should not be hot and should be soft enough to be swallowed without chewing. Any bead/food mixture should be used immediately and not stored for future use. Subdividing the contents of a capsule is not recommended.

Taking theophylline extended-release capsules immediately after a high-fat meal may alter its rate of absorption. However, the differences are usually small, and theophylline extended-release capsules may normally be administered without regard to meals.

Theochron and other 12-hour extended-release tablets – When dosing on a once-daily basis, tablets should be taken whole and not split. Administration with a high-fat meal does not result in a significantly different rate or extent of absorption of theophylline compared with administration in the fasting state.

Uniphyl – *Uniphyl* can be taken once a day in the morning or evening. Patients should be advised that, if they choose to take *Uniphyl* with food, they should take it consistently with food and, if they take it in a fasted condition, they should routinely take it in a fasted state. It is important that the medication, whenever dosed, be dosed consistently with or without food.

Uniphyl is not to be chewed or crushed because this may lead to a rapid release of theophylline, with the potential for toxicity. The scored tablet may be split. Infrequently, patients receiving this controlled-release tablet may pass an intact matrix tablet in the stool or via colostomy. These matrix tablets usually contain little or no residual theophylline.

Stabilized patients 12 years of age and older who are taking an immediate- or extended-release theophylline product may be transferred to once-daily administration of *Uniphyl* 400 or 600 mg tablets on a mg-for-mg basis.

It must be recognized that the peak and trough serum theophylline levels produced by the once-daily dosing may vary from those produced by the previous product and/or regimen.

Extended-release tablets – Extended-release tablets administered with a high-fat meal do not result in a significantly different rate or extent of absorption of theophylline compared with administration in the fasting state.

➤*Storage/Stability:*

Controlled-release tablets and 12-hour extended-release capsules – Store at 25°C (77°F); excursions are permitted between 15° and 30°C (59° and 86°F). Dispense in a tight, light-resistant container.

Elixir and extended-release tablets – Store at controlled room temperature, 15° to 30°C (59° to 86°F). Dispense in tight container.

24-hour extended-release capsules – Store below 25°C (77°F).

THEOPHYLLINE — INJECTION

For complete and comparative prescribing information, refer to the Xanthine Derivative group monograph.

Indications

➤*Reversible airflow obstruction:* Indicated as an adjunct to inhaled beta-2 selective agonists and systemically administered corticosteroids for the treatment of acute exacerbations of the symptoms and reversible airflow obstruction associated with asthma and other chronic lung diseases (eg, chronic bronchitis, emphysema).

Administration and Dosage

➤*General dosing considerations:* Theophylline distributes poorly into body fat; therefore, the mg/kg dose should be calculated on the basis of ideal body weight.

The steady-state serum theophylline concentration is a function of the infusion rate and the rate of theophylline clearance in the individual patient. Because of marked individual differences in the rate of clearance, the dose required to achieve a serum concentration in the 10 to 20 mcg/mL range varies 4-fold among otherwise similar patients in the absence of factors known to alter theophylline clearance. For a given population, there is no single dose that will provide both safe and effective serum concentrations for all patients. Administration of the median dose required to achieve a therapeutic serum concentration in a given population may result in subtherapeutic or potentially toxic serum concentrations in individual patients.

Many intravenous (IV) theophylline products are supplied as aminophylline in which ethylenediamine is added to solubilize theophylline. Ethylenediamine is not required for solubility of premixed theophylline and dextrose 5% injection. Each milligram of aminophylline dihydrate contains approximately 0.8 mg of theophylline anhydrous. Equivalent doses of premixed theophylline and dextrose 5% injection can be determined by multiplying those doses specified as aminophylline dihydrate by 0.8.

When theophylline is used as an acute bronchodilator, the goal of obtaining a therapeutic serum concentration is best accomplished with an IV loading dose.

Prior to initiation of theophylline therapy and prior to increases in theophylline dose, carefully consider the various interacting drugs and physiologic conditions that can alter theophylline clearance and require dosage adjustment.

➤*Adults:*

Reversible airflow obstruction –

Maximum dose: 900 mg/day, unless serum levels indicate the need for a larger dose.

Loading dose: Because of rapid distribution into body fluids, the serum concentration (C) obtained from an initial loading dose (LD) is related primarily to the volume of distribution (V), the apparent space into which the drug diffuses: C = LD/V. If a mean volume of distribution of about 0.5 L/kg is assumed (actual range, 0.3 to 0.7 L/kg), each mg/kg (ideal body weight) of theophylline administered as a loading dose over 30 minutes results in an average 2 mcg/mL increase in serum theophylline concentration.

A serum concentration obtained 30 minutes after an IV loading dose, when distribution is complete, can be used to assess the need for and size of subsequent loading doses, if clinically indicated, and for guidance of continuing therapy.

• *Patients who have not received theophylline in the previous 24 hours* – A loading dose of 4.6 mg/kg IV, calculated on the basis of ideal body weight and administered over 30 minutes, on average, will produce a maximum postdistribution serum concentration of 10 mcg/mL, with a range of 6 to 16 mcg/mL.

• *Patients who have already received theophylline* – A loading dose should not be given before obtaining a serum theophylline concentration if the patient has received any theophylline in the previous 24 hours.

Estimation of the serum concentration based upon the history is unreliable, and an immediate serum level determination is indicated. The loading dose can then be determined as follows: D = (Desired C − Measured C)(V), where D is the loading dose, C is the serum theophylline concentration, and V is the volume of distribution. The mean volume of distribution can be assumed to be 0.5 L/kg, and the desired serum concentration should be conservative (eg, 10 mcg/mL) to allow for the variability in the volume of distribution.

Maintenance dosage: Once a serum concentration of 10 to 15 mcg/mL has been achieved with the use of a loading dose(s), a constant IV infusion is started. For otherwise healthy nonsmoking adults, the initial infusion following an appropriate loading dose is 0.4 mg/kg/h, not to exceed 900 mg/day unless serum levels indicate the need for a larger dose.

Because there is large interpatient variability in theophylline clearance, serum concentrations will rise or fall when the patient's clearance is significantly different from the mean population value used to calculate the initial infusion rate. Therefore, a second serum concentration should be obtained 1 expected half-life after starting the constant infusion (eg, approximately 8 hours for nonsmoking adults) to determine if the concentration is accumulating or declining from the postloading dose level. If the level is declining as a result of a higher than average clearance, an additional loading dose can be administered and/or the infusion rate increased. In contrast, if the second sample demonstrates a higher level, accumulation of the drug can be assumed, and the infusion rate should be decreased before the concentration exceeds 20 mcg/mL. An additional sample is obtained 12 to 24 hours later to determine if further adjustments are required, and then at 24-hour intervals to adjust for changes, if they occur. This empiric method, based on mean pharmacokinetic parameters, will prevent large fluctuations in serum concentration during the most critical period of the patient's course.

Dosage adjustment:

Theophylline Final Dosage Adjustment Guided by Serum Concentration

Peak serum concentration	Dosage adjustment
< 9.9 mcg/mL	If symptoms are not controlled and current dosage is tolerated, increase infusion rate about 25%. Recheck serum concentration after 24 hours in adults for further dosage adjustment.
10 to 14.9 mcg/mL	If symptoms are controlled and current dosage is tolerated, maintain infusion rate and recheck serum concentration at 24-hour intervals.[a] If symptoms are not controlled and current dosage is tolerated, consider adding additional medication(s) to treatment regimen.
15 to 19.9 mcg/mL	Consider 10% decrease in infusion rate to provide greater margin of safety even if current dosage is tolerated.[a]

THEOPHYLLINE — INJECTION

Theophylline Final Dosage Adjustment Guided by Serum Concentration

Peak serum concentration	Dosage adjustment
20 to 24.9 mcg/mL	Decrease infusion rate by 25%, even if no adverse reactions are present. Recheck serum concentration after 24 hours in adults to guide further dosage adjustment.
25 to 30 mcg/mL	Stop infusion for 24 hours in adults and decrease subsequent infusion rate at least 25%, even if no adverse reactions are present. Recheck serum concentration after 24 hours in adults to guide further dosage adjustment. If symptomatic, stop infusion and consider whether overdose treatment is indicated.
> 30 mcg/mL	Stop the infusion and treat overdose as indicated. If theophylline is subsequently resumed, decrease infusion rate by at least 50% and recheck serum concentration after 24 hours in adults to guide further dosage adjustment.

[a] Dose reduction and/or serum theophylline concentration measurement is indicated whenever adverse reactions are present, physiologic abnormalities that can reduce theophylline clearance occur (eg, sustained fever), or a drug that interacts with theophylline is added or discontinued.

➤*Children:*

Reversible airflow obstruction –

Loading dose: See Adults for more information.

Maintenance dosage: Once a serum concentration of 10 to 15 mcg/mL has been achieved with the use of a loading dose(s), a constant IV infusion is started. The rate of administration is based on mean pharmacokinetic parameters for the population and calculated to achieve a target serum concentration of 10 mcg/mL. The mean and range of steady-state serum concentrations when the average child (1 to 9 years of age) is given a loading dose of theophylline 4.6 mg/kg followed by a constant IV infusion of 0.8 mg/kg/h.

Because there is large interpatient variability in theophylline clearance, serum concentrations will rise or fall when the patient's clearance is significantly different from the mean population value used to calculate the initial infusion rate. Therefore, a second serum concentration should be obtained 1 expected half-life after starting the constant infusion (eg, approximately 4 hours for children 1 to 9 years of age) to determine if the concentration is accumulating or declining from the postloading dose level. If the level is declining as a result of a higher than average clearance, an additional loading dose can be administered and/or the infusion rate increased. In contrast, if the second sample demonstrates a higher level, accumulation of the drug can be assumed, and the infusion rate should be decreased before the concentration exceeds 20 mcg/mL. An additional sample is obtained 12 to 24 hours later to determine if further adjustments are required and then at 24-hour intervals to adjust for changes, if they occur. This empiric method, based on mean pharmacokinetic parameters, will prevent large fluctuations in serum concentration during the most critical period of the patient's course.

Initial Theophylline Infusion Rates Following an Appropriate Loading Dose

Patient population	Age	Theophylline infusion rate (mg/kg/h)[a,b]
Neonates	Postnatal age ≤ 24 days	1 mg/kg every 12 h[c]
	Postnatal age > 24 days	1.5 mg/kg every 12 h[c]
Infants	6 to 52 weeks	mg/kg/h = (0.008) (age in weeks) + 0.21
Young children	1 to 9 years	0.8
Older children	9 to 12 years	0.7

Initial Theophylline Infusion Rates Following an Appropriate Loading Dose

Patient population	Age	Theophylline infusion rate (mg/kg/h)[a,b]
Adolescents (cigarette or marijuana smokers)	12 to 16 years	0.7
Adolescents (nonsmokers)	12 to 16 years	0.5[d]
Older adolescents (otherwise healthy nonsmokers)	16 years and older	0.4[d]

[a] To achieve a target concentration of 10 mcg/mL, use ideal body weight for obese patients.
[b] Lower initial dosage may be required for patients receiving other drugs that decrease theophylline clearance (eg, cimetidine).
[c] To achieve a target concentration of 7.5 mcg/mL for neonatal apnea.
[d] Not to exceed 900 mg/day, unless serum levels indicate the need for a larger dose.

Dosage adjustment: See Adults for more information.

➤*Elderly:* The maximum infusion rate in patients older than 60 years of age ordinarily should not exceed 17 mg/h, unless the patient continues to be symptomatic, and the steady-state serum concentration is less than 10 mcg/mL. Theophylline infusion rates of more than 17 mg/h should be prescribed with caution in elderly patients.

For adults older than 60 years of age, the initial infusion following an appropriate loading dose is 0.3 mg/kg/h, not to exceed 400 mg/day unless serum levels indicate the need for a larger dose.

➤*Hepatic function impairment:* The initial theophylline infusion rate should not exceed 17 mg/h unless serum concentrations can be monitored at 24-hour intervals. In these patients, 5 days may be required before steady state is reached.

For patients with hepatic impairment, the initial infusion following an appropriate loading dose is 0.2 mg/kg/h, not to exceed 400 mg/day unless serum levels indicate the need for a larger dose.

➤*Patients with cor pulmonale, cardiac decompensation, multiorgan failure, or shock:* For patients with cor pulmonale or cardiac decompensation, the initial theophylline infusion rate should not exceed 17 mg/h, unless serum concentrations can be monitored at 24-hour intervals. In these patients, 5 days may be required before steady state is reached.

For patients with cor pulmonale, cardiac decompensation, multiorgan failure, or shock, the initial infusion following an appropriate loading dose is 0.2 mg/kg/h, not to exceed 400 mg/day unless serum levels indicate the need for a larger dose.

➤*Patients taking drugs that markedly reduce theophylline clearance (eg, cimetidine):* The initial theophylline infusion rate should not exceed 17 mg/h, unless serum concentrations can be monitored at 24-hour intervals. In these patients, 5 days may be required before steady state is reached.

➤*Therapeutic drug monitoring:* The therapeutic serum concentration range for theophylline is 10 to 20 mcg/mL. Serum theophylline concentration measurements are readily available and should be used to determine whether the dosage is appropriate. Specifically, measure the serum concentration as follows:

1.) Before making a dose increase to determine whether the serum concentration is subtherapeutic in a patient who continues to be symptomatic.
2.) Whenever signs or symptoms of theophylline toxicity are present.
3.) Whenever there is a new illness, worsening of an existing concurrent illness, or a change in the patient's treatment regimen that may alter theophylline clearance (eg, fever above 38.9°C [102°F] sustained for 24 hours or more, hepatitis, or drugs listed in the Drug Interactions table are added or discontinued).

➤*Admixture compatibility:* Because dosages of this drug are titrated to response, no additives should be made to theophylline and dextrose 5% injections.

➤*Storage/Stability:* Avoid excessive heat. Protect from freezing. Store at room temperature (25°C [77°F]). Brief exposure up to 40°C (104°F) does not adversely affect the product.

AMINOPHYLLINE (Theophylline Ethylenediamine) – 79% theophylline

Rx	**Aminophylline** (Various, eg, URL, West-Ward)	**Tablets; oral:** 100 mg	Equiv. to theophylline 79 mg. In 100s and UD 100s.
Rx	**Aminophylline** (Various, eg, Balan, Moore, Searle, URL)	**Tablets; oral:** 200 mg	Equiv. to theophylline 158 mg. In 100s and UD 100s.
Rx	**Aminophylline** (Various, eg, American Regent, Hospira)	**Injection:** 25 mg/mL	Equiv. to theophylline 19.75 mg. In 10 and 20 mL amps and vials.

AMINOPHYLLINE — ORAL

For complete and comparative prescribing information, refer to the Xanthine Derivatives group monograph.

Indications

➤*Reversible airflow obstruction:* For the treatment of the symptoms and reversible airflow obstruction associated with chronic asthma and other chronic lung diseases (eg, chronic bronchitis, emphysema).

Administration and Dosage

➤*General dosing considerations:* The following information is based on theophylline except where noted. Aminophylline is approximately 79% of anhydrous theophylline by weight. Therefore, to convert a theophylline dose to aminophylline, divide the theophylline dose by 0.8.

AMINOPHYLLINE — ORAL

Theophylline distributes poorly into body fat; therefore, mg-per-kg doses should be calculated on the basis of ideal body weight.

The dose of theophylline must be individualized on the basis of peak serum theophylline concentration measurements in order to achieve a dose that will provide maximum potential benefit with minimal risk of adverse reactions.

Carefully consider the various interacting drugs and physiologic conditions that can alter theophylline clearance and require dosage adjustment prior to initiation of theophylline therapy, prior to increases in theophylline dose, and during follow-up. Instruct patients and caregivers to discontinue any dosage that causes adverse reactions, to withhold the medication until these symptoms are gone, and to then resume therapy at a lower, previously tolerated dosage.

➤*Adults:*

Acute bronchodilation – Theophylline 5 mg/kg in a patient who has not received any theophylline in the previous 24 hours will produce an average peak serum theophylline concentration of 10 mcg/mL (range, 5 to 15 mcg/mL). If dosing with theophylline is to be continued beyond the loading dose, the guidelines for reversible airflow obstruction should be used and serum theophylline concentration monitored at 24-hour intervals to adjust final dosage.

Reversible airflow obstruction –

Maximum dose: 400 mg/day (equivalent to aminophylline 507 mg) in the presence of risk factors for reduced theophylline clearance or if it is not feasible to monitor serum theophylline concentrations.

Initial dosage: 300 mg/day (equivalent to aminophylline 380 mg) divided every 6 to 8 h. After 3 days, if tolerated, increase dosage to 400 mg/day (equivalent to aminophylline 507 mg) divided every 6 to 8 h. After 3 more days, if tolerated, increase dosage to 600 mg/day (equivalent to aminophylline 760 mg) divided every 6 to 8 h.

Dosage adjustment: Dosage adjustment should be guided by serum theophylline concentration measurement.

Because the rate of theophylline clearance may be dose dependent (ie, steady-state serum concentrations may increase disproportionately to the increase in dose), an increase in dose based upon a subtherapeutic serum concentration measurement should be conservative. In general, limiting dose increases to about 25% of the previous total daily dose will reduce the risk of unintended excessive increases in serum theophylline concentration.

Transient caffeine-like adverse reactions and excessive serum concentrations in slow metabolizers can be avoided in most patients by starting with a sufficiently low dose and slowly increasing the dose, if judged to be clinically indicated, in small increments. Dose increases should only be made if the previous dosage is well tolerated and at intervals of no less than 3 days to allow serum theophylline concentrations to reach the new steady state.

Do not make increases in the dose of theophylline in response to an acute exacerbation of symptoms of chronic lung disease because theophylline provides little added benefit to inhaled beta-2 selective agonists and systemically administered corticosteroids in this circumstance and increases the risk of adverse reactions. Measure a peak steady-state serum theophylline concentration before increasing the dose in response to persistent chronic symptoms to ascertain whether an increase in dose is safe. Before increasing the theophylline dose on the basis of a low serum concentration, consider whether the blood sample was obtained at an appropriate time in relationship to the dose and whether the patient has adhered to the prescribed regimen.

Dosage Adjustment Based on Serum Theophylline Concentration

Peak serum concentration	Dosage adjustment
< 9.9 mcg/mL	If symptoms are not controlled and current dosage is tolerated, increase dose about 25%. Recheck serum concentration after 3 days for further dosage adjustment.
10 to 14.9 mcg/mL	If symptoms are controlled and current dosage is tolerated, maintain dose and recheck serum concentration at 6- to 12-month intervals.[a] If symptoms are not controlled and current dosage is tolerated, consider adding additional medication(s) to treatment regimen.
15 to 19.9 mcg/mL	Consider 10% decrease in dose to provide greater margin of safety even if current dosage is tolerated.[a]
20 to 24.9 mcg/mL	Decrease dose by 25% even if no adverse reactions are present. Recheck serum concentration after 3 days to guide further dosage adjustment.
25 to 30 mcg/mL	Skip next dose and decrease subsequent doses at least 25% even if no adverse reactions are present. Recheck serum concentration after 3 days to guide further dosage adjustment. If symptomatic, consider whether overdose treatment is indicated.
> 30 mcg/mL	Treat overdose as indicated. If theophylline is subsequently resumed, decrease dose by at least 50% and recheck serum concentration after 3 days to guide further dosage adjustment.

[a] Dose reduction and/or serum theophylline concentration measurement is indicated whenever adverse reactions are present, physiologic abnormalities that can reduce theophylline clearance occur (eg, sustained fever), or a drug that interacts with theophylline is added or discontinued.

➤*Children:*

Children 16 years of age and older – See Adults for dosing.

Children 1 to 15 years of age –

Maximum dose: 16 mg/kg/day (equivalent to aminophylline 20.3 mg) up to a maximum of 400 mg/day (equivalent to aminophylline 507 mg) in the presence of risk factors for reduced theophylline clearance or if it is not feasible to monitor serum theophylline concentrations.

Initial dosage:

- *Children weighing less than 45 kg* – 12 to 14 mg/kg/day (equivalent to aminophylline 15.2 to 17.7 mg) up to a maximum of 300 mg/day (equivalent to aminophylline 380 mg) divided every 4 to 6 h. After 3 days, if tolerated, increase dosage to 16 mg/kg/day (equivalent to aminophylline 20.3 mg) up to a maximum of 400 mg/day (equivalent to aminophylline 507 mg) divided every 4 to 6 h. After 3 more days, if tolerated, increase dosage to 20 mg/kg/day (equivalent to aminophylline 25.3 mg) up to a maximum of 600 mg/day (equivalent to aminophylline 760 mg) divided every 4 to 6 h.
- *Children weighing more than 45 kg* – 300 mg/day (equivalent to aminophylline 380 mg) divided every 6 to 8 h. After 3 days, if tolerated, increase dosage to 400 mg/day (equivalent to aminophylline 507 mg) divided every 6 to 8 h. After 3 more days, if tolerated, increase dosage to 600 mg/day (equivalent to aminophylline 760 mg) divided every 6 to 8 h.

Children younger than 1 year of age – Carefully consider the benefits and risks of theophylline use and the need for more intensive monitoring of serum theophylline concentrations in neonates (term and premature) and children younger than 1 year of age.

➤*Elderly:* Elderly patients are at significantly greater risk of experiencing serious toxicity from theophylline than younger patients because of pharmacokinetic and pharmacodynamic changes associated with aging. The maximum daily dose of theophylline in patients older than 60 years of age ordinarily should not exceed 400 mg/day unless the patient continues to be symptomatic and the peak steady-state serum theophylline concentration is less than 10 mcg/mL. Prescribe theophylline doses greater than 400 mg daily with caution in elderly patients.

➤*Renal function impairment:* Careful attention to dose reduction and frequent monitoring of serum theophylline concentrations are required in neonates with renal impairment.

➤*Hepatic function impairment:* Careful attention to dose reduction and frequent monitoring of serum theophylline concentrations are required in patients with hepatic impairment.

➤*Special risk patients:* Patients with more rapid metabolism, clinically identified by higher than average dose requirements, should receive a smaller dose more frequently to prevent breakthrough symptoms resulting from low trough concentrations before the next dose. A reliably absorbed slow-release formulation will decrease fluctuations and permit longer dosing intervals.

➤*Therapeutic drug monitoring:* If the patient's symptoms are well controlled, there are no apparent adverse reactions, and no intervening factors that might alter dosage requirements, serum theophylline concentrations should be monitored at 6-month intervals for rapidly growing children and at yearly intervals for all others. In acutely ill patients, serum theophylline concentrations should be monitored at frequent intervals (eg, every 24 hours).

➤*Storage/Stability:* Store between 15° and 30°C (59° and 86°F). Protect from light and moisture.

AMINOPHYLLINE — INJECTION

For complete and comparative prescribing information, refer to the Xanthine Derivatives group monograph.

Indications

➤*Reversible airflow obstruction:* As an adjunct to inhaled beta-2 selective agonists and systemically administered corticosteroids for the treatment of acute exacerbations of the symptoms and reversible airflow obstruction associated with asthma and other lung diseases (eg, emphysema and bronchitis).

Administration and Dosage

➤*General dosing considerations:* The following information is based on theophylline except where noted. Aminophylline is approximately 79% of anhydrous theophylline by weight; therefore, to convert a theophylline dose to aminophylline, divide the theophylline dose by 0.8.

Theophylline distributes poorly into body fat; therefore, mg-per-kg doses should be calculated on the basis of ideal body weight.

AMINOPHYLLINE — INJECTION

The dose of theophylline must be individualized on the basis of peak serum theophylline concentration measurements in order to achieve a dose that will provide maximum potential benefit with minimal risk of adverse reactions.

A serum concentration obtained 30 minutes after an IV loading dose, when distribution is complete, can be used to assess the need for and size of subsequent loading doses, if clinically indicated, and for guidance of continuing therapy. (See Therapeutic drug monitoring.)

➤*Adults:*

Reversible airflow obstruction –

Loading dose: Because of rapid distribution into body fluids, the serum concentration (C) obtained from an initial loading dose (LD) is related primarily to the volume of distribution (V), the apparent space into which the drug diffuses: C = LD/V.

• *Patients not currently receiving theophylline –* The mean volume of distribution can be assumed to be 0.5 L/kg, and the desired serum concentration should be conservative (eg, 10 mcg/mL) to allow for the variability in the volume of distribution.

If a mean volume of distribution of approximately 0.5 L/kg is assumed (actual range is 0.3 to 0.7 L/kg), each mg/kg (ideal body weight) of theophylline administered as a loading dose over 30 minutes results in an average 2 mcg/mL increase in serum theophylline concentration.

• *Patients who received a dose in the last 24 hours –* When a loading dose becomes necessary in the patient who has already received theophylline, estimation of the serum concentration based upon the history is unreliable, and an immediate serum level determination is indicated, the loading dose can then be determined as follows: LD = (desired C − measured C)(V). A loading dose should not be given before obtaining a serum theophylline concentration if the patient has received any theophylline in the previous 24 hours.

Maintenance dosage: Once a serum concentration of 10 to 15 mcg/mL has been achieved with the use of a loading dose(s), a constant IV infusion is started. The rate of administration is based upon mean pharmacokinetic parameters for the population and calculated to achieve a target serum concentration of 10 mcg/mL.

Dosage adjustment:

If the level, obtained from the second sample one expected half-life after starting the constant infusion, is declining as a result of a higher than average clearance, an additional loading dose can be administered and/or the infusion rate increased. In contrast, if the second sample demonstrates a higher level, accumulation of the drug can be assumed, and the infusion rate should be decreased before the concentration exceeds 20 mcg/mL.

Do not make increases in the dose of IV theophylline in response to an acute exacerbation of symptoms unless the steady-state serum theophylline concentration is less than 10 mcg/mL.

Because the rate of theophylline clearance may be dose dependent (ie, steady-state serum concentrations may increase disproportionately to the increase in dose), an increase in dose based upon a subtherapeutic serum concentration measurement should be conservative. In general, limiting infusion rate increases to about 25% of the previous infusion rate will reduce the risk of unintended excessive increases in serum theophylline concentration.

Final Dosage Adjustment Based on Serum Theophylline Concentration

Peak serum concentration	Dosage adjustment
< 9.9 mcg/mL	If symptoms are not controlled and current dosage is tolerated, increase infusion rate by approximately 25%. Recheck serum concentration after 12 hours in children and 24 hours in adults for further dosage adjustments.
10 to 14.9 mcg/mL	If symptoms are controlled and current dosage is tolerated, maintain infusion rate and recheck serum concentration at 24-hour intervals.[a] If symptoms are not controlled and current dosage is tolerated, consider adding additional medication(s) to treatment regimen.
15 to 19.9 mcg/mL	Consider 10% decrease in infusion rate to provide greater margin of safety even if current dosage is tolerated.[a]
20 to 24.9 mcg/mL	Decrease infusion rate by 25% even if no adverse reactions are present. Recheck serum concentration after 12 hours in children and 24 hours in adults to guide further dosage adjustment.
25 to 30 mcg/mL	Stop infusion for 12 hours in children and 24 hours in adults and decrease subsequent infusion rate at least 25% even if no adverse reactions are present. Recheck serum concentration after 12 hours in children and 24 hours in adults to guide further dosage adjustment. If symptomatic, stop infusion and consider whether overdose treatment is indicated.
> 30 mcg/mL	Stop the infusion and treat overdose as indicated. If theophylline is subsequently resumed, decrease infusion rate by at least 50% and recheck serum concentration after 12 hours in children and 24 hours in adults to guide further dosage adjustment.

[a] Dose reduction and/or serum theophylline concentration measurement is indicated whenever adverse reactions are present, physiologic abnormalities that can reduce theophylline clearance occur (eg, sustained fever), or a drug that interacts with theophylline is added or discontinued.

➤*Children:*

Reversible airflow obstruction –

1 year of age or older: See Adults for dosing.

• *Dosage adjustment –*

If the level, obtained from the second sample one expected half-life after starting the constant infusion, is declining as a result of a higher than average clearance, an additional loading dose can be administered and/or the infusion rate increased. In contrast, if the second sample demonstrates a higher level, accumulation of the drug can be assumed, and the infusion rate should be decreased before the concentration exceeds 20 mcg/mL.

Do not make increases in the dose of IV theophylline in response to an acute exacerbation of symptoms unless the steady-state serum theophylline concentration is less than 10 mcg/mL.

Because the rate of theophylline clearance may be dose dependent (ie, steady-state serum concentrations may increase disproportionately to the increase in dose), an increase in dose based upon a subtherapeutic serum concentration measurement should be conservative. In general, limiting infusion rate increases to about 25% of the previous infusion rate will reduce the risk of unintended excessive increases in serum theophylline concentration.

Final Dosage Adjustment Based on Serum Theophylline Concentration

Peak serum concentration	Dosage adjustment
< 9.9 mcg/mL	If symptoms are not controlled and current dosage is tolerated, increase infusion rate by approximately 25%. Recheck serum concentration after 12 hours in children and 24 hours in adults for further dosage adjustments.
10 to 14.9 mcg/mL	If symptoms are controlled and current dosage is tolerated, maintain infusion rate and recheck serum concentration at 24-hour intervals.[a] If symptoms are not controlled and current dosage is tolerated, consider adding additional medication(s) to treatment regimen.
15 to 19.9 mcg/mL	Consider 10% decrease in infusion rate to provide greater margin of safety even if current dosage is tolerated.[a]
20 to 24.9 mcg/mL	Decrease infusion rate by 25% even if no adverse reactions are present. Recheck serum concentration after 12 hours in children and 24 hours in adults to guide further dosage adjustment.
25 to 30 mcg/mL	Stop infusion for 12 hours in children and 24 hours in adults and decrease subsequent infusion rate at least 25% even if no adverse reactions are present. Recheck serum concentration after 12 hours in children and 24 hours in adults to guide further dosage adjustment. If symptomatic, stop infusion and consider whether overdose treatment is indicated.
> 30 mcg/mL	Stop the infusion and treat overdose as indicated. If theophylline is subsequently resumed, decrease infusion rate by at least 50% and recheck serum concentration after 12 hours in children and 24 hours in adults to guide further dosage adjustment.

[a] Dose reduction and/or serum theophylline concentration measurement is indicated whenever adverse reactions are present, physiologic abnormalities that can reduce theophylline clearance occur (eg, sustained fever), or a drug that interacts with theophylline is added or discontinued.

Children younger than 1 year of age: Because of the immaturity of theophylline metabolic pathways in children younger than 1 year of age, pay particular attention to dosage selection and monitor serum theophylline concentrations frequently when prescribing theophylline to children in this age group.

➤*Elderly:* The maximum daily dose of theophylline in patients older than 60 years of age ordinarily should not exceed 400 mg/day unless the patient continues to be symptomatic and the peak steady-state serum theophylline concentration is less than 10 mcg/mL. Prescribe theophylline infusion rates greater than 17 mg/h (21 mg/h as aminophylline) with caution in elderly patients.

AMINOPHYLLINE — INJECTION

➤*Renal function impairment:* Careful attention to dose reduction and frequent monitoring of serum theophylline concentrations are required in neonates with renal impairment.

➤*Hepatic function impairment:* The initial theophylline infusion rate should not exceed 17 mg/h (21 mg/h as aminophylline) unless serum concentrations can be monitored at 24-hour intervals. In these patients, 5 days may be required before steady state is reached.

➤*Special risk patients:* In patients with cor pulmonale, cardiac decompensation, or in those taking drugs that markedly reduce theophylline clearance (eg, cimetidine), the initial theophylline infusion rate should not exceed 17 mg/h (21 mg/h as aminophylline) unless serum concentrations can be monitored at 24-hour intervals. In these patients, 5 days may be required before steady state is reached.

➤*Therapeutic drug monitoring:* Because there is large interpatient variability in theophylline clearance, serum concentrations will rise or fall when the patient's clearance is significantly different from the mean population value used to calculate the initial infusion rate. Therefore, a second serum concentration should be obtained one expected half-life after starting the constant infusion (eg, approximately 4 hours for children 1 to 9 years of age and 8 hours for nonsmoking adults) to determine if the concentration is accumulating or declining from the postloadingdose level. Obtain an additional sample 12 to 24 hours later to determine if further adjustments are required, and then at 24-hour intervals to adjust for changes, if they occur.

➤*Administration:*
Infusion rates –

Initial Theophylline Infusion Rates Following an Appropriate Loading Dose

Patient population	Age	Theophylline infusion rate (mg/kg/h)[a], [b]
Neonates	≤ 24 days (postnatal)	1 mg/kg every 12 h[c]
	> 24 days (postnatal)	1.5 mg/kg every 12 h[c]
Infants	6 to 52 wk	mg/kg/h = 0.008 × age in wk + 0.21
Young children	1 to 9 y	0.8
Older children	9 to 12 y	0.7
Adolescents (cigarette or marijuana smokers)	12 to 16 y	0.7
Adolescents (nonsmokers)	12 to 16 y	0.5[d]
Adults (otherwise healthy nonsmokers)	16 to 60 y	0.4[d]
Elderly patients	> 60 y	0.3[e]
Cardiac decompensation, cor pulmonale, hepatic function impairment, sepsis with multiorgan failure, or shock		0.2[e]

[a] To achieve a target concentration of 10 mcg/mL, aminophylline = theophylline divided by 0.8. Use ideal body weight for obese patients.
[b] Lower initial dosage may be required for patients receiving other drugs that decrease theophylline clearance (eg, cimetidine).
[c] To achieve a target concentration of 7.5 mcg/mL for neonatal apnea.
[d] Not to exceed 900 mg/day, unless serum levels indicate the need for a larger dose.
[e] Not to exceed 400 mg/day, unless serum levels indicate the need for a larger dose.

➤*Extravasation:* Extravasation may occur during administration of aminophylline. If signs or symptoms of extravasation occur, stop the infusion immediately. If possible, withdraw 3 to 5 mL of blood to remove some of the drug. Remove the infusion needle. Delineate the infiltrated area on the patient's skin with a felt-tip marker. Hyaluronidase is an effective antidote for hyperosmolar drug infiltrations; administer promptly within the first few minutes to 1 hour after extravasation. Higher doses (150 units) have primarily been used in adults while lower doses (15 units) have been used in children. Administer hyaluronidase according to the following steps. Dilute hyaluronidase to desired concentration, depending on the dose and product used. (Note: Some products do not require dilution.) For example, if the total dose is 15 units, make 15 units/mL dilution. If the total dose is 150 units, make 150 units/mL dilution. Cleanse area with povidone-iodine. Inject hyaluronidase locally, subcutaneously or intradermally, using a 25-gauge needle or smaller. The dose is given as five 0.2 mL injections at the leading edge of the extravasation site. Change needle after each injection. Elevate for 48 hours above heart level using a sling or stockinette dressing with an observation window cut in the dressing. Avoid pressure or friction. Do not rub area. Observe for signs of increased erythema, pain, or skin necrosis. If increased symptoms occur, consult a plastic surgeon. Ensure that no medication is given distally to extravasation site. After 48 hours, encourage the patient to use the extremity normally to promote full range of motion.

➤*Admixture compatibility:* Although there have been reports of aminophylline precipitating in acidic media, these reports do not apply to the diluted solutions found in IV infusions. Aminophylline injection should not be mixed in a syringe with other drugs but should be added separately to the IV solution.

When an IV solution containing aminophylline is given piggyback, the IV system already in place should be turned off while the aminophylline is infused if there is a potential problem with admixture incompatibility.

Because of the alkalinity of aminophylline-containing solutions, drugs known to be alkali labile should be avoided in admixtures. These include epinephrine, norepinephrine, isoproterenol, and penicillin G potassium. It is suggested that specialized literature be consulted before preparing admixtures with aminophylline and other drugs.

➤*Storage/Stability:* Store between 15° and 30°C (59° and 86°F). Protect from light. Store in carton until time of use. Discard unused portion.

DYPHYLLINE (Dihydroxypropyl Theophylline)

Rx	**Lufyllin** (MedPointe)	**Tablets; oral:** 200 mg	(Wallace 521). White, rectangular, scored. In 100s.
Rx	**Lufyllin-400** (MedPointe)	**Tablets; oral:** 400 mg	(Wallace 731). White, capsule shaped, scored. In 100s.
Rx	**Dylix** (Lunsco)	**Elixir; oral:** 100 mg per 15 mL	20% alcohol. In 437 mL.

DYPHYLLINE ORAL

For complete and comparative prescribing information, refer to the Xanthine Derivatives group monograph.

Indications

➤*Bronchial asthma/reversible bronchospasm:* For relief of acute bronchial asthma and for reversible bronchospasm associated with chronic bronchitis and emphysema.

Administration and Dosage

➤*Adults:*
Bronchial asthma –
Tablets: Up to 15 mg/kg every 6 hours.
Elixir: 30 to 60 mL every 6 hours.

Reversible bronchospasm – See Bronchial asthma for dosing.

➤*Elderly:* Use caution in dose selection for an elderly patient, usually starting at the low end of the dosing range, reflecting the greater frequency of decreased hepatic, renal, or cardiac function, and of concomitant disease or other drug therapy.

➤*Renal function impairment:* Appropriate dosage adjustments should be made in patients with renal impairment.

➤*Storage/Stability:*
Elixir – Store between 15° and 30°C (59° and 86°F).
Tablets – Store between 20° and 25°C (68° and 77°F).

IPRATROPIUM BROMIDE

Rx	**Ipratropium Bromide** (Dey)	**Solution for Inhalation**: 0.02% (500 mcg per vial)	Preservative free. In 25 and 60 unit-dose vials (2.5 ml each).
Rx	**Atrovent HFA** (Boehringer Ingelheim)	**Aerosol**: Each actuation delivers 17 mcg	In 12.9 g metered dose inhaler w/mouthpiece (200 inhalations).
Rx	**Ipratropium Bromide** (Various, eg, Bausch & Lomb, Roxane)	**Nasal spray**: 0.03%. Each spray delivers 21 mcg	In 30 mL with spray pump (345 sprays).
Rx	**Atrovent** (Boehringer Ingelheim)		In 30 mL bottles with spray pump (345 sprays).
Rx	**Ipratropium Bromide** (Various, eg, Bausch & Lomb, Roxane)	**Nasal spray**: 0.06%. Each spray delivers 42 mcg	In 15 mL with spray pump (165 sprays).
Rx	**Atrovent** (Boehringer Ingelheim)		In 15 mL bottles with spray pump (165 sprays).

IPRATROPIUM BROMIDE — INHALATION

Indications

➤*Chronic obstructive pulmonary disease (COPD):* Alone or with other bronchodilators, especially beta adrenergics, as a bronchodilator for maintenance treatment of bronchospasm associated with COPD, including chronic bronchitis and emphysema.

Administration and Dosage

➤*Maximum dose:*

Adults – 12 inhalations/day of ipratropium HFA according to the prescribing information. For ipratropium inhalation solution, there is no well-established maximum dose for the approved indication according to the prescribing information.

➤*Adults:*

Chronic obstructive pulmonary disease –

HFA aerosol: The usual starting dose is 2 inhalations 4 times a day. Patients may take additional inhalations as required; however, the total number of inhalations should not exceed 12 in 24 hours.

Solution: 500 mcg (1 unit-dose vial) administered 3 to 4 times a day by oral nebulization, with doses 6 to 8 hours apart.

➤*Children:*

HFA aerosol – Safety and efficacy in children have not been established.

Solution – See Adults for dosing for children 12 years of age and older.

➤*Preparation for administration:*

HFA aerosol – Prime or actuate the inhaler before using for the first time by releasing 2 test sprays into the air away from the face. In cases where the inhaler has not been used for more than 3 days, prime the inhaler again by releasing 2 test sprays into the air away from the face.

➤*Administration:*

HFA aerosol – The HFA inhalation aerosol canister is to be used only with the accompanying white mouthpiece that has a clear, colorless sleeve and green protective cap. Do not use this mouthpiece with other aerosol medications. Each 12.9 g canister provides sufficient medication for 200 inhalations. Discard the canister after the labeled number of actuations has been used. The amount of medication in each actuation cannot be ensured after this point, even though the canister is not completely empty.

Solution – Use of a nebulizer with mouthpiece rather than face mask may be preferable to reduce the likelihood of the nebulizer solution reaching the eyes. The solution should be used consistently, as prescribed throughout the course of therapy.

➤*Admixture compatibility:*

Compatibility – Ipratropium inhalation solution can be mixed in the nebulizer with albuterol or metaproterenol if used within 1 hour.

➤*Storage/Stability:*

HFA aerosol – Store at 25°C (77°F). Excursions permitted to 15° to 30°C (59° to 86°F). For optimal results, store the canister at room temperature before use.

Contents under pressure: Do not puncture. Do not use or store near heat or open flame. Exposure to temperatures above 49°C (120°F) may cause bursting. Never throw the inhaler into a fire or incinerator.

Solution – Store between 15° and 30°C (59° and 86°F). Protect from light. Retain in foil pouch until time of use.

Actions

➤*Pharmacology:* Ipratropium bromide is an anticholinergic (parasympathetic) agent that, based on animal studies, appears to inhibit vagally mediated reflexes by antagonizing the action of acetylcholine, the transmitter agent released at neuromuscular junctions in the lung. Anticholinergics prevent the increase in intracellular concentration of cyclic guanosine monophosphate (cyclic GMP), which are caused by interaction of acetylcholine with the muscarinic receptor on bronchial smooth muscle.

➤*Pharmacokinetics:*

Absorption – The bronchodilation following inhalation of ipratropium is primarily a local, site-specific effect, not a systemic one. Much of an administered dose is swallowed but not absorbed, as shown by fecal excretion studies. Ipratropium is a quaternary amine. Following nebulization of a 2 mg dose, a mean 7% of the dose was absorbed into the systemic circulation either from the surface of the lung or from the GI tract.

Distribution – Ipratropium is minimally bound (0% to 9% in vitro) to plasma albumin and α_1-acid glycoprotein. Its blood/plasma concentration ratio was estimated to be about 0.89. Autoradiographic studies in rats have shown that ipratropium does not penetrate the blood-brain barrier.

Metabolism/Excretion – Ipratropium is partially metabolized to inactive ester hydrolysis products. Following intravenous (IV) administration, approximately one half of the dose is excreted unchanged in the urine.

The half-life of elimination is about 2 hours after inhalation or IV administration. The total body clearance and renal clearance were estimated to be 2,505 and 1,019 mL/min, respectively. The amount of the total dose excreted unchanged in the urine (Ae) within 24 hours was approximately one half of the administered dose.

A pharmacokinetic study with 29 COPD patients (48 to 79 years of age) demonstrated that mean peak plasma ipratropium concentrations of 59 ± 20 pg/mL were obtained following a single administration of 4 inhalations of ipratropium HFA inhalation aerosol (84 mcg). Plasma ipratropium concentrations rapidly declined to 24 ± 15 pg/mL by 6 hours. When these patients were administered 4 inhalations 4 times daily (16 inhalations/day = 336 mcg) for 1 week, the mean peak plasma ipratropium concentration increased to 82 ± 39 pg/mL with a trough (6 hour) concentration of 28 ± 12 pg/mL at steady state.

Contraindications

Hypersensitivity to ipratropium or its components, or atropine or its derivatives.

Warnings/Precautions

➤*Acute bronchospasm:*

HFA aerosol – Ipratropium HFA inhalation aerosol is a bronchodilator for the maintenance treatment of bronchospasm associated with COPD and is not indicated for the initial treatment of acute episodes of bronchospasm where rescue therapy is required for rapid response.

Inhaled medicines, including ipratropium HFA inhalation aerosol, may cause paradoxical bronchospasm. If this occurs, stop treatment with ipratropium HFA inhalation aerosol and consider other treatments.

Solution – The use of ipratropium inhalation solution as a single agent for the relief of bronchospasm in acute COPD exacerbation has not been adequately studied. Drugs with faster onset of action may be preferable as initial therapy in this situation. Combination of ipratropium and beta agonists has not been shown to be more effective than either drug alone in reversing the bronchospasm associated with acute COPD exacerbation.

➤*Hypersensitivity reactions:* Immediate hypersensitivity reactions may occur after administration of ipratropium as demonstrated by rare cases of urticaria, angioedema, rash, bronchospasm, anaphylaxis, and oropharyngeal edema.

➤*Special risk:* Use ipratropium with caution in patients with narrow-angle glaucoma, prostatic hyperplasia, or bladder-neck obstruction, particularly if they are receiving an anticholinergic by another route. Cases of precipitation or worsening of narrow-angle glaucoma and acute eye pain have been reported with direct eye contact of ipratropium administered by oral inhalation.

➤*Pregnancy: Category B.* At oral doses of 90 mg/kg and above in rats in the aerosol HFA formulation (approximately 3,600 times the maximum recommended daily inhalation dose in adults on a mg/m^2 basis) embryotoxicity was observed as increased resorption. This effect is not considered relevant to human use due to the large doses at which it was observed and the difference in route of administration. There are, however, no adequate or well-controlled studies have been conducted in pregnant women. Because animal reproduction studies are not always predictive of human response, use ipratropium during pregnancy only if clearly needed.

➤*Lactation:* It is not known whether ipratropium inhalation solution or aerosol are excreted in human milk. Although lipid-soluble quaternary cations pass into breast milk, it is unlikely that the active component, ipratropium, would reach the infant to an important extent, especially when taken by inhalation. Ipratropium is not well absorbed systemically after inhalation or oral administration. However, because many drugs are excreted in human milk, exercise caution when ipratropium is administered to a breast-feeding woman.

➤*Children:*

HFA aerosol – Safety and efficacy in children have not been established.

Solution – Safety and efficacy in children younger than 12 years of age have not been established.

IPRATROPIUM BROMIDE — INHALATION

Drug Interactions

➤*Anticholinergic agents:* Although ipratropium is minimally absorbed into the systemic circulation, there is some potential for an additive interaction with concomitantly used anticholinergic medications. Caution is therefore advised in the coadministration of ipratropium inhalation with other anticholinergic-containing drugs.

Adverse Reactions

➤*HFA aerosol:*

Adverse Reactions Reported in any Ipratropium Bromide Group (≥ 3%)					
	Placebo-controlled 12-week study 244.1405 and active-controlled 12-week study 244.1408			Active-controlled 1-year study 244.2453	
Adverse reaction	Ipratropium HFA aerosol (n = 243)	Ipratropium CFC (n = 183)	Placebo (n = 128)	Ipratropium HFA aerosol (n = 305)	Ipratropium CFC (n = 151)
Total with any adverse reaction	63%	68%	72%	91%	87%
CNS					
Dizziness	3%	3%	2%	3%	1%
Headache	6%	9%	8%	7%	5%
GI					
Dry mouth	4%	2%	2%	2%	3%
Dyspepsia	1%	3%	1%	5%	3%
Nausea	4%	1%	2%	4%	4%
GU					
Urinary tract infection	2%	3%	1%	10%	8%
Respiratory					
Bronchitis	10%	11%	6%	23%	19%
COPD exacerbation	8%	14%	13%	23%	23%
Coughing	3%	4%	6%	5%	5%
Dyspnea	8%	8%	4%	7%	4%
Rhinitis	4%	2%	4%	6%	2%
Sinusitis	1%	4%	3%	11%	14%
Upper respiratory tract infection	9%	10%	16%	34%	34%
Miscellaneous					
Back pain	2%	3%	2%	7%	3%
Influenza-like symptoms	4%	2%	2%	8%	5%

Overall, in the above mentioned studies, 9.3% of the patients taking ipratropium 42 mcg HFA inhalation aerosol and 8.7% of the patients taking ipratropium 42 mcg inhalation aerosol CFC reported at least 1 adverse reaction that was considered by the investigator to be related to the study drug. The most common drug-related adverse reactions were dry mouth (1.6% of ipratropium HFA inhalation aerosol and 0.9% of ipratropium inhalation aerosol CFC patients) and taste perversion (bitter taste) (0.9% of ipratropium HFA inhalation aerosol and 0.3% of ipratropium inhalation aerosol CFC patients).

As an anticholinergic drug, cases of precipitation or worsening of narrow-angle glaucoma, mydriasis, acute eye pain, hypotension, urinary retention, tachycardia, constipation, and bronchospasm, including paradoxical bronchospasm, have been reported.

Allergic-type reactions such as skin rash; angioedema of tongue, lips, and face; urticaria (including giant urticaria); laryngospasm; and anaphylactic reaction have been reported.

Postmarketing experience –

HFA aerosol: Allergic-type reactions such as skin rash; angioedema of tongue, lips, and face; urticaria (including giant urticaria); laryngospasm; and anaphylactic reactions have been reported, with positive rechallenge in some cases. Many of the patients had a history of allergies to other drugs and/or foods, including soybean.

Additionally, urinary retention, mydriasis, and bronchospasm, including paradoxical bronchospasm, have been reported during the postmarketing period with use of ipratropium inhalation aerosol CFC.

➤*Solution:*

All Adverse Reactions from a Double-Blind, Parallel, 12-week Study of Patients With COPD Receiving Ipratropium[a]					
Adverse reaction	Ipratropium (500 mcg 3 times daily) (n = 219)	Metaproterenol (15 mg 3 times daily) (n = 212)	Ipratropium/ Metaproterenol (500 mcg 3 times daily/ 15 mg 3 times daily) (n = 108)	Albuterol (2.5 mg 3 times daily) (n = 205)	Ipratropium/ Albuterol (500 mcg 3 times daily/ 2.5 mg 3 times daily) (n = 100)
Cardiovascular					
Chest pain	3.2%	4.2%	5.6%	2%	1%
Hypertension/hypertension aggravated	0.9%	1.9%	0.9%	1.5%	4%
CNS					
Dizziness	2.3%	3.3%	1.9%	3.9%	4%
Headache	6.4%	5.2%	6.5%	6.3%	9%
Insomnia	0.9%	0.5%	4.6%	1%	1%
Nervousness	0.5%	4.7%	6.5%	1%	1%
Tremor	0.9%	7.1%	8.3%	1%	0%
GI					
Constipation	0.9%	0%	3.7%	1%	1%
Dry mouth	3.2%	0%	1.9%	2%	3%
Nausea	4.1%	3.8%	1.9%	2.9%	2%
Musculoskeletal					
Arthritis	0.9%	1.4%	0.9%	0.5%	3%
Respiratory					
Bronchitis	14.6%	24.5%	15.7%	16.6%	20%
Bronchospasm	2.3%	2.8%	4.6%	5.4%	5%
Coughing	4.6%	8%	6.5%	5.4%	6%
Dyspnea	9.6%	13.2%	16.7%	12.7%	9%
Pharyngitis	3.7%	4.2%	5.6%	2.9%	4%
Respiratory tract disorder	0%	6.1%	6.5%	2%	4%
Rhinitis	2.3%	4.2%	1.9%	2.4%	0%
Sinusitis	2.3%	2.8%	0.9%	5.4%	4%
Sputum increased	1.4%	1.4%	4.6%	3.4%	0%
Upper respiratory tract infection	13.2%	11.3%	9.3%	12.2%	16%
Miscellaneous					
Back pain	3.2%	1.9%	1.9%	2.4%	0%
Influenza-like symptoms	3.7%	4.7%	8.5%	0.5%	1%
Pain	4.1%	3.3%	0.9%	2.9%	5%

[a] All adverse reactions, regardless of drug relationship, reported by greater than or equal to 3% of patients in the 12-week controlled clinical trials.

IPRATROPIUM BROMIDE — INHALATION

Additional adverse reactions reported in less than 3% of the patients treated with ipratropium include tachycardia, palpitations, eye pain, urinary retention, urinary tract infection, and urticaria. Cases of precipitation or worsening of narrow-angle glaucoma and acute eye pain have been reported.

Lower respiratory tract adverse reactions (bronchitis, dyspnea, and bronchospasm) were the most common reactions leading to discontinuation of ipratropium therapy in the 12-week trials. Headache, mouth dryness, and aggravation of COPD symptoms are more common when the total daily dose of ipratropium equals or exceeds 2,000 mcg.

Hypersensitivity – Allergic-type reactions such as skin rash; angioedema of tongue, lips, and face; urticaria; laryngospasm; and anaphylactic reaction have been reported. Many of the patients had a history of allergies to other drugs and/or foods.

Overdosage

Acute overdose by inhalation is unlikely because ipratropium is not well absorbed systemically after inhalation or oral administration.

Patient Information

Advise patients that ipratropium inhalation is for the maintenance treatment of bronchospasm associated with COPD and is not indicated for the initial treatment of acute episodes of bronchospasm where rescue therapy is required for rapid response.

Do not use ipratropium inhalation more frequently than recommended. The dose or frequency of ipratropium inhalation aerosol should not be increased without patients consulting their doctors. If treatment with ipratropium inhalation aerosol becomes less effective for symptomatic relief, their symptoms become worse, and/or patients need to use the product more frequently than usual, seek medical attention immediately. Advise patients who are pregnant or breast-feeding to contact their doctors about the use of ipratropium inhalation. Appropriate use of ipratropium inhalation includes an understanding of the way it should be administered.

Instruct patients to avoid spraying ipratropium in or around the eyes. Caution patients to avoid spraying the aerosol into their eyes and advise them that this may result in precipitation or worsening of narrow-angle glaucoma, mydriasis, eye pain or discomfort, temporary blurring of vision, visual halos, or colored images in association with red eyes from conjunctival and corneal congestion. Advise patients that should any combination of these symptoms develop, they should consult their doctors immediately.

While taking ipratropium inhalation aerosol, other inhaled drugs should not be used unless prescribed.

Remind patients that ipratropium inhalation should be used consistently as prescribed throughout the course of therapy.

➤*HFA aerosol:* The action of ipratropium inhalation aerosol should last 2 to 4 hours. Advise patients that although the taste and inhalation sensation of ipratropium HFA inhalation aerosol may be slightly different from that of the CFC (chlorofluorocarbon) formulation of ipratropium inhalation aerosol, they are comparable in terms of safety and efficacy.

Do not shake the ipratropium HFA inhalation aerosol canister before using it.

"Prime" ipratropium HFA inhalation aerosol 2 times before taking the first dose from a new inhaler or when the inhaler has not been used for more than 3 days. To prime, push the canister against the mouthpiece, allowing the medicine to spray into the air. Avoid spraying the medicine into your eyes while priming ipratropium HFA inhalation aerosol.

Use ipratropium HFA inhalation aerosol exactly as prescribed by your doctor. Do not change your dose or how often you use ipratropium HFA inhalation aerosol without talking with your doctor. Talk to you doctor if you have questions about your medical condition or your treatment.

IPRATROPIUM BROMIDE — INTRANASAL

Indications

➤*Perennial rhinitis 0.03%:* For the symptomatic relief of rhinorrhea associated with allergic and nonallergic perennial rhinitis in adults and children 6 years of age and older. Ipratropium bromide nasal spray 0.03% does not relieve nasal congestion, sneezing, or postnasal drip associated with allergic or nonallergic perennial rhinitis.

➤*Common cold or seasonal allergic rhinitis 0.06%:* For the symptomatic relief of rhinorrhea associated with the common cold or seasonal allergic rhinitis for adults and children 5 years of age and older. Ipratropium bromide 0.06% nasal spray does not relieve nasal congestion or sneezing associated with the common cold or seasonal allergic rhinitis.

Administration and Dosage

➤*Adults:*

0.03% –

Perennial rhinitis: 2 sprays (42 mcg) per nostril 2 or 3 times daily (total dose 168 to 252 mcg/day).

0.06% –

Rhinorrhea associated with the common cold: 2 sprays (84 mcg) per nostril 3 or 4 times daily (total dose 504 to 672 mcg/day). The safety and effectiveness of using beyond 4 days have not been established.

Rhinorrhea associated with seasonal allergic rhinitis: 2 sprays (84 mcg) per nostril 4 times daily (total dose 672 mcg/day). The safety and efficacy of using beyond 3 weeks have not been established.

➤*Children:*

0.03% –

Perennial rhinitis: See Adults for dosing.

0.06% –

Rhinorrhea associated with the common cold:

• *12 years of age and older* – 2 sprays (84 mcg) per nostril 3 or 4 times daily (total dose 504 to 672 mcg/day). The safety and effectiveness of using beyond 4 days have not been established.

• *5 to 11 years of age* – 2 sprays (84 mcg) per nostril 3 times daily (total dose of 504 mcg/day). The safety and effectiveness of using beyond 4 days have not been established.

Rhinorrhea associated with seasonal allergic rhinitis:

• *5 years of age and older* – 2 sprays (84 mcg) per nostril 4 times daily (total dose 672 mcg/day). The safety and efficacy of using beyond 3 weeks have not been established.

➤*Preparation for administration:* Initial pump priming requires 7 sprays of the pump. If used regularly as recommended, no further priming is required. If not used for more than 24 hours, the pump will require 2 sprays, or if not used for more than 7 days, the pump will require 7 sprays to reprime.

➤*Storage/Stability:* Store tightly closed between 15° and 30°C (59° and 86°F). Avoid freezing.

Actions

➤*Pharmacology:* Ipratropium bromide is an anticholinergic agent that inhibits vagally mediated reflexes by antagonizing the action of acetylcholine at the cholinergic receptor. In humans, ipratropium bromide has antisecretory properties and, when applied locally, inhibits secretions from the serous and seromucous glands lining the nasal mucosa. Ipratropium bromide is a quaternary amine that minimally crosses the nasal and GI membranes and the blood-brain barrier, resulting in a reduction of the systemic anticholinergic effects (eg, neurologic, ophthalmic, cardiovascular, GI effects) that are seen with tertiary anticholinergic amines.

➤*Pharmacokinetics:*

Absorption – Ipratropium bromide is poorly absorbed into the systemic circulation following oral administration (2% to 3%). Less than 20% of an 84 mcg per nostril dose was absorbed from the nasal mucosa of healthy volunteers, induced-cold adult volunteers, naturally acquired common cold pediatric patients, or perennial rhinitis adult patients.

Distribution – Ipratropium bromide is minimally bound (0% to 9% in vitro) to plasma albumin and alpha-1-acid glycoprotein. Its blood/plasma concentration ratio was estimated to be approximately 0.89. Studies in rats have shown that ipratropium bromide does not penetrate the blood-brain barrier.

Metabolism – Ipratropium bromide is partially metabolized to ester hydrolysis products, tropic acid, and tropane. These metabolites appear to be inactive based on in vitro receptor affinity studies using rat brain tissue homogenates.

Excretion – After IV administration of 2 mg ipratropium bromide to 10 healthy volunteers, the terminal half-life of ipratropium was approximately 1.6 hours. The total body clearance and renal clearance were estimated to be 2,505 and 1,019 mL/min, respectively. The amount of the total dose excreted unchanged in the urine (Ae) within 24 hours was approximately one-half of the administered dose.

Special populations –

Children:

• *0.03%* – Following administration of 42 mcg of ipratropium bromide 0.03% nasal spray per nostril 2 or 3 times a day in perennial rhinitis patients 6 to 18 years old, the mean amounts of the total dose excreted unchanged in the urine (8.6% to 11.1%) were higher than those reported in adult volunteers or adult perennial rhinitis patients (3.7% to 5.6%). Plasma ipratropium concentrations were relatively low (ranging from undetectable up to 0.49 ng/mL). No correlation of the amount of the total dose excreted unchanged in the urine (Ae) with age or gender was observed in the pediatric population.

• *0.06%* – Following administration of 84 mcg of ipratropium bromide per nostril 3 times a day in patients 5 to 18 years old (n = 42) with a naturally acquired common cold, the mean amount of the total dose excreted unchanged in the urine of 7.8% was comparable to 84 mcg per nostril 4 times a day in an adult induced common cold population (n = 22) of 7.3% to 8.1%. Plasma ipratropium concentrations were relatively low (ranging from undetectable up to 0.62 ng/mL). No correlation of the amount of the total dose excreted unchanged in the urine (Ae) with age or gender was observed in the pediatric population.

Contraindications

History of hypersensitivity to atropine or its derivatives, or to any of the other ingredients.

Warnings/Precautions

➤*Hypersensitivity reactions:* Immediate hypersensitivity reactions may occur after administration of ipratropium bromide, as demonstrated by rare cases of urticaria, angioedema, rash, bronchospasm, and oropharyngeal edema.

➤*Special risk:* Ipratropium bromide nasal spray should be used with caution in patients with narrow-angle glaucoma, prostatic hypertrophy, or bladder neck obstruction, particularly if they are receiving an anticholinergic by another route. Cases of precipitation or worsening of narrow-angle glaucoma

IPRATROPIUM BROMIDE — INTRANASAL

and acute eye pain have been reported with direct eye contact of ipratropium bromide administered by oral inhalation.

➤*Pregnancy: Category B.* At oral doses greater than 90 mg/kg in rats (approximately 2,900 times for 0.03% ipratropium bromide and approximately 1,100 times for 0.06% ipratropium bromide the maximum recommended daily intranasal dose in adults on a mg/m^2 basis) embryotoxicity was observed as increased resorption. This effect is not considered relevant to human use due to the large doses at which it was observed and the difference in route of administration. However, no adequate or well-controlled studies have been conducted in pregnant women. Because animal reproduction studies are not always predictive of human response, ipratropium bromide nasal spray should be used during pregnancy only if clearly needed.

➤*Lactation:* It is known that some ipratropium bromide is systemically absorbed following nasal administration; however the portion that may be excreted in human milk is unknown. Although lipid-insoluble quaternary bases pass into breast milk, the minimal systemic absorption makes it unlikely that ipratropium bromide would reach the infant in an amount sufficient to cause a clinical effect. However, because many drugs are excreted in human milk, exercise caution when ipratropium bromide nasal spray is administered to a nursing woman.

➤*Children:*

0.03% – Safety and efficacy in patients younger than 6 years of age have not been established.

0.06% – Safety and efficacy in patients younger than 5 years of age have not been established.

Drug Interactions

No controlled clinical trials were conducted to investigate drug-drug interactions. Ipratropium bromide nasal spray is minimally absorbed into the systemic circulation; nonetheless, there is some potential for an additive interaction with other coadministered anticholinergic medications, including ipratropium bromide for oral inhalation.

Adverse Reactions

➤*0.03%:*

Ipratropium Intranasal Adverse Reactions[a]

Adverse reactions	Ipratropium bromide nasal spray 0.03% (n = 356) Incidence (%)	Ipratropium bromide nasal spray 0.03% (n = 356) Discontinued (%)	Vehicle control (n = 347) Incidence (%)	Vehicle control (n = 347) Discontinued (%)
Headache	9.8%	0.6%	9.2%	0%
Upper respiratory tract infection	9.8%	1.4%	7.2%	1.4%
Epistaxis[b]	9%	0.3%	4.6%	0.3%
Rhinitis[a]				
Nasal dryness	5.1%	0%	0.9%	0.3%
Nasal irritation[c]	2%	0%	1.7%	0.6%
Other nasal symptoms[d]	3.1%	1.1%	1.7%	0.3%
Pharyngitis	8.1%	0.3%	4.6%	0%
Nausea	2.2%	0.3%	0.9%	0%

[a] This table includes adverse events that occurred at an incidence rate of at least 2% in the ipratropium bromide group and more frequently in the ipratropium bromide group than in the vehicle group.All events are listed by their WHO term; rhinitis has been presented by descriptive terms for clarification.
[b] Epistaxis reported by 7% of ipratropium bromide patients and 2.3% of vehicle patients, blood-tinged mucus by 2% of ipratropium bromide patients and 2.3% of vehicle patients.
[c] Nasal irritation includes reports of nasal itching, nasal burning, nasal irritation, and ulcerative rhinitis.
[d] Other nasal symptoms include reports of nasal congestion, increased rhinorrhea, increased rhinitis, posterior nasal drip, sneezing, nasal polyps, and nasal edema.

Ipratropium bromide 0.03% nasal spray was well tolerated by most patients. The most frequently reported nasal adverse events were transient episodes of nasal dryness or epistaxis. These adverse events were mild or moderate in nature, none was considered serious, none resulted in hospitalization and most resolved spontaneously or following a dose reduction. Treatment for nasal dryness and epistaxis was required infrequently (less than or equal to 2%) and consisted of local application of pressure or a moisturizing agent (eg, petroleum jelly, saline nasal spray). Patient discontinuation for epistaxis or nasal dryness was infrequent in both the controlled (less than or equal to 0.3%) and 1-year, open-label (less than or equal to 2%) trials. There was no evidence of nasal rebound (ie, a clinically significant increase in rhinorrhea, posterior nasal drip, sneezing, or nasal congestion severity compared to baseline) upon discontinuation of double-blind therapy in these trials.

Adverse events reported by less than 2% of the patients receiving ipratropium bromide nasal spray 0.03% during the controlled clinical trials or during the open-label follow-up trial, which are potentially related to ipratropium bromide's local effects or systemic anticholinergic effects include the following: Dry mouth/throat, dizziness, ocular irritation, blurred vision, conjunctivitis, hoarseness, cough, and taste perversion.

Additional anticholinergic effects noted with other ipratropium bromide dosage forms (ipratropium bromide inhalation solution, ipratropium bromide inhalation aerosol, and ipratropium bromide 0.06% nasal spray) include the following: Precipitation or worsening of narrow-angle glaucoma, urinary retention, prostatic disorders, tachycardia, constipation, and bowel obstruction.

There were infrequent reports of skin rash in both the controlled and uncontrolled clinical studies. Allergic-type reactions such as skin rash, angioedema of the throat, tongue, lips and face, generalized urticaria, laryngospasm, and anaphylactic reactions have been reported with ipratropium bromide 0.03% nasal spray and other ipratropium bromide products.

➤*0.06%:*

Ipratropium Intranasal Adverse Reactions in Patients with Common Cold[a]

Adverse reactions	Ipratropium bromide 0.06% nasal spray (n = 352)	Vehicle control (n = 351)
Epistaxis[b]	8.2%	2.3%
Dry mouth/throat	1.4%	0.3%
Nasal congestion	1.1%	0%
Nasal dryness	4.8%	2.8%

[a] This table includes adverse events for which the incidence was greater than or equal to 1% in the ipratropium bromide group and higher in the ipratropium bromide group than in the vehicle group.
[b] Epistaxis was reported by 5.4% of ipratropium bromide patients and 1.4% of vehicle patients, blood-tinged nasal mucus by 2.8% of ipratropium bromide patients, and 0.9% of vehicle patients.

Ipratropium bromide 0.06% nasal spray was well tolerated by most patients. The most frequently reported adverse events were transient episodes of nasal dryness or epistaxis. The majority of these adverse events (96%) were mild or moderate in nature, none was considered serious, and none resulted in hospitalization. No patient required treatment for nasal dryness, and only 3 patients (less than 1%) required treatment for epistaxis, which consisted of local application of pressure or a moisturizing agent (eg, petroleum jelly). No patient receiving ipratropium bromide 0.06% nasal spray was discontinued from the trial due to either nasal dryness or bleeding.

Adverse events reported by less than 1% of patients receiving ipratropium bromide 0.06% nasal spray during the controlled clinical trials, which are potentially related to local effects or systemic anticholinergic effects of ipratropium bromide include taste perversion, nasal burning, conjunctivitis, coughing, dizziness, hoarseness, palpitation, pharyngitis, tachycardia, thirst, tinnitus, and blurred vision. No controlled trial was conducted to address the relative incidence of adverse events for 3-times-daily versus 4-times-daily therapy.

Ipratropium Intranasal Adverse Reactions in Patients with SAR[a]

Adverse reactions	Ipratropium bromide 0.06% nasal spray (n = 218)	Vehicle control (n = 211)
Epistaxis[b]	6%	3.3%
Pharyngitis	5%	3.8%
URI	5%	3.3%
Nasal dryness	4.6%	0.9%
Headache	4.1%	0.5%
Dry mouth/throat	4.1%	0%
Taste perversion	3.7%	1.4%
Sinusitis	2.8%	2.8%
Pain	1.8%	0.9%
Diarrhea	1.8%	0.5%

[a] This table includes adverse events for which the incidence was 1% or greater in the ipratropium bromide group and higher in the ipratropium bromide group than in the vehicle group.
[b] Epistaxis reported by 3.7% of ipratropium bromide and 2.4% of vehicle patients, blood-tinged nasal mucus by 2.3% of ipratropium bromide patients and 1.9% of vehicle patients.

Additional anticholinergic effects noted with other ipratropium bromide dosage forms (ipratropium bromide inhalation solution, ipratropium inhalation aerosol, and ipratropium bromide 0.03% nasal spray) include precipitation or worsening of narrow-angle glaucoma, urinary retention, prostate disorders, constipation, and bowel obstruction.

There were no reports of allergic-type reactions in the controlled clinical trials. Allergic-type reactions such as skin rash, angioedema of the throat, tongue, lips and face, generalized urticaria, laryngospasm, and anaphylactic reactions have been reported with ipratropium bromide 0.06% nasal spray and other ipratropium bromide products.

Overdosage

Acute overdosage by intranasal administration is unlikely since ipratropium bromide is not well absorbed systemically after intranasal or oral administration. Following administration of a 20 mg oral dose (equivalent to ingesting more than 4 bottles of ipratropium bromide 0.03% nasal spray or 2 bottles of ipratropium bromide 0.06% nasal spray) to 10 male volunteers, no change in heart rate or blood pressure was noted. Following a 2 mg IV infusion over 15 minutes to the same 10 male volunteers, plasma ipratropium concentrations of 22 to 45 ng/mL were observed (greater than 100 times the concentrations observed following intranasal administration). Following IV infusion these 10 volunteers had a mean increase of heart rate of 50 bpm and less than 20 mm Hg change in systolic or diastolic blood pressure at the time of peak ipratropium levels.

IPRATROPIUM BROMIDE — INTRANASAL

Patient Information

Advise patients that temporary blurring of vision, precipitation or worsening of narrow-angle glaucoma, or eye pain may result if ipratropium bromide nasal spray comes into direct contact with the eyes. Instruct patients to avoid spraying ipratropium bromide nasal spray in or around their eyes. Instruct patients who experience eye pain, to carefully read and follow the accompanying Patient's instructions for use.

TIOTROPIUM

Rx	**Spiriva** (Boehringer Ingelheim)	**Capsule, powder for administration; inhalation:** 18 mcg	Equiv. to tiotropium bromide 22.5 mcg. Lactose. (TI OI). Lt. green. In UD 5s, 30s, and 90s with *HandiHaler* device.

TIOTROPIUM BROMIDE — INHALATION

Indications

➤*Chronic obstructive pulmonary disease:* For the long-term, once-daily maintenance treatment of bronchospasm associated with chronic obstructive pulmonary disease (COPD), including chronic bronchitis and emphysema; to reduce exacerbations in COPD patients.

Administration and Dosage

➤*Adults:*

Chronic obstructive pulmonary disease – Two inhalations of the contents of 1 capsule once daily.

➤*Administration:* Capsules are for oral inhalation only and are to be used only with the *HandiHaler* device. Capsules must not be swallowed because the intended effects on the lungs will not be obtained.

For administration, a capsule is placed into the center chamber of the *HandiHaler* device. The capsule is pierced by pressing and releasing the green piercing button on the side of the *HandiHaler* device. The medication is dispersed into the air stream when the patient inhales through the mouth piece.

➤*Storage/Stability:* Store at 25°C (77°F); excursions are permitted between 15° and 30°C (59° and 86°F). The capsules should not be exposed to extreme temperature or moisture. Do not store capsules in the inhalation device. The drug should be used immediately after the packaging over an individual capsule is opened.

Actions

➤*Pharmacology:* Tiotropium is a long-acting, antimuscarinic agent, which is often referred to as an anticholinergic. It has similar affinity to the subtypes of muscarinic receptors, M_1 to M_5. In the airways, it exhibits pharmacological effects through inhibition of M_3-receptors at the smooth muscle leading to bronchodilation. The competitive and reversible nature of antagonism was shown with human and animal origin receptors and isolated organ preparations. In preclinical in vitro as well as in vivo studies, prevention of methacholine-induced bronchoconstriction effects were dose-dependent and lasted longer than 24 hours. The bronchodilation following inhalation of tiotropium is predominantly a site-specific effect.

➤*Pharmacokinetics:*

Absorption – Following dry powder inhalation by young healthy volunteers, the absolute bioavailability of 19.5% suggests that the fraction reaching the lung is highly bioavailable. It is expected from the chemical structure of the compound (quaternary ammonium compound) that tiotropium is poorly absorbed from the GI tract. Oral solutions of tiotropium have an absolute bioavailability of 2% to 3%. Maximum tiotropium plasma concentrations were observed 5 minutes after inhalation.

Distribution – Tiotropium shows a volume of distribution of 32 L/kg, indicating that the drug binds extensively to tissues. The human plasma protein binding for tiotropium is 72%. At steady state, peak tiotropium plasma levels in COPD patients were 17 to 19 pg/mL when measured 5 minutes after dry powder inhalation of an 18 mcg dose and decreased in a multicompartmental manner. Steady-state trough plasma concentrations were 3 to 4 pg/mL.

Metabolism – The extent of metabolism appears to be small. This is evident from a urinary excretion of 74% of unchanged substance after an intravenous (IV) dose to young healthy volunteers. Tiotropium, an ester, is nonenzymatically cleaved to the alcohol *N*-methylscopine and dithienylglycolic acid, neither of which bind to muscarinic receptors.

In vitro experiments with human liver microsomes and human hepatocytes suggest that a fraction of the administered dose (74% of an IV dose is excreted unchanged in the urine, leaving 25% for metabolism) is metabolized by cytochrome P450 (CYP-450)–dependent oxidation and subsequent glutathione conjugation to a variety of phase II metabolites. This enzymatic pathway can be inhibited by CYP-450 2D6 and 3A4 inhibitors, such as quinidine, ketoconazole, and gestodene. Thus, CYP-450 2D6 and 3A4 are involved in the metabolic pathway that is responsible for the elimination of a small part of the administered dose.

Excretion – The terminal elimination half-life of tiotropium is between 5 and 6 days following inhalation. Total clearance was 880 mL/min after an IV dose in young healthy volunteers with an inter-individual variability of 22%. IV-administered tiotropium is mainly excreted unchanged in urine (74%). After dry powder inhalation, urinary excretion is 14% of the dose, the remainder being mainly nonabsorbed drug in the gut that is eliminated via the feces. The renal clearance of tiotropium exceeds the creatinine clearance (CrCl), indicating active secretion into the urine. After chronic once-daily inhalation by COPD patients, pharmacokinetic steady state was reached after 2 to 3 weeks with no accumulation thereafter.

Special populations –

Renal function impairment: Because tiotropium is predominantly renally excreted, renal impairment is associated with increased plasma drug concentrations and reduced drug clearance after both IV infusion and dry powder inhalation. Mild renal impairment (CrCl 50 to 80 mL/min), which is often seen in elderly patients, increased tiotropium plasma concentrations (39% increase in area under the curve [$AUC_{0\text{-}4h}$] after IV infusion). In COPD patients with moderate to severe renal impairment (CrCl less than 50 mL/min), the IV administration of tiotropium resulted in doubling of the plasma concentrations (82% increase in $AUC_{0\text{-}4h}$), which was confirmed by plasma concentrations after dry powder inhalation.

See Warnings/Precautions for more information.

Elderly: As expected for drugs predominantly excreted renally, advanced age was associated with a decrease of tiotropium renal clearance (326 mL/min in COPD patients younger than 58 years of age to 163 mL/min in COPD patients older than 70 years of age), which may be explained by decreased renal function. Tiotropium excretion in urine after inhalation decreased from 14% (young healthy volunteers) to about 7% (COPD patients). Plasma concentrations were numerically increased with advancing age within COPD patients (43% increase in $AUC_{0\text{-}4h}$ after dry powder inhalation), which was not significant when considered in relation to inter- and intraindividual variability.

Contraindications

Hypersensitivity to ipratropium or tiotropium.

Warnings/Precautions

➤*Acute bronchospasm:* Tiotropium is intended as a once-daily maintenance treatment for COPD and is not indicated for the initial treatment of acute episodes of bronchospasm (ie, rescue therapy).

➤*Narrow-angle glaucoma:* Use tiotropium with caution in patients with narrow-angle glaucoma. Health care providers and patients should be alert for signs and symptoms of acute narrow-angle glaucoma (eg, eye pain or discomfort, blurred vision, visual halos, colored images in association with red eyes from conjunctival congestion, and corneal edema). Instruct patients to consult a health care provider immediately should any of these signs or symptoms develop.

➤*Urinary retention:* Use tiotropium with caution in patients with urinary retention. Health care providers and patients should be alert for signs and symptoms of prostatic hyperplasia or bladder-neck obstruction (eg, difficulty passing urine, painful urination). Instruct patients to consult a health care provider immediately should any of these signs or symptoms develop.

➤*Hypersensitivity reactions:* In clinical trials and postmarketing experience with tiotropium, immediate hypersensitivity reactions, including angioedema (eg, swelling of the lips, tongue, or throat), itching, or rash, have been reported. If such a reaction occurs, stop therapy with tiotropium at once and consider alternative treatments.

Inhaled medicines, including tiotropium, may cause paradoxical bronchospasm. If this occurs, treatment with tiotropium should be stopped and other treatments considered.

Given the similar structural formula of atropine to tiotropium, closely monitor patients with a history of hypersensitivity reactions to atropine for similar hypersensitivity reactions to tiotropium. In addition, use tiotropium with caution in patients with severe hypersensitivity to milk proteins.

➤*Renal function impairment:* As a predominantly renally excreted drug, closely monitor patients with moderate to severe renal impairment (CrCl less than or equal to 50 mL/min) treated with tiotropium for anticholinergic adverse reactions.

➤*Pregnancy: Category C.* There are no adequate and well-controlled studies in pregnant women. It is not known if tiotropium crosses the placenta. The drug's molecular weight (about 490 for the bromide monohydrate salt) is low enough for placental transfer. The peak plasma concentrations at steady state are very low (17 to 19 pg/mL), thus limiting the amount of drug at the maternal-fetal interface. Use tiotropium during pregnancy only if the potential benefit justifies the potential risk to the fetus.

In rats, fetal resorption, litter loss, decreases in the number of live pups at birth and the mean pup weights, and a delay in pup sexual maturation were observed at inhalation tiotropium doses of 0.078 mg/kg or more (approximately 35 times the recommended human daily dose on a mg/m² basis). In rabbits, an increase in postimplantation loss was observed at an inhalation dosage of 0.4 mg/kg/day (approximately 360 times the recommended human daily dose on a mg/m² basis).

➤*Lactation:* Clinical data from breast-feeding women exposed to tiotropium are not available. Based on lactating rodent studies, tiotropium is excreted into breast milk. It is not known whether tiotropium is excreted in human milk, but because many drugs are excreted in human milk and given these findings in rats, exercise caution if tiotropium is administered to a breast-feeding woman. Because of the very low amounts in plasma (steady-state peak plasma levels of 17 to 19 pg/mL) and the poor oral bioavailability (about 2% to 3%), maternal use of the drug during lactation probably would have no effect on a breast-feeding infant. However, close monitoring of the

TIOTROPIUM BROMIDE — INHALATION

infant for anticholinergic effects (such as dry mouth, constipation, urinary retention, and increased heart rate) is warranted.

➤*Children:* Safety and efficacy in children have not been established.

➤*Elderly:* See Administration and Dosage for more information.

➤*Monitoring:* Closely monitor patients with a history of hypersensitivity reactions to atropine for similar hypersensitivity reactions to tiotropium.

Monitor patients for signs and symptoms of narrow-angle glaucoma and urinary retention.

Drug Interactions

Tiotropium has been used concomitantly with other drugs commonly used in COPD without increases in adverse drug reactions. These include sympathomimetic bronchodilators, methylxanthines, and oral and inhaled steroids. However, the coadministration of tiotropium with other anticholinergic-containing drugs (eg, ipratropium) has not been studied and is therefore not recommended.

Adverse Reactions

➤*6- to 12-month trials:*

Common adverse reactions – The most commonly reported adverse drug reaction was dry mouth. Dry mouth was usually mild and often resolved during continued treatment. Other reactions reported in individual patients and consistent with possible anticholinergic effects included constipation, tachycardia, blurred vision, glaucoma (new onset or worsening), dysuria, and urinary retention.

Adverse reactions (3% or more) –

Tiotropium Adverse Reactions (≥ 3%)

	Placebo-controlled trials		Ipratropium-controlled trials	
Adverse reactions	Tiotropium (n = 550)	Placebo (n = 371)	Tiotropium (n = 356)	Ipratropium (n = 179)
GI				
Abdominal pain	5%	3%	6%	6%
Constipation	4%	2%	1%	1%
Dry mouth	16%	3%	12%	6%
Dyspepsia	6%	5%	1%	1%
Vomiting	4%	2%	1%	2%
Respiratory				
Epistaxis	4%	2%	1%	1%
Pharyngitis	9%	7%	7%	3%
Rhinitis	6%	5%	3%	2%
Sinusitis	11%	9%	3%	2%
Upper respiratory tract infection	41%	37%	43%	35%
Miscellaneous				
Accidents	13%	11%	5%	8%
Chest pain (nonspecific)	7%	5%	5%	2%
Dependent edema	5%	4%	3%	5%
Infection	4%	3%	1%	3%
Moniliasis	4%	2%	3%	2%
Myalgia	4%	3%	4%	3%
Rash	4%	2%	2%	2%
Urinary tract infection	7%	5%	4%	2%

Arthritis, coughing, and influenza-like symptoms occurred at a rate of 3% or more in the tiotropium treatment group, but were less than 1% in the placebo group.

Cardiovascular – Angina pectoris (including aggravated angina pectoris) (1% to 3%).

CNS – Depression, dysphonia, paresthesia (1% to 3%).

GI – GI disorder not otherwise specified (NOS), gastroesophageal reflux, stomatitis (including ulcerative stomatitis) (1% to 3%).

Metabolic/Nutritional – Hypercholesterolemia, hyperglycemia (1% to 3%).

Miscellaneous – Allergic reaction, cataract, herpes zoster, laryngitis, leg pain, skeletal pain (1% to 3%).

Adverse reactions (less than 1%) – In addition, among the adverse reactions observed in the clinical trials with an incidence of less than 1% were atrial fibrillation, supraventricular tachycardia, angioedema, and urinary retention.

Age – In the 1-year trials, the incidence of dry mouth, constipation, and urinary tract infection increased with age.

➤*Four-year trial:*

Adverse reactions (3% or more) – When the adverse reactions were analyzed with a frequency of 3% or more in the tiotropium group where the rates in the tiotropium group exceeded placebo by 1% or more, adverse reactions included the following (tiotropium, placebo): pharyngitis (12.5%, 10.8%), sinusitis (6.5%, 5.3%), headache (5.7%, 4.5%), constipation (5.1%, 3.7%), dry mouth (5.1%, 2.7%), depression (4.4%, 3.3%), insomnia (4.4%, 3%), and arthralgia (4.2%, 3.1%).

Additional adverse reactions – Other adverse reactions not previously listed that were reported more frequently in COPD patients treated with tiotropium than placebo include: dehydration, dry skin, gingivitis, joint swelling, oropharyngeal candidiasis, skin infection, skin ulcer, and stomatitis.

➤*Postmarketing:*

Cardiovascular – Palpitations, tachycardia.

Dermatologic – Pruritus, urticaria.

GI – Dysphagia; intestinal obstruction, including ileus paralytic.

Special senses – Hoarseness, intraocular pressure increased, oral candidiasis, throat irritation.

Miscellaneous – Application site irritation (glossitis, mouth ulceration, pharyngolaryngeal pain), dizziness.

Overdosage

➤*Symptoms:* High doses of tiotropium may lead to anticholinergic signs and symptoms. However, there were no systemic anticholinergic adverse reactions following a single inhaled tiotropium dose of up to 282 mcg in 6 healthy volunteers. In a study of 12 healthy volunteers, bilateral conjunctivitis and dry mouth were seen following repeated once-daily inhalation of tiotropium 141 mcg.

A case of overdose has been reported from postmarketing experience. A female patient was reported to have inhaled 30 capsules over a 2.5-day period and developed altered mental status, tremors, abdominal pain, and severe constipation. The patient was hospitalized, tiotropium bromide was discontinued, and the constipation was treated with an enema. The patient recovered and was discharged on the same day.

Patient Information

Instruct patients how to correctly administer tiotropium using the *HandiHaler* device. Tiotropium should only be administered via the *HandiHaler* device and the device should not be used for administering other medications.

Inform patients that the contents of the capsules are for oral inhalation only and must not be swallowed.

Inform patients that capsules should always be stored in sealed blisters and only removed immediately before use or the effectiveness may be reduced. Capsules that are inadvertently exposed to air (ie, not intended for immediate use) should be discarded.

Inform patients that tiotropium can produce paradoxical bronchospasm. If paradoxical bronchospasm occurs, patients should discontinue tiotropium.

Advise patients that difficulty passing urine and dysuria may be symptoms of new or worsening prostatic hyperplasia or bladder outlet obstruction. Instruct patients to consult a health care provider immediately should any of these signs or symptoms develop.

Inform patients that eye pain or discomfort, blurred vision, visual halos or colored images in association with red eyes from conjunctival congestion and corneal edema may be signs of acute narrow-angle glaucoma. Should any of these signs and symptoms develop, they should consult a health care provider immediately. Miotic eye drops alone are not considered to be effective treatment.

Inform patients that care must be taken not to allow the powder to enter into the eyes as this may cause blurring of vision and pupil dilation.

Inform patients that tiotropium is a once-daily maintenance bronchodilator and should not be used for immediate relief of breathing problems (ie, as a rescue medication).

IPRATROPIUM BROMIDE/ALBUTEROL SULFATE

Rx	**Combivent** (Boehringer Ingelheim)	**Aerosol; inhalation:** 18 mcg/103 mcg	Equiv. to 90 mcg albuterol base. In 14.7 g metered dose inhaler w/mouthpiece (200 inhalations).
Rx	**Ipratropium and Albuterol** (Sandoz)	**Solution; inhalation:** 0.5 mg/3 mg	Equiv. to 2.5 mg albuterol base. In 3 mL unit-dose vials. In 30s and 60s
Rx	**DuoNeb** (Dey)		Equiv. to 2.5 mg albuterol base. In 3 mL unit-dose vials. In 30s and 60s.

IPRATROPIUM BROMIDE/ALBUTEROL SULFATE — INHALATION

For complete and comparative prescribing information, refer to the individual Ipratropium Bromide and Albuterol monographs.

Indications

➤*Bronchospasm:* For use in patients with chronic obstructive pulmonary disease (COPD) on a regular aerosol bronchodilator who continue to have evidence of bronchospasm and require a second bronchodilator.

Administration and Dosage

➤*Maximum dose:*

Adults – 12 inhalations/day of the aerosol (*Combivent*) according to the prescribing information. For the solution for inhalation, there is no well-established maximum dose for the approved indication according to the prescribing information.

➤*General dosing considerations:* The use of these agents can be continued as medically indicated to control recurring bouts of bronchospasm. If a previously effective regimen fails to provide the usual relief, medical advice should be sought immediately, as this is often a sign of worsening COPD, which would require reassessment of therapy.

➤*Adults:*

Chronic obstructive pulmonary disease –

Combivent: 2 inhalations 4 times a day. Additional inhalations may be taken as required; not to exceed 12 in 24 hours.

DuoNeb: One 3 mL vial administered 4 times/day via nebulization with up to 2 additional 3 mL doses allowed per day, if needed.

➤*Preparation for administration:* Shake *Combivent* well before using. It is recommended to test spray 3 times before using for the first time and in cases where the aerosol has not be used for more than 24 hours.

➤*Administration:* Administer *DuoNeb* via jet nebulizer connected to an air compressor with an adequate air flow, equipped with mouthpiece or suitable face mask.

➤*Storage/Stability:* Store *Combivent* between 15° and 30°C (59° and 86°F). Avoid excessive humidity. For optimal results, the canister should be at room temperature before use. Store *DuoNeb* between 2° and 25°C (36° and 77°F). Protect from light.

Warnings/Precautions

➤*Pregnancy: Category C.* There are no adequate and well-controlled studies of ipratropium and albuterol in pregnant women. Albuterol has been shown to be teratogenic in mice. Like all beta sympathomimetics, albuterol may cause transient fetal and maternal hyperglycemia followed by an increase in serum insulin. Cord blood levels of insulin are about twice those of untreated control infants and are not dependent on the duration of exposure, gestational age, or birth weight. These effects are more pronounced in diabetic patients, especially in juvenile diabetics, with the occurrence of significant increases in glycogenolysis and lipolysis. Maternal blood glucose should be closely monitored and neonatal hypoglycemia prevented with adequate doses of glucose. Although human data in ipratropium is rare, there is no evidence that the drug is hazardous to the fetus. Use during pregnancy only if the potential benefit justifies the potential risk to the fetus.

➤*Lactation:* Ipratropium is lipid insoluble and, similar to other quarternary ammonium bases, may appear in milk. The amounts, although unknown, are probably clinically insignificant, however, especially after inhalation. No reports describing the use of albuterol during human lactation have been located. Because of the potential for tumorigenicity shown for albuterol in animal studies, a decision should be made whether to discontinue breast-feeding or to discontinue the drug, taking into account the importance of the drug to the mother.

LEUKOTRIENE RECEPTOR ANTAGONISTS

ZAFIRLUKAST

Rx	**Zafirlukast** (Various, eg, Dr. Reddy's, Par)	**Tablets; oral:** 10 mg	May contain lactose, PEG. In 30s, 60s, 100s, 500s, and UD 100s.
Rx	**Accolate** (AstraZeneca)		Lactose, povidone. (ACCOLATE 10 ZENECA). White. Film-coated. In 60s and UD 100s.
Rx	**Zafirlukast** (Various, eg, Dr. Reddy's, Par)	20 mg	May contain lactose, PEG. In 30s, 60s, 100s, 500s, and UD 100s.
Rx	**Accolate** (AstraZeneca)		Lactose, povidone. (ACCOLATE 20 ZENECA). White. Film-coated. In 60s and UD 100s.

ZAFIRLUKAST — ORAL

Indications

➤*Asthma:* Prophylaxis and chronic treatment of asthma in adults and children 5 years of age and older.

➤*Off-label uses:*

Chronic urticaria – [4] = Insufficient documentation. Data from a limited number of patients regarding the use of zafirlukast in the management of chronic urticaria are conflicting. (See Administration and Dosage.)

Administration and Dosage

➤*Adults:*

Asthma – 20 mg twice daily.

Off-label dosing –

Chronic urticaria: [4] = Insufficient documentation. 20 mg twice daily for 3 to 6 weeks. Follow-up assessments have indicated use for up to 24 months.

➤*Children:*

Asthma –

12 years of age and older: 20 mg twice daily.

5 through 11 years of age: 10 mg twice daily.

➤*Administration:* Take at least 1 hour before or 2 hours after meals.

➤*Storage/Stability:* Store at 20° to 25°C (68° to 77°F). Protect from light and moisture. Dispense in the original airtight container.

Actions

➤*Pharmacology:* Zafirlukast is a selective and competitive receptor antagonist of leukotriene D_4 and E_4 (LTD_4 and LTE_4), components of slow-reacting substance of anaphylaxis (SRSA). Cysteinyl leukotriene production and receptor occupation have been correlated with the pathophysiology of asthma, including airway edema, smooth muscle constriction, and altered cellular activity associated with the inflammatory process, which contribute to the signs and symptoms of asthma. Patients with asthma were found in 1 study to be 25 to 100 times more sensitive to the bronchoconstricting activity of inhaled LTD_4 than nonasthmatic subjects.

In vitro studies demonstrated that zafirlukast antagonized the contractile activity of 3 leukotrienes (LTC_4, LTD_4, and LTE_4) in conducting airway smooth muscle from laboratory animals and humans. Zafirlukast prevented intradermal LTD_4-induced increases in cutaneous vascular permeability and inhibited inhaled LTD_4-induced influx of eosinophils into animal lungs. Inhalational challenge studies in sensitized sheep showed that zafirlukast suppressed the airway responses to antigen; this included both the early- and late-phase response and the nonspecific hyperresponsiveness.

In humans, zafirlukast inhibited bronchoconstriction caused by several kinds of inhalational challenges. Pretreatment with single oral doses of zafirlukast inhibited the bronchoconstriction caused by sulfur dioxide and cold air in patients with asthma. Pretreatment with single doses of zafirlukast attenuated the early- and late-phase reaction caused by inhalation of various antigens such as grass, cat dander, ragweed, and mixed antigens in patients with asthma. Zafirlukast also attenuated the increase in bronchial hyperresponsiveness to inhaled histamine that followed inhaled allergen challenge.

➤*Pharmacokinetics:*

Mean (% Coefficient of Variation) Pharmacokinetic Parameters of Zafirlukast Following Single 20 mg Oral Dose Administration to Male Volunteers (n = 36)

C_{max} (ng/mL)	T_{max}[a] (h)	AUC (ng•h/mL)	t½ (h)	CL/f (L/h)
326 (31)	2 (0.5 to 5)	1,137 (34)	13.3 (75.6)	19.4 (32)

[a] Median and range.

Absorption – Zafirlukast is rapidly absorbed following oral administration. Peak plasma concentrations are generally achieved 3 hours after oral administration. The absolute bioavailability of zafirlukast is unknown. In 2 separate studies, 1 using a high-fat and the other a high-protein meal, administration of zafirlukast with food reduced the mean bioavailability by approximately 40%.

Distribution – Zafirlukast is more than 99% bound to plasma proteins, predominantly albumin. The degree of binding was independent of concentration in the clinically relevant range. The apparent steady-state volume of distribution (Vss/F) is approximately 70 L, suggesting moderate distribution into tissues. Studies in rats using radiolabeled zafirlukast indicate minimal distribution across the blood-brain barrier.

Metabolism – Zafirlukast is extensively metabolized. The most common metabolic products are hydroxylated metabolites, which are excreted in the feces. The metabolites of zafirlukast identified in plasma are at least 90 times less potent as LTD_4 receptor antagonists than zafirlukast in a standard in vitro test of activity. In vitro studies using human liver microsomes showed that the hydroxylated metabolites of zafirlukast excreted in the feces are formed through the cytochrome P450 2C9 (CYP2C9) pathway.

ZAFIRLUKAST — ORAL

Additional in vitro studies utilizing human liver microsomes show that zafirlukast inhibits the cytochrome P450 CYP3A4 and CYP2C9 isoenzymes at concentrations close to the clinically achieved total plasma concentrations.

Excretion – The apparent oral clearance (CL/f) of zafirlukast is approximately 20 L/h. Studies in the rat and dog suggest that biliary excretion is the primary route of excretion. Following oral administration of radiolabeled zafirlukast to volunteers, urinary excretion accounts for approximately 10% of the dose and the remainder is excreted in feces. Zafirlukast is not detected in urine.

In the pivotal bioequivalence study, the mean terminal half-life of zafirlukast is approximately 10 hours in both healthy adult subjects and patients with asthma. In other studies, the mean plasma half-life of zafirlukast ranged from approximately 8 to 16 hours in both healthy subjects and patients with asthma. The pharmacokinetics of zafirlukast are approximately linear over the range from 5 to 80 mg. Steady-state plasma concentrations of zafirlukast are proportional to the dose and predictable from single-dose pharmacokinetic data. Accumulation of zafirlukast in the plasma following twice-daily dosing is approximately 45%.

Special populations –

Renal function impairment:

Hepatic function impairment: In a study of patients with hepatic impairment (biopsy-proven cirrhosis), there was a reduced clearance of zafirlukast resulting in a 50% to 60% greater C_{max} and AUC compared with healthy subjects.

Elderly: The apparent oral clearance of zafirlukast decreases with age. In patients older than 65 years of age, there is an approximately 2- to 3-fold greater C_{max} and AUC compared with young adult patients.

Children: Following administration of 20 mg zafirlukast to 20 boys and girls between 7 and 11 years of age, and in a second study, to 29 boys and girls between 5 and 6 years of age, the following pharmacokinetic parameters were obtained:

Zafirlukast Pharmacokinetic Parameters in Children

Parameter	Mean (% coefficient of variation) Children 5 to 6 years of age	Children 7 to 11 years of age
C_{max} (ng/mL)	756 (39%)	601 (45%)
AUC (ng•h/mL)	2,458 (34%)	2,027 (38%)
T_{max} (h)	2.1 (61%)	2.5 (55%)
CL/f (L/h)	9.2 (37%)	11.4 (42%)

Weight unadjusted apparent clearance was 11.4 L/h (42%) in the 7- to 11-year-old children and 9.2 L/h (37%) in the 5- to 6-year-old children, which resulted in greater systemic drug exposures than that obtained in adults for an identical dose. To maintain similar exposure levels in children compared with adults, a dose of 10 mg twice daily is recommended in children 5 to 11 years of age.

Contraindications

Hypersensitivity to zafirlukast or any of its inactive ingredients.

Warnings/Precautions

➤*Acute asthma attacks:* Zafirlukast is not indicated for use in the reversal of bronchospasm in acute asthma attacks, including status asthmaticus. Therapy with zafirlukast can be continued during acute exacerbations of asthma.

➤*Hepatic effects:* Cases of life-threatening hepatic failure have been reported in patients treated with zafirlukast. Cases of liver injury without other attributable cause have been reported from postmarketing adverse reaction surveillance of patients who have received the recommended dosage of zafirlukast (40 mg/day). In most, but not all postmarketing reports, the patient's symptoms abated and the liver enzymes returned to normal or near normal after stopping zafirlukast. In rare cases, patients have either presented with fulminant hepatitis or progressed to hepatic failure, liver transplantation, and death.

Consider the value of liver function testing. Periodic serum transaminase testing has not proven to prevent serious injury but it is generally believed that early detection of drug-induced hepatic injury along with immediate withdrawal of the suspect drug enhances the likelihood for recovery.

Advise patients to be alert for signs and symptoms of liver dysfunction (eg, right upper quadrant abdominal pain, nausea, fatigue, lethargy, pruritus, jaundice, flu-like symptoms, anorexia) and to contact their health care provider immediately if they occur, Ongoing clinical assessment of patients should govern health care provider interventions, including diagnostic evaluations and treatment.

If liver dysfunction is suspected based upon clinical signs or symptoms (eg, right upper quadrant abdominal pain, nausea, fatigue, lethargy, pruritus, jaundice, and flu-like symptoms, anorexia, enlarged liver), discontinue zafirlukast. Liver function tests, in particular serum ALT, should be measured immediately and the patient managed accordingly. If liver function tests are consistent with hepatic dysfunction, do not resume zafirlukast therapy. Patients in whom zafirlukast was withdrawn because of hepatic dysfunction where no other attributable cause is identified should not be re-exposed to zafirlukast.

➤*Eosinophilic conditions:* In rare cases, patients on zafirlukast therapy may present with systemic eosinophilia, sometimes presenting with clinical features of vasculitis consistent with Churg-Strauss syndrome, a condition that is often treated with systemic steroid therapy. These events usually, but not always, have been associated with the reduction of oral steroid therapy. Be alert to eosinophilia, vasculitic rash, worsening pulmonary symptoms, cardiac complications, or neuropathy presenting in their patients. A causal association between zafirlukast and these underlying conditions has not been established.

➤*Hepatic function impairment:* See Pharmacokinetics for more information.

➤*Pregnancy: Category B.* According to the 2004 Working Group Report on Managing Asthma During Pregnancy, zafirlukast may be considered in those patients with asthma who had a favorable response to the drug prior to becoming pregnant. However, when initiating new asthma therapy during pregnancy, zafirlukast is considered an alternative (not preferred) treatment option for mild persistent asthma.

At an oral dosage of 2,000 mg/kg/day (approximately 410 times the maximum recommended daily oral dose in adults [on a mg/m^2 basis]) in rats, maternal toxicity and deaths were seen with increased incidence of early fetal resorption. Spontaneous abortions occurred in cynomolgus monkeys at a maternally toxic oral dosage of 2,000 mg/kg/day. There are no adequate and well-controlled trials in pregnant women. Because animal reproduction studies are not always predictive of human response, use zafirlukast during pregnancy only if clearly needed.

➤*Lactation:* Zafirlukast is excreted in breast milk. Following repeated 40 mg twice-a-day dosing in healthy women, average steady-state concentrations of zafirlukast in breast milk were 50 ng/mL compared with 255 ng/mL in plasma. Because of the potential for tumorigenicity shown for zafirlukast in mouse and rat studies and the enhanced sensitivity of neonatal rats and dogs to the adverse effects of zafirlukast, do not administer zafirlukast to mothers who are breastfeeding.

➤*Elderly:* See Actions for more information.

A total of 8,094 patients were exposed to zafirlukast in North American and European short-term placebo-controlled clinical trials. Of these, 243 patients were elderly (65 years of age and older). No overall difference in adverse reactions was seen in the elderly patients, except for an increase in the frequency of infections among zafirlukast-treated elderly patients compared with placebo-treated elderly patients (7% vs 2.9%). The infections were not severe, occurred mostly in the lower respiratory tract, and did not necessitate withdrawal of therapy.

An open-label, uncontrolled, 4-week trial of 3,759 asthma patients compared the safety and efficacy of 20 mg zafirlukast given twice daily in 3 patient age groups, adolescents (12 to 17 years of age), adults (18 to 65 years of age), and elderly (older than 65 years of age). A higher percentage of elderly patients (n = 384) reported adverse reactions when compared with adults and adolescents. These elderly patients showed less improvement in efficacy measures. In the elderly patients, adverse reactions occurring in greater than 1% of the population included headache (4.7%), diarrhea and nausea (1.8%), and pharyngitis (1.3%). The elderly reported the lowest percentage of infections of all 3 age groups in this study.

Drug Interactions

Because of zafirlukast's inhibition of cytochrome P450 2C9 and 3A4 isoenzymes, use caution with coadministration of drugs known to be metabolized by these isoenzymes.

Zafirlukast Drug Interactions

Precipitant drug	Object drug[a]		Description
Aspirin	Zafirlukast	↑	Coadministration of zafirlukast with aspirin results in mean increased plasma levels of zafirlukast by ≈ 45%.
Erythromycin	Zafirlukast	↓	Coadministration of a single dose of zafirlukast with erythromycin to steady state results in decreased mean plasma levels of zafirlukast by ≈ 40% because of decreased zafirlukast bioavailability.
Theophylline	Zafirlukast	↓	Coadministration of zafirlukast at steady state with a single dose of a liquid theophylline preparation results in decreased mean plasma levels of zafirlukast by ≈ 30%, but no effects on plasma theophylline levels were observed.
Zafirlukast	Warfarin	↑	Coadministration of zafirlukast with warfarin results in a clinically significant increase in prothrombin time (PT). Closely monitor PT and adjust anticoagulant dose accordingly.

[a] ↑ = Object drug increased. ↓ = Object drug decreased.

➤*Warfarin:* In a drug interaction study in 16 healthy male volunteers, coadministration of multiple doses of zafirlukast (160 mg/day) to steady state with a single 25 mg dose of warfarin resulted in a significant increase in the mean AUC (+63%) and half-life (+36%) of S-warfarin. The mean PT increased by approximately 35%. This interaction is probably due to an inhibition by zafirlukast of the cytochrome P450 2C9 isoenzyme system.

ZAFIRLUKAST — ORAL

Patients on oral warfarin anticoagulant therapy and zafirlukast should have their prothrombin times monitored closely and anticoagulant dose adjusted accordingly.

➤*Theophylline:* Rare cases of patients experiencing increased theophylline levels with or without clinical signs or symptoms of theophylline toxicity after the addition of zafirlukast to an existing theophylline regimen have been reported. The mechanism of the interaction between zafirlukast and theophylline in these patients is unknown.

Adverse Reactions

➤*Adults and children 12 years of age and older:* A comparison of adverse reactions reported by greater than or equal to 1% of zafirlukast-treated patients, and at rates numerically greater than in placebo-treated patients, is shown for all trials in the following table.

Zafirlukast Adverse Reactions

Adverse reaction	Zafirlukast (n = 4,058)	Placebo (n = 2,032)
Abdominal pain	1.8%	1.1%
Accidental injury	1.6%	1.5%
ALT elevation	1.5%	1.1%
Asthenia	1.8%	1.6%
Back pain	1.5%	1.2%
Diarrhea	2.8%	2.1%
Dizziness	1.6%	1.5%
Dyspepsia	1.3%	1.2%
Fever	1.6%	1.1%
Headache	12.9%	11.7%
Infection	3.5%	3.4%
Myalgia	1.6%	1.5%
Nausea	3.1%	2%
Pain (generalized)	1.9%	1.7%
Vomiting	1.5%	1.1%

The frequency of less common adverse reactions was comparable between zafirlukast and placebo.

➤*Miscellaneous:* Rarely, elevations of 1 or more liver enzymes have occurred in patients receiving zafirlukast in controlled clinical trials. In clinical trials, most of these have been observed in asymptomatic patients at doses 4 times higher than the recommended dose. The following hepatic events (which have occurred predominantly in females) have been reported from postmarketing adverse reaction surveillance of patients who have received the recommended dose of zafirlukast (40 mg/day): cases of symptomatic hepatitis (with or without hyperbilirubinemia) without other attributable cause; and rarely, hyperbilirubinemia without other elevated liver function tests. In most, but not all postmarketing reports, the patient's symptoms abated and the liver enzymes returned to normal or near normal after stopping zafirlukast. In rare cases, patients have presented with fulminant hepatitis or progressed to hepatic failure, liver transplantation, and death.

In clinical trials, an increased proportion of zafirlukast patients older than 55 years of age reported infections as compared with placebo-treated patients. A similar finding was not observed in other age groups studied. These infections were mostly mild or moderate in intensity and predominantly affected the respiratory tract. Infections occurred equally in both sexes, were dose-proportional to total milligrams of zafirlukast exposure, and were associated with coadministration of inhaled corticosteroids. The clinical significance of this finding is unknown.

See Warnings/Precautions for more information.

Hypersensitivity reactions, including urticaria, angioedema, and rashes, with or without blistering, have been reported in association with zafirlukast therapy. Additionally, there have been reports of patients experiencing agranulocytosis, bleeding, bruising, or edema, arthralgia, and myalgia in association with zafirlukast therapy.

➤*Pediatric patients 5 through 11 years of age:* In pediatric patients receiving zafirlukast in multidose clinical trials, the following reactions occurred with a frequency of greater than or equal to 2% and more frequently than in pediatric patients who received placebo, regardless of causality assessment: headache (4.5% vs 4.2%) and abdominal pain (2.8% vs 2.3%).

Overdosage

➤*Symptoms:* Overdosage with zafirlukast has been reported in 4 patients surviving reported doses as high as 200 mg. The predominant symptoms reported following zafirlukast overdose were rash and upset stomach. There were no acute toxic effects in humans that could be consistently ascribed to the administration of zafirlukast.

➤*Treatment:* It is reasonable to employ the usual supportive measures in the event of an overdose (eg, remove unabsorbed material from the GI, employ clinical monitoring, and institute supportive therapy) if required.

Patient Information

Zafirlukast is indicated for the chronic treatment of asthma; regularly as prescribed, even during symptom-free periods. Zafirlukast is not a bronchodilator; do not use to treat acute episodes of asthma. Do not decrease the dose or stop taking any other antiasthma medications unless instructed by your doctor. Women who are breastfeeding should not take zafirlukast. Alternative antiasthma medication should be considered in such patients.

The bioavailability of zafirlukast may be decreased when taken with food. Take zafirlukast at least 1 hour before or 2 hours after meals.

A rare side effect of zafirlukast is hepatic dysfunction; contact your doctor immediately if you experience signs or symptoms of hepatic dysfunction (eg, right upper quadrant abdominal pain, nausea, fatigue, lethargy, pruritus, jaundice, flu-like symptoms, anorexia). Liver failure resulting in liver transplantation and death has occurred in patients taking zafirlukast.

MONTELUKAST

Rx	**Singulair** (Merck)	**Tablets; oral:** 10 mg	Equiv. to montelukast sodium 10.4 mg. Lactose. (MRK 117 SINGULAIR). Beige, rounded square. Film-coated. In 30s, 90s, 8,000s, and UD 100s.
		Tablets, chewable; oral: 4 mg	Equiv. to montelukast sodium 4.2 mg. Mannitol, aspartame, phenylalanine 0.674 mg. (MRK 711 SINGULAIR). Pink, oval, scored. Cherry flavor. In 30s, 90s, and UD 100s.
		5 mg	Equiv. to montelukast sodium 5.2 mg. Mannitol, aspartame, phenylalanine 0.842 mg. (MRK 275 SINGULAIR). Pink, round, scored. Cherry flavor. In 30s, 90s, 1,000s, and UD 100s.
		Granules; oral: 4 mg/packet	Equiv. to montelukast sodium 4.2 mg. Mannitol. In unit-of-use 30 packets.

MONTELUKAST SODIUM — ORAL

Indications

➤*Allergic rhinitis:* For the relief of symptoms of allergic rhinitis (seasonal allergic rhinitis in patients 2 years of age and older, and perennial allergic rhinitis in patients 6 months of age and older).

➤*Asthma:* For the prophylaxis and chronic treatment of asthma in adults and children 12 months of age and older.

➤*Exercise-induced bronchoconstriction:* For the prevention of exercise-induced bronchoconstriction (EIB) in patients 15 years of age and older.

➤*Off-label uses:*

Atopic dermatitis – Although there are several studies evaluating the efficacy of montelukast in the treatment of atopic dermatitis, the majority of studies have not shown any significant improvement in disease severity. Montelukast may improve itching and help with sleep. Larger studies over longer time periods are needed to fully evaluate the benefit of montelukast in patients with atopic dermatitis.

Atopic dermatitis (adults): [4] = Insufficient documentation.

Atopic dermatitis (children/adolescents): [4] = Insufficient documentation.

Chronic urticaria – [4] = Insufficient documentation. Conflicting information exists regarding the usefulness of montelukast in the management of chronic urticaria. It may be beneficial when used in combination with an antihistamine but was not effective when used as monotherapy. Trials have been limited by small sample size and short duration (up to 6 weeks). Larger, controlled trials are needed to establish the use of montelukast in the treatment of chronic urticaria.

Eosinophilic esophagitis – [5] = Poor documentation. The minimum goal of therapy for eosinophilic esophagitis is to reduce symptoms. It is unknown whether any therapy can affect the long-term outcomes of the disease. The lack of evidence hinders decision making on choice and duration of treatment. Based on the lack of pathophysiologic rationale and the lack of improvement in histology observed during treatment, montelukast was not recommended by the American Gastroenterological Association and North American Society for Pediatric Gastroenterology, Hepatology and Nutrition for the treatment of eosinophilic esophagitis.

Urticaria (nonsteroidal anti-inflammatory drug–induced) – [4] = Insufficient documentation. In small, noncontrolled trials, montelukast was beneficial in the management of nonsteroidal anti-inflammatory drug (NSAID)–induced urticaria. Larger, controlled trials are needed to establish the role of this drug for the treatment of this condition.

Administration and Dosage

➤*Adults:*

Allergic rhinitis – 10 mg once daily.

Asthma – 10 mg once daily.

Exercise-induced bronchoconstriction – 10 mg once daily taken at least 2 hours before exercise.

Off-label dosing –

Atopic dermatitis (adults): [4] = Insufficient documentation. 10 mg once daily.

MONTELUKAST SODIUM — ORAL

Chronic urticaria: [4] = Insufficient documentation. 10 mg daily orally for up to 6 weeks.

Urticaria (NSAID-induced): [4] = Insufficient documentation. 10 mg daily orally for up to 6 weeks.

➤*Children:*

Allergic rhinitis (perennial) –

15 years of age and older: 10 mg once daily.

6 to 14 years of age: 5 mg once daily (1 chewable tablet).

2 to 5 years of age: 4 mg once daily (1 chewable tablet or 1 packet of oral granules).

6 to 23 months of age: 4 mg once daily (1 packet of oral granules).

Allergic rhinitis (seasonal) –

15 years of age and older: 10 mg once daily.

6 to 14 years of age: 5 mg once daily (1 chewable tablet).

2 to 5 years of age: 4 mg once daily (1 chewable tablet or 1 packet of oral granules).

Asthma –

15 years of age and older: 10 mg once daily.

6 to 14 years of age: 5 mg daily (chewable tablet).

2 to 5 years of age: 4 mg once daily (1 chewable tablet or 1 packet of oral granules).

12 to 23 months of age: 4 mg once daily (1 packet of oral granules).

Exercise-induced bronchoconstriction –

15 years of age and older: 10 mg once daily taken at least 2 hours before exercise.

Off-label dosing –

Allergic rhinitis (seasonal):

- *6 months to 2 years of age* – 4 mg once daily at bedtime (1 chewable tablet or 1 packet of oral granules).

Asthma:

- *6 to 12 months of age* – 4 mg once daily at bedtime (1 chewable tablet or 1 packet of oral granules).

Atopic dermatitis (children/adolescents): [4] = Insufficient documentation. 5 mg once daily for children 2 to 12 years of age and 10 mg once daily for children older than 12 years of age.

➤*Administration:* May be taken with or without food.

Asthma/allergic rhinitis – Patients with both asthma and allergic rhinitis should take only 1 tablet daily in the evening.

Exercise-induced bronchoconstriction – A single dose of montelukast should be taken at least 2 hours before exercise. An additional dose should not be taken within 24 hours of a previous dose. Patients already taking montelukast daily for another indication (including chronic asthma) should not take an additional dose to prevent EIB. All patients should have a short-acting beta-agonist available for rescue.

Daily administration of montelukast for the chronic treatment of asthma has not been established to prevent acute episodes of EIB.

Oral granules – Administer either directly in the mouth, dissolved in 1 teaspoonful (5 mL) of cold or room temperature baby formula or breast milk, or mixed with a spoonful of cold or room temperature soft foods; based on stability studies, only applesauce, carrots, rice, or ice cream should be used. The packet should not be opened until ready to use. After opening the packet, the full dose (with or without mixing with baby formula, breast milk, or food) must be administered within 15 minutes. If mixed with baby formula, breast milk, or food, montelukast oral granules must not be stored for future use. Discard any unused portion. Montelukast oral granules are not intended to be dissolved in any liquid other than baby formula or breast milk for administration. However, liquids may be taken subsequent to administration. Montelukast oral granules can be administered without regard to time of meals.

➤*Storage/Stability:* Store at 25°C (77°F); excursions are permitted between 15° and 30°C (59° and 86°F). Protect from moisture and light. Store in original package. When bulk bottle product container is subdivided, repackage into a well-closed, light-resistant container.

Actions

➤*Pharmacology:* Montelukast is a selective and orally active leukotriene receptor antagonist that inhibits the cysteinyl leukotriene ($CysLT_1$) receptor. The cysteinyl leukotrienes (LTC_4, LTD_4, LTE_4) are products of arachidonic acid metabolism and are released from various cells, including mast cells and eosinophils. These eicosanoids bind to CysLT receptors. The CysLT type-1 ($CysLT_1$) receptor is found in the human airway (including airway smooth muscle cells and airway macrophages) and on other proinflammatory cells (including eosinophils and certain myeloid stem cells). CysLTs have been correlated with the pathophysiology of asthma and allergic rhinitis.

Montelukast is an orally active compound that binds with high affinity and selectivity to the $CysLT_1$ receptor (in preference to other pharmacologically important airway receptors, such as the prostanoid, cholinergic, or beta-adrenergic receptor). Montelukast inhibits physiologic actions of LTD_4 at the $CysLT_1$ receptor without any agonist activity.

Asthma – Leukotriene-mediated effects include airway edema, smooth muscle contraction, and altered cellular activity associated with the inflammatory process.

Allergic rhinitis – CysLTs are released from the nasal mucosa after allergen exposure during early- and late-phase reactions and are associated with symptoms of allergic rhinitis.

➤*Pharmacokinetics:*

Absorption – Montelukast is absorbed rapidly following oral administration.

Food effects: After administration of the 10 mg film-coated tablet to fasted adults, the mean peak montelukast plasma concentration (C_{max}) is achieved in 3 to 4 hours (time to maximal concentration [T_{max}]). The mean oral bioavailability is 64%. The oral bioavailability and C_{max} are not influenced by a standard meal in the morning.

For the 5 mg chewable tablet, the mean C_{max} is achieved in 2 to 2.5 hours after administration to adults in the fasted state. The mean oral bioavailability is 73% in the fasted state versus 63% when administered with a standard meal in the morning.

For the 4 mg chewable tablet, the mean C_{max} is achieved 2 hours after administration in children 2 to 5 years of age in the fasted state.

The coadministration of the oral granule formulation with applesauce did not have a clinically significant effect on the pharmacokinetics of montelukast. A high-fat meal in the morning did not affect the area under the curve (AUC) of montelukast oral granules; however, the meal decreased C_{max} by 35% and prolonged T_{max} from 2.3 ± 1 hours to 6.4 ± 2.9 hours.

Bioequivalence: The 4 mg oral granule formulation is bioequivalent to the 4 mg chewable tablet when administered to adults in the fasted state.

Distribution – Montelukast is more than 99% bound to plasma proteins. The steady-state volume of distribution of montelukast averages 8 to 11 L.

Metabolism – Montelukast is metabolized extensively. In studies with therapeutic doses, plasma concentrations of metabolites of montelukast are undetectable at steady state in adults and children.

In vitro studies using human liver microsomes indicate that cytochromes P450 3A4 and 2C9 are involved in the metabolism of montelukast.

Excretion – The plasma clearance of montelukast averages 45 mL/min in healthy adults. Following an oral dose of radiolabeled montelukast, 86% of the radioactivity was recovered in 5-day fecal collections, and less than 0.2% was recovered in urine. Coupled with estimates of montelukast oral bioavailability, this indicates that montelukast and its metabolites are excreted almost exclusively via the bile.

In several studies, the mean plasma half-life of montelukast ranged from 2.7 to 5.5 hours in healthy young adults. The pharmacokinetics of montelukast are nearly linear for oral doses of up to 50 mg. During once-daily dosing with montelukast 10 mg, there is little accumulation of the parent drug in plasma (14%).

Special populations –

Hepatic function impairment: Patients with mild to moderate hepatic impairment and clinical evidence of cirrhosis had evidence of decreased metabolism of montelukast, resulting in 41% (90% confidence interval [CI], 7% to 85%) higher mean montelukast AUC following a single 10 mg dose. The elimination of montelukast was slightly prolonged compared with that in healthy subjects (mean half-life, 7.4 hours). No dosage adjustment is required in patients with mild to moderate hepatic impairment. The pharmacokinetics of montelukast in patients with more severe hepatic impairment or with hepatitis have not been evaluated.

Elderly: The plasma half-life of montelukast is slightly longer in elderly patients.

Children: In children 6 to 11 months of age, the systemic exposure to montelukast and the variability of plasma montelukast concentrations were higher than those observed in adults. Based on population analyses, the mean AUC (4,296 ng•h/mL [range, 1,200 to 7,153]) was 60% higher, and the mean C_{max} (667 ng/mL [range, 201 to 1,058]) was 89% higher than those observed in adults (mean AUC, 2,689 ng•h/mL [range, 1,521 to 4,595]) and mean C_{max} (353 ng/mL [range, 180 to 548]). The systemic exposure in children 12 to 23 months of age was less variable, but it was still higher than that observed in adults. The mean AUC (3,574 ng•h/mL [range, 2,229 to 5,408]) was 33% higher, and the mean C_{max} (562 ng/mL [range, 296 to 814]) was 60% higher than those observed in adults.

Contraindications

Hypersensitivity to any component of this product.

Warnings/Precautions

➤*Acute asthma attacks:* Montelukast is not indicated for use in the reversal of bronchospasm in acute asthma attacks, including status asthmaticus. Advise patients to have appropriate rescue medication available. Therapy with montelukast can be continued during acute exacerbations of asthma. Patients who have exacerbations of asthma after exercise should have a short-acting inhaled beta-agonist available for rescue.

➤*Concurrent corticosteroids:* While the dose of inhaled corticosteroid may be reduced gradually under medical supervision, do not abruptly substitute montelukast for inhaled or oral corticosteroids.

➤*Aspirin sensitivity:* Patients with known aspirin sensitivity should continue avoidance of aspirin or nonsteroidal anti-inflammatory drugs (NSAIDs) while taking montelukast. Although montelukast is effective in improving airway function in asthmatic patients with documented aspirin sensitivity, it has not been shown to truncate bronchoconstrictor response to aspirin and other NSAIDs in aspirin-sensitive asthmatic patients.

➤*Neuropsychiatric events:* Neuropsychiatric events have been reported in adults, adolescents, and children taking montelukast. Postmarketing reports with montelukast use include agitation, aggressive behavior or hostility, anxiousness, depression, disorientation, dream abnormalities, hallucinations, insomnia, irritability, restlessness, somnambulism, suicidal thinking and behavior (including suicide), and tremor. The clinical details of some postmarketing reports involving montelukast appear consistent with a drug-induced effect.

MONTELUKAST SODIUM — ORAL

Patients and health care provider should be alert for neuropsychiatric events. Instruct patients to notify their health care provider if these changes occur. Carefully evaluate the risks and benefits of continuing treatment with montelukast if such events occur.

➤*Eosinophilia:* Patients with asthma on therapy with montelukast may present with systemic eosinophilia, sometimes presenting with clinical features of vasculitis consistent with Churg-Strauss syndrome, a condition that is often treated with systemic corticosteroid therapy. These reactions usually, but not always, have been associated with the reduction of oral corticosteroid therapy. Be alert to the presentation of eosinophilia, vasculitic rash, worsening pulmonary symptoms, cardiac complications, and/or neuropathy in patients. A causal association between montelukast and these underlying conditions has not been established.

➤*Phenylketonurics:* Phenylketonuric patients should be informed that the 4 and 5 mg chewable tablets contain phenylalanine (a component of aspartame) 0.674 and 0.842 mg per 4 and 5 mg chewable tablet, respectively.

➤*Pregnancy: Category B.* According to the 2004 Working Group Report on Managing Asthma During Pregnancy, montelukast may be considered in those patients with asthma who had a favorable response to the drug prior to becoming pregnant. However, when initiating new asthma therapy during pregnancy, montelukast is considered an alternative (not preferred) treatment option for mild persistent asthma. There are, however, no adequate and well-controlled studies in pregnant women. Because animal reproduction studies are not always predictive of human response, use montelukast during pregnancy only if clearly needed.

Montelukast crosses the placenta following oral dosing in rats and rabbits.

During worldwide marketing experience, congenital limb defects have been rarely reported in the offspring of women being treated with montelukast during pregnancy. Most of these women were also taking other asthma medications during their pregnancy. A causal relationship between these events and montelukast has not been established.

Pregnancy registry – The manufacturer maintains a registry to monitor the pregnancy outcomes of women exposed to montelukast while pregnant. Patients and health care providers are encouraged to report any prenatal exposure by calling the pregnancy registry at 1-800-986-8999.

➤*Lactation:* Studies in rats have shown that montelukast is excreted in milk. It is not known if montelukast is excreted in human milk. The elimination half-life (2.7 to 5.5 hours) and molecular weight (approximately 608) suggest that the drug will be excreted into breast milk. However, exposure should be limited because of the high protein binding (greater than 99%) and extensive metabolism of montelukast. Because many drugs are excreted in human milk, exercise caution when montelukast is given to a breastfeeding mother.

➤*Children:* The safety and efficacy in children younger than 12 months of age with asthma and younger than 6 months of age with perennial allergic rhinitis have not been established. The safety and effectiveness in children below the age of 15 years with EIB have not been established.

➤*Elderly:* No overall differences in safety or efficacy were observed between these subjects and younger subjects, and other reported clinical experience has not identified differences in responses between elderly and younger patients, but greater sensitivity of some older individuals cannot be ruled out.

➤*Monitoring:* Monitor patients for mood or behavioral changes, including suicidal thoughts/behavior.

Drug Interactions

Montelukast Drug Interactions

Precipitant drug	Object drug[a]		Description
CYP-450 inducers (eg, phenobarbital, rifampin)	Montelukast	⬇	Montelukast plasma concentrations may be reduced, decreasing the pharmacologic effect. Monitor the clinical response and adjust the montelukast dose as needed.
Gemfibrozil	Montelukast	⬆	Montelukast plasma concentrations may be elevated, increasing the pharmacologic effects and risk of adverse reactions. Monitor the clinical response and adjust the montelukast dose as needed.
Montelukast	Prednisone	⬆	Adverse effects of prednisone (eg, edema) may be increased. Monitor the clinical response. If an interaction is suspected, consider discontinuing one or both agents.

[a] ⬆ = object drug increased; ⬇ = object drug decreased.

Adverse Reactions

➤*Common adverse reactions:* The most common adverse reactions (incidence at least 5% and greater than placebo; listed in descending order of frequency) in controlled clinical trials were: upper respiratory infection, fever, headache, pharyngitis, cough, abdominal pain, diarrhea, otitis media, influenza, rhinorrhea, sinusitis, otitis.

➤*Asthma:*

Adults and adolescents 15 years of age and older –

Montelukast Adverse Reactions (≥ 1%)

Adverse reactions	Montelukast 10 mg/day (n = 1,955)	Placebo (n = 1,180)
CNS		
Asthenia/Fatigue	1.8%	1.2%
Dizziness	1.9%	1.4%
Headache	18.4%	18.1%
GI		
Abdominal pain	2.9%	2.5%
Dyspepsia	2.1%	1.1%
Gastroenteritis, infectious	1.5%	0.5%
Pain, dental	1.7%	1%
Lab abnormalities[a]		
ALT increased	2.1%	2%
AST increased	1.6%	1.2%
Respiratory		
Congestion, nasal	1.6%	1.3%
Cough	2.7%	2.4%
Miscellaneous		
Fever	1.5%	0.9%
Influenza	4.2%	3.9%
Pyuria	1%	0.9%
Rash	1.6%	1.2%
Trauma	1%	0.8%

[a] Number of patients tested (montelukast and placebo, respectively): ALT and AST, 1,935 and 1,170; pyuria, 1,924 and 1,159.

Children 6 to 14 years of age –

GI: Diarrhea, dyspepsia, nausea (at least 2%).
Respiratory: Laryngitis, pharyngitis, sinusitis (at least 2%).
Miscellaneous: Fever, influenza, otitis, viral infection (at least 2%).

Children growth rate (6 to 8 years of age) – In studies evaluating growth rate, the safety profile in these children was consistent with the safety profile previously described for montelukast. In a 56-week double-blind study evaluating the growth rate in children 6 to 8 years of age receiving montelukast, the following reactions not previously observed with the use of montelukast in this age group occurred with a frequency of at least 2% and more frequently than in children who received placebo, regardless of causality assessment: headache, rhinitis (infective), varicella, gastroenteritis, atopic dermatitis, acute bronchitis, tooth infection, skin infection, and myopia.

Children 2 to 5 years of age –

Dermatologic: Dermatitis, eczema, rash, urticaria, varicella (at least 2%).
GI: Abdominal pain, diarrhea, gastroenteritis (at least 2%).
Respiratory: Cough, pneumonia, rhinorrhea, sinusitis (at least 2%).
Special senses: Conjunctivitis, ear pain, otitis (at least 2%).
Miscellaneous: Fever, headache, influenza (at least 2%).

Children 6 to 23 months of age –

Respiratory: Cough, pharyngitis, rhinitis, tonsillitis, upper respiratory tract infection, wheezing (at least 2%).
Special senses: Otitis media (at least 2%).

➤*Seasonal allergic rhinitis:*

Adults and adolescents 15 years of age and older –

Respiratory: In placebo-controlled clinical trials, the following reaction was reported with montelukast with a frequency of at least 1% and at an incidence greater than placebo: upper respiratory tract infection in 1.9% of patients receiving montelukast versus 1.5% of patients receiving placebo.

Children 2 to 14 years of age –

Respiratory: Pharyngitis, upper respiratory tract infection (at least 2%).
Miscellaneous: Headache, otitis media (at least 2%).

➤*Perennial allergic rhinitis:*

Adults and adolescents 15 years of age and older –

Lab test abnormalities: Increased ALT (at least 1%).
Respiratory: Cough, epistaxis, sinus headache, sinusitis, upper respiratory tract infection (at least 1%).

➤*Postmarketing:*

CNS – Agitation (including aggressive behavior or hostility, restlessness, tremor), anxiousness, depression, disorientation, dream abnormalities, drowsiness, hallucinations, hypesthesia, insomnia, paresthesia, irritability, seizures, suicidal thinking and behavior (including suicide).

GI – Diarrhea, dyspepsia, nausea, vomiting, pancreatitis.

Hematologic – Increased bleeding tendency.

In rare cases, patients with asthma on therapy with montelukast may present with systemic eosinophilia, sometimes presenting with clinical features of vasculitis consistent with Churg-Strauss syndrome, a condition that is often treated with systemic corticosteroid therapy. These reactions usually,

MONTELUKAST SODIUM — ORAL

but not always, have been associated with the reduction of oral corticosteroid therapy. Be alert to the presentation of eosinophilia, vasculitic rash, worsening pulmonary symptoms, cardiac complications, and/or neuropathy in patients.

Hepatic – Cholestatic hepatitis, hepatocellular liver injury, and mixed-pattern liver injury. Most of these occurred in combination with other confounding factors, such as use of other medications, or when montelukast was administered to patients who had underlying potential for liver disease such as alcohol use or other forms of hepatitis.

Musculoskeletal – Arthralgia, myalgia (including muscle cramps).

Miscellaneous – Bruising, edema, epistaxis, erythema nodosum, angioedema, pruritus, urticaria, and systemic eosinophilia), palpitations.

Overdosage

➤*Symptoms:* There have been reports of acute overdosage in postmarketing experience and clinical studies with montelukast. These include reports in adults and children with a dose as high as 1,000 mg. The clinical and laboratory findings observed were consistent with the safety profile in adults and older children. There were no adverse experiences reported in the majority of overdosage reports. The most frequently occurring adverse reactions were consistent with the safety profile of montelukast and included abdominal pain, somnolence, thirst, headache, vomiting, and psychomotor hyperactivity.

➤*Treatment:* No specific information is available on the treatment of overdosage with montelukast. In the event of overdose, it is reasonable to employ the usual supportive measures (eg, remove unabsorbed material from the GI tract, employ clinical monitoring, and institute supportive therapy, if required).

It is not known whether montelukast is removed by peritoneal dialysis or hemodialysis.

Patient Information

Advise patients to take montelukast daily as prescribed, even when they are asymptomatic, as well as during periods of worsening asthma, and to contact their health care provider if their asthma is not well controlled.

Advise patients that oral montelukast is not for the treatment of acute asthma attacks. They should have appropriate short-acting inhaled beta-agonist medication available to treat asthma exacerbations.

Advise patients that, while using montelukast, to seek medical attention if short-acting inhaled bronchodilators are needed more often than usual, or if more than the maximum number of inhalations of short-acting bronchodilator treatment prescribed for a 24-hour period are needed.

Instruct patients receiving montelukast not to decrease the dose or stop taking any other asthma medications unless instructed by a health care provider.

Instruct patients who have exacerbations of asthma after exercise to continue to have available for rescue a short-acting inhaled beta-agonist. Daily administration of montelukast for the chronic treatment of asthma has not been established to prevent acute episodes of EIB.

Advise patients with known aspirin sensitivity to continue avoidance of aspirin or NSAIDs while taking montelukast.

Inform phenylketonuric patients that the 4 and 5 mg chewable tablets contain phenylalanine (a component of aspartame) 0.674 and 0.842 mg, respectively.

Advise patients to notify their health care provider if neuropsychiatric events (eg, agitation, depression, insomnia, suicidal thinking and behavior) occur while using montelukast.

LEUKOTRIENE FORMATION INHIBITORS

ZILEUTON

Rx	**Zyflo** (Cornerstone Therapeutics)	**Tablets; oral:** 600 mg	(CT 1). White to off-white, ovaloid. Film-coated. In 120s.
Rx	**Zyflo CR** (Cornerstone Therapeutics)	**Tablets, extended-release; oral:** 600 mg	Mannitol. (CT 2). Red/White, oblong. Film-coated. In 120s.

ZILEUTON — ORAL

Indications

➤*Asthma:* For the prophylaxis and long-term treatment of asthma in adults and children 12 years of age and older.

Administration and Dosage

➤*Adults:*

Asthma –

Immediate-release tablets: One 600 mg tablet 4 times a day for a total daily dose of 2,400 mg.

Extended-release tablets: Two 600 mg tablets twice daily, within 1 hour of morning and evening meals, for a total daily dose of 2,400 mg.

➤*Children:*

Asthma –

12 years of age and older: See Adults for dosing.

➤*Hepatic function impairment:* Contraindicated in patients with active liver disease or persistent ALT elevations 3 times or more the upper limit of normal (ULN). Because treatment may result in increased hepatic transaminases and liver injury, use with caution in patients who consume substantial quantities of alcohol and/or have a history of liver disease.

➤*Administration:*

Immediate-release tablets – For ease of administration, zileuton immediate-release tablets may be taken with meals and at bedtime.

Extended-release tablets – Zileuton extended-release tablets should not be chewed, cut, or crushed. If a dose is missed, the patient should take the next dose at the scheduled time and not double the dose.

➤*Storage/Stability:* Store between 20° and 25°C (68° and 77°F). Protect from light.

Actions

➤*Pharmacology:* Zileuton is a specific inhibitor of 5-lipoxygenase and, thus, inhibits leukotriene (LTB_4, LTC_4, LTD_4, and LTE_4) formation. Both the R(+) and S(−) enantiomers are pharmacologically active as 5-lipoxygenase inhibitors in vitro and in vivo. Leukotrienes are substances that induce numerous biological effects, including augmentation of neutrophil and eosinophil migration, neutrophil and monocyte aggregation, leukocyte adhesion, increased capillary permeability, and smooth muscle contraction. These effects contribute to inflammation, edema, mucus secretion, and bronchoconstriction in the airways of asthmatic patients. Sulfido-peptide/cysteinyl leukotrienes (LTC_4, LTD_4, LTE_4, also known as the slow-releasing substances of anaphylaxis) and LTB_4, a chemo-attractant for neutrophils and eosinophils, can be measured in a number of biological fluids, including bronchoalveolar lavage fluid (BALF), blood, urine, and sputum from asthmatic patients.

➤*Pharmacokinetics:*

Absorption – Zileuton is rapidly absorbed upon oral administration with a mean time to peak plasma concentration (T_{max}) of 1.7 hours and a mean peak level (C_{max}) of 4.98 mcg/mL. The absolute bioavailability of zileuton is unknown. Systemic exposure (mean area under the curve [AUC]) following zileuton 600 mg administration is 19.2 mcg•h/mL. Plasma concentrations of zileuton are proportional to dose, and steady-state levels are predictable from single-dose pharmacokinetic data.

The relative bioavailability of zileuton extended-release to zileuton immediate-release with respect to C_{max} and AUC under fasted conditions was 0.39 (90% confidence interval [CI], 0.36 to 0.43) and 0.57 (90% CI, 0.52 to 0.62), respectively. Similarly, relative bioavailability of zileuton extended-release to zileuton immediate-release with respect to C_{max} and AUC under fed conditions was 0.45 (90% CI, 0.41 to 0.49) and 0.76 (90% CI, 0.7 to 0.83), respectively.

Effect of food:

• *Immediate-release tablets* – Administration of zileuton with food resulted in a small, but statistically significant increase (27%) in zileuton C_{max} without significant changes in the extent of absorption (AUC) or T_{max}. Therefore, zileuton can be administered with or without food.

• *Extended-release tablets* – A 3-way crossover study was conducted in healthy men and women (N = 23) with a mean age of 33 years (range, 20 to 55) following a single dose of zileuton 1,200 mg extended-release tablets (2 × 600 mg) under fasted and fed conditions, and 2 doses of zileuton 600 mg immediate-release tablets every 6 hours under fasted conditions. Food increased the C_{max} and the mean extent of absorption (AUC) of zileuton extended-release tablets by 18% and 34%, respectively, and prolonged T_{max} from 2.1 to 4.3 hours.

A 3-way crossover study was conducted in healthy men and women (n = 24) with a mean age of 35 (range, 19 to 56) following multiple doses of zileuton 1,200 mg extended-release tablets (2 × 600 mg) administered every 12 hours under fasted and fed conditions, and zileuton 600 mg immediate-release every 6 hours under fed conditions until steady-state zileuton levels were achieved. Food increased AUC and minimum concentration (C_{min}) of zileuton extended-release tablets by 43% and 170%, respectively, but had no effect on C_{max}. Therefore, it is recommended that zileuton extended-release tablets be administered with food. At steady state, relative bioavailability of zileuton extended-release to zileuton immediate-release tablets with respect to C_{max}, C_{min}, and AUC were 0.65 (90% CI, 0.6 to 0.71), 1.05 (90% CI, 0.88 to 1.25), and 0.85 (90% CI, 0.78 to 0.92), respectively. These data indicate that at steady state, under fed conditions, the C_{max} of zileuton extended-release tablets is about 35% lower than that of zileuton, but the C_{min} and AUC are similar for both formulations.

Distribution – The apparent volume of distribution of zileuton is approximately 1.2 L/kg. Zileuton is 93% bound to plasma proteins, primarily to albumin, with minor binding to alpha-1 acid glycoprotein.

Metabolism – Several zileuton metabolites have been identified in human plasma and urine. These include 2 diastereomeric O-glucuronide conjugates (major metabolites) and an N-dehydroxylated metabolite (A-66193) of zileuton. The urinary excretion of the inactive N-dehydroxylated metabolite and unchanged zileuton each accounted for less than 0.5% of the single radiolabeled dose. In vitro studies utilizing human liver microsomes have shown that zileuton and its N-dehydroxylated metabolite can be oxidatively metabolized by the CYP-450 isoenzymes 1A2, 2C9, and 3A4 (CYP1A2, CYP2C9, and CYP3A4).

ZILEUTON — ORAL

Multiple doses of zileuton 1,200 mg extended-release twice daily resulted in peak plasma levels of 4.9 mcg/mL of the inactive metabolite A-66193 with an AUC of 93 mcg•h/mL, showing large intersubject variability. This inactive metabolite was formed by the GI microflora prior to absorption of zileuton, and its formation increases with delayed absorption of zileuton.

Excretion – Elimination of zileuton is predominantly via metabolism with a mean terminal half-life of 2.5 and 3.2 hours (immediate-release and extended-release, respectively). Apparent oral clearance of zileuton is 7 mL/min/kg and 669 mL/min (immediate-release and extended-release, respectively). Zileuton activity is primarily due to the parent drug. Studies with radiolabeled drug demonstrated that orally administered zileuton is well absorbed into the systemic circulation with 94.5% and 2.2% of the radiolabeled dose recovered in urine and feces, respectively.

Special populations –

Hepatic function impairment: The pharmacokinetics of zileuton immediate-release were compared between subjects with mild and moderate chronic hepatic impairment. The mean apparent plasma clearance of total zileuton in subjects with hepatic impairment was approximately half the value of the healthy subjects. The percent binding of zileuton to plasma proteins after multiple dosing was significantly reduced in patients with moderate hepatic impairment. Zileuton is contraindicated in patients with active liver disease or persistent ALT elevations 3 times or more the ULN.

Contraindications

Active liver disease or persistent transaminase elevations at least 3 times the ULN; a history of allergic reaction (eg, rash, eosinophilia) to zileuton or any of its inactive ingredients.

Warnings/Precautions

➤*Acute asthma attacks:* Zileuton is not indicated for use in the reversal of bronchospasm in acute asthma attacks, including status asthmaticus. Therapy with zileuton can be continued during acute exacerbations of asthma.

➤*Hepatic effects:* Elevations of 1 or more liver function tests may occur during zileuton therapy. These laboratory abnormalities may progress to clinically significant injury, remain unchanged, or resolve with continued treatment, usually within 3 weeks. In a few cases, initial transaminase elevations were first noted after discontinuing treatment, usually within 2 weeks. The ALT test is considered the most sensitive indicator of liver injury. In placebo-controlled clinical trials, the frequency of ALT elevations of 3 or more times the ULN was 1.9% for zileuton-treated patients, compared with 0.2% for placebo-treated patients.

If clinical signs or symptoms of liver dysfunction (eg, fatigue, flu-like symptoms, jaundice, lethargy, nausea, pruritus, right upper quadrant pain) develop or transaminase elevations of 5 or more times the ULN occur, discontinue zileuton and follow transaminase levels until they return to normal.

➤*CNS effects:* Neuropsychiatric events have been reported in adult and adolescent patients taking zileuton. Postmarketing reports with zileuton include sleep disorders and behavior changes. The clinical details of some postmarketing reports involving zileuton appear consistent with a drug-induced effect. Patients and prescribers should be alert for neuropsychiatric events. Patients should be instructed to notify their prescriber if these changes occur. Prescribers should carefully evaluate the risks and benefits of continuing treatment with zileuton if such events occur.

➤*Renal function impairment:* Dosing adjustment in patients with renal dysfunction or patients undergoing hemodialysis is not necessary.

➤*Hepatic function impairment:* See Contraindications for more information.

Because treatment with zileuton may result in increased hepatic transaminases and liver injury, use zileuton with caution in patients who consume substantial quantities of alcohol and/or have a history of liver disease.

➤*Pregnancy: Category C.* According to the 2004 Working Group Report on Managing Asthma During Pregnancy, zileuton is to be avoided during pregnancy.

There are no adequate and well-controlled studies in pregnant women. Only use zileuton during pregnancy if the potential benefit justifies the potential risk to the fetus.

Developmental studies indicated adverse reactions (eg, increased skeletal variations, reduced body weight) in rats at an oral dosage of 300 mg/kg/day (providing approximately 18 or more than 10 times [zileuton immediate-release formulation and zileuton extended-release formulation, respectively] the AUC achieved at the MRHD oral dose). Comparative systemic exposure (AUC) is based on measurements in nonpregnant female rats at a similar dosage. Zileuton and/or its metabolites cross the placental barrier of rats. Three of 118 (2.5%) rabbit fetuses had cleft palates at an oral dosage of 150 mg/kg/day (equivalent to the MRHD oral dose on a mg/m^2 basis).

➤*Lactation:* Zileuton and/or its metabolites are excreted in rat milk. It is not known if zileuton is excreted in human milk. The molecular weight (approximately 236) is low enough that passage into human breast milk should be expected. Because many drugs are excreted in human milk and because of the potential for tumorigenicity shown for zileuton in animal studies, decide whether to discontinue breast-feeding or the drug, taking into account the importance of the drug to the mother.

➤*Children:* The safety and efficacy of zileuton in children younger than 12 years of age have not been established.

➤*Elderly:* Subgroup analysis of controlled and open-label clinical studies with zileuton immediate-release tablets suggests that women 65 years of age and older appear to be at increased risk of ALT elevations.

➤*Monitoring:* It is recommended that hepatic transaminases be evaluated at initiation of and during therapy with zileuton. Monitor serum ALT before treatment begins, once a month for the first 3 months, every 2 to 3 months for the remainder of the first year, and periodically thereafter for patients receiving long-term zileuton therapy.

Drug Interactions

Zileuton Drug Interactions			
Precipitant drug	Object drug[a]		Description
Zileuton	Alcohol	↑	Because zileuton treatment may result in increased hepatic function enzymes and liver injury, use with caution in patients who consume substantial quantities of alcohol.
Alcohol	Zileuton		
CYP3A4 agents (eg, calcium channel blockers, cisapride, cyclosporine, ketoconazole)	Zileuton	↔	No interaction studies have been conducted; however, since zileuton is metabolized by CYP3A4, an interaction cannot be ruled out. Use with caution and careful monitoring when these agents are coadministered with zileuton.
Zileuton	Beta adrenergic blocking agents (eg, propranolol)	↑	Coadministration of zileuton results in elevated propranolol concentrations. Closely monitor the patient and adjust dose of propranolol as needed. No drug interaction studies have been conducted with other beta-blocking agents; however, employ appropriate clinical monitoring when they are coadministered with zileuton.
Zileuton	Pimozide	↑	Zileuton may inhibit pimozide metabolism, which may increase the risk of life-threatening cardiac arrhythmias. Coadministration is contraindicated.
Zileuton	Theophylline	↑	Coadministration results in elevated theophylline concentrations. Reduce the theophylline dose by 50% when starting therapy with zileuton and monitor theophylline concentration. Adjust the theophylline dose as needed.
Zileuton	Warfarin	↑	Coadministration results in clinically important increases in prothrombin time. Monitor coagulation parameters and adjust the warfarin dose as needed.

[a] ↑ = object drug increased; ↔ = undetermined clinical effect.

Adverse Reactions

➤*Immediate-release tablets:*

Zileuton Immediate-Release Adverse Reactions (≥ 3%)		
Adverse reactions	Zileuton 600 mg 4 times daily (n = 475)	Placebo (n = 491)
CNS		
Asthenia	3.8%	2.4%
Headache	24.6%	24%
GI		
Abdominal pain	4.6%	2.4%
Dyspepsia	8.2%[a]	2.9%
Nausea	5.5%	3.7%
Miscellaneous		
Accidental injury	3.4%	2%
Myalgia	3.2%	2.9%
Pain (unspecified)	7.8%	5.3%

[a] $P \leq 0.05$ vs placebo.

Less common adverse reactions – Less common adverse events occurring at a frequency of greater than 1% and more commonly in zileuton-treated patients included: arthralgia, chest pain, conjunctivitis, constipation, dizziness, fever, flatulence, hypertonia, insomnia, lymphadenopathy, malaise, neck pain/rigidity, nervousness, pruritus, somnolence, urinary tract infection, vaginitis, and vomiting.

Discontinuation – The frequency of discontinuation from the asthma clinical studies due to any adverse reaction was comparable between zileuton (9.7%) and placebo-treated (8.4%) groups.

ZILEUTON — ORAL

Hematologic – Occurrences of low white blood cell count (less than or equal to 2.8×10^9/L) were observed in 1% of 1,678 patients taking zileuton and 0.6% of 1,056 patients taking placebo in placebo-controlled studies. These findings were transient, and the majority of cases returned toward normal or baseline with continued zileuton dosing. All remaining cases returned toward normal or baseline after discontinuation of zileuton. Similar findings were also noted in a long-term safety surveillance study of 2,458 patients treated with zileuton plus usual asthma care versus 489 patients treated only with usual asthma care for up to 1 year. The clinical significance of these observations is not known.

Hepatic – In placebo-controlled clinical trials, the frequency of ALT elevations at least 3 times ULN was 1.9% for zileuton-treated patients, compared with 0.2% for placebo-treated patients. In controlled and uncontrolled trials, 1 patient developed symptomatic hepatitis with jaundice, which resolved upon discontinuation of therapy. An additional 3 patients with transaminase elevations developed mild hyperbilirubinemia that was less than 3 times the ULN. There was no evidence of hypersensitivity or other alternative etiologies for these findings. Zileuton is contraindicated in patients with active liver disease or transaminase elevations 3 times ULN or more. It is recommended that hepatic transaminases be evaluated at initiation of and during therapy with zileuton.

➤*Extended-release tablets:*

Short-term use –

Most common adverse reactions: The most commonly occurring adverse reactions (at least 5%) are nausea, pharyngolaryngeal pain, and sinusitis.

Hepatic: See Warnings/Precautions for more information.

In the 12-week, placebo-controlled trial, the incidence of ALT elevations (3 or more times ULN) was 2.5% (5/199) in the zileuton extended-release group, compared with 0.5% (1/198) in the placebo group. In the zileuton extended-release group, the majority (60%) of ALT elevations occurred in the first month of treatment. In 2 of the 5 patients in the zileuton extended-release group, ALT elevations were detected 14 days after completion of the 3-month study treatment. The levels returned to less than 2 times the ULN or normal within 9 and 12 days, respectively. The ALT elevations in the other 3 patients were observed to return to less than 2 times the ULN or normal within 15, 19, and 31 days after zileuton extended-release discontinuation. There appeared to be no clinically relevant relationship between the time of onset and the magnitude of the first elevation or the magnitude of first elevation and time to resolution. The hepatic function enzyme elevations attributed to zileuton extended-release did not result in any cases of jaundice, development of chronic liver disease, or death in this clinical trial.

Long-term use –

Most common adverse reactions: The rate and type of adverse reactions observed in this study were comparable with the adverse reactions observed in the 12-week study. Other commonly reported adverse reactions (occurring at a frequency of 5% or more) in zileuton extended-release–treated patients and at a frequency greater than placebo-treated patients included the following: headache (23%), upper respiratory tract infection (9%), myalgia (7%), and diarrhea (5%), compared with 21%, 7%, 5%, and 2%, respectively, in the placebo-treated group.

Hepatic: ALT elevations (3 or more times the ULN) were observed in 1.8% of patients treated with zileuton extended-release tablets compared with 0.7% in patients treated with placebo. The majority (82%) of elevations were reported within the first 3 months of treatment and resolved within 21 days for most of these patients after discontinuation of the drug. The hepatic function enzyme elevations attributed to zileuton extended-release did not result in any cases of jaundice, development of chronic liver disease, or death in this clinical trial.

Hematologic: Occurrences of low white blood cell (WBC) count (less than 3×10^9/L) were observed in 2.6% (15/619) of the zileuton extended-release–treated patients and in 1.7% (5/307) of the placebo-treated patients. The WBC counts returned to normal or baseline following discontinuation of zileuton extended-release tablets. The clinical significance of these findings is not known.

➤*Postmarketing:* Cases of severe hepatic injury have been reported in patients taking zileuton immediate-release tablets. These cases included death, life-threatening liver injury with recovery, symptomatic jaundice, hyperbilirubinemia, and elevations of ALT of more than 8 times the ULN. Cases of behavior changes, rash, sleep disorders, and urticaria have also been reported.

Overdosage

➤*Symptoms:* Human experience of acute overdose with zileuton is limited. A patient in a clinical trial took between 6.6 and 9 g of zileuton in a single dose.

➤*Treatment:* Zileuton is not removed by dialysis. If an overdose occurs, treat the patient symptomatically and institute supportive measures as required. If indicated, attempt to eliminate unabsorbed drug by gastric lavage; observe usual precautions to maintain the airway. Consult a certified poison control center for up-to-date information on management of overdose with zileuton.

Patient Information

Inform the patients that zileuton is indicated for the chronic treatment of asthma and should be taken regularly as prescribed, even during symptom-free periods.

Inform the patients that zileuton is a leukotriene synthesis inhibitor, which works by inhibiting the formation of leukotrienes.

Advise the patients that zileuton is not a bronchodilator and should not be used to treat acute episodes of asthma.

Advise the patients not to decrease the dose or stop taking any other asthma medications when taking zileuton unless instructed by their health care provider.

Advise the patients that if a dose is missed to take the next dose at the scheduled time and the dose should not be doubled.

Advise the patients to take zileuton extended-release tablets within 1 hour after morning and evening meals.

Advise the patients not to cut, chew, or crush zileuton extended-release tablets.

Advise the patients to seek medical attention if short-acting bronchodilators are needed more often than usual or if more than the maximum number of inhalations of short-acting bronchodilator treatment prescribed for a 24-hour period are needed during treatment with zileuton.

Inform the patients that the most serious adverse reaction of zileuton is potential elevation of liver enzyme tests and that, while taking zileuton, they must return to their health care provider for liver enzyme test monitoring on a regular basis.

Inform the patients to contact their health care provider immediately if they experience signs and/or symptoms of liver dysfunction (eg, fatigue, flu-like symptoms, jaundice, lethargy, nausea, pruritus, right upper quadrant pain).

Advise the patients to consult their health care provider before starting or stopping any prescription or nonprescription medicines.

Instruct patients to notify their health care provider if neuropsychiatric events (eg, behavioral changes, sleep disorders) occur while using zileuton.

MONOCLONAL ANTIBODIES

OMALIZUMAB

Rx	**Xolair** (Genentech)	**Injection, lyophilized powder for solution:** 150 mg	Preservative free. Sucrose. In single-use vials.[a]

[a] Contains 202.5 mg of omalizumab , 145.5 mg of sucrose, 2.8 mg of L-histidine hydrochloride monohydrate, 1.8 mg of L-histidine, and 0.5 mg of polysorbate 20, and is designed to deliver 150 mg of omalizumab in 1.2 mL after reconstitution.

OMALIZUMAB — INJECTION

WARNING

Anaphylaxis, presenting as bronchospasm, hypotension, syncope, urticaria, and/or angioedema of the throat or tongue, has been reported to occur after administration of omalizumab. Anaphylaxis has occurred as early as after the first dose of omalizumab but also has occurred beyond 1 year after beginning regularly administered treatment. Because of the risk of anaphylaxis, closely observe patients for an appropriate period of time after omalizumab administration and be prepared to manage anaphylaxis, which can be life-threatening. Also inform patients of the signs and symptoms of anaphylaxis and instruct them to seek immediate medical care if symptoms occur.

Indications

➤*Asthma:* For adults and adolescents 12 years of age and older with moderate to severe persistent asthma who have a positive skin test or in vitro reactivity to a perennial aeroallergen and whose symptoms are inadequately controlled with inhaled corticosteroids.

Omalizumab has been shown to decrease the incidence of asthma exacerbations in these patients. Safety and efficacy have not been established in other allergic conditions.

➤*Off-label uses:* Seasonal allergic rhinitis.

Administration and Dosage

➤*Adults:*

Asthma –

Usual dosage: 150 to 375 mg administered subcutaneously every 2 or 4 weeks. Because the solution is slightly viscous, the injection may take 5 to 10 seconds to administer. Doses (mg) and dosing frequency are determined by serum total immunoglobulin E (IgE) level (units/mL), measured before the start of treatment, and body weight (kg). Doses of more than 150 mg are divided among more than 1 injection site to limit injections to not more than 150 mg per site.

Omalizumab Doses Administered Every 4 Weeks (mg)

Pretreatment serum IgE (units/mL)	Body weight (kg)			
	30 to 60	> 60 to 70	> 70 to 90	> 90 to 150
≥ 30 to 100	150	150	150	300
> 100 to 200	300	300	300	See the following table.
> 200 to 300	300	See the following table.	See the following table.	See the following table.

OMALIZUMAB — INJECTION

Omalizumab Doses Administered Every 2 Weeks (mg)				
Pretreatment serum IgE (units/mL)	Body weight (kg)			
	30 to 60	> 60 to 70	> 70 to 90	> 90 to 150
> 100 to 200	See previous table.	See previous table.	See previous table.	225
> 200 to 300	See previous table.	225	225	300
> 300 to 400	225	225	300	Do not dose.
> 400 to 500	300	300	375	Do not dose.
> 500 to 600	300	375	Do not dose.	Do not dose.
> 600 to 700	375	Do not dose.	Do not dose.	Do not dose.

Dosage adjustment: Total IgE levels are elevated during treatment and remain elevated for up to 1 year after discontinuation of treatment. Therefore, retesting of IgE levels during omalizumab treatment cannot be used as a guide for dose determination. Base dose determination after treatment interruptions lasting less than 1 year on serum IgE levels obtained at the initial dose determination. Total serum IgE levels may be retested for dose determination if treatment with omalizumab has been interrupted for 1 year or longer.

Adjust doses for significant changes in body weight.

Duration of therapy: Periodically reassess the need for continued therapy based on the patient's disease severity and level of asthma control.

➤*Children:*

Asthma –

12 years of age and older: See Adults for dosing for children 12 years of age and older.

➤*Preparation for administration:* Prepare omalizumab for subcutaneous administration by using sterile water for injection only.

The lyophilized product takes 15 to 20 minutes to dissolve. The fully reconstituted product will appear clear or slightly opalescent and may have a few small bubbles or foam around the edge of the vial. The reconstituted product is somewhat viscous; in order to obtain the full 1.2 mL dose, all of the product must be withdrawn from the vial before expelling any air or excess solution from the syringe.

1.) Draw sterile water for injection 1.4 mL into a 3 mL syringe equipped with a 1-inch 18-gauge needle.
2.) Place the vial upright on a flat surface and, using a standard aseptic technique, insert the needle and inject the sterile water for injection directly into the product.
3.) Keeping the vial upright, gently swirl the vial for approximately 1 minute to evenly wet the powder. Do not shake.
4.) After completing the preceding step, gently swirl the vial for 5 to 10 seconds approximately every 5 minutes to dissolve any remaining solids. There should be no visible gel-like particles in the solution. Do not use if foreign particles are present. Some vials may take longer than 20 minutes to dissolve completely. If this is the case, repeat this step until there are no visible gel-like particles in the solution. It is acceptable to have small bubbles or foam around the edge of the vial. Do not use if the contents do not dissolve completely by 40 minutes.
5.) Invert the vial for 15 seconds to allow the solution to drain toward the stopper. Using a new 3 mL syringe equipped with a 1-inch 18-gauge needle, insert the needle into the inverted vial. Position the needle tip at the very bottom of the solution in the vial stopper when drawing the solution into the syringe. Before removing the needle from the vial, pull the plunger all the way back to the end of the syringe barrel in order to remove all of the solution from the inverted vial.
6.) Replace the 18-gauge needle with a 25-gauge needle for subcutaneous injection.
7.) Expel air, large bubbles, and any excess solution in order to obtain the required 1.2 mL dose. A thin layer of small bubbles may remain at the top of the solution in the syringe. Because the solution is slightly viscous, the injection may take 5 to 10 seconds to administer.

A vial delivers omalizumab 1.2 mL (150 mg). For a 75 mg dose, draw up 0.6 mL into the syringe and discard the remaining product.

Number of Injections/Total Injection Volumes of Omalizumab		
Dose (mg)	Number of injections	Total volume injected (mL)[a]
150	1	1.2
225	2	1.8
300	2	2.4
375	3	3

[a] 1.2 mL maximum delivered volume per vial.

➤*Administration:* Administer subcutaneously. Because the solution is slightly viscous, the injection may take 5 to 10 seconds to administer. Doses of more than 150 mg are divided among more than 1 injection site to limit injections to not more than 150 mg per site.

➤*Storage/Stability:* Ship omalizumab at 30°C (86°F) or lower. Store omalizumab under refrigerated conditions, 2° to 8°C (36° to 46°F).

Omalizumab is for single use only and contains no preservatives. The solution may be used for subcutaneous administration within 8 hours following reconstitution when stored in the vial at 2° to 8°C (36° to 46°F), or within 4 hours of reconstitution when stored at room temperature. Protect reconstituted omalizumab vials from direct sunlight.

Actions

➤*Pharmacology:* Omalizumab is a recombinant DNA-derived humanized IgG1 κ monoclonal antibody that selectively binds to human IgE. Omalizumab inhibits the binding of IgE to the high-affinity IgE receptor (FcεRI) on the surface of mast cells and basophils. Reduction in surface-bound IgE on FcεRI-bearing cells limits the degree of release of mediators of the allergic response. Treatment with omalizumab also reduces the number of FcεRI receptors on basophils in atopic patients.

Pharmacodynamics – In clinical studies, serum-free IgE levels were reduced in a dose-dependent manner within 1 hour of the first dose and were maintained between doses. Mean serum-free IgE decrease was more than 96% using recommended doses. Serum total IgE levels (ie, bound and unbound) increased after the first because of the formation of omalizumab:IgE complexes, which have a slower elimination rate than free IgE. At 16 weeks after the first dose, average serum total IgE levels were 5-fold higher than during pretreatment when using standard assays. After discontinuation of omalizumab dosing, the omalizumab-induced increase in total IgE and decrease in free IgE were reversible, with no observed rebound in IgE levels after drug washout. Total IgE levels did not return to pretreatment levels for up to 1 year after discontinuation of omalizumab.

➤*Pharmacokinetics:*

Absorption/Distribution – After subcutaneous administration, omalizumab is absorbed, with an average absolute bioavailability of 62%. Following a single subcutaneous dose in adult and adolescent patients with asthma, omalizumab was absorbed slowly, reaching peak serum concentrations after an average of 7 to 8 days. The pharmacokinetics of omalizumab are linear at doses higher than 0.5 mg/kg. Following multiple doses of omalizumab, areas under the curve (AUCs) from days 0 to 14 at steady state were up to 6-fold of those after the first dose.

In vitro, omalizumab forms complexes of limited size with IgE. Precipitating complexes and complexes larger than 1 million daltons in molecular weight are not observed in vitro or in vivo. Tissue distribution studies in cynomolgus monkeys showed no specific uptake of ^{125}I-omalizumab by any organ or tissue. The apparent volume of distribution in patients following subcutaneous administration was 78 ± 32 mL/kg.

Metabolism/Excretion – Clearance of omalizumab involves IgG clearance processes as well as clearance via specific binding and complex formation with its target ligand, IgE. Liver elimination of IgG includes degradation in the liver reticuloendothelial system (RES) and endothelial cells. Intact IgG is also excreted in bile. In studies with mice and monkeys, omalizumab:IgE complexes were eliminated by interactions with Fc-gamma receptors within the RES at rates that were generally faster than IgG clearance. In asthma patients, omalizumab serum elimination half-life averaged 26 days, with apparent clearance averaging 2.4 ± 1.1 mL/kg/day. In addition, doubling body weight approximately doubled apparent clearance.

Contraindications

Severe hypersensitivity reaction to omalizumab.

Warnings/Precautions

➤*Hypersensitivity:* Anaphylaxis has been reported to occur after administration of omalizumab in premarketing clinical trials and postmarketing spontaneous reports. Signs and symptoms in these reported cases have included angioedema of the throat or tongue, bronchospasm, hypotension, syncope, and urticaria. Some of these reactions have been life-threatening. In premarketing clinical trials, the frequency of anaphylaxis attributed to omalizumab use was estimated to be 0.1%. In postmarketing spontaneous reports, the frequency of anaphylaxis attributed to omalizumab use was estimated to be at least 0.2% of patients based on an estimated exposure of approximately 57,300 patients from June 2003 through December 2006. Anaphylaxis has occurred as early as after the first dose of omalizumab but also has occurred beyond 1 year after beginning regularly scheduled treatment.

Only administer omalizumab in a health care setting and be prepared to manage anaphylaxis, which can be life-threatening. Closely observe patients for an appropriate period of time after administration of omalizumab, taking into account the time to onset of anaphylaxis seen in premarketing clinical trials and postmarketing spontaneous reports. Inform patients of the signs and symptoms of anaphylaxis, and instruct them to seek immediate medical care if signs or symptoms occur.

Discontinue omalizumab in patients who experience a severe hypersensitivity reaction.

➤*Malignancy:* Malignant neoplasms were observed in 20 of 4,127 (0.5%) omalizumab-treated patients compared with 5 of 2,236 (0.2%) control patients in clinical studies of asthma and other allergic disorders. The observed malignancies in omalizumab-treated patients were a variety of types, with breast, nonmelanoma skin, prostate, melanoma, and parotid occurring more than once, and 5 other types occurring once each. The majority of patients were observed for less than 1 year. The impact of longer exposure to omalizumab or use in patients at higher risk for malignancy (eg, current smokers, elderly patients) is not known.

➤*Acute asthma exacerbations:* Omalizumab has not been shown to alleviate asthma exacerbations acutely. Do not use for the treatment of acute bronchospasm or status asthmaticus.

➤*Corticosteroid reduction:* Do not abruptly discontinue systemic or inhaled corticosteroids upon initiation of omalizumab therapy. Perform decreases in corticosteroids under the direct supervision of a health care provider; decreases may need to be performed gradually.

➤*Eosinophilic conditions:* In rare cases, patients with asthma on omalizumab therapy may present with serious systemic eosinophilia, sometimes

OMALIZUMAB — INJECTION

presenting with clinical features of vasculitis consistent with Churg-Strauss syndrome, a condition that is often treated with systemic corticosteroid therapy. These events usually, but not always, have been associated with the reduction of oral corticosteroid therapy. Be alert to eosinophilia, vasculitic rash, worsening pulmonary symptoms, cardiac complications, and/or neuropathy presenting in patients. A causal association between omalizumab and these underlying conditions has not been established.

➤*Parasitic (helminth) infection:* In a 1-year clinical trial conducted in Brazil in patients at high risk for geohelminthic infections (eg, hookworm, roundworm, threadworm, whipworm), 53% (36/68) of omalizumab-treated patients experienced an infection, as diagnosed by standard stool examination, compared with 42% (29/69) of placebo controls. The point estimate of the odds ratio for infection was 1.96, with a 95% confidence interval (CI) of 0.88 to 4.36, indicating that in this study, a patient who had an infection was anywhere from 0.88 to 4.36 times as likely to have received omalizumab than a patient who did not have an infection. Response to appropriate anti-geohelminth treatment of infection, as measured by stool egg counts, was not different between treatment groups. Monitor patients at high risk of geohelminth infection for such infections while on omalizumab therapy. Insufficient data are available to determine the length of monitoring required for geohelminth infections after stopping omalizumab.

➤*Immunogenicity:* Low titers of antibodies to omalizumab were detected in approximately 1 of 1,723 (less than 0.1%) patients treated with omalizumab. The data reflect the percentage of patients whose test results were considered positive for antibodies to omalizumab in an enzyme-linked immunosorbent assay (ELISA) and are highly dependent on the sensitivity and specificity of the assay. Additionally, the observed incidence of antibody positivity in the assay may be influenced by several factors, including sample handling, timing of sample collection, concomitant medications, and underlying disease. Therefore, comparison of the incidence of antibodies to omalizumab with the incidence of antibodies to other products may be misleading.

➤*Pregnancy: Category B.* IgG molecules are known to cross the placental barrier. There are no adequate and well-controlled studies of omalizumab in pregnant women. Because animal reproduction studies are not always predictive of human response, use omalizumab during pregnancy only if clearly needed.

Pregnancy exposure registry – To monitor outcomes of pregnant women exposed to omalizumab, including women who are exposed to at least 1 dose of omalizumab within 8 weeks prior to conception or any time during pregnancy, a pregnancy exposure registry has been established. Encourage patients to call 1-866-496-5247 to enroll in the omalizumab pregnancy exposure registry. Health care providers can call this number to obtain further information about this registry.

➤*Lactation:* The excretion of omalizumab in milk was evaluated in female cynomolgus monkeys receiving subcutaneous doses of 75 mg/kg/week. Neonatal plasma levels of omalizumab after in utero exposure and 28 days of breast-feeding were between 11% and 94% of the maternal plasma level. Milk levels of omalizumab were 1.5% of maternal blood concentration. While omalizumab presence in human milk has not been studied, IgG is excreted in human milk and therefore it is expected that omalizumab will be present in human milk. The potential for omalizumab absorption or harm to a breast-feeding infant are unknown, but the potential for adverse reactions is probably low; exercise caution when administering omalizumab to a breast-feeding woman.

➤*Children:* Safety and efficacy in children younger than 12 years of age have not been established.

➤*Lab test abnormalities:* Serum total IgE levels increase following administration of omalizumab because of formation of omalizumab:IgE complexes. Elevated serum total IgE levels may persist for up to 1 year after discontinuation of omalizumab. Serum total IgE levels obtained less than 1 year following discontinuation may not reflect steady-state free IgE levels; do not use them to reassess the dosing regimen.

➤*Monitoring:* Closely monitor patients for anaphylaxis for an appropriate time after administration.

Monitor patients at high risk of geohelminth infection for such infections while they are on omalizumab therapy. Insufficient data are available to determine the length of monitoring required for geohelminth infections after stopping omalizumab.

Periodically reassess the need for continued therapy based on the patient's disease severity and level of asthma control.

Drug Interactions

None known.

Adverse Reactions

➤*Serious adverse reactions:* The most serious adverse reactions occurring in clinical studies with omalizumab are malignancies and anaphylaxis. Anaphylaxis was reported in 3 of 3,507 (0.1%) patients in clinical trials. Anaphylaxis occurred with the first dose of omalizumab in 2 patients and with the fourth dose in 1 patient. The time to onset of anaphylaxis was 90 minutes after administration in 2 patients and 2 hours after administration in 1 patient.

In clinical trials, the observed incidence of malignancy among omalizumab-treated patients (0.5%) was numerically higher than among patients in control groups (0.2%).

➤*Common adverse reactions:* The adverse reactions most commonly observed among patients treated with omalizumab included injection-site reaction (45%), viral infection (23%), upper respiratory tract infection (20%), sinusitis (16%), headache (15%), and pharyngitis (11%). These reactions were observed at similar rates in omalizumab-treated patients and control patients. These were also the most frequently reported adverse reactions resulting in clinical intervention (eg, discontinuation of omalizumab, the need for concomitant medication to treat an adverse reaction).

Omalizumab Adverse Reactions (≥ 1%)		
Adverse reaction	Omalizumab (n = 738)	Placebo (n = 717)
CNS		
Dizziness	3%	2%
Fatigue	3%	2%
Dermatologic		
Dermatitis	2%	1%
Pruritus	2%	1%
Musculoskeletal		
Arm pain	2%	1%
Arthralgia	8%	6%
Fracture	2%	1%
Leg pain	4%	2%
Miscellaneous		
Earache	2%	1%
Pain	7%	5%

➤*Injection-site reactions:* Injection-site reactions of any severity occurred at a rate of 45% in omalizumab-treated patients compared with 43% in placebo-treated patients. The types of injection-site reactions included bruising, burning, hive formation, indurations, inflammation, itching, mass, pain, redness, stinging, and warmth.

Severe injection-site reactions occurred more frequently in omalizumab-treated patients than in placebo-treated patients (12% vs 9%).

The majority of injection-site reactions occurred within 1 hour of injection, lasted less than 8 days, and generally decreased in frequency at subsequent dosing visits.

➤*Postmarketing:*

Dermatologic – Hair loss.

Eosinophilic conditions – See Warnings/Precautions for more information.

Hematologic – Severe thrombocytopenia.

Hypersensitivity – Based on spontaneous reports and an estimated exposure of about 57,300 patients from June 2003 through December 2006, the frequency of anaphylaxis attributed to omalizumab use was estimated to be at least 0.2% of patients. Diagnostic criteria of anaphylaxis were skin or mucosal tissue involvement, and, either airway compromise, and/or reduced blood pressure with or without associated symptoms, and a temporal relationship to omalizumab administration with no other identifiable cause. Signs and symptoms in these reported cases included angioedema of the throat or tongue, bronchospasm, chest tightness, cough, cutaneous angioedema, dyspnea, hypotension, syncope, and urticaria. Pulmonary involvement was reported in 89% of the cases. Hypotension or syncope was reported in 14% of cases. Fifteen percent of the reported cases resulted in hospitalization. A previous history of anaphylaxis unrelated to omalizumab was reported in 24% of the cases.

Of the reported cases of anaphylaxis attributed to omalizumab, 39% occurred with the first dose, 19% occurred with the second dose, 10% occurred with the third dose, and the rest after subsequent doses. One case occurred after 39 doses (after 19 months of continuous therapy, anaphylaxis occurred when treatment was restarted following a 3-month gap). The time to onset of anaphylaxis in these cases was up to 30 minutes in 35%, more than 30 and up to 60 minutes in 16%, more than 60 and up to 90 minutes in 2%, more than 90 and up to 120 minutes in 6%, more than 2 hours and up to 6 hours in 5%, more than 6 hours and up to 12 hours in 14%, more than 12 hours and up to 24 hours in 8%, and more than 24 hours and up to 4 days in 5%. In 9% of cases, the times to onset were unknown. Twenty-three patients who experienced anaphylaxis were rechallenged with omalizumab and 18 patients had a recurrence of similar symptoms of anaphylaxis. In addition, anaphylaxis occurred upon rechallenge with omalizumab in 4 patients who previously experienced only urticaria.

Overdosage

The maximum tolerated dose of omalizumab has not been determined. Single intravenous doses of up to 4,000 mg have been administered to patients without evidence of dose-limiting toxicities. The highest cumulative dose administered to patients was 44,000 mg over a 20-week period, which was not associated with toxicities.

Patient Information

Advise patients of the risk of life-threatening anaphylaxis with omalizumab; inform them that there have been reports of anaphylaxis up to 4 days after administration of omalizumab. Omalizumab should only be administered in a health care setting by a health care provider. Closely observe patients following administration. Inform patients of the signs and symptoms of anaphylaxis. Instruct patients to seek immediate medical care if such signs or symptoms occur.

Tell patients receiving omalizumab not to decrease the dose of or stop taking any other asthma medications unless otherwise instructed by their health care provider. Tell patients that they may not see immediate improvement in their asthma after beginning omalizumab therapy.

ROFLUMILAST

Rx	**Daliresp** (Forest Pharmaceuticals)	**Tablets; oral:** 500 mcg	Lactose. (D 500). White to off-white, round. In 30s and 90s.

ROFLUMILAST — ORAL

Indications

➤*Chronic obstructive pulmonary disease:* To reduce the risk of chronic obstructive pulmonary disease (COPD) exacerbations in patients with severe COPD associated with chronic bronchitis and a history of exacerbations.

Administration and Dosage

➤*Adults:*

Chronic obstructive pulmonary disease – 500 mcg/day.

➤*Hepatic function impairment:* Contraindicated in moderate to severe liver impairment.

➤*Administration:* Administer with or without food.

➤*Storage/Stability:* Store at 20° to 25°C (68° to 77°F); excursions are permitted between 15° and 30°C (59° and 86°F).

Actions

➤*Pharmacology:* Roflumilast and its active metabolite (roflumilast N-oxide) are selective inhibitors of phosphodiesterase 4 (PDE4). Roflumilast and roflumilast N-oxide inhibition of PDE4 (a major cyclic-3′,5′-adenosine monophosphate [cyclic AMP]–metabolizing enzyme in lung tissue) activity leads to accumulation of intracellular cyclic AMP. While the specific mechanism(s) by which roflumilast exerts its therapeutic action in COPD patients is not well defined, it is thought to be related to the effects of increased intracellular cyclic AMP in lung cells.

➤*Pharmacokinetics:*

Absorption – The absolute bioavailability of oral roflumilast following a 500 mcg dose is approximately 80%. Maximum plasma concentrations (C_{max}) of roflumilast typically occur approximately 1 hour after dosing (range, 0.5 to 2 hours) in the fasted state while plateau-like C_{max} of the N-oxide metabolite are reached in approximately 8 hours (range, 4 to 13 hours). Steady-state plasma concentrations of roflumilast and its N-oxide metabolite are reached after approximately 4 days for roflumilast and 6 days for roflumilast N-oxide following once-daily dosing.

While roflumilast is 3 times more potent than roflumilast N-oxide at the inhibition of the PDE4 enzyme in vitro, the plasma area under the curve (AUC) of roflumilast N-oxide on average is approximately 10-fold greater than the plasma AUC of roflumilast.

Effect of food: Food has no affect on total drug absorption, but delays time to maximum concentration (T_{max}) of roflumilast by 1 hour and reduces C_{max} by approximately 40%; however, C_{max} and T_{max} of roflumilast N-oxide are unaffected.

Distribution – Plasma protein binding of roflumilast and its N-oxide metabolite is approximately 99% and 97%, respectively. Volume of distribution for a single dose of roflumilast 500 mcg is approximately 2.9 L/kg. Studies in rats with radiolabeled roflumilast indicate low penetration across the blood-brain barrier.

Metabolism – Roflumilast is extensively metabolized via phase 1 (cytochrome P450 [CYP-450]) and phase 2 (conjugation) reactions. The N-oxide metabolite is the only major metabolite observed in human plasma. Together, roflumilast and roflumilast N-oxide account for the majority (87.5%) of total dose administered in plasma. In urine, roflumilast was not detectable, while roflumilast N-oxide was only a trace metabolite (less than 1%). Other conjugated metabolites, such as roflumilast N-oxide glucuronide and 4-amino-3,5-dichloropyridine N-oxide, were detected in urine.

In vitro studies and clinical drug-drug interaction studies suggest that the biotransformation of roflumilast to its N-oxide metabolite is mediated by CYP 1A2 and 3A4.

Excretion – The plasma clearance after short-term intravenous (IV) infusion of roflumilast is, on average, approximately 9.6 L/h. Following an oral dose, the median plasma effective half-life of roflumilast and its N-oxide metabolite are approximately 17 and 30 hours, respectively. Following IV or oral administration of radiolabeled roflumilast, approximately 70% of the radioactivity was recovered in the urine.

Special populations –

Renal function impairment: In 12 subjects with severe renal impairment administered a single dose of roflumilast 500 mcg, roflumilast and roflumilast N-oxide AUCs were decreased by 21% and 7%, respectively, and C_{max} was reduced by 16% and 12%, respectively. No dosage adjustment is necessary for patients with renal impairment.

Hepatic function impairment: Roflumilast 250 mcg once daily for 14 days was studied in subjects with mild to moderate hepatic impairment classified as Child-Pugh class A and B (n = 8 for each group). The AUC of roflumilast and roflumilast N-oxide were increased by 51% and 24%, respectively, in Child-Pugh class A subjects and by 92% and 41%, respectively, in Child-Pugh class B subjects, as compared with age-, weight-, and gender-matched healthy subjects. The C_{max} of roflumilast and roflumilast N-oxide was increased by 3% and 26%, respectively, in Child-Pugh class A subjects and by 26% and 40%, respectively, in Child-Pugh class B subjects, as compared with healthy subjects. Roflumilast 500 mcg has not been studied in hepatically impaired patients. Consider the risk-benefit of administering roflumilast to patients who have mild liver impairment (Child-Pugh class A). Roflumilast is not recommended for use in patients with moderate or severe liver impairment (Child-Pugh class B or C).

Elderly: Roflumilast 500 mcg once daily for 15 days was studied in healthy elderly subjects. The exposure in elderly patients (older than 65 years) was 27% higher in AUC and 16% higher in C_{max} for roflumilast and 19% higher in AUC and 13% higher in C_{max} for roflumilast-N-oxide than in that of younger volunteers (18 to 45 years of age). No dosage adjustment is necessary for elderly patients.

Gender: In a phase 1 study evaluating the effect of age and gender on the pharmacokinetics of roflumilast and roflumilast N-oxide, a 39% and 33% increase in roflumilast and roflumilast N-oxide AUC was noted in healthy women as compared with healthy men. No dosage adjustment is necessary based on gender.

Race: As compared with white subjects, black, Hispanic, and Japanese subjects showed a 16%, 41%, and 15% higher AUC, respectively, for roflumilast and 43%, 27%, and 16% higher AUC, respectively, for roflumilast N-oxide. As compared with white subjects, black, Hispanic, and Japanese subjects showed an 8%, 21%, and 5% higher C_{max}, respectively, for roflumilast, and a 43%, 27%, and 17% higher C_{max}, respectively, for roflumilast N-oxide. No dosage adjustment is necessary for race.

Smoking: The pharmacokinetics of roflumilast and roflumilast N-oxide were comparable in smokers as compared with nonsmokers. There was no difference in C_{max} between smokers and nonsmokers when roflumilast 500 mcg was administered as a single dose to 12 smokers and 12 nonsmokers. The AUC of roflumilast in smokers was 13% less than that in nonsmokers, while the AUC of roflumilast N-oxide in smokers was 17% more than that in nonsmokers.

Contraindications

Moderate to severe liver impairment (Child-Pugh class B or C).

Warnings/Precautions

➤*Acute bronchospasm:* Roflumilast is not a bronchodilator and should not be used for the relief of acute bronchospasm.

➤*CNS effects:* Treatment with roflumilast is associated with an increase in psychiatric adverse reactions. In 8 controlled clinical trials, 5.9% of patients treated with roflumilast 500 mcg daily reported psychiatric adverse reactions compared with 3.3% treated with placebo. The most commonly reported psychiatric adverse reactions were insomnia, anxiety, and depression, which were reported at higher rates in those treated with roflumilast 500 mcg daily (2.4%, 1.4%, and 1.2% for roflumilast vs 1%, 0.9%, and 0.9% for placebo, respectively). Instances of suicidal ideation and behavior, including completed suicide, have been observed in clinical trials. Three patients experienced suicide-related adverse reactions (1 completed suicide and 2 suicide attempts) while receiving roflumilast compared with 1 patient (suicidal ideation) who received placebo.

Before using roflumilast in patients with a history of depression and/or suicidal thoughts or behavior, carefully weigh the risks and benefits of treatment with roflumilast. Patients, their caregivers, and families should be advised of the need to be alert for the emergence or worsening of insomnia, anxiety, depression, suicidal thoughts, or other mood changes, and if such changes occur to contact their health care provider. Carefully evaluate the risks and benefits of continuing treatment with roflumilast if such events occur.

➤*Weight loss:* Weight loss was a common adverse reaction in roflumilast clinical trials and was reported in 7.5% of patients treated with roflumilast 500 mcg once daily compared with 2.1% treated with placebo. In addition to being reported as an adverse reaction, weight change was prospectively assessed in 2 placebo-controlled clinical trials of 1-year duration. In these studies, 20% of patients receiving roflumilast experienced moderate weight loss (defined as between 5% and 10% of body weight) compared with 7% of patients who received placebo. In addition, 7% of patients who received roflumilast compared with 2% of patients receiving placebo experienced severe (greater than 10% body weight) weight loss. During follow-up after treatment discontinuation, the majority of patients with weight loss regained some of the weight they had lost while receiving roflumilast. Regularly monitor weight of patients treated with roflumilast. If unexplained or clinically significant weight loss occurs, evaluate weight loss, and consider discontinuation of roflumilast.

➤*Hepatic function impairment:* Roflumilast is contraindicated for use in patients with moderate or severe liver impairment (Child-Pugh class B or C). Consider the risk-benefit of administering roflumilast to patients who have mild liver impairment (Child-Pugh class A). (See Actions.)

➤*Pregnancy: Category C.* There are no adequate and well controlled studies of roflumilast in pregnant women. Use roflumilast during pregnancy only if the potential benefit justifies the potential risk to the fetus.

Teratogenic – Roflumilast induced stillbirth and decreased pup viability in mice at doses corresponding to approximately 16 and 49 times, respectively, the maximum recommended human dose (MRHD) (on a mg/m^2 basis at maternal dosages greater than 2 mg/kg/day and 6 mg/kg/day, respectively). Roflumilast induced postimplantation loss in rats at doses approximately 10 times or more the MRHD (on a mg/m^2 basis at maternal dosages at least 0.6 mg/kg/day).

Nonteratogenic – Roflumilast has been shown to adversely affect pup postnatal development when dams were treated with the drug during pregnancy and lactation periods in mice. These studies found that roflumilast decreased pup rearing frequencies at approximately 49 times the MRHD (on a mg/mg^2 basis at a maternal dosage of 6 mg/kg/day) during pregnancy and lactation. Roflumilast also decreased survival and forelimb grip reflex and

ROFLUMILAST — ORAL

delayed pinna detachment in mouse pups at approximately 97 times the MRHD (on a mg/m² basis at a maternal dosage of 12 mg/kg/day) during pregnancy and lactation.

Labor and delivery – Roflumilast should not be used during labor and delivery. There are no human studies that have investigated effects of roflumilast on preterm labor or labor at term; however, animal studies showed that roflumilast disrupted the labor and delivery process in mice. Roflumilast induced delivery retardation in pregnant mice at doses approximately 16 times or more the MRHD (on a mg/m² basis at a maternal dosage greater than 2 mg/kg/day).

➤*Lactation:* Roflumilast and/or its metabolites are excreted into the breast milk of lactating rats. Excretion of roflumilast and/or its metabolites into human breast milk is probable. There are no human studies that have investigated effects of roflumilast on breast-fed infants. Roflumilast should not be used by breast-feeding women.

➤*Children:* COPD does not normally occur in children. The safety and effectiveness of roflumilast have not been established in children.

➤*Elderly:* Greater sensitivity of some older individuals cannot be ruled out.

➤*Monitoring:* Monitor weight regularly during therapy. Monitor for new or worsening depressive symptoms and/or development of suicidality.

Drug Interactions

Roflumilast Drug Interactions

Precipitant drug	Object drug[a]		Description
Strong CYP3A4 inducers (eg, carbamazepine, phenobarbital, phenytoin, rifampin)	Roflumilast	↓	Strong CYP3A4 inducers reduce roflumilast plasma concentrations, which decreases drug exposure and may result in decreased efficacy. Avoid coadministration.
Strong CYP3A4 inhibitors or drugs that inhibit both CYP3A4 and CYP1A2 (eg, cimetidine, erythromycin, fluvoxamine, ketoconazole)	Roflumilast	↑	Strong CYP3A4 inhibitors increase roflumilast plasma concentrations, increasing drug exposure and the risk of adverse reactions. The risk of concurrent use should be weighed carefully against the benefit.
Contraceptives, oral (eg, ethinyl estradiol, gestodene)	Roflumilast	↑	Coadministration of roflumilast with oral contraceptives containing gestodene and ethinyl estradiol may increase roflumilast systemic exposure and the risk of adverse effects. The risk of concurrent use should be weighed carefully against the benefit.

[a] ↑ = object drug increased; ↓ = object drug decreased.

➤*Drug/Food interaction:* See Actions for more information.

➤*Drug/Smoking interaction:* See Actions for more information.

Adverse Reactions

Discontinuation – The proportion of patients who discontinued treatment due to adverse reaction was 14.8% for roflumilast-treated patients and 9.9% for placebo-treated patients. The most common adverse reactions that led to discontinuation of roflumilast were diarrhea (2.4%) and nausea (1.6%).

Serious adverse reactions – Serious adverse reactions, whether considered drug-related or not by the investigators, occurred more frequently in roflumilast-treated patients and included acute pancreatitis, acute renal failure, atrial fibrillation, diarrhea, lung cancer, and prostate cancer.

Adverse reactions (2% or more) –

Roflumilast Adverse Reactions (≥ 2%)

Adverse reactions	Roflumilast (n = 4,438)	Placebo (n = 4,192)
CNS		
Dizziness	2.1%	1.1%
Headache	4.4%	2.1%
Insomnia	2.4%	1%
GI		
Decreased appetite	2.1%	0.4%
Diarrhea	9.5%	2.7%
Nausea	4.7%	1.4%
Weight decreased	7.5%	2.1%
Miscellaneous		
Back pain	3.2%	2.2%
Influenza	2.8%	2.7%

➤*Other adverse reactions (1% to 2%):*

CNS – Anxiety, depression, tremor.

GI – Abdominal pain, dyspepsia, gastritis, vomiting.

Respiratory – Rhinitis, sinusitis.

Miscellaneous – Muscle spasms, urinary tract infection.

Overdosage

➤*Symptoms:* No case of overdose has been reported in clinical studies with roflumilast. During the phase 1 studies of roflumilast, the following symptoms were observed at an increased rate after a single oral dose of 2,500 mcg and a single dose of 5,000 mcg: headache, GI disorders, dizziness, palpitations, light-headedness, clamminess, and arterial hypotension.

➤*Treatment:* In case of overdose, patients should seek immediate medical help. Appropriate supportive medical care should be provided. Because roflumilast is highly protein bound, hemodialysis is not likely to be an efficient method of drug removal. It is not known whether roflumilast is dialyzable by peritoneal dialysis.

Patient Information

Inform patients that roflumilast is not a bronchodilator and should not be used for the relief of acute bronchospasm.

Advise patients that treatment with roflumilast is associated with an increase in psychiatric adverse reactions (eg, insomnia, anxiety, depression). Instances of suicidal ideation and behavior, including completed suicide, have been observed.

Advise patients, their caregivers, and families of the need to be alert for the emergence or worsening of insomnia, anxiety, depression, suicidal thoughts, or other mood changes, and if such changes occur to contact their health care provider. Health care providers should carefully evaluate the risks and benefits of continuing treatment with roflumilast if such events occur.

Inform patients that weight loss was a common adverse reaction and that patients treated with roflumilast should have their weight monitored regularly. If unexplained or clinically significant weight loss occurs, weight loss should be evaluated, and discontinuation of roflumilast should be considered.

Advise patients that the use of strong CYP-P450 enzyme inducers (eg, rifampicin, phenobarbital, carbamazepine, phenytoin) with roflumilast is not recommended because the therapeutic effectiveness of roflumilast may be decreased.

RESPIRATORY INHALANT PRODUCTS

Corticosteroids

For additional information, refer to the general discussion of Systemic Glucocorticoids in the Endocrine and Metabolic Agents chapter.

WARNING

Adrenal insufficiency – Deaths caused by adrenal insufficiency have occurred in asthmatic patients during and after transfer from systemic corticosteroids to inhaled corticosteroids. After withdrawal from systemic corticosteroids, several months are required for recovery of hypothalamic-pituitary-adrenal (HPA) function. During this period of HPA suppression, patients may exhibit symptoms of adrenal insufficiency when exposed to trauma, surgery, or infections, particularly gastroenteritis or other conditions with acute electrolyte loss. Although inhaled glucocorticoids may control asthmatic symptoms during these episodes, they do not provide the necessary mineralocorticoid for the treatment of these emergencies. Patients previously maintained on at least 20 mg/day of prednisone (or equivalent) may be most susceptible, especially when their systemic corticosteroids have been almost completely withdrawn.

WARNING (cont.)

Stress/Severe asthma attack – During periods of stress or a severe asthmatic attack, have patients withdrawn from systemic corticosteroids resume them (in large doses) immediately and contact a physician. Have patients carry a warning card indicating that they may need supplementary systemic corticosteroids during such periods. To assess the risk of adrenal insufficiency in emergency situations, periodically perform routine adrenal cortical function tests, including measurement of early morning resting cortisol levels in all patients. An early morning resting cortisol level may be accepted as normal only if it falls at or near the normal mean level.

Indications

➤*Asthma, chronic:* Maintenance and prophylactic treatment of asthma; includes patients who require systemic corticosteroids and may benefit from systemic dose reduction/elimination.

For specific labeled indications, refer to individual drug monographs.

➤*Off-label uses:* Refer to individual monographs for further information.

Eosinophilic esophagitis –
Budesonide: [2] = Fair documentation.
Fluticasone: [2] = Fair documentation.

Lung cancer prevention –
Budesonide: [4] = Insufficient documentation.

Administration and Dosage

➤*Comparative efficacy:* Specific dosage guidelines for individual agents are included in the product listings. The relative anti-inflammatory potency of inhaled corticosteroids are in the following order: Flunisolide = triamcinolone acetonide < beclomethasone dipropionate = budesonide < fluticasone. Current data only supports a difference in potency, not efficacy, among the inhaled corticosteroids. The principle advantage of more potent inhaled corticosteroids may be in improved patient compliance and acceptance.

Estimated Comparative Daily Doses for Inhaled Corticosteroids (Adults)[a,b]

Drug	Low daily dose	Medium daily dose	High daily dose
Beclomethasone dipropionate (HFA)	80 to 240 mcg	240 to 480 mcg	> 480 mcg
40 mcg/inhalation	2 to 6 inhalations	6 to 12 inhalations	> 12 inhalations
80 mcg/inhalation	1 to 3 inhalations	3 to 6 inhalations	> 6 inhalations
Budesonide *Turbuhaler*	200 to 600 mcg	600 to 1,200 mcg	> 1,200 mcg
200 mcg/inhalation	1 to 3 inhalations	3 to 6 inhalations	> 6 inhalations
Flunisolide	500 to 1,000 mcg	1,000 to 2,000 mcg	> 2,000 mcg
250 mcg/inhalation	2 to 4 inhalations	4 to 8 inhalations	> 8 inhalations
Fluticasone			
MDI: 44, 110, 220 mcg/inhalation	88 to 264 mcg	264 to 660 mcg	> 660 mcg
DPI: 50, 100, 250 mcg/inhalation	100 to 300 mcg	300 to 600 mcg	> 600 mcg
Triamcinolone acetonide	400 to 1,000 mcg	1,000 to 2,000 mcg	> 2,000 mcg
100 mcg/inhalation	4 to 10 inhalations	10 to 20 inhalations	> 20 inhalations

[a] *Guidelines for the Diagnosis and Management of Asthma Update on Selected Topics 2002.* Expert Panel Report 2. National Institutes of Health. National Heart, Lung, and Blood Institute. June 2003. http://www.nhlbi.nih.gov/guidelines/asthma/asthmafullrpt.pdf

[b] MDI = metered dose inhaler; DPI = dry powder inhaler.

Estimated Comparative Daily Doses for Inhaled Corticosteroids (Children)[a]

Drug	Low daily dose	Medium daily dose	High daily dose
Beclomethasone dipropionate (HFA) (5 to 11 years of age)	80 to 160 mcg	160 to 320 mcg	> 320 mcg
40 mcg/inhalation	2 to 4 inhalations	4 to 8 inhalations	> 8 inhalations
80 mcg/inhalation	1 to 2 inhalations	2 to 4 inhalations	> 4 inhalations
Budesonide *Turbuhaler* (≥ 6 years of age)	200 to 400 mcg	400 to 800 mcg	> 800 mcg
200 mcg/inhalation	1 to 2 inhalations	2 to 4 inhalations	> 4 inhalations
Flunisolide (6 to 15 years of age)	500 to 750 mcg	1,000 to 1,250 mcg	> 1,250 mcg
250 mcg/inhalation	2 to 3 inhalations	4 to 5 inhalations	> 5 inhalations
Fluticasone (4 to 11 years of age)			
MDI: 44, 110, 220 mcg/inhalation	88 to 176 mcg	176 to 440 mcg	> 440 mcg
DPI: 50, 100, 250 mcg/inhalation	100 to 200 mcg	200 to 400 mcg	> 440 mcg
Triamcinolone acetonide (6 to 12 years of age)	400 to 800 mcg	800 to 1,200 mcg	> 1,200 mcg
100 mcg/inhalation	4 to 8 inhalations	8 to 12 inhalations	> 12 inhalations

[a] *Guidelines for the Diagnosis and Management of Asthma Update on Selected Topics 2002.* Expert Panel Report 2. National Institutes of Health. National Heart, Lung, and Blood Institute. June 2003. http://www.nhlbi.nih.gov/guidelines/asthma/asthmafullrpt.pdf

➤*Patients receiving concomitant systemic steroids:* Stabilize the patient's asthma before treatment is started. Initially, use inhaled corticosteroids concurrently with usual maintenance dose of systemic steroid. After ≈ 1 week, start gradual withdrawal of the systemic steroid by reducing the daily or alternate daily dose. Make the next reduction after 1 to 2 weeks, depending on response. These decrements should not exceed 2.5 mg prednisone or equivalent. A slow rate of withdrawal cannot be overemphasized.

During withdrawal, some patients may experience symptoms of steroid withdrawal (eg, joint or muscular pain, lassitude, depression) despite maintenance or even improvement of respiratory function. Encourage continuance with the inhaler, but observe for objective signs of adrenal insufficiency. If adrenal insufficiency occurs, increase the systemic steroid dose temporarily and continue further withdrawal more slowly.

During periods of stress or severe asthma attack, transfer patients may require supplementary systemic steroids (see Warning box).

Actions

➤*Pharmacology:* Corticosteroids may have direct inhibitory effects on many cells involved in airway inflammation in asthma (eg, macrophages, T-lymphocytes, eosinophils, airway epithelial cells). In vitro, corticosteroids decrease cytokine-mediated survival of eosinophils, reducing the number of eosinophils in the circulation and airways of patients with asthma during corticosteroid therapy. While corticosteroids may not inhibit the release of mast cells in an allergic reaction, they do reduce the number of mast cells within the airway. Corticosteroids may also inhibit plasma exudation and the secretion of mucous in inflamed airways.

Inhaled corticosteroids have anti-inflammatory effects of the bronchial mucosa of asthma patients. Treatment with inhaled corticosteroids for 1 to 3 months results in a reduction in mast cells, macrophages, T-lymphocytes, and eosinophils in the epithelium and submucosa in the bronchioles. By reducing airway inflammation, inhaled corticosteroids lessen airway hyperresponsiveness in asthmatic adults and children. Long-term therapy reduces airway responsiveness to histamine cholinergic agonists, and allergens. Treatment also lowers responsiveness to exercise, fog, cold air, bradykinin, adenosine, and irritants. Inhaled corticosteroids make the airways less sensitive to these spasmogens and limits the maximal narrowing of the airway. Maximal effects of inhaled corticosteroid treatment may not be seen for several months.

➤*Pharmacokinetics:*

Pharmacokinetics of Inhaled Corticosteroids

Parameters	Beclomethasone	Budesonide	Ciclesonide	Flunisolide	Fluticasone	Triamcinolone
Absorption						
Systemic bioavailability from lungs	≈ 20%	25%	22%	40%	20%	21.5%
Distribution						
Vd (L/kg)	NA	4.3	2.9	1.8	3.5	1.4
Protein binding	87%	85% to 90%	99%	NA	91%	≈ 68%

Corticosteroids

Pharmacokinetics of Inhaled Corticosteroids						
Parameters	Beclomethasone	Budesonide	Ciclesonide	Flunisolide	Fluticasone	Triamcinolone
Metabolism						
Site	liver (CYP3A)	liver (CYP3A)	liver (CYP3A4)	liver	liver (CYP3A4)	mostly from liver, less extensively from the kidneys
Metabolites (Activity)	beclomethasone 17-monopropionate (active), free beclomethasone (very weak anti-inflammatory effects)	16α-hydroxyprednisolone and 6β-hydroxybudesonide (< 1% of parent)	desciclesonide	6β-OH (low corticosteroid potency)	17β-carboxylic acid (negligible in animal studies)	6β-hydroxytriamcinolone acetonide, 21-carboxytriamcinolone acetonide, and 21-carboxy-6β-hydroxytriamcinolone acetonide (less active than parent)
Excretion						
Site	feces, urine (less than 10%)	urine (≈ 60%), feces	feces (66%), urine (20% or less)	renal (50%), feces (40%)	feces, urine (less than 0.02%)	urine (≈ 40%), feces (≈ 60%)
$T_{½}$	2.8 h	2.8 h	0.71 h	≈ 1.8 h	3.1 h	1.5 h

Contraindications

Relief of acute bronchospasm; primary treatment of status asthmaticus or other acute episodes of asthma when intensive measures are required; hypersensitivity to any ingredients.

➤*Vanceril:* Relief of asthma that can be controlled by bronchodilators and other nonsteroid medications; in patients who require systemic corticosteroid treatment infrequently; treatment of nonasthmatic bronchitis.

Warnings/Precautions

➤*Infections:* Localized fungal infections with *Candida albicans* or *Aspergillus niger* have occurred in the mouth, pharynx, and occasionally the larynx. Positive cultures for oral *Candida* may be present in up to 34% to 75% of patients. Incidence of clinically apparent infection is low and may require treatment with appropriate antifungal therapy or discontinuance of inhaled steroid treatment. Actions that may minimize the problem include dose reduction, decreasing dose frequency, rinsing mouth after use, and use of an add-on spacer device.

Use inhaled corticosteroids with caution, if at all, in patients with active or quiescent tuberculous infection of the respiratory tract; untreated systemic fungal, bacterial, parasitic, or viral infection; or ocular herpes simplex.

➤*Compromised immune systems:* People who are on drugs that suppress the immune system are more susceptible to infections than healthy individuals. For example, chickenpox and measles can have a more serious or even fatal course in nonimmune children or adults on corticosteroids. In such children or adults who have not had these diseases, take particular care to avoid exposure. How the dose, route, and duration of corticosteroid administration affect the risk of disseminated infection is unknown. The contribution of the underlying disease or prior corticosteroid treatment to the risk is also unknown. If exposed to chickenpox, prophylaxis with varicella-zoster immune globulin (VZIG) may be indicated. If exposed to measles, prophylaxis with pooled IM immunoglobulin (IG) may be indicated. If chickenpox develops, consider treatment with antiviral agents.

➤*Acute asthma:* These products are not bronchodilators and are not for rapid relief of bronchospasm. Contact a physician immediately when asthmatic episodes do not respond to bronchodilators. Patients may require systemic corticosteroids.

There is no evidence that control of asthma can be achieved by inhaled corticosteroids in amounts greater than recommended doses.

➤*Bronchospasm:* This may occur with an immediate increase in wheezing following dosing. If bronchospasm occurs following corticosteroid inhalation, treat immediately with a short-acting inhaled bronchodilator. Discontinue inhalation treatment, and institute an alternative treatment.

Instruct patients to contact their health care provider immediately when episodes of asthma do not respond to bronchodilators during treatment with corticosteroid inhalation. During such episodes, patients may require treatment with systemic corticosteroids.

➤*Combination with prednisone:* Combination therapy of inhaled corticosteroids with systemic corticosteroids may increase the risk of HPA suppression compared to a therapeutic dose of either one alone. Use inhaled corticosteroids with caution in patients already receiving prednisone.

➤*Replacement therapy:* Transfer from systemic steroid therapy may unmask allergic conditions previously suppressed (eg, rhinitis, conjunctivitis, eczema).

➤*Steroid withdrawal:* During withdrawal from oral steroids, some patients may experience symptoms of systemically active steroid withdrawal (eg, joint or muscular pain, lassitude, depression), despite maintenance or even improvement of respiratory function. Although steroid withdrawal effects are usually transient and not severe, severe and even fatal exacerbation of asthma can occur if the previous daily oral corticosteroid requirement had significantly exceeded 10 mg/day of prednisone or equivalent.

➤*HPA suppression:* In responsive patients, inhaled corticosteroids may permit control of asthmatic symptoms with less HPA suppression. Because these agents are absorbed and can be systemically active, the beneficial effects in minimizing or preventing HPA dysfunction may be expected only when recommended dosages are not exceeded. When administered in excessive doses or at recommended doses in a minority of susceptible patients, systemic corticosteroid effects (eg, hypercorticoidism, adrenal suppression) may occur. Slowly reduce or discontinue corticosteroid therapy when these events occur. Titrate patients to the lowest effective dose because of individual sensitivity to cortisol product effects. Carefully observe patients for evidence of systemic corticosteroid effects. Take particular care in observing patients postoperatively or during periods of stress for evidence of a decrease in adrenal function.

Flunisolide – Because of the possibility of higher systemic absorption, monitor patients using **flunisolide** for any evidence of systemic corticosteroid effect. If such changes occur, discontinue slowly, consistent with accepted procedures for discontinuing oral corticosteroids. When flunisolide is used chronically at 2 mg/day, monitor patients periodically for effects on the HPA axis.

➤*Bone mineral density:* Decreases in bone mineral density (BMD) have been observed.

➤*Glaucoma:* Rare instances of glaucoma, increased intraocular pressure, and cataracts have been reported following the inhaled administration of corticosteroids.

➤*Long-term effects:* The effects of long-term glucocorticoid inhalation are unknown. Although there is no clinical evidence of adverse effects, the local and systemic effects on developmental or immunologic processes in the mouth, pharynx, trachea, and lung are unknown.

There is no information about effects on acute, recurrent, or chronic pulmonary infection (including active or quiescent tuberculosis) or effects of long-term use on lung or other tissues. Use with caution (see Warnings).

➤*Pulmonary infiltrates:* Pulmonary infiltrates with eosinophilia may occur with **beclomethasone** or **flunisolide**. This may manifest because of systemic steroid withdrawal when inhalational agents are used, but a causative role for either agent or vehicle cannot be ruled out.

➤*Reduction in growth velocity:* A reduction in growth velocity in children may occur as a result of inadequate control of chronic diseases such as asthma or from corticosteroid use. Closely follow the growth of adolescents taking corticosteroids by any route, and weigh the benefits of corticosteroid therapy and asthma control against the possibility of growth suppression if an adolescent's growth appears slowed.

➤*Hypersensitivity reactions:* Rare cases of hypersensitivity reactions with manifestations such as angioedema have been reported.

➤*Pregnancy: Category C; Category B* (**budesonide** only).

According to the 2004 Working Group Report on Managing Asthma During Pregnancy, inhaled corticosteroids are considered the most effective antiinflammatory medications for the management of persistent asthma. They have been shown to reduce to the risk of asthma exacerbations associated with pregnancy and also improve lung function (FEV_1). Budesonide is now considered the preferred inhaled corticosteroid rather than beclomethasone.

In a position statement from a joint committee of the American College of Obstetricians and Gynecologists (ACOG) and the American College of Allergy, Asthma, and Immunology (ACAAI) published in 2000, either beclomethasone or budesonide were considered the inhaled steroids of choice for use during pregnancy.

Studies have not shown an increased risk of congenital malformations when low to moderate doses of inhaled corticosteroids were used by women in the first trimester of pregnancy. The results of a cohort study involving over 13,000 pregnant women with asthma showed that there may be an increased risk of congenital malformations when high doses are used. However, the authors stated that it is not possible to attribute the observed increased risk of congenital malformation entirely to a teratogenic effect of inhaled corticosteroids because the asthma severity itself may have confounding effects. The lowest dosage of an inhaled corticosteroid needed to control the asthma during pregnancy should be used.

Glucocorticoids are teratogenic in rodents. Findings include cleft palate, internal hydrocephaly, and axial skeletal defects; CNS and cranial malformations were observed in monkeys. There are no adequate and well-controlled studies in pregnant women. Use these agents during pregnancy only if the benefit clearly justifies the potential risk to the fetus. Infants born of mothers who received substantial doses during pregnancy should be observed for adrenal insufficiency.

Budesonide – Studies of pregnant women have not shown that *Pulmicort Turbuhaler* increases the risk of abnormalities when administered during pregnancy. The results from a large population-based prospective cohort epidemiological study indicate no increased risk for congenital malformations from the use of inhaled budesonide during early pregnancy. Congenital malformations were studied in 2014 infants born to mothers reporting the use of inhaled budesonide for asthma in early pregnancy (usually 10 to 12 weeks after the last menstrual period), the period when most major organ malformations occur. The rate of recorded congenital malformations was similar compared with the general population rate (3.8% vs 3.5%, respectively). In addition, after exposure to inhaled budesonide, the number of infants born with orofacial clefts was similar to the expected number in the normal population (4 children vs 3.3, respectively).

➤*Lactation:* Glucocorticoids are excreted in breast milk. It is unknown whether inhaled corticosteroids are excreted in breast milk. Decide whether to discontinue nursing or to discontinue the drug.

➤*Children:* Insufficient information is available to warrant use in children younger than 6 years of age or younger than 12 with **fluticasone**, **beclomethasone**, and **ciclesonide**. Monitor growth in children and adolescents because there is evidence that oral corticosteroids may suppress growth in a dose-related fashion, particularly in higher doses for extended periods.

➤*Monitoring:* Monitor lung function (FEV_1 or morning peak expiratory flow rate), beta-agonist use, and asthma symptoms during withdrawal of corticosteroids. Observe patients for signs and symptoms of adrenal insufficiency. Monitor patients with major risk factors for decreased BMD. Monitor growth of children regularly (via stadiometry). Close monitoring is warranted in patients with a change in vision or a history of glaucoma and/or cataracts.

Drug Interactions

➤*Delavirdine, protease inhibitors:* Plasma concentrations of **ciclesonide** may be increased.

➤*Ketoconazole:* A potent inhibitor of cytochrome P450 3A4 may increase plasma levels of **budesonide**, **ciclesonide**, and **fluticasone** during concomitant dosing. The clinical significance is unknown. Use caution.

Adverse Reactions

Suppression of HPA function (see Warning Box; Warnings).

Inhaled Corticosteroids Adverse Reactions (%)

Adverse reactions	Beclomethasone dipropionate	Budesonide inhalation powder	Budesonide inhalation suspension	Ciclesonide	Flunisolide	Fluticasone propionate aerosol	Fluticasone propionate inhalation powder	Triamcinolone acetonide
Cardiovascular								
Tachycardia	< 2				1 to 3	—	—	—
Chest pain	< 2	—	1 to 3	< 1	3 to 9	—	—	—
CNS								
Headache	12[a] 22 to 27[b]	13 to 14	—	5 to 11	25	17 to 22	9 to 15	7 to 21
Migraine	< 2	1 to 3	—		—	—	1 to 3	—
Insomnia	< 2	1 to 3	—		1 to 3	—		—
Dermatological								
Eczema	< 2[b]	—	1 to 3		3 to 9			
Pruritus	< 2[b]	—	1 to 3		3 to 9	—	—	—
Rash	Rare[a] < 2	—	< 1 to 4		3 to 9	1 to 3	—	1 to 3
GI								
Nausea	1[a] < 2	1 to 3	—	< 1	25	1 to 3	—	—
Dyspepsia	3 to 6[b]	1 to 4	—		1 to 3	1 to 3	—	—
Dry mouth	—	1 to 3	—		1 to 3	—	—	1 to 3
Oral candidiasis	—	2 to 4	—	< 1	3 to 9	2 to 5	3 to 11	1 to 3
Gastroenteritis	—	1 to 3	5		—	—	1 to 3	—
Vomiting	—	1 to 3	2 to 4	≥ 3	25	1 to 3	—	1 to 3
Diarrhea	< 2	—	2 to 4		10	1 to 3	< 4	1 to 3
Abdominal pain	—	1 to 3	2 to 3	≥ 3	3 to 9	—	1 to 3	1 to 3
Anorexia	—	—	1 to 3		3 to 9	—	—	—
GU								
Dysmenorrhea	1 to 3[a] [b]	—	—		—	1 to 3	1 to 3	—
Menstrual disturbance	—	—	—		3 to 9	—	1 to 3	—
Hypersensitivity								
Urticaria	Rare[a] < 2	—	—	≥ 3	1 to 3	Rare	1 to 3	Rare
Angioedema	Rare[a]	—	—		—	Rare	Rare	—
Respiratory								
Upper respiratory tract infections	9[a] < 2	19 to 24	34 to 38	4 to 9	25	15 to 22	16 to 22	—
Pharyngitis	8[a] 11 to 14[b]	5 to 10	—		1 to 3	10 to 14	6 to 13	7 to 25
Rhinitis	6[a]	—	7 to 12		3 to 9	1 to 3	2 to 9	—
Sinusitis	3[a] 3 to 4[b]	2 to 11	—	3 to 6	3 to 9	3 to 6	4 to 6	2 to 9
Nasal congestion	5 to 6[b]	—	—	2 to 6	15	8 to 16	4 to 7	—
Coughing	1 to 3[a] 7 to 9[b]	—	5 to 9	< 1	3 to 9	—	—	—
Dysphonia	1 to 3[a] [b]	—	1 to 3	< 1	—	3 to 8	< 1 to 6	—
Bronchospasm	Rare[a] < 2	—	—		—	Rare	—	—
Sneezing	2 to 3[b]	—	—		3 to 9	—	1 to 3	—
Epistaxis	—	2 to 4	—		1 to 3	—	1 to 3	—
Chest congestion	< 2	—	—		3 to 9	1 to 3	1 to 3	1 to 3

Corticosteroids

Inhaled Corticosteroids Adverse Reactions (%)

Adverse reactions	Beclomethasone dipropionate	Budesonide inhalation powder	Budesonide inhalation suspension	Ciclesonide	Flunisolide	Fluticasone propionate aerosol	Fluticasone propionate inhalation powder	Triamcinolone acetonide
Bronchitis	< 2	—	—		1 to 3	1 to 3	1 to 4	—
Special senses								
Taste alteration	< 2	1 to 3			10			
Otitis media	—	—	9 to 12		—	—	1 to 3	—
Ear infection	—	—	2 to 5		3 to 9		—	—
Conjunctivitis	—	—	< 1 to 4	≥ 3	—	—	1 to 3	—
Earache	< 2	—	1 to 3		1 to 3	—	1 to 3	—
Miscellaneous								
Infection, viral	5 to 8[b]	—	3 to 5		—	—	—	—
Weight changes	—	1 to 3	—		1 to 3			1 to 3
Back pain	1[a]	2 to 6	—	≥ 3	—	—	—	2 to 4
Influenza-like syndrome	< 1 to 3[b]	6 to 14	1 to 3	≥ 3	10	3 to 8	3 to 4	2 to 5
Pain	2[a] < 2	5	—		—	—	1 to 3	1 to 3
Fever	< 2	< 4	—		3 to 9	1 to 3	2 to 4	—
Infection	—	1 to 3	1 to 3		—	—		

[a] *QVAR*.

[b] *Vanceril* (both strengths).

➤*Beclomethasone:*

Miscellaneous – Fatigue (2% to 3%); increased asthma symptoms (less than 2% to 3%); rigors, rectal hemorrhage, lacrimation, arthralgia, depression, skin discoloration, UTI, lymphadenopathy, respiratory disorder (less than 2%).

➤*Budesonide inhalation powder:*

Musculoskeletal – Fracture, myalgia, neck pain (1% to 3%).

Miscellaneous – Voice alteration (1% to 6%); ecchymosis, syncope, hypertonia (1% to 3%).

➤*Budesonide inhalation suspension:*

CNS – Hyperkinesias, emotional lability (1% to 3%).

Dermatologic – Pustular rash, contact dermatitis (1% to 3%).

Musculoskeletal – Fracture, myalgia (1% to 3%).

Special senses – Eye infection, otitis externa (1% to 3%).

Miscellaneous – Moniliasis (3% to 4%); allergic reaction, fatigue, stridor, cervical lymphadenopathy, purpura, herpes simplex (1% to 3%).

Postmarketing: Hypersensitivity reactions, symptoms of hypocorticism/hypercorticism, psychiatric symptoms including depression, aggressive reactions, irritability, anxiety and psychosis, bone disorders including avascular necrosis of the femoral head and osteoporosis (less than 1%).

➤*Ciclesonide:*

CNS – Dizziness, fatigue (3% or more).

Musculoskeletal – Arthralgia (3% or more); pain in extremity (1% to 3%).

Respiratory – Nasopharyngitis (11%); pharyngolaryngeal pain (2% to 5%); pneumonia (3% or more).

Miscellaneous – Face edema, hoarseness, musculoskeletal chest pain (3% or more); dry throat (less than 1%).

Postmarketing – Immediate or delayed hypersensitivity reactions.

➤*Flunisolide:*

CNS – Dizziness, irritability, nervousness, shakiness (3% to 9%); anxiety, depression, faintness, fatigue, hyperactivity, hypoactivity, moodiness, numbness, vertigo (1% to 3%).

Dermatologic – Acne, hives (1% to 3%).

GI – Upset stomach (10%); heartburn (3% to 9%); constipation, gas, increased appetite (1% to 3%); abdominal fullness (less than 1%).

Hematologic – Capillary fragility, enlarged lymph nodes (1% to 3%).

Respiratory – Sore throat (20%); cold symptoms (15%); runny nose, sinus congestion, sinus drainage, sinus infection, hoarseness, sputum, wheezing (3% to 9%); glossitis, mouth/throat irritation, phlegm, chest tightness, dyspnea, head stuffiness, laryngitis, nasal irritation, pleurisy, pneumonia, sinus discomfort (1% to 3%); shortness of breath (less than 1%).

Special senses – Loss of smell (3% to 9%); blurred vision, eye discomfort, eye infection (1% to 3%).

Miscellaneous – Edema, palpitations (3% to 9%); chills, malaise, peripheral edema, sweating, weakness (1% to 3%).

➤*Fluticasone:*

CNS – Giddiness, nervousness (1% to 3%).

Respiratory – Nasal discharge (4% to 5%); allergic rhinitis (3% to 5%); pain in nasal sinus(es), laryngitis, acute nasopharyngitis, dyspnea, irritation caused by inhalant, tonsillitis (1% to 3%).

GI – Stomach disorder, gastroenteritis/colitis, abdominal discomfort, mouth/throat irritation (1% to 3%).

GU – Moniliasis, candidiasis of vagina, pelvic inflammatory disease, vaginitis/vulvovaginitis (1% to 3%).

Musculoskeletal – Back problems (less than 1% to 4%); joint pain, sprain/strain, aches and pains, limb pain, muscular soreness, disorder/symptoms of neck (1% to 3%).

Special senses – Eye irritation, dental disorder, conjunctivitis (1% to 3%).

Miscellaneous – Dermatitis, rash/skin eruption, injury (1% to 3%).

Postmarketing: Throat soreness and irritation; hoarseness; aphonia; Cushingoid features; growth velocity reduction in children/adolescents; weight gain; hyperglycemia; restlessness; aggression; depression; immediate bronchospasm; asthma exacerbation; dyspnea; wheezing; chest tightness; cough; pruritus; contusions; ecchymosis; laryngitis; bronchospasm.

➤*Triamcinolone:*

GU – Cystitis, urinary tract infection, vaginal monilia (1% to 3%).

Musculoskeletal – Bursitis, myalgia, tenosynovitis (1% to 3%).

Respiratory – Hoarseness; cough; increased wheezing; irritated throat; dry throat; dry mouth; oral candidiasis.

Miscellaneous – Facial edema, photosensitivity, toothache, easy bruisability, steroid withdrawal symptoms, voice alteration (1% to 3%).

Overdosage

The potential for acute toxic effects following overdose of inhaled corticosteroids is low. Chronic overdosage may result in signs/symptoms of hypercorticoidism.

Patient Information

Patient instructions are available with each product.

Rinse mouth with water without swallowing after each dose to reduce the risk of oral candidiasis. If the infection develops, treat with appropriate therapy. Corticosteroid therapy may need to be interrupted.

Instruct patients whose systemic corticosteroids have been reduced or withdrawn to carry a warning card indicating the need for supplemental systemic steroids in the event of stress or severe asthmatic attack that is unresponsive to bronchodilators.

Advise patients not to stop therapy abruptly. If discontinuation is necessary, contact the physician.

This medication is intended for treatment of asthma. It does not contain medication intended to provide rapid relief of breathing difficulties during an asthma attack. It is very important that the medication is used regularly at the intervals recommended by doctor, and not as an emergency measure.

Warn people who are on immunosuppressant doses of corticosteroids to avoid exposure to chickenpox or measles. Advise patients to seek medical advice without delay if they are exposed.

Advise patients receiving bronchodilators (eg, albuterol) by inhalation to use the bronchodilator several minutes before the corticosteroid inhalant to enhance penetration of the steroid into the bronchial tree and reduce potential toxicity from the inhaled fluorocarbon propellants in the 2 aerosols.

Notify physician if sore throat or sore mouth occurs.

➤*Administration technique:* The success of these agents is a function of proper administration technique. The following guidelines may be useful:

Aerosol – Thoroughly shake the inhaler with canister in place; breathe out to the end of a normal breath. Hold the inhaler system upright; place the mouthpiece into the mouth and close the lips tightly. While activating the inhaler, take a slow, deep breath for 3 to 5 seconds, hold the breath for approximately 10 seconds, and exhale slowly. Allow at least 1 minute between inhalations (inhalations). Rinse the mouth with water after each use to help reduce dry mouth and hoarseness.

Inhaled powder – Hold inhaler upright, and twist the cover off. Twist the grip fully to the right as far as it will go, then twist it back. You will hear a click. Exhale; then place the mouthpiece between lips, slightly tilt head back, and inhale deeply and forcefully. Remove inhaler from mouth, and hold breath for approximately 10 seconds. Allow at least 1 minute between inhalations (inhalations). Rinse the mouth with water after each use to help reduce dry mouth and hoarseness.

BECLOMETHASONE DIPROPIONATE

Rx	QVAR (IVAX)	**Aerosol:** 40 mcg/actuation	In 7.3 g canisters (100 actuations) with actuator.
		80 mcg/actuation	In 7.3 g canisters (100 actuations) with actuator.

BECLOMETHASONE DIPROPIONATE — INHALATION

For complete and comparative prescribing information, refer to the Corticosteroids Respiratory Inhalant group monograph.

Indications

➤*Asthma, chronic:* Maintenance treatment of asthma as prophylactic therapy in patients 5 years of age and older.

For asthma patients who require systemic corticosteroid administration, where adding beclomethasone dipropionate inhalation aerosol may reduce or eliminate the need for the systemic corticosteroids.

Beclomethasone dipropionate HFA inhalation aerosol is not indicated for the relief of acute bronchospasm.

Administration and Dosage

➤*General dosing considerations:* The recommended dosage of beclomethasone HFA inhalation aerosol relative to chlorofluorocarbon (CFC)-based beclomethasone (CFC-BDP) inhalation aerosol is lower due to differences in delivery characteristics between the products. Recognizing that a definitive comparative therapeutic ratio between beclomethasone HFA inhalation aerosol and CFC-BDP has not been demonstrated, any patient who is switched from CFC-BDP to beclomethasone HFA inhalation aerosol should be dosed appropriately, taking into account the dosing recommendations, and should be monitored to ensure that the dose of beclomethasone HFA inhalation aerosol selected is safe and efficacious.

Patients should be advised that beclomethasone HFA inhalation aerosol may have a different taste and inhalation sensation than that of an inhaler containing CFC propellant.

➤*Adults:*

Chronic asthma –

Maximum dose: 320 mcg twice daily.

Initial dosage:

• *Patients previously on bronchodilators alone* – 40 to 80 mcg twice daily.

• *Patients previously on inhaled corticosteroids* – 40 to 160 mcg twice daily.

Dosage adjustment: For patients who do not respond adequately to the starting dose after 3 to 4 weeks of therapy, higher doses may provide additional asthma control. Once the desired effect is achieved, consideration should be given to tapering to the lowest effective dose.

➤*Children:*

Chronic asthma –

12 years of age and older: See Adults for dosing.

5 to 11 years of age:

• *Maximum dose* – 80 mcg twice daily.

• *Initial dosage* – 40 mcg twice daily. (See also Off-Label Dosing for guideline dosing.)

• *Dosage adjustment* – For patients who do not respond adequately to the starting dose after 3 to 4 weeks of therapy, higher doses may provide additional asthma control. Once the desired effect is achieved, consideration should be given to tapering to the lowest effective dose. This is particularly important in children since a controlled study has shown that beclomethasone has the potential to affect growth in children.

Off-label dosing –

Chronic asthma: The following dosing is from National Asthma Education and Prevention guidelines.

• *5 to 11 years of age –*

Low-dose therapy: 80 to 160 mcg daily.

Medium-dose therapy: 160 to 320 mcg daily.

High-dose therapy: More than 320 mcg daily.

• *12 years of age and older –*

Low-dose therapy: 80 to 240 mcg daily.

Medium-dose therapy: More than 240 to 480 mcg daily.

High-dose therapy: More than 480 mcg daily.

➤*Conversion from systemic corticosteroids:* The patient's asthma should be reasonably stable before treatment with beclomethasone is started. Initially, beclomethasone should be used concurrently with the patient's usual maintenance dose of systemic corticosteroid. After approximately 1 week, gradual withdrawal of the systemic corticosteroid is started by reducing the daily or alternate daily dose. Reductions may be made after an interval of 1 or 2 weeks, depending on the response of the patient. A slow rate of withdrawal is strongly recommended. Generally, these decrements should not exceed 2.5 mg of prednisone or its equivalent. During withdrawal, some patients may experience symptoms of systemic corticosteroid withdrawal (eg, joint or muscular pain, lassitude, depression) despite maintenance or even improvement in pulmonary function. Such patients should be encouraged to continue with the inhaler but should be monitored for objective signs of adrenal insufficiency. If evidence of adrenal insufficiency occurs, the systemic corticosteroid doses should be increased temporarily, and, thereafter, withdrawal should continue more slowly. During periods of stress or a severe asthma attack, transfer patients may require supplementary treatment with systemic corticosteroids.

➤*Administration:* Administer by the oral inhaled route. Patients should prime by actuating into the air twice before using for the first time or if the aerosol has not been used for over 10 days. Avoid spraying in the eyes or face when priming. Beclomethasone is an aerosol solution, which does not require shaking. Beclomethasone HFA inhalation aerosol canister should only be used with the beclomethasone HFA inhalation aerosol actuator, and the actuator should not be used with any other inhalation drug product.

➤*Storage/Stability:* Store at 25°C (77°F). Excursions between 15° and 30°C (59° and 86°F) are permitted. Do not use or store near heat or open flame. Exposure to temperatures above 49°C (120°F) may cause bursting. Store aerosol when not being used so that the product rests on the concave end of the canister with the plastic actuator on top. For optimal results, the canister should be at room temperature when used. Do not puncture. Never throw container into fire or incinerator. The correct amount of medication in each inhalation cannot be ensured after 100 actuations from the 7.3 g canister, even though the canister will not be completely empty. The canister should be discarded when the labeled number of actuations have been used.

BUDESONIDE

Rx	**Pulmicort Flexhaler** (AstraZeneca)	**Powder; inhalation:** 90 mcg (each actuation delivers ≈ 80 mcg) per metered dose	Lactose. In 60 dose *Flexhaler*.
		180 mcg (each actuation delivers ≈ 160 mcg) per metered dose	Lactose. In 120 dose *Flexhaler*.
Rx	**Budesonide** (Teva Pharmaceutical)	**Suspension; inhalation:** 0.25 mg per 2 mL	Disodium edetate. In single-dose vials. In 30s.
Rx	**Pulmicort Respules** (AstraZeneca)		EDTA. In single-dose envelopes. In 30s.
Rx	**Budesonide** (Teva Pharmaceutical)	**Suspension; inhalation:** 0.5 mg per 2 mL	Disodium edetate. In single-dose vials. In 30s.
Rx	**Pulmicort Respules** (AstraZeneca)		EDTA. In single-dose envelopes. In 30s.
Rx	**Pulmicort Respules** (AstraZeneca)	**Suspension; inhalation:** 1 mg per 2 mL	EDTA. In single-dose envelopes. In 30s.

BUDESONIDE — INHALATION

For complete and comparative prescribing information, refer to the Corticosteroids Respiratory Inhalant group monograph.

WARNING

Particular care is needed for patients who are transferred from systemically active corticosteroids to inhaled corticosteroids (eg, budesonide) because deaths due to adrenal insufficiency have occurred in asthmatic patients during and after transfer from systemic corticosteroids to less systemically available inhaled corticosteroids. After withdrawal from systemic corticosteroids, a number of months are required for recovery of HPA-axis function.

Patients who have been previously maintained on greater than or equal to 20 mg/day of prednisone (or its equivalent) may be most susceptible, particularly when their systemic corticosteroids have been almost completely withdrawn.

During this period of HPA-axis suppression, patients may exhibit signs and symptoms of adrenal insufficiency when exposed to trauma, surgery, or infection (particularly gastroenteritis) or other conditions associated with severe electrolyte loss. Although budesonide may provide control of asthma symptoms during these episodes, in recommended doses it supplies less than normal physiological amounts of corticosteroid systemically and does not provide the mineralocorticoid activity that is necessary for coping with these emergencies.

During periods of stress or a severe asthma attack, patients who have been withdrawn from systemic corticosteroids should be instructed to resume oral corticosteroids (in large doses) immediately and to contact their physicians for further instruction. These patients should also be instructed to carry a medical identification card indicating that they may need supplementary systemic corticosteroids during periods of stress or a severe asthma attack.

Indications

➤*Powder for inhalation:* For the maintenance treatment of asthma as prophylactic therapy in adult and pediatric patients 6 years of age or older. It is also indicated for patients requiring oral corticosteroid therapy for asthma. Many of those patients may be able to reduce or eliminate their requirement for oral corticosteroids over time.

➤*Inhalation suspension:* For the maintenance treatment of asthma and as prophylactic therapy in children 12 months to 8 years of age.

➤*Off-label uses:*

Eosinophilic esophagitis (children) – [2] = Fair documentation. American Gastroenterological Association Institute and North American Society for Pediatric Gastroenterology, Hepatology and Nutrition guidelines recommend budesonide slurry administered orally, especially for younger or developmentally disabled children who might have difficulty using a metered-dose inhaler, as an alternative steroid administration method.

Lung cancer prevention – [4] = Insufficient documentation. American College of Chest Physicians (ACCP) guidelines evaluated the use of budesonide for chemoprevention of lung cancer. No agents were recommended by the ACCP for lung cancer prevention.

Administration and Dosage

➤*Maximum dose:*

Adults – 720 mcg twice daily (*Pulmicort Flexhaler*) according to the prescribing information.

Children – 1 mg/day (inhalation suspension); 360 mcg twice daily (*Pulmicort Flexhaler*) according to the prescribing information.

➤*General dosing considerations:* In all patients, it is desirable to downward-titrate to the lowest effective dose once asthma stability is achieved.

Inhalation suspension – Improvement in asthma control following inhaled administration can occur within 2 to 8 days of initiation of treatment, although maximum benefit may not be achieved for 4 to 6 weeks.

Powder for inhalation – Budesonide has a relatively rapid onset of action for an inhaled corticosteroid. Improvement in asthma control following inhaled administration can occur within 24 hours of initiation of treatment, although maximum benefit may not be achieved for 1 to 2 weeks or longer.

➤*Adults:*

Asthma –

Pulmicort Flexhaler:

- *Maximum dose* – 720 mcg twice daily.
- *Initial dosage* – 360 mcg twice daily. In some patients, a starting dose of 180 mcg twice daily may be adequate.
- *Maintenance dosage* – In well-controlled patients, a dosage of 180 mcg twice daily may be considered. If the 180 mcg twice-daily dose does not provide adequate control, the dose should be increased.

Off-label dosing –

Lung cancer prevention: [4] = Insufficient documentation. 800 mcg inhaled twice daily for 6 months.

➤*Children:*

Asthma –

Inhalation suspension:

See also Off-Label Dosing for guideline dosing.

- *12 months to 8 years of age* –

Budesonide Inhalation Suspension Recommended Dosages in Children		
Previous therapy	Recommended starting dose	Highest recommended dose
Bronchodilators alone	0.5 mg/day administered either once daily or twice daily in divided doses	0.5 mg/day
Inhaled corticosteroids	0.5 mg/day administered either once daily or twice daily in divided doses	1 mg/day
Oral corticosteroids	1 mg/day administered either as 0.5 mg twice daily or 1 mg once daily	1 mg/day

Maximum dose: 1 mg/day.

Dosage adjustment: If once-daily treatment does not provide adequate control of asthma symptoms, the total daily dose should be increased or administered as a divided dose.

Symptomatic children not responding to nonsteroidal therapy: A starting dose of 0.25 mg once daily may also be considered.

Patients not receiving systemic (oral) corticosteroids: Patients who require maintenance therapy of asthma may benefit from treatment with budesonide inhalation suspension at the doses previously recommended. For patients who do not respond adequately to the starting dose, consideration should be given to administering the total daily dose as a divided dose if a once-daily dosing schedule was followed. If necessary, higher doses, up to the maximum recommended doses, may provide additional asthma control.

Pulmicort Flexhaler:

- *6 years of age and older* –
  - *Maximum dose:* 360 mcg twice daily.
  - *Initial dosage:* 180 mcg twice daily. In some patients, a starting dose of 360 mcg twice daily may be appropriate.

Off-label dosing –

Chronic asthma: The following dosing is from National Asthma Education and Prevention guidelines. Dose may be administered 1 to 3 times per day.

- *Inhalation suspension* –
  - *4 years of age and younger:* 0.25 to 0.5 mg daily (low-dose therapy); more than 0.5 to 1 mg daily (medium-dose therapy); more than 1 mg daily (high-dose therapy).
  - *5 to 11 years of age:* 0.5 mg daily (low-dose therapy); 1 mg daily (medium-dose therapy); 2 mg daily (high-dose therapy).
- *Inhalation powder* –
  - *5 to 11 years of age:* 180 to 400 mcg daily (low-dose therapy); more than 400 to 800 mcg daily (medium-dose therapy); more than 800 mcg daily (high-dose therapy).
  - *12 years of age and older:* 180 to 600 mcg daily (low-dose therapy); more than 600 to 1,200 mcg daily (medium-dose therapy); more than 1,200 mcg daily (high-dose therapy).

Eosinophilic esophagitis (oral budesonide): [2] = Fair documentation.

- *Usual dose* – 1 to 2 mg orally as a viscous slurry each day, divided into 2 doses, for 3 to 4 months before repeat endoscopy.

Patients were instructed to avoid ingesting any solid or liquid food for 30 minutes after budesonide administration.

See Preparation for Administration for compounding information.

- *Initial dosage* –
  - *Older than 10 years of age:* 1 mg orally twice daily.
  - *Younger than 10 years of age:* 500 mcg orally twice daily, but may be increased to 1 mg twice daily if no response is observed.

➤*Concomitant therapy with oral corticosteroids:* For patients who are maintained on chronic oral corticosteroids, the usual maintenance dose should be used concurrently with the initial budesonide therapy. After approximately 1 week, gradual withdrawal of the systemic corticosteroid is started by reducing the daily or alternate daily dose. The next reduction is made after 1 or 2 weeks, depending on the response of the patient. Generally, these decrements should not exceed 25% of the prednisone dose or its equivalent. A slow rate of withdrawal is strongly recommended. During reduction of oral corticosteroids, patients should be carefully monitored for asthma instability, including objective measures of airway function, and for adrenal insufficiency. During withdrawal, some patients may experience symptoms of systemic corticosteroid withdrawal (eg, joint or muscular pain, lassitude, depression) despite maintenance or even improvement in pulmonary function. Such patients should be encouraged to continue with budesonide but should be monitored for objective signs of adrenal insufficiency. If evidence of adrenal insufficiency occurs, the systemic corticosteroid doses should be increased temporarily, and thereafter withdrawal should continue more slowly. During periods of stress or a severe asthma attack, transfer patients may require supplementary treatment with systemic corticosteroids.

➤*Preparation for administration:*

Inhalation suspension – Gently shake the inhalation suspension using a circular motion before use.

Powder for inhalation – Prime budesonide prior to its initial use.

BUDESONIDE — INHALATION

Extemporaneous compounding – Viscous budesonide for oral administration was made by mixing a 0.5 mg *Pulmicort Respule* with sucralose 5 g to provide a final volume of 8 to 12 mL.

➤*Administration:* Budesonide can be administered once daily either in the morning or in the evening.

Inhalation suspension – For inhalation use via compressed air driven jet nebulizers only (not for use with ultrasonic devices). Not for injection. Read patient instructions before using.

Pari-LC-Jet Plus Nebulizer (with face mask or mouthpiece) connected to a *Pari* compressor was used to deliver budesonide inhalation suspension to each patient. The safety and efficacy of budesonide inhalation suspension delivered by other nebulizers and compressors have not been established.

Administer via jet nebulizer connected to an air compressor with an adequate air flow, equipped with a mouthpiece or suitable face mask. Ultrasonic nebulizers are not suitable for adequate administration and, therefore, are not recommended.

Powder for inhalation – Inhale deeply and forcefully each time the unit is used. Rinsing the mouth after inhalation is also recommended.

➤*Admixture compatibility:* Budesonide suspension is compatible with albuterol, ipratropium, and levalbuterol nebulizer solutions in the same nebulizer.

➤*Storage/Stability:*

Inhalation suspension – Store upright at controlled room temperature, 20° to 25°C (68° to 77°F), and protect from light. When an envelope has been opened, the shelf life of the unused inhalation suspension is 2 weeks when protected. After opening the aluminum foil envelope, the unused inhalation suspension should be returned to the aluminum foil envelope to protect them from light. Any opened inhalation suspension must be used promptly. Do not freeze.

Powder for inhalation – Store with the cover tightened in a dry place at controlled room temperature, 20° to 25°C (68° to 77°F).

FLUNISOLIDE

Rx	**AeroBid** (Forest)	**Aerosol:** ≈ 250 mcg/actuation	In canisters (100 metered doses).
Rx	**AeroBid-M** (Forest)		Menthol flavor. In canisters (100 metered doses).

FLUNISOLIDE — INHALATION

For complete and comparative prescribing information, refer to the Corticosteroids Respiratory Inhalant group monograph.

WARNING

Particular care is needed in patients who are transferred from systemically active corticosteroids to flunisolide inhaler because deaths due to adrenal insufficiency have occurred in asthmatic patients during and after transfer from systemic corticosteroids to aerosol corticosteroids. After withdrawal from systemic corticosteroids, a number of months are required for recovery of hypothalamic-pituitary-adrenal (HPA) function. During this period of HPA suppression, patients may exhibit signs and symptoms of adrenal insufficiency when exposed to trauma, surgery or infections, particularly gastroenteritis. Although flunisolide inhaler may provide control of asthmatic symptoms during these episodes, it does not provide the systemic steroid that is necessary for coping with these emergencies. During periods of stress or a severe asthmatic attack, patients who have been withdrawn from systemic corticosteroids should be instructed to resume systemic steroids (in large doses) immediately and to contact their physician for further instruction. These patients should also be instructed to carry a warning card indicating that they may need supplementary systemic steroids during periods of stress or a severe asthma attack. To assess the risk of adrenal insufficiency in emergency situations, routine tests of adrenal cortical function, including measurement of early morning resting cortisol levels, should be performed periodically in all patients. An early morning resting cortisol level may be accepted as normal if it falls at or near the normal mean level.

Indications

➤*Asthma, chronic:* Maintenance treatment of asthma as prophylactic therapy. Flunisolide is also indicated for asthma patients who require systemic corticosteroid administration, where adding flunisolide may reduce or eliminate the need for the systemic corticosteroids.

Administration and Dosage

➤*General dosing considerations:* The patient's asthma should be reasonably stable before treatment with flunisolide is started.

May be used alone or in combination with systemic corticosteroids.

When the drug is used chronically at 2 mg/day, patients should be monitored periodically for effects on the hypothalamic-pituitary-adrenal (HPA) axis. With chronic use, children should be monitored for growth as well.

➤*Adults:*

Asthma, chronic –

Maximum dose: 4 inhalations twice daily.

Initial dosage: 2 inhalations twice daily.

Dosage adjustment: Once the desired effect is achieved, consideration should be given to tapering to the lowest effective dose.

➤*Children:*

Asthma, chronic –

16 years of age and older: See Adults for dosing.

6 to 15 years of age:

• *Usual dosage* – 2 inhalations twice daily. Higher doses have not been studied.

• *Dosage adjustment* – Once the desired effect is achieved, consideration should be given to tapering to the lowest effective dose.

➤*Conversion to flunisolide:* Initially, flunisolide should be used concurrently with the patient's usual maintenance dose of systemic corticosteroid. After approximately 1 week, gradual withdrawal of the systemic corticosteroid is started by reducing the daily or alternate daily dose. Reductions may be made after an interval of 1 or 2 weeks, depending on the response of the patient. A slow rate of withdrawal is strongly recommended. Generally, these decrements should not exceed 2.5 mg of prednisone or its equivalent. During withdrawal, some patients may experience symptoms of systemic corticosteroid withdrawal (eg, joint or muscular pain, lassitude and depression, despite maintenance or even improvement of pulmonary function). Such patients should be encouraged to continue with the inhaler but should be monitored for objective signs of adrenal insufficiency. If evidence of adrenal insufficiency occurs, the systemic corticosteroid doses should be increased temporarily and thereafter withdrawal should continue more slowly. During periods of stress or a severe asthma attack, transfer patients may require supplementary treatment with systemic corticosteroids.

➤*Administration:* For oral inhalation only. Shake well before use. Avoid spraying in eyes. Administer twice daily in the morning and evening. Rinse the mouth after inhalation.

➤*Storage/Stability:* Store at 59° to 86°F away from heat or open flame. Protect from freezing and prolonged exposure to sunlight. Do not puncture or discard pressurized canisters in incinerator.

FLUTICASONE PROPIONATE

Rx	**Flovent HFA** (GlaxoSmithKline)	**Aerosol; oral:** 44 mcg/actuation	In 10.6 g canister containing 120 metered inhalations. With actuator.
		110 mcg/actuation	In 12 g canister containing 120 metered inhalations. With actuator.
		220 mcg/actuation	In 12 g canister containing 120 metered inhalations. With actuator.
Rx	**Flovent Diskus** (GlaxoSmithKline)	**Powder; inhalation:** 50 mcg/actuation	Lactose. In inhalation device containing 60 blisters.
		100 mcg/actuation	Lactose. In inhalation device containing 60 blisters.
		250 mcg/actuation	Lactose. In inhalation device containing 60 blisters.

FLUTICASONE PROPIONATE — INHALATION

For complete and comparative prescribing information, refer to the Corticosteroids Respiratory Inhalant group monograph.

Indications

➤*Asthma, chronic:* For the maintenance treatment of asthma as prophylactic therapy in patients 4 years of age and older. Also indicated for patients requiring oral corticosteroid therapy for asthma. Many of these patients may be able to reduce or eliminate their requirement for oral corticosteroids over time.

Fluticasone is not indicated for relief of acute bronchospasm.

➤*Off-label uses:*

Eosinophilic esophagitis – [2] = Fair documentation. According to American Gastroenterological Association Institute and North American Society for Pediatric Gastroenterology, Hepatology and Nutrition guidelines, swallowed topical corticosteroids, such as fluticasone, delivered by metered-dose inhaler effectively resolve the acute clinicopathologic features of eosinophilic esophagitis; however, the disease tends to recur when the steroids are discontinued.

FLUTICASONE PROPIONATE — INHALATION

Administration and Dosage

➤*General dosing considerations:* Individual patients will experience a variable time to onset and degree of symptom relief. Maximum benefit may not be achieved for 1 to 2 weeks or longer after starting treatment.

After asthma stability has been achieved, titrate to the lowest effective dose to reduce adverse reaction possibility. For patients not responding adequately to the starting dose after 2 weeks, higher doses may provide additional asthma control.

➤*Adults:*

Asthma –

Fluticasone aerosol:

Recommended Adult Dosages for Fluticasone Aerosol

Previous therapy	Recommended starting dosage	Highest recommended dosage
Bronchodilators alone	88 mcg twice daily	440 mcg twice daily
Inhaled corticosteroids	88 to 220 mcg twice daily[a]	440 mcg twice daily
Oral corticosteroids[b]	440 mcg twice daily	880 mcg twice daily

[a] For patients currently receiving inhaled corticosteroid therapy, starting doses > 88 mcg twice daily may be considered for patients with poorer asthma control or those who have previously required doses of inhaled corticosteroids that are in the higher range for that specific agent.
[b] See Concomitant therapy with oral corticosteroids.

• *Maximum dose* – 880 mcg twice daily.

Fluticasone Diskus:

Recommended Adult Dosages for Fluticasone *Diskus*[a]

Previous therapy	Recommended starting dosage	Highest recommended dosage
Bronchodilators alone	100 mcg twice daily	500 mcg twice daily
Inhaled corticosteroids	100 to 250 mcg twice daily	500 mcg twice daily
Oral corticosteroids[b]	500 to 1,000 mcg twice daily	1,000 mcg twice daily

[a] Starting dosages > 100 mcg twice daily for adults may be considered for patients with poorer asthma control or those who have previously required doses of inhaled corticosteroids that are in the higher range for that specific agent.
[b] See Concomitant therapy with oral corticosteroids.

• *Maximum dose* – 1,000 mcg twice daily.

Off-label dosing –

Eosinophilic esophagitis: [2] = Fair documentation. 880 to 1,760 mcg/day. Doses may be divided for twice-daily or 4-times-daily administration.

Patients should be instructed to use the fluticasone metered-dose inhaler without a spacer, to insert the inhaler into the mouth, to spray the dose with lips sealed around the device, and then to swallow the powder and not rinse. Patients should avoid eating or drinking for at least 30 minutes. The regimen is continued for 6 to 8 weeks.

➤*Children:*

Asthma –

Fluticasone aerosol:

Recommended Pediatric Dosages for Fluticasone Aerosol

Previous therapy	Recommended starting dosage	Highest recommended dosage
≥ 12 years of age		
Bronchodilators alone	88 mcg twice daily	440 mcg twice daily
Inhaled corticosteroids	88 to 220 mcg twice daily[a]	440 mcg twice daily
Oral corticosteroids[b]	440 mcg twice daily	880 mcg twice daily
4 to 11 years of age[c]		
–	88 mcg twice daily	88 mcg twice daily

[a] For patients currently receiving inhaled corticosteroid therapy, starting doses > 88 mcg twice daily may be considered for patients with poorer asthma control or those who have previously required doses of inhaled corticosteroids that are in the higher range for that specific agent.
[b] See Concomitant therapy with oral corticosteroids.
[c] Recommended pediatric dosage is 88 mcg twice daily regardless of prior therapy.

• *Maximum dose* – 880 mcg twice daily for children 12 years of age and older; 88 mcg twice daily for children 4 to 11 years of age.

Fluticasone Diskus –

Recommended Pediatric Dosages for Fluticasone *Diskus*[a]

Previous therapy	Recommended starting dosage	Highest recommended dosage
≥ 12 years of age		
Bronchodilators alone	100 mcg twice daily	500 mcg twice daily
Inhaled corticosteroids	100 to 250 mcg twice daily	500 mcg twice daily
Oral corticosteroids[b]	500 to 1,000 mcg twice daily[c]	1,000 mcg twice daily
4 to 11 years of age[d]		
Bronchodilators alone	50 mcg twice daily	100 mcg twice daily
Inhaled corticosteroids	50 mcg twice daily	100 mcg twice daily

[a] Starting dosages > 100 mcg twice daily for children ≥ 12 years of age and > 50 mcg twice daily for children 4 to 11 years of age may be considered for patients with poorer asthma control or those who have previously required doses of inhaled corticosteroids that are in the higher range for that specific agent.
[b] See Concomitant therapy with oral corticosteroids.
[c] The choice of starting dosage should be made on the basis of individual patient assessment. A controlled clinical study of 111 oral corticosteroid–dependent patients with asthma showed few significant differences between the 2 doses of fluticasone *Diskus* on safety and efficacy end points. However, inability to decrease the dose of oral corticosteroids further during corticosteroid reduction may be indicative of the need to increase the dose of fluticasone *Diskus* up to the maximum of 1,000 mcg twice daily.
[d] Because individual responses may vary, children previously maintained on other inhaled corticosteroids may require dosage adjustments upon transfer to fluticasone *Diskus*.

Maximum dose: 1,000 mcg twice daily for children 12 years of age and older; 100 mcg twice daily for children 4 to 11 years of age.

Off-label dosing –

Eosinophilic esophagitis: [2] = Fair documentation. Patients should be instructed to use the fluticasone metered-dose inhaler without a spacer, to insert the inhaler into the mouth, to spray the dose with lips sealed around the device, and then to swallow the powder and not rinse. Patients should avoid eating or drinking for at least 30 minutes. The regimen is continued for 6 to 8 weeks.

• *Adolescents* – 880 to 1,760 mcg/day. Doses may be divided for twice-daily or 4-times-daily administration.

• *Children* – 440 to 880 mcg/day. Doses may be divided for twice-daily or 4-times-daily administration.

➤*Concomitant therapy with oral corticosteroids:* For patients currently receiving chronic oral corticosteroids, reduce prednisone no faster than 2.5 to 5 mg/day on a weekly basis, beginning after at least 1 week of fluticasone inhalation therapy. Monitor patients for signs of asthma instability, including serial objective measures of airflow, and for signs of adrenal insufficiency. Decrease fluticasone dosage to the lowest effective dose once prednisone reduction is complete.

➤*Preparation for administration:* Shake well before using.

Patients should rinse their mouth after inhalation.

Aerosol – For best results, the aerosol canister should be at room temperature before use. Prime inhaler before using for the first time by releasing 4 test sprays into the air away from the face, shaking well before each spray. In cases in which the inhaler has not been used for more than 7 days or when it has been dropped, prime again by shaking well and releasing 1 test spray into the air away from the face.

➤*Storage/Stability:* Store at 25°C (77°F); excursions are permitted from 15° to 30°C (59° to 86°F). Store with mouthpiece down. Do not spray in the eyes. Do not puncture or incinerate. Protect from freezing and direct heat or sunlight.

MOMETASONE FUROATE

Rx	Asmanex Twisthaler (Schering)	**Powder; inhalation:** 110 mcg (delivers mometasone furoate 100 mcg)/actuation	Lactose. In inhalation device of 7 and 30 units.
		220 mcg (delivers mometasone furoate 200 mcg)/actuation	Lactose. In inhalation device of 14, 30, 60, and 120 units.

MOMETASONE FUROATE — ORAL INHALATION

Indications

➤*Asthma:* For the maintenance treatment of asthma as prophylactic therapy in patients 4 years of age and older.

Mometasone is not indicated for the relief of acute bronchospasm or for children younger than 4 years of age.

Administration and Dosage

➤*Adults:*

Asthma –

Maximum dose: 440 mcg/day in patients who previously received bronchodilators alone or inhaled corticosteroids; 880 mcg/day in patients who previously received oral corticosteroids.

MOMETASONE FUROATE — ORAL INHALATION

Initial dosage:

• *Patients who previously received bronchodilators alone* – 220 mcg once daily in the evening.

• *Patients who previously received inhaled corticosteroids* – 220 mcg once daily in the evening.

• *Patients who previously received oral corticosteroids* – 440 mcg twice daily.

Dosage adjustment: In patients who do not respond adequately to the starting dose after 2 weeks of therapy, higher doses may provide additional asthma control. Titrate to the lowest effective dose once asthma stability is achieved to reduce the possibility of adverse reactions.

➤*Children:*

Asthma –

12 years of age and older: See Adults for dosing.

4 to 11 years of age:

• *Maximum dose* – 110 mcg/day.

• *Initial dosage* – 110 mcg once daily in the evening.

• *Dosage adjustment* – To minimize the systemic effects of mometasone, titrate each patient to the lowest effective dose.

➤*Conversion to mometasone:* For patients receiving chronic oral corticosteroid therapy, reduce prednisone no faster than 2.5 mg/day on a weekly basis, beginning after at least 1 week of mometasone therapy. Carefully monitor patients for signs of asthma instability, including serial objective measures of airflow, and adrenal insufficiency during steroid taper and following discontinuation of oral corticosteroid therapy.

➤*Administration:* For oral inhalation only. The 440 mcg daily dose may be administered in divided doses of 220 mcg twice daily or as 440 mcg once daily. When administered once daily, mometasone should only be taken in the evening. Instruct patients to inhale rapidly and deeply. Rinsing the mouth after inhalation is advised.

➤*Storage/Stability:* Store in a dry place at 25°C (77°F); excursions are permitted to 15° to 30°C (59° to 86°F). Discard the inhaler 45 days after opening the foil pouch or when the dose counter reads "00," whichever comes first.

CICLESONIDE

Rx	**Alvesco** (Sepracor)	**Solution; inhalation:** 80 mcg/actuation	In 6.1 g canister (60 actuations) with actuator.
		160 mcg/actuation	In 6.1 g canister (60 actuations) with actuator.

CICLESONIDE — INHALATION

For complete prescribing information, refer to the Corticosteroids Respiratory Inhalant class monograph.

Indications

➤*Asthma:* For the maintenance treatment of asthma as prophylactic therapy in adult and adolescent patients 12 years of age and older.

Administration and Dosage

➤*Adults:*

Asthma –

Patients who receive bronchodilators alone:

• *Maximum dose* – 160 mcg twice daily.

• *Initial dosage* – 80 mcg twice daily.

• *Dosage adjustment* – For patients who do not respond adequately to the starting dose after 4 weeks of therapy, higher doses may provide additional asthma control. After asthma stability has been achieved, titrate to the lowest effective dosage.

Patients who receive inhaled corticosteroids:

• *Maximum dose* – 320 mcg twice daily.

• *Initial dosage* – 80 mcg twice daily.

• *Dosage adjustment* – See Patients Who Receive Bronchodilators Alone for dosing.

Patients who receive oral corticosteroids:

• *Maximum dose* – 320 mcg twice daily.

• *Initial dosage* – 320 mcg twice daily.

• *Dosage adjustment –*

• *Concomitant therapy* – Prednisone should be reduced gradually, no sooner than 2.5 mg/day on a weekly basis, beginning after 1 week or more of therapy with ciclesonide.

➤*Children:*

Asthma –

12 years of age and older: See Adults for dosing.

➤*Preparation for administration:* The actuator should be primed before using for the first time by actuating 3 times prior to using the first dose from a new canister or when the inhaler has not been used for more than 10 days. Avoid spraying in the eyes or face while priming.

➤*Administration:* Administer by the orally inhaled route. The actuators are fitted with a dose indicator and should not be used with other inhalation aerosol medications.

➤*Storage/Stability:* Store at 25°C (77°F). Excursions are permitted between 15° and 30°C (59° and 86°F). The canister should be discarded when the dose indicator display window shows zero.

For optimal results, the canister should be at room temperature when used. Do not puncture. Do not use or store near heat or open flame. Exposure to temperatures higher than 49°C (120°F) may cause bursting. Never throw canister into fire or incinerator.

Intranasal Steroids

For information on the systemic use of corticosteroids, refer to the Adrenocortical Steroids (Glucocorticoids) monograph in the Endocrine and Metabolic Agents chapter.

Indications

See individual product listings for specific labeled indications.

Intranasal Steroids Summary of Indications

Indications ✓ = Approved uses X = Unlabeled uses	Beclomethasone	Budesonide	Ciclesonide	Flunisolide	Fluticasone	Mometasone	Triamcinolone
Nasal polyps	✓	X			X	✓	
Nonallergic (vasomotor) rhinitis	✓				✓		
Perennial allergic rhinitis	✓	✓	✓	✓	✓	✓	✓
Seasonal allergic rhinitis	✓	✓	✓	✓	✓	✓[a]	✓
Recurrent chronic sinusitis[b]		X			X	X	

[a] Treatment and prophylaxis.
[b] As adjunctive therapy with an antibiotic and/or decongestant.

Administration and Dosage

Refer to the individual monographs for specific dosing information.

Use intranasal steroids at regular intervals for optimal effect.

➤*Duration of therapy:* Although some symptomatic relief may be achieved sooner, maximum benefit may not be reached until at least 2 weeks of therapy. Generally do not continue use beyond 3 weeks in the absence of significant symptomatic improvement.

Actions

➤*Pharmacology:* These drugs have potent glucocorticoid and weak mineralocorticoid activity. The mechanisms responsible for the anti-inflammatory action of corticosteroids on the nasal mucosa are unknown. However, glucocorticoids have a wide range of inhibitory activities against multiple cell types (eg, mast cells, eosinophils, neutrophils, macrophages, lymphocytes) and mediators (eg, histamine, eicosanoids, leukotrienes, cytokines) involved in allergic and nonallergic/irritant-mediated inflammation. These agents, when administered topically in recommended doses, exert direct local anti-inflammatory effects with minimal systemic effects. Exceeding the recommended dose may result in systemic effects, including hypothalamic-pituitary-adrenal (HPA) function suppression.

➤*Pharmacokinetics:*

Intranasal Steroids: Pharmacokinetics

Parameters	Corticosteroids: Beclomethasone	Budesonide	Ciclesonide	Flunisolide	Fluticasone	Mometasone	Triamcinolone
Bioavailability	44%	≈ 34%	< 1%	50%	< 2%	< 1%	Minimal
Volume of distribution	20 L, 424 L[a]	2 to 3 L/kg	2.9 L/kg,[c] 12.1 L/kg[a]	NA[b]	4.2 L/kg[c]	NA	99.5 L[c]

Intranasal Steroids

Intranasal Steroids: Pharmacokinetics

Parameters	Corticosteroids						
	Beclomethasone	Budesonide	Ciclesonide	Flunisolide	Fluticasone	Mometasone	Triamcinolone
Protein binding	87%	85% to 90%[d]	99%	NA	91%[c]	98% to 99%[e]	NA
Site of metabolism		Liver (CYP3A)	Liver (CYP3A4)	Liver	Liver (CYP3A4)	Liver (CYP3A4)	Liver
Metabolites (activity)	17-monopropionate (active), free beclomethasone (very weak; prodrug)	16α-hydroxyprednisolone and 6β-hydroxybudesonide (< 1% of parent)	des-ciclesonide (active)	NA	17β-carboxylic acid (inactive)	6β-hydroxymometasone furoate	6β-hydroxytriamcinolone acetonide, 21-carboxytriamcinolone acetonide, and 21-carboxy-6β-hydroxytriamcinolone acetonide (substantially < parent)
Excretion site	Feces (≈ 60%), urine (≈ 12%)[f]	Feces, urine (≈ 66%)	Feces (66%) Urine (≤ 20%)[c]	Feces (≈ 50%), urine (≈ 50%)	Feces (> 95%), urine (< 5%)[c]	Feces, urine	Feces (≈ 60%), urine (≈ 40%)
Half-life	0.5 h, 2.7 h[a,c]	2 to 3 h[c]	NA	1 to 2 h	7.8 h[c]	5.8 h[c]	3.1 h

[a] Value for metabolite.
[b] Not available.
[c] Data from intravenous administration.
[d] Over a concentration range of 1 to 100 nmol/L.
[e] Over a concentration range of 5 to 500 ng/mL.
[f] Data from oral administration.

Special populations –

Hepatic function impairment: Reduced liver function may affect the elimination of corticosteroids. The systemic availability of oral **budesonide** was doubled by compromised liver function. The relevance of this finding to intranasal budesonide has not been established. The maximal drug concentration (C_{max}) and area under the curve (AUC) of **ciclesonide** increased in the range of 1.4- to 2.7-fold in patients with hepatic impairment. The systemic exposure (C_{max} and AUC) in patients with hepatic function impairment increased in the range of 1.4- to 2.7-fold.

Children: Children had **budesonide** plasma concentrations approximately twice that observed in adults after intranasal administration primarily because of differences in weight.

Contraindications

Untreated localized infections involving the nasal mucosa (**flunisolide**); hypersensitivity to the drug or any component of the product.

Warnings/Precautions

➤*Special senses:* Temporary or permanent loss of the sense of smell and taste has been reported with **flunisolide** use (see Adverse Reactions).

➤*Systemic corticosteroids:* The combined administration of alternate-day systemic prednisone with these products may increase the likelihood of HPA suppression. Therefore, use with caution in patients already on alternate-day prednisone.

Replacement of a systemic corticosteroid with intranasal corticosteroids can be accompanied by signs of adrenal insufficiency.

During withdrawal from oral corticosteroids, some patients may experience withdrawal symptoms (eg, joint or muscular pain, lassitude, depression). Carefully monitor patients previously treated with systemic corticosteroids for prolonged periods and then transferred to intranasal steroids to avoid acute adrenal insufficiency in response to stress. This is particularly important in patients who have asthma or other conditions where too rapid a decrease in systemic corticosteroids may cause a severe exacerbation of their symptoms.

➤*Hypercorticism:* If recommended doses of intranasal corticosteroids are exceeded or if individuals are particularly sensitive or predisposed by virtue of recent systemic steroid therapy, symptoms of hypercorticism may occur, including, very rarely, menstrual irregularities, acneiform lesions, cataracts, and cushingoid features. If such changes occur, discontinue slowly, consistent with accepted procedures for discontinuing oral steroids. Avoid doses greater than recommended.

➤*Nasopharyngeal irritation:* If persistent nasopharyngeal irritation occurs, it may be an indication to stop therapy.

➤*Epistaxis:* Observed more frequently in patients with allergic rhinitis treated with **mometasone** compared with those who received placebo in clinical studies.

➤*Ophthalmic effects:* Rare instances of cataracts, glaucoma, and increased intraocular pressure have been reported following intranasal application of corticosteroids. Close follow-up is warranted in patients with a change in vision and a history of glaucoma and/or cataracts.

➤*Infections:* Localized infections of the nose and pharynx with *Candida albicans* have developed only rarely. When such an infection occurs, it may require treatment with appropriate local or systemic therapy and/or discontinuation of steroid treatment.

Use with caution, if at all, in patients with active or quiescent tuberculosis infections of the respiratory tract; untreated fungal, bacterial, or systemic viral infections; or ocular herpes simplex.

Individuals receiving immunosuppressant agents are more susceptible to infections than healthy individuals. For example, chickenpox and measles can have a more serious or fatal course in susceptible children or adults receiving immunosuppressant doses of corticosteroids. Take particular care to avoid exposure in children or adults who have not had these diseases or who have not been properly immunized. Prophylaxis with varicella-zoster immune globulin may be indicated if exposed to chickenpox. If an individual is exposed to measles, prophylaxis with pooled immunoglobulin may be indicated. Consider treatment with antiviral agents if chickenpox develops.

➤*Nasal septum perforation:* Rare instances of nasal septum perforation have been reported following the intranasal application of corticosteroids.

➤*Wound healing:* Because of the inhibitory effect of corticosteroids on wound healing, do not use nasal steroids in patients who have experienced recent nasal septal ulcers, recurrent epistaxis, or nasal surgery or trauma until healing has occurred.

➤*Effect on growth:* Intranasal corticosteroids may cause a reduction in growth velocity when administered to children.

➤*Vasoconstrictors:* In the presence of excessive nasal mucosa secretion or edema of the nasal mucosa, the drug may fail to reach the site of intended action. In such cases, use a nasal vasoconstrictor during the first 2 to 3 days of therapy.

➤*Respiratory effects:* Rare instances of wheezing have been reported following intranasal application of corticosteroids.

➤*Systemic effects:* Although systemic effects are low when used in recommended dosage, HPA suppression and other systemic effects may occur, especially with excessive doses.

➤*Long-term treatment:* Examine patients periodically over several months or longer for possible changes in the nasal mucosa.

➤*Hypersensitivity reactions:* Rare cases of immediate and delayed hypersensitivity reactions, including angioedema, bronchospasm, rash, and urticaria, have been reported after intranasal administration of corticosteroids. Refer to Management of Acute Hypersensitivity Reactions.

➤*Hepatic function impairment:* Reduced liver function may affect the elimination of corticosteroids. The systemic availability of oral **budesonide** was doubled by compromised liver function. The relevance of this finding to intranasal budesonide has not been established. Concentrations of **mometasone** appear to increase with the severity of hepatic impairment.

➤*Pregnancy: Category C.* There are no adequately controlled trials in pregnant women. However, animal studies have demonstrated teratogenic, fetotoxic, and embryocidal effects. Topical administration of recommended doses is unlikely to achieve significant systemic levels; however, use these agents during pregnancy only if the potential benefits outweigh the potential hazards to the fetus.

Carefully observe infants born of mothers who have received substantial doses of corticosteroids during pregnancy for signs of adrenal insufficiency.

➤*Lactation:* It is not known whether these drugs are excreted in breast milk. Because other corticosteroids are excreted in human milk, use caution when administering to breast-feeding women.

➤*Children:*

Beclomethasone, budesonide, flunisolide, triamcinolone – Safety and efficacy for use in children younger than 6 years of age have not been established.

Ciclesonide – Safety and effectiveness for seasonal and perennial allergic rhinitis in children 12 years of age and older have been established.

Fluticasone – Safety and efficacy for use in children younger than 4 years of age have not been established.

Mometasone – Safety and efficacy for use in allergic rhinitis in children younger than 2 years of age and for nasal polyps in children younger than 18 years of age have not been established.

Controlled clinical studies have shown that intranasal corticosteroids may cause a reduction in growth velocity in children. This effect has been observed in the absence of laboratory evidence of HPA-axis suppression, suggesting that growth velocity is a more sensitive indicator of systemic corticosteroid exposure in children than some commonly used tests of HPA-axis function. The long-term effects of this reduction in growth velocity associated with intranasal corticosteroids, including the impact on final adult height, are unknown. The potential for "catch-up" growth following discontinuation of treatment with intranasal corticosteroids has not been adequately studied. Routinely monitor the growth of children receiving intranasal corticosteroids (eg, via stadiometry). Weigh the potential growth effects of prolonged treatment against the clinical benefits obtained and the risks/benefits of treatment alternatives. To minimize the systemic effects of intranasal corticosteroids, titrate each patient to the lowest dose that effectively controls his/her symptoms.

➤*Elderly:* In general, use caution in dose selection for an elderly patient, starting at the low end of the dosing range, reflecting greater frequency of decreased hepatic, renal, or cardiac function, and concomitant disease or other drug therapy.

➤*Monitoring:* Routinely monitor the growth of children receiving intranasal corticosteroids (eg, via stadiometry). Carefully monitor patients previously treated for prolonged periods with systemic corticosteroids and then transferred to topical corticosteroids for acute adrenal insufficiency in response to stress. Examine periodically for evidence of *Candida* infection or other signs of adverse effects on the nasal mucosa. Close follow-up is warranted in patients with a change in vision and with a history of glaucoma and/or cataracts.

Drug Interactions

Intranasal Steroids Drug Interactions

Precipitant drug	Object drug[a]		Description
Cimetidine	Budesonide	↑	Coadministration caused a slight decrease in budesonide clearance and a corresponding increase in its oral bioavailability.
Inhibitors of CYP3A4 (eg, ketoconazole, itraconazole, clarithromycin, erythromycin, cimetidine, ritonavir)	Budesonide Ciclesonide Fluticasone	↑	Coadministration may inhibit metabolism and increase systemic exposure of the intranasal steroid. After oral administration of ketoconazole, the mean plasma concentration of oral budesonide increased by more than 7-fold and 3.6-fold for des-ciclesonide. Coadministration of oral ritonavir and intranasal fluticasone resulted in a significant increase in fluticasone plasma concentrations resulting in possible Cushing syndrome and adrenal suppression. Use with caution.

[a] ↑ = object drug increased.

Adverse Reactions

Intranasal Steroids Adverse Reactions (%)[a]

Adverse reaction	Beclomethasone	Budesonide	Ciclesonide	Flunisolide (nasal solution)	Flunisolide (nasal spray)	Fluticasone	Mometasone	Triamcinolone
CNS								
Dizziness						1% to 3%		
Headache	< 5%		6.6%	≤ 5%		7% to 16%	26%	≥ 2%
Light-headedness	< 5%							
GI								
Abdominal pain						1% to 3%		
Diarrhea						1% to 3%	2% to < 5%	
Dyspepsia							2% to < 5%	
Nausea	< 5%			≤ 5%	> 1%	3% to 5%	2% to < 5%	
Vomiting				≤ 5		3% to 5%	5%	≥ 2%
Hypersensitivity								
Anaphylaxis						Rare[b]	✓[b,c]	
Angioedema	Rare	Rare[b]				Rare[b]	✓[b,c]	
Bronchospasm	Rare					Rare[b]		
Dyspnea						Rare[b]		
Edema of face/tongue						Rare[b]		
Pruritus						Rare[b]		
Rash	Rare					Rare[b]		
Wheezing	Rare	Rare				Rare[b]	2% to < 5%	
Urticaria	Rare					Rare[b]		
Respiratory								
Asthma symptoms						3% to 7%	2% to < 5%	≥ 2%
Bronchitis						1% to 3%	2% to < 5%	
Bronchospasm		2%						
Cough		2%			> 1%	4%	7%	2%
Epistaxis	< 3%	8%	4.9%	≤ 5%[d]	3% to 9%	6% to 7%[d]	1% to 13%[d]	3%
Mild nasopharyngeal irritation	24%							
Nasal burning/stinging				45%	13%	2% to 3%	✓[b]	
Nasal dryness	✓				> 1%			
Nasal irritation	✓	2%		≤ 5%		2% to 3%	2% to < 5%	
Nasal mucosal ulceration	Rare					Rare[b]	Rare	
Nasal septal perforation	Rare	Rare[b]		Rare	Rare	Rare[b]	Rare[b]	Rare

Intranasal Steroids

Intranasal Steroids Adverse Reactions (%)[a]								
Adverse reaction	Beclomethasone	Budesonide	Ciclesonide	Flunisolide (nasal solution)	Flunisolide (nasal spray)	Fluticasone	Mometasone	Triamcinolone
Nasal stuffiness/ congestion	< 3%			≤ 5%				
Nasopharyngitis			6.6%					
Pharyngitis		4%			> 1%	6% to 8%	12%	5%
Pharyngolaryngeal pain			3.4%					
Rhinitis							2% to < 5%	≥ 2%
Rhinorrhea	< 3%					1% to 3%		
Sinusitis					≤ 1%		5%	≥ 2%
Sneezing	4%			≤ 5%				
Throat discomfort (burning, itching, swelling, pain)		Rare[b]		≤ 5		Rare[b]		
Throat dryness/ irritation	✓	Rare[b]				Rare[b]		
Upper respiratory tract infection							5% to 6%	
Special senses								
Aftertaste					17%			
Blurred vision						✓[b]		
Cataracts	Rare					Rare[b]		
Conjunctivitis						✓[b]	2% to < 5%	
Dry/Irritated eyes						✓[b]		
Earache			2.2%				2% to < 5%	
Glaucoma	Rare					Rare[b]		
Hoarseness					≤ 1	Rare[b]		
Increased intraocular pressure	Rare	Rare				Rare[b]	Rare	
Loss of taste/smell	Rare	Rare[b]		≤ 5%	≤ 1%	✓[b]	Rare[b]	
Otitis media							2% to < 5%	≥ 2%
Unpleasant taste/ smell	✓							
Watery eyes	< 3%			≤ 5%				
Miscellaneous								
Aches and pains						1% to 3%		
Arthralgia							2% to < 5%	
Chest pain							2% to < 5%	
Dysmenorrhea							5%	
Fever						1% to 3%		
Flu-like symptoms						1% to 3%	2% to < 5%	
Growth suppression	✓	✓				✓[b]		
Infection	Rare[e]	Rare[e]		Rare[e]	Rare[e]	Rare[e]	Rare[e]	Rare[e]
Myalgia							2% to < 5%	
Palpitations		Rare[b]						
Viral infection							14%	
Voice changes						Rare[b]		

[a] Data pooled from all age groups and from separate studies and are not necessarily comparable.
[b] Occurred during postmarketing.
[c] ✓ = reported; no incidence given.
[d] Including bloody mucus.
[e] Localized infections of the nose and pharynx with *Candida albicans*.

Overdosage

Acute overdosage is unlikely with intranasal corticosteroids. However, chronic overdosage may occur and result in hypercorticism and adrenal suppression. If such symptoms occur, slowly discontinue intranasal corticosteroids consistent with accepted procedures for discontinuing oral steroid therapy.

Patient Information

Instruct patients to read the patient instructions provided with the product.

Advise patients that effects may not be immediate and not to exceed the recommended dosage. Benefit requires regular use and usually occurs within a few days. One to two weeks may pass before full effect is achieved.

Advise patients to contact their health care provider if symptoms worsen or do not improve by 3 weeks of treatment.

Instruct patients to clear nasal passages before use. If nasal passages are blocked, use of a topical nasal decongestant 5 to 10 minutes prior to administering the intranasal steroid may be beneficial.

Instruct patients to shake bottle gently before each use. Patients will also need to prime the pump the first time it is used and if it has not been used for more than a week.

Instruct patients to close the other nostril with a finger and tilt head slightly forward while using.

Advise patients to avoid blowing nose for at least 10 to 15 minutes after use.

Advise patients to avoid spraying into eyes or directly into nasal septum.

Advise patients not to use the bottle for more than the labeled number of sprays, even if the bottle is not completely empty.

Advise patients on immunosuppressant doses of corticosteroids to avoid exposure to chickenpox or measles, and to seek medical advice if exposed.

Inform patients that nasal corticosteroids may result in the development of glaucoma and/or cataracts.

Advise patients to contact their health care provider if they experience recurrent episodes of epistaxis or nasal septum discomfort.

FLUNISOLIDE

Rx	**Flunisolide** (Bausch & Lomb)	**Solution**: 0.025% (25 mcg/actuation)[a]	In 25 mL nasal pump dispenser (200 sprays/bottle).
Rx	**Flunisolide** (Apotex)	**Solution**: 0.025% (29 mcg/actuation)[b]	In 25 mL nasal pump dispenser (200 sprays/bottle).

[a] With propylene glycol, polyethylene glycol 3350, benzalkonium chloride, EDTA.

[b] With PEG 400, benzalkonium chloride, edetate disodium.

FLUNISOLIDE — INTRANASAL

For complete and comparative prescribing information, refer to the Intranasal Steroids group monograph.

Indications

➤*Allergic rhinitis:* For the relief and management of nasal symptoms of seasonal and perennial allergic rhinitis.

Administration and Dosage

➤*Adults:*

Allergic rhinitis –

Usual dosage: 2 sprays in each nostril 2 times per day. The dose may be increased to 2 sprays in each nostril 3 times per day.

Maximum dose: 8 sprays in each nostril per day.

➤*Children:*

Allergic rhinitis –

15 years of age and older: See adults for dosing.

6 to 14 years of age:

• *Usual dosage* – 1 spray in each nostril 3 times per day or 2 sprays in each nostril 2 times per day.

• *Maximum dose* – 4 sprays in each nostril per day.

➤*Maintenance dose:* After the desired clinical effect is obtained, reduce the maintenance dose to the smallest amount necessary to control symptoms. Some patients with perennial allergic rhinitis may be maintained on 1 spray in each nostril per day.

➤*Duration of therapy:* Improvement in symptoms usually becomes apparent within a few days. However, relief may not occur in some patients for as long as 2 weeks. Do not use for more than 3 weeks in absence of significant symptomatic improvement.

➤*Preparation for administration:* Before use, prime the nasal spray by pushing down on the pump 5 or 6 times until a fine mist appears. If the pump has not been used for 5 days or more, the spray must be primed again.

➤*Administration:* Encourage patients with blocked nasal passages to use a decongestant just before administration to ensure adequate penetration of the spray. Advise patients to clear their nasal passages of secretions prior to use.

➤*Storage/Stability:* Store between 15° and 30°C (59° and 86°F).

BECLOMETHASONE DIPROPIONATE

Rx	**Beconase AQ** (GlaxoSmithKline)	**Spray**: 0.042% (42 mcg/actuation)[a]	In 25 g bottles (180 metered doses per bottle) with metering atomizing pump and nasal adapter.

[a] With dextrose, polysorbate 80, benzalkonium chloride, 0.25% v/w phenylethyl alcohol.

BECLOMETHASONE DIPROPIONATE MONOHYDRATE — INTRANASAL

For complete and comparative prescribing information, refer to the Intranasal Steroids group monograph.

Indications

➤*Rhinitis:* For the relief of symptoms of seasonal or perennial allergic and nonallergic (vasomotor) rhinitis.

Results from 2 clinical trials have shown that significant symptom relief was obtained within 3 days. However, symptom relief may not occur in some patients for as long as 2 weeks.

➤*Nasal polyps:* For the prevention of recurrence of nasal polyps following surgical removal.

Administration and Dosage

➤*General dosing considerations:* The therapeutic effects of corticosteroids, unlike those of a decongestant on allergic rhinitis or on nasal polyps, are not immediate, this should be explained to the patient in advance in order to ensure cooperation and continuation of treatment with the prescribed dosage regimen.

A topical or oral nasal vasoconstrictor/decongestant may need to be used during the first 2-3 days of therapy. (See Concomitant Therapy.)

➤*Adults:*

Rhinitis – 1 or 2 nasal inhalations (42 to 84 mcg) in each nostril twice a day (total dose, 168 to 336 mcg/day).

Nasal polyps – 1 or 2 nasal inhalations (42 to 84 mcg) in each nostril twice a day (total dose, 168 to 336 mcg/day).

➤*Children:*

Rhinitis –

Children 12 years of age and older: See Adults for dosing.

Children 6 to 12 years of age:

• *Maximum dose* – 2 sprays in each nostril twice daily (336 mcg/day).

• *Initial dosage* – 1 nasal inhalation in each nostril twice daily (168 mcg/day). Patients with more severe symptoms may use 2 inhalations in each nostril twice daily (336 mcg/day).

• *Dosage adjustment* – Patients not adequately responding may use 2 inhalations in each nostril (336 mcg/day). Once adequate control is achieved, the dosage should be decreased to 1 spray in each nostril twice daily (168 mcg/day).

Nasal polyps – See Rhinitis.

➤*Concomitant therapy:* In the presence of excessive nasal mucus secretion or edema of the nasal mucosa, the drug may fail to reach the sites of intended action. In such cases it is advisable to use a topical or oral nasal vasoconstrictor/decongestant during the first 2 to 3 days of beclomethasone therapy.

➤*Duration of therapy:* Beclomethasone should not be continued beyond 3 weeks in the absence of significant symptom improvement.

➤*Administration:* Avoid spraying in eyes. The nasal spray should be shaken well before use.

➤*Storage/Stability:* Store between 15° and 30°C (59° and 86°F).

TRIAMCINOLONE ACETONIDE

Rx	**Triamcinolone Acetonide** (Barr Labs)	**Spray, suspension; intranasal**: 55 mcg/actuation	Benzalkonium chloride, dextrose, edetate disodium. In 16.5 g bottles (providing 120 actuations) with metered-dose pump unit and nasal adapter.
Rx	**Nasacort AQ** (Sanofi-Aventis)		Benzalkonium chloride, dextrose, polysorbate 80, edetate disodium. In 16.5 g bottles (providing 120 actuations) with metered-dose pump unit and nasal adapter.

TRIAMCINOLONE ACETONIDE — INTRANASAL

For complete and comparative prescribing information, refer to the Intranasal Steroids class monograph.

Indications

➤*Allergic rhinitis:* For the treatment of the nasal symptoms of seasonal and perennial allergic rhinitis in adults and children 2 years of age and older.

Administration and Dosage

➤*Adults:*

Allergic rhinitis –

Maximum dose: 220 mcg/day as 2 sprays in each nostril once daily.

Initial dosage: 220 mcg/day as 2 sprays in each nostril once daily.

Dosage adjustment: Titrate an individual patient to the minimum effective dose to reduce the possibility of side effects. When the maximum benefit has been achieved and symptoms have been controlled, reducing the dosage to 110 mcg/day (1 spray in each nostril once a day) has been shown to be effective in maintaining control of the allergic rhinitis symptoms.

➤*Children:*

Allergic rhinitis –

12 years of age and older: See Adults for dosing.

6 to 12 years of age:

• *Maximum dose* – 220 mcg/day as 2 sprays in each nostril once daily.

• *Initial dosage* – 110 mcg/day given as 1 spray in each nostril once daily.

• *Dosage adjustment* – Children not responding adequately to 110 mcg/day may use 220 mcg/day (2 sprays in each nostril once daily). Once symptoms have been controlled, the dosage may be decreased to 110 mcg once daily.

2 to 5 years of age:

• *Maximum dose* – 110 mcg/day as 1 spray in each nostril once daily.

TRIAMCINOLONE ACETONIDE — INTRANASAL

• *Initial dosage* – 110 mcg/day as 1 spray in each nostril once daily.

➤*Discontinuation of therapy:* If adequate relief of symptoms has not been obtained after 3 weeks of treatment, triamcinolone should be discontinued.

➤*Preparation for administration:* Prime the spray before using for the first time by shaking the contents well and releasing 5 sprays into the air, away from the face. It will remain adequately primed for 2 weeks. If the product is not used for more than 2 weeks, then it can be adequately reprimed with 1 spray.

➤*Administration:* For intranasal use only. Shake well before each use.

➤*Storage/Stability:* Store at 20° to 25°C (68° to 77°F). Discard the bottle when the labeled number of actuations (120) have been reached, even though the bottle is not completely empty.

BUDESONIDE

Rx	**Rhinocort Aqua** (AstraZeneca)	**Spray, suspension; intranasal**: 32 mcg/actuation[a]	In 8.6 g bottles (120 metered sprays) with metered-dose pump.

[a] Dextrose, polysorbate 80, EDTA.

BUDESONIDE — INTRANASAL

For complete and comparative prescribing information, refer to the Intranasal Steroids group monograph.

Indications

➤*Seasonal or perennial allergic rhinitis:* For the management of nasal symptoms of seasonal or perennial allergic rhinitis in adults and children 6 years of age and older.

Administration and Dosage

➤*Maximum dose:*

Adults and children 12 years of age and older – 256 mcg/day (4 sprays per nostril once daily).

Children 6 to younger than 12 years of age – 128 mcg/day (2 sprays per nostril once daily).

➤*General dosing considerations:* It is always desirable to titrate an individual patient to the minimum effective dose to reduce the possibility of side effects. Some patients who do not achieve symptom control at the recommended starting dose may benefit from an increased dose. When the maximum benefit has been achieved and symptoms have been controlled, reducing the dose may be effective in maintaining control of allergic rhinitis symptoms in patients who were initially controlled on higher doses.

An improvement in nasal symptoms may be noted in patients within 10 hours of first using budesonide nasal spray.

➤*Adults:*

Seasonal or perennial allergic rhinitis –

Maximum dose: 256 mcg/day (4 sprays per nostril once daily).
Initial dosage: 64 mcg/day (1 spray per nostril once daily).

➤*Children:*

Seasonal or perennial allergic rhinitis –

Maximum dose:
• *12 years of age and older* – 256 mcg/day (4 sprays per nostril once daily).
• *6 to 11 years of age* – 128 mcg/day (2 sprays per nostril once daily).

Initial dosage:
• *6 years of age and older* – 64 mcg/day (1 spray per nostril once daily).

➤*Preparation for administration:* Prior to initial use, shake the container gently and prime the pump by actuating 8 times. If used daily, the pump does not need to be reprimed. If not used for 2 consecutive days, reprime with 1 spray or until a fine spray appears. If not used for more than 14 days, rinse the applicator and reprime with 2 sprays or until a fine spray appears.

➤*Storage/Stability:* Store at controlled room temperature, 20° to 25°C (68° to 77°F), with the valve up. Do not freeze. Protect from light.

FLUTICASONE

Rx	**Fluticasone Propionate** (Par)	**Spray; intranasal**: 50 mcg/actuation[a] (as propionate)	In 16 g (120 actuations) amber glass bottles with metering atomizing pump and nasal adapter.
Rx	**Flonase** (GlaxoSmithKline)		In 16 g (120 actuations) amber glass bottles with metering atomizing pump and nasal adapter.
Rx	**Veramyst** (GlaxoSmithKline)	**Spray, suspension; intranasal**: 27.5 mcg/actuation[b] (as furoate)	In 10 g (120 actuations) brown glass bottles with metering atomizing pump and nasal adapter.

[a] With dextrose, polysorbate 80, 0.02% w/w benzalkonium chloride, 0.25% w/w phenylethyl alcohol.

[b] With dextrose, 0.015% w/w benzalkonium chloride, polysorbate 80, EDTA.

FLUTICASONE PROPIONATE — INTRANASAL

For complete and comparative prescribing information, refer to the Intranasal Steroids group monograph.

Indications

➤*Allergic and nonallergic rhinitis:* For the management of the nasal symptoms of seasonal and perennial allergic and nonallergic rhinitis in adults and pediatric patients 4 years of age and older.

Administration and Dosage

➤*General dosing considerations:* Greater symptom control may be achieved with scheduled regular use. Maximum effect may take several days.

➤*Adults:*

Allergic and nonallergic rhinitis –

Maximum dose: 2 sprays in each nostril daily (200 mcg/day).
Initial dosage: 2 sprays (50 mcg each) in each nostril once daily (total daily dose, 200 mcg). The same dosage divided into 100 mcg given twice daily (eg, 8 am and 8 pm) is also effective.
Maintenance dosage: After the first few days, patients may be able to reduce their dosage to 100 mcg (1 spray in each nostril) once daily.
Seasonal allergic rhinitis: May find as-needed use (not to exceed 200 mcg daily) effective for symptom control.

➤*Children:*

Allergic and nonallergic rhinitis –

4 years of age and older:
• *Maximum dose* – 2 sprays in each nostril (200 mcg/day).
• *Initial dosage* – 100 mcg (1 spray in each nostril once daily).
• *Dosage titration* – Patients not adequately responding to 100 mcg may use 200 mcg (2 sprays in each nostril once daily or 1 spray in each nostril twice daily).
• *Maintenance dosage* – Once adequate control is achieved, the dosage should be decreased to 100 mcg (1 spray in each nostril) daily.
• *Seasonal allergic rhinitis* – For children 12 years of age and older, some may find as-needed use (not to exceed 200 mcg daily) effective for symptom control.

➤*Preparation for administration:* Shake gently before use.

➤*Storage/Stability:* Store between 4° and 30°C (39° and 86°F).

FLUTICASONE FUROATE — INTRANASAL

For complete and comparative prescribing information, refer to the Intranasal Steroids group monograph.

Indications

➤*Allergic rhinitis:* For the treatment of the symptoms of seasonal and perennial allergic rhinitis in patients 2 years of age and older.

Administration and Dosage

➤*Adults:*

Allergic rhinitis –

Initial dosage: 110 mcg once daily administered as 2 sprays (27.5 mcg/spray) in each nostril.
Dosage adjustment: Titrate to the minimum effective dosage to reduce the possibility of adverse reactions. When the maximum benefit has been achieved and symptoms have been controlled, reducing the dose to 55 mcg (1 spray in each nostril) once daily might be effective in maintaining control of symptoms.

➤*Children:*

Allergic rhinitis –

12 years of age and older: See Adults for dosing.
2 to 11 years of age:
• *Initial dosage* – 55 mcg once daily administered as 1 spray (27.5 mcg/spray) in each nostril.
• *Dosage adjustment* – If response is not adequate, may increase to 110 mcg (2 sprays in each nostril) once daily. Once symptoms have been controlled, the dose may be decreased to 55 mcg once daily.

Intranasal Steroids

FLUTICASONE FUROATE — INTRANASAL

➤*Preparation for administration:* Prime before using for the first time by shaking the contents well and releasing 6 test sprays into the air away from the face. When fluticasone has not been used for more than 30 days or if the cap has been left off the bottle for 5 days or longer, prime the pump again until a fine mist appears. Shake well before each use.

➤*Storage/Stability:* Store the device between 15° and 30°C (59° and 86°F) in the upright position with the cap in place. Do not freeze or refrigerate. Discard the nasal device after 120 sprays have been used, even though the bottle is not completely empty.

MOMETASONE FUROATE

Rx	**Nasonex** (Schering)	**Spray, suspension; intranasal:** 0.05% (50 mcg/actuation)	In 17 g bottles (120 sprays) with metered-dose manual spray pump.

MOMETASONE FUROATE — INTRANASAL

For complete and comparative prescribing information, refer to the Intranasal Steroids class monograph.

Indications

➤*Allergic rhinitis:* For the treatment of the nasal symptoms of seasonal allergic and perennial allergic rhinitis in adults and children 2 years of age and older.

➤*Nasal congestion associated with seasonal rhinitis:* For the relief of nasal congestion associated with seasonal allergic rhinitis in adults and children 2 years of age and older.

➤*Nasal polyps:* For the treatment of nasal polyps in patients 18 years of age and older.

➤*Prophylaxis of seasonal allergic rhinitis:* For the prophylaxis of the nasal symptoms of seasonal allergic rhinitis in adults and children 12 years of age and older.

Administration and Dosage

➤*General dosing considerations:* Prophylaxis for seasonal allergic rhinitis with mometasone is recommended 2 to 4 weeks prior to the anticipated start of the pollen season.

➤*Adults:*

Allergic rhinitis – 2 sprays in each nostril once daily.

Nasal polyps –

Usual dosage: 2 sprays in each nostril twice daily.

Alternative dosage: 2 sprays in each nostril once daily is also effective in some patients.

➤*Children:*

Allergic rhinitis –

12 years of age and older: 2 sprays in each nostril once daily.

2 to 11 years of age: 1 spray in each nostril once daily.

Prophylaxis of seasonal allergic rhinitis –

12 years of age and older: 2 sprays in each nostril once daily 2 to 4 weeks prior to the anticipated start of the pollen season.

➤*Administration:* For intranasal use only. Prior to initial use, the pump must be primed by actuating 10 times or until a fine spray appears. The pump may be stored unused for up to 1 week without repriming. If unused for more than 1 week, reprime by actuating 2 times or until a fine spray appears. Shake well before each use.

➤*Storage/Stability:* Store at 25°C (77°F); excursions permitted between 15° and 30°C (59° and 86°F). Protect from light. When mometasone is removed from its cardboard container, avoid prolonged exposure of the product to direct light. Brief exposure to light, as with normal use, is acceptable.

CICLESONIDE

Rx	**Omnaris** (Sepracor)	**Spray, suspension; intranasal:** 50 mcg/actuation	Edetate sodium. In 12.5 g glass bottle (120 actuations) with metered-dose pump with oxygen absorber sachet.

CICLESONIDE — INTRANASAL

Indications

➤*Perennial allergic rhinitis:* For the treatment of nasal symptoms associated with perennial allergic rhinitis in adults and adolescents 12 years of age and older.

➤*Seasonal allergic rhinitis:* For the treatment of nasal symptoms associated with seasonal allergic rhinitis in adults and children 6 years of age and older.

Administration and Dosage

➤*Adults:*

Perennial allergic rhinitis –

Usual dosage: 200 mcg/day, administered as 2 sprays (50 mcg/spray) in each nostril once daily.

Maximum dose: 2 sprays in each nostril per day (200 mcg/day).

Seasonal allergic rhinitis –

Usual dosage: 200 mcg/day, administered as 2 sprays (50 mcg/spray) in each nostril once daily.

Maximum dose: 2 sprays in each nostril per day (200 mcg/day).

➤*Children:*

Perennial allergic rhinitis –

12 years of age and older: See Adults for dosing.

Seasonal allergic rhinitis –

6 years of age and older: See Adults for dosing.

➤*Preparation for administration:* Prior to initial use, ciclesonide must be shaken gently and then the pump must be primed by actuating 8 times. If the product is not used for 4 consecutive days, it should be shaken gently and reprimed with 1 spray or until a fine mist appears. Do not spray in eyes.

➤*Storage/Stability:* Store at 25°C (77°F); excursions are permitted between 15° and 30°C (59° and 86°F). Do not freeze.

Mucolytics

ACETYLCYSTEINE (N-Acetylcysteine)

Rx	**Acetylcysteine** (Various, eg, American Regent, Hospira, Mayne)	**Solution; inhalation:** 10%	May contain disodium edetate. In 4, 10 and 30 mL vials.
Rx	**Acetylcysteine** (Various, eg, American Regent, Hospira, Mayne)	**Solution, concentrate; inhalation:** 20%	May contain disodium edetate. In 4, 10, and 30 mL vials.

ACETYLCYSTEINE — INHALATION

Indications

➤*Mucolytic:* As adjuvant therapy for patients with abnormal, viscid, or inspissated mucous secretions in such conditions as: chronic bronchopulmonary disease (chronic emphysema, emphysema with bronchitis, chronic asthmatic bronchitis, tuberculosis, bronchiectasis and primary amyloidosis of the lung); acute bronchopulmonary disease (pneumonia, bronchitis, tracheobronchitis); pulmonary complications of cystic fibrosis; tracheostomy care; pulmonary complications associated with surgery; use during anesthesia; posttraumatic chest conditions; atelectasis due to mucous obstruction; diagnostic bronchial studies (bronchograms, bronchospirometry, and bronchial wedge catheterization).

➤*Off-label uses:*

Keratoconjunctivitis sicca (dry eye syndrome) – [4] = Insufficient documentation. Initial data from a limited number of trials suggest that ocular acetylcysteine may be of benefit in patients with keratoconjunctivitis sicca by reducing mucous production in the eye; however, these trials are dated. Larger trials are needed to establish the role of this agent in therapy. (See Administration and Dosage.)

Other possible off-label uses – Acetylcysteine has been used as an enema to treat bowel obstruction due to meconium ileus or its equivalent.

Administration and Dosage

➤*General dosing considerations:* The 20% solution may be diluted to a lesser concentration and the 10% solution may be used undiluted. (See Preparation for Administration.)

➤*Adults:*

Diagnostic bronchial studies – 2 or 3 administrations of 1 to 2 mL of the 20% solution or 2 to 4 mL of the 10% solution should be given by nebulization or by instillation intratracheally, prior to the procedure.

Abnormal, viscid, or inspissated mucous secretions – 1 to 2 mL of a 10% solution may be given as often as every hour.

Direct instillation into a particular segment of the bronchopulmonary tree: Insert (under local anesthesia and direct vision) a small plastic catheter into the trachea. 2 to 5 mL of the 20% solution may then be instilled by means of a syringe connected to the catheter.

ACETYLCYSTEINE — INHALATION

Direct instillation into percutaneous intratracheal catheter: 1 to 2 mL of the 20% or 2 to 4 mL of the 10% solution every 1 to 4 hours given by a syringe attached to the catheter.

Direct instillation for routine care of tracheostomy: 1 to 2 mL of a 10% or 20% solution given every 1 to 4 hours by instillation into the tracheostomy.

Nebulization with face mask, mouth piece, tracheostomy:

- *Usual dosage* – 3 to 5 mL of the 20% solution or 6 to 10 mL of the 10% solution 3 to 4 times a day.
- *Alternative dosage* – 1 to 10 mL of the 20% solution or 2 to 20 mL of the 10% solution may be given every 2 to 6 hours.

Nebulization with tent, croupette: Recommended dose is the volume of acetylcysteine (using 10% or 20%) that will maintain a very heavy mist in the tent or croupette for the desired period, occasionally as much as 300 mL during a single treatment period. Administration for intermittent or continuous prolonged periods, including overnight, may be desirable.

Off-label dosing –

Keratoconjunctivitis sicca (dry eye syndrome): [4] = Insufficient documentation. 1 drop of a 20% ophthalmic solution in each eye every 2 hours (while awake).

➤*Children:* See Adults for dosing.

Off-label dosing –

Mucolytic:

Acetylcysteine Inhalation Dosage in Children

Age	Acetylcysteine 10% dosage	Acetylcysteine 20% dosage	Frequency
13 to 17 years of age	5 to 10 mL	5 to 10 mL	3 or 4 times per day
1 to 12 years of age	6 to 10 mL	3 to 5 mL[a]	3 or 4 times per day
30 days to 1 year of age	2 to 4 mL	1 to 2 mL[a]	3 or 4 times per day

[a] Dilute with an equal volume of sterile water or sterile saline to a final concentration of 10%.

➤*Preparation for administration:* The 20% solution may be diluted to a lesser concentration with sodium chloride inhalation solution, sodium chloride injection, sterile water for injection, or sterile water for inhalation. The 10% solution may be used undiluted. If it is deemed advisable to prepare an admixture, it should be administered as soon as possible after preparation (within 1 hour). Do not store unused mixtures.

➤*Administration:* Acetylcysteine is usually administered as fine nebulae, and the nebulizer used should be capable of providing optimal quantities of a suitable range of particle sizes. The nebulized solution may be inhaled directly from the nebulizer. Nebulizers may also be attached to plastic face masks, plastic mouthpieces, plastic face tents, conventional plastic oxygen tents, or head tents. Suitable nebulizers may also be fitted for use with the various intermittent positive pressure breathing machines.

When three-fourths of the initial volume of acetylcysteine solution has been nebulized, a quantity of sterile water for injection (approximately equal to the volume of solution remaining), should be added to the nebulizer. This obviates any concentration of the agent in the residual solvent remaining after prolonged nebulization.

Acetylcysteine should not be placed directly into the chamber of a heated (hot pot) nebulizer. A heated nebulizer may be part of the nebulization assembly to provide a warm saturated atmosphere if the acetylcysteine aerosol is introduced by means of a separate unheated nebulizer. Usual precautions for administration of warm saturated nebulae should be observed.

➤*Admixture compatibility:*

Acetylcysteine Inhalation Solution Compatibility[a] Tests

Product or agent	Compatibility rating	Ratio tested[b]: Acetylcysteine	Ratio tested[b]: Product or agent
Anesthetic, gas			
Halothane	Compatible	20%	Infinite
Nitrous oxide	Compatible	20%	Infinite
Anesthetic, local			
Cocaine	Compatible	10%	5%
Lidocaine	Compatible	10%	2%
Tetracaine	Compatible	10%	1%
Antibacterials (a parenteral form of each antibiotic was used)			
Bacitracin[c,d] (mix and use at once)	Compatible	10%	5,000 U/mL
Chloramphenicol sodium succinate	Compatible	20%	20 mg/mL
Carbenicillin disodium[c] (mix and use at once)	Compatible	10%	125 mg/mL
Gentamicin sulfate[c]	Compatible	10%	20 mg/mL
Kanamycin sulfate[c] (mix and use at once)	Compatible	10%	167 mg/mL
	Compatible	17%	85 mg/mL
Lincomycin[c]	Compatible	10%	150 mg/mL
Neomycin sulfate[c]	Compatible	10%	100 mg/mL
Novobiocin sodium[c]	Compatible	10%	25 mg/mL
Penicillin G potassium[c] (mix and use at once)	Compatible	10%	25,000 U/mL
			100,000 U/mL
Polymyxin B sulfate[c]	Compatible	10%	50,000 U/mL
Cephalothin sodium	Compatible	10%	110 mg/mL
Colistimethate sodium[c] (mix and use at once)	Compatible	10%	37.5 mg/mL
Vancomycin[c]	Compatible	10%	25 mg/mL
Amphotericin B	Incompatible	4% to 15%	1 to 4 mg/mL
Chlortetracycline[c]	Incompatible	10%	12.5 mg/mL
Erythromycin lactobionate	Incompatible	10%	15 mg/mL
Oxytetracycline	Incompatible	10%	12.5 mg/mL
Ampicillin sodium	Incompatible	10%	50 mg/mL
Tetracycline	Incompatible	10%	12.5 mg/mL
Bronchodilators			
Isoproterenol[c]	Compatible	3%	0.5%
Isoproterenol[c]	Compatible	10%	0.05%
Isoproterenol[c]	Compatible	20%	0.05%
Isoproterenol	Compatible	13.3% (2 parts)	0.33% (1 part)
Isoetharine	Compatible	13.3% (2 parts)	(1 part)
Epinephrine	Compatible	13.3% (2 parts)	0.33% (1 part)
Contrast media			
Iodized oil	Incompatible	20%/20 mL	40%/10 mL
Decongestants			
Phenylephrine[c]	Compatible	3%	0.25%
Phenylephrine	Compatible	13.3% (2 parts)	0.17% (1 part)
Enzymes			
Chymotrypsin	Incompatible	5%	400 gamma/mL
Trypsin	Incompatible	5%	400 gamma/mL
Solvents			
Alcohol	Compatible	12%	10% to 20%
Propylene glycol	Compatible	3%	10%
Steroids			
Dexamethasone sodium phosphate	Compatible	16%	0.8 mg/mL
Prednisolone sodium phosphate[e]	Compatible	16.7%	3.3 mg/mL
Other agents			
Hydrogen peroxide	Incompatible	(All ratios)	
Sodium bicarbonate	Compatible	20% (1 part)	4.2% (1 part)

[a] The rating, incompatible, is based on the formation of a precipitate, a change in clarity, immiscibility or a rapid loss of potency of acetylcysteine or the active ingredient of the product or agent in the admixture. The rating, compatible, means that there was no significant physical change in the admixture when compared with a control solution of the product or agent, and that there was no predicted chemical incompatibility. All of the admixtures have been tested for short-term chemical compatibility by assaying for the concentration of acetylcysteine after mixing.

[b] Entries are final corrections. Values in parentheses relate volumes of acetylcysteine solution to volume of test solutions.

[c] The active ingredient in the product or agent was also assayed after mixing. Some of the admixtures developed minor physical changes, which were considered to be insufficient to rate the admixture incompatible. These are listed in footnotes d and e.

[d] A strong odor developed after storage for 24 hours at room temperature.

[e] A light tan color developed after storage for 24 hours at room temperature.

ACETYLCYSTEINE — INHALATION

➤*Storage/Stability:* Store unopened vials at 20° to 25°C (68° to 77°F); excursions are permitted between 15° and 30°C (59° and 86°F). Use freshly prepared solution within one hour. If only a portion of the solution in a vial is used, store the remainder in a refrigerator and use for inhalation only within 96 hours. The nebulizing equipment should be cleaned immediately after use because the residues may clog the smaller orifices or corrode metal parts.

Actions

➤*Pharmacology:* The viscosity of pulmonary mucous secretions depends on the concentrations of mucoprotein and to a lesser extent DNA. The latter increases with increasing purulence owing to the presence of cellular debris. The mucolytic action of acetylcysteine is related to the sulfhydryl group in the molecule. This group probably "opens" disulfide linkages in mucous, thereby lowering the viscosity. The mucolytic activity of acetylcysteine is unaltered by the presence of DNA, and increases with increasing pH. Significant mucolysis occurs between pH 7 and 9.

Acetylcysteine undergoes rapid deacetylation in vivo to yield cysteine or oxidation to yield diacetylcystine.

Occasionally, patients exposed to the inhalation of an acetylcysteine aerosol respond with the development of increased airway obstruction of varying and unpredictable severity. Those patients who are reactors cannot be identified a priori from a random patient population. Even when patients are known to have reacted previously to the inhalation of an acetylcysteine aerosol, they may not react during a subsequent treatment. The converse is also true; patients who have had inhalation treatments of acetylcysteine without incident may still react to a subsequent inhalation with increased airway obstruction. Most patients with bronchospasm are quickly relieved by the use of a bronchodilator given by nebulization. If bronchospasm progresses, the medication should be discontinued immediately.

➤*Pharmacokinetics:*

Distribution – The steady-state volume of distribution and the protein binding for acetylcysteine were reported to be 0.47 L/kg and 83%, respectively.

Metabolism/Excretion – Acetylcysteine may form cysteine, disulfides, and conjugates in vivo (eg, N, N'-diacetylcysteine, N-acetylcysteine-cysteine, N-acetylcysteine-glutathione, N-acetylcysteine-protein). Based on published data, it was reported that after an oral dose of ^{35}S-acetylcysteine, approximately 22% of total radioactivity was excreted in urine after 24 hours. No metabolites were identified.

After a single intravenous (IV) dose of acetylcysteine, the plasma concentration of total acetylcysteine declined in a polyexponential decay manner with a mean terminal half-life of 5.6 hours. The mean clearance for acetylcysteine was reported to be 0.11 L/h/kg and renal clearance constituted approximately 30% of total clearance.

Special populations –

Renal function impairment: Pharmacokinetic information is not available.

Hepatic function impairment: In subjects with severe liver damage (ie, cirrhosis caused by alcohol [with Child-Pugh score of 7 to 13]) or primary and/or secondary biliary cirrhosis (with Child-Pugh score of 5 to 7), mean half-life increased by 80%, while mean clearance decreased by 30% compared with control group.

Elderly: Adequate information on acetylcysteine pharmacokinetics in elderly patients is not available.

Children: The mean elimination half-life of acetylcysteine is longer in newborns (11 hours) than in adults (5.6 hours).

Gender: Adequate info is not available to assess if there are differences in pharmacokinetics between men and women.

Contraindications

Sensitivity to acetylcysteine.

Warnings/Precautions

➤*Bronchial secretions:* After proper administration of acetylcysteine, an increased volume of liquified bronchial secretions may occur. When cough is inadequate, the open airway must be maintained by mechanical suction if necessary. When there is a mechanical block due to foreign body or local accumulation, the airway should be cleared by endotracheal aspiration, with or without bronchoscopy. Asthmatics under treatment with acetylcysteine should be watched carefully. Most patients with bronchospasm are quickly relieved by the use of a bronchodilator given by nebulization. If bronchospasm progresses, this medication should be discontinued immediately.

➤*Administration:* With administration, the patient may initially notice a slight disagreeable odor that is soon not noticeable. With a face mask there may be a stickiness on the face after nebulization. This is easily removed by washing with water.

Under certain conditions, a color change may occur in the solution of acetylcysteine in the opened bottle. The light purple color is the result of a chemical reaction that does not significantly affect the safety or mucolytic effectiveness of acetylcysteine.

➤*Continued nebulization:* Continued nebulization of an acetylcysteine solution with a dry gas will result in an increased concentration of the drug in the nebulizer because of evaporation of the solvent. Extreme concentration may impede nebulization and efficient delivery of the drug. Dilution of the nebulizing solution with appropriate amounts of sterile water for injection, as a concentration occurs, will obviate this problem.

➤*Pregnancy:* *Category B.* There are no adequate and well-controlled studies in pregnant women. Consistent with its low molecular weight (approximately 163), acetylcysteine crosses the human placenta. Because animal reproduction studies may not always be predictive of human responses, this drug should be used during pregnancy only if clearly needed. A 1999 report concluded that acetaminophen overdose in pregnant women should be managed the same way as in nonpregnant patients and that acetylcysteine therapy was protective to both the mother and the fetus.

➤*Lactation:* It is not known whether this drug is excreted in human milk. The molecular weight of the drug (approximately 163) is low enough for excretion into breast milk. Because many drugs are excreted in human milk, caution should be exercised when acetylcysteine is administered to a breastfeeding woman. IV acetylcysteine has been administered directly to preterm neonates for therapeutic indications at doses far above those that would be obtained from milk, without causing toxicity.

➤*Monitoring:* Monitor for the development of airway obstruction.

Drug Interactions

None well documented.

Adverse Reactions

➤*GI:* Stomatitis, nausea, and vomiting.

➤*Hypersensitivity:* Acquired sensitization to acetylcysteine have been reported rarely.

➤*Respiratory:* Bronchoconstriction. Clinically overt acetylcysteine-induced bronchospasm occurs infrequently and unpredictably, even in patients with asthmatic bronchitis or bronchitis complicating bronchial asthma. Reports of irritation to the tracheal and bronchial tracts have been received, and although hemoptysis has occurred in patients receiving acetylcysteine, such findings are not uncommon in patients with bronchopulmonary disease and a causal relationship has not been established.

➤*Miscellaneous:* Chest tightness, clamminess, drowsiness, fever, rhinorrhea.

Patient Information

Advise the patient or caregiver that medication has a disagreeable odor (rotten eggs) but that this should become unnoticeable after continued use.

Advise the patient or caregiver that treatment is expected to increase volume of respiratory secretions and that effective coughing will be required to clear the secretions. Advise the patient or caregiver to immediately notify their health care provider if respiratory secretions cannot be adequately removed by coughing.

Advise the patient that medication may turn a light purple color after opening the bottle. Advise the patient that this is normal and does not alter the safety or effectiveness of the medication.

Caution the patient or caregiver to dilute the nebulizer solution to prevent the solution from becoming concentrated and plugging the nebulizer.

Caution the patient or caregiver not to add other medications or solutions to the nebulizer canister unless advised by their health care provider.

Advise the patient or caregiver to notify their health care provider if any of the following occur: rash or other signs or allergic reaction, new or worsening wheezing, chest tightness or difficulty breathing, persistent nausea or vomiting, coughing up blood, fever, or other signs of respiratory infection.

Advise the patient or caregiver that administration using a face mask may leave a sticky residue on the face that can be easily removed by washing with water.

DORNASE ALFA (Recombinant human deoxyribonuclease; DNase)

Rx	**Pulmozyme** (Genentech)	**Solution for inhalation:** 1 mg/ml	Preservative free. With 0.15 mg/ml calcium chloride dihydrate and 8.77 mg/ml sodium chloride. In 2.5 ml amps.

DORNASE ALFA — INHALATION

Indications

➤*Cystic fibrosis:* Daily administration of dornase alfa in conjunction with standard therapies is indicated in the management of cystic fibrosis patients to improve pulmonary function. In patients with an FVC greater than or equal to 40% of predicted, daily administration of dornase alfa has also been shown to reduce the risk of respiratory tract infections requiring parenteral antibiotics.

Safety and efficacy of daily administration have not been demonstrated in patients for longer than 12 months.

DORNASE ALFA — INHALATION

Administration and Dosage

➤*General dosing considerations:* Use only with a recommended nebulizer. (See Administration.)

Dornase alfa should be used in conjunction with standard therapies for cystic fibrosis.

➤*Adults:*

Cystic fibrosis –

Usual dosage: 2.5 mg inhaled once daily using a nebulizer. Some patients may benefit from twice daily administration.

➤*Children:*

Cystic fibrosis –

5 years of age and older:

• *Usual dosage* – 2.5 mg inhaled once daily using a nebulizer. Some patients may benefit from twice daily administration.

➤*Administration:* Patients should be advised to squeeze each ampule prior to use in order to check for leaks. Clinical trial results and laboratory information are only available to support use of the following nebulizer/compressor systems: *Hudson T Up-draft II* nebulizer with *Pulmo-Aide* compressor; *Marquest Acorn II* nebulizer with *Pulmo-Aide* compressor; *Pari LC Jet+* nebulizer with *Pari Proneb* compressor; *Pari Baby* nebulizer with *Pari Proneb* compressor; *Durable Sidestream* nebulizer with *Mobilaire* compressor; *Durable Sidestream* nebulizer with *Porta-Neb* compressor. Patients who are unable to inhale or exhale orally throughout the entire nebulization period may use the *Pari Baby* nebulizer.

Patients who use the *Sidestream* nebulizer with the *Mobilaire* compressor should turn the compressor control knob fully to the right and then turn on the compressor. At this setting, the needle on the pressure gauge should vibrate between 35 and 45 pounds per square inch (highest pressure output).

➤*Admixture compatibility:* Dornase alfa should not be diluted or mixed with other drugs in the nebulizer. Mixing of dornase alfa with other drugs could lead to adverse physicochemical or functional changes in dornase alfa or the admixed compound.

➤*Storage / Stability:* Store in foil packs at 2° to 8°C (36° to 46°F). Ampules should be protected from strong light.

Actions

➤*Pharmacology:* In cystic fibrosis patients, retention of viscous purulent secretions in the airways contributes both to reduced pulmonary function and to exacerbations of infection.

Purulent pulmonary secretions contain very high concentrations of extracellular DNA released by degenerating leukocytes that accumulate in response to infection. In vitro, dornase alfa hydrolyzes the DNA in sputum of cystic fibrosis patients and reduces sputum viscoelasticity.

➤*Pharmacokinetics:* When 2.5 mg dornase alfa was administered by inhalation to 18 cystic fibrosis patients, mean sputum concentrations of 3 mcg/mL DNase were measurable within 15 minutes. Mean sputum concentrations declined to an average of 0.6 mcg/mL 2 hours following inhalation. Inhalation of up to 10 mg three times a day of dornase alfa by 4 cystic fibrosis patients for 6 consecutive days, did not result in a significant elevation of serum concentrations of DNase above normal endogenous levels. After administration of up to 2.5 mg of dornase alfa twice daily for 6 months to 321 cystic fibrosis patients, no accumulation of serum DNase was noted.

Dornase alfa, 2.5 mg by inhalation, was administered daily to 98 patients aged 3 months to less than or equal to 10 years, and bronchoalveolar lavage (BAL) fluid was obtained within 90 minutes of the first dose. BAL DNase concentrations were detectable in all patients but showed a broad range, from 0.007 to 1.8 mcg/mL. Over an average of 14 days of exposure, serum DNase concentrations (mean ± SD) increased by 1.3 ± 1.3 ng/mL for the 3 months to less than 5 year age group and by 0.8 ± 1.2 ng/mL for the 5 to less than or equal to 10 year age group. The relationship between BAL or serum DNase concentration and adverse experiences and clinical outcomes is unknown.

Contraindications

Known hypersensitivity to dornase alfa, Chinese hamster ovary cell products, or any component of the product.

Warnings/Precautions

➤*Administration:* Dornase alfa should be used in conjunction with standard therapies for cystic fibrosis.

➤*Pregnancy:* Category B.

There are no adequate and well-controlled studies in pregnant women. Because animal reproductive studies are not always predictive of the human response, this drug should be used during pregnancy only if clearly needed.

➤*Lactation:* It is not known whether dornase alfa is excreted in human milk. Small amounts of dornase alfa were detected in maternal milk of cynomolgus monkeys when administered a bolus dose (100 mcg/kg) of dornase alfa followed by a 6 hour intravenous infusion (80 mcg/kg/hr). Little or no measurable dornase alfa would be expected in human milk after chronic aerosol administration of recommended doses. Because many drugs are excreted in human milk, caution should still be exercised when dornase alfa is administered to a nursing woman.

➤*Children:* Because of the limited experience with the administration of dornase alfa to patients younger than 5 years of age, its use should be considered only for those patients in whom there is a potential for benefit in pulmonary function or in risk of respiratory tract infection.

Drug Interactions

None known.

Adverse Reactions

In a randomized, placebo-controlled clinical trial in patients with FVC greater than or equal to 40% of predicted, over 600 patients received dornase alfa once or twice daily for 6 months; most adverse events were not more common on dornase alfa than on placebo and probably reflected the sequelae of the underlying lung disease. In most cases events that were increased were mild, transient in nature, and did not require alterations in dosing. Few patients experienced adverse events resulting in permanent discontinuation from dornase alfa, and the discontinuation rate was similar for placebo (2%) and dornase alfa (3%). Events that were more frequent (greater than 3%) in dornase alfa-treated patients than in placebo-treated patients are listed in the table below.

In a randomized, placebo-controlled trial of patients with advanced disease (FVC less than 40% of predicted) the safety profile for most adverse events was similar to that reported for the trial in patients with mild to moderate disease.

Adverse Reactions Increased ≥ 3% in Dornase Alfa-Treated Patients Over Placebo in Cystic Fibrosis Clinical Trials

Adverse event (of any severity or seriousness)	Trial in mild to moderate cystic fibrosis patients (FVC greater than or equal to 40% of predicted) treated for 24 weeks			Trial in advanced cystic fibrosis patients (FVC less than 40% of predicted) treated for 12 weeks	
	Placebo (n = 325)	Dornase alfa every day (n = 322)	Dornase alfa twice a day (n = 321)	Placebo (n = 159)	Dornase alfa every day (n = 161)
Voice alteration	7%	12%	16%	6%	18%
Pharyngitis	33%	36%	40%	28%	32%
Rash	7%	10%	12%	1%	3%
Laryngitis	1%	3%	4%	1%	3%
Chest pain	16%	18%	21%	23%	25%
Conjunctivitis	2%	4%	5%	0%	1%
Rhinitis	< 3%[a]	< 3%[a]	< 3%[a]	24%	30%
FVC decrease of ≥ 10% of predicted[b]	< 3%[a]	< 3%[a]	< 3%[a]	17%	22%
Fever	< 3%[a]	< 3%[a]	< 3%[a]	28%	32%
Dyspepsia	< 3%[a]	< 3%[a]	< 3%[a]	0%	3%
Dyspnea (when reported as serious)	< 3%[c]	< 3%[c]	< 3%[c]	12%[d]	17%[d]

[a] Differences were less than 3% for these adverse events in the trial in mild to moderate cystic fibrosis patients.
[b] Single measurement only, does not reflect overall FVC changes.
[c] Difference was less than 3% for this adverse event in the trial in mild to moderate cystic fibrosis patients.
[d] Total reports of dyspnea (regardless of severity or seriousness) had a difference of less than 3% for the trial in advanced cystic fibrosis patients.

➤*Events observed at similar rates in dornase alfa inhalation solution and placebo-treated patients with FVC greater than or equal to 40% of predicted:*

Allergic – There have been no reports of anaphylaxis attributed to the administration of dornase alfa to date. Urticaria, mild to moderate, and mild skin rash have been observed and have been transient. Within all of the studies, a small percentage (average of 2% to 4%) of patients treated with dornase alfa developed serum antibodies to dornase alfa. None of these patients developed anaphylaxis, and the clinical significance of serum antibodies to dornase alfa is unknown.

GI – Intestinal obstruction, gall bladder disease, liver disease, pancreatic disease.

Metabolic / Nutritional – Diabetes mellitus, hypoxia, weight loss.

Respiratory – Apnea, bronchiectasis, bronchitis, change in sputum, increased cough, dyspnea, hemoptysis, decreased lung function, nasal polyps, pneumonia, pneumothorax, rhinitis, sinusitis, increased sputum, wheeze.

Miscellaneous – Abdominal pain, asthenia, fever, flu syndrome, malaise, sepsis.

Mortality rates observed in controlled trials were similar for the placebo- and dornase alfa-treated patients. Causes of death were consistent with progression of cystic fibrosis and included apnea, cardiac arrest, cardiopulmonary arrest, cor pulmonale, heart failure, massive hemoptysis, pneumonia, pneumothorax, and respiratory failure.

The safety of dornase alfa, 2.5 mg by inhalation, was studied with 2 weeks of daily administration in 98 patients with cystic fibrosis (65 patients aged 3 months to less than 5 years, 33 patients aged 5 to less than or equal to 10 years). The *Pari Baby* reusable nebulizer (which uses a facemask instead of a mouthpiece) was utilized in patients unable to demonstrate the ability to inhale or exhale orally throughout the entire treatment period (54/65, 83% of the younger and 2/33, 6% of the older patients). The number of patients reporting cough was higher in the younger age group as compared to the older age group (29/65, 45% compared to 10/33, 30%) as was the number reporting moderate to severe cough (24/65, 37% as compared to 6/33, 18%). Other events tended to be of mild to moderate severity. The number of

Mucolytics

DORNASE ALFA — INHALATION

patients reporting rhinitis was higher in the younger age group as compared to the older age group (23/65, 35% compared to 9/33, 27%) as was the number reporting rash (4/65, 6% as compared to 0/33, 0%). The nature of adverse events was similar to that seen in the larger trials of dornase alfa inhalation solution.

Overdosage

Cystic fibrosis patients have received up to 20 mg twice daily for up to 6 days and 10 mg twice daily intermittently (2 weeks on/2 weeks off drug) for 168 days. These doses were well tolerated.

Patient Information

Store in the refrigerator at 2° to 8°C (36° to 46°F) and protect from strong light. It should be kept refrigerated during transport and should not be exposed to room temperatures for a total time of 24 hours. The solution should be discarded if it is cloudy or discolored. Dornase alfa contains no preservative and, once opened, the entire contents of the ampule must be used or discarded. Patients should be instructed in the proper use and maintenance of the nebulizer and compressor system used in its delivery.

Dornase alfa should not be diluted or mixed with other drugs in the nebulizer. Mixing of dornase alfa with other drugs could lead to adverse physicochemical and/or functional changes in dornase alfa or the admixed compound.

Mast Cell Stabilizers

CROMOLYN SODIUM (Disodium Cromoglycate)

Rx	**Cromolyn Sodium** (Various, eg, Alpharma, Dey)	**Solution for inhalation**: 20 mg per 2 mL	In 60 and 120 UD vials or amps.
Rx	**Intal** (King Pharm)	**Aerosol**: 800 mcg/actuation	In 8.1 g (≥ 112 metered sprays) and 14.2 g (≥ 200 metered sprays).
otc	**Nasalcrom** (Pharmacia)	**Nasal solution**: 40 mg/mL[a] (Each actuation delivers 5.2 mg)	In 13 mL or 26 mL metered spray device.
Rx	**Gastrocrom** (Celltech)	**Oral concentrate**: 100 mg/5 mL	In 8 UD amps/foil pouch.

[a] With benzalkonium chloride and EDTA.

CROMOLYN SODIUM— ORAL

Indications

➤*Mastocytosis:* In the management of mastocytosis.

➤*Off-label uses:*

Eosinophilic esophagitis – [5] = Poor documentation. The minimum goal of therapy for eosinophilic esophagitis is symptom reduction. It is unknown whether any therapy can affect the long-term outcomes of the disease. The lack of evidence hinders decision making on choice and duration of treatment. American Gastroenterological Association Institute and North American Society for Pediatric Gastroenterology, Hepatology and Nutrition guidelines concluded that the use of cromolyn sodium for the management of eosinophilic esophagitis was not supported by the literature.

Uremic pruritus – [4] = Insufficient documentation. Initial data from isolated case reports suggest that cromolyn may be beneficial in hemodialysis patients with uremic pruritus unresponsive to previous therapy.

Administration and Dosage

➤*General dosing considerations:* The recommended dose may need to be decreased in patients with renal or hepatic impairment.

➤*Adults:*

Mastocytosis –

Maximum dose: 40 mg/kg/day.

Initial dosage: 200 mg (2 ampules) orally 4 times per day.

Dosage titration: If satisfactory control of symptoms is not achieved within 2 to 3 weeks, the dosage may be increased; do not exceed 40 mg/kg/day.

Maintenance dosage: Once a therapeutic response has been achieved, the dosage may be reduced to the minimum required to maintain the patient with a lower degree of symptomatology. To prevent relapses, maintain the dosage.

Off-label dosing –

Uremic pruritus: The dosage in 2 patients was reported as 100 mg 4 times daily. The ampules were broken open, and the contents were dissolved in water and swallowed as an oral solution. The solution was administered half an hour prior to meals and at bedtime, preferably on an empty stomach. Although initial treatment was for 12 weeks, the complete duration of therapy at follow-up was 6 months.

➤*Children:*

Mastocytosis –

13 years of age and older: See Adults for dosing.

2 to 12 years of age:

- *Maximum dose* – 40 mg/kg/day.
- *Initial dosage* – 100 mg (1 ampule) orally 4 times per day.
- *Dosage titration* – If satisfactory control of symptoms is not achieved within 2 to 3 weeks, the dosage may be increased; do not exceed 40 mg/kg/day.
- *Maintenance dosage* – Once a therapeutic response has been achieved, the dosage may be reduced to the minimum required to maintain the patient with a lower degree of symptomatology. To prevent relapses, maintain the dosage.

Off-label dosing –

➤*Renal function impairment:* Decrease recommended dosage.

➤*Hepatic function impairment:* Decrease recommended dosage.

➤*Preparation for administration:* Break open and squeeze liquid contents of ampule(s) into a glass of water. Stir solution. Drink all of the liquid.

➤*Administration:* Not for inhalation or injection. For oral use only. Administer as a solution at least 30 minutes before meals and at bedtime.

➤*Storage/Stability:* Store between 15° and 30°C (59° and 86°F). Protect from light. Store ampules in foil pouch until ready for use.

Actions

➤*Pharmacology:* In vitro and in vivo animal studies have shown that cromolyn inhibits the release of mediators from sensitized mast cells. Cromolyn acts by inhibiting the release of histamine and leukotrienes (SRS-A) from the mast cell.

➤*Pharmacokinetics:*

Absorption/Distribution – Cromolyn is poorly absorbed from the GI tract. No more than 1% of an administered dose is absorbed after oral administration, the remainder being excreted in the feces. Very little absorption of cromolyn was seen after oral administration of 500 mg by mouth to each of 12 volunteers.

Metabolism/Excretion – From 0.28 to 0.5% of the administered dose was recovered in the first 24 hours of urinary excretion in 3 subjects. The mean urinary excretion of an administered dose over 24 hours in the remaining 9 subjects was 0.45%.

Contraindications

Hypersensitivity to cromolyn.

Warnings/Precautions

➤*Hypersensitivity reactions:* Severe anaphylactic reactions may occur rarely in association with cromolyn administration.

➤*Renal function impairment:* In view of the biliary and renal routes of excretion of cromolyn, consider decreasing the dosage of the drug in patients with impaired renal function.

➤*Hepatic function impairment:* Because the biliary and renal routes of excretion of cromolyn, consider decreasing the dosage of the drug in patients with impaired hepatic function.

➤*Pregnancy:* Category B. There are no adequate and well controlled studies in pregnant women. Although small amounts are absorbed systematically from the lungs, it is not known whether the drug crosses the placenta to the fetus.

Because animal reproduction studies are not always predictive of human response, use this drug during pregnancy only if clearly needed.

➤*Lactation:* It is not known whether this drug is excreted in human milk. Because cromolyn has an extremely low pKa, minimal levels would be expected to penetrate into human breastmilk. Because many drugs are excreted in human milk, exercise caution when cromolyn is administered to a breast-feeding woman. Less than 1% of this drug is absorbed from the maternal (and probably the infant's) GI tract, so it is unlikely to produce untoward effects in breast-feeding infants.

➤*Children:* Reserve the use of this product in children younger than 2 years of age for patients with severe disease in which the potential benefits clearly outweigh the risks.

➤*Elderly:* Use caution in selecting the dose for an elderly patient should be cautious, usually starting at the low end of the dosing range, reflecting the greater frequency of decreased hepatic, renal, or cardiac function, and of concomitant disease or other drug therapy.

Drug Interactions

None well documented.

Adverse Reactions

➤*Frequent adverse reactions:* Most of the adverse reactions reported in mastocytosis patients have been transient and could represent symptoms of the disease. The most frequently reported adverse reactions in mastocytosis patients who have received cromolyn during clinical studies were headache and diarrhea, each of which occurred in 4 of the 87 patients. Pruritus, nau-

CROMOLYN SODIUM— ORAL

sea, and myalgia were each reported in 3 patients, and abdominal pain, rash, and irritability in 2 patients each. One report of malaise was also recorded.

➤*Postmarketing:* Additional adverse reactions have been reported during studies in other clinical conditions and from worldwide postmarketing experience. In most cases, the available information is incomplete and attribution to the drug cannot be determined. The majority of these reports involve the GI system and include abdominal pain, constipation, diarrhea, dyspepsia, dysphagia, esophagospasm, flatulence, glossitis, nausea, stomatitis, vomiting.

➤*Less common adverse reactions (the majority representing only a single report):*

Cardiovascular – Palpitations, premature ventricular contractions, tachycardia.

CNS – Anxiety, behavior change, convulsions, depression, dizziness, fatigue, hallucinations, headache, hypoesthesia, insomnia, migraine, nervousness, paresthesia, postprandial lightheadedness and lethargy, psychosis.

Dermatologic – Erythema/burning, flushing, photosensitivity, pruritus, purpura, rash, urticaria/angioedema.

GU – Dysuria, urinary frequency.

Hematologic / Lymphatic – Neutropenia, pancytopenia.

Musculoskeletal – Arthralgia, myalgia, stiffness/weakness of legs.

Respiratory – Dyspnea, pharyngitis.

Special senses – Tinnitus, unpleasant taste.

Miscellaneous – Chest pain, edema, hepatic function test abnormal, lupus erythematosus syndrome, polycythemia.

Patient Information

Advise patients to take cromolyn as directed.

Advise patients to break open and squeeze liquid contents of ampules into a glass of water; stir and drink all of the liquid.

CROMOLYN SODIUM — ORAL INHALATION

Indications

➤*Asthma:* In the management of bronchial asthma.

➤*Prevention of acute bronchospasm:* In patients who develop acute bronchoconstriction in response to exposure to exercise, toluene diisocyanate, environmental pollutants, etc, give cromolyn shortly before exposure to the precipitating factor.

➤*Off-label uses:*

Uremic pruritus – [4] = Insufficient documentation. Initial data from isolated case reports suggest that cromolyn may be beneficial in hemodialysis patients with uremic pruritus unresponsive to previous therapy.

Administration and Dosage

➤*General dosing considerations:* Introduce cromolyn into the patient's therapeutic regimen when the acute episode has been controlled, the airway has been cleared, and the patient is able to inhale adequately.

➤*Adults:*

Asthma – 1 vial administered by nebulization 4 times per day at regular intervals.

Prevention of acute bronchospasm – 1 vial administered by nebulization shortly before exposure to the precipitating factor.

Off-label dosing –

Uremic pruritus: [4] = Insufficient documentation. The dosage in 2 hemodialysis patients was reported as 100 mg orally 4 times daily.

➤*Children:*

2 years of age and older – See Adults for dosing

➤*Concomitant therapy:*

Corticosteroids – In patients chronically receiving corticosteroids for the management of bronchial asthma, the dosage should be maintained following the introduction of cromolyn. If the patient improves, an attempt to decrease corticosteroids should be made. Even if the corticosteroid-dependent patient fails to show symptomatic improvement following cromolyn administration, the potential to reduce corticosteroids may be present. Thus, gradual tapering of corticosteroid dosage may be attempted. It is important that the dose be reduced slowly, maintaining close supervision of the patient to avoid an exacerbation of asthma.

Keep in mind that prolonged corticosteroid therapy frequently causes an impairment in the activity of the hypothalamic-pituitary-adrenal axis and a reduction in the size of the adrenal cortex. A potentially critical degree of impairment or insufficiency may persist asymptomatically for some time even after gradual discontinuation of adrenocortical steroids. Therefore, if a patient is subjected to significant stress, such as a severe asthmatic attack, surgery, trauma, or severe illness while being treated or within 1 year (occasionally up to 2 years) after corticosteroid treatment has been terminated, consider reinstituting corticosteroid therapy. When respiratory function is impaired, as may occur in severe exacerbation of asthma, a temporary increase in the amount of corticosteroids may be required to regain control of the patient's asthma.

It is particularly important that great care be exercised if, for any reason, cromolyn is withdrawn in cases where its use has permitted a reduction in the maintenance dose of corticosteroids. In such cases, continued close supervision of the patient is essential because there may be sudden reappearance of severe manifestations of asthma, which will require immediate therapy and possible reintroduction of corticosteroids.

Nonsteroidal agents – Cromolyn should be added to the patient's existing treatment regimen (eg, bronchodilators). When a clinical response to cromolyn is evident, usually within 2 to 4 weeks, and if the asthma is under good control, an attempt may be made to decrease concomitant medication usage gradually. If concomitant medications are eliminated or required on no more than an as-needed basis, the frequency of administration of cromolyn may be titrated downward to the lowest level consistent with the desired effect. The usual decrease is from 4 to 3 vials per day. It is important that the dosage be reduced gradually to avoid exacerbation of asthma. It is emphasized that in patients whose dosage has been titrated to fewer than 4 vials per day, an increase in the dose of cromolyn and the introduction of, or increase in, symptomatic medications may be needed if the patient's clinical condition deteriorates.

➤*Administration:* For oral inhalation use only. Not for injection. Cromolyn should be used in a power-driven nebulizer with an adequate airflow rate equipped with a suitable face mask or mouthpiece. Cromolyn inhalation solution is poorly absorbed when swallowed and is not effective by this route of administration.

➤*Admixture compatibility:* Drug stability and safety of cromolyn sodium inhalation solution when mixed with other drugs in a nebulizer have not been established.

➤*Storage / Stability:* Store at 20° to 25°C (68° to 77°F). Retain in foil pouch until time of use. Protect from light.

Actions

➤*Pharmacology:* In vitro and in vivo animal studies have shown that cromolyn inhibits sensitized mast cell degranulation that occurs after exposure to specific antigens. Cromolyn acts by inhibiting the release of mediators from mast cells. Studies show that cromolyn indirectly blocks calcium ions from entering the mast cell, thereby preventing mediator release.

Cromolyn inhibits both the immediate and nonimmediate bronchoconstrictive reactions to inhaled antigen. Cromolyn also attenuates bronchospasm caused by exercise, toluene diisocyanate, aspirin, cold air, sulfur dioxide, and environmental pollutants.

➤*Pharmacokinetics:*

Absorption – After administration by inhalation, approximately 8% of the total cromolyn dose is absorbed and rapidly excreted unchanged, approximately equally divided between urine and bile. The remainder of the dose is either exhaled or deposited in the oropharynx, swallowed, and excreted via the alimentary tract.

Contraindications

Hypersensitivity to cromolyn.

Warnings/Precautions

➤*Asthmaticus:* Cromolyn inhalation solution has no role in the treatment of status asthmaticus.

➤*Respiratory effects:* Occasionally, patients may experience cough and/or bronchospasm following inhalation of cromolyn. At times, patients who develop bronchospasm may not be able to continue cromolyn administration despite prior bronchodilator administration. Rarely, very severe bronchospasm has been encountered.

➤*Dosage reduction / discontinuation:* Symptoms of asthma may recur if cromolyn is reduced below the recommended dosage or discontinued.

➤*Hypersensitivity reactions:* Anaphylactic reactions with cromolyn administration have been reported rarely.

➤*Pregnancy:* *Category B.* According to the 2004 Working Group Report on Managing Asthma During Pregnancy, cromolyn is well tolerated and has an excellent safety profile. However, it is less effective than inhaled corticosteroids in reducing asthma signs and symptoms. The authors of the report consider cromolyn to be an alternative (not preferred) agent for the management of mild persistent asthma.

Because animal reproduction studies are not always predictive of human response, use this drug during pregnancy only if clearly needed.

Adverse fetal effects (increased resorption and decreased fetal weight) were noted only at the very high parenteral doses that produced maternal toxicity. There are no adequate and well-controlled studies in pregnant women. Although small amounts are absorbed systematically from the lungs, it is not known whether the drug crosses the placenta to the fetus.

➤*Lactation:* It is not known whether this drug is excreted in human milk. Cromolyn has an extremely low pKa; therefore, minimal levels would be expected to penetrate into human breast milk. Because many drugs are excreted in human milk, exercise caution when cromolyn is administered to a breast-feeding woman. Less than 1% of this drug is absorbed from the maternal (and probably the infant's) GI tract, so it is unlikely to produce untoward effects in breast-feeding infants.

➤*Children:* Safety and effectiveness in children younger than 2 years of age have not been established.

CROMOLYN SODIUM — ORAL INHALATION

Drug Interactions

None well documented.

Adverse Reactions

Clinical experience with the use of cromolyn suggests that adverse reactions are rare. The following adverse reactions have been associated with cromolyn: cough, nasal congestion, nausea, sneezing, and wheezing.

➤*Other adverse reactions:* Other reactions have been reported in clinical trials; however, a causal relationship could not be established: drowsiness, nasal itching, nose bleed, nose burning, serum sickness, and stomachache.

Overdosage

There is no clinical syndrome associated with an overdosage of cromolyn. Acute toxicity testing in a wide variety of species has demonstrated that toxicity with cromolyn occurs only with very high exposure levels, regardless of whether administration was parenteral, oral, or by inhalation.

Patient Information

Advise patients to take as directed. Because it is preventive medication, advise patients that it may take up to 4 weeks before they experience maximum benefit.

Instruct patients to use cromolyn sodium in a power-driven nebulizer with an adequate airflow rate equipped with a suitable face mask or mouthpiece.

Advise patients that drug stability and safety of cromolyn when mixed with other drugs in a nebulizer have not been established.

CROMOLYN SODIUM INTRANASAL

Indications

➤*Allergic rhinitis:* To prevent and relieve nasal symptoms of hay fever and other nasal allergies (runny/itchy nose, sneezing, allergic stuffy nose).

Administration and Dosage

➤*General dosing considerations:* Discontinue use if symptoms do not improve after 2 weeks.

➤*Adults:*

Allergic rhinitis –

Usual dosage: Spray once into each nostril. Repeat 3 to 4 times per day (every 4 to 6 hours). If needed, it may be used up to 6 times per day.

Maximum dose: 6 sprays per nostril/day.

➤*Children:*

Allergic rhinitis – See Adults for dosing.

2 years of age and older:

• *Usual dosage* – Spray once into each nostril. Repeat 3 to 4 times per day (every 4 to 6 hours). If needed, it may be used up to 6 times per day.

• *Maximum dose* – 6 sprays/day.

➤*Preparation for administration:* Prior to first use or if the pump has not been used in several days, spray into the air until a fine mist is produced.

➤*Administration:* For intranasal use only. Blow nose before using cromolyn. Use care when inserting the nozzle in the nostril to avoid injury.

➤*Storage/Stability:* Store between 20° and 25°C (68° and 77°F). Protect from light. To keep clean, wipe the nozzle after use. Put the plastic cap and safety clip back on the bottle.

Actions

➤*Pharmacology:* Cromolyn is a nasal mast cell stabilizer. In addition to treating nasal allergy symptoms, it decreases the allergic reaction by reducing the release of histamine, the trigger of allergy symptoms from mast cells.

➤*Pharmacokinetics:*

Onset – It may take up to 2 weeks to notice an effect.

Contraindications

Patients who are allergic to cromolyn.

Warnings/Precautions

➤*Pregnancy: Category B* (per Briggs' *Drugs in Pregnancy and Lactation*). Although small amounts are absorbed systemically from the lungs, it is not known whether the drug crosses the placenta to the fetus.

➤*Lactation:* Cromolyn has an extremely low pKa, and minimal levels would be expected to penetrate into human breast milk. Less than 1% of this drug is absorbed from maternal (and probably the infant's) GI tract, so it is unlikely to produce untoward effects in breast-feeding infants.

Drug Interactions

None well documented.

Adverse Reactions

Stinging or sneezing may occur right after use.

Patient Information

Advise patients that brief stinging and/or sneezing may occur right after use.

Advise patients to not use to treat sinus infection, asthma, or cold symptoms.

Instruct patients not to share this bottle with anyone else because this may spread germs.

Advise patients to discontinue cromolyn if the solution causes irritation to their nose.

Advise patients that full protection may take as long as 1 to 2 weeks with regular use.

Advise patients to contact their health care provider if their symptoms worsen, new symptoms occur, or symptoms do not begin to improve within 2 weeks or if they need to use cromolyn longer than 12 weeks.

Advise patients to contact their health care provider if shortness of breath, wheezing, chest tightness, hives, or swelling of the mouth or throat occurs while using this medication.

Advise patients to ask a health care provider before use if they have a fever, discolored nasal discharge, sinus pain, or wheezing.

Respiratory Gases

NITRIC OXIDE — INHALATION

Rx	INOmax (INO Therapeutics, Inc.)	Gas: 100 ppm	In 353 (delivered volume 344 L) and 1963 L (delivered volume 1918 L).
		800 ppm	In 353 (delivered volume 344 L) and 1963 L (delivered volume 1918 L).

NITRIC OXIDE — INHALATION

Indications

➤*Neonates with hypoxic respiratory failure:* Nitric oxide, in conjunction with ventilatory support and other appropriate agents, is indicated for the treatment of term and near-term (greater than 34 weeks) neonates with hypoxic respiratory failure associated with clinical or echocardiographic (ECG) evidence of pulmonary hypertension, where it improves oxygenation and reduces the need for extracorporeal membrane oxygenation.

➤*Off-label uses:* Reduce pulmonary artery pressure (PAP) and pulmonary vascular resistance during neonatal cardiac operations; symptomatic treatment of hypoxemia or pulmonary hypertension due to allograft dysfunction subsequent to lung transplantation.

Administration and Dosage

➤*General dosing considerations:* Nitric oxide must be discontinued slowly. (See Tapering.)

➤*Children:*

Hypoxic respiratory failure –

Neonates:

• *Usual dosage* – 20 ppm. Treatment should be maintained up to 14 days or until the underlying oxygen desaturation has resolved and the neonate is ready to be weaned from nitric oxide therapy. As the risk of methemoglobinemia and elevated NO_2 levels increases significantly when nitric oxide is administered at doses greater than 20 ppm, doses above this level ordinarily should not be used.

• *Concomitant therapy* – Additional therapies should be used to maximize oxygen delivery. In patients with collapsed alveoli, additional therapies might include surfactant and high-frequency oscillatory ventilation.

• *Tapering* – The nitric oxide dose should not be discontinued abruptly as it may result in an increase in pulmonary artery pressure (PAP) or worsening of blood oxygenation (PaO_2). Deterioration in oxygenation and elevation in PAP may also occur in children with no apparent response to nitric oxide. Discontinue/wean cautiously.

➤*Administration:* The nitric oxide delivery systems used in the clinical trials provided operator-determined concentrations of nitric oxide in the breathing gas, and the concentration was constant throughout the respiratory cycle. Nitric oxide must be delivered through a system with these characteristics and which does not cause generation of excessive inhaled nitrogen dioxide. The *INOvent* system and other systems meeting these criteria were used in the clinical trials. In the ventilated neonate, precise monitoring of inspired nitric oxide and NO_2 should be instituted, using a properly calibrated analysis device with alarms. The system should be calibrated using a precisely defined calibration mixture of nitric oxide and nitrogen dioxide, such as *INOcal*. Sample gas for analysis should be drawn before the Y-piece, proximal to the patient. Oxygen levels should also be measured.

Respiratory Gases

NITRIC OXIDE — INHALATION

In the event of a system failure or a wall-outlet power failure, a backup battery power supply and reserve nitric oxide delivery system should be available.

➤*Storage/Stability:* Store at 25°C (77°F) with excursions permitted between 15° to 30°C (59° to 86°F).

Occupational exposure – The exposure limit set by the Occupational Safety and Health Administration (OSHA) for nitric oxide is 25 ppm, and for NO_2 the limit is 5 ppm.

Actions

➤*Pharmacology:* Nitric oxide is a compound produced by many cells of the body. It relaxes vascular smooth muscle by binding to the heme moiety of cytosolic guanylate cyclase, activating guanylate cyclase and increasing intracellular levels of cyclic guanosine 3',5'-monophosphate, which then leads to vasodilation. When inhaled, nitric oxide produces pulmonary vasodilation.

Nitric oxide appears to increase the partial pressure of arterial oxygen (PaO_2) by dilating pulmonary vessels in better ventilated areas of the lung, redistributing pulmonary blood flow away from lung regions with low ventilation/perfusion (V/Q) ratios toward regions with normal ratios.

Effects on pulmonary vascular tone in PPHN – Persistent pulmonary hypertension of the newborn (PPHN) occurs as a primary developmental defect or as a condition secondary to other diseases such as meconium aspiration syndrome (MAS), pneumonia, sepsis, hyaline membrane disease, congenital diaphragmatic hernia (CDH), and pulmonary hypoplasia. In these states, pulmonary vascular resistance (PVR) is high, which results in hypoxemia secondary to right-to-left shunting of blood through the patent ductus arteriosus and foramen ovale. In neonates with PPHN, nitric oxide improves oxygenation (as indicated by significant increases in PaO_2).

➤*Pharmacokinetics:*

Metabolism – Methemoglobin disposition has been investigated as a function of time and nitric oxide exposure concentration in neonates with respiratory failure.

Methemoglobin concentrations increased during the first 8 hours of nitric oxide exposure. The mean methemoglobin level remained below 1% in the placebo group and in the 5 ppm and 20 ppm nitric oxide groups, but reached approximately 5% in the 80 ppm nitric oxide group. Methemoglobin levels greater than 7% were attained only in patients receiving 80 ppm, where they comprised 35% of the group. The average time to reach peak methemoglobin was 10 ± 9 (SD) hours (median, 8 hours) in these 13 patients; but 1 patient did not exceed 7% until 40 hours.

Excretion – Nitrate has been identified as the predominant nitric oxide metabolite excreted in the urine, accounting for greater than 70% of the nitric oxide dose inhaled. Nitrate is cleared from the plasma by the kidney at rates approaching the rate of glomerular filtration.

Contraindications

Nitric oxide should not be used in the treatment of neonates known to be dependent on right-to-left shunting of blood.

Warnings/Precautions

➤*Rebound:* Abrupt discontinuation of nitric oxide may lead to worsening oxygenation and increasing pulmonary artery pressure.

➤*Methemoglobinemia:* Methemoglobinemia increases with the dose of nitric oxide. In the clinical trials, maximum methemoglobin levels usually were reached approximately 8 hours after initiation of inhalation, although methemoglobin levels have peaked as late as 40 hours following initiation of nitric oxide therapy. In 1 study, 13 of 37 (35%) of neonates treated with nitric oxide 80 ppm had methemoglobin levels exceeding 7%. Following discontinuation or reduction of nitric oxide the methemoglobin levels returned to baseline over a period of hours.

➤*Elevated NO_2 levels:* In 1 study, NO_2 levels were less than 0.5 ppm when neonates were treated with placebo, 5 ppm, and 20 ppm nitric oxide over the first 48 hours. The 80 ppm group had a mean peak NO_2 level of 2.6 ppm.

➤*Pregnancy: Category C.* Animal reproduction studies have not been conducted with nitric oxide. It is not known if nitric oxide can cause fetal harm when administered to a pregnant woman or can affect reproductive capacity. Nitric oxide is not intended for adults.

➤*Lactation:* Nitric oxide is not indicated for use in the adult population, including nursing mothers. It is not known whether nitric oxide is excreted in human milk.

➤*Children:* Nitric oxide for inhalation has been studied in a neonatal population (up to 14 days of age).

Drug Interactions

No formal drug-interaction studies have been performed, and a clinically significant interaction with other medications used in the treatment of hypoxic respiratory failure cannot be excluded based on the available data. In particular, although there are no data to evaluate the possibility nitric oxide donor compounds, including sodium nitroprusside and nitroglycerin, may have an additive effect with nitric oxide on the risk of developing methemoglobinemia. Nitric oxide has been administered with tolazoline, dopamine, dobutamine, steroids, surfactant, and high-frequency ventilation.

Adverse Reactions

Controlled studies have included 325 patients on nitric oxide doses of 5 to 80 ppm and 251 patients on placebo. Total mortality in the pooled trials was 11% on placebo and 9% on nitric oxide, a result adequate to exclude nitric oxide mortality being more than 40% worse than placebo.

➤*Adverse reactions with an incidence of at least 5%:*

Nitric Oxide Adverse Reactions in the CINRGI trial

Adverse reaction	Placebo (n = 89)	Inhaled NO (n = 97)
Hypotension	9 (10%)	13 (13%)
Withdrawal	9 (10%)	12 (12%)
Atelectasis	8 (9%)	9 (9%)
Hematuria	5 (6%)	8 (8%)
Hyperglycemia	6 (7%)	8 (8%)
Sepsis	2 (2%)	7 (7%)
Infection	3 (3%)	6 (6%)
Stridor	3 (3%)	5 (5%)
Cellulitis	0 (0%)	5 (5%)

Overdosage

➤*Symptoms:* Overdosage with nitric oxide will be manifest by elevations in methemoglobin and NO_2. Elevated NO_2 may cause acute lung injury. Elevations in methemoglobinemia reduce the oxygen delivery capacity of the circulation. In clinical studies, NO_2 levels greater than 3 ppm or methemoglobin levels greater than 7% were treated by reducing the dose of, or discontinuing, nitric oxide.

➤*Treatment:* Methemoglobinemia that does not resolve after reduction or discontinuation of therapy can be treated with intravenous vitamin C, intravenous methylene blue, or blood transfusion, based upon the clinical situation.

Intranasal Antihistamines

AZELASTINE HYDROCHLORIDE

Rx	**Astelin** (Medpointe)	**Spray, solution; intranasal:** 0.1% (137 mcg/spray)	Equivalent to 125 mcg azelastine base. Benzalkonium chloride, edetate disodium. In 30 mg (1 mg/mL) (200 metered sprays) per bottle.
Rx	**Astepro** (MEDA Pharmaceuticals)	**Spray, solution; intranasal:** 0.15% (205.5 mcg/spray)	Equivalent to 187.6 mcg azelastine base. Benzalkonium chloride, edetate disodium. In 17 (106 metered sprays) and 30 mL (200 metered sprays).

AZELASTINE HYDROCHLORIDE — INTRANASAL

For complete and comparative prescribing information, refer to the Antihistamines group monograph.

Indications

➤*Perennial allergic rhinitis (Astepro only):* For the relief of symptoms of perennial allergic rhinitis in patients 12 years of age and older.

➤*Seasonal allergic rhinitis:* Such as rhinorrhea, sneezing, and nasal pruritus in adults and children 5 years of age and older (*Astelin*) or 12 years of age and older (*Astepro*).

➤*Vasomotor rhinitis (Astelin only):* Such as rhinorrhea, nasal congestion, and postnasal drip in adults and children 12 years of age and older.

Administration and Dosage

➤*Adults:*

Astelin –

Seasonal allergic rhinitis: 1 or 2 sprays per nostril twice daily.

Vasomotor rhinitis: 2 sprays per nostril twice daily.

Astepro 0.1% –

Seasonal allergic rhinitis: 1 or 2 sprays per nostril twice daily.

Astepro 0.15% –

Perennial allergic rhinitis: 2 sprays per nostril twice daily.

Seasonal allergic rhinitis: 1 or 2 sprays per nostril twice daily or 2 sprays per nostril once daily.

➤*Children:*

Astelin –

Seasonal allergic rhinitis:

- *12 years of age and older* – 1 or 2 sprays per nostril twice daily.
- *5 to 11 years of age* – 1 spray per nostril twice daily.

Vasomotor rhinitis:

- *12 years of age and older* – 2 sprays per nostril twice daily

AZELASTINE HYDROCHLORIDE — INTRANASAL

Astepro 0.1% –

Seasonal allergic rhinitis:

- *12 years of age and older* – 1 or 2 sprays per nostril twice daily.

Astepro 0.15% –

Perennial allergic rhinitis:

- *12 years of age and older* – 2 sprays per nostril twice daily.

Seasonal allergic rhinitis:

- *12 years of age and older* – 1 or 2 sprays per nostril twice daily or 2 sprays per nostril once daily.

➤*Preparation for administration:* Before initial use, replace the screw cap on the bottle with the pump unit and prime the delivery system with 4 sprays or until a fine mist appears. When 3 days or more have elapsed since last use, reprime the pump with 2 sprays or until a fine mist appears.

➤*Administration:* Administer by the intranasal route only. Avoid spraying in the eyes.

➤*Storage/Stability:* Store at 20° to 25°C (68° to 77°F). Protect from freezing.

Actions

➤*Pharmacology:* Azelastine HCl, a phthalazinone derivative, exhibits histamine H_1-receptor antagonist activity in isolated tissues, animal models, and humans. Azelastine HCl nasal spray is administered as a racemic mixture with no difference in pharmacologic activity noted between the enantiomers in in vitro studies. The major metabolite, desmethyl-azelastine, also possesses H_1-receptor antagonist activity.

➤*Pharmacokinetics:*

Absorption – After intranasal administration, the systemic bioavailability of azelastine HCl is approximately 40%. Maximum plasma concentrations (C_{max}) are achieved in 2 to 3 hours. Azelastine HCl administered intranasally at doses greater than 2 sprays per nostril twice daily for 29 days resulted in greater than proportional increases in C_{max} and area under the curve (AUC) for azelastine HCl. Studies in healthy subjects administered oral doses of azelastine HCl demonstrated linear responses in C_{max} and AUC.

Distribution – Based on IV and oral administration, the elimination half-life, steady-state volume of distribution, and plasma clearance are 22 hours, 14.5 L/kg, and 0.5 L/h/kg, respectively. After intranasal dosing of azelastine HCl to steady-state, plasma concentrations of desmethylazelastine range from 20% to 50% of azelastine HCl concentrations. In vitro studies with human plasma indicate that the plasma protein binding of azelastine HCl and desmethylazelastine are approximately 88% and 97%, respectively.

Metabolism – Azelastine HCl is oxidatively metabolized to the principal active metabolite, desmethylazelastine, by the cytochrome P450 enzyme system. The specific P450 isoforms responsible for the biotransformation of azelastine HCl have not been identified; however, clinical interaction studies with the known CYP3A4 inhibitor erythromycin failed to demonstrate a pharmacokinetic interaction. In a multiple-dose, steady-state drug interaction study in healthy volunteers, cimetidine (400 mg twice daily), a nonspecific P450 inhibitor, raised orally administered mean azelastine HCl (4 mg twice daily) concentrations by approximately 65%.

The major active metabolite, desmethylazelastine, was not measurable (below assay limits) after single-dose intranasal administration of azelastine HCl. Limited data indicate that the metabolite profile is similar when azelastine HCl is administered via the intranasal or oral route.

Excretion – Approximately 75% of an oral dose of radiolabeled azelastine HCl was excreted in the feces with less than 10% as unchanged azelastine HCl. When azelastine HCl is administered orally, desmethylazelastine has an elimination half-life of 54 hours.

Special populations –

Renal function impairment: Based on oral, single-dose studies, renal insufficiency (creatine clearance less than 50 mL/min) resulted in a 70% to 75% higher C_{max} and AUC compared to healthy subjects. Time to maximum concentration was unchanged.

Contraindications

Azelastine HCl nasal spray is contraindicated in patients with a known hypersensitivity to azelastine HCl or any of its components.

Warnings/Precautions

➤*Hazardous tasks:* In clinical trials, the occurrence of somnolence has been reported in some patients taking azelastine HCl nasal spray; due caution should therefore be exercised when driving a car or operating potentially dangerous machinery. Concurrent use of azelastine HCl nasal spray with alcohol or other CNS depressants should be avoided because additional reductions in alertness and additional impairment of CNS performance may occur.

➤*Pregnancy:* *Category C.* Azelastine has been shown to cause developmental toxicity. Azelastine HCl has been shown to be embryotoxic, fetotoxic, and teratogenic (external and skeletal abnormalities) in mice at an oral dose of 68.8 mg/kg/day (280 times the maximum recommended human daily intranasal dose in adults on a mg/m^2 basis)caused embryo-fetal death, malformations (cleft palate; short or absent tail; fused, absent or branched ribs), delayed ossification and decreased fetal weight. This dose also caused maternal toxicity as evidenced by decreased body weight. Neither fetal nor maternal effects occurred at a dose of 3 mg/kg (approximately 10 times the maximum recommended daily intranasal dose in adults on a mg/m^2 basis).

In rats, an oral dose of 30 mg/kg/day (approximately 240 times the maximum recommended human daily intranasal dose in adults on a mg/m^2 basis), caused malformations (oligo-and brachydactylia), delayed ossification, skeletal variations, in the absence of maternal toxicity. At 68.6 mg/kg/ (approximately 560 times the maximum recommended daily intranasal dose in adults on a mg/m^2 basis) azelastine HCl also caused embryo-fetal death and decreased fetal weight; however, the 68.6 mg/kg dose caused severe maternal toxicity. Neither fetal nor maternal effects occurred in a dose of 3 mg/kg (approximately 25 times the maximum recommended daily intranasal dose in adults on a mg/m^2 basis).

In rabbits, oral doses of greater than or equal to 30 mg/kg (approximately 500 times the maximum recommended daily intranasal dose in adults on a mg/m^2 basis) caused abortion, delayed ossification, and decreased fetal weight; however, these doses also resulted in severe maternal toxicity. Neither fetal nor maternal effects occurred at a dose of 0.3 mg/kg (approximately 5 times the maximum recommended daily intranasal dose in adults on a mg/m^2 basis).

There are no adequate and well-controlled clinical studies in pregnant women. Azelastine HCl nasal spray should be used during pregnancy only if the potential benefit justifies the potential risk to the fetus.

➤*Lactation:* It is not known whether azelastine HCl is excreted in human milk. Because many drugs are excreted in human milk, caution should be exercised when azelastine HCl nasal spray is administered to a nursing woman.

➤*Children:* The safety and efficacy of azelastine nasal spray at a dose of 1 spray per nostril twice daily has been established for patients 5 through 11 years of age for the treatment of symptoms of seasonal allergic rhinitis. The safety of this dosage of azelastine nasal spray was established in well-controlled studies of this dose in 176 patients 5 to 12 years of age treated for less than or equal to 6 weeks. The efficacy of azelastine nasal spray at this dose is based on an extrapolation of the finding of efficacy in adults, on the likelihood that the disease course, pathophysiology and response to treatment are substantially similar in children compared to adults, and on supportive data from controlled clinical trials in patients 5 to 12 years of age at the dose of 1 spray per nostril twice daily. The safety and efficacy of azelastine nasal spray in patients younger than 5 years of age have not been established.

➤*Elderly:* Clinical studies of azelastine nasal spray did not include sufficient numbers of subjects at least 65 years of age to determine whether they respond differently from younger subjects. Other reported clinical experience has not identified differences in responses between the elderly and younger patients. In general, dose selection for an elderly patient should be cautious, usually starting at the low end of the dosing range, reflecting the greater frequency of decreased hepatic, renal, or cardiac function, and of concomitant disease or other drug therapy.

Drug Interactions

➤*Alcohol or other CNS depressants:* Concurrent use of azelastine HCl nasal spray with alcohol or other CNS depressants should be avoided because additional reductions in alertness and additional impairment of CNS performance may occur.

➤*Cimetidine:* Cimetidine (400 mg twice daily) increased the mean C_{max} and AUC of orally administered azelastine HCl (4 mg twice daily) by approximately 65%.

Adverse Reactions

➤*Seasonal allergic rhinitis:* In these clinical studies, adverse events that occurred statistically significantly more often in patients treated with azelastine HCl nasal spray vs vehicle placebo included bitter taste (19.7% vs 0.6%), somnolence (11.5% vs 5.4%), weight increase (2% vs 0%), and myalgia (1.5% vs 0%).

The following adverse events were reported with frequencies at least 2% in the azelastine HCl nasal spray treatment group and more frequently than placebo in short-term (less than or equal to 2 days) and long-term (2 to 8 weeks) clinical trials.

Azelastine Nasal Spray Adverse Reactions (≥ 2%) in Patients With Seasonal Allergic Rhinitis

Adverse reaction	Azelastine HCl nasal spray (n = 391)	Vehicle placebo (n = 353)
Bitter taste	19.7	0.6
Headache	14.8	12.7
Somnolence	11.5	5.4
Nasal burning	4.1	1.7
Pharyngitis	3.8	2.8
Dry mouth	2.8	1.7
Paroxysmal sneezing	3.1	1.1
Nausea	2.8	1.1
Rhinitis	2.3	1.4
Fatigue	2.3	1.4
Dizziness	2	1.4
Epistaxis	2	1.4

AZELASTINE HYDROCHLORIDE — INTRANASAL

Azelastine Nasal Spray Adverse Reactions (≥ 2%) in Patients With Seasonal Allergic Rhinitis		
Adverse reaction	Azelastine HCl nasal spray (n = 391)	Vehicle placebo (n = 353)
Weight increase	2	0

A total of 176 patients 5 to 12 years of age were exposed to azelastine nasal spray at a dose of 1 spray each nostril twice daily in 3 placebo-controlled studies. In these studies, adverse events that occurred more frequently in patients with azelastine nasal spray than with placebo, and that were not represented in the adult adverse event information above include rhinitis/cold symptoms (17% vs 9.5%), cough (11.4% vs 8.3%), conjunctivitis (5.1% vs 1.8%), and asthma (4.5% vs 4.1%).

The following events were observed infrequently (less than 2% and exceeding placebo incidence) in patients who received azelastine HCl nasal spray (2 sprays/nostril twice daily) in US clinical trials.

Cardiovascular – Flushing; hypertension; tachycardia.

CNS – Hyperkinesia; hypoesthesia; vertigo.

Dermatologic – Contact dermatitis; eczema, hair and follicle infection, furunculosis.

GI – Constipation; gastroenteritis; glossitis; ulcerative stomatitis; vomiting; increased AST; aphthous stomatitis.

GU – Albuminuria; amenorrhea; breast pain; hematuria; increased urinary frequency.

Metabolic/Nutritional – Increased appetite.

Musculoskeletal – Myalgia; temporomandibular dislocation.

Psychiatric – Anxiety; depersonalization; depression; nervousness; sleep disorder; thinking abnormal.

Respiratory – Bronchospasm; coughing; throat burning; laryngitis.

Special senses – Conjunctivitis; eye abnormality; eye pain; watery eyes; taste loss.

Miscellaneous – Allergic reaction; back pain; herpes simplex; viral infection; malaise; pain in extremities; abdominal pain.

➤*Vasomotor rhinitis:* The following adverse events were reported with frequencies greater than or equal to 2% in the azelastine nasal spray treatment group and more frequently than placebo.

Azelastine Nasal Spray Adverse Reactions (≥ 2%) in Patients With Vasomotor Rhinitis		
Adverse reaction	Azelastine HCl nasal spray (n = 216)	Vehicle placebo (n = 210)
Bitter taste	19.4	2.4
Headache	7.9	7.6
Dysesthesia	7.9	3.3
Rhinitis	5.6	2.4
Epistaxis	3.2	2.4
Sinusitis	3.2	1.9
Somnolence	3.2	1

Events observed infrequently (less than 2% and exceeding placebo incidence) in patients who received azelastine nasal spray (2 sprays/nostril twice daily) in US clinical trials in vasomotor rhinitis were similar to those observed in US clinical trials in seasonal allergic rhinitis.

In controlled trials involving nasal and oral azelastine HCl formulations, there were infrequent occurrences of hepatic transaminase elevations. The clinical relevance of these reports has not been established.

In addition, the following spontaneous adverse events have been reported during the marketing of azelastine HCl nasal spray and causal relationship with the drug is unknown: anaphylactoid reaction, application site irritation, chest pain, nasal congestion, confusion, diarrhea, dyspnea, facial edema, involuntary muscle contractions, paresthesia, parosmia, pruritus, rash, tolerance, urinary retention, vision abnormal, and xerophthalmia.

Overdosage

➤*Symptoms:* There have been no reported overdosages with azelastine nasal spray. Acute overdosage by adults with this dosage form is unlikely to result in clinically significant adverse events, other than increased somnolence, since 1 bottle of azelastine nasal spray contains 17 mg of azelastine HCl. Clinical studies in adults with single doses of the oral formulation of azelastine HCl (less than or equal to 16 mg) have not resulted in increased incidence of serious adverse events.

➤*Treatment:* General supportive measures should be employed if overdosage occurs. There is no known antidote to azelastine nasal spray. Oral ingestion of antihistamines has the potential to cause serious adverse effects in young children. Accordingly, azelastine nasal spray should be kept out of the reach of children. Oral doses of greater than or equal to 120 mg/kg (approximately 460 times the maximum recommended daily intranasal dose in adults and children on a mg/m^2 basis) were lethal in mice. Responses seen prior to death were tremor, convulsions, decreased muscle tone, and salivation. In dogs, single oral doses as high as 10 mg/kg (approximately 260 times the maximum recommended daily intranasal dose in adults and children on a mg/m^2 basis) were well tolerated, but single oral doses of 20 mg/kg were lethal.

Patient Information

Patients should be instructed to use azelastine HCl nasal spray only as prescribed. For the proper use of the nasal spray and to attain maximum improvement, the patient should read and follow carefully the accompanying patient instructions. Patients should be instructed to prime the delivery system before initial use and after storage for greater than or equal to 3 days. Patients should also be instructed to store the bottle upright at room temperature with the pump tightly closed and out of the reach of children. In case of accidental ingestion by a young child, seek professional assistance or contact a poison control center immediately.

Patients should be advised against the concurrent use of azelastine HCl nasal spray with other antihistamines without consulting a physician. Patients who are, or may become, pregnant should be told that this product should be used in pregnancy or during lactation only if the potential benefit justifies the potential risks to the fetus or nursing infant. Patients should be advised to assess their individual responses to azelastine HCl nasal spray before engaging in any activity requiring mental alertness, such as driving a car or operating machinery. Patients should be advised that the concurrent use of azelastine HCl nasal spray with alcohol or other CNS depressants may lead to additional reductions in alertness and impairment of CNS performance and should be avoided (see Drug Interactions).

OLOPATADINE

Rx	**Patanase** (Alcon Labs)	**Spray, solution; intranasal:** 0.6% (600 mcg per spray)	Equiv. to olopatadine hydrochloride 665 mcg per spray. In 30.5 g (240 actuations) with metered-dose manual spray pump and applicator.[a]

[a] With benzalkonium chloride 0.01%, edetate disodium.

OLOPATADINE HYDROCHLORIDE — INTRANASAL

Indications

➤*Seasonal allergic rhinitis:* For the relief of the symptoms of seasonal allergic rhinitis in patients 6 years of age and older.

Administration and Dosage

➤*Adults:*

Seasonal allergic rhinitis – Two sprays per nostril twice daily.

➤*Children:*

Seasonal allergic rhinitis –

12 years of age and older: See Adults for dosing.

6 to 11 years of age: 1 spray per nostril twice daily.

➤*Preparation for administration:* Before initial use, prime the product by releasing 5 sprays or until a fine mist appears. When the product has not been used for more than 7 days, re-prime by releasing 2 sprays. The correct amount of medication cannot be assured before the initial priming and after 240 sprays have been used, even though the bottle is not completely empty.

➤*Administration:* Administer by the intranasal route only.

➤*Storage/Stability:* Store between 4° and 25°C (39° and 77°F). Discard after 240 sprays (enough for 30 days of dosing) have been used.

Actions

➤*Pharmacology:* Olopatadine is a histamine H_1-receptor antagonist. The antihistamine activity of olopatadine has been documented in isolated tissues, animal models, and humans.

➤*Pharmacokinetics:*

Absorption – Olopatadine was absorbed with individual peak plasma concentrations (C_{max}) observed between 30 minutes and 1 hour after twice-daily intranasal administration of olopatadine in healthy subjects. The mean steady-state C_{max} of olopatadine was 16 ± 8.99 ng/mL. Systemic exposure as indexed by area under the curve (AUC_{0-12}) averaged 66 ± 26.8 ng•h/mL. The average absolute bioavailability of intranasal olopatadine is 57%. The mean accumulation ratio following multiple intranasal administration of olopatadine was approximately 1.3.

Systemic exposure of olopatadine in patients with seasonal allergic rhinitis after twice-daily intranasal administration of olopatadine was comparable with that observed in healthy subjects. Olopatadine was absorbed with C_{max} observed between 15 minutes and 2 hours. The mean steady-state C_{max} was 23.3 ± 6.2 ng/mL and AUC_{0-12} averaged 78 ± 13.9 ng•h/mL.

OLOPATADINE HYDROCHLORIDE — INTRANASAL

Distribution – The protein binding of olopatadine was moderate, at approximately 55% in human serum, and independent of drug concentration over the range of 0.1 to 1,000 ng/mL. Olopatadine was bound predominately to human serum albumin.

Metabolism – Olopatadine is not extensively metabolized. Based on plasma metabolite profiles following oral administration of [^{14}C] olopatadine, at least 6 minor metabolites circulate in human plasma. Olopatadine accounts for 77% of peak plasma total radioactivity, and all metabolites amounted to less than 6% combined. Two of these have been identified as the olopatadine N-oxide and N-desmethyl olopatadine. In in vitro studies with cDNA-expressed human cytochrome P450 isoenzymes and flavin-containing monooxygenases (FMO), N-desmethyl olopatadine (M1) formation was catalyzed mainly by CYP3A4, while olopatadine N-oxide (M3) was primarily catalyzed by FMO1 and FMO3.

Excretion – The plasma elimination half-life of olopatadine is 8 to 12 hours. Olopatadine is mainly eliminated through urinary excretion. Approximately 70% of a [^{14}C] olopatadine oral dose was recovered in urine and 17% in the feces. Of the drug-related material recovered within the first 24 hours in the urine, 86% was unchanged olopatadine, with the balance comprised of olopatadine N-oxide and N-desmethyl olopatadine.

Special populations –

Renal function impairment: Mean plasma $AUC_{0\text{-}12}$ was 2-fold higher in patients with severe impairment (creatinine clearance [CrCl] less than 30 mL/min/1.73 m^2). In these patients, steady-state C_{max} of olopatadine are approximately 10-fold lower than those observed after higher 20 mg oral doses twice daily, which were well tolerated. These findings indicate that no adjustment of the dosing regimen of olopatadine is warranted in patients with renal impairment.

Children:

• *6 to 11 years of age* –

The mean C_{max} (15.4 ± 7.3 ng/mL) of olopatadine was approximately 2-fold less than was comparable with that observed in adults (78 ± 13.9 ng•h/mL). The C_{max} and $AUC_{0\text{-}12}$ of olopatadine N-oxide were comparable with that observed in adults. The C_{max} and $AUC_{0\text{-}12}$ of N-desmethyl olopatadine are approximately 18% and 37% higher than that observed in adults, respectively.

• *2 to 5 years of age* –

The mean C_{max} and $AUC_{0\text{-}12}$ of olopatadine were 13.4 ± 4.6 ng/mL and 75 ± 26.4 ng•h/mL, respectively. The mean C_{max} and $AUC_{0\text{-}12}$ of olopatadine N-oxide and N-desmethyl olopatadine were similar to that of patients 6 to 11 years of age.

Gender: The mean systemic exposure (C_{max} and $AUC_{0\text{-}12}$) in women with seasonal allergic rhinitis following multiple administrations of olopatadine was 40% and 27% higher, respectively, than those values observed in men with seasonal allergic rhinitis.

Contraindications

None well documented.

Warnings/Precautions

➤*Local nasal effects:*

Epistaxis and nasal ulceration – In placebo (vehicle)-controlled clinical trials of 2 weeks' to 12 months' duration, epistaxis and nasal ulcerations were reported.

Nasal septal perforation – Two placebo (vehicle)-controlled, long-term (12 months) safety trials were conducted. In the first safety trial, patients were treated with an investigational formulation of olopatadine containing povidone (not the commercially marketed formulation) or a vehicle nasal spray containing povidone. Nasal septal perforations were reported in 1 patient treated with the investigational formulation of olopatadine and 2 patients treated with the vehicle. In the second safety trial with olopatadine, which does not contain povidone, there were no reports of nasal septal perforation.

➤*Hazardous tasks:* In clinical trials, the occurrence of somnolence has been reported in some patients. Caution patients against engaging in hazardous occupations requiring complete mental alertness and motor coordination, such as driving or operating machinery, after administration of olopatadine.

➤*Pregnancy: Category C.* No adequate and well-controlled studies in pregnant women have been conducted. It is not known if olopatadine crosses the human placenta. The molecular weight (about 374) is low enough to cross the placenta, but the very small amounts in the systemic circulation suggest that clinically significant amounts will not reach the embryo and/or fetus. Animal reproductive studies in rats and rabbits revealed treatment-related effects on fetuses or pups. Because animal studies are not always predictive of human responses, use olopatadine in pregnant women only if the potential benefit to the mother justifies the potential risk to the embryo or fetus. Antihistamines, in general, are not thought to cause human developmental toxicity at recommended doses.

A decrease in the number of live fetuses was observed in rabbits and rats at oral olopatadine doses of approximately 88 times (25 mg/kg) and 100 times (60 mg/kg) the MRHD and above, respectively, for adults on a mg/m^2 basis. In rats, viability and body weights of pups were reduced on day 4 postpartum at the oral dose approximately 100 times (60 mg/kg) the MRHD for adults on a mg/m^2 basis, but no effect on viability was observed at the dose approximately 35 times (20 mg/kg) the MRHD for adults on a mg/m^2 basis.

➤*Lactation:* Olopatadine has been identified in the milk of nursing rats following oral administration. It is not known whether topical nasal administration could result in sufficient systemic absorption to produce detectable quantities in human breast milk. Use olopatadine in breast-feeding mothers only if the potential benefit to the patient outweighs the potential risk to the infant.

➤*Children:* Safety and effectiveness in children younger than 6 years of age has not been established.

See Adverse Reactions for more information.

➤*Elderly:* In general, use caution in dose selection for an elderly patient, reflecting the greater frequency of decreased hepatic, renal, or cardiac function and of concomitant disease or other drug therapy.

➤*Monitoring:* Before starting olopatadine, conduct a nasal examination to ensure that patients are free of nasal disease other than allergic rhinitis. Perform nasal examinations periodically for signs of adverse reactions on the nasal mucosa, and consider stopping olopatadine if patients develop nasal ulcerations.

Drug Interactions

➤*CNS depressants:* Advise patients to avoid concurrent use of alcohol or other CNS depressants with olopatadine because additional reductions in alertness and impairment of CNS function could occur.

Adverse Reactions

The safety data reflect exposure to olopatadine in 2,427 patients with seasonal or perennial allergic rhinitis in 9 controlled clinical trials of 2 weeks' to 12 months' duration.

➤*Children 6 to 11 years of age:*

Discontinuation –

Overall, 1.4% of the 870 children across all 3 studies treated with olopatadine and 1.3% of the 872 children treated with vehicle discontinued because of adverse reactions.

Olopatadine Adverse Reactions in Children 6 to 11 Years of Age (≥ 1%)

Adverse reactions	Olopatadine[a] (n = 298)	Vehicle[a] (n = 297)
Respiratory		
Epistaxis	5.7%	3.7%
Upper respiratory tract infection	2.6%	0%
Miscellaneous		
Bitter taste	1%	0%
Headache	4.4%	3.7%
Pyrexia	1.3%	1%
Rash	1.3%	0%

[a] 1 spray per nostril.

➤*Long-term trials:*

Adults and children 12 years of age and older – The most frequently reported adverse reaction was epistaxis, which occurred in 25% of patients treated with olopatadine and 28% of patients treated with vehicle. Epistaxis resulted in discontinuation of 0.9% of patients treated with olopatadine and 0.2% of patients treated with vehicle. Nasal ulcerations occurred in 10% of patients treated with olopatadine and 9% of patients treated with vehicle. Nasal ulcerations resulted in discontinuation of 0.4% of patents treated with olopatadine and 0.2% of patients treated with vehicle. There were no patients with nasal septal perforation in either treatment group. Somnolence was reported in 1 patient treated with olopatadine and 1 patient treated with vehicle. Weight increase was reported in 6 patients treated with olopatadine and 1 patient treated with vehicle. Depression or worsening of depression occurred in 9 patients treated with olopatadine and in 5 patients treated with vehicle. Three patients, 2 of whom had preexisting histories of depression, who received olopatadine were hospitalized for depression compared with none who received vehicle.

Nasal septal perforations were reported in 1 patient treated with the investigational formulation of olopatadine and 2 patients treated with the vehicle. Epistaxis was reported in 19% of patients treated with the investigational formulation of olopatadine and 12% of patients treated with vehicle. Somnolence was reported in 3 patients treated with the investigational formulation of olopatadine compared with 1 patient treated with vehicle. Fatigue was reported in 5 patients treated with the investigational formulation of olopatadine compared with 1 patient treated with vehicle.

Overdosage

➤*Symptoms:* Acute overdosage with this dosage form is unlikely because of the configuration of the primary container closure system. However, symptoms of antihistamine overdose may include drowsiness in adults and, initially, agitation and restlessness, followed by drowsiness in children.

➤*Treatment:* There is no known specific antidote to olopatadine overdose. Should overdose occur, symptomatic or supportive treatment is recommended, taking into account any concomitantly ingested medications.

For additional information about overdose treatment, call a poison control center (1-800-222-1222).

Patient Information

Inform patients that treatment with olopatadine may lead to adverse reactions, which include epistaxis and nasal ulcerations. Other common adverse reactions reported with the use of olopatadine include bitter taste, cough, headache, pharyngolaryngeal pain, postnasal drip, and urinary tract infection.

OLOPATADINE HYDROCHLORIDE — INTRANASAL

Somnolence has been reported in some patients taking olopatadine. Caution patients against engaging in hazardous occupations requiring complete mental alertness and motor coordination, such as driving or operating machinery, after administration of olopatadine.

Advise patients to avoid concurrent use with alcohol or other CNS depressants because additional reductions in alertness and additional impairment of CNS performance may occur.

Advise patients to avoid spraying olopatadine in their eyes.

RESPIRATORY INHALANT COMBINATIONS

BUDESONIDE/FORMOTEROL FUMARATE

Rx	**Symbicort** (AstraZeneca LP)	**Aerosol; inhalation:** budesonide 80 mcg/formoterol fumarate 4.5 mcg per actuation	PEG. In 6.9 g canisters (60 actuations) and 10.2 g canisters (120 actuations) with actuator.
		budesonide 160 mcg/formoterol fumarate 4.5 mcg per actuation	PEG. In 6 g canisters (60 actuations) and 10.2 g canisters (120 actuations) with actuator.

BUDESONIDE/FORMOTEROL FUMARATE — INHALATION

WARNING

Long-acting beta-2 adrenergic agonists (LABAs) such as formoterol, one of the active ingredients in budesonide/formoterol, increase the risk of asthma-related death. Data from a large placebo-controlled US study that compared the safety of another LABA (salmeterol) or placebo added to usual asthma therapy showed an increase in asthma-related deaths in patients receiving salmeterol. This finding with salmeterol is considered a class effect of the LABAs, including formoterol. Currently available data are inadequate to determine whether concurrent use of inhaled corticosteroids or other long-term asthma control drugs mitigates the increased risk of asthma-related death from LABAs. Available data from controlled clinical trials suggest that LABAs increase the risk of asthma-related hospitalization in pediatric and adolescent patients. Therefore, when treating patients with asthma, only use budesonide/formoterol for patients not adequately controlled on a long-term asthma control medication, such as an inhaled corticosteroid, or for patients whose disease severity clearly warrants initiation of treatment with both an inhaled corticosteroid and a LABA. Once asthma control is achieved and maintained, assess the patient at regular intervals and step down therapy (eg, discontinue budesonide/formoterol) if possible without loss of asthma control, and maintain the patient on a long-term asthma control medication such as an inhaled corticosteroid. Do not use budesonide/formoterol for patients whose asthma is adequately controlled on low- or medium-dose inhaled corticosteroids.

Indications

➤*Asthma:* For the treatment of asthma in patients 12 years of age and older.

➤*Chronic obstructive pulmonary disease:* For the twice-daily maintenance treatment of airflow obstruction in patients with chronic obstructive pulmonary disease (COPD), including chronic bronchitis and emphysema. Budesonide 160 mcg/formoterol 4.5 mcg is the only approved dosage for the treatment of airflow obstruction in COPD.

Administration and Dosage

➤*General dosing considerations:* Particular care is needed for patients who have been transferred from systemically active corticosteroids to inhaled corticosteroids because deaths due to adrenal insufficiency have occurred in patients with asthma during and after transfer from systemic corticosteroids to less systemically available inhaled corticosteroids. After withdrawal from systemic corticosteroids, a number of months are required for recovery of hypothalamic-pituitary-adrenal (HPA) function.

If a previously effective dosage regimen of budesonide/formoterol fails to provide adequate control of asthma, the therapeutic regimen should be reevaluated and additional therapeutic options (eg, adding additional inhaled corticosteroids, initiating oral corticosteroids, replacing the current strength of budesonide/formoterol with a higher strength) should be considered.

For all patients, it is desirable to titrate to the lowest effective strength after adequate asthma stability has been achieved.

Improvement in asthma control following inhaled administration of budesonide/formoterol can occur within 15 minutes of beginning treatment, although maximum benefit may not be achieved for 2 weeks or longer after beginning treatment. Individual patients may experience a variable time to onset and degree of symptom relief.

More frequent administration or a higher number of inhalations (more than 2 inhalations twice daily) of the prescribed strength of budesonide/formoterol is not recommended because some patients are more likely to experience adverse reactions with higher doses of formoterol. Patients using budesonide/formoterol should not use additional LABAs for any reason.

If asthma symptoms arise in the period between doses, an inhaled short-acting beta-2 agonist should be taken for immediate relief.

➤*Adults:*

Asthma –

Maximum dose: Budesonide 640 mcg/formoterol 18 mcg daily (given as 2 inhalations of budesonide 160 mcg/formoterol 4.5 mcg twice daily).

Initial dosage: 2 inhalations twice daily (morning and evening, approximately 12 hours apart).

Dosage titration: Titrate to the lowest effective strength after adequate asthma stability is achieved.

Dosage adjustment: For patients who do not respond adequately to the starting dose after 1 to 2 weeks of therapy with budesonide 80 mcg/formoterol 4.5 mcg, replacing the strength with budesonide 160 mcg/formoterol 4.5 mcg may provide additional asthma control.

Chronic obstructive pulmonary disease –

Initial dosage: Budesonide 160 mcg/formoterol 4.5 mcg, 2 inhalations twice daily.

If shortness of breath occurs in the period between doses, an inhaled short-acting beta-2 agonist should be taken for immediate relief.

➤*Children:*

Asthma –

12 years of age and older: See Adults for dosing.

Off-label dosing –

Asthma: The following dosing is from the National Asthma Education and Prevention guidelines.

• *5 to 11 years of age* – Budesonide 80 mcg/formoterol 4.5 mcg, 2 inhalations twice daily.

➤*Transferring patients from systemic corticosteroid therapy:* Patients requiring oral corticosteroids should be weaned slowly from systemic corticosteroid use after transferring to budesonide/formoterol. Prednisone reduction can be accomplished by reducing the daily prednisone dose by 2.5 mg on a weekly basis during therapy with budesonide/formoterol.

➤*Administration:* Budesonide/formoterol should be administered twice daily every day by the orally inhaled route only. The inhaler should be shaken well for 5 seconds right before each use. After inhalation, patients should rinse the mouth with water without swallowing. Advise patients to avoid spraying in eyes.

For best results, the canister should be at room temperature before use.

The correct amount of medication in each inhalation cannot be ensured after the labeled number of inhalations from the canister have been used, even though the inhaler may not feel completely empty and may continue to operate. The inhaler should be discarded when the labeled number of inhalations have been used or within 3 months of removal from the foil pouch. Never immerse the canister into water to determine the amount remaining in the canister ("float test").

Priming – Patients should prime before using for the first time by releasing 2 test sprays into the air away from the face, shaking well for 5 seconds before each spray. In cases in which the inhaler has not been used for more than 7 days or when it has been dropped, the inhaler should be primed again by shaking well before each spray and releasing 2 test sprays into the air, away from the face.

➤*Storage/Stability:* Store between 20° and 25°C (68° and 77°F). Store the inhaler with the mouthpiece down.

Contents are under pressure; do not puncture or incinerate. Do not store near heat or open flame. Exposure to temperatures higher than 49°C (120°F) may cause bursting. Never throw container into fire or incinerator.

FLUTICASONE PROPIONATE/SALMETEROL

Rx	**Advair Diskus** (GlaxoSmithKline)	**Powder; inhalation:** fluticasone propionate 100 mcg/salmeterol 50 mcg	Equiv. to salmeterol xinafoate 72.5 mcg. Lactose. In a disposable device of 14s and 60s.
		fluticasone propionate 250 mcg/salmeterol 50 mcg	Equiv. to salmeterol xinafoate 72.5 mcg. Lactose. In a disposable device of 14s and 60s.
		fluticasone propionate 500 mcg/salmeterol 50 mcg	Equiv. to salmeterol xinafoate 72.5 mcg. Lactose. In a disposable device of 14s and 60s.

FLUTICASONE PROPIONATE/SALMETEROL

Rx	**Advair HFA**[a] (GlaxoSmithKline)	**Aerosol; inhalation**: fluticasone propionate 45 mcg/salmeterol 21 mcg per actuation	Equiv. to salmeterol xinafoate 30.45 mcg. In 8 g (60 inhalations) and 12 g (120 inhalations) canisters.
		fluticasone propionate 115 mcg/salmeterol 21 mcg per actuation	Equiv. to salmeterol xinafoate 30.45 mcg. In 8 g (60 inhalations) and 12 g (120 inhalations) canisters.
		fluticasone propionate 230 mcg/salmeterol 21 mcg per actuation	Equiv. to salmeterol xinafoate 30.45 mcg. In 8 g (60 inhalations) and 12 g (120 inhalations) canisters.

[a] HFA = hydrofluoroalkane.

FLUTICASONE PROPIONATE/SALMETEROL XINAFOATE — INHALATION

For complete and comparative prescribing information, refer to the Corticosteroids and Sympathomimetics class monographs.

WARNING

Long-acting beta-2 adrenergic agonists such as salmeterol may increase the risk of asthma-related death. Data from a large placebo-controlled US study that compared the safety of salmeterol or placebo added to usual asthma therapy showed an increase in asthma-related deaths in patients receiving salmeterol (13 deaths of 13,176 patients treated for 28 weeks on salmeterol vs 3 deaths of 13,179 patients on placebo). Currently available data are inadequate to determine whether concurrent use of inhaled corticosteroids or other long-term asthma-control drugs mitigates the increased risk of asthma-related death from long-acting beta-2 adrenergic agonists. Available data from controlled clinical trials suggest that long-acting beta-2 adrenergic agonists increase the risk of hospitalization in children and adolescents.

Therefore, when treating patients with asthma, only prescribe fluticasone/salmeterol for patients not adequately controlled on a long-term asthma-control medication (eg, inhaled corticosteroids) or whose disease severity clearly warrants initiation of treatment with both an inhaled corticosteroid and long-acting beta-2 adrenergic agonist. Once asthma control is achieved and maintained, assess the patient at regular intervals and step down therapy (eg, discontinue fluticasone/salmeterol) if possible without loss of asthma control, and maintain the patient on a long-term asthma-control medication, such as an inhaled corticosteroid. Do not use fluticasone/salmeterol for patients whose asthma is adequately controlled on low- or medium-dose inhaled corticosteroids.

Indications

➤*Asthma:* For the treatment of asthma in patients 4 years of age and older (*Diskus*) and in patients 12 years of age and older (HFA).

➤*Chronic obstructive pulmonary disease (Diskus only)*: For the twice-daily maintenance treatment of airflow obstruction in patients with chronic obstructive pulmonary disease (COPD), including chronic bronchitis and/or emphysema. Fluticasone 250 mcg/salmeterol 50 mcg *Diskus* is also indicated to reduce exacerbations of COPD in patients with a history of exacerbations.

Administration and Dosage

➤*General dosing considerations:* Fluticasone/salmeterol should not be used for transferring patients from systemic corticosteroid therapy.

If symptoms arise in the period between doses, an inhaled, short-acting beta-2 agonist should be taken for immediate relief.

More frequent administration or a higher number of inhalations of the prescribed strength is not recommended because some patients are more likely to experience adverse effects with higher doses of salmeterol. The safety and efficacy of fluticasone/salmeterol when administered in excess of recommended dose have not been established.

Improvement in asthma control following administration of can occur within 30 minutes of beginning treatment, although maximum benefit may not be achieved for 1 week or longer after starting treatment. Individual patients will experience variable times to onset and degree of symptom relief.

See the Warning box for more information.

➤*Adults:*

Asthma –

Diskus:

• *Usual dosage* – 1 inhalation twice daily (morning and evening, approximately 12 hours apart). The recommended starting dosage is based on the patient's asthma severity.

• *Maximum dose* – 1 inhalation of fluticasone 500 mcg/salmeterol 50 mcg twice daily.

HFA:

• *Usual dosage* – 2 inhalations twice daily (morning and evening, approximately 12 hours apart). The recommended starting dosage is based on the patient's current asthma therapy.

• *Maximum dose* – 2 inhalations of fluticasone 230 mcg/salmeterol 21 mcg twice daily.

Chronic obstructive pulmonary disease –

Diskus: 1 inhalation (fluticasone 250 mcg/salmeterol 50 mcg) twice daily (morning and evening, approximately 12 hours apart).

➤*Children:*

Asthma –

Diskus:

• *12 years of age and older* – See Adults for dosing.

• *4 to 11 years of age* – 1 inhalation of fluticasone 100 mcg/salmeterol 50 mcg twice daily (morning and evening, approximately 12 hours apart).

HFA:

• *12 years of age and older* – See Adults for dosing.

➤*Hepatic function impairment:* May lead to accumulation of fluticasone and salmeterol in plasma. Closely monitor patients with hepatic impairment.

➤*Dosage adjustment:* For patients who do not respond adequately to the starting dosage after 2 weeks of therapy, replacing the current strength of fluticasone/salmeterol with a higher strength may provide additional improvement in asthma control.

If a previously effective dosage regimen of fluticasone/salmeterol fails to provide adequate improvement in asthma control, the therapeutic regimen should be reevaluated, and additional therapeutic options (eg, replacing the current strength of fluticasone/salmeterol with a higher strength, adding additional inhaled corticosteroids, initiating oral corticosteroids) should be considered.

➤*Concomitant therapy:* Patients receiving fluticasone/salmeterol twice daily should not use additional salmeterol or other inhaled, long-acting beta-2 agonists (eg, formoterol, arformoterol) for prevention of exercise-induced bronchospasm (EIB) or for any other reason.

➤*Administration:* Administer by the orally inhaled route only.

Diskus – After inhalation, rinse the mouth with water without swallowing.

HFA – Prime before using for the first time by releasing 4 test sprays into the air, away from the face, shaking well for 5 seconds before each spray. In cases in which the inhaler has not been used for more than 4 weeks or when it has been dropped, prime the inhaler again by shaking well before each spray and releasing 2 test sprays into the air, away from the face.

The purple actuator should not be used with any other product canisters, and actuators from other products should not be used with fluticasone/salmeterol HFA canisters.

The correct amount of medication in each actuation cannot be ensured after the counter reads "000," even though the canister is not completely empty and will continue to operate. The inhaler should be discarded when the counter reads "000."

➤*Storage/Stability:*

Diskus – Store at 20° to 25°C (68° to 77°F) in a dry place, away from direct heat or sunlight. The inhalation device is not reusable. Discard 1 month after removal from the moisture-protective foil pouch or after every blister has been used (when the dose indicator reads "0"), whichever comes first. Do not attempt to take the device apart.

HFA – Store at 25°C (77°F); excursions are permitted between 15° and 30°C (59° and 86°F). Contents are under pressure; do not puncture. Do not use or store near heat or open flame. Exposure to temperatures above 48.9°C (120°F) may cause bursting. Never throw the container into a fire or incinerator. Store inhaler with the mouthpiece down. For best results, the inhaler should be at room temperature before use.

MOMETASONE FUROATE/FORMOTEROL FUMARATE

Rx	**Dulera** (Schering)	**Aerosol; inhalation**: mometasone furoate 100 mcg/ formoterol fumarate 5 mcg per actuation	In 13 g canisters (120 inhalations) with actuator.
		mometasone furoate 200 mcg/formoterol fumarate 5 mcg per actuation	In 13 g canisters (120 inhalations) with actuator.

MOMETASONE FUROATE/FORMOTEROL FUMARATE — INHALATION

For complete and comparative prescribing information, refer to the Corticosteroids and Sympathomimetics class monographs.

WARNING

Asthma-related death – Long-acting beta$_2$-adrenergic agonists (LABAs), such as formoterol, one of the active ingredients in mometasone/formoterol, increase the risk of asthma-related death. Data from a large placebo-controlled US study that compared the safety of another LABA (salmeterol) with placebo added to usual asthma therapy showed an increase in asthma-related deaths in patients receiving salmeterol. This finding with salmeterol is considered a class effect of the LABAs, including formoterol. Currently available data are inadequate to determine whether concurrent use of inhaled corticosteroids or other long-term asthma control drugs mitigates the increased risk of asthma-related death from LABAs. Available data from controlled clinical trials suggest that LABAs increase the risk of asthma-related hospitalization in pediatric and adolescent patients. Therefore, when treating patients with asthma, use mometasone/formoterol only in patients not adequately controlled on a long-term asthma control medication, such as an inhaled corticosteroid, or in patients whose disease severity clearly warrants initiation of treatment with both an inhaled corticosteroid and a LABA. Once asthma control is achieved and maintained, assess the patient at regular intervals, step down therapy (eg, discontinue mometasone/formoterol) if possible without loss of asthma control, and maintain the patient on a long-term asthma control medication such as an inhaled corticosteroid. Do not use mometasone/formoterol for patients whose asthma is adequately controlled on low- or medium-dose inhaled corticosteroids.

Indications

➤*Asthma:* For the treatment of asthma in patients 12 years of age and older. Mometasone/formoterol is not indicated for the relief of acute bronchospasm.

Administration and Dosage

➤*General dosing considerations:* If symptoms arise between doses, an inhaled short-acting beta$_2$-adrenergic agonist should be taken for immediate relief.

If a previously effective dosage regimen of mometasone/formoterol fails to provide adequate control of asthma, the therapeutic regimen should be reevaluated and additional therapeutic options (eg, replacing the current strength of mometasone/formoterol with a higher strength, adding an additional inhaled corticosteroid, initiating oral corticosteroids) should be considered.

The maximum benefit may not be achieved for 1 week or longer after beginning treatment. Individual patients may experience a variable time to onset and degree of symptom relief.

➤*Adults:*

Asthma –

Maximum dose: 2 inhalations of mometasone 200 mcg/formoterol 5 mcg twice daily. Do not use more than 2 inhalations twice daily of the prescribed strength of mometasone/formoterol, because some patients are more likely to experience adverse effects with higher doses of formoterol.

Initial dosage: The recommended starting dosages for mometasone/formoterol treatment are based on prior asthma therapy.

Recommended Dosages for Mometasone/Formoterol		
Previous therapy	Recommended dosage	Maximum recommended daily dose
Inhaled medium-dose corticosteroids	Mometasone 100 mcg/formoterol 5 mcg, 2 inhalations twice daily	Mometasone 400 mcg/formoterol 20 mcg
Inhaled high-dose corticosteroids	Mometasone 200 mcg/formoterol 5 mcg, 2 inhalations twice daily	Mometasone 800 mcg/formoterol 20 mcg

Dosage adjustment: For patients who do not respond adequately after 2 weeks of therapy, a higher strength may provide additional asthma control.

➤*Children:*

Asthma –

12 years of age and older: See Adults for dosing.

➤*Transferring from systemic corticosteroid therapy:* Patients requiring systemic corticosteroids should be weaned slowly from systemic corticosteroid use after transferring to mometasone/formoterol.

➤*Preparation for administration:* Mometasone/formoterol should be primed before using for the first time by releasing 4 test sprays into the air, away from the face, shaking well before each spray. In cases in which the inhaler has not been used for more than 5 days, prime the inhaler again by releasing 4 test sprays into the air, away from the face, shaking well before each spray.

➤*Administration:* Administer as 2 inhalations twice daily every day (morning and evening) by the orally inhaled route. The canister should be at room temperature before use. Shake well prior to each inhalation. Avoid spraying in the eyes. After each dose, patients should rinse their mouth with water without swallowing.

The mometasone/formoterol canister should only be used with the mometasone/formoterol actuator. The mometasone/formoterol actuator should not be used with any other inhalation drug product. Actuators from other products should not be used with the mometasone/formoterol canister.

The correct amount of medication in each inhalation cannot be ensured after the labeled number of actuations from the canister has been used, even though the inhaler may not feel completely empty and may continue to operate. The inhaler should be discarded when the labeled number of actuations has been used (the dose counter will read "0").

➤*Storage / Stability:* Store at 20° to 25°C (68° to 77°F); excursions are permitted between 15° and 30°C (59° and 86°F).

Contents under pressure; do not puncture. Do not use or store near heat or open flame. Exposure to temperatures above 49°C (120°F) may cause bursting. Never throw the container into a fire or incinerator.

NASAL DECONGESTANTS

Indications

➤*Oral:* For temporary relief of nasal congestion due to the common cold, hay fever or other upper respiratory allergies, and nasal congestion associated with sinusitis; to promote nasal or sinus drainage.

➤*Topical:* Symptomatic relief of nasal and nasopharyngeal mucosal congestion due to the common cold, sinusitis, hay fever or other upper respiratory allergies.

Administration and Dosage

Recommended Dosage Guidelines for Oral and Topical Nasal Decongestants (Dosage Maximum/24 h)[a]

Drug and route	Adults ≥ 12 years of age	Children 6 to < 12 years of age	Children 2 to < 6 years of age
Naphazoline			
Topical			
Sprays	0.05%: 1 or 2 sprays in each nostril no more than q 6 h (4 doses/24 h)	not recommended	not recommended
Drops	0.05%: 1 or 2 drops in each nostril no more than q 6 h (4 doses/24 h)	not recommended	not recommended
Oxymetazoline HCl			
Topical			
Sprays	0.05%: 2 or 3 sprays in each nostril q 10 to 12 h (2 doses/24 h)	same as adults	not recommended
Phenylephrine HCl			
Oral	10-20 mg q 4 h (120 mg/24 h)	10 mg q 4 h (60 mg/24 h)	0.25% drops: 1 mL q 4 h (6 doses/24 h); (15 mg/24 h)
Topical			
Sprays	0.25%, 0.5%, 1%: 2 to 3 sprays in each nostril no more than q 4 h (6 doses/24 h)	0.25%: 2 to 3 sprays in each nostril no more than q 4 h (6 doses/24 h)	not recommended
Drops	0.25%, 0.5%, 1%: 2 to 3 drops in each nostril no more than q 4 h (6 doses/24 h)		0.125%: 2 to 3 drops in each nostril no more than q 4 h (6 doses/24 h)
Pseudoephedrine HCl			
Oral	60 mg q 4 to 6 h (240 mg/24 h)	30 mg q 4 to 6 h (120 mg/24 h)	15 mg q 4 to 6 h (60 mg/24 h)
Oral SR, CR	120 mg SR q 12 h or 240 mg CR q 24 h (240 mg/24 h)	not recommended	not recommended
Pseudoephedrine sulfate			
Oral ER	120 mg ER q 12 h (240 mg/24 h)	not recommended	not recommended
Tetrahydrozoline HCl			
Topical			
Sprays	0.1%: 3 to 4 sprays in each nostril prn, no more than q 3 h (8 doses/24 h)	same as adults	not recommended
Drops	0.1%: 2 to 4 drops in each nostril prn, no more than q 3 h (8 doses/24 h)	same as adults	0.05%: 2 to 3 drops in each nostril prn no more than q 3 h (8 doses/24 h)
Xylometazoline HCl			
Topical			

Recommended Dosage Guidelines for Oral and Topical Nasal Decongestants (Dosage Maximum/24 h)[a]

Drug and route	Adults ≥ 12 years of age	Children 6 to < 12 years of age	Children 2 to < 6 years of age
Sprays	0.1%: 1 to 3 sprays in each nostril q 8 to 10 h (3 doses/24 h)	0.05%: 1 spray in each nostril q 8 to 10 h (3 doses/24 h)	same dose for 2 to 12 years of age
Drops	0.1%: 2 to 3 drops in each nostril q 8 to 10 h (3 doses/24 h)	0.05%: 2 to 3 drops in each nostril q 8 to 10 h (3 doses/24 h)	same dose for 2 to 12 years of age

[a] Refer to manufacturer's directions.SR = sustained release; CR = controlled release; ER = extended release

Actions

➤*Pharmacology:* Drugs that cause vasoconstriction, such as decongestants, act on the adrenergic receptors in the nasal mucosa by affecting the blood vessels' sympathetic tone and provoking vasoconstriction. Available decongestants include noradrenaline releasers (eg, amphetamines, **pseudoephedrine**), alpha$_1$-adrenergic agonists (eg, **phenylephrine**), and alpha$_2$-adrenergic agonists (eg, **naphazoline**, **oxymetazoline**). Decongestants improve nasal ventilation by shrinking swollen nasal mucosa. Constriction in the mucous membranes results in their shrinkage; this promotes drainage, thus improving ventilation and the stuffy feeling.

Decongestants are sympathomimetic amines administered directly to swollen membranes (eg, via spray, drops) or systemically via the oral route. They are used in acute conditions such as hay fever, allergic rhinitis, vasomotor rhinitis, sinusitis, and the common cold to relieve membrane congestion.

Oral agents are not as effective as topical products, especially on an immediate basis, but generally have a longer duration of action, cause less local irritation, and are not associated with rebound congestion (rhinitis medicamentosa).

Contraindications

Monoamine oxidase inhibitor (MAOI) therapy; hypersensitivity.

➤*Oral:*

Sustained-release pseudoephedrine – Children younger than 12 years of age.

➤*Topical:*

Tetrahydrozoline – 0.1% solution in children younger than 6 years of age; 0.05% solution in infants younger than 2 years of age. Systemic effects are less likely from topical use, but use caution in the conditions listed for oral agents. Adverse reactions are more likely with excessive use, in the elderly, and in children.

Warnings/Precautions

➤*Special risk patients:* Administer with caution to patients with thyroid disease, diabetes, cardiovascular disease, coronary artery disease, hypertension, intraocular pressure, peripheral vascular disease, heart disease, or difficulty in urination due to enlargement of the prostate gland, unless directed by a physician. Rarely, some tablets may cause bowel obstruction or blockage, usually in people with severe narrowing of the bowel, esophagus, stomach, or intestine. If a patient has had obstruction or narrowing of the bowel, have him or her consult a physician before taking oral tablet products. Advise patients to contact their physician if they experience persistent abdominal pain or vomiting. As with any drug, if a patient is pregnant or nursing a baby, she should seek the advice of a health professional before using these products.

➤*Hypertension:* Hypertensive patients should use these products only with medical advice, as they may experience a change in blood pressure because of the added vasoconstriction. Studies suggest pseudoephedrine is the drug of choice. Sustained-action preparations may affect the cardiovascular system to a lesser degree.

➤*Excessive use:* Do not exceed recommended dosage. If nervousness, dizziness, or sleeplessness occur, discontinue use and have the patient consult a physician. Do not take topical products for greater than 3 days or oral products for greater than 7 days. If symptoms do not improve or are accompanied by a fever, the patient should consult a physician.

➤*Rebound congestion (rhinitis medicamentosa):* Following topical application, this may occur after the vasoconstriction subsides. Patients who increase the amount of drug and frequency of use may produce toxicity and perpetuate the rebound congestion.

Treatment – A simple but uncomfortable solution is to completely withdraw the topical medication. A more acceptable method is to gradually withdraw therapy by initially discontinuing the medication in one nostril, followed by total withdrawal. Substituting an oral decongestant for a topical one also may be useful.

➤*Acute use:* Use topical decongestants only in acute states and not longer than 3 days. Use sparingly (especially the imidazolines) in all patients, particularly infants, children, and patients with cardiovascular disease.

➤*Stinging sensation:* Some individuals may experience a mild, transient stinging sensation after topical application.

➤*Sulfite sensitivity:* Some of the nasal decongestant products contain sulfites that may cause allergic-type reactions including anaphylactic symptoms and life-threatening or less severe asthmatic episodes in certain susceptible people. The overall prevalence of sulfite sensitivity in the general population is unknown but is probably low. Sulfite sensitivity is seen more frequently in asthmatic than in nonasthmatic people. Products containing sulfites are identified in the product listings.

➤*Pregnancy:* (*Category C* – **tetrahydrozoline**, **pseudoephedrine**, **phenylephrine**, **oxymetazoline**). It is not known whether these agents can cause fetal harm or affect reproduction capacity. Give only when clearly needed.

➤*Lactation:*

Oral preparations – Consult a physician before using.

Topical – It is not known if these agents are excreted in breast milk. Exercise caution when administering to a nursing woman.

➤*Children:* Use in children is product-specific. Refer to individual product listings.

➤*Elderly:* Patients 60 years of age or older are more likely to experience adverse reactions to sympathomimetics. Overdosage may cause hallucinations, convulsions, CNS depression, and death. Demonstrate safe use of a short-acting sympathomimetic before use of a sustained-action formulation in elderly patients.

Drug Interactions

Most interactions listed apply to sympathomimetics when used as vasopressors; however, consider the interaction when using the nasal decongestants.

Nasal Decongestant Drug Interactions

Precipitant drug	Object drug[a]		Description
Furazolidone	Nasal decongestants	↑	The pressor sensitivity to mixed-acting agents may be increased. Direct-acting agents are not affected.
Guanethidine	Nasal decongestants		Guanethidine potentiates the effects of the direct-acting agents and inhibits the effects of the mixed-acting agents. Guanethidine's hypotensive action also may be reversed.
	Direct	↑	
	Mixed	↓	
Nasal decongestants	Guanethidine	↓	
Methyldopa	Nasal decongestants	↑	Coadministration may result in an increased pressor response.
MAO inhibitors	Nasal decongestants	↑	Concurrent use of MAOIs and mixed-acting agents may result in severe headache, hypertension, and hyperpyrexia, possibly resulting in hypertensive crisis. Direct-acting agents interact minimally, if at all.
Rauwolfia alkaloids	Nasal decongestants		Reserpine potentiates the pressor response of direct-acting agents, which may result in hypotension. The pressor response of mixed-acting agents is decreased.
	Direct	↑	
	Mixed	↓	
Tricyclic antidepressants (TCAs)	Nasal decongestants		TCAs potentiate the pressor response of direct-acting agents; dysrhythmias have occurred. The pressor response of mixed-acting agents is decreased.
	Direct	↑	
	Mixed	↓	
Urinary acidifiers	Nasal decongestants	↓	Acidification of the urine may increase the elimination of the nasal decongestant; therapeutic effects may be decreased. Conversely, urinary alkalinization may decrease the elimination of these agents, possibly increasing therapeutic or toxic effects.
Urinary alkalinizers		↑	

[a] ↑ = Object drug increased. ↓ = Object drug decreased.

Adverse Reactions

➤*Cardiovascular:* Arrhythmias; palpitations; tachycardia; transient hypertension; bradycardia.

➤*CNS:* Headache; lightheadedness; dizziness; drowsiness; tremor; insomnia; nervousness; restlessness; giddiness; psychological disturbances; prolonged psychosis (eg, paranoia, terror, delusions); weakness.

➤*GI:* Nausea; gastric irritation.

➤*Hypersensitivity:* Hypersensitivity reactions such as rash, urticaria, leukopenia, agranulocytosis, and thrombocytopenia may occur.

➤*Miscellaneous:* Orofacial dystonia; sweating; blepharospasm (eg, ocular irritation, tearing, photophobia); urinary retention may occur in patients with prostatic hypertrophy.

Topical use – Burning; stinging; sneezing; dryness; local irritation; rebound congestion.

Overdosage

➤*Symptoms:* Overdoses have caused hypertension, bradycardia, drowsiness, and rebound hypotension in adults; a shock-like syndrome with hypotension and bradycardia also may occur. In either case, the treatment of overdosage is usually that of watchful expectancy and general supportive measures. If possible, keep the patient warm and maintain fluid balance orally or parenterally, if necessary. Overdosage of **tetrahydrozoline** nasal solution may result in oversedation in young children.

➤*Treatment:* Treatment is supportive; in severe cases, IV phentolamine may be used. See General Management of Acute Overdosage.

Tetrahydrozoline – There is no known antidote. The use of stimulants is contraindicated. If respiratory rate drops to less than or equal to 10, administer oxygen and assist respiration. Monitor blood pressure to prevent hypotensive crisis.

Patient Information

Patients with hypertension, heart disease, or other cardiovascular diseases, thyroid disease, diabetes, or difficulty urinating due to an enlarged prostate should use these products only with medical advice.

➤*Topical:* Notify physician of insomnia, dizziness, weakness, tremor, or irregular heart beat.

Do not exceed recommended dosage and do not use longer than 3 days. If symptoms persist, contact the doctor. Frequent or prolonged use may cause nasal congestion to recur or worsen.

Stinging, burning, sneezing, increased nasal discharge, or drying of the nasal mucosa may occur.

Do not share container with other patients. Do not allow tip of container to touch the nasal passage. Discard after medication is no longer required.

Proper use – Spray – Keep head upright. Sniff hard for a few minutes after use.

Drops – Recline on a bed and hang your head over the edge; remain in this position for several minutes after using the drops, turning the head from side to side.

Inhalers – Warm in the hand before use. Wipe the inhaler after each use.

➤*Oral:* Do not exceed recommended dosage; higher doses may cause nervousness, dizziness, or sleeplessness.

If symptoms do not improve within 7 days or are accompanied by a high fever, consult physician before continuing use.

Arylalkylamines

PSEUDOEPHEDRINE

otc	**Pseudoephedrine Hydrochloride** (Various, eg, Geneva, Roxane)	**Tablets; oral:** 30 mg	As pseudoephedrine hydrochloride. In 24s, 100s, 1,000s, blister pack 100s.
otc	**Congestaid** (Zee Medical)		As pseudoephedrine hydrochloride. In 24s.
otc	**Genaphed** (Goldline)		As pseudoephedrine hydrochloride. Lactose. In 24s.
otc	**Simply Stuffy** (McNeil Consumer)		As pseudoephedrine hydrochloride. Lactose. In 24s.
otc	**Sudafed Non-Drowsy, Maximum Strength** (McNeil)		As pseudoephedrine hydrochloride. Lactose, sucrose. (SU). In 24s, and 96s.
Rx	**SudoGest Non-Drowsy** (Major)		As pseudoephedrine hydrochloride. PEG, sugar. In 100s.
otc	**Pseudoephedrine Hydrochloride** (Various, eg, Geneva, Roxane)	**Tablets; oral:** 60 mg	As pseudoephedrine hydrochloride. In 100s, 1,000s, and blister pack 100s.
otc	**Pseudoephedrine Hydrochloride** (OHM Labs)	**Tablets, extended-release; oral:** 120 mg	As pseudoephedrine hydrochloride. Castor oil. Capsule shape. In 10s.
otc	**Sudafed Non-Drowsy 12 Hour Long-Acting** (McNeil)		As pseudoephedrine hydrochloride. Capsule shape. (SUDAFED 12 HOUR). In 10s.
otc	**Dimetapp, Maximum Strength 12-Hour Non-Drowsy Extentabs** (Whitehall-Robins)		As pseudoephedrine hydrochloride. Capsule shape. In 10s.
otc	**Sudafed Non-Drowsy 24 Hour Long-Acting** (McNeil)	**Tablets, controlled-release; oral:** 240 mg (immediate-release 60 mg, controlled-release 180 mg).	As pseudoephedrine hydrochloride. (SU-24). In 10s.
otc	**Sinustop** (Nature's Way)	**Capsules; oral:** 60 mg	As pseudoephedrine hydrochloride. In 20s.
otc	**AllergyCare** (Nature's Way)		As pseudoephedrine hydrochloride. In 20s.
otc	**Nasal Decongestant, Children's Non-Drowsy** (Various, eg, AmerisourceBergen)	**Liquid; oral:** 15 mg per 5 mL	As pseudoephedrine hydrochloride. In 118 mL.
otc sf	**Sudafed, Children's Non-Drowsy** (McNeil)		As pseudoephedrine hydrochloride. EDTA, saccharin, sorbitol. Alcohol free. Grape flavor. In 118 mL.
otc	**Pseudoephedrine HCl** (Various)	**Liquid; oral:** 30 mg per 5 mL	As pseudoephedrine hydrochloride. In 120 and 473 mL.
otc	**Silfedrine, Children's** (Silarx)		As pseudoephedrine hydrochloride. Methylparaben, saccharin, sucrose. In 118 and 237 mL.
otc	**Unifed** (Altaire)		As pseudoephedrine hydrochloride. Methylparaben, glycerin, sorbitol, sucrose. In 118 mL.
otc	**ElixSure Children's Congestion** (Taro Consumer)	**Syrup; oral:** 15 mg per 5 mL	As pseudoephedrine hydrochloride. Glycerin, propylparaben. Grape and bubble gum flavors. In 118 mL.
otc	**Nasal Decongestant Oral** (Various, eg, ProMetic)	**Drops; oral:** 7.5 mg per 0.8 mL	As pseudoephedrine hydrochloride. In 15 and 30 mL w/dropper.
otc	**Kid Kare** (Rugby)		As pseudoephedrine hydrochloride. Alcohol free. Sorbitol, sugar. Cherry flavor. In 30 mL w/dropper.

[a] Contains phenylalanine 7 mg per 5 mL.

PSEUDOEPHEDRINE HYDROCHLORIDE — ORAL

For complete and comparative prescribing information, refer to the Nasal Decongestants class monograph.

Indications

➤*Nasal congestion:* Temporary relieves nasal congestion due to the common cold, hay fever, or other upper respiratory allergies, and nasal congestion associated with sinusitis; reduces swelling of nasal passages; relieves sinus pressure; promotes nasal or sinus drainage; restores freer breathing through the nose.

Administration and Dosage

➤*Adults:*

Nasal congestion –

Usual dosage: 60 mg every 4 to 6 hours (120 mg sustained-release every 12 hours, 240 mg controlled-release every 24 hours).

Maximum dose: 240 mg/day.

➤*Children:* Do not administer extended-release pseudoephedrine to children younger than 12 years of age.

Nasal congestion –

12 years of age and older: See Adults for dosing.

6 to 12 years of age:

- *Usual dosage* – 30 mg every 4 to 6 hours.
- *Maximum dose* – 120 mg/day.

2 to 5 years of age:

- *Usual dosage* – 15 mg every 4 to 6 hours.
- *Maximum dose* – 60 mg/day.

➤*Storage/Stability:* Store at room temperature 15° to 25°C (59° to 77°F).

PHENYLEPHRINE HYDROCHLORIDE

otc	**Sudafed PE** (McNeil)	**Tablets; oral:** 10 mg	Acesulfame K. In 18s.
otc	**Sudogest PE** (Major)		Dextrose. In 36s.
Rx	**AH-chew D** (WE Pharm)	**Tablets, chewable; oral:** 10 mg	(WE 07). Scored. Bubble gum flavor. In 100s.
Rx	**Lusonal** (WraSer)	**Liquid; oral:** 7.5 mg per 5 mL	Strawberry flavor. In 473 mL.[b]
otc	**Little Colds Decongestant Drops for Infants and Children** (Vetco)	**Solution, concentrate; oral:** 2.5 mg/mL	Alcohol free. Grape flavor. Glycerin, sorbitol and sucralose. In 30 mL.
otc	**Pedia Care Children's Decongestant** (Pfizer Cons Health)	**Solution; oral:** 2.5 mg per 5 mL	EDTA, sorbitol, sucralose. In 118 mL.
otc	**Little Noses Gentle Formula, Infants & Children** (Vetco[c])	**Solution; intranasal:** 0.125%	**Drops:** Alcohol free. In 15 mL w/dropper.[d]
otc	**Neo-Synephrine Mild Strength** (Bayer Corp.)	**Solution; intranasal:** 0.25%	**Spray:** In 15 mL.[e]
otc	**Rhinall** (Scherer)		**Spray:** In 40 mL.[f]
			Drops: In 30 mL.[f]
otc	**Neo-Synephrine Regular Strength** (Bayer Corp.)	**Solution; intranasal:** 0.5%	**Drops:** In 15 mL.[e]
			Spray: In 15 mL.[e]
otc	**Vicks Sinex Ultra Fine Mist** (Procter & Gamble Co.)		**Spray:** In 14.7 mL.[g]
otc	**Phenylephrine hydrochloride** (Various)	**Solution; intranasal:** 1%	In 480 mL.
otc	**4-Way Fast Acting** (Novartis Consumer Health)		**Spray:** In 30 mL.[h]
otc	**Neo-Synephrine Extra Strength** (Bayer Corp.)		**Drops:** In 15 mL.[e]
			Spray: In 15 mL.[e]
otc	**Triaminic Thin Strips Cold** (Novartis Consumer Health)	**Strip; oral:** 2.5 mg	Maltodextrin, sucralose. Raspberry flavor. In 16s.

[a] With phenylalanine 4 mg, aspartame, sorbitol.
[b] With aspartame, phenylalanine, parabens.
[c] Vetco, 105 Baylis Road, Melville, NY 11747; (631)755-1155.
[d] With EDTA, benzalkonium chloride.
[e] With benzalkonium chloride.
[f] With chlorobutanol, sodium bisulfite, benzalkonium chloride.
[g] With benzalkonium chloride, camphor, EDTA, eucalyptol, menthol, tyloxapol.
[h] With benzalkonium chloride, boric acid, sodium borate.

PHENYLEPHRINE HYDROCHLORIDE — ORAL

For complete and comparative prescribing information, refer to the Nasal Decongestants group monograph.

Indications

➤*Nasal congestion:* Phenylephrine is recommended for the temporary relief of nasal congestion due to the common cold, sinusitis, hay fever, or upper respiratory allergies.

➤*Lusonal*: For temporarily relief of symptoms of upper respiratory tract disorders such as sinusitis, vasomotor rhinitis, and hay fever, as well as for the temporary relief of coughs associated with respiratory tract infections and related conditions such as sinusitis, bronchitis, and asthma, when these conditions are complicated by tenacious mucus and/or mucus plugs and congestion.

Administration and Dosage

➤*General dosing considerations:* Do not take oral products for more than 7 days.

➤*Adults:*

Nasal congestion –

Maximum dose:
- *Liquid* – 40 mL (60 mg)/day.
- *Strips* – 6 strips (15 mg)/day.

Chewable tablets: 1 or 2 tablets (10 or 20 mg) every 4 hours.
Liquid: 10 mL (15 mg) every 6 hours.
Strips: 1 strip (2.5 mg) every 4 hours.
Tablets: 1 to 2 tablets (10 to 20 mg) every 4 hours.

➤*Children:*

Nasal congestion –

Maximum dose:
- *Liquid –*
  12 years of age and older: 40 mL (60 mg)/day.
  6 through 11 years of age: 20 mL (30 mg)/day.
  2 through 5 years of age: 10 mL (15 mg)/day.
- *Oral drops –*
  2 through 6 years of age: 6 mL (15 mg)/day.
- *Oral solution –*
  6 to younger than 12 years of age: 60 mL (30 mg)/day.
  2 to 5 years of age: 30 mL (15 mg)/day.
- *Strips –*
  12 years of age and older: 6 strips (15 mg)/day.

Chewable tablets:
- *12 years of age and older* – 1 or 2 tablets (10 or 20 mg) every 4 hours.
- *6 to 11 years of age* – 1 tablet (10 mg) every 4 hours.

Liquid:
- *12 years of age or older* – 10 mL (15 mg) every 6 hours.
- *6 through 11 years of age* – 5 mL (7.5 mg) every 6 hours.
- *2 through 5 years of age* – 2.5 mL (3.75 mg) every 6 hours.

Oral drops:
- *2 through 6 years of age* – 1 mL (2.5 mg) every 4 hours.

Oral solution:
- *6 to 11 years of age* – 10 mL (5 mg) every 4 hours.
- *2 to younger than 6 years of age* – 5 mL (2.5 mg) every 4 hours.

Strips:
- *12 years of age and older* – 1 strip (2.5 mg) every 4 hours.

Tablets:
- *12 years of age or older* – 1 to 2 tablets (10 to 20 mg) every 4 hours.
- *6 through 11 years of age* – 1 tablet (10 mg) every 4 hours.

➤*Administration:*

Chewable tablets – Tablets may be broken in half for ease of administration.

Strips – Place 1 film strip on tongue and allow it to dissolve.

➤*Storage/Stability:* Store at 15° to 30°C (59° to 86°F). Store strips in a dry place.

PHENYLEPHRINE HYDROCHLORIDE — INTRANASAL

For complete and comparative prescribing information, refer to the Nasal Decongestants group monograph.

Indications

➤*Nasal congestion:* For prompt, temporary relief of nasal congestion due to the common cold, sinusitis, hay fever, or other upper respiratory allergies, or associated with sinusitis.

Administration and Dosage

➤*Adults:*

Nasal congestion – 2 to 3 sprays or drops in each nostril every 3 to 4 hours as needed. The 1% solution should be repeated no more often than every 4 hours.

➤*Children:*

Nasal congestion –

0.5% and 1%:
- *12 years of age and older* – See Adults for dosing.

0.25%:
- *12 years of age and older* – 2 to 3 sprays or drops in each nostril every 3 to 4 hours as needed.
- *6 through 11 years of age* – 2 to 3 sprays or drops in each nostril not more often than every 4 hours.

0.125%:
- *2 through 5 years of age* – 2 or 3 drops into each nostril not more often than every 4 hours.

➤*Duration of therapy:* The patient should not use for more than 3 days.

➤*Administration:* For nasal inhalation only.

➤*Storage/Stability:* Store at room temperature and protect from light.

Imidazolines

NAPHAZOLINE HYDROCHLORIDE

otc	**Privine** (Insight[a])	**Solution:** 0.05%	**Drops:** In 25 mL w/dropper.[b]
			Spray: In 20 mL.[b]

[a] Insight Pharmaceuticals Corp., 1170 Wheeler Way, Suite 150, Langhorne, PA 19047-1749; 1-(267) 852-0505; fax 1-(267) 852-0515.
[b] With benzalkonium chloride, EDTA.

NAPHAZOLINE HYDROCHLORIDE — INTRANASAL

For complete and comparative prescribing information, refer to the Nasal Decongestants group monograph.

Indications

➤*Nasal congestion:* Temporary relief of nasal congestion due to the common cold, hay fever or other upper respiratory tract allergies, or associated with sinusitis.

Administration and Dosage

➤*Adults:*

Nasal congestion –

Usual dosage: 1 or 2 drops or sprays in each nostril not more often than every 6 hours.

Maximum dose: 8 drops or sprays/day in each nostril.

Duration of therapy: Do not use longer than 3 days

➤*Children:*

Nasal congestion –

12 years of age and older: See Adults for dosing.

➤*Administration:*

Drops – Recline on a bed and hang your head over the edge; remain in this position for several minutes after using the drops, turning the head from side to side.

Spray – Keep head upright. Sniff hard for a few minutes after use.

➤*Storage/Stability:* Store between 15° to 30°C (59° to 86°F).

OXYMETAZOLINE HYDROCHLORIDE

otc	**Oxymetazoline HCl** (Various, eg, Alpharma, Clay Park, Thames)	**Solution; intranasal:** 0.05%	**Spray:** In 15 and 30 mL.
otc	**12 Hour Nasal** (Various, eg, URL)		**Spray:** In 15 mL.
otc	**Twice-A-Day 12-Hour Nasal** (Major)		**Spray:** In 15 and 30 mL.[a]
otc	**Neo-Synephrine 12-Hour Extra Moisturizing** (Bayer Corp.)		**Spray:** In 15 mL.[i]
otc	**Duration** (Schering-Plough Healthcare)		**Spray:** In 30 mL.[b]
otc	**Afrin 12-Hour Original Pump Mist** (Schering-Plough Healthcare)		**Spray:** In 15 mL.[b]
otc	**Afrin 12-Hour Original** (Schering-Plough Healthcare)		**Spray:** In 15 mL.[b]
otc	**Afrin All Night No Drip** (Schering-Plough Healthcare)		**Spray:** In 15 mL.[q]
otc	**Afrin Severe Congestion with Menthol** (Schering-Plough Healthcare)		**Spray:** In 15 mL.[c]
otc	**Afrin No-Drip 12-Hour** (Schering-Plough Healthcare)		**Spray:** In 15 mL.[d]
otc	**Afrin No-Drip 12-Hour Extra Moisturizing** (Schering-Plough Healthcare)		**Spray:** In 15 mL.[e]
otc	**Afrin Extra Moisturizing 12 Hour Relief** (Schering-Plough Healthcare)		**Spray:** In 15 mL.[n]
otc	**Afrin Sinus 12 Hour Relief** (Schering-Plough Healthcare)		**Spray:** In 15 mL.[c]
otc	**Dristan 12-Hr Nasal** (Wyeth)		**Spray:** In 15 mL.[g]
otc	**Duramist Plus 12-Hr Decongestant** (Pfeiffer)		**Spray:** In 15 mL.[h]
otc	**Genasal** (Goldline)		**Spray:** In 15 and 30 mL.[b]
otc	**Nasal Decongestant, Maximum Strength** (Taro)		**Spray:** In 15 and 30 mL.
otc	**Nasal Relief** (Rugby)		**Spray:** In 15 and 30 mL.[j]
otc	**Nōstrilla 12-Hour** (Heritage)		**Spray:** In 15 mL metered pump spray.[k]
otc	**Nōstrilla Complete Congestion Relief 12-Hour** (Insight)		**Spray:** In 15 mL.[o]
otc	**Nōstrilla Conditioning Double-Moisture** (Insight)		**Spray:** In 15 mL.[p]
otc	**Vicks Sinex 12-Hour Long-Acting** (Procter & Gamble)		**Spray:** In 15 mL.[l]
otc	**Vicks Sinex 12-Hour Ultra Fine Mist for Sinus Relief** (Procter & Gamble)		**Spray:** In 15 mL.[m]

[a] With EDTA, benzalkonium chloride, benzyl alcohol.
[b] With benzalkonium chloride, edetate disodium, PEG 1450.
[c] With benzalkonium chloride, benzyl alcohol, camphor, EDTA, eucalyptol, menthol.
[d] With carboxymethylcellulose sodium, microcrystalline cellulose, benzalkonium chloride, benzyl alcohol, EDTA.
[e] With carboxymethylcellulose sodium, microcrystalline cellulose, benzalkonium chloride, benzyl alcohol, EDTA, glycerin.
[f] With carboxymethylcellulose sodium, microcrystalline cellulose, benzalkonium chloride, benzyl alcohol, camphor, EDTA, eucalyptol, menthol.
[g] With benzalkonium chloride, benzyl alcohol, edetate disodium, sodium chloride.
[h] With benzalkonium chloride, EDTA, sodium chloride.
[i] With benzalkonium chloride, glycerin, sorbitol, sodium chloride.
[j] With EDTA, sorbitol, sodium chloride.
[k] With benzalkonium chloride, sorbitol.
[l] With benzalkonium chloride, camphor, chlorhexidine gluconate, EDTA, eucalyptol, menthol, sodium chloride, tyloxapol.
[m] With aromatic vapors (camphor, eucalyptus, menthol), tyloxapol, EDTA, benzalkonium chloride, sodium chloride.
[n] With benzalkonium chloride, edetate disodium
[o] With benzalkonium chloride, camphor, edetate disodium, eucalyptol, menthol.
[p] With benzalkonium chloride, eucalyptol, sodium chloride, spearmint oil, winter green oil.
[q] With benzalkonium chloride, benzyl alcohol, edetate disodium, flower oil, glycerin, PEG.

OXYMETAZOLINE HYDROCHLORIDE — INTRANASAL

For complete and comparative prescribing information, refer to the Nasal Decongestants class monograph.

Indications

➤*Nasal congestion:* For the temporary relief of nasal congestion due to a cold, hay fever, or other upper respiratory allergies, or associated with sinusitis. Reduces swelling of nasal passages; shrinks swollen membranes. Temporarily restores freer breathing through the nose; temporarily relieves sinus congestion and pressure.

Administration and Dosage

➤*Adults:*

Nasal congestion –

Usual dosage: 2 or 3 sprays of 0.05% solution in each nostril twice daily, morning and evening, or every 10 to 12 hours.

Maximum dose: 2 doses per 24 hours.

Imidazolines

OXYMETAZOLINE HYDROCHLORIDE — INTRANASAL

➤*Children:*

Nasal congestion –

6 years of age or older: See Adults for dosing.

➤*Duration of therapy:* Do not exceed recommended dosage and do not use longer than 3 days. Frequent or prolonged use may cause nasal congestion to recur or worsen.

➤*Administration:* Do not allow tip of container to touch the nasal passage.

Drops – Lie down and tilt your head back. Place the correct number of drops in your nose. Continue to lie down with your head tilted back for 2 minutes.

Spray – Keep head upright. Press against the one nostril to close it off. Breathe gently through the open nostril and squeeze the spray container. If you are using more than 1 spray, wait for 1 to 2 minutes between sprays. Inhale deeply.

➤*Storage/Stability:* Store at room temperature. Discard after medication is no longer required.

TETRAHYDROZOLINE HYDROCHLORIDE

Rx	**Tyzine Pediatric** (Kenwood)	**Solution:** 0.05%	**Drops:** In 15 mL with dropper.[a]
Rx	**Tyzine** (Kenwood)	**Solution:** 0.1%	**Drops:** In 30 mL with dropper.[a]
			Spray: In 15 mL.[a]

[a] With benzalkonium chloride, EDTA.

TETRAHYDROZOLINE HYDROCHLORIDE — INTRANASAL

For complete and comparative prescribing information, refer to the Nasal Decongestants group monograph.

Indications

➤*Nasal congestion:* Decongestion of nasal and nasopharyngeal mucosa.

Administration and Dosage

➤*Adults:*

Nasal congestion –

0.1% solution: 2 to 4 drops or 3 to 4 sprays instilled in each nostril as needed, never more often than every 3 hours. Less frequent administration is usually sufficient because relief is maintained for 4 hours or longer in most cases, and often for as long as 8 hours.

➤*Children:*

Nasal congestion –

6 years and older: See Adults for dosing.

2 to 5 years of age:

• *0.05% solution* – 2 to 3 drops instilled in each nostril as needed, and never more often than every 3 hours. Relief usually lasts for several hours, so that instillation is usually needed only every 4 to 6 hours.

➤*Administration:* Bedtime instillation usually ensures sleep undisturbed by the need for remedication before morning, or by insomnia from central stimulation. Instillation of nose drops can be most conveniently accomplished with the patient in the lateral head-low position.

➤*Storage/Stability:* Store below 30°C (86°F).

XYLOMETAZOLINE HYDROCHLORIDE

otc	**Otrivin Pediatric Nasal** (Novartis Consumer)	**Solution; nasal:** 0.05%	**Drops:** In 25 mL dropper bottle.[a]
otc	**4–Way Nasal Decongestant Moisturizing Relief** (Novartis Consumer Health)	**Solution; nasal:** 0.1%	**Spray:** In 14.8 mL.[b]
otc	**Otrivin** (Novartis Consumer)	**Solution; nasal:** 0.1%	**Drops:** In 25 mL dropper bottle.[b]
			Spray: In 20 mL.[b]

[a] With benzalkonium chloride, EDTA.
[b] With benzalkonium chloride, sodium chloride, EDTA.

XYLOMETAZOLINE HYDROCHLORIDE — INTRANASAL

For complete and comparative prescribing information, refer to the Nasal Decongestants group monograph.

Indications

➤*Spray/Drops:* For the temporary relief of nasal congestion due to the common cold, hay fever, or other respiratory allergies.

➤*Pediatric drops:* For temporary relief of nasal and sinus congestion and pressure due to a cold.

Administration and Dosage

➤*Adults:*

Nasal and sinus congestion –

0.1% Spray:

• *Usual dosage* – 2 to 3 sprays in each nostril not more often than every 8 to 10 hours.

• *Maximum dose* – 3 doses in 24 hours.

➤*Children:*

Nasal and sinus congestion –

12 years of age or older: See Adults for dosing.

2 to 11 years of age:

• *0.05% Spray –*

Usual dosage: 1 to 2 sprays in each nostril not more often than every 8 to 10 hours.

Maximum dose: 3 doses in 24 hours.

➤*Administration:* For intranasal use only. Wipe nozzle clean after each use.

➤*Storage/Stability:* Store between 68° and 77°F (20° and 25°C).

NASAL DECONGESTANTS

NASAL DECONGESTANT INHALERS

otc	**Benzedrex** (B.F. Ascher)	**Inhaler:** 250 mg propylhexedrine	In single plastic inhalers.[a]
otc	**Vicks Vapor Inhaler** (Procter & Gamble Consumer)	**Inhaler:** 50 mg levmetamfetamine	In single plastic inhalers.[b]

[a] With menthol, lavender oil.
[b] With camphor, lavender oil, menthol.

NASAL DECONGESTANT INHALERS — INHALATION

For complete and comparative prescribing information, refer to the Nasal Decongestants group monograph.

Indications

➤*Nasal congestion:* For the temporary relief of nasal congestion due to the common cold, hay fever, upper respiratory allergies, or sinusitis.

Administration and Dosage

➤*Adults:*

Nasal congestion –

Usual dosage: 1 to 2 inhalations in each nostril (while blocking the other nostril) not more than every 2 hours.

Maximum dose: 24 inhalations in each nostril/day.

➤*Children:*

Nasal congestion –

6 years of age or older: See Adults for dosing.

➤*Duration of therapy:* Do not use these products for greater than 3 days. If symptoms persist beyond this time, consult physician.

➤*Storage/Stability:* Store at room temperature.

NASAL PRODUCTS

otc	**Nasal Spray** (Various, eg, Ivax)	**Solution; intranasal:** Sodium chloride	**Spray:** In 45 mL.
otc	**Entsol** (Kenwood Therapeutics)		**Spray:** In 29.6 mL.
otc	**Pretz Moisturizing** (Parnell)		**Spray:** In 50 mL.[a]
otc	**Simply Saline** (Blairex)		**Spray:** In 44 mL.
otc	**Pretz Irrigation** (Parnell)		**Spray:** In 237 mL.[c]
otc	**Rhinaris** (Pharma Science)	**Solution; intranasal:** 0.2% sodium chloride	**Spray:** In 30 mL.[p]
otc	**SalineX** (Muro)	**Solution; intranasal:** 0.4% sodium chloride	**Drops:** In 15 mL.[d]
			Mist: In 50 mL.[d]
otc	**Ayr Saline** (B.F. Ascher)	**Solution; intranasal:** 0.65% sodium chloride	**Drops:** In 50 mL.[b]
			Mist: In 50 mL.[b]
			Gel: In 14 g.[e]
otc	**Breathe Free** (Thompson Medical)		**Spray:** In 45 mL.[f]
otc	**HuMist Moisturizing Mist** (Scherer)		**Spray:** In 45 mL.[g]
otc	**NaSal** (Bayer Corp.)		**Drops:** Alcohol free. In 15 mL.[h]
			Spray: Alcohol free. In 30 mL.[h]
otc	**Nasal Moist** (Blairex)		**Spray:** Alcohol free, dye free. In 45 mL.
			Mist pump: Alcohol free, dye free. In 15 mL.
			Gel: Alcohol free, dye free. In 28.5 g and unit-of-use 2 mL.[i]
otc	**Ocean** (Fleming)		**Spray:** In 45 and 473 mL.[f]
otc	**Ocean for Kids** (Fleming)		**Spray:** Alcohol free. In 37.5 mL.[j]
otc	**Mycinaire Saline Mist** (Pfieffer)		**Spray:** In 45 mL.[f]
otc	**Rhinaris Lubricating Mist** (Pharmascience)	**Solution; intranasal:** 15% polyethylene glycol, 5% propylene glycol	**Spray:** In 30 mL.[k]
		Solution; intranasal: 15% polyethylene glycol, 20% propylene glycol	**Gel:** In 28.35 g.[k]
otc	**Nasal•Ease with Zinc** (Health Care Products)	**Solution; intranasal:** Zinc acetate	**Gel:** In 14.1 g.[l]
otc	**Nasal•Ease with Zinc Gluconate** (Health Care Products)	**Solution; intranasal:** Zinc gluconate	**Spray:** In 30 mL.[m]
otc	**Ayr Saline** (B.F. Ascher)	**Gel; intranasal:** methyl gluceth-10, propylene glycol, glycerin	**Swabs:** In 20s.[n]
otc	**Entsol** (Kenwood Therapeutics)	**Gel; intranasal:** Sodium chloride	**Gel:** Preservative free. In 20 g.[o]
otc	**Rhinaris** (PharmaScience)	**Gel; intranasal:** 0.2% sodium chloride	**Gel:** In 28.4 g[p]

[a] With glycerin, yerba santa.
[b] With benzalkonium chloride, EDTA.
[c] With yerba santa.
[d] With benzalkonium chloride, propylene glycol, polyethylene glycol, EDTA.
[e] With aloe vera gel, glycerin, parabens.
[f] With benzalkonium chloride.
[g] With chlorobutanol.
[h] With benzalkonium chloride, edetate disodium.
[i] With aloe vera.
[j] With benzalkonium chloride, EDTA, glycerin.
[k] With benzalkonium chloride, sodium chloride.
[l] With aloe vera, calendula extract, parabens, glycerin, tocopherol acetate, EDTA.
[m] With sodium chloride, benzalkonium chloride, glycerin.
[n] With glyceryl polymethacrylate, triethanolamine, aloe vera, PEG/PPG-18/18 dimethicone, carbomer, poloxamer 184, sodium chloride, xanthan gum, diazolidinyl urea, parabens, soybean oil, geranium maculatum oil, tocopheryl acetate, blue 1.
[o] With aloe, benzalkonium chloride, disodium EDTA, propylene glycol, glycerin, triethanolamine, vitamin E.
[p] With benzalkonium chloride, PEG, propylene glycol.

NASAL PRODUCTS — INTRANASAL

For complete and comparative prescribing information, refer to the Nasal Decongestants class monograph.

Indications

➤*Nasal dryness/congestion and inflammation:* Can be used as a nasal wash for sinuses and to restore moisture, thin nasal secretions, and relieve dry, crusted, and inflamed nasal membranes due to colds, low humidity, nasal decongestant overuse, allergies, minor nose bleeds, winter dryness, air travel, pregnancy, oxygen therapy, chronic sinusitis, asthma, intranasal and endoscopic sinus surgery, and other irritations.

Administration and Dosage

➤*Adults:*

Nasal moisturizer –

Drops: 2 to 6 drops in each nostril every 2 hours, as often as needed.

• *Nasal•Ease with Zinc Gluconate* – 1 to 2 sprays/drops in each nostril 2 to 4 times per day. Discontinue use after 5 days.

Gel: Use as needed to help relieve nasal discomfort.

• *Rhinaris* – Apply a small amount of gel into each nostril every 4 hours as needed.

Spray: 2 to 6 sprays in each nostril every 2 hours, as often as needed.

• *Nasal•Ease with Zinc Gluconate* – 1 to 2 sprays in each nostril 2 to 4 times per day. Discontinue use after 5 days.

• *Rhinaris* – 1 or 2 sprays into each nostril every 4 hours as needed.

➤*Children:*

Nasal moisturizer –

Drops: See Adults for dosing.

• *Nasal•Ease with Zinc Gluconate –*

4 years of age and older: 1 to 2 sprays/drops in each nostril 2 to 4 times per day. Discontinue use after 5 days.

Gel: See Adults for dosing.

Spray: See Adults for dosing.

• *Nasal•Ease with Zinc Gluconate –*

4 years of age and older: 1 to 2 sprays in each nostril 2 to 4 times per day. Discontinue use after 5 days.

• *Rhinaris –*

2 years of age and older: 1 or 2 sprays into each nostril every 4 hours as needed.

➤*Administration:*

Drops – Tilt head back and hold bottle upside down.

Gel – Apply around nostrils, under nose, or in nostrils as needed to help relieve discomfort. Use at bedtime to prevent drying and crusting.

Spray – Hold head in upright position and give short, firm squeezes in each nostril. Sniff deeply.

➤*Storage/Stability:* Store at 15° to 30°C (59° to 86°F). Wipe nozzle clean after use.

ALPHA$_1$-PROTEINASE INHIBITOR, HUMAN

Rx	**Aralast NP** (Baxter Healthcare)	**Injection, lyophilized powder for solution:** 0.5 g	Preservative free. In single-dose vials with 25 mL of diluent.[a]
		1 g	Preservative free. In single-dose vials with 50 mL of diluent.[a]
Rx	**Glassia** (Kamada)	**Injection, solution:** 1 g per 50 mL	Preservative, latex free. In single-use vials.
Rx	**Prolastin** (Talecris)	**Injection, lyophilized powder for solution:** 500 mg (≥ 20 mg of alpha$_1$-proteinase inhibitor/mL when reconstituted)	Preservative free. In single-dose vial[b] with 20 mL of diluent.
		1,000 mg (≥ 20 mg of alpha$_1$-proteinase inhibitor/mL when reconstituted)	Preservative free. In single-dose vial[b] with 40 mL of diluent.
Rx	**Zemaira** (CSL Behring)	**Injection, lyophilized powder for solution:** 1,000 mg	Preservative free. In single-dose vial[c] with 20 mL of diluent.

[a] With polyethylene glycol, sodium, and albumin. The total alpha$_1$-proteinase inhibitor functional activity in milligrams is stated on the label of each vial.
[b] With polyethylene glycol, sucrose, sodium, and small amounts of other plasma proteins. The total alpha$_1$-proteinase inhibitor functional activity in milligrams is stated on the label of each vial.
[c] With sodium and mannitol. The specific activity is ≥ 0.7 mg of functional alpha$_1$-proteinase inhibitor/mg of total protein. The total alpha$_1$-proteinase inhibitor functional activity in milligrams is stated on the label of each vial.

ALPHA$_1$-PROTEINASE INHIBITOR, HUMAN — INJECTION

Indications

➤*Congenital alpha$_1$-proteinase inhibitor (alpha$_1$-antitrypsin) deficiency:* For chronic augmentation and maintenance therapy in patients having congenital deficiency of alpha$_1$-proteinase inhibitor (alpha$_1$-antitrypsin deficiency) with clinically evident emphysema.

Clinical data demonstrating the long-term effects of chronic augmentation or replacement therapy of individuals with alpha$_1$-proteinase inhibitor are not available. Only adult subjects have received alpha$_1$-proteinase inhibitor to date.

Alpha$_1$-proteinase inhibitor is not indicated as therapy for patients with lung disease in whom congenital alpha$_1$-proteinase inhibitor deficiency has not been established.

The effect of augmentation therapy with alpha$_1$-proteinase inhibitor on pulmonary exacerbations and on the progression of emphysema in alpha$_1$-proteinase inhibitor deficiency has not been demonstrated in randomized, controlled clinical trials.

Clinical and biochemical studies have demonstrated that with such therapy, alpha$_1$-proteinase inhibitor is effective in maintaining target serum alpha$_1$-proteinase inhibitor trough levels and increasing alpha$_1$-proteinase inhibitor levels in epithelial lining fluid. As some individuals with alpha$_1$-antitrypsin deficiency will not go on to develop panacinar emphysema, only those with evidence of such disease should be considered for chronic replacement therapy with alpha$_1$-proteinase inhibitor.

Administration and Dosage

➤*General dosing considerations:* Alpha$_1$-proteinase inhibitor is for intravenous (IV) use only.

Each bottle of alpha$_1$-proteinase inhibitor has the functional activity, as determined by inhibition of porcine pancreatic elastase, stated on the label of the bottle. *Zemaira* contains the labeled amount of functionally active alpha$_1$-proteinase inhibitor in milligrams as stated on the vial label, as determined by the capacity to neutralize human neutrophil elastase.

The maintenance of blood serum levels of alpha$_1$-proteinase inhibitor (antigenically measured) above 11 mcM is historically thought to provide therapeutically relevant antineutrophil elastase protection. However, the hypothesis that maintaining a serum level of antigenic alpha$_1$-proteinase inhibitor will restore protease-antiprotease balance and prevent further lung damage has never been tested in an adequately powered clinical trial. However, assays of alpha$_1$-proteinase inhibitor based on commercial standards measure antigenic activity of alpha$_1$-proteinase inhibitor, whereas the labeled potency value of alpha$_1$-proteinase inhibitor is expressed as actual functional activity (ie, actual capacity to neutralize porcine pancreatic elastase). As functional activity may be less than antigenic activity, serum levels of alpha$_1$-proteinase inhibitor determined using commercial immunologic assays may not accurately reflect actual functional alpha$_1$-proteinase inhibitor levels. Therefore, although it may be helpful to monitor serum levels of alpha$_1$-proteinase inhibitor in individuals receiving alpha$_1$-proteinase inhibitor, using currently available commercial assays of antigenic activity, results of these assays should not be used to determine the required therapeutic dosage.

➤*Adults:*

Usual dosage – 60 mg/kg body weight administered once weekly by IV infusion. The recommended dosage of 60 mg/kg takes approximately 15 to 30 minutes to infuse. *Glassia* takes approximately 60 to 80 minutes to infuse.

This dose is intended to increase and maintain a level of functional alpha$_1$-proteinase inhibitor in the epithelial lining of the lower respiratory tract, providing augmented antielastase activity in the lung of individuals with alpha$_1$-antitrypsin deficiency.

➤*Preparation for administration:*

Glassia – Inspect the vial. The solution should be clear and colorless to yellow-green and may contain a few protein particles. Do not use if the product is cloudy.

Infusion can be made directly from the vial or, alternatively, vials may be pooled in an empty, sterile IV container. When infusing directly from the vial, use a vented spike adapter and a 5 micron in-line filter (neither is supplied). When infusion from a sterile IV container, attach an appropriate IV administration set to the IV container. Use a vent filter (not supplied) to withdraw the material from the vial and then use the supplied 5 micron filter needle to transfer the product into the infusion container.

Reconstitution –

Aralast NP: Use aseptic technique.

Alpha$_1$-proteinase inhibitor and diluent should be at room temperature before reconstitution.

Remove caps from the diluent and product vials. Swab the exposed stopper surfaces with alcohol. Remove cover from one end of the double-ended transfer needle. Insert the exposed end of the needle through the center of the stopper in the diluent vial. Remove plastic cap from the other end of the double-ended transfer needle now seated in the stopper of the diluent vial. To reduce any foaming, invert the vial of diluent and insert the exposed end of the needle through the center of the stopper in the product vial at an angle, making certain that the diluent vial is always above the product vial. The angle of insertion directs the flow of diluent against the side of the product vial. The vacuum in the vial is sufficient to allow transfer of all of the diluent.

Disconnect the 2 vials by removing the transfer needle from the diluent vial stopper. Remove the double-ended transfer needle from the product vial and discard the needle into the appropriate safety container. Let the vial stand until most of the contents is in solution, then gently swirl until the powder is completely dissolved. Reconstitution requires no more than 5 minutes for a 0.5 g vial and no more than 10 minutes for a 1 g vial. Do not shake the contents of the vial. Do not invert the vial until ready to withdraw contents. Use within 3 hours of reconstitution. Parenteral drug products should be inspected visually for particulate matter and discoloration prior to administration. The reconstituted product should be a colorless or slightly yellow to yellowish-green solution. When reconstitution procedure is strictly followed, a few small visible particles may occasionally remain. These will be removed by the microaggregate filter. Reconstituted product from several vials may be pooled into an empty, sterile IV solution container by using aseptic technique. A sterile 20 micron filter is provided for this purpose.

Prolastin: Aseptic technique should be carefully followed. All needles and vial tops that will come into contact with the product to be administered via the IV route should not come in contact with any nonsterile surface. Any contaminated needles should be discarded by placing in a puncture-proof container, and new equipment should be used.

After removing all items from the box, warm the sterile water (diluent) to room temperature (25°C [77°F]). Remove the plastic flip tops from each vial. Cleanse vial tops (grey stoppers) with alcohol swab and allow surface to dry. After cleaning, do not allow anything to touch the latex (rubber) stopper. Carefully remove the plastic sheath from the short end of the transfer needle. Insert the exposed needle into the diluent vial to the hub.Carefully grip the sheath of the other end of the transfer needle and twist to remove it. Invert the diluent vial and insert the attached needle into the vial of concentrate at a 45 degree angle.This will direct the stream of diluent against the wall of the concentrate vial and minimize foaming. The vacuum will draw the diluent into the concentrate vial. Remove the diluent bottle and transfer needle.Gently swirl the concentrate bottle until the powder is completely dissolved.The vial should then be visually inspected for particulate matter and discoloration prior to administration. Clean the top of the vial of reconstituted alpha$_1$-proteinase inhibitor again with an alcohol swab and let surface dry. Attach the filter needle (from the package) to sterile syringe. Withdraw the alpha$_1$-proteinase inhibitor solution into the syringe through the filter needle.Remove the filter needle from the syringe and replace with an appropriate injection needle for administration. Discard filter needle into a puncture-proof container.

The contents of more than 1 bottle of alpha$_1$-proteinase inhibitor may be drawn into the same syringe before administration. If more than 1 bottle of alpha$_1$-proteinase inhibitor is used, withdraw contents from bottles using aseptic technique. Place contents into an administration container (plastic minibag or glass bottle) using a syringe (for a patient of average weight [approximately 70 kg], the volume needed will exceed the limit of 1 syringe). Avoid pushing an IV administration set spike into the product container stopper, as this has been known to force the stopper into the vial, with a resulting loss of sterility.

A number of factors could reduce the efficacy of this product or even result in an ill effect following its use. These include improper storage and handling of the product after it leaves the manufacturer, diagnosis, dosage, method of administration, and biological differences in individual patients. Because of these factors, it is important that this product be stored properly, that the directions be followed carefully during use, and that the risk of transmitting viruses be carefully weighed before the product is prescribed.

ALPHA$_1$-PROTEINASE INHIBITOR, HUMAN — INJECTION

Zemaira: Each product package contains 1 *Zemaira* single-use vial, one 20 mL vial of sterile water for injection (diluent), and 1 color-coded vented transfer device with air inlet filter. Administer within 3 hours after reconstitution.

Bring both product (green cap) vial and diluent (white cap) vial to room temperature prior to reconstitution. Remove the plastic flip-top caps from the vials. Aseptically cleanse the rubber stoppers with antiseptic solution and allow them to dry.The transfer device provided in the package is comprised of a white (diluent) end, which has a double orifice, and a green (product) end, which has a single orifice. Incorrect use of the transfer device will result in loss of vacuum and prevent transfer of the diluent, thereby preventing reconstitution of the product. Remove the protective cover from the white (diluent) end of the transfer device. Insert the white end of the transfer device into the center of the stopper of the upright diluent vial first. Remove the protective cover from the green (product) end of the transfer device. Invert the diluent vial with the attached transfer device and, using minimum force, insert the green end of the transfer device into the center of the rubber stopper of the upright vial (green top). The flange of the transfer device should rest on the surface of the stopper so that the diluent flows into the vial.

Allow the vacuum in the vial to pull the diluent into the vial. During diluent transfer, wet the lyophilized cake completely by gently tilting the vial. Do not allow the air inlet filter to face downward. Care should be taken not to lose the vacuum, as this will prolong reconstitution of the product. After diluent transfer is complete, the transfer device will allow filtered air into the vial through the air filter. Additional venting of the product vial after diluent transfer is complete is not required. When diluent transfer is complete, withdraw the transfer device and diluent vial and properly discard in accordance with biohazard procedures. Gently swirl the vial until the powder is completely dissolved. Do not shake. Parenteral drug preparations should be inspected visually for particulate matter and discoloration prior to administration. Administer at room temperature within 3 hours after reconstitution.

• *Pooling reconstituted vials* – If more than 1 vial of alpha$_1$-proteinase inhibitor is needed to achieve the required dose, use an aseptic technique to transfer the reconstituted solution from the vials into the administration container (eg, empty IV bag or glass bottle).

➤*Administration:* Alpha$_1$-proteinase inhibitor should be administered IV at a rate not exceeding 0.08 mL/kg/min (0.04 mL/kg/min for *Glassia*) as determined by the response and comfort of the patient. Monitor the infusion rate closely during administration and observe the patient for signs of infusion-related reactions. If adverse events occur, the rate should be reduced or the infusion interrupted until the symptoms subside. The infusion may then be resumed at a rate tolerated by the subject. Administer *Zemaira* reconstituted solution through a filter. During infusion of *Glassia*, it is recommended to use a 5 micron in-line filter (not supplied). The infusion should take approximately 15 to 30 minutes to complete (60 to 80 minutes for *Glassia*).

Administration of alpha$_1$-proteinase inhibitor within 3 hours after reconstitution (within 3 hours of entering the vial for *Glassia*) is recommended to avoid the potential ill effect of any inadvertent microbial contamination.

The reconstituted solution should be filtered during administration. To ensure proper filtration of alpha$_1$-proteinase inhibitor, use an IV administration set with a suitable 5 micron infusion filter (not supplied). Follow the appropriate procedure for IV administration.

After administration, any unused solution and administration equipment should be discarded in accordance with biohazard procedures.

➤*Admixture compatibility:* Administer alpha$_1$-proteinase inhibitor alone; do not mix with other agents or diluting solutions.

➤*Storage/Stability:* Administration within 3 hours after reconstitution or of entering the ready-to-use vial is recommended to avoid the potential ill effect of any inadvertent microbial contamination. Do not refrigerate after reconstitution. Refrigerate at 2° to 8°C (35° to 46°F) or at temperatures not to exceed 25°C (77°F). Avoid freezing, which may damage container for the diluent. Discard partially used vials; do not save for future use.

Aralast NP – Product removed from refrigeration must be used within 1 month.

Glassia – Stability data support short and moderate temperature excursions similar to those that may be encountered when using *Glassia*. Keep vial in carton until required for use.

Actions

➤*Pharmacology:* Alpha$_1$-PI functions in the lungs to inhibit serine proteases such as neutrophil elastase (NE), which is capable of degrading protein components of the alveolar walls and is chronically present in the lung. In the healthy lung, alpha$_1$-PI is thought to provide more than 90% of the anti-NE protection in the lower respiratory tract.

Alpha$_1$-PI deficiency is an autosomal, codominant, hereditary disorder characterized by low serum and lung levels of alpha$_1$-PI. Severe forms of the deficiency are frequently associated with slowly progressive, moderate to severe panacinar emphysema that most often manifests in the third to fourth decades of life, resulting in a significantly lower life expectancy. Individuals with alpha$_1$-PI deficiency have little protection against NE released by a chronic, low-level of neutrophils in their lower respiratory tract, resulting in a protease:protease inhibitor imbalance in the lung. The emphysema associated with alpha$_1$-PI deficiency is typically worse in the lower lung zones. It is believed to develop because there are insufficient amounts of alpha$_1$-PI in the lower respiratory tract to inhibit NE. This imbalance allows unopposed destruction of the connective tissue framework of the lung parenchyma.

➤*Pharmacokinetics:* In clinical studies of alpha$_1$-PI in 23 subjects with the PiZZ variant of congenital deficiency of alpha$_1$-antitrypsin deficiency and documented destructive lung disease, the mean in vivo recovery of alpha$_1$-PI was 4.2 mg (immunologic)/dL/mg (functional)/kg administered. Half-life of alpha$_1$-PI in vivo was approximately 4.5 days. Nineteen of the subjects received alpha$_1$-PI replacement therapy, 60 mg/kg/week for up to 26 weeks (average, 24 weeks). Blood levels of alpha$_1$-PI were maintained above 80 mg/dL. Within a few weeks, bronchoalveolar lavage studies demonstrated significantly increased levels of alpha$_1$-PI and functional antineutrophil elastase capacity in the epithelial lining fluid of the lower respiratory tract of the lungs.

In 18 subjects treated with a single dose (60 mg/kg) of *Zemaira*, the AUC and standard deviation (SD) were 144 mcM × day (SD 27), maximum serum concentration was 44.1 mcM (SD 10.8), clearance was 603 mL/day (SD 129), and terminal half-life was 5.1 days (SD 2.4).

Contraindications

In individuals with selective immunoglobulin A (IgA) deficiencies (IgA level less than 15 mg/dL) who have known antibody against IgA, because they may experience severe reactions, including anaphylaxis, to IgA that may be present.

➤*Zemaira*: Hypersensitivity to any of its components or a history of anaphylaxis or severe systemic response to alpha$_1$-PI products

Warnings/Precautions

➤*Infectious transmission:* Because alpha$_1$-PI is derived from pooled human plasma, it may carry a risk of transmitting infectious agents (eg, viruses and, theoretically, the Creutzfeldt-Jakob disease [CJD] agent).

There is also the possibility that unknown infectious agents may be present in such products. Individuals who receive infusions of blood or plasma products may develop signs and/or symptoms of some viral infections, particularly hepatitis C. All infections thought by a physician possibly to have been transmitted by these products should be reported by the physician or other health care provider to Bayer Corporation for *Prolastin* (1-800-228-8371) or to Aventis Behring for *Zemaira* (1-800-504-5434). Weigh the risks and benefits of the use of this product and discuss with the patient.

Prolastin has been heat-treated in solution at 60°C for 10 hours in order to reduce the potential for transmission of infectious disease. No cases of hepatitis B or hepatitis C have been recorded in individuals receiving *Prolastin*. However, as all individuals receive prophylaxis against hepatitis B, no conclusion can be drawn at this time regarding potential transmission of hepatitis B virus.

During clinical studies, no cases of hepatitis A, B, C, or HIV viral infections were reported with the use of *Zemaira*.

➤*Circulatory overload:* There will be an increase in plasma volume following IV administration of *Prolastin* and *Zemaira*. Use caution in patients at risk for circulatory overload.

➤*Hepatitis B immunization:* It is recommended that in preparation for receiving *Prolastin*, recipients be immunized against hepatitis B using a licensed hepatitis B vaccine. If it becomes necessary to treat an individual with *Prolastin*, and time is insufficient for adequate antibody response to vaccination, administer a single dose of hepatitis B immune globulin (human), 0.06 mL/kg/body weight, IM, at the time of administration of the initial dose of hepatitis B vaccine.

➤*Hypersensitivity reactions:* If anaphylactic or severe anaphylactoid reactions occur, discontinue infusion immediately. Epinephrine and other appropriate supportive therapy should be available for the treatment of any acute anaphylactic or anaphylactoid reaction.

➤*Pregnancy: Category C.* It is not known whether this drug can cause fetal harm when administered to a pregnant woman or can affect reproduction capacity. Use only when clearly needed and when the potential benefits outweigh the potential hazards to the fetus.

➤*Lactation:* It is not known whether alpha$_1$-PI is excreted in human milk. Because many drugs are excreted in human milk, exercise caution when administering alpha$_1$-PI to a nursing woman.

➤*Children:* Safety and efficacy in children have not been established.

➤*Monitoring:* The "threshold" level of *Prolastin* in the serum believed to provide adequate antielastase activity in the lung of individuals with alpha$_1$-antitrypsin deficiency is 80 mg/mL (based on commercial standards for alpha$_1$-PI immunologic assay). However, assays of alpha$_1$-PI based on commercial standards measure antigenic activity of alpha$_1$-PI is expressed as actual functional activity (ie, actual capacity to neutralize porcine pancreatic elastase). As functional activity may be less than antigenic activity, serum levels of alpha$_1$-PI determined using commercial immunologic assays may not accurately reflect actual functional alpha$_1$-PI levels. Therefore, although it may be helpful to monitor serum levels of alpha$_1$-PI in individuals receiving *Prolastin* using currently available commercial assays of antigenic activity, do not use results of these assays to determine the required therapeutic dosage.

Adverse Reactions

➤*Prolastin:* Delayed fever (maximum temperature rise was 38.9°C, resolving spontaneously over 24 hours) occurring up to 12 hours following treatment (0.77%); lightheadedness, dizziness (0.19%). Mild transient leukocytosis and dilutional anemia several hours after infusion have also been noted.

Postmarketing – Occasional reports of other flu-like symptoms, allergic-like reactions, chills, dyspnea, rash, tachycardia, and rarely, hypotension.

➤*Zemaira:* Asthenia, injection site pain, dizziness, headache, paresthesia, pruritus (1%).

ALPHA$_1$-PROTEINASE INHIBITOR, HUMAN — INJECTION

Alpha$_1$-Proteinase Inhibitor Adverse Reactions		
Adverse reactions	*Zemaira*	*Prolastin*
Subject treated	89	32
Subjects with adverse events regardless of causality (%)	78	63
Subjects with related adverse events (%)	6	13
Subjects with related serious adverse events	0	0
Number of infusions	1296	160
Adverse events regardless of causality (rates per infusion)	298 (0.230)	83 (0.519)
Related adverse events (rates per infusion)	6 (0.005)	5 (0.03)

The frequencies of adverse events per infusion that were at least 0.4% in *Zemaira*-treated subjects, regardless of causality, were: Headache (2.5%); upper respiratory tract infection (1.6%); sinusitis (1.5%); injection site hemorrhage, sore throat (0.9%); bronchitis (0.8%); asthenia, fever (0.6%); pain, rhinitis, bronchospasm, chest pain (0.5%); increased cough, rash, infection (0.4%).

The following adverse events, regardless of causality, occurred at a rate of 0.2% to less than 0.4% per infusion: Abnormal pain; diarrhea; dizziness; ecchymosis; myalgia; pruritus; vasodilation; accidental injury; back pain; dyspepsia; dyspnea; hemorrhage; injection site reaction; lung disorder; migraine; nausea; paresthesia.

Diffuse interstitial lung disease was noted on a routine chest x-ray of 1 subject at week 24. Causality could not be determined.

In a retrospective analysis, during the 10-week blinded portion of the 24-week clinical study, 6 subjects (20%) of the 30 treated with *Zemaira* had a total of 7 exacerbations of their COPD. Nine subjects (64%) of the 14 treated with *Prolastin* had a total of 11 exacerbations of their COPD. The observed difference between groups was 44% (95% confidence interval from 8% to 70%). Over the entire 24-week treatment period of the 30 subjects in the *Zemaira* treatment group, 7 subjects (23%) had a total of 11 exacerbations of their COPD.

Patient Information

Inform patients of the early signs of hypersensitivity reactions including hives, generalized urticaria, tightness of the chest, dyspnea, wheezing, faintness, hypotension, and anaphylaxis. Advise patients to discontinue use of the product and contact their physician and/or seek immediate emergency care, depending on the severity of the reaction, if these symptoms occur.

As with all plasma-derived products, some viruses, such as parvovirus B19, are particularly difficult to remove or inactivate at this time. Parvovirus B19 may most seriously affect pregnant women and immune-compromised individuals. Symptoms of parvovirus B19 include fever, drowsiness, chills, and runny nose followed 2 weeks later by a rash and joint pain. Encourage patients to consult their physician if such symptoms occur.

LUNG SURFACTANTS

BERACTANT (Natural Lung Surfactant)

Rx	**Survanta** (Ross Laboratories)	**Suspension:** 25 mg phospholipids per mL suspended in 0.9% sodium chloride solution.[a]	In single use vials containing 8 mL suspension.

[a] With 0.5 to 1.75 mg triglycerides, 1.4 to 3.5 mg free fatty acids and less than 1 mg protein per mL.

BERACTANT — INTRATRACHEAL

Indications

➤*Respiratory distress syndrome:* Beractant is indicated for prevention and treatment ("rescue") of respiratory distress syndrome (RDS) (hyaline membrane disease) in premature infants. Beractant significantly reduces the incidence of RDS, mortality due to RDS and air-leak complications.

In premature infants less than 1250 g birth weight or with evidence of surfactant deficiency, give beractant as soon as possible, preferably within 15 minutes of birth.

To treat infants with RDS confirmed by x-ray and requiring mechanical ventilation, give beractant as soon as possible, preferably by 8 hours of age.

Administration and Dosage

➤*General dosing considerations:* Marked improvements in oxygenation may occur within minutes of administration of beractant. Therefore, frequent and careful clinical observation and monitoring of systemic oxygenation are essential to avoid hyperoxia.

If an infant experiences bradycardia or oxygen desaturation during the dosing procedure, stop the dosing procedure and initiate appropriate measures to alleviate the condition. After the infant has stabilized, resume the dosing procedure.

Rales and moist breath sounds can occur transiently after administration. Endotracheal suctioning or other remedial action is unnecessary unless clear-cut signs of airway obstruction are present.

➤*Children:*

Respiratory distress syndrome –

Usual dosage: 100 mg of phospholipids/kg birth weight (4 mL/kg), as soon as possible, preferably within 15 minutes of birth (for prevention of respiratory distress syndrome) or 8 hours of age (for treatment of respiratory distress syndrome). Four doses can be administered in the first 48 hours of life, no more frequently than every 6 hours.

Beractant Dosing	
Weight (grams)	Total dose (mL)
600 to 650	2.6
651 to 700	2.8
701 to 750	3
751 to 800	3.2
801 to 850	3.4
851 to 900	3.6
901 to 950	3.8
951 to 1,000	4
1,001 to 1,050	4.2
1,051 to 1,100	4.4
1,101 to 1,150	4.6
1,151 to 1,200	4.8
1,201 to 1,250	5
1,251 to 1,300	5.2
1,301 to 1,350	5.4
1,351 to 1,400	5.6
1,401 to 1,450	5.8
1,451 to 1,500	6
1,501 to 1,550	6.2
1,551 to 1,600	6.4
1,601 to 1,650	6.6
1,651 to 1,700	6.8
1,701 to 1,750	7
1,751 to 1,800	7.2
1,801 to 1,850	7.4
1,851 to 1,900	7.6
1,901 to 1,950	7.8
1,951 to 2,000	8

Repeat dosage: Phospholipids 100 mg/kg birth weight. The infant should not be reweighed for determination of the beractant dosage.

The need for additional doses of beractant is determined by evidence of continuing respiratory distress. Using the following criteria for redosing, significant reductions in mortality because of respiratory distress syndrome were observed in the multiple-dose clinical trials with beractant: Dose no sooner than 6 hours after the preceding dose if the infant remains intubated and requires at least 30% inspired oxygen to maintain a PaO_2 less than or equal to 80 torr; radiographic confirmation of respiratory distress syndrome should be obtained before administering additional doses to those who received a prevention dose.

➤*Preparation for administration:* If settling occurs during storage, swirl the vial gently (do not shake) to redisperse. Some foaming at the surface may occur during handling and is inherent in the nature of the product. The color of beractant is off-white to light brown. Beractant does not require reconstitution or sonication before use. Before administration, beractant should be warmed by standing at room temperature for at least 20 minutes or warmed in the hand for at least 8 minutes. Artificial warming methods should not be used. If a prevention dose is to be given, preparation of beractant should begin before the infant's birth.

➤*Administration:* Beractant is administered intratracheally by instillation through a 5 French end-hole catheter. The catheter can be inserted into the infant's endotracheal tube without interrupting ventilation by passing the catheter through a neonatal suction valve attached to the endotracheal tube. Alternatively, beractant can be instilled through the catheter by briefly disconnecting the endotracheal tube from the ventilator.

The neonatal suction valve used for administering beractant should be a type that allows entry of the catheter into the endotracheal tube without interrupting ventilation and also maintains a closed airway circuit system by sealing the valve around the catheter. If the neonatal suction valve is used, the catheter should be rigid enough to pass easily into the endotracheal tube. A very soft and pliable catheter may twist or curl within the neonatal suction valve. The length of the catheter should be shortened so that the tip of the catheter protrudes just beyond the end of the endotracheal tube above the infant's carina. Beractant should not be instilled into a mainstem bronchus.

The dosing procedure is facilitated if 1 person administers the dose while another person positions and monitors the infant.

To ensure homogenous distribution of beractant throughout the lungs, each dose is divided into 4 quarter doses. Each quarter dose is administered with the infant in a different position. The recommended positions are as follows: Head and body inclined 5° to 10° down, head turned to the right; Head and

BERACTANT — INTRATRACHEAL

body inclined 5° to 10° down, head turned to the left; Head and body inclined 5° to 10° up, head turned to the right; Head and body inclined 5° to 10° up, head turned to the left.

First dose – Determine the total dose of beractant from the beractant dosing information, based on the infant's birth weight. Slowly withdraw the entire contents of the vial into a plastic syringe through a large-gauge needle (eg, at least 20 gauge). Do not filter beractant and avoid shaking

Attach the premeasured 5 French end-hole catheter to the syringe. Fill the catheter with beractant. Discard excess beractant through the catheter so that only the total dose to be given remains in the syringe.

Before administering beractant, ensure proper placement and patency of the endotracheal tube. At the discretion of the clinician, the endotracheal tube may be suctioned before administering beractant. The infant should be allowed to stabilize before proceeding with dosing.

Prevention – In the prevention strategy, weigh, intubate, and stabilize the infant. Administer the dose as soon as possible after birth, preferably within 15 minutes. Position the infant appropriately and gently inject the first quarter dose through the catheter over 2 to 3 seconds. After administration of the first quarter dose, remove the catheter from the endotracheal tube. Manually ventilate with a handbag with sufficient oxygen to prevent cyanosis, at a rate of 60 breaths/minute, and sufficient positive pressure to provide adequate air exchange and chest wall excursion.

Treatment – In the rescue strategy, the first dose should be given as soon as possible after the infant is placed on a ventilator for management of respiratory distress syndrome. In the clinical trials, immediately before instilling the first quarter dose, the infant's ventilator settings were changed to rate 60 breaths/minute, inspiratory time 0.5 second, and FiO_2. Position the infant appropriately and gently inject the first quarter dose through the catheter over 2 to 3 seconds. After administration of the first quarter dose, remove the catheter from the endotracheal tube and continue mechanical ventilation.

In both strategies, ventilate the infant for at least 30 seconds or until stable. Reposition the infant for instillation of the next quarter dose. Instill the remaining quarter doses using the same procedures. After instillation of each quarter dose, remove the catheter and ventilate for at least 30 seconds or until the infant is stabilized. After instillation of the final quarter dose, remove the catheter without flushing it. Do not suction the infant for 1 hour after dosing unless signs of significant airway obstruction occur. After completion of the dosing procedure, resume usual ventilator management and clinical care.

Repeat doses – Prepare beractant and position the infant for administration of each quarter dose as previously described. After instillation of each quarter dose, remove the dosing catheter from the endotracheal tube and ventilate the infant for at least 30 seconds or until stable.

In the clinical studies, ventilator settings used to administer repeat doses were different than those used for the first dose. For repeat doses, the FiO_2 was increased by 0.2 or an amount sufficient to prevent cyanosis. The ventilator delivered a rate of 30 breaths/minute with an inspiratory time less than 1 second. If the infant's pretreatment rate was 30 or more, it was left unchanged during beractant instillation.

Manual handbag ventilation should not be used to administer repeat doses. During the dosing procedure, ventilator settings may be adjusted at the discretion of the clinician to maintain appropriate oxygenation and ventilation. After completion of the dosing procedure, resume usual ventilator management and clinical care.

➤*Storage/Stability:* Store between 2° and 8°C (35.6° and 46.4°F). Protect from light. Store vials in carton until ready for use. Date and time need to be recorded in the box on the front of the carton or vial whenever beractant is removed from the refrigerator. Unopened, unused vials that have been warmed to room temperature may be returned to the refrigerator within 24 hours of warming and stored for future use. Beractant should not be removed from the refrigerator for longer than 24 hours. Beractant should not be warmed and returned to the refrigerator more than once. Each single-use vial should be entered only once. Used vials with residual drug should be discarded.

Actions

➤*Pharmacology:* Endogenous pulmonary surfactant lowers surface tension on alveolar surfaces during respiration and stabilizes the alveoli against collapse at resting transpulmonary pressures. Deficiency of pulmonary surfactant causes RDS in premature infants. Beractant replenishes surfactant and restores surface activity to the lungs of these infants.

In vitro, beractant reproducibly lowers minimum surface tension to less than 8 dynes/cm as measured by the pulsating bubble surfactometer and Wilhelmy Surface Balance. In situ, beractant restores pulmonary compliance to excised rat lungs artificially made surfactant-deficient. In vivo, single beractant doses improve lung pressure-volume measurements, lung compliance, and oxygenation in premature rabbits and sheep.

Animal pharmacology – Beractant is administered directly to the target organ, the lungs, where biophysical effects occur at the alveolar surface. In surfactant-deficient premature rabbits and lambs, alveolar clearance of radiolabeled lipid components of beractant is rapid. Most of the dose becomes lung associated within hours of administration, and the lipids enter endogenous surfactant pathways of reutilization and recycling. In surfactant-sufficient adult animals, beractant clearance is more rapid than in premature and young animals. There is less reutilization and recycling of surfactant in adult animals.

Contraindications

None known.

Warnings/Precautions

➤*Administration:* Beractant is intended for intratracheal use only.

➤*Oxygenation/Lung compliance:* Beractant can rapidly affect oxygenation and lung compliance. Therefore, its use should be restricted to a highly supervised clinical setting with immediate availability of clinicians experienced with intubation, ventilator management, and general care of premature infants. Infants receiving beractant should be frequently monitored with arterial or transcutaneous measurement of systemic oxygen and carbon dioxide.

➤*Transient effects:* During the dosing procedure, transient episodes of bradycardia and decreased oxygen saturation have been reported. If these occur, stop the dosing procedure and initiate appropriate measures to alleviate the condition. After stabilization, resume the dosing procedure.

➤*Rales and moist breath sounds:* Rales and moist breath sounds can occur transiently after administration. Endotracheal suctioning or other remedial action is not necessary unless clear-cut signs of airway obstruction are present.

➤*Nosocomial sepsis:* Increased probability of posttreatment nosocomial sepsis in beractant-treated infants was observed in the controlled clinical trials (see information below). The increased risk for sepsis among beractant-treated infants was not associated with increased mortality among these infants. The causative organisms were similar in treated and control infants. There was no significant difference between groups in the rate of posttreatment infections other than sepsis.

➤*Usage:* Use of beractant in infants less than 600 g birth weight or greater than 1750 g birth weight has not been evaluated in controlled trials. There is no controlled experience with use of beractant in conjunction with experimental therapies for RDS (eg, high-frequency ventilation, extracorporeal membrane oxygenation).

No information is available on the effects of doses other than 100 mg phospholipids/kg, greater than 4 doses, dosing more frequently than every 6 hours, or administration after 48 hours of age.

➤*Pregnancy: Category: Undetermined.* Beractant is not approved for use in adults.

➤*Lactation:* Beractant is not approved for use in adults.

Adverse Reactions

The most commonly reported adverse reactions were associated with the dosing procedure. In the multiple-dose, controlled clinical trials, each dose of beractant was divided into 4 quarter doses which were instilled through a catheter inserted into the endotracheal tube by briefly disconnecting the endotracheal tube from the ventilator. Transient bradycardia occurred with 11.9% of doses. Oxygen desaturation occurred with 9.8% of doses.

Other reactions during the dosing procedure occurred with less than 1% of doses, and included endotracheal tube reflux, pallor, vasoconstriction, hypotension, endotracheal tube blockage, hypertension, hypocarbia, hypercarbia, and apnea. No deaths occurred during the dosing procedure, and all reactions resolved with symptomatic treatment.

The occurrence of concurrent illnesses common in premature infants was evaluated in the controlled trials. The rates in all controlled studies are in the following table:

Concurrent Illnesses in Controlled Studies During Beractant Treatment

Concurrent event	All controlled studies		
	Beractant (%)	Control (%)	P-value [a]
Patent ductus arteriosus	46.9%	47.1%	0.814
Intracranial hemorrhage	48.1%	45.2%	0.241
Severe intracranial hemorrhage	24.1%	23.3%	0.693
Pulmonary air leaks	10.9%	24.7%	< 0.001
Pulmonary interstitial emphysema	20.2%	38.4%	< 0.001
Necrotizing enterocolitis	6.1%	5.3%	0.427
Apnea	65.4%	59.6%	0.283
Severe apnea	46.1%	42.5%	0.114
Posttreatment sepsis	20.7%	16.1%	0.019
Posttreatment infection	10.2%	9.1%	0.345
Pulmonary hemorrhage	7.2%	5.3%	0.166

[a] P-value comparing groups in controlled studies.

When all controlled studies were pooled, there was no difference in intracranial hemorrhage. However, in 1 of the single-dose rescue studies and 1 of the multiple-dose prevention studies, the rate of intracranial hemorrhage was significantly higher in beractant patients than control patients (63.3% vs 30.8%, P = 0.001; and 48.8% vs 34.2%, P = 0.047, respectively). The rate in a treatment IND involving approximately 8100 infants was lower than in the controlled trials.

➤*Complications reported in controlled clinical studies in premature infants:*

Cardiovascular – Hypotension, hypertension, tachycardia, ventricular tachycardia, aortic thrombosis, cardiac failure, cardiorespiratory arrest, increased apical pulse, persistent fetal circulation, air embolism, total anomalous pulmonary venous return.

CNS – Seizures.

Endocrine – Adrenal hemorrhage, inappropriate antidiuretic hormone (ADH) secretion, hyperphosphatemia.

GI – Abdominal distention, hemorrhage, intestinal perforations, volvulus, bowel infarct, feeding intolerance, hepatic failure, stress ulcer.

BERACTANT — INTRATRACHEAL

Hematologic – Coagulopathy, thrombocytopenia, disseminated intravascular coagulation.

Musculoskeletal – Inguinal hernia.

Renal – Renal failure, hematuria.

Respiratory – Lung consolidation, blood from the endotracheal tube, deterioration after weaning, respiratory decompensation, subglottic stenosis, paralyzed diaphragm, respiratory failure.

Systemic – Fever, deterioration.

➤*Follow-up evaluations:*

Multiple-dose studies: Six-month, age-adjusted, follow-up evaluations have been completed in 631 (345 treated) of 916 surviving infants. There were significantly less cerebral palsy and need for supplemental oxygen in beractant infants than controls. Wheezing at the time of examination was significantly more frequent among beractant infants, although there was no difference in bronchodilator therapy.

Final, 12-month, follow-up data from the multiple-dose studies are available from 521 (272 treated) of 909 surviving infants. There was significantly less wheezing in beractant infants than controls, in contrast to the 6-month results. There was no difference in the incidence of cerebral palsy at 12 months.

Twenty-four-month, age-adjusted evaluations were completed in 429 (226 treated) of 906 surviving infants. There were significantly fewer beractant infants with rhonchi, wheezing, and tachypnea at the time of examination. No other differences were found.

Overdosage

Rales and moist breath sounds can transiently occur after beractant is given, and do not indicate overdosage. Endotracheal suctioning or other remedial action is not required unless clear-cut signs of airway obstruction are present.

➤*Symptoms:* Overdosage with beractant has not been reported. Based on animal data, overdosage might result in acute airway obstruction.

➤*Treatment:* Treatment should be symptomatic and supportive.

CALFACTANT

Rx	**Infasurf** (Forest Pharmaceuticals)	**Suspension, intratracheal:** 35 mg phospholipids per mL suspended in 0.9% sodium chloride solution[a] and 0.65 mg proteins[b]	In single-use vials, containing 6 mL suspension.

[a] Including 26 mg phosphatidylcholine of which 16 mg is desaturated phosphatidylcholine.

[b] Including 0.26 mg of SP-B.

CALFACTANT — INTRATRACHEAL

Indications

➤*Respiratory distress syndrome:* Calfactant is indicated for the prevention of respiratory distress syndrome (RDS) in premature infants at high risk for RDS and for the treatment ("rescue") of premature infants who develop RDS. Calfactant decreases the incidence of RDS, mortality due to RDS, and air leaks associated with RDS.

Prophylaxis therapy at birth with calfactant is indicated for premature infants younger than 29 weeks of gestational age at significant risk for RDS. Calfactant prophylaxis should be administered as soon as possible, preferably within 30 minutes after birth.

Calfactant therapy is indicated for infants 72 hours of age or younger with RDS (confirmed by clinical and radiologic findings) and requiring endotracheal intubation.

Administration and Dosage

➤*General dosing considerations:* Rapid and substantial increases in blood oxygenation and improved lung compliance often follow calfactant instillation. Close clinical monitoring and surveillance following administration may be needed to adjust oxygen therapy and ventilator pressures appropriately.

During administration of calfactant liquid suspension into the airway, infants often experience bradycardia, reflux of calfactant into the endotracheal tube, airway obstruction, cyanosis, dislodgment of the endotracheal tube, or hypoventilation. If any of these events occur, the administration should be interrupted and the infant's condition should be stabilized using appropriate interventions before the administration of calfactant is resumed. Endotracheal suctioning or reintubation is sometimes needed when there are signs of airway obstruction during the administration of the surfactant.

➤*Children:*

Prevention of respiratory distress syndrome –

Infants younger than 29 weeks of gestational age: 3 mL/kg body weight at birth every 12 hours for a total of up to 3 doses as soon as possible after birth.

Treatment of respiratory distress syndrome –

Infants 72 hours of age or younger: 3 mL/kg body weight at birth every 12 hours for a total of up to 3 doses. Repeat doses have been given in the calfactant controlled clinical trials if the patient was still intubated.

➤*Preparation for administration:* Calfactant is a suspension that settles during storage. Gentle swirling or agitation of the vial is often necessary for redispersion. Do not shake. Visible flecks in the suspension and foaming at the surface are normal for calfactant. Calfactant does not require reconstitution. Do not dilute or sonicate. Warming of calfactant before administration is not necessary.

➤*Administration:* Administer intratracheally through a side-port adapter into the endotracheal tube. The dose is drawn into a syringe from the single-use vial using a 20 gauge or larger needle with care taken to avoid excessive foaming.

Two attendants, one to instill the calfactant, the other to monitor the patient and assist in positioning, facilitate the dosing. The dose (3 mL/kg) should be administered in 2 aliquots of 1.5 mL/kg each. After each aliquot is instilled, the infant should be positioned with either the right or the left side dependent. Administration is made while ventilation is continued over 20 to 30 breaths for each aliquot, with small bursts timed only during the inspiratory cycles. A pause followed by evaluation of the respiratory status and repositioning should separate the 2 aliquots.

➤*Storage/Stability:* Store at 2° to 8°C (36° to 46°F) and protect from light. Each single-use vial should be entered only once and the vial with any unused material should be discarded after the initial entry. Unopened, unused vials that have warmed to room temperature can be returned to refrigerated storage within 24 hours for future use. Repeated warming to room temperature should be avoided.

Actions

➤*Pharmacology:* Endogenous lung surfactant is essential for effective ventilation because it modifies alveolar surface tension thereby stabilizing the alveoli. Lung surfactant deficiency is the cause of respiratory distress syndrome (RDS) in premature infants. Calfactant restores surface activity to the lungs of these infants.

Calfactant absorbs rapidly to the surface of the air:liquid interface and modifies surface tension similarly to natural lung surfactant. A minimum surface tension of less than or equal to 3 mN/m is produced in vitro by calfactant as measured on a pulsating bubble surfactometer. Ex vivo, calfactant restores the pressure volume mechanics and compliance of surfactant-deficient rat lungs. In vivo, calfactant improves lung compliance, respiratory gas exchange, and survival in preterm lambs with profound surfactant deficiency.

➤*Pharmacokinetics:* Calfactant is administered directly to the lung lumen surface, its site of action. No human studies of absorption, biotransformation or excretion of calfactant have been performed. The administration of calfactant with radiolabeled phospholipids into the lungs of adult rabbits results in the persistence of 50% of radioactivity in the lung alveolar lining and 25% of radioactivity in the lung tissue 24 hours later. Less than 5% of the radioactivity is found in other organs. In premature lambs with lethal surfactant deficiency, less than 30% of instilled calfactant is present in the lung lining after 24 hours.

Warnings/Precautions

➤*Administration:* Calfactant is intended for intratracheal use only.

➤*Oxygenation/Lung compliance:* The administration of exogenous surfactants, including calfactant, often rapidly improves oxygenation and lung compliance. Following administration of calfactant, patients should be carefully monitored so that oxygen therapy and ventilatory support can be modified in response to changes in respiratory status.

➤*Transient effects:* Transient episodes of reflux of calfactant into the endotracheal tube, cyanosis, bradycardia, or airway obstruction have occurred during the dosing procedures. These events require stopping calfactant administration and taking appropriate measures to alleviate the condition. After the patient is stable, dosing can proceed with appropriate monitoring.

➤*Intensive care:* Calfactant therapy is not a substitute for neonatal intensive care. Optimal care of premature infants at risk for RDS and newborn infants with RDS who need endotracheal intubation requires an acute care unit organized, staffed, equipped, and experienced with intubation, ventilator management, and general care of these patients.

➤*Usage:* No data are available on the use of calfactant in conjunction with experimental therapies of RDS, eg, high-frequency ventilation.

Data from controlled trials on the efficacy of calfactant are limited to doses of approximately 100 mg phospholipid/kg body weight and up to a total of 4 doses.

➤*Special risk:* When repeat dosing was given at fixed 12-hour intervals in the calfactant vs colfosceril palmitate trials, transient episodes of cyanosis, bradycardia, reflux of surfactant into the endotracheal tube, and airway obstruction were observed more frequently among infants in the calfactant-treated group.

An increased proportion of patients with both intraventricular hemorrhage (IVH) and periventricular leukomalacia (PVL) was observed in calfactant-treated infants in the calfactant-colfosceril palmitate controlled trials. These observations were not associated with increased mortality.

➤*Pregnancy: Category: Undetermined.* Calfactant is not indicated for use in adults.

CALFACTANT — INTRATRACHEAL

➤*Lactation:* Calfactant is not indicated for use in adults.

Adverse Reactions

The most common adverse reactions associated with calfactant dosing procedures in the controlled trials were cyanosis (65%), airway obstruction (39%), bradycardia (34%), reflux of surfactant into the endotracheal tube (21%), requirement for manual ventilation (16%), and reintubation (3%). These events were generally transient and not associated with serious complications or death.

➤*Follow-up evaluations:* Two-year follow-up data of neurodevelopmental outcomes in 415 infants enrolled in 5 centers that participated in the calfactant vs colfosceril palmitate controlled trials demonstrated significant developmental delays in equal percentages of calfactant and colfosceril palmitate patients.

➤*Common complications:* The incidence of common complications of prematurity and RDS in the 4 controlled calfactant trials are presented below. Prophylaxis and treatment study results for each surfactant are combined.

Common Complications of Prematurity and RDS in Controlled Calfactant Trials

Complication	Calfactant (n = 1001)	Colfosceril palmitate (n = 978)	Calfactant (n = 553)	Colfosceril palmitate (n = 566)
Apnea	61%	61%	76%	76%
Patent ductus arteriosus	47%	48%	45%	48%
Intracranial hemorrhage	29%	31%	36%	36%
Severe intracranial hemorrhage[a]	12%	10%	9%	7%
IVH and PVL	7%	3%	5%	5%

Common Complications of Prematurity and RDS in Controlled Calfactant Trials

Complication	Calfactant (n = 1001)	Colfosceril palmitate (n = 978)	Calfactant (n = 553)	Colfosceril palmitate (n = 566)
Sepsis	20%	22%	28%	27%
Pulmonary air leaks	12%	22%	15%	15%
Pulmonary interstitial emphysema	7%	17%	10%	10%
Pulmonary hemorrhage	7%	7%	7%	6%
Necrotizing enterocolitis	5%	5%	17%	18%

[a] Grade III and IV by the method of Papile.

Overdosage

There have been no reports of overdosage with calfactant. While there are no known adverse effects of excess lung surfactant, overdosage would result in overloading the lungs with an isotonic solution. Ventilation should be supported until clearance of the liquid is accomplished.

PORACTANT ALFA (PORCINE ORIGIN)

Rx	**Curosurf** (Cornerstone Biopharma)	**Suspension, intratracheal:** 80 mg/mL phospholipids[a]	Preservative free. In 1.5 or 3 mL single-use vials.

[a] Includes 54 mg of phosphatidylcholine, of which 30.5 mg is dipalmitoyl phosphatidylcholine and 1 mg of protein, including 0.3 mg of SP-B.

PORACTANT ALFA — INTRATRACHEAL

Indications

➤*Respiratory distress syndrome (RDS):* Poractant alfa is indicated for the treatment (rescue) of respiratory distress syndrome (RDS) in premature infants. Poractant alfa reduces mortality and pneumothoraces associated with RDS.

➤*Off-label uses:* Severe meconium aspiration syndrome in term infants; respiratory failure caused by group B streptococcal infection in neonates.

Administration and Dosage

➤*General dosing considerations:* Correction of acidosis, hypotension, anemia, hypoglycemia, and hypothermia is recommended prior to poractant alfa administration.

Transient episodes of bradycardia, decreased oxygen saturation, reflux of the surfactant into the endotracheal tube, and airway obstruction have occurred during the dosing procedure of poractant alfa. These events require interrupting the administration of poractant alfa and taking the appropriate measures to alleviate the condition. After stabilization, dosing may resume with appropriate monitoring.

➤*Children:*

Respiratory distress syndrome –

Premature infants:

• *Maximum dose* – 5 mL/kg, total dose (sum of the initial and up to 2 repeat doses).

• *Initial dosage* – 2.5 mL/kg birth weight.

Poractant Alfa Dosing

Weight (g)	Initial dose 2.5 mL/kg — Each dose (mL)	Repeat dose 1.25 mL/kg — Each dose (mL)	Weight (g)	Initial dose 2.5 mL/kg — Each dose (mL)	Repeat dose 1.25 mL/kg — Each dose (mL)
600 to 650	1.6	0.8	1,301 to 1,350	3.3	1.65
651 to 700	1.7	0.85	1,351 to 1,400	3.5	1.75
701 to 750	1.8	0.9	1,401 to 1,450	3.6	1.8
751 to 800	2	1	1,451 to 1,500	3.7	1.85
801 to 850	2.1	1.05	1,501 to 1,550	3.8	1.9
851 to 900	2.2	1.1	1,551 to 1,600	4	2
901 to 950	2.3	1.15	1,601 to 1,650	4.1	2.05
951 to 1,000	2.5	1.25	1,651 to 1,700	4.2	2.1
1,001 to 1,050	2.6	1.3	1,701 to 1,750	4.3	2.15
1,051 to 1,100	2.7	1.35	1,751 to 1,800	4.5	2.25
1,101 to 1,150	2.8	1.4	1,801 to 1,850	4.6	2.3
1,151 to 1,200	3	1.5	1,851 to 1,900	4.7	2.35
1,201 to 1,250	3.1	1.55	1,901 to 1,950	4.8	2.4
1,251 to 1,300	3.2	1.6	1,951 to 2,000	5	2.5

• *Repeat doses* – Up to 2 repeat doses of 1.25 mL/kg birth weight may be administered at approximately 12-hour intervals in infants who remain intubated and in whom RDS is considered responsible for their persisting or deteriorating respiratory status.

➤*Preparation for administration:* Before use, slowly warm the vial to room temperature and gently turn upside-down in order to obtain a uniform suspension. Do not shake.

➤*Administration:* For intratracheal use only. Before administering, ensure proper placement and patency of the endotracheal tube. At the discretion of the clinician, the endotracheal tube may be suctioned before administering poractant alfa. Allow the infant to stabilize before proceeding with dosing.

For endotracheal tube instillation using a 5 French end-hole catheter – Slowly withdraw the entire contents of the vial into a 3 or 5 mL plastic syringe through a large-gauge needle (eg, at least 20 gauge). Attach the precut 8-centimeter 5 French end-hole catheter to the syringe. Fill the catheter with poractant alfa. Discard excess through the catheter so that only the total dose to be given remains in the syringe.

Immediately before poractant alfa administration, change the infant's ventilator settings to a rate of 40 to 60 breaths/minute, inspiratory time of 0.5 seconds, and supplemental oxygen sufficient to maintain SaO_2 greater than 92%. Keep the infant in a neutral position (head and body in alignment without inclination). Briefly disconnect the endotracheal tube from the ventilator. Insert the precut 5 French catheter into the endotracheal tube and instill the first aliquot (1.25 mL/kg birth weight). Position the infant so that either the right or left side is dependent for this aliquot. After the first aliquot is instilled, remove the catheter from the endotracheal tube and manually ventilate the infant with 100% oxygen at a rate of 40 to 60 breaths/minute for 1 minute. When the infant is stable, reposition the infant so that the other side is dependent and administer the remaining aliquot using the same procedures. Do not suction airways for 1 hour after surfactant instillation unless signs of significant airway obstruction occur.

After completion of the dosing procedure, resume usual ventilator management and clinical care. In the clinical trials, ventilator management was modified to maintain a PaO_2 of approximately 55 mm Hg, $PaCO_2$ of 35 to 45, and pH greater than 7.3.

For endotracheal instillation using the secondary lumen of a dual lumen endotracheal tube – Slowly withdraw the entire contents of the vial into a 3 or 5 mL plastic syringe through a large-gauge needle (eg, at least 20 gauge). Do not attach the 5 French end-hole catheter. Keep the infant in a neutral position (head and body in alignment without inclination). Administer poractant alfa through the proximal end of the secondary lumen of the endotracheal tube as a single dose given over 1 minute and without interrupting mechanical ventilation. After completion of this dosing procedure, ventilatory management may require transient increases in FiO_2 ventilatory rate or peak inspiratory pressure.

➤*Storage/Stability:* Store in a refrigerator at 2° to 8°C (36° to 46°F). Unopened vials may be warmed to room temperature for up to 24 hours prior to use. Unopened, unused vials that have warmed to room temperature may be returned to refrigerated storage within 24 hours for future use. Do not warm to room temperature or return it to the refrigerator more than

PORACTANT ALFA — INTRATRACHEAL

once. Protect from light. Enter each single-use vial only once, and discard the vial with any unused material after the initial entry.

Actions

➤*Pharmacology:* Endogenous pulmonary surfactant reduces surface tension at the air-liquid interface of the alveoli during ventilation and stabilizes the alveoli against collapse at resting transpulmonary pressures. A deficiency of pulmonary surfactant in preterm infants results in RDS, characterized by poor lung expansion, inadequate gas exchange, and a gradual collapse of the lungs (atelectasia). Poractant alfa compensates for the deficiency of surfactant and restores surface activity to the lungs of these infants.

In vitro, poractant alfa lowers minimum surface tension to less than or equal to 4 mN/m as measured by the Wilhelmy Balance System.

In vivo, in several pharmacodynamic studies, poractant alfa improved lung compliance, pulmonary gas exchange, or survival in premature rabbits.

➤*Pharmacokinetics:*

Absorption / Distribution – Poractant alfa is administered directly to the target organ, the lung, where biophysical effects occur at the alveolar surface. No human pharmacokinetic studies to characterize the absorption, biotransformation, or excretion of poractant alfa have been performed. Nonclinical studies have been performed to evaluate the disposition of phospholipids present in poractant alfa.

The concentration of ^{14}C-DPPC in alveolar macrophages was less than or equal to 2% of that in the lung in newborn and adult rabbits. Of the total ^{14}C-DPPC recovered in newborn rabbits, less than 0.6% was found in the serum, liver, kidneys, and brain, respectively, at 48 hours.

Metabolism / Excretion – In both adult and newborn rabbits, approximately 50% of the radiolabeled component rapidly was removed from the alveoli in the first 3 hours after single intratracheal administration of poractant alfa-^{14}C-DPPC (dipalmitoylphosphatidylcholine). Over a 24-hour period, approximately 45% of the labeled DPPC was cleared from the lungs of adult rabbits compared to approximately 20% in newborn rabbits. In newborn rabbits, poractant alfa-^{14}C-DPPC passed from the alveolar space into the lung parenchyma and then was secreted again into the alveoli, whereas in adult rabbits, most of the DPPC was not recycled. The $t_{½}$ in the lung appeared to be approximately 25 hours in adult rabbits and 67 hours in newborn rabbits.

Contraindications

None known.

Warnings/Precautions

➤*Administration:* Poractant alfa is intended for intratracheal use only. Administer poractant alfa only by those trained and experienced in the care, resuscitation, and stabilization of preterm infants.

➤*Dosing precautions:* Transient adverse effects seen with the administration of poractant alfa include bradycardia, hypotension, endotracheal tube blockage, and oxygen desaturation. These events require stopping poractant alfa administration and taking appropriate measures to alleviate the condition. After the patient is stable, dosing may proceed with appropriate monitoring.

➤*Prior to administration:* Correction of acidosis, hypotension, anemia, hypoglycemia, and hypothermia is recommended prior to poractant alfa administration.

➤*Complications of prematurity:* Surfactant administration can be expected to reduce the severity of RDS, but will not eliminate the mortality and morbidity associated with other complications of prematurity.

➤*Pregnancy: Category: Undetermined*. This drug is not indicated for use in adults.

➤*Lactation:* This drug is not indicated for use in adults.

➤*Monitoring:* The administration of exogenous surfactants, including poractant alfa, rapidly can affect oxygenation and lung compliance. Therefore, give infants receiving poractant alfa frequent clinical and laboratory assessments so oxygen and ventilatory support can be modified to respond to respiratory changes.

Adverse Reactions

Transient adverse effects seen with the administration of poractant alfa include bradycardia, hypotension, endotracheal tube blockage, and oxygen desaturation.

The rates of common complications of prematurity observed in study 1 are shown below.

Complications of Prematurity: Poractant Alfa vs Control (%)

Complications	Poractant alfa 2.5 mL/kg (200 mg/kg) (n = 78)	Control[a] (n = 66)
Acquired pneumonia	17%	21%
Acquired septicemia	14%	18%
Bronchopulmonary dysplasia	18%	22%
Intracranial hemorrhage	51%	64%
Patent ductus arteriosus	60%	48%
Pneumothorax	21%	36%
Pulmonary interstitial emphysema	21%	38%

[a] Controlled patients were disconnected from the ventilator and manually ventilated for 2 minutes. No surfactant was instilled.

➤*Follow-up:* Seventy-six infants (45 treated with poractant alfa) were evaluated at 1 year of age and 73 infants (44 treated with poractant alfa) at 2 years of age. Data from follow-up evaluations for weight and length, persistent respiratory symptoms, incidence of cerebral palsy, visual impairment, or auditory impairment were similar between treatment groups. In 16 patients (10 treated with poractant alfa and 6 controls) evaluated at 5.5 years of age, the developmental quotient, derived using the Griffiths Mental Developmental Scales, was similar between groups.

Overdosage

➤*Symptoms:* There have been no reports of overdosage following the administration of poractant alfa.

➤*Treatment:* In the event of accidental overdosage, and only if there are clear clinical effects on the infant's respiration, ventilation, or oxygenation, aspirate as much of the suspension as possible and manage the infant with supportive treatment, with particular attention to fluid and electrolyte balance.

ANTIHISTAMINES

Indications

➤*Allergic conditions:* As a group, these agents are used for the relief of manifestations of immediate-type hypersensitivity reactions.

➤*Sedation / Antiemetic / Antitussive / Antiparkinson / Analgesic / Motion sickness:* The varying degrees of anticholinergic, antihistaminic, and antimuscarinic activity make many antihistamines useful as sedatives, antiemetics, antitussives, antiparkinson agents, adjuncts to pre- or postoperative analgesic therapy, and agents to combat motion sickness.

➤*Off-label uses:* Refer to individual monographs for further information.

Appetite stimulation –

Cyproheptadine: [2] = Fair documentation.

Bronchial asthma –

Cetirizine: [2] = Fair documentation.

Nausea and vomiting of pregnancy – The recommended first-line treatment according to the American College of Obstetrics and Gynecology (ACOG) is pyridoxine alone or pyridoxine combined with doxylamine. Additional pharmacologic interventions were recommended only for refractory cases.

Doxylamine: [1] = Good documentation.

Promethazine: [2] = Fair documentation.

Nightmares (posttraumatic stress disorder) –

Cyproheptadine: [2] = Fair documentation.

Oral mucositis –

Diphenhydramine: [4] = Insufficient documentation.

Prevention of migraine (adults) –

Cyproheptadine: [4] = Insufficient documentation.

Prevention of migraine (children / adolescents) –

Cyproheptadine: [4] = Insufficient documentation.

Other possible off-label uses –

Cetirizine: To decrease the initial wheal response and pruritus associated with mosquito bites.

Cyproheptadine: Suppression of vascular headaches.

Diphenhydramine: Diphenhydramine has been used as an antianxiety agent in dosages of 25 to 200 mg/day, treatment or prophylaxis of chemotherapy-induced emesis, and drug-induced extrapyramidal reactions. For antipsychotic-induced dystonia, diphenhydramine 50 mg intramuscular or intravenous has been shown to be effective.

Actions

➤*Pharmacology:*

Antihistamine	Dose[b] (mg)	Dosing interval[c] (h)	Sedative effects	Antihistaminic activity	Anticholinergic activity	Antiemetic effects
Antihistamines: Dosage and Effects[a]						
First-generation (nonselective)						
Alkylamines						
Brompheniramine	4 mg	4 to 6 h	+	+++	++	—
Chlorpheniramine	4 mg	4 to 6 h	+	++	++	—
Dexchlorpheniramine	2 mg	4 to 6 h	+	+++	++	—
Pheniramine	15 to 30 mg	8 to 12 h	++	—	—	—
Triprolidine	2.5 mg	4 to 6 h	+	—	—	—
Ethanolamines						
Carbinoxamine	4 mg	6 h	+++		+++	
Clemastine	1 mg	12 h	++	+ to ++	+++	++ to +++
Diphenhydramine	25 to 50 mg	6 to 8 h	+++	+ to ++	+++	++ to +++
Ethylenediamine						
Pyrilamine	25 to 50 mg	6 to 8 h	+	—	±	—
Phenothiazines						
Promethazine	12.5 to 25 mg	6 to 24 h	+++	+++	+++	++++
Piperazines						
Hydroxyzine	25 to 100 mg	4 to 8 h	+++	++ to +++	++	+++
Piperidines						
Azatadine	1 to 2 mg	12 h	++	++	++	—
Cyproheptadine	4 mg	8 h	+	++	++	—
Phenindamine	25 mg	4 to 6 h	±	++	++	—
Second-generation (peripherally selective)						
Phthalazinone						
Azelastine[d]	0.5 mg	12 h	±	++ to +++	±	
Piperazine						
Cetirizine	5 to 10 mg	24 h	+	++ to +++	±	—
Levocetirizine	1.25 to 5 mg	24 h	±	++ to +++	±	—
Piperidines						
Desloratadine	5 mg	24 h	±	—		—
Fexofenadine	60 mg	12 h	±	—		—
Loratadine	10 mg	24 h	±	++ to +++		—

[a] ++++ = very high; +++ = high; ++ = moderate; + = low; ± = low to none.
[b] Usual single adult dose.
[c] For conventional dosage forms.
[d] Some effects may be enhanced or reduced as a result of administration via the nasal route.

Antihistamines are reversible, competitive H_1 receptor antagonists that reduce or prevent most of the physiologic effects that histamine normally induces at the H_1 receptor site. They do not prevent histamine release nor bind with histamine that already has been released. Antihistaminic effects include inhibition of respiratory, vascular, and GI smooth muscle constriction; decreased capillary permeability, which reduces the wheal, flare, and itch response; and decreased histamine-activated exocrine secretions (eg, salivary, lacrimal). Antihistamines with strong anticholinergic (atropine-like) properties also may potentiate the drying effect by suppressing cholinergically innervated exocrine glands. **First-generation antihistamines** bind nonselectively to central and peripheral H_1 receptors and may result in CNS stimulation or depression. CNS depression, which usually occurs with higher therapeutic doses, allows some of these agents to be used clinically for sedation. However, **second-generation antihistamines** are selective for peripheral H_1 receptors and, as a group, are less sedating. Several first-generation agents (eg, diphenhydramine, some piperazines, promethazine) with strong anticholinergic properties bind to central muscarinic receptors and produce antiemetic effects, decreasing nausea, vomiting, and motion sickness (seeAntiemetic/Antivertigo Agents). At doses much higher than that needed to antagonize histamine, a few agents (especially promethazine) exhibit local anesthetic effects. Some agents (eg, cyproheptadine, azatadine) also have antiserotonergic effects.

Switching from one class of antihistamines to another may restore responsiveness when a patient becomes refractory to the effects of a particular agent.

➤*Pharmacokinetics:*

First-generation agents – Pharmacokinetics of first-generation agents have not been studied extensively. With a few exceptions, these agents are well absorbed following oral administration, have an onset of action within 15 to 30 minutes, are maximal within 1 to 2 hours, and have a duration of action of approximately 4 to 6 hours, although some are much longer acting (see Pharmacology table). Most are metabolized by the liver. Antihistamine metabolites and small amounts of unchanged drug are excreted in urine. Small amounts may be excreted in breast milk.

Second-generation agents – Intranasal administration of **azelastine** yields peak levels in 2 to 3 hours, with an elimination half-life of 22 hours. Metabolism by the cytochrome P450 (CYP-450) system results in steady-state peak levels of a major active metabolite (desmethylazelastine), which are 20% to 50% of azelastine levels. The elimination half-life of the metabolite is predicted to be 54 hours. The major route of excretion is via feces.

In therapeutic doses, second-generation antihistamines do not significantly cross the blood-brain barrier and thus produce significantly less sedation (if any) compared to first-generation antihistamines.

Levocetirizine is the active enantiomer of cetirizine. **Cetirizine** is a metabolite of **hydroxyzine**. **Desloratadine** is a metabolite of **loratadine**. The pharmacokinetics of the second-generation agents have been studied more thoroughly and are provided in the following table.

Pharmacokinetics of Peripherally Selective H_1 Antagonists[a]

Antihistamine	Onset of action	T_{max} (h)	Elimination t½ (h)	Protein binding (%)	CYP-450 metabolism	Food effect on absorption
Cetirizine	rapid	1	8.3	93	↓; 50% excreted unchanged	delayed 1.7 h
Desloratadine	≤ 1 h	3	27	82 to 87	—	None
Fexofenadine	rapid	2.6	14.4	60 to 70	↓↓; 95% excreted unchanged	—
Levocetirizine	rapid	0.9	8 to 9	91 to 92	↓↓; 3A4	delayed 1.25 h
Loratadine	rapid	1.3 to 2.5[b]	8.4 to 28[b]	97 (75)[c]	↑; 3A4, 2D6	delayed 1 h

[a] T_{max} = time to maximal concentration; t½ = elimination half-life; ↑ = high; ↓ = low; ↓↓ = very low.
[b] All active constituents (parent drug and active metabolites).
[c] Active metabolite.

Contraindications

➤*First-generation antihistamines:* Hypersensitivity to specific or structurally related antihistamines, newborns or premature infants (see Warnings/Precautions), breast-feeding mothers (see Warnings/Precautions), monoamine oxidase inhibitor (MAOI) therapy (see Drug Interactions), pregnancy (**hydroxyzine**), angle-closure glaucoma, stenosing peptic ulcer, symptomatic prostatic hypertrophy, bladder neck obstruction, pyloroduodenal obstruction, elderly patients, debilitated patients (**cyproheptadine**).

➤*Second-generation antihistamines:* Hypersensitivity to specific or structurally related antihistamines. **Desloratadine** is contraindicated in those who are hypersensitive to **loratadine**. **Cetirizine** is contraindicated in those who are hypersensitive to **hydroxyzine**. **Levocetirizine** is contraindicated in those who are hypersensitive to cetirizine; end-stage renal disease (creatinine clearance less than 10 mL/min); patients undergoing hemodialysis; children 6 months to 11 years of age with renal impairment.

Warnings/Precautions

➤*Neuroleptic malignant syndrome:* A potentially fatal symptom complex sometimes referred to as neuroleptic malignant syndrome (NMS) has been reported in association with **promethazine** alone or in combination with antipsychotic drugs. Clinical manifestations of NMS are hyperpyrexia, muscle rigidity, altered mental status, and evidence of autonomic instability (eg, irregular pulse or blood pressure, tachycardia, diaphoresis, cardiac dysrhythmias).

➤*CNS depression:* Antihistamines may impair the mental and/or physical abilities required for the performance of potentially hazardous tasks, such as driving a vehicle or operating machinery. The impairment may be amplified by concomitant use of other CNS depressants such as alcohol, sedatives/hypnotics (including barbiturates), narcotics, narcotic analgesics, general anesthetics, tricyclic antidepressants, and tranquilizers. Therefore, such agents should be eliminated or given in reduced dosage in the presence of certain antihistamines with strong CNS-depressant effects.

When given concomitantly with **promethazine**, reduce the dose of barbiturates by at least one-half, and reduce the dose of the narcotics by one-fourth to one-half. Individualize dosage. Excessive amounts of promethazine relative to a narcotic may lead to restlessness and motor hyperactivity in patients experiencing pain.

➤*Special risk patients:* Use antihistamines with caution in patients with narrow-angle glaucoma, stenosing peptic ulcer, pyloroduodenal obstruction, symptomatic prostatic hypertrophy, bladder neck obstruction, bronchial asthma, increased intraocular pressure, hyperthyroidism, cardiovascular disease, and hypertension.

➤*Carcinogenesis:* Mice and rats given **loratadine** had a higher incidence in hepatocellular tumors (combined adenomas and carcinomas) than controls.

➤*Respiratory disease:* In general, antihistamines are not recommended to treat lower respiratory tract symptoms (eg, emphysema, chronic bronchitis, asthma) because their anticholinergic (drying) effects may thicken secretions and impair expectoration. However, several reports indicate antihistamines may be used safely in asthmatic patients with severe perennial allergic rhinitis without exacerbating the asthma.

➤*Seizure threshold:* **Promethazine** may lower the seizure threshold; consider this when giving to people with known seizure disorders or when giving in combination with narcotics or local anesthetics that also may affect seizure threshold.

➤*Respiratory depression:* Avoid sedatives and CNS depressants in patients with compromised respiratory function (eg, chronic obstructive pulmonary disease, sleep apnea).

➤*Hematologic:* Use **promethazine** with caution in bone marrow depression. Leukopenia and agranulocytosis have been reported, usually when used with other marrow-toxic agents.

➤*Anticholinergic effects:* Antihistamines have varying degrees of atropine-like actions; use with caution in patients with a predisposition to urinary retention, history of bronchial asthma, increased intraocular pressure, hyperthyroidism, cardiovascular disease, or hypertension. Antihistamines may thicken bronchial secretions caused by anticholinergic properties and may inhibit expectoration and sinus drainage.

➤*Phenothiazines:* Use phenothiazines with caution in patients with cardiovascular disease, liver dysfunction, or ulcer disease. **Promethazine** has been associated with cholestatic jaundice.

Use cautiously in patients with acute or chronic respiratory impairment, particularly children, because phenothiazines may suppress the cough reflex. If hypotension occurs, epinephrine is not recommended because phenothiazines may reverse its usual pressor effect and cause a paradoxical further lowering of blood pressure. Because these drugs have an antiemetic action, they may obscure signs of intestinal obstruction, brain tumor, or overdosage of toxic drugs.

Phenothiazines elevate prolactin levels, which persist through chronic administration. Approximately one-third of breast cancers are prolactin-dependent in vitro, an important factor if these drugs are prescribed for a patient with a history of breast cancer. Although galactorrhea, amenorrhea, gynecomastia, and impotence have been reported, the clinical significance of elevated serum prolactin levels is unknown.

➤*Phenylketonurics:* Inform phenylketonuric patients that some of these products contain phenylalanine.

➤*Tartrazine sensitivity:* Some of these products contain tartrazine (FD&C yellow No.5), which may cause allergic-type reactions (including bronchial asthma) in susceptible individuals. Although the incidence of sensitivity is low, it is frequently seen in patients who also have aspirin hypersensitivity. Specific products containing tartrazine are identified in the product listings.

➤*Hypersensitivity reactions:* Hypersensitivity reactions may occur, and any of the usual manifestations of drug allergy may develop. Have epinephrine 1:1000 immediately available. Refer to Management of Acute Hypersensitivity Reactions.

➤*Renal/Hepatic function impairment:* Use a lower initial dose of **loratadine**, **desloratadine**, and **cetirizine** in patients with renal or hepatic impairment. Dosage adjustment of **levocetirizine** is required in patients with mild, moderate, or severe renal impairment, and is contraindicated in patients with end-stage renal disease or those on dialysis.

➤*Hazardous tasks:* Antihistamines have varying degrees of sedative effects and may cause drowsiness and reduce mental alertness; instruct patients not to drive or perform other tasks requiring alertness, coordination, or physical dexterity. Supervise children who are taking antihistamines when they engage in potentially hazardous activities (eg, bicycle riding).

➤*Photosensitivity:* Photosensitization may occur; therefore, caution patients to take protective measures (eg, sunscreens, protective clothing) against exposure to ultraviolet light or sunlight until tolerance is determined.

➤*Pregnancy:* Category B (**azatadine**, **cetirizine**, **chlorpheniramine** [per Briggs' *Drugs in Pregnancy and Lactation*], **clemastine**, **cyproheptadine**, **dexchlorpheniramine**, **diphenhydramine**, **levocetirizine**, **loratadine**); *Category C* (**brompheniramine**, **carbinoxamine**, **chlorpheniramine** [per manufacturers' prescribing information], **desloratadine**, **fexofenadine**, **hydroxyzine**, **pheniramine**, **phenytoloxamine**, **promethazine**, **pyrilamine**, **triprolidine**). Safety for use during pregnancy has not been established. Several possible associations with malformations have been found, but the significance is unknown. Use only when clearly needed and when the potential benefits outweigh the potential hazards to the fetus. Do not use during the third trimester; newborn and premature infants may have severe reactions (eg, convulsions) to some antihistamines.

Reports of jaundice, hyperreflexia, and prolonged extrapyramidal symptoms occurred in infants whose mothers received phenothiazines during pregnancy. Promethazine, when taken within 2 weeks of delivery, may inhibit newborn platelet aggregation.

➤*Lactation:* The following antihistamines have been reported to be excreted in breast milk: **cetirizine**, **clemastine**, **desloratadine**, **diphenhydramine**, **loratadine**, **triprolidine**. **Levocetirizine** is expected to be excreted in breast milk. The use of cetirizine or **levocetirizine** in breast-feeding mothers is not recommended. The American Academy of Pediatrics considers triprolidine to be compatible with breast-feeding. Loratadine and its metabolite pass easily into breast milk and achieve concentrations that are equivalent to plasma levels with an area under the curve (AUC) milk/AUC plasma ratio of 1.17 and 0.85, respectively. Because of the higher risk of adverse effects for infants in general, and for newborns and prematures in particular, antihistamine therapy is contraindicated in breast-feeding mothers.

Although there are no quantitative measures, the molecular weight for **fexofenadine**, **hydroxyzine**, and **promethazine** is low enough that excretion into breast milk should be expected.

➤*Children:* Antihistamines may diminish mental alertness; conversely, they may produce excitation occasionally, particularly in young children.

Promethazine is not recommended in children younger than 2 years of age. Exercise caution when administering promethazine to children because of the potential for fatal respiratory depression. Limit antiemetics to prolonged vomiting of known etiology. The extrapyramidal symptoms that may occur secondary to promethazine may be confused with the CNS signs of undiagnosed primary disease (eg, encephalopathy, Reye syndrome). Avoid use in children whose signs and symptoms may suggest Reye syndrome or other hepatic diseases. In children who are acutely ill associated with dehydration, there is an increased susceptibility to dystonias with the use of promethazine.

➤*Elderly:* Antihistamines are more likely to cause dizziness, excessive sedation, syncope, toxic confusional states, and hypotension in elderly patients, and also may cause paradoxical stimulation. Dosage reduction may be required.

The phenothiazine adverse effects (extrapyramidal signs, especially parkinsonism, akathisia, and persistent dyskinesia) are more prone to develop in elderly patients.

According to the Beers list, **chlorpheniramine**, **cyproheptadine**, **dexchlorpheniramine**, **diphenhydramine**, **hydroxyzine**, and **promethazine** may have potent anticholinergic properties. Nonanticholinergic antihistamines are preferred in elderly patients when treating allergic reactions. Diphenhydramine may cause confusion and sedation. It should not be used as a hypnotic, and when used to treat emergency allergic reactions, it should be used in the smallest possible dose.Diphenhydramine, hydroxyzine, cyproheptadine, promethazine, and dexchlorpheniramine are also considered high-risk medications for elderly patients according to the Centers of Medicare and Medicaid Services.

Drug Interactions

Antihistamine Drug Interactions

Precipitant drug	Object drug[a]		Description
Antacids, aluminum/magnesium containing	Antihistamines Fexofenadine	↓	Administration of fexofenadine within 15 minutes of an aluminum- and magnesium-containing antacid decreased fexofenadine AUC by 41% and C_{max}[b] by 43%. Fexofenadine should not be taken closely in time to these antacids.
Cimetidine	Antihistamines Azelastine Desloratadine Loratadine	↑	Concomitant use resulted in substantially increased plasma levels of loratadine and desloratadine and an increase of approximately 65% in levels of orally administered azelastine.
Erythromycin	Antihistamines Desloratadine Fexofenadine Loratadine	↑	Plasma levels (including metabolites) may be increased. There are no clinically relevant changes in safety profile.
Ketoconazole	Antihistamines Desloratadine Fexofenadine Loratadine	↑	Plasma levels (including metabolites) may be increased. There are no clinically relevant changes in safety profile.
MAOIs	Antihistamines	↑	MAOIs may prolong and intensify the anticholinergic and sedative effects of antihistamines. MAOIs may cause hypotension and extrapyramidal reactions with phenothiazines and severe hypotension with dexchlorpheniramine.
Antihistamines	MAOIs		
Rifamycins (eg, rifampin)	Antihistamines Fexofenadine	↓	Rifampin may reduce the absorption of fexofenadine, thereby decreasing the pharmacologic effect.
Ritonavir	Antihistamines Cetirizine Levocetirizine	↑	Ritonavir increased the AUC and half-life and decreased the clearance of cetirizine. Risk of adverse reactions may be increased.
Theophylline	Antihistamines Cetirizine Levocetirizine	↑	Theophylline 400 mg led to a small decrease (approximately 16%) in the clearance of cetirizine. Higher theophylline doses may have a greater effect.
Antihistamines	Alcohol, CNS depressants	↑	Additive CNS-depressant effects may occur (see Warnings/Precautions). This may be less likely with second-generation agents.
Antihistamines Cyproheptadine	Metyrapone	↓	Cyproheptadine may diminish the expected pituitary adrenal response to metyrapone. Avoid concurrent use or discontinue cyproheptadine before metyrapone is used.
Antihistamines Cyproheptadine	SSRIs[c] Nefazodone Venlafaxine	↓	SSRIs have serotonergic activity and cyproheptadine is a serotonin antagonist. If a loss of the antidepressant effectiveness occurs, consider discontinuing cyproheptadine.
Antihistamine Diphenhydramine	Beta-blockers	↑	Diphenhydramine may inhibit the CYP2D6-mediated metabolism of certain beta-blockers (eg, metoprolol), producing increased plasma concentrations and cardiovascular effects. Monitor closely.

[a] ↑ = object drug increased; ↓ = object drug decreased.
[b] C_{max} = maximal drug concentration.
[c] SSRIs = selective serotonin reuptake inhibitors.

See the Antipsychotic Agents monograph for a complete discussion of the drug interactions that relate to the phenothiazine antihistamine, promethazine.

➤*Drug/Lab test interactions:* Diagnostic pregnancy tests based on human chorionic gonadotropin (hCG) and anti-hCG may result in false-negative or false-positive interpretations in patients taking **promethazine**. Increased blood glucose has occurred in patients taking promethazine.

Phenothiazines may increase serum cholesterol, spinal fluid protein, and urinary urobilinogen levels; decrease protein bound iodine; yield false-positive urine bilirubin tests; and interfere with urinary ketone and steroid determinations.

Discontinue antihistamines approximately 4 days prior to **skin testing procedures**; these drugs may prevent or diminish otherwise positive reactions to dermal reactivity indicators.

➤*Drug/Food interactions:* Food increased the AUC of **loratadine** by approximately 40% and the metabolite by approximately 15%; absorption was delayed by 1 hour; peak levels were unaffected. Although not expected to be clinically important, take on an empty stomach. The AUC of loratadine rapidly disintegrating tablets was increased by 26% when administered without water compared with water; peak levels were not affected significantly. Bioavailability was unaffected; dissolved remnants may be swallowed with or without water.

Systemic absorption of **cetirizine** was delayed by 1.7 hours, and peak plasma levels were decreased by 23%. However, cetirizine may be taken with or without food.

In one study of **desloratadine** orally disintegrating tablets, administration with food shifted the median T_{max} from 2.5 to 4 hours.

Certain fruit juices (ie, apple, orange, grapefruit) administered with **fexofenadine** significantly reduced the AUC and C_{max} of fexofenadine. Therefore, fexofenadine's clinical effect may be decreased. It would be prudent for patients to take fexofenadine with a liquid other than these juices.

Adverse Reactions

➤*Allergic:* Anaphylactic shock; angioneurotic, laryngeal, and peripheral edema; asthma; dermatitis; drug rash; lupus erythematosus-like syndrome; urticaria.

➤*Cardiovascular:* Bradycardia; cardiac arrest; electrocardiogram (ECG) changes, including blunting of T-waves and prolongation of the QT interval; extrasystoles; faintness; hypertension; hypotension; palpitations; postural hypotension; reflex tachycardia; syncope; tachycardia; venous thrombosis at injection site (intravenous [IV] **promethazine**).

➤*CNS:* Disturbed coordination, dizziness, drowsiness (often transient), faintness, sedation (most frequent); acute labyrinthitis, blurred vision, catatonic-like states, confusion, convulsions, diplopia, disorientation, disturbing dreams/nightmares, euphoria, excitation, fatigue, tonic-clonic seizures, hallucinations, headache, hysteria, insomnia, lassitude, neuritis, oculogyric crisis, paresthesias, pseudoschizophrenia, restlessness, tinnitus, tongue protrusion (usually in association with IV administration or excessive dosage), torticollis, tremor, vertigo, weakness. Extrapyramidal reactions may occur with high doses; these reactions usually respond to dose reduction.

➤*GI:* Epigastric distress (most frequent, especially ethylenediamines), anorexia, constipation, diarrhea, increased appetite, nausea, stomatitis, vomiting, weight gain.

Nasal spray – Glossitis, increased ALT, ulcerative and aphthous stomatitis.

➤*GU:* Dysuria, early menses, gynecomastia, induced lactation, inhibition of ejaculation, urinary frequency, urinary retention.

➤*Hematologic:* Agranulocytosis, aplastic anemia, hemolytic anemia, hypoplastic anemia, leukopenia, pancytopenia, thrombocytopenia.

➤*Respiratory:* Thickening of bronchial secretions (most frequent); chest tightness; dry mouth, nose, and throat; nasal stuffiness; respiratory depression; sore throat; wheezing.

Nasal spray – Epistaxis, paroxysmal sneezing, rhinitis.

➤*Special senses:*

Nasal spray – Bitter taste (most frequent), conjunctivitis, eye abnormality, eye pain, nasal burning, taste loss, watery eyes.

➤*Miscellaneous:* Chills; elevated spinal fluid proteins; elevation of plasma cholesterol levels; erythema; excessive perspiration; glycosuria; heaviness, tingling, and weakness of the hands; high or prolonged glucose tolerance curves; obstructive jaundice (usually reversible upon drug discontinuation); photosensitivity; thrombocytopenic purpura; tissue necrosis following subcutaneous administration of IV **promethazine**.

Nasal spray – Temporomandibular dislocation.

Adverse Reactions for Peripherally Selective H_1 Antagonists[a]

Adverse reactions	Azelastine (n = 391)	Cetirizine (n = 2,034)	Desloratadine (n = 1,866)	Fexofenadine (n = 679)	Levocetirizine (n = 1,491)	Loratadine (n = 1,926)
CNS						
Dizziness	2%	2%	4%	—	—	—
Drowsiness/Somnolence	11.5%	13.7%	2.1%	1.3%	5% to 6%	8%
Fatigue	2.3%	5.9%	2.1% to 5%	1.3%	1% to 4%	4%
Headache	14.8%	> 2%	14%	> 1%	—	12%
Weight gain	2%	—	—	—	—	—

Adverse Reactions for Peripherally Selective H_1 Antagonists[a]

Adverse reactions	Azelastine (n = 391)	Cetirizine (n = 2,034)	Desloratadine (n = 1,866)	Fexofenadine (n = 679)	Levocetirizine (n = 1,491)	Loratadine (n = 1,926)
Ear, nose, throat						
Dry mouth, nose, throat	2.8%	5%	3%	—	2% to 3%	3%
Epistaxis	2%	—	—		—	—
Nasopharyngitis	—	—	—	—	4% to 6%	—
Pharyngitis	3.8%	2%	3% to 4.1%	> 1%	1% to 2%	—
GI						
Nausea, vomiting, abdominal distress, bowel changes	2.8%	> 2%	3% to 4%	1.3% to 1.6%	—	
Miscellaneous						
Dysmenorrhea	—	—	2.1%	1.5%	—	—
Myalgia	—	—	2.1% to 3%	—	—	—

[a] Data pooled from several studies and are not necessarily comparable.

➤*Phenothiazines:* These antihistamines infrequently cause typical phenothiazine adverse reactions. See the Antipsychotic Agents monograph for a complete discussion.

Overdosage

➤*Symptoms:* Effects may vary from CNS depression (eg, sedation, apnea, diminished mental alertness) and cardiovascular collapse to stimulation (eg, insomnia, hallucinations, tremors, convulsions), especially in children and elderly patients. Profound hypotension, respiratory depression, unconsciousness, coma, and death may occur, particularly in infants and children. Convulsions occur rarely and indicate a poor prognosis. The convulsant dose lies near the lethal dose.

Toxic effects are seen within 30 minutes to 2 hours and result in drowsiness, dizziness, ataxia, tinnitus, blurred vision, and hypotension. Anticholinergic effects result in fixed dilated pupils, flushing, dry mouth, hyperthermia (especially in children), and fever. GI symptoms also may occur. Hyperpyrexia to 41.8°C (107°F) and acute oral and facial dystonic reactions have been reported.

Children often manifest CNS stimulation and may have hallucinations, toxic psychosis, delirium tremens, excitement, ataxia, incoordination, muscle twitching, athetosis, hyperthermia, cyanosis, convulsions, and hyperreflexia followed by postictal depression and cardiorespiratory arrest. Seizures resistant to therapy may follow and may be preceded by mild depression. A paradoxical reaction has been reported in children receiving single doses of 75 to 125 mg of oral **promethazine,** characterized by hyperexcitability and nightmares. CNS stimulation in adults usually manifests as seizures. Marked cerebral irritation, resulting in jerking of muscles and possible convulsions, may be followed by deep stupor. Occasionally, respiratory depression, cardiovascular collapse, and death follows a latent period.

Less common findings include ECG changes, such as wandering pacemaker, prolonged QT interval, and nonspecific ST-T wave changes that disappear quickly. The electroencephalogram may show general cerebral dysrhythmia and diffuse delta wave activity that may persist after clinical recovery.

➤*Treatment:* Take adequate precautions to protect against aspiration, especially in infants and children. Administer activated charcoal as a slurry with water and a cathartic to minimize absorption. Correct acidosis and electrolyte imbalances. Do not induce emesis in unconscious patients. Gastric lavage is indicated within 3 hours after ingestion and even later if large amounts were taken. Continue therapy directed at reversing the effects of timed-release medication and supporting the patient. Hemoperfusion may be used in severe cases. **Cetirizine, fexofenadine, levocetirizine,** and **loratadine** do not appear to be dialyzable. Refer to General Management of Acute Overdosage.

Hypotension is an early sign of impending cardiovascular collapse; treat vigorously using general supportive measures or specific vasopressor treatment (eg, norepinephrine, phenylephrine, dopamine). Avoid epinephrine; it may worsen hypotension. Propranolol may be used for refractory ventricular arrhythmias.

Administer diazepam 0.1 mg/kg IV slowly for convulsions; repeat as needed. IV physostigmine may reverse central anticholinergic effects. Use with caution. Avoid analeptics; they may cause convulsions. Depressant effects of **promethazine** are not reversed by naloxone.

Ice packs and cooling sponge baths, not alcohol, may help reduce a child's fever.

Patient Information

Instruct patients to inform a physician of a history of glaucoma, peptic ulcer, urinary retention, or pregnancy before starting antihistamine therapy.

Some antihistamines may cause nervousness, insomnia, and dry mouth.

Some antihistamines may cause drowsiness or dizziness; advise patients to observe caution while driving or performing other tasks requiring alertness, coordination, or physical dexterity and to avoid alcohol and other CNS depressants (eg, sedatives, hypnotics, tranquilizers, antianxiety agents).

Some antihistamines may cause GI upset; instruct patients to take with food.

Advise patients to avoid prolonged exposure to sunlight; some agents may cause photosensitivity.

Instruct patients not to crush or chew sustained-release preparations.

➤*Phenothiazines:* Advise patients to report any involuntary muscle movements or unusual sensitivity to sunlight.

Alkylamines, Nonselective

BROMPHENIRAMINE

Rx	**Brompheniramine** (Various, eg, Ani Pharmaceuticals, Brighton)	**Tablets, chewable; oral:** 12 mg brompheniramine tannate	Sugar. Oval, scored. In 60s.
Rx	**BrōveX CT** (Athlon)		Sucrose. (273). Yellow, oval, scored. Banana flavor. In 60s.
Rx	**LoHist 12 Hour** (Larken)	**Tablets, extended release; oral:** 6 mg brompheniramine tannate	(LH 12). White, oval, scored. In 100s.
Rx sf	**Brompheniramine Maleate** (Kylemore)	**Drops; oral:** 1 mg/mL brompheniramine maleate	Alcohol free, dye free, sugar free. Saccharin. Strawberry-banana flavor. In 30 mL.
Rx	**Lodrane 24** (ECR Pharmaceuticals)	**Capsules, extended release; oral:** 12 mg brompheniramine maleate	(Lodrane 24). White. In 100s.
Rx	**VaZol** (WraSer)	**Liquid; oral:** 2 mg/5 mL brompheniramine tannate	Bubble gum flavor. In 472 mL.
Rx	**J-Tan** (Jaymac Pharmaceuticals)	**Suspension; oral:** 4 mg/5 mL brompheniramine tannate	Strawberry cream flavor. In 473 mL.
Rx sf	**Lodrane XR** (ECR Pharmaceuticals)	**Suspension; oral:** 8 mg/5 mL brompheniramine tannate	Alcohol free. Strawberry flavor. In pints and 10 mL.
Rx sf	**P-tex** (Poly Pharmaceuticals)	**Suspension; oral:** 10 mg/5 mL brompheniramine tannate	Alcohol free. Peach flavor. In 480 mL.
Rx	**Brompheniramine** (Ani Pharmaceuticals)	**Suspension; oral:** 12 mg/5 mL brompheniramine tannate	Methylparaben, sucrose, tartrazine. Banana flavor. In 118 mL.
Rx	**BrōveX** (MCR/American Pharmaceutical)		Equiv. to 5.4 mg/5 mL brompheniramine. Saccharin, tartrazine. Banana flavor. In 20 and 118 mL.

Alkylamines, Nonselective

BROMPHENIRAMINE — ORAL

For complete and comparative prescribing information, refer to the Antihistamines group monograph.

Indications

➤*Allergies:* For the temporary relief of sneezing, itchy, watery eyes, itchy nose or throat, and runny nose caused by hay fever (allergic rhinitis), or other respiratory allergies.

VaZol also is indicated for the temporary relief of runny nose and sneezing caused by the common cold; treatment of allergic and nonallergic pruritic symptoms; temporary relief of mild, uncomplicated urticaria and angioedema; amelioration of allergic reactions to blood or plasma; adjunctive therapy in anaphylactic reactions.

Administration and Dosage

➤*Adults:*

Allergies –

Usual dosage:

- *Capsules, extended release* – 1 or 2 capsules (12 to 24 mg) once daily.
- *Oral liquid* – 10 mL (4 mg) 4 times daily.
- *Oral suspension* – 5 to 10 mL (12 to 24 mg) every 12 hours.
- *Tablets, chewable* – 1 or 2 tablets (12 to 24 mg) every 12 hours.
- *Tablets, extended release* – 1 or 2 tablets (6 to 12 mg) every 12 hours.

Maximum dose:

- *Oral suspension* – 20 mL (48 mg) in 24 hours.
- *Tablets, chewable* – 4 tablets (48 mg) in 24 hours.

➤*Administration:*

Capsules, extended release and tablets, extended release – Take with food, water or milk to minimize gastric irritation. Swallow whole; do not crush capsules or tablets.

Oral suspension – Shake well before use. Measure and administer prescribed dose using dosing syringe, dosing spoon, or dosing cup.

Tablets, chewable – Chew tablet before swallowing and do not swallow tablet whole. Drink small amount of water or juice after administering chewable tablet.

➤*Storage/Stability:* Store between 15° and 30°C (59° to 86°F).

CHLORPHENIRAMINE

otc	**Chlorpheniramine Maleate** (Various, eg, Contract Pharmacal, URL)	**Tablets; oral:** 4 mg	As maleate. In 24s, 100s, and 1,000s.
otc	**Aller-Chlor** (Rugby)		As maleate. In 24s, 100s, and 1,000s.
otc	**Allergy** (Major)		As maleate. Lactose. In 24s and 100s.
otc	**Allergy Relief** (Zee Medical)		As maleate. In 12s.
otc	**Allergy-Time** (Time-Cap Labs)		As maleate. Lactose. In 1,000s.
otc	**Chlo-Amine** (Hollister-Stier)	**Tablets, chewable; oral:** 2 mg	As maleate. Sugar. Orange flavor. In 96s.
otc	**Chlor-Trimeton Allergy 8 Hour** (Schering-Plough Healthcare)	**Tablets, extended-release; oral:** 8 mg	As maleate. 374). In 15s.
otc	**Chlorpheniramine** (KVK Tech)	**Tablets, extended-release; oral:** 12 mg	As maleate. Calcium 28 mg, lactose, propyl parahydroxybenzoate, sodium benzoate, sucrose, sugar. In 24s and 60s.
otc	**Chlor-Trimeton Allergy 12 Hour** (Schering-Plough Healthcare)		As maleate. 009). In 10s.
otc	**Efidac 24**[a] (Hogil)	**Tablets, extended-release; oral:** 16 mg	As maleate. Mannitol. In 6s.
Rx	**QDALL AR**[b] (Atley)	**Capsules, extended-release; oral:** 12 mg	As maleate. Sucrose. (QD 111). Blue/White. In 100s.
Rx	**Chlorpheniramine Maleate** (Various, eg, Qualitest)	**Capsules, extended-release; oral:** 8 mg	As maleate. In 100s and 1,000s.
Rx	**Chlorpheniramine Maleate** (Various, eg, Qualitest)	**Capsules, extended-release; oral:** 12 mg	As maleate. In 100s and 1,000s.
Rx	**ED-CHLOR-TAN** (Edwards Pharmaceuticals)	**Caplets; oral:** 8 mg	As tannate. In 100s.
Rx	**Tanahist-PD** (Larken Labs)	**Drops; oral:** 2 mg/mL	As tannate. Glycerin, methylparaben, saccharin, sodium benzoate, sorbitol. Cotton candy flavor. In 59 mL with dropper.
otc	**Aller-Chlor** (Rugby)	**Syrup; oral:** 2 mg/5 mL	As maleate. 5% alcohol, parabens, sugar. In 118 mL.
Rx	**Pediox-S** (Atley)	**Suspension; oral:** 4 mg/5 mL	As maleate. Acesulfame K, aspartame, methylparaben, 8.419 mg phenylalanine per 5 mL, sucralose. Cotton candy flavor. In 118 mL.

[a] 4 mg immediate release, 12 mg controlled release.

[b] 2 mg immediate release, 10 mg sustained release.

CHLORPHENIRAMINE — ORAL

For complete and comparative prescribing information, refer to the Antihistamines group monograph.

Indications

➤*Allergic rhinitis:* For the temporary relief of sneezing, itchy, watery eyes, itchy throat, and runny nose caused by hay fever, other upper respiratory allergies, and the common cold.

Administration and Dosage

➤*Adults:*

Allergic rhinitis –

Usual dosage:

- *Caplets* – 8 mg every 12 hours.
- *Capsules, extended-release* – 12 mg once daily.
- *Capsules, sustained-release* – 8 or 12 mg every 12 hours.
- *Efidac 24* – 16 mg with liquid every 24 hours.
- *Suspension* – 5 to 10 mL every 12 hours.
- *Tablets or syrup* – 4 mg every 4 to 6 hours.
- *Tablets, extended-release* – 8 mg every 8 to 12 hours or 12 mg every 12 hours.

Maximum dose:

- *Caplets* – 16 to 24 mg/day.
- *Capsules, extended-release* – 24 mg in 24 hours.
- *Capsules, sustained-release* – 16 to 24 mg/day.
- *Efidac 24* – 16 mg in 24 hours.
- *Suspension* – 20 mL/day.
- *Tablets or syrup* – 24 mg in 24 hours.
- *Tablets, extended-release* – 24 mg in 24 hours.

➤*Children:*

Allergic rhinitis –

Caplets:

- *Usual dosage –*
  12 years of age and older: 8 mg every 12 hours.
- *Maximum dose –*
  12 years of age and older: 16 to 24 mg/day.

Capsules, extended-release:

- *Usual dosage –*
  12 years of age and older: 12 mg once daily.
- *Maximum dose –*
  12 years of age and older: 24 mg in 24 hours.

Capsules, sustained-release:

- *Usual dosage –*
  12 years of age and older: 8 or 12 mg every 12 hours.
  6 to 12 years of age: 8 mg at bedtime or during the day as indicated.
- *Maximum dose –*
  12 years of age and older: 16 to 24 mg/day.

Drops:

- *Usual dosage –*
  6 years of age and older: 2 mL every 12 hours
  18 months to 6 years of age: 1 mL every 12 hours
  9 to 18 months of age: 0.5 to 0.75 mL every 12 hours
  6 to 9 months of age: 0.5 mL every 12 hours
  3 to 6 months of age: 0.25 mL every 12 hours

Efidac 24:

- *Usual dosage –*
  12 years of age and older: 16 mg with liquid every 24 hours.
- *Maximum dose –*
  12 years of age and older: 16 mg in 24 hours.

Alkylamines, Nonselective

CHLORPHENIRAMINE — ORAL

Suspension:
- *Usual dosage –*
  12 years of age and older: 5 to 10 mL every 12 hours.
  6 to younger than 12 years of age: 2.5 to 5 mL every 12 hours.
  2 to younger than 6 years of age: 1.25 mL every 12 hours.
- *Maximum dose –*
  12 years of age and older: 20 mL/day.
  6 to younger than 12 years of age: 10 mL/day.
  2 to younger than 6 years of age: 5 mL/day.

Tablets or syrup:
- *Usual dosage –*
  12 years of age and older: 4 mg every 4 to 6 hours.
  6 to 12 years of age: 2 mg (break 4 mg tablets in half) every 4 to 6 hours.
- *Maximum dose –*
  12 years of age and older: 24 mg in 24 hours.
  6 to 12 years of age: 12 mg in 24 hours.

Tablets, extended-release:
- *Usual dosage –*
  12 years of age and older: 8 mg every 8 to 12 hours or 12 mg every 12 hours.
- *Maximum dose –*
  12 years of age and older: 24 mg in 24 hours.

➤*Administration:* Administer without regard to meals. Administer with food if GI upset occurs. Measure and administer prescribed dose of oral syrup using dosing syringe, dosing spoon, or dosing cup.

Extended-release or sustained-release capsules and tablets – Swallow whole; do not divide, crush, chew, or dissolve.

➤*Storage/Stability:* Store between 15° and 30°C (59° and 86°F).

DEXCHLORPHENIRAMINE MALEATE

Rx	**Dexchlorpheniramine Maleate** (Various, eg, Amide, Breckenridge, URL)	**Tablets, extended-release:** 4 mg	In 100s and 1,000s.
Rx	**Dexchlorpheniramine Maleate** (Various, eg, Amide, Breckenridge, URL)	**Tablets, extended-release:** 6 mg	In 100s and 1,000s.
Rx	**Dexchlorpheniramine Maleate** (Morton Grove)	**Syrup:** 2 mg/5 mL	Alcohol, orange flavor. In 473 mL.

DEXCHLORPHENIRAMINE MALEATE — ORAL

For complete and comparative prescribing information, refer to the Antihistamines group monograph.

Indications

➤*Hypersensitivity reactions, type I:* For the treatment of perennial and seasonal allergic rhinitis; vasomotor rhinitis; allergic conjunctivitis; mild, uncomplicated allergic skin manifestations of urticaria and angioedema; amelioration of allergic reactions to blood or plasma; dermatographism; and adjunctive anaphylactic therapy.

Administration and Dosage

➤*Adults:*

Hypersensitivity reactions – 4 or 6 mg at bedtime or every 8 to 10 hours.

➤*Children:* Safety and efficacy of the 4 and 6 mg timed-release tablets in children younger than 6 and 12 years of age, respectively, have not been established.

Hypersensitivity reactions –
12 years of age and older: See Adults for dosing.
6 to 12 years of age: 4 mg/day, preferably taken at bedtime.
Younger than 6 years of age: Safety and efficacy in children younger than 2 years of age have not been established. Do not use in newborn or premature infants because of the possibility of severe reactions, such as convulsions.

➤*Storage/Stability:* Store between 2° and 30°C (36° and 86°F).

TRIPROLIDINE

Rx sf	**Triprolidine** (Centurion Labs)	**Liquid; oral:** 1.25 mg per 5 mL	Alcohol free. Apple flavor. In 473 mL.
Rx sf	**Zymine** (Vindex)		As hydrochloride. Alcohol free. Apple flavor. In 15 and 473 mL.
Rx sf	**Zymine XR** (Vindex)	**Suspension; oral:** 2.5 mg per 5 mL	As tannate. Alcohol free. Aspartame,[a] parabens. Red. Apple flavor. In 10 and 473 mL.

[a] 7 mg phenylalanine per 5 mL.

TRIPROLIDINE HYDROCHLORIDE — ORAL

For complete and comparative prescribing information, refer to the Antihistamines class monograph.

Indications

➤*Allergies:* For the symptomatic relief of perennial and seasonal allergic rhinitis, vasomotor rhinitis, allergic conjunctivitis caused by inhalant allergens and foods, and mild, uncomplicated allergic skin manifestations of urticaria and angioedema.

Administration and Dosage

➤*Adults:*

Allergies –
Usual dosage: 10 mL every 4 to 6 hours.
Maximum dose: Do not exceed 40 mL in 24 hours.

➤*Children:*

Allergies –
12 years of age and older: See Adults for dosing.
6 to 12 years of age:
- *Usual dosage –* 5 mL every 4 to 6 hours.
- *Maximum dose –* Do not exceed 20 mL in 24 hours.

4 to 6 years of age:
- *Usual dosage –* 3.75 mL every 4 to 6 hours.
- *Maximum dose –* Do not exceed 15 mL in 24 hours.

2 to 4 years of age:
- *Usual dosage –* 2.5 mL every 4 to 6 hours.
- *Maximum dose –* Do not exceed 10 mL in 24 hours.

4 months to 2 years of age:
- *Usual dosage –* 1.25 mL every 4 to 6 hours.
- *Maximum dose –* Do not exceed 5 mL in 24 hours.

➤*Elderly:* Antihistamines are more likely to cause dizziness, excessive sedation, syncope, toxic confusional states, and hypotension in elderly patients and also may cause paradoxical stimulation. Dosage reduction may be required.

➤*Storage/Stability:* Store between 15° and 30°C (59° and 86°F).

Warnings/Precautions

➤*Pregnancy: Category C.* Animal reproduction studies have not been conducted with this product. It is not known whether it can cause fetal harm when administered to a pregnant woman.

➤*Lactation:* Because of the possible passage of the ingredients into breast milk, do not give this product to breast-feeding mothers. However, the American Academy of Pediatrics classifies triprolidine as compatible with breast-feeding.

TRIPROLIDINE TANNATE — ORAL

Indications

➤*Allergies:* For the symptomatic relief of perennial and seasonal allergic rhinitis, vasomotor rhinitis, allergic conjunctivitis due to inhalant allergens and foods, and mild uncomplicated allergic skin manifestations of urticaria and angioedema.

Administration and Dosage

➤*Adults:*

Allergies – 10 mL every 12 hours.

➤*Children:*

Allergies –
12 years of age and older: 10 mL every 12 hours.
6 to younger than 12 years of age: 5 mL every 12 hours.
2 to younger than 6 years of age: 2.5 mL every 12 hours.

➤*Elderly:* Antihistamines are more likely to cause dizziness, excessive sedation, syncope, toxic confusional states, and hypotension in elderly patients and also may cause paradoxical stimulation. Dosage reduction may be required.

➤*Administration:* Shake well before use.

Alkylamines, Nonselective

TRIPROLIDINE TANNATE — ORAL

➤*Storage/Stability:* Store at 15° to 30°C (59° to 86°F).

Warnings/Precautions

➤*Pregnancy: Category C.* Animal reproduction studies have not been conducted with this product. It is not known whether it can cause fetal harm when administered to a pregnant woman.

➤*Lactation:* Because of the possible passage of the ingredients into breast milk, do not give this product to breast-feeding mothers. However, the American Academy of Pediatrics classifies triprolidine as compatible with breast-feeding.

DEXBROMPHENIRAMINE MALEATE

Rx	**Ala-Hist IR** (Poly Pharmaceuticals)	**Tablets; oral:** 2 mg	In 60s.

DEXBROMPHENIRAMINE MALEATE — ORAL

Indications

➤*Hay fever/respiratory allergies:* For the temporary relief of runny nose, sneezing, itching of the nose or throat, and itchy, watery eyes due to hay fever or other respiratory allergies.

Administration and Dosage

➤*Maximum dose:*

Adults – 6 tablets per day.

Children 6 to 12 years of age – 3 tablets per day.

➤*Adults and children 12 years of age and older:*

Usual dosage – 1 tablet every 4 to 6 hours.

Maximum dose – Not to exceed 6 tablets in a 24 hour period.

➤*Children 6 to 12 years of age:*

Usual dosage – Half tablet every 4 to 6 hours.

Maximum dose – Not to exceed 3 tablets in a 24 hour period.

➤*Children 6 years of age and younger:* Consult a health care provider.

➤*Storage/Stability:* Store at 15° to 30°C (59° to 86°F).

Ethanolamines, Nonselective

CARBINOXAMINE

Rx	**Carbinoxamine Maleate** (Boca)	**Tablets; oral:** 4 mg	Lactose. (BP 605). Scored. In 100s.
Rx	**Palgic** (Pamlab)		Lactose. (PAL 4). White, scored. In 100s and 500s.
Rx	**Histex CT** (Teamm Pharm[a])	**Tablets, timed release; oral:** 8	(258). Blue, scored. Film-coated. In 30s and 100s.
Rx	**Histex I/E** (Teamm Pharm[a])	**Capsules, extended release; oral:** 10 mg[b]	(050 HISTEX I/E). Green and white. In 60s.
Rx sf	**Pediatex** (Zyber)	**Liquid; oral:** 1.67 mg per 5 mL	Saccharin, sorbitol. Alcohol and dye-free. Cotton candy flavor. In 15 and 473 mL.
Rx	**Carbinoxamine Maleate** (Boca)	**Solution; oral:** 4 mg per 5 mL	Parabens, sorbitol. Banana bubble gum flavor. In 120 and 473 mL.
Rx sf	**Histex Pd** (Teamm Pharm[a])		Saccharin, sorbitol. Alcohol and dye free. Gum fruit flavor. In 473 mL.
Rx sf	**Palgic** (Pamlab)		Parabens. Clear. Bubble gum flavor. In 118 and 473 mL.
Rx	**Pediatex 12** (Zyber)	**Suspension; oral:** 3.2 mg per 5 mL	Methylparaben, saccharin, sucrose. Candy apple flavor. In 20 and 473 mL.

[a] Teamm Pharmaceuticals, 3000 Aerial Center Parkway, Suite 110, Morrisville, NC 27560; 919-481-9020, 866-481-9020, fax 919-481-9311.

[b] 2 mg immediate-release and 8 mg extended-release.

CARBINOXAMINE MALEATE — ORAL

For complete and comparative prescribing information, refer to the Antihistamines group monograph.

Indications

➤*Allergies:* For relief of nasal and nonnasal symptoms of seasonal and perennial allergic rhinitis. *Palgic* tablets also are indicated for the symptomatic treatment of vasomotor rhinitis; allergic conjunctivitis caused by inhalant allergens and foods; mild, uncomplicated allergic skin manifestations of urticaria and angioedema; dermatographism; as therapy for anaphylactic reactions adjunctive to epinephrine and other standard measures after the acute manifestations have been controlled; amelioration of the severity of allergic reactions to blood or plasma.

Administration and Dosage

➤*Adults:*

Allergies –

Maximum dose:
- *Histex I/E* – 2 capsules (20 mg) in 24 hours.

Histex CT: 1 tablet (8 mg) every 12 hours.
Histex I/E: 1 capsule (10 mg) every 12 hours.
Histex Pd: 5 mL (4 mg) 4 times daily.
Pediatex liquid: 10 mL (3.34 mg) 4 times daily.
Palgic solution: 5 or 10 mL (4 to 8 mg) 3 to 4 times daily.
Palgic tablets: 1 or 2 tablets (4 to 8 mg) 3 to 4 times daily.
Pediatex 12 suspension: 10 to 20 mL (6.4 to 12.8 mg) every 12 hours.

➤*Children:*

Allergies –

Histex CT:
- *12 years of age and older* – 1 tablet (8 mg) every 12 hours.
- *6 to 12 years of age* – ½ tablet (4 mg) every 12 hours.

Histex I/E:
- *12 years of age and older* –
  Usual dosage: 1 capsule (10 mg) every 12 hours.
  Maximum dose: 2 capsules (20 mg) in 24 hours.

Histex Pd:
- *6 years of age and older* – 5 mL (4 mg) 4 times daily.
- *18 months to 6 years of age* – 2.5 mL (2 mg) 4 times daily.
- *9 to 18 months of age* – 1.25 to 2.5 mL (1 to 2 mg) 4 times daily.

Pediatex liquid:
- *6 years of age and older* – 10 mL (3.34 mg) 4 times daily.
- *18 months to 6 years of age* – 5 mL (1.67 mg) 4 times daily.
- *9 to 18 months of age* – 3.75 to 5 mL (1.25 to 1.67 mg) 4 times daily.
- *6 to 9 months of age* – 3.75 mL (1.25 mg) 4 times daily.
- *3 to 6 months of age* – 2.5 mL (0.835 mg) 4 times daily.
- *1 to 3 months of age* – 1.25 mL (0.412 mg) 4 times daily.

Palgic solution:
- *Older than 6 years of age* – 5 to 7.5 mL (4 to 6 mg) 3 or 4 times daily.
- *3 to 6 years of age* – 2.5 to 5 mL (2 to 4 mg) 3 or 4 times daily.
- *1 to 3 years of age* – 2.5 mL (2 mg) 3 or 4 times daily.

Pediatex 12 suspension:
- *12 years of age and older* – 10 to 20 mL (6.4 to 12.8 mg) every 12 hours.
- *6 to 12 years of age* – 5 to 10 mL (3.2 to 6.4 mg) every 12 hours.
- *2 to 6 years of age* – 2.5 to 5 mL (1.6 to 3.2 mg) every 12 hours.

Palgic tablets:
- *6 years of age and older* – 1 to 1½ tablets (4 to 6 mg) 3 or 4 times daily.
- *3 to 6 years of age* – ½ to 1 tablet (2 to 4 mg) 3 or 4 times daily.
- *1 to 3 years of age* – ½ tablet (2 mg) 3 or 4 times daily.

➤*Administration:* Administer without regards to meals. Administer with food if GI upset occurs. Swallow capsules whole and not to crush, chew, or open. Shake suspension well before administering the dose. Tablets may be broken in half for ease of administration without affecting release of the medication, but should not be crushed or chewed prior to swallowing.

➤*Storage/Stability:* Store between 15° and 30°C (59° and 86°F). Protect suspension from freezing.

CLEMASTINE FUMARATE

otc	**Clemastine Fumarate** (Various, eg, Geneva)	**Tablets:** 1.34 mg as fumarate (equivalent to 1 mg clemastine)	In 100s.
otc	**Dayhist-1** (Major)		Lactose. In 8s.
otc	**Tavist Allergy** (Novartis Consumer Health)		Lactose. (TAVIST ALLERGY). In 8s.
Rx	**Clemastine Fumarate** (Various, eg, Teva)	**Tablets:** 2.68 mg (equivalent to 2 mg clemastine)	In 100s.
Rx	**Clemastine Fumarate** (Various, eg, Qualitest, Teva)	**Syrup:** 0.67 mg /5 mL (equivalent to 0.5 mg clemastine)	May contain alcohol. In 118 and 120.

CLEMASTINE FUMARATE — ORAL

For complete and comparative prescribing information, refer to the Antihistamines group monograph.

Indications

➤*Allergic rhinitis:* For the relief of symptoms associated with allergic rhinitis or other upper respiratory allergies, such as sneezing, rhinorrhea, pruritus, and lacrimation, in adults (tablets and syrup) and in children 6 to 12 years of age (syrup only).

➤*Urticaria/Angioedema:* For the relief of mild, uncomplicated allergic skin manifestations of urticaria and angioedema in adults (tablets and syrup) and in children 6 to 12 years of age (syrup only).

Administration and Dosage

➤*Adults:*

Allergic rhinitis –

Usual dosage: 1.34 mg every 12 hours or twice daily.

Maximum dose: 8.04 mg/day for the syrup or 2.68 mg in 24 hours for the tablets.

Angioedema –

Usual dosage: 2.68 mg twice daily.

Maximum dose: 8.04 mg/day.

Urticaria – See angioedema.

➤*Children:*

6 to 12 years of age (syrup only) –

Allergic rhinitis:
- *Usual dosage* – 0.67 mg twice daily.
- *Maximum dose* – 4.02 mg/day.
- *Single dose* – Single doses of up to 2.25 mg have been well tolerated.

Angioedema:
- *Usual dosage* – 1.34 mg twice daily.
- *Maximum dose* – 4.02 mg/day.

Urticaria: See angioedema.

➤*Dosage adjustment:* Dosage may be increased as needed.

➤*Administration:* Safety and effectiveness of the tablets have not been established in children younger than 12 years of age.

➤*Storage/Stability:* Store between 15° and 30°C (59° to 86°F).

DIPHENHYDRAMINE

otc	**Diphenhydramine** (Various, eg, Eon, Marlex)	**Tablets; oral:** 25 mg	As hydrochloride. In 24s and 100s.
otc	**Banophen** (Major)		As hydrochloride. In 24s and 100s.
otc	**Benadryl Allergy Ultratabs** (Pfizer)		As hydrochloride. In 24s, 48s, and 100s.
otc	**Diphenhist Captabs** (Rugby)		As hydrochloride. Capsule shape. In 100s.
otc	**Dormin** (Randob)		As hydrochloride. In 32s.
otc	**Miles Nervine** (Miles)		As hydrochloride. (Nervine). In 12s and 30s.
otc	**Nytol** (Block)		As hydrochloride. Lactose. (N). In 16s, 32s and 72s.
otc	**Simply Sleep** (McNeil)		As hydrochloride. In 24s and 48s.
otc	**Sleep-eze 3** (Whitehall)		As hydrochloride. In 12s and 24s.
otc	**Sleepwell 2-nite** (Rugby)		As hydrochloride. Sucrose. In 72s.
otc	**Sominex** (SmithKline Beecham)		As hydrochloride. (S). In 16s, 32s and 72s.
otc	**Diphenhydramine Hydrochloride** (Rugby)	**Tablets; oral:** 50 mg	As hydrochloride. Blue. In 50s.
otc	**AllerMax Maximum Strength Caplets** (Pfeiffer)		As hydrochloride. Lactose. In 24s.
otc	**Compoz Nighttime Sleep Aid** (Medtech)		As hydrochloride. Lactose. In 12s and 24s.
otc	**40 Winks** (Roberts Med)		As hydrochloride. In 30s.
otc	**Maximum Strength Nytol** (Block)		As hydrochloride. Lactose. (N). In 8s and 16s.
otc	**Midol PM** (Sterling Health)		As hydrochloride. In 16s.
otc	**Snooze Fast** (BDI)		As hydrochloride. In 36s.
otc	**Sominex** (SmithKline-Beecham)		As hydrochloride. (S). In 8s, 16s and 32s.
otc	**Twilite** (Pfeiffer)		As hydrochloride. Lactose. In 20s.
otc	**Benadryl Allergy** (Pfizer)	**Tablets, chewable; oral:** 12.5 mg	As hydrochloride. Aspartame, 4.2 mg phenylalanine. Grape flavor. In 24s.
Rx	**Dytan** (Hawthorn)	**Tablets, chewable; oral:** 25 mg	As tannate. Phenylalanine. (HAW 571). Oval-shape, scored. Strawberry flavor. In 60s.
otc	**Children's Benadryl Allergy Fastmelt** (Pfizer)	**Tablets, disintegrating; oral:** 12.5 mg	Equiv. to 19 mg diphenhydramine citrate. Aspartame, mannitol, 4.5 mg phenylalanine. In 20s.
otc/Rx[a]	**Diphenhydramine HCl** (Various, eg, Eon, Marlex, Major)	**Capsules; oral:** 25 mg	As hydrochloride. In 24s, 100s, and 1,000s.
otc	**Banophen** (Major)		As hydrochloride. In 24s and 100s.
otc	**Benadryl Allergy Kapseals** (Pfizer)		As hydrochloride. Lactose. In 24s and 48s.
otc	**Benadryl Dye-Free Allergy Liqui Gels** (Pfizer)		As hydrochloride. Sorbitol. In 24s.
otc	**Compoz Gel Caps** (Medtech)		As hydrochloride. In 16s.
otc	**Dormin** (Randob)		As hydrochloride. Lactose. In 32s and 72s.
otc	**Diphenhist** (Rugby)		As hydrochloride. Benzyl alcohol, butylparaben, EDTA, lactose, parabens. In 100s.
otc	**Genahist** (Goldline)		As hydrochloride. Lactose, parabens. In 100s.
otc/Rx[a]	**Diphenhydramine HCl** (Various, eg, Eon, Major)	**Capsules; oral:** 50 mg	As hydrochloride. In 100s and 1,000s.
otc	**Maximum Strength Sleepinal** Capsules and Soft Gels (Thompson)		**Capsules:** As hydrochloride. Lactose. In 16s. **Soft Gels:** As hydrochloride. Sorbitol. (Sleepinal). In 16s.
otc	**Maximum Strength Unisom SleepGels** (Pfizer)		As hydrochloride. Sorbitol. (UNISOM). In 8s.

DIPHENHYDRAMINE

otc	**Triaminic Children's Allergy** (Novartis Consumer Health)	**Strips, disintegrating; oral:** 12.5 mg	As hydrochloride. Alcohol less than 5%, maltodextrin, PEG, propylene glycol, sorbitol, sucralose. Grape flavor. In 14s.
otc	**Triaminic Cough & Runny Nose** (Novartis Consumer Health)		As hydrochloride. Alcohol less than 5%, sorbitol, sucralose. Grape flavor. In 16s.
otc	**Benadryl Allergy Quick Dissolve Strips** (Pfizer)	**Strips, disintegrating; oral:** 25 mg	As hydrochloride. Sucralose. Vanilla mint flavor. In 10s and 20s.
otc	**Triaminic MultiSymptom** (Novartis Consumer Health)		As hydrochloride. Alcohol less than 5%, sorbitol, sucralose. Cherry flavor. In 12s.
otc	**AllerMax** (Pfeiffer)	**Liquid; oral:** 12.5 mg per 5 mL	As hydrochloride. 0.5% alcohol, glucose, saccharin, sorbitol, sucrose, menthol. Raspberry flavor. In 118 mL.
otc	**Altaryl Children's Allergy** (Altaire)		As hydrochloride. Alcohol free. Glycerin, saccharin, sugar, 9 mg sodium. Cherry flavor. In 118 mL.
otc	**Benadryl Children's Allergy** (Pfizer)		As hydrochloride. Sugar. Alcohol free. Cherry flavor. In 118 and 236 mL.
otc sf	**Benadryl Children's Dye-Free Allergy** (Pfizer)		As hydrochloride. Saccharin, sorbitol. Alcohol free. Bubble gum flavor. In 118 mL.
otc	**Diphen AF** (Morton Grove)		As hydrochloride. Saccharin, sugar. Alcohol free. Cherry flavor. In 118, 237, and 473 mL.
otc sf	**Genahist** (Goldline)		As hydrochloride. Alcohol free. Cherry flavor. In 118 mL.
otc	**Q-dryl** (Qualitest Pharmaceuticals)		As hydrochloride. Alcohol free. Sodium 5 mg, glycerin, saccharin, sucrose. Cherry flavor. In 237 mL.
otc sf	**Scot-Tussin Allergy Relief Formula Clear** (Scot-Tussin)		As hydrochloride. Menthol, parabens. Alcohol and dye free. Cherry-strawberry flavor. In 118 mL.
otc	**Diphenhist** (Rugby)	**Solution; oral:** 12.5 mg per 5 mL	As hydrochloride. Glycerin, saccharin, sucrose. Alcohol free. In 473 mL.
otc	**PediaCare Children's Nighttime Cough** (Pfizer)		As hydrochloride. Alcohol free. Sucrose. Cherry flavor. In 120 mL.
otc	**Banophen Allergy** (Major)	**Elixir; oral:** 12.5 mg per 5 mL	As hydrochloride. Sugar. In 118 mL.
otc	**Siladryl** (Silarx)		As hydrochloride. 5.6% alcohol. Cherry flavor. In 118 mL.
otc/ Rx[a]	**Hydramine Cough** (Various, eg, Alpharma)	**Syrup; oral:** 12.5 mg/5 mL	May contain alcohol. In 473 mL.
otc	**Silphen Cough** (Silarx)		Menthol, parabens, sucrose, 5% alcohol. Strawberry flavor. In 118 mL.
Rx	**Tusstat** (Century)	**Syrup; oral:** 12.5 mg per 5 mL	As hydrochloride. 5% alcohol. In 30, 118, and 473 mL, and 3.8 L.
Rx	**Dytan** (Hawthorn)	**Suspension; oral:** 25 mg per 5 mL	As tannate. Phenylalanine. Strawberry flavor. In 118 mL.
Rx	**Diphenhydramine** (Various, eg, Abbott)	**Injection:** 50 mg/mL	As hydrochloride. In 1 mL fill in 2 mL cartridges.
Rx	**Benadryl** (Parke-Davis)		As hydrochloride. In 1 mL amps, 1 and 10 mL *Steri-vials*,[b] and 1 mL *Steri-dose* syringe.

[a] Products are available OTC or *Rx*, depending on product labeling.

[b] With benzethonium chloride.

DIPHENHYDRAMINE HYDROCHLORIDE — ORAL

For complete and comparative prescribing information, refer to the Antihistamines class monograph. For a complete listing of diphenhydramine sleep aids, see Nonprescription Sleep Aids in the CNS Agents chapter. Also refer to the general discussion in the Antiparkinson Agents introduction and the Antiparkinson Agent Anticholinergics group monograph.

Indications

➤*Hypersensitivity reactions, type I:* Perennial and seasonal allergic rhinitis; vasomotor rhinitis and sneezing caused by the common cold; allergic conjunctivitis caused by inhalant allergens and foods; mild, uncomplicated allergic skin manifestations of urticaria and angioedema; amelioration of allergic reactions to blood or plasma in patients with a known history of such reactions; dermatographism; as adjunctive anaphylactic therapy; for uncomplicated allergic conditions of the immediate type. Parenteral therapy also is indicated when oral therapy is impossible or contraindicated.

➤*Antiparkinsonism:* Parkinsonism in the elderly who are unable to tolerate more potent agents; mild cases of parkinsonism in other age groups; in other cases of parkinsonism in combination with centrally acting anticholinergic agents. Parenteral therapy also is indicated when oral therapy is impossible or contraindicated.

➤*Antitussive (syrup and liquid only):* For control of coughs caused by colds or allergy.

➤*Insomnia:* Aid in the relief of insomnia.

➤*Off-label uses:*

Oral mucositis – [4] = Insufficient documentation. Diphenhydramine is commonly used in mouthwashes for relief of oral mucositis symptoms in patients undergoing treatment for cancer, though empiric evidence to support the use of these mouthwashes is sparse and inconsistent. Other therapies (eg, allopurinol, granulocyte-macrophage colony-stimulating factor) have been found to be effective in improving and resolving oral mucositis. More randomized clinical trials are needed to determine the role of diphenhydramine in the prevention and management of oral mucositis.

Other possible off-label uses – Diphenhydramine also has been used as an antianxiety agent in doses of 25 to 200 mg/day.

Treatment or prophylaxis of chemotherapy-induced emesis; drug-induced extrapyramidal reactions.

Administration and Dosage

➤*Adults:*

Antihistamine –

Usual dosage: 25 to 50 mg every 4 to 6 hours.

Maximum dose: 300 mg/day.

Antitussive –

Liquid: 25 to 50 mg every 4 hours; do not exceed 300 mg/day.

Syrup: 25 mg every 4 hours; do not exceed 150 mg/day.

Insomnia – 50 mg orally at bedtime.

Motion sickness –

Usual dosage: 25 to 50 mg every 4 to 6 hours.

Maximum dose: 300 mg/day.

Off-label dosing –

Oral mucositis: [4] = Insufficient documentation. 20 mL swished and spit out 4 to 6 times per day as needed. In 1 controlled trial, the solution contained diphenhydramine 0.25 mL per dose.

➤*Children:*

Antihistamine –

12 years of age and older: 25 to 50 mg every 4 to 6 hours; do not exceed 300 mg/day.

6 to younger than 12 years of age: 12.5 to 25 mg every 4 to 6 hours; do not exceed 150 mg/day.

DIPHENHYDRAMINE HYDROCHLORIDE — ORAL

Antitussive –

12 years of age and older:

- *Liquid* – 25 to 50 mg every 4 hours; do not exceed 300 mg/day.
- *Syrup* – 25 mg every 4 hours; do not exceed 150 mg/day.

6 to 12 years of age:

- *Liquid* – 12.5 to 25 mg every 4 hours; do not exceed 150 mg/day.
- *Syrup* – 12.5 mg every 4 hours; do not exceed 75 mg/day.

2 to 6 years of age: 6.25 mg (syrup) every 4 hours; do not exceed 25 mg/day.

Insomnia –

12 years of age and older: 50 mg orally at bedtime.

Motion sickness –

12 years of age and older: 25 to 50 mg every 4 to 6 hours; do not exceed 300 mg/day.

6 to younger than 12 years of age: 12.5 to 25 mg every 4 to 6 hours; do not exceed 150 mg/day.

➤*Storage/Stability:* Store at 15° to 30°C (59° to 86°F).

DIPHENHYDRAMINE CITRATE — ORAL

For complete and comparative prescribing information, refer to the Antihistamines class monograph. For a complete listing of diphenhydramine sleep aids, see Nonprescription Sleep Aids in the CNS Agents chapter. Also refer to the general discussion in the Antiparkinson Agents introduction and the Antiparkinson Agent Anticholinergics group monograph.

Indications

➤*Antihistamine:* Temporarily relieves symptoms due to hay fever or other upper respiratory allergies, including runny nose; sneezing; itchy, watery eyes; itching of the nose or throat.

Temporarily relieves runny nose and sneezing symptoms due to the common cold.

➤*Insomnia:* Aid in the relief of insomnia.

➤*Off-label uses:*

Oral mucositis – [4] = Insufficient documentation. Diphenhydramine is commonly used in mouthwashes for relief of oral mucositis symptoms in patients undergoing treatment for cancer, although empiric evidence to support the use of these mouthwashes is sparse and inconsistent. Other therapies (eg, allopurinol, granulocyte-macrophage colony-stimulating factor) have been found to be effective in improving and resolving oral mucositis. More randomized clinical trials are needed to determine the role of diphenhydramine in the prevention and management of oral mucositis.

Other possible off-label uses – Treatment or prophylaxis of chemotherapy-induced emesis; drug-induced extrapyramidal reactions.

Administration and Dosage

➤*Adults:*

Antihistamine –

Usual dosage: 38 to 76 mg (2 to 4 tablets) every 4 to 6 hours.

Maximum dose: 6 doses in 24 hours.

Insomnia – 38 to 76 mg (2 to 4 tablets) before bedtime.

Off-label dosing –

Oral mucositis: [4] = Insufficient documentation. 20 mL swished and spit out 4 to 6 times per day as needed. In 1 controlled trial, the solution contained diphenhydramine 0.25 mL per dose.

➤*Children:* Do not use as a sleep aid in children younger than 12 years of age.

Antihistamine –

12 years of age and older:

- *Usual dosage* – 38 to 76 mg (2 to 4 tablets) every 4 to 6 hours.
- *Maximum dose* – 6 doses in 24 hours.

6 to younger than 12 years of age:

- *Usual dosage* – 19 to 38 mg (1 to 2 tablets) every 4 to 6 hours.
- *Maximum dose* – 6 doses in 24 hours.

Nonprescription sleep aid –

12 years of age and older: 38 to 76 mg (2 to 4 tablets) before bedtime.

➤*Elderly:* Dosage reduction may be needed.

➤*Storage/Stability:* Store at 15° to 25°C (59° to 77°F) in a dry place. Protect from heat, humidity, and light.

DIPHENHYDRAMINE TANNATE — ORAL

For complete and comparative prescribing information, refer to the Antihistamines group monograph. Also refer to the general discussion in the Antiparkinson Agents introduction and the Antiparkinson Agent Anticholinergics group monograph.

Indications

➤*Allergic conditions:* For amelioration of allergic reactions in the absence of acute symptoms or after acute symptoms have been controlled, and for other uncomplicated allergic conditions when oral therapy is indicated.

➤*Off-label uses:*

Oral mucositis – [4] = Insufficient documentation. Diphenhydramine is commonly used in mouthwashes for relief of oral mucositis symptoms in patients undergoing treatment for cancer, though empiric evidence to support the use of these mouthwashes is sparse and inconsistent. Other therapies (eg, allopurinol, granulocyte-macrophage colony-stimulating factor) have been found to be effective in improving and resolving oral mucositis. More randomized clinical trials are needed to determine the role of diphenhydramine in the prevention and management of oral mucositis.

Other possible off-label uses – Treatment or prophylaxis of chemotherapy-induced emesis; drug-induced extrapyramidal reactions.

Administration and Dosage

➤*Adults:*

Allergic conditions – 25 to 50 mg every 12 hours.

Off-label dosing –

Oral mucositis: [4] = Insufficient documentation. 20 mL swished and spit out 4 to 6 times per day as needed. In 1 controlled trial, the solution contained diphenhydramine 0.25 mL per dose.

➤*Children:*

Allergic conditions –

Oral suspension:

- *2 to 6 years of age* – 6.25 to 12.5 mg (1.25 to 2.5 mL) every 12 hours.

Tablets:

- *12 years of age and older* – 25 to 50 mg every 12 hours.
- *6 to younger than 12 years of age* – 12.5 to 25 mg every 12 hours.

➤*Storage/Stability:* Store at controlled room temperature, 15° to 30°C (59° to 86°F).

DIPHENHYDRAMINE HYDROCHLORIDE — INJECTION

For complete and comparative prescribing information, refer to the Antihistamines group monograph. Also refer to the general discussion in the Antiparkinson Agents introduction and the Antiparkinson Agent Anticholinergics group monograph.

Indications

➤*General information:* Diphenhydramine in the injectable form is effective in adults and pediatric patients, other than premature infants and neonates, for the following conditions when diphenhydramine in the oral form is impractical.

➤*Allergic conditions:* For amelioration of allergic reactions to blood or plasma, in anaphylaxis as an adjunct to epinephrine and other standard measures after the acute symptoms have been controlled, and for other uncomplicated allergic conditions of the immediate type when oral therapy is impossible or contraindicated.

➤*Motion sickness:* For active treatment of motion sickness.

➤*Antiparkinsonism:* For use in parkinsonism, when oral therapy is impossible or contraindicated, as follows: parkinsonism in the elderly who are unable to tolerate more potent agents; mild cases of parkinsonism in other age groups, and in other cases of parkinsonism in combination with centrally acting anticholinergic agents.

➤*Off-label uses:* For antipsychotic-induced dystonia, diphenhydramine 50 mg IM or IV has been shown to be effective. Treatment or prophylaxis of chemotherapy-induced emesis; drug-induced extrapyramidal reactions; treatment of mucositis in combination with other drugs.

Administration and Dosage

➤*Adults:*

Usual dosage – 10 to 50 mg IV at a rate generally not exceeding 25 mg/min, or deep IM, 100 mg if required.

➤*Children:* Do not use in neonates and premature infants.

Usual dosage – 5 mg/kg per 24 hour or 150 mg/m^2 per 24 hour. Divide into 4 doses, administered IV at a rate generally not exceeding 25 mg/min, or deep IM.

➤*Administration:* This product is for IV or deep IM administration only. Administer at an IV rate generally not exceeding 25 mg/min.

➤*Storage/Stability:* Store at controlled room temperature 15° to 30°C (59° to 86°F). Protect from light and freezing. Retain in carton until time of use.

Ethanolamines, Nonselective

DOXYLAMINE SUCCINATE

otc	**Unisom Nighttime Sleep-Aid** (Pfizer)	**Tablets; oral:** 25 mg	(Unisom). Blue, scored. Oval. In 8s, 16s, 32s, 48s.
Rx	**Aldex AN** (Zyber)	**Tablets, chewable; oral:** 5 mg	Sucralose. (AN). Oval, scored. Orange flavor. In 100s.
Rx	**Aldex AN** (Zyber)	**Suspension; oral:** 1 mg/mL	Methylparaben, tartrazine, sucralose, sucrose. Apple-melon flavor. In 473 mL.
Rx sf	**Doxytex** (Centurion Labs)	**Liquid; oral:** 1 mg/mL	Alcohol free, sugar free. Apple sauce flavor. In 473 mL.

DOXYLAMINE SUCCINATE — ORAL

Indications

➤*Insomnia (Unisom only):* Aid in the relief of insomnia.

➤*Upper respiratory tract allergies:* For the relief of runny nose, sneezing, itching of the nose or throat, and itchy, watery eyes due to hay fever or other upper respiratory tract allergies.

➤*Off-label uses:*

Nausea and vomiting of pregnancy – [1] = Good documentation. Doxylamine is recommended as a first-line therapy in combination with pyridoxine by the American College of Obstetrics and Gynecology (ACOG) for the management of nausea and vomiting of pregnancy in its 2004 practice bulletin.

Although pyridoxine and doxylamine are recommended as a first-line nonprescription combination for the treatment of nausea and vomiting of pregnancy, the combination product is not commercially available in the United States.

Administration and Dosage

➤*Adults:*

Insomnia (Unisom only) – 25 mg orally 30 minutes before bedtime. If sleepiness persists for more than 2 weeks, the patient should contact their health care provider.

Upper respiratory tract allergies – 2 tablets 4 to 6 times per day.

Off-label dosing –

Nausea and vomiting of pregnancy: [1] = Good documentation. 12.5 mg (in combination with pyridoxine 10 to 25 mg) 3 to 4 times per day. The dose and schedule may be adjusted according to the severity of the patient's symptoms.

➤*Children:*

Insomnia (Unisom only) –

12 years of age and older: See Adults for dosing.

Upper respiratory tract allergies –

12 years of age and older: See Adults for dosing.

6 to younger than 12 years of age: 1 tablet 4 to 6 times per day.

2 to younger than 6 years of age:

- *Usual dosage* – 2.5 mL or ½ tablet every 4 to 6 hours.
- *Maximum dose* – Up to 6 doses per day (15 mL).

➤*Storage/Stability:* Store at 20° to 25°C (68° to 77°F). Store *Unisom* tablets at 15° to 30°C (59° to 86°F).

Phenothiazines, Nonselective

PROMETHAZINE HYDROCHLORIDE

Rx	**Promethazine Hydrochloride** (Able Labs)	**Tablets; oral:** 12.5 mg	May contain lactose. (A405). Lt. peach. In 30s, 100s, 500s, and 1,000s.
Rx	**Phenergan** (Wyeth Labs)		Lactose, saccharin. (WYETH 19). Orange, scored. In 100s.
Rx	**Promethazine Hydrochloride** (Various, eg, Able Labs, Geneva)	**Tablets; oral:** 25 mg	May contain lactose. In 30s, 100s, 500s, and 1,000s.
Rx	**Phenergan** (Wyeth Labs)		Lactose, saccharin. (WYETH 27). White, scored. In 100s and 10 blister strips of 10.
Rx	**Promethazine Hydrochloride** (Various, eg, Able Labs, Geneva)	**Tablets; oral:** 50 mg	May contain lactose. In 30s, 100s, 500s, and 1,000s.
Rx	**Phenergan** (Wyeth Labs)		Lactose. (WYETH 227). Pink. In 100s.
Rx	**Promethazine Hydrochloride** (Various, eg, Morton Grove)	**Syrup; oral:** 6.25 mg per 5 mL	Alcohol. In 473 mL.
Rx	**Promethazine Hydrochloride** (Ivax)	**Suppositories; rectal:** 12.5 mg	May contain hard fat. In 12s.
Rx	**Phenadoz** (Paddock)		Cocoa butter. In 12s.
Rx	**Phenergan** (Wyeth Labs)		Cocoa butter. In 12s.
Rx	**Promethegan** (G & W Labs)		In 12s and 1,000s.
Rx	**Promethazine Hydrochloride** (Various, eg, Alpharma, Ivax)	**Suppositories; rectal:** 25 mg	May contain hard fat. In 12s.
Rx	**Phenadoz** (Paddock)		Cocoa butter. In 12s.
Rx	**Phenergan** (Wyeth Labs)		Cocoa butter. In 12s.
Rx	**Promethegan** (G & W Labs)		In 12s and 1,000s.
Rx	**Promethazine Hydrochloride** (Various, eg, Ivax, Major)	**Suppositories; rectal:** 50 mg	In 12s.
Rx	**Promethegan** (G & W Labs)		In 12s and 1,000s.
Rx	**Promethazine Hydrochloride** (Various, eg, Abbott)	**Injection:** 25 mg/mL	May contain EDTA. In 1 mL amps.
Rx	**Phenergan** (Wyeth Labs)		EDTA, 0.25 mg/mL sodium metabisulfite. In 1 mL amps.
Rx	**Promethazine Hydrochloride** (Various, eg, Abbott)	**Injection:** 50 mg/mL	May contain EDTA. In 1 mL amps.
Rx	**Phenergan** (Wyeth Labs)		EDTA, 0.25 mg/mL sodium metabisulfite. In 1 mL amps.

PROMETHAZINE HYDROCHLORIDE — ORAL

For complete and comparative prescribing information, refer to the Antihistamines group monograph. For more information on promethazine as an antiemetic/antivertigo agent, see the Antiemetic/Antivertigo monograph in the CNS Agents chapter.

WARNING

Do not use promethazine in children younger than 2 years of age because of the potential for fatal respiratory depression.

Postmarketing cases of respiratory depression, including fatalities, have been reported with the use of promethazine in children younger than 2 years of age. A wide range of weight-based doses of promethazine have resulted in respiratory depression in these patients.

Exercise caution when administering promethazine to children 2 years of age and older. It is recommended that the lowest effective dose of promethazine be used in children 2 years of age and older and that coadministration of other drugs with respiratory-depressant effects be avoided.

Indications

➤*Allergic conditions:* For perennial and seasonal allergic rhinitis; vasomotor rhinitis; allergic conjunctivitis due to inhalant allergens and foods; mild, uncomplicated allergic skin manifestations of urticaria and angioedema; amelioration of allergic reactions to blood or plasma; dermographism; anaphylactic reactions, as adjunctive therapy to epinephrine and other standard measures, after the acute manifestations have been controlled.

➤*Pre and postoperative/obstetric sedation:* Preoperative, postoperative, or obstetric sedation.

➤*Nausea/vomiting:* Prevention and control of nausea and vomiting associated with certain types of anesthesia and surgery.

➤*Postoperative pain:* Therapy adjunctive to meperidine or other analgesics for control of postoperative pain.

➤*Sedation:* For sedation in both children and adults, as well as relief of apprehension and production of light sleep from which the patient can be easily aroused.

➤*Motion sickness:* For active and prophylactic treatment of motion sickness.

➤*Postoperative antiemetic:* For antiemetic therapy in postoperative patients.

➤*Off-label uses:*

Nausea and vomiting of pregnancy – [2] = Fair documentation. The American College of Obstetrics and Gynecology (ACOG) practice bulletin included promethazine among the therapies recommended for the management of nausea and vomiting of pregnancy. Promethazine use in this setting was also endorsed by the American Gastroenterological Association Institute (AGAI).

Administration and Dosage

➤*General dosing considerations:* Antiemetics should not be used in vomiting of unknown etiology in children and adolescents.

When oral medication cannot be tolerated, the dose should be given parenterally (eg, promethazine injection) or by rectal suppository.

➤*Adults:*

Allergy –

Usual dosage: 25 mg taken before retiring; however, 12.5 mg may be taken before meals or on retiring, if necessary. Single 25 mg doses at bedtime or 6.25 to 12.5 mg taken 3 times daily will usually suffice.

Dosage adjustment: After initiation of treatment, dosage should be adjusted to the smallest amount adequate to relieve symptoms.

Transfusion reactions: 25 mg doses will control minor transfusion reactions of an allergic nature.

Motion sickness –

Initial dosage: 25 mg taken one-half to 1 hour before anticipated travel and repeated 8 to 12 hours later, if necessary.

Maintenance dosage: 25 mg twice daily (on arising and before evening meal) on succeeding days of travel.

Nausea and vomiting –

Usual dosage: 12.5 to 25 mg every 4 to 6 hours as necessary.

Prophylactic dosage: 25 mg every 4 to 6 hours as necessary (given during surgery and the postoperative period).

Postoperative use – 25 to 50 mg with analgesics.

Preoperative use – 50 mg with an appropriately reduced dose of narcotic or barbiturate and the required amount of a belladonna alkaloid.

Sedation – 25 to 50 mg for nighttime, presurgical, or obstetrical sedation.

Off-label dosing –

Nausea and vomiting of pregnancy: [2] = Fair documentation. 12.5 to 25 mg every 4 hours orally, rectally, or IV.

➤*Children:* Promethazine is contraindicated for use in children younger than 2 years of age. Exercise caution when administering to children 2 years of age and older because of the potential for fatal respiratory depression.

Allergy –

2 years of age and older: See Adults for dosing.

Motion sickness –

2 years of age and older:

• *Initial dosage* – 12.5 to 25 mg taken one-half to 1 hour before anticipated travel and repeated 8 to 12 hours later, if necessary.

• *Maintenance dosage* – 12.5 to 25 mg twice daily (on arising and before evening meal) on succeeding days of travel.

Nausea and vomiting –

2 years of age and older:

• *Usual dosage* – 1.1 mg/kg, and the dose should be adjusted to the age and weight of the patient and the severity of the condition being treated.

• *Prophylactic dosage* – 25 mg every 4 to 6 hours as necessary (during surgery and the postoperative period).

Postoperative use –

2 years of age and older: 12.5 to 25 mg with analgesics.

Preoperative use –

2 years of age and older: 1.1 mg/kg in combination with an appropriately reduced dose of narcotic or barbiturate and the appropriate dose of an atropine-like drug.

Sedation –

2 years of age and older: 12.5 to 25 mg at bedtime for nighttime, presurgical, or obstetrical sedation.

Off-label dosing –

Allergy:

• *Children 2 years of age and older* –

Usual dosage: 0.1 mg/kg/dose every 6 hours during the day and 0.5 mg/kg/dose as needed at bed time.

Maximum dose: 12.5 mg/dose daytime; 25 mg/dose bedtime.

Motion sickness:

• *Children 2 years of age and older* –

Usual dosage: 0.5 mg/kg/dose every 12 hours as needed. Take the first dose one-half to 1 hour before departure.

Maximum dose: 25 mg/dose.

Nausea and vomiting:

• *Children 2 years of age and older* –

Usual dosage: 0.25 to 1 mg/kg/dose every 4 to 6 hours as needed.

Maximum dose: 25 mg/dose.

➤*Storage/Stability:*

Tablets – Store at controlled room temperature, 20° to 25°C (68° to 77°F). Keep tightly closed. Protect from light and dispense in a tight, light-resistant container. Use the carton to protect the contents from light.

Syrup – Store at controlled room temperature, 15° to 25°C (59° to 77°F). Protect from light. Dispense in a tight, light-resistant container.

PROMETHAZINE HYDROCHLORIDE — RECTAL

For complete and comparative prescribing information, refer to the Antihistamines group monograph. For more information on promethazine as an antiemetic/antivertigo agent, see the Antiemetic/Antivertigo monograph in the CNS Agents chapter.

WARNING

Do not use promethazine in children younger than 2 years of age because of the potential for fatal respiratory depression.

Postmarketing cases of respiratory depression, including fatalities, have been reported with use of promethazine suppositories in children younger than 2 years of age. A wide range of weight-based doses of promethazine suppositories have resulted in respiratory depression in these patients.

Exercise caution when administering promethazine in children 2 years of age and older. It is recommended that the lowest effective dose of promethazine be used in children 2 years of age and older and that coadministration of other drugs with respiratory-depressant effects be avoided.

Indications

➤*Allergic conditions:* For perennial and seasonal allergic rhinitis; vasomotor rhinitis; allergic conjunctivitis due to inhalant allergens and foods;

PROMETHAZINE HYDROCHLORIDE — RECTAL

mild, uncomplicated allergic skin manifestations of urticaria and angioedema; amelioration of allergic reactions to blood or plasma; dermographism; anaphylactic reactions, as adjunctive therapy to epinephrine and other standard measures, after the acute manifestations have been controlled.

➤*Pre and postoperative/obstetric sedation:* Preoperative, postoperative, or obstetric sedation.

➤*Nausea/vomiting:* Prevention and control of nausea and vomiting associated with certain types of anesthesia and surgery.

➤*Postoperative pain:* Therapy adjunctive to meperidine or other analgesics for control of postoperative pain.

➤*Sedation:* For sedation in both children and adults, as well as relief of apprehension and production of light sleep from which the patient can be easily aroused.

➤*Motion sickness:* For active and prophylactic treatment of motion sickness.

➤*Postoperative antiemetic:* For antiemetic therapy in postoperative patients.

➤*Off-label uses:*

Nausea and vomiting of pregnancy – [2] = Fair documentation. The American College of Obstetrics and Gynecology (ACOG) practice bulletin included promethazine among the therapies recommended for the management of nausea and vomiting of pregnancy. Promethazine use in this setting was also endorsed by the American Gastroenterological Association Institute (AGAI).

Administration and Dosage

➤*General dosing considerations:* Antiemetics should not be used in vomiting of unknown etiology in children and adolescents.

When oral medication cannot be tolerated, the dose should be given parenterally (eg, promethazine injection) or by rectal suppository.

➤*Adults:*

Allergy –

Usual dosage: 25 mg taken before retiring; however, 12.5 mg may be taken before meals or on retiring, if necessary. Single 25 mg doses at bedtime or 6.25 to 12.5 mg taken 3 times daily will usually suffice.

Dosage adjustment: After initiation of treatment, dosage should be adjusted to the smallest amount adequate to relieve symptoms.

Transfusion reactions: 25 mg doses will control minor transfusion reactions of an allergic nature.

Motion sickness –

Initial dosage: 25 mg taken one-half to 1 hour before anticipated travel and be repeated 8 to 12 hours later, if necessary.

Maintenance dosage: 25 mg taken twice daily (on arising and before evening meal) on succeeding days of travel.

Nausea and vomiting –

Usual dosage: 12.5 to 25 mg every 4 to 6 hours as necessary.

Prophylactic dosage: 25 mg every 4 to 6 hours as necessary (given during surgery and the postoperative period).

Postoperative use – 25 to 50 mg with analgesics.

Preoperative use – 50 mg the night before surgery with an appropriately reduced dose of narcotic or barbiturate and the required amount of a belladonna alkaloid.

Sedation – 25 to 50 mg for nighttime, presurgical, or obstetrical sedation.

Off-label dosing –

Nausea and vomiting of pregnancy: [2] = Fair documentation. 12.5 to 25 mg every 4 hours orally, rectally, or IV.

➤*Children:* Promethazine is contraindicated for use in children younger than 2 years of age. Exercise caution when administering to children 2 years of age and older because of the potential for fatal respiratory depression.

Allergy –

2 years of age and older: See Adults for dosing.

Motion sickness –

2 years of age and older:

• *Initial dosage* – 12.5 to 25 mg one-half to 1 hour before anticipated travel and repeated 8 to 12 hours later, if necessary.

• *Maintenance dosage* – 12.5 to 25 mg twice daily (on arising and before evening meal) on succeeding days of travel.

Nausea and vomiting –

2 years of age and older:

• *Usual dosage* – 1.1 mg/kg, and the dose should be adjusted to the age and weight of the patient and the severity of the condition being treated.

• *Prophylactic dosage* – 25 mg every 4 to 6 hours as necessary (during surgery and the postoperative period).

Postoperative use –

2 years of age and older: 12.5 to 25 mg with analgesics.

Preoperative use –

2 years of age and older:

• *Usual dosage* – 1.1 mg/kg the night before surgery in combination with an appropriately reduced dose of narcotic or barbiturate and the appropriate dose of an atropine-like drug.

• *Single dose* – 12.5 to 25 mg the night before surgery.

Sedation –

2 years of age and older: 12.5 to 25 mg at bedtime for nighttime, presurgical, or obstetrical sedation.

Off-label dosing –

Motion sickness:

• *2 years of age and older* –

Usual dosage: 0.5 mg/kg every 12 hours as needed. Take the first dose 30 to 60 minutes before departure.

Maximum dose: 25 mg/dose.

Nausea and vomiting:

• *2 years of age and older* –

Usual dosage: 0.25 to 1 mg/kg every 4 to 6 hours as needed.

Maximum dose: 25 mg/dose.

➤*Storage/Stability:* Store refrigerated between 2° to 8°C (36° to 46°F). Dispense in a well-closed container.

PROMETHAZINE HYDROCHLORIDE — INJECTION

For complete and comparative prescribing information, refer to the Antihistamines group monograph. For more information on promethazine as an antiemetic/antivertigo agent, see the Antiemetic/Antivertigo monograph in the CNS Agents chapter.

WARNING

Do not use promethazine in children younger than 2 years of age because of the potential for fatal respiratory depression.

Postmarketing cases of respiratory depression, including fatalities, have been reported with use of promethazine in children younger than 2 years of age. A wide range of weight-based doses of promethazine have resulted in respiratory depression in these patients.

Exercise caution when administering promethazine to children 2 years of age and older. It is recommended that the lowest effective dose of promethazine be used in children 2 years of age and older, and that concomitant administration of other drugs with respiratory depressant effects be avoided.

Indications

➤*Analgesia:* Adjunctive therapy for control of postoperative pain.

➤*Antiemetic:* Prevention and control of nausea and vomiting associated with certain types of anesthesia and surgery and in postoperative patients.

➤*Hypersensitivity reactions, type I:* Perennial and seasonal allergic rhinitis; vasomotor rhinitis; allergic conjunctivitis caused by inhalant allergens and foods; mild, uncomplicated allergic skin manifestations of urticaria and angioedema; amelioration of allergic reactions to blood or plasma; dermatographism; adjunctive anaphylactic therapy. Parenteral therapy is indicated when oral therapy is impossible or contraindicated.

➤*Sedation:* Preoperative, postoperative, or obstetric sedation; relief of apprehension and production of light sleep.

➤*Off-label uses:*

Nausea and vomiting of pregnancy – [2] = Fair documentation. The American College of Obstetrics and Gynecology (ACOG) practice bulletin included promethazine among the therapies recommended for the management of nausea and vomiting of pregnancy. Promethazine use in this setting was also endorsed by the American Gastroenterological Association Institute (AGAI).

Administration and Dosage

➤*General dosing considerations:* Individualize dosage; after initiation, adjust to smallest effective dose.

Antiemetics are not recommended for treatment of uncomplicated vomiting in children; limit use to prolonged vomiting of known etiology.

➤*Adults:*

Antiemetic – 12.5 to 25 mg deep IM (preferred route) or IV; may repeat every 4 hours as needed. If used postoperatively, reduce doses of concomitant analgesics or barbiturates accordingly.

Hypersensitivity reactions, type I – 25 mg deep IM (preferred route) or IV; may repeat dose within 2 hours if needed. Resume oral therapy as soon as patient's circumstances permit.

Nighttime sedation – 25 to 50 mg deep IM (preferred route) or IV at bedtime.

Obstetric sedation –

Usual dosage: 50 mg deep IM (preferred route) or IV provides sedation and relieves apprehension during early stages of labor. When labor is definitely established, 25 to 75 mg (average dose, 50 mg) IM or IV with an appropriately reduced dose of any desired narcotic. If necessary, promethazine injection with a reduced dose of analgesic may be repeated once or twice at 4-hour intervals.

Maximum dose: 100 mg per 24 hours for patients in labor.

Pre- and postoperative use – 25 to 50 mg deep IM (preferred route) or IV in combination with appropriately reduced doses of analgesics, hypnotics, and atropine-like drugs as appropriate.

PROMETHAZINE HYDROCHLORIDE — INJECTION

Off-label dosing –

Nausea and vomiting of pregnancy: [2] = Fair documentation. 12.5 to 25 mg every 4 hours orally, rectally, or IV.

Opioid-induced nausea and vomiting: 6.25 mg IV every 6 hours as needed. May repeat once in 15 minutes if symptoms do not resolve. Administer slowly, using a large vein or preferably a central line (if available). Discontinue if patient complains of pain related to the IV administration.

➤*Children:* Promethazine injection is not recommended for use in children younger than 2 years of age. Exercise caution when administering to children 2 years of age and older because of the potential for fatal respiratory depression.

Antiemetic –

Older than 12 years of age: See Adults for dosing.

2 to 12 years of age: Do not exceed half the adult dose. (See also Off-Label Dosing.)

Hypersensitivity reactions, type I –

2 years of age and older: Dose should not exceed half the adult dose of 25 mg.

Nighttime sedation –

Older than 12 years of age: See Adults for dosing.

2 to 12 years of age: Do not exceed half the adult dose.

Obstetric sedation –

Older than 12 years of age: See Adults for dosing.

Pre- and postoperative use –

Older than 12 years of age: See Adults for dosing.

2 to 12 years of age: 1.1 mg/kg deep IM (preferred) or IV in combination with an appropriately reduced dose of narcotic or barbiturate and the appropriate dose of an atropine-like drug.

Off-label dosing –

Antiemetic:

• *2 years of age and older –*

Usual dosage: 0.25 to 1 mg/kg administered IM (preferred route) or IV every 4 to 6 hours.

Maximum dose: 25 mg/dose.

➤*Elderly:* Dosage reduction may be required.

➤*Administration:* The preferred parenteral route of administration is deep IM injection. Avoid subcutaneous and intra-arterial injection because tissue necrosis and gangrene can result.

Properly administered IV doses are well tolerated, but this method is associated with increased hazard. Dilute promethazine 25 mg/mL (eg, in 10 to 20 mL normal saline) to reduce vesicant effects. Check patency of the access site before giving promethazine. Use a large vein or central line if available; do not use hand or wrist veins. Give slowly over 10 to 15 minutes; if patient complains of pain, stop IV. IV administration should be at a concentration not to exceed 25 mg/mL at a rate no greater than 25 mg/min. Avoid subcutaneous and intra-arterial injection because tissue necrosis and gangrene can result.

➤*Storage/Stability:*

Injection – Store at controlled room temperature 20° to 25°C (68° to 77°F). Protect from light. Keep covered in carton until time of use. Do not use if solution has developed color or contains a precipitate.

HYDROXYZINE

Rx	**Hydroxyzine** (Various, eg, Sidmak)	**Tablets:** 10 mg	In 100s, 500s, and 1,000s.
Rx	**Hydroxyzine** (Various, eg, Sidmak)	**Tablets:** 25 mg	In 100s, 500s, and 1,000s.
Rx	**Hydroxyzine** (Various, eg, Sidmak)	**Tablets:** 50 mg	In 100s, 500s, and 1,000s.
Rx	**Hydroxyzine Pamoate** (Various, eg, Barr, IVAX)	**Capsules:** 25 mg (as pamoate)[a]	In 100s, 500s, 1,000s, and UD 100s.
Rx	**Vistaril** (Pfizer)		Sucrose. Two-tone green. In 100s.
Rx	**Hydroxyzine Pamoate** (Various, eg, Barr, IVAX)	**Capsules:** 50 mg (as pamoate)[a]	In 100s, 500s, 1,000s, and UD 100s.
Rx	**Vistaril** (Pfizer)		Sucrose. Green/white. In 100s.
Rx	**Hydroxyzine Pamoate** (Various, eg, Barr)	**Capsules:** 100 mg (as pamoate)[a]	In 100s, 500s, and 1,000s.
Rx	**Vistaril** (Pfizer)		Sucrose. Green/gray. In 100s.
Rx	**Hydroxyzine** (Various, eg, Alpharma, Hi-Tech Pharmacal, Morton Grove, URL)	**Syrup:** 10 mg/5 mL	May contain alcohol. In 118 and 473 mL.
Rx	**Vistaril** (Pfizer)	**Oral suspension:** 25 mg/5 mL (as pamoate)[a]	Sorbitol. Lemon flavor. In 120 and 473 mL.
Rx	**Hydroxyzine HCl** (Various, eg, Abbott, American Pharmaceutical Partners, American Regent)	**Injection:** 25 mg/mL	May contain benzyl alcohol. In 1 and 2 mL vials.
Rx	**Hydroxyzine HCl** (Various, eg, Abbott, American Pharmaceutical Partners, American Regent)	**Injection:** 50 mg/mL	May contain benzyl alcohol. In 1, 2, and 10 mL vials.

[a] Hydroxyzine pamoate is equivalent to hydroxyzine hydrochloride.

HYDROXYZINE — ORAL

For complete and comparative prescribing information, refer to the Antihistamines group monograph.

Indications

➤*Pruritus:* Caused by allergic conditions such as chronic urticaria and atopic or contact dermatoses and in histamine-mediated pruritus.

➤*Sedation:* When used as premedication and following general anesthesia.

➤*Anxiety and tension:* Associated with psychoneurosis and as an adjunct in organic disease states in which anxiety is manifested.

Administration and Dosage

➤*Adults:*

Anxiety and tension – 50 to 100 mg 4 times daily.

Pruritus – 25 mg 3 or 4 times daily.

Sedation – 50 to 100 mg as premedication or following general anesthesia.

➤*Children:*

Anxiety and tension –

6 years of age and older: 50 to 100 mg/day in divided doses.

Younger than 6 years of age: 50 mg/day in divided doses.

Pruritus –

6 years of age and older: 50 to 100 mg/day in divided doses.

Younger than 6 years of age: 50 mg/day in divided doses.

Sedation – 0.6 mg/kg as premedication or following general anesthesia.

➤*Concomitant therapy:* Hydroxyzine may potentiate concomitant narcotics (eg, meperidine), nonnarcotic analgesics, and barbiturates; reduce dosages accordingly. Atropine and other belladonna alkaloids may be given as appropriate.

➤*Storage/Stability:* Store oral dosage forms at controlled room temperature 15° to 30°C (59° to 86°F). Dispense in a tight, light-resistant container.

Actions

➤*Pharmacology:* Hydroxyzine hydrochloride is unrelated chemically to phenothiazines, reserpine, meprobamate or the benzodiazepines. Hydroxyzine is not a cortical depressant, but its action may be due to a suppression of activity in certain key regions of the subcortical area of the central nervous system (CNS).

Primary skeletal muscle relaxation has been demonstrated experimentally. Bronchodilator activity, and antihistaminic and analgesic effects have been demonstrated experimentally and confirmed clinically. An antiemetic effect, both by the apomorphine test and the veriloid test, has been demonstrated.

Pharmacological and clinical studies indicate that hydroxyzine in therapeutic dosage does not increase gastric secretion or acidity and in most cases has mild antisecretory activity.

➤*Pharmacokinetics:* Hydroxyzine is rapidly absorbed in the gastrointestinal tract and its clinical effects are usually noted within 15 to 30 minutes after oral administration.

Contraindications

Hydroxyzine, when administered to the pregnant mouse, rat and rabbit, induced fetal abnormalities in the rat and mouse at doses substantially above the human therapeutic range. Clinical data in human beings are inadequate to establish safety in early pregnancy. Until such data are available, hydroxyzine is contraindicated in early pregnancy.

Hydroxyzine is contraindicated for patients who have shown a previous hypersensitivity to it.

Warnings/Precautions

➤*Hazardous tasks:* Since drowsiness may occur with use of this drug, patients should be warned of this possibility and cautioned against driving a car or operating dangerous machinery while taking hydroxyzine. Patients

HYDROXYZINE — ORAL

should also be advised against the simultaneous use of other CNS depressant drugs, and cautioned that the effects of alcohol may be increased.

➤*Pregnancy: Category C.* Hydroxyzine, when administered to the pregnant mouse, rat and rabbit, induced fetal abnormalities in the rat and mouse at doses substantially above the human therapeutic range. Clinical data in human beings are inadequate to establish safety in early pregnancy. Until such data are available, hydroxyzine is contraindicated in early pregnancy.

➤*Lactation:* It is not known whether this drug is excreted in human milk. Since many drugs are so excreted, hydroxyzine should not be given to nursing mothers.

➤*Elderly:* A determination has not been made whether controlled clinical studies of hydroxyzine included sufficient numbers of subjects aged 65 years and over to define a difference in response from younger subjects. Other reported clinical experience has not identified differences in responses between the elderly and younger patients. In general, dose selection for an elderly patient should be cautious, usually starting at the low end of the dosing range, reflecting the greater frequency of decreased hepatic, renal or cardiac function, and of concomitant disease or other drug therapy.

The extent of renal excretion of hydroxyzine has not been determined. Because elderly patients are more likely to have decreased renal function, care should be taken in dose selections.

Sedating drugs may cause confusion and over sedation in the elderly; elderly patients generally should be started on low doses of hydroxyzine and observed closely.

Per the Beers list, hydroxyzine may have potent anticholinergic properties. Nonanticholinergic antihistamines are preferred in elderly patients when treating allergic reactions. Hydroxyzine is also considered a high risk medication for the elderly according to the Centers for Medicare and Medicaid Services.

Adverse Reactions

Side effects reported with the administration of hydroxyzine hydrochloride are usually mild and transitory in nature.

➤*CNS:* Drowsiness is usually transitory and may disappear in a few days of continued therapy or upon reduction of the dose. Involuntary motor activity including rare instances of tremor and convulsions have been reported, usually with doses considerably higher than those recommended. Clinically significant respiratory depression has not been reported at recommended doses.

➤*Miscellaneous:* Dry mouth.

Overdosage

➤*Symptoms:* The most common manifestation of hydroxyzine overdosage is hypersedation. As in the management of overdosage with any drug, it should be borne in mind that multiple agents may have been taken.

➤*Treatment:* Immediate gastric lavage is recommended. General supportive care, including frequent monitoring of the vital signs and close observation of the patient, is indicated. Hypotension, though unlikely, may be controlled with intravenous fluids and levarterenol, norepinephrine, or metaraminol. Do not use epinephrine as hydroxyzine counteracts its pressor action.

There is no specific antidote. It is doubtful that hemodialysis would be of any value in the treatment of overdosage with hydroxyzine. However, if other agents such as barbiturates have been ingested concomitantly, hemodialysis may be indicated. There is no practical method to quantitate hydroxyzine in body fluids or tissue after its ingestion or administration.

HYDROXYZINE HYDROCHLORIDE — INJECTION

For complete and comparative prescribing information, refer to the Antihistamines group monograph.

Indications

➤*Pruritus:* Caused by allergic conditions such as chronic urticaria and atopic or contact dermatoses and in histamine-mediated pruritus.

➤*Sedation:* When used as premedication and following general anesthesia.

➤*Anxiety and tension:* Associated with psychoneurosis and as an adjunct in organic disease states in which anxiety is manifested.

Administration and Dosage

➤*General dosing considerations:* Individualize dosage. Start patients on IM therapy only when indicated; maintain on oral therapy whenever possible.

➤*Adults:*

Anxiety and tension – 50 to 100 mg IM 4 times daily.

Pruritus – 25 mg IM 3 to 4 times daily.

Sedation – 50 to 100 mg IM as premedication or following general anesthesia.

➤*Children:*

Sedation – 0.6 mg/kg IM as premedication or following general anesthesia.

Off-label dosing –

Anxiety: 0.5 to 1 mg/kg IM every 4 to 6 hours as needed.

Pruritis: 0.5 to 1 mg/kg IM every 4 to 6 hours as needed.

➤*Concomitant therapy:* Hydroxyzine may potentiate concomitant narcotics (eg, meperidine), nonnarcotic analgesics, and barbiturates; reduce dosages accordingly. Atropine and other belladonna alkaloids may be given as appropriate.

➤*Administration:* Intended for deep IM administration only and may be given without further dilution. Avoid IV, subcutaneous, or intra-arterial administration. The preferred site of administration for adults is the upper, outer quadrant of the buttock or the mid-lateral thigh. For children, it is preferable to administer in the mid-lateral thigh; for infants and small children, use the periphery of the upper, outer quadrant of the gluteal region only when necessary, such as in burn patients, to minimize the possibility of damage to the sciatic nerve. The deltoid area should be used only if well developed such as in certain adults and older children, and then only with caution to avoid radial nerve injury. Do not make IM injections into the lower and mid-third of the upper arm.

➤*Storage/Stability:* Store injection below 30°C (86°F).

CYPROHEPTADINE

Rx	**Cyproheptadine** (Various, eg, IVAX, Par, Pliva)	**Tablets**: 4 mg	In 100s, 1,000s, and UD 100s.
Rx	**Cyproheptadine** (Various, eg, Alpharma)	**Syrup**: 2 mg/5 mL	May contain alcohol. In 473 mL.

CYPROHEPTADINE HYDROCHLORIDE — ORAL

For complete and comparative prescribing information, refer to the Antihistamines group monograph.

Indications

➤*Hypersensitivity reactions:* Perennial and seasonal allergic rhinitis; vasomotor rhinitis; allergic conjunctivitis caused by inhalant allergens and foods; mild, uncomplicated allergic skin manifestations of urticaria and angioedema; amelioration of allergic reactions to blood or plasma; cold urticaria; dermatographism; adjunctive anaphylactic therapy.

➤*Off-label uses:*

Appetite stimulation – [2] = Fair documentation. Clinical studies suggest that the effectiveness of cyproheptadine as an appetite stimulant may be dependent on disease and disease severity. It appears to be more effective in patients with mild to moderate disease than in patients in advanced disease states. The majority of weight gain seems to occur in the first few months of use.

Nightmares (posttraumatic stress disorder) – [2] = Fair documentation. Cyproheptadine has been studied in a small number of patients with posttraumatic stress disorder (PTSD) with varied results.

Prevention of migraine (adults) – [4] = Insufficient documentation. Controlled trials evaluating the use of cyproheptadine for migraine preventionhave shown inconsistent findings. American Academy of Neurology practice guidelines consider cyproheptadine to be clinically efficacious based on consensus and clinical experience, despite the lack of scientific evidence of efficacy.

Prevention of migraine (children/adolescents) – [4] = Insufficient documentation. Published data on the use of cyproheptadine for the prevention of migraine headaches in children and adolescents are limited, and the number of patients studied is small. Evidence was insufficient for current practice guidelines to recommend its use.

Tardive dyskinesia – [5] = Poor documentation. The use of cyproheptadine in neuroleptic-induced tardive dyskinesias showed variable results and no clear benefits. Its use in levodopa-induced tardive dyskinesias showed no benefit.

Other possible off-label uses – Suppression of vascular headaches; appetite stimulation.

Administration and Dosage

➤*Adults:*

Hypersensitivity reactions –

Usual dosage: 4 to 20 mg/day. Most patients require 12 to 16 mg/day and occasionally as much as 32 mg/day.

Maximum dose: 0.5 mg/kg/day.

Initial dosage: 4 mg 3 times/day.

Off-label dosing –

Appetite stimulation: [2] = Fair documentation. 4 mg orally 2 to 4 times per day for 1 week to 12 months. One study tested lower dosages of 2 to 6 mg/day for at least 7 days.

Piperidines, Nonselective

CYPROHEPTADINE HYDROCHLORIDE — ORAL

Nightmares (posttraumatic stress disorder): [2] = Fair documentation. 4 to 12 mg at bedtime; maximum is 32 mg.

Prevention of migraine (adults): [4] = Insufficient documentation. Dosages ranged from 2 mg twice daily to 4 to 8 mg 3 times daily.

➤*Children:*

Hypersensitivity reactions – Calculate total daily dosage as approximately 0.25 mg/kg/day or 8 mg/m^2/day.

15 years of age and older: See Adults for dosing.

7 to 14 years of age:

- *Usual dosage* – 4 mg 2 or 3 times/day.
- *Maximum dose* – 16 mg/day.

2 to 6 years of age:

- *Usual dosage* – 2 mg 2 or 3 times/day.
- *Maximum dose* – 12 mg/day.

Off-label dosing –

Appetite stimulation:

- *Older than 13 years of age* –
  Initial dosage: 2 mg every 6 hours.
  Dosage titration: May increase gradually over 3 weeks to 8 mg every 6 hours.
- *4 to 8 years of age* – Limited data suggest possible efficacy with 2 mg every 8 hours.

Prevention of migraine (children/adolescents): [4] = Insufficient documentation. Doses ranged from 2 to 8 mg daily in one study and 0.2 to 0.4 mg/kg/day in another.

➤*Elderly:* Use is contraindicated.

➤*Storage/Stability:* Store at 15° to 30°C (59° to 86°F).

Piperazine, Peripherally Selective

CETIRIZINE HYDROCHLORIDE

otc	**Cetirizine** (Apotex USA)	**Tablets; oral:** 5 mg	Lactose. In 100s.
otc	**Cetirizine** (Various, eg, Apotex USA, Perrigo, Sandoz)	**Tablets; oral:** 10 mg	May contain lactose and polydextrose. In 100s and 300s.
otc	**Zyrtec Hives Relief** (McNeil Consumer)		Lactose. In blister pack 14s.
otc	**Zyrtec Allergy** (McNeil Consumer)		Lactose. In 30s.
otc	**Zyrtec Children's Allergy** (McNeil Consumer)	**Tablets, chewable; oral:** 5 mg	Acesulfame K, lactose, maltodextrin, mannitol, sorbitol. Grape flavor. In 5s.
otc	**All Day Allergy Children's** (Major)	**Tablets, chewable; oral:** 10 mg	Acesulfame K, benzyl alcohol, lactose, maltodextrin, propylene glycol. Tutti frutti flavor. In 24s.
otc	**Zyrtec Children's Allergy** (McNeil Consumer)		Acesulfame K, lactose, maltodextrin, mannitol, sorbitol. Grape flavor. In 12s.
otc	**Zyrtec** (McNeil Consumer)	**Capsules, liquid-filled; oral:** 10 mg	Glycerin, mannitol, PEG-400, sorbitan, sorbitol. In 10s, 25s, and 40s.
otc	**Cetirizine Hydrochloride** (Various, eg, Ohm, Teva)	**Syrup; oral:** 1 mg/mL	May contain parabens, saccharin, sucrose. In 118 and 473 mL.
otc	**Zyrtec Children's Hives Relief** (McNeil Consumer)		Parabens, sugar. Grape flavor. In 118 mL.
otc	**Zyrtec Children's Allergy** (McNeil Consumer)		Parabens, sugar. Grape flavor. In 118 mL.

CETIRIZINE HYDROCHLORIDE — ORAL

For complete and comparative prescribing information, refer to the Antihistamines group monograph.

Indications

➤*Urticaria:* Relieves itching due to hives (urticaria). This product will not prevent hives or an allergic skin reaction from occurring.

➤*Allergies/hay fever:* Temporarily relieves runny nose, sneezing, itching of the nose or throat and/or itchy, watery eyes due to hay fever or other upper respiratory allergies.

➤*Off-label uses:*

Bronchial asthma – [2] = Fair documentation. Studies show that cetirizine, at a dose 10 to 20 mg daily, may have a positive impact on asthma-related symptoms in patients with allergy-related asthma. Larger studies, for longer durations, may be necessary to confirm these results. Further study may clarify the impact of cetirizine on additional outcomes, such as overall lung function or global evaluations, for allergy-related asthma. (See Administration and Dosage.)

Other possible off-label uses – To decrease the initial wheal response and pruritus associated with mosquito bites.

Administration and Dosage

➤*Adults:*

Usual dosage – 5 to 10 mg once daily depending upon the severity of symptoms.

Off-label dosing –

Bronchial asthma: [2] = Fair documentation. 10 to 20 mg/day. Study durations reviewed ranged from 4 to 26 weeks.

➤*Children:*

Usual dosage –

6 years of age and older: 5 to 10 mg once daily depending upon the severity of symptoms.

2 to younger than 6 years of age: 2.5 mg once daily of the oral solution. Dose can be increased to a maximum of 5 mg once daily or 2.5 mg every 12 hours of the oral solution.

Off-label dosing –

6 months of younger than 12 months: 2.5 mg once daily.

12 months to younger than 2 years of age:

- *Usual dose* – 2.5 mg once daily. Dose may be increased to 2.5 mg every 12 hours.
- *Maximum dose* – 2.5 mg every 12 hours.

Bronchial asthma: [2] = Fair documentation. Therapy represents rational use as evidenced by consistent favorable clinical reports/trials, but further study is needed because of at least 1 of the following factors:

1.) Appropriate candidates for therapy have not been clearly identified.
2.) Optimal dosage and duration of therapy have not been consistently studied or determined.
3.) Some safety issues require further investigation (eg, bacterial resistance).

- *Children 12 years of age and older* – 10 to 20 mg/day. Study durations reviewed ranged from 4 to 26 weeks.

➤*Elderly:*

Usual dosage – 5 mg once daily.

➤*Renal function impairment:* Dosing adjustment is necessary in patients with moderate or severe renal impairment and in patients on dialysis.

➤*Hepatic function impairment:* Consider dosage adjustment in patients with hepatic impairment.

➤*Administration:* May be given with or without water.

➤*Storage/Stability:* Store at 20° to 25°C (68° to 77°F).

LEVOCETIRIZINE DIHYDROCHLORIDE

Rx	**Levocetirizine** (Various, eg, Perrigo, Winthrop US)	**Tablets; oral:** 5 mg	May contain lactose. In 30s and 90s.
Rx	**Xyzal** (UCB)		Lactose. (Y Y). White, oval shape, scored. Film-coated. In 90s and UD 30s.
Rx	**Levocetirizine** (Winthrop US)	**Solution; oral:** 0.5 mg/mL	Glycerin, maltitol, parabens, saccharin. In 150 mL.
Rx	**Xyzal** (UCB)		Maltitol, parabens, saccharin. In 150 mL.

Piperazine, Peripherally Selective

LEVOCETIRIZINE DIHYDROCHLORIDE — ORAL

For complete and comparative prescribing information, refer to the Antihistamines class monograph.

Indications

➤*Chronic idiopathic urticaria:* For the treatment of the uncomplicated skin manifestations of chronic idiopathic urticaria in adults and children 6 months of age and older.

➤*Perennial allergic rhinitis:* For the relief of symptoms associated with perennial allergic rhinitis in adults and children 6 months of age and older.

➤*Seasonal allergic rhinitis:* For the relief of symptoms associated with seasonal allergic rhinitis in adults and children 2 years of age and older.

Administration and Dosage

➤*Adults:*

Chronic idiopathic urticaria –
Usual dosage: 5 mg (1 tablet or 10 mL oral solution) once daily in the evening. Some patients may be adequately controlled by 2.5 mg (½ tablet or 5 mL oral solution) once daily in the evening.
Maximum dose: 5 mg once daily.

Perennial allergic rhinitis – See Chronic Idiopathic Urticaria for dosing.
Maximum dose: 5 mg once daily.

Seasonal allergic rhinitis – See Chronic Idiopathic Urticaria for dosing.
Maximum dose: 5 mg once daily.

➤*Children:*

Chronic idiopathic urticaria –
12 years of age and older:
• *Usual dosage* – 5 mg (1 tablet or 10 mL oral solution) once daily in the evening. Some patients may be adequately controlled by 2.5 mg (½ tablet or 5 mL oral solution) once daily in the evening.
• *Maximum dose* – 5 mg once daily.
6 to 11 years of age:
• *Usual dosage* – 2.5 mg (½ tablet or 5 mL oral solution) once daily in the evening.
• *Maximum dose* – The 2.5 mg dose should not be exceeded because the systemic exposure with 5 mg is approximately twice that of adults.
6 months to 5 years of age:
• *Usual dosage* – 1.25 mg (2.5 mL oral solution) once daily in the evening.
• *Maximum dose* – The 1.25 mg once-daily dose should not be exceeded based on comparable exposure to adults receiving 5 mg.

Perennial allergic rhinitis –
12 years of age and older: See Chronic Idiopathic Urticaria for dosing.
6 to 11 years of age: See Chronic Idiopathic Urticaria for dosing.
6 months to 5 years of age: See Chronic Idiopathic Urticaria for dosing.

Seasonal allergic rhinitis –
12 years of age and older: See Chronic Idiopathic Urticaria for dosing.
6 to 11 years of age: See Chronic Idiopathic Urticaria for dosing.
2 to 5 years of age: See Chronic Idiopathic Urticaria for dosing.

➤*Renal function impairment:* The following applies to adults and children 12 years of age and older.

Mild renal impairment (creatinine clearance [CrCl] 50 to 80 mL/min) – 2.5 mg once daily.

Moderate renal impairment (CrCl 30 to 50 mL/min) – 2.5 mg once every other day.

Severe renal impairment (CrCl 10 to 30 mL/min) – 2.5 mg twice weekly (administered once every 3 to 4 days).

End-stage renal disease (CrCl less than 10 mL/min) and patients undergoing hemodialysis – These patients should not receive levocetirizine.

➤*Administration:* Can be taken without regard to food consumption.

➤*Storage/Stability:* Store at 20° to 25°C (68° to 77°F); excursions are permitted between 15° and 30°C (59° and 86°F).

Piperidines, Peripherally Selective

DESLORATADINE

Rx	**Clarinex** (Schering)	**Tablets:** 5 mg	Lactose. (C5). Lt. blue. Film-coated. In 100s, 500s, unit-of-use 30s, and UD hospital pack 100s.
Rx	**Clarinex RediTabs** (Schering)	**Tablets, rapidly disintegrating:** 2.5 mg	Mannitol, aspartame, 1.4 mg phenylalanine. (K). Speckled, light red. Tutti frutti flavor. In blister packages of 30.
		5 mg	Mannitol, aspartame, 2.9 mg phenylalanine. (A). Speckled, light red. Tutti frutti flavor. In blister packages of 30.
Rx	**Clarinex** (Schering)	**Syrup:** 2.5 mg per 5 mL	Sugar, EDTA. Bubble gum flavor. In 480 mL.

DESLORATADINE — ORAL

For complete and comparative prescribing information, refer to the Antihistamines group monograph.

Indications

➤*Chronic idiopathic urticaria:* Symptomatic relief of pruritus and reduction in the number and size of hives in patients 6 months of age and older.

➤*Perennial allergic rhinitis:* For the relief of the nasal and nonnasal symptoms of perennial allergic rhinitis in patients 6 months of age and older.

➤*Seasonal allergic rhinitis:* For the relief of the nasal and nonnasal symptoms of seasonal allergic rhinitis in patients 2 years of age and older.

Administration and Dosage

➤*General dosing considerations:* Reduced doses recommended for hepatic impairment (see Hepatic function impairment).

➤*Adults:*

Chronic idiopathic urticaria – 5 mg once daily.

Perennial allergic rhinitis – 5 mg once daily.

Seasonal allergic rhinitis – 5 mg once daily.

➤*Children:*

Chronic idiopathic urticaria –
12 years of age and older: 5 mg once daily.
6 to 11 years of age: 2.5 mg once daily.
12 months to 5 years of age: 1.25 mg once daily.
6 to 11 months of age: 1 mg once daily.

Perennial allergic rhinitis – See Chronic idiopathic urticaria.

Seasonal allergic rhinitis –
12 years of age and older: 5 mg once daily.
6 to 11 years of age: 2.5 mg once daily.
2 to 5 years of age: 1.25 mg once daily.

➤*Renal function impairment:*
Adults – 5 mg every other day.

➤*Hepatic function impairment:*
Adults – 5 mg every other day.

➤*Administration:* May be taken without regard to meals.

Rapidly disintegrating tablets – Place on the tongue immediately after opening the blister; tablet disintegration occurs rapidly. Administer with or without water.

➤*Storage/Stability:* Store at 15° to 30°C (59° to 86°F). Protect tablet unit-of-use packaging and UD hospital packs from excessive moisture. Heat-sensitive; avoid exposure at or above 30°C (86°F). Store syrup and disintegrating tablets at 25°C (77°F); excursions permitted between 15° to 30°C (59° to 86°F). Protect syrup from light.

FEXOFENADINE HYDROCHLORIDE

Rx	**Fexofenadine Hydrochloride** (Various, eg, Dr. Reddy's, Teva)	**Tablets; oral:** 30 mg	May contain lactose. In 30s, 100s, 500s, and UD 100s.
Rx	**Fexofenadine Hydrochloride** (Various, eg, Dr. Reddy's, Teva, UDL Laboratories)	**Tablets; oral:** 60 mg	May contain lactose. In 30s, 60s, 100s, 500s, and UD 100s.
Rx	**Allegra** (Sanofi-Aventis)		(06 E). Peach. Film-coated. In 100s, 500s, and blister pack 100s.
Rx	**Fexofenadine Hydrochloride** (Various, eg, Dr. Reddy's, Teva)	**Tablets; oral:** 180 mg	May contain lactose. In 30s, 100s, 500s, and UD 100s.
Rx	**Allegra** (Sanofi-Aventis)		(018 E). Peach. Film-coated. In 100s and 500s.

Piperidines, Peripherally Selective

FEXOFENADINE HYDROCHLORIDE

Rx	**Allegra ODT** (Sanofi-Aventis)	**Tablets, orally disintegrating; oral:** 30 mg	Aspartame, mannitol, 5.3 mg phenylalanine. (E 311AV). Orange-cream flavor. In UD 60s.
Rx	**Allegra** (Sanofi-Aventis)	**Suspension; oral:** 6 mg/mL	Sucrose, xylitol, parabens, EDTA. Raspberry cream flavor. In 30 and 300 mL.

FEXOFENADINE HYDROCHLORIDE — ORAL

For complete and comparative prescribing information, refer to the Antihistamines group monograph.

Indications

➤*Chronic idiopathic urticaria:* For the treatment of uncomplicated skin manifestations of chronic idiopathic urticaria in adults and children 6 months of age and older.

➤*Seasonal allergic rhinitis:* For the relief of symptoms associated with seasonal allergic rhinitis in adults and children 2 years of age and older.

Administration and Dosage

➤*Adults:*
Usual dosage – 60 mg twice daily or 180 mg once daily.

➤*Children:*
Chronic idiopathic urticaria –
12 years of age and older: 60 mg twice daily or 180 mg once daily.
6 to 11 years of age: 30 mg twice daily.
2 to 11 years of age: 30 mg (5 mL of oral suspension) twice daily.
6 months to younger than 2 years of age: 15 mg (2.5 mL of oral suspension) twice daily.

Seasonal allergic rhinitis –
12 years of age and older: 60 mg twice daily or 180 mg once daily.
6 to 11 years of age: 30 mg twice daily.
2 to 11 years of age: 30 mg (5 mL of oral suspension) twice daily.

➤*Renal function impairment:*
Adults and children 12 years of age and older – Starting dosage is 60 mg once daily.

Children 2 to 11 years of age – Starting dosage is 30 mg once daily.

Children 6 months to younger than 2 years of age – Starting dosage is 15 mg once daily for the treatment of chronic idiopathic urticaria.

➤*Administration:*
Tablets – Take with water.

Orally disintegrating tablets – The orally disintegrating tablet is designed to disintegrate on the tongue, followed by swallowing with or without water, and should be taken on an empty stomach. The orally disintegrating tablet is not intended to be chewed. The orally disintegrating tablet should not be removed from the original blister package until time of administration.

Suspension – Shake oral suspension well before each use.

➤*Storage/Stability:* Store at controlled room temperature, between 20° and 25°C (68° and 77°F). Foil-backed blister packs containing tablets or orally disintegrating tablets should be protected from excessive moisture.

LORATADINE

otc	**Loratadine** (Various, eg, Geneva)	**Tablets; oral:** 10 mg	May contain lactose. In 30s and 100s.
otc	**Claritin 24 Hour Allergy** (Schering-Plough)		Lactose. (Claritin 10 458). 1s, 2s, 5s, 10s, 20s, 30s, and 40s.
otc	**Claritin Hives Relief** (Schering)		Lactose. In 10s.
otc	**Non-Drowsy Allergy** (Major)		Lactose. In 30s.
otc	**Children's Claritin Allergy** (Schering-Plough Healthcare)	**Tablets, chewable; oral:** 5 mg	Aspartame, mannitol, 1.4 mg phenylalanine. Grape flavor. In 5s and 10s.
otc	**Claritin RediTabs** (Schering-Plough)	**Tablets, orally disintegrating; oral:** 5 mg	Mannitol. Mint flavor. In 10s, 30s, and 40s.
otc	**Alavert** (Wyeth Consumer)	**Tablets, orally disintegrating; oral:** 10 mg	Lactose. In 6s, 12s, 15s, 30s, and 48s.
otc	**Claritin Reditabs** (Schering)		Mannitol. (C). White to off-white. Mint flavor. In 4s, 10s, 20s, and 30s.
otc	**Dimetapp Children's ND Non-Drowsy Allergy** (Wyeth)		Aspartame, corn syrup, mannitol, phenylalanine 8.4 mg. In 6s and 12s.
otc	**Non-drowsy Allergy Relief** (Major)		Phenylalanine 0.9 mg. Aspartame, lactose, mannitol. Cherry flavor. In 10s.
otc	**Triaminic Allerchews** (Novartis)		Mannitol. In 8s.
otc	**Claritin Non-Drowsy Liqui-Gels** (Schering-Plough)	**Capsules, liquid-filled; oral:** 10 mg	Sorbitol. In 70s.
otc	**Loratadine** (Ranbaxy)	**Syrup; oral:** 5 mg per 5 mL	Sucrose. Fruit flavor. In 480 mL.
otc sf	**Loratadine Hives Relief** (Silarx)		Alcohol free, dye free, sugar free. Glycerin, propylene glycol, sodium benzoate, sucralose. Grape flavor. In 120 mL.
otc	**Claritin** (Schering)		Sucrose, sugar, EDTA. Fruit flavor. In 120 mL.
otc	**Children's Claritin Allergy** (Schering)		Maltitol, sorbitol, sucralose. Grape flavor. In 60 and 120 mL.
otc	**Clear-Atadine Children's** (Major)		Alcohol free. Sucrose. Fruit flavor. In 120 mL.
otc	**Dimetapp Children's ND Non-Drowsy Allergy** (Wyeth)		Sucrose. In 118 mL.
otc	**Alavert Children's** (Wyeth)		
otc	**Non-Drowsy Allergy Relief for Kids** (Major)		Sucrose, glycerin. Fruit flavor. In 120 mL.
otc	**Children's Loratadine Syrup** (Taro)		Fruit flavor. In 120 mL.

LORATADINE — ORAL

For complete prescribing information, refer to the Antihistamines class monograph.

Indications

➤*Allergic rhinitis:* For the relief of nasal and nonnasal symptoms of seasonal allergic rhinitis.

➤*Off-label uses:* For the treatment of chronic idiopathic urticaria in patients 2 years of age and older.

Administration and Dosage

➤*Maximum dose:*
Adults and children 6 years of age and older – 10 mg/day according to the prescribing information.

Children 2 to 5 years of age – 5 mg/day according to the prescribing information.

➤*Adults:*
Allergic rhinitis –
Usual dosage: 10 mg once daily or 5 mg every 12 hours (*RediTabs*).
Maximum dose: 10 mg/day.

➤*Children:*
Allergic rhinitis –
6 years of age and older:
- *Usual dosage* – 10 mg once daily or 5 mg every 12 hours (*RediTabs*).
- *Maximum dose* – 10 mg/day.

2 to 5 years of age:
- *Usual dosage* – 5 mg (chewable tablets, syrup) once daily.
- *Maximum dose* – 5 mg/day.

➤*Renal function impairment:* Hemodialysis does not have an effect on the pharmacokinetics of loratadine or descarboethoxyloratadine in subjects with chronic renal function impairment.

6 years of age and older (glomerular filtration rate less than 30 mL/min) – 10 mg every other day as the starting dose.

Piperidines, Peripherally Selective

LORATADINE — ORAL

2 to 5 years of age (glomerular filtration rate less than 30 mL/min) – 5 mg every other day as the starting dose.

➤*Hepatic function impairment:*

6 years of age and older – 10 mg every other day as the starting dose.

2 to 5 years of age – 5 mg every other day as the starting dose.

➤*Administration:*

Orally disintegrating tablets – Place tablets on the tongue immediately upon opening the individual tablet blister. Tablet disintegration occurs rapidly. Administer with or without water.

➤*Storage/Stability:* Protect unit dose packs, unit-of-use packs, and rapidly disintegrating tablets from excessive moisture. Store the tablets between 2° and 30°C (36° and 86°F). Store the syrup and rapidly disintegrating tablets between 2° and 25°C (36° and 77°F).

Orally disintegrating tablets – Use within 6 months of opening laminated foil pouch.

ANTIHISTAMINES

ANTIHISTAMINE COMBINATIONS

Content given per 5 mL.

	Product & Distributor	Antihistamine	Average Dose	Excipients & How Supplied
Rx sf	**Carbinoxamine Maleate and Carbinoxamine Tannate Oral Suspension** (Brighton)	2 mg carbinoxamine maleate, 6 mg carbinoxamine tannate	**6 yr of age or older** - 5 mL q 12 h **18 mo to 6 yr of age** - 2.5 mL q 12 h **9 to 18 mo of age** - 1.25 mL q 12 h **younger than 9 mo of age** - only as directed by physician	Alcohol free, dye free. Saccharin, sorbitol, parabens. Bubble-gum flavor. In 118 and 473 mL.

For complete prescribing information, refer to the Antihistamine group monograph.

NONNARCOTIC ANTITUSSIVES

BENZONATATE

Rx	**Benzonatate Softgels** (Various, eg, Inwood, Sidmak)	**Capsules; oral:** 100 mg	In 100s and 500s.
Rx	**Tessalon Perles** (Forest)		Parabens. (T). Yellow. In 100s and 500s.
Rx	**Zonatuss** (Atley)	**Capsules; oral:** 150 mg	(150 ZON). Opaque white/opaque lt. blue. In 100s.
Rx	**Benzonatate Softgels** (Various, eg, Inwood)	**Capsules; oral:** 200 mg	In 100s and 500s.
Rx	**Tessalon** (Forest)		Parabens. (0698). Yellow. In 100s and 500s.

BENZONATATE — ORAL

Indications

➤*Cough:* Benzonatate is indicated for the symptomatic relief of cough.

Administration and Dosage

➤*Adults:*

Cough – One 100 mg, 150 mg, or 200 mg capsule 3 times daily as required. If necessary, up to 600 mg daily may be given.

➤*Children:*

Cough –

Older than 10 years of age: See Adults for dosing.

➤*Administration:* Instruct patients to swallow capsules whole and not to suck or chew the capsule, because benzonatate can produce a temporary local anesthesia of the oral mucosa and choking could occur. Administer without regard to meals but administer with food or milk if GI upset occurs.

➤*Storage/Stability:*

Capsules – Store at 15° to 30°C (59° to 86°F). The softgels should be protected from light, moisture, and humidity.

Actions

➤*Pharmacology:* Benzonatate acts peripherally by anesthetizing the stretch receptors located in the respiratory passages, lungs, and pleura by dampening their activity and thereby reducing the cough reflex at its source. It begins to act within 15 to 20 minutes and its effect lasts for 3 to 8 hours. Benzonatate has no inhibitory effect on the respiratory center in recommended dosage.

Contraindications

Hypersensitivity to benzonatate or related compounds.

Warnings/Precautions

➤*CNS effects:* Benzonatate is chemically related to anesthetic agents of the paraaminobenzoic acid class (eg, procaine, tetracaine) and has been associated with adverse CNS effects possibly related to a prior sensitivity to related agents or interaction with concomitant medication.

➤*Hypersensitivity reactions:* Severe hypersensitivity reactions (including bronchospasm, laryngospasm, and cardiovascular collapse) have been reported, which are possibly related to local anesthesia from sucking or chewing the capsule or softgel capsule instead of swallowing it. Severe reactions have required intervention with vasopressor agents and supportive measures.

➤*Pregnancy: Category C.* Animal reproduction studies have not been conducted with benzonatate. It is also not known whether benzonatate can cause fetal harm when administered to a pregnant woman or can affect reproduction capacity. Benzonatate should be given to a pregnant woman only if clearly needed.

➤*Lactation:* It is not known whether this drug is excreted in human milk. Because many drugs are excreted in human milk caution should be exercised when benzonatate is administered to a nursing woman.

➤*Children:* Safety and efficacy in children younger than 10 years of age have not been established.

Drug Interactions

Isolated instances of bizarre behavior, including mental confusion and visual hallucinations, have also been reported in patients taking benzonatate in combination with other prescribed drugs.

Adverse Reactions

Potential adverse reactions to benzonatate may include the following:

➤*CNS:* Sedation, headache, dizziness, mental confusion, and visual hallucinations.

➤*Dermatologic:* Pruritus and skin eruptions.

➤*GI:* Constipation, nausea, and GI upset.

➤*Hypersensitivity:* Hypersensitivity reactions including bronchospasm, laryngospasm, cardiovascular collapse possibly related to local anesthesia from chewing or sucking the capsule or softgel capsules.

➤*Miscellaneous:* Nasal congestion; sensation of burning in the eyes; vague "chilly" sensation; numbness of the chest. Rare instances of deliberate or accidental overdose have resulted in death.

Overdosage

➤*Symptoms:* If capsules or softgel capsules are chewed or dissolved in the mouth, oropharyngeal anesthesia will develop rapidly. CNS stimulation may cause restlessness and tremors, which may proceed to clonic convulsions followed by profound CNS depression.

Overdose may result in death. The drug is chemically related to tetracaine and other topical anesthetics and shares various aspects of their pharmacology and toxicology. Drugs of this type are generally well absorbed after ingestion.

➤*Treatment:* Evacuate gastric contents and administer copious amounts of activated charcoal slurry. Even in the conscious patient, cough and gag reflexes may be so depressed as to necessitate special attention to protection against aspiration of gastric contents and orally administered materials. Convulsions should be treated with a short-acting barbiturate given intravenously and carefully titrated for the smallest effective dosage. Intensive support of respiration and cardiovascular-renal function is an essential feature of the treatment of severe intoxication from overdosage.

Do not use CNS stimulants.

Patient Information

Release of benzonatate from the capsule in the mouth can produce a temporary local anesthesia of the oral mucosa and choking could occur. Therefore, the capsules and softgel capsules should be swallowed without chewing.

DEXTROMETHORPHAN HBr

otc	**Robitussin CoughGels** (Wyeth)	**Capsule, liquid-filled; oral:** 15 mg	Sorbitol. In 20s.
otc	**DexAlone** (DexGen)	**Capsule, liquid-filled; oral:** 30 mg	Sorbitol. In 30s.
otc	**Hold DM** (B. F. Ascher)	**Lozenges; oral:** 5 mg	Sucrose, corn syrup. Original and cherry flavor. In 10s.
otc sf	**Scot-Tussin DM Cough Chasers** (Scot-tussin)		Peppermint oil, sorbitol. Dye-free. In 20s.
otc	**Trocal** (Textilease)	**Lozenges; oral:** 7.5 mg	Cherry flavor. In 10s, 50s, and 500s.
otc	**Sucrets DM Cough Suppressant** (Insight Pharmaceuticals)	**Lozenges; oral:** 10 mg	Corn syrup, menthol, sucrose. Cherry flavor. In 6s.
otc	**Sucrets DM Cough Formula** (Insight Pharmaceuticals)		Corn syrup, hydrogenated palm oil (honey lemon flavor only), menthol, sucrose (cherry flavor only) sugar (honey lemon flavor only). Cherry and honey lemon flavors. In 18s.
otc	**Triaminic Thin Strips Long Acting Cough** (Novartis Consumer Health)	**Strips, orally disintegrating; oral:** 7.5 mg	Alcohol (less than 5%), sorbitol, sucralose. Cherry flavor. In 16s.
otc	**Theraflu Thin Strips Long Acting Cough** (Novartis Consumer Health)	**Strips, orally disintegrating; oral:** 15 mg	Alcohol (less than 5%), sorbitol, sucralose. Cherry flavor. In 12s.
otc	**Simply Cough** (McNeil-PPC)	**Liquid; oral:** 5 mg/5 mL	Corn syrup, sucralose. Alcohol free. Cherry berry flavor. In 120 mL.
otc	**Creo-Terpin** (Lee)	**Liquid; oral:** 10 mg/15 mL (3.33 mg/5 mL)	Tartrazine, 25% alcohol, corn syrup, saccharin. In 120 mL.
otc	**Robitussin Maximum Strength Cough** (Whitehall-Robins)	**Liquid; oral:** 15 mg/5 mL	1.4% alcohol, glucose, corn syrup, saccharin. Cherry flavor. In 118 and 237 mL.
otc	**Vicks 44 Cough Relief** (Procter and Gamble Co.)	**Liquid; oral:** 10 mg/5 mL	31 mg sodium/15 mL, alcohol, corn syrup, saccharin. In 118 mL.
otc sf	**Buckley's Cough Mixture** (Novartis Consumer Health)	**Liquid; oral:** 12.5 mg/5 mL	Alcohol free. Parabens, pine needle oil, menthol. In 118 mL.
otc	**Creomulsion for Children** (Summit)	**Syrup; oral:** 5 mg/5 mL	Alcohol free. Sucrose. Cherry flavor. In 118 mL.
otc sf	**Robitussin Pediatric Cough** (Whitehall-Robins)	**Syrup; oral:** 7.5 mg/5 mL	Alcohol free. Saccharin, sorbitol. Cherry flavor. In 118 mL.
otc	**ElixSure Children's Cough** (Taro Consumer)		Propylparaben, sorbitol. Cherry and bubble gum flavors. In 118 mL.
otc	**Triaminic Long Acting Cough** (Novartis Consumer Health)		Dye free. EDTA, sorbitol, sucrose. Berry punch flavor. In 118 mL.
otc	**Silphen DM** (Silarx)	**Syrup; oral:** 10 mg/5 mL	5% alcohol, menthol, methylparaben, sucrose. In 118 mL.
otc	**Vicks DayQuil Cough** (P & G Health)	**Syrup; oral:** 15 mg/15 mL	Fructose, saccharin, sodium 15 mg/15 mL. In 180 mL.
otc	**Creomulsion Adult Formula** (Summit)	**Syrup; oral:** 20 mg/15 mL	Alcohol free. Sucrose. In 118 mL.
Rx	**AeroTuss 12** (Aero Pharmaceuticals, Inc.)	**Suspension; oral:** 30 mg/5 mL	Methylparaben, sodium saccharin, sucrose. Grape flavor. In 237 mL.
otc	**Delsym** (Adams Respiratory Therapeutics)	**Suspension, extended-release; oral:** 30 mg/ 5 mL	As dextromethorphan polistirex. Corn syrup, EDTA, sucrose, parabens. Orange and grape flavors. In 89 and 148 mL.
otc	**PediaCare Infants' Long-Acting Cough** (Pfizer Consumer Health)	**Solution, concentrate; oral:** 3.75 mg/0.8 mL	Alcohol free. Glycerin, sorbitol. Grape flavor. In 15 mL.
otc	**Little Colds Cough Formula** (Vetco)	**Solution. concentrate; oral:** 7.5 mg/mL	Glycerin, corn syrup. Natural grape flavor. In 30 mL.
otc sf	**Children's PediaCare Long-Acting Cough** (Pfizer)	**Solution; oral:** 7.5 mg/5 mL	Alcohol free. Saccharin, sorbitol. Grape flavor. In 120 mL.
otc	**PediaCare Infants' Long-Acting Cough** (Pfizer Consumer Health)	**Freezer pops; oral:** 7.5 mg/25 mL (per pop)	Benzyl alcohol, corn syrup, ethyl maltol, sucralose. Berry flavor. In 8s.

DEXTROMETHORPHAN HYDROBROMIDE — ORAL

Indications

➤*Cough:* Temporarily relieves cough caused by minor throat and bronchial irritation as may occur with the common cold or inhaled irritants.

➤*Off-label uses:*

Neuropathy – [5] = Poor documentation. Based on the limited data available, the analgesic effects of dextromethorphan have not been proven. In addition, CNS effects at high doses may not be tolerable for long-term management of neuropathic syndromes.

Postherpetic neuralgia – [5] = Poor documentation. Use of dextromethorphan for treatment of postherpetic neuralgia (PHN) has been studied in 2 controlled trials, neither of which showed any benefit. American Academy of Neurology clinical practice guidelines state that the efficacy of dextromethorphan is not better than that of placebo for patients with PHN.

Administration and Dosage

➤*Adults:*

Cough –

Usual dosage:

- *Extended-release liquid* – 60 mg every 12 hours up to 120 mg/day.
- *Gelcaps* – 30 mg every 6 to 8 hours. Do not exceed 120 mg in 24 hours.
- *Liquid and syrup* – 10 to 20 mg every 4 hours or 30 mg every 6 to 8 hours up to 120 mg/day.
- *Lozenges* – 5 to 15 mg every 1 to 4 hours up to 120 mg/day.
- *Strips* – 30 mg every 6 to 8 hours up to 120 mg/day.

Maximum dose: 120 mg/day.

➤*Children:*

Cough –

Usual dosage:

- *Drops* –
  - *2 to 3 years of age:* 7.5 mg (one dropperful [2 dropperfuls *PediaCare*]) every 6 to 8 hours, if needed, up to 30 mg/day.
- *Extended-release liquid* –
  - *12 years of age and older:* 60 mg every 12 hours up to 120 mg/day.
  - *6 to younger than 12 years of age:* 30 mg every 12 hours up to 60 mg/day.
  - *2 to younger than 6 years of age:* 15 mg every 12 hours up to 30 mg/day.
- *Gelcaps* –
  - *12 years of age and older:* 30 mg every 6 to 8 hours. Do not exceed 120 mg in 24 hours.
- *Liquid and syrup* –
  - *12 years of age and older:* 10 to 20 mg every 4 hours or 30 mg every 6 to 8 hours up to 120 mg/day.
  - *6 to younger than 12 years of age:* 15 mg every 6 to 8 hours up to 60 mg/day.
  - *2 to younger than 6 years of age:* 7.5 mg every 6 to 8 hours up to 30 mg/day.
- *Lozenges* –
  - *12 years of age and older:* 5 to 15 mg every 1 to 4 hours up to 120 mg/day.

DEXTROMETHORPHAN HYDROBROMIDE — ORAL

6 to younger than 12 years of age: 5 to 10 mg every 1 to 4 hours up to 60 mg/day.

- *Oral solution –*

6 to younger than 12 years of age: 15 mg (10 mL) every 6 to 8 hours. Do not exceed 4 doses in 24 hours.

2 to younger than 6 years of age: 7.5 mg (5 mL) every 6 to 8 hours. Do not exceed 4 doses in 24 hours.

- *Strips –*

12 years of age and older: 30 mg every 6 to 8 hours up to 120 mg/day.

6 to younger than 12 years of age: 15 mg every 6 to 8 hours up to 60 mg/day.

Maximum dose:

- *12 years of age and older –* 120 mg/day.
- *6 to younger than 12 years of age –* 60 mg/day.
- *2 to younger than 6 years of age –* 30 mg/day.

➤*Administration:*

Strips – Allow the strip to dissolve on the tongue.

➤*Storage/Stability:* Store at controlled room temperature 15° to 30°C (59° to 86°F).

Actions

➤*Pharmacology:* Dextromethorphan is the d-isomer of the codeine analog of levorphanol; it lacks analgesic and addictive properties. Its cough suppressant action is due to a central action on the cough center in the medulla. Dextromethorphan 15 to 30 mg equals codeine 8 to 15 mg as an antitussive.

➤*Pharmacokinetics:*

Absorption – Dextromethorphan is rapidly absorbed in the GI tract.

Metabolism/Excretion – It undergoes metabolism in the liver and is then excreted in the urine as unchanged drug and demethylated metabolites.

Contraindications

Hypersensitivity to any component.

Warnings/Precautions

➤*Persistent cough:* Do not take this product for persistent or chronic cough such as occurs with smoking, asthma or emphysema, or if cough is accompanied by excessive phlegm (mucus) unless directed by a health care provider. A persistent cough may be a sign of a serious condition. If cough persists for more than 1 week, tends to recur, or if it is accompanied by fever, rash, or persistent headache, consult a health care provider. These could be signs of a serious condition.

➤*Tartrazine sensitivity:* Some dextromethorphan-containing products contain tartrazine, which may cause allergic-type reactions (including bronchial asthma) in certain susceptible people. Although the overall incidence of tartrazine sensitivity in the general population is low, it is frequently seen in patients who also have aspirin hypersensitivity.

➤*Special risk:*

Asthma, chronic bronchitis, emphysema, or mucus with cough – Because dextromethorphan decreases coughing, it makes it difficult to get rid of the mucus that collects in the lungs and airways with some diseases.

Diabetes – Some products contain sugar and may affect control of blood glucose monitoring.

Slowed breathing – Dextromethorphan may slow the rate or breathing even further.

➤*Drug abuse and dependence:* Anecdotal reports of abuse of dextromethorphan-containing cough/cold products have increased, especially among teenagers. Additional data are needed before determining the abuse and dependency potential of dextromethorphan.

➤*Pregnancy: Category C.* It is not known if dextromethorphan can cause fetal harm or affect reproduction capacity when administered to a pregnant woman. Give to a pregnant woman only if clearly needed.

The molecular weight (about 271) of dextromethorphan is low enough that transfer to the fetus should be expected. The available human data on the reproductive effects of dextromethorphan does not demonstrate a major teratogenic risk. In a study of 184 pregnant women who were exposed to dextromethorphan during pregnancy, an increased rate of major malformations (above the baseline rate of 1% to 3%) was not observed. The authors of the study concluded that dextromethorphan does not pose a risk to the fetus; however, the authors were unable to rule out an increased risk of rare malformations due to the sample size of the study.

Use of liquid preparations of dextromethorphan that contain ethanol, however, should be avoided during pregnancy because ethanol is a known teratogen.

➤*Lactation:* Dextromethorphan is probably safe to use during breastfeeding. The low molecular weight (about 271) of dextromethorphan suggests that passage into milk probably occurs. However, it is unlikely that with usual maternal doses amounts in milk are as large as those given directly to infants or that breastfed infants would be harmed by the drug in breast milk, especially in infants over 1 month of age. Preparations containing ethanol should be avoided.

➤*Children:*

Gelcaps – Do not give to children younger than 12 years of age.

Lozenges – Do not give to children younger than 6 years of age unless directed by a health care provider.

Liquid, syrup, and pediatric liquid – Do not give to children younger than 2 years of age unless directed by a health care provider.

Drug Interactions

Dextromethorphan Drug Interactions

Precipitant drug	Object drug[a]		Description
MAOIs	Dextromethorphan	↑	Hyperpyrexia, abnormal muscle movement, hypotension, coma, and death have been associated with concurrent use. Avoid coadministration and avoid use for 2 weeks after stopping the MAOI.
Quinidine	Dextromethorphan	↑	Plasma dextromethorphan levels may be elevated because of quinidine inhibiting the metabolism of dextromethorphan (via CYP 2D6). Increased toxic effects may develop. Reduce dose if needed.
Sibutramine	Dextromethorphan	↑	A "serotonin syndrome," including CNS irritability, motor weakness, shivering, myoclonus, and altered consciousness, may occur because of additive serotonergic effects. Coadministration is not recommended.

[a] ↑ = object drug increased.

Adverse Reactions

Adverse reactions may include dizziness, drowsiness, and GI disturbances.

Overdosage

➤*Symptoms:*

Adults – Altered sensory perception, ataxia, dysphoria, slurred speech.

Children – Ataxia, convulsions, respiratory depression.

Patient Information

Do not use if you are currently taking a prescription monoamine oxidase (MAO) inhibitor (certain drugs for depression, psychiatric, or emotional conditions, or Parkinson disease), or for 2 weeks after stopping the MAO inhibitor drug. If you are uncertain whether your prescription drug contains an MAO inhibitor, consult your doctor before taking this product.

Do not use dextromethorphan for persistent or chronic cough, such as with smoking, asthma, or emphysema, or if cough is accompanied by excessive phlegm (mucus), unless directed by your doctor. Contact your doctor if cough lasts for more than 1 week, comes back, or is accompanied by fever, rash, or persistent headache. These could be signs of a serious condition.

If you are pregnant or breast-feeding, seek the advice of your doctor before using this product.

DEXTROMETHORPHAN POLISTIREX — ORAL

Indications

➤*Cough:* Temporary relief of cough due to minor throat and bronchial irritation that may occur with the common cold or inhaled irritants.

Administration and Dosage

➤*Adults:*

Cough –

Usual dosage: 60 mg (2 teaspoonfuls) every 12 hours, not to exceed 120 mg (4 teaspoonfuls) in 24 hours.

Maximum dose: 120 mg/day.

➤*Children:*

Cough –

12 years of age and older:

- *Usual dosage –* 60 mg (2 teaspoonfuls) every 12 hours, not to exceed 120 mg (4 teaspoonfuls) in 24 hours.
- *Maximum dose –* 120 mg/day.

6 to younger than 12 years of age:

- *Usual dosage –* 30 mg (1 teaspoonful) every 12 hours, not to exceed 60 mg (2 teaspoonfuls) in 24 hours.
- *Maximum dose –* 60 mg/day.

2 to younger than 6 years of age:

- *Usual dosage –* 15 mg (1/2 teaspoonful) every 12 hours, not to exceed 30 mg (1 teaspoonful) in 24 hours.
- *Maximum dose –* 30 mg/day.

➤*Preparation for administration:* Shake bottle well before using.

➤*Storage/Stability:* Store at 15° to 30°C (59° to 86°F).

Warnings/Precautions

➤*Persistent cough:* Do not take this product for persistent or chronic cough such as occurs with smoking, asthma, or emphysema, or if cough is accompanied by excessive phlegm (mucus) unless directed by a physician. A persistent cough may be a sign of a serious condition. If cough persists for

DEXTROMETHORPHAN POLISTIREX — ORAL

more than 1 week, tends to recur, or is accompanied by fever, rash, or persistent headache, consult a physician.

➤*Pregnancy: Category C.* The molecular weight (about 271) of dextromethorphan is low enough that transfer to the fetus should be expected. The available human data on the reproductive effects of dextromethorphan does not demonstrate a major teratogenic risk. In a study of 184 pregnant women who were exposed to dextromethorphan during pregnancy, an increased rate of major malformations (above the baseline rate of 1% to 3%) was not observed. The authors of the study concluded that dextromethorphan does not pose a risk to the fetus; however, the authors were unable to rule out an increased risk of rare malformations due to the sample size of the study.

Use of liquid preparations of dextromethorphan that contain ethanol, however, should be avoided during pregnancy because ethanol is a known teratogen.

➤*Lactation:* Dextromethorphan is probably safe to use during breastfeeding. The low molecular weight (about 271) of dextromethorphan suggests that passage into milk probably occurs. However, it is unlikely that with usual maternal doses amounts in milk are as large as those given directly to infants or that breastfed infants would be harmed by the drug in breast milk, especially in infants over 1 month of age. Preparations containing ethanol should be avoided.

Drug Interactions

➤*Monoamine oxidase inhibitor (MAOI):* Do not use this product if you are now taking a prescription MAOI (certain drugs for depression, psychiatric or emotional conditions, or Parkinson's disease), or for 2 weeks after stopping the MAOI drug. If you are uncertain whether your prescription drug contains an MAOI, consult a health professional before taking this product.

Overdosage

In case of accidental overdose, seek professional assistance or contact a poison control center immediately.

DIPHENHYDRAMINE HYDROCHLORIDE

For complete prescribing information, refer to the Diphenhydramine monograph in the Antihistamines section.

DEXTROMETHORPHAN HBr/BENZOCAINE

otc	**Cepacol Ultra Sore Throat Plus Cough** (Combe)	**Lozenges; oral:** 7.5 mg benzocaine, 5 mg dextromethorphan hydrobromide	Glucose, sucrose. Mixed berry flavor. In 18s.
otc	**Tetra-Formula** (Reese Pharm.)	**Lozenges; oral:** 10 mg dextromethorphan HBr and 15 mg benzocaine	Sucrose, glucose, dextrose. In 10s.
otc sf	**Cēpacol Dual Relief Sore Throat + Cough** (Combe)	**Spray, solution; oral:** 5% benzocaine, 5 mg dextromethorphan hydrobromide, 30% glycerin	Sugar free. SD alcohol 38B, sucralose. Cherry flavor. In 20.2 mL.

DEXTROMETHORPHAN HBr/BENZOCAINE — ORAL

For complete and comparative prescribing information, refer to the Dextromethorphan HBr and Benzocaine individual monographs.

Indications

➤*Cough:* Temporarily suppresses cough caused by minor throat and bronchial irritants as may occur with the common cold.

➤*Sore throat:* For the temporary relief of occasional minor irritation and sore throat.

Administration and Dosage

➤*Adults:*

Cough –

Lozenge:

- *Cepacol –*
  Usual dosage: 2 lozenges (1 immediately after the other); may repeat every 4 hours.
  Maximum dose: 12 lozenges/day.
- *Tetra-Formula* – 1 lozenge; may repeat every 4 hours.

Spray:

- *Usual dosage* – Two sprays every 4 hours.
- *Maximum dose* – 8 sprays/day.

➤*Children:*

Cough –

Lozenge:

- *Cepacol –*
  12 years of age and older: See adults for dosing.
  6 to 12 years of ageUsual dosage: 1 lozenge; may repeat every 4 hours-.Maximum dose 6 lozenges/day.
- *Tetra-Formula –*
  6 years of age and older: See adults for dosing.

Spray:

- *12 years of age or older* – See Adults for dosing.
- *6 to 12 years of age –*
  Usual dosage: One spray every 4 hours.
  Maximum dose: 4 sprays/day.

➤*Duration of therapy:* Do not use for more than 2 days for sore throat or for more than 7 days for cough unless directed by a health care provider.

➤*Administration:*

Lozenge – Allow lozenge to dissolve slowly in the mouth; do not chew.

Spray – Spray into throat or onto affected area and then swallow.

➤*Storage/Stability:* Store below 86°F and protect from moisture.

EXPECTORANTS

GUAIFENESIN (Glyceryl Guaiacolate)

Rx	**Guaifenesin** (Various, eg, URL)	**Tablets; oral:** 200 mg	In 100s.
Rx	**Organidin NR** (Medpointe)		Rose, scored. In 100s.
Rx	**Liquibid** (Capellon)	**Tablets; oral:** 400 mg	In 100s.
otc	**Mucinex** (Reckitt Benckiser)	**Tablets, extended-release; oral:** 600 mg	Bi-layered. In 20s, 40s, and 500s.
otc	**Humibid Maximum Strength** (Adams)	**Tablets, extended-release; oral:** 1,200 mg	Bi-layered. In 100s.
otc	**Mucinex Maximum Strength** (Reckitt Benckiser)		Bi-layered. In 28s.
otc	**Mucinex Mini-Melts for Kids** (Reckitt Benckiser)	**Granules; oral:** 50 mg per packet	Aspartame, 0.6 mg phenylalanine, sorbitol. Grape flavor. In 12s.
otc	**Mucinex Mini-Melts for Kids** (Reckitt Benckiser)	**Granules; oral:** 100 mg per packet	Aspartame, 1 mg phenylalanine, sorbitol. Bubble gum flavor. In 12s.
otc	**Guaifenesin** (Various, eg, URL)	**Syrup; oral:** 100 mg per 5 mL	In 473 mL.
otc	**Altarussin** (Altaire)		Alcohol-free. Corn syrup, menthol, saccharin. In 118 mL.
otc	**Guiatuss** (Various, eg, Goldline)		May contain corn syrup, saccharin, and menthol. In 118 mL.

GUAIFENESIN (Glyceryl Guaiacolate)

otc sf	**Buckley's Chest Congestion Mixture** (Novartis Consumer Health)	**Liquid; oral:** 100 mg per 5 mL	Alcohol free. Acesulfame K, parabens, pine needle oil, menthol. In 118 mL.
otc	**Mucinex for Kids** (Reckitt Benckiser)		Alcohol free. Parabens, saccharin. Grape flavor. In 118 mL.
otc sf	**Diabetic Tussin** (Health Care Products)		Alcohol- and dye-free. 8.4 mg per 5 mL phenylalanine. Aspartame, menthol, methylparaben. In 118 mL.
Rx	**Ganidin NR** (Cypress)		In 473 mL.
Rx	**Guaifenesin NR** (Silarx)		Raspberry flavor. In 473 mL.
otc	**Robitussin** (Wyeth)		Alcohol-free. Glucose, corn syrup, saccharin, menthol. In 118 and 237 mL.
otc	**Siltussin DAS** (Silarx)		Strawberry flavor. In 118 mL.
otc sf	**Scot-Tussin Expectorant** (Scot-Tussin)		Alcohol- and dye-free. Contains phenylalanine.[a] Aspartame, parabens, menthol. Grape flavor. In 118 mL.
otc	**Siltussin SA** (Silarx)		Strawberry flavor. In 118, 237, and 473 mL.
otc sf	**Naldecon Senior EX** (Sandoz)	**Liquid; oral:** 200 mg per 5 mL	Alcohol-free. Sorbitol, saccharin. In 120 mL.

[a] Amount not specified.

GUAIFENESIN — ORAL

Indications

➤*100 mg tablets:* Guaifenesin 100 mg tablets relieve bronchial drainage, and dry, nonproductive coughs become more productive and less frequent. This medication relieves irritated membranes in the respiratory tract by preventing dryness through increased mucous flow.

➤*200 mg tablets, 200 mg capsules, granules, and 100 mg per 5 mL syrup and liquid:* Guaifenesin help loosen phlegm (mucus) and thin bronchial secretions to rid the bronchial passageways of bothersome mucus, drain bronchial tubes, and make coughs more productive. This medication helps loosen phlegm and thin bronchial secretions in patients with stable chronic bronchitis.

➤*400 and 600 mg tablets:* For the temporary relief of coughs associated with respiratory tract infections and related conditions such as sinusitis, pharyngitis, bronchitis, and asthma, when these conditions are complicated by tenacious mucus or mucus plugs and congestion.

Administration and Dosage

➤*Adults:*

Expectorant –

Usual dosage: 200 to 400 mg (immediate-release) every 4 hours or 600 to 1,200 mg (extended-release) every 12 hours.

Maximum dose: 2,400 mg/day.

➤*Children:*

Expectorant –

12 years of age and older: See Adults for dosing.

6 to younger than 12 years of age:
- *Usual dosage* – 100 to 200 mg (immediate-release) every 4 hours or 600 mg (extended-release) every 12 hours.
- *Maximum dose* – 1,200 mg/day.

2 to younger than 6 years of age:
- *Usual dosage* – 50 to 100 mg (immediate-release) every 4 hours.
- *Maximum dose* – 600 mg/day.

➤*Administration:* Take with a full glass of water.

For granules, empty entire contents of packet onto tongue and swallow. For best taste, do not chew granules.

For the extended-release tablets, do not crush, chew, or break the tablet.

➤*Storage/Stability:* Store at controlled room temperature, 15° to 30°C (59° to 86°F). Dispense in tight, light-resistant containers.

Actions

➤*Pharmacology:* Guaifenesin is an expectorant which increases respiratory tract fluid secretions and helps to loosen phlegm and bronchial secretions. By reducing the viscosity of secretions and increasing sputum volume, guaifenesin increases the efficiency of the cough reflex and of ciliary action in removing accumulated secretions from the trachea and bronchi. As a result, bronchial drainage is improved and less frequent.

➤*Pharmacokinetics:*

Absorption – Guaifenesin is readily absorbed from the gastrointestinal tract.

Metabolism/Excretion – Guaifenesin is rapidly metabolized and excreted in the urine. Guaifenesin has a plasma half-life of 1 hour. The major urinary metabolite is β-(2-methoxyphenoxy) lactic acid.

Contraindications

These products are contraindicated in patients with hypersensitivity to guaifenesin.

Warnings/Precautions

➤*Kidney stone formation:* Reports in the literature have suggested that consumption of large quantities of guaifenesin-containing medications may be associated with an increased risk of drug-induced kidney stone formation.

➤*Evaluation:* Before prescribing medication to suppress or modify cough, it is important to ascertain that the underlying cause of cough is identified, that modification of cough does not increase the risk of clinical or physiological complications, and that appropriate therapy for the primary disease is instituted.

➤*Pregnancy: Category C.* Animal reproduction studies have not been conducted. Safe use in pregnancy has not been established relative to possible adverse effects on fetal development. It is not known whether guaifenesin tablets can cause fetal harm when administered to a pregnant woman or can affect reproduction capacity. Therefore, this product should not be used in pregnant patients, unless in the judgment of the physician, the potential benefits outweigh possible hazards. Guaifenesin tablets should be given to a pregnant woman only if clearly needed.

➤*Lactation:* It is not known whether guaifenesin is excreted in human milk. Because many drugs are excreted in human milk, caution should be exercised when guaifenesin is administered to a nursing woman, and a decision should be made whether to discontinue nursing or to discontinue the drug, taking into account the importance of the drug to the mother.

➤*Children:*

400 mg tablets – Guaifenesin 400 mg tablets are not recommended to children under 6 years of age.

600 mg sustained-release tablets – Safety and efficacy of 600 mg sustained-release tablets in pediatric patients under the age of 12 years have not been established.

Drug Interactions

➤*Drug/Lab test interactions:* Guaifenesin may increase renal clearance for urate and thereby lower serum uric acid levels. Guaifenesin may produce an increase in urinary 5-hydroxyindoleacetic (5-HIAA) acid and may therefore interfere with the interpretation of this test for the diagnosis of carcinoid syndrome. It may also falsely elevate the vanillylmandelic acid (VMA) test for catechols. Administration of this drug should be discontinued 48 hours prior to the collection of urine specimens for such tests.

Adverse Reactions

Guaifenesin is well tolerated and has a wide margin of safety. Products containing guaifenesin have been associated with nausea, vomiting, GI discomfort, dizziness, headache, skin rash, and urticaria.

Overdosage

➤*Symptoms:* Overdosage with guaifenesin is unlikely to produce toxic effects since its toxicity is low. Guaifenesin, when administered by stomach tube to test animals in doses up to 5 g/kg, produced no signs of toxicity.

➤*Treatment:* In severe cases of overdosage, treatment should be aimed at reducing further absorption of the drug. Gastric emptying (emesis or gastric lavage) is recommended as soon as possible after ingestion. Treatment is symptomatic and supportive.

Patient Information

Do not give this product to children under 2 years of age, unless directed by a physician. Do not take guaifenesin for persistent or chronic cough such as occurs with smoking, asthma, chronic bronchitis, emphysema, or if cough is accompanied by excessive phlegm (mucus), unless directed by a physician. A persistent cough may be a sign of a serious condition. If cough persists for more than 1 week, tends to recur, or is accompanied by fever, rash, or persistent headache, consult a physician.

Combination products are frequently used in respiratory conditions. These products present two problems: (1) The patient may not need the components of the product; (2) the patient may need the components, but in different strengths or intervals.

➤Product Selection Guidelines: When recommending a respiratory combination product, consider the following guidelines.

Patient's data –

Symptoms: Pain, fever, congestion, runny nose, productive/nonproductive cough.

Patient's medical history/health: Age, allergy history, pregnancy, heart disease, hypertension, asthma, bronchitis, glaucoma, hyperthyroidism, diabetes, depression.

Drugs patient is currently taking: Other cold or allergy medications; medications for hypertension, diabetes, etc.

Do not exceed the recommended dosage. Do not take an *otc* product for greater than 7 days. If symptoms do not improve or are accompanied by fever, consult a physician.

Humidification of room air and adequate fluid intake (6 to 8 glasses/day) are important in treating cold symptoms.

Sulfite/Tartrazine sensitivity – Some of these products contain sulfites or tartrazine, which may cause allergic-type reactions (eg, hives, itching, wheezing, anaphylaxis) in certain susceptible persons. Although overall prevalence of sensitivity in general population is probably low, it is seen more frequently in asthmatics or in atopic nonasthmatic persons (sulfites) or in those with aspirin hypersensitivity (tartrazine).

Sugar free liquid products (sf) – The small amount of sugar in usual doses of medication is probably insignificant to the well controlled diabetic. However, consider the effects of alcohol and sympathomimetics in addition to the sugar content.

Sustained release formulations – Products with identical active ingredients are listed together. Due to formulation differences, do not consider them bioequivalent.

Dosage – Usually average adult dose. For children, consult package literature or physician.

➤Groups: These combination products are presented in groups based on the components of their formulations. Products with identical or similar ingredients are listed adjacent to each other, regardless of therapeutic claims, which may differ even for identical formulations. Pediatric preparations (those products intended mainly or exclusively for children) are grouped at the end of each respective section.

Antiasthmatic Combinations – These contain xanthine derivatives and sympathomimetics for bronchodilation. Many products also contain expectorants to facilitate mobilization of mucus.

- Xanthine Combinations
- Xanthine-Sympathomimetic Combinations

Upper Respiratory Combinations – These are used primarily for relief of symptoms associated with colds, upper respiratory tract infections and allergic conditions (eg, acute rhinitis, sinusitis).

- Decongestant Combinations
- Antihistamine and Analgesic Combinations
- Decongestant and Antihistamine Combinations
- Decongestant, Antihistamine and Analgesic Combinations
- Decongestant, Antihistamine and Anticholinergic Combinations

Cough Preparations – These include an antitussive or expectorant, but may also contain ingredients for relief of associated symptoms.

- Antitussive Combinations
- Expectorant Combinations
- Narcotic Antitussives with Expectorants
- Nonnarcotic Antitussives with Expectorants
- Antitussive and Expectorant Combinations

➤Ingredients: An FDA advisory review panel has proposed monographs for all *otc* cold, cough, allergy, bronchodilator and antihistamine products. In addition, the FDA proposes to classify *otc* drugs as "monograph conditions" (old Category I) and "nonmonograph conditions" (old Categories II and III). When using these combination products, consider the prescribing information for each ingredient.

Antihistamines – (See individual monograph). These are used for symptomatic relief from allergic rhinitis (hay fever) including runny nose, sneezing, itching of the nose or throat, and itchy and watery eyes. The anticholinergic effects of antihistamines may cause a thickening of bronchial secretions; therefore, these agents may be counterproductive in respiratory conditions characterized by congestion. Antihistamines may cause drowsiness.

Xanthines – (See individual monograph). These, primarily theophylline, relieve bronchial spasm by direct action on the bronchial smooth muscle in bronchospastic conditions such as asthma and chronic bronchitis. Product listings include anhydrous theophylline dosage equivalents. Some xanthine-containing combination products are available *otc,* but asthmatic patients should use them only under physician supervision.

Sympathomimetics – These are used for their α-adrenergic (vasoconstrictor/decongestant) or β_2-adrenergic (bronchodilator) effects.

Decongestants: Used for temporary relief of nasal congestion due to colds or allergy. Given orally, they are less effective than topical nasal decongestants, and they have a potential for systemic side effects. Frequent or prolonged topical use may lead to local irritation and rebound congestion.

Bronchodilators: Ephedrine common in these combinations, stimulates cardiac (β_1) receptors. Bronchodilation is weaker than with catecholamines; α-adrenergic effects may decrease congestion of mucous membranes. Other β-active agents are effective bronchodilators, but pseudoephedrine is not.

Narcotic antitussives – The antitussive dose is lower than that required for analgesia. Consider general precautions for the use of narcotics, including the potential for abuse, when using these products. See Narcotic Antitussive monograph for complete prescribing information. See also the Narcotic Agonist Analgesics monograph for complete information on the narcotics.

Codeine: 10 to 20 mg every 4 to 6 hours.
Hydrocodone (dihydrocodeinone): 5 to 10 mg every 6 to 8 hours.
Hydromorphone HCl: 2 mg every 4 hours.

Nonnarcotic antitussives – These decrease the cough reflex without inducing many of the common characteristics of narcotic preparations.

Dextromethorphan: 10 to 30 mg every 4 to 8 hours.
Diphenhydramine: 25 mg every 4 hours.

Carbetapentane: This has atropine-like and local anesthetic actions and suppresses cough reflex through selective depression of the medullary cough center.

- *Dose –* 15 to 30 mg, 3 or 4 times daily.

Caramiphen edisylate: A weak anticholinergic and centrally acting antitussive.

- *Dose –*
  - *Adults:* 10 to 20 mg every 4 to 6 hours.
  - *Children (6 to 12):* 5 to 10 mg q 4 to 6 h.
  - *Children (2 to 6):* 2.5 to 5 mg q 4 to 6 h.

Expectorants – In the FDA's final monograph for *otc* expectorants, guaifenesin (see individual monograph) is the only agent approved for use as an expectorant. Guaifenesin may help loosen phlegm and thin bronchial secretions to rid the bronchial passageways of bothersome mucus, drain bronchial tubes or make coughs more productive. Humidification of room air and adequate fluid intake (6 to 8 glasses/day) are important therapeutic measures as well.

Dose:

- *Adults –* 200 to 400 mg every 4 hours, not to exceed 2400 mg in 24 hours.
- *Children –* Lower dosages are specified on labeling. Consult a physician for children younger than 2 years of age.

Other ingredients not upgraded by the FDA include: Ammonium chloride, beechwood creosote, benzoin preparations, camphor, eucalyptol/eucalyptus oil, iodines, ipecac syrup, menthol/peppermint oil, pine tar preparations, potassium guaiacolsulfonate, sodium citrate, squill preparations, terpin hydrate preparations, tolu preparations and turpentine oil. Products containing these ingredients must be reformulated.

Analgesics – These (eg, acetaminophen, aspirin, ibuprofen, sodium salicylate) are frequently included to treat headache, fever, muscle aches, pain. See individual monographs.

Anticholinergics – (See individual monograph). These are included for their drying effects on mucus secretions. This action may be beneficial in acute rhinorrhea; however, drying of respiratory secretions may lead to thickened mucus and more difficult expectoration. Traditionally, anticholinergics have been avoided in patients with asthma or chronic obstructive pulmonary disease (COPD); however, some patients respond well to these agents. Caution is still advised in this group.

An anticholinergic for oral inhalation is available as a bronchodilator for maintenance of bronchospasm associated with COPD, including chronic bronchitis and emphysema (see Ipratropium monograph).

The FDA has ruled that no anticholinergic product for *otc* use is recognized as safe and effective. Therefore, the products must be reapproved by new drug application (NDA) before November 10, 1986, or be regarded as misbranded (*Federal Register* 1985 Nov 8; 50:46582-87).

Papaverine HCl – (See individual monograph). This relaxes the smooth muscle of the bronchial tree.

Barbiturates – (See individual monograph). These are included for sedative effects as "correctives" with xanthines or sympathomimetics which may cause CNS stimulation. The sedative efficacy of low doses (eg, 8 mg phenobarbital) is questionable.

Caffeine – (See individual monograph). This is included for CNS stimulation to counteract antihistamine depression and to enhance concomitant analgesics.

XANTHINE COMBINATIONS

Content given per tablet or 5 mL.

	Product & Distributor	Xanthine[a]	Expectorant	Average Dose	Excipients & How Supplied
Rx	**Dyphylline-GG Elixir** (Various, eg, Breckenridge, Qualitest, Silarx)	33.3 mg dyphylline	33.3 mg guaifenesin	**Adults** - 30 mL qid; **Children > 6 y** - 15 to 30 mL tid or qid	17% alcohol, saccharin, sucrose. In 473 mL.
Rx	**Lufyllin-GG Elixir** (Medpointe)				17% alcohol, saccharin, sucrose. Wine flavor. In 473 and 3,785 mL.
Rx sf	**Jay-Phyl Syrup** (JayMac)	100 mg dyphylline	50 mg guaifenesin	**> 12 y** - 10 mL tid or qid; **6 to 12 y** – lowest dose possible, not to exceed 10 mg/kg/day	Vanilla flavor. Alcohol free. In 473 mL.
Rx	**Difil-G Forte Liquid** (Stewart-Jackson)	100 mg dyphylline	100 mg guaifenesin	**Adults** - 5 to 10 mL tid or qid; **Children > 6 y** - 2 to 3 mg dyphylline per lb of body weight	Menthol flavor. In 237 mL.
Rx	**Dilex-G Syrup** (Poly)			**Adults** - 5 to 10 mL tid or qid	Alcohol free. Parabens, saccharin, sucrose, sorbitol. Menthol flavor. In 473 mL.
Rx	**Dy-G Liquid** (Cypress)			**Adults** - 5 to 10 mL tid or qid; **Children > 6 y** - 2 to 3 mg dyphylline per lb of body weight	Alcohol free. Mint flavor. In 473 mL.
Rx sf	**Dilex-G 200 Syrup** (Poly)	100 mg dyphylline	200 mg guaifenesin	**Adults** - 5 to 10 mL tid or qid; **Children > 6 y** - 80 to 100 lbs: ⅔ to ¾ tsp tid 60 to 80 lbs: ½ to ⅔ tsp tid; 40 to 60 lbs: ¼ to ⅓ tsp qid	In 473 mL.
Rx	**Dyphylline & Guaifenesin Tablets** (Various, eg, Breckenridge, Cypress)	200 mg dyphylline	200 mg guaifenesin	**Adults** - 1 qid; **Children** - > 6 y - ½ to 1 tid or qid	May contain dextrose. In 100s.
Rx	**Dyflex-G Tablets** (Econo Med)			1 or 2 qid	In 100s and 1,000s.
Rx	**Difil-G Tablets** (Stewart-Jackson)	200 mg dyphylline	300 mg guaifenesin	**Adults** - 1 tid or qid	(SJ/647). Capsule shape. In 100s.
Rx	**Difil-G 400 Tablets** (SJ Pharmaceuticals)	200 mg dyphylline	400 mg guaifenesin	**Adults** - 1 tid or qid; in severe cases, dosage may be doubled	Maltodextrin. (SJP/226). White, capsule shape. In 100s.
Rx	**Dilex-G 400 Tablets** (Poly)			**Adults** - 1 tid or qid	(Dilex/G Poly 400). Gold, oblong, scored. In 100s.
Rx sf	**Ed-Bron G Liquid** (Edwards)	50 mg theophylline	33.3 mg guaifenesin	**> 12 y** - 15 to 30 mL tid or qid; **6 to 12 y** - 10 to 15 mL tid or qid; **3 to 6 y** - 5 to 7.5 mL tid or qid; **1 to 3 y** - 2.5 to 5 mL tid or qid	In 473 mL.

[a] Theophylline content given as anhydrous unless otherwise specified.

Refer to the general discussion of these products in the Respiratory Combinations Introduction.

DECONGESTANT AND ANALGESIC COMBINATIONS

Content given per capsule, tablet, 5 mL, or 1 mL (oral drops).

	Product & Distributor	Decongestant	Analgesic	Average Dose	Excipients & How Supplied
otc	**Tylenol Infants' Drops Plus Cold** (McNeil Consumer)	1.56 mg phenylephrine HCl	100 mg acetaminophen	**2 to 3 y** – 1.6 mL q 4 h, up to 8 mL/day	Sorbitol, sucralose. Bubble-gum flavor. In 15 mL w/ dropper.
otc	**Alka-Seltzer Plus Sinus Tablets** (Bayer Consumer)	5 mg phenylephrine HCl	250 mg acetaminophen	≥ **12 y** – 2 tablets dissolved in 120 mL (4 oz) water q 4 h, up to 8/day	Acesulfame K, 4.2 mg phenylalanine, saccharin, 477 mg sodium, sorbitol. In 20s.
otc	**Dilotab II Tablets** (Zee Medical)	5 mg phenylephrine HCl	325 mg acetaminophen	≥ **12 y** – 2 q 4 h, up to 12/day	In 100s and 250s.
otc	**Excedrin Sinus Headache Tablets** (Novartis Consumer Health)				Film-coated. In 24s, 50s, and 100s.
otc	**Māpap Sinus Congestion and Pain Maximum Strength Tablets** (Major)				Acesulfame K. Capsule shape. In 24s.
otc	**Sinutab Sinus Maximum Strength Tablets** (McNeil)				PEG. Capsule shape. In 24s.
otc	**Sudafed PE Sinus Headache Maximum Strength Tablets** (McNeil)				PEG. Capsule shape. In 24s.
otc	**Tylenol Sinus Congestion & Pain Daytime Caplets** and **Gelcaps** (McNeil Consumer Healthcare)				**Caplets:** PEG, sucralose. Cool burst flavor. In 24s and 48s. **Gelcaps:** EDTA, parabens. In 24s and 48s.
otc	**Vicks DayQuil Sinex Liqui-caps** (Proctor & Gamble)			≥ **12 y** – 2 q 4 h, up to 8/day	Glycerin, PEG, sorbitol. In 20s.
otc	**Sine-Off Non-Drowsy Maximum Strength Tablets** (Hogil)	5 mg phenylephrine HCl	500 mg acetaminophen	≥ **12 y** – 2 q 6 h, up to 8/day	In 24s.
otc	**Ornex No Drowsiness Tablets** (B.F. Ascher)	30 mg pseudoephedrine HCl	325 mg acetaminophen	≥ **12 y** – 2 q 4 to 6 h, up to 8/day; **6 to < 12 y** – 1 q 4 to 6 h, up to 4/day	Lactose, PEG. Capsule shape. In 24s and 48s.
otc	**Māpap Sinus Maximum Strength Tablets** (Major)	30 mg pseudoephedrine HCl	500 mg acetaminophen	≥ **12 y** – 2 q 4 to 6 h, up to 8/day	PEG. In 24s.
otc	**Ornex No Drowsiness Maximum Strength Tablets** (BF Ascher)			≥ **12 y** – 2 q 6 h, up to 8/day	PEG. Capsule shape. In 24s.
otc	**Tylenol Sinus Non-Drowsy Maximum Strength Geltabs, Tablets,** and **Gelcaps** (McNeil)			2 q 4 to 6 h up to 8/day[a]	**Tablets:** (TYLENOL Sinus). Capsule shape. In 24s. **Geltabs:** Parabens. (TYLENOL SINUS). In 24s, 48s, and 60s. **Gelcaps:** Parabens. (TYLENOL SINUS). In 24s, 48s, and 60s.

DECONGESTANT AND ANALGESIC COMBINATIONS

	Product & Distributor	Decongestant	Analgesic	Average Dose	Excipients & How Supplied
otc	**Ibuprofen Children's Cold Suspension** (Major)	15 mg pseudoephedrine HCl	100 mg ibuprofen	**6 to 11 y** – 10 mL q 6 h, up to 40 mL/day; **2 to 5 y** – 5 mL q 6 h, up to 20 mL/day	Alcohol free. Acesulfame K, corn syrup. Berry flavor. In 120 mL.
otc	**Advil Children's Cold Suspension** (Pfizer Consumer Healthcare)				Edetate disodium, glycerin, polysorbate 80, sodium 3 mg, sodium benzoate, sorbitol, sucrose. Grape flavor. In 120 mL.
otc	**Motrin Children's Cold Suspension** (McNeil)				Dye free. Acesulfame K, sucralose, sucrose. Berry, grape, or tropical punch flavors. In 118 mL.
otc	**Advil Cold & Sinus Tablets** and **Liqui-gels** (Wyeth Consumer)	30 mg pseudoephedrine HCl	200 mg ibuprofen	**≥ 12 y** – 1 to 2 q 4 to 6 h, up to 6/day	Tablets: Parabens, sucrose. Oval. In 20s. Liqui-gels: Liquid filled. PEG, sorbitol. In 16s.
otc	**Aleve Cold & Sinus Tablets** (Bayer Consumer)	120 mg pseudoephedrine HCl (extended release)	220 mg naproxen sodium (equiv to 200 mg naproxen) (immediate release)	**≥ 12 y** – 1 q 12 h, up to 2/day	Extended release. Lactose, 20 mg sodium. Capsule shape. In 10s, 20s, 24s, and 30s.
otc	**Aleve Sinus & Headache Tablets** (Bayer Consumer)				Extended release. Lactose, PEG, 20 mg sodium. Capsule shape. In 10s and 20s.

[a] Children's dosing could not be verified. Please refer to the manufacturer's prescribing information for more information.

For complete and comparative prescribing information, refer to the Respiratory Combinations Introduction.

DECONGESTANT AND EXPECTORANT COMBINATIONS

Content given per capsule, tablet, 1 mL (oral drops), or 5 mL.

	Product & Distributor	Decongestant	Expectorant	Other	Average Dose	Excipients & How Supplied
Rx	**Broncholate Syrup** (Sanofi-Aventis)	6.25 mg ephedrine HCl	100 mg guaifenesin		≥ **12 y** - 10 to 20 mL q 4 h, up to 120 mL/day	Orange flavor. In 473 mL.
otc	**Primatene Asthma Tablets** (Wyeth Consumer)	12.5 mg ephedrine HCl	200 mg guaifenesin		≥ **12 y** -1 to 2 q 4 h, up to 12/day	In 24s and 60s.
otc	**Bronkaid Dual Action Tablets** (Bayer)	25 mg ephedrine sulfate	400 mg guaifenesin		≥ **12 y** - 1 q 4 h up to 6/day	Capsule shape. In 24s.
Rx sf	**Donatussin Drops** (Laser)	1.5 mg phenylephrine HCl	20 mg guaifenesin		**6 to < 12 y** - 2 mL q 4 to 6 h, up to 8 mL/day; **2 to < 6 y** - 1 mL q 4 to 6 h, up to 4 mL/day	Sugar free, alcohol free. Saccharin, sorbitol. Raspberry flavor. In 30 mL with dropper.
Rx sf	**PE-GUAI Drops** (Palmetto)				**6 to < 12 y** - 2 mL q 4 to 6 h, up to 8 mL/day; **2 to < 6 y** - 1 mL q 4 to 6 h, up to 4 mL/day	Sugar free, alcohol free. Saccharin, sorbitol. Raspberry flavor. In 30 mL with dropper.
otc	**Supress-PE Pediatric Drops** (Kramer-Novis)	2.5 mg phenylephrine HCl	50 mg guaifenesin		**2 to < 6 y** - 1 mL q 4 h, up to 6 mL/day	Parabens, sucralose, sucrose. Grape flavor. In 30 mL.
otc	**Triaminic Chest & Nasal Congestion Liquid** (Novartis Consumer)				**6 to < 12 y** - 10 mL q 4 h, up to 60 mL/day; **2 to < 6 y** - 5 mL q 4 h, up to 30 mL/day	Tropical flavor. In 118 mL.
otc	**Mucinex Cold for Kids Liquid** (Reckitt Benckiser)	2.5 mg phenylephrine HCl	100 mg guaifenesin		**6 to < 12 y** - 10 mL q 4 h, up to 60 mL/day; **4 to < 6 y** - 5 mL q 4 h, up to 30 mL/day	Alcohol free. Dextrose, parabens, saccharin, sorbitol, sucralose. Mixed berry flavor. In 118 mL.
otc sf	**Despec Liquid** (International Ethical)	5 mg phenylephrine HCl	100 mg guaifenesin		≥ **12 y** - 5 to 10 mL q 4 to 6 h, up to 60 mL/day; **6 to < 12 y** - 5 mL q 4 to 6 h, up to 30 mL/day	Alcohol free, dye free, sugar free. Glycerin, maltitol, propylene glycol, saccharin, sorbitol. Grape flavor. In 473 mL.
otc sf	**ED Bron GP Liquid** (Edwards Pharmaceuticals)				≥ **12 y** - 10 mL q 4 h, up to 60 mL/day; **6 to < 12 y** - 5 mL q 4 h, up to 30 mL/day	Alcohol free, dye free, sugar free. Parabens, potassium citrate, potassium sorbate, propylene glycol, sorbitol, sucralose. Orange flavor. In 473 mL.
otc	**Rescon-GG Liquid** (Capellon)				≥ **12 y** -10 mL q 4 to 6 h, up to 40 mL/day; **6 to < 12 y** - 5 mL q 4 to 6 h, up to 20 mL/day; **2 to < 6 y** - 2.5 mL q 4 to 6 h, up to 10 mL/day	Alcohol free, dye free. Parabens, sorbitol, sugar. Cherry flavor. In 118 and 473 mL.
otc	**Robitussin PE Head and Chest Congestion Liquid** (Wyeth Consumer)				≥ **12 y** - 10 mL q 4 h, up to 60 mL/day; **6 to < 12 y** - 5 mL q 4 h, up to 30 mL/day; **2 to < 6 y** - 2.5 mL q 4 h, up to 15 mL/day	Menthol, sorbitol, sucralose. In 118 mL.

DECONGESTANT AND EXPECTORANT COMBINATIONS

	Product & Distributor	Decongestant	Expectorant	Other	Average Dose	Excipients & How Supplied
Rx	**Guaifenesin/Phenylephrine Hydrochloride Syrup** (Kylemore)	5 mg phenylephrine HCl	200 mg guaifenesin		≥ **12 y** - 5 to 10 mL q 4 to 6 h, up to 60 mL/day; **6 to < 12 y** - 5 mL q 4 to 6 h, up to 30 mL/day; **2 to < 6 y** - 2.5 mL q 4 to 6 h, up to 15 mL/day	Edetate disodium, parabens, sucralose, sucrose. Strawberry vanilla flavor. In 473 mL.
Rx *sf*	**Guiatex PE Syrup** (Breckenridge)				**> 12 y** - 5 to 10 mL q 4 to 6 h, up to 60 mL/day; **6 to 12 y** - 2.5 to 5 mL q 4 to 6 h, up to 30 mL/day	Sugar free, alcohol free. PEG, saccharin, sorbitol, sucralose. Strawberry flavor. In 473 mL.
Rx	**J-Max Syrup** (Jaymac)				≥ **12 y** - 5 to 10 mL q 4 to 6 h, up to 60 mL/day; **6 to < 12 y** - 5 mL q 4 to 6 h, up to 30 mL/day; **2 to < 6 y** - 2.5 mL q 4 to 6 h, up to 15 mL/day	Dye free, gluten free. Aspartame, parabens. Strawberry cream flavor. In 473 mL.
otc	**Liquibid PD-R Tablets** (Capellon)				≥ **12 y** - 2 q 4 h; **6 to < 12 y** - 1 q 4 h	In 90s.
otc	**Sinutab Non-Drying Capsules** (McNeil)				≥ **12 y** - 2 q 4 h, up to 12/day	Capsule shape. In 24s.
otc	**Sudafed PE Non-Drying Sinus Caplets** (McNeil)					Capsule shape. In 24s.
Rx	**Sitrex PD Liquid** (Vindex)	7.5 mg phenylephrine HCl	75 mg guaifenesin		**> 12 y** - 5 to 10 mL q 4 to 6 h, up to 40 mL/day; **6 to 12 y** - 5 mL q 4 to 6 h, up to 20 mL/day; **2 to 6 y** - 2.5 mL q 4 to 6 h, up to 10 mL/day	Alcohol free, dye free. Punch flavor. In 473 mL.
Rx	**PE/GG Liquid** (Kylemore)	7.5 mg phenylephrine HCl	100 mg guaifenesin		≥ **12 y** - 5 to 10 mL q 4 to 6 h, up to 40 mL/day; **6 to 12 y** - 2.5 to 5 mL q 4 to 6 h, up to 20 mL/day	Propylene glycol, propylparaben, saccharin, sodium benzoate, sorbitol. Orange flavor. In 473 mL.
Rx	**Crantex Liquid** (Breckenridge)				≥ **12 y** - 5 to 10 mL q 4 to 6 h, up to 40 mL/day; **6 to 12 y** - 5 mL q 4 to 6 h, up to 20 mL/day; **2 to 6 y** - 2.5 mL q 4 to 6 h, up to 10 mL/day	Alcohol free, dye free. Saccharin, sorbitol. In 473 mL.
Rx	**Entex Liquid** (Andrx)					Alcohol free, dye free. Punch flavor. In 15 and 473 mL.
Rx	**Sil-Tex Liquid** (Silarx)					Alcohol free, dye free. Saccharin, sorbitol. Punch flavor. In 473 mL.

DECONGESTANT AND EXPECTORANT COMBINATIONS

	Product & Distributor	Decongestant	Expectorant	Other	Average Dose	Excipients & How Supplied
Rx	**Guaifed-PD Capsules** (Victory)	7.5 mg phenylephrine HCl	200 mg guaifenesin		**≥ 12 y** - 1 to 2 q 12 h; **6 to < 12 y** - 1 q 12 h	Extended-release. Parabens, sucrose. (GUAIFED-PD). Purple/White. In 30s and 100s.
Rx sf	**Lusair Liquid** (Centurion)				**≥ 12 y** - 10 mL q 4 to 6 h, up to 40 mL/day; **6 to 12 y** - 5 mL q 4 to 6 h, up to 20mL/day; **2 to 6 y** - 2.5 mL q 4 to 6 h, up to 10 mL/day	Sugar free, alcohol free. Strawberry flavor. In 473 mL.
Rx	**Nariz Liquid** (Hawthorn)				**≥ 12 y** - 10 mL q 4 to 6 h, up to 40 mL/day; **6 to 12 y** - 5 mL q 4 to 6 h, up to 20 mL/day; **2 to 6 y** - 2.5 mL q 4 to 6 h, up to 10 mL/day	Saccharin, sorbitol. Bubble gum flavor. In 473 mL.
Rx	**Tussbid PD Capsules** (Breckenridge)				**≥ 12 y** - 1 or 2 q 12 h; ***6 to < 12 y*** - 1 q 12 h	Extended-release. (B 089). In 100s.
Rx sf	**Zyrphen Liquid** (Akyma)				**≥ 12 y** - 10 mL q 4 to 6 h, up to 40 mL/day; **6 to < 12 y** - 5 mL q 4 to 6 h, up to 20 mL/day; **2 to < 6 y** - 2.5 mL q 4 to 6 h, up to 10 mL/day	Sugar free, alcohol free. Saccharin, sorbitol. Bubble gum flavor. In 473 mL.
Rx	**Zotex GPX Tablets** (Vertical[b])	8.5 mg phenylephrine HCl	550 mg guaifenesin		**≥ 12 y** - 1 or 2 q 12 h, up to 4/day; **6 to < 12 y** - ½ or 1 q 12 h, up to 2/day	Extended-release. (VP 020). Capsule shape. In 100s.
otc sf	**Entex LQ Liquid** (WraSer)	10 mg phenylephrine HCl	100 mg guaifenesin		**> 12 y** - 5 mL q 4 h, up to 30 mL/day; **6 to < 12 y** - 2.5 mL q 4 h, up to 15 mL/day; **2 to < 6 y** - 1.25 mL q 4 h, up to 7.5 mL/day	Alcohol free, sugar free. Benzoic acid, edetate disodium, glycerin, propylene glycol, sorbitol. Strawberry flavor. In 473 mL.
otc	**Deconex IR Tablets** (Poly)	10 mg phenylephrine HCl	380 mg guaifenesin		**≥ 12 y** - 1 q 4 h, up to 6/day	Maltodextrin. (POLY 716). Green, oval, scored. In 60s.
Rx	**Gilphex TR Tablets** (Gil Pharmaceutical[d])	10 mg phenylephrine HCl	388 mg guaifenesin		**≥ 12 y** - 1 q 6 h up to 4/day; **6 to < 12 y** - ½ q 6 h up to 4/day	Dye free, preservative free. Lactose, maltodextrin, mineral oil. (GIL 304). Capsule shape, scored. Film-coated. In 100s and 500s.
Rx	**Deconex Capsules** (Poly Pharmaceuticals)	10 mg phenylephrine HCl	390 mg guaifenesin		**≥ 12 y** - 1 q 4 h, up to 6/day	(Deconex 582). Blue/Orange. In 60s.
Rx	**AMBI 10PEH/400GFN Tablets** (Ambi Pharmaceuticals)	10 mg phenylephrine HCl	400 mg guaifenesin		**> 12 y** - 1 q 4 h, up to 6/day; **6 to 12 y** - ½ to q 4 h, up to 3/day	(AMBI 402). White, capsule shape, scored. In 100s.
otc	**Liquibid D-R Tablets** (Capellon)				**≥ 12 y** - 1 q 4 h; **6 to 12 y** - ½ q 4 h	In 90s.
otc	**Medent-PEI Tablets** (SJP)				**≥ 12 y** - 1 q 4 to 6, up to 4/day	Maltodextrin. In 100s.
otc	**MucusRelief Sinus Tablets** (Major)				**≥ 12 y** - 1 q 4 h, up to 6/day	In 60s.
Rx	**ExeFen-PD Tablets** (Larken)	10 mg phenylephrine HCl	600 mg guaifenesin		**≥ 12 y** - 1 or 2 q 12 h; **6 to 12 y** - ½ to 1 q 12 h	Extended-release. (LL50). Blue, capsule shape, scored. In 100s.
Rx	**Medent-PE Tablets** (SJP[c])	12.5 mg phenylephrine HCl	600 mg guaifenesin		**> 12 y** - 1 q 8 h or 1 to 2 q 12 h, up to 4/day	Extended-release. Dye free. (SJP 224). Oval. In 100s.

DECONGESTANT AND EXPECTORANT COMBINATIONS

	Product & Distributor	Decongestant	Expectorant	Other	Average Dose	Excipients & How Supplied
Rx	**Guaifed Capsules** (Victory)	15 mg phenylephrine HCl	400 mg guaifenesin		≥ **12 y** - 1 q 12 h	Extended-release. Parabens, sucrose. (GUAIFED 400-15 VICTORY). Purple/White. In 30s and 100s.
Rx	**Tussbid Capsules** (Breckenridge)	15 mg phenylephrine HCl	400 mg guaifenesin			Extended-release. Sugar. (B 088). In 100s.
Rx	**Phenylephrine HCl/Guaifenesin Tablets** (Brighton)	15 mg phenylephrine HCl	600 mg guaifenesin		2 bid q 12 h[a]	Extended-release. (BP 300). Capsule shape, scored. In 100s.
Rx	**SINUvent PE Tablets** (WE Pharm)				≥ **12 y** - 2 bid q 12 h; **6 to 12 y** - 1 bid q 12 h	Extended-release. (WE 35). Lt. green, capsule shape, scored. In 100s.
Rx	**Liquibid-PD Tablets** (Capellon)	20 mg phenylephrine HCl (5 mg immediate-release/ 15 mg extended-release)	315 mg guaifenesin (120 mg immediate-release/195 mg extended-release)		≥ **12 y** - 2 q 12 h; **6 to 12 y** - 1 q 12 h	Extended-release. (Star 2). Blue/White, triangular, scored. In 90s.
Rx	**GFN 600/Phenylephrine 20 Tablets** (Cypress)	20 mg phenylephrine HCl	600 mg guaifenesin		≥ **12 y** - 1 to 2 q 12 h, up to 2/day; **6 to 12 y** - ½ to 1 q 12 h, up to 1/day	Extended-release. Dye free. (CYP 269). Oval, scored. In 100s.
Rx	**Xedec Tablets** (Cypress)	20 mg phenylephrine HCl	800 mg guaifenesin		≥ **12 y** - 1 q 8 h, up to 3/day; **6 to 12 y** - ½ q 8 h, up to 1½/day	Extended-release. Dye free. (CYP 324). Oval, scored. In 100s.
Rx	**Sitrex Tablets** (Vindex)	20 mg phenylephrine HCl	1,200 mg guaifenesin		≥ **12 y** - 1 q 12 h, up to 2/day; **6 to < 12 y** - ½ q 12 h, up to 1/day	Extended-release. Dye free. (VX 076). Capsule shape, scored. In 100s.
Rx	**Gentex LA Tablets** (Gentex)	23.75 mg phenylephrine HCl	650 mg guaifenesin		**> 12 y** - 1 q 12 h, up to 2/day; **6 to 12 y** - ½ q 12 h, up to 1/day	Extended-release. (GENTEX LA). Capsule shape, scored. In 100s.
Rx	**Deconsal II Tablets** (Cornerstone)	25 mg phenylephrine HCl	275 mg guaifenesin		≥ **12 y** - 1 to 2 q 12 h, up to 3/day; **6 to 12 y** - 1/day	Extended-release. (CBP). Blue/White, bilayered. In 100s.
Rx	**Guaifen PE Tablets** (Breckenridge)	25 mg phenylephrine HCl	800 mg guaifenesin		**> 12 y** - 1 q 12 h, up to 2/day; **6 to 12 y** - ½ q 12 h, up to 1/day	Extended-release. Dye free. (B428). Oval, scored. In 100s.
Rx	**Guaifenesin 900 mg/Phenylephrine HCl 25 mg Tablets** (Brighton)	25 mg phenylephrine HCl	900 mg guaifenesin		≥ **12 y** - 1 q 12 h; **6 to < 12 y** - ½ q 12 h, up to 1/day	Extended-release. Dye free. (100/100). Capsule shape. In 100s.
Rx	**Duratuss Tablets** (Victory)					Extended-release. (900/25). In 100s.
Rx	**ExeTuss Tablets** (Larken)				≥ **12 y** - 1 q 12 h, up to 2/day; **6 to < 12 y** - ½ q 12 h, up to 1/day	Extended-release. (LL 80). Capsule shape. In 100s.
Rx	**Phenylephrine HCl/Guaifenesin Tablets** (Brighton)	25 mg phenylephrine HCl	1,200 mg guaifenesin		1 q 12 h, up to 2/day[a]	Extended-release. Dye free. (200/200). In 100s.
Rx	**Duratuss GP Tablets** (Victory)				≥ **12 y** - 1 q 12 h, up to 2/day	Extended-release. (1200/25). In 100s.
Rx	**ExeTuss GP Tablets** (Larken)					Extended-release. (LL 81). Capsule shape, scored. In 100s.
Rx	**Simuc-GP Tablets** (Cypress)					Extended-release. (CYP 327). Capsule shape, scored. In 100s.
Rx	**Guaphenyl LA Capsules** (River's Edge)	30 mg phenylephrine HCl (extended-release)	400 mg guaifenesin (immediate-release)		≥ **12 y** - 1 q 12 h, up to 2/day	Extended-release. Sucrose. (RE 140). Blue/White. In 100s.
Rx	**Dynex LA Tablets** (Athlon)	30 mg phenylephrine HCl	800 mg guaifenesin (400 mg extended-release/400 mg immediate-release)		≥ **12 y** - 1 q 12 h, up to 2/day; **6 to 12 y** - ½ q 12 h, up to 1/day	Extended-release. (DYN). Lt green/yellow, bilayered, capsule shape, scored. In 100s.
Rx	**Entex LA Tablets** (Andrx)				≥ **12 y** - 1 q 12 h, up to 2/day	Extended-release. Dye free. (ENTEX LA 330/330). Oval, scored. In 100s.

DECONGESTANT AND EXPECTORANT COMBINATIONS

	Product & Distributor	Decongestant	Expectorant	Other	Average Dose	Excipients & How Supplied
Rx	**Guaifenesin/Phenylephrine HCl Tablets** (Various, eg, River's Edge, Prasco)	30 mg phenylephrine HCl	900 mg guaifenesin		≥ **12 y** - 1 q 12 h, up to 2/day; **6 to 12 y** - ½ q 12 h, up to 1/day	Extended-release. Oval, scored. In 100s.
Rx	**MyDex Tablets** (Larken)					Extended-release. (LL 32). Capsule shape, scored. In 100s.
Rx	**Visonex Tablets** (Vision)					Extended-release. (VP 9). Oval, scored. Film-coated. In 100s.
Rx	**D-Phen 1000 Tablets** (Midlothian)	30 mg phenylephrine HCl	1,000 mg guaifenesin		**> 12 y** - 1 q 12 h, up to 2/day; **6 to 12 y** - ½ q 12 h, up to 1/day	Extended-release. (ML 174). Capsule shape, scored. In 100s.
Rx	**Extendryl G Tablets** (Auriga)				≥ **12 y** - 1 q 12 h; **6 to < 12 y** - ½ q 12 h, up to 1/day	Extended-release. Dye free. (AP 204). In 100s.
Rx	**Zinx GP Tablets** (Auriga)					Extended-release. (AP 204). Capsule shape. In 100s.
Rx	**Xedec II Tablets** (Cypress)	30 mg phenylephrine HCl	1,100 mg guaifenesin		≥ **12 y** - 1 q 12 h, up to 2/day; **6 to 12 y** - ½ q 12 h, up to 1/day	Extended-release. Dye free. (CYP 358). Oval, scored. In 100s.
Rx	**Phenylephrine HCl/Guaifenesin Tablets** (Prasco)	30 mg phenylephrine HCl	1,200 mg guaifenesin		≥ **12 y** - 1 q 12 h, up to 2/day; **6 to 12 y** - ½ q 12 h, up to 1/day	Extended-release. Dye free. (Prasco 328). Oval, scored. In 100s.
Rx	**Reluri Tablets** (Cypress)					Extended-release. Dye free. (CYP 355). Capsule shape, scored. In 100s.
Rx	**J-Max Tablets** (Jaymac)	35 mg phenylephrine HCl	1,200 mg guaifenesin		≥ **12 y** - 1 q 12 h, up to 2/day	Extended-release. (JMAX). In 100s.
Rx	**Phenylephrine HCl/Guaifenesin Tablets** (River's Edge)	40 mg phenylephrine HCl	600 mg guaifenesin		≥ **12 y** - 1 q 12 h; **6 to 12 y** - ½ q 12 h	Extended-release. (α 088). Oval, scored. In 100s.
Rx	**Liquibid-D Tablets** (Capellon)	40 mg phenylephrine HCl (extended-release)	650 mg guaifenesin (250 mg immediate release/400 mg extended-release)		≥ **12 y** - 1 q 12 h; **6 to 12 y** - ½ q 12 h	Extended-release. Lactose. (LIQUIBID D). Blue/White, capsule shape, scored. In 90s.
Rx	**Norel EX Tablets** (US Pharmaceutical)	40 mg phenylephrine HCl (extended-release)	800 mg guaifenesin (400 mg immediate-release/400 mg extended-release)		**> 12 y** - 1 q 12 h, up to 2/day	Extended-release. Lactose. (US 440). Lt blue/dk blue, bilayered, capsule shape. In 100s.
Rx	**D-Tab Tablets** (Palm)	40 mg phenylephrine HCl	1,200 mg guaifenesin		≥ **12 y** - 1 q 12 h; **6 to 12 y** - ½ q 12 h	Extended-release. (Palm). Lt green, capsule shape, scored. Film-coated. In 100s.
Rx	**PhenaVent D Tablets** (Ethex)					Extended-release. (ETHEX 444).Capsule shape. Film-coated. In 100s.
Rx	**Sina-12X Suspension** (MedPointe)	5 mg phenylephrine tannate	100 mg guaifenesin		**6 y** - 5 to 10 mL q 12 h; **2 to 6 y** - 2.5 to 5 mL q 12 h; titrate individually	Methylparaben, saccharin, sucrose. Grape flavor. In 118 mL.
Rx	**Sina-12X Tablets** (MedPointe)	25 mg phenylephrine tannate	200 mg guaifenesin		≥ **12 y** - 1 or 2 q 12 h; **6 to 11 y** - ½ or 1 q 12 h	(SINA 6301). Purple, capsule shape, scored. In 30s.
otc	**Coldonyl Tablets** (Dover)	5 mg phenylephrine HCl	100 mg guaifenesin	325 mg acetaminophen	≥ **12 y** - 2 q 4 h	In UD 500s.
otc	**Tylenol Sinus Congestion and Pain Severe Caplet** (McNeil Consumer Health)	5 mg phenylephrine HCl	200 mg guaifenesin	325 mg acetaminophen	≥ **12 y** - 2 q 4 h up to 12/day	Sucralose. Cool burst flavor. In 24s.
Rx	**Duratuss A Tablets** (Victory Pharma)	20 mg phenylephrine HCl	600 mg guaifenesin	650 mg acetaminophen	≥ **12 y** - 1 q 8 h, up to 3/day; **6 to < 12 y** - ½ q 8 h, up to 1½/day	Extended-release. (650 600). Capsule shape. In 100s.
otc	**Triacting Liquid** (Various, eg, Amerisource, Bergen, Topco)	15 mg pseudoephedrine HCl	50 mg guaifenesin		**6 to < 12 y** - 10 mL q 4 to 6 h, up to 40 mL/day; **2 to < 6 y** - 5 mL q 4 to 6 h, up to 20 mL/day	May contain EDTA, sorbitol, or sucrose. In 118 mL.

DECONGESTANT AND EXPECTORANT COMBINATIONS

	Product & Distributor	Decongestant	Expectorant	Other	Average Dose	Excipients & How Supplied
Rx	**Ambifed-G Tablets** (MCR American)	20 mg pseudoephedrine HCl	400 mg guaifenesin		**> 12 y** - 1 q 4 to 6 h, up to 6/day; **6 to < 12 y** - ½ q 4 to 6 h, up to 3/day	(AMBIFED-G). White, capsule shape, scored. In 100s.
otc	**Altarussin-PE Liquid** (Altaire Pharmaceuticals)	30 mg pseudoephedrine HCl	100 mg guaifenesin		10 mL q 4 h, up to 40 mL/day[a]	Alcohol free. Corn syrup, saccharin. In 118 mL.
otc	**Q-Tussin PE Syrup** (Qualitest)				**≥ 12 y** - 10 mL q 4 h, up to 40 mL/day; **6 to < 12 y** - 5 mL q 4 h, up to 20 mL/day; **2 to < 6 y** - 2.5 mL q 4 h, up to 10 mL/day	Alcohol free. Glucose, high fructose corn syrup, saccharin. In 188 mL.
Rx	**Respaire-30 Capsules** (Laser)	30 mg pseudoephedrine HCl	150 mg guaifenesin		**> 12 y** - 1 or 2 q 4 to 6 h, up to 8/day; **6 to 12 y** - 1 q 4 to 6 h, up to 4/day	Sugar. (LASER 360). Clear/Opaque lt green. In 100s.
otc	**Severe Congestion Tussin Softgels** (AmerisourceBergen)	30 mg pseudoephedrine HCl	200 mg guaifenesin		2 q 4 h up to 8/day[a]	Sorbitol. In 12s.
Rx	**Ambifed Tablets** (MCR American)	30 mg pseudoephedrine HCl	400 mg guaifenesin		**> 12 y** - 1 q 4 to 6 h, up to 6/day; **6 to < 12 y** - ½ q 4 to 6 h, up to 3/day	(AMBIFED). White, capsule shape, scored. In 100s.
Rx	**Tenar PSE Liquid** (Centrix)	40 mg pseudoephedrine HCl	200 mg guaifenesin		**≥ 12 y** - 10 mL, up to 4 times/day; **6 to 12 y** - 5 mL, up to 4 times/day, not to exceed 4 mg/kg of body weight of pseudoephedrine HCl/day; **2 to 6 y** - 2.5 mL, up to 4 times/day, not to exceed 4 mg/kg of body weight of pseudoephedrine HCl/day	Sorbitol, sucralose. Grape flavor. In 20 and 473 mL.
Rx	**AMBI 40PSE/400GFN Tablets** (Ambi Pharmaceuticals)	40 mg pseudoephedrine HCl	400 mg guaifenesin		**> 12 y** - 1 q 4 to 6 h, up to 6/day; **6 to < 12 y** - ½ q 4 to 6 h, up to 3/day	(AMBI 408). White, capsule shape, scored. In 100s.
Rx	**Despec-Tab Tablets** (International Ethical Labs)				**≥ 12 y** - 1 q 6 h, up to 4/day	Maltodextrin. (DESPEC TAB 400/40). White, oval, scored. In 60s.
otc	**SudaTex-G** (Larken)					Maltodextrin. (LL 243). White, oval, scored. In 100s.
otc	**Poly-Vent IR Tablets** (Poly)	45 mg pseudoephedrine HCl	400 mg guaifenesin		**≥ 12 y** - 1 q 6 h, up to 4/day	Maltodextrin. (POLY 561). Blue, oval, scored. In 60s.
Rx	**Stamoist E Tablets** (Magna)	45 mg pseudoephedrine HCl	600 mg guaifenesin		**> 12 y** - 1 bid; **6 to 12 y** - ½ bid	Extended-release. (17). Capsule shape, scored. In 100s.
Rx	**Poly-Vent JR Tablets** (Poly)	45 mg pseudoephedrine HCl	650 guaifenesin		**≥ 12 y** - 1 q 12 h; **6 to < 12 y** - ½ q 12 h	Extended-release. Maltodextrin. (POLY-VENT JR 650 45). White, scored. In 25s and 100s.
Rx	**Pseudoephedrine HCl/Guaifenesin Tablets** (Various, eg URL)	45 mg pseudoephedrine HCl	800 mg guaifenesin		1 to 1½ q 12 h, up to 3/day[a]	Scored. In 100s.
Rx	**Pseudoephedrine HCl/Guaifenesin Tablets** (River's Edge)				**> 12 y** -1 to 1½ q 12 h, up to 3/day; **6 to 12 y** -½ q 12 h, up to 1/day	Extended-release. (NL 705). Scored. In 100s.
Rx	**Pseudoephedrine HCl/Guaifenesin SR Tablets** (URL)	48 mg pseudoephedrine HCl	595 mg guaifenesin		1 or 2 q 12 h up to 4/day[a]	Extended-release. (α 1891). Capsule shape. In 100s.
Rx	**Coldmist JR Tablets** (Breckenridge)					Extended-release. (B 368). Scored. In 100s.

DECONGESTANT AND EXPECTORANT COMBINATIONS

	Product & Distributor	Decongestant	Expectorant	Other	Average Dose	Excipients & How Supplied
Rx	**Entex PSE Tablets** (Athlon)	50 mg pseudoephedrine HCl	525 mg guaifenesin		≥ **12 y** - 1 or 2 q 12 h	Extended-release. Dye free. (P525). Scored. White, capsule shape. In 100s.
Rx	**Pseudoephedrine HCl/Guaifenesin Tablets** (River's Edge)	50 mg pseudoephedrine HCl	1,200 mg guaifenesin		1 q 12 h[a]	Extended-release. (NL 732). Capsule shape. In 30s and 100s.
Rx	**Respa-1st Tablets** (Respa)	58 mg pseudoephedrine HCl	600 mg guaifenesin		≥ **12 y** - 1 or 2 q 12 h; **6 to < 12 y** - 1 q 12 h	Extended-release. (RESPA 87). Scored. In 100s.
Rx	**Nomuc-PE Capsules** (Cypress)	60 mg pseudoephedrine HCl	200 mg guaifenesin		**> 12 y** - 2 q 12 h, up to 4/day; **6 to 12 y** - 1 q 12 h, up to 2/day	Extended-release. Parabens. (CYP 353). Blue/Natural. In 100s.
Rx	**Respaire-60 SR Capsules** (Laser)					Extended-release. Corn starch, sugar. (LASER 0174). Green/ Clear. In 100s.
Rx	**AMBI 60PSE/400GFN Tablets** (AMBI)	60 mg pseudoephedrine HCl	400 mg guaifenesin		**> 12 y** - 1 q 4 to 6 h, up to 4/day; **6 to < 12 y** - ½ q 4 to 6 h, up to 2/day	(AMBI 406). White, capsule shape, scored. In 100s.
otc	**Congestac Tablets** (B.F. Ascher)					In 12s and 24s.
Rx	**Exefen-IR Tablets** (Larken)					Maltodextrin. (LL 154). White, oval. In 100s.
Rx	**Maxifed Tablets** (MCR American)					(MAXIFED). Green, capsule shape, scored. In 100s.
otc	**Medent-LDI Tablets** (SJP)				≥ **12 y** - 1 q 4 to 6 h, up to 4/day	In 100s.
Rx	**Pseudoephedrine HCl/Guaifenesin SR Tablets** (River's Edge)	60 mg pseudoephedrine HCl	500 mg guaifenesin		≥ **12 y** - 1 to 2 q 12 h; **6 to < 12 y** - ½ to 1 q 12 h	Extended-release. (NL 717). Capsule shape. In 100s.
Rx	**AMBI 60/580 Tablets** (AMBI)	60 mg pseudoephedrine HCl	580 mg guaifenesin		**> 12 y** - 1 or 2 q 12 h, up to 4/day; **6 to < 12 y** - ½ q 12 h, up to 1/day	(AMBI 121). Capsule shape. In 100s.
Rx	**Maxifed-G Tablets** (MCR American)				**> 12 y** - 1 to 2 q 12 h, up to 4/day; **6 to < 12 y** - 1 q 12 h, up to 2/day; **2 to < 6 y** - ½ q 12 h, up to 1/day	Extended-release. (MAXIFED-G). Capsule shape, scored. In 100s.
Rx	**SudaTex-G Tablets** (Larken)				**> 12 y** - 1 to 2 q 12 h, up to 4/day; **6 to < 12 y** - 1 q 12 h, up to 2/day	Extended-release. Dye free. (LL 41). Scored. White, capsule shape. In 100s.
otc	**Mucinex D Tablets** (Reckitt Benckiser)	60 mg pseudoephedrine HCl	600 mg guaifenesin		≥ **12 y** - 2 q 12 h, up to 4/day	Extended-release. In 18s.
Rx	**Guaifenex PSE 60 Tablets** (Ethex)				**> 12 y** - 1 or 2 q 12 h, up to 4/day; **6 to 12 y** - 1 q 12 h, up to 2/day; **2 to 6 y** - ½ q 12 h, up to 1/day	Extended-release. Lactose. (ETHEX 214). Blue, capsule shape, scored. In 100s.
Rx	**Iosal II Tablets** (Iopharm)				1 or 2 q 12 h, up to 4/day[a]	Extended-release. In 100s.
Rx	**AMBI 60/1,000 Caplets** (AMBI)	60 mg pseudoephedrine HCl	1,000 mg guaifenesin		**> 12 y** - 1 q 12 h, up to 2/day; **6 to 12 y (47 to 90 pounds)** - ½ q 12 h, up to 1/day	Extended-release. (AMBI 60/1,000). White, capsule shape, scored. In 100s.
Rx	**Ambifed-G Caplets** (MCR American)					Extended-release. (AMBI/G AMBIfED G). White, capsule shape, scored. In 100s.
Rx	**Maxifed Tablets** (MCR American)	80 mg pseudoephedrine	400 mg guaifenesin		**> 12 y** - 1 to 1 ½ q 12 h, up to 3/day; **6 to < 12 y** - ½ q 12 h, up to 1/day	(MAXIFED). Green, capsule shape, scored. In 100s.
Rx	**ExeFen Tablets** (Larken)	80 mg pseudoephedrine	780 guaifenesin		≥ **12 y** - 1 q 12 h, up to 2/day	(LL 52). White, capsule shape. In 100s.

DECONGESTANT AND EXPECTORANT COMBINATIONS

	Product & Distributor	Decongestant	Expectorant	Other	Average Dose	Excipients & How Supplied
Rx	**Pseudoephedrine HCl/Guaifenesin LA Tablets** (URL)	85 mg pseudoephedrine HCl	795 mg guaifenesin		1 q 12 h, up to 3/day[a]	Extended-release. (NL 734). Capsule shape. In 100s.
Rx	**Coldmist LA Tablets** (Breckenridge)				1 q 12 h, up to 2/day[a]	Extended-release. (B-367). Scored. In 100s.
Rx	**Guaifenex PSE 85 Tablets** (Ethex)				**> 12 y** - 1 q 12 h, up to 3/day; **6 to 12 y** - ½ q 12 h, up to 1/day	Extended-release. Lactose. (ETHEX 478). Capsule shape. In 100s.
Rx	**LEV/PSE/GG Capsules** (Varsity)	90 mg pseudoephedrine HCl	400 mg guaifenesin		**≥ 12 y** - 1 q 12 h, up to 2/day; **6 to 12 y** - 1/day	Extended-release. (035). Orange. In 100s.
Rx	**Poly-Vent Tablets** (Poly)	90 mg pseudoephedrine HCl	650 guaifenesin		**≥ 12 y** - 1 q 12 h; **6 to < 12 y** - ½ q 12 h	Extended-release. Maltodextrin. (POLY-VENT 650 90). White, scored. In 25s and 100s.
Rx	**Pseudoephedrine HCl/Guaifenesin Tablets** (River's Edge)	90 mg pseudoephedrine HCl	800 mg guaifenesin		1 q 12 h, up to 2/day[a]	Extended-release. White, oval, scored. In 100s.
Rx	**Dynex Tablets** (Athlon)	90 mg pseudoephedrine HCl	1,200 mg guaifenesin		1 q 12 h[a]	Extended-release. Dye free. (DG 033). Capsule shape, scored. In 30s and 100s.
Rx	**Respaire-120 SR Capsules** (Laser)	120 mg pseudoephedrine HCl (extended-release)	250 mg guaifenesin (immediate-release)		**> 12 y** - 1 q 12 h, up to 2/day	Extended-release. Corn starch, sugar. (LASER 0169). Orange/Clear. In 100s.
Rx	**Nasatab LA Tablets** (ECR Pharm)	120 mg pseudoephedrine HCl	500 mg guaifenesin		**> 12 y** - 1 bid; **6 to 12 y** - ½ bid	Extended-release. (MX 225). Capsule shape, scored. In 100s.
Rx	**Touro LA Tablets** (Dartmouth)	120 mg pseudoephedrine HCl	525 mg guaifenesin		**> 12 y** - 1 q 12 h; **6 to 12 y** - ½ q 12 h	Extended-release. (TOURO LA DP636). White, capsule shape. In 100s.
Rx	**Guaifenex PSE 120 Tablets** (Ethex)	120 mg pseudoephedrine HCl	600 mg guaifenesin		**≥ 12 y** - 1 q 12 h; **6 to < 12 y** -½ q 12 h	Extended-release. Dye free. (Ethex 208). Capsule shape, scored. In 100s.
Rx	**GuaiMAX-D Tablets** (Schwarz)					Extended-release. (GUAIMAX-D SP 2055). White to off-white, capsule shape, scored. In 100s.
Rx	**GFN/PSE Tablets** (Cypress)	120 mg pseudoephedrine HCl	1,200 mg guaifenesin		1 q 12 h, up to 2/day[a]	Extended-release. (CYP 266). In 100s.
Rx	**Guaifenex GP Tablets** (Ethex)				**≥ 12 y** - 1 q 12 h, up to 2/day	Extended-release. Dye free. Lactose. (ETHEX 373). Oval, scored. Film-coated. In 100s.
otc	**Maximum Strength Mucinex D** (Reckitt Benckiser)				**≥ 12 y** - 1 q 12 h, up to 2/day	Extended-release. (120/1200 MUCINEX). White/Red, oval. In 24s.
otc	**Tylenol Sinus Severe Congestion Tablets** (McNeil Consumer)	30 mg pseudoephedrine HCl	200 mg guaifenesin	325 mg acetaminophen	**≥ 12 y** - 2 q 4 to 6 h, up to 8/day	Mannitol, sucralose. Capsule shape. In 24s.
otc	**Poly-Vent Plus Tablets** (Poly Pharmaceuticals)	45 mg pseudoephedrine HCl	200 mg guaifenesin	500 mg acetaminophen	**≥ 12 y** - 1 q 6 h, up to 4/day	(POLY 500). White, capsule shape, scored. In 100s.

[a] Pediatric dosing could not be verified.
[b] Vertical Pharmaceuticals Inc, 3 Kellogg Court Suite #19, Edison, NJ 08817, Phone: 732-287-0044 http://www.verticalpharma.com.
[c] Stewart-Jackson Pharmacal Inc, 4587 Damascus Road, Memphis TN 38118, Phone: 800-367-1395 http://www.sjpharma.com.
[d] Gil Pharmaceutical Corporation, P.O. Box 10489, Ponce, Puerto Rico 00733-0489, Phone: 787-848-9114 http://www.gilpharmaceutical.com/pages/2/index.htm.

Refer to the general discussion of these products in the Respiratory Combinations Introduction.

ANTIHISTAMINE AND ANALGESIC COMBINATIONS

Content given per tablet or 5 mL.

	Product & Distributor	Antihistamine	Analgesic	Average Dose	Excipients & How Supplied
otc	**Coricidin HBP Cold & Flu Tablets** (Schering-Plough)	2 mg chlorpheniramine maleate	325 mg acetaminophen	**> 12 y** - 2 q 4 to 6 h up to 12/day **6 to 12 y** - 1 q 4 to 6 h up to 5/day	In 12s.
otc	**Tylenol Sore Throat Nighttime Liquid** (McNeil Consumer)	8.3 mg diphenhydramine hydrochloride	166.6 mg acetaminophen	≥ **12 y** - 30 mL q 4 to 6 h up to 120 mL/day	Sodium 3.6 mg/5 mL, sorbitol, sucralose, sucrose. Cool burst flavor. In 240 mL.
otc	**Tylenol Severe Allergy Tablets** (McNeil)	12.5 mg diphenhydramine hydrochloride	500 mg acetaminophen	≥ **12 y** - 2 q 4 to 6 h up to 8/day	Capsule shape. In 24s.

For complete and comparative prescribing information, refer to the Respiratory Combinations Introduction.

DECONGESTANT, ANTIHISTAMINE, AND EXPECTORANT COMBINATIONS

Content given per tablet, 1 mL, or 5 mL.

	Product & Distributor	Decongestant	Antihistamine	Expectorant	Other	Average Dose	Excipients & How Supplied
Rx	**P Chlor GG Drops** (Boca)	2 mg phenylephrine HCl	1 mg chlorpheniramine maleate	20 mg guaifenesin		≥ **1 to 2 y** - 1 to 2 mL q 4 to 6 h up to 4 doses/day ≥ **6 mo to < 1 y** - 0.6 to 1 mL q 4 to 6 h up to 4 doses/day ≥ **3 mo to < 6 mo** - 0.3 to 0.6 mL q 4 to 6 h up to 4 doses/day **< 3 mo** - 2 to 3 drops/mo of age q 4 to 6 h up to 4 doses/day	Peach flavored. In 30 mL with dropper.
Rx	**Qual-Tussin Pediatric Drops** (Pharmaceutical Associates)						Parabens, saccharin, sucrose. Peach flavored. In 30 mL with dropper.
Rx	**Ryna-12X Suspension** (MedPointe)	5 mg phenylephrine tannate	30 mg pyrilamine tannate	100 mg guaifenesin		≥ **6 y** -5 to 10 mL q 12 h **2 y to < 6 y** - 2.5 to 5 mL q 12 h titrate dose individually	Methylparaben, saccharin, sucrose. Grape flavor. In 120 mL.
Rx	**SymPak Tablets** (Dexo LLC)	*Day:* 15 mg phenylephrine HCl		600 mg guaifenesin		≥ **12 y** - 2 in a.m.; **6 to 12 y** - 1 in a.m.	In cartons with 2 blister cards of 14 day dosing regimen of day/night tablets).
		Night: 25 mg phenylephrine HCl	8 mg chlorpheniramine maleate		2.5 mg methscopolamine nitrate	≥ **12 y** - 1 in p.m.; **6 to 12 y** - ½ in p.m.	
Rx	**Ryna-12X Tablets** (MedPointe)	25 mg phenylephrine tannate	60 mg pyrilamine tannate	200 mg guaifenesin		≥ **12 y** - 1 to 2 q 12 h; **6 to < 12 y** - ½ to 1 q 12 h	(RYNA 1708). Blue, oval, scored. In 30s.

Refer to the general discussion of these products in the Respiratory Combinations Introduction.

DECONGESTANTS AND ANTIHISTAMINES

Content given per capsule, tablet, 5 mL or 1 mL oral drops.

	Product & Distributor	Decongestant	Antihistamine	Average Dose	Excipients & How Supplied
Rx	**Alacol Oral Drops** (Ballay)	1 mg phenylephrine HCl	0.4 mg brompheniramine maleate	**2 to < 6 y** - 2.5 mL q 4 h, up to 15 mL/day	Saccharin, sorbitol. In 30 mL w/dropper.
otc	**Dimetapp Children's Cold & Allergy Elixir** (Wyeth)	2.5 mg phenylephrine HCl	1 mg brompheniramine maleate	**≥ 12 y** - 20 mL q 4 h, up to 120 mL/day; **6 to < 12 y** - 10 mL q 4 h up, to 60 mL/day	Alcohol free. Sorbitol, sucralose. Grape flavor. In 237 mL w/dosage cup.
Rx *sf*	**Alacol Syrup** (Ballay)	5 mg phenylephrine HCl	2 mg brompheniramine maleate	**> 12 y** -10 mL q 4 h, up to 60 mL/day; **6 to 12 y** - 5 mL q 4 h, up to 30 mL/day; **2 to < 6 y** - 2.5 mL q 4 h, up to 15 mL/day	Alcohol free. Saccharin, sorbitol. Black raspberry flavor. In 473 mL.
Rx	**Alenaze-D Liquid** (Cypress)	7.5 mg phenylephrine HCl	2 mg brompheniramine maleate	**≥ 12 y** – 10 mL q 6 h, up to 40 mL/day; **6 to 12 y** - 5 mL q 6 h, up to 20 mL/day; **2 to 6 y** - 2.5 mL q 6 h, up to 10 mL/day	Saccharin, sorbitol. Bubble gum flavor. In 473 mL.
Rx	**Alenaze-D NR Liquid** (Cypress)	7.5 mg phenylephrine HCl	4 mg brompheniramine maleate	**≥ 12 y** - 5 mL q 6 h, up to 30 mL/day; **6 to 12 y** - 2.5 mL q 6 h, up to 15 mL/day; **2 to 6 y** - 1.25 mL q 6 h, up to 7.5 mL/day	Saccharin, sorbitol. Bubble gum flavor. In 474 mL.
Rx	**VaZol-D Liquid** (Wraser)				Maltitol, saccharin, sorbitol. Bubble gum flavor. In 474 mL.
Rx	**Phenylephrine HCl 7.5 mg/ Brompheniramine Maleate 6 mg Capsules** (Brighton Pharmaceuticals)	7.5 mg phenylephrine HCl	6 mg brompheniramine maleate	**≥ 12 y** - 1 to 2 q 12 h; **6 to < 12 y** - 1 q 12 h	Parabens, sucrose. Extended release. (BP-500). Purple, opaque. In 100s.
Rx	**Brovex PB Tablets** (MCR American)	10 mg phenylephrine HCl	4 mg brompheniramine maleate	**> 12 y** - 1 q 4 to 6 h, up to 6/day; **6 to < 12 y** - ½ q 4 to 6 h, up to 3/day	(BROVEX PB). White, capsule shape, scored. In 100s.
Rx	**V-Hist Suspension** (Macoven Pharmaceuticals)	10 mg phenylephrine HCl	6 mg brompheniramine maleate	**> 12 y** - 5 to 10 mL qid; **6 to 12 y** - 5 mL qid; **2 to 6 y** - 2.5 mL qid	Acesulfame, aspartame, glycerin, methylparaben, phenylalanine 5.863 mg per 5 mL, sodium benzoate. Bubble gum flavor. In 118 mL.
Rx	**Entre-B Suspension** (Acella Pharmaceuticals)			**> 12 y** - 5 to 10 mL q 12 h, **6 to 12 y** - 5 mL q 12 h	Benzoic acid, glycerin, parabens, propylene glycol, saccharin. Bubble gum flavor. In 118 mL.
Rx	**Vazotab Chewable Tablets** (Wraser Pharmaceutical)	15 mg phenylephrine HCl	6 mg brompheniramine maleate	**> 12 y** - 1 q 12 h; **6 to 12 y** - ½ q 12 h	Saccharin, sucralose. (V T). Purple, scored. Grape flavor. In 60s.
Rx	**Phenylephrine HCl 15 mg/ Brompheniramine Maleate 12 mg Capsules** (Brighton Pharmaceuticals)	15 mg phenylephrine HCl	12 mg brompheniramine maleate	**≥ 12 y** - 1 q 12 h	Sugar. (12/15). Clear. In 100s.
Rx	**Respahist-II Tablets** (Respa Pharmaceuticals)	19 mg phenylephrine HCl	6 mg brompheniramine maleate	**> 12 y** - 1 or 2 q 12 h	Extended release. (RESPA 694). White, capsule shape. In 100s.
Rx	**Seradex-LA Tablets** (Allegis)				Extended release. (E0110). Capsule shape. In 100s.
Rx	**Tanabid SR Tablets** (Portal Pharmaceutical)	30 mg phenylephrine HCl	6 mg brompheniramine maleate	**> 12 y** - 1 q 12 h	(JTD). Pink, oval, scored. In 100s.
Rx	**Zotex-PE Tablets** (Vertical Pharmaceutical)				(JTD). Pink, oval, scored. In 100s.
Rx	**Histamax D Drops** (Laser)	1.5 mg phenylephrine HCl	1.5 mg carbinoxamine maleate	**12 to 24 mo** - 1 mL qid; **6 to 12 mo** - 0.75 mL qid; **3 to 6 mo** - 0.5 mL qid; **1 to 3 mo** - 2 to 3 drops per mo of age qid	Cotton candy flavor. In 30 mL w/dropper.
Rx *sf*	**XiraHist Pediatric Drops** (Hawthorn)	2 mg phenylephrine HCl	2 mg carbinoxamine maleate	**12 to 24 mo** - 1 mL qid **6 to 12 mo** - 0.75 mL qid **3 to 6 mo** - 0.5 mL qid	Alcohol and dye free. Saccharin, sorbitol. Strawberry flavor. In 30 mL w/dropper.

DECONGESTANTS AND ANTIHISTAMINES

	Product & Distributor	Decongestant	Antihistamine	Average Dose	Excipients & How Supplied
Rx	**Centergy Pediatric Drops** (Centurion)	2 mg phenylephrine HCl	1 mg chlorpheniramine maleate	**6 to < 12 y** - 2 mL every 4 to 6 h up to 8 mL/day; **2 to < 6 y** -1 mL every 4 to 6 h up to 4 mL/day.	Glycerin, sodium benzoate, sorbitol. Strawberry flavor. In 30 mL w/ dropper.
Rx	**Dallergy Drops** (Laser)			**12 to 24 mo** - 1 to 2 mL q 4 to 6 h up to 8 mL/day; **6 to 12 mo** - 0.6 to 1 mL q 4 to 6 h up to 4 mL/day; **3 to 6 mo** - 0.3 to 0.6 mL q 4 to 6 h up to 2.4 mL/day; **1 to 3 mo** - 2 to 3 drops per month of age q 4 to 6 h up to 9 drops/day.	Peach/Tangerine flavor. In 30 mL w/dropper.
Rx	**Nasohist Drops** (Hawthorn)			**6 to < 12** - 2 mL q 4 to 6 h; **2 to < 6 y** - 1 mL q 4 to 6 h.	Saccharin, sorbitol. Orange-vanilla flavor. In 30 mL.
Rx	**Sonahist Drops** (Kylemore Pharmaceuticals)				Parabens, saccharin, sorbitol. Orange-vanilla flavor. In 30 mL.
otc	**Triaminic Cold & Allergy Children's Syrup** (Novartis)	2.5 mg phenylephrine HCl	1 mg chlorpheniramine maleate	**6 to < 12 y** - 10 mL q 4 h up to 60 mL/day.	Acesulfame K, benzoic acid, edetate disodium, malitol, tartrazine. Orange flavor. In 118 mL.
Rx *sf*	**C-Phen Drops** (Boca)	3.5 mg phenylephrine HCl	1 mg chlorpheniramine maleate	**12 to 24 mo** - 1 mL 4 times daily; **6 to 12 mo** - 0.75 mL 4 times daily.	Alcohol, sugar free. Sorbitol. In 30 mL w/dropper.
Rx	**R-Tanna Pediatric Suspension** (Prasco Labs)	5 mg phenylephrine tannate	4.5 mg chlorpheniramine tannate	**≥ 6 y** - 5 to 10 mL q 12 h; **2 to < 6 y** - 2.5 to 5 mL q 12 h; **< 2 y** - Titrate dose individually.	Benzoic acid, glycerin, kaolin, pectin, methylparaben, saccharin, sucrose, tartrazine. In 473 mL.
Rx	**Rynatan Pediatric Chewable Tablets** (MedaPharm)			**≥ 6 y** - 1 to 2 q 12 h; **2 to < 6 y** -½ to 1 q 12 h.	Maltodextrin, saccharin, sucrose. (RYNATAN 712). Purple, capsule shape, scored. In 30s.
Rx	**Rynatan Pediatric Suspension** (MedaPharm)			**> 6 y** - 5 to 10 mL q 12 h; **2 to 6 y** - 2.5 to 5 mL q 12 h; Titrate dose individually.	Benzoic acid, glycerin, kaolin, pectin, methylparaben, saccharin, sucrose, tartrazine. Strawberry-currant flavor. In 473 mL.
otc	**Ed-A-Hist Tablets** (Edwards)	10 mg phenylephrine HCl	3 mg chlorpheniramine maleate	**≥ 12 y** — 1 q 4 h up to 6/day; **6 to < 12 y** — ½ q 4 h up to 3/day.	PEG, tartrazine. (E). Wheat, capsule shape, scored. In 100s.

DECONGESTANTS AND ANTIHISTAMINES

	Product & Distributor	Decongestant	Antihistamine	Average Dose	Excipients & How Supplied
otc	**Actifed Cold & Allergy Tablets** (McNeil Consumer)	10 mg phenylephrine HCl	4 mg chlorpheniramine maleate	**≥ 12 y** - 1 q 4 h up to 6/day; **6 to < 12 y** - ½ tablet q 4 h up to 3/day.	(A). In 12s.
otc	**Allerest PE Tablets** (Insight)				In 18s.
otc	**AMBI 10PEH/4CPM Tablets** (Ambi)			**≥ 12 y** - 1 q 4 to 6 h up to 6/day; **6 to < 12 y** - ½ q 4 to 6 h up to 3/day.	(AMBI 444). White, capsule shape, scored. In 100s.
otc	**Cold & Allergy Tablets** (Various, eg, Leader, Perrigo)			**≥ 12 y** - 1 q 4 to 6 h up to 6/day.	PEG. In 24s.
otc *sf*	**Ed A-Hist Liquid** (Edwards)			**≥ 12 y** - 5 mL q 4 h up to 30 mL/day; **6 to < 12 y** - 2.5 mL q 4 h up to 15 mL/day.	Gluten free and sugar free. Alcohol 5%, grape flavoring, propylene glycol, saccharin, sodium benzoate, sorbitol. In 473 mL.
Rx	**Maxichlor PEH Tablets** (MCR American)			**≥ 12 y** - 1 q 4 to 6 h up to 6/day; **6 to < 12 y** - ½ q 4 to 6 h up to 3/day.	(MOXICHLOR PEH). White, capsule shape, scored. In 100s.
otc	**Sudafed PE Sinus & Allergy Maximum Strength Tablets** (McNeil)			**≥ 12 y** - 1 q 4 h up to 6/day.	PEG. In 24s.
Rx *sf*	**C-Phen Syrup** (Boca)	12.5 mg phenylephrine HCl	4 mg chlorpheniramine maleate	**≥ 12 y** - 5 mL q 4 to 6 h up to 30 mL/day; **6 to < 12 y** - 2.5 mL q 4 to 6 h up to 15 mL/day; **2 to < 6 y** - 1.25 mL q 4 to 6 h up to 7.5 mL/day.	Alcohol free and sugar free. Sorbitol. In 118 and 473 mL.
Rx *sf*	**Ceron Syrup** (Cypress)				Alcohol free and sugar free. Saccharin, sorbitol. Raspberry flavor. In 473 mL.
Rx *sf*	**Sildec-PE Syrup** (Silarx)			**≥ 12 y** - 5 mL q 4 to 6 h up to 30 mL/day; **6 to < 12 y** - 2.5 mL q 4 to 6 h up to 15 mL/day.	Alcohol free and sugar free. Glycerin, saccharin, sodium benzoate, sorbitol. Raspberry flavor. In 118 and 473 mL.
Rx	**Rescon-Jr. Tablets** (Capellon)	20 mg phenylephrine HCl	3 mg chlorpheniramine maleate	**> 12 y** - 1 or 2 q 12 h; **6 to 12 y** - 1 q 12 h.	Extended release. (RESCON JR). Yellow/White, bilayered, capsule shape, scored. In 100s.
Rx	**Dallergy-JR Capsules** (Laser)	20 mg phenylephrine HCl	4 mg chlorpheniramine maleate	**> 12 y** - 2 q 12 h up to 4/day; **6 to 12 y** - 1 q 12 h up to 2/day.	Extended release. Sucrose. (Dallergy JR Laser 176). Maize/Clear. In 100s.
Rx	**NoHist Tablets** (Larken)	20 mg phenylephrine HCl	8 mg chlorpheniramine maleate	**≥ 12 y** -1 q 12 h; **6 to < 12 y** - ½ q 12 h.	Extended release. (LL 60). Capsule shape, scored. In 100s.
Rx *sf*	**Phenabid Tablets** (Gil)			**≥ 12 y** - 1 or 2 q 12 h; **6 to 12 y** - ½ to 1 q 12 h; **2 to 6 y** - ½ q 12 h.	Extended release. Dye free and sugar free. Scored. In 100s.
Rx	**R-Tanna Tablets** (Prasco Labs)	25 mg phenylephrine tannate	9 mg chlorpheniramine tannate	**Adults** - 1 or 2 q 12 h.	Extended release. (PRASCO 534). Buff, capsule shape, scored. In 100s.
Rx	**Rynatan Tablets** (MedaPharm)			**Adults** - 1 or 2 q 12 h.	Extended release. (RYNATAN 707). Buff, capsule shape, scored. In 100s.

DECONGESTANTS AND ANTIHISTAMINES

	Product & Distributor	Decongestant	Antihistamine	Average Dose	Excipients & How Supplied
Rx *sf*	**Nalex-A Liquid** (Blansett)	5 mg phenylephrine HCl	2.5 mg chlorpheniramine maleate, 7.5 mg phenyltoloxamine citrate	**> 12 y** - 10 mL q 4 to 6 h; **6 to 12 y** - 5 mL q 4 to 6 h; **2 to 6 y** - 1.25 to 2.5 mL q 4 to 6 h	Alcohol free. Cotton candy flavor. In 473 mL.
Rx *sf*	**NoHist-A Liquid** (Larken)				Alcohol free. Saccharin, sorbitol. Cotton candy flavor. In 473 mL.
Rx *sf*	**Phenyltoloxamine PE CPM Liquid** (Boca)			**> 12 y** - 10 mL q 4 to 6 h; **6 to 12 y** - 5 mL q 4 to 6 h; **2 to < 6 y** - 1.25 to 2.5 mL q 4 to 6 h	Alcohol free. Cotton candy flavor. In 473 mL.
Rx	**Rhinacon A Tablets** (Breckenridge)	20 mg phenylephrine HCl	4 mg chlorpheniramine maleate, 40 mg phenyltoloxamine citrate	**> 12 y** - 1 q 8 to 12 h, up to 3/day	Extended release. (B 138). White to off-white, capsule shape, scored. In 100s.
Rx	**Nalex-A Tablets** (Blansett)			**> 12 y** - 1 bid or tid; **6 to 12 y** - ½ bid or tid	Lactose. (Blansett 3 08). Beige, capsule shape, scored. In 100s.
Rx *sf*	**Polyhist PD Suspension** (Poly Pharmaceuticals, Inc.)	7.5 mg phenylephrine HCl	2 mg chlorpheniramine maleate, 12.5 mg pyrilamine maleate	**6 to 12 y** - 5 mL q 4 to 6 h; **2 to 6 y** - 2.5 mL q 4 to 6 h[a]	Alcohol and dye free. Saccharin, sorbitol. Bubble gum flavor. In 473 mL.
Rx *sf*	**MyHist-PD Liquid** (Larken)			**> 12 y** - 5 to 10 mL q 4 to 6 h, up to 50 mg phenylephrine/day; **6 to 12 y** - 5 mL q 4 to 6 h, up to 30 mg phenylephrine/day; **2 to 6 y** - 2.5 mL q 4 to 6 h, up to 15 mg phenylephrine/day	Alcohol and dye free. Parabens, saccharin, sorbitol. Bubble gum flavor. In 473 mL.
Rx	**NalDex Tablets** (Blansett Pharmacal)	18.5 mg phenylephrine HCl	3.5 mg dexbrompheniramine maleate	**≥ 12 y** - 1 q 12 h; **6 to 12 y** - ½ q 12 h	(NALDEX). Capsule shape. Scored. In 100s.
Rx	**Ala-Hist PE Tablets** (Poly Pharmaceuticals)	10 mg phenylephrine HCl	2 mg dexchlorpheniramine maleate	**≥ 12 y** - 1 q 4 to 6 h, up to 6/day; **6 to 12 y** - ½ q 4 to 6 h, up to 3/day	(Poly 782). Purple, capsule shape, scored. In 60s.
Rx	**Rescon-Jr. Tablets** (Capellon)	20 mg phenylephrine HCl	3 mg dexchlorpheniramine maleate	**≥ 12 y** - 1 to 2 q 12 h; **6 to 12 y** - 1 q 12 h	Extended release. (RES JR). Yellow/white, capsule shape, scored. In 90s.
otc	**Triaminic Night Time Cold & Cough Liquid** (Novartis)	2.5 mg phenylephrine HCl	6.25 mg diphenhydramine HCl	**6 to < 12 y** - 10 mL q 4 h up to 60 mL/day	Alcohol free. Acesulfame K, EDTA, maltitol. Grape flavor. In 118 mL w/dosage cup.
Rx	**Aldex-CT Chewable Tablets** (Zyber)	5 mg phenylephrine HCl	12.5 mg diphenhydramine HCl	**≥ 12 y** - 1 to 2 q 6 h; **6 to < 12 y** - ½ to 1 q 6 h	Magnasweet, mannitol, saccharin. (ZYBER M012). Blue, capsule shape, scored. Strawberry flavor. In 100s.
otc	**Pedia Care Children's NightRest Multi-Symptom Cold Liquid** (J & J)			**6 to < 12 y** - 5 mL q 4 h up to 30 mL/day	EDTA, sorbitol, sucralose. Grape flavor. In 118 mL.
Rx	**Pediatex-CT Tablets** (Zyber)			**≥ 12 y** - 1 to 2 q 12 h; **6 to < 12 y** - 0.5 to 1 q 12 h	Chewable. Saccharin. (ZYBER M012). Blue, scored. Strawberry flavor. In 100s.
otc	**Triaminic Children's Night Time Cold & Cough Thin Strips** (Novartis Consumer Health)			**6 to < 12 y** - 1 strip q 4 h up to 6/day	Maltodextrin, mannitol, sucralose. Grape flavor. In 14s.
Rx *sf*	**Alahist LQ Liquid** (Poly Pharmaceutical)	7.5 mg phenylephrine HCl	25 mg diphenhydramine HCl	**≥ 12 y** - 5 mL q 4 to 6 h up to 30 mL/day; **6 to 12 y** - 2.5 mL q 4 to 6 h up to 15 mL/day	Alcohol free, sugar free. Saccharin, sorbitol. Fruit candy flavor. In 473 mL.
otc	**Benadryl-D Allergy & Sinus Tablets** (J & J)	10 mg phenylephrine HCl	25 mg diphenhydramine HCl	**≥ 12 y** - 1 q 4 h up to 6/day	PEG. In 24s.
otc	**Sudafed PE Nighttime Nasal Decongestant Tablets** (McNeil)				PEG. In 12s.
otc	**Theraflu Nighttime Cold & Cough Thin-Strips** (Novartis Consumer Health)	10 mg phenylephrine HCl	25 mg diphenhydramine HCl	**≥ 12 y** - 1 strip q 4 h up to 6/day	Mannitol, sucralose. Peppermint flavor. In 12s.

DECONGESTANTS AND ANTIHISTAMINES

	Product & Distributor	Decongestant	Antihistamine	Average Dose	Excipients & How Supplied
otc	**Sudafed PE Day & Night Tablets** (McNeil Consumer)	*Day:* 10 mg phenylephrine HCl		≥ **12 y** - 1 q 4 h, up to 6/day	PEG. (PE). Round. In 18s.
		Night: 10 mg phenylephrine HCl	25 mg diphenhydramine HCl	≥ **12 y** - 1 q 4 h, up to 6/day	PEG. (PE). Capsule shape. In 12s.
Rx	**Promethazine HCl and Phenylephrine HCl Syrup** (Various, eg, Alpharma)	5 mg phenylephrine HCl	6.25 mg promethazine HCl	5 mL q 4 to 6 h up to 30 mL/day[b]	7% alcohol. May contain sorbitol, sugar, parabens. In 118 and 473 mL and 3.8 L.
Rx	**Promethazine VC Syrup** (Various, eg, Qualitest)			≥ **12 y** - 5 mL q 4 to 6 h up to 30 mL/day; **6 to < 12 y** - 2.5 to 5 mL q 4 to 6 h up to 30 mL/day; **2 to < 6 y** - 1.25 to 2.5 mL q 4 to 6 h	May contain alcohol 7%, menthol, parabens, saccharin, sucrose. In 118, 237, and 473 mL.
Rx	**Prometh VC Plain Syrup** (Alpharma)			5 mL q 4 to 6 h up to 30 mL/day[b]	7% alcohol. In 3.8 L.
Rx	**Pyril D Suspension** (Macoven Pharmaceuticals)	5 mg phenylephrine HCl	16 mg pyrilamine maleate	**> 12 y** - 5 to 10 mL q 6 h; **6 to 12 y** - 5 mL q 6 h; **2 to 6 y** - 2.5 mL q 6 h	Glycerin, methylparabens, saccharin, sodium benzoate, sucrose. Grape flavored. In 473 mL.
Rx	**Deconsal CT Chewable Tablets** (Cornerstone)	10 mg phenylephrine HCl	16 mg pyrilamine maleate	≥ **12 y** - up to 4/day; **6 to 12 y** - up to 2/day	Dye free. Saccharin, sugar. (CC). Mottled brown, round, scored. Grape flavor. In 100s.
otc	**Poly Hist Forte Tablets** (Poly Pharmaceuticals)	10 mg phenylephrine HCl	25 mg pyrilamine maleate	≥ **12 y** - 1 q 4 to 6 h, up to 6/day; **6 to 12 y** - ½ q 4 to 6 h, up to 3/day	(Poly 210). White, capsule shape, scored. In 100s.
Rx	**J-Tan D Suspension** (Jaymac)	1.58 mg phenylephrine tannate	2.2 mg brompheniramine tannate	≥ **12 y** - 5 to 10 mL q 12 h up to 20 mL/day; **6 to < 12 y** - 5 mL q 12 h, up to 10 mL/day; **4 to < 6 y** - 2.5 mL q 12 h, up to 5 mL/day	5 mg per 5 mL phenylalanine. Strawberry cream flavor. In 473 mL.
Rx	**C-Tan D Plus Oral Suspension** (Centurion Labs)	5 mg phenylephrine tannate	5 mg brompheniramine tannate	≥ **12 y** - 5 to 10 mL q 12 h up to 20 mL/day; **6 to < 12 y** - 5 mL q 12 h up to 10 mL/day	Raspberry flavor. In 473 mL.
Rx	**Relhist Chewable Tablets** (Burel Pharmaceuticals)	15 mg phenylephrine tannate	6 mg brompheniramine tannate	**> 12 y** - 1 q 6 to 8 h, up to 4/day; **6 to 12 y** - ½ q 6 to 8 h, up to 2/day	(C L). White, scored. Orange flavor. In 60s.
Rx	**Brompheniramine Phenylephrine Tannate Suspension** (ANI)	20 mg phenylephrine tannate	12 mg brompheniramine tannate	≥ **12 y** - 5 to 10 mL q 12 h up to 20 mL/day; **6 to < 12 y** - 5 mL q 12 h up to 10 mL/day; **2 to < 6 y** - 2.5 mL q 12 h up to 5 mL/day	Acesulfame K, aspartame, methylparaben, phenylalanine 6 mg/mL. Bubble gum flavor. In 473 mL.
Rx	**Phenyl Chlor-Tan Pediatric Suspension** (Hi-Tech)	5 mg phenylephrine tannate	4.5 mg chlorpheniramine tannate	**> 6 y** - 5 to 10 mL q 12 h; **2 to 6 y** - 2.5 to 5 mL q 12 h; titrate dose individually	Methylparaben, saccharin, sucrose. In 473 mL.
Rx	**Rynatan Pediatric Suspension** (MedPointe)				Methylparaben, saccharin, sucrose, tartrazine. Strawberry-currant flavor. In 473 mL.
Rx	**Rynatan Pediatric Chewable Tablets** (MedPointe)			**> 6 y** - 1 or 2 q 12 h; **2 to 6 y** - ½ to 1 q 12 h	Maltodextrin, saccharin, sucrose. (Rynatan 712). Purple, capsule shape, scored. Grape flavor. In 30s.
Rx	**Ed Chlor-PED D Suspension Drops** (Edwards)	6 mg phenylephrine tannate	2 mg chlorpheniramine tannate	**> 6 y** - 2 mL q 12 h; **2 to 6 y** - 1 mL q 12 h	Extended release. Methylparaben, saccharin. Apple sauce flavor. In 60 mL w/dropper.

DECONGESTANTS AND ANTIHISTAMINES

	Product & Distributor	Decongestant	Antihistamine	Average Dose	Excipients & How Supplied
Rx	**AllerX Suspension** (Cornerstone)	7.5 mg phenylephrine tannate	3 mg chlorpheniramine tannate	**≥ 12 y** - 15 mL q 12 h; **6 to 12 y** - 2.5 to 5 mL q 12 h; **2 to 6 y** - 1.25 to 2.5 mL q 12 h	Methylparaben, saccharin, sucrose. Raspberry flavor. In 473 mL.
Rx sf	**PediaPhyl D Suspension** (River's Edge)	10 mg phenylephrine tannate	8 mg chlorpheniramine tannate	**≥ 12 y** - 5 to 10 mL bid up to 20 mL/day; **6 to < 12 y** - 2.5 to 5 mL bid up to 10 mL/day; **2 to < 6 y** - 1.25 mL bid up to 5 mL/day	Aspartame, methylparaben, phenylalanine, saccharin, sorbitol. Bubble gum flavor. In 473 mL.
Rx sf	**PediaTan D Suspension** (ProEthic)				Magnasweet, methylparaben, saccharin, sorbitol. Bubble gum flavor. In 473 mL.
Rx sf	**P-Tann D Suspension** (Midlothian)				Magnasweet, methylparaben, saccharin, sorbitol. Bubble gum flavor. In 473 mL.
Rx	**BP Allergy Junior Suspension** (Brookstone)	20 mg phenylephrine tannate	4 mg chlorpheniramine tannate	**> 12 y** - 10 mL q 12 h up to 20 mL/day; **6 to < 12 y** - 5 mL q 12 h up to 10 mL/day; **2 to < 6 y** - 2.5 mL q 12 h up to 5 mL/day	Alcohol free. Aspartame, methylparaben, phenylalanine 5 mg per 5 mL, prosweet, saccharin, sorbitol. Bubble gum flavor. In 473 mL.
Rx	**Dallergy-JR Suspension** (Laser)				Alcohol free. Magnasweet, methylparaben, saccharin, sucrose. Peaches and cream flavor. In 473 mL.
Rx	**PE Tann/CP Tann Suspension** (Brighton)				Alcohol free. Aspartame, methylparaben, phenylalanine 5 mg/5 mL, saccharin. sorbitol. Bubble gum flavor. In 473 mL.
Rx	**Ny-Tannic Tablets** (Allegis)	25 mg phenylephrine tannate	9 mg chlorpheniramine tannate	**Adults** - 1 or 2 q 12 h	(KL 142). Tan, capsule shape. In 100s.
Rx	**Rynatan Tablets** (MedPointe)				(Rynatan 707). Buff, capsule shape, scored. In 100s.
Rx	**R-Tanna Tablets** (Prasco)				(Prasco 534). Buff, capsule shape, scored. In 100s.
Rx	**Phenylephrine Tannate/Chlorpheniramine Tannate/Pyrilamine Tannate Pediatric Suspension** (Duramed)	5 mg phenylephrine tannate	2 mg chlorpheniramine tannate, 12.5 mg pyrilamine tannate	**> 6 y** - 5 to 10 mL q 12 h; **2 to 6 y** - 2.5 to 5 mL q 12 h; titrate dose individually	Methylparaben, saccharin, sucrose. Strawberry-blackberry-currant flavor. In 118 mL unit of use and 473 mL.
Rx	**Nalex-A 12 Suspension** (Blansett)			**≥ 12 y** - 30 mL q 12 h; **6 to < 12 y** - 5 to 10 mL q 12 h; **2 to** 2.5 to 5 mL q 12 h	Methylparaben, sucrose, saccharin. Raspberry flavor. In 120 mL.
Rx	**Triotann Pediatric Suspension** (Prasco)			**> 6 y** - 5 to 10 mL q 12 h; **2 to 6 y** - 2.5 to 5 mL q 12 h; titrate dose individually	Methylparaben, saccharin, sucrose. Strawberry-blackberry-currant flavor. In 473 mL.
Rx	**Triple Tannate Pediatric Suspension** (Hi-Tech)				Methylparaben, saccharin, sucrose. In 473 mL.
Rx	**Conal Suspension** (Cypress)	15 mg phenylephrine tannate	8 mg chlorpheniramine tannate, 12.5 mg pyrilamine tannate	**≥ 12 y** - 5 to 10 mL every 12 h up to 20 mL/day; **6 to < 12 y** - 5 mL q 12 h up to 10 mL/day; **2 to < 6 y** - 2.5 mL q 12 h up to 5 mL/day	Aspartame, parabens, phenylalanine 7 mg/5 mL. Raspberry flavor. In 473 mL.
Rx	**D-Tann Suspension** (Midlothian)	7.5 mg phenylephrine tannate	25 mg diphenhydramine tannate	**≥ 12 y** - 5 to 10 mL q 12 h; **6 to < 12 y** - 2.5 to 5 mL q 12 h; **2 to < 6 y** - 1.25 to 2.5 mL q 12 h	Methylparaben, saccharin, sucrose. Bubble gum flavor. In 118 mL.
Rx	**Dytan-D Suspension** (Hawthorn)				Phenylalanine. Bubble gum flavor. In 118 mL.
Rx	**D-Tann Chewable Tablets** (Midlothian)	10 mg phenylephrine tannate	25 mg diphenhydramine tannate	**≥ 12 y** - 1 to 2 q 12 h; **6 to < 12 y** - ½ to 1 q 12 h	Phenylalanine. (ML 526). Blue, triangular. Berry flavor. In 60s.
Rx	**R-Tanna 12 Suspension** (Duramed)	5 mg phenylephrine tannate	30 mg pyrilamine tannate	**> 6 y** - 5 to 10 mL q 12 h; **2 to 6 y** - 2.5 to 5 mL q 12 h; titrate dose individually	Methylparaben, saccharin, sucrose. Strawberry-currant flavor. In 118 mL unit-of-use with syringe.
Rx	**Ryna-12 S Suspension** (MedPointe)				Methylparaben, saccharin, sucrose. Strawberry-currant flavor. In 118 mL unit-of-use with syringe.
Rx	**Rynesa 12S Suspension** (Amneal)				Methylparaben, saccharin, sucrose. Cherry berry flavor. In 118 and 473 mL.
Rx	**RY-T-12 Suspension** (Hi-Tech)				Methylparaben, saccharin, sucrose. Strawberry-currant flavor. In 118 and 473 mL.

DECONGESTANTS AND ANTIHISTAMINES

	Product & Distributor	Decongestant	Antihistamine	Average Dose	Excipients & How Supplied
Rx	**AllanVan-S B.I.D. Suspension** (Allan)	12.5 mg phenylephrine tannate	30 mg pyrilamine tannate	**> 12 y** - 5 to 10 mL q 12 h; **6 to 12 y** - 5 mL q 12 h; **2 to 6 y** - 2.5 mL q 12 h	Parabens, saccharin, sucrose. Grape flavor. In 480 mL.
Rx	**K-Tan Tablets** (Prasco)	25 mg phenylephrine tannate	60 mg pyrilamine tannate	**≥ 12 y** - 1 or 2 q 12 h; **6 to 11 y** - ½ or 1 q 12 h	(Prasco 525). Buff, capsule shape, scored. In 100s.
Rx	**Ryna-12 Tablets** (MedPointe)				(Wallace 673). Buff, capsule shape, scored. In 100s.
Rx	**Semprex-D Capsules** (Celltech)	60 mg pseudoephedrine HCl	8 mg acrivastine	**≥ 12 y** - 1 q 4 to 6 h up to 4/day	Lactose. (404 Semprex-D). Dark green/white. In 100s.
Rx *sf*	**Brompheniramine Maleate/ Pseudoephedrine HCl Drops** (Kylemore)	7.5 mg pseudoephedrine HCl	1 mg brompheniramine maleate	**12 to 24 mo** - 1 mL qid up to 4 mL/day; **6 to 12 mo** - 0.75 mL qid up to 3 mL/day; **3 to 6 mo** - 0.5 mL qid up to 2 mL/day; **1 to 3 mo** - 0.25 mL qid up to 1 mL/day	Alcohol free, dye free, sugar free. Glycerin, parabens, propylene glycol, saccharin, sorbitol. Cotton candy flavor. In 30 mL w/dropper.
Rx *sf*	**J-Tan D PD Drops** (Jaymac)				Alcohol and dye free. Saccharin, sorbitol. Strawberry-banana flavor. In 30 mL w/dropper.
Rx *sf*	**Bromhist-NR Drops** (Cypress)	12.5 mg pseudoephedrine HCl	1 mg brompheniramine maleate	**12 to 24 mo** - 1 mL qid up to 4 mL/day; **6 to 12 mo** - 0.75 mL qid up to 3 mL/day; **3 to 6 mo** - 0.5 mL qid up to 2 mL/day; **1 to 3 mo** - 0.25 mL qid up to 1 mL/day	Alcohol free. Saccharin, sorbitol. Cherry flavor. In 30 mL w/dropper.
otc	**Bromaline Solution** (Rugby)	15 mg pseudoephedrine HCl	1 mg brompheniramine maleate	**≥ 12 y** - 20 mL q 4 to 6 h, up to 80 mL/day; **6 to < 12 y** - 10 mL q 4 to 6 h, up to 40 mL/day	Alcohol free. Corn syrup, glycerin, propylene glycol, saccharin, sodium benzoate, sorbitol. Grape flavor. In 473 mL.
Rx *sf*	**Bromhist Pediatric Drops** (Cypress)			**12 to 24 mo** - 1 mL qid; **6 to 12 mo** - 0.75 mL qid; **3 to 6 mo** - 0.5 mL qid; **1 to 3 mo** - 0.25 mL qid	Alcohol and dye free. Saccharin, sorbitol. Cherry flavor. In 30 mL w/dropper.
otc	**Q-Tapp Elixir** (Qualitest)			**≥ 12 y** - 20 mL q 4 h up to 80 mL/day; **6 to < 12 y** - 10 mL q 4 h up to 40 mL/day	Alcohol free. Corn syrup, saccharin, sorbitol. Grape flavor. In 237 mL.
Rx	**Brovex PSB Liquid** (MCR American Pharmaceutical)	20 mg pseudoephedrine HCl	4 mg brompheniramine maleate	**> 12 y** - 5 to 10 mL q 4 to 6 h up to 40 mL/day; **6 to < 12 y** - 5 mL q 4 to 6 h up to 20 mL/day; **2 to < 6 y** - 2.5 mL q 4 to 6 h up to 10 mL/day	Saccharin, sorbitol. Cotton candy flavor. In 473 mL.
Rx	**TG 40PSE/4BRM Tablets** (TG United)	40 mg pseudoephedrine HCl	4 mg brompheniramine maleate	**> 12 y** - 1 q 4 to 6 h, up to 6/day; **6 to < 12 y** - ½ q 4 to 6 h, up to 3/day	(TG 704). White, capsule shape, scored. In 100s.
Rx	**Sildec Syrup** (Silarx)	45 mg pseudoephedrine HCl	4 mg brompheniramine maleate	**≥ 6 y** - 5 mL qid; **2 to 6 y** - 2.5 mL qid	Saccharin, sorbitol. Raspberry flavor. In 120 and 480 mL.
Rx	**BPM Pseudo 6/45 mg Tablets** (Boca)	45 mg pseudoephedrine HCl	6 mg brompheniramine maleate	**> 12 y** - 1 or 2 q 12 h; **6 to 12 y** - 1 q 12 h	Extended release. (BP 544). Oval, scored. In 30s and 100s.
Rx	**Bidhist-D Tablets** (Cypress)				Extended release. (CYP 470). Oval. In 100s.
Rx	**Lodrane 12 D Tablets** (ECR)				Extended release. Dye free. (ECR 645). Oval, scored. In 100s.
Rx	**LoHist 12D Tablets** (Larken)				Extended release. Dye free. (LH 12D). Scored. In 100s.
Rx	**Sinuhist Tablets** (Airpharma)				Dye free. (DX 114). White, oval. In 100s.

DECONGESTANTS AND ANTIHISTAMINES

	Product & Distributor	Decongestant	Antihistamine	Average Dose	Excipients & How Supplied
Rx	**Brompheniramine Maleate/ Pseudoephedrine HCl Syrup** (Cypress)	60 mg pseudoephedrine HCl	4 mg brompheniramine maleate	**> 6 y** - 5 mL qid; **2 to 6 y** - 2.5 mL qid	Saccharin, sorbitol. Raspberry flavor. In 473 mL.
Rx sf	**Lodrane Liquid** (ECR)			**> 12 y** - 5 mL q 4 to 6 h up to 20 mL/day; **6 to 12 y** - 2.5 mL q 4 to 6 h up to 10 mL/day; **2 to 6 y** - 1.25 mL q 4 to 6 h up to 5 mL/day; **< 2 y** - titrate dose individually	Alcohol and dye free. Cherry flavor. In 473 mL.
Rx sf	**LoHist-LQ Liquid** (Larken)				Alcohol and dye free. Saccharin, sorbitol. Cherry flavor. In 473 mL.
Rx sf	**PSE-BPM Liquid** (Boca)				Alcohol and dye free. Cherry flavor. In 473 mL.
Rx	**Touro Allergy Capsules** (Dartmouth)	60 mg pseudoephedrine HCl	5.75 mg brompheniramine maleate	1 or 2 q 12 h[b]	Extended release. Sucrose. (Touro Allergy). Orange/Clear. In 100s.
Rx	**Respahist Capsules** (Respa)	60 mg pseudoephedrine HCl	6 mg brompheniramine maleate	**> 12 y** - 1 to 2 q 12 h; **6 to 12 y** - 1 q 12 h	Extended release. Sucrose. In 100s.
Rx	**Brovex SR Capsules** (MCR American)	90 mg pseudoephedrine HCl	9 mg brompheniramine maleate	1 q 12 h up to 2/day[b]	Extended release. Sucrose. (271 9/90). Blue/Yellow. In 100s.
Rx	**Histex SR Capsules** and **Tablets** (Tiber)	120 mg pseudoephedrine HCl	10 mg brompheniramine maleate	**> 12 y** - 1 q 12 h	**Capsules:** Extended release. Sucrose. (NL 738). Peach/Clear. In 100s. **Tablets:** Extended release. Lactose. (TL). Peach, capsule shape. In 100s.
Rx	**Lodrane 24 D Capsules** (ECR)	90 mg pseudoephedrine HCl	12 mg brompheniramine maleate	**> 12 y** - 1 or 2/day; **6 to 12 y** - 1/day	Extended release. (ECR 24 D). Blue. In 60s.
Rx	**ULTRAbrom Capsules** (WE Pharm)	120 mg pseudoephedrine HCl	12 mg brompheniramine maleate	1 q 12 h	Extended release. In 100s and dispenser pack 10s.
Rx sf	**Cordron-D NR Liquid** (Cypress)	12.5 mg pseudoephedrine HCl	2 mg carbinoxamine maleate	**≥ 6 y** - 10 mL qid; **18 mo to 6 y** - 5 mL qid; **9 to 18 mo** - 3.75 to 5 mL qid; **6 to 9 mo** - 3.75 mL qid; **3 to 6 mo** - 2.5 mL qid; **1 to 3 mo** - 1.25 mL qid	Alcohol and dye free. Saccharin, sorbitol. In 473 mL.
Rx sf	**Pseudo Carb Pediatric Liquid** (Boca)			**≥ 6 y** - 10 mL q 4 to 6 h; **18 mo to 6 y** - 5 mL q 4 to 6 h; **9 to 18 mo** - 3.75 to 5 mL q 4 to 6 h; **6 to 9 mo** - 3.75 mL q 4 to 6 h; **3 to 6 mo** - 2.5 mL q 4 to 6 h; **1 to 3 mo** - 1.25 mL q 4 to 6 h	Alcohol and dye free. In 118 and 473 mL.
Rx	**Sildec Oral Drops** (Silarx)	15 mg pseudoephedrine HCl	1 mg carbinoxamine maleate	**12 to 24 mo** - 1 mL qid; **6 to 12 mo** - 0.75 mL qid; **3 to 6 mo** - 0.5 mL qid; **1 to 3 mo** - 0.25 mL qid	Saccharin, sorbitol. In 30 mL w/dropper.
Rx sf	**Cordron-D Liquid** (Cypress)	17.5 mg pseudoephedrine HCl	2 mg carbinoxamine maleate	**≥ 6 y** - 10 mL qid; **18 mo to < 6 y** - 5 mL qid; **9 to < 18 mo** - 3.75 to 5 mL qid; **6 to < 9 mo** - 3.75 mL qid; **3 to < 6 mo** - 2.5 mL qid; **1 to < 3 mo** - 1.25 mL qid	Alcohol and dye free. Saccharin, sorbitol. In 473 mL.

DECONGESTANTS AND ANTIHISTAMINES

	Product & Distributor	Decongestant	Antihistamine	Average Dose	Excipients & How Supplied
Rx	**Hydro-Tussin CBX Syrup** (Ethex)	25 mg pseudoephedrine HCl	2 mg carbinoxamine maleate	≥ **6 y** - 10 mL qid; **18 mo to 6 y** - 5 mL qid; **9 to 18 mo** - 3.75 to 5 mL qid; **6 to 9 mo** - 3.75 mL qid; **3 to 6 mo** - 2.5 mL qid; **1 to 3 mo** - 1.25 mL qid	In 473 mL.
otc	**Allergy-D Tablets** (Major)	120 mg pseudoephedrine HCl	5 mg cetirizine HCl	≥ **12 y** - 1 q 12 h up to 2/day	Extended release. Lactose. In 12s.
otc	**Zyrtec-D Tablets** (McNeil Consumer)				Extended release. Lactose. In 12s.
Rx	**AccuHist Drops** (Tiber)	9 mg pseudoephedrine HCl	0.8 mg chlorpheniramine maleate	**24 to 36 mo** - 1 mL qid up to 4 mL/day; **12 to 24 mo** - 0.75 mL qid up to 3 mL/day; **6 to 12 mo** - 0.5 mL qid up to 2 mL/day	Saccharin, sorbitol. Cherry flavor. In 30 mL w/dropper.
Rx	**Neutrahist Drops** (Cypress)				Saccharin, sorbitol. Cherry flavor. In 30 mL w/dropper.
Rx	**PSE CPM Chewable Tablets** (Boca)	15 mg pseudoephedrine HCl	2 mg chlorpheniramine maleate	≥ **12 y** - 2 q 4 to 6 h; **6 to 12 y** - 1 q 4 to 6 h	Aspartame, mannitol, phenylalanine, sugar. (BOCA 133). Purple, capsule shape, scored. Grape flavor. In 100s.
Rx	**PSE 15/CPM 2 Chewable Tablets** (Cypress)			≥ **12 y** - 2 q 4 to 6 h; **6 to < 12 y** - 1 q 4 to 6 h	Aspartame, 1.7 mg phenylalanine. (CYP 295). Red. In 100s.
otc	**Allerest Maximum Strength Tablets** (Insight)	30 mg pseudoephedrine HCl	2 mg chlorpheniramine maleate	≥ **12 y** - 2 q 4 to 6 h up to 8/day; **6 to < 12 y** - 1 q 4 to 6 h up to 4/day	In 24s.
Rx	**CPM PSE Syrup** (Boca Pharmacal)			≥ **12 y** - 5 to 10 mL 3 or 4 times/day; **6 to 12 y** - 2.5 mL to 5 mL 3 or 4 times/day up to 20 mL/day; **2 to 6 y** - 2.5 mL 3 or 4 times/day up to 10 mL/day	Alcohol free, dye free. Sorbitol. Grape flavor. In 473 mL.
otc	**Dicel Chewable Tablets** (Centrix)			≥ **12 y** - 2 q 4 to 6 h, up to 8/day; **6 to < 12 y** - 1 q 4 to 6 h, up to 4/day	Fructose, glycyrrhizate, maltodextrin, PEG, soy lecithin, sucralose, sugar, vegetable oil. In 20s.
Rx	**Histex Liquid** (Tiber)			**> 12 y** - 10 mL q 4 to 6 h; **6 to 12 y** - 5 mL q 4 to 6 h; **2 to 6 y** - 2.5 mL q 4 to 6 h	Peach flavor. In 473 mL.
Rx	**LoHist D Liquid** (Larken Labs)			**> 12 y** - 10 mL q 4 to 6 h, up to 40 mL/day; **6 to < 12 y** - 5 mL q 4 to 6 h, up to 20 mL/day; **2 to < 6 y** - 2.5 mL q 4 to 6 h, up to 10 mL/day	Alcohol free, dye free. Saccharin, sorbitol. Peach flavor. In 473 mL.
Rx	**RE2+30 Syrup** (River's Edge)			**> 12 y** - 5 to 10 mL tid or qid; **6 to 12 y** - 2.5 to 5 mL tid or qid up to 20 mL/day; **2 to 6 y** - 2.5 mL tid or qid up to 10 mL/day	Saccharin, sorbitol. Grape flavor. In 118 mL.

DECONGESTANTS AND ANTIHISTAMINES

	Product & Distributor	Decongestant	Antihistamine	Average Dose	Excipients & How Supplied
Rx	**Deconamine Syrup** (Kenwood)	30 mg pseudoephedrine HCl (as d-pseudoephedrine)	2 mg chlorpheniramine maleate	**> 12 y** -5 to 10 mL tid or qid; **6 to 12 y** - 2.5 to 5 mL tid or qid up to 20 mL/day; **2 to 6 y** - 2.5 mL tid or qid up to 10 mL/day	Alcohol and dye free. Sorbitol, sucrose. Grape flavor. In 473 mL.
Rx	**Sudal-12 Tannate Chewable Tablets** (Atley)	30 mg pseudoephedrine HCl	4 mg chlorpheniramine maleate	**> 12 y** - 1 to 2 q 12 h; **6 to 12 y** - ½ to 1 q 12 h; **2 to 6 y** - ½ q 12 h	Acesulfame K, aspartame, magnasweet, mannitol, 25 mg phenylalanine, sucralose. (S/12 4/30). Purple. Grape flavor. In 100s.
otc	**AMBI 60PSE/4CPM Tablets** (Ambi)	60 mg pseudoephedrine HCl	4 mg chlorpheniramine maleate	≥ **12 y** - 1 q 4 to 6 h up to 4/day; **6 to < 12 y** - ½ q 4 to 6 h up to 2/day	(AMBI 442). White, capsule shape, scored. In 100s.
otc	**Genaphed Plus Tablets** (Ivax)				Lactose. In 24s.
Rx	**Pseudoephedrine HCl/ Chlorpheniramine Maleate Capsules** (Brighton Pharmaceuticals)	100 mg pseudoephedrine HCl	12 mg chlorpheniramine maleate	≥ **12 y** - 1/day up to 2/day	Extended release. Sugar. (BP 950). Clear. In 100s.
Rx	**Chlorpheniramine Maleate/ Pseudoephedrine HCl ER Capsules** (Various, eg, Kremers Urban)	120 mg pseudoephedrine HCl	8 mg chlorpheniramine maleate	1 q 12 h	Extended release. May contain parabens and sucrose. In 100s, 250s, 500s, and 1,000s.
Rx	**Deconomed SR Capsules** (Iopharm)				Extended release. Parabens, sucrose. Blue/Clear. In 100s and 500s.
Rx	**Chlorpheniramine Maleate/ Pseudoephedrine Hydrochloride LA Tablets** (River's Edge)	120 mg pseudoephedrine HCl	12 mg chlorpheniramine maleate	**> 12 y** - ½ to 1 q 12 h; **6 to 12 y** - ½ q 12 h	Extended release. Lactose. In 100s.
otc	**Benadryl Children's Allergy & Cold Fastmelt Tablets** (J & J)	30 mg pseudoephedrine HCl	19 mg diphenhydramine citrate (equiv to 12.5 mg diphenhydramine HCl)	≥ **12 y** - 2 q 4 h up to 8/day; **6 to < 12 y** - 1 q 4 h up to 4/day	Aspartame, lactitol, mannitol, 4.6 mg phenylalanine. In 20s.
otc *sf*	**Benadryl-D Children's Allergy & Sinus Liquid** (J & J)	30 mg pseudoephedrine HCl	12.5 mg diphenhydramine HCl	≥ **12 y** - 10 mL q 4 to 6 h up to 40 mL/day; **6 to < 12 y** - 5 mL q 4 to 6 h up to 20 mL/day	Alcohol free. Saccharin, sorbitol. Grape flavor. In 118 mL.
Rx	**Tekral Tablets** (Capellon Pharmaceutical)	120 mg pseudoephedrine HCl	100 mg diphenhydramine HCl	≥ **12 y** - 1 q 12 h, up to 2/day	Lactose. (TEKRAL). Lt. green/Lt. yellow, capsule shape. Scored. In 90s.
Rx	**Allegra-D 12 Hour Tablets** (Sanofi-Aventis)	120 mg pseudoephedrine HCl (extended release)	60 mg fexofenadine HCl (immediate release)	≥ **12 y** - 1 bid	Extended release. PEG. (06/012D). White/Tan, layered. Film coated. In 100s.
Rx	**Allegra-D 24 Hour Tablets** (Sanofi-Aventis)	240 mg pseudoephedrine HCl (extended release)	180 mg fexofenadine HCl (immediate release)	≥ **12 y** - 1 q 24 h	Extended release. PEG, isopropyl and methyl alcohols. (308A V). Film coated. In 100s.
Rx	**Viravan-P Suspension** (Tiber)	15 mg pseudoephedrine HCl	15 mg pyrilamine maleate	**> 12 y** – 5 to 10 mL q 12 h; **6 to 12 y** - 5 mL q 12 h; **2 to 6 y** - 2.5 mL q 12 h	Methylparaben, sucralose, sucrose. Cherry bubble gum flavor. In 473 mL.
otc *sf*	**Hist-PSE Drops** (Cypress)	10 mg pseudoephedrine HCl	0.938 mg triprolidine HCl	≥ **12 y** - 2.67 mL q 4 to 6 h, up to 10.68 mL/day; **6 to < 12 y** - 1.33 mL q 4 to 6 h, up to 5.32 mL/day	Alcohol free, sugar free. Glycerin, propylene glycol, saccharin, sorbitol. Cotton candy flavor. In 30 mL.
otc	**Allerfrim Syrup** (Rugby)	30 mg pseudoephedrine HCl	1.25 mg triprolidine HCl	≥ **12 y** - 10 mL q 4 to 6 h, up to 40 mL/day; **6 to < 12 y** - 5 mL q 4 to 6 h, up to 20 mL/day	In 118 mL.
otc	**Altafed Syrup** (Altaire)			≥ **12 y** - 10 mL q 4 to 6 h up to 40 mL/day; **6 to < 12 y** - 5 mL q 4 to 6 h up to 20 mL/day	Methylparaben, sorbitol. In 118 mL.
otc	**Aprodine Syrup** (Major)			≥ **12 y** - 10 mL q 4 to 6 h; **6 to < 12 y** - 5 mL q 4 to 6 h	Methylparaben, saccharin, sucrose. In 118 mL.
otc	**Silafed Syrup** (Silarx)				Methylparaben, saccharin, sucrose. In 118 mL.

DECONGESTANTS AND ANTIHISTAMINES

	Product & Distributor	Decongestant	Antihistamine	Average Dose	Excipients & How Supplied
Rx *sf*	**Tripohist D Liquid** (Breckenridge Pharmaceutical)	45 mg pseudoephedrine HCl	1.25 mg triprolidine HCl	**> 12 y** - 5 to 10 mL q 4 to 6 h up to 240 mg pseudoephedrine/day; **6 to 12 y** - 2.5 to 5 mL q 4 to 6 h up to 120 mg pseudoephedrine/day	Alcohol free. Saccharin, sorbitol. Blueberry flavor. In 473 mL.
otc	**Allerfrim Tablets** (Rugby)	60 mg pseudoephedrine HCl	2.5 mg triprolidine HCl	**≥ 12 y** - 1 q 4 to 6 h up to 4/day; **6 to < 12 y** - ½ q 4 to 6 h up to 2/day	Film coated. In 24s.
otc	**Aprodine Tablets** (Major)				Lactose, PEG. In 24s.
otc	**Genac Tablets** (Ivax)				In 24s and 48s.
Rx	**Clarinex-D 12 Hour Tablets** (Schering)	120 mg pseudoephedrine sulfate	2.5 mg desloratadine	**≥ 12 y** - 1 q 12 h	Extended release. Edetate disodium. (D12). Blue, oval. In 100s.
Rx	**Clarinex-D 24 Hour Tablets** (Schering-Plough)	240 mg pseudoephedrine sulfate	5 mg desloratadine	**≥ 12 y** - 1 q 24 h	Extended release. Edetate disodium. (D24). Lt. blue, oval. In 100s.
otc	**Drixoral Cold & Allergy Maximum Strength Tablets** (Schering-Plough Healthcare)	120 mg pseudoephedrine sulfate	6 mg dexbrompheniramine maleate	**≥ 12 y** - 1 q 12 h up to 2/day	Extended release. Lactose, sucrose. In 20s.
otc	**Claritin-D 12 Hour Tablets** (Schering-Plough)	120 mg pseudoephedrine sulfate	5 mg loratadine	**≥ 12 y** - 1 q 12 h up to 2/day	Extended release. Lactose. In 10s, 20s, and 30s.
otc	**Alavert Allergy & Sinus D-12 Hour Tablets** (Wyeth)				Extended release. Lactose. In 12s and 24s.
otc	**Claritin-D 24 Hour Tablets** (Schering-Plough)	240 mg pseudoephedrine sulfate	10 mg loratadine	**≥ 12 y** - 1 q 24 h	Extended release. PEG, sugar. Oval. In 15s.
otc	**Clear-Atadine D Tablets** (Major)				Extended release. Lactose, PEG. Oval. In 10s and 15s.
otc	**Loratadine D Tablets** (Major)				Extended release. Lactose, PEG, sodium 10 mg. In 10s and 15s.
Rx	**Brovex PD Suspension** (MCR American Pharmaceutical)	30 mg pseudoephedrine tannate	6 mg brompheniramine tannate	**> 12 y** - 5 to 20 mL q 12 h up to 40 mL/day; **6 to 12 y** - 5 to 10 mL q 12 h up to 20 mL/day	Aspartame, parabens, phenylalanine 7 mg per 5 mL. Cotton candy flavor. In 480 mL.
Rx *sf*	**Lodrane D Suspension** (ECR)	90 mg pseudoephedrine tannate	8 mg brompheniramine tannate	**> 12 y** - 5 mL q 12 h up to 10 mL/day; **6 to 12 y** - 2.5 mL q 12 h up to 5 mL/day; **2 to 6 y** - 1.25 mL q 12 h up to 2.5 mL/day; Titrate dose individually	Alcohol free. Strawberry flavor. In 473 mL.
Rx	**Dicel Suspension** (Centrix)	75 mg pseudoephedrine tannate	5 mg chlorpheniramine tannate	**> 12 y** - 10 to 20 mL q 12 h up to 40 mL/day; **6 to 12 y** - 5 to 10 mL q 12 h up to 20 mL/day; **2 to < 6 y** - 2.5 to 5 mL q 12 h up to 10 mL/day	Methylparaben, saccharin, sucrose. Strawberry-banana flavor. In 473 mL.
Rx	**Bi-Tann DP Suspension** (Midland Healthcare)	75 mg pseudoephedrine tannate	2.5 mg dexchlorpheniramine tannate	**≥ 12 y** -10 to 20 mL q 12 h up to 40 mL/day; **6 to < 12 y** - 5 to 10 mL q 12 h up to 20 mL/day; **2 to < 6 y** - 2.5 to 5 mL q 12 h up to 10 mL/day	Methylparaben, saccharin, sucrose. Strawberry-banana flavor. In 118 and 473 mL.
Rx *sf*	**Zymine DXR Suspension** (Vindex)	45 mg pseudoephedrine tannate	2.5 mg triprolidine tannate	**≥ 12 y** - 10 mL q 12 h; **6 to < 12 y** - 5 mL q 12 h; **2 to < 6 y** - 2.5 mL q 12 h	Alcohol free. Aspartame, parabens, phenylalanine 7 mg/5 mL. Berry flavor. In 473 mL.

[a] Adult dosing could not be verified. Please consult manufacturer prescribing information.

[b] Pediatric dosing could not be verified. Please consult manufacturer prescribing information.

Refer to the general discussion of these products in the Respiratory Combinations Introduction.

DECONGESTANT, ANTIHISTAMINE, AND ANALGESIC COMBINATIONS

Content given per capsule, tablet, packet, or 5 mL.

	Product & Distributor	Decongestant	Antihistamine	Analgesic/Other	Average Dose	Excipients & How Supplied
otc	**Pain-gesic Tablets** (Mason Remedies[a])		30 mg phenyltoloxamine citrate	325 mg acetaminophen	**≥ 12 y** - 1 to 2 q 4 h, up to 8/day **6 to < 12 y**- 1 q 4 h, up to 4/day	Lactose. In 100s.
otc	**Alka-Seltzer Plus Cold Effervescent Tablets** (Bayer)	7.8 mg phenylephrine bitartrate	2 mg chlorpheniramine maleate	325 mg aspirin	**≥ 12 y** - 2 dissolved in water q 4 h, up to 8/day	Acesulfame K, aspartame, mannitol, phenylalanine 8.4 mg, sodium 474 mg. Orange, cherry, and original flavors. In 12s, 20s, 36s, and 48s.
otc	**Tylenol Plus Children's Cold Suspension** (McNeil Consumer)	2.5 mg phenylephrine HCl	1 mg chlorpheniramine maleate	160 mg acetaminophen	**6 to < 12 y (21.8 to 43.2 kg)** - 10 mL q 4 h, up to 50 mL/day	Sorbitol, sucrose. Grape flavor. In 118 mL.
otc	**Onset Forte Micro-Coated Tablets** (Medique)	5 mg phenylephrine HCl	2 mg chlorpheniramine maleate	162.5 mg acetaminophen	**≥ 12 y** - 2 q 4 h, up to 12/day	In 100s and 500s.
otc	**Alka-Seltzer Multi-Symptom Cold Relief Effervescent Tablets** (Bayer Consumer)	5 mg phenylephrine HCl	2 mg chlorpheniramine maleate	250 mg acetaminophen	**≥ 12 y** - 2 tablets dissolved in 120 mL (4 oz) water q 4 h, up to 8/day	Maltodextrin. 503 mg sodium per tablet. In 20s.
otc	**Comtrex Maximum Strength Day and Night Flu Therapy Tablets** (Novartis Consumer)	*Day:* 5 mg phenylephrine HCl		325 mg acetaminophen	**≥ 12 y** - *Day:* 2 q 4 h, up to 8/day *Night:* 2 q 4 h (after last day dose), up to 4/night	*Day:* PEG. Orange, capsule shape. *Night:* PEG. Green, capsule shape. In 20s (10 day; 10 night).
otc	**Comtrex Maximum Strength Day and Night Severe Cold and Sinus Tablets** (Novartis Consumer)	*Night:* 5 mg phenylephrine HCl	2 mg chlorpheniramine maleate	325 mg acetaminophen		*Day:* PEG. Orange, capsule shape. *Night:* PEG. Green, capsule shape. In 20s (10 day; 10 night).
otc	**Tylenol Sinus Congestion & Pain Nighttime Cool Burst Caplet** (McNeil Consumer Health)	5 mg phenylephrine HCl	2 mg chlorpheniramine maleate	325 mg acetaminophen	**≥ 12 y** - 2 q 4 h, up to 12/day	Corn starch, PEG, sucralose. In 24s.
otc	**Contac Cold + Flu Maximum Strength Caplets** (GlaxoSmithKline)	5 mg phenylephrine HCl	2 mg chlorpheniramine maleate	500 mg acetaminophen	**≥ 12 y** - 2 q 6 h, up to 8/day	PEG. In 24s and 36s.
otc	**Contac Cold + Flu Day & Night Tablets** (GlaxoSmithKline Consumer)	*Day:* 5 mg phenylephrine HCl		500 mg acetaminophen	**≥ 12 y** - 2 q 6 h, up to 8/day	PEG, polyvinyl alcohol. Capsule shape. In 28s (16 day, 12 night).
		Night: 5 mg phenylephrine HCl	2 mg chlorpheniramine maleate	500 mg acetaminophen		
otc	**Tylenol Allergy Multi-Symptom Convenience Pack Tablets** (McNeil Consumer)	*Day:* 5 mg phenylephrine HCl	2 mg chlorpheniramine maleate	325 mg acetaminophen	**≥ 12 y** - 2 q 4 h, up to 12/day	*Day and Night:* Sucralose. Capsule shape. In 24s.
		Night: 5 mg phenylephrine HCl	25 mg diphenhydramine HCl	325 mg acetaminophen		
otc	**Coricidin 'D' Cold, Flu, & Sinus Tablets** (Schering-Plough Healthcare)	5 mg phenylephrine HCl	2 mg chlorpheniramine maleate	325 mg acetaminophen	**≥ 12 y** - 2 q 4 h, up to 12/day	PEG. In 24s.
otc	**Dristan Cold Multi-Symptom Formula Tablets** (Wyeth Consumer)					PEG. In 20s.
otc	**Dryphen Multi-Symptom Formula Tablets** (Major)					In 40s.
otc	**Medicidin-D Tablets** (Medique)					Sucrose. In 100s, 200s, and 500s.
otc	**Tylenol Allergy Multi-Symptom Tablets and Gelcaps** (McNeil Consumer)					**Tablets**: PEG, sucralose. (TY C1076). Off white, capsule shape. In 24s. **Gelcaps**: Benzyl alcohol, parabens. (TY C1077). Green/Yellow, capsule shape. In 24s.
otc	**Tylenol Sinus Congestion & Pain Nighttime Cool Burst Tablets** (McNeil Consumer)					PEG, sucralose. Capsule shape. Cool burst flavor. In 24s.
otc	**Sine Off Sinus/Cold Tablets** (Hogil)	5 mg phenylephrine HCl	2 mg chlorpheniramine maleate	500 mg acetaminophen	**≥ 12 y** - 2 q 6 h, up to 8/day	Capsule shape. In 24s.

DECONGESTANT, ANTIHISTAMINE, AND ANALGESIC COMBINATIONS

	Product & Distributor	Decongestant	Antihistamine	Analgesic/Other	Average Dose	Excipients & How Supplied
otc	**Pyrroxate Extra-Strength Tablets** (Lee)	10 mg phenylephrine HCl	4 mg chlorpheniramine maleate	650 mg acetaminophen	**≥ 12 y** - 1 q 4 to 6 h, up to 6/day	PEG. Capsule shape. In 24s.
otc	**Alka-Seltzer Plus Fast Crystal Packs** (Bayer Healthcare)				**≥ 12 y** - Dissolve 1 packet in 180 to 240 mL of hot or cold beverage q 4 h, up to 6 packets/day	Acesulfame K, aspartame, phenylalanine 6 mg, sucralose, sucrose. Taste free. In 10s.
Rx	**Norel SR Tablets** (US Pharm. Corp.)	40 mg phenylephrine HCl	8 mg chlorpheniramine maleate 50 mg phenyltoloxamine citrate	325 mg acetaminophen	**> 12 y** - 1 q 12 h, up to 2/day	Extended release. (0420/US). Yellow/White, triangular, scored. In 100s.
Rx	**Trital SR** (Breckenridge)				**> 12 y** - 1 q 12 h, up to 2/day	Tartrazine. (B529). Yellow, triangle shape, scored. In 100s.
otc	**Theraflu Warming Relief Flu & Sore Throat Liquid** (Novartis)	1.67 mg phenylephrine HCl	4.16 mg diphenhydramine HCl	108.3 mg acetaminophen	**≥ 12 y** - 30 mL q 4 h, up to 180 mL/day	Acesulfame K, alcohol 10%, edetate disodium, glycerin, maltitol, propylene glycol, sodium 2.3 mg, sodium benzoate. Cherry flavor. In 245.5 mL.
otc	**Tylenol Plus Children's Cold & Allergy Suspension** (McNeil Consumer)	2.5 mg phenylephrine HCl	12.5 mg diphenhydramine HCl	160 mg acetaminophen	**6 to 11 y (21.8 to 43.1 kg)** - 10 mL q 4 h, up to 50 mL/day	Sorbitol, sucralose, sucrose. Bubble gum flavor. In 118.3 mL.
otc	**Benadryl Allergy & Cold Tablets** (J&J)	5 mg phenylephrine HCl	12.5 mg diphenhydramine HCl	325 mg acetaminophen	**≥ 12 y** - 2 q 4 h, up to 12/day **6 to < 12 y** – 1 q 4 h, up to 5/day	Capsule shape. In 24s.
otc	**Benadryl Allergy Plus Sinus Headache Tablets** (J&J)					PEG. Capsule shape. In 24s and 48s.
otc	**Sudafed PE Multi-Symptom Severe Cold Tablets** (McNeil)					PEG. Capsule shape. In 12s and 24s.
otc	**Benadryl Severe Allergy & Sinus Headache Maximum Strength Tablets** (J&J)	5 mg phenylephrine HCl	25 mg diphenhydramine HCl	325 mg acetaminophen	**≥ 12 y** - 2 q 4 h, up to 12/day	PEG. Capsule shape. In 20s.
otc	**Sudafed PE Nighttime Cold Maximum Strength Tablets** (McNeil)					Capsule shape. In 20s.
otc	**Tylenol Allergy Multi-Symptom Nighttime Tablets** (McNeil Consumer)					Sucralose. Capsule shape. In 24s.
otc	**Theraflu Nighttime Severe Cold & Cough Powder** (Novartis)	10 mg phenylephrine HCl	25 mg diphenhydramine HCl	650 mg acetaminophen	**≥ 12 y** - 1 packet dissolved in 240 mL (8 oz) hot water q 4 h, up to 6/day	Acesulfame K, aspartame, maltodextrin, 13 mg phenylalanine, sucrose. Honey lemon flavor infused with chamomile and white tea. In 6s.
otc *sf*	**Theraflu Sugar-Free Nighttime Severe Cold & Cough Powder** (Novartis)				**≥ 12 y** - 1 packet dissolved in 240 mL (8 oz) hot water q 4 h, up to 6/day	Sugar free. Acesulfame K, aspartame, maltodextrin, 13 mg phenylalanine. Honey lemon flavor. In 6s.
otc	**Vicks NyQuil Sinex LiquiCaps** (Procter & Gamble)	5 mg phenylephrine HCl	6.25 mg doxylamine succinate	325 mg acetaminophen	**≥ 12 y** - 2 q 4 h, up to 8/day	Glycerin, PEG, sorbitol. In 20s.
otc	**Theraflu Cold & Sore Throat Powder** (Novartis)	10 mg phenylephrine HCl	20 mg pheniramine maleate	325 mg acetaminophen	**≥ 12 y** - 1 packet dissolved in 240 mL (8 oz) hot water q 4 h, up to 6/day	Acesulfame K, sucrose, 44 mg sodium. Lemon flavor. In 6s.
otc	**Theraflu Flu & Sore Throat Powder** (Novartis)	10 mg phenylephrine HCl	20 mg pheniramine maleate	650 mg acetaminophen	**≥ 12 y** - 1 packet dissolved in 240 mL (8 oz) hot water q 4 h, up to 6/day	Acesulfame K, sucrose, 51 mg sodium. Apple cinnamon flavor. In 6s.
otc *sf*	**Scot-Tussin Original Clear 5-Action Cold and Allergy Formula Liquid** (Scot-Tussin)	4.2 mg phenylephrine HCl	13.3 mg pheniramine maleate	83.3 mg Na citrate, 83.3 mg Na salicylate, 25 mg caffeine citrate	**≥ 12 y**- 5 mL q 3 to 4 h, up to qid **6 to < 12 y**- 2.5 mL q 3 to 4 h, up to qid	Alcohol and dye free. Parabens, saccharin. Cherry-strawberry flavor. In 118 and 473 mL and 3.8 L.
otc	**Scot-Tussin Original 5-Action Cold and Allergy Formula Syrup** (Scot-Tussin)					Alcohol free. Parabens, sorbitol, sugar. Grape flavor. In 118 and 473 mL and 3.8 L.

DECONGESTANT, ANTIHISTAMINE, AND ANALGESIC COMBINATIONS

	Product & Distributor	Decongestant	Antihistamine	Analgesic/Other	Average Dose	Excipients & How Supplied
otc	**Sinadrin PE Capsules** (Reese)	10 mg phenylephrine	2 mg dexbrompheniramine	650 mg acetaminophen	**≥ 12 y** - 1 q 4 h, up to 6/day **6 to < 12 y** - ½ q 4 h, up to 3/day	Dye free. (RC/SPE). White, capsule shape. In 30s.
otc	**Alka-Seltzer Plus Cold Medicine Liqui-Gel Capsules** (Bayer Consumer)	30 mg pseudoephedrine HCl	2 mg chlorpheniramine maleate	325 mg acetaminophen	2 q 4 h, up to 8/day[b]	Liquid filled. Sorbitol. (AS+ COLD). In 12s and 20s.
otc	**Sinutab Sinus Allergy, Maximum Strength Tablets** (J&J)	30 mg pseudoephedrine HCl	2 mg chlorpheniramine maleate	500 mg acetaminophen	**≥ 12 y** - 2 q 6 h, up to 8/day	Capsule shape. In 24s.
otc	**Advil Allergy Sinus Tablets** (Pfizer Consumer Healthcare)	30 mg pseudoephedrine HCl	2 mg chlorpheniramine maleate	200 mg ibuprofen	**≥ 12 y** - 1 q 4 to 6 h, up to 6/day	PEG. Capsule shape. In 20s and 40s.
otc	**BC Allergy, Sinus, Headache Powder** (GlaxoSmithKline Consumer)	60 mg pseudoephedrine HCl	4 mg chlorpheniramine maleate	650 mg acetaminophen	**≥ 12 y** - 1 q 6 h, up to 4/day	In 6s and 12s.

[a] Mason Remedies, 5105 NW 159th Street, Miami Lakes, FL 33014; 1-888-860-5376; http://www.masonvitamins.com.
[b] Pediatric dosing could not be verified.

Refer to the general discussion of these products in the Respiratory Combinations Introduction.

DECONGESTANT, ANTIHISTAMINE, AND ANTICHOLINERGIC COMBINATIONS

Content given per tablet, capsule, or 5 mL.

	Product & Distributor	Decongestant	Antihistamine	Anticholinergic	Average Dosage	Excipients & How Supplied
Rx	**Dexodryl Suspension** (Dexo Pharma)		2 mg chlorpheniramine maleate (as chlorpheniramine tannate)	1.5 mg methscopolamine nitrate	**≥ 12 y** - 5 to 10 mL q 12 h, up to 20 mL/day; **6 to 12 y** - 2.5 to 5 mL q 12 h, up to 10 mL/day	Parabens, sucralose. In 118 mL.
Rx	**Dexodryl Chewable Tablets** (Dexo Pharma)				**≥ 12 y** - 1 to 2 q 12 h; **6 to 12 y** - ½ to 1 q 12 h	Saccharin, sugar. (P3 171). Dark purple, capsule shape, scored. In 100s.
Rx	**AlleRx DF Dose Pack Tablets** (Cornerstone Biopharma)	*Day:*	4 mg chlorpheniramine maleate	2.5 mg methscopolamine nitrate	**≥ 12 y** - 1 q AM	*Day:* Lactose. (CBP 03). Elongated, scored. *Night:* Lactose. (CBP 02). Blue, elongated, scored. In 20s (10 day, 10 night) and 60s (30 day, 30 night).
		Night:	8 mg chlorpheniramine maleate	2.5 mg methscopolamine nitrate	**≥ 12 y** - 1 q PM	
Rx	**RespiVent DF Dose Pack Tablets** (Aristos Pharmaceuticals)					*Day:* (CBP 03). White, elongated, scored. *Night:* (CBP 02). Blue, elongated, scored. In 20s (10 day, 10 night) and 60s (30 day, 30 night).
Rx	**Aerohist Tablets** (Aero)		8 mg chlorpheniramine maleate	2.5 mg methscopolamine nitrate	**> 12 y** - 1 q 12 h, up to 2/day	Extended-release. (AERO). Blue, scored. In 100s.
Rx	**NoHist EXT Tablets** (Larken)				**> 12 y** - 1 q 12 h, up to 2/day; **6 to < 12 y** - ½ q 12 h, up to 1/day	Extended-release. (LL 61). Blue, scored. In 100s.
Rx	**RelCof CPM Tablets** (Burel Pharmaceuticals)				**> 12 y** - 1 q 12 h, up to 2/day	Extended-release. (RELCOF CPM). Blue, capsule shape. In 10s and 100s.
Rx *sf*	**Ryneze Liquid** (SJ Pharmaceuticals)		4 mg chlorpheniramine maleate	1.25 mg scopolamine methyl nitrate	**≥ 12 y** - 5 mL q 4 to 6 h, up to 30 mL/day; **6 to < 12 y** - 2.5 mL q 4 to 6 h, up to 15 mL/day	Alcohol free, dye free, gluten free, sugar free. Saccharin, sorbitol. Grape flavor. In 473 mL.
Rx	**Bellahist-D LA Tablets** (Cypress)	20 mg phenylephrine HCl	8 mg chlorpheniramine maleate	0.19 mg hyoscyamine sulfate, 0.04 mg atropine sulfate, 0.01 mg scopolamine HBr	1 q 12 h, up to 2/day[a]	Extended-release. Alcohol and dye free. (CYP 449). Capsule shape, scored. In 100s.

DECONGESTANT, ANTIHISTAMINE, AND ANTICHOLINERGIC COMBINATIONS

	Product & Distributor	Decongestant	Antihistamine	Anticholinergic	Average Dosage	Excipients & How Supplied
Rx	**Dallergy Syrup** (Laser)	8 mg phenylephrine HCl	2 mg chlorpheniramine maleate	0.75 mg methscopolamine nitrate	≥ **12 y** - 10 mL q 4 to 6 h, up to 40 mL/day; **6 to < 12 y** - 5 mL q 4 to 6 h, up to 20 mL/day	In 473 mL.
Rx	**ScopoHist Syrup** (Larken)					Sorbitol, sugar. Grape flavor. In 473 mL.
Rx	**Triall Syrup** (Breckenridge)				**> 12 y** - 10 mL q 4 to 6 h, up to 40 mL/day; **6 to 12 y** - 5 mL q 4 to 6 h, up to 20 mL/day	Alcohol free. Sorbitol. Grape flavor. In 473 mL.
Rx	**PE-CPM-MSN 8-2-0.75 Syrup** (Kylemore)				≥ **12 y** - 10 mL q 4 to 6 h, up to 40 mL/day; **6 to < 12 y** - 5 mL q 4 to 6 h, up to 20 mL	Glycerin, parabens, PEG, potassium sorbate, Prosweet, sucrose, saccharin, sorbitol, sucralose. Grape flavor. In 473 mL.
Rx	**QV-Allergy Syrup** (Pharmaceutical Associates)	10 mg phenylephrine HCl	2 mg chlorpheniramine maleate	0.625 mg methscopolamine nitrate	≥ **12 y** - 10 mL q 4 to 6 h, up to 40 mL/day; **6 to < 12 y** - 5 mL q 4 to 6 h, up to 20 mL/day	Sucrose. Grape flavor. In 473 mL.
Rx	**PE HCL-CPM-MSN 10-2-0.75 Syrup** (Kylemore)	10 mg phenylephrine HCl	2 mg chlorpheniramine maleate	0.75 mg methscopolamine nitrate	≥ **12 y** - 10 mL q 4 to 6 h, up to 40 mL/day; **6 to < 12 y** - 5 mL q 4 to 6 h, up to 20 mL/day	Glycerin, parabens, propylene glycol, sodium benzoate, sucrose. Grape flavor. In 473 mL.
Rx	**Dallergy Chewable Tablets** (Palmetto Pharmaceuticals)	10 mg phenylephrine HCl	2 mg chlorpheniramine maleate	1.25 mg methscopolamine nitrate	≥ **12 y** - 1 to 2 q 4 to 6 h, up to 8/day; **6 to < 12 y** - ½ to 1 q 4 to 6 h, up to 4/day	Mannitol, saccharin, sugar. (LAS 152). Purple, capsule shape, scored. Grape flavor. In 100s.
Rx	**Dehistine Syrup** (Cypress)				≥ **12 y** - 5 to 10 mL q 4 to 6 h, up to 40 mL/day; **6 to < 12 y** - 5 mL q 4 to 6 h, up to 20 mL/day	Alcohol free. Root beer flavor. In 473 mL.
Rx	**Duradryl Syrup** (Breckenridge)				≥ **12 y** - 5 to 10 mL q 3 to 4 h; **6 to < 12 y** - 2.5 to 5 mL q 4 h	Alcohol free. Sorbitol. Cherry flavor. In 473 mL.
Rx	**Duravent Chewable Tablets** (Auriga)				≥ **12 y** - 2 q 4 to 6 h, up to 8/day; **6 to 12 y** - 1 q 4 to 6 h, up to 4/day	Mannitol, sugar. (CBP). Brown. Root beer flavor. In 100s.
Rx	**Extendryl Chewable Tablets** (Auriga)					Mannitol, sugar. (CBP). Brown. Root beer flavor. In 100s.
Rx	**NoHist-Plus Chewable Tablets** (Larkin Labs)				≥ **12 y** – 2 q 4 to 6 h up to 8/day; **6 to 12 y** – 1 q 4 to 6 h up to 4/day	Chewable. Mannitol, saccharin. (LL 166). Purple, capsule shape. Grape flavor. In 100s.
Rx	**PCM Chewable Tablets** (Boca Pharmacal)				≥ **12 y** - 1 to 2 q 4 h, up to 8/day; **6 to 12 y** - 1 q 4 h, up to 4/day	Lactose, mannitol, sugar. (BOCA 131). Mottled purple, capsule shape, scored. In 100s.
Rx	**Zinx PCM Oral Solution** (Auriga)				**> 12 y** - 10 mL q 4 to 6 h, up to 40 mL/day; **6 to 12 y** - 5 mL q 4 to 6 h, up to 20 mL/day	Alcohol free, dye free. Saccharin, sorbitol. Berry flavor. In 118 mL.
Rx	**AH-chew Suspension** (Dexo Pharma)	10 mg phenylephrine HCl (as phenylephrine tannate)	2 mg chlorpheniramine maleate (as chlorpheniramine tannate)	1.5 mg methscopolamine nitrate	≥ **12 y** - 5 to 10 mL q 12 h; **6 to 12 y** - 2.5 to 5 mL q 12 h	Parabens, sucralose. In 20 and 118 mL.
Rx	**AH-chew Ultra Chewable Tablets** (Dexo Pharma)				≥ **12 y** - 1 to 2 q 12 h; **6 to 12 y** - ½ to 1 q 12 h	Saccharin, sugar. (P3 115). Dark purple, capsule shape, scored. In 100s.

DECONGESTANT, ANTIHISTAMINE, AND ANTICHOLINERGIC COMBINATIONS

	Product & Distributor	Decongestant	Antihistamine	Anticholinergic	Average Dosage	Excipients & How Supplied
Rx	**SymPak PDX Chewable Tablets** (Airpharma)	*Day:* 10 mg phenylephrine HCl (as phenylephrine tannate)	2 mg chlorpheniramine maleate (as chlorpheniramine tannate)	1.5 mg methscopolamine nitrate	≥ **12 y** - 1 q AM; **6 to 12 y** - ½ to 1 q AM	Saccharin, sugar. In 2 blister cards for 14-day dosing regimen.
		Night:	2 mg chlorpheniramine maleate (as chlorpheniramine tannate)	1.5 mg methscopolamine nitrate	≥ **12 y** - 1 q PM; **6 to 12 y** - 1 q PM	Saccharin, sugar. In 2 blister cards for 14-day dosing regimen.
Rx	**AeroKid Syrup** (Aero)	10 mg phenylephrine HCl	4 mg chlorpheniramine maleate	1.25 mg methscopolamine nitrate	≥ **12 y** - 5 to 10 mL q 3 to 4 h; **6 to < 12 y** - 2.5 to 5 mL q 4 h	Saccharin, sorbitol. Blue raspberry flavor. In 20, 120, and 473 mL.
Rx	**Dallergy Tablets** (Laser)				≥ **12 y** - 1 q 4 to 6 h, up to 2/day; **6 to < 12 y** - ½ q 4 to 6 h, up to 2/day	(Laser Dallergy). Scored. In 100s.
Rx	**Denaze Liquid** (Cypress)				≥ **12 y** - 5 to 10 mL q 3 or 4 h; **6 to < 12 y** - 2.5 to 5 mL q 4 h	Alcohol free, dye free. Saccharin, sorbitol. Blue raspberry flavor. In 473 mL.
Rx	**NoHist-Plus JR Tablets** (Larken)				≥ **12 y** - 1 to 2 q 12 h, up to 4/day	Extended-release. (LL 165). White, capsule shape. In 100s.
Rx	**CPM 8/PE 20/MSC 1.25 Tablets** (Cypress)	20 mg phenylephrine HCl	8 mg chlorpheniramine maleate	1.25 mg methscopolamine nitrate	≥ **12 y** - 1 q 12 h, up to 2/day; **6 to < 12 y** - ½ q 12 h, up to 1/day	Extended-release. Lactose. (CYP 250). Capsule shape, scored. In 100s.
Rx	**ScopoHist-PE Tablets** (Larken)				≥ **12 y** - 1 q 12 h, up to 2/day	Extended-release. Lactose. (LL 291). Capsule shape. In 100s.
Rx	**AeroHist Plus Tablets** (Aero)	20 mg phenylephrine HCl	8 mg chlorpheniramine maleate	2.5 mg methscopolamine nitrate	≥ **12 y** - 1 q 12 h, up to 2/day; **6 to < 12 y** - ½ q 12 h, up to 1/day	Extended-release. (2376 aero). Capsule shape, scored. In 100s.
Rx	**Dallergy PE Caplets** (Palmetto Pharmaceuticals)				≥ **12 y** - 1 q 12 h, up to 2/day	Extended-release. (LAS 154). White, capsule shape. In 100s.
Rx	**DriHist SR Tablets** (Prasco)				≥ **12 y** - 1 q 12 h; **6 to < 12 y** - ½ q 12 h	Extended-release. (110). Capsule shape, scored. In 100s.
Rx	**Drysec Tablets** (A.G. Marin)				≥ **12 y** - 1 q 12 h, up to 2/day; **6 to < 12 y** - ½ q 12 h, up to 1/day	Extended-release. (CPM M/D). Scored. In 100s.
Rx	**Duradryl SR Tablets** (Breckenridge)				≥ **12 y** - 1 q 12 h	Extended-release. (B 592). White, oral, scored. In 100s.
Rx	**Duravent-DA Tablets** (Auriga)				≥ **12 y** - 1 q 8 to 12 h	Extended-release. (AP 101). White, capsule shape, scored. In 100s.
Rx	**NoHist-Plus Tablets** (Larken)					Extended-release. (LL 163). White, capsule shape. In 100s.
Rx	**RelCof PE Tablets** (Burel Pharmaceuticals)				≥ **12 y** - 1 q 8 to 12 h	(RELCOF PE). White, capsule shape. In 10s and 100s.
Rx	**OMNIhist II LA Tablets** (Dexo Pharma)	25 mg phenylephrine HCl	8 mg chlorpheniramine maleate	2.5 mg methscopolamine nitrate	≥ **12 y** - 1 q 12 h, up to 2/day; **6 to < 12 y** - ½ q 12 h, up to 1/day	Dye free. (WE 32). Capsule shape, scored. In 100s.

DECONGESTANT, ANTIHISTAMINE, AND ANTICHOLINERGIC COMBINATIONS

	Product & Distributor	Decongestant	Antihistamine	Anticholinergic	Average Dosage	Excipients & How Supplied
Rx	**Phenylephrine CM Tablets** (Boca Pharmacal)	40 mg phenylephrine HCl	8 mg chlorpheniramine maleate	2.5 mg methscopolamine nitrate	**> 12 y** - 1 q 12 h; **6 to 12 y** - ½ q 12 h	Extended-release. (BP 546). Green/White, capsule shape, scored. In 30s and 100s.
Rx	**Ralix Tablets** (Cypress)					Extended-release. (CYP 232). In 100s.
Rx	**Rescon-MX Tablets** (Capellon)				**≥ 12 y** - 1 q 12 h; **6 to 12 y** - ½ q 12 h	Extended-release. (PHE). Green/White, capsule shape, scored. In 100s.
Rx	**Rescon Tablets** (Capellon)	40 mg phenylephrine HCl	12 mg chlorphenir-amine maleate	1.25 mg methscopolamine nitrate	**≥ 12 y** - 1 q 12 h; **6 to < 12 y** - ½ q 12 h	Sustained-release. Lactose. (RESCON). Purple/Yellow, capsule shape, scored. In 90s.
Rx	**Dexphen M Oral Solution** (Boca)	10 mg phenylephrine HCl	1 mg dexchlorphenir-amine maleate	1.25 mg methscopolamine nitrate	**≥ 12 y** - 10 mL q 4 to 6 h, up to 40 mL/day; **6 to 12 y** - 5 mL q 4 to 6 h, up to 20 mL/day	Sorbitol. Root beer flavor. In 473 mL.
Rx	**Extendryl Syrup** (Auriga)					Sorbitol, sugar. Root beer flavor. In 473 mL.
Rx	**Re-Drylex Syrup** (River's Edge)					Sorbitol, sugar. Root beer flavor. In 473 mL.
Rx	**Extendryl PEM Tablets** (Auriga)	30 mg phenylephrine HCl		1.25 mg methscopolamine nitrate	**≥ 12 y** - 1 q 8 to 12 h	Extended-release. (AP 205). Oval. In 100s.
Rx	**AlleRx-D Tablets** (Cornerstone)	120 mg pseudoephed-rine HCl		2.5 mg methscopolamine nitrate	**≥ 12 y** - 1 q 12 h, up to 2/day	Extended-release. (CBP 01). Yellow, elongated. In 60s.
Rx	**Amdry-D Tablets** (Prasco Laboratories)					Extended-release (120). Yellow, capsule shape, scored. In 60s.
Rx	**PSE 120/MSC 2.5 Tablets** (Cypress)				**> 12 y** - 1 q 12 h, up to 2/day	Extended-release. (CYP281). Dye free. Scored. In 60s.
Rx	**RespiVent-D Tablets** (Aristos Pharmaceuti-cals)				**≥ 12 y** - 1 q 12 h, up to 2/day	(CBP 01). Yellow, capsule shape, scored. In 60s.
Rx	**SudaTrate Tablets** (Larken)					Extended-release. (LL 245). Capsule shape. In 100s.
Rx	**SymPak II Tablets** (Airpharma)	*Day:* 45 mg pseudoephedrine HCl	6 mg bromphenir-amine maleate		**≥ 12 y** - 1 q AM; **6 to 12 y** - 1 q AM	In 2 blister cards for 14-day dosing regimen.
		Night: 25 mg phenylephrine HCl	8 mg chlorpheniramine maleate	2.5 mg methscopolamine nitrate	**≥ 12 y** - 1 q PM; **6 to 12 y** - ½ q PM	In 2 blister cards for 14-day dosing regimen.
Rx	**DryMax Syrup** (Jaymac Pharma-ceutical)	30 mg pseudoephedrine HCl	4 mg chlorpheniramine maleate	1.25 mg methscopolamine nitrate	**≥ 12 y** - 5 to 10 mL q 4 to 6 h up to 40 mL/day; **6 to < 12 y** - 5 mL q 4 to 6 h up to 20 mL/day	Alcohol free, gluten free. Glycerin, propylene glycol, saccharin, sucrose. Grape flavor. In 118 mL.
Rx	**Dallergy PSE Tablets** (Laser)	60 mg pseudoephedrine HCl	4 mg chlorpheniramine maleate	1.25 mg methscopolamine nitrate	**≥ 12 y** - 1 to 2 q 12 h, up to 4/day; **6 to < 12 y** - 1 q 12 h, up to 2/day	Extended-release. (LAS 146). White, scored. In 100s.
Rx	**Histatab Tablets** (Breckenridge)	60 mg pseudoephedrine HCl	8 mg chlorpheniramine maleate	1.25 mg methscopolamine nitrate	**> 12 y** - 1 q 12 h, up to 2/day	Extended-release. (B 423). White, scored. In 100s.
Rx	**ScopoHist Tablets** (Larken)				**≥ 12 y** - 1 q 12 h, up to 2/day	Extended-release. (LL 290). Capsule shape. In 100s.
Rx *sf*	**Respa A.R. Tablets** (Respa Pharm)	90 mg pseudoephedrine HCl	8 mg chlorpheniramine maleate	0.24 mg belladonna alkaloids (atropine, hyoscyamine, scopolamine)	**> 12 y** - 1 q 12 h, up to 2/day	Extended-release. Dye free. (RESPA 177). Scored. In 100s.

DECONGESTANT, ANTIHISTAMINE, AND ANTICHOLINERGIC COMBINATIONS

	Product & Distributor	Decongestant	Antihistamine	Anticholinergic	Average Dosage	Excipients & How Supplied
Rx	**Stahist Tablets** (Magna)	90 mg pseudoephedrine HCl	8 mg chlorpheniramine maleate	0.19 mg hyoscyamine sulfate, 0.04 mg atropine sulfate, 0.01 mg scopolamine hydrobromide	**> 12 y** - 1 q 12 h, up to 2/day	Extended-release. Dye free. (27). Scored. In 100s.
Rx	**CPM 8/PSE 90/MSC 2.5 Tablets** (Cypress)	90 mg pseudoephedrine HCl	8 mg chlorpheniramine maleate	2.5 mg methscopolamine nitrate	**> 12 y** - 1 q 12 h, up to 2/day; **6 to 12 y** - ½ q 12 h, up to 1/day	Extended-release. Dye free. (CYP282). Scored. In 100s.
Rx	**Time-Hist QD Tablets** (AMBI)	120 mg pseudoephedrine HCl	6 mg chlorpheniramine maleate	2.5 mg methscopolamine nitrate	**> 12 y** - 1/day	Extended-release. PEG. (TH/701). In 100s.
Rx	**Relcof PSE Tablets** (Burel Pharmaceuticals)	120 mg pseudoephedrine HCl	8 mg chlorpheniramine maleate	2.5 mg methscopolamine nitrate	**> 12 y** - 1 q 12 h, up to 2/day	Extended-release. Lactose. (Relcof PSE). Mottled green, scored. In 10s and 100s.
Rx	**Allergy DN Tablets** (Breckenridge)	*Day*: 120 mg pseudoephedrine HCl		2.5 mg methscopolamine nitrate	≥ **12 y** - 1 AM	*Day*: (B 488). Elongated, scored. *Night*: Tartrazine. (B 489). Green, elongated, scored. In 20s (10 day, 10 night).
Rx	**AlleRx Dose Pack Tablets** (Cornerstone Biopharma)	*Night*: 10 mg phenylephrine HCl	8 mg chlorpheniramine maleate	2.5 mg methscopolamine nitrate	≥ **12 y** - 1 PM	*Day*: Controlled-release. (CPB 01). Yellow, elongated, scored. *Night*: Controlled-release. Lactose. (CPB 05). Blue, elongated, scored. In 20s (10 day, 10 night) and 60s (30 day, 30 night).
Rx	**VisRx Dose Pack Tablets** (Vision Pharma)	*Day:* 120 mg pseudoephedrine HCl		2.5 mg methscopolamine nitrate	≥ **12 y** - 1 q AM	*Day:* Controlled-release. (VP 7). Oval, scored. *Night:* Controlled-release. (VP 6). Green, oval, scored. In 20s (10 day, 10 night) and 60s (30 day, 30 night).
		Night:	8 mg chlorpheniramine maleate	2.5 mg methscopolamine nitrate	≥ **12 y** - 1 q PM	
Rx	**CoryZa-D Tablets** (Larken)	45 mg pseudoephedrine HCl	3.5 mg dexchlorpheniramine maleate	1 mg methscopolamine nitrate	≥ **12 y** - 1 q 12 h, up to 2/day	Extended-release. Lactose. (LL 271). White, capsule shape. In 100s.
Rx	**D-Hist D Tablets** (Midlothian)				≥ **12 y** - 1 q 12 h, up to 2/day; **6 to 12 y** - ½ q 12 h, up to 1/day	Extended-release. PEG. (ML/180n). Capsule shape, scored. In 100s.
Rx	**Histatab D Tablets** (Breckenridge)				≥ **12 y** - 1 q 12 h, up to 2/day	Extended-release. (B 583). Scored. In 100s.

[a] Dosing could not be verified. Please refer to the manufacturer's prescribing information for more information.

Refer to the general discussion of these products in the Respiratory Combinations Introduction.

ANTITUSSIVE COMBINATIONS

Content given per tablet, capsule, packet, pouch, strip, 1 mL (oral drops), or 5 mL.

	Product & Distributor	Antitussive	Antihistamine	Decongestant	Other	Average Dose	Excipients & How Supplied
Rx	**Respi-Tann Pd Suspension** (Teamm)	7.5 mg carbetapentane citrate (as 15 mg carbetapentane tannate)		30 mg pseudoephedrine HCl (as 60 mg pseudoephedrine tannate)		≥ **12 y** - 10 mL q 12 h, up to 40 mL/day; **4 to 12 y** - 5 mL q 12 h, up to 20 mL/day; **2 to 4 y** - 2.5 mL q 12 h, up to 10 mL/day	*Magnasweet*, methylparaben, sucrose. Grape bubble gum flavor. In 15 and 473 mL.

ANTITUSSIVE COMBINATIONS

	Product & Distributor	Antitussive	Antihistamine	Decongestant	Other	Average Dose	Excipients & How Supplied
Rx	**Respi-Tann Chewable Tablet** (Teamm)	20 mg carbetapentane citrate (as 25 mg carbetapentane tannate)		30 mg pseudoephedrine HCl (as 75 mg pseudoephedrine tannate)		**> 12 y** - 2 q 12 h, up to 8/day; **6 to 12 y** - 1 q 12 h, up to 4/day; **2 to 6 y** - ½ q 12 h, up to 2/day	Dye free. Saccharin, sugar. Cherry flavor. In 1s and 100s.
Rx	**Respi-Tann Suspension** (Teamm)					**> 12 y** - 10 mL q 12 h, up to 40 mL/day; **6 to 12 y** - 5 mL q 12 h, up to 20 mL/day; **2 to 6 y** - 2.5 mL q 12 h, up to 10 mL/day	Dye free. Methylparaben, saccharin, sucrose. Cherry flavor. In 473 mL.
Rx sf	**Corzall Liquid** (Hawthorn)	20 mg carbetapentane citrate		30 mg pseudoephedrine HCl		**≥ 12 y** - 5 to 10 mL q 4 to 6 h, up to 60 mL/day; **6 to 12 y** - 2.5 to 5 mL q 4 to 6 h, up to 30 mL/day	Alcohol free, dye free, sugar free. Saccharin, sorbitol. Grape flavor. In 473 mL.
Rx sf	**Zotex-D Syrup** (Vertical Pharmaceuticals)	20 mg carbetapentane citrate	7.5 mg pyrilamine maleate	8 mg pseudoephedrine HCl		**> 12 y** - 5 to 10 mL q 4 to 6 h, up to 60 mL/day; **6 to 12 y** - 2.5 to 5 mL q 4 to 6 h, up to 30 mL/day	Alcohol free, dye free, sugar free. Saccharin, sorbitol. Cherry flavor. In 473 mL.
Rx sf	**Corzall Plus Liquid** (Hawthorn)	20 mg carbetapentane citrate	7.5 mg pyrilamine maleate	30 mg pseudoephedrine HCl		**≥ 12 y** - 5 to 10 mL q 4 to 6 h, up to 60 mL/day; **6 to 12 y** - 2.5 to 5 mL q 4 to 6 h, up to 30 mL/day	Alcohol free, dye free, sugar free. Saccharin, sorbitol. Fruit gum flavor. In 473 mL.
Rx	**Vazotan Tannate Suspension** (Gentex Pharma)	25 mg carbetapentane citrate	6 mg brompheniramine maleate	10 mg phenylephrine HCl		**> 12 y** - 5 to 10 mL up to 4 times/day; **6 to 12 y** - 5 mL up to 4 times/day	Acesulfame K, aspartame, glycerin, methylparaben, 8.419 mg phenylalanine per 5 mL, sodium benzoate. Bubble gum flavor. In 118 mL.
Rx sf	**Seradex Liquid** (Gentex Pharma)	30 mg carbetapentane citrate	6 mg brompheniramine maleate	10 mg phenylephrine HCl		**≥ 12 y** - 5 mL q 6 h, up to 20 mL/day; **6 to 12 y** - 2.5 mL q 6 h, up to 10 mL/day	Alcohol free. Edetate disodium, saccharin, sorbitol. Bubble gum flavor. In 120 mL.
Rx sf	**Carbaphen 12 Suspension** (Gil Pharmaceutical)	27.5 mg carbetapentane citrate	4 mg chlorpheniramine maleate	10 mg phenylephrine HCl		**Adults** - 5 mL q 6 to 8 h	Alcohol free, sugar free. Parabens, saccharin. Blueberry banana flavor. In 473 mL.
Rx sf	**Corzall-PE Liquid** (Hawthorn)	20 mg carbetapentane citrate	1 mg dexchlorpheniramine maleate	10 mg phenylephrine HCl		**> 12 y** - 5 mL q 4 to 6 h, up to 30 mL/day; **6 to 12 y** - 2.5 mL q 4 to 6 h, up to 15 mL/day	Alcohol free, dye free, sugar free. Glycerin, propylene glycol, saccharin, sorbitol. Cherry flavor. In 473 mL.

ANTITUSSIVE COMBINATIONS

	Product & Distributor	Antitussive	Antihistamine	Decongestant	Other	Average Dose	Excipients & How Supplied
Rx	**Levall 12 Suspension** (Auriga)	30 mg carbetapentane tannate		25 mg phenylephrine tannate		**> 12 y** - 5 to 10 mL q 12 h, up to 20 mL/day; **6 to 12 y** - 5 mL q 12 h, up to 10 mL/day; **2 to 6 y** - 2.5 mL q 12 h, up to 5 mL/day	Aspartame, parabens, 7 mg phenylalanine per 5 mL. Strawberry flavor. In 118 mL.
Rx	**Zinx D-Tuss Suspension** (Auriga)						Aspartame, parabens, 7 mg phenylalanine per 5 mL. Strawberry flavor. In 118 mL.
Rx sf	**Carbetaplex TS Suspension** (Breckenridge)	30 mg carbetapentane tannate		30 mg phenylephrine tannate		**> 12 y** - 5 to 10 mL q 12 h, up to 20 mL/day; **6 to 12 y** - 5 mL q 12 h, up to 10 mL/day	Alcohol free. Saccharin. Strawberry flavor. In 118 mL.
Rx	**L-All 12 Suspension** (Midlothian)					**> 12 y** - 5 to 10 mL q 12 h, up to 20 mL/day; **6 to 12 y** - 5 mL q 12 h, up to 10 mL/day; **2 to 6 y** - 2.5 mL q 12 h, up to 5 mL/day	Methylparaben, phenylalanine, saccharin. Strawberry flavor. In 118 mL.
Rx	**Carb Pseudo-Tan Suspension** (Hi-Tech)	25 mg carbetapentane tannate		75 mg pseudoephedrine tannate		**> 12 y** - 10 mL q 12 h, up to 40 mL/day; **6 to 12 y** - 5 mL q 12 h, up to 20 mL/day; **2 to 6 y** - 2.5 mL q 12 h, up to 10 mL/day	Dye free. Methylparaben, saccharin, sucrose. Cherry flavor. In 473 mL.
Rx	**Pseudacarb Chewable Tablets** (Breckenridge)					**≥ 12 y** - 2 q 12 h, up to 4/day	Dye free. Saccharin, sucrose, xylitol. (B 108). Grape flavor. In 100s.
Rx	**Tannic-12 S Suspension** (Cypress)	30 mg carbetapentane tannate	4 mg chlorpheniramine tannate			**> 6 y** - 5 to 10 mL q 12 h; **2 to 6 y** - 2.5 to 5 mL q 12 h; **< 2 y** - titrate individually	Methylparaben, saccharin, sucrose. Strawberry flavor. In 118 mL.
Rx	**Tussi-12 S Suspension** (MedPointe)					**> 6 y** - 5 to 10 mL q 12 h; **2 to 6 y** - 2.5 to 5 mL q 12 h	Methylparaben, saccharin, sucrose, tartrazine. Strawberry-currant flavor. In 118 mL w/syringe.
Rx	**Tustan 12S Suspension** (Amneal Pharmaceutical)					**> 6 y** - 5 to 10 mL q 12 h; **2 to 6 y** - 2.5 to 5 mL q 12 h	Methylparaben, saccharin, sucrose. Grape flavor. In 118 and 473 mL.

ANTITUSSIVE COMBINATIONS

	Product & Distributor	Antitussive	Antihistamine	Decongestant	Other	Average Dose	Excipients & How Supplied
Rx	**Tannic-12 Tablets** (Cypress)	60 mg carbetapentane tannate	5 mg chlorpheniramine tannate			**Adults** - 1 to 2 q 12 h[a]	(CYP 303). Tan, capsule shape, scored. In 100s.
Rx	**Trionate Tablets** (Breckenridge)						(B072). Off-white, capsule shape. In 100s.
Rx	**Tussi-12 Tablets** (MedPointe)						(Wallace 0681). Mauve, capsule shape, scored. In 100s.
Rx	**Tussizone-12 RF Tablets** (Mallinckrodt)						(0037 0681). Mauve, capsule shape, scored. In 100s.
Rx	**D-Tann AT Suspension** (Midlothian)	30 mg carbetapentane tannate	25 mg diphenhydramine tannate			≥ **12 y** - 5 to 10 mL q 12 h; **6 to < 12 y** - 2.5 to 5 mL q 12 h; **2 to < 6 y** - 1.25 to 2.5 mL q 12 h	Aspartame, parabens, 7 mg phenylalanine per 5 mL. Cotton candy flavor. In 118 mL.
Rx	**Quad-Tuss Tannate Pediatric Suspension** (Hi-Tech)	30 mg carbetapentane tannate	4 mg chlorpheniramine tannate	5 mg phenylephrine tannate 5 mg ephedrine tannate		**> 6 y** - 5 to 10 mL q 12 h; **2 to 6 y** - 2.5 to 5 mL q 12 h; **< 2 y** - titrate individually	Methylparaben, saccharin, sucrose. In 473 mL.
Rx	**Rynatuss Pediatric Suspension** (MedPointe)					**> 6 y** - 5 to 10 mL q 12 h; **2 to 6 y** - 2.5 to 5 mL q 12 h	Methylparaben, saccharin, sucrose, tartrazine. Strawberry-currant flavor. In 237 and 473 mL.
Rx	**XiraTuss Tablets** (Hawthorn)	60 mg carbetapentane tannate	5 mg chlorpheniramine tannate	10 mg phenylephrine tannate		**> 12 y** - 1 to 2 q 12 h, up to 4/day	(HAW 551). Mottled tan/brown, capsule shape, scored. In 60s.
Rx	**Rynatuss Tablets** (MedPointe)	60 mg carbetapentane tannate	5 mg chlorpheniramine tannate	10 mg phenylephrine tannate, 10 mg ephedrine tannate		**Adults** - 1 to 2 q 12 h[a]	(Rynatuss 717). Mauve, capsule shape, scored. In 100s.
Rx *sf*	**Carbaphen 12 Liquid** (GIL)	60 mg carbetapentane tannate	8 mg chlorpheniramine tannate	20 mg phenylephrine tannate		**Adults** - 5 to 10 mL q 12 h, up to 20 mL/day[a]	Alcohol free. Acesulfame K, aspartame, methylparaben, 1 mg phenylalanine. Blueberry-banana flavor. In 473 mL.
Rx	**D-Tann CT Suspension** (Midlothian)	30 mg carbetapentane tannate	25 mg diphenhydramine tannate	7.5 mg phenylephrine tannate		≥ **12 y** - 5 to 10 mL q 12 h; **6 to < 12 y** - 2.5 to 5 mL q 12 h; **2 to < 6 y** - 1.25 to 2.5 mL q 12 h	Methylparaben, saccharin, sucrose. Strawberry-banana flavor. In 118 mL.
Rx	**Dytan-CS Suspension** (Hawthorn)						Aspartame, parabens, phenylalanine. Strawberry-banana flavor. In 118 mL.
Rx	**D-Tann CT Tablets** (Midlothian)	30 mg carbetapentane tannate	25 mg diphenhydramine tannate	10 mg phenylephrine tannate		≥ **12 y** - 1 to 2 q 12 h; **6 to < 12 y** - ½ to 1 q 12 h	Lactose. (NL 755). Tan, oval. In 60s.
Rx	**Dytan-CS Tablets** (Hawthorn)						(HAW 581). Tan, triangular. In 60s.
Rx	**D-Tann CD Suspension** (Midlothian)	30 mg carbetapentane tannate	25 mg diphenhydramine tannate	15 mg phenylephrine tannate		≥ **12 y** - 5 to 10 mL q 12 h; **6 to < 12 y** - 2.5 to 5 mL q 12 h	PEG, parabens, saccharin. Strawberry flavor. In 118 mL.

ANTITUSSIVE COMBINATIONS

	Product & Distributor	Antitussive	Antihistamine	Decongestant	Other	Average Dose	Excipients & How Supplied
Rx	**C-Tanna 12D Suspension** (Prasco)	30 mg carbetapentane tannate	30 mg pyrilamine tannate	5 mg phenylephrine tannate		**> 6 y** - 5 to 10 mL q 12 h; **2 to 6 y** - 2.5 to 5 mL q 12 h; **< 2 y** - titrate individually	Methylparaben, saccharin, sucrose, tartrazine. Strawberry-currant flavor. In 118 mL.
Rx	**Tannate-12D S Suspension** (Hi-Tech)						Methylparaben, saccharin, sucrose. 118 mL.
Rx	**Tussi-12D S Suspension** (MedPointe)					**> 6 y** - 5 to 10 mL q 12 h; **2 to 6 y** - 2.5 to 5 mL q 12 h	Methylparaben, saccharin, sucrose, tartrazine. Strawberry-currant flavor. In 118 mL w/oral syringe.
Rx	**Tannihist-12 D Suspension** (Morton Grove)						Methylparaben, saccharin, tartrazine. Strawberry-black currant flavor. In 118 and 473 mL.
Rx	**Tussi-12D Tablets** (MedPointe)	60 mg carbetapentane tannate	40 mg pyrilamine tannate	10 mg phenylephrine tannate		**≥ 12 y** - 1 to 2 q 12 h; **6 to 11 y** - ½ to 1 q 12 h	(WALLACE 0692). Pink, capsule shape, scored. In 100s.
otc sf	**Clofera Liquid** (Centrix)	12.5 mg chlophedianol HCl		30 mg pseudoephedrine HCl		**≥ 12 y** - 10 mL q 6 to 8 h, up to 40 mL/day; **6 to < 12 y** - 5 mL q 6 to 8 h, up to 20 mL/day	Alcohol free, dye free, gluten free, sugar free. Saccharin, sorbitol. Grape flavor. In 473 mL.
otc sf	**Dicel CD Liquid** (Centrix)	12.5 mg chlophedianol HCl	2 mg brompheniramine maleate	30 mg pseudoephedrine HCl		**≥ 12 y** - 10 mL q 6 to 8 h, up to 40 mL/day; **6 to < 12 y** - 5 mL q 6 to 8 h, up to 20 mL/day	Alcohol free, dye free, sugar free. Glycerin, grape flavoring, propylene glycol, saccharin, sorbitol. In 473 mL.
otc sf	**Vanacof Liquid** (GM Pharmaceuticals)	12.5 mg chlophedianol HCl	1 mg dexchlorpheniramine maleate	30 mg pseudoephedrine HCl		**≥ 12 y** – 10 mL q 6 to 8 h, up to 40 mL/day; **6 to < 12 y** – 5 mL q 6 to 8 h, up to 20 mL/day	Alcohol free, dye free, sugar free. Glycerin, propylene glycol, saccharin, sorbitol. Tutti fruitti flavor. In 473 mL.
c-v	**M-END PE Liquid** (R.A. McNeil)	6.33 mg codeine phosphate	1.33 mg brompheniramine maleate	3.33 mg phenylephrine HCl		**≥ 12 y** – 15 mL q 4 to 6 h, up to 90 mL/day; **6 to < 12 y** – 7.5 mL q 4 to 6 h, up to 45 mL/day	Saccharin, sorbitol. Cotton candy flavor. In 354 mL.
c-v	**TL-Hist CD Liquid** (Trigen Labs)	10 mg codeine phosphate	4 mg brompheniramine maleate	7.5 mg phenylephrine HCl		**> 12 y** – 5 mL q 4 to 6 h, up to 30 mL/day; **6 to < 12 y** – 2.5 mL q 4 to 6 h, up to 15 mL/day	Parabens, potassium citrate, potassium sorbate, propylene glycol, sorbitol, sucralose. Cotton candy flavor. In 473 mL.

ANTITUSSIVE COMBINATIONS

	Product & Distributor	Antitussive	Antihistamine	Decongestant	Other	Average Dose	Excipients & How Supplied
c-v	**M-END WC Liquid** (R.A. McNeil)	6.3 mg codeine phosphate	1.3 mg brompheniramine maleate	10 mg pseudoephedrine HCl		**≥ 12 y** – 15 mL q 4 to 6 h, up to 90 mL/day; **6 to < 12 y** – 7.5 mL q 4 to 6 h, up to 45 mL/day	Saccharin, sorbitol. Cherry flavor. In 473 mL.
c-v	**CPB WC Liquid** (Elge)						Saccharin, sorbitol. Cherry flavor. In 473 mL.
c-v *sf*	**Mesehist WC Liquid** (Trigen)					**> 12 y** – 15 mL q 4 to 6 h, up to 90 mL/day; **6 to < 12 y** – 7.5 mL q 4 to 6 h, up to 45 mL/day	Alcohol free, sugar free. Cherry flavoring, parabens, potassium citrate, potassium sorbate, propylene glycol, sorbitol, sucralose. In 473 mL.
c-v *sf*	**Rydex Liquid** (Centurion Labs)					**6 to < 12 y** – 7.5 mL q 4 to 6 h, up to 45 mL/day	Alcohol free, sugar free. Glycerin, propylene glycol, saccharin, sorbitol. Cotton candy flavor. In 473 mL.
c-v *sf*	**Mar-Cof BP Liquid** (Marnel Pharmaceutical)	7.5 mg codeine phosphate	2 mg brompheniramine maleate	30 mg pseudoephedrine HCl		**≥ 12 y** – 10 mL q 4 to 6 h, up to 60 mL/day; **6 to < 12 y** – 5 mL q 4 to 6 h, up to 30 mL/day	Alcohol free, sugar free. *Magnasweet*, saccharin, sorbitol. In 473 mL.
c-v *sf*	**Notuss-PE Liquid** (SJ Pharmaceuticals)	10 mg codeine phosphate		10 mg phenylephrine HCl		**≥ 12 y** – 5 mL q 4 h, up to 30 mL/day; **6 to < 12 y** – 2.5 mL q 4 h, up to 15 mL/day	Alcohol free, dye free, gluten free, sugar free. Saccharin, sorbitol. Cotton candy flavor. In 473 mL.
c-v *sf*	**EndaCof-AC Syrup** (Larken)	10 mg codeine phosphate	2 mg brompheniramine maleate			**> 12 y** – 5 to 10 mL q 4 to 6 h, up to 30 mL/day **6 to 12 y** – 5 mL q 4 to 6 h, up to 15 mL/day	Alcohol free, sugar free. *Magnasweet*, saccharin, sorbitol. Cotton candy flavor. In 118 mL.
c-v	**Nalex AC Syrup** (Blansett Pharmacal)					**> 12 y** – 5 to 10 mL q 4 to 6 h up to 30 mL/day **6 to 12 y** – 5 mL q 4 to 6 h up to 15 mL/day	Alcohol free. Saccharin, sorbitol. Blueberry flavor. In 118 mL.
c-iii	**Brōvex CB Tablets** (MCR American)	10 mg codeine phosphate	4 mg brompheniramine maleate			**> 12 y** – 1 q 4 to 6 h, up to 6/day; **6 to < 12 y** – ½ q 4 to 6 h, up to 3/day	(BROVEX CB). White, capsule shape, scored. In 100s.
c-iii	**Brōvex CBX Tablets** (MCR American)	20 mg codeine phosphate	4 mg brompheniramine maleate			**> 12 y** – 1 q 4 to 6 h, up to 6/day; **6 to < 12 y** – ½ q 4 to 6 h, up to 3/day	(BROVEX CBX). White, capsule shape, scored. In 100s.

ANTITUSSIVE COMBINATIONS

	Product & Distributor	Antitussive	Antihistamine	Decongestant	Other	Average Dose	Excipients & How Supplied
c-v	**Poly-Tussin AC Liquid** (Poly Pharmaceutical)	10 mg codeine phosphate	2 mg brompheniramine maleate	7.5 mg phenylephrine HCl		**> 12 y** – 5 mL q 4 to 6 h up to 30 mL/day **6 to < 12 y** – 2.5 mL q 4 to 6 h up to 15 mL/day	Alcohol free. Saccharin, sorbitol. Raspberry bubble gum flavor. In 473 mL.
c-v sf	**Pluratuss Liquid** (Creekwood Pharmaceuticals)	10 mg codeine phosphate	4 mg brompheniramine maleate	7.5 mg phenylephrine HCl		**> 12 y** – 5 mL q 4 to 6 h, up to 30 mL/day; **6 to < 12 y** – 2.5 mL q 4 to 6 h, up to 15 mL/day	Alcohol free, dye free, sugar free. Glycerin, propylene glycol, saccharin, sorbitol. Raspberry-bubble gum flavor. In 473 mL.
c-iii	**Brōvex PB C Tablets** (MCR American)	10 mg codeine phosphate	4 mg brompheniramine maleate	10 mg phenylephrine HCl		**> 12 y** – 1 q 4 to 6 h, up to 6/day; **6 to < 12 y** – ½ q 4 to 6 h, up to 3/day	(BROVEX PB C). White, capsule shape, scored. In 100s.
c-iii	**Brōvex PB CX Tablets** (MCR American)	20 mg codeine phosphate	4 mg brompheniramine maleate	10 mg phenylephrine HCl		**> 12 y** – 1 q 4 to 6 h, up to 6/day; **6 to < 12 y** – ½ q 4 to 6 h, up to 3/day	(BROVEX PB CX). White, capsule shape, scored. In 100s.
c-v	**Zodryl AC 25 Liquid** (CodaDOSE)	5 mg codeine phosphate	1.665 mg chlorpheniramine maleate			**2 to < 6 y (> 10.5 to 13 kg)** — 3 mL q 4 to 6 h up to 12 mL/day	Methylparaben, sucralose. Grape flavor. In 118 mL with oral dispenser.
c-v	**Zodryl AC 30 Liquid** (CodaDOSE)	5 mg codeine phosphate	1.43 mg chlorpheniramine maleate			**2 to < 6 y (> 13 to 15 kg)** — 3.5 mL q 4 to 6 h up to 14 mL/day	Methylparaben, sucralose. Grape flavor. In 118 mL with oral dispenser.
c-v	**Zodryl AC 35 Liquid** (CodaDOSE)	5 mg codeine phosphate	1.25 mg chlorpheniramine maleate			**2 to < 6 y (> 15 to 17 kg)** — 4 mL q 4 to 6 h up to 16 mL/day	Methylparaben, sucralose. Grape flavor. In 118 mL with oral dispenser.
c-v	**Zodryl AC 40 Liquid** (CodaDOSE)	5 mg codeine phosphate	1.11 mg chlorpheniramine maleate			**2 to < 6 y (> 17 to 19 kg)** — 4.5 mL q 4 to 6 h up to 18 mL/day	Methylparaben, sucralose. Grape flavor. In 118 mL with oral dispenser.
c-v	**Zodryl AC 50 Liquid** (CodaDOSE)	5 mg codeine phosphate	2 mg chlorpheniramine maleate			**6 to < 12 y (> 19 to 25.5 kg)** — 5 mL q 4 to 6 h up to 30 mL/day	Methylparaben, sucralose. Grape flavor. In 236 mL with oral dispenser.
c-v	**Zodryl AC 60 Liquid** (CodaDOSE)	5 mg codeine phosphate	1.335 mg chlorpheniramine maleate			**6 to < 12 y (> 25.5 to 32 kg)** — 7.5 mL q 4 to 6 h up to 45 mL/day	Methylparaben, sucralose. Grape flavor. In 236 mL with oral dispenser.
c-v	**Zodryl AC 80 Liquid** (CodaDOSE)	5 mg codeine phosphate	1 mg chlorpheniramine maleate			**6 to < 12 y (> 32 to 40 kg)** — 10 mL q 4 to 6 h up to 60 mL/day	Methylparaben, sucralose. Grape flavor. In 236 mL with oral dispenser.

ANTITUSSIVE COMBINATIONS

	Product & Distributor	Antitussive	Antihistamine	Decongestant	Other	Average Dose	Excipients & How Supplied
c-v *sf*	**Z-Tuss AC Liquid** (Magna)	9 mg codeine phosphate	2 mg chlorpheniramine maleate			**≥ 12 y** - 10 mL q 4 to 6 h, up to 60 mL/day; **6 to < 12 y** - 5 mL q 4 to 6 h, up to 30 mL/day	Alcohol free, gluten free, sugar free. Cherry flavoring, propylene glycol, saccharin, sodium benzoate, sorbitol. In 473 mL.
c-v *sf*	**Lexuss 210 Liquid** (Centurion)	10 mg codeine phosphate	2 mg chlorpheniramine maleate			**≥ 12 y** - 5 to 10 mL q 4 to 6 h, up to 40 mL/day; **6 to < 12 y** - 2.5 to 5 mL q 4 to 6 h, up to 20 mL/day	Sugar free. Alcohol 0.1%, parabens, potassium citrate, potassium sorbate, sucralose, sorbitol. Vanilla cream flavor. In 473 mL.
c-v *sf*	**Z-Tuss AC Liquid** (Magna)					**≥ 12 y** - 10 mL q 4 to 6 h, up to 60 mL/day; **6 to < 12 y** - 5 mL q 4 to 6 h, up to 30 mL/day	Alcohol free, sugar free. Saccharin, sorbitol. Cherry flavor. In 473 mL.
c-v *sf*	**EndaCof-C Liquid** (Larken Labs)	10 mg codeine phosphate	2 mg chlorpheniramine maleate			**≥ 12 y** - 5 to 10 mL q 4 to 6 h, up to 40 mL/day; **6 to < 12 y** - 2.5 to 5 mL q 4 to 6 h, up to 20 mL/day	Alcohol free, dye free, sugar free. Saccharin, sodium benzoate, sorbitol. Cotton candy flavor. In 473 mL.
c-v *sf*	**Notuss-AC Liquid** (SJ Pharmaceuticals)					**≥ 12 y** - 5 to 10 mL q 4 to 6 h up to 40 mL/day; **6 to < 12 y** - 2.5 to 5 mL q 4 to 6 h up to 20 mL/day	Alcohol free, dye free, gluten free. Saccharin, sorbitol. Cotton candy flavor. In 473 mL.
c-iii	**Cotab A Tablets** (MCR American)	10 mg codeine phosphate	4 mg chlorpheniramine maleate			**> 12 y** - 1 q 4 to 6 h, up to 6/day; **6 to < 12 y** - ½ q 4 to 6 h, up to 3/day	(COTAB A). White, capsule shape, scored. In 100s.
c-iii	**Cotab AX Tablets** (MCR American)	20 mg codeine phosphate	4 mg chlorpheniramine maleate			**≥ 12 y** - 1 q 4 to 6 h, up to 6/day; **6 to < 12 y** - ½ q 4 to 6 h, up to 3/day	(COTAB AX). Capsule shape, scored. In 100s.
c-v	**Zodryl DAC 25 Suspension** (CodaDOSE)	5 mg codeine phosphate	1.665 mg chlorpheniramine maleate	25 mg pseudoephedrine HCl		**2 to < 6 y (> 10.5 to 13 kg)** – 3 mL q 4 to 6 h, up to 12 mL/day	Methylparaben, sucralose. Grape flavor. In 118 mL.
c-v	**Zodryl DAC 30 Suspension** (CodaDOSE)	5 mg codeine phosphate	1.43 mg chlorpheniramine maleate	21.43 mg pseudoephedrine HCl		**2 to < 6 y (> 13 to 15 kg)** – 3.5 mL q 4 to 6 h, up to 14 mL/day	Methylparaben, sucralose. Grape flavor. In 118 mL.

ANTITUSSIVE COMBINATIONS

	Product & Distributor	Antitussive	Antihistamine	Decongestant	Other	Average Dose	Excipients & How Supplied
c-v	**Zodryl DAC 35 Suspension** (CodaDOSE)	5 mg codeine phosphate	1.25 mg chlorpheniramine maleate	18.75 mg pseudoephedrine HCl		**2 to < 6 y (> 15 to 17 kg)** – 4 mL q 4 to 6 h, up to 16 mL/day	Methylparaben, sucralose. Grape flavor. In 118 mL.
c-v	**Zodryl DAC 40 Suspension** (CodaDOSE)	5 mg codeine phosphate	1.11 mg chlorpheniramine maleate	16.665 mg pseudoephedrine HCl		**2 to < 6 y (> 17 to 19 kg)** – 4.5 mL q 4 to 6 h, up to 18 mL/day	Methylparaben, sucralose. Grape flavor. In 118 mL.
c-v	**Zodryl DAC 50 Suspension** (CodaDOSE)	5 mg codeine phosphate	2 mg chlorpheniramine maleate	30 mg pseudoephedrine HCl		**6 to < 12 y (> 19 to 25.5 kg)** – 5 mL q 4 to 6 h, up to 20 mL/day	Methylparaben, sucralose. Grape flavor. In 236 mL.
c-v	**Zodryl DAC 60 Suspension** (CodaDOSE)	5 mg codeine phosphate	1.43 mg chlorpheniramine maleate	20 mg pseudoephedrine HCl		**6 to < 12 y (> 25.5 to 32 kg)** – 7.5 mL q 4 to 6 h, up to 30 mL/day	Methylparaben, sucralose. Grape flavor. In 236 mL.
c-v	**Zodryl DAC 80 Suspension** (CodaDOSE)	5 mg codeine phosphate	1 mg chlorpheniramine maleate	15 mg pseudoephedrine HCl		**6 to < 12 y (> 32 to 40 kg)** – 10 mL q 4 to 6 h, up to 40 mL/day	Methylparaben, sucralose. Grape flavor. In 236 mL.
c-v	**Phenylhistine DH Liquid** (Qualitest)	10 mg codeine phosphate	2 mg chlorpheniramine maleate	30 mg pseudoephedrine HCl		**≥ 12 y** - 10 mL q 4 to 6 h up to 40 mL/day; **6 to < 12 y** - 5 mL q 4 to 6 h, up to 20 mL/day	5% alcohol, saccharin, sorbitol, sucrose. In 118 and 473 mL.
c-v	**Promethazine HCl w/Codeine Syrup** (Various, eg, Actavis Mid Atlantic,[b] Major, Morton Grove, URL)	10 mg codeine phosphate	6.25 mg promethazine HCl			**≥ 16 y** - 5 mL q 4 to 6 h, up to 30 mL/day	May contain corn syrup, parabens, saccharin. In 118 and 473 mL.
c-v *sf*	**EndaCof-DC Liquid** (Larken Labs)	10 mg codeine phosphate		30 mg pseudoephedrine HCl		**≥ 12 y** - 5 to 10 mL q 4 to 6 h, up to 40 mL/day; **6 to < 12 y** - 2.5 to 5 mL q 4 to 6 h, up to 20 mL/day	Alcohol free, dye free, sugar free. Saccharin, sodium benzoate, sorbitol. Fruit gum flavor. In 473 mL.
c-v *sf*	**Notuss-DC Liquid** (SJ Pharmaceuticals)					**≥ 12 y** - 5 to 10 mL q 4 to 6 h, up to 40 mL/day; **6 to < 12 y** - 2.5 to 5 mL q 4 to 6 h, up to 20 mL/day	Alcohol free, dye free, gluten free. Saccharin, sorbitol. Bubble gum flavor. In 473 mL.
c-iii	**Nucofed Capsules** (Monarch)	20 mg codeine phosphate		60 mg pseudoephedrine HCl		**≥ 12 y** - 1 q 6 h, up to 4/day	Lactose. (M 018). Green/Clear. In 60s.
c-iii	**Cotabflu Tablets** (MCR American)	20 mg codeine phosphate	4 mg chlorpheniramine maleate		500 mg acetaminophen	**≥ 12 y** - 1 q 4 to 6 h, up to 6/day; **6 to < 12 y** - ½ q 4 to 6 h, up to 3/day	(COTABFLU). Capsule shape, scored. In 100s.

ANTITUSSIVE COMBINATIONS

	Product & Distributor	Antitussive	Antihistamine	Decongestant	Other	Average Dose	Excipients & How Supplied
c-v	**Ala-Hist AC Liquid** (Ploy Pharmaceuticals)	10 mg codeine phosphate		7.5 mg phenylephrine HCl		**≥ 12 y** - 5 mL q 4 to 6 h, up to 30 mL/day; **6 to < 12 y** - 2.5 to 5 mL q 4 to 6 h, up to 30 mL/day	Alcohol free. Fruit flavor. In 473 mL.
c-v sf	**Dexphen w/C Liquid** (Breckenridge Pharmaceuticals)	10 mg codeine phosphate	1 mg dexchlorpheniramine maleate	5 mg phenylephrine HCl		**≥ 12 y** - 10 mL q 4 h, up to 60 mL/day; **6 to < 12 y** - 5 mL q 4 h, up to 30 mL/day	Alcohol free, dye free, gluten free, sugar free. Grape flavoring, propylene glycol, saccharin, sodium benzoate, sorbitol. In 473 mL.
c-v sf	**Endal CD Syrup** (Kylemore Pharmaceuticals)	7.5 mg codeine phosphate	12.5 mg diphenhydramine HCl	7.5 mg phenylephrine HCl		**≥ 12 y** - 10 mL q 4 h, up to 40 mL/day; **6 to < 12 y** - 5 mL q 4 h, up to 20 mL/day	Alcohol free, dye free, sugar free. Glycerin, saccharin, sorbitol. Cherry flavor. In 473 mL.
c-v	**Promethazine Hydrochloride, Phenylephrine Hydrochloride and Codeine Phosphate Syrup** (Alpharma)	10 mg codeine phosphate	6.25 mg promethazine HCl	5 mg phenylephrine HCl		**≥ 12 y** - 5 mL q 4 to 6 h, up to 30 mL/day; **6 to < 12 y**- 2.5 to 5 mL q 4 to 6 h, up to 30 mL/ day.	7% alcohol, parabens, saccharin, sucrose, sugar. Strawberry flavor. In 118, 237, and 473 mL.
c-v	**Promethazine VC W/Codeine Syrup** (Qualitest)					**≥ 12 y** - 5 mL q 4 to 6 h, up to 30 mL/day; **6 to < 12 y**- 2.5 to 5 mL q 4 to 6 h, up to 30 mL/ day.	7% alcohol, menthol, parabens, saccharin, sucrose. Strawberry flavor. In 118 mL
c-v sf	**Pro-Red AC Syrup** (Pro-Pharma)	9 mg codeine phosphate	8.33 mg pyrilamine maleate	5 mg phenylephrine HCl		**≥ 12 y** - 5 to 10 mL q 4 to 6 h, up to 40 mL/day; **6 to 12 y** - 2.5 to 5 mL q 4 to 6 h, up to 20 mL/day	Alcohol free, sugar free. Glycerin, saccharin, sorbitol. Cotton candy flavor. In 473 mL.
c-v sf	**Zotex-C Syrup** (Vertical Pharmaceuticals)	10 mg codeine phosphate	5 mg pyrilamine maleate	5 mg phenylephrine HCl		**≥ 12 y** - 5 to 10 mL q 4 to 6 h, up to 60 mL/day; **6 to < 12 y**- 2.5 to 5 mL q 4 to 6 h, up to 30 mL/day	Alcohol free, sugar free. Saccharin, sorbitol. Cherry flavor. In 473 mL.
c-v	**Codimal PH Syrup** (Victory Pharma)	10 mg codeine phosphate		5 mg phenylephrine HCl		**Adults** - 10 mL q 4 to 6 h, up to 60 mL/day[a]	Alcohol free. Sucrose. In 118 and 473 mL.
c-v sf	**Notuss-NX Liquid** (SJ Pharmaceuticals)	10 mg codeine phosphate	9.375 mg chlorcyclizine HCl			**≥ 12 y** – 10 mL q 6 to 8 h, up to 40 mL/day	Alcohol free, dye free, gluten free, sugar free. Glycerin, propylene glycol, saccharin, sorbitol. Cherry flavor. In 473 mL.
c-v sf	**Notuss-NXD Liquid** (SJ Pharmaceuticals)	10 mg codeine phosphate	9.375 mg chlorcyclizine HCl	30 mg pseudoephedrine HCl		**≥ 12 y** – 10 mL q 6 to 8 h, up to 40 mL/day	Alcohol free, dye free, gluten free, sugar free. Glycerin, propylene glycol, saccharin, sorbitol. Berry vanilla flavor. In 473 mL.
Rx sf	**Neo AC Syrup** (Laser)	10 mg codeine phosphate	15 mg pyrilamine maleate	30 mg pseudoephedrine HCl		**≥ 12 y** – 5 to 10 mL q 4 to 6 h, up to 40 mL/day **6 < 12 y** – 2.5 to 5 mL q 4 to 6 h, up to 20 mL/day	Alcohol free, dye free, sugar free. Saccharin, sorbitol. Orange vanilla flavor. In 473 mL.

ANTITUSSIVE COMBINATIONS

	Product & Distributor	Antitussive	Antihistamine	Decongestant	Other	Average Dose	Excipients & How Supplied
c-v sf	**Poly Hist NC Liquid** (Poly Pharmaceuticals)	10 mg codeine phosphate	1.25 mg triprolidine HCl	15 mg pseudoephedrine HCl		**≥ 12 y** – 5 to 10 mL q 4 to 6 h, up to 40 mL/day; **6 to < 12 y** – 2.5 to 5 mL q 4 to 6 h, up to 20 mL/day	Alcohol free, dye free, sugar free. Glycerin, propylene glycol, saccharin, sorbitol. Cotton candy flavor. In 473 mL.
otc	**Triaminic Infant Decongestant Plus Cough Thin Strips** (Novartis Consumer)	1.83 mg dextromethorphan (equivalent to 2.5 mg dextromethorphan HBr)		1.25 phenylephrine HCl		**2 to 3 y** - 2 q 4 h, up to 12/day	Alcohol, sucralose. Berry flavor. In 16s.
otc	**Triaminic Day Time Cold & Cough Thin Strips** (Novartis Consumer Health)	3.67 mg dextromethorphan (equivalent to 5 mg dextromethorphan HBr)		2.5 mg phenylephrine HCl		**6 to < 12 y** – 2 strips q 4 h, up to 12/day **4 to < 6 y** – 1 strip q 4 h, up to 6/day	Alcohol < 5%, PEG, propylene glycol, sucralose. Wild berry flavor. In 14s.
otc	**Theraflu Daytime Cold & Cough Thin Strips** Novartis Consumer Health)	14.8 mg dextromethorphan (equivalent to 20 mg dextromethorphan HBr)		10 mg phenylephrine HCl		**≥ 12 y** – 1 strip q 4 h up to 6/day	Alcohol, mannitol, sucralose. Cherry menthol flavor. In 12s.
otc	**Tylenol Plus Children's Cough & Sore Throat Oral Suspension** (McNeil Consumer)	5 mg dextromethorphan HBr			160 mg acetaminophen	**6 to 11 y (21.8 to 43.18 kg)** - 10 mL q 4 h, up to 50 mL/day; **2 to 5 y (10.9 to 21.36 kg)** - 5 mL q 4 h, up to 25 mL/day	Acesulfame K, corn syrup, sorbitol. Cherry flavor. In 120 mL.
otc	**Triaminic Cough & Sore Throat Liquid** (Novartis Consumer)					**6 to < 12 y** - 10 mL q 4 h, up to 50 mL/day **2 to < 6 y** - 5 mL q 4 h, up to 25 mL/day	Alcohol free. EDTA, 5 mg sodium per 5 mL, sorbitol, sucrose. Grape flavor. In 118 mL.
otc	**Triaminic Cough & Sore Throat Softchews** (Novartis Consumer)					**6 to < 12 y** - 2 q 4 h, up to 10/day; **2 to < 6 y** - 1 q 4 h, up to 5/day	Aspartame, mannitol, 28.1 mg phenylalanine, 8 mg sodium per 5 mL, sorbitol, sucrose. Grape flavor. In 18s.
otc	**Tylenol Cough & Sore Throat Daytime Liquid** (McNeil Consumer)	5 mg dextromethorphan HBr			166.67 mg acetaminophen	**≥ 12 y** - 30 mL q 6 h, up to 120 mL/day	3.67 mg sodium per 5 mL, sorbitol, sucralose, sucrose. In 240 mL.
otc sf	**PediaCare Infant Decongestant & Cough (PE) Oral Drops** (Johnson & Johnson)	3.125 mg dextromethorphan HBr		1.56 mg phenylephrine HCl		**2 to < 6 y** - 1.6 mL q 4 h, up to 9.6 mL/day	Alcohol free. EDTA, 3 mg sodium per dropperful, sorbitol, sucralose. Grape flavor. In 15 mL.
otc	**Dimetapp Toddler's Decongestant Plus Cough Drops** (Wyeth Consumer)						Alcohol free. Sorbitol. Grape flavor. In 15 mL.

ANTITUSSIVE COMBINATIONS

	Product & Distributor	Antitussive	Antihistamine	Decongestant	Other	Average Dose	Excipients & How Supplied
otc	**PediaCare Children's Multi-Symptom Cold Liquid** (McNeil Consumer)	5 mg dextromethorphan HBr		2.5 mg phenylephrine HCl		**6 to 11 y** - 10 mL q 4 h, up to 60 mL/day **4 to 5 y** - 5 mL q 4 h, up to 30 mL/day	Edetate disodium, glycerin, sodium benzoate, sorbitol, sucralose. Grape flavor. In 118 mL.
otc	**Triaminic Daytime Cold & Cough Liquid** (Novartis Consumer)					**6 to < 12 y** - 10 mL q 4 h, up to 60 mL/day; **2 to < 6 y** - 5 mL q 4 h, up to 30 mL/day	Alcohol free. Sorbitol, sucrose. Cherry flavor. In 118 mL.
otc	**Triaminic Daytime Cold & Cough Strips** (Novartis Consumer)					**6 to < 12 y** - 2 q 4 h, up to 12/day; **2 to < 6 y** - 1 q 4 h, up to 6/day	Alcohol. Wild fruit flavor. In 14s.
otc	**Vicks Formula 44D Cough & Head Congestion Relief Liquid** (Procter & Gamble Co.)	6.67 mg dextromethorphan HBr		3.33 mg phenylephrine HCl		**≥ 12 y** - 15 mL q 4 h, up to 90 mL/day; **6 to < 12 y** - 7.5 mL q 4 h, up to 45 mL/day	Alcohol, saccharin, 11 mg sodium per 5 mL, sorbitol, sucrose. In 118 and 236 mL.
otc	**Safetussin CD Liquid** (Kramer)	15 mg dextromethorphan HBr		2.5 mg phenylephrine HCl		**≥ 12 y** - 10 mL q 6 h, up to 40 mL/day; **6 to 12 y** - 5 mL q 6 h, up to 20 mL/day; **2 to 6 y** - 2.5 mL q 6 h, up to 10 mL/day	Menthol, parabens. In 120 mL.
otc	**PediaCare Infant Decongestant & Cough (PSE) Oral Drops** (Johnson & Johnson)	3.125 mg dextromethorphan HBr		9.375 mg pseudoephedrine HCl		**2 to < 6 y** - 1.6 mL q 4 h, up to 6.4 mL/day	Alcohol free. Sorbitol. Cherry flavor. In 15 mL.
otc *sf*	**Sudafed Children's Non-Drowsy Cold & Cough Liquid** (Johnson & Johnson)	5 mg dextromethorphan HBr		15 mg pseudoephedrine HCl		**≥ 12 y** - 20 mL q 4 h, up to 80 mL/day; **6 to < 12 y** - 10 mL q 4 h, up to 40 mL/day; **2 to < 6 y** - 5 mL q 4 h, up to 20 mL/day	Alcohol free. Saccharin, sorbitol. Cherry-berry flavor. In 118 mL.
otc	**Tylenol Plus Infants' Cold & Cough Concentrated Drops** (McNeil Consumer)	3.125 mg dextromethorphan HBr		1.56 mg phenylephrine HCl	100 mg acetaminophen	**2 to 3 y (10.9 to 15.9 kg)** - 1.6 mL q 4 h, up to 8 mL/day	Sorbitol, sucralose. Cherry flavor. In 15 mL w/syringe.

ANTITUSSIVE COMBINATIONS

	Product & Distributor	Antitussive	Antihistamine	Decongestant	Other	Average Dose	Excipients & How Supplied
otc	**Tylenol Cold Multi-Symptom Daytime Citrus Burst Liquid** (McNeil Consumer)	3.33 mg dextromethorphan HBr		1.67 mg phenylephrine HCl	108.33 mg acetaminophen	**≥ 12 y** - 30 mL q 4 h, up to 180 mL/day	Ethanol, 1.67 mg sodium per 5 mL, sorbitol, sucralose. In 240 mL.
otc	**Vicks DayQuil Multi-Symptom Cold/Flu Relief Liquid** (Procter & Gamble Co.)					**≥ 12 y** - 30 mL q 4 h, up to 120 mL/day; **6 to < 12 y** - 15 mL q 4 h, up to 60 mL/day	Alcohol free. Disodium EDTA, glycerin, propylene glycol, saccharin, sodium 50 mg sorbitol, sucralose. In 177 mL.
otc	**Alka-Seltzer Plus Day Non-Drowsy Cold Liquid** (Bayer)	5 mg dextromethorphan HBr		2.5 mg phenylephrine HCl	162.5 mg acetaminophen	**≥ 12 y** - 20 mL q 4 h, up to 120 mL/day	Alcohol free. Edetate disodium, PEG-400, sorbitol, sucralose. In 180 mL.
otc	**Comtrex Maximum Strength Non-Drowsy Cold & Cough Tablets** (Novartis Consumer)	10 mg dextromethorphan HBr		5 mg phenylephrine HCl	325 mg acetaminophen	**≥ 12 y** - 2 q 4 h, up to 12/day	Capsule shape. In 20s.
otc	**GNP Cold Head Congestion Daytime Tablets** (Amerisource Bergen)						Acesulfame K, polyvinyl alcohol. Capsule shape. In 24s.
otc	**Mapap Cold Formula Multi-Symptom Tablets** (Major)						Polyvinyl alcohol, sucralose. Capsule shape. In 24s.
otc	**Theraflu Daytime Severe Cold & Cough Tablets** (Novartis Consumer Health)						PEG. Capsule shape. In 24s.
otc	**Theraflu Warming Relief Daytime Multi-Symptom Cold Caplets** (Novartis)						Benzoic acid, menthol, PEG, sucralose. In 24s.
otc	**Tylenol Cold Head Congestion Daytime Cool Burst Tablets** (McNeil Consumer)						Sucralose. Capsule shape. In 24s.
otc	**Tylenol Cold Multi-Symptom Daytime Cool Burst Tablets** (McNeil Consumer)						Sucralose. Capsule shape. In 24s.
otc	**Tylenol Cold Multi-Symptom Daytime Gelcaps** (McNeil Consumer)						Benzyl alcohol, edetate calcium disodium, parabens. In 24s.
otc	**Vicks DayQuil Multi-Symptom Cold/Flu Relief LiquiCaps** (Procter & Gamble Co.)						Sorbitol. In 12s, 20s, 40s, and 60s.
otc	**666 Cold Preparation, Maximum Strength Liquid** (Monticello)	3.3 mg dextromethorphan HBr		30 mg pseudoephedrine HCl	108.33 mg acetaminophen	**≥ 12 y** - 30 mL q 4 h, up to 120 mL/day; **6 to 11 y** - 15 mL q 4 h, up to 60 mL/day	Saccharin, 23.5 mg sodium per 5 mL, sucrose. In 118 and 177 mL.
otc	**Children's Dimaphen DM Elixir** (Major)	5 mg dextromethorphan HBr	1 mg brompheniramine maleate	2.5 mg phenylephrine HCl		**≥ 12 y** - 20 mL q 4 h, up to 120 mL/day; **6 to < 12 y** - 10 mL q 4 h, up to 60 mL/day	Alcohol free. 3 mg sodium, sorbitol, sucralose. Grape flavor. In 118 mL.
otc	**Dimetapp Cold & Cough, Children's Liquid** (Wyeth)						Alcohol free. Sorbitol, sucralose. Grape flavor. In 118 mL.

ANTITUSSIVE COMBINATIONS

	Product & Distributor	Antitussive	Antihistamine	Decongestant	Other	Average Dose	Excipients & How Supplied
Rx *sf*	**Balacall DM Syrup** (Centurion Labs)	10 mg dextromethorphan HBr	2 mg brompheniramine maleate	5 mg phenylephrine HCl		**≥ 12 y** - 10 mL q 4 h, up to 60 mL/day; **6 to < 12 y** - 5 mL q 4 h, up to 30 mL/day	Alcohol and dye free. Saccharin. In 473 mL.
Rx *sf*	**BPM PE DM Syrup** (Boca)					**≥ 12 y** - 10 mL q 4 h, up to 60 mL/day; **6 to < 12 y** - 5 mL q 4 h, up to 30 mL/day; **2 to < 6 y** - 2.5 mL q 4 h, up to 15 mL/day	Alcohol free, sugar free. Glycerin, saccharin, sodium benzoate, sorbitol. Raspberry flavor. In 473 mL.
Rx	**BROM/PE/DM Syrup** (Brighton)					**≥ 12 y** - 10 mL q 4 h, up to 60 mL/day; **6 to < 12 y** - 5 mL q 4 h, up to 30 mL/day; **2 to < 6 y** - 2.5 mL q 4 h, up to 15 mL/day	Glycerin, prosweet, saccharin, sodium benzoate, sorbitol. Strawberry flavor. In 473 mL.
Rx	**LoHist-DM Syrup** (Larken Labs)					**> 12 y** - 10 mL q 4 h, up to 60 mL/day; **6 to 12 y** - 5 mL q 4 h, up to 30 mL/day	Parabens, saccharin, sorbitol. Strawberry flavor. In 473 mL.
Rx *sf*	**Tusdec-DM Liquid** (Cypress)	15 mg dextromethorphan HBr	2 mg brompheniramine maleate	7.5 mg phenylephrine HCl		**≥ 12 y** - 10 mL q 6 h, up to 40 mL/day; **6 to 12 y** - 5 mL q 6 h, up to 20 mL/day	Alcohol and dye free. Saccharin, sorbitol. Strawberry flavor. In 473 mL.

ANTITUSSIVE COMBINATIONS

	Product & Distributor	Antitussive	Antihistamine	Decongestant	Other	Average Dose	Excipients & How Supplied
Rx *sf*	**Alahist DM Liquid** (Poly Pharmaceuticals)	15 mg dextromethorphan HBr	4 mg brompheniramine maleate	7.5 mg phenylephrine HCl		**≥ 12 y** - 5 mL q 4 to 6 h, up to 30 mL/day; **6 to 12 y** - 2.5 mL q 4 to 6 h, up to 15 mL/day	Alcohol free, dye free, sugar free. Saccharin, sorbitol. Strawberry flavor. In 473 mL.
Rx *sf*	**Phenylephrine Complex Liquid** (Breckenridge)					**≥ 12 y** - 5 mL q 6 h, up to 30 mL/day; **6 to 12 y** - 2.5 mL q 6 h, up to 15 mL/day	Alcohol free, dye free, sugar free. Glycerin, saccharin, sodium benzoate, sorbitol. Strawberry flavor. In 473 mL.
Rx	**TGQ 7.5PEH/4BRM/15DM Liquid** (TG United)					**≥ 12 y** - 5 mL q 4 h, up to 30 mL/day; **6 to < 12 y** - 2.5 mL q 4 h, up to 15 mL/day	Parabens, potassium citrate, potassium sorbate, propylene glycol, sorbitol, sucralose. Strawberry flavor. In 473 mL.
Rx	**TL-Hist DM Liquid** (Trigen Labs)					**≥ 12 y** - 5 mL q 4 to 6 h, up to 30 mL/day; **6 to < 12 y** - 2.5 mL q 4 to 6 h, up to 15 mL/day	Parabens, potassium citrate, potassium sorbate, propylene glycol, sorbitol, sucralose. Strawberry flavor. In 473 mL
Rx	**Brompheniramine/Phenylephrine/DM Liquid** (Various, eg, Macoven Pharmaceuticals, River's Edge Pharmaceuticals)	20 mg dextromethorphan HBr	4 mg brompheniramine maleate	10 mg phenylephrine HCl		**> 12 y** - 5 to 10 mL q 4 to 6 h, up to 40 mL/day; **6 to < 12 y** - 5 mL q 4 to 6 h, up to 20 mL/day	May be alcohol free. May contain parabens, potassium citrate, potassium sorbate, sorbitol, sucralose. In 473 mL.
Rx	**Brōvex PEB DM Liquid** (Zyber Pharmaceutical)						Alcohol free. Parabens, sorbitol, sucralose. Bubble gum flavor. In 473 mL.
Rx	**Brōvex PB DM Tablets** (MCR American)					**> 12 y** - 1 q 4 to 6 h, up to 6/day; **6 to < 12 y** - ½ q 4 to 6 h, up to 3/day	(BROVEX PB DM). White, capsule shape, scored. In 100s.
Rx *sf*	**Neo DM Suspension** (Laser)	30 mg dextromethorphan tannate	10 mg brompheniramine maleate	25 mg phenylephrine tannate		**> 12 y** - 10 mL q 12 h, up to 20 mL/day; **6 to 12 y** - 5 mL q 12 h, up to 10 mL/day **2 to 6 y** - 2.5 mL q 12 h, up to 5 mL/day	Alcohol free, sugar free. Aspartame, phenylalanine 7 mg/5 mL, parabens. Cherry flavor. In 473 mL.
otc	**Theraflu Daytime Severe Cold & Cough Powder** (Novartis)	20 mg dextromethorphan HBr		10 mg phenylephrine HCl	650 mg acetaminophen	**≥ 12 y** - 1 packet dissolved in 8 oz hot water q 4 h, up to 6 packets/day	Acesulfame K, aspartame, maltodextrin, 14 mg phenylalanine per packet, sucrose. Berry infused with menthol and green tea flavor. In 6s.
Rx *sf*	**P Chlor DM Drops** (SDA Labs)	3 mg dextromethorphan HBr	1 mg chlorpheniramine maleate	3.5 mg phenylephrine HCl		**12 to 24 mo** - 1 mL, up to 4 mL/day	Alcohol free, sugar free. Glycerin, sodium benzoate, sorbitol. Grape flavor. In 30 mL.

ANTITUSSIVE COMBINATIONS

	Product & Distributor	Antitussive	Antihistamine	Decongestant	Other	Average Dose	Excipients & How Supplied
otc	**Comtrex Maximum Strength Nighttime Cold & Cough Caplets** (Novartis Consumer)	10 mg dextromethorphan HBr	2 mg chlorpheniramine maleate	5 mg phenylephrine HCl	325 mg acetaminophen	**≥ 12 y** - 2 q 4 h, up to 12/day	PEG. In 20s.
Rx	**AccuHist DM Pediatric Drops** (Tiber)	4 mg dextromethorphan HBr	1 mg brompheniramine maleate	15 mg pseudoephedrine HCl		**12 to 24 mo** - 1 mL qid, up to 4 mL/day; **6 to 12 mo** - 0.75 mL qid, up to 3 mL/day; **3 to 6 mo** - 0.5 mL qid, up to 2 mL/day; **1 to 3 mo** - 0.25 mL qid, up to 1 mL/day	Saccharin, sorbitol. Grape flavor. In 38 mL w/dropper.
Rx	**Pediahist DM Drops** (Boca)					**9 to 18 mo** - 1 mL qid; **6 to 9 mo** - 0.75 mL qid; **3 to 6 mo** 0.5 mL qid; **1 to 3 mo** - 0.25 mL qid	Sorbitol. Grape flavor. In 30 mL w/dropper.
Rx	**Resperal-DM Drops** (Cypress)	5 mg dextromethorphan HBr	1 mg brompheniramine maleate	12 mg pseudoephedrine HCl		**6 to < 12 y** - 2 mL q 4 to 6 h, up to 8 mL/day; **2 to < 6 y** - 1 mL q 4 to 6 h, up to 4 mL/day	Alcohol and dye free. Saccharin, sorbitol, sucrose. Grape flavor. In 30 mL w/dropper.
otc	**Bromaline DM Elixir** (Rugby)	5 mg dextromethorphan HBr	1 mg brompheniramine maleate	15 mg pseudoephedrine HCl		**≥ 12 y** - 20 mL q 6 h, up to 80 mL/day; **6 to < 12 y** - 10 mL q 6 h, up to 40 mL/day	Alcohol free. Fructose, saccharin, sorbitol. Grape flavor. In 473 mL.
otc *sf*	**Brotapp-DM Liquid** (Silarx)					**≥ 12 y** - 20 mL q 6 h, up to 80 mL/day; **6 to < 12 y** - 10 mL q 6 h, up to 40 mL/day	Alcohol free, sugar free. Saccharin, sorbitol. Grape flavor. In 118 and 237 mL.
otc *sf*	**Q-Tapp DM Elixir** (Qualitest)					**≥ 12 y** - 20 mL q 4 to 6 h, up to 80 mL/day; **6 to < 12 y** - 10 mL q 4 to 6 h, up to 40 mL/day	Alcohol free, sugar free. Saccharin, sorbitol. Grape flavor. In 118 mL.

ANTITUSSIVE COMBINATIONS

	Product & Distributor	Antitussive	Antihistamine	Decongestant	Other	Average Dose	Excipients & How Supplied
Rx	**Bromfed DM Cough Syrup** (Wockhardt)	10 mg dextromethorphan HBr	2 mg brompheniramine maleate	30 mg pseudoephedrine HCl		≥ **12 y** - 10 mL q 4 h, up to 60 mL/day; **6 to < 12 y** - 5 mL q 4 h, up to 30 mL/day; **2 to < 6 y** - 2.5 mL q 4 h, up to 15 mL/day	0.95% alcohol, methylparaben, sugar. Butterscotch flavor. In 118 and 473 mL.
Rx *sf*	**Dimetane DX Liquid** (Creekwood Pharmaceuticals)						Alcohol free, dye free, gluten free, sugar free. Berry flavoring, glycerin, propylene glycol, saccharin, sorbitol. In 118 mL.
Rx *sf*	**Dallergy DM Syrup** (Laser)	15 mg dextromethorphan HBr	3 mg brompheniramine maleate	30 mg pseudoephedrine HCl		**> 12 y** – 5 to 10 mL q 4 to 6 h, up to 40 mL/day **6 to < 12 y**– 2.5 to 5 mL q 4 to 6 h, up to 20 mL/day	Alcohol free, sugar free. Saccharin, sorbitol. Berry vanilla flavor. In 473 mL.
Rx *sf*	**PBM Allergy Syrup** (Boca Pharmacal)						Alcohol free. Saccharin, sorbitol. Berry-vanilla flavor. In 473 mL.
Rx	**Sildec-DM Syrup** (Silarx)	15 mg dextromethorphan HBr	4 mg brompheniramine maleate	45 mg pseudoephedrine HCl		≥ **6 y** - 5 mL qid; **2 to 6 y** - 2.5 mL qid	Saccharin, sorbitol. Grape flavor. In 118 and 473 mL.
Rx	**BPM Mal 4/PSE HCl 20/DM HBr 20 Liquid** (River's Edge Pharmaceuticals)	20 mg dextromethorphan HBr	4 mg brompheniramine maleate	20 mg pseudoephedrine HCl		**> 12 y** - 5 to 10 mL q 4 to 6 h, up to 40 mL/day; **6 to < 12 y** - 5 mL q 4 to 6 h, up to 20 mL/day; **2 to < 6 y** - 2.5 mL q 4 to 6 h, up to 10 mL/day	Alcohol free. Cotton candy flavoring, glycerin, propylene glycol, sorbitol, saccharin. Cotton candy flavor. In 473 mL.
Rx	**Brōvex PSB DM Liquid** (Zyber Pharmaceuticals)						Alcohol free. Sorbitol. Cotton candy flavor. In 473 mL.
Rx	**Brōvex PSE DM Tablets** (Zyber Pharmaceutical)	20 mg dextromethorphan HBr	4 mg brompheniramine maleate	40 mg pseudoephedrine HCl		**> 12 y** - 1 q 4 to 6 h, up to 6/day; **6 to < 12 y** - ½ q 4 to 6 h, up to 3/day	(BROVEX PSE DM). Capsule shape, white, scored. In 100s.
Rx	**TG 40PSE/4BRM/20DM Tablets** (TG United)					**> 12 y** - 1 q 4 to 6 h, up to 6/day; **6 to < 12 y** - ½ q 4 to 6 h, up to 3/day	(TG 705). White, capsule shape, scored. In 100s.

ANTITUSSIVE COMBINATIONS

	Product & Distributor	Antitussive	Antihistamine	Decongestant	Other	Average Dose	Excipients & How Supplied
Rx *sf*	**Bromdex D Syrup** (Breckenridge)	30 mg dextromethorphan HBr	3 mg brompheniramine maleate	50 mg pseudoephedrine HCl		≥ **12 y** - 5 mL q 6 h, up to 20 mL/day; **6 to < 12 y** - 2.5 mL q 6 h, up to 10 mL/day	Alcohol free, sugar free. Saccharin, sorbitol. Berry vanilla flavor. In 473 mL
Rx	**Neo DM Syrup** (Laser)						Saccharin, sorbitol. Berry vanilla flavor. In 473 mL.
Rx	**TGQ 50PSE/3BRM/30DM Syrup** (TG United)					≥ **12 y** - 5 mL q 4 to 6 h, up to 20 mL/day; **6 to < 12 y** - 2.5 mL q 4 to 6 h, up to 10 mL/day	Parabens, potassium sorbate, propylene glycol, sorbitol, sucralose. Berry-vanilla flavor. In 473 mL.
Rx	**DM/PSE/BPM Syrup** (Kylemore)					≥ **12 y** - 5 mL q 6 h, up to 20 mL/day; **6 to < 12 y** - 2.5 mL q 6 h, up to 10 mL/day	Glycerin, parabens, propylene glycol, saccharin, sorbitol. Berry-vanilla flavor. In 473 mL.
Rx *sf*	**Anaplex-DM Cough Syrup** (ECR)	30 mg dextromethorphan HBr	4 mg brompheniramine maleate	60 mg pseudoephedrine HCl		≥ **12 y** - 5 mL q 4 to 6 h, up to 20 mL/day; **6 to 12 y** - 2.5 mL q 4 to 6 h, up to 10 mL/day;	Alcohol and dye free. Fruit flavor. In 473 mL.
Rx *sf*	**Bromphenex DM Liquid** (Breckenridge)					≥ **12 y** - 5 mL q 4 to 6 h, up to 20 mL/day	Alcohol and dye free. Saccharin, sorbitol. Fruit flavor. In 473 mL.
Rx *sf*	**PSE Brom DM Syrup** (Boca)					≥ **12 y** - 5 mL q 4 to 6 h, up to 20 mL/day; **6 to 12 y** - 2.5 mL q 4 to 6 h, up to 10 mL/day; **2 to 6 y** - 1.25 mL q 4 to 6 h, up to 5 mL/day	Alcohol free. Sorbitol. In 473 mL.
Rx *sf*	**XiraHist DM Pediatric Drops** (Hawthorn)	3 mg dextromethorphan HBr	2 mg carbinoxamine maleate	2 mg phenylephrine HCl		**12 to 24 mo** - 1 mL qid; **6 to 12 mo** - 0.75 mL qid; **3 to 6 mo** - 0.5 mL qid	Alcohol and dye free. Saccharin, sorbitol. Peach flavor. In 30 mL w/dropper.
Rx	**Balamine DM Oral Drops** (Ballay)	3.5 mg dextromethorphan HBr	2 mg carbinoxamine maleate	25 mg pseudoephedrine HCl		**9 to 18 mo** - 1 mL qid; **6 to 9 mo** - 0.75 mL qid; **3 to 6 mo** - 0.5 mL qid; **1 to 3 mo** - 0.25 mL qid	Menthol. Grape flavor. In 30 mL w/dropper.
Rx	**Balamine DM Syrup** (Ballay)	12.5 mg dextromethorphan HBr	4 mg carbinoxamine maleate	60 mg pseudoephedrine HCl		≥ **6 y** - 5 mL qid; **18 mo to 6 y** - 2.5 mL qid	Menthol. Grape flavor. In 473 mL.

ANTITUSSIVE COMBINATIONS

	Product & Distributor	Antitussive	Antihistamine	Decongestant	Other	Average Dose	Excipients & How Supplied
Rx *sf*	**Cordron-DM NR Liquid** (Cypress)	15 mg dextromethorphan HBr	3 mg carbinoxamine maleate	12.5 mg pseudoephedrine HCl		≥ **12 y** - 10 mL qid; **6 to 12 y** - 5 mL qid; **18 mo to 6 y** - 2.5 mL qid	Alcohol and dye free. Saccharin, sorbitol. In 473 mL.
Rx *sf*	**Pseudo Carb DM Pediatric Liquid** (Boca)						Alcohol and dye free. In 118 and 473 mL.
otc	**Vicks Children's NyQuil Cold & Cough Relief Liquid** (Procter & Gamble Co.)	5 mg dextromethorphan HBr	0.67 mg chlorpheniramine maleate			≥ **12 y** - 30 mL q 6 h, up to 120 mL/day; **6 to < 12 y** - 15 mL q 6 h, up to 60 mL/day	Alcohol free. 23.7 mg sodium per 5 mL, sucrose. Cherry flavor. In 118 mL.
otc	**Vicks Formula 44m Pediatric Cough & Cold Relief Liquid** (Procter & Gamble Co.)						Corn syrup, saccharin, 9 mg sodium per 5 mL. In 118 mL.
otc	**Triaminic Cough & Runny Nose Soft Chews** (Novartis Consumer Health)	5 mg dextromethorphan HBr	1 mg chlorpheniramine maleate			**6 to < 12 y** 2 q 4 to 6 h, up to 12/day	Aspartame, maltodextrin, mannitol, 17.6 mg phenylalanine, 5 mg sodium, sorbitol, sucrose. Cherry flavor. In 18s.
otc	**Dimetapp Long Acting Cough Plus Cold Syrup** (Wyeth)	7.5 mg dextromethorphan HBr	1 mg chlorpheniramine maleate			≥ **12 y** - 20 mL q 6 h, up to 80 mL/day; **6 to < 12 y** - 10 mL q 6 h, up to 40 mL/day	3 mg sodium per 5 mL, sorbitol, sucralose. Fruit punch flavor. In 118 mL.
otc	**Robitussin Pediatric Cough & Cold Long-Acting Liquid** (Wyeth)					≥ **12 y** (≥ **43.6 kg**) - 20 mL q 6 h, up to 80 mL/day; **6 to < 12 y** - 10 mL q 6 h, up to 40 mL/day	3 mg sodium per 5 mL, sorbitol, sucralose. In 118 mL.
otc *sf*	**Tricodene Sugar Free Cough & Cold Liquid** (Pfeiffer)	10 mg dextromethorphan HBr	2 mg chlorpheniramine maleate			≥ **12 y** - 10 mL q 4 to 6 h, up to 60 mL/day; **6 to < 12 y** - 5 mL q 4 to 6 h, up to 30 mL/day	Alcohol free. Mannitol, menthol, saccharin, 12 mg sodium per 5 mL, sorbitol. In 120 mL.
otc *sf*	**Scot-Tussin DM Liquid** (Scot-Tussin)	15 mg dextromethorphan HBr	2 mg chlorpheniramine maleate			≥ **12 y** - 10 mL q 6 to 8 h, up to 40 mL/day; **6 to < 12 y** - 5 mL q 6 to 8 h, up to 20 mL/day; **2 to < 6 y** - 2.5 mL q 6 to 8 h, up to 10 mL/day	Alcohol free. *Magnasweet*, menthol, parabens. In 118 mL.
Rx	**AMBI 20DM/4CPM Tablets** (AMBI)	20 mg dextromethorphan HBr	4 mg chlorpheniramine maleate			**> 12 y** - 1 q 4 to 6 h up to 6/day; **6 to < 12 y** - ½ q 4 to 6 h up to 3/day	(AMBI 448). White, capsule shape, scored. In 100s.
otc	**Coricidin HBP Cough & Cold Tablets** (Schering-Plough)	30 mg dextromethorphan HBr	4 mg chlorpheniramine maleate			≥ **12 y** - 1 q 6 h, up to 4/day	Sugar. (C C + C). Red. In 16s.

ANTITUSSIVE COMBINATIONS

	Product & Distributor	Antitussive	Antihistamine	Decongestant	Other	Average Dose	Excipients & How Supplied
otc	**Tylenol Plus Children's Cough & Runny Nose Oral Suspension** (McNeil Consumer)	5 mg dextromethorphan HBr	1 mg chlorpheniramine maleate		160 mg acetaminophen	**6 to 11 y (21.8 to 43.18 kg)** - 10 mL q 4 h, up to 50 mL/day	Acesulfame K, corn syrup, sorbitol. Cherry flavor. In 120 mL.
otc	**Triaminic Flu, Cough & Fever Liquid** (Novartis Consumer)	7.5 mg dextromethorphan HBr	1 mg chlorpheniramine maleate		160 mg acetaminophen	**6 to < 12 y** - 10 mL q 6 h, up to 40 mL/day	EDTA, 6 mg sodium per 5 mL, sorbitol, sucrose. Bubble gum flavor. In 118 mL.
otc	**Coricidin HBP Maximum Strength Flu Tablets** (Schering-Plough)	15 mg dextromethorphan HBr	2 mg chlorpheniramine maleate		500 mg acetaminophen	**≥ 12 y** - 2 q 6 h, up to 8/day	Lactose. (Coricidin HBP Flu). Red, oval. In 20s.
otc	**Alka-Seltzer Plus Flu Formula Effervescent Tablets** (Bayer)	15 mg dextromethorphan HBr	2 mg chlorpheniramine maleate		500 mg aspirin	**≥ 12 y** - 2 dissolved in 4 oz of water q 6 h, up to 8/day	Acesulfame K, aspartame, mannitol, 6.7 mg phenylalanine per tablet, saccharin, 381 mg sodium per tablet. In 20s.
Rx	**Extendryl DM Tablets** (Auriga)	30 mg dextromethorphan HBr	8 mg chlorpheniramine maleate		2.5 methscopolamine nitrate	**≥ 12 y** - 1 bid, up to 2/day; **6 to 12 y** - ½ bid, up to 1/day	Extended release. (AP 202). Scored. In 100s.
otc	**Father John's Medicine Plus Liquid** (Oakhurst)	1.67 mg dextromethorphan HBr	0.67 mg chlorpheniramine maleate	1.67 mg phenylephrine HCl		**≥ 12 y** - 30 mL q 4 h, up to 180 mL/day	Alcohol free. In 118 mL.
Rx sf	**Bronkids Oral Drops** (Portal Pharmaceuticals)	2.75 mg dextromethorphan HBr	0.6 mg chlorpheniramine maleate	1.5 mg phenylephrine HCl		**1 to 2 y** - 1 mL q 4 h **6 to 12 mo** - ¾ mL q 4 h	Alcohol free. Saccharin, sorbitol. Bubble gum flavor. In 30 mL w/ dropper.
Rx sf	**Neo DM Drops** (Laser)	2.75 mg dextromethorphan HBr	0.75 mg chlorpheniramine maleate	1.75 mg phenylephrine HCl		**6 to < 12 y** - 2 mL q 4 to 6 h, up to 8 mL/day; **2 to < 6 y** - 1 mL q 4 to 6 h, up to 4 mL/day	Alcohol free. Saccharin, sorbitol. Black cherry flavor. In 30 mL w/dropper.
Rx sf	**NoHist-PDX Drops** (Larken)						Alcohol free. Saccharin, sorbitol. Cherry flavor. In 30 mL w/dropper.
Rx sf	**RE DCP Drops** (River's Edge)						Alcohol free, sugar free. Saccharin, sorbitol. Cherry flavor. In 30 mL w/dropper.

ANTITUSSIVE COMBINATIONS

	Product & Distributor	Antitussive	Antihistamine	Decongestant	Other	Average Dose	Excipients & How Supplied
Rx *sf*	**DM/PE/CPM Drops** (Kylemore)	3 mg dextromethorphan HBr	1 mg chlorpheniramine maleate	1.5 mg phenylephrine HCl		**6 to < 12 y** - 2 mL q 4 to 6 h, up to 8 mL/ day; **2 to < 6 y**- 1 mL q 4 to 6 h, up to 4 mL/day	Alcohol free, sugar free. Glycerin, parabens, propylene glycol, saccharin, sorbitol. Fruit gum flavor. In 30 mL w/dropper.
Rx *sf*	**DM-PE-CHLOR Drops** (Palmetto)						Alcohol free. Saccharin, sorbitol. Bubble gum flavor. In 30 mL w/dropper.
Rx *sf*	**Donatussin DM Drops** (Laser)						Alcohol free. Saccharin, sorbitol. Bubble gum flavor. In 30 mL w/dropper.
Rx *sf*	**Quartuss DM Drops** (Breckenridge)					**12 to 24 mo** - 1 to 2 mL 4 times daily, up to 8 mL/day; **6 to 12 mo** - 0.6 to 1 mL 4 times daily, up to 4 mL/day; **3 to 6 mo** - 0.3 to 0.6 mL 4 times daily, up to 2.4 mL/day; **1 to 3 mo** - 2 to 3 drops/month of age 4 times daily	Alcohol and dye free. Bubble gum flavor. In 30 mL w/dropper.
Rx	**Centergy DM Drops** (Centurion)	3 mg dextromethorphan HBr	1 mg chlorpheniramine maleate	2 mg phenylephrine HCl		**6 to < 12 y** - 2 mL q 4 to 6 h up to 8 mL/ day; **2 to > 6 y** – 1 mL q 4 to 6 h up to 4 mL/ day	Sorbitol. Strawberry flavor. In 30 mL.
Rx	**Nasohist DM Drops** (Hawthorn)						Saccharin, sorbitol. Orange-vanilla flavor. In 30 mL.
Rx	**Sonahist DM Drops** (Kylemore)						Parabens, saccharin, sorbitol. Orange-vanilla flavor. In 30 mL.
Rx *sf*	**C-Phen DM Oral Drops** (Boca)	3 mg dextromethorphan HBr	1 mg chlorpheniramine maleate	3.5 mg phenylephrine HCl		**12 to 24 mo** - 1 mL q 4 to 6 h, up to 4 mL/day; **6 to 12 mo** - 0.75 mL q 4 to 6 h, up to 3 mL/ day	Alcohol free. Sorbitol. Grape flavor. In 30 mL w/dropper.
Rx	**PE-Hist DM Syrup** (Larkin)	15 mg dextromethorphan HBr	2 mg chlorpheniramine maleate	5 mg phenylephrine HCl		**> 12 y** - 10 mL q 6 h, up to 40 mL/day; **6 to < 12 y** - 5 mL q 6 h, up to 20 mL/day; **2 to < 6 y** - 2.5 mL q 6 h, up to 10 mL/day	Alcohol free. Methylparaben, saccharin, sucrose. In 473 mL.
Rx *sf*	**Reme Tussin DM Syrup** (River's Edge)						Saccharin, sorbitol. Strawberry flavor. In 473 mL.

ANTITUSSIVE COMBINATIONS

	Product & Distributor	Antitussive	Antihistamine	Decongestant	Other	Average Dose	Excipients & How Supplied
Rx *sf*	**De-Chlor DR Liquid** (Cypress)	15 mg dextromethorphan HBr	2 mg chlorpheniramine maleate	6 mg phenylephrine HCl		**> 12 y** - 10 mL q 6 h, up to 40 mL/day; **6 to < 12 y** - 5 mL q 6 h, up to 20 mL/day	Alcohol free, dye free. Saccharin, sorbitol. Strawberry flavor. In 473 mL.
Rx	**Dex PC Syrup** (Boca)					**> 12 y** - 10 mL q 6 h, up to 40 mL/day; **6 to < 12 y** - 5 mL q 6 h, up to 20 mL/day; **2 to < 6 y** - 2.5 mL q 6 h, up to 10 mL/day	Alcohol free. Corn syrup. Strawberry flavor. In 473 mL.
Rx *sf*	**Mintuss DR Syrup** (Breckenridge)					**> 12 y** - 10 mL q 6 h, up to 40 mL/day; **6 to < 12 y** - 5 mL q 6 h, up to 20 mL/day	Alcohol free. Sorbitol. Strawberry flavor. In 473 mL.
Rx *sf*	**De-Chlor DM Liquid** (Cypress)	15 mg dextromethorphan HBr	2 mg chlorpheniramine maleate	10 mg phenylephrine HCl		**> 12 y** - 5 mL q 4 h, up to 30 mL/day; **6 to 12 y** - 2.5 mL q 4 h, up to 15 mL/day	Alcohol free, dye free. Saccharin, sorbitol. Strawberry flavor. In 473 mL.
Rx *sf*	**Corfen-DM Liquid** (Cypress)	15 mg dextromethorphan HBr	4 mg chlorpheniramine maleate	10 mg phenylephrine HCl		**≥ 12 y** - 5 mL q 4 to 6 h, up to 30 mL/day; **6 to < 12 y** - 2.5 mL q 4 to 6 h, up to 15 mL/day	Alcohol free, dye free. Saccharin, sorbitol. Grape flavor. In 473 mL.
Rx *sf*	**Ed-A-Hist DM Liquid** (Edwards)					**> 12 y** - 5 mL q 6 h, up to 30 mL/day; **6 to 12 y** - 2.5 mL q 6 h, up to 15 mL/day;	Saccharin, sorbitol. Banana flavor. In 473 mL.
Rx *sf*	**Trital DM Liquid** (Breckenridge Pharmaceutical)					**≥ 12 y** - 5 mL q 4 h, up to 30 mL/day; **6 to < 12 y** - 2.5 mL q 4 h, up to 15 mL/day	Alcohol free, dye free. Sorbitol. Grape flavor. In 473 mL.

ANTITUSSIVE COMBINATIONS

	Product & Distributor	Antitussive	Antihistamine	Decongestant	Other	Average Dose	Excipients & How Supplied
Rx *sf*	**C-Phen DM Syrup** (Boca)	15 mg dextromethorphan HBr	4 mg chlorpheniramine maleate	12.5 mg phenylephrine HCl		≥ **12 y** - 5 mL q 4 to 6 h, up to 20 mL/day; **6 to < 12 y** - 2.5 mL q 4 to 6 h, up to 10 mL/day; **2 to < 6 y** - 1.25 mL q 4 to 6 h, up to 5 mL/day	Alcohol free. Sorbitol. Grape flavor. In 118 and 473 mL.
Rx *sf*	**Ceron-DM Syrup** (Cypress)					≥ **12 y** - 5 mL q 6 h, up to 20 mL/day; **6 to < 12 y** - 2.5 mL q 4 to 6 h, up to 10 mL/day	Alcohol free. Saccharin, sorbitol. Grape flavor. In 118 and 473 mL.
Rx	**TGQ 15DM/5PEH/2CPM Liquid** (TG United)	15 mg dextromethorphan HBr	2 mg chlorpheniramine maleate	5 mg phenylephrine HCl		**> 12 y** - 5 to 10 mL q 4 to 6 h, up to 40 mL/day; **6 to < 12 y** - 2.5 to 5 mL q 4 to 6 h, up to 20 mL/day	Parabens, potassium citrate, potassium sorbate, propylene glycol, sorbitol, sucralose. Strawberry flavor. In 473 mL.
Rx	**AMBI 10PEH/4CPM/20DM Tablets** (AMBI)	20 mg dextromethorphan HBr	4 mg chlorpheniramine maleate	10 mg phenylephrine HCl		**> 12 y** - 1 q 4 to 6 h up to 6/day; **6 to < 12 y** - ½ q 4 to 6 h up to 3/day	(AMBI 445). White, capsule shape, scored. In 100s.
Rx	**Maxichlor PEH DM Tablets** (MCR American)						(MAXICHLOR PEH DM). White, capsule shape, scored. In 100s.
Rx *sf*	**NeoTuss Plus Liquid** (A.G. Marin)	30 mg dextromethorphan HBr	4 mg chlorpheniramine maleate	7.5 mg phenylephrine HCl		**> 12 y** - 5 mL q 6 to 8 h, up to 20 mL/day; **6 to 12 y** - 2.5 mL q 6 to 8 h, up to 10 mL/day	Alcohol free, dye free. Parabens, sorbitol, sucralose. Cherry flavor. In 474 mL.
Rx	**NoHist DMX Tablets** (Larkin Laboratories)	30 mg dextromethorphan HBr	8 mg chlorpheniramine maleate	20 mg phenylephrine HCl		**> 12 y** - 1 or 2 q 12 h, up to 3/day	Extended release. (LL 167). Capsule shape. In 100s.
Rx *sf*	**Phenabid DM Timed-Release Tablets** (GIL)					≥ **12 y** - 1 or 2 q 12 h, up to 4/day; **6 to < 12 y** - ½ or 1 q 12 h, up to 2/day; **2 to < 6 y** - ½ q 12 h, up to 1/day	Extended release. Dye free, preservative free. (GIL 306). Capsule shape, scored. In 100s, 500s and 1,000s.
Rx	**Zotex-12D Tablets** (Vertical)					**> 12 y** - 1 or 2 q 12 h, up to 3/day	Extended release. (VP 033). Capsule shape. In 100s.

ANTITUSSIVE COMBINATIONS

	Product & Distributor	Antitussive	Antihistamine	Decongestant	Other	Average Dose	Excipients & How Supplied
Rx *sf*	**AccuHist PDX Drops** (PediaMed)	3 mg dextromethorphan HBr	0.8 mg chlorpheniramine maleate	9 mg pseudoephedrine HCl		**24 to 36 mo** - 1 mL qid, up to 4 mL/day; **12 to 24 mo** - 0.75 mL qid, up to 3 mL/day ; **6 to 12 mo** - 0.5 mL qid, up to 2 mL/day;	Alcohol free. Saccharin, sorbitol. Grape flavor. In 30 mL w/dropper.
Rx	**CPM/PSE DM Drops** (Trigen Labs)					**6 to < 12 y** - 2 mL q 4 to 6 h, up to 8 mL/day	Glycerin, parabens, potassium citrate, potassium sorbate, propylene glycol, sorbitol, sucralose. Grape flavor. In 30 mL w/dropper.
Rx *sf*	**Neutrahist PDX Drops** (Cypress)						Alcohol free. Grape flavor. In 30 mL.
otc	**KidKare Children's Cough/Cold Liquid** (Rugby)	5 mg dextromethorphan HBr	1 mg chlorpheniramine maleate	15 mg pseudoephedrine HCl		**6 to < 12 y** - 10 mL q 4 to 6 h, up to 40 mL/day	Alcohol free. Corn syrup, sorbitol. Cherry flavor. In 118 mL.
otc	**Pedia Relief Cough-Cold Liquid** (Major)					**6 to < 12 y** - 10 mL q 6 h, up to 40 mL/day	Alcohol free. Cherry flavor. In 118 mL.
otc	**Pediatric Cough & Cold Medicine Liquid** (Silarx)					**6 to < 12 y** - 10 mL q 4 to 6 h, up to 40 mL/day	Alcohol free. Sorbitol. In 120 mL.
otc	**Triaminic-D Multi-Symptom Cold Syrup** (Novartis)	7.5 mg dextromethorphan HBr	1 mg chlorpheniramine maleate	15 mg pseudoephedrine HCl		**6 to < 12 y** - 10 mL q 6 h, up to 40 mL/day	Alcohol free. Benzoic acid, disodium edetate, propylene glycol, sodium 6 mg per 5 mL, sorbitol, sucrose. Grape flavor. In 118 mL.
otc	**Dicel DM Chewable Tablets** (Centrix)	10 mg dextromethorphan HBr	2 mg chlorpheniramine maleate	30 mg pseudoephedrine HCl		**≥ 12 y** - 2 q 4 to 6 h, up to 8/day; **6 to < 12 y** - 1 q 4 to 6 h, up to 4/day	Alcohol free. Glycyrrhizate, maltodextrin, PEG, soy lecithin, sucralose, sugar, vegetable oil. Cotton candy flavor. In 20s.
otc *sf*	**Rescon DM Liquid** (Capellon)					**≥ 12 y** - 10 mL q 4 to 6 h, up to 40 mL/day; **6 to < 12 y** - 5 mL q 4 to 6 h, up to 20 mL/day	Alcohol free, corn allergen free, dye free. Parabens, PEG, saccharin, sorbitol. Fruit punch flavor. In 118 and 473 mL.
Rx	**Dicel DM Suspension** (Centrix)	10.5 mg dextromethorphan (as dextromethorphan tannate)	2.25 mg chlorpheniramine (as chlorpheniramine tannate)	21.75 mg pseudoephedrine (as pseudoephedrine tannate)		**≥ 12 y** - 5 to 10 mL up to 4 times daily (40 mL/day); **6 to < 12 y** - 2.5 to 5 mL up to 4 times daily (20 mL/day)	Methylparaben, saccharin, sucrose. Cotton candy flavor. In 473 mL.
Rx *sf*	**M-End DM Liquid** (R.A. McNeil)	15 mg dextromethorphan HBr	2 mg chlorpheniramine maleate	15 mg pseudoephedrine HCl		**≥ 12 y** - 10 mL q 6 h, up to 40 mL/day; **6 to < 12 y** - 5 mL q 6 h, up to 20 mL/day	Alcohol free. Sucrose. In 473 mL.

ANTITUSSIVE COMBINATIONS

	Product & Distributor	Antitussive	Antihistamine	Decongestant	Other	Average Dose	Excipients & How Supplied
Rx	**Maxichlor PSE DM** (MCR American)	20 mg dextromethorphan HBr	4 mg chlorpheniramine maleate	60 mg pseudoephedrine HCl		≥ **12 y** - 1 q 4 to 6 h, up to 4/day; **6 to < 12 y** - ½ q 4 to 6 h, up to 2/day	(MAXICHLOR PSE DM). White, capsule shape, scored. In 100s.
Rx	**Atuss DS Tannate Suspension** (Atley)	30 mg dextromethorphan HBr (as 60 mg dextromethorphan tannate)	4 mg chlorpheniramine maleate (as 8 mg chlorpheniramine tannate)	30 mg pseudoephedrine (as 60 mg pseudoephedrine tannate)		≥ **12 y** - 5 to 10 mL q 12 h; **6 to < 12 y** - 2.5 to 5 mL q 12 h; **2 to < 6 y** - 2.5 mL q 12 h	Acesulfame K, aspartame, methylparaben, 25.25 mg phenylalanine per 5 mL, sucralose. Grape bubble gum flavor. In 473 mL.
otc	**Robitussin Cough, Cold & Flu Nighttime Syrup** (Wyeth Consumer)	5 mg dextromethorphan HBr	1 mg chlorpheniramine maleate	2.5 mg phenylephrine HCl	160 mg acetaminophen	≥ **12 y** - 20 mL q 4 h, up to 100 mL/day; **6 to < 12 y** - 10 mL q 4 h, up to 50 mL/day	Alcohol free. Menthol, 2 mg sodium per 5 mL, sorbitol, sucralose. In 118 mL.
otc	**Tylenol Plus Children's Flu Suspension** (McNeil Consumer)					**6 to 11 y (21.8 to 43.18 kg)** - 10 mL q 4 h, up to 50 mL/day	Sorbitol, sucrose. Bubble gum flavor. In 120 mL.
otc	**Tylenol Plus Children's Multi-Symptom Cold Suspension** (McNeil Consumer)						Sorbitol, sucrose. Grape flavor. In 120 mL.
otc	**Alka-Seltzer Plus Cold & Cough Liqui-Gels** (Bayer)	10 mg dextromethorphan HBr	2 mg chlorpheniramine maleate	5 mg phenylephrine HCl	325 mg acetaminophen	≥ **12 y** - 2 q 4 h, up to 12/day	Liquid filled. Sorbitol. In 12s.
otc	**Comtrex Maximum Strength Nighttime Cold & Cough Tablets** (Novartis Consumer)						Benzoic acid, PEG. Film-coated, capsule shape. In 20s.
otc	**Theraflu Nightime Severe Cold Caplets** (Novartis Consumer Health)						Acesulfame K. In 24s.
otc	**Tylenol Cold Head Congestion Nighttime Cool Burst Tablets** (McNeil Consumer)						PEG, sucralose. Capsule shape. In 24s.
otc	**Tylenol Cold Multi-Symptom Nighttime Cool Burst Tablets** (McNeil Consumer)						PEG, sucralose. Capsule shape. In 24s.
Rx	**Respa C & C Tablets** (Respa Pharmaceuticals)	30 mg dextromethorphan HBr	37.5 diphenhydramine HCl	18 mg phenylephrine HCl	575 mg acetaminophen	**> 12 y** 1 to 2 q 12 h, up to 4/day; **6 to 12 y** ½ to 1 q 12 h, up to 2/day	(RESPA C & C 531). White, capsule shape. Scored. In 100s.
otc	**Alka-Seltzer Day & Night Cold Formula Effervescent Tablets** (Bayer)	*Day:* 10 mg dextromethorphan HBr		5 mg phenylephrine HCl	250 mg acetaminophen	≥ **12 y** - *Day*: 2 dissolved in water q 4 h *Night*: 2 dissolved in 120 mL of water at bedtime, up to 8/day	*Day:* Acesulfame K, aspartame, maltodextrin, mannitol, phenylalanine 5.6 mg per tablet, saccharin, sodium 416 mg per tablet. In 10s. *Night:* Acesulfame K, aspartame, maltodextrin, phenylalanine 5.6 mg per tablet, saccharin, sodium 477 mg per tablet, sorbitol. In 10s.
		Night: 10 mg dextromethorphan HBr	6.25 mg doxylamine succinate	5 mg phenylephrine HCl	250 mg acetaminophen		
otc	**Alka-Seltzer Day & Night Cold Formula Liquid Gels** (Bayer)	*Day:* 10 mg dextromethorphan HBr		5 mg phenylephrine HCl	325 mg acetaminophen	**> 12 y** - *Day*: 2 q 4 h, up to 12/day; *Night*: 2 q 6 h	*Day:* Mannitol, PEG 400, PEG 600, sorbitol. In 10s. *Night:* Mannitol, PEG 400, PEG 600, sorbitol. In 10s.
		Night: 15 mg dextromethorphan HBr	6.25 mg doxylamine succinate		325 mg acetaminophen		

ANTITUSSIVE COMBINATIONS

	Product & Distributor	Antitussive	Antihistamine	Decongestant	Other	Average Dose	Excipients & How Supplied
otc	**Comtrex Day & Night Cold & Cough Maximum Strength Tablets** (Novartis Consumer)	*Day:* 10 mg dextromethorphan HBr		5 mg phenylephrine HCl	325 mg acetaminophen	**> 12 y** - *Day:* 2 q 4 h, up to 8/day;	Capsule shape. *Day:* Orange. In 10s. *Night:* Blue. In 10s.
		Night: 10 mg dextromethorphan HBr	2 mg chlorpheniramine maleate	5 mg phenylephrine HCl	325 mg acetaminophen	*Night:* 2 no sooner than 4 h after last daytime tablet, up to 4/day	
Rx	**Panatuss DXP Syrup** (Seyer)	20 mg dextromethorphan HBr	2 mg dexbrompheniramine maleate	10 mg phenylephrine HCl		**≥ 12 y** - 5 mL q 4 to 6 h, up to 30 mL/day; **6 to < 12 y** - 2.5 mL q 4 to 6 h, up to 15 mL/day	Alcohol free. Aspartame, parabens, PEG, 15 mg per 5 mL phenylalanine, propylene glycol, sucrose. Raspberry flavor. In 118 mL.
Rx	**Tussall Syrup** (Everett)						EDTA, saccharin, sorbitol. Strawberry flavor. In 473 mL.
Rx	**Tussall-ER Extended-Release Tablets** (Everett)	30 mg dextromethorphan HBr	6 mg dexbrompheniramine maleate	20 mg phenylephrine HCl		**≥ 12 y** - 1 q 12 h, up to 2/day; **6 to < 12 y** - ½ q 12 h, up to 1/day	Extended release. (EV 0471). Capsule shape, scored. In 100s.
otc *sf*	**Diabetic Tussin Night Time Formula Cold/Flu Liquid** (Health Care Products)	10 mg dextromethorphan HBr	12.5 mg diphenhydramine		325 mg acetaminophen	**≥ 12 y** - 10 mL q 4 to 6 h, up to 60 mL/day; **6 to < 12 y** - 5 mL q 4 to 6 h, up to 30 mL/day	Alcohol free, dye free, sugar free. Acesulfame K, aspartame, menthol, methylparaben, PEG, phenylalanine 8.4 mg per 5 mL. In 118 mL.
otc *sf*	**Diabetic Tussin Cold & Flu Liquid** (Health Care Products)						Alcohol free, dye free, sugar free. Acesulfame K, aspartame, menthol, methylparaben, orange flavoring, PEG, phenylalanine 8.4 mg per 5 mL, potassium sorbate, propylene glycol. In 118 and 237 mL.
otc	**Vicks NyQuil Cough Syrup** (Procter & Gamble Co.)	5 mg dextromethorphan HBr	2.08 mg doxylamine succinate			**≥ 12 y** - 30 mL q 6 h, up to 120 mL/day	Alcohol, corn syrup, saccharin, 9.33 mg sodium per 5 mL. In 177 and 295 mL.
otc	**All-Nite Liquid** (Major)	5 mg dextromethorphan HBr	2.08 mg doxylamine succinate		166.7 mg acetaminophen	**≥ 12 y** - 30 mL q 6 h, up to 120 mL/day	10% alcohol, saccharin. In 177 mL.
otc	**Tylenol Cough & Sore Throat Nighttime Liquid** (McNeil Consumer)						3.67 mg sodium per 5 mL, sorbitol, sucralose, sucrose. In 240 mL.
otc	**Vicks NyQuil Multi-Symptom Cold/Flu Relief Liquid** (Procter & Gamble Co.)						10% alcohol, corn syrup, saccharin, 6 mg sodium per 5 mL. Regular and cherry flavors. In 180, 300, and 420 mL.
otc	**Alka-Seltzer Plus Night Cold Softgels** (Bayer)	15 mg dextromethorphan HBr	6.25 mg doxylamine succinate		325 mg acetaminophen	**≥ 12 y** - 2 q 6 h, up to 8/day	Liquid filled. Sorbitol. In 12s.
otc	**Vicks NyQuil Multi-Symptom Cold/Flu Relief LiquiCaps** (Procter & Gamble Co.)						Sorbitol. In 12s, 20s, and 40s.
otc	**Tylenol Cold Multi-Symptom Nighttime Cool Burst Liquid** (McNeil Consumer)	3.33 mg dextromethorphan HBr	2.08 mg doxylamine succinate	1.67 mg phenylephrine HCl	108.33 mg acetaminophen	**≥ 12 y** - 30 mL q 4 h, up to 180 mL/day	1.67 mg sodium per 5 mL, sorbitol, sucralose. In 240 mL.
otc	**Alka-Seltzer Plus Night Cold Formula Liquid** (Bayer)	5 mg dextromethorphan HBr	3.125 mg doxylamine succinate	2.5 mg phenylephrine HCl	162.5 mg acetaminophen	**≥ 12 y** - 20 mL q 4 h, up to 120 mL/day	Alcohol free. Edetate disodium, PEG 400, sorbitol, sucralose. In 180 mL.

ANTITUSSIVE COMBINATIONS

	Product & Distributor	Antitussive	Antihistamine	Decongestant	Other	Average Dose	Excipients & How Supplied
otc	**Alka-Seltzer Plus Night Cold Effervescent Tablets** (Bayer)	10 mg dextromethorphan HBr	6.25 mg doxylamine succinate	5 mg phenylephrine HCl	250 mg acetaminophen	**≥ 12 y** - 2 dissolved in 118 mL water at bedtime or q 4 h, up to 8/day	Acesulfame K, aspartame, 5.6 mg phenylalanine, saccharin, 477 mg sodium, sorbitol. In 20s.
otc	**Night Time Multi-Symptom Cold/Flu Relief Liquid Caps** (Major)	15 mg dextromethorphan HBr	6.25 mg doxylamine succinate	30 mg pseudoephedrine HCl	325 mg acetaminophen	**≥ 12 y** - 2 q 6 h, up to 8/day	PEG, sorbitol. In 12s.
otc	**Theraflu Cold & Cough Powder** (Novartis Consumer)	20 mg dextromethorphan HBr	20 mg pheniramine maleate	20 mg phenylephrine HCl		**≥ 12 y** - 1 packet dissolved in 236 mL hot water q 4 h, up to 6 packets/day	Acesulfame K, maltodextrin, 46 mg sodium. In 6 packets.
Rx	**Promethazine w/Dextromethorphan Cough Syrup** (Morton Grove)	15 mg dextromethorphan HBr	6.25 mg promethazine HCl			**≥ 12 y** - 5 mL q 4 to 6 h, up to 30 mL/day; **6 to < 12 y** - 2.5 to 5 mL q 4 to 6 h, up to 20 mL/day; **2 to < 6 y** - 1.25 to 2.5 mL q 4 to 6 h, up to 10 mL/day	7.1% alcohol, EDTA, methylparaben, sugar. In 118 and 473 mL.
Rx	**P-Hist Syrup** (Midlothian)	5 mg dextromethorphan HBr	5 mg pyrilamine maleate, 1.25 mg dexchlorpheniramine maleate	5 mg phenylephrine HCl		**≥ 12 y** - 10 mL q 4 to 6 h; **6 to < 12 y** - 5 mL q 4 to 6 h; **2 to < 6 y** - 2.5 mL q 4 to 6 h	Saccharin, sorbitol. Grape flavor. In 473 mL.
Rx sf	**Resperal Syrup** (Cypress)						Alcohol, dye, and gluten free. Saccharin, sorbitol. Grape flavor. In 473 mL.
otc sf	**Codal-DM Syrup** (Cypress)	10 mg dextromethorphan HBr	8.33 mg pyrilamine maleate	5 mg phenylephrine HCl		**≥ 12 y** - 10 mL q 4 h, up to 60 mL/day; **6 to < 12 y** - 5 mL q 4 h, up to 30 mL/day	Alcohol and dye free. In 473 mL.
otc sf	**Codimal DM Syrup** (Victory Pharma)						Alcohol and dye free. Menthol, saccharin, sorbitol. In 118 and 473 mL.
otc sf	**Albutussin**(A. J. Bart)	15 mg dextromethorphan HBr	12.5 pyrilamine maleate	5 mg phenylephrine HCl		**≥ 12 y** - 10 mL q 6 to 8 h, up to 40 mL/day **6 to 12 y** - 5 mL q 6 to 8 h, up to 20 mL/day **2 to 6 y** - 2.5 mL q 6 to 8 h, up to 10 mL/day	Alcohol free and sugar free. Menthol, saccharin, sorbitol. Peppermint flavor. In 118 mL.

ANTITUSSIVE COMBINATIONS

	Product & Distributor	Antitussive	Antihistamine	Decongestant	Other	Average Dose	Excipients & How Supplied
Rx *sf*	**MyHist-DM Liquid** (Larken)	15 mg dextromethorphan HBr	12.5 pyrilamine maleate	7.5 mg phenylephrine HCl		**> 12 y** - 5 to 10 mL q 4 to 6 h, up to 40 mL/day; **6 to 12 y** - 5 mL q 4 to 6 h, up to 20 mL/day; **2 to 6 y** - 2.5 mL q 4 to 6 h, up to 10 mL/day	Alcohol and dye free. EDTA, parabens, saccharin, sorbitol. Grape flavor. In 473 mL.
Rx *sf*	**Poly Hist DM Liquid** (Poly)						Alcohol and dye free. Saccharin, sorbitol. Grape flavor. In 20 mL and 473 mL.
Rx *sf*	**Reme Hist DM Liquid** (River's Edge)						Alcohol and dye free. Saccharin, sorbitol. Grape flavor. In 473 mL.
Rx *sf*	**Triplex DM Liquid** (Breckenridge)					**≥ 12 y** - 5 to 10 mL q 4 to 6 h, not to exceed 60 mg phenylephrine HCl /day; **6 to 12 y** - 5 mL q 4 to 6 h, not to exceed 30 mg phenylephrine HCl/day	Alcohol and dye free. Saccharin, sorbitol. Grape flavor. In 473 mL.
Rx	**Aldex DM Tannate Suspension** (Zyber)	15 mg dextromethorphan HBr	16 mg pyrilamine maleate	5 mg phenylephrine HCl		**> 12 y** - 5 to 10 mL q 12 h; **6 to 12 y** - 5 mL q 12 h; **2 to 6 y** - 2.5 mL q 12 h	Methylparaben, sucralose, sucrose. Grape flavor. In 473 mL.
Rx	**Pyril DM Suspension** (Macoven)					**> 12 y** - 5 to 10 mL q 8 h; **6 to 12 y** - 5 mL q 8 h; **2 to 6 y** - 2.5 mL q 8 h	Glycerin, methylparaben, sucrose, sucralose. Grape flavor. In 473 mL.
Rx	**Viravan-PDM Suspension** (Tiber)	15 mg dextromethorphan HBr	15 mg pyrilamine maleate	15 mg pseudoephedrine HCl		**> 12 y** - 5 to 10 mL q 12 h; **6 to 12 y** - 5 mL q 12 h; **2 to 6 y** - 2.5 mL q 12 h	Methylparaben, sucralose, sucrose. Grape flavor. In 473 mL.
Rx	**Dur-Tann DM Suspension** (Midlothian)	20 mg dextromethorphan tannate	8 mg brompheniramine tannate	20 mg phenylephrine tannate		**≥ 12 y** - 10 mL q 12 h, up to 20 mL/day; **6 to < 12 y** - 5 mL q 12 h, up to 10 mL/day; **2 to < 6 y** - 2.5 mL q 12 h, up to 5 mL/day	Alcohol free. Methylparaben, phenylalanine, saccharin. Bubble gum flavor. In 473 mL.
Rx	**DuraTan DM Suspension** (ProEthic)						Methylparaben, saccharin. Bubble gum flavor. In 473 mL.

ANTITUSSIVE COMBINATIONS

	Product & Distributor	Antitussive	Antihistamine	Decongestant	Other	Average Dose	Excipients & How Supplied
Rx *sf*	**BP New Allergy DM Suspension** (Brookstone)	30 mg dextromethorphan tannate	10 mg brompheniramine tannate	25 mg phenylephrine tannate		**> 12 y** - 10 mL q 12 h, up to 20 mL/day; **6 to < 12 y** - 5 mL q 12 h, up to 10 mL/day; **2 to < 6 y** - 2.5 mL q 12 h, up to 5 mL/day	Alcohol free, sugar free. Methylparaben, 5 mg phenylalanine per 5 mL, saccharin, sorbitol. In 473 mL.
Rx *sf*	**Neo DM Suspension** (Laser)						Alcohol free. Aspartame, parabens, 7 mg phenylalanine per 5 mL. Cherry flavor. In 473 mL.
Rx	**Carb PSE 12 DM Suspension** (River's Edge)	27.5 mg dextromethorphan tannate	3.2 mg carbinoxamine tannate	45.2 mg pseudoephedrine tannate		≥ **12 y** - 10 to 20 mL q 12 h; **6 to 12 y** - 5 to 10 mL q 12 h; **2 to 6 y** - 2.5 to 5 mL q 12 h	Methylparaben, saccharin, sorbitol. Candy apple flavor. In 473 mL bottles.
Rx	**Dicel DM Suspension** (Centrix)	25 mg dextromethorphan tannate	5 mg chlorpheniramine tannate	75 mg pseudoephedrine tannate		**> 12 y** - 10 to 20 mL q 12 h, up to 40 mL/day; **6 to 12 y** - 5 to 10 mL q 12 h, up to 20 mL/day; **2 to** - 2.5 to 5 mL q 12 h, up to 10 mL/day	Methylparaben, saccharin, sucrose. Cotton candy flavor. In 473 mL.
Rx *sf*	**Dextromethorphan Tannate, Phenylephrine Tannate, Dexchlorpheniramine Tannate Oral Suspension** (River's Edge)	30 mg dextromethorphan tannate	2 mg dexchlorpheniramine tannate	20 mg phenylephrine tannate		**> 12 y** - 10 mL q 12 h, up to 20 mL/day; **6 to 12 y** - 5 mL q 12 h, up to 10 mL/day; **2 to 6 y** - 2.5 mL q 12 h, up to 5 mL/day	Alcohol free, sugar free. Saccharin. Cotton candy, strawberry flavor. In 473 mL.
Rx	**Indamix DM Suspension** (Centurion Labs	27.5 dextromethorphan tannate	3 mg dexchlorpheniramine tannate	50 mg pseudoephedrine tannate		≥ **12 y** – 5 to 15 mL q 12 h up to 30 mL/day **6 to < 12 y** – 2.5 to 5 mL q 12 h up to 10 mL/day	Grape flavor. In 473 mL.
Rx	**SuTan-DM Suspension** (Cypress)					≥ **12 y** - 5 to 15 mL q 12 h, up to 30 mL/day; **6 to < 12 y** - 2.5 to 5 mL q 12 h, up to 10 mL/day; **2 to < 6 y** - 1.25 to 2.5 mL q 12 h, up to 5 mL/day	Aspartame, 7 mg phenylalanine per 5 mL, parabens. Grape flavor. In 473 mL.
Rx	**Tannate PD-DM Suspension** (Hi-Tech)						Methylparaben, saccharin, sucrose. Grape flavor. In 473 mL.
Rx	**Bromatan Plus Suspension** (Cypress)	30 mg dextromethorphan tannate	3.5 mg dexchlorpheniramine tannate	45 mg pseudoephedrine tannate		≥ **12 y** - 5 to 15 mL q 12 h, up to 30 mL/day; **6 to < 12 y**- 2.5 to 5 mL q 12 h, up to 10 mL/day; **2 to < 6 y** - 1.25 to 2.5 mL q 12 h, up to 5 mL/day	Aspartame, parabens, 7 mg phenylalanine per 5 mL. Orange-pineapple flavor. In 473 mL.
Rx	**DuraTan Forte Suspension** (ProEthic)						Methylparaben, saccharin, sucrose. Grape flavor. In 473 mL.

ANTITUSSIVE COMBINATIONS

	Product & Distributor	Antitussive	Antihistamine	Decongestant	Other	Average Dose	Excipients & How Supplied
Rx	**D-Tann DM Suspension** (Midlothian)	75 mg dextromethorphan tannate	25 mg diphenhydramine tannate	7.5 phenylephrine tannate		**≥ 12 y** - 5 to 10 mL q 12 h; **6 to < 12 y** - 2.5 to 5 mL q 12 h; **2 to < 6 y** - 1.25 to 2.5 mL q 12 h	Aspartame, parabens, 7 mg phenylalanine per 5 mL, saccharin. Black cherry flavor. In 118 mL.
Rx *sf*	**Dextromethorphan Tannate, Phenylephrine Tannate, Pyrilamine Tannate Oral Suspension** (River's Edge)	25 mg dextromethorphan tannate	15.5 mg pyrilamine tannate	15.5 mg phenylephrine tannate		**> 12 y** - 5 to 10 mL q 12 h, up to 20 mL/day; **6 to 12 y** - 5 mL q 12 h, up to 10 mL/day; **2 to 6 y** - 2.5 mL q 12 h, up to 5 mL/day	Alcohol free, sugar free. Saccharin. Cherry flavored. In 473 mL.
Rx	**AllanVan-DM B.I.D. Suspension** (Allan)	25 mg dextromethorphan tannate	30 mg pyrilamine tannate	12.5 mg phenylephrine tannate		**> 12 y** - 5 to 10 mL q 12 h; **6 to 12 y** - 5 mL q 12 h; **2 to 6 y** - 2.5 mL q 12 h	Methylparaben, saccharin, sucrose. Grape flavor. In 473 mL.
Rx	**ViraTan-DM Suspension B.I.D.** (Ani[c])						Dye free. Methylparaben, sucralose, sucrose. Grape flavor. In 473 mL.
Rx	**ViraTan-DM Chewable Tablets B.I.D.** (Ani[c])	25 mg dextromethorphan tannate	30 mg pyrilamine tannate	25 mg phenylephrine tannate		**> 12 y** - 1 to 2 q 12 h; **6 to 12 y** - ½ to 1 q 12 h; **2 to 6 y** - ½ q 12 h	Dye free. Mannitol, sucralose, sugar. (Λ 11). Mottled brown, scored. Grape flavor. In 100s.
c-v	**Alahist DHC Liquid** (Poly Pharmaceuticals)	3 mg dihydrocodeine bitartrate		7.5 mg phenylephrine HCl		**≥ 12 y** - 5 mL q 4 to 6 h, up to 30 mL/day; **6 to 12 y** - 2.5 mL q 4 to 6 h, up to 15 mL/day	Saccharin, sorbitol. Mango flavor. In 473 mL.
c-v	**Dihydrocodeine 3 mg/BPM 4 mg/ Phenylephrine HCl 7.5 mg Liquid** (Kylemore)	3 mg dihydrocodeine bitartrate	4 mg brompheniramine maleate	7.5 mg phenylephrine HCl		**≥ 12 y** - 5 mL q 4 to 6 h, up to 30 mL/day; **6 to 12 y** - 2.5 mL q 4 to 6 h, up to 15 mL/day	Glycerin, propylene glycol, saccharin, sorbitol. Grape flavor. In 473 mL.
c-v	**Poly-Tussin DHC Liquid** (Great Southern)					**≥ 12 y** - 5 mL q 4 to 6 h, up to 30 mL/day; **6 to < 12 y** - 2.5 mL q 4 to 6 h, up to 15 mL/day	PEG, saccharin. Grape flavor. In 473 mL.

ANTITUSSIVE COMBINATIONS

	Product & Distributor	Antitussive	Antihistamine	Decongestant	Other	Average Dose	Excipients & How Supplied
c-v	**DiHydro-PE Syrup** (Cypress)	3 mg dihydrocodeine bitartrate	2 mg chlorpheniramine maleate	7.5 mg phenylephrine HCl		**> 12 y** - 5 to 10 mL q 4 to 6 h, up to 40 mL/day; **6 to 12 y** - 2.5 to 5 mL q 4 to 6 h, up to 20 mL/day;	Saccharin, sorbitol. Grape flavor. In 118 mL.
c-iii sf	**Pancof PD Syrup** (Pan American)					**> 12 y** - 5 to 10 mL q 4 to 6 h, up to 40 mL/day; **6 to 12 y** - 2.5 to 5 mL q 4 to 6 h, up to 20 mL/day; **2 to 6 y** - 1.25 to 2.5 mL q 4 to 6 h, up to 10 mL/day	Alcohol free. In 120 mL.
c-v sf	**Despec PDC Liquid** (International Ethical Labs)	3 mg dihydrocodeine bitartrate	2.5 mg chlorpheniramine maleate	7.5 mg phenylephrine HCl		**> 12 y** - 5 to 10 mL q 4 to 6 h, up to 40 mL/day; **6 to 12 y** - 2.5 to 5 mL q 4 to 6 h, up to 20 mL/day	Alcohol free, dye free, sugar free. Glycerin, propylene glycol, saccharin, sorbitol. Grape flavor. In 118 mL.
c-iii sf	**Tusscough DHC Syrup** (Breckenridge Pharmaceuticals)	3 mg dihydrocodeine bitartrate	5 mg chlorpheniramine maleate	20 mg phenylephrine HCl		**≥ 12 y** - 5 mL q 4 to 6 h	Alcohol free, dye free, sugar free. Benzoic acid, glycerin, parabens, propylene glycol, saccharin, sorbitol. Grape flavor. In 473 mL.
c-iii sf	**Duohist DH Liquid** (Breckenridge)	7.25 mg dihydrocodeine bitartrate	2 mg chlorpheniramine maleate	5 mg phenylephrine HCl		**> 12 y** - 5 to 10 mL q 4 to 6 h, up to 40 mL/day; **6 to 12 y** - 2.5 to 5 mL q 4 to 6 h, up to 20 mL/day	Alcohol and dye free. Saccharin, sorbitol. Strawberry flavor. In 473 mL.
c-iii sf	**J-Cof DHC Liquid** (Great Southern)	7.5 mg dihydrocodeine bitartrate	3 mg brompheniramine maleate	15 mg pseudoephedrine HCl		**> 12 y** - 5 to 10 mL q 4 to 6 h; **6 to 12 y** - 2.5 to 5 mL q 4 to 6 h	Alcohol free, dye free, sugar free. Saccharin, sorbitol. Grape flavor. In 473 mL.
c-iii sf	**DiHydro-CP Syrup** (Cypress)	7.5 mg dihydrocodeine bitartrate	2 mg chlorpheniramine maleate	15 mg pseudoephedrine HCl		**> 12 y** - 5 to 10 mL q 4 to 6 h; **6 to 12 y** - 2.5 to 5 mL q 4 to 6 h; **2 to 6 y** -1.25 to 2.5 mL q 4 to 6 h	Alcohol free, dye free, sugar free. Saccharin, sorbitol. Grape flavor. In 473 mL.
c-iii sf	**Poly Hist DHC Liquid** (Poly Pharmaceuticals)	7.5 mg dihydrocodeine bitartrate	7.5 mg pyrilamine maleate	5 mg phenylephrine		**> 12 y** - 5 mL q 4 to 6 h, up to 30 mL/day; **6 to 12 y** - 2.5 mL q 4 to 6 h, up to 15 mL/day	Alcohol free, dye free, gluten free, sugar free. Fruit gum flavoring, glycerin, propylene glycol, saccharin, sorbitol. In 473 mL.

ANTITUSSIVE COMBINATIONS

	Product & Distributor	Antitussive	Antihistamine	Decongestant	Other	Average Dose	Excipients & How Supplied
c-iii	**Hydrocodone Bitartrate and Homatropine Methylbromide Tablets** (Actavis)	5 mg hydrocodone bitartrate			1.5 mg homatropine MBr	**> 12 y** - 1 q 4 to 6 h, up to 6/day; **6 to 12 y** - ½ q 4 to 6 h, up to 3/day	Lactose. (A 140). Scored. In 100s and 500s.
c-iii	**Hycodan Tablets** (Endo)						Lactose. (HYCODAN). Scored. In 100s.
c-iii	**Hycodan Syrup** (Endo)					**> 12 y** - 5 mL q 4 to 6 h, up to 30 mL/day; **6 to 12 y** - 2.5 mL q 4 to 6 h, up to 15 mL/day	Parabens, sorbitol, sugar. Cherry flavor. In 473 mL.
c-iii	**Tussigon Tablets** (Monarch)					**> 12 y** - 1 q 4 to 6 h, up to 6/day; **6 to 12 y** - ½ q 4 to 6 h, up to 3/day	Blue, scored. In 100s and 500s.
c-iii	**Hydrocodone Bitartrate/Homatropine Methylbromide Syrup** (Pharmaceutical Associates)	5 mg hydrocodone bitartrate			1.5 mg homatropine MBr	**≥ 12 y** - 5 mL q 4 to 6 h, up to 30 mL/day; **6 to 12 y** - 2.5 mL q 4 to 6 h, up to 15 mL/day	Alcohol < 0.1%, glycerin, parabens, sorbitol, sugar. Cherry flavor. In UD 5 mL.
c-iii	**Hydromet Syrup** (Actavis)						Methylparaben, saccharin, sucrose. Cherry flavor. In 473 mL.
c-iii *sf*	**Nalex DH Liquid** (Blansett)	2.5 mg hydrocodone bitartrate		5 mg phenylephrine HCl		**> 12 y** - 10 mL q 4 to 6 h, up to 40 mL/day; **6 to 12 y** - 5 mL q 4 to 6 h, up to 20 mL/day; **2 to 6 y** - 2.5 mL q 4 to 6 h, up to 10 mL/day	Alcohol free. Cherry flavor. In 15 and 437 mL.
c-iii *sf*	**Lortuss HC Liquid** (ProEthic)	3.75 mg hydrocodone bitartrate		7.5 mg phenylephrine HCl		**≥ 12 y** - 5 mL q 4 h, up to 30 mL/day; **6 to < 12 y** - 2.5 mL q 4 h, up to 15 mL/day	Alcohol free. Saccharin, sorbitol. Grape flavor. In 20 and 473 mL.
c-iii	**P-V-Tussin Tablets** (Numark)	5 mg hydrocodone bitartrate		60 mg pseudoephedrine HCl		**Adults** - 1 q 4 to 6 h, up to 4/day[a]	Lactose. (NUMARK 10/91). Orange, capsule shape, scored. In 100s.
c-iii *sf*	**FluTuss HC Liquid** (Wraser)	2.5 mg hydrocodone bitartrate	4 mg brompheniramine maleate	7.5 mg phenylephrine HCl		**≥ 12 y** - 5 mL q 4 to 6 h, up to 30 mL/day; **6 to 12 y** - 2.5 mL q 4 to 6 h, up to 15 mL/day; **2 to 6 y** - 1.25 mL q 4 to 6 h, up to 7.5 mL/day	Alcohol free. Saccharin, sorbitol, tartrazine. Peach flavor. In 15 and 474 mL.
c-iii *sf*	**Tusnel-HC Liquid** (LLorens)						Alcohol free. Saccharin. Peach flavor. In 473 mL.

ANTITUSSIVE COMBINATIONS

	Product & Distributor	Antitussive	Antihistamine	Decongestant	Other	Average Dose	Excipients & How Supplied
c-iii	**M-End Max Liquid** (R.A. McNeil)	5 mg hydrocodone bitartrate	2 mg brompheniramine maleate	7.5 mg phenylephrine HCl		**≥ 12 y** - 5 to 10 mL q 4 to 6 h, up to 30 mL/day; **6 to < 12 y** - 2.5 mL q 4 to 6 h, up to 15 mL/day	Methylparaben, sucrose. Grape flavor. In 473 mL.
c-iii *sf*	**Anaplex HD Liquid** (ECR)	1.7 mg hydrocodone bitartrate	2 mg brompheniramine maleate	30 mg pseudoephedrine HCl		**> 12 y** - 10 mL tid or qid, up to 40 mL/day; **6 to 12 y** - 5 mL tid or qid, up to 20 mL/day	Alcohol and dye free. Strawberry flavor. In 118 and 473 mL.
c-iii *sf*	**Bromphenex HD Liquid** (Breckenridge)						Alcohol and dye free. Saccharin, sorbitol. Strawberry flavor. In 473 mL.
c-iii	**M-End Liquid** (R.A. McNeil)	2.5 mg hydrocodone bitartrate	2 mg brompheniramine maleate	15 mg pseudoephedrine HCl		**≥ 12 y** - 10 mL q 4 to 6 h; **6 to < 12 y** - 5 mL q 4 to 6 h	Saccharin, sorbitol. Cherry flavor. In 473 mL.
c-iii *sf*	**J-Tan D HC Liquid** (JayMac)	2.5 mg hydrocodone bitartrate	3 mg brompheniramine maleate	15 mg pseudoephedrine HCl		**≥ 12 y** - 5 to 10 mL q 4 to 6 h, up to 40 mL/day; **6 to 12 y** - 5 mL q 4 to 6 h, up to 20 mL/day; **2 to 6 y** - 2.5 mL q 4 to 6 h, up to 10 mL/day	Alcohol free. Saccharin, sorbitol. Strawberry-banana flavor. In 473 mL.
c-iii *sf*	**Brompheniramine/Hydrocodone/PSE Liquid** (Varsity)	2.5 mg hydrocodone bitartrate	3 mg brompheniramine maleate	30 mg pseudoephedrine HCl		**≥ 12 y** - 5 to 10 mL q 4 to 6 h, up to 40 mL/day; **6 to 12 y** - 5 mL q 4 to 6 h, up to 20 mL/day; **2 to 6 y** - 2.5 mL q 4 to 6 h, up to 10 mL/day; **18 mo to 2 y** - 1.25 mL q 4 to 6 h, up to 5 mL/day	Alcohol free. Saccharin, sorbitol. Bubble gum flavor. In 473 mL.
c-iii	**TussiCaps Half Strength Extended-Release Capsules** (Mallinckrodt)	5 mg hydrocodone bitartrate (as hydrocodone polistirex)	4 mg chlorpheniramine maleate (as chlorpheniramine polistirex)			**6 to 12 y** - 1 q 12 h, up to 2/day	Extended release. Butyl, dehydrated, isopropyl, SD-45, and SDA 3A alcohol. (M HP/CP 5/4). Ivory, capsule shape. In 20s and 100s.
c-iii	**HyTan Suspension** (Prasco)	5 mg hydrocodone bitartrate (as hydrocodone tannate)	4 mg chlorpheniramine maleate (as chlorpheniramine tannate)			**> 12 y** - 10 mL q 12 h, up to 20 mL/day; **6 to 12 y** - 5 mL q 12 h, up to 10 mL/day	Aspartame, parabens, phenylalanine. Tropical fruit flavor. In 118 mL.

ANTITUSSIVE COMBINATIONS

	Product & Distributor	Antitussive	Antihistamine	Decongestant	Other	Average Dose	Excipients & How Supplied
c-iii	**Chlorpheniramine Polistirex/ Hydrocodone Polistirex Extended-Release Suspension** (Various, eg, Kremers Urban, Par)	10 mg hydrocodone bitartrate (as hydrocodone polistirex)	8 mg chlorpheniramine maleate (as chlorphenir-amine polistirex)			**≥ 12 y** - 5 mL q 12 h, up to 10 mL/day; **6 to 11 y** - 2.5 mL q 12 h, up to 5 mL/day	Extended release. May contain corn syrup, parabens, polysorbate 80, propylene glycol, sucrose. In 473 mL.
c-iii	**TussiCaps Full Strength Extended-Release Capsules** (Mallinckrodt)					**> 12 y** - 1 q 12 h, up to 2/day	Extended release. Butyl, dehy-drated, isopropyl, SD-45, and SDA 3A alcohol. (M HP/CP 10/8). Ivory, capsule shape. In 20s and 100s.
c-iii	**Tussionex Pennkinetic Extended-Release Suspension** (UCB Pharma)					**> 12 y** - 5 mL q 12 h, up to 10 mL/day; **6 to 12 y** - 2.5 mL q 12 h, up to 5 mL/day	Extended release. Corn syrup, parabens, PEG, sucrose. In 473 mL.
c-iii *sf*	**Histinex HC Syrup** (Ethex)	2.5 mg hydrocodone bitartrate	2 mg chlorpheniramine maleate	5 mg phenylephrine HCl		**> 12 y** - 10 mL q 4 h, up to 40 mL/day; **6 to 12 y** - 5 mL q 4 h, up to 20 mL/day	Alcohol free. Saccharin, sorbitol. In 473 and 946 mL.
c-iii *sf*	**Rindal HD Plus Syrup** (Breckenridge)	3.5 mg hydrocodone bitartrate	2 mg chlorpheniramine maleate	7.5 mg phenylephrine HCl		**> 12 y** - 10 mL q 4 h, up to 40 mL/day;	Alcohol free. Saccharin, sorbitol. Black raspberry flavor. In 473 mL.
c-iii *sf*	**Endal HD Plus Syrup** (Tiber)					**6 to 12 y** - 5 mL q 4 h, up to 20 mL/day	Alcohol free. Saccharin, sorbitol. Black raspberry flavor. In 473 mL.
c-iii *sf*	**Coughtuss Liquid** (Breckenridge)	5 mg hydrocodone bitartrate	2 mg chlorpheniramine maleate	5 mg phenylephrine HCl		**> 12 y** - 10 mL q 4 to 6 h, up to 40 mL/day; **6 to 12 y** - 5 mL q 4 to 6 h, up to 20 mL/day	Alcohol free. Saccharin, sorbitol. Candy apple flavor. In 473 mL.
c-iii *sf*	**Neo HC Syrup** (Laser)	5 mg hydrocodone bitartrate	3 mg chlorpheniramine maleate	7.5 mg phenylephrine HCl		**> 12 y** - 5 to 10 mL q 4 to 6 h, up to 40 mL/day; **6 to < 12 y** - 2.5 to 5 mL q 4 to 6 h, up to 20 mL/day **3 to < 6 y** - 1.25 to 2.5 mL q 4 to 6 h, up to 10 mL/day	Alcohol free, sugar free. Glycerin, saccharin, sorbitol. Orange cream flavor. In 473 mL.
c-iii	**P-V-Tussin Syrup** (Numark)	2.5 mg hydrocodone bitartrate	2 mg chlorpheniramine maleate	30 mg pseudoephedrine HCl		**> 12 y** - 10 mL q 4 to 6 h, up to 40 mL/day; **6 to 12 y** - 5 mL q 4 to 6 h, up to 20 mL/day; **2 to 6 y** - 2.5 mL q 4 to 6 h, up to 10 mL/day	5% alcohol, glucose, parabens, saccharin, sorbitol, sucrose. Banana flavor. In 473 mL.

ANTITUSSIVE COMBINATIONS

	Product & Distributor	Antitussive	Antihistamine	Decongestant	Other	Average Dose	Excipients & How Supplied
c-iii *sf*	**WellTuss HC Liquid** (Prasco)	3 mg hydrocodone bitartrate	2 mg chlorpheniramine maleate	15 mg pseudoephedrine HCl		**> 12 y** - 5 to 10 mL qid; **6 to 12 y** - 2.5 to 5 mL qid; **2 to 6 y** - 1.25 to 2.5 mL qid	Alcohol and dye free. Saccharin, sorbitol. Grape flavor. In 473 mL.
c-iii *sf*	**Notuss-Forte Syrup** (SJ Pharmaceutical)	5 mg hydrocodone bitartrate	4 mg chlorpheniramine maleate	40 mg pseudoephedrine HCl		**> 12 y** - 5 mL 3 or 4 times daily, up to 20 mL/day	Alcohol free, dye free, gluten free, sugar free. Saccharin, sorbitol. Vanilla flavor. In 473 mL.
c-iii *sf*	**Rindal HPD Syrup** (Breckenridge)	2 mg hydrocodone bitartrate	12.5 mg diphenhydramine HCl	7.5 mg phenylephrine HCl		**> 12 y** - 10 mL q 4 h, up to 40 mL/day; **6 to 12 y** - 5 mL q 4 h, up to 20 mL/day	Alcohol free. Saccharin. Cherry flavor. In 473 mL.
c-iii *sf*	**Novasus Suspension** (SJ Pharmaceutical)	5 mg hydrocodone tannate	4 mg chlorpheniramine tannate			**≥ 12 y** - 10 mL q 12 h, up to 20 mL/day; **6 to < 12 y** - 5 mL q 12 h, up to 10 mL/day	Alcohol free, sugar free. Aspartame, parabens, 7 mg phenylalanine per 5 mL. Tropical fruit flavor. In 473 mL.
c-iii	**Vazotuss HC Tannate Suspension** (WraSer)	10 mg hydrocodone tannate (equivalent to 5 mg hydrocodone bitartrate)	12 mg brompheniramine tannate (equivalent to 6 mg brompheniramine maleate)	20 mg phenylephrine tannate (equivalent to 10 mg phenylephrine HCl)		**Adults** - 5 to 10 mL q 12 h; **6 to 12 y** - 5 mL q 12 h	Acesulfame K, aspartame, methylparaben, 42 mg phenylalanine per 5 mL. Grape flavor. In 473 mL.
c-iii	**Atuss HS Suspension** (Atley)	10 mg hydrocodone tannate (equivalent to 5 mg hydrocodone bitartrate)	8 mg chlorpheniramine tannate (equivalent to 4 mg chlorpheniramine maleate)	60 mg pseudoephedrine tannate (equivalent to 30 mg pseudoephedrine HCl)		**> 12 y** - 5 to 10 mL q 12 h; **6 to 12 y** - 2.5 to 5 mL q 12 h	Acesulfame K, aspartame, methylparaben, 25.25 mg phenylalanine per 5 mL. Cherry bubble gum flavor. In 473 mL.

[a] Pediatric dosing could not be verified. Refer to the manufacturer's prescribing information for more information.
[b] Actavis Mid Atlantic, 7205 Windsor Blvd, Baltimore, MD 21244; 1-800-432-8534; http://www.actavis.com.
[c] Ani, 1302 Concourse Dr, Suite 101, Linthicum, MD 21090; 1-800-434-1121; http://anipharmaceuticals.com.

For complete and comparative prescribing information, refer to the Respiratory Combinations Introduction.

ANTITUSSIVE AND EXPECTORANT COMBINATIONS

Content given per tablet, 5 mL, 1 mL (oral drops), or packet.

	Product & Distributor	Antitussive	Expectorant	Decongestant	Antihistamine/Other	Average Dose	Excipients & How Supplied
Rx	**Levall Liquid** (Auriga)	15 mg carbetapentane citrate	100 mg guaifenesin	5 mg phenylephrine HCl		**> 12 y** - 10 mL q 4 to 6 h, up to 60 mL/day; **6 to 12 y** - 5 mL q 4 to 6 h, up to 30 mL/day; **2 to 6 y** - 2.5 mL q 4 to 6 h, up to 15 mL/day	Alcohol free. Maltitol, saccharin, sorbitol. Strawberry flavor. In 473 mL.
Rx	**Zinx GCP Solution** (Auriga)						Alcohol free. Maltitol, saccharin, sorbitol. Strawberry flavor. In 118 mL.
Rx	**Extendryl GCP Solution** (Auriga)	15 mg carbetapentane citrate	100 mg guaifenesin	5 mg phenylephrine HCl		**> 12 y** - 10 mL q 4 to 6 h up to 60 mL/day; **6 to 12 y** - 5 mL q 4 to 6 h up to 30 mL/day; **2 to 6 y** - 2.5 mL q 4 to 6 h up to 15 mL/day	Alcohol free. Maltitol, saccharin, sorbitol. Strawberry flavor. In 473 mL.
Rx	**Phencarb GG Syrup** (Boca Pharmacal)	20 mg carbetapentane citrate	100 mg guaifenesin	10 mg phenylephrine HCl		**> 12 y** - 5 to 10 mL q 4 to 6 h; **6 to 12 y** - 5 mL q 4 to 6 h; **2 to 6 y** - 2.5 mL q 4 to 6 h	EDTA, sorbitol, sugar. Spearmint flavor. In 473 mL.
Rx	**Albatussin Capsules** (Baroli)	25 mg carbetapentane citrate	400 mg guaifenesin	10 mg phenylephrine HCl		**> 12 y** - 1 to 2 q 6 to 8 h, up to 4/day	In 100s.
Rx	**Gentex 30 Liquid** (Gentex Pharma)	30 mg carbetapentane citrate	200 mg guaifenesin	8 mg phenylephrine HCl		**> 12 y** - 5 or 10 mL q 4 to 6 h; **6 to 12 y** - 5 mL q 4 to 6 h	EDTA, parabens, saccharin. Cherry flavor. In 118 mL.

ANTITUSSIVE AND EXPECTORANT COMBINATIONS

	Product & Distributor	Antitussive	Expectorant	Decongestant	Antihistamine/Other	Average Dose	Excipients & How Supplied
Rx	**Aquatab C Tablets** (Deston)	30 mg carbetapentane citrate	400 mg guaifenesin	10 mg phenylephrine HCl		**> 12 y** - 1 q 4 to 6 h, up to 6/day.	(C-620). White, oval. In 100s.
Rx	**Carbatab-12 Tablets** (GM)	60 mg carbetapentane citrate	600 mg guaifenesin	15 mg phenylephrine HCl		**> 12 y** - 1 to 2 q 12 h, up to 4/day; **6 to 12 y** - ½ to 1 q 12 h, up to 2/day	Extended release. (GMP/12). Scored. In 100s.
Rx *sf*	**Exall-D Liquid** (Hawthorn)	10 mg carbetapentane citrate	100 mg guaifenesin	30 mg pseudoephedrine HCl		**≥ 12 y** - 5 to 10 mL q 4 to 6 h, up to 40 mL/day; **6 to 12 y** - 5 mL q 4 to 6 h, up to 20 mL/day	Alcohol free, dye free, sugar free. Saccharin, sorbitol. Fruit gum flavor. In 473 mL.
otc *sf*	**VanaCof DX Liquid** (GM Pharmaceuticals)	12.5 mg chlophedianol HCl	100 mg guaifenesin	30 mg pseudoephedrine HCl		**≥ 12 y** - 10 mL q 6 to 8 h, up to 40 mL/day; **6 to < 12 y** - 5 mL q 6 to 8 h, up to 20 mL/day	Sugar free, alcohol free, dye free. Glycerin, propylene glycol, saccharin, sorbitol. Raspberry flavor. In 473 mL.
c-v	**Zodryl DEC 80 Suspension** (Codadose)	5 mg codeine phosphate	100 mg guaifenesin	15 mg pseudoephedrine HCl		**6 to < 12 y** - 10 mL q 4 to 6 h, up to 40 mL/day	Methylparaben, sucralose. Grape flavor. In 236 mL.
c-v	**Zodryl DEC 40 Suspension** (Codadose)	5 mg codeine phosphate	100 mg guaifenesin	16.665 mg pseudoephedrine HCl		**2 to < 6 y** - 4.5 mL q 4 to 6 h, up to 18 mL/day	Methylparaben, sucralose. Grape flavor. In 118 mL.
c-v	**Zodryl DEC 35 Suspension** (Codadose)	5 mg codeine phosphate	100 mg guaifenesin	18.75 mg pseudoephedrine HCl		**2 to < 6 y** - 4 mL q 4 to 6 h, up to 16 mL/day	Methylparaben, sucralose. Grape flavor. In 118 mL.
c-v	**Zodryl DEC 60 Suspension** (Codadose)	5 mg codeine phosphate	100 mg guaifenesin	20 mg pseudoephedrine HCl		**6 to < 12 y** - 7.5 mL q 4 to 6 h, up to 30 mL/day	Methylparaben, sucralose. Grape flavor. In 236 mL.
c-v	**Zodryl DEC 30 Suspension** (Codadose)	5 mg codeine phosphate	100 mg guaifenesin	21.43 mg pseudoephedrine HCl		**2 to < 6 y** - 3.5 mL q 4 to 6 h, up to 14 mL/day	Methylparaben, sucralose. Grape flavor. In 118 mL.
c-v	**Zodryl DEC 25 Suspension** (Codadose)	5 mg codeine phosphate	100 mg guaifenesin	25 mg pseudoephedrine HCl		**2 to < 6 y** - 3 mL q 4 to 6 h, up to 12 mL/day	Methylparaben, sucralose. Grape flavor. In 118 mL.
c-v	**Zodryl DEC 50 Suspension** (Codadose)	5 mg codeine phosphate	100 mg guaifenesin	30 mg pseudoephedrine HCl		**6 to < 12 y** - 5 mL q 4 to 6 h, up to 20 mL/day	Methylparaben, sucralose. Grape flavor. In 236 mL.
c-v *sf*	**Cheratussin DAC Liquid** (Qualitest)	10 mg codeine phosphate	100 mg guaifenesin	30 mg pseudoephedrine HCl		**≥ 12 y** - 10 mL q 4 h, up to 40 mL/day; **6 to < 12 y** - 5 mL q 4 h, up to 20 mL/day	Sugar free. 2.1% alcohol, menthol, saccharin, sorbitol. In 473 mL.
c-v *sf*	**Guiatuss DAC Syrup** (Various, eg, Ivax)						1.9% alcohol, menthol, saccharin, sodium 4 mg/5 mL, sorbitol. In 473 mL.
c-v *sf*	**Mytussin DAC Liquid** (Morton Grove)						Menthol, saccharin, sorbitol. In 118 mL.
c-v *sf*	**Tusnel C Syrup** (LLorens)						1.9% alcohol, menthol, saccharin, sorbitol. In 473 mL.
c-v *sf*	**Tussirex Sugar Free Liquid** (Scot-Tussin)	10 mg codeine phosphate	83.3 mg sodium citrate	4.17 mg phenylephrine HCl	13.33 mg pheniramine maleate, 83.33 mg sodium salicylate, 25 mg caffeine citrate	**Adult** - 5 mL tid[c]	Alcohol and dye free. Menthol 0.17 mg. In 30 and 473 mL.
otc	**Robitussin Pediatric Cough/Cold CF Drops** (Wyeth Consumer)	2 mg dextromethorphan HBr	40 mg guaifenesin	1 mg phenylephrine HCl		**2 to < 6 y** - 2.5 mL q 4 h, up to 15 mL/day[b]	Alcohol free. PEG, sorbitol, sucralose. In 30 mL with oral dosing device.
Rx *sf*	**Zotex Pediatric Drops** (Vertical)	3 mg dextromethorphan HBr	35 mg guaifenesin	2.5 mg phenylephrine HCl		**9 to 18 mo** - 1 mL qid; **6 to 9 mo** - 0.75 mL qid[b]	Alcohol free. Parabens, saccharin. Grape flavor. In 30 mL with dropper.
Rx *sf*	**Z-Dex Pediatric Drops** (Trigen)						Alcohol free. Parabens, saccharin. Grape flavor. In 30 mL with dropper.

ANTITUSSIVE AND EXPECTORANT COMBINATIONS

	Product & Distributor	Antitussive	Expectorant	Decongestant	Antihistamine/Other	Average Dose	Excipients & How Supplied
Rx	**Despec NR Drops** (Great Southern Labs)	4 mg dextromethorphan HBr	20 mg guaifenesin	1.5 mg phenylephrine HCl		**12 to 24 mo** - 1 mL q 4 to 6 h up to 4 mL/day; **6 to 12 mo** - ¾ mL q 4 to 6 h up to 3 mL/day; **3 to 6 mo** - ½ mL q 4 to 6 h up to 2 mL/day; **1 to 3 mo** - ¼ mL q 4 to 6 h up to 1 mL/day	Saccharin, sorbitol. Grape flavor. In 15 and 30 mL with dropper.
Rx	**Robitussin Children's Cough & Cold CF Liquid** (Pfizer Consumer Healthcare)	5 mg dextromethorphan HBr	50 mg guaifenesin	2.5 mg phenylephrine HCl		**≥ 12 y** - 20 mL q 4 h, up to 120 mL/day; **6 to < 12 y** - 10 mL q 4 h, up to 60 mL/day; **4 to < 6 y** - 5 mL q 4 h, up to 30 mL/day	Sodium 3 mg. Glycerin, propylene glycol, sodium benzoate, sorbitol, sucralose. In 118 mL.
Rx sf	**Tussi-Pres Pediatric Liquid** (Kramer-Novis)	5 mg dextromethorphan HBr	75 mg guaifenesin	2.5 mg phenylephrine HCl		**> 12 y (> 43 kg)** - 20 mL q 6 h, up to 80 mL/day; **6 to 12 y (20 to 43 kg)** - 10 mL q 6 h, up to 40 mL/day; **2 to 6 y (11 to 20 kg)** - 5 mL q 6 h, up to 20 mL/day	Alcohol and dye free. Aspartame, parabens, phenylalanine 14 mg/5 mL. Orange flavor. In 473 mL.
otc	**Q-Tussin CF Liquid** (Qualitest)	10 mg dextromethorphan HBr	100 mg guaifenesin	5 mg phenylephrine		**≥ 12 y** - 10 mL q 4 h, up to 60 mL/day; **6 to < 12 y** - 5 mL q 4 h, up to 30 mL/day; **2 to < 6 y** - 2.5 mL q 4 h, up to 15 mL/day	Alcohol free. Corn syrup, glucose, saccharin. In 118 mL.
otc	**Robafen CF Liquid** (Major)						Alcohol free. Saccharin, sorbitol. In 237 mL.
Rx sf	**Zotex-D Syrup** (Vertical Pharmaceuticals)	15 mg dextromethorphan HBr	100 mg guaifenesin	8.5 mg phenylephrine HCl		**≥ 12 y** - 5 to 10 mL q 4 to 6 h, up to 60 mL/day; **6 to 12 y** - 2.5 to 5 mL q 4 to 6 h, up to 30 mL/day	Alcohol free, dye free, sugar free. Glycerin, propylene glycol, saccharin, sodium benzoate, sorbitol. Cherry flavor. In 473 mL.
Rx sf	**Tussi-Pres Liquid** (Kramer-Novis)	15 mg dextromethorphan HBr	200 mg guaifenesin	5 mg phenylephrine HCl		**> 12 y** - 10 mL q 6 h, up to 40 mL/day; **6 to 12 y** - 5 mL q 6 h, up to 20 mL/day	Alcohol free. Aspartame, parabens, phenylalanine 1.5 mg/5 mL. Cherry flavor. In 474 mL.
Rx sf	**Biogil Liquid** (Advanced Generic)	15 mg dextromethorphan HBr	300 mg guaifenesin	10 mg phenylephrine HCl		**≥ 12 y** - 5 mL q 4 h, up to 30 mL/day; **6 to < 12 y** - 2.5 mL q 4 h, up to 15 mL/day	Alcohol free, sugar free. Parbens, sorbitol. Grape flavor. In 473 mL.
Rx	**Zotex-Ex Caplets** (Vertical Pharmaceuticals)	15 mg dextromethorphan HBr	350 mg guaifenesin	10 mg phenylephrine HCl		**≥ 12 y** - 1 q 6 h, up to 4/day	(VP 035). White, capsule shape. In 100s.
otc	**Deconex DMX Tablets** (Poly Pharmaceuticals)	15 mg dextromethorphan HBr	380 mg guaifenesin	10 mg phenylephrine HCl		**≥ 12 y** - 1 q 4 to 6 h, up to 6/day	Maltodextrin. (POLY 730). Orange, capsule shape, scored. In 60s.
otc	**Deconex DM Capsules** (Poly Pharmaceuticals)	15 mg dextromethorphan HBr	390 mg guaifenesin	10 mg phenylephrine HCl		**≥ 12 y** - 1 q 4 h, up to 6/day	Yellow #5. (Deconex 583). Purple/orange. In 60s.

ANTITUSSIVE AND EXPECTORANT COMBINATIONS

	Product & Distributor	Antitussive	Expectorant	Decongestant	Antihistamine/Other	Average Dose	Excipients & How Supplied
Rx *sf*	**Endacon Liquid** (Allegis)	20 mg dextromethorphan HBr	100 mg guaifenesin	10 mg phenylephrine HCl		**≥ 12 y** - 5 to 10 mL q 4 h up to 60 mL/day	Alcohol free, sugar free. Benzoic acid, edetate disodium, glycerin, propylene glycol, sorbitol. Strawberry flavor. In 473 mL.
Rx	**Tusso XR Suspension** (Everett)					**> 12 y** - 10 mL bid; **6 to 12 y** - 5 mL bid; **3 to 6 y** - 2.5 mL bid	Acesulfame K, aspartame, methylparaben, phenylalanine 25.26 mg/5 mL. Grape flavor. In 473 mL.
Rx *sf*	**Z-Dex Syrup** (Trigen Labs)					**≥ 12 y** - 5 mL q 4 to 6 h, up to 30 mL/day; **6 to 12 y** - 2.5 mL q 4 to 6 h, up to 15 mL/day; **2 to 6 y** - 1.25 mL q 4 to 6 h, up to 7.5 mL/day	Alcohol free, sugar free. Edetate disodium, glycerin, sorbitol. Strawberry flavor. In 473 mL.
Rx *sf*	**Zotex Syrup** (Vertical Pharmaceuticals)					**≥ 12 y** - 5 mL q 4 to 6 h, up to 30 mL/day; **6 to 12 y** - 2.5 mL q 4 to 6 h, up to 15 mL/day; **2 to 6 y** - 1.25 mL q 4 to 6 h, up to 7.5 mL/day	Alcohol free, sugar free. Parabens, saccharin, Strawberry flavor. In 10 and 473 mL.
otc *sf*	**Broncotron-D Suspension** (Seyer Pharmatec)	20 mg dextromethorphan HBr	200 mg guaifenesin	5 mg phenylephrine HCl		**≥ 12 y** - 10 mL q 4 h, up to 40 mL/day; **6 to < 12 y** - 5 mL q 4 h, up to 20 mL/day; **2 to < 6 y** - 2.5 mL q 4 h, up to 10 mL/day	Alcohol and dye free. Aspartame, phenylalanine, sorbitol. Cherry flavor. In 118.3 mL.
otc *sf*	**Brontuss DX Liquid** (Portal)	20 mg dextromethorphan HBr	200 mg guaifenesin	10 mg phenylephrine HCl		**≥ 12 y** - 10 mL q 6 h, up to 40 mL/day; **6 to < 12 y** - 5 mL q 6 h, up to 20 mL/day	Alcohol free, dye free, gluten free, sugar free. Cherry flavoring, maltitol, propylene glycol, saccharin, sorbitol. In 118 mL.
Rx	**AMBI 10PEH/400GFN/20DM Tablets** (AMBI Pharmaceuticals)	20 mg dextromethorphan HBr	400 mg guaifenesin	10 mg phenylephrine HCl		**> 12 y** - 1 q 4 to 6 h, up to 6/day; **6 to < 12 y** - ½ q 4 to 6 h, up to 3/day	(AMBI 403). White, capsule shape, scored. In 100s.
Rx	**Maxiphen DM Tablets** (MCR American)					**> 12 y** - 1 q 4 to 6 h, up to 4/day; **6 to < 12 y** - ½ q 4 to 6 h, up to 2/day	(MAXIPHEN DM). Capsule shape, scored. In 100s.
Rx	**Phlemex-PE Tablets** (Cypress)	20 mg dextromethorphan HBr	800 mg guaifenesin	20 mg phenylephrine HCl		**≥ 12 y** - 1 to 1½ q 12 h, up to 3/day; **6 to 12 y** - ½ q 12 h, up to 1/day	Extended release. (CYP 321). Purple, scored. In 100s.
Rx	**GFN 1,200/DM 20/PE 40 Tablets** (Cypress)	20 mg dextromethorphan HBr	1,200 guaifenesin	40 mg phenylephrine HCl		**≥ 12 y** - 1 bid, up to 2/day; **6 to < 12 y** - ½ q 12 h, up to 1/day	Extended release. Dye free. (CYP 252). Scored. In 100s.
Rx	**Guaifen DM Tablets** (Breckenridge)					**≥ 12 y** - 1 bid, up to 2/day; **6 to 12 y** - ½ bid, up to 1/day	Extended release. Dye free. (B429). Capsule shape, scored. In 100s.
Rx	**Tusso DM Tablets** (Everett)	23 mg dextromethorphan HBr (8 mg immediate release/ 15 mg extended release)	600 mg guaifenesin (200 mg immediate release/400 mg extended release)	9 mg phenylephrine HCl (extended release)		**> 12 y** - 1 to 2 bid, up to 4/day; **6 to 12 y** - ½ bid, up to 1/day	Extended release. Lactose. (EV 0630). White/blue, capsule shape, scored. In 100s.

ANTITUSSIVE AND EXPECTORANT COMBINATIONS

	Product & Distributor	Antitussive	Expectorant	Decongestant	Antihistamine/Other	Average Dose	Excipients & How Supplied
Rx sf	**Dacex DM Syrup** (Cypress)	25 mg dextromethorphan HBr	175 mg guaifenesin	12.5 mg phenylephrine HCl		**≥ 12 y** - 5 mL q 6 h, up to 20 mL/day; **6 to < 12 y** - 2.5 mL q 6 h, up to 10 mL/day; **2 to < 6 y** - 1.25 mL q 6 h, up to 5 mL/day	Alcohol free. Saccharin, sorbitol. Strawberry flavor. In 473 mL.
Rx sf	**ExeTuss-DM Tablets** (Larken)	25 mg dextromethorphan HBr	600 mg guaifenesin	20 mg phenylephrine HCl		**≥ 12 y** - 1 or 2 q 12 h	Extended release. Dye free. (LL183). Oval. In 100s.
Rx sf	**NeoTuss-D** (A.G. Marin Pharmaceuticals)	30 mg dextromethorphan HBr	200 mg guaifenesin	7.5 mg phenylephrine HCl		**> 12 y** - 5 mL q 6 to 8 h, up to 20 mL/day; **6 to 12 y** - 2.5 mL q 6 to 8 h, up to 10 mL/day	Alcohol free, dye free, sugar free. Glycerin, parabens, propylene glycol, sucralose. Raspberry flavor. In 474 mL.
Rx	**Dynatuss EX Syrup** (Breckenridge)	30 mg dextromethorphan HBr	200 mg guaifenesin	10 mg phenylephrine HCl		**≥ 6 y** - 5 mL qid; **18 mo to 6 y** - 2.5 mL qid	PEG, saccharin, sorbitol. In 473 mL.
Rx sf	**Dacex PE Tablets** (Cypress)	30 mg dextromethorphan HBr	600 mg guaifenesin	10 mg phenylephrine HCl		**≥ 12 y** - 1 to 2 q 12 h, up to 4/day; **6 to < 12 y** - 1 q 12 h, up to 2/day	Extended release. Dye and gluten free. (CYP 248). Capsule shape. In 100s.
Rx	**TriTuss ER Tablets** (Everett)					**> 12 y** - 1 to 2 q 12 h, up to 4/day; **6 to 12 y** - 1 q 12 h, up to 2/day	Extended release. (EV/0661). Capsule shape, scored. In 100s.
Rx	**SINUtuss DM Tablets** (Dexo Pharma)	30 mg dextromethorphan HBr	600 mg guaifenesin	15 mg phenylephrine HCl		**≥ 12 y** - 2 q 12 h; **6 to 12 y** - 1 q 12 h	(WE 45). Scored. In 100s.
Rx	**SymPak DM Tablets** (Dexo LLC)	*Day:* 30 mg dextromethorphan HBr	600 mg guaifenesin	15 mg phenylephrine HCl		**≥ 12 y** - 2 in a.m.; **6 to 12 y** - 1 in a.m.	In carton with 2 blister cards of 14 day dosing regimen of day/night tablets.
		Night:		25 mg phenylephrine HCl	8 mg chlorpheniramine maleate, 2.5 mg methscopolamine nitrate	**≥ 12 y** - 1 in p.m.; **6 to 12 y** - ½ in p.m.	
Rx sf	**Endacon DM Tablets** (Allegis)	30 mg dextromethorphan HBr	600 mg guaifenesin	20 mg phenylephrine HCl		**≥ 12 y** - 1 or 2 bid	Dye and preservative free. (ENDACON). White, oval. In 100s.
Rx	**Deconex DM Tablets** (Poly)	30 mg dextromethorphan HBr	900 mg guaifenesin	30 mg phenylephrine HCl		**≥ 12 y** - 1 q 12 h, up to 2/day; **6 to 12 y** - ½ q 12 h, up to 1/day	Extended release. (DECONEX DM DM GP). Orange, scored. In 100s.
Rx	**Phlemex Forte Tablets** (Cypress)	30 mg dextromethorphan HBr	1,200 mg guaifenesin	30 mg phenylephrine HCl		**≥ 12 y** - 1 bid, up to 2/day; **6 to 12 y** - ½ q 12 h, up to 1/day	Extended release. Dye free. (CYP 323). Scored. In 100s.
Rx	**ExeCof Tablets** (Larken)	60 mg dextromethorphan HBr	1,000 mg guaifenesin	40 mg phenylephrine HCl		**≥ 12 y** - 1 bid; **6 to 12 y** - ½ bid	Extended release. Dye free. (LL 70). Capsule shape, scored. In 100s.
otc	**Tusnel-DM Pediatric Drops** (LLorens)	2.5 mg dextromethorphan HBr	25 mg guaifenesin	7.5 mg pseudoephedrine HCl		**2 to < 6 y** - 2 mL q 4 to 6 h, up to 8 mL/day	Glycerin, propylene glycol, saccharin, sodium benzoate. In 60 mL.
Rx	**Bionel Pediatric Liquid** (Advanced Generic)	5 mg dextromethorphan HBr	50 mg guaifenesin	15 mg pseudoephedrine HCl		**6 to < 12 y** - 10 mL q 4 to 6 h, up to 40 mL/day; **2 to < 6 y** - 5 mL q 4 to 6 h, up to 20 mL/day	Alcohol free. Aspartame, parabens, 14 mg phenylalanine per 5 mL. In 473 mL.
Rx	**Tusnel Pediatric Liquid** (LLorens)					**≥ 12 y** - 20 mL q 6 h, up to 80 mL/day; **6 to < 12 y** - 10 mL q 6 h, up to 40 mL/day; **2 to < 6 y** - 5 mL q 6 h, up to 20 mL/day	Alcohol free. Aspartame, corn syrup, parabens, phenylalanine. In 118 and 3,780 mL.

ANTITUSSIVE AND EXPECTORANT COMBINATIONS

	Product & Distributor	Antitussive	Expectorant	Decongestant	Antihistamine/Other	Average Dose	Excipients & How Supplied
Rx *sf*	**Maxifed DM Liquid** (MCR American)	10 mg dextromethorphan HBr	200 mg guaifenesin	20 mg pseudoephedrine HCl		**> 12 y** - 5 mL q 4 to 6 h, up to 30 mL/day; **6 to < 12 y** - 2.5 mL q 4 to 6 h, up to 15 mL/day	Sugar free. 0.1% alcohol, parabens, sorbitol, sucralose. Orange cream flavor. In 473 mL.
otc	**Robitussin Cold, Cold & Congestion Tablets** (Wyeth Consumer)	10 mg dextromethorphan HBr	200 mg guaifenesin	30 mg pseudoephedrine HCl		**≥ 12 y** - 2 q 4 h, up to 8/day; **6 to < 12 y** - 1 q 4 h, up to 4/day	PEG. Capsule shape. In 20s.
Rx *sf*	**Donatussin DM Syrup** (Great Southern Labs)	15 mg dextromethorphan HBr	150 mg guaifenesin	30 mg pseudoephedrine HCl		**≥ 12 y** - 5 to 10 mL q 4 to 6 h up to 4 doses/day **6 to < 12 y** - 2.5 to 5 mL q 4 to 6 h up to 4 doses/day	Alcohol free. Saccharin, sorbitol. Mint flavor. In 30 and 473 mL.
Rx	**TGQ 30PSE/150GFN/15DM Liquid** (TG United Pharmaceuticals)					**> 12 y** - 5 to 10 mL q 6 h, up to 40 mL/day; **6 to < 12 y** - 2.5 to 5 mL q 6 h, up to 20 mL/day.	Parabens, potassium sorbate, propylene glycol, sorbitol, sucralose. In cool mint flavor. In 473 mL.
Rx	**Z-Cof 8 DM Suspension** (Zyber Pharmaceuticals)	15 mg dextromethorphan HBr	175 mg guaifenesin	30 mg pseudoephedrine HCl		**≥ 12 y** - 10 mL, tid; **6 to 12 y** - 5 mL, tid; **2 to 6 y** - 2.5 mL, tid	Alcohol free. Acesulfame K, aspartame, methylparaben, 25.26 mg/mL phenylalanine. Grape flavor. In 473 mL.
Rx	**Z-Cof 12 DM Suspension** (Zyber)	15 mg dextromethorphan HBr (as 30 mg dextromethorphan tannate)	175 mg guaifenesin	30 mg pseudoephedrine HCl (as 60 mg pseudoephedrine tannate)		**≥ 12 y** - 10 mL bid, up to 20 mL/day; **6 to 12 y** - 5 mL bid, up to 10 mL/day; **2 to 6 y** - 2.5 mL bid, up to 5 mL/day	Alcohol free. Acesulfame K, aspartame, methylparaben, Grape flavor. In 473 mL.
Rx *sf*	**Liquicough DM Liquid** (Breckenridge)	15 mg dextromethorphan HBr	175 mg guaifenesin	32 mg pseudoephedrine HCl		**≥ 12 y** - 10 mL bid or tid, up to 3 doses/day; **6 to 12 y** - 5 mL bid or tid, up to 3 doses/day; **2 to 6 y** - 2.5 mL bid or tid, up to 3 doses/day	Alcohol free. Acesulfame K, saccharin, sorbitol. Grape flavor. In 473 mL.
Rx	**Pseudo Cough Liquid** (Boca Pharmacal)						Alcohol free. Acesulfame K, saccharin, sorbitol. Grape flavor. In 118 and 473 mL.
Rx	**Relasin DM Liquid** (Cypress)						Alcohol free. Menthol, saccharin, sorbitol. Grape flavor. In 473 mL.
Rx	**Donatuss XP Suspension** (Laser)	15 mg dextromethorphan HBr	180 mg guaifenesin	30 mg pseudoephedrine HCl		**≥ 12 y** - 10 mL 3 times/day, up to 30 mL/day; **6 to 12 y** - 5 mL 3 times/day, up to 15 mL/day	Alcohol free, gluten free. Benzoic acid, glycerin, grape flavoring, parabens, propylene glycol, saccharin, sorbitol. Grape flavor. In 473 mL.
otc *sf*	**Bionel Liquid** (Advanced Generic)	15 mg dextromethorphan HBr	200 mg guaifenesin	30 mg pseudoephedrine HCl		**≥ 12 y** - 10 mL q 6 h, up to 40 mL/day; **6 to 12 y** - 5 mL q 6 h, up to 20 mL/day	Alcohol free, dye free, sugar free. Aspartame, glycerin, parabens, 19 mg phenylalanine per 5 mL. In 473 mL.
otc	**Robitussin Cough & Cold D Liquid** (Wyeth Consumer Healthcare)					**≥ 12 y** - 10 mL q 4 h, up to 40 mL/day	Menthol, PEG, 4 mg sodium, sorbitol, sucralose. In 118 mL.
Rx *sf*	**Tusnel Liquid** (Llorens)					**≥ 12 y** - 10 mL q 6 h, up to 40 mL/day; **6 to < 12 y** - 5 mL q 6 h, up to 20 mL/day	Alcohol free, dye free, sugar free. Aspartame, parabens, phenylalanine 16.9 mg/5 mL. In 178 mL.
Rx	**Relacon DM NR Liquid** (Cypress)	15 mg dextromethorphan HBr	200 mg guaifenesin	32 mg pseudoephedrine HCl		**≥ 12 y** - 10 mL bid or tid, up to 3 doses/day; **6 to 12 y** - 5 mL bid or tid, up to 3 doses/day; **2 to 6 y** - 2.5 mL bid or tid, up to 3 doses/day	Alcohol free. Saccharin, sorbitol. Grape flavor. In 473 mL.

ANTITUSSIVE AND EXPECTORANT COMBINATIONS

	Product & Distributor	Antitussive	Expectorant	Decongestant	Antihistamine/Other	Average Dose	Excipients & How Supplied
Rx	**Z-Cof DMX Liquid** (Zyber)	15 mg dextromethorphan HBr	200 mg guaifenesin	36 mg pseudoephedrine HCl		**≥ 12 y** - 10 mL bid or tid, up to 3 doses/day; **6 to 12 y** - 5 mL bid or tid, up to 3 doses/day; **2 to 6 y** - 2.5 mL bid or tid, up to 3 doses/day	Alcohol free. Glucose, menthol, PEG, saccharin, sorbitol. Grape flavor. In 473 mL.
Rx	**AMBI 40PSE/400GFN/ 20DM Tablets** (AMBI Pharmaceuticals)	20 mg dextromethorphan HBr	400 mg guaifenesin	40 mg pseudoephedrine HCl		**> 12 y** - 1 q 4 to 6 h, up to 6/day; **6 to < 12 y** - ½ q 4 to 6 h, up to 3/day	(AMBI 409). White, capsule shape, scored. In 100s.
Rx	**Maxifed DM Tablets** (MCR American)						(MAXIFED DM). Capsule shape, scored. In 100s.
Rx	**AMBI 60PSE/400GFN/ 20DM Tablets** (AMBI Pharmaceuticals)	20 mg dextromethorphan HBr	400 mg guaifenesin	60 mg pseudoephedrine HCl		**> 12 y** - 1 q 4 to 6 h, up to 4/day; **6 to < 12 y** - ½ q 4 to 6 h, up to 2/day	(AMBI 407). White, capsule shape, scored. In 100s.
otc	**ExeFen DMX Tablets** (Larken)					**≥ 12 y** - 1 q 6 h, up to 4/day	Maltodextrin. (LL 155). White, oval, scored. In 100s.
otc	**Capmist DM Tablets** (Capital Pharmaceutical)	30 mg dextromethorphan HBr	400 mg guaifenesin	30 mg pseudoephedrine HCl		**≥ 12 y** - 1 q 6 h, up to 4/day	Maltodextrin. (CAP DM). Green, capsule shape, scored. In 30s.
Rx	**Touro CC-LD Tablets** (Dartmouth)	30 mg dextromethorphan HBr	575 mg guaifenesin	25 mg pseudoephedrine HCl		**> 12 y** - 1 or 2 q 12 h, up to 4/day; **6 to 12 y** - 1 q 12 h, up to 2/day; **2 to < 6 y** - ½ q 12 h, up to 1/day	Extended release. Dye free. (TOURO CC-LD DP 445). Capsule shape, scored. In 100s.
Rx	**AMBI 60/580/30 Tablets** (AMBI)	30 mg dextromethorphan HBr	580 mg guaifenesin	60 mg pseudoephedrine HCl		**> 12 y** - 1 to 2 q 12 h, up to 4/day; **6 to < 12 y** - ½ q 12 h, up to 1/day	Extended release. Dye free. (AMBI/122). Capsule shape, scored. In 100s.
Rx	**GFN 600/PSE 60/DM 30 Tablets** (Cypress)	30 mg dextromethorphan HBr	600 mg guaifenesin	60 mg pseudoephedrine HCl		**> 12 y** - 1 to 2 q 12 h, up to 4/day; **6 to 12 y** - 1 q 12 h, up to 2/day; **2 to 6 y** - ½ q 12 h, up to 1/day	Extended release. Dye free. (CYP 264). Capsule shape, scored. In 100s.
Rx	**GUAI 800/PSE 60/DM 30 Tablets** (Brighton)	30 mg dextromethorphan HBr	800 mg guaifenesin	60 mg pseudoephedrine HCl		**> 12 y** - 1 to 1½ q 12 h or 1 q 8 h, up to 3/day; **6 to 12 y** - ½ q 12 h, up to 1/day	Extended release. Dye free. (BP 971). Capsule shape, scored. In 100s.
Rx	**Medent-DM Tablets** (Stewart-Jackson)						Extended release. Dye free. (SJ 641). Oval, scored. In 100s.
Rx	**Ambifed-G DM Tablets** (MCR American)	30 mg dextromethorphan HBr	1,000 guaifenesin	60 mg pseudoephedrine HCl		**> 12 y** - 1 q 12 h, up to 2/day; **6 to 12 y** - ½ q 12 h, up to 1/day	Extended release. (AMBI/G DM AMBIFED G). Capsule shape, scored. In 100s.
Rx	**Maxifed DMX Tablets** (MCR American)	20 mg dextromethorphan HBr	400 mg guaifenesin	60 mg pseudoephedrine HCl		**> 12 y** - 1 q 4 to 6 h, up to 4/day; **6 to < 12 y** - ½ q 4 to 6 h, up to 2/day	(MAXIFED DMX). Capsule shape, scored. In 100s.
Rx	**Tidafen DM Tablets** (Tiber)[d]	60 mg dextromethorphan HBr	800 mg guaifenesin	90 mg pseudoephedrine HCl		**> 12 y** - 1 q 12 h, up to 2/day; **6 to 12 y** - ½ q 12 h, up to 1/day	Extended release. (NL 719). Capsule shape, scored. In 100s.

ANTITUSSIVE AND EXPECTORANT COMBINATIONS

	Product & Distributor	Antitussive	Expectorant	Decongestant	Antihistamine/Other	Average Dose	Excipients & How Supplied
otc	**Tylenol Cold Multi-Symptom Severe Daytime Citrus Burst Liquid** (McNeil Consumer)	3.33 mg dextromethorphan HBr	66.66 mg guaifenesin	1.66 mg phenylephrine HCl	108.33 mg acetaminophen	≥ **12 y** - 30 mL q 4 h, up to 180 mL/day	Ethyl alcohol, 1.66 mg sodium per 5 mL, sorbitol, sucralose. Citrus burst flavor. In 237 mL.
otc	**Sudafed PE Multi-Symptom Cold and Cough Tablets** (Johnson & Johnson)	10 mg dextromethorphan HBr	100 mg guaifenesin	5 mg phenylephrine HCl	325 mg acetaminophen	≥ **12 y** - 2 q 4 h, up to 12/day[c]	PEG. Capsule shape. In 20s.
otc	**Tylenol Cold Head Congestion Severe Cool Burst Tablets** (McNeil Consumer)	10 mg dextromethorphan HBr	200 mg guaifenesin	5 mg phenylephrine HCl	325 mg acetaminophen	≥ **12 y** - 2 q 4 h, up to 12/day	Mannitol, 3 mg sodium, sucralose. Capsule shape. Cool burst flavor. In 24s and 50s.
otc	**Tylenol Cold Multi-Symptom Severe Cool Burst Tablets** (McNeil Consumer)						Mannitol, 3 mg sodium, sucralose. Capsule shape. Cool burst flavor. In 24s.
otc	**Sine-Off Cough/Cold Tablets** (Hogil)	15 mg dextromethorphan HBr	200 mg guaifenesin	5 mg phenylephrine HCl	325 mg acetaminophen	≥ **12 y** - 2 q 6 to 8 h, up to 8/day[c]	In 24s.
otc	**Sine-Off Multi Symptom Relief Tablets** (Hogil)						In 24s.
otc	**Tylenol Cold Severe Congestion Tablets** (McNeil Consumer)	15 mg dextromethorphan HBr	200 mg guaifenesin	30 mg pseudoephedrine HCl	325 mg acetaminophen	≥ **12 y** - 2 q 6 h, up to 8/day[c]	Mannitol, sodium 3 mg, sucralose. In 100s.
Rx	**Duraflu Tablets** (Kowa Pharm)	20 mg dextromethorphan HBr	200 mg guaifenesin	60 mg pseudoephedrine HCl	500 mg acetaminophen	≥ **12 y** - 1 qid, up to 4/day; **6 to 12 y** - ½ qid, up to 2/day	Dye free. (PE 723). Scored. In 100s.
Rx	**Flutabs Tablets** (Breckenridge)						Dye free. (B 442). Capsule shape, scored. In 100s.
Rx	**AccuHist PDX Syrup** (Tiber)[d]	5 mg dextromethorphan HBr	50 mg guaifenesin	5 mg phenylephrine HCl	2 mg brompheniramine maleate	≥ **12 y** - 10 mL q 4 to 6 h, up to 60 mL/day; **6 to < 12 y** - 5 mL q 4 to 6 h, up to 30 mL/day; **2 to < 6 y** - 2.5 mL q 4 to 6 h, up to 15 mL/day	Alcohol free. Corn syrup, sucrose. Grape flavor. In 473 mL.
Rx	**Bromhist-PDX Syrup** (Cypress)						Alcohol free. Parabens, sugar. Grape flavor. In 473 mL.
Rx	**Bromhist DM Pediatric Syrup** (Cypress)	5 mg dextromethorphan HBr	50 mg guaifenesin	30 mg pseudoephedrine HCl	2 mg brompheniramine maleate	≥ **12 y** - 10 mL q 6 h, up to 40 mL/day; **6 to < 12 y** - 5 mL q 6 h, up to 20 mL/day; **2 to < 6 y** - 2.5 mL q 6 h, up to 10 mL/day	Alcohol and dye free. Saccharin, sorbitol. Grape flavor. In 473 mL.
Rx	**Pediahist DM Syrup** (Boca Pharmacal)						Alcohol free. Corn syrup. Grape flavor. In 473 mL.
Rx *sf*	**Chlordex GP Syrup** (Cypress)	7.5 mg dextromethorphan HBr	100 mg guaifenesin	10 mg phenylephrine HCl	2 mg chlorpheniramine maleate	≥ **12 y** - 10 mL q 4 to 6 h, up to 40 mL/day; **6 to 12 y** - 5 mL q 4 to 6 h, up to 20 mL/day; **2 to 6 y** - 2.5 mL q 4 to 6 h, up to 10 mL/day	Alcohol free. Saccharin, sorbitol. Grape flavor. In 473 mL.
Rx	**DM/CPM/PE/GG Syrup** (Kylemore)	15 mg dextromethorphan HBr	100 mg guaifenesin	10 mg phenylephrine HCl	2 mg chlorpheniramine maleate	≥ **12 y** - 10 mL q 6 h, up to 40 mL/day; **6 to < 12 y** - 5 mL q 6 h, up to 20 mL/day; **2 to < 6 y** - 2.5 mL q 6 h, up to 10 mL/day	Fruit gum flavoring, glycerin, parabens, propylene glycol, saccharin, sorbitol. In 473 mL.
Rx	**Donatussin Syrup** (Laser)						In 473 mL.

ANTITUSSIVE AND EXPECTORANT COMBINATIONS

	Product & Distributor	Antitussive	Expectorant	Decongestant	Antihistamine/Other	Average Dose	Excipients & How Supplied
c-iii	**Donatuss DC Syrup** (Laser)	7.5 mg dihydrocodeine bitartrate	50 mg guaifenesin	7.5 mg phenylephrine HCl		**≥ 12 y** - 5 to 10 mL q 4 to 6 h; **6 to < 12 y** - 2.5 to 5 mL q 4 to 6 h	Alcohol free, gluten free. Saccharin, sucrose. Grape flavor. In 473 mL.
c-iii *sf*	**Poly-Tussin EX Liquid** (Poly Pharmaceuticals)					**> 12 y** - 5 to 10 mL q 4 to 6 h; **6 to < 12 y** - 2.5 to 5 mL q 4 to 6 h	Alcohol free, dye free, gluten free, sugar free. Glycerin, propylene glycol, saccharin, sorbitol. Grape flavor. In 473 mL.

[b] Adult dosing could not be verified. Refer to the manufacturer's prescribing information for more information.
[c] Pediatric dosing could not be verified. Refer to the manufacturer's prescribing information for more information.
[d] Tiber Laboratories, 5400 Laurel Springs Pkwy, Suite 503, Suwanee, GA 30024; (866) 507-4837, http://www.tiberlabs.com.
[e] Pai Pharmaceutical Associates, 1700 Perimeter Rd, Greenville, SC 29605; (800) 845-8210, http://www.pa-inc.net.

Refer to the general discussion of these products in the Respiratory Combinations Introduction.

ANTITUSSIVES WITH EXPECTORANTS

Content given per tablet or 5 mL.

	Product & Distributor	Antitussive	Expectorant	Average Dose	Excipients & How Supplied
Rx	**AMBI 1000/5 Tablets** (AMBI)	5 mg carbetapentane citrate	1,000 mg guaifenesin	**> 12 y** - 1 q 12 h, up to 2/day; **6 to 12 y** - ½ q 12 h, up to 1/day	(AMBI 713). Capsule shape. In 100s.
Rx	**Tusso-ZR Syrup** (Everett Labs)	7.5 mg carbetapentane citrate	150 mg guaifenesin	**> 12 y** - 10 mL q 4 to 6 h; **6 to 12 y** - 5 mL q 4 to 6 h	Saccharin, sorbitol, sucralose. Grape flavor. In 473 mL.
Rx	**Tusso-ZMR Capsules** (Everett)	8 mg carbetapentane citrate	200 mg guaifenesin	**> 12 y** - 2 q 4 to 6 h; **6 to 12 y** - 1 q 4 to 6 h	Maltodextrin, tartrazine. (EV0647). White/green, oval. In 100s.
Rx	**BetaVent Syrup** (Wraser)	20 mg carbetapentane citrate	100 mg guaifenesin	**≥ 12 y** - 10 mL q 4 to 6 h; **6 to 12 y** - 5 mL q 4 to 6 h; **2 to 6 y** - 2.5 mL q 4 to 6 h	Alcohol free. Grape flavor. In 473 mL.
Rx	**Dynex VR Capsules** (Athlon)	30 mg carbetapentane citrate (extended release)	400 mg guaifenesin (immediate release)	**> 12 y** - 1 to 2 q 12 h, up to 4/day; **6 to 12 y** - 1/day	Extended release. (Dynex VR). Blue/Gray. In 100s.
Rx	**XPect-AT Tablets** (Hawthorn)	60 mg carbetapentane citrate	600 mg guaifenesin	**> 12 y** - 1 to 2 q 12 h, up to 4/day; **6 to 12 y** - ½ to 1 q 12 h, up to 2/day	Extended release. (HAW/240). Capsule shape. In 100s.
Rx	**Duratuss CS Tablets** (Victory)	60 mg carbetapentane citrate	900 mg guaifenesin	**≥ 12 y** - 1 q 12 h, up to 2/day; **6 to 12 y** - ½ q 12, up to 1/day	Extended release. (60 900). Capsule shape, scored. In 100s.
c-v *sf*	**CGU WC Liquid** (Elge)	6.3 mg codeine phosphate	100 mg guaifenesin	**≥ 12 y** - 15 mL q 4 to 6 h, up to 90 mL/day; **6 to < 12 y** - 7.5 mL q 4 to 6 h, up to 45 mL/day	Alcohol free. Saccharin, sorbitol, PEG. In 473 mL.
c-v *sf*	**M-Clear WC Liquid** (R.A. McNeil)				Alcohol free. Saccharin, sorbitol, PEG. In 473 mL.
c-v *sf*	**Mar-Cof-CG**(Marnel)	7.5 mg codeine phosphate	225 mg guaifenesin	**≥ 12 y** - 5 to 7.5 mL q 4 h, up to 45 mL/day; **6 to < 12 y** - 2.5 to 3.75 mL q 4 h, up to 22.5 mL/day	Alcohol free, sugar free. PEG, saccharin, sorbitol. In 473 mL.
c-v	**M-Clear Capsules** (R.A. McNeil)	9 mg codeine phosphate	200 mg guaifenesin	**≥ 12 y** - 2 q 4 h, up to 12/day; **6 to < 12 y** - 1 q 4 h, up to 6/day	Maltodextrin, tartrazine. (CLR). Green/yellow. In 100s.
c-v	**Pro-Clear Capsules** (ProPharma)				Maltodextrin, tartrazine. (CLR). Green/yellow. In 100s.
c-v *sf*	**Cheratussin AC Expectorant Cough Suppressant Liquid** (Qualitest)	10 mg codeine phosphate	100 mg guaifenesin	**≥ 12 y** - 10 mL q 4 h, up to 60 mL/day; **6 to < 12 y** - 5 mL q 4 h, up to 30 mL/day	Alcohol 3.5%, saccharin, sorbitol. In 118, 236, 473, and 3,785 mL.
c-v *sf*	**Gani-Tuss NR Liquid** (Cypress)			**Adults** - 10 mL q 4 h, up to 60 mL/day[a]	Alcohol free. Raspberry flavor. In 120 and 473 mL.
c-v *sf*	**Guiatuss AC Syrup** (Ivax)			**≥ 12 y** - 10 mL q 4 h, up to 60 mL/day; **6 to < 12 y** - 5 mL q 4 h, up to 30 mL/day	3.5% alcohol, saccharin, sodium 4 mg per 5 mL, sorbitol. In 118 and 473 mL.
c-v *sf*	**Mytussin AC Syrup** (Morton Grove Pharmaceuticals)			**≥ 12 y** - 10 mL q 4 to 6 h, up to 60 mL/day; **6 to < 12 y** - 2.5 to 5 mL q 4 to 6 h, up to 30 mL/day	3.5% alcohol, saccharin, sodium, menthol. Apricot peach flavor. In 473 mL.
c-v *sf*	**Romilar AC Syrup** (Scot-Tussin)			**≥ 12 y** - 10 mL q 4 h, up to 60 mL/day; **6 to < 12 y** - 5 mL q 4 h, up to 30 mL/day	Alcohol free, sugar free, aspartame, parabens, menthol. Clear grape flavor. In 473 mL.

ANTITUSSIVES WITH EXPECTORANTS

	Product & Distributor	Antitussive	Expectorant	Average Dose	Excipients & How Supplied
c-v	**Tusso-C Syrup** (Everett)	10 mg codeine phosphate	200 mg guaifenesin	≥ **12 y** - 10 mL q 4 to 6 h, up to 60 mL/day; **6 to < 12 y** - 5 mL q 4 to 6 h, up to 30 mL/day; **5 to < 6 y** - 2.5 mL q 4 to 6 h, up to 10 mL/day; **3 to < 5 y** - 1.25 mL q 4 to 6 h, up to 5 mL/day	Acesulfame K, aspartame, menthol, phenylalanine 0.03 mcg per 5 mL. Cherry vanilla flavor. In 473 mL.
c-v	**ExeClear-C Syrup** (Larken Laboratories)			≥ **12 y** - 10 mL q 4 to 6 h, up to 60 mL/day; **6 to < 12 y** - 5 mL q 4 to 6 h, up to 30 mL/day; **5 to < 6 y** - 2.5 mL q 4 to 6 h, up to 10 mL/day; **3 to < 5 y** -1.25 mL q 4 to 6 h, up to 5 mL/day	Alcohol free, sugar free, dye free, antihistamine free. Sodium, saccharin, *magnasweet*, sorbitol. Clear grape flavor. In 473 mL.
c-v *sf*	**Dex-Tuss Liquid** (Cypress)	10 mg codeine phosphate	300 mg guaifenesin	≥ **12 y** - 5 mL q 4 h, up to 40 mL/day; **6 to < 12 y** - 2.5 mL q 4 h, up to 20 mL/day; **5 y** - 2.25 mL q 4 to 6 h, up to 9 mL/day; **4 y** - 2 mL q 4 to 6 h, up to 8 mL/day; **3 y** - 1.75 mL q 4 to 6 h, up to 7 mL/day; **2 y** - 1.5 mL q 4 to 6 h, up to 6 mL/day	Alcohol and gluten free. Saccharin, sorbitol. Grape flavor. In 473 mL.
c-v *sf*	**Tussi-Organidin NR Liquid** (Victory Pharma)				Alcohol free. PEG, saccharin, sorbitol. In 473 mL.
c-v *sf*	**Tussi-Organidin-S NR Liquid** (Victory Pharma)				Alcohol free. PEG, saccharin, sorbitol. In 118 mL w/ dosing syringe.
c-v	**Brontex Tablets** (PharmaDerm)			≥ **12 y** - 1 q 4 h, up to 6/day;	(BRONTEX). Sugar, sodium. Red, capsule shape. In 100s.
c-iii	**Allfen CDX Liquid** (MCR American)	20 mg codeine phosphate	200 mg guaifenesin	> **12 y** - 5 mL q 4 to 6 h, up to 30 mL/day; **6 to < 12 y** - 2.5 mL q 4 to 6 h, up to 15 mL/day	Parabens, sorbitol, sucralose. Orange cream flavor. In 473 mL.
c-iii	**Allfen CDX Tablets** (MCR American)	20 mg codeine phosphate	400 mg guaifenesin	> **12 y** - 1 q 4 to 6 h, up to 6/day; **6 to < 12 y** - ½ q 4 to 6 h, up to 3/day	(ALLFEN CDX). White, scored, capsule shape. In 100s.
otc	**Vicks Formula 44e Pediatric Cough & Chest Congestion Relief Syrup** (Procter & Gamble Co.)	3.3 mg dextromethorphan HBr	33.3 mg guaifenesin	≥ **12 y** - 30 mL q 4 h, up to 180 mL/day; **6 to < 12 y** - 15 mL q 4 h, up to 90 mL/day; **2 to < 6 y** - 7.5 mL q 4 h, up to 45 mL/day	Alcohol free. Corn syrup, saccharin, sodium 27 mg per 15 mL. Cherry flavor. In 118 mL.
otc	**Mucinex Cough for Kids Liquid** (Reckitt Benckiser)	5 mg dextromethorphan HBr	100 mg guaifenesin	**6 to < 12 y** - 5 to 10 mL q 4 h, up to 60 mL/day; **2 to < 6 y** - 2.5 to 5 mL q 4 h, up to 30 mL/day	Alcohol free. Dextrose, parabens, saccharin, sucralose. Cherry flavor. In 118 mL.
otc	**Mucinex Cough Mini-Melts for Kids Granules** (Reckitt Benckiser)	5 mg dextromethorphan HBr	100 mg guaifenesin	≥ **12 y** - 2 to 4 packets q 4 h up to 24/day; **6 to < 12 y** - 1 to 2 packets q 4 h up to 12/day; **4 to < 6 y** - 1 packet q 4 h up to 6/day	Aspartame, phenylalanine 2 mg, sorbitol. Orange cream flavor. In 12s.
otc	**Vicks 44E Cough & Chest Congestion Relief Liquid** (Procter & Gamble Co.)	6.67 mg dextromethorphan HBr	66.7 mg guaifenesin	≥ **12 y** - 15 mL q 4 h, up to 90 mL/day; **6 to < 12 y** - 7.5 mL q 4 h, up to 45 mL/day	Alcohol, corn syrup, saccharin. In 118 and 236 mL.

ANTITUSSIVES WITH EXPECTORANTS

	Product & Distributor	Antitussive	Expectorant	Average Dose	Excipients & How Supplied
otc	**Cheracol D Cough Formula Syrup** (Lee)	10 mg dextromethorphan HBr	100 mg guaifenesin	**≥ 12 y** - 10 mL q 4 h, up to 60 mL/day; **6 to < 12 y** - 5 mL q 4 h, up to 30 mL/day	4.75% alcohol, fructose, sucrose. In 118 and 180 mL.
otc	**Cheracol Plus Syrup** (Lee)				4.75% alcohol, fructose, sucrose. In 118 mL.
Rx *sf*	**Gani-Tuss DM NR Liquid** (Cypress)			**≥ 12 y** - 10 mL q 4 h, up to 60 mL/day; **6 to < 12 y** - 5 mL q 4 h, up to 30 mL/day; **2 to < 6 y** - 2.5 mL q 4 h, up to 15 mL/day; **6 mo to < 2 y** - 0.6 to 1.25 mL q 4 h or 2.5 mL q 6 to 8 h, up to 7.5 mL/day	Alcohol free. Raspberry flavor. In 473 mL.
Rx *sf*	**Dex-Tuss DM Liquid** (Cypress)			**≥ 12 y** - 10 mL q 4 h, up to 60 mL/day; **6 to < 12 y** - 5 mL q 4 h, up to 30 mL/day; **2 to < 6 y** - 2.5 mL q 4 h, up to 15 mL/day	Alcohol and gluten free. Saccharin, sorbitol. Grape flavor. In 473 mL.
otc *sf*	**Diabetic Tussin DM Liquid** (Health Care Products)				Alcohol and dye free. Aspartame, phenylalanine 8.4 mg/5 mL, methylparaben, menthol. In 118 mL.
otc	**Genatuss DM Syrup** (Ivax)				Alcohol free. Corn syrup, menthol, saccharin, sodium 3 mg/mL. In 118 mL.
otc	**Geri-Tussin DM Liquid** (Geri-Care)			**≥ 12 y** - 10 mL q 4 h, up to 60 mL/day	Alcohol free. Fructose, glucose, saccharin. In 473 mL.
Rx *sf*	**Guaifenesin-DM NR Liquid** (Silarx)			**≥ 12 y** - 10 mL q 4 h, up to 60 mL/day; **6 to < 12 y** - 5 mL q 4 h, up to 30 mL/day; **2 to < 6 y** - 2.5 mL q 4 h, up to 15 mL/day	Alcohol free. Methylparaben, saccharin, sorbitol. Raspberry flavor. In 118, 473, and 3,785 mL.
otc	**Guiatuss DM Syrup** (Ivax)				Alcohol free. Corn syrup, menthol, saccharin. In 118, 473, and 3,785 mL.
otc *sf*	**Robitussin Cough Sugar-Free DM Liquid** (Wyeth Consumer)				Alcohol free. Acesulfame K, methylparaben, PEG, saccharin. In 118 mL.
otc	**Robitussin-DM Liquid** (Wyeth Consumer)				Alcohol free. Glucose, corn syrup, menthol, saccharin. In 118, 237, and 473 mL.
otc	**Siltussin-DM Liquid** (Silarx)				Alcohol free. Sucrose, saccharin, menthol, methylparaben. In 118, 237, and 473 mL.
otc	**Tussin DM Liquid** (ANI)				Alcohol free. Corn syrup, dextrose, menthol, saccharin. In 473 mL.
otc *sf*	**Tussin DM Sugar Free Liquid** (ANI)				Alcohol free. Acesulfame K, methylparaben, PEG, phenylalanine, saccharin. In 118 mL.
otc	**Guaifenesin DM Syrup** (UDL)			**Adults** - 10 mL q 4 h, up to 60 mL/day[a]	Alcohol free. Saccharin, sorbitol. In UD 5 and 10 mL.
otc	**Kolephrin GG/DM Liquid** (Pfeiffer)	10 mg dextromethorphan HBr	150 mg guaifenesin	**≥ 12 y** - 10 mL q 4 h, up to 60 mL/day; **6 to** - 5 mL q 4 h, up to 30 mL/day; **2 to < 6 y** - 2.5 mL q 4 h, up to 15 mL/day	Alcohol free. Glucose, saccharin, sodium 0.9 mg/5 mL, sucrose. Cherry flavor. In 118 mL.
otc	**Coricidin HBP Chest Congestion & Cough Softgel Capsules** (Schering-Plough)	10 mg dextromethorphan HBr	200 mg guaifenesin	**≥ 12 y** - 1 or 2 q 4 h, up to 12/day	In 20s.
otc *sf*	**Diabetic Tussin Maximum Strength DM Liquid** (Health Care Products)			**≥ 12 y** - 10 mL q 4 h, up to 60 mL/day	Alcohol and dye free. Aspartame, menthol, methylparaben, PEG, phenylalanine 8.4 mg/5 mL. In 237 mL.
otc *sf*	**Robafen DM Max Liquid** (Major)				Alcohol free, sugar free. Glycerin, menthol, PEG, propylene glycol, saccharin, sorbitol. In 118 mL.
otc	**Robitussin Cough & Congestion Liquid** (Wyeth Consumer)			**≥ 12 y** - 10 mL q 4 h, up to 60 mL/day; **6 to < 12 y** - 5 mL q 4 h, up to 30 mL/day; **2 to < 6 y** - 2.5 mL q 4 h, up to 15 mL/day	Alcohol free. Corn syrup, menthol, PEG, saccharin, sorbitol. In 118 mL.
Rx *sf*	**Tussi-Organidin DM-S NR Liquid** (Victory)	10 mg dextromethorphan HBr	300 mg guaifenesin	**≥ 12 y** - 5 mL q 4 h, up to 30 mL/day; **6 to < 12 y** - 2.5 mL q 4 h, up to 15 mL/day; **2 to < 6 y** - 1.25 mL q 4 h, up to 7.5 mL/day; **6 mo to < 2 y** - 0.6 mL q 4 h, up to 3.75 mL/day	Alcohol free. *Magnasweet*, PEG, saccharin, sorbitol. Grape flavor. In 118 mL w/ dosing syringe.
otc	**Biospec DMX Liquid** (Deliz Pharmaceutical)	15 mg dextromethorphan HBr	25 mg guaifenesin	**≥ 12 y** - 5 mL q 4 h, up to 30 mL/day; **6 to < 12 y** - 2.5 mL q 4 h, up to 15 mL/day; **4 to < 6 y** - 1.25 mL q 4 h, up to 7.5 mL/day	Alcohol free. Glucose, saccharin. Cherry flavor. In 473 mL.
otc	**Safe Tussin DM Liquid** (Kramer)	15 mg dextromethorphan HBr	100 mg guaifenesin	**≥ 12 y** - 10 mL q 6 h, up to 40 mL/day; **6 to 12 y** - 5 mL q 6 h, up to 20 mL/day; **2 to 6 y** - 2.5 mL q 6 h, up to 10 mL/day	Aspartame, menthol, parabens, phenylalanine 4.2 mg/5 mL. Mint flavor. In 120 mL.
otc *sf*	**Scot-Tussin Senior Clear Liquid** (Scot-tussin)	15 mg dextromethorphan HBr	200 mg guaifenesin	**Adults** - 5 mL q 4 h, up to 30 mL/day[a]	Alcohol free. Aspartame, menthol, parabens, phenylalanine. In 118 mL.

ANTITUSSIVES WITH EXPECTORANTS

	Product & Distributor	Antitussive	Expectorant	Average Dose	Excipients & How Supplied
otc	**Fenesin DM IR** (Pharma Medica)	15 mg dextromethorphan HBr	400 mg guaifenesin	**≥ 12 y**-1 tablet q 4 h up to 6/day. **6 to < 12 y**-1/2 tablet q 4 h up to 3/day.	In 100s.
Rx *sf*	**SU-TUSS DM Liquid** (Cypress)	20 mg dextromethorphan HBr	200 mg guaifenesin	**> 12 y** - 5 mL q 4 h, up to 30 mL/day; **6 to 12 y** - 2.5 mL q 4 h, up to 15 mL/day; **2 to 6 y** - 1.25 mL q 4 h, up to 7.5 mL/day	5% alcohol, saccharin, sorbitol. Fruit flavor. In 473 mL.
otc	**Congesta DM Tablets** (Trimarc Labs)	20 mg dextromethorphan HBr	400 mg guaifenesin	**≥ 12 y** - 1 q 4 h, up to 6/day	Maltodextrin. In 90s.
Rx	**Duratuss DM Elixir** (Victory)	25 mg dextromethorphan HBr	225 mg guaifenesin	**> 12 y** - 5 mL q 4 h, up to 30 mL/day; **6 to 12 y** - 2.5 mL q 4 h, up to 15 mL/day; **2 to 6 y** - 1.25 mL q 4 h, up to 7.5 mL/day	Saccharin, sorbitol. Grape flavor. In 473 mL.
Rx	**Bidex-A Tablets** (SJ[b])	25 mg dextromethorphan HBr	600 mg guaifenesin	**≥ 12 y** - 1 q 8 h, or 1 to 2 q 12 h, up to 4/day	Extended release. Dye free. (SJP 223). Oval. In 100s.
Rx	**Respa-DM Tablets** (Respa)	28 mg dextromethorphan HBr	600 mg guaifenesin	**> 12 y** - 1 or 2 q 12 h, up to 4/day; **6 to 12 y** - 1 q 12 h, up to 2/day; **2 to 5 y** - ½ q 12 h, up to 1/day	Extended release. Dye free. (RESPA 78). Scored. In 100s.
otc *sf*	**NeoTuss Liquid** (A.G. Marin Pharmaceuticals)	30 mg dextromethorphan HBr	200 mg guaifenesin	**> 12 y** - 5 mL q 6 to 8 h; **6 to < 12 y** - 2.5 mL q 6 to 8 h	Alcohol free, dye free, sugar free. Glycerin, menthol, parabens, propylene glycol, sorbitol, sucralose. Grape menthol flavor. In 473 mL.
Rx	**Dextromethorphan HBr/ Guaifenesin Tablets** (URL)	30 mg dextromethorphan HBr	500 mg guaifenesin	**Adults** - 1 or 2 q 12 h, up to 4/day[a]	Extended release. Dye free. (NL 736). Capsule shape, scored. In 100s.
Rx	**Touro DM Tablets** (Dartmouth)	30 mg dextromethorphan HBr	575 mg guaifenesin	**Adults** - 1 or 2 q 12 h, up to 4/day[a]	Extended release. (TOURO DM/DP311). Lt. blue, scored. In 100s.
Rx	**Guaifenex DM Tablets** (Ethex)	30 mg dextromethorphan HBr	600 mg guaifenesin	**> 12 y** - 1 or 2 q 12 h, up to 4/day; **6 to 12 y** - 1 q 12 h, up to 2/day; **2 to 6 y** - ½ q 12 h, up to 1/day.	Extended release. (Ethex 213). Green, capsule shape, scored. In 100s.
Rx	**Iobid DM Tablets** (Iopharm)			**Adults** - 1 or 2 q 12 h, up to 4/day[a]	Extended release. In 100s.
otc	**Mucinex DM Tablets** (Reckitt Benckiser)			**≥ 12 y** - 1 or 2 q 12 h, up to 4/day	Extended release. In 20s.
Rx *sf*	**GUAI 800 mg/DM 30 mg Tablets** (Brighton)	30 mg dextromethorphan HBr	800 mg guaifenesin	**≥ 12 y** - 1 to 1½ q 12 h or 1 q 8 h, up to 3/day; **6 to 12 y** - ½ q 12 h, up to 1/day	Extended release. Dye free. Scored. (BP 150). In 100s.
Rx	**AMBI 1000/55 Tablets** (AMBI)	55 mg dextromethorphan HBr	1000 mg guaifenesin	**> 12 y** - 1 to 1½ q 12 h or 1 q 8 h, up to 3/day; **6 to < 12 y** - ½ q 12 h, up to 1/day	Extended release. Dye free. (AMBI 120). Capsule shape, scored. In 100s.
Rx	**Allfen DM Tablets** (MCR American)	58 mg dextromethorphan HBr	1000 mg guaifenesin	**> 12 y** - 1 q 12 h, up to 2/day; **6 to 12 y** - ½ q 12 h, up to 1/day	Dye free. (ALLFEN DM). Scored. In 100s.
Rx	**GFN 1000/DM 60 Tablets** (Cypress)	60 mg dextromethorphan HBr	1,000 mg guaifenesin	**≥ 12 y** - 1 q 12 h, up to 2/day	Extended release. Dye free. (CYP 267). Capsule shape, scored. In 100s.
Rx	**Guaifenesin DM 1000/60 Tablets** (Prasco)			**> 12 y** - 1 q 12 h, up to 2/day; **6 to 12 y** - ½ q 12 h, up to 1/day	Extended release. Dye free. (312). Capsule shape, scored. In 100s.
Rx	**GFN 1200/DM 60 Tablets** (Cypress)	60 mg dextromethorphan HBr	1,200 mg guaifenesin	**≥ 12 y** - 1 q 12 h, up to 2/day	Extended release. Dye free. (CYP 263). Capsule shape, scored. In 100s.
otc	**Mucinex DM Maximum Strength Tablets** (Reckitt Benckiser)			**≥ 12 y** - 1 q 12 h, up to 2/day	Extended release. In 14s.
Rx	**TUSSI-bid Tablets** (Capellon)			**Adults** - 1 q 12 h, up to 2/day[a]	Extended release. (L/DM). Mottled pink, capsule shape, scored. In 100s.
Rx *sf*	**Prolex DMX Liquid** (Blansett Pharmacal)	15 mg dextromethorphan HBr	100 mg potassium guaiacolsulfonate	**≥ 12 y** - 5 to 7.5 mL q 4 to 6 h, up to 4/day; **6 to < 12 y** - 2.5 to 5 mL q 4 to 6 h, up to 4/day	Alcohol free, sugar free. Benzoic acid, menthol, propylene glycol, saccharin, sorbitol. Pineapple-orange flavor. In 473 mL.
Rx *sf*	**Prolex DM Liquid** (Blansett Pharmacal)	15 mg dextromethorphan HBr	300 mg potassium guaiacolsulfonate	**> 12 y** - 5 to 7.5 mL, up to 4/day; **6 to 12 y** - 2.5 to 5 mL, up to 4/day; **3 to 6 y** - 1.25 to 2.5 mL, up to 4/day	Alcohol free, sugar free. Pineapple-orange flavor. In 473 mL.
c-iii *sf*	**Hydron EX Liquid** (Cypress)	2.5 mg hydrocodone bitartrate	120 mg potassium guaiacolsulfonate	**> 12 y** - 10 to 15 mL q 4 to 6 h, up to 60 mL/day; **6 to 12 y** - 5 to 10 mL q 4 to 6 h, up to 40 mL/day; **2 to 6 y** - 2.5 to 5 mL q 4 to 6 h, up to 20 mL/day	Alcohol free. Menthol, saccharin, sorbitol. Cherry flavor. In 473 mL.
c-iii *sf*	**De-Chlor NX Liquid** (Cypress)	3 mg hydrocodone bitartrate	150 mg potassium guaiacolsulfonate	**> 12 y** - 10 to 15 mL q 4 to 6 h, up to 4 doses/day; **6 to 12 y** - 5 to 7.5 mL q 4 to 6 h, up to 4 doses/day; **2 to < 6 y** - 2.5 to 5 mL q 4 to 6 h, up to 4 doses/day	Alcohol and dye free. Cherry flavor. In 473 mL.

ANTITUSSIVES WITH EXPECTORANTS

	Product & Distributor	Antitussive	Expectorant	Average Dose	Excipients & How Supplied
c-iii *sf*	**Hy-KXP Liquid** (Cypress)	4.5 mg hydrocodone bitartrate	300 mg potassium guaiacolsulfonate	**> 12 y** - 5 to 7.5 mL q 4 h, up to 4 doses/day; **6 to 12 y** - 2.5 to 5 mL q 4 h, up to 4 doses/day	Alcohol free. Saccharin, sorbitol. In 473 mL.
c-iii *sf*	**Prolex DH Liquid** (Blansett Pharmacal)			**> 12 y** - 5 to 7.5 mL, up to 4 doses/day; **6 to 12 y** - 2.5 to 5 mL, up to 4 doses/day; **3 to 6 y** - 1.25 to 2.5 mL, up to 4 doses/day	Alcohol free. Saccharin, sorbitol, menthol. Tropical fruit punch flavor. In 118 and 473 mL.
c-iii *sf*	**Hydron KGS Liquid** (Cypress)	5 mg hydrocodone bitartrate	300 mg potassium guaiacolsulfonate	**> 12 y** - 5 to 7.25 mL, up to 4 doses/day; **6 to 12 y** - 2.5 to 5 mL, up to 4 doses/day; **3 to 6 y** - 1.25 to 2.5 mL, up to 4 doses/day	Alcohol free. Saccharin, sorbitol. Cherry flavor. In 473 mL.
c-iii *sf*	**Marcof Expectorant Syrup** (Marnel)	5 mg hydrocodone bitartrate	350 mg potassium guaiacolsulfonate	**Adult**: 5 mL after meals and at bedtime, not less than 4 h apart, up to 30 mL/day; **Pediatric**: **> 12 y** - 5 mL after meals and at bedtime, not less than 4 h apart; **6 to 12 y** - 2.5 mL after meals and at bedtime, not less than 4 h apart.	Alcohol and dye free. Menthol, PEG, saccharin, sorbitol. In 473 mL.

[a] Pediatric dosing could not be verified. Refer to manufacturer's prescribing information.

[b] SJ Pharmaceuticals, 4587 Damascus Rd, Memphis, TN 38118; (800) 367-1395; http://www.sjpharma.com.

Refer to the general discussion of these products in the Respiratory Combinations Introduction.

EXPECTORANTS WITH ANALGESICS COMBINATIONS

Content given per tablet, packet, or 5 mL.

	Product & Distributor	Expectorant	Analgesic	Average Dose	Excipients & How Supplied
otc	**Tylenol Chest Congestion Liquid** (McNeil)	66.67 mg guaifenesin	166.67 mg acetaminophen	≥ **12 y** - 30 mL q 4 to 6 h up to 120 mL/day	PEG, sorbitol, sucralose, sucrose. In 240 mL.
otc	**Comtrex Multi-Symptom Deep Chest Cold Tablets** (Novartis)	200 mg guaifenesin	325 mg acetaminophen	≥ **12 y** - 2 q 4 h up to 12/day	PEG, polyvinyl alcohol. Capsule shape. In 24s.
otc	**Tylenol Chest Congestion Tablets** (McNeil)			≥ **12 y** - 2 q 4 to 6 h up to 12/day	Mannitol, PEG, polyvinyl alcohol, sucralose. Capsule shape. In 24s.
otc	**Theraflu Flu & Chest Congestion Powder** (Novartis)	400 mg guaifenesin	1,000 mg acetaminophen	≥ **12 y** - Dissolve contents of one packet into 240 mL (8 oz) hot water	Acesulfame K, aspartame, maltodextrin, 24 mg phenylalanine/packet, 15 mg sodium/packet, sucrose. Citrus flavor. In 6s.

TOPICAL COMBINATIONS

	Product & Distributor	Ingredients	Excipients & How Supplied
otc	**Nose Better Gel** (Oakhurst)	0.5% allantoin, 0.75% camphor, 0.5% menthol	Lanolin, methylparaben. In 12.9 g.
otc	**Mentholatum Cherry Chest Rub for Kids** (Mentholatum Co.)	4.7% camphor, 2.6% menthol, 1.2% eucalyptus oil	Petrolatum. In 28 g.
otc	**Vicks VapoRub Cream** (Procter & Gamble)	5.2% camphor, 2.8% menthol, 1.2% eucalyptus oil	Cedarleaf, nutmeg, and turpentine oils, cetyl and stearyl alcohol, EDTA, glycerin, parabens. In 85 g.
otc	**Vicks VapoRub Ointment** (Procter & Gamble)	4.8% camphor, 2.6% menthol, 1.2% eucalyptus oil.	Cedarleaf, nutmeg, and turpentine oils, petrolatum. In 50 g.
otc	**Mentholatum Ointment** (Mentholatum Co.)	9% camphor, 1.3% menthol	Petrolatum. In 28 and 84 g.
otc	**Breathe Right Colds Nasal Strips** (GlaxoSmithKline)	Menthol	In 10s.
otc	**Ayr Mentholated Vapor Inhaler** (B.F. Ascher)	0.5 mL mixture of eucalyptus oil, menthol, lavender oil	In 1s.

CAFFEINE

otc	**Caffedrine** (Various, eg, Blairex)	**Tablets; oral:** 200 mg	In 16s.
otc	**Maximum Strength NoDoz** (Novartis Consumer Health)		Mineral oil, sucrose. Capsule shape. Coated. In 16s, 36s and 60s.
otc	**Vivarin** (GlaxoSmithKline)		Dextrose, (V). In 16s, 24s, 40s, and 80s.
otc	**Keep Alert** (Magno-Humphries Labs.)		Caplet shape. In 60s.
otc	**357 HR Magnum** (BDI)		In 36s, 100s, and 500s.
otc	**Overtime** (BDI)		In 100s and 500s.
otc	**20-20** (BDI)		In 100s and 500s.
otc	**Valentine** (BDI)		In 100s and 500s.
otc	**Keep Going** (Block Drug Co.)		Capsule shape. In 4s.
otc	**44 Magnum** (BDI)	**Capsules; oral:** 200 mg	In 100s and 500s.
otc	**Molie** (BDI)		In 100s and 500s.
otc	**Fastlene** (BDI)		In 100s and 500s.
otc	**Enerjets** (Chilton Labs)	**Lozenges; oral:** 75 mg	Sugar. Coffee, mocha mint, and "butterscotch" flavors. In 10s.
Rx	**Caffeine Citrate** (Paddock)	**Solution; oral:** 20 mg/mL	As caffeine citrate.[a] Preservative free. In 3 mL vials.
Rx	**Cafcit** (Bedford)		As caffeine citrate.[a] Preservative free. In 3 mL vials.
Rx	**Caffeine Citrate** (Paddock)	**Injection:** 20 mg/mL	As caffeine citrate.[a] Preservative free. In 3 mL vials.
Rx	**Cafcit** (Bedford)		As caffeine citrate.[a] Preservative free. In 3 mL vials.
Rx	**Caffeine and Sodium Benzoate** (Bedford)	**Injection:** 250 mg/mL	121 mg caffeine, 129 mg sodium benzoate. In 2 mL single-use vials.
Rx	**Caffeine and Sodium Benzoate** (American Regent)	**Injection:** 250 mg/mL	125 mg caffeine, 125 mg sodium benzoate. In 2 mL single-dose vials.

[a] 2 mg of caffeine citrate is equivalent to 1 mg caffeine base.

CAFFEINE — ORAL

Indications

➤*Fatigue/drowsiness:* Helps restore mental alertness or wakefulness when experiencing fatigue or drowsiness.

➤*Analgesia:* As an adjuvant in analgesic formulations.

➤*Off-label uses:*

Obesity – In combination with ephedrine, caffeine causes a modest, but significant, weight loss in obese individuals when energy intake is restricted over an extended period. This reflects a synergistic interaction as not seen with either agent alone.

Headache – Caffeine enhances the effect of ergotamine and may have direct actions on the extracranial vasculature or on trigeminal afferents in the treatment of migraine. Caffeine has been shown to effectively relieve headache resulting from lumbar puncture, and appears to produce an intrinsic analgesic effect in headaches of nonvascular origin.

Alcohol intoxication – For the treatment of excited or comatose alcoholic patients.

Postprandial hypotension – Postprandial decreases in blood pressure occur in elderly individuals, particularly after meals high in carbohydrates. Caffeine 250 mg, attenuated postprandial hypotension in a small number of patients. Analeptic use of caffeine is strongly discouraged by clinicians.

Administration and Dosage

➤*Adults:*

Drowsiness or fatigue – 100 to 200 mg by mouth not more often than every 3 to 4 hours, as needed.

➤*Children:*

Drowsiness or fatigue –

12 years of age and older: See Adults for dosing.

Younger than 12 years of age: Not recommended for children younger than 12 years of age.

➤*Storage/Stability:* Store at room temperature. Avoid excessive heat (greater than 37.7°C [100°F]) or humidity.

Actions

➤*Pharmacology:* Caffeine, a methylxanthine, exerts its pharmacological effects by increasing calcium permeability in sarcoplasmic reticulum, inhibiting phosphodiesterase promoting accumulation of cyclic AMP, and is a competitive, nonselective antagonist at adenosine A_1 and A_{2A} receptors. Evidence suggests that adenosine receptor antagonism is the most important factor responsible for most pharmacological effects of methylxanthines in doses that are administered therapeutically or consumed in xanthine-containing beverages.

Caffeine is a potent stimulant of the CNS. Its cortical effects are milder and of shorter duration than those of the amphetamines. In slightly larger doses, it stimulates medullary, vagal, vasomotor, and respiratory centers, promoting bradycardia, vasoconstriction, and increased respiratory rate. Caffeine produces a positive inotropic effect on the myocardium and a positive chronotropic effect at the sinoatrial node, causing transient increases in heart rate, force of contraction, cardiac output, and heart work. In doses greater than 250 mg, the centrally mediated vagal effects of caffeine may be masked by increased sinus rates, tachycardia, extrasystoles, or other major ventricular arrhythmias. Caffeine constricts cerebral vasculature, but directly peripheral blood vessels, decreasing peripheral vascular resistance. The latter effect (and possibly vagal cardiac stimulation) on blood pressure is offset by increased cardiac output (and possibly stimulation of the medullary vasomotor area). The overall effect of caffeine on heart rate and blood pressure depends on whether CNS or peripheral effects predominate.

Caffeine stimulates voluntary skeletal muscle, increasing the force of contraction and decreasing muscular fatigue. It also stimulates gastric acid secretion from parietal cells. Caffeine increases renal blood flow and glomerular filtration rate and decreases proximal tubular reabsorption of sodium and water, resulting in mild diuresis. It also stimulates glycogenolysis and lipolysis.

Long-term administration of caffeine results in an upregulation of A_1 receptors in the brain, as well as an enhanced sensitivity to adenosine analogs that have an affinity for A_1 receptors. Tolerance to the cardiovascular, CNS, and diuretic effects may develop. Differences in effects of caffeine on various organ systems may be observed in nonusers of caffeine vs habitual consumers. Acute ingestion of caffeine produces increases in systolic blood pressure, plasma catecholamines, plasma renin activity, and heart rate; chronic ingestion has little or no effect on these hemodynamic variables.

➤*Pharmacokinetics:*

Absorption/Distribution – Caffeine is well absorbed orally (99%) and is widely distributed throughout the body. Peak plasma levels of 5 to 25 mcg/mL are achieved 15 to 120 minutes after 250 mg. Protein binding is approximately 17%. Caffeine readily crosses the blood-brain barrier and placenta; low concentrations are also present in breast milk. Therapeutic plasma concentrations are approximately 6 to 13 mcg/mL; those greater than 20 mcg/mL may produce adverse effects. The lethal concentration is greater than 100 mcg/mL.

Metabolism/Excretion – Caffeine is metabolized in the liver and is excreted in the urine as methyluric acid, methylxanthine, and other metabolites with only approximately 1% excreted unchanged. In the adult, plasma half-life ranges from 3 to 7 hours. Half-life is increased with smoking and is prolonged in pregnancy (less than or equal to 18 hours), cirrhosis, and with concomitant use of some drugs.

Contraindications

Hypersensitivity to any components.

Warnings/Precautions

➤*GI effects:* Theophylline derivatives tend to relax the lower esophageal sphincter and increase gastric acid secretion. Caffeine-containing products may exacerbate duodenal ulcers. Caffeine may also considerably aggravate diarrhea in patients with irritable colon.

➤*Seizure disorder:* Caffeine is a CNS stimulant and in cases of caffeine overdose, seizures have been reported.

➤*Cardiovascular disease:* Although no cases of cardiac toxicity were reported in the placebo-controlled trial, caffeine has been shown to increase heart rate, left ventricular output, and stroke volume in published studies.

➤*Metabolic effects:* Caffeine stimulates glycogenolysis and lipolysis which increases free fatty acids and produces hyperglycemia. Caffeine also causes a release of catecholamines and increased metabolic activity.

CAFFEINE — ORAL

➤*Bone mineral density:* Lifetime caffeinated coffee intake equivalent to 2 cups/day is associated with decreased bone density in older women (mean age, 72.7 years) who do not drink milk on a daily basis. In elderly women whose calcium balance was impaired (less than 800 mg of calcium/day), high caffeine intake predisposed them to bone loss of the hip. However, caffeine or coffee-induced calcium loss and bone loss are insignificant in the face of adequate calcium intake.

➤*Withdrawal:* Symptoms occur within 12 to 24 hours following cessation of chronic caffeine ingestion (as little as 100 mg of caffeine/day) and may endure up to 7 days. The most common symptom is headache, but other frequently reported reactions include fatigue, depression, anxiety, and insomnia.

➤*Pregnancy: Category C.* Safety for use in pregnancy has not been established. Caffeine crosses the placenta and achieves fetal blood and tissue levels similar to maternal concentrations. Excessive caffeine intake (greater than 600 mg/day) has been weakly associated with increased fetal loss, low birth weight, premature deliveries, an increase in the incidence of fetal breathing activity, and a significant fall in baseline fetal heart rate. Three cases of fetal arrhythmia have also been reported. However, when used in moderation, there is no association with these effects or congential manifestations. Caffeine causes birth defects in animals when administered at doses toxic to the mother.

➤*Lactation:* Caffeine appears in the breast milk of nursing mothers. Milk:plasma rations of 0.5 and 0.76 have been reported. Approximately 1.3 to 3.1 mg of caffeine would be ingested by a nursing infant whose mother had 35 to 336 mg of oral caffeine.

➤*Children:* Do not use in children under 12 years old.

Drug Interactions

Caffeine Drug Interactions

Precipitant drug	Object drug[a]		Description
Allopurinol	Caffeine	↔	Allopurinol inhibits the conversion of caffeine metabolite methylxanthine to methyluric acid.
Cimetidine Contraceptives, oral Disulfiram Fluoroquinolones	Caffeine	↑	Caffeine hepatic metabolism may be impaired, resulting in decreased clearance and increased half-life. Consider avoiding caffeine consumption if excessive CNS or cardiovascular effects occur.
Mexiletine	Caffeine	↑	Concomitant administration reduced the elimination of caffeine by 30% to 50%.
Phenytoin	Caffeine	↓	Phenytoin decreases the half-life of caffeine and increases clearance. Concomitant administration results in lower caffeine levels.
Smoking	Caffeine	↓	Smoking induces hepatic metabolism and increases caffeine clearance.
Caffeine	Aspirin	↑	Caffeine appears to increase the GI absorption of aspirin, but does not appear to affect salicylate elimination.
Caffeine	Clozapine	↑	Caffeine may inhibit clozapine metabolism (P450 1A2), resulting in elevation of clozapine levels; possible increase in side effects may occur.
Caffeine	Lithium	↓	Caffeine may reduce serum lithium concentrations and may enhance renal clearance. Monitoring of serum lithium concentrations and adjustments in lithium dose may be necessary.
Caffeine	Theophylline	↑	Ingestion of caffeine (120 to 630 mg daily) can reduce theophylline clearance 23% and increase the elimination half-life. Serum theophylline levels may be increased. Advise patients to avoid drastic changes in daily caffeine intake.

[a] ↑ = Object drug increased. ↓ = Object drug decreased. ↔ = Undetermined clinical effect.

➤*Drug/Lab test interactions:* Caffeine produces false-positive elevations of serum urate as measured by the Bittner method. Caffeine also produces slight increases in urine levels of vanillylmandelic acid (VMA), catecholamines, and 5-hydroxyindoleacetic acid. Because high urine levels of VMA or catecholamines may result in false-positive diagnosis of pheochromocytoma or neuroblastoma, avoid caffeine intake during tests for these disorders.

➤*Drug/Food interactions:* Coffee and tea consumed with a meal or 1 hour after meal significantly inhibits the absorption of dietary iron. Clinical significance has not been determined.

Adverse Reactions

➤*Cardiovascular:* Tachycardia, extrasystoles, palpitations, other cardiac arrhythmias.

➤*CNS:* Insomnia, restlessness, excitement, nervousness, tinnitus, scintillating scotoma, muscular tremor, headache, lightheadedness.

Large doses of caffeine also may produce agitation, a condition resembling anxiety neurosis, hyperesthesia, and muscle twitches.

➤*GI:* Nausea, vomiting, diarrhea, stomach pain.

➤*Miscellaneous:* Hypersensitivity (eg, dermatitis, rhinitis, bronchial asthma), urticaria, hyperglycemia, diuresis.

Overdosage

➤*Symptoms:* Ingestion of 15 to 30 mg/kg results in significant toxicity (vomiting, myoclonus, myocardial irritability, hematemesis). Oral doses of 5 to 50 g (mean, 10 g) have produced fatalities; the lethal dose is estimated to be 100 to 200 mg/kg. In adults, IV doses of 57 mg/kg have been fatal. Toxicity correlates to serum caffeine levels. Several cups of coffee may produce caffeine concentrations of 5 to 10 mcg/mL. Symptoms of agitation and myoclonus develop at levels of 5 to 10 mcg/mL; cardiac arrythmias and seizures may develop at 50 to 100 mcg/mL. Caffeine concentrations as low as 80 mcg/mL to up to 1560 mcg/mL have been associated with death, although patients with concentrations up to 200 mcg/mL have survived. Fatalities have also been observed after the use of coffee enemas as a homeopathic therapy. Other symptoms of caffeine overdose that may develop include opisthotonus, decerebrate posturing, generalized muscular hypertonicity, rhabdomyolysis with resultant renal failure, pulmonary edema, hyperglycemia, hypokalemia, leukocytosis, ketosis, and metabolic acidosis.

Infants and children – In one 5-year-old patient, death occurred following oral ingestion of approximately 3 g. Signs and symptoms reported in the literature after caffeine overdose in preterm infants include fever, tachypnea, jitteriness, fine tremor of the extremities, hypertonia, opisthotonos, tonic-clonic movements, nonpurposeful jaw and lip movements, vomiting, hyperglycemia, elevated blood urea nitrogen, and elevated total leukocyte concentration. Seizures have also been reported. One case of caffeine overdose complicated by development of intraventricular hemorrhage and long-term neurological sequelae has been reported. No deaths associated with caffeine overdose have been reported in preterm infants.

➤*Treatment:* Primarily symptomatic and supportive. GI decontamination should include gastric lavage followed by activated charcoal. Control seizures with IV diazepam and phenobarbital. Caffeine levels have been shown to decrease after exchange transfusions. Even though not clearly established, indications for hemodialysis should include a caffeine serum concentration greater than 100 mcg/mL and life-threatening seizures or cardiac arrhythmias, regardless of serum concentration.

Patient Information

Limit the use of caffeine-containing medications, foods, or beverages while taking caffeine products because too much caffeine may cause nervousness, irritability, sleeplessness, and occasionally, rapid heart beat. Discontinue use if increased or abnormal heart rate, dizziness, or palpitations occur.

For occasional use only. Not intended for use as a substitute for sleep. If fatigue or drowsiness persists or continues to recur, consult a doctor.

Do not give to children under 12 years of age. Keep this and all drugs out of the reach of children.

As with any drug, if you are pregnant or nursing a baby, seek the advice of a health professional before using this product. Pregnant women should limit their intake of caffeine and caffeine-containing beverages.

In case of accidental overdose, seek professional assistance or contact a poison control center immediately.

Do not exceed recommended dosage.

CAFFEINE CITRATE — ORAL

Indications

➤*Apnea of prematurity:* For the short-term treatment of apnea of prematurity in infants between 28 and younger than 33 weeks gestational age.

Administration and Dosage

➤*General dosing considerations:* Prior to initiation of caffeine citrate, baseline serum levels of caffeine should be measured in infants previously treated with theophylline because preterm infants metabolize theophylline to caffeine. Likewise, baseline serum levels of caffeine should be measured in infants born to mothers who consumed caffeine prior to delivery because caffeine readily crosses the placenta.

➤*Children:*

Apnea of prematurity –

Infants between 28 and younger than 33 weeks gestational age:

• *Loading dose –* See the following table and Caffeine Citrate Injection monograph.

• *Maintenance dosage –* See the following table.

Recommended Loading and Maintenance Doses of Caffeine Citrate				
	Dose of caffeine citrate volume	Dose of caffeine citrate mg/kg	Route	Frequency
Loading dose	1 mL/kg	20 mg/kg	IV[a] (over 30 minutes)	One time
Maintenance dose	0.25 mL/kg	5 mg/kg	IV[a] (over 10 minutes) or orally	Every 24 hours[b]

[a] Using a syringe infusion pump.
[b] Beginning 24 hours after the loading dose.

Note that the dose of caffeine base is one-half the dose when expressed as caffeine citrate (eg, 20 mg of caffeine citrate is equivalent to 10 mg of caffeine base).

➤*Therapeutic drug monitoring:* Serum concentrations of caffeine may need to be monitored periodically throughout treatment to avoid toxicity. Serious toxicity has been associated with serum levels greater than 50 mg/L.

➤*Duration of therapy:* The duration of treatment of apnea of prematurity in the placebo-controlled trial was limited to 10 to 12 days. The safety and efficacy of caffeine citrate for longer periods of treatment have not been established.

➤*Administration:* Maintenance dose of caffeine citrate solution may be administered orally.

➤*Storage/Stability:* Store at 15° to 30°C (59° to 86°F).

This product is preservative free and is therefore for single use only. Discard unused portion.

Actions

➤*Pharmacology:*

Mechanism of action – Caffeine is structurally related to other methylxanthines, theophylline and theobromine. It is a bronchial smooth muscle relaxant, a CNS stimulant, a cardiac muscle stimulant and a diuretic.

Although the mechanism of action of caffeine in apnea of prematurity is not known, several mechanisms have been hypothesized. These include the following: Stimulation of the respiratory center; increased minute ventilation; decreased threshold to hypercapnia; increased response to hypercapnia; increased skeletal muscle tone; decreased diaphragmatic fatigue; increased metabolic rate; increased oxygen consumption.

Most of these effects have been attributed to antagonism of adenosine receptors, both A_1 and A_2 subtypes, by caffeine, which has been demonstrated in receptor binding assays and observed at concentrations approximating those achieved therapeutically.

➤*Pharmacokinetics:*

Absorption – Caffeine is well absorbed orally and is widely distributed throughout the body. After oral administration of 10 mg caffeine base/kg to preterm neonates, the peak plasma level (C_{max}) for caffeine ranged from 6 to 10 mg/L and the mean time to reach peak concentration (T_{max}) ranged from 30 minutes to 2 hours. The T_{max} was not affected by formula feeding. The absolute bioavailability, however, was not fully examined in preterm neonates.

Distribution – Caffeine is rapidly distributed into the brain across the blood-brain barrier. Caffeine levels in the cerebrospinal fluid of preterm neonates approximate their plasma levels. The mean volume of distribution of caffeine in infants (0.8 to 0.9 L/kg) is slightly higher than that in adults (0.6 L/kg). Plasma protein binding data are not available for neonates or infants. In adults, the mean plasma protein binding in vitro is reported to be approximately 36%.

Metabolism – Hepatic cytochrome P450 1A2 (CYP1A2) is involved in caffeine biotransformation. Caffeine metabolism in preterm neonates is limited due to their immature hepatic enzyme systems.

Interconversion between caffeine and theophylline has been reported in preterm neonates; caffeine levels are approximately 25% of theophylline levels after theophylline administration and approximately 3% to 8% of caffeine administered would be expected to convert to theophylline.

Excretion – In young infants, the elimination of caffeine is much slower than that in adults due to immature hepatic or renal function. Mean half-life ($T_{1/2}$) and fraction excreted unchanged in urine (A_e) of caffeine in infants have been shown to be inversely related to gestational/postconceptual age. In neonates, the $T_{1/2}$ is approximately 3 to 4 days and the A_e is approximately 86% (within 6 days). By 9 months of age, the metabolism of caffeine approximates that seen in adults ($T_{1/2}$ = 5 hours and A_e = 1%).

Contraindications

Hypersensitivity to any of its components.

Warnings/Precautions

➤*Necrotizing enterocolitis:* During the double-blind, placebo-controlled clinical trial, 6 cases of necrotizing enterocolitis developed among the 85 infants studied (caffeine = 46, placebo = 39), with 3 cases resulting in death. Five of the 6 patients with necrotizing enterocolitis were randomized to or had been exposed to caffeine citrate.

Reports in the published literature have raised a question regarding the possible association between the use of methylxanthines and development of necrotizing enterocolitis, although a causal relationship between methylxanthine use and necrotizing enterocolitis has not been established. Therefore, as with all preterm infants, patients being treated with caffeine citrate should be carefully monitored for the development of necrotizing enterocolitis.

➤*Apnea:* Apnea of prematurity is a diagnosis of exclusion. Other causes of apnea (eg, central nervous system disorders, primary lung disease, anemia, sepsis, metabolic disturbances, cardiovascular abnormalities, or obstructive apnea) should be ruled out or properly treated prior to initiation of caffeine citrate.

➤*Seizures:* Caffeine is a central nervous system stimulant and in cases of caffeine overdose, seizures have been reported. Caffeine citrate should be used with caution in infants with seizure disorders.

➤*Duration of use:* The duration of treatment of apnea of prematurity in the placebo-controlled trial was limited to 10 to 12 days. The safety and efficacy of caffeine citrate for longer periods of treatment have not been established. Safety and efficacy of caffeine citrate for use in the prophylaxis treatment of sudden infant death syndrome (SIDS) or prior to extubation in mechanically ventilated infants have also not been established.

➤*Cardiovascular effects:* Although no cases of cardiac toxicity were reported in the placebo-controlled trial, caffeine has been shown to increase heart rate, left ventricular output, and stroke volume in published studies. Therefore, caffeine citrate should be used with caution in infants with cardiovascular disease.

➤*Renal/Hepatic function impairment:* Caffeine citrate should be administered with caution in infants with impaired renal or hepatic function.

➤*Pregnancy: Category C* (per manufacturer's prescribing information). *Category B* (per Briggs' *Drugs in Pregnancy and Lactation*). Concern for the teratogenicity of caffeine is not relevant when administered to infants. In studies performed in adult animals, caffeine (as caffeine base) administered to pregnant mice as sustained release pellets at 50 mg/kg (less than the maximum recommended intravenous loading dose for infants on a mg/m^2 basis), during the period of organogenesis, caused a low incidence of cleft palate and exencephaly in the fetuses. There are no adequate and well-controlled studies in pregnant women.

➤*Lactation:* Caffeine is excreted into breast milk. Milk:plasma ratios of 0.5 and 0.76 have been reported. The American Academy of Pediatrics classifies caffeine as compatible with breast-feeding.

➤*Monitoring:* Prior to initiation of caffeine citrate, baseline serum levels of caffeine should be measured in infants previously treated with theophylline, since preterm infants metabolize theophylline to caffeine. Likewise, baseline serum levels of caffeine should be measured in infants born to mothers who consumed caffeine prior to delivery, since caffeine readily crosses the placenta.

In the placebo-controlled clinical trial, caffeine levels ranged from 8 to 40 mg/L. A therapeutic plasma concentration range of caffeine could not be determined from the placebo-controlled clinical trial. Serious toxicity has been reported in the literature when serum caffeine levels exceed 50 mg/L.

In clinical studies reported in the literature, cases of hypoglycemia and hyperglycemia have been observed. Therefore, serum glucose may need to be periodically monitored in infants receiving caffeine citrate.

Drug Interactions

Few data exist on drug interactions with caffeine in preterm neonates. Based on adult data, lower doses of caffeine may be needed following coadministration of drugs which are reported to decrease caffeine elimination (eg, cimetidine and ketoconazole) and higher caffeine doses may be needed following coadministration of drugs that increase caffeine elimination (eg, phenobarbital and phenytoin).

➤*CYP450 system:* Cytochrome P450 1A2 (CYP1A2) is known to be the major enzyme involved in the metabolism of caffeine. Therefore, caffeine has the potential to interact with drugs that are substrates for CYP1A2, inhibit CYP1A2, or induce CYP1A2.

➤*Ketoprofen:* Caffeine administered concurrently with ketoprofen reduced the urine volume in 4 healthy volunteers. The clinical significance of this interaction in preterm neonates is not known.

➤*Theophylline:* Interconversion between caffeine and theophylline has been reported in preterm neonates. The concurrent use of these drugs is not recommended.

CAFFEINE CITRATE — ORAL

Adverse Reactions

➤*Adverse events that occurred more frequently in caffeine citrate treated patients than placebo during double-blind therapy:*

Caffeine Citrate Adverse Reactions

Adverse reaction	Caffeine citrate (n = 46); n (%)	Placebo (n = 39); n (%)
Cardiovascular		
Hemorrhage	1 (2.2%)	0 (0%)
CNS		
Cerebral hemorrhage	1 (2.2%)	0 (0%)
Dermatologic		
Dry skin	1 (2.2%)	0 (0%)
Rash	4 (8.7%)	3 (7.7%)
Skin breakdown	1 (2.2%)	0 (0%)
GI		
Necrotizing enterocolitis	2 (4.3%)	1 (2.6%)
Gastritis	1 (2.2%)	0 (0%)
Gastrointestinal hemorrhage	1 (2.2%)	0 (0%)
GU		
Kidney failure	1 (2.2%)	0 (0%)
Hemic/Lymphatic		
Disseminated intravascular coagulation	1 (2.2%)	0 (0%)
Metabolic/Nutritional		
Acidosis	1 (2.2%)	0 (0%)
Healing abnormal	1 (2.2%)	0 (0%)
Respiratory		
Dyspnea	1 (2.2%)	0 (0%)
Lung edema	1 (2.2%)	0 (0%)
Special senses		
Retinopathy of prematurity	1 (2.2%)	0 (0%)
Miscellaneous		
Accidental injury	1 (2.2%)	0 (0%)
Feeding intolerance	4 (8.7%)	2 (5.1%)
Sepsis	2 (4.3%)	0 (0%)

In addition to the cases above, three cases of necrotizing enterocolitis were diagnosed in patients receiving caffeine citrate during the open-label phase of the study.

Three of the infants who developed necrotizing enterocolitis during the trial died. All had been exposed to caffeine. Two were randomized to caffeine, and 1 placebo patient was "rescued" with open-label caffeine for uncontrolled apnea.

Adverse events described in the published literature include: central nervous system stimulation (ie, irritability, restlessness, jitteriness), cardiovascular effects (ie, tachycardia, increased left ventricular output, and increased stroke volume), gastrointestinal effects (ie, increased gastric aspirate, gastrointestinal intolerance), alterations in serum glucose (hypoglycemia and hyperglycemia) and renal effects (increased urine flow rate, increased creatinine clearance, and increased sodium and calcium excretion). Published long-term follow-up studies have not shown caffeine to adversely affect neurological development or growth parameters.

Overdosage

➤*Symptoms:* Following overdose, serum caffeine levels have ranged from approximately 50 mg/L to 350 mg/L. Signs and symptoms reported in the literature after caffeine overdose in preterm infants include fever, tachypnea, jitteriness, fine tremor of the extremities, hypertonia, opisthotonos, tonic-clonic movements, nonpurposeful jaw and lip movements, vomiting, hyperglycemia, elevated blood urea nitrogen, and elevated total leukocyte concentration. Seizures have also been reported in cases of overdose. One case of caffeine overdose complicated by development of intraventricular hemorrhage and long-term neurological sequelae has been reported. No deaths associated with caffeine overdose have been reported in preterm infants.

➤*Treatment:* Treatment of caffeine overdose is primarily symptomatic and supportive. Caffeine levels have been shown to decrease after exchange transfusions. Convulsions may be treated with intravenous administration of diazepam or a barbiturate such as pentobarbital sodium.

Patient Information

Caffeine citrate does not contain any preservatives and each vial is for single use only. Any unused portion of the medication should be discarded. It is important that the dose of caffeine citrate be measured accurately, ie, with a 1 cc or other appropriate syringe.

Consult your physician if the baby continues to have apnea events; do not increase the dose of caffeine citrate without medical consultation. Consult your physician if the baby begins to demonstrate signs of gastrointestinal intolerance, such as abdominal distention, vomiting, or bloody stools, or seems lethargic.

Caffeine citrate should be inspected visually for particulate matter and discoloration prior to its administration. Vials containing discolored solution or visible particulate matter should be discarded.

CAFFEINE CITRATE — INJECTION

Indications

➤*Apnea of prematurity:* For the short-term treatment of apnea of prematurity in infants between 28 and younger than 33 weeks gestational age.

Administration and Dosage

➤*General dosing considerations:* Prior to initiation of caffeine citrate, baseline serum levels of caffeine should be measured in infants previously treated with theophylline because preterm infants metabolize theophylline to caffeine. Likewise, baseline serum levels of caffeine should be measured in infants born to mothers who consumed caffeine prior to delivery because caffeine readily crosses the placenta.

➤*Children:*

Apnea of prematurity –

Infants between 28 and younger than 33 weeks gestational age:

- *Loading dose* – See the following table.
- *Maintenance dosage* – See the following table.

Recommended Loading and Maintenance Doses of Caffeine Citrate

	Dose of caffeine citrate volume	Dose of caffeine citrate mg/kg	Route	Frequency
Loading dose	1 mL/kg	20 mg/kg	IV[a] (over 30 minutes)	One time
Maintenance dose	0.25 mL/kg	5 mg/kg	IV[a] (over 10 minutes) or orally	Every 24 hours[b]

[a] Using a syringe infusion pump.
[b] Beginning 24 hours after the loading dose.

Note that the dose of caffeine base is one-half the dose when expressed as caffeine citrate (eg, 20 mg of caffeine citrate is equivalent to 10 mg of caffeine base).

➤*Therapeutic drug monitoring:* Serum concentrations of caffeine may need to be monitored periodically throughout treatment to avoid toxicity. Serious toxicity has been associated with serum levels greater than 50 mg/L.

➤*Duration of therapy:* The duration of treatment of apnea of prematurity in the placebo-controlled trial was limited to 10 to 12 days.

➤*Preparation for administration:* Dissolve caffeine citrate 10 g powder (caffeine 5 g) in 250 mL Sterile Water for Injection, add sufficient quantity of sterile water to reach 500 mL, filter, and autoclave. Final concentration is caffeine base 10 mg/mL (caffeine citrate 20 mg/mL). Stable in glass vials for up to 342 days when refrigerated (22°C; 73.4°F) or frozen (4°C; 39.2°F) and protected from light.

➤*Administration:* Administer dose of caffeine citrate injection solution using a syringe infusion pump.

Caffeine citrate injection for IV administration is available as a clear, colorless, sterile, non-pyrogenic, preservative-free, aqueous solution adjusted to pH 4.7. Each mL contains caffeine citrate 20 mg (equivalent to caffeine base 10 mg).

➤*Admixture compatibility:* Based on testing, caffeine citrate injection 60 mg/3 mL is chemically stable for 24 hours at room temperature when combined with the following test products: Dextrose Injection, 5%; 50% Dextrose Injection, *Intralipid* 20% IV Fat Emulsion; *Aminosyn* 8.5% Crystalline Amino Acid Solution; Dopamine Hydrochloride Injection 40 mg/mL diluted to 0.6 mg/mL with Dextrose Injection 5%; Calcium Gluconate Injection 10% (0.465 mEq/Ca^{+2}/mL); Heparin Sodium Injection 1,000 units/mL diluted to 1 unit/mL with Dextrose Injection 5%; Fentanyl Citrate Injection 50 mcg/mL diluted to 10 mcg/mL with Dextrose Injection 5%.

➤*Storage / Stability:* Store at 15° to 30°C (59° to 86°F). Preservative free. For single use only; discard unused portion.

Actions

➤*Pharmacology:* Caffeine is structurally related to other methylxanthines, theophylline and theobromine. It is a bronchial smooth muscle relaxant, a CNS stimulant, a cardiac muscle stimulant and a diuretic.

CAFFEINE CITRATE — INJECTION

Although the mechanism of action of caffeine in apnea of prematurity is not known, several mechanisms have been hypothesized. These include: Stimulation of the respiratory center; increased minute ventilation; decreased threshold to hypercapnia; increased response to hypercapnia; increased skeletal muscle tone; decreased diaphragmatic fatigue; increased metabolic rate; increased oxygen consumption.

Most of these effects have been attributed to antagonism of adenosine receptors, both A_1 and A_2 subtypes, by caffeine, which has been demonstrated in receptor binding assays and observed at concentrations approximating those achieved therapeutically.

➤*Pharmacokinetics:*

Distribution – Caffeine is rapidly distributed into the brain. Caffeine levels in the cerebrospinal fluid of preterm neonates approximate their plasma levels. The mean volume of distribution of caffeine in infants (0.8 to 0.9 L/kg) is slightly higher than that in adults (0.6 L/kg). Plasma protein binding data are not available for neonates or infants. In adults, the mean plasma protein binding in vitro is reported to be approximately 36%.

Metabolism – Hepatic cytochrome P450 1A2 (CYP1A2) is involved in caffeine biotransformation. Caffeine metabolism in preterm neonates is limited due to their immature hepatic enzyme systems.

Interconversion between caffeine and theophylline has been reported in preterm neonates; caffeine levels are approximately 25% of theophylline levels after theophylline administration and approximately 3% to 8% of caffeine administered would be expected to convert to theophylline.

Excretion – In young infants, the elimination of caffeine is much slower than that in adults due to immature hepatic or renal function. Mean half-life ($T_{½}$) and fraction excreted unchanged in urine (A_e) of caffeine in infants have been shown to be inversely related to gestational/postconceptual age. In neonates, the $T_{½}$ is approximately 3 to 4 days and the A_e is approximately 86% (within 6 days). By 9 months of age, the metabolism of caffeine approximates that seen in adults ($T_{½}$ = 5 hours and A_e = 1%).

Contraindications

Hypersensitivity to any of its components.

Warnings/Precautions

➤*Necrotizing enterocolitis:* During the double-blind, placebo-controlled clinical trial, 6 cases of necrotizing enterocolitis developed among the 85 infants studied (caffeine = 46, placebo = 39), with 3 cases resulting in death. Five of the 6 patients with necrotizing enterocolitis were randomized to or had been exposed to caffeine citrate.

Reports in the published literature have raised a question regarding the possible association between the use of methylxanthines and development of necrotizing enterocolitis, although a causal relationship between methylxanthine use and necrotizing enterocolitis has not been established. Therefore, as with all preterm infants, patients being treated with caffeine citrate should be carefully monitored for the development of necrotizing enterocolitis.

➤*Apnea:* Apnea of prematurity is a diagnosis of exclusion. Other causes of apnea (eg, central nervous system disorders, primary lung disease, anemia, sepsis, metabolic disturbances, cardiovascular abnormalities, or obstructive apnea) should be ruled out or properly treated prior to initiation of caffeine citrate.

➤*Seizures:* Caffeine is a central nervous system stimulant and in cases of caffeine overdose, seizures have been reported. Caffeine citrate should be used with caution in infants with seizure disorders.

➤*Use:* The duration of treatment of apnea of prematurity in the placebo-controlled trial was limited to 10 to 12 days. The safety and efficacy of caffeine citrate for longer periods of treatment have not been established. Safety and efficacy of caffeine citrate for use in the prophylaxis treatment of sudden infant death syndrome (SIDS) or prior to extubation in mechanically ventilated infants have also not been established.

➤*Cardiovascular:* Although no cases of cardiac toxicity were reported in the placebo-controlled trial, caffeine has been shown to increase heart rate, left ventricular output, and stroke volume in published studies. Therefore, caffeine citrate should be used with caution in infants with cardiovascular disease.

➤*Renal/Hepatic function impairment:* Caffeine citrate should be administered with caution in infants with impaired renal or hepatic function.

➤*Pregnancy: Category C* (per manufacturer's prescribing information). *Category B* (per Briggs' *Drugs in Pregnancy and Lactation*). Concern for the teratogenicity of caffeine is not relevant when administered to infants. In studies performed in adult animals, caffeine (as caffeine base) administered to pregnant mice as sustained release pellets at 50 mg/kg (less than the maximum recommended intravenous loading dose for infants on a mg/m^2 basis), during the period of organogenesis, caused a low incidence of cleft palate and exencephaly in the fetuses. There are no adequate and well-controlled studies in pregnant women.

➤*Lactation:* Caffeine is excreted into breast milk. Milk:plasma ratios of 0.5 and 0.76 have been reported. The American Academy of Pediatrics classifies caffeine as compatible with breast-feeding.

➤*Monitoring:* Prior to initiation of caffeine citrate, baseline serum levels of caffeine should be measured in infants previously treated with theophylline, since preterm infants metabolize theophylline to caffeine. Likewise, baseline serum levels of caffeine should be measured in infants born to mothers who consumed caffeine prior to delivery, since caffeine readily crosses the placenta.

In the placebo-controlled clinical trial, caffeine levels ranged from 8 to 40 mg/L. A therapeutic plasma concentration range of caffeine could not be determined from the placebo-controlled clinical trial. Serious toxicity has been reported in the literature when serum caffeine levels exceed 50 mg/L.

In clinical studies reported in the literature, cases of hypoglycemia and hyperglycemia have been observed. Therefore, serum glucose may need to be periodically monitored in infants receiving caffeine citrate.

Drug Interactions

Few data exist on drug interactions with caffeine in preterm neonates. Based on adult data, lower doses of caffeine may be needed following coadministration of drugs which are reported to decrease caffeine elimination (eg, cimetidine and ketoconazole) and higher caffeine doses may be needed following coadministration of drugs that increase caffeine elimination (eg, phenobarbital and phenytoin).

➤*CYP450 system:* Cytochrome P450 1A2 (CYP1A2) is known to be the major enzyme involved in the metabolism of caffeine. Therefore, caffeine has the potential to interact with drugs that are substrates for CYP1A2, inhibit CYP1A2, or induce CYP1A2.

➤*Ketoprofen:* Caffeine administered concurrently with ketoprofen reduced the urine volume in 4 healthy volunteers. The clinical significance of this interaction in preterm neonates is not known.

➤*Theophylline:* Interconversion between caffeine and theophylline has been reported in preterm neonates. The concurrent use of these drugs is not recommended.

Adverse Reactions

➤*Adverse events that occurred more frequently in caffeine citrate treated patients than placebo during double-blind therapy:*

Caffeine Citrate Adverse Reactions		
Adverse reaction	Caffeine citrate (n = 46); n (%)	Placebo (n = 39); n (%)
Cardiovascular		
Hemorrhage	1 (2.2%)	0 (0%)
CNS		
Cerebral hemorrhage	1 (2.2%)	0 (0%)
Dermatologic		
Dry skin	1 (2.2%)	0 (0%)
Rash	4 (8.7%)	3 (7.7%)
Skin breakdown	1 (2.2%)	0 (0%)
GI		
Necrotizing enterocolitis	2 (4.3%)	1 (2.6%)
Gastritis	1 (2.2%)	0 (0%)
Gastrointestinal hemorrhage	1 (2.2%)	0 (0%)
GU		
Kidney failure	1 (2.2%)	0 (0%)
Hemic/Lymphatic		
Disseminated intravascular coagulation	1 (2.2%)	0 (0%)
Metabolic/Nutritional		
Acidosis	1 (2.2%)	0 (0%)
Healing abnormal	1 (2.2%)	0 (0%)
Respiratory		
Dyspnea	1 (2.2%)	0 (0%)
Lung edema	1 (2.2%)	0 (0%)
Special senses		
Retinopathy of prematurity	1 (2.2%)	0 (0%)
Miscellaneous		
Accidental injury	1 (2.2%)	0 (0%)
Feeding intolerance	4 (8.7%)	2 (5.1%)
Sepsis	2 (4.3%)	0 (0%)

In addition to the cases above, 3 cases of necrotizing enterocolitis were diagnosed in patients receiving caffeine citrate during the open-label phase of the study.

Three of the infants who developed necrotizing enterocolitis during the trial died. All had been exposed to caffeine. Two were randomized to caffeine, and 1 placebo patient was "rescued" with open-label caffeine for uncontrolled apnea.

Adverse events described in the published literature include: central nervous system stimulation (ie, irritability, restlessness, jitteriness), cardiovascular effects (ie, tachycardia, increased left ventricular output, and increased stroke volume), gastrointestinal effects (ie, increased gastric aspirate, gastrointestinal intolerance), alterations in serum glucose (hypoglycemia and hyperglycemia) and renal effects (increased urine flow rate,

CAFFEINE CITRATE — INJECTION

increased creatinine clearance, and increased sodium and calcium excretion). Published long-term follow-up studies have not shown caffeine to adversely affect neurological development or growth parameters.

Overdosage

➤*Symptoms:* Following overdose, serum caffeine levels have ranged from approximately 50 mg/L to 350 mg/L. Signs and symptoms reported in the literature after caffeine overdose in preterm infants include fever, tachypnea, jitteriness, fine tremor of the extremities, hypertonia, opisthotonos, tonic-clonic movements, nonpurposeful jaw and lip movements, vomiting, hyperglycemia, elevated blood urea nitrogen, and elevated total leukocyte concentration. Seizures have also been reported in cases of overdose. One case of caffeine overdose complicated by development of intraventricular hemorrhage and long-term neurological sequelae has been reported. No deaths associated with caffeine overdose have been reported in preterm infants.

➤*Treatment:* Treatment of caffeine overdose is primarily symptomatic and supportive. Caffeine levels have been shown to decrease after exchange transfusions. Convulsions may be treated with intravenous administration of diazepam or a barbiturate such as pentobarbital sodium.

Patient Information

➤*What are the possible side effects of caffeine citrate?:* Your baby may or may not develop side effects from taking caffeine citrate. Each baby is different. If your baby develops 1 or more of the following symptoms, speak with your baby's doctor right away:
- Restlessness, jitteriness or shakiness.
- Faster heart beat.
- Increased urination (increased diaper wetting).The following symptoms may be caused by serious bowel or stomach problems. Call your baby's doctor right away if your baby develops:
- Bloated abdomen (stomach area).
- Vomiting.
- Bloody stools (bloody bowel movements).
- Loss of energy, lethargy (acting sluggish).

CAFFEINE AND SODIUM BENZOATE — INJECTION

Indications

➤*Respiratory depression:* Caffeine and sodium benzoate injection has been used in conjunction with supportive measure to treat respiratory depression associated with overdosage with CNS-depressant drugs (eg, narcotic analgesics, alcohol). However, because of questionable benefit and transient action, most authorities believe caffeine and other analeptics should not be used in these conditions and recommend other supportive therapy.

➤*Off-label uses:*

Postprandial hypotension – Postprandial decreases in blood pressure occur in elderly individuals, particularly after meals high in carbohydrates. Caffeine 250 mg attenuated postprandial hypotension in a small number of patients. Analeptic use of caffeine is strongly discouraged by most clinicians.

Administration and Dosage

➤*General dosing considerations:* Analeptic use of caffeine is strongly discouraged by most clinicians. However, the manufacturer of caffeine and sodium benzoate injection recommends intramuscular (IM), or in emergency respiratory failure, intravenous (IV) injection of 500 mg of the drug (about 250 mg of anhydrous caffeine) or a maximum single dose of 1 g (about 500 mg of anhydrous caffeine) for the treatment of respiratory depression associated with overdosage of CNS depressants, including narcotic analgesics and alcohol, and with electric shock.

➤*Adults:*

Respiratory depression –

Usual dosage: 0.5 g (7½ grains) IM or IV as frequently directed by the health care provider; however most clinicians strongly discourage analeptic use of caffeine.

Maximum dose: The maximum safe dose is 0.5 g and the total dose in 24 hours should rarely exceed 2.5 g. The maximum single dose is 1 g (about 500 mg of anhydrous caffeine).

➤*Administration:* Caffeine and sodium benzoate injection may be administered by IM or slow IV injection.

Administer caffeine and sodium benzoate injection IV in emergency respiratory failure.

➤*Storage/Stability:* Store at controlled room temperature between 15° to 30°C (59° to 86°F).

Actions

➤*Pharmacology:* Caffeine is pharmacologically similar to the other xanthine drugs, such as theobromine and theophylline; however, these 3 agents differ in the intensity of their actions on various structures. Caffeine's CNS and skeletal muscle effects are greater than those of other xanthines. In all other areas, theophylline has greater activity than caffeine, although some studies report that caffeine has greater diuretic effect than theobromine. The increased levels of intracellular cyclic-AMP mediate most of caffeine's pharmacologic actions. Caffeine competitively inhibits phosphodiesterase, the enzyme that degrades cyclic 3'-5' adenosine monophosphate. Caffeine stimulates all levels of the CNS. Caffeine's cortical effects are milder and of shorter duration than those of amphetamines. In slightly larger doses, caffeine stimulates medullary vagal, vasomotor and respiratory centers, promoting bradycardia, vasoconstriction, and increased respiratory rate.

Caffeine produces a positive inotropic effect on the myocardium and a positive chronotropic effect at the sinoatrial node, causing transient increases in heart rate, force of contraction, cardiac output and heart work. In doses greater than 250 mg, the centrally mediated vagal effects of caffeine may be masked by increased sinus rates, tachycardia, extrasystoles, or other major ventricular arrhythmias may result.

Caffeine constricts cerebral vasculature. In contrast, the drug directly dilates peripheral blood vessels, decreasing peripheral vascular resistance. The effect of this decrease in peripheral vascular resistance (and possibly that of vagal cardiac stimulation) on blood pressure is offset by increased cardiac output (and possibly stimulation of the medullary vasomotor area). The overall effect of caffeine on heart rate and blood pressure depends on whether CNS or peripheral effects predominate. Therapeutic doses of caffeine increase blood pressure only slightly.

Caffeine stimulates voluntary skeletal muscle, increasing the force of contraction and decreasing muscular fatigue. The drug also stimulates gastric acid secretion from parietal cells. Caffeine increases renal blood flow and glomerular filtration rate and decreases proximal tubular reabsorption of sodium and water, resulting in mild diuresis.

Caffeine stimulates glycogenolysis and lipolysis, but increase in blood glucose and in plasma lipids are insignificant in healthy patients. Tolerance may develop to the diuretic, cardiovascular, and CNS effects of caffeine.

➤*Pharmacokinetics:*

Distribution – Caffeine is rapidly distributed throughout the body tissues, readily crossing the placenta and blood-brain barrier. Approximately 17% of the drug is bound to plasma proteins. Caffeine has approximately a half-life ($t_{½}$) of 3 to 4 hours in adults.

Metabolism/Excretion – In adults, the drug is rapidly metabolized in the liver to 1-methyluric acid, 1-methylxanthine and 7-methylxanthine. Caffeine and its metabolites are excreted primarily by the kidneys.

Warnings/Precautions

➤*Toxicities:* Large doses of caffeine may produce headache, excitement, agitation, a condition resembling anxiety neurosis, scintillating scotoma, hyperesthia, tinnitus, muscle tremors or twitches, diuresis, tachycardia, extrasystoles, and other cardiac arrhythmias. Further CNS depression may occur when already depressed patients are too vigorously treated with caffeine and sodium benzoate injection.

➤*Pregnancy: Category C.* Animal reproduction studies have not been conducted. It is also not known whether this medication can cause fetal harm when administered to a pregnant woman or can affect reproduction capacity. Give to a pregnant woman only if clearly needed.

➤*Lactation:* Caffeine appears in breast milk. The American Academy of Pediatrics classifies caffeine as compatible with breast-feeding.

Drug Interactions

Caffeine and other xanthines may enhance the cardiac inotropic effects of beta-adrenergic-stimulating agents. Caffeine has also been reported to increase its own metabolism and that of other drugs, including phenobarbital and aspirin.

➤*Drug/Lab test interactions:* Caffeine produces false-positive elevations of serum urate as measured by the Bittner method. The drug also produces slight increases in urine levels of vanilamandelic acid (VMA), catecholamines, and 5-hydrocyindoleacetic acid. Because high urine levels of VMA or catecholamines may result in false-positive diagnosis of pheochromocytoma or neuroblastoma, caffeine intake should be avoided during tests for these disorders.

Overdosage

➤*Symptoms:* Acute toxicity involving caffeine has been reported rarely. Mild delirium, insomnia, diuresis, dehydration, and fever commonly occur with overdosage. More serious symptoms of overdosage include cardiac arrhythmias and clonic-tonic convulsions. In adults, IV doses of 57 mg/kg of body weight and oral doses of 18.5 g have been fatal. In one 5-year-old patient, death occurred following oral ingestion of ≈ 3 g of caffeine.

➤*Treatment:* Convulsions may be treated with IV administration of diazepam or a barbiturate such as phenobarbital sodium.

DOXAPRAM HYDROCHLORIDE

Rx	**Doxapram Hydrochloride** (Bedford)	**Injection:** 20 mg/mL	0.9% benzyl alcohol. In 20 mL multiple-dose vials.
Rx	**Dopram** (Baxter Healthcare Corp.)		0.9% benzyl alcohol. In 20 mL multiple-dose vials.

DOXAPRAM HYDROCHLORIDE — INJECTION

Indications

➤*Postanesthesia:* When the possibility of airway obstruction and/or hypoxia have been eliminated, doxapram may be used to stimulate respiration in patients with drug-induced postanesthesia respiratory depression or apnea other than that caused by muscle relaxants.

To pharmacologically stimulate deep breathing in the postoperative patient, a quantitative method of assessing oxygenation, such as pulse oximetry, is recommended.

➤*Drug-induced CNS depression:* To stimulate respiration, hasten arousal, and encourage return of laryngopharyngeal reflexes in patients with mild to moderate respiratory and CNS depression caused by overdosage. Exercise care to prevent vomiting and aspiration.

Controlled ventilation and standard supportive care for respiratory depression caused by CNS overdose is safer, more reliable, and more effective than doxapram therapy.

➤*Chronic obstructive pulmonary disease associated with acute hypercapnia:* As a temporary measure in hospitalized patients with acute respiratory insufficiency superimposed on chronic obstructive pulmonary disease (COPD). Use for a short period of time (approximately 2 hours) to prevent elevation of arterial CO_2 tension during the administration of oxygen. Do not use in conjunction with mechanical ventilation.

➤*Off-label uses:*

Neonatal apnea (apnea of prematurity) – Doxapram has been used when methylxanthines have failed.

Administration and Dosage

➤*General dosing considerations:*

Drug-induced CNS depression – Watch for relapse into unconsciousness or development of respiratory depression, because doxapram does not affect the metabolism of CNS depressant drugs.

➤*Adults:*

Chronic obstructive pulmonary disease associated with acute hypercapnia –

Maximum dose: 3 mg/min.

Initial dosage: Start infusion at 1 to 2 mg/min (0.5 to 1 mL/min); if indicated, increase to maximum of 3 mg/min.

Determine arterial blood gases prior to administration and at least every 30 minutes during the 2 hours of infusion to ensure against development of CO_2 retention and acidosis. Altering oxygen concentration or flow rate may necessitate adjustment in doxapram infusion rate. Predictable blood gas patterns are more readily established with continuous infusion.

Duration of therapy: Additional infusions beyond the maximum 2-hour administration period are not recommended.

Discontinuation of therapy: If the blood gases deteriorate, discontinue infusion.

Drug-induced CNS depression –

Doxapram Dosage for Drug-Induced CNS Depression

Level of depression	Method 1 Priming dose single/ repeat IV injection (mg/kg)	Method 2 Rate of intermittent IV infusion (mg/kg/h)
Mild[a]	1	1 to 2
Moderate[b]	2	2 to 3

[a] Class 0: Asleep, but can be aroused and can answer questions; Class 1: Comatose, will withdraw from painful stimuli, reflexes intact.

[b] Class 2: Comatose, will not withdraw from painful stimuli, reflexes intact; Class 3: Comatose, reflexes absent, no depression of circulation or respiration.

Single and/or repeat single IV injections (Method 1):

• *Usual dosage* – See previous table.

Give priming IV dose and repeat in 5 minutes. The priming dose for moderate depression is 2 mg/kg IV and the priming dose for mild depression is 1 mg/kg IV. Repeat every 1 to 2 hours until patient awakens. If relapse occurs, resume every 1 to 2 hours until arousal is sustained, or total maximum daily dose (3 g) is given. After maximum dose has been given, allow patient to sleep until 24 hours has elapsed from first injection, using assisted or automatic respiration if necessary.

Repeat procedure the following day until patient breathes spontaneously and sustains desired level of consciousness, or until maximum dosage (3 g) is given. After maximum dose has been given, administer repetitive doses only to patients who have shown response to the initial dose. Failure to respond appropriately indicates the need for neurologic evaluation for a possible CNS source of sustained coma.

• *Maximum dose* – 3 g/day.

Intermittent IV Infusion (Method 2):

• *Usual dosage* – See previous table.

Give priming dose as in Method 1. If patient awakens, watch for relapse; if no response, continue general supportive treatment for 1 to 2 hours and repeat priming dose. If some respiratory stimulation occurs, prepare IV infusion of doxapram 250 mg (12.5 mL) in 250 mL of saline or dextrose solution. Deliver at a rate of 1 to 3 mg/min (60 to 180 mL/h) according to size of patient and depth of coma. Discontinue use at end of 2 hours or if patient begins to awaken.

Continue supportive treatment for 0.5 to 2 hours and repeat the steps following the priming dose as above.

• *Maximum dose* – 3 g/day.

Postanesthetia –

Infusion:

• *Usual dosage* – See the following table.

Prepare the solution by adding doxapram 250 mg (12.5 mL) to 250 mL of dextrose 5% or 10% in water or normal saline solution. Initiate infusion at a rate of approximately 5 mg/min until a satisfactory respiratory response is observed, and maintained at a rate of 1 to 3 mg/min. Adjust the rate of infusion to sustain the desired level of respiratory stimulation with a minimum of side effects.

• *Maximum dose* – The maximum total dosage by infusion is 4 mg/kg, or approximately 300 mg for the average adult. Dose not to exceed 3 g/day.

IV injection:

• *Usual dosage* – See the following table. Slow administration of the drug and careful observation of the patient during administration and for some time subsequently are advisable.

Doxapram Dosage for Postanesthetic Use (IV)

IV administration	Recommended dosage (mg/kg)	Maximum dose per single injection (mg/kg)	Maximum total dose (mg/kg)[a]
Single injection	0.5 to 1	1.5	1.5
Repeat injections (5-min intervals)	0.5 to 1	1.5	2
Infusion	0.5 to 1	—	4

[a] Dose not to exceed 3 g per 24 hours.

• *Maximum dose* – 1.5 mg/kg as total dose for single injection; 2 mg/kg total dose for repeated injections (5-minute intervals). Dose not to exceed 3 g/day.

➤*Children:* See Adults for dosing in children 12 years of age and older.

➤*Preparation for administration:*

COPD associated with acute hypercapnia – Mix doxapram 400 mg in 180 mL of dextrose 5% or 10% or normal saline solution (concentration of 2 mg/mL).

Postanesthetia (infusion) – Prepare the solution by adding doxapram 250 mg (12.5 mL) to 250 mL of dextrose 5% or 10% in water or normal saline solution.

➤*Administration:* Avoid vascular extravasation or use of a single injection site over an extended period; thrombophlebitis or local skin irritation may occur. Rapid infusion may result in hemolysis.

Do not use doxapram in conjunction with mechanical ventilation.

IV short-acting barbiturates, oxygen, and resuscitative equipment should be readily available to manage overdosage manifested by excessive CNS stimulation. Slow administration and careful observation of the patient during and following administration are advisable to ensure that the protective reflexes have been restored and to prevent possible posthyperventilation or hypoventilation.

➤*Admixture compatibility:*

Compatibility – Doxapram is compatible with dextrose 5% and 10% in water or normal saline.

Incompatibility – Admixture of doxapram with alkaline solutions such as thiopental 2.5%, sodium bicarbonate, furosemide, or aminophylline will result in precipitation or gas formation.

Doxapram is also not compatible with ascorbic acid, cefoperazone, cefotaxime, cefotetan, cefuroxime, folic acid, dexamethasone disodium phosphate, diazepam, hydrocortisone sodium phosphate, methylprednisolone, or hydrocortisone sodium succinate.

Admixture of doxapram and ticarcillin results in an 18% loss of doxapram in 3 hours. When doxapram is mixed with minocycline, there is a loss of 8% of doxapram in 3 hours and a 13% loss of doxapram in 6 hours.

➤*Storage/Stability:* Store at 20° to 25°C (68° to 77°F).

Actions

➤*Pharmacology:* Doxapram produces respiratory stimulation mediated through the peripheral carotid chemoreceptors. The respiratory stimulant action is manifested by an increase in tidal volume associated with a slight increase in respiratory rate. As the dosage is increased, the central respiratory centers in the medulla are stimulated with progressive stimulation of other parts of the brain and spinal cord.

A pressor response caused by improved cardiac output rather than peripheral vasoconstriction may occur. If there is no cardiac impairment, the pressor effect is greater in hypovolemic than in normovolemic states. Following administration, an increased release of catecholamines has occurred.

DOXAPRAM HYDROCHLORIDE — INJECTION

Although opiate-induced respiratory depression is antagonized by doxapram, the analgesic effect is not affected.

➤*Pharmacokinetics:* The onset of respiratory stimulation following the recommended single IV injection usually occurs in 20 to 40 seconds, with peak effect at 1 to 2 minutes. The duration of effect varies from 5 to 12 minutes.

Contraindications

Hypersensitivity to the drug or any of the injection components; epilepsy or other convulsive states; mechanical disorders of ventilation such as mechanical obstruction, muscle paresis (including neuromuscular blockage), flail chest, pneumothorax, acute bronchial asthma, pulmonary fibrosis, or other conditions resulting in restriction of chest wall, muscles of respiration or alveolar expansion; head injury; cerebrovascular accident; cerebral edema; significant cardiovascular impairment; uncompensated heart failure; severe coronary artery disease; severe hypertension, including that associated with hyperthyroidism or pheochromocytoma; proven or suspected pulmonary embolism.

Warnings/Precautions

➤*CNS effects:* There is a risk that doxapram will produce adverse effects, including seizures, caused by general CNS stimulation. Muscle involvement may range from fasciculation to spasticity.

➤*Postanesthetic use:* Exercise the same consideration to preexisting disease states as in non-anesthetized individuals. Doxapram is neither an antagonist to muscle relaxant drugs nor a specific narcotic antagonist. More specific tests (eg, peripheral nerve stimulation, airway pressures, head lift, pulse oximetry, end-tidal carbon dioxide) to assess adequacy of ventilation are recommended before administering doxapram. Ensure adequacy of airway and oxygenation prior to use. Administer carefully and only under careful supervision to patients with hypermetabolic states such as hyperthyroidism or pheochromocytoma. Narcosis may recur after stimulation with doxapram, take care to maintain close observation until the patient has been fully alert for 0.5 to 1 hour.

➤*General anesthesia:* In patients who have received general anesthesia utilizing a volatile agent known to sensitize the myocardium to catecholamines, delay administration of doxapram until the volatile agent has been excreted in order to lessen the potential for arrhythmias, including ventricular tachycardia and ventricular fibrillation.

➤*Drug-induced CNS and respiratory depression:* Doxapram alone may not stimulate adequate spontaneous breathing or provide sufficient arousal in patients who are severely depressed either due to respiratory failure or to CNS depressant drugs. May be used as an adjunct to established supportive measures and resuscitative techniques.

➤*COPD:* In an attempt to lower pCO_2, do not increase rate of infusion in severely ill patients because of the associated increased work in breathing. Do not use in conjunction with mechanical ventilation.

In some patients, arrhythmias in acute respiratory failure secondary to COPD are probably the result of hypoxia. Use with caution in these patients.

Obtain arterial blood gases prior to the initiation of doxapram infusion and oxygen administration, then at least every 30 minutes during the infusion period to prevent development of CO_2 retention and acidosis in patients with COPD with acute hypercapnia. Doxapram administration does not diminish the need for careful patient monitoring or the need for supplemental oxygen in acute respiratory failure. Discontinue use if the arterial blood gases deteriorate and initiate mechanical ventilation.

➤*Administration:* Avoid vascular extravasation or use of a single injection site over an extended period; thrombophlebitis or local skin irritation may occur. Rapid infusion may result in hemolysis.

Do not use doxapram in conjunction with mechanical ventilation.

IV short-acting barbiturates, oxygen, and resuscitative equipment should be readily available to manage overdosage manifested by excessive CNS stimulation. Slow administration and careful observation of the patient during and following administration are advisable to ensure that the protective reflexes have been restored and to prevent possible posthyperventilation or hypoventilation. Administer cautiously to patients receiving sympathomimetics or monoamine oxidase inhibitors (MAOIs), as an additive pressor effect may occur. An adequate airway is essential and airway protection should be considered, as doxapram may stimulate vomiting. Employ recommended dosages; do not exceed maximum total dosages. Use the minimum effective dosage to avoid side effects.

➤*Cardiovascular/Respiratory effects:* Blood pressure increases are generally modest, but significant increases have occurred. Not recommended for use in severe hypertension. If sudden hypotension or dyspnea develop, discontinue use. Cardiovascular effects may include various dysrhythmias. Monitor patients receiving doxapram for disturbance of their cardiac rhythm. Monitor blood pressure, pulse rate, and deep tendon reflexes to prevent overdosage.

➤*Lowered pCO_2:* Lowered pCO_2 induced by hyperventilation produces cerebral vasoconstriction and slowing of the cerebral circulation. In certain patients, a pressor effect of doxapram on the pulmonary circulation may result in a fall of the arterial pO_2 probably caused by a worsening of ventilation perfusion-matching in the lungs despite an overall improvement in alveolar ventilation and a fall in pCO_2. Carefully supervise patients, taking into account available blood gas measurements.

➤*Benzyl alcohol:* Doxapram products may contain benzyl alcohol, which has been associated with a fatal "gasping syndrome" in premature infants. Exposure to excessive amounts of benzyl alcohol has been associated with toxicity (hypotension, metabolic acidosis), particularly in neonates, and an increased incidence of kernicterus, particularly in small preterm infants. There have been rare reports of deaths, primarily in preterm infants, associated with exposure to excessive amounts of benzyl alcohol. Administration of high dosages of medications containing this preservative must take into account the total amount of benzyl alcohol administered. The amount of benzyl alcohol at which toxicity may occur is not known. If the patient requires more than the recommended dosages or other medications containing this preservative, consider the daily metabolic load of benzyl alcohol from these combined sources (see Warnings).

➤*Renal/Hepatic function impairment:* Administer with caution to patients with significant renal or hepatic impairment, as a reduction in the rate of metabolism or excretion of metabolites may alter the response.

➤*Pregnancy: Category B.* There are no adequate and well-controlled studies in pregnant women. Use during pregnancy only when clearly needed.

➤*Lactation:* It is not known whether this drug is excreted in breast milk. Exercise caution when administering to a nursing mother.

➤*Children:* Safety and effectiveness in pediatric patients younger than 12 years of age have not been established. This product contains benzyl alcohol as a preservative. Benzyl alcohol, a component of this product, has been associated with serious adverse events and death, particularly in pediatric patients. The "gasping syndrome," (characterized by central nervous system depression, metabolic acidosis, gasping respirations, and high levels of benzyl alcohol and its metabolites found in the blood and urine) has been associated with benzyl alcohol dosages higher than 99 mg/kg/day in neonates and low birth weight neonates. Additional symptoms may include gradual neurological deterioration, seizures, intracranial hemorrhage, hematological abnormalities, skin breakdown, hepatic and renal failure, hypotension, bradycardia, and cardiovascular collapse. Premature and low-birthweight infants, as well as patients receiving high dosages, may be more likely to develop toxicity.

Premature neonates – Premature neonates given doxapram have developed hypertension, irritability, jitteriness, hyperglycemia, glucosuria, abdominal distension, increased gastric residuals, vomiting, bloody stools, necrotizing enterocolitis, erratic limb movements, excessive crying, disturbed sleep, premature eruption of teeth, and QT prologizing that has resulted in heart block. In premature neonates with risk factors such as a previous seizure, perinatal asphyxia, or intracerebral hemorrhage, seizures have occurred. In many instances, doxapram was administered following administration of xanthine derivatives such as caffeine, aminophylline, or theophylline.

➤*Monitoring:* Monitor blood pressure, pulse rate, and deep tendon reflexes to prevent overdosage. Monitor for disturbance in cardiac rhythm.

Drug Interactions

Doxapram Drug Interactions

Precipitant drug	Object drug[a]		Description
Doxapram	Anesthetics	⬆	In patients who have received general anesthesia utilizing a volatile agent known to sensitize the myocardium to catecholamines, delay administration of doxapram until the volatile agent has been excreted in order to lessen the potential for arrhythmias, including ventricular tachycardia and ventricular fibrillation.
Doxapram	MAOIs	⬆	Administer cautiously to patients receiving these drugs because an additive pressor effect may occur.
Doxapram	Neuromuscular blocking agents	⬇	Doxapram may temporarily mask residual effects of neuromuscular blocking agents.
Doxapram	Sympathomimetics	⬆	Administer cautiously to patients receiving these drugs because an additive pressor effect may occur.
Aminophylline Theophylline	Doxapram	⬆	Administer cautiously, as increased skeletal muscle activity, agitation, and hyperactivity may occur.

[a] ⬆ = Object drug increased. ⬇ = Object drug decreased.

Adverse Reactions

➤*Cardiovascular:* Arrhythmias (including ventricular tachycardia and ventricular fibrillation); chest pain; lowered T-waves; phlebitis; tightness in chest; variations in heart rate. A mild to moderate increase in blood pressure is commonly noted and may be of concern in patients with severe cardiovascular diseases (see Precautions).

➤*CNS:* Apprehension; bilateral Babinski; clonus; convulsions; disorientation; dizziness; hallucinations; headache; hyperactivity; involuntary movements; paresthesia (eg, feeling of warmth, burning or hot sensation), especially in the area of the genitalia and perineum.

➤*GI:* Desire to defecate; diarrhea; nausea; vomiting.

DOXAPRAM HYDROCHLORIDE — INJECTION

➤*GU:* Albuminuria; elevation of BUN; stimulation of urinary bladder with spontaneous voiding; urinary retention.

➤*Hematologic / Lymphatic:* A decrease in hemoglobin, hematocrit, or red blood cell count has occurred in postoperative patients. In the presence of preexisting leukopenia, a further decrease in WBC has occurred following anesthesia and treatment with doxapram; hemolysis with rapid infusion.

➤*Respiratory:* Bronchospasm; cough; dyspnea; hiccoughs; hyperventilation; laryngospasm; rebound hypoventilation; tachypnea.

➤*Miscellaneous:* Flushing; increased deep tendon reflexes; muscle fistulization; muscle spasticity; pruritus; pupillary dilatation; pyrexia; sweating.

Overdosage

➤*Symptoms:* Excessive pressor effect, hypertension, tachycardia, skeletal muscle hyperactivity, and enhanced deep tendon reflexes may be early signs of overdosage. Other effects may include agitation, confusion, sweating, cough, and dyspnea. Evaluate blood pressure, pulse rate, and deep tendon reflexes periodically and adjust dosage or infusion rate accordingly.

➤*Treatment:* There is no specific antidote. Management should be symptomatic. Refer to General Management of Acute Overdosage. Convulsive seizures are unlikely at recommended dosages, but anticonvulsants, oxygen, and resuscitative equipment should be available. There is no evidence that doxapram is dialyzable. Because of the half-life of doxapram, it is unlikely that dialysis would be appropriate treatment for overdosage.

MODAFINIL

c-iv	**Provigil** (Cephalon)	**Tablets ; oral:** 100 mg	Lactose. (PROVIGIL 100 MG). Capsule shape. In 100s.
		200 mg	Lactose. (PROVIGIL 200 MG). Capsule shape, scored. In 100s.

MODAFINIL — ORAL

Indications

➤*Sleep disorder:* To improve wakefulness in patients with excessive sleepiness associated with narcolepsy, obstructive sleep apnea (OSA)/ hypopnea syndrome, and shift work sleep disorder.

In OSA/hypopnea syndrome, as an adjunct to standard treatment(s) for the underlying obstruction. If continuous positive airway pressure is the treatment of choice for a patient, make a maximal effort to treat with continuous positive airway pressure for an adequate period of time prior to initiating modafinil. If modafinil is used adjunctively with continuous positive airway pressure, the encouragement of and periodic assessment of continuous positive airway pressure compliance is necessary.

➤*Off-label uses:*

Attention deficit hyperactivity disorder (adults) – [4] = Insufficient documentation. The role, if any, of modafinil in the treatment of attention deficit hyperactivity disorder (ADHD) has not been established. Studies have been limited by inadequate controls and small numbers of patients. Additional information is needed for this drug to be considered effective in the treatment of ADHD. (See Administration and Dosage.)

Attention deficit hyperactivity disorder (children and adolescents) – [2] = Fair documentation. The role, if any, of modafinil for the treatment of ADHD has not been established. Additional information comparing modafinil with conventional management is needed for this drug to be considered an alternative for the treatment of ADHD. (See Administration and Dosage.)

Multiple sclerosis–related fatigue – [2] = Fair documentation. Variable results from a limited number of trials indicate that the role, if any, of modafinil in the treatment of multiple sclerosis (MS)-related fatigue has not been established. Studies have been limited by inadequate controls (single-blind controls), small numbers of patients, varied titration schedules, and short duration of treatment. Larger, controlled trials with longer treatment periods are needed. (See Administration and Dosage.)

Multiple sclerosis–related nocturnal enuresis – [4] = Insufficient documentation. Beneficial results from case report data indicate that the role, if any, of modafinil in the treatment of primary nocturnal enuresis in patients with MS has not been established. Larger, controlled trials with longer treatment periods are needed. (See Administration and Dosage.)

Parkinson-related fatigue – [4] = Insufficient documentation. The role of modafinil in the treatment of Parkinson disease has not been established. Studies to date have been limited by small study populations and variable data, demonstrating improvements in some scales but not others (see Administration and Dosage). (See Administration and Dosage.)

Postpoliomyelitis syndrome–related fatigue – [5] = Poor documentation. Evidence from controlled studies suggests that the use of modafinil in the treatment of postpoliomyelitis syndrome–related fatigue is not beneficial.

Sedation (drug induced) – [4] = Insufficient documentation. The role, if any, of modafinil in the treatment of drug-induced sedation has not been established. Currently, there is limited information in only a small number of patients, varied titration schedules, and short duration of treatment (see Administration and Dosage). (See Administration and Dosage.)

Underarousal, fatigue related to brain injury – [4] = Insufficient documentation. To date, the utility of modafinil in the management of underarousal in patients with brain injury has been evaluated and published fully in only a small patient sample (approximately 10 patients). Initial data suggest a beneficial effect, increasing cognition, facilitating rehabilitation, and increasing the quality of life (see Administration and Dosage). (See Administration and Dosage.)

Administration and Dosage

➤*Adults:*

Hypopnea syndrome –

Usual dosage: 200 mg as a single dose in the morning.

Narcolepsy –

Usual dosage: 200 mg as a single dose in the morning.

Obstructive sleep apnea –

Usual dosage: 200 mg as a single dose in the morning.

Shift-work sleep disorder –

Usual dosage: 200 mg approximately 1 hour prior to the start of the work shift.

Off-label dosing –

Attention deficit hyperactivity disorder (adults): [4] = Insufficient documentation. 50 mg twice daily titrated to tolerated effects to a maximum of 400 mg daily.

Multiple sclerosis–related fatigue: [2] = Fair documentation. An initial dosage of 100 mg once daily in the morning, titrated by 100 mg weekly to tolerated effects to a maximum of 400 mg daily.

Multiple sclerosis–related nocturnal enuresis: [4] = Insufficient documentation. Oral dosing of 50 mg twice daily for up to 3 months.

Parkinson-related fatigue: [4] = Insufficient documentation. 100 to 200 mg once daily in the morning; titrate by 100 mg weekly to tolerated effects to a maximum of 400 mg/day (in divided doses).

Sedation (drug induced): [4] = Insufficient documentation. 50 to 300 mg daily.

Underarousal, fatigue related to brain injury: [4] = Insufficient documentation. Initiate at 100 mg daily (in the morning), and increase weekly by 100 mg to optimal response or maximal dosage of 400 mg daily (as 200 mg twice daily).

Duration of therapy ranged from 4 weeks to 13 months.

➤*Children:* See Adults for dosing for children 16 years of age and older.

Off-label dosing –

Attention deficit hyperactivity disorder (children and adolescents): [2] = Fair documentation. Initial doses ranged from 85 to 425 mg daily (depending on weight). In studies using lower doses, titration to tolerated effects to a maximum of 400 or 425 mg daily was employed. Treatment duration ranged from 2 to 9 weeks.

➤*Elderly:* In elderly patients, elimination of modafinil and its metabolites may be reduced as a consequence of aging. Therefore, consider using lower doses in this population.

➤*Hepatic function impairment:* In patients with severe hepatic function impairment, reduce the dose of modafinil to one-half that recommended for patients with healthy hepatic function.

➤*Concomitant medications:* Consider dosage adjustment for concomitant medications that are substrates for CYP3A4, such as triazolam and cyclosporine.

Drugs that are largely eliminated via CYP2C19 metabolism, such as diazepam, propranolol, phenytoin (also via CYP2C9), or S-mephenytoin, may have prolonged elimination when coadministered with modafinil and may require dosage reduction and monitoring for toxicity.

➤*Duration of therapy:* The efficacy of modafinil in long-term use (more than 9 weeks in narcolepsy clinical trials and 12 weeks in obstructive sleep apnea/hypopnea syndrome and shift-work sleep disorder clinical trials) has not been systematically evaluated in placebo-controlled trials. Periodically reevaluate long-term usefulness for the individual patient if prescribing modafinil for an extended time.

➤*Storage / Stability:* Store at 20° to 25°C (68° to 77°F).

Actions

➤*Pharmacology:* The precise mechanism(s) through which modafinil promotes wakefulness is unknown. Modafinil has wake-promoting actions like sympathomimetic agents, including amphetamine and methylphenidate, although the pharmacologic profile is not identical to that of sympathomimetic amines.

Modafinil has weak to negligible interactions with receptors for norepinephrine, serotonin, dopamine, gamma-aminobutyric acid (GABA), adenosine, histamine-3, melatonin, and benzodiazepines. Modafinil also does not inhibit the activities of monoamine oxidase type B (MAO-B) or phosphodiesterases II to V. Modafinil-induced wakefulness can be attenuated by the alpha-1 adrenergic receptor antagonist prazosin; however, modafinil is inactive in other in vitro assay systems known to be responsive to alpha-1 adrenergic agonists, such as the rat vas deferens preparation.

Modafinil is not a direct- or indirect-acting dopamine receptor agonist. However, in vitro, modafinil binds to the dopamine transporter and inhibits dopamine reuptake. This activity has been associated in vivo with increased

MODAFINIL — ORAL

extracellular dopamine levels in some brain regions of animals. In genetically engineered mice lacking the dopamine transporter (DAT), modafinil lacked wakefulness-promoting activity, suggesting that this activity was DAT-dependent. However, the wakefulness-promoting effects of modafinil, unlike those of amphetamine, were not antagonized by the dopamine receptor antagonist haloperidol in rats. In addition, alpha-methyl-p-tyrosine, a dopamine synthesis inhibitor, blocks the action of amphetamine but does not block locomotor activity induced by modafinil.

➤*Pharmacokinetics:* Modafinil is a racemic compound whose enantiomers have different pharmacokinetics (eg, the half-life of the L-isomer is approximately 3 times that of the d-isomer in adults). The enantiomers do not interconvert. At steady state, total exposure to the L-isomer is approximately 3 times that for the d-isomer. The trough concentration (C_{minss}) of circulating modafinil after once-daily dosing consists of 90% of the L-isomer and 10% of the d-isomer. The enantiomers of modafinil exhibit linear kinetics upon multiple dosing of 200 to 600 mg/day once daily in healthy volunteers. Apparent steady states of total modafinil and L-(-)-modafinil are reached after 2 to 4 days of dosing.

Absorption – Absorption of modafinil is rapid, with peak plasma concentrations occurring at 2 to 4 hours. The bioavailability of modafinil tablets is approximately equal to that of an aqueous suspension. The absolute oral bioavailability was not determined because of the aqueous insolubility (less than 1 mg/mL) of modafinil, which precluded intravenous (IV) administration.

Effect of food: Food has no effect on overall modafinil bioavailability; however, its absorption (T_{max}) may be delayed by approximately 1 hour if taken with food.

Distribution – Modafinil is well distributed in body tissue, with an apparent volume of distribution (approximately 0.9 L/kg) that is larger than the volume of total body water (0.6 L/kg). In human plasma, in vitro, modafinil is moderately bound to plasma protein (approximately 60%, mainly to albumin). Modafinil acid at concentrations higher than 500 mcM decreases the extent of warfarin binding, but these concentrations are more than 35 times those achieved therapeutically.

Metabolism/Excretion – The effective elimination half-life of modafinil after multiple doses is about 15 hours. The major route of elimination (approximately 90%) is metabolism, primarily by the liver, with subsequent renal elimination of the metabolites. Urine alkalinization has no effect on the elimination of modafinil.

Metabolism occurs through hydrolytic deamidation, S-oxidation, aromatic ring hydroxylation, and glucuronide conjugation. Less than 10% of an administered dose is excreted as the parent compound. In a clinical study using radiolabeled modafinil, a total of 81% of the administered radioactivity was recovered in 11 days postdose, predominantly in the urine (80% vs 1% in the feces). The largest fraction of the drug in urine was modafinil acid, but at least 6 other metabolites were present in lower concentrations. Only 2 metabolites reach appreciable concentrations in plasma (ie, modafinil acid, modafinil sulfone). In preclinical models, modafinil acid, modafinil sulfone, 2-]acetic acid and 4-hydroxy modafinil were inactive or did not appear to mediate the arousal effects of modafinil.

In adults, decreases in trough levels of modafinil have sometimes been observed after multiple weeks of dosing, suggesting auto-induction, but the magnitude of the decreases and the inconsistency of their occurrence suggest that their clinical significance is minimal. Significant accumulation of modafinil sulfone has been observed after multiple doses because of its long elimination half-life of 40 hours. Induction of metabolizing enzymes, most importantly CYP-450 3A4, has also been observed in vitro after incubation of primary cultures of human hepatocytes with modafinil and in vivo after extended administration of modafinil 400 mg/day.

Special populations –

Renal function impairment: In a single-dose, modafinil 200 mg study, severe long-term renal failure (creatinine clearance [CrCl] of 20 mL/min or less) did not significantly influence the pharmacokinetics of modafinil, but exposure to modafinil acid (an inactive metabolite) was increased 9-fold.

Hepatic function impairment: Pharmacokinetics and metabolism were examined in patients with cirrhosis of the liver (6 men and 3 women). Three patients had stage B or B+ cirrhosis (per the Child criteria), and 6 patients had stage C or C+ cirrhosis. Clinically, 8 of 9 patients were icteric and all had ascites. In these patients, the oral clearance of modafinil was decreased by about 60%, and the steady-state concentration was doubled compared with healthy patients. Reduce the dose of modafinil in patients with severe hepatic function impairment.

Elderly: A slight decrease (approximately 20%) in the oral clearance of modafinil was observed in a single-dose study at 200 mg in 12 subjects with a mean age of 63 years (range, 53 to 72 years), but the change was considered unlikely to be clinically significant.

Contraindications

Known hypersensitivity to modafinil, armodafinil, or its inactive ingredients.

Warnings/Precautions

➤*Dermatologic effects:* Serious rash requiring hospitalization and discontinuation of treatment has been reported in adults and children in association with the use of modafinil.

In clinical trials of modafinil, the incidence of rash resulting in discontinuation was approximately 0.8% (13/1,585) in children (younger than 17 years of age); these rashes included one case of possible Stevens-Johnson Syndrome and one case of apparent multiorgan hypersensitivity reaction. Several of the cases were associated with fever and other abnormalites (eg, vomiting, leukopenia). The median time to rash that resulted in discontinuation was 13 days. No such cases were observed among 380 children who received placebo. No serious skin rashes have been reported in adult clinical trials (0/4,264) of modafinil.

Rare cases of serious or life-threatening rash, including Stevens-Johnson syndrome, toxic epidermal necrolysis (TEN), and drug rash with eosinophilia and systemic symptoms have been reported in adults and children in worldwide postmarketing experience. The reporting rate of TEN and Stevens-Johnson syndrome associated with modafinil use, which is generally accepted to be an underestimate because of underreporting, exceeds the background incidence rate. Estimates of the background incidence rate for these serious skin reactions in the general population range between 1 to 2 cases per million person-years.

There are no factors that are known to predict the risk of occurrence or the severity of rash associated with modafinil. Nearly all cases of serious rash associated with modafinil occurred within 1 to 5 weeks of treatment initiation. However, isolated cases have been reported after prolonged treatment (eg, 3 months). Accordingly, duration of therapy cannot be relied upon as a means to predict the potential risk heralded by the first appearance of a rash.

Although benign rashes also occur with modafinil use, it is not possible to reliably predict which rashes will prove to be serious. Accordingly, modafinil should ordinarily be discontinued at the first sign of rash, unless the rash is clearly not drug related. Discontinuation of treatment may not prevent a rash from becoming life-threatening or permanently disabling or disfiguring.

➤*Persistent sleepiness:* Advise patients with abnormal levels of sleepiness who take modafinil that their level of wakefulness may not return to normal. Frequently reassess patients with excessive sleepiness, including those taking modafinil, for their degrees of sleepiness and, if appropriate, advise them to avoid driving or any other potentially dangerous activity. Be aware that patients may not acknowledge sleepiness or drowsiness until directly questioned about drowsiness or sleepiness during specific activities.

➤*Psychiatric effects:* There have been reports of psychiatric adverse experiences in patients treated with modafinil. Postmarketing adverse reactions associated with the use of modafinil have included, mania, delusions, hallucinations, and suicidal ideation, some resulting in hospitalization. Many, but not all, patients had a psychiatric history. One healthy male volunteer developed ideas of reference, paranoid delusions, and auditory hallucinations in association with multiple daily doses of modafinil 600 mg and sleep deprivation. There was no evidence of psychosis 36 hours after drug discontinuation.

In the adult modafinil controlled trials database, psychiatric symptoms resulting in treatment discontinuation (at a frequency of 0.3% or more) and reported more often in patients treated with modafinil compared with those treated with placebo were anxiety (1%), nervousness (1%), insomnia (less than 1%), confusion (less than 1%), agitation (less than 1%), and depression (less than 1%). Exercise caution when modafinil is given to patients with a history of psychosis, depression, or mania. Consider the possible emergence or exacerbation of psychiatric symptoms in patients treated with modafinil. If psychiatric symptoms develop in association with modafinil administration, consider discontinuing modafinil.

➤*Diagnosis of sleep disorders:* Use modafinil only in patients who have had complete evaluations of their excessive sleepiness and in whom a diagnosis of either narcolepsy, OSA/hypopnea syndrome, and/or shift work sleep disorder has been made in accordance with ICSD or DSM-IV diagnostic criteria. Such an evaluation usually consists of a complete history and physical examination, and it may be supplemented with laboratory testing. Some patients may have more than 1 sleep disorder contributing to their excessive sleepiness (eg, OSA/hypopnea syndrome and shift work sleep disorder coincident in the same patient).

➤*Continuous positive airway pressure use in patients with OSA/hypopnea syndrome:* In OSA/hypopnea syndrome, modafinil is indicated as an adjunct to standard treatment(s) for the underlying obstruction. If continuous positive airway pressure use is the treatment of choice for a patient, make a maximal effort to treat with continuous positive airway pressure for an adequate period of time prior to initiating modafinil. If modafinil is used adjunctively with continuous positive airway pressure, the encouragement of and periodic assessment of continuous positive airway pressure compliance is necessary.

➤*Cardiovascular effects:* In clinical studies of modafinil, signs and symptoms, including chest pain, palpitations, dyspnea, and transient ischemic T-wave changes on electrocardiogram (ECG), were observed in 3 subjects in association with mitral valve prolapse or left ventricular hypertrophy. It is recommended that modafinil not be used in patients with histories of left ventricular hypertrophy or in patients with mitral valve prolapse who have experienced the mitral valve prolapse syndrome when previously receiving CNS stimulants. Such signs may include, but are not limited to, arrhythmia, chest pain, or ischemic ECG changes. If new onset of any of these symptoms occurs, consider cardiac evaluation.

Modafinil has not been evaluated or used to any appreciable extent in patients with recent histories of myocardial infarction or unstable angina. Treat such patients with caution.

Blood pressure monitoring in short-term (less than 3 months) controlled trials showed no clinically significant changes in mean systolic and diastolic blood pressure in patients receiving modafinil as compared to placebo. However, a retrospective analysis of the use of antihypertensive medication in these studies showed that a greater proportion of patients on modafinil required new or increased use of antihypertensive medications (2.4%) compared with patients on placebo (0.7%). The differential use was slightly larger when only studies in OSA/hypopnea syndrome were included, with 3.4% of patients on modafinil and 1.1% of patients on placebo requiring such

MODAFINIL — ORAL

alterations in the use of antihypertensive medication. Increased monitoring of blood pressure may be appropriate in patients on modafinil.

➤*Hypersensitivity reactions:*

Angioedema/Anaphylactoid reactions – One serious case of angioedema and one case of hypersensitivity (with bronchospasm, dysphagia, rash) were observed among 1,595 patients treated with armodafinil, the R-enantiomer of modafinil (which is the racemic mixture). No such cases were observed in modafinil clinical trials. However, angioedema has been reported in postmarketing experience with modafinil use. Advise patients should be to discontinue therapy and immediately report to their health care provider any signs or symptoms suggesting angioedema or anaphylaxis (eg, difficulty in swallowing or breathing; hoarseness; swelling of the face, eyes, lips, tongue, or larynx).

Multiorgan hypersensitivity reactions – Multiorgan hypersensitivity reactions, including at least one fatality in postmarketing experience, have occurred in close temporal association (median time to detection, 13 days; range, 4 to 33) to the initiation of modafinil.

Although there have been a limited number of reports, multiorgan hypersensitivity reactions may be life-threatening or result in hospitalization. There are no factors that are known to predict the risk of occurrence or the severity of multiorgan hypersensitivity reactions associated with modafinil. Signs and symptoms of this disorder were diverse; however, patients typically, although not exclusively, presented with fever and rash associated with other organ system imvolvement. Other associated manifestations included myocarditis, hepatitis, liver function test abnormalities, hematological abnormalities (eg, eosinophilia, leukopenia, thrombocytopenia), pruritis, and asthenia. Because multiorgan hypersensitivity is variable in its expression, other organ system symptoms and signs, not noted here, may occur.

If a multiorgan hypersensitivity reaction is suspected, discontinue modafinil. Although there are no case reports to indicate cross-sensitivity with other drugs that produce this syndrome, the experience with drugs associated with multiorgan hypersensitivity would indicate this to be a possibility.

➤*Hepatic function impairment:* See Administration and Dosage for more information.

➤*Drug abuse and dependence:*

Controlled substance class – Modafinil is listed in Schedule IV of the Controlled Substances Act.

Abuse potential and dependence – In addition to its wakefulness-promoting effect and increased locomotor activity in animals, in humans, modafinil produces psychoactive and euphoric effects, and alterations in mood, perception, thinking, and feelings typical of other CNS stimulants. In in vitro binding studies, modafinil binds to the dopamine reuptake site and causes an increase in extracellular dopamine, but no increase in dopamine release. Modafinil is reinforcing, as evidenced by its self-administration in monkeys previously trained to self-administer cocaine. In some studies, modafinil was also partially discriminated as stimulant-like. Follow patients closely, especially those with a history of drug or stimulant (eg, amphetamine, cocaine, methylphenidate) abuse. Observe patients for signs of misuse or abuse (eg, incrementation of doses, drug-seeking behavior).

The abuse potential of modafinil (200, 400, and 800 mg) was assessed relative to methylphenidate (45 and 90 mg) in an inpatient study in individuals experienced with drugs of abuse. Results from this clinical study demonstrated that modafinil produced psychoactive and euphoric effects and feelings consistent with other scheduled CNS stimulants (methylphenidate).

Withdrawal – The effects of modafinil withdrawal were monitored following 9 weeks of modafinil use in one US phase 3 controlled clinical trial. No specific symptoms of withdrawal were observed during 14 days of observation, although sleepiness returned in narcoleptic patients.

➤*Hazardous tasks:* Although modafinil has not been shown to produce functional impairment, any drug affecting the CNS may alter judgment, motor skills, or thinking. Caution patients about operating an automobile or other hazardous machinery until they are reasonably certain that modafinil therapy will not adversely affect their abilities to engage in such activities.

➤*Pregnancy: Category C.* In studies conducted in rats and rabbits, developmental toxicity was observed at clinically relevant exposures.

Oral administration of armodafinil (the R-enantiomer of modafinil; 60, 200, or 600 mg/kg/day) to pregnant rats throughout the period of organogenesis resulted in increased incidences of fetal visceral and skeletal variations at the intermediate dose or greater and decreased fetal body weights at the highest dose. The no-effect dose for rat embryofetal developmental toxicity was associated with a plasma armodafinil exposure (AUC) approximately one-tenth times the AUC for armodafinil in humans treated with modafinil at the recommended daily dose.

There are no adequate and well-controlled studies in pregnant women. Two cases of inrauterine growth retardation and one case of spontaneous abortion have been reported in association with armodafinil and modafinil. Although the pharmacology of modafinil and armodafinil is not identical to that of the sympathomimetic amines, they do share some pharmacologic properties with this class. Certain of these drugs have been associated with intrauterine growth retardation and spontaneous abortions. Whether the cases reported are drug-related is unknown.

Use modafinil during pregnancy only if the potential benefit justifies the potential risk to the fetus.

Labor and delivery – The effect of modafinil on labor and delivery in humans has not been systematically investigated.

➤*Lactation:* It is not known whether modafinil or its metabolites are excreted in human milk. Because many drugs are excreted in human milk, exercise caution when modafinil is administered to a breast-feeding woman.

➤*Children:* Modafinil is not approved for use in children for any indication. Safety and efficacy in individuals younger than 16 years of age have not been established. Serious skin rashes, including erythema multiforme major and Stevens-Johnson syndrome, have been associated with modafinil use in children.

In a controlled 6-week study, 165 children (5 to 17 years of age) with narcolepsy were treated with modafinil (n = 123) or placebo (n = 42). There were no statistically significant differences favoring modafinil over placebo in prolonging sleep latency as measured by Multiple Sleep Latency Test (MSLT) or in perceptions of sleepiness as determined by the Clinical Global Impression of Change (CGIC).

In the controlled and open-label clinical studies, treatment-emergent adverse reactions of the psychiatric and nervous system included hostility, increased cataplexy, increased hypnagogic hallucinations, insomnia, suicidal ideation, and Tourette syndrome. Transient leukopenia, which resolved without medical intervention, was also observed. In the controlled clinical study, 3 of 28 girls (12 years of age and older) treated with modafinil experienced dysmenorrhea compared with 0 of 10 girls who received placebo.

➤*Monitoring:* Monitor prothrombin time/international normalized ratio more frequently with warfarin coadministration. Increased monitoring of blood pressure may be appropriate in patients on modafinil.

Drug Interactions

Modafinil Drug Interactions

Precipitant drug	Object drug[a]		Description
CYP3A4 inducers (eg, carbamazepine, phenobarbital, rifampin)	Modafinil	⬇	Because of the partial involvement of CYP3A4 in the metabolic elimination of modafinil, coadministration with potent inducers or inhibitors of CYP3A4 could alter the plasma levels of modafinil.
CYP3A4 inhibitors (eg, itraconazole, ketoconazole)	Modafinil	⬆	
MAOIs[b] (eg, phenelzine)	Modafinil	⬌	Interaction studies have not been performed. Use caution when administering MAOIs and modafinil.
Methylphenidate Dextroamphetamine	Modafinil	⬌	Modafinil absorption may be delayed by approximately 1 hour.
Modafinil	Alcohol	⬌	Avoid coadministration.
Modafinil	Clozapine	⬆	Based on a single case report, clozapine serum levels may be elevated, increasing the pharmacologic and toxic effects. Closely observe the clinical response of the patient when starting or stopping modafinil.
Modafinil	Contraceptives, hormonal Estrogens	⬇	The effectiveness of hormonal contraceptives and estrogens may be reduced when used with modafinil. Alternative or concomitant methods of contraception are recommended for patients treated with modafinil and for 1 month after discontinuation of modafinil.
Modafinil	Cyclosporine	⬇	After 1 month of modafinil 200 mg/day, cyclosporine blood levels were decreased by 50% in 1 patient. Cyclosporine dosage adjustment may be needed.
Modafinil	CYP2C9/2C19 (eg, diazepam, propranolol, phenytoin, SSRIs, certain tricyclic antidepressants [eg, clomipramine, desipramine])	⬆	Coadministration with drugs that are eliminated via CYP2C19 or CYP2C9 metabolism may have prolonged elimination upon coadministration with modafinil and may require dosage reduction and monitoring for toxicity.
Modafinil	CYP1A2, CYP2B6, and CYP3A4 substrates	⬇	In vitro, modafinil was shown to slightly induce CYP1A2, CYP2B6, and CYP3A4 in a concentration-dependent manner. Use caution when modafinil is coadministered with drugs that depend on these 3 enzymes for their clearance.

MODAFINIL — ORAL

Modafinil Drug Interactions			
Precipitant drug	Object drug[a]		Description
Modafinil	Triazolam	↓	Triazolam C_{max}, AUC, and half-life may be decreased.

[a] ↑ = object drug increased; ↓ = object drug decreased; ↔ = undetermined clinical effect.
[b] MAOIs = monoamine oxidase inhibitors.

➤*Drug/Food interactions:* See Actions for more information.

Adverse Reactions

➤*Common adverse reactions:* The most commonly observed adverse reactions (5% or more) associated with the use of modafinil more frequently than placebo-treated patients in the placebo-controlled clinical studies in primary disorders of sleep and wakefulness were anxiety, back pain, diarrhea, dizziness, dyspepsia, headache, insomnia, nausea, nervousness, and rhinitis. The adverse reaction profile was similar across these studies.

➤*Discontinuation:* In the placebo-controlled clinical trials, 74 of the 934 (8%) patients who received modafinil discontinued because of an adverse experience compared with 3% of patients that received placebo. The most frequent reasons for discontinuation that occurred at a higher rate for modafinil than placebo patients were headache (2%), nausea, anxiety, dizziness, insomnia, chest pain, and nervousness (each 1% or less). In a Canadian clinical trial, an obese narcoleptic man 35 years of age with a history of syncopal episodes experienced a 9-second episode of asystole after 27 days of modafinil treatment (300 mg/day in divided doses).

➤*Incidence in controlled trials:*

Modafinil Adverse Reactions[a] (≥ 1%)[b]		
Adverse reaction	Modafinil (n = 934)	Placebo (n = 567)
Cardiovascular		
Hypertension	3%	1%
Palpitation	2%	1%
Tachycardia	2%	1%
Vasodilatation	2%	0%
CNS		
Anxiety	5%	1%
Agitation	1%	0%
Confusion	1%	0%
Depression	2%	1%
Dizziness	5%	4%
Dyskinesia (orofacial)	1%	0%
Emotional lability	1%	0%
Headache	34%	23%
Hyperkinesia	1%	0%
Hypertonia	1%	0%
Insomnia	5%	1%
Nervousness	7%	3%
Paresthesia	2%	0%
Somnolence	2%	1%
Tremor	1%	0%
Vertigo	1%	0%
Dermatologic		
Herpes simplex	1%	0%
Sweating	1%	0%
GI		
Abnormal liver function[c]	2%	1%
Anorexia	4%	1%
Constipation	2%	1%
Diarrhea	6%	5%
Dry mouth	4%	2%
Dyspepsia	5%	4%
Flatulence	1%	0%
Mouth ulceration	1%	0%
Nausea	11%	3%
Thirst	1%	0%
GU		
Hematuria	1%	0%
Pyuria	1%	0%
Urine abnormality	1%	0%
Hematologic/Lymphatic		
Eosinophilia	1%	0%
Metabolic/Nutritional		
Edema	1%	0%
Respiratory		
Asthma	1%	0%
Epistaxis	1%	0%
Lung disorder	2%	1%
Pharyngitis	4%	2%
Rhinitis	7%	6%
Special senses		
Abnormal vision	1%	0%
Amblyopia	1%	0%
Eye pain	1%	0%
Taste perversion	1%	0%
Miscellaneous		
Back pain	6%	5%
Chest pain	3%	1%
Chills	1%	0%
Flu syndrome	4%	3%
Neck rigidity	1%	0%

[a] Six double-blind, placebo-controlled clinical studies in narcolepsy, OSA/hypopnea syndrome, and shift work sleep disorder.
[b] Reactions reported by at least 1% of patients treated with modafinil that were more frequent than in the placebo group are included; incidence is rounded to the nearest 1%. The adverse reaction terminology is coded using a standard modified Coding Symbols for Thesaurus of Adverse Reaction Terms dictionary.
[c] Elevated liver enzymes.

Reactions for which the modafinil incidence was at least 1% but equal to or less than placebo are not listed in the table. These reactions included the following: abdominal pain, abnormal ECG, accidental injury, allergic reaction, arthritis, asthenia, bronchitis, cataplexy, conjunctivitis, dysmenorrhea (incidence adjusted for gender), dyspnea, ear pain, ecchymosis, fever, hyperglycemia, hypotension, hypothermia, increased appetite, increased cough, infection, leg cramps, migraine, myalgia, neck pain, pain, periodontal abscess, peripheral edema, rash, sinusitis, sleep disorder, thinking abnormality, tooth disorder, urinary tract infection, viral infection, vomiting, weight gain, and weight loss.

➤*Dose-related adverse reactions:* In the adult placebo-controlled clinical trials, which compared doses of modafinil 200, 300, and 400 mg/day and placebo, the only adverse reactions that were clearly dose related were headache and anxiety.

➤*Vital sign changes:* See Warnings/Precautions for more information.

➤*Lab test abnormalities:* Clinical chemistry, hematology, and urinalysis parameters were monitored in phase 1, 2, and 3 studies. In these studies, mean plasma levels of gamma-glutamyl transferase (GGT) and alkaline phosphatase (AP) were found to be higher following administration of modafinil but not placebo. Few subjects had GGT or AP elevations outside of the normal range. Shifts to higher, but not clinically significantly abnormal, GGT and AP values appeared to increase with time in the population treated with modafinil in the phase 3 clinical trials.

➤*Postmarketing:*

Hematologic – Agranulocytosis.

Overdosage

➤*Symptoms:* Adverse reactions that were reported included agitation or excitation, insomnia, and slight or moderate elevations in hemodynamic parameters. Other observed high-dose effects in clinical studies have included aggressiveness, anxiety, confusion, decreased prothrombin time, diarrhea, irritability, nausea, nervousness, palpitations, sleep disturbances, and tremor.

From postmarketing experience, there have been no reports of fatal overdoses involving modafinil alone (doses of up to 12 g). Overdoses involving multiple drugs, including modafinil, have resulted in fatal outcomes. Symptoms most often accompanying modafinil overdose, alone or in combination with other drugs have included the following: cardiovascular changes such as bradycardia, chest pain, hypertension, tachycardia; CNS symptoms such as confusion, disorientation, excitation, hallucination, restlessness; digestive changes such as diarrhea and nausea; and insomnia.

➤*Treatment:* No specific antidote to the toxic effects of modafinil overdose has been identified. Manage such overdoses with primarily supportive care, including cardiovascular monitoring. If there are no contraindications, consider gastric lavage. There are no data to suggest the utility of dialysis or urinary acidification or alkalinization in enhancing drug elimination. Consider contacting a poison control center on the treatment of any overdose.

MODAFINIL — ORAL

Patient Information

Modafinil is indicated for patients who have abnormal levels of sleepiness. Modafinil has been shown to improve, but not eliminate this abnormal tendency to fall asleep. Therefore, patients should not alter their previous behavior with regard to potentially dangerous activities (eg, driving, operating machinery), or other activities requiring appropriate levels of wakefulness, until and unless treatment with modafinil has been shown to produce levels of wakefulness that permit such activities. Advise patients that modafinil is not a replacement for sleep.

Inform patients that it may be critical that they continue to take their previously prescribed treatments (eg, patients with OSA/hypopnea syndrome receiving continuous positive airway pressure should continue to do so).

Advise patients to contact their health care provider if they experience anxiety, chest pain, depression, rash, or sign of psychosis or mania.

Advise patients to stop taking modafinil and to notify their health care provider if they develop blisters, hives, mouth sores, peeling skin, rash, trouble swallowing or breathing, or a related allergic phenomenon.

Advise patients to notify their health care providers if they become pregnant, intend to become pregnant during therapy, or are breast-feeding an infant. Caution patients regarding the potentially increased risk of pregnancy when using steroidal contraceptives (including depot or implantable contraceptives) with modafinil and for 1 month after discontinuation of therapy.

Advise patients to inform their health care providers if they are taking, or planning to take, any prescription or nonprescription drugs because of the potential for interactions between modafinil and other drugs.

Advise patients that the use of modafinil in combination with alcohol has not been studied. Advise patients that it is prudent to avoid alcohol while taking modafinil.

ARMODAFINIL

c-iv	**Nuvigil** (Cephalon)	**Tablets; oral:** 50 mg		Lactose. (C 205). In 60s.
			150 mg	Lactose. Oval. (C 215). In 60s.
			250 mg	Lactose. Oval. (C 225). In 60s.

ARMODAFINIL — ORAL

Indications

➤*Narcolepsy:* To improve wakefulness in patients with excessive sleepiness associated with narcolepsy.

➤*Obstructive sleep apnea-hypopnea syndrome:* To improve wakefulness in patients with excessive sleepiness associated with obstructive sleep apnea-hypopnea syndrome (OSAHS).

In OSAHS, armodafinil is indicated as an adjunct to standard treatment(s) for the underlying obstruction. If continuous positive airway pressure (CPAP) is the treatment of choice for a patient, a maximal effort to treat with CPAP for an adequate period of time should be made prior to initiating armodafinil. If armodafinil is used adjunctively with CPAP, the encouragement of and periodic assessment of CPAP compliance is necessary.

➤*Shift-work sleep disorder:* To improve wakefulness in patients with excessive sleepiness associated with shift-work sleep disorder.

Administration and Dosage

➤*General dosing considerations:* In all cases, careful attention to the diagnosis and treatment of the underlying sleep disorder(s) is of the utmost importance. Health care providers should be aware that some patients may have more than 1 sleep disorder contributing to their excessive sleepiness.

➤*Adults:*

Narcolepsy – 150 or 250 mg given as a single dose in the morning.

Obstructive sleep apnea-hypopnea syndrome – 150 or 250 mg given as a single dose in the morning.

Shift-work sleep disorder – 150 mg given daily approximately 1 hour prior to the start of the patient's work shift.

➤*Elderly:* In elderly patients, elimination of armodafinil and its metabolites may be reduced as a consequence of aging. Therefore, consideration should be given to the use of lower doses in this population.

➤*Hepatic function impairment:* In patients with severe hepatic function impairment, armodafinil should be administered at a reduced dose.

➤*Duration of therapy:* The efficacy of armodafinil in long-term use (more than 12 weeks) has not been systematically evaluated in placebo-controlled trials. The health care provider who elects to prescribe armodafinil for an extended period of time should periodically reevaluate the long-term usefulness for the individual patient.

➤*Storage/Stability:* Store at 20° to 25°C (68° to 77°F).

Actions

➤*Pharmacology:* The precise mechanism(s) through which armodafinil (R-enantiomer) or modafinil (mixture of R- and S-enantiomers) promote wakefulness is unknown. Both armodafinil and modafinil have shown similar pharmacological properties in nonclinical animal and in vitro studies, to the extent tested.

Modafinil-induced wakefulness can be attenuated by the alpha$_1$-adrenergic receptor antagonist, prazosin; however, modafinil is inactive in other in vitro assay systems known to be responsive to alpha-adrenergic agonists such as the rat vas deferens preparation.

Armodafinil is not a direct- or indirect-acting dopamine receptor agonist. However, in vitro, both armodafinil and modafinil bind to the dopamine transporter and inhibit dopamine reuptake. For modafinil, this activity has been associated in vivo with increased extracellular dopamine levels in some brain regions of animals. In genetically engineered mice lacking the dopamine transporter, modafinil lacked wake-promoting activity, suggesting that this activity was dopamine transporter–dependent. However, the wake-promoting effects of modafinil, unlike those of amphetamine, were not antagonized by the dopamine receptor antagonist haloperidol in rats. In addition, alpha-methyl-p-tyrosine, a dopamine synthesis inhibitor, blocks the action of amphetamine, but does not block locomotor activity induced by modafinil.

Armodafinil and modafinil have wake-promoting actions similar to sympathomimetic agents including amphetamine and methylphenidate, although their pharmacologic profile is not identical to that of the sympathomimetic amines. In addition to its wake-promoting effects and ability to increase locomotor activity in animals, modafinil produces psychoactive and euphoric effects and alterations in mood, perception, thinking, and feelings typical of other CNS stimulants in humans. Modafinil has reinforcing properties, as evidenced by its self-administration in monkeys previously trained to self-administer cocaine; modafinil was also partially discriminated as stimulant-like.

➤*Pharmacokinetics:*

Absorption – Armodafinil, the longer-lived enantiomer of modafinil, is readily absorbed after oral administration. Armodafinil exhibits linear time-independent kinetics following single and multiple oral dose administration. Peak plasma concentrations are attained at approximately 2 hours in the fasted state. Increase in systemic exposure is proportional over the dose range of 50 to 400 mg. No time-dependent change in kinetics was observed through 12 weeks of dosing. Apparent steady state for armodafinil was reached within 7 days of dosing. At steady state, the systemic exposure for armodafinil is 1.8 times the exposure observed after a single dose. The concentration-time profiles of the pure R-enantiomer following administration of armodafinil 50 mg or modafinil 100 mg are nearly superimposable.

The absolute oral bioavailability was not determined because of the aqueous insolubility of armodafinil, which precluded intravenous administration.

Food effects: Food effect on the overall bioavailability of armodafinil is considered minimal; however, time to reach peak concentration (T_{max}) may be delayed by approximately 2 to 4 hours in the fed state. Since the delay in T_{max} is also associated with elevated plasma levels later in time, food can potentially affect the onset and time course of pharmacologic action for armodafinil.

Distribution – Armodafinil has an apparent volume of distribution of approximately 42 L. Data specific to armodafinil protein binding are not available. However, modafinil is moderately bound to plasma protein (approximately 60%), mainly to albumin.

Metabolism/Excretion – In vitro and in vivo data show that armodafinil undergoes hydrolytic deamidation, S-oxidation, and aromatic ring hydroxylation, with subsequent glucuronide conjugation of the hydroxylated products. Amide hydrolysis is the single most prominent metabolic pathway, with sulfone formation by CYP-450 3A4/5 being next in importance. The other oxidative products are formed too slowly in vitro to enable identification of the enzyme(s) responsible. Only 2 metabolites reach appreciable concentrations in plasma (ie, R-modafinil acid and modafinil sulfone).

Data specific to armodafinil disposition are not available. However, modafinil is mainly eliminated via metabolism, predominantly in the liver, with less than 10% of the parent compound excreted in the urine. A total of 81% of the administered radioactivity was recovered in 11 days postdose, predominantly in the urine (80% vs 1% in the feces).

After oral administration, armodafinil exhibits an apparent monoexponential decline from the peak plasma concentration. The apparent terminal elimination half-life ($t_{½}$) is approximately 15 hours. The oral clearance of armodafinil is approximately 33 mL/min.

Special populations –

Hepatic function impairment: The pharmacokinetics and metabolism of modafinil were examined in patients with cirrhosis of the liver (6 men and 3 women). Three patients had stage B or B+ cirrhosis and 6 patients had stage C or C+ cirrhosis (per the Child-Pugh score criteria). Clinically 8 of 9 patients were icteric and all had ascites. In these patients, the oral clearance of modafinil was decreased by about 60% and the steady-state concentration was doubled compared with healthy patients. Reduce the dose of armodafinil in patients with severe hepatic function impairment.

Elderly: A slight decrease (approximately 20%) in the oral clearance of modafinil was observed in a single dose study at 200 mg in 12 subjects with a mean age of 63 years (range, 53 to 72 years of age), but the change was considered not likely to be clinically significant. In a multiple-dose study (300 mg/day) in 12 patients with a mean age of 82 years (range, 67 to 87 years of age), the mean levels of modafinil in plasma were approximately

ARMODAFINIL — ORAL

2 times those historically obtained in matched younger subjects. Because of potential effects from the multiple concomitant medications with which most of the patients were being treated, the apparent difference in modafinil pharmacokinetics may not be attributable solely to the effects of aging. However, the results suggest that the clearance of modafinil may be reduced in elderly patients.

Contraindications

Known hypersensitivity to modafinil and armodafinil or its inactive ingredients.

Warnings/Precautions

➤*Serious rash:* Serious rash, including Stevens-Johnson syndrome, requiring hospitalization and discontinuation of treatment has been reported in adults and children in association with the use of modafinil, a racemic mixture of S and R modafinil (the latter is armodafinil).

Armodafinil has not been studied in children in any setting and is not approved for use in children for any indication.

No serious skin rashes have been reported in adult clinical trials (0/1,595) of armodafinil. However, because armodafinil is the R isomer of racemic modafinil, a similar risk of serious rash with armodafinil cannot be ruled out.

There are no factors that are known to predict the risk of occurrence or the severity of rash associated with modafinil or armodafinil. Nearly all cases of serious rash associated with modafinil occurred within 1 to 5 weeks after treatment initiation. However, isolated cases have been reported after prolonged treatment (eg, 3 months). Accordingly, duration of therapy cannot be relied upon as a means to predict the potential risk heralded by the first appearance of a rash.

Although benign rashes also occur with armodafinil, it is not possible to reliably predict which rashes will prove to be serious. Accordingly, armodafinil should ordinarily be discontinued at the first sign of rash, unless the rash is clearly not drug-related. Discontinuation of treatment may not prevent a rash from becoming life-threatening or permanently disabling or disfiguring.

➤*Persistent sleepiness:* Advise patients with abnormal levels of sleepiness who take armodafinil that their level of wakefulness may not return to normal. Frequently reassess patients with excessive sleepiness, including those taking armodafinil, for their degree of sleepiness and, if appropriate, advise them to avoid driving or any other potentially dangerous activity. Be aware that patients may not acknowledge sleepiness or drowsiness until directly questioned about drowsiness or sleepiness during specific activities.

➤*Psychiatric effects:* Psychiatric adverse reactions have been reported in patients treated with modafinil. Modafinil and armodafinil are very closely related. Therefore, the incidence and type of psychiatric symptoms associated with armodafinil are expected to be similar to the incidence and type of these events with modafinil.

Postmarketing adverse reactions associated with the use of modafinil have included mania, delusions, hallucinations, and suicidal ideation, some resulting in hospitalization. Many, but not all, patients had a prior psychiatric history. One healthy male volunteer developed ideas of reference, paranoid delusions, and auditory hallucinations in association with multiple daily doses of modafinil 600 mg and sleep deprivation. There was no evidence of psychosis 36 hours after drug discontinuation.

Exercise caution when armodafinil is given to patients with a history of psychosis, depression, or mania. If psychiatric symptoms develop in association with armodafinil administration, consider discontinuing armodafinil.

➤*Diagnosis of sleep disorders:* Use armodafinil only in patients who have had a complete evaluation of their excessive sleepiness, and in whom a diagnosis of either narcolepsy, OSAHS, and/or shift-work sleep disorder has been made in accordance with ICSD or DSM diagnostic criteria. Such an evaluation usually consists of a complete history and physical examination, and it may be supplemented with testing in a laboratory setting. Some patients may have more than one sleep disorder contributing to their excessive sleepiness (eg, OSAHS and shift-work sleep disorder coincident in the same patient).

➤*CPAP use in patients with OSAHS:* See Indications for more information.

➤*Cardiovascular effects:* Armodafinil has not been evaluated or used to any appreciable extent in patients with a recent history of myocardial infarction or unstable angina; treat such patients with caution.

In clinical studies of modafinil, signs and symptoms including chest pain, palpitations, dyspnea and transient ischemic T-wave changes on electrocardiogram (ECG) were observed in 3 subjects in association with mitral valve prolapse or left ventricular hypertrophy. It is recommended that armodafinil not be used in patients with a history of left ventricular hypertrophy or in patients with mitral valve prolapse who have experienced the mitral valve prolapse syndrome when previously receiving CNS stimulants. Signs of mitral valve prolapse syndrome include but are not limited to ischemic ECG changes, chest pain, or arrhythmia. If new onset of any of these symptoms occurs, consider cardiac evaluation.

Blood pressure monitoring in short-term (at least 3 months) controlled trials showed only small average increases in mean systolic and diastolic blood pressure in patients receiving armodafinil, compared with placebo (1.2 to 4.3 mm Hg in the various experimental groups). There was also a slightly greater proportion of patients on armodafinil requiring new or increased use of antihypertensive medications (2.9%) compared with patients on placebo (1.8%). Increased monitoring of blood pressure may be appropriate in patients on armodafinil.

➤*Hypersensitivity reactions:*

Angioedema and anaphylactoid reactions – One serious case of angioedema and one case of hypersensitivity (with rash, dysphagia, and bronchospasm), were observed among 1,595 patients treated with armodafinil. Advise patients to discontinue therapy and immediately report any signs or symptoms suggesting angioedema or anaphylaxis (eg, swelling of face, eyes, lips, tongue or larynx; difficulty in swallowing or breathing; hoarseness) to their health care provider.

Multiorgan hypersensitivity reactions – Multiorgan hypersensitivity reactions, including at least one fatality in postmarketing experience, have occurred in close temporal association (median time to detection, 13 days; range, 4 to 33) to the initiation of modafinil. A similar risk of multiorgan hypersensitivity reactions with armodafinil cannot be ruled out.

Although there have been a limited number of reports, multiorgan hypersensitivity reactions may result in hospitalization or be life-threatening. There are no factors that are known to predict the risk of occurrence or the severity of multiorgan hypersensitivity reactions associated with modafinil. Signs and symptoms of this disorder were diverse; however, patients typically, although not exclusively, presented with fever and rash associated with other organ system involvement. Other associated manifestations included myocarditis, hepatitis, liver function test abnormalities, hematological abnormalities (eg, eosinophilia, leukopenia, thrombocytopenia), pruritis, and asthenia. Because multiorgan hypersensitivity is variable in its expression, other organ system symptoms and signs, not noted here, may occur.

If a multiorgan hypersensitivity reaction is suspected, discontinue armodafinil. Although there are no case reports to indicate cross-sensitivity with other drugs that produce this syndrome, the experience with drugs associated with multiorgan hypersensitivity would indicate this to be a possibility.

➤*Hepatic function impairment:* See Actions for more information.

➤*Drug abuse and dependence:*

Controlled substance class – Armodafinil is a Schedule IV controlled substance.

Abuse potential and dependence – Although the abuse potential of armodafinil has not been specifically studied, its abuse potential is likely to be similar to that of modafinil. In humans, modafinil produces psychoactive and euphoric effects and alterations in mood, perception, thinking, and feelings typical of other CNS stimulants. In in vitro binding studies, modafinil binds to the dopamine reuptake site and causes an increase in extracellular dopamine but no increase in dopamine release. Modafinil is reinforcing, as evidenced by its self administration in monkeys previously trained to self-administer cocaine. In some studies, modafinil was also partially discriminated as stimulant-like. Follow patients closely, especially those with a history of drug and/or stimulant (eg, methylphenidate, amphetamine, cocaine) abuse. Observe patients for signs of misuse or abuse (eg, incrementation of doses, drug-seeking behavior).

The abuse potential of modafinil (200, 400, and 800 mg) was assessed relative to methylphenidate (45 and 90 mg) in an inpatient study in individuals experienced with drugs of abuse. Results from this clinical study demonstrated that modafinil produced psychoactive and euphoric effects and feelings consistent with other scheduled CNS stimulants (methylphenidate).

➤*Hazardous tasks:* Although armodafinil has not been shown to produce functional impairment, any drug affecting the CNS may alter judgment, thinking, or motor skills. Caution patients about operating an automobile or other hazardous machinery until they are reasonably certain that armodafinil therapy will not adversely affect their ability to engage in such activities.

➤*Pregnancy: Category C.* In studies conducted in rats (armodafinil, modafinil) and rabbits (modafinil), developmental toxicity was observed at clinically relevant exposures.

Oral administration of armodafinil (60, 200, or 600 mg/kg/day) to pregnant rats throughout the period of organogenesis resulted in increased incidences of fetal visceral and skeletal variations at the intermediate dose or greater and decreased fetal body weights at the highest dose. The no-effect dose for rat embryofetal developmental toxicity was associated with a plasma armodafinil exposure (AUC) approximately 0.03 times the AUC in humans at the maximum recommended daily dose of 250 mg.

Modafinil administration to rats throughout gestation and lactation at oral doses of up to 200 mg/kg/day resulted in decreased viability in the offspring at doses greater than 20 mg/kg/day (plasma modafinil AUC approximately 0.1 times the AUC in humans at the recommended daily dose). No effects on postnatal developmental and neurobehavioral parameters were observed in surviving offspring.

There are no adequate and well-controlled studies of either armodafinil or modafinil in pregnant women. Two cases of intrauterine growth retardation and one case of spontaneous abortion have been reported in association with armodafinil and modafinil. Although the pharmacology of armodafinil is not identical to that of the sympathomimetic amines, it does share some pharmacologic properties with this class. Certain of these drugs have been associated with intrauterine growth retardation and spontaneous abortions. Whether the cases reported with armodafinil are drug-related is unknown.

Use armodafinil or modafinil during pregnancy only if the potential benefit justifies the potential risk to the fetus.

➤*Lactation:* It is not known whether armodafinil or its metabolites are excreted in human milk. Because many drugs are excreted in human milk, exercise caution when armodafinil tablets are administered to a breast-feeding woman.

➤*Children:* Safety and efficacy of armodafinil use in patients younger than 17 years of age have not been established. Serious rash has been seen in children receiving modafinil.

ARMODAFINIL — ORAL

➤*Elderly:* See Actions for more information.

➤*Monitoring:* Increased monitoring of blood pressure may be appropriate in patients on armodafinil.

Drug Interactions

Armodafinil Drug Interactions			
Precipitant drug	Object drug[a]		Description
CYP 3A4/5 inducers (eg, carbamazepine, phenobarbital, rifampin)	Armodafinil	↓	Possible decrease in armodafinil plasma levels due to increased metabolism.
CYP 3A4/5 inhibitors (eg, erythromycin, ketoconazole)	Armodafinil	↑	Possible increase in armodafinil plasma levels due to decreased metabolism.
Monoamine oxidase inhibitors (MAOIs) (eg, phenelzine)	Armodafinil	↔	Use caution when administering MAOIs and armodafinil.
Armodafinil	Alcohol	↑	Avoid concomitant use.
Armodafinil	Benzodiazepines (eg, diazepam, midazolam, triazolam)	↓↑	Armodafinil can decrease systemic exposure to midazolam and triazolam through CYP3A4/5 induction. Armodafinil may increase systemic exposure to diazepam through inhibition of CYP2C19. Dose adjustment may be required.
Armodafinil	Clomipramine	↑	Armodafinil may increase systemic exposure to clomipramine through inhibition of CYP2C19. A dose reduction may be required.
Armodafinil	Cyclosporine	↓	Blood levels of cyclosporine may be reduced. Monitor circulating cyclosporine levels and adjust dose.
Armodafinil	Ethinyl estradiol	↓	Armodafinil can decrease systemic exposure of ethinyl estradiol. Dose adjustment may be required.
Armodafinil	Omeprazole	↑	Armodafinil may increase systemic exposure through inhibition of CYP2C19. Dose reduction may be required.
Armodafinil	Phenytoin	↑	Armodafinil may increase systemic exposure through inhibition of CYP2C19. Dose reduction may be required.
Armodafinil	Propranolol	↑	Armodafinil may increase systemic exposure through inhibition of CYP2C19. Dose reduction may be required.
Armodafinil	Steroidal contraceptives	↓	The efficacy of steroidal contraceptives may be reduced during and for 1 month after armodafinil coadministration. Use of alternative or concomitant methods of contraception are recommended during and for 1 month after coadministration with armodafinil.
Armodafinil	Warfarin	↔	A pharmacodynamic interaction cannot be ruled out. Monitor prothrombin times and international normalization ratios more frequently when armodafinil is coadministered with warfarin.

[a] ↑ = object drug increased; ↓ = object drug decreased; ↔ = undetermined clinical effects.

➤*Drug/Food interactions:* See Actions for more information.

Adverse Reactions

In the placebo-controlled clinical studies, the most commonly observed adverse reactions (at least 5%) associated with the use of armodafinil occurring more frequently than in the placebo-treated patients were headache, nausea, dizziness, and insomnia. The adverse reaction profile was similar across the studies.

In the placebo-controlled clinical trials, 44 of 645 patients (7%) who received armodafinil discontinued because of an adverse reaction, compared with 16 of 445 (4%) of patients who received placebo. The most frequent reason for discontinuation was headache (1%).

➤*Incidence in controlled trials:*

Armodafinil Adverse Reactions (> 1%)[a]		
Adverse reaction	Armodafinil (n = 645)	Placebo (n = 445)
CNS		
Agitation	1%	0%
Anxiety	4%	1%
Depressed mood	1%	0%
Depression	2%	0%
Disturbance in attention	1%	0%
Dizziness	5%	2%
Fatigue	2%	1%
Headache	17%	9%
Insomnia	5%	1%
Migraine	1%	0%
Nervousness	1%	0%
Paresthesia	1%	0%
Tremor	1%	0%
Cardiovascular		
Heart rate increased	1%	0%
Palpitations	2%	1%
Dermatologic		
Contact dermatitis	1%	0%
Hyperhidrosis	1%	0%
Rash	2%	0%
GI		
Constipation	1%	0%
Diarrhea	4%	2%
Dry mouth	4%	1%
Dyspepsia	2%	0%
Loose stools	1%	0%
Nausea	7%	3%
Upper abdominal pain	2%	1%
Vomiting	1%	0%
Metabolic/Nutritional		
Anorexia	1%	0%
Decreased appetite	1%	0%
Miscellaneous		
Dyspnea	1%	0%
Gamma-glutamyltransferase (GGT) increased	1%	0%
Influenza-like illness	1%	0%
Pain	1%	0%
Polyuria	1%	0%
Pyrexia	1%	0%
Seasonal allergy	1%	0%
Thirst	1%	0%

[a] Four double-blind, placebo-controlled clinical studies in shift-work sleep disorder, OSAHS, and narcolepsy; incidence is rounded to the nearest whole percent. Included are only those reactions for which armodafinil incidence is greater than that of placebo.

➤*Dose dependency of adverse reactions:*

Armodafinil Dose-Dependent Adverse Reactions[a]				
Adverse reaction	Armodafinil 250 mg (n = 198)	Armodafinil 150 mg (n = 447)	Armodafinil combined (n = 645)	Placebo (n = 445)
CNS				
Depression	3%	1%	2%	< 1%
Headache	23%	14%	17%	9%
Insomnia	6%	4%	5%	1%
Dermatologic				
Rash	4%	1%	2%	< 1%

ARMODAFINIL — ORAL

Armodafinil Dose-Dependent Adverse Reactions[a]				
Adverse reaction	Armodafinil 250 mg (n = 198)	Armodafinil 150 mg (n = 447)	Armodafinil combined (n = 645)	Placebo (n = 445)
GI				
Dry mouth	7%	2%	4%	< 1%
Nausea	9%	6%	7%	3%

[a] Four double-blind, placebo-controlled clinical studies in shift-work sleep disorder, OSAHS, and narcolepsy.

➤*Vital sign changes:* There were small but consistent increases in average values for mean systolic and diastolic blood pressure in controlled trials. There was a small but consistent average increase in pulse rate over placebo in controlled trials. This increase varied from 0.9 to 3.5 beats per minute.

➤*Lab test abnormalities:* Clinical chemistry, hematology, and urinalysis parameters were monitored in the studies. Mean plasma levels of GGT and alkaline phosphatase were found to be higher following administration of armodafinil, but not placebo. Few subjects, however, had GGT or alkaline phosphatase elevations outside of the normal range. No differences were apparent in ALT, AST, total protein, albumin, or total bilirubin, although there were rare cases of isolated elevations of AST and/or ALT. A single case of mild pancytopenia was observed after 35 days of treatment and resolved with drug discontinuation. A small mean decrease from baseline in serum uric acid compared with placebo was seen in clinical trials. The clinical significance of this finding is unknown.

Overdosage

➤*Symptoms:* Symptoms of armodafinil overdose are likely to be similar to those of modafinil. Overdose in modafinil clinical trials included excitation or agitation, insomnia, and slight or moderate elevations in hemodynamic parameters. From postmarketing experience with modafinil, there have been no reports of fatal overdoses involving modafinil alone (doses up to 12). Overdoses involving multiple drugs, including modafinil, have resulted in fatal outcomes. Symptoms most often accompanying modafinil overdose, alone or in combination with other drugs, have included insomnia; CNS symptoms such as restlessness, disorientation, confusion, excitation, and hallucination; digestive changes such as nausea and diarrhea; and cardiovascular changes such as tachycardia, bradycardia, hypertension, and chest pain.

➤*Treatment:* No specific antidote exists for the toxic effects of a armodafinil overdose. Manage such overdoses with primarily supportive care, including cardiovascular monitoring. If there are no contraindications, consider gastric lavage. There are no data to suggest the utility of dialysis or urinary acidification or alkalinization in enhancing drug elimination. The health care provider should consider contacting a poison control center for advice in the treatment of any overdose.

Patient Information

Armodafinil is indicated for patients who have abnormal levels of sleepiness. Armodafinil has been shown to improve, but not eliminate, this abnormal tendency to fall asleep. Therefore, patients should not alter their previous behavior with regard to potentially dangerous activities (eg, driving, operating machinery) or other activities requiring appropriate levels of wakefulness, until and unless treatment with armodafinil has been shown to produce levels of wakefulness that permit such activities. Advise patients that armodafinil is not a replacement for sleep.

Inform patients that it may be critical that they continue to take their previously prescribed treatments (eg, patients with OSAHS receiving CPAP should continue to do so).

Inform patients of the availability of a patient information leaflet, and instruct them to read the leaflet prior to taking armodafinil.

Advise patients to contact their health care provider if they experience rash, depression, anxiety, or signs of psychosis or mania.

Advise patients to inform their health care provider if they are taking, or plan to take, any prescription or over-the-counter drugs, because of the potential for interactions between armodafinil and other drugs.

Advise patients that the use of armodafinil in combination with alcohol has not been studied. Advise patients that it is prudent to avoid alcohol while taking armodafinil.

Advise patient to notify their health care provider if they become pregnant or intend to become pregnant during therapy. Caution patients regarding the potential increased risk of pregnancy when using steroidal contraceptives (including depot or implantable contraceptives) with armodafinil and for one month after discontinuation of therapy.

Advise patients to notify their health care provider if they are breast-feeding an infant.

Advise patients to stop taking armodafinil and notify their health care provider if they develop a rash, hives, mouth sores, blisters, peeling skin, trouble swallowing or breathing or a related allergic phenomenon.

Amphetamines

WARNING

Amphetamines have a high potential for abuse. Use in weight reduction programs only when alternative therapy has been ineffective. Administration for prolonged periods may lead to drug dependence and must be avoided. Pay particular attention to the possibility of subjects obtaining amphetamines for nontherapeutic use or distribution to others. Prescribe or dispense sparingly.

Misuse of amphetamines may cause sudden death and serious cardiovascular adverse reactions.

Indications

➤*Narcolepsy (amphetamine mixture, dextroamphetamine):* To improve wakefulness in patients with excessive day-time sleepiness associated with narcolepsy.

➤*Attention deficit disorder with hyperactivity:* Indicated as an integral part of a total treatment program that includes other remedial measures (psychological, educational, social) for a stabilizing effect in children 3 to 16 years of age with a behavioral syndrome characterized by moderate to severe distractibility, short attention span, hyperactivity, emotional lability, and impulsivity. Do not diagnose this syndrome with finality when these symptoms are only of comparatively recent origin. Nonlocalizing (soft) neurological signs, learning disability, and abnormal EEG may be present and a diagnosis of CNS dysfunction may be warranted.

➤*Exogenous obesity (methamphetamine):* As a short-term adjunct in a regimen of weight reduction based on caloric restriction, for patients refractory to alternative therapy (eg, repeated diets, group programs, other drugs). Weigh the limited usefulness against the possible risks inherent in use.

➤*Off-label uses:*

Traumatic brain injury –

Dextroamphetamine: [3] = Safety concerns.

Other possible off-label uses – Cocaine dependence treatment (**dextroamphetamine**), autism (**dextroamphetamine**).

Administration and Dosage

Administer at the lowest effective dosage and adjust individually. Avoid late evening doses, particularly with the long-acting form, because of the resulting insomnia.

When treating attention deficit disorder in children, occasionally interrupt drug administration to determine if there is a recurrence of behavioral symptoms sufficient to require continued therapy.

Actions

➤*Pharmacology:* Amphetamines are sympathomimetic amines with CNS stimulant activity. CNS effects are mediated by release of norepinephrine from central noradrenergic neurons. At higher doses, dopamine may be released in the mesolimbic system. Amphetamines are thought to block the reuptake of norepinephrine and dopamine into the presynaptic neuron and increase the release of these monoamines into the extraneuronal space.

Peripheral alpha and beta activity includes elevation of systolic and diastolic blood pressures and weak bronchodilator and respiratory stimulant action. At therapeutic doses, the heart rate may be reflexly slowed; large doses may produce cardiac arrhythmias.

There is neither specific evidence that clearly establishes the mechanism whereby amphetamines produce mental and behavioral effects in children, nor conclusive evidence regarding how these effects relate to the condition of the CNS.

The site of action for appetite suppression is thought to be the lateral hypothalamic feeding center.

➤*Pharmacokinetics:* Amphetamine is metabolized in the liver by aromatic hydroxylation, N-dealkylation, and deamination.

Amphetamines are effective after oral administration and effects last for several hours.

Amphetamine mixture – Following administration of immediate-release amphetamine mixture tablets, the peak plasma concentrations occurred in ≈ 3 hours for d-amphetamine and l-amphetamine.

The time to reach maximum plasma concentration (T_{max}) for extended-release amphetamine mixture capsules is ≈ 7 hours, which is ≈ 4 hours longer compared with the immediate-release formulation.

A single dose of 20 mg extended-release amphetamine mixture capsules provided comparable plasma concentration profiles of d-amphetamine and l-amphetamine with 10 mg immediate-release amphetamine mixture tablets twice daily administered 4 hours apart.

The mean elimination half-life is 1 hour shorter for d-amphetamine and 2 hours shorter for l-amphetamine in children 6 to 12 years of age compared with that of adults ($t_{1/2}$ is 10 hours for d-amphetamine and 13 hours for l-amphetamine in adults and 9 and 11 hours, respectively, for children). Extended-release amphetamine mixture capsules demonstrate linear pharmacokinetics over the dose range of 10 to 30 mg. There is no unexpected accumulation at steady state.

Food does not affect the extent of absorption of extended-release amphetamine mixture capsules, but prolongs T_{max} by 2.5 hours (from 5.2 hours at fasted state to 7.7 hours after a high-fat meal). Opening the capsule and sprinkling the contents on applesauce results in comparable absorption to the intact capsule taken in the fasted state.

Dextroamphetamine – Following administration of three 5 mg tablets, average maximal dextroamphetamine plasma concentrations (C_{max}) of 36.6 ng/mL were achieved at ≈ 3 hours. Following administration of one 15 mg sustained-release capsule, maximal dextroamphetamine plasma concentrations were obtained ≈ 8 hours after dosing. The average C_{max} was 23.5 ng/mL. The average plasma half-life was similar for the tablet and sustained-release capsule and was approximately 12 hours.

Lisdexamfetamine – Lisdexamfetamine is rapidly absorbed from the GI tract. The time to reach maximum concentration (T_{max}) of dextroamphetamine is approximately 3.5 hours following single-dose oral administration of lisdexamfetamine 30, 50, or 70 mg after an 8-hour overnight fast. The T_{max} of lisdexamfetamine was approximately 1 hour.

Food prolongs T_{max} by approximately 1 hour (from 3.8 hours at fasted state to 4.7 hours after a high-fat meal.)

Lisdexamfetamine is converted to dextroamphetamine and L-lysine, which is believed to occur by first-pass intestinal and/or hepatic metabolism. Approximately 96% of the oral dose radioactivity was recovered in the urine and only 0.3% recovered in the feces over a period of 120 hours. The plasma elimination half-life of lisdexamfetamine typically averaged less than 1 hour in studies of lisdexamfetamine in volunteers.

Methamphetamine – Methamphetamine is rapidly absorbed from the GI tract. The biological half-life has been reported in the range of 4 to 5 hours. Excretion occurs primarily in the urine and is dependent on urine pH. Alkaline urine will increase the drug half-life significantly. Approximately 62% of an oral dose is eliminated in the urine within the first 24 hours with ≈ 33% as intact drug and the remainder as metabolites.

Special populations –

Children: Children eliminated amphetamine faster than adults.

Gender: Systemic exposure to amphetamine was 20% to 30% higher in women than in men because of the higher dose administered to women on a mg/kg body weight basis.

Contraindications

Advanced arteriosclerosis; symptomatic cardiovascular disease; moderate to severe hypertension; hyperthyroidism; known hypersensitivity or idiosyncrasy to the sympathomimetic amines; glaucoma; agitated states; history of drug abuse; during or within 14 days following administration of MAO inhibitors (hypertensive crises may result).

Warnings/Precautions

➤*Cardiovascular effects:*

Sudden death and preexisting structural cardiac abnormalities or other serious heart problems –

Children and adolescents: Sudden death has been reported in association with CNS stimulant treatment at usual doses in children and adolescents with structural cardiac abnormalities or other serious heart problems. In general, do not use stimulant products in children or adolescents with known serious structural cardiac abnormalities, cardiomyopathy, serious heart rhythm abnormalities, or other serious cardiac problems that may place them at increased vulnerability to the sympathomimetic effects of a stimulant drug.

Adults: Sudden deaths, stroke, and myocardial infarction have been reported in adults taking stimulant drugs at usual doses for ADHD. Adults have a greater likelihood than children of having serious structural cardiac abnormalities, cardiomyopathy, serious heart rhythm abnormalities, coronary artery disease, or other serious cardiac problems. In general, do not treat adults with such abnormalities with stimulant drugs.

Assessing cardiovascular status: Perform a careful history (including assessment for a family history of sudden death or ventricular arrhythmia) and physical exam to assess for the presence of cardiac disease in children, adolescents, or adults who are being considered for treatment with stimulant medications.

➤*CNS effects:*

Preexisting psychosis – Administration of stimulants may exacerbate symptoms of behavior disturbance and thought disorder in patients with preexisting psychotic disorder.

Bipolar illness – Take particular care in using stimulants to treat patients with ADHD with comorbid bipolar disorder because of concern for possible induction of mixed/manic episodes in such patients.

Emergence of new psychotic or manic symptoms – Treatment-emergent psychotic or manic symptoms (eg, hallucinations, delusional thinking, mania) in children and adolescents without a history of psychotic illness or mania can be caused by stimulants at usual doses. If such symptoms occur, consider a possible causal role of the stimulant; discontinuation of treatment may be appropriate.

Aggression – Aggressive behavior or hostility is often observed in children and adolescents with ADHD and has been reported in clinical trials and postmarketing experience of some medications indicated for the treatment of ADHD. Monitor patients beginning treatment for ADHD for the appearance or worsening of aggressive behavior or hostility.

➤*Tolerance:* When tolerance to the anorectic effect develops, do not exceed recommended dose in an attempt to increase the effect; rather, discontinue the drug.

➤*Drug dependence:* Amphetamines have been extensively abused. Tolerance, extreme psychological dependence, and severe social disability have occurred. Patients may increase the dosage to many times that recommended. Abrupt cessation following prolonged high dosage results in extreme fatigue, mental depression, and changes on the sleep EEG.

Manifestations of chronic intoxication – Severe dermatoses, marked insomnia, irritability, hyperactivity, and personality changes have occurred. Disorganization of thoughts, poor concentration, visual hallucinations, and compulsive behavior often occur. The most severe manifestation of chronic intoxication is psychosis, often clinically indistinguishable from paranoid schizophrenia. This is rare with oral amphetamines.

➤*Growth inhibition:* Decrements in the predicted growth (ie, weight gain or height) rate have been reported with the long-term use of stimulants in children. Therefore, carefully monitor patients requiring long-term therapy.

➤*Hypertension:* Exercise caution in prescribing amphetamines for patients with even mild hypertension.

➤*Prescribe or dispense:* Prescribe or dispense the least amount feasible at one time to minimize the possibility of overdosage.

➤*Potentially hazardous tasks:* Amphetamines may impair the ability of the patient to engage in potentially hazardous activities such as operating machinery or vehicles; caution the patient accordingly.

➤*Tics:* Amphetamines have been reported to exacerbate motor and phonic tics and Tourette syndrome. Therefore, precede use of stimulant medications with clinical evaluation for tics and Tourette syndrome in children and their families.

➤*Attention deficit disorders:* Drug treatment is not indicated in all cases and should be considered only in light of the complete history and evaluation of the child. Amphetamine use should depend on the chronicity and severity of the child's symptoms and appropriateness for his/her age. Use should not depend solely on the presence of 1 or more of the behavioral characteristics.

When these symptoms are associated with acute stress reactions, amphetamine treatment is usually not indicated.

➤*Seizures:* There is some clinical evidence that stimulants may lower the convulsive threshold in patients with a history of seizures, in patients with prior electroencephalogram (EEG) abnormalities in the absence of seizures, and, very rarely, in patients without a history of seizures and no prior EEG evidence of seizures. In the presence of seizures, discontinue the drug.

➤*Fatigue:* Do not use **methamphetamine** to combat fatigue or replace rest in normal people.

➤*Visual disturbance:* Difficulties with accommodation and blurring of vision have been reported with stimulant treatment.

➤*Tartrazine sensitivity:* Some of these products contain tartrazine, which may cause allergic-type reactions (including bronchial asthma) in susceptible individuals. Although the incidence of tartrazine sensitivity in the general population is low, it is frequently seen in patients who also have aspirin hypersensitivity. Specific products containing tartrazine are identified in the product listings.

➤*Pregnancy:* *Category C.* Safety for use during pregnancy has not been established. Reproduction studies in mammals at many times the human dose have suggested an embryotoxic and teratogenic potential. Congenital defects associated with amphetamine use include cardiac abnormalities, bifidexencephaly, and biliary atresia.

Methamphetamine has been shown to have teratogenic and embryocidal effects in mammals given high multiples of the human dose.

Fetal malformations and death have been reported in mice following parenteral administration of **dextroamphetamine** doses of 50 mg/kg/day or more to pregnant animals. Administration of these doses was also associated with severe maternal toxicity.

A number of studies in rodents indicate that prenatal or early postnatal exposure to amphetamine (d- or d,l-) at doses similar to those used clinically can result in long-term neurochemical and behavioral alterations. Reported behavioral effects include learning and memory deficits, altered locomotor activity, and changes in sexual function.

There are no adequate and well-controlled studies in pregnant women. Use in women who are or who may become pregnant (especially those in the first trimester) only when clearly needed and when the potential benefits outweigh the potential hazards to the fetus.

Infants born to mothers dependent on amphetamines have an increased risk of premature delivery and low birth weight. Also, these infants may experience symptoms of withdrawal as demonstrated by dysphoria, including agitation and significant lassitude.

➤*Lactation:* Amphetamines are excreted in breast milk. Advise patients to discontinue breast-feeding while taking amphetamines.The American Academy of Pediatrics classifies amphetamines as contraindicated during breast-feeding.

➤*Children:* Safety and efficacy have not been established for the use of amphetamines as anorectic agents in children younger than 12 years of age.

Lisdexamfetamine is indicated for use in children 6 to 12 years of age.

Amphetamine and **dextroamphetamine** are not recommended in children younger than 3 years of age for attention deficit disorder with hyperactivity. In psychotic children, amphetamines may exacerbate symptoms of behavior disturbance and thought disorder. Amphetamines may exacerbate motor and phonic tics and Tourette's syndrome. Therefore, clinical evaluation for tics and Tourette's syndrome in children and their families should precede use of stimulants.

Data are inadequate to determine whether chronic administration of amphetamines may be associated with growth inhibition; therefore, monitor growth during treatment and interrupt treatment in patients who are not growing or gaining weight as expected.

Long-term effects in children have not been well established.

Extended-release amphetamine mixture – Extended-release amphetamine mixture capsules are indicated for children ≥ 6 years of age. Effects in children 3 to 5 years of age have not been studied.

➤*Elderly:* Per the Beers list, amphetamines have the potential for causing dependence, hypertension, angina, myocardial infarction, and CNS stimulant adverse reactions. Amphetamines are also considered high risk medications for the elderly according to the Centers of Medicare and Medicaid Services.

➤*Monitoring:* Monitor all patients for larger changes in heart rate and blood pressure. Monitor patients beginning treatment for ADHD for the appearance or worsening of aggressive behavior or hostility. Monitor growth during treatment with stimulants; patients who are not growing or gaining weight as expected may need to have their treatment interrupted.

Drug Interactions

Insulin requirements in diabetes mellitus may be altered in association with the use of **methamphetamine** and the concomitant dietary regimen.

Amphetamine Drug Interactions

Precipitant drug	Object drug[a]		Description
Furazolidone	Amphetamines	↑	Increased sensitivity to amphetamines may occur. If an interaction is suspected, monitor patient for signs and symptoms of amphetamine toxicity and reduce the amphetamine dose accordingly.
Haloperidol	Amphetamines	↓	Haloperidol blocks dopamine receptors, inhibiting the central stimulant effects of amphetamines.
Lithium	Amphetamines	↓	The anorectic and stimulatory effects of amphetamines may be inhibited by lithium.
MAO inhibitors	Amphetamines	↑	Coadministration is contraindicated during or within 14 days following the administration of MAOIs; hypertensive crisis may result. MAOI antidepressants slow amphetamine metabolism, which may increase their effect on the release of norepinephrine and other monoamines from adrenergic nerve endings; this can cause headaches and other signs of hypertensive crisis. A variety of toxic neurologic effects and malignant hyperpyrexia, sometimes fatal, can occur.
Methenamine	Amphetamines	↓	Urinary excretion of amphetamines is increased, and efficacy is reduced by acidifying agents used in methenamine therapy.
Phenothiazines (eg, chlorpromazine, thioridazine)	Amphetamines	↓	The pharmacologic effects of amphetamines and congeners may be diminished. Do not use amphetamines or related substances for weight reduction in patients receiving phenothiazines.
Amphetamines	Phenothiazines		Amphetamines may exacerbate psychotic symptoms. Chlorpromazine can be used to treat amphetamine poisoning.
Propoxyphene	Amphetamines	↑	In cases of propoxyphene overdosage, amphetamine CNS stimulation is potentiated and fatal seizures can occur.
SSRIs (eg, citalopram, fluoxetine, venlafaxine)	Amphetamines	↑	Increased sensitivity to effect of sympathomimetics and increased risk of "serotonin syndrome" may occur.
Amphetamines	SSRIs (eg, citalopram, fluoxetine, venlafaxine)		If these agents must be given concurrently, monitor the patient for increased signs and symptoms of CNS effects. Adjust therapy as needed.

Amphetamine Drug Interactions

Precipitant drug	Object drug[a]		Description
Urinary acidifying agents (eg, ammonium chloride, sodium acid phosphate)	Amphetamines	↓	The elimination of amphetamines is hastened with a concomitant reduction in their duration of action. No special precautions appear necessary. This interaction has been exploited therapeutically in the management of amphetamine overdose.
Urinary alkalinizers (eg, sodium bicarbonate)	Amphetamines	↑	Alkalinized urine may prolong the effects of amphetamines. Avoid agents that may alkalinize urine, particularly in overdose situations.
Amphetamines	Adrenergic blockers	↓	Adrenergic blockers are inhibited by amphetamines.
Amphetamines	Antihistamines	↔	Amphetamines may counteract the sedative effects of antihistamines.
Amphetamines	Antihypertensive agents	↓	Amphetamines may antagonize the hypotensive effects of antihypertensives.
Amphetamines	Ethosuximide	↔	Amphetamines may delay intestinal absorption of ethosuximide.
Amphetamines	Guanethidine	↓	Amphetamines may reverse the hypotensive effects of guanethidine. Monitor patients. If there is a loss of blood pressure control, stop the amphetamine or switch to alternative hypotensive therapy.
Amphetamines	Meperidine	↑	Amphetamines may potentiate the analgesic effect of meperidine.
Amphetamines	Norepinephrine	↑	Amphetamines enhance the adrenergic effect of norepinephrine.
Amphetamines	Phenobarbital, phenytoin	↑	Amphetamines may delay intestinal absorption of phenobarbital and phenytoin; coadministration may produce a synergistic anticonvulsant action.
Amphetamines	Tricyclic antidepressants	↑	Amphetamine may enhance the activity of tricyclic antidepressants. d-Amphetamine with desipramine or protriptyline and possibly other tricyclics cause striking and sustained increases in the concentration of d-amphetamine in the brain. Cardiovascular effects may be potentiated.
Tricyclic antidepressants (ie, desipramine, protriptyline)	Amphetamines		
Amphetamines	Veratrum alkaloids	↓	Amphetamines may inhibit the hypotensive effect of veratrum alkaloids.

[a] ↑ = object drug increased; ↓ = object drug decreased; ↔ = undetermined clinical effect.

➤*Drug/Lab test interactions:* Plasma **corticosteroid** levels may be increased. This increase is greatest in the evening. This should be considered if determination of plasma corticosteroid levels is desired in a person receiving amphetamines. **Urinary steroid** determinations may be altered by amphetamines.

➤*Drug/Food interactions:* Food does not affect the extent of absorption of **amphetamine** mixtures extended-release, but prolongs T_{max} by 2.5 hours (from 5.2 hours at fasted state to 7.7 hours after a high-fat meal). **Lisdexamfetamine** 70 mg taken with food prolongs T_{max} by approximately 1 hour (from 3.8 hours at fasted state to 4.7 hours after a high-fat meal). Fruit juices may lower the absorption of **dextroamphetamine**, thereby decreasing its efficacy.

Adverse Reactions

➤*Cardiovascular:* Palpitations; stroke; myocardial infarction; sudden death; tachycardia; elevation of blood pressure; reflex decrease in heart rate; arrhythmias (at larger doses). There have been isolated reports of cardiomyopathy associated with chronic amphetamine use.

➤*CNS:* Overstimulation; restlessness; seizure; dizziness; insomnia; irritability; somnolence; affect lability; dyskinesia; euphoria; dysphoria; tremor; headache; changes in libido; psychotic episodes at recommended doses (rare). CNS stimulants have exacerbated Tourette's disorder and have exacerbated motor and phonic tics.

➤*GI:* Dry mouth; unpleasant taste; diarrhea; constipation; nausea; vomiting; abdominal pain; other GI disturbances. Anorexia and weight loss may occur as undesirable effects when amphetamines are used other than for their anorectic effect.

➤*Hypersensitivity:* Hypersensitivity reactions, including anaphylaxis and angioedema; urticaria. Serious skin rashes, including Stevens-Johnson syndrome and toxic epidermal necrolysis, have been reported.

➤*Miscellaneous:* Urticaria; impotence; pyrexia; rash;suppression of growth in children with long-term stimulant use.

Overdosage

➤*Symptoms:* Individual patient response to amphetamines varies widely. Manifestations of acute overdosage with amphetamines include the following: Restlessness; irritability; insomnia; tremor; hyperreflexia; rhabdomyolysis; rapid respiration; hyperpyrexia; assaultiveness; hallucinations; panic states; diaphoresis; mydriasis; flushing; hyperactivity; confusion; hypertension or hypotension; extrasystoles; tachypnea; fever; delirium; self-injury; marked hypertension; arrhythmias. Fatigue and depression usually follow the central stimulation. Cardiovascular effects include arrhythmias, hypertension or hypotension, and circulatory collapse. GI symptoms include nausea, vomiting, diarrhea, and abdominal cramps. Fatal poisoning usually is preceded by convulsions and coma.

➤*Treatment:* Consult with a certified poison control center for up-to-date guidance and advice. Treatment is largely symptomatic and includes gastric evacuation, although this is usually ineffective more than 4 hours after ingestion. After emptying the stomach, administer activated charcoal and a cathartic. Acidification of the urine increases amphetamine excretion. Experience with hemodialysis and peritoneal dialysis is inadequate to permit recommendations.

If acute, severe hypertension complicates amphetamine overdosage, administration of IV phentolamine has been suggested. However, a gradual drop in blood pressure usually results from sufficient sedation. Chlorpromazine antagonizes the central stimulant effects of amphetamines and can be used to treat amphetamine intoxication.

Because much of the long-acting form of medication is coated for gradual release, direct therapy at reversing the effects of the ingested drug and at supporting the patient; continue until overdosage symptoms subside. Use saline cathartics to hasten the evacuation of pellets that have not released medication.

Amphetamine mixture – Consider the prolonged release of mixed amphetamine salts from extended-release amphetamine mixture capsules when treating patients with overdose.

Patient Information

Regardless of indication, administer amphetamines at the lowest effective dosage and individually adjust dosage. Avoid late evening doses because of the resulting insomnia.

Do not chew or crush sustained-release or long-acting tablets.

Do not increase dosage, except on physician's advice.

Amphetamines may impair the ability of the patient to engage in potentially hazardous activities such as operating machinery or vehicles; caution the patient accordingly.

May cause nervousness, restlessness, insomnia, dizziness, anorexia, dry mouth, and GI disturbances. Notify physician if these effects become pronounced.

DEXTROAMPHETAMINE SULFATE

c-ii	**Dextroamphetamine** (Various, eg, Barr)	**Tablets; oral:** 5 mg	In 100s. May contain sucrose.
c-ii	**DextroStat** (Shire Richwood)		Tartrazine, lactose, sucrose. (RP 51). Yellow, scored. In 100s.
c-ii	**Dextroamphetamine** (Various, eg, Barr)	**Tablets; oral:** 10 mg	In 100s. May contain sucrose.
c-ii	**DextroStat** (Shire Richwood)		Tartrazine, lactose, sucrose. (RP 52). Yellow, scored. In 100s.
c-ii	**Dextroamphetamine** (Various, eg, Barr)	**Capsules, extended-release; oral:** 5 mg	In 100s. May contain sucrose.
c-ii	**Dexedrine Spansules** (Amedra)		Sugar spheres. (5 mg 3512/5 mg SB). Clear and brown. In 100s.
c-ii	**Dextroamphetamine** (Various, eg, Barr)	**Capsules, extended-release; oral:** 10 mg	In 100s. May contain sucrose.
c-ii	**Dexedrine Spansules** (Amedra)		Sugar spheres. (10 mg 3513/10 mg SB). Clear and brown. In 100s.
c-ii	**Dextroamphetamine** (Various, eg, Barr)	**Capsules, extended-release; oral:** 15 mg	In 100s. May contain sucrose.
c-ii	**Dexedrine Spansules** (Amedra)		Sugar spheres. (15 mg 3514/15 mg SB). Clear and brown. In 100s.
c-ii	**LiQuadd** (Auriga)	**Solution; oral:** 5 mg per 5 mL	Saccharin, sorbitol. Bubble gum flavor. In 473 mL.
c-ii	**ProCentra** (FSC Laboratories)		Benzoic acid, saccharin, sorbitol. Bubble gum flavor. In 473 mL.

DEXTROAMPHETAMINE SULFATE — ORAL

Complete and comparative prescribing information for these products begins in the Amphetamines group monograph.

WARNING

Amphetamines have a high potential for abuse. Administration of amphetamines for prolonged periods of time may lead to drug dependence and must be avoided. Pay particular attention to the possibility of subjects obtaining amphetamines for nontherapeutic use or distribution to others; prescribe and dispense the drugs sparingly.

Misuse of amphetamines may cause sudden death and serious cardiovascular adverse reactions.

Indications

➤*Attention deficit hyperactivity disorder (ADHD):* For the treatment of ADHD.

Dextroamphetamine is indicated in ADHD, as an integral part of a total treatment program that typically includes other remedial measures (psychological, educational, social) for a stabilizing effect in children 3 to 16 years of age with a behavioral syndrome characterized by the following group of developmentally inappropriate symptoms: emotional lability, hyperactivity, impulsivity, moderate to severe distractibility, and a short attention span. Do not make the diagnosis of this syndrome with finality when these symptoms are only of comparatively recent origin. Nonlocalizing (soft) neurological signs, learning disability, and abnormal electroencephalogram (EEG) may or may not be present, and a diagnosis of CNS dysfunction may or may not be warranted.

➤*Narcolepsy:* For the treatment of narcolepsy.

➤*Off-label uses:*

Traumatic brain injury – [3] = Safety concerns. The Neurobehavioral Guidelines Working Group assigned different levels to their recommendations for drug therapy of neurobehavioral sequelae of traumatic brain injury (TBI). They ranged from options to guidelines to the highest level of standards, based on the quality of evidence available and the extent of efficacy observed. Dextroamphetamine was considered an option level recommendation by the guideline authors because of the limited number of studies conducted to date and their less than optimal quality. In addition, there is a black box warning regarding the risk of dependence with amphetamines and the potential for serious adverse effects from misuse. Therefore, dextroamphetamine may be considered, but is not recommended, for all cases of problems of attention, processing speed, or working memory following a TBI. Weigh the risks and benefits of therapy for each patient.

Other possible off-label uses – Cocaine dependence treatment; autism.

Administration and Dosage

➤*General dosing considerations:* Amphetamines should be administered at the lowest effective dosage and dosage should be individually adjusted.

➤*Adults:*

Attention deficit hyperactivity disorder –

Initial dosage: 5 mg once or twice daily.

Dosage adjustment: The daily dose may be raised in increments of 5 mg at weekly intervals until optimal response is obtained. Only in rare cases will it be necessary to exceed a total of 40 mg/day.

Duration of therapy: When possible, drug administration should be interrupted occasionally to determine if there is a recurrence of behavioral symptoms sufficient to require continued therapy.

Narcolepsy – 5 to 60 mg/day in divided doses, depending on the individual patient response.

Off-label dosing –

Traumatic brain injury: [3] = Safety concerns. 5 to 30 mg/day orally.

➤*Children:*

Attention deficit hyperactivity disorder –

6 years of age and older:

- *Initial dosage* – 5 mg once or twice daily.
- *Dosage adjustment* – The daily dose may be raised in increments of 5 mg at weekly intervals until optimal response is obtained. Only in rare cases will it be necessary to exceed a total of 40 mg/day.
- *Duration of therapy* – When possible, drug administration should be interrupted occasionally to determine if there is a recurrence of behavioral symptoms sufficient to require continued therapy.

DEXTROAMPHETAMINE SULFATE — ORAL

3 to 5 years of age:
• *Initial dosage* – 2.5 mg daily, by tablet.
• *Dosage adjustment* – The daily dose may be raised in increments of 2.5 mg at weekly intervals until optimal response is obtained.

Narcolepsy –
12 years of age and older:
• *Initial dosage* – 10 mg daily.
• *Dosage adjustment* – The daily dose may be raised in increments of 10 mg at weekly intervals until optimal response is obtained. If bothersome adverse reactions appear (eg, anorexia, insomnia), dosage should be reduced.
6 to 12 years of age:
• *Initial dosage* – 5 mg daily.
• *Dosage adjustment* – The daily dose may be raised in increments of 5 mg at weekly intervals until optimal response is obtained. If bothersome adverse reactions appear (eg, anorexia, insomnia), dosage should be reduced.

Off-label dosing –
Attention deficit hyperactivity disorder:
• *3 years of age and older* –
Maximum dose: 40 mg/day given once per day or up to 3 divided doses.
Narcolepsy:
• *6 years of age and older* –
Maximum dose: 60 mg daily.

➤*Administration:* Late evening doses, particularly with the extended-release capsule forms, should be avoided because of the resulting insomnia. Extended-release capsules may be used for once-daily dosage whenever appropriate. With tablets, give first dose on awakening; give additional doses (1 or 2) at intervals of 4 to 6 hours.

➤*Storage/Stability:* Store at controlled room temperature, 15° to 30°C (59° to 86°F). Dispense in a tight, light- and child-resistant container.

METHAMPHETAMINE HYDROCHLORIDE (Desoxyephedrine Hydrochloride)

c-ii	**Methamphetamine** (Mylan)	**Tablets; oral:** 5 mg	Lactose. (115). White, round. In 100s.
c-ii	**Desoxyn** (Ovation Pharm)		Lactose. (OV 12). White. In 100s.

METHAMPHETAMINE HYDROCHLORIDE — ORAL

For complete and comparative prescribing information for these products, refer to the Amphetamines general monograph.

WARNING

Methamphetamine has a high potential for abuse. It should thus be tried only in weight reduction programs for patients in whom alternative therapy has been ineffective. Administration of methamphetamine for prolonged periods of time in obesity may lead to drug dependence and must be avoided. Particular attention should be paid to the possibility of subjects obtaining methamphetamine for nontherapeutic use or distribution to others, and the drug should be prescribed or dispensed sparingly.

Indications

➤*Attention deficit disorder with hyperactivity:* As an integral part of a total treatment program that typically includes other remedial measures (psychological, educational, social) for a stabilizing effect in children greater than 6 years of age with a behavioral syndrome characterized by the following group of developmentally inappropriate symptoms: Moderate to severe distractibility, short attention span, hyperactivity, emotional lability, and impulsivity. The diagnosis of this syndrome should not be made with finality when these symptoms are only of comparatively recent origin. Nonlocalizing (soft) neurological signs, learning disability, and abnormal EEG may or may not be present, and a diagnosis of CNS dysfunction may or may not be warranted.

➤*Exogenous obesity:* As a short-term (ie, a few weeks) adjunct in a regimen of weight reduction based on caloric restriction, for patients in whom obesity is refractory to alternative therapy (eg, repeated diets, group programs, other drugs). The limited usefulness of methamphetamine hydrochloride tablets should be weighed against possible risks inherent in use.

Administration and Dosage

➤*General dosing considerations:* Methamphetamine should be administered at the lowest effective dosage, and dosage should be individually adjusted. Late evening medication should be avoided because of the resulting insomnia.

➤*Adults:*
Attention-deficit disorder with hyperactivity –
Initial dosage: 5 mg once or twice a day is recommended.
Maintenance dosage: The usual effective dose is 20 to 25 mg daily. The total daily dose may be given in 2 divided doses daily.
Dosage adjustment: Daily dosage may be raised in increments of 5 mg at weekly intervals until an optimal clinical response is achieved.
Duration of therapy: When possible, drug administration should be interrupted occasionally to determine if there is a recurrence of behavioral symptoms sufficient to require continued therapy.

Obesity –
Usual dosage: 5 mg tablet should be taken 30 minutes before each meal.
Alternative dosage: Total daily dose may be given as conventional tablets in 2 divided doses or once daily using the long-acting form. Do not use the long-acting form for initiation of dosage or until the titrated daily dose is equal to or greater than the dosage provided in a long-acting tablet.
Duration of therapy: Treatment should not exceed a few weeks in duration. Intermittent or interrupted courses of therapy may be useful. A 3- to 6-week course of therapy followed by a discontinuation period of half the original treatment length has been suggested.

➤*Children:*
Attention-deficit disorder with hyperactivity – See Adults for dosing in children 6 years of age and older.

Obesity – See Adults for dosing in children 12 years of age and older.

➤*Administration:* The total daily dose for attention-deficit disorder with hyperactivity may be given in 2 divided doses daily.

For obesity, take methamphetamine 30 minutes before each meal.

Taking the medication during the late evening should be avoided because of the resulting insomnia.

➤*Storage/Stability:* Store below 30°C (86°F).

LISDEXAMFETAMINE DIMESYLATE

c-ii	**Vyvanse** (Shire US)	**Capsules; oral:** 20 mg	(20 mg). Ivory. In 100s.
		30 mg	(30 mg). White/Orange. In 100s.
		40 mg	(40 mg). White/Blue-green. In 100s.
		50 mg	(50 mg). White/Blue. In 100s.
		60 mg	(60 mg). Aqua blue. In 100s.
		70 mg	(70 mg). Blue/Orange. In 100s.

LISDEXAMFETAMINE DIMESYLATE — ORAL

WARNING

Potential for abuse – Amphetamines have a high potential for abuse. Administration of amphetamines for prolonged periods of time may lead to drug dependence. Pay particular attention to the possibility of patients obtaining amphetamines for nontherapeutic use or distribution to others; prescribe or dispense amphetamines sparingly.

Misuse of amphetamines may cause sudden death and serious cardiovascular adverse reactions. (See also Warnings/Precautions.)

Indications

➤*Attention deficit hyperactivity disorder:* For the treatment of attention deficit hyperactivity disorder (ADHD).

The efficacy of lisdexamfetamine in the treatment of ADHD was established on the basis of 2 controlled trials in children 6 to 12 years of age, 1 controlled trial in adolescents 13 to 17 years of age, and 2 controlled trials in adults who met *Diagnostic and Statistical Manual of Mental Disorders* (Fourth Edition, Text Revision) (*DSM-IV-TR*) criteria for ADHD.

A diagnosis of ADHD implies the presence of hyperactive-impulsive and/or inattentive symptoms that cause impairment and were present before the age of 7 years. The symptoms must cause clinically significant impairment (eg, in social, academic, or occupational functioning) and be present in 2 or more settings (eg, school, work, and at home). The symptoms must not be better accounted for by another mental disorder. For the inattentive type, at least 6 of the following symptoms must have persisted for at least 6 months: lack of attention to details/careless mistakes, lack of sustained attention, poor listener, failure to follow through on tasks, poor organization, avoids tasks requiring sustained mental effort, loses things, easily distracted, forgetful. For the hyperactive-impulsive type, at least 6 of the following symptoms (or adult equivalent symptoms) must have persisted for at least 6 months: fidgeting/squirming, leaving seat, inappropriate running/climbing, difficulty with quiet activities, on the go, excessive talking, blurt-

LISDEXAMFETAMINE DIMESYLATE — ORAL

ing answers, cannot wait turn, intrusive. The combined type requires both inattentive and hyperactive-impulsive criteria to be met.

Administration and Dosage

➤*Adults:*

Attention deficit hyperactivity disorder –
Maximum dose: 70 mg/day.
Initial dosage: 30 mg once daily in the morning.
Dosage adjustment: Dosage may be adjusted in increments of 10 or 20 mg/day at approximately weekly intervals, up to a maximum of 70 mg/day.

➤*Children:*

Attention deficit hyperactivity disorder –
6 years of age and older: See Adults for dosing.

➤*Duration of therapy:* The effectiveness of lisdexamfetamine for long-term use (longer than 4 weeks) has not been systematically evaluated in controlled trials. Therefore, the health care provider who elects to use lisdexamfetamine for extended periods should periodically reevaluate the long-term usefulness of the drug for the individual patient.

When possible, drug administration should be interrupted occasionally to determine if there is a recurrence of behavioral symptoms sufficient to require continued therapy.

➤*Administration:* Should be taken once a day in the morning with or without food. Afternoon doses should be avoided because of the potential for insomnia.

Lisdexamfetamine may be taken whole, or the capsule may be opened and the entire contents dissolved in a glass of water. If the patient is using the solution administration method, the solution should be consumed immediately; it should not be stored. The dose of a single capsule should not be divided. The contents of the entire capsule should be taken, and patients should not take anything less than 1 capsule per day.

➤*Storage/Stability:* Store at 25°C (77°F); excursions are permitted to 15° to 30°C (59° to 86°F). Dispense in a tight, light-resistant container.

AMPHETAMINE MIXTURES

c-ii	**Amphetamine Salt Combo** (Various, eg, Barr)	**Tablets; oral:** 5 mg (1.25 mg dextroamphetamine sulfate, 1.25 mg dextroamphetamine saccharate, 1.25 mg amphetamine aspartate, 1.25 mg amphetamine sulfate)	In 50s, 100s, and 500s.
c-ii	**Adderall** (Teva)		Lactose, sucrose. (AD 5). Blue, scored. In 100s.
c-ii	**Adderall** (Teva)	**Tablets; oral:** 7.5 mg (1.875 mg dextroamphetamine sulfate, 1.875 mg dextroamphetamine saccharate, 1.875 mg amphetamine aspartate, 1.875 mg amphetamine sulfate)	Lactose, sucrose. (AD 7.5). Blue, scored. In 100s.
c-ii	**Amphetamine Salt Combo** (Various, eg, Barr)	**Tablets; oral:** 10 mg (2.5 mg dextroamphetamine sulfate, 2.5 mg dextroamphetamine saccharate, 2.5 mg amphetamine aspartate, 2.5 mg amphetamine sulfate)	In 50s, 100s, and 500s.
c-ii	**Adderall** (Teva)		Lactose, sucrose. (AD 10). Blue, scored. In 100s.
c-ii	**Adderall** (Teva)	**Tablets; oral:** 12.5 mg (3.125 mg dextroamphetamine sulfate, 3.125 mg dextroamphetamine saccharate, 3.125 mg amphetamine aspartate, 3.125 mg amphetamine sulfate)	Lactose, sucrose. (AD 12.5). Orange, scored. In 100s.
c-ii	**Adderall** (Teva)	**Tablets; oral:** 15 mg (3.75 mg dextroamphetamine sulfate, 3.75 mg dextroamphetamine saccharate, 3.75 mg amphetamine aspartate, 3.75 mg amphetamine sulfate)	Lactose, sucrose. (AD 15). Orange, scored. In 100s.
c-ii	**Amphetamine Salt Combo** (Various, eg, Barr)	**Tablets; oral:** 20 mg (5 mg dextroamphetamine sulfate, 5 mg dextroamphetamine saccharate, 5 mg amphetamine aspartate, 5 mg amphetamine sulfate)	In 50s, 100s, and 500s.
c-ii	**Adderall** (Teva)		Lactose, sucrose. (AD 20). Orange, scored. In 100s.
c-ii	**Amphetamine Salt Combo** (Various, eg, Barr)	**Tablets; oral:** 30 mg (7.5 mg dextroamphetamine sulfate, 7.5 mg dextroamphetamine saccharate, 7.5 mg amphetamine aspartate, 7.5 mg amphetamine sulfate)	In 50s, 100s, and 500s.
c-ii	**Adderall** (Teva)		Lactose, sucrose. (AD 30). Orange, scored. In 100s.
c-ii	**Dextroamphetamine Saccharate/Amphetamine Aspartate/Dextroamphetamine Sulfate/Amphetamine Sulfate** (Barr)	**Capsules, extended release; oral:** 5 mg (1.25 mg dextroamphetamine saccharate, 1.25 mg amphetamine aspartate monohydrate, 1.25 mg dextroamphetamine sulfate, 1.25 mg amphetamine sulfate)	In 100s.
c-ii	**Adderall XR** (Shire)		Sugar spheres, talc. (ADDERALL XR 5 mg). Clear/Blue. In 100s.
c-ii	**Dextroamphetamine Saccharate/Amphetamine Aspartate/Dextroamphetamine Sulfate/Amphetamine Sulfate** (Barr)	**Capsules, extended release; oral:** 10 mg (2.5 mg dextroamphetamine saccharate, 2.5 mg amphetamine aspartate monohydrate, 2.5 mg dextroamphetamine sulfate, 2.5 mg amphetamine sulfate)	In 100s.
c-ii	**Adderall XR** (Shire)		Sugar spheres. (SHIRE 381 10 mg). Blue. In 100s.
c-ii	**Dextroamphetamine Saccharate/Amphetamine Aspartate/Dextroamphetamine Sulfate/Amphetamine Sulfate** (Barr)	**Capsules, extended release; oral:** 15 mg (3.75 mg dextroamphetamine saccharate, 3.75 mg amphetamine aspartate monohydrate, 3.75 mg dextroamphetamine sulfate, 3.75 mg amphetamine sulfate)	In 100s.
c-ii	**Adderall XR** (Shire)		Sugar spheres, talc. (ADDERALL XR 15 mg). Blue/White. In 100s.
c-ii	**Dextroamphetamine Saccharate/Amphetamine Aspartate/Dextroamphetamine Sulfate/Amphetamine Sulfate** (Barr)	**Capsules, extended release; oral:** 20 mg (5 mg dextroamphetamine saccharate, 5 mg amphetamine aspartate monohydrate, 5 mg dextroamphetamine sulfate, 5 mg amphetamine sulfate)	In 100s.
c-ii	**Adderall XR** (Shire)		Sugar spheres. (SHIRE 381 20 mg). Orange. In 100s.
c-ii	**Dextroamphetamine Saccharate/Amphetamine Aspartate/Dextroamphetamine Sulfate/Amphetamine Sulfate** (Barr)	**Capsules, extended release; oral:** 25 mg (6.25 mg dextroamphetamine saccharate, 6.25 mg amphetamine aspartate monohydrate, 6.25 mg dextroamphetamine sulfate, 6.25 mg amphetamine sulfate)	In 100s.
c-ii	**Adderall XR** (Shire)		Sugar spheres, talc. (ADDERALL XR 25 mg). Orange/White. In 100s.
c-ii	**Dextroamphetamine Saccharate/Amphetamine Aspartate/Dextroamphetamine Sulfate/Amphetamine Sulfate** (Barr)	**Capsules, extended release; oral:** 30 mg (7.5 mg dextroamphetamine saccharate, 7.5 mg amphetamine aspartate monohydrate, 7.5 mg dextroamphetamine sulfate, 7.5 mg amphetamine sulfate)	In 100s.
c-ii	**Adderall XR** (Shire)		Sugar spheres. (SHIRE 381 30 mg). Natural/Orange. In 100s.

AMPHETAMINE MIXTURES — ORAL

For complete and comparative prescribing information for these products, refer to the Amphetamines group monograph.

WARNING

Amphetamines have a high potential for abuse. Administration of amphetamines for prolonged periods of time may lead to drug dependence and must be avoided. Particular attention should be paid to the possibility of subjects obtaining amphetamines for non-therapeutic use or distribution to others, and the drugs should be prescribed or dispensed sparingly.

Indications

➤*Attention deficit disorder with hyperactivity:* As an integral part of a total treatment program that typically includes other remedial measures (psychological, educational, social) for a stabilizing effect in children with behavioral syndrome characterized by the following group of developmentally inappropriate symptoms: Moderate to severe distractibility, short attention span, hyperactivity, emotional lability, and impulsivity. The diagnosis of this syndrome should not be made with finality when these symptoms are only of comparatively recent origin. Nonlocalizing (soft) neurological signs, learning disability and abnormal EEG may or may not be present, and a diagnosis of central nervous system dysfunction may or may not be warranted.

➤*Narcolepsy:* Amphetamines tablets are also indicated in narcolepsy.

Administration and Dosage

➤*General dosing considerations:* Regardless of indication, amphetamines should be administered at the lowest effective dosage, and the dosage should be individually adjusted. Late evening doses should be avoided because of the resulting insomnia.

➤*Adults:*

Tablets –

Attention deficit disorder with hyperactivity:

• *Maximum dose* – 40 mg/day.

• *Initial dosage* – Start with 5 mg once or twice daily.

• *Dosage titration* – Daily dosage may be raised in increments of 5 mg at weekly intervals until optimal response is obtained. Only in rare cases will it be necessary to exceed a total of 40 mg/day.

Narcolepsy:

• *Usual dosage* – 5 to 60 mg/day in divided doses, depending on individual patient response.

• *Initial dosage* – Start with 10 mg daily.

• *Dosage adjustment* – Daily dosage may be raised in increments of 10 mg at weekly intervals until optimal response is obtained. If bothersome adverse reactions appear (eg, anorexia, insomnia), dosage should be reduced.

Extended-release capsule –

Attention deficit disorder with hyperactivity:

• *Maximum dose* – 30 mg/day. Doses more than 30 mg/day of amphetamine extended-release have not been studied.

• *Initial dosage* – 10 mg once daily in the morning if starting treatment for the first time or switching from another medication.

• *Dosage titration* – Daily dosage may be raised in increments of 10 mg at weekly intervals.

• *Conversion* – Based on bioequivalence data, patients taking divided doses of immediate-release amphetamine, for example twice a day, may be switched to amphetamine extended-release at the same total daily dose taken once daily. Titrate at weekly intervals to appropriate efficacy and tolerability as indicated.

➤*Children:*

Tablets –

Attention deficit disorder with hyperactivity:

• *6 years of age and older* – See Adults for dosing.

• *3 to 5 years of age –*

Initial dosage: 2.5 mg daily.

Dosage titration: Daily dosage may be raised in increments of 2.5 mg at weekly intervals until optimal response is obtained.

Narcolepsy:

• *12 years of age and older* – See Adults for dosing.

• *6 to 12 years of age* – Narcolepsy seldom occurs in children younger than 12 years of age; however, when it does, dextroamphetamine sulfate may be used.

Initial dosage: 5 mg daily.

Dosage titration: Daily dose may be raised in increments of 5 mg at weekly intervals until optimal response is obtained.

Extended-release capsule:

• *Attention deficit disorder with hyperactivity –*

6 years of age and older: See Adults for dosing.

Off-label dosing –

Attention deficit disorder with hyperactivity:

• *3 years of age and older –*

Maximum dose: 40 mg/day administered in 1 to 3 divided doses per day.

• *Narcolepsy –*

6 years of age and older: 60 mg/day.

➤*Duration of therapy:* Where possible, drug administration should be interrupted occasionally to determine if there is a recurrence of behavioral symptoms sufficient to require continued therapy.

➤*Administration:*

Tablets – Give first dose on awakening; give additional doses (1 or 2) at intervals of 4 to 6 hours.

Extended-release capsule – Amphetamine extended-release capsules may be taken whole, or the capsule may be opened and the entire contents sprinkled on applesauce. If the patient is using the sprinkle administration method, the sprinkled applesauce should be consumed immediately; it should not be stored. Patients should take the applesauce with sprinkled beads in its entirety, without chewing. The dose of a single capsule should not be divided. The contents of the entire capsule should be taken, and patients should not take anything less than 1 capsule per day.

Amphetamine extended-release capsules should be given upon awakening. Afternoon doses should be avoided because of the potential for insomnia.

➤*Storage/Stability:* Store at 15° to 30°C (59° to 86°F). Dispense in a tight, light-resistant container.

DEXMETHYLPHENIDATE HYDROCHLORIDE

c-ii	**Dexmethylphenidate Hydrochloride** (Teva)	**Tablets; oral:** 2.5 mg	Lactose. (93 5275). Blue. In 100s.
c-ii	**Focalin** (Novartis)		Lactose. (D 2.5). Blue. In 100s.
c-ii	**Dexmethylphenidate Hydrochloride** (Teva)	**Tablets; oral:** 5 mg	Lactose. (93 5276). Yellow. In 100s.
c-ii	**Focalin** (Novartis)		Lactose. (D 5). Yellow. In 100s.
c-ii	**Dexmethylphenidate Hydrochloride** (Teva)	**Tablets; oral:** 10 mg	Lactose. (93 5277). White to off-white. In 100s.
c-ii	**Focalin** (Novartis)		Lactose. (D 10). White. In 100s.
c-ii	**Focalin XR** (Novartis)	**Capsules, extended-release[a]; oral:** 5 mg	Sugar spheres. (NVR D5). Lt. blue. In 100s.
		10 mg	PEG, sugar spheres. (NVR D10). Lt. caramel. In 100s.
		15 mg	PEG, sugar spheres. (NVR D15). Green. In 100s.
		20 mg	PEG, sugar spheres. (NVR D20). White. In 100s.
		30 mg	PEG, sugar spheres. (NVR D30). Lt. caramel and white. In 100s.
		40 mg	PEG, sugar spheres. (NVR D40). Green/White. In 100s.

[a] Contains half the dose as immediate-release beads and half as much as enteric-coated, delayed-release beads.

DEXMETHYLPHENIDATE HYDROCHLORIDE — ORAL

WARNING

Drug dependence – Give dexmethylphenidate cautiously to patients with a history of drug dependence or alcoholism. Long-term, abusive use can lead to marked tolerance and psychological dependence with varying degrees of abnormal behavior. Frank psychotic episodes can occur, especially with parenteral abuse. Careful supervision is required during drug withdrawal from abusive use because severe depression may occur. Withdrawal following long-term therapeutic use may unmask symptoms of the underlying disorder that may require follow-up.

Indications

➤*Attention deficit hyperactivity disorder:* For the treatment of attention deficit hyperactivity disorder (ADHD) in patients 6 years of age and older.

The efficacy of dexmethylphenidate for more than 6 weeks (immediate-release) or for more than 7 weeks (extended-release [ER]) has not been systematically evaluated in controlled trials. Therefore, the health care provider who elects to use dexmethylphenidate immediate release or ER for extended periods should periodically reevaluate the long-term usefulness of the drug for the individual patient.

Administration and Dosage

➤*General dosing considerations:* Individualize dosage according to the needs and responses of the patient.

The health care provider who elects to use dexmethylphenidate for extended periods in patients with ADHD should periodically reevaluate the long-term usefulness of the drug for the individual patient with periods off medication to assess the patient's functioning without pharmacotherapy. Improvement may be sustained when the drug is either temporarily or permanently discontinued.

➤*Adults:*

Attention deficit hyperactivity disorder –

Maximum dose:

• *Immediate-release tablets* – 20 mg/day (10 mg twice daily).

• *ER capsules* – 40 mg/day.

Initial dosage: The recommended starting dose of dexmethylphenidate for patients who are not currently taking racemic methylphenidate or for patients who are on stimulants other than methylphenidate is the following:

• *Immediate-release tablets* – 2.5 mg twice daily (5 mg/day).

• *ER capsules* – 10 mg/day.

Dosage adjustment: In general, dosage adjustments may proceed at approximate weekly intervals. The patient should be observed for a sufficient duration at a given dose to ensure that a maximal benefit has been achieved before a dose increase is considered. (See also Dose Reduction and Discontinuation of Therapy.)

• *Immediate-release tablets* – Dosage may be adjusted in 2.5 to 5 mg increments at weekly intervals to a maximum of 20 mg/day (10 mg twice daily).

• *ER capsules* – Dosage may be adjusted in 10 mg/day increments at weekly intervals to a maximum of 40 mg/day.

Conversion: Patients currently using dexmethylphenidate immediate release may be switched to the same daily dose of dexmethylphenidate ER.

• *Patients currently using methylphenidate* – The recommended starting dose of dexmethylphenidate immediate release or ER is half the dose of racemic methylphenidate.

➤*Children:*

Attention deficit hyperactivity disorder –

6 years of age and older:

• *Maximum dose –*

Immediate-release tablets: 20 mg/day (10 mg twice daily).

ER capsules: 30 mg/day.

• *Initial dosage* – The recommended starting dose of dexmethylphenidate for patients who are not currently taking racemic methylphenidate or for patients who are on stimulants other than methylphenidate is the following:

Immediate-release tablets: 2.5 mg twice daily (5 mg/day).

ER capsules: 5 mg/day.

• *Dosage adjustment* – In general, dosage adjustments may proceed at approximate weekly intervals. (See also Dose Reduction and Discontinuation of Therapy.)

Immediate-release tablets: Dosage may be adjusted in 2.5 to 5 mg increments to a maximum of 20 mg/day (10 mg twice daily).

ER capsules: Dosage may be adjusted in 5 mg increments to a maximum of 30 mg/day.

• *Conversion –*

Patients currently using methylphenidate: The recommended starting dose of dexmethylphenidate immediate release or ER is half the dose of racemic methylphenidate.

➤*Dose reduction and discontinuation of therapy:* If paradoxical aggravation of symptoms or other adverse reactions occur, reduce the dosage, or, if necessary, discontinue the drug. If improvement is not observed after appropriate dosage adjustment over a 1-month period, discontinue the drug.

➤*Administration:*

Immediate-release tablets – 1 tablet twice daily administered at least 4 hours apart with or without food.

ER capsules – 1 capsule once daily in the morning.

Capsules may be swallowed whole or alternatively administered by sprinkling the capsule contents on a small amount of applesauce. The capsules and/or their contents should not be crushed, chewed, or divided. The capsules should be opened carefully and the beads sprinkled over a spoonful of applesauce. The mixture of drug and applesauce should be consumed immediately in its entirety. The drug and applesauce mixture should not be stored for future use.

➤*Storage/Stability:* Store at 25°C (77°F); excursions are permitted to 15° to 30°C (59° to 86°F). Protect the tablets from light and moisture. Dispense in a tight container.

Actions

➤*Pharmacology:* Dexmethylphenidate is a CNS stimulant. Dexmethylphenidate, the more pharmacologically active enantiomer of the d- and l-enantiomers (racemic methylphenidate), is thought to block the reuptake of norepinephrine and dopamine into the presynaptic neuron and increase the release of these monoamines into the extraneuronal space. The mode of therapeutic action in ADHD is not known.

➤*Pharmacokinetics:*

Absorption –

Immediate-release tablets: Dexmethylphenidate immediate release is readily absorbed following oral administration. In patients with ADHD, plasma dexmethylphenidate concentrations increase rapidly, reaching a maximum in the fasted state at about 1 to 1.5 hours postdose. No differences in the pharmacokinetics of dexmethylphenidate were noted following single and repeated twice-daily dosing, thus indicating no significant drug accumulation in children with ADHD.

When given to children as capsules in single doses of 2.5, 5, and 10 mg, maximum plasma concentration (C_{max}) and area under the curve (AUC_{0-inf}) of dexmethylphenidate were proportional to dose. In the same study, plasma dexmethylphenidate levels were comparable with those achieved following single dl-threo-methylphenidate doses given as capsules in twice the total milligram amount (equimolar with respect to dexmethylphenidate).

ER capsules: Dexmethylphenidate ER produces a bimodal plasma concentration-time profile (ie, 2 distinct peaks approximately 4 hours apart) when orally administered to healthy adults. The initial rate of absorption for dexmethylphenidate ER is similar to that of dexmethylphenidate immediate-release tablets as shown by the similar rate parameters between the 2 formulations (ie, first peak concentration [C_{max1}], and time to first peak [T_{max1}], which is reached in 1.5 hours [typical range, 1 to 4 hours]). The mean time to the interpeak minimum (T_{minip}) is slightly shorter, and time to the second peak (T_{max2}) is slightly longer for dexmethylphenidate ER given once daily (about 6.5 hours; range, 4.5 to 7 hours) compared with dexmethylphenidate immediate-release tablets given in 2 doses 4 hours apart, although the ranges observed are greater for dexmethylphenidate ER.

Dexmethylphenidate ER given once daily exhibits a lower second peak concentration (C_{max2}), higher interpeak minimum concentrations (C_{minip}), and less peak and trough fluctuations than dexmethylphenidate tablets given in 2 doses given 4 hours apart. This is because of an earlier onset and more prolonged absorption from the delayed-release beads.

The AUC (exposure) after administration of dexmethylphenidate ER given once daily is equivalent to the same total dose of dexmethylphenidate tablets given in 2 doses 4 hours apart. The variability in C_{max}, C_{min}, and AUC is similar between dexmethylphenidate ER and dexmethylphenidate immediate release, with approximately a 3-fold range in each.

Radiolabeled racemic methylphenidate is well absorbed after oral administration, with approximately 90% of the radioactivity recovered in urine. However, because of first-pass metabolism, the mean absolute bioavailability of dexmethylphenidate when administered in various formulations was 22% to 25%.

• *Dose proportionality* – Dose proportionality of dexmethylphenidate ER was evaluated in a randomized, single-dose, 5-period, crossover study with administration of single doses of 5, 10, 20, 30, and 40 mg to healthy adults. Results confirmed dose proportionality within this range.

Food effects:

• *Immediate-release tablets* – In a single-dose study conducted in adults, coadministration of 2 × 10 mg of dexmethylphenidate with a high-fat breakfast resulted in a dexmethylphenidate T_{max} of 2.9 hours postdose as compared with 1.5 hours postdose when given in a fasting state. C_{max} and AUC_{0-inf} were comparable in both the fasted and nonfasted states.

• *ER capsules* – Administration times relative to meals and meal composition may need to be individually titrated.

No food-effect study was performed with dexmethylphenidate ER. However, the effect of food has been studied in adults with racemic methylphenidate in the same type of ER formulation. The findings of that study are considered applicable to dexmethylphenidate ER. After a high-fat breakfast, there was a longer lag time until absorption began and variable delays in the time until the first peak concentration, the time until the interpeak minimum, and the time until the second peak. The first peak concentration and the extent of absorption were unchanged after food relative to the fasting state, although the second peak was approximately 25% lower. The effect of a high-fat lunch was not examined. There is no evidence of dose dumping in the presence or absence of food. There were no differences in the plasma concentration-time profile when administered with applesauce compared with administration in the fasting condition. The results are expected not to differ for dexmethylphenidate ER.

For patients unable to swallow the capsule, the contents may be sprinkled on applesauce and administered.

Distribution – The plasma protein binding of dexmethylphenidate is not known; racemic methylphenidate is bound to plasma proteins by 12% to 15%, independent of concentration. Dexmethylphenidate shows a volume of

DEXMETHYLPHENIDATE HYDROCHLORIDE — ORAL

distribution of 2.65 ± 1.11 L/kg. Plasma dexmethylphenidate concentrations decline monophasically following oral administration of dexmethylphenidate ER.

Immediate-release tablets: Plasma dexmethylphenidate concentrations in children decline exponentially following oral administration of dexmethylphenidate immediate release.

Metabolism/Excretion – In humans, dexmethylphenidate is metabolized primarily to d-alpha-phenyl-piperindine acetic acid (also known as d-ritalinic acid) by de-esterification. This metabolite has little or no pharmacological activity. There is little or no in vivo interconversion to the l-threo-enantiomer, based on a finding of minute or no levels of l-threo-methylphenidate being detectable after administration in adults and children. After oral dosing of radiolabeled racemic methylphenidate in humans, approximately 90% of the radioactivity was recovered in urine. The main urinary metabolite of racemic (d,l-)methylphenidate was d,l-ritalinic acid, accountable for approximately 80% of the dose. Urinary excretion of parent compound accounted for 0.5% of an intravenous (IV) dose.

IV dexmethylphenidate was eliminated with a mean clearance of 0.4 ± 0.12 L/kg•h-1 corresponding to 0.56 ± 0.18 L/min. The mean terminal elimination half-life of dexmethylphenidate was just over 3 hours in healthy adults and typically varied between 2 and 4.5 hours, with an occasional subject exhibiting a terminal half-life between 5 and 7 hours. Children tend to have slightly shorter half-lives, with means of 2 to 3 hours.

Special populations –

Gender:

• *Immediate-release tablets* – In a single-dose study conducted in adults, the mean dexmethylphenidate $AUC_{0\text{-}inf}$ values (adjusted for body weight) following single 2 × 10 mg doses of dexmethylphenidate were 25% to 35% higher in adult women (n = 6) compared with men (n = 9). Both T_{max} and $t_{1/2}$ were comparable for men and women.

• *ER capsules* – After administration of dexmethylphenidate ER, the first peak (C_{max1}) was on average 45% higher in women. The interpeak minimum and the second peak also tended to be slightly higher in women, although the difference was not statistically significant and these patterns remained even after weight normalization.

Age:

• *Immediate-release tablets* – The pharmacokinetics of dexmethylphenidate immediate release administration have not been studied in children younger than 6 years of age. When single doses of dexmethylphenidate were given to children between 6 and 12 years of age and healthy adult volunteers, C_{max} of dexmethylphenidate was similar; however, children showed somewhat lower AUCs compared with the adults.

• *ER capsules* – The pharmacokinetics of dexmethylphenidate ER administration have not been studied in children younger than 18 years of age. When a similar formulation of racemic methylphenidate was examined in 15 children between 10 and 12 years of age and 3 children with ADHD between 7 and 9 years of age, the time to the first peak was similar, although the time until the between peak minimum and the time until the second peak were delayed and more variable in children compared with adults. After administration of the same dose to children and adults, concentrations in children were approximately twice the concentrations observed in adults. This higher exposure is almost completely because of smaller body size, as no relevant age-related differences in dexmethylphenidate pharmacokinetic parameters (ie, clearance and volume of distribution) are observed after normalization to dose and weight.

Contraindications

Marked anxiety, tension, and agitation because the drug may aggravate these symptoms; hypersensitivity to methylphenidate or other components of the product; glaucoma; motor tics or with a family history or diagnosis of Tourette syndrome; during treatment with monoamine oxidase inhibitors (MAOIs), and also within a minimum of 14 days following discontinuation of an MAOI (hypertensive crises may result).

Warnings/Precautions

➤*Cardiovascular effects:*

Sudden death and preexisting structural cardiac abnormalities –

Children and adolescents: Sudden death has been reported in association with CNS stimulant treatment at usual doses in children and adolescents with structural cardiac abnormalities or other serious heart problems. Although some serious heart problems alone carry an increased risk of sudden death, in general, do not use stimulant products in children or adolescents with known serious structural cardiac abnormalities, cardiomyopathy, serious heart rhythm abnormalities, or other serious cardiac problems that may place them at increased vulnerability to the sympathomimetic effects of a stimulant drug.

Adults: Sudden death, stroke, and myocardial infarction have been reported in adults taking stimulant drugs at the usual doses for ADHD. Although the role of stimulants in these adult cases is also unknown, adults have a greater likelihood than children of having serious structural cardiac abnormalities, cardiomyopathy, serious heart rhythm abnormalities, coronary artery disease, or other serious cardiac problems. In general, do not treat adults with such abnormalities with stimulant drugs.

Hypertension and other cardiovascular conditions – Stimulant medications cause a modest increase in average blood pressure (approximately 2 to 4 mm Hg) and average heart rate (approximately 3 to 6 bpm), and patients may have larger increases. While the mean changes alone would not be expected to have short-term consequences, monitor all patients for larger changes in heart rate and blood pressure. Caution is indicated in treating patients whose underlying medical conditions might be compromised by increases in blood pressure or heart rate (eg, those with preexisting hypertension, heart failure, recent myocardial infarction, ventricular arrhythmia).

Assessing cardiovascular status – Children, adolescents, or adults who are being considered for treatment with stimulant medications should have a careful history (including assessment for family history of sudden death or ventricular arrhythmia) and physical exam to assess for the presence of cardiac disease, and should receive further cardiac evaluation if findings suggest such disease (eg, echocardiogram, electrocardiogram). Patients who develop symptoms such as exertional chest pain, unexplained syncope, or other symptoms suggestive of cardiac disease during stimulant treatment should undergo a prompt cardiac evaluation.

➤*Psychiatric effects:*

Preexisting psychosis – Administration of stimulants may exacerbate symptoms of behavior disturbance and thought disorder in patients with a preexisting psychotic disorder.

Bipolar illness – Take particular care in using stimulants to treat ADHD in patients with comorbid bipolar disorder because of concern for possible induction of a mixed/manic episode in such patients. Prior to initiating treatment with a stimulant, adequately screen patients with comorbid depressive symptoms to determine if they are at risk for bipolar disorder; include in such screening a detailed psychiatric history, including a family history of bipolar disorder, depression, and suicide.

Emergence of new psychotic or manic symptoms – Treatment-emergent psychotic or manic symptoms (eg, delusional thinking, hallucinations, mania) in children and adolescents without a history of psychotic illness or mania can be caused by stimulants at usual doses. If such symptoms occur, consider a possible causal role of the stimulant, and discontinuation of treatment may be appropriate. In a pooled analysis of multiple short-term, placebo-controlled studies, such symptoms occurred in about 0.1% (4 patients with reactions out of 3,482 exposed to methylphenidate or amphetamine for several weeks at usual doses) of stimulant-treated patients compared with 0 in placebo-treated patients.

Aggression – Aggressive behavior or hostility is often observed in children and adolescents with ADHD and has been reported in clinical trials and the postmarketing experience of some medications indicated for the treatment of ADHD. Although there is no systematic evidence that stimulants cause aggressive behavior or hostility, monitor patients beginning treatment for ADHD for the appearance or worsening of aggressive behavior or hostility.

➤*Long-term suppression of growth:* Careful follow-up of weight and height in children 7 to 10 years of age who were randomized to methylphenidate or nonmedication treatment groups over 14 months, as well as in naturalistic subgroups of newly methylphenidate-treated and nonmedication-treated children (10 to 13 years of age) over 36 months, suggests that consistently medicated children (ie, treatment for 7 days/week throughout the year) have a temporary slowing in growth rate (on average, a total of about 2 cm less growth in height and 2.7 kg less growth in weight over 3 years), without evidence of growth rebound during this period of development. In the 7-week, double-blind, placebo-controlled study of dexmethylphenidate ER capsules, the mean weight gain was greater for patients receiving placebo (+0.4 kg) than for patients receiving dexmethylphenidate ER (−0.5 kg). Published data are inadequate to determine whether long-term use of amphetamines may cause a similar suppression of growth; however, it is anticipated that they likely have this effect as well. Therefore, monitor growth during treatment with stimulants, and patients who are not growing or gaining height or weight as expected may need to have their treatment interrupted.

➤*Seizures:* There is some clinical evidence that stimulants may lower the convulsive threshold in patients with history of seizures, in patients with prior electroencephalogram (EEG) abnormalities in absence of seizures, and, very rarely, in patients without a history of seizures and no prior EEG evidence of seizures. In the presence of seizures, discontinue the drug.

➤*Visual disturbance:* Difficulties with accommodation and blurring of vision have been reported with stimulant treatment.

➤*Pregnancy: Category C.* Adequate and well-controlled studies in pregnant women have not been conducted. Use during pregnancy only if the potential benefit justifies the potential risk to the fetus. No reports describing the use of dexmethylphenidate in human pregnancy have been located. Until human data are available for dexmethylphenidate, the safest course is to avoid the drug in pregnancy. If the mother's condition requires the drug, the lowest effective dose, avoiding the first trimester if possible, should be used. Long-term follow-up of exposed offspring may be warranted.

In studies conducted in rats and rabbits, dexmethylphenidate was administered orally at dosages of up to 20 and 100 mg/kg/day, respectively, during the period of organogenesis. No evidence of teratogenic activity was found in either the rat or rabbit study; however, delayed fetal skeletal ossification was observed at the highest dose level in rats. When dexmethylphenidate was administered to rats throughout pregnancy and lactation at dosages of up to 20 mg/kg/day, postweaning body-weight gain was decreased in male offspring at the highest dose, but no other effects on postnatal development were observed. At the highest doses tested, plasma levels (AUCs) of dexmethylphenidate in pregnant rats and rabbits were approximately 5 and 1 times, respectively, those in adults dosed with the maximum recommended human dosage of 20 mg/day.

Racemic methylphenidate has been shown to have teratogenic effects in rabbits when given in dosages of 200 mg/kg/day throughout organogenesis.

➤*Lactation:* It is not known whether dexmethylphenidate is excreted in human milk. Exercise caution if dexmethylphenidate is administered to a breast-feeding woman. The molecular weight (approximately 234 for the free base) is low enough that excretion into breast milk should be expected. However, the relatively short plasma elimination half-life should limit the amount of the drug in milk. The effects of this exposure on a breast-feeding infant are unknown. If a mother chooses to breast-feed while taking dexmethylphenidate, the infant should be monitored for adverse effects observed in children and adults (eg, abdominal pain, fever, anorexia, nau-

DEXMETHYLPHENIDATE HYDROCHLORIDE — ORAL

sea). Information from 4 published case reports on the use of racemic methylphenidate during breast-feeding suggest that at maternal dosages of 35 to 80 mg/day, milk concentrations of methylphenidate range from undetectable to 15.4 ng/mL. Based on these limited data, the calculated infant daily dose for an exclusively breast-fed infant would be about 0.4 to 2.9 mcg/kg/day or approximately 0.2% to 0.7% of the maternal weight adjusted dose.

➤*Children:* The safety and efficacy of dexmethylphenidate in children younger than 6 years of age have not been established. Long-term effects of dexmethylphenidate in children have not been well established.

In a study conducted in young rats, racemic methylphenidate was administered orally at dosages of up to 100 mg/kg/day for 9 weeks, starting early in the postnatal period (postnatal day 7) and continuing through sexual maturity (postnatal week 10). When these animals were tested as adults (postnatal weeks 13 through 14), decreased spontaneous locomotor activity was observed in males and females previously treated with 50 mg/kg/day (approximately 6 times the maximum recommended human dose [MRHD] of racemic methylphenidate on a mg/m² basis) or greater, and a deficit in the acquisition of a specific learning task was seen in females exposed to the highest dose (12 times the MRHD on a mg/m² basis). The no-effect level for juvenile neurobehavioral development in rats was 5 mg/kg/day (half the racemic MRHD on a mg/m² basis). The clinical significance of the long-term behavioral effects observed in rats is unknown.

➤*Elderly:* Per the Beers list, amphetamines have the potential for causing dependence, hypertension, angina, and myocardial infarction. Dexmethylphenidate is also considered a high-risk medication for elderly patients according to the Centers of Medicare and Medicaid Services.

➤*Monitoring:* Periodic complete blood cell, differential, and platelet counts are advised during prolonged therapy. In children and adolescents, monitor for the appearance or worsening of aggressive behavior or hostility. Monitor growth in children during treatment with stimulants, and patients who are not growing or gaining height or weight as expected may need to have their treatment interrupted.

Drug Interactions

Dexmethylphenidate Drug Interactions

Precipitant drug	Object drug[a]		Description
Antacids/Acid suppressants	Dexmethylphenidate ER	↑↓	Because the modified-release characteristics of dexmethylphenidate ER are pH-dependent, the coadministration of antacids or acid suppressants could alter the release of dexmethylphenidate.
Halogenated anesthetics	Dexmethylphenidate	↑	Coadministration may cause a sudden increase in blood pressure during surgery. Methylphenidate is contraindicated on the day of the planned surgery with halogenated anesthetics.
MAOIs (eg, isocarboxazid, phenelzine, selegiline)	Dexmethylphenidate	↑	Dexmethylphenidate use is contraindicated during treatment with MAOIs and also within a minimum of 14 days following discontinuation of treatment with an MAOI. Hypertensive crisis may result.
Methylphenidate (racemic)	Anticonvulsants (eg, phenobarbital, phenytoin, primidone)	↑	Downward dose adjustments of anticonvulsant therapy may be required when it is given concomitantly with dexmethylphenidate.
Methylphenidate (racemic)	Antihypertensive agents	↓	Antihypertensive effectiveness may be decreased.
Methylphenidate (racemic)	Clonidine	↔	Serious adverse reactions have been reported in concomitant use with clonidine; however, no causality for the combination has been established.
Methylphenidate (racemic)	Coumarin anticoagulants (eg, warfarin)	↑	Dexmethylphenidate may inhibit the metabolism of warfarin-like drugs. It may be necessary to adjust the dosage or monitor coagulation times when starting or stopping therapy.
Methylphenidate (racemic)	SSRIs[b] (eg, fluoxetine)	↑	Pharmacologic effects of SSRIs may be increased by dexmethylphenidate, resulting in development of serotonin syndrome. However, methylphenidate and SSRIs have been used concurrently in an attempt to enhance the antidepressant response to the SSRI. Use with caution.
Methylphenidate (racemic)	Tricyclic antidepressants (eg, clomipramine, desipramine, imipramine)	↑	It may be necessary to adjust the dosage of antidepressant therapy when these agents are given concurrently.
Dexmethylphenidate	Vasopressor agents (eg, dopamine, epinephrine, phenylephrine)	↑	Because of possible effects on blood pressure, use dexmethylphenidate cautiously with pressor agents.

[a] ↑ = object drug increased; ↓ = object drug decreased; ↔ = undetermined clinical effect; ↑↓ = object drug moth increased and decreased.
[b] SSRIs = selective serotonin reuptake inhibitors.

Adverse Reactions

➤*Immediate-release tablets:*

Discontinuation of treatment – No dexmethylphenidate-treated patients discontinued because of adverse reactions in 2 placebo-controlled trials. Overall, 50 of 684 (7.3%) children treated with dexmethylphenidate experienced an adverse reaction that resulted in discontinuation. The most common reasons for discontinuation were anorexia, insomnia, tachycardia, and twitching (described as motor or vocal tics) (approximately 1% each).

Adverse reactions (5% or more) –

Dexmethylphenidate Immediate Release Adverse Reactions (≥ 5%)[a]

Adverse reactions	Dexmethylphenidate immediate release (n = 79)	Placebo (n = 82)
GI		
Abdominal pain	15%	6%
Anorexia	6%	1%
Nausea	9%	1%
Miscellaneous		
Fever	5%	1%

[a] Events, regardless of causality, for which the incidence for patients treated with dexmethylphenidate was at least 5% and twice the incidence among placebo-treated patients. Incidence has been rounded to the nearest whole number.

➤*ER capsules:*

Discontinuation of treatment in children – None of the 53 dexmethylphenidate ER–treated children discontinued treatment because of adverse reactions in the 7-week, placebo-controlled study.

Adverse reactions in children (5% or more) –

Dexmethylphenidate ER (Flexible Doses) Adverse Reactions[a] in Children (≥ 5%)

Adverse reactions	Dexmethylphenidate ER (n = 53)	Placebo (n = 47)
Number of patients with adverse reactions (total)	76%	57%
CNS, NOS[b]	30%	13%
Headache	25%	11%
GI, NOS	38%	19%
Dyspepsia	8%	4%
Metabolic/Nutritional, NOS	34%	11%
Decreased appetite	30%	9%
Psychiatric, NOS	26%	15%
Anxiety	6%	0%

[a] Reactions, regardless of causality, for which the incidence of patients treated with dexmethylphenidate ER was at least 5% and twice the incidence among placebo-treated patients. Incidence has been rounded to the nearest whole number.
[b] NOS = not otherwise specified.

The following table enumerates the incidence of dose-related adverse reactions that occurred during a fixed-dose, double-blind, placebo-controlled trial of dexmethylphenidate ER up to 30 mg/day versus placebo in children and adolescents with ADHD.

Dexmethylephenidate ER (Fixed Doses) Adverse Reactions in Children

Adverse reactions	Dexmethylphenidate ER 10 mg/day (n= 64)	Dexmethylphenidate ER 20 mg/day (n= 60)	Dexmethylphenidate ER 30 mg/day (n= 58)	Placebo (n = 63)
GI, NOS	22%	23%	29%	24%
Vomiting	2%	8%	9%	0%
Metabolic/Nutritional, NOS	16%	17%	22%	5%

DEXMETHYLPHENIDATE HYDROCHLORIDE — ORAL

Dexmethylephenidate ER (Fixed Doses) Adverse Reactions in Children				
Adverse reactions	Dexmethyl-phenidate ER 10 mg/day (n= 64)	Dexmethyl-phenidate ER 20 mg/day (n= 60)	Dexmethyl-phenidate ER 30 mg/day (n= 58)	Placebo (n = 63)
Anorexia	5%	5%	7%	0%
Psychiatric, NOS	19%	20%	38%	8%
Insomnia	5%	8%	17%	3%
Depression	0%	0%	3%	0%
Mood swings	0%	0%	3%	2%
Miscellaneous				
Irritability	0%	2%	5%	0%
Nasal congestion	0%	0%	5%	0%
Pruritus	0%	0%	3%	0%

Discontinuation of treatment in adults – In the adult placebo-controlled study, 10.7% of dexmethylphenidate ER–treated patients and 7.5% of placebo-treated patients discontinued for adverse reactions. Among dexmethylphenidate ER–treated patients, anorexia (1.2%, n = 2), anxiety (1.2%, n = 2), feeling jittery (1.8%, n = 3), and insomnia (1.8%, n = 3) were the reasons for discontinuation reported by more than 1 patient.

Adverse reactions in adults (5% or more) –

Dexmethylphenidate ER Adverse Reactions in Adults (≥ 5%)[a]				
Adverse reactions	Dexmethyl-phenidate ER 20 mg (n = 57)	Dexmethyl-phenidate ER 30 mg (n = 54)	Dexmethyl-phenidate ER 40 mg (n = 54)	Placebo (n = 53)
Number of patients with adverse reactions (total)	84%	94%	85%	68%
CNS, NOS	37%	39%	50%	28%
Headache	26%	30%	39%	19%
GI, NOS	28%	32%	44%	19%
Dry mouth	7%	20%	20%	4%
Dyspepsia	5%	9%	9%	2%
Psychiatric, NOS	40%	43%	46%	30%
Anxiety	5%	11%	11%	2%
Respiratory, NOS	16%	9%	15%	8%
Pharyngo-laryngeal pain	4%	4%	7%	2%

[a] Reactions, regardless of causality, for which the incidence was at least 5% in a dexmethylphenidate ER group and that appeared to increase with randomized dose. Incidence has been rounded to the nearest whole number.

Two other adverse reactions occurring in clinical trials with dexmethylphenidate ER at a frequency greater than placebo, but which were not dose related, were feeling jittery (12% and 2%, respectively) and dizziness (6% and 2%, respectively).

The following table summarizes changes in vital signs and weight that were recorded in the adult study (N = 218) of dexmethylphenidate ER in the treatment of ADHD.

Dexmethylphenidate ER Changes in Adult Vital Signs and Weight				
	Dexmethyl-phenidate ER 20 mg (n = 57)	Dexmethyl-phenidate ER 30 mg (n = 54)	Dexmethyl-phenidate ER 40 mg (n = 54)	Placebo (n = 53)
Pulse (bpm)	3.1 ± 11.1	4.3 ± 11.7	6 ± 10.1	−1.4 ± 9.3
Diastolic BP[a] (mm Hg)	−0.2 ± 8.2	1.2 ± 8.9	2.1 ± 8	0.3 ± 7.8
Weight (kg)	−1.4 ± 2	−1.2 ± 1.9	−1.7 ± 2.3	−0.1 ± 3.9

[a] BP = blood pressure.

➤*Adverse reactions with other methylphenidate forms:* Nervousness and insomnia are the most common adverse reactions reported with other methylphenidate products. In children, abdominal pain, insomnia, loss of appetite, tachycardia, and weight loss during prolonged therapy may occur more frequently; however, any of the other following adverse reactions also may occur.

Cardiovascular – Angina, arrhythmia, blood pressure increased or decreased, cerebral arteritis and/or occlusion, palpitations, pulse increased or decreased, tachycardia.

CNS – Dizziness, drowsiness, dyskinesia, headache, rare reports of Tourette syndrome, toxic psychosis.

GI – Abdominal pain, anorexia, nausea.

Hypersensitivity – Hypersensitivity reactions, including arthralgia, erythema multiforme with histopathological findings of necrotizing vasculitis, exfoliative dermatitis, fever, skin rash, thrombocytopenic purpura, and urticaria.

Metabolic/Nutritional – Weight loss during prolonged therapy.

➤*Other adverse reactions reported in patients taking methylphenidate (causal relationship not established):* Although a definite causal relationship has not been established, the following have been reported in patients taking methylphenidate:

CNS – Aggressive behavior, transient depressed mood.

Dermatologic – Scalp hair loss.

Hematologic/Lymphatic – Anemia and/or leukopenia.

Hepatic – Abnormal liver function, ranging from transaminase elevation to hepatic coma.

Neuroleptic malignant syndrome – Very rare reports of neuroleptic malignant syndrome (NMS) have been received, and, in most of these, patients were concurrently receiving therapies associated with NMS. In a single report, a 10-year-old boy who had been taking methylphenidate for approximately 18 months experienced an NMS-like reaction within 45 minutes of ingesting his first dose of venlafaxine. It is uncertain whether this case represented a drug-drug interaction, a response to either drug alone, or some other cause.

Overdosage

➤*Symptoms:* Signs and symptoms of acute methylphenidate overdosage, resulting principally from overstimulation of the CNS and from excessive sympathomimetic effects, may include the following: agitation, cardiac arrhythmias, confusion, convulsions (may be followed by coma), delirium, dryness of mucous membranes, euphoria, flushing, hallucinations, headache, hyperpyrexia, hyperreflexia, hypertension, muscle twitching, mydriasis, palpitations, sweating, tachycardia, tremors, and vomiting.

➤*Treatment:* Treatment consists of appropriate supportive measures. The patient must be protected against self-injury and against external stimuli that would aggravate overstimulation already present. Gastric contents may be evacuated by gastric lavage as indicated. Before performing gastric lavage, control agitation and seizures if present and protect the airway. Other measures to detoxify the gut include administration of activated charcoal and a cathartic. Intensive care must be provided to maintain adequate circulation and respiratory exchange; external cooling procedures may be required for hyperpyrexia.

When treating overdose, practitioners should bear in mind that there is a prolonged release of dexmethylphenidate from dexmethylphenidate ER capsules.

Efficacy of peritoneal dialysis for dexmethylphenidate overdosage has not been established.

As with the management of all overdosage, consider the possibility of multiple drug ingestion. Consider contacting a poison control center (1-800-222-1222) for up-to-date information on the management of overdosage with methylphenidate.

Patient Information

Advise patients that the dexmethylphenidate ER capsules may be swallowed as whole capsules or the capsule may be opened and sprinkled on a small amount of applesauce. Do not crush, chew, or divide the capsule.

Advise patients that dexmethylphenidate ER is to be taken once a day in the morning.

Advise patient to take dexmethylphenidate immediate release twice daily, at least 4 hours apart. May be taken with or without food.

Advise patients to report to their health care provider any changes in vision.

METHYLPHENIDATE HYDROCHLORIDE

c-ii	**Methylphenidate Hydrochloride** (Various, eg, Sandoz, Watson)	**Tablets; oral:** 5 mg	In 100s and 1,000s.
c-ii	**Methylin** (Mallinckrodt)		Lactose. (5 M). In 100s and 1,000s. Color-additive free.
c-ii	**Ritalin** (Novartis)		Lactose, sucrose. (CIBA 7). Yellow. In 100s.
c-ii	**Methylphenidate Hydrochloride** (Various, eg, Sandoz, Watson)	**Tablets; oral:** 10 mg	In 100s and 1,000s.
c-ii	**Methylin** (Mallinckrodt)		Lactose. (10 M). Scored. In 100s and 1,000s. Color-additive free.
c-ii	**Ritalin** (Novartis)		Lactose, sucrose. (CIBA 3). Pale green, scored. In 100s.

METHYLPHENIDATE HYDROCHLORIDE

c-ii	**Methylphenidate Hydrochloride** (Various, eg, Sandoz, Watson)	**Tablets; oral:** 20 mg	In 100s and 1,000s.
c-ii	**Methylin** (Mallinckrodt)		Lactose. (20 M). Scored. In 100s and 1,000s. Color-additive free.
c-ii	**Ritalin** (Novartis)		Sucrose, lactose. (CIBA 34). Pale yellow, scored. In 100s.
c-ii	**Methylin** (Shionogi Pharma)	**Tablets, chewable; oral:** 2.5 mg	Aspartame, phenylalanine 0.42 mg. Maltose. (2.5 CHEW). White to cream color, rounded square. Grape flavor. In 100s.
		5 mg	Aspartame, phenylalanine 0.84 mg. Maltose. (5 CHEW). White to cream color, rounded square. Grape flavor. In 100s.
		10 mg	Aspartame, phenylalanine 1.68 mg. Maltose. (10 CHEW). White to cream color, rounded square. Grape flavor. In 100s.
c-ii	**Metadate ER** (UCB)	**Tablets, extended-release; oral:** 10 mg	Lactose. Color-additive free. (561 MD). Oval. In 100s.
c-ii	**Methylin ER** (Mallinckrodt)		Color-additive free. (1423 M). White to off-white. In 100s.
c-ii	**Concerta**[a] (Janssen)	**Tablets, extended-release; oral:** 18 mg	Lactose. (alza 18). Yellow. In 100s.
c-ii	**Methylphenidate Hydrochloride** (Various, eg, Sandoz, Watson)	**Tablets, extended-release; oral:** 20 mg	In 100s.
c-ii	**Metadate ER** (UCB)		Lactose. Color-additive free. (562 MD). In 100s.
c-ii	**Methylin ER** (Mallinckrodt)		Color-additive free. (1451 M). White to off-white. In 100s.
c-ii	**Concerta**[a] (Janssen)	**Tablets, extended-release; oral:** 27 mg	Lactose. (alza 27). Gray. In 100s.
c-ii	**Concerta**[a] (Janssen)	**Tablets, extended-release; oral:** 36 mg	Lactose. (alza 36). In 100s.
c-ii	**Concerta**[a] (Janssen)	**Tablets, extended-release; oral:** 54 mg	Lactose. (alza 54). Brownish-red. In 100s.
c-ii	**Ritalin-SR** (Novartis)	**Tablets, sustained-release; oral:** 20 mg	Lactose. Color-additive free. (CIBA 16). Coated. In 100s.
c-ii	**Metadate CD**[b] (UCB)	**Capsules, extended-release; oral:** 10 mg	Sugar spheres. (UCB 579 10 mg). Green/White. In 100s.
c-ii	**Ritalin LA**[c] (Novartis)		Sugar spheres. (NVR R10). White/Lt. brown. In 100s.
c-ii	**Metadate CD**[b] (UCB)	**Capsules, extended-release; oral:** 20 mg	Sugar spheres. (UCB 580 20 mg). Blue/White. In 100s.
c-ii	**Ritalin LA**[c] (Novartis)		Sugar spheres. (NVR R20). In 100s.
c-ii	**Metadate CD**[b] (UCB)	**Capsules, extended-release; oral:** 30 mg	Sugar spheres. (UCB 581 30 mg). Reddish-brown/white. In 100s.
c-ii	**Ritalin LA**[c] (Novartis)		Sugar spheres. (NVR R30). Yellow. In 100s.
c-ii	**Metadate CD**[b] (UCB)	**Capsules, extended-release; oral:** 40 mg	Sugar spheres. (UCB 582 40 mg). Yellow-ivory/white. In 100s.
c-ii	**Ritalin LA**[c] (Novartis)		Sugar spheres. (NVR R40). Lt. brown. In 100s.
c-ii	**Metadate CD**[b] (UCB)	**Capsules, extended-release; oral:** 50 mg	Sugar spheres. (UCB 583 50 mg). Purple/white. In 100s.
c-ii	**Metadate CD**[b] (UCB)	**Capsules, extended-release; oral:** 60 mg	Sugar spheres. (UCB 584 60 mg). In 100s.
c-ii	**Methylphenidate** (Breckenridge)	**Solution; oral:** 5 mg per 5 mL	Glycerin, PEG. Grape flavor. In 500 mL.
c-ii	**Methylin** (Shionogi Pharma)		Grape flavor. In 500 mL.
c-ii	**Methylphenidate** (Breckenridge)	**Solution; oral:** 10 mg per 5 mL	Glycerin, PEG. Grape flavor. In 500 mL.
c-ii	**Methylin** (Shionogi Pharma)		Grape flavor. In 500 mL.
c-ii	**Daytrana** (Shire)	**Patch; transdermal:** 10 mg per 9 h[d] (1.1 mg/h)	27.5 mg of total methylphenidate per patch. 12.5 cm^2. In 10s and 30s.
		15 mg per 9 h[d] (1.6 mg/h)	41.3 mg of total methylphenidate per patch. 18.75 cm^2. In 10s and 30s.
		20 mg per 9 h[d] (2.2 mg/h)	55 mg of total methylphenidate per patch. 25 cm^2. In 10s and 30s.
		30 mg per 9 h[d] (3.3 mg/h)	82.5 mg of total methylphenidate per patch. 37.5 cm^2. In 10s and 30s.

[a] The initial dose of *Concerta* is released from the outer coating within 1 hour, and the remainder is released at a controlled rate over 5 to 9 hours. Therefore, the total methylphenidate dose is released over 6 to 10 hours.

[b] The immediate-release beads comprise 30% of the total methylphenidate dose (ie, 6 mg of a 20 mg capsule) and provide the initial phase, rapid release of methylphenidate. The second set of beads provides the second extended-release phase of methylphenidate, and comprises 70% of the total methylphenidate dose (ie, 14 mg from a 20 mg capsule).

[c] Extended-release formulation using *Spheroidal Oral Drug Absorption System* (*SODAS*) technology, a bimodal release delivery system. Fifty percent of the contents are immediate-release beads to provide rapid onset. The second half of the contents consists of delayed-release beads that are released approximately 4 hours after administration. This delivery system mimics twice-daily administration of immediate-release methylphenidate.

[d] Nominal in vivo delivery rate per hour in children 6 to 12 years of age when applied to the hip, based on a 9-hour wear period.

METHYLPHENIDATE HYDROCHLORIDE — ORAL

WARNING

Drug dependence – Give methylphenidate cautiously to emotionally unstable patients such as those with a history of drug dependence or alcoholism, because such patients may increase dosage at their own initiative.

Long-term abusive use can lead to marked tolerance and psychological dependence with varying degrees of abnormal behavior. Frank psychotic episodes can occur, especially with parenteral abuse. Careful supervision is required during withdrawal, because severe depression as well as the effects of chronic overactivity can be unmasked. Withdrawal following long-term therapeutic use may unmask symptoms of the underlying disorder that may require follow-up. Long-term follow-up may be required because of the patient's basic personality disturbances.

Indications

➤*Attention deficit disorders/attention deficit hyperactivity disorder:* For the treatment of attention deficit disorders (ADD) and attention deficit hyperactivity disorder (ADHD) (previously known as minimal brain dysfunction in children).

➤*Narcolepsy (except Concerta, Metadate CD,* and *Ritalin LA)*: For the treatment of narcolepsy.

➤*Off-label uses:*

Traumatic brain injury – [3] = Safety concerns. The Neurobehavioral Guidelines Working Group assigned different levels to their recommendations for drug therapy of neurobehavioral sequelae of traumatic brain injury (TBI). They ranged from "options" to "guidelines" to the highest level of "standards," based on the quality of evidence available and the extent of efficacy observed. Methylphenidate was recommended at the guideline level for improving attentional function and speed of cognitive function. Methylphenidate was recommended at the option level for improving general cognitive functioning, learning, memory, and aggression in patients with moderate to severe TBI. Methylphenidate should be considered a therapeu-

METHYLPHENIDATE HYDROCHLORIDE — ORAL

tic option for all patients with TBI and problems with attention and cognitive function speed. For patients with TBI and problems with general cognition, learning, memory, or aggression, methylphenidate may be considered a treatment option, but the risks and benefits of therapy should be weighed for each patient.

Other possible off-label uses – Depression in medically ill (including stroke) elderly persons; improvement in pain control, sedation, or both in patients receiving opiates.

Administration and Dosage

➤*General dosing considerations:* Individualize dosage according to the needs and responses of the patient.

➤*Adults:*

Attention deficit disorders/attention deficit hyperactivity disorder –

Concerta:

• *18 to 65 years of age* –

Maximum dose: 72 mg/day.

Initial dosage: 18 or 36 mg/day for patients who are not currently taking methylphenidate or for patients who are on stimulants other than methylphenidate.

Dosage titration: Doses may be increased in 18 mg increments at weekly intervals for patients who have not achieved an optimal response at a lower dosage.

Maintenance dosage: 18 to 72 mg/day.

Extended-release capsules (Metadate CD and *Ritalin LA*):

• *Maximum dose* – 60 mg/day.

• *Initial dosage* – 20 mg once daily in the morning before breakfast. When in the judgement of the health care provider a lower initial dose is appropriate, patients may begin treatment with *Ritalin LA* 10 mg.

• *Dosage titration* – Dosage may be adjusted in weekly 10 to 20 mg increments (10 mg increments for *Ritalin LA*), depending on tolerability and degree of efficacy observed.

ER and SR tablets (Metadate ER, Methylin ER, and *Ritalin SR*): Methylphenidate ER and SR tablets have a duration of action of approximately 8 hours. Therefore, methylphenidate ER and SR tablets may be used in place of methylphenidate immediate-release tablets when the 8-hour dosage of methylphenidate ER and SR tablets corresponds to the titrated 8-hour dosage of methylphenidate IR.

Immediate-release tablets, chewable tablets, and oral solution:

• *Usual dosage* – 20 to 30 mg daily, administered in divided doses 2 or 3 times daily.

• *Dosage adjustment* – Some patients may require 40 to 60 mg daily. In others, 10 to 15 mg daily will be adequate.

Narcolepsy (except Concerta, Metadate CD, and *Ritalin LA)* –

Immediate-release tablets, chewable tablets, and oral solution:

• *Usual dosage* – 20 to 30 mg daily in divided doses, 2 or 3 times daily.

• *Dosage adjustment* – Some patients may require 40 to 60 mg daily. In others, 10 to 15 mg daily will be adequate.

Extended-release and sustained-release tablets (Metadate ER, Methylin ER, and *Ritalin SR*): See ADHD in Adults for dosing.

Off-label dosing –

Traumatic brain injury: [3] = Safety concerns. 0.25 to 0.3 mg/kg orally twice daily, continued through subacute or chronic periods of recovery if response is adequate.

➤*Children:*

Attention deficit disorders/attention deficit hyperactivity disorder –

Concerta:

• *13 to 17 years of age* –

Maximum dose: 72 mg/day, not to exceed 2 mg/kg/day.

Initial dosage: 18 mg/day for patients who are not currently taking methylphenidate or for patients who are on stimulants other than methylphenidate.

Dosage titration: Doses may be increased in 18 mg increments at weekly intervals for patients who have not achieved an optimal response at a lower dosage.

Maintenance dosage: 18 to 72 mg/day.

• *6 to 12 years of age* –

Maximum dose: 54 mg/day.

Initial dosage: 18 mg/day for patients who are not currently taking methylphenidate or for patients who are on stimulants other than methylphenidate.

Dosage titration: Doses may be increased in 18 mg increments at weekly intervals for patients who have not achieved an optimal response at a lower dose.

Maintenance dosage: 18 to 54 mg/day.

Extended-release capsules (Metadate CD and *Ritalin LA*):

• *6 years of age and older* – See ADHD in Adults for dosing.

Extended-release and sustained-release tablets (Metadate ER, Methylin ER, and *Ritalin SR*):

• *6 years of age and older* – See ADHD in Adults for dosing.

Immediate-release tablets, chewable tablets, and oral solution:

• *6 years of age and older* –

Maximum dose: 60 mg/day.

Initial dosage: 5 mg twice daily (before breakfast and lunch).

Dosage titration: Initiate methylphenidate in small doses, with gradual increments of 5 to 10 mg weekly.

Discontinuation of therapy: If improvement is not observed after appropriate dosage adjustment over a 1-month period, discontinue the drug.

Narcolepsy (except Concerta, Metadate CD, and *Ritalin LA)* –

Extended-release and sustained-release tablets (Metadate ER, Methylin ER, and *Ritalin SR*):

• *6 years of age and older* – See ADHD in Adults for dosing.

Immediate-release tablets, chewable tablets, and oral solution:

• *6 years of age and older* – See ADHD in Children for dosing.

Off-label dosing –

Attention deficit disorders/attention deficit hyperactivity disorder:

• *6 years of age and older* –

Maximum dose: 2 mg/kg/day or 60 mg/day.

Initial dosage: 0.3 mg/kg/dose (or 2.5 to 5 mg/dose) administered before breakfast and lunch.

Dosage titration: May increase by 0.1 mg/kg/dose (or 5 to 10 mg/day) weekly until maintenance dose is achieved. May give an extra afternoon dose if needed.

Maintenance dosage: 0.3 to 1 mg/kg/day.

➤*Conversion:*

Methylphenidate to Concerta – The recommended dosage of *Concerta* for patients who are currently taking methylphenidate 2 or 3 times daily at dosages of 10 to 60 mg/day is provided in the following table. Dosing recommendations are based on current dose regimen and clinical judgment. Conversion dosage should not exceed 72 mg daily.

Recommended Dosage Conversion from Methylphenidate Regimens to *Concerta*

Previous methylphenidate daily dosage	Recommended *Concerta* starting dosage
Methylphenidate 5 mg, 2 or 3 times daily	18 mg every morning
Methylphenidate 10 mg, 2 or 3 times daily	36 mg every morning
Methylphenidate 15 mg, 2 or 3 times daily	54 mg every morning
Methylphenidate 20 mg, 2 or 3 times daily	72 mg every morning

For other methylphenidate regimens, use clinical judgment when selecting the starting dose. A 27 mg strength is available for health care providers who wish to prescribe between the 18 and 36 mg doses.

Methylphenidate to Ritalin LA – The recommended dosage of *Ritalin LA* for patients currently taking methylphenidate twice daily or SR is provided in the following table.

Recommended Dosage Conversion From Methylphenidate Regimens to *Ritalin LA*

Previous methylphenidate dosage	Recommended *Ritalin LA* dosage
Methylphenidate 5 mg twice daily	10 mg once daily
Methylphenidate 10 mg twice daily, or methylphenidate SR 20 mg	20 mg once daily
Methylphenidate 15 mg twice daily	30 mg once daily
Methylphenidate 20 mg twice daily, or methylphenidate SR 40 mg	40 mg once daily
Methylphenidate 30 mg twice daily, or methylphenidate SR 60 mg	60 mg once daily

For other methylphenidate regimens, use clinical judgment when selecting a starting dosage. *Ritalin LA* dosage may be adjusted at weekly intervals in 10 mg increments.

➤*Dosage adjustment:* In general, dosage adjustment may proceed at approximately weekly intervals.

➤*Duration of therapy:* The efficacy of methylphenidate extended-release products (*Concerta, Metadate CD, Ritalin LA*) for long-term use (ie, for more than 4 weeks [*Concerta*], 3 weeks [*Metadate CD*], or 2 weeks [*Ritalin LA*]) has not been systematically evaluated in controlled trials.

There is no body of evidence available from controlled trials to indicate how long the patient with ADHD should be treated with methylphenidate. It is generally agreed, however, that pharmacological treatment of ADHD may be needed for extended periods. Nevertheless, the health care provider who elects to use methylphenidate for extended periods in patients with ADHD should periodically reevaluate the long-term usefulness of the drug for the individual patient with trials off the medication to assess the patient's functioning without pharmacotherapy.

➤*Discontinuation of therapy:* If improvement is not observed after appropriate dosage adjustment over a 1-month period, discontinue the drug.

If paradoxical aggravation of symptoms or other adverse reactions occur, reduce the dosage or, if necessary, discontinue the drug.

Drug treatment should not and need not be indefinite, and usually may be discontinued after puberty.

➤*Administration:*

Immediate-release tablets, chewable tablets, and oral solution – Administer IR tablets, chewable tablets, and oral solution in divided doses 2 or 3 times daily, preferably 30 to 45 minutes before meals. Patients who are unable to sleep if medication is taken late in the day should take the last dose before 6 pm.

Instruct patients to take methylphenidate chewable tablets with at least 240 mL (8 ounces) of water or other fluid. Taking this product without enough liquid may cause choking.

METHYLPHENIDATE HYDROCHLORIDE — ORAL

Extended-release and sustained-release tablets (Metadate ER, Methylin ER, and Ritalin SR) – Methylphenidate ER and SR tablets must be swallowed whole with the aid of liquids and never crushed, chewed, or divided.

Extended-release capsules (Metadate CD and Ritalin LA) – Methylphenidate ER capsules may be swallowed whole with the aid of liquids or, alternatively, may be administered by opening the capsule and sprinkling the capsule contents onto a small amount (tablespoon) of applesauce. The applesauce should not be warm because it could affect the modified-release properties of *Ritalin LA*. The mixture of drug and applesauce should be consumed immediately in its entirety. Drinking some fluids (eg, water) should follow the intake of the sprinkles with applesauce. The drug and applesauce mixture should not be stored for future use. Methylphenidate ER capsules and/or their contents should not be crushed, chewed, or divided.

Methylphenidate ER capsules are administered once daily in the morning before breakfast.

Concerta – Administer orally once daily in the morning, with or without food. *Concerta* must be swallowed whole with the aid of liquids and must not be chewed, divided, or crushed.

➤*Storage/Stability:*

Methylin IR, ER, chewable tablets, and oral solution – Store at 20° to 25°C (68° to 77°F). Protect tablets from moisture and light.

Concerta, Metadate CD, Ritalin, Ritalin LA, and *Ritalin SR* – Store at 25°C (77°F); excursions are permitted between 15° and 30°C (59° and 86°F). Protect from light, humidity, and moisture.

Metadate ER – Store at controlled room temperature between 15° and 30°C (59° and 86°F). Protect from moisture.

Actions

➤*Pharmacology:* Methylphenidate is a mild CNS stimulant. The mode of action in humans is not completely understood, but methylphenidate presumably activates the brain stem arousal system and cortex to produce its stimulant effect. Methylphenidate is thought to block the reuptake of norepinephrine and dopamine into the presynaptic neuron and increase the release of these monoamines into the extraneuronal space.

There is neither specific evidence that clearly establishes the mechanism whereby methylphenidate produces its mental and behavioral effects in children, nor conclusive evidence regarding how these effects relate to the condition of the CNS.

Methylphenidate is a racemic mixture comprised of the d- and l-threo enantiomers. The d-threo enantiomer is more pharmacologically active than the l-threo enantiomer.

➤*Pharmacokinetics:*

Absorption –

Methylphenidate Pharmacokinetic Parameters[a]							
Pharmacokinetic parameter	IR tablets	SR tablets	Chewable tablets	Oral Solution	*Metadate CD*	*Concerta*	ER tablets
T_{max}			1 to 2 h	1 to 2 h		6 to 10 h	
Adults	6.5 h					6.8 h	
Children	1.9 h	4.7 h			1.5 to 4.5 h		4.7 h
C_{max}	4.2 ng/mL		10 ng/mL	9 ng/mL	8.6 to 16.8 ng/mL	3.7 ng/mL	
AUC	38 ng•h/mL				63 to 120 ng•h/mL	41.8 ng•h/mL	
Half-life							
Adults	2.8 to 3.5 h	3.4 h	3 h	2.7 h	6.8 h	3.5 h	
Children	2.5 h						

[a] T_{max} = time of maximal concentration; C_{max} = maximal drug concentration; AUC = area under the curve.

Methylphenidate is rapidly absorbed. Methylphenidate in the ER and SR tablets is more slowly but as extensively absorbed as in the IR tablets. Relative bioavailability of the SR tablet compared with the IR tablet, measured by the urinary excretion of methylphenidate major metabolite (α-phenyl-2-piperidine acetic acid), was 105% (49% to 168%) in children and 101% (85% to 152%) in adults.

Concerta: *Concerta* once daily minimizes the fluctuations between peak and trough concentrations associated with methylphenidate IR 3 times daily. The relative bioavailability of *Concerta* once daily and methylphenidate 3 times daily in adults is comparable.

Metadate ER and *Methylin ER*: Pharmacokinetic and statistical analyses for a multiple-dose study demonstrated that 3 times daily administration of two *Metadate ER* and *Methylin ER* 10 mg tablets met the requirements for bioequivalence to one methylphenidate SR 20 mg tablet when administered every 8 hours. Pharmacokinetic parameters (ie, $AUC_{0-\infty}$, T_{max}, C_{max}, minimum plasma drug concentration [C_{min}], and average concentration [C_{av}]) demonstrated achievement of steady state following 3-times-daily administration of two *Metadate ER* and *Methylin ER* 10 mg tablets was confirmed. Bioavailability of *Metadate ER* and *Methylin ER* 20 mg tablets was compared with an SR reference product and an IR product. The extent of absorption for the 3 products was similar, and the rate of absorption of the 2 SR products was not statistically different.

Chewable tablets and oral solution: Methylphenidate chewable tablets and oral solution have been shown to be bioequivalent to methylphenidate IR tablets.

Metadate CD: *Metadate CD* capsules have a plasma/time concentration profile showing 2 phases of drug release with a sharp initial slope similar to a methylphenidate IR tablet, and a second rising portion approximately 3 hours later, followed by a gradual decline.

Ritalin LA: *Ritalin LA* produces a bimodal plasma concentration-time profile (ie, 2 distinct peaks approximately 4 hours apart) when orally administered to children diagnosed with ADHD and to healthy adults.

Food effects:

• *Chewable tablets and oral solution* – In a study in adult volunteers investigating the effects of a high-fat meal on the bioavailability of methylphenidate chewable tablets and oral solution at a dose of 20 mg, the presence of food delayed the peak concentrations by approximately 1 hour (chewable tablets: 1.5 hours fasted, 2.4 hours fed; oral solution: 1.7 hours fasted, 2.7 hours fed). Overall, a high-fat meal increased the C_{max} of methylphenidate oral solution by approximately 13%, and increased the AUC of methylphenidate chewable tablets and oral solution by approximately 20% and 25% on average, respectively. Through a cross-study comparison, the magnitude of food effect is found to be comparable between methylphenidate chewable tablets, oral solution, and the IR tablet.

• *Metadate CD* – In a study in adult volunteers to investigate the effects of a high-fat meal on the bioavailability of a dose of *Metadate CD* 40 mg, the presence of food delayed the early peak by approximately 1 hour (range, −2 to 5 hours of delay). The plasma levels rose rapidly following the food-induced delay in absorption. Overall, a high-fat meal increased the C_{max} of *Metadate CD* capsules by approximately 30% and AUC by approximately 17%, on average.

• *Metadate ER* and *Methylin ER* – The administration of the methylphenidate ER tablets with food resulted in a greater C_{max} and $AUC_{0-\infty}$ than when administered in a fasting condition.

• *Ritalin LA* – When *Ritalin LA* was administered with a high-fat breakfast to adults, *Ritalin LA* had a longer lag time until absorption began and variable delays in the time until the first peak concentration, the time until interpeak minimum, and the time until the second peak. The first peak concentration and the extent of absorption were unchanged after food, relative to the fasting state, although the second peak was approximately 25% lower.

Distribution – Binding to plasma proteins is low (10% to 33%), and the apparent distribution volume at steady state with intravenous (IV) administration has been reported to be approximately 6 L/kg.

Concerta: Plasma methylphenidate concentrations in adults and adolescents decline bioexponentially following oral administration.

Metabolism – In humans, methylphenidate is metabolized rapidly primarily via de-esterification to alpha-phenyl-piperidine acetic acid (PPA or ritalinic acid). The metabolite has little or no pharmacologic activity; therapeutic activity is principally due to the parent compound. Only small amounts of hydroxylated metabolites (eg, hydroxymethylphenidate and hydroxyritalinic acid) are detectable in plasma.

Ritalin LA: The absolute bioavailability of methylphenidate in children has been reported to be approximately 30% (range, 10% to 52%), suggesting pronounced presystemic metabolism.

Excretion – After oral dosing of radiolabeled methylphenidate in humans, approximately 90% of the radioactivity was recovered in urine. The main urinary metabolite was ritalinic acid, accounting for approximately 80% of the dose.

ER and SR tablets: An average of 67% of ER and SR tablet dose was excreted in children as compared with 86% in adults.

Metadate CD: The elimination process observed for *Metadate CD* is controlled by the release rate of methylphenidate from the ER formulation, and that the drug absorption is the rate-limiting process.

Ritalin LA: The rapid half-life of methylphenidate IR in both children and adults may result in unmeasurable concentrations between the morning and midday doses. No accumulation of methylphenidate is expected following multiple once-daily dosing with *Ritalin LA*. The half-life of ritalinic acid is approximately 3 to 4 hours.

After oral administration of an IR formulation of methylphenidate, 78% to 97% of the dose is excreted in the urine and 1% to 3% in the feces in the form of metabolites within 48 to 96 hours. Only small quantities (less than 1%) of unchanged methylphenidate appear in the urine. Most of the dose is excreted in the urine as ritalinic acid (60% to 86%), with the remainder being accounted for by minor metabolites.

Contraindications

Marked anxiety, tension, and agitation; glaucoma; patients with motor tics or a family history or diagnosis of Tourette syndrome; during treatment with a monoamine oxidase inhibitor (MAOI) and within a minimum of 14 days following discontinuation of an MAOI; patients known to be hypersensitive to methylphenidate or other components of the product(s).

Metadate CD, Metadate ER, and *Methylin ER* are contraindicated in patients with severe hypertension, angina pectoris, cardiac arrhythmias, heart failure, recent myocardial infarction (MI), hyperthyroidism, or thyrotoxicosis.

Warnings/Precautions

➤*Serious cardiovascular effects:*

Children and adolescents – Sudden death has been reported in association with CNS stimulant treatment at usual doses in children and adolescents with structural cardiac abnormalities or other serious heart problems. Although some serious heart problems alone carry an increased risk of sudden death, stimulant products generally should not be used in children or adolescents with known serious structural cardiac abnormalities, cardiomy-

METHYLPHENIDATE HYDROCHLORIDE — ORAL

opathy, serious heart rhythm abnormalities, or other serious cardiac problems that may place them at increased vulnerability to the sympathomimetic effects of a stimulant drug.

Adults – Sudden death, stroke, and MI have been reported in adults taking stimulant drugs at usual doses for ADHD. Although the role of stimulants in these adult cases is also unknown, adults have a greater likelihood than children of having serious structural cardiac abnormalities, cardiomyopathy, serious heart rhythm abnormalities, coronary artery disease, or other serious cardiac problems. Adults with such abnormalities should also generally not be treated with stimulant drugs.

Hypertension and other cardiovascular conditions – Stimulant medications cause a modest increase in average blood pressure (about 2 to 4 mm Hg) and average heart rate (about 3 to 6 beats/min), and patients may have larger increases. While the mean changes alone would not be expected to have short-term consequences, monitor all patients for larger changes in heart rate and blood pressure. Caution is indicated in treating patients whose underlying medical conditions might be compromised by increases in blood pressure or heart rate (eg, those with preexisting hypertension, heart failure, recent MI, or ventricular arrhythmia).

Assessing cardiovascular status – Ensure children, adolescents, or adults who are being considered for treatment with stimulant medications have a careful history (including assessment for a family history of sudden death or ventricular arrhythmia) and physical exam to assess for the presence of cardiac disease, and that they receive further cardiac evaluation if findings suggest such disease (eg, electrocardiogram [ECG] and echocardiogram). Ensure that patients who develop symptoms such as exertional chest pain, unexplained syncope, or other symptoms suggestive of cardiac disease during stimulant treatment undergo a prompt cardiac evaluation.

➤*Depression:* Do not use methylphenidate to treat severe depression of either exogenous or endogenous origin.

➤*Fatigue:* Do not use methylphenidate for the prevention or treatment of healthy fatigue states.

➤*Long-term suppression of growth:* Sufficient data on safety and efficacy of long-term use of methylphenidate in children are not yet available. Although a causal relationship has not been established, suppression of growth (ie, weight gain and/or height) has been reported with the long-term use of stimulants in children. Therefore, carefully monitor growth in patients requiring long-term therapy. Patients who are not growing or gaining height or weight as expected may need to have their treatment interrupted.

Careful follow-up of weight and height in children ages 7 to 10 years who were randomized to either methylphenidate or nonmedication treatment groups for more than 14 months, as well as in naturalistic subgroups of newly methylphenidate-treated and nonmedication-treated children for more than 36 months (to the ages of 10 to 13 years), suggests that consistently medicated children (ie, treatment for 7 days per week throughout the year) have a temporary slowing in growth rate (on average, a total of about 2 cm less growth in height and 2.7 kg less growth in weight over 3 years), without evidence of growth rebound during this period of development.

➤*Psychiatric effects:*

Preexisting psychosis – Administration of methylphenidate may exacerbate symptoms of behavior disturbance and thought disorder in patients with a preexisting psychotic disorder.

Bipolar illness – Particular care should be taken in using stimulants to treat ADHD in patients with comorbid bipolar disorder because of concern for possible induction of a mixed/manic episode in such patients. Prior to initiating treatment with a stimulant, adequately screen patients with comorbid depressive symptoms to determine if they are at risk for bipolar disorder; such screening includes a detailed psychiatric history, including a family history of suicide, bipolar disorder, and depression.

Emergence of new psychotic or manic symptoms – Treatment-emergent psychotic or manic symptoms (eg, hallucinations, delusional thinking, or mania in children and adolescents without a history of psychotic illness or mania) can be caused by stimulants at usual doses. If such symptoms occur, consider a possible causal role of the stimulant; discontinuation of treatment may be appropriate.

Aggression – Aggressive behavior or hostility is often observed in children and adolescents with ADHD, and has been reported in clinical trials and the postmarketing experience of some medications indicated for the treatment of ADHD. Although there is no systematic evidence that stimulants cause aggressive behavior or hostility, monitor patients beginning treatment for ADHD for the appearance of or worsening of aggressive behavior or hostility.

➤*Seizures:* There is some clinical evidence that methylphenidate may lower the convulsive threshold in patients with a history of seizures, with prior electroencephalogram (EEG) abnormalities in absence of seizures, and, very rarely, in absence of a history of seizures and no prior EEG evidence of seizures. In the presence of seizures, discontinue the drug.

➤*Visual disturbances:* Symptoms of visual disturbances have been encountered in rare cases. Difficulties with accommodation and blurring of vision have been reported with stimulant treatment.

➤*GI obstruction (Concerta only):* Because the *Concerta* tablet is nondeformable and does not appreciably change in shape in the GI tract, it should not be ordinarily administered to patients with preexisting severe GI narrowing (pathologic or iatrogenic) (eg, esophageal motility disorders, small bowel inflammatory disease, "short gut" syndrome caused by adhesions or decreased transit time, history of peritonitis, cystic fibrosis, chronic intestinal pseudo-obstruction, Meckel diverticulum). There have been rare reports of obstructive symptoms in patients with known strictures in association with the ingestion of drugs in nondeformable controlled-release formulations. Because of the controlled-release design of the tablet, only use *Concerta* in patients who are able to swallow the tablet whole.

➤*Prescribing methylphenidate:* Drug treatment is not indicated in all cases of this behavioral syndrome and should be considered only in light of the complete history and evaluation of the child. The decision to prescribe methylphenidate should depend on the health care provider's assessment of the chronicity and severity of the child's symptoms and the appropriateness for the child's age. Prescription should not depend solely on the presence of one or more of the behavioral characteristics.

➤*Acute stress reactions:* Treatment with methylphenidate is usually not indicated when symptoms are associated with an acute stress reaction.

➤*Phenylketonurics:* Phenylalanine is a component of aspartame. Each methylphenidate 2.5 mg chewable tablet contains phenylalanine 0.42 mg, each 5 mg chewable tablet contains phenylalanine 0.84 mg, and each 10 mg chewable tablet contains phenylalanine 1.68 mg.

➤*Agitation:* Patients with an element of agitation may react adversely; discontinue therapy if necessary.

➤*Drug abuse and dependence:* Methylphenidate is classified as a Schedule II controlled substance by federal regulation.

➤*Pregnancy: Category C.* Methylphenidate has been shown to have teratogenic effects in rabbits when given in dosages of 200 mg/kg/day.

In studies conducted in rats and rabbits, methylphenidate was administered orally at dosages of up to 75 and 200 mg/kg/day, respectively, during the period of organogenesis. Teratogenic effects (increased incidence of fetal spina bifida) were observed in rabbits at the highest dose, which is approximately 40 times the MRHD on a mg/m^2 basis. The no-effect level for embryo-fetal development in rabbits was 60 mg/kg/day (11 times the MRHD on a mg/m^2 basis). There was no evidence of specific teratogenic activity in rats, although increased incidences of fetal skeletal variations were seen at the highest dose level (7 times the MRHD on a mg/m^2 basis), which was also maternally toxic. The no-effect level for embryo-fetal development in rats was 25 mg/kg/day (2 times the MRHD on a mg/m^2 basis). When methylphenidate was administered to rats throughout pregnancy and lactation at dosages of up to 45 mg/kg/day, offspring body weight gain was decreased at the highest dosage (4 times the MRHD on a mg/m^2 basis), but no other effects on postnatal development were observed. The no-effect level for pre- and postnatal development in rats was 15 mg/kg/day (equal to the MRHD on a mg/m^2 basis).

A reproduction study in rats revealed no evidence of teratogenicity at oral doses of up to 30 mg/kg/day (approximately 15- and 3-fold the MRHD of *Concerta* on a mg/kg and mg/m^2 basis, respectively), 58 mg/kg/day (approximately 30- and 6-fold the MRHD of *Metadate CD* on a mg/kg and mg/m^2 basis, respectively), or 75 mg/kg/day (which is 62.5 and 13.5 times the MRHD of chewable tablets and oral solution on a mg/kg and mg/m^2 basis, respectively). However, this dose, which caused some maternal toxicity, resulted in decreased postnatal pup weights and survival when given to the dams from day 1 of gestation through the lactation period. The approximate plasma exposure to *Metadate CD* plus its main metabolite ritalinic acid in pregnant rats was 2 times that seen in trials in volunteers and patients with the maximum recommended dose of *Concerta* based on the AUC.

Therefore, until more information is available, do not prescribe methylphenidate for women of childbearing age, unless, in the opinion of the health care provider, the potential benefits outweigh the possible risks.

There are no adequate and well-controlled studies in pregnant women. Use methylphenidate during pregnancy only if the potential benefit justifies the potential risk to the fetus.

➤*Lactation:* It is not known whether methylphenidate is excreted in human milk. Because many drugs are excreted in human milk, exercise caution if methylphenidate is administered to a breast-feeding woman.

➤*Children:* Do not use methylphenidate in children younger than 6 years of age because safety and efficacy in this age group have not been established. Long-term effects of methylphenidate in children have not been well established.

➤*Elderly:* Per the Beers list, amphetamines have the potential for causing dependence, hypertension, angina, and myocardial infarction. Methylphenidate is also considered a high-risk medication for the elderly population according to the Centers of Medicare and Medicaid Services.

➤*Monitoring:* Periodic complete blood cell, differential, and platelet counts are advised during prolonged therapy.

Monitor blood pressure and heart rate at appropriate intervals in all patients taking methylphenidate, especially those with hypertension. Carefully monitor weight gain and/or height in children requiring long-term therapy. Also, monitor patients beginning treatment for the appearance of or worsening of aggressive behavior or hostility.

Drug Interactions

Methylphenidate Drug Interactions

Precipitant drug	Object drug[a]		Description
Antacids/Acid suppressants	Methylphenidate	⬇	Because the modified-release characteristics of *Ritalin LA* are pH dependent, the coadministration of antacids or acid suppressants could alter the release of methylphenidate.

METHYLPHENIDATE HYDROCHLORIDE — ORAL

Methylphenidate Drug Interactions			
Precipitant drug	Object drug[a]		Description
MAOIs (eg, isocarboxazid, phenelzine)	Methylphenidate	↑	Methylphenidate is contraindicated during treatment with an MAOI and also within a minimum of 14 days following discontinuation of an MAOI.
Methylphenidate	Anticonvulsants (eg, phenytoin, phenobarbital, primidone)	↑	Anticonvulsant levels may be increased, resulting in increased pharmacologic and toxic effects of the anticonvulsant.
Methylphenidate	Antidepressants (eg, SSRIs, tricyclics[b])	↑	Coadministration may cause an increased serum concentration of the tricyclic antidepressants and SSRIs, resulting in increased pharmacologic effects and adverse reactions of the antidepressants.
Methylphenidate	Antihypertensives (eg, guanethidine)	↓	Coadministration may cause decreased efficacy of antihypertensives.
Methylphenidate	Clonidine	↑	Serious adverse reactions have been reported with coadministration.
Methylphenidate	Coumarin anticoagulants	↑	Human pharmacologic studies have shown that methylphenidate may inhibit the metabolism of coumarin anticoagulants. Monitor coagulation times when initiating or discontinuing methylphenidate.
Methylphenidate	Vasopressor agents (eg, norepinephrine, dobutamine)	↑	Because of possible adverse effects upon blood pressure, use cautiously with pressor agents.

[a] ↑ = object drug increased; ↓ = object drug decreased.
[b] SSRIs = selective serotonin reuptake inhibitors.

➤*Drug/Food interactions:*

Chewable tablets and oral solution – See Actions for more information.

Metadate CD – See Actions for more information.

Metadate ER and *Methylin ER* – See Actions for more information.

Ritalin LA – See Actions for more information.

Adverse Reactions

➤*Concerta:*

Concerta Adverse Reactions[a] in Children (≥ 1%)		
Adverse reaction	*Concerta* (n = 106)	Placebo (n = 99)
CNS		
Dizziness	2%	0%
Headache	14%	10%
Insomnia	4%	1%
GI		
Abdominal pain (stomachache)	7%	1%
Anorexia (loss of appetite)	4%	0%
Vomiting	4%	3%
Respiratory		
Cough increased	4%	2%
Pharyngitis	4%	3%
Sinusitis	3%	0%
Upper respiratory tract infection	8%	5%

[a] Reactions, regardless of causality, for which the incidence for patients treated with *Concerta* was at least 1% and greater than the incidence among placebo-treated patients. Incidence has been rounded to the nearest whole number.

Concerta Adverse Reactions[a] in Adolescents (≥ 2%)		
Adverse reaction	*Concerta* (n = 87)	Placebo (n = 90)
CNS		
Headache	9%	8%
Insomnia	5%	0%
GI		
Anorexia	2%	0%
Diarrhea	2%	0%
Vomiting	3%	0%
GU		
Dysmenorrhea	2%	0%
Respiratory		
Pharyngitis	2%	1%
Rhinitis	3%	2%
Miscellaneous		
Accidental injury	6%	3%
Fever	3%	0%

[a] Reactions, regardless of causality, for which the incidence for patients treated with *Concerta* was at least 2% and greater than the incidence among placebo-treated patients. Incidence has been rounded to the nearest whole number.

Tics – In a long-term uncontrolled study (N = 432 children), the cumulative incidence of new-onset tics was 9% after 27 months of treatment with *Concerta*. In a second uncontrolled study (N = 682 children), the cumulative incidence of new-onset tics was 1% (9/682 children). The treatment period was up to 9 months with mean treatment duration of 7.2 months.

Hypertension – In the laboratory classroom clinical trials in children (studies 1 and 2), both *Concerta* once daily and methylphenidate IR 3 times daily increased resting pulse by an average of 2 to 6 beats/min and produced average increases of systolic and diastolic blood pressure of roughly 1 to 4 mm Hg during the day, relative to placebo.

In the placebo-controlled adolescent trial (study 4), mean increases from baseline in resting pulse rate were observed with *Concerta*and placebo at the end of the double-blind phase (5 and 3 beats/min, respectively). Mean increases from baseline in blood pressure at the end of the double-blind phase for *Concerta* and placebo-treated patients were 0.7 and 0.7 mm Hg (systolic) and 2.6 and 1.4 mm Hg (diastolic), respectively.

➤*Metadate CD:*

Metadate CD Adverse Reactions (≥ 5%)[a]		
Adverse reaction	*Metadate CD* (n = 188)	Placebo (n = 190)
CNS		
Headache	12%	8%
Insomnia	5%	2%
GI		
Abdominal pain (stomachache)	7%	4%
Anorexia (loss of appetite)	9%	2%

[a] Reactions, regardless of causality, for which the incidence for patients treated with *Metadate CD* was at least 5% and more than the incidence among placebo-treated patients. Incidence has been rounded to the nearest whole number.

➤*Ritalin LA:* Adverse reactions with an incidence of more than 5% during the initial 4-week, single-blind *Ritalin LA* titration period of this study were anorexia, decreased appetite, headache, insomnia, and upper abdominal pain.

Ritalin LA Adverse Reactions (≥ 2%)		
Adverse reaction	*Ritalin LA* (n = 65)	Placebo (n = 71)
Anorexia	3.1%	0%
Insomnia	3.1%	0%

➤*Adverse reactions associated with discontinuation of treatment:*

Concerta – In the 4-week, placebo-controlled, parallel-group trial in children (study 3), 1 *Concerta*-treated patient (0.9% [1/106]) and 1 placebo-treated patient (1% [1/99]) discontinued because of an adverse reaction (sadness and increase in tics, respectively).

In the 2-week, placebo-controlled phase of a trial in adolescents (study 4), no *Concerta*-treated patients (0% [0/87]) and 1 placebo-treated patient (1.1% [1/90]) discontinued because of an adverse reaction (increased mood irritability).

In the 2 open-label, long-term safety trials (studies 5 and 6; one 24-month study in children 6 to 13 years of age and one 9-month study in child, adolescent, and adult patients treated with *Concerta*), 6.7% (101/1,514) of patients discontinued because of adverse reactions. These reactions with an incidence of more than 0.5% included the following: abdominal pain (0.7%), anorexia (0.7%), insomnia (1.5%), emotional lability (0.7%), nervousness (0.7%), and twitching (1%), .

Metadate CD – In the 3-week, placebo-controlled, parallel-group trial, 2 *Metadate CD*–treated patients (1%) and no placebo-treated patients discontinued because of an adverse reaction (pruritus and rash; abdominal pain, dizziness, and headache, respectively).

Ritalin LA – In the 2-week, double-blind treatment phase of a placebo-controlled, parallel-group study in children with ADHD, only 1 *Ritalin LA*–treated subject (1/65 [1.5%]) discontinued because of an adverse reaction (depression).

METHYLPHENIDATE HYDROCHLORIDE — ORAL

In the single-blind titration period of this study, subjects received *Ritalin LA* for up to 4 weeks. During this period a total of 6 subjects (6/161 [3.7%]) discontinued because of adverse reactions. The adverse reactions leading to discontinuation were anger (in 2 patients), anxiety, depressed mood, fatigue, hypomania, lethargy, and migraine.

➤*IR/ER/SR tablets, chewable tablets, and oral solution:*

Most common – Nervousness and insomnia are the most common adverse reactions but are usually controlled by reducing dosage and omitting the drug in the afternoon or evening.

Other reactions include the following:

Cardiovascular – Angina, blood pressure increased/decreased, cardiac arrhythmia, palpitations, pulse increased/decreased, tachycardia.

CNS – Dizziness, drowsiness, dyskinesia, headache, Tourette syndrome (rare), toxic psychosis.

GI – Abdominal pain, anorexia, nausea.

Hypersensitivity – Hypersensitivity (including skin rash, urticaria, fever, arthralgia, exfoliative dermatitis, erythema multiforme with histopathological findings of necrotizing vasculitis, and thrombocytopenic purpura).

Miscellaneous – Weight loss during prolonged therapy.

Children – In children, abdominal pain, insomnia, loss of appetite, weight loss during prolonged therapy, and tachycardia may occur more frequently; however, any of the other adverse reactions previously listed may also occur.

Other (causal relationship not established) – Aggressive behavior; anemia and/or leukopenia; isolated cases of cerebral arteritis and/or occlusion; transient depressed mood; a few instances of scalp hair loss; instances of abnormal liver function (ranging from transaminase elevation to hepatic coma).

Neuroleptic malignant syndrome: Very rare reports of neuroleptic malignant syndrome (NMS) of have been received, and, in most of these, patients were concurrently receiving therapies associated with NMS. In a single report, a boy 10 years of age who had been taking methylphenidate for approximately 18 months experienced an NMS-like event within 45 minutes of ingesting his first dose of venlafaxine. It is uncertain whether this case represented a drug-drug interaction, a response to either drug alone, or some other cause.

➤*Postmarketing:*

Cardiovascular – Cardiac arrest.

CNS – Abnormal behavior, aggression, anxiety, depression, hyperactivity, irritability, suicidal behavior (including complete suicide).

Miscellaneous – Fixed drug eruption, sudden death, thrombocytopenia.

Concerta – Postmarketing experiences with *Concerta* have revealed spontaneous reports of the following adverse reactions: abnormal liver function tests (eg, transaminase elevation), alopecia, arrhythmia, arthralgia, blood alkaline phosphatase increased; blood bilirubin increased, blurred vision, bradycardia, chest discomfort, confusional state, difficulties in visual accommodation, disorientation, drug effect decreased, erythema, hyperhidrosis, hyperpyrexia, hypersensitivity reactions (eg, angioedema, anaphylactic reactions, auricular swelling, bullous conditions, exfoliative conditions, urticarias, pruritus [not elsewhere classified], rashes, eruptions, and exanthemas [not elsewhere classified]), leukopenia, myalgia, muscle twitching, mydriasis, palpitations, pancytopenia, platelet count decreased, Raynaud phenomenon, restlessness, therapeutic response decreased, thrombocytopenia, weight decreased, white blood cell count abnormal.

Overdosage

➤*Symptoms:* Signs and symptoms of acute overdosage, resulting principally from overstimulation of the CNS and from excessive sympathomimetic effects, may include the following: agitation, cardiac arrhythmias, confusion, convulsions (may be followed by coma), delirium, dryness of mucous membranes, euphoria, flushing, hallucinations, headache, hyperpyrexia, hyperreflexia, hypertension, muscle twitching, mydriasis, palpitations, sweating, tachycardia, tremors, vomiting.

➤*Treatment:* Consult with a certified poison control center for up-to-date guidance and advice regarding treatment. As with the management of all overdosage, consider the possibility of multiple drug ingestion.

Treatment consists of appropriate supportive measures. The patient must be protected against self-injury and against external stimuli that would aggravate overstimulation already present. Gastric contents may be evacuated by gastric lavage. In the presence of severe intoxication, use a carefully titrated dosage of a short-acting barbiturate before performing gastric lavage. Before performing gastric lavage, control agitation and seizures, if present, and protect the airway. Other measures to detoxify the gut include administration of activated charcoal and a cathartic. Intensive care must be provided to maintain adequate circulation and respiratory exchange; external cooling procedures may be required for hyperpyrexia.

Efficacy of peritoneal dialysis or extracorporeal hemodialysis for methylphenidate overdosage has not been established; also, dialysis is considered unlikely to be of benefit because of the large volume of distribution of methylphenidate.

Consider the prolonged release of methylphenidate from *Concerta*, *Metadate CD*, and *Ritalin LA* when treating patients with overdose.

Patient Information

Inform patients, their families, and their caregivers about the benefits and risks associated with treatment with methylphenidate and counsel them in its appropriate use. Instruct patients to read the provided Medication Guide and assist them in understanding its contents. Give patients the opportunity to discuss the contents of the Medication Guide and answer any questions they may have.

Instruct patients to swallow methylphenidate ER/SR tablets whole with the aid of liquids. Tablets should not be chewed, divided, or crushed.

Concerta is contained within a nonabsorbable shell designed to release the drug at a controlled rate. The tablet shell, along with insoluble core components, is eliminated from the body; instruct patients not be concerned if they occasionally notice something that looks like a tablet in their stool.

Instruct patients using *Ritalin LA/Metadate CD* to take 1 dose in the morning before breakfast. Instruct them that the capsule may be swallowed whole, or, alternatively, the capsule may be opened and the capsule contents sprinkled onto a small amount (1 tablespoon) of applesauce and given immediately, and not stored for future use. The capsules and the capsule contents must not be crushed or chewed.

Taking methylphenidate chewable tablets without adequate fluid may cause them to swell and block the throat or esophagus and may cause choking. Instruct patients to take methylphenidate chewable tablets (child or adult dose) with at least 8 ounces (a full glass) of water or other fluid. Advise patients not to take this product if they have difficulty swallowing. Instruct patients to seek immediate medical attention if they experience chest pain, vomiting, or difficulty in swallowing or breathing after taking this product.

Each methylphenidate 2.5 mg chewable tablet contains phenylalanine 0.42 mg, each 5 mg chewable tablet contains phenylalanine 0.84 mg, and each 10 mg chewable tablet contains phenylalanine 1.68 mg.

It is very important that ADHD be accurately diagnosed and that the need for medication be carefully assessed. It is important to remember that methylphenidate is only part of the overall management of ADHD. Parents, teachers, health care providers, and other professionals are part of a team that must work together.

Abuse of methylphenidate can lead to dependence. Advise patients to inform the health care provider of any abuse or dependence on alcohol or drugs, or if they are now abusing or dependent on alcohol or drugs. Misuse of stimulants may be associated with sudden death and serious cardiovascular adverse reactions.

METHYLPHENIDATE — TRANSDERMAL

WARNING

Drug dependence – Give methylphenidate cautiously to patients with a history of drug dependence or alcoholism.

Chronic abusive use can lead to marked tolerance and psychological dependence, with varying degrees of abnormal behavior. Frank psychotic episodes can occur, especially with parenteral abuse. Careful supervision is required during withdrawal from abusive use because severe depression may occur. Withdrawal following chronic therapeutic use may unmask symptoms of the underlying disorder that may require follow-up

Indications

➤*Attention deficit hyperactivity disorder (ADHD):* For the treatment of ADHD.

Administration and Dosage

➤*General dosing considerations:* Dose titration, final dosage, and wear time should be individualized according to the needs and response of the patient. Individualization of wear time may help manage some of the adverse reactions caused by methylphenidate.

Residual methylphenidate remains in patches that have been used when they are worn as recommended.

➤*Adults:*

Attention deficit hyperactivity disorder –

Usual dosage: Dosage should be titrated to effect. The recommended dose titration schedule is shown in the following table. It is recommended that methylphenidate transdermal be applied to the hip area 2 hours before an effect is needed and be removed 9 hours after application. The patch may be removed earlier than 9 hours if a shorter duration of effect is desired or late day adverse effects appear.

Methylphenidate Transdermal Recommended Titration Schedule (Patients New to Methylphenidate)

	Upward titration, if response is not maximized			
	Week 1	Week 2	Week 3	Week 4
Patch size	12.5 cm^2	18.75 cm^2	25 cm^2	37.5 cm^2
Nominal delivered dose[a] (mg per 9 h)	10 mg	15 mg	20 mg	30 mg
Delivery rate[a]	1.1 mg/h[a]	1.6 mg/h[a]	2.2 mg/h[a]	3.3 mg/h[a]

[a] Nominal in vivo delivery rate in children 6 to 12 years of age when applied to the hip, based on a 9-hour wear period.

Dosage adjustment: If aggravation of symptoms or other adverse reactions occur, the dosage or wear time should be reduced, or, if necessary, the drug should be discontinued.

Duration of therapy: The health care provider who elects to use methylphenidate for extended periods in patients with attention deficit hyperactiv-

METHYLPHENIDATE — TRANSDERMAL

ity disorder (ADHD) should periodically reevaluate the long-term usefulness of the drug for the individual patient with periods off medication to assess the patient's functioning without pharmacotherapy. Improvement may be sustained when the drug is either temporarily or permanently discontinued.

Conversion: Patients converting from another formulation of methylphenidate should follow the previous titration schedule.

➤*Children:* See Adults for dosing for children 6 years of age and older.

➤*Administration:* For transdermal use only.

Apply the patch immediately on removal from the protective pouch.

Application – The parent or caregiver should be encouraged to use the administration chart included with each carton of transdermal methylphenidate to monitor application and removal time and method of disposal. If a patch was removed without the parent or caregiver's knowledge, or if a patch is missing from the tray, the parent or caregiver should be encouraged to ask the child when and how the patch was removed.

The adhesive side of the patch should be placed on a clean, dry area of the hip. The area selected should not be oily, damaged, or irritated. Apply patch to the hip area. Avoid the waistline because clothing may cause the patch to rub off. When applying the patch, place on the opposite hip at a new site if possible.

The patch should be applied immediately after opening the pouch and removing the protective liner. Do not use if the pouch seal is broken. The patch should then be pressed firmly in place with the palm of the hand for approximately 30 seconds, making sure that there is good contact of the patch with the skin, especially around the edges. After proper application, bathing, swimming, or showering have not been shown to affect patch adherence. In the unlikely event that a patch should fall off, a new patch may be applied at a different site, but the total recommended wear time for that day should remain 9 hours.

Disposal – Upon removal, used patches should be folded so that the adhesive side of the patch adheres to itself and should be flushed down the toilet or disposed of in an appropriate lidded container. If the patient stops using the prescription, each unused patch should be removed from its pouch, separated from the protective liner, folded onto itself, and flushed down the toilet or disposed of in an appropriate lidded container.

➤*Storage/Stability:* Do not store patches unpouched. Store at 25°C (77°F); excursions are permitted to 15° to 30°C (59° to 86°F). Once the tray is opened, use contents within 2 months.

Anorexiants

Indications

➤*Obesity:* In addition to the nonamphetamine anorexiants included in this section, amphetamines are also used for short-term obesity therapy.

➤*Exogenous obesity:* As a short-term adjunct in a regimen of weight reduction based on caloric restriction. Measure the limited usefulness of these agents against their inherent risks. Refer to individual monographs for extended indications.

Actions

➤*Pharmacology:* Adrenergic agents (eg, **diethylpropion**, **benzphetamine**, **phendimetrazine**, **phentermine**) act by modulating central norepinephrine and dopamine receptors through the promotion of catecholamine release. Aside from phentermine, other adrenergic agents are infrequently used, perhaps because of the lack of long-term, well-controlled data or the fear of their potential abuse. Older adrenergic weight-loss drugs (eg, amphetamine, methamphetamine, phenmetrazine), which strongly engage in dopamine pathways, are no longer recommended because of the risk of their abuse.

➤*Pharmacokinetics:*

Distribution – **Diethylpropion** is rapidly absorbed from the GI tract after oral administration and is extensively metabolized through a complex pathway of biotransformation involving N-dealkylation and reduction. Many of these metabolites are biologically active and may participate in the therapeutic action of diethylpropion. Diethylpropion and its active metabolites are believed to cross the blood-brain barrier and the placenta, and are excreted mainly by the kidneys with 75% to 106% of the dose recovered in the urine within 48 hours after dosing. The plasma half-life of the aminoketone metabolites is ≈ 4 to 6 hours.

Excretion – Most of the drugs and their metabolites are excreted via the kidneys. The average half-lives for **phendimetrazine** are ≈ 1.9 hours for *Bontril PDM*, 9.8 hours for *Bontril*, and 3.7 hours for *Prelu-2*.

Contraindications

Advanced arteriosclerosis; symptomatic cardiovascular disease; moderate-to-severe hypertension; hyperthyroidism; known hypersensitivity or idiosyncrasy to sympathomimetic amines; glaucoma; highly nervous or agitated states; history of drug abuse; during or within 14 days following the administration of MAO inhibitors (hypertensive crises may result); coadministration with other CNS stimulants.

➤*Pregnancy:* *Category X*. **Benzphetamine hydrochloride** is contraindicated during pregnancy (see Warnings).

Warnings/Precautions

➤*Tolerance:* Tolerance to the anorectic effects may develop within a few weeks. If tolerance to the anorectic effect develops, do not exceed the recommended dose in an attempt to increase the effect; rather, discontinue the drug.

➤*Other drugs:* These agents should not be used in combination with other anorectic agents, including prescribed drugs (eg, SSRIs [eg, fluoxetine, sertraline, fluvoxamine, paroxetine]), *otc* preparations, and herbal products. When using CNS-active agents, consider the possibility of adverse interactions with alcohol.

➤*Primary pulmonary hypertension (PPH):* PPH, a rare, frequently fatal disease of the lungs, has been reported to occur in patients receiving certain anorectic agents. The initial symptom of PPH is usually dyspnea. Other initial symptoms include the following: Angina pectoris, syncope, or lower extremity edema. Advise patients to report immediately any deterioration in exercise tolerance. Discontinue treatment in patients who develop new, unexplained symptoms of dyspnea, angina pectoris, syncope, or lower extremity edema.

➤*Valvular heart disease:* Serious regurgitant cardiac valvular disease, primarily affecting the mitral, aortic, or tricuspid valves, has been reported in otherwise healthy people who had taken certain anorectic agents in combination for weight loss. The etiology of these valvulopathies has not been established and their course in individuals after the drugs are stopped is not known.

➤*Psychological disturbances:* Psychological disturbances occurred in patients who received an anorectic agent together with a restrictive diet.

➤*Cardiovascular disease:* Exercise caution in prescribing amphetamines for patients with even mild hypertension.

➤*Dispensing:* The least amount feasible should be prescribed or dispensed at one time in order to minimize the possibility of overdosage.

➤*Convulsions:* Convulsions may increase in some epileptics receiving **diethylpropion**. Dose titration or drug discontinuance may be necessary.

➤*Diabetes:* Insulin requirements in diabetes mellitus may be altered in association with the use of anorexigenic drugs and the concomitant dietary restrictions.

➤*Tartrazine sensitivity:* Some of these products contain tartrazine, which may cause allergic-type reactions (including bronchial asthma) in susceptible individuals. Although the incidence of tartrazine sensitivity in the general population is low, it is frequently seen in patients who also have aspirin hypersensitivity. Specific products containing tartrazine are identified in the product listings.

➤*Drug abuse and dependence:* These drugs are chemically and pharmacologically related to the amphetamines, and have abuse potential. Intense psychological dependence and severe social dysfunction may occur. If this occurs, gradually reduce the dosage to avoid withdrawal symptoms (eg, extreme fatigue, sleep EEG changes, mental depression). Chronic intoxication is manifested by severe dermatoses, marked insomnia, irritability, hyperactivity, and personality changes. Psychosis, often clinically indistinguishable from schizophrenia, is the most severe manifestation.

➤*Hazardous tasks:* May produce dizziness, extreme fatigue, and depression after abrupt cessation of prolonged high-dosage therapy; patients should observe caution while driving or performing other tasks requiring alertness.

➤*Pregnancy:* (*Category X* - Benzphetamine hydrochloride. *Category B* - Diethylpropion. *Category C* - Phentermine, phendimetrazine). Safety for use during pregnancy has not been established. Use in women who are or who may become pregnant (especially those in the first trimester) only when clearly needed and when the potential benefits outweigh the potential hazards to the fetus.

In animal studies with **phendimetrazine**, conception rate was adversely affected, as well as survival and body weight of pups. Congenital malformations are associated with phendimetrazine use, but a causal relationship has not been proven. Animal and clinical studies have not shown a teratogenic potential for **diethylpropion**. Abuse of diethylpropion during pregnancy may result in withdrawal symptoms in the human neonate.

➤*Lactation:* Safety for use in the nursing mother has not been established. Amphetamines are excreted in human milk. Advise mothers taking amphetamines to refrain from nursing.

Diethylpropion and its metabolites are excreted in breast milk. Exercise caution when administering to a nursing woman.

➤*Children:* **Phendimetrazine** and **benzphetamine** are not recommended for use in children less than 12 years of age. **Diethylpropion** is not recommended for use in pediatric patients less than 16 years of age.

Phentermine – Safety and efficacy have not been established for *Adipex-P*, *Pro-Fast SA*, *ProFast HS*, and *Pro-Fast SR* are not recommended in patients less than 12 years of age. *Ionamin* is not recommended in children less than 16 years of age.

➤*Elderly:* Per the Beers list, anorexic agents have the potential for causing dependence, hypertension, angina, and myocardial infarction. **Benzphetamine**, **diethylpropion**, **phendimetrazine**, and **phentermine** are also considered high risk medications for the elderly according to the Centers of Medicare and Medicaid Services.

Drug Interactions

Phentermine may decrease the hypotensive effect of adrenergic neuron blocking drugs.

Precipitant drug	Object drug[b]		Description
	Anorexiant Drug Interactions[a]		
CNS stimulants (eg, amphetamine)	Anorexiants	↑	Additive CNS effects. Anorexiants should not be used with other CNS stimulants.
Anorexiants	CNS stimulants (eg, amphetamine)		
MAO inhibitors (eg, phenelzine)	Anorexiants	↑	Hypertensive crisis has resulted when sympathomimetic amines have been used concomitantly or within 14 days following use of MAO inhibitors. Coadministration is contraindicated.
Urinary acidifying agents (ie, ammonia chloride)	Anorexiants (ie, benzphetamine)	↓	Benzphetamine concentrations may be reduced and urinary excretion may be decreased, increasing the pharmacologic effects. Avoid agents that may acidify the urine, except in the treatment of overdosage.
Urinary alkalinizing agents (eg, sodium bicarbonate)	Anorexiants (ie, benzphetamine)	↑	Benzphetamine concentrations may be elevated and urinary excretion may be decreased, increasing the pharmacologic effects. Avoid agents that may alkalinize the urine, especially in overdose situations.
SSRIs	Anorexiants	↑	Increased sensitivity to effect of sympathomimetics and increased risk of "serotonin syndrome" may occur. Monitor patient for increased signs/symptoms of CNS effects.
Anorexiants	SSRIs		
Anorexiants	Guanethidine	↓	Anorexiants may decrease the hypotensive effect of guanethidine.
Anorexiants	Insulin	↔	Insulin requirements in diabetes mellitus may be altered in association with use of anorexigenic drugs and the concomitant dietary restrictions.
Anorexiants	TCAs	↑	Amphetamines may enhance the effects of tricyclic antidepressants.

[a] SSRIs = selective serotonin reuptake inhibitors; TCAs = tricyclic antidepressants.
[b] ↑ = object drug increased; ↓ = object drug decreased.

➤*Drug/Lab test interactions:* **Benzphetamine** may reduce retention and diagnostic efficacy of iobenguane, resulting in a false-negative iobenguane imaging test. Discontinuation of benzphetamine approximately 5 biological half-lives (approximately 72 hours) prior to iobenguane administration is recommended.

Adverse Reactions

➤*Cardiovascular:* Palpitations; tachycardia; arrhythmias (including ventricular); precordial pain; primary pulmonary hypertension or regurgitant cardiac valvular disease; elevation of blood pressure. ECG changes have been reported with **diethylpropion**; valvulopathy has been reported with diethylpropion very rarely, but the causal relationship is unknown. Isolated reports of cardiomyopathy have been associated with chronic amphetamine use.

➤*CNS:* Overstimulation; cerebrovascular accident; nervousness; restlessness; dizziness; insomnia; malaise; anxiety; euphoria; drowsiness; depression; agitation; dysphoria; dyskinesia; tremor; headache; psychotic episodes (rare); agitation; jitteriness; depression following withdrawal of the drug. An increase in convulsive episodes occurred in a few epileptics.

➤*GI:* Dry mouth; unpleasant taste; nausea; vomiting; abdominal discomfort; diarrhea; GI disturbances; constipation; stomach pain.

➤*GU:* Dysuria; polyuria; urinary frequency; impotence; menstrual upset; gynecomastia; changes in libido.

➤*Hematologic:* Bone marrow depression; agranulocytosis; leukopenia.

➤*Hypersensitivity:* Urticaria; rash; erythema.

➤*Ophthalmic:* Mydriasis; blurred vision.

➤*Miscellaneous:* Hair loss; muscle pain; excessive sweating; ecchymosis; flushing; dyspnea.

Overdosage

➤*Symptoms:*

CNS – Restlessness; tremor; tachypnea; hyperreflexia; hyperpyrexia; rhabdomyolysis; confusion; belligerence; assaultiveness; hallucinations; panic states. Depression and fatigue usually follow central stimulation.

Convulsions, coma, and death may result.

Cardiovascular – Arrhythmias (tachycardia); hypertension or hypotension; circulatory collapse.

GI – Nausea; vomiting; diarrhea; abdominal cramps.

➤*Treatment:* Includes symptomatic and supportive therapy. Refer to Management of Acute Overdosage.

Sedate patient with a barbiturate or another sedative, and employ gastric lavage. Give activated charcoal if ingestion was recent.

Experience with hemodialysis or peritoneal dialysis is inadequate to permit recommendations.

Patient Information

May cause insomnia; avoid taking medication late in the day.

Caution patients about concomitant use of alcohol or other CNS-active drugs and anorectic agents.

Weight reduction requires strict adherence to dietary restriction.

Do not take more frequently than prescribed.

Notify physician if palpitations, nervousness, or dizziness occurs.

Medication may cause dry mouth and constipation; notify physician if these become pronounced.

May produce dizziness or blurred vision; observe caution while driving or performing other tasks requiring alertness.

These drugs should generally be taken on an empty stomach.

Do not crush or chew sustained-release products.

BENZPHETAMINE HYDROCHLORIDE

c-iii	**Benzphetamine** (Various, eg, Boca, CorePharma, Paddock)	**Tablets; oral:** 50 mg	May contain lactose, PEG, sorbitol. In 30s, 90s, 100s, and 500s.
c-iii	**Didrex** (Pharmacia)		Lactose, sorbitol. (DIDREX 50). Peach, round, scored. In 100s and 500s.

BENZPHETAMINE HYDROCHLORIDE — ORAL

Complete and comparative prescribing information begins in the Anorexiants class monograph.

Indications

➤*Obesity:* Management of exogenous obesity as a short-term adjunct (a few weeks) in a regimen of weight reduction based on caloric restriction in patients with an initial body mass index of 30 kg/m^2 or higher who have not responded to appropriate weight-reducing regimen (diet and/or exercise) alone. Benzphetamine is indicated for use as monotherapy only.

Administration and Dosage

➤*Adults:*

Obesity –

Usual dosage: 25 to 50 mg 1 to 3 times daily.

Initial dosage: 25 to 50 mg once daily with subsequent increase in individual dose or frequency according to response.

➤*Children:*

Obesity – See Adults for dosing in children 12 years of age and older.

➤*Administration:* A single daily dose is preferably given mid-morning or mid-afternoon, according to the patient's eating habits.

In an occasional patient, it may be desirable to avoid late afternoon administration.

➤*Storage/Stability:* Store at 20° to 25°C (68° to 77°F).

DIETHYLPROPION HYDROCHLORIDE

c-iv	**Diethylpropion Hydrochloride** (Various, eg, Schein, Watson)	**Tablets**: 25 mg	In 100s.
c-iv	**Diethylpropion Hydrochloride** (Various, eg, Watson)	**Tablets, controlled release**: 75 mg	In 100s.

DIETHYLPROPION HYDROCHLORIDE — ORAL

Complete and comparative prescribing information begins in the Anorexiants group monograph.

Indications

➤*Obesity:* Management of exogenous obesity as a short-term adjunct (a few weeks) in a regimen of weight reduction based on caloric restriction in patients with an initial body mass index (BMI) of 30 kg/m^2 or higher and who have not responded to appropriate weight reducing regimen (diet and/or exercise) alone.

Administration and Dosage

➤*Adults:*

Obesity –

Immediate-release: 25 mg 3 times daily, 1 hour before meals, and in midevening if desired to overcome night hunger.

Controlled-release: 75 mg daily, swallowed whole, in midmorning.

➤*Children:* See Adults for dosing in patients 16 years of age and older.

➤*Storage/Stability:* Keep tightly closed. Store at room temperature, below 30°C (86°F).

PHENDIMETRAZINE TARTRATE

c-iii	**Phendimetrazine** (Various, eg, Eon, Major, Schein)	**Tablets; oral**: 35 mg	In 100s, 1000s, and 5000s.
c-iii	**Bontril PDM** (Valeant)		Sugar, isopropyl alcohol, lactose. (B 35 V). Green, white, and yellow layered; scored. In 100s and 1,000s.
c-iii	**Phendimetrazine** (Sandoz)	**Capsules, extended release; oral**: 105 mg	Sucrose. (E 5254). Brown/clear. In 100s and 1,000s.
c-iii	**Bontril Slow-Release** (Valeant)		(A 047). Green/Yellow. In 100s.
c-iii	**Melfiat-105 Unicelles** (Numark)		Sucrose. (NUMARK 1082). Orange/Clear. In 100s.
c-iii	**Prelu-2** (Roxane)		Sucrose. Celery/Green. In 100s.

PHENDIMETRAZINE TARTRATE — ORAL

Complete and comparative prescribing information begins in the Anorexiants group monograph.

Indications

➤*Obesity:* Management of exogenous obesity as a short-term adjunct (a few weeks) in a regimen of weight reduction based on caloric restriction.

Administration and Dosage

➤*Adults:*

Obesity –

Tablets:

• *Usual dosage* – 35 mg 2 or 3 times a day, 1 hour before meals.

Dosage should be individualized to obtain an adequate response with the lowest effective dosage. In some cases, one-half tablet (17.5 mg) per dose may be adequate.

• *Maximum dose* – Dosage should not exceed 2 tablets 3 times a day.

Capsules, sustained-release: 105 mg in the morning, taken 30 to 60 minutes before the morning meal.

➤*Children:* See Adults for dosing in patients 12 years of age and older.

➤*Administration:*

Tablets – Administer 2 or 3 times a day, 1 hour before meals.

Capsules, sustained-release – Administer 30 to 60 minutes before the morning meal.

➤*Storage/Stability:* Store at controlled room temperature, 15° to 30°C (59° to 86°F). Protect from moisture.

PHENTERMINE HYDROCHLORIDE

c-iv	**Phentermine Hydrochloride** (Various, eg, Eon)	**Capsules**: 15 mg phentermine resin	In 100s and 1000s.
c-iv	**Ionamin** (Celltech)		Lactose. (Ionamin 15). Yellow/gray. In 100s and 400s.
c-iv	**Phentermine Hydrochloride** (Various)	**Capsules**: 18.75 mg (equivalent to 15 mg phentermine base)	In 1000s.
c-iv	**Pro-Fast HS** (MCR American)		EDTA, benzyl alcohol, parabens. Gray/Yellow. In 100s.
c-i	**Phentermine Hydrochloride** (Various, eg, Amide, Eon)	**Capsules**: 30 mg (equivalent to 24 mg phentermine base)	In 100s and 1000s.
c-iv	**Ionamin** (Celltech)	**Capsules**: 30 mg phentermine resin	Lactose. (Ionamin 30). Yellow. In 100s.
c-iv	**Phentermine Hydrochloride** (Various, eg, Amide, Purepac)	**Tablets**: 37.5 mg (equivalent to 30 mg phentermine base)	In 100s and 1000s.
c-iv	**Adipex-P** (Gate)		Lactose, sucrose. (ADIPEX-P 9 9). Blue/White, oblong, scored. In 30s, 100s, and 1000s.
c-iv	**Phentermine Hydrochloride** (Various, eg, Amide, Geneva, Ivax, URL)	**Capsules**: 37.5 mg (equivalent to 30 mg phentermine base)	In 100s and 1000s.
c-iv	**Adipex-P** (Gate)		Lactose. (ADIPEX-P 37.5). Blue/White. In 100s.
c-iv	**Pro-Fast SR** (MCR American)		Sugar, tartrazine, EDTA, benzyl alcohol, parabens. Black/Yellow. In 100s.

PHENTERMINE HYDROCHLORIDE — ORAL

Complete and comparative prescribing information begins in the Anorexiants group monograph.

Indications

➤*Obesity:* Short-term (a few weeks) adjunct in a regimen of weight reduction based on exercise, behavioral modification and caloric restriction in the management of exogenous obesity for patients with an initial body mass index greater than or equal to 30 kg/m^2, or greater than or equal to 27 kg/m^2 in the presence of other risk factors (eg, hypertension, diabetes, hyperlipidemia).

Administration and Dosage

➤*General dosing considerations:* Dosage should be individualized to obtain an adequate response with the lowest effective dose.

➤*Adults:*

Obesity –

Usual dosage:

• *Capsules* – 15 to 30 mg at approximately 2 hours after breakfast for appetite control.

Administration of 1 capsule daily has been found to be adequate in suppression of the appetite for 12 to 14 hours.

• *Tablets* – 1 tablet daily, administered before breakfast or 1 to 2 hours after breakfast.

Dosage adjustment: The dosage may be adjusted to the patient's need. For some patients ½ tablet (18.75 mg) daily may be adequate, while in some cases it may be desirable to give ½ tablet (18.75 mg) 2 times a day.

➤*Children:*

Obesity – See Adults for dosing in children 17 years of age and older.

➤*Administration:* Administer capsules 2 hours after breakfast and tablets either before breakfast or 1 to 2 hours after breakfast.

PHENTERMINE HYDROCHLORIDE — ORAL

Late evening medication should be avoided because of the possibility of resulting insomnia.

➤*Storage/Stability:* Store at 15° to 30°C (59° to 86°F). Protect from moisture. Keep tightly closed.

PHENTERMINE RESIN — ORAL

Complete and comparative prescribing information begins in the Anorexiants group monograph.

Indications

➤*Obesity:* Short-term (a few weeks) adjunct in a regimen of weight reduction based on exercise, behavioral modification, and caloric restriction in the management of exogenous obesity for patients with an initial body mass index greater than or equal to 30 kg/m^2, or greater than or equal to 27 kg/m^2 in the presence of other risk factors (eg, hypertension, diabetes, hyperlipidemia).

Administration and Dosage

➤*Adults:*

Obesity – One capsule daily, before breakfast or 10 to 14 hours before bedtime. For individuals exhibiting greater drug responsiveness, phentermine resin 15 mg capsules will usually suffice. Phentermine resin 30 mg capsules are recommended for less responsive patients.

➤*Children:* See Adults for dosing in children 16 years of age and older.

➤*Administration:* Phentermine resin capsules should be swallowed whole.

Take capsule before breakfast or 10 to 14 hours before bedtime.

➤*Storage/Stability:* Store at 25°C (77°F); excursions permitted to 15° to 30°C (59° to 86°F). Keep out of the reach of children.

SIBUTRAMINE HYDROCHLORIDE

c-iv	**Meridia** (Abbott)	**Capsules; oral:** 5 mg	Lactose. (MERIDIA -5-). Blue/yellow. In 30s.
		10 mg	Lactose. (MERIDIA -10-). Blue/white. In 30s.
		15 mg	Lactose. (MERIDIA -15-). Yellow/white. In 30s.

SIBUTRAMINE HYDROCHLORIDE MONOHYDRATE — ORAL

Indications

➤*Obesity:* For the management of obesity, including weight loss and maintenance of weight loss; should be used in conjunction with a reduced-calorie diet.

Sibutramine is recommended for obese patients with an initial body mass index (BMI) greater than or equal to 30 kg/m^2, or greater than or equal to 27 kg/m^2 in the presence of other risk factors (eg, controlled hypertension, diabetes, dyslipidemia).

BMI is calculated by taking the patient's weight in kg and dividing by the patient's height in m^2. Metric conversions are as follows: lb ÷ 2.2 = kg; inches × 0.0254 = meters.

Administration and Dosage

➤*General dosing considerations:* If a patient has not lost at least 4 pounds in the first 4 weeks of treatment, consider reevaluation of therapy, which may include increasing the dose or discontinuing sibutramine.

➤*Adults:*

Obesity –

Maximum dose: Dosages above 15 mg daily are not recommended.

Initial dosage: 10 mg administered once daily with or without food.

Dosage titration: If there is inadequate weight loss, the dosage may be titrated after 4 weeks to a total of 15 mg once daily.

Blood pressure and heart rate changes should be taken into account when making decisions regarding dose titration.

Alternative dosage: The 5 mg dose should be reserved for patients who do not tolerate the 10 mg dose.

➤*Children:* See Adults for dosing in patients 16 years of age and older.

➤*Renal function impairment:* Use sibutramine with caution in patients with mild to moderate renal impairment. Do not use sibutramine in patients with severe renal function impairment, including those with end-stage renal disease on dialysis.

➤*Hepatic function impairment:* Do not use sibutramine in patients with severe hepatic dysfunction.

➤*Administration:* Sibutramine is administered once daily with or without food. In most clinical trials, sibutramine was given in the morning.

➤*Storage/Stability:* Store at 25°C (77°F); excursions are permitted to 15° to 30°C (59° to 86°F). Protect from heat and moisture.

Actions

➤*Pharmacology:* Sibutramine produces its therapeutic effects by norepinephrine, serotonin, and dopamine reuptake inhibition. Sibutramine and its major pharmacologically active metabolites (M_1 and M_2) do not act via release of monoamines.

Sibutramine exerts its pharmacological actions predominantly via its secondary (M_1) and primary (M_2) amine metabolites. The parent compound, sibutramine, is a potent inhibitor of serotonin (5-hydroxytryptamine [5-HT]) and norepinephrine reuptake in vivo, but not in vitro. However, metabolites M_1 and M_2 inhibit the reuptake of these neurotransmitters both in vitro and in vivo.

In human brain tissue, M_1 and M_2 also inhibit dopamine reuptake in vitro, but with approximately 3-fold lower potency than for the reuptake inhibition of serotonin or norepinephrine.

Potencies of Sibutramine, M_1 and M_2 as In Vitro Inhibitors of Monoamine Reuptake in Human Brain (Ki;nM)

	Serotonin	Norepinephrine	Dopamine
Sibutramine	298	5,451	943
M_1	15	20	49
M_2	20	15	45

A study using plasma samples taken from sibutramine-treated volunteers showed monoamine reuptake inhibition of norepinephrine was greater than serotonin, which was greater than dopamine; maximum inhibitions were 73% (norepinephrine), 54% (serotonin), and 16% (dopamine).

➤*Pharmacokinetics:*

Sibutramine Special Population Pharmacokinetic Parameters (15 mg Dose)

Study population	C_{max} (ng/mL)	T_{max} (h)	AUC[a] (ng•h/mL)	t½[b] (h)
Metabolite M_1				
Target population:				
Obese subjects (n = 18)	4 (42)	3.6 (28)	25.5 (63)	—
	3.2 to 4.8	3.1 to 4.1	18.1 to 32.9	
Special population:				
Moderate hepatic function impairment (n = 12)	2.2 (36)	3.3 (33)	18.7 (65)	—
	1.8 to 2.7	2.7 to 3.9	11.9 to 25.5	
Metabolite M_2				
Target population:				
Obese subjects (n = 18)	6.4 (28)	3.5 (17)	92.1 (26)	17.2 (58)
	5.6 to 7.2	3.2 to 3.8	81.2 to 103	12.5 to 21.8
Special population:				
Moderate hepatic function impairment (n = 12)	4.3 (37)	3.8 (34)	90.5 (27)	22.7 (30)
	3.4 to 5.2	3.1 to 4.5	76.9 to 104	18.9 to 26.5

[a] Calculated only up to 24 hours for M_1.
[b] t½ = reaction half-time.

Absorption – Sibutramine is rapidly absorbed from the GI tract (time to maximum concentration [T_{max}] of 1.2 hours) following oral administration and undergoes extensive first-pass metabolism in the liver (oral clearance of 1,750 L/h and half-life of 1.1 hour) to form the pharmacologically active mono- and didesmethyl metabolites M_1 and M_2. Peak plasma concentrations of M_1 and M_2 are reached within 3 to 4 hours. On the basis of mass balance studies, on average, at least 77% of a single oral dose of sibutramine is absorbed. The absolute bioavailability of sibutramine has not been determined.

Effect of food: Administration of a single dose of sibutramine 20 mg with a standard breakfast resulted in reduced peak M_1 and M_2 concentrations (27% and 32%, respectively) and delayed the time to peak by approximately 3 hours. However, the area under the curve (AUC) of M_1 and M_2 were not significantly altered.

Distribution – Radiolabeled studies in animals indicated rapid and extensive distribution into tissues: highest concentrations of radiolabeled material were found in the eliminating organs, liver, and kidney. In vitro, sibutramine, M_1, and M_2 are extensively bound (97%, 94%, and 94%, respectively) to human plasma proteins at plasma concentrations seen following therapeutic doses.

Metabolism – Sibutramine is metabolized in the liver, principally by the CYP-450 3A4 isoenzyme, to desmethyl metabolites, M_1 and M_2. These active metabolites are further metabolized by hydroxylation and conjugation to pharmacologically inactive metabolites, M_5 and M_6. Following oral administration of radiolabeled sibutramine, essentially all of the peak radiolabeled material in plasma was accounted for by unchanged sibutramine (3%), M_1 (6%), M_2 (12%), M_5 (52%), and M_6 (27%).

M_1 and M_2 plasma concentrations reached steady-state within 4 days of dosing and were approximately 2-fold higher than following a single dose. The

SIBUTRAMINE HYDROCHLORIDE MONOHYDRATE — ORAL

elimination half-lives of M_1 and M_2, 14 and 16 hours, respectively, were unchanged following repeated dosing.

Excretion – Approximately 85% (range, 68% to 95%) of a single orally administered radiolabeled dose was excreted in urine and feces over a 15-day collection period, with the majority of the dose (77%) excreted in the urine. Major metabolites in urine were M_5 and M_6; unchanged sibutramine, M_1, and M_2 were not detected. The primary route of excretion for M_1 and M_2 is hepatic metabolism, and for M_5 and M_6 is renal excretion.

Special populations –

Renal function impairment: The disposition of sibutramine metabolites (M_1, M_2, M_5, and M_6) was studied in patients with varying degrees of renal function. Sibutramine itself was not measurable.

In patients with moderate and severe renal function impairment, the AUC values of the active metabolite M_1 were 24% to 46% higher and the AUC values of M_2 were similar, as compared with healthy subjects. Cross-study comparison showed that the patients with end-stage renal disease on dialysis had similar AUC values of M_1 but approximately half of the AUC values of M_2 measured in healthy subjects (creatinine clearance [Ccr] 80 mL/min or more). The AUC values of inactive metabolites M_5 and M_6 increased 2- to 3-fold (range, 1- to 7-fold) in patients with moderate impairment (30 mL/min to less than Ccr = 60 mL/min) and 8- to 11-fold (range, 5- to 15-fold) in patients with severe impairment (Ccr 30 mL/min or less), as compared with healthy subjects. Cross-study comparison showed that the AUC values of M_5 and M_6 increased 22- to 33-fold in patients with end-stage renal disease on dialysis, as compared with healthy subjects. Approximately 1% of the oral dose was recovered in the dialysate as a combination of M_5 and M_6 during hemodialysis process, while M_1 and M_2 were not measurable in the dialysate.

Do not use sibutramine in patients with severe renal function impairment, including those with end-stage renal disease on dialysis.

Hepatic function impairment: In 12 patients with moderate hepatic function impairment receiving a single oral dose of sibutramine 15 mg, the combined AUCs of M_1 and M_2 were increased 24% compared with healthy subjects, while M_5 and M_6 plasma concentrations were unchanged. The observed differences in M_1 and M_2 concentrations do not warrant dosage adjustment in patients with mild to moderate hepatic function impairment. Do not use sibutramine in patients with severe hepatic function impairment.

Contraindications

History of coronary artery disease (eg, angina, history of myocardial infarction), congestive heart failure, tachycardia, peripheral arterial occlusive disease, arrhythmia or cerebrovascular disease (stroke or transient ischemic attack (TIA); patients with inadequately controlled hypertension more than 145/90 mm Hg; patients who are older than 65 years of age; patients receiving monoamine oxidase inhibitors (MAOIs); hypersensitivity to sibutramine or any of the inactive ingredients of sibutramine; a major eating disorder (anorexia nervosa or bulimia nervosa); patients taking other centrally acting weight-loss drugs.

Warnings/Precautions

➤*Blood pressure and pulse:* Sibutramine substantially increases blood pressure and/or pulse rate in some patients. Regular monitoring of blood pressure and pulse rate is required when prescribing sibutramine.

➤*Concomitant cardiovascular disease:* Sibutramine substantially increases blood pressure and/or pulse rate in some patients. Therefore, do not use sibutramine in patients with a history of coronary artery disease, congestive heart failure, arrhythmias, or stroke.

➤*Glaucoma:* Because sibutramine can cause mydriasis, use it with caution in patients with narrow-angle glaucoma.

➤*Causes of obesity:* Exclude organic causes of obesity (eg, untreated hypothyroidism) before prescribing sibutramine.

➤*Bleeding:* There have been reports of bleeding in patients taking sibutramine. While a causal relationship is unclear, caution is advised in patients predisposed to bleeding events and those taking concomitant medications known to affect hemostasis or platelet function.

➤*Gallstones:* Weight loss can precipitate or exacerbate gallstone formation.

➤*Pulmonary hypertension:* Certain centrally acting weight-loss agents that cause release of serotonin from nerve terminals have been associated with pulmonary hypertension, a rare but lethal disease. In premarketing clinical studies, no cases of pulmonary hypertension have been reported with sibutramine. Because of the low incidence of this disease in the underlying population, however, it is not known whether sibutramine may cause this disease.

➤*Seizures:* During premarketing testing, seizures were reported in less than 0.1% of sibutramine-treated patients. Use sibutramine with caution in patients with a history of seizures. Discontinue sibutramine in any patient who develops seizures.

➤*Renal function impairment:* Use sibutramine with caution in patients with mild to moderate renal function impairment. Do not use sibutramine in patients with severe renal function impairment, including those with end-stage renal disease on dialysis.

➤*Hepatic function impairment:* Patients with severe hepatic function impairment have not been systematically studied; therefore, do not use sibutramine in such patients.

➤*Drug abuse and dependence:*

Controlled substance – Sibutramine is a controlled substance in Schedule IV of the Controlled Substances Act.

Abuse and physical and psychological dependence – Carefully evaluate patients for history of drug abuse and follow such patients closely, observing them for signs of misuse or abuse (eg, development of tolerance, incrementation of doses, drug-seeking behavior).

➤*Hazardous tasks:* Although sibutramine did not affect psychomotor or cognitive performance in healthy volunteers, any CNS active drug has the potential to impair judgment, thinking, or motor skills.

➤*Pregnancy: Category C.* Radiolabeled studies in animals indicated that tissue distribution was unaffected by pregnancy, with relatively low transfer to the fetus. In rats, there was no evidence of teratogenicity at doses of 1, 3, or 10 mg/kg/day, generating combined plasma AUCs of the 2 major active metabolites up to approximately 32 times those following the human dose of 15 mg. In rabbits dosed at 3, 15, or 75 mg/kg/day, plasma AUCs greater than approximately 5 times those following the human dose of 15 mg caused maternal toxicity. At markedly toxic doses, Dutch Belted rabbits had a slightly higher than control incidence of pups with a broad, short snout; short, rounded pinnae; short tail; and, in some, shorter, thickened long bones in the limbs. At comparably high doses in New Zealand white rabbits, 1 study showed a slightly higher than control incidence of pups with cardiovascular anomalies, while a second study showed a lower incidence than in the control group.

No adequate and well-controlled studies with sibutramine have been conducted in pregnant women. The use of sibutramine during pregnancy is not recommended. Instruct women of childbearing potential to employ adequate contraception while taking sibutramine. Advise patients to notify their health care provider if they become pregnant or intend to become pregnant during therapy.

➤*Lactation:* It is not known whether sibutramine or its metabolites are excreted in human milk. Sibutramine is not recommended for use in breastfeeding women. Advise patients to notify their health care provider if they are breast-feeding.

➤*Children:* The efficacy of sibutramine in obese adolescents has not been adequately studied.

Sibutramine's mechanism of action inhibiting the reuptake of serotonin and norepinephrine is similar to the mechanism of action of some antidepressants. Pooled analyses of short-term, placebo-controlled trials of antidepressants in children and adolescents with major depressive disorder (MDD), obsessive compulsive disorder (OCD), and other psychiatric disorders have revealed a greater risk of adverse reactions representing suicidal behavior of thinking during the first few months of treatment in those receiving antidepressants. The average risk of such reactions in patients receiving antidepressants was 4%, twice the placebo risk of 2%.

The data are inadequate to recommend the use of sibutramine for the treatment of obesity in children.

➤*Elderly:* Clinical studies of sibutramine did not include sufficient numbers of patients 65 years of age and older to determine whether they respond differently from younger patients. In general, dose selection for an elderly patient should be cautious, reflecting the greater frequency of decreased hepatic, renal, or cardiac function, and of concomitant disease or other drug therapy.

➤*Monitoring:* Monitor blood pressure and pulse prior to starting therapy and at regular intervals during treatment.

Drug Interactions

Sibutramine Drug Interactions

Precipitant drug	Object drug[a]		Description
Alcohol	Sibutramine	⬆	Concomitant use of sibutramine and excess alcohol is not recommended.
Cimetidine	Sibutramine	⟷	Coadministration resulted in small increases in combined sibutramine metabolites (M_1 and M_2), plasma C_{max} (3.4%), and AUC (7.3%); these differences are unlikely to be of clinical significance.
Erythromycin	Sibutramine	⟷	Concomitant erythromycin resulted in small increases in sibutramine metabolites' AUC (less than 14%) for M_1 and M_2. A small reduction (11%) in C_{max} for M_1 and a slight increase (10%) in C_{max} for M_2 were observed.
Ketoconazole	Sibutramine	⟷	Coadministration resulted in moderate increases in sibutramine metabolites' AUC and C_{max} of 58% and 36% for M_1 and of 20% and 19% for M_2, respectively.

SIBUTRAMINE HYDROCHLORIDE MONOHYDRATE — ORAL

Sibutramine Drug Interactions			
Precipitant drug	Object drug[a]		Description
Sibutramine	Agents that may raise blood pressure or increase heart rate (eg, ephedrine, pseudoephedrine, other decongestants)	↑	These agents include decongestants, and cough, cold, and allergy products that contain agents such as ephedrine or pseudoephedrine. Use caution when using concurrently with sibutramine.
Sibutramine	CNS active drugs	↑	Caution is advised if the coadministration of sibutramine with other centrally acting drugs is indicated.
Sibutramine	MAOIs (eg, phenelzine, selegiline)	↑	In patients receiving MAOIs in combination with serotonergic agents (eg, fluoxetine, fluvoxamine, paroxetine, sertraline, venlafaxine), there have been reports of serious, sometimes fatal, reactions ("serotonin syndrome"). Because sibutramine inhibits serotonin reuptake, do not use concomitantly with an MAOI. Allow at least 2 weeks to elapse between discontinuation of an MAOI and initiation of treatment with sibutramine. Similarly, allow ≥ 2 weeks to elapse between discontinuation of therapy and initiation of treatment with an MAOI.
Sibutramine	SSRIs, ergot alkaloids (eg, dihydroergotamine), lithium, certain opioids (eg, dextromethorphan, meperidine, pentazocine, fentanyl), 5-HT_1 receptor agonists (eg, sumatriptan, zolmitriptan), tryptophan	↑	The serotonergic effects of these agents may be additive. A "serotonin syndrome" may occur. Coadministration of these agents is not recommended. Carefully monitor patients if concurrent use cannot be avoided.

[a] ↑ = object drug increased; ↔ = undetermined clinical effect.

➤*Drug/Food interactions:* Administration of a single dose of sibutramine 20 mg with a standard breakfast resulted in reduced peak M_1 and M_2 concentrations (27% and 32%, respectively), and delayed the time to peak by approximately 3 hours. However, the AUCs of M_1 and M_2 were not significantly altered.

Adverse Reactions

In placebo-controlled studies, the most common reactions were dry mouth, anorexia, insomnia, constipation, and headache. Adverse reactions in these studies occurring in greater than or equal to 1% of sibutramine-treated patients and more frequently than in the placebo group are shown in the following table.

Sibutramine Adverse Reactions (≥ 1%)		
Adverse reaction	Sibutramine (n = 2,068) % incidence	Placebo (n = 884) % incidence
Cardiovascular		
Hypertension/Increased blood pressure	2.1%	0.9%
Migraine	2.4%	2%
Palpitation	2%	0.8%
Tachycardia	2.6%	0.6%
Vasodilation	2.4%	0.9%
CNS		
Anxiety	4.5%	3.4%
CNS stimulation	1.5%	0.5%
Depression	4.3%	2.5%
Dizziness	7%	3.4%
Emotional lability	1.3%	0.6%
Headache	30.3%	18.6%
Insomnia	10.7%	4.5%
Nervousness	5.2%	2.9%
Paresthesia	2%	0.5%
Somnolence	1.7%	0.9%
Dermatologic		
Acne	1%	0.8%
Cough increased	3.8%	3.3%
Herpes simplex	1.3%	1%
Rash	3.8%	2.5%
Sweating	2.5%	0.9%
GI		
Abdominal pain	4.5%	3.6%
Anorexia	13%	3.5%
Constipation	11.5%	6%
Dry mouth	17.2%	4.2%
Dyspepsia	5%	2.6%
Gastritis	1.7%	1.2%
Increased appetite	8.7%	2.7%
Nausea	5.9%	2.8%
Rectal disorder	1.2%	0.5%
Vomiting	1.5%	1.4%
GU		
Dysmenorrhea	3.5%	1.4%
Metrorrhagia	1%	0.8%
Urinary tract infection	2.3%	2%
Vaginal monilia	1.2%	0.5%
Metabolic/Nutritional		
Generalized edema	1.2%	0.8%
Thirst	1.7%	0.9%
Musculoskeletal		
Arthralgia	5.9%	5%
Joint disorder	1.1%	0.6%
Myalgia	1.9%	1.1%
Tenosynovitis	1.2%	0.5%
Respiratory		
Laryngitis	1.3%	0.9%
Pharyngitis	10%	8.4%
Rhinitis	10.2%	7.1%
Sinusitis	5%	2.6%
Special senses		
Ear disorder	1.7%	0.9%
Ear pain	1.1%	0.7%
Taste perversion	2.2%	0.8%
Miscellaneous		
Allergic reaction	1.5%	0.8%
Asthenia	5.9%	5.3%
Back pain	8.2%	5.5%
Chest pain	1.8%	1.2%
Flu syndrome	8.2%	5.8%
Injury accident	5.9%	4.1%
Neck pain	1.6%	1.1%

➤*Premarketing studies:* The following adverse reactions were reported in greater than or equal to 1% of all patients who received sibutramine in controlled and uncontrolled premarketing studies.

CNS – Abnormal thinking, agitation, hypertonia, leg cramps (at least 1%).

GI – Diarrhea, flatulence, gastroenteritis, tooth disorder (at least 1%).

Respiratory – Bronchitis, dyspnea (at least 1%).

Miscellaneous – Amblyopia, arthritis, fever, menstrual disorder, peripheral edema, pruritus (at least 1%).

➤*Hematologic:* Ecchymosis (bruising) was observed in 0.7% of sibutramine-treated patients and in 0.2% of placebo-treated patients in premarketing placebo-controlled obesity studies. One patient had prolonged

SIBUTRAMINE HYDROCHLORIDE MONOHYDRATE — ORAL

bleeding of a small amount, which occurred during minor facial surgery. Sibutramine may have an effect on platelet function as a result of its effect on serotonin uptake.

➤*Renal:* Acute interstitial nephritis (confirmed by biopsy) was reported in 1 obese patient receiving sibutramine during premarketing studies. After discontinuation of the medication, dialysis and oral corticosteroids were administered; renal function normalized. The patient made a full recovery.

➤*Seizures:* Convulsions were reported in 3 of 2,068 (0.1%) sibutramine-treated patients and in none of 884 placebo-treated patients in placebo-controlled premarketing obesity studies. Two of the 3 patients with seizures had potentially predisposing factors (1 had a history of epilepsy; 1 had a subsequent diagnosis of brain tumor). The incidence in all subjects who received sibutramine was less than 0.1% (3/4,588 subjects).

➤*Lab test abnormalities:* Abnormal liver function tests, including increases in AST, ALT, gamma-glutamyltransferase (GGT), lactate dehydrogenase (LDH), alkaline phosphatase, and bilirubin, were reported as adverse reactions in 1.6% of sibutramine-treated obese patients in placebo-controlled trials, compared with 0.8% of placebo patients. In these studies, potentially clinically significant values (total bilirubin greater than or equal to 2 mg/dL; ALT, AST, GGT, LDH, or alkaline phosphatase greater than or equal to 3 times the upper limit of normal) occurred in 0% (alkaline phosphatase) to 0.6% (ALT) of the sibutramine-treated patients and in none of the placebo-treated patients. Abnormal values tended to be sporadic, often diminished with continued treatment, and did not show a clear dose-response relationship.

➤*Postmarketing:* Voluntary reports of adverse reactions temporally associated with the use of sibutramine are listed in the following sections. It is important to emphasize that although these reactions occurred during treatment with sibutramine, they may have no causal relationship with the drug. Obesity itself, concurrent disease states/risk factors, or weight reduction may be associated with an increased risk for some of these reactions.

Cardiovascular – Angina pectoris, atrial fibrillation, congestive heart failure, heart arrest, heart rate decreased, myocardial infarction, supraventricular tachycardia, syncope, torsades de pointes, vascular headache, ventricular extrasystoles, ventricular fibrillation, ventricular tachycardia.

CNS – Cases of depression, suicidal ideation, and suicide have been reported rarely in patients on sibutramine treatment. However, a relationship has not been established between the occurrence of depression and/or suicidal ideation and the use of sibutramine. If depression occurs during treatment with sibutramine, further evaluation may be necessary.

Abnormal dreams, abnormal gait, amnesia, anger, cerebrovascular accident, concentration impaired, confusion, depression aggravated, hypesthesia, libido decreased, libido increased, manic reaction, mood changes, nightmares, serotonin syndrome, short-term memory loss, speech disorder, Tourette syndrome, transient ischemic attack, tremor, twitch, vertigo.

Dermatologic – Alopecia, dermatitis, photosensitivity (skin), urticaria.

Endocrine – Goiter, hyperthyroidism, hypothyroidism.

GI – Cholecystitis, cholelithiasis, duodenal ulcer, GI hemorrhage, eructation, increased salivation, intestinal obstruction, mouth ulcer, stomach ulcer, tongue edema.

GU – Abnormal ejaculation, hematuria, impotence, increased urinary frequency, micturition difficulty, urinary retention.

Hematologic/Lymphatic – Anemia, leukopenia, lymphadenopathy, petechiae, thrombocytopenia.

Hypersensitivity – Allergic hypersensitivity reactions ranging from mild skin eruptions and urticaria to angioedema and anaphylaxis have been reported.

Metabolic – Hyperglycemia, hypoglycemia.

Musculoskeletal – Arthrosis, bursitis.

Respiratory – Epistaxis, nasal congestion, respiratory disorder, yawn.

Special senses – Abnormal vision, blurred vision, dry eye, eye pain, increased intraocular pressure, otitis externa, otitis media, photosensitivity (eyes), tinnitus.

Miscellaneous – Anaphylactic shock, anaphylactoid reaction, chest pressure, chest tightness, facial edema, limb pain, sudden unexplained death.

Overdosage

➤*Symptoms:* There is limited experience of overdose with sibutramine. The most frequently noted adverse reactions associated with overdose are tachycardia, hypertension, headache, and dizziness.

➤*Treatment:* Treatment should consist of general measures employed in the management of overdosage: Establish an airway as needed; cardiac and vital sign monitoring is recommended; institute general symptomatic and supportive measures. Cautious use of beta-blockers may be indicated to control elevated blood pressure or tachycardia. The results from a study in patients with end-stage renal disease on dialysis showed that sibutramine metabolites were not eliminated to a significant degree with hemodialysis.

Patient Information

Advise patients to notify their health care provider if they develop a rash, hives, or other allergic reactions.

Advise patients to inform their health care provider if they are taking or planning to take any prescription or nonprescription drugs, especially weight-reducing agents, decongestants, antidepressants, cough suppressants, lithium, dihydroergotamine, sumatriptan, or tryptophan, because there is a potential for interactions.

Remind patients of the importance of having their blood pressure and pulse monitored at regular intervals.

OPIOID ANALGESICS

WARNING

Fentanyl transmucosal – Oral transmucosal fentanyl is indicated only for the management of breakthrough cancer pain in patients with malignancies who are already receiving and tolerant of opioid therapy for their underlying persistent cancer pain. Patients considered opioid tolerant are those who are taking morphine 60 mg/day or more, transdermal fentanyl 50 mcg/h, or an equianalgesic dose of another opioid for a week or longer. It is contraindicated in the management of acute or postoperative pain. Because life-threatening hypoventilation could occur at any dose in patients not taking long-term opiate therapy, do not use in nonopioid-tolerant patients. Use only in the care of cancer patients and only by oncologists and pain specialists who are knowledgeable of and skilled in the use of schedule II opioids to treat cancer pain. Instruct patients and their caregivers that this drug contains medicine in an amount that can be fatal to a child. Keep all units out of the reach of children, and discard opened units properly.

Fentanyl transdermal system – Fentanyl transdermal systems contain a high concentration of the potent schedule II opioid agonist, fentanyl. Schedule II opioid substances have the highest potential for abuse and associated risk of fatal overdose due to respiratory depression. Fentanyl can be abused and is subject to criminal diversion. The high content of fentanyl in the patches may be a particular target for abuse and diversion.

Fentanyl transdermal system is indicated for management of persistent, moderate to severe chronic pain that requires continuous around-the-clock opioid administration for an extended period of time, and cannot be managed by other means, such as nonsteroidal analgesics, opioid combination products, or immediate-release (IR) opioids.

Use fentanyl transdermal system only in patients who are already receiving opioid therapy, who have demonstrated opioid tolerance, and who require a total daily dose at least equivalent to fentanyl transdermal system 25 mcg/h. Patients who are considered opioid tolerant are those who have been taking, for a week or longer, morphine 60 mg/day or more, oral oxycodone 30 mg/day or more, oral hydromorphone 8 mg/day or more, or an equianalgesic dose of another opioid.

WARNING (cont.)

Because serious or life-threatening hypoventilation could occur, fentanyl transdermal is contraindicated:

- in patients who are not opioid tolerant,
- in the management of acute pain or in patients who require opioid analgesia for a short period of time,
- in the management of postoperative pain, including use after outpatient or day surgeries (eg, tonsillectomies),
- in the management of mild pain, and
- in the management of intermittent pain (eg, use on an as-needed basis).

Because peak fentanyl levels occur between 24 and 72 hours of treatment, serious or life-threatening hypoventilation may occur, even in opioid-tolerant patients, during the initial application period. The concomitant use of fentanyl transdermal system with potent CYP3A4 inhibitors (clarithromycin, itraconazole, ketoconazole, nefazodone, nelfinavir, ritonavir, troleandomycin) may result in an increase in fentanyl plasma concentrations, which could increase or prolong adverse drug effects and may cause potentially fatal respiratory depression. Carefully monitor patients receiving fentanyl transdermal system and potent CYP3A4 inhibitors for an extended period of time and make dosage adjustments if warranted.

Do not administer fentanyl transdermal system to children younger than 2 years of age. Administer to children only if they are opioid tolerant and 2 years of age and older.

Fentanyl transdermal system is only for use in patients who are already tolerant to opioid therapy of comparable potency. Use in nonopioid-tolerant patients may lead to fatal respiratory depression. Overestimating the fentanyl transdermal system dose when converting patients from another opioid medication can result in fatal overdose with the first dose. Because of the 17-hour mean elimination half-life of fentanyl transdermal system, patients who are thought to have had a serious adverse event, including overdose, will require monitoring and treatment for at least 24 hours.

Fentanyl transdermal system can be abused in a manner similar to other opioid agonists, legal or illicit. Consider this risk when administering, prescribing, or dispensing fentanyl transdermal system in situations in which there is concern about increased risk of misuse, abuse, or diversion.

WARNING (cont.)

Fentanyl transdermal patches are intended for transdermal use (on intact skin) only. Using damaged or cut fentanyl transdermal patches can lead to the rapid release of the contents of the fentanyl transdermal patch and absorption of a potentially fatal dose of fentanyl.

Hydromorphone –

High-potency injection: High-potency injection is a highly concentrated solution of hydromorphone intended for use in opioid-tolerant patients. Do not confuse high potency injection with standard parenteral formulations of injection or other opioids. Overdose and death could result.

Extended-release capsules: Hydromorphone extended-release (ER) capsules are indicated for the management of persistent moderate to severe pain in patients requiring continuous, around-the-clock analgesia with a high-potency opioid for an extended period of time (weeks to months) or longer. Use ER capsules only in patients who are already receiving opioid therapy, have demonstrated opioid tolerance, and require a minimum total daily dose of opiate medication equivalent to oral hydromorphone 12 mg. Patients considered opioid tolerant are those taking, for a week or longer, oral morphine 60 mg/day or more, oral oxycodone 30 mg/day or more, oral hydromorphone 8 mg/day or more, or an equianalgesic dose of another opioid. Administer ER capsules once every 24 hours.

Appropriate patients for treatment with ER capsules include patients who require high doses of potent opioids on an around-the-clock basis to improve pain control, and patients who have difficulty attaining adequate analgesia with IR opioid formulations. ER capsules are contraindicated for use on an as-needed basis.

ER capsules are not intended to be used as the first opioid product prescribed for a patient or in patients who require opioid analgesia for a short period of time.

ER capsules are for opioid-tolerant patients only. Use in nonopioid-tolerant patients may lead to fatal respiratory depression. Overestimating the ER capsule dose when converting patients from another opioid medication can result in fatal overdose with the first dose. Because of the mean apparent 18-hour elimination half-life of ER capsules, patients who receive an overdose will require an extended period of monitoring and treatment that may go beyond 18 hours. Even in the face of improvement, continued medical monitoring is required because of the possibility of extended effects.

Schedule II opioid agonists (eg, fentanyl, hydromorphone, methadone, morphine, oxycodone, oxymorphone) have the highest risk of fatal overdoses because of respiratory depression, as well as the highest potential for abuse. ER capsules can be abused in a manner similar to other opioid agonists, legal or illicit. Consider these risks when administering, prescribing, or dispensing ER capsules in situations in which there is concern about increased risk of misuse, abuse, or diversion.

People at increased risk for opioid abuse include those with a personal or family history of substance abuse (ie, drug or alcohol abuse or addiction) or mental illness (eg, major depression). Assess patients for clinical risks for opioid abuse or addiction prior to prescribing opioids. Routinely monitor all patients receiving opioids for signs of misuse, abuse, and addiction. Patients at increased risk of opioid abuse may still be appropriately treated with modified-release opioid formulations; however, these patients will require intensive monitoring for signs of misuse, abuse, or addiction.

ER capsules are to be swallowed whole and not broken, chewed, opened, dissolved, or crushed. Taking broken, chewed, dissolved, or crushed ER capsules or capsule contents can lead to the rapid release and absorption of a potentially fatal dose of hydromorphone. Overestimating the ER capsule dose when converting the patient from another opioid medication can result in fatal overdose with the first dose. With the long half-life of ER capsules (18 hours), patients who receive the wrong dose will require an extended period of monitoring and treatment that may go beyond 18 hours. Even in the face of improvement, continued medical monitoring is required because of the possibility of extended effects.

Methadone – To treat narcotic addiction in detoxification or maintenance programs, methadone should be dispensed only by hospitals, community pharmacies, and maintenance programs approved by the Food and Drug Administration (FDA) and designated state authorities. Approved maintenance programs shall dispense and use methadone in oral form only and according to treatment requirements stipulated in *Federal Methadone Regulations*. Failure to abide by the requirements in these regulations may result in criminal prosecution, seizure of drug supply, revocation of program approval, and injunction precluding program operation.

Methadone, used as an analgesic, may be dispensed in any licensed pharmacy.

Methadone dispersible tablets are for oral administration only. This preparation contains insoluble excipients and therefore must not be injected. It is recommended that methadone dispersible tablets, if dispensed, be packaged in child-resistant containers and kept out of the reach of children to prevent accidental ingestion.

Cardiac conduction effects: Laboratory studies, in vivo and in vitro, have demonstrated that methadone inhibits cardiac potassium channels and prolongs the QT interval. Cases of QT interval prolongation and serious arrhythmia (torsades de pointes) have been observed during treatment with methadone. These cases appear to be more commonly associated with, but not limited to, higher dose treatment (more than 200 mg/day). Most cases involve patients being treated for pain with large, multiple daily doses of methadone, although cases have been reported in patients receiving doses commonly used for maintenance treatment of opioid addiction.

WARNING (cont.)

Morphine –

Avinza: *Avinza* capsules are a modified-release formulation of morphine sulfate indicated for once-daily administration for the relief of moderate to severe pain requiring continuous, around-the-clock opioid therapy for an extended period of time. *Avinza* capsules are to be swallowed whole or the contents of the capsules sprinkled on applesauce. The capsule beads are not to be chewed, crushed, or dissolved because of the risk of rapid release and absorption of a potentially fatal dose of morphine.

Astramorph PF, Duramorph, Infumorph: Because of the risk of severe adverse effects when the epidural or intrathecal route of administration is employed, patients must be observed in a fully equipped and staffed environment for at least 24 hours after the initial dose.

Infumorph: Infumorph is not recommended for single-dose intravenous (IV), intramuscular (IM), or subcutaneous administration because of the very large amount of morphine in the ampul and the associated risk of overdosage.

Oxycodone – Controlled-release (CR) oxycodone is an opioid agonist and a schedule II controlled substance with an abuse liability similar to morphine.

Oxycodone can be abused in a manner similar to other opioid agonists, legal or illicit. Consider this when prescribing or dispensing oxycodone CR tablets in situations in which there is concern about an increased risk of misuse, abuse, or diversion.

Oxycodone CR tablets are indicated for the management of moderate to severe pain when a continuous, around-the-clock analgesic is needed for an extended period of time.

Oxycodone CR tablets are not intended for use as an as-needed analgesic.

Oxycodone 80 and 160 mg CR tablets are for use in opioid-tolerant patients only. These tablet strengths may cause fatal respiratory depression when administered to patients not previously exposed to opioids.

Oxycodone CR tablets are to be swallowed whole and are not to be broken, chewed, or crushed. Taking broken, chewed, or crushed oxycodone CR tablets leads to rapid release and absorption of a potentially fatal dose of oxycodone.

Propoxyphene –

Fatalities: Do not prescribe propoxyphene for patients who are suicidal or addiction-prone. Prescribe propoxyphene with caution to patients taking tranquilizers or antidepressant drugs and patients who use alcohol in excess. Tell patients not to exceed the recommended dose and to limit alcohol intake.

Propoxyphene products in excessive doses, either alone or in combination with other CNS depressants (including alcohol), are a major cause of drug-related deaths. Fatalities within the first hour of overdosage are not uncommon. In 1975, a survey was conducted of deaths due to overdosage; in approximately 20% of fatal cases, death occurred within the first hour (5% within 15 minutes). Propoxyphene should not be taken in higher doses than those recommended by the health care provider. Judicious prescribing of propoxyphene is essential for safety. Consider nonnarcotic analgesics for depressed or suicidal patients. Do not prescribe propoxyphene for suicidal or addiction-prone patients. Caution patients about the concomitant use of propoxyphene products and alcohol because of potentially serious CNS-additive effects of these agents. Because of added CNS depressant effects, cautiously prescribe with concomitant sedatives, tranquilizers, muscle relaxants, antidepressants, or other CNS-depressant drugs. Advise patients of the additive depressant effects of these combinations.

Many propoxyphene-related deaths have occurred in patients with histories of emotional disturbances, suicidal ideation or attempts, or misuse of tranquilizers, alcohol, and other CNS-active drugs. Deaths have occurred as a consequence of the accidental ingestion of excessive quantities of propoxyphene alone or in combination with other drugs. Do not exceed the recommended dosage.

Indications

Opioid Analgesic Indications

Drug	Analgesia	Anesthesia	Cough	Detoxification	Diarrhea	Relief of anxiety in patients with dyspnea associated with pulmonary edema
Alfentanil	✓	✓				
Codeine	✓		✓[a]			
Fentanyl injection	✓	✓				
Fentanyl transdermal	✓					
Fentanyl transmucosal	✓					
Hydrocodone	✓[a]		✓[a]			
Hydromorphone	✓					
Levorphanol	✓					
Meperidine	✓	✓				

Opioid Analgesic Indications						
Drug	Analgesia	Anesthesia	Cough	Detoxification	Diarrhea	Relief of anxiety in patients with dyspnea associated with pulmonary edema
Methadone	✓			✓		
Morphine sulfate	✓	✓				
Opium					✓	
Oxycodone	✓					
Oxymorphone	✓	✓				b
Propoxyphene	✓					
Remifentanil	✓	✓				
Sufentanil	✓	✓				
Tapentadol	✓					
Tramadol	✓					

[a] Currently only available for this indication when part of a multi-ingredient product.
[b] Pulmonary edema secondary to acute left ventricular dysfunction.

Refer to individual product listings for specific indications.

➤*Off-label uses:*

Postherpetic neuralgia –

Morphine (epidural): [5] = Poor documentation.

Premature ejaculation –

Tramadol: [2] = Fair documentation.

Restless legs syndrome –

Tramadol: [4] = Insufficient documentation.

Administration and Dosage

With any potent opioid drug product, it is critical to adjust the dosing regimen for each patient individually, taking into account the patient's prior analgesic treatment experience. Although it is clearly impossible to enumerate every consideration that is important to the selection of initial dose and dosing interval, consider the following:

- the daily dose, potency, and precise characteristics of the opioid the patient has been taking previously (eg, whether it is a pure agonist or mixed agonist/antagonist, the elimination half-life);
- the reliability of the relative potency estimate used to calculate the dose of morphine needed (potency estimates may vary with the route of administration);
- the degree of opioid tolerance, if any; and
- the general condition and medical status of the patient.

The following equianalgesic dosing table is based on parenteral **morphine** 10 mg. Dosage adjustments may be needed if the elimination half-life of the new opioid differs from the current opioid (see Pharmacokinetics).

Approximate Equianalgesic Dosing of Opioid Analgesics in Adults[a,b]			
	Equianalgesic dose		
Opioid	Oral	Parenteral (IM, subcutaneous, IV)	Rectal
Codeine	200 mg	120 to 130 mg	NA[c]
Fentanyl[d]	NA	0.1 mg	NA
Hydrocodone	30 mg	NA	NA
Hydromorphone	7.5 mg	1.5 mg	3 mg
Levorphanol	4 mg	2 mg	NA
Meperidine	300 mg	75 mg	NA
Methadone	10 to 20 mg	5 to 10 mg	NA
Morphine	60 mg single dose, 30 mg repeated doses	10 mg	ND[e]
Oxycodone	20 to 30 mg	NA	NA
Oxymorphone	10 mg	1 mg	10 mg

[a] Table is to be used for estimation only. Data are compiled from multiple references and may be based on single-dose studies.
[b] Caution: Recommended doses do not apply for adult patients with body weight less than 50 kg. Recommended doses do not apply to patients with renal or hepatic insufficiency or other conditions affecting drug metabolism and kinetics. Starting doses should be lower for elderly patients.
[c] NA = not available commercially for this route of administration.
[d] Refer to Fentanyl Transdermal monograph for dosing conversion.
[e] ND = no data.

➤*Patient-controlled analgesia:*

Adults – The following patient-controlled analgesia (PCA) dosing parameters are for opioid-naive adults.

PCA: Dosing Parameters for Opioid-Naive Adults			
Dosing parameter	Fentanyl 10 mcg/mL	Hydromorphone 0.2 mg/mL	Morphine 1 mg/mL
Maximum dose	The total amount of drug over time and the maximum number of patient demand doses per hour will vary.	The total amount of drug over time and the maximum number of patient demand doses per hour will vary.	The total amount of drug over time and the maximum number of patient demand doses per hour will vary.
Loading dose	20 mcg bolus	0.4 mg (400 mcg) bolus	2 mg bolus
Clinician dose	20 mcg bolus. One clinician bolus may be given each hour.	0.4 mg (400 mcg) bolus. One clinician bolus may be given each hour.	2 mg bolus. One clinician bolus may be given each hour.
PCA dose	10 mcg with a lockout time of 10 minutes	0.2 mg (200 mcg) with a lockout time of 10 minutes	1 mg with a lockout time of 10 minutes
Basal dose	Not recommended for starting PCA		

Children: Prior to starting PCA, assess the child's developmental age and cognitive ability. If the patient requires more than 3 patient-demand doses over 2 hours, the health care provider should be contacted and the patient reassessed.

The following PCA dosing parameters are for opioid-naive children.

PCA: Dosing Parameters for Opioid-Naive Children			
Dosing parameter	Fentanyl 10 mcg/mL	Hydromorphone 0.2 mg/mL	Morphine 1 mg/mL
Maximum dose	The total amount of drug over time should not exceed 3 mcg/kg/h.	The total amount of drug over time should not exceed 20 mcg/kg/h.	The total amount of drug over time should not exceed 100 mcg/kg/h (0.1 mg/kg/h).
Loading dose	0.5 mcg/kg bolus	8 mcg/kg bolus	40 mcg/kg (0.04 mg/kg) bolus
Clinician dose	0.5 mcg/kg bolus. Two clinician bolus doses may be given each hour.	8 mcg/kg bolus. Two clinician bolus doses may be given each hour.	40 mcg/kg (0.04 mg/kg) bolus. Two clinician bolus doses may be given each hour.
PCA dose	0.25 mcg with a lockout time of 10 minutes	2 mcg/kg with a lockout time of 10 minutes	10 mcg/kg (0.01 mg/kg) with a lockout time of 10 minutes
Basal dose/ continuous infusion	0.25 mcg/kg/h	1 mcg/kg/h	5 mcg/kg/h (0.005 mg/kg/h)

Actions

➤*Pharmacology:* The precise mechanism of analgesic action of narcotic or opioid analgesics is unknown. They have affinity for the opioid mu-receptor located in the brain, spinal cord, and smooth muscle.

Narcotic analgesics are classified as full agonists, mixed agonist-antagonists, or partial agonists by their activity at opioid receptors. There are 3 major classes of opioid receptors in the CNS, designated mu, kappa, and delta. Opiate receptors in the CNS mediate analgesic activity. Narcotic agonists occupy the same receptors as endogenous opioid peptides (enkephalins or endorphins), and both may alter the central release of neurotransmitters from afferent nerves sensitive to noxious stimuli.

Consequences of the mu-receptor activation include analgesia, respiratory depression, miosis, reduced GI motility, and euphoria. Kappa receptors act primarily in the spinal cord and cause analgesia, dysphoria, and psychotomimetic effects. They also cause less intense miosis and respiratory depression than mu-receptor activation. The consequence of delta-receptor stimulation in human beings is unclear. Morphine-like narcotic agonists have activity at the mu, kappa, and delta receptors. Opioid agonists include natural opium alkaloids (eg, **codeine**, **morphine**), semisynthetic analogs (eg, **hydromorphone**, **oxycodone**, **oxymorphone**), and synthetic compounds (eg, **fentanyl**, **levorphanol**, **methadone**, **sufentanil**, **tapentadol**, **tramadol**).

Tapentadol and tramadol and its active metabolite (M1) appear to bind to mu-opioid receptors and weakly inhibit reuptake of norepinephrine and serotonin.

Mixed *agonist-antagonist* drugs (eg, nalbuphine, pentazocine) have agonist activity at some receptors and antagonist activity at other receptors; also included are the *partial agonists* (eg, buprenorphine, butorphanol) (see the Narcotic Agonist-Antagonist Analgesics group monograph).

Narcotic antagonists – Narcotic antagonists (eg, naloxone) do not have agonist activity at any of the opioid receptor sites (see individual monographs). Antagonists block the opiate receptor, inhibit pharmacological activity of the agonist, and precipitate withdrawal in dependent patients.

Secondary pharmacological effects – The narcotics have a variety of secondary pharmacological effects, including the following:

Cardiovascular: Peripheral vasodilation, reduced peripheral resistance, and inhibition of baroreceptors. Orthostatic hypotension and fainting may occur when the patient sits up.

CNS: Alterations in mood, apathy, drowsiness, dysphoria, euphoria, feelings of relaxation, mental confusion, pupillary constriction, reduction in body temperature. Nausea and vomiting are caused by direct stimulation of the emetic chemoreceptors located in the medulla. **Hydromorphone** increases cerebrospinal (CSF) pressure.

Dermatologic: Flushing, histamine release, pruritus, and red eyes.

Endocrine: Opioid agonists have a variety of effects on the secretion of hormones. Opioids inhibit the secretion of adrenocorticotropic hormone, cortisol, and luteinizing hormone in humans. They also stimulate prolactin, growth hormone secretion, and pancreatic secretion of insulin and glucagon in humans, rats, dogs, and other species. Thyroid-stimulating hormone is both inhibited and stimulated by opioids.

GI:

• *Stomach* – Decreases gastric motility, thus prolonging gastric emptying time. This may lead to esophageal reflux.

• *Small intestine* – Decreases biliary, pancreatic, and intestinal secretions and delays digestion of food in the small intestine. Resting tone increases and periodic spasms occur.

• *Large intestine* – Propulsive peristaltic waves in the colon are diminished and tone increases until it spasms. This, along with the inattention to the normal stimuli for defecation reflex, contribute to constipation.

• *Biliary tract* – The sphincter of Oddi constricts, leading to epigastric distress or biliary colic.

GU: Increases smooth muscle tone in the urinary tract and can induce spasms. Urinary urgency and difficulty with urination may result.

Respiratory: Depressant effects first diminish tidal volume, then respiratory rate, because of reduced sensitivity of the respiratory center to carbon dioxide.

• *Cough* – Suppresses cough reflex by direct effect on cough center in the medulla.

Miscellaneous: **Hydromorphone** causes transient hyperglycemia; **codeine** causes release of antidiuretic hormone.

Comparative pharmacology is summarized as follows. Consider these comparisons as approximations that may vary widely among patients.

Opioid Analgesics Comparative Pharmacology[a,b]

Drug	Analgesic	Antitussive	Constipation	Respiratory depression	Sedation	Emesis	Physical dependence
Phenanthrenes							
Codeine	+	+++	+	+	+	+	+
Hydrocodone	++	+++	nd	nd	nd	nd	++
Hydromorphone	++	++	+	++	+	+	++
Levorphanol	++	++	nd	++	++	+	++
Morphine	++	++	++	++	++	++	++
Oxycodone	++	+++	++	++	++	++	++
Oxymorphone	++	+	+++	+++	nd	+++	+++
Phenylpiperidines							
Fentanyl	++	nd	nd	+	nd	+	nd
Meperidine	++	nd	+	++	+	nd	++
Diphenylheptanes							
Methadone	++	++	+	++	+	+	+
Propoxyphene	+	nd	nd	+	+	+	+

[a] + = degree of activity from the least (+) to the greatest (+++); nd = no data available.

[b] Table adapted from: Catalano RB. The medical approach to management of pain caused by cancer. *Semin Oncol.* 1975;2(4):379-392.

➤**Pharmacokinetics** Administration IV is most reliable and rapid; IM or subcutaneous use may delay absorption and peak effect. Many agents undergo a significant first-pass effect.

Opioid Analgesic Pharmacokinetics[a]

Drug	Onset of effect	Peak effect	Duration of effect	Elimination t½	Vd (L/kg)	Protein binding (%)	Metabolism pathway	Active metabolites	Major excretion pathway
Alfentanil	immediate	1.5 to 2 min	< 10 min	1.5 to 1.85 h	0.4 to 1	92%	liver	—	urine
Codeine	Oral: 10 to 30 min, IV: 15 min	0.5 to 1 h	Oral: 4 to 6 h, IV: 5 h	2.5 to 3 h	—	—	liver	morphine	urine
Fentanyl injection	IV: immediate, IM: 7 to 8 min	—	IV: 0.5 to 1 h, IM: 1 to 2 h	3.65 h	4	alters with increasing ionization	liver		urine
Fentanyl transdermal	—	24 to 72 h	72 h	≈ 17 h	6	decreases with increasing ionization	liver: CYP3A4	—	urine
Fentanyl transmucosal	—	—	—	7 h	4	80% to 85%	liver: CYP3A4	—	urine
Hydromorphone	IM/Subcutaneous: 15 min, Oral: 30 min	0.5 to 1 h	IR: 4 to 5 h, ER: 24 h, IM/Subcutaneous: 4 to 5 h	IR: 2.3 h, ER: 18.6 h, IM/Subcutaneous: 2.6 h	≈ 4	8% to 20%	liver: glucuronidation	—	urine
Levorphanol	IM: 15 to 30 min	Oral: 1 h	—	IV: 11 to 16 h	IV: 10 to 13	40%	—	—	—
Meperidine	—	—	2 to 4 h	3 to 6 (parent), < 20 h (normeperidine)		60% to 80%	liver	normeperidine	—
Methadone	Parenteral: 10 to 20 min, Oral: 30 to 60 min	—	4 h	8 to 59 h	2 to 6	85% to 90%	liver: primarily CYP3A4 and to lesser extent CYP2D6	—	urine and fecal
Morphine sulfate	IM/Subcutaneous: 10 to 30 min	Epidural: 10 to 15 min, Oral: 1 h	Subcutaneous/IM: 4 to 5 h	1.5 to 2 h	1 to 6	20% to 35%	liver: glucuronidation	morphine-6-glucuronide	urine
Oxycodone	within 60 min	—	IR: 3 to 4 h, CR: 12 h	IR: 3.2 h, CR: 4.5 h	2.6	45%	liver: somewhat involves CYP2D6	noroxycodone and oxymorphone	urine
Oxymorphone	Parenteral: 5 to 10 min	—	Parenteral: 3 to 6 h	1.3 h	≈ 3	—	liver	—	urine
Propoxyphene	—	2 to 2.5 h	—	6 to 12 h (parent), 30 to 36 h (norpropoxyphene)	—	80%	liver	norpropoxyphene	urine
Remifentanil	rapid	—	—	10 to 20 min	0.35	70%	hydrolysis by esterases	—	urine

Opioid Analgesic Pharmacokinetics[a]									
Drug	Onset of effect	Peak effect	Duration of effect	Elimination t½	Vd (L/kg)	Protein binding (%)	Metabolism pathway	Active metabolites	Major excretion pathway
Sufentanil	IV: immediate, Epidural: 10 min[b]	—	Epidural: 1.7 h[b]	2.7 h	—	91% to 93%, 79% in neonates	liver and small intestine	—	—
Tapentadol	—	1.25 h	—	—	—	20%	conjugation with glucuronic acid; CYP2C9 and CYP2C19	Tapentadol-O-glucuronide	urine
Tramadol	—	—	2 h (tramadol), 3 h (M1, active metabolite)	6.3 h (tramadol), 7.4 h (M1, active metabolite)	2.6 to 2.9	20%	liver: CYP2D6 and CYP3A4	O-desmethyl-tramadol (M1) via CYP2D6	urine

[a] t½ = half-life; Vd = volume of distribution.

[b] With bupivacaine.

Special populations –

Elderly:

• *Alfentanil* – Patients older than 65 years of age have reduced plasma clearance and increased elimination half-life, which may prolong postoperative recovery.

• *Fentanyl* – Clearance may be greatly decreased.

• *Hydromorphone* – Age-related increases in exposure have been observed. Greater sensitivity of older individuals cannot be excluded. Adjust dosages according to clinical situation.

• *Meperidine* – Elderly patients have a slower elimination rate compared with younger patients.

• *Morphine* – Elderly patients may have reduced clearance.

• *Oxycodone* – Plasma levels are approximately 15% greater in elderly patients than in young patients.

• *Remifentanil* – The clearance of remifentanil is reduced (approximately 25%) in elderly patients (older than 65 years of age) compared with younger adults (average, 25 years of age). However, remifentanil blood concentrations fall as rapidly after termination of administration in elderly patients as in younger adults.

• *Tapentadol* – Maximum plasma concentration (C_{max}) is 16% lower in elderly patients.

• *Tramadol* – In subjects older than 75 years of age, maximum serum concentrations are elevated (208 vs 162 ng/mL) and the elimination half-life is prolonged (7 vs 6 hours) compared with subjects 65 to 75 years of age. Adjustment of the daily dose is recommended for patients older than 75 years of age.

Gender:

• *Oxycodone* – Women exhibit plasma levels up to 25% higher than men on a body weight–adjusted basis. The cause of this difference is unknown.

• *Tramadol* – The absolute bioavailability of tramadol was 73% in men and 79% in women. The plasma clearance was 6.4 mL/min/kg in men and 5.7 mL/min/kg in women following an IV dose of tramadol 100 mg. Following a single oral dose and after adjusting for body weight, women had a 12% higher peak tramadol concentration and a 35% higher area under the curve (AUC) compared with men. The clinical significance of this difference is unknown.

Renal function impairment:

• *Hydromorphone* – Possible accumulation with severe impairment. Use with caution.

• *Meperidine* – Accumulation of meperidine and/or normeperidine may occur in patients with renal impairment.

• *Methadone* – Methadone pharmacokinetics have not been extensively evaluated in patients with renal insufficiency. Unchanged methadone and its metabolites are excreted in urine to a variable degree. Methadone is a basic (pKa = 9.2) compound, and the luminal pH of the urinary tract can affect its extraction from plasma. Urine acidification increases renal elimination of methadone. Forced diuresis, peritoneal dialysis, hemodialysis, and charcoal hemoperfusion have not been established as beneficial for increasing methadone or metabolite elimination.

• *Morphine* – Clearance is decreased and plasma levels increased in patients with renal failure.

• *Oxycodone* – Patients with mild to severe renal impairment (creatinine clearance [CrCl] less than 60 mL/min) show peak plasma oxycodone and noroxycodone concentrations 50% and 20% higher, respectively, and AUC values for oxycodone, noroxycodone, and oxymorphone 60%, 50%, and 40% higher than healthy subjects, respectively. This is accompanied by increased sedation but not by differences in respiratory rate, pupillary constriction, or several other measures of drug effect. There was an increase in the elimination half-life for oxycodone of 1 hour.

• *Remifentanil* – In anephric patients, the half-life of the carboxylic acid metabolite increases from 90 minutes to 30 hours. The metabolite is removed by hemodialysis with a dialysis extraction ratio of approximately 30%.

• *Tapentadol* – Increased exposure (AUC) to tapentadol-O-glucuronide with increasing degree of renal impairment (1.5-, 2.5-, and 5.5-fold higher in mild, moderate, and severe renal impairment, respectively).

• *Tramadol* – Impaired renal function results in a decreased rate and extent of excretion of tramadol and its active metabolite, M1. In patients with CrCl less than 30 mL/min, adjustment of the dosing regimen is recommended. The total amount of tramadol and M1 removed during a 4-hour dialysis period is less than 7% of the administered dose.

Hepatic function impairment:

• *Alfentanil* – Patients with compromised liver function have reduced plasma clearance and an extended elimination half-life, which may prolong postoperative recovery.

• *Hydromorphone* – Possible accumulation with severe impairment; use with caution.

• *Meperidine* – Accumulation of meperidine and/or normeperidine may occur in patients with hepatic impairment.

• *Methadone* – Methadone is metabolized in the liver, and patients with liver impairment may be at risk of accumulating methadone after multiple dosing.

• *Morphine* – Clearance is decreased and half-life is increased in patients with cirrhosis. The 3- and 6-glucuronide metabolites to morphine plasma AUC ratios are also decreased, indicating diminished metabolic activity.

• *Oxycodone* – Patients with mild to moderate hepatic dysfunction show peak plasma oxycodone and noroxycodone concentrations 50% and 20% higher, respectively, and AUC values are 95% and 65% higher, respectively, than healthy subjects. Oxymorphone peak plasma levels and AUC values are lower by 30% and 40%. The elimination half-life for oxycodone increased by 2.3 hours.

• *Tapentadol* – Higher exposure to and increased serum levels of tapentadol may occur in patients with hepatic impairment; the rate of formation of tapentadol-O-glucuronide is lower in patients with increased liver impairment.

• *Tramadol* – Metabolism of tramadol and M1 is reduced in patients with advanced cirrhosis of the liver, resulting in both a larger AUC for tramadol and longer tramadol and M1 elimination half-lives (13 hours for tramadol and 19 hours for M1). In cirrhotic patients, adjustment of the dosing regimen is recommended.

Children:

• *Meperidine* – Meperidine has a slower elimination rate in neonates and young children compared with older children and adults.

• *Morphine* – Infants younger than 1 month of age have a prolonged elimination half-life and decreased clearance relative to older infants and pediatric patients. The clearance and half-life begin to approach adult values by the second month of life. Children old enough to take capsules should have pharmacokinetic parameters similar to adults, dosed on a per kilogram basis.

• *Remifentanil* – Clearance and volume of distribution of remifentanil were increased in younger children and declined to young, healthy adult values by 17 years of age. The average clearance of remifentanil in neonates (younger than 2 months of age) was approximately 90.5 mL/min/kg, while in adolescents (13 to 16 years of age) this value was approximately 57.2 mL/min/kg. The total (steady-state) volume of distribution in neonates was approximately 452 mL/kg versus 223 mL/kg in adolescents. The half-life of remifentanil was the same in neonates and adolescents.

Cardiopulmonary bypass:

• *Remifentanil* – Remifentanil clearance is reduced by approximately 20% during hypothermic cardiopulmonary bypass.

Race:

• *Morphine* – In 1 study, Chinese subjects given IV morphine had a higher clearance compared with white subjects (1,852 mL/min compared with 1,495 mL/min).

Contraindications

Hypersensitivity to the drug or known intolerance to other opioids or any components of the products.

➤*Fentanyl:*

Transmucosal – Management of acute or postoperative pain; nonopioid-tolerant patients.

Transdermal – Nonopioid-tolerant patients; management of acute pain or in patients who require opioid analgesia for a short period of time; management of postoperative pain, including use after outpatient day surgeries; management of mild or intermittent pain (eg, use on an as-needed basis); respiratory depression; acute or severe bronchial asthma; paralytic ileus; doses exceeding 25 mcg/h at initiation of opioid therapy.

➤*Hydromorphone:*

Oral / Suppositories – Use on an as-needed basis; respiratory depression; acute or severe bronchial asthma; paralytic ileus; obstetrical analgesia; intracranial lesion associated with increased intracranial pressure (2 and 4 mg tablets only).

Injection – Patients not already receiving large amounts of parenteral narcotics (high potency injection only); respiratory depression; status asthmaticus; obstetrical analgesia.

➤*Meperidine:* In patients taking monoamine oxidase inhibitors (MAOIs) or in those who have received such agents within 14 days.

➤*Methadone:*

Injection – Respiratory depression; acute bronchial asthma; hypercarbia.

➤*Morphine:*

IR concentrated oral solution and tablets / suppositories – Respiratory insufficiency or depression; severe CNS depression; attack of bronchial asthma; heart failure secondary to chronic lung disease; cardiac arrhythmias; increased intracranial or CSF pressure; head injuries; brain tumor; acute alcoholism; delirium tremens; convulsive disorders; after biliary tract surgery; suspected surgical abdomen; surgical anastomosis; concomitantly with MAOIs or within 14 days of such treatment; paralytic ileus.

Injection – Heart failure secondary to chronic lung disease; cardiac arrhythmias; brain tumor; acute alcoholism; delirium tremens; idiosyncrasy to the drug; increased intracranial or CSF pressure; head injuries; acute bronchial asthma; upper airway obstruction. Because of its stimulating effect on the spinal cord, morphine should not be used in convulsive states (eg, status epilepticus, tetanus, strychnine poisoning); concomitantly with MAOIs or within 14 days of such treatment.

Epidural / Intrathecal – Presence of infection at the injection microinfusion site; concomitant anticoagulant therapy; uncontrolled bleeding diathesis; parenterally administered corticosteroids within a 2-week period, or other concomitant drug therapy or medical condition that would contraindicate the technique of epidural or intrathecal analgesia; acute bronchial asthma; upper airway obstruction.

Soluble tablets for injection – Convulsive states such as those occurring in status epilepticus, tetanus, and strychnine poisoning.

DepoDur – Respiratory depression; acute or severe bronchial asthma; upper airway obstruction; paralytic ileus; head injury; increased intracranial pressure; circulatory shock.

Sustained-release (SR) / ER / CR – Respiratory depression; acute or severe bronchial asthma; paralytic ileus.

➤*Opium:* Diarrhea caused by poisoning until the toxic material is eliminated from the GI tract; use in children (opium tincture only); convulsive states such as those occurring in status epilepticus, tetanus, and strychnine poisoning (*Paregoric* only).

➤*Oxycodone:*

CR / IR tablets (15 and 30 mg) / IR capsules (5 mg) / ER / Concentrated solution – Significant respiratory depression; acute or severe bronchial asthma; hypercarbia; paralytic ileus.

➤*Oxymorphone:* Hypersensitivity to morphine analogs; acute asthma attack; severe respiratory depression or upper airway obstruction; paralytic ileus; pulmonary edema secondary to a chemical respiratory irritant.

➤*Remifentanil:* For epidural or intrathecal administration; hypersensitivity to fentanyl analogs.

➤*Tapentadol:* Significant respiratory depression in unmonitored settings or the absence of resuscitative equipment; acute or severe bronchial asthma or hypercapnia in unmonitored settings or the absence of resuscitative equipment; paralytic ileus; concurrent MAOI use or within 14 days of such treatment.

➤*Tramadol:* Acute intoxication with alcohol, hypnotics, narcotics, centrally acting analgesics, opioids, or psychotropic drugs.

Warnings/Precautions

➤*Suicide:* Do not prescribe **propoxyphene** for patients who are suicidal or addiction prone. Many of the propoxyphene-related deaths have occurred in patients with histories of emotional disturbances, suicidal ideation, or suicide attempts, as well as misuse of tranquilizers, alcohol, and other CNS-active drugs. Some deaths were a consequence of accidental ingestion of excessive quantities of propoxyphene alone or in combination with other drugs. Warn patients not to exceed the dosage recommended by their health care provider (see Black Box Warning).

➤*Respiratory depression:* Narcotics may be expected to produce serious or potentially fatal respiratory depression if given in an excessive dose, too frequently, or in full dosage to compromised or vulnerable patients because the doses required to produce analgesia in the general clinical population may cause serious respiratory depression in vulnerable patients. Safe use of opioids requires that the dose and dosage interval be individualized to each patient based on the severity of the pain, weight, age, diagnosis, and physical status of the patient, and the type and dose of coadministered medication.

Respiratory depression caused by opioid analgesics can be reversed by opioid antagonists, such as naloxone. Because the duration of respiratory depression may last longer than the duration of the opioid antagonist action, maintain appropriate surveillance.

Certain forms of conduction anesthesia, such as spinal anesthesia and some peridural anesthetics, can alter respiration by blocking intercostal nerves. Through other mechanisms, **fentanyl** injection also can alter respiration. Therefore, when fentanyl injection is used to supplement these forms of anesthesia, the anesthetist needs to be aware of the physiological alterations involved and manage them appropriately. Profound analgesia is accompanied by respiratory depression and diminished sensitivity to CO_2 stimulation, which may persist or recur in the postoperative period. Respiratory depression secondary to chest wall rigidity has been reported in the postoperative period. Intraoperative hyperventilation may further alter postoperative response to CO_2. Employ appropriate postoperative monitoring to ensure that adequate spontaneous breathing is established and maintained in the absence of stimulation prior to discharging the patient from the recovery area.

Fentanyl transdermal – Because significant amounts of fentanyl are absorbed from the skin for 17 hours or more after the system is removed, hypoventilation may persist beyond the removal. Consequently, observe patients with hypoventilation carefully for degree of sedation, and monitor their respiratory rate until respiration has stabilized.

Levorphanol – Reduce the initial levorphanol dose by 50% or more when the drug is given to patients with any condition affecting respiratory reserve or in conjunction with other drugs affecting the respiratory center. Then, individually titrate subsequent doses according to patient response. Respiratory depression produced by levorphanol can be reversed by naloxone, a specific antagonist.

Remifentanil – Respiratory depression in spontaneously breathing patients is generally managed by decreasing the rate of infusion of remifentanil by 50% or by temporarily discontinuing the infusion.

➤*CNS depressants:* Use with caution and in reduced dosage in patients concurrently receiving other opioid narcotic analgesics, general anesthetics, phenothiazines, other tranquilizers, sedative-hypnotics (including barbiturates), tricyclic antidepressants, and/or other CNS depressants (including alcohol). Respiratory depression, hypotension, and profound sedation or coma may result.

If **fentanyl** is administered with a tranquilizer such as droperidol, pulmonary arterial pressure may be decreased. Be familiar with the special properties of each drug, particularly the widely differing durations of action, and have available fluids and other countermeasures to manage hypotension when such a combination is used.

➤*Head injury and increased intracranial pressure:* Narcotics may obscure the clinical course of patients with head injuries. The respiratory-depressant effects and the capacity to elevate CSF pressure may be markedly exaggerated in the presence of head injury, brain tumor, other intracranial lesions, impaired consciousness, or preexisting elevated intracranial pressure. Use with extreme caution, and use only if deemed essential. Pupillary changes (miosis) from narcotics may obscure the existence, extent, and course or intracranial pathology. High doses of neuraxial **morphine** may produce myoclonic events.

➤*QT prolongation:* Administer **methadone** with particular caution to patients already at risk for development of prolonged QT interval (eg, cardiac hypertrophy, concomitant diuretic use, hypokalemia, hypomagnesemia). Careful monitoring is recommended when using methadone in patients with a history of cardiac conduction abnormalities, those taking medications affecting cardiac conduction, and in other cases in which history or physical exam suggest an increased risk of dysrhythmia. QT prolongation also has been reported in patients with no prior cardiac history who have received high doses of methadone. Evaluate patients developing QT prolongation while on methadone treatment for the presence of modifiable risk factors, such as concomitant medications with cardiac effects, drugs that might cause electrolyte abnormalities, and drugs that might act as inhibitors of methadone metabolism. When using methadone to treat pain, weigh the risk of QT prolongation and development of dysrhythmias against the benefit of adequate pain management and the availability of alternative therapies. In using methadone, carry out an individualized benefit-to-risk assessment and include evaluation of patient presentation and complete medical history. For patients judged to be at risk, perform careful monitoring of cardiovascular status, including QT prolongation and dysrhythmias and those conditions described previously.

➤*Seizures:* Seizures may be aggravated or may occur in patients with or without a history of convulsive disorders when the dosage is substantially increased above recommended levels because of tolerance. Closely observe patients with known seizure disorders for **meperidine**- or **morphine**-induced seizure activity. Reports of mild to severe seizures and myoclonus have been reported in severely compromised patients administered high doses of parenteral **hydromorphone** in treating cancer and severe pain. Opioid administration at very high doses is associated with seizures and myoclonus in a variety of diseases when pain control is the primary focus.

Seizures have been reported in patients receiving **tramadol** within the recommended dosage range. Spontaneous postmarketing reports indicate the seizure risk is increased with doses above the recommended range. Concomitant use with selective serotonin reuptake inhibitors (SSRIs or anorectics), tricyclic compounds (eg, cyclobenzaprine, promethazine, tricyclic antidepressants [TCAs]), or other opioids also increases the risk of seizures. Administration of tramadol with neuroleptics, MAOIs (see Warnings), or other drugs that reduce the seizure threshold may also enhance the seizure risk. Risk of convulsions may increase in patients with epilepsy, with a history of seizures, or with a recognized risk for seizure (eg, head trauma, metabolic disorders, alcohol and drug withdrawal, CNS infections). In a tramadol overdose, naloxone administration may increase the risk of seizure (see Overdosage).

➤*Administration:* **Alfentanil**, **fentanyl**, **morphine**, **remifentanil**, and **sufentanil** should be administered only by personnel specifically trained in the use of IV and epidural anesthetics and the management of potent opioid respiratory effects.

An opioid antagonist, resuscitative and intubation equipment, and oxygen should be readily available.

Administer continuous infusions only by an infusion device. Use IV bolus administration of remifentanil only during the maintenance of general anesthesia. In nonintubated patients, administer remifentanil doses over 30 to 60 seconds.

Interruption of infusion – Interruption of an infusion of **remifentanil** will result in rapid offset of effect. Rapid clearance and lack of drug accumulation will result in rapid dissipation of respiratory-depressant and analgesic effects upon discontinuation of remifentanil at recommended doses. Precede discontinuation of an infusion of remifentanil with the establishment of adequate postoperative analgesia.

IV tubing – Make injections of **remifentanil** into IV tubing at or close to the venous cannula. Upon discontinuation of remifentanil, clear the IV tubing to prevent the inadvertent administration of remifentanil at a later point in time. Failure to adequately clear the IV tubing to remove residual remifentanil has been associated with respiratory depression, apnea, and muscle rigidity upon the administration of additional fluids or medications through the same IV tubing.

Do not administer remifentanil into the same IV tubing with blood because of potential inactivation by nonspecific esterases in blood products.

➤*ER, SR, CR products:* These dosage forms must not be chewed, crushed, or dissolved because of the risk of rapid release and absorption of a potentially fatal dose.

➤*Parenteral therapy:* Give by very slow IV injection, preferably as a diluted solution. The patient should be lying down. Rapid IV injection increases the incidence of adverse reactions; respiratory depression, hypotension, apnea, circulatory collapse, cardiac arrest, and anaphylactoid reactions have occurred. Do not administer IV unless a narcotic antagonist and facilities for assisted or controlled respiration are available.

Smooth muscle hypertonicity may result in biliary colic, difficulty in urination, and possible urinary retention requiring catheterization. Consider inherent risks in urethral catheterization (eg, sepsis) when epidural or intrathecal administration is considered, especially in the perioperative period.

➤*Epidural/Intrathecal administration:* Limit epidural or intrathecal administration of preservative-free **morphine** and **sufentanil** to the lumbar area. Intrathecal use has been associated with a higher incidence of respiratory depression than epidural use. Prior to any epidural or intrathecal drug administration, the health care provider should be familiar with patient conditions (eg, infection at the injection site, bleeding diathesis, anticoagulant therapy) that call for special evaluation of the benefit-versus-risk potential.

Thoracic administration dramatically increases the incidence of early and late respiratory depression even with morphine 1 to 2 mg. Administer narcotics by or under the direction of a health care provider experienced in the technique of epidural administration who is thoroughly familiar with the drug labeling. Administer only in settings where adequate patient monitoring is possible. Have resuscitative equipment and a specific antagonist (naloxone injection) immediately available for the management of respiratory depression as well as complications that might result from inadvertent intrathecal or intravascular injection. (Note: intrathecal morphine dosage is usually one-tenth that of epidural dosage.) Continue patient monitoring for at least 24 hours after each dose because delayed respiratory depression may occur.

Verify proper placement of the needle or catheter in the epidural space before injection of sufentanil or preservative-free morphine to ensure that unintentional intravascular or intrathecal administration does not occur. Unintentional intravascular injection of sufentanil could result in a potentially serious overdose, including acute truncal muscular rigidity and apnea. Unintentional intrathecal injection of the full sufentanil/bupivacaine epidural doses and volume could produce effects of high spinal anesthesia, including prolonged paralysis and delayed recovery. If analgesia is inadequate, verify the placement and integrity of the catheter prior to the administration of any additional epidural medications. Administer sufentanil epidurally by slow injection.

➤*Asthma and other respiratory conditions:* The use of bisulfites is contraindicated in asthmatic patients. Bisulfites and **morphine** may potentiate each other, preventing use by causing severe adverse reactions. Use with extreme caution in patients having an acute asthmatic attack, bronchial asthma, chronic obstructive pulmonary disease (COPD) or cor pulmonale, a substantially decreased respiratory reserve, and preexisting respiratory depression, hypoxia, hypercapnia, or upper airway obstruction. Even usual therapeutic doses of narcotics may decrease respiratory drive while simultaneously increasing airway resistance to the point of apnea. Reserve use for those whose conditions require endotracheal intubation and respiratory support or control of ventilation. In these patients, consider alternative nonopioid analgesics, and employ only under careful medical supervision at the lowest effective dose.

➤*Hypotensive effect:* Opioid analgesics may cause severe hypotension in the postoperative patient or in individuals whose ability to maintain blood pressure has been compromised by a depleted blood volume or coadministration of drugs such as phenothiazines or general anesthetics. In ambulatory patients, orthostatic hypotension may occur.

Carefully observe patients with reduced circulating blood volume, impaired myocardial function, or those on sympatholytic drugs for orthostatic hypotension, particularly in transport.

➤*Renal toxicity:* *Avinza* dosages of more than 1,600 mg/day contain a quantity of fumaric acid that has not been demonstrated to be safe, and which may result in serious renal toxicity. Daily dosage of *Avinza* must be limited to a maximum of 1,600 mg/day.

➤*Acute abdominal conditions:* Narcotics may obscure diagnosis or clinical course. Do not give SR **morphine** to patients with GI obstruction, particularly paralytic ileus, because there is a risk of the product remaining in the stomach for an extended period and the risk of subsequent release of a bolus of morphine when normal gut motility is restored. As with other solid morphine formulations, diarrhea may reduce morphine absorption. Opioids decrease bowel motility. Ileus is a common postoperative complication, especially after intra-abdominal surgery with opioid analgesia. Use with caution and monitor for decreased bowel motility in postoperative patients receiving opioids. Implement standard supportive therapy.

➤*Special risk patients:* Use caution and reduce the initial dose in elderly or debilitated patients and in those suffering from conditions accompanied by hypoxia or hypercapnia when even moderate therapeutic doses may dangerously decrease pulmonary ventilation. Also exercise caution in patients sensitive to CNS depressants, including those with cardiovascular, pulmonary, renal, or hepatic disease; myxedema; CNS depression; coma; convulsive disorders; increased intracranial or ocular pressure; acute alcoholism; delirium tremens; cerebral arteriosclerosis; fever; decreased respiratory reserve (eg, emphysema, severe obesity, asthma, COPD or cor pulmonale, sleep apnea syndrome); inflammatory bowel disease; diarrhea secondary to poisoning until the toxin is eliminated; diarrhea secondary to pseudomembranous colitis; GI hemorrhage; bronchial asthma; hypothyroidism; kyphoscoliosis; Addison disease; prostatic hypertrophy; urethral stricture; gallbladder disease or gallstones; recent GI or GU tract surgery; toxic psychosis; alcohol or drug abuse; sickle cell anemia; bradyarrhythmias; paralysis of the phrenic nerve; inability to swallow.

In obese patients (more than 20% above ideal body weight), determine the **alfentanil**, **remifentanil**, and **sufentanil** dosage on the basis of ideal body weight.

Use **fentanyl transmucosal** with caution in patients with diabetes because it contains approximately 2 g of sugar per unit.

In patients with pheochromocytoma, **meperidine** has been reported to provoke hypertension.

Bradycardia – **Fentanyl**, **sufentanil**, **remifentanil**, and **alfentanil** may produce bradycardia, which may be treated with ephedrine or anticholinergic drugs, such as atropine or glycopyrrolate. Use caution when administering to patients with bradyarrhythmias.

➤*Serotonin syndrome:* The development of a potentially life-threatening serotonin syndrome may occur with the use of **tapentadol** and serotonergic drugs, such as SSRIs, serotonin-norepinephrine reuptake inhibitors (SNRIs), TCAs, MAOIs, and triptans, and with drugs that impair the metabolism of serotonin. Serotonin syndrome may include mental status changes (eg, agitation, hallucinations, coma), autonomic instability (eg, tachycardia, hyperthermia), neuromuscular aberrations (eg, hyperreflexia, incoordination), and/or GI symptoms.

➤*Skeletal muscle rigidity:* **Alfentanil**, **fentanyl**, and **sufentanil** may cause skeletal muscle rigidity, particularly of the truncal muscles. The incidence and severity of muscle rigidity are usually dose related. Alfentanil, fentanyl, and sufentanil may produce muscular rigidity that involves all skeletal muscles, including those of the neck, external eye, and extremities. The incidence may be reduced by the following:

1.) routine methods of administration of neuromuscular-blocking agents for balanced opioid anesthesia;
2.) administration of up to ¼ of the full paralyzing dose of a nondepolarizing neuromuscular-blocking agent just prior to administration of alfentanil, fentanyl, or sufentanil; following loss of consciousness or eyelash reflex, administer a full paralyzing dose of a neuromuscular-blocking agent; or
3.) simultaneous administration of alfentanil, fentanyl, or sufentanil and a full paralyzing dose of a neuromuscular-blocking agent when alfentanil, fentanyl, or sufentanil is used in rapidly administered anesthetic dosages. The neuromuscular-blocking agent should be compatible with the patient's cardiovascular status.

Alfentanil administration at anesthetic dosages (more than 130 mcg/kg) will consistently produce muscular rigidity with an immediate onset.

Skeletal muscle rigidity can be caused by **remifentanil** and is related to the dose and speed of administration. Remifentanil may cause chest wall rigidity (inability to ventilate) after single doses of greater than 1 mcg/kg administered over 30 to 60 seconds, or after infusion rates of 0.1 mcg/kg/min or greater. Single doses of less than 1 mcg/kg may cause chest wall rigidity when given concurrently with a continuous infusion of remifentanil.

Muscle rigidity seen during the use of remifentanil in spontaneously breathing patients may be treated by stopping or decreasing the rate of administration of remifentanil. Resolution of muscle rigidity after discontinuing the infusion of remifentanil occurs within minutes. In the case of life-threatening muscle rigidity, a rapid-onset neuromuscular blocker or naloxone may be administered.

➤*Fever/External heat:* Serum **fentanyl** concentrations may increase by approximately one-third for patients with a body temperature of 40°C (104°F) because of temperature-dependent increases in fentanyl release from the transdermal system and increased skin permeability. Therefore, monitor patients wearing fentanyl transdermal systems who develop fever for opioid adverse effects and adjust the dose as necessary. Similar increases also may be observed if the fentanyl transdermal system is exposed to external heat (eg, heating pads, electric blankets, saunas, hot tubs). Therefore, advise patients to avoid exposing the patch application site to direct external heat.

➤*Supraventricular tachycardias:* Use **meperidine** with caution in atrial flutter and other supraventricular tachycardias; vagolytic action may increase the ventricular response rate.

➤*Cardiovascular effects:* Limit use of **levorphanol** in acute myocardial infarction (MI) or in cardiac patients with myocardial dysfunction or coronary insufficiency because the effects of levorphanol on the heart are unknown.

Administer opioids with caution to patients in circulatory shock because vasodilation produced by the drug may further reduce cardiac output and blood pressure.

➤*Pancreatitis/Biliary tract disease:* Use opioids with caution in patients with biliary tract disease, including acute pancreatitis, and in those about to undergo surgery of the biliary tract because it may cause spasm of the sphincter of Oddi and diminish biliary and pancreatic secretions. **Levorphanol** has been shown to cause moderate to marked rises in pressure in the common bile duct when given in analgesic doses; it is not recommended for use in biliary surgery. Opioids may cause increases in serum amylase concentration.

➤*Urinary system disorders:* Initiation of neuraxial opiate analgesia is frequently associated with disturbances of micturition, especially in men with prostatic enlargement. Early recognition of difficulty in urination and prompt intervention in cases of urinary retention is indicated.

➤*Cough reflex:* Cough reflex is suppressed. Exercise caution when using opioid analgesics postoperatively and in patients with pulmonary disease.

➤*Intraoperative awareness:* Intraoperative awareness has been reported in patients younger than 55 years of age when **remifentanil** has been administered with propofol infusion rates of 75 mcg/kg/min or less.

➤*Tolerance:* Tolerance, in which increasingly large doses are required in order to produce the same degree of analgesia, is manifested initially by a shortened duration of analgesic effect, and subsequently by decreases in the intensity of analgesia. The rate of development of tolerance varies among patients. In patients with long-term pain, and in opioid-tolerant cancer patients, guide the dose of opioids by the degree of tolerance manifested.

➤*Hypersensitivity reactions:* Although extremely rare, cases of anaphylaxis have been reported.

Serious and rarely fatal anaphylactoid reactions have been reported in patients receiving therapy with **tramadol**. When these events do occur, it is often following the first dose. Other reported allergic reactions include pruritus, hives, bronchospasm, angioedema, toxic epidermal necrolysis, and Stevens-Johnson syndrome. Patients with a history of anaphylactoid reactions to **codeine** and other opioids may be at increased risk and therefore should not receive tramadol (see Contraindications).

➤*Sulfite sensitivity:* May cause allergic-type reactions (eg, hives, itching, wheezing, anaphylaxis) in certain susceptible patients. Although the overall prevalence of sulfite sensitivity in the general population is probably low, it is seen more frequently in asthmatic patients or in atopic nonasthmatic patients. Specific products containing sulfites are identified in the product listings.

➤*Renal/Hepatic function impairment:* Renal and hepatic dysfunction may cause a prolonged duration and cumulative effect. Administer with caution; smaller doses may be necessary (see Pharmacokinetics).

Meperidine – In patients with renal or hepatic dysfunction, normeperidine (an active metabolite of meperidine) may accumulate, resulting in increased CNS adverse reactions.

Tapentadol – Tapentadol has not been studied in patients with severe renal or hepatic impairment; use in this population is not recommended.

➤*Drug abuse and dependence:* Psychological dependence, physical dependence, and tolerance may develop upon repeated administration of opioids; therefore, prescribe and administer opioids with caution. However, psychological dependence is unlikely to develop when opioids are used for a short time for the treatment of pain. Physical dependence, the condition in which continued administration of the drug is required to prevent the appearance of a withdrawal syndrome, usually assumes clinically significant proportions only after several weeks of continued opioid use, although some mild degree of physical dependence may develop after a few days of opioid therapy. Withdrawal symptoms also may be precipitated in the patient with physical dependence by the administration of a drug with opioid-antagonist activity (eg, naloxone).

Use opioids with caution in patients with alcoholism or other drug dependencies because of the increased frequency of opioid tolerance, dependence, and the risk of addiction observed in these patient populations. Abuse of opioids in combination with other CNS depressants can result in serious risk to the patient.

Abuse of ER doseforms by crushing, chewing, snorting, or injecting the dissolved product will result in the immediate release of the entire daily dose of the opioid and pose a significant risk to the abuser that could result in overdose and death.

Acute abstinence syndrome (withdrawal) – In patients with long-term pain in whom opioid analgesics are abruptly discontinued, anticipate a severe abstinence syndrome. This may be similar to the abstinence syndrome noted in patients who withdraw from heroin. Severity is related to the degree of dependence, the abruptness of withdrawal, and the drug used. Generally, withdrawal symptoms develop at the time the next dose would ordinarily be given.

Symptoms of withdrawal – The opioid agonist abstinence syndrome is characterized by some or all of the following: restlessness, lacrimation, rhinorrhea, yawning, perspiration, gooseflesh, restless sleep or "yen," and mydriasis during the first 24 hours. These symptoms often increase in severity and, over the next 72 hours, may be accompanied by increasing irritability, anxiety, weakness, twitching, and spasms of muscles; kicking movements; severe backache; severe abdominal and leg pains; abdominal and muscle cramps; hot and cold flashes, insomnia; nausea, anorexia, vomiting, intestinal spasm, diarrhea; coryza and repetitive sneezing; and increase in body temperature, blood pressure, respiratory rate, and heart rate. Because of excessive loss of fluids through sweating, vomiting, and diarrhea, there is usually marked weight loss, dehydration, ketosis, and disturbances in acid-base balance. Cardiovascular collapse can occur. Without treatment, most observable symptoms disappear in 5 to 14 days; however, there appears to be a phase of secondary or chronic abstinence, which may last for 2 to 6 months and is characterized by insomnia, irritability, and muscular aches.

Treatment – Primarily symptomatic and supportive; maintain proper fluid and electrolyte balance and administer a tranquilizer to suppress anxiety. Severe withdrawal symptoms may require narcotic replacement. Gradual withdrawal using successively smaller doses will minimize symptoms.

Methadone is not a tranquilizer; patients maintained on this drug may react to problems and stresses with the same anxiety symptoms as others do. Do not confuse such symptoms with narcotic abstinence; do not treat anxiety by increasing the methadone dose.

➤*Hazardous tasks:* May produce drowsiness or dizziness. Patients should use caution while driving or performing other tasks requiring alertness, coordination, or physical dexterity.

➤*Pregnancy:* *Category C* – hydromorphone, opium, oxymorphone, codeine, oxycodone, paregoric, and tapentadol (per manufacturer prescribing information). *Category B* – hydromorphone, methadone (per Briggs' *Drugs in Pregnancy and Lactation*), opium (per Briggs' *Drugs in Pregnancy and Lactation*), **oxycodone**, oxymorphone (per Briggs' *Drugs in Pregnancy and Lactation*), paregoric (per Briggs' *Drugs in Pregnancy and Lactation*). *Category D* if used for prolonged periods or in high doses at term (except tramadol). Safety for use during pregnancy has not been established. There are no adequate and well-controlled studies in pregnant women. Use in pregnant women only if the potential benefits outweigh the possible risks.

The placental transfer of narcotics is rapid. Maternal addiction and neonatal withdrawal occur following use. Withdrawal symptoms include irritability, excessive crying, yawning, sneezing, increased respiratory rate, tremors, convulsions, hyperreflexia, fever, vomiting, increased stools, diarrhea, hyperactivity, abnormal sleep patterns, high-pitched crying, weight loss, and failure to gain weight. Symptoms usually appear during the first days of life, but may be delayed for 2 to 4 weeks.

Alfentanil and **sufentanil** have an embryocidal effect in rats and rabbits when given in doses 2.5 times the upper human dose for 10 days to more than 30 days.

Fentanyl reproduction studies in rats revealed a significant decrease in the pregnancy rate. This decrease was most pronounced in the high-dose group (1.25 mg/kg) in which 1 in 20 animals became pregnant. Female rats were treated with fentanyl 0, 0.025, 0.1, or 0.4 mg/kg/day via IV infusion from day 6 of pregnancy through 3 weeks of lactation. Fentanyl treatment (0.4 mg/kg/day) significantly decreased body weight in male and female pups and also decreased survival in pups at day 4.

In a rat pre- and postnatal study, an increase in pup mortality and a decrease in pup body weight that was associated with maternal toxicity was observed at dosages of **hydromorphone** 2 and 5 mg/kg/day. Hydromorphone administration to pregnant hamsters and mice during major organ development revealed teratogenicity likely the result of maternal toxicity associated with sedation and hypoxia. In hamsters given single subcutaneous doses from 14 to 278 mg/kg during organogenesis (gestation days 8 to 10), doses of 19 mg/kg or more of hydromorphone produced skull malformations (exencephaly and cranioschisis). Continuous infusion of hydromorphone (5 mg/kg, subcutaneously) via implanted osmotic mini pumps during organogenesis (gestation days 7 to 10) produced soft tissue malformations (cryptochidism, cleft palate, malformed ventricals and retina) and skeletal variations (supraoccipital, checkerboard and split sternebrae, delayed ossification of the paws and ectopic ossification sites). The malformations and variations observed in the hamsters and mice were at doses approximately 3-fold higher and less than 1-fold lower, respectively, than a 32 mg human daily oral dose on a body surface area basis.

Levorphanol was teratogenic in mice when given as a single oral dose of 25 mg/kg. The tested dose caused a near 50% mortality of the mouse embryos.

Meperidine should not be used in pregnant women prior to the labor period because safe use in pregnancy prior to labor has not been established relative to possible adverse effects on fetal development. Meperidine is known to cross the placental barrier.

In humans, the frequency of congenital anomalies has been reported to be no greater than expected among the children of 70 women who were treated with **morphine** during the first 4 months of pregnancy or in 448 women treated with this drug any time during pregnancy. Furthermore, no malformations were observed in the infant of a woman who attempted suicide by taking an overdose of morphine and other medication during the first trimester of pregnancy. In animals, several reports indicate that morphine administered subcutaneously during the early gestational period in mice and hamsters produced neurological, soft tissue, and skeletal abnormalities. With one exception, the effects that have been reported were following doses that were maternally toxic and the abnormalities noted were characteristic of those observed when maternal toxicity is present. In 1 study, following subcutaneous infusion of doses 0.15 mg/kg or more to mice, exencephaly, hydronephrosis, intestinal hemorrhage, split supraoccipital, malformed sternebrae, and malformed xiphoid were noted in the absence of maternal toxicity. In the hamster, morphine given subcutaneously on gestation day 8 produced exencephaly and cranioschisis.

Oxymorphone was reported to produce malformations in offspring of hamsters that received 1,500 times the recommended human dose on day 8 of gestation.

Tapentadol produced evidence of embryofetal toxicity at the 40 mg/kg/day dosage in pregnant rats and rabbits, which includes transient delays in skeletal maturation (ie, reduced ossification). Treatment-related developmental delays were observed in rats administered 150 mg/kg/day and higher. These included incomplete ossification, and significant reductions in pup body weights and body weight gains. A dose-related increase in pup mortality was observed through postnatal day 4.

Tramadol is embryotoxic and fetotoxic in mice (360 mg/m^2), rats (150 mg/m^2), and rabbits (900 mg/m^2) at maternally toxic doses. Embryo and fetal toxicity consisted primarily of decreased fetal weights, skeletal ossification, and increased supernumerary ribs at maternally toxic dose levels. Transient delays in developmental or behavioral parameters also were seen in pups from rat dams allowed to deliver. Embryo and fetal lethality were reported in only 1 rabbit study at 300 mg/kg (3,600 mg/m^2). In peri- and postnatal studies in rats, progeny of dams receiving oral (gavage) dose levels of 50 mg/kg or more had decreased weights, and pup survival was decreased early in lactation at 80 mg/kg.

Methadone – An expert review of published data on experiences with methadone use during pregnancy by Teratogen Information System (TERIS) concluded that maternal use of methadone during pregnancy as part of a supervised, therapeutic regimen is unlikely to pose a substantial teratogenic risk (quantity and quality of data assessed as "limited to fair"); however, the data are insufficient to state that there is no risk (TERIS, last reviewed October 2002). Pregnant women involved in methadone maintenance programs have been reported to have significantly improved prenatal care, improved fetal outcomes, and reduced mortality when compared with pregnant women using illicit drugs. Several factors complicate the interpretation of investigations of the children of women who took methadone during pregnancy. These include the maternal use of illicit drugs; other maternal factors, such as nutrition, infection, and psychosocial circumstances; limited information regarding dose and duration of methadone use during pregnancy; and the fact that most maternal exposure appears to occur after the first trimester of pregnancy. In addition, reported studies generally compare the benefit of methadone with the risk of untreated addiction to illicit drugs; the relevance of these findings to pain patients prescribed methadone during pregnancy is unclear.

Methadone has been detected in amniotic fluid and cord plasma at concentrations proportional to maternal plasma and in newborn urine at lower concentrations than corresponding maternal urine. Several studies suggested that infants born to narcotic-addicted women treated with methadone during all or part of pregnancy had decreased fetal growth with reduced birth weight, length, and/or head circumference compared with controls. The growth deficit does not appear to persist into later childhood. However, children born to women treated with methadone during pregnancy demonstrated mild but persistent deficits in performance on psychometric and behavioral tests.

Following large doses, methadone produced teratogenic effects in the guinea pig, hamster, and mouse. One published study found that in hamster fetuses, subcutaneous methadone doses of 31 mg/kg or more (estimated exposure was approximately 2 times a human daily oral dosage of 120 mg/day on a mg/m^2 basis, or equivalent to a human daily IV dosage of 120 mg/day) on day 8 of gestation produced exencephaly and neurological effects. Some of the reported effects were observed at doses that were maternally toxic. In another study, a single subcutaneous dose of methadone 22 to 24 mg/kg (estimated exposure was approximately equivalent to a human daily oral dosage of 120 mg/day on a mg/m^2 basis, or half a human daily IV dosage of 120 mg/day) on day 9 of gestation in mice also produced exencephaly in 11% of the embryos.

There are conflicting reports on whether the risk of sudden infant death syndrome (SIDS) is increased in infants born to women treated with methadone during pregnancy.

Labor – Narcotics cross the placenta and can produce respiratory depression and psychophysiologic effects in the neonate. Resuscitation may be required; have naloxone available. The use of epidurally administered **sufentanil** in combination with bupivacaine 0.125% with or without epinephrine is indicated for labor and delivery. Sufentanil is not recommended for IV use or in larger epidural doses during labor and delivery because of potential risks to the newborn after delivery. In a human clinical trial, the average maternal **remifentanil** concentrations were approximately twice those seen in the fetus. However, in some cases, fetal concentrations were similar to those in the mother. The umbilical arteriovenous ratio of remifentanil concentrations was approximately 30%, suggesting metabolism of remifentanil in the neonate. The use of **alfentanil**, **levorphanol**, **meperidine**, **morphine**, **oxycodone**, and **fentanyl** is not recommended. Do not use **methadone** for obstetrical analgesia. Its long duration of action increases the probability of neonatal respiratory depression. It has also been associated with low infant birth weight.

Opioid analgesics in therapeutic doses may prolong labor. Generally, the effect of opioids on the pregnant uterus appears to depend on the time of administration; administration of the drugs during the latent phase of the first stage of labor, or before cervical dilation of 4 to 5 cm has occurred, may hamper the progress of labor.

Do not use narcotics with mixed agonist-antagonist properties for pain control during labor in patients on long-term methadone treatment because they may precipitate acute withdrawal.

Oral hydromorphone is not recommended to be initiated prior to or during labor or in the immediate postpartum period. Hydromorphone injection is contraindicated in labor and delivery.

Use **oxymorphone** with caution during labor. Sinusoidal fetal heart rate patterns may occur with the use of opioid analgesics.

Tapentadol is not recommended for use in women during and immediately prior to labor and delivery.

Tramadol has been shown to cross the placenta; do not use prior to or during labor unless the potential benefits outweigh the risks. The mean ratio of serum tramadol in the umbilical veins compared with maternal veins was 0.83 for 40 women given tramadol during labor.

➤*Lactation:* Most of these agents appear in breast milk, but effects on the infant may not be significant. Some recommend waiting 4 to 6 hours after use before breast-feeding. Withdrawal symptoms can occur in breast-feeding infants when maternal administration of an opioid-analgesic is stopped. Decide whether to discontinue breast-feeding or the drug, taking into account the importance of the drug to the mother.

Alfentanil – Significant levels of alfentanil were found in breast milk 4 hours after administration of 60 mcg/kg. No detectable levels were found after 28 hours.

Codeine – Codeine passes into breast milk in very small amounts that are probably insignificant. The American Academy of Pediatrics considers codeine to be compatible with breast-feeding.

Fentanyl – Fentanyl (transmucosal, transdermal) is excreted in human milk; therefore, it is not recommended for use in breast-feeding women because of the possibility of the effects in infants. It is not known whether fentanyl injection is excreted in breast milk; use with caution.

Hydromorphone, oxymorphone – It is not known whether oxymorphone and hydromorphone are excreted in human milk.

Hydrocodone – It is not known if hydrocodone is excreted into human milk; however, because of its small molecular weight, passage into milk should be expected. Monitor infant for GI effects, sedation, and changes in feeding patterns.

Levorphanol – Levorphanol is not recommended for use in breast-feeding mothers because it is not known if levorphanol is secreted in pharmacologically active amounts in human milk.

Meperidine, oxycodone – Concentrations of these drugs have been detected in breast milk. Meperidine achieves an average milk:plasma ratio of greater than 1 (peak milk levels of 0.13 mcg/mL occur 2 hours after a 50 mg IM dose). Breast-feeding should not be undertaken during administration of these drugs because of the possibility of sedation and/or respiratory depression in the infant.

Methadone – Methadone is secreted into human milk. There is no information on use of parenteral methadone in breast-feeding or on the safety of the high doses of methadone typically used in chronic pain treatment. The safety of breast-feeding while taking oral methadone is also controversial. At maternal oral dosages of 10 to 80 mg/day, methadone concentrations from 50 to 570 mcg/L in milk have been reported, which, in the majority of samples, were lower than maternal serum drug concentrations at steady state. Peak methadone levels in milk occur approximately 4 to 5 hours after an oral dose. Based on an average milk consumption of 150 mL/kg/day, an infant would consume approximately 17.4 mcg/kg/day, which is approximately 2% to 3% of the oral maternal dose. Methadone has been detected in very low plasma concentrations in some infants whose mothers were taking methadone. Counsel women on high-dose methadone maintenance who are already breast-feeding to wean breast-feeding gradually in order to prevent neonatal abstinence syndrome. Inform methadone-treated mothers considering breast-feeding an opioid-naive infant of the presence of methadone in breast milk.

Morphine – Low levels of morphine have been detected in maternal milk. The milk:plasma morphine AUC ratio is about 2.5:1.

Propoxyphene – Low levels of propoxyphene have been detected in human milk. In postpartum studies, no adverse effects were seen in infants receiving breast milk from mothers who were given propoxyphene.

Remifentanil, sufentanil – It is not known whether these drugs are excreted in human milk. Because fentanyl analogs are excreted in human milk, use with caution.

Tapentadol – Physiochemical and available pharmacodynamic/toxicological data point to excretion in breast milk.

Tramadol – Following a single IV 100 mg dose, the cumulative excretion in breast milk within 16 hours postdose was tramadol 100 mcg (0.1% of the maternal dose) and 27 mcg of the active metabolite (M1).

➤*Children:*

Alfentanil – There are no adequate data to support the use of alfentanil in children younger than 12 years of age. Hypotension has occurred in neonates with respiratory distress syndrome receiving alfentanil 20 mcg/kg.

Codeine – Safe dosage of codeine has not been established for children younger than 3 years of age.

Fentanyl – Safety and efficacy of fentanyl (transdermal and injection) in children younger than 2 years of age have not been established. Administer transdermal fentanyl only to children 2 years of age and older if they are opioid tolerant. Safety and efficacy of fentanyl transmucosal have not been established in patients younger than 16 years of age. Methemoglobinemia has occurred rarely in premature neonates undergoing emergency anesthesia and surgery including combined use of fentanyl injection, pancuronium, and atropine; a cause-and-effect relationship has not been established.

Meperidine – Meperidine has a slower elimination rate in neonates and young infants compared with older children and adults. Neonates and young infants also may be more susceptible to the effects, especially the respiratory depressant effects. Use with caution in neonates and young infants, and weigh any potential benefits against the relative risk.

Oxycodone – Do not use oxycodone in children; safety and efficacy have not been established.

Remifentanil – Safety and efficacy have been established in patients from birth to 12 years of age for use in the maintenance of general anesthesia in outpatient and inpatient pediatric surgery. Remifentanil has not been studied in children for use as a postoperative analgesic or as an analgesic component of monitored anesthesia care.

Sufentanil – Safety and efficacy of IV sufentanil in children younger than 2 years of age undergoing cardiovascular surgery have been documented in a limited number of cases.

Tapentadol – Safety and effectiveness in children younger than 18 years of age have not been established.

Tramadol – Safety and efficacy in patients younger than 16 years of age have not been established.

Hydromorphone / Levorphanol / Methadone / Morphine / Opium / Oxymorphone / Propoxyphene – Safety and efficacy have not been established in children.

➤*Elderly:* Appropriately reduce the initial dose in elderly and debilitated patients. Consider the effect of the initial dose in determining supplemental doses. Use caution because opioids have the ability to depress respiration and reduce ventilatory drive to a clinically significant event.

In 1 clinical trial, the dose of **alfentanil** required to produce anesthesia, as determined by appearance of delta waves in electroencephalogram, was 40% lower in elderly patients than that needed in healthy young patients.

Because elderly, cachectic, or debilitated patients may have altered pharmacokinetics due to poor fat stores, muscle wasting, or altered clearance, do not start them on **transdermal fentanyl** doses higher than 25 mcg/h unless they are already taking oral **morphine** 135 mg/day or more or an equivalent dose of another opioid.

In studies with **transmucosal fentanyl**, patients older than 65 years of age were titrated to a mean dose that was about 200 mcg less than the mean dose titrated to by younger patients. Studies with **IV fentanyl** showed that elderly patients are twice as sensitive to the effects of fentanyl as the younger population. The clearance of IV fentanyl may be greatly decreased in patients older than 60 years of age.

Elderly patients have a slower elimination rate compared with younger patients, and they may be more susceptible to the effects of **meperidine**; a reduction in total daily dose may be required. Per the Beers list, meperidine is not an effective oral analgesic in doses commonly used. It may cause confusion and has many disadvantages to other narcotic drugs. Meperidine is also considered a high-risk medication for elderly patients according to the Centers of Medicare and Medicaid Services.

The pharmacodynamic effects of neuraxial **morphine** in elderly patients are more variable than in the younger population. Base initial doses on careful clinical observation following "test doses," after making due allowances for the effects of the patient's age and infirmity on his/her ability to clear the drug, particularly in patients receiving epidural morphine. Elderly patients may be more susceptible to respiratory depression and/or respiratory arrest following administration of morphine.

In elderly patients, the clearance of **oxycodone** appears to be slightly reduced. Compared with younger adults, the plasma concentrations of oxycodone were increased approximately 15%.

The rate of **propoxyphene** metabolism may be reduced in some patients. Consider increased dosing intervals.

After termination of **remifentanil** administration, blood concentrations fell as rapidly in elderly patients as in younger adults. While the effective biological half-life of remifentanil is unchanged, elderly patients were twice as sensitive to the pharmacodynamic effects as younger patients. Decrease the recommended starting dose by 50% in patients older than 65 years of age.

Daily doses greater than **tramadol** 300 mg are not recommended in patients older than 75 years of age (see Administration and Dosage). Patients older than 75 years of age had slightly elevated serum concentrations and a slightly prolonged elimination half-life (see Actions). Patients older than 75 years of age also experienced more treatment-limiting adverse events during clinical trials, as compared with those younger than 65 years of age. Constipation resulted in the discontinuation of treatment in 10% of those older than 75 years of age.

➤*Monitoring:* Because of the possibility of delayed respiratory depression, continue monitoring patients well after surgery. Monitor vital signs routinely.

Patients receiving monitored anesthesia care (MAC) should be continuously monitored by people not involved in the conduct of the surgical or diagnostic procedure. Oxygen supplementation should be immediately available and provided where clinically indicated. Continuously monitor oxygen saturation. Observe the patient for early signs of hypotension, apnea, upper airway obstruction, or oxygen desaturation.

Drug Interactions

➤*CYP-450 system:* **Fentanyl** is metabolized mainly via CYP3A4; therefore, potential interactions may occur when fentanyl is given concurrently with agents that affect CYP3A4 activity. Coadministration with CYP3A4 inducers may reduce the efficacy of fentanyl while coadministration with CYP3A4 inhibitors may increase fentanyl plasma concentration. Carefully monitor patients receiving fentanyl and potent CYP3A4 inhibitors (eg, clarithromycin, ketoconazole, ritonavir) for an extended period of time and adjust dosage as needed.

Oxycodone is metabolized in part by CYP2D6 to **oxymorphone**. The interaction between oxycodone and CYP2D6 inhibitors (eg, amiodarone, amitriptyline, fluoxetine, paroxetine, quinidine) has not been shown to be of clinical significance.

Tramadol is extensively metabolized by a number of pathways including CYP2D6 and CYP3A4. The formation of M1 (active metabolite) is dependent upon CYP2D6 and as such is subject to inhibition, which may affect the therapeutic response. Therefore, coadministration of tramadol with a CYP2D6 inhibitor (eg, fluoxetine, paroxetine, quinidine) may increase concentrations of tramadol and reduce concentrations of M1. Coadministration of tramadol with CYP3A4 inhibitors (eg, azole antifungals, macrolide antibiotics, protease inhibitors) may decrease tramadol clearance, and CYP3A4 inducers (eg, carbamazepine, phenytoin, rifampin) may increase tramadol clearance.

Opioid Analgesics Drug Interactions

Precipitant drug	Object drug[a]		Description
Acyclovir	Opioid analgesics	↑	Plasma concentrations of meperidine and normeperidine may be increased; use with caution.
Amiodarone	Opioid analgesics Fentanyl	↑	Profound bradycardia, sinus arrest, and hypotension have occurred with coadministration. Monitor hemodynamic function and administer inotropic, chronotropic, and pressor support as necessary. Bradycardia is usually unresponsive to atropine; large doses of vasopressors have been used.
Anticholinergics	Opioid analgesics	↑	Coadministration may result in increased risk of urinary retention and/or severe constipation, which may lead to paralytic ileus.
Azole antifungals	Opioid analgesics Alfentanil Fentanyl Methadone	↑	Coadministration may lead to increased pharmacological and adverse effects of the narcotic. Use with caution, and monitor for prolonged or recurrent respiratory depression. A lower dose of the narcotic may be necessary.
Barbiturate anesthetics	Opioid analgesics	↑	Barbiturate anesthetics may increase the respiratory and CNS depressant effects of the narcotics because of additive pharmacologic activity.
Opioid analgesics	Barbiturate anesthetics		
Barbiturates	Opioid analgesics Methadone	↓	Coadministration may reduce methadone action. Patients receiving long-term methadone treatment may experience withdrawal symptoms. A higher dose of methadone may be required during coadministration of barbiturates.
Benzodiazepines	Opioid analgesics Sufentanil	↑	Coadministration may result in decreased mean arterial pressure and systemic vascular resistance (also see CNS depressant interaction).
Benzodiazepines Diazepam	Opioid analgesics Alfentanil Fentanyl	↑	Diazepam may produce cardiovascular depression when given with high doses of fentanyl and alfentanil. Administration prior to or following high doses of alfentanil decreases blood pressure secondary to vasodilation; recovery may be prolonged.
Beta-blockers Calcium channel blockers	Opioid analgesics Sufentanil	↑	Increased incidence and degree of bradycardia and hypotension during induction of sufentanil in patients on long-term calcium channel or beta-blocker therapy.
Opioid analgesics Sufentanil	Beta-blockers Calcium channel blockers		
Carbamazepine	Opioid analgesics Tramadol	↓	Because carbamazepine increases tramadol metabolism and because of the seizure risk associated with tramadol, coadministration is not recommended.
Cigarette smoking	Opioid analgesics Propoxyphene	↓	Cigarette smoking may induce liver enzymes responsible for the metabolism of propoxyphene; efficacy is reportedly decreased in smokers. Patients may increase the dosage to obtain adequate pain relief.
Cimetidine	Opioid analgesics	↑	The actions of opioid analgesics may be enhanced, resulting in toxicity. Alfentanil clearance may be reduced; therefore, smaller alfentanil doses may be needed.
CNS depressants (eg, barbiturates, ethanol, inhalation anesthetics, tranquilizers)	Opioid analgesics	↑	Both the magnitude and duration of CNS and cardiovascular effects may be enhanced. Reduce the dose of one or both agents during concomitant use.
CYP2D6 inhibitors (eg, amitriptyline, fluoxetine, paroxetine, quinidine)	Opioid analgesics Oxycodone Tramadol	↑	Inhibition of the metabolism of tramadol or oxycodone may occur.

Opioid Analgesics Drug Interactions

Precipitant drug	Object drug[a]		Description
CYP3A4 inducers (eg, phenytoin, rifampin)	Opioid analgesics Fentanyl Tramadol	↓	May produce increased clearance of fentanyl and tramadol; use with caution.
CYP3A4 inhibitors (eg, certain protease inhibitors, erythromycin, ketoconazole)	Opioid analgesics Fentanyl Tramadol	↑	Coadministration may produce increased fentanyl and tramadol concentrations. Carefully monitor patients receiving fentanyl and potent CYP3A4 inhibitors (eg, clarithromycin, ketoconazole, ritonavir) for an extended period of time and adjust the dosage as needed.
Droperidol	Opioid analgesics Fentanyl	↑	Pulmonary arterial pressure may be depressed and hypotension may occur.
Erythromycin	Opioid analgesics Alfentanil Fentanyl Methadone	↑	Erythromycin may inhibit the metabolism of the narcotic. Coadministration may result in increased pharmacologic effects of the narcotic. Monitor for prolonged or recurrent respiratory depression and sedation. Consider a lower dose of the narcotic or an alternate narcotic.
Ethanol	Opioid analgesics Alfentanil	↓	Chronic ethanol consumption may produce a pharmacodynamic tolerance to alfentanil. Chronic ethanol consumers may need higher doses of alfentanil (see also CNS depressants interaction).
Hydantoins (eg, phenytoin)	Opioid analgesics Meperidine Methadone	↓	Hydantoins may decrease the pharmacologic effects of meperidine and methadone, possibly because of increased hepatic metabolism of the narcotic.
Lidocaine	Opioid analgesics Morphine	↑	Respiratory depression and loss of consciousness may occur.
Opioid analgesics Morphine	Lidocaine		
MAOIs	Opioid analgesics	↑	Severe and unpredictable potentiation by MAOIs has been reported with certain opioid analgesics. Opioids are not recommended for use in patients who have received MAOIs within 14 days. Meperidine is contraindicated in patients who have recently received an MAOI. Coadministration could result in adverse reactions that may include agitation, seizures, diaphoresis, and fever, which may progress to coma, apnea, and death. Reactions may occur several weeks following withdrawal of MAOIs. Meperidine, morphine, and tapentadol are contraindicated in patients receiving an MAOI or who have taken an MAOI in the last 14 days.
Opioid analgesics	MAOIs		
Neostigmine	Opioid analgesics Morphine	↑	Increases the intensity and duration of the analgesic action.
Nitrous oxide	Opioid analgesics Fentanyl Sufentanil	↑	Nitrous oxide may cause cardiovascular depression with high-dose sufentanil and fentanyl.
NNRTIs[b] (eg, efavirenz, nevirapine)	Opioid analgesics Methadone	↓	Coadministration may result in reduced methadone action and opiate withdrawal symptoms. Anticipate an increase in the methadone dose when starting an NNRTI and monitor for withdrawal symptoms. Monitor for signs of methadone overdose when an NNRTI is discontinued and adjust the methadone dose accordingly.
NRTIs[b] Abacavir	Opioid analgesics Methadone	↓	When coadministered with abacavir, methadone clearance increased 22%. Methadone dosage adjustment may be needed in a small number of patients. Coadministration may decrease AUC and C_{max} of didanosine and stavudine; however, coadministration may increase zidovudine concentration. Monitor zidovudine effects closely; a lower dosage may be needed.
Opioid analgesics Methadone	NRTIs Didanosine Stavudine Zidovudine	↑↓	
Opioid agonist/antagonist analgesics, opioid partial agonist analgesics	Opioid analgesics	↓	Do not administer opioid agonist/antagonist analgesics (eg, butorphanol, nalbuphine, pentazocine) or partial agonists (eg, buprenorphine) to a patient who has received or is receiving a course of therapy with a pure agonist opioid analgesic. In opioid-dependent patients, mixed agonist/antagonist analgesics and partial agonists may precipitate withdrawal symptoms.
Phenothiazines	Opioid analgesics	↑	Although the analgesic effect of narcotics may be potentiated, a higher incidence of toxic effects may occur. Reduce the dose of meperidine.
Propofol	Opioid analgesics Oxycodone	↑	Increased risk of bradycardia with concomitant use.
Protease inhibitors (eg, nelfinavir, ritonavir, saquinavir)	Opioid analgesics Fentanyl Meperidine Methadone Propoxyphene	↑↓	Plasma concentrations of propoxyphene and fentanyl may be increased, possibly causing toxicity. The pharmacologic effects of methadone may be decreased. Meperidine levels may decrease and normeperidine levels may increase, possibly decreasing efficacy but increasing neurologic toxicity. Concurrent use of propoxyphene or meperidine with a protease inhibitor is contraindicated.
Quinidine	Opioid analgesics Codeine	↓	The analgesic effects of codeine may be decreased. It may be necessary to use an alternative analgesic.
Reserpine	Opioid analgesics Morphine	↓	Inhibits analgesic action.
Rifamycins (eg, rifampin)	Opioid analgesics Methadone Morphine	↓	Rifampin appears to stimulate methadone metabolism. Coadministration may result in reduced methadone action and opiate withdrawal symptoms. A higher dosage of methadone may be required during coadministration of rifampin. The analgesic effects of morphine may be decreased with coadministration. An alternative analgesic may be necessary.
Sibutramine	Opioid analgesics Meperidine	↑	Serotonergic effects of these agents may be additive, resulting in a serotonin syndrome. Coadministration is not recommended.
Opioid analgesics Meperidine	Sibutramine		
SSRIs Nefazodone Venlafaxine	Opioid analgesics Methadone Tapentadol Tramadol	↑	Fluvoxamine may inhibit methadone metabolism, therefore increasing toxicity. Use with caution. The serotonergic effects of tapentadol and tramadol, and serotonin reuptake effects of tapentadol, tramadol, and serotonin reuptake inhibitors may be additive, increasing the risk for adverse effects (eg, seizures, serotonin syndrome).
Opioid analgesics Tramadol	SSRIs Nefazodone Venlafaxine		

Opioid Analgesics Drug Interactions			
Precipitant drug	Object drug[a]		Description
Tricyclic antidepressants Amitriptyline Clomipramine Nortriptyline	Opioid analgesics Morphine Tapentadol	⬆	Monitor for increased CNS and respiratory depression when administered with morphine. A serotonin syndrome may occur when tricyclic antidepressants are used with tapentadol.
Urinary acidifiers	Opioid analgesics Methadone	⬇	Urinary acidifiers increase the renal clearance of methadone.
Opioid analgesics Propoxyphene	Carbamazepine	⬆	Propoxyphene may inhibit the metabolism of carbamazepine, thereby increasing carbamazepine serum concentrations and toxicity.
Opioid analgesics Methadone	Desipramine	⬆	Desipramine blood levels have increased with concurrent methadone therapy.
Opioid analgesics Tramadol	Digoxin	⬆	Rare reports of digoxin toxicity have been reported in postmarketing surveillance.
Opioid analgesics Morphine	Diuretics	⬇	Reduces efficacy by inducing the release of antidiuretic hormone.
Opioid analgesics Remifentanil	Opioid analgesics Morphine	⬇	The analgesic effect of morphine may be decreased with coadministration. It may be necessary to titrate morphine to higher levels than expected.
Opioid analgesics	Skeletal muscle relaxants	⬆	Coadministration may enhance the neuromuscular blocking action and produce an increased degree of respiratory depression.
Opioid analgesics Morphine Propoxyphene Tramadol	Warfarin	⬆	The oral anticoagulant effect of warfarin may be increased. Monitor coagulation tests and adjust dose as needed.

[a] ⬆ = object drug increased; ⬇ = object drug decreased; ⬆⬇ = object drug increased and decreased.

[b] NNRTIs = nonnucleoside reverse transcriptase inhibitors; NRTIs = nucleoside reverse transcriptase inhibitors.

➤*Drug/Food interactions:* Grapefruit juice may increase **methadone** serum concentrations, thereby increasing the pharmacologic and adverse effects.

Adverse Reactions

Opioid Analgesic Adverse Reactions (%)[a,b]

System	Adverse reactions	Alfentanil	Codeine	Fentanyl injection	Fentanyl transdermal: Adults	Fentanyl transdermal: Children (2 to 18 years of age)	Fentanyl transmucosal	Hydromorphone ER[c]	Hydromorphone IR[c]	Levorphanol	Meperidine	Methadone	Morphine	Oxycodone CR[c]	Oxycodone IR[c]	Oxymorphone	Propoxyphene	Remifentanil: Adults	Remifentanil: Children (≤ 12 years of age)	Sufentanil	Tapentadol	Tramadol
Cardiovascular	Abnormal electrocardiogram							< 1				✓										PM
	Angina pectoris						< 1	< 1														
	Arrhythmia	14			≥ 1			< 1		✓		✓								0.3-1		
	Atrial fibrillation							< 1					✓					< 1				
	Bradycardia	14	✓	✓	< 1			< 1	✓	✓	✓	✓	✓			✓		1-7		3-9	≤ 1	
	Cardiac arrest		✓	✓							✓	✓	✓		✓							PM
	Cardiomegaly							< 1														
	Chest pain				≥ 1		≥ 1	≥ 1					✓	< 1				< 1				
	Circulatory depression/collapse		✓	✓							✓	✓	✓	✓	✓							
	Congestive Heart failure/heart failure							< 1				✓			< 3							
	Deep thrombophlebitis						≥ 1	< 1							< 3							
	Extrasystoles									✓												
	Faintness		✓								✓	✓	✓									
	Flushing		✓	✓		≥ 1		✓	✓	✓	✓	✓	✓			✓		1				
	Hemorrhage						< 1	< 1							< 3							
	Hypertension	18	✓	✓		≥ 1	0-1	< 1	✓				✓					1-2		3-9		PM
	Hypotension	10	✓ (orthostatic)	✓			< 1	< 1	✓	✓	✓	✓	✓	1-5	< 3	✓		4-19		3-9	≤ 1	< 1
	Migraine						≥ 1	≥ 1						< 1	< 3							PM
	MI							< 1														
	Myocardial ischemia																					PM
	Palpitation		✓				≥ 1	< 1	✓		✓	✓	✓		< 3	✓						PM
	Pallor							< 1					✓									
	Peripheral vascular disorder						< 1															
	Phlebitis										✓	✓	✓ (IV)									
	QT interval prolongation							< 1				✓										
	ST depression													< 1								
	Supraventricular tachycardia							< 1														
	Syncope		✓		≥ 1	≥ 1	< 1	< 1	✓		✓	✓	✓	< 1				< 1			≤ 1	< 1
	Tachycardia	12	✓		PM	≥ 1	< 1	≥ 1	✓	✓	✓	✓	✓		< 3	✓		< 1		0.3-1	≤ 1	< 1
	Thrombosis							< 1														
	Vascular disorder						≥ 1															
	Vasodilation						0-4	≥ 1					✓	< 1	< 3							1-5

Opioid Analgesic Adverse Reactions (%)[a,b]

System	Adverse reactions	Alfentanil	Codeine	Fentanyl injection	Fentanyl transdermal		Fentanyl transmucosal	Hydromorphone ER[c]	Hydromorphone IR[c]	Levorphanol	Meperidine	Methadone	Morphine	Oxycodone CR[c]	Oxycodone IR[c]	Oxymorphone	Propoxyphene	Remifentanil		Sufentanil	Tapentadol	Tramadol
					Adults	Children (2 to 18 years of age)												Adults	Children (≤ 12 years of age)			
CNS	Abnormal coordination				≥1																≤ 1	
	Abnormal dreams				≥ 1		0-1	< 1		✓			✓	1-5							1	
	Abnormal gait				≥1		0-5	≥ 1					✓	< 1								< 1
	Abnormal thinking				≥ 1		0-2	≥ 1		✓			✓	1-5							≤ 1	< 1
	Acute brain syndrome						< 1															
	Addiction							< 1														
	Agitation		✓		≥ 1	≥ 1	< 1	≥ 1			✓	✓	✓		< 1			< 1			≤ 1	
	Amnesia				≥1		< 1	≥ 1		✓			✓	< 1				< 1				< 1
	Anxiety		✓		3-10	≥ 1	0-15	≥ 1	✓				✓	1-5	< 3			< 1			1	1-5
	Apathy							< 1														
	Aphasia				< 1			< 1														
	Asthenia				≥ 10	3-10	0-38	3.2					✓	6								6-12
	Ataxia							< 1					✓								≤ 1	
	Cerebral ischemia						< 1															
	Cerebrovascular accident							< 1														
	CNS stimulation									✓						✓						7-14
	Coma									✓			✓					< 1				
	Confusion				≥ 10	≥ 1	0-13	≥ 1		✓		✓	✓	1-5	< 3	✓		< 1			1	1-5
	Convulsion/Seizure		✓			≥ 1	0-2	< 1		✓	✓, severe	✓	✓	< 1								< 1
	Delirium							< 1					✓									
	Dementia							< 1														
	Depersonalization				< 1			< 1						< 1								
	Depressed level of consciousness																				≤ 1	
	Depression				3-10	≥ 1	2-9	≥ 1		✓			✓	< 1		✓						< 1
	Disorientation		✓						✓		✓	✓	✓					< 1			≤ 1	
	Disturbance in attention																				≤ 1	
	Dizziness	3-9	✓	✓	3-10	≥ 1	0-17	≥ 1	✓	✓		✓	✓	13	✓		< 1	< 5			24	26-33
	Drowsiness							< 1	✓				✓			✓						
	Dysarthria																				≤ 1	
	Dyskinesia									✓												
	Dysphoria		✓					< 1	✓		✓	✓			✓	✓	< 1	< 1				
	Emotional lability						< 1	< 1						< 1								
	Euphoria	0.3-1	✓		3-10		< 1	< 1	✓		✓	✓	✓	1-5	✓	✓	< 1				≤ 1	1-5
	Facial paralysis						< 1															
	Fatigue																				3	
	Fear		✓						✓													
	Feeling drunk																				≤ 1	
	Foot drop						< 1															
	Hallucinations				3-10	≥ 1	≤ 2	≥ 1	✓		✓		✓	< 1		✓	< 1	< 1				< 1
	Headache	0.3-1	✓		3-10	3-10	3-20	4.7	✓		✓	✓	✓	7		✓	< 1	≤ 18				18-32
	Hemiplegia						< 1															
	Hostility				< 1			< 1														
	Hyperkinesia									✓				< 1								
	Hypertonia				< 1			≥ 1							< 3							1-5

System	Adverse reactions	Alfentanil	Codeine	Fentanyl injection	Fentanyl transdermal		Fentanyl transmucosal	Hydromorphone ER[c]	Hydromorphone IR[c]	Levorphanol	Meperidine	Methadone	Morphine	Oxycodone CR[c]	Oxycodone IR[c]	Oxymorphone	Propoxyphene	Remifentanil		Sufentanil	Tapentadol	Tramadol
					Adults	Children (2 to 18 years of age)												Adults	Children (≤ 12 years of age)			
CNS (cont.)	Hypesthesia						≥ 1	≥ 1						< 1							≤ 1	
	Hypokinesia						≥ 1	< 1		✓												
	Hypotonia				< 1									< 1								
	Impairment of mental and physical performance		✓						✓													
	Incoordination						< 1	< 1	✓		✓		✓									1-5
	Increased intracranial pressure								✓				✓									
	Insomnia		✓		≥ 1	3-10	≤ 8	≥ 1	✓	✓		✓	✓	1-5		✓					2	
	Irritability																				≤ 1	
	Lethargy		✓						✓	✓			✓								1	
	Light-headedness		✓						✓		✓	✓	✓		✓	✓	< 1					
	Memory impairment																				≤ 1	
	Mental clouding		✓						✓				✓			✓						
	Mood changes		✓						✓				✓									
	Myoclonic movements	PM					0-4	< 1			✓											
	Nervousness				3-10	3-10	0-4	≥ 1		✓			✓	1-5	< 3	✓					≤ 1	1-5
	Neuralgia							< 1							< 3							
	Neuropathy						≥ 1															
	Paranoid reaction				≥ 1	≥ 1		< 1														
	Paresthesia				≥ 1		≥ 1	≥ 1	✓				✓	< 1				< 1			≤ 1	< 1
	Personality disorder									✓					< 3							
	Postoperative confusion	0.3-1																				
	Psychosis							< 1														
	Restlessness															✓					≤ 1	
	Sedation																				≤ 1	
	Seizure																				≤ 1	
	Serotonin syndrome																					< 1
	Shivering	0.3-1			≥ 1													1-5	3			
	Sleep disorder euphoria							< 1														
	Sleepiness/sedation/ Somnolence	1-3	✓		≥ 10	3-10	7-20	4.7	✓		✓	✓	✓	23	✓	✓	< 1			3-9		16-25
	Somnolence																				15	
	Speech disorder				≥ 1	≥ 1	≥ 1	≥ 1						< 1				< 1				PM
	Stupor				< 1	≥ 1	0-4	< 1						< 1								
	Subdural hematoma						< 1															
	Suicide attempt/Tendency									✓												
	Tremor				≥ 1	≥ 1	0-2	≥ 1	✓		✓		✓	< 1	< 3			< 1			1	< 1
	Twitching							< 1			✓			1-5				< 1				
	Vertigo				< 1		0-4	< 1					✓	< 1								26-33
	Weakness		✓						✓		✓	✓	✓			✓	< 1					
	Withdrawal syndrome							< 1		✓			✓	< 1							≤ 1	

Opioid Analgesic Adverse Reactions (%)[a,b]

Opioid Analgesic Adverse Reactions (%)[a,b]

System	Adverse reactions	Alfentanil	Codeine	Fentanyl injection	Fentanyl transdermal: Adults	Fentanyl transdermal: Children (2 to 18 years of age)	Fentanyl transmucosal	Hydromorphone ER[c]	Hydromorphone IR[c]	Levorphanol	Meperidine	Methadone	Morphine	Oxycodone CR[c]	Oxycodone IR[c]	Oxymorphone	Propoxyphene	Remifentanil: Adults	Remifentanil: Children (≤ 12 years of age)	Sufentanil	Tapentadol	Tramadol
Dermatological	Alopecia						≥ 1	< 1														
	Application-site reactions				> 1	3-10																
	Dry skin												✓	< 1								
	Erythema																			0.3-1		
	Erythematous rash					≥ 1																
	Exfoliative dermatitis				< 1		< 1							< 1								
	Herpes simplex														< 3							
	Herpes zoster						< 1															
	Hyperhidrosis																				3	
	Itching/pruritus	0.3-1	✓		3-10	3-10	0-5	2.6	✓	✓		✓	✓	13	✓	✓		≤ 18		25	5	8-11
	Localized skin reaction					≥ 1												< 1				
	Maculopapular rash						< 1	< 1														
	Photosensitivity reaction							< 1							< 3							
	Pustules				< 1																	
	Rash				≥ 1	≥ 1	0-8	≥ 1	✓	✓		✓	✓	1-5	< 3		< 1	< 1			1	1-5
	Skin discoloration						< 1															
	Skin ulcer						≥ 1															
	Stevens-Johnson syndrome/ Toxic epidermal necrolysis																					< 1
	Sweating		✓	✓	≥ 10	≥ 1	0-4	≥ 1	✓	✓	✓	✓	✓	5	< 3	✓		6				6-9
	Urticaria	0.3-1					< 1	< 1	✓	✓		✓	✓	< 1	< 3			< 1			≤ 1	< 1
	Vesicles																					< 1
	Vesiculobullous						< 1															

Opioid Analgesic Adverse Reactions (%)[a,b]

System	Adverse reactions	Alfentanil	Codeine	Fentanyl injection	Fentanyl transdermal		Fentanyl transmucosal	Hydromorphone ER[c]	Hydromorphone IR[c]	Levorphanol	Meperidine	Methadone	Morphine	Oxycodone CR[c]	Oxycodone IR[c]	Oxymorphone	Propoxyphene	Remifentanil		Sufentanil	Tapentadol	Tramadol
					Adults	Children (2 to 18 years of age)												Adults	Children (≤ 12 years of age)			
GI	Abdominal distention				< 1		≥ 1															
	Abdominal pain				3-10	≥ 1	≥ 1	≥ 1		✓		✓		1-5	< 3	✓	< 1				≤ 1	1-5
	Abnormal liver function tests							< 1					✓				< 1					PM
	Abnormal stools							< 1														
	Anorexia		✓		3-10	≥ 1		≥ 1	✓			✓	✓	1-5	< 3	✓						1-5
	Appetite increased							< 1						< 1								
	Biliary tract spasm		✓					< 1	✓	✓	✓	✓	✓		✓	✓						
	Cheilitis						< 1															
	Cholangitis							< 1														
	Cholecystitis							< 1														
	Colitis							< 1														
	Colon hemorrhage						< 1															
	Colonic motility increased												✓									
	Constipation		✓		≥ 10	3-10	0-20	15.8	✓		✓	✓	✓	23	✓	✓	< 1	< 1			8	24-46
	Cramps								✓			✓		✓								
	Diarrhea				3-10	≥ 1	≥ 1	≥ 1	✓				✓	1-5	< 3			< 1				5-10
	Dry mouth		✓		≥ 10	≥ 1	0-4	≥ 1	✓	✓	✓	✓	✓	6	< 3	✓					4	5-10
	Dyspepsia				3-10		≥ 1	≥ 1		✓			✓	1-5	< 3						2	5-13
	Dysphagia						≥ 1	≥ 1					✓	< 1	< 3			< 1				
	Enterocolitis							< 1														
	Eructation						≥ 1	< 1						< 1								
	Esophageal stenosis						< 1															
	Esophagitis						< 1	< 1														
	Fecal impaction						< 1	< 1														
	Fecal incontinence						< 1	< 1														
	Flatulence				≥ 1		≥ 1	≥ 1						< 1								1-5
	Gastritis													1-5								
	Gastroenteritis						< 1						✓									
	GI disorder						< 1							< 1								
	GI hemorrhage						≥ 1	< 1														PM
	Gingivitis						≥ 1								< 3							
	Glossitis						≥ 1	< 1				✓			< 3							
	Gum hemorrhage						< 1															
	Gum line erosion						PM															
	Hepatic failure							< 1														PM
	Hepatitis																					PM
	Hepatomegaly							< 1														
	Hepatorenal syndrome						< 1															
	Ileus							< 1	✓				✓	< 1		✓		< 1				
	Impaired gastric emptying																				≤ 1	

Opioid Analgesic Adverse Reactions (%)[a,b]

System	Adverse reactions	Alfentanil	Codeine	Fentanyl injection	Fentanyl transdermal		Fentanyl transmucosal	Hydromorphone ER[c]	Hydromorphone IR[c]	Levorphanol	Meperidine	Methadone	Morphine	Oxycodone CR[c]	Oxycodone IR[c]	Oxymorphone	Propoxyphene	Remifentanil		Sufentanil	Tapentadol	Tramadol
					Adults	Children (2 to 18 years of age)												Adults	Children (≤ 12 years of age)			
GI (cont.)	Increased pressure in the biliary tract		✓																			
	Intestinal obstruction						0-4	< 1					✓									
	Jaundice						≥ 1	< 1									< 1					
	Liver tenderness						< 1															
	Melena							< 1														
	Mouth ulceration						≥ 1	< 1														
	Nausea	28	✓	✓	≥ 10	≥ 10	11-45	10.5	✓	✓	✓	✓	✓	23	< 3	✓	< 1	1-4.4	6-8	3-9	30	24-40
	Oral moniliasis						≥ 1															
	Periodontal abscess						≥ 1															
	Rectal disorder						≥ 1						✓									
	Rectal hemorrhage						≥ 1	< 1														
	Salivation increased							< 1														
	Stomatitis						≥ 1							< 1								PM
	Thirst						< 1	< 1					✓	< 1								
	Tongue edema							< 1														
	Tooth caries						< 1															
	Tooth disorder						< 1															
	Tooth loss						PM															
	Toxic megacolon															✓[d]						
	Vomiting	18	✓	✓	≥ 10	≥ 10	6-31	3.2	✓	✓	✓	✓	✓	12	< 3	✓	< 1	≤ 22	12-16	3-9	18	9-17
	Weight loss				PM		≥ 1	≥ 1					✓									< 1
GU	Abnormal ejaculation				PM								✓									
	Amenorrhea											✓		< 1								
	Antidiuretic effect		✓						✓		✓	✓	✓	< 1		✓						
	Bladder pain				< 1																	
	Breast neoplasm						≥ 1															
	Breast pain						≥ 1															
	Creatinine increased							< 1														PM
	Decreased libido/Potency		✓		PM		< 1					✓	✓	< 1								
	Dysmenorrhea							< 1														
	Dysuria						≥ 1	≥ 1					✓	< 1				< 1				< 1
	Hematuria						≥ 1	< 1						< 1								
	Hydronephrosis						≥ 1															
	Impotence							< 1					✓		✓							
	Kidney failure						≥ 1			✓												
	Kidney pain						< 1															
	Menopausal symptoms																					1-5
	Menstrual disorder																					< 1
	Nocturia						< 1															
	Oliguria				< 1		< 1						✓					< 1				
	Pollakiuria																				≤ 1	
	Polyuria						< 1							< 1								
	Proteinuria																					PM
	Pyelonephritis						< 1															
	Scrotal edema						≥ 1															
	Spasm of vesical sphincters		✓						✓				✓									
	Ureteral spasm		✓						✓				✓			✓						
	Urinary frequency				< 1			< 1														1-5
	Urinary hesitancy		✓						✓			✓	✓			✓					≤ 1	
	Urinary incontinence						≥ 1	≥ 1										< 1				
	Urinary retention		✓		3-10	≥ 1	0-2	< 1	✓	✓	✓	✓	✓	< 1		✓		< 1		✓		1-5
	Urinary tract infection						≥ 1	< 1					✓		< 3						1	
	Urinary urgency						≥ 1	< 1														
	Urination impaired						≥ 1	< 1		✓				< 1								
	Vaginal hemorrhage						≥ 1															
	Vaginitis						≥ 1															

Opioid Analgesic Adverse Reactions (%)[a,b]

System	Adverse reactions	Alfentanil	Codeine	Fentanyl injection	Fentanyl transdermal Adults	Fentanyl transdermal Children (2 to 18 years of age)	Fentanyl transmucosal	Hydromorphone ER[c]	Hydromorphone IR[c]	Levorphanol	Meperidine	Methadone	Morphine	Oxycodone CR[c]	Oxycodone IR[c]	Oxymorphone	Propoxyphene	Remifentanil Adults	Remifentanil Children (≤ 12 years of age)	Sufentanil	Tapentadol	Tramadol
Hematologic/Lymphatic	Agranulocytosis							< 1														
	Anemia						≥ 1	≥ 1					✓		< 3							
	Bleeding time increased						< 1															
	Ecchymosis						≥ 1	< 1														
	Hemoglobin decrease																					PM
	Leukocytosis							< 1														
	Leukopenia						≥ 1	≥ 1							< 3							
	Lymphadenopathy						≥ 1	< 1						< 1								
	Lymphedema						≥ 1															
	Lymphoma-like reaction							< 1														
	Pancytopenia						≥ 1	< 1														
	Petechia							< 1														
	Thrombocytopenia						≥ 1	< 1				✓	✓									
Hypersensitivity	Allergic reaction		✓			≥ 1	< 1	< 1	✓						< 3	✓[e]					≤ 1	< 1
	Allergic bronchospastic reaction															✓						
	Allergic laryngeal edema															✓						
	Allergic laryngospasm															✓						
	Anaphylaxis/ Anaphylactoid	PM		✓								✓	✓	< 1				< 1		PM		< 1
	Edema											✓	✓									
	Hemorrhagic urticaria		Rare									✓	✓									
	Pruritus		✓								✓	✓	✓			✓						
	Skin rash		✓								✓	✓	✓			✓						
	Urticaria		✓								✓	✓	✓			✓						
	Wheal and flare over vein with IV injection								✓		✓	✓	✓									
Metabolic	Acidosis						< 1	< 1														
	Adrenal cortex insufficiency							< 1														
	Cachexia							< 1														
	Cyanosis							< 1			✓											
	Decreased appetite																				2	
	Diabetes mellitus							< 1														
	Gout							< 1							< 3							
	Hypercalcemia						≥ 1															
	Hyperglycemia						≥ 1	< 1							< 3			< 1				
	Hypocalcemia						< 1			< 1												
	Hypoglycemia						< 1															
	Hypokalemia						≥ 1	≥ 1				✓										
	Hypomagnesemia						≥ 1	< 1				✓										
	Hyponatremia						< 1	< 1						< 1								
	Hypoproteinemia						< 1															
Musculoskeletal	Arthralgia						≥ 1	≥ 1							< 3						1	
	Arthritis						< 1								< 3							
	Bone disorder						≥ 1															
	Chest wall rigidity	17		✓																3-9		
	Joint disorder						≥ 1															
	Leg cramps						≥ 1	≥ 1														
	Muscle atrophy						< 1															
	Muscle rigidity			✓					✓				✓					2-11		✓		
	Muscle tremor								✓													
	Myalgia						≥ 1	≥ 1							< 3							
	Myasthenia						< 1	< 1														
	Myopathy						< 1															
	Neck and extremity rigidity	PM																		PM		
	Pathological fracture						≥ 1								< 3							
	Skeletal muscle movement	3-9																				
	Synovitis						< 1															
	Tendon disorder						< 1															

Opioid Analgesic Adverse Reactions (%)[a,b]

System	Adverse reactions	Alfentanil	Codeine	Fentanyl injection	Fentanyl transdermal		Fentanyl transmucosal	Hydromorphone ER[c]	Hydromorphone IR[c]	Levorphanol	Meperidine	Methadone	Morphine	Oxycodone CR[c]	Oxycodone IR[c]	Oxymorphone	Propoxyphene	Remifentanil		Sufentanil	Tapentadol	Tramadol
					Adults	Children (2 to 18 years of age)												Adults	Children (≤ 12 years of age)			
Respiratory	Apnea	1-3		✓	3-10			< 1	✓	✓			✓	✓				≤ 30		0.3-1		
	Asthma				< 1		≥ 1	< 1														
	Atelectasis							< 1								✓						
	Bronchitis				≥ 1		≥ 1								< 3			< 1				
	Bronchospasm	< 1							✓									< 1		0.3-1		
	Cough					≥ 1	≥ 1	≥ 1						< 1	< 3			< 1	1		≤ 1	
	Dyspnea				3-10	≥ 1	2-22	≥ 1					✓	1-5	< 3			< 1			≤ 1	< 1
	Epistaxis						≥ 1	≥ 1							< 3							
	Hemoptysis				≥ 1		≥ 1	< 1														
	Hiccoughs				≥ 1		< 1	≥ 1					✓	1-5				< 1				
	Hypercarbia	0.3-1																				
	Hyperventilation						< 1	< 1														
	Hypoventilation				3-10			< 1		✓			✓									
	Hypoxia							≥ 1										< 1				
	Laryngismus							< 1							< 3							
	Laryngospasm	0.3-1		✓					✓				✓					< 1				
	Lung disorder						< 1								< 3							
	Nasopharyngitis																				1	
	Oxygen saturation decreased																				≤ 1	
	Pharyngitis				3-10		≥ 1	≥ 1						< 1	< 3			< 1				
	Pleural effusion						< 1	≥ 1										< 1				
	Pneumonia						≥ 1	≥ 1														
	Pneumothorax						< 1															
	Pulmonary edema											✓						< 1				PM
	Pulmonary embolus							< 1														PM
	Respiratory arrest		✓	✓			✓		✓		✓	✓	✓	✓	✓							
	Respiratory depression	3-9 (postop)	✓	✓		≥ 1			✓		✓	✓	✓	✓	✓	✓		< 1		0.3-1	≤ 1	
	Respiratory disorder				< 1																	
	Respiratory insufficiency						< 1															
	Rhinitis					≥ 1	≥ 1	≥ 1							< 3							
	Sinusitis						≥ 1								< 3							
	Sputum increased						≥ 1															
	Stertorous breathing				< 1																	
	Suppressed cough reflex		✓																			
	Upper respiratory tract infection																				1	
	Voice alteration						< 1						✓	< 1								
Special senses	Abnormal vision						0-3	< 1		✓				< 1								
	Amblyopia				< 1			≥ 1							< 3							
	Blurred vision	1-3		✓	PM			< 1	✓							✓						
	Cataracts																					PM
	Conjunctivitis						≥ 1															
	Diplopia							< 1	✓	✓			✓			✓						
	Dry eyes							< 1														
	Dysgeusia																					< 1
	Ear disorder						≥ 1															
	Ear pain						< 1															
	Eye hemorrhage						< 1															
	Hyperacusis							< 1														
	Lacrimation disorder						< 1	< 1														
	Miosis		✓				< 1		✓				✓			✓						
	Nystagmus							< 1	✓													
	Partial permanent/ transitory deafness						< 1															PM
	Taste perversion						≥ 1	≥ 1	✓				✓	< 1								
	Tinnitus						≥ 1	≥ 1						< 1								PM
	Visual disturbances		✓						✓		✓	✓	✓				✓				≤ 1	1-5

Opioid Analgesic Adverse Reactions (%)[a,b]

System	Adverse reactions	Alfentanil	Codeine	Fentanyl injection	Fentanyl transdermal		Fentanyl transmucosal	Hydromorphone ER[c]	Hydromorphone IR[c]	Levorphanol	Meperidine	Methadone	Morphine	Oxycodone CR[c]	Oxycodone IR[c]	Oxymorphone	Propoxyphene	Remifentanil		Sufentanil	Tapentadol	Tramadol
					Adults	Children (2 to 18 years of age)												Adults	Children (≤ 12 years of age)			
Miscellaneous	Abscess						< 1															
	Accidental injury				≥ 1		0-9	≥ 1					✓	< 1	< 3							< 1
	Ascites						≥ 1	< 1														
	Back pain				≥ 1		≥ 1								< 3							
	Bone pain						≥ 1	≥ 1							< 3							
	Carcinoma							≥ 1														
	Cellulitis						≥ 1	< 1														
	Chills						≥ 1	≥ 1	✓				✓	1-5	< 3			1				
	Dehydration						≥ 1	≥ 1					✓	< 1								
	Edema				PM		≥ 1	≥ 1				✓	✓	< 1	< 3						≤ 1	
	Face edema							< 1						< 1								
	Feeling hot																				1	
	Fever				≥ 1	≥ 1	≥ 1	≥ 1					✓	< 1	< 3							
	Flank pain							< 1										< 10				
	Flu syndrome				3-10		≥ 1						✓		< 3							
	Fungal infection						≥ 1															
	Hot flush																				1	
	Hypothermia							< 1														
	Infection				3-10		≥ 1	5.3					✓									
	Injection-site pain/ reaction	0.3-1							✓	✓								1				
	Intraoperative muscle movement																			0.3-1		
	Malaise						≥ 1	≥ 1					✓	< 1								1-5
	Neck pain						≥ 1	≥ 1						< 1	< 3							
	Neoplasm							< 1														
	Pain					3-10	≥ 1	≥ 1						< 1	< 3							
	Pelvic pain						≥ 1															
	Sepsis						≥ 1	< 1					✓		< 3							
	Shock		✓						✓	✓	✓	✓	✓	✓	✓							
	Viral infection						≥ 1															

[a] IR = immediate-release; ER = extended-release; CR = controlled-release; PM = postmarketing.
[b] Data pooled from separate studies and are not necessarily comparable.
[c] ✓ = occurs, but the incidence is unknown.
[d] In patients with inflammatory bowel disease.
[e] Including erythema, papules, itching, and edema.

➤*Lab test abnormalities:*

Tapentadol – Increased gamma glutamyl transferase, AST, ALT (less than 1%).

Management of adverse reactions – Most patients receiving opioids, especially those who are opioid-naive, will experience adverse reactions. Frequently the adverse reactions from opioids are transient, but may require evaluation and management. Anticipate adverse events such as constipation. Treat constipation aggressively and prophylactically with a stimulant laxative and/or stool softener. Patients do not usually become tolerant to the constipating effects of opioids.

Other opioid-related adverse reactions such as sedation and nausea are usually self-limited and often do not persist beyond the first few days. If nausea persists and is unacceptable to the patient, consider treatment with antiemetics or other modalities because they may relieve these symptoms.

Patients receiving some opioids may pass an intact matrix "ghost" in the stool or via colostomy. These ghosts contain little or no residual drug and are of no clinical consequence.

Overdosage

In general, the shorter the onset and duration of action of the opiate, the greater the intensity and rapidity of symptom onset. Infants and children may be relatively more sensitive on a body weight basis. Elderly patients are comparatively intolerant.

➤*Symptoms:* In severe overdosage, mainly by the IV route, apnea, circulatory collapse, convulsions, cardiac arrest, pulmonary edema, and death may occur. The less severely poisoned patient often has a triad of CNS depression, miosis, and respiratory depression. Serious overdosage is characterized by respiratory depression, extreme somnolence progressing to stupor or coma, constricted pupils, skeletal muscle flaccidity, and cold and clammy skin. Hypotension, bradycardia, hypothermia, pulmonary edema, pneumonia, or shock occurs in 40% or less of patients.

➤*Treatment:* Employ supportive measures as indicated. Refer to General Management of Acute Overdosage. Give primary attention to reestablishment of adequate respiratory exchange; provide a patent airway and institute assisted or controlled ventilation.

Administer a narcotic antagonist (eg, naloxone). The duration of respiratory depression following overdosage may be longer than the duration of the opioid antagonist, so repeated administration of the antagonist may be necessary; keep the patient under surveillance. Do not give an antagonist in the absence of clinically significant respiratory or cardiovascular depression. Naloxone is the antagonist of choice (see individual monograph). If it is necessary to give an antagonist to an opioid-tolerant patient, administer with extreme caution and by titration with smaller than usual doses.

While naloxone will reverse some, but not all, symptoms caused by **tramadol** overdose, the risk of seizures is also increased with naloxone administration. In animals, convulsions following the administration of toxic doses of tramadol were suppressed with barbiturates or benzodiazepines but were increased with naloxone. Hemodialysis is not expected to be helpful in a tramadol overdose because it removed less than 7% of the administered dose in a 4-hour dialysis period.

IV fluids and vasopressors for the treatment of hypotension and other supportive measures may be employed.

In painful conditions, reversal of narcotic effect may result in acute onset of pain and release of catecholamines. Careful administration of naloxone may permit reversal of adverse reactions without affecting analgesia. Parenteral administration of narcotics in patients receiving epidural or intrathecal **morphine** may result in overdosage.

In cases of overdose from the **fentanyl transdermal** patch, remove the patch immediately.

In cases of oral overdose, evacuate the stomach by emesis or gastric lavage if treatment can be instituted within 2 hours following ingestion. Do not induce emesis. Absorption of drugs from the GI tract may be decreased by giving activated charcoal which, in many cases, is more effective than lavage. Observe the patient for a rise in temperature or pulmonary complications that may require antibiotic therapy.

Forced diuresis, peritoneal dialysis, hemodialysis, or charcoal hemoperfusion have not been established as beneficial for a **codeine** or **methadone** overdosage. Dialysis is of little value in poisoning due to **propoxyphene**.

Patient Information

Advise patients to swallow SR, CR, and ER products whole and not to break, crush, chew, open, or dissolve them because doing so may lead to rapid release and absorption of a potentially fatal dose. ER and SR **morphine** capsules may be opened and the beads sprinkled on a small amount of applesauce immediately prior to ingestion; advise patients not to chew, crush, or dissolve the beads.

Instruct patients and caregivers to keep used and unused **fentanyl transdermal** systems out of the reach of children. Used systems should be folded so that the adhesive side of the system adheres to itself and should be flushed down the toilet immediately upon removal. Advise patients to dispose of any systems remaining from a prescription as soon as they are no longer needed. Unused systems should be removed from their pouches and flushed down the toilet.

Keep **fentanyl** lozenges out of the reach of children. Dispose of properly (see individual monograph). Advise diabetic patients that each lozenge contains 2 g of sugar. Consumption of sugar-containing products may increase dental caries. Consult a dentist to ensure proper oral hygiene.

Advise patients that narcotics may cause drowsiness, dizziness, or blurring of vision and to use caution while driving or performing other tasks requiring alertness, coordination, or physical dexterity.

Orthostatic hypotension may occur with the use of this medication, especially in ambulatory patients. Advise patients to get up slowly from a sitting or lying position.

Instruct patients to avoid alcohol and other CNS depressants.

Instruct patients to notify their health care provider if nausea, vomiting, or constipation become prominent.

If GI upset occurs, these agents may be taken with food.

Instruct patients to notify their health care provider if shortness of breath or difficulty in breathing occurs.

Advise patients not to adjust the dose without consulting their health care provider.

Instruct patients to inform their health care provider if pregnant or planning to become pregnant.

Because of the potential for these drugs to be abused, advise patients to protect them from theft and not to give them to anyone else.

Advise the patient not to discontinue the drug abruptly if therapy has lasted more than a few weeks. Instruct them to consult their health care provider.

Instruct patients to avoid exposing the **fentanyl transdermal** system application site to a direct external heat source. There is a potential for temperature-dependent increases in fentanyl release from the system.

ALFENTANIL

c-ii	**Alfentanil hydrochloride** (Abbott)	**Injection:** 500 mcg (as base)/mL	Preservative free. In 2, 5, and 10 mL amps.

ALFENTANIL — INJECTION

For complete and comparative prescribing information, refer to the Narcotic Agonist Analgesics group monograph.

Indications

➤*Analgesia:* Analgesic adjunct given in incremental doses in the maintenance of anesthesia with barbiturate/nitrous oxide/oxygen.

As an analgesic administered by continuous infusion with nitrous oxide/oxygen in the maintenance of general anesthesia.

➤*Anesthetic:* Primary anesthetic for induction of anesthesia in general surgery when endotracheal intubation and mechanical ventilation are required.

➤*Monitored anesthesia care (MAC):* Analgesic component for MAC.

Administration and Dosage

➤*General dosing considerations:* Individualize dosage and titrate to desired effect in each patient according to body weight, physical status, underlying pathological conditions, use of other drugs, and type and duration of surgical procedure and anesthesia.

Monitor vital signs routinely.

In patients administered anesthetic (induction) dosages, qualified personnel and adequate facilities are essential for the management of intraoperative and postoperative respiratory depression.

➤*Adults:*

General anesthesia – See the following table for the use of alfentanil, such as by the following:

1.) by incremental injection as an analgesic adjunct to anesthesia with barbiturate/nitrous oxide/oxygen for short surgical procedures (expected duration of less than 1 hour);
2.) by continuous infusion as a maintenance analgesic with nitrous oxide/oxygen for general surgical procedures; and
3.) by intravenous (IV) injection in anesthetic doses for the induction of anesthesia for general surgical procedures with a minimum expected duration of 45 minutes; and
4.) by IV injection as the analgesic component for MAC.

Alfentanil Dosage Range for Use During General Anesthesia

Clinical status	Induction[a]	Maintenance	Total dose
Spontaneously breathing/Assisted ventilation	8 to 20 mcg/kg	3 to 5 mcg/kg every 5 to 20 min or 0.5 to 1 mcg/kg/min	8 to 40 mcg/kg
Assisted or controlled ventilation			
Incremental injection (to attenuate response to laryngoscopy and intubation)	20 to 50 mcg/kg	5 to 15 mcg/kg every 5 to 20 min	up to 75 mcg/kg
Continuous infusion[b] (to provide attenuation of response to intubation and incision)	50 to 75 mcg/kg	0.5 to 3 mcg/kg/min. Average infusion rate 1 to 1.5 mcg/kg/min	dependent on duration of procedure
Anesthetic induction (give slowly [over 3 min]).[c] Reduce concentration of inhalation agents by 30% to 50% for initial hour	130 to 245 mcg/kg	0.5 to 1.5 mcg/kg/min or general anesthetic	dependent on duration of procedure
MAC[d] (for sedated and responsive spontaneously breathing patients)	3 to 8 mcg/kg	3 to 5 mcg/kg every 5 to 20 min or 0.25 to 1 mcg/kg/min	3 to 40 mcg/kg

[a] Administer induction doses of alfentanil slowly (over 3 minutes). Administration may produce loss of vascular tone and hypotension. Consider fluid replacement prior to induction.
[b] 0.5 to 3 mcg/kg/min with nitrous oxide/oxygen in general surgery. Following anesthetic induction dose, reduce infusion rate requirements by 30% to 50% for the first hour of maintenance.Vital sign changes that indicate response to surgical stress or lightening of anesthesia may be controlled by increasing rate to a maximum of 4 mcg/kg/min or administering bolus doses of 7 mcg/kg. If changes are not controlled after 3 bolus doses given over 5 minutes, use a barbiturate, vasodilator, and/or inhalation agent. Always adjust infusion rates downward in the absence of these signs until there is some response to surgical stimulation.Rather than an increase in infusion rate, administer 7 mcg/kg bolus doses of alfentanil or a potent inhalation agent in response to signs of lightening of anesthesia within the last 15 minutes of surgery. Discontinue infusion at least 10 to 15 minutes prior to the end of surgery.
[c] At these doses, expect truncal rigidity and use a muscle relaxant.
[d] During administration of alfentanil for MAC, infusions may be continued to the end of the procedure.

➤*Children:* See Adults for dosing in children 12 years of age and older.

➤*Elderly:* The initial dose of alfentanil should be appropriately reduced in elderly patients. The effect of the initial dose should be considered when determining supplemental doses.

➤*Debilitated patients:* The initial dose of alfentanil should be appropriately reduced in debilitated patients. The effect of the initial dose should be considered when determining supplemental doses.

➤*Obesity:* In obese patients (more than 20% above ideal total body weight), determine dosage on the basis of lean body weight.

➤*Concomitant therapy:* Individualize the selection of preanesthetic medications.

Neuromuscular-blocking agents should be compatible with the patient's condition.

➤*Administration:* Give by incremental injection, continuous IV infusion, or intravenous (IV) injection.

Use a tuberculin syringe or equivalent for accuracy when administering small volumes.

➤*Admixture compatibility:* Physical and chemical compatibilities of alfentanil have been demonstrated in solution with normal saline, 5% dextrose in normal saline, 5% dextrose in water, and Ringer's lactate.

➤*Storage/Stability:* Protect from light. Store at room temperature (15° to 25°C [59° to 77°F]).

CODEINE

c-ii	**Codeine Sulfate** (Various, eg, Roxane)	**Tablets:** 15 mg (as sulfate)	In UD 100s.
		30 mg (as sulfate)	In 100s and UD 100s.
		60 mg (as sulfate)	In 100s
c-ii	**Codeine Phosphate** (Various, eg, Hospira)	**Injection:** 15 mg/mL (as phosphate)	May contain sulfites. In 2 mL *Carpuject* syringe system.
		30 mg/mL (as phosphate)	May contain sulfites. In 2 mL *Carpuject* syringe system.

CODEINE SULFATE — ORAL

For complete and comparative prescribing information, refer to the Opioid Analgesicsgroup monograph.

Indications

➤*Antitussive:* In combination with other respiratory agents for the treatment of cough (seeUpper Respiratory Combinations in the Respiratory chapter).

➤*Pain:* For the relief of mild to moderate pain.

Administration and Dosage

➤*Adults:*

Analgesic –

Usual dosage: 15 to 60 mg every 4 to 6 hours.

Dosage adjustment: Adjust dosage according to the severity of the pain and the response of the patient. It may occasionally be necessary to exceed the usual dosage recommended in cases of more severe pain or in those patients who have become tolerant to the analgesic effect of narcotics.

➤*Children:*

Off-label dosing –

Analgesic:

- *Maximum dose* – 60 mg/dose.
- *Initial dosage* – 0.5 to 1 mg/kg every 4 to 6 hours.

➤*Storage/Stability:* Store at 25°C (77°F); excursions permitted to 15° to 30°C (59° to 86°F) and protect from moisture.

CODEINE PHOSPHATE — INJECTION

For complete and comparative prescribing information, refer to the Opioid Analgesics group monograph.

Indications

➤*Antitussive:* In combination with other respiratory agents for the treatment of cough (see Upper Respiratory Combinations in the Respiratory chapter).

➤*Pain:* For the relief of mild to moderate pain.

Administration and Dosage

➤*Adults:*

Analgesic –

Usual dosage: 30 mg subcutaneously or intramuscularly (IM) every 4 hours as needed. The usual range is 15 to 60 mg.

Dosage adjustment: Adjust dosage according to the severity of the pain and the response of the patient. It may occasionally be necessary to exceed the usual dosage recommended in cases of more severe pain or in those patients who have become tolerant to the analgesic effect of narcotics.

➤*Children:* Narcotic analgesics, including codeine, should not be used in premature infants. Narcotic analgesics should be administered to infants and small children only with great caution and in carefully monitored dosage. Safety and effectiveness of codeine in newborn infants have not been established.

See Warnings/Precautions.

Analgesic – 500 mcg/kg or 15 mg/m² subcutaneously or IM every 4 hours as necessary.

➤*Admixture compatibility:* Codeine is incompatible with soluble barbiturates.

➤*Storage/Stability:* Store below 40°C (104°F) and protect from light and freezing.

FENTANYL

c-ii	**Fentora** (Cephalon)	**Tablets; buccal:** 100 mcg	Mannitol. (1). In blister card 28s with blue carton blister packs.
		200 mcg	Mannitol. (2). In blister card 28s with orange carton blister packs.
		400 mcg	Mannitol (4). In blister card 28s with green carton blister packs.
		600 mcg	Mannitol (6). In blister card 28s with pink carton blister packs.
		800 mcg	Mannitol. (8). In blister card 28s with yellow carton blister packs.
c-ii	**Abstral** (ProStrakan)	**Tablets; sublingual:** 100 mcg	Mannitol. (1). White, round. In light-blue carton blister packs of 12s and 32s.
		200 mcg	Mannitol. (2). White, oval. In dark-orange carton blister packs of 12s and 32s.
		300 mcg	Mannitol. (3). White, triangle. In brown carton blister packs of 12s and 32s.
		400 mcg	Mannitol. (4). White, diamond. In violet carton blister packs of 12s and 32s.
		600 mcg	Mannitol. (6). White, D-shaped. In turquoise carton blister packs of 32s.
		800 mcg	Mannitol. (8). White, capsule-shaped. In indigo carton blister packs of 32s.
c-ii	**Fentanyl Citrate** (Various, eg, Barr)	**Lozenge on a stick; transmucosal:** 200 mcg (as base)	Sugar. Berry flavor. In 30s with gray carton blister packs.
c-ii	**Actiq**[a] (Cephalon)		Sugar. Berry flavor. In 30s with gray carton blister packs.
c-ii	**Fentanyl Citrate** (Various, eg, Barr)	**Lozenge on a stick; transmucosal:** 400 mcg (as base)	Sugar. Berry flavor. In 30s with blue carton blister packs.
c-ii	**Actiq** (Cephalon)		Sugar. Berry flavor. In 30s with blue carton blister packs.
c-ii	**Fentanyl Citrate** (Various, eg, Barr)	**Lozenge on a stick; transmucosal:** 600 mcg (as base)	Sugar. Berry flavor. In 30s with orange carton blister packs.
c-ii	**Actiq** (Cephalon)		Sugar. Berry flavor. In 30s with orange carton blister packs.
c-ii	**Fentanyl Citrate** (Various, eg, Barr)	**Lozenge on a stick; transmucosal:** 800 mcg (as base)	Sugar. Berry flavor. In 30s with purple carton blister packs.
c-ii	**Actiq** (Cephalon)		Sugar. Berry flavor. In 30s with purple carton blister packs.
c-ii	**Fentanyl Citrate** (Various, eg, Barr)	**Lozenge on a stick; transmucosal:** 1,200 mcg (as base)	Sugar. Berry flavor. In 30s with green carton blister packs.
c-ii	**Actiq** (Cephalon)		Sugar. Berry flavor. In 30s with green carton blister packs.
c-ii	**Fentanyl Citrate** (Various, eg, Barr)	**Lozenge on a stick; transmucosal:** 1,600 mcg (as base)	Sugar. Berry flavor. In 30s with burgundy carton blister packs.
c-ii	**Actiq** (Cephalon)		Sugar. Berry flavor. In 30s with burgundy carton blister packs.

FENTANYL

c-ii	**Onsolis** (Meda Pharmaceuticals)	**Film, soluble; buccal**: 200 mcg per film	As fentanyl citrate. Saccharin, parabens, peppermint oil. (2). Bilayer with one white and one pink side. In bright blue aqua foil packages of 30.
		400 mcg per film	As fentanyl citrate. Saccharin, parabens, peppermint oil. (4). Bilayer with one white and one pink side. In bright magenta foil packages of 30.
		600 mcg per film	As fentanyl citrate. Saccharin, parabens, peppermint oil. (6). Bilayer with one white and one pink side. In bright lime green foil packages of 30.
		800 mcg per film	As fentanyl citrate. Saccharin, parabens, peppermint oil. (8). Bilayer with one white and one pink side. In bright orange foil packages of 30.
		1,200 mcg per film	As fentanyl citrate. Saccharin, parabens, peppermint oil. (12). Bilayer with one white and one pink side. In bright purple foil packages of 30.
c-ii	**Fentanyl** (Various, eg, Baxter)	**Injection**: 50 mcg (as base)/mL	In 2, 5, 10, and 20 mL amps; 30 and 50 mL single-dose vials.

[a] Each unit contains approximately 2 g of sugar.

FENTANYL CITRATE — TRANSMUCOSAL

For complete and comparative prescribing information, refer to the Opioid Analgesics group monograph.

WARNING

Fentanyl is an opioid agonist and a schedule II controlled substance with an abuse liability similar to other opioid analgesics. Fentanyl can be abused in a manner similar to other opioid agonists, legal or illicit. This should be considered when prescribing or dispensing fentanyl in situations in which the health care provider or pharmacist is concerned about in increased risk of misuse, abuse, or diversion. Schedule II opioid substances, which include morphine, oxycodone, hydromorphone, oxymorphone, and methadone, have the highest potential for abuse and risk of fatal overdose due to respiratory depression.

Serious adverse events, including deaths, in patients treated with oral transmucosal fentanyl products have been reported. Deaths occurred as a result of improper patient selection (eg, use in opioid-nontolerant patients) and/or improper dosing. The substitution of fentanyl buccal soluble film or sublingual tablets for any other fentanyl product may result in fatal overdose.

The fentanyl lozenge, buccal and sublingual tablets, and buccal soluble film are indicated only for the management of breakthrough cancer pain in patients with cancer already receiving and tolerant to opioid therapy for their underlying persistent cancer pain. Patients considered opioid-tolerant are those who are taking oral morphine 60 mg/day or more, transdermal fentanyl 25 mcg/h or more, oral oxycodone 30 mg/day or more, oral hydromorphone 8 mg/day or more, oral oxymorphone 25 mg/day or more, or an equianalgesic dose of another opioid for a week or longer.

Because life-threatening respiratory depression could occur at any dose in patients not on long-term opiates, it is contraindicated in the management of acute or postoperative pain, including headache/migraine, dental pain, or use in the emergency department. This product is not indicated for use in opioid-nontolerant patients, including those using opioids intermittently, on an as-needed basis. Deaths have occurred in opioid-nontolerant patients treated with other fentanyl products.

Instruct patients and their caregivers that this drug contains a medicine in an amount that can be fatal to children, in individuals for whom it is not prescribed, and in those who are not opioid tolerant. Keep all units out of the reach of children, and discard opened units properly.

This medicine should be used only in the care of opioid-tolerant cancer patients and only by health care providers who are knowledgeable of and skilled in the use of schedule II opioids to treat cancer pain.

Buccal tablet – Because of the higher bioavailability of fentanyl in the buccal tablet, when converting patients from other oral fentanyl products (including the fentanyl lozenge) to the buccal tablet, do not substitute the buccal tablet on a mcg per mcg basis. Adjust dosage as appropriate.

Buccal soluble film and sublingual tablet – When prescribing, do not convert patients on a mcg per mcg basis from any other oral transmucosal fentanyl product to fentanyl buccal soluble film or sublingual tablet. Patients beginning treatment with fentanyl buccal soluble film must begin with titration from the 200 mcg dose. Patients beginning treatment with sublingual tablets must begin with titration from the 100 mcg dose.

When dispensing, do not substitute an fentanyl buccal soluble film or sublingual tablet prescription for any other fentanyl product. Substantial differences exist in the pharmacokinetic profile of fentanyl buccal soluble film and sublingual tablets compared with other fentanyl products that result in clinically important differences in the extent of absorption of fentanyl. As a result of these differences, the substitution of fentanyl buccal soluble film or sublingual tablet for any other fentanyl product may result in fatal overdose.

Special care must be used when dosing fentanyl buccal soluble film or sublingual tablet. If the breakthrough pain episode is not relieved, patients should wait at least 2 hours before taking another dose.

The concomitant use of fentanyl buccal soluble film or sublingual tablet with CYP3A4 inhibitors may result in an increase in fentanyl plasma concentrations and may cause potentially fatal respiratory depression.

WARNING (cont.)

Because of the risk for misuse, abuse, and overdose, fentanyl buccal soluble film is available only through a restricted distribution program, called the FOCUS Program, and the fentanyl sublingual tablets are available only through a restricted program, required by the Food and Drug Administration, called the Risk Evaluation and Mitigation Strategy (REMS). Under the FOCUS Program, only prescribers, pharmacies, and patients registered with the program are able to prescribe, dispense, and receive fentanyl buccal soluble film. To enroll in the FOCUS Program, call 1-877-466-7654 or visit http://www.onsolisfocus.com. Under the REMS, health care providers who prescribe to outpatients, outpatients, pharmacies, and distributors must enroll in the program to prescribe, receive, dispense, and distribute fentanyl sublingual tablets, respectively. Further information is available at http://www.abstralrems.com or by calling 1-888-227-8725.

Indications

➤*Breakthrough cancer pain:* For the management of breakthrough cancer pain in patients with cancer who are already receiving and are tolerant of opioid therapy for their underlying persistent cancer pain. Patients considered opioid tolerant are those who are taking around-the-clock medicine consisting of oral morphine 60 mg/day or more, transdermal fentanyl 25 mcg/h or more, oral oxycodone 30 mg/day or more, oral hydromorphone 8 mg/day or more, or oral oxymorphone 25 mg/day or more, or an equianalgesic dose of another opioid for 1 week or longer.

See the Warning box for more information.

➤*Off-label uses:* For pain and anxiety management in pediatric burn patients undergoing dressing change and tubbing; for reduction of postoperative anxiety and excitement in ambulatory children.

Administration and Dosage

➤*General dosing considerations:* Fentanyl should be individually titrated to a dose that provides adequate analgesia and minimizes adverse reactions.

Dosage adjustment of both the fentanyl and the maintenance opioid analgesic may be required in some patients to continue to provide adequate relief of breakthrough cancer pain.

The fentanyl buccal and sublingual tablets, transmucosal lozenge, and buccal soluble film are supplied in individually sealed, child-resistant blister packages. The amount of fentanyl contained in the tablet, lozenge, and film can be lethal to a child. Keep out of the reach of children.

Patients and members of their household must be advised to dispose of any tablets remaining from a prescription as soon as they are no longer needed. Partially consumed units represent a special risk because they are no longer protected by the child-resistant pouch, yet may contain enough medicine to be fatal to a child. A temporary storage bottle is provided to be used in the event that a partially consumed unit cannot be disposed of promptly.

Patients and members of their household must be instructed to dispose of any unneeded fentanyl buccal soluble films remaining from a prescription as soon as they are no longer needed. The film should be removed from its foil package and dropped into the toilet. This should be repeated for each film. Flush the toilet after all unneeded films have been put into the toilet. Do not flush the foil packages or cartons down the toilet.

Patients should record their use of the tablet over several episodes of breakthrough pain and discuss their experience with their health care provider to determine if a dosage adjustment is warranted.

➤*Adults:*

Breakthrough cancer pain –

Buccal tablet:

- *Initial dosage* – 100 mcg.
- *Dosage titration* – To reduce the risk of overdose during titration, patients should have only one strength of the buccal tablet available at any one time. Initiate titration using multiples of the 100 mcg buccal tablets. Follow patients closely and change the dosage level until the patient reaches a dose that provides adequate analgesia with tolerable adverse reactions.

Dosing may be repeated once during a single episode of breakthrough pain if pain is not adequately relieved by 1 dose. Redosing may occur 30 minutes after the start of administration, and the same dosage strength should be used.

FENTANYL CITRATE — TRANSMUCOSAL

• *Dosage adjustment* – If several consecutive breakthrough cancer pain episodes require more than 1 buccal tablet per episode, consider an increase in dose. Patients needing to titrate above 100 mcg can be instructed to use two 100 mcg tablets (1 on each side of the mouth in the buccal cavity). If this dose is not successful in controlling the breakthrough pain episode, the patient may be instructed to place two 100 mcg tablets on each side of the mouth in the buccal cavity (total of four 100 mcg tablets).

Titrate above 400 mcg by 200 mcg increments, bearing in mind that using more than 4 tablets simultaneously has not been studied and that it is important to minimize the number of strengths available to patients at any time to prevent confusion and possible overdose.

Once a successful dose has been established (ie, an average episode is treated with a single unit), if the patient experiences more than 4 breakthrough pain episodes per day, reevaluate the dose of the maintenance (around-the-clock) opioid used for persistent pain.

• *Conversion* –

Fentanyl Transmucosal Dosing Conversion Recommendations	
Current lozenge fentanyl	Initial buccal tablet dose
200 mcg	100 mcg
400 mcg	100 mcg
600 mcg	200 mcg
800 mcg	200 mcg
1,200 mcg	400 mcg
1,600 mcg	400 mcg

Sublingual tablet:

• *Initial dosage* – A single 100 mcg tablet.

Because of differences in the pharmacokinetic properties and individual variability, even patients switching from other fentanyl containing products to fentanyl sublingual tablet must start with the 100 mcg dose. The sublingual tablet is not equivalent on a mcg per mcg basis with all other fentanyl products, therefore, do not switch patients on a mcg per mcg basis from any other fentanyl product. Fentanyl sublingual tablet is not a generic version of any other fentanyl product.

• *Dosage titration* –

Individually titrate fentanyl sublingual tablet to a dose that provides adequate analgesia with tolerable adverse effects.

If adequate analgesia is obtained within 30 minutes of administration of the 100 mcg tablet, continue to treat subsequent episodes of breakthrough pain with this dose. If adequate analgesia is not obtained after fentanyl sublingual tablet, the patient may use a second fentanyl sublingual tablet dose (after 30 minutes) as directed by their health care provider. No more than 2 doses of fentanyl sublingual tablet may be used to treat an episode of breakthrough pain. Patients must wait at least 2 hours before treating another episode of breakthrough pain with fentanyl sublingual tablet.

If adequate analgesia was not obtained with the first 100 mcg dose, continue dose escalation in a stepwise manner over consecutive breakthrough episodes until adequate analgesia with tolerable adverse effects is achieved. Increase the dose by 100 mcg multiples up to 400 mcg as needed. If adequate analgesia is not obtained with a 400 mcg dose, the next titration step is 600 mcg. If adequate analgesia is not obtained with a 600 mcg dose, the next titration step is 800 mcg. During titration, patients can be instructed to use multiples of 100 mcg tablets and/or 200 mcg tablets for any single dose. Instruct patients not to use more than 4 tablets at one time. If adequate analgesia is not obtained 30 minutes after the use of fentanyl sublingual tablet, the patient may repeat the same dose of fentanyl sublingual tablet. No more than 2 doses of fentanyl sublingual tablet may be used to treat an episode of breakthrough pain.

• *Maintenance dosage* – Once an appropriate dose for pain management has been established, instruct patients to use only one sublingual tablet of the appropriate strength per dose. Maintain patients on this dose.

If adequate analgesia is not obtained after use of fentanyl sublingual tablet, the patient may use a second sublingual dose (after 30 minutes) as directed by their health care provider. No more than 2 doses of sublingual tablets may be used to treat an episode of breakthrough pain.

Patients must wait at least 2 hours before treating another episode of breakthrough pain with fentanyl sublingual tablet.

• *Dosage adjustment* – If the response (analgesia or adverse reactions) to the titrated fentanyl sublingual tablet dose markedly changes, an adjustment of dose may be necessary to ensure that an appropriate dose is maintained.

If more than 4 episodes of breakthrough pain are experienced per day, reevaluate the dose of the long-acting opioid used for persistent underlying cancer pain. If the long-acting opioid or dose of long-acting opioid is changed, reevaluate and retitrate the fentanyl sublingual dose as necessary to ensure the patient is on an appropriate dose.

Limit the use of fentanyl sublingual tablets to treat 4 or fewer episodes of breakthrough pain per day.

It is imperative that any dose retitration is monitored carefully by a health care provider.

• *Concomitant therapy* – Rescue medication as directed by the health care provider can be used if adequate analgesia is not achieved after use of fentanyl sublingual tablet.

• *Discontinuation of therapy* – For patients no longer requiring opioid therapy, consider discontinuing fentanyl sublingual tablets along with a gradual downward titration of other opioids to minimize possible withdrawal effects.

In patients who continue to take their long-term opioid therapy for persistent pain but no longer require treatment for breakthrough pain, fentanyl sublingual therapy can usually be discontinued immediately.

Lozenge:

• *Maximum dose* – 4 units/day.

• *Initial dosage* – 200 mcg. Prescribe 6 units and advise patients to use all units before increasing to a higher dose.

• *Dosage titration* – Follow patients closely and change the dosage level until the patient reaches a dose that provides adequate analgesia using a single lozenge unit per breakthrough cancer pain episode.

Until the appropriate dose is reached, it may be necessary to use an additional unit during a single episode. Redosing may start 15 minutes after the previous unit has been completed (30 minutes after the start of the previous unit). While patients are in the titration phase and consuming units that individually may be subtherapeutic, do not give more than 2 units for each individual breakthrough cancer pain episode.

• *Dosage adjustment* – If several consecutive breakthrough cancer pain episodes require more than 1 lozenge per episode, consider an increase in dose to the next higher available strength. At each new dose during titration, prescribe 6 units of the titration dose. Evaluate each new dose used in the titration period over several episodes of breakthrough cancer pain (generally 1 to 2 days) to determine whether it provides adequate efficacy with acceptable adverse reactions. The incidence of adverse reactions is likely to be greater during this initial titration period compared with later, after the effective dose is determined.

Once a successful dose has been established (ie, an average episode is treated with a single unit), limit consumption to 4 units/day or less. If consumption increases to more than 4 units/day, reevaluate the dose of the long-acting opioid.

If the patient experiences more than 4 breakthrough pain episodes per day, reevaluate the dose of the maintenance (around-the-clock) opioid used for persistent pain.

• *Discontinuation of therapy* – A gradual downward titration is recommended because it is not known at what dose level the opioid may be discontinued without producing the signs and symptoms of abrupt withdrawal.

Buccal soluble film: Only prescribers enrolled in the FOCUS Program may prescribe fentanyl buccal soluble film.

• *Dosage titration* –

Starting dose: The goal of dose titration is to find the individual patient's effective and tolerable dose. The dose of fentanyl buccal soluble film is not predicted from the daily maintenance dose of opioid used to manage the persistent cancer pain and must be determined by dose titration.

Individually titrate fentanyl buccal soluble film to a dose that provides adequate analgesia with tolerable adverse reactions. All patients must begin treatment using one fentanyl 200 mcg buccal soluble film. Because of differences in pharmacokinetic properties and individual variability, patients switching from another oral transmucosal fentanyl product must be started on no greater than fentanyl 200 mcg buccal soluble film. When prescribing, do not switch patients on a mcg per mcg basis from any other oral transmucosal fentanyl product to fentanyl buccal soluble film as fentanyl buccal soluble film is not equivalent on a mcg per mcg basis with any other fentanyl product. Fentanyl buccal soluble film is not a generic version of any other oral transmucosal fentanyl product.

From the initial dose, closely follow patients and change the dosage level until the patient reaches a dose that provides adequate analgesia.

If adequate pain relief is not achieved after one fentanyl 200 mcg buccal soluble film, titrate using multiples of the fentanyl 200 mcg buccal soluble film (for doses of 400, 600, or 800 mcg). Increase the dose by 200 mcg in each subsequent episode until the patient reaches a dose that provides adequate analgesia with tolerable adverse reactions. Do not use more than 4 of the fentanyl 200 mcg buccal soluble films simultaneously. When multiple fentanyl 200 mcg buccal soluble films are used, they should not be placed on top of each other and may be placed on both sides of the mouth.

If adequate pain relief is not achieved after fentanyl 800 mcg buccal soluble film (four fentanyl 200 mcg buccal soluble films), and the patient has tolerated the 800 mcg dose, treat the next episode by using one fentanyl 1,200 mcg buccal soluble film. Doses above fentanyl 1,200 mcg buccal soluble film should not be used.

Once adequate pain relief is achieved with a dose between fentanyl 200 and 800 mcg buccal soluble film, the patient should use or safely dispose of all remaining fentanyl 200 mcg buccal soluble films. Patients who require fentanyl 1,200 mcg buccal soluble film should dispose of all remaining unused fentanyl 200 mcg buccal soluble films. The patient should then get a prescription for fentanyl buccal soluble films of the dose determined by titration (200, 400, 600, 800, or 1,200 mcg) to treat subsequent episodes.

Single doses should be separated by at least 2 hours. Fentanyl buccal soluble film should only be used once per breakthrough cancer pain episode; fentanyl buccal soluble film should not be redosed within an episode.

During any episode of breakthrough cancer pain, if adequate pain relief is not achieved after fentanyl buccal soluble film, the patient may use a rescue medication (after 30 minutes) as directed by their health care provider.

• *Dosage adjustment* – During maintenance treatment, if the prescribed dose no longer adequately manages the breakthrough cancer pain episode for several consecutive episodes, increase the dose of fentanyl buccal soluble film as described in Dose Titration. Once a successful dose has been found, each episode is treated with a single film. Fentanyl buccal soluble film should be limited to 4 or fewer doses per day. Consider increasing the dose of the around-the-clock opioid medicine used for persistent cancer pain in patients experiencing more than 4 breakthrough cancer pain episodes daily.

➤*Elderly:* Exercise caution in individually titrating fentanyl in elderly patients to provide adequate efficacy while minimizing risk.

➤*Renal function impairment:* Use with caution in these patients and use the lowest possible dose.

FENTANYL CITRATE — TRANSMUCOSAL

➤*Hepatic function impairment:* Use with caution in these patients and use the lowest possible dose.

➤*Current CYP3A4 inhibitor use:* Particular caution should be exercised for patients receiving CYP3A4 inhibitors, and the lowest possible dose should be used in these patients.

➤*Administration:*

Buccal tablet – Do not open the blister until ready to administer. A single blister unit should be separated from the blister card by tearing it apart at the perforations. The blister unit should then be bent along the line where indicated. The blister backing should then be peeled back to expose the tablet. Patients should not attempt to push the tablet through the blister, as this may cause damage to the tablet. The tablet should not be stored once it has been removed from the blister package, as the tablet's integrity may be compromised, and because this increases the risk of accidental exposure to the tablet.

Remove the tablet from the blister unit and immediately place the entire fentanyl buccal tablet in the buccal cavity (above a rear molar, between the upper cheek and gum). Patients should not attempt to split the tablet. The buccal tablet should not be sucked, chewed, or swallowed, as this will result in lower plasma concentrations than when taken as directed. The buccal tablet should be left between the cheek and gum until it has disintegrated, which usually takes approximately 14 to 25 minutes. After 30 minutes, if remnants from the buccal tablet remain, they may be swallowed with a glass of water.

Sublingual tablet – Place sublingual tablets on the floor of the mouth directly under the tongue immediately after removal from the blister unit. Do not chew, suck, or swallow sublingual tablets. Allow the tablets to completely dissolve in the sublingual cavity. Advise patients not to eat or drink anything until the tablet is completely dissolved.

In patients who have a dry mouth, water may be used to moisten the buccal mucosa before taking the sublingual tablets.

Lozenge – Open the blister package with scissors immediately prior to product use. Place the unit in the patient's mouth between the cheek and lower gum, moving it from one side to the other using the handle. Instruct the patient to suck, not chew, the lozenge. A unit dose, if chewed and swallowed, might result in lower peak concentrations (C_{max}) and lower bioavailability.

Instruct the patient to consume the lozenge over a 15-minute period. Longer or shorter consumption times may produce less efficacy than reported in clinical trials. If signs of excessive opioid effects appear before the unit is consumed, remove the drug matrix from the patient's mouth immediately and decrease future doses.

Buccal film – Use the tongue to wet the inside of the cheek or rinse the mouth with water to wet the area for placement of fentanyl buccal soluble film. Open the fentanyl buccal soluble film package immediately prior to product use. Place the entire fentanyl buccal soluble film near the tip of a dry finger with the pink side facing up and hold in place. Place the pink side of the fentanyl buccal soluble film against the inside of the cheek. Press and hold the fentanyl buccal soluble film in place for 5 seconds. The fentanyl buccal soluble film should stay in place on its own after this period. Liquids may be consumed after 5 minutes.

An fentanyl buccal soluble film, if chewed and swallowed, might result in lower peak concentrations and lower bioavailability than when used as directed.

The fentanyl buccal soluble film should not be cut or torn prior to use.

The fentanyl buccal soluble film will dissolve within 15 to 30 minutes after application. The film should not be manipulated with the tongue or finger(s) and eating food should be avoided until the film has dissolved.

➤*Storage/Stability:* Store at 20° to 25°C (68° to 77°F), with excursions permitted between 15° and 30°C (59° and 86°F), until ready to use. Protect from freezing and moisture. Do not use if the package has been tampered with or has been opened.

FENTANYL CITRATE — INJECTION

For complete prescribing information, refer to the Opioid Analgesics group monograph.

Indications

➤*Pain:* For analgesic action of short duration during anesthesia (premedication, induction, maintenance), and in the immediate postoperative period (recovery room) as needed.

For use as an opioid analgesic supplement in general or regional anesthesia.

For administration with a neuroleptic such as droperidol (see monograph in the General Anesthetics section) as an anesthetic premedication, for induction of anesthesia, and as an adjunct in maintenance of general and regional anesthesia.

For use as an anesthetic agent with oxygen in selected high-risk patients (open heart surgery or certain complicated neurological or orthopedic procedures).

Administration and Dosage

➤*General dosing considerations:* Individualize dosage. Monitor vital signs routinely.

Concomitant anesthesia – Certain forms of conduction anesthesia, such as spinal anesthesia and some peridural anesthetics, can alter respiration by blocking intercostal nerves. Fentanyl can also alter respiration through other mechanisms.

Concomitant narcotic administration – The respiratory depressant effect of fentanyl may persist longer than the analgesic effect. Consider the total dose of all opioid analgesics used before ordering narcotic analgesics during recovery from anesthesia. Use opioids in reduced doses initially, one fourth to one third those usually recommended.

➤*Adults:*

Adjunct to general anesthesia –

Initial dosage: 2 to 20 mcg/kg. In addition to adequate analgesia, some abolition of the stress response should occur. Respiratory depression necessitates artificial ventilation and careful observation of postoperative ventilation. 20 to 50 mcg/kg for "stress-free" anesthesia. Use during open heart surgery and complicated neurosurgical and orthopedic procedures where surgery is prolonged and the stress response is detrimental. Inject with nitrous oxide/oxygen to attenuate the stress response. Postoperative ventilation and observation are required.

Maintenance dosage: 2 to 50 mcg/kg. Additional doses are needed infrequently in minor procedures. Use 25 to 100 mcg intravenously (IV) or intramuscularly (IM) when movement and/or changes in vital signs indicate surgical stress or lightening of analgesia.

Adjunct to regional anesthesia – 50 to 100 mcg IM or slowly IV over 1 to 2 minutes as required.

General anesthetic – 50 to 100 mcg/kg with oxygen and a muscle relaxant when attenuation of the responses to surgical stress is especially important. Up to 150 mcg/kg may be necessary. It has been used for open heart surgery and other major surgical procedures to protect the myocardium from excess oxygen demand and for complicated neurological and orthopedic procedures.

Postoperative – 50 to 100 mcg IM, repeat dose in 1 to 2 hours as needed.

Premedication – 50 to 100 mcg IM, 30 to 60 minutes prior to surgery.

Off-label dosing –

Patient-controlled analgesia: The following patient-controlled analgesia (PCA) dosing parameters for fentanyl (10 mcg/mL) are for opioid-naive adults.

- *Maximum dose* – The total amount of drug over time and the maximum number of patient-demand doses per hour will vary.
- *Loading dose* – 20 mcg bolus.
- *Clinician dose* – 20 mcg bolus. One clinician bolus may be given each hour.
- *Patient-controlled analgesia dose* – 10 mcg, with a lockout time of 10 minutes.
- *Basal dose* – Not recommended for starting PCA.

➤*Children:*

General anesthesia –

2 to 12 years of age: A dose as low as 2 to 3 mcg/kg is recommended.

Off-label dosing –

Analgesia:

- *Intermittent dosing* –
  - *30 days of age and older:* 1 to 3 mcg/kg every ½ to 1 hour.
  - *29 days of age or younger:* 1 to 4 mcg/kg every 2 to 4 hours.
- *Continuous infusion* – 1 to 5 mcg/kg loading dose followed by continuous infusion of 1 to 20 mcg/kg/hour; titrate by 0.5 mcg/kg/hour until desired effect occurs (usually 1 to 3 mcg/kg/hour).

Anesthesia:

- *Usual dose* – 5 to 50 mcg/kg/dose.
- *Maximum dose* – 75 to 100 mcg/kg/dose.

Sedation: See Analgesia.

Patient-controlled analgesia: Prior to starting a PCA, a child's developmental age and cognitive ability should be assessed. The following PCA dosing parameters for fentanyl (10 mcg/mL) are for opioid-naive children.

- *Maximum dose* – The total amount of drug over time should not exceed 3 mcg/kg/hour. If the patient requires more than 3 patient-demand doses over 2 hours, the health care provider should be contacted and the patient reassessed.
- *Loading dose* – 0.5 mcg/kg bolus.
- *Clinician dose* – 0.5 mcg/kg bolus. Two clinician bolus doses may be given each hour.
- *Patient-controlled analgesia dose* – 0.25 mcg/kg with a lockout time of 10 minutes.
- *Basal/continuous infusion* – 0.25 mcg/kg/hour.

➤*Elderly:* Reduce initial dose.

➤*Renal function impairment:* Fentanyl should be administered with caution. Reduce initial dose.

➤*Hepatic function impairment:* Fentanyl should be administered with caution. Reduce initial dose.

➤*Storage/Stability:* Store at 15° to 25°C (59° to 77°F). Protect from light.

FENTANYL TRANSDERMAL SYSTEM

	Product/Distributor	Dose (mcg/h)	System size (cm²)	Fentanyl content (mg)	How supplied
c-ii	**Fentanyl Transdermal System** (Sandoz)	12.5	5	1.25	In cartons containing 5 individually packaged systems.
c-ii	**Duragesic-12** (Janssen)	12.5	5	1.25	In cartons containing 5 individually packaged systems.[a]
c-ii	**Fentanyl Transdermal System** (Various, eg, Mylan, Sandoz)	25	6.25 to 10	2.5 to 2.55	In cartons containing 5 individually packaged systems.
c-ii	**Duragesic-25** (Janssen)	25	10	2.5	In cartons containing 5 individually packaged systems.[a]
c-ii	**Fentanyl Transdermal System** (Various, eg, Mylan, Sandoz)	50[b]	12.5 to 20	5 to 5.1	In cartons containing 5 individually packaged systems.
c-ii	**Duragesic-50** (Janssen)	50[b]	20	5	In cartons containing 5 individually packaged systems.[a]
c-ii	**Fentanyl Transdermal System** (Various, eg, Mylan, Sandoz)	75[b]	18.75 to 30	7.5 to 7.65	In cartons containing 5 individually packaged systems.
c-ii	**Duragesic-75** (Janssen)	75[b]	30	7.5	In cartons containing 5 individually packaged systems.[a]
c-ii	**Fentanyl Transdermal System** (Various, eg, Mylan, Sandoz)	100[b]	25 to 40	10 to 10.2	In cartons containing 5 individually packaged systems.
c-ii	**Duragesic-100** (Janssen)	100[b]	40	10	In cartons containing 5 individually packaged systems.[a]

[a] Less than 0.2 mL alcohol is released during use.

[b] For use only in opioid-tolerant patients.

FENTANYL — TRANSDERMAL

For complete prescribing information, refer to the Opioid Analgesics group monograph.

WARNING

Fentanyl transdermal systems contain a high concentration of the potent Schedule II opioid agonist, fentanyl. Schedule II opioid substances, which include fentanyl, hydromorphone, methadone, morphine, oxycodone, and oxymorphone, have the highest potential for abuse and associated risk of fatal overdose caused by respiratory depression. Fentanyl can be abused and is subject to criminal diversion. The high content of fentanyl in the patches may be a particular target for abuse and diversion.

Fentanyl transdermal system is indicated for management of persistent, moderate to severe chronic pain (such as that of malignancy) that:

- requires continuous, around-the-clock opioid administration for an extended period of time, and
- cannot be managed by other means such as acetaminophen-opioid combinations, nonsteroidal analgesics, opioid combination products, or immediate-release opioids, or as-needed dosing with short-acting opioids.

Only use the 50, 75, and 100 mcg/h dosages in patients who are already on and are tolerant of opioid therapy.

Only use fentanyl transdermal system in patients who are already receiving opioid therapy, who have demonstrated opioid tolerance, and who require a total daily dose at least equivalent to fentanyl 25 mcg/h transdermal system. Patients who are considered opioid tolerant are those who have been taking, for a week or longer, morphine 60 mg/day or more, or oral oxycodone 30 mg/day or more, or oral hydromorphone 8 mg/day or more, or an equianalgesic dose of another opioid.

Because serious or life-threatening hypoventilation could occur, fentanyl transdermal is contraindicated:

- in patients who are not opioid tolerant
- in the management of acute pain or in patients who require opioid analgesia for a short period of time
- in the management of acute or postoperative pain, including use after outpatient or day surgeries (eg, tonsillectomies)
- in the management of mild pain
- in the management of intermittent pain responsive to as-needed therapy or nonopioid therapy
- in doses exceeding 25 mcg/h at the initiation of opioid therapy.

Because the peak fentanyl levels occur between 24 and 72 hours of treatment, be aware that serious or life-threatening hypoventilation may occur, even in opioid-tolerant patients, during the initial application period.

The concomitant use of fentanyl transdermal system with potent CYP-450 3A4 inhibitors (ie, ritonavir, ketoconazole, itraconazole, troleandomycin, clarithromycin, nelfinavir, nefazodone) may result in an increase in fentanyl plasma concentrations, which could increase or prolong adverse drug reactions and may cause potentially fatal respiratory depression. Carefully monitor patients receiving fentanyl transdermal system and potent CYP3A4 inhibitors for an extended period of time and make dosage adjustments if warranted.

The safety of fentanyl has not been established in children younger than 2 years of age. Only administer fentanyl to children if they are opioid tolerant and 2 years of age and older.

Fentanyl transdermal system is only for use in patients who are already tolerant to opioid therapy of comparable potency. Use in nonopioid-tolerant patients may lead to fatal respiratory depression. Overestimating the fentanyl transdermal system dose when converting patients from another opioid medication can result in fatal overdose with the first dose. Because of the 17-hour mean elimination half-life of fentanyl transdermal system, patients who are thought to have had a serious adverse reaction, including overdose, will require monitoring and treatment for at least 24 hours.

WARNING (cont.)

Fentanyl transdermal system can be abused in a manner similar to other opioid agonists, legal or illicit. Consider this risk when administering, prescribing, or dispensing in situations in which there is concern about increased risk of misuse, abuse, or diversion.

Persons at increased risk for opioid abuse include those with a personal or family history of substance abuse (including drug or alcohol abuse or addiction) or mental illness (eg, major depression). Assess patients for their clinical risks for opioid abuse or addiction prior to prescribing opioids. Routinely monitor all patients receiving opioids for signs of misuse, abuse, and addiction. Patients at increased risk of opioid abuse may still be appropriately treated with modified-release opioid formulations; however, these patients will require intensive monitoring for signs of misuse, abuse, or addiction.

Fentanyl transdermal patches are intended for transdermal use (on intact skin) only. Using damaged or cut fentanyl transdermal patches can lead to the rapid release of the contents of the fentanyl transdermal patch and absorption of a potentially fatal dose of fentanyl.

Indications

➤*Pain:* Management of persistent, moderate to severe chronic pain that requires continuous, around-the-clock opioid administration for an extended period of time and that cannot be managed by other means, such as nonsteroidal analgesics, opioid combination products, immediate-release opioids, acetaminophen-opioid combinations, or as-needed dosing with short-acting opioids.

Only use fentanyl transdermal systems in patients who are already receiving opioid therapy, who have demonstrated opioid tolerance, and who require a total daily dose at least equivalent to fentanyl 25 mcg/h transdermal system. Patients who are considered opioid tolerant are those who have been taking, for a week or longer, morphine 60 mg/day or more, oral oxycodone 30 mg/day or more, oral hydromorphone 8 mg/day or more, or an equianalgesic dose of another opioid.

Administration and Dosage

➤*General dosing considerations:* Prescribers should individualize treatment using a progressive plan of pain management such as outlined by the WHO, the Agency for Health Research and Quality, the Federation of State Medical Boards Model policy, or the American Pain Society. The most important factor to be considered in determining the appropriate dose is the extent of preexisting opioid tolerance.

➤*Adults:*

Pain –

Initial dosage: There has been no systematic evaluation of fentanyl as an initial opioid analgesic in the management of chronic pain because most patients in the clinical trials were converted to fentanyl from other narcotics. The efficacy of fentanyl 12 mcg/h as an initiating dose has not been determined. In addition, patients who are not opioid tolerant have experienced hypoventilation and death during use of fentanyl. Therefore, fentanyl should be used only in patients who are opioid tolerant.

Overestimating the fentanyl dose when converting patients from another opioid medication can result in fatal overdose with the first dose. Because of the mean elimination half-life of 17 hours of fentanyl, patients who are thought to have had a serious adverse reaction, including overdose, will require monitoring and treatment for at least 24 hours.

In selecting an initial dose, give attention to the following:

1.) the daily dose, potency, and characteristics of the opioid the patient has been taking previously (eg, whether it is a pure agonist or mixed agonist-antagonist);
2.) the reliability of the relative potency estimates used to calculate the dose needed (potency estimates may vary with the route of administration);
3.) the degree of opioid tolerance, if any; and
4.) the general condition and medical status of the patient. Maintain each patient at the lowest dose providing acceptable pain control.

FENTANYL — TRANSDERMAL

The majority of patients are adequately maintained with fentanyl administered every 72 hours. Some patients may not achieve adequate analgesia using this dosing interval and may require systems to be applied every 48 hours rather than every 72 hours. An increase in the fentanyl dose should be evaluated before changing dosing intervals in order to maintain patients on a 72-hour regimen. Dosing intervals less than every 72 hours were not studied in children and adolescents and are not recommended.

Because of the increase in serum fentanyl concentration over the first 24 hours following initial system application, the initial evaluation of the maximum analgesic effect cannot be made before 24 hours of wearing.

Dosage titration: The recommended initial transdermal dose based upon the daily oral morphine dose is conservative, and 50% of patients are likely to require a dose increase after initial application of fentanyl. The initial dosage may be increased after 3 days, based on the daily dose of supplemental opioid analgesics required by the patient in the second or third day of the initial application.

It may take up to 6 days after increasing the dose for the patient to reach equilibrium on the new dose. Therefore, patients should wear a higher dose through 2 applications before any further increase in dosage is made on the basis of the average daily use of a supplemental analgesic.

Appropriate dosage increments should be based on the daily dose of supplementary opioids, using the ratio of 45 mg per 24 hours of oral morphine to a 12.5 mcg/h increase in transdermal fentanyl dose.

Concomitant therapy: During the initial application, patients should use short-acting analgesics as needed until analgesic efficacy with the transdermal system is attained. Thereafter, some patients may still require periodic supplemental doses of other short-acting analgesics for breakthrough pain.

➤*Children:*

2 years of age and older – Administer to children only if they are opioid tolerant receiving at least oral morphine 60 mg/day and 2 years of age and older with chronic pain.

See Adults for dosing.

➤*Elderly:* Reduced doses of fentanyl are suggested for elderly patients. Elderly, cachectic, or debilitated patients should not be started on fentanyl transdermal system doses higher than 25 mcg/h unless they are already tolerating an around-the-clock opioid at a dose and potency comparable with fentanyl 25 mcg/h transdermal system.

➤*Conversion:*

Fentanyl Transdermal Dose Conversion Guidelines[a]

Current analgesic	Daily dose (mg/day)			
Oral morphine	60 to 134	135 to 224	225 to 314	315 to 404
IM/IV[b] morphine	10 to 22	23 to 37	38 to 52	53 to 67
Oral oxycodone	30 to 67	67.5 to 112	112.5 to 157	157.5 to 202
IM/IV oxycodone	15 to 33	33.1 to 56	56.1 to 78	78.1 to 101
Oral codeine	150 to 447	448 to 747	748 to 1,047	1,048 to 1,347
Oral hydromorphone	8 to 17	17.1 to 28	28.1 to 39	39.1 to 51
IV hydromorphone	1.5 to 3.4	3.5 to 5.6	5.7 to 7.9	8 to 10
IM meperidine	75 to 165	166 to 278	279 to 390	391 to 503
Oral methadone	20 to 44	45 to 74	75 to 104	105 to 134
IM methadone	10 to 22	23 to 37	38 to 52	53 to 67
Recommended fentanyl transdermal system dose				
Fentanyl transdermal system	25 mcg/h	50 mcg/h	75 mcg/h	100 mcg/h

[a] This table should not be used to convert fentanyl transdermal system to other therapies because this conversion to fentanyl transdermal system is conservative. Use of this table for conversion to other analgesic therapies can overestimate the dose of the new analgesic agent. Overdosage of the new analgesic agent is possible.

[b] IM = intramuscular; IV = intravenous. Alternatively, for adults and children taking other opioids or doses, use the following methodology:

1.) Calculate the previous 24-hour analgesic requirement.
2.) Convert this amount to the equianalgesic oral morphine dose using the fentanyl equianalgesic potency conversion table.
3.) The table titled Recommended Initial Fentanyl Dose Based Upon Daily Oral Morphine Dose displays the range of 24-hour oral morphine doses that are recommended for conversion to each fentanyl dose. Use this table to find the calculated 24-hour morphine dose and the corresponding fentanyl dose. Initiate fentanyl treatment using the recommended dose and titrate patients upwards (no more frequently than every 3 days after the initial dose or than every 6 days thereafter) until analgesic efficacy is attained. The recommended starting dose when converting from other opioids to fentanyl is likely too low for 50% of patients. The starting dose is recommended to minimize the potential for overdosing patients with the first dose. For delivery rates in excess of 100 mcg/h, multiple systems may be used.

Fentanyl Equianalgesic Potency Conversion[a,b]

Drug name	Equianalgesic dose (mg) IM[c,d]	Equianalgesic dose (mg) Oral
Morphine	10	60 (30)[e]
Hydromorphone	1.5	7.5
Methadone	10	20
Oxycodone	15	30
Levorphanol	2	4
Oxymorphone	1	10 (rectal)
Meperidine	75	
Codeine	130	200

[a] This table should not be used to convert from fentanyl to other therapies because this conversion to fentanyl is conservative. Use of this table for conversion to other analgesic therapies can overestimate the dose of the new agent. Overdosage of the new analgesic agent is possible.

[b] All IM and oral doses in this chart are considered equivalent to 10 mg of IM morphine in analgesic effect.

[c] Based on single-dose studies in which an IM dose of each drug listed was compared with morphine to establish the relative potency. Oral doses are those recommended when changing from parenteral to an oral route. Reference: Foley KM. The treatment of cancer pain. *N Engl J Med.* 1985;313:84-95.

[d] Although controlled studies are not available, in clinical practice it is customary to consider the doses of opioid given IM, IV, or subcutaneously to be equivalent. There may be some differences in pharmacokinetic parameters such as maximal drug concentration (C_{max}) and time of maximal concentration (T_{max}).

[e] The conversion ratio of parenteral morphine 10 mg = oral morphine 30 mg is based on clinical experience in patients with chronic pain. The conversion ratio of parenteral morphine 10 mg = oral morphine 60 mg is based on a potency study in acute pain. Reference: Ashburn MA, and Lipman AG. Management of pain in the cancer patient. *Anesth Analg.* 1993;76:402-416.

Recommended Initial Fentanyl Dose Based Upon Daily Oral Morphine Dose[a,b]

Oral 24-hour morphine (mg/day)	Fentanyl dose (mcg/h)
60 to 134[c]	25
135 to 224	50
225 to 314	75
315 to 404	100
405 to 494	125
495 to 584	150
585 to 674	175
675 to 764	200
765 to 854	225
855 to 944	250
945 to 1,034	275
1,035 to 1,124	300

[a] Note: In clinical trials, these ranges of daily oral morphine doses were used as a basis for conversion to fentanyl.

[b] This table should not be used to convert from fentanyl to other therapies because the conversion to fentanyl is conservative. Use of this table for conversion to other analgesic therapies can overestimate the dose of the new agent. Overdosage of the new analgesic agent is possible.

[c] Children initiating therapy on a 25 mcg/h fentanyl system should be opioid tolerant and receiving at least oral morphine 60 mg equivalents per day.

➤*Discontinuation of therapy:* To convert patients to another opioid, remove fentanyl and titrate the dose of the new analgesic based upon the patient's report of pain until adequate analgesia has been attained. Upon system removal, 17 hours or more are required for a 50% decrease in serum fentanyl concentrations. Opioid withdrawal symptoms (eg, anxiety, diarrhea, nausea, shivering, vomiting) are possible in some patients after conversion or dose adjustment. For patients requiring discontinuation of opioids, a gradual downward titration is recommended because it is not known at what dose level the opioid may be discontinued without producing the signs and symptoms of abrupt withdrawal.

Do not use the tables to convert from fentanyl to other therapies. Because the conversion to fentanyl is conservative, use of the tables for conversion to other analgesic therapies can overestimate the dose of the new agent. Overdosage of the new analgesic agent is possible.

➤*Administration:* Apply fentanyl to intact, nonirritated, and nonirradiated skin on a flat surface, such as the chest, back, flank, or upper arm. Monitor adhesion in young children and persons with cognitive impairment. The upper back is the preferred location to minimize the potential of inappropriate patch removal. Clip (not shave) hair at the application site prior to system application. If the site of fentanyl application must be cleansed prior to the application of the patch, do so with clear water. Do not use soaps, oils, lotions, alcohol, or any other agents that might irritate the skin or alter its characteristics. Allow the skin to dry completely prior to patch application.

Apply fentanyl immediately upon removal from the sealed package. Do not use if the seal is broken. Do not alter the patch (eg, cut) in any way prior to application and do not use cut or damaged patches. If the fentanyl system is cut or damaged, controlled drug delivery will not be possible, which can lead to the rapid release and absorption of a potentially fatal dose of fentanyl.

Firmly press the transdermal system in place with the palm of the hand for 30 seconds, making sure the contact is complete, especially around the edges. If the gel from the drug reservoir accidentally contacts the skin of the patient or caregiver, the skin should be washed with copious amounts of water. Do not use soap, alcohol, or other solvents to remove the gel because they may enhance the drug's ability to penetrate the skin.

FENTANYL — TRANSDERMAL

Wear each system continuously for 72 hours. Apply the next patch to a different skin site after removal of the previous transdermal system.

Keep fentanyl out of the reach of children. Fold used systems so that the adhesive side of the system adheres to itself, then flush the system down the toilet immediately upon removal. Dispose of any patches remaining from a prescription as soon as they are no longer needed. Remove unused patches from their pouches, fold so that the adhesive side of the patch adheres to itself, and flush down the toilet.

Fentanyl is supplied in sealed transdermal systems that pose little risk of exposure to health care workers. If the gel from the drug reservoir accidentally contacts the skin, the area should be washed with copious amounts of water. Do not use soap, alcohol, or other solvents to remove the gel because they may enhance the drug's ability to penetrate the skin.

➤*Storage / Stability:* Do not store above 25°C (77°F).

HYDROCODONE

Hydrocodone is only available in combination with other ingredients for the treatment of pain and cough. See Upper Respiratory Combinations in the Respiratory chapter or the Opioid Analgesic Combinations.

HYDROMORPHONE HYDROCHLORIDE

c-ii	**Hydromorphone Hydrochloride** (Various, eg, Ethex, Lannett, Roxane)	**Tablets; oral:** 2 mg	In 100s and UD 25s and 100s.
c-ii	**Dilaudid** (Purdue Phrama)		Lactose. (2). Orange. In 100s, 500s, and UD 100s.
c-ii	**Hydromorphone Hydrochloride** (Various, eg, Ethex, Lannett, Roxane)	**Tablets; oral:** 4 mg	In 100s, and UD 25s and 100s.
c-ii	**Dilaudid** (Purdue Phrama)		Lactose. (4). Yellow. In 100s, 500s, and UD 100s.
c-ii	**Hydromorphone Hydrochloride** (Various, eg, Ethex, Mallinckrodt, Roxane)	**Tablets; oral:** 8 mg	In 100 and UD 100s.
c-ii	**Dilaudid** (Purdue Pharma)		Lactose. May contain sodium metabisulfite. (8). Scored, triangular. In 100s.
c-ii	**Exalgo** (Alza)	**Tablets, extended-release; oral:** 8 mg	Lactose, PEG. (EXH 8). Red, round. In 100s.
		12 mg	Lactose, PEG. (EXH 12). Dark yellow, round. In 100s.
		16 mg	Lactose, PEG. (EXH 16). Yellow, round. In 100s.
c-ii	**Hydromorphone Hydrochloride** (Various, eg, Roxane)	**Liquid; oral:** 1 mg per 1 mL	In 4 and 8 mL UD patient cups and 250 mL bottles.
c-ii	**Dilaudid** (Purdue Pharma)		Glycerin, parabens, sucrose. May contain sodium metabisulfite. In 473 mL.
c-ii	**Hydromorphone Hydrochloride** (Various, eg, Hospira)	**Injection, solution:** 1 mg/mL	In 1 mL prefilled syringes.
c-ii	**Dilaudid** (Purdue Pharma)		In 1 mL amps.
c-ii	**Hydromorphone Hydrochloride** (Various, eg, Hospira)	**Injection, solution:** 2 mg/mL	In 1 and 20 mL vials and 1 mL prefilled syringes.
c-ii	**Dilaudid** (Purdue Pharma)		In 1 mL amps and 20 mL multiple-dose vials.[a]
c-ii	**Hydromorphone Hydrochloride** (Various, eg, Hospira)	**Injection, solution:** 4 mg/mL	In 1 mL prefilled syringes.
c-ii	**Dilaudid** (Purdue Pharma)		In 1 mL amps.
c-ii	**Hydromorphone Hydrochloride** (Various, eg, Faulding, Hospira)	**Injection, solution, concentrate:** 10 mg/mL	In 1, 5, and 50 mL single-dose vials.
c-ii	**Dilaudid-HP** (Purdue Pharma)		In 1 and 5[b] mL amps and 50 mL single-dose vials.[b]
c-ii	**Dilaudid-HP** (Purdue Pharma)	**Injection, lyophilized powder for solution, concentrate:** 250 mg (10 mg/mL after reconstitution)	Preservative free. In single-dose vials.[b]
c-ii	**Hydromorphone Hydrochloride** (Paddock)	**Suppositories; rectal:** 3 mg	In 6s.
c-ii	**Dilaudid** (Abbott)		Cocoa butter. In 6s.

[a] With EDTA, methylparabens, and propylparabens. Vial stopper contains latex.

[b] For use in the preparation of large-volume parenteral solutions.

HYDROMORPHONE HYDROCHLORIDE — ORAL

For complete and comparative prescribing information, refer to the Opioid Analgesics group monograph.

WARNING

Exalgo –

Potential for abuse: Hydromorphone is an opioid agonist and a schedule II controlled substance with an abuse liability similar to other opioid analgesics. Hydromorphone can be abused in a manner similar to other opioid agonists, legal or illicit. These risks should be considered when administering, prescribing, or dispensing hydromorphone in situations where the health care provider is concerned about increased risk of misuse, abuse, or diversion. Schedule II opioid substances, which include hydromorphone, morphine, oxycodone, fentanyl, oxymorphone, and methadone, have the highest potential for abuse and risk of fatal overdose due to respiratory depression.

Proper patient selection: Hydromorphone is an extended-release (ER) formulation of hydromorphone hydrochloride indicated for the management of moderate to severe pain in opioid-tolerant patients when a continuous around-the-clock opioid analgesic is needed for an extended period of time. Patients considered opioid-tolerant are those who are taking at least oral morphine 60 mg per day, transdermal fentanyl 25 mcg/h, oral oxycodone 30 mg/day, oral hydromorphone 8 mg/day, oral oxymorphone 25 mg/day, or an equianalgesic dose of another opioid, for a week or longer.

Hydromorphone ER is for use in opioid-tolerant patients only.

Fatal respiratory depression could occur in patients who are not opioid tolerant.

WARNING (cont.)

Accidental consumption of hydromorphone ER, especially in children, can result in a fatal overdose of hydromorphone.

Limitations of use: Hydromorphone ER is not indicated for the management of acute or postoperative pain.

Hydromorphone ER is not intended for use as an as-needed analgesic.

Hydromorphone ER tablets are to be swallowed whole and are not to be broken, chewed, dissolved, crushed, or injected. Taking broken, chewed, dissolved, or crushed hydromorphone ER or its contents leads to rapid release and absorption of a potentially fatal dose of hydromorphone ER.

Indications

➤*Pain:* Relief of moderate to severe pain, such as that caused by biliary colic, burns, cancer, myocardial infarction, renal colic, surgery, and trauma (soft tissue and bone).

Exalgo – For the management of moderate to severe pain in opioid-tolerant patients requiring continuous, around-the-clock opioid analgesia for an extended period of time.

Patients considered opioid tolerant are those who are taking at least oral morphine 60 mg per day, transdermal fentanyl 25 mcg/h, oral oxycodone 30 mg/day, oral hydromorphone 8 mg/day, oral oxymorphone 25 mg/day, or an equianalgesic dose of another opioid, for a week or longer.

Hydromorphone is not intended for use as an as-needed analgesic.

Hydromorphone is not indicated for the management of acute or postoperative pain.

HYDROMORPHONE HYDROCHLORIDE — ORAL

Administration and Dosage

➤*General dosing considerations:*

Exalgo – Selection of patients for treatment with hydromorphone ER is governed by the same principles that apply to the use of similar opioid analgesics. Health care providers should individualize treatment in every case, using nonopioid analgesics, opioids on an as-needed basis and/or combination products, and long-term opioid therapy in a progressive plan of pain management such as outlined by the World Health Organization and Federation of State Medical Boards Model Guidelines. Safe and effective administration of opioid analgesics to patients with acute or chronic pain depends upon a comprehensive assessment of the patient. The nature of the pain (eg, etiology, frequency, pathophysiology, severity) and the concurrent medical status of the patient will affect selection of the starting dosage.

In patients receiving opioids, the dose and the duration of analgesia will vary substantially, depending on the patient's opioid tolerance. The dose should be selected and adjusted so that at least 3 to 4 hours of pain relief may be achieved.

Use caution to avoid medication errors when prescribing or dispensing hydromorphone ER 8 mg tablets because 8 mg tablets are also available as hydromorphone immediate-release tablets.

➤*Adults:*

Pain –

Usual dosage:

• *Tablets* – The usual starting dose is 2 to 4 mg every 4 to 6 hours as necessary. More severe pain may require 4 mg or more every 4 to 6 hours.

For chronic pain, doses should be administered around the clock. A supplemental dose of 5% to 15% of the total daily usage may be administered every 2 hours on an as-needed basis.

• *Liquid* – 2.5 to 10 mg (2.5 to 10 mL) every 3 to 6 hours as directed by the clinical situation. Oral dosages higher than the usual dosages may be required in some patients.

Dosage titration: Dose titration should be guided more by the need for analgesia than by the absolute dose of opioid employed.

Dosage adjustment: The dose must be individually adjusted according to severity of pain, patient response, and patient size. If the pain increases in severity, analgesia is not adequate, or tolerance occurs, a gradual increase in dosage may be required.

Periodic reassessment after the initial dosing is always required. If pain management is not satisfactory, and in the absence of significant opioid-induced adverse reactions, the hydromorphone dose may be increased gradually. If excessive opioid adverse reactions are observed early in the dosing interval, the hydromorphone dose should be reduced. If this results in breakthrough pain at the end of the dosing interval, the dosing interval may need to be shortened.

Conversion:

• *Conversion to hydromorphone ER in opioid-tolerant patients* – The dose range of hydromorphone ER studied in clinical trials is 8 to 64 mg. The tablets are to be administered every 24 hours with or without food. Discontinue all other ER opioids when beginning hydromorphone ER therapy. As hydromorphone ER is only for use in opioid-tolerant patients, do not begin any patient on hydromorphone ER as the first opioid.

It is critical to initiate the dosing regimen individually for each patient. Overestimating the hydromorphone ER dose when converting patients from another opioid medication can result in fatal overdose with the first dose.

In the selection of the initial dose of hydromorphone, give attention to the following:

- the daily dose, potency, and specific characteristics of the opioid the patients has been taking previously;
- the reliability of the relative potency estimate used to calculate the equivalent hydromorphone dose needed;
- the patient's degree of opioid tolerance;
- the age, general condition, and medical status of the patient;
- concurrent nonopioid analgesics and other medications, such as those with CNS activity;
- the type and severity of the patient's pain;
- the balance between pain control and adverse reactions;
- risk factors for abuse, addiction, or diversion, including a history of abuse, addiction, or diversion.

The following dosing recommendations, therefore, can only be considered as suggested approaches to what is actually a series of clinical decisions over time in the management of the pain of each individual patient.

Maintenance therapy: During long-term therapy with hydromorphone ER, assess the continued need for around-the-clock opioid therapy periodically. Continue to assess patients for their clinical risks for opioid abuse, addiction, or diversion particularly with high-dose formulations.

Conversion from other oral hydromorphone formulations to hydromorphone: Patients receiving oral immediate-release hydromorphone may be converted to hydromorphone ER by administering a starting dose equivalent to the patient's total daily oral hydromorphone ER dose, taken once daily. The dose of hydromorphone ER can be titrated every 3 to 4 days until adequate pain relief with tolerable adverse reactions has been achieved.

Conversion from oral opioids to hydromorphone: For conversion from other opioids to hydromorphone ER, refer to published relative potency information, keeping in mind that conversion ratios are only approximate. In general, start hydromorphone ER therapy by administering 50% of the calculated total daily dose of hydromorphone ER (see conversion ratio table) every 24 hours. The initial dose of hydromorphone ER can be titrated until adequate pain relief with tolerable adverse reactions has been achieved. The opioid conversion provides approximate equivalent doses, which may be used as a guideline for conversion.

- The conversion ratios and approximate equivalent doses in this conversion table are only to be used for the conversion from current oral opioid therapy to hydromorphone ER. No fixed conversion ratio is likely to be satisfactory in all patients, especially in patients receiving large opioid doses.
- For patients on a regimen of mixed opioids, calculate the approximate oral hydromorphone dose for each opioid and sum the totals.
- For patients on a regimen of fixed-ratio opioid/nonopioid analgesic medications, only the opioid component of these medications should be used in the conversion. The nonopioid component may be continued as a separate drug, or a different nonopioid analgesic may be selected.
- There is substantial patient variation in the relative potency of different opioid drugs and formulations.
- It is extremely important to monitor all patients closely when converting from methadone to other opioid agonists. The ratio between methadone and other opioid agonists may vary widely as a function of previous dose exposure. Methadone has a long half-life and tends to accumulate in the plasma.
- The recommended doses are only a starting point, and close observation and titration is indicated until a satisfactory dose is obtained on the new therapy.

Conversion Ratios to Hydromorphone ER[a,b]

Previous opioid	Approximate equivalent oral dose	Oral conversion ratio[c]
Hydromorphone	12 mg	1
Codeine	200 mg	0.06
Hydrocodone	30 mg	0.4
Methadone[d]	20 mg	0.6
Morphine	60 mg	0.2
Oxycodone	30 mg	0.4
Oxymorphone	20 mg	0.6

[a] Select opioid, sum the total daily dose, and then multiply the dose by the conversion ratio to calculate the approximate oral hydromorphone equivalent.
[b] The conversion ratios and approximate equivalent doses in this conversion table are only to be used for the conversion from current opioid therapy to hydromorphone ER.
[c] Ratio for conversion of oral opioid dose to approximate hydromorphone equivalent dose.
[d] It is extremely important to monitor all patients closely when converting from methadone to other opioid agonists. The ratio between methadone and other opioid agonists may vary widely as a function of previous dose exposure. Methadone has a long half-life and tends to accumulate in the plasma.

Conversion from transdermal fentanyl to hydromorphone ER: Eighteen hours following the removal of the transdermal fentanyl patch, hydromorphone ER treatment can be initiated. For each fentanyl transdermal 25 mcg/h dose the equianalgesic dose of hydromorphone is 12 mg every 24 hours. An appropriate starting dose of hydromorphone ER is 50% of the calculated total daily dose every 24 hours.

Individualization of dosage:

- Once therapy is initiated, assess pain relief and other opioid adverse reactions frequently.
- Titrate patients to adequate analgesia with dose increases not more often than every 3 to 4 days, in order to attain steady-state plasma concentrations of hydromorphone at each dose.
- As a guideline, consider dosage increases of 25% to 50% of the current daily dose of hydromorphone ER for each titration step.
- If more than 2 doses of rescue medication are needed within a 24 hour period for 2 consecutive days, the dose of hydromorphone ER may need to be titrated upward.
- Administer hydromorphone ER no more frequently than every 24 hours.

During periods of changing analgesic requirements, including initial titration, maintain frequent contact between physician, other members of the health care team, the patient, and the caregiver/family. In patients taking opioid analgesics, the starting dose of hydromorphone should be based upon prior opioid usage. This should be done by converting the total daily usage of the previous opioid to an equivalent total daily dosage of oral hydromorphone, using an equianalgesic table (see the following table). For opioids not in the table, first estimate the equivalent total daily usage of oral morphine, then use the table to find the equivalent total daily dosage of hydromorphone.

Opioid Analgesic Equivalents With Approximately Equianalgesic Potency[a]

Drug name	Intramuscular or subcutaneous dose	Oral dose
Morphine	10 mg	40 to 60 mg
Hydromorphone	1.3 to 2 mg	6.5 to 7.5 mg
Oxymorphone	1 to 1.1 mg	6.6 mg
Levorphanol	2 to 2.3 mg	4 mg
Meperidine, pethidine	75 to 100 mg	300 to 400 mg
Methadone	10 mg	10 to 20 mg

[a] Dosages and ranges of dosages represented are a compilation of estimated equipotent dosages from published references comparing opioid analgesics in cancer and severe pain.

HYDROMORPHONE HYDROCHLORIDE — ORAL

Once the total daily dosage of hydromorphone has been estimated, it should be divided into the desired number of doses. Because there is individual variation in response to different opioid drugs, only half to two-thirds of the estimated dose of hydromorphone calculated from equivalence tables should be given for the first few doses, then the dose may be increased, as needed, according to the patient's response.

➤*Elderly:* In general, give opioids with caution, and reduce the initial dose in elderly patients.

➤*Renal function impairment:*

ER – Start patients with moderate renal impairment on a reduced dose and closely monitor during dose titration. As hydromorphone is only intended for once-daily administration, consider use of an alternate analgesic that may permit more flexibility with the dosing interval in patients with severe renal impairment.

Patients with renal function impairment should be started on a lower starting dose.

➤*Hepatic function impairment:*

ER – Start patients with moderate and severe hepatic impairment on a reduced dose and closely monitor during dose titration.

Patients with hepatic function impairment should be started on a lower starting dose.

➤*Debilitated patients:* In general, give opioids with caution, and reduce the initial dose in debilitated patients.

➤*Discontinuation of therapy:* When the patient no longer requires therapy with hydromorphone ER, taper doses gradually, by 25% to 50% every 2 or 3 days down to a dose of 8 mg before discontinuation of therapy, to prevent signs and symptoms of withdrawal in the physically dependent patient.

➤*Administration:* Hydromorphone ER should be swallowed whole and should not be broken, crushed, dissolved, or chewed before swallowing.

➤*Storage/Stability:* Store at 25°C (77°F); excursions are permitted to 15° to 30°C (59° to 86°F). Protect from light.

HYDROMORPHONE HYDROCHLORIDE — INJECTION

For complete and comparative prescribing information, refer to the Opioid Analgesics group monograph.

WARNING

High-potency hydromorphone injection is a highly concentrated solution of hydromorphone, a potent schedule II controlled opioid agonist intended for use in opioid-tolerant patients. Do not confuse high-potency hydromorphone injection with standard parenteral formulations of hydromorphone or other opioids. Overdose and death could result.

Indications

➤*Pain:* Relief of moderate to severe pain, such as that caused by biliary colic, burns, cancer, myocardial infarction, renal colic, surgery, and trauma (soft tissue and bone). High-potency hydromorphone is recommended for opioid-tolerant patients who require larger than usual doses of opioids to provide adequate pain relief.

Because hydromorphone high-potency injection contains hydromorphone 10 mg/mL, a smaller injection volume can be used than with other parenteral opioid formulations. Discomfort associated with the intramuscular (IM) or subcutaneous injection of an unusually large volume of solution can, therefore, be avoided.

Administration and Dosage

➤*General dosing considerations:* The packaging (vial stopper) may contain rubber latex, which may cause allergic reactions.

Individualization of dosage – The dosage of hydromorphone should be individualized for each patient because adverse reactions can occur at doses that may not provide complete freedom from pain.

Safe and effective administration of opioid analgesics to patients with acute or chronic pain depends upon a comprehensive assessment of the patient. The nature of the pain (eg, etiology, frequency, pathophysiology, severity) and the concurrent medical status of the patient will affect selection of the starting dosage.

A gradual increase in dose may be required if analgesia is inadequate, tolerance occurs, or pain severity increases. The first sign of tolerance is usually a reduced duration of effect.

High-potency hydromorphone (10 mg/mL) – High-potency hydromorphone is indicated for relief of moderate to severe pain in opioid-tolerant patients; thus, these patients will already have been treated with other opioid analgesics.

High-potency hydromorphone should be given only to patients who are already receiving large doses of opioids.

Because of its high concentration, the delivery of precise doses of high-potency hydromorphone may be difficult if low doses of hydromorphone are required. Therefore, use high-potency hydromorphone only if the amount of hydromorphone required can be delivered accurately with this formulation.

➤*Adults:*

Pain –

Usual dosage:

• *Regular-strength injection (1, 2, and 4 mg/mL)* – 1 to 2 mg subcutaneously or IM every 4 to 6 hours as needed. For opioid-naive patients, a lower dose should be considered to prevent oversedation.

Patients with terminal cancer may be tolerant to opioid analgesics and may, therefore, require higher doses for adequate pain relief.

• *High-potency (10 mg/mL)* – In open clinical trials with high-potency hydromorphone in patients with terminal cancer, doses ranged from 1 to 14 mg subcutaneously or IM; 1 patient received 30 mg subcutaneously on 2 occasions. In these trials, both subcutaneous and IM injections of high-potency hydromorphone were well tolerated, with minimal pain and/or burning at the injection site. Mild erythema was rarely noted after IM injection. There was no induration after IM or subcutaneous administration of high-potency hydromorphone.

Dosage adjustment: The dose should be adjusted according to the severity of pain, as well as the patient's underlying disease, age, and size.

Conversion:

• *From regular to high-potency hydromorphone* – If the patient is being changed from regular hydromorphone to high-potency hydromorphone, similar doses should be used, depending on the patient's clinical response to the drug.

• *From other opioid analgesics to high-potency hydromorphone* – If high-potency hydromorphone is substituted for a different opioid analgesic, the following equivalency table should be used as a guide to determine the appropriate dose of high-potency hydromorphone.

Approximate Equianalgesic Dosing of Opioid Analgesics (IM or Subcutaneous Administration)

Drug	Dose (mg)[a]	Duration compared with morphine
Butorphanol	1.5 to 2.5	Same
Heroin	4 to 5	Slightly shorter
Hydromorphone	1.3	Slightly shorter
Levorphanol	2.3	Same
Meperidine, pethidine	80	Shorter
Methadone	10	Same
Morphine	10	Same
Nalbuphine	12	Same
Oxymorphone	1.1	Slightly shorter
Pentazocine	60	Shorter

[a] Equianalgesic to morphine 10 mg IM in terms of the area under the analgesic time-effect curve.

Off-label dosing –

Patient controlled analgesia (PCA): The following PCA dosing parameters for hydromorphone (0.2 mg/mL) are for opioid naive adults:

• *Maximum dose* – The total amount of drug over time and the maximum number of patient demand doses per hour will vary.

• *Loading dose* – 0.4 mg (400 mcg) bolus.

• *Clinician dose* – 0.4 mg (400 mcg) bolus. One clinician bolus may be given each hour.

• *PCA dose* – 0.2 mg (200 mcg) with a lockout time of 10 minutes.

• *Basal dose* – Not recommended for starting PCA.

➤*Elderly:* Elderly patients should be started on a lower starting dose.

➤*Renal function impairment:* Patients with renal function impairment should be started on a lower starting dose.

➤*Hepatic function impairment:* Patients with hepatic function impairment should be started on a lower starting dose.

➤*Debilitated patients:* In general, give opioid analgesics with caution and reduce the initial dose in debilitated patients.

➤*Preparation for administration:*

High-potency injection (10 mg/mL) – Reconstitute immediately prior to use with sterile water for injection 25 mL to provide a sterile solution containing 10 mg/mL.

500 mg per 50 mL vial: To use this single-dose presentation, do not penetrate the stopper with a syringe. Instead, remove both the aluminum flipseal and rubber stopper in a suitable work area, such as under a laminar flow hood (or equivalent clean air compounding area). The contents may then be withdrawn for preparation of a single, large-volume parenteral solution. Any unused portion should be discarded in an appropriate manner.

➤*Administration:*

Regular strength injection – If intravenous (IV) administration is necessary, the injection should be given slowly over at least 2 to 3 minutes, depending on the dose. IV or subcutaneous injection is usually not painful.

High-potency injection (10 mg/mL) – Experience with administration of high-potency hydromorphone by the IV route is limited. If IV administration is necessary, the injection should be given slowly over at least 2 to 3 minutes. The IV route is usually painless.

Subcutaneous injections of high-potency hydromorphone were particularly well accepted when administered with a short 30-gauge needle.

➤*Storage/Stability:* Store at 25°C (77°F); excursions are permitted to 15° to 30°C (59° to 86°F). Protect from light. High-potency hydromorphone is physically compatible and chemically stable for at least 24 hours at 25°C (77°F) protected from light in most common large-volume parenteral solutions.

HYDROMORPHONE HYDROCHLORIDE — RECTAL

For complete and comparative prescribing information, refer to the Opioid Analgesics group monograph.

Indications

➤*Pain:* Relief of moderate to severe pain such as that caused by biliary colic, burns, cancer, myocardial infarction, renal colic, surgery, and trauma (soft tissue and bone).

Administration and Dosage

➤*General dosing considerations:* Hydromorphone suppositories may provide longer duration of relief, which could obviate additional medication during the sleeping hours.

Individualization of dosage – Safe and effective administration of opioid analgesics to patients with acute or chronic pain depends upon a comprehensive assessment of the patient. The nature of the pain (eg, etiology, frequency, pathophysiology, severity) and the concurrent medical status of the patient will affect selection of the starting dosage.

In patients receiving opioids, the dose and duration of analgesia will vary substantially, depending on the patient's opioid tolerance. The dose should be selected and adjusted so that at least 3 to 4 hours of pain relief may be achieved. In patients taking opioid analgesics, the starting dose of hydromorphone should be based upon prior opioid usage.

Once the total daily dosage of hydromorphone has been estimated, it should be divided into the desired number of doses. Because there is individual variation in response to different opioid drugs, only half to two-thirds of the estimated dose of hydromorphone should be given for the first few doses, then increase as needed, according to the patient's response.

➤*Adults:*

Moderate to severe pain –

Usual dosage: 3 mg (1 suppository) inserted rectally every 6 to 8 hours or as directed by a health care provider.

In chronic pain, doses should be administered around the clock. A supplemental dose of 5% to 15% of the total daily usage may be administered every 2 hours on an as-needed basis.

Dosage titration: Dose titration should be guided more by the need for analgesia than by the absolute dose of opioid employed.

Dosage adjustment: Periodic reassessment after the initial dosing is always required.

If pain management is not satisfactory and significant opioid-induced adverse reactions are absent, the hydromorphone dose may be increased gradually.

If excessive opioid adverse reactions are observed early in the dosing interval, the hydromorphone dose should be reduced. If this results in breakthrough pain at the end of the dosing interval, the dosing interval may need to be shortened.

➤*Elderly:* Give hydromorphone with caution and reduce the initial dose in elderly patients.

➤*Renal function impairment:* Give hydromorphone with caution and reduce the initial dose in patients with renal function impairment.

➤*Hepatic function impairment:* Give hydromorphone with caution and reduce the initial dose in patients with hepatic function impairment.

➤*Debilitated patients:* Give hydromorphone with caution and reduce the initial dose in debilitated patients.

➤*Administration:* Administer rectally.

➤*Storage/Stability:* Store in a refrigerator between 2° to 8°C (36° to 46°F).

LEVORPHANOL TARTRATE

c-ii	**Levorphanol Tartrate** (Roxane)	**Tablets**: 2 mg	(54 410). Lactose. White, scored. In 100s.

[a] Contains parabens.

[b] Contains phenol 14.5 mg/mL.

LEVORPHANOL TARTRATE — ORAL

For complete prescribing information, refer to the Opioid Analgesics group monograph.

Indications

➤*Pain:* Management of moderate to severe pain where an opioid analgesic is appropriate.

➤*Preoperative medication (Levo-Dromoran* only): As a preoperative medication where an opioid analgesic is appropriate.

Administration and Dosage

➤*General dosing considerations:* Levo-Dromoran has been used for analgesic action during premedication and the postoperative period. Factors to be considered in determining the dosage include age, body weight, physical status, underlying pathological condition, use of other drugs, type of anesthesia used, the surgical procedure involved, and the severity of pain.

➤*Adults:*

Levo-Dromoran –

Chronic pain:

• *Usual dosage* – Individualize dosage for chronic pain. When converting a patient from morphine to levorphanol, begin the total daily dose of oral levorphanol at approximately one-fifteenth to one-twelfth of the previously required total daily dose of oral morphine, and then adjust the dose to the patient's clinical response.

• *Dosage adjustment* – If a patient is to be placed on fixed-schedule dosing (round-the-clock) with this drug, take care to allow adequate time after each dose change (approximately 72 hours) for the patient to reach a new steady state before a subsequent dose adjustment to avoid excessive sedation because of drug accumulation.

Pain (moderate to severe):

• *Maximum dose* – Total oral daily doses of more than 16 mg in 24 hours are generally not recommended as starting doses in nonopioid-tolerant patients.

• *Initial dosage* – 2 mg, repeat in 6 to 8 hours as needed, provided the patient is assessed for signs of hypoventilation and excessive sedation.

• *Dosage adjustment* – If necessary, increase the dose to up to 3 mg every 6 to 8 hours, after adequate evaluation of the patient's response. Higher doses may be appropriate in opioid-tolerant patients. Adjust dosage according to the severity of pain; the patient's age, weight, physical status, and underlying diseases; use of concomitant medications; and other factors.

Preoperative medication: See Pain (moderate to severe) for dosing.

Levorphanol tartrate –

Pain (moderate to severe):

• *Maximum dose* – Total oral daily doses of more than 16 mg in 24 hours are generally not recommended as starting doses in nonopioid-tolerant patients.

• *Initial dosage* – 2 mg, repeat in 3 to 6 hours as needed, provided the patient is assessed for signs of hypoventilation and excessive sedation. The effective daily dosage range, depending on the severity of the pain, is 8 to 16 mg in 24 hours in the nontolerant patient.

➤*Elderly:* The initial doses of levorphanol should be reduced by 50% or more when the drug is given to elderly patients. Subsequent doses should then be individually titrated according to the patient's response.

➤*Renal function impairment:* Levorphanol should be administered with caution, and the initial dose should be reduced in patients with severe impairment of renal function.

➤*Hepatic function impairment:* Levorphanol should be administered with caution, and the initial dose should be reduced in patients with severe impairment of hepatic function.

➤*Patients with any condition or other drugs affecting respiratory reserve:* The initial doses of levorphanol should be reduced by 50% or more when the drug is given to patients with any condition affecting respiratory reserve or in conjunction with other drugs affecting the respiratory center. Subsequent doses should then be individually titrated according to the patient's response. Respiratory depression produced by levorphanol can be reversed by naloxone, a specific antagonist.

➤*Storage/Stability:* Store at 15° to 30°C (59° to 86°F).

LEVORPHANOL TARTRATE — INJECTION

For complete prescribing information, refer to the Opioid Analgesics group monograph.

Indications

➤*Pain:* Management of moderate to severe pain where an opioid analgesic is appropriate.

➤*Preoperative medication (Levo-Dromoran* only): As a preoperative medication where an opioid analgesic is appropriate.

Administration and Dosage

➤*General dosing considerations:* Levorphanol 2 mg is approximately equivalent to morphine 10 to 15 mg or meperidine 100 mg.

➤*Adults:*

Acute pain (moderate to severe) –

Usual dosage:

• *Intravenous* – Up to 1 mg given in divided doses by slow injection. This may be repeated in 3 to 6 hours as needed, provided the patient is assessed for signs of hypoventilation or excessive sedation.

• *Intramuscular or subcutaneous* – 1 to 2 mg. This may be repeated in 6 to 8 hours as needed, provided the patient is assessed for signs of hypoventilation or excessive sedation.

Maximum dose:

• *Intravenous* – 4 to 8 mg IV in 24 hours in nonopioid tolerant patients.

• *Intramuscular* – 3 to 8 mg IM in 24 hours in nonopioid-tolerant patients.

Dosage adjustment: Adjust dosage according to the severity of the pain; age, weight, and physical status of the patient; the patient's underlying diseases; use of concomitant medications; and other factors.

LEVORPHANOL TARTRATE — INJECTION

Chronic pain –

Usual dosage: For chronic pain, individualize the dosage.

Conversion from morphine: Levorphanol is 4 to 8 times as potent as morphine and has a longer half-life. Because there is incomplete cross-tolerance among opioids, when converting a patient from morphine to levorphanol, begin the total daily dose of oral levorphanol at approximately 1/15 to 1/12 of the total daily dose of oral morphine that such patients had previously required, and then adjust the dose to the patient's clinical response. If a patient is to be placed on fixed-schedule dosing (round-the-clock) with this drug, take care to allow adequate time after each dose change (approximately 72 hours) for the patient to reach a new steady state before a subsequent dose adjustment to avoid excessive sedation because of drug accumulation.

Premedication (Levo-Dromoran only) – 1 to 2 mg IM or subcutaneously, administered 60 to 90 minutes before surgery. Individualize the preoperative medication dose.

Levorphanol has been used for analgesic action during premedication and the postoperative period. Factors to be considered in determining the dosage include age, body weight, physical status, underlying pathological condition, use of other drugs, type of anesthesia used, the surgical procedure involved, and the severity of pain.

➤*Elderly:* Reduce the initial doses of levorphanol by 50% or more when the drug is given to elderly patients. Subsequent doses should then be individually titrated according to the patient's response

➤*Debilitated patients:* Debilitated patients usually require less drug.

➤*Preexisting pulmonary disease:* Reduce the initial doses of levorphanol by 50% or more when the drug is given to patients with any condition affecting respiratory reserve or in conjunction with other drugs affecting the respiratory center. Subsequent doses should then be individually titrated according to the patient's response.

➤*Administration:*

Pain – Administer IM, IV, or subcutaneously.

Premedication (Levo-Dromoran only) – IM or subcutaneously, administered 60 to 90 minutes before surgery.

➤*Admixture compatibility:* Levorphanol injection has been reported to be physically incompatible with solutions containing aminophylline, ammonium chloride, amobarbital sodium, chlorothiazide sodium, heparin sodium, methicillin sodium, nitrofurantoin sodium, novobiocin sodium, pentobarbital sodium, perphenazine, phenobarbital sodium, phenytoin sodium, secobarbital sodium, sodium bicarbonate, sodium iodide, sulfadiazine sodium, sulfisoxazole diethanolamine, and thiopental sodium.

➤*Storage/Stability:* Store at 15° to 30°C (59° to 86°F).

Safety and handling – Levorphanol injection is packaged in sealed systems that have a low risk of accidental exposure to health care workers. Take ordinary care to avoid aerosol generation while preparing a syringe for use. Significant absorption from accidental dermal exposure is unlikely, and wash spilled levorphanol from the skin by rinsing with cool water. As with all controlled substances, abuse by health care personnel is possible and handle the drug accordingly.

MEPERIDINE HYDROCHLORIDE

c-ii	**Meperidine Hydrochloride** (Various, eg, Amide, Barr, Roxane, Watson)	**Tablets**: 50 mg	In 100s, 500s, 1,000s, and UD 25s.
c-ii	**Demerol** (Sanofi-Synthelabo)		White, scored, convex. In 100s, 500s, and UD 25s.
c-ii	**Meperidine Hydrochloride** (Various, eg, Amide, Barr, Roxane, Watson)	**Tablets**: 100 mg	In 100s, 500s, and 1,000s, and UD 25s.
c-ii	**Demerol** (Sanofi-Synthelabo)		White, convex. In 100s.
c-ii	**Demerol** (Sanofi-Synthelabo)	**Syrup**: 50 mg per 5 mL	Glucose, saccharin. Alcohol free. Banana flavor. In 473 mL.
c-ii	**Meperidine Hydrochloride** (Roxane)	**Oral solution**: 50 mg per 5 mL	Sorbitol. In 500 mL.
c-ii	**Meperidine Hydrochloride** (Hospira)	**Injection**: 10 mg/mL	In 30 mL single-dose container.[a]
c-ii	**Meperidine Hydrochloride** (Various, eg, Baxter)	**Injection**: 25 mg/mL	In 1 mL amps and 1 mL vials.
c-ii	**Demerol** (Abbott)		In 1 mL *Carpuject* syringes.[b]
c-ii	**Meperidine Hydrochloride** (Various, eg, Baxter)	**Injection**: 50 mg/mL	In 1 mL amps and 1 mL vials.
c-ii	**Demerol** (Abbott)		In 0.5, 1, 1.5, and 2 mL amps,[c] 30 mL multidose vials,[c] and 1 mL *Carpuject* syringes.[b]
c-ii	**Meperidine Hydrochloride** (Various, eg, Baxter)	**Injection**: 75 mg/mL	In 1 mL vials and 1 mL amps
c-ii	**Demerol** (Abbott)		In 1 mL *Carpuject* syringes.[b]
c-ii	**Meperidine Hydrochloride** (Various, eg, Baxter)	**Injection**: 100 mg/mL	In 1 mL vials and 1 mL amps.
c-ii	**Demerol** (Abbott)		In 1 mL amp,[c] 20 mL multidose vials,[c] and 1 mL *Carpuject* syringes.[b]

[a] This vial is only for use with a compatible Hospira *PCA* pump set with injector and a compatible Hospira infusion device (see directions for use supplied with the set or infuser).

[b] Ampuls and *Carpuject* syringes are preservative free.

[c] Multidose vials contain metacresol as preservative.

MEPERIDINE HYDROCHLORIDE — ORAL

For complete prescribing information, refer to the Opioid Analgesics group monograph.

Indications

➤*Moderate to severe pain:* Relief of moderate to severe pain.

Administration and Dosage

➤*Adults:*

Moderate to severe pain –

Usual dosage: 50 to 150 mg orally every 3 to 4 hours as necessary.

Dosage adjustment: Adjust dosage according to the severity of the pain and the response of the patient.

➤*Children:*

Moderate to severe pain –

Usual dosage: 1.1 to 1.75 mg/kg (0.5 to 0.8 mg/lb) up to the adult dose, every 3 to 4 hours, as necessary.

Dosage adjustment: Adjust dosage according to the severity of the pain and the response of the patient.

➤*Elderly:* Give meperidine with caution and reduce the initial dose in elderly patients.

➤*Renal function impairment:* Give meperidine with caution and reduce the initial dose in certain patients, such as those with severe impairment of renal function.

➤*Hepatic function impairment:* Give meperidine with caution and reduce the initial dose in certain patients, such as those with severe impairment of hepatic function.

➤*Debilitated patients:* Give meperidine with caution and reduce the initial dose in certain patients, such as debilitated patients.

➤*Concomitant therapy:* Proportionately reduce the dose (usually by 25% to 50%) when administered concomitantly with phenothiazines and many other tranquilizers because they potentiate the action of meperidine.

➤*Storage/Stability:* Store at 25°C (77°F); excursions are permitted to 15° to 30°C (59° to 86°F).

MEPERIDINE HYDROCHLORIDE — INJECTION

For complete prescribing information, refer to the Opioid Analgesics group monograph.

Indications

➤*Relief of moderate to severe pain:* Relief of moderate to severe pain.

➤*Preoperative medication:* For preoperative medication.

➤*Anesthesia support:* For support of anesthesia.

➤*Obstetrical analgesia:* For obstetrical analgesia (except for meperidine 10 mg/mL).

Administration and Dosage

➤*General dosing considerations:* Reduced dosage is indicated in poor-risk patients, in the very young or very old, in patients with impaired renal or hepatic function, and in patients receiving other CNS depressants.

For surgical patients, dosage should be based on response of the patient, other premedications and concomitant medications, the anesthetic being used, and the nature and duration of the operation.

➤*Adults:*

Obstetrical analgesia (except for meperidine 10 mg/mL) – Administer 50 to 100 mg IM or subcutaneously; may repeat at 1- to 3-hour intervals, when pain becomes regular.

MEPERIDINE HYDROCHLORIDE — INJECTION

Pain (moderate to severe) –

Usual dosage: 50 to 150 mg IM or subcutaneously every 3 to 4 hours as necessary.

Occasionally, it may be necessary to exceed the usual dosage recommended in cases of exceptionally severe pain or in those patients who become tolerant.

• *10 mg/mL strength (via Hospira infusion device)* – 10 mg IV, with a range of 1 to 5 mg per incremental dose. The recommended lockout interval is 6 to 10 minutes. The minimum recommended lockout interval is 5 minutes.

For continuous infusion, the usual adult dose is 15 to 35 mg per hour administered IV as required.

Dosage adjustment: Adjust dosage according to the severity of the pain and the response of the patient.

• *10 mg/mL strength (via Hospira infusion device)* – The health care provider may adjust the dosage either upward or downward, or increase or decrease the lockout interval, depending on patient response.

Preoperative medication – 50 to 100 mg IM or subcutaneously, 30 to 90 minutes before beginning anesthesia.

Support of anesthesia – Meperidine may be administered by repeated slow IV injections of fractional doses (eg, 10 mg/mL) or by a continuous IV infusion of a more dilute solution (eg, 1 mg/mL). Individualize dosage.

➤*Children:*

Pain (moderate to severe) –

Usual dosage: 1.1 to 1.75 mg/kg (0.5 to 0.8 mg/lb) IM or subcutaneously up to the adult dose, every 3 to 4 hours, as necessary.

Dosage adjustment: Adjust dosage according to the severity of the pain and the response of the patient.

Preoperative medication – 1.1 to 2.2 mg/kg (0.5 to 1 mg/lb) IM or subcutaneously, up to the adult dose, 30 to 90 minutes before beginning anesthesia.

➤*Elderly:* For moderate to severe pain and for use as a preoperative medication, elderly patients should usually be given meperidine at the lower end of the dosage range and observed closely.

➤*Renal function impairment:* Meperidine should be given with caution and the initial dose should be reduced in patients with severe impairment of renal function.

CrCl 10 to 50 mL/min – 75% of normal dose.

CrCl less than 10 mL/min – 25 to 50% of normal dose.

Hemodialysis – Not recommended.

Peritoneal dialysis – Not recommended.

➤*Hepatic function impairment:* Meperidine should be given with caution and the initial dose should be reduced in patients with severe impairment of hepatic function.

➤*Concomitant therapy:* The dose should be proportionately reduced (usually by 25% to 50%) when coadministered with phenothiazines and many other tranquilizers because they potentiate the action of meperidine.

➤*Administration:* While subcutaneous administration is suitable for occasional use, IM administration is preferred when repeated doses are required. If IV administration is required, the dosage should be decreased and the injection given very slowly, preferably utilizing a diluted solution.

10 mg/mL strength – When administered IV, meperidine should be given very slowly. Rapid IV injection increases the incidence of adverse reactions; severe respiratory depression, apnea, hypotension, peripheral circulatory collapse, and cardiac arrest have occurred. This drug should be administered IV only if a narcotic antagonist (naloxone) and the facilities for assisted or controlled respiration are immediately available. When meperidine is given parenterally, especially IV, the patient should be lying down.

For use as a single-dose unit to provide analgesia via the IV route using a compatible *Hospira* infusion device. Each vial is intended for single dose only. When the dosing requirement is complete, the unused portion should be discarded in an appropriate manner. Do not autoclave.

Health care providers should completely familiarize themselves with a compatible *Hospira* infusion device before deciding to administer meperidine injection via the infuser.

➤*Admixture compatibility:* Meperidine is incompatible with soluble barbiturates, aminophylline, heparin, morphine sulfate, methicillin, phenytoin, sodium bicarbonate, iodide, sulfadiazine, and sulfisoxazole.

➤*Storage/Stability:* Store at room temperature, up to 25°C (77°F).

10 mg/mL – Store at 20° to 25°C (68° to 77°F).

METHADONE HYDROCHLORIDE

c-ii	**Methadone Hydrochloride** (Various, eg, Mallinckrodt, Roxane, VistaPharm)	**Tablets; oral:** 5 mg	In 100s and UD 100s.
c-ii	**Dolophine Hydrochloride** (Roxane)		(54 162). White, scored. In 100s.
c-ii	**Methadose** (Mallinckrodt)		(Methadose 5). White, scored. In 100s.
c-ii	**Methadone Hydrochloride** (Various, eg, Mallinckrodt, Roxane, VistaPharm)	**Tablets; oral:** 10 mg	In 100s and UD 100s.
c-ii	**Dolophine Hydrochloride** (Roxane)		(54 549). White, scored. In 100s.
c-ii	**Methadose** (Mallinckrodt)		(Methadose 10). White, scored. In 100s.
c-ii	**Methadone Hydrochloride**[a] (Various, eg, Cebert, VistaPharm)	**Tablets for suspension, dispersible; oral:** 40 mg	In 100s.
c-ii	**Methadose**[a] (Mallinckrodt)		(Methadose 40). White, quadrisected. In 100s.
c-ii	**Diskets** (Cebert)		(54 883). Peach, scored. Orange-pineapple flavor. In 100s.
c-ii	**Methadone Hydrochloride** (Roxane)	**Solution; oral:** 5 mg per 5 mL	May contain alcohol, sorbitol. In 500 mL.
		10 mg per 5 mL	May contain alcohol, sorbitol. In 500 mL.
c-ii	**Methadone Hydrochloride**[a] (Various, eg, Cebert, VistaPharm)	**Liquid concentrate; oral:** 10 mg/mL	In 946 mL and 1 L.
c-ii	**Methadone Hydrochloride Intensol** (Roxane)		In 30 mL with calibrated dropper.
c-ii	**Methadose**[a] (Mallinckrodt)		Sucrose. Red. Cherry flavor. In 1 and 15 L. Also available as sugar free, dye free, unflavored.
c-ii	**Methadone Hydrochloride** (AAIPharma)	**Injection:** 10 mg/mL	In 20 mL multidose vials.[b]

[a] For detoxification and maintenance only.
[b] With 0.5% chlorobutanol.

METHADONE HYDROCHLORIDE — ORAL

For complete prescribing information, refer to the Opioid Analgesics group monograph.

WARNING

Deaths have been reported during initiation of methadone treatment for opioid dependence. In some cases, drug interactions with other drugs, both licit and illicit, have been suspected. However, in other cases, deaths appear to have occurred because of the respiratory or cardiac effects of methadone and too-rapid titration without appreciation for the accumulation of methadone over time. It is critical to understand the pharmacokinetics of methadone and to exercise vigilance during treatment initiation and dose titration. Patients must also be strongly cautioned against self-medicating with CNS depressants during initiation of methadone treatment.

Respiratory depression is the chief hazard associated with methadone administration. Methadone's peak respiratory depressant effects typically occur later and persist longer than its peak analgesic effects, particularly in the early dosing period. These characteristics can contribute to the cases of iatrogenic overdose, particularly during treatment initiation and dose titration.

WARNING (cont.)

Cases of QT interval prolongation and serious arrhythmia (torsades de pointes) have been observed during treatment with methadone. Most cases involve patients being treated for pain with large, multiple daily doses of methadone, although cases have been reported in patients receiving doses commonly used for maintenance treatment of opioid addiction.

Conditions for distribution and use of methadone products for the treatment of opioid addiction – Methadone products, when used for the treatment of opioid addiction in detoxification or maintenance programs, shall be dispensed only by opioid treatment programs (and agencies, practitioners, or institutions by formal agreement with the program sponsor) certified by the Substance Abuse and Mental Health Services Administration and approved by the designated state authority. Certified treatment programs shall dispense and use methadone in oral form only and according to the treatment requirements stipulated in the Federal Opioid Treatment Standards (42 CFR 8.12). See the following information for important regulatory exceptions to the general requirement for certification to provide opioid agonist treatment.

METHADONE HYDROCHLORIDE — ORAL

WARNING (cont.)

Failure to abide by the requirements in these regulations may result in criminal prosecution, seizure of the drug supply, revocation of the program approval, and injunction precluding operation of the program.

Regulatory exceptions to the general requirement for certification to provide opioid agonist treatment include the following:

- During inpatient care, when the patient was admitted for any condition other than concurrent opioid addiction (pursuant to 21 CFR 1306.07[c]), to facilitate the treatment of the primary admitting diagnosis.
- During an emergency period of no longer than 3 days while definitive care for the addiction is being sought in an appropriately licensed facility (pursuant to 21 CFR 1306.07[b]).

Indications

➤*Detoxification:* For detoxification treatment of opioid addiction (heroin or other morphine-like drugs).

For maintenance treatment of opioid addiction (heroin or other morphine-like drugs), in conjunction with appropriate social and medical services.

Note – Outpatient maintenance and detoxification treatment may be provided only by Opioid Treatment Programs (OTPs) certified by the Federal Substance Abuse and Mental Health Services Administration (SAMHSA) and registered by the Drug Enforcement Administration (DEA). This does not preclude the maintenance treatment of a patient with concurrent opioid addiction who is hospitalized for conditions other than opioid addiction and who requires temporary maintenance during the critical period of his/her stay, or of a patient whose enrollment has been verified in a program which has been certified for maintenance treatment with methadone.

➤*Pain (except oral concentrate and tablets for suspension):* For the treatment of moderate to severe pain not responsive to nonnarcotic analgesics.

Administration and Dosage

➤*General dosing considerations:* Methadone differs from many other opioid agonists in several important ways. Methadone's pharmacokinetic properties, coupled with high interpatient variability in its absorption, metabolism, and relative analgesic potency, necessitate a cautious and highly individualized approach to prescribing. Particular vigilance is necessary during treatment initiation, conversion from one opioid to another, and dose titration.

While methadone's duration of analgesic action (typically 4 to 8 hours) in the setting of single-dose studies approximates that of morphine, methadone's plasma elimination half-life is substantially longer than that of morphine (typically 8 to 59 hours vs 1 to 5 hours, respectively). Methadone's peak respiratory depressant effects typically occur later and persist longer than its peak analgesic effects. Also, with repeated dosing, methadone may be retained in the liver and then slowly released, prolonging the duration of action despite low plasma concentrations. For these reasons, steady-state plasma concentrations and full analgesic effects are usually not attained until 3 to 5 days of dosing. Additionally, incomplete cross-tolerance between mu-opioid agonists makes determination of dosing during opioid conversion complex.

The complexities associated with methadone dosing can contribute to cases of iatrogenic overdose, particularly during treatment initiation and dose titration. A high degree of opioid tolerance does not eliminate the possibility of methadone overdose, iatrogenic or otherwise. Deaths have been reported during conversion to methadone from chronic, high-dose treatment with other opioid agonists and during initiation of methadone treatment of addiction in subjects previously abusing high doses of other agonists.

➤*Adults:*

Detoxification – For detoxification and maintenance of opiate dependence, administer methadone in accordance with the treatment standards cited in the Federal Opioid Treatment Standards (42 CFR 8.12), including limitations on unsupervised administration.

Initial dosage: A single dose of methadone 20 to 30 mg will often be sufficient to suppress withdrawal symptoms. The initial dose should not exceed 30 mg. Administer the initial dose under supervision, when there are no signs of sedation or intoxication and the patient shows symptoms of withdrawal.

Initial doses should be lower for patients whose tolerance is expected to be low at treatment entry. Consider loss of tolerance in any patient who has not taken opioids for more than 5 days. Initial doses should not be determined by previous treatment episodes or dollars spent per day on illicit drug use.

If same-day dosing adjustments are to be made, the patient should be asked to wait 2 to 4 hours for further evaluation, when peak levels have been reached. An additional 5 to 10 mg of methadone may be provided if withdrawal symptoms have not been suppressed or if symptoms reappear. The total daily dose of methadone on the first day of treatment should not ordinarily exceed 40 mg.

Short-term therapy: For patients preferring a brief course of stabilization followed by a period of medically supervised withdrawal, it is generally recommended that the patient be titrated to a total daily dose of approximately 40 mg in divided doses to achieve an adequate stabilizing level. Stabilization can be continued for 2 to 3 days, after which the dose of methadone should be gradually decreased. The rate at which methadone is decreased should be determined separately for each patient. The dose of methadone can be decreased on a daily basis or at 2-day intervals, but the amount of intake should remain sufficient to keep withdrawal symptoms at a tolerable level. In hospitalized patients, a daily reduction of 20% of the total daily dose may be tolerated. In ambulatory patients, a somewhat slower schedule may be needed.

Dosage adjustment: Make dosage adjustments over the first week of treatment based on control of withdrawal symptoms at the time of expected peak activity (eg, 2 to 4 hours after dosing). Dose adjustment should be cautious; deaths have occurred in early treatment because of the cumulative effects of the first several days' dosing.

Remind patients that the dose will hold for a longer period of time as tissue stores of methadone accumulate.

Maintenance treatment of opioid addiction –

Usual dosage: Most commonly, clinical stability is achieved at doses of between 80 and 120 mg/day.

Dosage titration: Titrate patients in maintenance treatment to a dose at which opioid symptoms are prevented for 24 hours, drug hunger or craving is reduced, the euphoric effects of self-administered opioids are blocked or attenuated, and the patient is tolerant to the sedative effects of methadone.

Tapering: There is considerable variability in the appropriate rate of methadone taper in patients choosing medically supervised withdrawal from methadone treatment. It is generally suggested that dose reductions should be less than 10% of the established tolerance or maintenance doses, and 10- to 14-day intervals should elapse between dose reductions. Apprise patients of the high risk of relapse to illicit drug use associated with discontinuation of methadone maintenance treatment.

Pain – The oral concentrate and tablets for suspension are not indicated for pain.

Optimal methadone initiation and dose titration strategies for the treatment of pain have not been determined. Published equianalgesic conversion ratios between methadone and other opioids are imprecise, providing at best only population averages that cannot be applied consistently to all patients. It should be noted that many commonly cited equianalgesic tables only present relative analgesic potencies of single opioid doses in nontolerant patients, thus greatly underestimating methadone's analgesic potency and its potential for adverse reactions in repeated dose settings. Regardless of the dose-determination strategy employed, methadone is most safely initiated and titrated using small initial doses and gradual dose adjustments.

As with all opioid drugs, it is necessary to adjust the dosing regimen for each patient individually, taking into account the patient's prior analgesic treatment experience. The dosing recommendations should only be considered as suggested approaches to what is actually a series of clinical decisions over time in the management of the pain of each individual patient. Prescribers should always follow appropriate management principles of careful assessment and ongoing monitoring.

In the selection of an initial dose of methadone, pay attention to:

1.) The total daily dose, potency, and specific characteristics of the opioid the patient had been taking previously, if any;
2.) The relative potency estimate used to calculate an equianalgesic starting methadone dose; in particular, whether it is intended for use in acute or chronic methadone dosing;
3.) The patients degree of opioid tolerance;
4.) The age, general condition, and medical status of the patient;
5.) Concurrent medications, particularly other CNS and respiratory depressants;
6.) The type, severity, and expected duration of the patient's pain;
7.) The acceptable balance between pain control and adverse reactions.

Initial dosage: When oral methadone is used as the first analgesic in patients who are not already being treated with and tolerant to opioids, the usual methadone starting dose is 2.5 to 10 mg every 8 to 12 hours, slowly titrated to effect. More frequent administration may be required during methadone initiation in order to maintain adequate analgesia, and extreme caution is necessary to avoid overdosage, taking into account methadone's long half-life.

Conversion:

- *Parenteral to oral methadone* – Conversion from parenteral to oral methadone should initially use a 1:2 dose ratio (eg, parenteral methadone 5 mg to oral methadone 10 mg).
- *Switching from other chronic opioids* – Switching a patient from another chronically administered opioid to methadone requires caution because of the uncertainty of dose-conversion ratios and incomplete cross-tolerance. Deaths have occurred in opioid-tolerant patients during conversion to methadone.

Conversion ratios in many commonly used equianalgesic dosing tables do not apply in the setting of repeated methadone dosing. Although the onset and duration of analgesic action, as well as the analgesic potency of methadone and morphine, are similar with single-dose administration, methadone's potency increases over time with repeated dosing. Furthermore, the conversion ratio between methadone and other opiates varies dramatically depending on baseline opiate (morphine equivalent) use.

The morphine to methadone conversion scheme is derived from various consensus guidelines for converting chronic pain patients to methadone from morphine. Health care providers should consult published conversion guidelines to determine the equivalent morphine dose for patients converting from other opioids.

Oral Morphine to Oral Methadone Conversion for Chronic Administration

Total daily baseline oral morphine dose	Estimated daily oral methadone requirement as percent of total daily morphine dose
< 100 mg	20% to 30%
100 to 300 mg	10% to 20%
300 to 600 mg	8% to 12%
600 to 1,000 mg	5% to 10%
1,000 mg	< 5%

METHADONE HYDROCHLORIDE — ORAL

The total daily methadone dose derived from the conversion table may then be divided to reflect the intended dosing schedule (eg, for administration every 8 hours, divide total daily dose by 3).

Note: Equianalgesic methadone dosing varies not only among patients, but also within the same patient, depending on baseline morphine (or other opioid) dose. The conversion table has been included in order to illustrate this concept and to provide a safe starting point for opioid conversion. Methadone dosing should not be based solely on these tables. Methadone conversion and dose titration methods should always be individualized to account for the patient's achievement of adequate pain relief and balanced against tolerability of opioid adverse reactions. If a patient develops intolerable opioid-related adverse reactions, the methadone dose, or dosing interval, may need to be adjusted.

➤*Children:*

Off-label dosing – See also Preparation for Administration.

Opiate withdrawal:

• *Neonates* –

Initial dosage: 0.05 to 0.2 mg/kg every 12 to 24 hours.

Tapering: Reduce dose by 10% to 20% per week over 4 to 6 weeks. Adjust tapering schedule on signs and symptoms of withdrawal.

Pain:

• *Usual dose* – 0.7 mg/kg daily in divided doses every 4 to 6 hours, as needed.

• *Maximum dose* – 10 mg per dose.

➤*Pregnancy:* Methadone clearance may be increased during pregnancy. Several small studies have demonstrated significantly lower trough methadone plasma concentrations and shorter methadone half-lives in women during pregnancy compared with after delivery. During pregnancy, a woman's methadone dose may need to be increased or their dosing interval decreased. Use methadone in pregnancy only if the potential benefit justifies the potential risk to the fetus.

➤*Preparation for administration:* For preparation of a 0.5 mg/mL oral solution, mix 1 mL of methadone 10 mg/mL concentrated solution with 19 mL of sterile water. Solution is stable for 24 hours if refrigerated.

➤*Administration:*

Dispersible tablets – Methadone dispersible tablets have been formulated with insoluble excipients to deter the use of this drug by injection. Dissolve each tablet in approximately 1 oz of liquid (other than grapefruit juice) and swallow. Do not swallow tablets whole or chew tablets.

Diskets – *Diskets* are intended for dispersion in a liquid immediately prior to oral administration of the prescribed dose. The tablets should not be chewed or swallowed before dispersing in liquid. The tablets are cross-scored, allowing for flexible dosing adjustment. Each tablet may be broken or cut in half to yield two 20 mg doses or in quarters to yield four 10 mg doses.

Prior to administration, dispense the desired dose in approximately 120 mL (4 oz) of water, orange juice, *Tang*, citrus flavors of *Kool-Aid*, or other acidic fruit beverage prior to taking. Methadone is very soluble in water, but there are some insoluble excipients that will not entirely dissolve. If residue remains in the cup after initial administration, a small amount of liquid should be added and the resulting mixture administered to the patient.

Because *Diskets* can be administered only in 10 mg increments, they may not be the appropriate product for initial dosing or gradual dose reduction in many patients.

➤*Storage/Stability:* Store at 25°C (77°F); excursions are permitted between 15° and 30°C (59° and 86°F). Dispense in a tight, light-resistant container.

Diskets, if dispensed, must be packaged in child-resistant containers and kept out of the reach of children to prevent accidental ingestion.

METHADONE HYDROCHLORIDE — INJECTION

For complete prescribing information, refer to the Opioid Analgesics group monograph.

WARNING

To treat narcotic addiction in detoxification or maintenance programs, methadone should be dispensed only by hospitals, community pharmacies, and maintenance programs approved by the FDA and designated state authorities. Approved maintenance programs shall dispense and use methadone in oral form only and according to treatment requirements stipulated in *Federal Methadone Regulations*. Failure to abide by the requirements in these regulations may result in criminal prosecution, seizure of drug supply, revocation of program approval, and injunction precluding program operation.

Methadone, used as an analgesic, may be dispensed in any licensed pharmacy.

Cardiac conduction effects – Laboratory studies, in vivo and in vitro, have demonstrated that methadone inhibits cardiac potassium channels and prolongs the QT interval. Cases of QT interval prolongation and serious arrhythmia (torsades de pointes) have been observed during treatment with methadone. These cases appear to be more commonly associated with, but not limited to, higher dose treatment (greater than 200 mg/day). Most cases involve patients being treated for pain with large, multiple daily doses of methadone, although cases have been reported in patients receiving doses commonly used for maintenance treatment of opioid addiction.

Indications

➤*Pain/Detoxification:* For relief of severe pain; detoxification and temporary maintenance treatment of narcotic addiction.

Note – If used to treat heroin dependence for longer than 3 weeks, the procedure passes from treatment of acute withdrawal syndrome (detoxification) to maintenance therapy. Maintenance may be undertaken only by approved methadone programs. This does not preclude maintenance treatment of addicts hospitalized for other conditions and who require temporary maintenance during the critical period of their stays or whose enrollment has been verified in a program approved for maintenance treatment with methadone.

Administration and Dosage

➤*General dosing considerations:* Oral methadone is about one-half as potent as parenteral methadone. Oral administration results in a delay of onset, lower peak, and increased duration of analgesic effect.

Duration of effect increases with repeated use because of cumulative effects.

➤*Adults:*

Detoxification and maintenance treatment of narcotic addiction – Oral administration is preferred. However, if the patient is unable to ingest oral methadone, the parenteral form may be used. The patient's oral methadone dose should be converted to an equivalent parenteral dose.

Injectable methadone products are not approved for the outpatient treatment of opioid dependence. Parenteral methadone should be used only for patients who are unable to take oral medication, such as during hospitalization.

For a complete description of detoxification and maintenance regulations and dosage protocols, consult a local approved methadone program.

Duration of therapy: Detoxification treatment should not exceed 21 days and may not be repeated earlier than 4 weeks after the completion of the preceding course. If methadone is administered longer than 3 weeks, the procedure is considered to have progressed from detoxification or treatment of the acute withdrawal syndrome to maintenance treatment, even though the goal and intent may be eventual, total withdrawal.

Pain – As with all opioid drugs, it is necessary to adjust the dosing regimen for each patient individually, taking into account the patient's prior analgesic treatment experience. The dosing recommendations should only be considered as suggested approaches to what is actually a series of clinical decisions over time in the management of each individual patient's pain. Health care providers should always follow appropriate pain management principles of careful assessment and ongoing monitoring.

In the selection of an initial dose of methadone injection, pay attention to:

1.) The total daily dose, potency, and specific characteristics of the opioid the patient had been taking previously, if any;
2.) The relative potency estimate used to calculate an equianalgesic starting methadone dose; in particular, whether it is intended for use in acute or chronic methadone dosing;
3.) The patient's degree of opioid tolerance;
4.) The age, general condition, and medical status of the patient;
5.) Concurrent medications, particularly other CNS and respiratory depressants;
6.) The type, severity, and expected duration of the patient's pain;
7.) The acceptable balance between pain control and adverse reactions.

Initial dosage: In opioid-nontolerant patients, 2.5 to 10 mg every 8 to 12 hours intravenously (IV), intramuscularly (IM), or subcutaneously, slowly titrated to effect. More frequent administration may be required during methadone initiation in order to maintain adequate analgesia. Extreme caution is necessary to avoid overdosage, taking into account methadone's long elimination half-life.

Conversion:

• *Conversion from oral to parenteral methadone* – Initially use a 2:1 dose ratio to go from oral to parenteral (eg, oral methadone 10 mg to parenteral methadone 5 mg).

• *Switching patients to parenteral methadone from other chronic opioids* – Switching a patient from another chronically administered opioid to methadone requires caution because of the uncertainty of dose conversion ratios and incomplete cross-tolerance. Deaths have occurred in opioid-tolerant patients during conversion to methadone.

Conversion ratios in many commonly used equianalgesic dosing tables do not apply for repeated methadone dosing. Although the onset and duration of analgesic action and the analgesic potency of methadone and morphine are similar with single-dose administration, methadone's potency increases over time with repeated dosing. Furthermore, the conversion ratio between methadone and other opiates varies dramatically, depending on baseline opiate (morphine equivalent) use.

Oral Morphine to IV Methadone Conversion for Chronic Administration

Total daily baseline oral morphine dose	Estimated daily oral methadone as percent of total daily morphine dose	Estimated daily IV methadone as percent of total daily oral morphine dose[a]
< 100 mg	20% to 30%	10% to 15%
100 to 300 mg	10% to 20%	5% to 10%
300 to 600 mg	8% to 12%	4% to 6%
600 to 1,000 mg	5% to 10%	3% to 5%
> 1,000 mg	< 5%	< 3%

[a] The total daily methadone dose derived from the previous table may then be divided to reflect the intended dosing schedule (ie, for administration every 8 hours, divide total daily methadone dose by 3).

METHADONE HYDROCHLORIDE — INJECTION

Parenteral Morphine to IV Methadone Conversion for Chronic Administration[a]	
Total daily baseline parenteral morphine dose	Estimated daily parenteral methadone requirement as percent of total daily morphine dose[b]
10 to 30 mg	40% to 66%
30 to 50 mg	27% to 66%
50 to 100 mg	22% to 50%
100 to 200 mg	15% to 34%
200 to 500 mg	10% to 20%

[a] Derived from previous table assuming a 3:1 oral:parenteral morphine ratio.
[b] The total daily methadone dose derived from the previous table may then be divided to reflect the intended dosing schedule (ie, for administration every 8 hours, divide total daily methadone dose by 3).

Note: Equianalgesic methadone dosing varies among patients and within a single patient, depending on baseline morphine (or other opioid) dose. The conversion tables have been included in order to illustrate this concept and to provide a safe starting point for opioid conversion. Methadone dosing should not be based solely on these tables. Methadone conversion and dose-titration methods should always be individualized to account for the patient's prior opioid exposure, general medical condition, concomitant medication, and anticipated breakthrough medication use.

Acute pain – Maintenance patients on a stable methadone dose who experience physical trauma, postoperative pain, or other causes of acute pain cannot be expected to derive analgesia from their stable dose of methadone regimens. Give such patients analgesics, including opioids that would be indicated in other patients experiencing similar nociceptive stimulation. When opioids are required for the management of acute pain in patients receiving methadone, somewhat higher and/or more frequent doses will often be required than would be the case for other, nontolerant patients because of the opioid tolerance induced by methadone.

➤*Children:*

Off-label dosing –

Pain:

• *Usual dose* – 0.7 mg/kg daily divided every 4 to 6 hours as needed for pain given IM, IV, or subcutaneously.

• *Maximum dose* – 10 mg/dose.

➤*Pregnancy:* Methadone clearance may be increased during pregnancy. Several small studies have demonstrated significantly lower trough methadone plasma concentrations and shorter methadone half-lives in women during pregnancy compared with after delivery. During pregnancy, a woman's methadone dose may need to be increased or the dosing interval decreased. Keep dosage as low as possible. Use methadone in pregnancy only if the potential benefit justifies the potential risk to the fetus.

➤*Administration:* Methadone injection may be administered IV, subcutaneously, or IM. The absorption of subcutaneous and IM methadone has not been well characterized and appears to be unpredictable. Local tissue reactions may occur.

➤*Storage/Stability:* Store at controlled room temperature, 15° to 30°C (59° to 86°F). Protect from light.

MORPHINE SULFATE

c-ii	**Morphine Sulfate** (Various, eg, Ethex, Roxane)	**Tablets; oral:** 15 mg	In 100s and UD 100s.
c-ii	**Morphine Sulfate** (Various, eg, Ethex, Roxane)	**Tablets; oral:** 30 mg	In 100s and UD 100s.
c-ii	**Morphine Sulfate** (Watson)	**Tablets, controlled-release; oral:** 15 mg	Lactose. (ABG 15). Blue. Film-coated. In 100s.
c-ii	**MS Contin** (Purdue Frederick)		Lactose. (PF M15). Blue. In 100s, 500s, and UD 25s.
c-ii	**Oramorph SR** (aaiPharma)		Lactose. (15). White. In 100s and 500s, and UD 100s.
c-ii	**Morphine Sulfate** (Watson)	**Tablets, controlled-release; oral:** 30 mg	Lactose. (ABG 30). Lavender. Film-coated. In 100s.
c-ii	**MS Contin** (Purdue Frederick)		Lactose. (PF M30). Lavender. In 100s, 500s, and UD 25s.
c-ii	**Oramorph SR** (aaiPharma)		Lactose. (30). White. In 50s, 100s, 250s, and UD 100s.
c-ii	**Morphine Sulfate** (Watson)	**Tablets, controlled-release; oral:** 60 mg	Lactose. (ABG 60). Orange. Film-coated. In 100s.
c-ii	**MS Contin** (Purdue Frederick)		Lactose. (PF M 60). Orange. In 100s, 500s, and UD 25s.
c-ii	**Oramorph SR** (aaiPharma)		Lactose. (60). White. In 100s and UD 25s.
c-ii	**Morphine Sulfate** (Watson)	**Tablets, controlled-release; oral:** 100 mg[a]	(ABG 100). Gray. Film-coated. In 100s.
c-ii	**MS Contin** (Purdue Frederick)		(PF 100). Gray. In 100s, 500s, and UD 25s.
c-ii	**Oramorph SR** (aaiPharma)		Lactose. (100). White. In 100s and UD 25s.
c-ii	**Morphine Sulfate** (Watson)	**Tablets, controlled-release; oral:** 200 mg[a]	(ABG 200). Green. Capsule shape. Film-coated. In 100s.
c-ii	**MS Contin** (Purdue Frederick)		(PFM 200). Green. Capsule shape. In 100s.
c-ii	**Morphine Sulfate** (Various, eg, Endo, Mallinckrodt)	**Tablets, extended-release; oral:** 15 mg	In 100s, 500s, UD 100s, and 150 punch cards.
		30 mg	In 50s, 100s, 500s, UD 100s, and 150 punch cards.
		60 mg	In 100s, 500s, UD 100s, and 150 punch cards.
c-ii	**Morphine Sulfate** (Various, eg, Endo, Mallinckrodt, Watson)	**Tablets, extended-release; oral:** 100 mg	In 100s, 500s, and UD 100s.
c-ii	**Morphine Sulfate** (Various, eg, Endo, Mallinckrodt)	**Tablets, extended-release; oral:** 200 mg[a]	In 100s.
c-ii	**Morphine Sulfate** (Ranbaxy)	**Tablets for solution; injection:** 10 mg	Lactose and sucrose. In 100s.
		15 mg	Lactose and sucrose. In 100s.
		30 mg	Lactose and sucrose. In 100s.
c-ii	**Avinza** (King Pharmaceuticals)	**Capsules, extended-release pellets; oral:** 30 mg	Sugar starch spheres, fumaric acid. Yellow/white. (30 mg 505). In 100s.
		45 mg[a]	Sugar starch spheres, fumaric acid. Lt. blue/white. (45 mg 509). In 100s.
		60 mg[a]	Sugar starch spheres, fumaric acid. Bluish-green/white. (60 mg 506). In 100s.
		75 mg[a]	Sugar starch spheres, fumaric acid. Orange/white. (75 mg 510). In 100s.
		90 mg[a]	Sugar starch spheres, fumaric acid. Red/white. (90 mg 507). In 100s.
		120 mg[a]	Sugar starch spheres, fumaric acid. Blue-violet/white. (120 mg 508). In 100s.

MORPHINE SULFATE

c-ii	**Kadian** (Actavis)	**Capsules, extended-release pellets; oral:** 10 mg	Sucrose. (KADIAN 10 mg). Lt. blue. In 100s.
		20 mg	Sucrose. (KADIAN 20 mg). Yellow. In 100s.
		30 mg	Sucrose. (KADIAN 30 mg). Blue-violet. In 100s.
		50 mg	Sucrose. (KADIAN 50 mg). Blue. In 100s.
		60 mg	Sucrose. (KADIAN 60 mg). Pink. In 100s.
		80 mg	Sucrose. (KADIAN 80 mg). Light orange. In 100s.
		100 mg[a]	Sucrose. (KADIAN 100 mg). Green. In 100s.
		200 mg[a]	Sucrose. (KADIAN 200 mg). Lt. brown. In 100s.
c-ii	**Morphine Sulfate** (Roxane)	**Solution; oral:** 10 mg per 5 mL	May contain edetate disodium, glycerin, sorbitol. In 100 and 500 mL and UD 5 and 10 mL.
c-ii	**MSIR** (Purdue Frederick)		Sugar, sucrose, EDTA. In 120 mL.
c-ii	**Morphine Sulfate** (Roxane)	**Solution; oral:** 20 mg per 5 mL	May contain edetate disodium, glycerin, parabens, sorbitol. In 100 and 500 mL.
c-ii	**MSIR** (Purdue Frederick)		Sugar, sucrose, EDTA. In 120 mL.
c-ii	**Morphine Sulfate** (Roxane)	**Solution, concentrate; oral:** 100 mg per 5 mL	May contain edetate disodium, glycerin, sorbitol. In 30 and 120 mL with oral syringe.
c-ii	**Morphine Sulfate** (Abbott[b])	**Injection:** 0.5 mg/mL	In 10 mL amps and vials.
c-ii	**Astramorph PF**[b] (APP Pharmaceutical)		In 2 and 10 mL amps and 10 mL single-use vials.
c-ii	**Duramorph**[b] (Baxter)		In single-use 10 mL amps.
c-ii	**Morphine Sulfate** (Various, eg, Abbott[b], International Medication Systems)	**Injection:** 1 mg/mL	In 10 mL amps and vials and 30 mL vials.
c-ii	**Morphine Sulfate in 5% Dextrose** (Hospira)		100 and 250 mL.
c-ii	**Astramorph PF**[b] (APP Pharmaceutical)		In 2 and 10 mL amps and 10 mL single-use vials.
c-ii	**Duramorph**[b] (Baxter)		In 10 mL single-use amps.
c-ii	**Morphine Sulfate** (Various, eg, Abbott, Hospira)	**Injection:** 2 mg/mL	In 30 mL vials, and 1 mL syringes, *Carpuject*, and *Tubex*.
c-ii	**Morphine Sulfate** (Various, eg, Abbott, Hospira)	**Injection:** 4 mg/mL	In 1 and 2 mL disposable syringes, and 1 mL *Carpuject* and *Tubex*.
c-ii	**Morphine Sulfate** (Various, eg, Faulding)	**Injection:** 5 mg/mL	In 1 mL vials.
c-ii	**Morphine Sulfate** (Various, eg, Hospira)	**Injection:** 8 mg/mL	In 1 mL *Carpuject*, vials, and amps.
c-ii	**Morphine Sulfate** (Various, eg, Hospira)	**Injection:** 10 mg/mL	In 1 mL *Carpuject*, vials, and amps and 10 mL multidose vials.
c-ii	**Infumorph 200**[b] (Baxter)		In 20 mL (200 mg) amps.
c-ii	**DepoDur**[b] (Endo)	**Injection, extended-release liposomal:** 10 mg/mL	In 1 mL, 1.5 mL, and 2 mL single-use vials in cartons of 5.
c-ii	**Morphine Sulfate** (Various, eg, Hospira)	**Injection:** 15 mg/mL	In 1 mL *Carpuject*, amps, and vials and 20 mL multidose vials.
c-ii	**Morphine Sulfate** (Various, eg, Faulding, International Medication Systems)	**Injection, solution:** 25 mg/mL[c]	In 4, 10, 20, and 40 mL syringes[b] and single-use vials.[d]
c-ii	**Infumorph 500**[b] (Baxter)		In 20 mL (500 mg) amps.
c-ii	**Morphine Sulfate** (Various, eg, Faulding, International Medication Systems)	**Injection, solution:** 50 mg/mL[c]	In 10, 20, 40, 50 mL syringes[b] and single-use vials.[d]
c-ii	**Morphine Sulfate in 5% Dextrose** (Hospira)	**Injection:** 1 mg/mL	In 100 and 250 mL.
c-ii	**Morphine Sulfate** (Various, eg, G & W, Paddock)	**Suppositories; rectal:** 5 mg	In 12s.
c-ii	**RMS** (Upsher-Smith)		In 12s.
c-ii	**Morphine Sulfate** (Various, eg, G & W, Paddock)	**Suppositories; rectal:** 10 mg	In 12s
c-ii	**RMS** (Upsher-Smith)		In 12s.
c-ii	**Morphine Sulfate** (Various, eg, G & W, Paddock)	**Suppositories; rectal:** 20 mg	In 12s.
c-ii	**RMS** (Upsher-Smith)		In 12s.
c-ii	**Morphine Sulfate** (Various, eg, G & W, Paddock)	**Suppositories; rectal:** 30 mg	In 12s.
c-ii	**RMS** (Upsher-Smith)		In 12s.

[a] For use only in opioid-tolerant patients.
[b] Some preparations are preservative free.
[c] For IV use after dilution. Not for direct injection.
[d] May contain sulfites; for IV use only.

MORPHINE SULFATE — ORAL

For complete prescribing information, refer to the Opioid Analgesics group monograph.

WARNING

Avinza – *Avinza* capsules are a modified-release formulation of morphine indicated for once-daily administration for the relief of moderate to severe pain requiring continuous, around-the-clock opioid therapy for an extended period of time. *Avinza* capsules are to be swallowed whole or the contents of the capsules sprinkled on a small amount of applesauce immediately prior to ingestion. The capsule beads are not to be chewed, crushed, or dissolved because of the risk of rapid release and absorption of a potentially fatal dose of morphine. Patients must not consume alcoholic beverages while on *Avinza* therapy. Additionally, patients must not use prescription or nonprescription medications containing alcohol while on *Avinza* therapy. Consumption of alcohol while taking *Avinza* may result in the rapid release and absorption of a potentially fatal dose of morphine.

WARNING (cont.)

Kadian – Morphine, an opioid agonist and a Schedule II controlled substance, has an abuse liability similar to other opioid analgesics. Morphine can be abused in a manner similar to other opioid agonists, legal or illicit. Consider this when prescribing or dispensing *Kadian* in situations in which the health care provider or pharmacist is concerned about an increased risk of misuse, abuse, or diversion.

Kadian capsules are an extended-release oral formulation of morphine indicated for the management of moderate to severe pain requiring a continuous, around-the-clock opioid analgesic for an extended period of time. .

MORPHINE SULFATE — ORAL

WARNING (cont.)

Kadian capsules are NOT for use as an as-needed analgesic. *Kadian* 100 and 200 mg capsules are for use in opioid-tolerant patients only. Ingestion of these capsules or of the pellets within the capsules may cause fatal respiratory depression when administered to patients not already tolerant to high doses of opioids. *Kadian* capsules are to be swallowed whole or the contents of the capsules sprinkled on applesauce. The pellets in the capsules are not to be chewed, crushed, or dissolved because of the risk of rapid release and absorption of a potentially fatal dose of morphine

Oral solution – Morphine oral solution is available in 10 mg per 5 mL, 20 mg per 5 mL, and 100 mg per 5 mL (20 mg/mL) concentrations.

The 100 mg per 5 mL (20 mg/mL) concentration is indicated for use in opioid-tolerant patients only.

Take care when prescribing and administering morphine oral solution to avoid dosing errors due to confusion between different concentrations and between mg and mL, which could result in accidental overdose and death. Take care to ensure the proper dose is communicated and dispensed.

Keep morphine oral solution out of the reach of children. In case of accidental ingestion, seek emergency medical help immediately.

Indications

➤*Controlled-release/extended-release tablets/capsules:* Relief of moderate to severe pain in patients requiring continuous, around-the-clock opioid therapy for an extended period of time. Not intended for use as an as-needed analgesic.

➤*Immediate-release tablets/oral solution:* For the relief of moderate to severe acute and chronic pain where use of an opioid analgesic is appropriate.

Morphine oral solution 100 mg per 5 mL (20 mg/mL) is for the relief of moderate to severe acute and chronic pain in opioid-tolerant patients.

Administration and Dosage

➤*Maximum dose:*

Adults – 1,600 mg/day (*Avinza*) according to the prescribing information.

➤*General dosing considerations:* Morphine may suppress respiration in the elderly, patients taking other CNS depressants, very ill patients, and patients with respiratory problems; therefore, lower doses may be required.

There has been no evaluation of controlled-release (CR)/ER morphine as an initial opioid analgesic in the management of pain. Because it may be more difficult to titrate a patient to adequate analgesia using a CR/ER morphine, it is ordinarily advisable to begin treatment using an immediate-release (IR) morphine formulation.

The best use of opioid analgesics in the management of chronic malignant and nonmalignant pain is challenging, and is well described in materials published by the World Health Organization (WHO) and the Agency for Health Care Policy and Research.

Take care when prescribing and administering morphine oral solution to avoid dosing errors due to confusion between different concentrations and between milligrams and milliliters, which could result in accidental overdose and death. Take care to ensure the proper dose is communicated and dispensed. When writing prescriptions, include both the total dose in milligrams and the total dose in volume. Always use the enclosed calibrated oral syringe when administering morphine oral solution 100 mg per 5 mL (20 mg/mL) to ensure the dose is measured and administered accurately.

Selection of patients for treatment with morphine should be governed by the same principles that apply to the use of similar opioid analgesics. Individualize treatment in every case, using nonopioid analgesics, opioids on an as-needed basis and/or combination products, and chronic opioid therapy in a progressive plan of pain management such as outlined by the WHO, the Agency for Healthcare Research and Quality, and the American Pain Society.

Morphine 100 mg per 5 mL (20 mg/mL) oral solution is a concentrated oral solution. Use in opioid-tolerant patients only who have already been receiving opioid therapy.

Morphine oral solution 100 mg per 5 mL (20 mg/mL) may cause fatal respiratory depression when administered to patients not previously exposed to opioids. Patients considered to be opioid tolerant are those who are taking at least oral morphine 60 mg/day, or at least of oral oxycodone 30 mg/day, or at least hydromorphone 12 mg/day, or an equianalgesic dose of another opioid, for a week or longer.

As with any opioid drug product, adjust the dosing regimen for each patient individually, taking into account the patient's prior analgesic treatment experience. In the selection of the initial dose of morphine, give attention to the following: the total daily dose, potency and specific characteristics of the opioid the patient has been taking previously; the reliability of the relative potency estimate used to calculate the equivalent morphine dose needed; the patient's degree of opioid tolerance; the general condition and medical status of the patient; concurrent medications; the type and severity of the patients pain; risk factors for abuse, addiction, or diversion, including a prior history of abuse, addiction, or diversion.

The following dosing recommendations, therefore, can only be considered suggested approaches to what is actually a series of clinical decisions over time in the management of the pain of each individual patient.

Continual re-evaluation of the patient receiving morphine is important, with special attention to the maintenance of pain control and the relative incidence of adverse effects associated with therapy. During chronic therapy, especially for non–cancer-related pain, periodically re-assess the continued need for the use of opioid analgesics.

During periods of changing analgesic requirements, including initial titration, frequent contact is recommended between the health care provider, other members of the health care team, the patient, and the caregiver/family.

➤*Adults:*

Moderate to severe pain –

Extended release:

• *Avinza* – The 60, 90, and 120 mg capsules are for use only in opioid-tolerant patients. All doses are intended to be administered once daily.

Maximum dose: 1,600 mg daily.

Initial dosage: 30 mg once daily for patients who do not have a proven tolerance to opioids.

Dosage titration: For opioid-naive patients increase dose conservatively. Adjusted in increments not greater than 30 mg every 4 days.

Dosage adjustment: Some degree of tolerance may occur, requiring dosage adjustment until the achievement of a balance between analgesia and opioid adverse reactions. When necessary, the total daily dose of *Avinza* should be increased until pain relief is reached or clinically significant opioid-related adverse reactions occur. The dose may be titrated as frequently as every other day to control analgesia.

Concomitant therapy: In the event that breakthrough pain occurs, *Avinza* may be supplemented with a small dose (5% to 15% of the total daily dose of morphine) of a short-acting analgesic.

• *Kadian* – 100 and 200 mg capsules are for use only in opioid-tolerant patients.

Kadian is a third step drug that is most useful when the patient requires a constant level of opioid analgesia as a floor or platform from which to manage breakthrough pain. When a patient has reached the point where comfort cannot be provided with a combination of nonopioid medications (nonsteroidal anti-inflammatory drugs and acetaminophen) and intermittent use of moderate or strong opioids, the patient's total opioid therapy should be converted into a 24-hour oral morphine equivalent.

Administer one half of the estimated total daily oral morphine dose every 12 hours (twice a day) or administer the total daily oral morphine dose every 24 hours (once a day). To avoid accumulation, the dosing interval should not be reduced below 12 hours.

Initial dosage: 10 or 20 mg in patients who do not have a proven tolerance to opioids.

Dosage titration: Increase at a rate of up to 20 mg every other day. The dose should be titrated no more frequently than every other day to allow the patient to stabilize before escalating the dose. Individualize dosage.

Dosage adjustment: Patients who are excessively sedated after a once daily dose or who regularly experience inadequate analgesia before the next dose should be switched to a twice daily dosing. Most patients will rapidly develop some degree of tolerance, requiring dosage adjustment until they have achieved their individual best balance between baseline analgesia and opioid adverse reactions such as confusion, sedation, and constipation. No guidance can be given as to the recommended maximal dose, especially in patients with chronic pain of malignancy. In such cases the total dose of *Kadian* should be advanced until the desired therapeutic end point is reached or clinically significant opioid-related adverse reactions intervene.

Concomitant therapy: If breakthrough pain occurs, the dose may be supplemented with a small dose (less than 20% of the total daily dose) of a short-acting analgesic.

• *MS Contin* – The *MS Contin* 200 mg tablet is for use only in opioid-tolerant patients requiring daily morphine-equivalent doses of 400 mg or more. Reserve this strength for patients who have already been titrated to a stable analgesic regimen using lower strengths of *MS Contin* or other opioids.

• *Dosage reduction* – If signs of excessive opioid effects are observed early in a dosing interval, the next dose should be reduced. If this adjustment leads to inadequate analgesia (ie, breakthrough pain occurs late in the dosing interval) the dosing interval may be shortened.

Immediate-release:

• *Tablets* –

Usual dosage: 5 to 30 mg every 4 hours or as directed by the health care provider. For control of severe chronic pain in patients with certain terminal diseases, this drug should be administered on a regularly scheduled basis every 4 hours at the lowest dosage level that will achieve adequate analgesia.

Dosage reduction: During the first 2 to 3 days of effective pain relief, the patient may sleep for many hours. This can be misinterpreted as the effect of excessive analgesic dosing rather than the first sign of relief in a pain-exhausted patient. The dose, therefore, should be maintained for at least 3 days before reduction, if respiratory activity and other vital signs are adequate. Following successful relief of severe pain, periodic attempts to reduce the narcotic dose should be made. Smaller doses or complete discontinuation of the narcotic analgesic may become feasible due to a physiologic change or the improved mental state of the patient.

• *Oral solution* –

Initial dosage:

➤*Opiate-naive patients:* 10 to 20 mg every 4 hours as needed for pain using the 10 mg/mL or 20 mg/mL strengths.

➤*Opioid-tolerant patients:* The 100 mg per 5 mL (20 mg/mL) oral solution is for use in opioid-tolerant patients only who have already been receiving opioid therapy. Use this strength only for patients that have already been titrated to a stable analgesic regimen using lower strengths of morphine and who can benefit from use of a smaller volume of oral solution.

Dosage titration: Titrate the dose based upon the individual patients response to their initial dose of morphine.

MORPHINE SULFATE — ORAL

Maintenance dosage: Continual re-evaluation of the patient receiving morphine is important, with special attention to the maintenance of pain control and the relative incidence of adverse effects associated with therapy. If the level of pain increases, effort should be made to identify the source of increased pain, while adjusting the dose to decrease the level of pain. During chronic therapy, especially for non–cancer-related pain (or pain associated with other terminal illnesses), periodically reassess the continued need for the use of opioid analgesics.

Dosage adjustment: Adjust the dose to an acceptable level of analgesia taking into account the improvement in pain intensity and the tolerability of the morphine by the patient.

Conversion: There is interpatient variability in the potency of opioid drugs and opioid formulations. Therefore, a conservative approach is advised when determining the total daily dose of morphine. It is better to underestimate a patient's 24-hour oral morphine dose and make available rescue medication than to overestimate the 24-hour oral morphine dose and manage an adverse experience of overdose.

• *Conversion from conventional IR oral morphine formulations to CR/ER oral morphine* –

Extended-release tablets: A patient's daily morphine requirement is established using IR oral morphine (dosing every 4 to 6 hours). The patient is then converted to ER morphine in either of 2 ways: by administering one-half of the patient's 24-hour requirement as ER morphine on an every-12-hour schedule; or by administering one-third of the patient's daily requirement as ER morphine on an every-8-hour schedule.

With either method, dose and dosing interval is then adjusted as needed. The 15 mg ER tablet should be used for initial conversion if the patient's total daily requirement is expected to be less than 60 mg. Morphine 30 mg ER tablets are recommended for patients with a daily morphine requirement of 60 to 120 mg. When the total daily dose is expected to be greater than 120 mg, the appropriate tablet strength should be employed.

Extended-release capsules: Patients receiving other oral morphine formulations may be converted to *Avinza* or *Kadian* by administering the patient's total daily oral morphine dose as *Avinza* or *Kadian* once daily or by administering one-half of the patient's total daily oral morphine dose as *Kadian* every 12 hours. *Avinza* should not be given more frequently than every 24 hours, and *Kadian* should not be given more frequently than every 12 hours. The first dose of *Kadian* may be taken with the last dose of any IR opioid medication because of the long delay until the peak effect after administration of *Kadian*. Supplemental pain medication may be required until the response to the patient's daily *Avinza* dosage has stabilized (up to 4 days).

Controlled-release tablets: The patient may convert in 1 of 2 ways: by administering one-half of the patient's 24-hour requirement as *MS Contin* or *Oramorph SR* on an every-12-hour schedule; or by administering one-third of the patient's daily requirement as *MS Contin* on an every-8-hour schedule.

The 15 mg tablet of *MS Contin* should be used for initial conversion, for patients whose total daily requirement is expected to be less than 60 mg. The 30 mg tablet is recommended for patients with a daily morphine requirement of 60 to 120 mg. When the total daily dose is expected to be greater than 120 mg, the appropriate combination of tablet strength should be employed. The *Oramorph SR* 30 mg tablet for initial conversion is recommended for patients with a daily morphine requirement of 120 mg or less.

• *Conversion from parenteral morphine or other opioids (parenteral or oral) to controlled-release/extended-release oral morphine* – Particular care must be exercised in the conversion process. Because of uncertainty about, and intersubject variation in, relative estimates of opioid potency and cross-tolerance, initial dosing regimens should be conservative; that is, an underestimation of the 24-hour oral morphine requirement is preferred to an overestimate. To this end, initial individual doses should be estimated conservatively. In patients whose daily morphine requirements are expected to be no more than 120 mg, the 30 mg tablet is recommended for the initial titration period. Once a stable dose regimen is reached, the patient can be converted to the 60 or 100 mg tablet or appropriate combination of tablet strengths.

The following general points should be considered regarding opioid conversions:

Parenteral to oral morphine ratio: It may take anywhere from 2 to 6 mg of oral morphine to provide analgesia equivalent to 1 mg of parenteral morphine. A dose of oral morphine 3 times the daily parenteral morphine requirement may be sufficient in chronic use settings. A reasonable starting dose of *Avinza* would be approximately 3 times the previous daily parenteral morphine requirement.Other parenteral or oral nonmorphine opioids to oral morphine In general, it is safest to administer half of the estimated daily morphine requirement as the initial dose, and to manage inadequate analgesia by supplementation with IR morphine.

• *Conversion from controlled-release/extended-release oral morphine to parenteral opioids* – It is best to assume that the parenteral-to-oral potency is high. For example, to estimate the required 24-hour dose of morphine for intramuscular (IM) use, the health care provider could employ a conversion of 1 mg of morphine IM for every 6 mg of morphine as CR tablet. The IM 24-hour dose would have to be divided by 6 and administered on an every-4-hour regimen. This approach is recommended because it is least likely to cause overdose.

Avinza/Kadian: When converting from *Avinza* or *Kadian* to parenteral opioids, it is best to calculate an equivalent parenteral dose and then initiate treatment at half of this calculated value. As an example, an estimated total 24-hour parenteral morphine requirement of a patient receiving *Avinza* or *Kadian* is one-third of the dose of *Avinza* or *Kadian*. This estimated dose should then be divided in half, and this last calculated dose is the total daily dose. This value should be further divided by 6 if the desire is to dose with parenteral morphine every 4 hours.

Consider a patient taking 360 mg of *Avinza* or *Kadian* daily. First, divide by 3 to account for differences in bioavailability between oral and parenteral morphine. This new figure, 120 mg, is the estimated total 24-hour requirement of parenteral morphine. Dividing by 2, the result gives the total daily dose of 60 mg. If it is decided to administer the drug at 4-hour intervals, then administer 10 mg (60 divided by 6) every 4 hours.

Although this approach may require a dosage increase in the first 24 hours for many patients, this method is recommended, as it is less likely to result in overdose. Overdose is more likely to occur when administering an equivalent dose of parenteral morphine without titration. Provision for breakthrough pain should be made.

• *Conversion of extended-release (Avinza or Kadian) to other controlled-release/extended-release oral morphine formulations* – *Kadian* is not bioequivalent to other ER morphine preparations. For a given dose, the same total amount of morphine is available from *Avinza* or *Kadian* as from oral morphine solution or CR/ER morphine tablets. However, the slower release of morphine from *Kadian* results in reduced maximum and increased minimum plasma morphine concentrations than with shorter-acting morphine products.

Conversion from *Kadian* or *Avinza* to the same total daily dose of another CR/ER morphine formulation may lead to either excessive sedation at peak or inadequate analgesia at trough. Close observation and appropriate dosage adjustments are recommended.

• *Conversion from Avinza to other pain control therapies* – It is important to remember that the persistence of *Avinza*-derived plasma morphine concentrations may be in excess of 36 hours when making a conversion to other pain control therapies.

• *Conversion from parenteral morphine to immediate-release oral morphine* – For conversion from parenteral to oral morphine, anywhere from 3 to 6 mg of oral morphine may be required to provide pain relief equivalent to 1 mg of parenteral morphine.

• *Conversion from parenteral oral nonmorphine opioids to immediate-release oral morphine* – In converting patients from other opioids to morphine, close observation and adjustment of dosage based upon the patient's response to morphine is imperative. Health care providers and other health care professionals are advised to refer to published relative potency information, keeping in mind that conversion ratios are only approximate.

• *Conversion from controlled-release/extended-release oral morphine to immediate-release oral morphine* – For a given dose, the same total amount of morphine is available from morphine oral solution, morphine tablets, and CR and ER morphine capsules. The extended duration of release of morphine from CR tablets or ER tablets results in reduced maximum and increased minimum plasma morphine concentrations than with shorter acting morphine products. Conversion from oral solution or IR tablets to the same total daily dose of CR tablets or ER tablets could lead to excessive sedation at peak serum levels. Therefore, dosage adjustment with close observation is necessary.

➤*Children:*

Off-label dosing –

Narcotic abstinence, opiate withdrawal, severe pain:

Morphine Off-Label Dosing in Children

Condition	Dosage	
	Neonates[a]	Infants and children[b]
Narcotic abstinence	0.03 to 0.1 mg/kg/dose every 3 to 4 h. Wean dose by 10% to 20% every 2 to 3 days based on abstinence scoring.	
Opiate withdrawal	0.08 to 0.2 mg/dose every 3 to 4 h as needed.	
Severe pain		
Immediate release		0.02 to 0.5 mg/kg/dose every 4 to 6 h as needed
CR/ER		0.3 to 0.6 mg/kg/dose every 12 h as needed

[a] Neonates < 30 days of age.
[b] Infants and children 30 days to 18 years of age.

➤*Discontinuation of therapy:* When the patient no longer requires therapy, doses should be tapered gradually to prevent signs and symptoms of withdrawal in the physically dependent patient.

➤*Administration:*

Avinza – Capsules may be opened and the entire bead contents sprinkled on a small amount of applesauce immediately prior to ingestion. The applesauce should be at room temperature or cooler. Patients should ingest the mixture immediately. Patients must swallow the mixture without chewing or crushing beads, then rinse their mouths and swallow to ensure all beads have been ingested. Patients should consume the entire portion and not divide the applesauce into separate doses.

CR/ER tablets/capsules – Must be swallowed whole (not chewed, crushed, or dissolved) because of the risk of acute overdose. Ingesting

MORPHINE SULFATE — ORAL

chewed or crushed beads or pellets will lead to the rapid release and absorption of a potentially fatal dose of morphine.

Kadian – Patients who have difficulty swallowing whole capsules or tablets may open the capsule and sprinkle the entire contents on a small amount of applesauce immediately prior to ingestion. Applesauce should be at room temperature or cooler. The patient must be cautioned not to chew the pellets which could result in the immediate release of a potentially dangerous, even fatal dose of morphine. Patients should rinse their mouths to ensure all pellets have been swallowed. Patients should consume the entire portion and not divide the applesauce into separate doses.

Alternatively, administer the entire capsule contents through a 16-French gastrostomy tube. Flush the gastrostomy tube with water to ensure that it is wet. Sprinkle the *Kadian* pellets into 10 mL of water. Use a swirling motion to pour the pellets and water into the gastrostomy tube through a funnel. Rinse the beaker with a further 10 mL of water and pour this into the funnel. Repeat rinsing until no pellets remain in the beaker. The administration of *Kadian* pellets through a nasogastric tube should not be attempted.

Concentrate oral solution – Administer with caution because the solution is a highly concentrated solution of morphine. Error in dosage or confusion between milligrams of morphine and milliliters of solution may cause significant overdosage. Dosing instructions should be clearly prescribed in milligrams of morphine and milliliters of solution. Verify correct dose and volume before administration to patient.

➤*Storage/Stability:* Store oral solutions, tablets, and capsules at 15° to 30°C (59° to 86°F). Protect from light and moisture.

MORPHINE SULFATE — INJECTION

For complete prescribing information, refer to the Opioid Analgesics group monograph.

WARNING

Astramorph PF, Infumorph, Duramorph – Because of the risk of severe adverse effects when the epidural or intrathecal route of administration is employed, patients must be observed in a fully equipped and staffed environment for at least 24 hours after the initial dose.

Infumorph – Infumorph is not recommended for single-dose intravenous (IV), intramuscular (IM), or subcutaneous administration because of the very large amount of morphine in the ampul and the associated risk of overdosage.

Indications

➤*IV:* Relief of severe pain (eg, pain of myocardial infarction [MI], severe injuries, severe chronic pain associated with terminal cancer after all nonnarcotic analgesics have failed); used preoperatively to sedate the patient and allay apprehension, facilitate anesthesia induction, and reduce anesthetic dosage; control postoperative pain; relieve anxiety and reduce left ventricular work by reducing preload pressure; treatment of dyspnea associated with acute left ventricular failure and pulmonary edema; produce anesthesia for open-heart surgery.

➤*Subcutaneous/IM:* Relief of moderate to severe pain; relieve preoperative apprehension; preoperative sedation; control postoperative pain; supplement to anesthesia; analgesia during labor; acute pulmonary edema; allay anxiety.

➤*Epidural/Intrathecal:* Management of pain not responsive to nonnarcotic analgesics. For the treatment of intractable chronic pain (*Infumorph* only).

➤*ER epidural: DepoDur* is an ER liposome injection of morphine intended for single-dose administration by the epidural route, at the lumbar level, for the treatment of pain following major surgery. *DepoDur* is administered prior to surgery or after clamping the umbilical cord during cesarean section.

➤*Off-label uses:*

Postherpetic neuralgia (epidural) – [5] = Poor documentation. The results from a trial evaluating the efficacy of epidural morphine for the treatment of postherpetic neuralgia (PHN) showed no benefit. American Academy of Neurology clinical practice guidelines state that the epidural morphine is of no benefit for the treatment of PHN (level B, class II). Because of safety concerns and the lack of favorable data, epidural morphine should not be used for pain associated with PHN.

Administration and Dosage

➤*General dosing considerations:* Morphine may suppress respiration in elderly patients, patients taking other CNS depressants, the very ill, and patients with respiratory problems; therefore, lower doses may be required.

Do not administer intravenously (IV) unless an opioid antagonist is immediately available.

➤*Adults:*

Analgesia –

Subcutaneous/IM: 10 mg per 70 kg of body weight (range, 5 to 20 mg) subcutaneous or intramuscular (IM) every 4 hours as needed.

IV: 10 mg every 4 hours IV, depending on the severity of the condition and the patient's response. The usual individual dose range is 5 to 15 mg IV. The usual daily dose range is 12 to 120 mg IV.

Analgesia during labor – 10 mg is usually administered subcutaneous or IM.

Intractable chronic pain –

Infumorph:

• *Initial dosage* – The starting dose must be individualized. The recommended initial epidural dose in patients who are not tolerant to opioids ranges from 3.5 to 7.5 mg/day. The usual starting dose for continuous epidural infusion, based upon limited data in patients who have some degree of opioid tolerance, is 4.5 to 10 mg/day.

• *Dosage adjustment* – The dose requirements may increase significantly during treatment, frequently to 20 to 30 mg/day.

Myocardial infarction pain – 8 to 15 mg administered IV. For very severe pain, additional smaller doses may be given every 3 to 4 hours as needed.

Open heart surgery – Administer large doses (0.5 to 3 mg/kg) of morphine IV as the sole anesthetic or with a suitable anesthetic agent. The patients are given oxygen and cardiovascular function is not depressed by morphine, as long as adequate ventilation is maintained.

Pain following major surgery –

ER epidural: Patient monitoring should be continued for at least 48 hours after dosing, as delayed respiratory depression may occur.

• *Cesarean section* – 10 mg. *DepoDur* should not be administered to women for vaginal labor and delivery.

• *Lower abdominal or pelvic surgery* – 10 to 15 mg. Some patients may benefit from a 20 mg dose of *DepoDur*, but the incidence of serious adverse respiratory events was dose-related in clinical trials.

• *Major orthopedic surgery* – Major orthopedic surgery of the lower extremity is dosed at 15 mg.

Pain not responsive to nonnarcotic analgesics –

Epidural: Intrathecal dosage is usually one-tenth that of epidural dosage.

• *Maximum dose* – 10 mg in 24 hours.

• *Initial dosage* – Injection of 5 mg in the lumbar region may provide satisfactory pain relief for up to 24 hours.

For continuous infusion, an initial dose of 2 to 4 mg per 24 hours is recommended.

• *Dosage titration* – If adequate pain relief is not achieved within 1 hour, carefully administer incremental doses of 1 to 2 mg at intervals sufficient to assess effectiveness. Give no more than 10 mg per 24 hours.

For continuous infusion further doses of 1 to 2 mg may be given if pain relief in not achieved initially.

• *Monitoring* – Thoracic administration has been shown to dramatically increase the incidence of early and late respiratory depression even at doses of 1 to 2 mg. Patient monitoring should be continued for at least 24 hours after each dose because delayed respiratory depression may occur.

Intrathecal: Intrathecal dosage is usually one-tenth that of epidural dosage.

• *Usual dosage* – A single injection of 0.2 to 1 mg may provide satisfactory pain relief for up to 24 hours. (Caution: This is only 0.4 to 2 mL of the 0.5 mg/mL potency or 0.2 to 1 mL of the 1 mg/mL potency.) Do not inject intrathecally more than 2 mL of the 0.5 mg/mL potency or 1 mL of the 1 mg/mL potency. Use in lumbar area only.

• *Concomitant therapy* – A constant IV infusion of naloxone 0.6 mg/h for 24 hours after intrathecal injection may reduce incidence of potential adverse reactions.

• *Repeat dosage* – If pain recurs, consider alternative administration routes because experience with repeated doses by this route is limited. Repeated intrathecal injections are not recommended.

• *Monitoring* – Patient monitoring should be continued for at least 24 hours after each dose, because delayed respiratory depression may occur.

Infumorph:

• *Usual dosage* – The published range of doses for individuals who have some degree of opioid tolerance varies from 1 to 10 mg/day.

• *Initial dosage* – Individualize the starting dose. The recommended initial lumbar intrathecal dose range in patients with no tolerance to opioids is 0.2 to 1 mg/day.

• *Alternative dosage* – Limited experience with continuous intrathecal infusion of morphine has shown that the daily doses have to be increased over time. Employ doses greater than 20 mg/day with caution because they may be associated with a higher likelihood of serious adverse reactions.

Preanesthetic medication –

Subcutaneous/IM: 10 mg per 70 kg of body weight (range, 5 to 20 mg).

IV: 10 mg every 4 hours IV, depending on the severity of the condition and the patient's response. The usual individual dose range is 5 to 15 mg IV. The usual daily dose range is 12 to 120 mg IV.

Severe chronic pain associated with terminal cancer –

Usual dosage: The infusion dosage range is 0.8 to 80 mg/h, though doses up to 144 mg/h have been used. Thus, for the 1 mg/mL solution, the infusion may be run from 0.8 to 80 mL/h, and for a 0.5 mg/mL solution, the infusion may be run from 1.6 to 160 mL/h.

A constant infusion rate must be maintained with an infusion pump in order to assure proper dosage control. Take care to avoid overdosage (respiratory depression) or abrupt cessation of therapy, which may give rise to withdrawal symptoms.

Loading dose: Prior to initiation of the morphine infusion (in concentrations between 0.2 to 1 mg/mL), a loading dose of 15 mg or more of morphine may be administered by IV push to alleviate pain.

Off-label dosing –

Patient-controlled analgesia: The following patient-controlled analgesia (PCA) dosing parameters for morphine (1 mg/mL) are for opioid-naive adults.

• *Maximum dose* – The total amount of drug over time and the maximum number of patient demand doses per hour will vary.

• *Loading dose* – 2 mg bolus.

• *Clinician dose* – 2 mg bolus. One clinician bolus may be given each hour.

• *PCA dose* – 1 mg with a lockout time of 10 minutes.

• *Basal dose* – Not recommended for starting PCA.

MORPHINE SULFATE — INJECTION

➤*Children:*

Analgesic –

IV:

- *Usual dosage* – 50 to 100 mcg IV (0.05 to 0.1 mg) per kg of body weight, administered very slowly.
- *Maximum dose* – Not to exceed 10 mg per dose.

Subcutaneous/IM:

- *Usual dosage* – 0.1 to 0.2 mg/kg every 4 hours.
- *Maximum dose* – 15 mg.

Preanesthetic medication –

1 year of age and older:

- *Usual dosage* – 0.1 mg/kg subcutaneous or IM.
- *Maximum dose* – 10 mg.

Off-label dosing –

Patient-controlled analgesia: Prior to starting PCA, a child's developmental age and cognitive ability should be assessed. The following PCA dosing parameters for morphine (1 mg/mL) are for opioid-naive children.

- *Maximum dose* – The total amount of drug over time should not exceed 100 mcg/kg/h (0.1 mg/kg/h). If the patient requires more than 3 patient-demand doses over 2 hours, the health care provider should be contacted and the patient reassessed.
- *Loading dose* – 40 mcg/kg (0.04 mg/kg) bolus.
- *Clinician dose* – 40 mcg/kg (0.04 mg/kg) bolus. Two clinician bolus doses may be given each hour.
- *PCA dose* – 10 mcg/kg (0.01 mg/kg) with a lockout time of 10 minutes.
- *Basal/Continuous infusion* – 5 mcg/kg/h (0.005 mg/kg/h).

30 days old to 12 years of age:

- *Analgesia –*
  IM/IV/subcutaneous: 0.05 to 0.2 mg/kg/dose every 2 to 4 hours as needed. 15 mg/dose.
- *Postoperative pain –*
  Continuous IV infusion: 0.01 to 0.04 mg/kg/h.
- *Sickle cell cancer –*
  Continuous IV infusion: 0.04 to 0.07 mg/kg/h.

Younger than 30 days of age:

- *Analgesia –*
  Continuous IV infusion: 0.005 to 0.03 mg/kg/h.
- *IM/IV/subcutaneous* – 0.05 to 0.2 mg/kg every 4 hours.

➤*Elderly:* Use extreme caution. Lower dose is usually satisfactory.

Epidural – Doses less than 5 mg may provide satisfactory pain relief for up to 24 hours.

DepoDur should be administered to elderly patients (older than 65 years of age) after careful evaluation of their underlying medical condition and consideration of the risks associated with *DepoDur*. Vigilant perioperative monitoring should be exercised for elderly patients receiving *DepoDur*. In general, as with all opiates, the dose for elderly or debilitated patients should be at the low end of the dosing range.

➤*Discontinuation of therapy:* When the patient no longer requires therapy, doses should be tapered gradually to prevent signs and symptoms of withdrawal in the physically dependent patient.

➤*Preparation for administration:*

IV – A strength of 2.5 to 15 mg of morphine may be diluted in 4 to 5 mL of sterile water for injection.

Subcutaneous/IM –

Soluble tablets: Prepare soluble tablets in sterile water and filter through a 0.22 micron membrane filter.

➤*Administration:*

DepoDur – Not intended for intrathecal, IV, or IM administration. Administration of *DepoDur* into the thoracic epidural space or higher has not been evaluated and therefore is not recommended. *DepoDur* may be administered via needle or catheter at the lumbar level. *DepoDur* may be administered undiluted or may be diluted up to 5 mL total volume with preservative-free 0.9% normal saline. Do not use an in-line filter during administration of *DepoDur*.

Infumorph – Familiarization with the continuous microinfusion device is essential. To minimize risk from glass or other particles, the product must be filtered through not more than a 5 micron microfilter before injecting into the microinfusion device. If dilution is required, 0.9% sodium chloride injection is recommended.

IV – Administer slowly over 4 to 5 minutes. Rapid IV use increases the incidence of adverse reactions. Do not administer IV unless an opioid antagonist is immediately available.

➤*Admixture compatibility:* Morphine has been reported to be physically or chemically incompatible with various drug products. Specialized references should be consulted for specific compatibility information.

➤*Storage/Stability:*

DepoDur – Store in the refrigerator at 2° to 8°C (36° to 46°F). *DepoDur* may be held at 15° to 30°C (59° to 86°F) for up to 7 days in sealed, intact (unopened) vials.

Although *DepoDur* is a sterile agent, it does not contain any bacteriostatic agents. Therefore, *DepoDur* must be administered within 4 hours after withdrawal from the vial. Do not heat or gas sterilize. Following withdrawal from the vial, *DepoDur* may be held at 15° to 30°C (59° to 86°F) for up to 4 hours prior to administration. Protect from freezing; do not administer if it is suspected that the vial has been frozen.

Infumorph, Duramorph, Astramorph PF injections – Protect from light. Store at 20° to 25°C (68° to 77°F), excursions are permitted between 15° to 30°C (59° to 86°F) until ready to use. Do not freeze. Contains no preservative or antioxidant. Discard any unused portion. Do not heat sterilize.

Injection – Store injections at 15° to 30°C (59° to 86°F). Solutions may darken with age. Do not use if injection is darker than pale yellow, discolored in any way, or contains a precipitate.

Soluble tablets for injection – Store at 15° to 30°C (59° to 86°F). Protect from light and moisture.

Solutions may darken with age. Do not use if the solution is darker than pale yellow, is discolored in any other way, or contains a precipitate.

MORPHINE SULFATE — RECTAL

For complete prescribing information, refer to the Opioid Analgesics group monograph.

Indications

➤*Severe pain:* Morphine is indicated for the relief of severe chronic and acute pain.

Administration and Dosage

➤*General dosing considerations:* Morphine may suppress respiration in the elderly, the very ill, and those patients with respiratory problems; therefore, lower doses may be required.

➤*Adults:*

Severe pain –

Usual dosage: 10 to 20 mg every 4 hours or as directed by a health care provider.

Dosage is a patient-dependent variable; therefore, increased dosage may be required to achieve adequate analgesia.

Dosage adjustment: During the first 2 to 3 days of effective pain relief, the patient may sleep for many hours. This can be misinterpreted as the effect of excessive analgesic dosing rather than the first sign of relief of a pain-exhausted patient. The dose, therefore, should be maintained for at least 3 days before reduction, if respiratory activity and other vital signs are adequate.

Discontinuation of therapy: Following successful relief of severe pain, periodic attempts to reduce the narcotic dose should be made. Smaller doses or complete discontinuation of the narcotic analgesic may become feasible because of a physiologic change or the improved mental state of the patient.

➤*Elderly:* Morphine may suppress respiration in the elderly therefore, lower doses may be required.

➤*Renal function impairment:* Give morphine with caution and reduce the initial dose in those with severe renal impairment. (See Warnings/Precautions.)

➤*Hepatic function impairment:* Give morphine with caution and reduce the initial dose in those with severe hepatic impairment. (See Warnings/Precautions.)

➤*Storage/Stability:* Store at temperatures below 25°C (77°F).

OPIUM

c-ii	**Opium Tincture, Deodorized** (Ranbaxy)	**Liquid:** anhydrous morphine equiv. 10 mg per mL	19% alcohol. In 120 and 473 mL.
c-iii	**Paregoric** (Various, eg, Barre-National)	**Liquid:** anhydrous morphine equiv. 2 mg per 5 mL	45% alcohol.[a] In 473 mL.

[a] May also contain benzoic acid.

OPIUM TINCTURE — ORAL

For complete prescribing information, refer to the Opioid Analgesics group monograph.

Indications

➤*Diarrhea:* For treatment of diarrhea. This preparation should not be used in diarrhea caused by poisoning until the toxic material is eliminated from the GI tract.

Administration and Dosage

➤*General dosing considerations:* Opium tincture contains 25 times more morphine than paregoric. Do not confuse opium tincture with paregoric; this may lead to a potentially fatal overdose of morphine.

OPIUM TINCTURE — ORAL

➤*Adults:*

Diarrhea –

Opium tincture: 0.6 mL 4 times daily.
Paregoric: 5 to 10 mL 1 to 4 times daily.

➤*Children:*

Diarrhea –

Paregoric: 0.25 to 0.5 mL/kg 1 to 4 times daily.

➤*Storage/Stability:* Store at controlled room temperature 15° to 30°C (59° to 86°F). Protect from light.

OXYCODONE HYDROCHLORIDE

c-ii	**Oxycodone Hydrochloride** (Various, eg, Amide, Ethex, Mallinckrodt)	**Tablets; oral:** 5 mg	In 100s, 500s, and UD 100s.
c-ii	**M-oxy** (Mallinckrodt)		(M-OXY 5). White, scored. In 100s.
c-ii	**Roxicodone** (aaiPharma)		(54 582). White, scored. In 100s and UD 100s.
c-ii	**Oxycodone Hydrochloride** (Ethex)	**Tablets; oral:** 10 mg	In 100s and UD 100s.
c-ii	**Oxycodone Hydrochloride** (Various, eg, Amide, Ethex)	**Tablets; oral:** 15 mg	In 100s and UD 100s.
c-ii	**Roxicodone** (aaiPharma)		Lactose. (54 710). Green, scored. In 100s and UD 100s.
c-ii	**Oxycodone Hydrochloride** (Ethex)	**Tablets; oral:** 20 mg	In 100s and UD 100s.
c-ii	**Oxycodone Hydrochloride** (Various, eg, Amide, Ethex)	**Tablets; oral:** 30 mg	In 100s and UD 100s.
c-ii	**Roxicodone** (aaiPharma)		Lactose. (54 199). Blue, scored. In 100s and UD 100s.
c-ii	**Oxycodone Hydrochloride** (Endo)	**Tablets, controlled-release; oral:** 10 mg	(E702 10). White. In 30s and 500s.
c-ii	**OxyContin** (Purdue Pharma LP)		Butylated hydroxytoluene, polyethylene glycol 400. (OP 10). White, round. In 100s.
c-ii	**OxyContin** (Purdue Pharma LP)	**Tablets, controlled-release; oral:** 15 mg	Butylated hydroxytoluene, polyethylene glycol 400. (OP 15). Gray, round. In 100s.
c-ii	**Oxycodone Hydrochloride** (Endo)	**Tablets, controlled-release; oral:** 20 mg	(E703 20). Pink. In 30s and 500s.
c-ii	**OxyContin** (Purdue Pharma LP)		Butylated hydroxytoluene, polyethylene glycol 400. (OP 20). Pink, round. In 100s.
c-ii	**OxyContin** (Purdue Pharma LP)	**Tablets, controlled-release; oral:** 30 mg	Butylated hydroxytoluene, polyethylene glycol 400. (OP 30). Brown, round. In 100s.
c-ii	**Oxycodone Hydrochloride** (Endo)	**Tablets, controlled-release; oral:** 40 mg	(E705 40). Yellow. In 30s and 500s.
c-ii	**OxyContin** (Purdue Pharma LP)		Butylated hydroxytoluene, polyethylene glycol 400. (OP 40). Yellow, round. In 100s.
c-ii	**OxyContin** (Purdue Pharma LP)	**Tablets, controlled-release; oral:** 60 mg[a]	Butylated hydroxytoluene, polyethylene glycol 400. (OP 60). Red, round. In 100s.
c-ii	**Oxycodone Hydrochloride** (Various, eg, Global, Teva)	**Tablets, controlled-release; oral:** 80 mg[a]	Lactose. In 100s, 500s, and 1,000s.
c-ii	**OxyContin** (Purdue Pharma LP)		Butylated hydroxytoluene, polyethylene glycol 400. (OP 80). Green, round. In 100s and UD 25s.
c-ii	**Oxycodone Hydrochloride** (Ethex)	**Capsules; oral:** 5 mg	Lactose. (Ethex 041). Buff/white. In 100s and UD 100s.
c-ii	**OxyIR** (Purdue Pharma)		Sucrose. (O-IR PF5mg). Beige/orange. In 100s.
c-ii	**Oxycodone Hydrochloride** (Various, eg, Mallinckrodt)	**Solution; oral:** 5 mg per 5 mL	In 500 mL.
c-ii	**Roxicodone** (aaiPharma)		Sorbitol. In 500 mL and UD 5 mL.
c-ii	**Oxycodone Hydrochloride** (Various, eg, Mallinckrodt)	**Solution, concentrate; oral:** 20 mg/mL	In 30 mL.
c-ii	**Roxicodone Intensol** (aaiPharma)		In 30 mL with calibrated dropper.
c-ii	**OxyFAST** (Purdue Pharma LP)		Saccharin. In 30 mL with dropper.

[a] For use in opioid-tolerant patients only.

OXYCODONE — ORAL

For complete prescribing information, refer to the Opioid Analgesics group monograph.

WARNING

Controlled-release (CR) oxycodone is an opioid agonist and a schedule II controlled substance with an abuse liability similar to morphine.

Oxycodone can be abused in a manner similar to other opioid agonists, legal or illicit. This should be considered when prescribing or dispensing oxycodone CR tablets in situations where the health care provider or pharmacist is concerned about an increased risk of misuse, abuse, or diversion.

OxyContin is a CR oral formulation of oxycodone hydrochloride. Oxycodone CR tablets are indicated for the management of moderate to severe pain when a continuous, around-the-clock opioid analgesic is needed for an extended period of time. Oxycodone CR tablets are not intended for use as as-needed analgesics.

Patients considered opioid tolerant are those who are taking at least oral morphine 60 mg/day, transdermal fentanyl 25 mcg/h, oral oxycodone 30 mg/day, oral hydromorphone 8 mg/day, oral oxymorphone 25 mg/day, or an equianalgesic dose of another opioid for 1 week or longer.

Oxycodone 60 and 80 mg tablets, a single dose greater than 40 mg, or a total daily dose greater than 80 mg are only for use in opioid-tolerant patients, as they may cause fatal respiratory depression when administered to patients who are not tolerant to the respiratory-depressant or sedating effects of opioids.

WARNING (cont.)

People at increased risk for opioid abuse include those with a personal or family history of substance abuse (including drug or alcohol abuse or addiction) or mental illness (eg, major depression). Patients should be assessed for their clinical risks for opioid abuse or addiction prior to being prescribed opioids. All patients receiving opioids should be routinely monitored for signs of misuse, abuse, and addiction.

Oxycodone 60 and 80 mg CR tablets are for use in opioid-tolerant patients only. These tablet strengths may cause fatal respiratory depression when administered to patients not previously exposed to opioids.

Oxycodone CR tablets are to be swallowed whole and are not to be cut, broken, chewed, crushed, or dissolved. Taking cut, broken, chewed, crushed, or dissolved oxycodone CR tablets leads to rapid release and absorption of a potentially fatal dose of oxycodone.

The concomitant use of oxycodone with all CYP3A4 inhibitors, such as macrolide antibiotics (eg, erythromycin), azole-antifungal agents (eg, ketoconazole), and protease inhibitors (eg, ritonavir), may result in an increase in oxycodone plasma concentrations, which could increase or prolong adverse effects and may cause potentially fatal respiratory depression. Patients receiving oxycodone and a CYP3A4 inhibitor should be carefully monitored for an extended period of time and dosage adjustments should be made if warranted.

Indications

➤*Pain:*

Immediate-release tablets – Management of moderate to severe pain where use of an opioid analgesic is appropriate.

OXYCODONE — ORAL

Oral solution and concentrate solution – Relief of moderate to moderately severe pain.

CR tablets – Management of moderate to severe pain when a continuous, around-the-clock analgesic is needed for an extended period of time. Not intended for use as an as-needed analgesic.

Oxycodone CR is not intended for use on an as-needed basis; not indicated for pain in the immediate postoperative period (the first 12 to 24 hours following surgery), or if the pain is mild or not expected to persist for an extended period of time. Oxycodone CR tablets are only indicated for postoperative use if the patient is already receiving the drug prior to surgery or if the postoperative pain is expected to be moderate to severe and persist for an extended period of time. Individualize treatment, moving from parenteral to oral analgesics as appropriate. Oxycodone CR is not indicated for preemptive analgesia (preoperative administration for the management of postoperative pain) and is not indicated for rectal administration.

Administration and Dosage

➤*General dosing considerations:*

Initiation of therapy – It is critical to initiate the dosing regimen for each patient individually. Attention should be given to the following:

1.) risk factors for abuse or addiction, including whether the patient has a previous or current substance abuse problem, a family history of substance abuse, or a history of mental illness or depression;
2.) the age, general condition, and medical status of the patient;
3.) the balance between pain control and adverse reactions;
4.) the daily dose, potency, and kind of the analgesic(s) the patient has been taking;
5.) the patient's opioid exposure and opioid tolerance (if any);
6.) the reliability of the conversion estimate used to calculate the dose of oxycodone;
7.) the special instructions for oxycodone 60 and 80 mg tablets, a single dose greater than 40 mg, or total daily doses greater than 80 mg.

CR tablets – Most patients given around-the-clock therapy with CR opioids may need to have immediate release medication available for "rescue" from breakthrough pain or to prevent pain that occurs predictably during certain patient activities (incident pain).

During periods of changing analgesic requirements, including initial titration, frequent contact is recommended between the health care provider, other members of the health care team, the patient, and the caregiver/family.

In treating pain, it is vital to assess the patient regularly and systematically. Regularly review therapy and adjust it based upon the patient's own reports of pain and adverse reactions and the health care provider's clinical judgment.

If the level of pain increases, make efforts to identify the source of increased pain, while adjusting the dose to decrease the level of pain.

During long-term therapy, especially for noncancer-related pain (or pain associated with other terminal illnesses), the continued need for the use of opioid analgesics should be reassessed as appropriate.

Instruct patients not to share or permit use by individuals other than the patient for whom oxycodone was prescribed, as such inappropriate use may have severe medical consequences, including death.

During periods of changing analgesic requirements, including initial titration, maintain frequent contact between the health care provider, other members of the health care team, the patient and, with proper consent, the caregiver/family.

➤*Adults:*

Management of moderate to severe pain –

Immediate-release tablets:

• *Usual dosage* – 10 to 30 mg every 4 hours, as needed. Individualize dosage. For control of severe chronic pain, administer on a regularly scheduled basis, every 4 to 6 hours, at the lowest dosage level that will achieve adequate analgesia.

Patients not currently on opioid therapy (opioid naive): Start in the dosing range of 5 to 15 mg every 4 to 6 hours as needed for pain. Titrate the dose based upon the response. For control of chronic pain, administer on a regularly scheduled basis to prevent the reoccurrence of pain rather than treating the pain after it has occurred.

Patients currently on opioid therapy: The potency of the prior opioid relative to oxycodone should be factored into the selection of the total daily dose of oxycodone.

• *Dosage adjustment* – If the pain increases in severity, analgesia is not adequate, or tolerance occurs, a gradual increase in dosage may be required. More severe pain may require 30 mg or more every 4 hours.

• *Conversion* – In converting patients from other opioids to immediate-release tablets, close observation and adjustment of dosage based upon the patient's response to immediate-release tablets is imperative. Administration of supplemental analgesia for breakthrough or incident pain and titration of the total daily dose of immediate-release tablets may be necessary, especially in patients who have disease states that are changing rapidly.

Conversion from fixed-ratio opioid/acetaminophen, opioid/aspirin, or opioid/nonsteroidal combination drugs: When converting patients from fixed-ratio opioid/nonopioid drug regimens, a decision should be made whether or not to continue the nonopioid analgesic. If a decision is made to discontinue the use of the nonopioid analgesic, it may be necessary to titrate the dose of the immediate-release tablets in response to the level of analgesia and adverse effects afforded by the dosing regimen. If the nonopioid regimen is continued as a separate single entity agent, base the starting dose upon the most recent dose of opioid as a baseline for further titration of oxycodone. Gauge incremental increases according to adverse effects to an acceptable level of analgesia.

• *Discontinuation of therapy* – It is important that therapy be gradually discontinued over time to prevent the development of an opioid abstinence syndrome (narcotic withdrawal). In general, decrease by 25% to 50% per day with careful monitoring for signs and symptoms of withdrawal. If the patient develops these signs or symptoms, the dose should be raised to the previous level and titrated down more slowly, either by increasing the interval between decreases, decreasing the amount of change in dose, or both.

Immediate-release capsules: 5 mg every 6 hours, as needed. Individualize dosage.

Oral concentrate solution: 5 mg every 6 hours as needed for pain. Individualize dosage.

Oral solution:

• *Usual dosage* – 10 to 30 mg every 4 hours, as needed. For control of severe chronic pain, administer on a regularly scheduled basis, every 4 to 6 hours, at the lowest dosage level that will achieve adequate analgesia.

• *Dosage adjustment* – If the pain increases in severity, analgesia is not adequate, or tolerance occurs, a gradual increase in dosage may be required. More severe pain may require 30 mg or more every 4 hours.

Management of moderate to severe pain when a continuous, around-the-clock analgesic is needed for an extended period of time (not intended for use as an as-needed analgesic) –

CR tablets:

• *Initial dosage* – Take care to use low initial doses of CR tablets in patients who are not already opioid tolerant, especially those who are receiving concurrent treatment with muscle relaxants, sedatives, or other CNS-active medications. A reasonable starting dose for patients who are taking nonopioid analgesics and require continuous around-the-clock therapy for an extended period of time is 10 mg every 12 hours.

Patients not already taking opioids (opioid naive): Do not begin treatment with oxycodone 60 and 80 mg tablets, a single dose greater than 40 mg, or a total daily dose greater than 80 mg in patients who are not already tolerant to the respiratory-depressant and sedating effects of opioids. Use of these doses in patients who are not opioid tolerant may cause fatal respiratory depression. These doses are only for use in opioid-tolerant patients.

Patients considered opioid tolerant: Patients considered opioid tolerant are those who are taking at least oral morphine 60 mg/day, transdermal fentanyl 25 mcg/h, oral oxycodone 30 mg/day, oral hydromorphone 8 mg/day, oral oxymorphone 25 mg/day, or an equianalgesic dose of another opioid for 1 week or longer.

• *Dosage adjustment* – Once therapy is initiated, assess pain relief and other opioid effects frequently. Patients who experience breakthrough pain require dosage adjustment or rescue medication. Because steady-state plasma concentrations are approximated within 24 to 36 hours, dosage adjustment may be carried out every 1 to 2 days.

There are no well-controlled clinical studies evaluating the safety and efficacy with dosing more frequently than every 12 hours. Increase the oxycodone dose by increasing the total daily dose, not by changing the 12-hour dosing interval. As a guideline, the total daily oxycodone dose usually can be increased by 25% to 50% of the current dose, each time an increase is clinically indicated.

If signs of excessive opioid-related adverse reactions are observed, the next dose may be reduced. If this adjustment leads to inadequate analgesia, a supplemental dose of immediate release oxycodone may be given. Alternatively, nonopioid analgesic adjuvants may be employed. Make dose adjustments to obtain an appropriate balance between pain relief and opioid-related adverse reactions.

• *Duration of therapy* – During long-term therapy, especially for noncancer pain syndromes, the continued need for around-the-clock opioid therapy should be reassessed periodically (eg, every 6 to 12 months) as appropriate.

• *Concomitant therapy* – Use low initial doses of oxycodone in patients who are not already opioid-tolerant, especially those who are receiving concurrent treatment with muscle relaxants, sedatives, or other CNS-active medications.

• *Conversion* –

Patients currently on opioid therapy: For initiation of oxycodone therapy for patients previously taking opioids, the conversion ratios found in the following table are a reasonable starting point, although not verified in well-controlled, multiple-dose trials. No fixed conversion ratio is likely to be satisfactory in all patients, especially patients receiving large opioid doses. A reasonable approach for converting from existing opioid therapy to oxycodone is as follows:

- Discontinue all other around-the clock opioid drugs when oxycodone therapy is initiated.
- Using standard conversion ratio estimates (see the following table), multiply the mg/day of each of the current opioids to be converted by their appropriate multiplication factor to obtain the equivalent total daily dose of oral oxycodone.
- Divide the calculated 24-hour oxycodone dose in half to approximate the every 12-hour dose of oxycodone.
- Round down, if necessary, to the appropriate oxycodone tablet strengths available.
- Close observation and frequent titration are indicated until patients are stable on the new therapy.

OXYCODONE — ORAL

Multiplication Factors for Converting the Daily Dose of Prior Opioids to the Daily Dose of Oral Oxycodone[a]		
mg/day prior opioid × factor = mg/day oral oxycodone		
	Oral prior opioid	Parenteral prior opioid
Oxycodone	1	—
Codeine	0.15	—
Fentanyl transdermal therapeutic system	see next section	see next section
Hydrocodone	0.9	—
Hydromorphone	4	20
Levorphanol	7.5	15
Meperidine	0.1	0.4
Methadone	1.5	3
Morphine	0.5	3

[a] To be used only for conversion to oral oxycodone. For patients receiving high-dose parenteral opioids, a more conservative conversion is warranted. For example, for high-dose parenteral morphine, use 1.5 instead of 3 as a multiplication factor.

Transdermal fentanyl to CR tablets: Eighteen hours after the removal of the transdermal fentanyl patch, treatment with CR tablets can be initiated. Although there has been no systemic assessment of such conversion, a conservative oxycodone dose, approximately 10 mg every 12 hours of CR tablets, should be initially substituted for each fentanyl 25 mcg/h transdermal patch. Closely follow the patient during conversion from transdermal fentanyl to oxycodone, as there is very limited clinical experience with this conversion.

CR tablets to parenteral opioids: To avoid overdose, follow conservative dose conversion ratios. When converting from oxycodone to parenteral opioids, it is advisable to calculate an equivalent parenteral dose and then initiate treatment at half of this calculated value.

• *Discontinuation of therapy* – Taper doses gradually to prevent signs and symptoms of withdrawal in the physically dependent patient.

➤*Children:*

Off-label dosing –

Analgesia: 0.05 mg to 0.15 mg/kg/dose orally every 4 to 6 hours as needed up to 5 mg/dose.

➤*Elderly:* Use of oxycodone is associated with increased potential risks and should be used only with caution in elderly patients.

➤*Renal function impairment:* Dose initiation should follow a conservative approach. Dosages should be adjusted according to the clinical situation.

➤*Hepatic function impairment:* The initiation of therapy at one-third to one-half the usual doses and careful dose titration is warranted.

➤*Managing expected opioid adverse reactions:* Most patients receiving oxycodone, especially those who are opioid-naive, will experience adverse reactions. Patients do not usually become tolerant to the constipating effects of opioids, therefore, anticipate constipation and treat aggressively and prophylactically with a stimulant laxative with or without a stool softener. If nausea persists and is unacceptable to the patient, consider treatment with antiemetics or other modalities to relieve these symptoms.

➤*Administration:*

Immediate-release tablets/oral solution – For control of severe chronic pain, administer on a regularly scheduled basis, every 4 to 6 hours, at the lowest dosage level that will achieve adequate analgesia.

CR tablets – Swallow tablets whole; do not cut, break, chew, crush, or dissolve. Taking cut, broken, chewed, crushed, or dissolved tablets could lead to the rapid release and absorption of a potentially fatal dose of oxycodone. *OxyContin* is not indicated for rectal administration.

Oral concentrate solution – *Roxicodone Intensol, OxyFAST*, and *ETH-Oxydose* 20 mg/mL solution are highly concentrated solutions. Take care in prescribing and dispensing this solution strength. Fill dropper to the level of the prescribed dose (1 mL = 20 mg; 0.75 mL = 15 mg; 0.5 mL = 10 mg; 0.25 mL = 5 mg). For ease of administration, add dose to approximately 30 mL (1 fluid oz) or more of juice or other liquid. May also be added to applesauce, pudding, or other semi-solid foods. The drug-food mixture should be used immediately and not stored for future use.

➤*Storage/Stability:* Store at 25°C (77°F); excursions permitted between 15° and 30°C (59° and 86°F). Discard open bottles of oral solution after 90 days. Dispense in tight, light-resistant container.

OXYMORPHONE HYDROCHLORIDE

c-ii	**Oxymorphone** (Endo Pharmaceuticals)	**Tablets; oral:** 5 mg	Lactose. (E794 5). Blue, round. In 100s and UD 100s.
	Opana (Endo)		Lactose. (E612 5). Blue. In 100s and UD 100s.
c-ii	**Oxymorphone** (Endo Pharmaceuticals)	**Tablets; oral:** 10 mg	Lactose. (E795 10). Red, round. In 100s and UD 100s.
c-ii	**Opana** (Endo)		Lactose. (E613 10). Red. In 100s and UD 100s.
c-ii	**Opana ER** (Endo)	**Tablets, extended-release; oral:** 5 mg	Methylparaben. (5). Pink, octagon shape. Film-coated. In 100s and UD 100s.
		7.5 mg	Methylparaben. (7½). Gray, octagon shape. Film-coated. In 100s and UD 100s.
		10 mg	Methylparaben. (10). Lt. orange, octagon shape. Film-coated. In 100s and UD 100s.
		15 mg	Methylparaben. (15). Octagon shape. Film-coated. In 100s and UD 100s.
		20 mg	Methylparaben. (20). Lt. green, octagon shape. Film-coated. In 100s and UD 100s.
		30 mg	Methylparaben. (30). Red, octagon shape. Film-coated. In 100s and UD 100s.
		40 mg	Lactose, methylparaben. (40). Yellow, octagon shape. Film-coated. In 100s and UD 100s.
c-ii	**Opana** (Endo)	**Injection, solution:** 1 mg/mL	In 1 mL amps.

OXYMORPHONE HYDROCHLORIDE — ORAL

For complete prescribing information, refer to the Opioid Analgesics group monograph.

WARNING

Oxymorphone extended-release – Oxymorphone extended-release (ER) is a morphine-like opioid agonist and a Schedule II controlled substance with an abuse liability similar to other opioid analgesics. Oxymorphone can be abused in a manner similar to other opioid agonists, legal or illicit. Consider this when prescribing or dispensing oxymorphone ER in situations in which the health care provider or pharmacist is concerned about an increased risk of misuse, abuse, or diversion.

Oxymorphone ER oral formulation is indicated for the management of moderate to severe pain when a continuous, around-the-clock opioid analgesic is needed for an extended period of time. Oxymorphone ER is not intended for use on an as-needed basis.

Oxymorphone ER tablets are to be swallowed whole and not broken, chewed, dissolved, or crushed. Taking broken, chewed, dissolved, or crushed oxymorphone ER tablets leads to rapid release and absorption of a potentially fatal dose of oxymorphone.

Patients must not consume alcoholic beverages or prescription or nonprescription medications containing alcohol while on oxymorphone ER therapy. The coingestion of alcohol with oxymorphone ER may result in increased plasma levels and a potentially fatal overdose of oxymorphone.

Indications

➤*Moderate to severe pain:*

Oxymorphone immediate-release – For the relief of moderate to severe acute pain when the use of an opioid is appropriate.

Oxymorphone ER – For the relief of moderate to severe pain in patients requiring continuous, around-the-clock opioid treatment for an extended period of time; not intended for use as an as-needed analgesic.

Administration and Dosage

➤*General dosing considerations:*

Individualization of dosage – Selection of patients for treatment with oxymorphone should be governed by the same principles that apply to the use of other similar opioid analgesics. Health care providers should individualize treatment in every case, using nonopioid analgesics, as-needed opioids and/or combination products, and chronic opioid therapy in a progressive plan of pain management such as that outlined by the World Health Organization, the Agency for Healthcare Research and Quality, the Federation of State Medical Boards model guidelines, and the American Pain Society. Health care providers should follow appropriate pain management principles of careful assessment and ongoing monitoring.

OXYMORPHONE HYDROCHLORIDE — ORAL

As with any opioid drug product, it is necessary to adjust the dosing regimen for each patient individually, taking into account the patient's prior analgesic treatment experience. In the selection of the initial dose of oxymorphone, attention should be given to the following: the total daily dose, potency, and specific characteristics of the opioid the patient has been taking previously; the relative potency estimate used to calculate the equivalent oxymorphone dose needed; the patient's degree of opioid tolerance; the age, general condition, and medical status of the patient; concurrent nonopioid analgesic and other medications; the type and severity of the patient's pain; the balance between pain control and adverse reactions; and risk factors for abuse, addiction, or diversion, including a history of abuse, addiction, or diversion.

Once therapy is initiated, pain relief and other opioid effects should be frequently assessed.

In clinical practices, titration of the total daily oxymorphone ER dose should be based upon the amount of supplemental opioid utilization, the severity of the patient's pain, and the patient's ability to tolerate the opioid. Patients should be titrated to generally mild or no pain (with the regular use of no more than 2 doses of supplemental analgesia [ie, rescue] per 24 hours for oxymorphone ER).

➤Adults:

Moderate to severe pain –

Opioid-naive patients:

- *Extended-release tablets –*
  - *Initial dosage:* It is suggested that patients who are not opioid-experienced and initiated on chronic, around-the-clock opioid therapy be started with oxymorphone ER 5 mg every 12 hours.
  - *Dosage titration:* Individually titrate, preferably at increments of 5 to 10 mg every 12 hours every 3 to 7 days, to a level that provides adequate analgesia and minimizes adverse reactions under the close supervision of the prescribing health care provider.
- *Immediate-release tablets –*
  - *Initial dosage:* 10 to 20 mg every 4 to 6 hours, depending on the initial pain intensity. If deemed necessary to initiate therapy at a lower dose, patients may be started with oxymorphone immediate-release 5 mg.

  Initiation of therapy with doses of more than 20 mg is not recommended because of potential serious adverse reactions.

  - *Dosage titration:* Titrate dose based upon the individual patient's response to the initial dose of oxymorphone. This dose can then be adjusted to an acceptable level of analgesia, taking into account the pain intensity and adverse reactions experienced by the patient.

Opioid-experienced patients:

- *Immediate-release tablets –*
  - *Conversion from parenteral to oxymorphone immediate release:* Given the absolute oral bioavailability of approximately 10%, patients receiving parenteral oxymorphone may be converted to oxymorphone immediate-release tablets by administering 10 times the patient's total daily parenteral oxymorphone dose as oxymorphone immediate-release tablets, in 4 or 6 equally divided doses (eg, intravenous [IV] dose × 10/4). For example, approximately 10 mg of oxymorphone immediate-release every 4 to 6 hours may be required to provide pain relief equivalent to a total daily dose of intramuscular (IM) oxymorphone 4 mg. The dose can be titrated to optimal pain relief or combined with acetaminophen/nonsteroidal anti-inflammatory drugs (NSAIDs) for optimal pain relief. Because of patient variability with regard to opioid analgesic response, upon conversion, patients should be closely monitored to ensure adequate analgesia and to minimize adverse reactions.
  - *Conversion from other oral opioids to oxymorphone immediate-release:* For conversion from other oral opioids to oxymorphone immediate-release, health care providers are advised to refer to published relative potency information, keeping in mind that conversion ratios are only approximate. In general, it is safest to start the oxymorphone immediate-release therapy by administering half of the calculated total daily dose of oxymorphone immediate-release in 4 to 6 equally divided doses every 4 to 6 hours. The initial dose of oxymorphone immediate-release can be gradually adjusted until adequate pain relief and acceptable adverse reactions have been achieved.
- *Extended-release tablets –*
  - *Conversion from oxymorphone immediate-release to ER:* Patients receiving oxymorphone immediate-release may be converted to ER by administering half the patient's total daily oral oxymorphone immediate-release dose as ER every 12 hours. For example, a patient receiving oxymorphone immediate-release 40 mg/day may require oxymorphone ER 20 mg every 12 hours.
  - *Conversion from parenteral oxymorphone to oxymorphone ER:* Given the absolute oral bioavailability of approximately 10%, patients receiving parenteral oxymorphone may be converted to oxymorphone ER by administering 10 times the patient's total daily parenteral oxymorphone dose as oxymorphone ER in 2 equally divided doses (eg, IV dose × 10/2). For example, approximately 20 mg of oxymorphone ER every 12 hours may be required to provide pain relief equivalent to a total daily dose of parenteral oxymorphone 4 mg. Because of patient variability with regard to opioid analgesic response, upon conversion, patients should be closely monitored to ensure adequate analgesia and to minimize adverse reactions.
  - *Conversion from other oral opioids to oxymorphone ER:* For conversion from other opioids to oxymorphone ER, advise health care providers to refer to published relative potency information, keeping in mind that conversion ratios are only approximate. In general, it is safest to start oxymorphone therapy by administering half of the calculated total daily dose of oxymorphone ER (see the following table) in 2 divided doses every 12 hours. The initial dose of oxymorphone ER can be gradually adjusted until adequate pain relief and acceptable adverse reactions have been achieved. The following table provides approximate equivalent doses, which may be used as a guideline for conversion. The conversion ratios and approximate equivalent doses in this conversion table are only to be used for the conversion from current opioid therapy to oxymorphone ER. In a phase 3 clinical trial with an open-label titration period, patients were converted from their current opioid to oxymorphone ER using the following table as a guide. In general, patients were able to successfully titrate to a stabilized dose of oxymorphone ER within 4 weeks. There is substantial patient variation in the relative potency of different opioid drugs and formulations.

Conversion Ratios to Oxymorphone ER

Opioid	Approximate equivalent dose (oral)	Oral conversion ratio[a]
Oxymorphone	10 mg	1
Hydrocodone	20 mg	0.5
Oxycodone	20 mg	0.5
Methadone[b]	20 mg	0.5
Morphine	30 mg	0.333

[a] Ratio for conversion of oral opioid dose to approximate oxymorphone equivalent dose. Select opioid and multiply the dose by the conversion ratio to calculate the approximate oral oxymorphone equivalent.

- The conversion ratios and approximate equivalent doses in this conversion table are only to be used for the conversion from current opioid therapy to oxymorphone ER.
- Sum the total daily dose for the opioid and multiply by the conversion ratio to calculate the oxymorphone total daily dose.
- For patients on a regimen of mixed opioids, calculate the approximate oral oxymorphone dose for each opioid and sum the totals to estimate the total daily oxymorphone dose.
- The dose of oxymorphone ER can be gradually adjusted, preferably at increments of 10 mg every 12 hours every 3 to 7 days, until adequate pain relief and acceptable adverse reactions have been achieved.

[b] It is extremely important to monitor all patients closely when converting from methadone to other opioid agonists. The ratio between methadone and other opioid agonists may vary widely as a function of previous dose exposure. Methadone has a long half-life and tends to accumulate in the plasma.

➤Renal function impairment: In patients with a creatinine clearance (CrCl) rate less than 50 mL/min, oxymorphone should be started with the lowest dose and titrated slowly, while carefully monitoring adverse reactions.

➤Hepatic function impairment: Patients with mild hepatic function impairment should be started with the lowest dose, titrated slowly, and monitored carefully for adverse reactions.

Oxymorphone is contraindicated in patients with moderate and severe hepatic function impairment.

➤Maintenance therapy:

Immediate-release – During therapy, continual reevaluation of the patient receiving oxymorphone is important, with special attention to the maintenance of pain control and the relative incidence of adverse reactions associated with therapy. If the level of pain increases, effort should be made to identify the source of increased pain, while adjusting the dose and/or using adjuvant analgesics, such as acetaminophen or NSAIDs.

Extended-release – The intent of the titration period is to establish a patient-specific, every-12-hour dose that will maintain adequate analgesia with acceptable adverse reactions for as long as pain relief is necessary. During titration and before a stable dose is achieved, oxymorphone immediate-release or other immediate-release medications can be used as supplemental analgesia between dosings. Should pain recur, the dose can be incrementally increased to reestablish pain control. The method of therapy adjustment outlined previously should be employed to reestablish pain control.

During chronic therapy with oxymorphone ER, the continued need for around-the-clock opioid therapy should be reassessed periodically.

➤Dosage adjustment: Patients who experience breakthrough pain on oxymorphone immediate-release may require dosage adjustment or nonopioid therapy, such as acetaminophen or NSAIDs.

If signs of excessive opioid-related adverse reactions are observed, the next dose may be reduced. If this adjustment leads to inadequate analgesia with oxymorphone ER, a supplemental dose of oxymorphone immediate-release, another immediate-release opioid, or a nonopioid analgesic may be administered.

Dose adjustments should be made to obtain an appropriate balance between pain relief and opioid-related adverse reactions. If significant adverse reactions occur before the therapeutic goal of mild or no pain is achieved, the reactions should be treated aggressively. Once adverse reactions are under control, upward titration should continue to an acceptable level of pain control.

OXYMORPHONE HYDROCHLORIDE — ORAL

➤*Concomitant medications:*

CNS depressants – Oxymorphone, like all opioid analgesics, should be started at one-third to one-half of the usual dose in patients who are concurrently receiving other CNS depressants, including sedatives or hypnotics, general anesthetics, phenothiazines, tranquilizers, and alcohol, because respiratory depression, hypotension, and profound sedation or coma may result. No specific interaction between oxymorphone and monoamine oxidase inhibitors (MAOIs) has been observed, but caution in the use of any opioid in patients taking this class of drugs is appropriate.

Alcohol – Patients must not consume alcoholic beverages or prescription or nonprescription medications containing alcohol while taking oxymorphone ER therapy. The coingestion of alcohol with oxymorphone ER may result in increased plasma levels and a potentially fatal overdose of oxymorphone.

➤*Discontinuation of therapy:* When the patient no longer requires therapy with oxymorphone, doses should be tapered gradually to prevent signs and symptoms of withdrawal in the physically-dependent patient.

➤*Administration:* Oxymorphone should be administered on an empty stomach at least 1 hour prior to or 2 hours after eating.

Oxymorphone ER tablets are to be swallowed whole and not broken, chewed, dissolved, or crushed. Taking broken, chewed, dissolved, or crushed oxymorphone ER tablets leads to rapid release and absorption of a potentially fatal dose of oxymorphone.

➤*Storage / Stability:* Store at 25°C (77°F); excursions are permitted to 15° to 30°C (59° to 86°F).

OXYMORPHONE HYDROCHLORIDE — INJECTION

For complete prescribing information, refer to the Opioid Analgesics group monograph.

Indications

➤*Anxiety:* For relief of anxiety in patients with dyspnea associated with pulmonary edema secondary to acute left ventricular dysfunction.

➤*Pain:* Relief of moderate to severe pain.

➤*Preoperative medication / anesthesia / analgesia:* For preoperative medication, support of anesthesia, and obstetrical analgesia.

Administration and Dosage

➤*General dosing considerations:*

Individualization of dosage – Selection of patients for treatment with oxymorphone should be governed by the same principles that apply to the use of similar opioid analgesics. The health care provider should individualize treatment in every case, using nonopioid analgesics, as-needed opioids and/or combination products, and chronic opioid therapy in a progressive plan of pain management such as that outlined by the World Health Organization, the Agency for Healthcare Research and Quality, and the American Pain Society.

As with any opioid drug product, it is necessary to adjust the dosing regimen for each patient individually, taking into account the patient's prior analgesic treatment experience. In the selection of the initial dose of oxymorphone, attention should be given to the total daily dose, potency, and specific characteristics of the opioid the patient has been taking previously; the relative potency estimate used to calculate the equivalent oxymorphone dose needed; the patient's degree of opioid tolerance; the age, general condition, and medical status of the patient; concurrent nonopioid analgesic and other medications; the type and severity of the patient's pain; the balance between pain control and adverse experiences; and risk factors for abuse, addiction, or diversion, including a prior history of abuse, addiction, or diversion.

Once therapy is initiated, pain relief and other opioid effects should be frequently assessed. Patients should be titrated to adequate pain relief (generally mild or no pain).

During periods of changing analgesic requirements, including initial titration, frequent contact is recommended among the health care provider, other members of the health care team, the patient, and the caregiver/family. Advise patients and family members of the potential common adverse reactions to decrease fear of the use of opioids and promote their optimal use.

➤*Adults:*

Anxiety –

Initial dosage:

• *Intravenous* – Initially, 0.5 mg. In nondebilitated patients, the dose can be cautiously increased until satisfactory pain relief is obtained.

• *Subcutaneous or intramuscular* – Initially, 1 to 1.5 mg every 4 to 6 hours as needed.

Labor analgesia – For analgesia during labor, give 0.5 to 1 mg intramuscularly (IM).

Pain (moderate to severe) –

Initial dosage:

• *Intravenous* – Initially, 0.5 mg. In nondebilitated patients, the dose can be cautiously increased until satisfactory pain relief is obtained.

• *Subcutaneous or intramuscular* – Initially, 1 to 1.5 mg every 4 to 6 hours as needed.

Dosage adjustment: Patients who experience breakthrough pain may require dosage adjustment or nonopioid therapy such as acetaminophen or nonsteroidal anti-inflammatory drugs (NSAIDs).

If signs of excessive opioid-related adverse experiences are observed, the next dose may be reduced. Make dose adjustments to obtain an appropriate balance between pain relief and opioid-related adverse reactions. If significant adverse reactions occur before the therapeutic goal of mild or no pain is achieved, treat the reactions aggressively. Once adverse reactions are under control, continue upward titration to an acceptable level of pain control.

Maintenance therapy: Oxymorphone is intended as an opioid analgesic for the management of moderate to severe pain when the use of an opioid analgesic is appropriate. During therapy, continual reevaluation of the patient receiving oxymorphone is important, giving special attention to the maintenance of pain control and the relative incidence of adverse reactions associated with therapy. If the level of pain increases, effort should be made to identify the source of increased pain, while adjusting the dose and/or using adjuvant analgesics, such as acetaminophen or NSAIDs.

Preoperative medication / anesthesia / analgesia –

Initial dosage:

• *Intravenous* – Initially, 0.5 mg. In nondebilitated patients, the dose can be cautiously increased until satisfactory pain relief is obtained.

• *Subcutaneous or intramuscular* – Initially, 1 to 1.5 mg every 4 to 6 hours as needed.

➤*Renal function impairment:* Administer oxymorphone cautiously and in reduced dosages to patients with a creatinine clearance rate less than 50 mL/min.

➤*Hepatic function impairment:* Use oxymorphone with caution in patients with mild hepatic function impairment. Patients with mild hepatic function impairment should be started with the lowest dose and titrated slowly while carefully monitoring adverse reactions.

Oxymorphone injection is contraindicated in patients with moderate and severe hepatic function impairment.

➤*Concomitant therapy:* Oxymorphone, like all opioid analgesics, should be started at one-third to one-half of the usual dose in patients who are concurrently receiving other CNS depressants, including sedatives or hypnotics, general anesthetics, phenothiazines, tranquilizers, and alcohol because respiratory depression, hypotension, and profound sedation or coma may result. No specific interaction between oxymorphone and monoamine oxidase inhibitors has been observed, but use appropriate caution in the use of any opioid in patients taking this class of drugs.

➤*Conversion (oral to injection):* Given an absolute oral bioavailability of approximately 10%, patients receiving oral oxymorphone may be converted to oxymorphone injection by administering one-tenth the patient's total daily oral oxymorphone dose as oxymorphone injection in 4 or 6 equally divided doses (eg, total daily oral dose/[10 × 4]). For example, approximately oxymorphone 1 mg IM every 6 hours (4 mg IM total dose) may be required to provide pain relief equivalent to a total daily dose of oxymorphone 40 mg orally. The dose can be titrated to optimal pain relief or combined with acetaminophen/NSAIDs for optimal pain relief. Because of patient variability with regard to opioid analgesic response, upon conversion, closely monitor patients to ensure adequate analgesia and minimize adverse reactions.

➤*Discontinuation of therapy:* When the patient no longer requires therapy with oxymorphone, taper doses gradually to prevent signs and symptoms of withdrawal in the physically dependent patient.

➤*Storage / Stability:* Store at 25°C (77°F); excursions are permitted to 15° to 30°C (59° to 86°F). Protect from light.

PROPOXYPHENE (Dextropropoxyphene)

c-iv	**Propoxyphene Hydrochloride** (Various, eg, Ivax)	**Capsules; oral:** 65 mg (as hydrochloride)	In 100s.

PROPOXYPHENE NAPSYLATE — ORAL

For complete prescribing information, refer to the Opioid Analgesics monograph.

WARNING

Fatalities –

- Do not prescribe propoxyphene for patients who are suicidal or addiction prone.
- Prescribe propoxyphene with caution for patients taking tranquilizers or antidepressant drugs and patients who use alcohol in excess.
- Tell patients not to exceed the recommended dose and to limit alcohol intake.

Propoxyphene products in excessive doses, either alone or in combination with other CNS depressants (including alcohol), are a major cause of drug-related deaths. Fatalities within the first hour of overdosage are not uncommon. In a survey of deaths due to overdosage conducted in 1975, in approximately 20% of fatal cases, death occurred within the first hour (5% within 15 minutes). Propoxyphene should not be taken in higher doses than those recommended by the health care provider. Judicious prescribing of propoxyphene is essential for safety. Consider nonopioid analgesics for depressed or suicidal patients. Caution patients about the concomitant use of propoxyphene products and alcohol because of potentially serious CNS-additive effects of these agents. Because of added CNS depressant effects, cautiously prescribe with concomitant sedatives, tranquilizers, muscle relaxants, antidepressants, or other CNS-depressant drugs. Advise patients of the additive depressant effects of these combinations.

WARNING (cont.)

Many propoxyphene-related deaths have occurred in patients with histories of emotional disturbances, suicidal ideation or attempts, or misuse of tranquilizers, alcohol, and other CNS-active drugs. Deaths have occurred as a consequence of the accidental ingestion of excessive quantities of propoxyphene alone or in combination with other drugs. Do not exceed the recommended dosage.

Indications

➤*Mild to moderate pain:* For the relief of mild to moderate pain.

Administration and Dosage

➤*General dosing considerations:* Because of differences in molecular weight, 100 mg of propoxyphene napsylate is required to supply propoxyphene equivalent to 65 mg of the hydrochloride.

➤*Adults:*

Mild to moderate pain –

Usual dosage: 100 mg every 4 hours as needed.
Maximum dose: 600 mg/day.

➤*Elderly:* Propoxyphene metabolism rate may be reduced in some patients. Consider increased dosing interval.

➤*Renal function impairment:* Consider a reduced total daily dosage in patients with renal impairment.

➤*Hepatic function impairment:* Consider a reduced total daily dosage in patients with hepatic impairment.

➤*Storage/Stability:* Store at controlled room temperature, 15° to 30°C (59° to 86°F).

PROPOXYPHENE HYDROCHLORIDE — ORAL

For complete prescribing information, refer to the Opioid Analgesics monograph.

WARNING

Fatalities –

- Do not prescribe propoxyphene for patients who are suicidal or addiction prone.
- Prescribe propoxyphene with caution for patients taking tranquilizers or antidepressant drugs and patients who use alcohol in excess.
- Tell patients not to exceed the recommended dose and to limit alcohol intake.

Propoxyphene products in excessive doses, either alone or in combination with other CNS depressants (including alcohol), are a major cause of drug-related deaths. Fatalities within the first hour of overdosage are not uncommon. In a survey of deaths due to overdosage conducted in 1975, in approximately 20% of fatal cases, death occurred within the first hour (5% within 15 minutes). Propoxyphene should not be taken in higher doses than those recommended by the health care provider. Judicious prescribing of propoxyphene is essential for safety. Consider nonopioid analgesics for depressed or suicidal patients. Caution patients about the concomitant use of propoxyphene products and alcohol because of potentially serious CNS-additive effects of these agents. Because of added CNS depressant effects, cautiously prescribe with concomitant sedatives, tranquilizers, muscle relaxants, antidepressants, or other CNS-depressant drugs. Advise patients of the additive depressant effects of these combinations.

WARNING (cont.)

Many propoxyphene-related deaths have occurred in patients with histories of emotional disturbances, suicidal ideation or attempts, or misuse of tranquilizers, alcohol, and other CNS-active drugs. Deaths have occurred as a consequence of the accidental ingestion of excessive quantities of propoxyphene alone or in combination with other drugs. Do not exceed the recommended dosage.

Indications

➤*Pain:* Relief of mild to moderate pain.

Administration and Dosage

➤*General dosing considerations:* Because of differences in molecular weight, 100 mg of propoxyphene napsylate is required to supply propoxyphene equivalent to 65 mg of the hydrochloride.

➤*Adults:*

Pain –

Usual dosage: 65 mg every 4 hours as needed.
Maximum dose: 390 mg/day.

➤*Elderly:* Propoxyphene metabolism rate may be reduced in some patients. Consider increased dosing interval.

➤*Renal function impairment:* Consider a reduced total daily dosage in patients with renal impairment.

➤*Hepatic function impairment:* Consider a reduced total daily dosage in patients with hepatic impairment.

➤*Storage/Stability:* Store at 15° to 30°C (59° to 86°F).

REMIFENTANIL

c-ii	**Ultiva** (Bioniche Pharma Group)	**Injection, lyophilized powder for solution:** 1 mg	As remifentanil hydrochloride. Preservative free. Glycine 15 mg. In 3 mL vials.
		2 mg	As remifentanil hydrochloride. Preservative free. Glycine 15 mg. In 5 mL vials.
		5 mg	As remifentanil hydrochloride. Preservative free. Glycine 15 mg. In 10 mL vials.

REMIFENTANIL HYDROCHLORIDE — INJECTION

For complete prescribing information, refer to the Opioid Analgesics group monograph.

Indications

➤*Analgesia:* An analgesic agent for use during the induction and maintenance of general anesthesia for inpatient and outpatient procedures and for continuation as an analgesic into the immediate postoperative period under the direct supervision of an anesthesia practitioner in a postoperative anesthesia care unit or intensive care setting. As an analgesic component of monitored anesthesia care.

Administration and Dosage

➤*General dosing considerations:* Individualize dosage.

Remifentanil infusions may be continued into the immediate postoperative period for select patients for whom later transition to longer-acting analgesics may be desired. The use of bolus injections of remifentanil to treat pain during the postoperative period is not recommended.

General anesthesia – Remifentanil is not recommended as the sole agent in general anesthesia because loss of consciousness cannot be assured and because of a high incidence of apnea, muscle rigidity, and tachycardia.

Analgesic component of monitored anesthesia care (MAC) – It is strongly recommended that supplemental oxygen be supplied whenever remifentanil is administered.

➤*Adults:*

Analgesia –

Coronary artery bypass surgery: The table below summarizes the recommended doses for induction, maintenance, and continuation as an analgesic into the intensive care unit (ICU) in adult patients, predominantly ASA

REMIFENTANIL HYDROCHLORIDE — INJECTION

physical status III or IV. To avoid hypotension during the induction phase, it is important to consider the concomitant medication regimens used.

Remifentanil Dosing Recommendations—Coronary Artery Bypass Surgery			
Phase	Continuous IV infusion (mcg/kg/min)	Infusion dose range (mcg/kg/min)	Supplemental IV bolus dose (mcg/kg)
Induction of anesthesia (through intubation)	1	—	—
Maintenance of anesthesia	1	0.125 to 4	0.5 to 1
Continuation as an analgesic into ICU	1	0.05 to 1	—

General anesthesia:

Remifentanil Dosing Guidelines—General Anesthesia and Continuing as an Analgesic into the Postoperative Care Unit or Intensive Care Setting			
Phase	Continuous IV infusion (mcg/kg/min)	Infusion dose range (mcg/kg/min)	Supplemental IV bolus dose (mcg/kg)
Induction of anesthesia (through intubation)	0.5 to 1[a]	NA[b]	NA[b]
Maintenance of anesthesia with:			
Nitrous oxide (66%)	0.4	0.1 to 2	1
Isoflurane (0.4 to 1.5 MAC[c])	0.25	0.05 to 2	1
Propofol (100 to 200 mcg/kg/min)	0.25	0.05 to 2	1
Continuation as an analgesic into the immediate postoperative period	0.1	0.025 to 0.2	Not recommended

[a] An initial dose of 1 mcg/kg may be administered over 30 to 60 seconds.
[b] No data available.
[c] MAC = monitored anesthesia care.

• *Induction of general anesthesia* – Administer at an infusion rate of 0.5 to 1 mcg/kg/min with a hypnotic or volatile agent for the induction of anesthesia. If endotracheal intubation is to occur less than 8 minutes after the start of infusion of remifentanil, then an initial dose of 1 mcg/kg may be administered over 30 to 60 seconds.

• *Maintenance of general anesthesia* –

Continuous IV dose: After endotracheal intubation, decrease the infusion rate of remifentanil in accordance with the dosing guidelines in the table above. Because of the rapid onset and short duration of action of remifentanil, the rate of administration during anesthesia can be titrated upward in 25% to 100% increments or downward in 25% to 50% decrements every 2 to 5 minutes to attain the desired level of mu-opioid effect.

Supplemental IV bolus dose: In response to light anesthesia or transient episodes of intense surgical stress, supplemental bolus doses of 1 mcg/kg may be administered every 2 to 5 minutes. At infusion rates greater than 1 mcg/kg/min, consider increases in the concomitant anesthetic agents to increase the depth of anesthesia.

• *Continuation as an analgesic into the immediate postoperative period* – Administer remifentanil initially by continuous infusion at a rate of 0.1 mcg/kg/min. The infusion rate may be adjusted every 5 minutes in 0.025 mcg/kg/min increments to balance the patient's level of analgesia and respiratory rate. Infusion rates more than 0.2 mcg/kg/min are associated with respiratory depression (respiratory rate less than 8 breaths/min).

Monitored anesthesia care (MAC):

Remifentanil Dosing Guidelines for Adults—Monitored Anesthesia Care			
Method	Timing	Remifentanil alone	Remifentanil + midazolam 2 mg
Single IV dose	Given 90 seconds before local anesthetic	1 mcg/kg over 30 to 60 seconds	0.5 mcg/kg over 30 to 60 seconds
Continuous IV infusion	Beginning 5 minutes before local anesthetic	0.1 mcg/kg/min	0.05 mcg/kg/min
	After local anesthetic	0.05 mcg/kg/min (range: 0.025 to 0.2 mcg/kg/min)	0.025 mcg/kg/min (range: 0.025 to 0.2 mcg/kg/min)

• *Single IV dose* – See table above.

A single IV dose of 0.5 to 1 mcg/kg over 30 to 60 seconds may be given 90 seconds before the placement of the local or regional anesthetic block.

• *Continuous IV infusion* – See table above.

Administer initially by continuous infusion at a rate of 0.1 mcg/kg/min beginning 5 minutes before placement of the local or regional anesthetic block.

Because of the risk for hypoventilation, decrease the infusion rate of remifentanil to 0.05 mcg/kg/min following placement of the block. Thereafter, rate adjustments of 0.025 mcg/kg/min at 5-minute intervals may be used to balance the patient's level of analgesia and respiratory rate. Rates greater than 0.2 mcg/kg/min are generally associated with respiratory depression (respiratory rates less than 8 breaths/min).

Bolus doses of remifentanil administered simultaneously with a continuous infusion of remifentanil to spontaneously breathing patients are not recommended.

➤*Children:*

Analgesia –

Maintenance of general anesthesia:

• *1 year of age and older* – The table below summarizes the recommended doses in children, predominantly American Society of Anesthesiologists (ASA) physical status I, II, or III. In children, remifentanil was administered with nitrous oxide or nitrous oxide in combination with halothane, sevoflurane, or isoflurane.

Remifentanil Dosing Guidelines in Children—Maintenance of Anesthesia			
Phase	Continuous IV infusion[a] (mcg/kg/min)	Infusion dose range (mcg/kg/min)	Supplemental IV bolus dose (mcg/kg)
Maintenance of anesthesia with:			
Halothane (0.3 to 1.5 MAC)	0.25	0.05 to 1.3	1
Sevoflurane (0.3 to 1.5 MAC)	0.25	0.05 to 1.3	1
Isoflurane (0.4 to 1.5 MAC)	0.25	0.05 to 1.3	1

[a] An initial dose of 1 mcg/kg may be administered over 30 to 60 seconds.

Continuous IV dose: After endotracheal intubation, decrease the infusion rate of remifentanil in accordance with the dosing guidelines in the table above. Because of the rapid onset and short duration of action of remifentanil, the rate of administration during anesthesia can be titrated upward up to 50% increments or downward in 25% to 50% decrements every 2 to 5 minutes to attain the desired level of mu-opioid effect.

Supplemental IV bolus dose: In response to light anesthesia or transient episodes of intense surgical stress, supplemental bolus doses of 1 mcg/kg may be administered every 2 to 5 minutes. At infusion rates greater than 1 mcg/kg/min, consider increases in the concomitant anesthetic agents to increase the depth of anesthesia.

➤*Elderly:* Decrease the starting doses of remifentanil by 50% in elderly patients (older than 65 years of age). Cautiously titrate to effect.

➤*Obesity:* Base the starting dose of remifentanil on ideal body weight (IBW) in obese patients (more than 30% over their IBW).

➤*Concomitant therapy:* The need for premedication and the choice of anesthetic agents must be individualized. In clinical studies, patients who received remifentanil frequently received a benzodiazepine premedication.

Adults – Remifentanil is synergistic with other anesthetics, and doses of thiopental, propofol, isoflurane, and midazolam may need to be reduced by up to 75% with the coadministration of remifentanil.

Children – In children, remifentanil was administered with nitrous oxide or nitrous oxide in combination with halothane, sevoflurane, or isoflurane.

➤*Discontinuation of therapy:* Upon discontinuation of remifentanil, clear the IV tubing to prevent inadvertent administration at a later time. Because of the rapid offset of action, no residual analgesic activity will be present within 5 to 10 minutes after discontinuation. For patients undergoing surgical procedures where postoperative pain is generally anticipated, administer alternative analgesics prior to discontinuation of remifentanil. The choice of analgesic should be appropriate for the patient's surgical procedure and the level of follow-up care.

➤*Preparation for administration:* To reconstitute solution, add 1 mL of diluent per mg of remifentanil. Shake well to dissolve. When reconstituted as directed, the solution contains approximately 1 mg of remifentanil activity per mL. Remifentanil should be diluted to a recommended final concentration of 20, 25, 50, or 250 mcg/mL prior to administration. Do not administer remifentanil without dilution.

Reconstitution and Dilution of Remifentanil		
Final concentration	Amount of remifentanil in each vial	Final volume after reconstitution and dilution
20 mcg/mL	1 mg 2 mg 5 mg	50 mL 100 mL 250 mL
25 mcg/mL	1 mg 2 mg 5 mg	40 mL 80 mL 200 mL
50 mcg/mL	1 mg 2 mg 5 mg	20 mL 40 mL 100 mL
250 mcg/mL	5 mg	20 mL

➤*Administration:* For intravenous (IV) use only. The injection site should be close to the venous cannula.

Single dose – Administer single IV dose over 30 to 60 seconds, beginning 90 seconds before the placement of the local or regional anesthetic block.

Continuous infusion – Administer over 30 to 60 seconds.

Administer continuous infusions of remifentanil only by an infusion device.

REMIFENTANIL HYDROCHLORIDE — INJECTION

Supplemental IV bolus – Use IV bolus administration of remifentanil only during the maintenance of general anesthesia.

➤*Admixture compatibility:*

Compatibility – Remifentanil is stable for 24 hours at room temperature after reconstitution and further dilution to concentrations of 20 to 250 mcg/mL with the following IV fluids: sterile water for injection; 5% dextrose injection; 5% dextrose and 0.9% sodium chloride injection; 0.9% sodium chloride injection; 0.45% sodium chloride injection; lactated Ringer's and 5% dextrose injection.

Remifentanil is stable for 4 hours at room temperature after reconstitution and further dilution to concentrations of 20 to 250 mcg/mL with lactated Ringer's injection.

Remifentanil has been shown to be compatible with propofol when coadministered into a running IV administration set.

Incompatibility – Nonspecific esterases in blood products may lead to the hydrolysis of remifentanil to its carboxylic acid metabolite. Therefore, administration of remifentanil into the same IV tubing with blood is not recommended.

➤*Storage/Stability:* Store at 2° to 25°C (36° to 77°F).

SUFENTANIL CITRATE

c-ii	**Sufentanil Citrate** (Various, eg, Baxter)	**Injection:** 50 mcg (as base)/mL	In 1, 2, and 5 mL amps and 1, 2, and 5 mL vials.
c-ii	**Sufenta** (Akorn)		Preservative free. In 1, 2, and 5 mL amps.

SUFENTANIL CITRATE — INJECTION

For complete prescribing information, refer to the Opioid Analgesics group monograph.

Indications

➤*Analgesia:* Analgesic adjunct for the maintenance of balanced general anesthesia in patients who are intubated and ventilated.

➤*Anesthetic:* As a primary anesthetic agent for the induction and maintenance of anesthesia with 100% oxygen in patients undergoing major surgical procedures. In patients who are intubated and ventilated, such as cardiovascular surgery or neurosurgical procedures in the sitting position, to provide favorable myocardial and cerebral oxygen balance or when extended postoperative ventilation is anticipated.

➤*Epidural analgesic:* For epidural administration as an analgesic combined with low-dose bupivacaine, usually 12.5 mg per administration, during labor and vaginal delivery.

Administration and Dosage

➤*General dosing considerations:* Individualize dosage.

Monitor vital signs routinely.

➤*Adults:*

Analgesia and anesthesia – See chart below.

Sufentanil Adult Dosage Range Chart — Analgesic Component to General Anesthesia (Total Dosage Requirements of 1 mcg/kg/h or Less are Recommended)

Total dosage	Maintenance dosage
Analgesic dosages	
Incremental or infusion: 1 to 2 mcg/kg (expected duration of anesthesia is 1 to 2 hours). Approximately ≥ 75% of total sufentanil dosage may be administered prior to intubation by either slow injection or infusion titrated to individual patient response. Dosages in this range are generally administered with nitrous oxide/oxygen in patients undergoing general surgery ≤ 8 hours in which endotracheal intubation and mechanical ventilation are required.	*Incremental:* 10 to 25 mcg (0.2 to 0.5 mL) may be administered in increments as needed when movement and/or changes in vital signs indicate surgical stress or lightening of analgesia. *Infusion:* Sufentanil may be administered as an intermittent or continuous infusion as needed in response to signs of lightening of analgesia. In absence of signs of lightening of analgesia, always adjust infusion rates downward until there is some response to surgical stimulation. Individualize supplemental dosages. Adjust maintenance infusion rates based upon the induction dose of sufentanil so that the total dose does not exceed 1 mcg/kg/h of expected surgical time. Individualize dosage and adjust to remaining operative time anticipated.
Analgesic dosages	
Incremental or infusion: 2 to 8 mcg/kg (expected duration of anesthesia is 2 to 8 hours). Approximately ≤ 75% of the total calculated sufentanil dosage may be administered by slow injection or infusion prior to intubation, titrated to individual patient response. Dosages in this range are generally administered with nitrous oxide/oxygen in more complicated major surgical procedures in which endotracheal intubation and mechanical ventilation are required. Provides some attenuation of sympathetic reflex activity in response to surgical stimuli, hemodynamic stability, and relatively rapid recovery.	*Incremental:* 10 to 50 mcg (0.2 to 1 mL) may be administered in increments as needed when movement and/or changes in vital signs indicate stress or lightening of analgesia. Individualize supplemental dosages. *Infusion:* Sufentanil may be administered as an intermittent or continuous infusion as needed in response to signs of lightening of analgesia. In the absence of signs of lightening of analgesia, infusion rates should always be adjusted downward until there is some response to surgical stimulation. Maintenance infusion rates should be adjusted based upon the induction dose of sufentanil so that the total dose does not exceed 1 mcg/kg/h of expected surgical time. Individualize dosage and adjust to remaining operative time anticipated.
Anesthetic dosages	
Incremental or infusion: 8 to 30 mcg/kg (anesthetic doses). At this anesthetic dosage range, sufentanil is generally administered as a slow injection, as an infusion, or as an injection followed by an infusion. Sufentanil with 100% oxygen and a muscle relaxant produces sleep at doses ≥ 8 mcg/kg and maintains a deep level of anesthesia without additional agents. The addition of N_2O to these dosages will reduce systolic blood pressure. At doses of up to 25 mcg/kg, catecholamine release is attenuated; dosages of 25 to 30 mcg/kg block sympathetic responses including catecholamine release. Use high doses in patients undergoing major surgical procedures in which endotracheal intubation and mechanical ventilation are required (eg, cardiovascular surgery and neurosurgery in the sitting position with maintenance of favorable myocardial and cerebral oxygen balance). Postoperative observation is essential and postoperative mechanical ventilation may be required at the higher dosage range because of extended postoperative respiratory depression. Titrate dosage to individual patient response.	*Incremental:* Depending on the initial dose, maintenance doses of 0.5 to 10 mcg/kg may be administered by slow injection in anticipation of surgical stress, such as incision, sternotomy, or cardiopulmonary bypass. *Infusion:* Sufentanil may be administered by continuous or intermittent infusion as needed in response to signs of lightening of anesthesia. In the absence of lightening of anesthesia, infusion rates should always be adjusted downward until there is some response to surgical stimulation. Base the maintenance infusion rate for sufentanil upon the induction dose so that the total dose for the procedure does not exceed 30 mcg/kg.

Epidural analgesic – 10 to 15 mcg administered with bupivacaine 0.125% 10 mL with or without epinephrine by slow injection. Mix sufentanil and bupivacaine together before administration. Doses can be repeated twice (for a total of 3 doses) at not less than 1-hour intervals until delivery. Closely monitor respiration following each administration of an epidural injection of sufentanil.

➤*Children:*

Anesthesia (undergoing cardiovascular surgery) –

2 to younger than 12 years of age:

• *Initial dosage* – 10 to 25 mcg/kg administered with 100% oxygen is recommended for induction of anesthesia.

• *Maintenance dosage* – Supplemental doses of up to 25 to 50 mcg are recommended for maintenance of anesthesia.

➤*Elderly:* Dosage should be reduced.

➤*Debilitated patients:* Dosage should be reduced.

➤*Obesity:* In obese patients (more then 20% above ideal body weight), the dosage of sufentanil should be determined on the basis of lean body weight.

➤*Concomitant medication:* If benzodiazepines, barbiturates, inhalation agents, other opioids, or CNS depressants are used concomitantly, the dose of sufentanil and/or these agents should be reduced. In all cases, dosage should be titrated to individual patient response.

The selection of preanesthetic medications should be based upon the needs of the individualized patient.

➤*Administration:* Administer by slow intravenous (IV) injection or IV infusion.

Epidural analgesic – Mix sufentanil and bupivacaine together before administration.

➤*Storage/Stability:* Store at 15° to 25°C (59° to 77°F). Protect from light.

TAPENTADOL

c-ii	**Nucynta** (PriCara)	**Tablets; oral:** 50 mg	As tapentadol hydrochloride. Lactose. (O-M 50). Yellow, round. Film-coated. In 100s and UD 10s.
		75 mg	As tapentadol hydrochloride. Lactose. (O-M 75). Yellow-orange, round. Film-coated. In 100s and UD 10s.
		100 mg	As tapentadol hydrochloride. Lactose. (O-M 100). Orange, round. Film-coated. In 100s and UD 10s.

TAPENTADOL HYDROCHLORIDE — ORAL

Indications

➤*Acute pain:* For the relief of moderate to severe acute pain in patients 18 years of age and older.

Administration and Dosage

➤*Adults:*

Acute pain –

Usual dosage: 50 to 100 mg every 4 to 6 hours. On the first day of dosing, the second dose may be administered as soon as 1 hour after the first dose if adequate pain relief is not attained with the first dose. Subsequent dosing is 50 to 100 mg every 4 to 6 hours.

Maximum dose: Daily doses greater than 700 mg on the first day of therapy and 600 mg on subsequent days have not been studied and are not recommended.

Dosage adjustment: Dosage should be adjusted to maintain adequate analgesia with acceptable tolerability.

Discontinuation of therapy: Withdrawal symptoms may occur if tapentadol is discontinued abruptly. These symptoms may include anxiety, sweating, insomnia, rigors, pain, nausea, tremors, diarrhea, upper respiratory tract symptoms, piloerection, and, rarely, hallucinations. Withdrawal symptoms may be reduced by tapering tapentadol.

➤*Children:* Not recommended for use in children younger than 18 years of age.

➤*Elderly:* Consider starting elderly patients with the lower range of recommended doses because elderly patients are more likely to have impaired renal or hepatic function.

➤*Renal function impairment:* Tapentadol has not been studied in patients with severe renal impairment. The use in this population is not recommended.

➤*Hepatic function impairment:*

Moderate hepatic function impairment – Initiate treatment at 50 mg with the interval between doses no less than every 8 hours. Further treatment should reflect maintenance of analgesia with acceptable tolerability, to be achieved by either shortening or lengthening the dosing interval.

Maximum dose: 3 doses in 24 hours.

Severe hepatic function impairment – Tapentadol has not been studied in patients with severe hepatic impairment; use in this population is not recommended.

➤*Administration:* May be given with or without food.

➤*Storage/Stability:* Store up to 25°C (77°F); excursions are permitted between 15° and 30°C (59° and 86°F). Protect from moisture.

TRAMADOL HYDROCHLORIDE

Rx	**Tramadol Hydrochloride** (Various, eg, Caraco, Eon, Mallinckrodt)	**Tablets; oral:** 50 mg	In 100s, 500s, and 1,000s.
Rx	**Ultram** (Janssen)		Lactose, PEG. (Ultram 0659). Capsule shape, scored. Film-coated. In 100s.
Rx	**Tramadol Hydrochloride** (Various, eg, Par, Patriot Pharmaceuticals)	**Tablets, extended-release; oral:** 100 mg	In 30s, 90s, and 500s.
Rx	**Ryzolt** (Purdue Pharma)		(PP 100). White, round. In 30s and 90s.
Rx	**Ultram ER** (Ortho-McNeil)		Polyvinyl alcohol. (100ER). White to off-white. In 30s.
Rx	**Tramadol Hydrochloride** (Various, eg, Par, Patriot Pharmaceuticals)	**Tablets, extended-release; oral:** 200 mg	In 30s, 90s, and 500s.
Rx	**Ryzolt** (Purdue Pharma)		(PP 200). White, round. In 30s and 90s.
Rx	**Ultram ER** (Ortho-McNeil)		Polyvinyl alcohol. (200ER). White to off-white. In 30s.
Rx	**Tramadol Hydrochloride** (Patriot Pharmaceuticals)	**Tablets, extended-release; oral:** 300 mg	In 30s and 90s.
Rx	**Ryzolt** (Purdue Pharma)		(PP 300). White, round. In 30s and 90s.
Rx	**Ultram ER** (Ortho-McNeil)		Polyvinyl alcohol. (300ER). White to off-white. In 30s.
Rx	**Rybix ODT** (Victory Pharma)	**Tablets, disintegrating; oral:** 50 mg	Aspartame, mannitol. (T 50). White. Mint flavor. In UD 30s.

TRAMADOL HYDROCHLORIDE — ORAL

For complete prescribing information, refer to the Opioid Analgesics group monograph.

Indications

➤*Immediate-release and orally disintegrating tablets:* Management of moderate to moderately severe pain in adults.

➤*Extended-release tablets:* Management of moderate to moderately severe chronic pain in adults who require around-the-clock treatment of pain for an extended period of time.

➤*Off-label uses:*

Premature ejaculation – [2] = Fair documentation. In a small, placebo-controlled trial, the use of tramadol in the management of premature ejaculation demonstrated significant improvements compared with placebo. Larger, controlled trials are needed before this agent can be recommended.

Restless legs syndrome – [4] = Insufficient documentation. Limited evidence is available regarding use of tramadol as a reasonable alternative in patients with restless legs syndrome (RLS) who have not responded to other drug therapies. In addition, adverse events or possible RLS augmentation have been reported with its use, and RLS guidelines include conflicting statements regarding its benefits. Larger, controlled trials are needed before the therapeutic benefits of tramadol can be established in RLS treatment.

Administration and Dosage

➤*General dosing considerations:* Good pain management practice dictates that the dose be individualized according to patient need using the lowest beneficial dose. Starting at the lowest possible dose and titrating upward as needed has resulted in increased tolerability and fewer discontinuations.

Concomitant therapy – The concomitant use of tramadol extended-release (ER) tablets with other tramadol products is not recommended.

➤*Adults:*

Immediate-release tablets –

Moderate to moderately severe chronic pain:

• *Maximum dose* – 400 mg/day.

• *Initial dosage* – 25 mg/day in the morning.

• *Dosage titration* – Titrate in 25 mg increments as separate doses every 3 days to reach 100 mg/day (25 mg 4 times/day). Thereafter, increase the total daily dose by 50 mg as tolerated every 3 days to reach 200 mg/day (50 mg 4 times/day).

• *Maintenance dosage* – After titration, administer 50 to 100 mg every 4 to 6 hours as needed for pain relief.

• *Alternative dosage* – For the subset of patients for whom rapid onset of analgesic effect is required and for whom the benefits outweigh the risk of discontinuation because of adverse reactions associated with higher initial doses, administer 50 to 100 mg every 4 to 6 hours as needed for pain relief.

Extended-release tablets –

Moderate to moderately severe chronic pain:

• *Maximum dose* – 300 mg/day.

• *Initial dosage* – For patients not currently treated with tramadol immediate-release products, tramadol ER tablets should be initiated at a dosage of 100 mg once daily.

• *Dosage titration* – Titrate as necessary by 100 mg increments every 5 days to relieve pain, depending upon tolerability.

• *Conversion* – For patients maintained on tramadol immediate-release products, calculate the 24-hour tramadol immediate-release dose and initiate a total daily dose of tramadol ER rounded down to the next lowest 100 mg increment. The dose may subsequently be individualized according to patient need. Because of limitations in flexibility of dose selection with tramadol ER, some patients maintained on tramadol immediate-release products may not be able to convert to tramadol ER.

TRAMADOL HYDROCHLORIDE — ORAL

Orally disintegrating tablets –

Moderate to moderately severe chronic pain:

• *Usual dosage* – 50 to 100 mg as needed for pain relief every 4 to 6 hours.

• *Maximum dose* – 400 mg/day.

• *Dosage titration* – For patients not requiring rapid onset of analgesic effect, the tolerability of tramadol can be improved by initiating therapy with a titration regimen. The total daily dose may be increased by 50 mg as tolerated every 3 days to reach 200 mg/day (50 mg 4 times daily). After titration, 50 to 100 mg can be administered as needed for pain relief every 4 to 6 hours not to exceed 400 mg/day.

• *Alternative dosage* – For patients for whom rapid onset of analgesic effect is required and for whom the benefits outweigh the risk of discontinuation due to adverse events associated with higher initial doses, 50 to 100 mg can be administered as needed for pain relief every 4 to 6 hours, not to exceed 400 mg/day.

Off-label dosing –

Premature ejaculation: [2] = Fair documentation. 50 mg administered 2 hours prior to sexual activity.

Restless legs syndrome: [4] = Insufficient documentation. 50 to 100 mg/day for up to 24 months. One patient received 150 mg daily. A summary of current guidelines and standards of practice recommends 50 to 400 mg daily to treat daily RLS symptoms.

➤*Elderly:* Use caution; start at the low end of the dosing range, reflecting the greater frequency of decreased hepatic, renal, or cardiac function, and of concomitant disease or other drug therapy.

Immediate-release and orally disintegrating tablets – Do not exceed 300 mg/day of tramadol immediate-release or orally disintegrating tablets in patients 75 years of age and older.

Extended-release tablets – ER tablets should be administered with even greater caution in patients older than 75 years of age because of the greater frequency of adverse reactions seen in this population.

➤*Renal function impairment:*

Maximum dose –

Immediate-release and orally disintegrating tablets: 200 mg/day.

Immediate-release and orally disintegrating tablets – In patients with a creatinine clearance (CrCl) less than 30 mL/min, increase the dosing interval to 12 hours.

Hemodialysis: Because hemodialysis only removes 7% of an administered dose, dialysis patients can receive their regular dose on the day of dialysis.

Extended-release tablets – ER tablets should not be used in patients with CrCl less than 30 mL/min.

➤*Hepatic function impairment:*

Immediate-release and orally disintegrating tablets – For adults with cirrhosis, the usual dosage is 50 mg every 12 hours.

Extended-release tablets – ER tablets should not be used in patients with severe hepatic function impairment (Child-Pugh class C).

➤*Administration:* Tramadol can be administered without regard to meals. ER tablets must be swallowed whole and must not be chewed, crushed, or split.

Do not chew, break, or split the orally disintegrating tablet. Place the orally disintegrating tablet on the tongue until it completely disintegrates and then swallow it. It may take approximately 1 minute for the tablet to disintegrate on the tongue. The orally disintegrating tablet may be taken with or without water.

➤*Storage / Stability:* Store at 25°C (77°F); excursions are permitted to 15° to 30°C (59° to 86°F).

OPIOID ANALGESIC COMBINATIONS

Content given per tablet; capsule; 5 mL oral solution, suspension, elixir; or suppository.

	Product and Distributor	Narcotic	Acetaminophen	Aspirin	Other Content	Average Adult Dose	How Supplied
c-v	**Acetaminophen and Codeine Oral Solution** (Various, eg, Morton Grove, Roxane)	12 mg codeine phosphate	120 mg			15 mL q 4 h	May contain alcohol. In 120 mL, pt and gal.
c-v	**Capital w/Codeine Suspension** (Carnrick)						Fruit punch flavor. In 473 mL.
c-v	**Tylenol w/Codeine Elixir** (McNeil)						7% alcohol, saccharin, sucrose. Cherry flavor. In 480 mL.
c-iii	**Acetaminophen and Codeine Tablets** (Various, eg, Lemmon)	15 mg codeine phosphate	300 mg			1 to 4 q 4 h	In 100s and 1000s.
c-iii	**Tylenol w/Codeine No. 2 Tablets** (McNeil)						Sodium metabisulfite. (McNeil Tylenol Codeine 2). White. In 100s and UD 500s.
c-iii	**Acetaminophen and Codeine Tablets** (Various, eg, Lemmon, Moore, Purepac, Roxane)	30 mg codeine phosphate	300 mg			0.5 to 2 q 4 h	In 100s, 1000s, and UD 100s.
c-iii	**Aceta w/Codeine Tablets** (Century)					1 tid	In 100s and 1000s.
c-iii	**Tylenol w/Codeine No. 3 Tablets** (McNeil)					0.5 to 2 q 4 h	Sodium metabisulfite. (McNeil Tylenol Codeine 3). White. In 100s, 500s, 1000s, and UD 500s.
c-iii	**Butalbital, Acetaminophen, Caffeine, and Codeine Phosphate Capsules** (Breckenridge)	30 mg codeine phosphate	325 mg		40 mg caffeine, 50 mg butalbital	1 or 2 q 4 h up to 6/day	May contain tartrazine. In 100s and 500s.
c-iii	**Fioricet w/Codeine Capsules** (Watson)						(Fioricet codeine). Dark blue/gray. In 100s and *ControlPak* 25s.
c-iii	**Phrenilin w/Caffeine and Codeine Capsules** (Valeant)						(A 061). Opaque lavender/opaque white. In 100s.
c-iii	**Cocet Tablets** (Poly Pharms)	30 mg codeine phosphate	650 mg			1 q 4 h up to 6/day	(POLY 316). White, scored, capsule shape. In 100s and 500s.
c-iii	**Vopac Tablets** (Athlon)					½ to 2 q 4 h up to 6/day	(CM 650). White, scored, capsule-shape. In 100s and 500s.
c-iii	**Aspirin and Codeine Phosphate Tablets** (Vintage)	15 mg codeine phosphate		325 mg		1 or 2 q 4 h as needed	In 100s, 500s, and 1000s.
c-iii	**Aspirin and Codeine No. 3 Tablets** (Various, eg, Goldline, Moore, Schein, URL, Zenith)	30 mg codeine phosphate		325 mg		1 or 2 q 4 h	In 100s, 500s, and 1000s.
c-iii	**Empirin w/Codeine No. 3 Tablets** (GlaxoWellcome)						(Empirin 3). White. In 100s, 500s, 1000s and *Dispenserpak* 25s.
c-iii	**Butalbital, Aspirin, Caffeine and Codeine Phosphate Capsules** (Watson)	30 mg codeine phosphate		325 mg	40 mg caffeine, 50 mg butalbital	1 or 2 q 4 h up to 6/day	(WATSON 3456). Blue/yellow. In 100s and 500s.
c-iii	**Ascomp with Codeine Capsules** (Breckenridge)						In 100s and 500s.
c-iii	**Fiorinal w/Codeine Capsules** (Watson)						(FIORINAL CODEINE WATSON 956). Blue/yellow. In 100s.
c-iii	**Acetaminophen and Codeine Tablets** (Various, eg, Lemmon, Moore, Purepac)	60 mg codeine phosphate	300 mg			1 q 4 h	In 100s, 500s, 1000s.
c-iii	**Tylenol w/Codeine No. 4 Tablets** (McNeil)						Sodium metabisulfite. (McNeil Tylenol Codeine 4). White. In 100s, 500s, and UD 500s.
c-iii	**Cocet Plus Tablets** (Poly Pharmaceuticals)	60 mg codeine phosphate	650 mg			1 q 4 h up to 6/day	(POLY 312 COCET PLUS). White, capsule shape. In 100s and 500s.

OPIOID ANALGESIC COMBINATIONS

	Product and Distributor	Narcotic	Acetaminophen	Aspirin	Other Content	Average Adult Dose	How Supplied
c-iii	**Aspirin and Codeine No. 4 Tablets** (Various, eg, Goldline, Major, Moore, URL, Zenith)	60 mg codeine phosphate		325 mg		1 q 4 h	In 100s, 500s, and 1000s.
c-iii	**Empirin w/Codeine No. 4 Tablets** (Glaxo-Wellcome)						(Empirin 4). White. In 100s, 500s, and *Dispenserpak* 25s.
c-iii	**Reprexain Tablets** (Hawthorn Pharm)	2.5 mg hydrocodone bitartrate			200 mg ibuprofen	1 q 4 to 6 h, up to 5/day	PEG, polydextrose. (IP 116). White, capsule shape. Film-coated. In 100s.
c-iii	**Ibudone Tablets** (Kowa Pharm)	5 mg hydrocodone bitartrate			200 mg ibuprofen	1 q 4 to 6, h up to 5/day	PEG. (3584 V). White, oval, scored. Film-coated. In 100s.
c-iii	**Reprexain Tablets** (Hawthorn Pharm)						PEG. (IP 146). White, oval. Film-coated. In 60s.
c-iii	**Hydrocodone Bitartrate and Ibuprofen Tablets** (Qualitest)	7.5 mg hydrocodone bitartrate			200 mg ibuprofen	1 q 4 to 6 h up to 5/day	Film-coated. In 10s, 100s, 500s, and 1000s.
c-iii	**Vicoprofen Tablets** (Abbott)						(VP). White. Film-coated. In 100s, 500s, and UD 100s.
c-iii	**Hydrocodone Bitartrate and Ibuprofen Tablets** (Qualitest)	10 mg hydrocodone bitartrate			200 mg ibuprofen	1 q 4 to 6, h up to 5/day	Film-coated. In 10s, 100s, and 1000s.
c-iii	**Ibudone Tablets** (Kowa Pharm)						PEG. (3586 V). Purple, scored, oval. Film-coated. In 100s.
c-iii	**Reprexain Tablets** (Hawthorn Pharm)						PEG. (IP 117). Yellow, round. Film-coated. In 100s.
c-iii	**Hycet Oral Solution** (Xanodyne)	2.5 mg hydrocodone bitartrate	108 mg			15 mL q 4 to 6 h up to 120 mL/day.	7% alcohol, glycerin, parabens, saccharin, sorbitol, sucrose. In 473 mL.
c-iii	**Hydrocodone Bitartrate and Acetaminophen Oral Solution** (Various, eg, Pharmaceutical Associates)	2.5 mg hydrocodone bitartrate	167 mg			15 mL q 4 to 6 h up to 90 mL/day	May contain 7% alcohol. In 473 mL.
c-iii	**Lortab Elixir** (UCB Pharma)						7% alcohol, saccharin, sorbitol, sucrose, parabens. Tropical fruit punch flavor. In 473 mL.
c-iii	**Hydrocodone Bitartrate and Acetaminophen Tablets** (Various, eg, Qualitest, Vintage Pharm)	2.5 mg hydrocodone bitartrate	500 mg			1 or 2 q 4 to 6 h up to 8/day	May contain sucrose. In 100s, 500s, and 1,000s.
c-iii	**Zolvit Liquid** (Atley Pharmaceuticals)	3.3 mg hydrocodone bitartrate	100 mg			11.25 mL q 4 to 6 h, up to 67.5 mL/day	Alcohol 7%, glycerin, parabens, propylene glycol, saccharin, sorbitol, sucrose. Tropical fruit punch flavor. In 473 mL.
c-iii	**Zamicet Oral Solution** (Hawthorn Pharm)	3.3 mg hydrocodone bitartrate	108.3 mg			15 mL q 4 to 6 h, up to 90 mL/day	6.7% alcohol, edetate disodium, glycerin, methylparaben, saccharin, sorbitol, sucrose. Fruit flavor. In 473 mL.
c-iii	**Liquicet Oral Solution** (Mallinckrodt)	3.3 mg hydrocodone bitartrate	167 mg			15 mL q 4 to 6 h up to 90 mL/day	Saccharin, sorbitol, sucrose. Raspberry flavor. In 473 mL.
c-iii	**Xodol Tablets** (Victory Pharma)	5 mg hydrocodone bitartrate	300 mg			1 or 2 q 4 to 6 h	(5 300 TP). White, scored, capsule shape. In 100s and 500s.

OPIOID ANALGESIC COMBINATIONS

	Product and Distributor	Narcotic	Acetaminophen	Aspirin	Other Content	Average Adult Dose	How Supplied
c-iii	**Hydrocodone Bitartrate and Acetaminophen Tablets** (Various, eg, Mallinckrodt, Watson)	5 mg hydrocodone bitartrate	325 mg			1 or 2 q 4 to 6 h up to 12/day	In 100s, 500s, 1000s, and UD 100s.
c-iii	**Anexsia Tablets** (Andrx)					1 or 2 q 4 to 6 h as needed up to 12/day	(M365). White, scored, capsule shape. In 100s and 1000s.
c-iii	**Norco 5/325 Tablets** (Watson)					1 to 2 q t to 6 h	Sucrose. (Watson 913). White with orange specks, scored, capsule shape. In 100s and 500s.
c-iii	**Zydone Tablets** (Endo)	5 mg hydrocodone bitartrate	400 mg			1 or 2 q 4 to 6 h up to 8/day	(E5). Yellow, octagonal. In 100s, 500s, and UD 100s.
c-iii	**Hydrocodone Bitartrate and Acetaminophen Capsules** (Various, eg, Goldline)	5 mg hydrocodone bitartrate	500 mg			1 or 2 q 4 to 6 h up to 8/day	In 100s and 500s.
c-iii	**Hydrocodone Bitartrate and Acetaminophen Tablets** (Various, eg, Geneva, Goldline, Moore, Watson, Vintage Pharm)						In 100s and 500s.
c-iii	**Ceta-Plus Capsules** (Seatrace)						(Seatrace). White. In 100s.
c-iii	**Co-Gesic Tablets** (Schwarz Pharma)						(500 5/SP 2104) White, scored, oval. In 100s.
c-iii	**Hydrocet Capsules** (Carnrick)						(C 8657). Blue/white. In 100s.
c-iii	**Hydrogesic Capsules** (Edwards)	5 mg hydrocodone bitartrate	500 mg			1 or 2 q 4 to 6 h up to 8/day	In 100s.
c-iii	**Hy-Phen Tablets** (B.F. Ascher)						(225-450). White, scored. Capsule shape. In 100s.
c-iii	**Margesic H Capsules** (Marnel)						(Margesic H). Gray/lavender. In 100s.
c-iii	**Lortab 5/500 Tablets** (UCB Pharma)						Sugar. (UCB 902). White w/blue specks, scored, capsule shape. In 100s, 500s, and UD 100s.
c-iii	**Anexsia 5/500 Tablets** (Mallinckrodt)						(BMP 207). White, scored. In 100s.
c-iii	**Stagesic Capsules** (Huckaby)	5 mg hydrocodone bitartrate	500 mg			1 to 2 q 4 to 6 h up to 8/day	Parabens. (Stagesic). White. In 100s.
c-iii	**T-Gesic Capsules** (T.E. Williams)					1 to 2 q 6 to 8 h	(T-Gesic/TEW). White. In 100s.
c-iii	**Vicodin Tablets** (Abbott)					1 to 2 q 4 to 6 h up to 8/day	(Vicodin). White, scored, capsule shape. In 100s, 500s, and UD 100s.
c-iii	**Xodol Tablets** (Victory Pharma)	7.5 mg hydrocodone bitartrate	300 mg			1 q 4 to 6 h up to 6/day.	(7.5 300 TP). White, capsule shape. In 100s.
c-iii	**Hydrocodone Bitartrate and Acetaminophen Tablets** (Various, eg, Mallinckrodt, Watson)	7.5 mg hydrocodone bitartrate	325 mg			1 q 4 to 6 h as needed up to 8/day	In 100s, 500s, 1000s, and UD 100s.
c-iii	**Anexsia Tablets** (Andrx)						(M366). White, oval. In 100s and 1000s.
c-iii	**Zydone Tablets** (Endo)	7.5 mg hydrocodone bitartrate	400 mg			1 q 4 to 6 h up to 6/day	(E 7.5). Blue, octagonal. In 100s and 500s.
c-iii	**Hydrocodone and Acetaminophen Tablets** (Various, eg, Watson, Vintage Pharm)	7.5 mg hydrocodone bitartrate	500 mg			1 q 4 to 6 h	In 100s and 500s.
c-iii	**Lortab 7.5/500 Tablets** (UCB Pharma)						Sucrose. (UCB/903). White w/green specks, scored, capsule shape. In 100s and 500s.

OPIOID ANALGESIC COMBINATIONS

	Product and Distributor	Narcotic	Acetaminophen	Aspirin	Other Content	Average Adult Dose	How Supplied
c-iii	**Hydrocodone Bitartrate and Acetaminophen Tablets** (Various, eg, King Pharm, Vintage Pharm)	7.5 mg hydrocodone bitartrate	650 mg			1 q 4 to 6 h up to 6/day	In 100s and 500s.
c-iii	**Anexsia 7.5/650 Tablets** (Mallinckrodt)						(BMP 188). Peach, scored, capsule shape. In 100s.
c-iii	**Lorcet Plus Tablets** (Forest)						(U 201). White, scored, capsule shape. In 100s and 500s.
c-iii	**Hydrocodone and Acetaminophen Tablets** (Various, eg, Barr, Geneva, Mallinckrodt, Royce, URL, Zenith Goldline, Vintage Pharm)	7.5 mg hydrocodone bitartrate	750 mg			1 q 4 to 6 h up to 6/day	In 100s, 500s, and 1000s.
c-iii	**Vicodin ES Tablets** (Abbott)					1 q 4 to 6 h up to 5/day	(Vicodin ES). White, scored, oval. In 100s and UD 100s.
c-iii	**Xodol Tablets** (Victory Pharma)	10 mg hydrocodone bitartrate	300 mg			1 q 4 to 6 h up to 6/day	(10 300 TP). White, capsule shape. In 100s and 500s.
c-iii	**Hydrocodone Bitartrate and Acetaminophen Tablets** (Various, eg. Mallinckrodt, Vintage Pharm)	10 mg hydrocodone bitartrate	325 mg			1 q 4 to 6 h up to 6/day	In 100s, 500s, and UD 100s.
c-iii	**Norco Tablets** (Watson Labs)						(NORCO 539). Yellow, scored, capsule shape. In 100s and 500s.
c-iii	**Zydone Tablets** (Endo)	10 mg hydrocodone bitartrate	400 mg			1 q 4 to 6 h up to 6/day	(E 10). Red, octagonal. In 100s, 500s, and UD 100s.
c-iii	**Hydrocodone Bitartrate and Acetaminophen Tablets** (Various, eg, Barr, Mallinckrodt, Qualitest, Watson, Vintage Pharm)	10 mg hydrocodone bitartrate	500 mg			1 q 4 to 6 h up to 6/day	In 30s, 60s, 90s, 100s, 120s, 180s, 500s, and 1000s.
c-iii	**Liquicet Oral Solution** (Mallinckrodt)					15 mL q 4 to 6 h up to 90 mL/day	Saccharin, sorbitol, sucrose. Raspberry flavor. In 473 mL.
c-iii	**Lortab 10/500 Tablets** (UCB Pharma)					1 q 4 to 6 h up to 6/day	(UCB/910). Pink, capsule shape. In 100s, 500s, and UD 100s.
c-iii	**Hydrocodone Bitartrate and Acetaminophen Tablets** (Various, eg, Major, Vintage Pharm)	10 mg hydrocodone bitartrate	650 mg			1 q 4 to 6 h up to 6/day	In 500s.
c-iii	**Lorcet 10/650 Tablets** (Forest)						(UAD 6350). Light blue, scored, capsule shape. In 100s and 500s.
c-iii	**Hydrocodone Bitartrate and Acetaminophen Tablets** (Various, eg, Inwood, Mallinckrodt, Vintage Pharm)	10 mg hydrocodone bitartrate	660 mg			1 q 4 to 6 h up to 6/day	In 100s and 500s.
c-iii	**Anexsia 10/660 Tablets** (Mallinckrodt)					1 q 4 to 6 h	(KPI 3). White, scored, capsule shape. In 100s and 1000s.
c-iii	**Vicodin HP Tablets** (Abbott)						(Vicodin HP). White, scored, oval. In 100s.
c-iii	**Hydrocodone Bitartrate and Acetaminophen Tablets** (Various, eg, Mallinckrodt, Watson)	10 mg hydrocodone bitartrate	750 mg			1 q 4 to 6 h, as needed up to 5/day.	In 100s, 500s, and UD 100s.
c-iii	**Maxidone Tablets** (Watson)					1 q 4 to 6 h, up to 5/day.	Lactose. (Maxidone 634). Yellow, scored, capsule shape. In 100s and 500s.
c-iii	**Trezix Capsules** (Wraser Pharm)	16 mg dihydrocodeine bitartrate	356.4 mg		30 mg caffeine	2 q 4 h, up to 10/day	(TREZIX). Red. In 100s.
c-iii	**Synalgos-DC Capsules** (Leitner)	16 mg dihydrocodeine bitartrate		356.4 mg	30 mg caffeine	2 q 4 h	(Wyeth 4191). Blue/gray. In 100s and 500s.

OPIOID ANALGESIC COMBINATIONS

OPIOID ANALGESIC COMBINATIONS

	Product and Distributor	Narcotic	Acetaminophen	Aspirin	Other Content	Average Adult Dose	How Supplied
c-iii	**Acetaminophen, Caffeine, and Dihydrocodeine Bitartrate Tablets** (Boca)	32 mg dihydrocodeine bitartrate	712.8 mg		60 mg caffeine	1 q 4 h, up to 5/day	(Boca 611). Oval, scored. In 30s.
c-iii	**Panlor SS Tablets** (Pan American Labs)						(PAL 032). Lavender, scored, oval. in 100s.
c-ii	**Percocet Tablets** (Endo)	2.5 mg oxycodone hydrochloride	325 mg			1 or 2 q 6 h, up to 12/day	(PERCOCET 2.5). Pink, oval. In 100s.
c-ii	**Primlev Tablets** (Atley Pharm)	5 mg oxycodone hydrochloride	300 mg			1 q 6 h, up to 12/day	(AP 681). Yellow, capsule shape. In 100s.
c-ii	**Acetaminophen and Oxycodone Tablets** (Various, eg, Goldline, Major)	5 mg oxycodone hydrochloride	325 mg			1 q 6 h	In 100s, 500s, 1000s, and UD 25s.
c-ii	**Endocet Tablets** (Endo Labs)						(Endo 602). White. In 100s and 500s.
c-ii	**Percocet Tablets** (Du Pont)						(Percocet 5). In 100s, 500s, and UD 100s.
c-ii	**Roxicet Tablets** (Roxane)						(54 543). White, scored. In 100s, 500s, and UD 100s.
c-ii	**Roxicet Oral Solution** (Roxane)					5 mL q 6 h	0.4% alcohol, EDTA, saccharin, sucrose. In 500 mL and UD 5 mL.
c-ii	**Magnacet Tablets** (Victory Pharma)	5 mg oxycodone hydrochloride	400 mg			1 q 6 h, up to 10/day	(ADG 5/400). Capsule shape. In 100s.
c-ii	**Oxycodone and Acetaminophen Capsules** (Various, eg, Goldline, Major, Schein)	5 mg oxycodone hydrochloride	500 mg			1 q 6 h	In 100s, 500s, 1000s, and UD 25s.
c-ii	**Roxicet 5/500 Tablets** (Roxane)						(54 730). White, scored. In 100s and UD 100s.
c-ii	**Roxilox Capsules** (Roxane)						(HD532). In 100s.
c-ii	**Tylox Capsules** (McNeil)						Sodium metabisulfite. (Tylox McNeil). Red. In 100s and UD 100s.
c-ii	**Primlev Tablets** (Atley Pharm)	7.5 mg oxycodone hydrochloride	300 mg			1 q 6 h, up to 8/day	(A P 682). Red, capsule shape. In 100s.
c-ii	**Oxycodone Hydrochloride and Acetaminophen Tablets** (Mallinckrodt)	7.5 mg oxycodone hydrochloride	325 mg			1 q 6 h prn, not to exceed 8 tablets/day	(M522 7.5/325). White to off-white, capsule shape. In 20s, 100s, 500s, 1000s, and UD 100s.
c-ii	**Endocet Tablets** (Endo)						(E700 7.5/325). Peach, capsule shape. In 100s and 500s.
c-ii	**Percocet Tablets** (Endo)						(PERCOCET 7.5/325). Peach, oval. In 100s.
c-ii	**Magnacet Tablets** (Victory Pharma)	7.5 mg oxycodone hydrochloride	400 mg			1 q 6 h, up to 8/day	(ADG 7.5/400). Capsule shape. In 100s.
c-ii	**Oxycodone Hydrochloride and Acetaminophen Tablets** (Mallinckrodt)	7.5 mg oxycodone hydrochloride	500 mg			1 q 6 h prn, not to exceed 8 tablets/day	(M582). White to off-white, oval. In 20s, 100s, 500s, 1000s, and UD 100s.
c-ii	**Endocet Tablets** (Endo)						(E796 7.5). Peach, capsule shape. In 100s and 500s.
c-ii	**Percocet Tablets** (Endo)					1 q 6 h	(PERCOCET 7.5). Peach, capsule shape. In 100s and 500s.
c-ii	**Primlev Tablets** (Atley Pharm)	10 mg oxycodone hydrochloride	300 mg			1 q 6 h up to 6/day	(A P 683). Orange, oval. In 100s.

OPIOID ANALGESIC COMBINATIONS

	Product and Distributor	Narcotic	Acetaminophen	Aspirin	Other Content	Average Adult Dose	How Supplied
c-ii	**Oxycodone Hydrochloride and Acetaminophen Tablets** (Mallinckrodt)	10 mg oxycodone hydrochloride	325 mg			1 q 6 h prn, not to exceed 6 tablets/day	(M523 10/325). White to off-white, capsule shape. In 20s, 100s, 500s, 1000s, and UD 100s.
c-ii	**Endocet Tablets** (Endo)						(E712 10/325). Yellow, oval. In 100s and 500s.
c-ii	**Percocet Tablets** (Endo)					1 q 6 h	In 100s, 500s, and UD 100s.
c-ii	**Magnacet Tablets** (Victory Pharma)	10 mg oxycodone hydrochloride	400 mg			1 q 6 h, up to 6/day	(ADG 10/400). Capsule shape. In 100s.
c-ii	**Xolox Tablets** (WraSer Pharm)	10 mg oxycodone hydrochloride	500 mg			1 q 6 h, up to 6/day	(10/500 WraSer). White, capsule shape. In 50s and 100s.
c-ii	**Oxycodone Hydrochloride and Acetaminophen Tablets** (Mallinckrodt)	10 mg oxycodone hydrochloride	650 mg			1 q 6 h prn, not to exceed 6 tablets/day	(M562). White to off-white, capsule shape. In 20s, 100s, 500s, 1000s, and UD 100s.
c-ii	**Endocet Tablets** (Endo)						(E797 10). Yellow, oval. In 100s and 500s.
c-ii	**Percocet Tablets** (Endo)					1 q 6 h	(PERCOCET 10). Yellow, oval. In 100s and 500s.
c-ii	**Oxycodone and Ibuprofen Tablets** (Various, eg, Watson, Barr)	5 mg oxycodone hydrochloride			400 mg ibuprofen	1 tablet, up to 4 per 24 h not to exceed 7 days	May contain lactose, polydextrose. In 30s, 100s, and 500s.
c-ii	**Oxycodone and Aspirin Tablets** (Various, eg, Goldline)	4.5 mg oxycodone hydrochloride, 0.38 mg oxycodone terephthalate		325 mg		1 q 6 h	In 100s, 500s, 1000s, and UD 25s.
c-ii	**Percodan Tablets** (Endo)						Yellow, scored. In 500s, 1000s, and UD 250s.
c-ii	**Roxiprin Tablets** (Roxane)						(54 902). White, scored. In 100s, 1000s, and UD 100s.
c-iv	**Propoxyphene Napsylate and Acetaminophen Tablets** (Various, eg, Moore)	50 mg propoxyphene napsylate	325 mg			2 q 4 h	In 100s, 500s, 550s, 1000s, and UD 100s.
c-iv	**Propoxyphene Napsylate and Acetaminophen Tablets** (Aristos)	100 mg propoxyphene napsylate	325 mg			1 q 4 h up to 6/day	Lactose, PEG. (P325). Violet, capsule shape. Film-coated. In 100s.
c-iv	**Trycet Tablets** (Auriga)						Lactose. (P325). Violet, capsule shape. Film-coated. In 100s.
c-iv	**Propoxyphene Napsylate and Acetaminophen Tablets** (Pliva)	100 mg propoxyphene napsylate	500 mg			1 q 4 h up to 6/day	Lactose. (P500). Pink. Film-coated. In 100s.
c-iv	**Darvocet A500 Tablets** (Xanodyne Pharm)						Film-coated. In 100s.
c-iv	**Propoxyphene Napsylate and Acetaminophen Tablets** (Various, eg, Zenith)	100 mg propoxyphene napsylate	650 mg			1 q 4 h	In 30s, 50s, 100s, 500s, 1,000s, and UD 100s.
c-iv	**Propoxyphene Hydrochloride and Acetaminophen Tablets** (Various, eg, Moore, Mylan)	65 mg propoxyphene hydrochloride	650 mg			1 q 4 h	In 500s.
c-ii	**Opium and Belladonna Suppositories** (Various, eg, Paddock)	30 mg powdered opium			16.2 mg powdered belladonna extract	1 or 2/day	May have a cocoa butter or polyethylene glycol/polysorbate 60 base. In 12s.
c-ii	**B & O Supprettes No. 15A Suppositories** (Amerifit)						Polyethylene glycol/polysorbate 60 base. Scored. In 12s.

OPIOID ANALGESIC COMBINATIONS

	Product and Distributor	Narcotic	Acetaminophen	Aspirin	Other Content	Average Adult Dose	How Supplied
c-ii	**Opium and Belladonna Suppositories** (Wyeth-Ayerst)	60 mg powdered opium			15 mg belladonna extract. Cocoa butter base	1 or 2/day	In 20s.
c-ii	**Opium and Belladonna Suppositories** (Various, eg, Paddock)				16.2 mg powdered belladonna extract	1 or 2/day	May have a cocoa butter or polyethylene glycol/polysorbate 60 base. In 12s and 20s.
c-ii	**B & O Supprettes No.16A Suppositories** (Amerifit)						Polyethylene glycol/polysorbate 60 base. Scored. In 12s.
c-ii	**Meperidine Hydrochloride and Promethazine Hydrochloride Capsules** (Ethex)	50 mg meperidine hydrochloride, 25 mg promethazine hydrochloride				1 every 4 to 6 hours	Lactose. (ETHEX 027). Opaque maroon. In 100s.
c-ii	**Meprozine Capsules** (Qualitest)						Lactose. (4206/V). Red. In 100s.
Rx	**Tramadol and Acetaminophen Tablets** (Par)	37.5 mg tramadol hydrochloride	325 mg			2 every 4 to 6 hours up to 8/day	(083 KALI). Orange, capsule shape. Film-coated. In 20s, 100s, and 500s.
Rx	**Ultracet Tablets** (Janssen Ortho)						(O-M 650). Lt. yellow, capsule shape. Film-coated. In 100s and UD 100s.

Mixed opioid agonist-antagonists (pentazocine, butorphanol, and nalbuphine) are primarily κ-opioid receptor agonists and μ-opioid receptor antagonists. They produce analgesia in nontolerant patients but may precipitate withdrawal in those dependent on morphine-like drugs.

A partial agonist analgesic (buprenorphine) is an antagonist at the κ-opioid receptor but is a partial agonist at the μ-opioid receptor. It may also precipitate withdrawal effects in those dependent on morphine-like drugs, but to a lesser degree than mixed agonist-antagonists. Partial agonists also produce less psychotomimetic effects that are seen with mixed agonist-antagonists.

Opioid Agonist-Antagonist Pharmacokinetics

Agonist/Antagonist		Onset (min)	Peak (min)	Duration (h)	Equivalent dose[a] (mg)	Relative antagonist activity
Buprenorphine	IM	15	60	≥ 6	0.3	Equipotent with naloxone
	IV[b]	-				
Butorphanol	IM	≤ 15	30-60	3-4	2	More potent than pentazocine, but less than naloxone
	IV	Few min	30-60	3-4		
	Nasal	≤ 15	60-120	4-5		
Nalbuphine	SC/IM	< 15	60	3-6	10	10 times that of pentazocine
	IV	2-3	nd[c]			
Pentazocine	SC/IM	15-20	15-60	4-6	30	Weak
	IV	2-3	nd	nd		
	Oral	15-30	nd	≥ 3		

[a] Parenteral dose equivalent to 10 mg morphine.
[b] When given IV, the time to onset and peak effect are shortened
[c] nd – no data

BUPRENORPHINE

c-iii	**Buprenorphine** (Various, eg, Roxane Labs, Teva)	**Tablets; sublingual:** 2 mg	As buprenorphine hydrochloride. May contain lactose, mannitol. In 30s.
c-iii	**Subutex** (Reckitt Benckiser)		As buprenorphine hydrochloride. Lactose, mannitol. White, oval. In 30s.
c-iii	**Buprenorphine** (Various, eg, Roxane Labs, Teva)	**Tablets; sublingual:** 8 mg	As buprenorphine hydrochloride. May contain lactose, mannitol. In 30s.
c-iii	**Subutex** (Reckitt Benckiser)		As buprenorphine hydrochloride. Lactose, mannitol. White, oval. In 30s.
c-iii	**Buprenorphine Hydrochloride** (Hospira)	**Injection, solution:** 0.3 mg/mL	Equiv. to buprenorphine hydrochloride 0.324 mg/mL. In 1 mL *Carpuject*.
c-iii	**Buprenex** (Reckitt Benckiser)		Equiv. to buprenorphine hydrochloride 0.324 mg/mL. Dextrose 50 mg. In 1 mL amps.
c-iii	**Butrans** (Purdue)	**Patch; transdermal:** 5 mcg/h[a]	In cartons of 4.
		10 mcg/h[b]	
		20 mcg/h[c]	

[a] Patch contains a total of buprenorphine 5 mg.
[b] Patch contains a total of buprenorphine 10 mg.
[c] Patch contains a total of buprenorphine 20 mg.

BUPRENORPHINE HYDROCHLORIDE — ORAL

Refer to the general discussion in the Opioid Agonist-Antagonist Analgesic introduction.

Indications

➤*Opioid dependence:* For the treatment of opioid dependence.

Administration and Dosage

➤*General dosing considerations:* Following induction, buprenorphine/naloxone is preferred when clinical use includes unsupervised administration because of the presence of naloxone. The use of buprenorphine for unsupervised administration should be limited to patients who cannot tolerate buprenorphine/naloxone, for example, those patients who have been shown to be hypersensitive to naloxone.

Induction – Buprenorphine sublingual tablets contain no naloxone and are preferred for use during induction. Prior to induction, consider the type of opioid dependence (ie, long- or short-acting opioid), the time since last opioid use, and the degree or level of opioid dependence. To avoid precipitating withdrawal, induction with buprenorphine should be undertaken when objective and clear signs of withdrawal are evident.

➤*Adults:*

Opioid dependence –

Initial dosage: 8 mg on day 1 and 16 mg on day 2. From day 3 onward, patients received buprenorphine/naloxone at the same buprenorphine dose as day 2.

In some studies, gradual induction over several days led to a high dropout rate of buprenorphine patients during the induction period. Therefore, it is recommended that an adequate maintenance dose, titrated to clinical effectiveness, should be achieved as rapidly as possible to prevent undue opioid withdrawal symptoms.

Maintenance dosage: 12 to 16 mg/day.

Buprenorphine/naloxone is the preferred medication for maintenance treatment because of the presence of naloxone in the formulation.

Discontinuation of therapy: The decision to discontinue therapy with buprenorphine after a period of maintenance or brief stabilization should be made as part of a comprehensive treatment plan. Both gradual and abrupt discontinuations have been used, but no controlled trials have been undertaken to determine the best method of dose tapering at the end of treatment.

➤*Children:*

Opioid dependence –

16 years of age and older: See Adults for dosing.

➤*Patients taking heroin or other short-acting opioids:* At treatment initiation, the dose of buprenorphine should be administered at least 4 hours after the patient last used opioids, or preferably when early signs of opioid withdrawal appear.

➤*Patients taking methadone or other long-acting opioids:* There is little controlled experience with the transfer of methadone-maintained patients to buprenorphine. Available evidence suggests that withdrawal symptoms are possible during induction to buprenorphine treatment. Withdrawal appears more likely in patients maintained on higher doses of methadone (more than 30 mg) and when the first buprenorphine dose is administered shortly after the last methadone dose.

➤*Administration:* Administer sublingually as a single daily dose.

Buprenorphine tablets should be placed under the tongue until they are dissolved. For doses requiring the use of more than 2 tablets, patients are advised to either place all the tablets under the tongue at once or, alternatively, if they cannot comfortably fit in more than 2 tablets, place 2 tablets at a time under the tongue. Either way, the patients should continue to hold the tablets under the tongue until they dissolve; swallowing the tablets reduces the bioavailability of the drug.

➤*Storage/Stability:* Store at 25°C (77°F); excursions are permitted between 15° and 30°C (59° and 86°F).

Actions

➤*Pharmacology:* Buprenorphine is a partial agonist at the mu-opioid receptor and an antagonist at the kappa-opioid receptor.

Pharmacodynamics –

Subjective effects: Comparisons of buprenorphine with full agonists, such as methadone and hydromorphone, suggest that sublingual buprenorphine produces typical opioid agonist effects, which are limited by a ceiling effect.

In nondependent subjects, short-term sublingual doses of buprenorphine/naloxone produced opioid agonist effects, which reached a maximum between doses of buprenorphine 8 and 16 mg. The effects of buprenorphine/naloxone 16 mg were similar to those produced by buprenorphine 16 mg (buprenorphine alone).

Opioid agonist ceiling effects were also observed in a double-blind, parallel group, dose-ranging comparison of single doses of buprenorphine sublingual solution (1, 2, 4, 8, 16, or 32 mg), placebo, and a full agonist control at various doses. The treatments were given in ascending dose order at intervals of at least 1 week to 16 opioid-experienced, nondependent subjects. Both drugs

BUPRENORPHINE HYDROCHLORIDE — ORAL

produced typical opioid agonist effects. For all the measures for which the drugs produced an effect, buprenorphine produced a dose-related response; however, in each case, there was a dose that produced no further effect. In contrast, the highest dose of the full agonist control always produced the greatest effects. Agonist objective rating scores remained elevated longer for the higher doses of buprenorphine (8 to 32 mg) than for the lower doses and did not return to baseline until 48 hours after drug administrations. The onset of effects appeared more rapidly with buprenorphine than with the full agonist control, with most doses nearing peak effect after 100 minutes for buprenorphine compared with 150 minutes for the full agonist control.

➤*Pharmacokinetics:*

Absorption – Plasma levels of buprenorphine increased with the dose. There was a wide inter-patient variability in the sublingual absorption of buprenorphine, but within subjects, the variability was low. Both maximal drug concentration (C_{max}) and area under the curve (AUC) of buprenorphine increased in a linear fashion with the dose increase (range, 4 to 16 mg), although the increase was not directly dose-proportional.

Buprenorphine Oral Mean (% CV[a]) Pharmacokinetic Parameters	
Pharmacokinetic parameter	Buprenorphine 16 mg
C_{max} (ng/mL)	5.47 (23)
AUC_{0-48} (ng•hr/mL)	32.63 (25)

[a] CV = coefficient of variation.

Distribution – Buprenorphine is approximately 96% protein bound, primarily to alpha- and beta-globulin.

Metabolism – Buprenorphine undergoes N-dealkylation to norbuprenorphine and glucuronidation. The N-dealkylation pathway is mediated by cytochrome P450 3A4 isozyme. Norbuprenorphine, an active metabolite, can further undergo glucuronidation.

Excretion – A mass balance study of buprenorphine showed complete recovery of radiolabel in urine (30%) and feces (69%) collected up to 11 days after dosing. Almost all of the dose was accounted for in terms of buprenorphine, norbuprenorphine, and 2 unidentified buprenorphine metabolites. In urine, most of the buprenorphine and norbuprenorphine was conjugated (buprenorphine, 1% free, 9.4% conjugated; norbuprenorphine, 2.7% free, and 11% conjugated). In feces, almost all of the buprenorphine and norbuprenorphine were free (buprenorphine, 33% free, and 5% conjugated; norbuprenorphine, 21% free, 2% conjugated).

Buprenorphine has a mean elimination half-life from plasma of 37 hours.

Special populations –

Hepatic function impairment: The effect of hepatic impairment on the pharmacokinetics of buprenorphine is unknown. Because it is extensively metabolized, the plasma levels will be expected to be higher in patients with moderate and severe hepatic impairment. Therefore, adjust dosage in patients with hepatic impairment and observe patients for symptoms of precipitated opioid withdrawal.

Contraindications

Hypersensitivity to buprenorphine.

Warnings/Precautions

➤*Respiratory depression:* Significant respiratory depression has been associated with buprenorphine, particularly by the intravenous (IV) route. A number of deaths have occurred when addicts have misused buprenorphine IV, usually when coadministered with benzodiazepines. Deaths have also been reported in association with coadministration of buprenorphine with other depressants, such as alcohol or other opioids. Warn patients of the potential danger of the self-administration of benzodiazepines or other depressants while under treatment with buprenorphine.

In the case of overdose, the primary management should be the reestablishment of adequate ventilation with mechanical assistance of respiration, if required. Naloxone may not be effective in reversing any respiratory depression produced by buprenorphine.

Use buprenorphine with caution in patients with compromised respiratory function (eg, chronic obstructive pulmonary disease, cor pulmonale, decreased respiratory reserve, hypoxia, hypercapnia, preexisting respiratory depression).

➤*Hepatic effects:* Cases of cytolytic hepatitis and hepatitis with jaundice have been observed in the addict population receiving buprenorphine in clinical trials and in postmarketing adverse event reports. The spectrum of abnormalities ranges from transient asymptomatic elevations in hepatic transaminases to case reports of hepatic failure, hepatic necrosis, hepatorenal syndrome, and hepatic encephalopathy. In many cases, the presence of preexisting liver enzyme abnormalities, infection with hepatitis B or C virus, concomitant usage of other potentially hepatotoxic drugs, and ongoing IV drug use may have played a causative or contributory role. In other cases, insufficient data were available to determine the cause of the abnormality. The possibility exists that buprenorphine had a causative or contributory role in the development of the hepatic abnormality in some cases. Measurements of liver function tests prior to initiation of treatment is recommended to establish a baseline. Periodic monitoring of liver function tests during treatment is also recommended. A biological and causal evaluation is recommended when a hepatic event is suspected. Depending on the case, carefully discontinue the drug to prevent withdrawal symptoms and a return to illicit drug use, and initiate strict monitoring of the patient.

➤*Hypotensive effects:* Like other opioids, buprenorphine may produce orthostatic hypotension.

➤*Head injury and increased intracranial pressure:* Buprenorphine, like other potent opioids, may elevate cerebrospinal fluid pressure; use with caution in patients with head injury, intracranial lesions, and other circumstances where cerebrospinal pressure may be increased. Buprenorphine can produce miosis and changes in the level of consciousness that may interfere with patient evaluation.

➤*GI conditions:* Buprenorphine has been shown to increase intracholedochal pressure, as do other opioids; therefore, administer with caution to patients with dysfunction of the biliary tract.

As with other mu-opioid receptor agonists, the administration of buprenorphine may obscure the diagnosis or clinical course of patients with acute abdominal conditions.

➤*Hypersensitivity reactions:* Cases of short- and long-term hypersensitivity to buprenorphine have been reported in clinical trials and in the postmarketing experience. The most common signs and symptoms include rashes, hives, and pruritus. Cases of bronchospasm, angioneurotic edema, and anaphylactic shock have been reported. A history of hypersensitivity to buprenorphine is a contraindication to buprenorphine.

➤*Renal function impairment:* Use with caution in patients with severe renal impairment.

➤*Hepatic function impairment:* Buprenorphine is extensively metabolized; therefore, the plasma levels will be expected to be higher in patients with moderate and severe hepatic impairment. Adjust dosage and watch patients for symptoms of precipitated opioid withdrawal. Use with caution in patients with severe hepatic impairment.

➤*Special risk:* Administer buprenorphine with caution in elderly or debilitated patients and those with severe impairment of pulmonary function, myxedema or hypothyroidism, adrenal cortical insufficiency (eg, Addison disease), CNS depression or coma, toxic psychoses, prostatic hypertrophy or urethral stricture, acute alcoholism, delirium tremens, or kyphoscoliosis.

➤*Drug abuse and dependence:* Buprenorphine is controlled as a schedule III narcotic under the Controlled Substances Act.

Buprenorphine is a partial-agonist at the mu-opioid receptor and long-term administration produces dependence of the opioid type, characterized by moderate withdrawal upon abrupt discontinuation or rapid taper. The withdrawal syndrome is milder than that seen with full agonists, and may be delayed in onset.

Neonatal withdrawal has been reported in the infants of women treated with buprenorphine during pregnancy.

➤*Hazardous tasks:* Buprenorphine may impair the mental or physical abilities required for the performance of potentially dangerous tasks, such as driving a car or operating machinery, especially during drug induction and dose adjustment. Caution patients about operating hazardous machinery, including automobiles, until they are reasonably certain that buprenorphine therapy does not adversely affect their ability to engage in such activities.

➤*Pregnancy:* Category C. There are no adequate and well-controlled studies of buprenorphine in pregnant women. Use buprenorphine only during pregnancy if the potential benefit justifies the potential risk to the fetus.

Neonatal withdrawal – Neonatal withdrawal has been reported in the infants of women treated with buprenorphine during pregnancy. From postmarketing reports, the time to onset of neonatal withdrawal symptoms ranged from days 1 to 8 of life, with most occurring on day 1. Adverse reactions associated with neonatal withdrawal syndrome included hypertonia, neonatal tremor, neonatal agitation, and myoclonus. There have been rare reports of convulsions and in 1 case, apnea and bradycardia were also reported.

Teratogenic – Significant increases in skeletal abnormalities (eg, extra thoracic vertebra, thoraco-lumbar ribs) were noted in rats after subcutaneous administration of 1 mg/kg/day and up (estimated exposure was approximately 0.6 times the recommended human daily sublingual dose of 16 mg on a mg/m^2 basis), but were not observed at oral dosages of up to 160 mg/kg/day. Increases in skeletal abnormalities in rabbits after IM administration of 5 mg/kg/day (estimated exposure was approximately 6 times the recommended human daily sublingual dose of 16 mg on a mg/m^2 basis) or oral administration of 1 mg/kg/day or greater (estimated exposure was approximately equal to the recommended human daily sublingual dose of 16 mg on a mg/m^2 basis) were not statistically significant.

In rabbits, buprenorphine produced statistically significant preimplantation losses at oral dosages of 1 mg/kg/day or greater and postimplantation losses that were statistically significant at IV dosages of 0.2 mg/kg/day or greater (estimated exposure was approximately 0.3 times the recommended human daily sublingual dose of 16 mg on a mg/m^2 basis).

Nonteratogenic – Dystocia was noted in pregnant rats treated with buprenorphine 5 mg/kg/day intramuscularly (IM) (approximately 3 times the recommended human daily sublingual dose of 16 mg on a mg/m^2 basis). Both fertility and peri- and postnatal development studies with buprenorphine in rats indicated increases in neonatal mortality after oral dosages of 0.8 mg/kg/day and up (approximately 0.5 times the recommended human daily sublingual dose of 16 mg on a mg/m^2 basis), after IM dosages of 0.5 mg/kg/day and up (approximately 0.3 times the recommended human daily sublingual dose of 16 mg on a mg/m^2 basis), and after subcutaneous dosages of 0.1 mg/kg/day and up (approximately 0.06 times the recommended human daily sublingual dose of 16 mg on a mg/m^2 basis). Delays in the occurrence of righting reflex and startle response were noted in rat pups at an oral dosage of 80 mg/kg/day (approximately 50 times the recommended human daily sublingual dose of 16 mg on a mg/m^2 basis).

➤*Lactation:* An apparent lack of milk production during general reproduction studies with buprenorphine in rats caused decreased viability and lac-

BUPRENORPHINE HYDROCHLORIDE — ORAL

tation indices. Use of high doses of sublingual buprenorphine in pregnant women showed that buprenorphine passes into the mother's milk. Because depression of the breast-feeding infant resulting in lower weight gain is a possibility, breast-feeding is not advised in mothers treated with buprenorphine.

➤*Children:* Buprenorphine is not recommended for use in children. The safety and effectiveness of buprenorphine in patients younger than 16 years of age have not been established.

➤*Monitoring:* Monitor all patients receiving opioids for signs of abuse, misuse, and addiction.

Measurements of liver function tests prior to initiation of treatment is recommended to establish a baseline. Periodic monitoring of liver function tests during treatment is also recommended.

Drug Interactions

➤*QT prolongation:* An additive effect of buprenorphine with other drugs that prolong the QT interval cannot be excluded. The following drugs may prolong the QT interval and increase the risk of life-threatening cardiac arrhythmias, including torsades de pointes: antiarrhythmic agents (eg, amiodarone, bretylium, disopyramide, dofetilide, procainamide, quinidine, sotalol), arsenic trioxide, chlorpromazine, cisapride, dolasetron, droperidol, gatifloxacin, halofantrine, levomethadyl, mefloquine, mesoridazine, moxifloxacin, pentamidine, pimozide, probucol, sparfloxacin, thioridazine, ziprasidone.

Buprenorphine Drug Interactions

Precipitant drug	Object drug[a]		Description
Barbiturate anesthetics (eg, thiopental)	Buprenorphine	⬆	Barbiturate anesthetics may increase the respiratory and CNS depression of buprenorphine because of additive pharmacologic activity. Monitor the patient and adjust the buprenorphine dose as needed.
Buprenorphine	Barbiturate anesthetics (eg, thiopental)		
Benzodiazepines (eg, diazepam)	Buprenorphine	⬆	Coma and death have been associated with the concomitant IV misuse of buprenorphine and benzodiazepines by addicts. Use with caution. Warn patients of the potential danger of self-administration of benzodiazepines while receiving treatment with buprenorphine.
Cimetidine	Buprenorphine	⬆	The risk of buprenorphine CNS toxicity may be increased. Monitor the patient. If excessive CNS or respiratory depression occurs, discontinue both drugs. Give a narcotic antagonist (eg, naloxone) if needed.
CNS depressants (eg, alcohol, benzodiazepines, general anesthetics, opioid analgesics, phenothiazines, other tranquilizers, sedative/hypnotics, other CNS depressants)	Buprenorphine	⬆	Patients receiving both agents may exhibit increased CNS depression. When combined therapy is contemplated, consider reduction of the dose of one or both agents.
CYP3A4 inducers (eg, carbamazepine, phenobarbital, phenytoin, rifampin)	Buprenorphine	⬇	Although not investigated, it is recommended to closely monitor patients when buprenorphine is coadministered with a CYP3A4 inducer. May cause possible increased clearance. Adjust the buprenorphine dose as needed.
CYP3A4 inhibitors (ie, azole antifungals [eg, ketoconazole, voriconazole], macrolide antibiotics [eg, erythromycin], protease inhibitors [eg, indinavir, ritonavir])	Buprenorphine	⬆	Coadministration may increase buprenorphine plasma concentrations and the risk of adverse reactions. Closely monitor the patient. Buprenorphine dosage adjustment may be required.
MAOIs[b] (eg, phenelzine)	Buprenorphine	⬌	Exercise caution. Specific information is not available.
Naltrexone	Buprenorphine	⬇	Naltrexone may decrease or attenuate the pharmacologic effects of buprenorphine. Precipitation of withdrawal symptoms may occur. Closely monitor for signs of buprenorphine withdrawal or reduced efficacy. Detoxify buprenorphine-dependent patients before starting treatment with naltrexone. If there is any question of occult buprenorphine dependence, perform a naltrexone challenge test and defer treatment until the naltrexone challenge is negative. Make cardiopulmonary resuscitation staff and equipment available for patients receiving naltrexone extended-release injection requiring emergency pain management with opioids.
Sodium oxybate (GHB)	Buprenorphine	⬆	Concurrent use may result in increased sleep duration and CNS depression because of additive pharmacologic activity. Coadministration of sodium oxybate is contraindicated with other sedative-hypnotics.
Buprenorphine	Sodium oxybate (GHB)		
Buprenorphine	Methadone	⬇	Buprenorphine may decrease or attenuate the pharmacologic effects of methadone. Precipitation of withdrawal symptoms may occur. Closely monitor for signs of opioid withdrawal or reduced opioid efficacy. Do not administer buprenorphine to patients with dependence on methadone.
Buprenorphine	Nondepolarizing muscle relaxants (eg, tubocurarine)	⬆	Concurrent use may enhance neuromuscular blocking action and increase respiratory depression. If coadministration cannot be avoided, monitor respiratory function and be prepared to provide life support if needed.

[a] ⬆ = object drug increased; ⬇ = object drug decreased; ⬌ = undetermined clinical effect.

[b] MAOIs = monoamine oxidase inhibitors.

Adverse Reactions

➤*Adverse reactions (5% or more):*

Buprenorphine Oral Adverse Reactions (≥ 5%) in a 4-Week Study

Adverse reactions	Buprenorphine 16 mg/day (n = 103)	Buprenorphine/ Naloxone 16 mg/day (n = 107)	Placebo (n = 107)
CNS			
Asthenia	4.9%	6.5%	6.5%
Chills	7.8%	7.5%	7.5%
Headache	29.1%	36.4%	22.4%
Insomnia	21.4%	14%	15.9%
GI			
Abdominal pain	11.7%	11.2%	6.5%
Constipation	7.8%	12.1%	2.8%
Diarrhea	4.9%	3.7%	15%
Nausea	13.6%	15%	11.2%
Vomiting	7.8%	7.5%	4.7%
Miscellaneous			
Back pain	7.8%	3.7%	11.2%
Infection	11.7%	5.6%	6.5%
Pain	18.4%	22.4%	18.7%
Rhinitis	9.7%	4.7%	13.1%
Sweating	12.6%	14%	10.3%
Vasodilation	3.9%	9.3%	6.5%
Withdrawal syndrome	18.4%	25.2%	37.4%

BUPRENORPHINE HYDROCHLORIDE — ORAL

Buprenorphine Oral Solution Adverse Reactions (≥ 5%) in a 16-Week Study					
	Buprenorphine dose[a]				
Adverse reactions	Very low[a] (n = 184)	Low[a] (n = 180)	Moderate[a] (n = 186)	High[a] (n = 181)	Total[a] (n = 731)
CNS					
Anxiety	12%	13%	11%	14%	12%
Asthenia	14%	16%	14%	13%	14%
Chills	6%	7%	5%	6%	6%
Depression	13%	9%	13%	10%	11%
Dizziness	2%	5%	4%	6%	4%
Headache	28%	34%	29%	29%	30%
Insomnia	23%	28%	23%	28%	25%
Nervousness	7%	6%	5%	7%	6%
Somnolence	3%	7%	5%	6%	5%
GI					
Constipation	5%	13%	12%	14%	11%
Diarrhea	10%	4%	5%	2%	5%
Dyspepsia	3%	6%	2%	2%	3%
Nausea	7%	12%	12%	10%	10%
Vomiting	4%	3%	5%	8%	5%
Respiratory					
Cough increase	3%	6%	3%	2%	4%
Pharyngitis	3%	4%	3%	5%	4%
Rhinitis	15%	9%	8%	12%	11%
Miscellaneous					
Abscess	5%	1%	2%	1%	2%
Accidental injury	3%	6%	3%	3%	3%
Back pain	10%	16%	15%	15%	14%
Fever	4%	1%	1%	6%	3%
Flu syndrome	2%	7%	10%	4%	6%
Infection	17%	22%	20%	22%	20%
Pain	26%	21%	26%	24%	24%
Runny eyes	7%	5%	3%	3%	5%
Sweat	13%	12%	11%	13%	12%
Withdrawal syndrome	24%	22%	22%	20%	22%

[a] Sublingual solution. Doses in this table cannot necessarily be delivered in tablet form, but for comparison purposes: "very low" dose (1 mg solution) would be less than a tablet dose of 2 mg; "low" dose (4 mg solution) approximates a 6 mg tablet dose; "moderate" dose (8 mg solution) approximates a 12 mg tablet dose; "high" dose (16 mg solution) approximates a 24 mg tablet dose.

Overdosage

➤*Symptoms:* Manifestations of acute overdose include death, hypotension, pinpoint pupils, respiratory depression, and sedation.

➤*Treatment:* Carefully monitor the respiratory and cardiac status of the patient. In the event of depression of respiratory or cardiac function, give primary attention to the reestablishment of adequate respiratory exchange through provision of a patent airway and institution of assisted or controlled ventilation. Employ oxygen, IV fluids, vasopressors, and other supportive measures as indicated.

In the case of overdose, the primary management should be the reestablishment of adequate ventilation with mechanical assistance of respiration, if required. Naloxone may not be effective in reversing any respiratory depression produced by buprenorphine.

High doses of naloxone (10 to 35 mg per 70 kg) may be of limited value in the management of buprenorphine overdose. Doxapram, a respiratory stimulant, also has been used.

Patient Information

Inform patients and their family members to inform the treating health care provider or emergency room staff in the event of an emergency that the patient is physically dependent on opioids and that the patient is being treated with buprenorphine.

Advise patients that a serious overdose may occur if benzodiazepines, sedatives, tranquilizers, antidepressants, or alcohol are taken at the same time as buprenorphine.

Advise patients that buprenorphine may impair the mental or physical abilities required for the performance of potentially dangerous tasks, such as driving a car or operating machinery, especially during drug induction and dose adjustment. Advise patients not to drive or operate complex machinery until they know how buprenorphine affects their ability to function in these circumstances.

Advise patients to consult their health care provider if other prescription medications are currently being used or are prescribed for future use.

Advise patients that buprenorphine may cause orthostatic hypotension and to use caution when rising from a sitting or lying position.

BUPRENORPHINE HYDROCHLORIDE — INJECTION

Refer to the general discussion in the Opioid Agonist-Antagonist Analgesic introduction.

Indications

➤*Moderate to severe pain:* For the relief of moderate to severe pain.

Administration and Dosage

➤*Adults:*

Moderate to severe pain –

Usual dosage: 0.3 mg given by deep intramuscular (IM) or slow (over at least 2 minutes) intravenous (IV) injection at up to 6-hour intervals, as needed. Repeat once (up to 0.3 mg), if required, 30 to 60 minutes after initial dosage, taking the previous dose's pharmacokinetics into consideration, and thereafter only as needed.

Alternative dosage: Occasionally, it may be necessary to administer single doses of up to 0.6 mg IM, depending on the severity of the pain and the response of the patient. This dose should only be given IM and only to adult patients not in a high-risk category.

➤*Children:*

Moderate to severe pain –

13 years of age and older: See Adults for dosing.

2 to 12 years of age:

• *Usual dosage* – 2 to 6 mcg/kg of body weight IM or slow IV (over at least 2 minutes) given every 4 to 6 hours.

There is insufficient experience to recommend the use of a repeat or second dose at 30 to 60 minutes (such as is used in adults).

Because there is some evidence that not all children excrete buprenorphine faster than adults, fixed-interval or 24-hour dosing should not be undertaken until the proper interdose interval has been established by clinical observation of the child. Health care providers should recognize that, as with adults, some children may not need to be remedicated for 6 to 8 hours.

• *Maximum dose* – There is insufficient experience to recommend single doses greater than 6 mcg/kg of body weight.

➤*Elderly:* Reduce the dose by approximately one-half. Exercise extra caution with the IV route of administration, particularly with the initial dose.

➤*High-risk patients:* Reduce the dose by approximately one-half in high-risk patients (eg, in the presence of respiratory disease, debilitated patients) and/or in patients in whom other CNS depressants are present, such as in the immediate postoperative period. Exercise extra caution with the IV route of administration, particularly with the initial dose.

➤*Administration:* For deep IM or slow IV (over at least 2 minutes) administration only.

➤*Storage/Stability:* Avoid excessive heat (greater than 40°C [104°F]). Protect from prolonged exposure to light.

Actions

➤*Pharmacology:* Buprenorphine, a parenteral opioid analgesic, exerts its analgesic effect via high affinity binding to mu subclass opiate receptors in the CNS. Although buprenorphine may be classified as a partial agonist, under the conditions of recommended use it behaves very much like classical mu-agonists, such as morphine. One unusual property of buprenorphine observed in in vitro studies is its very slow rate of dissociation from its receptor. This could account for its longer duration of action than morphine, the unpredictability of its reversal by opioid antagonists, and its low level of manifest physical dependence.

Buprenorphine 0.3 mg is approximately equivalent to morphine 10 mg in analgesic and respiratory depressant effects in adults.

Narcotic antagonist activity – Buprenorphine demonstrates narcotic antagonist activity and has been shown to be equipotent with naloxone as an antagonist of morphine in the mouse tail flick test.

Pharmacodynamics –

Cardiovascular effects: Buprenorphine may cause a decrease or, rarely, an increase in pulse rate and blood pressure in some patients.

Effects on respiration: Under usual conditions of use in adults, buprenorphine and morphine show similar dose-related respiratory depressant effects. At adult therapeutic doses, buprenorphine 0.3 mg can decrease respiratory rate in an equivalent manner to an equianalgesic dose of morphine 10 mg.

➤*Pharmacokinetics:*

Absorption – Pharmacological effects occur as soon as 15 minutes after IM injection and persist for 6 hours or longer. Peak pharmacologic effects usually are observed at 1 hour. When used IV, the times to onset and peak effect are shortened.

Metabolism/Excretion – Buprenorphine, like morphine and other phenolic opioid analgesics, is metabolized by the liver and has a clearance

BUPRENORPHINE HYDROCHLORIDE — INJECTION

related to hepatic blood flow. Studies in patients anesthetized with halothane 0.5% have shown that this anesthetic decreases hepatic blood flow by approximately 30%.

In postoperative adults, pharmacokinetic studies have shown elimination half-lives ranging from 1.2 to 7.2 hours (mean 2.2 hours) after IV administration of buprenorphine 0.3 mg.

Special populations –

Children: A single 10-patient pharmacokinetic study of doses of 3 mcg/kg in children 5 to 7 years of age showed high interpatient variability, but suggests that the clearance of the drug may be higher in children than in adults. This is supported by at least 1 repeat-dose study in postoperative pain that showed an optimal interdose interval of 4 to 5 hours in children as opposed to the recommended 6 to 8 hours in adults.

Contraindications

Known hypersensitivity to the drug.

Warnings/Precautions

➤*Respiratory depression:* As with other potent opioids, clinically significant respiratory depression may occur within the recommended dose range in patients receiving therapeutic doses of buprenorphine. Use buprenorphine with caution in patients with compromised respiratory function (eg, chronic obstructive pulmonary disease, cor pulmonale, decreased respiratory reserve, hypoxia, hypercapnia, preexisting respiratory depression). Particular caution is advised if buprenorphine is administered to patients taking or recently receiving drugs with CNS/respiratory depressant effects. In patients with the physical and/or pharmacological risk factors above, reduce the dose by approximately one-half.

Naloxone may not be effective in reversing the respiratory depression produced by buprenorphine. Therefore, as with other potent opioids, reestablish the primary management of overdose of adequate ventilation with mechanical assistance of respiration, if required.

➤*Head injury and increased intracranial pressure:* Buprenorphine, like other potent analgesics, may elevate cerebrospinal fluid pressure. Use with caution in patients with head injury, intracranial lesions, and other circumstances where cerebrospinal pressure may be increased. Buprenorphine can produce miosis and changes in the level of consciousness, which may interfere with patient evaluation.

➤*GI conditions:* Buprenorphine has been shown to increase intracholedochal pressure to a similar degree as other opioid analgesics; administer with caution to patients with dysfunction of the biliary tract.

➤*Narcotic-dependent patients:* Because of the narcotic antagonist activity of buprenorphine, use in the physically dependent individual may result in withdrawal effects.

➤*Renal function impairment:* Use with caution in patients with severe renal impairment.

➤*Hepatic function impairment:* Because buprenorphine is metabolized by the liver, the activity of buprenorphine may be increased and/or extended in those individuals with impaired hepatic function or those receiving other agents known to decrease hepatic clearance. Use with caution in patients with severe hepatic impairment.

➤*Special risk:* Administer buprenorphine with caution in elderly patients; debilitated patients; children; patients with severe pulmonary impairment; myxedema, hypothyroidism, adrenal cortical insufficiency (eg, Addison disease), CNS depression or coma, toxic psychoses, prostatic hypertrophy or urethral stricture, acute alcoholism, delirium tremens, or kyphoscoliosis.

➤*Drug abuse and dependence:* Buprenorphine is a partial agonist of the morphine type (ie, it has certain opioid properties that may lead to psychic dependence of the morphine type because of an opiate-like euphoric component of the drug). Direct dependence studies have shown little physical dependence upon withdrawal of the drug. However, use caution in prescribing to individuals who are known to be drug abusers or ex-narcotic addicts. The drug may not be a substitute in acutely dependent narcotic addicts because of its antagonist component, and may induce withdrawal symptoms.

➤*Hazardous tasks:* Buprenorphine may impair the mental or physical abilities required for the performance of potentially dangerous tasks, such as driving a car or operating machinery. Therefore, administer buprenorphine with caution to ambulatory patients and warn them to avoid such hazards.

➤*Pregnancy:* *Category C.* There are no adequate and well-controlled studies in pregnant women. Use buprenorphine during pregnancy only if the potential benefit justifies the potential risk to the fetus.

Teratogenic – Significant increases in skeletal abnormalities (eg, extra thoracic vertebra, thoraco-lumbar ribs) were noted in rats after subcutaneous administration of 1 mg/kg/day and up (approximately 9.5 times the recommended human daily dose of 1.2 mg on a mg/m^2 basis) and in rabbits after IM administration of 5 mg/kg/day (approximately 95 times the recommended human daily dose of 1.2 mg on a mg/m^2 basis), but these increases were not statistically significant. Increases in skeletal abnormalities after oral administration were not observed in rats, and increases in rabbits (1 to 25 mg/kg/day) were not statistically significant.

➤*Lactation:* An apparent lack of milk production during general reproduction studies with buprenorphine in rats caused decreased viability and lactation indices. Use of high doses of sublingual buprenorphine in pregnant women showed that buprenorphine passes into the mother's milk. Breastfeeding is not advised in women treated with buprenorphine because depression of the breast-feeding infant resulting in lower weight is a possibility.

➤*Children:* The safety and efficacy of buprenorphine have been established for children between 2 and 12 years of age. Use of buprenorphine in children is supported by evidence from adequate and well-controlled trials of buprenorphine in adults, with additional data from studies of 960 children ranging from 9 months to 18 years of age. Data are available from a pharmacokinetic study, several controlled clinical trials, and several large postmarketing studies and case series. The available information provides reasonable evidence that buprenorphine may be used safely in children ranging from 2 to 12 years of age, and that it is of similar effectiveness in children as in adults.

➤*Monitoring:* Monitor all patients receiving opioids for signs of abuse, misuse, and addiction.

Drug Interactions

➤*QT prolongation:* An additive effect of buprenorphine with other drugs that prolong the QT interval cannot be excluded. The following drugs may prolong the QT interval and increase the risk of life-threatening cardiac arrhythmias, including torsades de pointes: antiarrhythmic agents (eg, amiodarone, bretylium, disopyramide, dofetilide, procainamide, quinidine, sotalol), arsenic trioxide, chlorpromazine, cisapride, dolasetron, droperidol, gatifloxacin, halofantrine, levomethadyl, mefloquine, mesoridazine, moxifloxacin, pentamidine, pimozide, probucol, sparfloxacin, thioridazine, ziprasidone.

Buprenorphine Drug Interactions

Precipitant drug	Object drug[a]		Description
Barbiturate anesthetics (eg, thiopental)	Buprenorphine	↑	Barbiturate anesthetics may increase respiratory and CNS depression because of additive pharmacologic activity. Monitor the patient and adjust the buprenorphine dose as needed.
Buprenorphine	Barbiturate anesthetics (eg, thiopental)		
Benzodiazepines (eg, diazepam)	Buprenorphine	↑	Coma and death have been associated with the concomitant IV misuse of buprenorphine and benzodiazepines by addicts. There have been reports of respiratory and cardiovascular collapse in patients who received therapeutic doses of diazepam and buprenorphine. Use with caution. Warn patients of the potential danger of self-administration of benzodiazepines while receiving treatment with buprenorphine.
Cimetidine	Buprenorphine	↑	The risk of buprenorphine CNS toxicity may be increased. Monitor the patient. If excessive CNS or respiratory depression occurs, discontinue both drugs. Give a narcotic antagonist (eg, naloxone) if needed.
CNS depressants (eg, alcohol, benzodiazepines, general anesthetics, opioid analgesics, phenothiazines, other tranquilizers, sedative/hypnotics, other CNS depressants)	Buprenorphine	↑	Patients receiving both agents may exhibit increased CNS depression. When combined therapy is contemplated, consider reduction of the dose of 1 or both agents. Caution patients about risks associated with concurrent use of buprenorphine and CNS depressants.
CYP3A4 inducers (eg, carbamazepine, phenobarbital, phenytoin, rifampin)	Buprenorphine	↓	Although not investigated, it is recommended to closely monitor patients when buprenorphine is coadministered with a CYP3A4 inducer. May cause possible increased clearance. Adjust the buprenorphine dose as needed.
CYP3A4 inhibitors (ie, azole antifungals [eg, ketoconazole, voriconazole], macrolide antibiotics [eg, erythromycin], protease inhibitors [eg, ritonavir])	Buprenorphine	↑	Coadministration may increase buprenorphine plasma concentrations and the risk of adverse reactions. Closely monitor the patient. Buprenorphine dosage adjustment may be required.
MAOIs[b] (eg, phenelzine)	Buprenorphine	↔	Exercise caution. Specific information is not available.

BUPRENORPHINE HYDROCHLORIDE — INJECTION

Buprenorphine Drug Interactions

Precipitant drug	Object drug[a]		Description
Naltrexone	Buprenorphine	⬇	Naltrexone may decrease or attenuate the pharmacologic effects of buprenorphine. Precipitation of withdrawal symptoms may occur. Closely monitor for signs of buprenorphine withdrawal or reduced efficacy. Detoxify buprenorphine-dependent patients before treatment with naltrexone. If there is any question of occult buprenorphine dependence, perform a naltrexone challenge test and defer treatment until the naltrexone challenge is negative. Make cardiopulmonary resuscitation staff and equipment available for patients receiving naltrexone extended-release injection requiring emergency pain management with opioids.
Sodium oxybate (GHB)	Buprenorphine	⬆	Concurrent use may result in increased sleep duration and CNS depression because of additive pharmacologic activity. Coadministration of sodium oxybate is contraindicated with other sedative-hypnotics.
Buprenorphine	Sodium oxybate (GHB)		
Buprenorphine	Methadone	⬇	Buprenorphine may decrease or attenuate the pharmacologic effects of methadone. Precipitation of withdrawal symptoms may occur. Closely monitor for signs of opioid withdrawal or reduced opioid efficacy. Do not administer buprenorphine to patients with dependence on methadone.
Buprenorphine	Nondepolarizing muscle relaxants (eg, tubocurarine)	⬆	Concurrent use may enhance neuromuscular blocking action and increase respiratory depression. If coadministration cannot be avoided, monitor respiratory function and be prepared to provide life support if needed.

[a] ⬆ = object drug increased; ⬇ = object drug decreased; ⟷ = undetermined clinical effect.
[b] MAOIs = monoamine oxidase inhibitors.

Adverse Reactions

➤*Most common adverse reaction:* The most frequent adverse reaction in clinical studies involving 1,133 patients was sedation, which occurred in approximately two-thirds of the patients. Although sedated, these patients could easily be aroused to an alert state.

➤*Cardiovascular:* Hypotension (1% to 5%); bradycardia, hypertension, tachycardia, Wenckebach block (less than 1%).

➤*CNS:* Dizziness/vertigo (5% to 10%); headache (1% to 5%); chills/cold, confusion, depression, dreaming, euphoria, fatigue, nervousness, paresthesia, psychosis, slurred speech, weakness (less than 1%).

➤*Dermatologic:* Sweating (1% to 5%); pruritus (less than 1%).

➤*GI:* Nausea (5% to 10%); nausea/vomiting, vomiting (1% to 5%); constipation, dry mouth (less than 1%).

➤*Hypersensitivity:* Cases of short- and long-term hypersensitivity to buprenorphine have been reported in clinical trials and in postmarketing reports of buprenorphine and other buprenorphine-containing products. The most common signs and symptoms include hives, pruritus, and rashes. Cases of anaphylactic shock, angioneurotic edema, and bronchospasm have been reported. A history of hypersensitivity to buprenorphine is a contraindication to buprenorphine.

➤*Respiratory:* Hypoventilation (1% to 5%); cyanosis, dyspnea (less than 1%).

➤*Special senses:* Miosis (1% to 5%); blurred vision, conjunctivitis, diplopia, tinnitus, visual abnormalities (less than 1%).

➤*Miscellaneous:* Flushing/warmth, injection-site reaction, and urinary retention (less than 1%).

➤*Other adverse reactions:* Other adverse reactions observed infrequently include amblyopia, apnea, coma, depersonalization, dyspepsia, flatulence, hallucination, malaise, pallor, rash, and tremor.

The following adverse reactions have been reported to occur rarely: convulsions/lack of muscle coordination, diarrhea, dysphoria/agitation, loss of appetite, and urticaria.

Overdosage

➤*Symptoms:* Clinical experience with buprenorphine overdosage has been insufficient to define the signs of this condition at this time. Although the antagonist activity of buprenorphine may become manifest at doses somewhat above the recommended therapeutic range, doses in the recommended therapeutic range may produce clinically significant respiratory depression in certain circumstances.

➤*Treatment:* Carefully monitor the respiratory and cardiac status of the patients. Give primary attention to the reestablishment of adequate respiratory exchange through provision of a patent airway and institution of assisted or controlled ventilation. Employ oxygen, IV fluids, vasopressors, and other supportive measures as indicated. Doxapram, a respiratory stimulant, may be used.

Naloxone may not be effective in reversing the respiratory depression produced by buprenorphine. Therefore, as with other potent opioids, the primary management of overdose should be the reestablishment of adequate ventilation with mechanical assistance of respiration, if required.

Patient Information

Advise patients that the effects of buprenorphine, particularly drowsiness, may be potentiated by other centrally acting agents, such as alcohol or benzodiazepines. It is particularly important that patients not drive or operate machinery in these circumstances.

Inform patients that buprenorphine has some pharmacologic effects similar to morphine, which may lead to self-administration of the drug when pain no longer exists in susceptible patients. Patients must not exceed the dosage of buprenorphine prescribed by their health care provider.

Advise patients to consult their health care provider if other prescription medications are currently being used or are prescribed for future use.

BUPRENORPHINE — TRANSDERMAL

Refer to the general discussion in the Opioid Agonist-Antagonist Analgesics introduction.

WARNING

Proper patient selection – The transdermal formulation of buprenorphine is indicated for the management of moderate to severe chronic pain in patients requiring a continuous, around-the-clock opioid analgesic for an extended period of time.

Potential for abuse – Buprenorphine is a mu opioid partial agonist and a schedule III controlled substance. Buprenorphine can be abused in a manner similar to other opioid agonists, legal or illicit. Consider the abuse potential when prescribing or dispensing buprenorphine in situations in which the health care provider or pharmacist is concerned about an increased risk of misuse, abuse, or diversion.

People at increased risk of opioid abuse include those with a personal or family history of substance abuse (including drug or alcohol abuse or addiction) or mental illness (eg, major depression). Assess patients for their clinical risks of opioid abuse or addiction prior to prescribing opioids. Routinely monitor all patients receiving opioids for signs of misuse, abuse, and addiction.

Limitations of use – Do not exceed a dose of 1 buprenorphine 20 mcg/h system because of the risk of QTc interval prolongation.

Avoid exposing the buprenorphine system application site and surrounding area to direct external heat sources. Temperature-dependent increases in buprenorphine release from the system may result in overdose and death.

Indications

➤*Moderate to severe chronic pain:* Management of moderate to severe chronic pain in patients requiring a continuous, around-the-clock opioid analgesic for an extended period of time.

Administration and Dosage

➤*General dosing considerations:*

Each buprenorphine system is intended to be worn for 7 days.

➤*Adults:*

Moderate to severe chronic pain –

Maximum dose: One 20 mcg/h transdermal system.

Initial dosage: It is critical to initiate the dosing regimen individually for each patient. Overestimating the buprenorphine dose when converting patients from another opioid medication can result in fatal overdose with the first dose.

• *Opioid-naive patients* – Initiate treatment with 5 mcg/h.

Dosage titration: Based on the patient's requirement for supplemental short-acting analgesics, upward titration may be instituted with a minimum buprenorphine titration interval of 72 hours, based on the pharmacokinetic profile and time to reach steady-state levels. Individually titrate the dose, under close supervision, to a level that provides adequate analgesia with tolerable adverse effects.

Duration of therapy: During long-term opioid analgesic therapy with buprenorphine, reassess the continued need for around-the-clock opioid analgesic therapy periodically.

Discontinuation of therapy: When the patient no longer requires therapy with buprenorphine, taper the dose gradually to prevent signs and symp-

BUPRENORPHINE — TRANSDERMAL

toms of withdrawal in the physically dependent patient; consider introduction of an appropriate immediate-release opioid medication. Undertake discontinuation of therapy as part of a comprehensive treatment plan.

Supplemental analgesia: The intent of the titration period is to establish a patient-specific weekly buprenorphine dose that will maintain adequate analgesia with tolerable adverse reactions for as long as pain management is necessary. Immediate-release opioid and non-opioid medications can be used as supplemental analgesia during buprenorphine therapy.

➤*Hepatic function impairment:*

Mild to moderate hepatic impairment – Start patients with mild to moderate hepatic impairment with the buprenorphine 5 mcg/h dosage. Thereafter, individually titrate the dosage to a level that provides adequate analgesia and tolerable adverse effects under the close supervision of the health care provider.

Severe hepatic impairment – Buprenorphine has not been evaluated in patients with severe hepatic impairment. Because buprenorphine is only intended for 7-day application, consider use of an alternate analgesic that may permit more flexibility with the dosing in patients with severe hepatic impairment.

➤*Administration:* Buprenorphine is for transdermal use (on intact skin) only and should be applied to the upper outer arm, upper chest, upper back, or the side of the chest. These 4 sites (each present on both sides of the body) provide 8 possible application sites. Rotate buprenorphine among the 8 described skin sites. After buprenorphine removal, wait a minimum of 21 days before reapplying to the same skin site.

Apply buprenorphine to a hairless or nearly hairless skin site. If none are available, the hair at the site should be clipped, not shaven. Do not apply buprenorphine to irritated skin. If the application site must be cleaned, clean the site with water only. Do not use soaps, alcohol, oils, lotions, or abrasive devices. Allow the skin to dry before applying buprenorphine.

Apply immediately after removal from the individually sealed pouch. Do not use buprenorphine if the pouch seal is broken or the patch is cut, damaged, or changed in any way. Do not cut the transdermal system.

If problems with adhesion of buprenorphine occur, the edges may be taped with first aid tape.

If buprenorphine falls off during the 7-day dosing interval, dispose of the transdermal system properly and place a new buprenorphine system at a different skin site.

If the buprenorphine-containing adhesive matrix accidentally contacts the skin, wash the area with water. Do not use soap, alcohol, or other solvents to remove the adhesive because they may enhance the absorption of the drug.

When changing the system, remove buprenorphine, fold it over on itself, and flush it down the toilet. Alternatively, buprenorphine can be sealed in the patch-disposal unit provided and then disposed of in the trash. Never throw buprenorphine away in the trash without sealing it in the patch-disposal unit.

➤*Storage/Stability:* Store at 25°C (77°F); excursions are permitted between 15° and 30°C (59° and 86°F).

Actions

➤*Pharmacology:* Buprenorphine is a partial agonist at mu-opioid receptors. Buprenorphine is also an antagonist at kappa-opioid receptors, an agonist at delta-opioid receptors, and a partial agonist at ORL-1 (nociceptin) receptors. Its clinical actions result from binding to the opioid receptors.

Pharmacodynamics –

Cardiovascular effects: Buprenorphine may cause a reduction in blood pressure.

CNS effects: Buprenorphine binds to and dissociates from the mu-opioid receptor slowly.

Electrophysiology: There was no clinically meaningful effect on mean QTc with a buprenorphine transdermal system dose of 10 mcg/h. A buprenorphine dose of 40 mcg/h (given as 2 buprenorphine 20 mcg/h) prolonged mean QTc by a maximum of 9.2 msec (90% confidence interval, 5.2 to 13.3) across the 13 assessment time points.

Endocrine effects: Opioids may influence the hypothalamic-pituitary-adrenal or -gonadal axes. Some changes that can be seen include an increase in serum prolactin, and decreases in plasma cortisol and testosterone. Clinical symptoms may be manifest from these hormonal changes.

Other effects: Buprenorphine causes dose-related miosis and produces urinary retention in some patients.

➤*Pharmacokinetics:*

Absorption – Transdermal delivery studies showed that intact human skin is permeable to buprenorphine. In clinical pharmacology studies, the median time for buprenorphine 10 mcg/h to deliver quantifiable buprenorphine concentrations (at least 25 pg/mL) was approximately 17 hours. The absolute bioavailability of buprenorphine transdermal system relative to intravenous (IV) administration, following a 7-day application, is approximately 15% for all doses (buprenorphine 5, 10, and 20 mcg/h).

Each buprenorphine transdermal system provides delivery of buprenorphine for 7 days. Steady state was achieved during the first application by day 3.

Buprenorphine transdermal system 5, 10, and 20 mcg/h provide dose-proportional total buprenorphine exposures (area under the curve [AUC]) following 7-day applications. Plasma buprenorphine concentrations after titration showed no further change over the 60-day period studied.

Buprenorphine Transdermal System Pharmacokinetic Parameters (Single 7-day Application) Mean (CV%[a])

Dose	AUC_{inf} (pg•h/mL)	C_{max}[a] (pg/mL)
Buprenorphine transdermal system 5 mcg/h	12,087 (37)	176 (67)
Buprenorphine transdermal system 10 mcg/h	27,035 (29)	191 (34)
Buprenorphine transdermal system 20 mcg/h	54,294 (36)	471 (49)

[a] CV = coefficient of variation; C_{max} = maximal drug concentration.

Distribution – Buprenorphine is approximately 96% bound to plasma proteins, mainly to alpha- and beta-globulin.

Studies of IV buprenorphine have shown a large volume of distribution (approximately 430 L), implying extensive distribution of buprenorphine.

Following IV administration, buprenorphine and its metabolites are secreted into bile and excreted in urine. Cerebrospinal fluid (CSF) buprenorphine concentrations appear to be approximately 15% to 25% of concurrent plasma concentrations.

Metabolism – Buprenorphine metabolism in the skin following buprenorphine application is negligible. Following transdermal application, buprenorphine is eliminated via hepatic metabolism, with subsequent biliary excretion and renal excretion of soluble metabolites.

Buprenorphine primarily undergoes N-dealkylation by cytochrome P450 3A4 (CYP3A4) to norbuprenorphine and glucuronidation by UGT-isoenzymes (mainly UGT1A1 and 2B7) to buprenorphine 3-O-glucuronide. Norbuprenorphine, the major metabolite, is also glucuronidated (mainly UGT1A3) prior to excretion.

Norbuprenorphine is the only known active metabolite of buprenorphine. It has been shown to be a respiratory depressant in rats, but only at concentrations at least 50-fold greater than those observed following application to humans of buprenorphine 20 mcg/h.

Because metabolism and excretion of buprenorphine occur mainly via hepatic elimination, reductions in hepatic blood flow induced by some general anesthetics (eg, halothane) and other drugs may result in a decreased rate of hepatic elimination of the drug, resulting in increased plasma concentrations.

Excretion – Following intramuscular administration of buprenorphine 2 mcg/kg, approximately 70% of the dose was excreted in feces within 7 days. Approximately 27% was excreted in urine. The total clearance of buprenorphine is approximately 55 L/h in postoperative patients.

After removal of buprenorphine transdermal system, mean buprenorphine concentrations decrease approximately 50% within 10 to 24 hours, followed by decline with an apparent terminal half-life of approximately 26 hours.

Special populations –

Elderly: Following a single application of buprenorphine 10 mcg/h to 12 healthy young adults (mean, 32 years of age) and 12 healthy elderly subjects (mean, 72 years of age), the pharmacokinetic profile of buprenorphine was similar in healthy elderly and healthy young adult subjects, though the elderly subjects showed a trend toward higher plasma concentrations immediately after buprenorphine removal. Both groups eliminated buprenorphine at similar rates after system removal.

Application site: A study in healthy subjects demonstrated that the pharmacokinetic profile of buprenorphine delivered by buprenorphine transdermal system 10 mcg/h is similar when applied to the upper outer arm, upper chest, upper back, or the side of the chest.

The reapplication of buprenorphine 10 mcg/h after various rest periods to the same application site in healthy subjects showed that the minimum rest period needed to avoid variability in drug absorption is 3 weeks (21 days).

External heat: In a study of healthy subjects, application of a heating pad directly on the buprenorphine transdermal 10 mcg/h system caused a 26% to 55% increase in blood concentrations of buprenorphine. Concentrations returned to normal within 5 hours after the heat was removed. For this reason, avoid applying heating pads directly to the buprenorphine transdermal system during system.

Endotoxin challenge: Fever may increase the permeability of the skin, leading to increased buprenorphine concentrations during buprenorphine transdermal system treatment. As a result, febrile patients are at increased risk of the possibility of buprenorphine transdermal system–related reactions during treatment with buprenorphine. Monitor patients with febrile illness for adverse effects and consider dose adjustment. In a crossover study of healthy subjects receiving endotoxin or placebo challenge during buprenorphine 10 mcg/h wear, the AUC and C_{max} were similar despite a physiologic response of mild fever to endotoxin.

Flux determination: Buprenorphine flux for the 7-day application period was established to be 5, 10, and 20 mcg/h for buprenorphine transdermal system containing buprenorphine 5, 10, and 20 mg, respectively.

Contraindications

Patients who have significant respiratory depression; severe bronchial asthma; paralytic ileus or suspected paralytic ileus; known hypersensitivity to any of its components or the active ingredient, buprenorphine; management of acute pain or in patients who require opioid analgesia for a short period of time; management of postoperative pain, including use after outpatient or day surgeries; management of mild pain; management of intermittent pain (eg, use on an as-needed basis).

BUPRENORPHINE — TRANSDERMAL

Warnings/Precautions

➤*Respiratory depression:* Respiratory depression is the chief hazard of buprenorphine. Respiratory depression occurs more frequently in elderly or debilitated patients, as well as those suffering from conditions accompanied by hypoxia or hypercapnia when even moderate therapeutic doses may dangerously decrease pulmonary ventilation, and when opioids, including buprenorphine, are given in conjunction with other agents that depress respiration.

Profound sedation, unresponsiveness, infrequent deep (sighing) breaths, or atypical snoring frequently accompany opioid-induced respiratory depression.

Use buprenorphine with extreme caution in patients with any of the following: significant chronic obstructive pulmonary disease or cor pulmonale; other risk of substantially decreased respiratory reserve, such as asthma, severe obesity, sleep apnea, myxedema, clinically-significant kyphoscoliosis, and CNS depression; hypoxia; hypercapnia; or preexisting respiratory depression.

➤*CNS effects:* Buprenorphine may cause somnolence, dizziness, alterations in judgment, and alterations in levels of consciousness, including coma.

➤*Cardiovascular effects:*

QTc prolongation – A positive-controlled study of the effects of buprenorphine on the QTc interval in healthy subjects demonstrated no clinically meaningful effect at a buprenorphine dose of 10 mcg/h; however, a buprenorphine dose of 40 mcg/h (given as 2 buprenorphine 20 mcg/h) was observed to prolong the QTc interval.

Consider these observations in clinical decisions when prescribing buprenorphine to patients with hypokalemia or clinically unstable cardiac disease, including unstable atrial fibrillation, symptomatic bradycardia, unstable congestive heart failure, or active myocardial ischemia. Avoid the use of buprenorphine in patients with a history of long QT syndrome or an immediate family member with this condition, or those taking class IA antiarrhythmic medications (eg, quinidine, procainamide, disopyramide) or class III antiarrhythmic medications (eg, sotalol, amiodarone, dofetilide).

Hypotensive effects – Buprenorphine may cause severe hypotension. There is an added risk to individuals whose ability to maintain blood pressure has been compromised by a depleted blood volume, or after coadministration with drugs such as phenothiazines or other agents that compromise vasomotor tone. Buprenorphine may produce orthostatic hypotension in ambulatory patients. Administer buprenorphine with caution to patients in circulatory shock because vasodilation produced by the drug may further reduce cardiac output and blood pressure.

➤*Head injury and increased intracranial pressure:* The respiratory depressant effects of opioids, including buprenorphine, include carbon dioxide retention, which can lead to an elevation of CSF pressure. This effect may be exaggerated in the presence of head injury, intracranial lesions, or other sources of preexisting increased intracranial pressure. Buprenorphine may produce miosis that is independent of ambient light, and altered consciousness, either of which may obscure neurologic signs associated with increased intracranial pressure in people with head injuries.

➤*Hepatic effects:* Although not observed in buprenorphine transdermal system chronic pain clinical trials, cases of cytolytic hepatitis and hepatitis with jaundice have been observed in individuals receiving sublingual buprenorphine for the treatment of opioid dependence, both in clinical trials and through postmarketing adverse event reports. The spectrum of abnormalities ranges from transient asymptomatic elevations in hepatic transaminases to case reports of hepatic failure, hepatic necrosis, hepatorenal syndrome, and hepatic encephalopathy. In many cases, the presence of preexisting liver enzyme abnormalities, infection with hepatitis B or hepatitis C virus, concomitant usage of other potentially hepatotoxic drugs, and ongoing injection drug abuse may have played a causative or contributory role. In other cases, insufficient data were available to determine the cause of the abnormality. The possibility exists that buprenorphine had a causative or contributory role in the development of the hepatic abnormality in some cases. For patients at increased risk of hepatotoxicity (eg, history of excessive alcohol intake, IV drug abuse, liver disease), baseline and periodic monitoring of liver function during treatment with buprenorphine is recommended. A biological and etiological evaluation is recommended when a hepatic event is suspected.

➤*Application-site reactions:* In rare cases, severe application-site skin reactions with signs of marked inflammation, including burn, discharge, and vesicles, have occurred. Time of onset varies, ranging from days to months following the initiation of buprenorphine transdermal system treatment. Instruct patients to promptly report the development of severe application-site reactions and discontinue therapy.

➤*Application of external heat:* Advise patients and their caregivers to avoid exposing the buprenorphine transdermal system application site and surrounding area to direct external heat sources (eg, heating pads or electric blankets, heat or tanning lamps, saunas, hot tubs, heated water beds) while wearing the system because an increase in absorption of buprenorphine may occur. Advise patients against exposure of the buprenorphine application site and surrounding area to hot water or prolonged exposure to direct sunlight. There is a potential for temperature-dependent increases in buprenorphine released from the system resulting in possible overdose and death.

➤*Fever/Increased body temperature:* Monitor patients wearing buprenorphine system who develop fever or increased core body temperature due to strenuous exertion for opioid adverse reactions, and adjust the buprenorphine dose if necessary.

➤*Seizures:* Buprenorphine, as with other opioids, may aggravate seizure disorders and lower seizure threshold, and therefore, may induce seizures in some clinical settings. Use buprenorphine with caution in patients with a history of seizure disorders.

➤*GI conditions:* Buprenorphine may cause spasm of the sphincter of Oddi. Use with caution in patients with biliary tract disease, including acute pancreatitis. Opioids, including buprenorphine, may cause increased serum amylase.

The administration of buprenorphine may obscure the diagnosis or clinical course in patients with acute abdominal conditions. Use buprenorphine with caution in patients who are at risk of developing ileus.

➤*Addictive disorders:* Buprenorphine has not been studied and is not approved for use in the management of addictive disorders.

➤*Hypersensitivity reactions:* Cases of acute and chronic hypersensitivity to buprenorphine have been reported both in clinical trials and in the postmarketing experience. The most common signs and symptoms include rashes, hives, and pruritus. Cases of bronchospasm, angioneurotic edema, and anaphylactic shock have been reported. A history of hypersensitivity to buprenorphine is a contraindication to the use of buprenorphine transdermal system.

➤*Hepatic function impairment:* Buprenorphine has not been evaluated in patients with severe hepatic impairment; administer with caution.

➤*Special risk:* Use buprenorphine with caution in the following conditions because of an increased risk of adverse reactions: alcoholism; delirium tremens; adrenocortical insufficiency; CNS depression; debilitation; kyphoscoliosis associated with respiratory compromise; myxedema or hypothyroidism; prostatic hypertrophy or urethral stricture; severe impairment of hepatic, pulmonary, or renal function; and toxic psychosis.

➤*Drug abuse and dependence:*

Controlled substance – Buprenorphine transdermal system contains buprenorphine, a mu-opioid partial agonist and schedule III controlled substance. Buprenorphine can be abused in a manner similar to other opioid agonists, legal or illicit, and is subject to misuse, abuse, addiction, and criminal diversion. Consider this potential for abuse when prescribing or dispensing buprenorphine in situations where the prescriber or pharmacist is concerned about an increased risk of misuse, abuse, or diversion. Monitor all patients receiving opioids for signs of abuse, misuse, and addiction.

Abuse – Abuse of buprenorphine poses a hazard of overdose and death. This risk is increased with compromise of the buprenorphine transdermal system and with concurrent abuse of alcohol or other substances. Buprenorphine has been diverted for nonmedical use.

All patients treated with opioids, including buprenorphine, require careful monitoring for signs of abuse and addiction, because use of opioid analgesic products carries the risk of addiction even under appropriate medical use. Assess patients for their potential for opioid abuse prior to being prescribed opioid therapy. Persons at increased risk of opioid abuse include those with a personal or family history of substance abuse (including drug or alcohol abuse) or mental illness (eg, depression). Opioids may still be appropriate for use in these patients; however, they will require intensive monitoring for signs of abuse. Data are not available to establish the true incidence of addiction in patients with chronic pain treated with opioids.

Addiction is a primary, chronic, neurobiologic disease with genetic, psychosocial, and environmental factors influencing its development and manifestations. It is characterized by behaviors that include 1 or more of the following: impaired control over drug use, compulsive use, continued use despite harm, and craving. Opioid drugs are sought by people with substance use disorders (abuse or addiction, the latter of which is also called substance dependence) and criminals who supply them by diverting medicines out of legitimate distribution channels. Buprenorphine is a target for theft and diversion.

"Drug-seeking behavior" is very common in people with substance use disorders. Drug-seeking tactics include, but are not limited to, emergency calls or visits near the end of office hours; refusal to undergo appropriate examination, testing, or referral; repeated loss of prescriptions; altering or forging of prescriptions; and reluctance to provide prior medical records or contact information for other treating health care providers. Doctor-shopping to obtain additional prescriptions is common among people with untreated substance use disorders and criminals who divert controlled substances.

Abuse and addiction are separate and distinct from physical dependence and tolerance. Health care providers should be aware that addiction may not be accompanied by concurrent tolerance and symptoms of physical dependence in all addicts. In addition, abuse of opioids can occur in the absence of true addiction and is characterized by misuse for nonmedical purposes, often in combination with other psychoactive substances. Because buprenorphine may be diverted for nonmedical use, careful record keeping of prescribing information, including quantity, frequency, and renewal requests, is strongly advised.

Consider the risks of misuse and abuse when prescribing or dispensing buprenorphine transdermal system. However, concerns about abuse and addiction should not prevent the proper management of pain. Individualize treatment of pain, balancing the potential benefits and risks of each patient.

Buprenorphine transdermal system is intended for transdermal use only. Compromising the transdermal delivery system will result in the uncontrolled delivery of buprenorphine and pose a significant risk to the abuser that could result in overdose and death. The risk of fatal overdose is further increased when buprenorphine is abused concurrently with alcohol or other CNS depressants, including other opioids and benzodiazepines. Abuse may occur by applying the transdermal system in the absence of legitimate purpose, or by swallowing, snorting, or injecting buprenorphine extracted from the transdermal system.

BUPRENORPHINE — TRANSDERMAL

Proper assessment of the patient, proper prescribing practices, periodic reevaluation of therapy, proper dispensing, and correct storage and handling are appropriate measures that help to limit misuse and abuse of opioid drugs. Careful record keeping of prescribing information, including quantity, frequency, and renewal requests, is strongly advised.

Health care providers should contact their state Professional Licensing Board or state Controlled Substances Authority for information on how to prevent and detect abuse or diversion of this product.

Physical dependence and tolerance – Tolerance is a state of adaptation in which exposure to a drug induces changes that result in a diminution of 1 or more of the drug's effects over time. Tolerance could occur to both the desired and undesired effects of drugs, and may develop at different rates for different effects.

Physical dependence to an opioid is manifested by characteristic withdrawal signs and symptoms after abrupt discontinuation of a drug, significant dose reduction, or upon administration of an antagonist. Physical dependence and tolerance are not unusual during long-term opioid analgesic therapy.

The opioid abstinence or withdrawal syndrome in adults is characterized by some or all of the following: restlessness, lacrimation, rhinorrhea, yawning, perspiration, chills, piloerection, myalgia, mydriasis, irritability, anxiety, backache, joint pain, weakness, abdominal cramps, insomnia, nausea, anorexia, vomiting, diarrhea, or increased blood pressure, respiratory rate, or heart rate.

Infants born to mothers physically dependent on opioids will also be physically dependent and may exhibit respiratory difficulties and withdrawal symptoms.

In general, opioids should not be abruptly discontinued.

➤*Hazardous tasks:* Buprenorphine may impair the mental and physical abilities needed to perform potentially hazardous activities, such as driving a car or operating machinery. Caution patients accordingly.

➤*Pregnancy: Category C.* There are no adequate and well-controlled studies with buprenorphine in pregnant women. Use buprenorphine during pregnancy only if the potential benefit justifies the potential risk to the mother and the fetus. In animal studies, buprenorphine caused an increase in the number of stillborn offspring, reduced litter size, and reduced offspring growth in rats at maternal exposure levels that were approximately 10 times that of human subjects who received one buprenorphine 20 mcg/h, the MRHD.

Teratogenic – Studies in rats and rabbits demonstrated no evidence of teratogenicity following buprenorphine transdermal system or subcutaneous administration of buprenorphine during the period of major organogenesis. Rats were administered up to 1 buprenorphine transdermal system 20 mcg/h every 3 days (gestation days 6, 9, 12, and 15) or received daily subcutaneous buprenorphine up to 5 mg/kg (gestation days 6 to 17). Rabbits were administered 4 buprenorphine transdermal systems 20 mcg/h every 3 days (gestation days 6, 9, 12, 15, 18, and 19) or received daily subcutaneous buprenorphine up to 5 mg/kg (gestation days 6 to 19). No teratogenicity was observed at any dose. AUC values for buprenorphine with buprenorphine transdermal system application and subcutaneous injection were approximately 140 and 110 times that of human subjects who received the MRHD of 1 buprenorphine transdermal system 20 mcg/h.

Nonteratogenic – In a peri- and postnatal study conducted in pregnant and lactating rats, administration of buprenorphine either as buprenorphine transdermal system or subcutaneous buprenorphine was associated with toxicity to offspring. Buprenorphine was present in maternal milk. Pregnant rats were administered 1/4 of 1 buprenorphine transdermal system 5 mcg/h every 3 days or received daily subcutaneous buprenorphine at doses of 0.05, 0.5, or 5 mg/kg from gestation day 6 to lactation day 21 (weaning). Administration of buprenorphine transdermal system or subcutaneous buprenorphine at 0.5 or 5 mg/kg caused maternal toxicity and an increase in the number of stillborns, reduced litter size, and reduced offspring growth at maternal exposure levels that were approximately 10 times that of human subjects who received the MRHD of 1 buprenorphine transdermal system 20 mcg/h. Maternal toxicity was also observed at the no observed adverse effect level for offspring.

Labor and delivery – Opioids cross the placenta and may produce respiratory depression and psychophysiologic effects in neonates. Buprenorphine is not recommended for use in women immediately prior to and during labor, when use of shorter acting analgesics or other analgesic techniques are more appropriate. Occasionally, opioid analgesics may prolong labor through actions that temporarily reduce the strength, duration, and frequency of uterine contractions. However, this effect is not consistent and may be offset by an increased rate of cervical dilatation, which tends to shorten labor.

Closely observe neonates whose mothers received opioid analgesics during labor for signs of respiratory depression. Have a specific opioid antagonist, such as naloxone or nalmefene, available for reversal of opioid-induced respiratory depression in the neonate.

Neonates whose mothers have been taking opioids chronically may also exhibit withdrawal signs at birth and/or in the nursery because they have developed physical dependence. This is not, however, synonymous with addiction. Neonatal opioid withdrawal syndrome, unlike opioid withdrawal syndrome in adults, may be life-threatening. Treat according to protocols developed by neonatology experts.

➤*Lactation:* Buprenorphine has been detected in low concentrations in human milk. Breast-feeding is not advised in women treated with buprenorphine because depression of the breast-feeding infant may result in lower weight gain.

➤*Children:* The safety and efficacy of buprenorphine in patients younger than 18 years of age has not been established. Buprenorphine is not recommended for use in children.

➤*Elderly:* In the clinical program, the incidences of selected buprenorphine-related adverse reactions were higher in older subjects. The incidences of application-site adverse reactions were slightly higher among subjects younger than 65 years of age than those at least 65 years of age or older for both buprenorphine and placebo treatment groups.

In the elderly groups evaluated, adverse reaction rates were similar to or lower than rates in healthy young adult subjects, except for constipation and urinary retention, which were more common in the elderly. Although specific dose adjustments on the basis of advanced age are not required for pharmacokinetic reasons, use caution in the elderly population to ensure safe use.

➤*Monitoring:* Monitor all patients receiving opioids for signs of abuse, misuse, and addiction.

For patients at increased risk of hepatotoxicity (eg, history of excessive alcohol intake, IV drug abuse, liver disease), baseline and periodic monitoring of liver function during treatment with buprenorphine is recommended.

Drug Interactions

➤*QT prolongation:* An additive effect of buprenorphine with other drugs that prolong the QT interval cannot be excluded. The following drugs may prolong the QT interval and increase the risk of life-threatening cardiac arrhythmias, including torsades de pointes: antiarrhythmic agents (eg, amiodarone, bretylium, disopyramide, dofetilide, procainamide, quinidine, sotalol), arsenic trioxide, chlorpromazine, cisapride, dolasetron, droperidol, gatifloxacin, halofantrine, levomethadyl, mefloquine, mesoridazine, moxifloxacin, pentamidine, pimozide, probucol, sparfloxacin, thioridazine, ziprasidone.

Buprenorphine Transdermal Drug Interactions

Precipitant drug	Object drug[a]		Description
Antiarrhythmic agents, class IA (eg, disopyramide, procainamide, quinidine) or class III (eg, amiodarone, dofetilide, sotalol)	Buprenorphine	↑	Avoid concurrent use.
Buprenorphine	Antiarrhythmic agents, class IA (eg, disopyramide, procainamide, quinidine) or class III (eg, amiodarone, dofetilide, sotalol)		
Barbiturate anesthetics (eg, thiopental)	Buprenorphine	↑	Barbiturate anesthetics may increase respiratory and CNS depression because of additive pharmacologic activity. Monitor the patient and adjust the buprenorphine dose as needed.
Buprenorphine	Barbiturate anesthetics (eg, thiopental)		
Benzodiazepines (eg, diazepam)	Buprenorphine	↑	Coma and death have been associated with the concomitant IV misuse of buprenorphine and benzodiazepines by addicts. Use with caution. Warn patients of the potential danger of self-administration of benzodiazepines while receiving treatment with buprenorphine.
Cimetidine	Buprenorphine	↑	The risk of buprenorphine CNS toxicity may be increased. Monitor the patient. If excessive CNS or respiratory depression occurs, discontinue both drugs. Give a narcotic antagonist (eg, naloxone) if needed.
CNS depressants (eg, alcohol, anxiolytics, hypnotics, muscle relaxants, neuroleptics, other opioids, sedatives)	Buprenorphine	↑	Hypotension, profound sedation, coma, or respiratory depression may occur. Use with caution. Consider giving a lower initial dose of the CNS depressant.
CYP3A4 inducers (eg, carbamazepine, phenobarbital, phenytoin, rifampin)	Buprenorphine	↓	Although not investigated, it is recommended to closely monitor patients when buprenorphine is coadministered with a CYP3A4 inducer. Buprenorphine clearance may be increased. Adjust the buprenorphine dose as needed.

BUPRENORPHINE — TRANSDERMAL

Buprenorphine Transdermal Drug Interactions			
Precipitant drug	Object drug[a]		Description
MAOIs[b] (eg, phenelzine)	Buprenorphine	↔	Buprenorphine transdermal is not recommended for use in patients who have received MAOIs within 14 days.
Naltrexone	Buprenorphine	⬇	Naltrexone may decrease or attenuate the pharmacologic effects of buprenorphine. Precipitation of withdrawal symptoms may occur. Closely monitor for signs of buprenorphine withdrawal or reduced efficacy. Detoxify buprenorphine-dependent patients before treatment with naltrexone. If there is any question of occult buprenorphine dependence, perform a naltrexone challenge test and defer treatment until the naltrexone challenge is negative. Make cardiopulmonary resuscitation staff and equipment available for patients receiving naltrexone extended-release injection requiring emergency pain management with opioids.
Sodium oxybate (GHB)	Buprenorphine	⬆	Concurrent use may result in increased sleep duration and CNS depression because of additive pharmacologic activity. Coadministration of sodium oxybate is contraindicated with other sedative-hypnotics.
Buprenorphine	Sodium oxybate (GHB)		
Buprenorphine	Methadone	⬇	Buprenorphine may decrease or attenuate the pharmacologic effects of methadone. Precipitation of withdrawal symptoms may occur. Closely monitor for signs of opioid withdrawal or reduced opioid efficacy. Do not administer buprenorphine to patients with dependence on methadone.
Buprenorphine	Nondepolarizing muscle relaxants (eg, tubocurarine)	⬆	Concurrent use may enhance neuromuscular blocking action and increase respiratory depression. If coadministration cannot be avoided, monitor respiratory function and be prepared to provide life support if needed.

[a] ⬆ = object drug increased; ⬇ = object drug decreased; ↔ = undetermined clinical effect.
[b] MAOIs = monoamine oxidase inhibitors.

Adverse Reactions

➤*Adverse reactions (more than 5%):*

Opioid-naive patients –

Buprenorphine Transdermal Adverse Reactions: Opioid-Naive Patients (≥ 5%)			
	Open-label titration period	Double-blind treatment period	
Adverse reactions	Buprenorphine (n = 1,024)	Buprenorphine (n = 256)	Placebo (n = 283)
CNS			
Dizziness	10%	4%	1%
Headache	10%	5%	5%
Somnolence	8%	2%	2%
GI			
Constipation	7%	4%	1%
Nausea	23%	13%	11%
Vomiting	8%	4%	2%
Miscellaneous			
Application-site pruritus	8%	4%	7%

Opioid-experienced patients –

Buprenorphine Transdermal Adverse Reactions: Opioid-Experienced Patients (≥ 5%)			
	Open-label titration period	Double-blind treatment period	
Adverse reactions	Buprenorphine (n = 1,160)	Buprenorphine 20 mcg/h (n = 219)	Buprenorphine 5 mcg/h (n = 221)
CNS			
Dizziness	5%	5%	2%
Headache	11%	11%	5%
Somnolence	6%	5%	2%
GI			
Constipation	4%	6%	3%
Nausea	15%	12%	8%
Vomiting	5%	5%	2%
Local			
Application-site erythema	3%	10%	5%
Application-site irritation	2%	5%	3%
Application-site pruritus	9%	13%	5%
Application-site rash	3%	9%	6%

➤*Adverse reactions (2% or more):*

Buprenorphine Transdermal Adverse Reactions Reported in Titration-to-Effect (≥ 2%)		
Adverse reactions	Buprenorphine (n = 392)	Placebo (n = 261)
CNS		
Confusional state	2%	3%
Dizziness	16%	8%
Fatigue	5%	1%
Headache	16%	11%
Hypoesthesia	2%	1%
Insomnia	3%	2%
Paraesthesia	2%	1%
Somnolence	14%	5%
Tremor	2%	< 1%
Dermatologic		
Application-site erythema	7%	2%
Application-site pruritus	15%	12%
Application-site rash	6%	6%
Hyperhidrosis	4%	1%
Pruritus	4%	1%
Rash	2%	1%
GI		
Anorexia	2%	1%
Constipation	14%	5%
Diarrhea	3%	2%
Dry mouth	7%	2%
Dyspepsia	3%	3%
Nausea	23%	8%
Stomach discomfort	2%	1%
Vomiting	11%	2%
Musculoskeletal		
Arthralgia	2%	2%
Back pain	3%	2%
Joint swelling	3%	1%
Pain in extremity	3%	2%
Miscellaneous		
Dyspnea	3%	1%
Fall	4%	2%
Peripheral edema	7%	3%
Urinary tract infection	3%	2%

BUPRENORPHINE — TRANSDERMAL

➤*Other adverse reactions:*

Cardiovascular – Hypertension (1% to less than 5%); angina pectoris, bradycardia, hot flush, hypotension, orthostatic hypotension, palpitations, syncope, tachycardia, vasodilatation (less than 1%).

CNS – Dizziness, headache, somnolence (5% or more); anxiety, asthenia, depression, fatigue, hypoesthesia, insomnia, migraine, paresthesia, tremor (1% to less than 5%); affect lability, agitation, apathy, chills, confusional state, coordination abnormal, depersonalization, depressed level of consciousness, depressed mood, disorientation, disturbance in attention, dysarthria, euphoric mood, gait disturbance, hallucination, insomnia, libido decreased, loss of consciousness, malaise, memory impairment, mental impairment, mental status changes, nervousness, nightmare, psychotic disorder, restlessness, sedation (less than 1%).

Dermatologic – Generalized pruritus, hyperhidrosis, pruritus, rash (1% to less than 5%); contact dermatitis, dry skin, urticaria (less than 1%).

GI – Constipation, dry mouth, nausea, vomiting (5% or more); anorexia, diarrhea, dyspepsia, upper abdominal pain (1% to less than 5%); abdominal distention, abdominal pain, diverticulitis, dysgeusia, dysphagia, flatulence, ileus (less than 1%).

GU – Urinary tract infection (1% to less than 5%); dysmenorrhea, sexual dysfunction, urinary hesitation, urinary incontinence, urinary retention (less than 1%).

Local – Application-site erythema, application-site pruritus, application-site rash (5% or more); application-site irritation (1% to less than 5%); application-site dermatitis (less than 1%).

Metabolic/Nutritional – Peripheral edema (1% to less than 5%); dehydration, face edema, weight decreased (less than 1%).

Musculoskeletal – Arthralgia, back pain, joint swelling, muscle spasms, musculoskeletal pain, myalgia, neck pain, pain in extremity (1% to less than 5%); muscle weakness (less than 1%).

Respiratory – Bronchitis, cough, dyspnea, nasopharyngitis, pharyngolaryngeal pain, sinusitis, upper respiratory tract infection (1% to less than 5%); asthma aggravated, hyperventilation, hypoventilation, respiration abnormal, respiratory depression, respiratory distress, respiratory failure, rhinitis, wheezing (less than 1%).

Special senses – Dry eye, miosis, tinnitus, vertigo, vision blurred, visual disturbance (less than 1%).

Miscellaneous – Chest pain, fall, influenza, pain, pyrexia (1% to less than 5%); accidental injury, ALT increased, angioedema, drug hypersensitivity, drug withdrawal syndrome, flushing, hiccups (less than 1%).

Overdosage

➤*Symptoms:* Acute overdosage with buprenorphine can be manifested by atypical snoring, bradycardia, cold and clammy skin, constricted pupils, death, hypotension, partial or complete airway obstruction, respiratory depression, skeletal muscle flaccidity, and somnolence progressing to stupor or coma.

Deaths due to overdose have been reported with abuse and misuse of buprenorphine. Review of case reports has indicated that the risk of fatal overdose is further increased when buprenorphine is abused concurrently with alcohol or other CNS depressants, including other opioids.

➤*Treatment:* In cases of overdose, remove buprenorphine transdermal system immediately. It is important to take the pharmacokinetic profile of buprenorphine into account when treating overdose. Even in the face of improvement, continued medical monitoring is required because of the possibility of extended effects as the opioid continues to be absorbed from the skin. After removal of buprenorphine, the mean buprenorphine concentrations decrease approximately 50% in 12 hours (range, 10 to 24 hours) with an apparent terminal half-life of approximately 26 hours. Because of this long apparent terminal half-life, patients may require monitoring and treatment for at least 24 hours.

In the treatment of buprenorphine overdosage, give primary attention to the maintenance of a patent airway, and effective ventilation (clearance of oxygen) and oxygenation, whether by spontaneous, assisted, or controlled respiration. Employ supportive measures (including oxygen and vasopressors) in the management of circulatory shock and pulmonary edema accompanying overdose as indicated. Cardiac arrest or arrhythmias may require cardiac massage or defibrillation.

Naloxone may not be effective in reversing any respiratory depression produced by buprenorphine. High doses of naloxone (10 to 35 mg per 70 kg) may be of limited value in the management of buprenorphine overdose. The onset of naloxone effect may be delayed by 30 minutes or more. Doxapram (a respiratory stimulant) has also been used. Because the duration of action of buprenorphine may exceed that of the antagonist, keep the patient under continued surveillance and administer repeated doses of the antagonist according to the antagonist labeling as needed to maintain adequate respiration. Maintenance of adequate ventilation is essential when managing buprenorphine overdose and more important than specific antidote treatment with an opioid antagonist, such as naloxone.

Do not administer opioid antagonists in the absence of clinically significant respiratory or circulatory depression secondary to buprenorphine overdose. In patients who are physically dependent on any opioid agonist, including buprenorphine, an abrupt partial or complete reversal of opioid effects may precipitate an acute abstinence or withdrawal syndrome. The severity of the withdrawal syndrome produced will depend on the degree of physical dependence and the dose of the antagonist administered. See the monograph for the specific opioid antagonist for details of its proper use.

Patient Information

Advise patients to carefully follow instructions for the application, removal, and disposal of buprenorphine transdermal system. Instruct patients to apply buprenorphine to a different site each week based on the 8 described skin sites, with a minimum of 3 weeks between applications to a previously used site.

Advise patients to apply buprenorphine to a hairless or nearly hairless skin site. If none are available, instruct patients to clip the hair at the site and not to shave the area. Instruct patients not to apply to irritated skin. If the application site must be cleaned, use clear water only. Do not use soaps, alcohol, oils, lotions, or abrasive devices. Advise patients to allow the skin to dry before applying buprenorphine.

Advise the patient to wear the buprenorphine transdermal system continuously for 7 days.

Advise patients to talk to their health care provider if they have any pain or bothersome adverse reactions while they are using buprenorphine. Their dose may have to be changed.

Advise patients not to increase or decrease the buprenorphine dose they are using without first speaking to their health care provider.

Advise patients that buprenorphine may impair mental and/or physical ability required for the performance of potentially hazardous tasks (eg, driving, operating heavy machinery).

Advise patients who are taking buprenorphine not to drink alcohol and to avoid taking sleep aids and CNS depressants unless a health care provider prescribes them.

Advise patients to avoid exposing the buprenorphine transdermal system site to external heat sources (eg, heating pads, electric blankets, heat lamps, saunas, hot tubs, heated water beds) while wearing buprenorphine because an increase in absorption of buprenorphine may occur that could lead to an overdose or death.

Advise women who become pregnant or who plan to become pregnant to ask their health care provider about the effects buprenorphine may have on themselves and their pregnancy.

Advise patients that buprenorphine is a drug that some people may abuse. They should use buprenorphine only as directed, and not give it to anyone other than the individual for whom it was prescribed. Protect it from theft. Be especially careful to keep this medication away from children and pets.

Advise patients to tell their health care provider if they have a history of serious skin reactions to adhesives because they may not be able to use the buprenorphine transdermal system.

Advise patients who must stop using buprenorphine to speak with their health care provider to manage the transition to other pain medications.

BUPRENORPHINE HYDROCHLORIDE/NALOXONE HYDROCHLORIDE

c-iii	**Suboxone** (Reckitt Benckiser)	**Film; sublingual:** 2 mg buprenorphine base/ 0.5 mg naloxone	As buprenorphine hydrochloride and naloxone hydrochloride. Acesulfame potassium. Orange. In 30s.
		8 mg buprenorphine base/2 mg naloxone	As buprenorphine hydrochloride and naloxone hydrochloride. Acesulfame potassium. In 30s.
		Tablets; sublingual: 2 mg buprenorphine base/ 0.5 mg naloxone	Acesulfame K, lactose. Orange, hexagonal. Lemon/Lime flavor. In 30s.
		8 mg buprenorphine base/2 mg naloxone	Acesulfame K, lactose. Orange, hexagonal. Lemon/Lime flavor. In 30s.

BUPRENORPHINE HYDROCHLORIDE/NALOXONE HYDROCHLORIDE — ORAL

Refer to the general discussion in the Opioid Agonist-Antagonist Analgesic introduction and the Buprenorphine and Naloxone monographs.

Indications

➤*Opioid dependence:* Treatment of opioid dependence.

Administration and Dosage

➤*General dosing considerations:* Buprenorphine/naloxone sublingual film should be used in patients who have been initially inducted using buprenorphine sublingual tablets.

When taken sublingually, buprenorphine and buprenorphine/naloxone tablets have similar clinical effects and are interchangeable.

Following induction, buprenorphine/naloxone (because of the presence of naloxone) is preferred when clinical use includes unsupervised administration. Limit the use of buprenorphine for unsupervised administration to those patients who cannot tolerate buprenorphine/naloxone (eg, those patients who have been shown to be hypersensitive to naloxone).

Induction – Buprenorphine tablets contain no naloxone and are preferred for use during induction. Prior to induction, consider the type of opioid dependence (ie, long- or short-acting opioid), the time since last opioid use, and the degree or level of opioid dependence. To avoid precipitating withdrawal, undertake induction with buprenorphine when objective and clear signs of withdrawal are evident.

➤*Adults:*

Opioid dependence –

Sublingual film:

• *Initial dosage* – Target dosage is buprenorphine 16 mg/naloxone 4 mg as a single daily dose. The maintenance dose is generally in the range of buprenorphine 4 mg/naloxone 1 mg to buprenorphine 24 mg/naloxone 6 mg per day depending on the individual patient. Dosages higher than this have not been demonstrated to provide any clinical advantage.

• *Dosage adjustment* – The dosage should be progressively adjusted in increments/decrements of buprenorphine 2 mg/naloxone 0.5 mg or buprenorphine 4 mg/naloxone 1 mg to a level that holds the patient in treatment and suppresses opioid withdrawal signs and symptoms.

• *Discontinuation of therapy* – The decision to discontinue therapy after a period of maintenance should be made as part of a comprehensive treatment plan. Both gradual and abrupt discontinuation of buprenorphine has been used, but the data are insufficient to determine the best method of dose taper at the end of treatment.

Sublingual tablets:

• *Initial dosage* – Buprenorphine 8 mg on day 1 and buprenorphine 16 mg on day 2. From day 3 onward, patients received buprenorphine/naloxone tablets at the same buprenorphine dose as day 2.

Induction in the studies of buprenorphine solution was accomplished over 3 to 4 days, depending on the target dose. In some studies, gradual induction over several days led to a high rate of drop-out of buprenorphine patients during the induction period. Therefore, it is recommended that an adequate maintenance dose, titrated to clinical effectiveness, should be achieved as rapidly as possible to prevent undue opioid withdrawal symptoms.

• *Maintenance dosage* – 12 to 16 mg/day administered sublingually as a single daily dose. The recommended target dose of buprenorphine/naloxone is 16 mg/day. Clinical studies have shown that buprenorphine or buprenorphine/naloxone 16 mg is a clinically effective dose compared with placebo and indicate that doses as low as 12 mg may be effective in some patients.

Buprenorphine/naloxone is the preferred medication for maintenance treatment because of the presence of naloxone in the formulation.

• *Dosage adjustment* – Adjust the dosage in increments/decrements of 2 or 4 mg to a level that holds the patient in treatment and suppresses opioid withdrawal effects. This is likely to be in the range of 4 to 24 mg per day, depending on the individual.

• *Discontinuation of therapy* – Make the decision to discontinue therapy with buprenorphine/naloxone after a period of maintenance or brief stabilization as part of a comprehensive treatment plan. Gradual and abrupt discontinuation have been used, but no controlled trials have been undertaken to determine the best method of dose taper at the end of treatment.

Conversion: Patients being switched between buprenorphine/naloxone sublingual tablets and sublingual film should be started on the same dosage as the previously administered product. However, dosage adjustments may be necessary when switching between products. Because of the potentially greater relative bioavailability of sublingual film compared to sublingual tablets, patients switching from sublingual tablets to sublingual film should be monitored for over-medication. Those switching from sublingual film to sublingual tablets should be monitored for withdrawal or other indications of under-dosing. In clinical studies, pharmacokinetics of sublingual film was similar to the respective dosage strengths of sublingual tablets, although not all doses and dose combinations met bioequivalence criteria.

➤*Children:*

Opioid dependence –

Sublingual tablets:

• *16 years and older* – See Adults for dosing.

➤*Elderly:* Use with caution. See Adults for dosing.

➤*Patients taking heroin or other short-acting opioids:* At treatment initiation, administer the dose of buprenorphine at least 4 hours after the patient last used opioids or, preferably, when early signs of withdrawal appear.

➤*Patients on methadone or other long-acting narcotics:* There is little controlled experience with the transfer of methadone-maintained patients to buprenorphine. Available evidence suggests that withdrawal symptoms are possible during induction of buprenorphine treatment. Withdrawal appears more likely in patients maintained on higher doses of methadone (more than 30 mg) and when the first buprenorphine dose is administered shortly after the last methadone dose.

➤*Administration:* Buprenorphine /naloxone sublingual film and tablets are administered sublingually as a single daily dose.

Sublingual film – Place the sublingual film under the tongue. If an additional sublingual film is necessary to achieve the prescribed dose, place the additional sublingual film sublingually on the opposite side from the first film. Place the sublingual film in a manner to minimize overlapping as much as possible. The sublingual film must be kept under the tongue until the film is completely dissolved. The sublingual film should not be chewed, swallowed, or moved after placement.

Sublingual tablets – Place tablets under the tongue until they are dissolved. For doses requiring the use of more than 2 tablets, patients are advised to place all the tablets at once or, alternatively (if they cannot fit in more than 2 tablets comfortably), place 2 tablets at a time under the tongue. Either way, the patient should continue to hold the tablets under the tongue until they dissolve; swallowing the tablets reduces the bioavailability of the drug.

To ensure consistency in bioavailability, patients should follow the same manner of dosing with continued use of the product.

➤*Storage/Stability:* Store at 25°C (77°F). Excursions are permitted to 15° to 30°C (59° to 86°F).

Contraindications

Do not administer to patients who have been shown to be hypersensitive to buprenorphine or naloxone.

Warnings/Precautions

➤*Opioid withdrawal effects:* Because it contains naloxone, buprenorphine/naloxone is highly likely to produce marked and intense withdrawal symptoms if misused parenterally by individuals dependent on opioid agonists (eg, heroin, morphine, methadone). Sublingually, buprenorphine/naloxone may cause opioid withdrawal symptoms in these people if administered before the agonist effects of the opioid have subsided.

➤*Pregnancy:* Category C. There are no adequate and well-controlled studies in pregnant women. Use during pregnancy only if the potential benefit justifies the potential risk to the fetus.

Neonatal withdrawal – Neonatal withdrawal has been reported in the infants of women treated with buprenorphine during pregnancy. From postmarketing reports, the time to onset of neonatal withdrawal symptoms ranged from day 1 to day 8 of life, with most occurring on day 1. Adverse events associated with neonatal withdrawal syndrome included hypertonia, neonatal tremor, neonatal agitation, and myoclonus. There have been rare reports of convulsions and in one case, apnea and bradycardia were also reported.

Teratogenic – Effects on embryofetal development were studied in Sprague-Dawley rats and Russian white rabbits following oral (1:1) and intramuscular (3:2) administration of mixtures of buprenorphine and naloxone. Following oral administration to rats and rabbits, no teratogenic effects were observed at doses up to 250 mg/kg/day and 40 mg/kg/day, respectively (estimated exposure was approximately 150 times and 50 times, respectively, the recommended human daily sublingual dose of 16 mg on a mg/m^2 basis). No definitive, drug-related teratogenic effects were observed in rats and rabbits at IM doses up to 30 mg/kg/day (estimated exposure was approximately 20 times and 35 times, respectively, the recommended human daily dose of 16 mg on a mg/m^2 basis). Acephalus was observed in 1 rabbit fetus from the low-dose group and omphacele was observed in 2 rabbit fetuses from the same litter in the mid-dose group; no findings were observed in fetuses from the high-dose group. Following oral administration to the rat, dose-related postimplantation losses, evidenced by increases in the number of early resorptions with consequent reductions in the numbers of fetuses, were observed at doses of 10 mg/kg/day or greater (estimated exposure was approximately 6 times the recommended human

BUPRENORPHINE HYDROCHLORIDE/NALOXONE HYDROCHLORIDE — ORAL

daily sublingual dose of 16 mg on a mg/m² basis). In the rabbit, increased postimplantation losses occurred at an oral dose of 40 mg/kg/day. Following IM administration in the rat and the rabbit, postimplantation losses, as evidenced by decreases in live fetuses and increases in resorptions, occurred at 30 mg/kg/day.

Nonteratogenic – Dystocia was noted in pregnant rats treated IM with buprenorphine 5 mg/kg/day (approximately 3 times the recommended human daily sublingual dose of 16 mg on a mg/m² basis). Both fertility and peri- and postnatal development studies with buprenorphine in rats indicated increases in neonatal mortality after oral doses of 0.8 mg/kg/day and up (approximately 0.5 times the recommended human daily sublingual dose of 16 mg on a mg/m² basis), after IM doses of 0.5 mg/kg/day and up (approximately 0.3 times the recommended human daily sublingual dose of 16 mg on a mg/m² basis) and after subcutaneous doses of 0.1 mg/kg/day and up (approximately 0.06 times the recommended human daily sublingual dose of 16 mg on a mg/m² basis). Delays in the occurrence of righting reflex and startle response were noted in rat pups at an oral dose of 80 mg/kg/day (approximately 50 times the recommended human daily sublingual dose of 16 mg on a mg/m² basis).

➤*Lactation:* An apparent lack of milk production during general reproduction studies with buprenorphine in rats caused decreased viability and lactation indices. Use of high doses of sublingual buprenorphine in pregnant women showed that buprenorphine passes into the mother's milk. Breastfeeding is, therefore, not advised.

➤*Children:* Buprenorphine/naloxone is not recommended for use in children. The safety and effectiveness in patients younger than 16 years of age have not been established.

BUTORPHANOL TARTRATE

c-iv	**Butorphanol Tartrate** (Various, eg, Bedford, Bertek, Hospira, Novaplus)	**Injection:** 1 mg/mL[a]	In 2 mL vials.
c-iv	**Stadol** (Bristol-Myers Squibb)		In 1 mL vials.
c-iv	**Butorphanol Tartrate** (Various, eg, Bedford, Bertek, Hospira, Novaplus)	**Injection:** 2 mg/mL[a]	In 1 and 2 mL vials.
c-iv	**Stadol** (Bristol-Myers Squibb)		In 1, 2 and 10[b] mL vials.
c-iv	**Butorphanol Tartrate** (Various, eg, Mylan, Roxane)	**Nasal spray:** 10 mg/mL	In 2.5 mL.

[a] 1 mg of tartrate salt is equal to 0.68 mg base.

[b] With 0.1 mg/mL benzethonium chloride.

BUTORPHANOL TARTRATE — INJECTION

Refer to the general discussion in the Opioid Agonist-Antagonist Analgesic introduction.

Indications

➤*Pain:* For the management of pain when the use of an opioid analgesic is appropriate.

➤*Preoperative/Preanesthetic medication:* For use as a preoperative or preanesthetic medication.

➤*Balanced anesthesia supplement:* As a supplement to balanced anesthesia.

➤*Labor pain:* For the relief of pain during labor.

Administration and Dosage

➤*General dosing considerations:* Factors to be considered in determining the dose are age, body weight, physical status, underlying pathological condition, use of other drugs, type of anesthesia to be used, and surgical procedure involved.

➤*Adults:*

Balanced anesthesia – 2 mg intravenously (IV) shortly before induction and/or 0.5 to 1 mg IV in increments during anesthesia. The increment may be higher, up to 0.06 mg/kg (4 mg per 70 kg), depending on previous sedative, analgesic, and hypnotic drugs administered. The total dose of butorphanol injection will vary; however, patients seldom require less than 4 mg or more than 12.5 mg (approximately 0.06 to 0.18 mg/kg).

Labor (full-term patients 37 weeks or beyond and without signs of fetal distress in early labor) –

Usual dosage: 1 to 2 mg dose IV or intramuscularly (IM), may be repeated after 4 hours.

Dosage adjustment: A dose should not be repeated in less than 4 hours nor administered less than 4 hours prior to the anticipated delivery. Dosage adjustments in labor should be based on initial response with consideration given to concomitant analgesic or sedative drugs and the expected time of delivery.

Concomitant therapy: If concomitant use of butorphanol with drugs that may potentiate its effects is deemed necessary, the lowest effective dose should be employed.

Pain –

IM: 2 mg IM every 3 to 4 hours, as necessary in patients who will be able to remain recumbent, in the event drowsiness or dizziness occurs. The effective dosage range, depending on the severity of pain, is 1 to 4 mg IM repeated every 3 to 4 hours. There are insufficient clinical data to recommend single doses greater than 4 mg.

IV: 1 mg IV every 3 to 4 hours as necessary. The effective dosage range, depending on the severity of pain, is 0.5 to 2 mg repeated every 3 to 4 hours.

Preoperative/preanesthetic medication – 2 mg IM 60 to 90 minutes before surgery. The preoperative medication dosage should be individualized.

➤*Elderly:* The initial dose should generally be half the recommended adult dose (0.5 mg IV and 1 mg IM). Repeat doses in these patients should be determined by the patient's response rather than at fixed intervals, but will generally be no less than 6 hours.

➤*Renal function impairment:* The initial dose should generally be half the recommended adult dose (0.5 mg IV and 1 mg IM). Repeat doses in these patients should be determined by the patient's response rather than at fixed intervals, but will generally be no less than 6 hours.

CrCl less than 30 mL/min – 50% normal dose not less than every 6 hours.

➤*Hepatic function impairment:* See Elderly for dosing.

➤*Administration:* Give by IV or IM.

➤*Storage/Stability:* Store at 25°C (77°F) (controlled room temperature).

Actions

➤*Pharmacology:* Butorphanol is a mixed agonist-antagonist with low intrinsic activity at receptors of the μ-opioid type (morphine-like). It is also an agonist against at K-opioid receptors.

Its interactions with these receptors in the central nervous system apparently mediate most of its pharmacologic effects, including analgesia.

In addition to analgesia, CNS effects include depression of spontaneous respiratory activity and cough, stimulation of the emetic center, miosis, and sedation. Effects possibly mediate by non-CNS mechanisms include alteration in cardiovascular resistance and capacitance, bronchomotor tone, gastrointestinal secretory and motor activity, and bladder sphincter activity.

In an animal model, the dose of the butorphanol tartrate required to antagonize morphine analgesia by 50% was similar to that for nalorphine, less than that for pentazocine and more than that for naloxone.

In human studies of butorphanol, sedation is commonly noted at doses of 0.5 mg or more. Narcosis is produced by 10 to 12 mg doses of butorphanol administered over 10 to 15 minutes intravenously.

Butorphanol, like other mixed agonist-antagonists with a high affinity for the kappa receptor, may produce unpleasant psychotomimetic effects in some individuals.

Nausea and/or vomiting may be produced by doses of 1 mg or more administered by any route.

In human studies involving individuals without significant respiratory dysfunction, 2 mg of butorphanol IV and 10 mg of morphine sulfate IV depressed respiration to a comparable degree. At higher doses, the magnitude of respiratory depression with butorphanol is not appreciably increased; however, the duration of respiratory depression is longer. Respiratory depression noted after administration of butorphanol to humans by any route is reversed by treatment with naloxone, a specific opioid antagonist.

Butorphanol tartrate demonstrates antitussive effects in animals at doses less than those required for analgesia.

Hemodynamic changes noted during cardiac catheterization in patients receiving single 0.025 mg/kg IV doses of butorphanol have included increases in pulmonary artery pressure, wedge pressure and vascular resistance, increases in left ventricular and diastolic pressure, and in systemic arterial pressure.

Pharmacodynamics – The analgesic effect of butorphanol is influenced by the route of administration. Onset of analgesia is within a few minutes for intravenous administration and within 15 minutes for IM injection.

Peak analgesic activity occurs within 30 to 60 minutes following IV and IM administration.

The duration of analgesia varies depending on the pain model as well as the route of administration, but is generally 3 to 4 hours with IM and IV doses as defined by the time 50% of patients required remedication. In postoperative studies, the duration of analgesia with IV or IM butorphanol was similar to morphine, meperidine, and pentazocine when administered in the same fashion at equipotent doses.

➤*Pharmacokinetics:*

Absorption/Distribution – Butorphanol tartrate injectable is rapidly absorbed after IM injection, and peak plasma levels are reached in 20 to 40 minutes. Following its initial absorption/distribution phase, the single-dose pharmacokinetics of butorphanol by the IV, IM, and nasal routes of administration are similar. Serum protein binding is independent of concentration over the range achieved in clinical practice (up to 7 ng/mL), with a bound fraction of approximately 80%. The drug is transported across the blood:brain and placental barriers and into human milk.

BUTORPHANOL TARTRATE — INJECTION

Metabolism/Excretion – Butorphanol is extensively metabolized in the liver. Metabolism is qualitatively and quantitatively similar following IV, IM, or nasal administration. Oral bioavailability is only 5% to 17% because of extensive first-pass metabolism of butorphanol.

The major metabolite of butorphanol is hydroxybutorphanol, while norbutorphanol is produced in small amounts. Both have been detected in plasma following administration of butorphanol, with norbutorphanol present at trace levels at most time points. The elimination half-life of hydroxybutorphanol is about 18 hours and, as a consequence, considerable accumulation (approximately 5-fold) occurs when butorphanol is dosed to steady-state (1 mg transnasally every 6 hours for 5 days).

Elimination occurs by urine and fecal excretion. When ^{3}H-labeled butorphanol is administered to healthy subjects, most (70% to 80%) of the dose is recovered in the urine, while approximately 15% is recovered in the feces.

About 5% of the dose is recovered in the urine as butorphanol. Forty-nine percent (49%) is eliminated in the urine as hydroxybutorphanol. Less than 5% is excreted in the urine as norbutorphanol.

Special populations –

Renal function impairment: In renally impaired patients with creatinine clearances less than 30 mL/min the elimination half-life is approximately doubled and the total body clearance is approximately one half (10.5 hours [clearance 150 L/hr] as compared to 5.8 hours [clearance 260 L/hr] in healthy subjects). No effect was observed on C_{max} or t_{max} after a single dose.

Hepatic function impairment: After IV administration to patients with hepatic impairment, the elimination half-life of butorphanol was approximately tripled and total body clearance was approximately one-half (half-life 16.8 hours, clearance 92 L/hr) compared to healthy subjects (half-life 4.8 hours, clearance 175 L/hr). The exposure of hepatically impaired patients to butorphanol was significantly greater (about 2-fold) than that in healthy subjects.

Pharmacokinetic parameters based on age:

Mean Pharmacokinetic Parameters of Butorphanol IV in Younger and Elderly Subjects[a]

Parameters	Younger	Elderly
AUC (inf)[b] (ng•h/mL)	7.24 (1.57) (4.4 to 9.77)	8.71 (2.02) (4.76 to 13.03)
Half-life (h)	4.56 (1.67) (2.06 to 8.7)	5.61 (1.36) (3.25 to 8.79)
Volume of distribution[c] (L)	487 (155) (305 to 901)	552 (124) (305 to 737)
Total body clearance (L/h)	99 (23) (70 to 154)	82 (21) (52 to 143)

[a] Younger subjects (n = 24) are from 20 to 40 years old and elderly (n = 24) are greater than 65 years of age.
[b] Area under the plasma concentration time curve after a 1 mg dose.
[c] Derived from IV data.

Contraindications

Hypersensitivity to butorphanol tartrate or the preservative benzethonium chloride.

Warnings/Precautions

➤*Patients dependent on narcotics:* Because of its opioid antagonist properties, butorphanol is not recommended for use in patients dependent on narcotics. Such patients should have an adequate period of withdrawal from opioid drugs prior to beginning butorphanol therapy. In patients taking opioid analgesics chronically, butorphanol has precipitated withdrawal symptoms such as anxiety, agitation, mood changes, hallucinations, dysphoria, weakness and diarrhea.

Because of the difficulty in assessing opioid tolerance in patients who have recently received repeated doses of narcotic analgesic medication, caution should be used in the administration of butorphanol to such patients.

➤*Head injury and increased intracranial pressure:* As with other opioids, the use of butorphanol in patients with head injury may be associated with carbon dioxide retention and secondary elevation of cerebrospinal fluid pressure, drug-induced miosis, and alterations in mental state that would obscure the interpretation of the clinical course of patients with head injuries. In such patients, butorphanol should be used only if the benefits of use outweigh the potential risks.

➤*Respiratory depression:* Butorphanol may produce respiratory depression, especially in patients receiving other CNS active agents, or patients suffering from CNS diseases or respiratory impairment.

➤*Cardiovascular effects:* Because butorphanol may increase the work of the heart, especially the pulmonary circuit, the use of butorphanol in patients with acute myocardial infarction, ventricular dysfunction, or coronary insufficiency should be limited to those situations where the benefits clearly outweigh the risk.

Severe hypertension has been reported rarely during butorphanol therapy. In such cases, butorphanol should be discontinued and the hypertension treated with antihypertensive drugs. In patients who are not opioid dependent, naloxone has also been reported to be effective.

➤*Renal/Hepatic function impairment:* See Administration and Dosage for more information.

➤*Drug abuse and dependence:* Butorphanol is one of a class of drugs known to be abused and thus should be handled accordingly. Butorphanol tartrate, by all routes of administration, has been associated with episodes of abuse. Of the cases received, there were more reports of abuse with the nasal spray formulation than with the injectable formulation.

Physical dependence, tolerance, and withdrawal – Prolonged, continuous use of butorphanol tartrate may result in physical dependence or tolerance (a decrease in response to a given dose). Abrupt cessation of use by patients with physical dependence may result in symptoms of withdrawal.

➤*Hazardous tasks:* Opioid analgesics, including butorphanol, impair the mental and physical abilities required for the performance of potentially dangerous tasks such as driving a car or operating machinery. Effects such as drowsiness or dizziness can appear, usually within the first hour after dosing. These effects may persist for varying periods of time after dosing. Patients who have taken butorphanol should not drive or operate dangerous machinery for at least 1 hour and until the effects of the drug are no longer present.

➤*Pregnancy:* *Category C.* Pregnant rats treated subcutaneously with butorphanol at 1 mg/kg (5.9 mg/m^2) had a higher frequency of stillbirths than controls. Butorphanol at 30 mg/kg/oral (360 mg/m^2) and 60 mg/kg/oral (720 mg/m^2) also showed higher incidences of post-implantation loss in rabbits.

There are no adequate and well-controlled studies of butorphanol tartrate in pregnant women before 37 weeks of gestation. Butorphanol tartrate should be used during pregnancy only if the potential benefit justifies the potential risk to the infant.

Labor and delivery – There have been rare reports of infant respiratory distress/apnea following the administration of butorphanol tartrate injectable during labor. The reports of respiratory distress/apnea have been associated with administration of a dose within 2 hours of delivery, use of multiple doses, use with additional analgesic or sedative drugs, or use in preterm pregnancies.

In a study of 119 patients, the administration of 1 mg of IV butorphanol tartrate injectable during labor was associated with transient (10 to 90 minutes) sinusoidal fetal heart rate patterns, but was not associated with adverse neonatal outcomes. In the presence of an abnormal fetal heart rate pattern, butorphanol tartrate injectable should be used with caution.

➤*Lactation:* Butorphanol has been detected in milk following administration of butorphanol tartrate injectable to nursing mothers. The amount an infant would receive is probably clinically insignificant (estimated 4 mcg/L of milk in a mother receiving 2 mg IM 4 times a day).

➤*Children:* Butorphanol is not recommended for use in patients below 18 years of age because safety and efficacy have not been established in the population.

➤*Elderly:* See Administration and Dosage for more information.

Due to changes in clearance, the mean half-life of butorphanol is increased by 25% (to over 6 hours) in patients over the age of 65 years. Elderly patients may be more sensitive to the side effects of butorphanol. In clinical studies of butorphanol nasal spray, elderly patients had an increased frequency of headache, dizziness, drowsiness, vertigo, constipation, nausea and/or vomiting, and nasal congestion compared with younger patients. There are insufficient efficacy data for patients 65 years to determine whether they respond differently from younger patients.

Butorphanol and its metabolites are known to be substantially excreted by the kidney, and the risk of toxic reactions to this drug may be greater in patients with impaired renal function. Because elderly patients are more likely to have decreased renal function, care should be taken in dose selection.

Drug Interactions

➤*CNS depressants:* Concurrent use of butorphanol with central nervous system depressants (eg, alcohol, barbiturates, tranquilizers, antihistamines) may result in increased central nervous system depressant effects. When used concurrently with such drugs, the dose of butorphanol should be the smallest effective dose and the frequency of dosing reduced as much as possible when administered concomitantly with drugs that potentiate the action of opioids.

Adverse Reactions

The most frequently reported adverse experiences across all clinical trials with butorphanol tartrate were somnolence (43%), dizziness (19%), nausea and/or vomiting (13%).

The following adverse experiences were reported at a frequency of 1% or greater, and were considered to be probably related to the use of butorphanol:

➤*Cardiovascular:* Vasodilation, palpitations.

➤*CNS:* Anxiety, confusion, dizziness, euphoria, floating feeling, insomnia, nervousness, paresthesia, somnolence, tremor.

➤*Dermatologic:* Sweating/clammy, pruritus.

➤*GI:* Anorexia, constipation, dry mouth, nausea or vomiting, stomach pain.

➤*Respiratory:* Bronchitis, cough, dyspnea, epistaxis, nasal congestion, nasal irritation, pharyngitis, rhinitis, sinus congestion, sinusitis, upper respiratory tract infection.

➤*Special senses:* Blurred vision, ear pain, tinnitus, unpleasant taste.

➤*Miscellaneous:* Asthenia/lethargy, headache, sensation of heat.

➤*The following adverse experiences were reported with a frequency of less than 1% in clinical trials and were considered to be probably related to the use of butorphanol:*

Cardiovascular – Hypotension, syncope.

BUTORPHANOL TARTRATE — INJECTION

CNS – Abnormal dreams, agitation, dysphoria, hallucinations, hostility, withdrawal symptoms.

Dermatologic – Rash/hives.

GU – Impaired urination.

➤*Postmarketing:* Postmarketing experience with butorphanol tartrate injection and nasal spray has shown an adverse event profile similar to that seen during the premarketing evaluation of butorphanol by all routes of administration. Adverse experiences that were associated with the use of butorphanol tartrate and that are not listed above have been chosen for inclusion below because of their seriousness, frequency of reporting, or probably relationship to butorphanol. Because they are reported voluntarily from a population of unknown size, estimates of frequency cannot be made. These adverse experiences include apnea, convulsion, delusion, drug dependence, excessive drug effect associated with transient difficulty speaking or executing purposeful movements, overdose, and vertigo. Reports of butorphanol overdose with fatal outcomes have usually but not always been associated with ingestion of multiple drugs.

Overdosage

➤*Symptoms:* The clinical manifestations of overdose are those of opioid drugs in general. Consequences of overdose vary with the amount of butorphanol ingested and individual response to the effects of opiates. The most serious symptoms are hypoventilation, cardiovascular insufficiency, coma, and death. Butorphanol overdose may be associated with ingestion of multiple drugs.

Overdose can occur due to accidental or intentional misuse of butorphanol, especially in young children who may gain access to the drug in the home.

➤*Treatment:* The management of suspected butorphanol overdosage includes maintenance of adequate ventilation, peripheral perfusion, normal body temperature, and protection of the airway. Patients should be under continuous observation with adequate serial measures of mental state, responsiveness and vital signs. Oxygen and ventilatory assistance should be available with continual monitoring by pulse oximetry if indicated. In the presence of coma, placement of an artificial airway may be required. An adequate intravenous portal should be maintained to facilitate treatment of hypotension associated with vasodilation.

The use of a specific opioid antagonist such as naloxone should be considered. As the duration of butorphanol action usually exceeds the duration of action of naloxone, repeated dosing with naloxone may be required.

In managing cases of suspected butorphanol overdose, the possibility of multiple drug ingestion should always be considered.

Patient Information

Drowsiness and dizziness related to the use of butorphanol may impair mental and/or physical abilities required for the performance of potentially hazardous tasks (eg, driving, operating machinery).

Alcohol should not be consumed while using butorphanol. Concurrent use of butorphanol with drugs that affect the central nervous system (eg, alcohol, barbiturates, tranquilizers, antihistamines) may result in increased central nervous system depressant effects such as drowsiness, dizziness and impaired mental function.

BUTORPHANOL TARTRATE — INTRANASAL

Refer to the general discussion in the Opioid Agonist-Antagonist Analgesic introduction.

Indications

➤*Pain:* Management of pain when the use of an opioid analgesic is appropriate.

Administration and Dosage

➤*General dosing considerations:* Factors to be considered in determining the dose are age, body weight, physical status, underlying pathological condition, use of other drugs, type of anesthesia to be used, and surgical procedure involved.

➤*Adults:*

Management of pain –

Usual dosage: 1 mg (1 spray in 1 nostril). If adequate pain relief is not achieved within 60 to 90 minutes, an additional 1 mg dose may be given. The initial 2-dose sequence may be repeated in 3 to 4 hours as required after the second dose of the sequence.

Alternative dosage: An initial dose of 2 mg (1 spray in each nostril), depending on the severity of the pain, may be used in patients who will be able to remain recumbent in the event drowsiness or dizziness occur. In such patients, single additional 2 mg doses should not be given for 3 to 4 hours.

➤*Elderly:* The initial dose sequence should be limited to 1 mg followed, if needed, by 1 mg in 90 to 120 minutes. The repeat dose sequence in these patients should be determined by the patient's response rather than at fixed times, but will generally be no less than at 6-hour intervals.

➤*Renal function impairment:* See Elderly for dosing.

➤*Hepatic function impairment:* See Elderly for dosing.

➤*Storage/Stability:* Store at 25°C (77°F) controlled room temperature.

Actions

➤*Pharmacology:* Butorphanol is a mixed agonist-antagonist with low intrinsic activity at receptors of the μ-opioid type (morphine-like). It is also an agonist at κ-opioid receptors.

Its interactions with these receptors in the central nervous system apparently mediate most of its pharmacologic effects, including analgesia.

In addition to analgesia, CNS effects include depression of spontaneous respiratory activity and cough, stimulation of the emetic center, miosis and sedation. Effects possibly mediate by non-CNS mechanisms include alteration in cardiovascular resistance and capacitance, bronchomotor tone, gastrointestinal secretory and motor activity and bladder sphincter activity.

In an animal model, the dose of the butorphanol tartrate required to antagonize morphine analgesia by 50% was similar to that for nalorphine, less than that for pentazocine and more than that for naloxone.

In human studies of butorphanol, sedation is commonly noted at doses of 0.5 mg or more. Narcosis is produced by 10 to 12 mg doses of butorphanol administered over 10 to 15 minutes intravenously.

Butorphanol, like other mixed agonist-antagonists with a high affinity for the kappa receptor, may produce unpleasant psychotomimetic effects in some individuals.

Nausea and/or vomiting may be produced by doses of 1 mg or more administered by any route.

In human studies involving individuals without significant respiratory dysfunction, 2 mg of butorphanol IV and 10 mg of morphine sulfate IV depressed respiration to a comparable degree. At higher doses, the magnitude of respiratory depression with butorphanol is not appreciably increased; however, the duration of respiratory depression is longer. Respiratory depression noted after administration of butorphanol to humans by any route is reversed by treatment with naloxone, a specific opioid antagonist. As the duration of butorphanol action usually exceeds the duration of action of naloxone, repeated dosing with naloxone may be required.

Butorphanol tartrate demonstrates antitussive effects in animals at doses less than those required for analgesia.

Hemodynamic changes noted during cardiac catheterization in patients receiving single 0.025 mg/kg intravenous doses of butorphanol have included increases in pulmonary artery pressure, wedge pressure and vascular resistance, increases in left ventricular and diastolic pressure and in systemic arterial pressure.

Pharmacodynamics – The analgesic effect of butorphanol is influenced by the route of administration. Onset of analgesia is within 15 minutes for the nasal spray dose.

Peak analgesic activity occurs within 1 to 2 hours following the nasal spray administration.

The duration of analgesia varies depending on the pain model as well as the route of administration. Compared to the injectable form and other drugs in this class, butorphanol tartrate nasal spray has a longer duration of action (4 to 5 hours).

➤*Pharmacokinetics:*

Absorption/Distribution – After nasal administration, mean peak blood levels of 0.9 to 1.04 ng/mL occur at 30 to 60 minutes after a 1 mg dose (see below). The absolute bioavailability of butorphanol tartrate is 60% to 70% and is unchanged in patients with allergic rhinitis. In patients using a nasal vasoconstrictor (oxymetazoline) the fraction of the dose absorbed was unchanged, but the rate of absorption was slowed. The peak plasma concentrations were approximately half those achieved in the absence of the vasoconstrictor.

Serum protein binding is independent of concentration over the range achieved in clinical practice (up to 7 ng/mL) with a bound fraction of approximately 80%.

Mean Pharmacokinetic Parameters of Butorphanol in Younger and Elderly Subjects[a]

	IV		Nasal	
Parameters	Younger	Elderly	Younger	Elderly
t_{max}[b] (h)			0.62 (0.32)[e] (0.15 to 1.5)[g]	1.03 (0.74) (0.25 to 3)
C_{max}[c] (ng/mL)			1.04 (0.4) (0.35 to 1.97)	0.9 (0.57) (0.1 to 2.68)
AUC (inf)[d] (ng•h/mL)	7.24 (1.57) (4.4 to 9.77)	8.71 (2.02) (4.76 to 13.03)	4.93 (1.24) (2.16 to 7.27)	5.24 (2.27) (0.3 to 10.34)
Half-life (h)	4.56 (1.67) (2.06 to 8.7)	5.61 (1.36) (3.25 to 8.79)	4.74 (1.57) (2.89 to 8.79)	6.56 (1.51) (3.75 to 9.17)
Absolute bioavailability (%)			69 (16) (44 to 113)	61 (25) (3 to 121)
Volume of distribution[f] (L)	487 (155) (305 to 901)	552 (124) (305 to 737)		
Total body clearance (L/h)	99 (23) (70 to 154)	82 (21) (52 to 143)		

[a] Younger subjects (n = 24) are from 20 to 40 years old and elderly (n = 24) are greater than 65 years of age.
[b] Time to peak plasma concentration.
[c] Peak plasma concentration normalized to 1 mg dose.
[d] Area under the plasma concentration time curve after a 1 mg dose.
[e] Mean (1 SD).
[f] Derived from IV data.
[g] (range of observed values)

Dose proportionality for butorphanol tartrate nasal spray has been determined at steady state in doses up to 4 mg at 6-hour intervals. Steady state is achieved within 2 days. The mean peak plasma concentration at steady state was 1.8-fold (maximal 3-fold) following a single dose.

BUTORPHANOL TARTRATE — INTRANASAL

The drug is transported across the blood:brain and placental barriers and into human milk.

Metabolism / Excretion – Butorphanol is extensively metabolized in the liver. Metabolism is qualitatively and quantitatively similar following intravenous, intramuscular, or nasal administration. Oral bioavailability is only 5% to 17% because of extensive first-pass metabolism of butorphanol.

The major metabolite of butorphanol is hydroxybutorphanol, while norbutorphanol is produced in small amounts. Both have been detected in plasma following administration of butorphanol, with norbutorphanol present at trace levels at most time points. The elimination half-life of hydroxybutorphanol is about 18 hours and, as a consequence, considerable accumulation (approximately 5-fold) occurs when butorphanol is dosed to steady state (1 mg transnasally every 6 hours for 5 days).

Elimination occurs by urine and fecal excretion. When 3H labeled butorphanol is administered to healthy subjects, most (70% to 80%) of the dose is recovered in the urine, while approximately 15% is recovered in the feces.

About 5% of the dose is recovered in the urine as butorphanol. Forty-nine percent is eliminated in the urine as hydroxybutorphanol. Less than 5% is excreted in the urine as norbutorphanol.

Special populations –

Renal function impairment: In renally impaired patients with creatinine clearances less than 30 mL/min, the elimination half-life is approximately doubled and the total body clearance is approximately one half (10.5 hours [clearance 150 L/hr] as compared to 5.8 hours [clearance 260 L/hr] in healthy subjects). No effect was observed on C_{max} or t_{max} after a single dose.

Hepatic function impairment: After intravenous administration to patients with hepatic impairment, the elimination half-life of butorphanol was approximately tripled and total body clearance was approximately one-half (half-life 16.8 hours, clearance 92 L/hr) compared to healthy subjects (half-life 4.8 hours, clearance 175 L/hr). The exposure of hepatically impaired patients to butorphanol was significantly greater (about 2-fold) than that in healthy subjects. Similar results were seen after nasal administration. No effect on C_{max} or t_{max} was observed after a single intranasal dose.

Elderly: Butorphanol pharmacokinetics in the elderly differ from younger patients. The mean absolute bioavailability of butorphanol tartrate in elderly women (48%) was less than that in elderly men (75%), younger men (68%) or younger women (70%). Elimination half-life is increased in the elderly (6.6 hours as opposed to 4.7 hours in younger subjects).

Contraindications

Hypersensitivity to butorphanol tartrate or the preservative benzethonium chloride.

Warnings/Precautions

➤*Patients dependent on narcotics:* Because of its opioid antagonist properties, butorphanol is not recommended for use in patients dependent on narcotics. Such patients should have an adequate period of withdrawal from opioid drugs prior to beginning butorphanol therapy. In patients taking opioid analgesics chronically, butorphanol has precipitated withdrawal symptoms such as anxiety, agitation, mood changes, hallucinations, dysphoria, weakness and diarrhea.

Because of the difficulty in assessing opioid tolerance in patients who have recently received repeated doses of narcotic analgesic medication, caution should be used in the administration of butorphanol to such patients.

➤*Head injury and increased intracranial pressure:* As with other opioids, the use of butorphanol in patients with head injury may be associated with carbon dioxide retention and secondary elevation of cerebrospinal fluid pressure, drug-induced miosis, and alterations in mental state that would obscure the interpretation of the clinical course of patients with head injuries. In such patients, butorphanol should be used only if the benefits of use outweigh the potential risks.

➤*Respiratory depression:* Butorphanol may produce respiratory depression, especially in patients receiving other CNS active agents, or patients suffering from CNS diseases or respiratory impairment.

➤*Cardiovascular effects:* Because butorphanol may increase the work of the heart, especially the pulmonary circuit, the use of butorphanol in patients with acute myocardial infarction, ventricular dysfunction, or coronary insufficiency should be limited to those situations where the benefits clearly outweigh the risk.

Hypotension associated with syncope during the first hour of dosing with butorphanol tartrate nasal spray has been reported rarely, particularly in patients with a history of similar reactions to opioid analgesics. Therefore, patients should be advised to avoid activities with potential risks.

Severe hypertension has been reported rarely during butorphanol therapy. In such cases, butorphanol should be discontinued and the hypertension treated with antihypertensive drugs. In patients who are not opioid dependent, naloxone has also been reported to be effective.

➤*Hazardous tasks:* Opioid analgesics, including butorphanol, impair the mental and physical abilities required for the performance of potentially dangerous tasks such as driving a car or operating machinery. Effects such as drowsiness or dizziness can appear, usually within the first hour after dosing. These effects may persist for varying periods of time after dosing. Patients who have taken butorphanol should not drive or operate dangerous machinery for at least 1 hour and until the effects of the drug are no longer present.

Alcohol should not be consumed while using butorphanol. Concurrent use of butorphanol with drugs that effect the central nervous system (eg, alcohol, barbiturates, tranquilizers, antihistamines) may result in increased central nervous system depressant effects such as drowsiness, dizziness, and impaired mental function.

Butorphanol is one of a class of drugs known to be abused and thus should be handled accordingly.

Patients should be instructed on the proper use of butorphanol tartrate.

➤*Renal / Hepatic function impairment:* In patients with hepatic or renal impairment, the initial dose sequence of butorphanol tartrate nasal spray should be limited to 1 mg followed, if needed, by 1 mg in 90 to 120 minutes. The repeat dose sequence in these patients should be determined by the patient's response rather than at fixed times but will generally be at intervals of no less than 6 hours.

➤*Drug abuse and dependence:* Butorphanol tartrate, by all routes of administration, has been associated with episodes of abuse. Of the cases received, there were more reports of abuse with the nasal spray formulation than with the injectable formulation.

Physical dependence, tolerance, and withdrawal – Prolonged, continuous use of butorphanol tartrate may result in physical dependence or tolerance (a decrease in response to a given dose). Abrupt cessation of use by patients with physical dependence may result in symptoms of withdrawal.

Clinical trial experience – In all clinical trials, less than 1% of patients using butorphanol tartrate nasal spray had experiences that suggested the development of physical dependence or tolerance. Much of this information is based on experience with patients who did not have prolonged continuous exposure to butorphanol tartrate nasal spray. However, in 1 controlled clinical trial where patients with chronic pain from nonmalignant disease were treated with butorphanol tartrate nasal spray (n = 303) or placebo (n = 99) for up to 6 months, overuse (which may suggest the development of tolerance) was reported in nine (2.9%) patients receiving butorphanol tartrate nasal spray and no patients receiving placebo. Probable withdrawal symptoms were reported in eight (2.6%) patients using butorphanol tartrate nasal spray and no patients receiving placebo in the chronic nonmalignant pain study. Most of these patients abruptly discontinued butorphanol tartrate nasal spray after extended use or high doses. Symptoms suggestive of withdrawal included anxiety, agitation, tremulousness, diarrhea, chills, sweats, insomnia, confusion, incoordination, and hallucinations.

Postmarketing experience – Butorphanol tartrate has been associated with episodes of abuse and dependence. Of the cases received, there were more reports of abuse with the nasal spray formulation than with the injectable formulation.

➤*Pregnancy: Category C.* Pregnant rats treated subcutaneously with butorphanol at 1 mg/kg (5.9 mg/m^2) had a higher frequency of stillbirths than controls. Butorphanol at 30 mg/kg/oral (360 mg/m^2) and 60 mg/kg/oral (720 mg/m^2) also showed higher incidences of post-implantation loss in rabbits.

There are no adequate and well controlled studies of butorphanol tartrate in pregnant women before 37 weeks of gestation. Butorphanol tartrate should be used during pregnancy only if the potential benefit justifies the potential risk to the infant.

Labor and delivery – Butorphanol tartrate nasal spray is not recommended during labor or delivery because there is no clinical experience with its use in this setting.

➤*Lactation:* Although there is no clinical experience with the use of butorphanol tartrate nasal spray in nursing mothers, it should be assumed that butorphanol will appear in the milk following the nasal route of administration.

➤*Children:* Butorphanol is not recommended for use in patients below 18 years of age because safety and efficacy have not been established in the population.

➤*Elderly:* See Administration and Dosage for more information.

Due to changes in clearance, the mean half-life of butorphanol is increased by 25% (to over 6 hours) in patients over the age of 65 years. Elderly patients may be more sensitive to the side effects of butorphanol. In clinical studies of butorphanol tartrate nasal spray, elderly patients had an increased frequency of headache, dizziness, drowsiness, vertigo, constipation, nausea and/or vomiting, and nasal congestion compared with younger patients. There are insufficient efficacy data for patients greater than or equal to 65 years to determine whether they respond differently from younger patients.

Butorphanol and its metabolites are known to be substantially excreted by the kidney, and the risk of toxic reactions to this drug may be greater in patients with impaired renal function. Because elderly patients are more likely to have decreased renal function, care should be taken in dose selection.

Drug Interactions

➤*CNS depressants:* Concurrent use of butorphanol with central nervous system depressants (eg, alcohol, barbiturates, tranquilizers, and antihistamines) may result in increased central nervous system depressant effects. When used concurrently with such drugs, the dose of butorphanol should be the smallest effective dose and the frequency of dosing reduced as much as possible when administered concomitantly with drugs that potentiate the action of opioids.

➤*Sumatriptan:* In healthy volunteers, the pharmacokinetics of a 1 mg dose of butorphanol administered as butorphanol tartrate nasal spray were not affected by the coadministration of a single 6 mg subcutaneous dose of sumatriptan. However, in another study in healthy volunteers, the pharmacokinetics of butorphanol were significantly altered (29% decrease in AUC and 38% decrease in C_{max}) when a 1 mg dose of butorphanol tartrate nasal spray was administered 1 minute after a 20 mg dose of sumatriptan nasal spray. (The 2 drugs were administered in opposite nostrils.) When the butor-

BUTORPHANOL TARTRATE — INTRANASAL

phanol tartrate nasal spray was administered 30 minutes after the sumatriptan nasal spray, the AUC of butorphanol increased 11% and C_{max} decreased 18%.

In neither case were the pharmacokinetics of sumatriptan affected by coadministration with butorphanol tartrate nasal spray. These results suggest that the analgesic effect of butorphanol tartrate nasal spray may be diminished when it is administered shortly after sumatriptan nasal spray, but by 30 minutes any such reduction in effect should be minimal.

The safety of using butorphanol tartrate nasal spray and sumatriptan nasal spray during the same episode of migraine has not been established. However, it should be noted that both products are capable of producing transient increases in blood pressure.

➤*Nasal vasoconstrictors:* The fraction of butorphanol tartrate absorbed is unaffected by the concomitant administration of a nasal vasoconstrictor (oxymetazoline), but the rate of absorption is decreased. Therefore, a slower onset can be anticipated if butorphanol tartrate is administered concomitantly with, or immediately following, a nasal vasoconstrictor.

Adverse Reactions

The most frequently reported adverse experiences across all clinical trials with butorphanol tartrate injection and nasal spray were somnolence (43%), dizziness (19%), nausea and/or vomiting (13%). In long-term trials with butorphanol tartrate nasal spray only, nasal congestion (13%) and insomnia (11%) were frequently reported.

The following adverse experiences were reported at a frequency of 1% or greater, and were considered to be probably related to the use of butorphanol.

➤*Cardiovascular:* Vasodilation, palpitations.

➤*CNS:* Anxiety, confusion, dizziness, euphoria, floating feeling, insomnia, nervousness, paresthesia, somnolence, tremor.

➤*Dermatologic:* Sweating/clammy, pruritus.

➤*GI:* Anorexia, constipation, dry mouth, nausea and/or vomiting, stomach pain.

➤*Respiratory:* Bronchitis, cough, dyspnea, epistaxis, nasal congestion, nasal irritation, pharyngitis, rhinitis, sinus congestion, sinusitis, upper respiratory tract infection.

➤*Special senses:* Blurred vision, ear pain, tinnitus, unpleasant taste.

➤*Miscellaneous:* Asthenia/lethargy, headache, sensation of heat.

➤*Adverse experiences reported with a frequency of less than 1%:* The following adverse experiences were reported with a frequency of less than 1%, in clinical trials or from postmarketing experience, and were considered to be probably related to the use of butorphanol.

Cardiovascular – Hypotension, syncope.

CNS – Abnormal dreams, agitation, dysphoria, hallucinations, hostility, withdrawal symptoms.

Dermatologic – Rash/hives.

GU – Impaired urination.

➤*Adverse reactions (less than 1% frequency and postmarketing experiences):* The following infrequent additional adverse experiences were reported in a frequency of less than 1% of the patients studied in short-term butorphanol tartrate nasal spray trials and under circumstances where the association between these events and butorphanol administration is unknown. They are being listed as altering information for the physician.

Cardiovascular – Chest pain, hypertension, tachycardia.

CNS – Depression.

Respiratory – Shallow breathing.

Miscellaneous – Edema.

➤*Postmarketing experience:* Postmarketing experience with butorphanol tartrate nasal spray and butorphanol tartrate injection has shown an adverse event profile similar to that seen during the premarketing evaluation of butorphanol by all routes of administration. Adverse experiences that were associated with the use of butorphanol tartrate nasal spray or butorphanol tartrate injection and that are not listed above have been chosen for inclusion below because of their seriousness, frequency of reporting, or probable relationship to butorphanol. Because they are reported voluntarily from a population of unknown size, estimates of frequency cannot be made. These adverse experiences include apnea, convulsion, delusion, drug dependence, excessive drug effect associated with transient difficulty speaking and/or executing purposeful movements, overdose, and vertigo. Reports of butorphanol overdose with a fatal outcome have usually but not always been associated with ingestion of multiple drugs.

Overdosage

➤*Symptoms:* The clinical manifestations of overdose are those of opioid drugs, the most serious of which are hypoventilation, cardiovascular insufficiency, coma, and death. Butorphanol overdose may be associated with ingestion of multiple drugs.

Consequences of overdose vary with the amount of butorphanol ingested and individual response to the effects of opiates.

Overdose can occur due to accidental or intentional misuse of butorphanol, especially in young children who may gain access to the drug in the home.

➤*Treatment:* The management of suspected butorphanol overdosage includes maintenance of adequate ventilation, peripheral perfusion, normal body temperature, and protection of the airway. Patients should be under continuous observation with adequate serial measures of mental state, responsiveness and vital signs. Oxygen and ventilatory assistance should be available with continual monitoring by pulse oximetry if indicated. In the presence of coma, placement of an artificial airway may be required. An adequate intravenous portal should be maintained to facilitate treatment of hypotension associated with vasodilation.

The use of a specific opioid antagonist such as naloxone should be considered. As the duration of butorphanol action usually exceeds the duration of action of naloxone, repeated dosing with naloxone may be required.

In managing cases of suspected butorphanol overdosage, the possibility of multiple drug ingestion should always be considered.

Patient Information

Drowsiness and dizziness related to the use of butorphanol may impair mental and/or physical abilities required for the performance of potentially hazardous tasks (eg, driving, operating machinery).

Alcohol should not be consumed while using butorphanol. Concurrent use of butorphanol with drugs that affect the central nervous system (eg, alcohol, barbiturates, tranquilizers, antihistamines) may result in increased central nervous system depressant effects such as drowsiness, dizziness and impaired mental function.

Patients should be instructed on the proper use of butorphanol tartrate.

NALBUPHINE HYDROCHLORIDE

Rx	**Nalbuphine Hydrochloride** (Various, eg, Hospira)	**Injection:** 10 mg/mL	In 1 and 10 mL vials.
Rx	**Nubain** (Endo)		In 1 mL amps[a] and 10 mL vials. Parabens.
Rx	**Nalbuphine Hydrochloride** (Various, eg, Hospira)	**Injection:** 20 mg/mL	In 1 and 10 mL vials.
Rx	**Nubain** (Endo)		In 1 mL amps[a] and 10 mL vials. Parabens.

[a] Available as sulfite/paraben-free.

NALBUPHINE HYDROCHLORIDE — INJECTION

Refer to the general discussion in the Opioid Agonist-Antagonist Analgesic introduction.

Indications

➤*Pain:* For the relief of moderate to severe pain.

➤*Anesthesia:* For use as a supplement to balanced anesthesia, for preoperative and postoperative analgesia, and for obstetrical analgesia during labor and delivery.

➤*Off-label uses:* For the prevention and treatment of intrathecal morphine-induced pruritus after cesarean delivery.

Administration and Dosage

➤*General dosing considerations:* Patients who have been taking opioids chronically may experience withdrawal symptoms upon the administration of nalbuphine. If unduly troublesome, opioid withdrawal symptoms may be controlled by the slow IV administration of small increments of morphine until relief occurs.

➤*Adults:*

Pain –

Nonopioid tolerant patients:

- *Usual dosage* – 10 mg for a 70 kg individual administered subcutaneously, intramuscularly, or IV. May repeat the dose every 3 to 6 hours as necessary.
- *Maximum dose* – Recommended single maximum dose is 20 mg with a maximum total daily dose of 160 mg.

Patients dependent on opioids: If the previous analgesic was morphine, meperidine, codeine, or another opioid with similar duration of activity, 25% of the anticipated dose of nalbuphine may be administered initially and the patient observed for signs of withdrawal (ie, abdominal cramps, nausea and vomiting, lacrimation, rhinorrhea, anxiety, restlessness, elevation of temperature, piloerection). If untoward symptoms do not occur, progressively larger doses may be tried at appropriate intervals until the desired level of analgesia is obtained.

Supplement to anesthesia –

Initial dosage: 0.3 to 3 mg/kg IV administered over a 10- to 15-minute period.

Maintenance dosage: 0.25 to 0.5 mg/kg in a single IV administration.

➤*Renal function impairment:* Use nalbuphine with caution in patients with renal dysfunction and administer in reduced amounts.

NALBUPHINE HYDROCHLORIDE — INJECTION

➤*Hepatic function impairment:* Use nalbuphine with caution in patients with liver dysfunction and administer in reduced amounts.

➤*Administration:* Administer subcutaneously, intramuscularly, or IV.

➤*Admixture compatibility:* Nalbuphine is physically incompatible with nafcillin and ketorolac.

➤*Storage/Stability:* Store at 25°C (77°F); excursions permitted to 15° to 30°C (59° to 86°F). Protect from excessive light. Store in carton until contents have been used.

Actions

➤*Pharmacology:* Nalbuphine is a synthetic opioid agonist-antagonist analgesic of the phenanthrene series. It is related chemically to both the widely used opioid antagonist, naloxone, and the potent opioid analgesic, oxymorphone.

Nalbuphine is a potent analgesic. Its analgesic potency is essentially equivalent to that of morphine on a milligram basis. The opioid antagonist activity of nalbuphine is one-fourth as potent as nalorphine and 10 times that of pentazocine. Receptor studies show that nalbuphine binds to mu, kappa, and delta receptors, but not to sigma receptors. Nalbuphine is primarily a kappa agonist/partial mu antagonist analgesic.

Nalbuphine may produce the same degree of respiratory depression as equianalgesic doses of morphine. However, nalbuphine exhibits a ceiling effect such that increases in dose greater than 30 mg do not produce further respiratory depression.

Nalbuphine by itself has potent opioid antagonist activity at doses equal to or lower than its analgesic dose. When administered following or concurrent with mu agonist opioid analgesics (eg, morphine, oxymorphone, fentanyl), nalbuphine may partially reverse or block opioid-induced respiratory depression from the mu agonist analgesic. Nalbuphine may precipitate withdrawal in patients dependent on opioid drugs. Use nalbuphine with caution in patients who have been receiving mu opioid analgesics on a regular basis.

➤*Pharmacokinetics:* The onset of action of nalbuphine occurs within 2 to 3 minutes after IV administration, and in less than 15 minutes following subcutaneous or intramuscular injection. The plasma half-life of nalbuphine is 5 hours, and in clinical studies the duration of analgesic activity has been reported to range from 3 to 6 hours. Nalbuphine is metabolized in the liver and excreted by the kidneys.

Contraindications

Hypersensitivity to nalbuphine, or to any of the other ingredients in the product.

Warnings/Precautions

➤*Administration:* Nalbuphine should be given as a supplement to general anesthesia only by persons specifically trained in the use of IV anesthetics and management of the respiratory effects of potent opioids. Naloxone, resuscitative and intubation equipment, and oxygen should be readily available.

➤*Head injury and increased intracranial pressure:* The possible respiratory depressant effects and the potential of potent analgesics to elevate cerebrospinal fluid pressure (resulting from vasodilation following CO_2 retention) may be exaggerated markedly in the presence of head injury, intracranial lesions, or a preexisting increase in intracranial pressure. Furthermore, potent analgesics may produce effects that may obscure the clinical course of patients with head injuries. Therefore, use nalbuphine in these circumstances only when essential, and then administer with extreme caution.

➤*Respiratory depression:* At the usual adult dose of 10 mg/70 kg, nalbuphine causes some respiratory depression approximately equal to that produced by equal doses of morphine. However, in contrast to morphine, respiratory depression is not increased appreciably with higher doses of nalbuphine. Respiratory depression induced by nalbuphine may be reversed by naloxone when indicated. Administer nalbuphine with caution at low doses to patients with impaired respiration (eg, from other medication, uremia, bronchial asthma, severe infection, cyanosis, or respiratory obstructions).

➤*Myocardial infarction:* Use with caution in patients with myocardial infarction who have nausea or vomiting.

➤*Biliary tract surgery:* Use with caution in patients about to undergo surgery of the biliary tract since it may cause spasm of the sphincter of Oddi.

➤*Cardiovascular effects:* During evaluation of nalbuphine in anesthesia, a higher incidence of bradycardia has been reported in patients who did not receive atropine preoperatively.

➤*Renal/Hepatic function impairment:* Because nalbuphine is metabolized in the liver and excreted by the kidneys, use nalbuphine with caution in patients with renal or liver dysfunction and administer in reduced amounts.

➤*Drug abuse and dependence:* Observe caution in prescribing nalbuphine to emotionally unstable patients or to individuals with a history of opioid abuse. Closely supervise such patients when long-term therapy is contemplated.

There have been reports of abuse and dependence associated with nalbuphine among health care providers, patients, and bodybuilders. There have been reported instances of psychological and physical dependence and tolerance in patients abusing nalbuphine. Individuals with a prior history of opioid or other substance abuse or dependence may be at greater risk in responding to reinforcing properties of nalbuphine.

Opioid withdrawal effects – Abrupt discontinuation of nalbuphine following prolonged use has been followed by symptoms of opioid withdrawal (ie, abdominal cramps, nausea and vomiting, rhinorrhea, lacrimation, restlessness, anxiety, elevated temperature, piloerection).

➤*Hazardous tasks:* Nalbuphine may impair the mental or physical abilities required for the performance of potentially dangerous tasks such as driving a car or operating machinery. Therefore, administer nalbuphine with caution to ambulatory patients who should be warned to avoid such hazards.

➤*Pregnancy:* *Category B*. (*Category D* in prolonged use or in high doses at term). Safe use of nalbuphine in pregnancy has not been established. Although animal reproductive studies have not revealed teratogenic or embryotoxic effects, administer nalbuphine to pregnant women only if clearly needed, if the potential benefit outweighs the risk to the fetus, and if appropriate measures such as fetal monitoring are taken to detect and manage any potential adverse effect on the fetus.

Neonatal body weight and survival rates were reduced at birth and during lactation when nalbuphine was administered subcutaneously to female and male rats prior to mating and throughout gestation and lactation or to pregnant rats during the last third of the gestation period and throughout lactation at doses approximately 4 times the maximum recommended human dose.

Severe fetal bradycardia has been reported when nalbuphine is administered during labor. Naloxone may reverse these effects. Although there are no reports of fetal bradycardia earlier in pregnancy, it is possible that this may occur.

Labor and delivery – The placental transfer of nalbuphine is high, rapid, and variable with a maternal to fetal ratio ranging from 1:0.37 to 1:6. Fetal and neonatal adverse effects that have been reported following the administration of nalbuphine to the mother during labor include fetal bradycardia, respiratory depression at birth, apnea, cyanosis, and hypotonia. Maternal administration of naloxone during labor has normalized these effects in some cases. Severe and prolonged fetal bradycardia has been reported. Permanent neurological damage attributed to fetal bradycardia has occurred. A sinusoidal fetal heart rate pattern associated with the use of nalbuphine also has been reported. Use nalbuphine during labor and delivery only if clearly indicated and only if the potential benefit outweighs the risk to the infant. Monitor newborns for respiratory depression, apnea, bradycardia, and arrhythmias if nalbuphine has been used.

➤*Lactation:* Limited data suggest that nalbuphine is excreted in maternal milk but only in a small amount (less than 1% of the administered dose) and with a clinically insignificant effect. Exercise caution when nalbuphine is administered to a nursing woman.

➤*Children:* Safety and effectiveness in pediatric patients below the age of 18 years have not been established.

Drug Interactions

Nalbuphine Drug Interactions

Precipitant drug	Object drug[a]		Description
Cimetidine	Nalbuphine	⬆	The actions of nalbuphine may be enhanced, resulting in toxicity. If significant CNS depression develops, withdraw the drugs.
Nalbuphine	Barbiturate anesthetics (ie, thiopental)	⬆	The dose required to induce anesthesia may need to be reduced in the presence of nalbuphine. Monitor for additive pharmacologic effects such as respiratory depression.
Nalbuphine	CNS depressants (ie, opioid analgesics, general anesthetics, phenothiazines, tranquilizers, sedatives, hypnotics, alcohol)	⬆	Concomitant use may exhibit additive CNS depression. When such combined therapy is used, reduce the dose of one or both agents.
CNS depressants (ie, opioid analgesics, general anesthetics, phenothiazines, tranquilizers, sedatives)	Nalbuphine		

[a] ⬆ = object drug increased.

➤*Drug/Lab test interactions:* Nalbuphine may interfere with enzymatic methods for the detection of opioids depending on the specificity/sensitivity of the test. Please consult the test manufacturer for specific details.

Adverse Reactions

➤*Hypersensitivity:* Anaphylactic/anaphylactoid and other serious hypersensitivity reactions have been reported. These reactions may include shock, respiratory distress, respiratory arrest, bradycardia, cardiac arrest, hypotension, or laryngeal edema. Other allergic-type reactions reported include stridor, bronchospasm, wheezing, edema, rash, pruritus, nausea, vomiting, diaphoresis, weakness, and shakiness.

NALBUPHINE HYDROCHLORIDE — INJECTION

➤*Cardiovascular:* Bradycardia, hypertension, hypotension, tachycardia (1% or less).

➤*CNS:* Sedation (36%); dizziness/vertigo (5%); headache (3%); confusion, crying, depression, dysphoria, euphoria, faintness, feeling of heaviness, floating, hallucinations, hostility, nervousness, numbness, restlessness, tingling, unreality, unusual dreams (1% or less). The incidence of psychotomimetic effects, such as delusions, depersonalization, dysphoria, hallucinations, and unreality, has been shown to be less than that which occurs with pentazocine.

➤*Dermatologic:* Sweaty/clammy (9%); burning, itching, urticaria (1% or less).

➤*GI:* Nausea/vomiting (6%); dry mouth (4%); bitter taste, cramps, dyspepsia (1% or less).

➤*Respiratory:* Asthma, depression, dyspnea (1% or less).

➤*Miscellaneous:* Blurred vision, flushing and warmth, speech difficulty, urinary urgency (1% or less).

Postmarketing – Other reports include agitation; injection-site reactions such as burning, hot sensations, pain, redness, and swelling; pulmonary edema; seizures.

Overdosage

➤*Symptoms:* The administration of single doses of 72 mg nalbuphine subcutaneously to 8 healthy subjects has been reported to have resulted primarily in symptoms of sleepiness and mild dysphoria.

➤*Treatment:* The immediate IV administration of an opiate antagonist such as naloxone or nalmefene is a specific antidote. Use oxygen, IV fluids, vasopressors, and other supportive measures as indicated.

Patient Information

Nalbuphine is associated with sedation and may impair mental and physical abilities required for the performance of potentially dangerous tasks such as driving a car or operating machinery.

Nalbuphine is to be used as prescribed by a physician. Do not increase dose or frequency without first consulting with a physician since nalbuphine may cause psychological or physical dependence.

The use of nalbuphine with other narcotics may cause signs and symptoms of withdrawal.

Abrupt discontinuation of nalbuphine after prolonged usage may cause signs and symptoms of withdrawal.

PENTAZOCINE

c-iv	**Talwin** (Abbott Hospital Products)	**Injection:** 30 mg (as lactate)/mL	In 10 mL vials[a], 1 mL *Uni-Amps*, 1 mL *Uni-Nest* amps and 1 and 2 mL fill in 2 mL *Carpuject*.[b]

[a] With 2 mg acetone sodium bisulfite and 1 mg methylparaben per mL.

[b] With 1 mg acetone sodium bisulfite.

PENTAZOCINE LACTATE — INJECTION

Refer to the general discussion in the Opioid Agonist-Antagonist Analgesic introduction.

Indications

➤*Moderate to severe pain:* For the relief of moderate to severe pain.

➤*Preoperative or preanesthetic/supplement to surgical anesthesia:* For use as a preoperative or preanesthetic medication and as a supplement to surgical anesthesia.

Administration and Dosage

➤*Adults:*

Labor pain –

Usual dosage: 30 mg as a single IM dose.

Alternative dosage: 20 mg IV dose has given adequate pain relief to some patients in labor when contractions become regular, and this dose may be given 2 or 3 times at 2- to 3-hour intervals, as needed.

Moderate to severe pain –

Usual dosage: 30 mg by IM, subcutaneous, or IV route. This may be repeated every 3 to 4 hours.

Maximum dose: 30 mg IV or 60 mg IM or subcutaneously. Total daily dosage should not exceed 360 mg.

Preoperative or preanesthetic/supplement to surgical anesthesia – See Moderate to severe pain for dosing.

➤*Children:*

12 years of age and older – See Adults for dosing for patients 12 years of age and older.

➤*Administration:* The subcutaneous route of administration should be used only when necessary because of possible severe tissue damage at injection sites.

When frequent injections are needed, the drug should be administered IM. In addition, constant rotation of injection sites (eg, the upper outer quadrants of the buttocks, mid-lateral aspects of the thighs, and the deltoid areas) is essential.

➤*Admixture compatibility:* Pentazocine should not be mixed in the same syringe with soluble barbiturates because precipitation will occur.

Actions

➤*Pharmacology:* Pentazocine lactate is a potent analgesic and 30 mg is usually as effective an analgesic as morphine 10 mg or meperidine 75 mg to 100 mg; however, a few studies suggest the pentazocine lactate to morphine ratio may range from 20 mg to 40 mg pentazocine lactate to 10 mg morphine. The duration of analgesia may sometimes be less than that of morphine. Analgesia usually occurs within 15 to 20 minutes after IM or subcutaneous injection and within 2 to 3 minutes after IV injection. Pentazocine lactate weakly antagonizes the analgesic effects of morphine, meperidine, and phenazocine; in addition, it produces incomplete reversal of cardiovascular, respiratory, and behavioral depression induced by morphine and meperidine. Pentazocine lactate has about 1/50 the antagonistic activity of nalorphine. It also has sedative activity.

Contraindications

Hypersensitivity to pentazocine lactate.

Warnings/Precautions

➤*General information:* In prescribing parenteral pentazocine lactate for chronic use, particularly if the drug is to be self-administered, the physician should take precautions to avoid increases in dose and frequency of injection by the patient.

Just as with all medication, the oral form of pentazocine lactate is preferable for chronic administration.

➤*Tissue damage at injection sites:* Severe sclerosis of the skin, subcutaneous tissues, and underlying muscle have occurred at the injection sites of patients who have received multiple doses of pentazocine lactate. Constant rotation of injection sites is, therefore, essential. In addition, animal studies have demonstrated that pentazocine lactate is not tolerated as well subcutaneously as it is intramuscularly (see Administration and Dosage).

➤*Head injury and increased intracranial pressure:* As in the case of other potent analgesics, the potential of pentazocine lactate injection for elevating cerebrospinal fluid pressure may be attributed to CO_2 retention due to the respiratory depressant effects of the drug. These effects may be markedly exaggerated in the presence of head injury, other intracranial lesions, or a preexisting increase in intracranial pressure. Furthermore, pentazocine lactate can produce effects which may obscure the clinical course of patients with head injuries. In such patients, pentazocine lactate must be used with extreme caution and only if its use is deemed essential.

➤*Acute CNS manifestations:* Patients receiving therapeutic doses of pentazocine have experienced hallucinations (usually visual), disorientation, and confusion which have cleared spontaneously within a period of hours. The mechanism of this reaction is not known. Such patients should be closely observed and vital signs checked. If the drug is reinstituted, it should be done with caution since these acute CNS manifestations may recur.

➤*Myocardial infarction:* Caution should be exercised in the IV use of pentazocine for patients with acute myocardial infarction accompanied by hypertension or left ventricular failure. Data suggest that intravenous administration of pentazocine increases systemic and pulmonary arterial pressure and systemic vascular resistance in patients with acute myocardial infarction.

➤*Biliary surgery:* Narcotic drug products are generally considered to elevate biliary tract pressure for varying periods following their administration. Some evidence suggests that pentazocine may differ from other marketed narcotics in this respect (ie, it causes little or no elevation in biliary tract pressures). The clinical significance of these findings, however, is not yet known.

➤*Respiratory depression:* The possibility that pentazocine lactate may cause respiratory depression should be considered in treatment of patients with bronchial asthma. Pentazocine lactate should be administered only with caution and in low dosage to patients with respiratory depression (eg, from other medication, uremia, or severe infection), severely limited respiratory reserve, obstructive respiratory conditions, or cyanosis.

➤*CNS effect:* Caution should be used when pentazocine lactate is administered to patients prone to seizures; seizures have occurred in a few such patients in association with the use of pentazocine lactate although no cause and effect relationship has been established.

➤*Sulfite sensitivity:* Some of these products may contain acetone sodium bisulfite, a sulfite that may cause allergic-type reactions including anaphylactic symptoms and life-threatening or less severe asthmatic episodes in certain susceptible people. The overall prevalence of sulfite sensitivity in the general population is unknown and probably low. Sulfite sensitivity is seen more frequently in asthmatic than in nonasthmatic people.

➤*Renal/Hepatic function impairment:* Although laboratory tests have not indicated that pentazocine lactate causes or increases renal or hepatic impairment, the drug should be administered with caution to patients with such impairment. Extensive liver disease appears to predispose to greater side effects (eg, marked apprehension, anxiety, dizziness, sleepiness) from the usual clinical dose, and may be the result of decreased metabolism of the drug by the liver.

➤*Drug abuse and dependence:* Special care should be exercised in prescribing pentazocine for emotionally unstable patients and for those with a history of drug misuse. Such patients should be closely supervised when

PENTAZOCINE LACTATE — INJECTION

more than 4 or 5 days of therapy is contemplated. There have been instances of psychological and physical dependence on pentazocine lactate in patients with such a history and, rarely, in patients without such a history. Extended use of parenteral pentazocine lactate may lead to physical or psychological dependence in some patients. When pentazocine lactate is abruptly discontinued, withdrawal symptoms such as abdominal cramps, elevated temperature, rhinorrhea, restlessness, anxiety, and lacrimation may occur. However, even when these have occurred, discontinuance has been accomplished with minimal difficulty. In the rare patient in whom more than minor difficulty has been encountered, reinstitution of parenteral pentazocine lactate with gradual withdrawal has ameliorated the patient's symptoms. Substituting methadone or other narcotics for pentazocine lactate in the treatment of the pentazocine abstinence syndrome should be avoided. There have been rare reports of possible abstinence syndromes in newborns after prolonged use of pentazocine lactate during pregnancy.

➤*Hazardous tasks:* Since sedation, dizziness, and occasional euphoria have been noted, ambulatory patients should be warned not to operate machinery, drive cars, or unnecessarily expose themselves to hazards.

➤*Pregnancy: Category C. Category D* if used for prolonged periods or in high doses at term (per Briggs' *Drugs in Pregnancy and Lactation*).

Safe use of pentazocine during pregnancy (other than labor) has not been established. Animal reproduction studies have not demonstrated teratogenic or embryotoxic effects. Pentazocine rapidly crosses the placenta, resulting in cord blood levels of 40% to 70% of maternal serum. However, pentazocine should be administered to pregnant patients (other than labor) only when, in the judgment of the physician, the potential benefits outweigh the possible hazards. Patients receiving pentazocine during labor have experienced no adverse effects other than those that occur with commonly used analgesics. Pentazocine should be used with caution in women delivering premature infants.

➤*Lactation:* No reports describing the use of pentazocine during lactation have been located. The molecular weight (about 285) suggests that the drug will be excreted into breast milk. The effects of this exposure on a breastfeeding infant are unknown, but small infrequent doses most likely present a minimal risk.

➤*Children:* Because clinical experience in children under 12 years of age is limited, the use of pentazocine lactate in this age group is not recommended.

➤*Elderly:* Per the Beers list, pentazocine is a narcotic analgesic that causes more CNS adverse reactions, including confusion and hallucinations, more commonly than other narcotic drugs. Additionally, it is a mixed agonist and antagonist. Pentazocine is also considered a high-risk medication for the elderly according to the Centers for Medicare and Medicaid Services.

Avoid long-term use of pentazocine for treatment of pain in elderly patients because of the risk of falls, fractures, confusion, dependency, and withdrawal. Consider using a stepped approach starting with nondrug therapy, followed by acetaminophen, and then codeine, morphine, or hydromorphone, if needed.

Drug Interactions

Pentazocine Drug Interactions

Precipitant drug	Object drug[a]		Description
Pentazocine	Alcohol	↑	Due to the potential for increased CNS depressant effects, use cautiously in patients currently receiving pentazocine.
Barbiturate anesthetics	Pentazocine	↑	Barbiturate anesthetics may increase the respiratory and CNS depression of pentazocine because of additive pharmacologic activity.

[a] ↑ = object drug increased.

➤*CNS depressants:* Concomitant use of CNS depressants with parenteral pentazocine lactate may produce additive CNS depression. Adequate equipment and facilities should be available to identify and treat systemic emergencies should they occur.

➤*Patients receiving narcotics:* Pentazocine lactate is a mild narcotic antagonist. Some patients previously given narcotics, including methadone for the daily treatment of narcotic dependence, have experienced withdrawal symptoms after receiving pentazocine lactate.

Adverse Reactions

The most commonly occurring reactions are nausea, dizziness or lightheadedness, vomiting, and euphoria.

➤*Dermatologic:* Soft tissue induration, nodules, and cutaneous depression can occur at injection sites. Ulceration (sloughing) and severe sclerosis of the skin and subcutaneous tissues (and, rarely, underlying muscle) have been reported after multiple doses. Other reported dermatologic reactions include diaphoresis, sting on injection, flushed skin including plethora, dermatitis including pruritus.

➤*Infrequent reactions:*

Cardiovascular – Circulatory depression, shock, hypertension.

CNS – Dizziness, lightheadedness, hallucinations, sedation, euphoria, headache, confusion, disorientation; infrequently weakness, disturbed dreams, insomnia, syncope, visual blurring and focusing difficulty, depression; and rarely tremor, irritability, excitement, tinnitus.

GI – Constipation, dry mouth.

Respiratory – Respiratory depression, dyspnea, transient apnea in a small number of newborn infants whose mothers received pentazocine lactate during labor.

Miscellaneous – Urinary retention, headache, paresthesia, alterations in rate or strength of uterine contractions during labor.

➤*Rare reactions:*

CNS – Muscle tremor, insomnia, disorientation, hallucinations.

GI – Taste alteration, diarrhea and cramps.

Hematologic – Depression of white blood cells (especially granulocytes), which is usually reversible, moderate transient eosinophilia.

Ophthalmic – Blurred vision, nystagmus, diplopia, miosis.

Miscellaneous – Tachycardia, weakness or faintness, chills, allergic reactions including edema of the face, toxic epidermal necrolysis (see Acute CNS manifestations and Drug abuse under Warnings/Precautions).

Overdosage

➤*Symptoms:* Clinical experience with pentazocine lactate overdosage has been insufficient to define the signs of this condition.

➤*Treatment:* Oxygen, IV fluids, vasopressors, and other supportive measures should be employed as indicated. Assisted or controlled ventilation should also be considered. For respiratory depression due to overdosage or unusual sensitivity to pentazocine lactate, parenteral naloxone is a specific and effective antagonist.

PENTAZOCINE COMBINATIONS

c-iv	**Pentazocine Hydrochloride/Acetaminophen** (Watson)	**Tablets**: 25 mg (as hydrochloride) and 650 mg acetaminophen	(396 25 650). Aqua, capsule shape. In 100s, 500s, and 1000s.
c-iv	**Pentazocine/Naloxone Hydrochloride** (Royce)	**Tablets**: 50 mg (as hydrochloride) and 0.5 mg naloxone hydrochloride	In 100s, 500s and 1000s.

PENTAZOCINE COMBINATIONS — ORAL

Refer to the general discussion in the Opioid Agonist-Antagonist Analgesic introduction. For complete prescribing information, refer to the Pentazocine monograph.

Administration and Dosage

➤*Adults:*

Pain –

Pentazocine and acetaminophen: 1 tablet every 4 hours, up to 6 tablets per day.

Pentazocine and naloxone:

• *Usual dosage* – 50 mg every 3 or 4 hours; increase to 100 mg if necessary.

• *Maximum dose* – 600 mg/day.

• *Concomitant therapy* – When anti-inflammatory or antipyretic effects are desired in addition to analgesia, aspirin can be administered concomitantly.

➤*Children:* See Adults for dosing in patients 12 years of age and older.

➤*Administration:* Pentazocine tablets are intended for oral use only. Severe, potentially lethal reactions may result from misuse by injection or when combined with other substances. Oral pentazocine tablets contain 0.5 mg naloxone, an opioid antagonist, to aid in elimination of the abuse potential.

Warnings/Precautions

➤*Pregnancy: Category C.* Animal reproduction studies have not been conducted. It is also not known whether these drugs can cause fetal harm when administered to pregnant women or can affect reproduction capacity. Give to pregnant women only if clearly needed. However, animal reproduction studies with pentazocine have not demonstrated teratogenic or embryotoxic effects.

Nonteratogenic – There has been no experience in this regard with the combination pentazocine and acetaminophen. However, there have been rare reports of possible abstinence syndrome in newborns after prolonged use of pentazocine during pregnancy.

PENTAZOCINE COMBINATIONS — ORAL

➤*Lactation:* It is not known whether this drug is excreted in human milk. Because many drugs are excreted in human milk, exercise caution when administering to a breast-feeding woman.

➤*Elderly:* Per the Beers list, pentazocine is a narcotic analgesic that causes more CNS adverse reactions, including confusion and hallucinations, more commonly than other narcotic drugs. Additionally, it is a mixed agonist and antagonist. Pentazocine is also considered a high risk medication for the elderly according to the Centers for Medicare and Medicaid Services.

Avoid long-term use of pentazocine for treatment of pain in elderly patients because of the risk of falls, fractures, confusion, dependency, and withdrawal. Consider using a stepped approach starting with nondrug therapy, followed by acetaminophen, and then codeine, morphine, or hydromorphone, if needed.

MORPHINE SULFATE/NALTREXONE HYDROCHLORIDE

c-ii	**Embeda** (King Pharmaceuticals)	**Capsules, extended-release; oral:** Morphine sulfate 20 mg/naltrexone hydrochloride 0.8 mg	Gluten free. PEG, sugar spheres. (EMBEDA/20). Yellow opaque. In 100s.
		Morphine sulfate 30 mg/naltrexone hydrochloride 1.2 mg	Gluten free. PEG, sugar spheres. (EMBEDA/30). Blue-violet opaque. In 100s.
		Morphine sulfate 50 mg/naltrexone hydrochloride 2 mg	Gluten free. PEG, sugar spheres. (EMBEDA/50). Blue opaque. In 100s.
		Morphine sulfate 60 mg/naltrexone hydrochloride 2.4 mg	Gluten free. PEG, sugar spheres. (EMBEDA/60). Pink opaque. In 100s.
		Morphine sulfate 80 mg/naltrexone hydrochloride 3.2 mg	Gluten free. PEG, sugar spheres. (EMBEDA/80). Light peach opaque. In 100s.
		Morphine sulfate 100 mg/naltrexone hydrochloride 4 mg	Gluten free. PEG, sugar spheres. (EMBEDA/100). Green opaque. In 100s.

MORPHINE SULFATE/NALTREXONE HYDROCHLORIDE — ORAL

WARNING

Morphine/naltrexone capsules contain morphine, an opioid agonist and a schedule II controlled substance with an abuse liability similar to other opioid agonists. Morphine/naltrexone can be abused in a manner similar to other opioid agonists, legal or illicit. This should be considered when prescribing or dispensing morphine/naltrexone in situations where the health care provider or pharmacist is concerned about an increase risk of misuse, abuse, or diversion.

Morphine/naltrexone contains pellets of an extended-release (ER) oral formulation of morphine, an opioid receptor agonist, surrounding an inner core of naltrexone, an opioid receptor antagonist indicated for the management of moderate to severe pain when a continuous, around-the-clock opioid analgesic is needed for an extended period of time.

Morphine/naltrexone is not intended for use as an as-needed analgesic.

Morphine 100 mg/naltrexone 4 mg is for use in opioid-tolerant patients only. Ingestion of these capsules or the pellets within the capsules may cause fatal respiratory depression when administered to patients not already tolerant to high doses of opioids.

Patients should not consume alcoholic beverages while on morphine/naltrexone therapy. Additionally, patients must not use prescription or nonprescription medications containing alcohol while on morphine/naltrexone therapy. The coingestion of alcohol with morphine/naltrexone may result in an increase of plasma levels and a potentially fatal overdose of morphine. Morphine/naltrexone is to be swallowed whole or the contents of the capsules sprinkled over applesauce. The pellets in the capsules are not to be crushed, dissolved, or chewed because of the risk of rapid release and absorption of a potentially fatal dose of morphine.

Crushing, chewing, or dissolving morphine/naltrexone will also result in the release of naltrexone, which may precipitate withdrawal in opioid-tolerant patients.

Indications

➤*Moderate to severe pain:* For the management of moderate to severe pain when a continuous, around-the-clock opioid analgesic is needed for an extended period of time.

Administration and Dosage

➤*General dosing considerations:* Care should be taken to use low initial doses of morphine/naltrexone in patients who are not already opioid-tolerant, especially those who are receiving concurrent treatment with muscle relaxants, sedatives, or other CNS-active medications.

Do not give more frequently than every 12 hours.

The morphine 100 mg/naltrexone 4 mg capsules are for use only in opioid-tolerant patients.

➤*Adults:*

Moderate to severe pain –

Initial dosage: The lowest dose of should be used. Do not dose more frequently than every 12 hours.

Dosage titration: Patients may subsequently be titrated to a once- or twice-daily dosage that adequately manages their pain. It is critical to adjust the dosing regimen for each patient individually, taking into account the patient's prior analgesic treatment experience. Patients may develop some degree of tolerance, requiring dosage adjustment until they have achieved their individual balance between effective analgesia and opioid adverse effects such as confusion, sedation, and constipation.

Titrate no more frequently than every other day to allow patients to stabilize before escalating the dose.

During periods of changing analgesic requirements, including initial titration, frequent communication is recommended between health care provider, other members of the health care team, the patient, and the caregiver/family.

Maintenance dosage: Continual reevaluation of the patient receiving morphine is important, with special attention to the maintenance of pain control and the relative incidence of adverse effects associated with therapy. If the level of pain increases, effort should be made to identify the source of increased pain, while adjusting the dose as previously described to decrease the level of pain. During long-term therapy, especially for noncancer-related pain (or pain associated with other terminal illnesses), the continued need for the use of opioid analgesics should be reassessed as appropriate.

Dosage adjustment: Patients who exhibit signs of excessive opioid adverse effects such as sedation should have their dose reduced.

Patients who experience inadequate analgesia on once-daily dosing should be switched to twice-a-day.

Concomitant therapy: If breakthrough pain occurs, the dose may be supplemented with a small dose (less than 20% of the total daily dose) of a short-acting analgesic.

Conversion: The first dose of morphine/naltrexone may be taken with the last dose of any immediate-release (short-acting) opioid medication because of the extended-release characteristics of morphine/naltrexone.

• *Oral morphine* – Patients on other oral morphine formulations may be converted to morphine/naltrexone by administering one-half of the patient's total daily oral morphine dose as morphine/naltrexone every 12 hours (twice a day) or by administering the total daily oral morphine dose as morphine/naltrexone every 24 hours (once a day).

• *Other opioids or parenteral morphine* – While there are useful tables of oral and parenteral equivalents in cancer analgesia, there is substantial interpatient variation in the relative potency of different opioid drugs and formulations. For these reasons, it is better to underestimate the patient's 24-hour oral morphine requirement and provide rescue medication than to overestimate and manage an adverse reaction. The following general points should be considered:

Parenteral to oral morphine: It may take anywhere from 2 to 6 mg of oral morphine to provide analgesia equivalent to 1 mg of parenteral morphine. A dose of oral morphine 3 times the daily parenteral morphine requirement may be sufficient in long-term use settings.

Other oral or parenteral opioids to oral morphine:

In general, it is safest to give half of the estimated daily morphine demand as the initial dose and to manage inadequate analgesia by supplementation with immediate-release morphine.

Discontinuation of therapy: In general, morphine/naltrexone should not be abruptly discontinued. However, morphine/naltrexone, like other opioids, can be safely discontinued without the development of withdrawal symptoms by slowly tapering the daily dose.

➤*Elderly:* Administer with caution and in reduced doses.

➤*Renal function impairment:* Administer with caution and in reduced doses in patients with severe renal insufficiency.

➤*Hepatic function impairment:* Administer with caution and in reduced doses in patients with severe hepatic insufficiency.

➤*Administration:* Do not dose more frequently than every 12 hours.

Morphine/naltrexone is to be swallowed whole or the contents of the capsules sprinkled onto a small amount of applesauce and taken by mouth immediately. Patients should consume entire portion and should not divide applesauce into separate doses. Rinse mouth to ensure all pellets have been swallowed. Other foods have not been tested and should not be substituted for applesauce. The pellets in the capsules are not to be crushed, dissolved, or chewed before swallowing.

Do not administer through a nasogastric or gastric tube.

➤*Storage/Stability:* Store at 25°C (77°F); excursions are permitted between 15° and 30°C (59° and 86°F). Protect from light.

Actions

➤*Pharmacology:*

Morphine – Morphine, a pure opioid agonist, is relatively selective for the mu receptor, although it can interact with other opioid receptors at higher doses. In addition to analgesia, the widely diverse effects of morphine include analgesia, dysphoria, euphoria, somnolence, respiratory depression,

MORPHINE SULFATE/NALTREXONE HYDROCHLORIDE — ORAL

diminished GI motility, altered circulatory dynamics, histamine release, physical dependence, and alterations of the endocrine and autonomic nervous systems.

Morphine produces both its therapeutic and its adverse effects by interaction with one or more classes of specific opioid receptors located throughout the body. Morphine acts as a pure agonist, binding with and activating opioid receptors at sites in the periaqueductal and periventricular grey matter, the ventromedial medulla, and the spinal cord to produce analgesia.

Naltrexone – Naltrexone is a pure, centrally acting mu-opioid antagonist that reverses the subjective and analgesic effects of mu-opioid receptor agonists by competitively binding at mu-opioid receptors.

➤*Pharmacokinetics:*

Absorption – Morphine/naltrexone capsules contain ER pellets of morphine that release morphine slowly compared with an oral morphine solution. Following the administration of oral morphine solution, approximately 50% of the morphine absorbed reaches the systemic circulation within 30 minutes. However, following the administration of an equal amount of morphine/naltrexone to healthy volunteers, this occurs, on average, after 8 hours. As with most forms of oral morphine, because of presystemic elimination, only about 20% to 40% of the administered dose reaches the systemic circulation.

Morphine/naltrexone is bioequivalent to a similar morphine ER capsules product with regard to rate and extent of plasma morphine absorption. The median time to peak plasma morphine levels was shorter for morphine/naltrexone (7.5 hours) compared with *Kadian* (morphine sulfate ER capsules) (10 hours). Dose-related increase in steady-state predose plasma concentrations of morphine were noted following multiple dose administration of morphine/naltrexone in patients.

When taken as directed, the sequestered naltrexone in morphine/naltrexone is not consistently absorbed into systemic circulation following single-dose administration. In some subjects, a limited number (approximately 2%) of blood samples had low and highly variable plasma naltrexone levels (median, 7.74 pg/mL; range, 4.05 to 132 pg/mL) following single-dose administration of morphine/naltrexone 60 to 120 mg compared with oral naltrexone solution. In patients titrated up to 60 to 80 mg of twice a day morphine/naltrexone, naltrexone levels (4 to 25.5 pg/mL) were detected in 13 out of 67 patients at steady state. In a long-term safety study where an average dose of morphine/naltrexone was up to 860 mg administered twice a day for 12 months, 11% of blood samples at predose time points at steady state had detectable plasma naltrexone concentrations ranging from 4.03 to 145 pg/mL.

Compared with naltrexone 2.4 mg oral solution, which produced mean (standard deviation [SD]) naltrexone plasma levels of 689 (± 429 pg/mL) and mean (SD) 6-beta-naltrexol plasma levels of 3,920 (± 1,350 pg/mL), administration of intact morphine/naltrexone 60 mg produced no naltrexone plasma levels and mean (SD) 6-beta-naltrexol plasma levels of 16.7 (± 13.5 pg/mL). Trough levels of plasma naltrexone and 6-beta-naltrexol did not accumulate upon repeated administration of morphine/naltrexone.

Tampering with the morphine/naltrexone formulation by crushing or chewing the pellets results in the rapid release and absorption of both morphine and naltrexone comparable with an oral solution; this has not been shown to reduce the abuse liability of morphine/naltrexone.

Distribution – Once absorbed, morphine is distributed to skeletal muscle, kidneys, liver, intestinal tract, lungs, spleen, and brain. The volume of distribution of morphine is approximately 3 to 4 L/kg. Morphine is 30% to 35% reversibly bound to plasma proteins. Although the primary site of action of morphine is in the CNS, only small quantities pass the blood-brain barrier. Morphine also crosses the placental membranes and has been found in breast milk.

Metabolism – Major pathways of morphine metabolism include glucuronidation and sulfation in the liver to produce morphine-3-glucuronide (M3G) (approximately 50%) and morphine-6-glucuronide (M6G) (approximately 5% to 15%) or morphine-3-etheral sulfate. A small fraction (less than 5%) of morphine is demethylated. M3G has no significant contribution to the analgesic activity. Although M6G does not readily cross the blood-brain barrier, it has been shown to have opioid agonist and analgesic activity in humans.

Naltrexone is extensively metabolized into 6-beta-naltrexol.

Excretion – Approximately 10% of the morphine dose is excreted unchanged in the urine. Elimination of morphine is primarily via hepatic metabolism to glucuronide metabolites M3G and M6G (55% to 65%), which are then renally excreted. A small amount of the glucuronide metabolites is excreted in the bile and there is some minor enterohepatic cycling. The mean adult plasma clearance is about 20 to 30 mL/min/kg. The effective half-life of morphine after IV administration is reported to be approximately 2 hours. The terminal elimination half-life of morphine following single-dose morphine/naltrexone administration is approximately 29 hours.

Special populations –

Renal function impairment: The pharmacokinetics of morphine is altered in patients with renal failure. Area under the curve (AUC) is increased and clearance is decreased. The metabolites, M3G and M6G, accumulate several-fold in patients with renal failure compared with healthy subjects. Adequate studies of naltrexone in patients with severe renal impairment have not been conducted.

Hepatic function impairment: The pharmacokinetics of morphine were found to be significantly altered in individuals with alcoholic cirrhosis. The clearance was found to decrease with a corresponding increase in half-life. The M3G and M6G to morphine plasma AUC ratios also decreased in these patients, indicating a decrease in metabolic activity. Adequate studies of naltrexone in patients with severe hepatic impairment have not been conducted.

Race: Pharmacokinetic differences because of race may exist. Additionally, Chinese subjects given IV morphine in one study had a higher clearance when compared with white subjects (1,852 ± 116 mL/min vs 1,495 ± 80 mL/min).

Contraindications

Known hypersensitivity to morphine, morphine salts, naltrexone, or in any situation where opioids are contraindicated; significant respiratory depression in unmonitored settings or the absence of resuscitative equipment; acute or severe bronchial asthma or hypercapnia in unmonitored settings or the absence of resuscitative equipment; any patient who has or is suspected of having paralytic ileus.

Warnings/Precautions

➤*Administration:* Morphine/naltrexone is to be swallowed whole or the contents of the capsules sprinkled on applesauce. The pellets in the capsules are not to be crushed, dissolved, or chewed. The resulting morphine dose may be fatal, particularly in opioid-naive individuals. In opioid-tolerant individuals, the absorption of naltrexone may increase the risk of precipitating withdrawal.

See the Warning box for more information.

➤*Respiratory depression:* Respiratory depression is the chief hazard of all morphine preparations, including morphine/naltrexone. Respiratory depression occurs more frequently and is more dangerous in elderly and debilitated patients and those suffering from conditions accompanied by hypoxia, hypercapnia, or upper airway obstruction (when even moderate therapeutic doses may significantly decrease pulmonary ventilation).

Use morphine/naltrexone with extreme caution in patients with chronic obstructive pulmonary disease or cor pulmonale, and in patients having a substantially decreased respiratory reserve (eg, severe kyphoscoliosis), hypoxia, hypercapnia, or preexisting respiratory depression. In such patients, even usual therapeutic doses of morphine may increase airway resistance and decrease respiratory drive to the point of apnea. In these patients, consider alternative nonopioid analgesics, and employ opioids only under careful medical supervision at the lowest effective dose.

➤*Head injury/increased intracranial pressure:* The respiratory depressant effects of morphine with carbon dioxide retention and secondary elevation of cerebrospinal fluid pressure may be markedly exaggerated in the presence of head injury, other intracranial lesions, or a preexisting increase in intracranial pressure. Morphine/naltrexone can produce effects on pupillary response and consciousness, which may obscure neurologic signs of further increases in pressure in patients with head injuries. Only administer morphine/naltrexone under such circumstances when considered essential and then with extreme care.

➤*Hypotensive effect:* Morphine/naltrexone may cause severe hypotension. There is an added risk to individuals whose ability to maintain blood pressure has already been compromised by a reduced blood volume or a coadministration of drugs such as phenothiazines or general anesthetics. Morphine/naltrexone may produce orthostatic hypotension and syncope in ambulatory patients.

Administer morphine/naltrexone with caution to patients in circulatory shock, as vasodilation produced by the drug may further reduce cardiac output and blood pressure.

➤*GI effects:* Do not give morphine/naltrexone to patients with GI obstruction, particularly paralytic ileus, as there is a risk of the product remaining in the stomach for an extended period and the subsequent release of a bolus of morphine when normal gut motility is restored. As with other solid morphine formulations, diarrhea may reduce morphine absorption.

The administration of morphine may obscure the diagnosis or clinical course in patients with acute abdominal condition.

➤*Cordotomy:* In patients who are scheduled for cordotomy or other interruption of pain transmission pathways, cease morphine/naltrexone 24 hours prior to the procedure and control the pain by parenteral short-acting opioids. In addition, individualize the postprocedure titration of analgesics for such patients to avoid oversedation or withdrawal syndromes.

➤*Pancreatic/Biliary tract disease:* Morphine/naltrexone may cause spasm of the sphincter of Oddi; use with caution in patients with biliary tract disease, including acute pancreatitis. Opioids may cause increases in the serum amylase level.

➤*Accidentally precipitated withdrawal:* Consuming morphine/naltrexone that has been tampered by crushing, chewing, or dissolving the ER formulation can release sufficient naltrexone to precipitate withdrawal in opioid-dependent individuals. Symptoms of withdrawal usually appear within 5 minutes of ingestion of naltrexone and can last for up to 48 hours. Mental status changes can include confusion, somnolence, and visual hallucinations. Significant fluid losses from vomiting and diarrhea can require IV fluid administration. Closely monitor patients and tailor therapy with nonopioid medications to meet individual requirements.

➤*Hypersensitivity reactions:* Although extremely rare, cases of anaphylaxis have been reported with the use of a similar ER morphine formulation.

➤*Renal function impairment:* See Administration and Dosage for more information.

➤*Hepatic function impairment:* See Administration and Dosage for more information.

➤*Special risk:* Administer morphine/naltrexone with caution and in reduced dosages in debilitated patients and patients with Addison disease, hypothyroidism, myxedema, prostatic hypertrophy, or urethral stricture.

MORPHINE SULFATE/NALTREXONE HYDROCHLORIDE — ORAL

Exercise caution in the administration of morphine/naltrexone to patients with acute alcoholism, CNS depression, delirium tremens, or toxic psychosis.

All opioids may aggravate convulsions in patients with convulsive disorders, and all opioids may induce or aggravate seizures in some clinical settings.

➤*Drug abuse and dependence:*

Controlled substance – Morphine/naltrexone contains morphine, a mu-opioid agonist, and is a schedule II controlled substance. Morphine/naltrexone can be abused and is subject to criminal diversion.

Abuse – Opioid agonists have the potential for being abused, are sought by drug abusers and people with addiction disorders, and are subject to criminal diversion.

Morphine can be abused in a manner similar to other opioid agonists, legal or illicit. This should be considered when prescribing or dispensing morphine/naltrexone in situations where the health care provider or pharmacist is concerned about an increased risk of misuse, abuse, or diversion.

Morphine/naltrexone is intended for oral use only. Misuse or abuse of morphine/naltrexone by crushing or chewing the pellets, or snorting or injecting the dissolved product, will result in the uncontrolled release of both morphine and naltrexone, posing the risk of overdose and death. In opioid-tolerant individuals, the absorption of naltrexone may increase the risk of precipitating withdrawal. The risk of overdose and death is increased with concurrent abuse of alcohol and other CNS depressants. The sequestered naltrexone is intended to have no clinical effect when morphine/naltrexone is taken as directed; however, if crushed or chewed, up to 100% of the sequestered naltrexone dose could be released, bioequivalent to an immediate-release naltrexone oral solution of the same dose.

Because of the presence of talc as one of the excipients in morphine/naltrexone, parenteral abuse can be expected to result in local tissue necrosis, infection, pulmonary granulomas, and increased risk of endocarditis and valvular heart injury. Parenteral drug abuse is commonly associated with transmission of infectious diseases such as hepatitis and HIV.

Dependence and tolerance – Tolerance is the need for increasing doses of opioids to maintain a defined effect such as analgesia (in the absence of disease progression or other external factors). Physical dependence is manifested by withdrawal symptoms after abrupt discontinuation of a drug or upon administration of an antagonist. Physical dependence and tolerance are common during long-term opioid therapy.

Withdrawal – Opioid abstinence or withdrawal syndrome is characterized by some or all of the following: chills, lacrimation, myalgia, mydriasis, perspiration, restlessness, rhinorrhea, and/or yawning. Other symptoms also may develop, including abdominal cramps; anorexia; anxiety; backache; diarrhea; increased blood pressure, respiratory rate, or heart rate; insomnia; irritability; joint pain; nausea; vomiting; or weakness.

Morphine/naltrexone should not be abruptly discontinued.

➤*Hazardous tasks:* Morphine/naltrexone may impair the mental and/or physical abilities needed to perform potentially hazardous activities such as driving a car or operating machinery. Caution patients accordingly. Also warn patients about the potential combined effects of morphine/naltrexone with other CNS depressants, including other opioids, phenothiazines, sedative/hypnotics, and alcohol.

➤*Pregnancy: Category C.*

Neonatal withdrawal syndrome – Long-term maternal use of opiates or opioids during pregnancy coexposes the fetus. The newborn may experience subsequent neonatal withdrawal syndrome (NWS). Manifestations of NWS include abnormal sleep pattern, diarrhea, failure to gain weight, high-pitched cry, hyperactivity, irritability, tremor, weight loss, and vomiting. The onset, duration, and severity of the disorder differ based on such factors as the addictive drug used, time and amount of mother's last dose, and rate of elimination of the drug from the newborn. Approaches to the treatment of this syndrome have included supportive care and, when indicated, drugs such as paregoric or phenobarbital.

Teratogenic – Teratogenic effects of morphine have been reported in the animal literature. High parental doses during the second trimester were teratogenic in neurological, soft, and skeletal tissue. The abnormalities included encephalopathy and axial skeletal fusions. These doses were often maternally toxic and were 0.3- to 3-fold the maximum recommended human dose (MRHD) on a mg/m^2 basis. The relative contribution of morphine-induced maternal hypoxia and malnutrition, each of which can be teratogenic, has not been clearly defined. Treatment of male rats with approximately 3-fold the MRHD for 10 days prior to mating decreased litter size and viability.

Nonteratogenic – Morphine given subcutaneously at nonmaternally toxic doses to rats during the third trimester at approximately 0.15-fold the MRHD caused reversible reductions in brain and spinal cord volume, testes size, and body weight in the offspring, and decreased fertility in female offspring. The offspring of rats and hamsters treated orally or intraperitoneally throughout pregnancy with 0.04- to 0.3-fold the MRHD of morphine have demonstrated delayed growth, motor, and sexual maturation, and decreased male fertility. Chronic morphine exposure of fetal animals resulted in mild withdrawal, altered reflex and motor skill development, and altered responsiveness to morphine that persisted into adulthood.

There are no well-controlled studies of chronic in utero exposure to morphine in human subjects. However, uncontrolled retrospective studies of human neonates chronically exposed to other opioids in utero demonstrated reduced brain volume, which normalized over the first month of life. Infants born to opioid-abusing mothers are more often small for gestational age, have a decreased ventilatory response to CO_2, and are at an increased risk of sudden infant death syndrome.

Morphine/naltrexone should only be used during pregnancy if the need for strong opioid analgesia justifies the potential risk to the fetus.

Labor and delivery – Morphine/naltrexone is not recommended for use in women during and immediately prior to labor when shorter-acting analgesics or other analgesic techniques are more appropriate. Occasionally, opioid analgesics may prolong labor through actions that temporarily reduce the strength, duration, and frequency of uterine contractions. However, this effect is not consistent and may be offset by an increased rate of cervical dilatation, which tends to shorten labor. Closely observe for signs of respiratory depression in neonates whose mothers received opioid analgesics during labor. A specific opioid antagonist, such as naloxone or nalmefene, should be available for reversal of opioid-induced respiratory depression in the neonate.

➤*Lactation:* Morphine is excreted in the maternal milk, and the milk to plasma morphine AUC ratio is about 2.5:1. The amount of morphine received by the infant depends on the maternal plasma concentration, amount of milk ingested by the infant, and the extent of first-pass metabolism. Naltrexone and its metabolite, 6-beta-naltrexol, are excreted into the milk of lactating rats. The molecular weight (about 378) is low enough that excretion into human breast milk should be expected.

Withdrawal symptoms can occur in breast-feeding infants when maternal administration of morphine is stopped. Because of the potential for adverse reactions in breast-feeding infants from morphine/naltrexone, decide whether to discontinue breast-feeding or the drug, taking into account the importance of the drug to the mother.

➤*Children:* Safety and efficacy of morphine/naltrexone in children younger than 18 years of age have not been established.

➤*Elderly:* In general, use caution in dose selection for an elderly patient, usually starting at the low end of the dosing range, reflecting the greater frequency of decreased hepatic, renal, or cardiac function, and of concomitant disease or other drug therapy. Respiratory depression occurs more frequently and is more dangerous in elderly patients. Administer with caution and in reduced doses in elderly patients.

➤*Monitoring:* Assess pain type and intensity prior to administration. Assess efficacy of pain relief during therapy and monitor for adverse reactions, such as confusion, constipation, and sedation.

Drug Interactions

Morphine/Naltrexone Drug Interactions

Precipitant drug	Object drug[a]		Description
Alcohol	Morphine/ Naltrexone	⬆	Additive CNS depressant effects, including respiratory depression, hypotension, and profound sedation and coma, may occur. In addition, morphine plasma concentrations may be elevated, increasing the risk of a potentially fatal overdose. Avoid coingestion of alcohol and morphine/ naltrexone.
Morphine/ Naltrexone	Alcohol		
Anticholinergic agents (eg, atropine, benztropine)	Morphine/ Naltrexone	⬆	Risk of urinary retention and/or severe constipation leading to paralytic ileus may be increased. Use with caution. If an interaction is suspected, it may be necessary to stop one or both drugs and treat the complication.
Morphine/ Naltrexone	Anticholinergic agents (eg, atropine, benztropine)		
Cimetidine	Morphine/ Naltrexone	⬆	Confusion and respiratory depression has been reported in a dialysis patient receiving morphine and cimetidine. Monitor patients. If excessive CNS or respiratory depression occurs, discontinue both drugs. Administer a narcotic antagonist, if needed.
CNS depressants (eg, antiemetics, general anesthetics, hypnotics or sedatives, other opioids, phenothiazines, tranquilizers)	Morphine/ Naltrexone	⬆	Additive CNS depressant effects, including respiratory depression, hypotension, and profound sedation and coma, may occur. If coadministered, consider reducing the dose of one or both agents by at least 50%.
Morphine/ Naltrexone	CNS depressants (eg, antiemetics, general anesthetics, hypnotics or sedatives [eg, barbiturates], other opioids, phenothiazines, tranquilizers)		

MORPHINE SULFATE/NALTREXONE HYDROCHLORIDE — ORAL

Morphine/Naltrexone Drug Interactions			
Precipitant drug	Object drug[a]		Description
Mixed agonist/antagonist opioid analgesics (eg, butorphanol, nalbuphine, pentazocine)	Morphine/Naltrexone	↓	The analgesic effect of morphine/naltrexone may be reduced. In addition, withdrawal symptoms may occur. Use with caution.
MAOIs[b] (eg, phenelzine)	Morphine/Naltrexone	↑	The effects of morphine may be potentiated, resulting in anxiety, confusion, respiratory depression, and coma. Do not administer morphine/naltrexone in patients receiving MAOIs or within 14 days of stopping an MAOI.
P-glycoprotein inhibitors (eg, quinidine)	Morphine/Naltrexone	↑	Morphine exposure may be increased about 2-fold, increasing the pharmacologic effects and risk of adverse reactions. Use with caution.
Rifamycins (eg, rifampin)	Morphine/Naltrexone	↓	Morphine plasma concentrations may be reduced, decreasing the analgesic effect. Monitor the response of the patient. It may be necessary to increase the morphine/naltrexone dose or administer alternative treatment.
Morphine/Naltrexone	Diuretics (eg, furosemide)	↓	Morphine may decrease diuretic efficacy by inducing the release of antidiuretic hormone. In addition, morphine may cause spasm of the bladder sphincter, causing acute urinary retention, especially in men with prostatism. Use with caution and monitor diuretic response. Be prepared to stop one or both agents and to treat the complication.
Morphine/Naltrexone	Skeletal muscle relaxants (eg, cyclobenzaprine)	↑	Neuromuscular blocking action of skeletal muscle relaxants may be increased, producing respiratory depression. If coadministration is necessary, monitor neuromuscular function; titrate the muscle relaxant dose and be prepared to provide mechanical respiratory support when needed.

[a] ↑ = object drug increased; ↓ = object drug decreased.
[b] MAOIs = monoamine oxidase inhibitors.

➤*Drug/Lab test interactions:* Naltrexone may or may not interfere with enzymatic methods for the detection of opioids, depending on the specificity of the test. Consult the test manufacturer for specific details.

Adverse Reactions

➤*Serious adverse reactions:* Serious adverse reactions that may be associated with morphine/naltrexone therapy in clinical use include apnea, cardiac arrest, circulatory depression, hypotension, respiratory arrest, respiratory depression, and/or shock.

➤*Common adverse reactions:* The most frequent adverse reactions include constipation, dizziness, drowsiness, and nausea.

➤*Short-term study:*

Discontinuation – The most common adverse reactions leading to study discontinuation were constipation, dizziness, fatigue, nausea, pruritus, somnolence, and vomiting.

Morphine/Naltrexone Adverse Reactions (≥ 2%): Short-Term Study			
	Titration	Maintenance	
Adverse reactions	Morphine/Naltrexone (n = 547)	Morphine/Naltrexone (n = 171)	Placebo (n = 173)
Subjects with ≥1 treatment-related adverse reaction	57.2%	32.7%	26%
CV, NOS[a]	0.7%	2.9%	1.2%
Flushing	0%	2.3%	0.6%
CNS, NOS	24.7%	7%	6.4%
Dizziness	7.7%	1.2%	1.2%
Fatigue	2.9%	0.6%	1.2%
Headache	4%	2.3%	1.2%
Insomnia	1.3%	2.9%	2.3%
Psychiatric disorders	6.2%	5.8%	5.2%
Somnolence	13.9%	1.2%	2.9%
Dermatologic, NOS	8.4%	4.1%	4%
Pruritus	6.2%	0%	0.6%
GI, NOS	47.5%	24%	16.2%
Abdominal pain upper	1.1%	2.3%	1.7%
Constipation	30.2%	7%	4%
Diarrhea	1.1%	7%	6.9%
Dry mouth	5.7%	1.8%	1.2%
Nausea	19.4%	11.1%	6.4%
Vomiting	8.4%	4.1%	1.2%
Miscellaneous, NOS	7.1%	5.3%	5.8%

[a] NOS = not otherwise specified.

➤*Long-term study:*

Morphine/Naltrexone Adverse Reactions (≥ 2%): Long-Term Study	
Adverse reactions	Morphine/Naltrexone (N = 465)
Any related adverse reaction	61.9%
CNS, NOS	21.3%
Anxiety	2.2%
Dizziness	4.1%
Fatigue	4.1%
Headache	6.9%
Insomnia	2.8%
Psychiatric disorders, NOS	9%
Somnolence	7.3%
Dermatologic, NOS	11.2%
Hyperhidrosis	3.4%
Pruritus	5.6%
GI, NOS	47.1%
Constipation	31.2%
Diarrhea	2.2%
Dry mouth	3.7%
Nausea	22.2%
Vomiting	8%
Miscellaneous, NOS	11%

➤*Other adverse reactions:*

Cardiovascular – Hot flush (1% to less than 10%); flushing, hypotension, orthostatic hypotension (less than 1%).

CNS – Somnolence (at least 10%); anxiety, depression, dizziness, fatigue, headache, insomnia, irritability, lethargy, restlessness, sedation, tremor (1% to less than 10%); abnormal dreams, confusional state, coordination abnormal, depressed level of consciousness, disorientation, disturbance in attention, euphoric mood, hallucination, memory impairment, mental impairment, mental status changes, mood swings, nervousness, paraesthesia, stupor, thinking abnormal (less than 1%).

Dermatologic – Hyperhidrosis, pruritus (1% to less than 10%); cold sweat, night sweat, piloerection, rash (less than 1%).

GI – Constipation, nausea (at least 10%); abdominal pain, diarrhea, dry mouth, dyspepsia, flatulence, stomach discomfort, vomiting (1% to less than 10%); abdominal discomfort, abdominal distension, abdominal pain lower, abdominal tenderness, fecaloma, pancreatitis (less than 1%).

GU – Dysuria, erectile dysfunction, urinary retention (less than 1%).

Hepatic – ALT increased, AST increased, cholecystitis (less than 1%).

Metabolic/Nutritional – Anorexia, decreased appetite (1% to less than 10%).

Musculoskeletal – Arthralgia, muscle spasms (1% to less than 10%); myalgia, muscular weakness (less than 1%).

Respiratory – Dyspnea, rhinorrhoea (less than 1%).

Miscellaneous – Chills, peripheral edema (1% to less than 10%); asthenia, drug withdrawal syndrome, feeling jittery, malaise, vision blurred (less than 1%).

Overdosage

➤*Symptoms:* Acute overdosage with morphine is manifested by cold and clammy skin, constricted pupils, respiratory depression, skeletal muscle flaccidity, somnolence progressing to stupor or coma, and, sometimes, bra-

MORPHINE SULFATE/NALTREXONE HYDROCHLORIDE — ORAL

dycardia, hypotension, pulmonary edema, and death. Marked mydriasis rather than miosis may be seen because of severe hypoxia in overdose situations.

➤*Treatment:* Give primary attention to the reestablishment of a patent and protected airway, and institute assisted or controlled ventilation if needed. Employ other supportive measures (eg, oxygen, vasopressors) in the management of circulatory shock and pulmonary edema accompanying overdose as indicated. Cardiac arrest or arrhythmias will require advanced life support techniques.

The pure opioid antagonists, naloxone or nalmefene, are specific antidotes to respiratory depression that results from opioid overdose. Because the duration of reversal would be expected to be less than the duration of action of morphine in morphine/naltrexone, monitor the patient carefully until spontaneous respiration is reliably reestablished. Morphine/naltrexone will continue to release and add to the morphine load for up to 24 hours after administration; monitor the management of an overdose accordingly. If the response to opioid antagonists is suboptimal or not sustained, give additional antagonist as directed by the manufacturer of the product.

Do not administer opioid antagonists in the absence of clinically significant respiratory or circulatory depression secondary to morphine overdose. Administer such agents cautiously to persons who are known or suspected to be physically dependent on morphine/naltrexone. In such cases, an abrupt or complete reversal of opioid effects may precipitate an acute withdrawal syndrome.

In an individual physically dependent on opioids, administration of an opioid receptor antagonist may precipitate an acute withdrawal. The severity of the withdrawal produced will depend on the degree of physical dependence and the dose of the antagonist administered. Reserve use of an opioid antagonist for cases where such treatment is clearly needed. If it is necessary to treat serious respiratory depression in the physically dependent patient, begin administration of the antagonist with care and titrate with smaller than usual doses of the antagonist.

Patient Information

Advise patients that this product contains morphine and naltrexone and to take only as directed.

Advise patients not to adjust the dose without consulting with a health care provider. Inform patients to swallow morphine/naltrexone whole (not to crush, dissolve, or chew) because of a risk of fatal morphine overdose or naltrexone-precipitated withdrawal symptoms. Alternately, morphine/naltrexone capsules may be opened and the entire contents sprinkled on a small amount of applesauce immediately prior to ingestion.

Tell patient not to consume alcoholic beverages while on morphine/naltrexone therapy. Additionally, tell patient not to use prescription or nonprescription medications containing alcohol while on morphine/naltrexone therapy. The coingestion of alcohol with morphine/naltrexone may result in an increase of plasma levels and potentially fatal overdose of morphine.

Advise patients of the following most common adverse reactions that may occur while taking morphine/naltrexone: constipation, dizziness, headache, nausea, pruritus, somnolence, and vomiting.

Advise patients that morphine/naltrexone may cause drowsiness, dizziness, or light-headedness and may impair mental and/or physical ability required for the performance of potentially hazardous tasks (eg, driving, operating machinery). Tell patients started on morphine/naltrexone or patients whose dose has been adjusted to refrain from any potentially dangerous activity until it is established that they are not adversely affected.

Advise patients not to combine morphine/naltrexone with CNS depressants (sleep aids, tranquilizers) except by the orders of the prescribing health care provider because dangerous additive effects may occur, resulting in serious injury or death.

Advise patients that morphine/naltrexone is a potential drug of abuse and to protect it from theft.

Special care must be taken to avoid accidental ingestion or use by individuals (including children) other than the patient for whom it was originally prescribed, as such unsupervised use may have severe, even fatal, consequences.

Advise patients that morphine 100 mg/naltrexone 4 mg is for use only in opioid-tolerant patients.

Tell women of childbearing potential who become pregnant or are planning to become pregnant to consult a health care provider prior to initiating or continuing therapy with morphine/naltrexone.

Advise patients that safe use in pregnancy has not been established. Prolonged use of opioid analgesics during pregnancy may cause fetal neonatal physical dependence, and neonatal withdrawal may occur.

As with other opioids, advise patients taking morphine/naltrexone of the potential for severe constipation; initiate appropriate laxatives and/or stool softeners as well as other appropriate treatments from the onset of opioid therapy.

Advise patients to seek medical attention immediately if signs of a serious allergic reaction, such as swelling of the face, throat, or tongue, trouble breathing, feeling dizzy or faint, pounding heartbeat, chest pain or feeling of doom, occur.

Advise patients to report episodes of breakthrough pain and adverse experiences occurring during therapy. Individualization of dosage is essential to make optimal use of this medication.

Advise patients that if they have been receiving treatment with morphine/naltrexone for more than a few weeks and cessation of therapy is indicated, it may be appropriate to taper the morphine/naltrexone dose rather than abruptly discontinue it because of the risk of precipitating withdrawal symptoms. Provide a dose schedule to accomplish a gradual discontinuation of the medication.

Instruct patients to keep morphine/naltrexone in a secure place out of the reach of children. When morphine/naltrexone is no longer needed, instruct patient to destroy unused capsules by flushing down the toilet.

CENTRAL ANALGESICS

CLONIDINE HYDROCHLORIDE

Rx	**Clonidine** (American Regent)	**Injection, solution**: 100 mcg/mL	Preservative free. In single-dose 10 ml vials.
Rx	**Duraclon** (Bioniche Pharma)		Preservative free. In 10 ml vials.
Rx	**Clonidine** (American Regent)	**Injection, solution**: 500 mcg/mL	Preservative free. In 10 single-dose ml vials.
Rx	**Duraclon** (Bioniche Pharma)		Preservative free. In 10 ml vials.

CLONIDINE HYDROCHLORIDE — INJECTION

WARNING

The 500 mcg/mL strength product should be diluted prior to use in an appropriate solution.

Note – Epidural clonidine is not recommended for obstetrical, postpartum, or perioperative pain management. The risk of hemodynamic instability, especially hypotension and bradycardia, from epidural clonidine may be unacceptable in these patients. However, in a rare obstetrical, postpartum or perioperative patient, potential benefits may outweigh the possible risks.

Indications

➤*Severe pain in cancer patients:* For the treatment of severe pain in cancer patients that is not adequately relieved by opioid analgesics alone. Epidural clonidine is more likely to be effective in patients with neuropathic pain than somatic or visceral pain.

➤*Off-label uses:*

Postanesthetic shivering – [2] = Fair documentation. Data regarding the use of single-dose clonidine indicate that it is as effective as meperidine and superior to placebo in preventing postanesthetic shivering.

Postherpetic neuralgia – [2] = Fair documentation. Although guidelines do not list clonidine as a preferred treatment for postherpetic neuralgia, published data indicate patient received benefit from oral doses of clonidine 0.2 mg or repetitive paravertebral block injections of combination bupivacaine and clonidine. All patients had failed other treatment options but found pain relief with clonidine treatment. Reports showed a high tolerability and significant effect on pain with clonidine treatment.

Prevention of migraine (children/adolescents) – [5] = Poor documentation. In studies evaluating clonidine use for the prevention of migraine headaches in children (published in 1977 and 1982), it was no more effective than placebo; it has not been studied further. Current practice guidelines state that clonidine is not effective for the prevention of migraine in children and its use is not recommended.

Administration and Dosage

➤*General dosing considerations:* Familiarization with the continuous epidural infusion device is essential. Closely monitor patients receiving epidural clonidine from a continuous infusion device for the first few days to assess their response.

➤*Adults:*

Severe pain in cancer patients –

Initial dosage: 30 mcg/h continuous epidural infusion.

Dosage titration: Titrate up or down depending on pain relief and occurrence of adverse reactions; experience with dosage rates above 40 mcg/h is limited.

Off-label dosing –

Postanesthetic shivering: [2] = Fair documentation. Single IV doses of clonidine administered at induction of anesthesia, end of surgery, or upon return of laryngeal reflexes and spontaneous breathing. The most common regimen was 3 mcg/kg as a single dose. Isolated studies have also used single doses of 2 mcg/kg or 150 mcg.

Postherpetic neuralgia: [2] = Fair documentation. 20 mL repetitive paravertebral block injections of bupivacaine 0.5% and clonidine 150 mcg/mL have been used.

➤*Children:*

Severe pain in cancer patients –

Initial dosage: 0.5 mcg/kg/h.

Dosage titration: Cautiously adjust dose based on clinical response.

CLONIDINE HYDROCHLORIDE — INJECTION

➤*Renal function impairment:* Adjust dosage according to the degree of renal function impairment and carefully monitor patients. Because only a minimal amount of clonidine is removed during routine hemodialysis, there is no need to give supplemental clonidine following dialysis.

➤*Discontinuation of therapy:* When discontinuing therapy, reduce the dose gradually over 2 to 4 days to avoid withdrawal symptoms.

If therapy is to be discontinued in patients receiving a beta-blocker and clonidine concurrently, the beta-blocker should be withdrawn several days before the gradual discontinuation of clonidine.

➤*Preparation for administration:* Prior to use, dilute the 500 mcg/mL (0.5 mg/mL) strength product in sodium chloride 0.9% for injection to a final concentration of 100 mcg/mL.

To obtain a final clonidine concentration of 100 mcg/mL, the addition of 4, 8, 12, 16, 20, 24, 28, 32, 36, and 40 mL of sodium chloride 0.9% for injection to 1, 2, 3, 4, 5, 6, 7, 8, 9, and 10 mL of clonidine 500 mcg/mL for injection results in a final concentration of 100 mcg per mL or 500 mcg per 5 mL, 1,000 mcg per 10 mL, 1,500 mcg per 15 mL, 2,000 mcg per 20 mL, 2,500 mcg per 25 mL, 3,000 mcg per 30 mL, 4,000 mcg per 40 mL, 4,500 mcg per 45 mL, and 5,000 mcg per 50 mL, respectively.

➤*Admixture compatibility:* Clonidine must not be used with a preservative.

➤*Storage/Stability:* Store at 25°C (77°F). Discard unused portion.

Actions

➤*Pharmacology:* Epidurally administered clonidine produces dose-dependent analgesia not antagonized by opiate antagonists. The analgesia is limited to the body regions innervated by the spinal segments where analgesic concentrations of clonidine are present. Clonidine is thought to produce analgesia at presynaptic and postjunctional alpha-2-adrenoceptors in the spinal cord by preventing pain signal transmission to the brain.

➤*Pharmacokinetics:*

Absorption/Distribution – Clonidine is highly lipid soluble and readily distributes into extravascular sites including the central nervous system. Clonidine's volume of distribution is 2.1 ± 0.4 L/kg. The binding of clonidine to plasma protein is primarily to albumin and varies between 20% and 40% in vitro. Epidurally administered clonidine readily partitions into plasma via the epidural veins and attains systemic concentrations (0.5 to 2 ng/mL) that are associated with a hypotensive effect mediated by the central nervous system.

Following a 700 mcg clonidine hydrochloride epidural dose given over 5 minutes to 4 male and 5 female volunteers, peak clonidine plasma levels (4.4 ± 1.4 ng/mL) were obtained in 19 ± 27 minutes. The plasma elimination half-life was determined to be 22 ± 15 hours following sample collection for 24 hours. CL was 190 ± 70 mL/min.

Metabolism – In humans, clonidine metabolism follows minor pathways with the major metabolite, p-hydroxyclonidine, being present at less than 10% of the concentration of unchanged drug in urine.

Excretion – Following an intravenous dose of ^{14}C-clonidine, 72% of the administered dose was excreted in urine in 96 hours of which 40% to 50% was unchanged clonidine. Renal clearance for clonidine was determined to be 133 ± 66 mL/min. In a study where ^{14}C-clonidine was given to subjects with varying degrees of kidney function, elimination half-lives varied (17.5 to 41 hours) as a function of creatinine clearance. In subjects undergoing hemodialysis only 5% of body clonidine stores was removed.

Following a 10 minute intravenous infusion of 300 mcg clonidine hydrochloride to five male volunteers, plasma clonidine levels showed an initial rapid distribution phase (mean ± SD $t_{1/2}$ = 11 ± 9 minutes) followed by a slower elimination phase ($t_{1/2}$ = 9 ± 2 hours) over 24 hours. Clonidine's total body clearance (CL) was 219 ± 92 mL/min.

Following a 700 mcg clonidine hydrochloride epidural dose given over 5 minutes to 4 male and 5 female volunteers, in cerebral spinal fluid (CSF), peak clonidine levels (418 ± 255 ng/mL) were achieved in 26 ± 11 minutes. The clonidine CSF elimination half-life was 1.3 ± 0.5 hours when samples were collected for 6 hours.

Special populations –

Renal function impairment: The pharmacokinetics of epidurally administered clonidine has not been studied in patients with renal disease.

Hepatic function impairment: The pharmacokinetics of epidurally administered clonidine has not been studied in patients with hepatic disease.

Children: The pharmacokinetics of epidurally administered clonidine has not been studied in the pediatric population.

Gender: Following a 700 mcg clonidine hydrochloride epidural dose given over 5 minutes to 4 male and 5 female volunteers, compared with men, women had a lower mean plasma clearance, longer mean plasma half-life, and higher mean peak level of clonidine in both plasma and CSF.

Cancer patients: In cancer patients who received 14 days of clonidine hydrochloride epidural infusion (rate = 30 mcg/hr) plus morphine by patient-controlled analgesia (PCA), steady state clonidine plasma concentrations of 2.2 ± 1.1 and 2.4 ± 1.4 ng/mL were obtained on dosing days 7 and 14, respectively. CL was 279 ± 184 and 272 ± 163 mL/min on these days. CSF concentrations were not determined in these patients.

Contraindications

History of sensitization or allergic reactions to clonidine. Epidural administration is contraindicated in the presence of an injection site infection, in patients on anticoagulant therapy, and in those with a bleeding diathesis. Administration of clonidine hydrochloride above the C4 dermatome is contraindicated.

Warnings/Precautions

➤*Use in postoperative or obstetrical analgesia:* Epidural clonidine is not recommended for obstetrical, postpartum, or perioperative pain management. The risk of hemodynamic instability, especially hypotension and bradycardia, from epidural clonidine may be unacceptable in these patients.

➤*Hypotension:* Because severe hypotension may follow the administration of clonidine, it should be used with caution in all patients. It is not recommended in most patients with severe cardiovascular disease or in those who are otherwise hemodynamically unstable. The benefit of its administration in these patients should be carefully balanced against the potential risks resulting from hypotension.

Vital signs should be monitored frequently, especially during the first few days of epidural clonidine therapy. When clonidine is infused into the upper thoracic spinal segments, more pronounced decreases in the blood pressure may be seen.

Clonidine decreases sympathetic outflow from the central nervous system resulting in decreases in peripheral resistance, renal vascular resistance, heart rate, and blood pressure. However, in the absence of profound hypotension, renal blood flow and glomerular filtration rate remain essentially unchanged.

In the pivotal double-blind, randomized study of cancer patients, where 38 subjects were administered epidural clonidine hydrochloride at 30 mcg/hr in addition to epidural morphine, hypotension occurred in 45% of subjects. Most episodes of hypotension occurred within the first 4 days after beginning epidural clonidine. However, hypotensive episodes occurred throughout the duration of the trial. There was a tendency for these episodes to occur more commonly in women, and in those with higher serum clonidine levels. Patients experiencing hypotension also tended to weigh less than those who did not experience hypotension. The hypotension usually responded to intravenous fluids and, if necessary, parenteral ephedrine.

Published reports on the use of epidural clonidine for intraoperative or postoperative analgesia also show a consistent and marked hypotensive response to clonidine. Severe hypotension may occur even if intravenous fluid pretreatment is given.

➤*Withdrawal:* Sudden cessation of clonidine treatment, regardless of the route of administration, has, in some cases, resulted in symptoms such as nervousness, agitation, headache, and tremor, accompanied or followed by a rapid rise in blood pressure. The likelihood of such reactions appears to be greater after administration of higher doses or with concomitant beta blocker treatment. Special caution is therefore advised in these situations. Rare instances of hypertensive encephalopathy, cerebrovascular accidents and death have been reported after abrupt clonidine withdrawal. Patients with a history of hypertension or other underlying cardiovascular conditions may be at particular risk of the consequences of abrupt discontinuation of clonidine. In the pivotal double-blind, randomized cancer pain study, 4 of 38 subjects receiving 720 mcg of clonidine per day experienced rebound hypertension following abrupt withdrawal. One of these patients with rebound hypertension subsequently experienced a cerebrovascular accident.

Careful monitoring of infusion pump function and inspection of catheter tubing for obstruction or dislodgement can help reduce the risk of inadvertent abrupt withdrawal of epidural clonidine. Patients should notify their physician immediately if clonidine administration is inadvertently interrupted for any reason. Patients should also be instructed not to discontinue therapy without consulting their physician.

When discontinuing therapy with epidural clonidine, the physician should reduce the dose gradually over 2 to 4 days to avoid withdrawal symptoms.

An excessive rise in blood pressure following discontinuation of epidural clonidine can be treated by administration of clonidine or by IV phentolamine. If therapy is to be discontinued in patients receiving a beta blocker and clonidine concurrently, the beta blocker should be withdrawn several days before the gradual discontinuation of epidural clonidine.

➤*Infections:* Infections related to implantable epidural catheters pose a serious risk. Evaluation of fever in a patient receiving epidural clonidine should include the possibility of a catheter-related infection such as meningitis or epidural abscess.

➤*Special risk:*

Cardiac effects – Epidural clonidine frequently causes decreases in heart rate. Symptomatic bradycardia can be treated with atropine. Rarely, atrioventricular block greater than first degree has been reported. Clonidine does not alter the hemodynamic response to exercise, but may mask the increase in heart rate associated with hypovolemia.

Respiratory depression and sedation – Clonidine administration may result in sedation through the activation of alpha-adrenoceptors in the brainstem. High doses of clonidine cause sedation and ventilatory abnormalities that are usually mild. Tolerance to these effects can develop with chronic administration. These effects have been reported with bolus doses that are significantly larger than the infusion rate recommended for treating cancer pain.

Depression – Depression has been seen in a small percentage of patients treated with oral or transdermal clonidine. Depression commonly occurs in cancer patients and may be exacerbated by treatment with clonidine. Patients, especially those with a known history of affective disorders, should be monitored for the signs and symptoms of depression.

Pain of visceral or somatic origin – In the clinical investigations, at doses tested, clonidine hydrochloride was most effective in well-localized, "neuropathic" pain that was characterized as electrical, burning, or shooting in nature, and which was localized to a dermatomal or peripheral nerve distribution. Clonidine hydrochloride may be less effective, or possibly ineffective in the treatment of pain that is diffuse, poorly localized, or visceral in origin.

CLONIDINE HYDROCHLORIDE — INJECTION

➤*Pregnancy: Category C.*

Teratogenic – Reproduction studies in rabbits at clonidine hydrochloride doses up to approximately the MRDHD revealed no evidence of teratogenic or embryotoxic potential. In rats, however, doses as low as one-third the MRDHD were associated with increased resorptions in a study in which dams were treated continuously from 2 months prior to mating. Increased resorptions were not associated with treatment with the same or higher doses up to 0.5 times the MRDHD when dams were treated on days 6 to 15 of gestation. Increased resorptions were observed at higher levels (7 times the MRDHD) in rats and mice treated on days 1 to 14 of gestation.

Clonidine readily crosses the placenta and its concentrations are equal in maternal and umbilical cord plasma; amniotic fluid concentrations can be 4 times those found in serum. There are no adequate and well-controlled studies in pregnant women during early gestation when organ formation takes place. Studies using epidural clonidine during labor have demonstrated no apparent adverse effects on the infant at the time of delivery. However, these studies did not monitor the infants for hemodynamic effects in the days following delivery. Clonidine hydrochloride injection should be used during pregnancy only if the potential benefits justify the potential risk to the fetus.

Labor and delivery – There are no adequate controlled clinical trials evaluating the safety, efficacy, and dosing of clonidine hydrochloride in obstetrical settings. Because maternal perfusion of the placenta is critically dependent on blood pressure, use of clonidine hydrochloride as an analgesic during labor and delivery is not indicated.

➤*Lactation:* Concentrations of clonidine in human breast milk are approximately twice those found in maternal plasma. Caution should be exercised when clonidine is administered to a nursing woman. Because of the potential for severe adverse reactions in nursing infants, a decision should be made to either discontinue nursing or to discontinue clonidine.

➤*Children:* The safety and effectiveness of clonidine hydrochloride in this limited indication and clinical population have been established in patients old enough to tolerate placement and management of an epidural catheter, based on evidence from adequate and well controlled studies in adults and experience with the use of clonidine in the pediatric age group for other indications. The use of clonidine hydrochloride should be restricted to pediatric patients with severe intractable pain from malignancy that is unresponsive to epidural or spinal opiates or other more conventional analgesic techniques. The starting dose of clonidine hydrochloride should be selected on per kilogram basis (0.5 mcg/kg/hr) and cautiously adjusted based on the clinical response.

Drug Interactions

Clonidine Drug Interactions

Precipitant drug	Object drug[a]		Description
Beta blockers	Clonidine	↑	Beta blockers may exacerbate the hypertensive response seen with clonidine withdrawal. Also, because of the potential for additive effects such as bradycardia and AV block, use caution in patients receiving clonidine with agents known to affect sinus node function or AV nodal conduction (eg, digitalis, calcium channel blockers, beta blockers).
Fluphenazine	Clonidine	↑	There is one reported case of a patient with acute delirium associated with the simultaneous use of fluphenazine and oral clonidine. Symptoms resolved when clonidine was withdrawn and recurred when the patient was rechallenged with clonidine.
Narcotic analgesics	Clonidine	↑	Narcotic analgesics may potentiate the hypotensive effects of clonidine.
Tricyclic antidepressants	Clonidine	↓	Tricyclic antidepressants may antagonize the hypotensive effects of clonidine. The effects of tricyclic antidepressants on clonidine's analgesic actions are not known.
Clonidine	Alcohol/ barbiturates	↑	Clonidine may potentiate the CNS-depressive effect of alcohol, barbiturates or other sedating drugs.
Clonidine	Local anesthetics	↑	Epidural clonidine may prolong the duration of pharmacologic effects of epidural local anesthetics, including sensory and motor blockade.

[a] ↑ = object drug increased. ↓ = object drug decreased.

➤*CNS depressants:* Clonidine may potentiate the CNS-depressive effect of alcohol, barbiturates or other sedating drugs. Narcotic analgesics may potentiate the hypotensive effects of clonidine. Tricyclic antidepressants may antagonize the hypotensive effects of clonidine. The effects of tricyclic antidepressants on clonidine's analgesic actions are not known.

➤*Cardiac agents:* Beta-blockers may exacerbate the hypertensive response seen with clonidine withdrawal. Also, due to the potential for additive effects such as bradycardia and AV block, caution is warranted in patients receiving clonidine with agents known to affect sinus node function or AV nodal conduction (eg, digitalis, calcium channel blockers, and beta blockers).

➤*Fluphenazine:* There is one reported case of a patient with acute delirium associated with the simultaneous use of fluphenazine and oral clonidine. Symptoms resolved when clonidine was withdrawn and recurred when the patient was rechallenged with clonidine.

➤*Anesthetics:* Epidural clonidine may prolong the duration of pharmacologic effects of epidural local anesthetics, including both sensory and motor blockade.

Adverse Reactions

The following adverse events may be related to administration of either clonidine or morphine.

Clonidine Adverse Reactions

Adverse Events	Clonidine (%)	Placebo (%)
Total number of patients who experienced ≥ 1 adverse event	97.4	80.5
Hypotension	44.8	10.6
Postural hypotension	31.6	0
Dry mouth	13.2	8.5
Nausea	13.2	21.3
Somnolence	13.2	21.3
Dizziness	13.2	4.3
Confusion	13.2	10.6
Vomiting	10.5	14.9
Nausea/Vomiting	7.9	2.1
Sweating	5.3	0
Anxiety	11	2
Chest pain	5.3	0
Hallucination	5.3	2.1
Tinnitus	5.3	0
Constipation	6	4.3
Tachycardia	2.6	4.3
Hypoventilation	2.6	4.3
Urinary tract infection	22	nd[a]
Dyspnea	6	nd
Infection	6	nd
Asthenia	5	nd
Hyperesthesia	5	nd
Pain	5	nd
Skin ulcer	5	nd
Decreased heart rate	†[b]	nd
Rebound hypertension	11	nd

[a] nd = No data.
[b] † = Occurs, but the incidence is unknown.

Adverse reactions seen during continuous epidural clonidine infusion are dose-dependent and typical for a compound of this pharmacologic class. The adverse events most frequently reported in the pivotal controlled clinical trial of continuous epidural clonidine administration consisted of hypotension, postural hypotension, decreased heart rate, rebound hypertension, dry mouth, nausea, confusion, dizziness, somnolence, and fever. Hypotension is the adverse event that most frequently requires treatment. The hypotension is usually responsive to intravenous fluids and, if necessary, parenterally-administered ephedrine. Hypotension was observed more frequently in women and in lower weight patients, but no dose-related response was established.

The inadvertent intrathecal administration of clonidine has not been associated with a significantly increased risk of adverse events, but there are inadequate safety and efficacy data to support the use of intrathecal clonidine. Epidural clonidine was compared to placebo in a 2 week double-blind study of 85 terminal cancer patients with intractable pain receiving epidural morphine. The following adverse events were reported in 2 or more patients and may be related to administration of either clonidine hydrochloride or morphine.

CLONIDINE HYDROCHLORIDE — INJECTION

Incidence of Clonidine Adverse Events in the 2-week Trial		
Adverse events	Clonidine (n = 38), n (%)	Placebo (n = 47), n (%)
Total number of patients who experienced at least 1 adverse event	37 (97.4)	38 (80.5)
Hypotension	17 (44.8)	5 (10.6)
Postural hypotension	12 (31.6)	0 (0)
Dry mouth	5 (13.2)	4 (8.5)
Nausea	5 (13.2)	10 (21.3)
Somnolence	5 (13.2)	10 (21.3)
Dizziness	5 (13.2)	2 (4.3)
Confusion	5 (13.2)	5 (10.6)
Vomiting	4 (10.5)	7 (14.9)
Nausea/vomiting	3 (7.9)	1 (2.1)
Sweating	2 (5.3)	0 (0)
Chest pain	2 (5.3)	0 (0)
Hallucinations	2 (5.3)	1 (2.1)
Tinnitus	2 (5.3)	0 (0)
Constipation	1 (2.6)	2 (4.3)
Tachycardia	1 (2.6)	2 (4.3)
Hypoventilation	1 (2.6)	2 (4.3)

➤*Long-term extension of the above trial:* An open-label long-term extension of the above trial was performed. Thirty-two subjects received epidural clonidine and morphine for up to 94 weeks a median dosing period of 10 weeks. The following adverse events (and percent incidence) were reported: Hypotension/postural hypotension (47%); nausea (13%); anxiety/confusion (38%); somnolence (25%); urinary tract infection (22%); constipation, dyspnea, fever, infection (6% each); asthenia, hyperesthesia, pain, skin ulcer, and vomiting (5% each). Eighteen percent of subjects discontinued this study as a result of catheter-related problems (eg, infections, accidental dislodging), and one subject developed meningitis, possibly as a result of a catheter-related infection. In this study, rebound hypertension was not assessed, and ECG and laboratory data were not systematically sought.

The following adverse reactions have also been reported with the use of any dosage form of clonidine. In many cases, patients were receiving concomitant medication and a causal relationship has not been established:

Cardiovascular – Palpitations and tachycardia, and bradycardia, each 0.5%. Syncope, Raynaud's phenomenon, congestive heart failure, and electrocardiographic abnormalities (ie, sinus node arrest, functional bradycardia, high degree AV block) have been reported rarely. Rare cases of sinus bradycardia and atrioventricular block have been reported, both with and without the use of concomitant digitalis.

CNS – Nervousness and agitation, 3%; mental depression, 1%; insomnia, 0.5%. Cerebrovascular accidents, other behavioral changes, vivid dreams or nightmares, restlessness, and delirium have been reported rarely.

Dermatologic – Rash, 1%; pruritus, 0.7%; hives, angioneurotic edema and urticaria, 0.5%; alopecia, 0.2%.

GI – Anorexia and malaise, each 1%; mild transient abnormalities in liver function tests, 1%; hepatitis, parotitis, ileus and pseudo obstruction, and abdominal pain, rarely.

GU – Decreased sexual activity, impotence, and libido, 3%; nocturia, about 1%; difficulty in micturition, about 0.2%; urinary retention, about 0.1%.

Hematologic – Thrombocytopenia, rarely.

Metabolic – Weight gain, 0.1%; gynecomastia, 1%; transient elevation of glucose or serum phosphatase, rarely.

Musculoskeletal – Muscle or joint pain, about 0.6%; leg cramps, 0.3%.

Ophthalmic – Dryness of the eyes, burning of the eyes and blurred vision were rarely reported.

Special senses – Dryness of the nasal mucosa was rarely reported.

Miscellaneous – Weakness, 10%; fatigue, 4%; headache and withdrawal syndrome, each 1%. Also reported were pallor, a weakly positive Coomb's test, and increased sensitivity to alcohol.

Overdosage

➤*Symptoms:* Hypertension may develop early and may be followed by hypotension, bradycardia, respiratory depression, hypothermia, drowsiness, decreased or absent reflexes, irritability, and miosis. With large oral overdoses, reversible cardiac conduction defects or arrhythmias, apnea, coma, and seizures have been reported. As little as 100 mcg of oral clonidine has produced signs of toxicity in pediatric patients.

The largest overdose reported to date involved a 28-year old white male who ingested 100 mg of clonidine hydrochloride powder. This patient developed hypertension followed by hypotension, bradycardia, apnea, hallucinations, semicoma, and premature ventricular contractions. The patient fully recovered after intensive treatment. Plasma clonidine levels were 60 ng/mL after 1 hour, 190 ng/mL after 1.5 hours, 370 ng/mL after 2 hours, and 120 ng/mL after 5.5 and 6.5 hours. In mice and rats, the oral LD_{50} of clonidine is 206 and 465 mg/kg, respectively.

➤*Treatment:* There is no specific antidote for clonidine overdosage. Supportive care may include atropine sulfate for bradycardia, intravenous fluids or vasopressor agents for hypotension. Hypertension associated with overdosage has been treated with intravenous furosemide, diazoxide or alpha-blocking agents such as phentolamine. Naloxone may be a useful adjunct in the treatment of clonidine-induced respiratory depression, hypotension, or coma; blood pressure should be monitored since the administration of naloxone has occasionally resulted in paradoxical hypertension. Tolazoline administration has yielded inconsistent results and is not recommended as first-line therapy. Dialysis is not likely to significantly enhance the elimination of clonidine.

Patient Information

Patients should be instructed about the risks of rebound hypertension and warned not to discontinue clonidine except under the supervision of a physician. Patients should notify their physician immediately if clonidine administration is inadvertently interrupted for any reason. Patients who engage in potentially hazardous activities, such as operating machinery or driving, should be advised of the potential sedative and hypotensive effects of epidural clonidine. They should also be informed that sedative effects may be increased by CNS-depressing drugs such as alcohol and barbiturates, and that hypotensive effects may be increased by opiates.

ACETAMINOPHEN

ACETAMINOPHEN (N-Acetyl-P-Aminophenol; APAP)

otc	**Acetaminophen** (Various, eg, Akyma, Moore, Plus, URL)	**Tablets; oral:** 325 mg	In 50s, 100s, and 1,000s.
otc	**Aminofen** (Dover)		In 500s.
otc	**Apap** (Medique)		Film-coated. In 150s.
otc sf	**Cetafen** (Hart Health & Safety)		Film-coated. In UD 100s and 250s.
otc	**Genapap** (Ivax)		In 100s.
otc	**Mapap Regular Strength** (Major)		In 100s, 1,000s, and UD 100s.
otc	**Masophen** (Mason)		In 100s.
otc	**Pain and Fever** (Rugby)		In 100s.
otc	**Pain Reliever** (Magno-Humphries)		In 100s, 250s, and 1,000s.
otc	**Q-Pap** (Qualitest)		In 100s.
otc	**Tylenol Regular Strength** Tablets (McNeil Consumer)		(TYLENOL 325). In 100s.
otc sf	**Valorin** (Otis Clapp)		In 300s.

ACETAMINOPHEN (N-Acetyl-P-Aminophenol; APAP)

otc	**Acetaminophen** (Various, eg, Akyma, Marlex, Moore, Plus)	**Tablets; oral:** 500 mg	In 100s, 1,000s, and UD 100s.
otc	**Acetaminophen** Caplets (Various, eg, Akyma, Moore, Plus, UDL, URL)		In 25s, 100s, 700s, and 1,000s.
otc	**Acetaminophen Extra Strength Caplets** (Akyma)		In 100s, 700s, and 1,000s.
otc	**Aminofen Max Extra Strength** (Dover)		In 500s.
otc	**Anacin Aspirin Free** (Insight)		Parabens. Film-coated. In 100s.
otc	**Apap** (Medique)		Film-coated. In UD 100s.
otc sf	**Cetafen Extra** (Hart Health & Safety)		Film-coated. In UD 100s.
otc	**Mapap Caplets** (Major)		In 24s, 50s, 100s, 175s, 500s, and 1,000s.
otc	**Masophen** (Mason)		Tablets and caplets: In 100s.
otc	**Non-Aspirin Extra Strength Caplets** (Mason)		In 100s.
otc	**Pain and Fever** (Rugby)		Tablets and caplets: In 100s and 1,000s.
otc	**Pain Relief Extra Strength Caplets** (Basic)		In 100s.
otc	**Pain Reliever Extra Strength** (Magno-Humphries)		In 100s, 250s, and 1,000s.
otc	**Q-Pap Extra Strength** (Qualitest)		In 100s.
otc	**Tylenol Extra Strength EZ Tabs** (McNeil Consumer)		Sucralose. In 50s, 100s, and 225s.
otc	**Tylenol Extra Strength Caplets** (McNeil Consumer)		Castor oil, sucralose. Regular and cool flavors. In 50s and 100s.
otc	**UN-Aspirin Extra Strength** (Zee Medical)		Castor oil. Capsule shape. In 250s.
otc sf	**Valorin** (Otis Clapp)		In UD 300s.
otc	**Acetaminophen Children's** (Geri-care)	**Tablets, chewable; oral:** 80 mg	Aspartame, dextrose, mannitol, phenylalanine, sugar. Fruit flavor. In 30s.
otc	**Genapap Children's** (Ivax)		Grape flavor. In 30s.
otc	**Mapap Children's** (Major)		Aspartame, mannitol, phenylalanine 3 mg, sucrose. Grape, fruit, and bubble gum flavors. In 30s.
otc	**Pain and Fever Children's** (Rugby)		Aspartame, dextrose, phenylalanine, sugar. Fruit flavor. In 30s.
otc	**Mapap Junior Strength** (Major)	**Tablets, chewable; oral:** 160 mg	Grape flavor. In 24s.
otc	**Tylenol Extra Strength Go Tabs** (McNeil Consumer)	**Tablets, chewable; oral:** 500 mg	Acesulfame potassium, dextrose, sucralose. Spearmint ice flavor. In 6s.
otc	**Mapap Arthritis Pain** (Major)	**Tablets, extended-release; oral:** 650 mg	In 100s.
otc	**Tylenol 8 Hour Caplets** (McNeil Consumer)		Polyvinyl alcohol, sucralose. In 24s, 50s, 100s, and 150s.
otc	**Tylenol Arthritis Pain** (McNeil Consumer)		Caplets: In 24s, 50s, 100s, 150s, and 225s. Geltabs: Parabens. In 20s, 40s, and 80s.
otc	**Quick Melts Children's Non-Aspirin** (Marlex)	**Tablets, disintegrating; oral:** 80 mg	Bubble gum flavor: Gluten free. Mannitol, sorbitol, sucralose, sugar. Grape flavor: Gluten free and sugar free. Corn syrup, mannitol, sorbitol, sucralose. Watermelon flavor: Gluten free and sugar free. Mannitol, sorbitol, sucralose. In 30s.
otc	**Quick Melts Jr. Strength Non-Aspirin** (Marlex)	**Tablets, disintegrating; oral:** 160 mg	Bubble gum flavor: Gluten free. Mannitol, sorbitol, sucralose, sugar. Grape flavor: Gluten free and sugar free. Corn syrup, mannitol, sorbitol, sucralose. In 30s.
otc	**Tylenol Children's Meltaways** (McNeil Consumer)	**Tablets, chewable/dispersible; oral:** 80 mg	Dextrose, sucralose. Bubble gum, grape, and watermelon flavors. In 30s.
otc	**Tylenol Jr. Meltaways** (McNeil Consumer)	**Tablets, chewable/dispersible; oral:** 160 mg	Dextrose, sucralose. Bubble gum, grape, and punch flavors. In 24s.
otc	**Genapap Extra Strength Gelcaps** (Ivax)	**Tablets, rapid-release; oral:** 500 mg	In 100s.
otc	**Mapap Gelcaps** (Major)		In 24s, 50s, 100s, 175s, 500s, and 1,000s.
otc	**Tylenol Extra Strength Rapid Release Gels** (McNeil Consumer)		Benzyl alcohol, parabens. In 24s, 50s, 100s, and 225s.
otc	**Acetaminophen** (Various, eg, URL)	**Capsules; oral:** 500 mg	In 100s.
otc	**Mapap** (Major)		In 24s, 50s, 100s, 175s, 500s, and 1,000s.
otc	**Masophen Extra Strength** (Mason)		In 100s.
otc	**Acetaminophen** (Various, eg, Ivax, URL)	**Liquid; oral:** 160 mg per 5 mL	May contain methylparaben, saccharin, sorbitol, sucrose. In 118, 120, 473, and 500 mL.
otc	**Q-Pap Children's** (Qualitest)		Alcohol free. Sorbitol, sucrose. Cherry and grape flavors. In 118, 473, and 3,785 mL.
otc sf	**Silapap Children's** (Silarx)		Alcohol free. Methylparaben, saccharin. In 118, 237, and 473 mL.
otc	**Acetaminophen** (Various, eg, Ivax)	**Liquid; oral:** 166.6 mg per 5 mL	In 237 mL.
otc	**Tylenol Extra Strength** (McNeil Consumer)		Corn syrup, saccharin, sorbitol. In 240 mL with dosage cup.
otc	**Tylenol Sore Throat Daytime** (McNeil Consumer)		Sorbitol, sucralose, sucrose. Cool burst flavor. In 240 mL.
otc sf	**Apap 500** (Cypress)	**Liquid; oral:** 500 mg per 5 mL	Alcohol free. In 237 mL.

ACETAMINOPHEN (N-Acetyl-P-Aminophenol; APAP)

otc	**Apra Children's** (Altaire)	**Elixir; oral:** 160 mg per 5 mL	Alcohol free. Sorbitol, sucrose. Grape and cherry flavors. In 118 mL.
otc	**Mapap Children's** (Major)		Alcohol free. Sorbitol, sucrose. Cherry flavor. In 118 mL.
otc	**Q-Pap Children's** (Qualitest)		Alcohol free. Sorbitol, sucrose. Grape flavor. In 118 and 3,785 mL.
otc	**Silapap Children's** (Silarx)		Alcohol free. In 237 mL.
otc	**Acetaminophen** (Various, eg, Ivax)	**Solution; oral:** 160 mg per 5 mL	May contain sorbitol, sucrose. In 118 and 473 mL.
otc	**Ed-Apap Children's** (Edwards)		Alcohol free. Sorbitol. Cherry flavor. In 236 mL.
otc	**ElixSure Children's Fever Reducer/Pain Reliever** (Alterna)		Butylparaben, sucralose. Cherry flavor. In 120 mL.
otc	**Pain and Fever Relief Children's** (Rugby)		Sorbitol, sucrose. Cherry flavor. In 118 mL.
otc	**Little Fevers Fever/Pain Reliever** (Medtech)	**Solution, concentrate; oral:** 80 mg/mL	Gluten free, alcohol free, dye free. Corn syrup, glycerin, PEG, propylene glycol, , sodium benzoate, sucralose. Berry flavor. In 30 mL with dropper.
otc	**Apap Infant's Drops** (Various, eg, Actavis, Ivax)	**Solution, concentrate; oral:** 100 mg/mL	May contain butylparaben, saccharin. In 15 mL.
otc	**Infantaire Drops** (Altaire)		In 15 and 30 mL w/0.8 mL dropper.
otc	**Mapap Infant Drops** (Major)		Alcohol free. Cherry flavor. In 15 and 30 mL.
otc	**Pain and Fever Relief Children's Drops** (Rugby)		Alcohol free. Butylparaben, corn syrup, sorbitol. Cherry flavor. In 15 mL.
otc	**Q-Pap Infants Drops** (Qualitest)		Alcohol free. Butylparaben, saccharin. Fruit flavor. In 15 mL.
otc	**Silapap Infants** (Silarx)		Alcohol free. In 15 and 30 mL.
otc	**Triaminic Infants' Fever Reducer/Pain Reliever** (Novartis)		Alcohol free. Butylparaben, corn syrup, glycerin, propylene glycol, sodium benzoate, sorbitol. Cherry and grape flavor. In 15 mL w/dropper.
otc	**Tylenol Infants' Drops** (McNeil Consumer)		Cherry and grape flavors: Corn syrup, sorbitol. Cherry flavor: Dye free. Parabens, sorbitol, sucralose. In 15 and 30 mL w/0.8 mL dropper.
otc	**Nortemp Children's** (Ballay)	**Suspension; oral:** 160 mg per 5 mL	Alcohol free. Butylparaben, corn syrup, sorbitol. Cotton candy flavor. In 118 mL.
otc	**Q-Pap Children's** (Qualitest)		Alcohol free. Butylparaben, corn syrup, sorbitol. Grape and bubble gum flavors. In 118 mL.
otc	**Tylenol Children's** (McNeil Consumer)		2 mg sodium per 5 mL. Cherry, grape, and bubble gum flavors: Alcohol free and dye free. Butylparaben, corn syrup, sorbitol. Strawberry flavor: Butylparaben, corn syrup, sorbitol, sucrose. Cherry flavor: Dye free. Parabens, sorbitol, sucralose, sucrose. In 60 and 120 mL.
otc sf	**Tylenol with Flavor Creator Children's** (McNeil Consumer)		Butylparaben, corn syrup, sorbitol, sucralose. Apple, bubble gum, chocolate, and strawberry flavors. In 120 mL.
otc	**FeverAll Infants** (Actavis)	**Suppositories; rectal:** 80 mg	Hydrogenated vegetable oil. In 6s and 50s.
otc	**Acetaminophen** (Various, eg, Ivax, Moore, Rugby)	**Suppositories; rectal:** 120 mg	Hydrogenated vegetable oil. In 12s.
otc	**Acephen** (G & W Labs)		Glyceryl stearate, vegetable oil. In 6s, 12s, and UD 12s, 50s, and 100s.
otc	**FeverAll Children's** (Actavis)		Hydrogenated vegetable oil. In 6s and 50s.
otc	**Acetaminophen** (Various, eg, Ivax, Moore, Rugby)	**Suppositories; rectal:** 325 mg	Hydrogenated vegetable oil. In 12s.
otc	**Acephen** (G & W Labs)		Hydrogenated vegetable oil. In 12s, 50s, 100s, and 1,000s and UD 6s and 12s.
otc	**FeverAll Junior Strength** (Actavis)		Hydrogenated vegetable oil. In 12s and 50s.
otc	**Acetaminophen** (Various, eg, Ivax, Moore, Rugby)	**Suppositories; rectal:** 650 mg	Hydrogenated vegetable oil. In 12s.
otc	**Acephen** (G & W Labs)		Hydrogenated vegetable oil. In 12s, 50s, 100s, 500s, and 1,000s.
otc	**FeverAll** (Actavis)		Hydrogenated vegetable oil. In 50s.
Rx	**Ofirmev** (Cadence Pharmaceuticals)	**Injection, solution:** 10 mg/mL	Mannitol. In 100 mL single-use vials.

ACETAMINOPHEN — ORAL

Indications

➤*Adults and children at least 12 years of age:* For the temporary reduction of fever and temporary relief of minor aches and pains caused by backache, the common cold, headache, menstrual cramps, minor arthritis pain, muscular aches, and toothache.

➤*Children:* Children 2 to 11 years of age: For the temporary reduction of fever and temporary relief of minor aches and pains caused by the common cold, flu, headache, sore throat, and toothache.

➤*Off-label uses:*

Prevention of adverse reactions with diphtheria, tetanus toxoids, and pertussis vaccination – [2] = Fair documentation. The published data are conflicting. While acetaminophen was consistently shown to be effective in reducing fever and local and systemic reactions when whole-cell pertussis vaccine was used, one trial evaluating its efficacy at reducing local reactions after the fifth dose of the acellular product failed to show any benefit. Published data and current Advisory Committee on Immunization Practices (ACIP) recommendations do not support routine use of acetaminophen prophylaxis with diphtheria, tetanus, and pertussis vaccination. (See Administration and Dosage.)

Prevention of adverse reactions with diphtheria, tetanus toxoids, and pertussis vaccination in patients at risk for seizures – [1] = Good documentation. The published data are conflicting (see previous section). However, consider acetaminophen prophylaxis in patients at high risk for seizures. (See Administration and Dosage.)

Administration and Dosage

➤*Maximum dose:* 4 g in 24 hours for adults and children older than 12 years of age. Varies by patient population and age.

➤*General dosing considerations:* Caution chronic alcoholics to limit acetaminophen intake to 2 g or less per day.

Patients should not use oral acetaminophen with any other product containing acetaminophen.

➤*Adults:*

Antipyretic / Analgesic –

Usual dosage: 325 to 650 mg every 4 to 6 hours (immediate release) or 1,300 mg every 8 hours (extended release).

Maximum dose: 4 g in 24 hours.

ACETAMINOPHEN — ORAL

➤*Children:*

Antipyretic/Analgesic –

Older than 12 years of age: See Adults for dosing in children older than 12 years of age.

2 to 12 years of age: If possible, use the patient's weight to determine the dose; otherwise, use age. For children, a dosage of 10 mg/kg also has been used.

General Acetaminophen Dosing

Age	Weight		Dose and frequency	Maximum daily amount
	lb	kg		
12 years	≥ 96	≥ 43.6	640 mg every 4 to 6 h	5 doses per day (3.2 g in 24 h)
11 years	72 to 95	32.7 to 42.3	480 mg every 4 to 6 h	5 doses per day (2.4 g)
9 to 10 years	60 to 71	27.3 to 32.3	400 mg every 4 to 6 h	5 doses per day (2 g in 24 h)
6 to 8 years	48 to 59	21.8 to 26.8	320 mg every 4 to 6 h	5 doses per day (1.6 g in 24 h)
4 to 5 years	36 to 47	16.4 to 21.4	240 mg every 4 h	5 doses per day (1.2 g in 24 h)
2 to 3 years	24 to 35	10.9 to 15.9	160 mg every 4 h	5 doses per day (800 mg in 24 h)

See Off-label dosing for children younger than 2 years of age.

Children's Acetaminophen Dosing by Formulation

Age	Weight		Dose given every 4 h up to 5 times per day	Acetaminophen formulation			
	lb	kg		Jr. strength chewable and disintegrating tablets (160 mg)	Children's chewable and disintegrating tablets (80 mg)	Children's liquid, solution, and suspension (160 mg per 5 mL)	Infants' concentrated drops (80 mg per 0.8 mL)
12 years	≥ 96	≥ 43.6	640 mg	4 tablets	—	—	—
11 years	72 to 95	32.7 to 42.3	480 mg	3 tablets	6 tablets	15 mL (3 tsp)	—
9 to 10 years	60 to 71	27.3 to 32.3	400 mg	2.5 tablets	5 tablets	12.5 mL (2.5 tsp)	—
6 to 8 years	48 to 59	21.8 to 26.8	320 mg	2 tablets	4 tablets	10 mL (2 tsp)	—
4 to 5 years	36 to 47	16.4 to 21.4	240 mg	—	3 tablets	7.5 mL (1.5 tsp)	—
2 to 3 years	24 to 35	10.9 to 15.9	160 mg	—	2 tablets	5 mL (1 tsp)	1.6 mL (2 droppersful)

See Off-label dosing for children younger than 2 years of age.

Off-label dosing –

Antipyretic/Analgesic:

Off-Label Acetaminophen Dosing

Age	Weight		Dose and frequency	Maximum daily amount
	lb	kg		
1 to 2 years	18 to 23	8.2 to 10.5	120 mg every 4 h	5 doses per day (600 mg in 24 h)
4 to 11 months	12 to 17	5.5 to 7.7	80 mg every 4 h	5 doses per day (400 mg in 24 h)
0 to 3 months	6 to 11	2.7 to 5	40 mg every 4 h	5 doses per day (200 mg in 24 h)

Off-Label Children's Acetaminophen Dosing by Formulation

Age	Weight		Dose given every 4 h up to 5 times per day	Acetaminophen formulation			
	lb	kg		Jr. strength chewable and disintegrating tablets (160 mg)	Children's chewable and disintegrating tablets (80 mg)	Children's liquid, solution, and suspension (160 mg per 5 mL)	Infants' concentrated drops (80 mg per 0.8 mL)
1 to 2 years	18 to 23	8.2 to 10.5	120 mg	—	—	3.75 mL (¾ tsp)	1.2 mL (1.5 droppersful)
4 to 11 months	12 to 17	5.5 to 7.7	80 mg	—	—	2.5 mL (½ tsp)	0.8 mL (1 dropperful)
0 to 3 months	6 to 11	2.7 to 5	40 mg	—	—	—	0.4 mL (½ dropperful)

• *Neonates* – 10 to 15 mg/kg/dose orally every 6 to 8 hours. Some suggest oral loading doses of 20 to 25 mg/kg/dose may be used.

Prevention of adverse reactions with diphtheria, tetanus toxoids, and pertussis vaccination: [2] = Fair documentation. 10 to 15 mg/kg given with or prior to the vaccination and continued for several doses after vaccination. One study evaluated a single acetaminophen 75 mg dose given 4 hours after vaccination.

Prevention of adverse reactions with diphtheria, tetanus toxoids, and pertussis vaccination in patients at risk for seizures: [1] = Good documentation. 10 to 15 mg/kg given with or prior to the vaccination and continued for several doses after vaccination. One study evaluated a single acetaminophen 75 mg dose given 4 hours after vaccination.

➤*Hepatic function impairment:* Use with caution in patients with any type of liver disease.

➤*Administration:*

Chewable tablets – Chew tablets before swallowing.

Chewable/Dispersible tablets – Dissolve in the mouth or chew before swallowing.

Elixirs, suspensions, and concentrated infants' drops – Shake well before using.

Extended-release tablets – Swallow whole; do not crush, chew, or dissolve.

Orally disintegrating tablets – Put tablet on the tongue and allow tablet to dissolve. Do not chew or swallow the tablet whole.

➤*Storage/Stability:* Store at 15° to 30°C (59° to 86°F). Avoid high humidity and excessive heat. Protect from freezing.

Actions

➤*Pharmacology:* Acetaminophen is the active metabolite of phenacetin and has antipyretic and analgesic activities. In peripheral tissues, acetaminophen is a weak COX-1 and COX-2 inhibitor. Acetaminophen appears to be equivalent to aspirin as an analgesic and antipyretic agent. However, acetaminophen lacks anti-inflammatory properties, does not affect uric acid levels, and does not inhibit platelet function.

➤*Pharmacokinetics:*

Absorption/Distribution – Immediate-release acetaminophen is absorbed rapidly, and peak plasma levels are reached in 30 to 60 minutes. Acetaminophen is distributed throughout most body fluids and is slightly bound to plasma proteins.

Metabolism/Excretion – Approximately 90% of acetaminophen usually undergoes hepatic conjugation with glucuronide (40% to 67%) and sulfate (20% to 46%) to form inactive metabolites that are excreted in the urine. A small amount (5% to 15%) of acetaminophen is metabolized to N-acetyl-p-benzoquinoneimine (NAPQI), a highly reactive intermediate. Normally, glutathione combines with NAPQI, and the resulting complex is rendered harmless and excreted. After a large ingestion of acetaminophen, these pathways become saturated, and glutathione stores become depleted. Therefore, NAPQI concentrations increase, which may cause hepatotoxicity.

The elimination half-life of acetaminophen is about 2 to 3 hours. Less than 5% of acetaminophen is excreted unchanged.

Special populations –

Hepatic function impairment: The half-life may increase 2-fold or more in patients with liver disease.

Contraindications

Hypersensitivity to acetaminophen or any other ingredient in the product.

Warnings/Precautions

➤*Alcohol warning:* Patients who consume 3 or more alcoholic drinks every day should ask their health care provider whether they should take acetaminophen or other pain relievers/fever reducers. Acetaminophen may cause liver damage. Caution chronic alcoholics to limit acetaminophen intake to 2 g or less per day.

➤*Hepatic effects:* Acetaminophen may cause liver damage (see Adverse Reactions and Overdosage).

➤*Sore throat:* If sore throat is severe, persists for more than 2 days, is accompanied by fever, headache, nausea, rash, or vomiting, tell patients to consult a health care provider promptly.

ACETAMINOPHEN — ORAL

➤*Usage:* Patients should not use oral acetaminophen with any other product containing acetaminophen.

Advise patients to stop use and ask a health care provider if pain gets worse or lasts for more than 5 days (children) or more than 10 days (adults), fever gets worse or lasts for more than 3 days, redness or swelling is present, or new symptoms occur. These could be signs of a serious condition.

➤*Hepatic function impairment:* Use with caution in patients with any type of liver disease.

➤*Pregnancy:* Category B. Acetaminophen crosses the placenta. It is routinely used during all stages of pregnancy; when used in therapeutic doses, it appears to be safe for short-term use. Continuous high daily dosage probably caused severe anemia in a mother, and the neonate had fatal kidney disease. Although there is no evidence of a relationship between acetaminophen ingestion and congenital malformations, 3 cases of congenital hip dislocation may have been associated with acetaminophen.

➤*Lactation:* Acetaminophen is excreted in breast milk in low concentrations with reported milk:plasma ratios of 0.91 to 1.42 at 1 and 12 hours, respectively. No adverse reactions in breast-feeding infants were reported, except for a single case of maculopapular rash on a breast-feeding infant. Acetaminophen is compatible with breast-feeding, according to the American Academy of Pediatrics.

➤*Children:* For children younger than 2 years of age (or less than 24 pounds), instruct patients to consult their health care provider.

Drug Interactions

Acetaminophen Drug Interactions

Precipitant drug	Object drug[a]		Description
Barbiturates (eg, phenobarbital)	Acetaminophen	↑↓	The potential hepatotoxicity of acetaminophen may be increased when large or chronic doses of barbiturates are coadministered. The therapeutic effects of acetaminophen may be reduced with barbiturate therapy.
Charcoal, activated	Acetaminophen	↓	Charcoal can reduce the GI absorption of acetaminophen when administered as soon as possible after overdose.
Ethanol	Acetaminophen	↑	Chronic consumption of ethanol may increase the risk of acetaminophen-induced liver damage.
Hydantoins (eg, phenytoin)	Acetaminophen	↑↓	The potential hepatotoxicity of acetaminophen may be increased when chronic doses of hydantoins are coadministered. The therapeutic effects of acetaminophen may be reduced with hydantoin therapy.
Sulfinpyrazone	Acetaminophen	↑↓	The potential hepatotoxicity of acetaminophen may be increased when coadministered with sulfinpyrazone. The therapeutic effects of acetaminophen may be reduced with sulfinpyrazone therapy.
Acetaminophen	Lamotrigine	↓	Serum lamotrigine concentrations may be reduced, producing a decrease in therapeutic effects. A clinically important interaction is unlikely to occur with a single dose or several doses of acetaminophen. With chronic administration of acetaminophen, if an interaction is suspected, adjust the dose of lamotrigine if needed.
Acetaminophen	Warfarin	↑	Acetaminophen appears to increase the antithrombotic effect of warfarin in a dose-dependent manner. The interaction may not be clinically important with low-dose, infrequent use (no more than 1,950 mg per week) of acetaminophen. Limit acetaminophen use and monitor coagulation parameters 1 to 2 times per week when starting or stopping acetaminophen, particularly if more than 2,275 mg per week are consumed. Adjust warfarin dose as needed.

[a] ↑ = object drug increased; ↓ = object drug decreased.

Adverse Reactions

Acetaminophen is usually well tolerated.

➤*CNS:* Dizziness, disorientation, and excitement have been seen with large doses.

➤*Hematologic:* Anecdotal reports of neutropenia, pancytopenia, and thrombocytopenia. Very rare reports of hemolytic anemia and methemoglobinemia.

➤*Hepatic:* Mild increases in liver enzymes (reversible after drug is withdrawn); liver damage, especially in overdose.

➤*Hypersensitivity:* Rash (usually erythematous or urticarial). It may be more serious and accompanied by drug fever and mucosal lesions.

➤*Renal:* Cases of renal damage (without hepatic damage) have been reported.

Overdosage

➤*Symptoms:* In adults, an acute ingestion of more than 7.5 g of acetaminophen is capable of causing toxicity. Patients taking supratherapeutic doses over an extended period of time are also at risk for toxicity. The course of acetaminophen poisoning is divided into 4 stages:

Stage 1 – Onset may be within a few hours of ingestion and may resolve within 24 hours. Symptoms include abdominal pain, diaphoresis, malaise, nausea, pallor, and vomiting. Liver function tests may be normal.

Stage 2 – Onset is 24 to 36 hours post acute ingestion. Liver injury develops and is noted by right upper quadrant pain and elevations of liver function tests (eg, ALT, AST, bilirubin, prothrombin time [PT]).

Stage 3 – Onset is 72 to 96 hours post acute ingestion. Hepatotoxicity peaks and is evident by fulminant hepatic failure, encephalopathy, coma, AST and ALT levels of more than 10,000 units/L, and abnormal PT, bilirubin, glucose, lactate, and phosphate. Fatalities caused by hepatic failure generally occur 3 to 5 days after an acute ingestion.

Stage 4 – Recovery stage for those patients who survive stage 3.

Acetaminophen levels – The optimal time to draw an acetaminophen level is 4 hours after an acute ingestion or as soon as possible after 4 hours. Plot serum levels drawn between 4 and 24 hours after an acute ingestion on the Rumack-Matthew nomogram to determine the risk of acetaminophen-induced hepatotoxicity and the need for n-acetylcysteine treatment (see the Acetylcysteine monograph for the nomogram). The Rumack-Matthew nomogram cannot be used when 1) the time of ingestion is unknown; 2) the ingestion occurred more than 24 hours before the serum sample was taken; or 3) repeated ingestion occurred. Once a toxic acetaminophen level has been determined, a repeat level is not useful and does not need to be done.

➤*Treatment:* For recent acetaminophen ingestions, administer activated charcoal to limit GI absorption. Provide general supportive care. N-acetylcysteine is the specific antidote for acetaminophen. See the acetylcysteine monographs (oral and injection) for more information. Contact a poison control center (1-800-222-1222) for further information, especially in cases of chronic ingestions and ingestions of extended-release acetaminophen.

Patient Information

Tell patients that if they consume 3 or more alcoholic drinks every day, they should ask their health care provider whether they should take acetaminophen or other pain relievers/fever reducers. Acetaminophen may cause liver damage.

If sore throat is severe, persists for more than 2 days, or is accompanied or followed by fever, headache, nausea, rash, or vomiting, tell patients to consult a health care provider promptly.

Tell patients to stop use and ask a health care provider if pain gets worse or lasts for more than 5 days (children) or 10 days (adults), fever gets worse or lasts for more than 3 days, redness or swelling is present, or new symptoms occur. These could be signs of a serious condition.

Tell patients not to use with any other products containing acetaminophen.

Tell patients not to exceed the recommended dose. In case of accidental overdose, patients should contact a health care provider or poison control center immediately. Prompt medical attention is critical for adults as well as for children, even if no signs or symptoms are noted. Acetaminophen should be kept out of the reach of children.

Patients should not use if the carton is opened or the neck wrap or the foil inner seal imprinted "safety seal" is broken or missing.

As with any drug, inform patients that if they are pregnant or breast-feeding, they should seek the advice of a health care provider before using this product.

ACETAMINOPHEN — RECTAL

Indications

➤*Antipyretic/analgesic:* For the temporary reduction of fever and the temporary relief of occasional aches and pains, and headaches.

➤*Off-label uses:* Prophylactic acetaminophen use in children receiving diphtheria, tetanus toxoid, and acellular pertussis vaccination appears to decrease incidence of fever and injection-site pain. A dose immediately following vaccination every 4 to 6 hours thereafter for 48 to 72 hours is suggested.

Administration and Dosage

➤*General dosing considerations:* Caution chronic alcoholics to limit acetaminophen intake to 2 g or less per day.

Patients should not use rectal acetaminophen with any other product containing acetaminophen.

➤*Adults:*

Antipyretic/Analgesic –

Usual dosage: 650 mg (given as two 325 mg suppositories or one 650 mg suppository) every 4 to 6 hours.

Maximum dose: 3,900 mg in 24 hours.

➤*Children:*

Antipyretic/Analgesic –

Older than 12 years of age: See Adults for dosing in children older than 12 years of age.

6 to 12 years of age:
- *Usual dosage* – 325 mg every 4 to 6 hours.
- *Maximum dose* – 1,950 mg in 24 hours.

3 to 6 years of age:
- *Usual dosage* – 120 mg every 4 to 6 hours.
- *Maximum dose* – 720 mg in 24 hours.

12 to 36 months of age:
- *Usual dosage* – 80 mg every 4 hours.
- *Maximum dose* – 480 mg in 24 hours.

3 to 11 months of age: 80 mg every 6 hours.

Off-label dosing –

Antipyretic/Analgesic:
- *Neonates* – 10 to 15 mg/kg/dose rectally every 6 to 8 hours. Some suggest loading doses of 30 mg/kg/dose rectally may be used.

➤*Hepatic function impairment:* Use with caution in patients with any type of liver disease.

➤*Administration:* For rectal use only. Remove the wrapper and carefully insert the suppository well into the rectum.

➤*Storage/Stability:* Store at 2° to 27°C (36° to 80°F). Do not use if imprinted suppository wrapper is opened or damaged.

Actions

➤*Pharmacology:* Acetaminophen is the active metabolite of phenacetin and has antipyretic and analgesic activities. In peripheral tissues, acetaminophen is a weak COX-1 and COX-2 inhibitor. Acetaminophen appears to be equivalent to aspirin as an analgesic and antipyretic agent. However, acetaminophen lacks anti-inflammatory properties, does not affect uric acid levels, and does not inhibit platelet function.

➤*Pharmacokinetics:*

Absorption/Distribution – In children, acetaminophen rectal suppositories were shown to reach peak levels in between 107 and 288 minutes, and bioavailability ranged from 30% to 40%. Acetaminophen is distributed throughout most body fluids and is slightly bound to plasma proteins.

Metabolism/Excretion – Approximately 90% of acetaminophen usually undergoes hepatic conjugation with glucuronide (40% to 67%) and sulfate (20% to 46%) to form inactive metabolites that are excreted in the urine. A small amount (5% to 15%) of acetaminophen is metabolized to N-acetyl-p-benzoquinoneimine (NAPQI), a highly reactive intermediate. Normally, glutathione combines with NAPQI, and the resulting complex is rendered harmless and excreted. After a large ingestion of acetaminophen, these pathways become saturated, and glutathione stores become depleted. Therefore, NAPQI concentrations increase, which may cause hepatotoxicity.

The elimination half-life of acetaminophen is about 2 to 3 hours. Less than 5% of acetaminophen is excreted unchanged.

Special populations –

Hepatic function impairment: The half-life may increase 2-fold or more in patients with liver disease.

Contraindications

Hypersensitivity to acetaminophen or any other ingredient in the product.

Warnings/Precautions

➤*Alcohol warning:* Patients who consume 3 or more alcoholic drinks every day should ask their health care providers whether they should take acetaminophen or other pain relievers/fever reducers. Acetaminophen may cause liver damage. Caution chronic alcoholics to limit acetaminophen intake to 2 g or less per day.

➤*Hepatic effects:* Acetaminophen may cause liver damage (see Adverse Reactions and Overdosage).

➤*Usage:* For rectal use only. Patients should not use rectal acetaminophen with any other product containing acetaminophen.

Advise patients to stop use and ask a health care provider if pain gets worse or lasts for more than 3 days (children 3 to 36 months of age), 5 days (children 3 to 6 years of age), or 10 days (adults and children 6 years of age and older); fever lasts for more than 3 days (72 hours) or recurs; redness or swelling is present in the painful area; or new symptoms occur. These could be signs of a serious condition.

➤*Hepatic function impairment:* Use with caution in patients with any type of liver disease.

➤*Pregnancy: Category B.* Acetaminophen crosses the placenta. It is routinely used during all stages of pregnancy; when used in therapeutic doses, it appears to be safe for short-term use. Continuous high daily dosage probably caused severe anemia in a mother, and the neonate had fatal kidney disease. Although there is no evidence of a relationship between acetaminophen ingestion and congenital malformations, 3 cases of congenital hip dislocation may have been associated with acetaminophen.

➤*Lactation:* Acetaminophen is excreted in breast milk in low concentrations with reported milk:plasma ratios of 0.91 to 1.42 at 1 and 12 hours, respectively. No adverse reactions in breast-feeding infants were reported, except for a single case of maculopapular rash on a breast-feeding infant. Acetaminophen is compatible with breast-feeding, according to the American Academy of Pediatrics.

➤*Children:* For children younger than 3 months of age, instruct patients to consult their health care provider. For children 3 to 36 months of age, use 80 mg suppositories. For children 3 to 6 years of age, use 120 mg suppositories. For children 6 to 12 years of age, use 325 mg suppositories. For adults and children 12 years of age and older, use the 325 or 650 mg suppositories.

Drug Interactions

Acetaminophen Drug Interactions

Precipitant drug	Object drug[a]		Description
Barbiturates (eg, phenobarbital)	Acetaminophen	↑↓	The potential hepatotoxicity of acetaminophen may be increased when large or chronic doses of barbiturates are coadministered. The therapeutic effects of acetaminophen may be reduced with barbiturate therapy.
Ethanol	Acetaminophen	↑	Chronic consumption of ethanol may increase the risk of acetaminophen-induced liver damage.
Hydantoins (eg, phenytoin)	Acetaminophen	↑↓	The potential hepatotoxicity of acetaminophen may be increased when chronic doses of hydantoins are coadministered. The therapeutic effects of acetaminophen may be reduced with hydantoin therapy.
Sulfinpyrazone	Acetaminophen	↑↓	The potential hepatotoxicity of acetaminophen may be increased when coadministered with sulfinpyrazone. The therapeutic effects of acetaminophen may be reduced with sulfinpyrazone therapy.
Acetaminophen	Lamotrigine	↓	Serum lamotrigine concentrations may be reduced, producing a decrease in therapeutic effects. A clinically important interaction is unlikely to occur with a single dose or several doses of acetaminophen. With chronic administration of acetaminophen, if an interaction is suspected, adjust the dose of lamotrigine if needed.
Acetaminophen	Warfarin	↑	Acetaminophen appears to increase the antithrombotic effect of warfarin in a dose-dependent manner. The interaction may not be clinically important with low-dose, infrequent use (no more than 1,950 mg per week) of acetaminophen. Limit acetaminophen use and monitor coagulation parameters 1 to 2 times per week when starting or stopping acetaminophen, particularly if more than 2,275 mg per week are consumed. Adjust warfarin dose as needed.

[a] ↑ = object drug increased; ↓ = object drug decreased.

Adverse Reactions

Acetaminophen is usually well tolerated.

ACETAMINOPHEN — RECTAL

➤*CNS:* Dizziness, disorientation, and excitement have been seen with large doses.

➤*Hematologic:* Anecdotal reports of neutropenia, pancytopenia, and thrombocytopenia. Very rare reports of hemolytic anemia and methemoglobinemia.

➤*Hepatic:* Increases in liver enzymes (reversible after drug is withdrawn); liver damage, especially in overdose.

➤*Hypersensitivity:* Rash (usually erythematous or urticarial). It may be more serious and accompanied by drug fever and mucosal lesions.

➤*Renal:* Cases of renal damage (without hepatic damage) have been reported.

Overdosage

➤*Symptoms:* In adults, an acute ingestion of more than 7.5 g of acetaminophen is capable of causing toxicity. Patients taking supratherapeutic doses over an extended period of time are also at risk for toxicity. The course of acetaminophen poisoning is divided into 4 stages:

Stage 1 – Onset may be within a few hours of ingestion and may resolve within 24 hours. Symptoms include abdominal pain, diaphoresis, malaise, nausea, pallor, and vomiting. Liver function tests may be normal.

Stage 2 – Onset is 24 to 36 hours post acute ingestion. Liver injury develops and is noted by right upper quadrant pain and elevations of liver function tests (eg, aspartate aminotransferase [AST], alanine aminotransferase [ALT], prothrombin time [PT], bilirubin).

Stage 3 – Onset is 72 to 96 hours post acute ingestion. Hepatotoxicity peaks and is evident by fulminant hepatic failure, encephalopathy, coma, AST and ALT levels of more than 10,000 units/L, and abnormal PT, bilirubin, glucose, lactate, and phosphate. Fatalities caused by hepatic failure generally occur 3 to 5 days after an acute ingestion.

Stage 4 – Recovery stage for those patients who survive stage 3.

Acetaminophen levels – The optimal time to draw an acetaminophen level is 4 hours after an acute ingestion or as soon as possible after 4 hours. Plot serum levels drawn between 4 and 24 hours post acute ingestion on the Rumack-Matthew nomogram to determine the risk of acetaminophen-induced hepatotoxicity and the need for n-acetylcysteine treatment (see the Acetylcysteine monograph for the nomogram). The Rumack-Matthew nomogram cannot be used when 1) the time of ingestion is unknown; 2) the ingestion occurred more than 24 hours before the serum sample was taken; or 3) repeated ingestion occurred. Once a toxic acetaminophen level has been determined, a repeat level is not useful and does not need to be done.

➤*Treatment:* For recent acetaminophen ingestions, administer activated charcoal to limit GI absorption. Provide general supportive care. N-acetylcysteine is the specific antidote for acetaminophen. See the acetylcysteine monographs (oral and injection) for more information. Contact a poison control center (1-800-222-1222) for further information, especially in cases of chronic ingestions and ingestions of extended-release acetaminophen.

Patient Information

Tell patients that if they consume 3 or more alcoholic drinks every day, they should ask their health care provider whether they should take acetaminophen or other pain relievers/fever reducers. Acetaminophen may cause liver damage.

Tell patients to stop use and ask a health care provider if pain gets worse or lasts for more than 3 days (children 3 to 36 months of age), 5 days (children 3 to 6 years of age), or 10 days (adults and children 6 years of age and older); fever lasts for more than 3 days (72 hours) or recurs; redness or swelling is present in the painful area; or new symptoms occur. These could be signs of a serious condition.

Tell patients not to use with any other products containing acetaminophen.

Tell patients not to exceed the recommended dose. In case of accidental overdose, patients should contact a health care provider or poison control center immediately. Prompt medical attention is critical for adults as well as for children, even if no signs or symptoms are noted. Acetaminophen should be kept out of the reach of children.

Patients should not use if the imprinted suppository wrapper is opened or damaged.

ACETAMINOPHEN — INJECTION

Indications

➤*Fever:* For the reduction of fever.

➤*Pain:* For the management of mild to moderate pain and the management of moderate to severe pain with adjunctive opioid analgesics.

Administration and Dosage

➤*General dosing considerations:* No dose adjustment is required when converting between oral acetaminophen and acetaminophen injection dosing in adults and adolescents.

Acetaminophen injection may be given as a single or repeated dose for the treatment of acute pain or fever. Minimum recommended dosing interval is 4 hours.

The maximum daily dose of acetaminophen is based on all routes of administration (ie, intravenous [IV], oral, and rectal) and all products containing acetaminophen.

➤*Adults:*

Fever/Pain –
Usual dosage: 1,000 mg every 6 hours or 650 mg every 4 hours IV.
Maximum dose: 1,000 mg as a single dose and 4,000 mg/day.

➤*Children:*

Fever/Pain –
13 years of age and older:
- *50 kg or more* – See Adults for dosing.
- *Less than 50 kg* –
  Usual dosage: 15 mg/kg every 6 hours or 12.5 mg/kg every 4 hours IV.
  Maximum dose: 15 mg/kg (up to 750 mg) as a single dose and 75 mg/kg (up to 3,750 mg) per day.

2 to 12 years of age:
- *Usual dosage* – 15 mg/kg every 6 hours or 12.5 mg/kg every 4 hours IV.
- *Maximum dose* – 15 mg/kg as a single dose and 75 mg/kg per day.

➤*Renal function impairment:* Longer dosing intervals and a reduced total daily dose may be warranted in patients with severe renal impairment (creatinine clearance [CrCl] 30 mL/min or less).

➤*Hepatic function impairment:* Use with caution in patients with hepatic impairment or active liver disease; a reduced total daily dose may be warranted.

Contraindicated in patients with severe hepatic impairment or sever active liver disease.

➤*Administration:* Administer IV over 15 minutes. Acetaminophen may be administered without further dilution.

For patients requiring acetaminophen 1,000 mg, administer the dose by inserting a vented IV set through the septum of the 100 mL vial. Administer contents of the vial IV over 15 minutes.

For acetaminophen doses of less than 1,000 mg, the appropriate dose must be withdrawn from the vial and placed into a separate container prior to administration. Withdraw the appropriate dose (650 mg or weight-based) from an intact sealed vial and place the measured dose in a separate empty, sterile container (eg, glass bottle, plastic IV container, syringe) for IV infusion to avoid the inadvertent delivery and administration of the total volume of the commercially available container. Place small-volume pediatric doses of up to 60 mL in volume in a syringe and administer over 15 minutes using a syringe pump.

Monitor the end of the infusion in order to prevent the possibility of an air embolism, especially in cases where the acetaminophen infusion is the primary infusion.

➤*Admixture compatibility:* Do not add other medications to the acetaminophen vial or infusion device. Diazepam and chlorpromazine hydrochloride are physically incompatible with acetaminophen; therefore, do not administer simultaneously.

➤*Storage/Stability:* Store at 20° to 25°C (68° to 77°F). Use within 6 hours after the vacuum seal of the vial has been penetrated, or the contents transferred to another container. Do not refrigerate or freeze. Vials are for single use; discard unused portion.

Actions

➤*Pharmacology:* Acetaminophen is a non-salicylate antipyretic and non-opioid analgesic agent. The precise mechanism of the analgesic and antipyretic properties of acetaminophen is not established but is thought to primarily involve central actions.

➤*Pharmacokinetics:* The pharmacokinetics of acetaminophen injection have been studied in patients and healthy subjects from premature neonates up to adults 60 years old. The pharmacokinetic profile of acetaminophen injection has been demonstrated to be dose proportional in adults following administration of single doses of 500, 650, and 1,000 mg.

Absorption – The maximum concentration (C_{max}) occurs at the end of the 15-minute IV infusion of acetaminophen. Compared with the same dose of oral acetaminophen, the C_{max} following administration of acetaminophen injection is up to 70% higher, while overall exposure (area under the concentration-time curve) is very similar.

Distribution – At therapeutic levels, binding of acetaminophen to plasma proteins is low (ranging from 10% to 25%). Acetaminophen appears to be widely distributed throughout most body tissues except fat.

Metabolism/Excretion – Acetaminophen is primarily metabolized in the liver by first-order kinetics and involves 3 principal separate pathways: conjugation with glucuronide, conjugation with sulfate, and oxidation via the cytochrome P450 (CYP-450) enzyme pathway, primarily CYP2E1, to form a reactive intermediate metabolite (N-acetyl-p-benzoquinone imine [NAPQI]). With therapeutic doses, NAPQI undergoes rapid conjugation with glutathione and is then further metabolized to form cysteine and mercapturic acid conjugates.

Acetaminophen metabolites are mainly excreted in the urine. Less than 5% is excreted in the urine as unconjugated (free) acetaminophen, and more than 90% of the administered dose is excreted within 24 hours.

Special populations –
Children: The pharmacokinetic exposure of acetaminophen injection observed in children and adolescents is similar to adults, but higher in neonates and infants. Dosing simulations from pharmacokinetic data in infants and neonates suggest that dose reductions of 33% in infants 1 month to younger than 2 years of age, and 50% in neonates up to 28 days of age, with a minimum dosing interval of 6 hours, will produce a pharmacokinetic exposure similar to that observed in children 2 years of age and older.

ACETAMINOPHEN — INJECTION

Contraindications

Hypersensitivity to acetaminophen or to any of the excipients in the IV formulation; severe hepatic impairment or severe active liver disease.

Warnings/Precautions

➤*Hepatic effects:* Administration of acetaminophen in doses higher than recommended may result in hepatic injury, including the risk of severe hepatotoxicity and death. Do not exceed the maximum recommended daily dose of acetaminophen.

Use caution when administering acetaminophen in patients with the following conditions: hepatic impairment or active hepatic disease, alcoholism, chronic malnutrition, severe hypovolemia (eg, due to dehydration or blood loss), or severe renal impairment (CrCl 30 mL/min or less).

➤*Hypersensitivity reactions:* There have been postmarketing reports of hypersensitivity and anaphylaxis associated with the use of acetaminophen. Clinical signs included swelling of the face, mouth, and throat; respiratory distress; urticaria; rash; and pruritus. There were infrequent reports of life-threatening anaphylaxis requiring emergent medical attention. Discontinue acetaminophen immediately if symptoms associated with allergy or hypersensitivity occur. Do not use acetaminophen injection in patients with acetaminophen allergy.

➤*Renal function impairment:* See Administration and Dosage for more information.

➤*Hepatic function impairment:* See Administration and Dosage for more information.

➤*Pregnancy: Category C.* There are no studies of acetaminophen IV in pregnant women; however, epidemiological data on oral acetaminophen use in pregnant women show no increased risk of major congenital malformations. Animal reproduction studies have not been conducted with acetaminophen IV, and it is not known whether acetaminophen injection can cause fetal harm when administered to a pregnant woman. Give acetaminophen injection to a pregnant woman only if clearly needed.

The results from a large population-based prospective cohort study, including data from 26,424 women with live-born singletons who were exposed to oral acetaminophen during the first trimester, indicate no increased risk of congenital malformations compared with a control group of unexposed children. The rate of congenital malformations (4.3%) was similar to the rate in the general population. A population-based, case-control study from the National Birth Defects Prevention Study showed that 11,610 children with prenatal exposure to acetaminophen during the first trimester had no increased risk of major birth defects compared with 4,500 children in the control group. Other epidemiological data showed similar results.

Though animal reproduction studies have not been conducted with acetaminophen IV, studies in pregnant rats that received oral acetaminophen during organogenesis at doses of up to 0.85 times the MHDD (MHDD = 4 g/day, based on a BSA comparison) showed evidence of fetotoxicity (reduced fetal weight and length) and a dose-related increase in bone variations (reduced ossification and rudimentary rib changes). Offspring had no evidence of external, visceral, or skeletal malformations. When pregnant rats received oral acetaminophen throughout gestation at doses of 1.2 times the MHDD (based on a BSA comparison), areas of necrosis occurred in both the liver and kidney of pregnant rats and fetuses. These effects did not occur in animals that received oral acetaminophen at doses of 0.3 times the MHDD, based on a BSA comparison.

In a continuous breeding study, pregnant mice received 0.25%, 0.5%, or 1% acetaminophen via the diet (357, 715, or 1,430 mg/kg/day). These doses are approximately 0.43, 0.87, and 1.7 times the MHDD, respectively, based on a BSA comparison. A dose-related reduction in body weights of fourth and fifth litter offspring of the treated mating pair occurred during lactation and postweaning at all doses. Animals in the high-dose group had a reduced number of litters per mating pair, male offspring with an increased percentage of abnormal sperm, and reduced birth weights in the next generation pups.

Labor and delivery – There are no adequate and well-controlled studies with acetaminophen injection during labor and delivery; therefore, use in such settings only after a careful benefit-risk assessment.

➤*Lactation:* While studies with acetaminophen injection have not been conducted, acetaminophen is secreted in human milk in small quantities after oral administration. Based on data from more than 15 breast-feeding mothers, the calculated infant daily dose of acetaminophen is approximately 1% to 2% of the maternal dose. There is 1 well-documented report of a rash in a breast-fed infant that resolved when the mother stopped acetaminophen use and recurred when she resumed acetaminophen use. Exercise caution when acetaminophen injection is administered to a breast-feeding woman. The American Academy of Pediatrics classifies oral acetaminophen as compatible with breast-feeding.

➤*Children:* The safety and effectiveness of acetaminophen injection for the treatment of acute pain and fever in children 2 years of age and older is supported by evidence from adequate and well-controlled studies of acetaminophen injection in adults. Additional safety and pharmacokinetic data were collected in 355 patients across the full pediatric age strata, from premature neonates (at least 32 weeks post menstrual age) to adolescents. The effectiveness of acetaminophen injection for the treatment of acute pain and fever has not been studied in children younger than 2 years of age.

Drug Interactions

Acetaminophen Drug Interactions

Precipitant drug	Object drug[a]		Description
Alcohol	Acetaminophen	↑	Chronic alcohol consumption may increase the risk of acetaminophen-induced liver damage. Use with caution in patients with a history of chronic alcohol ingestion.
Barbiturates (eg, phenobarbital), carbamazepine, hydantoins (eg, phenytoin), sulfinpyrazone	Acetaminophen	↑↓	The risk of acetaminophen-induced hepatotoxicity may be increased when large or chronic doses of one of these agents is coadministered with acetaminophen. In addition, the therapeutic effects of acetaminophen may be reduced. At usual therapeutic doses, no special precautions are needed.
CYP2E1 inducers	Acetaminophen	↑	The metabolism of acetaminophen may be altered, increasing the risk of hepatotoxicity. Use with caution.
Acetaminophen	Warfarin	↑	Acetaminophen appears to increase the antithrombotic effect of warfarin in a dose-dependent manner. More frequent assessment of international normalized ratio is warranted. Adjust the warfarin dose as needed.

[a] ↑ = object drug increased; ↑↓ = object drug both increased and decreased.

Adverse Reactions

➤*Adults:*

Most common – The most common adverse events in adult patients treated with acetaminophen injection (incidence of at least 5% and greater than placebo) were headache, insomnia, nausea, and vomiting.

Adverse reactions (3% or more) –

Acetaminophen Injection Adverse Reactions (≥3%) in Placebo-Controlled, Repeated-Dose Studies

Adverse reactions	Acetaminophen injection (n = 402)	Placebo (n = 379)
CNS		
Headache	10%	9%
Insomnia	7%	5%
GI		
Nausea	34%	31%
Vomiting	15%	11%
Miscellaneous		
Pyrexia[a]	5%	14%

[a] Pyrexia adverse reaction frequency data are included in order to alert health care professionals that the antipyretic effects of acetaminophen injection may mask fever.

Other adverse reactions (1% or more) –

Cardiovascular: Hypertension, hypotension.
CNS: Anxiety, fatigue.
Metabolic/Nutritional: Edema peripheral, hypokalemia.
Musculoskeletal: Muscle spasms, trismus.
Respiratory: Breath sounds abnormal, dyspnea.
Miscellaneous: AST increased, infusion-site pain.

➤*Children:*

Most common – The most common adverse reactions (incidence of at least 5%) in children treated with acetaminophen injection were agitation, atelectasis, constipation, nausea, pruritus, and vomiting.

Adverse reactions (1% or more) –

Cardiovascular: Hypertension, hypotension, tachycardia.
CNS: Headache, insomnia.
Dermatologic: Periorbital edema, rash.
GI: Abdominal pain, diarrhea.
Metabolic/Nutritional: Hepatic enzyme increase, hypervolemia, hypoalbuminemia, hypokalemia, hypomagnesemia, hypophosphatemia, peripheral edema.
Musculoskeletal: Muscle spasm, pain in extremity.
Respiratory: Hypoxia, pleural effusion, pulmonary edema, stridor, wheezing.
Miscellaneous: Anemia, oliguria, injection-site pain, pyrexia.

Overdosage

➤*Symptoms:* In acute acetaminophen overdosage, dose-dependent, potentially fatal hepatic necrosis is the most serious adverse effect. Renal tubular necrosis, hypoglycemic coma, and thrombocytopenia may also occur. Plasma acetaminophen levels greater than 300 mcg/mL at 4 hours after oral ingestion were associated with hepatic damage in 90% of patients; minimal hepa-

ACETAMINOPHEN — INJECTION

tic damage is anticipated if plasma levels at 4 hours are less than 150 mcg/mL or less than 37.5 mcg/mL at 12 hours after ingestion. Early symptoms following a potentially hepatotoxic overdose may include: nausea, vomiting, diaphoresis, and general malaise. Clinical and laboratory evidence of hepatic toxicity may not be apparent until 48 to 72 hours postingestion.

➤*Treatment:* If an acetaminophen overdose is suspected, obtain a serum acetaminophen assay as soon as possible, but no sooner than 4 hours following oral ingestion. Obtain liver function studies initially and repeat at 24-hour intervals. Administer the antidote N-acetylcysteine (NAC) as early as possible. As a guide to treatment of acute ingestion, the acetaminophen level can be plotted against time since oral ingestion on a nomogram (Rumack-Matthew). The lower toxic line on the nomogram is equivalent to 150 mcg/mL at 4 hours and 37.5 mcg/mL at 12 hours. If serum level is above the lower line, administer the entire course of NAC treatment. Withhold NAC therapy if the acetaminophen level is below the lower line. For additional information, call a poison control center at 1-800-222-1222.

Patient Information

Advise patients that use in higher than recommended doses may result in hepatic injury, including the risk of severe hepatotoxicity and death. Advise patients not to exceed the maximum recommended daily dose and to avoid use with other products containing acetaminophen.

Instruct patients to inform their health care provider if swelling of the face, mouth, or throat; respiratory distress; urticaria; rash; and/or pruritus occur.

SALICYLATES

WARNING

Children and teenagers should not use salicylates for chickenpox or flu symptoms before a doctor is consulted about Reye's syndrome, a rare but serious illness.

Indications

➤*Mild to moderate pain:* For the treatment of mild to moderate pain.

➤*Antipyretic:* For the treatment of fever.

➤*Inflammatory conditions:* For the treatment of various inflammatory conditions such as rheumatic fever, rheumatoid arthritis and osteoarthritis.

➤*Vascular disease:*

Aspirin – Aspirin, for reducing the risk of recurrent transient ischemic attacks (TIAs) or stroke in men who have had transient ischemia of the brain due to fibrin platelet emboli. It has not been effective in women and is of no benefit for completed strokes.

Aspirin: Aspirin, to reduce the risk of death or nonfatal myocardial infarction (MI) in patients with previous infarction or unstable angina pectoris.

➤*Off-label uses:* Refer to individual monographs for further information.

Kawasaki disease –

Aspirin: [1] = Good documentation. Use of aspirin in the management of Kawasaki disease is recommended in American Heart Association and American College of Chest Physicians guidelines.

Postherpetic neuralgia –

Aspirin (topical): [4] = Insufficient documentation. Topical aspirin has shown benefit in patients with postherpetic neuralgia (PHN). However, American Academy of Neurology clinical practice guidelines consider the degree of pain relief from topical aspirin to be below the level considered clinically important for treatment of chronic pain.

Other possible off-label uses – Possible effect of long-term aspirin-like analgesics to prevent cataract formation is being studied. Dipyridamole is often added to aspirin to prevent MI and stroke, but data do not show improved antithrombotic aspirin efficacy during coadministration. Low-dose aspirin may help prevent toxemia of pregnancy and may be beneficial in pregnant women with inadequate uteroplacental blood flow (eg, systemic lupus erythematosus). Further studies are needed. See Warnings.

Actions

➤*Pharmacology:* The salicylates have analgesic, antipyretic and anti-inflammatory effects. **Aspirin** and other salicylic acid derivatives are hydrolyzed to salicylic acid. Salicylamide and **diflunisal** are structurally related, but are not true salicylates because they are not hydrolyzed to salicylic acid.

Salicylates have analgesic, antipyretic, anti-inflammatory and antirheumatic effects. The pharmacological effects of these agents are qualitatively similar. Salicylates lower elevated body temperature through vasodilation of peripheral vessels, thus enhancing dissipation of excess heat. The anti-inflammatory and analgesic activity may be mediated through inhibition of the prostaglandin synthetase enzyme complex.

Aspirin – Aspirin differs from the other agents in this group in that it more potently inhibits prostaglandin synthesis, has greater anti-inflammatory effects and irreversibly inhibits platelet aggregation. The aspirin molecule's acetyl group is believed to account for these differences. Aspirin inhibits prostaglandin production by acetylating cyclo-oxygenase, the initial enzyme in the prostaglandin biosynthesis pathway.

Irreversible inhibition of platelet aggregation (aspirin) – Single analgesic aspirin doses prolong bleeding time. Acetylation of platelet cyclo-oxygenase prevents synthesis of thromboxane A_2, a prostaglandin derivative, which is a potent vasoconstrictor and inducer of platelet aggregation and platelet release reaction. Aspirin (no other salicylates) inhibits platelet aggregation for the life of the platelet (7 to 10 days).

Aspirin has shown some success as an antiplatelet agent in patients with thromboembolic disease. Low doses of aspirin inhibit platelet aggregation and may be more effective than higher doses. Larger doses inhibit cyclo-oxygenase in arterial walls, interfering with prostacyclin production, a potent vasodilator and inhibitor of platelet aggregation. Combinations of dipyridamole or sulfinpyrazone with aspirin have been recommended for antithrombotic action for prophylaxis in various high risk situations (ie, coronary bypass graft patency, total hip replacement).

Myocardial infarction (MI) – **Aspirin** use in MI patients was associated with ≈ 20% reduction in risk of subsequent death and nonfatal reinfarction, a median absolute decrease of 3% from the 12% to 22% event rates with placebo. Daily aspirin dosage in post-MI studies was 300 mg in one and 900 to 1500 mg in five. In aspirin-treated unstable angina patients (325 mg/day), reduction in risk was about 50%, a reduction in event rate of 5% from the 10% rate with placebo over the 12-week study.

In the Aspirin Myocardial Infarction Study (AMIS) trial, 1 g/day was associated with small increases in systolic BP (average, 1.5 to 2.1 mmHg) and diastolic BP (0.5 to 0.6 mmHg). Uric acid levels and BUN increased by < 1 mg/dl.

In the Second International Study of Infarct Survival (ISIS-2) trial, patients who received a combination of aspirin (160 mg/day) and streptokinase after the onset of suspected acute MI had significantly fewer reinfarctions, strokes and deaths than those patients who received placebo. Also, the combination was significantly better than either drug alone; their separate effects on vascular deaths appeared additive.

Other pharmacological actions – Inhibition of prothrombin synthesis and prolonged prothrombin time are clinically significant only after large doses (≥ 6 g/day). Doses > 3 to 5 g/day have a uricosuric effect; low doses (< 2 g/day) decrease uric acid secretion.

➤*Pharmacokinetics:*

Absorption/Distribution – Salicylates are rapidly and completely absorbed after oral use. Bioavailability is dependent on the dosage form, presence of food, gastric emptying time, gastric pH, presence of antacids or buffering agents and particle size. Bioavailability of some enteric coated products may be erratic. Food slows the absorption of salicylates. Absorption from rectal suppositories is slower, resulting in lower salicylate levels. **Aspirin** is partially hydrolyzed to salicylic acid during absorption and is distributed to all body tissues and fluids, including fetal tissues, breast milk and CNS. Highest concentrations are found in plasma, liver, renal cortex, heart and lungs. Protein binding of salicylates is concentration-dependent. At low therapeutic concentrations (100 mcg/ml), ≈ 90% is bound; at higher plasma concentrations (400 mcg/ml), 76% is bound. Signs of salicylism (eg, tinnitus) occur at serum levels > 200 mcg/ml; severe toxic effects may occur at levels > 400 mcg/ml (see Adverse Reactions).

Metabolism/Excretion – Salicylic acid is eliminated by renal excretion and by oxidation and conjugation of metabolites. **Aspirin** has a half-life of ≈ 15 to 20 minutes. Salicylic acid has a half-life of 2 to 3 hours at low doses; at higher doses, it may exceed 20 hours. In therapeutic anti-inflammatory doses, half-life ranges from 6 to 12 hours. Plasma salicylate levels increase disproportionately as dosage is increased. Elimination is determined by zero order kinetics. Renal excretion of unchanged drug depends upon urine pH. As urinary pH changes from 5 to 8, renal clearance of free ionized salicylate increases from 2% to 3% of amount excreted to > 80%.

Contraindications

Hypersensitivity to salicylates or nonsteroidal anti-inflammatory drugs (NSAIDs). Use extreme caution in patients with history of adverse reactions to salicylates. Cross-sensitivity may exist between aspirin and other NSAIDs which inhibit prostaglandin synthesis, and aspirin and tartrazine. Aspirin cross-sensitivity does not appear to occur with sodium salicylate, or salicylamide. Aspirin hypersensitivity is more prevalent in those with asthma, nasal polyposis, chronic urticaria.

In hemophilia, bleeding ulcers and hemorrhagic states.

➤*Magnesium salicylate:* Magnesium salicylate in advanced chronic renal insufficiency due to magnesium retention.

Warnings/Precautions

➤*Reye's syndrome:*

Salicylate association – Use of salicylates, particularly **aspirin**, in children or teenagers with influenza or chickenpox may be associated with development of Reye's syndrome. This rare, acute, life-threatening condition is characterized by vomiting, lethargy and belligerence that may progress to delirium and coma. Mortality rate is 20% to 30%; permanent brain damage has been reported in survivors.

A causal relationship is controversial, but CDC, FDA, American Academy of Pediatrics' Committee on Infectious Diseases and Surgeon General advise against salicylate use in children and teens with influenza or chickenpox. (See Warning Box.)

➤*Otic effects:* Discontinue use if dizziness, ringing in ears (tinnitus) or impaired hearing occurs. Tinnitus probably represents blood salicylic acid levels reaching or exceeding the upper limit of the therapeutic range. It is a helpful guide to dose titration. Temporary hearing loss disappears gradually upon discontinuation of the drug.

➤*Use in surgical patients:* Avoid **aspirin**, if possible, for 1 week prior to surgery because of the possibility of postoperative bleeding.

➤*Renal effects:* Use with caution in chronic renal insufficiency; **aspirin** may cause a transient decrease in renal function, and may aggravate chronic kidney diseases (rare).

In patients with renal impairment, take precautions when administering **magnesium salicylate**. Discontinue other drugs containing magnesium and monitor serum magnesium levels if dosage levels of magnesium salicylate are high.

➤*GI effects:* Use caution in those intolerant to salicylate because of GI irritation, and in gastric ulcers, peptic ulcer, mild diabetes, gout, erosive gastritis or bleeding tendencies. **Salsalate** may cause less GI irritation than **aspirin**.

Although fecal blood loss is less with enteric coated aspirin than with uncoated, give enteric coated aspirin with caution to patients with GI distress, ulcer or bleeding problems. Occult GI bleeding occurs in many patients but is not correlated with gastric distress. The amount of blood lost is usually clinically insignificant (average, 2.5 ml), but with prolonged use, it may result in iron deficiency anemia. Patients developing peptic ulcers while taking salicylates for rheumatic disease have healed during treatment with cimetidine and antacids despite continued salicylate use. In addition, although acute aspirin use results in mucosal lesions, only 20% to 25% of those on chronic aspirin for rheumatism develop mucosal injury.

➤*Hematologic effects:* **Aspirin** interferes with hemostasis. Avoid use if patients have severe anemia, history of blood coagulation defects, or take anticoagulants (see Drug Interactions).

➤*Long-term therapy:* To avoid potentially toxic concentrations, warn patients on long-term therapy not to take other salicylates (nonprescription analgesics, etc).

Periodically monitor plasma salicylic acid concentrations during long-term treatment to aid maintenance of therapeutic levels (100 to 300 mcg/ml). Toxic manifestations are not usually seen until concentrations exceed 300 mcg/ml. Monitor urinary pH regularly; sudden acidification, as from pH 6.5 to 5.5, can double the plasma level, resulting in toxicity.

➤*Salicylism:* Salicylism may require dosage adjustment.

➤*Controlled release aspirin:* Controlled release aspirin, because of its relatively long onset of action, is not recommended for antipyresis or short-term analgesia. Not recommended in children younger than 12; contraindicated in all children with fever accompanied by dehydration.

➤*Benzyl alcohol:* Some of these products contain the preservative benzyl alcohol, which has been associated with a fatal "gasping syndrome" in premature infants.

➤*Hypersensitivity reactions:* **Aspirin** intolerance, manifested by acute bronchospasm, generalized urticaria/angioedema, severe rhinitis or shock occurs in 4% to 19% of asthmatics. Symptoms occur within 3 hours after ingestion. The aspirin triad consists of the association of asthma, nasal polyps and aspirin intolerance. Have epinephrine 1:1000 immediately available. Refer to Management of Acute Hypersensitivity Reactions.

Foods – Foods may contribute to a reaction. Some foods with 6 mg/100 g salicylate include curry powder, paprika, licorice, Benedictine liqueur, prunes, raisins, tea, gherkins. A typical American diet contains 10 to 200 mg/day salicylate.

Desensitization – Desensitization has been successfully induced and maintained. Perform in hospital; generally maintain with one **aspirin**/day. Any NSAID can maintain desensitization. However, if maintenance is interrupted, sensitivity will reappear (2 to 5 days).

➤*Tartrazine sensitivity:* Some of these products contain tartrazine, which may cause allergic-type reactions (including bronchial asthma) in susceptible individuals. Although the incidence of tartrazine sensitivity in the general population is low, it is frequently seen in patients who also have aspirin hypersensitivity. Specific products containing tartrazine are identified in the product listings.

➤*Hepatic function impairment:* Use caution in liver damage, preexisting hypoprothrombinemia and vitamin K deficiency. Reversible hepatic encephalopathy occurred in a chronic alcoholic with cirrhosis who took ASA 5 g/day for osteoarthritis. Aspirin-induced hepatotoxicity occurred after therapeutic doses for rheumatoid arthritis.

➤*Pregnancy: Category D* (aspirin); *Category C* (salsalate, magnesium salicylate). **Aspirin** may produce adverse maternal effects: Anemia, ante- or postpartum hemorrhage, prolonged gestation and labor. Salicylates readily cross the placenta. By inhibiting prostaglandin synthesis, salicylates may cause constriction of ductus arteriosus, and, possibly, other untoward fetal effects. Maternal aspirin use during later stages of pregnancy may cause adverse fetal effects: Low birth weight, increased incidence of intracranial hemorrhage in premature infants, stillbirths, neonatal death. Salicylates may be teratogens. Avoid use during pregnancy, especially in third trimester.

➤*Lactation:* Salicylates are excreted in breast milk in low concentrations, producing peak milk levels ranging from 1.1 to 10 mcg/ml. Adverse effects on platelet function in the nursing infant have not been reported, but are a potential risk.

➤*Children:* Safety and efficacy of **magnesium salicylate** or **salsalate** have not been established. Administration of **aspirin** to children (including teenagers) with acute febrile illness has been associated with the development of Reye's syndrome. Dehydrated febrile children appear more prone to salicylate intoxication.

Drug Interactions

Salicylate Drug Interactions

Precipitant drug	Object drug[a]		Description
Alcohol	Salicylates	↑	The risk of GI ulceration increases when salicylates are given concomitantly. Ingestion of alcohol during salicylate therapy may also prolong bleeding time.
Ammonium chloride	Salicylates	↑	Urinary acidifiers decrease salicylate excretion.
Ascorbic acid			
Methionine			
Antacids	Salicylates	↓	Antacids and urinary alkalinizers may decrease the pharmacologic effects of salicylates. Urinary alkalinization increases the renal excretion of salicylic acid due to decreased tubular reabsorption of un-ionized drug. The magnitude of the antacid interaction depends on the agent, dose and pretreatment urine pH.
Urinary alkalinizers			
Carbonic anhydrase inhibitors	Salicylates	↑	Salicylate intoxication has occurred after coadministration of these agents. However, salicylic acid renal elimination may be increased if urine is kept alkaline. Conversely, salicylates may displace acetazolamide from protein binding sites resulting in toxicity. Further study is needed.
Salicylates	Carbonic anhydrase inhibitors		
Charcoal, activated	Aspirin	↓	Coadministration decreases aspirin absorption, depending on charcoal dose and interval between ingestion. May be useful (see Overdosage).
Corticosteroids	Salicylates	↓	Corticosteroids increase salicylate clearance and decrease serum levels.
Nizatidine	Salicylates	↑	Increased serum salicylate levels have occurred in patients receiving high dose aspirin (3.9 g/day) and concurrent nizatidine.
Aspirin	Anticoagulants, oral	↑	Therapeutic aspirin has an additive hypoprothrombinemic effect. Impaired platelet function may prolong bleeding time. Use caution.
Anticoagulants, oral	Aspirin		
Aspirin	Heparin	↑	Aspirin can increase bleeding risk in heparin anticoagulated patients.
Aspirin	Nitroglycerin	↑	Nitroglycerin, when taken with aspirin, may result in unexpected hypotension. Data are limited. If hypotension occurs, reduce the nitroglycerin dose.
Aspirin	NSAIDs	↓	Aspirin may decrease NSAID serum concentrations. Concomitant use offers no advantage and may significantly increase incidence of GI effects.
Aspirin	Valproic acid	↑	Aspirin displaces the drug from its protein-binding sites and may decrease its total body clearance, thus increasing the pharmacologic effects.
Salicylates	Angiotensin-converting enzyme inhibitors	↓	Antihypertensive effectiveness of these agents may be decreased by concurrent salicylate administration, possibly due to prostaglandin inhibition. Consider discontinuing salicylates if problems occur.
Salicylates	Beta-adrenergic blockers	↓	Beta-adrenergic blockers may have their antihypertensive action blunted by concurrent salicylate administration, possibly due to prostaglandin inhibition. Consider discontinuing salicylates if problems occur.
Salicylates	Loop diuretics	↓	Loop diuretics may be less effective when given with salicylates in patients with compromised renal function or with cirrhosis with ascites; however, data conflict.

Precipitant drug	Object drug[a]		Description
			Salicylate Drug Interactions
Salicylates	Methotrexate	↑	Salicylates increase drug levels causing toxicity by interfering with protein binding and renal elimination of the antimetabolite.
Salicylates	Probenecid	↓	Salicylates antagonize the uricosuric effect of probenecid and sulfinpyrazone. While salicylates in large doses (> 3 g/day) have a uricosuric effect, smaller amounts may reduce the uricosuric effect of these agents.
	Sulfinpyrazone		
Salicylates	Spironolactone	↓	Salicylates may inhibit the diuretic effects; antihypertensive action does not appear altered. Effects depend on the dose of spironolactone.
Salicylates	Sulfonylureas	↑	Salicylates in doses > 2 g/day have a hypoglycemic action, perhaps by altering pancreatic beta cell function. They may potentiate the glucose-lowering effect of these drugs.
	Insulin		

[a] ↑ = object drug increased; ↓ = object drug decreased.

➤*Drug/Lab test interactions:* Salicylates compete with thyroid hormone for binding sites on thyroid binding pre-albumin and possibly thyroid-binding globulin resulting in increases in **protein bound iodine (PBI)**. Salicylates probably do not interfere with T_3 resin uptake.

Serum uric acid – Serum uric acid levels are elevated by salicylate levels **phenylbutazone** and salicylates decrease uric acid excretion and may increase serum uric acid by an average of 2 mg/dl.

Salicylates in moderate to large (anti-inflammatory) doses cause false-negative readings for **urine glucose** by the glucose oxidase method and false-positive readings by the copper reduction method.

Salicylates in the urine interfere with 5-HIAA determinations by fluorescent methods, but not by the nitrosonaphthol colorimetric method.

Salicylates in the urine interact with **urinary ketone** determinations by the ferric chloride (Gerhardt) method producing a reddish color.

Large doses may decrease urinary excretion of **PSP (phenolsulfonphthalein)**.

Salicylates in the urine result in falsely elevated **VMA (vanillylmandelic acid)** with most tests, but falsely decrease VMA determinations by the Pisano method.

Adverse Reactions

➤*Dermatologic:* Hives, rashes and angioedema may occur, especially in patients suffering from chronic urticaria.

➤*GI:* Nausea, dyspepsia (5% to 25%), heartburn, epigastric discomfort, anorexia, acute reversible hepatotoxicity, massive GI bleeding and occult blood loss may occur. Aspirin may potentiate peptic ulcer.

Chronic aspirin use may cause persistent iron deficiency anemia.

➤*Hematologic:* Prolongation of bleeding time, leukopenia, thrombocytopenia, purpura, decreased plasma iron concentration, shortened erythrocyte survival time.

➤*Hepatic:* High aspirin doses reportedly produced reversible hepatic dysfunction.

➤*Miscellaneous:* Fever, thirst, dimness of vision.

Allergic reactions – Allergic and anaphylactic reactions were noted when hypersensitive individuals took aspirin. Fatal anaphylactic shock, while not common, has been reported.

Aspirin intolerance – Aspirin intolerance, manifested by exacerbation of bronchospasm and rhinitis, may occur in patients with a history of nasal polyps, asthma or rhinitis. The mechanism of this intolerance may be the result of aspirin-induced shunting of prostaglandin synthesis to the lipoxygenase pathway and liberation of leukotrienes, ie, slow-reacting substance of anaphylaxis.

Salicylism – Mild "salicylism" may occur after repeated use of large doses and consists of dizziness, tinnitus (manifested as musical perceptions in one patient), difficulty hearing, nausea, vomiting, diarrhea, mental confusion, CNS depression, headache, sweating, hyperventilation and lassitude. Salicylate serum concentrations correlate with pharmacological actions and adverse effects observed. See table below:

Serum Salicylate: Clinical Correlations

Serum salicylate concentration (mcg/ml)	Desired effects	Adverse effects/ intoxication
≈ 100	Antiplatelet Antipyresis Analgesia	GI intolerance and bleeding, hypersensitivity, hemostatic defects
150-300	Anti-inflammatory	Mild salicylism
250-400	Treatment of rheumatic fever	Nausea/vomiting, hyperventilation, salicylism, flushing, sweating, thirst, headache, diarrhea, and tachycardia
> 400-500		Respiratory alkalosis, hemorrhage, excitement, confusion, asterixis, pulmonary edema, convulsions, tetany, metabolic acidosis, fever, coma, cardiovascular collapse, renal and respiratory failure

Overdosage

➤*Symptoms:*

Acute lethal dose (approximate) –

Adults: 10 to 30 g.

Children: 4 g. Respiratory alkalosis is seen initially in acute salicylate ingestions. Hyperpnea and tachypnea occur as a result of increased CO_2 production and a direct stimulatory effect of salicylate on the respiratory center. Other symptoms may include nausea, vomiting, hypokalemia, tinnitus, neurologic abnormalities (eg, disorientation, irritability, hallucinations, lethargy, stupor, coma, seizures), dehydration, hyperthermia, hyperventilation, hyperactivity, thrombocytopenia, platelet dysfunction, hypoprothrombinemia, increased capillary fragility and other hematologic abnormalities. Symptoms may progress quickly to depression, coma, respiratory failure and collapse. Although blood glucose is usually normal or slightly elevated, hypoglycemia may occur with chronic toxicity or in late acute toxicity. A mixed respiratory alkalosis and metabolic acidosis may also develop. Chronic salicylate toxicity may occur when > 100 mg/kg/day is ingested for 2 or more days. It is more difficult to recognize and is associated with increased morbidity and mortality. Compared to acute poisoning, hyperventilation, dehydration, systemic acidosis and severe CNS manifestations occur more frequently.

➤*Treatment:* Initial treatment includes induction of emesis or gastric lavage to remove any unabsorbed drug from the stomach. Activated charcoal diminishes salicylate absorption, most effectively if given within 2 hours after ingestion. Monitor salicylate levels, acid-base and fluid and electrolyte balance. Further therapy is largely supportive. Refer to General Management of Acute Overdosage. Reduce hyperthermia; treat severe convulsions with diazepam. Forced alkaline diuresis will enhance renal excretion of salicylates. Hemodialysis is very efficient in eliminating salicylate, but use only in patients who are severely poisoned, and in those with noncardiogenic pulmonary edema, severe CNS symptoms, renal failure, acidosis refractory to conservative therapy or clinical deterioration despite other therapies. Rarely, IV vitamin K may be indicated to correct hypoprothrombinemia.

Patient Information

May cause GI upset; take with food or after meals.

Do not crush or chew sustained release preparations.

Take with a full glass of water (240 ml) to reduce the risk of lodging medication in the esophagus.

Patients allergic to tartrazine dye should avoid **aspirin**.

Notify physician if ringing in ears or persistent GI pain occurs.

Do not use **aspirin** if it has a strong vinegar-like odor.

ASPIRIN (Acetylsalicylic Acid; ASA)

otc	**Bayer Heart Advantage** (Bayer)	**Tablets; oral:** 81 mg	Lactose, phytosterols 400 mg, tartrazine. Capsule shape. In 60s.
otc	**Aspirin** (Various, eg, Moore, Parmed, URL, Warner-C)	**Tablets; oral:** 325 mg	In 100s, 200s, 250s, 500s, and 1,000s.
otc	**Genuine Bayer Aspirin** (Bayer)		(BAYER BAYER BAYER BAYER). Film-coated. Capsule shape. In 50s, 100s, and 200s.
otc	**Empirin** (GlaxoWellcome)		(Tabloid brand). White. In 50s, 100s, and 250s.
otc	**Norwich Regular Strength** (Lee)		Coated. In 100s.

ASPIRIN (Acetylsalicylic Acid; ASA)

otc	**Aspirin** (Various, eg, URL)	**Tablets; oral:** 500 mg	In 100s.
otc	**Arthritis Foundation Pain Reliever** (McNeil-CPC)		In 50s.
otc	**Maximum Bayer Aspirin Tablets and Caplets** (Bayer)		**Tablets**: Film-coated. In 30s, 60s, and 100s. **Caplets**: Film-coated. In 30s and 60s.
otc	**Norwich Extra-Strength** (Lee)		In 150s.
otc	**Tri-Buffered Bufferin Tablets and Caplets** (Bristol-Myers Squibb)	**Tablets, buffered; oral:** 325 mg with calcium carbonate, magnesium oxide, and magnesium carbonate	**Tablets**: (B). White. In 12s, 36s, 60s, 100s, 200s, 275s, 1,000s. **Caplets**: (B). White, scored. In 36s, 60s, and 100s.
otc	**Adprin-B** (Pfeiffer)		Coated. In 130s.
otc	**Bufferin** (Novartis Consumer Health)		(B). Mineral oil. In 12s, 36s, 39s, 60s, 65s, 100s, 200s, and UD 150s.
otc	**Ascriptin** (Novartis)	**Tablets, buffered; oral:** 325 mg with magnesium hydroxide, aluminum hydroxide, and calcium carbonate	(Ascriptin). Coated. In 60s.
otc	**Buffered Aspirin** (Various, eg, Geneva, Goldline, Major, Moore, UDL, URL)	**Tablets, buffered; oral:** 325 mg	In 100s, 500s, 1,000s, and UD 100s and 200s.
otc	**Bayer Buffered Aspirin** (Bayer Consumer)		(Bayer Buffered). In 100s.
otc	**Bayer Plus Extra Strength** (Bayer Consumer)	**Tablets, buffered; oral:** 500 mg with calcium carbonate	Capsule shape. In 30s and 60s.
otc	**Bufferin Extra Strength** (Novartis Consumer)		In 130s.
otc	**Ascriptin Maximum Strength** (Novartis)	**Tablets, buffered; oral:** 500 mg with calcium carbonate 237 mg, magnesium hydroxide 33 mg, and aluminum hydroxide 33 mg	Capsule shape. In 85s.
otc	**Arthritis Pain Formula** (Whitehall)	**Tablets, buffered; oral:** 500 mg with magnesium hydroxide 100 mg and aluminum hydroxide 27 mg	Capsule shape. In 40s, 100s, and 175s.
otc	**Bayer Children's Aspirin** (Bayer)	**Tablets, chewable; oral:** 81 mg	Saccharin. (BAYER BAYER BAYER BAYER). Orange flavor. In 36s.
otc	**St. Joseph Adult Aspirin** (Schering-Plough)		Saccharin. (SJ). Orange flavor. In 36s.
otc	**Aspir Low** (Major)	**Tablets, enteric-coated; oral:** 81 mg	PEG, polydextrose. (L). Yellow, round. In 1,000s.
otc	**Ecotrin** (GlaxoSmithKline Consumer Healthcare)		EDTA, parabens. (ECOTRIN LOW). In 45s.
otc	**Halfprin 81** (Kramer)		In 90s.
otc	**Heartline** (BDI)		In 36s.
otc	**½ Halfprin** (Kramer)	**Tablets, enteric-coated; oral:** 162 mg	Red. In 60s and 200s.
otc	**Aspirin** (Various, eg, Geneva, Major, Moore, Parmed, URL)	**Tablets, enteric-coated; oral:** 325 mg	In 30s, 60s, 90s, 100s, 1,000s, and UD 100s.
otc	**Ecotrin Tablets and Caplets** (SmithKline Beecham)		**Tablets**: (Ecotrin Reg). In 100s, 250s, and 1,000s. **Caplets**: (Ecotrin Reg). In 100s.
otc	**Ecotrin Maximum Strength Caplets** (SmithKline Beecham)	**Tablets, enteric-coated; oral:** 500 mg	**Caplets**: (Ecotrin Max). In 60s.
otc	**Bayer Enteric 500 Aspirin Extra Strength** (Bayer)		(Bayer 500). In 60s.
otc	**Aspirin** (Various, eg, Moore)	**Tablets, enteric-coated; oral:** 650 mg	In 100s and 1,000s.
otc	**Bayer Extended Release 8-Hour** (Bayer)	**Tablets, extended-release; oral:** 650 mg	White, capsule shape, scored. In 50s.
Rx	**ZORprin** (PAR)	**Tablets, controlled-release; oral:** 800 mg	(57). White, elongated. In 100s.
otc	**Bayer Low Adult Strength** (Bayer)	**Tablets, delayed-release; oral:** 81 mg	Lactose. (81). In 120s.
otc	**Alka-Seltzer with Aspirin** (Bayer Consumer)	**Tablets, effervescent, buffered; oral:** 325 mg with sodium bicarbonate 1.9 g and citric acid 1 g	Sodium 567 mg/tablet. In 12s, 24s, 36s, 72s, 96s, and 100s.
otc	**Alka-Seltzer with Aspirin (Flavored)** (Bayer Consumer)	**Tablets, effervescent, buffered; oral:** 325 mg with sodium bicarbonate 1.7 g and citric acid 1.2 g	Sodium 506 mg/tablet, saccharin. In 12s, 24s, and 36s.
otc	**Alka-Seltzer Extra Strength with Aspirin** (Bayer Consumer)	**Tablet, effervescent, buffered; oral:** 500 mg with sodium bicarbonate 1.9 g and citric acid 1 g	In 12s and 24s.
otc	**Aspirin** (Various, eg, Goldline, Moore, URL)	**Suppositories**[a]**; rectal:** 120 mg	In 12s.
		200 mg	In 12s.
		300 mg	In 12s.
		600 mg	In 12s and 100s.

[a] Refrigerate.

ASPIRIN — ORAL

For complete and comparative prescribing information, refer to the Salicylates class monograph.

Indications

➤*Analgesic/Antipyretic:* For the temporary relief of headache, pain, and fever caused by colds, muscle aches and pains, menstrual pain, toothache pain, and minor aches and pains of arthritis.

➤*Revascularization procedures (coronary artery bypass graft, percutaneous transluminal coronary angioplasty, and carotid endarterectomy):* In patients who have undergone revascularization procedures (ie, coronary artery bypass graft, percutaneous transluminal coronary angioplasty, or carotid endarterectomy) when there is a preexisting condition for which aspirin is already indicated.

➤*Rheumatoid disease:* For the relief of the signs and symptoms of rheumatoid arthritis (RA), juvenile RA, osteoarthritis, spondyloarthropathies, and arthritis and pleurisy associated with systemic lupus erythematosus.

➤*Vascular indication (ischemic stroke, transient ischemic attack, acute myocardial infarction, prevention of recurrent myocardial infarction, unstable angina pectoris, and chronic stable angina pectoris):* To reduce the combined risk of death and nonfatal stroke in patients who have had ischemic stroke or transient ischemia of the brain due to fibrin platelet emboli; to reduce the risk of vascular mortality in patients with a suspected acute myocardial infarction (MI); to reduce the combined risk of death and nonfatal MI in patients with a previous MI or unstable angina pectoris; to reduce the combined risk of MI and sudden death in patients with chronic stable angina pectoris.

➤*Off-label uses:*

Kawasaki disease – [1] = Good documentation. Use of aspirin in the management of Kawasaki disease is recommended in the American Heart Association and American College of Chest Physicians guidelines. (See Administration and Dosage.)

Postherpetic neuralgia (topical) – [4] = Insufficient documentation. Topical aspirin has shown benefit in patients with postherpetic neuralgia. However, the American Academy of Neurology clinical practice guidelines consider the degree of pain relief from topical aspirin to be below the level considered clinically important for the treatment of chronic pain. (See Administration and Dosage.)

Other possible off-label uses – Prophylaxis against thromboembolic events in patients with atrial fibrillation, mitral valve prolapse, peripheral arterial disease, bioprosthetic or mechanical heart valves, and in pregnant patients with prosthetic heart valves; antithrombotic therapy in children with Blalock-Taussig shunt, ischemic stroke, Kawasaki disease, and in children after Fontan surgery.

Administration and Dosage

➤*General dosing considerations:* Do not use in children or teenagers with chickenpox or flu symptoms because of the possibility of Reye syndrome.

The addition of small amounts of antacids may decrease GI irritation and increase the dissolution and absorption rates of buffered products.

➤*Adults:*

Acute myocardial infarction –
Initial dosage: 160 to 325 mg as soon as a MI is suspected.
Maintenance dosage: See also Off-Label Dosing recommendations from the American College of Chest Physicians.
Continue the maintenance dosage of 160 to 325 mg/day for 30 days postinfarction. After 30 days, consider further therapy based on dosage and administration for prevention of recurrent MI.

Analgesic/Antipyretic –
Tablets:
- *Usual dosage* – 324 to 1,000 mg every 4 to 6 hours as needed.
- *Maximum dose* – 4,000 mg per 24 hours or as directed by a health care provider.

Tablets (controlled-, extended-, and delayed-release products):
- *Usual dosage* – 1,300 mg followed by 650 to 1,300 mg every 8 hours. For maximum nighttime and early-morning relief from stiffness upon arising, administer 1,300 mg at bedtime.
- *Maximum dose* – 3,900 mg per 24 hours or as directed by a health care provider.

Arthritis and pleurisy of systemic lupus erythematosus –
Initial dosage: 3 g/day in divided doses.
Dosage adjustment: Increase as needed for anti-inflammatory efficacy with target plasma salicylate levels of 150 to 300 mcg/mL. At high doses (ie, plasma levels of more than 200 mcg/mL), the incidence of toxicity increases.

Carotid endarterectomy –
Usual dosage: 80 mg once daily to 650 mg twice daily started presurgery.
Duration of therapy: Continue therapy indefinitely.

Chronic stable angina pectoris –
Usual dosage: 75 to 325 mg once daily.
Duration of therapy: Continue therapy indefinitely.

Coronary artery bypass graft – See also Off-Label Dosing recommendations from the American College of Chest Physicians.
Usual dosage: 325 mg daily starting 6 hours postprocedure.
Duration of therapy: Continue therapy for 1 year postprocedure.

Ischemic stroke and transient ischemic attack – See also Off-Label Dosing recommendations from the American College of Chest Physicians.
Usual dosage: 50 to 325 mg once daily.
Duration of therapy: Continue therapy indefinitely.

Myocardial infarction, prophylaxis – See Chronic Stable Angina Pectoris for dosing.

See also Off-Label Dosing recommendations from the American College of Chest Physicians.

Osteoarthritis – Up to 3 g/day in divided doses.

Percutaneous transluminal coronary angioplasty –
Initial dosage: 325 mg 2 hours presurgery.
Maintenance dosage: 160 to 325 mg daily.
Duration of therapy: Continue therapy indefinitely.

Rheumatoid arthritis –
Initial dosage: 3 g/day in divided doses.
Dosage adjustment: Increase as needed for anti-inflammatory efficacy with target plasma salicylate levels of 150 to 300 mcg/mL. At high doses (ie, plasma levels of more than 200 mcg/mL), the incidence of toxicity increases.

Spondyloarthropathies – Up to 4 g/day in divided doses.

Unstable angina pectoris – See Chronic Stable Angina Pectoris for dosing.

Off-label dosing –
Acute myocardial infarction:
- *Non–ST-segment elevation* –
  Initial dosage: 162 to 325 mg once daily.
  Maintenance dosage: 75 to 100 mg once daily.
- *ST-segment elevation* –
  Initial dosage: 160 to 325 once daily at initial elevation.
  Maintenance dosage: 75 to 162 mg once daily.
- *Primary prophylaxis* – 75 to 100 mg once daily.

Atrial fibrillation (including paroxysmal atrial fibrillation): 75 to 325 mg once daily.

Coronary artery bypass graft: 75 to 100 mg once daily, started 6 hours after surgery or as soon as possible if bleeding prevents administration at 6 hours postoperatively.

Infrainguinal arterial reconstruction or bypass: 75 to 100 mg once daily begun preoperatively.

Internal mammary artery bypass grafting:
- *Usual dose* – 75 to 162 mg once daily.
- *Duration of therapy* – Indefinitely.

Ischemic stroke and transient ischemic attack:
- *Cardioembolic stroke, anticoagulation contraindicated* – 75 to 325 mg once daily.
- *Noncardioembolic stroke or transient ischemic attack* – 50 to 100 mg once daily.

Mitral annular calcification with systemic embolism, stroke, or transient ischemic attack: 50 to 100 mg once daily.

Mitral valve prolapse with documented transient ischemic attack or stroke: 50 to 100 mg once daily.

Percutaneous coronary intervention:
- *Initial dosage* –
  Patients on daily aspirin therapy: 75 to 325 mg before percutaneous coronary intervention (PCI) is performed.
  Patients not on daily aspirin therapy: 300 to 325 mg at least 2 hours, and preferably 24 hours, before PCI is performed.
  Bare metal stent: 162 to 325 mg once daily for 1 month.
  Sirolimus-eluting stent: 162 to 325 mg once daily for 3 months.
  Tacrolimus-eluting stent: 162 to 325 mg once daily for 6 months.
- *Maintenance dosage* – 75 to 162 mg once daily indefinitely.
- *Duration of therapy* – Duration varies by stent type.

Peripheral arterial disease: 75 to 100 mg once daily.

Kawasaki disease: [1] = Good documentation. 80 to 100 mg/kg/day in 4 divided doses for up to 14 days within 10 days of symptom onset, followed by 1 to 5 mg/kg/day for a minimum of 6 to 8 weeks. Aspirin therapy may continue indefinitely in patients with significant cardiac sequelae from Kawasaki disease.

Postherpetic neuralgia (topical): [4] = Insufficient documentation. Aspirin (median dose, 1,000 mg) in diethyl ether applied as a single dose. Other trials used multiple doses of different topical applications (1,200 mg in 20 to 30 mL of chloroform; 750 mg in 100 g of washable ointment).

Prophylaxis of thromboembolism in pregnant women with prosthetic heart valves: 75 to 100 mg/day.

Prosthetic heart valves:
- *Bioprosthetic aortic valve* – 50 to 100 mg once daily.
- *Bioprosthetic mitral valve* – 50 to 100 mg once daily after 3 months of anticoagulation.
- *Mechanical heart valve* – 50 to 100 mg once daily in addition to anticoagulation.

➤*Children:*

Analgesic/Antipyretic –
12 years of age and older:
- *Tablets* –
  Usual dosage: 324 to 1,000 mg every 4 to 6 hours as needed.
  Maximum dose: 4,000 mg per 24 hours or as directed by a health care provider.
- *Tablets (controlled-, extended-, and delayed-release products)* –
  Usual dosage: 1,300 mg followed by 650 to 1,300 mg every 8 hours. For maximum nighttime and early-morning relief from stiffness upon arising, administer 1,300 mg at bedtime.
  Maximum dose: 3,900 mg per 24 hours or as directed by a health care provider.

ASPIRIN — ORAL

Younger than 12 years of age:

• *Tablets* – 10 to 15 mg/kg/dose every 4 hours, up to 60 to 80 mg/kg/day.

Aspirin Dosage in Children				
Age (years)	Weight (kg)	Dosage (every 4 hours)	Number of 81 mg tablets (every 4 hours)	Number of 325 mg tablets (every 4 hours)
2 to 3	10.6 to 15.9	162 mg	2	0.5
4 to 5	16 to 21.4	243 mg	3	
6 to 8	21.5 to 26.8	324 mg	4	1
9 to 10	26.9 to 32.3	405 mg	5	
11	32.4 to 43.2	486 mg	6	1.5
12 to 14	≥ 43.3	648 mg	8	2

Juvenile rheumatoid arthritis –

Tablets:

• *Initial dosage* – 90 to 130 mg/kg/day in divided doses.

• *Dosage adjustment* – Increase as needed for anti-inflammatory efficacy with target plasma salicylate levels of 150 to 300 mcg/mL. At high doses (ie, plasma levels more than 200 mcg/mL), the incidence of toxicity increases.

Off-label dosing –

Blalock-Taussig shunt: 1 to 5 mg/kg/day.

Fontan surgery: 1 to 5 mg/kg/day.

Ischemic stroke:

• *Usual dose* – 1 to 5 mg/kg/day

• *Duration of therapy* – 2 years minimum.

Kawasaki disease:

• *Initial dosage* – 80 to 100 mg/kg/day in 4 divided doses until 48 to 72 hours after fever defervescence.

• *Maintenance dosage* – 3 to 5 mg/kg/day for 6 to 8 weeks or until erythrocyte sedimentation rate and platelet count are normal and if no coronary artery abnormalities present, or indefinitely if coronary artery abnormalities persist.

➤*Renal function impairment:* Avoid aspirin in patients with severe renal failure (glomerular filtration rate less than 10 mL/min).

➤*Hepatic function impairment:* Avoid aspirin in patients with severe hepatic insufficiency.

➤*Administration:* Administer each dose of aspirin with a full glass of water, unless the patient is fluid restricted.

For acute MI, have patient chew tablet.

➤*Storage/Stability:* Store in a cool, dry place at 15° to 30°C (59° to 86°F).

ASPIRIN — RECTAL

For complete and comparative prescribing information, refer to the Salicylates group monograph.

Indications

➤*Analgesic/Antipyretic:* For the relief of minor aches, pains, and headache and for reduction of fever.

Administration and Dosage

➤*Adults:*

Fever reduction, relief of minor aches, pains, and headache – Insert 1 suppository rectally every 4 hours for no more than 10 days or as directed by a health care provider.

➤*Children:* See Adults for dosing in children 12 years of age and older.

➤*Renal function impairment:* Avoid aspirin in patients with severe renal failure (ie, glomerular filtration rate less than 10 mL/min).

➤*Hepatic function impairment:* Avoid aspirin in patients with severe hepatic impairment.

➤*Administration:* Remove suppository from plastic packet and insert into the rectum as far as possible.

➤*Storage/Stability:* Store in a cool place 8° to 15°C (46° to 59°F) or refrigerate.

DIFLUNISAL

Rx	**Diflunisal** (Teva)	**Tablets; oral:** 500 mg	In 100s, 500s, and unit-of-use 60s.

DIFLUNISAL — ORAL

WARNING

Cardiovascular (CV) risk – Nonsteroidal anti-inflammatory drugs (NSAIDs) may cause an increased risk of serious CV thrombotic reactions, myocardial infarction (MI), and stroke, which can be fatal. This risk may increase with duration of use. Patients with CV disease or risk factors for CV disease may be at greater risk.

Diflunisal is contraindicated for the treatment of perioperative pain in the setting of coronary artery bypass graft (CABG) surgery.

GI risk – NSAIDs cause an increased risk of serious GI adverse reactions, including bleeding, ulceration, and perforation of the stomach or intestines, which can be fatal. These reactions can occur at any time during use and without warning symptoms. Elderly patients are at greater risk for serious GI reactions.

Indications

➤*Mild to moderate pain:* For acute or long-term use for symptomatic treatment of mild to moderate pain.

➤*Osteoarthritis/Rheumatoid arthritis (RA):* For acute or long-term use for symptomatic treatment of osteoarthritis and rheumatoid arthritis (RA).

Administration and Dosage

➤*General dosing considerations:* Carefully consider the potential benefits and risks of diflunisal and other treatment options before deciding to use diflunisal. Use the lowest effective dose for the shortest duration consistent with individual patient treatment goals.

Concentration-dependent pharmacokinetics prevail when diflunisal is administered; a doubling of dosage produces a greater than doubling of drug accumulation. The effect becomes more apparent with repetitive doses.

➤*Adults:*

Mild to moderate pain –

Initial dosage: 1,000 mg followed by 500 mg every 12 hours is recommended for most patients. Following the initial dose, some patients may require 500 mg every 8 hours.

Dosage adjustment: A lower dosage may be appropriate depending on such factors as pain severity, patient response, weight, or advanced age; for example, 500 mg initially, followed by 250 mg every 8 to 12 hours.

Osteoarthritis –

Usual dosage: 250 to 1,000 mg daily in 2 divided doses is the suggested dosage range.

Maintenance dosage: Doses more than 1,500 mg/day are not recommended.

Dosage adjustment: The dosage of diflunisal may be increased or decreased according to patient response.

Rheumatoid arthritis – See osteoarthritis for dosing.

➤*Children:*

12 years of age and older – See Adults for dosing.

➤*Renal function impairment:* Treatment in patients with advanced renal disease with diflunisal is not recommended. If diflunisal therapy must be initiated, close monitoring of the patient's renal function is advisable.

➤*Administration:* Tablets should be swallowed whole, not crushed or chewed.

➤*Storage/Stability:* Store at 20° to 25°C (68° to 77°F). Dispense is a well-closed container with a child-resistant closure.

Actions

➤*Pharmacology:* Diflunisal is a nonsteroidal drug with analgesic, anti-inflammatory, and antipyretic properties. It is a peripherally acting nonnarcotic analgesic drug. Habituation, tolerance, and addiction have not been reported.

Diflunisal is a difluorophenyl derivative of salicylic acid. Chemically, diflunisal differs from aspirin (acetylsalicylic acid) in two respects. The first of these two is the presence of a difluorophenyl substituent at carbon 1. The second difference is the removal of the 0-acetyl group from the carbon 4 position. Diflunisal is not metabolized to salicylic acid, and the fluorine atoms are not displaced from the difluorophenyl ring structure.

The precise mechanism of the analgesic and anti-inflammatory actions of diflunisal is not known. Diflunisal is a prostaglandin synthetase inhibitor. In animals, prostaglandins sensitize afferent nerves and potentiate the action of bradykinin in inducing pain. Since prostaglandins are known to be among the mediators of pain and inflammation, the mode of action of diflunisal may be caused by a decrease of prostaglandins in peripheral tissues.

➤*Pharmacokinetics:*

Absorption/Distribution – Diflunisal is rapidly and completely absorbed following oral administration, with peak plasma concentrations occurring between 2 and 3 hours.

As is the case with salicylic acid, concentration-dependent pharmacokinetics prevail when diflunisal is administered; a doubling of dosage produces a greater than doubling of drug accumulation. The effect becomes more apparent with repetitive doses.

Following single doses, peak plasma concentrations of 41 ± 11 mcg/mL (mean ± standard deviation) were observed following 250 mg doses, 87 ± 17 mcg/mL were observed following 500 mg, and 124 ± 11 mcg/mL following single 1,000 mg doses. However, following administration of 250 mg twice daily, a mean peak level of 56 ± 14 mcg/mL was observed on day 8, while the mean peak level after 500 mg twice a day for 11 days was 190 ± 33 mcg/mL.

DIFLUNISAL — ORAL

Several days are required for diflunisal plasma levels to reach steady state following multiple doses because of its long half-life and nonlinear pharmacokinetics. For this reason, an initial loading dose is necessary to shorten the time to reach steady-state levels, and 2 to 3 days of observation are necessary for evaluating changes in treatment regimens if a loading dose is not used.

Studies in baboons to determine passage across the blood-brain barrier have shown that only small quantities of diflunisal, under normal or acidotic conditions, are transported into the cerebrospinal fluid (CSF). The ratio of blood per CSF concentrations after intravenous doses of 50 mg/kg or oral doses of 100 mg/kg of diflunisal was 100:1. In contrast, oral doses of 500 mg/kg of aspirin resulted in a blood per CSF ratio of 5:1.

Diflunisal appears in human milk in concentrations of 2% to 7% of those in plasma. More than 99% of diflunisal in plasma is bound to proteins.

Metabolism/Excretion – In contrast with salicylic acid, which has a plasma half-life of 2.5 hours, the plasma half-life of diflunisal is 3 to 4 times longer (8 to 12 hours) because of a difluorophenyl substituent at carbon 1.

The drug is excreted in the urine as 2 soluble glucuronide conjugates accounting for about 90% of the administered dose. Little or no diflunisal is excreted in the feces.

Contraindications

Known hypersensitivity to diflunisal or the excipients; the treatment of perioperative pain in the setting of coronary artery bypass graft (CABG) surgery; patients who have experienced asthma, urticaria, or allergic-type reactions after taking aspirin or other NSAIDs.

Warnings/Precautions

➤*CV effects:*

CV thrombotic events – Clinical trials of several cyclooxygenase-2 (COX-2) selective and nonselective NSAIDs of up to 3 years' duration have shown an increased risk of serious CV thrombotic events, MI, and stroke, which can be fatal. All NSAIDs, both COX-2 selective and nonselective, may have a similar risk. Patients with known CV disease or risk factors for CV disease may be at greater risk. To minimize the potential risk for an adverse CV reaction in patients treated with an NSAID, use the lowest effective for the shortest duration possible. Health care providers and patients should remain alert for the development of such reactions, even in the absence of previous CV symptoms. Inform patients about the signs and/or symptoms of serious CV reactions and the steps to take if they occur.

There is no consistent evidence that concurrent use of aspirin mitigates the increased risk of serious CV thrombotic reactions associated with NSAID use. The concurrent use of aspirin and an NSAID does increase the risk of serious GI reactions.

Two large, controlled clinical trials of a COX-2 selective NSAID for the treatment of pain in the first 10 to 14 days following CABG surgery found an increased incidence of MI and stroke.

Hypertension – NSAIDs, including diflunisal, can lead to onset of new hypertension or worsening of preexisting hypertension, either of which may contribute to the increased incidence of CV events. Patients taking thiazides or loop diuretics may have impaired response to these therapies when taking NSAIDs. Use NSAIDs, including diflunisal, with caution in patients with hypertension. Closely monitor blood pressure during the initiation of NSAID treatment and throughout the course of therapy.

Fluid retention/edema – Fluid retention and edema have been observed in some patients taking NSAIDs. Use diflunisal with caution in patients with fluid retention or heart failure.

➤*GI effects:* NSAIDs, including diflunisal, can cause serious GI adverse reactions, including inflammation, bleeding, ulceration, and perforation of the stomach, small intestine, or large intestine, which can be fatal. These serious adverse reactions can occur at any time, with or without warning symptoms, in patients treated with NSAIDS. Only 1 in 5 patients who develop a serious upper GI adverse reaction on NSAID therapy is symptomatic. Upper GI ulcers, gross bleeding, or perforation caused by NSAIDs occur in approximately 1% of patients treated for 3 to 6 months, and in about 2% to 4% of patients treated for 1 year. These trends continue with longer duration of use, increasing the likelihood of developing a serious GI reaction at some time during the course of therapy. However, even short-term therapy is not without risk.

Prescribe NSAIDs with extreme caution in those with a history of ulcer disease or GI bleeding. Patients with a history of peptic ulcer disease and/or GI bleeding who use NSAIDs have a more than 10-fold increased risk for developing a GI bleed compared with patients with neither of these risk factors. Other factors that increase the risk for GI bleeding in patients treated with NSAIDs include concomitant use of oral corticosteroids or anticoagulants, longer duration of NSAID therapy, smoking, use of alcohol, older age, and poor general health status. Most spontaneous reports of fatal GI reactions are in elderly or debilitated patients; therefore, take special care in treating this population.

To minimize the potential risk for an adverse GI reaction in patients treated with an NSAID, use the lowest effective dose for the shortest possible duration. Patients and health care providers should remain alert for signs and symptoms of GI ulceration and bleeding during NSAID therapy. Promptly initiate additional evaluation and treatment if a serious GI adverse reaction is suspected. This should include discontinuation of the NSAID until a serious GI adverse reaction is ruled out. For high risk patients, consider alternate therapies that do not involve NSAIDs.

➤*Renal effects:* Long-term administration of NSAIDs has resulted in renal papillary necrosis and other renal injury. Renal toxicity has also been seen in patients in whom renal prostaglandins have a compensatory role in the maintenance of renal perfusion. In these patients, administration of a NSAID may cause a dose-dependent reduction in prostaglandin formation and, secondarily, in renal blood flow, which may precipitate overt renal decompensation. Patients at greatest risk of this reaction are those with renal function impairment, heart failure, liver dysfunction, those taking diuretics and angiotensin-converting enzyme (ACE) inhibitors, patients who are volume depleted, and elderly patients. Discontinuation of NSAID therapy is usually followed by recovery to the pretreatment site.

No information is available from controlled clinical studies regarding the use of diflunisal in patients with advanced renal disease; therefore, treatment with diflunisal is not recommended in these patients. If diflunisal therapy must be initiated, close monitoring of the patient's renal function is advisable.

➤*Skin reactions:* NSAIDs, including diflunisal, can cause serious skin adverse reactions such as exfoliative dermatitis, Stevens-Johnson syndrome, and toxic epidermal necrolysis, which can be fatal. These serious reactions may occur without warning. Inform patients about the signs and symptoms of serious skin manifestations and discontinue use of the drug at the first appearance of skin rash or any other sign of hypersensitivity.

➤*Corticosteroid use:* Diflunisal cannot be expected to substitute for corticosteroids or to treat corticosteroid insufficiency. Abrupt discontinuation of corticosteroids may lead to disease exacerbation. If a decision is made to discontinue corticosteroids, slowly taper therapy for patients on prolonged corticosteroid therapy.

➤*Fever/Inflammation:* The pharmacological activity of diflunisal in reducing fever and inflammation may diminish the utility of these diagnostic signs in detecting complications of presumed noninfectious, painful conditions.

➤*Hepatic effects:* Borderline elevations of one or more liver tests may occur in up to 15% of patients taking NSAIDs, including diflunisal. These abnormalities may progress, may remain unchanged, or may be transient with continued therapy. Notable (approximately 3 or more times the upper limit of normal) elevations of ALT or AST have been reported in clinical trials with NSAIDs in approximately 1% of patients. In addition, rare cases of severe hepatic reactions, including jaundice and fatal fulminant hepatitis, liver necrosis, and hepatic failure, some of them with fatal outcomes, have been reported.

Evaluate a patient with symptoms and/or signs suggesting liver dysfunction, or in whom an abnormal liver test has occurred, for evidence of the development of more severe hepatic reactions while on therapy with diflunisal. If clinical signs and symptoms consistent with liver disease develop, or if systemic manifestations occur (eg, eosinophilia, rash), discontinue diflunisal.

➤*Hematologic effects:*

Anemia – Anemia is sometimes seen in patients receiving NSAIDs, including diflunisal. This may be caused by fluid retention, occult or gross GI blood loss, or an incompletely described effect upon erythropoiesis. Check the hemoglobin or hematocrit of patients on long-term treatment with NSAIDs, including diflunisal, if they exhibit any signs or symptoms of anemia.

Platelet aggregation – NSAIDs inhibit platelet aggregation and have been shown to prolong bleeding time in some patients. Unlike aspirin, their effect on platelet function is quantitatively less, of shorter duration, and reversible. Carefully monitor patients receiving diflunisal who may be adversely affected by alterations in platelet function, such as those with coagulation disorders or patients receiving anticoagulants.

➤*Ophthalmic effects:* It is recommended that patients who develop eye complaints during treatment with diflunisal have ophthalmologic studies because of reports of adverse eye findings with agents of this class.

➤*Preexisting asthma:* Patients with asthma may have aspirin-sensitive asthma. The use of aspirin in patients with aspirin-sensitive asthma has been associated with severe bronchospasm, which can be fatal. Because cross-reactivity, including bronchospasm, between aspirin and other NSAIDs has been reported in such aspirin-sensitive patients, do not administer diflunisal to patients with this form of aspirin sensitivity and use caution in patients with preexisting asthma.

➤*Reye syndrome:* Acetylsalicylic acid has been associated with Reye syndrome. Because diflunisal is a derivative of salicylic acid, the possibility of its association with Reye syndrome cannot be excluded.

➤*Hypersensitivity reactions:* As with other NSAIDs, anaphylactic/anaphylactoid reactions may occur in patients without known prior exposure to diflunisal. Do not give diflunisal to patients with the aspirin triad. This symptom complex typically occurs in asthmatic patients who experience rhinitis with or without nasal polyps, or who exhibit severe, potentially fatal bronchospasm after taking aspirin or other NSAIDs. Seek emergency help in cases where an anaphylactic/anaphylactoid reaction occurs.

A potentially life-threatening, apparent hypersensitivity syndrome has been reported. This multisystem syndrome includes constitutional symptoms (fever, chills) and cutaneous findings. It may also include involvement of major organs (changes in liver function, jaundice, leukopenia, thrombocytopenia, eosinophilia, disseminated intravascular coagulation, renal function impairment, including renal failure), and less specific findings (eg, adenitis, anorexia, arthralgia, arthritis, disorientation, malaise, myalgia). If evidence of hypersensitivity occurs, discontinue therapy with diflunisal.

➤*Pregnancy: Category C.*

Teratogenic – A dose of 60 mg/kg/day of diflunisal (equivalent to 2 times the maximum human dose) was maternotoxic, embryotoxic, and teratogenic in rabbits. In 3 of 6 studies in rabbits, evidence of teratogenicity was observed at doses ranging from 40 to 50 mg/kg/day. Aspirin and other salicylates have been shown to be teratogenic in a wide variety of species, including the rat and rabbit, at doses ranging from 50 to 400 mg/kg/day (approximately 1 to 8 times the human dose). Animal reproduction studies

DIFLUNISAL — ORAL

are not always predictive of human response. There are no adequate and well-controlled studies with diflunisal in pregnant women. Only use diflunisal in pregnancy if the potential benefit justifies the potential risk to the fetus.

Nonteratogenic – Avoid use during pregnancy (particularly late pregnancy) because of the known effects of NSAIDs on the fetal CV system (closure of ductus arteriosus).

The known effects of drugs of this class on the human fetus during the third trimester of pregnancy include the following: constriction of the ductus arteriosus prenatally, tricuspid incompetence, and pulmonary hypertension; nonclosure of the ductus arteriosus postnatally, which may be resistant to medical management; myocardial degenerative changes, platelet dysfunction with resultant bleeding, intracranial bleeding, renal dysfunction or failure, renal injury/dysgenesis, which may result in prolonged or permanent renal failure, oligohydramnios, GI bleeding or perforation, and increased risk of necrotizing enterocolitis.

In rats at a dose of 1.5 times the maximum human dose, there was an increase in the average length of gestation. Similar increases in the length of gestation have been observed with aspirin, indomethacin, and phenylbutazone, and may be related to inhibition of prostaglandin synthetase.

Labor and delivery – In rat studies with NSAIDs, as with other drugs known to inhibit prostaglandin synthesis, an increased incidence of dystocia, delayed parturition, and decreased pup survival occurred. The effects of diflunisal on labor and delivery in pregnant women are unknown.

➤*Lactation:* Diflunisal is excreted in human milk in concentrations of 2% to 7% of those in plasma. Because of the potential for serious adverse reactions in breast-feeding infants from diflunisal, make a decision whether to discontinue breast-feeding or the drug, taking into account the importance of the drug to the mother.

➤*Children:* Safety and efficacy of diflunisal in children younger than 12 years of age have not been established. Use of diflunisal in children younger than 12 years of age is not recommended.

➤*Elderly:* As with any NSAID, exercise caution in treating elderly patients (65 years of age and older) because advancing age appears to increase the possibility of adverse reactions. Elderly patients seem to tolerate ulceration or bleeding less well than other individuals, and many spontaneous reports of fatal GI reactions are in this population.

This drug is known to be substantially excreted by the kidney, and the risk of toxic reactions to this drug may be greater in patients with renal function impairment. Because elderly patients are more likely to have decreased renal function, take care in dose selection. It may be useful to monitor renal function.

➤*Monitoring:* Because serious GI tract ulceration and bleeding can occur without warning symptoms, monitor for the signs and symptoms of GI bleeding. Periodically perform a complete blood cell count and check the chemistry profile of patients on long-term treatment with NSAIDs. Carefully monitor patients receiving diflunisal who may be adversely affected by alterations in platelet function, such as those with coagulation disorders or patients receiving anticoagulants. If clinical signs and symptoms consistent with liver or renal disease develop, systemic manifestations occur (eg, eosinophilia, rash), or if abnormal liver tests persist or worsen, discontinue diflunisal. Closely monitor blood pressure during the initiation of NSAID treatment and throughout the course of therapy.

Drug Interactions

Diflunisal Drug Interactions

Precipitant drug	Object drug[a]		Description
Antacids	Diflunisal	↓	Concomitant therapy may reduce plasma levels of diflunisal, which may be clinically significant when antacids are used regularly.
Aspirin	Diflunisal	↑↓	Coadministration may reduce diflunisal protein binding; the clinical significance is unknown. Coadministration is not recommended because of the potential of increased adverse reactions. A small decrease in diflunisal levels was observed when multiple doses of diflunisal and aspirin were coadministered.
Probenecid	Diflunisal	↑	The pharmacologic and toxic effects of diflunisal may be increased. Observe patients for diflunisal toxicity.
Diflunisal	Acetaminophen	↑	Administration of diflunisal resulted in ≈ 50% increased acetaminophen plasma levels. Acetaminophen had no effect on diflunisal plasma levels. Use with caution and monitor patients carefully.
Diflunisal	ACE inhibitors; Angiotensin II antagonists	↓	Coadministration may diminish the antihypertensive effect. In patients with renal function impairment, coadministration may result in further deterioration of renal function. Monitor patients carefully.
Diflunisal	Anticoagulants, oral	↑	Coadministration of diflunisal may increase hypoprothrombinemic effects of anticoagulants. Diflunisal competitively displaces coumarins from protein-binding sites. Monitor prothrombin time during and for several days after coadministration. Adjust dosage of oral anticoagulants as required.
Diflunisal	Cyclosporine	↑	Coadministration may be associated with an increase in cyclosporine-induced toxicity, possibly caused by decreased synthesis of renal prostacyclin. Use with caution and monitor renal function.
Diflunisal	Diuretics (eg, furosemide, hydrochlorothiazide)	↔	Diflunisal may reduce the natriuretic effect of furosemide and thiazides in some patients. Coadministration of diflunisal resulted in significantly increased plasma levels of hydrochlorothiazide. Diflunisal decreased the hyperuricemic effects of hydrochlorothiazide.
Diflunisal	Indomethacin	↑	Administration of diflunisal decreased renal clearance and significantly increased plasma levels of indomethacin. The combined use has been associated with fatal GI hemorrhage. Avoid coadministration.
Diflunisal	Lithium	↑	NSAIDs have produced an elevation of plasma lithium levels and a reduction in renal lithium clearance. Monitor patient for lithium toxicity with coadministration of lithium and diflunisal.
Diflunisal	Methotrexate	↑	Coadministration may enhance the toxicity of methotrexate. Use with caution.
Diflunisal	Naproxen	↔	Diflunisal significantly decreased the urinary excretion of naproxen and its glucuronide metabolite, but had no effect on the plasma levels of naproxen.
Diflunisal	NSAIDs	↑	Coadministration of diflunisal and other NSAIDs is not recommended because of the increased possibility of GI toxicity, with little or no increase in efficacy.
Diflunisal	Sulindac	↓	Administration of diflunisal resulted in lowering of the plasma levels of the active sulindac sulfide metabolite by ≈ one-third.

[a] ↑ = object drug increased; ↓ = object drug decreased; ↔ = undetermined clinical effect; ↑↓ = object drug is both increased and decreased.

➤*Drug/Lab test interactions:* Use caution when interpreting the results of serum salicylate assays when diflunisal is present. Salicylate levels have been found to be falsely elevated with some assay methods.

Adverse Reactions

The following adverse reactions were reported in the 1,314 of these patients who received treatment in studies of 2 weeks or longer. Five hundred thirteen patients were treated for at least 24 weeks, 255 patients were treated for at least 48 weeks, and 46 patients were treated for 96 weeks. In general, the following adverse reactions were 2 to 14 times less frequent in the 1,113 patients who received short-term treatment for mild to moderate pain.

➤*Cardiovascular:* Palpitation, syncope (rare).

➤*CNS:* Headache (3% to 9%); dizziness, fatigue/tiredness, insomnia, somnolence (1% to 3%); asthenia, confusion, depression, disorientation, hallucinations, light-headedness, nervousness, paresthesias, vertigo (less than 1%).

DIFLUNISAL — ORAL

➤*Dermatologic:* Rash (3% to 9%); dry mucous membranes, erythema multiforme, exfoliative dermatitis, photosensitivity, pruritus, Stevens-Johnson syndrome, stomatitis, sweating, toxic epidermal necrolysis, urticaria (less than 1%).

➤*GI:* Diarrhea, dyspepsia, GI pain, nausea (3% to 9%); constipation, flatulence, vomiting (1% to 3%); anorexia, eructation, gastritis, GI bleeding, GI perforation, peptic ulcer (less than 1%).

➤*GU:* Dysuria, hematuria, interstitial nephritis, proteinuria, renal function impairment, including renal failure (less than 1%); nephrotic syndrome (rare).

➤*Hematologic:* Agranulocytosis, hemolytic anemia, thrombocytopenia (less than 1%).

➤*Hepatic:* Cholestasis, hepatitis, jaundice (sometimes with fever), liver function abnormalities (less than 1%).

➤*Hypersensitivity:* Acute anaphylactic reaction with bronchospasm, angioedema, flushing, hypersensitivity syndrome, hypersensitivity vasculitis (less than 1%).

➤*Special senses:* Tinnitus (1% to 3%); transient visual disturbances, including blurred vision (less than 1%); hearing loss (rare).

➤*Miscellaneous:* Edema (less than 1%); chest pain, dyspnea, muscle cramps (rare).

A rare occurrence of fulminant necrotizing fasciitis, particularly in association with group A β-hemolytic streptococcus, has been described in persons treated with NSAIDs, including diflunisal, sometimes with fatal outcome.

➤*Other NSAID adverse reactions:* In addition, a variety of adverse reactions not observed with diflunisal in clinical trials or in marketing experience, but reported with other nonsteroidal analgesic/anti-inflammatory agents, should be considered potential adverse reactions of diflunisal.

Overdosage

➤*Symptoms:* Cases of overdosage have occurred and deaths have been reported. Most patients recovered without evidence of permanent sequelae. The most common signs and symptoms observed with overdosage were drowsiness, vomiting, nausea, diarrhea, hyperventilation, tachycardia, sweating, tinnitus, disorientation, stupor, and coma. Diminished urine output and cardiorespiratory arrest have also been reported. The lowest dosage of diflunisal at which a death has been reported was 15 grams without the presence of other drugs. In a mixed drug overdose, ingestion of diflunisal 7.5 g resulted in death.

➤*Treatment:* In the event of overdosage, empty the stomach by gastric lavage, and carefully observe the patient and give symptomatic and supportive treatment. Because of the high degree of protein binding, hemodialysis may not be effective.

Patient Information

Diflunisal, like other NSAIDs, can cause GI discomfort and, rarely, serious GI side effects, such as ulcers and bleeding, which may result in hospitalization and even death. Although serious GI tract ulcerations and bleeding can occur without warning symptoms, alert patients to the signs and symptoms of ulcerations and bleeding, and inform patients to ask for medical advice when observing any indicative signs or symptoms, including epigastric pain, dyspepsia, melena, and hematemesis. Apprise patients of the importance of this follow-up.

Diflunisal, like other NSAIDs, can cause serious skin side effects, such as exfoliative dermatitis, Stevens Johnson syndrome, and toxic epidermal necrosis, which may result in hospitalizations and even death. Although serious skin reactions may occur without warning, alert patients to the signs and symptoms of skin rash and blisters, fever, or other signs of hypersensitivity, such as itching, and inform patients to ask for medical advice when observing any indicative signs or symptoms. Advise patients to stop the drug immediately if they develop any type of rash and to contact their health care provider as soon as possible.

Inform patients to promptly report signs or symptoms of unexplained weight gain or edema to their physicians.

Inform patients of the warning signs and symptoms of hepatotoxicity (eg, nausea, fatigue, lethargy, pruritus, jaundice, right upper quadrant tenderness, "flu-like" symptoms). If these occur, instruct patients to stop therapy and seek immediate medical therapy.

Inform patients of the signs of an anaphylactic/anaphylactoid reaction (eg, difficulty breathing, swelling of the face or throat). If these occur, instruct patients to seek immediate emergency help.

In late pregnancy, as with other NSAIDs, avoid diflunisal because it may cause premature closure of the ductus arteriosus.

MAGNESIUM SALICYLATE

otc	**Doan's** (Novartis Consumer Health)	**Tablets**: 377 mg (as tetrahydrate, equivalent to 303.7 mg magnesium salicylate anhydrous)	In 24s.
otc	**DeWitt's Pain Reliever** (Monticello)	**Tablets**: 406 mg (equivalent to 325 mg magnesium salicylate anhydrous)	In 12s and 24s.
otc	**Doan's Extra Strength** (Novartis Consumer Health)	**Tablets**: 580 mg (as tetrahydrate, equivalent to 467 mg magnesium salicylate anhydrous)	(DOAN'S). In 24s and 48s.
otc	**Momentum Backache Relief** (Medtech)	**Tablets**: 580 mg (as tetrahydrate, equivalent to 467 mg magnesium salicylate anhydrous)	(MSM). In 48s.
Rx	**MST 600** (Cypress)	**Tablets**: 600 mg (as tetrahydrate)	(CYP 106). Yellow, scored. In 100s.

MAGNESIUM SALICYLATE TETRAHYDRATE — ORAL

Complete prescribing information for these products begins in the Salicylates monograph.

Indications

➤*Pain and inflammation:*

Rx – For the relief of pain and inflammation and the daily management of rheumatoid arthritis, osteoarthritis, and related diseases.

OTC – For temporary relief of minor aches and pains associated with backache and muscular aches; back pain caused by muscle strain or spasm; muscle stiffness.

Administration and Dosage

➤*Adults:*

OTC –

Minor aches and pains associated with backache and muscular aches:

• *Usual dosage* – 2 tablets with a full glass of water every 4 to 6 hours while symptoms persist, or as directed by a health care provider. See labeling information for specific dosing information.

• *Maximum dose* – Patients should not take more than 8 to 12 tablets in any 24-hour period.

Rx –

Osteoarthritis and related diseases: 600 mg 3 or 4 times per day.

Rheumatoid arthritis and related diseases: 600 mg 3 or 4 times per day.

➤*Children:* See Adults for dosing of OTC magnesium salicylate in children 12 years of age and older.

➤*Elderly:* A reduced dosage, lower than the recommended schedules, should always be considered for patients 65 years of age and older. See Adults for dosing.

➤*Renal function impairment:* Magnesium salicylate is contraindicated in patients with advanced chronic renal insufficiency. Take appropriate precautions in administering magnesium salicylate to patients with any impairment of renal function, including discontinuing other drugs containing magnesium and monitoring serum magnesium levels if dosage levels of magnesium salicylate tetrahydrate are high.

➤*Storage/Stability:* Store at 15° to 30°C (59° to 86°F).

SALICYLATE COMBINATIONS

Rx	**Choline Magnesium Trisalicylate** (Various, eg, Sidmak, Zenith Goldline)	**Tablets**: 500 mg salicylate (as 293 mg choline salicylate, 362 mg Mg salicylate)	(SL 528). Yellow, scored. Film coated, capsule shape. In 100s and 500s.
		750 mg salicylate (as 440 mg choline salicylate, 544 mg Mg salicylate)	(SL 529). Blue, scored. Film coated, capsule shape. In 100s and 500s.
		1000 mg salicylate (as 587 mg choline salicylate, 725 mg Mg salicylate)	(SL 530). Pink, scored. Capsule shape, film coated. In 100s and 500s.
Rx	**Choline Magnesium Trisalicylate** (Various, eg, Cypress)	**Liquid**: 500 mg salicylate (as 293 mg choline salicylate, 362 mg Mg salicylate)/5 ml	In 237 ml.

Complete prescribing information for these products begins in the Salicylates monograph.

SALSALATE (Salicylsalicylic Acid)

Rx	**Salsalate** (Various, eg, Geneva, Goldline, Major, Moore, URL, Vitarine)	**Tablets**: 500 mg	In 100s, 500s and UD 100s.
Rx	**Amigesic** (Amide)		(A 019). Yellow or blue. Film coated. In 100s and 500s.
Rx	**Argesic-SA** (Econo Med)		In 100s.
Rx	**Salflex** (Carnrick)		Dye free. (C 8671). White. Film coated. In 100s.
Rx	**Salsitab** (Upsher-Smith)		(500). Blue. Film coated. In 100s, 500s and UD 100s.
Rx	**Salsalate** (Various, eg, Copley, Geneva, Goldline, Major, Moore, URL, Vitarine)	**Tablets**: 750 mg	In 100s, 500s and UD 100s.
Rx	**Amigesic Caplets** (Amide)		(A0 10). Yellow or blue, scored. Film coated, Capsule shaped. In 100s and 500s.
Rx	**Artha-G** (T.E. Williams)		(Artha-G). Lavender, scored. In 120s.
Rx	**Marthritic** (Marnel)		In 100s.
Rx	**Salsitab** (Upsher-Smith)		(750). Blue, scored. Film coated. In 100s, 500s and UD 100s.
Rx	**Salflex** (Carnrick)		Dye free. (C 8672). White, scored. Film coated. In 100s and 500s.

SALSALATE — ORAL

Complete prescribing information for these products begins in the Salicylates monograph.

Administration and Dosage

➤*General dosing considerations:* Alleviation of symptoms is gradual, and full benefit may not be evident for 3 to 4 days when plasma salicylate levels have achieved steady state. There is no evidence for development of tissue tolerance (tachyphylaxis), but salicylate therapy may induce increased activity of metabolizing liver enzymes, causing a greater rate of salicyluric acid production and excretion, with a resultant increase in dosage requirement for maintenance of therapeutic serum salicylate levels.

➤*Adults:*

Osteoarthritis –

Usual dosage: 3,000 mg daily, given in divided doses, such as 2 tablets twice daily or 1 tablet 4-times daily.

Dosage adjustment: Dosage should be adjusted according to the severity of the disease and the response of the patient.

Rheumatoid arthritis – See Osteoarthritis for dosing.

Rheumatic disorders – See Osteoarthritis for dosing.

➤*Elderly:* Elderly patients may require a lower dosage to achieve therapeutic blood concentrations and to avoid the more common side effects such as auditory disturbances.

➤*Renal function impairment:* This drug is known to be substantially excreted by the kidney and the risk of toxic reactions to this drug may be greater in patients with impaired renal function.

➤*Therapeutic drug monitoring:* To avoid potentially toxic concentrations, plasma salicylic acid levels should be monitored periodically during long-term treatment to maintain therapeutically effective levels of 10 to 30 mg/100 mL. Toxic manifestations are not usually seen until plasma concentrations exceed 30 mg/100 mL. Urinary pH should also be periodically monitored. Sudden acidification, as from pH 6.5 to 5.5, can double the plasma level, resulting in toxicity, while an increase in urinary pH will increase renal clearance and urinary excretion of salicylic acid, thus lowering plasma levels.

➤*Storage/Stability:* Store at controlled room temperature 15° to 30°C (59° to 86°F).

NONNARCOTIC ANALGESIC COMBINATIONS

Content given per capsule, tablet, or packet.

	Product and Distributor	Acetaminophen	Aspirin	Other Analgesics	Caffeine	Other Content	How Supplied
otc	**Painaid BRF Back Relief Formula Tablets** (Zee Medical)			250 mg magnesium salicylate tetrahydrate			In 24s.
otc	**Pamprin Maximum Pain Relief Caplets** (Chattem)			250 mg magnesium salicylate		25 mg pamabrom	In 16s and 32s.
c-iv	**Equagesic Tablets** (Leitner)		325 mg			200 mg meprobamate	(WFHC 91). Pink/Yellow, layered, scored. In 100s.
otc	**Painaid ESF Extra-Strength Formula Tablets** (Zee Medical)		250 mg		65 mg		In 24s.
otc	**Summit Extra Strength Caplets** (Pfeiffer)						In 50s.
otc	**Anacin Regular Strength Tablets** (Insight Pharmaceuticals)		400 mg		32 mg		**Caplets**: In 100s. **Tablets**: In 30s, 50s, 100s, 200s, and 300s.
otc	**P-A-C Tablets** (Lee)						In 100s and 1,000s.
otc	**Anacin Maximum Strength Tablets** (Insight Pharmaceuticals)		500 mg		32 mg		In 20s, 40s, and 75s.
otc	**Bayer Extra Strength Back & Body Pain** (Bayer)		500 mg		32.5 mg		Capsule shape. In 50s and 100s.
otc	**Alka-Seltzer Wake-Up Call Effervescent Tablets** (Bayer)		500 mg		65 mg		Acesulfame potassium, aspartame, mannitol, phenylalanine 9 mg. In 16s.
otc	**BC Powder Arthritis Strength** (GlaxoSmithKline)		742 mg	222 mg salicylamide	38 mg		Lactose. In 50s.
otc	**BC Fast Pain Relief Powder** (Glaxo Consumer Healthcare)		845 mg		65 mg		Lactose, potassium 55 mg per packet. In 2s, 6s, and 24s.
otc	**Stanback Headache Powder** (Glaxo Consumer Healthcare)						Lactose, potassium 55 mg per packet. In 2s, 6s, and 50s.
otc	**Bayer Quick Release Crystals** (Bayer Consumer)		850 mg		65 mg		Acesulfame K, aspartame, phenylalanine 6 mg per packet, sucralose. In 20s.
otc	**BC Fast Pain Relief Arthritis Powder** (Glaxo Consumer Healthcare)		1,000 mg		65 mg		Lactose, potassium 65 mg per packet. In 2s, 6s, and 50s.
otc	**Relagesic Liquid** (International Ethical Lab)	160 mg				5 mg phenyltoloxamine citrate	Alcohol free, dye free, sugar free. Parabens, sucralose. Grape flavor. In 118 mL.
otc	**Aceta-Gesic Tablets** (Rugby)	325 mg				30 mg phenyltoloxamine citrate	In 24s, 100s, and 1000s.
otc	**Phenagesic Tablets** (Major)						In 80s.
otc	**Phenylgesic Tablets** (Goldline)						In 100s and 1000s.
otc	**Percogesic Tablets** (Medtech)	325 mg				12.5 mg diphenhydramine HCl	Mineral oil, PEG. In 90s.
otc	**Percogesic Extra Strength Tablets** (Medtech)	500 mg				12.5 mg diphenhydramine HCl	Capsule shape. In 60s.
otc	**Midol Teen Maximum Strength Caplets** (Bayer)	500 mg				25 mg pamabrom	(Midol TEEN). In 24s.
otc	**Painaid PMF Premenstrual Formula Tablets** (Zee Medical)						In 24s.
otc	**Women's Tylenol Multi-Symptom Menstrual Relief Caplets** (McNeil Consumer)						In 24s.
otc	**Vitelle Lurline PMS Tablets** (Fielding)	500 mg				25 mg pamabrom, 50 mg pyridoxine hydrochloride	In 50s.
otc	**Prēmsyn PMS Caplets** (Chattem)	500 mg				25 mg pamabrom, 15 mg pyrilamine maleate	In 20s and 40s.
otc	**Midol Maximum Strength PMS Caplets and Gelcaps** (Bayer Consumer)						**Caplets**: (MIDOL). In 24s. **Gelcaps**: EDTA. In 24s.
otc	**Pamprin Multi-Symptom Maximum Strength Caplets and Tablets** (Chattem)						**Caplets**: (PAMPRIN). In 24s and 48s. **Tablets**: (PAMPRIN). In 12s, 24s, and 48s.
Rx	**Flextra-DS Tablets** (Poly Pharm)	500 mg				50 mg phenyltoloxamine citrate	In 100s.
Rx	**Staflex Tablets** (Magna)	500 mg				55 mg phenyltoloxamine citrate	(07). Orange, capsule shape, scored. In 100s.
Rx	**Zflex Tablets** (Huckaby Pharmaceuticals)						(ZFLEX). Red, capsule shape, scored. In 100s.
Rx	**Lagesic Tablets** (Laser)	600 mg				66 mg phenyltoloxamine citrate	Extended release. Lactose. (LASER 01 87). Scored, capsule shape. In 100s.
Rx	**PB Poly-650 Tablets** (Brookstone)	650 mg				60 mg phenyltoloxamine citrate	(BP 650). Reddish orange, scored. In 100s.

NONNARCOTIC ANALGESIC COMBINATIONS

	Product and Distributor	Acetaminophen	Aspirin	Other Analgesics	Caffeine	Other Content	How Supplied
otc	**Excedrin Tension Headache Geltabs, Caplets,** and **Tablets** (Novartis Consumer Health)	500 mg			65 mg		**Geltabs**: Parabens. In 50s and 100s. **Caplets**: Parabens. Capsule shape. In 24s, 50s, 100s and 250s. **Tablets**: Parabens. In 24s, 100s and 250s.
otc	**Excedrin Aspirin Free Geltabs and Caplets** (Bristol-Myers Squibb)						**Geltabs**: (AF Excedrin). In 24s, 50s, and 100s. **Caplets**: Saccharin, parabens. (AFE). In 24s, 50s, and 100s.
otc	**APAP-Plus Tablets** (Textilease Medique)						In 100s, 200s, and 500s.
otc	**Midol Maximum Strength Menstrual Caplets and Gelcaps** (Bayer Consumer)	500 mg			60 mg	15 mg pyrilamine maleate	**Caplets**: (Midol MENSTRUAL). In 8s and 24s. **Gelcaps**: EDTA. In 24s.
Rx	**Be-Flex Plus Capsules** (Larken)	300 mg		200 mg salicylamide		20 mg phenyltoloxamine citrate	(LL 16). Orange. In 100s.
Rx	**Ed-Flex Plus Capsules** (Edwards)						(ED-FLEX). Red. In 100s.
Rx	**Duraxin Capsules** (Portal)	325 mg		200 mg salicylamide		25 mg phenyltoloxamine citrate	In 30s.
Rx	**Durabac Capsules** (Poly Pharmaceuticals)	325 mg		250 mg salicylamide	50 mg	20 mg phenyltoloxamine citrate	(PE 826). Red and white. In 100s.
Rx	**Durabac Forte Tablets** (Poly Pharm)	500 mg		500 mg magnesium salicylate	50 mg	20 mg phenyltoloxamine citrate	(PE 827). Off-white, scored. In 100s.
otc	**Excedrin Back & Body Extra Strength Caplets** (Novartis Consumer Health)	250 mg	250 mg				Mineral oil. In 24s.
otc	**Goody's Body Pain Powder** (Glaxo Consumer)	325 mg	500 mg				Lactose. In 6s and 24s.
otc	**Vanquish Caplets** (Bayer Consumer)	194 mg	227 mg		33 mg	50 mg magnesium hydroxide, 25 mg aluminum hydroxide	(Vanquish). In 60s and 100s.
otc	**Anacin Advanced Headache Tablets** (Insight)	250 mg	250 mg		65 mg		In 75s.
otc	**Excedrin Extra Strength Caplets, Tablets,** and **Geltabs** (Novartis Consumer Health)						**Caplets**: Mineral oil. (E). In 24s, 50s, 100s and 250s. **Tablets**: Mineral oil. (E). In 24s, 50s, 100s and 250s. **Geltabs**: Mineral oil. In 24s, 50s, and 100s.
otc	**Excedrin Migraine Caplets and Tablets** (Novartis Consumer Health)						**Caplets**: (E). Mineral oil. In 24s, 50s, 100s and 250s. **Tablets**: (E). Mineral oil. In 24s, 50s, 100s, and 250s.
otc	**Goody's Extra Strength Headache Powders** (Glaxo Consumer)	260 mg	520 mg		32.5 mg		Lactose. In 2s, 6s, 24s, and 50s.
otc	**Goody's Extra Strength Fast Pain Relief Powders** (Glaxo Consumer)	325 mg	500 mg		65 mg		Mannitol, sucralose. Orange flavor. In 4s and 24s.
otc	**Medi-First Extra Strength Pain Relief Tablets** (Medique Products)	110 mg	162 mg	152 mg salicylamide	32.4 mg		In 100s, 250s, and 500s.
otc	**Painaid Tablets** (Zee Medical)						In 24s.
Rx	**Levacet Caplets** (Gentex)	250 mg	500 mg	150 mg salicylamide	32.5 mg		(LEVACET). White, capsule shape. In 50s.
otc	**Saleto Tablets** (Mallard)	115 mg	210 mg	65 mg salicylamide	16 mg		Pink. In 100s, 1000s, and *Sani-Pak* 1000s.
Rx	**Levacet Tablets** (Pharmakon)	400 mg	400 mg	150 mg salicylamide	40 mg	50 mg phenyltoloxamine citrate	(LEVACET). Yellow, capsule shape. In 50s.

NONNARCOTIC ANALGESIC COMBINATIONS — ORAL

Indications

Components of these combinations include the following (see individual monographs):

➤*Nonnarcotic analgesics:* Acetaminophen, aspirin, salicylates, salicylamide.

Barbiturates, meprobamate, and antihistamines – (eg, pyrilamine, diphenhydramine, phenyltoloxamine). Used for their sedative effects.

Antacids – (eg, calcium carbonate, magnesium hydroxide, aluminum hydroxide). Used to minimize gastric upset from salicylates.

Caffeine – A traditional component of many analgesic formulations, may be beneficial in certain vascular headaches.

Pamabrom – Used as a diuretic.

Aminobenzoate – Retards the conjugation of salicylic acid and prolongs the action of salicylates.

Another component listed, but not contributing to the analgesic properties of these products includes pyridoxine hydrochloride.

Administration and Dosage

➤*Adults:*

Analgesia – The average adult dose is 1 or 2 capsules or tablets or 1 powder packet every 2 to 6 hours as needed for pain. Each product varies; for complete prescribing information, refer to the product label/packaging information.

Warnings/Precautions

➤*Pregnancy: Category C.*

➤*Lactation:* Meprobamate is present in breast milk of lactating mothers at concentrations 2 to 4 times that of maternal plasma.

Acetaminophen, aspirin and other salicylates, and caffeine are excreted into breast milk (per Briggs' *Drugs in Pregnancy and Lactation*).

NONNARCOTIC ANALGESICS WITH BARBITURATES

Rx	**Butalbital, Acetaminophen, and Caffeine Tablets** (Various, eg, Major, Schein, Teva, Zenith Goldline)	**Tablets; oral:** 325 mg acetaminophen, 40 mg caffeine, 50 mg butalbital	In 30s, 50s, 100s, 500s, 1000s, and UD 100s.
Rx	**Americet** (MCR American)		In 100s.
Rx	**Esgic** (Forest)		(535-11). White, scored. Capsule shape. In 100s.
Rx	**Fioricet** (Novartis)		(Fioricet). Light blue. In 100s, 500s, and UD 100s.
Rx	**Repan** (Everett)		(162E305). White. In 100s.
Rx	**Orbivan** (Atley)	**Capsules; oral:** 300 mg acetaminophen, 40 mg caffeine, 50 mg butalbital	(AP 661). Green/yellow. In 100s.
Rx	**Margesic** (Marnel)	**Capsules; oral:** 325 mg acetaminophen, 40 mg caffeine, 50 mg butalbital	(Margesic/Mar). White. In 100s.
Rx	**Triad** (UAD Laboratories)		(TRIAD/UAD 905). White. In 100s.
Rx	**Esgic** (Forest)		(535-12). White. In 100s.
c-iii	**Butalbital, Aspirin, and Caffeine Capsules** (Various, eg, Lannett, Major)	**Capsules; oral:** 325 mg aspirin, 40 mg caffeine, 50 mg butalbital	In 100s and 1000s.
c-iii	**Butalbital Compound** (Various, eg, Qualitest)		In 100s.
c-iii	**Fiorinal** (Novartis)		Benzyl alcohol, EDTA, parabens. (Fiorinal 78-103). Lime green/green. In 100s, 500s, and UD 25s.
c-iii	**Butalbital, Aspirin, and Caffeine Tablets** (Various, eg, Purepac, Schein, Zenith Goldline)		In 30s, 50s, 100s, 500s, 1000s, and UD 100s.
c-iii	**Butalbital Compound** (Various, eg, Qualitest)		In 100s and 1000s.
Rx	**Phrenilin** (Valeant)	**Tablets; oral:** 325 mg acetaminophen, 50 mg butalbital	(C 8650). Violet, scored. In 100s and 500s.
Rx	**Marten-Tab** (Marnel)		(MIA/106). White. Capsule shape. In 100s.
Rx	**Butalbital, Acetaminophen, and Caffeine Tablets** (Various, eg, Able, Inwood, Major, Qualitest, URL, West-Ward)	**Tablets; oral:** 500 mg acetaminophen, 40 mg caffeine, 50 mg butalbital	In 100s and 500s.
Rx	**Esgic-Plus** (Forest)		(Forest 678). White, scored. Capsule shape. In 100s and 500s.
Rx	**Esgic-Plus** (Forest)	**Capsules; oral:** 500 mg acetaminophen, 40 mg caffeine, 50 mg butalbital	(Forest 0372/Esgic Plus). Red. In 20s, 100s, and 500s.
Rx	**Axocet** (Savage)	**Tablets; oral:** 650 mg acetaminophen, 50 mg butalbital	(0389). Blue, capsule shape. In 100s.
Rx	**Bupap** (ECR Pharmaceuticals)		(59010/240). Blue, scored. Capsule shape. In 100s.
Rx	**Cephadyn** (Atley Pharmaceuticals)		(A P 110). Blue, capsule shape. In 100s and 500s.
Rx	**Dolgic** (Athlon[a])		(MIA/112). Blue. Capsule shape. In 100s.
Rx	**Promacet** (MCR American)		In 100s.
Rx	**Repan CF** (Everett Labs)		(EVERETT 166). Blue, scored. Capsule shape. In 100s.
Rx	**Sedapap** (Merz Pharmaceuticals)		(MP 392). White. Capsule shape. In 100s.
Rx	**Tencon** (International Ethical Labs)		(Tencon 029). White, capsule shape. In 100s.
Rx	**Phrenilin Forte** (Valeant)	**Capsules; oral:** 650 mg acetaminophen, 50 mg butalbital	Benzyl alcohol, parabens, EDTA. (C 8656). Amethyst. In 100s and 500s.
Rx	**Butex Forte** (Athlon[a])		Benzyl alcohol, EDTA, parabens. (Butex Forte/070). White. In 100s.
Rx	**Dolgic Plus** (Victory Pharma)	**Tablets; oral:** 750 mg acetaminophen, 40 mg caffeine, 50 mg butalbital	(A 074). Dark pink, oval. Film-coated. In 100s.
Rx	**Alagesic LQ** (Poly Pharmaceuticals)	**Solution; oral:** 325 mg acetaminophen, 50 mg butalbital, 40 mg caffeine per 15 mL	Alcohol 7.368%, glucose, parabens, saccharin, sorbitol, sucrose. Tropical fruit punch flavor. In 473 mL.

[a] Athlon Pharmaceuticals, Inc., P. O. Box 3181, Ridgeland, MS 39158; (601) 899–5714.

BUTALBITAL/ASPIRIN/CAFFEINE — ORAL

The following is an abbreviated monograph. For additional information, refer to the Aspirin and Caffeine individual monographs.

Indications

➤*Tension or muscle contraction headache:* Relief of symptom complex of tension (or muscle contraction) headache.

Administration and Dosage

➤*Adults:*

Tension or muscle contraction headache –

Usual dosage:

- *Capsules* – 1 to 2 capsules every 4 hours.

Maximum dose: 6 capsules per day.

➤*Children:*

Tension or muscle contraction headache –

12 years of age and older: See Adults for dosing.

➤*Storage/Stability:* Store in airtight, light-resistant container at room temperature.

Actions

➤*Pharmacology:* Butalbital has generalized depressant effect on CNS and, in very high doses, has peripheral effects. Aspirin has analgesic, antipyretic, anti-inflammatory, and antirheumatic effects; its analgesic and anti-inflammatory effects may be mediated through inhibition of prostaglandin synthetase enzyme complex. Aspirin also irreversibly inhibits platelet aggregation. Caffeine is thought to produce constriction of cerebral blood vessels.

Contraindications

Hypersensitivity to salicylates, aspirin, caffeine, or barbiturates; porphyria; bleeding disorders; syndrome of nasal polyps, angioedema, and bronchospastic reactivity to aspirin or other NSAIDs; peptic ulcer.

Warnings/Precautions

➤*Drug dependency:* Prolonged use may produce drug dependency (psychologic and physical) and tolerance.

➤*Peptic ulcer, coagulation abnormalities and preoperative states:* Use with extreme caution because of increased bleeding time.

➤*Reye syndrome:* May occur in children because of aspirin component; do not use for chickenpox or flu symptoms.

➤*Renal function impairment:* Use with caution because of decreased elimination.

➤*Hepatic function impairment:* Use with caution because of decreased elimination.

➤*Pregnancy:* *Category C.*

➤*Lactation:* Undetermined.

➤*Children:* Safety and efficacy in children under the age of 12 has not been established.

➤*Elderly:* Per the Beers list, butalbital is highly addictive and cause more adverse effects than most sedative or hypnotic drugs in elderly patients.

Drug Interactions

➤*Beta-blockers (eg, propranolol), doxycycline, estrogens (including oral contraceptives), felodipine, griseofulvin, nifedipine, phenylbutazone, quinidine, theophylline:* Effects of these drugs may be increased.

➤*Corticosteroids:* May enhance renal clearance of aspirin; sudden discontinuation of corticosteroids may result in symptoms of salicylism; effects of corticosteroids may be decreased.

BUTALBITAL/ASPIRIN/CAFFEINE — ORAL

➤*Insulin, oral antidiabetic agents:* Hypoglycemic effects may be increased.

➤*MAO inhibitors:* May increase CNS effects.

➤*Methotrexate, 6-mercaptopurine:* Bone marrow toxicity may occur.

➤*NSAIDs:* Increased GI ulceration or bleeding may occur.

➤*Other CNS depressants (ethanol, narcotics, general anesthetics, tranquilizers, sedative-hypnotics):* Increased drowsiness, dizziness and other CNS depressive effects may occur.

➤*Sulfinpyrazone, probenecid:* Uricosuric effects may be decreased.

➤*Tricyclic antidepressants:* Antidepressant levels/effect may decrease.

➤*Warfarin:* Anticoagulant effects may be increased or decreased.

➤*Drug/Lab test interactions:*

Blood tests – Serum amylase; fasting blood glucose; cholesterol; protein; serum hepatic aminotransferase (ALT); uric acid; prothrombin time.

Urine tests – Glucose, 5-hydroxyindoleacetic acid; Gerhardt ketone, vanillylmandelic acid; uric acid; diacetic acid; spectrophotometric detection of barbiturates.

Adverse Reactions

➤*Cardiovascular:* Tachycardia.

➤*CNS:* Drowsiness; dizziness; lightheadedness; confusion; mental depression; unusual excitement; nervousness.

➤*Dermatologic:* Rash.

➤*GI:* Nausea; vomiting; flatulence; heartburn; abdominal pains; constipation.

Overdosage

➤*Symptoms:* Hyperthermia, tachycardia, respiratory depression, bleeding, drowsiness, confusion, coma, hypotension, hypovolemic shock, nausea, vomiting, tremor, tinnitus, fluid and electrolyte abnormalities, insomnia, restlessness.

Patient Information

Caution patient that dependency/tolerance may result from long-term use.

Tell patient to take with food or full glass of water.

Instruct patient not to discontinue abruptly after long-term regular use.

Caution patient to avoid intake of alcoholic beverages and other CNS depressants without health care provider approval.

Warn patient to avoid any hazardous activity (eg, driving, smoking) if dizziness, drowsiness, or decrease in mental acuity occurs.

Instruct patient to avoid sudden position changes to avoid orthostatic hypotension.

Advise patient to notify health care provider if any surgical procedures are required. Discontinue aspirin therapy 5 days prior to surgery to reduce potential for bleeding problems.

Instruct patient not to take *otc* medications without consulting health care provider.

Advise patient to report these symptoms to health care provider: persistent or recurrent pain before next scheduled dose, difficulty breathing, buzzing in ears, increased drowsiness, vomiting, abdominal pain, tarry stools, unusual bruising or bleeding.

BUTALBITAL/ACETAMINOPHEN/CAFFEINE — ORAL

The following is an abbreviated monograph. For additional information, refer to the Acetaminophen and Caffeine individual monographs.

Indications

➤*Tension or muscle contraction headache:* Relief of symptom complex of tension or muscle contraction headache.

Administration and Dosage

➤*Adults:*

Tension or muscle contraction headache –

Usual dosage:

- *Capsules/tablets* – 1 to 2 tablets or capsules every 4 hours.
- *Oral solution* – 15 or 30 mL every 4 hours.

Maximum dose: 6 tablets/capsules or 180 mL per day.

➤*Children:*

Tension (or muscle contraction) headache –

12 years of age and older: See Adults for dosing.

➤*Storage/Stability:* Store in airtight, light-resistant container at room temperature.

Actions

➤*Pharmacology:* Butalbital has generalized depressant effect on CNS and, in very high doses, has peripheral effects. Acetaminophen has analgesic and antipyretic effects; its analgesic effects may be mediated through inhibition of prostaglandin synthetase enzyme complex. Caffeine is thought to produce constriction of cerebral blood vessels.

Contraindications

Standard considerations.

Warnings/Precautions

➤*Drug dependency:* Prolonged use may produce drug tolerance and dependency (psychologic and physical).

➤*Pregnancy: Category C.*

➤*Lactation:* Undetermined.

➤*Children:* Safety and efficacy in children under 12 yr not established.

➤*Elderly:* Per the Beers list, butalbital is highly addictive and causes more adverse effects than most sedative or hypnotic drugs in elderly patients.

Drug Interactions

➤*Beta-blockers (eg, propranolol), corticosteroids, doxycycline, estrogens (including oral contraceptives), felodipine, griseofulvin, nifedipine, phenylbutazone, quinidine, theophylline, warfarin:* Effects of these drugs may be decreased.

➤*Carbamazepine, sulfinpyrazone:* May increase risk of hepatotoxicity.

➤*MAO inhibitors:* May increase CNS effects.

➤*Other CNS depressants (ethanol, narcotics, general anesthetics, tranquilizers, sedative-hypnotics):* Increased drowsiness, dizziness and other CNS depressive effects may occur.

➤*Tricyclic antidepressants:* Antidepressant effect may decrease.

➤*Drug/Lab test interactions:* With *Chemstrip bG* and *Dextrostix* home blood glucose systems, may cause false decrease in mean glucose values; may give false-positive urinary 5-hydroxyindoleacetic acid test result.

Adverse Reactions

➤*CNS:* Drowsiness; dizziness; lightheadedness; confusion.

➤*Dermatologic:* Rash.

➤*GI:* Nausea; vomiting; flatulence.

Overdosage

➤*Symptoms:* Blood dyscrasias, respiratory depression, hepatic damage, drowsiness, confusion, coma, hypotension, tachycardia, hypovolemic shock, nausea, vomiting, insomnia, restlessness, tremor.

Patient Information

Caution patient that dependency/tolerance may result from regular long-term use.

Tell patient to take drug with full glass of water.

Instruct patient not to discontinue drug abruptly after long-term regular use.

Caution patient to avoid intake of alcoholic beverages and other CNS depressants without health care provider approval.

Advise patient to avoid any hazardous activity (driving or smoking) if dizziness, drowsiness or a decrease in mental acuity occurs.

Warn patient that orthostatic hypotension may occur. Instruct patient to change positions slowly and to sit or lie down if symptoms occur.

Instruct patient not to take OTC or other medications unless directed by health care provider.

Inform patient to report the following symptoms to health care provider: persistent or recurrent pain before next scheduled dose, difficulty breathing, increased drowsiness, vomiting or yellowing of skin or gums.

DICLOFENAC SODIUM/MISOPROSTOL

Rx	**Arthrotec** (Searle)	**Tablets; oral**[a]: diclofenac sodium 50 mg/misoprostol 200 mcg	Lactose, hydrogenated castor oil. (AAAA50 SEARLE 1411). White to off-white, round. Film-coated. In 60s, 90s, and UD 100s.
		diclofenac sodium 75 mg/misoprostol 200 mcg	Lactose, hydrogenated castor oil. (AAAA75 SEARLE 1421). White to off-white, round. Film-coated. In 60s and UD 100s.

[a] Each tablet consists of an enteric-coated core containing diclofenac sodium surrounded by an outer mantle containing misoprostol.

DICLOFENAC SODIUM/MISOPROSTOL — ORAL

For complete and comparative prescribing information, refer to the NSAIDs class monograph and the misoprostol monograph.

WARNING

Pregnancy – This product contains diclofenac and misoprostol. The administration of misoprostol to women who are pregnant can cause abortion, premature birth, or birth defects.

Uterine rupture has been reported when misoprostol was administered to pregnant women to induce labor or abortion beyond the eighth week of pregnancy. This drug should not be taken by pregnant women.

Advise patients of the abortifacient property and warn them not to give the drug to others. Do not use in women of childbearing potential unless the patient requires nonsteroidal anti-inflammatory drug (NSAID) therapy and is at high risk of developing gastric or duodenal ulceration or of developing complications from gastric or duodenal ulcers associated with the use of the NSAID. In such patients, this drug may be prescribed if the patient:

- had a negative serum pregnancy test within 2 weeks prior to beginning therapy;
- is capable of complying with effective contraceptive measures;
- has received both oral and written warnings of the hazards of misoprostol, risk of possible contraception failure, and danger to other women of childbearing potential if the drug is taken by mistake; and
- will begin using this product only on the second or third day of the next normal menstrual period.

Cardiovascular risk – NSAIDs may cause an increased risk of serious cardiovascular thrombotic events, myocardial infarction (MI), and stroke, which can be fatal. This risk may increase with duration of use. Patients with cardiovascular disease or risk factors for cardiovascular disease may be at greater risk.

Diclofenac/misoprostol is contraindicated for treatment of perioperative pain in the setting of coronary artery bypass graft (CABG) surgery.

GI risk – NSAIDs cause an increased risk of serious GI adverse reactions, including bleeding, ulceration, and perforation of the stomach or intestines, which can be fatal. These reactions can occur at any time during use and without warning symptoms. Elderly patients are at greater risk for serious GI reactions.

Indications

➤*Arthritis:* For treatment of the signs and symptoms of osteoarthritis or rheumatoid arthritis in patients at high risk of developing NSAID-induced gastric and duodenal ulcers and their complications.

Administration and Dosage

➤*General dosing considerations:* Carefully consider the potential benefits and risks of diclofenac/misoprostol and other treatment options before deciding to use diclofenac/misoprostol.

Use the lowest effective dose for the shortest duration consistent with individual patient treatment goals.

Dosages may be individualized using the separate products (misoprostol and diclofenac), after which the patient may be changed to the appropriate combination diclofenac/misoprostol dose.

If clinically indicated, misoprostol cotherapy with diclofenac/misoprostol or use of the individual components to optimize the misoprostol dose and/or frequency of administration may be appropriate.

Misoprostol – This product contains misoprostol, which provides protection against gastric and duodenal ulcers. For gastric ulcer prevention, 200 mcg 3 and 4 times daily are therapeutically equivalent but more protective than the twice-daily regimen. For duodenal ulcer prevention, 4 times daily is more protective than the 2- or 3-times-daily regimens. However, the 4-times-daily regimen is less tolerated than the 3-times-daily regimen because of usually self-limited diarrhea related to the misoprostol dose, and the 2-times-daily regimen may be better tolerated than the 3-times-daily regimen in some patients.

➤*Adults:*

Osteoarthritis –

Usual dosage: Diclofenac 50 mg/misoprostol 200 mcg 3 times daily for maximal GI mucosal protection.

For patients who experience intolerance, doses of 50 mg/200 mcg or 75 mg/200 mcg 2 times daily can be used, but they are less effective in preventing ulcers.

Maximum dose:

- *Diclofenac* – 150 mg/day.
- *Misoprostol* – 800 mcg/day. Do not administer more than misoprostol 200 mcg at any one time.

Dosage adjustment: After observing the response to initial therapy with diclofenac/misoprostol, adjust the dosage and frequency according to the needs of the individual patient.

Rheumatoid arthritis –

Usual dosage: Diclofenac 50 mg/misoprostol 200 mcg 3 or 4 times daily.

For patients who experience intolerance, dosages of 50 mg/200 mcg or 75 mg/200 mcg 2 times daily can be used, but they are less effective in preventing ulcers.

Maximum dose:

- *Diclofenac* – 225 mg/day.
- *Misoprostol* – 800 mcg/day. Do not administer more than misoprostol 200 mcg at any one time.

Dosage adjustment: After observing the response to initial therapy with diclofenac/misoprostol, adjust the dosage and frequency according to the needs of the individual patient.

➤*Elderly:* Because elderly patients are more likely to have decreased renal function, take care in dosage selection and consider monitoring renal function.

➤*Renal function impairment:* Treatment with diclofenac/misoprostol is not recommended in patients with advanced renal disease. If diclofenac/misoprostol therapy must be initiated, closely monitor the patient's renal function.

➤*Administration:* Swallow tablets whole; do not chew, crush, or dissolve. May be taken with meals to minimize GI effects.

➤*Storage/Stability:* Store at or below 25°C (77°F) in a dry area.

Actions

➤*Pharmacology:*

Diclofenac – Diclofenac is an NSAID. In pharmacologic studies, diclofenac has shown anti-inflammatory, analgesic, and antipyretic properties. The mechanism of action of diclofenac, like other NSAIDs, is not completely understood, but may be related to prostaglandin synthetase inhibition.

Misoprostol – Misoprostol is a synthetic prostaglandin E_1 analog with gastric antisecretory and, in animals, mucosal protective properties. NSAIDs inhibit prostaglandin synthesis. A deficiency of prostaglandins within the gastric and duodenal mucosa may lead to diminishing bicarbonate and mucus secretion, and may contribute to the mucosal damage caused by NSAIDs.

Misoprostol can increase bicarbonate and mucus production, but in humans it has been shown that doses of 200 mcg and above are also antisecretory. It is, therefore, not possible to tell whether the ability of misoprostol to reduce the risk of gastric and duodenal ulcers is the result of its antisecretory effect, its mucosal protective effect, or both.

Misoprostol produces a moderate decrease in pepsin concentrations during basal conditions, but not during histamine stimulation. It has no significant effect on fasting or postprandial gastrin or intrinsic factor output.

Effects on gastric acid secretion: Misoprostol doses over the range of 50 to 200 mcg inhibit basal and nocturnal gastric acid secretion and acid secretion in response to a variety of stimuli, including meals, histamine, pentagastrin, and coffee. Activity is apparent 30 minutes after oral administration and persists for at least 3 hours. In general, the effects of 50 mcg were modest and shorter lived, and only the 200 mcg dose had substantial effects on nocturnal secretion or on histamine- and meal-stimulated secretion.

➤*Pharmacokinetics:*

Absorption/Distribution –

Diclofenac: Diclofenac is completely absorbed from the GI tract after fasting oral administration. The diclofenac sodium in diclofenac/misoprostol is in a pharmaceutical formulation that resists dissolution in the low pH of gastric fluid, but allows a rapid release of drug in the higher pH environment of the duodenum. Only 50% of the absorbed dose is systemically available because of first-pass metabolism. Peak plasma levels (C_{max}) are achieved in 2 hours (range, 1 to 4 hours), and the area under the curve (AUC) is dose-proportional within the range of 25 to 150 mg. C_{max} is less than dose-proportional and is approximately 1.5 and 2 mcg/mL for 50 and 75 mg doses, respectively.

Plasma concentrations of diclofenac decline from peak levels in a biexponential fashion, with the terminal phase having a half-life of approximately 2 hours. Clearance and volume of distribution are about 350 mL/min and 550 mL/kg, respectively. More than 99% of diclofenac is reversibly bound to human plasma albumin.

Misoprostol: Orally administered misoprostol is rapidly and extensively absorbed, and it undergoes rapid metabolism to its biologically active metabolite, misoprostol acid. Misoprostol acid in diclofenac/misoprostol reaches C_{max} in about 20 minutes. There is high variability in plasma levels of misoprostol acid between and within studies, but mean values after single doses show a linear relationship with doses of misoprostol over the range of 200 to 400 mcg. No accumulation of misoprostol acid was found in multiple-dose studies, and plasma steady state was achieved within 2 days. The serum protein binding of misoprostol acid is less than 90% and is concentration-independent in the therapeutic range.

Diclofenac/Misoprostol: The pharmacokinetics following oral administration of a single dose or multiple doses of diclofenac/misoprostol to healthy subjects under fasted conditions are similar to the pharmacokinetics of the 2 individual components.

Misoprostol Acid Mean (SD[a])			
Treatment (N = 36)	C_{max} (pg/mL)	T_{max}[b] (h)	AUC (0 to 4 h) (pg•h/mL)
Diclofenac 50 mg/ misoprostol 200 mcg	441 (137)	0.3 (0.13)	266 (95)
Misoprostol	478 (201)	0.3 (0.1)	295 (143)
Diclofenac 75 mg/ misoprostol 200 mcg	304 (110)	0.26 (0.09)	177 (49)
Misoprostol	290 (130)	0.35 (0.12)	176 (58)

[a] Standard deviation (SD) of the mean.
[b] T_{max} = time to C_{max}.

DICLOFENAC SODIUM/MISOPROSTOL — ORAL

Treatment (N = 36)	Diclofenac Mean (SD[a])		
	C_{max} (ng/mL)	T_{max} (h)	AUC (0 to 12 h) (ng•h/mL)
Diclofenac 50 mg/ misoprostol 200 mcg	1,207 (364)	2.4 (1)	1,380 (272)
Diclofenac	1,298 (441)	2.4 (1)	1,357 (290)
Diclofenac 75 mg/ misoprostol 200 mcg	2,025 (2,005)	2 (1.4)	2,773 (1,347)
Diclofenac	2,367 (1,318)	1.9 (0.7)	2,609 (1,185)

[a] SD of the mean.

The rate and extent of absorption of diclofenac and misoprostol acid from diclofenac 50 mg/misoprostol 200 mcg and diclofenac 75 mg/misoprostol 200 mcg are similar to those from diclofenac sodium and misoprostol formulations administered alone.

• *Effect of food* – Neither diclofenac nor misoprostol acid accumulated in plasma following repeated doses of diclofenac/misoprostol given every 12 hours under fasted conditions. Food decreases the multiple-dose bioavailability profile of diclofenac 50 mg/misoprostol 200 mcg and diclofenac 75 mg/misoprostol 200 mcg.

The C_{max} of misoprostol acid is diminished when the dose is taken with food, and total availability of misoprostol acid is reduced by use of a concomitant antacid. Clinical trials were conducted with concomitant antacid; this effect does not appear to be clinically important.

Metabolism / Excretion –

Diclofenac: Diclofenac metabolism is predominantly mediated via cytochrome P450 enzyme 2C9 (CYP2C9) in the liver. Administer diclofenac with caution to patients who are known or suspected to be poor CYP2C9 metabolizers based on previous history/experience with other CYP2C9 substrates because they may have abnormally high plasma levels caused by reduced metabolic clearance.

Diclofenac is eliminated through metabolism and subsequent urinary and biliary excretion of the glucuronide and the sulfate conjugates of the metabolites. Approximately 65% of the dose is excreted in the urine and 35% in the bile.

Conjugates of unchanged diclofenac account for 5% to 10% of the dose excreted in the urine and for less than 5% excreted in the bile. Little or no unchanged unconjugated drug is excreted. Conjugates of the principal metabolite account for 20% to 30% of the dose excreted in the urine and for 10% to 20% of the dose excreted in the bile.

Conjugates of 3 other metabolites together account for 10% to 20% of the dose excreted in the urine and for small amounts excreted in the bile. The elimination half-life values for these metabolites are shorter than those for the parent drug. Urinary excretion of an additional metabolite (half-life = 80 hours) accounts for only 1.4% of the oral dose. The degree of accumulation of diclofenac metabolites is unknown. Some of the metabolites may have activity.

Misoprostol: Misoprostol undergoes rapid metabolism to its biologically active metabolite, misoprostol acid. Misoprostol is quickly eliminated, with an elimination half-life of about 30 minutes. After oral administration of radiolabeled misoprostol, about 70% of detected radioactivity appears in the urine.

Special populations –

Renal function impairment: Pharmacokinetic studies with misoprostol in patients with varying degrees of renal impairment showed an approximate doubling of half-life, C_{max}, and AUC compared with healthy subjects. In patients older than 64 years of age, the AUC for misoprostol acid is increased.

Hepatic function impairment: In a study of patients with mild to moderate hepatic impairment, mean misoprostol acid AUC and C_{max} showed approximately double the mean values obtained in healthy subjects. Three patients who had the lowest antipyrine and lowest indocyanine green clearance values had the highest misoprostol acid AUC and C_{max} values.

Lactation: After a single oral dose of misoprostol to breast-feeding mothers, misoprostol acid was excreted in breast milk. The maximum concentration of misoprostol acid in expressed breast milk was achieved within 1 hour after dosing and was 7.6 pg/mL (coefficient of variation [CV], 37%) and 20.9 pg/mL (CV, 77%) after single misoprostol 200 and 600 mcg administration, respectively. The misoprostol acid concentrations in breast milk declined to less than 1 pg/mL at 5 hours postdose.

Contraindications

Hypersensitivity to diclofenac, misoprostol, or other prostaglandins; patients who have experienced asthma, urticaria, or other allergic-type reactions after taking aspirin or other NSAIDs; pregnancy; for the treatment of perioperative pain in the setting of CABG surgery.

Warnings/Precautions

➤*Cardiovascular effects:*

Cardiovascular thrombotic events – Clinical trials of several COX-2 selective and nonselective NSAIDs of up to 3 years' duration increased the risk of serious cardiovascular thrombotic reactions, MI, and stroke, which can be fatal. All NSAIDs, both COX-2 selective and nonselective, may have a similar risk. Patients with known cardiovascular disease or risk factors for cardiovascular disease may be at greater risk. To minimize the potential risk for an adverse cardiovascular reaction in patients treated with an NSAID, use the lowest effective dose for the shortest duration possible. Remain alert for the development of such reactions, even in the absence of previous cardiovascular symptoms. Inform patients about the signs and/or symptoms of serious cardiovascular reactions and the steps to take if they occur.

Two large, controlled clinical trials of a COX-2 selective NSAID for the treatment of pain in the first 10 to 14 days following CABG surgery found an increased incidence of MI and stroke.

Hypertension – NSAIDs, including diclofenac/misoprostol, can lead to onset of new hypertension or worsening of preexisting hypertension, either of which may contribute to the increased incidence of cardiovascular reactions. Patients taking thiazides or loop diuretics may have impaired response to these therapies when taking NSAIDs. Use NSAIDs, including diclofenac/misoprostol, with caution in patients with hypertension. Closely monitor blood pressure during the initiation of NSAID treatment and throughout the course of therapy.

Congestive heart failure and edema – Fluid retention and edema have been observed in some patients taking NSAIDs. Use diclofenac/misoprostol with caution in patients with fluid retention or heart failure.

➤*GI effects:*

Risk of ulceration, bleeding, and perforation – NSAIDs, including diclofenac/misoprostol, can cause serious GI adverse reactions, including inflammation, bleeding, ulceration, and perforation of the stomach, small intestine, or large intestine, which can be fatal. These serious adverse reactions can occur at any time, with or without warning symptoms, in patients treated with NSAIDs.

Only 1 in 5 patients who develop a serious upper GI adverse reaction on NSAID therapy is symptomatic. Upper GI ulcers, gross bleeding, or perforation caused by NSAIDs occur in approximately 1% of patients treated for 3 to 6 months and in about 2% to 4% of patients treated for 1 year. These trends continue with longer duration of use, increasing the likelihood of developing a serious GI reaction at some time during the course of therapy. However, even short-term therapy is not without risk. Prescribe NSAIDs with extreme caution in patients with a prior history of ulcer disease or GI bleeding. Patients with a prior history of peptic ulcer disease and/or GI bleeding who use NSAIDs have a more than 10-fold increased risk for developing a GI bleed compared with patients treated with neither of these risk factors. Other factors that increase the risk of GI bleeding in patients treated with NSAIDs include concomitant use of oral corticosteroids or anticoagulants, longer duration of NSAID therapy, smoking, alcohol use, older age, and poor general health status. Most spontaneous reports of fatal GI reactions are in elderly or debilitated patients; therefore, take special care in treating this population.

To minimize the potential risk for an adverse GI reaction in patients treated with an NSAID, use the lowest effective dosage for the shortest possible duration. Remain alert for signs and symptoms of GI ulcerations and bleeding during NSAID therapy and promptly initiate additional evaluation and treatment if a serious GI reaction is suspected. This includes discontinuation of the NSAID until a serious GI adverse reaction is ruled out. For high-risk patients, consider alternate therapies that do not involve NSAIDs.

➤*Renal effects:* Long-term administration of NSAIDs has resulted in renal papillary necrosis and other renal injury. Renal toxicity has also been seen in patients in whom renal prostaglandins have a compensatory role in the maintenance of renal perfusion. In these patients, administration of an NSAID may cause a dose-dependent reduction in prostaglandin formation and, secondarily, in renal blood flow, which may precipitate overt renal decompensation. Patients at greatest risk of this reaction are those with impaired renal function, heart failure, or liver dysfunction; those taking diuretics and angiotensin-converting enzyme (ACE) inhibitors; and elderly patients. Discontinuation of NSAID therapy is usually followed by recovery to the pretreatment state.

Advanced renal disease – Diclofenac metabolites are eliminated primarily by the kidneys. The extent to which the metabolites may accumulate in patients with renal failure has not been studied. Therefore, treatment with diclofenac is not recommended in patients with advanced renal disease. If diclofenac therapy must be initiated, closely monitor the patient's renal function.

➤*Hepatic effects:* Elevations of one or more liver tests may occur during therapy with diclofenac. These laboratory abnormalities may progress, remain unchanged, or be transient with continued therapy. Borderline elevations (less than 3 times the upper limits of normal [ULN] range) or greater elevations of transaminases occurred in about 15% of diclofenac-treated patients. Of the hepatic enzymes, ALT is the one recommended for the monitoring of liver injury.

Almost all meaningful elevations in transaminases were detected before patients became symptomatic. Abnormal tests occurred during the first 2 months of therapy with diclofenac in 42 of the 51 patients in all trials who developed marked transaminase elevations.

In postmarketing reports, cases of drug-induced hepatoxicity have been reported in the first month and, in some cases, the first 2 months of therapy, but can occur at any time during treatment with diclofenac. Postmarketing surveillance has reported cases of severe hepatic reactions, including liver necrosis, jaundice, fulminant fatal hepatitis with and without jaundice, and liver failure. Some of these reported cases resulted in fatalities or liver transplantation.

Measure transaminases periodically in patients receiving long-term therapy with diclofenac because severe hepatotoxicity may develop without a prodrome of distinguishing symptoms. The optimum times for making the first and subsequent transaminase measurements are not known. Based on clinical trial data and postmarketing experiences, monitor transaminases within 4 to 8 weeks after initiating treatment with diclofenac. However, severe hepatic reactions can occur at any time during treatment with diclofenac.

If abnormal liver tests persist or worsen, if clinical signs and/or symptoms consistent with liver disease develop, or if systemic manifestations occur (eg, eosinophilia, rash , abdominal pain, diarrhea, dark urine), discontinue diclofenac/misoprostol immediately.

Exercise caution when prescribing diclofenac with concomitant drugs that are known to be potentially hepatotoxic (eg, antibiotics, antiepileptics).

➤*Corticosteroid use:* Diclofenac/misoprostol is not a substitute for corticosteroids or corticosteroid insufficiency treatment. Abrupt discontinuation of corticosteroids may lead to disease exacerbation. If a decision is made to discontinue corticosteroids, slowly taper the therapy of patients on prolonged corticosteroids.

➤*Fever and/or inflammation:* The pharmacological activity of diclofenac/misoprostol in reducing fever and inflammation may diminish the utility of these diagnostic signs in detecting complications of presumed noninfectious, painful conditions.

➤*Hematological effects:*

Anemia – Anemia is sometimes seen in patients receiving NSAIDs, including diclofenac/misoprostol. This may be caused by fluid retention, occult or gross GI blood loss, or an incompletely described effect upon erythropoiesis. Check the hemoglobin or hematocrit of patients on long-term treatment with NSAIDs, including diclofenac/misoprostol, if they exhibit any signs or symptoms of anemia.

Platelet aggregation – NSAIDs inhibit platelet aggregation and have been shown to prolong bleeding time in some patients. Unlike aspirin, their effect on platelet function is quantitatively less, is of shorter duration, and is reversible.

Diclofenac impairs platelet aggregation but does not affect bleeding time, plasma thrombin clotting time, plasma fibrinogen, or factors V and VII to XII. Statistically significant changes in prothrombin and partial thromboplastin times have been reported in healthy volunteers. The mean changes were less than 1 second in both instances and are unlikely to be clinically important. Diclofenac is a prostaglandin synthetase inhibitor, and all drugs that inhibit prostaglandin synthesis interfere with platelet function to some degree; therefore, carefully observe patients who may be adversely affected by such an action. Misoprostol has not been shown to exacerbate the effects of diclofenac on platelet activity.

Carefully monitor patients receiving diclofenac/misoprostol who may be adversely affected by alterations in platelet function, such as those with coagulation disorders or patients receiving anticoagulants.

➤*Preexisting asthma:* Patients with asthma may have aspirin-sensitive asthma. The use of aspirin in patients with aspirin-sensitive asthma has been associated with severe bronchospasm that can be fatal. Because cross-reactivity, including bronchospasm, between aspirin and other NSAIDs has been reported in these aspirin-sensitive patients, do not administer diclofenac/misoprostol to patients with this form of aspirin sensitivity. Use this drug with caution in patients with preexisting asthma.

➤*Aseptic meningitis:* As with other NSAIDs, aseptic meningitis with fever and coma has been observed on rare occasions in patients on diclofenac therapy. Although it is probably more likely to occur in patients with systemic lupus and related connective tissue diseases, it has been reported in patients who do not have an underlying chronic disease. If signs or symptoms of meningitis develop in a patient on diclofenac, consider the possibility that it may be related to diclofenac.

➤*Porphyria:* Avoid the use of diclofenac/misoprostol in patients with hepatic porphyria. One patient has been described in whom diclofenac probably triggered a clinical attack of porphyria.

➤*Hypersensitivity reactions:*

Anaphylactoid reactions – As with other NSAIDs, anaphylactoid reactions may occur in patients without known prior exposure to diclofenac/misoprostol. Do not give diclofenac/misoprostol to patients with the aspirin triad. This symptom complex typically occurs in asthmatic patients who experience rhinitis, with or without nasal polyps, or patients who exhibit severe, potentially fatal bronchospasm after taking aspirin or other NSAIDs. Seek emergency help in cases in which an anaphylactoid reaction occurs. Allergic reactions have been reported by less than 0.1% of patients who received diclofenac/misoprostol in clinical trials, and there have been rare reports of anaphylaxis in the marketed use of diclofenac/misoprostol outside of the United States.

Skin reactions – NSAIDs, including diclofenac/misoprostol, can cause serious skin adverse reactions, such as exfoliative dermatitis, Stevens-Johnson syndrome, and toxic epidermal necrolysis, which can be fatal. These serious reactions may occur without warning.

➤*Renal function impairment:* Diclofenac metabolites are eliminated primarily by the kidneys. The extent to which the metabolites may accumulate in patients with renal failure has not been studied. Therefore, treatment with diclofenac/misoprostol is not recommended in patients with advanced renal disease. If diclofenac/misoprostol therapy must be initiated, closely monitor the patient's renal function.

➤*Pregnancy: Category X.* Contraindicated in pregnancy. There are no adequate and well-controlled studies in pregnant women (see Black Box Warning).

As with other NSAIDs, avoid diclofenac/misoprostol in late pregnancy because it may cause premature closure of the ductus arteriosus.

Teratogenic – Congenital anomalies, sometimes associated with fetal death, have been reported subsequent to the unsuccessful use of misoprostol as an abortifacient, but the drug's teratogenic mechanism has not been demonstrated. Several reports in the literature associate the use of misoprostol during the first trimester of pregnancy with skull defects, cranial nerve palsies, facial malformations, and limb defects.

Nonteratogenic – Misoprostol may endanger pregnancy (may cause abortion) and thereby cause harm to the fetus when administered to a pregnant woman. Misoprostol may produce uterine contractions, uterine bleeding, and expulsion of the products of conception. Misoprostol has been used to ripen the cervix, induce labor, and treat postpartum hemorrhage outside of its approved indication. A major adverse reaction of these uses is hyperstimulation of the uterus. Uterine rupture, amniotic fluid embolism, severe genital bleeding, shock, fetal bradycardia, and fetal and maternal death have been reported. Higher doses of misoprostol, including the 100 mcg tablet, may increase the risk of complications from uterine hyperstimulation. Diclofenac/misoprostol, which contains misoprostol 200 mcg, is likely to have a greater risk of uterine hyperstimulation than the misoprostol 100 mcg tablet. Abortions caused by misoprostol may be incomplete. If a woman is or becomes pregnant while taking this drug, discontinue the drug and apprise the patient of the potential hazard to the fetus.

Cases of amniotic fluid embolism that resulted in maternal and fetal death have been reported with use of misoprostol during pregnancy. Severe vaginal bleeding, retained placenta, shock, fetal bradycardia, and pelvic pain also have been reported. These women were administered misoprostol vaginally and/or orally over a range of dosages.

➤*Lactation:* Diclofenac/misoprostol is not recommended for breast-feeding women. Diclofenac is found in the milk of breast-feeding mothers. Misoprostol is rapidly metabolized in the mother to misoprostol acid, which is biologically active and excreted in breast milk. There are no published reports of adverse effects of misoprostol in breast-feeding infants of women taking misoprostol. Because of the low levels of misoprostol in breast milk, amounts ingested by the infant are small and would not be expected to cause any adverse effects in the breast-fed infant. Exercise caution when diclofenac/misoprostol is administered to a breast-feeding woman.

➤*Children:* Safety and efficacy in children have not been established.

➤*Elderly:* No overall differences in safety or efficacy were observed between elderly subjects and younger subjects, but greater sensitivity of some older individuals cannot be ruled out.

Diclofenac is known to be substantially excreted by the kidneys, and the risk of toxic reactions to diclofenac/misoprostol may be greater in patients with renal impairment. Because elderly patients are more likely to have decreased renal function, take care in dosage selection and consider monitoring renal function.

➤*Monitoring:* Because serious GI tract ulcerations and bleeding can occur without warning symptoms, monitor for signs and symptoms of GI bleeding. Perform complete blood cell counts and periodically check chemistry profiles for patients on long-term treatment with NSAIDs. If clinical signs and symptoms consistent with hepatic or renal disease develop, systemic manifestations occur (eg, eosinophilia, rash), or abnormal liver tests persist or worsen, discontinue diclofenac/misoprostol. Monitor blood pressure during the initiation of NSAID treatment and throughout the course of therapy. Monitor for fluid retention and edema in patients taking NSAIDs. Measure hepatic transaminases periodically in patients receiving long-term therapy with diclofenac and for 4 to 8 weeks after initiating therapy.

Carefully monitor patients receiving diclofenac/misoprostol who may be adversely affected by alterations in platelet function, such as those with coagulation disorders or patients receiving anticoagulants.

Drug Interactions

Diclofenac/Misoprostol Drug Interactions

Precipitant drug	Object drug[a]		Description
Alcohol	Diclofenac/ Misoprostol	↑	The risk of GI bleeding may be increased. Monitor for signs of GI bleeding.
Antacids	Diclofenac/ Misoprostol	↓↑	Antacids reduce the bioavailability of misoprostol acid. Antacids may delay the absorption of diclofenac. Magnesium-containing antacids exacerbate misoprostol-associated diarrhea.
Antiplatelet agents (eg, clopidogrel, prasugrel)	Diclofenac/ Misoprostol	↑	The risk of bleeding may be increased. Use with caution.
Diclofenac/ Misoprostol	Antiplatelet agents (eg, clopidogrel, prasugrel)		
Aspirin	Diclofenac/ Misoprostol	↓↑	Plasma concentrations of diclofenac may be reduced by aspirin, possibly because of reduced protein binding. These agents are also gastric irritants. In addition, the cardioprotective effect of aspirin may be reduced. Concurrent use of diclofenac and aspirin is not generally recommended.
Diclofenac/ Misoprostol	Aspirin		

DICLOFENAC SODIUM/MISOPROSTOL — ORAL

Diclofenac/Misoprostol Drug Interactions

Precipitant drug	Object drug[a]		Description
Azole antifungals (eg, fluconazole, voriconazole)	Diclofenac/ Misoprostol	↑	NSAID plasma concentrations may be elevated, increasing the pharmacologic and adverse reactions. Monitor the clinical response and adjust the dose of diclofenac/misoprostol as needed.
Bile acid sequestrants (eg, cholestyramine, colestipol)	Diclofenac/ Misoprostol	↓	The effects of diclofenac may be decreased.
Bisphosphonates (eg, alendronate)	Diclofenac/ Misoprostol	↑	Risk of gastric ulceration may be increased. Use with caution. Monitor for signs of GI adverse reactions, especially gastric ulceration.
Corticosteroids	Diclofenac/ Misoprostol	↑	The risk of GI bleeding may be increased. Monitor for signs of GI bleeding.
Probenecid	Diclofenac/ Misoprostol	↑	Diclofenac plasma concentrations may be elevated, increasing the risk of toxicity. Monitor for signs of diclofenac toxicity and adjust treatment as needed.
Selective serotonin reuptake inhibitors (eg, citalopram, fluoxetine, paroxetine)	Diclofenac/ Misoprostol	↑	The risk of upper GI bleeding may be increased. If coadministration cannot be avoided, close clinical monitoring for signs of GI bleeding is warranted. Consider shortening diclofenac/misoprostol treatment duration, decreasing the diclofenac/misoprostol dose, or using alternative therapy (eg, acetaminophen, tricyclic antidepressants).
Serotonin-norepinephrine reuptake inhibitors (eg, venlafaxine)	Diclofenac/ Misoprostol	↑	The risk of upper GI bleeding may be increased. If coadministration cannot be avoided, close clinical monitoring for signs of GI bleeding is warranted. Consider using alternative therapy (eg, acetaminophen, tricyclic antidepressants).
Smoking	Diclofenac/ Misoprostol	↑	The risk of GI bleeding may be increased. Monitor for signs of GI bleeding.
Sucralfate	Diclofenac/ Misoprostol	↓	The effects of diclofenac may be decreased, possibly because of decreased absorption. Monitor the clinical response and adjust treatment as needed.
Diclofenac/ Misoprostol	ACE inhibitors (eg, captopril, enalapril)	↓↑	NSAIDs may diminish the antihypertensive effect of ACE inhibitors. In addition, the risk of nephrotoxicity may be increased. Closely monitor blood pressure. If blood pressure control deteriorates, consider stopping diclofenac/misoprostol. Periodic measurement of renal function and potassium concentrations is warranted.
Diclofenac/ Misoprostol	Aminoglycosides (eg, amikacin, gentamicin, tobramycin)	↑	Aminoglycoside plasma concentrations may be elevated in premature infants because NSAIDs reduce the glomerular filtration rate. Avoid this combination if possible, or reduce the aminoglycoside dose prior to NSAID initiation or stop diclofenac/ misoprostol before starting aminoglycoside therapy. Monitor aminoglycoside levels and renal function.
Diclofenac/ Misoprostol	Anticoagulants (eg, warfarin)	↑	Coadministration may increase anticoagulant activity and risk of bleeding. Also consider the effects NSAIDs have on platelet function and gastric mucosa. Closely monitor coagulation status and adjust the anticoagulant dose as needed. Monitor for signs of GI bleeding.
Diclofenac/ Misoprostol	Barbiturates (eg, phenobarbital)	↑	Phenobarbital toxicity has been reported in patients on chronic phenobarbital treatment following initiation with diclofenac. Monitor for barbiturate toxicity.
Diclofenac/ Misoprostol	Cyclosporine	↑	Nephrotoxicity of both agents may be increased. Closely monitor renal function and cyclosporine concentrations. If an interaction is suspected, consider decreasing cyclosporine dosage or stopping diclofenac/ misoprostol.
Cyclosporine	Diclofenac/ Misoprostol		
Diclofenac/ Misoprostol	Digoxin	↑	Elevated levels of digoxin have been reported during coadministration with diclofenac. Monitor for possible digoxin toxicity.
Diclofenac/ Misoprostol	Heparins (eg, dalteparin, enoxaparin, heparin)	↑	The risk of hemorrhagic adverse reactions may be increased. If concurrent use cannot be avoided, close clinical and laboratory monitoring are warranted.
Diclofenac/ Misoprostol	Lithium	↑	Serum lithium levels may be increased and renal clearance decreased. Monitor for signs of lithium toxicity. Additional lithium plasma concentration monitoring is warranted. Adjust the lithium dose as needed.
Diclofenac/ Misoprostol	Loop diuretics (eg, furosemide)	↓	The natriuretic effect of furosemide may be reduced. Acute renal failure may occur during concomitant therapy; monitor closely for signs of renal failure and to ensure diuretic efficacy.
Diclofenac/ Misoprostol	Methotrexate	↑	NSAIDs have been reported to increase the risk of methotrexate toxicity. If coadministration cannot be avoided, use with caution. Monitor for signs of methotrexate toxicity. Monitoring methotrexate concentrations may be useful in managing treatment.
Diclofenac/ Misoprostol	Oral hypoglycemic agents	↑↓	There are rare reports of changes in the effect of oral hypoglycemic agents in the presence of diclofenac. Hypoglycemic and hyperglycemic effects have been reported. Monitor blood glucose and adjust the oral hypoglycemic dose as needed.
Diclofenac/ Misoprostol	Potassium-sparing diuretics (eg, triamterene)	↑	Coadministration with potassium-sparing diuretics may be associated with increased serum potassium levels. The risk of renal failure may be increased. If renal failure occurs, stop both drugs and treat this complication.
Diclofenac/ Misoprostol	Quinolones (eg, norfloxacin)	↑	Quinolone plasma concentrations may be elevated. The risk of CNS stimulation and seizures from quinolones may be increased. Use with caution.
Diclofenac/ Misoprostol	Thiazide diuretics (eg, hydrochlorothiazide)	↓	The natriuretic effect of thiazides can be reduced. Acute renal failure may occur during concomitant therapy; monitor closely for signs of renal failure and to ensure diuretic efficacy. Monitor blood pressure.

[a] ↑ = object drug increased; ↓ = object drug decreased; ↑↓ = object both increased and decreased.

DICLOFENAC SODIUM/MISOPROSTOL — ORAL

➤*Drug/Food interactions:* Maximum plasma concentrations of misoprostol acid are diminished when the dose is taken with food; food decreases the multiple-dose bioavailability profile of diclofenac/misoprostol.

Adverse Reactions

➤*GI:* GI disorders had the highest reported incidence of adverse reactions for patients receiving diclofenac/misoprostol. These reactions were generally minor but led to discontinuation of therapy in 9% of patients on diclofenac/misoprostol and in 5% on diclofenac.

Diclofenac/Misoprostol vs Diclofenac GI Adverse Reactions

GI disorder	Diclofenac/Misoprostol	Diclofenac
Abdominal pain	21%	15%
Diarrhea	19%	11%
Dyspepsia	14%	11%
Flatulence	9%	4%
Nausea	11%	6%

Diclofenac/misoprostol can cause more abdominal pain, diarrhea, and other GI symptoms than diclofenac alone. Diarrhea and abdominal pain developed early in the course of therapy and were usually self-limited (resolved after 2 to 7 days). Rare instances of profound diarrhea leading to severe dehydration have been reported in patients receiving misoprostol. Carefully monitor patients with an underlying condition, such as inflammatory bowel disease, or those in whom dehydration, were it to occur, would be dangerous if this product is prescribed. The incidence of diarrhea can be minimized by administering diclofenac/misoprostol with food and by avoiding coadministration with magnesium-containing antacids.

➤*GU:* Gynecological disorders previously reported with misoprostol use have also been reported for women receiving diclofenac/misoprostol. Postmenopausal vaginal bleeding may be related to administration of diclofenac/misoprostol. If it occurs, undertake diagnostic workup to rule out gynecological pathology.

➤*Other adverse reactions:* Other adverse experiences have been reported occasionally or rarely with diclofenac/misoprostol, diclofenac, misoprostol, or other NSAIDs.

Cardiovascular – Arrhythmia, atrial fibrillation, congestive heart failure, hypertension, hypotension, MI, palpitations, phlebitis, premature ventricular contractions, syncope, tachycardia, vasculitis.

CNS – Anxiety, asthenia, coma, concentration impaired, confusion, convulsions, depression, disorientation, dizziness, dream abnormalities, drowsiness, fatigue, hallucinations, headache, hyperesthesia, hypertonia, hypoesthesia, insomnia, irritability, malaise, meningitis, migraine, nervousness, neuralgia, paranoia, paresthesia, psychotic reaction, somnolence, tremor, vertigo.

Dermatologic – Acne, alopecia, bruising, eczema, erythema multiforme, exfoliative dermatitis, pemphigoid reaction, photosensitivity, pruritus, pruritus ani, rash, skin ulceration, Stevens-Johnson syndrome, sweating increased, toxic epidermal necrolysis.

GI – Anorexia, appetite changes, constipation, dry mouth, dysphagia, enteritis, eructation, esophageal ulceration, esophagitis, gastritis, gastroesophageal reflux, GI bleeding, GI neoplasm benign, glossitis, heartburn, hematemesis, hemorrhoids, intestinal perforation, peptic ulcer, rectal bleeding, stomatitis and ulcerative stomatitis, tenesmus, vomiting.

GU – Breast pain, cystitis, dysmenorrhea, dysuria, hematuria, impotence, intermenstrual bleeding, interstitial nephritis, leukorrhea, menorrhagia, menstrual disorder, micturition frequency, nephrotic syndrome, nocturia, oliguria/polyuria, papillary necrosis, perineal pain, proteinuria, renal failure, urinary tract infection, vaginal hemorrhage.

Hematologic/Lymphatic – Agranulocytosis, anemia, aplastic anemia, coagulation time increased, ecchymosis, eosinophilia, epistaxis, hemolytic anemia, leukocytosis, leukopenia, lymphadenopathy, melena, pancytopenia, purpura, thrombocythemia, thrombocytopenia.

Hepatic – Abnormal hepatic function, bilirubinemia, hepatitis, jaundice, liver failure, pancreatitis.

Hypersensitivity – Angioedema, laryngeal/pharyngeal edema, urticaria.

Metabolic/Nutritional – Alkaline phosphatase increased, dehydration, glycosuria, gout, hypercholesterolemia, hyperglycemia, hyperuricemia, hypoglycemia, hyponatremia, periorbital edema, porphyria, serum urea nitrogen increased, weight changes.

Musculoskeletal – Arthralgia, myalgia.

Ophthalmic – Amblyopia, blurred vision, conjunctivitis, diplopia, glaucoma, iritis, lacrimation abnormal, night blindness, vision abnormal.

Respiratory – Asthma, coughing, dyspnea, hyperventilation, pneumonia, pulmonary embolism, respiratory depression.

Special senses – Hearing impairment, taste loss, taste perversion, tinnitus.

Miscellaneous – Chills, death, fever, increased creatine phosphokinase, increased lactate dehydrogenase, infection, sepsis.

Overdosage

➤*Symptoms:*

Diclofenac – Clinical signs that may suggest diclofenac overdose include confusion, drowsiness, general hypotonia, or GI complaints. Reports of overdosage with diclofenac include 66 cases. In approximately 50% of these reports of overdosage, concomitant medications were also taken. The highest dose of diclofenac was 5 g in a man 17 years of age who suffered loss of consciousness, increased intracranial pressure, and aspiration pneumonitis, and died 2 days after overdose. A woman 24 years of age who took 4 g, and women 28 and 42 years of age, each of whom took 3.75 g, did not develop any clinically significant signs or symptoms. However, there was a report of a woman 17 years of age who experienced vomiting and drowsiness after an overdose of diclofenac 2.37 g.

Misoprostol – The toxic dose of misoprostol in humans has not been determined. Cumulative total daily doses of 1,600 mcg have been tolerated, with only symptoms of GI discomfort reported. In animals, the acute toxic effects are diarrhea, GI lesions, focal cardiac necrosis, hepatic necrosis, renal tubular necrosis, testicular atrophy, respiratory difficulties, and CNS depression. Clinical signs that may indicate an overdose are abdominal pain, bradycardia, convulsions, diarrhea, dyspnea, fever, hypotension, palpitations, sedation, or tremor.

➤*Treatment:* Treat symptoms of overdosage with diclofenac/misoprostol with supportive therapy. In case of acute overdosage, gastric lavage is recommended. Induced diuresis may be beneficial because diclofenac and misoprostol metabolites are excreted in the urine. The effect of dialysis or hemoperfusion on the elimination of diclofenac sodium (99% protein bound) and misoprostol acid remains unproven. The use of oral activated charcoal may help to reduce the absorption of diclofenac and misoprostol.

Patient Information

Tell women of childbearing potential using diclofenac/misoprostol to treat arthritis that they must not be pregnant when therapy with diclofenac/misoprostol is initiated and that they must use effective contraception while taking diclofenac/misoprostol.

Advise the patient not to give diclofenac/misoprostol to anyone else. Diclofenac/misoprostol that has been prescribed for a patient's specific condition may not be the correct treatment for another person and may be dangerous to a woman if she were to become pregnant. Special note for women: this drug contains diclofenac and misoprostol. Misoprostol may cause abortion (sometimes incomplete, which could lead to dangerous bleeding requiring hospitalization and surgery), premature labor, or birth defects if given to pregnant women. Inform women that they must avoid pregnancy while on this medication and for at least 1 month or through 1 menstrual cycle after stopping the medication.

Inform patients that diclofenac/misoprostol, like other NSAIDs, may cause serious adverse reactions, such as MI or stroke, that may result in hospitalization and even death. The risk may increase with duration of use; patients with heart disease or risk factors for heart disease are at greater risk. Although serious cardiovascular reactions can occur without warning symptoms, ensure that patients are alert for the signs and symptoms of chest pain, shortness of breath, weakness, and slurring of speech, and that they ask for medical advice when observing any indicative sign or symptom. Apprise patients of the importance of this follow-up.

Inform patients that diclofenac/misoprostol, like other NSAIDs, can cause GI discomfort and, rarely, serious GI reactions, such as ulcers and bleeding, that may result in hospitalizations and even death. Although serious GI tract ulcerations and bleeding can occur without warning symptoms, ensure that patients are alert for the signs and symptoms of ulceration and bleeding, and that they ask for medical advice when observing any indicative sign or symptom, including epigastric pain, dyspepsia, melena, and hematemesis. Apprise patients of the importance of this follow-up.

Tell patients that diclofenac/misoprostol may cause diarrhea, abdominal pain, upset stomach, and/or nausea in some people. In most cases, these problems develop during the first few weeks of therapy and stop after about a week with continued treatment. If patients have difficulty (more than 7 days) or have severe diarrhea, cramping, and/or nausea, advise them to call their health care provider. Inform patients that they can minimize possible diarrhea by making sure to take diclofenac/misoprostol with meals and by avoiding the use of antacids containing magnesium (if needed, use one containing aluminum or calcium instead). Advise patients to swallow diclofenac/misoprostol tablets whole and not to chew, crush, or dissolve.

Inform patients that diclofenac/misoprostol, like other NSAIDs, can cause serious skin adverse reactions, such as exfoliative dermatitis, Stevens-Johnson syndrome, and toxic epidermal necrolysis that may result in hospitalization and even death. Although serious skin reactions may occur without warning, ensure that patients are alert for the signs and symptoms of skin rash and blisters, fever, or other signs of hypersensitivity, such as itching, and that they ask for medical advice when observing any indicative sign or symptom. Advise patients to stop the drug immediately if they develop any type of rash and to contact their health care provider as soon as possible.

Advise patients to promptly report signs or symptoms of unexplained weight gain or edema to their health care provider.

Inform patients of the warning signs and symptoms of hepatotoxicity (eg, nausea, fatigue, lethargy, pruritus, jaundice, right upper quadrant tenderness, flu-like symptoms). Instruct patients to stop taking the drug and seek immediate medical therapy if these occur.

Inform patients of the signs of an anaphylactoid reaction (eg, difficulty breathing, swelling of the face or throat). Instruct patients to seek immediate emergency help if these occur.

Advise women in late pregnancy, as with other NSAIDs, to avoid diclofenac/misoprostol because it may cause premature closure of the ductus arteriosus.

Instruct women not to take diclofenac if they are breast-feeding.

NAPROXEN/ESOMEPRAZOLE

Rx	**Vimovo** (AstraZeneca)	**Tablets, delayed-release; oral:** naproxen 375 mg/esomeprazole 20 mg	As esomeprazole magnesium 22.3 mg. Parabens, PEG, polydextrose. (375/20). Yellow, oval. Enteric-coated. In 60s and 500s.
		naproxen 500 mg/esomeprazole 20 mg	As esomeprazole magnesium trihydrate 22.3 mg. Parabens, PEG, polydextrose. (500/20). Yellow, oval. Enteric-coated. In 60s, 500s, and UD 100s.

NAPROXEN/ESOMEPRAZOLE MAGNESIUM — ORAL

WARNING

Cardiovascular risk – Naproxen may cause an increased risk of serious cardiovascular thrombotic events, myocardial infarction (MI), and stroke, which can be fatal. This risk may increase with duration of use. Patients with cardiovascular disease or risk factors for cardiovascular disease may be at a greater risk.

Naproxen/esomeprazole is contraindicated for the treatment of perioperative pain in the setting of coronary artery bypass graft surgery (CABG).

GI risk – Nonsteroidal anti-inflammatory drugs (NSAIDs), including naproxen, cause an increased risk of serious GI adverse events, including bleeding, ulceration, and perforation of the stomach or intestines, which can be fatal. These events can occur at any time during use and without warning symptoms. Elderly patients are at a greater risk for serious GI events.

Indications

➤*Ankylosing spondylitis/osteoarthritis/rheumatoid arthritis:* For the relief of signs and symptoms of osteoarthritis, rheumatoid arthritis, and ankylosing spondylitis and to decrease the risk of developing gastric ulcers in patients at risk of developing NSAID-associated gastric ulcers.

Administration and Dosage

➤*General dosing considerations:* Use the lowest effective dose for the shortest duration consistent with individual patient treatment goals.

Naproxen/esomeprazole does not allow for administration of a lower daily dose of esomeprazole. If a dose of esomeprazole lower than a total daily dose of 40 mg is more appropriate, a different treatment should be considered.

➤*Adults:*

Ankylosing spondylitis/osteoarthritis/rheumatoid arthritis – *Usual dosage:* 1 tablet twice daily taken at least 30 minutes before meals.

➤*Elderly:* Use caution when high doses are required; some dosage adjustment may be required. Use the lowest effective dose.

➤*Renal function impairment:* Naproxen-containing products are not recommended for use in patients with moderate to severe or severe renal impairment (creatinine clearance [CrCl] less than 30 mL/min).

➤*Hepatic function impairment:* Monitor patients with mild to moderate hepatic impairment closely, and consider a possible dose reduction based on the naproxen component of naproxen/esomeprazole.

Naproxen/esomeprazole is not recommended in patients with severe hepatic impairment (Child-Pugh class C) because esomeprazole dosages should not exceed 20 mg daily in these patients.

➤*Administration:* The tablets are to be swallowed whole with liquid. Do not split, chew, crush, or dissolve the tablet. Administer at least 30 minutes before meals.

➤*Storage/Stability:* Store at 25°C (77°F); excursions are permitted between 15° and 30°C (59° and 86°F). Store in the original container and keep the bottle tightly closed to protect from moisture. Dispense in a tight container if package is subdivided.

NONSTEROIDAL ANTI-INFLAMMATORY AGENTS

WARNING

All nonsteroidal anti-inflammatory drugs –

Cardiovascular risk: Nonsteroidal anti-inflammatory drugs (NSAIDs) may cause an increased risk of serious cardiovascular thrombotic events, myocardial infarction (MI), and stroke, which can be fatal. This risk may increase with duration of use. Patients with cardiovascular disease or risk factors for cardiovascular disease may be at greater risk.

NSAIDs are contraindicated for treatment of perioperative pain in the setting of coronary artery bypass graft (CABG) surgery.

GI risk: NSAIDs cause an increased risk of serious GI adverse reactions, including bleeding, inflammation, ulceration, and perforation of the stomach or intestines, which can be fatal. These events can occur at any time during use and without warning symptoms. Elderly patients are at greater risk for serious GI events.

Ketorolac only – Ketorolac is indicated for the short-term (up to 5 days) management of moderately severe acute pain that requires analgesia at the opioid level in adults. It is not indicated for minor or chronic painful conditions. Ketorolac is a potent NSAID analgesic, and its administration carries many risks. The resulting NSAID-related adverse reactions can be serious in certain patients for whom ketorolac is indicated, especially when the drug is used inappropriately. Increasing the dose of ketorolac beyond the label recommendations will not provide better efficacy but will result in increasing the risk of developing serious adverse reactions.

GI effects: Ketorolac can cause peptic ulcers, GI bleeding, or perforation. Therefore, it is contraindicated in patients with active peptic ulcer disease, in patients with recent GI bleeding or perforation, and in patients with a history of peptic ulcer disease or GI bleeding.

Renal effects: Ketorolac is contraindicated in patients with advanced renal function impairment or in patients at risk for renal failure due to volume depletion.

Risk of bleeding: Ketorolac inhibits platelet function and is, therefore, contraindicated in patients with suspected or confirmed cerebrovascular bleeding, hemorrhagic diathesis, or incomplete hemostasis, and those at high risk of bleeding.

WARNING (cont.)

Ketorolac is contraindicated as prophylactic analgesic before any major surgery and is contraindicated intraoperatively when hemostasis is critical because of the increased risk of bleeding.

Hypersensitivity: Hypersensitivity reactions ranging from bronchospasm to anaphylactic shock have occurred and appropriate counteractive measures must be available when administering the first dose of ketorolac intravenous (IV)/intramuscular (IM). Ketorolac is contraindicated in patients who have previously demonstrated hypersensitivity to ketorolac or allergic manifestations to aspirin or other NSAIDs.

Intrathecal or epidural administration: Ketorolac is contraindicated for neuraxial (epidural or intrathecal) administration because of its alcohol content.

Labor, delivery, and breast-feeding: Ketorolac is contraindicated in labor and delivery because, through its prostaglandin synthesis inhibitory effect, it may adversely affect fetal circulation and inhibit uterine contractions.

The use of ketorolac is contraindicated in breast-feeding mothers because of the potential adverse effects of prostaglandin-inhibiting drugs on neonates.

Concomitant use with NSAIDs: Ketorolac is contraindicated in patients currently receiving aspirin or NSAIDs because of the cumulative risks of inducing serious NSAID-related adverse reactions.

Dosage and administration: Oral ketorolac is indicated only as continuation therapy to ketorolac IV/IM, and the combined duration of use of ketorolac IV/IM and oral ketorolac is not to exceed 5 days because of the increased risk of adverse reactions.

The recommended total daily dose of ketorolac oral (maximum 40 mg) is significantly lower than that for ketorolac IV/IM (maximum 120 mg).

Special populations: Ketorolac dosage should be adjusted for patients 65 years of age and older, for patients less than 50 kg (110 lb) of body weight, and for patients with moderately elevated serum creatinine. Doses of ketorolac IV/IM are not to exceed 60 mg (total dose per day) in these patients. Ketorolac is indicated as a single-dose therapy in pediatric patients, not to exceed 30 mg for IM administration and 15 mg for IV administration.

Indications

NSAIDs: Summary of Indications

Indications (✓-Labeled; X- Unlabeled)	Celecoxib	Diclofenac potassium	Diclofenac sodium/ Diclofenac sodium ER	Etodolac	Fenoprofen	Flurbiprofen	Ibuprofen injection	Ibuprofen oral	Indomethacin	Indomethacin sustained release	Ketoprofen	Ketoprofen sustained release	Ketorolac	Meclofenamate	Mefenamic acid	Meloxicam	Nabumetone	Naproxen	Oxaprozin	Piroxicam	Sulindac	Tolmetin
Rheumatoid arthritis (RA)	✓	✓[o]	✓	✓	✓	✓		✓	✓	✓	✓	✓		✓		✓	✓	✓	✓	✓	✓	✓
Osteoarthritis (OA)	✓	✓[o]	✓	✓	✓	✓		✓	✓	✓	✓	✓		✓		✓	✓	✓	✓	✓	✓	✓
Ankylosing spondylitis			✓[a]	X[k]		X[k]			✓	✓								✓			✓	
Mild to moderate pain				✓	✓			✓						✓	✓[b]							
Pain	✓	✓[p]					✓[l]				✓		✓[c]					✓				
Primary dysmenorrhea	✓	✓				X[k]		✓			✓			✓	✓			✓		X[k]		
Juvenile idiopathic arthritis (JIA)		X[k]	X[j]		X[k]						X[j]							✓		X[k]	X[k]	✓
Tendinitis				X[k]					✓	✓								✓			✓	
Bursitis				X[k]					✓	✓								✓			✓	
Acute painful shoulder			X[k]	X[k]					✓	✓								✓			✓	
Acute gout				X[k]		X[k]			✓									✓			✓	
Fever							✓[l]	✓[d]														
Familial adenomatous polyposis (FAP)	✓																					
Sunburn									X[e]													
Migraine		✓[q]																				
Abortive (acute attack)						X[k]		X[k]					X (IV/IM)[j]	X[k]	X[k]			X[k]				
Prophylactic					X[k]			X[k]	X[k]		X[k]			X[k]				X[k]				
Menstrual					X[k]				X[k]		X[k]			X[k]	X[k]			X[k]				
Cluster headache									X[k]													
Polyhydramnios									X[k]													
Acne vulgaris, resistant								X[k]														
Menorrhagia														X[k]								
Premenstrual syndrome															X[k]			X[k]				
Cystoid macular edema									X[e]													
Closure of persistent patent ductus arteriosus							✓[m]		✓[f]													
DTP[n] adverse reaction prevention								X[h]														
DTP adverse reaction prevention in patients at risk for seizures								X[g]														
Lung cancer prevention	X[j]																					
Patent ductus arteriosus								X[j]														
Preterm labor									X[i]													
Prevention of colorectal cancer	X[i]																					
Schizophrenia (adjunctive therapy)	X[i]																					

[a] Sodium only, not sodium ER.
[b] Therapy not to exceed 1 week.
[c] Therapy not to exceed 5 days.
[d] In children only.
[e] Topical formulation.
[f] IV formulation only.
[g] Good documentation.
[h] Fair documentation.
[i] Safety concerns.
[j] Insufficient documentation.
[k] Not rated.
[l] Excluding ibuprofen lysine injection.
[m] Ibuprofen lysine injection only.
[n] DTP = diphtheria and tetanus toxoids and pertussis.
[o] Tablets only.
[p] Capsules/tablets only.
[q] Oral solution only.

➤*Concomitant therapy:* Concomitant therapy with other second-line drugs (eg, gold salts) demonstrates additional therapeutic benefit. Whether they can be used with partially effective doses of corticosteroids for a "steroid-sparing" effect and result in greater improvement is not established.

Use with salicylates is not recommended; greater benefit is not achieved, and the potential for adverse reactions is increased. The use of aspirin with NSAIDs may cause a decrease in blood levels of the nonaspirin drug.

➤*Idiopathic heavy menstrual blood loss:* For the treatment of idiopathic heavy menstrual blood loss (**meclofenamate** only).

➤*Off-label uses:* Refer to individual monographs for further information.

Juvenile idiopathic arthritis –
Diclofenac (oral): [4] = Insufficient documentation.
Indomethacin: [5] = Poor documentation.
Ketoprofen: [4] = Insufficient documentation.

Lung cancer prevention –
Celecoxib: [4] = Insufficient documentation.

Patent ductus arteriosus –
Ibuprofen (oral): [4] = Insufficient documentation.

Postherpetic neuralgia –
Indomethacin (topical): [5] = Poor documentation.
Piroxicam (topical): [5] = Poor documentation.

Preterm labor –
Celecoxib: [5] = Poor documentation.
Indomethacin: [3] = Safety concerns.

Prevention of adverse reactions with DTP vaccination –
Ibuprofen: [2] = Fair documentation.

Prevention of adverse reactions with DTP vaccination in patients at risk for seizures –
Ibuprofen: [1] = Good documentation.

Prevention of colorectal cancer –
Celecoxib: [3] = Safety concerns.

Schizophrenia (adjunctive therapy) –
Celecoxib: [3] = Safety concerns.

Treatment of migraine (adults) –

Ketorolac (IM): [4] = Insufficient documentation.

Ketorolac (IV): [4] = Insufficient documentation.

Actions

➤*Pharmacology:* Clinically, there are no clear guidelines to assist in selecting the most appropriate agent. Base selection on clinical experience, patient convenience, adverse effects, and cost.

NSAIDs exhibit antipyretic, analgesic, and anti-inflammatory activities. The major mechanism of therapeutic effects is believed to result from inhibition of prostaglandin synthesis. NSAIDs inhibit cyclooxygenase (COX), the enzyme that catalyzes the synthesis of cyclic endoperoxides from arachidonic acid to form prostaglandins. In the gastric mucosa, prostaglandins decrease gastric acid synthesis, stimulate the production of glutathione that scavenges superoxides, promote the generation of a protective barrier of mucus and bicarbonate, and promote adequate blood flow to the gastric mucosal cells. Prostaglandin in the kidneys modulates intrarenal plasma flow and electrolyte balance.

Two COX isoenzymes have been identified: COX-1 and COX-2. COX-1, expressed constitutively, is synthesized continuously and is present in all tissues and cell types, most notably in platelets, endothelial cells, the GI tract, renal microvasculature, glomerulus, and collecting ducts. COX-1 is important for homeostatic maintenance, such as platelet aggregation, the regulation of blood flow in the kidney and stomach, and the regulation of gastric acid secretion. Inhibition of COX-1 activity is considered a major contributor to NSAID GI toxicity. COX-2 is considered an inducible isoenzyme, although there is some constitutive expression in the kidney, brain, bone, female reproductive system, neoplasias, and GI tract. The function of the COX-2 isoenzyme is induced during pain and inflammatory stimuli.

Many NSAIDs inhibit both COX-1 and COX-2. Most NSAIDs are mainly COX-1 selective (eg, **aspirin**, **ketoprofen**, **indomethacin**, **piroxicam**, **sulindac**). Others are considered slightly selective for COX-1 (eg, **ibuprofen**, **naproxen**, **diclofenac**) and others may be considered slightly selective for COX-2 (eg, **etodolac**, **nabumetone**, **meloxicam**). The mechanism of action of **celecoxib** is primarily selective inhibition of COX-2; at therapeutic concentrations, the COX-1 isoenzyme is not inhibited, thus GI toxicity may be decreased.

Other mechanisms that may contribute to NSAID anti-inflammatory activity include the reduction of superoxide radicals, induction of apoptosis, inhibition of adhesion molecule expression, decrease of nitric oxide synthase, decrease of proinflammatory cytokine levels (tumor necrosis factor-alpha, interleukin-1), modification of lymphocyte activity, and alteration of cellular membrane functions.

Central analgesic activity has been demonstrated in animal pain models by some NSAIDs, such as diclofenac, ibuprofen, indomethacin, and ketoprofen. This may be because of the interference of prostaglandin formation or with transmitters or modulators in the nociceptive system. Other proposals include the central action mediated by opioid peptides, inhibition of serotonin release, or inhibition of excitatory amino acids or N-methyl-D-aspartate receptors. Antipyretic activity of NSAIDs is because of the inhibition of prostaglandin E_2 (PGE_2) synthesis in circumventricular organs in and near the preoptic hypothalamic area. Infections, tissue damage, inflammation, graft rejection, malignancies, and other disease states enhance the formation of cytokines that increase PGE_2 production. PGE_2 triggers the hypothalamus to promote increases in heat generation and decreases in heat loss.

Rheumatoid arthritis – No one NSAID has demonstrated a clear advantage for the treatment of RA. Individual patients have demonstrated variability in response to certain NSAIDs. Anti-inflammatory activity is shown by reduced joint swelling, reduced pain, reduced duration of morning stiffness and disease activity, increased mobility, and by enhanced functional capacity (demonstrated by an increase in grip strength, delay in time to onset of fatigue, and a decrease in time to walk 50 feet).

Osteoarthritis – Improvement is demonstrated by increased range of motion and a reduction in the following: Tenderness with pressure, pain in motion and at rest, night pain, stiffness and swelling, overall disease activity, and by increased range of motion. There are no data to suggest superiority of one NSAID over another as therapy for OA in terms of efficacy and toxicity. NSAIDs for OA are to be used intermittently if possible during painful episodes and prescribed at the minimum effective dose to reduce the potential of renal and GI toxicities. Do not use **indomethacin** long term because of its greater toxicity profile and its potential for accelerating progression of OA.

Acute gouty arthritis, ankylosing spondylitis – Relief of pain; reduced fever, swelling, redness, and tenderness; and increased range of motion have occurred with treatment of NSAIDs.

Dysmenorrhea – Excess prostaglandins may produce uterine hyperactivity. These agents reduce elevated prostaglandin levels in menstrual fluid and reduce resting and active intrauterine pressure, as well as frequency of uterine contractions. Probable mechanism of action is to inhibit prostaglandin synthesis rather than provide analgesia.

➤*Pharmacokinetics:*

Absorption/Distribution – NSAIDs are rapidly and almost completely absorbed. **Naproxen sodium** is more rapidly absorbed than the **naproxen** formulation and is used when more prompt relief is desired. **Diclofenac potassium** is formulated to release diclofenac in the stomach. **Diclofenac sodium** resists dissolution in the low pH of gastric fluid but allows a rapid release of the drug in the higher-pH environment in the duodenum. In general, food delays absorption but does not significantly affect total amount absorbed. However, the rate of absorption of **meclofenamic acid** decreased by 26% and maximum plasma concentration was delayed by 3 hours when administered 0.5 hours after a meal. In general, administer NSAIDs with meals to minimize GI effects. Some NSAIDs can be given with an aluminum and magnesium hydroxide antacid, which does not affect absorption. All NSAIDs are highly protein bound (more than 90%). Because **diclofenac** is enteric coated, its time to peak levels are delayed despite its relatively short half-life.

Metabolism/Excretion – Most NSAIDs have negligible hepatic metabolism, except for **etodolac**, **ketorolac**, **nabumetone**, **oxaprozin**, and **meloxicam**. **Celecoxib** and **mefenamic acid** undergo metabolism via cytochrome P450 2C9 isoenzymes. Excretion is via the kidney, primarily as metabolites. **Sulindac** and **nabumetone** are inactive prodrugs converted by the liver to active metabolites.

NSAID Pharmacokinetic Parameters

NSAID	Bioavailability	Half-life	Volume of distribution	Clearance	Peak	Protein binding	Renal elimination	Fecal elimination
Acetic acids								
Diclofenac	50 to 60%	2 h	1.3 to 1.4 L/kg	350 mL/min	2 h	> 99%	65%	—
Indomethacin	98%	4.5 h	0.29 L/kg	0.084 L/h/kg	2 h	90%	60%	33%
Sulindac	90%	7.8 h	NS[a]	≈ 2.71 L/h	2 to 4 h	> 93%	50%	25%
Tolmetin	NS[a]	2 to 7 h	NS[a]	NS[a]	0.5 to 1 h	NS [a]	≈ 100%	—
COX-2 inhibitor								
Celecoxib	NS[a]	11 h	400 L	27.7 L/h	3 h	97%	27%	57%
Fenamates								
Meclofenamate	≈ 100%	1.3 h	23 L	206 mL/min	0.5 to 2 h	> 99%	70%	30%
Mefenamic acid	NS[a]	2 h	1.06 L/kg	21.23 L/h	2 to 4 h	> 90%	52%	20%
Naphthylalkanones								
Nambumetone	> 80%	22.5 h	0.1 to 0.2 L/kg	26.1 mL/min	9 to 12 h	> 99%	80%	9%
Oxicams								
Piroxicam	NS[a]	50 h	0.15 L/kg	0.002 to 0.003 L/kg/h	3 to 5 h	98.5%	NS[a]	NS[a]
Meloxicam	89%	15 to 20 h	10 L	7 to 9 mL/min	4 to 5 h	99.4%	50%	50%
Propionic acids								
Fenoprofen	NS[a]	3 h	NS[a]	NS[a]	2 h	99%	90%	—
Flurbiprofen	NS[a]	5.7 h	0.1 to 0.2 L/kg	1.13 L/h	≈ 1.5 h	> 99%	> 70%	—
Ibuprofen injection	—	2.22 to 2.44 h	—	—	—	> 99%	—	—
Ibuprofen oral	> 80%	1.8 to 2 h	0.15 L/kg	≈ 3 to 3.5 L/h	1 to 2 h	99%	45 to 79%	—
Ketoprofen	90%	2.1 h	0.1 L/kg	6.9 L/h	0.5 to 2 h	> 99%	80%	—

NSAID Pharmacokinetic Parameters								
NSAID	Bioavailability	Half-life	Volume of distribution	Clearance	Peak	Protein binding	Renal elimination	Fecal elimination
Ketoprofen ER	90%	5.4 h	0.1 L/kg	6.8 L/h	6 to 7 h	> 99%	80%	—
Naproxen	95%	12 to 17 h	0.16 L/kg	0.13 mL/min/kg	2 to 4 h	> 99%	95%	—
Oxaprozin	95%	42 to 50 h	10 to 12.5 L	0.25 to 0.34 L/h	3 to 5 h	> 99%	65%	35%
Pyranocarboxylic acid								
Etodolac	≥ 80%	7.3 h	0.362 L/kg	47 mL/h/kg	≈ 1.5 h	> 99%	72%	16%
Pyrrolizine carboxylic acid								
Ketorolac	100%	5 to 6 h	≈ 0.2 L/kg	≈ 0.025 L/h/kg	2 to 3 h	99%	91%	6%

[a] NS = not studied.

Contraindications

Hypersensitivity to the drug or any components; for the treatment of perioperative pain in the setting of CABG surgery; patients in whom aspirin or other NSAIDs have induced symptoms of asthma, rhinitis, urticaria, nasal polyps, angioedema, bronchospasm, and other symptoms of allergic or anaphylactoid reactions.

➤*Fenoprofen or mefenamic acid:* Preexisting renal disease.

➤*Mefenamic acid:* Active ulceration or chronic inflammation of either the upper or lower GI tract.

➤*Indomethacin suppositories:* History of proctitis or recent rectal bleeding.

➤*Celecoxib:* Hypersensitivity to sulfonamides.

➤*Ketorolac:* Active peptic ulcer disease; recent GI bleeding or perforation; a history of peptic ulcer disease or GI bleeding; advanced renal impairment or patients at risk for renal failure because of volume depletion; labor and delivery because, through its prostaglandin synthesis inhibitory effect, it may adversely affect fetal circulation and inhibit uterine contractions, thus increasing the risk of uterine hemorrhage; breast-feeding mothers because of the potential adverse effects of prostaglandin-inhibiting drugs on neonates; previously demonstrated hypersensitivity to ketorolac tromethamine, allergic manifestations to aspirin or other NSAIDs; as prophylactic analgesic before any major surgery; intraoperatively when hemostasis is critical because of the increased risk of bleeding; suspected or confirmed cerebrovascular bleeding, hemorrhagic diathesis, incomplete hemostasis and those at high risk of bleeding; patients currently receiving acetaminophen or NSAIDs because of the cumulative risks of inducing serious NSAID-related adverse events; for neuraxial (epidural or intrathecal) administration because of its alcohol content; concomitant use with probenecid.

Warnings/Precautions

➤*Cardiovascular thrombotic events:* Clinical trials of several COX-2 selective and nonselective NSAIDs of up to 3 years' duration have shown an increased risk of serious cardiovascular thrombotic events, MI, and stroke, which can be fatal. All NSAIDs, both COX-2 selective and nonselective, may have similar risk. Patients with known cardiovascular disease or risk factors for cardiovascular disease may be at greater risk. To minimize the potential risk for adverse cardiovascular events in patients treated with an NSAID, use the lowest effective dose for the shortest duration possible. Health care providers and patients should remain alert for the development of these events, even in the absence of previous cardiovascular symptoms.

➤*GI effects:* Serious GI toxicity such as inflammation, bleeding, ulceration and perforation of the stomach, small, or large intestine, can occur at any time, with or without warning symptoms, in patients treated long term with NSAID therapy. Although minor upper GI problems (eg, dyspepsia) are common, usually developing early in therapy, remain alert for ulceration and bleeding in patients treated long term with NSAIDs even in the absence of previous GI tract symptoms. In patients observed in clinical trials of several months to 2 years duration, symptomatic upper GI ulcers, gross bleeding, or perforation occurred in approximately 1% of patients treated for 3 to 6 months, and in approximately 2% to 4% of patients treated for 1 year. These trends continue, thus increasing the likelihood of developing a serious GI event at some time during the course of therapy. However, even short-term therapy is not without risk. In patients receiving **nabumetone**, the incidence of peptic ulcers was 0.3% at 3 to 6 months, 0.5% at 1 year, and 0.8% at 2 years. Only 1 in 5 patients who develop a serious upper GI adverse event on NSAID therapy is symptomatic. Inform patients about the signs or symptoms of serious GI toxicity and what steps to take if they occur.

Studies have shown that patients with a history of peptic ulcer disease or GI bleeding and who use NSAIDs, have a greater than 10-fold risk for developing a GI bleed than patients with neither of these risk factors. In addition, treatment with oral corticosteroids or anticoagulants, longer duration of NSAID therapy, smoking, alcoholism, older age, and poor general health status contribute to an increased risk for a GI bleed. High-dose NSAIDs probably carry a greater risk of these reactions, although controlled clinical trials generally do not show this. In considering the use of relatively large doses (within the recommended dosage range), sufficient benefit should offset the potential increased risk of GI toxicity. To minimize the potential risk for an adverse GI event, use the lowest effective dose for the shortest possible duration. For high-risk patients, consider alternate therapies that do not involve NSAIDs.

Ketorolac is contraindicated in patients with previously documented peptic ulcers and GI bleeding. In patients with active peptic ulcer and active RA, attempt to treat the arthritis with nonulcerogenic drugs. Deaths have occurred. GI bleeding is associated with higher morbidity and mortality in patients acutely ill with other conditions, elderly patients, and patients with hemorrhagic disorders. In patients with active GI bleeding or an active peptic ulcer, institute an appropriate ulcer regimen, and weigh the benefits of therapy with the NSAID against possible hazards, and carefully monitor the patient's progress. When the NSAID is given to patients with a history of upper or lower GI tract disease, it should be given under close supervision and only after consulting the Adverse Reactions section.

Do not give **indomethacin** to patients with active GI lesions or a history of recurrent GI lesions unless the high risk is warranted and patients can be monitored closely. To reduce GI effects, give NSAIDs after meals, with food, or with antacids (does not apply to enteric-coated **diclofenac**).

Higher doses of **meloxicam** (eg, long-term daily 30 mg doses) were associated with increased risk of serious GI effects. Do not exceed daily doses of 15 mg.

If diarrhea occurs with **mefenamic acid**, or diarrhea, GI irritation, and abdominal pain occur with **meclofenamate**, reduce dosage or temporarily discontinue use. Some patients may be unable to tolerate further therapy with these agents.

➤*CNS effects:* **Indomethacin** may aggravate depression or other psychiatric disturbances, epilepsy, and parkinsonism; use with considerable caution. If severe CNS adverse reactions develop, discontinue the drug. Some of these agents also may cause headaches (highest incidence with **fenoprofen**, **indomethacin**, **ketorolac**, and **celecoxib**). If headache persists despite dosage reduction, discontinue use.

➤*Corticosteroid use:* NSAIDs cannot be expected to be a substitute for corticosteroids or to treat corticosteroid insufficiency. Abrupt discontinuation of corticosteroids may lead to disease exacerbation.

➤*Functional class IV rheumatoid arthritis patients (incapacitated, largely or wholly bedridden, confined to wheelchair):* Safety and efficacy are not established.

➤*Steroid dosage:* If corticosteroid dosage is reduced or eliminated during NSAID therapy, reduce dosage slowly and observe patient closely for evidence of adverse effects, including adrenal insufficiency and exacerbation of symptoms (see Glucocorticoids monograph).

➤*Porphyria:* Avoid the use of NSAIDs in patients with hepatic porphyria. To date, 1 patient has been described in whom **diclofenac** probably triggered a clinical attack of porphyria. The postulated mechanism demonstrated in rats for causing such attacks by diclofenac, as well as some other NSAIDs, is through stimulation of the porphyria precursor delta-aminolevulinic acid (ALA).

➤*Aseptic meningitis:* Aseptic meningitis with fever and coma has been observed on rare occasions in patients on NSAIDs therapy. Although it is probably more likely to occur in patients with systemic lupus erythematosus (SLE) and related connective tissue diseases, it has been reported in patients who do not have an underlying chronic disease. If signs or symptoms of meningitis develop in a patient on NSAID therapy, consider the possibility of it being related to the NSAID.

➤*Platelet aggregation:* NSAIDs can inhibit platelet aggregation; the effect is reversible, quantitatively less, and of shorter duration than that seen with aspirin. These agents prolong bleeding time (within normal range) in healthy subjects. This may be exaggerated in patients with underlying hemostatic defects; use with caution and carefully monitor in patients with intrinsic coagulation defects and in those on anticoagulant therapy.

➤*Preexisting asthma:* Approximately 10% of patients with asthma may have aspirin-sensitive asthma. The use of aspirin in patients with aspirin-sensitive asthma has been associated with severe bronchospasm, which can be fatal. Because cross-reactivity, including bronchospasm, between aspirin and other NSAIDs has been reported in such aspirin-sensitive patients, do not administer NSAIDs to patients with this form of aspirin sensitivity, and use the drug with caution in patients with preexisting asthma.

➤*Hematologic effects:* Decreased hemoglobin or hematocrit levels have rarely required discontinuation. Anemia may be because of fluid retention, GI blood loss, or an incompletely described effect upon erythropoiesis. If anemia is suspected in patients on long-term therapy, determine hemoglobin and hematocrit values. Frequently determine hemoglobin values in patients with initial values 10 g/dL or less who are to receive long-term therapy.

Patients on long-term treatments should have their complete blood cell count and a chemistry profile checked periodically. Low white blood cell counts occur rarely, are transient, and usually return to normal while therapy continues. Persistent leukopenia, granulocytopenia, or thrombocytopenia warrants further evaluation and may require discontinuing the drug.

Postoperative hematomas and other signs of wound bleeding have occurred with perioperative IM use of **ketorolac**. Exercise caution when administering pre- or intraoperatively and when administering perioperatively if strict hemostasis is critical.

➤*Cardiovascular effects:* May cause fluid retention and peripheral edema. Use caution in compromised cardiac function, hypertension, in patients on long-term diuretic therapy, or other conditions predisposing to fluid retention. Agents may be associated with significant deterioration of circulatory hemodynamics in severe heart failure and hyponatremia, presumably because of inhibition of prostaglandin-dependent compensatory mechanisms.

NSAIDs can lead to onset of new hypertension or worsening or preexisting hypertension, either of which may contribute to the increased incidence of cardiovascular events. Use NSAIDs with caution in patients with hypertension. Monitor blood pressure closely during the initiation of NSAID treatment and throughout the course of therapy.

➤*Ophthalmologic effects:* Perform ophthalmological studies in patients who develop eye complaints during therapy. Effects include blurred or diminished vision, scotomata, changes in color vision, corneal deposits, and retinal disturbances, including maculas. Discontinue therapy if ocular changes are noted. Blurred vision may be significant and warrants thorough examination, including central visual fields and color vision testing. These changes may be asymptomatic; perform periodic examinations in patients on prolonged therapy.

➤*Infection:* NSAIDs may mask the usual signs of infection. Use with extra care in the presence of existing controlled infection. The pharmacologic activity of NSAIDs in reducing inflammation and possibly fever may diminish the utility of these diagnostic signs in detecting complications of presumed noninfectious, painful conditions.

➤*Renal effects:* Acute renal insufficiency, interstitial nephritis with hematuria, nephrotic syndrome, proteinuria, hyperkalemia, hyponatremia, renal papillary necrosis, and other renal medullary changes may occur.

Long-term administration of NSAIDs has resulted in renal papillary necrosis and other renal medullary changes. Renal toxicity also has been seen in patients in whom renal prostaglandins have a compensatory role in the maintenance of renal perfusion. In these patients, administration of NSAIDs may cause dose-dependent reduction in prostaglandin formation and, secondarily, in renal blood flow, which may precipitate overt renal decompensation. Patients at greatest risk of this reaction are those with impaired renal function, heart failure, liver dysfunction, those taking diuretics and angiotensin-converting enzyme (ACE) inhibitors, and elderly patients. Discontinuation of NSAID therapy is usually followed by recovery to the pretreatment state.

Exercise caution when initiating treatment with NSAIDs in patients with considerable dehydration. It is advisable to rehydrate patients first and then start therapy with NSAIDs. Correct hypovolemia before treatment with **ketorolac** is initiated. They are not recommended in patients with preexisting kidney disease.

Acute renal insufficiency – Patients with preexisting renal disease or compromised renal perfusion are at greatest risk for acute renal insufficiency. A form of renal toxicity seen in patients with prerenal conditions leads to reduced renal blood flow or blood volume. NSAID use may cause a dose-dependent reduction in prostaglandin formation and precipitate overt renal decompensation. Patients at greatest risk are elderly patients; premature infants; those with heart failure, renal, or hepatic dysfunction, SLE, chronic glomerulonephritis, dehydration, diabetes mellitus, or impaired renal function; those taking ACE inhibitors; septicemia; pyelonephritis; concomitant use of any nephrotoxic drug; extracellular volume depletion from any cause; and those on diuretics. Recovery usually follows discontinuation.

Those patients at high risk who take NSAIDs long term should have renal function monitored if they have signs or symptoms that may be consistent with mild azotemia (eg, malaise, fatigue, loss of appetite). Patients occasionally may develop some elevation of serum creatinine and serum urea nitrogen (BUN) levels without any signs and symptoms. There may also be substantial proteinuria and, on renal biopsy, electron microscopy has shown foot process fusion and T-lymphocyte infiltration in the renal interstitium.

Interstitial nephritis – Interstitial nephritis has occurred with increased frequency in patients receiving NSAIDs and may be due to altered prostaglandin metabolism.

GU tract problems have occurred in patients taking **fenoprofen**, most frequently, dysuria, cystitis, hematuria, interstitial nephritis, and nephrotic syndrome. This may be preceded by fever, rash, arthralgia, oliguria, and azotemia, and may progress to anuria. Rapid recovery followed early recognition and drug withdrawal.

Hyperkalemia – Another potentially serious NSAID-induced renal electrolyte abnormality is hyperkalemia. NSAIDs tend to blunt prostaglandin-mediated renin release, leading to diminished aldosterone formation and, hence, decreased potassium excretion. NSAIDs can augment sodium and chloride reabsorption within the renal tubule in the setting of diminished glomerular filtration rate by opposing natriuretic and diuretic prostaglandins. This decreases the delivery of intraluminal sodium for sodium-potassium exchange at the distal nephron.

Papillary necrosis – Papillary necrosis may present as an acute or chronic form of NSAID nephropathy in the setting of massive NSAID overdose in a dehydrated patient with preexisting normal renal function. The chronic form is associated with analgesic-abuse nephropathy.

➤*Hepatic effects:* Borderline liver function test elevations may occur in approximately 15% of patients and may progress, remain essentially unchanged, or become transient with continued therapy. The ALT test is probably the most sensitive indicator of liver dysfunction. Meaningful (at least 3 times the upper limit of normal) AST or ALT elevations occurred in approximately 1% of patients. If symptoms or signs suggesting liver dysfunction or an abnormal test occurs, evaluate for more severe hepatic reactions. Severe reactions, including jaundice and fatal fulminant hepatitis, liver necrosis, and hepatic failure have occurred rarely, some with fatal outcomes. Evaluate a patient with symptoms and signs suggesting liver dysfunction, or in whom an abnormal liver test has occurred, for evidence of the development of more severe hepatic reactions while on therapy with NSAIDs. If an NSAID is to be used in the presence of impaired liver function, it must be done under strict observation. Discontinue treatment if abnormal tests persist or worsen, if clinical signs and symptoms consistent with liver disease develop, or if systemic manifestations occur (eg, eosinophilia, rash).

➤*Pancreatitis:* Pancreatitis has occurred in patients receiving **sulindac**. If pancreatitis is suspected, discontinue the drug, start supportive therapy, and monitor closely (eg, serum and urine amylase, amylase/creatinine clearance ratio, electrolytes, serum calcium, glucose, lipase). Check for other causes of pancreatitis as well as for conditions that mimic pancreatitis.

➤*Auditory effects:* Perform periodic auditory function tests during long-term **fenoprofen** therapy in patients with impaired hearing.

➤*Heavy menstrual blood loss evaluation:* Prior to prescribing **meclofenamate** for heavy blood flow and primary dysmenorrhea, make a thorough risk/benefit assessment that takes into account the results described in the clinical pharmacology section. It is recommended that meclofenamate treatment not be prescribed for heavy menstrual flow without establishing its idiopathic nature. Fully evaluate spotting or bleeding between cycles and do not treat with meclofenamate. Worsening of menstrual blood loss or excessive blood loss failing to respond to meclofenamate should also be evaluated by an appropriate workup and not treated with meclofenamate.

➤*Dermatologic effects:* NSAIDs can cause serious skin adverse reactions, such as exfoliative dermatitis, Stevens-Johnson syndrome, and toxic epidermal necrolysis, which can be fatal. These serious events may occur without warning.

A combination of dermatologic and allergic signs and symptoms suggestive of serum sickness have occasionally occurred in conjunction with the use of **piroxicam**. These include arthralgias, pruritus, fever, fatigue, and rash including vesiculobullous reactions and exfoliative dermatitis.

➤*Concomitant NSAID therapy:* Do not use **naproxen sodium** and **naproxen** concomitantly; both drugs circulate as naproxen anion.

Do not use **diclofenac** immediate-release, delayed-release, and extended-release tablets concomitantly with other diclofenac-containing products because they also circulate in plasma as diclofenac anion.

➤*Hypersensitivity reactions:* A potentially fatal apparent hypersensitivity syndrome has occurred with **sulindac**; this syndrome may include constitutional symptoms, cutaneous findings, involvement of major organs, conjunctivitis, or other less specific findings. The clinical picture of hypersensitivity reactions may vary from vasomotor rhinitis, urticaria, and angioedema to serious bronchoconstriction and, in some cases, anaphylactic shock. This may be because of an allergic immunological hypersensitivity reaction or a pseudoallergic reaction characterized by mast-cell degranulation by complement components, histamine liberation by drugs, and interference with endogenous eicosanoid biosynthesis. The former mechanism appears to be responsible for the anaphylactic shock or urticaria that may develop after taking amidopyrine or noramidopyrine, the latter for the bronchoconstriction encountered after ingestion of aspirin, noramidopyrine, or of aminophenazone and other pyrazole drugs.

Rarely, fever and other evidence of hypersensitivity, including abnormalities in 1 or more liver function tests and severe skin reactions, have occurred during therapy with sulindac. Fatalities have occurred in these patients. Hepatitis, jaundice, or both, with or without fever, may occur usually within the first 1 to 3 months of therapy. Consider determination of liver function whenever a patient on therapy with sulindac develops unexplained fever, rash, or other dermatologic reactions or constitutional symptoms. If unexplained fever or other evidence of hypersensitivity occurs, discontinue therapy with sulindac. The elevated temperature and abnormalities in liver function caused by sulindac characteristically have reverted to normal after discontinuation of therapy. Administration of sulindac should not be reinstituted in such patients.

Anaphylactoid reactions – Anaphylactoid reactions have occurred in patients without known exposure to NSAIDs, but they typically occur in asthmatic patients who experience rhinitis with or without nasal polyps, or who exhibit severe, potentially fatal bronchospasm after taking aspirin or other NSAIDs. Anaphylactoid reactions have occurred in patients with aspirin hypersensitivity and in patients who discontinued **tolmetin**, and then restarted it. These reactions appear to occur more often with tolmetin than other NSAIDs not structurally related but data conflict. Refer to Management of Acute Hypersensitivity Reactions.

➤*Renal function impairment:* NSAID metabolites are eliminated primarily by kidneys; use with caution in those with renal function impairment. Assess renal function before and during therapy. Monitor serum creatinine or creatinine clearance. Reduce dosage to avoid excessive accumulation.

In cases of advanced kidney disease, treatment with **diclofenac**, **piroxicam** and **meloxicam** is not recommended. However, if NSAID therapy must be initiated, close monitoring of the patient's kidney function is advisable. **Sulindac** metabolites have been reported rarely as the major or a minor component in renal stones in association with other calculus components. Use sulindac with caution in patients with a history of renal lithiasis and keep patients well hydrated while receiving the drug.

➤*Hepatic function impairment:* **Naproxen** may exhibit an increase in unbound fraction and a reduced clearance of free drug in cirrhotic liver patients, suggesting an increased potential for toxicity in this group; consider reducing the dose. Also, **sulindac** AUC may increase in patients with cirrhosis because of altered sulfide formation/metabolism. Disposition of total and free **etodolac** is not altered in patients with compensated hepatic cirrhosis. Effects of hepatic disease on other NSAIDs is unknown. Use caution in patients with impaired hepatic function or history of liver disease.

In patients treated with a single 15 mg dose of **meloxicam**, there was no marked difference in plasma concentrations in patients with mild and moderate hepatic impairment compared with healthy subjects. Protein binding of meloxicam was not affected by hepatic insufficiency. No dose adjustment is needed in patients with mild to moderate hepatic insufficiency; patients with severe hepatic impairment have not been adequately studied.

➤*Photosensitivity:* Photosensitivity may occur; caution patients to take protective measures (ie, sunscreens, protective clothing) against ultraviolet (UV) or sunlight until tolerance is determined.

➤*Pregnancy: Category B* – **ketoprofen**, **naproxen**, **naproxen sodium**, **ibuprofen**, **meclofenamate**; per Briggs' *Drugs in Pregnancy and Lactation*: **flurbiprofen**, **diclofenac**, **fenoprofen**, **indomethacin**, **sulindac**. *Category C* – **etodolac**, **ketorolac**, **mefenamic acid**, **meloxicam**, **nabumetone**, **oxaprozin**, **tolmetin**, **piroxicam**, **celecoxib**; per manufacturer's prescribing information: **diclofenac**, **flurbiprofen**, **fenoprofen**, **indomethacin**, **sulindac**. All NSAIDs are *Category D* if used in the third trimester or near delivery.

Safety for use during pregnancy has not been established; use is not recommended. There are no adequate and well-controlled studies in pregnant women. An increased incidence of dystocia, increased postimplantation loss, decreased pup survival, increased length of delivery time, embryolethality, septal heart defects, stillbirth, and delayed parturition occurred in animals. Agents that inhibit prostaglandin synthesis may cause closure of the ductus arteriosus and other untoward effects to the fetus. GI tract toxicity increased in pregnant women in the last trimester. Some NSAIDs may prolong pregnancy if given before onset of labor.

The known effects of drugs of this class on the human fetus during the third trimester of pregnancy include the following: constriction of the ductus arteriosus prenatally, tricuspid incompetence, and pulmonary hypertension; nonclosure of the ductus arteriosus postnatally, which may be resistant to medical management; myocardial degenerative changes, platelet dysfunction with resultant bleeding, intracranial bleeding, renal dysfunction or failure, renal injury/dysgenesis that may result in prolonged or permanent renal failure, oligohydramnios, GI bleeding or perforation, and increased risk of necrotizing enterocolitis. Avoid during pregnancy, especially in the third trimester.

➤*Lactation:* Most NSAIDs are excreted in breast milk. **Naproxen** appears at approximately 1% of maternal serum concentration. In 10 healthy women, recovery of **flurbiprofen** in breast milk accounted for 0.05% (range, 0.03% to 0.07%) of a 100 mg dose; average peak concentration in milk was 0.09 mcg/mL. **Ketorolac** was detected in breast milk at a maximum milk-to-plasma ratio of 0.037. In general, do not use in breast-feeding mothers because of effects on the infant's cardiovascular system.

➤*Children:* **Mefenamic acid** and **meclofenamate** are not recommended in children younger than 14 years of age. Safety and efficacy of ibuprofen injection have not been established in children younger than 17 years of age; for use of ibuprofen lysine injection and indomethacin IV in premature infants see Agents for Patent Ductus Arteriosus. Safety and efficacy of **meloxicam** use have not been established in children younger than 18 years of age. **Indomethacin's** safety is not established in children; not recommended in children 14 years of age and younger, except in circumstances that warrant the risk. When using indomethacin in children 2 years of age and older, closely monitor liver function. Hepatotoxicity, including fatalities, has occurred in children with juvenile RA. Suggested starting dose is 2 mg/kg/day in divided doses. Do not exceed 4 mg/kg/day or 150 to 200 mg/day, whichever is less. As symptoms subside, reduce dosage or discontinue drug. **Tolmetin** and **naproxen** are the only agents labeled for juvenile RA, although studies are being conducted with other agents. Safety and efficacy of tolmetin and naproxen in infants younger than 2 years of age are not established. Safety and efficacy of other NSAIDs in children are not established.

➤*Elderly:* Age appears to increase the possibility of adverse reactions to NSAIDs. The risk of serious ulcer disease is increased in elderly patients (older than 65 years of age) taking NSAIDs; this risk appears to increase with the dose. Use with greater care and begin with reduced dosages. In **nabumetone**-treated patients, no differences in overall efficacy and safety were observed between older and younger patients. **Ketorolac** is cleared more slowly by elderly patients; use caution and reduce dosage.

Per the Beers list, avoid immediate and long-term use of **ketorolac** in elderly patients because a significant number have asymptomatic GI pathologic conditions. Ketorolac is also considered a high-risk medication for elderly patients according to the Centers for Medicare and Medicaid Services.

Per the Beers list, long-term use of full-dosage, longer half-life non–COX-selective NSAIDs (eg, **naproxen**, **oxaprozin**, **piroxicam**) have the potential to produce GI bleeding, renal failure, high blood pressure, and heart failure.

➤*Monitoring:* Monitor patients treated long term for signs and symptoms of ulceration and bleeding.

Monitor transaminases and other hepatic enzymes in patients treated with NSAIDs. For patients on **diclofenac** therapy, it is recommended that a determination from lab results be made within 4 to 8 weeks of initiating therapy and at intervals thereafter. If clinical signs and symptoms consistent with liver disease develop, or if systemic manifestations occur (eg, eosinophilia, rash) and abnormal liver tests are detected, persist, or worsen, discontinue diclofenac immediately.

Monitor blood pressure closely during the initiation of NSAID treatment and throughout the course of therapy. Carefully monitor patients who may be adversely affected by alterations in platelet function, such as those with coagulation disorders or patients receiving anticoagulants.

Drug Interactions

➤*Cytochrome P450:* Exercise caution when coadministering **celecoxib** and **mefenamic acid** with drugs known to inhibit the isoenzyme 2C9.

NSAID Drug Interactions

Precipitant drug	Object drug[a]		Description
ACE inhibitors (eg, enalapril)	NSAIDs	↑↓	NSAIDs may decrease the antihypertensive effects of ACE inhibitors. Antihypertensive effects of captopril may be blunted or completely abolished by indomethacin. The risk of nephrotoxicity may be increased. Consider discontinuation of NSAID if blood pressure control decreases. Periodically measure renal function during concomitant use.
NSAIDs	ACE inhibitors (eg, enalapril)		
Alcohol	NSAIDs	↑	Risk of GI bleeding may be increased. Use with caution.
Azole antifungals (eg, fluconazole, voriconazole)	NSAIDs (eg, celecoxib, ibuprofen)	↑	Increase in celecoxib, diclofenac, or ibuprofen plasma concentration may occur, increasing the pharmacologic effects and adverse reactions.
Bisphosphonates	NSAIDs	↑	Risk of gastric ulceration may be increased. Use cautiously.
Cholestyramine	NSAIDs	↓	The effects of NSAIDs may be decreased. Cholestyramine has enhanced piroxicam and meloxicam plasma clearance and decreased the GI absorption of NSAIDs.
Cimetidine	NSAIDs	↔	NSAID plasma concentrations may be increased or decreased by cimetidine; some studies report no effect. Also, indomethacin and sulindac have increased ranitidine and cimetidine bioavailability.
Colestipol	NSAIDs	↓	The effects of diclofenac may be decreased because colestipol may interfere with the absorption of diclofenac, thereby reducing bioavailability.
Corticosteroids, oral (eg, prednisone)	NSAIDs	↑	The risk of GI bleeding may be increased. Use with caution. Instruct patients to report any signs or symptoms of bleeding.
Diflunisal	NSAIDs Indomethacin	↑	Diflunisal may decrease the renal clearance and significantly increase indomethacin plasma concentrations that may produce toxicity.
Dimethyl sulfoxide (DMSO)	NSAIDs Sulindac	↓	DMSO may decrease the formation of the active metabolite of sulindac, possibly resulting in a decreased therapeutic effect. Also, topical DMSO with sulindac has resulted in severe peripheral neuropathy.
Hepatotoxic agents (eg, acetaminophen, certain antibiotics, and antiepileptic agents)	NSAIDs	↑	Risk of hepatotoxicity may be increased. Use with caution and closely monitor for signs and symptoms of hepatotoxicity.
Phenobarbital	NSAIDs Fenoprofen	↓	Phenobarbital, an enzyme inducer, may decrease fenoprofen half-life. Dosage adjustments of fenoprofen may be required if phenobarbital is added or withdrawn.
Phenylbutazone	NSAIDs Etodolac	↑	Phenylbutazone can increase by approximately 80% the free fraction of etodolac. Coadministration is not recommended.
Probenecid	NSAIDs	↑	Probenecid may increase the concentrations and possibly the toxicity of NSAIDs. Do not use ketorolac and probenecid concomitantly.

NSAID Drug Interactions			
Precipitant drug	Object drug[a]		Description
Ritonavir	NSAIDs Piroxicam	↑	Ritonavir may increase the concentrations and possibly the toxicity of piroxicam by inhibiting its metabolism.
Salicylates	NSAIDs	↓	Plasma concentrations of NSAIDs may be decreased by salicylates. Avoid concurrent use because it offers no therapeutic advantage and may significantly increase the incidence of GI effects.
Salicylates	NSAIDs Ketorolac	↑	Increased risk of serious ketorolac-related adverse effects may occur. Salicylates may displace ketorolac from protein binding sites and may produce possible synergistic adverse effects. Ketorolac is contraindicated in patients receiving aspirin.
Serotonin reuptake inhibitors (eg, fluoxetine, venlafaxine)	NSAIDs	↑	The risk of upper GI bleeding may be increased. Close clinical monitoring is warranted if coadministration cannot be avoided. Use of acid suppression therapy may be considered. Instruct patient to report any signs or symptoms of bleeding.
Sucralfate	NSAIDs	↓	The effects of diclofenac may be decreased, possibly because of decreased absorption. Sucralfate does not appear to alter ketoprofen or naproxen bioavailability.
Thienopyridines (eg, clopidogrel, prasugrel)	NSAIDs	↑	The risk of bleeding may be increased. Use with caution. Instruct patient to report any signs or symptoms of bleeding.
NSAIDs	Aminoglycosides	↑	Aminoglycoside plasma concentrations may be elevated. Reduce aminoglycoside dose prior to NSAID initiation and monitor serum aminoglycoside levels and renal function.
NSAIDs	Anticoagulants	↑	Coadministration may prolong prothrombin time (PT). Also consider the effects NSAIDs have on platelet function and gastric mucosa. Monitor PT and patients closely, especially the first few days, and instruct patients to watch for signs and symptoms of bleeding.
NSAIDs	Beta-blockers	↓	The antihypertensive effect of beta-blockers may be impaired, possibly because of NSAID inhibition of renal prostaglandin synthesis, thereby allowing unopposed pressor systems to produce hypertension. Avoid using this combination if possible. Monitor blood pressure and adjust beta-blocker dose as needed. Consider using a noninteracting NSAID (eg, sulindac).
NSAIDs	Cyclosporine, tacrolimus	↑	Nephrotoxicity of both agents may be increased.
Cyclosporine, tacrolimus	NSAIDs		
NSAIDs Ibuprofen Indomethacin	Digoxin	↑	Ibuprofen and indomethacin may increase digoxin serum levels.
NSAIDs Indomethacin	Dipyridamole	↑	Indomethacin and dipyridamole coadministration may augment water retention.
NSAIDs	Diuretics (eg, thiazides, potassium-sparing diuretics, triamterene)	↑	The effects of diuretics may be decreased. The risk of acute renal failure may be increased. Avoid coadministration with triamterene. Closely monitor renal function if coadministration cannot be avoided. If renal function decreases, consider stopping one or both drugs. Sulindac may enhance the effects of thiazides.
NSAIDs	Hydantoins	↑	Serum phenytoin levels may be increased, resulting in an increase in pharmacologic and toxic effects of phenytoin.
NSAIDs	Lithium	↑	Serum lithium levels may be increased; however, sulindac has no effect or may decrease lithium levels. Monitor for signs of lithium toxicity.
NSAIDs	Methotrexate	↑	The risks of methotrexate toxicity (eg, stomatitis, bone marrow suppression, nephrotoxicity) may be increased. Celecoxib and meloxicam did not have a significant effect on methotrexate pharmacokinetics.
NSAIDs Indomethacin	Penicillamine	↑	Indomethacin may increase the bioavailability of penicillamine.
NSAIDs Indomethacin Diclofenac	Potassium-sparing diuretics	↓	Effects of potassium-sparing diuretics may be decreased. Coadministration may increase serum potassium levels.
NSAIDs	Quinolones (eg, ciprofloxacin)	↑	Risk of CNS stimulation and seizures from quinolones may be increased. In addition, quinolone plasma concentrations may be increased. Use with caution.
NSAIDs	Tenofovir	↑	Pharmacologic and toxic effects (eg, nephrotoxicity) of tenofovir may be increased. Use with caution.
NSAIDs	Thiazide diuretics	↔	Decreased antihypertensive and diuretic action of thiazides may occur with concurrent indomethacin. Naproxen also has been implicated. Sulindac may enhance the effects of thiazides.
NSAIDs	Triamterene	↑	Coadministration may cause sudden onset of nephrotoxicity.

[a] ↑ = object drug increased; ↓ = object drug decreased; ↔ = undetermined clinical effect.

➤*Drug/Lab test interactions:* **Naproxen** use may result in increased urinary values for 17-ketogenic steroids because of an interaction between **naproxen** or its metabolites with m-dinitro-benzene used in this assay. Although 17-hydroxycorticosteroid measurements (Porter-Silber test) do not appear to be artificially altered, temporarily discontinue naproxen therapy 72 hours before adrenal function tests are performed. **Naproxen** may interfere with some urinary assays of 5-hydroxy indoleacetic acid.

Tolmetin metabolites in urine give positive tests for proteinuria using acid precipitation tests (eg, sulfosalicylic acid). Use commercially available dye-impregnated reagent strips.

A false-positive reaction for urinary bile, using the diazo tablet test, may result with **mefenamic acid**. If biliuria is suspected, use other procedures (ie, the Harrison spot test).

Amerlex-M kit assay values of total and free triiodothyronine in patients on **fenoprofen** have been reported as falsely elevated on the basis of a chemical cross-reaction that directly interferes with the assay. Thyroid-stimulating hormone, total thyroxine, and thyrotropin-releasing hormone response are not affected.

False-positive urine immunoassay screening tests for benzodiazepines have been reported in patients taking **oxaprozin**. This is because of the lack of specificity of the screening tests. False-positive test results may be expected for several days following discontinuation of **oxaprozin** therapy. Confirmatory tests, such as gas chromatography/mass spectrometry, will distinguish **oxaprozin** from benzodiazepines.

NSAIDs, by decreasing platelet adhesion and aggregation, can prolong bleeding time approximately 3 to 4 minutes.

➤*Drug/Food interactions:* Administration of **tolmetin** with milk had no effect on peak plasma **tolmetin** concentration, but decreased total **tolmetin** bioavailability by 16%. When **tolmetin** was taken immediately after a meal, peak plasma concentrations were reduced by 50%, while total bioavailability was again decreased by 16%. Peak concentration of **etodolac** is reduced by approximately 50% and the time to peak is increased by 1.4 to 3.8 hours following administration with food; however, the extent of absorption is not affected. Food may reduce the rate of absorption of **oxaprozin**, but the extent is unchanged.

Adverse Reactions

NSAIDs Adverse Reactions[a]

	Adverse reaction	Celecoxib	Diclofenac	Etodolac	Fenoprofen	Flurbiprofen	Ibuprofen injection	Ibuprofen oral	Indomethacin	Ketoprofen	Ketorolac	Meclofenamate	Mefenamic acid	Meloxicam	Nabumetone	Naproxen	Oxaprozin	Piroxicam	Sulindac	Tolmetin
Cardiovascular	Angina/Angina pectoris	< 2%				< 1%								< 2%	< 1%					
	Arrhythmia		< 1	< 1		< 1%		< 1%[b]	< 1%	< 1%			< 1%	< 2%	< 1%			< 1%	< 1%	
	CHF	< 0.1%	< 1%	< 1%				< 1%	< 1%				< 1%			< 1%		< 1%	< 1%	< 1%
	CVA	< 0.1%		< 1%		< 1%														
	Flushing			< 1%					< 1%											
	Hypertension		< 1%	< 1%		< 1%	10%	< 1%	< 1%	< 1%	1-3%		< 1%	< 2%	< 1%			< 1%	< 1%	3-9%
	Hypotension		< 1%				7-10%		< 1%				< 1%	< 2%				< 1%		
	MI	< 2%	< 1%	< 1%		< 1%			< 1%				< 1%	< 2%	< 1%			< 1%		
	Palpitations	< 2%	< 1%	< 1%	2.5%			< 1%	< 1%	< 1%	< 1%	< 1%	< 1%	< 2%	< 1%	1-3%	< 1%	< 1%	< 1%	
	Pulmonary embolism	< 0.1%				< 1%														
	Syncope	< 0.1%	< 1%	< 1%					< 1%		< 1%		< 1%	< 2%	< 1%			< 1%	< 1%	
	Tachycardia	< 2%	< 1%		< 1%				< 1%	< 1%			< 1%	< 2%				< 1%		
	Vasculitis	< 0.1%	< 1%	< 1%[c]									< 1%	< 2%	< 1%	< 1%				
CNS	Abnormal dreams/ dream abnormalities		< 1%					< 1%			< 1%		< 1%	< 2%		< 1%		< 1%		
	Aseptic meningitis		< 1%					< 1%[g]		< 1%						< 1%			< 1%	
	Anxiety	< 2%	< 1%						< 1%				< 1%	< 2%	< 1%			< 1%		
	Asthenia/Malaise	< 2%	< 1%	3-9%	1-5.4%						< 1%	< 1%	< 1%	< 2%	< 1%	< 1%	< 1%	< 1%		3-9%
	CNS inhibition[d]																1-3%			
	CNS inhibition or excitation					1-3%[e]				3-9%[f]										
	Confusion		< 1%	< 1%	1.4%	< 1%		< 1%	< 1%	< 1%			< 1%	< 2%	< 1%			< 1%		
	Convulsions		< 1%			< 1%			< 1%				< 1%	< 2%				< 1%	< 1%	
	Depression	< 2%	< 1%	1-3%	< 1%			< 1%	1-3%		< 1%	< 1%	< 1%	< 2%	< 1%	< 1%		< 1%	< 1%	1-3%
	Dizziness	2%	1-10%	3-9%	6.5%	1-3%	4-6%	3-9%	3-9%	1-3%	7%	3-9%	1-10%	1.1-3.8%	3-9%	3-9%		1-10%	3-9%	3-9%
	Drowsiness		< 1%						< 1%		6%		< 1%			3-9%		< 1%		1-3%
	Fatigue	< 2%			1.7%				1-3%			< 1%		< 2%	1-3%					
	Hallucinations		< 1%					< 1%		< 1%	< 1%		< 1%					< 1%		
	Headache	15.8%	1-10%	< 1%	8.7%	3-9%	9-12%	1-3%	11.7%	3-9%	17%	3-9%	1-10%	2.4-8.3%	3-9%	3-9%		1-10%	3-9%	3-9%
	Hypertonia	< 2%				< 1%														
	Hypesthesia	< 2%																		
	Insomnia	2.3%	< 1%	< 1%	< 1%			< 1%	< 1%		< 1%	< 1%	< 1%	≤ 3.6%	1-3%	< 1%		< 1%	< 1%	
	Light-headedness								< 1%							1-3%				
	Migraine	< 2%								< 1%										
	Nervousness	< 2%	< 1%	1-3%	5.7%	1-3%		1-3%	< 1%		< 1%		< 1%	< 2%	1-3%			< 1%	1-3%	
	Paresthesia	< 2%	< 1%	< 1%		< 1%		< 1%	< 1%	< 1%	< 1%	< 1%	< 1%	< 2%	< 1%			< 1%	< 1%	
	Somnolence	< 2%	< 1%	< 1%	8.5%			< 1%	1-3%				< 1%	< 2%	1-3%			< 1%	< 1%	
	Tremor		< 1%		2.2%						< 1%		< 1%	< 2%	< 1%			< 1%		
	Vertigo	< 2%	< 1%						1-3%	< 1%	< 1%		< 1%	2%	< 1%	1-3%		< 1%	< 1%	
Dermatologic	Alopecia/ Loss of hair	< 2%	< 1%	< 1%	< 1%	< 1%		< 1%	< 1%	< 1%		< 1%	< 1%	< 2%	< 1%	< 1%	< 1%	< 1%	< 1%	
	Bullous eruption/rash									< 1%			< 1%	< 2%	< 1%					
	Eczema					< 1%				< 1%										
	Erythema multiforme	< 0.1%	< 1%	< 1%				< 1%	< 1%	< 1%		< 1%	< 1%	< 0.1%	< 1%	< 1%	< 1%	< 1%	< 1%	< 1%
	Exfoliative dermatitis	< 0.1%	< 1%		< 1%	< 1%			< 1%	< 1%		< 1%	< 1%				< 1%	< 1%	< 1%	
	Increased sweating	< 2%	< 1%	< 1%	4.6%	< 1%			< 1%	< 1%	1-3%		< 1%	< 2%	1-3%	1-3%		< 1%		
	Photosensitivity/ Photosensitivity reaction	< 2%	< 1%	< 1%		< 1%				< 1%			< 1%	< 2%	< 1%	< 1%[h]	< 1%	< 1%	< 1%	
	Pruritus	< 2%	1-10%	1-3%	4.2%	< 1%		1-3%	< 1%	< 1%	1-3%	1-3%	1-10%	≤ 2.4%	3-9%	3-9%	< 1%	1-10%	1-3%	
	Rash	2.2%	1-10%	1-3%	3.7%	1-3%		3-9%	< 1%	1-3%	1-3%	3-9%	1-10%	0.3-3%	3-9%	< 1%	3-9%	1-10%	3-9%	
	Skin eruptions															3-9%				
	Skin irritation																			1-3%
	Stevens-Johnson syndrome	< 0.1%	< 1%	< 1%	< 1%			< 1%	< 1%	< 1%		< 1%	< 1%	< 0.1%	< 1%	< 1%	< 1%	< 1%	< 1%	
	Toxic epidermal necrolysis/ Lyell syndrome	< 0.1%	< 1%		< 1%	< 1%		< 1%	< 1%	< 1%				< 0.1%	< 1%		< 1%		< 1%	< 1%
	Urticaria	< 2%	< 1%	< 1%	< 1%	< 1%		< 1%	< 1%	< 1%	< 1%	1-3%	< 1%	< 2%	< 1%	< 1%	< 1%	< 1%		< 1%

NSAIDs Adverse Reactions[a]

	Adverse reaction	Celecoxib	Diclofenac	Etodolac	Fenoprofen	Flurbiprofen	Ibuprofen injection	Ibuprofen oral	Indomethacin	Ketoprofen	Ketorolac	Meclofenamate	Mefenamic acid	Meloxicam	Nabumetone	Naproxen	Oxaprozin	Piroxicam	Sulindac	Tolmetin
GI	Abdominal discomfort						< 1-3%													
	Abdominal distension								< 1%											
	Abdominal/ GI distress							1-3%	1-3%								1-3%			3-9%
	Abdominal pain or cramps	4.1%	1-10%	3-9%	2%	3-9%		1-3%	1-3%	3-9		3-9%	1-10%	1.9-4.7%	12%	3-9%	1-3%	1-10%	10% (pain) 1-3 (cramps)	3-9%
	Anorexia/ Decreased appetite	< 2%		< 1%	< 1%			1-3%	< 1%	1-3%	< 1%	1-3%			< 1%		1-3%	1-10%	1-3%	
	Appetite change		< 1%			< 1%							< 1%					< 1%		
	Appetite increase	< 2%								< 1%	< 1%			< 2%	< 1%					
	Bloating							1-3%	< 1%											
	Colitis		< 1%	< 1%		< 1%						< 1%		< 2%		< 1%			< 1%	
	Constipation	< 2%	1-10%	1-3%	7%	1-3%		1-3%	1-3%	3-9%	1-3%	1-3	1-10%	0.8-2.6%	3-9%	3-9%	3-9%	1-10%	3-9%	1-3%
	Diarrhea	5.6%	1-10%	3-9%	1.8%	3-9%	7-10%	1-3%	1-3%	3-9%	7%	10-33%	1-10%	1.9-7.8%	14%	1-3%	3-9%	1-10%	3-9%	3-9%
	Dry mouth	< 2%	< 1%	< 1%	< 1%	< 1%		< 1%		< 1%	< 1%		< 1%	< 2%	1-3%			< 1%		
	Dyspepsia/ Indigestion	8.8%	1-10%	10%	10.3%	3-9%	1-4%	1-3%	3-9%	11%	12%		1-10%	3.8-9.5%	13%	1-3%	3-9%	1-10%	3-9%	3-9%
	Epigastric discomfort																			
	Epigastric/ GI pain							3-9%			13%									
	Eructation	< 2%	< 1%	< 1%						< 1%	< 1%		< 1%	< 2%	< 1%			< 1%		
	Esophagitis	< 2%	< 1%	< 1%[l]									< 1%	< 2%				< 1%		
	Flatulence	2.2%	1-10%	3-9%	< 1%	1-3%	7-16%	1-3%	< 1%	3-9%	1-3%	3-9%	1-10%	0.4-3.2%	3-9%		1-3%	1-10%	1-3%	3-9%
	Gastritis	< 2%	< 1%	1-3%	< 1%	< 1%		< 1%		< 1%	< 1%		< 1%	< 2%	1-3%			< 1%	< 1%	1-3%
	Gastroenteritis	< 2%							< 1%						< 1%				< 1%	
	GI bleeding	< 0.1%	< 1%		< 1%	1-3%		< 1%					< 1%	< 2%	< 1%	< 1%	< 1%		< 1%	< 1%
	GI fullness							1-3%			1-3%									
	Glossitis		< 1%										< 1%		< 1%			< 1%	< 1%	< 1%
	Gross bleeding/ perforation		1-10%										1-10%					1-10%		
	Heartburn		1-10%					3-9%				3-9%	1-10%			3-9%		1-10%		
	Hematemesis		< 1%			< 1%				< 1%			< 1%	< 2%		< 1		< 1		
	Hepatitis	< 0.1%	< 1%	< 1%		< 1%		< 1%		< 1%			< 1%	< 2%			< 1%	< 1%	< 1%	< 1%
	Jaundice	< 0.1%	< 1%	< 1%	< 1%			< 1%		< 1%			< 1%	< 0.1%	< 1%	< 1%		< 1%	< 1%[j]	
	Liver failure	< 0.1%	< 1%	< 1%									< 1%	< 0.1%	< 1%			< 1%	< 1%	
	Melena	< 2%	< 1%	1-3%				< 1%		< 1%			< 1%	< 2%	< 1%	< 1%		< 1%		
	Nausea	3.5%	1-10%	3-9%	7.7%	3-9%	53-57%	3-9%	3-9%	3-9%	12%	11%	1-10%	2.4-7.2%	3-9%	3-9%	3-9%	1-10%	3-9%	11%
	Nausea and vomiting							1-3%	1-3%			11%							1-3%	
	Pancreatitis	< 0.1%	< 1%[k]	< 1%	< 1%			< 1%		< 1%			< 1%	< 2%	< 1%	< 1%	< 1%	< 1%	< 1%	
	Peptic ulcer		< 1%	< 1%	< 1%	< 1%			< 1%	< 1%		1-3%	1-10%	< 2%	< 1%		< 1%	1-10%	< 1%	1-3%
	Peptic ulcer bleed			< 1%				< 1%						< 2%			< 1%			
	Positive stool guaiac				< 1%										3-9%					
	Rectal bleeding/ hemorrhage		< 1%						< 1%	< 1%	< 1%		< 1%		< 1%		< 1%	< 1%		
	Stomatitis	< 2%				< 1%				1-3%	1-3%	1-3%	< 1%		1-3%	1-3%	< 1%	< 1%	< 1%	< 1%
	Vomiting	< 2%	1-10%	1-3%	2.6%	1-%3	15-22%			1-3%	1-3%		1-10%	0.6-2.6%	1-3%	< 1%	1-3%	1-10%		3-9%

NSAIDs Adverse Reactions[a]

	Adverse reaction	Celecoxib	Diclofenac	Etodolac	Fenoprofen	Flurbiprofen	Ibuprofen injection	Ibuprofen oral	Indomethacin	Ketoprofen	Ketorolac	Meclofenamate	Mefenamic acid	Meloxicam	Nabumetone	Naproxen	Oxaprozin	Piroxicam	Sulindac	Tolmetin
GU	Acute renal failure	< 0.1%	< 1%					< 1%									< 1%			
	Albuminuria	< 2%												< 2%	< 1%					
	Azotemia		< 1%		< 1%			< 1%							< 1%					
	Cystitis	< 2%	< 1%	< 1%	< 1%			< 1%					< 1%					< 1%		
	Dysuria	< 2%	< 1%	1-3%	< 1%								< 1%		< 1%		1-3%	< 1%	< 1%	< 1%
	Gynecomastia							< 1%	< 1%	< 1%									< 1%	
	Hematuria	< 2%	< 1%	< 1%	< 1%	< 1%		< 1%	< 1%	< 1%	< 1%		< 1%	< 2%	< 1%	< 1%	< 1%	< 1%	< 1%	< 1%
	Impotence		< 1%							< 1%					< 1%					
	Interstitial nephritis/ acute interstitial nephritis	< 0.1%	< 1%	< 1%	< 1%	< 1%			< 1%	< 1%			< 1%	< 0.1%	< 1%	< 1%	< 1%	< 1%	< 1%	
	Menstrual disorder/ disturbance	< 2%				< 1%										< 1%				
	Nephrotic syndrome								< 1%	< 1%					< 1%	< 1%	< 1%	< 1%	< 1%	
	Oliguria		< 1%		< 1%						< 1%		< 1%					< 1%		
	Papillary necrosis/ renal papillary necrosis			< 1%	< 1%			< 1%								< 1%				
	Proteinuria		< 1%						< 1%		< 1%		< 1%					< 1%	< 1%	< 1%
	Renal calculi/stones	< 2%		< 1%											< 1%				< 1%	
	Renal failure		< 1%	< 1%	< 1%	< 1%			< 1%	< 1%		< 1%	< 1%	< 2%	< 1%	< 1%		< 1%	< 1%	< 1%
	Renal function impairment/ insufficiency/ abnormal		1-10%	< 1%					< 1%	3-9%			1-10%				< 1%	1-10%	< 1%	
	Urinary frequency/ Polyuria	< 2%	< 1%	1-3%				< 1%	< 1%		< 1%		< 1%	0.1-2.4%			1-3%	< 1%		
	Urinary retention						3-5%													
	Urinary tract infection/ symptoms	< 2%				3-9				1-3%				0.3-6.9%						1-3%
	Vaginal bleeding/ hemorrhage	< 2%				< 1%			< 1%%						< 1%				< 1%	
Hematologic/Lymphatic	Agranulocytosis	< 0.1%	< 1%	< 1%	< 1%			< 1%	< 1%	< 1%		< 1%	< 1%	< 0.1%		< 1%	< 1%	< 1%	< 1%	< 1%
	Anemia	< 2%	1-10%	< 1%			2-36%			< 1%	< 1%		1-10%	≤ 4.1%	< 1%		< 1%	1-10%		
	Aplastic anemia	< 0.1%	< 1%		< 1%	< 1%		< 1%	< 1%				< 1%			< 1%		< 1%	< 1%	
	Ecchymoses	< 2%	< 1%	< 1%		< 1%			< 1%				< 1%			3-9%	< 1%	< 1%	< 1%	
	Eosinophilia		< 1%			< 1%	23-26%	< 1%			< 1%	< 1%	< 1%			< 1%		< 1%		
	Hemolytic anemia		< 1%	< 1%	< 1%	< 1%		< 1%	< 1%			< 1%	< 1%			< 1%		< 1%	< 1%	< 1%
	Hemorrhage						4-10%													
	Leukopenia	< 0.1%	< 1%	< 1%		< 1%			< 1%			< 1%	< 1%	< 2%	< 1%	< 1%	< 1%	< 1%	< 1%	
	Lymphadenopathy		< 1%		< 1%	< 1%							< 1%					< 1%		< 1%
	Neutropenia			< 1%			7-13%	< 1%				< 1%							< 1%	
	Pancytopenia	< 0.1%	< 1%	< 1%	< 1%								< 1%				< 1%	< 1%		
	Purpura		< 1%		< 1%					< 1%	1-3%		< 1%	< 2%		1-3%		< 1%	< 1%	< 1%
	Thrombocythemia						3-10%													
	Thrombocytopenia	< 0.1%	< 1%	< 1%	< 1%	< 1%		< 1%[m]		< 1%			< 1%	< 2%	< 1%	< 1%	< 1%	< 1%	< 1%	< 1%
	Wound hemorrhage						1-3%													
Hypersensitivity	Allergy/ Allergic reaction	< 2%		< 1%						< 1%				< 2%						
	Anaphylaxis or anaphylactic/ anaphylactoid reaction	< 0.1%	< 1%	< 1%[n]	< 1%	< 1%		< 1%	< 1%	< 1%			< 1%	< 0.1%[o]	< 1%	< 1%	< 1%	< 1%	< 1%	< 1%
	Angioedema/ Angioneurotic edema	< 0.1%	< 1%	< 1%	< 1%	< 1%		< 1%	< 1%				< 1%	< 2%	< 1%	< 1%		< 1%	< 1%	
	Serum sickness							< 1%									< 1%	< 1%		< 1%

NSAIDs Adverse Reactions[a]

	Adverse reaction	Celecoxib	Diclofenac	Etodolac	Fenoprofen	Flurbiprofen	Ibuprofen injection	Ibuprofen oral	Indomethacin	Ketoprofen	Ketorolac	Meclofenamate	Mefenamic acid	Meloxicam	Nabumetone	Naproxen	Oxaprozin	Piroxicam	Sulindac	Tolmetin
Lab test abnormalities	ALT or AST elevations	< 2%	2%		< 1%									< 2%						
	Bleeding time increased		1-10%	< 1%									1-10%					1-10%		
	BUN increased	< 2%		< 1%			0-10%		< 1%	3-9%				< 2%						1-3%
	Creatinine increase	< 2%		< 1%										< 2%						
	Hemoglobin and hematocrit decreases		< 1%			< 1%	2-3% (hemoglobin)	< 1%				< 1%								1-3%
	LDH[s] increased						3-10%													
	Liver test abnormalities/ elevations		1-10%	< 1%		1-3%		< 1%				< 1%	1-10%		< 1%	< 1%	< 1%	1-10%	< 1%	< 1%
	Body weight changes		< 1%	< 1%		1-3%				< 1%			< 1%	< 2%			< 1%	< 1%		3-9%
	Edema	< 2%	1-10%	< 1%		3-9%		1-3%	< 1%	3-9%	4%	1-3%	1-10	0.5-4.5%[p]	3-9%	3-9%	< 1%	1-10%	1-3%	3-9%
Metabolic/Nutritional	Fluid retention							1-3%	< 1%											
	Hyperglycemia	< 2%	< 1%	< 1%[q]					< 1%				< 1%		< 1%	< 1%		< 1%	< 1%	
	Hyperkalemia					< 1%			< 1%							< 1%		< 1%	< 1%	
	Hypernatremia						0-10%													
	Hypoalbuminemia						3-10%													
	Hypokalemia	< 2%					< 1-19%								< 1%					
	Hypoproteinemia						0-13%													
	Lower extremity edema																			
	Peripheral edema	2.1%			5%		< 1-3%													
	Thirst			< 1%						< 1%						1-3%				
	Weight gain	< 2%							< 1%		< 1%				< 1%					
Musculoskeletal	Arthralgia	< 2%												≤ 5.3%						
	Muscle weakness								< 1%							< 1%			< 1%	
	Myalgia	< 2%								< 1%						< 1%				
Respiratory	Asthma		< 1%	< 1%		< 1%			< 1%				< 1%	< 2%	< 1%			< 1%		
	Bacterial pneumonia						3-10%													
	Bronchitis	< 2%		< 1%		< 1%														
	Bronchospasm	< 2%						< 1%		< 1%				< 2%					< 1%	
	Coughing	< 2%					< 1-3%				< 1%			0.2-2.4%	< 1%					
	Dyspnea	< 2%	< 1%	< 1%	2.8%	< 1%			< 1%	< 1%	< 1%		< 1%	< 2%	< 1%	3-9%		< 1%	< 1%	
	Epistaxis	< 2%		< 1%		< 1%			< 1%	< 1%	< 1%							< 1%	< 1%	< 1%
	Pharyngitis	2.3%		< 1%						< 1%				0.6-3.2%						
	Pneumonia	< 2%	< 1%										< 1%					< 1%		
	Pulmonary edema				< 1%				< 1%		< 1%									
	Rhinitis	2%		< 1%		1-3%		< 1%		< 1%	< 1%									
	Sinusitis	5%		< 1%													< 1%			
	Upper respiratory infection	8.1%			1.5%									≤ 8.3%			< 1%			
Special senses	Blurred vision	< 2%	< 1%	1-3%	2.2%				< 1%		< 1%	< 1%	< 1%				< 1%	< 1%	< 1%	
	Conjunctivitis	< 2%	< 1%	< 1%		< 1%		< 1%		< 1%		< 1%	< 1%	2%			< 1%	< 1%		
	Diplopia				< 1%			< 1%	< 1%											
	Hearing disturbances								< 1%							1-3%				
	Hearing loss/ impairment		< 1%[r]		1.6%			< 1%		< 1%	< 1%		< 1%			< 1%	< 1%	< 1%	< 1%	
	Taste disorder/ perversion/ disturbance/ alteration/ changes	< 2%		< 1%		< 1%				< 1%		< 1%		< 2%	< 1%		< 1%			
	Tinnitus	< 2%	1-10%	1-3%	4.5%	1-3%		1-3%	1-3%	1-3%	< 1%	1-3%	1-10%	< 2%	3-9%	3-9%	1-3%	1-10%	1-3%	1-3%
	Visual disturbances/ changes			< 1%		1-3%				1-3%					< 1%	1-3%			< 1%	1-3%

NSAIDs Adverse Reactions[a]

	Adverse reaction	Celecoxib	Diclofenac	Etodolac	Fenoprofen	Flurbiprofen	Ibuprofen injection	Ibuprofen oral	Indomethacin	Ketoprofen	Ketorolac	Meclofenamate	Mefenamic acid	Meloxicam	Nabumetone	Naproxen	Oxaprozin	Piroxicam	Sulindac	Tolmetin
Miscellaneous	Accident, household													3.2-4.5%						
	Back pain	2.8%												0.4-3%						
	Bacteremia						0-13%													
	Chest pain	< 2%							< 1%											1-3%
	Chills			1-3%		< 1%				< 1%					< 1%	< 1%				
	Face edema	< 2%								< 1%				< 2%						
	Fall													≤ 2.6%						
	Fever	< 2%	< 1%	1-3%	< 1%	< 1%			< 1%		< 1%		< 1%	< 2%	< 1%	< 1%		< 1%		< 1%
	Infection			< 1%						< 1%	< 1%		< 1%					< 1%		
	Influenza-like disease/ symptoms	< 2%												4.5-5.8%				< 1%		
	Injury, accidental	2.9%																		
	Pain	< 2%								< 1%				0.9-5.2%						

[a] Data are pooled from separate studies and are not necessarily comparable.
[b] Sinus tachycardia, sinus bradycardia.
[c] Including necrotizing and allergic.
[d] CNS inhibition (depression, sedation, somnolence, or confusion).
[e] CNS stimulation (eg, anxiety, insomnia, reflexes increased, tremor) or CNS inhibition (eg, amnesia, asthenia, somnolence, malaise, depression).
[f] CNS inhibition (eg, somnolence, malaise, depression) or CNS excitation (eg, insomnia, nervousness, dreams).
[g] With fever and coma.
[h] Resembling porphyria cutanea tarda.
[i] Erythema multiforme major.
[j] Sometimes with fever.
[k] With or without concomitant hepatitis.
[l] With or without stricture or cardiospasm.
[m] With or without purpura.
[n] Anaphylactic/Anaphylactoid reaction (including shock).
[o] Including shock.
[p] Edema, dependent edema, peripheral edema, and leg edema combined.
[q] In previously uncontrolled diabetes.
[r] Reversible and irreversible.
[s] LDH = lactate dehydrogenase.

➤*Cardiovascular:*

Celecoxib – Aggravated hypertension, coronary artery disorder (less than 2%); peripheral gangrene, thrombophlebitis, ventricular fibrillation (less than 0.1%).

Fenoprofen – Atrial fibrillation, electrocardiogram changes, supraventricular tachycardia (less than 1%).

Flurbiprofen – Cerebrovascular ischemia, heart failure, vascular diseases, vasodilation (less than 1%).

Indomethacin – Thrombophlebitis (less than 1%).

Ketoprofen – Peripheral vascular disease, vasodilation (less than 1%).

Meloxicam – Cardiac failure (less than 2%).

Nabumetone – Thrombophlebitis (less than 1%).

Oxaprozin – Blood pressure changes (less than 1%).

Piroxicam – Exacerbation of angina (less than 1%).

➤*CNS:*

Celecoxib – Leg cramps, neuralgia, neuropathy (less than 2%); ataxia (less than 0.1%).

Diclofenac – Coma (less than 1%).

Fenoprofen – Disorientation, personality change, seizures, trigeminal neuralgia (less than 1%).

Flurbiprofen – Ataxia, emotional lability, meningitis, subarachnoid hemorrhage, twitching (less than 1%).

Ibuprofen – Emotional lability, pseudotumor cerebri (less than 1%).

Indomethacin – Aggravation of epilepsy and parkinsonism, coma, depersonalization, dysarthria, peripheral neuropathy, psychic disturbances (including psychotic episodes) (less than 1%).

Ketoprofen – Amnesia, dysphoria, libido disturbances, nightmares, personality disorder (less than 1%).

Ketorolac – Abnormal thinking, euphoria, excessive thirst, extrapyramidal symptoms, hyperkinesis, inability to concentrate, stupor (less than 1%).

Mefenamic acid – Coma, meningitis (less than 1%).

Nabumetone – Agitation, nightmares (less than 1%).

Naproxen – Cognitive dysfunction, inability to concentrate (less than 1%).

Oxaprozin – Sleep disturbance (1% to 3%); weakness (less than 1%).

Piroxicam – Akathisia, coma, meningitis, mood alterations (less than 1%).

Sulindac – Neuritis, psychic disturbances (including acute psychosis) (less than 1%).

➤*Dermatologic:*

Celecoxib – Cellulitis, contact dermatitis, dermatitis, dry skin, herpes simplex, herpes zoster, injection site reaction, nail disorder, rash erythematous, rash maculopapular, skin disorder, skin nodule (less than 2%).

Etodolac – Cutaneous vasculitis with purpura, hyperpigmentation, maculopapular rash, skin peeling, vesiculobullous rash (less than 1%).

Flurbiprofen – Dry skin, herpes simplex zoster, nail disorder (less than 1%).

Ibuprofen – Photoallergic skin reactions, vesiculobullous eruptions (less than 1%).

Indomethacin – Erythema nodosum, petechiae (less than 1%).

Ketoprofen – Onycholysis, purpuric rash, skin discoloration (less than 1%).

Ketorolac – Pallor (less than 1%).

Meclofenamate – Erythema nodosum (less than 1%).

Mefenamic acid – Toxic epidermal necrosis (less than 1%).

Nabumetone – Acne, pseudoporphyria cutanea tarda (less than 1%).

Naproxen – Epidermal necrolysis, epidermolysis bullosa, photosensitive dermatitis (less than 1%).

Oxaprozin – Pseudoporphyria (less than 1%).

Piroxicam – Bruising, desquamation, erythema, onycholysis, petechial rash, toxic epidermal necrosis, vesiculobullous reaction (less than 1%).

Sulindac – Sore or dry mucous membranes (less than 1%).

➤*GI:*

Celecoxib – Diverticulitis, dysphagia, gastroesophageal reflux, hemorrhoids, hepatic function abnormal, hiatal hernia, tenesmus (less than 2%); cholelithiasis, colitis with bleeding, esophageal perforation, ileus, intestinal obstruction, intestinal perforation (less than 0.1%).

Diclofenac – GI ulcers (1% to 10%).

Etodolac – Cholestatic hepatitis, cholestatic jaundice, duodenitis, intestinal ulceration, liver necrosis, peptic ulcer with or without bleeding and/or perforation, ulcerative stomatitis (less than 1%).

Fenoprofen – Aphthous ulceration of the buccal mucosa, cholestatic hepatitis, metallic taste, peptic ulcer without perforation (less than 1%).

Flurbiprofen – Bloody diarrhea, cholecystitis, cholestatic and noncholestatic jaundice, esophageal disease, exacerbation of inflammatory bowel disease, periodontal abscess, small intestine inflammation with loss of blood and protein (less than 1%).

Ibuprofen – Gastric or duodenal ulcer with bleeding and/or perforation, gingival ulcer (less than 1%).

Indomethacin – Development of ulcerative colitis and regional ileitis, ulcerative stomatitis, toxic hepatitis and jaundice (some fatal cases have been reported), intestinal strictures (diaphragms), GI bleeding without obvious ulcer formation and perforation of preexisting sigmoid lesions (eg, diverticulum, carcinoma), intestinal ulceration associated with stenosis and obstruction, proctitis, single or multiple ulcerations (including perforation and hemorrhage of the esophagus, stomach, duodenum, or small and large intestines) (less than 1%).

Ketoprofen – Buccal necrosis, cholestatic hepatitis, fecal occult blood, hepatic dysfunction, intestinal ulceration, microvesicular steatosis, GI perforation, salivation, ulcerative colitis (less than 1%).

Meclofenamate – Bleeding and/or perforation with or without obvious ulcer formation, cholestatic jaundice, paralytic ileus (less than 1%).

Meloxicam – Gastroesophageal reflux, intestinal perforation, perforated duodenal ulcer, perforated gastric ulcer, stomatitis ulcerative (less than 2%).

Nabumetone – Duodenitis, dysphagia, gallstones, gingivitis (less than 1%).

Naproxen – GI perforation, nonpeptic GI ulceration, ulcerative stomatitis (less than 1%).

Oxaprozin – Hemorrhoidal bleeding (less than 1%).

Piroxicam – Pain (colic) (less than 1%).

Sulindac – Ageusia, bile duct sludging, biliary calculi, cholestasis, GI perforation, intestinal strictures (diaphragm) (less than 1%).

Tolmetin – GI bleeding without evidence of peptic ulcer, perforation (less than 1%).

➤*GU:*

Celecoxib – Breast fibroadenosis, breast neoplasm, breast pain, dysmenorrhea, moniliasis genital, prostatic disorder, urinary incontinence, vaginitis (less than 2%).

Etodolac – Leukorrhea, uterine bleeding irregularities (less than 1%).

Fenoprofen – Anuria, mastodynia, nephrosis (less than 1%).

Flurbiprofen – Prostate disease, uterine hemorrhage, vulvovaginitis (less than 1%).

Indomethacin – Breast changes (including enlargement and tenderness, or gynecomastia) (less than 1%).

Ketoprofen – Menometrorrhagia (less than 1%).

Ketorolac – Urinary retention (less than 1%).

Meclofenamate – Nocturia (less than 1%).

Nabumetone – Bilirubinuria, hyperuricemia (less than 1%).

Naproxen – Glomerular nephritis, renal disease (less than 1%).

Oxaprozin – Decreased menstrual flow, increased menstrual flow (less than 1%).

Sulindac – Crystalluria, urine discoloration (less than 1%).

➤*Hematologic/Lymphatic:*

Celecoxib – Thrombocythemia (less than 2%).

Fenoprofen – Bruising, hemorrhage (less than 1%).

Flurbiprofen – Iron deficiency anemia (less than 1%).

Ibuprofen – Bleeding episodes (less than 1%).

Indomethacin – Anemia secondary to obvious or occult GI bleeding, bone marrow depression, disseminated intravascular coagulation, leukemia, thrombocytopenic purpura (less than 1%).

Ketoprofen – Hemolysis, hypocoagulability (less than 1%).

Meclofenamate – Thrombocytopenic purpura (less than 1%).

Meloxicam – Bilirubinemia (less than 2%).

Nabumetone – Granulocytopenia (less than 1%).

Naproxen – Granulocytopenia (less than 1%).

Sulindac – Bone marrow depression (including aplastic anemia) (less than 1%).

Tolmetin – Granulocytopenia (less than 1%).

➤*Hypersensitivity:*

Ibuprofen – Henoch-Schönlein vasculitis, lupus erythematosus syndrome, syndrome of abdominal pain, fever, chills, nausea, and vomiting (less than 1%).

Indomethacin – Acute respiratory distress, angiitis, purpura, rapid fall in blood pressure resembling a shock-like state (less than 1%).

Meclofenamate – Lupus, serum sickness-like syndrome (less than 1%).

Piroxicam – Positive antinuclear antibody test (less than 1%).

Sulindac – Hypersensitivity vasculitis, potentially fatal hypersensitivity syndrome (less than 1%).

➤*Metabolic/Nutritional:*

Celecoxib – Diabetes mellitus, hypercholesterolemia, nonprotein nitrogen increase (less than 2%); hypoglycemia (less than 0.1%).

Flurbiprofen – Hyperuricemia (less than 1%).

Ibuprofen – Acidosis, hypoglycemic reactions (less than 1%).

Indomethacin – Glycosuria (less than 1%).

Ketoprofen – Diabetes mellitus (aggravated), hyponatremia (less than 1%).

Meloxicam – Dehydration (less than 2%).

Naproxen – Hypoglycemia (less than 1%).

Piroxicam – Hypoglycemia (less than 1%).

➤*Lab test abnormalities:*

Celecoxib – Alkaline phosphatase increased, creatine phosphokinase increased (less than 2%).

Fenoprofen – Increase in alkaline phosphatase and LDH (less than 1%).

Ibuprofen – Decreased creatinine clearance (less than 1%).

Meloxicam – Gamma-glutamyl transferase increased (less than 2%).

Sulindac – Increased prothrombin time (patients taking oral anticoagulants) (less than 1%).

➤*Musculoskeletal:*

Celecoxib – Arthrosis, bone disorder, fracture accidental, neck stiffness, synovitis, tendinitis (less than 2%).

Flurbiprofen – Myasthenia (less than 1%).

Indomethacin – Involuntary muscle movement (less than 1%).

➤*Respiratory:*

Celecoxib – Bronchospasm aggravated, laryngitis (less than 2%).

Diclofenac – Respiratory depression (less than 1%).

Etodolac – Pulmonary infiltration with eosinophilia (less than 1%).

Fenoprofen – Nasopharyngitis (1.2%).

Flurbiprofen – Hyperventilation, laryngitis, pulmonary infarct (less than 1%).

Ketoprofen – Hemoptysis, laryngeal edema (less than 1%).

Mefenamic acid – Respiratory depression (less than 1%).

Nabumetone – Eosinophilic pneumonia, hypersensitivity pneumonitis, idiopathic interstitial pneumonitis (less than 1%).

Naproxen – Eosinophilic pneumonitis (less than 1%).

Oxaprozin – Pulmonary infections (less than 1%).

Piroxicam – Respiratory depression (less than 1%).

➤*Special senses:*

Celecoxib – Cataract, deafness, ear abnormality, earache, eye pain, glaucoma, otitis media (less than 2%).

Etodolac – Deafness, photophobia (less than 1%).

Fenoprofen – Burning tongue, optic neuritis (less than 1%).

Flurbiprofen – Corneal opacity, ear disease, glaucoma, parosmia, retinal hemorrhage, retrobulbar neuritis, transient hearing loss (less than 1%).

Ibuprofen – Amblyopia, cataracts, dry eyes, optic neuritis (less than 1%).

Indomethacin – Corneal deposits and retinal disturbances (including those of the macula), deafness (less than 1%).

Ketoprofen – Conjunctivitis sicca, eye pain, retinal hemorrhage and pigmentation change (less than 1%).

Ketorolac – Abnormal taste, abnormal vision (less than 1%).

Meclofenamate – Decreased visual acuity, iritis, macular and perimacular edema, retinal changes including macular fibrosis, reversible loss of color vision, temporary loss of vision (less than 1%).

Meloxicam – Abnormal vision (less than 2%).

Piroxicam – Swollen eyes (less than 1%).

Sulindac – Bitter taste, disturbances of retina and vasculature of retina, metallic taste (less than 1%).

Tolmetin – Optic neuropathy, retinal and macular changes (less than 1%).

➤*Miscellaneous:*

Celecoxib – Allergy aggravated, cyst NOS, hot flushes, infection bacterial/fungal/viral, infection soft tissue, moniliasis, peripheral pain, tooth disorder (less than 2%); sepsis, sudden death (less than 0.1%), suicide.

Diclofenac – Death, infection, sepsis (less than 1%).

Ketoprofen – Septicemia, shock (less than 1%).

Ketorolac – Injection site pain (2%).

Mefenamic acid – Death, sepsis (less than 1%).

Meloxicam – Hot flushes (less than 2%).

Piroxicam – Death, sepsis (less than 1%).

Sulindac – Fulminant necrotizing fasciitis (less than 1%).

Overdosage

➤*Symptoms:* The incidence of acute NSAID overdoses result in minimal or no toxicity. Most reports of toxic signs and symptoms are mild to moderate and include GI distress, nausea, vomiting, lethargy, tinnitus, confusion, headache, and blurred vision. More severe symptoms may include seizures, metabolic acidosis, hypotension, hypothermia, hepatic and renal injury, coma, anaphylactoid reactions, and respiratory depression. Severe poisoning may result in hypertension, acute renal failure, hepatic dysfunction, cardiovascular collapse, and cardiac arrest. Anaphylactoid reactions have been reported with therapeutic ingestion of NSAIDs and may occur following an overdose. Acute overdose studies of **ibuprofen** report approximately 60% of adults remaining asymptomatic, 30% to 40% suffer mild to moderate symptoms, and less than 3% experience severe symptoms. Those at risk for toxicity associated with long-term use include elderly patients and those with pre-existing renal, cardiovascular, or hepatic disease. Most organ systems are involved; however, the majority of deaths from long-term use are related to GI effects.

Symptoms may include the following: drowsiness; dizziness; mental confusion; disorientation; lethargy; paresthesia; numbness; vomiting; gastric irritation; nausea; abdominal pain; intense headache; tinnitus; convulsions; blurred vision; respiratory depression; GI bleeding; hypertension; dyspepsia; ataxia; tremor; hyperpyrexia; epigastric pain; metabolic acidosis; anaphylactoid reactions; heartburn; indigestion; elevations in serum creatinine and BUN; renal impairment, coma, seizures, status epilepticus (**mefenamic acid**); hypotension and tachycardia (acute ingestion of **fenoprofen**); stupor, coma, diminished urine output and hypotension (**sulindac**; deaths have occurred); metabolic acidosis (acute **ibuprofen** overdosage); acute renal failure (**diclofenac** 2 g; **fenoprofen**, **oxaprozin** [rare]).

➤*Treatment:* Treatment of NSAID toxicity is primarily supportive and symptomatic. In addition to supportive measures, the use of oral activated charcoal may help to reduce the absorption and reabsorption of the NSAID. Refer to General Management of Acute Overdosage. Syrup of ipecac and gastric lavage have been recommended, but effectiveness has not been studied in NSAID overdose. Gastric lavage performed more than 1 hour after overdosage has little benefit. Take care in administering syrup of ipecac to a child who has ingested 100 to 400 mg/kg of **ibuprofen** because ibuprofen at this dose range mimics the symptoms produced by ipecac. Because NSAIDs are rapidly absorbed, decontamination may not benefit more than 2- to 4-hour postingestion. Do not give syrup of ipecac to overdose patients at high risk of seizures, especially those who have ingested **mefenamic acid** or high amounts of other NSAIDs.

Because most NSAIDs are highly protein bound, extensively metabolized, and essentially excreted unchanged, elimination enhancement (hemodialysis, forced diuresis, alkalinization of urine, hemoperfusion, and peritoneal dialysis) may be of little value. However, hemodialysis may be necessary in cases of NSAID-induced prolonged or severe renal failure. Multiple doses of activated charcoal for elimination enhancement have been reported in **indomethacin** and **piroxicam** ingestions and, therefore, may be applied to **sulindac**, **diclofenac**, **meloxicam**, and **ibuprofen** to interrupt enterohepatic or enteroenteric recirculation. Use this therapy only in severely symptomatic overdoses.

Meclofenamate – Dialysis may be required to correct serious azotemia or electrolyte imbalance.

Meloxicam – In a clinical trial, 4 g of oral cholestyramine 3 times daily accelerated meloxicam clearance.

Patient Information

Adverse effects of NSAIDs can cause discomfort and, rarely, more serious adverse effects, such as GI bleeding, may occur, which may result in hospitalization and even death. NSAIDs are often essential in the management of arthritis and have a major role in treating pain, but they also may be commonly employed for less serious conditions. Apprise patients of potential risks.

Photosensitivity may occur; caution patients to take protective measures (ie, sunscreens, protective clothing) against UV or sunlight until tolerance is determined.

Avoid **aspirin** and alcoholic beverages while taking medication.

Although serious GI tract ulcerations and bleeding can occur without warning symptoms, alert patients for the signs and symptoms of ulcerations and bleeding, and have patients ask for medical advice when observing any indicative sign or symptoms. Apprise patients of the importance of this follow-up.

Inform patients that NSAIDs may cause serious cardiovascular events, such as MI or stroke, which may result in hospitalization and even death. Advise patients to be alert for the signs and symptoms of chest pain, shortness of breath, weakness, and slurring of speech, and to ask for medical advice when observing any indicative signs or symptoms.

Inform patients that NSAIDs can cause serious skin reactions, which may result in hospitalization and even death. Advise patients to be alert for the signs and symptoms of skin rash and blisters, fever, or other signs of hypersensitivity, such as itching, and to notify their health care provider if any of these occur.

Inform patients of the warning signs and symptoms of hepatotoxicity (eg, nausea, fatigue, lethargy, pruritus, jaundice, right upper quadrant tenderness, flu-like symptoms). If these occur, instruct patients to stop therapy and seek immediate medical therapy.

Instruct patients to seek immediate emergency help in the case of an anaphylactoid reaction.

Advise patients to avoid NSAIDs in late pregnancy because it may cause premature closure of the ductus arteriosus.

If GI upset occurs, advise patients to take with food, milk, or antacids. For GI upset with **tolmetin**, use antacids other than sodium bicarbonate; bioavailability is affected by food and milk. If GI symptoms persist, patient should notify health care provider.

Advise women who are taking **meclofenamate** for heavy menstrual flow to consult their doctor if they have spotting or bleeding between cycles or worsening of their menstrual blood flow. These symptoms may be signs of the development of a more serious condition that is not appropriately treated with meclofenamate.

Health care providers may wish to discuss the potential risks and likely benefits of NSAID treatment with their patients, particularly when the drugs are used for less serious conditions where treatment without NSAIDs may represent an acceptable alternative to both the patient and the health care provider.

Health care providers may want to make specific recommendations to patients about when they should take NSAIDs in relation to food and what patients should do if they experience minor GI symptoms associated with them.

May cause drowsiness, vertigo, depression, dizziness, or blurred vision; patients should use caution while driving or performing other tasks requiring alertness.

Advise patient to notify health care provider if skin rash, GI ulceration, bleeding, visual disturbances, weight gain, edema, black stools, or persistent headache occurs.

Advise patients taking mefenamic acid and meclofenamate that if rash, diarrhea, or other digestive problems occur, discontinue use and consult a health care provider.

Inform patients not to take nonprescription ibuprofen for more than 3 days for fever, or more than 10 days for pain. If symptoms persist, worsen, or if new symptoms develop, patients should contact a health care provider.

DICLOFENAC

Rx	**Cataflam** (Novartis)	**Tablets; oral**: 50 mg	As diclofenac potassium. Polyethylene glycol, sucrose. (CATAFLAM 50). Lt. brown, round. In 100s.
Rx	**Diclofenac Potassium** (Various, eg, Geneva, Mylan, Teva)		As diclofenac potassium. In 100s and 500s.
Rx	**Diclofenac Sodium** (Various, eg, Geneva, Roxane, Watson)	**Tablets, delayed-release**; **oral**: 25 mg	As diclofenac sodium. May be enteric-coated. In 60s and 100s.
Rx	**Diclofenac Sodium** (Various, eg, Geneva, Martec, Purepac)	**Tablets, delayed-release**; **oral**: 50 mg	As diclofenac sodium. May be enteric-coated. In 42s, 60s, 100s, 500s, 1,000s, and UD 100s.
Rx	**Diclofenac Sodium** (Various, eg, Geneva, Martec, Purepac)	**Tablets, delayed-release**; **oral**: 75 mg	As diclofenac sodium. May be enteric-coated. In 42s, 60s, 100s, 500s, 1,000s.
Rx	**Voltaren** (Novartis)		As diclofenac sodium. Enteric-coated. Lactose, polyethylene glycol. (VOLTAREN 75). Lt. pink, triangular. In 100s.
Rx	**Diclofenac Sodium** (Various, eg, Geneva, Purepac, Teva)	**Tablets, extended-release**; **oral**: 100 mg	As diclofenac sodium. May contain cetyl alcohol, polyethylene glycol, sucrose. In 100s.
Rx	**Voltaren-XR** (Novartis)		As diclofenac sodium. Film-coated. Cetyl alcohol, polyethylene glycol, sucrose. (Voltaren-XR 100). Lt. pink, round. In 100s.
Rx	**Zipsor** (Xanodyne)	**Capsules; oral**: 25 mg	As diclofenac potassium. Isopropyl alcohol, mineral oil, PEG, sorbitol. (X592). Pale yellow. In 100s.
Rx	**Cambia** (Mipharm)	**Powder for solution**; **oral**: 50 mg	As diclofenac potassium. Aspartame, mannitol, phenylalanine 25 mg, saccharin. In UD 1s, 3s, and 9s.

DICLOFENAC POTASSIUM — ORAL

For complete and comparative prescribing information, refer to the NSAIDs class monograph.

WARNING

Cardiovascular risk – Nonsteroidal anti-inflammatory drugs (NSAIDs) may cause an increased risk of serious cardiovascular thrombotic events, myocardial infarction (MI), and stroke, which can be fatal. This risk may increase with duration of use. Patients with cardiovascular disease or risk factors of cardiovascular disease may be at greater risk.

Diclofenac is contraindicated for treatment of perioperative pain in the setting of coronary artery bypass graft (CABG) surgery.

GI risk – NSAIDs cause an increased risk of serious GI adverse reactions, including bleeding, inflammation, ulceration, and perforation of the stomach or intestines, which can be fatal. These events can occur at any time during use and without warning symptoms. Elderly patients are at greater risk of serious GI events.

Indications

➤*Analgesia (capsules/tablets):* For the relief of mild to moderate acute pain in adults.

➤*Arthritis (tablets):* For the relief of signs and symptoms of osteoarthritis and rheumatoid arthritis.

➤*Dysmenorrhea (tablets):* For the treatment of primary dysmenorrhea.

➤*Migraine (oral solution):* For the acute treatment of migraine attacks with or without aura in adults.

Administration and Dosage

➤*General dosing considerations:* After observing the response to initial therapy with diclofenac, the dose and frequency should be adjusted to suit an individual patient's needs.

Different formulations of oral diclofenac are not bioequivalent, even if the milligram strength is the same.

Diclofenac capsules are not indicated for long-term treatment.

➤*Adults:*

Analgesia –

Capsules: 25 mg 4 times daily.

Tablets:

- *Usual dosage* – 50 mg 3 times daily.
- *Alternative dosage* – An initial dose of 100 mg followed by 50 mg doses may provide better relief.

Migraine – 50 mg (1 packet) as a single dose.

Osteoarthritis – 100 to 150 mg/day given as 50 mg 2 or 3 times daily.

Primary dysmenorrhea –

Tablets: See Analgesia for dosing.

Rheumatoid arthritis – 150 to 200 mg/day given as 50 mg 3 or 4 times daily.

➤*Renal function impairment:* In patients with advanced kidney disease, treatment with diclofenac is not recommended. However, if NSAID therapy must be initiated, close monitoring of the patient's kidney function is advisable.

➤*Hepatic function impairment:* Hepatic metabolism accounts for almost 100% of diclofenac elimination, so patients with hepatic disease may require reduced doses of diclofenac compared with patients with healthy hepatic function. There is insufficient information available to support specific dosing recommendations for diclofenac in patients with hepatic insufficiency.

➤*Administration:*

Oral solution – Advise patients to empty the contents of 1 packet into a cup containing 1 to 2 ounces (30 to 60 mL) of water, mix well, and drink immediately. Instruct them not to use liquids other than water. Administration of diclofenac oral solution with food may cause a reduction in effectiveness compared with administration on an empty stomach.

➤*Storage/Stability:* Do not store tablets at temperatures higher than 30°C (86°F). Dispense in a tight container.

Store capsules and powder for oral solution at 25°C (77°F); excursions are permitted between 15° and 30°C (59° and 86°F). Protect capsules from moisture and dispense in a tight container.

DICLOFENAC SODIUM — ORAL

For complete and comparative prescribing information, refer to the NSAIDs class monograph.

WARNING

Cardiovascular risk – Nonsteroidal anti-inflammatory drugs (NSAIDs) may cause an increased risk of serious cardiovascular thrombotic events, myocardial infarction (MI), and stroke, which can be fatal. This risk may increase with duration of use. Patients with cardiovascular disease or risk factors of cardiovascular disease may be at greater risk.

Diclofenac is contraindicated for treatment of perioperative pain in the setting of coronary artery bypass graft (CABG) surgery.

GI risk – NSAIDs cause an increased risk of serious GI adverse events, including inflammation, bleeding, ulceration, and perforation of the stomach or intestines, which can be fatal. These events can occur at any time during use and without warning symptoms. Elderly patients are at greater risk of serious GI events.

Indications

➤*Ankylosing spondylitis (delayed-release tablets only):* For acute or long-term use in the relief of signs and symptoms of ankylosing spondylitis.

➤*Osteoarthritis:* For relief of signs and symptoms of osteoarthritis.

➤*Rheumatoid arthritis:* For relief of signs and symptoms of rheumatoid arthritis.

➤*Off-label uses:*

Juvenile idiopathic arthritis – [4] = Insufficient documentation. Data evaluating the safety and efficacy of diclofenac for the treatment of juvenile idiopathic arthritis (JIA) are limited to 2 small controlled trials that were conducted more than 20 years ago. Results from these trials show that diclofenac is equivalent to other NSAIDs (aspirin, tolmetin, naproxen), with a good tolerability profile with short-term use. Currently, there are no national guidelines for the management of JIA. A review of treatment options for JIA notes that, while not all are Food and Drug Administration–labeled for use in JIA, many NSAIDs, including diclofenac, are commonly used.

Administration and Dosage

➤*General dosing considerations:* After observing the response to initial therapy with diclofenac, the dose and frequency should be adjusted to suit the individual patient's needs.

Different formulations of diclofenac (diclofenac sodium delayed-release tablets; diclofenac sodium extended-release [ER]) tablets; diclofenac potassium immediate-release tablets) are not necessarily bioequivalent, even if the milligram strength is the same.

➤*Adults:*

Ankylosing spondylitis –

Delayed-release tablets: 100 to 125 mg/day administered as 25 mg 4 times daily with an extra 25 mg dose at bedtime if necessary.

Osteoarthritis –

Delayed-release tablets: 100 to 150 mg/day in divided doses (50 mg twice daily or 3 times daily, or 75 mg twice daily).

ER tablets: 100 mg/day.

Rheumatoid arthritis –

Delayed-release tablets: 150 to 200 mg/day in divided doses (50 mg 3 times daily or 4 times daily, or 75 mg twice daily).

ER tablets: 100 mg/day. In the rare patient for whom diclofenac 100 mg/day ER tablets are unsatisfactory, the dose may be increased to 100 mg twice daily if the benefits outweigh the clinical risks of increased adverse reactions.

➤*Children:*

Off-label dosing –

Juvenile idiopathic arthritis: [4] = Insufficient documentation.

- *3 to 16 years of age* – 2 to 3 mg/kg given daily for up to 4 weeks.

➤*Renal function impairment:* In cases with advanced kidney disease, treatment with diclofenac is not recommended. If NSAID therapy must be initiated, close monitoring of the patient's kidney function is advisable.

➤*Hepatic function impairment:* Hepatic metabolism accounts for almost 100% of diclofenac elimination, so patients with hepatic disease may require reduced doses of diclofenac compared with patients with healthy hepatic function.

➤*Storage/Stability:* Do not store at temperatures higher than 30°C (86°F). Protect from moisture. Dispense in a tight container.

ETODOLAC

Rx	**Etodolac** (Various, eg, Eon, Par, Purepac, Ranbaxy, Taro, Teva, Watson, Zenith Goldline)	**Tablets**: 400 mg	In 100s and 500s.
Rx	**Etodolac** (Various, eg, Eon, Par, Purepac, Ranbaxy, Taro, Teva, Watson, Zenith Goldline)	**Tablets**: 500 mg	In 100s, 500s, and 1000s.
Rx	**Etodolac** (Various, eg, Purepac, Teva)	**Tablets, extended-release**: 400 mg	In 100s and 500s.
Rx	**Etodolac** (Various, eg, Teva)	**Tablets, extended-release**: 500 mg	In 100s.
Rx	**Etodolac** (Various, eg, Teva)	**Tablets, extended-release**: 600 mg	In 100s.

ETODOLAC

Rx	**Etodolac** (Various, eg, Mylan, Par, Taro, Teva, Watson)	**Capsules:** 200 mg	In 100s, 500s, and 1000s.
Rx	**Etodolac** (Various, eg, Mylan, Par, Taro, Teva, Watson)	**Capsules:** 300 mg	In 100s, 500s, and 1000s.

ETODOLAC — ORAL

For complete and comparative prescribing information, refer to the NSAIDs group monograph.

WARNING

Cardiovascular risk – NSAIDs may cause an increased risk of serious cardiovascular thrombotic events, myocardial infarction, and stroke, which can be fatal. This risk may increase with duration of use. Patients with cardiovascular disease or risk factors for cardiovascular disease may be at greater risk.

Mefenamic acid is contraindicated for treatment of perioperative pain in the setting of coronary artery bypass graft (CABG) surgery.

GI risk – NSAIDs cause an increased risk of serious GI adverse events including bleeding, ulceration, and perforation of the stomach or intestines, which can be fatal. These events can occur at any time during use and without warning symptoms. Elderly patients are at greater risk for serious GI events.

Indications

➤*Arthritis:* For the relief of the signs and symptoms of osteoarthritis, rheumatoid arthritis, juvenile rheumatoid arthritis.

➤*Analgesia:* For the management of other types of pain.

Administration and Dosage

➤*General dosing considerations:* As with other nonsteroidal anti-inflammatory drugs (NSAIDs), the lowest dose and longest dosing interval should be sought for each patient. Therefore, after observing the response to initial therapy with etodolac, the dose and frequency should be adjusted to suit an individual patient's needs.

In chronic conditions, a therapeutic response to therapy with etodolac is sometimes seen within 1 week of therapy, but most often is observed by 2 weeks. After a satisfactory response has been achieved, the patient's dose should be reviewed and adjusted as required.

If a decision is made to use etodolac extended-release tablets for patients 6 years of age and older, as with other NSAIDs, such patients should be monitored periodically.

➤*Adults:*

Analgesia –

Usual dosage:

• *Capsules and tablets* – 200 to 400 mg every 6 to 8 hours; up to 1,000 mg as a total daily dose.

Dosage adjustment: In some patients, if the potential benefits outweigh the risks; the dose may be increased to 1,200 mg/day in order to achieve a therapeutic benefit that might not have been achieved with 1,000 mg/day.

Osteoarthritis –

Maximum dose: 1,200 mg/day of extended-release tablets.

Initial dosage:

• *Capsules and tablets* – 300 mg 2 or 3 times daily, 400 mg 2 times daily, or 500 mg 2 times daily.

• *Tablets, extended release* – 400 to 1,000 mg, given once daily.

Dosage adjustment:

• *Capsules and tablets* – During long-term administration, the dose of etodolac may be adjusted up or down, depending on the clinical response of the patient. A lower dose of 600 mg/day may suffice for long-term administration.

In patients who tolerate 1,000 mg/day, the dose may be increased to 1,200 mg/day when a higher level of therapeutic activity is required.

• *Tablets, extended-release* – During long-term administration, the dose of etodolac extended-release tablets may be adjusted up or down, depending on the patient's clinical response, up to a maximum dose of 1,200 mg/day.

Rheumatoid arthritis – See Osteoarthritis for dosing.

➤*Children:*

Juvenile rheumatoid arthritis –

6 to 16 years of age:

• *Usual dosage* –

Tablets, extended-release: The recommended dose given orally once per day should be based on body weight, according to the following information:

Etodolac Recommended Dosage (Based on Body Weight)

Body weight range (kg)	Dose
20 to 30 kg	400 mg tablet × 1
31 to 45 kg	600 mg tablet × 1
46 to 60 kg	400 mg tablet × 2
> 60 kg	500 mg tablet × 2

➤*Storage/Stability:*

Capsules and tablets – Store at 15° to 30°C (59° to 86°F). Keep tightly closed. Preserve in tight, light-resistant container.

Tablets, extended-release – Store at 20° to 25°C (68° to 77°F). Protect from excessive heat and humidity.

FENOPROFEN CALCIUM

Rx	**Fenoprofen** (Various, eg, Geneva, Par, Watson)	**Capsules; oral:** 200 mg	In 100s.
Rx	**Nalfon** (Pedinol)		(RX681). Yellow/White opaque. In 100s.
Rx	**Fenoprofen** (Various, eg, Geneva, Par, Watson)	**Capsules; oral:** 300 mg	In 100s.
Rx	**Nalfon** (Pedinol)	**Capsules; oral:** 400 mg	(Nalfon 400 EP 123). Green/Blue opaque. In 90s and 500s.
Rx	**Fenoprofen** (Various, eg, Watson, Zenith Goldline)	**Tablets; oral:** 600 mg	In 100s, 500s, and 1000s, UD 100s, unit-of-use 30s, 60s, 90s, and 120s.

FENOPROFEN CALCIUM — ORAL

For complete and comparative prescribing information, refer to the NSAIDs class monograph.

WARNING

Cardiovascular risk – Nonsteroidal anti-inflammatory drugs (NSAIDs) may cause an increased risk of serious cardiovascular thrombotic events, myocardial infarction, and stroke, which can be fatal. This risk may increase with duration of use. Patients with cardiovascular disease or risk factors for cardiovascular disease may be at greater risk.

Fenoprofen is contraindicated for treatment of perioperative pain in the setting of coronary artery bypass graft (CABG) surgery.

GI risk – NSAIDs cause an increased risk of serious GI adverse events, including bleeding, ulceration, and perforation of the stomach or intestines, which can be fatal. These events can occur at any time during use and without warning symptoms. Elderly patients are at greater risk for serious GI events.

Indications

➤*Mild to moderate pain:* For the relief of mild to moderate pain.

➤*Osteoarthritis/Rheumatoid arthritis:* For relief of the signs and symptoms of rheumatoid arthritis (RA) and osteoarthritis.

➤*Off-label uses:* Selected NSAIDs have been used in the treatment of juvenile RA, symptomatic treatment of sunburn, and for various migraine headaches.

Administration and Dosage

➤*General dosing considerations:* Patients with RA generally seem to require larger doses of fenoprofen than do those with osteoarthritis. The smallest dose that yields acceptable control should be employed.

➤*Adults:*

Pain – 200 mg every 4 to 6 hours as needed for the treatment of mild to moderate pain.

Osteoarthritis –

Usual dosage: 400 to 600 mg 3 or 4 times a day.

Maximum dose: Total daily dose should not exceed 3,200 mg.

Dosage adjustment: The dose should be tailored to the needs of the patient and may be increased or decreased depending on the severity of the symptoms. Dosage adjustments may be made after initiation of drug therapy or during exacerbations of the disease.

Duration of therapy: Although improvement may be seen in a few days in many patients, an additional 2 to 3 weeks may be required to gauge the full benefits of therapy.

Rheumatoid arthritis – See Osteoarthritis for dosing.

FENOPROFEN CALCIUM — ORAL

➤*Elderly:* Because fenoprofen is primarily eliminated by the kidneys, patients with possibly compromised renal function (such as elderly patients) should be monitored periodically, especially during long-term therapy. For such patients, it may be anticipated that a lower daily dosage will avoid excessive drug accumulation.

➤*Renal function impairment:* For such patients, it may be anticipated that a lower daily dosage will avoid excessive drug accumulation.

➤*Administration:* If GI complaints occur, fenoprofen may be administered with meals or with milk. Although the total amount absorbed is not affected, peak blood levels are delayed and diminished.

➤*Storage/Stability:* Store at controlled room temperature, 20° to 25°C (68° to 77°F).

FLURBIPROFEN

Rx	**Flurbiprofen** (Various, eg, Mylan, Teva)	**Tablets; oral:** 50 mg	In 100s.
Rx	**Flurbiprofen** (Various, eg, Mylan, Teva)	**Tablets; oral:** 100 mg	In 100s and 500s.

FLURBIPROFEN — ORAL

For complete and comparative prescribing information, refer to the Nonsteroidal Anti-inflammatory Agents (NSAIDs) group monograph in this chapter.

WARNING

Cardiovascular (CV) risk – Nonsteroidal anti-inflammatory drugs (NSAIDs) may cause an increased risk of serious CV thrombotic events, myocardial infarction, and stroke, which can be fatal. This risk may increase with duration of use. Patients with CV disease or risk factors for CV disease may be at greater risk.

Flurbiprofen is contraindicated for treatment of perioperative pain in the setting of coronary artery bypass graft (CABG) surgery.

GI risk – NSAIDs cause an increased risk of serious GI adverse reactions including bleeding, ulceration, and perforation of the stomach or intestines, which can be fatal. These reactions can occur at any time during use and without warning symptoms. Elderly patients are at greater risk for serious GI reactions.

Indications

➤*Rheumatoid arthritis (RA) and osteoarthritis (OA):* For the relief of the signs and symptoms of RA and OA.

Administration and Dosage

➤*General dosing considerations:* Use the lowest effective dose for the shortest duration consistent with individual patient treatment goals.

After observing the response to initial therapy with flurbiprofen, adjust the dose and frequency to suit an individual patient's needs.

➤*Adults:*

Osteoarthritis

Usual dosage: 200 to 300 mg per day administered 2, 3, or 4 times a day.
Maximum dose: 100 mg as a single dose in a multiple-dose daily regimen.

Rheumatoid arthritis – See Osteoarthritis for dosing.

➤*Renal function impairment:* Treatment with flurbiprofen is not recommended in these patients with advanced renal disease. If flurbiprofen therapy must be initiated, close monitoring of the patient's renal function is advisable.

➤*Hepatic function impairment:* Patients with hepatic function impairment may require reduced doses of flurbiprofen.

➤*Storage/Stability:* Store at 20° to 25°C (68° to 77°F).

IBUPROFEN

otc	**Junior Strength Motrin** (McNeil)	**Tablets; oral:** 100 mg	(M 100). Yellow. In 24s.
otc	**Ibuprofen** (Various, eg, Geneva, Goldline, Major, UDL)	**Tablets; oral:** 200 mg	In 24s, 50s, 100s, 250s, 1,000s, and UD 100s.
otc	**Advil** (Whitehall-Robins)		Sucrose. (Advil). In 8s, 24s, 50s, 72s, 100s, 165s, and 250s.
otc	**Ibutab** (Zee Medical)		In 24s.
otc	**Midol Maximum Strength Cramp Formula** (Bayer)		(BAYER BAYER BAYER BAYER). In 24s.
otc	**Motrin IB** (McNeil)		**Tablets:** (Motrin IB). In 100s. **Gelcaps:** (Motrin IB). In 8s.
otc	**Motrin Migraine Pain** (McNeil Consumer)		(IB). White, capsule shape. In 24s, 50s, and 100s.
Rx	**Ibuprofen** (Various, eg, Geneva, Major, Schein, UDL, Zenith Goldline)	**Tablets; oral:** 400 mg	In 100s, 360s, 500s, UD 100s, UD 300s, unit-of-use 100s, *Robot ready* 25s, and *Emergi-script* 60s.
Rx	**Ibuprofen** (Various, eg, Geneva, Major, Schein, URL, Zenith Goldline)	**Tablets; oral:** 600 mg	In 100s, 270s, 500s, UD 100s, UD 300s, unit-of-use 100s, *Robot* ready 25s, and *Emergi-script* 60s.
Rx	**Ibuprofen** (Various, eg, Geneva, Major, Schein, UDL, URL, Zenith Goldline)	**Tablets; oral:** 800 mg	In 100s, 270s, 500s, UD 100s, UD 300s, unit-of-use 100s, *Robot* ready 25s, and *Emergi-script* 60s.
otc	**Children's Motrin** (McNeil)	**Tablets, chewable; oral:** 50 mg	Aspartame, phenylalanine 3 mg. Orange flavor. In 24s.
otc	**Motrin, Junior Strength** (McNeil)	**Tablets, chewable; oral:** 100 mg	Aspartame, phenylalanine 6 mg. (MOTRIN 100). Orange flavor. In 24s.
otc	**Advil Liqui-Gels** (Whitehall-Robins)	**Capsules; oral:** 200 mg	Sorbitol. (Advil). Green. In 4s, 20s, 40s, and 80s.
otc	**Advil Migraine** (Whitehall-Robins)		Sorbitol. (Advil). Brown, oval. In 20s.
otc	**Ibuprofen** (Various, eg, Alpharma, Major, Perrigo)	**Suspension; oral:** 100 mg per 5 mL	In 118 mL.
otc	**Children's Advil** (Wyeth-Ayerst)		Sorbitol, sucrose, EDTA. Fruit flavor. In 119 and 473 mL.
otc	**Children's Motrin** (McNeil-CPC)		Sucrose. Grape and bubble gum flavor. In 60 and 120 mL.
otc	**PediaCare Fever** (Pharmacia & Upjohn)		Sucrose. Berry flavor. In 120 mL.
otc	**Ibuprofen** (Perrigo)	**Drops; oral:** 40 mg/mL	In 15 mL.
otc	**Advil Pediatric Drops** (Whitehall-Robins)		Sorbitol, sucrose, EDTA, glycerin. Grape flavor. In 7.5 mL.
otc	**Motrin Infants'** (McNeil)		Sorbitol, sucrose. Berry flavor. In 30 mL with dropper.
otc	**PediaCare Fever** (Pharmacia & Upjohn)		Sorbitol, sucrose. Berry flavor. In 15 mL.
Rx	**Caldolor** (Cumberland Pharmaceuticals)	**Injection, solution, concentrate:** 100 mg/mL	Arginine 78 mg/mL. In 4 and 8 mL single-dose vials.

IBUPROFEN — ORAL

For complete and comparative prescribing information, refer to the NSAIDs group monograph.

> **WARNING**
>
> *Cardiovascular risk* – NSAIDs may cause an increased risk of serious cardiovascular thrombotic events, myocardial infarction, and stroke, which can be fatal. This risk may increase with duration of use. Patients with cardiovascular disease or risk factors for cardiovascular disease may be at greater risk.
>
> Ibuprofen is contraindicated for treatment of perioperative pain in the setting of coronary artery bypass graft (CABG) surgery.
>
> *GI risk* – NSAIDs cause an increased risk of serious GI adverse events including bleeding, ulceration, and perforation of the stomach or intestines, which can be fatal. These events can occur at any time during use and without warning symptoms. Elderly patients are at greater risk for serious GI events.

Indications

➤*OTC:*

Adults –

Liquid-filled capsules: Treats migraine.

Gelcaps and tablets: Temporarily relieves minor aches and pains due to the common cold, headache, toothache, muscular aches, backache, minor pain of arthritis, menstrual cramps.

Temporarily reduces fever.

Children –

Chewable tablets, junior strength tablets, oral suspension, and oral drops: For the temporary reduction of fever and relief of minor aches and pains due to colds, flu, sore throat, headaches, and toothaches. One dose lasts 6 to 8 hours. Ibuprofen children's chewable tablets are recommended for children 4 to 11 years of age. Ibuprofen junior strength tablets are recommended for children 6 to 11 years of age. Ibuprofen oral suspension is recommended for children 2 to 11 years of age. Ibuprofen oral drops are recommended for children 6 months to 3 years of age (varies by manufacturer).

➤*Rx:* Prescription strength ibuprofen tablets are indicated for relief of mild-to-moderate pain, for relief of the signs and symptoms of rheumatoid arthritis and osteoarthritis, and in the treatment of primary dysmenorrhea.

➤*Off-label uses:*

Patent ductus arteriosus – [4] = Insufficient documentation. Oral ibuprofen for the prophylaxis and management of patent ductus arteriosus has been limited to only 2 small studies. However, the success of intravenous (IV) data and initial beneficial results with oral administration of the drug suggested that this agent may be a useful and safer alternative to IV indomethacin. (See Administration and Dosage.)

Prevention of adverse reactions with diphtheria and tetanus toxoids and pertussis (DTP) vaccination – [2] = Fair documentation. The published data evaluating the safety and efficacy of ibuprofen for the prevention of adverse reactions associated with DTP vaccination are limited and conflicting. Ibuprofen was shown to be effective at reducing local and systemic reactions when whole-cell pertussis vaccine was used, but was not shown to be effective at reducing the incidence of fever. One trial evaluating its efficacy at reducing local reactions after the fifth dose of acellular product failed to show any benefit. Published data and current Advisory Committee on Immunization Practices (ACIP) recommendations do not support routine use of ibuprofen prophylaxis with DTP vaccination. However, ibuprofen prophylaxis should be considered in patients at high risk for seizures. (See Administration and Dosage.)

Prevention of adverse reactions with DTP vaccination in patients at risk for seizures – [1] = Good documentation. The published data evaluating the safety and efficacy of ibuprofen for the prevention of adverse reactions associated with DTP vaccination are limited and conflicting. Ibuprofen was shown to be effective at reducing local and systemic reactions when whole-cell pertussis vaccine was used, but was not shown to be effective at reducing the incidence of fever. One trial evaluating its efficacy at reducing local reactions after the fifth dose of acellular product failed to show any benefit. Published data and current ACIP recommendations do not support routine use of ibuprofen prophylaxis with DTP vaccination. However, ibuprofen prophylaxis should be considered in patients at high risk for seizures. (See Administration and Dosage.)

Administration and Dosage

➤*General dosing considerations:* The smallest dose of ibuprofen that yields acceptable control should be employed. A linear blood-level, dose-response relationship exists with single doses up to 800 mg.

In chronic conditions, a therapeutic response to therapy with ibuprofen is sometimes seen in a few days to a week but most often is observed by 2 weeks. After a satisfactory response has been achieved, the patient's dose should be reviewed and adjusted as required.

➤*Adults:*

OTC –

Migraine:

- *Capsules* – 2 capsules with a glass of water. If migraine symptoms persist or worsen, the patient should refer to his/her health care provider. Taking more than 2 capsules in 24 hours is not recommended, unless directed by a health care provider.

Analgesic/Antipyretic:

- *Gelcaps and tablets* – 1 gelcap or tablet every 4 to 6 hours while symptoms persist. If pain or fever does not respond to 1 gelcap or tablet, 2 gelcaps or tablets may be used, not to exceed 6 gelcaps or tablets in 24 hours, unless directed by a health care provider. The smallest effective dose should be used.

RX –

Dysmenorrhea: Beginning with the earliest onset of such pain, ibuprofen should be given in a dose of 400 mg every 4 hours as necessary for the relief of pain.

Mild to moderate pain: 400 mg every 4 to 6 hours as necessary for relief of pain.

Osteoarthritis, including flareups of chronic disease:

- *Usual dosage* – 1,200 mg to 3,200 mg daily (300 mg 4 times daily; 400, 600, or 800 mg 3 or 4 times daily).
- *Dosage adjustment* – The dose should be tailored to each patient, and may be decreased or increased depending on the severity of symptoms either at the time of initiating drug therapy or as the patient responds or fails to respond.

Rheumatoid arthritis, including flareups of chronic disease:

- *Usual dosage* – 1,200 mg to 3,200 mg daily (300 mg 4 times daily; 400, 600, or 800 mg 3 or 4 times daily).

In general, patients with rheumatoid arthritis seem to require higher doses of ibuprofen than do patients with osteoarthritis.

- *Dosage adjustment* – The dose should be tailored to each patient, and may be decreased or increased depending on the severity of symptoms either at the time of initiating drug therapy or as the patient responds or fails to respond.

➤*Children:*

OTC –

Analgesic/Antipyretic:

- *12 years of age and older* – See Adults for dosing.
- *6 months to 11 years of age* – If possible, use weight to dose; otherwise, use age. If needed, the dose may be repeated every 6 to 8 hours. The dose should not be taken more than 4 times a day.

Children's Ibuprofen Dosing

		Doseform			
Weight	Age	50 mg chewable tablet (every 6 to 8 h, up to 4 times/ day)[a]	100 mg chewable tablet (every 6 to 8 h, up to 4 times/ day)[b]	Oral suspension (every 6 to 8 h, up to 4 times/ day)[c]	Oral drops (every 6 to 8 h, up to 4 times/ day)[d]
12 to 17 lb	6 to 11 mo	—	—	—	1.25 mL (50 mg)
18 to 23 lb	12 to 23 mo	—	—	—	1.875 mL (75 mg)
24 to 35 lb	2 to 3 y	—	—	5 mL (100 mg)	—
36 to 47 lb	4 to 5 y	3 tablets (150 mg)	—	7.5 mL (150 mg)	—
48 to 59 lb	6 to 8 y	4 tablets (200 mg)	2 tablets (200 mg)	10 mL (200 mg)	—
60 to 71 lb	9 to 10 y	5 tablets (250 mg)	2.5 tablets (250 mg)	12.5 mL (250 mg)	—
72 to 95 lb	11 y	6 tablets (300 mg)	3 tablets (300 mg)	15 mL (300 mg)	—

[a] A health care provider should be consulted before giving 50 mg ibuprofen chewable tablets to children younger than 4 years of age or who weigh less than 36 lbs.
[b] A health care provider should be consulted before giving 100 mg ibuprofen chewable tablets to children younger than 6 years of age or who weigh less than 48 lbs.
[c] A health care provider should be consulted before giving 50 mg ibuprofen oral suspension to children younger than 2 years of age or who weigh less than 24 lbs.
[d] Dose at 7.5 mg/kg of body weight. A health care provider should be consulted before giving 50 mg ibuprofen oral drops to infants younger than 6 months of age or who weigh less than 12 lbs.

Off-label dosing –

Juvenile rheumatoid arthritis:

- *Usual dose* – 30 to 50 mg/kg/day orally administered in divided doses every 6 hours.
- *Maximum dose* – 2,400 mg/day.

Patent ductus arteriosus: [4] = Insufficient documentation. Initial dose of 10 mg/kg, then 2 doses of 5 mg/kg administered at 12- or 24-hour intervals.

Prevention of adverse reactions with DTP vaccination: [2] = Fair documentation. Oral ibuprofen was administered as prophylactic or rescue therapy to minimize fever and other adverse reactions associated with DTP vaccination. Doses ranged from 7 to 10 mg/kg/dose.

Prevention of adverse reactions with DTP vaccination in patients at risk for seizures: [1] = Good documentation. Oral ibuprofen was administered as prophylactic or rescue therapy to minimize fever and other adverse reactions associated with DTP vaccination. Doses ranged from 7 to 10 mg/kg/dose.

➤*Renal function impairment:* Because ibuprofen is eliminated primarily by the kidneys, patients with significantly impaired renal function should be closely monitored; a reduction in dosage should be anticipated to avoid drug accumulation.

IBUPROFEN — ORAL

➤*Administration:* Ibuprofen should be taken with food or milk if occasional and mild heartburn, upset stomach, or stomach pain occurs with use. A health care provider should be consulted if these symptoms are more than mild or if they persist.

Oral suspension and oral drops should be shaken well before using.

The administration of ibuprofen tablets either under fasting conditions or immediately before meals yields quite similar serum ibuprofen concentration-time profiles. When ibuprofen is administered immediately after a meal, there is a reduction in the rate of absorption but no appreciable decrease in the extent of absorption. The bioavailability of the drug is minimally altered by the presence of food.

➤*Storage/Stability:*

Capsules, gelcaps, and tablets – Store at 20° to 25°C (68° to 77°F). Avoid excessive heat greater than 40°C (104°F).

Oral suspension and oral drops – Store at 15° to 30°C (59° to 86°F).

IBUPROFEN — INJECTION

For complete and comparative prescribing information, refer to the NSAIDs group monograph.

WARNING

Cardiovascular risk – Nonsteroidal anti-inflammatory drugs (NSAIDs) may increase the risk of serious cardiovascular thrombotic events, myocardial infarction (MI), and stroke, which can be fatal. This risk may increase with duration of use. Patients with cardiovascular disease or risk factors for cardiovascular disease may be at greater risk.

Ibuprofen is contraindicated for the treatment of perioperative pain in the setting of coronary artery bypass graft (CABG) surgery.

GI risk – NSAIDs increase the risk of serious GI adverse events, including bleeding, ulceration, and perforation of the stomach or intestines, which can be fatal. These events can occur at any time during use and without warning symptoms. Elderly patients are at greater risk of serious GI events.

Indications

➤*Pain:* For the management of mild to moderate pain and the management of moderate to severe pain as an adjunct to opioid analgesics in adults.

➤*Fever:* For the reduction of fever in adults.

Administration and Dosage

➤*General dosing considerations:* To reduce the risk of renal adverse reactions, patients must be well hydrated prior to administration of ibuprofen.

➤*Adults:*

Fever –

Usual dosage: 400 mg intravenously (IV) followed by 400 mg IV every 4 to 6 hours or 100 to 200 mg IV every 4 hours as necessary.

Maximum dose: 3,200 mg/day.

Pain –

Usual dosage: 400 to 800 mg IV every 6 hours as necessary.

Maximum dose: 3,200 mg/day.

➤*Preparation for administration:* Must be diluted before administration. Infusion of the drug product without dilution can cause hemolysis. Dilute to a final concentration of 4 mg/mL or less. Appropriate diluents include sodium chloride 0.9% injection (normal saline), dextrose 5% injection, or Ringer's lactate solution. For an 800 mg dose, dilute 8 mL of ibuprofen in no less than 200 mL of diluent; for a 400 mg dose, dilute 4 mL of ibuprofen in no less than 100 mL of diluent.

➤*Administration:* For IV administration only. Infusion time must be no less than 30 minutes.

➤*Storage/Stability:* Store at 20° to 25°C (68° to 77°F). Diluted solutions are stable for up to 24 hours at 20° to 25°C (68° to 77°F).

INDOMETHACIN

Rx	**Indomethacin** (Various, eg, UDL, URL, Zenith Goldline)	**Capsules:** 25 mg	In 50s, 100s, 500s, 1,000s, UD 100s, and *Robot* ready 25s.
Rx	**Indomethacin** (Various, eg, Lederle, UDL, URL, Zenith Goldline)	**Capsules:** 50 mg	In 100s, 500s, 1,000s, UD 100s, and *Robot* ready 25s.
Rx	**Indomethacin Extended-Release** (Inwood)	**Capsules, sustained-release:** 75 mg	Sucrose, parabens. (IL-3607). Lavender/clear. In 60s and 100s.
Rx	**Indomethacin SR** (Various, eg, Endo, Eon, Inwood, Sandoz, Zenith Goldline)		In 60s, 100s, and 500s.
Rx	**Indocin** (Iroko)	**Suspension, oral:** 25 mg per 5 mL	1% alcohol, sorbitol. Pineapple coconut mint flavor. In 237 mL.
Rx	**Indomethacin** (G & W Laboratories)	**Suppositories:** 50 mg	In 30s.
Rx	**Indocin** (Iroko)		In 30s.

INDOMETHACIN — ORAL

For complete and comparative prescribing information, refer to the NSAIDs group monograph. For information on parenteral indomethacin, see Agents for Patent Ductus Arteriosus.

WARNING

Cardiovascular (CV) risk – Nonsteroidal anti-inflammatory drugs (NSAIDs) may cause an increased risk of serious CV thrombotic reactions, myocardial infarction, and stroke, which can be fatal. This risk may increase with duration of use. Patients with CV disease or risk factors for CV disease may be at a greater risk.

Indomethacin is contraindicated for the treatment of perioperative pain in the setting of coronary artery bypass graft (CABG) surgery.

GI risks – NSAIDs cause an increased risk of serious GI adverse reactions, including bleeding, ulceration, and perforation of the stomach or intestines, which can be fatal. These reactions can occur at any time during use and without warning symptoms. Elderly patients are at greater risk for serious GI reactions.

Indications

➤*Arthritis:* Moderate to severe rheumatoid arthritis (RA), including acute flares of chronic disease; moderate to severe osteoarthritis (OA); acute gouty arthritis (except extended-release [ER] capsules).

➤*Inflammatory conditions:* Moderate to severe ankylosing spondylitis; acute painful shoulder (bursitis and/or tendinitis).

➤*Off-label uses:*

Juvenile idiopathic arthritis – [5] = Poor documentation. Data evaluating the safety and efficacy of indomethacin for the treatment of juvenile idiopathic arthritis (JIA) are limited to a small, controlled trial that was conducted more than 30 years ago. While results from this trial showed some benefit, there are significant safety concerns that have been reported in patients with JIA. Currently, there are no national guidelines for the management of JIA. A review of treatment options for JIA notes that, while not all NSAIDs are Food and Drug Administration (FDA)–labeled for use in JIA, many NSAIDs are commonly used. Based on safety concerns and the availability of safer alternatives, indomethacin should not be used for the management of JIA.

Postherpetic neuralgia – [5] = Poor documentation. Use is not recommended. Indomethacin has only been studied in patients with postherpetic neuralgia (PHN) in 1 controlled trial that applied a single dose. American Academy of Neurology clinical practice guidelines state that the efficacy of topical indomethacin is not any better than that of placebo in patients with PHN.

Premature labor – [3] = Safety concerns. Several randomized, controlled trials involving tocolytic agents have been published; however, most are small and have limitations in study design. Because of a lack of substantive evidence, long-term maintenance therapy with tocolytics is not recommended. Tocolytic therapy is recommended only as a method to prevent delivery long enough for a course of corticosteroids to be administered and for the patient to be transferred to an appropriate facility with the ability to care for a premature infant. No one agent is preferred for tocolytic therapy for the treatment of premature labor. Because of the risk for serious adverse effects, all courses of tocolytic therapy should be individualized to reduce the risk to the mother and fetus. Indomethacin has demonstrated moderate efficacy in delaying premature labor; however, significant concerns regarding potential neonatal and fetal effects exist. Larger, controlled trials are needed to determine the efficacy and risks of indomethacin use for treatment of premature labor.

Administration and Dosage

➤*General dosing considerations:* Carefully consider the potential benefits and risks of indomethacin and other treatment options before deciding to use indomethacin. Use the lowest effective dose for the shortest duration consistent with individual patient treatment goals. After observing the response to initial therapy with indomethacin, the dose and frequency should be adjusted to suit an individual patient's needs.

INDOMETHACIN — ORAL

Adverse reactions appear to correlate with the size of the dose of indomethacin (particularly in doses higher than 150 to 200 mg/day, without a corresponding increase in clinical benefits) in most patients, but not all. Therefore, every effort should be made to determine the smallest effective dosage for the individual patient.

Indomethacin ER capsules are available for oral use. Indomethacin ER capsules can be administered once a day and can be substituted for indomethacin 25 mg capsules 3 times a day. However, there will be significant differences between the 2 dosage regimens in indomethacin blood levels, especially after 12 hours. In addition, indomethacin 75 mg ER capsules twice a day can be substituted for indomethacin 50 mg capsules 3 times a day. Indomethacin ER capsules may be substituted for all the indications of indomethacin capsules except acute gouty arthritis.

➤*Adults:*

Acute gouty arthritis (except ER capsules) – 50 mg 3 times a day until pain is tolerable. The dose should then be rapidly reduced to complete cessation of the drug.

Acute painful shoulder (bursitis and/or tendinitis) –

Usual dosage:

- *Capsules/suspension* – 75 to 150 mg daily (in 3 or 4 divided doses).
- *Capsule, extended-release* – 150 mg twice daily.

Duration of therapy: The usual course of therapy is 7 to 14 days.

Discontinuation of therapy: Discontinue after the signs and symptoms of inflammation have been controlled for several days.

Ankylosing spondylitis (moderate to severe) –

Maximum dose: 200 mg daily of immediate release capsules and suspension; 75 mg/day is the maximum recommended starting dose and 150 mg/day for extended-release capsules.

Initial dosage:

- *Capsules/suspension* – 25 mg 2 or 3 times a day.
- *Capsules, extended-release* – 1 capsule daily should be the usual starting dose in order to observe patient tolerance since 75 mg/day is the maximum recommended starting dose.

Dosage titration:

- *Capsules/suspension* – Increase the daily dosage by 25 or 50 mg, if required by continuing symptoms, at weekly intervals until a satisfactory response is obtained or until a total daily dose of 150 to 200 mg is reached. Doses above this amount generally do not increase the efficacy of the drug.

If minor adverse reactions develop as the dosage is increased, reduce the dosage rapidly to a tolerated dose and observe the patient closely.

- *Capsules, extended-release* – If indomethacin ER capsules are used to increase the daily dose, patients should be observed for possible signs and symptoms of intolerance since the daily increment will exceed the daily increment recommended for other dosage forms. For patients who require 150 mg/day and have demonstrated acceptable tolerance, indomethacin ER may be prescribed as 1 capsule twice daily.

Dosage adjustment: After the acute phase of the disease is under control, an attempt to reduce the daily dose should be made repeatedly until the patient is receiving the smallest effective dose or the drug is discontinued. Careful instructions to and observations of the individual patient are essential to the prevention of serious, irreversible (including fatal) adverse reactions.

Alternative dosage: In patients who have persistent night pain and/or morning stiffness, giving a large portion, up to a maximum of 100 mg (immediate release), of the total daily dose at bedtime, may be helpful in affording relief.

Discontinuation of therapy: If severe adverse reactions occur, stop the drug.

Osteoarthritis (moderate to severe) – See Ankylosing spondylitis (moderate to severe) for dosing.

Rheumatoid arthritis (moderate to severe [including acute flares of chronic disease]) – See Ankylosing spondylitis (moderate to severe) for dosing.

Off-label dosing –

Premature labor: [3] = Safety concerns. Several randomized, controlled trials involving more than 500 patients have evaluated the safety and efficacy of indomethacin as a tocolytic agent to delay premature labor. In addition, the American College of Obstetricians and Gynecologists (ACOG) provided a practice bulletin on management of premature labor.

➤*Children:*

15 years of age and older – See Adults for dosing.

2 to 14 years of age –

Do not prescribe indomethacin for children 14 years of age and younger unless toxicity or lack of efficacy associated with other drugs warrants the risk.

If a decision is made to use indomethacin for children 2 years of age and older, such patients should be monitored closely, and periodic assessment of liver function is recommended. There have been cases of hepatotoxicity reported in children with juvenile RA, including fatalities.

Juvenile rheumatoid arthritis:

- *Maximum dose* – 4 mg/kg/day or 150 to 200 mg/day, whichever is less.
- *Initial dosage* – 2 mg/kg/day given in divided doses.
- *Maintenance dosage* – As symptoms subside, the total daily dosage should be reduced to the lowest level required to control symptoms, or the drug should be discontinued.

Off-label dosing –

➤*Administration:* Always give indomethacin capsules, oral suspension, and ER capsules with food, immediately after meals, or with antacids to reduce gastric irritation.

➤*Storage/Stability:*

Capsules – Store at controlled room temperature, 15° to 30°C (59° to 86°F). Protect from light. Dispense in a tight, light-resistant container using a child-resistant closure.

Oral suspension – Store below 30°C (86°F). Avoid temperatures above 50°C (122°F). Protect from freezing.

ER capsules – Store at controlled room temperature, 15° to 30°C (59° to 86°F). Protect from moisture.

INDOMETHACIN — RECTAL

For complete and comparative prescribing information, refer to the NSAIDs group monograph. For information on parenteral indomethacin, see Agents for Patent Ductus Arteriosus.

WARNING

Cardiovascular (CV) risk – Nonsteroidal anti-inflammatory drugs (NSAIDs) may cause an increased risk of serious CV thrombotic reactions, myocardial infarction, and stroke, which can be fatal. This risk may increase with duration of use. Patients with CV disease or risk factors for CV disease may be at greater risk.

Indomethacin is contraindicated for treatment of perioperative pain in the setting of coronary artery bypass graft (CABG) surgery.

GI risk – NSAIDs cause an increased risk of serious GI adverse reactions, including bleeding, ulceration, and perforation of the stomach or intestines, which can be fatal. These reactions can occur at any time during use and without warning symptoms. Elderly patients are at greater risk for serious GI reactions.

Indications

➤*Arthritis:* Moderate to severe rheumatoid arthritis (RA), including acute flares of chronic disease; moderate to severe osteoarthritis (OA); acute gouty arthritis.

➤*Inflammatory conditions:* Moderate to severe ankylosing spondylitis; acute painful shoulder (bursitis and/or tendinitis).

➤*Off-label uses:*

Postherpetic neuralgia – [5] = Poor documentation. Use is not recommended. Indomethacin has only been studied in patients with postherpetic neuralgia (PHN) in 1 controlled trial that applied a single dose. American Academy of Neurology clinical practice guidelines state that the efficacy of topical indomethacin is not any better than that of placebo in patients with PHN.

Premature labor – [3] = Safety concerns. Several randomized, controlled trials involving tocolytic agents have been published; however, most are small and have limitations in study design. Because of a lack of substantive evidence, long-term maintenance therapy with tocolytics is not recommended. Tocolytic therapy is recommended only as a method to prevent delivery long enough for a course of corticosteroids to be administered and for the patient to be transferred to an appropriate facility with the ability to care for a premature infant. No one agent is preferred for tocolytic therapy for the treatment of premature labor. Because of the risk for serious adverse effects, all courses of tocolytic therapy should be individualized to reduce the risk to the mother and fetus. Indomethacin has demonstrated moderate efficacy in delaying premature labor; however, significant concerns regarding potential neonatal and fetal effects exist. Larger, controlled trials are needed to determine the efficacy and risks of indomethacin use for treatment of premature labor. (See Administration and Dosage.)

Administration and Dosage

➤*General dosing considerations:* Carefully consider the potential benefits and risks of indomethacin and other treatment options before deciding to use indomethacin. Use the lowest effective dose for the shortest duration consistent with individual patient treatment goals. After observing the response to initial therapy with indomethacin, adjust the dose and frequency to suit an individual patient's needs.

Adverse reactions appear to correlate with the size of the dose of indomethacin in most patients, but not all. Therefore, every effort should be made to determine the smallest effective dosage for the individual patient.

After the acute phase of the disease is under control, an attempt to reduce the daily dose should be made repeatedly until the patient is receiving the smallest effective dose or the drug is discontinued. Careful instructions to and observations of the individual patient are essential to the prevention of serious, irreversible (including fatal) adverse reactions.

➤*Adults:*

Acute gouty arthritis – 50 mg rectally 3 times a day until pain is tolerable. Then rapidly reduce the dose to complete cessation of the drug.

Bursitis –

Usual dosage: 75 to 150 mg rectally daily in 3 or 4 divided doses.

Duration of therapy: The usual course of therapy is 7 to 14 days.

Discontinuation of therapy: The drug should be discontinued after the signs and symptoms of inflammation have been controlled for several days.

Moderate to severe ankylosing spondylitis –

Usual dosage: 25 mg rectally 2 or 3 times a day.

Maximum dose: 200 mg per day.

INDOMETHACIN — RECTAL

Dosage adjustment: If the usual dosage is well tolerated, increase the daily dosage by 25 or 50 mg, if required by continuing symptoms, at weekly intervals until a satisfactory response is obtained or until a total daily dose of 150 to 200 mg is reached. Doses higher than this amount generally do not increase the efficacy of the drug.

If minor adverse reactions develop as the dosage is increased, reduce the dosage rapidly to a tolerated dose and observe the patient closely.

In patients who have persistent night pain and/or morning stiffness, giving a large portion, up to a maximum of 100 mg, of the total daily dose at bedtime, may be helpful in affording relief.

Discontinuation of therapy: If severe adverse reactions occur, stop the drug.

Moderate to severe osteoarthritis – See moderate to severe ankylosing spondylitis for dosing.

Moderate to severe rheumatoid arthritis, including acute flares of chronic disease – See Moderate to Severe Ankylosing Spondylitis for dosing.

Tendinitis – See Bursitis for dosing.

Off-label dosing –

Premature labor: [3] = Safety concerns. Several randomized, controlled trials involving more than 500 patients have evaluated the safety and efficacy of indomethacin as a tocolytic agent to delay premature labor. In addition, the American College of Obstetricians and Gynecologists (ACOG) provided a practice bulletin on management of premature labor.

➤*Children:*

15 years of age and older – See Adults for dosing.

2 to 14 years of age –

If a decision is made to use indomethacin for children 2 years of age and older, monitor such patients closely and periodic assessment of liver function is recommended. There have been cases of hepatotoxicity reported in children with juvenile rheumatoid arthritis, including fatalities.

Juvenile rheumatoid arthritis:

- *Maximum dose* – 4 mg/kg/day or 150 to 200 mg/day, whichever is less.
- *Initial dosage* – 2 mg/kg/day, given in divided doses.
- *Maintenance dosage* – As symptoms subside, reduce the total daily dosage to the lowest level required to control symptoms, or discontinue the drug.

➤*Elderly:* See Adults for dosing.

➤*Renal function impairment:* Because indomethacin is eliminated primarily by the kidneys, closely monitor patients with significant renal function impairment; anticipate a lower daily dosage to avoid excessive drug accumulation.

➤*Administration:* Administer rectally.

➤*Storage/Stability:* Store indomethacin suppositories below 30°C (86°F). Avoid transient temperatures above 40°C (104°F).

KETOPROFEN

Rx	**Ketoprofen** (Various, eg, Teva)	**Capsules**: 50 mg	In 100s.
Rx	**Ketoprofen** (Various, eg, Qualitest, Teva)	**Capsules**: 75 mg	In 100s and 500s.
Rx	**Ketoprofen** (Andrx Pharmaceuticals)	**Capsules, extended-release**: 100 mg	In 100s and 1000s.
Rx	**Ketoprofen** (Andrx Pharmaceuticals)	**Capsules, extended-release**: 150 mg	In 100s and 1000s.
Rx	**Ketoprofen** (Andrx Pharmaceuticals)	**Capsules, extended-release**: 200 mg	In 100s and 1000s.

KETOPROFEN — ORAL

For complete and comparative prescribing information, refer to the NSAIDs group monograph.

WARNING

Cardiovascular risk – NSAIDs may cause an increased risk of serious cardiovascular thrombotic events, myocardial infarction (MI), and stroke, which can be fatal. This risk may increase with duration of use. Patients with cardiovascular disease or risk factors for cardiovascular disease may be at greater risk.

NSAIDs are contraindicated for the treatment of perioperative pain in the setting of coronary artery bypass graft (CABG) surgery.

GI risk – NSAIDs cause an increased risk of serious GI adverse reactions, including bleeding, ulceration, and perforation of the stomach or intestines, which can be fatal. These reactions can occur at any time during use and without warning symptoms. Elderly patients are at greater risk for serious GI reactions.

Indications

➤*Rheumatoid arthritis:* For the management of the signs and symptoms of rheumatoid arthritis.

➤*Osteoarthritis:* For the management of the signs and symptoms of osteoarthritis.

➤*Pain:* Immediate-release ketoprofen is indicated for the management of pain. Ketoprofen extended-release is not recommended for treatment of acute pain because of its sustaine-release characteristics.

➤*Primary dysmenorrhea:* For the treatment of primary dysmenorrhea.

➤*Off-label uses:*

Juvenile idiopathic arthritis – [4] = Insufficient documentation. Data evaluating the safety and efficacy of ketoprofen for the treatment of juvenile idiopathic arthritis (JIA) are limited to 2 small trials that enrolled 65 patients and were conducted more than 25 years ago, both of which showed some benefit. Currently, there are no national guidelines for the management of JIA. A review of treatment options for JIA notes that, while not all are Food and Drug Administration (FDA)–labeled for use in JIA, many nonsteroidal anti-inflammatory drugs (NSAIDs) are commonly used.

Administration and Dosage

➤*General dosing considerations:* Because of its typical nonsteroidal anti-inflammatory drug adverse-effect profile, including, as its principal adverse reaction, GI adverse effects, higher doses of immediate-release ketoprofen should be used with caution, and patients receiving them should be observed carefully.

Smaller doses of ketoprofen should be used initially in small individuals.

Concomitant use of immediate-release capsules and sustained-release capsules is not recommended.

➤*Adults:*

Dysmenorrhea –

Usual dosage:

- *Immediate-release* – 25 to 50 mg every 6 to 8 hours as necessary.

Maximum dose: 300 mg/day.

Osteoarthritis –

Usual dosage:

- *Immediate-release* – 75 mg 3 times a day or 50 mg 4 times a day.
- *Extended-release* – 200 mg administered once a day.

Maximum dose:

- *Immediate-release* – 300 mg/day.
- *Extended-release* – 200 mg/day.

Dosage adjustment: If minor adverse effects appear, they may disappear at a lower dose, which may still have an adequate therapeutic effect. If well tolerated but not optimally effective, the dosage may be increased.

Pain management – See Dysmenorrhea for dosing.

Rheumatoid arthritis – See Osteoarthritis for dosing.

➤*Children:*

Off-label dosing –

Juvenile idiopathic arthritis: [4] = Insufficient documentation.

- *3 to 16 years of age* – Ketoprofen was given in 2 different dosing regimens: 25 to 50 mg twice daily for 2 weeks (dose determined by patient weight) and 100 to 200 mg/m^2/day given in 4 divided doses for 4 weeks.

➤*Elderly:* In elderly patients, renal function may be reduced with apparently normal serum creatinine or serum urea nitrogen (BUN) levels. Therefore, it is recommended that the initial dosage of immediate-release or extended-release should be reduced for patients older than 75 years of age.

➤*Renal function impairment:*

Mild renal function impairment – In patients with mildly impaired renal function, the maximum recommended total daily dose of ketoprofen is 150 mg.

Severe renal function impairment – In patients with a more severe renal impairment (GFR less than 25 mL/min per 1.73 m^2 or end-stage renal impairment), the maximum total daily dose should not exceed 100 mg.

➤*Hepatic function impairment:* It is recommended that for patients with impaired liver function and serum albumin concentration less than 3.5 g/dL, the maximum initial total daily dose of ketoprofen should be 100 mg.

➤*Debilitated patients:* Smaller doses should be used initially in debilitated patients.

➤*Hypoalbuminemia and renal function impairment:* Because hypoalbuminemia and reduced renal function both increase the fraction of free drug (biologically active form), patients who have both conditions may be at greater risk of adverse effects. Therefore, it is recommended that such patients also be started on lower doses of this medicine and closely monitored.

The dosage may be increased to the range recommended for the general population, if necessary, only after good individual tolerance has been ascertained.

➤*Administration:* As with other nonsteroidal anti-inflammatory drugs, the predominant adverse effects of ketoprofen are GI effects. To attempt to minimize these effects, health care providers may wish to prescribe that this agent be taken with antacids, food, or milk.

➤*Storage/Stability:* Store at room temperature 15° to 30°C (59° to 86°F). Dispense in a tight, light-resistant container using a child-resistant closure. Protect from direct light and excessive heat and humidity.

KETOROLAC TROMETHAMINE

Rx	**Ketorolac Tromethamine** (Various, eg, Ethex, Teva)	**Tablets; oral:** 10 mg	In 100s and 500s.
Rx	**Ketorolac Tromethamine** (Bedford)	**Injection:** 15 mg/mL	In 1 mL vials.
		30 mg/mL	In 1 and 2 mL single-dose vials and 10 mL multiple-dose vials.
Rx	**Sprix** (Roxro)	**Spray, solution; intranasal:** 15.75 mg/spray	Preservative free. Edetate disodium. In 1 single-day or 5 single-day 1.7 g bottles.[a]

[a] Delivers 8 sprays for a total of 126 mg of ketorolac.

KETOROLAC TROMETHAMINE — ORAL

For complete prescribing information, refer to the NSAIDs group monograph.

WARNING

Ketorolac tromethamine is indicated for the short-term (up to 5 days in adults) management of moderately severe acute pain that requires analgesia at the opioid level. It is not indicated for minor or chronic painful conditions. Ketorolac tromethamine is a potent NSAID analgesic, and its administration carries many risks. The resulting NSAID-related adverse events can be serious in certain patients for whom ketorolac tromethamine is indicated, especially when the drug is used inappropriately. Increasing the dose of ketorolac tromethamine beyond the label recommendations will not provide better efficacy but will result in increasing the risk of developing serious adverse events.

GI effects – Ketorolac tromethamine is contraindicated in patients with active peptic ulcer disease, in patients with recent GI bleeding or perforation, and in patients with a history of peptic ulcer disease or GI bleeding.

Renal effects – Ketorolac tromethamine is contraindicated in patients with advanced renal impairment or in patients at risk for renal failure due to volume depletion.

Risk of bleeding – Ketorolac tromethamine inhibits platelet function and is, therefore, contraindicated in patients with suspected or confirmed cerebrovascular bleeding, hemorrhagic diathesis, incomplete hemostasis, and those at high risk of bleeding.

Ketorolac tromethamine is contraindicated as prophylactic analgesic before any major surgery and is contraindicated intraoperatively when hemostasis is critical because of the increased risk of bleeding.

Hypersensitivity – Ketorolac tromethamine is contraindicated in patients with previously demonstrated hypersensitivity to ketorolac tromethamine or allergic manifestations to aspirin or other NSAIDs.

Labor, delivery, and nursing – Ketorolac tromethamine is contraindicated in labor and delivery because, through its prostaglandin synthesis inhibitory effect, it may adversely affect fetal circulation and inhibit uterine contractions.

The use of ketorolac tromethamine is contraindicated in nursing mothers because of the potential adverse effects of prostaglandin-inhibiting drugs on neonates.

Concomitant use with NSAIDs – Ketorolac tromethamine is contraindicated in patients currently receiving aspirin or NSAIDs because of the cumulative risks of inducing serious NSAID-related adverse events.

Dosage and administration – Ketorolac tromethamine oral is indicated only as continuation therapy to ketorolac tromethamine IV/IM, and the combined duration of use of ketorolac tromethamine IV/IM and ketorolac tromethamine oral is not to exceed 5 days because the increased risk of serious adverse events.

The recommended total daily dose of ketorolac tromethamine oral (maximum 40 mg) is significantly lower than that for ketorolac tromethamine IV/IM (maximum 120 mg).

Special populations – Dosage should be adjusted for patients 65 years of age and older, for patients less than 50 kg (110 lbs) of body weight, and for patients with moderately elevated serum creatine.

Indications

➤*Adult patients:* For the short-term (less than or equal to 5 days) management of moderately severe acute pain that requires analgesia at the opioid level, usually in a postoperative setting. Therapy should always be initiated with ketorolac tromethamine IV/IM, and ketorolac tromethamine oral is to be used only as continuation treatment, if necessary. Combined use of ketorolac tromethamine IV/IM and ketorolac tromethamine oral is not to exceed 5 days of use because of the potential of increasing the frequency and severity of adverse reactions associated with the recommended doses. Patients should be switched to alternative analgesics as soon as possible, but ketorolac tromethamine therapy is not to exceed 5 days.

Administration and Dosage

➤*General dosing considerations:* The use of ketorolac tromethamine oral is only indicated as continuation therapy to ketorolac tromethamine IV or IM.

In adults, the combined duration of use of ketorolac tromethamine IV or IM and ketorolac tromethamine oral is not to exceed 5 days.

Shortening the recommended dosing intervals may result in increased frequency and severity of adverse reactions.

➤*Adults:*

Moderate to severe acute pain –
Maximum dose: 40 mg in 24 hours.
Initial dosage: 20 mg orally as a first dose following IV or IM therapy.
Maintenance dosage: 10 mg orally every 4 to 6 hours.

➤*Children:*

16 years of age and older – See Adults for dosing.

➤*Elderly:*

Moderate to severe acute pain –
Maximum dose: 40 mg in 24 hours.
Initial dosage: 10 mg orally as a first dose following IV or IM therapy.
Maintenance dosage: 10 mg orally every 4 to 6 hours.

➤*Renal function impairment:* See Elderly for dosing.

➤*Patients weighing less than 50 kg (110 lb) of body weight:* See Elderly for dosing.

➤*Duration of therapy:* The combined duration of use of ketorolac IV or IM and ketorolac oral is not to exceed 5 days.

➤*Storage/Stability:* Store bottles at 15° to 30°C (59° to 86°F).

KETOROLAC TROMETHAMINE — INJECTION

For complete and comparative prescribing information, refer to the NSAIDs group monograph.

WARNING

Ketorolac tromethamine is indicated for the short-term (up to 5 days) management of moderately severe acute pain that requires analgesia at the opioid level in adults. It is not indicated for minor or chronic painful conditions. Ketorolac tromethamine is a potent NSAID analgesic, and its administration carries many risks. The resulting NSAID-related adverse reactions can be serious in certain patients for whom ketorolac tromethamine is indicated, especially when the drug is used inappropriately. Increasing the dose of ketorolac tromethamine beyond the label recommendations will not provide better efficacy but will result in increasing the risk of developing serious adverse reactions.

GI effects – Ketorolac tromethamine can cause peptic ulcers, GI bleeding or perforation. Therefore, it is contraindicated in patients with active peptic ulcer disease, in patients with recent GI bleeding or perforation, and in patients with a history of peptic ulcer disease or GI bleeding.

Renal effects – Ketorolac tromethamine is contraindicated in patients with advanced renal impairment and in patients at risk for renal failure due to volume depletion.

WARNING (cont.)

Risk of bleeding – Ketorolac tromethamine inhibits platelet function and is, therefore, contraindicated in patients with suspected or confirmed cerebrovascular bleeding, hemorrhagic diathesis, incomplete hemostasis, and those at high risk of bleeding.

Ketorolac tromethamine is contraindicated as prophylactic analgesic before any major surgery and is contraindicated intraoperatively when hemostasis is critical because of the increased risk of bleeding.

Hypersensitivity – Hypersensitivity reactions ranging from bronchospasm to anaphylactic shock, have occurred and appropriate counteractive measures must be available when administering the first dose of ketorolac tromethamine intravenously (IV)/intramuscularly (IM). Ketorolac tromethamine is contraindicated in patients who have previously demonstrated hypersensitivity to ketorolac tromethamine or allergic manifestations to aspirin or other NSAIDs.

Intrathecal or epidural administration – Ketorolac tromethamine is contraindicated for neuraxial (epidural or intrathecal) administration due to its alcohol content.

Labor, delivery, and nursing – Ketorolac tromethamine is contraindicated in labor and delivery because it may adversely affect fetal circulation and inhibit uterine contractions.

KETOROLAC TROMETHAMINE — INJECTION

WARNING (cont.)

The use of ketorolac tromethamine is contraindicated in nursing mothers because of the potential adverse effects of prostaglandin-inhibiting drugs on neonates.

Concomitant use with NSAIDs – Ketorolac tromethamine is contraindicated in patients currently receiving aspirin or NSAIDs because of the cumulative risks of inducing serious NSAID-related adverse reactions.

Special populations – Dosage should be adjusted for patients greater than or equal to 65 years of age, for patients less than 50 kg (110 lbs) of body weight and for patients with moderately elevated serum creatine. Doses of ketorolac tromethamine IV/IM are not to exceed 60 mg (total dose per day) in these patients. Ketorolac tromethamine is indicated as a single dose therapy in pediatric patients; not to exceed 30 mg for IM administration and 15 mg for IV administration.

Indications

➤*Adult patients:* For the short-term (less than or equal to 5 days) management of moderately severe acute pain that requires analgesia at the opioid level, usually in a postoperative setting.

See Administration and Dosage for more information.

➤*Pediatric patients:* The safety and effectiveness of single doses of ketorolac tromethamine IV/IM have been established in pediatric patients between 2 and 16 years of age. Ketorolac tromethamine, as a single injectable dose, has been shown to be effective in the management of moderately severe acute pain that requires analgesia at the opioid level, usually in the postoperative setting. There is limited data available to support the use of multiple doses of ketorolac tromethamine in pediatric patients. Safety and effectiveness have not been established in pediatric patients younger than 2 years of age. Use of ketorolac tromethamine in pediatric patients is supported by evidence from adequate and well-controlled studies of ketorolac tromethamine in adults with additional pharmacokinetic, efficacy and safety data on its use in pediatric patients available in the published literature.

➤*Off-label uses:*

Treatment of migraine (IM) (adults) – [4] = Insufficient documentation. Data evaluating the efficacy of IM ketorolac for the treatment of an acute migraine attack consistently show favorable results. American Academy of Neurology clinical practice guidelines for the pharmacologic treatment of migraine headache in adults consider IM ketorolac to be an option in a health care provider–supervised setting (eg, emergency department). They further state that while data support moderate benefit, conclusions about efficacy are uncertain (grade C evidence). (See Administration and Dosage.)

Treatment of migraine (IV) (adults) – [4] = Insufficient documentation. Data evaluating the efficacy of IV ketorolac for the treatment of an acute migraine attack show favorable results. While American Academy of Neurology clinical practice guidelines for the pharmacologic treatment of migraine headache in adults make no mention of IV ketorolac, they do consider IM ketorolac to be an option in a health care provider–supervised setting (eg, emergency department). They further state that conclusions about the efficacy of IM ketorolac are uncertain, despite data supporting moderate benefit (grade C evidence). (See Administration and Dosage.)

Administration and Dosage

➤*General dosing considerations:* Hypovolemia should be corrected prior to the administration of ketorolac.

Children should receive only a single dose of ketorolac injection. (See Children).

Because ketorolac may be cleared more slowly by elderly patients who are also more sensitive to the adverse reactions of NSAIDs, extra caution and reduced dosages must be used when treating elderly patients with ketorolac tromethamine IV or IM. (See Elderly).

Because patients with underlying renal insufficiency are at increased risk of developing acute renal failure, the risks and benefits should be assessed prior to giving ketorolac to these patients.

➤*Adults:*

Moderately severe acute pain –

Usual dosage:

- *Single-dose treatment (IV or IM)* – Ketorolac 60 mg IM or ketorolac 30 mg IV.
- *Multiple-dose treatment (IV or IM)* – Ketorolac 30 mg IV or IM every 6 hours.

Maximum dose: 120 mg/day.

Conversion:

- *Following a single 60 mg IM dose, single 30 mg IV dose, or multiple doses of ketorolac 30 mg IV or IM* –
  - *Maximum dose:* 40 mg orally in 24 hours.
  - *Initial dosage:* 20 mg orally as a first dose.
  - *Maintenance dosage:* 10 mg orally every 4 to 6 hours.

Off-label dosing –

Treatment of migraine (IM) (adults): [4] = Insufficient documentation. 30 to 60 mg IM as a single dose.

Treatment of migraine (IV) (adults): [4] = Insufficient documentation. 30 mg IV as a single dose.

➤*Children:*

Moderately severe acute pain –

17 years of age and older: See Adults for dosing.

2 to 16 years of age:

- *Usual dosage* –
  - *Single-dose treatment (IV or IM):* 1 mg/kg IM or 0.5 mg/kg IV.
- *Maximum dose* – 30 mg IM; 15 mg IV.

➤*Elderly:*

Moderately severe acute pain –

Usual dosage:

- *Single-dose treatment (IV or IM)* – Ketorolac 30 mg IM or ketorolac 15 mg IV.
- *Multiple-dose treatment (IV or IM)* – Ketorolac 15 mg IV or IM every 6 hours.

Maximum dose: 60 mg/day.

Conversion:

- *Following a single 30 mg IM dose, single 15 mg IV dose, or multiple doses of ketorolac 15 mg IV or IM* –
  - *Maximum dose:* 40 mg orally in 24 hours.
  - *Initial dose:* 10 mg orally as a first dose.
  - *Maintenance dose:* 10 mg orally every 4 to 6 hours.

➤*Renal function impairment:* See Elderly for dosing.

➤*Patients weighing less than 50 kg (110 lb):* See Elderly for dosing.

Maximum dose – 60 mg/day.

Conversion –

Following a single 30 mg IM dose, single 15 mg IV dose, or multiple doses of ketorolac 15 mg IV or IM:

- *Maximum dose* – 40 mg orally in 24 hours.
- *Initial dose* – 10 mg orally as a first dose.
- *Maintenance dose* – 10 mg orally every 4 to 6 hours.

➤*Concomitant therapy:* Ketorolac tromethamine IV or IM have been used concomitantly with morphine and meperidine and has shown an opioid-sparing effect. For breakthrough pain, it is recommended to supplement the lower end of the ketorolac IV or IM dosage range with low doses of narcotics as needed, unless otherwise contraindicated.

For breakthrough pain, do not increase the dose or the frequency of ketorolac.

➤*Duration of therapy:* In adults, the combined duration of use of IV or IM ketorolac and oral ketorolac is not to exceed 5 days.

➤*Administration:* Ketorolac IV or IM may be used as a single or multiple dose on a regular or as needed schedule for the management of moderately severe acute pain that requires analgesia at the opioid level, usually in a postoperative setting.

The analgesic effect begins in approximately 30 minutes with maximum effect in 1 to 2 hours after dosing IV or IM. Duration of analgesic effect is usually 4 to 6 hours.

IV dose – When administering ketorolac IV, the IV bolus must be given over no less than 15 seconds.

IM dose – The IM administration should be given slowly and deeply into the muscle.

➤*Admixture compatibility:* Ketorolac IV or IM should not be mixed in a small volume (eg, in a syringe) with morphine sulfate, meperidine hydrochloride, promethazine hydrochloride, or hydroxyzine hydrochloride; this will result in precipitation of ketorolac from solution.

➤*Storage/Stability:* Store at 15° to 30°C (59° to 86°F). Protect from light.

KETOROLAC TROMETHAMINE — INTRANASAL

WARNING

Limitations of use – Ketorolac nasal spray, a nonsteroidal anti-inflammatory drug (NSAID), is indicated for short-term (up to 5 days in adults) management of moderate to moderately severe pain that requires analgesia at the opioid level. Do not exceed a total combined duration of use of ketorolac nasal spray and other ketorolac formulations (intramuscular [IM]/intravenous [IV] or oral) of 5 days.

Ketorolac is not indicated for use in children, and it is not indicated for minor or chronic painful conditions.

GI risk – Ketorolac can cause peptic ulcers, GI bleeding, and/or perforation of the stomach or intestines, which can be fatal. These events can occur at any time during use and without warning symptoms. Therefore, ketorolac is contraindicated in patients with active peptic ulcer disease, in patients with recent GI bleeding or perforation, and in patients with a history of peptic ulcer disease or GI bleeding. Elderly patients are at greater risk for serious GI events.

Bleeding risk – Ketorolac inhibits platelet function and is, therefore, contraindicated in patients with suspected or confirmed cerebrovascular bleeding, hemorrhagic diathesis, or incomplete hemostasis, and those at high risk of bleeding.

Cardiovascular risk – NSAIDs may cause an increased risk of serious cardiovascular thrombotic events, myocardial infarction, and stroke, which can be fatal. This risk may increase with duration of use. Patients with cardiovascular disease or risk factors for cardiovascular disease may be at greater risk.

Ketorolac nasal spray is contraindicated for treatment of perioperative pain in the setting of coronary artery bypass graft (CABG) surgery.

Renal risk – Ketorolac is contraindicated in patients with advanced renal impairment and in patients at risk for renal failure due to volume depletion.

Indications

➤*Moderate to moderately severe pain:* For the short-term (up to 5 days) management of moderate to moderately severe pain that requires analgesia at the opioid level.

Administration and Dosage

➤*General dosing considerations:* Treat patients for the shortest duration possible.

➤*Adults:*

Moderate to moderately severe pain –

Usual dosage:

• *Weighing more than 50 kg* – 1 spray (15.75 mg/spray) in each nostril (total dose of 31.5 mg) every 6 to 8 hours.

• *Weighing less than 50 kg* – 1 spray (15.75 mg/spray) in only 1 nostril every 6 to 8 hours.

Maximum dose:

• *Weighing more than 50 kg* – 4 doses (total 126 mg/day) for no more than 5 days.

• *Weighing less than 50 kg* – 4 doses (total 63 mg/day) for no more than 5 days.

➤*Elderly:*

Moderate to moderately severe pain –

Usual dosage: 1 spray (15.75 mg/spray) in only 1 nostril every 6 to 8 hours.

Maximum dose: 4 doses (total 63 mg/day) for no more than 5 days.

➤*Renal function impairment:* One spray (15.75 mg/spray) in only 1 nostril every 6 to 8 hours, not to exceed 4 doses per day (total 63 mg/day) for no more than 5 days. Ketorolac is contraindicated in patients with advanced renal impairment and in patients at risk for renal failure due to volume depletion.

➤*Concomitant therapy:* Do not use concomitantly with other formulations of ketorolac or other NSAIDs.

➤*Duration of therapy:* Do not exceed 5 days of therapy.

➤*Administration:* Do not use any single bottle for more than 1 day as it will not deliver the intended dose after 24 hours. Therefore, the bottle must be discarded no more than 24 hours after taking the first dose, even if the bottle still contains some liquid.

➤*Storage/Stability:* Protect bottles from light and freezing. Store unopened bottles between 2° and 8°C (36° and 46°F). During use, keep between 15° and 30°C (59° and 86°F) and out of direct sunlight. Bottles should be discarded within 24 hours of priming.

MECLOFENAMATE SODIUM

Rx	**Meclofenamate Sodium** (Various, eg, Mylan, Schein)	**Capsules:** 50 mg[a]	In 100s, 500s, and 1000s.
Rx	**Meclofenamate Sodium** (Various, eg, Mylan, Schein)	**Capsules:** 100 mg[a]	In 100s, 500s, and 100s.

[a] Meclofenamic acid equivalent, as meclofenamate sodium.

MECLOFENAMATE SODIUM — ORAL

For complete and comparative prescribing information, refer to the NSAIDs group monograph.

WARNING

Cardiovascular risk – NSAIDs may cause an increased risk of serious cardiovascular thrombotic events, myocardial infarction (MI), and stroke, which can be fatal. This risk may increase with duration of use. Patients with cardiovascular disease or risk factors for cardiovascular disease may be at greater risk.

NSAIDs are contraindicated for the treatment of perioperative pain in the setting of coronary artery bypass graft (CABG) surgery.

GI risk – NSAIDs cause an increased risk of serious GI adverse reactions, including bleeding, ulceration, and perforation of the stomach or intestines, which can be fatal. These reactions can occur at any time during use and without warning symptoms. Elderly patients are at greater risk for serious GI reactions.

Indications

➤*Mild to moderate pain:* For the relief of mild to moderate pain.

➤*Primary dysmenorrhea/Excessive menstrual blood loss:* For the treatment of primary dysmenorrhea and idiopathic heavy menstrual blood loss.

➤*Rheumatoid arthritis:* For relief of the signs and symptoms of acute and chronic rheumatoid arthritis.

➤*Osteoarthritis:* For relief of the signs and symptoms of acute and chronic osteoarthritis.

Administration and Dosage

➤*General dosing considerations:* As with all nonsteroidal anti-inflammatory drugs, selection of meclofenamate sodium requires a careful assessment of the benefit/risk ratio.

➤*Adults:*

Excessive menstrual blood loss and primary dysmenorrhea –

Usual dosage: 100 mg 3 times a day, for up to 6 days, starting at the onset of menstrual flow.

Maximum dose: 400 mg per day.

Mild to moderate pain –

Usual dosage: 50 mg every 4 to 6 hours. Doses of 100 mg may be needed in some patients for optimal pain relief.

Maximum dose: 400 mg per day.

Osteoarthritis –

Usual dosage: For osteoarthritis, including acute exacerbations of chronic disease, the dosage is 200 to 400 mg per day, administered in 3 or 4 equal doses.

Maximum dose: 400 mg per day.

Rheumatoid arthritis –

Usual dosage: For rheumatoid arthritis, including acute exacerbations of chronic disease, the dosage is 200 to 400 mg per day, administered in 3 or 4 equal doses.

Maximum dose: 400 mg per day.

➤*Elderly:* Adverse reactions are seen more commonly in elderly patients; therefore, a lower starting dose and careful follow-up are advised.

➤*Renal function impairment:* Because meclofenamate sodium metabolites are eliminated primarily by the kidneys, patients with significantly impaired renal function should be closely monitored; a lower daily dosage should be employed to avoid excessive drug accumulation.

➤*Dosage adjustment:* Therapy should be initiated at the lower dosage, then increased as necessary to improve clinical response. The dosage should be individually adjusted for each patient, depending on the severity of the symptoms and the clinical response. The smallest dosage of meclofenamate sodium that yields clinical control should be employed.

If intolerance occurs, the dosage may need to be reduced.

After a satisfactory response has been achieved, the dosage should be adjusted as required. A lower dosage may suffice for long-term administration.

➤*Duration of therapy:* Although improvement may be seen in some patients in a few days, 2 to 3 weeks of treatment may be required to obtain the optimum therapeutic benefit.

➤*Discontinuation of therapy:* Therapy should be terminated if any severe adverse reactions occur.

➤*Administration:* If GI complaints occur, meclofenamate sodium may be administered with meals or with milk.

➤*Storage/Stability:* Store at controlled room temperature 15° to 30°C (59° to 86°F). Protect from light and moisture.

MEFENAMIC ACID

Rx	**Mefenamic Acid** (Paddock)	**Capsules; oral:** 250 mg	Lactose. (PAD 195). Yellow. In 100s.
Rx	**Ponstel** (Sciele Pharma)		Lactose. (FHPC 400). Ivory. In 100s.

MEFENAMIC ACID — ORAL

For complete and comparative prescribing information, refer to the NSAIDs group monograph.

WARNING

Cardiovascular risk – NSAIDs may cause an increased risk of serious cardiovascular thrombotic events, myocardial infarction, and stroke, which can be fatal. This risk may increase with duration of use. Patients with cardiovascular disease or risk factors for cardiovascular disease may be at greater risk.

Mefenamic acid is contraindicated for treatment of perioperative pain in the setting of coronary artery bypass graft (CABG) surgery.

GI risk – NSAIDs cause an increased risk of serious GI adverse events including bleeding, ulceration, and perforation of the stomach or intestines, which can be fatal. These events can occur at any time during use and without warning symptoms. Elderly patients are at greater risk for serious GI events.

Indications

➤*Mild to moderate pain:* For relief of mild to moderate pain in patients 14 years of age or older, when therapy will not exceed 1 week (7 days).

➤*Primary dysmenorrhea:* For treatment of primary dysmenorrhea.

Administration and Dosage

➤*General dosing considerations:* As with other NSAIDs, the lowest dose should be sought for each patient. Therefore, after observing the response to initial therapy with mefenamic acid, the dose and frequency should be adjusted to suit the individual patient's needs.

➤*Adults:*

Acute pain –

Initial dosage: 500 mg as an initial dose.

Maintenance dosage: Follow initial dose by 250 mg every 6 hours as needed, usually not to exceed 1 week.

Dosage adjustment: The dose and frequency should be adjusted to suit the individual patient's needs.

Duration of therapy: 1 week.

Primary dysmenorrhea –

Initial dosage: 500 mg as an initial dose.

Maintenance dosage: Follow initial dose by 250 mg every 6 hours, starting with the onset of bleeding and associated symptoms.

Clinical studies indicate that effective treatment can be initiated with the start of menses and should not be necessary for more than 2 to 3 days.

Duration of therapy: 2 to 3 days with the start of menses.

➤*Children:*

14 years of age and older – See Adults for dosing.

➤*Renal function impairment:* Mefenamic acid should not be administered to patients with preexisting renal disease or in patients with significantly impaired renal function.

➤*Hepatic function impairment:* Patients with acute and chronic hepatic disease may require reduced doses of mefenamic acid compared with patients with healthy hepatic function.

➤*Administration:* Administration is by the oral route, preferably with food.

➤*Storage/Stability:* Store at 15° to 30°C (59° to 86°F). Protect from moisture.

MELOXICAM

Rx	**Meloxicam** (Various, eg, Dr. Reddy, Genpharm, Mutual)	**Tablets:** 7.5 mg	In 30s, 60s, 100s, 250s, 500s, and 1000s.
Rx	**Mobic** (Boehringer Ingelheim/Abbott)		Lactose. (M). Pastel, yellow, biconvex. In 100s.
Rx	**Meloxicam** (Various, eg, Dr. Reddy, Genpharm, Mutual)	15 mg	In 30s, 60s, 100s, 250s, 500s, and 1000s.
Rx	**Mobic** (Boehringer Ingelheim/Abbott)		Lactose. (15 M). Pastel, yellow, oblong. In 100s.
Rx	**Meloxicam** (Roxane)	**Oral suspension:** 7.5 mg per 5 mL	Saccharin sodium. Raspberry flavor. In 100 mL.
Rx	**Mobic** (Boehringer Ingelheim/Abbott)		Sorbitol, saccharin. Raspberry flavor. In 100 mL.

MELOXICAM — ORAL

For complete and comparative prescribing information, refer to the nonsteroidal anti-inflammatory drugs (NSAIDs) group monograph.

WARNING

Cardiovascular risk – Nonsteroidal anti-inflammatory drugs (NSAIDs) may cause an increased risk of serious cardiovascular thrombotic events, myocardial infarction (MI), and stroke, which can be fatal. This risk may increase with duration of use. Patients with cardiovascular disease or risk factors for cardiovascular disease may be at higher risk.

Meloxicam is contraindicated for the treatment of perioperative pain in the setting of coronary artery bypass graft (CABG) surgery)

GI risk – NSAIDs cause an increased risk of serious GI adverse reactions, including bleeding, ulceration, and perforation of the stomach or intestines, which can be fatal. These reactions can occur at any time during use and without warning symptoms. Elderly patients are at highest risk for serious GI reactions.

Indications

➤*Osteoarthritis (OA)/Rheumatoid arthritis (RA):* For relief of the signs and symptoms of OA and RA.

➤*Pauciarticular/Polyarticular course juvenile rheumatoid arthritis (JRA):* For relief of the signs and symptoms of pauciarticular or polyarticular course JRA in patients 2 years of age and older.

➤*Off-label uses:* For the treatment of ankylosing spondylitis and acute shoulder pain.

Administration and Dosage

➤*General dosing considerations:* Meloxicam 7.5 mg per 5 mL or 15 mg per 10 mL oral suspension may be substituted for meloxicam 7.5 or 15 mg tablets, respectively.

To improve dosing accuracy in lesser-weight children, the use of meloxicam oral suspension is recommended.

➤*Adults:*

Osteoarthritis –

Maximum dose: 15 mg per day.

Initial dosage: 7.5 mg once daily.

Maintenance dosage: 7.5 mg once daily. Some patients may receive additional benefit by increasing the dosage to 15 mg once daily.

Rheumatoid arthritis – See dosing for osteoarthritis.

➤*Children:* Indicated in patients 2 years of age and older. To improve dosing accuracy in lesser-weight children, the use of meloxicam oral suspension is recommended.

Pauciarticular/Polyarticular course juvenile rheumatoid arthritis –

Usual dosage: 0.125 mg/kg once daily. Individualize dosage based on the weight of the child.

JRA Dosing With Meloxicam Oral Suspension

Weight	0.125 mg/kg Dose (1.5 mg/mL)	Delivered dose
12 kg (26 lbs)	1 mL	1.5 mg
24 kg (54 lbs)	2 mL	3 mg
36 kg (80 lbs)	3 mL	4.5 mg
48 kg (106 lbs)	4 mL	6 mg
≥ 60 kg (132 lbs)	5 mL	7.5 mg

Maximum dose: 7.5 mg per day.

Off-label dosing –

Juvenile idiopathic arthritis: [4] = Insufficient documentation.

• *Children 2 to 19 years of age* – Meloxicam was given in doses of 0.125 to 0.25 mg/kg administered as a once-daily dose.

➤*Renal function impairment:* Caution is recommended in patients with preexisting kidney disease. Treatment with meloxicam is not recommended in patients with advanced renal disease.

➤*Duration of therapy:* Use the lowest effective dose for the shortest duration consistent with individual patient treatment goals.

➤*Administration:* May be taken without regard to meals. Shake the oral suspension gently before using.

➤*Storage/Stability:* Store at 25°C (77°F); excursions are permitted to 15° to 30°C (59° to 86°F). Keep tablets in a dry place.

Dispense tablets in a tight container. Keep oral suspension container tightly closed.

NABUMETONE

Rx	**Nabumetone** (Various, eg, Eon, Teva, UDL)	**Tablets**: 500 mg	In 100s, 500s, and 1,000s.
Rx	**Nabumetone** (Various, eg, Eon, Teva)	**Tablets**: 750 mg	In 100s, 500s, and 1,000s.

NABUMETONE — ORAL

For complete and comparative prescribing information, refer to the Nonsteroidal Anti-inflammatory Agents group monograph.

WARNING

Cardiovascular risk – Nonsteroidal anti-inflammatory drugs (NSAIDs) may cause an increased risk of serious cardiovascular thrombotic events, myocardial infarction (MI), and stroke, which can be fatal. This risk may increase with duration of use. Patients with cardiovascular disease or risk factors for cardiovascular disease may be at greater risk.

Nabumetone tablets are contraindicated for the treatment of perioperative pain in the setting of coronary artery bypass graft (CABG) surgery.

GI risk – NSAIDs cause an increased risk of serious GI adverse reactions, including bleeding, ulceration, and perforation of the stomach or intestines, which can be fatal. These reactions can occur at any time during use and without warning symptoms. Elderly patients are at greater risk for serious GI reactions.

Indications

➤*Arthritis:* For acute and chronic treatment of signs and symptoms of osteoarthritis (OA) and rheumatoid arthritis (RA).

Administration and Dosage

➤*General dosing considerations:* Carefully consider the potential benefits and risks of nabumetone and other treatment options before deciding to use nabumetone.

Use the lowest effective dose for the shortest duration consistent with individual patient treatment goals.

➤*Adults:*

Osteoarthritis –

Maximum dose: 2,000 mg/day.

Initial dosage: 1,000 mg taken as a single dose.

Maintenance dosage: Some patients may obtain more symptomatic relief from 1,500 to 2,000 mg/day. Use the lowest effective dose for chronic treatment.

Rheumatoid arthritis – See Osteoarthritis for dosing.

➤*Renal function impairment:* Use caution in prescribing nabumetone to patients with moderate or severe renal insufficiency. The maximum starting dosage of nabumetone in patients with moderate or severe renal insufficiency should not exceed 750 or 500 mg, respectively, once daily. Following careful monitoring of renal function in patients with moderate or severe renal insufficiency, daily doses may be increased to a maximum of 1,500 and 1,000 mg, respectively.

➤*Administration:* Nabumetone can be given in either a single or twice-daily dose, with or without food.

➤*Storage/Stability:* Store at 20° to 25°C (68° to 77°F).

NAPROXEN

otc	**Naproxen Sodium** (Various, eg, Goldline)	**Tablets; oral**: 200 mg	Equiv to 220 mg naproxen sodium. In 24s and 50s.
otc	**Aleve** (Bayer Consumer)		**Tablets**: Equiv to 220 mg naproxen sodium. (ALEVE). In 24s, 50s, 100s, and 150s. **Capsules**: Equiv to 220 mg naproxen sodium. In 24s, 50s, 100s, 150s, and 200s. **Gelcaps**: Equiv to 220 mg naproxen sodium. (ALEVE). In 20s, 40s, and 80s.
otc	**Midol Extended Relief** (Bayer Consumer)		Equiv to 220 mg naproxen sodium. Sodium 20 mg. Capsule shape. In 24s.
Rx	**Naproxen Sodium** (Various, eg, Sidmak)	**Tablets; oral**: 250 mg	Equiv to 275 mg naproxen sodium. In 100s, 500s, 1,000s, and UD 100s.
Rx	**Anaprox** (Roche)		Equiv to 275 mg naproxen sodium. (Roche 274). Lt. blue, biconvex, oval. In 100s.
Rx	**Naproxen Sodium** (Various, eg, Sidmak)	**Tablets; oral**: 500 mg	Equiv to 550 mg naproxen sodium. In 100s, 500s, 1,000s, and UD 100s.
Rx	**Anaprox DS** (Roche)		Equiv to 550 mg naproxen sodium. (Roche/Anaprox DS). Dark blue, capsule shape. Film-coated. In 100s and 500s.
Rx	**Naproxen** (Various, eg, Lederle, Qualitest, Sidmak, UDL)	**Tablets; oral**: 250 mg	In 30s, 100s, 500s, 1,000s, UD 100s, unit-of-use 30s, 60s, 90s, and 120s, and *Robot ready* 25s.
Rx	**Naprosyn** (Roche)		(Roche/Naprosyn 250). Yellow. In 100s and 500s.
Rx	**Naproxen** (Various, eg, Lederle, Qualitest, Sidmak, UDL)	**Tablets; oral**: 375 mg	In 30s, 100s, 500s, 1,000s, UD 100s, and unit-of-use 30s, 60s, 90s, and 120s.
Rx	**Naprosyn** (Roche)		(Naprosyn 375). Peach. In 100s and 500s.
Rx	**Naproxen** (Various, eg, Lederle, Qualitest, Sidmak, UDL)	**Tablets; oral**: 500 mg	In 30s, 100s, 500s, 1,000s, UD 100s, UD 300s, unit-of-use 30s, 60s, 90s, and 120s, and *Robot ready* 25s.
Rx	**Naprosyn** (Roche)		(Naprosyn 500). Yellow. In 100s and 500s.
Rx	**Naproxen** (Various, eg, Apothecon, Purepac, Roxane, Teva)	**Tablets, delayed-release; oral**: 375 mg	In 100s and 500s.
Rx	**EC-Naprosyn** (Roche)		(EC-Naprosyn 375). White, capsule shape. Enteric-coated. In 100s.
	Naproxen (Various, eg, Apothecon, Purepac, Roxane, Teva)	**Tablets, delayed-release; oral**: 500 mg	In 100s and 500s.
Rx	**EC-Naprosyn** (Roche)		(EC-Naprosyn 500). White, capsule shape. Enteric-coated. In 100s.
Rx	**Naprelan** (Victory Pharma)	**Tablets, controlled-release; oral**: 375 mg	Equiv to 412.5 mg naproxen sodium. (N375). White, capsule shape. In 100s.
		500 mg	Equiv to 550 mg naproxen sodium. (N500). White, capsule shape. In 75s.
		750 mg	Equiv to 825 mg naproxen sodium. PEG. (N 750). White, capsule shape. In 30s and 60s.
Rx	**Naprosyn** (Roche)	**Suspension; oral**: 125 mg/5 mL	Sorbitol, sucrose, parabens. Orange-pineapple flavor. In 473 mL.
Rx	**Naproxen** (Various, eg, Roxane)		Methylparaben, sorbitol, sucrose. Pineapple-orange flavor. In 15, 20, and 500 mL.

NAPROXEN — ORAL

For complete and comparative prescribing information, refer to the NSAIDs group monograph.

WARNING

Cardiovascular risk – NSAIDs may cause an increased risk of serious cardiovascular thrombotic events, myocardial infarction, and stroke, which can be fatal. This risk may increase with duration of use. Patients with cardiovascular disease or risk factors for cardiovascular disease may be at greater risk.

Naproxen (except controlled-release tablets) is contraindicated for the treatment of perioperative pain in the setting of coronary artery bypass graft (CABG) surgery.

Gastrointestinal risk – NSAIDs cause an increased risk of serious gastrointestinal adverse events including bleeding, ulceration, and perforation of the stomach or intestines, which can be fatal. These events can occur at any time during use and without warning symptoms. Elderly patients are at greater risk for serious gastrointestinal events.

Indications

➤*Ankylosing spondylitis/Juvenile arthritis/Osteoarthritis/Rheumatoid arthritis:* Naproxen tablets, naproxen delayed-release tablets, naproxen sodium tablets and naproxen suspension are indicated for the treatment of rheumatoid arthritis, osteoarthritis, ankylosing spondylitis and juvenile arthritis.

➤*Juvenile rheumatoid arthritis:* Naproxen suspension is recommended for juvenile rheumatoid arthritis in order to obtain the maximum dosage flexibility based on the patient's weight.

➤*Acute gout/Bursitis/Tendonitis/Pain/Primary dysmenorrhea:* Naproxen tablets, naproxen sodium tablets, and naproxen suspension are also indicated for the treatment of tendonitis, bursitis, acute gout, and for the management of pain and primary dysmenorrhea. Naproxen delayed-release tablets is not recommended for initial treatment of acute pain because the absorption of naproxen is delayed compared to absorption from other naproxen-containing products.

➤*Off-label uses:* Analgesia in children. (See Administration and Dosage).

Administration and Dosage

➤*General dosing considerations:* Although naproxen tablets, naproxen suspension, naproxen delayed-release tablets, and naproxen sodium tablets all circulate in the plasma as naproxen; they have pharmacokinetic differences that may affect onset of action. Onset of pain relief can begin within 30 minutes in patients taking naproxen sodium and within 1 hour in patients taking naproxen. Because naproxen delayed-release tablets dissolve in the small intestine rather than in the stomach, the absorption of the drug is delayed compared to the other naproxen formulations.

Naproxen delayed-release tablets are not recommended for initial treatment of acute pain because absorption of naproxen is delayed compared to other naproxen-containing products.

The recommended strategy for initiating therapy is to choose a formulation and a starting dose likely to be effective for the patient and then adjust the dosage based on observation of benefit and/or adverse events.

The use of naproxen suspension allows for more flexible dose titration.

Naproxen suspension is recommended for juvenile rheumatoid arthritis in order to obtain the maximum dosage flexibility based on the patient's weight.

➤*Adults:*

Acute gout –

Usual dosage:
- *Naproxen tablets* – 250 mg every 8 hours until the attack has subsided.
- *Naproxen sodium tablets* – 275 mg every 8 hours.

Initial dosage:
- *Naproxen tablets* – 750 mg as a starting dose.
- *Naproxen sodium tablets* – 825 mg as a starting dose.

Acute tendinitis –

Usual dosage:
- *Naproxen sodium tablet* – 550 mg every 12 hours or 275 mg every 6 to 8 hours as required.

Maximum dose: The initial total daily dose should not exceed 1,375 mg of naproxen sodium. Thereafter, the total daily dose should not exceed 1,100 mg of naproxen sodium.

Initial dosage: 550 mg as a starting dose.

Ankylosing spondylitis –

Usual dosage:
- *Naproxen tablet/suspension* – 250 to 500 mg twice/day.
- *Naproxen sodium tablet* – 275 mg to 550 mg twice/day (250 mg naproxen with 25 mg sodium to 500 mg naproxen with 50 mg sodium twice daily).
- *Naproxen controlled-release/delayed-release tablet* – 375 or 500 mg twice/day.

Dosage adjustment: During long-term administration, the dose of naproxen may be adjusted up or down depending on the clinical response of the patient. A lower daily dose may suffice for long-term administration. In patients who tolerate lower doses well, the dose may be increased to 1,500 mg/day when a higher level of anti-inflammatory/analgesic activity is required. When treating patients with naproxen 1,500 mg/day (as naproxen tablets or 1,650 mg of naproxen sodium tablets), the health care provider should observe sufficient increased clinical benefit to offset the potential increased risk. The morning and evening doses do not have to be equal in size and administration of the drug more frequently than twice daily does not generally make a difference in response.

Bursitis –

Usual dosage:
- *Naproxen sodium tablet* – 550 mg every 12 hours or 275 mg every 6 to 8 hours as required.

Maximum dose: The initial total daily dose should not exceed 1,375 mg of naproxen sodium. Thereafter, the total daily dose should not exceed 1,100 mg of naproxen sodium.

Initial dosage: 550 mg as a starting dose

Management of pain –

Usual dosage:
- *Naproxen sodium tablet* – 550 mg every 12 hours or 275 mg every 6 to 8 hours as required.

Maximum dose: The initial total daily dose should not exceed 1,375 mg of naproxen sodium. Thereafter, the total daily dose should not exceed 1,100 mg of naproxen sodium.

Initial dosage: 550 mg as a starting dose.

Osteoarthritis –

Usual dosage:
- *Naproxen tablet/suspension* – 250 to 500 mg twice/day.
- *Naproxen sodium tablet* – 275 to 550 mg twice/day (250 mg naproxen with 25 mg sodium to 500 mg naproxen with 50 mg sodium twice daily).
- *Naproxen controlled-release/delayed-release tablet* – 375 or 500 mg twice/day.

Dosage adjustment: During long-term administration, the dose of naproxen may be adjusted up or down depending on the clinical response of the patient. A lower daily dose may suffice for long-term administration. In patients who tolerate lower doses well, the dose may be increased to 1,500 mg/day when a higher level of anti-inflammatory/analgesic activity is required. When treating patients with naproxen 1,500 mg/day (as naproxen tablets or 1,650 mg of naproxen sodium tablets), the health care provider should observe sufficient increased clinical benefit to offset the potential increased risk. The morning and evening doses do not have to be equal in size and administration of the drug more frequently than twice daily does not generally make a difference in response.

Primary dysmenorrhea –

Usual dosage:
- *Naproxen sodium tablet* – 550 mg every 12 hours or 275 mg every 6 to 8 hours as required.

Maximum dose: The initial total daily dose should not exceed 1,375 mg of naproxen sodium. Thereafter, the total daily dose should not exceed 1,100 mg of naproxen sodium.

Initial dosage: 550 mg as a starting dose.

Rheumatoid arthritis –

Usual dosage:
- *Naproxen tablet/suspension* – 250 to 500 mg twice/day.
- *Naproxen sodium tablet* – 275 to 550 mg twice/day (250 mg naproxen with 25 mg sodium to 500 mg naproxen with 50 mg sodium twice daily).
- *Naproxen controlled-release/delayed-release tablet* – 375 or 500 mg twice/day.

Dosage adjustment: During long-term administration, the dose of naproxen may be adjusted up or down depending on the clinical response of the patient. A lower daily dose may suffice for long-term administration. In patients who tolerate lower doses well, the dose may be increased to 1,500 mg/day when a higher level of anti-inflammatory/analgesic activity is required. When treating patients with naproxen 1,500 mg/day (as naproxen tablets or 1,650 mg of naproxen sodium tablets), the health care provider should observe sufficient increased clinical benefit to offset the potential increased risk. The morning and evening doses do not have to be equal in size and administration of the drug more frequently than twice daily does not generally make a difference in response.

➤*Children:*

Juvenile arthritis –

2 years of age and older:
- *Usual dosage* – The recommended total daily dose of naproxen suspension is approximately 10 mg/kg given in 2 divided doses (ie, 5 mg/kg given twice a day).

Dosing of Naproxen Suspension in Children

Patient's Weight	Dose	Administered As
13 kg (29 lb)	62.5 mg twice daily	2.5 mL (0.5 tsp) twice daily
25 kg (55 lb)	125 mg twice daily	5 mL (1 tsp) twice daily
38 kg (84 lb)	187.5 mg twice daily	7.5 mL (1.5 tsp) twice daily

- *Maximum dose* – 15 mg/kg/day as a total daily dose should not be exceeded.

Off-label dosing –

Analgesia:
- *Older than 2 years of age* – 5 to 7 mg/kg per dose orally every 8 to 12 hours.

➤*Elderly:* A lower dose should be considered in elderly patients. Caution is advised when high doses are required and some adjustment of dosage may be required.

➤*Renal function impairment:* A lower dose should be considered in patients with renal function impairment.

NAPROXEN — ORAL

➤*Hepatic function impairment:* A lower dose should be considered in patients with hepatic impairment.

➤*Administration:* To maintain the integrity of the enteric coating, the naproxen delayed-release tablets should not be broken, crushed or chewed during ingestion.

Naproxen suspension should be shaken gently before use.

➤*Storage/Stability:* Store at 15° to 30°C (59° to 86°F) in well-closed containers; dispense in light-resistant containers. Avoid excessive heat (more than 40°C; 104°F).

OXAPROZIN

Rx	**Oxaprozin** (Eon Labs)	**Tablets**: 600 mg	(141). White, capsule shape. Film-coated. In 100s, 500s, 1000s, and blister 100s.
Rx	**Daypro** (Searle)	**Caplets**: 600 mg	(Daypro 1381). White, capsule shape. Scored. Film-coated. In 100s, 500s, and UD 100s.
Rx	**Daypro ALTA** (Pharmacia)	**Tablets**: 678 oxaprozin potassium (equivalent to 600 mg oxaprozin)	(Searle 1391). Blue, capsule shape. Film-coated. In 100s, 500s, and UD 100s.

OXAPROZIN — ORAL

For complete and comparative prescribing information, refer to the NSAIDs group monograph.

WARNING

Cardiovascular risk – NSAIDs may cause an increased risk of serious cardiovascular thrombotic events, myocardial infarction, and stroke, which can be fatal. This risk may increase with duration of use. Patients with cardiovascular disease or risk factors for cardiovascular disease may be at greater risk.

Oxaprozin is contraindicated for treatment of perioperative pain in the setting of coronary artery bypass graft (CABG) surgery.

GI risk – NSAIDs cause an increased risk of serious GI adverse events including bleeding, ulceration, and perforation of the stomach or intestines, which can be fatal. These events can occur at any time during use and without warning symptoms. Elderly patients are at greater risk for serious GI events.

Indications

➤*Osteoarthritis:* For acute and long-term use in the management of the signs and symptoms of osteoarthritis.

➤*Rheumatoid arthritis:* For acute and long-term use in the management of the signs and symptoms of rheumatoid arthritis.

Administration and Dosage

➤*General dosing considerations:* Oxaprozin, like other NSAIDs, shows considerable interindividual differences in both pharmacokinetics and clinical response (pharmacodynamics). Therefore, the dosage for each patient should be individualized according to the patient's response to therapy.

As with all drugs of this class, the frequency and severity of adverse reactions will depend on the dose of the drug, the age and physical condition of the patient, any concurrent medical diagnoses, individual vulnerability, and the duration of therapy.

Regardless of the indication, the dosage should be individualized to the lowest effective dose of oxaprozin to minimize adverse reactions.

Health care providers should ensure that patients are tolerating doses in the 600 to 1,200 mg/day range without gastroenterologic, renal, hepatic, or dermatologic adverse reactions before advancing to the larger doses.

Experience with other NSAIDs has shown that starting therapy with maximal doses in patients at increased risk due to renal or hepatic disease, low body weight, advanced age, a known ulcer diathesis, or known sensitivity to NSAID effects is likely to increase the frequency of adverse reactions and is not recommended.

➤*Adults:* Doses greater than 1,200 mg/day should be reserved for patients who weigh more than 50 kg, have normal renal and hepatic function, are at low risk of peptic ulcer, and whose severity of disease justifies maximal therapy.

Osteoarthritis –

Usual dosage: 1,200 mg (two 600 mg tablets) once a day for the management of the signs and symptoms of moderate to severe osteoarthritis.

For patients of low body weight or with milder disease, an initial dosage of one 600 mg caplet once a day may be appropriate.

Maximum dose: 1,800 mg/day or 26 mg/kg, whichever is lower; in divided doses.

Initial dosage: 600 mg once a day for healthy weight patients with mild to moderate osteoarthritis.

Loading dose: 1,200 to 1,800 mg (not to exceed 26 mg/kg) may be used as a one-time loading dose in cases in which a quick onset of action is important.

Rheumatoid arthritis –

Usual dosage: 1,200 mg (two 600 mg tablets) once a day. Both smaller and larger doses may be required in individual patients.

Maximum dose: 1,800 mg/day or 26 mg/kg, whichever is lower; in divided doses.

Loading dose: 1,200 to 1,800 mg (not to exceed 26 mg/kg) may be used as a one-time loading dose in cases in which a quick onset of action is important.

➤*Elderly:* No adjustment of the dose of oxaprozin is necessary in elderly patients for pharmacokinetic reasons, although many elderly patients may need to receive a reduced dose because of low body weight or disorders associated with aging.

➤*Renal function impairment:* 600 mg/day, with cautious dosage increases if the desired effect is not obtained. The pharmacokinetics of oxaprozin may be significantly altered in patients with renal insufficiency or in patients who are undergoing hemodialysis.

Hemodialysis – 600 mg/day, with cautious dosage increases if the desired effect is not obtained. Oxaprozin is not dialyzed because of its high degree of protein binding.

➤*Administration:* Most patients will tolerate once-a-day dosing with oxaprozin, although divided doses may be tried in patients unable to tolerate single doses.

➤*Storage/Stability:* Keep bottles tightly closed and store below 25°C (77°F). Dispense in a tight, light-resistant container with a child-resistant closure. Protect the unit dose from light.

PIROXICAM

Rx	**Piroxicam** (Various, eg, Mylan, Ranbaxy, Teva)	**Capsules; oral**: 10 mg	In 100s, 500s, and UD 100s.
Rx	**Feldene** (Pfizer)		Lactose. (Feldene Pfizer 322). Blue/maroon. In 100s.
Rx	**Piroxicam** (Various, eg, Mylan, Ranbaxy, Teva, UDL Labs)	**Capsules; oral**: 20 mg	In 100s, 500s, and UD 100s.
Rx	**Feldene** (Pfizer)		Lactose. (Feldene Pfizer 323). Maroon. In 100s.

PIROXICAM — ORAL

For complete and comparative prescribing information, refer to the Nonsteroidal Antiinflammatory Drugs (NSAIDs) group monograph.

WARNING

Cardiovascular (CV) risk – NSAIDs may cause an increased risk of serious CV thrombotic reactions, myocardial infarction (MI), and stroke, which can be fatal. This risk may increase with duration of use. Patients with CV disease or risk factors for CV disease may be at greater risk.

Piroxicam is contraindicated for treatment of perioperative pain in the setting of coronary artery bypass graft (CABG) surgery.

GI risk – NSAIDs cause an increased risk of serious GI adverse reactions, including bleeding, ulceration, and perforation of the stomach or intestines, which can be fatal. These reactions can occur at any time during use and without warning symptoms. Elderly patients are at greater risk for serious GI reactions.

Indications

➤*Arthritis:* For relief of signs and symptoms of osteoarthritis and rheumatoid arthritis.

➤*Off-label uses:*

Postherpetic neuralgia (topical) – [5] = Poor documentation. Piroxicam has only been studied in patients with postherpetic neuralgia in 1 case series. American Academy of Neurology clinical practice guidelines state that the efficacy of topical piroxicam for the treatment of postherpetic neuralgia is unproven.

Other possible off-label uses – Primary dysmenorrhea, juvenile rheumatoid arthritis.

Administration and Dosage

➤*General dosing considerations:* Carefully consider the potential benefits and risks of piroxicam and other treatment options before deciding to use piroxicam. Use the lowest effective dose for the shortest duration consistent with individual patient treatment goals.

Because of the long half-life of piroxicam, steady-state blood levels are not reached for 7 to 12 days.

PIROXICAM — ORAL

➤*Adults:*

Osteoarthritis –

Usual dosage: 20 mg given orally once per day. If desired, the daily dose may be divided. Although the therapeutic effects of piroxicam are evident early in treatment, there is a progressive increase in response over several weeks, and the effect of therapy should not be assessed for 2 weeks.

Dosage adjustment: After observing the response to initial therapy with piroxicam, the dose and frequency should be adjusted to suit the individual's needs.

Rheumatoid arthritis – See Osteoarthritis for dosing.

➤*Elderly:* To minimize the potential risk of adverse GI reaction, use the lowest effective dose for the shortest possible duration.

In general, dose selection for an elderly patient should be cautious, usually starting at the low end of the dosing range, reflecting a greater frequency of impaired drug elimination and of concomitant disease or other drug therapy.

➤*Renal function impairment:* Treatment with piroxicam is not recommended in patients with advanced renal function impairment. If piroxicam therapy must be initiated, close monitoring of the patient's renal function is advisable.

➤*Storage/Stability:* Store at 20° to 25°C (68° to 77°F).

SULINDAC

Rx	**Sulindac** (Various, eg, Major, Mutual, Mylan, UDL, Watson)	**Tablets; oral:** 150 mg	In 100s, 500s, 1,000s, and UD 100s.
Rx	**Sulindac** (Various, eg, Mutual, Mylan, UDL, Watson)	**Tablets; oral:** 200 mg	In 100s, 500s, 1,000s, and UD 100s.
Rx	**Clinoril** (Merck)		(MSD 942). Yellow, hexagonal, scored. In 100s.

SULINDAC — ORAL

For complete and comparative prescribing information, refer to the NSAIDs group monograph.

WARNING

Cardiovascular (CV) risk – Nonsteroidal anti-inflammatory drugs (NSAIDs) may cause an increased risk of serious CV thrombotic reactions, myocardial infarction (MI), and stroke, which can be fatal. This risk may increase with duration of use. Patients with CV disease or risk factors for CV disease may be at greater risk.

Sulindac is contraindicated for the treatment of perioperative pain in the setting of coronary artery bypass graft (CABG) surgery.

GI risk – NSAIDs cause an increased risk of serious GI adverse reactions, including bleeding, ulceration, and perforation of the stomach or intestines, which can be fatal. These reactions can occur at any time during use and without warning symptoms. Elderly patients are at greater risk for serious GI reactions.

Indications

➤*Ankylosing spondylitis:* Acute or long-term use in the relief of signs and symptoms of ankylosing spondylitis.

➤*Arthritis:* Acute or long-term use in the relief of signs and symptoms of osteoarthritis, rheumatoid arthritis (RA), and acute gouty arthritis.

➤*Pain:* Acute or long-term use in the relief of signs and symptoms of acute painful shoulder (acute subacromial bursitis/supraspinatus tendinitis).

➤*Off-label uses:* Juvenile RA.

Administration and Dosage

➤*General dosing considerations:* Carefully consider the potential benefits and risks of sulindac and other treatment options before deciding whether to use sulindac. Use the lowest effective dose for the shortest duration consistent with individual patient treatment goals.

➤*Adults:*

Acute gouty arthritis –

Usual dosage: 200 mg twice daily with food.

Maximum dose: 400 mg/day.

Dosage adjustment: After observing the response to initial therapy with sulindac, the dose and frequency should be adjusted to suit an individual patient's needs.

Acute shoulder pain – See Acute Gouty Arthritis for dosing.

Duration of therapy: Therapy for 7 to 14 days is usually adequate.

Ankylosing spondylitis –

Maximum dose: 400 mg/day.

Initial dosage: 150 mg twice daily with food. The dosage may be lowered or raised, depending on response. A prompt response (within 1 week) can be expected in approximately one-half of patients. Others may require longer to respond.

Dosage adjustment: After observing the response to initial therapy with sulindac, the dose and frequency should be adjusted to suit an individual patient's needs.

Osteoarthritis – See Ankylosing Spondylitis for dosing.

Rheumatoid arthritis – See Ankylosing Spondylitis for dosing.

➤*Renal function impairment:* In patients with renal impairment, a reduction in daily dosage may be required.

➤*Hepatic function impairment:* In patients with hepatic impairment, a reduction in daily dosage may be required.

➤*Administration:* Administer twice daily with food.

➤*Storage/Stability:* Store in a tightly-closed container at 15° to 30°C (59° to 86°F).

TOLMETIN SODIUM

Rx	**Tolmetin Sodium** (Various, eg, Mutual, URL)	**Tablets:** 200 mg tolmetin (as sodium)	In 100s.
Rx	**Tolmetin Sodium** (Various, eg, Mylan, Purepac)	**Tablets:** 600 mg tolmetin (as sodium)	In 100s, 500s, and UD 100s.
Rx	**Tolmetin Sodium** (Various, eg, Allscripts, Mylan, Purepac, Teva)	**Capsules:** 400 mg tolmetin (as sodium)	In 100s, 500s, 1000s, and UD 100s.

TOLMETIN SODIUM — ORAL

For complete and comparative prescribing information, refer to the NSAIDs group monograph.

WARNING

Cardiovascular risk – Nonsteroidal anti-inflammatory agents (NSAIDs) may cause an increased risk of serious cardiovascular thrombotic events, myocardial infarction, and stroke, which can be fatal. This risk may increase with duration of use. Patients with cardiovascular disease or risk factors for cardiovascular disease may be at greater risk.

Tolmetin sodium is contraindicated for the treatment of perioperative pain in the setting of coronary artery bypass graft (CABG) surgery.

GI risk – NSAIDs cause an increased risk of serious GI adverse events including bleeding, ulceration, and perforation of the stomach or intestines, which can be fatal. These events can occur at any time during use and without warning symptoms. Elderly patients are at greater risk for serious GI events.

Indications

➤*Osteoarthritis/Rheumatoid arthritis/Juvenile rheumatoid arthritis:* For the relief of signs and symptoms of rheumatoid arthritis and osteoarthritis; in the treatment of acute flares and the long-term management of the chronic disease; for treatment of juvenile rheumatoid arthritis. The safety and efficacy of tolmetin sodium have not been established in children younger than 2 years of age.

Administration and Dosage

➤*General dosing considerations:* A therapeutic response to tolmetin can be expected in a few days to a week. Progressive improvement can be anticipated during succeeding weeks of therapy.

➤*Adults:*

Osteoarthritis –

Maximum dose: 1,800 mg/day.

Initial dosage: 400 mg 3 times daily (1,200 mg daily), preferably including a dose on arising and a dose at bedtime. To achieve optimal therapeutic effect, the dose should be adjusted according to the patient's response after 1 to 2 weeks.

Maintenance dosage: 600 to 1,800 mg daily in divided doses (generally 3 times daily).

Rheumatoid arthritis – See Osteoarthritis for dosing.

➤*Children:*

Juvenile rheumatoid arthritis –

2 years of age and older:

- *Maximum dose* – 30 mg/kg/day.
- *Initial dosage* – 20 mg/kg/day in divided doses (3 or 4 times daily).
- *Maintenance dosage* – 15 to 30 mg/kg/day.

➤*Elderly:* See Adults for dosing.

➤*Renal function impairment:* Since tolmetin sodium and its metabolites are eliminated primarily by the kidneys, patients with impaired renal function should be closely monitored, and it should be anticipated that they will require lower doses.

TOLMETIN SODIUM — ORAL

➤*Administration:* If GI symptoms occur, tolmetin can be administered with antacids other than sodium bicarbonate.

Tolmetin bioavailability and pharmacokinetics are not significantly affected by acute or chronic administration of magnesium and aluminum hydroxides; however, bioavailability is affected by food or milk.

➤*Storage/Stability:* Store at controlled room temperature (15° to 30°C; 59° to 86°F). Protect from light.

Selective COX-2 Inhibitors

CELECOXIB

Rx	Celebrex (Pfizer)	Capsules; oral: 50 mg	Lactose. (7767 50). White. In 60s.
		100 mg	Lactose. (7767 100). White. In 100s, 500s, and UD 100s.
		200 mg	Lactose. (7767 200). White. In 100s, 500s, and UD 100s.
		400 mg	Lactose. (7767 400). White. In 60s and UD 100s.

CELECOXIB — ORAL

For complete and comparative prescribing information, refer to the Nonsteroidal Anti-Inflammatory Agents class monograph.

WARNING

Cardiovascular risk – Celecoxib may cause an increased risk of serious cardiovascular thrombotic events, myocardial infarction (MI), and stroke, which can be fatal. All nonsteroidal anti-inflammatory drugs (NSAIDs) may have a similar risk. This risk may increase with duration of use. Patients with cardiovascular disease or risk factors for cardiovascular disease may be at higher risk.

Celecoxib is contraindicated for the treatment of perioperative pain in the setting of coronary artery bypass graft (CABG) surgery.

GI risk – NSAIDs, including celecoxib, cause an increased risk of serious GI adverse events, including bleeding, ulceration, and perforation of the stomach or intestines, which can be fatal. These events can occur at any time during use and without warning symptoms. Elderly patients are at higher risk for serious GI events.

Indications

➤*Acute pain:* For the management of acute pain in adults.

➤*Ankylosing spondylitis:* For the relief of signs and symptoms of ankylosing spondylitis.

➤*Familial adenomatous polyposis:* To reduce the number of adenomatous colorectal polyps in familial adenomatous polyposis (FAP), as an adjunct to usual care (eg, endoscopic surveillance, surgery).

➤*Juvenile rheumatoid arthritis:* For relief of the signs and symptoms of juvenile rheumatoid arthritis (RA) in patients 2 years of age and older.

➤*Osteoarthritis:* For relief of the signs and symptoms of osteoarthritis.

➤*Primary dysmenorrhea:* For the treatment of primary dysmenorrhea.

➤*Rheumatoid arthritis:* For relief of the signs and symptoms of RA in adults.

➤*Off-label uses:*

Lung cancer prevention – [4] = Insufficient documentation. According to American College of Chest Physicians (ACCP) guidelines, there are inadequate data to support the routine use of celecoxib for the prevention of lung cancer. However, several additional studies are underway evaluating celecoxib in this setting. Other candidate molecules are also being studied. The ACCP recommends that individuals with a high risk for lung cancer or history of lung cancer be encouraged to participate in lung cancer chemoprevention trials.

Preterm labor – [5] = Poor documentation. Preliminary data from a very small controlled trial suggest that celecoxib may be as effective as indomethacin in the treatment of preterm labor and may offer a better safety profile.

Prevention of colorectal cancer – [3] = Safety concerns. Current data with cyclooxygenase-2 (COX-2) inhibitors are not consistent in observational studies. Controlled prospective trials are needed; however, the role of these drugs, specifically celecoxib, in the prevention of colorectal cancer is compromised by recent data indicating significant or increased cardiovascular risk.

Schizophrenia (adjunctive therapy) – [3] = Safety concerns. The use of celecoxib as adjunctive treatment for schizophrenia is limited to 1 short-term (5 weeks), small, controlled trial enrolling 50 adult patients. These patients were hospitalized for acute exacerbation of schizophrenic psychosis and randomized to receive either risperidone with placebo or risperidone with celecoxib. Initial published data are not specific enough to justify the use of combination therapy at this time.

Administration and Dosage

➤*Adults:*

Acute pain –

Usual dosage: 200 mg twice daily as needed.

Initial dosage: 400 mg followed by an additional 200 mg dose if needed on the first day.

Ankylosing spondylitis –

Usual dosage: 200 mg daily as a single dose or as 100 mg twice daily.

Alternative dosage: If no effect is observed after 6 weeks, a trial of 400 mg daily may be worthwhile. If no effect is observed after 6 weeks on 400 mg daily, a response is not likely, and consideration should be given to alternate treatment options.

Familial adenomatous polyposis –

Usual dosage: 400 mg twice daily taken with food.

Concomitant therapy: Usual medical care for FAP patients should be continued while they are on celecoxib.

Osteoarthritis – 200 mg daily administered as a single dose or as 100 mg twice daily.

Primary dysmenorrhea –

Usual dosage: 200 mg twice daily as needed.

Initial dosage: 400 mg followed by an additional 200 mg dose if needed on the first day.

Rheumatoid arthritis – 100 to 200 mg twice daily.

Off-label dosing –

Lung cancer prevention: [4] = Insufficient documentation. 400 mg orally twice daily for 6 months.

Prevention of colorectal cancer: [3] = Safety concerns. 400 mg twice daily.

Schizophrenia (adjunctive therapy): [3] = Safety concerns. As adjunctive therapy to risperidone, celecoxib 200 mg twice daily for 5 weeks.

➤*Children:*

Juvenile rheumatoid arthritis –

2 years of age and older:

- *10 to 25 kg* – 50 mg twice daily.
- *More than 25 kg* – 100 mg twice daily.

➤*Elderly:* Dose adjustment is not generally necessary. However, for patients less than 50 kg body weight, initiate therapy at the lowest recommended dose.

➤*Renal function impairment:* Not recommended in patients with severe renal impairment.

➤*Hepatic function impairment:* In patients with moderate hepatic impairment (Child-Pugh class B), the daily dose should be reduced by approximately 50%. The use of celecoxib in patients with severe hepatic impairment is not recommended.

➤*Poor metabolizers of CYP2C9:* Use with caution. Consider starting treatment at half the lowest recommended dose. Consider using alternate management in juvenile RA patients who are poor metabolizers.

➤*Administration:* For patients who have difficulty swallowing capsules, the contents of a celecoxib capsule can be added to applesauce. The entire capsule contents can be carefully emptied onto a level teaspoon of cool or room temperature applesauce and ingested immediately with water.

Celecoxib can be given without regard to timing of meals. Patients with FAP should take celecoxib with food. Higher dosages (400 mg twice daily) should be administered with food to improve absorption.

➤*Storage/Stability:* Store at 25°C (77°F); excursions are permitted to 15° to 30°C (59° to 86°F). The sprinkled capsule contents on applesauce are stable for up to 6 hours under refrigerated conditions (2° to 8°C [35° to 45°F]).

ZICONOTIDE

Rx	**Prialt** (Azur Pharma)	**Solution; intrathecal:** 25 mcg/mL[a]	Preservative free. In 20 mL single-use vials.
		100 mcg/mL	Preservative free. In 1 and 5 mL single-use vials.

[a] Only use the diluted 25 mcg/mL formulation for the ziconotide-naive pump priming.

ZICONOTIDE — INTRATHECAL

WARNING

Severe psychiatric symptoms and neurological impairment may occur during treatment with ziconotide. Do not treat patients with a preexisting history of psychosis with ziconotide. Monitor all patients frequently for evidence of cognitive impairment, hallucinations, or changes in mood or consciousness. Ziconotide therapy can be interrupted or discontinued abruptly without evidence of withdrawal effects in the event of serious neurological or psychiatric signs or symptoms.

Indications

➤*Analgesia:* For the management of severe chronic pain in patients for whom intrathecal (IT) therapy is warranted, and who are intolerant of or refractory to other treatment, such as systemic analgesics, adjunctive therapies, or IT morphine.

Administration and Dosage

➤*Adults:*

Analgesia –

Maximum dose: Because of the frequency of adverse reactions, 19.2 mcg/day (0.8 mcg/h) is the maximum recommended dose.

Initial dosage: Initiate ziconotide intrathecal at no more than 2.4 mcg/day (0.1 mcg/h) and titrate to patient response.

Dosage titration: Doses may be titrated upward by up to 2.4 mcg/day (0.1 mcg/h) at intervals of no more than 2 to 3 times per week, up to a recommended maximum of 19.2 mcg/day (0.8 mcg/h) by day 21.

Dose increases in increments of less than 2.4 mcg/day (0.1 mcg/h) and increases in dose less frequently than 2 to 3 times per week may be used. For each dose titration, assess the dosing requirements and adjust the pump infusion flow rate as required to achieve the new dosing.

The average dose level at the end of the 21-day titration used in the slow titration clinical trial was 6.9 mcg/day (0.29 mcg/h), and the maximum dose was 19.2 mcg/day (0.8 mcg/h) on day 21.

Because of the lower incidence of serious adverse reactions and discontinuation for adverse reactions associated with the slower titration, use a faster titration schedule only if there is an urgent need for analgesia that outweighs the risk to the patient's safety.

Dosage adjustment: Adjust the dose of ziconotide intrathecal according to the patient's severity of pain, his response to therapy, and the occurrence of adverse reactions. The effective dose of ziconotide for analgesia is variable.

➤*Preparation for administration:* Ziconotide is used for therapy, undiluted (25 mcg/mL in 20 mL vial) or diluted (100 mcg/mL in 1, 2, or 5 mL vials).

Dilution – Diluted ziconotide is prepared with sodium chloride 0.9% injection using aseptic procedures to the desired concentration prior to placement in the microinfusion pump.

The 100 mcg/mL formulation may be administered undiluted once an appropriate dose has been established.

Refrigerate (but do not freeze) all ziconotide solutions after preparation, and begin infusion within 24 hours.

➤*Administration:* Ziconotide is intended for intrathecal delivery using a programmable implanted variable-rate microinfusion device or an external microinfusion device and catheter. Refer to the manufacturer's manual for specific instructions and precautions for programming the microinfusion device and/or refilling the reservoir.

Administer ziconotide intrathecal under the direction of a health care provider who is experienced in the technique of intrathecal administration and familiar with the drug and device labeling.

Ziconotide is not intended for intravenous (IV) administration.

➤*Admixture compatibility:* Saline solutions containing preservatives are not appropriate for intrathecal drug administration and should not be used.

➤*Storage/Stability:* Refrigerate ziconotide during transit.

Store ziconotide at 2° to 8°C (36° to 46°F). Ziconotide, once diluted aseptically with saline, may be stored at 2° to 8°C (36° to 46°F) for 24 hours. Do not freeze ziconotide. Protect from light.

Discard any ziconotide solution with observed particulate matter or discoloration and any unused portion left in the vial.

Actions

➤*Pharmacology:* Ziconotide binds to N-type calcium channels located on the primary nociceptive (A-δ and C) afferent nerves in the superficial layers (Rexed laminae I and II) of the dorsal horn in the spinal cord. Although the mechanism of action of ziconotide has not been established in humans, results in animals suggest that its binding blocks N-type calcium channels, which leads to a blockade of excitatory neurotransmitter release in the primary afferent nerve terminals and antinociception.

➤*Pharmacokinetics:*

Absorption – The cerebrospinal fluid (CSF) pharmacokinetics (PK) of ziconotide have been studied after 1-hour IT infusions of ziconotide 1 to 10 mcg to patients with chronic pain. The plasma PK following IV infusion (0.3 to 10 mcg/kg/day) have also been studied. Both IT and IV data are shown in the following table.

Ziconotide PK Parameters (Mean ± SD)					
Route	Fluid	N	CL (mL/min)	Vd (mL)	t½ (h)
IT	CSF	23	0.38 ± 0.56	155 ± 263	4.6 ± 0.9
IV	Plasma	21	270 ± 44	30,460 ± 6,366	1.3 ± 0.3

Following 1-hour IT administration of ziconotide 1 to 10 mcg, both total exposure (AUC; range: 83.6 to 608 ng•h/mL) and peak exposure (C_{max}; range: 16.4 to 132 ng/mL) values in the CSF were variable and dose-dependent, but appeared approximately dose-proportional. During 5 or 6 days of continuous IT infusions of ziconotide at infusion rates ranging from 0.1 to 7 mcg/h in patients with chronic pain, plasma ziconotide levels could not be quantified in 56% of patients using an assay with a lower limit of detection of approximately 0.04 ng/mL. Predictably, patients requiring higher IT infusion dose rates were more likely to have quantifiable ziconotide levels in plasma. Plasma ziconotide levels, when detectable, remain constant after many months of ziconotide IT infusion in patients followed for up to 9 months.

Distribution – Ziconotide is about 50% bound to human plasma proteins. The mean CSF volume of distribution (Vd) of ziconotide following IT administration approximates the estimated total CSF volume (140 mL).

Metabolism – Ziconotide is cleaved by endopeptidases and exopeptidases at multiple sites on the peptide. Following passage from the CSF into the systemic circulation during continuous IT administration, ziconotide is expected to be susceptible to proteolytic cleavage by various ubiquitous peptidases/proteases present in most organs (eg, kidney, liver, lung muscle), and thus readily degraded to peptide fragments and their individual constituent free amino acids. Human and animal CSF and blood exhibit minimal hydrolytic activity toward ziconotide in vitro. The biological activity of the various expected proteolytic degradation products of ziconotide has not been assessed.

Excretion – Minimal amounts of ziconotide (less than 1%) were recovered in human urine following IV infusion. The terminal half-life of ziconotide in CSF after an IT administration was around 4.6 hours (range, 2.9 to 6.5 hours). Mean CSF clearance (CL) of ziconotide approximates adult human CSF turnover rate (0.3 to 0.4 mL/min).

Contraindications

Hypersensitivity to ziconotide or any of its formulation components and in patients with any other concomitant treatment or medical condition that would render IT administration hazardous; preexisting history of psychosis with ziconotide; presence of infection at the microinfusion injection site; uncontrolled bleeding diathesis; spinal canal obstruction that impairs circulation of CSF.

Warnings/Precautions

➤*Psychiatric symptoms:* Severe psychiatric symptoms and neurological impairment may occur during treatment with ziconotide. Do not treat patients with a preexisting history of psychosis with ziconotide. Monitor all patients frequently for evidence of cognitive impairment, hallucinations, or changes in mood or consciousness. Ziconotide therapy can be interrupted or discontinued abruptly without evidence of withdrawal effects in the event of serious neurological or psychiatric signs or symptoms.

➤*Opiate withdrawal:* Ziconotide is not an opiate and cannot prevent or relieve the symptoms associated with the withdrawal of opiates. To avoid withdrawal syndrome when opiate withdrawal is necessary, patients must not be abruptly withdrawn from opiates. For patients being withdrawn from IT opiates, gradually taper the IT opiate infusion over a few weeks and replace with a pharmacologically equivalent dose of oral opiates. Ziconotide does not interact with opiate receptors and does not potentiate opiate-induced respiratory depression.

➤*Meningitis and other infections:* Meningitis can occur because of inadvertent contamination of the microinfusion device and other means, such as CSF seeding caused by hematogenous or direct spread from an infected pump pocket or catheter tract. While meningitis is rare with an internal microinfusion device and surgically implanted catheter, the incidence increases substantially with external devices. In the 1,254 patients in ziconotide clinical trials with an exposure of 662 patient years, meningitis occurred in 3% (40 cases) of the ziconotide group using either internal or external microinfusion devices and 1% (1 case) in the placebo group with an exposure of only 5 patient-years. The risk of meningitis with external microinfusion devices and catheters was higher, with 93% cases (38/41) occurring with external infusion systems (37 ziconotide, 1 placebo).

Patients, caregivers, and health care providers must be particularly vigilant for the signs and symptoms of meningitis, including but not limited to fever, headache, stiff neck, altered mental status (eg, lethargy, confusion, disorientation), nausea or vomiting, and occasionally seizures. Serious infection or meningitis can occur within 24 hours of a breach in sterility such as a disconnected catheter, the most common cause of meningitis with external microinfusion devices. The patient and health care provider should be familiar with the handling of the external microinfusion device and care of the catheter skin exit site at risk of infection. Strict aseptic procedures must be

ZICONOTIDE — INTRATHECAL

used during the preparation of the ziconotide solution or refilling of the microinfusion device to prevent accidental introduction of any contaminants or other environmental pathogens into the reservoir. In suspected cases (especially in immunocompromised patients) or in confirmed cases of meningitis, CSF cultures must be obtained and appropriate antibiotic therapy must be promptly instituted. Treatment of meningitis usually requires removal of the microinfusion system, catheter, and any other foreign body materials within the IT space and, therefore, discontinuation of ziconotide therapy.

➤*Cognitive and neuropsychiatric effects:* Use of ziconotide has been associated with CNS-related adverse reactions, including psychiatric symptoms, cognitive impairment, and decreased alertness/unresponsiveness. For the 1,254 patients treated, the following cognitive adverse event rates were reported: confusion (33%), memory impairment (22%), speech disorder (14%), aphasia (12%), thinking abnormal (8%), and amnesia (1%). Cognitive impairment may appear gradually after several weeks of treatment. Reduce or discontinue the ziconotide dose if signs or symptoms of cognitive impairment develop, but also consider other contributing causes. The various cognitive effects of ziconotide are generally reversible within 2 weeks after drug discontinuation. The medians for time to reversal of the individual cognitive effects ranged from 3 to 15 days. The elderly (65 years of age and older) are at higher risk for confusion.

Reactions of acute psychiatric disturbances such as hallucinations (12%), paranoid reactions (3%), hostility (2%), delirium (2%), psychosis (1%), and manic reactions (0.4%) have been reported in patients treated with ziconotide. Patients with pretreatment psychiatric disorders may be at an increased risk. Ziconotide may cause or worsen depression with the risk of suicide in susceptible patients. If appropriate, management of psychiatric complications should include discontinuation of ziconotide, treatment with psychotherapeutic agents if appropriate, and/or short-term hospitalization. Before drug is reinitiated, careful evaluation must be performed on an individual basis.

➤*Suicide:* In placebo-controlled trials, there was a higher incidence of suicide, suicide attempts, and suicide ideations in ziconotide-treated patients (N = 3) than in the placebo group (N = 1). The incidence was 0.1/patient-year for placebo patients and 0.27/patient-year for ziconotide patients.

➤*Reduced level of consciousness:* Patients have become unresponsive or stuporous while receiving ziconotide. The incidence of unresponsiveness or stupor in clinical trials was 2%. During these episodes, the patient sometimes appears to be conscious and breathing is not depressed. If reduced levels of consciousness occur, discontinue ziconotide until the event resolves, and consider other etiologies (eg, meningitis). There is no known pharmacologic antagonist for this effect. Patients taking concomitant antiepileptics, neuroleptics, sedatives, or diuretics may be at higher risk of depressed levels of consciousness. If altered consciousness occurs, discontinue other CNS-depressant drugs as clinically appropriate.

➤*Serum CK-muscle isoenzyme (CK-MM) elevation:* In clinical studies (mostly open label), 40% of patients had serum CK levels above the upper limit of normal (ULN), and 11% had CK levels that were at least 3 times the ULN. In cases where CK was fractionated, only the muscle isoenzyme (MM) was elevated. The time to occurrence was sporadic, but the greatest incidence of CK elevation was during the first 2 months of treatment. Elevated CKs were more often seen in men, in patients who were being treated with antidepressants or antiepileptics, and in patients treated with IT morphine. Most patients who experienced elevations in CK, even for prolonged periods of time, did not have limiting side effects. However, 1 case of symptomatic myopathy with EMG findings, and 2 cases of acute renal failure associated with rhabdomyolysis and extreme CK elevations (17,000 to 27,000 units/L) have been reported.

Therefore, it is recommended that physicians monitor serum CK in patients undergoing treatment with ziconotide periodically (eg, every other week for the first month and monthly as appropriate thereafter). Clinically evaluate patients and obtain CK measurements in the setting of new neuromuscular symptoms (eg, myalgias, myasthenia, muscle cramps, asthenia) or a reduction in physical activity. If these symptoms continue and CK levels remain elevated or continue to rise, it is recommended that the physician consider ziconotide dose reduction or discontinuation.

➤*Hazardous tasks:* Caution patients against engaging in hazardous activity requiring complete mental alertness or motor coordination, such as operating machinery or driving a motor vehicle, during treatment with ziconotide. Also caution patients about possible combined effects with other CNS-depressant drugs. Dosage adjustments may be necessary when ziconotide is administered with such agents because of the potentially additive effects.

➤*Pregnancy: Category C.* Ziconotide was embryolethal in rats when given as a continuous IV infusion during the major period of organogenesis as evidenced by significant increases in postimplantation loss caused by an absence or a reduced number of live fetuses. Estimated exposure for embryolethality in the rat was approximately 700-fold above the expected exposure resulting from the maximum recommended human daily IT dose of 0.8 mcg/h (19.2 mcg/day). Ziconotide was not teratogenic in female rats when given as a continuous IV infusion at doses up to 30 mg/kg/day or in female rabbits up to 5 mg/kg/day during the major period of organ development. Estimated exposures in the female rat and rabbit were approximately 26,000- and 940-fold higher than the expected exposure resulting from the maximum recommended human daily IT dose of 0.8 mcg/h (19.2 mcg/day) based on plasma exposure. Maternal toxicity in the rat and rabbit, as evidenced by decreased body weight gain and food consumption, was present at all dose levels. Maternal toxicity in the rat led to reduced fetal weights and transient, delayed ossification of the pubic bones at doses 15 mg/kg/day or higher, which is approximately 8,900-fold higher than the expected exposure resulting from the maximum recommended human daily IT dose of 0.8 mcg/h (19.2 mcg/day) based on plasma exposure. The no observable adverse effect level (NOAEL) for embryo-fetal development in rats was 0.5 mg/kg/day and in rabbits was 5 mg/kg/day. Estimated NOAEL exposures in the rat and rabbit were approximately 400- and 940-fold higher, respectively, than the expected exposure resulting from the maximum recommended human daily IT dose of 0.8 mcg/h (19.2 mcg/day) based on plasma exposure.

In a prenatal and postnatal study in rats, ziconotide given as a continuous IV infusion did not affect pup development or reproductive performance up to a dose of 10 mg/kg/day, which is approximately 3,800-fold higher than the expected exposure resulting from the maximum recommended human daily IT dose of 0.8 mcg/h (19.2 mcg/day) based on plasma exposure. Maternal toxicity as evidenced by clinical observations, and decreases in body weight gain and food consumption were observed at all doses.

No adequate and well-controlled studies have been conducted in pregnant women. Because animal studies are not always predictive of human response, use ziconotide during pregnancy only if the potential benefit justifies the risk to the fetus.

➤*Lactation:* It is not known whether ziconotide is excreted in human breast milk. Because many drugs are excreted in human milk, and because of the potential for serious adverse reactions in breast-feeding infants from ziconotide, decide whether to discontinue breast-feeding or to discontinue the drug, taking into account the importance of the drug to the mother.

➤*Children:* Safety and effectiveness in children have not been established.

➤*Elderly:* Of the total number of subjects in clinical studies of ziconotide, 22% were 65 years of age and older, while 7% were 75 years of age and older. In all trials, there was a higher incidence of confusion in older patients (42% of patients 65 years of age and older vs 29% of patients younger than 65 years of age). Other reported clinical experience has not identified differences in responses between the elderly and younger patients. In general, the dose selection for an elderly patient should be cautious, usually starting at the low end of the dosing range, reflecting the greater frequency of decreased hepatic, renal, or cardiac function, and of concomitant disease or other drug therapy.

➤*Lab test abnormalities:* In clinical studies (mostly open label), up to 40% of patients had serum CK levels above the ULN, and 11% had CK levels that were at least 3 times the ULN. Most cases of CK elevation were not associated with muscle weakness, however 1 case of myopathy with EMG findings and 2 cases of acute renal failure associated with rhabdomyolysis and extreme CK elevations (17,000 to 27,000 units/L) were reported.

Drug Interactions

Formal PK drug-drug interaction studies have not been performed with ziconotide. As ziconotide is a peptide, it is expected to be completely degraded by endopeptidases and exopeptidases (Phase I hydrolytic enzymes) widely located throughout the body, and not by other Phase I biotransformation processes (including the cytochrome P450 system) or by Phase II conjugation reactions. Thus, IT administration, low plasma ziconotide concentrations, and metabolism by ubiquitous peptidases make metabolic interactions of other drugs with ziconotide unlikely. Further, as ziconotide is not highly bound in plasma (approximately 50%) and has low plasma exposure following IT administration, clinically relevant plasma protein displacement reactions involving ziconotide and coadministered medications are unlikely.

➤*CNS depressants:* Almost all patients in the ziconotide clinical trials received concomitant non-IT medication. Of the 1,254 patients treated, most received several concomitant drugs, including antidepressants (66%), anxiolytics (52%), antiepileptics (47%), neuroleptics (46%), and sedatives (34%). The use of drugs with CNS-depressant activities may be associated with an increased incidence of CNS adverse reactions such as dizziness and confusion.

➤*Opioids:* Ziconotide does not bind to opioid receptors and its pharmacological effects are not blocked by opioid antagonists. In animal models, ziconotide IT potentiated opioid-induced reduction in GI motility, but did not potentiate morphine-induced respiratory depression. In rats receiving ziconotide IT, additive analgesic effects were observed with concurrent administration of morphine, baclofen, or clonidine. Concurrent administration of ziconotide IT and morphine did not prevent the development of morphine tolerance in rats.

More than 90% of patients treated with ziconotide IT used systemic opiates and in the slow titration study, 98% of patients received opioids.

Combination of ziconotide with IT opiates has not been studied in placebo-controlled clinical trials and is not recommended.

Adverse Reactions

The most frequently reported adverse reactions (25% or more) in the 1,254 patients (662 patient years) in clinical trials were dizziness, nausea, confusion, headache, somnolence, nystagmus, asthenia, and pain. Serious adverse reactions and discontinuation of ziconotide for adverse reactions are less frequent when the drug is slowly titrated over 21 days, than with a faster titration schedule.

The following table summarizes the treatment-emergent adverse reactions with a frequency of 5% or greater in the ziconotide-treated group from the 1 placebo-controlled trial using the slow titration schedule in patients with severe chronic pain. All reactions reported during the initial placebo-controlled period of the studies (21 days in the slow titration schedule) are tabulated, regardless of relationship to ziconotide.

ZICONOTIDE — INTRATHECAL

Ziconotide Adverse Reactions in Slow Titration Placebo-Controlled Trial (Reactions that Occurred in ≥ 5% of Patients)		
Adverse reaction	Ziconotide (n = 112)	Placebo (n = 108)
CNS	81%	51%
Abnormal gait	15%	2%
Anxiety	9%	5%
Aphasia	8%	1%
Ataxia	16%	2%
Confusion	18%	5%
Dizziness	47%	13%
Dysesthesia	7%	2%
Hallucinations	7%	0%
Headache	15%	12%
Hypertonia	11%	5%
Memory impairment	12%	1%
Nervousness	7%	4%
Nystagmus	8%	0%
Paresthesia	7%	3%
Somnolence	22%	15%
Speech disorder	9%	2%
Vertigo	7%	0%
GI	60%	51%
Anorexia	10%	5%
Diarrhea	19%	17%
Nausea	41%	31%
Vomiting	15%	13%
GU	22%	12%
Urinary retention	9%	0%
Special senses	20%	11%
Abnormal vision	10%	4%
Miscellaneous	57%	42%
Asthenia	22%	12%
Fever	7%	3%
Pain	11%	7%

The following adverse reactions assessed as related to ziconotide have been reported in 2% or greater of patients participating in the clinical studies (COSTART terms, by body system):

➤*Cardiovascular:* Hypertension, hypotension, postural hypotension, syncope, tachycardia, vasodilation.

➤*CNS:* Abnormal dreams, abnormal gait, agitation, anxiety, aphasia, ataxia, CSF abnormal, confusion, depression, difficulty concentrating, dizziness, dry mouth, dysesthesia, emotional lability, headache, hostility, hyperesthesia, hypertonia, incoordination, insomnia, memory impairment, mental slowing, meningitis, nervousness, neuralgia, nystagmus, paranoid reaction, paresthesia, reflexes decreased, somnolence, speech disorder, stupor, thinking abnormal, tremor, twitching, vertigo.

➤*Dermatologic:* Cutaneous surgical complication, dry skin, pruritus, rash, skin disorder, sweating.

➤*GI:* Anorexia, constipation, diarrhea, dyspepsia, gastrointestinal disorder, nausea, nausea and vomiting, vomiting.

➤*GU:* Dysuria, urinary incontinence, urinary retention, urinary tract infection, urination impaired.

➤*Hematologic:* Anemia, ecchymosis.

➤*Metabolic/Nutritional:* Creatine phosphokinase increased, dehydration, edema, hypokalemia, peripheral edema, weight loss.

➤*Musculoskeletal:* Arthralgia, arthritis, leg cramps, myalgia, myasthenia.

➤*Respiratory:* Bronchitis, cough increased, dyspnea, lung disorder, pharyngitis, pneumonia, rhinitis, sinusitis.

➤*Special senses:* Abnormal vision, diplopia, photophobia, taste perversion, tinnitus.

➤*Miscellaneous:* Abdominal pain, accidental injury, asthenia, back pain, catheter complication, catheter-site pain, cellulitis, chest pain, chills, fever, flu syndrome, infection, malaise, neck pain, neck rigidity, pain, pump-site complication, pump-site mass, pump-site pain, viral infection.

At less than 2%, the following reactions were assessed by the clinical investigators as related to ziconotide: acute kidney failure, atrial fibrillation, cerebrovascular accident, electrocardiogram abnormal, grand mal convulsion, meningitis, myoclonus, psychosis, respiratory distress, rhabdomyolysis, sepsis, and suicidal ideations. Rare instances of fatal aspiration pneumonia and suicide were reported (less than 1%).

Overdosage

➤*Symptoms:* The maximum recommended ziconotide IT dose is 19.2 mcg/day. The maximum IT dose of ziconotide in clinical trials was 912 mcg/day. In some patients who received IT doses greater than the maximum recommended dose, exaggerated pharmacological effects (eg, ataxia, nystagmus, dizziness, stupor, unresponsiveness, spinal myoclonus, confusion, sedation, hypotension, word-finding difficulties, garbled speech, nausea, vomiting) were observed. There was no indication of respiratory depression. Overdoses may occur because of pump programming errors or incorrect drug concentration preparations. In these cases, patients were observed and ziconotide was either temporarily discontinued or permanently withdrawn. Most patients recovered within 24 hours after withdrawal of drug.

➤*Treatment:* In the event of an IT overdose, elimination of ziconotide from CSF is expected to remain constant (CSF $t_{1/2}$ = 4.6 hours). Therefore, within 24 hours of stopping therapy, the ziconotide CSF concentration should be less than 5% of peak levels.

There is no known antidote to ziconotide. Administer general medical supportive measures to patients who receive an overdose until the exaggerated pharmacological effects of the drug have resolved. Treatment for an overdose is hospitalization, when needed, and symptom-related supportive care. Ziconotide does not bind to opiate receptors, and its pharmacological effects are not blocked by opioid antagonists.

In the event of an inadvertent IV or epidural administration, adverse reactions could include hypotension, which can be treated with a recumbent posture and blood pressure support as required. The half-life of ziconotide in serum is 1.3 hours.

Patient Information

Caution patients against engaging in hazardous activity requiring complete mental alertness or motor coordination such as operating machinery or driving a motor vehicle during treatment with ziconotide.

Caution patients about possible combined effects with other CNS-depressant drugs. Dosage adjustments may be necessary when ziconotide is administered with such agents because of the potentially additive effects.

Advise patients to contact their physician if they experience new or worsening muscle pain, soreness, or weakness with or without darkened urine.

Advise patients to contact their doctor immediately if they experience:
- A change in mental status (eg, lethargy, confusion, disorientation, decreased alertness)
- A change in mood or perception (eg, hallucinations, including unusual tactile sensations in the oral cavity)
- Symptoms of depression or suicidal ideation
- Nausea, vomiting, seizures, fever, headache, and/or stiff neck, as these may be symptoms of developing meningitis.

AGENTS FOR MIGRAINE

In addition to the agents on the following pages, propranolol and timolol are indicated for migraine prophylaxis (see Beta-Adrenergic Blocking Agents monograph).

Serotonin 5-HT_1 Receptor Agonists (Triptans)

Indications

➤*Migraine treatment:* For the acute treatment of migraine with or without aura in adults.

➤*Cluster headache (sumatriptan injection only):* For the acute treatment of cluster headache episodes.

➤*Off-label uses:* Refer to individual monographs for further information.

Migraines in children/adolescents –

Rizatriptan: 4 = Insufficient documentation.

Sumatriptan (injection): 4 = Insufficient documentation.

Sumatriptan (intranasal): 1 = Good documentation.

Sumatriptan (oral): 4 = Insufficient documentation.

Migraines in adolescents –

Zolmitriptan (oral): 4 = Insufficient documentation.

Zolmitriptan (intranasal): 4 = Insufficient documentation.

Postdural puncture headache –

Sumatriptan (injection): 4 = Insufficient documentation.

Actions

➤*Pharmacology:* **Sumatriptan**, **naratriptan**, **zolmitriptan**, **rizatriptan**, **frovatriptan**, **eletriptan**, and **almotriptan** are selective 5-hydroxytryptamine$_1$ (5-HT_1 or serotonin) receptor agonists.

Serotonin 5-HT_1 Receptor Agonists (Triptans)

Serotonin 5-HT_1 Receptor Agonists Receptor Site Affinity			
Drug	High	Weak	None
Almotriptan	5-HT_{1D}, 5-HT_{1B}, 5-HT_{1F}	5-HT_{1A}, 5-HT_7	5-HT_{2-4}, 5-HT_6, α-adrenergic, β-adrenergic, adenosine (A_1, A_2), angiotensin (AT_1, AT_2), dopaminergic D_1 or D_2, endothelin (ET_A, ET_B), tachykinin receptor sites
Eletriptan	5-HT_{1B}, 5-HT_{1D}, 5-HT_{1F}	5-HT_{1A}, 5-HT_{1E}, 5-HT_{2B}, 5-HT_7	5-HT_{2A}, 5-HT_{2C}, 5-HT_3, 5-HT_4, 5-HT_{5A}, 5-HT_6, α-adrenergic, and β-adrenergic, dopaminergic D_1 or D_2, muscarinic, or opioid receptors
Frovatriptan	5-HT_{1B}, 5-HT_{1D}	none	Benzodiazepine receptor sites
Naratriptan	5-HT_{1D}	none	5-HT_{2-4}, α-adrenergic, β-adrenergic, dopaminergic, muscarinic, benzodiazepine receptor sites
Rizatriptan	5-HT_{1B}, 5-HT_{1D}	5-HT_{1A}, 5-HT_{1E}, 5-HT_{1F}, 5-HT_7	5-HT_2, 5-HT_3, α-adrenergic, β-adrenergic, dopaminergic, muscarinic, benzodiazepine receptor sites
Sumatriptan	5-HT_1	5-HT_{1A}, 5-HT_{5A}, 5-HT_7	5-HT_{2-4}, α-adrenergic, β-adrenergic, dopaminergic, muscarinic, benzodiazepine receptor sites
Zolmitriptan	5-HT_{1D}, 5-HT_{1B}	5-HT_{1A}	5-HT_{2-4}, α-adrenergic, β-adrenergic, dopaminergic, muscarinic, histaminic receptor sites

The vascular 5-HT_1 receptor subtype is present on the human basilar artery and in the vasculature of isolated human dura mater. Current theories on the etiology of migraine headaches suggest that symptoms are caused by local cranial vasodilation or the release of vasoactive and proinflammatory peptides from sensory nerve endings in an activated trigeminal system. The therapeutic activity of the serotonin 5-HT_1 receptor agonists in migraine most likely can be attributed to agonist effects at 5-$HT_{1B/1D}$ receptors on the extracerebral, intracranial blood vessels that become dilated during a migraine attack and on nerve terminals in the trigeminal system. Activation of these receptors results in cranial vessel constriction, inhibition of neuropeptide release, and reduced transmission in trigeminal pain pathways.

➤*Pharmacokinetics:*

Pharmacokinetic Parameters of Triptans in Healthy Volunteers and in Patients with Migraine							
Drug	Dose and route of administration	T_{max} (h)	C_{max} (mcg/L)	Bioavailability (%)	t½ (h)	AUC (mcg/L•h)	Plasma protein binding (%)
Almotriptan	12.5 mg PO	2.5	49.5	80	3.1	266	≈ 35
	25 mg PO	2.7	64	69	3.6	443	
Eletriptan	20 mg PO	2		≈ 50	≈ 4	–	≈ 85
Frovatriptan	2.5 mg PO	3	4.2/7[a]	29.6	25.7	94	≈ 15
	40 mg PO	5	24.7/53.4[a]	17.5	29.7	881	
Naratriptan	2.5 mg PO	2	12.6	74	5.5	98	≈ 28
Rizatriptan	10 mg PO	1, 1.6 to 2.5[b]	19.8	40	2	50	14
Sumatriptan	6 mg SC	0.17	72	96	2	90	14 to 21
	100 mg PO	1.5	54	14	2	158	
	20 mg NAS	1.5	13	15.8	1.8	48	
	25 mg PR	1.5	27	19.2	1.8	78	
Zolmitriptan	2.5 mg PO	1.5, 3[b]	3.3/3.8[a]	39	2.3/2.6[a]	18/21[a]	≈ 25
	5 mg PO	1.5, 3[b]	10	46	3	42	
	5 mg NAS	3	3.93[c]	102[d]	≈ 3	22.4[c]	

[a] Value for men and women, respectively.
[b] Orally-disintegrating tablets.
[c] Values based on 2.5 mg dose.
[d] Compared with oral tablet.

Renal function impairment – Clearance of **zolmitriptan** was reduced by 25% in patients with severe renal impairment (CrCl approximately 5 to 25 mL/min); no significant change was observed in those with moderate renal impairment.

Clearance of **naratriptan** was reduced by 50% in patients with moderate renal impairment (CrCl 18 to 39 mL/min), resulting in an increase in mean half life from 6 hours (healthy) to 11 hours (range, 7 to 20 hours). The mean C_{max} increased by approximately 40%. The effects of severe renal impairment have not been assessed (see Contraindications and Administration and Dosage).

In hemodialysis patients (CrCl less than 2 mL/min/1.73 m^2), the AUC for **rizatriptan** was approximately 44% greater than that in patients with normal renal function.

The clearance of **almotriptan** was approximately 65% lower in patients with severe renal impairment (CrCl between 10 and 30 mL/min) and approximately 40% lower in patients with moderate renal impairment (CrCl between 31 and 71 mL/min).

Because less than 10% of **frovatriptan** is excreted in urine after an oral dose, it is unlikely that the exposure to frovatriptan will be affected by renal impairment. The pharmacokinetics of frovatriptan following a single oral dose of 2.5 mg was not different in patients with renal impairment (5 males and 6 females, CrCl 16 to 73 mL/min) vs subjects with normal renal function.

Hepatic function impairment – The liver plays an important role in the presystemic clearance of oral 5-HT_1 agonists. Accordingly, the bioavailability may be markedly increased in patients with liver disease.

Oral: In a small study of hepatically impaired patients, **sumatriptan** AUC and C_{max} increased by approximately 70%, and T_{max} decreased by 40 minutes.

In severely hepatically impaired patients, the mean C_{max}, T_{max}, and AUC of **zolmitriptan** were increased 1.5-, 2-, and 3-fold, respectively. Seven of 27 patients experienced 20 to 80 mm Hg elevations in systolic or diastolic blood pressure after a 10 mg dose. Administer zolmitriptan with caution in patients with liver disease, generally using doses less than 2.5 mg.

Clearance of **naratriptan** was decreased by 30% in patients with moderate hepatic impairment (Child-Pugh grade A or B). This resulted in an approximately 40% increase in the half life (range, 8 to 16 hours). The effects of severe hepatic impairment (Child-Pugh grade C) have not been assessed (see Contraindications).

Following oral administration in patients with hepatic impairment caused by mild to moderate alcoholic cirrhosis of the liver, plasma concentrations of **rizatriptan** were similar in patients with mild hepatic insufficiency compared with a control group of healthy subjects; plasma concentrations of rizatriptan were approximately 30% greater in patients with moderate hepatic insufficiency.

The pharmacokinetics of **almotriptan** have not been assessed in this population. Based on the mechanisms of almotriptan clearance, the maximum decrease expected because of hepatic impairment would be 60%.

The effects of severe hepatic impairment on **eletriptan** metabolism have not been evaluated. Subjects with mild or moderate hepatic impairment demonstrated an increase in AUC (34%) and half life. C_{max} was increased by 18% (see Contraindications).

Elderly – There is a statistically significant increase in **eletriptan** half life (from approximately 4.4 to 5.7 hours) between elderly (65 to 93 years of age) and younger adult subjects (18 to 45 years of age).

Contraindications

Injectable preparations used IV, because of the potential to cause coronary vasospasm; patients with ischemic heart disease (angina pectoris, history of MI, strokes, transient ischemic attacks [TIAs], or documented silent ischemia); Prinzmetal variant angina or other significant underlying cardiovascular disease (see Warnings); patients with signs or symptoms consistent with ischemic heart disease or coronary artery vasospasm; patients with uncontrolled hypertension; concurrent use of (or use within 24 hours of) ergotamine-containing preparations or ergot-type medications such as dihydroergotamine or methysergide; concurrent monoamine oxidase inhibitor (MAOI) therapy (or within 2 weeks of discontinuing an MAOI [except for **eletriptan**]; see Drug Interactions); within 24 hours of another 5-HT_1 agonist; hypersensitivity to the product or any of its ingredients; management of hemiplegic or basilar migraine; ischemic bowel disease.

➤*Naratriptan and sumatriptan:* Cerebrovascular or peripheral vascular syndromes, severe hepatic impairment (Child-Pugh grade C); severe renal impairment (CrCl less than 15 mL/min) (naratriptan only).

➤*Frovatriptan and eletriptan:* Peripheral vascular disease.

➤*Eletriptan:* Severe hepatic impairment.

Warnings/Precautions

➤*Migraine diagnosis:* Use 5-HT_1 agonists only when a clear diagnosis of migraine has been established.

➤*Risk of myocardial ischemia or MI and other adverse cardiac events:* Because of the potential of this class of compounds to cause coronary vasospasm, do not give these agents to patients with documented ischemic or vasospastic coronary artery disease (see Contraindications). It is strongly recommended that 5-HT_1 agonists not be given to patients in whom unrecognized coronary artery disease (CAD) is predicted by the presence of risk factors (eg, hypertension, hypercholesterolemia, smoking, obesity, diabetes, strong family history of CAD, female with surgical or physiological menopause, or male older than 40 years of age) unless a cardiovascular evaluation provides satisfactory clinical evidence that the patient is reasonably free of coronary artery and ischemic myocardial disease or other significant underlying cardiovascular disease. The sensitivity of cardiac diagnostic procedures to detect cardiovascular diseases or predisposition to coronary artery vasospasm is modest at best. If, during the cardiovascular evaluation, the patient's medical history, electrocardiogram (ECG), or other investigations reveal findings indicative of, or consistent with, coronary artery vasospasm or myocardial ischemia, do not administer 5-HT_1 agonists (see Contraindications). For patients with risk factors predictive of CAD who are determined to have a satisfactory cardiovascular evaluation, it is strongly recommended that administration of the first dose take place in the setting of a physician's office or similar medically staffed and equipped facility, unless the patient has previously received 5-HT_1 agonists. Because cardiac ischemia can occur in the absence of clinical symptoms, consider obtaining an ECG during the interval immediately following the first use in a patient with risk factors.

It is recommended that patients who are intermittent long-term users of 5-HT_1 agonists who have or acquire risk factors predictive of CAD, as described above, undergo periodic interval cardiovascular evaluation as they continue use.

The systematic approach described above is intended to reduce the likelihood that patients with unrecognized cardiovascular disease will be inadvertently exposed to 5-HT_1 agonists.

Zolmitriptan – There is a report of at least 1 patient experiencing coronary vasospasm without history of cardiac disease and with documented absence of CAD.

Patients with symptomatic Wolff-Parkinson-White syndrome or arrhythmias associated with other cardiac accessory conduction pathway disorders should not receive zolmitriptan.

➤*Cardiac events and fatalities associated with 5-HT_1 agonists:* Serious adverse cardiac events, including acute MI, life-threatening disturbances of cardiac rhythm, and death have been reported within a few hours following the administration of 5-HT_1 agonists. Considering the extent of use of 5-HT_1 agonists in patients with migraine, the incidence of these events is extremely low.

➤*Cerebrovascular events and fatalities with 5-HT_1 agonists:* Cerebral hemorrhage, subarachnoid hemorrhage, stroke, and other cerebrovascular events have been reported in patients treated with 5-HT_1 agonists, and some have resulted in fatalities. In a number of cases, it appears possible that the cerebrovascular events were primary, the agonist having been administered in the incorrect belief that the symptoms experienced were a consequence of migraine, when they were not. It should be noted that patients with migraine may be at increased risk of certain cerebrovascular events (eg, stroke, hemorrhage, TIA).

➤*Other vasospasm-related events:* 5-HT_1 agonists may cause vasospastic reactions other than coronary artery vasospasm. Peripheral vascular ischemia and colonic ischemia with abdominal pain and bloody diarrhea have been reported with 5-HT_1 agonists.

➤*Increases in blood pressure:* Significant elevations in systemic blood pressure, including hypertensive crisis, have been reported on rare occasions in patients with and without a history of hypertension treated with 5-HT_1 agonists. 5-HT_1 agonists are contraindicated in patients with uncontrolled hypertension.

➤*Local irritation:* Approximately 5% of patients noted irritation in the nose and throat after using **sumatriptan** nasal spray. Irritative symptoms such as burning, numbness, paresthesia, discharge, and pain or soreness were noted to be severe in approximately 1% of patients treated. The symptoms were transient and, in approximately 60% of the cases, resolved in less than 2 hours. Limited examinations of the nose and throat did not reveal any clinically noticeable injury in these patients. Adverse events of any kind perceived in the nasopharynx were severe in approximately 1% of patients, and approximately 60% resolved in 1 hour. Nasopharyngeal examinations failed to demonstrate any clinically significant changes with repeated use of sumatriptan nasal spray.

➤*CYP3A4 inhibitors:* In vitro studies have shown that **eletriptan** is metabolized by the CYP3A4 enzyme. A clinical study has shown that coadministration of eletriptan with ketoconazole, erythromycin, verapamil, and fluconazole increased the C_{max} and AUC of eletriptan 3- and 6-fold, 2- and 4-fold, 2- and 3-fold, and 1.4- and 2-fold, respectively. Do not use eletriptan within 72 hours of taking drugs that have demonstrated potent CYP3A4 inhibition (ketoconazole, itraconazole, nefazodone, troleandomycin, clarithromycin, ritonavir, nelfinavir).

➤*Chest, jaw, or neck tightness:* Chest, jaw, or neck tightness have occurred after 5-HT_1 agonist administration, and atypical sensations over the precordium (pain, tightness, pressure, heaviness) have occurred, but these rarely have been associated with arrhythmias or ischemic ECG changes. Evaluate patients who experience signs or symptoms suggestive of angina for the presence of CAD or a predisposition to Prinzmetal variant angina before receiving additional doses. Monitor ECG if dosing is resumed and similar symptoms recur.

Similarly, patients who experience other symptoms or signs suggestive of decreased arterial flow, such as ischemic bowel syndrome or Raynaud syndrome, following the use of any 5-HT_1 agonist are candidates for further evaluation.

➤*Seizures:* There have been rare reports of seizures following **sumatriptan** use.

➤*Ophthalmic effects:*

Binding to melanin-containing tissues – Because 5-HT_1 agonists bind to melanin, accumulation in melanin-rich tissues (eg, the eye) could occur over time, raising the possibility of toxicity in these tissues after extended use. Be aware of the possibility of long-term ophthalmologic effects.

Corneal effects – **Sumatriptan**, **naratriptan**, and **almotriptan** cause corneal opacities and defects in dogs; naratriptan also caused transient changes in precorneal tear film. These changes may occur in humans. **Eletriptan** caused transient corneal opacities in dogs receiving 5 mg/kg and above.

➤*Phenylketonurics:* Inform phenylketonuric patients that **rizatriptan** and **zolmitriptan** orally-disintegrating tablets contain phenylalanine (a component of aspartame). Each 5 mg rizatriptan orally-disintegrating tablet contains 1.05 mg phenylalanine, and each 10 mg orally-disintegrating tablet contains 2.1 mg phenylalanine. Each 2.5 mg zolmitriptan orally-disintegrating tablet contains 2.81 mg phenylalanine.

➤*Hypersensitivity reactions:* Hypersensitivity reactions have occurred on rare occasions, and severe anaphylaxis/anaphylactoid reactions have occurred. Such reactions can be life-threatening or fatal. Refer to Management of Acute Hypersensitivity Reactions.

➤*Renal function impairment:* Use **rizatriptan** and **sumatriptan** with caution in dialysis patients because of a decrease in the clearance (see Pharmacokinetics). After **eletriptan** administration, there was no significant change in clearance observed in subjects with mild, moderate, or severe renal impairment, although blood pressure elevations were observed in this population.

➤*Hepatic function impairment:* Administer with caution to patients with diseases that may alter the absorption, metabolism, or excretion of drugs. The liver plays an important role in the presystemic clearance of oral 5-HT_1 agonists. Accordingly, the bioavailability may be markedly increased in patients with liver disease (see Pharmacokinetics). No dosage adjustment is necessary when **frovatriptan** or **eletriptan** is given to patients with mild to moderate hepatic impairment. Do not use eletriptan in severe hepatic impairment.

➤*Photosensitivity:* Photosensitization (photoallergy or phototoxicity) may occur; therefore, caution patients to take protective measures (ie, sunscreens, protective clothing) against exposure to sunlight or ultraviolet light (eg, tanning beds) until tolerance is determined.

➤*Pregnancy: Category C.* In rats and rabbits, 5-HT_1 agonist administration is associated with embryolethality, fetal abnormalities, and pup mortality. There are no adequate and well-controlled studies in pregnant women. Use during pregnancy only if the potential benefit justifies the potential risk to the fetus.

In reproductive toxicity studies in rats and rabbits, oral administration of **eletriptan** was associated with developmental toxicity (decreased fetal and pup weights and an increased incidence of fetal structural abnormalities). Effects on fetal and pup weights were observed at doses that were 6 to 12 times greater than the clinical MRDD of 80 mg.

When pregnant rats were administered **frovatriptan** during the period of organogenesis at oral doses of 100, 500, and 1000 mg/kg/day (equivalent to 130, 650, and 1300 times the MRHD on a mg/m^2 basis), there were dose-related increases in incidences of both litters and total numbers of fetuses with dilated ureters, unilateral and bilateral pelvic cavitation, hydronephrosis, and hydroureters.

The manufacturer maintains a **sumatriptan** and **naratriptan** pregnancy registry. Register patients by calling (800) 336-2176.

➤*Lactation:* **Sumatriptan** and **eletriptan** are excreted in human breast milk. In one study of 8 women given a single 80 mg dose of eletriptan, the mean total amount in breast milk over 24 hours was approximately 0.02% of the administered dose. The resulting eletriptan concentration-time profile was similar to that seen in the plasma over 24 hours, with very low concentrations of drug (mean, 1.7 ng/mL) still present in the milk 18 to 24 hours postdose. Lactating rats dosed with **zolmitriptan** had milk levels equivalent to maternal plasma levels at 1 hour and 4 times higher than plasma levels at 4 hours. **Naratriptan**-related material is excreted in the milk of rats. **Rizatriptan** is extensively excreted in rat milk, at a level of 5-fold or greater than maternal plasma levels. Lactating rats dosed with **almotriptan** had milk levels equivalent to maternal plasma levels at 0.5 hours and 7 times higher than plasma levels at 6 hours after dosing. **Frovatriptan** and its metabolites are excreted in the milk of lactating rats with the maximum concentration being 4-fold higher than that seen in blood. Exercise caution when administering to a nursing woman.

➤*Children:* Safety and efficacy have not been established.

Clinical trials have evaluated 25 to 100 mg oral **sumatriptan** in 701 pediatric patients, 0.25 to 2.5 mg **naratriptan** in 300 adolescents 12 to 17 years of age, and 40 mg **eletriptan** in 274 adolescents 11 to 17 years of age. These studies did not establish efficacy. Adverse events observed in these clinical trials were similar in nature to those reported in clinical trials in adults. The frequency of all adverse events in sumatriptan patients appeared to be dose- and age-dependent, with younger patients reporting events more commonly than older adolescents.

The use of 5-HT$_1$ receptor agonists is not recommended in patients younger than 18 years of age.

➤*Elderly:* Pharmacokinetic disposition of 5-HT$_1$ agonists in the elderly is similar to that seen in younger adults.

The risk of adverse reactions to **naratriptan** and **sumatriptan** may be greater in elderly patients who have reduced renal function and who are more likely to have decreased hepatic function; they are at higher risk for CAD, and blood pressure increases may be more pronounced. Therefore, the use of naratriptan and sumatriptan in elderly patients is not recommended.

Dose selection of **almotriptan** for an elderly patient should be cautious, usually starting at the low end of the dosing range, reflecting the greater frequency of decreased hepatic, renal, or cardiac function, and of concomitant disease or other drug therapy. The recommended dose for elderly patients with normal renal function for their age is the same as that recommended for younger adults.

Mean blood concentrations of **frovatriptan** in elderly subjects were 1.5 to 2 times higher than those seen in younger adults. Because migraine occurs infrequently in the elderly, clinical experience with frovatriptan is limited to such patients.

Eletriptan has been given to only 50 patients older than 65 years of age. Blood pressure was increased to a greater extent in elderly subjects than in younger subjects. There is no information about the safety and efficacy of zolmitriptan in this population because patients older than 65 years of age were excluded from the controlled clinical trials.

Drug Interactions

Serotonin 5-HT$_1$ Receptor Agonist Drug Interactions

Precipitant drug	Object drug[a]		Description
Cimetidine	Zolmitriptan	↑	Following coadministration with cimetidine, the half life and AUC of a 5 mg dose of zolmitriptan and its active metabolite were approximately doubled.
Ergot alkaloids (dihydroergotamine, methysergide)	5-HT$_1$ agonists	↑↓	The risk of vasospastic reactions may be increased. Use of 5-HT$_1$ agonists within 24 hours of treatment with an ergot-containing medication is contraindicated. The AUC and C_{max} of frovatriptan (2 × 2.5 mg dose) were reduced by ≈ 25% when coadministered with ergotamine tartrate.
Potent CYP3A4 inhibitors (eg, ketoconazole, itraconazole, nefazodone, troleandomycin, clarithromycin, ritonavir, nelfinavir)	Almotriptan Eletriptan	↑	Coadministration of almotriptan and ketoconazole (400 mg/day for 3 days) resulted in an ≈ 60% increase in AUC and maximal plasma concentration of almotriptan. The AUC and C_{max} of eletriptan are increased with coadministration. Do not use eletriptan within 72 hours of treatment with a potent CYP3A4 inhibitor (see Warnings).
5-HT$_1$ agonists	5-HT$_1$ agonists		The risk of vasospastic reactions may be increased. Coadministration of two 5-HT$_1$ agonists within 24 hours of each other is contraindicated.
MAOIs	Almotriptan Rizatriptan Sumatriptan Zolmitriptan	↑	Use of certain 5-HT$_1$ agonists concomitantly with or within 2 weeks following the discontinuation of an MAOI is contraindicated. If it is necessary to use such agents together, naratriptan, eletriptan, and frovatriptan appear to be less likely to interact with MAOIs.
Oral contraceptives	Frovatriptan	↑	Mean C_{max} and AUC of frovatriptan are 30% higher in those subjects taking oral contraceptives compared with those not taking oral contraceptives.
Propranolol	Zolmitriptan	↔	C_{max} and AUC of zolmitriptan increased 1.5-fold but decreased for the N-desmethyl metabolite by 30% and 15%, respectively. No effects on blood pressure or pulse rate were observed.
	Rizatriptan	↑	In a study of coadministration of 240 mg/day propranolol and a single dose of 10 mg rizatriptan in healthy subjects, mean plasma AUC for rizatriptan was increased by 70% during propranolol administration, and a 4-fold increase was observed in 1 subject.
	Frovatriptan	↑	Propranolol increased the AUC of 2.5 mg frovatriptan in males by 60% and in females by 29%. The C_{max} of frovatriptan was increased 23% in males and 16% in females in the presence of propranolol.
	Eletriptan	↑	C_{max} and AUC of eletriptan were increased by 10% and 33%, respectively, in the presence of propranolol. No interactive increases in blood pressure were observed.
Sibutramine	Naratriptan Rizatriptan Sumatriptan Zolmitriptan	↑	A "serotonin syndrome," including CNS irritability, motor weakness, shivering, myoclonus, and altered consciousness may occur. Coadministration is not recommended. Monitor the patient for adverse effects if concurrent use cannot be avoided.
Almotriptan Frovatriptan Naratriptan Rizatriptan Sumatriptan Zolmitriptan	SSRIs Fluoxetine Fluvoxamine Paroxetine Sertraline SNRIs Duloxetine	↑	There have been rare reports of weakness, hyperreflexia, and incoordination with combined use of SSRIs or SNRIs. If concomitant treatment is clinically warranted, observe the patient carefully. No interaction was observed when rizatriptan was administered with paroxetine. Fluoxetine had no effect on almotriptan clearance, but C_{max} increased 18%.

[a] ↑ = object drug increased; ↓ = object drug decreased; ↔ = undetermined clinical effect.

➤*Drug/Food interactions:* Food has no significant effect on oral 5-HT$_1$ agonist bioavailability, but delays sumatriptan's T_{max} by approximately 30 minutes and **rizatriptan's** time to reach peak concentration by 1 hour. AUC and C_{max} of **eletriptan** are increased approximately 20% to 30% following oral administration with a high-fat meal.

Adverse Reactions

Serious coronary artery vasospasm, transient myocardial ischemia, ventricular fibrillation/tachycardia, and MI have been associated with 5-HT$_1$ agonists.

Oral – These agents are generally well tolerated. Across all doses, most adverse reactions were mild and transient and did not lead to long-lasting effects. In patients being treated for multiple migraine attacks for 1 year or less with **naratriptan**, **zolmitriptan**, **eletriptan**, or **frovatriptan**, 3.6%, 8%, 8.3%, and 5% withdrew from the trial because of adverse experiences, respectively. The most common events were asthenia, dizziness, nausea, paresthesia, fatigue, pain, chest tightness or heaviness, neck tightness or heaviness, somnolence, warm sensation, dry mouth, headache, flushing, hot or cold sensation, and chest pain.

Frovatriptan: Frovatriptan is generally well tolerated. The incidence of adverse events in clinical trials did not increase when up to 3 doses were used within 24 hours. The majority of adverse events were mild or moderate and transient. The incidence of adverse events in 4 placebo-controlled clinical trials was not affected by gender, age, or concomitant medications commonly used by migraine patients. There were insufficient data to assess the impact of race on the incidence of adverse events.

Serotonin 5-HT$_1$ Receptor Agonists (Triptans)

Oral 5-HT$_1$ Agonist Adverse Reactions (%)[a]

Adverse reaction	Almotriptan 6.25 mg (n = 527)	Almotriptan 12.5 mg (n = 1313)	Eletriptan 20 mg (n = 431)	Eletriptan 40 mg (n = 1774)	Eletriptan 80 mg (n = 1932)	Frovatriptan 2.5 mg (n = 1554)	Naratriptan 1 mg (n = 627)	Naratriptan 2.5 mg (n = 627)	Rizatriptan 5 mg (n = 977)	Rizatriptan 10 mg (n = 1167)	Sumatriptan 25 mg (n = 417)	Sumatriptan 50 mg (n = 771)	Sumatriptan 100 mg (n = 437)	Zolmitriptan 1 mg (n = 163)	Zolmitriptan 2.5 mg (n = 498)	Zolmitriptan 5 mg (n = 1012)
Atypical sensations																
Hot/Cold sensation	—	—	—	—	—	3	—	—	—	—	—	—	—	—	—	—
Hypesthesia	—	—	—	—	—	—	—	—	—	—	—	—	—	1	1	2
Miscellaneous sensations	—	—	—	—	—	—	2	4	4	5	—	—	—	—	—	—
Paresthesia	1	1	3	3	4	4	1	2	3	4	3	5	3	5	7	9
Warm/Cold sensation	—	—	—	—	—	—	—	—	—	—	3	2	3	—	—	—
Warm/Hot sensation	—	—	2	2	2	—	—	—	—	—	—	—	—	6	5	7
CNS																
Asthenia	—	—	4	5	10	—	—	—	—	—	—	—	—	5	3	9
Dizziness	—	—	3	6	7	8	1	2	4	9	> 1	> 1	> 1	6	8	10
Drowsiness	—	—	—	—	—	—	1	2	—	—	> 1	> 1	> 1	—	—	—
Fatigue	—	—	—	—	—	5	2	2	4	7	2	2	3	—	—	—
Headache	—	—	4	3	4	4	—	—	< 2	2	> 1	> 1	> 1	—	—	—
Myasthenia	—	—	—	—	—	—	—	—	—	—	—	—	—	0	1	2
Somnolence	—	—	3	6	7	—	—	—	4	8	—	—	—	5	6	8
Vertigo	—	—	—	—	—	—	—	—	—	—	< 1	< 1	2	0	0	2
Miscellaneous CNS effects	—	—	—	—	—	—	4	7	—	—	—	—	—	—	—	—
GI																
Abdominal pain/discomfort/stomach pain/cramps/pressure	—	—	1	2	2	—	—	—	—	—	—	—	—	—	—	—
Dry mouth	1	1	2	3	4	3	—	—	3	3	> 1	> 1	> 1	5	3	3
Dyspepsia	—	—	1	2	2	2	—	—	—	—	—	—	—	3	2	1
Dysphagia (including throat tightness/difficulty swallowing)	—	—	1	2	2	—	—	—	—	—	—	—	—	0	0	2
Nausea	4	5	4	6	—	—	—	4	9	6	1	2	—	4	5	8
Pain/Pressure sensations																
Chest tightness pressure, and/or heaviness	—	—	1	2	4	2	—	—	< 2	3	1	2	2	2	3	4
Heaviness	—	—	—	—	—	—	—	—	—	—	< 1	< 1	2	1	2	5
Neck pain or pressure/Throat pain or pressure/Jaw pain or pressure	—	—	—	—	—	—	1	2	< 2	2	< 1	2	3	4	7	10
Pain, location specified/unspecified	—	—	—	—	—	—	—	—	6	9	2	1	1	2	2	3
Pressure	—	—	—	—	—	—	—	—	—	—	< 1	2	2	—	—	—
Regional pain	—	—	—	—	—	—	—	—	< 1	2	—	—	—	—	—	—
Tightness	—	—	—	—	—	—	—	—	—	—	< 1	2	2	—	—	—
Skeletal	—	—	—	—	—	3	—	—	—	—	—	—	—	—	—	—
Other	2	4	3	3	1	1	3	2	2	3	—	—	—	—	—	—
Miscellaneous																
Flushing	—	—	2	2	2	4	—	—	—	—	—	—	—	—	—	—
Myalgia	—	—	—	—	—	—	—	—	—	—	—	—	—	1	1	2
Other	—	—	—	—	—	—	6	7	—	—	—	—	—	—	—	—
Palpitations	—	—	—	—	—	—	—	—	—	—	> 1	> 1	> 1	0	< 1	2
Sweating	—	—	—	—	—	—	—	—	—	—	—	—	—	0	2	3

[a] Data are pooled from separate studies and are not necessarily comparable.

➤*Almotriptan:*

Cardiovascular – Palpitations, tachycardia, vasodilation (0.1% to 1%); hypertension, syncope (less than 0.1%).

CNS – Dizziness, somnolence (1% or more); anxiety, CNS stimulation, hypesthesia, insomnia, restlessness, shakiness, tremor, vertigo (0.1% to 1%); abnormal coordination, change in dreams, depressive symptoms, euphoria, hyperreflexia, hypertonia, impaired concentration, nervousness, neuropathy, nightmares (less than 0.1%).

Dermatologic – Dermatitis, diaphoresis, erythema, pruritus, rash (0.1% to 1%); photosensitivity reaction (less than 0.1%).

GI – Diarrhea, dyspepsia, vomiting (0.1% to 1%); abdominal cramp or pain, colitis, esophageal reflux, gastritis, gastroenteritis, increased salivation, increased thirst (less than 0.1%).

Metabolic – Hyperglycemia, increased serum CPK (0.1% to 1%); hypercholesterolemia, increased GGT (less than 0.1%).

Musculoskeletal – Muscular weakness, myalgia (0.1% to 1%); arthralgia, arthritis, myopathy (less than 0.1%).

Respiratory – Bronchitis, dyspnea, epistaxis, laryngismus, pharyngitis, rhinitis, sinusitis (0.1% to 1%); hyperventilation, laryngitis, sneezing (less than 0.1%).

Special senses – Conjunctivitis, ear pain, eye irritation, hyperacusis, taste alteration (0.1% to 1%); diplopia, dry eyes, eye pain, nystagmus, otitis media, parosmia, scotoma, tinnitus (less than 0.1%).

Miscellaneous – Headache (1% or more); asthenia, back pain, chest pain, chills, dysmenorrhea, fatigue, neck pain, rigid neck (0.1% to 1%); fever (less than 0.1%).

➤*Eletriptan:*

Cardiovascular – Palpitation (1% or more); hypertension, migraine, peripheral vascular disorder, tachycardia (0.1% to 1%); angina pectoris, arrhythmia, atrial fibrillation, AV block, bradycardia, cerebrovascular disorder, hypotension, syncope, thrombophlebitis, vasospasm, ventricular arrhythmia (less than 0.1%).

CNS – Hypertonia, hypesthesia, vertigo (1% or more); abnormal dreams, agitation, anxiety, apathy, ataxia, confusion, depersonalization, depression, emotional lability, euphoria, hyperesthesia, hyperkinesia, incoordination, insomnia, nervousness, speech disorder, stupor, thinking abnormal, tremor (0.1% to 1%); abnormal gait, amnesia, aphasia, catatonic reaction, dementia, diplopia, dystonia, hallucinations, hemiplegia, hyperalgesia, hypokinesia, hysteria, manic reaction, neuropathy, neurosis, oculogyric crisis, paralysis, psychotic depression, sleep disorder, twitching (less than 0.1%).

Dermatologic – Sweating (1% or more); pruritus, rash, skin disorder (0.1% to 1%); alopecia, dry skin, eczema, exfoliative dermatitis, maculopapular rash, psoriasis, skin discoloration, skin hypertrophy, urticaria (less than 0.1%).

Endocrine – Goiter, thyroid adenoma, thyroiditis (less than 0.1%).

GI – Anorexia, constipation, diarrhea, eructation, esophagitis, flatulence, gastritis, GI disorder, glossitis, increased salivation, liver function tests abnormal (0.1% to 1%); gingivitis, hematemesis, increased appetite, rectal disorder, stomatitis, tongue disorder, tongue edema, tooth disorder (less than 0.1%).

GU – Impotence, polyuria, urinary frequency, urinary tract disorder (0.1% to 1%); breast pain, kidney pain, leukorrhea, menorrhagia, menstrual disorder, vaginitis (less than 0.1%).

Hematologic/Lymphatic – Anemia, cyanosis, leukopenia, lymphadenopathy, monocytosis, purpura (less than 0.1%).

Metabolic – CPK increased, edema, peripheral edema, thirst (0.1% to 1%); alkaline phosphatase increased, bilirubinemia, hyperglycemia, weight gain, weight loss (less than 0.1%).

Musculoskeletal – Arthralgia, arthritis, arthrosis, bone pain, myalgia, myasthenia (0.1% to 1%); bone neoplasm, joint disorder, myopathy, tenosynovitis (less than 0.1%).

Respiratory – Pharyngitis (1% or more); asthma, dyspnea, respiratory disorder, respiratory tract infection, rhinitis, voice alteration, yawn (0.1% to 1%); bronchitis, choking sensation, cough increased, epistaxis, hiccough, hyperventilation, laryngitis, sinusitis, sputum increased (less than 0.1%).

Special senses – Abnormal vision, conjunctivitis, ear pain, eye pain, lacrimation disorder, photophobia, taste perversion, tinnitus (0.1% to 1%); abnormality of accommodation, dry eyes, ear disorder, eye hemorrhage, otitis media, parosmia, ptosis (less than 0.1%).

Miscellaneous – Back pain, chills, pain (1% or more); face edema, malaise (0.1% to 1%); abdomen enlarged, abscess, accidental injury, allergic reaction, fever, flu syndrome, halitosis, hernia, hypothermia, lab test abnormal, moniliasis, rheumatoid arthritis, shock (less than 0.1%).

➤*Frovatriptan:*

Cardiovascular – Palpitation (1% or more); abnormal ECG, tachycardia (0.1% to 1%); bradycardia (less than 0.1%).

CNS – Anxiety, dysesthesia, hypesthesia, insomnia (1% or more); abnormal gait, agitation, amnesia, asthenia, ataxia, confusion, depersonalization, depression, emotional lability, euphoria, hyperesthesia, impaired concentration, involuntary muscle contractions, migraine aggravated, nervousness, rigors, speech disorder, thinking abnormal, tremor, vertigo (0.1% to 1%); abnormal dreaming, abnormal reflexes, depression aggravated, hypertonia, hypotonia, personality disorder, tongue paralysis (less than 0.1%).

Dermatologic – Sweating increased (1% or more); bullous eruption, pruritus (0.1% to 1%).

GI – Abdominal pain, diarrhea, vomiting (1% or more); anorexia, constipation, dysphagia, esophagospasm, flatulence, saliva increased (0.1% to 1%); change in bowel habits, cheilitis, eructation, gastroesophageal reflux, hiccough, peptic ulcer, salivary gland pain, stomatitis, toothache (less than 0.1%).

GU – Micturition frequency, polyuria (0.1% to 1%); abnormal urine, nocturia, renal pain (less than 0.1%).

Hematologic – Epistaxis (0.1% to 1%); purpura (less than 0.1%).

Metabolic/Nutritional – Dehydration, thirst (0.1% to 1%); hypocalcemia, hypoglycemia (less than 0.1%).

Musculoskeletal – Arthralgia, arthrosis, back pain, leg cramps, muscle weakness, myalgia (0.1% to 1%).

Respiratory – Rhinitis, sinusitis (1% or more); pharyngitis, dyspnea, hyperventilation, laryngitis (0.1% to 1%).

Special senses – Tinnitus, vision abnormal (1% or more); abnormal lacrimation, conjunctivitis, earache, eye pain, hyperacusis, taste perversion (0.1% to 1%).

Miscellaneous – Pain (1% or more); fever, hot flushes, malaise, (0.1% to 1%); feeling of relaxation, leg pain, mouth edema, syncope (less than 0.1%).

➤*Naratriptan:*

Atypical sensations – Warm/cold temperature sensations (1% or more); strange feeling and burning/stinging sensation (0.1% to 1%).

Cardiovascular – Abnormal ECG (PR prolongation, QT prolongation, ST/T wave abnormalities, premature ventricular contractions, atrial flutter/fibrillation), increased blood pressure, palpitations, syncope, tachyarrhythmias (0.1% to 1%); bradycardia, heart murmurs, hypotension, varicosities (less than 0.1%).

CNS – Vertigo (1% or more); anxiety, cognitive function disorders, depressive disorders, detachment, equilibrium disorders, sleep disorders, tremors (0.1% to 1%); aggression, agitation, compressed nerve syndromes, confusion, convulsions, coordination disorders, decreased consciousness, dreams, hallucinations, hostility, hyperactivity, hyperesthesia, hypesthesia, motor retardation, muscle twitching/fasciculation, neuralgia, neuritis, panic, paralysis of cranial nerves, psychomotor restlessness, sedation (less than 0.1%).

Dermatologic – Pruritus, skin rashes, sweating, urticaria (0.1% to 1%); acne, allergic skin reactions, dermatitis/dermatosis, folliculitis, hair loss, macular skin/rashes, photodermatitis, photosensitivity, pruritic skin rashes, skin erythema, skin flakiness/dryness (less than 0.1%).

GI – Hyposalivation, vomiting (1% or more); constipation, diarrhea, discomfort/pain, dyspeptic symptoms, gastroenteritis (0.1% to 1%); abnormal bilirubin levels, abnormal liver function tests, altered sense of taste, esophagitis, gastric ulcers, gastritis, hemorrhoids, oral itching and irritation, regurgitation and reflux, salivary gland inflammation (less than 0.1%).

GU – Bladder inflammation, diuresis, polyuria (0.1% to 1%); breast discharge, breast inflammation, decreased libido, endometrium disorders, fallopian tube inflammation, lumps in breast, lumps in female reproductive tract, pyelitis, urinary incontinence, urinary tract hemorrhage, urinary urgency, vaginal inflammation (less than 0.1%).

Hematologic – Increased white cells (0.1% to 1%); anemia, purpura, quantitative red cell or hemoglobin defects, thrombocytopenia (less than 0.1%).

Metabolic/Nutritional – Dehydration, fluid retention, polydipsia, thirst (0.1% to 1%); glycosuria, hypercholesterolemia, hyperglycemia, hyperlipidemia, hypothyroidism, ketonuria, parathyroid neoplasm (less than 0.1%).

Musculoskeletal – Pressure/tightness/heaviness sensations (1% or more); arthralgia, articular rheumatism, joint/muscle stiffness, muscle cramps/spasms, muscle pain, rigidity, tightness (0.1% to 1%); bone/skeletal pain (less than 0.1%).

Respiratory – Bronchitis, cough, pneumonia (0.1% to 1%); airway obstruction/constriction, asthma, pleuritis, tracheitis (less than 0.1%).

Special senses – Photophobia (1% or more); blurred vision (0.1% to 1%); aphasia, difficulty focusing, dry eyes, eye hemorrhage, eye pain/discomfort, scotoma, sensation of eye pressure (less than 0.1%).

Ear, nose, and throat: Ear, nose, and throat infections (1% or more); phonophobia, sinusitis, tinnitus, upper respiratory tract inflammation (0.1% to 1%); allergic rhinitis, ear/nose/throat hemorrhage, hearing difficulty, labyrinthitis (less than 0.1%).

Miscellaneous – Allergic reactions, allergies, chills, descriptions of odor or taste, edema, fever, swelling (0.1% to 1%); mobility disorders, spasms (less than 0.1%).

Postmarketing reports: These events do not include those already listed in the adverse reactions section above. Because the reports cite events reported spontaneously from worldwide postmarketing experience, frequency of events and the role of naratriptan in their causation cannot be reliably determined.

- *Cardiovascular* – Angina, MI.
- *CNS* – Cerebral vascular accident, including transient ischemic attack, subarachnoid hemorrhage, and cerebral infarction.
- *Miscellaneous* – Dyspnea, hypersensitivity including anaphylaxis/anaphylactoid reactions, in some cases severe (eg, circulatory collapse).

➤*Rizatriptan:*

Cardiovascular – Palpitation (1% or more); arrhythmia, bradycardia, cold extremities, hypertension, tachycardia (0.1% to 1%); angina pectoris (less than 0.1%).

CNS – Euphoria, hypesthesia, mental acuity decreased, tremor (1% or more); agitation, anxiety, ataxia, confusion, depression, disorientation, dream abnormality, dysarthria, gait abnormality, hyperesthesia, insomnia, irritability, memory impairment, nervousness, vertigo (0.1% to 1%); akinesia/bradykinesia, apprehension, depersonalization, dysesthesia, hyperkinesia, hypersomnia, hyporeflexia (less than 0.1%).

Dermatologic – Flushing (1% or more); pruritus, rash, sweating, urticaria (0.1% to 1%); acne, erythema, photosensitivity (less than 0.1%).

GI – Diarrhea, vomiting (1% or more); acid regurgitation, constipation, dyspepsia, dysphagia, flatulence, thirst, tongue edema (0.1% to 1%); anorexia, appetite increased, eructation, gastritis, paralysis (tongue) (less than 0.1%).

GU – Hot flashes (1% or more); menstruation disorder, polyuria, urinary frequency (0.1% to 1%); dysuria (less than 0.1%).

Musculoskeletal – Arthralgia, muscle cramp, muscle spasm, muscle weakness, musculoskeletal pain, myalgia, stiffness (0.1% to 1%).

Respiratory – Dyspnea (1% or more); congestion (nasal), dry nose, dry throat, epistaxis, irritation (nasal), pharyngitis, respiratory congestion (nasal), sinus disorder, upper respiratory tract infection, yawning (0.1% to 1%); cough, hiccough, hoarseness, pharyngeal edema, rhinorrhea, sneezing, tachypnea (less than 0.1%).

Special senses – Blurred vision, burning eye, dry eyes, ear pain, eye irritation, eye pain, tearing, tinnitus (0.1% to 1%); eye swelling, hyperacusis, itching eye, photophobia, photopsia, smell perversion (less than 0.1%).

Miscellaneous – Warm/cold sensations (1% or more); abdominal distention, chills, dehydration, facial edema, hangover effect, heat sensitivity (0.1% to 1%); edema/swelling, fever, orthostatic effects, syncope (less than 0.1%).

Postmarketing reports: The following additional adverse reactions have been reported very rarely and most have been reported in patients with risk factors predictive of CAD: Cerebrovascular accident; MI; myocardial ischemia. The following also have been reported: Dysgeusia; toxic epidermal necrolysis.

Serotonin 5-HT_1 Receptor Agonists (Triptans)

➤*Sumatriptan:*

Sumatriptan Adverse Reactions (%)

Adverse reaction	Tablets	Nasal	Injection
Atypical sensations			
Burning sensation	> 1	0.1 to 1	—
Cold sensation	—	0.1 to 1	—
Dysesthesia	< 0.1	< 0.1	< 0.1
Feeling of heaviness	—	0.1 to 1	—
Feeling strange	—	0.1 to 1	—
Numbness	> 1	0.1 to 1	—
Paresthesia	—	0.1 to 1	0.1 to 1
Pressure sensation	—	0.1 to 1	—
Prickling sensation	—	< 0.1	0.1 to 1
Simultaneous hot/cold sensation	—	—	< 0.1
Stinging sensations	—	—	0.1 to 1
Tickling sensations	—	—	< 0.1
Tight feeling in head	0.1 to 1	0.1 to 1	—
Tingling	—	0.1 to 1	—
Cardiovascular			
Abdominal aortic aneurysm	—	< 0.1	—
Abnormal pulse	—	—	< 0.1
Angina	< 0.1	—	—
Arrhythmia	0.1 to 1	0.1 to 1	0.1 to 1
Atherosclerosis	< 0.1	—	—
Bradycardia	< 0.1	< 0.1	0.1 to 1
Cerebral ischemia	< 0.1	—	—
Cerebrovascular lesion	< 0.1	—	—
ECG changes	0.1 to 1	0.1 to 1	0.1 to 1
Flushing	—	0.1 to 1	—
Heart block	< 0.1	—	—
Hypertension	> 1	0.1 to 1	0.1 to 1
Hypotension	> 1	< 0.1	0.1 to 1
Pallor	0.1 to 1	< 0.1	< 0.1
Palpitations	> 1	0.1 to 1	0.1 to 1
Peripheral cyanosis	< 0.1	—	—
Phlebitis	—	< 0.1	—
Pulsating sensations	0.1 to 1	—	0.1 to 1
Raynaud syndrome	—	—	< 0.1
Syncope	> 1	—	0.1 to 1
Tachycardia	0.1 to 1	0.1 to 1	0.1 to 1
Thrombosis	< 0.1	—	—
Transient myocardial ischemia	< 0.1	—	—
Vasodilation	< 0.1	—	< 0.1
CNS			
Aggressiveness	< 0.1	—	—
Agitation	< 0.1	0.1 to 1	0.1 to 1
Anxiety	< 0.1	0.1 to 1	—
Apathy	< 0.1	< 0.1	—
Bradylogia	< 0.1	—	—
Chills	—	0.1 to 1	0.1 to 1
Cluster headache	< 0.1	—	—
Confusion	0.1 to 1	0.1 to 1	0.1 to 1
Convulsions	< 0.1	—	—
Depression	0.1 to 1	0.1 to 1	< 0.1
Depressive disorders	< 0.1	—	—
Detachment	< 0.1	—	—
Difficulty concentrating	0.1 to 1	< 0.1	< 0.1
Disturbances of emotion	—	< 0.1	—
Drowsiness/Sedation	—	0.1 to 1	—
Dysarthria	0.1 to 1	< 0.1	< 0.1
Dystonic reaction	< 0.1	—	< 0.1
Euphoria	0.1 to 1	< 0.1	0.1 to 1
Facial pain	0.1 to 1	< 0.1	< 0.1
Facial paralysis	< 0.1	—	—
Globus hystericus	—	—	< 0.1
Hallucinations	< 0.1	—	—
Heat sensitivity	0.1 to 1	—	—
Hunger	< 0.1	< 0.1	—
Hyperesthesia	< 0.1	—	< 0.1
Hysteria	< 0.1	—	< 0.1
Incoordination	0.1 to 1	< 0.1	—
Increased alertness	< 0.1	—	—
Intoxication	—	< 0.1	< 0.1
Memory disturbance	< 0.1	< 0.1	—
Monoplegia	0.1 to 1	< 0.1	< 0.1

Sumatriptan Adverse Reactions (%)

Adverse reaction	Tablets	Nasal	Injection
Motor dysfunction	< 0.1	—	—
Myoclonia	—	—	< 0.1
Neoplasm of pituitary	—	< 0.1	—
Neuralgia	< 0.1	—	—
Neurotic disorders	< 0.1	—	—
Paralysis	< 0.1	—	—
Personality change	< 0.1	—	—
Phobia	< 0.1	—	—
Phonophobia	> 1	—	—
Photophobia	> 1	—	0.1 to 1
Psychomotor disorders	< 0.1	—	—
Radiculopathy	< 0.1	—	—
Raised intracranial pressure	< 0.1	—	—
Relaxation	—	—	0.1 to 1
Rigidity	< 0.1	—	—
Sensation of lightness	—	0.1 to 1	0.1 to 1
Shivering	0.1 to 1	0.1 to 1	0.1 to 1
Sleep disturbance	0.1 to 1	0.1 to 1	< 0.1
Stress	—	< 0.1	—
Suicide	< 0.1	—	—
Syncope	0.1 to 1	0.1 to 1	—
Transient hemiplegia	—	—	< 0.1
Tremor	0.1 to 1	0.1 to 1	0.1 to 1
Twitching	< 0.1	—	—
Yawning	—	—	< 0.1
Dermatologic			
Dry/Scaly skin	< 0.1	—	—
Eczema	< 0.1	—	—
Erythema	0.1 to 1	0.1 to 1	0.1 to 1
Herpes	—	—	< 0.1
Peeling of skin	—	—	< 0.1
Pruritus	0.1 to 1	0.1 to 1	0.1 to 1
Rash	0.1 to 1	0.1 to 1	0.1 to 1
Seborrheic dermatitis	< 0.1	—	—
Skin nodules	< 0.1	—	—
Skin tenderness	0.1 to 1	—	< 0.1
Sweating	> 1	< 0.1	—
Swelling of face	—	—	< 0.1
Tightness of the skin	< 0.1	—	—
Wrinkling of the skin	< 0.1	—	—
Endocrine/Metabolic			
Dehydration	—	—	< 0.1
Elevated TSH levels	< 0.1	—	—
Endocrine cysts	< 0.1	—	—
Fluid disturbances	< 0.1	—	—
Galactorrhea	< 0.1	< 0.1	—
Hyperglycemia	< 0.1	—	—
Hypoglycemia	< 0.1	< 0.1	—
Hypothyroidism	< 0.1	—	—
Polydipsia	< 0.1	—	< 0.1
Thirst	0.1 to 1	0.1 to 1	0.1 to 1
Weight gain	< 0.1	—	—
Weight loss	< 0.1	< 0.1	—
GI			
Abdominal discomfort	—	0.1 to 1	—
Abdominal distention	< 0.1	—	—
Colitis	—	< 0.1	—
Constipation	0.1 to 1	< 0.1	—
Decreased appetite	< 0.1	< 0.1	< 0.1
Diarrhea	> 1	0.1 to 1	0.1 to 1
Dry mouth	—	< 0.1	—
Dyspeptic symptoms	< 0.1	—	—
Dysphagia	0.1 to 1	0.1 to 1	—
Feelings of GI pressure	< 0.1	—	—
Flatulence/Eructation	—	< 0.1	< 0.1
Gallstones	—	—	< 0.1
Gastritis	< 0.1	—	—
Gastroenteritis	< 0.1	< 0.1	—
GERD	0.1 to 1	0.1 to 1	0.1 to 1
GI bleeding	< 0.1	—	—
GI pain	< 0.1	—	—
GI tract hemorrhage	—	< 0.1	—
Hematemesis	< 0.1	< 0.1	—
Hypersalivation	< 0.1	—	—
Intestinal obstruction	—	< 0.1	—

Serotonin 5-HT_1 Receptor Agonists (Triptans)

Sumatriptan Adverse Reactions (%)			
Adverse reaction	Tablets	Nasal	Injection
Melena	< 0.1	< 0.1	—
Oral itching/irritation	< 0.1	—	—
Pancreatitis	—	< 0.1	—
Peptic ulcer	< 0.1	—	< 0.1
Retching	—	—	< 0.1
Salivary gland swelling	< 0.1	—	—
Swallowing disorders	< 0.1	—	—
Taste disturbances	< 0.1	0.1 to 1	0.1 to 1
GU			
Breast cysts	< 0.1	—	—
Breast lumps	< 0.1	—	—
Breast masses	< 0.1	—	—
Breast swelling	< 0.1	—	—
Breast tenderness	0.1 to 1	—	—
Dysuria	—	—	< 0.1
Dysmenorrhea	—	—	< 0.1
Nipple discharge	< 0.1	—	—
Primary malignant breast neoplasm	< 0.1	—	—
Renal calculus	—	—	< 0.1
Urinary frequency	—	—	< 0.1
Musculoskeletal			
Acquired musculoskeletal deformity	< 0.1	—	—
Arthralgia	< 0.1	—	—
Arthritis	—	< 0.1	—
Articular rheumatitis	< 0.1	—	—
Backache	—	< 0.1	< 0.1
Intervertebral disc disorder	—	< 0.1	—
Joint symptoms	—	< 0.1	0.1 to 1
Muscle atrophy	< 0.1	—	—
Muscle cramps	0.1 to 1	< 0.1	—
Muscle stiffness	< 0.1	< 0.1	< 0.1
Muscle tightness	< 0.1	—	—
Muscle tiredness	< 0.1	—	< 0.1
Muscle weakness	< 0.1	0.1 to 1	—
Musculoskeletal inflammation	< 0.1	—	—
Myalgia	> 1	0.1 to 1	—
Neck pain/stiffness	—	< 0.1	—
Need to flex calf muscles	—	—	< 0.1
Tetany	< 0.1	< 0.1	—
Respiratory			
Allergic rhinitis	> 1	—	—
Asthma	0.1 to 1	< 0.1	—
Breathing disorders	< 0.1	—	—
Bronchitis	< 0.1	—	—
Coughing	< 0.1	—	—
Dyspnea	> 1	0.1 to 1	0.1 to 1
Hiccoughs	< 0.1	—	< 0.1
Lower respiratory tract infections	—	0.1 to 1	< 0.1
Sinusitis	> 1	—	—
Upper respiratory tract inflammation	> 1	—	—
Special senses			
Accommodation disorders	< 0.1	—	—
Blindness/Low vision	< 0.1	—	—
Burning/Numbness of tongue	—	< 0.1	—
Conjunctivitis	< 0.1	—	—
Disturbance of smell	0.1 to 1	< 0.1	< 0.1
Ear infection	—	0.1 to 1	—
Ear, nose, throat hemorrhage	> 1	—	—
External ocular disorders	< 0.1	—	—
External otitis	> 1	—	—
Eye edema	< 0.1	—	—
Eye hemorrhage	< 0.1	—	—
Eye irritation	< 0.1	0.1 to 1	0.1 to 1
Eye pain	< 0.1	—	—
Feeling of fullness in ears	< 0.1	—	—
Hearing loss	> 1	0.1 to 1	—
Keratitis	< 0.1	—	—
Lacrimation	0.1 to 1	< 0.1	0.1 to 1
Meniere disease	—	< 0.1	—
Mydriasis	< 0.1	—	—
Nasal inflammation	> 1	—	—
Noise sensitivity	> 1	—	—
Otalgia	0.1 to 1	< 0.1	—
Sclera disorders	< 0.1	—	—
Tinnitus	> 1	—	—
Visual disturbances	< 0.1	< 0.1	—
Miscellaneous			
Anemia	< 0.1	—	—
Chest tightness/discomfort/pressure/heaviness	—	0.1 to 1	—
Dental pain	< 0.1	—	—
Drug abuse	< 0.1	—	—
Fever	—	—	< 0.1
Hypersensitivity	—	—	0.1 to 1
Liver function test disturbance	—	—	0.1 to 1
Serotonin agonist effect	—	—	0.1 to 1

Postmarketing reports (oral, injection): The events enumerated include all except those already listed in the adverse reactions section above or those too general to be informative. Because the reports cite events reported spontaneously from worldwide postmarketing experience, frequency of events and the role of sumatriptan injection in their causation cannot be reliably determined. Systemic reactions following sumatriptan use are likely to be similar regardless of route of administration.

- *Cardiovascular* – Atrial fibrillation, cardiomyopathy, colonic ischemia, Prinzmetal variant angina, pulmonary embolism, shock, thrombophlebitis.
- *CNS* – Cerebrovascular accident, CNS vasculitis, dysphasia, panic disorder, subarachnoid hemorrhage.
- *Dermatologic* – Exacerbation of sunburn, hypersensitivity reactions (allergic vasculitis, erythema, pruritus, rash, shortness of breath, urticaria; in addition, severe anaphylaxis/anaphylactoid reactions have been reported), photosensitivity.

  Injection only: Following SC administration of sumatriptan, contusion, induration, pain, redness, SC bleeding, stinging, swelling, and on rare occasions, lipoatrophy (depression in the skin) or lipohypertrophy (enlargement or thickening of tissue) have been reported.
- *GI* – Ischemic colitis with rectal bleeding, xerostomia.
- *Hematologic* – Hemolytic anemia, pancytopenia, thrombocytopenia.
- *Special senses* – Deafness, ischemic optic neuropathy, loss of vision, retinal artery occlusion, retinal vein thrombosis.
- *Miscellaneous* – Acute renal failure, angioneurotic edema, bronchospasm in patients with and without a history of asthma, cyanosis, death, elevated liver function tests, temporal arteritis.

➤*Zolmitriptan:*

Cardiovascular – Arrhythmias, hypertension, syncope (0.1% to 1%); bradycardia, extrasystoles, postural hypotension, QT prolongation, tachycardia, thrombophlebitis (less than 0.1%).

CNS – Agitation, anxiety, depression, emotional lability, hyperesthesia, insomnia (0.1% to 1%); akathisia, amnesia, apathy, ataxia, cerebral ischemia, dystonia, euphoria, hallucinations, hyperkinesia, hypertonia, hypotonia, irritability (less than 0.1%).

Dermatologic – Pruritus, rash, urticaria (0.1% to 1%).

GI – Esophagitis, gastroenteritis, increased appetite, liver function abnormality, thirst, tongue edema (0.1% to 1%); anorexia, constipation, gastritis, hematemesis, melena, pancreatitis, ulcer (less than 0.1%).

GU – Cystitis, hematuria, polyuria, urinary frequency/urgency (0.1% to 1%); dysmenorrhea, miscarriage (less than 0.1%).

Hematologic – Ecchymosis (0.1% to 1%); cyanosis, eosinophilia, leukopenia, thrombocytopenia (less than 0.1%).

Metabolic – Edema (0.1% to 1%); alkaline phosphatase increased, hyperglycemia (less than 0.1%).

Musculoskeletal – Back pain, leg cramps, tenosynovitis (0.1% to 1%); arthritis, tetany, twitching (less than 0.1%).

Respiratory – Bronchitis, bronchospasm, epistaxis, hiccough, laryngitis, yawn (0.1% to 1%); apnea, voice alteration (less than 0.1%).

Special senses – Dry eye, ear pain, eye pain, hyperacusis, parosmia, tinnitus (0.1% to 1%); diplopia, lacrimation (less than 0.1%).

Miscellaneous – Allergic reaction, chills, facial edema, fever, malaise, photosensitivity (0.1% to 1%).

Postmarketing reports: The events enumerated include all except those already listed in the adverse reactions section above or those too general to be informative. Because the reports cite events reported spontaneously from worldwide postmarketing experience, frequency of events and the role of zolmitriptan in their causation cannot be reliably determined: Anaphylaxis/anaphylactoid reactions; angina pectoris; coronary artery vasospasm; headache; hypersensitivity reactions including angioedema, ischemic colitis, GI infarction, GI necrosis; MI; transient myocardial ischemia.

➤*Zolmitriptan Nasal spray:*

Zolmitriptan Nasal Spray Adverse Reactions (%)		
Adverse reaction	Zolmitriptan nasal spray 5 mg (n = 236)	Placebo (n = 228)
Atypical sensations		
Hyperesthesia	5	0
Paresthesia	10	6
CNS		
Dizziness	3	4
Somnolence	4	2
GI		
Dry mouth	2	0
Nausea	4	1
Unusual taste	21	3
Pain and pressure sensations		
Pain, location specified	4	1
Pain, throat	4	1
Tightness, throat	2	1
Miscellaneous		
Asthenia	3	1
Disorder/discomfort of nasal cavity	3	2

Other adverse events reported with zolmitriptan nasal spray are are included in the following sections.

Cardiovascular – Palpitation (1% or more to less than 2%); arrhythmias, hypertension, syncope, tachycardia, thrombophlebitis (0.01%); angina pectoris, atrial fibrillation, bradycardia, MI, vascular disorder, vasodilation (0.001%).

CNS – Headache, insomnia (1% or more to less than 2%); abnormal coordination, abnormal thinking, agitation, amnesia, anxiety, ataxia, circumoral paresthesia, confusion, depersonalization, depression, hypertonia, insomnia, nervousness, speech disorder, tremor, vertigo (0.01%); abnormal dreams, apathy, convulsions, euphoria, hypertonia, irritability, manic reaction, neuropathy, psychosis, tardive dyskinesia (0.001%).

Dermatologic – Pruritus, rash, skin disorder, sweating (0.01%); eczema, erythema, erythema multiforme, hair disorder, neoplasm.

Endocrine – Hyperthyroidism, thyroid edema (0.001%).

GI – Abdominal pain, dysphagia, vomiting (1% or more to less than 2%); diarrhea, dyspepsia, GI disorder, increased saliva, tongue edema, thirst (0.01%); colitis, constipation, eructation, gastritis, GI carcinoma, gingivitis, hepatic neoplasia, increased appetite, intestinal obstruction, jaundice, sialadenitis, stomatitis (0.001%).

GU – Menorrhagia, polyuria (0.01%); breast carcinoma, breast neoplasm, cystitis, dysmenorrhea, enlarged uterine fibroids, fibrocystic breast, kidney pain, metrorrhagia, pyelonephritis, suspicious PAP smear, unintended pregnancy, urinary frequency, urinary tract disorder, urinary tract infection, urine impaired, urogenital neoplasm, uterine disorder, vaginitis (0.001%).

Hematologic – Cyanosis (0.01%); ecchymosis, leukopenia, lymphadenopathy (0.001%).

Metabolic/Nutritional – Dehydration, increased weight, peripheral edema (0.001%).

Musculoskeletal – Arthralgia, joint disorder, myalgia (0.01%); bone pain, osteoporosis, tenosynovitis, twitching (0.001%).

Respiratory – Bronchitis, dyspnea, epistasis, increased cough, laryngeal edema, pharyngitis, rhinitis, sinusitis, throat discomfort, voice alteration (0.01%); hiccough, hyperventilation, increased sputum, laryngitis, yawning (0.001%).

Special senses – Amblyopia, disorder of lacrimation, ear pain, eye pain, parosmia, tinnitus (0.01%); conjunctivitis, dry eye, photophobia, pneumonia, visual field defect (0.001%).

Miscellaneous – Chest tightness, reaction aggravation (1% or more to less than 2%); abnormal laboratory test, allergic reaction, back pain, chest heaviness, chest pain, chest pressure, chills, cyst, edema of the face, flu syndrome, infection, jaw pain, jaw tightening, neck pain, neck tightness, neoplasm, pressure other (0.01%); cellulitis, fever, jaw pressure, neck heaviness (0.001%).

Overdosage

➤*Symptoms:* Based on the pharmacology of serotonin agonists, hypertension and other more serious cardiovascular symptoms can occur. Overdosage in animals has been fatal; possible symptoms include seizure, tremor, inactivity, extremity erythema, reduced respiratory rate, cyanosis, ataxia, mydriasis, injection-site reaction, and paralysis.

➤*Treatment:* There is no specific antidote. Consider GI decontamination (ie, gastric lavage followed by activated charcoal) in patients with suspected overdose. Institute standard supportive care. If chest pain or other symptoms of angina are present, perform ECG monitoring for evidence of ischemia. Based on the elimination half life, continue monitoring patients after overdose for at least 10 hours (**sumatriptan**), 12 hours (**rizatriptan**), 15 hours (**zolmitriptan**), 20 hours (**almotriptan**), 24 hours (**naratriptan**), 48 hours (**frovatriptan**), or 20 hours or more (**eletriptan**).

It is unknown what effect hemodialysis or peritoneal dialysis has on the serum concentrations of these agents.

Patient Information

A patient information leaflet is provided for patients.

➤*Injection (sumatriptan):* Instruct patients who are advised to self-administer sumatriptan in medically unsupervised situations on the proper use of the product prior to doing so for the first time, including loading the auto-injector and discarding the empty syringes.

For adults, the usual dose is a single injection given just below the skin. Administer as soon as migraine symptoms appear, but it may be given at any time during an attack. A second injection may be given if symptoms of migraine return. Do not use more than 2 injections/24 hours, and allow at least 1 hour between each dose.

Instruct patients using the needle-free injection (*Sumavel*) that a loud burst of air will be heard and a sensation felt at the time the dose is delivered. Advise patients not to use the device if the tip is tilted or broken off upon removal from packaging. Administration sites on the abdomen or thigh with adequate subcutaneous thickness to accommodate penetration of the drug into the subcutaneous space should be used. Advise patients not to administer to the arms or other areas of the body, or within 2 inches of the navel.

The patient may experience pain or redness at the site of injection, but this usually lasts less than 1 hour.

➤*Intranasal:* For adults, the usual dose is a single nasal spray into 1 nostril. If headache returns, a second nasal spray may be given 2 hours after the first spray. For any attack where the patient has no response to the first nasal spray, do not use a second nasal spray without first consulting a physician. Do not administer more than 40 mg **sumatriptan** or 10 mg **zolmitriptan** nasal spray in any 24-hour period.

➤*Oral:* Take a single dose with fluids as soon as symptoms of migraine appear; a second dose may be taken if symptoms return, but no sooner than 2 hours (**sumatriptan**, **zolmitriptan**, **eletriptan**) or 4 hours (**naratriptan**) following the first dose. For a given attack, if there is no response to the first dose, do not take a second dose without first consulting a physician. Do not take more than 200 mg sumatriptan, more than 5 mg naratriptan, more than 10 mg zolmitriptan, or more than 80 mg eletriptan in any 24-hour period.

Tell a physician if the patient has risk factors for heart disease (eg, high blood pressure, high cholesterol, obesity, diabetes, smoking, strong family history of heart disease or stroke, a male over 40 years of age, postmenopausal woman).

These agents are intended to relieve migraine but not to prevent or reduce the number of attacks. Use only to treat an actual migraine attack or cluster headache (sumatriptan injection only).

Instruct patients not to use these agents if they are pregnant, think they might be pregnant, are trying to become pregnant, or are not using adequate contraception, unless they have discussed this with a physician. The manufacturer maintains a sumatriptan and naratriptan pregnancy registry. Register patients by calling (800) 336-2176.

If pain, tightness, pressure, or heaviness in the chest, throat, neck, or jaw occurs when using these agents, instruct patients to discuss it with a physician before using more. If the chest pain is severe or does not go away, instruct patients to immediately call a physician.

If sudden or severe abdominal pain occurs following naratriptan or sumatriptan administration, instruct patients to immediately call a physician.

If shortness of breath, wheezing, heart throbbing, swelling of eyelids, face, or lips, skin rash, skin lumps, or hives occur, advise patients to immediately tell a physician. Instruct patients not to take additional doses unless directed by the physician.

If feelings of tingling, heat, flushing (redness of face lasting a short time), heaviness, pressure, drowsiness, dizziness, tiredness, or sickness develop, instruct patients to tell a physician.

Migraine or treatment with **rizatriptan** may cause somnolence in some patients; dizziness also has been reported. Evaluate ability to perform complex tasks during migraine attacks and after administration of rizatriptan.

Instruct patients not to remove the blister from the outer pouch until just prior to dosing zolmitriptan or rizatriptan orally-disintegrating tablets. Instruct patients to peel blister packs open with dry hands and to place the orally-disintegrating tablet on the tongue, where it will dissolve and be swallowed with the saliva.

Inform phenylketonuric patients that rizatriptan and zolmitriptan orally-disintegrating tablets contain phenylalanine (a component of aspartame). Each 5 mg rizatriptan orally-disintegrating tablet contains 1.05 mg phenylalanine and each 10 mg orally-disintegrating tablet contains 2.1 mg phenylalanine. Each 2.5 mg zolmitriptan orally-disintegrating tablet contains 2.81 mg phenylalanine.

Photosensitization (photoallergy or phototoxicity) may occur; therefore, caution patients to take protective measures (ie, sunscreens, protective clothing) against exposure to sunlight or ultraviolet light (eg, tanning beds) until tolerance is determined.

FROVATRIPTAN SUCCINATE

Rx	Frova (Elan)	Tablets: 2.5 mg (as base)	Lactose. (77). Film-coated. In blister card 9s.

FROVATRIPTAN SUCCINATE — ORAL

For complete and comparative prescribing information, refer to the Serotonin 5-HT$_1$ Receptor Agonists group monograph.

Indications

➤*Migraines:* For the acute treatment of migraine attacks with or without aura in adults.

Frovatriptan succinate is not intended for the prophylactic therapy of migraine or for use in the management of hemiplegic or basilar migraine. The safety and effectiveness of frovatriptan succinate have not been established for cluster headache, which is present in an older, predominately male population.

Administration and Dosage

➤*General dosing considerations:* There is no evidence that a second dose of frovatriptan is effective in patients who do not respond to a first dose of the drug for the same headache.

➤*Adults:*

Migraines –

Usual dosage: Single tablet taken orally with fluids. If the headache recurs after initial relief, a second tablet may be taken, providing there is an interval of at least 2 hours between doses.

The safety of treating an average of more than 4 migraine attacks in a 30-day period has not been established.

Maximum dose: 3 tablets (3 × 2.5 mg/day).

➤*Storage/Stability:* Store at controlled room temperature, 25°C (77°F) excursions permitted to 15° to 30°C (59° to 86°F) (see USP controlled room temperature). Protect from moisture and light.

ELETRIPTAN HYDROBROMIDE

Rx	Relpax (Pfizer)	Tablets: 24.2 mg eletriptan HBr (equivalent to 20 mg base)	Lactose. (REP20 Pfizer). Orange. Film-coated. In blister card 12s.
		48.5 mg eletriptan HBr (equivalent to 40 mg base)	Lactose. (REP40 Pfizer). Orange. Film-coated. In blister card 12s.

ELETRIPTAN HYDROBROMIDE — ORAL

For complete prescribing information, refer to the Serotonin 5-HT$_1$ Receptor Agonists group monograph.

Indications

➤*Migraines:* For the acute treatment of migraine with or without aura in adults.

Eletriptan hydrobromide is not intended for the prophylactic therapy of migraine or for use in the management of hemiplegic or basilar migraine. Safety and efficacy of eletriptan hydrobromide tablets have not been established for cluster headache, which is present in an older, predominantly male population.

Administration and Dosage

➤*General dosing considerations:* Individuals may vary in response to doses of eletriptan, therefore the choice of dose should be made on an individual basis.

The safety of treating an average of more than 3 headaches in a 30-day period has not been established.

An 80 mg dose, although also effective, was associated with an increased incidence of adverse reactions.

➤*Adults:*

Migraines –

Maximum dose: 40 mg as a single dose; 80 mg as a total daily dose.

Initial dosage: Single doses of 20 and 40 mg were effective for the acute treatment of migraines. If after the initial dose, headache improves but then returns, a repeat dose may be beneficial. If a second dose is required, it should be taken at least 2 hours after the initial dose.

If the initial dose is ineffective, controlled clinical trials have not shown a benefit of a second dose to treat the same attack.

Concomitant therapy: Eletriptan is metabolized by the CYP3A4 enzyme. Eletriptan should not be used within at least 72 hours of treatment with the following potent CYP3A4 inhibitors: ketoconazole, itraconazole, nefazodone, troleandomycin, clarithromycin, ritonavir, and nelfinavir. Eletriptan should not be used within 72 hours with drugs that have demonstrated potent CYP3A4 inhibition and have this potent effect described in the contraindications, warnings, or precautions sections of their labeling (ie, ketoconazole, itraconazole, nefazodone, troleandomycin, clarithromycin, ritonavir, nelfinavir).

➤*Hepatic function impairment:* The drug should not be given to patients with severe hepatic impairment because the effect of severe hepatic impairment on eletriptan metabolism was not evaluated.

➤*Storage/Stability:* Store at 25°C (77°F); excursions permitted to 15° to 30°C (59° to 86°F).

RIZATRIPTAN BENZOATE

Rx	Maxalt (Merck)	Tablets: 5 mg (as base)	Lactose. (MRK 266). Pale pink, capsule shape. In unit-of-use carrying case of 6 tablets.
		10 mg (as base)	Lactose. (MAXALT MRK 267). Pale pink, capsule shape. In unit-of-use carrying case of 6 tablets.
Rx	Maxalt-MLT (Merck)	Tablets, orally disintegrating: 5 mg (as base)	Lyophilized. 1.05 mg phenylalanine, mannitol, aspartame. White to off-white. Peppermint flavor. In 2 unit-of-use carrying case of 3 tablets (6 tablets total).
		10 mg (as base)	Lyophilized. 2.1 mg phenylalanine, mannitol, aspartame. White to off-white. Peppermint flavor. In 2 unit-of-use carrying case of 3 tablets (6 tablets total).

RIZATRIPTAN BENZOATE — ORAL

For complete and comparative prescribing information, refer to the Serotonin 5-HT$_1$ Receptor Agonists group monograph.

Indications

➤*Migraines:* For the acute treatment of migraine attacks with or without aura in adults.

Rizatriptan benzoate is not intended for the prophylactic therapy of migraine or for use in the management of hemiplegic or basilar migraine (such use is contraindicated). Safety and efficacy of rizatriptan benzoate has not been established for cluster headache, which is present in an older, predominantly male population.

➤*Off-label uses:*

Migraines in children/adolescents – [4] = Insufficient documentation. Rizatriptan has been studied for the treatment of migraine headaches in a limited number of pediatric patients with conflicting results. American Academy of Neurology guidelines consider there to be insufficient evidence to make a recommendation for the use of oral triptans in children or adolescents. Additional data are needed to determine the optimal dosing regimen and the patient population that would most benefit from therapy. (See Administration and Dosage.)

Administration and Dosage

➤*General dosing considerations:* The safety of treating, on average, greater than 4 headaches in a 30-day period has not been established.

For a given attack, if a patient has no response to the first dose of rizatriptan, the diagnosis of migraine should be reconsidered before administration of a second dose.

➤*Adults:*

Migraines –

Usual dosage: Single doses of 5 or 10 mg per headache attack.

There is evidence that the 10 mg dose may provide a greater effect than the 5 mg dose. Individuals may vary in response to doses of rizatriptan tablets. The choice of dose should therefore be made on an individual basis, weighing the possible benefit of the 10 mg dose with the potential risk for increased adverse events.

Maximum dose: 30 mg/day per 24-hour period.

Concomitant therapy: In patients receiving propranolol, the 5 mg dose of rizatriptan should be used, up to a maximum of 3 doses in any 24-hour period.

RIZATRIPTAN BENZOATE — ORAL

➤*Children:*

Off-label dosing –

Migraines in children/adolescents: [4] = Insufficient documentation. Oral rizatriptan 5 to 10 mg per headache attack.

➤*Elderly:* See Adults for dosing.

➤*Administration:* Doses should be separated by at least 2 hours.

Orally disintegrating tablets – Administration with liquid is not necessary. The orally disintegrating tablet is packaged in a blister within an outer aluminum pouch. Patients should be instructed not to remove the blister from the outer pouch until just prior to dosing. The blister pack should then be peeled open with dry hands and the orally disintegrating tablet placed on the tongue, where it will dissolve and be swallowed with the saliva.

➤*Storage/Stability:* Store tablets at 15° to 30°C (59° to 86°F). Dispense in a tight container, if product is subdivided.

NARATRIPTAN

Rx	**Amerge** (GlaxoSmithKline)	**Tablets; oral:** 1 mg	As naratriptan hydrochloride. Lactose. (GX CE3). White, D-shaped. Film-coated. In blister pack 9s.
Rx	**Naratriptan Hydrochloride** (Various, eg, Paddock, Sandoz, Teva)		Equiv. to 1.11 mg naratriptan hydrochloride. May contain lactose, PEG, polyvinyl alcohol. In blister pack 9s.
Rx	**Amerge** (GlaxoSmithKline)	**Tablets; oral:** 2.5 mg	As naratriptan hydrochloride. Lactose. (GX CE5). Green, D-shaped. Film-coated. In blister pack 9s.
Rx	**Naratriptan Hydrochloride** (Various, eg, Paddock, Sandoz, Teva)		Equiv. to 2.78 mg naratriptan hydrochloride. May contain lactose, PEG, polyvinyl alcohol. In blister pack 9s.

NARATRIPTAN HYDROCHLORIDE — ORAL

For complete and comparative prescribing information, refer to the Serotonin 5-HT_1 Receptor Agonists class monograph.

Indications

➤*Migraines:* For the acute treatment of migraine attacks with or without aura in adults.

Naratriptan is not intended for the prophylactic therapy of migraine or for use in the management of hemiplegic or basilar migraine. Safety and effectiveness have not been established for cluster headache, which is present in an older, predominantly male population.

Administration and Dosage

➤*General dosing considerations:* The safety of treating, on average, more than 4 headaches in a 30-day period has not been established.

➤*Adults:*

Migraines –

Usual dosage: Single doses of 1 and 2.5 mg taken with fluid. If the headache returns or if the patient has only partial response, the dose may be repeated once after 4 hours.

Maximum dose: 5 mg in a 24-hour period.

➤*Elderly:* The use of naratriptan in elderly patients is not recommended. Naratriptan is known to be substantially excreted by the kidney, and the risk of adverse reactions to this drug may be greater in elderly patients who have reduced renal function. In addition, elderly patients are more likely to have decreased hepatic function.

➤*Renal function impairment:* The use of naratriptan is contraindicated in patients with severe renal impairment (creatinine clearance less than 15 mL/min) because of decreased clearance of the drug. In patients with mild to moderate renal impairment, the maximum daily dose should not exceed 2.5 mg over a 24-hour period, and a lower starting dose should be considered.

➤*Hepatic function impairment:* The use of naratriptan is contraindicated in patients with severe hepatic impairment (Child-Pugh grade C) because of decreased clearance. In patients with mild or moderate hepatic impairment, the maximum daily dose should not exceed 2.5 mg over a 24-hour period, and a lower starting dose should be considered.

➤*Storage/Stability:* Store at controlled room temperature, 20° to 25°C (68° to 77°F).

SUMATRIPTAN

Rx	**Sumatriptan** (Various, eg, American Health, Greenstone, Ranbaxy, Teva)	**Tablets; oral:** 25 mg	Equiv. to sumatriptan succinate 35 mg. May contain lactose, PEG. In 9s, 100s, and UD 9s.
Rx	**Imitrex** (GlaxoSmithKline)		Equiv. to sumatriptan succinate 35 mg. (I 25). White, triangular shape. Film-coated. In UD 9s.
Rx	**Sumatriptan** (Various, eg, Greenstone, Ranbaxy, Teva)	**Tablets; oral:** 50 mg	Equiv. to sumatriptan succinate 70 mg. May contain lactose, PEG. In 9s, 100s, and UD 9s.
Rx	**Imitrex** (GlaxoSmithKline)		Equiv. to sumatriptan succinate 70 mg. (IMITREX 50). White, triangular shape. Film-coated. In UD 9s.
Rx	**Sumatriptan** (Various, eg, Greenstone, Ranbaxy, Teva)	**Tablets; oral:** 100 mg	Equiv. to sumatriptan succinate 140 mg. May contain lactose, PEG. In 9s, 100s, and UD 9s.
Rx	**Imitrex** (GlaxoSmithKline)		Equiv. to sumatriptan succinate 140 mg. (IMITREX 100). Pink, triangular shape. Film-coated. In UD 9s.
Rx	**Sumatriptan** (Various, eg, Par, Sandoz)	**Injection, solution:** 4 mg per 0.5 mL	As sumatriptan succinate. May contain sodium chloride. In single-dose vials.
Rx	**Imitrex** (GlaxoSmithKline)		As sumatriptan succinate. Sodium chloride 3.8 mg. In *STATdose* system (2 prefilled single-dose syringe cartridges, 1 *STATdose* pen, and instructions for use) injection cartridge pack.[a]
Rx	**Sumatriptan Succinate** (Various, eg, APP, Bedford, Cura, Sandoz, Sicor)	**Injection, solution:** 6 mg per 0.5 mL	As sumatriptan succinate. May contain sodium chloride. In single-dose vials and packs containing 6 mg single-dose prefilled syringe cartridges.
Rx	**Alsuma** (US Worldmeds)		As sumatriptan succinate. Sodium chloride 3.5 mg. In packs containing 6 mg single-dose prefilled auto injectors.
Rx	**Imitrex** (GlaxoSmithKline)		As sumatriptan succinate. Sodium chloride 3.5 mg. In single-dose vials and *STATdose* system (2 prefilled single-dose syringe cartridges, 1 *STATdose* pen, and instructions for use) injection cartridge pack.[a]
Rx	**Sumavel** (Zogenix)		As sumatriptan succinate. Sodium chloride 3.5 mg. In single-dose prefilled, needle-free *DosePro* system.
Rx	**Sumatriptan** (Sandoz)	**Solution; intranasal:** 5 mg	In 100 mcL unit-dose spray device. In 6s.
Rx	**Imitrex** (GlaxoSmithKline)		In 100 mcL unit-dose spray device. In 6s.
Rx	**Sumatriptan** (Sandoz)	**Solution; intranasal:** 20 mg	In 100 mcL unit-dose spray device. In 6s.
Rx	**Imitrex** (GlaxoSmithKline)		In 100 mcL unit-dose spray device. In 6s.

[a] Also available as 2 single-dose prefilled syringe cartridges for refill of *STATdose* system.

SUMATRIPTAN SUCCINATE — ORAL

For complete and comparative prescribing information, refer to the Serotonin 5-HT_1 Receptor Agonists class monograph.

Indications

➤*Migraines:* For the acute treatment of migraine attacks, with or without aura, in adults.

➤*Off-label uses:*

Migraines in children/adolescents – [4] = Insufficient documentation. All 3 dosage forms of sumatriptan have been studied for the treatment of migraine headaches in pediatric patients. The data for sumatriptan nasal spray are consistently positive. However, the published data for the oral dosage form are limited to a single controlled trial of fewer than 25 patients. American Academy of Neurology guidelines consider there to be insufficient evidence to make a recommendation for the use of any oral triptans in children or adolescents. (See Administration and Dosage.)

Administration and Dosage

➤*Adults:*

Migraines –

Maximum dose: 200 mg/day.

Initial dosage: Single dose of 25, 50, or 100 mg.

• *Repeat dosing* – If the headache returns or the patient has a partial response to the initial dose, the dose may be repeated after 2 hours, not to exceed a total daily dose of 200 mg.

Conversion: If a headache returns following an initial treatment with sumatriptan injection, additional single sumatriptan tablets (up to 100 mg/day) may be given with an interval of at least 2 hours between tablet doses.

➤*Children:*

Off-label dosing –

Migraines in children/adolescents: [4] = Insufficient documentation.

• *Adolescents* –

Older than 12 years of age: 100 mg. 200 mg daily; 100 mg as a single dose. Initiate dose at 25 mg orally as soon as possible after onset of headache. If no relief in 2 hours, give 25 to 100 mg every 2 hours up to a maximum daily dose of 200 mg.

• *Children* –

12 years of age and younger: 50 mg.

➤*Elderly:* Use is not recommended.

➤*Hepatic function impairment:* Contraindicated in severe hepatic impairment.

Maximum dose – 50 mg (single dose).

➤*Concomitant monoamine oxidase inhibitor therapy:* Because of the potential of monoamine oxidase (MAO)-A inhibitors to cause unpredictable elevations in the bioavailability of oral sumatriptan, their combined use is contraindicated.

➤*Storage/Stability:* Store between 2° and 30°C (36° and 86°F).

SUMATRIPTAN SUCCINATE — INJECTION

For complete and comparative prescribing information, refer to the Serotonin 5-HT_1 Receptor Agonists class monograph.

Indications

➤*Cluster headaches:* For acute treatment of cluster headache episodes.

➤*Migraines:* For acute treatment of migraine attacks with or without aura.

➤*Off-label uses:*

Migraines in children/adolescents – [4] = Insufficient documentation. All 3 dosage forms of sumatriptan have been studied for the treatment of migraine headaches in pediatric patients. The data for intranasal sumatriptan are consistently positive. However, the published data for the subcutaneous dosage form are limited by the small sample size and study design. American Academy of Neurology guidelines consider there to be insufficient evidence to make a recommendation for the use of any oral triptans in children or adolescents and further state that there are insufficient data to make an assessment of subcutaneous sumatriptan. (See Administration and Dosage.)

Postdural puncture headache – [4] = Insufficient documentation. There have been varying results with the use of sumatriptan in the management of postdural puncture headache. It is unclear if the efficacy of the drug may be related to the severity of the headache or is affected by other variables. Until further controlled studies demonstrate a clear benefit, the routine use of sumatriptan to manage postdural puncture headache cannot be recommended. However, this agent may be a useful alternative in cases in which epidural patches are contraindicated. (See Administration and Dosage.)

Administration and Dosage

➤*Adults:*

Cluster headaches –

Maximum dose: 6 mg (single dose); 12 mg (total daily dose).

Initial dosage: 6 mg injected subcutaneously.

Repeat dosing: The dose may be repeated once after 1 hour, not to exceed 12 mg in 24 hours.

Migraines – See Cluster Headaches for dosing.

Off-label dosing –

Postdural puncture headache: [4] = Insufficient documentation. 6 mg single dose given subcutaneously. In isolated cases, second doses have been administered when recurrent headache occurs.

➤*Children:*

Off-label dosing –

Migraines in children/adolescents: [4] = Insufficient documentation.

• *Usual dose* – The doses of sumatriptan subcutaneous injection were either fixed (3 mg for patients weighing less than 30 kg; 6 mg for patients weighing more than 30 kg) or weight-based (0.06 mg/kg).

• *Maximum dose* – 12 mg per 24 hour.

• *Alternative dosage* – 6 mg subcutaneously for 1 dose as soon as possible after the onset of headache, then may give an additional 6 mg or less subcutaneous dose 1 hour later if no response.

➤*Elderly:* Use is not recommended.

➤*Hepatic function impairment:* Contraindicated in severe hepatic impairment.

➤*Concomitant monoamine oxidase inhibitor therapy:* In patients receiving an monoamine oxidase inhibitor (MAOI), decreased doses of sumatriptan should be considered.

➤*Administration:* For subcutaneous use only. Sumatriptan is not to be administered intramuscularly or intravenously (IV). In patients receiving doses other than 4 or 6 mg, only the 6 mg single-dose vial dosage form should be used.

Needle-based injection – An autoinjection device is available for use with the 4 or 6 mg prefilled syringe cartridges to facilitate self-administration in patients using the 4 or 6 mg dose. With this device, the needle penetrates approximately one-fourth of an inch (5 to 6 mm). Patients should be directed to use injection sites with an adequate skin and subcutaneous thickness to accommodate the length of the needle.

Needle-free injection – Patients should be instructed to use administration sites on the abdomen or the thigh with an adequate subcutaneous thickness to accommodate penetration of sumatriptan injection into the subcutaneous space. Do not administer to other areas of the body, including the arm. Administration should not be made within 2 inches of the navel. Patients should be instructed not to use sumatriptan needle-free injection if the tip of the device is tilted or broken off upon removal from packaging.

➤*Storage/Stability:* Store vials/cartridges between 2° and 30°C (36° and 86°F). Protect from light. Store needle-free injection at 20° to 25°C (68° to 77°F), with excursions permitted between 15° and 30°C (59° and 86°F). Do not freeze. Sumatriptan prefilled injection is for single-use only. Discard after use.

SUMATRIPTAN — INTRANASAL

For complete and comparative prescribing information, refer to the Serotonin 5-HT_1 Receptor Agonists class monograph.

Indications

➤*Migraines:* For the acute treatment of migraine attacks with or without aura in adults.

➤*Off-label uses:*

Migraines in children/adolescents – [1] = Good documentation. Sumatriptan nasal spray has been studied for the treatment of migraine headaches in pediatric patients in several controlled trials. The published data show consistently favorable results. The current practice guidelines state that sumatriptan nasal spray should be considered an effective treatment option in pediatric patients. (See Administration and Dosage.)

Administration and Dosage

➤*Adults:*

Migraines –

Maximum dose: 40 mg/day.

Initial dosage: A single dose of 5, 10, or 20 mg administered into 1 nostril.

Repeat dosing: The dose may be repeated once after 2 hours, not to exceed a total daily dose of 40 mg.

➤*Children:*

Off-label dosing –

Migraines in children/adolescents: [1] = Good documentation. Sumatriptan nasal spray was administered in doses of 5, 10, and 20 mg. May repeat dose in 2 hours up to a maximum daily dose of 40 mg per 24 hours.

➤*Elderly:* Use is not recommended.

SUMATRIPTAN — INTRANASAL

➤*Hepatic function impairment:* Contraindicated in severe hepatic impairment.

➤*Concomitant monoamine oxidase inhibitor therapy:* Coadministration of sumatriptan nasal spray and an monoamine oxidase (MAO)-A inhibitor is contraindicated.

➤*Administration:* For intranasal administration only.

A 10 mg dose may be achieved by the administration of a single 5 mg dose in each nostril.

➤*Storage/Stability:* Store between 2° and 30°C (36° and 86°F). Protect from light.

ZOLMITRIPTAN

Rx	Zomig (AstraZeneca)	Tablets; oral: 2.5 mg	Lactose. (Zomig 2.5). Yellow, scored. Film-coated. In blister pack 6s.
		5 mg	Lactose. (Zomig 5). Pink. Film-coated. In blister pack 3s.
		Spray; intranasal: 5 mg	In 100 mcL unit-dose spray device. In 6s.
Rx	Zomig ZMT (AstraZeneca)	Tablets, disintegrating; oral: 2.5 mg	Phenylalanine 2.81 mg, mannitol, aspartame. (Z). White, bevelled. Orange flavor. In UD 6s.
		5 mg	Phenylalanine 5.62 mg, aspartame, mannitol, . (Z 5). White, round. Orange flavor. In UD 3s.

ZOLMITRIPTAN — ORAL

For complete prescribing information, refer to the Serotonin 5-HT$_1$ Receptor Agonists group monograph.

Indications

➤*Migraines:* For the acute treatment of migraine with or without aura in adults.

Zolmitriptan is not intended for the prophylactic therapy of migraine or for use in the management of hemiplegic or basilar migraine. Safety and efficacy of zolmitriptan have not been established for cluster headache, which is present in an older, predominantly male population.

➤*Off-label uses:*

Migraines in adolescents – [4] = Insufficient documentation. Published data on the use of zolmitriptan for prevention of migraine in adolescents are limited. Oral zolmitriptan did not offer any benefit over placebo. American Academy of Neurology guidelines state that there is insufficient evidence to make a recommendation for the use of oral triptans in children or adolescents. Additional data are needed to determine whether zolmitriptan formulations are of benefit to pediatric patients. (See Administration and Dosage.)

Administration and Dosage

➤*General dosing considerations:* The safety of treating an average of more than 3 headaches in a 30-day period has not been established.

Controlled trials have not adequately established the effectiveness of a second dose if the initial dose is ineffective.

➤*Adults:*

Migraine –

Orally disintegrating tablets:

- *Usual dosage* – Single dose of 2.5 mg per headache attack. If headache returns, the dose may be repeated after 2 hours.
- *Maximum dose* – 10 mg within a 24-hour period.

Tablets:

- *Usual dosage* – 2.5 mg as a single dose. Single doses of 1, 2.5, or 5 mg are effective. If the headache returns, the dose may be repeated after 2 hours.
- *Maximum dose* – 10 mg within a 24-hour period.

➤*Children:*

Off-label dosing –

Migraines in adolescents: [4] = Insufficient documentation. Zolmitriptan oral doses ranged from 2.5 to 10 mg per headache attack.

➤*Hepatic function impairment:* Zolmitriptan should be administered with caution in patients with liver disease, generally using doses less than 2.5 mg. Use of a low dose with blood pressure monitoring is recommended.

➤*Administration:*

Orally disintegrating tablet – Administration with liquid is not necessary. The orally disintegrating tablet is packaged in a blister. Patients should be instructed not to remove the tablet from the blister until just prior to dosing. The blister pack should then be peeled open and the orally disintegrating tablet placed on the tongue where it will dissolve and be swallowed with the saliva. It is not recommended to break the orally disintegrating tablet.

➤*Storage/Stability:* Store at controlled room temperature between 20° and 25°C (68° and 77°F). Protect from light and moisture.

ZOLMITRIPTAN — INTRANASAL

For complete and comparative prescribing information, refer to the Serotonin 5-HT$_1$ Receptor Agonists group monograph.

Indications

➤*Migraines:* For the acute treatment of migraine with or without aura in adults.

Zolmitriptan is not intended for the prophylactic therapy of migraine or for use in the management of hemiplegic or basilar migraine. Safety and effectiveness of zolmitriptan have not been established for cluster headache, which is present in an older, predominantly male population.

➤*Off-label uses:*

Migraines in adolescents – [4] = Insufficient documentation. Published data on the use of zolmitriptan for prevention of migraine in adolescents are limited. Zolmitriptan nasal spray showed a significant benefit over placebo, but the results are from a trial using a design that attempted to select out placebo responders. American Academy of Neurology guidelines state that there is insufficient evidence to make a recommendation for the use of oral triptans in children or adolescents. Additional data are needed to determine whether zolmitriptan formulations are of benefit to pediatric patients. (See Administration and Dosage.)

Administration and Dosage

September 30, 2003.

➤*General dosing considerations:* Individual response may vary to zolmitriptan nasal spray. The pharmacokinetics of a 5 mg nasal spray dose is similar to the 5 mg oral formulations. Doses lower than 5 mg can only be achieved through the use of an oral formulation. The choice of dose and route of administration should, therefore, be made on an individual basis.

The safety of treating an average of more than 4 headaches in a 30-day period has not been established.

➤*Adults:*

Acute migraine –

Usual dosage: 5 mg (1 spray) for the treatment of acute migraine. If the headache returns, the dose may be repeated after 2 hours.

Maximum dose: 10 mg (2 sprays) in any 24-hour period.

➤*Children:*

Off-label dosing –

Migraines in adolescents: [4] = Insufficient documentation. Zolmitriptan oral doses ranged from 2.5 to 10 mg per headache attack. One spray of zolmitriptan nasal spray (5 mg), with a second dose allowed 2 hours after the first dose if the headache pain persisted, was also studied.

➤*Hepatic function impairment:* Patients with moderate to severe hepatic impairment have decreased clearance of zolmitriptan and significant elevation in blood pressure was observed in some patients. Use of a lower dose of an alternate formulation with blood pressure monitoring is recommended.

➤*Storage/Stability:* Store at controlled room temperature, 20° to 25°C (68° to 77°F).

Serotonin 5-HT$_1$ Receptor Agonists (Triptans)

ALMOTRIPTAN

Rx	Axert (Ortho-McNeil)	**Tablets; oral:** 6.25 mg	As almotriptan malate. Mannitol, PEG. (2080). Round, white. Coated. In UD 6s.
		12.5 mg	As almotriptan malate. Mannitol, PEG. (A). Round, white. Coated. In UD 12s.

ALMOTRIPTAN MALATE — ORAL

For complete and comparative prescribing information, refer to the Serotonin 5-HT$_1$ Receptor Agonists class monograph.

Indications

➤*Migraine attacks:* For the acute treatment of migraine attacks in adults with a history of migraine with or without aura; for the acute treatment of migraine headache pain in children 12 years of age and older with a history of migraine attacks with or without aura usually lasting 4 hours or more (when untreated).

Administration and Dosage

➤*Adults:*

Migraine attacks –

Usual dosage: 6.25 to 12.5 mg, with the 12.5 mg dose tending to be a more effective dose in adults. If the headache is relieved after the initial almotriptan dose but returns, the dose may be repeated after 2 hours.

Maximum dose: 25 mg daily.

Duration of therapy: The safety of treating an average of more than 4 migraines in a 30-day period has not been established.

➤*Children:*

Migraine attacks –

12 to 17 years of age: See Adults for dosing.

• *Usual dosage* – 6.25 to 12.5 mg, with the 12.5 mg dose tending to be a more effective dose in adults. If the headache is relieved after the initial almotriptan dose but returns, the dose may be repeated after 2 hours.

• *Maximum dose* – 25 mg daily.

• *Duration of therapy* – The safety of treating an average of more than 4 migraines in a 30-day period has not been established.

➤*Elderly:* Dose selection for an elderly patient should be cautious, usually starting at the low end of the dosing range, reflecting the greater frequency of decreased hepatic, renal, or cardiac function, and of concomitant disease or other drug therapy.

➤*Renal function impairment:* The maximum daily dose should not exceed 12.5 mg over a 24-hour period, and a starting dose of 6.25 mg should be used in patients with severe renal impairment. Avoid concomitant use of almotriptan and potent CYP3A4 inhibitors in patients with renal impairment.

➤*Hepatic function impairment:* The maximum daily dose should not exceed 12.5 mg over a 24-hour period, and a starting dose of 6.25 mg should be used. Avoid concomitant use of almotriptan and potent CYP3A4 inhibitors in patients with hepatic impairment.

➤*Concomitant therapy with potent CYP3A4 inhibitors:* The recommended starting dose is 6.25 mg. The maximum daily dose should not exceed 12.5 mg within 24 hours. Avoid concomitant use of almotriptan and potent CYP3A4 inhibitors in patients with renal or hepatic impairment.

➤*Storage/Stability:* Store at 25°C (77°F); excursions are permitted between 15° and 30°C (59° and 86°F).

Ergotamine Derivatives

WARNING

Serious and/or life-threatening peripheral ischemia has been associated with the coadministration of dihydroergotamine with potent CYP3A4 inhibitors, including protease inhibitors and macrolide antibiotics. Because CYP3A4 inhibition elevates the serum levels of dihydroergotamine, the risk for vasospasm leading to cerebral ischemia and/or ischemia of the extremities is increased. Hence, concomitant use of these medications is contraindicated.

Indications

➤*Ergotamine:* To abort or prevent vascular headaches such as migraine, migraine variant, and histaminic cephalalgia.

➤*Dihydroergotamine:* For the acute treatment of migraine headaches with or without aura and the acute treatment of cluster headache episodes (injection only). Dihydroergotamine nasal spray is not intended for the prophylactic therapy of migraine or for the management of hemiplegic or basilar migraine.

Administration and Dosage

➤*Ergotamine sublingual:* Initiate therapy as soon as possible after the first symptoms of an attack. Place one 2 mg tablet under the tongue; take another tablet at 30-minute intervals thereafter, if necessary. Do not exceed 3 tablets in any 24-hour period. Do not exceed 5 tablets (10 mg) in any 1 week.

➤*Dihydroergotamine nasal spray:* Start with 1 spray (0.5 mg) in each nostril; repeat in 15 minutes for a total dosage of 4 sprays (2 mg). Studies have shown no additional benefit from acute doses greater than 2 mg for a single migraine administration. The safety of doses greater than 3 mg in a 24-hour period and 4 mg in a 7-day period has not been established. Do not use for chronic daily administration.

➤*Dihydroergotamine injection:* Administer in a dose of 1 mL IV, IM, or SC; may be repeated as needed at 1-hour intervals to a total dose of 3 mL for IM or SC delivery or 2 mL for IV delivery in a 24-hour period. Do not exceed a total weekly dosage of 6 mL. Do not use for chronic daily administration.

Actions

➤*Pharmacology:* Ergotamine has partial agonist or antagonist activity against tryptaminergic, dopaminergic, and alpha-adrenergic receptors, depending upon their site; it is a highly active uterine stimulant. It constricts peripheral and cranial blood vessels and depresses central vasomotor centers.

Ergotamine reduces extracranial blood flow, causes a decline in the amplitude of pulsation in the cranial arteries, and decreases hyperperfusion of the basilar artery territory. It does not reduce cerebral hemispheric blood flow. Small doses increase force and frequency of uterine contractions; larger doses increase resting uterine tone. The gravid uterus is more sensitive to these effects.

Ergotamine is hydrogenated in the 9, 10 position as the mesylate salt. Dihydroergotamine binds with high affinity to 5-HT$_{1D\alpha}$ and 5-HT$_{1D\beta}$ receptors. It also binds with high affinity to serotonin 5-HT$_{1A}$, 5-HT$_{2A}$, and 5-HT$_{2C}$ receptors; noradrenaline α_{2A}, α_{2B}, and α_1 receptors; and dopamine D_{2L} and D_3 receptors. The therapeutic activity of dihydroergotamine in migraine generally is attributed to the agonist effect at 5-HT$_{1D}$ receptors. Activation of 5-HT$_{1D}$ receptors located on intracranial blood vessels, including those on arteriovenous anastomoses, leads to vasoconstriction, which correlates with the relief of migraine headache. Dihydroergotamine also possesses oxytocic properties.

➤*Pharmacokinetics:*

Absorption/Distribution – GI and sublingual absorption of ergotamine is poor. Following intranasal administration, however, the mean bioavailability of dihydroergotamine mesylate is 32% relative to the injectable administration. Absorption is variable, probably reflecting intersubject differences of absorption and the technique used for self-administration.

Dihydroergotamine mesylate is 93% plasma protein bound. The apparent steady-state volume of distribution is approximately 800 L.

Metabolism/Excretion – Ergotamine is metabolized by the liver; 90% of the metabolites are excreted in the bile. Unmetabolized drug is erratically secreted in saliva, and only trace amounts of unmetabolized drug are excreted in the feces and urine. Although plasma half-life is about 2 hours, ergotamine has long-lasting effects that may be caused by tissue storage.

Following nasal administration, total metabolites represent only 20% to 30% of plasma AUC. The major metabolite, 8′-β-hydroxydihydroergotamine, exhibits affinity equivalent to its parent for adrenergic and 5-HT receptors and demonstrates equivalent potency in several venoconstrictor activity models. The systemic clearance of dihydroergotamine mesylate following IV and IM administration is 1.5 L/min, which mainly reflects hepatic clearance. After intranasal administration, the urinary recovery of parent drug amounts to about 2% of the administered dose compared with 6% after IM administration. The renal clearance (0.1 L/min) is unaffected by the route of dihydroergotamine administration. The decline of plasma dihydroergotamine is biphasic with a terminal half-life of about 9 to 10 hours.

Contraindications

Pregnancy, women who may become pregnant (powerful uterine stimulant actions of ergotamine and dihydroergotamine may cause fetal harm; see Warnings); hypersensitivity to ergot alkaloids or any component of the formulation; peripheral vascular disease (eg, thromboangiitis obliterans, luetic arteritis, severe arteriosclerosis, thrombophlebitis, Raynaud's disease); hepatic or renal impairment; severe pruritus; coronary artery disease (CAD); hypertension; sepsis.

There have been reports of serious adverse events associated with the coadministration of dihydroergotamine and potent CYP3A4 inhibitors (eg, protease inhibitors, macrolide antibiotics), resulting in vasospasm that led to cerebral ischemia and/or ischemia of the extremities. The use of potent CYP3A4 inhibitors (ritonavir, nelfinavir, indinavir, erythromycin, clarithromycin, troleandomycin, ketoconazole, itraconazole) with dihydroergotamine is, therefore, contraindicated.

Do not give dihydroergotamine to patients with ischemic heart disease (angina pectoris, history of MI, documented silent ischemia) or to patients who have clinical symptoms or findings consistent with coronary artery vasospasm, including Prinzmetal variant angina.

Dihydroergotamine may increase blood pressure; do not give to patients with uncontrolled hypertension.

Do not use dihydroergotamine, 5-HT$_1$ agonists (eg, sumatriptan), ergotamine-containing or ergot-type medications, or methysergide within 24 hours of each other.

Do not administer dihydroergotamine to patients with hemiplegic or basilar migraine.

Dihydroergotamine should not be used by nursing mothers.

Do not use dihydroergotamine with peripheral and central vasoconstrictors because the combination may result in additive or synergistic elevation of blood pressure.

Warnings/Precautions

➤*CYP3A4 inhibitors (eg, macrolide antibiotics, protease inhibitors):* There have been rare reports of serious adverse events in connection with the coadministration of dihydroergotamine and potent CYP3A4 inhibitors, such as protease inhibitors and macrolide antibiotics, resulting in vasospasm that led to cerebral ischemia and/or ischemia of the extremities. Avoid the use of potent CYP3A4 inhibitors with dihydroergotamine. Examples of some of the more potent CYP3A4 inhibitors include: Antifungals ketoconazole and itraconazole, protease inhibitors ritonavir, nelfinavir, and indinavir, and macrolide antibiotics erythromycin, clarithromycin, and troleandomycin. Administer other less potent CYP3A4 inhibitors with caution. Less potent inhibitors include the following: Saquinavir, nefazodone, fluconazole, grapefruit juice, fluoxetine, fluvoxamine, zileuton, clotrimazole. These lists are not exhaustive; consider the effects on CYP3A4 of other agents being considered for concomitant use with dihydroergotamine.

➤*Fibrotic complications:* There have been reports of pleural and retroperitoneal fibrosis in patients following prolonged daily use of injectable dihydroergotamine. Rarely, prolonged daily use of other ergot alkaloid drugs has been associated with cardiac valvular fibrosis. Rare cases also have been reported in association with the use of injectable dihydroergotamine; however, in those cases, patients also received drugs known to be associated with cardiac valvular fibrosis.

➤*Risk of myocardial ischemia and/or MI and other adverse cardiac events:* Do not use dihydroergotamine in patients with documented ischemic or vasospastic coronary artery disease. It is strongly recommended that dihydroergotamine not be given to patients in whom unrecognized CAD is predicted by the presence of risk factors (eg, hypertension, hypercholesterolemia, smoking, obesity, diabetes, strong family history of CAD, females who are surgically or physiologically postmenopausal, or males who are over 40 years of age) unless a cardiovascular evaluation provides satisfactory clinical evidence that the patient is reasonably free of coronary artery and ischemic myocardial disease or other significant underlying cardiovascular disease. The sensitivity of cardiac diagnostic procedures to detect cardiovascular disease or predisposition to coronary artery vasospasm is modest, at best. If during the cardiovascular evaluation, the patient's medical history or electrocardiographic investigations reveal findings indicative of or consistent with coronary artery vasospasm or myocardial ischemia, do not administer dihydroergotamine.

For patients with risk factors predictive of CAD who are shown to have a satisfactory cardiovascular evaluation, it is strongly recommended that administration of the first dose of dihydroergotamine take place in the setting of a physician's office or similar medically staffed and equipped facility unless the patient has previously received dihydroergotamine. Because cardiac ischemia can occur in the absence of clinical symptoms, consider obtaining, on the first occasion of use, an electrocardiogram during the interval immediately following dihydroergotamine in these patients with risk factors.

It is recommended that patients who are intermittent long-term users of dihydroergotamine and who have or acquire risk factors predictive of CAD, as described above, undergo periodic interval cardiovascular evaluation as they continue to use dihydroergotamine.

The systematic approach described above is currently recommended as a method to identify patients in whom dihydroergotamine may be used to treat migraine headaches with an acceptable margin of cardiovascular safety.

➤*Cardiac events and fatalities:* No deaths have been reported in patients using dihydroergotamine. The potential for adverse cardiac events exists. Serious adverse cardiac events, including acute MI, life-threatening disturbances of cardiac rhythm, and death have been reported following the administration of dihydroergotamine. Considering the extent of use of dihydroergotamine in patients with migraine, the incidence of these events is extremely low.

➤*Drug-associated cerebrovascular events and fatalities:* Cerebral hemorrhage, subarachnoid hemorrhage, stroke, and other cerebrovascular events have been reported in patients treated with dihydroergotamine; some have resulted in fatalities. It should be noted that patients with migraine may be at increased risk of certain cerebrovascular events (eg, stroke, hemorrhage, transient ischemic attack).

➤*Other vasospasm-related events:* Dihydroergotamine, like other ergot alkaloids, may cause vasospastic reactions other than coronary artery vasospasm. Myocardial and peripheral vascular ischemia have been reported with dihydroergotamine.

Dihydroergotamine associated vasospastic phenomena may also cause muscle pains, numbness, coldness, pallor, and cyanosis of the digits. In patients with compromised circulation, persistent vasospasm may result in gangrene or death. Immediately discontinue dihydroergotamine if signs or symptoms of vasoconstriction develop.

➤*Increase in blood pressure:* Significant elevation in blood pressure has been reported on rare occasions in patients with and without a history of hypertension treated with dihydroergotamine. Dihydroergotamine is contraindicated in patients with uncontrolled hypertension.

➤*Local irritation:* Approximately 30% of patients using dihydroergotamine nasal spray (compared with 9% of placebo patients) have reported irritation in the nose or throat and/or disturbance in taste. Irritative symptoms include congestion, burning sensation, dryness, paresthesia, discharge, epistaxis, pain, or soreness. The symptoms were predominantly mild to moderate in severity and transient. In approximately 70% of the above mentioned cases, the symptoms resolved within 4 hours after dosing with dihydroergotamine.

➤*Coronary artery vasospasm:* Dihydroergotamine may cause coronary artery vasospasm; patients who experience signs or symptoms suggestive of angina following its administration should, therefore, be evaluated for the presence of CAD or a predisposition to variant angina before receiving additional doses. Similarly, patients who experience other symptoms or signs suggestive of decreased arterial flow, such as ischemic bowel syndrome or Raynaud's syndrome following the use of any 5-HT agonist are candidates for further evaluation.

➤*Ergotism:* Although signs and symptoms of ergotism rarely develop even after long-term intermittent use of ergotamine, exercise care to remain within the limits of recommended dosage.

➤*Drug abuse and dependence:* Patients who take ergotamine for extended periods of time may become dependent upon it and require progressively increasing doses for relief of vascular headaches and for prevention of dysphoric effects that follow withdrawal.

➤*Pregnancy: Category X.* Although no specific teratogenic effects have been found, the fetus suffers if ergotamine is given to the mother. Retarded fetal growth, increased intrauterine death, and resorption occurred in animals, possibly resulting from drug-induced uterine motility and increased vasoconstriction in the placental vascular bed.

Dihydroergotamine possesses oxytocic properties and, therefore, should not be administered during pregnancy. If this drug is used during pregnancy or if the patient becomes pregnant while taking this drug, apprise the patient of the potential hazard to the fetus. There are no adequate studies of dihydroergotamine in human pregnancy, but developmental toxicity has been demonstrated in experimental animals.

➤*Lactation:* Ergotamine is secreted into breast milk and has caused symptoms of ergotism (eg, vomiting, diarrhea) in the infant. Exercise caution when administering to a nursing woman. Excessive dosing or prolonged administration may inhibit lactation. It is likely that dihydroergotamine is excreted in human milk, but there are no data on the drug concentration excreted. Because of the potential for these serious adverse events in nursing infants exposed to dihydroergotamine, nursing should not be undertaken while on this medication.

➤*Children:* Safety and efficacy for use in children have not been established.

Drug Interactions

Ergot Alkaloid Drug Interactions

Precipitant drug	Object drug[a]		Description
Beta-blockers	Ergot alkaloids	↑	Peripheral ischemia manifested by cold extremities, possible peripheral gangrene may occur.
CYP3A4 inhibitors (eg, protease inhibitors, macrolide antibiotics, ketoconazole, itraconazole, nefazodone, fluconazole, fluoxetine, fluvoxamine, delavirdine, efavirenz)	Ergot alkaloids	↑	The risk of ergot toxicity (ie, peripheral vasospasm/ischemia) may be increased. Coadministration with a potent CYP3A4 inhibitor is contraindicated. Use with caution with less potent CYP3A4 inhibitors (see Warnings and Contraindications).
Nicotine	Ergot alkaloids	↑	Nicotine may provoke vasoconstriction in some patients, predisposing them to a greater ischemic response to ergot therapy.
Sibutramine	Ergot alkaloids	↑	A serotonin syndrome may occur. Coadministration is not recommended. Carefully monitor patients if concurrent use cannot be avoided.
Dihydroergotamine	Nitrates	↓	Functional antagonism between these agents, decreasing the antianginal effects may occur.
Ergot alkaloids	$5\text{-}HT_1$ receptor agonists (eg, sumatriptan, frovatriptan, naratriptan, rizatriptan, zolmitriptan)	↑	Risk of vasospastic reactions may be increased. Administration of a $5\text{-}HT_1$ receptor agonist or ergot alkaloid within 24 hours of each other is contraindicated.
Ergot alkaloids	Vasoconstrictors	↑	The pressor effects of concurrent use can combine to cause dangerous hypertension.

[a] ↑ = object drug increased; ↓ = object drug decreased.

➤*Drug/Food interactions:* Administration with grapefruit juice may increase the serum levels of the ergotamine derivative. Use with caution.

Adverse Reactions

➤*Ergotamine tartrate:* Nausea and vomiting occur in up to 10% of patients. Numbness and tingling of fingers and toes; muscle pain in the extremities; pulselessness; weakness in the legs; precordial pain; transient tachycardia or bradycardia; localized edema; itching.

➤*Dihydroergotamine injection:* Serious cardiac events, including some that have been fatal, have occurred following use of dihydroergotamine injection but are extremely rare. Events reported have included coronary artery vasospasm, transient myocardial ischemia, MI, ventricular tachycardia, and ventricular fibrillation. Fibrotic complications have been reported in association with long-term use of injectable dihydroergotamine.

➤*Dihydroergotamine nasal spray:* During clinical studies and the foreign postmarketing experience with dihydroergotamine nasal spray, there have been no fatalities caused by cardiac events.

Dihydroergotamine Nasal Spray Adverse Reactions (≥ 1%) in the Migraine Placebo-Controlled Trials		
Adverse reaction	Dihydroergotamine (N = 597)	Placebo (N = 631)
CNS		
Dizziness	4	2
Somnolence	3	2
Paresthesia	2	2
GI		
Nausea	10	4
Altered sense of taste	8	1
Vomiting	4	1
Diarrhea	2	< 1
Respiratory		
Rhinitis	26	7
Pharyngitis	3	1
Sinusitis	1	1
Miscellaneous		
Application site reaction	6	2
Dry mouth	1	1
Fatigue	1	1
Asthenia	1	0
Hot flushes	1	< 1
Stiffness	1	< 1

Overdosage

➤*Symptoms:* Some cases of ergotamine poisoning have occurred in patients who have taken less than 5 mg. Usually, however, toxicity is seen at doses in excess of about 15 mg in 24 hours or 40 mg in a few days. Overdosage causes nausea, vomiting, weakness of the legs, pain in limb muscles, numbness and tingling of fingers and toes, precordial pain, tachycardia or bradycardia, hypertension or hypotension, and localized edema and itching with signs and symptoms of ischemia caused by vasoconstriction of peripheral arteries and arterioles. The feet and hands become cold, pale, and numb. Muscle pain occurs while walking and also later at rest. Gangrene may ensue. Confusion, depression, drowsiness, and convulsions are occasional signs of ergotamine toxicity. Overdosage is particularly likely to occur in patients with sepsis or impaired renal or hepatic function. Patients with peripheral vascular disease are especially at risk of developing peripheral ischemia following treatment with ergotamine.

➤*Treatment:* Treatment consists of the withdrawal of the drug followed by symptomatic measures, including attempts to maintain adequate circulation in the affected parts. Anticoagulant drugs, low molecular weight dextran, and potent vasodilators all may be beneficial. IV infusion of sodium nitroprusside has been successful. Vasodilators must be used with special care in the presence of hypotension. Ergotamine is dialyzable.

Patient Information

Once the nasal spray applicator has been prepared, discard it (with any remaining drug) after 8 hours.

Dosage is individualized. Take exactly as prescribed.

Do not exceed the dosing guidelines. Do not use for chronic daily administration.

Do not stop taking or change the dose unless directed by your physician.

Take at the first sign or hint of a migraine attack.

Stop taking the drug and notify your physician if you experience the following: Numbness, tingling, coldness, or paleness in fingers or toes; muscle pain in arms or legs; weakness in legs; chest pain; heart rate changes; sudden worsening of headache; swelling; itching.

DIHYDROERGOTAMINE MESYLATE

Rx	**Migranal** (Valeant)	**Spray, nasal:** 4 mg/mL (0.5 mg per spray)[a]	In 3.5 mL vials with nasal sprayer.
Rx	**D.H.E. 45** (Xcel[b])	**Injection:** 1 mg/mL[c]	In 1 mL amps.
Rx	**Dihydroergotamine Mesylate** (Various, eg, Bedford, Paddock)		6% alcohol. In 1 mL vials.

[a] With 10 mg caffeine and 50 mg dextrose.
[b] Xcel Pharmaceuticals, 6363 Greenwich Drive, Suite 100, San Diego, CA 92122; (858) 202-2700, fax (858) 202-2799.
[c] With 6.2% alcohol and 15% glycerin.

DIHYDROERGOTAMINE MESYLATE — INTRANASAL

For complete and comparative prescribing information, refer to the Ergotamine Derivatives group monograph.

WARNING

Serious or life-threatening peripheral ischemia has been associated with the coadministration of dihydroergotamine with potent CYP3A4 inhibitors, including protease inhibitors and macrolide antibiotics. Because CYP3A4 inhibition elevates the serum levels of dihydroergotamine, the risk for vasospasm leading to cerebral ischemia or ischemia of the extremities is increased. Hence, concomitant use of these medications is contraindicated.

Indications

➤*Migraines:* For the acute treatment of migraine headaches with or without aura.

Dihydroergotamine mesylate is not intended for the prophylactic therapy of migraine or for the management of hemiplegic or basilar migraine.

Administration and Dosage

➤*General dosing considerations:* Dihydroergotamine nasal spray should not be used for chronic daily administration.

➤*Adults:*

Migraines – One spray (0.5 mg) should be administered in each nostril. Fifteen minutes later, an additional 1 spray (0.5 mg) may be administered in each nostril, for a total dosage of 4 sprays (2 mg).

➤*Renal function impairment:* Dihydroergotamine is contraindicated in patients with severely impaired renal function.

➤*Hepatic function impairment:* Dihydroergotamine is contraindicated in patients with severely impaired hepatic function.

➤*Administration:* The solution used in dihydroergotamine nasal spray (4 mg/mL) is intended for intranasal use and must not be injected.

Prior to administration, the pump must be primed (ie, squeeze 4 times) before use.

Once the nasal spray applicator has been prepared, it should be discarded (with any remaining drug in opened ampul) after 8 hours.

➤*Storage/Stability:* Store below 25°C (77°F). Do not refrigerate or freeze.

Ergotamine Derivatives

DIHYDROERGOTAMINE MESYLATE — INJECTION

For complete and comparative prescribing information, refer to the Ergotamine Derivatives group monograph.

WARNING

Serious and life-threatening peripheral ischemia have been associated with the coadministration of dihydroergotamine with potent CYP3A4 inhibitors including protease inhibitors and macrolide antibiotics. Because CYP3A4 inhibition elevates the serum levels of dihydroergotamine, the risk for vasospasm leading to cerebral ischemia and ischemia of the extremities is increased. Hence, concomitant use of these medications is contraindicated.

Indications

➤*Migraines:* For the acute treatment of migraine headaches with or without aura and cluster headache episodes.

Administration and Dosage

➤*General dosing considerations:* Dihydroergotamine injection should not be used for chronic daily administration.

➤*Adults:*

Migraines –

Usual dosage: Administer a dose of 1 mL intravenously (IV), intramuscularly (IM), or subcutaneous. The dose can be repeated, as needed, at 1-hour intervals to a total dose of 3 mL for IM or subcutaneous delivery or 2 mL for IV delivery in a 24-hour period.

Maximum dose: The total weekly dosage should not exceed 6 mL.

➤*Renal function impairment:* Dihydroergotamine is contraindicated in patients with severely impaired renal function.

➤*Hepatic function impairment:* Dihydroergotamine is contraindicated in patients with severely impaired hepatic function.

➤*Administration:* Administer by IV, IM, or subcutaneous.

➤*Storage/Stability:* Store at 20° to 25°C (68° to 77°F) in light-resistant containers. Do not refrigerate or freeze. To ensure constant potency, protect the vials and ampules from light and heat.

ERGOTAMINE TARTRATE

Rx	**Ergomar** (Rosedale Therapeutics)	**Tablets; sublingual:** 2 mg	Saccharin. (LB2). Green, round. Peppermint flavor. In 20s.

ERGOTAMINE TARTRATE — ORAL

For complete and comparative prescribing information, refer to the Ergotamine Derivatives class monograph.

WARNING

Serious and/or life-threatening peripheral ischemia has been associated with the coadministration of ergotamine with potent CYP 3A4 inhibitors, including protease inhibitors and macrolide antibiotics. Because CYP3A4 inhibition elevates the serum levels of ergotamine, the risk for vasospasm leading to cerebral ischemia and/or ischemia of the extremities is increased. Therefore, concomitant use of these medications is contraindicated.

Indications

➤*Vascular headaches:* As therapy to abort or prevent vascular headache (eg, migraine, migraine variants or a so-called "histaminic cephalalgia").

Administration and Dosage

➤*General dosing considerations:* Do not use for chronic daily administration.

For best results, dosage should start at the first sign of an attack; early administration gives maximum effectiveness.

Place tablet under the tongue and allow to dissolve; do not crush, chew, or swallow whole.

➤*Adults:*

Vascular headaches –

Usual dosage: One 2 mg tablet placed under the tongue at the first sign of an attack or to relieve symptoms after onset of an attack. Another tablet should be taken at 30-minute intervals thereafter, if necessary.

Maximum dose: Dosage must not exceed 3 tablets in any 24-hour period or 10 mg in any 1 week.

➤*Renal function impairment:* Administration of ergotamine to patients with renal impairment is contraindicated.

➤*Hepatic function impairment:* Administration of ergotamine to patients with hepatic impairment is contraindicated.

➤*Storage/Stability:* Store at 20° to 25°C (68° to 77°F); excursions are permitted to 15° to 30°C (59° to 86°F). Protect from light and heat.

Migraine Combinations

MIGRAINE COMBINATIONS

Content given per tablet, capsule, or suppository.

	Product & Distributor	Content and Dosage	How Supplied
Rx	**Ergotamine Tartrate/ Caffeine** (West-Ward)	**Tablets; oral:** Ergotamine tartrate 1 mg, caffeine 100 mg *Dosage: Adults* – 2 tablets at first sign of an attack; follow with 1 tablet every ½ hour, if needed. Max dose is 6 tablets/attack. Do not exceed 10 tablets/week.	Sugar. (WW 120). Buff. Film-coated. In 30s, 100s, and 500s.
Rx	**Cafergot** (Sandoz)		Parabens, sugar. (SZ 183). Beige. Sugar-coated. In 100s.
Rx	**Migergot** (G & W)	**Suppositories; rectal:** Ergotamine tartrate 2 mg, caffeine 100 mg *Dosage: Adults* – Insert 1 suppository rectally at the first sign of an attack; may follow with an additional suppository 1 hour later if needed. Max dose is 2 suppositories per attack; 5 suppositories per week.	Cocoa butter. In 12s.
c-iv	**Isometheptene/ Dichloralphenazone/ Acetaminophen** (Various, eg, URL)	**Capsules; oral:** Isometheptene mucate 65 mg, acetaminophen 325 mg, dichloralphenazone 100 mg *Dosage: Adults – Migraine headache*: 2 capsules at once followed by 1 capsule every hour until headache is relieved, up to 5 capsules within a 12-hour period. *Tension headache*: 1 or 2 capsules every 4 hours, up to 8 capsules per day.	In 50s, 100s, 250s, and 500s.
c-iv	**Epidrin** (Excellium)		(EPI 101). Red and white. In 100s and 250s.
c-iv	**Midrin** (Caraco)		(MIDRIN). Red. In 100s.
c-iv	**Migrazone** (Breckenridge)		(B395). Dark red-orange. In 100s.
Rx	**Prodrin Caplets** (Gentex Pharma)	**Tablets; oral:** Isometheptene mucate 130 mg, acetaminophen 500 mg, caffeine 20 mg *Dosage:* 2 caplets at once, followed by 1 caplet every hour until relieved, up to 5 caplets within a 12-hour period.	(PRODRIN). White, scored. In 50s.
Rx	**Treximet** (GlaxoSmith-Kline)	**Tablets; oral:** Sumatriptan 85 mg, naproxen sodium 500 mg *Dosage: Adults* – 1 tablet at first sign of attack; may follow with 1 tablet 2 hours later. Max dose is 2 tablets per 24 hours.	Equiv to sumatriptan succinate 119 mg. Dextrose, sodium 61.2 mg. (GS YYG). Blue. Film-coated. In 9s.

Indications

Recommended Uses for Antiemetic/Antivertigo Agents

Class	Drug	Indications: Nausea and Vomiting	Indications: Motion Sickness	Indications: Vertigo
ANTIDOPAMINERGICS				
Phenothiazines	Chlorpromazine[a]	✓		
	Perphenazine[a]	✓		
	Prochlorperazine	✓		
	Promethazine	✓	✓	
	Thiethylperazine	✓		
Other	Metoclopramide	✓		
ANTICHOLINERGICS				
Antihistamines	Buclizine	✓	✓	
	Cyclizine	✓	✓	
	Dimenhydrinate	✓	✓	✓
	Diphenhydramine	✓	✓	
	Meclizine	✓	✓	✓[b]
Other	Scopolamine	✓	✓	
	Trimethobenzamide	✓		
MISCELLANEOUS				
Miscellaneous	Benzquinamide	✓		
	Cannabinoids	✓		
	Corticosteroids	✓[c]		
	Hydroxyzine HCl	✓[c]		
	Diphenidol	✓		✓
	Phosphorated Carbohydrate Solution	✓		

[a] Also indicated for relief of intractable hiccoughs.
[b] Classified "possibly effective" by the FDA.
[c] This is an *unlabeled* use.

Actions

➤*Pharmacology:* Drug-induced vomiting (eg, drugs, radiation, metabolic disorders) is generally stimulated through the chemoreceptor trigger zone (CTZ), which in turn stimulates the vomiting center (VC) in the brain. Nausea of motion sickness is initiated by stimulation of labyrinthine mechanism of the ear, which sends impulses to CTZ. VC may also be stimulated directly (by GI irritation, motion sickness, vestibular neuritis, etc). Increased activity of central neurotransmitters, dopamine in CTZ or acetylcholine in VC appears to be a major mediator for inducing vomiting.

Patients undergoing cancer chemotherapy often experience nausea and vomiting so intolerable that they may refuse further treatment. Some antineoplastic agents are more emetogenic than others. Prophylaxis with an antiemetic drug before the patient receives chemotherapy and treatment afterward may enable the patient to overcome this unpleasant side effect and continue a potentially curative protocol.

Vertigo is a feeling of whirling or rotation accompanied by involuntary swaying, weakness and lightheadedness. Motion sickness, a functional disorder, is caused by repetitive angular, linear or vertical motion. Both of these conditions are characterized by pallor, sweating, hyperventilation, nausea and vomiting.

The drugs that are effective as antiemetics are the **antidopaminergic** agents (phenothiazines, metoclopramide) which are especially effective for drug-induced emesis. **Anticholinergic agents** (antihistamines, trimethobenzamide, scopolamine) may be more appropriate in motion sickness, labyrinthine disorders, etc. Other agents, whose mechanisms are not known or that may act differently (eg, hydroxyzine, corticosteroids, cannabinoids), are effective in various types of emesis.

The preceding table indicates manufacturers' recommended uses for agents in this group. Several of these are indicated for uses other than as antiemetic/antivertigo agents. For a full discussion, see individual drug monographs.

Warnings/Precautions

➤*Benzyl alcohol:* Some of these products contain benzyl alcohol, which has been associated with a fatal "gasping syndrome" in premature infants.

➤*Severe emesis:* Severe emesis should not be treated with an antiemetic drug alone; where possible, establish cause of vomiting. Direct primary emphasis toward restoration of body fluids and electrolyte balance, and relief of fever and causative disease process. Avoid overhydration which may result in cerebral edema. Antiemetic effects may impede diagnosis of such conditions as brain tumors, intestinal obstruction and appendicitis, and may obscure signs of toxicity from overdosage of other drugs.

➤*Tartrazine sensitivity:* Some of these products contain tartrazine, which may cause allergic-type reactions (including bronchial asthma) in susceptible individuals. Although the incidence of sensitivity is low, it is frequently seen in patients who also have aspirin hypersensitivity. Specific products containing tartrazine are identified in the product listings.

➤*Sulfite sensitivity:* Some of these products contain sulfites which may cause allergic-type reactions (eg, hives, itching, wheezing, anaphylaxis) in certain susceptible people. Although the overall prevalence of sulfite sensitivity in the general population is probably low, it is seen more frequently in asthmatics or in atopic nonasthmatic people. Specific products containing sulfites are identified in the product listings.

➤*Children:* Not recommended for uncomplicated vomiting in children; limit use to prolonged vomiting of known etiology for three principal reasons:

1.) Although there is no confirmatory evidence, centrally-acting antiemetics may contribute, in combination with viral illnesses (a possible cause of vomiting in children), to the development of Reye's syndrome, a potentially fatal acute childhood encephalopathy. This syndrome follows a nonspecific febrile illness, and is characterized by an abrupt onset of persistent, severe vomiting, lethargy, irrational behavior, visceral fatty degeneration (especially involving the liver), progressive encephalopathy leading to coma, convulsions and death.
2.) The extrapyramidal symptoms that can occur secondary to some drugs may be confused with the CNS signs of an undiagnosed primary disease responsible for the vomiting, eg, Reye's syndrome or other encephalopathy.
3.) Drugs with hepatotoxic potential may unfavorably alter the course of Reye's syndrome. Avoid such drugs in children whose signs and symptoms (vomiting) could represent Reye's syndrome. It should also be noted that salicylates and acetaminophen are hepatotoxic at large doses. Although it is not known whether at usual doses they would represent a hazard in patients with the underlying hepatic disorder of Reye's syndrome, these drugs, too, should be avoided in children whose signs and symptoms could represent Reye's syndrome, unless alternative methods of controlling fever are not successful.

Children with acute illnesses (eg, chickenpox, CNS infections, measles, gastroenteritis) or dehydration seem to be much more susceptible to neuromuscular reactions, particularly dystonias, than are adults. In such patients, use antiemetics only under close supervision. Do not use dimenhydrinate in children less than 2 years of age unless directed by a doctor.

➤*Elderly:* **Scopolamine** is considered a high risk medication for the elderly according to the Centers of Medicare and Medicaid Services.

Patient Information

These agents may cause drowsiness; patients should observe caution while driving or performing other tasks requiring alertness.

Avoid alcohol and other CNS depressants.

Anticholinergics

CYCLIZINE

otc	**Bonine For Kids** (Insight Pharmaceuticals)	**Chewable, tablets; oral:** 25 mg	Mannitol, sorbitol, and sucralose. Berry blast flavor. In 8s.
otc	**Marezine** (Himmel)	**Tablets:** 50 mg (as HCl)	(Marezine T4A). Scored. In 12s and 100s.

CYCLIZINE — ORAL

For complete prescribing information, refer to the Antiemetic/Antivertigo Agents group monograph.

Indications

➤*Motion sickness:* For the prevention and treatment of the nausea, vomiting or dizziness associated with motion sickness.

Administration and Dosage

➤*General dosing considerations:* For prevention of motion sickness, take the first dose one-half hour before departure.

➤*Adults:*

Motion sickness –
Usual dosage: 50 mg every 4 to 6 hours.
Maximum dose: 200 mg/day.

➤*Children:*

Motion sickness – See Adults for dosing for children 12 years of age and older.

12 years of age and over:
- *Usual dose* – 50 mg every 4 to 6 hours.
- *Maximum dose* – 200 mg/day.

6 to younger than 12 years of age:
- *Usual dose* – 25 mg every 6 to 8 hours.
- *Maximum dose* – 75 mg/day.

➤*Storage/Stability:*

Marezine – Store at 15° to 25°C (59° to 77°F) in a dry place and protect from light.

Bonine – Store below 30°C (86°F).

CYCLIZINE — ORAL

Actions

➤*Pharmacology:* Cyclizine has antiemetic, anticholinergic, and antihistaminic properties. It reduces the sensitivity of the labyrinthine apparatus. The action may be mediated through nerve pathways to the vomiting center (VC) from the chemoreceptor trigger zone (CTZ), peripheral nerve pathways, the VC, or other CNS centers.

Cyclizine has an onset of action of 30 to 60 minutes, depending on dosage; the duration of action is 4 to 6 hours.

Contraindications

Contraindicated in patients with a hypersensitivity to cyclizine.

Do not use in patients with asthma, glaucoma, emphysema, chronic pulmonary disease, shortness of breath, difficulty in breathing or difficulty in urination due to enlargement of the prostate gland unless directed by a doctor. Cyclizine should not be used concurrently with sedatives, tranquilizers, or anticholinergic medications.

Warnings/Precautions

➤*Hypotension:* This drug may have a hypotensive action, which may be confusing or dangerous in postoperative patients.

➤*Special risk:* Do not take this product if you have asthma, glaucoma, emphysema, chronic pulmonary disease, shortness of breath, difficulty in breathing or difficulty in urination due to enlargement of the prostate gland unless directed by a doctor.

➤*Hazardous tasks:* May produce drowsiness; patients should observe caution while driving or performing other tasks requiring alertness.

➤*Pregnancy: Category B.* Cyclizine has been teratogenic in rodents, but large scale human studies have not demonstrated adverse fetal effects. Use only when clearly needed and when the potential benefits outweigh the potential hazards to the fetus.

➤*Lactation:* Safety for use in the nursing mother has not been established.

Drug Interactions

➤*CNS depressants:* May have additive effects with alcohol and other CNS depressants (eg, hypnotics, sedatives, tranquilizers, antianxiety agents); use with caution.

Overdosage

➤*Symptoms:* Moderate overdosage may cause hyperexcitability alternating with drowsiness. Massive overdosage may cause convulsions, hallucinations, and respiratory paralysis.

➤*Treatment:* Includes appropriate supportive and symptomatic treatment. Dialysis may be considered.

Caution – Do not use morphine or other respiratory depressants.

Patient Information

Do not take this product if you are taking sedatives, tranquilizers or anticholinergic drugs without first consulting with your doctor.

May cause drowsiness; alcohol, sedatives and tranquilizers may increase the drowsiness effect. Avoid alcoholic beverages while taking this product. Use caution when driving a motor vehicle or operating machinery.

As with any drug, if you are pregnant or nursing a baby, seek the advice of a health professional before using this product.

Not for frequent or prolonged use except on the advice of a doctor.

DIMENHYDRINATE

otc	**Dimenhydrinate** (Various)	**Tablets; oral:** 50 mg	In 12s, 100s, 300s, 500s, 1000s and UD 100s.
Rx	**Dimetabs** (Jones Medical)		In 1000s.
otc	**Dramamine** (McNeil Consumer)		(DRAMAMINE). White, scored. In UD 100s.
otc	**Triptone** (Del Pharmaceuticals)		Scored. In 12s.
otc	**Dramamine** (McNeil Consumer)	**Tablets, chewable; oral:** 50 mg	(DRAMAMINE).Tartrazine. Aspartame, sorbitol. Orange, scored. Orange flavor. In 8s and 24s.
otc	**Dimenhydrinate** (Various)	**Liquid; oral:** 12.5 mg per 4 ml	In pt and gal.
Rx	**Dimenhydrinate** (Abraxis)	**Injection:** 50 mg/ml	In 1 mL in 2 mL and 10 mL vials.[a]
Rx	**Dramanate** (Pasadena)		In 10 ml vials.[a]
Rx	**Dymenate** (Keene)		In 10 ml vials.[a]

[a] In benzyl alcohol and propylene glycol.

DIMENHYDRINATE — ORAL

Refer to the general discussion of these products beginning in the Antiemetic/Antivertigo group monograph.

Indications

➤*Motion sickness:* For the prevention and treatment of nausea, vomiting, and dizziness associated with motion sickness.

➤*Off-label uses:*

Nausea and vomiting of pregnancy – [2] = Fair documentation. The American College of Obstetricians and Gynecologists (ACOG) practice bulletin included dimenhydrinate among the recommended therapies for the management of nausea and vomiting of pregnancy. The recommended first-line treatment according to the ACOG is pyridoxine alone or pyridoxine combined with doxylamine. Additional pharmacologic interventions were recommended only for refractory cases.

Administration and Dosage

➤*General dosing considerations:* To prevent motion sickness, the first dose should be taken one-half to 1 hour before starting activity.

➤*Adults:*

Motion sickness –

Usual dosage: 50 to 100 mg every 4 to 6 hours.

Maximum dose: 400 mg/day.

Off-label dosing –

Nausea and vomiting of pregnancy: [2] = Fair documentation. 50 to 100 mg every 4 to 6 hours, not to exceed 400 mg/day, in patients refractory to pyridoxine and doxylamine. In patients taking concurrent doxylamine, the maximum recommended daily dose is 200 mg.

➤*Children:*

Motion sickness – See Adults for dosing for children 12 years of age and older.

6 years of age to younger than 12 years of age:
- *Usual dosage* – 25 to 50 mg every 6 to 8 hours.
- *Maximum dose* – 150 mg/day.

2 years of age to younger than 6 years of age:
- *Usual dosage* – 12.5 to 25 mg every 6 to 8 hours.
- *Maximum dose* – 75 mg/day.

➤*Storage/Stability:* Stored at room temperature. Patients should not use if the blister card is broken.

Actions

➤*Pharmacology:* Dimenhydrinate consists of equimolar proportions of diphenhydramine and chlorotheophylline.

➤*Pharmacokinetics:* Dimenhydrinate has a depressant action of hyperstimulated labyrinthine function. The precise mode of action is not known. The antiemetic effects are believed to be due to the diphenhydramine, an antihistamine also used as an antiemetic agent.

Warnings/Precautions

➤*Special risk:* Patients or parents of patients should ask a doctor before use if they or their children have breathing problems such as emphysema or chronic bronchitis, glaucoma, or difficulty in urination due to enlargement of the prostate gland.

➤*Use:* This medication is not for frequent or prolonged use except on advice of a doctor. Do not exceed recommended dosage.

➤*Benzyl alcohol:* Some of these products contain the preservative benzyl alcohol, which has been associated with a fatal "gasping syndrome" in premature infants.

➤*Tartrazine sensitivity:*

Chewable tablets – Dimenhydramine chewable tablets contain FD&C Yellow No. 5 (tartrazine) as a color additive.

➤*Hazardous tasks:* Patients should use caution when driving a motor vehicle or operating machinery.

➤*Pregnancy: Category B.* The ACOG practice bulletin included dimenhydrinate among the recommended therapies for the management of nausea and vomiting of pregnancy. (See Indications and Administration and Dosage.)

Safety for use during pregnancy has not been established. Patients should use only when clearly needed and when the potential benefits outweigh the potential hazards to the fetus.

➤*Lactation:* If breastfeeding, the patient should ask a health professional before use.

Small amounts of dimenhydrinate are excreted in breast milk. Because of the potential for adverse reactions in nursing infants, it should be decided whether to discontinue nursing or to discontinue the drug, taking into account the importance of the drug to the mother.

DIMENHYDRINATE — ORAL

➤*Children:* This medication should not be given to children under 2 years of age unless directed by a doctor.

Drug Interactions

Dimenhydrinate Drug Interactions

Precipitant drug	Object drug[a]		Description
Dimenhydrinate	Alcohol, CNS depressants	⬆	Concomitant use of alcohol or other CNS depressants with dimenhydrinate may have an additive effect.
Dimenhydrinate	Antibiotics	⬆	Use caution when given in conjunction with certain antibiotics that may cause ototoxicity; dimenhydrinate is capable of masking ototoxic symptoms, and irreversible damage may result.

[a] ⬆ = object drug increased.

Patients should ask a doctor or pharmacist before use if they are taking sedatives or tranquilizers.

Overdosage

➤*Symptoms:* Drowsiness is the usual side effect. Convulsions, coma, and respiratory depression may occur with massive overdosage.

➤*Treatment:* No specific antidote is known. If respiratory depression occurs, initiate mechanically assisted respiration and administer oxygen. Treat convulsions with appropriate doses of diazepam. Give phenobarbital (5 to 6 mg/kg) to control convulsions in children.

Patient Information

Do not use in children under 2 years of age unless directed by a doctor.

Ask a doctor before use if you have:
- A breathing problem such as emphysema or chronic bronchitis.
- Glaucoma.
- Difficulty in urination due to enlargement of the prostate gland.

Ask a doctor or pharmacist before use if you are taking sedatives or tranquilizers.

When using this product:
- Marked drowsiness may occur.
- Avoid alcoholic drinks.
- Alcohol, sedatives, and tranquilizers may increase drowsiness.
- Be careful when driving a motor vehicle or operating machinery.

DIMENHYDRINATE — INJECTION

Refer to the general discussion of these products beginning in the Antiemetic/Antivertigo group monograph.

Indications

➤*Motion sickness:* For the prevention and treatment of nausea, vomiting, or vertigo of motion sickness.

➤*Off-label uses:*

Nausea and vomiting of pregnancy – [2] = Fair documentation. The American College of Obstetricians and Gynecologists (ACOG) practice bulletin included dimenhydrinate among the recommended therapies for the management of nausea and vomiting of pregnancy. The recommended first-line treatment according to the ACOG is pyridoxine alone or pyridoxine combined with doxylamine. Additional pharmacologic interventions were recommended only for refractory cases.

Administration and Dosage

➤*General dosing considerations:* Dimenhydrinate in the injectable form is indicated when the oral form is impractical.

➤*Adults:*

Nausea, vomiting, or vertigo of motion sickness – 50 mg intravenously (IV) over 2 minutes or intramuscularly (IM) every 4 hours. Its administration may be attended by some degree of drowsiness in some patients.

100 mg IV over 2 minutes or IM every 4 hours may be given in conditions in which drowsiness is not objectionable or even desirable.

Off-label dosing –

Nausea and vomiting of pregnancy: [2] = Fair documentation. 50 mg in 50 mL of normal saline, administered IV over 20 minutes every 4 to 6 hours for women with refractory nausea and vomiting and dehydration.

➤*Children:* Some of these products contain benzyl alcohol. Benzyl alcohol has been associated with a fatal "gasping syndrome" in premature infants and infants of low birth weight.

Nausea, vomiting, or vertigo of motion sickness –

Children:
- *Usual dosage* – For IM administration, 1.25 mg/kg of body weight or 37.5 mg/m^2 of body surface area administered 4 times daily.
- *Maximum dose* – 300 mg/day.

Neonates: Do not treat neonates with dimenhydrinate.

➤*Preparation for administration:* For IV administration, each milliliter (50 mg) of solution must be diluted in 10 mL of sodium chloride 0.9% injection.

➤*Administration:* For IM administration, each milliliter (50 mg) of solution is injected as needed. For IV administration, inject diluted solution over a period of 2 minutes.

➤*Storage/Stability:* Store at 20° to 25°C (68° to 77°F). Protect from light.

Actions

➤*Pharmacology:* While the precise mode of action of dimenhydrinate is not known, it has a depressant action on hyperstimulated labyrinthine function.

Contraindications

Do not treat neonates or patients with a history of hypersensitivity to dimenhydrinate or its components (diphenhydramine or 8-chlorotheophylline).

Warnings/Precautions

➤*Drowsiness:* Drowsiness may be experienced by some patients, especially with high dosage. This effect frequently is not undesirable in conditions for which the drug is used.

➤*Administration:* Do not inject the preparation intra-arterially.

➤*Special risk:* Use caution when dimenhydrinate is given in conjunction with certain antibiotics that may cause ototoxicity because dimenhydrinate is capable of masking ototoxic symptoms, and an irreversible state may be reached.

Use dimenhydrinate with caution in patients with conditions that might be aggravated by anticholinergic therapy (eg, prostatic hypertrophy, stenosing peptic ulcer, pyloroduodenal obstruction, bladder neck obstruction, narrow-angle glaucoma, bronchial asthma, cardiac arrhythmias).

➤*Hazardous tasks:* This drug may impair the mental and/or physical abilities required for the performance of potentially hazardous tasks, such as driving a vehicle or operating machinery. The concomitant use of alcohol or other CNS depressants may have an additive effect. Warn patients accordingly.

➤*Pregnancy: Category B.* The ACOG practice bulletin included dimenhydrinate among the recommended therapies for the management of nausea and vomiting of pregnancy (See Indications and Administration and Dosage).

Reproduction studies have been performed in rats at doses up to 20 times the human dose, and in rabbits at doses up to 25 times the human dose (on a mg/kg basis), and have revealed no evidence of impaired fertility or harm to the fetus due to dimenhydrinate.

There are no adequate and well-controlled studies in pregnant women. However, clinical studies in pregnant women have not indicated that dimenhydrinate increases the risk of abnormalities when administered in any trimester of pregnancy. It would appear that the possibility of fetal harm is remote when the drug is used during pregnancy. Nevertheless, because the studies in humans cannot rule out the possibility of harm, use dimenhydrinate during pregnancy only if clearly needed.

Labor and delivery – The safety of dimenhydrinate given during labor and delivery has not been established. Reports have indicated dimenhydrinate may have an oxytocic effect. Caution is advised when this effect is unwanted or in situations where it may prove detrimental.

➤*Lactation:* Small amounts of dimenhydrinate are excreted in breast milk. Because of the potential for adverse reactions in breast-feeding infants from dimenhydrinate, decide whether to discontinue breast-feeding or discontinue the drug, taking into account the importance of the drug to the mother.

➤*Children:* As in adults, antihistamines may diminish mental alertness in pediatric patients. Particularly in the young child, they may produce excitation, hallucinations, convulsions, or death in overdose situations. Do not treat neonates with dimenhydrinate.

Note – Some of these products contain benzyl alcohol. Benzyl alcohol has been associated with a fatal "gasping syndrome" in premature infants and infants of low birth weight.

Adverse Reactions

The most frequent adverse reaction to dimenhydrinate is drowsiness. Dizziness may also occur. Symptoms of dry mouth, nose, and throat; blurred vision; difficult or painful urination; headache; anorexia; nervousness, restlessness, or insomnia (especially in pediatric patients); skin rash; thickening of bronchial secretions; tachycardia; epigastric distress; lassitude; excitation; and nausea have been reported.

Overdosage

➤*Symptoms:* Drowsiness is the usual clinical side effect. Convulsions, coma, and respiratory depression may occur with massive overdosage.

➤*Treatment:* No specific antidote is known. If respiratory depression occurs, initiate mechanically assisted respiration and administer oxygen. Treat convulsions with appropriate doses of diazepam. Phenobarbital (5 to 6 mg/kg) may be given to control convulsions in pediatric patients.

Patient Information

Because of the potential for drowsiness, caution patients taking dimenhydrinate against operating automobiles or dangerous machinery.

Anticholinergics

DIPHENHYDRAMINE

Refer to the general discussion of these products beginning in the Antiemetic/Antivertigo group monograph. Refer to the diphenhydramine monographs in the CNS chapter for information on antihistamines.

MECLIZINE

Rx	**Meclizine HCl** (Various)	**Tablets; oral:** 12.5 mg	In 30s, 60s, 100s, 500s, 1,000s, and UD 100s.
Rx	**Antivert** (Pfizer US)		(Antivert 210). In 100s, 1,000s, and UD 100s.
Rx	**Antrizine** (Major)		In 100s, 500s, and 1,000s.
otc/ Rx[a]	**Meclizine HCl** (Various)	**Tablets; oral:** 25 mg	In 12s, 20s, 30s, 60s, 100s, 500s, 1,000s, and UD 32s and 100s.
Rx	**Antivert/25** (Pfizer US)		(Antivert 211). In 100s, 1,000s, and UD 100s.
otc	**Dramamine Less Drowsy Formula** (McNeil Consumer)		Lactose. In 8s.
otc/ Rx[a]	**Meclizine HCl** (Various, eg, Goldline)	**Tablets, chewable; oral:** 25 mg	In 20s, 30s, 60s, 100s, 1,000s, and UD 100s.
otc	**Bonine** (Pfizer)		Lactose, saccharin. Raspberry flavor. In 8s.
Rx	**Meclizine HCl** (Various)	**Tablets; oral:** 50 mg	In 100s.
Rx	**Antivert/50** (Pfizer US)		(Antivert 214). Scored. In100s.

[a] Products are available *otc* or *Rx*, depending on product labeling.

MECLIZINE — ORAL

For complete prescribing information, refer to the Antiemetic/Antivertigo Agents group monograph.

Indications

➤*Motion sickness:* For the prevention and treatment of nausea, vomiting, or dizziness associated with motion sickness.

➤*Vertigo:* Meclizine is "possibly effective" for the management of vertigo associated with diseases affecting the vestibular system.

Administration and Dosage

➤*General dosing considerations:* For prevention of motion sickness, take the first dose 1 hour before departure.

➤*Adults:*

Motion sickness –

Maximum dose: 2 tablets daily.

Initial dosage: 25 to 50 mg taken 1 hour prior to travel for protection against motion sickness.

Maintenance dosage: The dose may be repeated every 24 hours for the duration of the journey.

Vertigo – 25 to 100 mg daily in divided doses.

➤*Children:* See Adults for dosing for children 12 years of age and older.

➤*Administration:* Chewable tablets may be chewed or swallowed with water.

➤*Storage/Stability:*

Tablets – Store at 15° to 30°C (59° to 86°F). Dispense in tight, light-resistant containers.

Chewable tablets – Store below 30°C (86°F).

Actions

➤*Pharmacology:* Meclizine HCl is an antihistamine which shows marked protective activity against nebulized histamine and lethal doses of IV injected histamine in guinea pigs. It has a marked effect in blocking the vasopressor response to histamine but only a slight blocking action against acetylcholine. Its activity is relatively weak in inhibiting the spasmogenic action of histamine on isolated guinea pig ileum.

➤*Pharmacokinetics:* Meclizine tablets have an onset of action of 30 to 60 minutes, depending on dosage; their duration of action is 4 to 6 hours and 12 to 24 hours, respectively.

Contraindications

Hypersensitivity to meclizine.

Warnings/Precautions

➤*Tartrazine sensitivity:* The meclizine HCl 25 mg and 50 mg tablets may contain FD&C Yellow No. 5 (tartrazine), which may cause allergic-type reactions (including bronchial asthma) in certain susceptible individuals. Although the overall incidence of FD&C Yellow No. 5 (tartrazine) sensitivity in the general population is low, it is frequently seen in patients who also have aspirin hypersensitivity.

➤*Special risk:* Due to its potential anticholinergic action, this drug should be used with caution in patients with asthma, emphysema, chronic bronchitis, glaucoma, or enlargement of the prostate gland.

➤*Hazardous tasks:* Since drowsiness may, on occasion, occur with use of this drug, patients should be warned of this possibility and cautioned against driving a car or operating dangerous machinery.

➤*Pregnancy: Category B.* Reproduction studies in rats have shown cleft palates at 25 to 50 times the human dose. Epidemiological studies in pregnant women, however, do not indicate that meclizine HCl increases the risk of abnormalities when administered during pregnancy. Despite the animal findings, it would appear that the possibility of fetal harm is remote. Nevertheless, meclizine HCl, or any other medication, should be used during pregnancy only if clearly necessary.

Patients should contact a health professional before using this medication if they are pregnant.

➤*Lactation:* Patients should contact a health professional before using this medication if they are breastfeeding.

➤*Children:* Clinical studies establishing safety and effectiveness in children have not been done; therefore, use is not recommended in children under 12 years of age.

Drug Interactions

Patients should avoid alcoholic beverages while taking this drug. Alcohol, sedatives, and tranquilizers may increase drowsiness.

Adverse Reactions

➤*Cardiovascular:* Hypotension; palpitations; tachycardia.

➤*CNS:* Drowsiness; restlessness; excitation; nervousness; insomnia; euphoria; blurred vision; diplopia; vertigo; tinnitus; auditory and visual hallucinations (particularly when dosage recommendations are exceeded).

➤*Dermatologic:* Urticaria; rash.

➤*GI:* Dry mouth; anorexia; nausea; vomiting; diarrhea; constipation; cholestatic jaundice (cyclizine).

➤*GU:* Urinary frequency; difficult urination; urinary retention.

➤*Miscellaneous:* Dry nose and throat.

Overdosage

➤*Symptoms:* Moderate overdosage may cause hyperexcitability alternating with drowsiness. Massive overdosage may cause convulsions, hallucinations and respiratory paralysis.

➤*Treatment:* Includes appropriate supportive and symptomatic treatment. In case of accidental overdose, seek professional assistance or contact a poison control center immediately.

Do not use morphine or other respiratory depressants.

Patient Information

➤*Chewable tablets:* Do not give this medication to children under 12 years of age unless directed by a doctor. Keep this medication out of the reach of children.

Ask a doctor before use if you have:
- Glaucoma.
- Breathing problems such as emphysema or chronic bronchitis.
- Trouble in urination due to enlargement of the prostate gland.

Ask a doctor or pharmacist before use if you are taking tranquilizers or sedatives.

When using this product:
- You may get drowsy.
- Avoid alcoholic beverages.
- Alcohol, sedatives, and tranquilizers may increase drowsiness.
- Do not drive or operate dangerous machinery.

If you are pregnant or breastfeeding, ask a health professional before use.

In case of overdose, get medical help or contact a poison control center right away.

SCOPOLAMINE — ORAL

For complete prescribing information, refer to the oral Scopolamine monograph in the GI Anticholinergics section.

SCOPOLAMINE — TRANSDERMAL

Rx	Transderm-Scōp (Baxter)	Transdermal patch: 1.5 mg scopolamine (delivers approximately 1 mg scopolamine over 3 days)	In 10s and 24s.

SCOPOLAMINE — TRANSDERMAL

Refer to the general discussion of these products beginning in the Antiemetic/Antivertigo group monograph.

Indications

➤*Motion sickness:* Prevention of nausea and vomiting associated with motion sickness.

Prevention of postoperative nausea and vomiting – Prevention of nausea and vomiting associated with recovery from anesthesia and surgery in adults.

➤*Off-label uses:*

Sialorrhea (drooling) – [1] = Good documentation. Although the cause of sialorrhea should be considered when selecting treatment options (ie, behavioral vs pharmacological), scopolamine transdermal patch appears to be an effective option in the disabled population or in those patients who have swallowing difficulties. (See Administration and Dosage.)

Administration and Dosage

➤*General dosing considerations:* Approximately scopolamine 1 mg will be delivered over 3 days. Wear only one disc at a time. Do not cut the patch.

➤*Adults:*

Prevention of nausea and vomiting – Apply one system to the postauricular skin (ie, behind the ear) at least 4 hours before the antiemetic effect is required.

Prevention of postoperative nausea and vomiting – Apply the patch the evening before scheduled surgery. To minimize exposure of the newborn to the drug, apply the patch 1 hour prior to cesarean section.

Perioperative use – Keep the patch in place for 24 hours following surgery; then remove and discard.

➤*Children:*

Off-label dosing –

Sialorrhea (drooling): [1] = Good documentation. 1.5 mg patch every 3 days.

➤*Elderly:* Use with caution in the elderly because of the increased likelihood of CNS effects.

➤*Renal function impairment:* Use with caution in individuals with impaired kidney function because of the increased likelihood of CNS effects.

➤*Hepatic function impairment:* Use with caution in individuals with impaired liver function because of the increased likelihood of CNS effects.

➤*Administration:* Wear only one disc at a time. Do not cut the patch.

For motion sickness, if therapy is required for more than 3 days, discard the first disc and place a fresh one on the hairless area behind the other ear.

If the disc is displaced, discard it and place a fresh one on the hairless area behind the other ear.

Handling – After applying the disc on dry skin behind the ear, wash hands thoroughly with soap and water and then dry them. Discard the removed disc and wash the hands and application site thoroughly with soap and water to prevent any traces of scopolamine from coming into direct contact with the eyes.

➤*Storage/Stability:* Store at 20° to 25°C (68° to 77°F).

Actions

➤*Pharmacology:* The sole active agent is scopolamine, a belladonna alkaloid with well-known pharmacological properties. It is an anticholinergic agent which acts as a competitive inhibitor at postganglionic muscarinic receptor sites of the parasympathetic nervous system, and on smooth muscles that respond to acetylcholine but lack cholinergic innervation. It has been suggested that scopolamine acts in the CNS by blocking cholinergic transmission from the vestibular nuclei to higher centers in the CNS and from the reticular formation to the vomiting center. Scopolamine can inhibit the secretion of saliva and sweat, decrease GI secretions and motility, cause drowsiness, dilate the pupils, increase heart rate, and depress motor function.

➤*Pharmacokinetics:*

Absorption – Scopolamine's activity is due to the parent drug. The pharmacokinetics of scopolamine delivered via the system are due to the characteristics of both the drug and dosage form. The system is programmed to deliver in vivo ≈ 1 mg of scopolamine at an approximately constant rate to the systemic circulation over 3 days. Upon application to the postauricular skin, an initial priming dose of scopolamine is released from the adhesive layer to saturate skin binding sites. The subsequent delivery of scopolamine to the blood is determined by the rate-controlling membrane and is designed to produce stable plasma levels in a therapeutic range. Following removal of the used system, there is some degree of continued systemic absorption of scopolamine bound in the skin layers.

Scopolamine is well absorbed percutaneously. Following application to the skin behind the ear, circulating plasma levels are detected within 4 hours with peak levels being obtained, on average, within 24 hours. The average plasma concentration produced is 87 pg/mL for free scopolamine and 354 pg/mL for total scopolamine (free + conjugates).

Distribution – The distribution of scopolamine is not well characterized. It crosses the placenta and the blood-brain barrier and may be reversibly bound to plasma proteins.

Metabolism – Although not well characterized, scopolamine is extensively metabolized and conjugated with less than 5% of the total dose appearing unchanged in the urine.

Excretion – The exact elimination pattern of scopolamine has not been determined. Following patch removal, plasma levels decline in a log linear fashion with an observed half-life of 9.5 hours; less than 10% of the total dose is excreted in the urine as parent and metabolites over 108 hours.

Contraindications

Hypersensitivity to scopolamine or other belladonna alkaloids, or any ingredient or component in the formulation or delivery system, or in patients with angle-closure (narrow angle) glaucoma.

Warnings/Precautions

➤*Ophthalmic effects:* Glaucoma therapy in patients with chronic open-angle (wide-angle) glaucoma should be monitored and may need to be adjusted during scopolamine use, as the mydriatic effect of scopolamine may cause an increase in intraocular pressure.

➤*Idiosyncratic reactions:* Rarely, idiosyncratic reactions may occur with ordinary therapeutic doses of scopolamine. The most serious of these that have been reported are acute toxic psychosis, including confusion, agitation, rambling speech, hallucinations, paranoid behaviors, and delusions.

➤*Special risk:* Scopolamine should be used with caution in patients with pyloric obstruction or urinary bladder neck obstruction. Caution should be exercised when administering an antiemetic or antimuscarinic drug to patients suspected of having intestinal obstruction.

Scopolamine should be used with caution in the elderly or in individuals with impaired liver or kidney functions because of the increased likelihood of CNS effects.

Caution should be exercised in patients with a history of seizures or psychosis, since scopolamine can potentially aggravate both disorders.

➤*Hazardous tasks:* Since drowsiness, disorientation, and confusion may occur with the use of scopolamine, patients should be warned of the possibility and cautioned against engaging in activities that require mental alertness, such as driving a motor vehicle or operating dangerous machinery.

➤*Pregnancy: Category C.* Scopolamine hydrobromide has been shown to have a marginal embryotoxic effect in rabbits when administered by daily IV injection at doses producing plasma levels ≈ 100 times the level achieved in humans using a transdermal system. During a clinical study among women undergoing cesarean section treated with scopolamine in conjunction with epidural anesthesia and opiate analgesia, no evidence of CNS depression was found in the newborns. There are no other adequate and well-controlled studies in pregnant women. Other than in the adjunctive use for delivery by cesarean section, scopolamine should be used in pregnancy only if the potential benefit justifies the potential risk to the fetus.

Teratogenic – Teratogenic studies were performed in pregnant rats and rabbits with scopolamine hydrobromide administered by daily IV injection. No adverse effects were recorded in rats.

➤*Lactation:* Because scopolamine is excreted in human milk, caution should be exercised when scopolamine is administered to a nursing woman.

➤*Children:* The safety and effectiveness of scopolamine in children has not been established. Children are particularly susceptible to the side effects of belladonna alkaloids. Scopolamine should not be used in children because it is not known whether this system will release an amount of scopolamine that could produce serious adverse effects in children.

➤*Elderly:* Scopolamine should be used with caution in the elderly.

Scopolamine is considered a high risk medication for the elderly according to the Centers of Medicare and Medicaid Services.

Drug Interactions

The absorption of oral medications may be decreased during the concurrent use of scopolamine because of decreased gastric motility and delayed gastric emptying.

Scopolamine should be used with care in patients taking other drugs that are capable of causing CNS effects such as sedatives, tranquilizers, or alcohol. Special attention should be paid to potential interactions with drugs having anticholinergic properties (eg, other belladonna alkaloids, antihistamines, (including meclizine) tricyclic antidepressants, and muscle relaxants).

➤*Drug/Lab test interactions:* Scopolamine will interfere with the gastric secretion test.

Adverse Reactions

➤*Motion sickness:* In motion sickness clinical studies of scopolamine, the most frequent adverse reaction was dryness of the mouth. This occurred in about two-thirds of patients on the drug. A less frequent adverse drug reaction was drowsiness, which occurred in less than one-sixth of patients on the

SCOPOLAMINE — TRANSDERMAL

drug. Transient impairment of eye accommodation, including blurred vision and dilation of the pupils, was also observed.

➤*Postoperative nausea and vomiting:* In a total of 5 clinical studies in which scopolamine was administered perioperatively to a total of 461 patients and safety was assessed, dry mouth was the most frequently reported adverse drug experience, which occurred in ≈ 29% of patients on the drug. Dizziness was reported by ≈ 12% of patients on the drug.

➤*Postmarketing:* In addition to the adverse experiences reported during clinical testing of scopolamine, the following are spontaneously reported adverse events from postmarketing experience. Because the reports cite events reported spontaneously from worldwide postmarketing experience, frequency of events and the role of scopolamine in their causation cannot be reliably determined: Acute angle-closure (narrow-angle) glaucoma; confusion; difficulty urinating; dry, itchy, or conjunctival injection of eyes; restlessness; hallucinations; memory disturbances; rashes and erythema; and transient changes in heart rate.

➤*Drug withdrawal/postremoval symptoms:* Symptoms such as dizziness, nausea, vomiting, and headache occur following abrupt discontinuation of antimuscarinics. Similar symptoms, including disturbances of equilibrium, have been reported in some patients following discontinuation of use of the scopolamine system. These symptoms usually do not appear until 24 hours or more after the patch has been removed. Some symptoms may be related to adaptation from a motion environment to a motion-free environment. More serious symptoms including muscle weakness, bradycardia and hypotension may occur following discontinuation of scopolamine.

Overdosage

➤*Symptoms:* The signs and symptoms of anticholinergic toxicity include lethargy, somnolence, coma, confusion, agitation, hallucinations, convulsion, visual disturbance, dry flushed skin, dry mouth, decreased bowel sounds, urinary retention, tachycardia, hypertension, and supraventricular arrhythmias.

The symptoms of overdose/toxicity due to scopolamine should be carefully distinguished from the occasionally observed syndrome of withdrawal (see Adverse Reactions). Although mental confusion and dizziness may be observed with both acute toxicity and withdrawal, other characteristic findings differ: Tachyarrhythmias, dry skin, and decreased bowel sounds suggest anticholinergic toxicity, while bradycardia, headache, nausea and abdominal cramps, and sweating suggest post-removal withdrawal. Obtaining a careful history is crucial to making the correct diagnosis.

➤*Treatment:* Because strategies for the management of drug overdose continually evolve, it is strongly recommended that a poison control center be contacted to obtain up-to-date information regarding the management of scopolamine patch overdose. The prescriber should be mindful that antidotes used routinely in the past may no longer be considered optimal treatment. For example, physostigmine, used more or less routinely in the past, is seldom recommended for the routine management of anticholinergic syndromes.

Until up-to-date authoritative advice is obtained, routine supportive measures should be directed to maintaining adequate respiratory and cardiac function.

Most cases of toxicity involving the use of the product will resolve with simple removal of the patch. Serious symptomatic cases of overdosage involving multiple patch applications or ingestion may be managed by initially ensuring the patient has an adequate airway, and supporting respiration and circulation. This should be rapidly followed by removal of all patches from the skin and the mouth. If there is evidence of patch ingestion, gastric lavage, endoscopic removal of swallowed patches, or administration of activated charcoal should be considered, as indicated by the clinical situation. In any case where there is serious overdosage or signs of evolving acute toxicity, continuous monitoring of vital signs and ECG, establishment of IV access, and administration of oxygen are all recommended.

Patient Information

Since scopolamine can cause temporary dilation of the pupils and blurred vision if it comes in contact with the eyes, patients should be strongly advised to wash their hands thoroughly with soap and water immediately after handling the patch. In addition, it is important that used patches be disposed of properly to avoid contact with children or pets.

Patients should be advised to remove the patch immediately and promptly and to contact a physician in the unlikely event that they experience symptoms of acute narrow-angle glaucoma (pain and reddening of the eyes, accompanied by dilated pupils). Patients should also be instructed to remove the patch if they develop any difficulties in urinating.

Patients who expect to participate in underwater sports should be cautioned regarding the potentially disorienting effects of scopolamine. A patient brochure is available.

TRIMETHOBENZAMIDE HYDROCHLORIDE

Rx	**Trimethobenzamide** (Various, eg, Amide, Mutual)	**Capsules; oral:** 300 mg	In 100, 250s, 500s, 1000s, UD 30s, and UD 60s.
Rx	**Tigan** (Monarch)		(Tigan MO79). Purple. In 100s.
Rx	**Trimethobenzamide HCl** (Various)	**Injection:** 100 mg/mL	In 2 mL amps and 20 mL vials.
Rx	**Tigan** (JHP Pharm)		In 2 mL amps[a], 20 mL vials,[b] and 2 mL syringe.[c]

[a] With methyl- and propylparabens.
[b] With phenol.
[c] With phenol and EDTA.

TRIMETHOBENZAMIDE HYDROCHLORIDE — ORAL

Refer to the general discussion of these products beginning in the Antiemetic/Antivertigo monograph.

Indications

➤*Nausea/Vomiting:* For the treatment of postoperative nausea and vomiting and for nausea associated with gastroenteritis.

Administration and Dosage

➤*Adults:*

Nausea and vomiting – 300 mg 3 or 4 times daily.

➤*Children:* Use with caution. Antiemetics are not recommended for the treatment of uncomplicated vomiting in children. See Warnings/Precautions.

➤*Storage/Stability:* Store at 20° to 25°C (68° to 77°F). Dispense in a tight, light-resistant container.

Actions

➤*Pharmacology:* The mechanism of action of trimethobenzamide as determined in animals is obscure, but may involve the chemoreceptor trigger zone (CTZ), an area in the medulla oblongata through which emetic impulses are conveyed to the vomiting center; direct impulses to the vomiting center apparently are not similarly inhibited. In dogs pretreated with trimethobenzamide, the emetic response to apomorphine is inhibited, while little or no protection is afforded against emesis induced by intragastric copper sulfate.

➤*Pharmacokinetics:*

Absorption – The pharmacokinetics of trimethobenzamide have been studied in healthy adult subjects. Following administration of 200 mg (100 mg/mL) trimethobenzamide IM injection, the time to reach maximum plasma concentration (t_{max}) was about 30 minutes, about 15 minutes longer for 300 mg trimethobenzamide oral capsule than an IM injection. A single dose of 300 mg trimethobenzamide oral capsule provided a plasma concentration profile of trimethobenzamide similar to 200 mg trimethobenzamide IM. The relative bioavailability of the capsule formulation compared to the solution is 100%.

Excretion – The mean elimination half-life of trimethobenzamide is 7 to 9 hours.

Contraindications

Hypersensitivity to trimethobenzamide.

Warnings/Precautions

➤*Special risk:* During the course of acute febrile illness, encephalitides, gastroenteritis, dehydration and electrolyte imbalance, especially in children and the elderly or debilitated, CNS reactions such as opisthotonos, convulsions, coma and extrapyramidal symptoms have been reported with and without use of trimethobenzamide or other antiemetic agents. In such disorders, exercise caution in administering trimethobenzamide, particularly to patients who recently received other CNS-acting agents (phenothiazines, barbiturates, belladonna derivatives). It is recommended that severe emesis not be treated with an antiemetic drug alone; where possible the cause of vomiting should be established. Direct primary emphasis toward the restoration of body fluids and electrolyte balance, the relief of fever and relief of the causative disease process. Avoid overhydration because it may result in cerebral edema.

The antiemetic effects of trimethobenzamide may render diagnosis more difficult in such conditions as appendicitis and obscure signs of toxicity due to overdosage of other drugs.

Reye's syndrome – Reye's syndrome has been associated with the use of trimethobenzamide and other drugs, including antiemetics, although their contribution, if any, to the cause and course of the disease has not been established. This syndrome is characterized by an abrupt onset shortly following a non-specific febrile illness, with persistent, severe vomiting, lethargy, irrational behavior, progressive encephalopathy leading to coma, convulsions, and death.

➤*Hazardous tasks:* Trimethobenzamide may produce drowsiness. Patients should not operate motor vehicles or other dangerous machinery until their individual responses have been determined.

➤*Pregnancy: Category C.* Trimethobenzamide was studied in reproduction experiments in rats and rabbits and no teratogenicity was suggested. The only effects observed were an increased percentage of embryonic resorptions or stillborn pups in rats administered 20 mg and 100 mg/kg and increased resorptions in rabbits receiving 100 mg/kg. In each study these adverse effects were attributed to 1 or 2 dams. The relevance to humans is not known. Since there is no adequate experience in pregnant women who have received this drug, safety in pregnancy has not been established.

TRIMETHOBENZAMIDE HYDROCHLORIDE — ORAL

➤*Lactation:* Since there is no adequate experience in lactating women who have received this drug, safety in nursing mothers has not been established.

➤*Children:* Exercise caution when administering trimethobenzamide to children for the treatment of vomiting. Antiemetics are not recommended for treatment of uncomplicated vomiting in children. Limit their use to prolonged vomiting of known etiology. There are 2 principal reasons for caution:

1.) The extrapyramidal symptoms which can occur secondary to trimethobenzamide may be confused with the central nervous system signs of an undiagnosed primary disease responsible for the vomiting (eg, Reye's syndrome or other encephalopathy).
2.) It has been suspected that drugs with hepatotoxic potential, such as trimethobenzamide, may unfavorably alter the course of Reye's syndrome. Therefore, avoid such drugs in children whose signs and symptoms (vomiting) could represent Reye's syndrome.

➤*Elderly:* Per the Beers list, trimethobenzamide is one of the least effective antiemetic drugs, yet it can cause extrapyramidal adverse effects. Trimethobenzamide is also considered a high risk medication for the elderly according to the Centers of Medicare and Medicaid Services.

Drug Interactions

➤*Use with alcohol:* Concomitant use of alcohol with trimethobenzamide may result in an adverse drug interaction.

Adverse Reactions

There have been reports of hypersensitivity reactions and Parkinson-like symptoms. There have been instances of hypotension reported following parenteral administration to surgical patients. There have been reports of blood dyscrasias, blurring of vision, coma, convulsions, depression of mood, diarrhea, disorientation, dizziness, drowsiness, headache, jaundice, muscle cramps and opisthotonos. If these occur, discontinue the administration of the drug. Allergic-type skin reactions have been observed; therefore, discontinue the drug at the first sign of sensitization. While these symptoms will usually disappear spontaneously, symptomatic treatment may be indicated in some cases.

Patient Information

Trimethobenzamide may produce drowsiness. Do not operate motor vehicles or other dangerous machinery until their individual responses have been determined.

TRIMETHOBENZAMIDE HYDROCHLORIDE — INJECTION

Refer to the general discussion of these products beginning in the Antiemetic/Antivertigo monograph.

Indications

➤*Nausea/Vomiting:* For the treatment of postoperative nausea and vomiting and for nausea associated with gastroenteritis.

Administration and Dosage

➤*Adults:*

Nausea and vomiting –

Postoperative: 200 mg intramuscular (IM), followed 1 hour later by a second 200 mg IM injection.

Secondary to gastritis: 200 mg IM.

➤*Children:* Use with caution. See Warnings/Precautions.

➤*Administration:* The injectable form is intended for IM administration only; it is not recommended for intravenous (IV) use.

IM administration may cause pain, stinging, burning, redness, and swelling at the injection site. Such effects may be minimized by deep injection into the upper-outer quadrant of the gluteal region and by avoiding the escape of solution along the route.

➤*Storage/Stability:* Store at room temperature up to 30°C (86°F).

Actions

➤*Pharmacology:* The mechanism of action of trimethobenzamide hydrochloride as determined in animals is obscure, but may be the chemoreceptor trigger zone (CTZ), an area in the medulla oblongata through which emetic impulses are conveyed to the vomiting center; direct impulses to the vomiting center apparently are not similarly inhibited. In dogs pretreated with trimethobenzamide hydrochloride, the emetic response to apomorphine is inhibited, while little or no protection is afforded against emesis induced by intragastric copper sulfate.

➤*Pharmacokinetics:*

Absorption – Oral and parenteral trimethobenzamide are not bioequivalent. An oral dose of 400 mg of trimethobenzamide yields plasma levels approximately equivalent to a 200 mg IM dose.

The pharmacokinetics of trimethobenzamide have been studied in healthy adult subjects. Following administration of 200 mg (100 mg/mL) trimethobenzamide hydrochloride IM injection, the time to reach maximum plasma concentration (t_{max}) was about half an hour, about 15 minutes longer for trimethobenzamide hydrochloride 300 mg oral capsule than an IM injection. A single dose of trimethobenzamide hydrochloride 300 mg oral capsule provided a plasma concentration profile of trimethobenzamide similar to trimethobenzamide hydrochloride 200 mg IM. The relative bioavailability of the capsule formulation compared to the solution is 100%. The mean elimination half-life of trimethobenzamide is 7 to 9 hours.

Contraindications

Pediatric patients; hypersensitivity to trimethobenzamide.

Warnings/Precautions

➤*Reye's syndrome:* Reye's syndrome has been associated with the use of trimethobenzamide hydrochloride and other drugs, including antiemetics, although their contribution, if any, to the cause and course of the disease has not been established. This syndrome is characterized by an abrupt onset shortly following a nonspecific febrile illness, with persistent, severe vomiting, lethargy, irrational behavior, progressive encephalopathy leading to coma, convulsions, and death.

➤*Special risk:* The antiemetic effects of trimethobenzamide hydrochloride may render diagnosis more difficult in such conditions as appendicitis and obscure signs of toxicity due to overdosage of other drugs.

During the course of acute febrile illness, encephalitides, gastroenteritis, dehydration and electrolyte imbalance, especially in children and the elderly or debilitated, CNS reactions such as opisthotonos, convulsions, coma and extrapyramidal symptoms have been reported with and without use of trimethobenzamide hydrochloride or other antiemetic agents. In such disorders, caution should be exercised in administering trimethobenzamide hydrochloride, particularly to patients who recently received other CNS-acting agents (phenothiazines, barbiturates, belladonna derivatives). It is recommended that severe emesis should not be treated with an antiemetic drug alone; where possible the cause of vomiting should be established. Primary emphasis should be directed toward the restoration of body fluids and electrolyte balance, the relief of fever and relief of the causative disease process. Overhydration should be avoided since it may result in cerebral edema.

➤*Hazardous tasks:* Trimethobenzamide hydrochloride may produce drowsiness. Patients should not operate motor vehicles or other dangerous machinery until their individual responses have been determined.

➤*Pregnancy: Category C.* Trimethobenzamide hydrochloride was studied in reproduction experiments in rats and rabbits and no teratogenicity was suggested. The only effects observed were an increased percentage of embryonic resorptions or stillborn pups in rats administered 20 mg and 100 mg/kg and increased resorptions in rabbits receiving 100 mg/kg. In each study these adverse effects were attributed to 1 or 2 dams. The relevance to humans is not known. Since there is no adequate experience in pregnant women who have received this drug, safety in pregnancy has not been established.

➤*Lactation:* Since there is no adequate experience in lactating women who have received this drug, safety in nursing mothers has not been established.

➤*Children:* Caution should be exercised when administering trimethobenzamide hydrochloride to children for the treatment of vomiting. Antiemetics are not recommended for treatment of uncomplicated vomiting in children and their use should be limited to prolonged vomiting of known etiology. There are 3 principal reasons for caution:

1.) There has been some suspicion that centrally acting antiemetics may contribute, in combination with viral illnesses (a possible cause of vomiting in pediatric patients), to development of Reye's syndrome, a potentially fatal acute childhood encephalopathy with visceral fatty degeneration, especially involving the liver. Although there is no confirmation of this suspicion, caution is nevertheless recommended.
2.) The extrapyramidal symptoms which can occur secondary to trimethobenzamide hydrochloride may be confused with the central nervous system signs of an undiagnosed primary disease responsible for the vomiting (eg, Reye's syndrome or other encephalopathy).
3.) It has been suspected that drugs with hepatotoxic potential, such as trimethobenzamide hydrochloride, may unfavorably alter the course of Reye's syndrome. Such drugs should therefore be avoided in pediatric patients whose signs and symptoms (vomiting) could represent Reye's syndrome. It should also be noted that salicylates and acetaminophen are hepatotoxic at large doses. Although it is not known that at usual doses they would represent a hazard in patients with the underlying hepatic disorder of Reye's syndrome, these drugs, too, should be avoided in pediatric patients whose signs and symptoms could represent Reye's syndrome, unless alternative methods of controlling fever are not successful.

➤*Elderly:* Per the Beers list, trimethobenzamide is one of the least effective antiemetic drugs, yet it can cause extrapyramidal adverse effects. Trimethobenzamide is also considered a high risk medication for the elderly according to the Centers of Medicare and Medicaid Services.

Drug Interactions

➤*Use with alcohol:* Concomitant use of alcohol with trimethobenzamide hydrochloride may result in an adverse drug interaction.

Adverse Reactions

There have been reports of hypersensitivity reactions and Parkinson-like symptoms. There have been instances of hypotension reported following parenteral administration to surgical patients. There have been reports of blood dyscrasias, blurring of vision, coma, convulsions, depression of mood, diarrhea, disorientation, dizziness, drowsiness, headache, jaundice, muscle cramps and opisthotonos. If these occur, the administration of the drug should be discontinued. Allergic-type skin reactions have been observed; therefore, the drug should be discontinued at the first sign of sensitization. While these symptoms will usually disappear spontaneously, symptomatic treatment may be indicated in some cases.

WARNING

Alosetron – Infrequent but serious GI adverse reactions have been reported with the use of alosetron. These reactions, including ischemic colitis and serious complications of constipation, have resulted in hospitalization and, rarely, blood transfusion, surgery, and death.

- The prescribing program for alosetron was implemented to help reduce risks of serious GI adverse reactions. Only health care providers who have enrolled in the manufacturer's prescribing program for alosetron, based on their understanding of the benefits and risks, should prescribe alosetron.
- Alosetron is indicated only for women with severe diarrhea–predominant irritable bowel syndrome (IBS) who have not responded adequately to conventional therapy. Before receiving the initial prescription for alosetron, the patient must read and sign the patient-physician agreement for alosetron.
- Discontinue alosetron immediately in patients who develop constipation or symptoms of ischemic colitis. Patients should immediately report constipation or symptoms of ischemic colitis to their health care provider. Do not resume alosetron in patients who develop ischemic colitis. Patients who have constipation should immediately contact their health care provider if the constipation does not resolve after alosetron is discontinued. Patients with resolved constipation should resume alosetron only on the advice of their treating health care provider.

Indications

➤*Antiemetic (except alosetron):* Prevention of nausea and vomiting associated with initial and repeat courses of emetogenic cancer therapy, including high-dose cisplatin; prevention of postoperative nausea or vomiting (**ondansetron**, **dolasetron**, and **granisetron** intravenous [IV]); prevention of nausea and vomiting associated with radiotherapy, including total body irradiation, fractionated abdominal radiation, or daily fractions to the abdomen (oral ondansetron, oral granisetron); treatment of postoperative nausea or vomiting (dolasetron IV, granisetron IV); prevention of acute and/or delayed nausea and vomiting associated with initial and repeat courses of emetogenic cancer chemotherapy (**palonosetron**).

➤*IBS (alosetron only):* For women with severe diarrhea–predominant IBS who have chronic IBS symptoms (generally lasting 6 months or longer), have had anatomic or biochemical abnormalities of the GI tract excluded, and have not responded adequately to conventional therapy.

➤*Off-label uses:* Refer to individual monographs for further information.

Alcohol consumption/effects –
Ondansetron: [4] = Insufficient documentation.

Bulimia –
Ondansetron: [4] = Insufficient documentation.

Cancer-related pruritus –
Granisetron: [4] = Insufficient documentation.

Cholestatic pruritus (adults) –
Ondansetron: [4] = Insufficient documentation.

Cholestatic pruritus (pregnancy) –
Ondansetron: [4] = Insufficient documentation.

Cholestatic pruritus (children) –
Ondansetron: [4] = Insufficient documentation.

Hyperemesis gravidarum –
Ondansetron: [4] = Insufficient documentation.

Melanocytic nevi–related pruritus (children) –
Ondansetron: [4] = Insufficient documentation.

Nausea and vomiting of pregnancy –
Ondansetron: [2] = Fair documentation.

Postanesthetic shivering –
Dolasetron: [5] = Poor documentation.
Granisetron: [4] = Insufficient documentation.
Ondansetron: [2] = Fair documentation.

Prevention of spinal opioid–related pruritus –
Dolasetron: [4] = Insufficient documentation.
Granisetron: [5] = Poor documentation.

Rectal administration –
Ondansetron: [2] = Fair documentation.

Tardive dyskinesia –
Ondansetron: [4] = Insufficient documentation.

Treatment of migraine (adults) –
Granisetron: [5] = Poor documentation.

Treatment of migraine –
Ondansetron: [5] = Poor documentation.

Uremic pruritus (adults) –
Granisetron: [4] = Insufficient documentation.
Ondansetron: [4] = Insufficient documentation.

Uremic pruritus (children/adolescents) –
Ondansetron: [4] = Insufficient documentation.

Other possible off-label uses –
Dolasetron: Prevention of radiation-induced nausea and vomiting; radiotherapy-induced nausea and vomiting (40 mg IV or 0.3 mg/kg IV).
Ondansetron: Treatment of vomiting associated with N-acetylcysteine use; treatment of radiation-induced nausea and vomiting.

Actions

➤*Pharmacology:* Selective 5-hydroxytryptamine3 (5-HT_3) receptor antagonists are antinauseant, antiemetic, and anti-IBS (**alosetron** only) agents with little or no affinity for other serotonin receptors, alpha- or beta-adrenoreceptors, or for dopamine D_2, histamine H_1, benzodiazepine, picrotoxin, or opioid receptors.

Serotonin receptors of the 5-HT_3 are located peripherally on vagal nerve terminals, enteric neurons in the GI tract, and centrally in the chemoreceptor trigger zone. During chemotherapy, mucosal enterochromaffin cells from the small intestine release serotonin, which stimulates the 5-HT_3 receptors. This evokes vagal afferent discharge, inducing vomiting.

Activation of the 5-HT_3 receptors and the resulting neuronal depolarization affect the regulation of visceral pain, colonic transit, and GI secretions, processes that relate to the pathophysiology of IBS. In IBS, it is presumed the pain, distension, and exaggerated motor response are at least in part caused by stimulation of the 5-HT_3 receptors.

➤*Pharmacokinetics:*

Absorption – **Alosetron** is rapidly absorbed, with a mean absolute bioavailability of approximately 50% to 60%. Oral **dolasetron** is well absorbed. **Dolasetron's** most clinically relevant species, hydrodolasetron, appears rapidly in plasma, with a maximum concentration occurring approximately 1 hour after oral dosing and 0.6 hours after IV dosing. The apparent bioavailability of dolasetron is 75%. Oral **ondansetron** is well absorbed from the GI tract, with a mean bioavailability of approximately 56%. **Palonosetron's** mean area under the curve (AUC) is 35.8 ng•h/mL.

Distribution – Plasma protein binding is 65% for **granisetron**, 70% to 76% for **ondansetron**, 82% for **alosetron**, and 62% for **palonosetron**. Sixty-nine percent to 77% of **hydrodolasetron** is bound to plasma proteins.

Metabolism – **Alosetron** is extensively metabolized by cytochrome P-450 (CYP), 2C9 (30%), 3A4 (18%), and 1A2 (10%) with at least 13 metabolites detected; the predominant product in the urine was 6-hydroxy metabolite. The reduction of **dolasetron** to hydrodolasetron is mediated by carbonyl reductase. CYP-450 2D6 is primarily responsible for the subsequent hydroxylation of hydrodolasetron and both CYP3A and flavin monooxygenase are responsible for the N-oxidation of hydrodolasetron. Oral **ondansetron** is extensively metabolized and undergoes some first-pass metabolism. The primary metabolic pathway is hydroxylation on the indole ring followed by subsequent glucuronide or sulfate conjugation. Ondansetron is a substrate for CYP-450 enzymes, with CYP3A4 playing the predominant role. **Granisetron** metabolism involves N-demethylation and aromatic ring oxidation followed by conjugation. In vitro liver microsomal studies show that granisetron's major route of metabolism is inhibited by ketoconazole, suggestive of metabolism mediated by the CYP-450 3A subfamily. Approximately 50% of **palonosetron** is metabolized to form 2 primary metabolites: N-oxide-palonosetron and 6-S-hydroxy-palonosetron. In vitro metabolism studies suggest that CYP2D6 and, to a lesser extent, CYP3A and CYP1A2 are involved in the metabolism of palonosetron.

Excretion – Renal elimination of unchanged **alosetron** accounts for only 6% of the dose. Hydrodolasetron is excreted unchanged in the urine (61% for oral dosing and 53% for IV dosing). **Granisetron** clearance is predominantly by hepatic metabolism. Approximately 11% of oral granisetron and 12% of granisetron IV is eliminated unchanged in the urine in 48 hours. The remainder of the dose is excreted as metabolites, 48% in the urine and 38% in the feces for the oral dose and 49% in the urine and 34% in the feces for the IV dose. After a single IV dose of ^{14}C-**palonosetron** 10 mcg/kg, approximately 40% of the dose was recovered within 144 hours in the urine.

Special populations –

Renal function impairment:

- *Ondansetron* – Ondansetron oral mean plasma clearance was reduced about 50% in patients with severe renal function impairment (creatinine clearance [Ccr] less than 30 mL/min).
- *Palonosetron* – Total systemic exposure increased approximately 28% in severe renal function impairment relative to healthy patients.

Hepatic function impairment:

- *Alosetron* – Patients with severe hepatic function impairment displayed higher systemic exposure to alosetron. Do not use alosetron in women with severe hepatic function impairment.
- *Granisetron* – In patients with hepatic function impairment due to neoplastic liver involvement, total clearance was approximately halved compared with patients without hepatic function impairment.
- *Ondansetron* – In patients with mild to moderate hepatic function impairment, clearance is reduced 2-fold and mean half-life is increased to 11.6 hours, compared with 5.7 hours in healthy patients. In patients with severe hepatic function impairment (Child-Pugh score of 10 or greater), clearance is reduced 2- to 3-fold and apparent volume of distribution (Vd) is increased with a resultant increase in half-life to 20 hours. Do not exceed a total daily dose of 8 mg in patients with severe hepatic function impairment.

Elderly:

- *Alosetron* – In some studies in healthy men and women, plasma concentrations were elevated approximately 40% in individuals 65 years and older compared with younger adults. However, this effect was not consistently observed in men.

Children:

• *Granisetron* – After a single 40 mcg/kg IV dose, children 2 to 16 years of age showed that Vd and total clearance increased with age.

• *Ondansetron (injection)* –

Pediatric cancer patients:

Ondansetron Injection Pharmacokinetics in Pediatric Cancer Patients 1 Month to 18 Years of Age				
Subjects and age group	n	Clearance (L/h/kg) Geometric mean	Vd at steady state (L/kg) Geometric mean	Half-life mean
Pediatric cancer patients 4 to 18 years of age	n = 21	0.599	1.9	2.8
Population PK patients[a] 1 to 48 months of age	n = 115	0.582	3.65	4.9

[a] Population PK (pharmacokinetic) patients: 64% cancer patients and 36% surgery patients.

Pediatric surgery patients:

Ondansetron Injection Pharmacokinetics in Pediatric Surgery Patients 1 Month to 12 Years of Age				
Subjects and age group	n	Clearance (L/h/kg) Geometric mean	Vd at steady state (L/kg) Geometric mean	Half-life mean
Pediatric surgery patients 3 to 12 years of age	n = 21	0.439	1.65	2.9
Pediatric surgery patients 5 to 24 months of age	n = 22	0.581	2.3	2.9
Pediatric surgery patients 1 to 4 months of age	n = 19	0.401	3.5	6.7

In general, surgical and cancer children younger than 18 years of age tend to have a higher ondansetron clearance compared with adults, leading to a shorter half-life in most children. In patients 1 to 4 months of age, a longer half-life was observed because of the higher Vd in this age group.

Gender:

• *Granisetron* – Generally, men had a higher maximal drug concentration (C_{max}).

Race:

• *Palonosetron* – Total body clearance was 25% higher in Japanese patients compared with white patients.

Pharmacokinetics –

5-HT$_3$ Antagonist Pharmacokinetics	Mean C_{max} (ng/mL)	Half-life (h)	Mean clearance (L/h/kg)	Mean Vd (L/kg)
Alosetron				
Adults (men)	5	1.5		65 to 95
Adults (women)	9	1.5		65 to 95
IV dolasetron				
Adults	320	7.3	0.564	5.8
Elderly	620	6.9	0.498	
Cancer patients				
Adults	505	7.5	0.612	
Elderly	562	5.5	0.75	
Children	505	4.4	1.15	
Pediatric surgery patients	255	4.8	0.786	
Severe renal function impairment (Ccr ≤ 10 mL/min)	867	10.9	0.3	
Severe hepatic function impairment	396	11.7	0.576	
Oral dolasetron				
Adults	556	8.1	0.804	5.8
Elderly	662	7.2	0.57	
Cancer patients				
Adults		7.9	0.774	
Adolescents	374	6.4	1.59	
Children	217	5.5	2.65	
Pediatric surgery patients	159	5.9	1.25	
Severe renal function impairment (Ccr ≤ 10 mL/min)	701	10.7	0.432	
Severe hepatic function impairment	410	11	0.528	

5-HT$_3$ Antagonist Pharmacokinetics	Mean C_{max} (ng/mL)	Half-life (h)	Mean clearance (L/h/kg)	Mean Vd (L/kg)
IV granisetron				
Adults (3-minute infusion)	64.3	4.9	0.79	3
Elderly (3-minute infusion)	57	7.7	0.44	4
Cancer patients (5-minute infusion)	63.8	9	0.38	3.1
Oral granisetron				
Adults (single 1 mg dose)	3.6	6.2	0.41	3.9
Cancer patients (1 mg twice daily for 7 days)	6		0.52	
IV ondansetron				
Adults	104	4.1	0.35	
Elderly	170	5.5	0.262	
Oral ondansetron				
Adults, men (single 8 mg dose)	25.2	3.6	0.394	
Adults, women (single 8 mg dose)	47.6	4.2	0.305	
Elderly ≥ 75 years of age, men	37	4.5	0.277	
Elderly ≥ 75 years of age, women	46.1	6.2	0.249	
Palonosetron				
Adults		40	0.16	8.3
Cancer patients	5.6			

Contraindications

➤*Alosetron:* Do not initiate in patients with constipation or patients who are unable to comply with or understand the patient-physician agreement for alosetron.

Coadministration with fluvoxamine.

In patients with a history of the following: chronic or severe constipation or sequelae from constipation; intestinal obstruction, stricture, toxic megacolon, GI perforation, and/or adhesions; ischemic colitis, impaired intestinal circulation, thrombophlebitis, or hypercoagulable state; Crohn disease or ulcerative colitis; diverticulitis; severe hepatic function impairment; hypersensitivity to any component of the product.

➤*Dolasetron, granisetron, ondansetron, palonosetron:* Hypersensitivity to the drug or any of its components.

Warnings/Precautions

➤*Constipation:* Serious complications of constipation, including obstruction, ileus, impaction, toxic megacolon, and secondary bowel ischemia, have been reported with **alosetron** use. Rare cases of perforation and death have been reported from postmarketing clinical practice. In some cases, complications of constipation required intestinal surgery, including colectomy. Patients who are elderly, debilitated, or taking additional medications that decrease GI motility may be at greater risk for complications of constipation. Discontinue immediately in patients who develop constipation.

➤*Ischemic colitis:* Ischemic colitis has been reported in **alosetron** patients. Discontinue immediately in patients with signs of ischemic colitis, such as rectal bleeding, bloody diarrhea, or new or worsening abdominal pain. Do not resume alosetron treatment in patients who develop ischemic colitis.

➤*Cardiac effects:* **Dolasetron** can cause electrocardiogram (ECG) interval changes (PR, QTc, JT prolongation, and QRS widening). These changes are related in magnitude and frequency to blood levels of the active metabolite and are self-limiting with declining blood levels. Some patients have interval prolongations for 24 hours or longer. Interval prolongation could lead to cardiovascular complications, including heart block or cardiac arrhythmias, but these have been rarely reported.

Rarely and predominantly with **ondansetron** IV, transient ECG changes, including QT interval prolongation have been reported.

Administer dolasetron and **palonosetron** with caution in patients who have or may develop cardiac conduction interval prolongation. These include patients with hypokalemia or hypomagnesemia, patients taking diuretics with potential for inducing electrolyte abnormalities, patients with congenital QT syndrome, patients taking antiarrhythmic drugs or other drugs that lead to QT prolongation, and cumulative high-dose anthracycline therapy.

➤*Peristalsis:* **Ondansetron** and **granisetron** do not stimulate gastric or intestinal peristalsis. They should not be used instead of nasogastric suction. Their use in patients following abdominal surgery or in patients with chemotherapy-induced nausea and vomiting may mask a progressive ileus and/or gastric distension.

➤*Phenylketonuric patients:* Inform phenylketonuric patients that **ondansetron** orally disintegrating tablets contain phenylalanine (a component of aspartame). Each 4 and 8 mg orally disintegrating tablet contains less than 0.03 mg of phenylalanine.

➤*Benzyl alcohol:* **Granisetron** 1 mg/mL injection contains benzyl alcohol as a preservative. Benzyl alcohol has been associated with a fatal gasping syndrome in premature infants and may cross the placenta of a pregnant woman and reach the fetus. Use granisetron injection in pregnancy only if the benefit outweighs the potential risk.

➤*Hypersensitivity reactions:* Hypersensitivity reactions may occur in patients who have exhibited hypersensitivity to other 5-HT_3 receptor antagonists.

➤*Hepatic function impairment:* Do not use **alosetron** in patients with severe hepatic function impairment and use alosetron with caution in patients with mild or moderate hepatic function impairment.

See Pharmacokinetics for more information.

➤*Pregnancy: Category B.* There are no adequate and well-controlled studies in pregnant women. Because animal reproduction studies are not always predictive of human response, only use 5-HT_3 receptor antagonists if the potential benefits justify the potential risk to the fetus.

➤*Lactation:* **Alosetron** and **ondansetron** are excreted in the breast milk of rats. It is not known whether 5-HT_3 receptor antagonists are excreted in human breast milk. Exercise caution when 5-HT_3 receptor antagonists are administered to a breast-feeding woman.

➤*Children:* Safety and efficacy of **alosetron**, **palonosetron**, and oral **granisetron** in children have not been established.

There is no experience with **dolasetron** in children younger than 2 years of age.

Safety and efficacy of granisetron injection have not been established in children younger than 2 years of age and have not been established in children for the prevention or treatment of postoperative nausea or vomiting.

Little information is available about oral **ondansetron** dosage in children 4 years of age or younger. Little information is known about the use of ondansetron injection in pediatric surgical patients younger than 1 month of age or in pediatric cancer patients younger than 6 months of age.

➤*Elderly:* Postmarketing experience suggests that elderly patients may be at greater risk for complications of constipation from **alosetron**. In general, dose selection for an elderly patient should be cautious, usually starting at the low end of the dosing range, reflecting the greater frequency of decreased hepatic, renal, or cardiac function, and of concomitant disease or other drug therapy.

Drug Interactions

5-HT_3 Antagonist Drug Interactions

Precipitant drug	Object drug[a]		Description
Atenolol	Dolasetron	⬆	Clearance of hydrodolasetron decreased by approximately 27% when dolasetron was administered IV concomitantly with atenolol.
Carbamazepine	Ondansetron	⬇	In patients treated with carbamazepine, the clearance of ondansetron was significantly increased and ondansetron blood levels were decreased.
Cimetidine	Dolasetron	⬆	Blood levels of hydrodolasetron increased 24% when dolasetron was coadministered with cimetidine for 7 days.
CYP1A2 inhibitors (eg, cimetidine, fluvoxamine, quinolone antibiotics)	Alosetron	⬆	Fluvoxamine increased mean alosetron AUC approximately 6-fold and prolonged the half-life by approximately 3-fold. Coadministration is contraindicated. Avoid coadministration of alosetron with other CYP1A2 inhibitors.
CYP3A4 inhibitors (eg, clarithromycin, ketoconazole, protease inhibitors)	Alosetron	⬆	Ketoconazole increased alosetron AUC 29%. Use caution when administering together. Undertake coadministration of alosetron with other CYP3A4 inhibitors with caution.
Phenobarbital	Granisetron	⬇	Hepatic enzyme induction with phenobarbital resulted in a 25% increase in total plasma clearance of IV granisetron.
Phenytoin	Ondansetron	⬇	In patients treated with phenytoin, the clearance of ondansetron was significantly increased and ondansetron blood levels were decreased.
Rifamycins	Dolasetron, Ondansetron	⬇	Plasma concentration of dolasetron and ondansetron may be reduced.

5-HT_3 Antagonist Drug Interactions

Precipitant drug	Object drug[a]		Description
Ziprasidone	Dolasetron	⬆	The risk of life-threatening cardiac arrhythmias, including torsades de pointes, may be increased. Ziprasidone is contraindicated in patients taking dolasetron.
Dolasetron	Ziprasidone		
Ondansetron	Cisplatin	⬇	Plasma cisplatin concentrations may be decreased, reducing the therapeutic effect. It may be necessary to increase the cisplatin dose.
Ondansetron	Cyclophosphamide	⬇	Plasma cyclophosphamide concentrations may be decreased, reducing the therapeutic effect. It may be necessary to increase the cyclophosphamide dose.

[a] ⬆ = Object drug increased. ⬇ = Object drug decreased.

➤*Drug/Food interactions:*

Alosetron – Alosetron absorption is decreased approximately 25% by coadministration with food, with a mean delay in time to peak concentration of 15 minutes.

Granisetron – When granisetron tablets were administered with food, AUC was decreased 5% and C_{max} increased 30% in nonfasted healthy volunteers who received a single 10 mg dose.

Ondansetron – Bioavailability is slightly enhanced by food.

Adverse Reactions

➤*Alosetron:*

Alosetron Adverse Reactions (≥ 1%)

Adverse reaction	Alosetron 1 mg twice daily (n = 8,328)	Placebo (n = 2,363)
GI		
Abdominal discomfort/pain	7%	4%
Abdominal distension	2%	1%
Constipation	29%	6%
GI discomfort/pain	5%	3%
Hemorrhoids	2%	1%
Nausea	6%	5%
Regurgitation and reflux	2%	2%

Cardiovascular – Tachyarrhythmias (0.1% to 1%); arrhythmias, extrasystoles, increased blood pressure (less than 0.1%).

CNS – Anxiety, hypnagogic effects (0.1% to 1%); cognitive function disorders, confusion, depressive moods, disorders of equilibrium, dreams, hypesthesia, memory effects, sedation, tremors (less than 0.1%).

Dermatologic – Sweating, urticaria (0.1% to 1%); acne, allergic skin reaction, alopecia, dermatitis, dermatosis, disorders of sweat and sebum, eczema, folliculitis, hair loss, nail disorders, skin infections (less than 0.1%).

GI – Dyspeptic symptoms, GI lesions, GI spasms, hyposalivation, ischemic colitis (0.1% to 1%); abnormal tenderness, colitis, decreased GI motility and ileus, disturbances of sense of taste, diverticulitis, gastritis, gastroduodenitis, gastroenteritis, GI intussusception, GI obstructions, GI signs and symptoms, hyperacidity, oral symptoms, positive fecal occult blood, proctitis, ulcerative colitis (less than 0.1%).

GU – Urinary frequency (0.1% to 1%); bladder inflammation, diuresis, female reproductive tract bleeding and hemorrhage, fungal reproductive infections, polyuria, reproductive infections, sexual function disorders, urinary tract hemorrhage (less than 0.1%).

Hematologic/Lymphatic – Hemorrhage, lymphatic signs and symptoms, quantitative red cell or hemoglobin defects (less than 0.1%).

Lab test abnormalities – Abnormal bilirubin levels, cholecystitis (0.1% to 1%).

Metabolic – Disorders of calcium and phosphate metabolism, fluid disturbances, hyperglycemia, hypoglycemia, hypothalamus/pituitary hypofunction (less than 0.1%).

Musculoskeletal – Bone and skeletal pain, muscle pain, stiffness, tightness, and rigidity (less than 0.1%).

Ophthalmic – Light sensitivity (less than 0.1%).

Respiratory – Breathing disorders (0.1% to 1%); ear, nose, and throat infections (including viral), laryngitis, viral respiratory infections (less than 0.1%).

Miscellaneous – Cramps, fatigue, malaise, pain, temperature regulation disturbances (0.1% to 1%); burning sensations, cold sensations, contusions, fungal infections, general signs and symptoms, hematoma, hot and cold sensations, nonspecific conditions (less than 0.1%).

➤*Postmarketing (alosetron):*
CNS – Headache.
Dermatologic – Rash.
GI – Constipation, ileus, impaction, ischemic colitis, obstruction, perforation, small bowel mesenteric ischemia, ulceration.

➤*Dolasetron (oral and injection):*

Dolasetron Tablets Adverse Reactions from Chemotherapy-Induced Nausea/Vomiting Studies (≥ 2%)

Adverse reaction	Dolasetron 25 mg tablets (n = 235)	Dolasetron 100 mg tablets (n = 227)
Cardiovascular		
Bradycardia	12 (5.1%)	9 (4%)
Tachycardia	7 (3%)	6 (2.6%)
CNS		
Dizziness	3 (1.3%)	7 (3.1%)
Fatigue	6 (2.6%)	13 (5.7%)
Headache	42 (17.9%)	52 (22.9%)
GI		
Diarrhea	5 (2.1%)	12 (5.3%)
Dyspepsia	7 (3%)	5 (2.2%)
Miscellaneous		
Chills/Shivering	3 (1.3%)	5 (2.2%)
Pain	0 (0%)	7 (3.1%)

Dolasetron Tablets Adverse Reactions from Postoperative Nausea/Vomiting Studies (≥ 2%)

Adverse reaction	Dolasetron 100 mg tablets (n = 228)	Placebo (n = 231)
Cardiovascular		
Hypertension	5 (2.2%)	7 (3%)
Hypotension	12 (5.3%)	15 (6.5%)
Tachycardia	5 (2.2%)	2 (0.9%)
CNS		
Dizziness	10 (4.4%)	0 (0%)
Headache	16 (7%)	11 (4.8%)
Miscellaneous		
Fever	8 (3.5%)	7 (3%)
Oliguria	6 (2.6%)	3 (1.3%)
Pruritus	7 (3.1%)	8 (3.5%)

Dolasetron Injection Adverse Reactions from Chemotherapy-Induced Nausea/Vomiting Studies (≥ 2%)

Adverse reaction	Dolasetron 1.8 mg/kg injection (n = 695)	Ondansetron/granisetron[a] (n = 356)
Cardiovascular		
Hypertension	20 (2.9%)	9 (2.5%)
CNS		
Dizziness	15 (2.2%)	7 (2%)
Fatigue	25 (3.6%)	12 (3.4%)
Headache	169 (24.3%)	73 (20.5%)
GI		
Abdominal pain	22 (3.2%)	7 (2%)
Diarrhea	86 (12.4%)	25 (7%)
Hepatic		
Abnormal hepatic function[b]	25 (3.6%)	12 (3.4%)
Miscellaneous		
Chills/Shivering	14 (2%)	6 (1.7%)
Fever	30 (4.3%)	18 (5.1%)
Pain	17 (2.4%)	7 (2%)

[a] Ondansetron 32 mg IV, granisetron 3 mg IV.
[b] Includes events coded as AST and/or ALT increased.

Dolasetron Injection Adverse Reactions from Postoperative Nausea/Vomiting Studies (≥ 2%)

Adverse reaction	Dolasetron 12.5 mg injection (n = 615)	Placebo (n = 739)
CNS		
Headache	58 (9.4%)	51 (6.9%)
Dizziness	34 (5.5%)	23 (3.1%)
Drowsiness	15 (2.4%)	18 (2.4%)
Miscellaneous		
Pain	15 (2.4%)	21 (2.8%)
Urinary retention	12 (2%)	16 (2.2%)

➤*Adverse reactions for dolasetron (oral and injection):*
Cardiovascular – Hypotension (infrequent); atrial flutter/fibrillation, bundle branch block (left and right), chest pain, edema, extrasystole (atrial premature complexes or ventricular premature complexes), hypotension, Mobitz I atrioventricular (AV) block, nodal arrhythmia, orthostatic myocardial infarction, palpitations, peripheral edema, peripheral ischemia, poor R-wave progression, severe bradycardia, sinus arrhythmia, ST-T wave change, syncope, T wave change, thrombophlebitis/phlebitis, U wave change. Bradycardia, severe hypotension, and syncope have been reported immediately or closely following IV administration.
CNS – Agitation, depersonalization, flushing, paresthesia, sleep disorder, tremor, vertigo (infrequent); abnormal dreaming, anxiety, ataxia, confusion, twitching (rare).
Dermatologic – Increased sweating, rash (infrequent).
GI – Abdominal pain, anorexia, constipation, dyspepsia (infrequent); pancreatitis (rare).
GU – Acute renal failure, dysuria, polyuria (rare).
Hematologic – Anemia, epistaxis, hematuria, partial thromboplastin time increased, prothrombin time prolonged, purpura/hematoma, thrombocytopenia (rare).
Hepatic – Transient increases in ALT and/or AST values (less than 1%); hyperbilirubinemia, increased gamma-glutamyltransferase (rare).
Metabolic – Alkaline phosphatase increased (rare).
Musculoskeletal – Arthralgia, myalgia (rare).
Ophthalmic – Abnormal vision (infrequent); photophobia (rare).
Respiratory – Bronchospasm, dyspnea (rare).
Special senses – Taste perversion (infrequent); tinnitus (rare).
Miscellaneous – Anaphylactic reaction, facial edema, local pain or burning on IV administration, urticaria (rare).

➤*Granisetron (oral):*

Granisetron Tablets Adverse Reactions (≥ 5%)

Adverse reaction	Granisetron[a] 1 mg tablets twice daily (n = 978)	Granisetron[a] 2 mg tablets daily (n = 1,450)	Comparator[b] (n = 599)	Placebo (n = 185)
CNS				
Asthenia	14%	18%	10%	4%
Headache[c]	21%	20%	13%	12%
GI				
Abdominal pain	6%	4%	6%	3%
Constipation	18%	14%	16%	8%
Diarrhea	8%	9%	10%	4%
Dyspepsia	4%	6%	5%	4%

[a] Adverse reactions were recorded for 7 days when granisetron tablets were given on a single day and for up to 28 days when granisetron tablets were administered for 7 to 14 days.
[b] Dexamethasone alone; metoclopramide/dexamethasone; phenothiazines/dexamethasone; prochlorperazine.
[c] Usually mild to moderate in severity.

Cardiovascular – Hypertension (1%); angina pectoris, atrial fibrillation, hypotension, syncope (rare).
CNS – Dizziness, insomnia (5%); anxiety (2%); somnolence (1%); extrapyramidal symptoms (rare).
GI – Nausea (20%); vomiting (12%).
Hepatic – Elevation of ALT (6%) and AST (5%) (greater than 2 times the upper limit of normal [ULN]).
Hypersensitivity – Hypersensitivity reactions (eg, anaphylaxis, shortness of breath, hypotension, urticaria) (rare).
Miscellaneous – Leukopenia (9%); decreased appetite (6%); fever (5%); anemia (4%); alopecia (3%); thrombocytopenia (2%).

➤*Granisetron (injection):*

Granisetron Injection Adverse Reactions in Single-Day Chemotherapy Studies (≥ 3%)

Adverse reaction	Granisetron 40 mcg/kg injection (n = 1,268)	Comparator[a] (n = 422)
CNS		
Asthenia	5%	6%
Headache	14%	6%
Somnolence	4%	15%
GI		
Constipation	3%	3%
Diarrhea	4%	6%

[a] Metoclopramide/dexamethasone and phenothiazines/dexamethasone.

Cardiovascular – Hypertension (2%); arrhythmias such as sinus bradycardia, atrial fibrillation, varying degrees of AV block, ventricular ectopy including nonsustained tachycardia, and ECG abnormalities, hypotension (rare).

CNS – Agitation, anxiety, CNS stimulation, insomnia (less than 2%); extrapyramidal syndrome (rare).

Hepatic – Elevations of ALT (3.3%) and AST (2.8%) (greater than 2 times the ULN).

Hypersensitivity – Hypersensitivity reactions (eg, anaphylaxis, hypotension, shortness of breath, urticaria) (rare).

Miscellaneous – Fever (3%), taste disorder (2%), skin rashes (1%).

Granisetron Injection Adverse Reactions (> 2%) in Postoperative Nausea/Vomiting Studies

Adverse reaction	Granisetron 1 mg injection (n = 267)	Placebo (n = 266)
Cardiovascular		
Bradycardia	4.5%	5.3%
Hypertension	2.6%	4.1%
Hypotension	3.4%	3.8%
CNS		
Anxiety	3.4%	3.8%
Dizziness	4.1%	3.4%
Headache	8.6%	7.1%
Insomnia	4.9%	6%
GI		
Abdominal pain	6%	6%
Constipation	9.4%	12%
Diarrhea	3.4%	1.1%
Dyspepsia	3%	1.9%
Flatulence	3%	3%
GU		
Oliguria	2.2%	1.5%
Urinary tract infection	2.6%	3.4%
Miscellaneous		
Anemia	9.4%	10.2%
Coughing	2.2%	1.1%
Fever	7.9%	4.5%
Hepatic enzymes increased	5.6%	4.1%
Infection	3%	2.3%
Leukocytosis	3.7%	4.1%
Pain	10.1%	8.3%

Japanese clinical trial – Fever (56% to 50%); increased sputum (2.7% to 1.7%); dermatitis (2.7% to 0%).

➤*Ondansetron (oral):*

Ondansetron Oral Adverse Reactions (≥ 5%): Single-Day Therapy with 24 mg Tablets (Highly Emetogenic Chemotherapy)

Adverse reaction	Ondansetron 24 mg daily (N = 300)	Ondansetron 8 mg twice daily (N = 124)	Ondansetron 32 mg daily (N = 117)
CNS			
Headache	33 (11%)	16 (13%)	17 (15%)
GI			
Diarrhea	13 (4%)	9 (7%)	3 (3%)

Ondansetron Oral Adverse Reactions (≥ 5%): 3 Days of Therapy with 8 mg Tablets (Moderately Emetogenic Chemotherapy)

Adverse reaction	Ondansetron 8 mg twice daily (N = 242)	Ondansetron 8 mg 3 times daily (N = 415)	Placebo (N = 262)
CNS			
Dizziness	13 (5%)	18 (4%)	12 (5%)
Headache	58 (24%)	113 (27%)	34 (13%)
Malaise/Fatigue	32 (13%)	37 (9%)	6 (2%)
GI			
Constipation	22 (9%)	26 (6%)	1 (< 1%)
Diarrhea	15 (6%)	16 (4%)	10 (4%)

Ondansetron Tablet Adverse Reactions (≥ 5%) in Postoperative Nausea and Vomiting Studies

Adverse reaction	Ondansetron 16 mg (N = 550)	Placebo (N = 531)
Cardiovascular		
Bradycardia	32 (6%)	30 (6%)
Hypotension	27 (5%)	32 (6%)
CNS		
Anxiety/Agitation	33 (6%)	29 (5%)
Drowsiness/Sedation	112 (20%)	122 (23%)
Dizziness	36 (7%)	34 (6%)
Headache	49 (9%)	27 (5%)
GU		
Gynecological disorder	36 (7%)	33 (6%)
Urinary retention	28 (5%)	18 (3%)
Miscellaneous		
Hypoxia	49 (9%)	35 (7%)
Pruritus	27 (5%)	20 (4%)
Pyrexia	45 (8%)	34 (6%)
Shivers	28 (5%)	30 (6%)
Wound problem	152 (28%)	162 (31%)

CNS – Extrapyramidal syndrome (rare).

Hepatic – AST (1%) and/or ALT (2%) have been reported to exceed twice the upper limit of normal.

Miscellaneous – Rash (1%); anaphylaxis, angina, bronchospasm, ECG alterations, grand mal seizures, hypokalemia, tachycardia, vascular occlusive events (rare).

➤*Postmarketing (ondansetron oral):*

Cardiovascular – Transient ECG changes including QT interval prolongation (rare). Observed predominantly with IV ondansetron.

CNS – Oculogyric crisis, appearing alone, as well with other dystonic reactions.

Dermatologic – Urticaria.

Hepatic – Liver enzyme abnormalities.

Hypersensitivity – Flushing. Rare cases of hypersensitivity reactions, sometimes severe (eg, anaphylaxis, angioedema, bronchospasm, shortness of breath, hypotension, laryngeal edema, stridor) have been reported. Laryngospasm, shock, and cardiopulmonary arrest have occurred during allergic reactions in patients receiving IV ondansetron.

Ophthalmic – Cases of transient blindness, predominantly during IV administration, have been reported.

Respiratory – Hiccups.

➤*Ondansetron (injection):*

Ondansetron Injection Adverse Reactions in Chemotherapy-Induced Nausea/Vomiting Studies

Adverse reaction	Ondansetron injection 0.15 mg/kg × 3 doses (n = 419)	Ondansetron injection 32 mg × 1 dose (n = 220)	Metoclopramide (n = 156)
CNS			
Acute dystonic reactions	0%	0%	5%
Headache	17%	25%	7%
GI			
Diarrhea	16%	8%	44%
Miscellaneous			
Akathisia	0%	0%	6%
Fever	8%	7%	5%

Ondansetron Injection Adverse Reactions (≥ 2%) in Postoperative Nausea/Vomiting Studies

Adverse reaction	Ondansetron 4 mg IV (n = 547)	Placebo (n = 547)
Cardiovascular		
Hypotension	10 (2%)	12 (2%)
CNS		
Anxiety/agitation	11 (2%)	16 (3%)
Dizziness	67 (12%)	88 (16%)
Drowsiness/sedation	44 (8%)	37 (7%)
Headache	92 (17%)	77 (14%)
Malaise/fatigue	25 (5%)	30 (5%)
GU		
Dysuria	11 (2%)	9 (2%)
Urinary retention	17 (3%)	15 (3%)
Musculoskeletal		
Musculoskeletal pain	57 (10%)	59 (11%)

Ondansetron Injection Adverse Reactions (≥ 2%) in Postoperative Nausea/Vomiting Studies		
Adverse reaction	Ondansetron 4 mg IV (n = 547)	Placebo (n = 547)
Miscellaneous		
Chest pain (unspecified)	12 (2%)	15 (3%)
Cold sensation	9 (2%)	8 (1%)
Fever	10 (2%)	6 (1%)
Injection-site reaction	21 (4%)	18 (3%)
Paresthesia	9 (2%)	2 (< 1%)
Postoperative carbon dioxide–related pain[a]	12 (2%)	16 (3%)
Pruritus	9 (2%)	3 (< 1%)
Shivers	38 (7%)	39 (7%)

[a] Sites of pain included abdomen, stomach, joints, rib cage, shoulder.

Cardiovascular – Angina (chest pain), ECG alterations, hypotension, tachycardia (rare).

CNS – Extrapyramidal reactions, grand mal seizure (rare).

GI – Constipation (11%).

Miscellaneous – Rash (1%); hypokalemia (rare).

Children –

Ondansetron Injection Adverse Reactions in Children 2 to 12 Years of Age		
Adverse reaction	Ondansetron (n = 755)	Placebo (n = 731)
CNS		
Anxiety/agitation	49 (6%)	47 (6%)
Drowsiness/sedation	41 (5%)	56 (8%)
Headache	44 (6%)	43 (6%)
Miscellaneous		
Pyrexia	32 (4%)	41 (6%)
Wound problem	80 (11%)	86 (12%)

Ondansetron Injection Adverse Reactions (≥ 2%) in Children 1 to 24 Months of Age		
Adverse reaction	Ondansetron (n = 366)	Placebo (n = 334)
GI		
Diarrhea	6 (2%)	3 (< 1%)
Respiratory		
Bronchospasm	2 (< 1%)	6 (2%)
Miscellaneous		
Postprocedural pain	4 (1%)	6 (2%)
Pyrexia	14 (4%)	14 (4%)

➤*Postmarketing (ondansetron injection):*

Cardiovascular – Arrhythmias (including ventricular and supraventricular tachycardia, premature ventricular contractions, and atrial fibrillation), bradycardia, ECG alterations (including second-degree heart block, QT interval prolongation, and ST segment depression), palpitations, syncope.

CNS – Oculogyric crisis, appearing alone, as well with other dystonic reactions.

Dermatologic – Urticaria.

Hypersensitivity – Flushing (rare). Rare cases of hypersensitivity reactions, sometimes severe (eg, anaphylaxis, angioedema, bronchospasm, hypotension, laryngeal edema, shortness of breath, stridor). Cardiopulmonary arrest, laryngospasm, and shock have been reported.

Hepatic – Liver enzyme abnormalities.

Respiratory – Hiccups.

Ophthalmic – Cases of transient blindness have been reported.

➤*Palonosetron:*

Palonosetron Adverse Reactions (≥ 2%) in Chemotherapy-Induced Nausea and Vomiting Studies			
Adverse reaction	Palonosetron 0.25 mg (n = 633)	Ondansetron 32 mg IV (n = 410)	Dolasetron 100 mg IV (n = 194)
CNS			
Dizziness	8 (1%)	9 (2%)	4 (2%)
Fatigue	3 (< 1%)	4 (1%)	4 (2%)
Headache	60 (9%)	34 (8%)	32 (16%)
Insomnia	1 (< 1%)	3 (1%)	3 (2%)
GI			
Abdominal pain	1 (< 1%)	2 (< 1%)	3 (2%)
Constipation	29 (5%)	8 (2%)	12 (6%)
Diarrhea	8 (1%)	7 (2%)	4 (2%)

Cardiovascular – Bradycardia, hypotension, nonsustained tachycardia (1%); extrasystoles, hypertension, myocardial ischemia, sinus arrhythmia, sinus tachycardia, supraventricular extrasystoles and QT prolongation, vein discoloration, vein distention (less than 1%).

CNS – Anxiety, dizziness (1%); euphoric mood, fatigue, hypersomnia, insomnia, paresthesia, somnolence (less than 1%).

Dermatologic – Allergic dermatitis, rash (less than 1%).

GI – Diarrhea (1%); abdominal pain, dry mouth, dyspepsia, flatulence, hiccups (less than 1%).

GU – Urinary retention (less than 1%).

Hepatic – Transient, asymptomatic increases in AST and/or ALT and bilirubin (less than 1%).

Metabolic – Hyperkalemia (1%); anorexia, appetite decrease, electrolyte fluctuations, glycosuria, hyperglycemia, metabolic acidosis (less than 1%).

Ophthalmic – Amblyopia, eye irritation (less than 1%).

Musculoskeletal – Arthralgia (less than 1%).

Miscellaneous – Weakness (1%); fever, flu-like syndrome, hot flash, motion sickness, tinnitus (less than 1%).

➤*Postmarketing (palonosetron):* Very rare cases (less than 0.01%) of hypersensitivity reactions and injection-site reactions (burning, discomfort, pain, and induration) were reported.

Overdosage

➤*Symptoms:* Labored respiration, subdued behavior, ataxia, tremors, convulsions, hypotension, dizziness, headache, transient second-degree heart block, gasping, pallor, cyanosis, collapse, death. Sudden blindness (amaurosis) of 2 to 3 minutes' duration plus severe constipation occurred in 1 patient administered ondansetron 72 mg IV.

➤*Treatment:* Manage with appropriate supportive therapy. Following a suspected overdose of **dolasetron** injection, a patient found to have second-degree or higher AV conduction block should undergo cardiac telemetry monitoring.

Patient Information

➤*Alosetron:* Counsel patients fully on and ensure that they understand the risks and benefits of **alosetron** before an initial prescription is written. The patient may be educated by the enrolled doctor or health care provider under a doctor's direction.

Health care providers must –

- Counsel patients for whom alosetron is appropriate about the benefits and risks of alosetron and discuss the impact of IBS symptoms on the patient's life.
- Give the patient a copy of the Medication Guide, which outlines the benefits and risks of alosetron, and instruct the patient to read it carefully. Answer all questions the patient may have about alosetron.
- Review the patient-physician agreement for alosetron with the patient, answer all questions, and give a copy of the signed agreement to the patient.
- Provide each patient with appropriate instructions for taking alosetron.

Copies of the patient-physician agreement for alosetron and additional copies of the Medication Guide are available by contacting the manufacturer at 1-888-825-5249 or visiting http://www.lotronex.com.

Instruct patients who are prescribed alosetron to –

- Read the Medication Guide before starting alosetron and each time they refill their prescription.
- Not start taking alosetron if they are constipated.
- Immediately discontinue alosetron and contact their health care provider if they become constipated, or have symptoms of ischemic colitis, such as new or worsening abdominal pain, bloody diarrhea, or blood in the stool. Contact their health care provider again if their constipation does not resolve after discontinuation of alosetron.
- Resume alosetron only if their constipation has resolved and after discussion with and the agreement of their treating health care provider.
- Stop taking alosetron and contact their health care provider if alosetron does not adequately control IBS symptoms after 4 weeks of taking 1 mg twice a day.

➤*Ondansetron:*

Phenylketonuric patients – Inform phenylketonuric patients that **ondansetron** orally disintegrating tablets contain phenylalanine (a component of aspartame). Each 4 and 8 mg orally disintegrating tablet contains less than 0.03 mg of phenylalanine.

Instruct patients not to remove ondansetron orally disintegrating tablets from the blister until just prior to dosing and not to push the tablet through the foil. Instruct patients to completely peel the blister backing off the blister with dry hands. Instruct patients to gently remove the tablet and immediately place it on the tongue to dissolve and be swallowed with the saliva. Peelable illustrated stickers are affixed to the product carton that can be provided with the prescription to ensure proper use and handling of the product.

ALOSETRON

Rx	**Lotronex** (Prometheus)	**Tablets; oral:** 0.5 mg	Equiv. to alosetron hydrochloride 0.562 mg. Lactose. (GX EX1). White, oval. Film-coated. In 30s.
		1 mg	Equiv. to alosetron hydrochloride 1.124 mg. Lactose. (GX CT1). Blue, oval. Film-coated. In 30s.

ALOSETRON HYDROCHLORIDE — ORAL

For complete and comparative prescribing information, refer to the 5-HT$_3$ Receptor Antagonists class monograph.

WARNING

Infrequent but serious GI adverse reactions have been reported with the use of alosetron. These reactions, including ischemic colitis and serious complications of constipation, have resulted in hospitalization, and, rarely, blood transfusion, surgery, and death.

- The prescribing program for alosetron was implemented to help reduce risks of serious GI adverse reactions. Only health care providers who have enrolled in the manufacturer's prescribing program for alosetron, based on their understanding of the benefits and risks, should prescribe alosetron.
- Alosetron is indicated only for women with severe diarrhea-predominant irritable bowel syndrome (IBS) who have failed to respond to conventional therapy. Before receiving the initial prescription for alosetron, the patient must read and sign the patient-physician agreement for alosetron.
- Discontinue alosetron immediately in patients who develop constipation or symptoms of ischemic colitis. Patients should immediately report constipation or symptoms of ischemic colitis to their health care provider. Do not resume alosetron in patients who develop ischemic colitis. Patients who have constipation should immediately contact their health care provider if the constipation does not resolve after alosetron is discontinued. Patients with resolved constipation should resume alosetron only on the advice of their treating health care provider.

Indications

➤*Irritable bowel syndrome:* For women with severe diarrhea-predominant IBS who have chronic IBS symptoms (generally lasting 6 months or longer), have had anatomic or biochemical abnormalities of the GI tract excluded, and who have not responded adequately to conventional therapy.

Because of infrequent but serious GI adverse reactions associated with alosetron, the indication is restricted to those patients for whom the benefit-to-risk balance is most favorable.

Clinical studies have not been performed to adequately confirm the benefits of alosetron in men.

Administration and Dosage

➤*General dosing considerations:* For safety reasons, only health care providers who enroll in the manufacturer's prescribing program for alosetron should prescribe alosetron.

Alosetron may be dispensed only on presentation of a prescription for alosetron with a sticker for the prescribing program for alosetron attached. A Medication Guide for alosetron must be given to the patient each time alosetron is dispensed, as required by law. No telephone, facsimile, or computerized prescriptions are permitted with this program. Refills are permitted to be written on prescriptions.

Alosetron may be taken with or without food.

➤*Adults:*

Irritable bowel syndrome –

Initial dosage: 0.5 mg twice a day. Patients who become constipated at this dosage should stop taking alosetron until the constipation resolves. They may be restarted at 0.5 mg once a day. If constipation recurs at the lower dose, alosetron should be discontinued immediately.

Maintenance dosage: 0.5 mg twice a day. May be increased up to 1 mg twice a day.

Dosage adjustment: Patients well controlled on 0.5 mg twice a day may be maintained on this regimen. If after 4 weeks the 0.5 mg twice-daily dosage is well tolerated but does not adequately control IBS symptoms, the dosage can be increased to up to 1 mg twice a day.

Discontinuation of therapy: Alosetron should be discontinued in patients who have not had adequate control of IBS symptoms after 4 weeks of treatment with 1 mg twice a day. Alosetron should be discontinued immediately in patients who develop constipation or signs of ischemic colitis. Alosetron should not be restarted in patients who develop ischemic colitis.

➤*Elderly:* Elderly patients may be at greater risk for complications from constipation; therefore, exercise appropriate caution and follow-up if alosetron is prescribed for these patients.

➤*Hepatic function impairment:* Alosetron is extensively metabolized by the liver, and increased exposure to alosetron is likely to occur in patients with hepatic impairment. Increased drug exposure may increase the risk of serious adverse reactions. Alosetron should be used with caution in patients with mild or moderate hepatic impairment and is contraindicated in patients with severe hepatic impairment.

➤*Special risk patients:* Debilitated patients or patients taking additional medications that decrease GI motility may be at greater risk for serious complications from constipation. Therefore, exercise appropriate caution and follow-up if alosetron is prescribed for these patients.

➤*Storage/Stability:* Store at 25°C (77°F); excursions are permitted to 15° to 30°C (59° to 86°F). Protect from light and moisture.

DOLASETRON MESYLATE

Rx	**Anzemet** (Aventis)	**Tablets, oral:** 50 mg	Lactose. (A 50). Pink. Film-coated. In 5s, blister-pack 5s, and UD 10s.
		100 mg	Lactose. (ANZEMET 100). Pink, oval. Film-coated. In 5s, blister-pack 5s, and UD 10s.
		Injection, solution: 20 mg/mL	Mannitol. In single-use 0.625 and 5 mL single-use vials, and 25 mL multidose vials.

DOLASETRON MESYLATE — ORAL

For complete and comparative prescribing information, refer to the 5-HT$_3$ Receptor Antagonists group monograph.

Indications

➤*Prevention of cancer chemotherapy-induced nausea and vomiting:* For the prevention of nausea and vomiting associated with moderately emetogenic cancer chemotherapy, including initial and repeat courses.

➤*Prevention of postoperative nausea and vomiting:* For the prevention of postoperative nausea and vomiting.

➤*Off-label uses:*

Other possible off-label uses – Prevention of radiation-induced nausea and vomiting.

Administration and Dosage

➤*General dosing considerations:* Dolasetron injection may also be given orally. See the dolasetron injection monograph for more information.

➤*Adults:*

Prevention of cancer chemotherapy–induced nausea and vomiting –

Usual dosage: 100 mg given within the 1 hour before chemotherapy.

Maximum dose: 100 mg.

Prevention of postoperative nausea and vomiting –

Usual dosage: 100 mg within the 2 hours before surgery.

Maximum dose: 100 mg.

➤*Children:*

Prevention of cancer chemotherapy–induced nausea and vomiting –

2 to 16 years of age:
- *Usual dose* – 1.8 mg/kg given within the 1 hour before chemotherapy.
- *Maximum dose* – 100 mg.

Prevention of postoperative nausea and vomiting –

2 to 16 years of age:
- *Usual dose* – 1.2 mg/kg given within the 2 hours before surgery.
- *Maximum dose* – 100 mg.

➤*Storage/Stability:* Store at controlled room temperature 20° to 25°C (68° to 77°F). Protect from light.

DOLASETRON MESYLATE — INJECTION

For complete and comparative prescribing information, refer to the 5-HT_3 Receptor Antagonists class monograph.

Indications

➤*Postoperative nausea or vomiting:* For the prevention and treatment of postoperative nausea and/or vomiting in adults and children 2 years of age and older.

➤*Off-label uses:*

Postanesthetic shivering – [5] = Poor documentation. Initial data regarding the use of single-dose dolasetron 12.5 mg indicate that this agent is not effective in preventing postanesthetic shivering. This treatment is not recommended based on the limited data available at this time.

Prevention of spinal opioid–related pruritus – [4] = Insufficient documentation. Initial data from a small controlled trial suggest that dolasetron may be beneficial in the prevention of spinal opioid–related pruritus.

Other possible off-label uses – Radiotherapy-induced nausea and vomiting (40 mg intravenously [IV] or 0.3 mg/kg IV).

Administration and Dosage

➤*Adults:*

Postoperative nausea or vomiting – 12.5 mg IV given as a single dose approximately 15 minutes before the cessation of anesthesia (prevention) or as soon as nausea or vomiting presents (treatment).

➤*Children:*

Postoperative nausea or vomiting –

2 to 16 years of age:

- *Usual dosage* – 0.35 mg/kg (up to 12.5 mg) IV given as a single dose approximately 15 minutes before the cessation of anesthesia or as soon as nausea or vomiting presents.
- *Maximum dose* – 12.5 mg (IV); 100 mg (oral).
- *Alternative dosage* – Also may be given orally as 1.2 mg/kg (up to 100 mg) within the 2 hours before surgery.

➤*Preparation for administration:* Dolasetron may be administered undiluted or may be diluted in a compatible IV solution to 50 mL (see Admixture Compatibility).

Dolasetron injection mixed in apple or apple-grape juice may be used for oral dosing of children.

➤*Administration:* Infuse IV as rapidly as 30 seconds or diluted in a compatible IV solution to 50 mL and infused over a period of up to 15 minutes. Flush the infusion line before and after administration.

Dolasetron injection mixed in apple or apple-grape juice may be used for oral dosing of children.

➤*Admixture compatibility:* Dolasetron is compatible with the following IV fluids: sodium chloride 0.9% injection, dextrose 5% injection, dextrose 5% and sodium chloride 0.45% injection, dextrose 5% and Ringer's lactate injection, Ringer's lactate injection, and mannitol 10% injection.

➤*Storage/Stability:* Store at 20° to 25°C (68° to 77°F), with excursions permitted to 15° to 30°C (59° to 86°F). Protect from light.

After dilution, IV dolasetron is stable under normal lighting conditions at room temperature for 24 hours or under refrigeration for 48 hours with compatible IV fluids (see Admixture Compatibility). Although dolasetron is chemically and physically stable when diluted as recommended, sterile precautions should be observed because diluents generally do not contain preservative. After IV dilution, do not use beyond 24 hours or 48 hours if refrigerated. After oral dilution with apple or apple-grape juice, store at room temperature and do not use beyond 2 hours.

GRANISETRON

Rx	**Granisetron Hydrochloride** (Various, eg, Corepharma LLC, Teva Pharmaceuticals)	**Tablets; oral:** 1 mg	Equiv. to granisetron hydrochloride 1.12 mg. May contain lactose. In blister packs of 2s, 20s, and bottles of 20s and 100s.
Rx	**Granisol** (PediatRx)	**Solution; oral:** 1 mg per 5 mL	Equiv. to granisetron hydrochloride 1.12 mg per 5 mL. Sorbitol. Orange flavor. In 30 mL.
Rx	**Kytril** (Roche)		Equiv. to granisetron hydrochloride 1.12 mg per 5 mL. Sorbitol. Orange flavor. In 30 mL.
Rx	**Granisetron Hydrochloride** (Various, eg, Apotex USA, Bedford Labs, Teva)	**Injection, solution:** 0.1 mg/mL	Equiv. to granisetron hydrochloride 0.112 mg per mL. Preservative free. May contain sodium chloride. In 1 mL single-use vials.
Rx	**Kytril** (Roche)		Equiv. to granisetron hydrochloride 0.112 mg per mL. Preservative free. Sodium chloride 9 mg. In 1 mL single-use vials
Rx	**Granisetron Hydrochloride** (Various, eg, Apotex USA, Baxter, Teva)	**Injection, solution:** 1 mg/mL	Equiv. to granisetron hydrochloride 1.12 mg per mL. May contain benzyl alcohol, parabens, and sodium chloride. In 1 mL single-dose, 1 mL preservative free, and 4 mL multi-dose vials.
Rx	**Kytril** (Roche)		Equiv. to granisetron hydrochloride 1.12 mg per mL. With benzyl alcohol 10 mg and sodium chloride 9 mg per mL. In 1 mL single-dose and 4 mL multi-dose vials.
Rx	**Sancuso** (ProStrakan[a])	**Patch; transdermal:** 3.1 mg per 24 h (34.3 mg per 52 cm^2)	(Granisetron 3.1 mg per 24 hours). In 1s.

[a] ProStrakan; 1430 US State Highway 206, Bedminster, NJ 07921-2652; (908) 234-1096.

GRANISETRON HYDROCHLORIDE — ORAL

For complete and comparative prescribing information, refer to the 5-HT_3 Receptor Antagonists group monograph.

Indications

➤*Antiemetic:* Prevention of nausea and/or vomiting associated with initial and repeat courses of emetogenic cancer therapy, including high-dose cisplatin.

Nausea and vomiting associated with radiation, including total body irradiation and fractionated abdominal radiation.

➤*Off-label uses:*

Uremic pruritus – [4] = Insufficient documentation. Initial data suggest that granisetron may be beneficial in hemodialysis patients with uremic pruritus unresponsive to previous therapy. However, these data are limited by a small population, and further study is required in larger, controlled settings to identify optimal dosage recommendations.

Administration and Dosage

➤*Adults:*

Prevention of chemotherapy-induced nausea and vomiting – 2 mg once daily (1 hour before chemotherapy), or 1 mg twice daily (give the first 1 mg dose up to 1 hour before chemotherapy and the second 1 mg dose 12 hours after the first dose). Either regimen is administered only on the day(s) chemotherapy is given.

Continued treatment while not on chemotherapy has not been found to be useful.

Prevention of radiation-induced nausea and vomiting – 2 mg once daily taken within 1 hour of radiation.

Off-label dosing –

Uremic pruritus: [4] = Insufficient documentation. The most common dosage was oral granisetron 1 mg once daily for 3 weeks or 1 mg twice daily for 4 weeks.

➤*Storage/Stability:* Keep tightly closed. Protect from light.

Tablets – Store between 15° and 30°C (59° and 86°F).

Oral solution – Store at 25°C (77°F); excursions are permitted to 15° to 30°C (59° to 86°F). Store bottle in an upright position.

GRANISETRON HYDROCHLORIDE — INJECTION

For complete and comparative prescribing information, refer to the 5-HT_3 Receptor Antagonists group monograph.

Indications

➤*Antiemetic:* For the prevention of nausea and vomiting associated with initial and repeat courses of emetogenic cancer therapy, including high-dose cisplatin.

➤*Postoperative nausea and vomiting:* For the prevention and treatment of postoperative nausea and vomiting. As with other antiemetics, routine prophylaxis is not recommended in patients in whom there is little expectation that nausea or vomiting will occur postoperatively. In patients where nausea or vomiting must be avoided during the postoperative period, granisetron injection is recommended even where the incidence of postoperative nausea or vomiting is low.

➤*Off-label uses:*

Cancer-related pruritus – [4] = Insufficient documentation. Initial data from case reports suggest that granisetron may be useful in the management of cancer-related pruritus not associated with cholestasis or opioid therapy.

Postanesthetic shivering – [4] = Insufficient documentation. Initial data regarding the use of single-dose granisetron indicate that this agent, when administered at 3 mg doses, is less effective than ketamine but more effective than placebo in the prevention of anesthetic-induced shivering. When administered at antiemetic doses (40 mcg/kg), it was comparable with meperidine or intravenous (IV) tramadol. More studies are needed to determine the appropriate and most effective dose for reducing postanesthetic shivering.

Prevention of spinal opioid–related pruritus – [5] = Poor documentation. Initial data from a small clinical trial suggest that granisetron is of no benefit in the prevention of spinal opioid–related pruritus.

Treatment of migraine (adults) – [5] = Poor documentation. The published data evaluating the efficacy of intravenous (IV) granisetron for the treatment of an acute migraine attack are limited to an open-label trial and a controlled trial, which show conflicting results. American Academy of Neurology clinical practice guidelines for the pharmacologic treatment of migraine headache in adults consider IV granisetron to be no better than placebo for aborting the acute attack (grade B evidence) but state it can be considered for controlling nausea when present.

Administration and Dosage

➤*General dosing considerations:* Granisetron injection 1 mg/mL may contain benzyl alcohol.

➤*Adults:*

Prevention of chemotherapy-induced nausea and vomiting – 10 mcg/kg administered intravenously (IV) within 30 minutes before initiation of chemotherapy, and only on the day(s) chemotherapy is given.

Prevention of postoperative nausea and vomiting – 1 mg (undiluted) administered IV over 30 seconds, before induction of anesthesia or immediately before reversal of anesthesia.

Treatment of postoperative nausea and vomiting – 1 mg (undiluted) administered IV over 30 seconds.

Off-label dosing –

Cancer-related pruritus: [4] = Insufficient documentation. Initial dosage of 3 mg IV followed by continuous subcutaneous infusion (3 mg per 24 hours) diluted in normal saline for up to 2.5 weeks.

Postanesthetic shivering: [4] = Insufficient documentation. Single IV bolus dose administered as 3 mg alone or as 1.5 mg in combination with ketamine (0.25 mg). Granisetron has also been studied for shivering at antiemetic doses (40 mcg/kg).

➤*Children:*

Prevention of chemotherapy-induced nausea and vomiting – See Adults for dosing for children 2 to 16 years of age.

➤*Administration:* For the prevention of chemotherapy-induced nausea and vomiting, granisetron may be administered IV undiluted over 30 seconds, or diluted with sodium chloride 0.9% or dextrose 5% and infused over 5 minutes.

For the prevention and treatment of postoperative nausea and vomiting, granisetron is given undiluted and administered IV over 30 seconds.

➤*Admixture compatibility:* As a general precaution, do not mix granisetron injection in a solution with other drugs. See also Storage/Stability.

➤*Storage/Stability:* Store at 20° to 25°C (68° to 77°F); excursions are permitted to 15° to 30°C (59° to 86°F). Once the multiuse vial is penetrated, use its contents within 30 days. Do not freeze. Protect from light.

Prepare IV infusion of granisetron injection at the time of administration. However, granisetron injection has been shown to be stable for at least 24 hours when diluted in sodium chloride 0.9% or dextrose 5% and stored at room temperature under normal lighting conditions.

GRANISETRON — TRANSDERMAL

For complete and comparative prescribing information, refer to the 5-HT_3 Receptor Antagonists group monograph.

Indications

➤*Antiemetic:* For the prevention of nausea and vomiting in patients receiving moderately and/or highly emetogenic chemotherapy regimens of up to 5 consecutive days' duration.

Administration and Dosage

➤*Adults:*

Prevention of chemotherapy-induced nausea and vomiting –

Usual dosage: Apply a single patch to the upper outer arm a minimum of 24 hours before chemotherapy. The patch may be applied up to a maximum of 48 hours before chemotherapy as appropriate.

Duration of therapy: The patch can be worn for up to 7 days, depending on the duration of the chemotherapy regimen. Remove the patch a minimum of 24 hours after completion of chemotherapy.

➤*Administration:* The transdermal system (patch) should be applied to clean, dry, intact, and healthy skin on the upper outer arm. Granisetron should not be placed on skin that is red, irritated, or damaged.

Each patch is packed in a pouch and should be applied directly after the pouch has been opened. The patch should not be cut into pieces.

➤*Storage/Stability:* Store at 20° to 25°C (68° to 77°F); excursions are permitted to between 15° and 30°C (59° and 86°F). Store in the original packaging.

ONDANSETRON

Rx	**Ondansetron Hydrochloride** (Various, eg, Dr. Reddy's, Sandoz)	**Tablets:** 4 mg	As hydrochloride. Lactose. Film-coated. In 30s, 500s, and UD 3s and 100s.
Rx	**Zofran** (GlaxoSmithKline)		As hydrochloride. Lactose. (Zofran 4). White, oval. Film-coated. In 30s, UD 100s, and 1 × 3 daily UD packs.
Rx	**Ondansetron Hydrochloride** (Various, eg, Dr. Reddy's, Sandoz)	**Tablets:** 8 mg	As hydrochloride. Lactose. Film-coated. In 30s, 100s, 500s, and UD 3s and 100s.
Rx	**Zofran** (GlaxoSmithKline)		As hydrochloride. Lactose. (Zofran 8). Yellow, oval. Film-coated. In 30s, UD 100s, and 1 × 3 daily UD packs.
Rx	**Ondansetron Hydrochloride** (Mylan)	**Tablets:** 16 mg	As hydrochloride. Lactose, polydextrose. (354 M). Orange. Film-coated. In 30s, 100s, 500s, and blister cards 1s.
Rx	**Ondansetron Hydrochloride** (Dr. Reddy's)	**Tablets:** 24 mg	As hydrochloride. Lactose. Film-coated. In 30s, 500s, and UD 1s and 100s.
Rx	**Zofran** (GlaxoSmithKline)		As hydrochloride. Lactose. (GX CF7/24). Pink, oval. Film-coated. In 1 × 1 daily UD packs.
Rx	**Ondansetron** (Sandoz)	**Tablets, orally disintegrating:** 4 mg	< 0.3 mg phenylalanine, aspartame, mannitol, parabens. Strawberry flavor. In UD 30s.
Rx	**Zofran ODT** (GlaxoSmithKline)		< 0.03 mg phenylalanine, aspartame, mannitol, parabens. (Z4). White. Strawberry flavor. In UD 30s.
Rx	**Ondansetron** (Sandoz)	**Tablets, orally disintegrating:** 8 mg	< 0.3 mg phenylalanine, aspartame, mannitol, parabens. Strawberry flavor. In UD 10s and 30s.
Rx	**Zofran ODT** (GlaxoSmithKline)		< 0.03 mg phenylalanine, aspartame, mannitol, parabens. (Z8). White. Strawberry flavor. In UD 10s and 30s.

ONDANSETRON

Rx	**Zuplenz** (Par)	**Film; oral:** 4 mg	Butylated hydroxytoluene, peppermint flavoring, sucralose. (4). White, rectangular, opaque. In 10s.
		8 mg	Butylated hydroxytoluene, peppermint flavoring, sucralose. (8). White, rectangular, opaque. In 10s.
Rx	**Ondansetron Hydrochloride** (Various, eg, Pliva, Roxane)	**Solution; oral:** 4 mg per 5 mL	As hydrochloride. May contain saccharin, sorbitol. Strawberry flavor. In 50 mL.
Rx	**Zofran** (GlaxoSmithKline)		As hydrochloride. Sorbitol. Strawberry flavor. In 50 mL.
Rx	**Ondansetron Hydrochloride** (Various, eg, Bedford, Sicor)	**Injection:** 2 mg/mL	As hydrochloride. Sodium chloride. May contain parabens. In single-dose and multi-dose vials.
Rx	**Ondansetron Hydrochloride** (Various, eg, Hospira, Sicor)	**Injection:** 32 mg per 50 mL (premixed)	As hydrochloride. Preservative free. 26 mg citric acid, 2,500 mg dextrose, 11.5 mg sodium citrate per 50 mL. In single-dose containers.
Rx	**Zofran** (GlaxoSmithKline)		As hydrochloride. Parabens. In 2 mL single-dose vials and 20 mL multidose vials (singles).

ONDANSETRON — ORAL

For complete prescribing information, refer to the 5-HT_3 Receptor Antagonists class monograph.

Indications

➤*Prevention of cancer chemotherapy-induced nausea and vomiting:* Prevention of nausea and vomiting associated with highly emetogenic cancer chemotherapy, including cisplatin greater than or equal to 50 mg/m^2.

Prevention of nausea and vomiting associated with initial and repeat courses of moderately emetogenic cancer chemotherapy.

➤*Prevention of nausea and vomiting associated with radiotherapy:* Prevention of nausea and vomiting associated with radiotherapy in patients receiving either total body irradiation, single high-dose fraction to the abdomen, or daily fractions to the abdomen.

➤*Prevention of postoperative nausea and/or vomiting:* Prevention of postoperative nausea and/or vomiting. As with other antiemetics, routine prophylaxis is not recommended for patients in whom there is little expectation that nausea and/or vomiting will occur postoperatively. In patients in whom nausea and/or vomiting must be avoided postoperatively, ondansetron tablets, ondansetron orally disintegrating tablets, and ondansetron oral solution are recommended, even when the incidence of postoperative nausea and/or vomiting is low.

➤*Off-label uses:*

Acute gastroenteritis vomiting (children) – Ondansetron orally disintegrating tablets have been used to treat vomiting in acute gastroenteritis.

Alcohol consumption/effects – [4] = Insufficient documentation. Initial data from controlled trials demonstrating the effects of ondansetron on alcohol consumption and/or cravings are promising.

Bulimia – [4] = Insufficient documentation. Based on a limited number of patients, ondansetron appears to have some benefit in controlling bulimic behavior in young women with severe chronic bulimia.

Cholestatic pruritus (adults) – [4] = Insufficient documentation. Initial data on the use of ondansetron in the management of cholestatic pruritus suggest that it may be of benefit based on mostly positive results in controlled trials. However, because 1 small trial showed no benefit, it is important that larger, controlled trials be conducted to establish the optimal candidates for treatment and to establish the role of this agent in the management of cholestatic pruritus.

Cholestatic pruritus (children) – [4] = Insufficient documentation. Initial data from an isolated case report suggest ondansetron may be of benefit in the management of cholestatic pruritus in children. However, before this drug can be recommended routinely, further controlled trials are needed.

Melanocytic nevi–related pruritus (children) – [4] = Insufficient documentation. Initial data suggest that ondansetron may be useful in the management of nevi-related pruritus. However, evidence is limited to case report data, and additional controlled studies are needed before the drug can be recommended in routine therapy.

Nausea and vomiting in palliative care (children) – Ondansetron has been used in palliative care of children for relief of nausea and vomiting.

Rectal administration – [2] = Fair documentation. Clinical data from large, multicenter studies suggest that the once-daily rectal administration of ondansetron may be effective in reducing the number of vomiting episodes and severity of nausea when used prior to chemotherapy and continued 2 days postchemotherapy.

Tardive dyskinesia – [4] = Insufficient documentation. Initial data suggest ondansetron may be beneficial in the management of tardive dyskinesia. However, larger, controlled trials in both tardive dyskinesia and psychosis are needed to identify the optimal lowest dose and patients who would be most responsive.

Uremic pruritus – [4] = Insufficient documentation. Data regarding ondansetron in the treatment of uremic pruritus are conflicting. However, in patients refractory to standard treatment, this drug may be a reasonable alternative.

Uremic pruritus (children/adolescents) – [4] = Insufficient documentation. Data from a single case report suggest that ondansetron may be beneficial in adolescent patients on dialysis with uremic pruritus unresponsive to previous therapy. However, further study is required in larger, controlled trials to identify optimal dosage recommendations.

Other possible off-label uses – Treatment of vomiting associated with N-acetylcysteine use.

Administration and Dosage

➤*Adults:*

Prevention of nausea and vomiting associated with highly emetogenic cancer chemotherapy – 24 mg orally, given 30 minutes before the start of single-day, highly emetogenic chemotherapy, including cisplatin 50 mg/m^2 or more.

Prevention of nausea and vomiting associated with moderately emetogenic cancer chemotherapy – 8 mg orally twice a day. The first dose should be administered 30 minutes before the start of emetogenic chemotherapy, with a subsequent dose 8 hours after the first dose; then give 8 mg twice a day (every 12 hours) for 1 to 2 days after completion of chemotherapy.

Prevention of nausea and vomiting associated with radiotherapy –

Usual dosage: 8 mg orally 3 times a day.

Total body irradiation: 8 mg orally 1 to 2 hours before each fraction of radiotherapy administered each day.

Single high-dose fraction to the abdomen: 8 mg orally administered 1 to 2 hours before radiotherapy, with subsequent doses every 8 hours after the first dose for 1 to 2 days after completion of radiotherapy.

Daily fractions to the abdomen: 8 mg orally administered 1 to 2 hours before radiotherapy, with subsequent doses every 8 hours after the first dose for each day radiotherapy is given.

Postoperative nausea and vomiting – 16 mg orally administered 1 hour before induction of anesthesia.

Off-label dosing –

Alcohol consumption/effects: [4] = Insufficient documentation.

• *Effect on alcohol consumption and cravings* – 1, 4, or 16 mcg/kg twice daily for 8 to 11 weeks. Alternative regimens have included a low-dose (0.25 mg twice daily) or high-dose (2 mg twice daily) regimen administered for a total of 6 weeks. In one study, ondansetron (4 mcg/kg twice daily) was coadministered with naltrexone (25 mg twice daily) for 8 weeks to evaluate effects on alcohol cravings.

• *Effect on alcohol intoxication effects* – In these studies, one-time oral ondansetron 4 or 8 mg doses were administered 60 to 90 minutes prior to acute alcohol ingestion.

Bulimia: [4] = Insufficient documentation. 4 mg 3 times/day as a base dose with as-needed usage during additional urges of binge-vomit episodes or 30 minutes prior to meals. Total daily dose did not exceed 24 mg. This regimen was administered for 4 weeks.

Cholestatic pruritus (adults): [4] = Insufficient documentation. 4 mg twice daily or 8 mg 2 to 3 times daily orally for 7 days up to 5 months.

Rectal administration: [2] = Fair documentation. 16 mg once daily administered rectally 2 hours prior to chemotherapy.

Tardive dyskinesia: [4] = Insufficient documentation. 4 to 12 mg orally daily. Lower doses have been used initially with an increase to higher doses by week 2 or 3. Dosages greater than 8 mg daily have been administered in divided doses (8 mg in the morning and 4 mg in the evening).

Uremic pruritus: [4] = Insufficient documentation. 4 mg twice daily or 8 mg 3 times/day for 14 days to 5 months.

➤*Children:*

Prevention of nausea and vomiting associated with moderately emetogenic cancer chemotherapy –

12 years of age and older: See Adults for dosing.

4 to 11 years of age: 4 mg orally 3 times a day. The first dose should be administered 30 minutes before the start of emetogenic chemotherapy, with subsequent doses 4 and 8 hours after the first dose. Then give 4 mg orally 3 times a day (every 8 hours) for 1 to 2 days after completion of chemotherapy.

Off-label dosing –

Acute gastroenteritis vomiting (children):

• *8 to 15 kg* – 2 mg orally disintegrating table for 1 dose.
• *Greater than 15 to 30 kg* – 4 mg orally disintegrating tablet for 1 dose.
• *Greater than 30 kg* – 8 mg orally disintegrating tablet for 1 dose.

ONDANSETRON — ORAL

Cholestatic pruritus (children): [4] = Insufficient documentation. 4 mg twice daily (0.8 mg/kg daily) orally for 5 months.

Melanocytic nevi–related pruritus (children): [4] = Insufficient documentation. 3.2 mg orally 3 times daily (0.46 mg/kg/day) for at least 6 months in a child 7 years of age; 0.6 mg orally twice daily for at least 6 weeks in a child 3 years of age.

Nausea and vomiting in palliative care (children): 0.15 mg/kg/dose orally every 6 to 8 hours.

Prevention of nausea and vomiting associated with chemotherapy: Dose is based on body surface area. Administer initial dose 30 minutes before chemotherapy.

- *Less than 0.3 m^2* – 1 mg orally 3 times daily as needed for nausea.
- *0.3 to 0.6 m^2* – 2 mg orally 3 times daily as needed for nausea.
- *0.6 to 1 m^2* – 3 mg orally 3 times daily as needed for nausea.
- *More than 1 m^2* – 4 to 8 mg orally 3 times daily as needed for nausea.

Uremic pruritus (children/adolescents): [4] = Insufficient documentation. Oral ondansetron was administered as 4 or 8 mg twice daily for approximately 10 weeks.

➤*Hepatic function impairment:* In patients with severe hepatic function impairment according to Child-Pugh criteria, clearance is reduced and apparent volume of distribution is increased, with a resultant increase in plasma half-life. In such patients, a total daily dose of 8 mg should not be exceeded.

➤*Administration:* Oral ondansetron should be administered 30 minutes before the start of emetogenic cancer chemotherapy; 1 to 2 hours before radiotherapy; or 1 hour before induction of anesthesia.

Do not attempt to push ondansetron orally disintegrating tablets through the foil backing. With dry hands, peel back the foil backing of 1 blister and gently remove the tablet. Immediately place the ondansetron orally disintegrating tablet on top of the tongue, where it will dissolve in seconds, then swallow with saliva. Administration with liquid is not necessary.

➤*Storage/Stability:*

Tablets/Orally disintegrating tablets – Store between 2° and 30°C (36° and 86°F). Protect the 4 mg tablets from light. Dispense in tight, light-resistant container. Store blisters in cartons.

Oral solution – Store upright between 15° and 30°C (59° and 86°F). Protect from light. Store bottles upright in cartons.

ONDANSETRON HYDROCHLORIDE — INJECTION

For complete and comparative prescribing information, refer to the 5-HT_3 Receptor Antagonists group monograph.

Indications

➤*Prevention of chemotherapy-induced nausea and vomiting:* Prevention of nausea and vomiting associated with initial and repeat courses of emetogenic cancer chemotherapy, including high-dose cisplatin. Efficacy of the 32 mg single dose beyond 24 hours in these patients has not been established.

➤*Prevention of postoperative nausea or vomiting:* As with other antiemetics, routine prophylaxis is not recommended for patients in whom there is little expectation that nausea and/or vomiting will occur postoperatively. In patients in whom nausea and/or vomiting must be avoided postoperatively, ondansetron injection is recommended even when the incidence of postoperative nausea and/or vomiting is low. For patients who do not receive prophylactic ondansetron injection and experience nausea and/or vomiting postoperatively, ondansetron injection may be given to prevent further episodes.

➤*Off-label uses:*

Acute gastroenteritis vomiting (children) – The oral route is preferred; however, the intravenous (IV) doseform may be used when oral administration is not possible.

Cholestatic pruritus (adults) – [4] = Insufficient documentation. Initial data on the use of ondansetron in the management of cholestatic pruritus suggest that it may be of benefit based on mostly positive results in controlled trials. However, because 1 small trial showed no benefit, it is important that larger, controlled trials be conducted to establish the optimal candidates for treatment and to establish the role of this agent in the management of cholestatic pruritus.

Cholestatic pruritus (pregnancy) – [4] = Insufficient documentation. Initial data on the use of ondansetron in the management of cholestatic pruritus of pregnancy suggest that this drug may be of benefit based on an isolated case report. However, before this drug can be routinely recommended, further controlled trials are needed.

Hyperemesis gravidarum – [4] = Insufficient documentation. In a very small number of patients (fewer than 20), ondansetron has been effective in treating severe hyperemesis gravidarum when administered in early pregnancy. However, optimal dosing and safety information have yet to be established.

Nausea and vomiting in palliative care (children) – Ondansetron has been used in palliative care of children for relief of nausea and vomiting.

Nausea and vomiting of pregnancy – [2] = Fair documentation. A position statement from the American Gastroenterological Association Institute (AGAI) noted that Food and Drug Administration safety categories for pregnancy may not reflect findings in the medical literature or clinical experience. The authors recommended using the lowest-risk drug possible when GI drugs are required during pregnancy and discussing all therapeutic decisions with the patient and her obstetrician.

The recommended first-line treatment for nausea and vomiting of pregnancy according to the American College of Obstetricians and Gynecologists (ACOG) is pyridoxine alone or pyridoxine combined with doxylamine. Additional pharmacologic interventions were recommended only for refractory cases.

Postanesthetic shivering – [2] = Fair documentation. Initial data regarding the use of single-dose ondansetron indicate that this agent, when administered in 8 mg doses, is effective and comparable with meperidine in preventing postanesthetic shivering.

Prevention of nausea and vomiting associated with highly emetogenic chemotherapy – Ondansetron has been used in prevention of nausea and vomiting associated with highly emetogenic chemotherapy.

Prevention of nausea and vomiting associated with moderately emetogenic chemotherapy – Ondansetron has been used in prevention of nausea and vomiting associated with moderately emetogenic chemotherapy.

Pruritus (opioid related) – [2] = Fair documentation. Ondansetron has been studied for the prevention and treatment of opioid-induced pruritus. It appears to be effective and may be less likely to interfere with pain control than naloxone or nalmefene.

Treatment of migraine (adults) – [5] = Poor documentation. Use is not recommended. The published data evaluating the efficacy of IV ondansetron for the treatment of an acute migraine attack are limited to 3 case reports. Clinical practice guidelines for the pharmacologic treatment of migraine headache in adults do not make a statement on ondansetron, likely because the available literature was published after the date of the guidelines.

Uremic pruritus (adults) – [4] = Insufficient documentation. Data from one case report suggest that IV ondansetron may be beneficial in hemodialysis patients with uremic pruritus unresponsive to previous therapy. However, larger, controlled trials are required to identify optimal dosage recommendations. Oral dosing may be a more preferable route.

Other possible off-label uses – Treatment of radiation-induced nausea and vomiting.

Administration and Dosage

➤*General dosing considerations:* Dilute ondansetron vial before use for prevention of chemotherapy-induced nausea and vomiting (See Preparation for administration).

➤*Adults:*

Prevention of chemotherapy-induced nausea and vomiting –

Usual dosage:

- *Single-dose regimen* – 32 mg single dose infused over 15 minutes beginning 30 minutes before the start of emetogenic chemotherapy. The recommended infusion rate should not be exceeded.
- *Three-dose regimen (3 doses of 0.15 mg/kg each)* – The first dose (0.15 mg/kg) is infused over 15 minutes beginning 30 minutes before the start of emetogenic chemotherapy. Subsequent doses (0.15 mg/kg) are administered 4 and 8 hours after the first dose of ondansetron.

Prevention of postoperative nausea and vomiting – While recommended as a fixed dose for patients weighing more than 40 kg, few patients above 80 kg have been studied.

Usual dosage: 4 mg undiluted administered IV in not less than 30 seconds, preferably over 2 to 5 minutes, immediately before induction of anesthesia, or postoperatively if the patient experiences nausea and/or vomiting occurring shortly after surgery.

In patients who do not achieve adequate control of postoperative nausea and/or vomiting following a single, prophylactic, preinduction, IV dose of ondansetron 4 mg, administration of a second IV dose of ondansetron 4 mg postoperatively does not provide additional control of nausea and/or vomiting.

Alternative dosage: 4 mg undiluted may be administered intramuscularly (IM) as a single injection for adults.

Off-label dosing –

Cholestatic pruritus (adults): [4] = Insufficient documentation. Intermittent short-term dosing with ondansetron 4 or 8 mg IV has been used.

Cholestatic pruritus (pregnancy): [4] = Insufficient documentation. Single dose of ondansetron 4 mg IV.

Hyperemesis gravidarum: [4] = Insufficient documentation. 10 mg IV every 8 hours as needed.

Nausea and vomiting of pregnancy: [2] = Fair documentation. 8 mg IV over 15 minutes every 12 hours.

Opioid-induced nausea and vomiting: 4 mg IV every 12 hours as needed if symptoms do not resolve in 30 to 60 minutes after IV administration of promethazine.

Postanesthetic shivering: [2] = Fair documentation. Single IV dose of 4 or 8 mg administered during induction of anesthesia.

Pruritus (opioid related): [2] = Fair documentation.

- *Prevention* – 4 or 8 mg IV administered 20 to 30 minutes prior to spina opioid administration. One study repeated dosing at 12, 24, 36, and 48 hours after spinal opioid dosing.
- *Treatment* – 4 or 8 mg IV.

ONDANSETRON HYDROCHLORIDE — INJECTION

Uremic pruritus (adults): [4] = Insufficient documentation. IV ondansetron was administered as an 8 mg single dose.

➤*Children:*

Prevention of chemotherapy-induced nausea and vomiting –

6 months to 18 years of age: On the basis of the limited available information, the dosage should be three 0.15 mg/kg IV doses. The first dose is to be administered 30 minutes before the start of moderately to highly emetogenic chemotherapy. Subsequent doses (0.15 mg/kg) are administered 4 to 8 hours after the first dose of ondansetron. The drug should be infused IV over 15 minutes. Little information is available about dosage in pediatric cancer patients younger than 6 months of age.

Prevention of postoperative nausea and vomiting –

1 month to 12 years of age: Single 0.1 mg/kg IV dose for children weighing less than 40 kg, or a single 4 mg dose for patients weighing more than 40 kg. The rate of administration should not be less than 30 seconds, preferably over 2 to 5 minutes, immediately prior to or following anesthesia induction, or postoperatively if the patient experiences nausea and/or vomiting occurring shortly after surgery.

Prevention of further nausea and/or vomiting was only studied in patients who had not received prophylactic ondansetron.

Off-label dosing –

Acute gastroenteritis vomiting (children):

• *Usual dose* – 0.1 to 0.5 mg/kg/dose IV for 1 dose.

• *Maximum dose* – 4 mg/dose IV.

Nausea and vomiting in palliative care (children): 0.15 mg/kg/dose IV every 6 to 8 hours.

Opioid-induced nausea and vomiting: 0.15 mg/kg IV every 6 hours as needed. Maximum dose is 4 mg. If ondansetron is unsuccessful, then consider metoclopramide IV.

Prevention of nausea and vomiting associated with highly emetogenic chemotherapy:

• *Usual dose* – 0.45 mg/kg/dose administered IV 30 minutes before emetogenic drugs, then administer 0.15 mg/kg/dose every 4 hours as needed.

• *Maximum dose* – 32 mg/dose IV.

Prevention of nausea and vomiting associated with moderately emetogenic chemotherapy: 0.15 mg/kg/dose administered IV 30 minutes before, 4 and 8 hours after emetogenic drugs; then administer the same dose every 4 hours as needed.

➤*Hepatic function impairment:* In patients with severe hepatic function impairment (Child-Pugh score of 10 or greater), a single maximal daily dose of 8 mg to be infused over 15 minutes beginning 30 minutes before the start of the emetogenic chemotherapy is recommended. There is no experience beyond first-day administration of ondansetron.

➤*Preparation for administration:*

Premixed in flexible plastic containers – To open, tear outer wrap at notch and remove solution container. Check for minute leaks by squeezing container firmly. If leaks are found, discard unit, as sterility may be impaired.

Use aseptic technique.

1.) Close flow control clamp of administration set.
2.) Remove cover from outlet port at bottom of container.
3.) Insert piercing pin of administration set into port with a twisting motion until the pin is firmly seated. See full directions on administration set carton.
4.) Suspend container from hanger.
5.) Squeeze and release the drip chamber to establish the proper fluid level in the chamber during infusion of ondansetron injection premixed.
6.) Open flow control clamp to expel air from set. Close clamp.
7.) Attach set to venipuncture device. If device is not indwelling, prime and make venipuncture.
8.) Perform venipuncture.

Dilution –

Prevention of chemotherapy-induced nausea and vomiting:

• *Vial* – Dilute before use for prevention of chemotherapy-induced nausea and vomiting. Ondansetron injection should be diluted in 50 mL of dextrose 5% injection or sodium chloride 0.9% injection before administration.

• *Flexible plastic container* – Ondansetron 32 mg premixed injection in 50 mL of dextrose 5% requires no dilution.

Prevention of postoperative nausea and vomiting:

• *Vial* – Ondansetron injection requires no dilution for administration for postoperative nausea and/or vomiting.

➤*Administration:* For prevention of chemotherapy-induced nausea and vomiting, administer the single-dose regimen (32 mg) and the 3-dose regimen (3 doses of 0.15 mg/kg each) by IV and infuse over 15 minutes.

For prevention of postoperative nausea and vomiting, administer 4 mg undiluted by IV in not less than 30 seconds, preferably over 2 to 5 minutes. As an alternative dosage, 4 mg undiluted may be administered IM as a single injection for adults.

Ondansetron injection premixed in flexible plastic containers is to be administered by IV drip infusion only. Do not administer unless solution is clear and container is undamaged. Do not use flexible plastic container in series connections.

Regulate rate of administration with flow control clamp.

Occasionally, ondansetron precipitates at the stopper/vial interface in vials stored upright. Potency and safety are not affected. If a precipitate is observed, resolubilize by shaking the vial vigorously.

➤*Admixture compatibility:* Ondansetron injection and premix injection should not be mixed with solutions for which physical and chemical compatibility has not been established. In particular, this applies to alkaline solutions, as a precipitate may form.

Premixed injection – If used with a primary IV fluid system, the primary solution should be discontinued during ondansetron injection premixed infusion.

➤*Storage/Stability:*

Injection – Store between 2° and 30°C (36° and 86°F). Protect from light.

Ondansetron injection is stable at room temperature under normal lighting conditions for 48 hours after dilution with the following IV fluids: sodium chloride 0.9% injection, dextrose 5% injection, dextrose 5% and sodium chloride 0.9% injection, dextrose 5% and sodium chloride 0.45% injection, and sodium chloride 3% injection.

Although ondansetron injection is chemically and physically stable when diluted as recommended, sterile precautions should be observed because diluents generally do not contain preservative. After dilution, do not use beyond 24 hours.

Premixed injection – Store between 2° and 30°C (36° and 86°F). Protect from light. Avoid excessive heat. Protect from freezing.

PALONOSETRON

Rx	**Aloxi** (Eisai)	**Injection, solution:** 0.05 mg/mL	As palonosetron hydrochloride. Disodium edetate. In 1.5[a] and 5 mL[b] single-use vials.

[a] With mannitol 83 mg.
[b] With mannitol 207.5 mg.

PALONOSETRON HYDROCHLORIDE — INJECTION

For complete and comparative prescribing information, refer to the 5-HT_3 Receptor Antagonists group monograph.

Indications

➤*Chemotherapy-induced nausea and vomiting:* For the prevention of acute and delayed nausea and vomiting associated with initial and repeat courses in patients treated with moderately emetogenic cancer chemotherapy; for the prevention of acute nausea and vomiting associated with initial and repeat courses in patients treated with highly emetogenic cancer chemotherapy.

➤*Postoperative nausea and vomiting:* For the prevention of postoperative nausea and vomiting for up to 24 hours following surgery. Efficacy beyond 24 hours has not been demonstrated.

Administration and Dosage

➤*Adults:*

Prevention of chemotherapy-induced nausea and vomiting – A single 0.25 mg intravenous (IV) dose administered over 30 seconds. Dosing should occur approximately 30 minutes before the start of chemotherapy.

Prevention of postoperative nausea and vomiting – A single 0.075 mg IV dose administered over 10 seconds immediately before the induction of anesthesia.

➤*Administration:* Palonosetron is supplied ready for IV injection. Flush the infusion line with isotonic sodium chloride solution before and after administration of palonosetron.

➤*Admixture compatibility:* Palonosetron should not be mixed with other drugs.

➤*Storage/Stability:* Store at 20° to 25°C (68° to 77°F). Excursions are permitted between 15° and 30°C (59° and 86°F). Protect from freezing and light.

APREPITANT

Rx	Emend (Merck)	Capsules; oral: 40 mg	Sucrose. (464 40 mg). White/Mustard Yellow. In unit-of-use 1s and UD 5s.
		80 mg	Sucrose. (461 80 mg). White. In 30s and UD 6s.
		125 mg	Sucrose. (462 125 mg). White/Pink. In 30s, UD 6s, and unit-of-use trifold pack containing one 125 mg capsule and two 80 mg capsules.

APREPITANT — ORAL

Indications

➤*Prevention of nausea/vomiting associated with highly emetogenic cancer chemotherapy:* In combination with other antiemetic agents for the prevention of acute and delayed nausea and vomiting associated with initial and repeat courses of highly emetogenic cancer chemotherapy, including high-dose cisplatin.

➤*Prevention of nausea/vomiting associated with moderately emetogenic cancer chemotherapy:* In combination with other antiemetic agents for the prevention of nausea and vomiting associated with initial and repeat courses of moderately emetogenic cancer chemotherapy.

➤*Prevention of postoperative nausea/vomiting:* For the prevention of postoperative nausea/vomiting.

Administration and Dosage

➤*Adults:*

Prevention of nausea/vomiting associated with cancer chemotherapy –

Usual dosage: 125 mg orally 1 hour prior to chemotherapy treatment on day 1 and 80 mg once daily in the morning on days 2 and 3.

Concomitant therapy: Aprepitant is given for 3 days as part of a regimen that includes a corticosteroid and a 5-HT_3 antagonist. (See also Concomitant corticosteroid therapy.)

Highly emetogenic cancer chemotherapy:

Aprepitant Dosage Regimen for Highly Emetogenic Cancer Chemotherapy

Treatment	Day 1	Day 2	Day 3	Day 4
Aprepitant[a]	125 mg	80 mg	80 mg	none
Dexamethasone[b]	12 mg orally	8 mg orally	8 mg orally	8 mg orally
Ondansetron[c]	32 mg IV[d]	none	none	none

[a] Aprepitant was administered orally 1 hour prior to chemotherapy treatment on day 1 and in the morning on days 2 and 3.
[b] Dexamethasone was administered 30 minutes prior to chemotherapy treatment on day 1 and in the morning on days 2 through 4. The dose of dexamethasone was chosen to account for drug interactions.
[c] Ondansetron was administered 30 minutes prior to chemotherapy treatment on day 1.
[d] IV = intravenous.

Moderately emetogenic cancer chemotherapy:

Aprepitant Dosage Regimen for Moderately Emetogenic Cancer Chemotherapy

Treatment	Day 1	Day 2	Day 3
Aprepitant[a]	125 mg	80 mg	80 mg
Dexamethasone[b]	12 mg orally	none	none
Ondansetron[c]	8 mg orally × 2	none	none

[a] Aprepitant was administered orally 1 hour prior to chemotherapy treatment on day 1 and in the morning on days 2 and 3.
[b] Dexamethasone was administered 30 minutes prior to chemotherapy treatment on day 1. The dexamethasone dose was chosen to account for drug interactions.
[c] One ondansetron 8 mg capsule was administered 30 to 60 minutes prior to chemotherapy treatment, and a second 8 mg capsule was administered 8 hours after the first dose on day 1.

Prevention of postoperative nausea/vomiting – 40 mg within 3 hours prior to induction of anesthesia.

➤*Concomitant corticosteroid therapy:*

Dexamethasone – The oral dexamethasone doses should be reduced approximately 50% when coadministered with aprepitant 125 mg/80 mg regimen.

Methylprednisolone – The IV methylprednisolone dose should be reduced approximately 25%, and the oral methylprednisolone dose should be reduced approximately 50% when coadministered with aprepitant 125 mg/80 mg regimen.

➤*Preparation for administration:* Aprepitant is not listed as potentially hazardous in the NIOSH Alert and many practitioners do not consider it hazardous. Safe handling precautions are not routinely required, although clinicians may consider using other special handling precautions to reduce risk for health care providers. Aprepitant was carcinogenic in rats at doses resulting in an area under the plasma concentration-time curve (AUC) equivalent to 0.7 to 1.6 times the usual human AUC with oral doses of aprepitant 125 mg/day.

➤*Administration:* May be taken with or without food.

➤*Storage/Stability:* Store at 20° to 25°C (68° to 77°F). The desiccant should remain in the original bottle.

Actions

➤*Pharmacology:* Aprepitant is a selective high-affinity antagonist of human substance P/neurokinin 1 (NK_1) receptors. Aprepitant has little or no affinity for serotonin (5-HT_3), dopamine, and corticosteroid receptors, the targets of existing therapies for chemotherapy-induced nausea/vomiting and postoperative nausea/vomiting.

Aprepitant has been shown in animal models to inhibit emesis induced by cytotoxic chemotherapeutic agents (eg, cisplatin), via central actions. Animal and human positron emission tomography (PET) studies with aprepitant have shown that it crosses the blood-brain barrier and occupies brain NK_1 receptors. Animal and human studies show that aprepitant augments the antiemetic activity of the 5-HT_3-receptor antagonist ondansetron and the corticosteroid dexamethasone and inhibits the acute and delayed phases of cisplatin-induced emesis.

➤*Pharmacokinetics:*

Absorption – Following oral administration of a single dose of aprepitant 40 mg in the fasted state, mean area under the curve ($AUC_{0-\infty}$) was 7.8 mcg•h/mL and mean peak plasma concentration (C_{max}) was 0.7 mcg/mL, occurring at approximately 3 hours postdose (T_{max}). The absolute bioavailability at the 40 mg dose has not been determined.

Following oral administration of a single aprepitant 125 mg dose on day 1 and 80 mg once daily on days 2 and 3, the AUC_{0-24h} was approximately 19.6 and 21.2 mcg•h/mL on day 1 and 3, respectively. The C_{max} of 1.6 and 1.4 mcg/mL were reached in approximately 4 hours (T_{max}) on day 1 and 3, respectively.

At the dose range of 80 to 125 mg, the mean absolute oral bioavailability of aprepitant is approximately 60% to 65%.

The pharmacokinetics of aprepitant are nonlinear across the clinical dose range. In healthy young adults, the increase in $AUC_{0-\infty}$ was 26% greater than dose proportional between 80 and 125 mg single doses administered in the fed state.

Effect of food: Oral administration of the capsule with a standard high-fat breakfast had no clinically meaningful effect on the bioavailability of aprepitant.

Distribution – Aprepitant is more than 95% bound to plasma proteins. The mean apparent volume of distribution at steady state is approximately 70 L in humans.

Aprepitant crosses the placenta in rats and rabbits and crosses the blood-brain barrier in humans.

Metabolism – Aprepitant undergoes extensive metabolism. In vitro studies using human liver microsomes indicate that aprepitant is metabolized primarily by CYP3A4 with minor metabolism by CYP1A2 and CYP2C19. Metabolism is largely via oxidation at the morpholine ring and its side chains. No metabolism by CYP2D6, CYP2C9, or CYP2E1 was detected. In healthy young adults, aprepitant accounts for approximately 24% of the radioactivity in plasma over 72 hours following a single oral dose of [^{14}C]-aprepitant 300 mg, indicating a substantial presence of metabolites in the plasma. Seven metabolites of aprepitant, which are only weakly active, have been identified in human plasma.

Excretion – Following administration of a single IV dose of [^{14}C]-aprepitant 100 mg prodrug to healthy subjects, 57% of the radioactivity was recovered in urine and 45% in feces. A study was not conducted with a radiolabeled capsule formulation. The results after oral administration may differ.

Aprepitant is eliminated primarily by metabolism; it is not renally excreted. The apparent plasma clearance of aprepitant ranged from approximately 62 to 90 mL/min. The apparent terminal half-life ranged from approximately 9 to 13 hours.

Special populations –

Renal function impairment: In patients with severe renal function impairment, the $AUC_{0-\infty}$ of total aprepitant (unbound and protein bound) decreased 21% and C_{max} decreased 32%, relative to healthy subjects. In patients with ESRD undergoing hemodialysis, the $AUC_{0-\infty}$ of total aprepitant decreased 42% and C_{max} decreased 32%.

Hepatic function impairment: Following administration of a single dose of aprepitant 125 mg on day 1 and 80 mg once daily on days 2 and 3 to patients with mild hepatic function impairment (Child-Pugh score 5 to 6), the AUC_{0-24h} of aprepitant was 11% lower on day 1 and 36% lower on day 3, compared with healthy subjects given the same regimen. In patients with moderate hepatic function impairment (Child-Pugh score 7 to 9), the AUC_{0-24h} of aprepitant was 10% higher on day 1 and 18% higher on day 3, as compared with healthy subjects given the same regimen.

Elderly: Following oral administration of a single dose of aprepitant 125 mg on day 1 and 80 mg once daily on days 2 through 5, the AUC_{0-24h} of aprepitant was 21% higher on day 1 and 36% higher on day 5 in elderly

APREPITANT — ORAL

(65 years of age and older) patients relative to younger adults. The C_{max} was 10% higher on day 1 and 24% higher on day 5 in elderly patients relative to younger adults.

Gender: The C_{max} for aprepitant is 16% higher in women compared with men. The half-life of aprepitant is 25% lower in women compared with men, and T_{max} occurs at approximately the same time.

Race: Following oral administration of a single dose of aprepitant 125 mg, the AUC_{0-24h} is approximately 25% and 29% higher in Hispanic subjects compared with white and black subjects, respectively. The C_{max} is 22% and 31% higher in Hispanic subjects compared with white and black subjects, respectively.

Contraindications

Hypersensitivity to any component of the product; concurrent use with pimozide, terfenadine, astemizole, or cisapride.

Warnings/Precautions

➤*Chronic therapy:* Chronic continuous use of aprepitant for prevention of nausea and vomiting is not recommended because it has not been studied and because the drug interaction profile may change during chronic continuous use.

➤*Hepatic function impairment:* There are no clinical or pharmacokinetic data in patients with severe hepatic function impairment (Child-Pugh score higher than 9). Therefore, exercise caution when aprepitant is administered in these patients.

➤*Pregnancy: Category B.* There are no adequate and well-controlled studies in pregnant women. Because animal reproduction studies are not always predictive of human response, use this drug during pregnancy only if clearly needed.

➤*Lactation:* Aprepitant is excreted in the milk of rats. It is not known whether this drug is excreted in human milk. Because many drugs are excreted in human milk, because of the potential for possible serious adverse reactions in breast-feeding infants from aprepitant, and because of the potential for tumorigenicity shown for aprepitant in rodent carcinogenicity studies, decide whether to discontinue breast-feeding or the drug, taking into account the importance of the drug to the mother.

➤*Children:* Safety and efficacy of aprepitant in children have not been established.

Drug Interactions

➤*CYP-450 system:* Aprepitant is a substrate, a weak to moderate (dose-dependent) inhibitor, and an inducer of CYP3A4. Aprepitant also is an inducer of CYP2C9. Use aprepitant with caution in patients receiving concomitant orally administered medicinal products, including chemotherapy agents that are primarily metabolized through CYP3A4.

Weak inhibition of CYP3A4 by a single aprepitant 40 mg is not expected to alter the plasma concentrations of concomitant medicinal products that are primarily metabolized through CYP3A4 to a clinically significant degree. However, higher aprepitant doses or repeated dosing at any aprepitant dose may have clinically significant effect.

➤*Chemotherapeutic agents:* Chemotherapy agents that are known to be metabolized by CYP3A4 include docetaxel, paclitaxel, etoposide, irinotecan, ifosfamide, imatinib, vinorelbine, vinblastine, and vincristine. In clinical studies, aprepitant (125 mg/80 mg regimen) was administered commonly with etoposide, vinorelbine, or paclitaxel. The doses of these agents were not adjusted to account for potential drug interactions. Because of the small number of patients in clinical studies who received CYP3A4 substrates vinblastine, vincristine, or ifosfamide, particular caution and careful monitoring are advised in patients receiving these agents or other chemotherapy agents metabolized primarily by CYP3A4 that were not studied.

Aprepitant Drug Interactions

Precipitant drug	Object drug[a]		Description
CYP3A4 inhibitors (eg, clarithromycin, diltiazem, itraconazole, ketoconazole, nefazodone, nelfinavir, ritonavir, troleandomycin)	Aprepitant	⬆	Concurrent use of CYP3A4 inhibitors with aprepitant may increase aprepitant plasma concentrations. Use with caution.
CYP3A4 inducers (eg, carbamazepine, phenytoin, rifampin)	Aprepitant	⬇	Coadministration may decrease aprepitant plasma concentrations and reduce efficacy.
Paroxetine	Aprepitant	⬇	Concurrent use decreased the AUC approximately 25% and C_{max} approximately 20% of both aprepitant and paroxetine.
Aprepitant	Paroxetine		
Aprepitant	Contraceptives, oral	⬇	The efficacy of oral contraceptives may be reduced during and for 28 days after administration of the last dose of aprepitant. Alternative or backup methods of contraception are recommended during treatment and for 1 month following the last dose of aprepitant.
Aprepitant	CYP2C9 substrates (eg, tolbutamide, warfarin)	⬇	Aprepitant is a CYP2C9 inducer and has been shown to induce the metabolism of warfarin and tolbutamide, resulting in lower plasma levels. In patients on chronic warfarin therapy, closely monitor the international normalized ratio in the 2-week period, particularly at 7 to 10 days, following the initiation of aprepitant.
Aprepitant	CYP3A4 substrates (eg, pimozide, cisapride[b], astemizole[c], terfenadine[c], dexamethasone, methylprednisolone, midazolam, alprazolam, triazolam, docetaxel, paclitaxel, etoposide, irinotecan, ifosfamide, imatinib, vinorelbine, vinblastine, vincristine)	⬆	Aprepitant is a moderate inhibitor of CYP3A4 and can increase plasma concentration of coadministered products that are metabolized through CYP3A4. Aprepitant is contraindicated with astemizole, terfenadine, pimozide, or cisapride. Reduce the oral dexamethasone dose approximately 50% when given with aprepitant (125 mg/80 mg regimen). Reduce the dose of methylprednisolone IV approximately 25% and the oral dose approximately 50% when given with aprepitant (125 mg/80 mg regimen). Dosage adjustment for IV midazolam may be necessary when it is coadministered with aprepitant for the chemotherapy-induced nausea/vomiting indication.

[a] ⬇ = object drug decreased; ⬆ = object drug increased.
[b] Available on a limited access basis only.
[c] No longer available in the United States.

Adverse Reactions

The overall safety of aprepitant was evaluated in approximately 4,400 individuals.

➤*Chemotherapy-induced nausea/vomiting highly emetogenic chemotherapy:*

Aprepitant Adverse Reactions in Patients Receiving Highly Emetogenic Chemotherapy (≥ 3%) (Cycle 1)

Adverse reaction	Aprepitant (n = 544)	Standard therapy (n = 550)
CNS		
Asthenia/fatigue	17.8%	11.8%
Dizziness	6.6%	4.4%
Headache	8.5%	8.7%
Insomnia	2.9%	3.1%
GI		
Abdominal pain	4.6%	3.3%
Anorexia	10.1%	9.5%
Constipation	10.3%	12.2%
Diarrhea	10.3%	7.5%
Epigastric discomfort	4%	3.1%
Gastritis	4.2%	3.1%
Heartburn	5.3%	4.9%
Nausea	12.7%	11.8%
Vomiting	7.5%	7.6%
Hematologic/Lymphatic		
Neutropenia	3.1%	2.9%
Respiratory		
Hiccups	10.8%	5.6%
Special senses		
Tinnitus	3.7%	3.8%

APREPITANT — ORAL

Aprepitant Adverse Reactions in Patients Receiving Highly Emetogenic Chemotherapy (≥ 3%) (Cycle 1)		
Adverse reaction	Aprepitant (n = 544)	Standard therapy (n = 550)
Miscellaneous		
Dehydration	5.9%	5.1%
Fever	2.9%	3.5%
Mucous membrane disorder	2.6%	3.1%

In addition, isolated cases of serious adverse reactions (regardless of causality) of bradycardia, disorientation, and perforating duodenal ulcer were reported in highly emetogenic chemotherapy-induced nausea/vomiting clinical studies.

➤*Chemotherapy-induced nausea/vomiting moderately emetogenic chemotherapy:*

Aprepitant Adverse Reactions in Patients Receiving Moderately Emetogenic Chemotherapy (≥ 3%) (Cycle 1)		
Adverse reaction	Aprepitant (n = 438)	Standard therapy (n = 428)
Cardiovascular		
Hot flush	3%	1.4%
CNS		
Asthenia	3.4%	3.7%
Dizziness	3.4%	4.2%
Fatigue	21.9%	21.5%
Headache	16.4%	16.4%
Insomnia	4.1%	5.6%
Dermatologic		
Alopecia	24%	22.2%
GI		
Anorexia	4.3%	5.8%
Constipation	12.3%	18%
Diarrhea	5.5%	6.3%
Dyspepsia	8.4%	4.9%
Nausea	7.1%	7.5%
Stomatitis	5.3%	4.4%
Hematologic/Lymphatic		
Neutropenia	8.9%	8.4%
Respiratory		
Pharyngolaryngeal pain	3%	2.3%
Miscellaneous		
Mucosal inflammation	2.5%	3.5%

Isolated cases of serious adverse reactions (regardless of causality) of dehydration, enterocolitis, febrile neutropenia, hypertension, hypesthesia, neutropenic sepsis, pneumonia, and sinus tachycardia were reported in the moderately emetogenic chemotherapy-induced nausea/vomiting clinical study.

➤*Chemotherapy-induced nausea/vomiting highly and moderately emetogenic chemotherapy:* The following additional clinical adverse reactions (incidence more than 0.5% and more than standard therapy), regardless of causality, were reported in patients treated with aprepitant regimen:

Cardiovascular – Deep venous thrombosis, flushing, hypertension, hypotension, myocardial infarction, palpitations, pulmonary embolism, tachycardia.

CNS – Anxiety disorder, confusion, depression, malaise, peripheral neuropathy, rigors, sensory neuropathy, taste disturbance, tremor.

Dermatologic – Acne, diaphoresis, rash.

GI – Acid reflux, deglutition disorder, dry mouth, dysgeusia, dysphagia, eructation, flatulence, increased salivation, obstipation.

GU – Dysuria, pelvic pain, urinary tract infection.

Hematologic/Lymphatic – Anemia, febrile neutropenia, thrombocytopenia.

Metabolic/Nutritional – Decreased appetite, diabetes mellitus, edema, hypokalemia, weight loss.

Musculoskeletal – Arthralgia, back pain, muscular weakness, musculoskeletal pain, myalgia, rigors.

Ophthalmic – Conjunctivitis.

Renal – Renal function impairment.

Respiratory – Cough, dyspnea, lower respiratory tract infection, nasal secretion, pharyngitis, pneumonitis, respiratory function impairment, upper respiratory tract infection, vocal disturbance.

Miscellaneous – Candidiasis, herpes simplex, malignant neoplasm, non-small cell lung carcinoma, septic shock.

➤*Lab test abnormalities:* The following table shows the percent of patients with laboratory adverse reactions reported at an incidence of 3% or more in patients receiving highly emetogenic chemotherapy.

Aprepitant Lab Test Abnormalities in Patients Receiving Highly Emetogenic Chemotherapy (≥ 3%) (Cycle 1)		
	Aprepitant (n = 544)	Standard therapy (n = 550)
ALT increased	6%	4.3%
AST increased	3%	1.3%
Proteinuria	6.8%	5.3%
Serum creatinine increased	3.7%	4.3%
Serum urea nitrogen (BUN) increased	4.7%	3.5%

The following additional laboratory adverse reactions (incidence more than 0.5% and more than standard therapy), regardless of causality, were reported in patients treated with aprepitant regimen: alkaline phosphatase increased, erythrocyturia, hyperglycemia, hyponatremia, leukocytes increased, and leukocyturia.

The adverse reactions of increased AST and ALT were generally mild and transient.

The following laboratory adverse reactions were reported at an incidence of 3% or more during cycle 1 of the moderately emetogenic chemotherapy study in patients treated with the aprepitant regimen or standard therapy, respectively: decreased hemoglobin (2.3%, 4.7%) and decreased white blood cell count (9.3%, 9%).

The adverse reaction profiles in the multiple-cycle extensions for up to 6 cycles of chemotherapy were generally similar to those observed in cycle 1.

Other adverse reactions – Stevens-Johnson syndrome was reported as a serious adverse reaction in a patient receiving aprepitant with cancer chemotherapy in another chemotherapy-induced nausea/vomiting study.

➤*Postoperative nausea/vomiting:*

Aprepitant Adverse Reactions in Postoperative Nausea/Vomiting Prevention Patients (≥ 3%)		
	Aprepitant 40 mg (n = 564)	Ondansetron (n = 538)
Cardiovascular		
Bradycardia	4.4%	3.9%
Hypertension	2.1%	3.2%
Hypotension	5.7%	4.6%
CNS		
Headache	5%	6.5%
Insomnia	2.1%	3.3%
Dermatologic		
Pruritus	7.6%	8.4%
GI		
Constipation	8.5%	7.6%
Flatulence	4.1%	5.8%
Nausea	8.5%	8.6%
Vomiting	2.5%	3.9%
Miscellaneous		
Anemia	3%	4.3%
Pyrexia	5.9%	10.6%
Urinary tract infection	2.3%	3.2%

Cardiovascular – Blood pressure decreased, syncope.

CNS – Dizziness, hypesthesia.

Dermatologic – Urticaria.

GI – Abdominal pain, abdominal pain upper, dry mouth, dyspepsia.

Metabolic/Nutritional – Hypokalemia, hypovolemia.

Respiratory – Dyspnea, hypoxia, respiratory depression.

Miscellaneous – Hematoma, hypothermia, operative hemorrhage, pain, postoperative infection, wound dehiscence.

CNS – Dysarthria, sensory disturbance.

GI – Bowel sounds abnormal, stomach discomfort.

Ophthalmic – Miosis, visual acuity reduced.

Respiratory – Wheezing.

Laboratory adverse reactions – One laboratory adverse reaction, hemoglobin decreased (aprepitant 40 mg 3.8%; ondansetron 4.2%), was reported at an incidence of 3% or more in a patient receiving general anesthesia.

APREPITANT — ORAL

The following additional laboratory adverse reactions (incidence more than 0.5% and greater than ondansetron), regardless of causality, were reported in patients treated with aprepitant 40 mg: blood albumin decreased, blood bilirubin increased, blood glucose increased, blood potassium decreased, and glucose urine present.

The adverse reactions of increased ALT occurred with similar incidence in patients treated with aprepitant 40 mg (1.1%) as in patients treated with ondansetron 4 mg (1%).

➤*Other studies:* Angioedema and urticaria were reported as serious adverse reactions in a patient receiving aprepitant in a non–chemotherapy-induced nausea and vomiting/non–postoperative nausea/vomiting study.

Overdosage

➤*Symptoms:* Single doses of aprepitant up to 600 mg were generally well tolerated in healthy subjects. Aprepitant was generally well tolerated when administered as 375 mg once daily for up to 42 days to patients in non–chemotherapy-induced nausea and vomiting studies. In 33 cancer patients, administration of a single dose of aprepitant 375 mg on day 1 and 250 mg once daily on days 2 to 5 was generally well tolerated.

Drowsiness and headache were reported in 1 patient who ingested aprepitant 1,440 mg.

➤*Treatment:* No specific information is available on the treatment of overdosage with aprepitant. In the event of overdose, discontinue aprepitant and provide general supportive treatment and monitoring. Because of the antiemetic activity of aprepitant, drug-induced emesis may not be effective.

Aprepitant cannot be removed by hemodialysis.

Patient Information

Instruct patients to take aprepitant only as prescribed. For the prevention of chemotherapy-induced nausea and vomiting, advise patients to take their first dose (125 mg) of aprepitant 1 hour prior to chemotherapy treatment. For the prevention of postoperative nausea/vomiting, advise patients to take their medication (aprepitant 40 mg capsule) within 3 hours prior to induction of anesthesia.

Aprepitant may interact with some drugs, including chemotherapy; therefore, advise patients to report to their health care providers the use of any other prescription or nonprescription medicines, vitamins, or herbal products.

Instruct patients on chronic warfarin therapy to have their clotting status closely monitored in the 2-week period, particularly at 7 to 10 days, following initiation of the 3-day regimen of aprepitant (125 mg/80 mg) with each chemotherapy cycle, or following administration of a single dose of aprepitant 40 mg for prevention of postoperative nausea/vomiting.

Administration of aprepitant may reduce the efficacy of hormonal contraceptives. Advise patients to use alternative or backup methods of contraception during treatment with aprepitant and for 1 month following the last dose of aprepitant.

FOSAPREPITANT

Rx	**Emend** (Merck)	**Injection, lyophilized powder for solution:** 115 mg	Equiv. to fosaprepitant dimeglumine 188 mg. Lactose, edetate disodium, polysorbate 80. In single-dose vials.
		Injection, lyophilized powder for solution: 150 mg	Equiv. to fosaprepitant dimeglumine 245.3 mg. Lactose, edetate disodium, polysorbate 80. In single-dose vials.

FOSAPREPITANT DIMEGLUMINE — INJECTION

Indications

➤*Prevention of chemotherapy-induced nausea and vomiting:* In combination with other antiemetic agents, for the prevention of acute and delayed nausea and vomiting associated with initial and repeat courses of highly and moderately emetogenic cancer chemotherapy, including high-dose cisplatin.

General information –

Long-term, continuous administration is not recommended.

Administration and Dosage

➤*Adults:*

Prevention of chemotherapy-induced nausea and vomiting –

Highly emetogenic cancer chemotherapy:

• *115 mg injection (3-day dosing regimen) –*

Fosaprepitant IV[a] and Aprepitant Oral 3-Day Dosing Regimen for Highly Emetogenic Cancer Chemotherapy

	Fosaprepitant[b]	Aprepitant	Dexamethasone[c]	Ondansetron[d]
Day 1	115 mg IV[e]	—	12 mg orally	32 mg IV
Day 2	—	80 mg orally	8 mg orally	—
Day 3	—	80 mg orally	8 mg orally once daily	—
Day 4	—	—	8 mg orally once daily	—

[a] IV = intravenous.
[b] Infuse over 15 min. Start 30 min prior to chemotherapy.
[c] Administer 30 min prior to chemotherapy treatment on day 1 and in the morning on days 2 through 4. The dose of dexamethasone was chosen to account for drug interactions.
[d] Administer 30 min prior to chemotherapy treatment on day 1.
[e] Aprepitant 125 mg orally may be substituted for fosaprepitant 115 mg IV on day 1.

• *150 mg injection (single-dose regimen) –*

Fosaprepitant 150 mg (Single-Dose) Dosing Regimen for Highly Emetogenic Cancer Chemotherapy

	Day 1	Day 2	Day 3	Day 4
Fosaprepitant[a]	150 mg IV	None	None	None
Dexamethasone[b]	12 mg orally	8 mg orally	8 mg orally twice daily	8 mg orally twice daily
Ondansetron[c]	32 mg IV	None	None	None

[a] Infuse over 20 to 30 min. Start 30 min prior to chemotherapy.
[b] Administer 30 min prior to chemotherapy treatment on day 1 and in the morning on days 2 through 4. The dose of dexamethasone accounts for drug interactions.
[c] Administer 30 min prior to chemotherapy treatment on day 1.

Moderately emetogenic cancer chemotherapy:

• *115 mg injection (3-day dosing regimen) –*

Fosaprepitant IV and Aprepitant Oral 3-Day Dosing Regimen for Moderately Emetogenic Cancer Chemotherapy

	Fosaprepitant	Aprepitant	Dexamethasone[a]	Ondansetron[b]
Day 1	115 mg IV[c]	—	12 mg orally	8 mg orally twice daily
Day 2	—	80 mg orally	—	—
Day 3	—	80 mg orally	—	—

[a] Administer 30 min prior to chemotherapy treatment on day 1. The dose of dexamethasone was chosen to account for drug interactions.
[b] Administer 30 to 60 min prior to chemotherapy treatment and 8 h after the first dose on day 1.
[c] Infuse over 15 min. Start 30 min prior to chemotherapy. Aprepitant 125 mg orally may be substituted for fosaprepitant 115 mg IV on day 1.

➤*Preparation for administration:* Aseptically inject 5 mL of sodium chloride 0.9% for injection into the vial; ensure that it is added to the vial along the vial wall in order to prevent foaming. Swirl the vial gently. Avoid shaking and jetting sodium chloride into the vial. Aseptically prepare an infusion bag filled with 110 mL (115 mg vial) or 145 mL (150 mg vial) of sodium chloride 0.9% injection. Aseptically withdraw the entire volume from the vial and transfer it into the infusion bag to yield a total volume of final concentration of 1 mg/mL. Gently invert the bag 2 to 3 times.

➤*Administration:* Administer IV as an infusion over 15 minutes for the 115 mg injection and over 20 to 30 minutes for the 150 mg injection. Infuse 30 minutes prior to chemotherapy. Aprepitant is available in capsules for oral administration. Long-term, continuous administration is not recommended.

➤*Admixture compatibility:* Fosaprepitant should not be mixed or reconstituted with solutions for which physical and chemical compatibility have not been established. Fosaprepitant is incompatible with any solutions containing divalent cations (eg, Ca^{2+}, Mg^{2+}), including Ringer's lactate solution and Hartmann solution.

To screen for specific compatibilities, see *Trissel's IV-Chek*.

➤*Storage/Stability:* Store vials at 2° to 8°C (36° to 46°F). The reconstituted final drug solution is stable for 24 hours at ambient room temperature (at or below 25°C [77°F]).

Actions

➤*Pharmacology:* Fosaprepitant is a prodrug of aprepitant and, accordingly, its antiemetic effects are attributable to aprepitant.

Aprepitant is a selective high-affinity antagonist of human substance NK1 receptors. Aprepitant has little or no affinity for serotonin (5-hydroxytryptamine [5-HT]), dopamine, and corticosteroid receptors, which are the targets of existing therapies for chemotherapy-induced nausea and vomiting. Animal and human positron emission tomography studies with aprepitant have shown that it crosses the blood-brain barrier and occupies brain NK1 receptors. Animal and human studies show that aprepitant augments the antiemetic activity of the 5-HT–receptor antagonist ondansetron and the corticosteroid dexamethasone, and inhibits the acute and delayed phases of cisplatin-induced emesis.

FOSAPREPITANT DIMEGLUMINE — INJECTION

➤*Pharmacokinetics:*

Absorption –

115 mg injection: Following a single dose of fosaprepitant 115 mg IV as a 15-minute infusion to healthy volunteers, the mean area under the curve ($AUC_{0-\infty}$) of aprepitant was 31.7 (± 14.3) mcg•h/mL, and the mean maximum aprepitant concentration (C_{max}) was 3.27 (± 1.16) mcg/mL. The mean aprepitant plasma concentration at 24 hours postdose was similar between the dose of oral aprepitant 125 mg and the dose of fosaprepitant 115 mg IV.

150 mg injection: Following a single IV dose of fosaprepitant 150 mg administered as a 20-minute infusion to healthy volunteers, the mean $AUC_{0-\infty}$ of aprepitant was 37.38 (± 14.75) mcg•h/mL and C_{max} was 4.15 (± 1.15) mcg/mL.

Distribution – Fosaprepitant is rapidly converted to aprepitant. Aprepitant is more than 95% bound to plasma proteins. The mean apparent volume of distribution at steady state is approximately 70 L in humans. Aprepitant crosses the placenta in rats and rabbits and crosses the blood-brain barrier in humans.

Metabolism – Fosaprepitant was rapidly converted to aprepitant in in vitro incubations with liver preparations from nonclinical species (rat and dog) and humans. Furthermore, fosaprepitant underwent rapid and nearly complete conversion to aprepitant in S9 preparations from multiple other human tissues, including kidney, lung, and ileum. Therefore, it appears that the conversion of fosaprepitant to aprepitant can occur in multiple extrahepatic tissues in addition to the liver. In humans, fosaprepitant IV was rapidly converted to aprepitant within 30 minutes following the end of infusion.

Aprepitant undergoes extensive metabolism. In vitro studies using human liver microsomes indicate that aprepitant is metabolized primarily by cytochrome P450 isoenzyme 3A4 (CYP3A4), with minor metabolism by CYP1A2 and CYP2C19. Metabolism is largely via oxidation at the morpholine ring and its side chains. No metabolism by CYP2D6, CYP2C9, or CYP2E1 was detected. In healthy young adults, aprepitant accounts for approximately 24% of the radioactivity in plasma over 72 hours following a single oral dose of ^{14}C-aprepitant 300 mg, indicating a substantial presence of metabolites in the plasma. Seven metabolites of aprepitant, which are only weakly active, have been identified in human plasma.

Excretion – Following administration of a single dose of ^{14}C-fosaprepitant 100 mg IV to healthy subjects, 57% of the radioactivity was recovered in urine and 45% in feces.

Aprepitant is eliminated primarily by metabolism; aprepitant is not renally excreted. The apparent terminal half-life of aprepitant ranged from approximately 9 to 13 hours.

Special populations –

Renal function impairment: In patients with severe renal impairment, the $AUC_{0-\infty}$ of total aprepitant (unbound and protein bound) decreased 21% and C_{max} decreased 32% compared with healthy subjects. In patients with end-stage renal disease (ESRD) undergoing hemodialysis, the $AUC_{0-\infty}$ of total aprepitant decreased 42% and C_{max} decreased 32%. Because of modest decreases in protein binding of aprepitant in patients with renal disease, the AUC of pharmacologically active, unbound drug was not significantly affected in patients with renal impairment compared with healthy subjects.

• *Hemodialysis* – Hemodialysis conducted 4 or 48 hours after dosing had no significant effect on the pharmacokinetics of aprepitant; less than 0.2% of the dose was recovered in the dialysate.

Hepatic function impairment: Following administration of a single dose of oral aprepitant 125 mg on day 1 and 80 mg once daily on days 2 and 3 to patients with mild hepatic impairment (Child-Pugh score 5 to 6), the AUC_{0-24h} of aprepitant was 11% lower on day 1 and 36% lower on day 3 compared with healthy subjects given the same regimen. In patients with moderate hepatic impairment (Child-Pugh score 7 to 9), the AUC_{0-24h} of aprepitant was 10% higher on day 1 and 18% higher on day 3 compared with healthy subjects given the same regimen. These differences in AUC_{0-24h} are not considered clinically meaningful.

Elderly: Following oral administration of a single dose of aprepitant 125 mg on day 1 and 80 mg once daily on days 2 through 5, the AUC_{0-24h} of aprepitant was 21% higher on day 1 and 36% higher on day 5 in elderly patients 65 years of age and older compared with younger adults. The C_{max} was 10% higher on day 1 and 24% higher on day 5 in elderly patients compared with younger adults. These differences are not considered clinically meaningful.

Gender: The C_{max} for aprepitant is 16% higher in women than in men. The half-life of aprepitant is 25% lower in women than in men, and time to C_{max} occurs at approximately the same time. These differences are not considered clinically meaningful.

Race: Following oral administration of a single dose of aprepitant 125 mg, the AUC_{0-24h} is approximately 25% and 29% higher in Hispanic patients compared with white and black patients, respectively. The C_{max} is 22% and 31% higher in Hispanic patients compared with white and black patients, respectively. These differences are not considered clinically meaningful.

Contraindications

Hypersensitivity to fosaprepitant, aprepitant, polysorbate 80, or any other component of the product; concurrent use with cisapride or pimozide.

Warnings/Precautions

➤*Long-term use:* Long-term, continuous use of fosaprepitant for prevention of nausea and vomiting is not recommended because it has not been studied and because the drug interaction profile may change during chronic continuous use.

➤*Hypersensitivity reactions:* Isolated reports of immediate hypersensitivity reactions, including flushing, erythema, dyspnea, and anaphylaxis, have occurred during infusion of fosaprepitant. These hypersensitivity reactions have generally responded to discontinuation of the infusion and administration of appropriate therapy. Reinitiation of the infusion is not recommended in patients who experience these symptoms during first-time use.

➤*Hepatic function impairment:* There are no clinical or pharmacokinetic data in patients with severe hepatic impairment (Child-Pugh score higher than 9); therefore, exercise caution when fosaprepitant or aprepitant is administered to these patients.

➤*Pregnancy: Category B.* There are no adequate and well-controlled studies in pregnant women. It is not known if aprepitant crosses the human placenta. The drug crosses the placenta in rats and rabbits, and crosses the blood-brain barrier in humans. Although protein binding is high, the molecular weight (about 534) and elimination half-life suggest that the drug will cross the human placenta to the embryo and/or fetus. Because animal reproduction studies are not always predictive of human response, use this drug during pregnancy only if clearly needed. The absence of human pregnancy experience prevents a full assessment of the embryo/fetal risk. Until additional data are available, the use of aprepitant, if indicated, should be restricted to the second and third trimesters. However, if inadvertent exposure does occur during organogenesis, the embryo/fetal risk appears to be low.

➤*Lactation:* Aprepitant is excreted in the milk of rats. It is not known whether this drug is excreted in human milk. The molecular weight (about 534) and elimination half-life (9 to 13 hours) suggest that the drug will be excreted into breast milk. However, the high plasma protein binding (more than 95%) should attenuate the amount excreted. Because many drugs are excreted in human milk and because of the potential for serious adverse reactions in breast-feeding infants from aprepitant and the potential for tumorigenicity shown for aprepitant in rodent carcinogenicity studies, decide whether the mother should discontinue breast-feeding or the drug, taking into account the importance of the drug to the mother.

➤*Children:* Safety and effectiveness in children have not been established.

➤*Elderly:* Greater sensitivity of some older individuals cannot be ruled out.

Drug Interactions

Drug interactions following administration of fosaprepitant are likely to occur with drugs that interact with oral aprepitant.

➤*Cytochrome P450 system:* Fosaprepitant is rapidly converted to aprepitant, which is a substrate, a moderate inhibitor, and an inducer of CYP3A4 when administered as a 3-day antiemetic dosing regimen for chemotherapy-induced nausea and vomiting. Aprepitant is also an inducer of CYP2C9. Use fosaprepitant with caution in patients receiving concomitant medications that are primarily metabolized through CYP3A4. Inhibition of CYP3A4 by aprepitant may result in elevated plasma concentrations of these concomitant medications. When fosaprepitant is used concomitantly with another CYP3A4 inhibitor, aprepitant plasma concentrations may be elevated.

➤*Chemotherapeutic agents:* Chemotherapy agents that are known to be metabolized by CYP3A4 include docetaxel, paclitaxel, etoposide, irinotecan, ifosfamide, imatinib, vinorelbine, vinblastine, and vincristine. In clinical studies, the oral aprepitant regimen was administered commonly with etoposide, vinorelbine, or paclitaxel. The doses of these agents were not adjusted to account for potential drug interactions. Because of the small number of patients in clinical studies who received the CYP3A4 substrates vinblastine, vincristine, or ifosfamide, particular caution and careful monitoring are advised in patients receiving these agents or other chemotherapy agents metabolized primarily by CYP3A4 that were not studied.

Fosaprepitant Drug Interactions

Precipitant drug	Object drug[a]		Description
CYP3A4 inducers (eg, carbamazepine, phenytoin, rifampin)	Fosaprepitant	⬇	Coadministration may decrease aprepitant plasma concentrations and reduce its efficacy. When a single dose of aprepitant 375 mg was administered on day 9 of a 14-day course of rifampin 600 mg daily, the AUC of aprepitant decreased ≈ 11-fold and mean terminal half-life decreased ≈ 3-fold. Use with caution and monitor the clinical response.
CYP3A4 inhibitors (eg, clarithromycin, itraconazole, ketoconazole, nefazodone, nelfinavir, ritonavir, troleandomycin[b])	Fosaprepitant	⬆	Concurrent use of CYP3A4 inhibitors may increase aprepitant plasma concentrations. When a single dose of aprepitant 125 mg was administered on day 5 of a 10-day course of ketoconazole 400 mg daily, the AUC of aprepitant increased ≈ 5-fold and the mean terminal half-life increased 3-fold. Use with caution.

FOSAPREPITANT DIMEGLUMINE — INJECTION

Fosaprepitant Drug Interactions			
Precipitant drug	Object drug[a]		Description
Diltiazem	Fosaprepitant	↑	Coadministration resulted in an increase of plasma concentrations of diltiazem and aprepitant. Closely monitor the clinical response.
Fosaprepitant	Diltiazem		
Paroxetine	Fosaprepitant	↓	Concurrent use decreased the AUC ≈ 25% and C_{max} ≈ 20% of aprepitant and paroxetine. Monitor the clinical response.
Fosaprepitant	Paroxetine		
Fosaprepitant	Cisapride,[c] pimozide	↑	Aprepitant is a moderate inhibitor of CYP3A4 and can increase concentrations of coadministered drugs that are metabolized through CYP3A4. The risk of life-threatening cardiac arrhythmias may be increased; therefore, fosaprepitant is contraindicated with cisapride or pimozide.
Fosaprepitant	Benzodiazepines (eg, alprazolam, midazolam, triazolam)	↑	Plasma concentrations of these drugs may be elevated, increasing the pharmacologic effects and adverse reactions. Closely monitor for increased benzodiazepine adverse reactions (eg, CNS depression) when fosaprepitant is coadministered.
Fosaprepitant	Chemotherapy agents (eg, docetaxel, etoposide, ifosfamide, imatinib, irinotecan, paclitaxel, vinblastine, vincristine, vinorelbine)	↑	Aprepitant is a moderate inhibitor of CYP3A4 and can increase plasma concentrations of chemotherapy drugs that are metabolized through CYP3A4. Use with caution.
Fosaprepitant	Colchicine	↑	Plasma concentrations of colchicine may be elevated, increasing the risk of toxicity. Use with caution and closely monitor for colchicine toxicity. Colchicine dosage adjustment may be required for patients receiving fosaprepitant.
Fosaprepitant	Contraceptives, hormonal	↓	The efficacy of hormonal contraceptives during and for 28 days following the last dose of aprepitant may be reduced. Use alternative or backup methods of contraception during treatment with aprepitant and for 1 month following the last dose of aprepitant.
Fosaprepitant	Corticosteroids (eg, dexamethasone, methylprednisolone)	↑	Reduce the oral dexamethasone dose ≈ 50% when coadministered with a regimen of fosaprepitant followed by aprepitant (125 and 80 mg regimen). Reduce the dose of methylprednisolone IV ≈ 25% and the oral dose ≈ 50% when coadministered with a regimen of fosaprepitant followed by aprepitant (125 mg and 80 mg regimen).
Fosaprepitant	CYP2C9 substrates (eg, tolbutamide, warfarin)	↓	Aprepitant is a CYP2C9 inducer and induces the metabolism of warfarin and tolbutamide, resulting in lower plasma levels. In patients on long-term warfarin therapy, monitor the international normalized ratio closely in the 2-week period, particularly at 7 to 10 days, following the initiation of the 3-day regimen of fosaprepitant followed by oral aprepitant with each chemotherapy cycle.
Fosaprepitant	Everolimus	↑	Everolimus plasma concentrations may be elevated, increasing the pharmacologic effects and risk of toxicity. Closely monitor everolimus concentrations and adjust the dose as needed.
Fosaprepitant	Fentanyl	↑	Fentanyl plasma concentrations may be elevated, increasing the pharmacologic effects and risk of toxicity. Closely monitor the patient for an extended period of time and increase the fentanyl dose conservatively.
Fosaprepitant	Ranolazine	↑	Ranolazine plasma concentrations may be elevated, increasing the pharmacologic effects and risk of toxicity. Closely monitor the patient for ranolazine toxicity, including QT prolongation. Limit the ranolazine dose to 500 mg twice daily.
Fosaprepitant	Tolvaptan	↑	Tolvaptan plasma concentrations may be elevated, increasing the pharmacologic effects and risk of toxicity. Avoid coadministration.

[a] ↑ = object drug increased; ↓ = object drug decreased.
[b] No longer marketed in the United States.
[c] Available from the manufacturer on a limited-access protocol.

➤*Minimally or noninteracting drugs:* In clinical studies, aprepitant did not have clinically important effects on the pharmacokinetics of granisetron, hydrodolasetron (the active metabolite of dolasetron), or ondansetron.

Adverse Reactions

➤*Aprepitant:*

Serious adverse reactions – In another chemotherapy-induced nausea and vomiting study, Stevens-Johnson syndrome was reported as a serious adverse reaction in a patient receiving aprepitant with cancer chemotherapy.

Two serious adverse reactions were reported in postoperative nausea and vomiting clinical studies in patients taking a higher dose of aprepitant, including 1 case of constipation and 1 case of sub-ileus.

Angioedema and urticaria were reported as serious adverse reactions in a patient receiving aprepitant in a non–chemotherapy-induced nausea and vomiting/non-postoperative nausea and vomiting study.

Highly emetogenic chemotherapy –

Aprepitant Highly Emetogenic Chemotherapy Adverse Reactions (≥ 1%)		
Adverse reactions	Aprepitant regimen[a] (n = 544)	Standard therapy (n = 550)
CNS		
Asthenia/Fatigue	2.9%	1.6%
Headache	2.2%	1.8%
GI		
Anorexia	2%	0.5%
Constipation	2.2%	2%
Diarrhea	1.1%	0.9%
Dyspepsia	1.5%	0.7%
Miscellaneous		
ALT increased	2.8%	1.5%
AST increased	1.1%	0.9%
Hiccups	4.6%	2.9%

[a] In combination with ondansetron and dexamethasone.

Discontinuation of therapy: Treatment was discontinued because of adverse reactions in 0.6% of patients treated with the aprepitant regimen compared with 0.4% of patients treated with standard therapy.

Moderately emetogenic chemotherapy –

Aprepitant Moderately Emetogenic Chemotherapy Adverse Reactions (≥ 1%)		
Adverse reaction	Aprepitant regimen[a] (n = 868)	Standard therapy (n = 846)
Eructation	1%	0.1%
Fatigue	1.4%	0.9%

[a] In combination with ondansetron and dexamethasone.

FOSAPREPITANT DIMEGLUMINE — INJECTION

Discontinuation of therapy: Treatment was discontinued because of adverse reactions in 0.7% of patients treated with the aprepitant regimen compared with 0.2% of patients treated with standard therapy.

Less common adverse reactions (less than 1%) –

Cardiovascular: Bradycardia, cardiovascular disorder, flushing, hot flush, palpitations.

CNS: Anxiety, chills, cognitive disorder, disorientation, dizziness, dream abnormality, euphoria, lethargy, somnolence.

Dermatologic: Acne, hyperhidrosis, oily skin, photosensitivity, pruritus, rash, skin lesion.

GI: Abdominal distention, abdominal pain, acid reflux, dry mouth, dysgeusia, epigastric discomfort, faeces hard, flatulence, gastroesophageal reflux disease, nausea, neutropenic colitis, obstipation, perforating duodenal ulcer, polydipsia, stomatitis, thirst, vomiting, weight gain, weight loss.

GU: Dysuria, microscopic hematuria, pollakiuria, polyuria.

Hematologic/Lymphatic: Anemia, febrile neutropenia, neutrophil count decreased.

Musculoskeletal: Muscle cramp, muscular weakness, myalgia.

Respiratory: Cough, pharyngitis, postnasal drip, sneezing, throat irritation.

Special senses: Conjunctivitis, tinnitus.

Miscellaneous: Alkaline phosphatase increased, candidiasis, chest discomfort, edema, gait disturbance, hyperglycemia, hyponatremia, malaise, *Staphylococcal* infection.

Postoperative nausea and vomiting –

Other adverse reactions:

- *CNS* – Dysarthria, hypoesthesia, insomnia, sensory disturbance (less than 1%).
- *GI* – Abdominal pain upper, bowel sounds abnormal, dry mouth, nausea, stomach discomfort (less than 1%).
- *Respiratory* – Dyspnea, wheezing (less than 1%).
- *Special senses* – Miosis, visual acuity reduced (less than 1%).
- *Miscellaneous* – Increased ALT (1.1%); bradycardia (less than 1%).

➤*Fosaprepitant:*

Infusion-site reactions – Infusion-site reactions occurred at a higher incidence in patients in the fosaprepitant group (3%) compared with those in the aprepitant group (0.5%). The reported infusion-site reactions included infusion-site erythema, infusion-site pruritus, infusion-site pain, infusion-site induration, and infusion-site thrombophlebitis.

Fosaprepitant 150 mg additional adverse reactions not reported with oral aprepitant –

Cardiovascular: Blood pressure increased, thrombophlebitis (predominantly infusion-site thrombophlebitis).

Dermatologic: Erythema.

Local: Infusion-site erythema, infusion-site induration, infusion-site pain, infusion-site pruritus.

➤*Postmarketing:*

Dermatologic – Pruritus, rash, urticaria.

Hypersensitivity – Hypersensitivity reactions, including anaphylactic reactions.

Overdosage

➤*Treatment:* In the event of overdose, discontinue fosaprepitant and/or oral aprepitant, provide general supportive treatment, and monitor patients. Aprepitant cannot be removed by hemodialysis.

Patient Information

Inform patients that allergic reactions, which may be sudden and/or serious, may include hives, rash, itching, redness of the face/skin, and may cause difficulty in breathing or swallowing, have been reported. Instruct patients to stop using fosaprepitant and call their health care provider right away if they experience an allergic reaction.

In patients who develop an infusion-site reaction, such as erythema, edema, pain, or thrombophlebitis, instruct them on how to care for the local reaction and when to seek further evaluation.

Fosaprepitant may interact with some drugs, including chemotherapy agents; therefore, advise patients to report to their health care provider the use of any other prescription or nonprescription medication or herbal products.

Instruct patients on long-term warfarin therapy to have their clotting status closely monitored in the 2-week period, particularly at 7 to 10 days following fosaprepitant.

Administration of fosaprepitant may reduce the efficacy of hormonal contraceptives. Advise patients to use alternative or backup methods of contraception during treatment with fosaprepitant and for 1 month following the last dose of aprepitant or fosaprepitant.

NABILONE

c-ii	**Cesamet** (Meda Pharmaceuticals)	**Capsules; oral:** 1 mg	(Valeant 0247). Purple/white. In 20s.

NABILONE — ORAL

Indications

➤*Antiemetic:* For the treatment of the nausea and vomiting associated with cancer chemotherapy in patients who have failed to respond adequately to conventional antiemetic treatments. This restriction is required because a substantial proportion of any group of patients treated with nabilone can be expected to experience disturbing psychotomimetic reactions not observed with other antiemetic agents.

Because of its potential to alter the mental state, nabilone is intended for use under circumstances that permit close supervision of the patient by a responsible individual, particularly during the initial use of nabilone and during dose adjustments.

Nabilone is not intended for use on an as-needed basis or as the first antiemetic product prescribed for a patient.

Administration and Dosage

➤*Adults:*

Antiemetic –

Usual dosage: 1 or 2 mg administered 2 or 3 times daily.

Maximum dose: 6 mg/day in divided doses 3 times a day.

Initial dosage: On the day of chemotherapy, the initial dose should be given 1 to 3 hours before the chemotherapeutic agent is administered. To minimize adverse reactions, it is recommended that the lower starting dose be used and that the dose be increased as necessary. A dose of 1 or 2 mg the night before may be useful.

Duration of therapy: May be administered during the entire course of each cycle of chemotherapy and, if needed, for 48 hours after the last dose of each cycle of chemotherapy.

➤*Elderly:* In general, be cautious in dose selection for an elderly patient, usually starting at the low end of the dosing range. Use nabilone with caution in elderly patients 65 years of age and older because they are generally more sensitive to the psychoactive effects of drugs and nabilone can elevate supine and standing heart rates and cause postural hypotension.

➤*Administration:* Clinical data suggest that the intake of food does not significantly affect either the rate or extent of absorption.

➤*Storage/Stability:* Store at 25°C (77°F); excursions permitted from 15° to 30°C (59° to 86°F).

Actions

➤*Pharmacology:* Nabilone is an orally active synthetic cannabinoid that, like other cannabinoids, has complex effects on the CNS. It has been suggested that the antiemetic effect of nabilone is caused by interaction with the cannabinoid receptor system (the CB 1 receptor), which has been discovered in neural tissues.

Nontherapeutic effects – Nabilone, a synthetic cannabinoid, has the potential to be abused and to produce psychological dependence. Nabilone has complex effects on the CNS. Its effects on the mental state ("inner mental life") are similar to those of cannabis. Subjects given nabilone may experience changes in mood (eg, anxiety, depression, detachment, euphoria, panic, paranoia), decrements in cognitive performance and memory, a decreased ability to control drives and impulses, and alterations in the experience of reality (eg, distortions in the perception of objects and the sense of time, hallucinations). These phenomena appear to be more common when larger doses of nabilone are administered; however, a full-blown picture of psychosis (psychotic organic brain syndrome) may occur in patients receiving doses within the lower portion of the therapeutic range. Tolerance to these effects develops rapidly and is readily reversible.

Data on the chronic use of nabilone are not available; experience with cannabis suggests that chronic use of cannabinoids may be associated with a variety of untoward effects on motivation, cognition, and judgment, as well as other mental status changes. Whether these phenomena reflect the underlying character of individuals chronically abusing cannabis or are a result of the use of cannabis is not known.

The simultaneous use of nabilone and alcohol or barbiturates may produce additive depressive effects on CNS function. Possible changes in mood and other adverse behavioral effects may occur in patients receiving nabilone. Patients should remain under the supervision of a responsible adult while using nabilone.

Nabilone has CNS activity. It produces relaxation, drowsiness, and euphoria in the recommended dosage range. Tolerance to these effects develops rapidly and is readily reversible.

In addition to effects on the mental state, nabilone has several systemic actions; the most prominent are dry mouth and hypotension. Nabilone has been observed to elevate supine and standing heart rates and to cause supine and orthostatic hypotension. In clinical studies, oral administration of nabilone 2 mg did produce some decrease in airway resistance in healthy controls but had no effect in patients with asthma. No other nontherapeutic effects of clinical significance due to nabilone have been reported.

➤*Pharmacokinetics:*

Absorption/Distribution – Nabilone appears to be completely absorbed from the human GI tract when administered orally. Following oral administration of a dose of radiolabeled nabilone 2 mg, peak plasma concentrations of approximately 2 ng/mL of nabilone and 10 ng equivalents/mL of total radioactivity are achieved within 2 hours. The initial rapid disappearance of radioactivity represents uptake and distribution of nabilone into tissue and the slower-phase elimination by metabolism and excretion. The apparent volume of distribution of nabilone is approximately 12.5 L/kg.

Nabilone exhibits dose linearity within its therapeutic range.

NABILONE — ORAL

Metabolism – Metabolism of nabilone is extensive, and several metabolites have been identified. Precise information concerning the metabolites that may accumulate is not available. The relative activities of the metabolites and the parent drug have not been established. There are at least 2 metabolic pathways involved in the biotransformation of nabilone. A minor pathway is initiated by the stereospecific enzymatic reduction of the 9-keto moiety of nabilone to produce the isomeric carbinol metabolite. The peak concentrations of nabilone and its carbinol metabolites are comparable, but their combined exposures in plasma do not account for more than 20% of that of total radioactivity. Secondly, a metabolite of nabilone in feces has been identified as a diol formed by reduction of the 9-keto group plus oxidation at the penultimate carbon of the dimethylheptyl side chain. In addition, there is evidence of extensive metabolism of nabilone by multiple P-450 enzyme isoforms. However, in clinical use, the very low nabilone plasma concentration is unlikely to interfere with the P-450–mediated degradation of coadministered drugs. Chronic oral administration of 1 mg 3 times daily for 14 days to 3 subjects gave no indication there was any significant accumulation of nabilone. Available evidence suggests that 1 or more of the metabolites has a terminal elimination half-life that exceeds that of nabilone. Consequently, in repeated use, the metabolites may accumulate at concentrations in excess of the parent drug.

Excretion – The plasma half-life ($t_{1/2}$) values for nabilone and total radioactivity of identified and unidentified metabolites are approximately 2 and 35 hours, respectively. The route and rate of the elimination of nabilone and its metabolites are similar to those observed with other cannabinoids, including delta-9-THC (dronabinol). When nabilone is administered intravenously, the drug and its metabolites are eliminated mainly in the feces (approximately 67%) and, to a lesser extent, in the urine (approximately 22%) within 7 days. Of the 67% recovered from the feces, 5% corresponded to the parent compound and 16% to its carbinol metabolite. Following oral administration, approximately 60% of nabilone and its metabolites were recovered in the feces and approximately 24% in urine. Therefore, it appears that the major excretory pathway is the biliary system.

Contraindications

History of hypersensitivity to any cannabinoid.

Warnings/Precautions

➤*Duration of effects:* The effects of nabilone may persist for a variable and unpredictable period of time following its oral administration. Adverse psychiatric reactions can persist for 48 to 72 hours following cessation of treatment.

➤*CNS effects:* Nabilone has the potential to affect the CNS and might manifest itself in dizziness, drowsiness, euphoria ("high"), ataxia, anxiety, disorientation, depression, hallucinations, and psychosis.

➤*Cardiovascular effects:* Nabilone can cause tachycardia and orthostatic hypotension.

➤*Close supervision:* Because of individual variation in response and tolerance to the effects of nabilone, patients should remain under the supervision of a responsible adult, especially during initial use of nabilone and during dose adjustments.

➤*Special risk:* Carefully evaluate the benefit/risk ratio of nabilone use in patients with the following medical conditions because of individual variation in response and tolerance to the effects of nabilone.

- Because nabilone can elevate supine and standing heart rates and cause postural hypotension, use it with caution in the elderly and in patients with hypertension or heart disease.
- Use nabilone with caution in patients with current or previous psychiatric disorders (eg, bipolar disorder, depression, schizophrenia) because the symptoms of these disease states may be unmasked by the use of cannabinoids.
- Use nabilone with caution in patients with a history of substance abuse, including alcohol abuse or dependence and marijuana use, because nabilone contains a similar active compound to marijuana.

➤*Drug abuse and dependence:* Nabilone, a synthetic cannabinoid pharmacologically related to *Cannabis sativa L*(Marijuana; delta-9-THC) is a highly abusable substance. Nabilone is controlled under schedule II of the Controlled Substances Act. Limit prescriptions for nabilone to the amount necessary for a single cycle of chemotherapy (ie, a few days). Nabilone may produce subjective adverse reactions that may be interpreted as a euphoria or marijuana-like "high" at therapeutic doses.

It is not known what proportion of individuals exposed chronically to nabilone or other cannabinoids will develop either psychological or physical dependence. Long-term use of these compounds has been associated with disorders of motivation, judgment, and cognition. However, it is not clear if these are a manifestation of the underlying personalities of chronic users of this class of drugs or if cannabinoids are directly responsible for these effects. An abstinence syndrome has been reported following discontinuation of delta-9-THC at high doses of 200 mg per day for 12 to 16 consecutive days. The acute phase was characterized by psychic distress, insomnia, and signs of autonomic hyperactivity (hiccups, loose stools, rhinorrhea, sweating). A protracted abstinence phase may have occurred in subjects who reported sleep disturbances for several weeks after delta-9-THC discontinuation.

Abuse – Nabilone was qualitatively and quantitatively similar to approved oral delta-9-THC in the production of cannabis-like effects, demonstrating its potential for abuse.

Preclinical studies performed in dogs and monkeys demonstrated that nabilone was cannabinoid-like. As with delta-9-THC, tolerance develops rapidly to the pharmacological effects in the dog and monkey. Cross-tolerance between nabilone and delta-9-THC was demonstrated in the monkey.

Dependence – The physical dependence capacity of nabilone is unknown at this time. Patients who participated in clinical trials of up to 5 days' duration evidenced no withdrawal symptoms upon cessation of dosing.

➤*Hazardous tasks:* Specifically warn patients receiving nabilone treatment not to drive, operate machinery, or engage in any hazardous activity while receiving nabilone.

➤*Pregnancy: Category C.* Teratology studies conducted in pregnant rats at dosages up to 12 mg/kg/day (about 16 times the human dose on a body surface area basis [BSA]) and pregnant rabbits at dosages up to 3.3 mg/kg/day (about 9 times the human dose on a BSA basis) did not disclose any evidence for a teratogenic potential of nabilone. However, there was dose-related developmental toxicity in both species which was displayed by increases in embryolethality, fetal resorptions, decreased fetal weights, and pregnancy disruptions. In rats, postnatal developmental toxicity was also observed. There are no adequate and well-controlled studies in pregnant women. Because animal studies cannot rule out the possibility of harm, only use nabilone during pregnancy if the potential benefit justifies the potential risk to the fetus.

➤*Lactation:* It is not known whether this drug is excreted in breast milk. Because many drugs, including some cannabinoids, are excreted in breast milk, it is not recommended that nabilone be given to breast-feeding mothers.

➤*Children:* Safety and efficacy have not been established in patients younger than 18 years of age. Caution is recommended in prescribing nabilone to children because of psychoactive effects.

➤*Elderly:* Clinical studies of nabilone did not include sufficient numbers of subjects 65 years of age and older to determine whether they respond differently than younger subjects. In general, be cautious in dose selection for an elderly patient, usually starting at the low end of the dosing range, reflecting the greater frequency of decreased hepatic, renal, or cardiac function, and of concomitant disease or other drug therapy. Use nabilone with caution in elderly patients 65 years of age and older because they are generally more sensitive to the psychoactive effects of drugs and nabilone can elevate supine and standing heart rates and cause postural hypotension.

➤*Monitoring:* As with all controlled drugs, monitor patients receiving nabilone for signs of excessive use, abuse, and misuse. Patients who may be at increased risk for substance abuse include those with a personal or family history of substance abuse (eg, drug, alcohol abuse) or mental illness.

Drug Interactions

➤*CYP-450 system:* In vitro P-450 inhibition studies using human liver microsomes showed that nabilone did not significantly inhibit CYP1A2, 2A6, 2C19, 2D6, and 3A4 (using midazolam and nifedipine as substrates). Nabilone had a weak inhibitory effect on CYP2E1 and 3A4 (using testosterone; IC_{50} greater than 50 mcM) and had a moderate inhibitory effect on CYP2C8 and 2C9 (IC_{50} greater than 10 mcM).

Cannabinoid Drug Interactions

Precipitant drug	Object drug[a]		Description
Amphetamines Cocaine Other sympathomimetic agents	Cannabinoids	↑	Additive hypertension, tachycardia, and possibly cardiotoxicity may occur.
Cannabinoids	Amphetamines Cocaine Other sympathomimetic agents		
Antihistamines Atropine Scopolamine Other anticholinergic agents	Cannabinoids	↑	Additive or super-additive tachycardia, or drowsiness may occur.
Cannabinoids	Antihistamines Atropine Scopolamine Other anticholinergic agents		

NABILONE — ORAL

Cannabinoid Drug Interactions			
Precipitant drug	Object drug[a]		Description
Barbiturates Benzodiazepines Buspirone Ethanol Lithium Muscle relaxants Opioids Other CNS depressants	Cannabinoids	⬆	Additive drowsiness and CNS-depressant effects. Psychomotor function was particularly impaired with concurrent use of nabilone and diazepam. Based on smoked marijuana, an increase in the positive subjective mood effects may occur when used with alcohol.
Cannabinoids	Barbiturates Benzodiazepines Buspirone Ethanol Lithium Muscle relaxants Opioids Other CNS depressants		
Naltrexone	Cannabinoids	⬆	Oral THC effects were enhanced by opioid receptor blockade.
Opioids	Cannabinoids	⬇	Cross-tolerance and mutual potentiation may occur.
Cannabinoids	Opioids		
Tricyclic antidepressants (eg, amitriptyline, amoxapine)	Cannabinoids	⬆	Additive tachycardia, hypertension, or drowsiness may occur.
Cannabinoids	Tricyclic antidepressants (eg, amitriptyline, amoxapine)		
Cannabinoids	Antipyrine Barbiturates	⬆	Decreased clearance of antipyrine and barbiturates, presumably via competitive inhibition of metabolism.
Cannabinoids	Disulfiram	⬇	A reversible hypomanic reaction was reported in a 28-year-old man who smoked marijuana; confirmed by dechallenge and rechallenge.
Cannabinoids	Fluoxetine	⬇	A 21-year-old woman with depression and bulimia receiving fluoxetine 20 mg/day for 4 weeks became hypomanic after smoking marijuana; symptoms resolved after 4 days.
Cannabinoids	Theophylline	⬇	Increased theophylline metabolism reported with smoking marijuana; effect similar to that following smoking tobacco.

[a] ⬆ = Object drug increased. ⬇ = Object drug decreased.

Adverse Reactions

During controlled clinical trials of nabilone, virtually all patients experienced at least 1 adverse reaction. The most commonly encountered reactions were ataxia, concentration difficulties, dry mouth, drowsiness, euphoria (feeling "high"), headache, and vertigo.

➤*Comparative incidence of reactions:* The following tables list the adverse reactions encountered by a substantial proportion of patients treated with nabilone participating in representative controlled clinical trials.

Incidence of Nabilone Adverse Reactions in Placebo-Controlled Studies				
	Nabilone (n = 132)		Placebo (n = 119)	
Adverse reaction	Patients	Percent	Patients	Percent
CNS				
Ataxia	19	14%	0	0%
Depersonalization	2	2%	1	1%
Disorientation	3	2%	0	0%
Drowsiness	69	52%	6	5%
Dysphoria	12	9%	0	0%
Euphoria	14	11%	1	1%
Headache	8	6%	0	0%
Sleep disturbance	14	11%	1	1%
Vertigo	69	52%	3	3%
GI				
Dry mouth	47	36%	2	2%
Nausea	5	4%	0	0%

Incidence of Nabilone Adverse Reactions in Active-Controlled Studies				
	Nabilone (n = 250)		Prochlorperazine (n = 232)	
Adverse reaction	Patients	Percent	Patients	Percent
Cardiovascular				
Hypotension	20	8%	3	1%
CNS				
Asthenia	19	8%	10	4%
Ataxia	32	13%	4	2%
Concentration difficulties	31	12%	3	1%
Depression	35	14%	37	16%
Drowsiness	165	66%	108	47%
Euphoria	95	38%	12	5%
Headache	18	7%	14	6%
Sedation	7	3%	2	1%
Vertigo/Dizziness	147	59%	53	23%
Visual disturbance	32	13%	9	4%
GI				
Anorexia	19	8%	22	9%
Dry mouth	54	22%	11	5%
Increased appetite	6	2%	2	1%

➤*Adverse reactions by body system:* The following list of adverse reactions is organized within body systems for patients treated with nabilone in controlled clinical trials. All reactions are listed regardless of causality assessment.

Cardiovascular – Arrhythmia, cerebral vascular accident, flushing, hypertension, hypotension, orthostatic hypotension, palpitation, syncope, tachycardia.

CNS – Abnormal dreams, akathisia, anxiety, apathy, asthenia, ataxia, confusion, convulsions, coordination disturbance, decreased concentration, depersonalization syndrome, depression, disorientation, dizziness, drowsiness, dysphoria, dystonia, emotional disorder, euphoria (feeling "high"), fatigue, hallucinations, headache, hyperactivity, inebriated feeling, inhibited walking, insomnia, irritability, light-headedness, malaise, memory disturbance, mood swings, nervousness, numbness, panic disorder, paranoia, paresthesia, perception disturbance, phobic neurosis, postural dizziness, sedation, sleep disturbance, speech disorder, thought disorder, toxic psychosis, tremor, twitch, unconsciousness, vertigo, withdrawal.

Dermatologic – Allergic reactions, anhidrosis, photosensitivity, pruritus, rash.

GI – Abdominal pain, anorexia, aphthous ulcer, constipation, diarrhea, dry mouth, dyspepsia, excessive appetite, gastritis, mouth irritation, nausea, taste change, vomiting.

GU – Decreased urination, frequency of micturition, hot flashes, impaired urination, increased urination, urinary retention.

Musculoskeletal – Back pain, joint pain, muscle pain, neck pain, unspecified pain.

Respiratory – Chest pain, cough, dry nose, dry throat, dyspnea, nasal congestion, nosebleed, pharyngitis, sinus headache, thick tongue, voice change, wheezing.

Special senses – Amblyopia, ear tightness, equilibrium dysfunction, eye disorder, eye dryness, eye irritation, eye swelling, eyelid diseases, photophobia, pupil dilation, tinnitus, vision disturbance, visual field defect.

Miscellaneous – Anemia, bacterial infection, chills, excessive sweating, fever, hypotonia, thirst.

➤*Postmarketing:* Nabilone has been marketed internationally since 1982. The following adverse reactions listed by body system have been reported since nabilone has been marketed. All reactions are listed regardless of causality assessment.

CNS – Abnormal thinking, anxiety, ataxia, circumoral paresthesia, CNS depression, CNS stimulation, confusion, convulsion, depersonalization, depression, dizziness, dysphoria, emotional lability, euphoria, hallucinations, headache, insomnia, psychosis, somnolence, stupor, vertigo.

GI – Constipation, dry mouth, nausea, vomiting.

Miscellaneous – Chest pain, face edema, hypotension, lack of effect, leukopenia, tachycardia, visual disturbances.

NABILONE — ORAL

Overdosage

➤*Symptoms:* Signs and symptoms of overdosage are an extension of the psychotomimetic and physiologic effects of nabilone. In overdose settings, pay attention to vital signs because hypertension and hypotension have been known to occur; tachycardia and orthostatic hypotension were most commonly reported. No cases of overdosage with more than 10 mg/day of nabilone were reported during clinical trials. Signs and symptoms that would be expected to occur in large overdose situations are psychotic episodes (eg, anxiety reactions, coma, hallucinations, respiratory depression).

➤*Treatment:* To obtain up-to-date information about the treatment of overdose, a good resource is your certified regional poison control center. In managing overdosage, consider the possibility of multiple drug overdoses, interaction among drugs, and unusual drug kinetics in the patient.

Overdosage may be considered to have occurred, even at prescribed dosages, if disturbing psychiatric symptoms are present. In these cases, observe the patient in a quiet environment and use supportive measures, including reassurance. Withhold subsequent doses until the patient has returned to baseline mental status; routine dosing may then be resumed if clinically indicated. In such instances, a lower initiating dose is suggested. In controlled clinical trials, alterations in mental status related to the use of nabilone resolved within 72 hours without specific medical therapy.

If psychotic episodes occur, manage the patient conservatively, if possible. For moderate psychotic episodes and anxiety reactions, verbal support and comforting may be sufficient. In more severe cases, antipsychotic drugs may be useful; however, the utility of antipsychotic drugs in cannabinoid psychosis has not been systematically evaluated. Support for their use is drawn from limited experience using antipsychotic agents to manage cannabis overdoses. Because of the potential for drug interactions (eg, additive CNS depressant effects due to nabilone and chlorpromazine), monitor such patients closely.

Protect the patient's airway and support ventilation and perfusion. Meticulously monitor and maintain, within acceptable limits, the patient's vital signs, blood gases, and serum electrolytes, as well as other laboratory values and physical assessments. Absorption of drugs from the GI tract may be decreased by giving activated charcoal, which, in many cases, is more effective than emesis or lavage; consider charcoal instead of or in addition to gastric emptying. Repeated doses of charcoal over time may hasten elimination of some drugs that have been absorbed. Safeguard the patient's airway when employing gastric emptying or charcoal.

The use of forced diuresis, peritoneal dialysis, hemodialysis, charcoal hemoperfusion, or cholestyramine has not been reported. In the presence of normal renal function, most of a dose of nabilone is eliminated through the biliary system.

Treatment for respiratory depression and comatose state consists of symptomatic and supportive therapy. Pay particular attention to the occurrence of hypothermia. If the patient becomes hypotensive, consider fluids, inotropes, and/or vasopressors.

The estimated oral median lethal dose in female mice is between 1,000 and 2,000 mg/kg; in the female rat, it is greater than 2,000 mg/kg.

Patient Information

Alert patients taking nabilone to the potential for additive CNS depression resulting from simultaneous use of nabilone and alcohol or other CNS depressants such as benzodiazepines and barbiturates. Avoid this combination. Specifically warn patients receiving treatment with nabilone not to drive, operate machinery, or engage in any hazardous activity. Make patients using nabilone aware of possible changes in mood and other adverse behavioral effects of the drug so as to avoid panic in the event of such manifestations. Tell patients to remain under the supervision of a responsible adult while using nabilone.

DRONABINOL

c-iii	**Dronabinol** (Watson)	**Capsules; oral:**[a] 2.5 mg	White. In 60s.
c-iii	**Marinol** (Unimed Pharmaceuticals, Inc.)		Parabens. (RL). White. In 25s, 60s, and 100s.
c-iii	**Dronabinol** (Watson)	**Capsules; oral:**[a] 5 mg	Dark brown. In 60s.
c-iii	**Marinol** (Unimed Pharmaceuticals, Inc.)		Parabens. (RL). Brown. In 25s and 100s.
c-iii	**Dronabinol** (Watson)	**Capsules; oral:**[a] 10 mg	Orange. In 60s.
c-iii	**Marinol** (Unimed Pharmaceuticals, Inc.)		Parabens. (RL). Orange. In 25s and 60s.

[a] In sesame oil.

DRONABINOL — ORAL

Refer to the general discussion of these products beginning in the Antiemetic/Antivertigo Agents monograph.

Indications

➤*Appetite stimulation in AIDS patients:* For the treatment of anorexia associated with weight loss in patients with acquired immune deficiency syndrome (AIDS).

➤*Cancer chemotherapy-induced nausea and vomiting:* For nausea and vomiting associated with cancer chemotherapy in patients who have failed to respond adequately to conventional antiemetic treatments.

➤*Off-label uses:*

Cholestatic pruritus (adults) – [4] = Insufficient documentation. The American Association for the Study of Liver Diseases practic guideline for the management of primary biliary cirrhosis recommends cholestyramine as the first-line drug for the treatment of pruritus associated with liver disease. In patients who are intolerant of or who fail therapy with cholestyramine, rifampin is recommended as a second-line agent. Dronabinol is not included in the guideline. Evidence for dronabinol use in the management of cholestatic pruritus is based on a limited number of case reports. Data from controlled trials are needed before this drug can be routinely recommended.

Marijuana cessation – [5] = Poor documentation. Studies have shown a reduction in marijuana withdrawal symptoms. One study that measured self-administration of marijuana found no benefit of dronabinol treatment, but the study population included research volunteers rather than patients with a desire to discontinue marijuana use. Although a range of possibly effective doses has been identified, no studies have identified the optimal dose or addressed the appropriate duration of treatment.

Administration and Dosage

➤*General dosing considerations:* The pharmacologic effects of dronabinol are dose-related and subject to considerable interpatient variability. Therefore, dosage individualization is critical in achieving the maximum benefit of dronabinol treatment.

Caution should be exercised in escalating the dosage of dronabinol because of the increased frequency of dose-related adverse experiences at higher dosages.

Dronabinol should be used with caution and careful psychiatric monitoring performed in patients with mania, depression, or schizophrenia because dronabinol may exacerbate these illnesses. The incidence of disturbing psychiatric symptoms increases significantly at maximum dose.

The pharmacologic effects of dronabinol are reversible upon treatment cessation.

➤*Adults:*

Antiemetic –

Usual dosage: Most patients respond to 5 mg given 3 or 4 times daily.

Maximum dose: 15 mg/m² per dose.

Initial dosage: Initial dose is 5 mg/m² given 1 to 3 hours prior to the administration of chemotherapy, then every 2 to 4 hours after chemotherapy is given, for a total of 4 to 6 doses/day.

Dosage titration: If the 5 mg/m² dose proves to be ineffective, and in the absence of significant side effects, the dose may be escalated by 2.5 mg/m² increments to a maximum of 15 mg/m² per dose. Dosage may be escalated during a chemotherapy cycle or at subsequent cycles, based upon initial results.

Concomitant therapy: Administration of dronabinol with phenothiazines, such as prochlorperazine, has resulted in improved efficacy as compared with either drug alone, without additional toxicity.

Appetite stimulation –

Usual dosage: 5 mg/day (range, 2.5 to 20 mg/day).

Maximum dose: 20 mg/day.

Initial dosage: 2.5 mg twice daily, before lunch and dinner. If CNS symptoms (feeling high, dizziness, confusion, somnolence) do occur, they usually resolve in 1 to 3 days with continued dosage.

Dosage adjustment: For patients unable to tolerate 5 mg/day, the dosage can be reduced to 2.5 mg/day, administered as a single dose in the evening or at bedtime.

When adverse effects are absent or minimal and further therapeutic effect is desired, increase the dose to 2.5 mg before lunch and 5 mg before dinner (or 5 mg at lunch and 5 mg after dinner). If clinically indicated, and in the absence of significant adverse effects, the dosage may be gradually increased to a maximum of 20 mg/day, administered in divided doses. Although most patients respond to 2.5 mg twice daily, 10 mg twice daily has been tolerated in approximately 50% of patients.

Off-label dosing –

Cholestatic pruritus: [4] = Insufficient documentation. 2.5 mg at night to 5 mg 3 times daily.

➤*Children:* Caution is recommended in prescribing dronabinol for children because of the psychoactive effects.

Antiemetic – See Adults for dosing.

➤*Storage/Stability:* Dronabinol should be packaged in a tightly closed container and stored in a cool environment between 8° and 15°C (46° and 59°F), and, alternatively, could be stored in a refrigerator. Protect from freezing.

DRONABINOL — ORAL

Actions

➤*Pharmacology:* Dronabinol is an orally active cannabinoid which, like other cannabinoids, has complex effects on the CNS, including central sympathomimetic activity. Cannabinoid receptors have been discovered in neural tissues. These receptors may play a role in mediating the effects of dronabinol and other cannabinoids. Dronabinol is the principal psychoactive substance present in *Cannabis sativa* L. (marijuana). Nontherapeutic effects of dronabinol are identical to those of marijuana and other centrally active cannabinoids. The mechanism of action is unknown.

Pharmacodynamics – Dronabinol-induced sympathomimetic activity may result in tachycardia or conjunctival injection. Its effects on blood pressure are inconsistent, but occasional subjects have experienced orthostatic hypotension and/or syncope upon abrupt standing.

Dronabinol also demonstrates reversible effects on appetite, mood, cognition, memory, and perception. These phenomena appear to be dose-related, increasing in frequency with higher dosages, and subject to great interpatient variability.

Patients may experience mood changes (eg, euphoria, detachment, depression, anxiety, panic, paranoia), decrements in cognitive performance and memory, a decreased ability to control drives and impulses, and alterations of reality (eg, distortions in perception of objects and sense of time, hallucinations). These latter phenomena are more common with larger doses; however, a full-blown picture of psychosis (psychotic organic brain syndrome) may occur in patients receiving doses in the lower portion of the therapeutic range.

After oral administration, dronabinol has an onset of action of approximately 0.5 to 1 hours and peak effect at 2 to 4 hours. Duration of action for psychoactive effects is 4 to 6 hours, but the appetite stimulant effect of dronabinol may continue for 24 hours or longer after administration.

Tachyphylaxis and tolerance develop to some of the pharmacologic effects of dronabinol and other cannabinoids with chronic use, suggesting an indirect effect on sympathetic neurons. In a study of the pharmacodynamics of chronic dronabinol exposure, healthy male volunteers (n = 12) received 210 mg/day dronabinol, administered orally in divided doses, for 16 days. An initial tachycardia induced by dronabinol was replaced successively by normal sinus rhythm and then bradycardia. A decrease in supine blood pressure, made worse by standing, was also observed initially. These volunteers developed tolerance to the cardiovascular and subjective adverse CNS effects of dronabinol within 12 days of treatment initiation. In 1 study, a slight but consistent decrease in oral temperature was recorded.

Tachyphylaxis and tolerance do not, however, appear to develop to the appetite stimulant effect of dronabinol. In studies involving patients with acquired immune deficiency syndrome (AIDS), the appetite stimulant effect of dronabinol has been sustained for up to 5 months in clinical trials, at dosages ranging from 2.5 mg/day to 20 mg/day.

➤*Pharmacokinetics:*

Absorption/Distribution – Dronabinol is almost completely absorbed (90% to 95%) after single oral doses. Due to the combined effects of first-pass hepatic metabolism and high lipid solubility, only 10% to 20% of the administered dose reaches the systemic circulation. Dronabinol has a large apparent volume of distribution, approximately 10 L/kg, because of its lipid solubility. The plasma protein binding of dronabinol and its metabolites is approximately 97%.

The elimination phase of dronabinol can be described using a 2 compartment model with an initial (alpha) half-life of about 4 hours and a terminal (beta) half-life of 25 to 36 hours. Because of its large volume of distribution, dronabinol and its metabolites may be excreted at low levels for prolonged periods of time.

Metabolism – Dronabinol undergoes extensive first-pass hepatic metabolism, primarily by microsomal hydroxylation, yielding both active and inactive metabolites. Dronabinol and its principal active metabolite, 11-OH-delta-9-THC, are present in approximately equal concentrations in plasma. Concentrations of both parent drug and metabolite peak at approximately 2 to 4 hours after oral dosing and decline over several days. Values for clearance average about 0.2 L/kg/hr, but are highly variable due to the complexity of cannabinoid distribution.

Excretion – Dronabinol and its biotransformation products are excreted in both feces and urine. Biliary excretion is the major route of elimination with about half of a radiolabeled oral dose being recovered from the feces within 72 hours as contrasted with 10% to 15% recovered from urine. Less than 5% of an oral dose is recovered unchanged in the feces.

Following single dose administration, low levels of dronabinol metabolites have been detected for more than 5 weeks in the urine and feces.

In a study of dronabinol involving AIDS patients, urinary cannabinoid/creatinine concentration ratios were studied biweekly over a 6-week period. The urinary cannabinoid/creatinine ratio was closely correlated with dose. No increase in the cannabinoid/creatinine ratio was observed after the first 2 weeks of treatment, indicating that steady-state cannabinoid levels had been reached. This conclusion is consistent with predictions based on the observed terminal half-life of dronabinol. Extended use at recommended doses may cause accumulation of toxic amounts of dronabinol and metabolites.

Contraindications

Hypersensitivity to any cannabinoid or sesame oil.

Warnings/Precautions

➤*Special risk:*

Dronabinol use should be carefully evaluated in patients with the following medical condition – The risk/benefit ratio of dronabinol use should be carefully evaluated in patients with the following medical conditions because of individual variation in response and tolerance to the effects of dronabinol:

Dronabinol should be used with caution in patients with cardiac disorders because of occasional hypotension, possible hypertension, syncope, or tachycardia.

Dronabinol should be used with caution in patients with a history of substance abuse, including alcohol abuse or dependence, because they may be more prone to abuse dronabinol as well. Multiple substance abuse is common and marijuana, which contains the same active compound, is a frequently abused substance.

Dronabinol should be used with caution and careful psychiatric monitoring in patients with mania, depression, or schizophrenia because dronabinol may exacerbate these illnesses.

Dronabinol should be used with caution in patients receiving concomitant therapy with sedatives, hypnotics, or other psychoactive drugs because of the potential for additive or synergistic CNS effects.

Dronabinol should be used with caution in pregnant patients, nursing mothers, or pediatric patients because it has not been studied in these patient populations.

➤*Drug abuse and dependence:* Dronabinol is one of the psychoactive compounds present in cannabis, and is abusable and controlled [Schedule III (CIII)] under the Controlled Substances Act. Both psychological and physiological dependence have been noted in healthy individuals receiving dronabinol, but addiction is uncommon and has only been seen after prolonged high dose administration. Limit prescriptions to the amount necessary for a single cycle of chemotherapy.

Chronic abuse of cannabis has been associated with decrements in motivation, cognition, judgement, and perception. The etiology of these impairments is unknown, but may be associated with the complex process of addiction rather than an isolated effect of the drug. No such decrements in psychological, social or neurological status have been associated with the administration of dronabinol for therapeutic purposes.

An abstinence syndrome has been reported after the abrupt discontinuation of dronabinol in volunteers receiving dosages of 210 mg/day for 12 to 16 consecutive days. Within 12 hours after discontinuation, these volunteers manifested symptoms such as irritability, insomnia, and restlessness. By approximately 24 hours post-dronabinol discontinuation, withdrawal symptoms intensified to include "hot flashes", sweating, rhinorrhea, loose stools, hiccoughs, and anorexia.

These withdrawal symptoms gradually dissipated over the next 48 hours. The syndrome was essentially complete within 96 hours. Electroencephalographic changes consistent with the effects of drug withdrawal (hyperexcitation) were recorded in patients after abrupt dechallenge. Patients also complained of disturbed sleep for several weeks after discontinuing therapy with high dosages of dronabinol.

➤*Hazardous tasks:* Patients receiving treatment with dronabinol should be specifically warned not to drive, operate machinery, or engage in any hazardous activity until it is established that they are able to tolerate the drug and to perform such tasks safely. Effects may persist for a variable and unpredictable period of time.

➤*Pregnancy:* *Category C.* Reproduction studies with dronabinol have been performed in mice at 15 to 450 mg/m^2, equivalent to 0.2 to 5 times maximum recommended human MRHD of 90 mg/m^2/day in cancer patients or 1 to 30 times MRHD of 15 mg/m^2/day in AIDS patients, and in rats at 74 to 295 mg/m^2 (equivalent to 0.8 to 3 times MRHD of 90 mg/m^2 in cancer patients or 5 to 20 times MRHD of 15 mg/m^2/day in AIDS patients). These studies have revealed no evidence of teratogenicity due to dronabinol. At these dosages in mice and rats, dronabinol decreased maternal weight gain and number of viable pups and increased fetal mortality and early resorptions. Such effects were dose dependent and less apparent at lower doses which produced less maternal toxicity. There are no adequate and well-controlled studies in pregnant women. Dronabinol should be used only if the potential benefit justifies the potential risk to the fetus.

➤*Lactation:* Use of dronabinol is not recommended in nursing mothers since, in addition to the secretion of HIV virus in breast milk, dronabinol is concentrated in and secreted in human breast milk and is absorbed by the nursing baby. The effects of chronic exposure to the drug and its metabolites on the infant are unknown.

➤*Children:* Dronabinol capsules are not recommended for AIDS-related anorexia in pediatric patients because it has not been studied in this population. The pediatric dosage for the treatment of chemotherapy-induced emesis is the same as in adults. Caution is recommended in prescribing dronabinol capsules for children because of the psychoactive effects.

➤*Elderly:* Caution is advised in prescribing dronabinol capsules in elderly patients because they are generally more sensitive to the psychoactive effects of drugs. In antiemetic studies, no difference in tolerance or efficacy was apparent in patients greater than 55 years of age.

➤*Monitoring:* Because of individual variation, clinically determine the period of time the patient needs to be supervised. Closely observe patients within an inpatient setting, if possible. This is especially important during treatment of patients with no prior experience with *Cannabis* or dronabinol. However, even patients experienced with these agents may have serious

DRONABINOL — ORAL

untoward responses not predicted by prior uneventful exposures. Closely observe any patient who has a psychotic experience with dronabinol until the mental state returns to normal. Do not give additional doses until the patient has been examined and the circumstances evaluated. If the situation warrants, give a lower dose under very close supervision.

Drug Interactions

In studies involving patients with AIDS and/or cancer, dronabinol has been coadministered with a variety of medications (eg, cytotoxic agents, anti-infective agents, sedatives, or opioid analgesics) without resulting in any clinically significant drug/drug interactions. Although no drug/drug interactions were discovered during the clinical trials of dronabinol, cannabinoids may interact with other medications through both metabolic and pharmacodynamic mechanisms. Dronabinol is highly protein bound to plasma proteins, and therefore, might displace other protein-bound drugs. Although this displacement has not been confirmed in vivo, practitioners should monitor patients for a change in dosage requirements when administering dronabinol to patients receiving other highly protein-bound drugs. Published reports of drug/drug interactions involving cannabinoids are summarized in the following table.

Dronabinol Drug Interactions

Precipitant drug	Object drug[a]		Description
Dronabinol	Amphetamines Cocaine Sympathomimetics	↑	Additive hypertension, tachycardia, possibly cardiotoxicity, may occur.
Dronabinol	Anticholinergics Antihistamines	↑	Additive or super-additive tachycardia, or drowsiness may occur.
Dronabinol	Antidepressants, tricyclic	↑	Additive tachycardia, hypertension, or drowsiness may occur.
Dronabinol	Alcohol Sedatives Hypnotics Psychomimetics	↑	Additive or synergistic CNS effects may occur. Also, clearance of barbiturates may be decreased, possibly because of inhibition of metabolism.
Cannabinoids	Disulfiram	↑	A reversible hypomanic reaction occurred in a patient who smoked marijuana; confirmed by rechallenge.
Cannabinoids	Fluoxetine	↑	A patient with depression and bulimia became hypomanic after smoking marijuana; symptoms resolved after 4 days.
Cannabinoids	Theophylline	↓	Increased theophylline metabolism was reported with marijuana smoking.

[a] ↑ = object drug increased. ↓ = object drug decreased.

Adverse Reactions

A cannabinoid dose-related "high" (easy laughing, elation, and heightened awareness) has been reported by patients receiving dronabinol in both the antiemetic (24%) and the lower dose appetite stimulant clinical trials (8%).

The most frequently reported adverse experiences in patients with AIDS during placebo-controlled clinical trials involved the CNS and were reported by 33% of patients receiving dronabinol. About 25% of patients reported a minor CNS adverse event during the first 2 weeks and about 4% reported such an event each week for the next 6 weeks thereafter.

➤*Probably causally related: Incidence greater than 1%:* Rates derived from clinical trials in AIDS-related anorexia (n = 157) and chemotherapy-related nausea (n = 317). Rates were generally higher in the antiemetic use (given in parentheses).

Cardiovascular – Palpitations, tachycardia, vasodilation/facial flush.

CNS – (Amnesia), anxiety/nervousness, (hallucination), (ataxia), confusion, depersonalization.

Incidence of events 3% to 10%: Dizziness, euphoria, paranoid reaction, somnolence, abnormal thinking.

GI –
Incidence of events 3% to 10%: Abdominal pain, nausea, vomiting.

Miscellaneous – Asthenia.

➤*Probably causally related: Incidence less than 1%:* Event rates derived from clinical trials in AIDS-related anorexia (n = 157) and chemotherapy-related nausea (n = 317).

Cardiovascular –
Incidence 0.3% to 1%: Hypotension.

CNS – Depression, nightmares, speech difficulties, tinnitus, emotional lability, tremors.

Dermatologic –
Incidence 0.3% to 1%: Flushing.

GI – Fecal incontinence.
Incidence 0.3% to 1%: Diarrhea.

Musculoskeletal – Myalgias.

Special senses –
Incidence 0.3% to 1%: Conjunctivitis. Vision difficulties.

➤*Causal relationship unknown: Incidence less than 1%:* The clinical significance of the association of these events with dronabinol treatment is unknown, but they are reported as alerting information for the clinician.

Dermatologic – Sweating.

GI – Anorexia, hepatic enzyme elevation.

Respiratory – Cough, rhinitis, sinusitis.

Miscellaneous – Chills, headache, malaise.

Overdosage

The estimated lethal human dose of intravenous dronabinol is 30 mg/kg (2100 mg/70 kg). Significant CNS symptoms in antiemetic studies followed oral doses of 0.4 mg/kg (28 mg/70 kg) of dronabinol.

➤*Symptoms:* Signs and symptoms following mild dronabinol intoxication include drowsiness, euphoria, heightened sensory awareness, altered time perception, reddened conjunctiva, dry mouth and tachycardia; following moderate intoxication include memory impairment, depersonalization, mood alteration, urinary retention, and reduced bowel motility; and following severe intoxication include decreased motor coordination, lethargy, slurred speech, and postural hypotension. Apprehensive patients may experience panic reactions, and seizures may occur in patients with existing seizure disorders.

➤*Treatment:* A potentially serious oral ingestion, if recent, should be managed with gut decontamination. In unconscious patients with a secure airway, instill activated charcoal (30 to 100 g in adults, 1 to 2 g/kg in infants) via a nasogastric tube. A saline cathartic or sorbitol may be added to the first dose of activated charcoal. Patients experiencing depressive, hallucinatory or psychotic reactions should be placed in a quiet area and offered reassurance. Benzodiazepines (5 to 10 mg diazepam by mouth) may be used for treatment of extreme agitation. Hypotension usually responds to Trendelenburg position and IV fluids. Pressors are rarely required.

Patient Information

Patients receiving treatment with dronabinol should be alerted to the potential for additive CNS depression if dronabinol is used concomitantly with alcohol or other CNS depressants such as benzodiazepines and barbiturates.

Patients receiving treatment with dronabinol should be specifically warned not to drive, operate machinery, or engage in any hazardous activity until it is established that they are able to tolerate the drug and to perform such tasks safely.

Patients using dronabinol should be advised of possible changes in mood and other adverse behavioral effects of the drug so as to avoid panic in the event of such manifestations. Patients should remain under the supervision of a responsible adult during initial use of dronabinol and following dosage adjustments.

PHOSPHORATED CARBOHYDRATE SOLUTION

otc	**Emetrol** (Pharmacia & Upjohn)	**Solution:** 1.87 g dextrose, 1.87 g fructose, 21.5 mg phosphoric acid per 5 mL	Methylparaben. Lemon mint or cherry flavor. In 118, 236, and 473 mL.
otc	**Formula EM** (Major)		Methylparaben. Cherry flavor. In 118 mL.
otc	**Nausea Relief** (Zenith Goldline)		Methylparaben. In 118 mL.
otc	**Nausetrol** (Walsh Dohmen)		Glycerin, methylparaben. Cherry flavor. In 118 mL.

PHOSPHORATED CARBOHYDRATE SOLUTION — ORAL

Refer to the general discussion beginning in the Antiemetic/Antivertigo Agents monograph.

Indications

➤*Antiemetic:* Relief of nausea caused by upset stomach from intestinal flu, stomach flu and food or drink indiscretions.

➤*Off-label uses:* Regurgitation in infants; morning sickness; motion sickness; nausea and vomiting caused by drug therapy or inhalation anesthesia.

Administration and Dosage

➤*Adults:*

Nausea –
Usual dosage: 15 or 30 mL. Dose may be repeated every 15 minutes until distress subsides.
Maximum dose: Do not take for more than 1 hour or more than 5 doses.

Miscellaneous Antiemetics

PHOSPHORATED CARBOHYDRATE SOLUTION — ORAL

Off-label dosing –

Morning sickness: 15 to 30 mL on arising; repeat every 3 hours or when nausea threatens.

Motion sickness: 15 mL doses.

Nausea and vomiting caused by drug therapy or inhalation anesthesia: 15 mL doses.

➤*Children:*

Nausea –

2 to 12 years of age:

• *Usual dosage* – 5 or 10 mL. Dose may be repeated every 15 minutes until distress subsides.

• *Maximum dose* – Do not take for more than 1 hour or more than 5 doses.

Off-label dosing –

Motion sickness: 5 mL doses.

Nausea and vomiting caused by drug therapy or inhalation anesthesia: 5 mL doses.

Regurgitation in infants: 5 or 10 mL given 10 to 15 minutes before each feeding; in refractory cases, 10 or 15 mL given 30 minutes before feeding.

➤*Administration:* Do not dilute. Do not take oral fluids immediately before the dose or for at least 15 minutes after the dose.

➤*Storage/Stability:* Store at room temperature.

Actions

➤*Pharmacology:* Hyperosmolar carbohydrate solutions with phosphoric acid relieve nausea and vomiting by a direct local action on the wall of the GI tract that reduces smooth muscle contraction.

Warnings/Precautions

➤*Nausea:* Nausea may signal a serious condition. If symptoms are not relieved or recur often, consult a physician.

➤*Diabetic patients:* Diabetic patients should avoid these preparations because they contain significant amounts of sugar.

➤*Hereditary fructose intolerance:* These preparations contain fructose and should be avoided by individuals with hereditary fructose intolerance.

➤*Pregnancy:* *Category: Undetermined.* Consult a health care provider before using in pregnant women.

➤*Lactation:* Consult a health care provider before using in breast-feeding women.

Adverse Reactions

Large doses of fructose can cause abdominal pain and diarrhea.

Antidopaminergics

CHLORPROMAZINE HYDROCHLORIDE

For complete prescribing information, refer to the Chlorpromazine Hydrochloride monograph in the Antipsychotic Agents section.

METOCLOPRAMIDE

For complete prescribing information, refer to the Metoclopramide monograph in the GI Stimulants.

PERPHENAZINE

For complete prescribing information, refer to the Perphenazine monograph in the Antipsychotic Agents section.

PROCHLORPERAZINE

For complete prescribing information, refer to the Prochlorperazine monograph in the Antipsychotic Agents section.

PROMETHAZINE

For complete prescribing information, refer to the Promethazine monograph in the Antihistamines section.

ANTIANXIETY AGENTS

Benzodiazepines

Indications

➤*Anxiety:* For the management of anxiety disorders or for the short-term relief of the symptoms of anxiety. Anxiety or tension associated with the stress of everyday life usually does not require treatment with an antianxiety agent.

Consult individual drug monographs for specific indications.

In addition to use as antianxiety agents, some benzodiazepines are also useful as hypnotics, anticonvulsants, and muscle relaxants. **Midazolam**, an injectable short-acting benzodiazepine, is used for induction of general anesthesia, preoperative sedation, conscious sedation for diagnostic procedures, and to supplement nitrous oxide and oxygen for short surgical procedures (see individual monograph).

➤*Off-label uses:* Refer to individual monographs for further information.

Bipolar disorder – Depressive episodes (adults) –

Clonazepam: [5] = Poor documentation.

Bipolar disorder – Manic or mixed episodes (adults) –

Clonazepam: [2] = Fair documentation.

Bipolar disorder – Rapid cycling (adults) –

Clonazepam: [5] = Poor documentation.

Postherpetic neuralgia –

Lorazepam: [5] = Poor documentation.

Premenstrual dysphoric disorders –

Alprazolam: [5] = Poor documentation.

Prevention of migraine (adults) –

Clonazepam: [5] = Poor documentation.

Restless legs syndrome –

Clonazepam: [4] = Insufficient documentation.

Smoking cessation –

Diazepam: [5] = Poor documentation.

Tardive dyskinesia –

Diazepam: [4] = Insufficient documentation.

Tic disorders –

Clonazepam: [2] = Fair documentation.

Other possible off-label uses – Management of irritable bowel syndrome (**alprazolam, chlordiazepoxide, clorazepate, diazepam, lorazepam, oxazepam**); panic attacks (alprazolam, diazepam); depression (alprazolam); status epilepticus, chemotherapy-induced nausea and vomiting, acute alcohol withdrawal syndrome, psychogenic catatonia (lorazepam injection); chronic insomnia (lorazepam).

Clonazepam: Parkinsonian (hypokinetic) dysarthria. Adjunct in the treatment of schizophrenia. Neuralgias (deafferentation pain syndromes).

Actions

➤*Pharmacology:* Benzodiazepines appear to potentiate the effects of gamma-aminobutyrate (GABA) (ie, they facilitate inhibitory GABA neurotransmission) and other inhibitory transmitters by binding to specific benzodiazepine receptor sites. Recent evidence suggest there are at least 2 benzodiazepine receptors, BZ_1 and BZ_2. BZ_1 is thought to be associated with sleep mechanisms; BZ_2 with memory, motor, sensory, and cognitive functions. The activity of the benzodiazepines may involve the following sites: spinal cord (muscle relaxation); brain stem (anticonvulsant properties); cerebellum (ataxia); limbic and cortical areas (emotional behavior). Anxiolytic effects are distinct from nonspecific consequences of CNS depression (ie, sedation and motor impairment). A distinctive feature of the benzodiazepines is the wide margin of safety between therapeutic and toxic doses. Ataxia and sedation occur only at doses beyond those needed for anxiolytic effects.

Clonazepam suppresses the spike and wave discharge in petit mal seizures and decreases frequency, amplitude, duration and spread of discharge in minor motor seizures.

➤*Pharmacokinetics:* There is little clinical evidence to suggest that one benzodiazepine is more effective than another. The major differences are reflected in their pharmacokinetic profiles and relative costs. The following table summarizes the major pharmacokinetic variables of these agents:

Benzodiazepine Pharmacokinetics						
Drug	Dosage range (mg/d)[a]	Peak plasma level (h)[a]	Elimination t½ (h)	Metabolites	Speed of onset[a]	Protein binding
Alprazolam	0.75 to 4	1 to 2	6.3 to 26.9	Alpha-hydroxy-alprazolam; Benzophenone	intermediate	80%
Chlordiazepoxide	15 to 100	0.5 to 4	5 to 30	Desmethylchlordiazepoxide[b]; Demoxepam; Desmethyl-diazepam	intermediate	96%
Clonazepam	1.5 to 20	1 to 2	18 to 50	Inactive 7–amino or 7–acetyl-amino derivatives[b]	intermediate	97%
Clorazepate	15 to 60	1 to 2	40 to 50	Desmethyl-diazepam	fast	97% to 98%[c]
Diazepam	4 to 40	0.5 to 2	20 to 80	Desmethyl-diazepam[b]; nordiazepam	very fast	98%
Lorazepam	2 to 4	2 to 4	10 to 20	Inactive glucuronide conjugate	intermediate	85%
Oxazepam	30 to 120	2 to 4	5 to 20	Inactive glucuronide conjugate	slow	87%

[a] Oral administration.
[b] Major metabolite.
[c] Nordiazepam (active metabolite).

Absorption – The major determinant of the onset and intensity of action of a single oral dose of a benzodiazepine is the rate of absorption from the GI tract. Benzodiazepines are readily absorbed following oral administration.

Intramuscular (IM) administration of **chlordiazepoxide** and **diazepam** results in slow erratic absorption and lower peak plasma levels than oral or intravenous (IV) administration. However, IM administration of diazepam into the deltoid muscle is more likely to be rapid and complete. **Lorazepam** IM is rapidly and completely absorbed.

Distribution – The highly lipid soluble benzodiazepines are widely distributed in the body tissues and highly bound to plasma proteins (70% to 99%). The duration of action is related to their lipid solubility. Highly lipophilic drugs, like **diazepam**, are rapidly taken into the brain and then rapidly redistributed throughout the body.

Metabolism – The effect of lipid solubility on duration of action is complicated by hepatic biotransformation to active metabolites. The benzophenone metabolite of **alprazolam** is inactive, while alpha-hydroxy-alprazolam is approximately 50% as active as the parent compound; both metabolites have the same half-life as alprazolam. Other benzodiazepines have active metabolites with very long half-lives; cumulative effects occur with chronic administration. Desmethyldiazepam is an active metabolite common to many of these agents (eg, **clorazepate, diazepam**); clorazepate is hydrolyzed in the stomach and absorbed as desmethyldiazepam. **Chlordiazepoxide** has several active intermediate metabolites. Five metabolites of clonazepam have been identified. Biotransformation of **clonazepam** is by oxidative hydroxylation and reduction.

Because hepatic biotransformation is the predominant route for benzodiazepine metabolism, the disposition of these drugs may be impaired in patients with chronic liver disease. **Oxazepam** and **lorazepam** are metabolized to inactive compounds and therefore have relatively short half-lives and duration of activity. Because of their simple 1-step inactivation, oxazepam or lorazepam may be preferred in patients with liver disease and in the elderly. Sustained clinical effects require multiple daily doses; significant accumulation does not occur. The other agents with prolonged half-lives may be administered as a single daily dose at bedtime. The elimination half-life of diazepam and desmethyldiazepam is prolonged in obese patients; total metabolic clearance does not change.

Excretion – Most benzodiazepines are excreted almost entirely in the urine and in the form of oxidized and glucuronide-conjugated metabolites.

Contraindications

Hypersensitivity to benzodiazepines; psychoses; acute narrow-angle glaucoma (may be used in patients with open-angle glaucoma and appropriate therapy); patients with clinical or biochemical evidence of significant liver disease (**clonazepam**); intra-arterial use (**lorazepam** injection); children younger than 6 months of age; lactation (**diazepam**); coadministration with ketoconazole and itraconazole due to inhibition of cytochrome P450 3A (see Warnings).

Warnings/Precautions

➤*Psychiatric disorders:* These agents are not intended for use in patients with a primary depressive disorder or psychosis, nor in those psychiatric disorders in which anxiety is not a prominent feature.

➤*Long-term use (longer than 4 months):* Effectiveness has not been assessed by systematic clinical studies. Periodically reassess the usefulness of the drug for the individual patient.

➤*Dependence:* Prolonged use of therapeutic doses can lead to dependence. Withdrawal syndrome has occurred after as little as 4 to 6 weeks treatment. It is more likely if the drug is short-acting (eg, **alprazolam**), taken regularly for longer than 3 months and abruptly discontinued.

After rapid decrease of dosage or abrupt discontinuation, withdrawal seizures were reported in alprazolam patients.

Onset is within 1 to 10 days; duration of reaction may be 5 days to 1 month depending on agent, dose, etc. Symptoms generally begin with anxiety-like manifestations; the following may occur in 50% or more of cases: anorexia; concentration difficulties; confusion; dizziness; dysphoria; fatigue; hallucinations; headache; increased anxiety; insomnia; memory impairment; muscle tension/cramps; muscle twitching; paranoid delusions; "psychosis"; seizures (generalized tonic-clonic); sensory disturbances (hypercusis, hypersomnia, metallic taste, paresthesias, photophobia); tremor; vomiting.

Abrupt withdrawal of **clonazepam**, particularly in those patients on long-term, high-dose therapy, may precipitate status epilepticus. While clonazepam is being gradually withdrawn, the simultaneous substitution of another anticonvulsant may be indicated. Other symptoms include diarrhea, sweating, and vomiting.

When discontinuing therapy in patients who have used these agents for prolonged periods, decrease dosage gradually over 4 to 8 weeks to avoid the possibility of withdrawal symptoms, especially in patients with a history of seizures or epilepsy, regardless of their concomitant anticonvulsant drug therapy. Patients on short-acting benzodiazepines may be switched to longer-acting drugs (eg, **diazepam**) which produce a gradual decrease in drug concentration and decrease the chance of withdrawal symptoms. Clonidine, propranolol, and carbamazepine have been used as adjuncts in the treatment of benzodiazepine withdrawal symptoms.

➤*Parenteral administration:* Parenteral (IM or IV) therapy is indicated primarily in acute states. Keep patients under observation, preferably in bed, for up to 3 hours.

Do not inject intra-arterially; this may produce arteriospasm, resulting in gangrene which may require amputation.

Administer parenterally with extreme care (particularly IV) to the elderly, very ill, and those with limited pulmonary reserve. Because of possible apnea or cardiac arrest, resuscitative facilities should be available. Not recommended for obstetric use. Do not administer to patients in shock, coma or in acute alcohol intoxication.

Hypotension or muscular weakness is possible, particularly when benzodiazepines are used with narcotics, barbiturates, or alcohol.

➤*Suicide:* In those patients in whom depression accompanies anxiety, suicidal tendencies may be present, and protective measures may be required. Dispense the least amount of drug feasible to the patient.

➤*Paradoxical reactions:* Excitement, stimulation, and acute rage have occurred in psychiatric patients and hyperactive aggressive children. These reactions may be secondary to relief of anxiety and usually appear in the first 2 weeks of therapy. Acute hyperexcited states, anxiety, hallucinations, increased muscle spasticity, insomnia, and sleep disturbances also have occurred. Should these occur, discontinue the drug. Minor EEG changes, usually low voltage fast activity, have been observed during and after therapy and are of no known significance. Anger, hostility and episodes of mania and hypomania have been reported with **alprazolam**.

➤*Multiple seizure type:* When used in patients in whom several different types of seizure disorders coexist, **clonazepam** may increase the incidence or precipitate the onset of generalized tonic-clonic (grand mal) seizures. This may require the addition of other anticonvulsants or an increase in their dosage.

Diazepam – If use in patients with seizure disorders results in an increase in the frequency or severity of grand mal seizures, there may be a need to increase the dosage of standard anticonvulsant medication.

➤*Chronic respiratory disease:* **Clonazepam** may produce an increase in salivation. Use with caution in patients if increased salivation causes respiratory difficulty. Due to the possibility of respiratory depression, use with caution in such patients.

➤*Benzyl alcohol:* Some of these products contain benzyl alcohol, which has been associated with a fatal "gasping syndrome" in premature infants.

➤*Tartrazine sensitivity:* Some of these products contain tartrazine, which may cause allergic-type reactions (including bronchial asthma) in susceptible individuals. Although the incidence of tartrazine sensitivity in the general population is low, it is frequently seen in patients who also have aspirin hypersensitivity. Specific products containing tartrazine are identified in the product listings.

➤*Renal function impairment:* Observe usual precautions in the presence of impaired renal or hepatic function to avoid accumulation of these agents. **Lorazepam** injection is not recommended in these patients. Metabolites of **clonazepam** are excreted by the kidneys; to avoid excess accumulation, exercise caution in patients with renal function impairment. Also, clonazepam is contraindicated in patients with significant liver disease.

➤*Hazardous tasks:* May produce drowsiness or dizziness; observe caution while driving or performing other tasks requiring alertness.

➤*Pregnancy: Category D* (No category designation for **clonazepam**). Benzodiazepines and their metabolites freely cross the placenta and accumulate in the fetal circulation. An increased risk of congenital malformations associated with the use of minor tranquilizers during the first trimester of pregnancy has been suggested. Malformations reported include cleft lip or palate. Recent studies suggest **diazepam** use in the first trimester does not cause an increased risk of this. Because use of these drugs is rarely a matter of urgency, avoid them during this period. Consider the possibility that a woman of childbearing potential may be pregnant at the time of institution of therapy. Advise patients that if they become pregnant, or plan to become pregnant, they should discuss the desirability of discontinuing the drug.

Labor and delivery – Benzodiazepines have been found in maternal and cord blood, indicating placental transfer of drug. Therefore, benzodiazepines are not recommended for obstetrical use.

Neonatal withdrawal consisting of severe tremulousness and irritability has been attributed to maternal ingestion of benzodiazepines as well as neonatal flaccidity and respiratory problems. Use during labor has resulted in a "floppy infant" syndrome, manifested by hypotonia, lethargy, and sucking difficulties.

Prolonged CNS depression has been observed in neonates, apparently due to inability to biotransform **diazepam** into inactive metabolites.

➤*Lactation:* Benzodiazepines are excreted in breast milk (**lorazepam** excretion is not known). Because neonates metabolize benzodiazepines at a slower rate than adults, accumulation of the drug and its metabolites to toxic levels is possible. Chronic **diazepam** use in breast-feeding mothers reportedly caused infants to become lethargic and to lose weight; do not give to breast-feeding mothers.

➤*Children:* The initial dose should be small and dosage increments made gradually, in accordance with the response of the patient, to preclude ataxia or excessive sedation. Hypotension is rare; however, use with caution if cardiac complications may result from a drop in blood pressure.

Alprazolam – Safety and efficacy for use in patients younger than 18 years of age have not been established.

Chlordiazepoxide – Chlordiazepoxide is not recommended in children younger than 6 years of age (oral) or 12 years of age (injectable).

Clorazepate – Not recommended for use in patients younger than 9 years of age.

Diazepam – Not for use in children younger than 6 months of age (oral); safety and efficacy have not been established in the neonate (30 days or less of age; injectable).

Lorazepam – Do not use in patients younger than 18 years of age (injection); safety and efficacy for use in patients younger than 12 years of age are not established (oral).

➤*Elderly:* The initial dose should be small and dosage increments made gradually, in accordance with the response of the patient, to preclude ataxia or excessive sedation. Hypotension is rare; however, use with caution if cardiac complications may result from a drop in blood pressure.

Per the Beers list, **alprazolam** doses greater than 2 mg, **lorazepam** doses greater than 3 mg, and **oxazepam** doses greater than 60 mg should not be used because of increased sensitivity to benzodiazepines in elderly patients. Smaller doses may be effective as well as safer. Total daily doses should rarely exceed the suggested maximums.

Per the Beers list, **chlordiazepoxide**, **diazepam**, and **clorazepate** have a long half-life in elderly patients (often several days), producing prolonged sedation and increasing the risk of falls and fractures. Short and intermediate acting benzodiazepines are preferred if a benzodiazepine is required. Chlordiazepoxide and diazepam are also considered a high risk medication for the elderly according to the Centers of Medicare and Medicaid services.

➤*Monitoring:* Because of isolated reports of neutropenia and jaundice, perform periodic blood counts and liver function tests during long-term therapy. There have been reports of abnormal liver and kidney function tests and of decrease in hematocrit.

Drug Interactions

Benzodiazepine Drug Interactions

Precipitant drug	Object drug[a]		Description
Alcohol/CNS depressants (eg, barbiturates, narcotics)	Benzodiazepines	↑	Increased CNS effects (eg, impaired psychomotor function, sedation) may occur.
Benzodiazepines	Alcohol/CNS depressants (eg, barbiturates, narcotics)		
Antacids	Benzodiazepines	↓	Antacids may alter the rate but generally not the extent of GI absorption. Staggering administration times may help avoid possible interaction.
Azole antifungals (itraconazole, ketoconazole, voriconazole)	Benzodiazepines	↑	Azole antifungals decrease the metabolism of benzodiazepines, leading to increased sedation and prolonged CNS depression. Triazolam is contraindicated with itraconazole and ketoconazole; midazolam is contraindicated with itraconazole.
Carbamazepine	Benzodiazepines	↓	May increase hepatic metabolism, resulting in decreased pharmacologic effects. Consider increased benzodiazepine dose.
Cimetidine Contraceptives, oral Disulfiram Fluoxetine Isoniazid Omeprazole Metoprolol Propoxyphene Propranolol Valproic acid	Alprazolam Chlordiazepoxide Clorazepate Diazepam	↑	The elimination of benzodiazepines that undergo oxidative hepatic metabolism (alprazolam, chlordiazepoxide, clorazepate, diazepam) may be decreased by the following drugs due to inhibition of hepatic metabolism. Pharmacologic effects of these benzodiazepines may be increased and excessive sedation/impaired psychomotor function may occur.
Clozapine	Benzodiazepines	↑	Delirium, sedation, sialorrhea, and ataxia may occur. Do not start simultaneously; it may be better to add clozapine to established clonazepam therapy than vice versa. Carefully monitor.
Contraceptives, oral	Lorazepam Oxazepam	↓	The clearance rate of benzodiazepines that undergo glucuronidation (lorazepam, oxazepam) may be increased.
Probenecid	Benzodiazepines	↑	Probenecid may interfere with benzodiazepine conjugation in the liver, possibly resulting in a more rapid onset or prolonged effect.
Protease inhibitors (eg, ritonavir, nelfinavir)	Benzodiazepines	↑	May decrease the oxidative metabolism of benzodiazepines, leading to severe sedation and respiratory depression. Midazolam and triazolam are contraindicated with atazanavir or darunavir.
Ranitidine	Diazepam	↓	Ranitidine may reduce the GI absorption of diazepam.
Rifampin	Benzodiazepines	↓	The oxidative metabolism of benzodiazepines may be increased due to microsomal enzyme induction. Pharmacologic effects of some benzodiazepines may be decreased.
St. John's Wort	Benzodiazepines	↓	May increase hepatic metabolism, resulting in decreased pharmacologic effects. Adjust benzodiazepine dose as needed.
Scopolamine	Lorazepam	↑	Scopolamine, used concomitantly with parenteral lorazepam, may increase the incidence of sedation, hallucinations, and irrational behavior.
Theophyllines	Benzodiazepines	↓	Theophyllines may antagonize the sedative effects of the benzodiazepines.
Benzodiazepines	Digoxin	↑	Digoxin's serum concentrations may be increased. Toxicity characterized by GI and neuropsychiatric symptoms and cardiac arrhythmias may occur. Monitor digoxin serum levels.
Benzodiazepines	Neuromuscular blocking agents	↔	Benzodiazepines may potentiate, counteract, or have no effect on the actions of these agents.
Benzodiazepines	Phenytoin	↑	Phenytoin serum concentrations may be increased, resulting in toxicity, but data are conflicting. Phenytoin may increase oxazepam clearance.

[a] ↑ = object drug increased; ↓ = object drug decreased; ↔ = undetermined clinical effect.

Adverse Reactions

Discontinuation of therapy due to undesirable effects is rare. Transient, mild drowsiness is commonly seen in the first few days of therapy. Drowsiness, ataxia and confusion have occurred, especially in elderly and debilitated patients. If these reactions are persistent, reduce dosage. Ataxia is rare with **oxazepam** and does not appear to be specifically related to dose or age. Other adverse reactions less frequently reported include:

➤*Cardiovascular:* Bradycardia; cardiovascular collapse; edema; hypertension; hypotension; palpitations; phlebitis and thrombosis at IV sites; tachycardia. Decrease in systolic blood pressure has been observed.

➤*CNS:* Agitation; akathisia; anterograde amnesia; apathy; aphonia; ataxia; coma; confusion; crying; delirium; depression; difficulty in concentration; disorientation; dizziness; dysarthria; dystonia; euphoria; extrapyramidal symptoms; fatigue; "glassy-eyed" appearance; headache; hemiparesis; hypoactivity; hypotonia; inability to perform complex mental functions; incoordination; irritability; lethargy; light-headedness; memory impairment; nervousness; paradoxical reactions (see Precautions); psychomotor retardation; restlessness; rigidity; sedation and sleepiness; seizures; slurred speech; sobbing; stupor; syncope; tremor; unsteadiness; vertigo; vivid dreams; weakness.

➤*Dermatologic:* Ankle and facial edema; dermatitis; hair loss; hirsutism; pruritus; urticaria; skin rash, including morbilliform, urticarial, and maculopapular.

➤*GI:* Anorexia; change in appetite; coated tongue; constipation; diarrhea; difficulty in swallowing; dry mouth; gastritis; increased salivation; nausea; sore gums; vomiting.

➤*GU:* Changes in libido; incontinence; menstrual irregularities; urinary retention.

➤*Ophthalmic:* Diplopia; nystagmus; visual disturbances.

➤*Psychiatric:* Behavior problems; hysteria; psychosis; suicidal tendencies.

➤*Miscellaneous:* Anemia; auditory disturbances; blood dyscrasias including agranulocytosis; depressed hearing; diaphoresis; dehydration; elevations of LDH, alkaline phosphatase, ALT, and AST; eosinophilia; fever; galactorrhea; gynecomastia; hepatic dysfunction (including hepatitis and jaundice); hiccups; increase or decrease in body weight; joint pain; leukopenia; lymphadenopathy; muscular disturbance; nasal congestion; pain, burning, and redness following IM injection; paresthesias; respiratory disturbances; thrombocytopenia. Partial airway obstruction has occurred and is believed to be due to excessive sedation at time of procedure (**lorazepam** injection).

Overdosage

There are no well-documented fatal overdoses resulting from oral ingestion of benzodiazepines alone. Most overdose-related fatalities implicate benzodiazepines only as a component in multiple drug ingestions.

➤*Symptoms:* Mild symptoms include confusion, diminished reflexes, drowsiness, impaired coordination, lethargy, and somnolence. These agents rarely cause significant respiratory or circulatory depression, particularly when they are the sole agents ingested. Serious symptoms may include ataxia, hypotonia, hypotension, hypnosis, stages 1 to 3 coma, and rarely, death. Consider multiple drug ingestion.

Unlike oral ingestions, IV administration of **diazepam** is associated with a 1.7% incidence of life-threatening reactions, including hypotension and respiratory or cardiac arrest.

➤*Treatment:* Induce vomiting if it has not occurred spontaneously. Employ general supportive measures, along with immediate gastric lavage or ipecac. Follow with activated charcoal administration and a saline cathartic. Monitor respiration, pulse, and blood pressure. Administer IV fluids and maintain an adequate airway. Treat hypotension with norepinephrine or metaraminol. With normal kidney function, forced diuresis with osmotic diuretics, IV fluids, and electrolytes may accelerate the elimination of benzodiazepines. Dialysis is of limited value; however, in more critical situations, renal dialysis and exchange blood transfusions may be indicated. Refer to General Management of Acute Overdosage.

Infusion of physostigmine 0.5 to 4 mg IV at the rate of 1 mg/min may reverse symptoms suggestive of central anticholinergic overdose (eg, confusion, delirium, hallucinations, memory disturbance, visual disturbances); however, weigh the hazards associated with the use of physostigmine (eg, induction of seizures) against its possible clinical benefit.

There have been occasional reports of excitation in patients following overdosage with **chlordiazepoxide**; if this occurs, do not give barbiturates.

Patient Information

Inform patients that these drugs may cause drowsiness and to avoid driving or other tasks requiring alertness.

Advise patients to avoid alcohol or other CNS depressants.

Inform patients that medication may be taken with food or water if stomach upset occurs.

Patients on long-term or high-dosage therapy may experience withdrawal symptoms on abrupt cessation of therapy; advise patients not to discontinue therapy abruptly or change dosage except on advice of the health care provider.

Inform patients that concomitant ingestion with antacids may alter the rate of absorption of these drugs (documented with **diazepam** and **chlordiazepoxide**).

➤*Clonazepam, clorazepate, and diazepam:* Patient should carry identification (*Medic Alert*) indicating medication usage and epilepsy.

ALPRAZOLAM

c-iv	**Alprazolam** (Various, eg, Geneva, Mylan, Purepac)	**Tablets:** 0.25 mg	In 100s, 500s, 1000s, and UD 100s.
c-iv	**Xanax** (Pfizer)		Lactose. (Xanax 0.25). White, oval, scored. In 100s, 500s, 1000s, and UD 100s.
c-iv	**Alprazolam** (Various, eg, Geneva, Mylan, Purepac)	**Tablets:** 0.5 mg	In 100s, 500s, 1000s, and UD 100s.
c-iv	**Xanax** (Pfizer)		Lactose. (Xanax 0.5). Peach, oval, scored. In 100s, 500s, 1000s, and UD 100s.
c-iv	**Alprazolam** (Various, eg, Geneva, Mylan, Purepac)	**Tablets:** 1 mg	In 100s, 500s, 1000s, and UD 100s.
c-iv	**Xanax** (Pfizer)		Lactose, FD & C Blue No. 2. (Xanax 1.0). Blue, oval, scored. In 100s, 500s, and 1000s.
c-iv	**Alprazolam** (Various, eg, Mylan, Purepac)	**Tablets:** 2 mg	In 100s and 500s.
c-iv	**Xanax** (Pfizer)		Lactose. (XANAX 2). White, oblong, multi-scored. In 100s and 500s.
c-iv	**Alprazolam Extended-Release** (Various, eg, Greenstone, Mylan)	**Tablets, extended-release:** 0.5 mg	May contain lactose. In 60s and 500s.
c-iv	**Xanax XR** (Pfizer)		Lactose. (X 0.5). White, pentagonal. In 60s.
c-iv	**Alprazolam Extended-Release** (Various, eg, Greenstone, Mylan)	**Tablets, extended-release:** 1 mg	May contain lactose. In 60s and 500s.
c-iv	**Xanax XR** (Pfizer)		Lactose. (X 1). Yellow, square. In 60s.
c-iv	**Alprazolam Extended-Release** (Various, eg, Greenstone, Mylan)	**Tablets, extended-release:** 2 mg	May contain lactose. In 60s and 500s.
c-iv	**Xanax XR** (Pfizer)		Lactose, FD & C Blue No. 2. (X 2). Blue. In 60s.
c-iv	**Alprazolam Extended-Release** (Various, eg, Greenstone, Mylan)	**Tablets, extended-release:** 3 mg	May contain lactose. In 60s and 500s.
c-iv	**Xanax XR** (Pfizer)		Lactose, FD & C Blue No. 2. (X 3). Green, triangular. In 60s.
c-iv	**Niravam** (Schwarz Pharma)	**Tablets, orally disintegrating:** 0.25 mg	Sucralose, sucrose. (SP 321 0.25). Yellow, scored. Orange flavor. In 100s.
		0.5 mg	Sucralose, sucrose. (SP 322 0.5). Yellow, scored. Orange flavor. In 100s.
		1 mg	Sucralose, sucrose. (SP 323 1). White, scored. Orange flavor. In 100s.
		2 mg	Sucralose, sucrose. (SP 324 2). White, scored. Orange flavor. In 100s.
c-iv	**Alprazolam Intensol** (Roxane)	**Oral solution:** 1 mg/mL	Flavorless. In 30 mL with calibrated dropper.

ALPRAZOLAM — ORAL

Complete and comparative prescribing information begins in the Benzodiazepines monograph.

Indications

➤*Panic disorder (Niravam, Xanax, Xanax XR)*: Treatment of panic disorder, with or without agoraphobia.

➤*Anxiety disorders (immediate-release tablets and intensol):* For the management of anxiety disorders or for the short-term relief of the symptoms of anxiety. Anxiety associated with depression is also responsive.

➤*Off-label uses:*

Premenstrual dysphoric disorders – [5] = Poor documentation. Data from a limited number of studies have not reported consistent benefits with the use of alprazolam in the treatment of premenstrual disorders. In addition, there is a risk of precipitating a withdrawal reaction with intermittent usage. In July 2000, fluoxetine was approved for the treatment of premenstrual dysphoric disorder. Based on these factors, it is recommended that alprazolam not be used to treat premenstrual disorders.

Administration and Dosage

➤*General dosing considerations:* Individualize dosage. Increase cautiously to avoid adverse effects.

Alprazolam given sublingually is absorbed as rapidly as after oral administration; completeness of absorption is comparable.

➤*Adults:*

Anxiety disorder –

Immediate-release tablets, oral disintegrating tablet, intensol oral solution:

- *Initial dosage* – 0.25 to 0.5 mg 3 times/day.
- *Dosage titration* – Titrate to a maximum total dose of 4 mg/day in divided doses at intervals of 3 to 4 days. If side effects occur with starting dose, decrease dose.

Panic disorder –

Immediate-release tablets and oral disintegrating tablet:

- *Initial dosage* – 0.5 mg 3 times/day
- *Dosage titration* – Depending on response, increase the dose at intervals of 3 to 4 days in increments of no more than 1 mg/day.
- *Maintenance dosage* – Successful treatment has required doses of more than 4 mg/day; in controlled studies, doses in the range of 1 to 10 mg/day were used. The mean dosage employed was approximately 5 to 6 mg/day.

Extended-release tablets:

- *Initial dosage* – 0.5 to 1 mg once daily.
- *Dosage titration* – Depending on response, increase the dose at intervals of 3 to 4 days in increments of no more than 1 mg/day.
- *Maintenance dosage* – The suggested total daily dose ranges between 3 and 6 mg/day. The suggested total daily dosages will meet the needs of most patients; however, there will be some who require doses greater than 6 mg/day. In controlled trials, a dose range of 1 to 10 mg/day was used. Occasionally as much as 10 mg/day was required to achieve successful response.

➤*Elderly:* Per the Beers list, alprazolam doses greater than 2 mg should not be used because of increased sensitivity to benzodiazepines in elderly patients. Smaller doses may be effective as well as safer. Total daily doses should rarely exceed the suggested maximums.

Immediate-release tablet, oral disintegrating tablet, intensol oral solution – 0.25 mg, given 2 or 3 times/day. Gradually increase if needed and tolerated.

Extended-release tablets – 0.5 mg once/day. Gradually increase if needed and tolerated.

➤*Hepatic function impairment:*

Advanced hepatic disease – See Elderly for dosing.

➤*Debilitated patients:* See Elderly for dosing.

➤*Conversion:* Patients currently treated with divided doses of immediate-release tablets (eg, 3 to 4 times/day) may be switched to extended-release tablets at the same total daily dose taken once daily. If the therapeutic response after switching is inadequate, dosage may be titrated.

➤*Discontinuation of therapy:* Because of the danger of withdrawal, avoid abrupt discontinuation. Gradually reduce dosage in all patients when discontinuing therapy or when decreasing the daily dosage. Although there are no systematically collected data to support a specific discontinuation schedule, it is suggested that the daily dosage be decreased by no more than 0.5 mg every 3 days.

Some patients may require an even slower dosage reduction. Some patients may prove resistant to all discontinuation regimens.

➤*Administration:*

Extended-release tablets – Administer once daily, preferably in the morning. Take the tablets intact; do not chew, crush, or break.

Intensol oral solution – Alprazolam intensol is a concentrated oral solution. It is recommended that the oral solution be mixed with liquids or semi-solid food, such as water, juices, soda or soda-like beverages, applesauce, and puddings. Use only the calibrated dropper provided with this product. Draw into the dropper the amount prescribed for a single dose. Then squeeze the dropper contents into a liquid or semi-solid food. Stir the liquid or food gently for a few seconds. The formulation blends quickly and completely. Consume the entire amount of the mixture of drug and liquid or drug and food immediately. Do not store for future use.

Orally disintegrating tablets – Just prior to administration, with dry hands, remove the tablet from the bottle. Immediately place the tablet on top of the tongue where it will disintegrate and be swallowed with saliva. Administration with liquid is not necessary. If only one-half of a scored tablet is used for dosing, discard the unused portion of the tablet immediately because it may not remain stable. Discard any cotton that was included in the bottle and reseal the bottle tightly to prevent introducing moisture that might cause the tablets to disintegrate.

➤*Storage/Stability:* Store at 15° to 30°C (59° to 86°F). Protect from moisture.

CLORAZEPATE DIPOTASSIUM

c-iv	**Clorazepate Dipotassium** (Various, eg, Able, Mylan, Taro, Watson)	**Tablets**: 3.75 mg	In 100s, 500s, 1000s, and UD 100s.
c-iv	**Tranxene T-tab** (Ovation)		FD & C Blue No. 2. (TL). Blue, scored. In 100s, 500s, and UD 100s.
c-iv	**Clorazepate Dipotassium** (Various, eg, Able, Mylan, Taro, Watson)	**Tablets**: 7.5 mg	In 20s, 100s, 500s, 1000s, and UD 100s and 500s.
c-iv	**Tranxene T-tab** (Ovation)		(TM). Peach, scored. In 100s, 500s, and UD 100s.
c-iv	**Clorazepate Dipotassium** (Various, eg, Able, Mylan, Taro, Watson)	**Tablets**: 15 mg	In 100s, 500s, 1000s, and UD 100s.
c-iv	**Tranxene T-tab** (Ovation)		(TN). Lavender, scored. In 100s, 500s, and UD 100s.

CLORAZEPATE DIPOTASSIUM — ORAL

Complete prescribing information begins in the Benzodiazepines monograph. Also see the Anticonvulsant monograph section.

Indications

➤*Anxiety:* For the management of anxiety disorders or for the short-term relief of the symptoms of anxiety. Anxiety or tension associated with the stress of everyday life usually does not require treatment with an anxiolytic.

➤*Seizures:* As adjunctive therapy in the management of partial seizures.

➤*Alcohol withdrawal:* For the symptomatic relief of acute alcohol withdrawal.

Administration and Dosage

➤*General dosing considerations:* Drowsiness may occur at the initiation of treatment and with dosage increment.

➤*Adults:*

Alcohol withdrawal –

Usual dosage:

- *First 24 hours (day 1)* – Clorazepate 30 mg initially, followed by 30 to 60 mg in divided doses.
- *Second 24 hours (day 2)* – 45 to 90 mg in divided doses.
- *Third 24 hours (day 3)* – 22.5 to 45 mg in divided doses.
- *Day 4* – 15 to 30 mg in divided doses.
- *Beyond day 4* – Gradually reduce the daily dose to 7.5 to 15 mg. Discontinue drug therapy as soon as the patient's condition is stable. Avoid excessive reductions in the total amount of drug administered on successive days.

Maximum dose: 90 mg/day.

Anxiety –

Usual dosage: 30 mg/day administered in divided doses. The dose should be adjusted gradually within the range of 15 to 60 mg/day in accordance with the patient's response.

Alternative dosage: When administered in a single daily dose at bedtime, the initial dosage is 15 mg. After the initial dose, the response of the patient may require subsequent dosage adjustment.

Partial seizures –

Maximum dose: 90 mg/day.

Initial dosage: 7.5 mg 3 times per day.

Dosage titration: Dosage should be increased by no more than 7.5 mg every week, up to 90 mg/day.

➤*Children:*

Partial seizures –

Older than 12 years of age: See Adults for dosing for children older than 12 years of age.

CLORAZEPATE DIPOTASSIUM — ORAL

9 to 12 years of age:
- *Maximum dose* – 60 mg/day.
- *Initial dosage* – 7.5 mg 2 times per day.
- *Dosage titration* – Dosage should be increased by no more than 7.5 mg every week, up to 60 mg/day.

➤*Elderly:* In elderly or debilitated patients, the initial dose should be small, and increments should be made gradually in accordance with the patient's response to preclude ataxia or excessive sedation.

Anxiety – Initiate treatment at 7.5 to 15 mg/day.

➤*Storage / Stability:* Store at 15° to 30°C (59° to 86°F). Protect from moisture and light. Dispense in a tight, light-resistant container using a child-resistant closure.

CHLORDIAZEPOXIDE HYDROCHLORIDE

c-iv	**Chlordiazepoxide HCl** (Various, eg, Barr, Geneva, Major, Watson)	**Capsules:** 5 mg	In 20s, 100s, 500s, 1000s, and UD 100s.
c-iv	**Chlordiazepoxide HCl** (Various, eg, Barr, Major, UDL, Watson)	**Capsules:** 10 mg	In 20s, 100s, 500s, 1000s, and UD 100s.
c-iv	**Chlordiazepoxide HCl** (Various, eg, Barr, Major, UDL, Watson)	**Capsules:** 25 mg	In 20s, 100s, 500s, 1000s, and UD 100s.

CHLORDIAZEPOXIDE HYDROCHLORIDE — ORAL

Complete and comparative prescribing information begins in the Benzodiazepines monograph.

Indications

➤*Anxiety disorders:* For the management of anxiety disorders or for short-term relief of anxiety symptoms.

➤*Acute alcohol withdrawal:* For the symptoms of acute alcohol withdrawal.

➤*Preoperative:* For preoperative apprehension and anxiety.

Administration and Dosage

➤*General dosing considerations:* Individualize dosage.

➤*Adults:*

Acute alcohol withdrawal – 50 to 100 mg; repeat as needed (up to 300 mg/day). Parenteral form usually used initially. Reduce to maintenance levels.

Anxiety –

Mild to moderate anxiety: 5 or 10 mg 3 to 4 times/day.

Severe anxiety: 20 or 25 mg 3 to 4 times/day.

Preoperative apprehension and anxiety: On days preceding surgery, 5 to 10 mg 3 or 4 times/day.

➤*Children:*

Anxiety –

6 Years of age and older:
- *Initial dosage* – 5 mg 2 to 4 times/day.
- *Dosage adjustment* – May be increased in some children to 10 mg 2 or 3 times/day.

➤*Elderly:* In elderly or debilitated patients, the usual dosage is 5 mg 2 to 4 times/day.

In elderly or debilitated patients, it is recommended that the dosage be limited to the smallest effective amount to preclude the development of ataxia or oversedation (10 mg/day or less initially, to be increased gradually as needed and tolerated).

➤*Storage / Stability:* Store at 15° to 30°C (59° to 86°F). Dispense in a tight, light-resistant container.

CLONAZEPAM

c-iv	**Clonazepam** (Various, eg, Mylan, PAR, Teva, TorPharm, UDL, Watson)	**Tablets:** 0.5 mg	May contain lactose. In 100s, 500s, 1000s, and UD 100s.
c-iv	**Klonopin** (Roche)		Lactose, FD&C Blue No. 1 and 2. (1/2 KLONOPIN ROCHE). Orange, scored. In 100s.
c-iv	**Clonazepam** (Various, eg, Mylan, PAR, Teva, TorPharm, UDL, Watson)	**Tablets:** 1 mg	May contain lactose. In 100s, 500s, 1000s, and UD 100s.
c-iv	**Klonopin** (Roche)		Lactose, FD&C Blue No. 1 and 2. (1 KLONOPIN ROCHE). Blue. In 100s.
c-iv	**Clonazepam** (Various, eg, Mylan, PAR, Teva, TorPharm, UDL)	**Tablets:** 2 mg	May contain lactose. In 100s, 500s, 1000s, and UD 100s.
c-iv	**Klonopin** (Roche)		Lactose, FD&C Blue No. 1 and 2. (2 KLONOPIN ROCHE). White. In 100s.
c-iv	**Clonazepam** (Barr)	**Tablets, orally disintegrating:** 0.125 mg	Aspartame, xylitol, mannitol, 2.4 mg phenylalanine. (b 94 1/8). Strawberry flavor. White to off-white. In blister packages of 60.
c-iv	**Clonazepam** (Barr)	**Tablets, orally disintegrating:** 0.25 mg	Aspartame, xylitol, mannitol, 2.4 mg phenylalanine. (b 95 1/4). Strawberry flavor. White to off-white. In blister packages of 60.
c-iv	**Clonazepam** (Barr)	**Tablets, orally disintegrating:** 0.5 mg	Aspartame, xylitol, mannitol, 2.4 mg phenylalanine. (b 96 1/2). Strawberry flavor. White to off-white. In blister packages of 60.
c-iv	**Clonazepam** (Barr)	**Tablets, orally disintegrating:** 1 mg	Aspartame, xylitol, mannitol, 2.4 mg phenylalanine. (b 97 1). Strawberry flavor. White to off-white. In blister packages of 60.
c-iv	**Clonazepam** (Barr)	**Tablets, orally disintegrating:** 2 mg	Aspartame, xylitol, mannitol, 2.4 mg phenylalanine. (b 98 2). Strawberry flavor. White to off-white. In blister packages of 60.

CLONAZEPAM — ORAL

For additional information, refer to the Benzodiazepines group monograph in the Antianxiety Agents section and to the Anticonvulsants introduction.

Indications

➤*Seizure disorders:* Alone or as an adjunct in the treatment of the Lennox-Gastaut syndrome (petit mal variant), akinetic and myoclonic seizures. In patients with absence seizures (petit mal) who have failed to respond to succinimides, clonazepam may be useful.

➤*Panic disorder:* For the treatment of panic disorder, with or without agoraphobia, as defined in DSM-IV.

➤*Off-label uses:*

Bipolar disorder – Depressive episodes (adults) – [5] = Poor documentation. Although clonazepam has demonstrated therapeutic efficacy in the management of unipolar depression, its benefit in bipolar depression appears to be limited based on data from small, noncontrolled trials. Clonazepam is not included in current guidelines and does not appear to have an established role in the management of depressive episodes of bipolar disorder.

Bipolar disorder – Manic or mixed episodes (adults) – [2] = Fair documentation. Results from clinical studies indicate that clonazepam may be effective in the treatment of the manic state of bipolar disorder as monotherapy or as adjunctive therapy. However, most clinical studies had very small sample sizes, and study doses differed from trial to trial, ranging from 2 to 16 mg/day. Few head to head trials have been conducted to evaluate the efficacy and safety of clonazepam monotherapy for the treatment of manic or mixed episodes of bipolar disorder. American Psychiatric Association guidelines for the treatment of patients with bipolar disorder suggest that the use of benzodiazepines, such as clonazepam, in sedative doses may be useful as adjunctive therapy.

Bipolar disorder– Rapid cycling (adults) – [5] = Poor documentation. Although clonazepam has demonstrated therapeutic efficacy in the management of acute mania associated with bipolar disorder, it is not included in the current guidelines and does not have an established role in the management of rapid cycling bipolar disorder. Dosage was not provided.

Prevention of migraine (adults) – [5] = Poor documentation. Data supporting efficacy of clonazepam for the prevention of migraine headaches in adults are limited and not favorable. A Cochrane review and American Academy of Neurology practice guidelines state that clonazepam is no more effective than placebo for the prevention of migraines.

CLONAZEPAM — ORAL

Rectal administration – [2] = Fair documentation. Clonazepam appears to be absorbed after rectal administration based upon 2 very small bioavailability studies in children and adults. After rectal administration time to peak concentrations in these studies ranged from 10 minutes to 2 hours. It is unclear what plasma concentrations are needed to reverse seizures after rectal administration. In addition, the degree of absorption was highly variable from patient to patient.

Restless legs syndrome – [4] = Insufficient documentation. Initial data suggest that clonazepam may be beneficial in patients with restless legs syndrome (RLS) and insomnia. Results are conflicting as to whether clonazepam reduces the frequency of periodic limb movement associated with RLS. Clonazepam may be beneficial in the treatment of patients with RLS who have difficulty sleeping or who only have a partial response to dopamine agonists. In guidelines, clonazepam is rated as probably effective when given in combination with other medications for the treatment of RLS.

Tic disorders – [2] = Fair documentation. Results from clinical studies suggest that clonazepam may be effective for some patients with multifocal tic disorder or Tourette syndrome. These studies were relatively small and not designed to demonstrate superiority. Therefore, further studies are needed to confirm the efficacy and safety of clonazepam for treatment of tic disorders.

Other possible off-label uses – Parkinsonian (hypokinetic) dysarthria. Adjunct in the treatment of schizophrenia. Neuralgias (deafferentation pain syndromes).

Administration and Dosage

➤*General dosing considerations:* The use of multiple anticonvulsants may result in an increase of depressant adverse reactions. Take this into account before adding clonazepam to an existing anticonvulsant regimen.

➤*Adults:*

Seizure disorders –

Maximum dose: 20 mg per day.

Initial dosage: Not to exceed 1.5 mg per day divided into 3 doses.

Dosage titration: Increase in increments of 0.5 to 1 mg every 3 days until seizures are adequately controlled or until adverse reactions preclude any further increase.

Panic disorder –

Usual dosage: 1 mg/day.

Maximum dose: 4 mg/day.

Initial dosage: 0.25 mg twice daily.

Dosage titration: An increase to the maintenance dose may be made after 3 days. It is possible that some individual patients may benefit from doses of up to a maximum dose of 4 mg/day, and in those instances, the dose may be increased in increments of 0.125 to 0.25 mg twice daily every 3 days until panic disorder is controlled or until adverse reactions make further increases undesired.

Maintenance dosage: 1 mg/day.

Duration of therapy: There is no body of evidence available to answer the question of how long patients treated with clonazepam should remain on it. Therefore, the health care provider who elects to use clonazepam for extended periods should periodically reevaluate the long-term usefulness of the drug for the individual patient.

Discontinuation of therapy: Discontinue treatment gradually, with a decrease of 0.125 mg twice daily every 3 days until the drug is completely withdrawn.

Off-label dosing –

Bipolar disorder – Manic or mixed episodes: [2] = Fair documentation. Monotherapy or adjunctive therapy in dosages ranging from 2 to 16 mg/day for up to 4 years.

Rectal administration: [2] = Fair documentation. Single doses administered rectally were 0.02 mg/kg.

Restless legs syndrome: [4] = Insufficient documentation. 0.5 to 2 mg 30 minutes before bedtime.

Tic disorders: [2] = Fair documentation. Doses of 0.5 to 12 mg after dose titration have been used for up to 48 weeks.

➤*Children:*

Seizure disorders –

Older than 10 years of age or more than 30 kg of body weight: See Adults for dosing.

- *Maximum dose* – 20 mg per day.
- *Initial dosage* – Not to exceed 1.5 mg per day divided into 3 doses.
- *Dosage titration* – Increase in increments of 0.5 to 1 mg every 3 days until seizures are adequately controlled or until adverse reactions preclude any further increase.
- *Maintenance dosage* – Must be individualized for each patient depending upon response.

10 years of age or younger or 30 kg of body weight or less:

- *Initial dosage* – 0.01 to 0.03 mg/kg/day given in 2 or 3 divided doses; not to exceed 0.05 mg/kg/day.
- *Dosage titration* – Increase the dosage by no more than 0.25 to 0.5 mg every third day until a daily maintenance dose of 0.1 to 0.2 mg/kg of body weight has been reached, unless seizures are controlled or adverse reactions preclude further increase. Whenever possible, the daily dose should be divided into 3 equal doses. If doses are not equally divided, give the largest dose before bedtime.
- *Maintenance dosage* – 0.1 to 0.2 mg/kg of body weight.

Off-label dosing –

Tic disorders: [2] = Fair documentation. Doses of 0.5 to 12 mg after dose titration have been used for up to 48 weeks.

Rectal administration: [2] = Fair documentation. Single doses administered rectally were 0.05 and 0.1 mg/kg.

➤*Therapeutic drug monitoring:* Therapeutic serum concentrations of clonazepam in children are 20 to 80 ng/mL.

➤*Administration:* To reduce the inconvenience of somnolence, administration of 1 dose at bedtime may be desirable.

Administer the tablets with water by swallowing the tablet whole.

Administer the orally disintegrating tablet as follows: After opening the pouch, peel back the foil on the blister. Do not push the tablet through the foil. Immediately upon opening the blister, using dry hands, remove the tablet and place it in the mouth. Tablet disintegration occurs rapidly in saliva so it can be easily swallowed with or without water.

➤*Storage/Stability:* Store at 25°C (77°F); excursions permitted to 15° to 30°C (59° to 86°F). Protect from moisture.

DIAZEPAM

c-iv	**Diazepam** (Various, eg, Barr, Danbury, Ivax, Mylan, Purepac, Zenith)	**Tablets; oral:** 2 mg	May contain lactose. In 100s, 500s, 1,000s, and 5,000s.
c-iv	**Valium** (Roche)		Lactose. (Roche 2 Valium). White, scored. In 100s and 500s.
c-iv	**Diazepam** (Various, eg, Barr, Danbury, Ivax, Mylan, Purepac, Zenith)	**Tablets; oral:** 5 mg	May contain lactose. In 100s, 500s, 1,000s, and 5,000s.
c-iv	**Valium** (Roche)		Lactose. (Roche 5 Valium). Yellow, scored. In 100s and 500s.
c-iv	**Diazepam** (Various, eg, Barr, Danbury, Ivax, Mylan, Purepac, Zenith)	**Tablets; oral:** 10 mg	May contain lactose, FD&C Blue No 1. In 100s, 500s, 1,000s, and 5,000s.
c-iv	**Valium** (Roche)		Lactose, FD&C Blue No 1. (Roche 10 Valium). Blue, scored. In 100s and 500s.
c-iv	**Diazepam** (Roxane)	**Solution; oral:** 5 mg per 5 mL	Sorbitol. Wintergreen-spice flavor. In 500 mL and 5 and 10 mg patient cups.
c-iv	**Diazepam Intensol** (Roxane)	**Solution, concentrate; oral:** 5 mg per mL	Alcohol. In 30 mL with dropper.
c-iv	**Diazepam** (Various, eg, Hospira)	**Injection:** 5 mg/mL[a]	In 2 mL *Carpuject* cartridges.
c-iv	**Diazepam** (Teva)	**Gel; rectal:** 2.5 mg	Benzyl alcohol 1.5%, ethyl alcohol 10%, benzoic acid, propylene glycol. In prefilled unit-dose rectal delivery system 2s. Includes lubricating jelly and plastic applicator with flexible, molded tip 4.4 cm in length.
c-iv	**Diastat** (Xcel)		Benzyl alcohol 1.5%, ethyl alcohol 10%. In twin packs. Includes lubricating jelly and plastic applicator with flexible, molded tip 4.4 cm in length.

Benzodiazepines

DIAZEPAM

c-iv	**Diazepam** (Teva)	**Gel; rectal:** 10 mg[b]	Benzyl alcohol 1.5%, ethyl alcohol 10%, benzoic acid, propylene glycol. In prefilled unit-dose rectal delivery system 2s. Includes lubricating jelly and plastic applicator with flexible, molded tip 4.4 cm in length.
c-iv	**Diastat** (Xcel)		Benzyl alcohol 1.5%, ethyl alcohol 10%. In twin packs. Includes lubricating jelly and plastic applicator with flexible, molded tip 4.4 cm in length.
c-iv	**Diazepam** (Teva)	**Gel; rectal:** 20 mg[d]	Benzyl alcohol 1.5%, ethyl alcohol 10%, benzoic acid, propylene glycol. In prefilled unit-dose rectal delivery system 2s. Includes lubricating jelly and plastic applicator with flexible, molded tip 6 cm in length.
c-iv	**Diastat** (Xcel)	**Gel; rectal:** 20 mg[c]	Benzyl alcohol 1.5%, ethyl alcohol 10%. In twin packs. Includes lubricating jelly and plastic applicator with flexible, molded tip 6 cm in length.

[a] With 40% propylene glycol, 10% ethyl alcohol, 5% sodium benzoate, benzoic acid, and 1.5% benzyl alcohol.
[b] The available doses from the 10 mg delivery system are 5, 7.5, and 10 mg.
[c] The available doses from the 20 mg delivery system are 10, 12.5, 15, 17.5, and 20 mg.
[d] The available doses from the 20 mg delivery system are 12.5, 15, 17.5, and 20 mg.

DIAZEPAM — ORAL

For complete and comparative prescribing information, refer to the Benzodiazepines monograph in the Antianxiety Agents section. Also refer to the general discussion beginning in the Anticonvulsants introduction.

Indications

➤*Anxiety disorders:* For the management of anxiety disorders or for the short-term relief of the symptoms of anxiety.

➤*Acute alcohol withdrawal:* May be useful in symptomatic relief of acute agitation, tremor, impending or acute delirium, tremens, and hallucinosis.

➤*Muscle relaxant:* As an adjunct for the relief of skeletal muscle spasm because of reflex spasm caused by local pathology (eg, inflammation of muscles or joints, secondary to trauma); spasticity caused by upper motor neuron disorders (eg, cerebral palsy, paraplegia); athetosis; stiff-man syndrome. Used parenterally in the treatment of tetanus.

➤*Anticonvulsant:* Oral diazepam may be used adjunctively in convulsive disorders.

➤*Off-label uses:*

Smoking cessation – [5] = Poor documentation. Information on the use of diazepam for smoking cessation is limited; the one trial to date found no benefit when diazepam was used in the management of tobacco dependence. Guidelines from the Veterans Administration specifically recommend against the use of benzodiazepines for the management of tobacco abuse. Use is not recommended.

Tardive dyskinesia – [4] = Insufficient documentation. The limited studies regarding the use of diazepam for tardive dyskinesia demonstrate conflicting results. Based on the available studies, diazepam may be an effective treatment option for tardive dyskinesia, but more studies are needed before it can be routinely recommended.

Administration and Dosage

➤*Adults:*

Acute alcohol withdrawal – 10 mg 3 or 4 times during first 24 hours; reduce to 5 mg 3 or 4 times/day, as needed.

Anticonvulsant – 2 to 10 mg 2 to 4 times/day as an adjunct.

Anxiety disorders – 2 to 10 mg 2 to 4 times/day.

Muscle relaxant – 2 to 10 mg 3 or 4 times/day as an adjunct.

Off-label dosing –

Tardive dyskinesia: [4] = Insufficient documentation. 5 to 40 mg daily for up to 24 weeks.

➤*Children:*

6 months of age and older – 1 to 2.5 mg 3 or 4 times/day initially; increase gradually as needed and tolerated.

Off-label dosing –

Muscle relaxant: 0.12 to 0.8 mg/kg/24 hours divided 3 to 4 times/day.
Sedation: 0.12 to 0.8 mg/kg/24 hours divided 3 to 4 times/day.

➤*Elderly:* 2 to 2.5 mg 1 or 2 times/day initially; increase gradually as needed and tolerated.

➤*Debilitated patient:* 2 to 2.5 mg 1 or 2 times/day initially; increase gradually as needed and tolerated.

➤*Administration:*

Oral solution – Diazepam intensol is a concentrated oral solution as compared with standard oral liquid medications. It is recommended that the intensol is mixed with liquid or semi-solid food such as water, juices, soda or soda-like beverages, applesauce, and puddings.

Use only the calibrated dropper provided with the product. Draw into the dropper the amount prescribed for a single dose. Then squeeze the dropper contents into a liquid or semi-solid food. Stir the liquid or food gently for a few seconds. Consume the entire amount of the mixture immediately. Do not store for future use.

➤*Storage/Stability:* Store at 15° to 30°C (59° to 86°F). Protect from light and moisture.

DIAZEPAM — INJECTION

For complete and comparative prescribing information, refer to the Benzodiazepine monograph in the Antianxiety Agents section. Also refer to the general discussion beginning in the Anticonvulsants introduction.

Indications

➤*Anxiety disorders:* For the management of anxiety disorders or for the short-term relief of the symptoms of anxiety.

➤*Acute alcohol withdrawal:* May be useful in symptomatic relief of acute agitation, tremor, impending or acute delirium, tremens, and hallucinosis.

➤*Muscle relaxant:* As an adjunct for the relief of skeletal muscle spasm because of reflex spasm caused by local pathology (eg, inflammation of muscles or joints, secondary to trauma); spasticity caused by upper motor neuron disorders (eg, cerebral palsy, paraplegia); athetosis; stiff-man syndrome. Used parenterally in the treatment of tetanus.

➤*Anticonvulsant:* Parenteral diazepam is a useful adjunct in status epilepticus and severe recurrent convulsive seizures.

➤*Preoperative:* Used parenterally for the relief of anxiety and tension in patients undergoing surgical procedures; IV prior to cardioversion for the relief of anxiety and tension and to diminish patient's recall; as an adjunct prior to endoscopic procedures for apprehension, anxiety, or acute stress reactions and to diminish patient's recall.

➤*Off-label uses:*

Tardive dyskinesia – [4] = Insufficient documentation. The limited studies regarding the use of diazepam for tardive dyskinesia demonstrate conflicting results. Based on the available studies, diazepam may be an effective treatment option for tardive dyskinesia, but more studies are needed before it can be routinely recommended.

Administration and Dosage

➤*Maximum dose:*

Adults – 30 mg intravenous (IV) or intramuscular (IM) for the treatment of status epilepticus and severe recurrent convulsive seizures according to the prescribing information. There are no well-established maximum doses for the other approved indications according to the prescribing information.

Children – The following maximum doses are according to the prescribing information:

Sedation or muscle relaxation: 0.6 mg/kg within an 8-hour period.
Status epilepticus and severe recurrent convulsive seizures:
- *5 years of age or older* – 10 mg.
- *30 days to younger than 5 years of age* – 5 mg.

There is no well-established maximum dose for the other approved indication according to the prescribing information.

➤*Adults:*

Acute alcohol withdrawal – 10 mg IM or IV initially; then 5 to 10 mg in 3 to 4 hours, if necessary.

Moderate anxiety – 2 to 5 mg IM or IV. Repeat in 3 to 4 hours, if necessary.

Severe anxiety – 5 to 10 mg IM or IV. Repeat in 3 to 4 hours, if necessary.

Cardioversion – 5 to 15 mg IV, 5 to 10 minutes prior to procedure.

Endoscopic procedures –

IM: 5 to 10 mg 30 minutes prior to procedure if IV route cannot be used.
IV: Titrate dosage to desired sedative response, such as slurring of speech. Administer slowly just prior to procedure. Reduce narcotic dosage by at least

DIAZEPAM — INJECTION

one-third, and in some cases, they may be omitted; 10 mg or less is usually adequate; up to 20 mg may be used, especially when concomitant narcotics are omitted.

Muscle relaxant – 5 to 10 mg IM or IV initially; then 5 to 10 mg in 3 to 4 hours if necessary.

Preoperative – 10 mg IM before surgery. If atropine, scopolamine, or other premedications are desired, administer in separate syringes.

Status epilepticus and severe recurrent convulsive seizures – Exercise extreme caution in patients with chronic lung disease or unstable cardiovascular status. Although seizures may be controlled promptly, many patients experience a return to seizure activity, presumably because of the short-lived effect of IV diazepam. The IV route is preferred; administer slowly. Use the IM route if IV administration is impossible.

Maximum dose: 30 mg.

Initial dosage: 5 to 10 mg IV or IM. Repeat if necessary at 10- to 15-minute intervals up to a maximum dose of 30 mg. If necessary, repeat therapy in 2 to 4 hours.

Maintenance dosage: Diazepam is not recommended for maintenance. Once seizures are controlled, consider other agents for long-term control.

Tetanus – 5 to 10 mg IM or IV initially; then 5 to 10 mg in 3 to 4 hours, if necessary. May require larger doses.

Off-label dosing –

Tardive dyskinesia: [4] = Insufficient documentation. 5 to 40 mg daily for up to 24 weeks.

➤*Children:*

Sedation or muscle relaxation –

Usual dosage: 0.04 to 0.2 mg/kg/dose every 2 to 4 hours.

Maximum dose: 0.6 mg/kg within an 8-hour period.

Status epilepticus and severe recurrent convulsive seizures –

5 years of age or older:

- *Usual dosage* – Inject 1 mg every 2 to 5 minutes up to a maximum of 10 mg. Repeat in 2 to 4 hours, if necessary. Electroencephalograph (EEG) monitoring of seizure may be helpful.
- *Maximum dose* – 10 mg.

30 days to younger than 5 years of age:

- *Usual dosage* – Inject 0.2 to 0.5 mg slowly every 2 to 5 minutes up to a maximum of 5 mg.
- *Maximum dose* – 5 mg.

Tetanus –

5 years of age or older: 5 to 10 mg repeated every 3 to 4 hours may be required.

30 days to younger than 5 years of age: 1 to 2 mg IM or IV slowly, repeated every 3 to 4 hours as necessary.

Off-label dosing –

Status epilepticus and severe recurrent convulsive seizures:

- *Children* – Diazepam injection has also been used rectally at a dosage of 0.5 mg/kg/dose followed by 0.25 mg/kg/dose in 10 minutes as needed.
- *Neonates* –
  Usual dosage: 0.3 to 0.75 mg/kg/dose IV every 15 to 30 minutes for 2 to 3 doses.
  Maximum dose: 2 mg.

➤*Elderly:* Use lower doses (2 to 5 mg) and more gradual increases in dosage.

➤*Debilitated patient:* Use lower doses (2 to 5 mg) and more gradual increases in dosage.

➤*Administration:* When used IV, to reduce the possibility of venous thrombosis, phlebitis, local irritation, swelling, and rarely, vascular impairment: Inject slowly, take at least 1 minute per 5 mg (1 mL); do not use small veins (ie, dorsum of hand or wrist); avoid intra-arterial administration or extravasation. Do not mix or dilute with other solutions or drugs in syringe or infusion flask. If not feasible to administer directly IV, inject slowly through infusion tubing as close as possible to the vein insertion. Once acute symptoms are controlled with injectable diazepam, place patient on oral therapy.

Children – To obtain maximum clinical effect with minimum amount of drug and to reduce the risk of hazardous adverse reactions such as apnea or prolonged periods of somnolence, administer slowly over 3 minutes. Do not exceed 0.25 mg/kg. After an interval of 15 to 30 minutes, the initial dose can be repeated. If relief of symptoms is not obtained after a third dose, appropriate adjunctive therapy is recommended. When IV use is indicated, facilities for respiratory assistance should be readily available.

➤*Admixture compatibility:* Because of the possibility of precipitation of diazepam in IV fluids and the instability of the drug in plastic (PVC [polyvinyl chloride]) bags and infusion tubing, IV infusion of diazepam is not recommended. Glass, polypropylene, polyethylene, or polyolefin solution bottles and infusion tubing have been used with negligible loss of diazepam.

➤*Storage/Stability:* Store at 15° to 30°C (59° to 86°F). Protect from light and moisture.

DIAZEPAM — RECTAL

For complete and comparative prescribing information, refer to the Benzodiazepines monograph in the Antianxiety Agents section. Also refer to the general discussion beginning in the Anticonvulsants introduction.

Indications

➤*Anticonvulsant:* For the management of selected refractory patients with epilepsy who are on stable regimens of antiepileptic drugs (AEDs) and require intermittent use of diazepam to control bouts of increased seizure activity.

Administration and Dosage

➤*General dosing considerations:* A decision to prescribe diazepam rectal gel involves more than the diagnosis and the selection of the correct dose for the patient.

First, the prescriber must be convinced from historical reports and/or personal observations that the patient exhibits the characteristic identifiable seizure cluster that can be distinguished from the patient's usual seizure activity by the caregiver who will be responsible for administering diazepam rectal gel.

Second, because diazepam rectal gel is only intended for adjunctive use, the prescriber must ensure that the patient is receiving an optimal regimen of standard AED treatment and is, nevertheless, continuing to experience these characteristic episodes.

Third, because a nonhealth care provider will be obliged to identify episodes suitable for treatment, make the decision to administer treatment upon that identification, administer the drug, monitor the patient, and assess the adequacy of the response to treatment; a major component of the prescribing process involves the necessary instruction of this individual.

Fourth, the prescriber and caregiver must have a common understanding of what is and is not an episode of seizures that is appropriate treatment, the timing of administration in relation to the onset of the episode, the mechanics of administering the drug, how and what to observe following administration, and what would constitute an outcome requiring immediate and direct medical attention.

➤*Adults:*

Anticonvulsant – Because diazepam rectal gel is provided as unit doses of 2.5, 5, 7.5, 10, 12.5, 15, 17.5, and 20 mg, the prescribed dose is obtained by rounding upward to the next available dose. The table provides acceptable weight ranges for each dose and age category, such that patients will receive between 90% and 180% of the calculated recommended dose. The safety of this strategy has been established in clinical trials.

Diazepam Rectal Dosing Based on Age and Weight	
12 years of age and older 0.2 mg/kg	
Weight (kg)	Dose
14 to 25	5 mg
26 to 37	7.5 mg
38 to 50	10 mg
51 to 62	12.5 mg
63 to 75	15 mg
76 to 87	17.5 mg
88 to 111	20 mg

Usual dosage: 0.2 mg/kg.

Dosage adjustment: Health care providers should adjust the dose periodically to reflect changes in the patient's age and weight.

Additional dose: The prescriber may wish to prescribe a second dose of diazepam rectal gel. A second dose, when required, may be given 4 to 12 hours after the first dose.

The diazepam rectal gel 2.5 mg dose may also be used as a partial replacement dose for patients who may expel a portion of the first dose.

Treatment frequency: It is recommended that diazepam rectal gel be used to treat no more than 5 episodes per month and no more than 1 episode every 5 days.

➤*Children:*

Anticonvulsant – Because diazepam rectal gel is provided as unit doses of 2.5, 5, 7.5, 10, 12.5, 15, 17.5, and 20 mg, the prescribed dose is obtained by rounding upward to the next available dose. The table provides acceptable weight ranges for each dose and age category, such that patients will receive between 90% and 180% of the calculated recommended dose. The safety of this strategy has been established in clinical trials.

Diazepam Rectal Dosing Based on Age and Weight			
2 to 5 years of age 0.5 mg/kg		6 to 11 years of age 0.3 mg/kg	
Weight (kg)	Dose	Weight (kg)	Dose
6 to 10	5 mg	10 to 16	5 mg
11 to 15	7.5 mg	17 to 25	7.5 mg
16 to 20	10 mg	26 to 33	10 mg
21 to 25	12.5 mg	34 to 41	12.5 mg
26 to 30	15 mg	42 to 50	15 mg

DIAZEPAM — RECTAL

Diazepam Rectal Dosing Based on Age and Weight			
2 to 5 years of age 0.5 mg/kg		6 to 11 years of age 0.3 mg/kg	
Weight (kg)	Dose	Weight (kg)	Dose
31 to 35	17.5 mg	51 to 58	17.5 mg
36 to 44	20 mg	59 to 74	20 mg

12 years of age and older: See adults for dosing for children 12 years of age and older.

6 to 11 years of age: 0.3 mg/kg.

2 to 5 years of age: 0.5 mg/kg.

Dosage adjustment: Health care providers should adjust the dose periodically to reflect changes in the patient's age and weight.

Additional dose: The prescriber may wish to prescribe a second dose of diazepam rectal gel. A second dose, when required, may be given 4 to 12 hours after the first dose.

The diazepam rectal gel 2.5 mg dose may also be used as a partial replacement dose for patients who may expel a portion of the first dose.

Treatment frequency: It is recommended that diazepam rectal gel be used to treat no more than 5 episodes per month and no more than 1 episode every 5 days.

Off-label dosing –

Status epilepticus:

• *Children –* Diazepam injection has also been used rectally as a dosage of 0.5 mg/kg/dose followed by 0.25 mg/kg/dose in 10 minutes as needed.

➤*Elderly:* Adjust dosage downward to reduce ataxia or over sedation.

➤*Debilitated patients:* Adjust dosage downward to reduce ataxia or oversedation.

➤*Administration:* The rectal delivery system includes a plastic applicator with a flexible, molded tip available in 2 lengths. The *Diastat AcuDial* 10 mg syringe is available with a 4.4 cm tip and the *Diastat AcuDial* 20 mg syringe is available with a 6 cm tip. *Diastat* 2.5 mg is also available with a 4.4 cm tip.

➤*Storage/Stability:* Store at 25°C (77°F); excursions are permitted to 15° to 30°C (59° to 86°F).

LORAZEPAM

c-iv	**Lorazepam** (Various, eg, Geneva, Major, Mylan, Squibb Mark, UDL)	**Tablets; oral:** 0.5 mg	In 100s, 500s, and 1000s.
		1 mg	In 100s, 500s, and 1000s.
		2 mg	In 100s, 500s, and 1000s.
c-iv	**Lorazepam** (Pharmaceutical Associates)	**Solution, concentrate; oral:** 2 mg/mL	PEG, propylene glycol. In 30 mL with dropper.
c-iv	**Lorazepam Intensol** (Roxane)		Alcohol and dye free. In 10 and 30 mL with dropper.
c-iv	**Lorazepam** (Hospira)	**Injection, solution:** 2 mg/mL	In 1 mL prefilled syringes, and 1 mL single and 10 mL multidose vials.[a]
c-iv	**Ativan** (Baxter)		In single and 10 mL multidose vials[a], in boxes of 10 *TUBEX*.
c-iv	**Lorazepam** (Hospira)	**Injection, solution:** 4 mg/mL	In 1 mL prefilled syringes, and 1 mL single and 10 mL multidose vials.[a]
c-iv	**Ativan** (Baxter)		In single and 10 mL multidose vials[a], in boxes of 10 *TUBEX*.

[a] With PEG 400, propylene glycol, and 2% benzyl alcohol.

LORAZEPAM — ORAL

Complete and comparative prescribing information begins in the Benzodiazepines group monograph. Also see the Anticonvulsant monograph.

Indications

➤*Anxiety:* For the management of anxiety disorders or for the short-term relief of the symptoms of anxiety or of anxiety associated with depressive symptoms.

The efficacy of lorazepam in long-term use (ie, greater than 4 months), has not been assessed by systematic clinical studies. Periodically reassess the usefulness of the drug for the individual patient.

➤*Off-label uses:*

Postherpetic neuralgia – [5] = Poor documentation. Use is not recommended. Use of lorazepam for the treatment of postherpetic neuralgia (PHN) has only been studied in 1 controlled trial that failed to show any benefit. American Academy of Neurology clinical practice guidelines state that the efficacy of lorazepam is not any better than that of placebo in patients with PHN.

Other possible off-label uses – Short-term improvement of chronic insomnia.

Administration and Dosage

➤*General dosing considerations:* For optimal results, individualize the dose, frequency of administration, and duration of therapy according to patient response.

➤*Adults:*

Anxiety –

Usual dosage: 2 to 6 mg daily given in divided doses, with the largest dose taken before bedtime. The daily dosage may vary from 1 to 10 mg/day.

Initial dosage: 2 to 3 mg daily, tablets or solution, given in divided doses 2 or 3 times daily.

Insomnia caused by anxiety or transient situational stress –

Usual dosage: Single 2 to 4 mg dose at bedtime.

➤*Children:*

Off-label dosing –

Anxiolytic/Sedation/Agitation:

• *Usual dose –* 0.05 mg/kg/dose every 4 to 8 hours.
• *Maximum dose –* 2 mg/dose.

➤*Elderly:* The recommended initial dosage is 1 to 2 mg daily in divided doses. Gradually increase the dosage as needed and tolerated to help avoid adverse reactions. When higher dosage is indicated, increase the evening dose before the daytime doses.

For elderly patients, the initial daily dose should not exceed 2 mg in order to avoid oversedation.

Per the Beers list, lorazepam doses greater than 3 mg should not be used because of increased sensitivity to benzodiazepines in elderly patients. Smaller doses may be effective as well as safer. Total daily doses should rarely exceed the suggested maximums.

➤*Debilitated patient:* The recommended initial dosage is 1 to 2 mg/day in divided doses. Gradually increase the dosage as needed and tolerated to help avoid adverse reactions. When higher dosage is indicated, increase the evening dose before the daytime doses.

For debilitated patients, the initial daily dose should not exceed 2 mg in order to avoid oversedation.

➤*Administration:*

Oral solution – It is recommended that an intensol, a concentrated oral solution, be mixed with liquid or semisolid food such as water, juice, soda or soda-like beverages, applesauce, and puddings.

Use only the calibrated dropper provided with this product. Draw the amount prescribed for a single dose into the dropper, and then squeeze the dropper contents into a liquid or semisolid food. Gently stir the liquid or food for a few seconds. The intensol formulation blends quickly and completely. Immediately consume the entire amount of the mixture (drug and liquid or drug and food). Do not store for future use.

➤*Storage/Stability:*

Oral solution – Refrigerate the solution. Store at 2° to 8°C (36° to 46°F). Protect from light.

Tablets – Store at 15° to 30°C (59° to 86°F). Protect from light. Dispense in a tight, light-resistant container using a child-resistant closure. Keep tightly closed.

LORAZEPAM — INJECTION

Complete and comparative prescribing information begins in the Benzodiazepines group monograph. Also see the Anticonvulsant monograph.

Indications

➤*Status epilepticus:* For the treatment of status epilepticus.

➤*Preanesthetic:* In adults for preanesthetic medication, producing sedation (sleepiness or drowsiness), relief of anxiety, and a decreased ability to recall events related to the day of surgery.

➤*Off-label uses:*

Rectal administration – [5] = Poor documentation. Because of the limited data available, potential kinetic issues, and the commercial availability of a rectal formulation of diazepam, this route of administration is not currently recommended.

Postherpetic neuralgia – [5] = Poor documentation. Use is not recommended. Use of lorazepam for the treatment of postherpetic neuralgia (PHN) has only been studied in 1 controlled trial that failed to show any

LORAZEPAM — INJECTION

benefit. American Academy of Neurology clinical practice guidelines state that the efficacy of lorazepam is not any better than that of placebo in patients with PHN.

Administration and Dosage

➤*Maximum dose:*

Adults – 4 mg for preanesthesia according to the prescribing information. There is no well-established maximum dose for the other approved indication according to the prescribing information.

Children – Not approved for use in children according to the prescribing information. However, maximum doses have been established off-label.

➤*General dosing considerations:* Lorazepam must never be used without individualization of dosage, particularly when used with other medications capable of producing CNS depression.

Equipment necessary to maintain a patent airway should be immediately available prior to intravenous (IV) administration of lorazepam.

➤*Adults:*

Preanesthetic – Doses of other injectable CNS-depressant drugs should ordinarily be reduced.

IM injection:

• *Usual dosage* – 0.05 mg/kg intramuscularly (IM) at least 2 hours before the anticipated operative procedure.

• *Maximum dose* – 4 mg IM.

IV injection:

• *Initial dosage* – 2 mg total or 0.044 mg/kg, whichever is smaller, 15 to 20 minutes before the anticipated operative procedure.

This dose will suffice for sedating most adults and should not ordinarily be exceeded in patients older than 50 years of age.

• *Alternative dosage* – Patients in whom a greater likelihood of lack of recall for perioperative events would be beneficial, larger doses as high as 0.05 mg/kg up to a total of 4 mg may be administered.

Status epilepticus –

General advice: Status epilepticus is a potentially life-threatening condition associated with a high risk of permanent neurological impairment, if inadequately treated. However, the treatment of status epilepticus requires far more than the administration of an anticonvulsant agent. It involves observation and management of all parameters critical to maintaining vital function and the capacity to provide support of those functions as required. Ventilatory support must be readily available. The use of benzodiazepines like lorazepam injection is ordinarily only an initial step of a complex and sustained intervention, which may require additional interventions (eg, concomitant IV administration of phenytoin). Because status epilepticus may result from a correctable acute cause such as hypoglycemia, hyponatremia, or other metabolic or toxic derangement, such an abnormality must be immediately identified and corrected. Furthermore, patients susceptible to further seizure episodes should receive adequate maintenance antiepileptic therapy.

Any health care professional who intends to treat a patient with status epilepticus should be familiar with this monograph and the pertinent medical literature concerning current concepts for the treatment of status epilepticus. A comprehensive review of the considerations that are critical to the informed and prudent management of status epilepticus cannot be provided in drug product labeling. The archival medical literature contains many informative references on the management of status epilepticus, including the report of the working group on status epilepticus of the Epilepsy Foundation of America (*JAMA*. 1993; 270[7]:854-859). As noted in the report just cited, it may be useful to consult with a neurologist if a patient fails to respond to therapy (eg, fails to regain consciousness).

IM injection: Lorazepam IM is not the preferred route of administration because therapeutic levels may not be reached as quickly as with IV administration. However, when an IV port is not available, the IM route may prove useful.

IV injection: Employ the usual precautions in treating status epilepticus. Start an IV infusion, monitor vital signs, maintain an unobstructed airway, and have artificial ventilation equipment available.

• *Usual dosage* – 4 mg given slowly (2 mg/min). May repeat in 10 to 15 minutes if seizures continue or recur.

• *Duration of therapy* – Experience with further doses of lorazepam is very limited.

➤*Children:*

Off-label dosing – Lorazepam injection may contain benzyl alcohol and propylene glycol, which may be toxic to newborns at high doses.

Antiemetic adjunct therapy:

• *Usual dose* – 0.02 to 0.08 mg/kg IV every 6 hours as needed.

• *Maximum dose* – 2 mg/dose.

Anxiolytic / Sedation / Agitation:

• *Usual dose* – 0.05 mg/kg IV every 4 to 8 hours. For procedural sedation, administer the IV dose 15 to 20 minutes prior to surgery, or alternatively administer the dose IM 2 hours prior to surgery.

• *Maximum dose* – 2 mg/dose.

Status epilepticus:

• *Neonates and children younger than 18 years of age* –

Usual dosage: 0.05 to 0.1 mg/kg given IV over 2 to 5 minutes. If needed, a dosage of 0.05 mg/kg may be repeated in 10 to 15 minutes.

Maximum dose: 4 mg/dose.

➤*Renal function impairment:* For acute dose administration, adjustment is not needed for patients with renal disease. However, in patients with renal disease, exercise caution if frequent doses are given over relatively short periods of time.

➤*Concomitant therapy:* Reduce the dose of lorazepam by 50% when coadministered with probenecid or valproate. It may be necessary to increase the dose of lorazepam in women who are concomitantly taking oral contraceptives.

➤*Preparation for administration:* Immediately prior to IV use, lorazepam injection must be diluted with an equal volume of compatible solution. Mix contents thoroughly by gently inverting the container repeatedly until a homogeneous solution results. Do not shake vigorously because this will result in air entrapment.

➤*Administration:*

IM – Lorazepam injection, undiluted, should be injected deep in the muscle mass.

IV – When properly diluted, the drug may be injected directly into a vein or into the tubing of an existing IV infusion. The rate of injection should not exceed 2 mg/min.

➤*Admixture compatibility:* Compatible for dilution purposes with the following solutions: sterile water for injection, sodium chloride injection, and dextrose 5% injection.

Injectable lorazepam can be used with atropine sulfate, narcotic analgesics, other parenterally used analgesics, commonly used anesthetics, and muscle relaxants.

➤*Storage / Stability:* Store in a refrigerator. Protect from light. Use carton to protect contents from light.

OXAZEPAM

c-iv	**Oxazepam** (Various, eg, Balan, Mark, Moore, Ivax, Squibb)	**Capsules:** 10 mg	In 100s, 500s, and UD 100s.
c-iv	**Oxazepam** (Various, eg, Balan, Mark, Moore, Ivax, Squibb)	**Capsules:** 15 mg	In 100s, 500s, and UD 100s.
c-iv	**Oxazepam** (Various, eg, Balan, Mark, Moore, Ivax, Squibb)	**Capsules:** 30 mg	In 100s, 500s, and UD 100s.

OXAZEPAM — ORAL

For complete prescribing information, refer to the Benzodiazepines class monograph.

Indications

➤*Anxiety:* For the management of anxiety disorders or for the short-term relief of the symptoms of anxiety. Anxiety associated with depression is also responsive to oxazepam therapy. This product has been found particularly useful in the management of anxiety, tension, agitation, and irritability in older patients.

➤*Alcohol withdrawal:* Alcoholics with acute tremulousness, inebriation, or with anxiety associated with alcohol withdrawal are responsive to therapy.

➤*Off-label uses:* Management of irritable bowel syndrome.

Administration and Dosage

➤*General dosing considerations:* Because of the flexibility of this product and the range of emotional disturbances responsive to it, dosage should be individualized for maximum beneficial effects.

➤*Adults:*

Alcohol withdrawal – 15 to 30 mg 3 or 4 times daily.

Anxiety –

Mild to moderate anxiety: 10 to 15 mg 3 or 4 times daily.

Severe anxiety syndromes, agitation, or anxiety associated with depression: 15 to 30 mg 3 or 4 times daily.

➤*Children:* See Adults for dosing for children older than 12 years of age.

➤*Elderly:* Per the Beers list, oxazepam doses greater than 60 mg should not be used because of increased sensitivity to benzodiazepines in elderly patients. Smaller doses may be effective as well as safer. Total daily doses should rarely exceed the suggested maximums.

Anxiety, tension, irritability, and agitation –

Initial dosage: 10 mg 3 times daily.

Dosage adjustment: If necessary, increase cautiously to 15 mg 3 or 4 times daily.

➤*Duration of therapy:* The effectiveness of oxazepam in long-term use, that is, more than 4 months, has not been assessed by systematic clinical studies. The physician should reassess periodically the usefulness of the drug for the individual patient.

➤*Storage / Stability:* Store at 25°C (77°F). Keep tightly closed and dispense in a tight container.

Miscellaneous Agents

BUSPIRONE HYDROCHLORIDE

Rx	**Buspirone HCl** (Various, eg, Amide, Ethex, PAR, Teva, UDL)	**Tablets:** 5 mg (4.6 mg as base)	May contain lactose. In 100s and 500s.
Rx	**Buspirone HCl** (Par)	**Tablets:** 7.5 mg (6.85 as base)	May contain lactose. In 100s and 500s.
Rx	**Buspirone HCl** (Various, eg, Amide, Ethex, PAR, Teva, UDL)	**Tablets:** 10 mg (9.1 mg as base)	May contain lactose. In 100s and 500s.
Rx	**Buspirone HCl** (Various, eg, Amide, Ethex, PAR, Teva, UDL)	**Tablets:** 15 mg (13.7 mg as base)	May contain lactose. In 100s and 500s.
Rx	**Buspirone HCl** (Mylan)	**Tablets:** 30 mg (27.4 mg as base)	Scored. In 60s, 100s, and 180s.

BUSPIRONE HYDROCHLORIDE — ORAL

Indications

➤*Anxiety:* For the management of anxiety disorders or the short-term relief of the symptoms of anxiety.

➤*Off-label uses:*

Smoking cessation – [5] = Poor documentation. One quality study has shown a positive effect of buspirone as an aid in smoking cessation, but the results were not replicated in other trials. Rational use cannot be established because of the inconsistent outcomes and availability of better established, Food and Drug Administration (FDA)-approved pharmacotherapy options. Guidelines from the Veterans Administration specifically recommend against the use of anxiolytics such as buspirone. If contraindications are present to all standard therapies and patient-specific factors provide a rationale for trying an antianxiety agent during smoking cessation, buspirone might be an acceptable alternative agent because of its benign safety profile.

Traumatic brain injury – [2] = Fair documentation. The appropriate use of buspirone in patients with traumatic brain injury (TBI) has been outlined in guidelines from the Neurobehavioral Guidelines Working Group. Given that buspirone was assigned the lowest level of recommendation (classification as an option rather than a standard or guideline), patients started on therapy should be closely monitored for response, and therapy should be continued only in those patients with sufficient benefit to outweigh the risks of therapy.

Other possible off-label uses – Decreasing the symptoms (eg, aches, pains, fatigue, cramps, irritability) of premenstrual syndrome.

Administration and Dosage

➤*Adults:*

Anxiety –

Usual dosage: In clinical trials allowing dose titration, divided doses of 20 to 30 mg/day were commonly employed.

Maximum dose: 60 mg/day.

Initial dosage: 15 mg daily (7.5 mg 2 times per day).

Dosage titration: To achieve an optimal therapeutic response, the dosage may be increased 5 mg/day, as needed, at intervals of 2 to 3 days.

Concomitant therapy: When buspirone is to be given with a potent inhibitor of cytochrome P450 3A4, a low dose of buspirone (eg, 2.5 mg twice daily) is recommended.

Off-label dosing –

Traumatic brain injury: [2] = Fair documentation. 10 to 60 mg once daily. In 1 series, patients received buspirone for 3 or more months.

➤*Renal function impairment:* The administration of buspirone to patients with severe renal impairment cannot be recommended.

➤*Hepatic function impairment:* The administration of buspirone to patients with severe hepatic impairment cannot be recommended.

➤*Administration:* Regarding the timing of dosing, patients should take buspirone consistently, either always with or always without food.

➤*Storage/Stability:* Store at 15° to 30°C (59° to 86°F). Protect from temperatures greater than 30°C (86°F).

Actions

➤*Pharmacology:* The mechanism of action of buspirone is unknown. Buspirone differs from typical benzodiazepine anxiolytics in that it does not exert anticonvulsant or muscle relaxant effects. It also lacks the prominent sedative effect that is associated with more typical anxiolytics. In vitro preclinical studies have shown that buspirone has a high affinity for serotonin ($5\text{-}HT_{1A}$) receptors. Buspirone has no significant affinity for benzodiazepine receptors and does not affect GABA binding in vitro or in vivo when tested in preclinical models.

Buspirone has moderate affinity for brain D_2-dopamine receptors. Some studies do suggest that buspirone may have indirect effects on other neurotransmitter systems.

➤*Pharmacokinetics:*

Absorption/Distribution – Buspirone is rapidly absorbed in man and undergoes extensive first-pass metabolism. In a radiolabeled study, unchanged buspirone in the plasma accounted for only about 1% of the radioactivity in the plasma. Following oral administration, plasma concentrations of unchanged buspirone are very low and variable between subjects. Peak plasma levels of 1 to 6 ng/mL have been observed 40 to 90 minutes after single oral doses of 20 mg. The single-dose bioavailability of unchanged buspirone when taken as a tablet is on the average about 90% of an equivalent dose of solution, but there is large variability.

The effects of food upon the bioavailability of buspirone have been studied in 8 subjects. They were given a 20 mg dose with and without food; the area under the plasma concentration-time curve (AUC) and peak plasma concentration (C_{max}) of unchanged buspirone increased by 84% and 116%, respectively, but the total amount of buspirone immunoreactive material did not change. This suggests that food may decrease the extent of presystemic clearance of buspirone, but the clinical significance of these findings is unknown.

A multiple-dose study conducted in 15 subjects suggests that buspirone has nonlinear pharmacokinetics. Thus, dose increases and repeated dosing may lead to somewhat higher blood levels of unchanged buspirone than would be predicted from results of single-dose studies.

An in vitro protein binding study indicated that approximately 86% of buspirone is bound to plasma proteins. It was also observed that aspirin increased the plasma levels of free buspirone by 23%, while flurazepam decreased the plasma levels of free buspirone by 20%. However, it is not known whether these drugs cause similar effects on plasma levels of free buspirone in vivo, or whether such changes, if they do occur, cause clinically significant differences in treatment outcome. An in vitro study indicated that buspirone did not displace highly protein-bound drugs such as phenytoin, warfarin, and propranolol from plasma protein, and that buspirone may displace digoxin.

Metabolism/Excretion – Buspirone is metabolized primarily by oxidation, which in vitro has been shown to be mediated by cytochrome P450 3A4 (CYP3A4). Several hydroxylated derivatives and a pharmacologically active metabolite, 1-pyrimidinylpiperazine (1-PP), are produced. In animal models predictive of anxiolytic potential, 1-PP has about one quarter of the activity of buspirone, but is present in up to 20-fold greater amounts. However, this is probably not important in humans: Blood samples from humans chronically exposed to buspirone HCl do not exhibit high levels of 1-PP; mean values are approximately 3 ng/mL and the highest human blood level recorded among 108 chronically dosed patients was 17 ng/mL, less than 1/200th of 1-PP levels found in animals given large doses of buspirone without signs of toxicity.

In a single-dose study using ^{14}C-labeled buspirone, 29% to 63% of the dose was excreted in the urine within 24 hours, primarily as metabolites; fecal excretion accounted for 18% to 38% of the dose. The average elimination half-life of unchanged buspirone after single doses of 10 to 40 mg is about 2 to 3 hours.

Special populations –

Renal function impairment: After multiple-dose administration of buspirone to renally impaired (Ccr = 10 to 70 mL/min/1.73 m^2) patients, steady-state AUC of buspirone increased 4-fold compared with healthy (Ccr greater than or equal to 80 mL/min/1.73 m^2) subjects. Therefore, administration of buspirone to patients with severe renal impairment cannot be recommended.

Hepatic function impairment: After multiple-dose administration of buspirone to patients with hepatic impairment, steady-state AUC of buspirone increased 13-fold compared with healthy subjects. Therefore, administration of buspirone to patients with severe hepatic impairment cannot be recommended.

Contraindications

Hypersensitivity to buspirone.

Warnings/Precautions

➤*Psychotic patients:* Because buspirone has no established antipsychotic activity, it should not be employed in lieu of appropriate antipsychotic treatment.

➤*Potential for withdrawal reactions in sedative/hypnotic/anxiolytic drug-dependent patients:* Because buspirone does not exhibit cross-tolerance with benzodiazepines and other common sedative/hypnotic drugs, it will not block the withdrawal syndrome often seen with cessation of therapy with these drugs. Therefore, before starting therapy with buspirone, it is advisable to withdraw patients gradually, especially patients who have been using a CNS-depressant drug chronically, from their prior treatment. Rebound or withdrawal symptoms may occur over varying time periods, depending in part on the type of drug, and its effective half-life of elimination.

The syndrome of withdrawal from sedative/hypnotic/anxiolytic drugs can appear as any combination of irritability, anxiety, agitation, insomnia, tremor, abdominal cramps, muscle cramps, vomiting, sweating, flu-like symptoms without fever, and occasionally, even as seizures.

➤*Possible concerns related to buspirone's binding to dopamine receptors:* Because buspirone can bind to central dopamine receptors, a question has been raised about its potential to cause acute and chronic

BUSPIRONE HYDROCHLORIDE — ORAL

changes in dopamine-mediated neurological function (eg, dystonia, pseudoparkinsonism, akathisia, tardive dyskinesia). Clinical experience in controlled trials has failed to identify any significant neuroleptic-like activity; however, a syndrome of restlessness, appearing shortly after initiation of treatment, has been reported in some small fraction of buspirone-treated patients. The syndrome may be explained in several ways. For example, buspirone may increase central noradrenergic activity; alternatively, the effect may be attributable to dopaminergic effects (ie, represent akathisia). Obviously, the question cannot be totally resolved at this point in time. Generally, long-term sequelae of any drug's use can be identified only after several years of marketing.

➤*Renal/Hepatic function impairment:* See Actions for more information.

➤*Drug abuse and dependence:* Although there is no direct evidence that buspirone causes physical dependence or drug-seeking behavior, it is difficult to predict from experiments the extent to which a CNS-active drug will be misused, diverted, or abused once marketed. Consequently, physicians should carefully evaluate patients for a history of drug abuse and follow such patients closely, observing them for signs of buspirone misuse or abuse (eg, development of tolerance, incrementation of dose, drug-seeking behavior).

➤*Hazardous tasks:* Studies indicate that buspirone is less sedating than other anxiolytics and that it does not produce significant functional impairment. However, its CNS effects in any individual patient may not be predictable. Therefore, patients should be cautioned about operating an automobile or using complex machinery until they are reasonably certain that buspirone treatment does not affect them adversely.

➤*Pregnancy: Category B.* In humans, however, adequate and well-controlled studies during pregnancy have not been performed. Because animal reproduction studies are not always predictive of human response, this drug should be used during pregnancy only if clearly needed.

➤*Lactation:* The extent of the excretion in human milk of buspirone or its metabolites is not known. In rats, however, buspirone and its metabolites are excreted in milk. Buspirone administration to nursing women should be avoided if clinically possible.

➤*Children:* The safety and efficacy of buspirone were evaluated in 2 placebo-controlled 6-week trials involving a total of 559 pediatric patients (ranging from 6 to 17 years of age) with GAD. Doses studied were 7.5 to 30 mg twice daily (15 to 60 mg/day). There were no significant differences between buspirone and placebo with regard to the symptoms of GAD following doses recommended for the treatment of GAD in adults. Pharmacokinetic studies have shown that, for identical doses, plasma exposure to buspirone and its active metabolite, 1-PP, are equal to or higher in pediatric patients than adults. No unexpected safety findings were associated with buspirone in these trials. There are no long-term safety or efficacy data in this population.

Drug Interactions

Buspirone Drug Interactions

Precipitant drug	Object drug[a]		Description
Cimetidine	Buspirone	↑	Coadministration increased buspirone C_{max} (40%) and T_{max} (2-fold), but had minimal effects on AUC.
CYP3A4 inhibitors (eg, itraconazole, ketoconazole, erythromycin, clarithromycin, diltiazem, verapamil, fluvoxamine, ritonavir)	Buspirone	↑	Plasma buspirone concentrations may be elevated because of inhibition of its metabolism (CYP3A4). Adjust buspirone dosage as needed. If given with erythromycin, a low dose of buspirone (eg, 2.5 mg twice/day) is recommended. If given with itraconazole, a low dose of buspirone (eg, 2.5 mg/day) is recommended.
CYP3A4 inducers (eg, rifampin, rifabutin, phenytoin, phenobarbital, carbamazepine, dexamethasone)	Buspirone	↓	Plasma buspirone concentrations may be decreased because of induction of its metabolism (CYP3A4). Adjust the buspirone dose as needed.
Fluoxetine	Buspirone	↓	Effects of buspirone may be decreased. Paradoxical worsening of OCD has occurred.
Nefazodone	Buspirone	↑	Coadministration increased plasma buspirone concentrations (up to 20-fold in C_{max} and up to 50-fold in AUC) and statistically significant decreases (≈ 50%) in plasma concentrations of the buspirone active metabolite. Slight increases (23%) in AUC were observed for nefazodone. If the 2 drugs are to be used in combination, a low dose of buspirone (eg, 2.5 mg/day) is recommended.
Buspirone	Nefazodone		
Buspirone	Diazepam	↑	Although coadministration produced no differences in diazepam kinetic parameters (C_{max}, AUC, and C_{min}), increases (about 15%) in nordiazepam kinetics were seen. Minor effects (dizziness, headache, and nausea) were observed.
Buspirone	Alcohol	↔	Formal studies of the interaction of buspirone with alcohol indicate that buspirone does not increase alcohol-induced impairment in motor and mental performance, but it is prudent to avoid concomitant use.
Buspirone	Haloperidol	↑	Haloperidol and buspirone coadministration may result in increased serum haloperidol concentrations.
Buspirone	MAO inhibitors	↑	There have been reports of elevated blood pressure when buspirone was added to a regimen including an MAOI. Therefore, do not use concomitantly.
Buspirone	Trazodone	↔	One report suggests that concomitant use may have caused 3- to 6-fold elevations of ALT in a few patients. In a similar study attempting to replicate this finding, no interactive effect on hepatic transaminases was identified.

[a] ↑ = object drug increased; ↓ = object drug decreased; ↔ = Undetermined clinical effect.

➤*Drug/Food interactions:*

Grapefruit juice – Coadministration of buspirone (10 mg as a single dose) with grapefruit juice (200 mL double strength 3 times daily for 2 days) increased plasma buspirone concentrations (4.3-fold increase in C_{max}; 9.2-fold increase in AUC). Patients receiving buspirone should be advised to avoid drinking such large amounts of grapefruit juice.

Adverse Reactions

Commonly observed – Dizziness, nausea, headache, nervousness, lightheadedness, and excitement.

Associated with discontinuation of treatment – Approximately 10% of the 2200 anxious patients who participated in the buspirone premarketing clinical efficacy trials in anxiety disorders lasting 3 to 4 weeks discontinued treatment due to an adverse reaction. The more common reactions causing discontinuation included central nervous system disturbances (3.4%), primarily dizziness, insomnia, nervousness, drowsiness, and lightheadedness; gastrointestinal disturbances (1.2%), primarily nausea; and miscellaneous disturbances (1.1%), primarily headache and fatigue. In addition, 3.4% of patients had multiple complaints, none of which could be characterized as primary.

Incidence in controlled clinical trials –

Buspirone Adverse Reactions (%)[a]

Adverse reaction	Buspirone HCl (n = 477)	Placebo (n = 464)
Cardiovascular		
Tachycardia/ palpitations	1%	1%
CNS		
Dizziness	12%	3%
Drowsiness	10%	9%
Nervousness	5%	1%
Insomnia	3%	3%
Lightheadedness	3%	< 1%
Decreased concentration	2%	2%
Excitement	2%	< 1%
Anger/hostility	2%	< 1%
Confusion	2%	< 1%
Depression	2%	2%
Special senses		
Blurred vision	2%	< 1%
Gastrointestinal		
Nausea	8%	5%

BUSPIRONE HYDROCHLORIDE — ORAL

Buspirone Adverse Reactions (%)[a]		
Adverse reaction	Buspirone HCl (n = 477)	Placebo (n = 464)
Dry mouth	3%	4%
Abdominal/gastric distress	2%	2%
Diarrhea	2%	< 1%
Constipation	1%	2%
Vomiting	1%	2%
Musculoskeletal		
Musculoskeletal aches/pains	1%	< 1%
Neurological		
Numbness	2%	< 1%
Paresthesia	1%	< 1%
Incoordination	1%	< 1%
Tremor	1%	< 1%
Dermatologic		
Skin rash	1%	< 1%
Miscellaneous		
Headache	6%	3%
Fatigue	4%	4%
Weakness	2%	< 1%
Sweating/clamminess	1%	< 1%

[a] Reactions reported by at least 1% of buspirone patients are included.

➤*Other reactions:* The following definitions of frequency are used: Frequent adverse reactions are defined as those occurring in at least 1/100 patients. Infrequent adverse reactions are those occurring in 1/100 to 1/1000 patients, while rare reactions are those occurring in less than 1/1000 patients.

Cardiovascular – Frequent was nonspecific chest pain; infrequent were syncope, hypotension, and hypertension; rare were cerebrovascular accident, congestive heart failure, myocardial infarction, cardiomyopathy, and bradycardia.

CNS – Frequent were dream disturbances; infrequent were depersonalization, dysphoria, noise intolerance, euphoria, akathisia, fearfulness, loss of interest, dissociative reaction, hallucinations, involuntary movements, slowed reaction time, suicidal ideation, and seizures; rare were feelings of claustrophobia, cold intolerance, stupor, and slurred speech and psychosis.

Dermatologic – Infrequent were edema, pruritus, flushing, easy bruising, hair loss, dry skin, facial edema, and blisters; rare were acne and thinning of nails.

Endocrine – Rare were galactorrhea and thyroid abnormality.

GI – Infrequent were flatulence, anorexia, increased appetite, salivation, irritable colon, and rectal bleeding; rare was burning of the tongue.

GU – Infrequent were decreased or increased libido, urinary frequency, urinary hesitancy, menstrual irregularity and spotting, and dysuria; rare were amenorrhea, delayed ejaculation, impotence, pelvic inflammatory disease, enuresis, and nocturia.

Lab test abnormalities – Infrequent were increases in hepatic aminotransferases (ALT, AST); rare were eosinophilia, leukopenia, and thrombocytopenia.

Musculoskeletal – Infrequent were muscle cramps, muscle spasms, rigid/stiff muscles, and arthralgias; rare was muscle weakness.

Respiratory – Infrequent were hyperventilation, shortness of breath, and chest congestion; rare was epistaxis.

Special senses – Frequent were tinnitus, sore throat, and nasal congestion; infrequent were redness and itching of the eyes, altered taste, altered smell, and conjunctivitis; rare were inner ear abnormality, eye pain, photophobia, and pressure on eyes.

Miscellaneous – Infrequent were weight gain, fever, roaring sensation in the head, weight loss, and malaise; rare were alcohol abuse, bleeding disturbance, loss of voice, and hiccoughs.

Overdosage

➤*Symptoms:* In clinical pharmacology trials, doses as high as 375 mg/day were administered to healthy male volunteers. As this dose was approached, the following symptoms were observed: Nausea, vomiting, dizziness, drowsiness, miosis, and gastric distress. A few cases of overdosage have been reported, with complete recovery as the usual outcome. No deaths have been reported following overdosage with buspirone alone. Rare cases of intentional overdosage with a fatal outcome were invariably associated with ingestion of multiple drugs or alcohol, and a causal relationship to buspirone could not be determined. Toxicology studies of buspirone yielded the following LD_{50} values: Mice, 655 mg/kg; rats, 196 mg/kg; dogs, 586 mg/kg; and monkeys, 356 mg/kg. These dosages are 160 to 550 times the recommended human daily dose.

➤*Treatment:* General symptomatic and supportive measures should be used along with immediate gastric lavage. Respiration, pulse, and blood pressure should be monitored as in all cases of drug overdosage. No specific antidote is known to buspirone, and dialyzability of buspirone has not been determined.

Patient Information

1.) Inform your physician of any medications, prescription or nonprescription, alcohol, or drugs that you are now taking or plan to take during your treatment with buspirone.
2.) Inform your physician if you are pregnant, or if you are planning to become pregnant, or if you become pregnant while you are taking buspirone.
3.) Inform your physician if you are breastfeeding an infant.
4.) Until you experience how this medication affects you, do not drive a car or operate potentially dangerous machinery.
5.) You should take buspirone consistently, either always with or always without food.
6.) During your treatment with buspirone, avoid drinking large amounts of grapefruit juice.

HYDROXYZINE

For complete prescribing information, refer to the Hydroxyzine monograph in the Antihistamines section.

ANTIANXIETY AGENTS

MEPROBAMATE

c-iv	**Meprobamate** (Various, eg, Watson)	**Tablets**: 200 mg	In 20s, 100s, and 1000s.
c-iv	**Miltown** (Wallace)		Sugar. (Wallace 37 1101). White. In 100s.
c-iv	**Meprobamate** (Various, eg, Watson)	**Tablets**: 400 mg	In 20s, 100s, 500s, 1000s, and UD 100s.
c-iv	**Miltown** (Wallace)		(Wallace 37 1001). White, scored. In 100s, 500s, and 1000s.

MEPROBAMATE — ORAL

Indications

➤*Anxiety:* For the management of anxiety disorders or for the short-term relief of the symptoms of anxiety. The effectiveness of meprobamate in long-term use, that is, more than 4 months, has not been assessed by systematic clinical studies. The physician should periodically reassess the usefulness of the drug for the individual patient.

Administration and Dosage

➤*Adults:*

Anxiety – 1,200 to 1,600 mg/day in 3 or 4 divided doses.

➤*Children:*

Anxiety – See Adults for dosing for children older than 12 years of age.

6 to 12 years of age: 100 to 200 mg 2 or 3 times daily.

➤*Elderly:* The lowest effective dose should be administered in order to preclude oversedation.

➤*Storage/Stability:* Store at 25°C (77°F). Keep tightly closed. Dispense in tight container.

Actions

➤*Pharmacology:* Meprobamate is a carbamate derivative which has been shown (in animal and human studies) to have effects at multiple sites in the central nervous system, including the thalamus and limbic system.

Contraindications

Acute intermittent porphyria as well as allergic or idiosyncratic reactions to meprobamate or related compounds such as carisoprodol, mebutamate, or carbromal.

Warnings/Precautions

➤*Additive effects:* Since the CNS-suppressant effects of meprobamate and alcohol or meprobamate and other CNS depressants or psychotropic drugs may be additive, appropriate caution should be exercised with patients who take more than 1 of these agents simultaneously.

➤*Renal/Hepatic function impairment:* Meprobamate is metabolized in the liver and excreted by the kidney; to avoid its excess accumulation, caution should be exercised in administration to patients with compromised liver or kidney function.

MEPROBAMATE — ORAL

➤*Special risk:* The lowest effective dose should be administered, particularly to elderly or debilitated patients, in order to preclude oversedation.

The possibility of suicide attempts should be considered and the least amount of drug feasible should be prescribed at any one time.

Meprobamate occasionally may precipitate seizures in epileptic patients.

➤*Drug abuse and dependence:* Physical dependence, psychological dependence, and abuse have occurred. When chronic intoxication from prolonged use occurs, it usually involves ingestion of greater than recommended doses and is manifested by ataxia, slurred speech, and vertigo. Therefore, careful supervision of dose and amounts prescribed is advised, as well as avoidance of prolonged administration, especially for alcoholics and other patients with a known propensity for taking excessive quantities of drugs.

Sudden withdrawal of the drug after prolonged and excessive use may precipitate recurrence of preexisting symptoms, such as anxiety, anorexia, or insomnia, or withdrawal reactions, such as vomiting, ataxia, tremors, muscle twitching, confusional states, hallucinosis, and, rarely, convulsive seizures. Such seizures are more likely to occur in persons with central nervous system damage or preexistent or latent convulsive disorders. Onset of withdrawal symptoms occurs usually within 12 to 48 hours after discontinuation of meprobamate; symptoms usually cease within the next 12 to 48 hours.

When excessive dosage has continued for weeks or months, dosage should be reduced gradually over a period of 1 or 2 weeks rather than abruptly stopped. Alternatively, a short-acting barbiturate may be substituted, then gradually withdrawn.

➤*Hazardous tasks:* Patients should be warned that meprobamate may impair the mental or physical abilities required for the performance of potentially hazardous tasks such as driving a motor vehicle or operating machinery.

➤*Pregnancy: Category D.* An increased risk of congenital malformations associated with the use of minor tranquilizers (meprobamate, chlordiazepoxide, and diazepam) during the first trimester of pregnancy has been suggested in several studies. Because use of these drugs is rarely a matter of urgency, their use during this period should almost always be avoided. The possibility that a woman of childbearing potential may be pregnant at the time of institution of therapy should be considered. Patients should be advised that if they become pregnant they should communicate with their physicians about the desirability of discontinuing the drug.

➤*Lactation:* Meprobamate passes the placental barrier. It is present both in umbilical cord blood at or near maternal plasma levels and in breast milk of lactating mothers at concentrations 2 to 4 times that of maternal plasma. When use of meprobamate is contemplated in breastfeeding patients, the drug's higher concentration in breast milk as compared to maternal plasma levels should be considered.

➤*Children:* See Administration and Dosage for more information.

➤*Elderly:* Per the Beers list, meprobamate is a highly additive and sedating anxiolytic. Those using meprobamate for prolonged periods may become addicted and may need to be withdrawn slowly. Meprobamate is also considered a high risk medication for the elderly according to the Centers of Medicare and Medicaid Services.

Drug Interactions

Meprobamate Drug Interactions

Precipitant drug	Object drug[a]		Description
Alcohol	Meprobamate	↑	Acute ingestion may result in a decreased clearance of meprobamate through inhibition of hepatic metabolic systems; enhanced CNS depressant effects may occur. Tolerance may occur with chronic alcohol ingestion, presumably due to enhanced metabolic capacity.
Meprobamate	CNS depressants (eg, barbiturates, narcotics)	↑	Anticipate additive CNS depressant effects.
CNS depressants (eg, barbiturates, narcotics)	Meprobamate		

[a] ↑ = object drug increased.

Adverse Reactions

➤*Allergic:* Milder reactions are characterized by an itchy, urticarial, or erythematous maculopapular rash which may be generalized or confined to the groin.

Other reactions have included leukopenia, acute nonthrombocytopenic purpura, petechiae, ecchymoses, eosinophilia, peripheral edema, adenopathy, fever, fixed drug eruption with cross reaction to carisoprodol, and cross-sensitivity between meprobamate/mebutamate and meprobamate/carbromal.

More severe hypersensitivity reactions, rarely reported, include hyperpyrexia, chills, angioneurotic edema, bronchospasm, oliguria, and anuria. Also, anaphylaxis, erythema multiforme, exfoliative dermatitis, stomatitis, and proctitis, Stevens-Johnson syndrome, and bullous dermatitis, including 1 fatal case of the latter following administration of meprobamate in combination with prednisolone have occurred.

➤*Cardiovascular:* Palpitations, tachycardia, various forms of arrhythmia, transient ECG changes, syncope, hypotensive crises.

➤*CNS:* Drowsiness, ataxia, dizziness, slurred speech, headache, vertigo, weakness, paresthesias, impairment of visual accommodation, euphoria, overstimulation, paradoxical excitement, fast EEG activity.

➤*GI:* Nausea, vomiting, diarrhea.

➤*Hematologic:* (See also Allergic.) Agranulocytosis and aplastic anemia have been reported, although no causal relationship has been established. These cases rarely were fatal. Rare cases of thrombocytopenic purpura have been reported.

➤*Miscellaneous:* Exacerbation of porphyric symptoms.

Overdosage

➤*Symptoms:* Suicidal attempts with meprobamate have resulted in drowsiness, lethargy, stupor, ataxia, coma, shock, vasomotor and respiratory collapse. Some suicidal attempts have been fatal. The following data on meprobamate tablets have been reported in the literature and from other sources. These data are not expected to correlate with each case (considering factors such as individual susceptibility and length of time from ingestion to treatment), but represent the usual ranges reported.

Acute simple overdose (meprobamate alone) – Death has been reported with ingestion of as little as 12 g meprobamate and survival with as much as 40 g.

Blood levels – Blood levels of 0.5 to 2 mg/dL represents the usual blood level range of meprobamate after therapeutic doses. The level may occasionally be as high as 3 mg%. Blood levels of 3 to 10 mg/dL usually corresponds to findings of mild to moderate symptoms of overdosage, such as stupor or light coma. Blood levels of 10 to 20 mg/dL usually corresponds to deeper coma, requiring more intensive treatment. Some fatalities occur. At levels greater than 20 mg/dL, more fatalities than survivals can be expected.

➤*Treatment:* In cases where excessive doses have been taken, sleep ensues rapidly and blood pressure, pulse, and respiratory rates are reduced to basal levels. Any drug remaining in the stomach should be removed and symptomatic therapy given. Should respiration or blood pressure become compromised, respiratory assistance, central nervous system stimulants and pressor agents should be administered cautiously as indicated. Meprobamate is metabolized in the liver and excreted by the kidney. Diuresis, osmotic (mannitol) diuresis, peritoneal dialysis, and hemodialysis have been used successfully. Careful monitoring of urinary output is necessary and caution should be taken to avoid overhydration. Relapse and death, after initial recovery, have been attributed to incomplete gastric emptying and delayed absorption.

ANTIDEPRESSANTS

Drugs with clinically useful antidepressant effects include the tricyclic antidepressants (TCAs), tetracyclic antidepressants, trazodone, bupropion, venlafaxine, nefazodone, selective serotonin reuptake inhibitors (SSRIs), and the monoamine oxidase inhibitors (MAOIs). The antidepressant agents all appear effective in the treatment of depression. "Major depressive episode" implies a prominent and relatively persistent (nearly every day for ≥ 2 weeks) depressed or dysphoric mood that usually interferes with daily functioning, and includes ≥ 5 of the following 9 symptoms: Depressed mood; markedly diminished interest or pleasure in all, for almost all activities; significant weight loss or gain when not dieting, or decrease or increase in appetite; insomnia or hypersomnia; psychomotor agitation or retardation; fatigue or loss of energy; feelings of worthlessness, or excessive or inappropriate guilt; diminished ability to think or concentrate, or indecisiveness; recurrent thoughts of death, suicidal ideation, or suicide attempt. These symptoms are not because of the direct physiologic effects of a substance or a general medical condition (eg, hypothyroidism). The symptoms are not better accounted for by bereavement (ie, after the loss of a loved one), persist for > 2 months, or are characterized by marked functional impairment, morbid preoccupation with worthlessness, suicidal ideation, psychotic symptoms, or psychomotor retardation.

➤*Mechanism of action:* Effective antidepressant activity has traditionally been associated with the "biogenic amine hypothesis of depression." The theory is that depression is due to reduced functional activity of ≥ 1 of the endogenous monoamines (norepinephrine, serotonin) in the brain. It was believed that certain types of depression were caused by brain neurotransmitter deficiency and that antidepressants relieved depression by inhibiting the reuptake of serotonin and norepinephrine, thereby correcting this deficiency and facilitating neurotransmission. This explanation is now being questioned for several reasons. First, several antidepressant agents lack any apparent effect on neurotransmitter reuptake. More importantly, the blockade of neurotransmitter reuptake occurs within minutes to hours of antidepressant drug initiation, while the antidepressant effects usually take 1 to 4 weeks to manifest.

The emphasis of research has shifted from acute reuptake effects to the slower adaptive changes in norepinephrine and serotonin receptor systems induced by chronic antidepressant therapy. Postsynaptic receptors participate in nerve impulse neurotransmission while the presynaptic receptors regulate neurotransmitter release and reuptake, an important mechanism of neurotransmitter inactivation. Long-term antidepressant treatment produces complex changes in the sensitivities of both presynaptic and postsynaptic receptor sites. The available antidepressant agents may increase the sensitivity of postsynaptic alpha (α_1) adrenergic and serotonin receptors and may decrease the sensitivity of presynaptic receptor sites. The net effect is the correction (re-regulation) of an abnormal receptor-neurotransmitter relationship. Clinically, this re-regulatory action speeds up the patient's natural recovery process from the depressive episode by normalizing neurotransmission efficacy.

➤*Drug selection:* The non-MAOIs are used more frequently than the MAOIs, mainly because of the perception that MAOIs are less effective than the non-MAOI antidepressants and the risk of hypertensive crisis from ingesting foods containing tyramine or from drug interactions (eg, sympathomimetics) with the MAOIs. However, when MAOIs are used in therapeutic doses, they are probably equally effective to non-MAOIs for the treatment of depression. In general, MAOIs are used for atypical depression.

Base antidepressant drug selection on the patient's history of drug response (if any), the specific drug's side effect profile relative to patient medical conditions and other factors, and clinician familiarity with specific antidepressants. Nortriptyline and desipramine are preferred TCAs in a patient without a history of favorable response to a specific antidepressant because they cause less sedation and have less anticholinergic activity than tertiary TCAs such as amitriptyline and, in the case of nortriptyline, are less likely to cause orthostatic hypotension. Trazodone has less anticholinergic activity than TCAs and causes fewer problems than TCAs when taken in overdose. SSRIs generally lack the adverse reactions (eg, sedation, anticholinergic effects) associated with TCAs, cause few cardiovascular side effects (including orthostasis), are associated with initial weight loss rather than weight gain as is the case with TCAs, and cause fewer problems than TCAs when taken in overdose. Newer information has shown that during long-term use, SSRIs cause similar weight gain as compared with TCAs. However, their use is associated with other side effects such as headache, nervousness, and insomnia. Fluoxetine and paroxetine are recommended to be taken in the morning; sertraline can be taken morning or evening. Use maprotiline, mirtazapine, and bupropion only when other antidepressants have not proven effective. In cases of mild depression, drug therapy and psychotherapy appear to be equally effective.

As a general guideline, continue treatment for 9 months after remission in patients who experience their first episode of depression; following a second episode, continue treatment for 5 years after remission; with a third episode, treat indefinitely.

➤*Actions:* The following table summarizes some of the important pharmacologic and pharmacokinetic data of these agents.

Antidepressant Pharmacologic and Pharmacokinetic Parameters

0 -none + -slight ++ -moderate +++ -high ++++ -very high +++++ -highest	Major side effects			Amine uptake blocking activity					
	Anticholinergic	Sedation	Orthostatic hypotension	Norepinephrine	Serotonin	Half-life (hours)	Therapeutic plasma level (ng/ml)	Time to reach steady state (days)	Dose range (mg/day)
Tricyclics - Tertiary Amines									
Amitriptyline	++++	++++	++	++	++++	31-46	110-250[a]	4-10	50-300
Clomipramine	+++	+++	++	++	+++++	19-37	80-100	7-14	25-250
Doxepin	++	+++	++	+	++	8-24	100-200[a]	2-8	25-300
Imipramine	++	++	+++	++[b]	++++	11-25	200-350[a]	2-5	30-300
Trimipramine	++	+++	++	+	+	7-30	180[a]	2-6	50-300
Tricyclics - Secondary Amines									
Amoxapine[c]	+++	++	+	+++	++	8[d]	200-500	2-7	50-600
Desipramine	+	+	+	++++	++	12-24	125-300	2-11	25-300
Nortriptyline	++	++	+	++	+++	18-44	50-150	4-19	30-100
Protriptyline	+++	+	+	++++	++	67-89	100-200	14-19	15-60
Tetracyclics									
Maprotiline	++	++	+	+++	0/+	21-25	200-300[a]	6-10	50-225
Mirtazapine	++	+++	++	+++	+++	20-40	-	5	15-45
Triazolopyridine									
Trazodone	+	++++	++	0	+++	4-9	800-1600	3-7	150-600
Aminoketone									
Bupropion[e]	++	++	+	0/+	0/+	8-24	-	1.5-8	200-450
Phenethylamine									
Venlafaxine	0	0	0	+++	+++	5-11 [a]	-	3-4	75-375
Phenylpiperazine									
Nefazodone	0/+	++	+	0/+	+++++	2-4	-	4-5	200-600
Selective Serotonin Reuptake Inhibitors									
Citalopram	0/+	0/+	0/+	0/+	++++	33	-	7	20-60
Escitalopram	0/+	0/+	0	0/+	++++	27-32	-	7	10-20
Fluoxetine	0/+	0/+	0/+	0/+	+++++	1-16 days[a]	-	2-4 weeks	20-80
Fluvoxamine	0/+	0/+	0	0/+	+++++	15.6	-	≈ 7	50-300
Paroxetine	0	0/+	0	0/+	+++++	10-24	-	7-14	10-50
Sertraline	0	0/+	0	0/+	+++++	1-4 days[a]	-	7	50-200
Monoamine Oxidase Inhibitors									
Isocarboxazid	0/+	0/+	+	-	-	-	-	-	10-60
Phenelzine	+	+	+	-	-	-	-	-	45-90
Tranylcypromine	+	+	0	-	-	2.4-2.8	-	-	30-60
Serotonin and Norepinephrine Reuptake Inhibitors									
Duloxetine	0/+	+	+	+++	+++	8-17	-	3	40-120
Desvenlafaxine	0	0	0	+++	+++	11-14	-	4-5	50-400

[a] Parent compound plus active metabolite.
[b] Via desipramine, the major metabolite.
[c] Also blocks dopamine receptors.
[d] 30 hours for major metabolite 8-hydroxyamoxapine.
[e] Inhibits dopamine uptake.

Refer to the Antidepressants introduction.

Indications

➤*Depression:* Relief of symptoms of depression (except **clomipramine**). The activating properties of **protriptyline** make it particularly suitable for withdrawn and anergic patients.

Agents with significant sedative action may be useful in depression associated with anxiety and sleep disturbances.

➤*Amoxapine:* Relief of depressive symptoms in patients with neurotic or reactive depressive disorders and endogenous and psychotic depression; depression accompanied by anxiety or agitation.

➤*Doxepin:* Treatment of psychoneurotic patients with depression or anxiety; depression or anxiety associated with alcoholism (not to be taken concomitantly with alcohol); depression or anxiety associated with organic disease (the possibility of drug interaction should be considered if the patient is receiving other drugs concomitantly); psychotic depressive disorders with associated anxiety including involutional depression and manic-depressive disorders. The target symptoms of psychoneurosis that respond particularly well to doxepin include anxiety, tension, depression, somatic symptoms and concerns, sleep disturbances, guilt, lack of energy, fear, apprehension, and worry.

➤*Imipramine:* Treatment of enuresis in children ≥ 6 years of age as temporary adjunctive therapy.

➤*Clomipramine:* Only for treatment of obsessive-compulsive disorder (OCD).

➤*Off-label uses:* Refer to individual monographs for further information.

Adult enuresis –
Amitriptyline: [4] = Insufficient documentation.

Alcoholism –
Desipramine: [4] = Insufficient documentation.
Imipramine: [4] = Insufficient documentation.

Attention deficit hyperactivity disorder (adults) –
Desipramine: [4] = Insufficient documentation.
Nortriptyline: [3] = Safety concerns.

Attention deficit hyperactivity disorder (children / adolescents) –
Desipramine: [3] = Safety concerns.
Imipramine: [1] = Good documentation.
Nortriptyline: [3] = Safety concerns.

Bulimia nervosa –
Amitriptyline: [4] = Insufficient documentation.
Desipramine: [2] = Fair documentation.
Imipramine: [3] = Safety concerns.

Cocaine dependence –
Imipramine: [4] = Insufficient documentation.

Diabetic neuropathy –
Desipramine: [4] = Insufficient documentation.

Fibromyalgia –
Amitriptyline: [2] = Fair documentation.

Irritable bowel syndrome –
Imipramine: [5] = Poor documentation.

Narcolepsy –
Imipramine: [3] = Safety concerns.

Neuropathic pain –
Amitriptyline: [5] = Poor documentation.
Imipramine: [3] = Safety concerns.

Nocturnal enuresis (children / adolescents) –
Desipramine: [3] = Safety concerns.

Panic disorder –
Clomipramine: [2] = Fair documentation.
Imipramine: [3] = Safety concerns.

Postherpetic neuralgia –
Amitriptyline (oral): [1] = Good documentation.
Amitriptyline (topical): [5] = Poor documentation.
Desipramine: [1] = Good documentation.
Nortriptyline: [1] = Good documentation.

Prevention of chronic headache (adults) –
Amitriptyline: [1] = Good documentation.

Prevention of migraine (adults) –
Amitriptyline: [1] = Good documentation.
Clomipramine: [5] = Poor documentation.
Doxepin: [2] = Fair documentation.
Imipramine: [2] = Fair documentation.
Nortriptyline: [4] = Insufficient documentation.
Protriptyline: [4] = Insufficient documentation.

Prevention of migraine (children / adolescents) –
Amitriptyline: [4] = Insufficient documentation.

Smoking cessation –
Nortriptyline: [3] = Safety concerns.

As evidenced by the black box warning for nortriptyline, this drug is not without risk. Additionally, it has a more bothersome adverse effect profile than therapeutic alternatives. Although there are data showing the efficacy of nortriptyline in smoking cessation, a recent large trial showed no significant difference over placebo. Clinicians must evaluate individual patient contraindications, treatment history, and comorbidities to determine if nortriptyline is the most appropriate cessation therapy choice.

Stuttering –
Clomipramine: [4] = Insufficient documentation.

Tourette syndrome with comorbid attention deficit hyperactivity disorder (children / adolescents) –
Desipramine: [3] = Safety concerns.

Traumatic brain injury –
Amitriptyline: [3] = Safety concerns.
Desipramine: [3] = Safety concerns.

Urinary incontinence –
Imipramine: [4] = Insufficient documentation.

Other possible off-label uses –
Pathologic laughing and weeping secondary to forebrain disease: Amitriptyline 30 to 75 mg/day.
Obstructive sleep apnea: Protriptyline.
Peptic ulcer disease: Doxepin 50 to 150 mg/day; trimipramine 25 to 50 mg/day.
Facilitation of cocaine withdrawal: Desipramine 50 to 200 mg/day; imipramine 150 to 300 mg/day.
Panic disorder: Imipramine; desipramine; nortriptyline. Other antidepressants may also be used.
Premenstrual symptoms: Clomipramine 25 to 75 mg/day for irritability and dysphoria; desipramine 100 to 150 mg/day for depression; nortriptyline 50 to 125 mg/day.
Dermatologic disorders (chronic urticaria and angioedema, nocturnal pruritus in atopic eczema): Amitriptyline 10 to 50 mg/day; desipramine 100 to 150 mg/day; doxepin 10 to 30 mg/day; nortriptyline 20 to 75 mg/day.
Desipramine: Tourette syndrome, anxiety.

Administration and Dosage

If minor side effects develop, reduce dosage. Discontinue treatment promptly if serious adverse effects or allergic manifestations occur.

➤*Plasma levels:* Determination of plasma levels may be useful in identifying patients who appear to have toxic effects and may have excessively high levels of the drug, or those in whom lack of absorption or noncompliance is suspected. Make adjustments in dosage according to patient's clinical response, not based on plasma levels.

➤*Adolescent, elderly, and outpatients:* Lower dosages are recommended. Initiate therapy at a low dosage and increase gradually, noting the clinical response and any evidence of intolerance. Most antidepressant drugs have a lag period of 10 days to 4 weeks before a therapeutic response is noted. Increasing the dose will not shorten this period but rather increase the incidence of adverse reactions. Following remission, maintenance medication may be required for a longer time at the lowest dose that will maintain remission. Continue maintenance therapy ≥ 3 months to decrease the possibility of relapse.

➤*Single daily dose:* A single daily dose may be used for maintenance therapy. A single daily dose at bedtime is convenient, will minimize daytime side effects (sedation and anticholinergic effects), and the sedative effect at bedtime may be beneficial in patients with sleep disorders. Because of increased risk of cardiovascular and other complications, the elderly may not tolerate single daily doses. **Protriptyline** may have a mild stimulant effect; it is generally not given as a single bedtime dose.

➤*Tricyclic / MAOI combined use:* Tricyclic/MAOI combined use is traditionally contraindicated because of the potential serious adverse reactions (see Drug Interactions). Such combinations may offer significant advantages in patients refractory to more conservative therapy. In conservative dosages, with observance of MAOI dietary restrictions, and under close medical observation, combined therapy has been safe. At least 7 to 10 days should elapse between MAOI discontinuation and TCA institution.

Specific dosage guidelines for individual agents are included in the product listings.

Actions

➤*Pharmacology:* The tricyclic antidepressants (TCAs), structurally related to the phenothiazine antipsychotic agents, possess 3 major pharmacologic actions in varying degrees: Blocking of the amine pump, sedation, and peripheral and central anticholinergic action. In contrast to phenothiazines, which act on dopamine receptors, TCAs inhibit reuptake of norepinephrine or serotonin (5-hydroxytryptamine, 5-HT) at the presynaptic neuron. **Amoxapine**, a metabolite of loxapine, retains some of the postsynaptic dopamine receptor-blocking action of neuroleptics.

Amine uptake inhibition – The amine hypothesis of depression proposes a relationship between depression and levels of CNS bioamines at postsynaptic adrenergic receptors in the brain. TCAs can be characterized by their ability to inhibit presynaptic reuptake of norepinephrine and serotonin (see table in Introduction).

Although amine pump blockade may be immediate, antidepressant response can take days to weeks.

Other pharmacologic effects – Inhibition of histamine and acetylcholine activity. Clinical effects, in addition to antidepressant effects, include sedation, anticholinergic effects, mild peripheral vasodilator effects, and possible "quinidine-like" actions.

Contraindications

Prior sensitivity to any tricyclic drug. Not recommended for use during the acute recovery phase following MI. Concomitant use of monoamine oxidase inhibitors (MAOIs) is generally contraindicated (see Warnings, Drug Interactions).

➤*Doxepin:* Patients with glaucoma or a tendency to have urinary retention.

Cross-sensitivity may occur among the dibenzazepines (**clomipramine**, **desipramine**, **imipramine**, **nortriptyline**, and **trimipramine**). In addition, dibenzoxepines (**doxepin**, **amoxapine**) may produce cross-sensitivity. **Amitriptyline** may block the antihypertensive action of guanethidine or similarly active compounds.

Warnings/Precautions

➤*Tardive dyskinesia:* Tardive dyskinesia, a syndrome consisting of potentially irreversible, involuntary, dyskinetic movements may develop in patients treated with neuroleptics (eg, antipsychotics). **Amoxapine** is not an antipsychotic, but it has substantive neuroleptic activity. Although the syndrome appears most often among the elderly, especially elderly women, it is impossible to determine which patients will develop the syndrome. Whether or not neuroleptic drugs differ in their potential to cause tardive dyskinesia is unknown. For a more complete discussion of tardive dyskinesia, see the Antipsychotic Agents group monograph.

➤*Neuroleptic malignant syndrome (NMS):* NMS is a potentially fatal condition reported in association with antipsychotic drugs and with **amoxapine**. Clinical manifestations of NMS are hyperpyrexia, muscle rigidity, altered mental status, and evidence of autonomic instability (irregular pulse or blood pressure, tachycardia, diaphoresis, and cardiac arrhythmias). The management of NMS should include the following: (1) Immediate discontinuation of antipsychotic drugs, amoxapine, and other drugs not essential to concurrent therapy, (2) intensive symptomatic treatment and medical monitoring, and (3) treatment of any concomitant serious medical problems for which specific treatments are available. There is no general agreement about specific pharmacologic treatment regimens for uncomplicated NMS.

Once the NMS is resolved, use a different antidepressant drug if the patient continues to require antidepressant treatment.

Hyperthermia has occurred with **clomipramine**; most cases occurred when it was used with other drugs (eg, neuroleptics) and may be an example of NMS.

➤*Seizure disorders:* Because TCAs lower the seizure threshold, use with caution in patients with a history of seizures or other predisposing factors (eg, brain damage of varying etiology, alcoholism, concomitant drugs known to lower the seizure threshold). However, seizures have occurred in patients with and without a history of seizure disorders. Seizure was identified as the most significant risk of **clomipramine** use in premarket evaluation.

➤*Anticholinergic effects:* Use with caution in patients with a history of urinary retention, narrow-angle glaucoma, or increased intraocular pressure. In angle-closure glaucoma, even average doses may precipitate an attack. In occasional susceptible patients or in those receiving anticholinergics (including antiparkinson agents), the atropine-like effects may become more pronounced (eg, paralytic ileus). See table in Introduction for relative anticholinergic actions.

➤*Cardiovascular disorders:* Use with extreme caution in patients with cardiovascular disorders because of the possibility of conduction defects, arrhythmias, CHF, sinus tachycardia, MI, strokes, and tachycardia. These patients require cardiac surveillance at all dose levels of the drug. In high doses, TCAs may produce arrhythmias, sinus tachycardia, conduction defects, and prolonged conduction time. Tachycardia and postural hypotension may occur more frequently with **protriptyline**.

➤*Hyperthyroid patients:* Hyperthyroid patients or those receiving thyroid medication require close supervision because of the possibility of cardiovascular toxicity, including arrhythmias.

➤*Psychiatric patients:* Schizophrenic or paranoid patients may exhibit a worsening of psychosis with TCA therapy. In overactive or agitated patients, increased anxiety or agitation may occur. Neuropsychiatric signs and symptoms (eg, delusions, hallucinations, psychotic episodes, confusion, paranoia) have been reported with **clomipramine** use. Paranoid delusions, with or without associated hostility, may be exaggerated. Reduction of TCA dosage and concomitant antipsychotic therapy (eg, perphenazine) may be necessary.

The possibility of suicide in depressed patients remains during treatment and until significant remission occurs. Patients should not have easy access to large quantities of the drug; advise the physician to prescribe small quantities of TCAs.

➤*Mania/Hypomania:* Hypomanic or manic episodes may occur, particularly in patients with cyclic disorders. Such reactions may necessitate discontinuation of the drug. If needed, **imipramine pamoate** may be resumed in lower doses when these episodes are relieved. Administration of a tranquilizer may be useful in controlling such episodes. Manic-depressive patients may experience a shift to a hypomanic or manic phase, which may necessitate discontinuation and possibly resuming at a lower dose when these episodes are relieved.

➤*MAOIs:* Do not give MAOIs with or immediately following TCAs. Such combinations can produce hyperpyretic crises, severe convulsions, sweating, coma, hyperexcitability, hyperthermia, tachycardia, tachypnea, headache, mydriasis, flushing, confusion, hypotension, disseminated intravascular coagulation, and death. Allow at least 14 days to elapse between MAOI discontinuation and TCA institution. Some TCAs have been used safely and successfully with MAOIs. Initiate TCA cautiously with gradual dosage increase until achieving optimum response. **Furazolidone** may interact similarly with TCAs.

➤*Rash:* Antidepressant drugs can cause skin rashes or "drug fever" in susceptible individuals. These allergic reactions may, in rare cases, be severe. They are more likely to occur during the first few days of treatment but may also occur later. Discontinue if rash or fever develop.

➤*Electroconvulsive therapy:* Electroconvulsive therapy with TCAs may increase the hazards of therapy.

➤*Elective surgery:* Discontinue therapy for as long as possible before elective surgery.

➤*Blood sugar levels:* Elevated and lowered blood sugar levels have occurred.

➤*Sexual dysfunction:* Sexual dysfunction was markedly increased in male patients with OCD taking **clomipramine** (42% ejaculatory failure, 20% impotence) compared with placebo.

➤*Weight changes:* Weight gain has been observed in clinical trials involving all TCAs. Weight gain occurred in 18% of patients receiving **clomipramine**. Some patients had weight gain in excess of 25% of their initial body weight.

➤*Serotonin syndrome:* Some TCAs inhibit neuronal reuptake of serotonin and can increase synaptic serotonin levels (eg, **clomipramine**, **amitriptyline**). Either therapeutic or excessive doses of these drugs, in combination with other drugs that also increase synaptic serotonin levels (such as MAOIs), can cause a serotonin syndrome consisting of tremor, agitation, delirium, rigidity, myoclonus, hyperthermia, and obtundation.

➤*Benzyl alcohol:* Some of these products contain benzyl alcohol, which has been associated with a fatal "gasping syndrome" in premature infants.

➤*Sulfite sensitivity:* Some of the injectable antidepressant products contain sulfites that may cause allergic-type reactions including anaphylactic symptoms and life-threatening or less-severe asthmatic episodes in certain susceptible people. The overall prevalence of sulfite sensitivity in the general population is unknown but is probably low. Sulfite sensitivity is seen more frequently in asthmatic than in non-asthmatic people. Products containing sulfites are identified in the product listings.

➤*Renal/Hepatic function impairment:* Use with caution and in reduced doses in patients with hepatic impairment; metabolism may be impaired, leading to drug accumulation. **Clomipramine** was occasionally associated with AST and ALT elevations (incidence of ≈ 1% and 3%, respectively) of potential clinical importance (values > 3 times the upper limit of normal) but was not associated with other clinical findings suggestive of hepatic injury. Rare reports of more severe liver injury, some fatal, have been reported. Use caution in treating patients with known liver disease, and periodic monitoring of hepatic enzyme levels is recommended in such patients. Use with caution in patients with significantly impaired renal function.

➤*Hazardous tasks:* May impair mental or physical abilities required for the performance of potentially hazardous tasks; have patients observe caution while driving or performing other tasks requiring alertness, coordination, or physical dexterity.

➤*Photosensitivity:* Photosensitization (photoallergy or phototoxicity) may occur; therefore, caution patients to take protective measures (ie, sunscreens, protective clothing) against exposure to ultraviolet light or sunlight until tolerance is determined.

➤*Pregnancy:* (*Category D* - imipramine (per manufacturer's prescribing information), nortriptyline (per manufacturer's prescribing information); *Category C* - amitriptyline, amoxapine, clomipramine, desipramine, doxepin, imipramine (per *Briggs' Drugs in Pregnancy and Lactation*), nortriptyline (per *Briggs' Drugs in Pregnancy and Lactation*), protriptyline, trimipramine). Clinical experience is limited. These agents have demonstrated teratogenicity and embryotoxicity in animals at doses greater than maximum human doses. There have been clinical reports of congenital malformations associated with **imipramine**. Limb reduction anomalies have been reported with **amitriptyline** and **nortriptyline**, and neonatal withdrawal symptoms have been seen with **clomipramine**, **desipramine**, and **imipramine**. All are isolated reports.

Safety for use during pregnancy has not been established; use only when clearly needed and when the potential benefits outweigh the potential hazards to the fetus.

➤*Lactation:* These agents are excreted into breast milk in low concentrations (approximate milk:plasma ratio of 0.4 to 1.5). Exercise caution when using in a nursing woman.

➤*Children:* Not recommended for patients < 12 years of age. Safety and efficacy have not been established for **amoxapine** in children **clomipramine** in children < 10 years of age. The safety and efficacy of **imipramine** as temporary adjunctive therapy for nocturnal enuresis in pediatric patients < 6 years of age have not been established. The safety of the drug for long-term, chronic use as adjunctive therapy for nocturnal enuresis in pediatric patients ≥ 6 years of age has not been established. Safety and efficacy are not established in the pediatric age group for **trimipramine**, **nortriptyline**, **protriptyline**, and **desipramine**.

Do not exceed 2.5 mg/kg/day of **imipramine**. ECG changes of unknown significance have occurred in pediatric patients with doses twice this amount. Effectiveness of imipramine in children for conditions other than nocturnal enuresis has not been established.

AMOXAPINE — ORAL

Administration and Dosage

➤*Adults:*

Depression –

Usual dosage: 200 to 300 mg/day.

Initial dosage: 50 mg 2 or 3 times daily.

Maintenance dosage: Maintenance dosage is the lowest dose that will maintain remission. If symptoms reappear, increase dosage to the earlier level until they are controlled. For maintenance therapy at doses of 300 mg or less, a single bedtime dose is recommended.

Dosage adjustment: Depending upon tolerance, increase dosage to 100 mg 2 or 3 times daily by the end of the first week. Initial dosage of 300 mg/day may cause sedation during the first few days of therapy. Increase above 300 mg/day only if 300 mg/day has been ineffective for at least 2 weeks. If no response is seen at 300 mg, increase dosage, depending upon tolerance, to 400 mg/day. Once an effective dosage is established, the drug may be given in a single bedtime dose (not to exceed 300 mg). If the total daily dosage exceeds 300 mg, give in divided doses.

Three weeks is an adequate trial period providing dosage has reached 300 mg/day (or a lower level of tolerance) for at least 2 weeks.

Hospitalized patients refractory to antidepressant therapy and who have no history of convulsive seizures may have dosage cautiously increased up to 600 mg/day in divided doses.

➤*Children:* Amoxapine is not recommended for patients younger than 16 years of age.

➤*Elderly:* Lower dosages are recommended. Initially, 25 mg 2 or 3 times/day. If tolerated, dosage may be increased by the end of the first week to 50 mg 2 or 3 times/day. Although 100 to 150 mg/day may be adequate for many elderly patients, some may require higher dosage; carefully increase up to 300 mg/day. Once an effective dosage is established, give amoxapine in a single bedtime dose, not to exceed 300 mg.

➤*Storage/Stability:* Store at 15° to 30°C (59° to 86°F). Dispense in a tight container.

CLOMIPRAMINE HYDROCHLORIDE

Rx	**Clomipramine Hydrochloride** (Various, eg, Teva, Watson)	**Capsules:** 25 mg	(Watson 594/25 mg). In 100s and 1,000s.
Rx	**Anafranil** (Novartis)		Parabens. (Anafranil 25 mg). Ivory and melon yellow. In 100s and UD 100s.
Rx	**Clomipramine HCl** (Various, eg, Teva, Watson)	**Capsules:** 50 mg	(Watson 595/50 mg). In 100s and 1,000s.
Rx	**Anafranil** (Novartis)		Parabens. (Anafranil 50 mg). Ivory and aqua blue. In 100s and UD 100s.
Rx	**Clomipramine HCl** (Various, eg, Teva, Watson)	**Capsules:** 75 mg	(Watson 596/75 mg). In 100s and 1,000s.
Rx	**Anafranil** (Novartis)		Parabens. (Anafranil 75 mg). Ivory and yellow. In 100s and UD 100s.

CLOMIPRAMINE HYDROCHLORIDE — ORAL

WARNING

Suicidality in children and adolescents – Antidepressants increased the risk of suicidal thinking and behavior (suicidality) in short-term studies in children and adolescents with major depressive disorder (MDD) and other psychiatric disorders. Anyone considering the use of clomipramine or any other antidepressant in a child or adolescent must balance the risk with the clinical need. Closely observe patients who are started on therapy for clinical worsening, suicidality, or unusual changes in behavior. Advise families and caregivers of the need for close observation and communication with the prescriber. Clomipramine is not approved for use in pediatric patients except for patients with obsessive compulsive disorder (OCD).

Pooled analysis of short-term (4 to 16 weeks) placebo-controlled trials of 9 antidepressant drugs (selective serotonin reuptake inhibitors [SSRIs] and others) in children and adolescence with MDD, OCD, or other psychiatric disorders (a total of 24 trials involving over 4,400 patients) have revealed a greater risk of adverse reactions representing suicidal thinking or behavior (suicidality) during the first few months of treatment in those receiving antidepressants. The average risk of such events in patients receiving antidepressants was 4%, twice the placebo risk of 2%. No suicides occurred in these trials.

Indications

➤*OCD:* Clomipramine is indicated for the treatment of obsessions and compulsions in patients with OCD. The obsessions or compulsions must cause marked distress, be time consuming, or significantly interfere with social or occupational functioning in order to meet the *Diagnostic and Statistical Manual of Mental Disorders, Third Edition, Revised* (*DSM-III-R*) (circa 1989) diagnosis of OCD.

➤*Off-label uses:*

Panic disorder – [2] = Fair documentation. Data from controlled trials suggest that clomipramine is as effective as monotherapy for the treatment of panic disorder. American Psychiatric Association guidelines state that SSRIs, tricyclic antidepressants, benzodiazepines, and monoamine oxidase inhibitors all have roughly comparable efficacy in the treatment of panic disorder, but that SSRIs are likely to have the most favorable balance of efficacy and adverse effects for most patients. (See Administration and Dosage.) (See Administration and Dosage.)

Prevention of migraine (adults) – [5] = Poor documentation. In 2 controlled trials, clomipramine failed to show efficacy for the prevention of migraine headaches in adult patients. American Academy of Neurology practice guidelines state that clomipramine is no more effective than placebo for the prevention of migraines. (See Administration and Dosage.)

Stuttering – [4] = Insufficient documentation. Published information regarding the use of clomipramine for the treatment of stuttering is limited to 2 small trials (less than 20 patients each) performed by the same group of investigators. The trials did not incorporate an adequate washout period between treatment phases. Alternatives are available in this drug class to treat stuttering and larger controlled studies are needed before clomipramine can be recommended for treatment of stuttering. (See Administration and Dosage for Adults and Children.) (See Administration and Dosage.)

Other possible off-label uses – Premenstrual symptoms.

Administration and Dosage

➤*General dosing considerations:* Because both clomipramine and its active metabolite, desmethylclomipramine, have long elimination half-lives, take into consideration the fact that steady-state plasma levels may not be achieved until 2 to 3 weeks after dosage change. Therefore, after initial titration, it may be appropriate to wait 2 to 3 weeks between further dosage adjustments.

➤*Adults:*

Obsessive compulsive disorder –

Maximum dose: 250 mg/day.

Initial dosage: 25 mg/day.

Dosage titration: Gradually increase, as tolerated, to approximately 100 mg/day during the first 2 weeks. During initial titration, clomipramine should be given in divided doses with meals to reduce GI side effects. Thereafter, the dosage may be increased gradually over the next several weeks, up to a maximum of 250 mg/day. After titration, the total daily dose may be given once daily at bedtime to minimize daytime sedation.

Off-label dosing –

Panic disorder: [2] = Fair documentation. Used as monotherapy in doses beginning at 10 mg and increased to a maximum dose of 150 mg given as multiple daily doses.

Stuttering: [4] = Insufficient documentation. Initial dosing was 25 mg twice daily with increases every 4 to 5 days until positive effect was realized, intolerance developed, or a maximum dose of 250 mg daily was reached. Duration of therapy was 5 weeks.

➤*Children:*

Obsessive compulsive disorder –

10 years of age and older:

- *Maximum dose* – 3 mg/kg or 200 mg/day, whichever is smaller.
- *Initial dosage* – 25 mg/day.
- *Dosage titration* – Gradually increase, as tolerated, to a daily maximum dose of 3 mg/kg or 100 mg, whichever is smaller. During initial titration, clomipramine should be given in divided doses with meals to reduce GI side effects. Thereafter, the dosage may be increased gradually over the next several weeks up to a daily maximum dose of 3 mg/kg or 200 mg, whichever is smaller. After titration, the total daily dose may be given once daily at bedtime to minimize daytime sedation.

Off-label dosing –

Stuttering: [4] = Insufficient documentation. In adolescents, initial dosing was 25 mg twice daily with increases every 4 to 5 days until a positive effect was realized, intolerance developed, or a maximum dose of 250 mg daily was reached. Duration of therapy was 5 weeks.

➤*Duration of therapy:* While there are no systematic studies that answer the question of how long to continue clomipramine, OCD is a chronic condition and it is reasonable to consider continuation for a responding patient. Although the efficacy of clomipramine after 10 weeks has not been documented in controlled trials, patients have been continued in therapy under double-blind conditions for up to 1 year without loss of benefit. However, dosage adjustments should be made to maintain the patient on the lowest effective dosage, and patients should be periodically reassessed to determine the need for treatment.

CLOMIPRAMINE HYDROCHLORIDE — ORAL

➤*Administration:* During initial titration, clomipramine should be given in divided doses with meals to reduce GI side effects. After titration, the total daily dose may be given once daily at bedtime to minimize daytime sedation.

The goal of this initial titration phase is to minimize side effects by permitting tolerance to side effects to develop, or allowing the patient time to adapt if tolerance does not develop.

➤*Storage/Stability:* Store at 20° to 25°C (68° to 77°F). Dispense in well-closed containers with a child-resistant closure. Protect from moisture.

DESIPRAMINE HYDROCHLORIDE

Rx	**Desipramine Hydrochloride** (Various, eg, Actavis Totowa, Sandoz)	**Tablets; oral:** 10 mg	May contain lactose, PEG. In 100s.
Rx	**Norpramin** (Sanofi-Aventis)		Mannitol, mineral oil, PEG 8000, soy oil, sucrose. (68-7). Blue. Film-coated. In 100s.
Rx	**Desipramine Hydrochloride** (Various, eg, Actavis Totowa, Sandoz)	**Tablets; oral:** 25 mg	May contain lactose, PEG. In 100s.
Rx	**Norpramin** (Sanofi-Aventis)		Mannitol, mineral oil, PEG 8000, soy oil, sucrose. (NORPRAMIN 25). Yellow. Film-coated. In 100s.
Rx	**Desipramine Hydrochloride** (Various, eg, Actavis Totowa, Sandoz)	**Tablets; oral:** 50 mg	May contain lactose, PEG. In 100s.
Rx	**Norpramin** (Sanofi-Aventis)		Mannitol, mineral oil, PEG 8000, soy oil, sucrose. (NORPRAMIN 50). Green. Film-coated. In 100s.
Rx	**Desipramine Hydrochloride** (Various, eg, Actavis Totowa, Sandoz)	**Tablets; oral:** 75 mg	May contain lactose, PEG. In 100s.
Rx	**Norpramin** (Sanofi-Aventis)		Mannitol, mineral oil, PEG 8000, soy oil, sucrose. (NORPRAMIN 75). Orange. Film-coated. In 100s.
Rx	**Desipramine Hydrochloride** (Various, eg, Actavis Totowa, Sandoz)	**Tablets; oral:** 100 mg	May contain lactose, PEG. In 100s.
Rx	**Norpramin** (Sanofi-Aventis)		Mannitol, mineral oil, PEG 8000, soy oil, sucrose. (NORPRAMIN 100). Peach. Film-coated. In 100s.
Rx	**Desipramine Hydrochloride** (Various, eg, Actavis Totowa, Sandoz)	**Tablets; oral:** 150 mg	May contain lactose, PEG. In 50s.
Rx	**Norpramin** (Sanofi-Aventis)		Mannitol, mineral oil, PEG 8000, soy oil, sucrose. (NORPRAMIN 150). White. Film-coated. In 50s.

DESIPRAMINE HYDROCHLORIDE — ORAL

For complete and comparative prescribing information, refer to the Tricyclic Compounds class monograph.

WARNING

Suicidality and antidepressant drugs – Antidepressants increased the risk of suicidal thinking and behavior (suicidality) in children, adolescents, and young adults in short-term studies of major depressive disorder (MDD) and other psychiatric disorders compared with placebo. Anyone considering the use of desipramine or any other antidepressant in a child, adolescent, or young adult must balance this risk with the clinical need. Short-term studies did not show an increase in the risk of suicidality with antidepressants compared with placebo in adults older than 24 years of age; there was a reduction in risk with antidepressants compared with placebo in adults 65 years of age and older. Depression and certain other psychiatric disorders are themselves associated with increases in the risk of suicide. Closely observe and appropriately monitor patients of all ages who are started on antidepressant therapy for clinical worsening, suicidality, or unusual changes in behavior. Advise families and caregivers of the need for close observation and communication with the prescribing health care provider. Desipramine is not approved for use in children.

Indications

➤*Depression:* For the treatment of depression.

➤*Off-label uses:*

Alcoholism – [4] = Insufficient documentation. Evidence-based guidelines suggest that desipramine may be used to treat alcoholism in adults who have failed treatment with a Food and Drug Administration (FDA)–approved medication. Desipramine may reduce the risk of drinking relapse in some patients with depression; however, no benefit has been reported in patients who have alcoholism in the absence of depression.

Attention deficit hyperactivity disorder (adults) – [4] = Insufficient documentation. Initial data suggest that tricyclic antidepressants (TCAs), such as desipramine, offer an alternative drug therapy option for patients who have an inadequate response to or who do not tolerate standard therapy for attention deficit hyperactivity disorder (ADHD) with stimulant medications. Larger, controlled trials are needed to fully define the efficacy of TCAs in the treatment of adult ADHD.

Attention deficit hyperactivity disorder (children/adolescents) – [3] = Safety concerns. Evidence-based guidelines suggest that desipramine may be used to treat ADHD in children and adolescents; however, it should only be used after a treatment failure with an FDA-approved therapy and other TCAs.

Bulimia nervosa – [2] = Fair documentation. Clinical trials have shown modest benefit with desipramine in past decades, although based on current guidelines, its use may be considered in combination with psychosocial therapy after other first-line medications have proven ineffective. According to American Psychiatric Association guidelines, selective serotonin reuptake inhibitors (SSRIs) are the preferred class of antidepressants for the initial treatment of bulimia nervosa. TCAs, including desipramine, and monoamine oxidase inhibitors (MAOIs) have been used rarely and are not recommended as initial treatments for bulimia nervosa.

Diabetic neuropathy – [4] = Insufficient documentation. Data from controlled trials suggest desipramine may be a treatment option for patients with diabetic neuropathy who cannot tolerate therapy with other tricyclic antidepressants, such as amitriptyline.

Nocturnal enuresis (children/adolescents) – [3] = Safety concerns. No data suggest that desipramine is more effective or better tolerated than imipramine, which has been studied extensively for the treatment of nocturnal enuresis. Although TCAs may reduce the number of nights per week with bedwetting and increase the rates of consistent "dry" sleep, benefits disappear with discontinuation of therapy. Short-term safety risks limit their use, and the long-term adverse effects of continuous TCA administration in children are unknown. American Academy of Child and Adolescent Psychiatry guidelines recommend that children undergo baseline electrocardiograms (ECGs) to evaluate for underlying rhythm disorders before starting a TCA for enuresis.

Postherpetic neuralgia – [1] = Good documentation. Studies have shown positive results with the use of desipramine for the management of pain associated with postherpetic neuralgia (PHN). American Academy of Neurology clinical practice guidelines consider desipramine to be effective for PHN and state that it should be used (level A, class I and II). The guidelines also state that desipramine may offer a reduced risk of cardiac adverse reactions in elderly patients compared with amitriptyline.

Tourette syndrome with comorbid attention deficit hyperactivity disorder (children/adolescents) – [3] = Safety concerns. Initial data from 2 randomized, controlled trials and 1 retrospective chart review suggest desipramine may have a role in the management of children and adolescents with comorbid Tourette syndrome and ADHD. Additional controlled trials are needed to validate these results.

Traumatic brain injury – [3] = Safety concerns. The appropriate use of desipramine in patients with traumatic brain injury has been outlined in Neurobehavioral Guidelines Working Group guidelines. Because desipramine was given the lowest level of recommendation, classification as an option rather than a standard or guideline, closely monitor patients started on therapy for response, and continue therapy only in those patients with sufficient benefit to outweigh the risks of therapy.

Other possible off-label uses – Alcohol dependence and major secondary depression, anxiety (eg, generalized anxiety disorder), enuresis, Tourette syndrome.

Administration and Dosage

➤*General dosing considerations:* Lower dosages are recommended for outpatients compared with hospitalized patients, who are closely supervised.

Following remission, maintenance medication may be required for a period of time and should be at the lowest dose that will maintain remission.

The best available evidence of impending toxicity from very high doses of desipramine is prolongation of the QRS or QT intervals on the ECG. Prolongation of the PR interval is also significant, but less closely correlated with plasma levels. Clinical symptoms of intolerance, especially drowsiness, diz-

DESIPRAMINE HYDROCHLORIDE — ORAL

ziness, and postural hypotension, should also alert the health care provider to the need for reduction in dosage.

➤*Adults:*

Depression –

Usual dosage: 100 to 200 mg/day.

Maximum dose: 300 mg/day.

Dosage titration: Dosage should be initiated at a lower level and increased according to tolerance and clinical response. In more severely ill patients, dosage may be increased gradually to 300 mg/day, if necessary.

Off-label dosing –

Alcoholism: [4] = Insufficient documentation. Desipramine has been titrated based on tolerability, clinical response, and plasma drug concentrations. Median oral dosages ranged from 200 to 275 mg daily.

Attention deficit hyperactivity disorder (adults): [4] = Insufficient documentation. Titrate dose over 2 weeks, up to 200 mg daily given orally; the mean dose reported in a retrospective chart review was 183 mg daily. FDA-approved dosing of desipramine in adults is 100 to 200 mg daily.

Bulimia nervosa: [2] = Fair documentation. 25 mg 3 times per day initially, titrated up to 200 to 300 mg/day, depending on response and adverse effects. Best results were seen with 24 weeks of therapy.

Diabetic neuropathy: [4] = Insufficient documentation. Desipramine 50 to 250 mg taken orally once daily as monotherapy. Study periods ranged from 2 to 6 weeks.

Postherpetic neuralgia: [1] = Good documentation. Mean dosages used were 94 to 167 mg daily for at least 6 weeks.

Traumatic brain injury: [3] = Safety concerns. 25 mg once daily at bedtime, rapidly increased over the first 3 days to 25 mg 3 times daily, followed by increases of 25 mg at 3-day intervals as needed, up to a maximum of 150 mg daily.

➤*Children:*

Depression –

Adolescents:

- *Usual dosage* – 25 to 100 mg/day.
- *Maximum dose* – 150 mg/day.
- *Dosage titration* – Dosage should be initiated at a lower level and increased according to tolerance and clinical response to a usual maximum of 100 mg/day. In more severely ill patients, dosage may be further increased to 150 mg/day.

Off-label dosing –

Attention deficit hyperactivity disorder (children/adolescents): [3] = Safety concerns. In the data reviewed, oral doses varied. The dosage studied in a randomized trial was 75 mg/day. Another trial reported an average daily dosage of 4.6 mg/kg/day. Desipramine should be initiated at the lowest dose and then increased according to tolerability and clinical response.

Nocturnal enuresis (children/adolescents): [3] = Safety concerns. 50 to 75 mg/day, depending on age. The duration of treatment in published studies was 60 days, but enuresis likely requires long-term treatment to maintain therapeutic effect.

Tourette syndrome with comorbid attention deficit hyperactivity disorder (children/adolescents): [3] = Safety concerns. Titrate to 3.5 mg/kg/day or 100 to 150 mg/day orally. The dosage studied in randomized trials ranged from 3.5 mg/kg/day to 100 to 150 mg/day given orally; 3.5 mg/kg/day was also the mean dosage reported in a retrospective chart review. FDA-approved dosing of desipramine in adolescents is 25 to 100 mg daily. Desipramine should be initiated at the lowest dose and then increased according to tolerability and clinical response.

➤*Elderly:*

Depression – See Children for dosing.

➤*Duration of therapy:* Following remission, maintenance medication may be required for a period of time and should be given at the lowest dose that will maintain remission.

➤*Administration:* Initial therapy may be administered in divided doses or a single daily dose. Maintenance therapy may be given on a once-daily schedule for patient convenience and compliance.

➤*Storage/Stability:* Store at 15° to 30°C (59° to 86°F), preferably below 30°C (86°F). Protect from excessive heat.

DOXEPIN

Rx	**Silenor** (Somaxon Pharmaceuticals)	**Tablets,oral** : 3 mg	Equiv to doxepin hydrochloride 3.39 mg. (3 SP). Blue, oval. In 30s, 100s, 500s, and UD 30s.
		6 mg	Equiv to doxepin hydrochloride 6.78 mg. (6 SP). Green, oval. In 30s, 100s, 500s, and UD 30s.
Rx	**Doxepin Hydrochloride** (Various, eg, Par, UDL, URL, Watson)	**Capsules, oral** : 10 mg	In 100s, 500s, 1,000s, and blister pack 100s.
Rx	**Sinequan** (Roerig)		As doxepin hydrochloride. (Sinequan Roerig 534). In 100s and 1,000s.
Rx	**Doxepin Hydrochloride** (Various, eg, Par, UDL, Watson)	**Capsules, oral** : 25 mg	In 100s, 500s, 1,000s, and blister pack 25s and 100s.
Rx	**Sinequan** (Roerig)		As doxepin hydrochloride. (Sinequan Roerig 535). In 100s, 1,000s, and 5000s.
Rx	**Doxepin Hydrochloride** (Various, eg, Par, UDL, Watson)	**Capsules, oral** : 50 mg	In 100s, 500s, 1,000s, and blister pack 25s and 100s.
Rx	**Sinequan** (Roerig)		As doxepin hydrochloride. (Sinequan Roerig 536). In 100s, 1,000s, and 5000s.
Rx	**Doxepin Hydrochloride** (Various, eg, Par, UDL)	**Capsules, oral** : 75 mg	In 100s, 500s, 1,000s, and blister pack 100s.
Rx	**Sinequan** (Roerig)		As doxepin hydrochloride. (Sinequan Roerig 539). In 100s and 1,000s.
Rx	**Doxepin Hydrochloride** (Various, eg, Par, UDL, URL)	**Capsules, oral** : 100 mg	In 100s, 500s, 1,000s, and blister pack 100s.
Rx	**Sinequan** (Roerig)		As doxepin hydrochloride. (Sinequan Roerig 538). In 100s and 1,000s.
Rx	**Doxepin hydrochloride** (Various, eg, Par)	**Capsules, oral** : 150 mg	In 50s, 100s, 500s, and 1,000s.
Rx	**Sinequan** (Roerig)		As doxepin hydrochloride. (Sinequan Roerig 537). In 50s and 500s.
Rx	**Doxepin Hydrochloride** (Various, eg, Copley, Morton Grove)	**Concentrate, oral** : 10 mg/mL	In 120 mL.

DOXEPIN HYDROCHLORIDE — ORAL

For complete and comparative prescribing information, refer to the Tricyclic Compounds group monograph.

WARNING

Suicidality in children and adolescents – Antidepressants increased the risk of suicidal thinking and behavior (suicidality) in short-term studies in children and adolescents with major depressive disorder (MDD) and other psychiatric disorders. Anyone considering the use of doxepin or any other antidepressant in a child or adolescent must balance this risk with the clinical need. Patients who are started on therapy should be observed closely for clinical worsening, suicidality, or unusual changes in behavior. Families and caregivers should be advised of the need for close observation and communication with the prescriber. Doxepin is not approved for use in pediatric patients.

WARNING (cont.)

Pooled analyses of short-term (4 to 16 weeks), placebo-controlled trials of 9 antidepressant drugs (selective serotonin reuptake inhibitor [SSRIs] and others) in children and adolescents with MDD, obsessive-compulsive disorder (OCD), or other psychiatric disorders (a total of 24 trials involving more than 4,400 patients) have revealed a greater risk of adverse reactions representing suicidal thinking or behavior (suicidality) during the first few months of treatment in those receiving antidepressants. The average risk of such reactions in patients receiving antidepressants was 4%, twice the placebo risk of 2%. No suicides occurred in these trials.

Indications

➤*Depression or anxiety:* Doxepin is recommended for the treatment of the following:

1.) Psychoneurotic patients with depression or anxiety.
2.) Depression or anxiety associated with alcoholism (not to be taken concomitantly with alcohol).
3.) Depression or anxiety associated with organic disease (consider the possibility of drug interaction if the patient is receiving other drugs concomitantly).
4.) Psychotic depressive disorders with associated anxiety including involutional depression and manic-depressive disorders.

DOXEPIN HYDROCHLORIDE — ORAL

The target symptoms of psychoneurosis that respond particularly well to doxepin include anxiety, tension, depression, somatic symptoms and concerns, sleep disturbances, guilt, lack of energy, fear, apprehension, and worry.

➤*Insomnia (Silenor only):* For the treatment of insomnia characterized by difficulty with sleep maintenance.

The clinical trials performed in support of efficacy were up to 3 months in duration.

➤*Off-label uses:*

Prevention of migraine (adults) – [2] = Fair documentation. There is a lack of published data on the use of doxepin for the prevention of migraines; the drug has been shown to be effective for the treatment of other types of headaches. American Academy of Neurology practice guidelines state that doxepin is clinically efficacious based on consensus and clinical experience, despite a lack of scientific evidence of efficacy. (See Administration and Dosage.)

Administration and Dosage

➤*General dosing considerations:* Although optimal antidepressant response may not be evident for 2 to 3 weeks, antianxiety activity is rapidly apparent.

The dose of *Silenor* should be individualized.

➤*Adults:*

Depression or anxiety –

Mild to moderate illness:

- *Maximum dose* – 150 mg/day.
- *Initial dosage* – 75 mg/day.
- *Maintenance dosage* – Individualize dosage. Usual optimum dosage is 75 to 150 mg/day. Alternatively, the total daily dosage, up to 150 mg, may be given at bedtime.

Mild symptomatology or emotional symptoms accompanying organic disease: 25 to 50 mg/day is often effective.

More severe illness: Higher dosages (eg, 50 mg 3 times/day) may be required; if necessary, gradually increase to 300 mg/day. Additional effectiveness is rarely obtained by exceeding 300 mg/day.

Insomnia (Silenor) –

Usual dosage: 6 mg once daily. A 3 mg once-daily dosage may be appropriate for some patients, if clinically indicated.

Maximum dose: 6 mg per day.

Off-label dosing –

Prevention of migraine (adults): [2] = Fair documentation. 75 to 150 mg daily, with dosages of up to 300 mg daily occasionally needed.

➤*Children:*

Depression or anxiety – See Adults for dosing for children 12 years of age and older.

Insomnia – Safety and effectiveness in children have not been evaluated.

➤*Elderly:* Carefully adjust the use of doxepin on a once-a-day dosage regimen in elderly patients based on the patient's condition. Sedating drug may cause confusion and oversedation in elderly patients; elderly patients generally should be started on low doses of doxepin and observed closely.

The recommended dosage of *Silenor* in elderly patients (at least 65 years of age) is 3 mg once daily. The daily dose can be increased to 6 mg, if clinically indicated.

➤*Preparation for administration:* Dilute oral concentrate with approximately 120 mL of water, milk, or fruit juice just prior to administration. The oral concentrate is not physically compatible with a number of carbonated beverages. Do not prepare or store bulk dilutions.

➤*Administration: Silenor* should be taken within 30 minutes of bedtime. To minimize the potential for next day effect, *Silenor* should not be taken within 3 hours of a meal.

➤*Storage/Stability:* Store at 20° to 25°C (68° to 77°F). Protect from light. Dispense tablets in a tight, light-resistant container. Preparation and storage of doxepin oral concentrate bulk dilutions are not recommended.

Store *Silenor* at controlled room temperature, 20° to 25°C (68° to 77°F), protected from light.

IMIPRAMINE

Rx	**Imipramine HCl** (Various, eg, Geneva, Mutual, Par, URL)	**Tablets:** 10 mg	In 100s, 250s, 500s, and 1,000s.
Rx	**Tofranil** (Novartis)		(Geigy 32). Coral. Sugar-coated. Triangular. In 100s.
Rx	**Imipramine HCl** (Various, eg, Geneva, Mutual, Par, URL)	**Tablets:** 25 mg	In 100s, 250s, 500s, and 1,000s.
Rx	**Tofranil** (Novartis)		(Geigy 140). Coral, biconvex. Sugar-coated. In 100s.
Rx	**Imipramine HCl** (Various, eg, Geneva, Mutual, Par, URL)	**Tablets:** 50 mg	In 50s, 100s, 250s, 500s, 1,000s, and UD 20s.
Rx	**Tofranil** (Novartis)		(Geigy 136). Coral, biconvex. Sugar-coated. In 100s.
Rx	**Imipramine Pamoate** (Mallinckrodt)	**Capsules:**[a] 75 mg	Parabens. (M 75). Coral. In 30s.
Rx	**Tofranil-PM** (Novartis)		Parabens. (Geigy 20). Coral. In 30s and 100s.
Rx	**Imipramine Pamoate** (Mallinckrodt)	**Capsules:**[a] 100 mg	Parabens. (M 100). Maize. In 30s.
Rx	**Tofranil-PM** (Novartis)		Parabens. (Geigy 40). Dark yellow/coral. In 30s and 100s.
Rx	**Imipramine Pamoate** (Mallinckrodt)	**Capsules:**[a] 125 mg	Parabens. (M 125). Ivory. In 30s.
Rx	**Tofranil-PM** (Novartis)		Parabens. (Geigy 45). Ivory/coral. In 30s and 100s.
Rx	**Imipramine Pamoate** (Mallinckrodt)	**Capsules:**[a] 150 mg	Parabens. (M 150). Coral. In 30s.
Rx	**Tofranil-PM** (Novartis)		Parabens. (Geigy 22). Coral. In 30s and 100s.

[a] Strengths are expressed as imipramine HCl equivalent.

IMIPRAMINE HYDROCHLORIDE — ORAL

For complete and comparative prescribing information, refer to the Tricyclic Compounds group monograph.

WARNING

Suicidality in children and adolescents – Antidepressants increased the risk of suicidal thinking and behavior (suicidality) in short-term studies in children and adolescents with major depressive disorder (MDD) and other psychiatric disorders. Anyone considering the use of imipramine or any other antidepressant in a child or adolescent must balance this risk with the clinical need. Patients who are started on therapy should be observed closely for clinical worsening, suicidality, or unusual changes in behavior. Families and caregivers should be advised of the need for close observation and communication with the prescriber. Imipramine is not approved for use in pediatric patients except for patients with nocturnal enuresis.

WARNING (cont.)

Pooled analyses of short-term (4 to 16 weeks) placebo-controlled trials of 9 antidepressant drugs (SSRIs and others) in children and adolescents with MDD, obsessive-compulsive disorder (OCD), or other psychiatric disorders (a total of 24 trials involving over 4,400 patients) have revealed a greater risk of adverse reactions representing suicidal thinking or behavior (suicidality) during the first few months of treatment in those receiving antidepressants. The average risk of such reactions in patients receiving antidepressants was 4%, twice the placebo risk of 2%. No suicides occurred in these trials.

Indications

➤*Depression:* For the relief of symptoms of depression. Endogenous depression is more likely to be alleviated than other depressive states. One to 3 weeks of treatment may be needed before optimal therapeutic effects are evident.

➤*Childhood enuresis:* May be useful as temporary adjunctive therapy in reducing enuresis in children aged 6 years and older, after possible organic causes have been excluded by appropriate tests. In patients having daytime symptoms of frequency and urgency, examination should include voiding cystourethrography and cystoscopy, as necessary. The effectiveness of treatment may decrease with continued drug administration.

➤*Off-label uses:*

Alcoholism – [4] = Insufficient documentation. Evidence-based guidelines suggest that imipramine may be used in the treatment of alcoholism in

IMIPRAMINE HYDROCHLORIDE — ORAL

patients with primary depression. No benefit has been shown with imipramine in treating alcoholism in the absence of depression.

Attention deficit hyperactivity disorder (children and adolescents) – [1] = Good documentation. Evidence-based guidelines suggest that imipramine may be used to treat attention deficit hyperactivity disorder (ADHD) in children and adolescents secondary to treatment failure with a Food and Drug Administration (FDA)–approved therapy.

Bulimia nervosa – [3] = Safety concerns. Evidence-based guidelines suggest that imipramine may be useful as second-line treatment of bulimia nervosa. Dose reductions or discontinuation of therapy may be necessary to alleviate adverse effects.

Cocaine dependence – [4] = Insufficient documentation. Initial data from 2 controlled trials indicate that imipramine may prolong time of cocaine abstinence in patients who have abused cocaine. Dose reductions or discontinuation of therapy may be necessary to alleviate adverse effects.

Irritable bowel syndrome – [5] = Poor documentation. Initial data from 1 small, noncontrolled trial suggest that imipramine is no better than placebo in affecting global irritable bowel syndrome (IBS) symptoms. The use of this drug is not recommended at this time for the treatment of IBS until further conclusive data suggest benefit.

Narcolepsy – [3] = Safety concerns. American Academy of Sleep Medicine guidelines suggest that tricyclic antidepressants (TCAs), including imipramine, may be used in the treatment of cataplexy in adults who do not respond adequately to sodium oxybate. Clinical trials evaluating imipramine for this use are necessary to clarify its benefit and place in therapy.

Neuropathic pain – [3] = Safety concerns. Evidence-based guidelines suggest that imipramine may be used in the treatment of neuropathic pain in adults if secondary amine TCAs are unavailable. Imipramine has been show to have comparable analgesic efficacy with secondary amine TCAs, but has been associated with an increased risk for adverse effects.

Panic disorder – [3] = Safety concerns. Evidence-based guidelines suggest that imipramine may be used in the treatment of panic disorder. This medication should be avoided in patients with acute narrow-angle glaucoma, significant prostatic hypertrophy, cardiac conduction abnormalities, suicidal ideation, and elderly patients who are likely to fall. Antipanic effects may be seen after 8 to 12 weeks of therapy.

Prevention of migraine (adults) – [2] = Fair documentation. Imipramine has not been formally studied for the prevention of migraine headaches; however, American Academy of Neurology practice guidelines state that imipramine is clinically efficacious based on consensus and clinical experience, despite a lack of scientific evidence of efficacy.

Urinary incontinence – [4] = Insufficient documentation. Initial data from a limited number of trials suggest imipramine may be beneficial for the treatment of urinary incontinence. Larger, controlled trials are needed to confirm these results and establish the role of imipramine in the treatment of urinary incontinence.

Other possible off-label uses – Imipramine has been used in children to treat depression and to augment analgesia in the treatment of chronic pain. (See also Administration and Dosage).

Administration and Dosage

➤*General dosing considerations:* Dosage should be initiated at a low level and increased gradually, carefully noting the clinical response and any evidence of intolerance.

➤*Adults:*

Depression –

Hospitalized patients:

- *Initial dosage* – 100 mg/day in divided doses.
- *Dosage titration* – Gradually increase to 200 mg/day as required. If no response after 2 weeks, increase to 250 to 300 mg/day.

Outpatients:

- *Maximum dose* – 200 mg/day.
- *Initial dosage* – 75 mg/day.
- *Dosage titration* – Increase to 150 mg/day.
- *Maintenance dosage* – 50 mg to 150 mg/day.

Off-label dosing –

Alcoholism: [4] = Insufficient documentation. 50 mg daily orally (initially), titrated by 50 mg every 3 to 5 days to a maximum daily dose of 300 mg.

Bulimia nervosa: [3] = Safety concerns. 50 mg daily (orally) titrated to 100 mg twice daily.

Cocaine dependence: [4] = Insufficient documentation. In controlled trials, an initial dosage of 50 mg daily orally, titrated gradually to 300 mg daily has been used.

Narcolepsy: [3] = Safety concerns. 100 to 200 mg orally daily.

Neuropathic pain: [3] = Safety concerns. Initially 25 mg orally daily at bedtime, titrated by 25 mg daily every 3 to 7 days as tolerated to a maximum dosage of 150 mg daily.

Panic disorder: [3] = Safety concerns. Initially 10 mg orally daily titrated up to 300 mg daily.

Prevention of migraine (adults): [2] = Fair documentation. 10 to 25 mg administered orally 3 times daily in patients with chronic tension headaches.

Urinary incontinence: [4] = Insufficient documentation. The oral dosage studied in an open-label clinical trial was 25 mg given 3 times daily. A second study found 25 mg given twice daily to be an effective dosage. A retrospective case series found doses ranging from 25 to 75 mg to be effective. The FDA-approved initial dosage of imipramine in adults is 25 to 50 mg daily and may be increased to 75 to 100 mg daily.

➤*Children:*

Depression –

Adolescents: Initially, 30 to 40 mg/day; it is generally not necessary to exceed 100 mg/day. (See Off-label dosing).

Nocturnal enuresis –

6 years of age and older: Evidence suggests that in early night bedwetters, the drug is more effective given earlier and in divided amounts (ie, 25 mg in midafternoon, repeated at bedtime). Consideration should be given to instituting a drug-free period following an adequate therapeutic trial with a favorable response.

- *Maximum dose* – 2.5 mg/kg/day. Electrocardiogram (ECG) changes of unknown significance have been reported in children with doses twice this amount. (See Off-label dosing).
- *Initial dosage* – 25 mg/day given 1 hour before bedtime. (See Off-label dosing).
- *Dosage titration* – If a satisfactory response does not occur within 1 week, increase the dose to 50 mg nightly in children younger than 12 years of age; children older than 12 years of age may receive up to 75 mg nightly. A daily dose more than 75 mg does not enhance efficacy and tends to increase adverse reactions.
- *Tapering* – Dosage should be tapered off gradually rather than abruptly discontinued; this may reduce the tendency to relapse. Children who relapse when the drug is discontinued do not always respond to a subsequent course of treatment.

Off-label dosing –

Attention deficit hyperactivity disorder (children and adolescents): [1] = Good documentation. 1 mg/kg/day (initial), titrated to a maximum dose of 4 mg/kg/day or 200 mg/day, whichever is smaller.

Perform an ECG upon initiation and following each dose increase of imipramine. Monitor plasma levels once the patient is on a stable dose to ensure that the level of imipramine is not toxic.

Augment analgesia for chronic pain:

- *Maximum dose* – 1 to 3 mg/kg/dose orally at bedtime.
- *Initial dosage* – 0.2 to 0.4 mg/kg/dose orally at bedtime.
- *Dosage adjustment* – May increase dose by 50% every 2 to 3 days.

Depression:

- *Adolescent* –
  Maximum dose: 200 mg/day.
  Initial dosage: 25 to 50 mg/day administered as a single dose or up to 3 divided doses.
- *Children* –
  Maximum dose: 5 mg/kg/day.
  Initial dosage: 1.5 mg/kg/day administered orally in 3 divided doses.
  Dosage adjustment: Increase by 1 to 1.5 mg/kg/day every 3 to 4 days.

Nocturnal enuresis:

- *6 years of age and older* –
  Maximum dose: 50 mg/day (6 to 12 years of age); 75 mg/day (12 to 14 years of age).
  Initial dosage: 10 to 25 mg at bedtime.
  Dosage titration: 10 to 25 mg/dose at 1 to 2 week intervals until the desired effect or the maximum dose for age is reached.
  Duration of therapy: Patient would then continue that dose for 2 or 3 months, then gradually taper.

➤*Elderly:*

Depression – Initially, 30 to 40 mg/day; it is generally not necessary to exceed 100 mg/day.

➤*Duration of therapy:* Following remission of depression, maintenance medication may be required for a longer period of time at the lowest dose that will maintain remission.

➤*Storage/Stability:* Store between 15° and 30°C (59° and 86°F). Dispense in tight container.

IMIPRAMINE PAMOATE — ORAL

For complete and comparative prescribing information, refer to the Tricyclic Compounds group monograph.

WARNING

Suicidality in children and adolescents – Antidepressants increased the risk of suicidal thinking and behavior (suicidality) in short-term studies in children and adolescents with major depressive disorder (MDD) and other psychiatric disorders. Anyone considering the use of imipramine pamoate or any other antidepressant in a child or adolescent must balance this risk with the clinical need. Patients who are started on therapy should be observed closely for clinical worsening, suicidality, or unusual changes in behavior. Families and caregivers should be advised of the need for close observation and communication with the prescriber. Imipramine pamoate is not approved for use in pediatric patients.

Pooled analyses of short-term (4 to 16 weeks) placebo-controlled trials of 9 antidepressant drugs (SSRIs and others) in children and adolescents with MDD, obsessive-compulsive disorder (OCD), or other psychiatric disorders (a total of 24 trials involving over 4,400 patients) have revealed a greater risk of adverse reactions representing suicidal thinking or behavior (suicidality) during the first few months of treatment in those receiving antidepressants. The average risk of such reactions in patients receiving antidepressants was 4%, twice the placebo risk of 2%. No suicides occurred in these trials.

Indications

➤*Depression:* For the relief of symptoms of depression. Endogenous depression is more likely to be alleviated than other depressive states. One to 3 weeks of treatment may be needed before optimal therapeutic effects are evident.

➤*Off-label uses:*

Alcoholism – [4] = Insufficient documentation. Evidence-based guidelines suggest that imipramine may be used in the treatment of alcoholism in patients with primary depression. No benefit has been shown with imipramine in treating alcoholism in the absence of depression.

Attention deficit hyperactivity disorder (children/adolescents) – [1] = Good documentation. Evidence-based guidelines suggest that imipramine may be used to treat attention deficit hyperactivity disorder (ADHD) in children and adolescents secondary to treatment failure with a Food and Drug Administration (FDA)–approved therapy.

Bulimia nervosa – [3] = Safety concerns. Evidence-based guidelines suggest that imipramine may be useful as second-line treatment of bulimia nervosa. Dose reductions or discontinuation of therapy may be necessary to alleviate adverse effects.

Cocaine dependence – [4] = Insufficient documentation. Initial data from 2 controlled trials indicate that imipramine may prolong time of cocaine abstinence in patients who have abused cocaine. Dose reductions or discontinuation of therapy may be necessary to alleviate adverse effects.

Irritable bowel syndrome – [5] = Poor documentation. Initial data from 1 small, noncontrolled trial suggest that imipramine is no better than placebo in affecting global irritable bowel syndrome (IBS) symptoms. The use of this drug is not recommended at this time for the treatment of IBS until further conclusive data suggest benefit.

Narcolepsy – [3] = Safety concerns. American Academy of Sleep Medicine guidelines suggest that tricyclic antidepressants (TCAs), including imipramine, may be used in the treatment of cataplexy in adults who do not respond adequately to sodium oxybate. Clinical trials evaluating imipramine for this use are necessary to clarify its benefit and place in therapy.

Neuropathic pain – [3] = Safety concerns. Evidence-based guidelines suggest that imipramine may be used in the treatment of neuropathic pain in adults if secondary amine TCAs are unavailable. Imipramine has been shown to have comparable analgesic efficacy with secondary amine TCAs, but has been associated with an increased risk for adverse effects.

Panic disorder – [3] = Safety concerns. Evidence-based guidelines suggest that imipramine may be used in the treatment of panic disorder. This medication should be avoided in patients with acute narrow-angle glaucoma, significant prostatic hypertrophy, cardiac conduction abnormalities, suicidal ideation, and elderly patients who are likely to fall. Antipanic effects may be seen after 8 to 12 weeks of therapy.

Prevention of migraine (adults) – [2] = Fair documentation. Imipramine has not been formally studied for the prevention of migraine headaches; however, American Academy of Neurology practice guidelines state that imipramine is clinically efficacious based on consensus and clinical experience, despite a lack of scientific evidence of efficacy.

Urinary incontinence – [4] = Insufficient documentation. Initial data from a limited number of trials suggest imipramine may be beneficial for the treatment of urinary incontinence. Larger, controlled trials are needed to confirm these results and establish the role of imipramine in the treatment of urinary incontinence.

Administration and Dosage

➤*Maximum dose:*

Adults and adolescents – There is no well-established maximum dose for the approved indication according to the prescribing information. However, maximum doses have been established off-label. (See Adults and Children.)

Children – Not approved for use in children according to the prescribing information. However, a maximum dose has been established off-label. (See Children.)

➤*General dosing considerations:* As with all tricyclics, the antidepressant effect of imipramine may not be evident for 1 to 3 weeks in some patients.

In cases of relapse because of premature withdrawal of the drug, the effective dosage of imipramine should be reinstituted.

Each capsule contains imipramine pamoate equivalent to imipramine hydrochloride 75, 100, 125, or 150 mg.

➤*Adults:*

Depression – The total daily dosage can be administered on a once-daily basis, preferably at bedtime. In some patients it may be necessary to employ a divided-dose schedule.

Initial dosage:

• *Hospitalized patients* – Initially, 100 to 150 mg/day and may be increased to 200 mg/day. If there is no response after 2 weeks, dosage should be increased to 250 to 300 mg/day.

Dosage higher than 150 mg/day may also be administered on a once-daily basis, after the optimum dosage and tolerance have been determined.

• *Outpatients* – Initially, 75 mg/day and may be increased to 150 mg/day, which is the dose level at which optimum response is usually obtained. If necessary, dosage may be increased to 200 mg/day.

Dosage higher than 75 mg/day may also be administered on a once-daily basis after the optimum dosage and tolerance have been determined.

Maintenance dosage: 75 to 150 mg/day.

Off-label dosing –

Alcoholism: [4] = Insufficient documentation. 50 mg daily orally (initially), titrated by 50 mg every 3 to 5 days to a maximum daily dose of 300 mg.

Bulimia nervosa: [3] = Safety concerns. 50 mg daily (orally) titrated to 100 mg twice daily.

Cocaine dependence: [4] = Insufficient documentation. In controlled trials, an initial dosage of 50 mg daily orally, titrated gradually to 300 mg daily has been used.

Narcolepsy: [3] = Safety concerns. 100 to 200 mg orally daily.

Neuropathic pain: [3] = Safety concerns. Initially 25 mg daily at bedtime, titrated by 25 mg daily every 3 to 7 days as tolerated to a maximum dosage of 150 mg daily.

Panic disorder: [3] = Safety concerns. Initially 10 mg orally daily titrated up to 300 mg daily.

Prevention of migraine (adults): [2] = Fair documentation. 10 to 25 mg administered orally 3 times daily in patients with chronic tension headaches.

Urinary incontinence: [4] = Insufficient documentation. The oral dosage studied in an open-label clinical trial was 25 mg given 3 times daily. A second study found 25 mg given twice daily to be an effective dosage. A retrospective case series found doses ranging from 25 to 75 mg to be effective. The FDA-approved initial dosage of imipramine in adults is 25 to 50 mg daily and may be increased to 75 to 100 mg daily.

➤*Children:*

Depression –

Adolescents: The total daily dosage can be administered on a once-daily basis, preferably at bedtime. In some patients it may be necessary to employ a divided-dose schedule.

• *Initial dosage* – Therapy should be initiated with imipramine hydrochloride tablets at a total daily dosage of 25 to 50 mg because imipramine pamoate capsules are not available in these strengths.

• *Dosage titration* – Dosage may be increased according to response and tolerance, but it is generally unnecessary to exceed 100 mg/day in these patients. Imipramine pamoate capsules may be used when total daily dosage is established at 75 mg or higher.

• *Maintenance dosage* – Adolescents can usually be maintained on a lower dosage.

Off-label dosing –

Attention deficit hyperactivity disorder (children/adolescents): [1] = Good documentation. 1 mg/kg/day (initial), titrated to a maximum dose of 4 mg/kg/day or 200 mg/day, whichever is smaller.

Upon initiation and following each dose increase of imipramine, perform an electrocardiogram. Monitor plasma levels once the patient is on a stable dose to ensure that the level of imipramine is not toxic.

➤*Elderly:*

Depression – The total daily dosage can be administered on a once-daily basis, preferably at bedtime. In some patients it may be necessary to employ a divided-dose schedule.

Initial dosage: Therapy should be initiated with imipramine hydrochloride tablets at a total daily dosage of 25 to 50 mg because imipramine pamoate capsules are not available in these strengths.

Dosage titration: Dosage may be increased according to response and tolerance, but it is generally unnecessary to exceed 100 mg/day in these patients. Imipramine pamoate capsules may be used when total daily dosage is established at 75 mg or higher.

Maintenance dosage: Elderly patients can usually be maintained at a lower dosage.

➤*Duration of therapy:* Following remission, maintenance medication may be required for a longer period of time at the lowest dose that will maintain remission, after which the dosage should gradually be decreased.

➤*Storage/Stability:* Do not store above 30°C (86°F). Dispense in tight container.

NORTRIPTYLINE HYDROCHLORIDE

Rx	**Nortriptyline HCl** (Various, eg, Geneva, Teva, UDL)	**Capsules; oral:** 10 mg	In 100s, 500s, 1,000s, blister pack 25s, 100s, and 600s, and UD 100s.
Rx	**Pamelor** (Mallinckrodt)		(PAMELOR 10 mg M). Orange/White. In 30s.[a]
Rx	**Nortriptyline HCl** (Various, eg, Geneva, Teva, UDL)	**Capsules; oral:** 25 mg	In 100s, 500s, 1,000s, blister pack 25s, 100s, and 600s, and UD 100s.
Rx	**Aventyl HCl Pulvules** (Eli Lilly)		(Lilly H19). White/yellow. In 100s and 500s.
Rx	**Pamelor** (Mallinckrodt)		(PAMELOR 25 mg M). Lt orange/white. In 30s.[a]
Rx	**Nortriptyline HCl** (Various, eg, Geneva, Teva)	**Capsules; oral:** 50 m	In 100s, 500s, 1,000s, blister pack 25s, 100s, and 600s, and UD 100s.
Rx	**Pamelor** (Mallinckrodt)		(Sandoz PAMELOR 50 mg M). White. In 30s.[a]
Rx	**Nortriptyline HCl** (Various, eg, Geneva, Teva)	**Capsules; oral:** 75 mg	In 100s, 500s, 1,000s, and blister pack 100s and 600s.
Rx	**Pamelor** (Mallinckrodt)		(PAMELOR 75 mg). Lt orange. In 30s.[a]
Rx	**Nortriptyline HCl** (Ranbaxy)	**Solution; oral:** 10 mg base/5 mL	In 480 mL.[b]

[a] With benzyl alcohol, sorbitol.
[b] With 4% alcohol, sorbitol.
[c] With 3.4% alcohol.

NORTRIPTYLINE HYDROCHLORIDE — ORAL

For complete and comparative prescribing information, refer to the Tricyclic Compounds group monograph.

WARNING

Suicidality in children and adolescents – Antidepressants increased the risk of suicidal thinking and behavior (suicidality) in short-term studies in children and adolescents with major depressive disorder (MDD) and other psychiatric disorders. Anyone considering the use of nortriptyline or any other antidepressant in a child or adolescent must balance this risk with the clinical need. Patients who are started on therapy should be observed closely for clinical worsening, suicidality, or unusual changes in behavior. Families and caregivers should be advised of the need for close observation and communication with the prescriber. Nortriptyline is not approved for use in pediatric patients.

Pooled analyses of short-term (4 to 16 weeks) placebo-controlled trials of 9 antidepressant drugs (SSRIs and others) in children and adolescents with MDD, obsessive-compulsive disorder (OCD), or other psychiatric disorders (a total of 24 trials involving over 4,400 patients) have revealed a greater risk of adverse reactions representing suicidal thinking or behavior (suicidality) during the first few months of treatment in those receiving antidepressants. The average risk of such reactions in patients receiving antidepressants was 4%, twice the placebo risk of 2%. No suicides occurred in these trials.

Indications

➤*Depression:* Nortriptyline HCl is indicated for the relief of symptoms of depression. Endogenous depressions are more likely to be alleviated than are other depressive states.

➤*Off-label uses:*

Attention deficit hyperactivity disorder (adults) – [3] = Safety concerns. Initial data suggest that tricyclic antidepressants (TCAs) may be an alternative drug therapy option for patients who have an inadequate response to or do not tolerate standard therapy for attention deficit hyperactivity disorder (ADHD) with stimulant medications. There are more data in the pediatric population than for adults; however, in the retrospective review available, nortriptyline was well tolerated and led to 42% of patients being improved or much improved, as measured by the Clinical Global Improvement scale. Larger, controlled trials are needed to fully define the efficacy of TCAs such as nortriptyline in the treatment of adult ADHD.

Attention deficit hyperactivity disorder (children and adolescents) – [3] = Safety concerns. Evidence-based guidelines confirm the use of nortriptyline in children and adolescents with ADHD as an acceptable second-line therapy for patients who did not respond or had a partial response to Food and Drug Administration (FDA)-approved medications.

Prevention of migraine (adults) – [4] = Insufficient documentation. Nortriptyline has not been formally studied for the prevention of migraine headache. American Academy of Neurology practice guidelines consider nortriptyline to be clinically efficacious based on consensus and clinical experience, despite a lack of scientific evidence of efficacy. No dosing was reported.

Postherpetic neuralgia – [1] = Good documentation. Studies have shown positive results with the use of nortriptyline for the management of pain associated with postherpetic neuralgia (PHN). American Academy of Neurology clinical practice guidelines state that nortriptyline is effective for PHN and that it should be used (level A, class I and II). They further state that, compared with amitriptyline, nortriptyline may offer a reduced risk of cardiac adverse effects in elderly patients.

Smoking cessation – [3] = Safety concerns. Most studies evaluating nortriptyline as an aid in smoking cessation have produced consistent data for its efficacy in this setting. Several randomized, placebo-controlled trials have shown a long-term benefit in using nortriptyline to improve cessation rates. Nortriptyline may be indicated if patients have failed first-line agents or have contraindications to them. Guidelines from the VA specify that treatment with the antidepressant nortriptyline is recommended as a second-line agent. Some clinicians have argued that the efficacy of nortriptyline coupled with its low cost should make it a first-line therapy in smoking cessation. Others have cited its poor adverse effect profile and the fact that fewer smokers have been exposed to nortriptyline in reliable trials as reasons to keep it as a second-line drug.

As evidenced by the black box warning for nortriptyline, this drug is not without risk. Additionally, it has a more bothersome adverse effect profile than therapeutic alternatives. Although there are data showing the efficacy of nortriptyline in smoking cessation, a recent large trial showed no significant difference over placebo. Clinicians must evaluate individual patient contraindications, treatment history, and comorbidities to determine if nortriptyline is the most appropriate cessation therapy choice.

Administration and Dosage

➤*Adults:*

Depression –

Usual dosage: 25 mg 3 to 4 times daily.
Maximum dose: 150 mg/day.
Alternative dosage: Total daily dose can be given at bedtime.

Off-label dosing –

Attention deficit hyperactivity disorder (adults): [3] = Safety concerns. The mean dose reported in a retrospective chart review was 91.7 ± 37.4 mg. FDA-approved dosing of nortriptyline in adults is 25 mg 3 to 4 times daily.

Postherpetic neuralgia: [1] = Good documentation. Oral nortriptyline (mean dosage, between 58 and 89 mg daily) for at least 5 weeks.

Smoking cessation: [3] = Safety concerns. 75 to 100 mg orally daily for at least 7 to 14 weeks, starting 1 to 2 weeks before the quit date. A single study has examined use for up to 52 weeks.

➤*Children:*

Depression –

Adolescents: 30 to 50 mg once daily or in divided doses.

Off-label dosing –

Attention deficit hyperactivity disorder (children and adolescents): [3] = Safety concerns. 0.5 mg/kg/day, titrated to a maximum dose of 2 mg/kg/day or 100 mg, whichever is less.

Depression:

• *6 to 12 years of age* – 1 to 3 mg/kg/day divided 3 to 4 times a day or 10 to 20 mg/day divided 3 to 4 times a day.

Nocturnal enuresis:

Nortriptyline Dosage for Children With Nocturnal Enuresis

Age	Dosage
> 11 years of age (36 to 54 kg)	25 to 35 mg at bedtime
8 to 11 years of age (26 to 35 kg)	10 to 20 mg at bedtime
6 to 7 years of age (20 to 25 kg)	10 mg at bedtime

➤*Elderly:* 30 to 50 mg once daily or in divided doses.

➤*Therapeutic drug monitoring:* When doses more than 100 mg/day are given, plasma levels of nortriptyline should be monitored and maintained in the optimum range of 50 to 150 ng/mL.

➤*Storage/Stability:* Store capsules below 30°C (86°F). Store solution at 25°C (77°F); excursions permitted to 15° to 30°C (59° to 86°F).

PROTRIPTYLINE HYDROCHLORIDE

Rx	**Protriptyline HCl** (Various, eg, Sidmak)	**Tablets:** 5 mg	In 100s and 1,000s.
Rx	**Vivactil** (Duramed)		Lactose. (MSD 26). Orange. Oval. Film coated. In 100s.
Rx	**Protriptyline HCl** (Various, eg, Sidmak)	**Tablets:** 10 mg	In 100s and 1,000s.
Rx	**Vivactil** (Duramed)		Lactose. (MSD 47). Yellow. Oval. Film coated. In 100s and UD 100s.

PROTRIPTYLINE HYDROCHLORIDE — ORAL

For complete and comparative prescribing information, refer to the Tricyclic Compounds group monograph.

WARNING

Suicidality in children and adolescents – Antidepressants increased the risk of suicidal thinking and behavior (suicidality) in short-term studies in children and adolescents with major depressive disorder (MDD) and other psychiatric disorders. Anyone considering the use of protriptyline or any other antidepressant in a child or adolescent must balance this risk with the clinical need. Closely observe patients who are started on therapy for clinical worsening, suicidality, or unusual changes in behavior. Advise families and caregivers of the need for close observation and communication with the prescriber. Protriptyline is not approved for use in pediatric patients.

Pooled analyses of short-term (4 to 16 weeks) placebo-controlled trials of 9 antidepressant drugs (selective serotonin reuptake inhibitors [SSRIs] and others) in children and adolescents with MDD, obsessive-compulsive disorder (OCD), or other psychiatric disorders (a total of 24 trials involving over 4,400 patients) have revealed a greater risk of adverse reactions representing suicidal thinking or behavior (suicidality) during the first few months of treatment in those receiving antidepressants. The average risk of such reactions in patients receiving antidepressants was 4%, twice the placebo risk of 2%. No suicides occurred in these trials.

Indications

➤*Depression:* Protriptyline is indicated for the treatment of symptoms of mental depression in patients who are under close medical supervision. Its activating properties make it particularly suitable for withdrawn and anergic patients.

➤*Off-label uses:*

Prevention of migraine (adults) – [4] = Insufficient documentation. Protriptyline has not been formally studied for the prevention of migraine headache; however, American Academy of Neurology practice guidelines state that protriptyline is clinically efficacious based on consensus and clinical experience, despite a lack of scientific evidence of efficacy. No dosing was reported.

Administration and Dosage

➤*General dosing considerations:* Dosage should be initiated at a low level and increased gradually, noting carefully the clinical response and any evidence of intolerance.

Minor adverse reactions require reduction in dosage. Major adverse reactions or evidence of hypersensitivity require prompt discontinuation of the drug.

➤*Adults:*

Depression –

Usual dosage: 15 to 40 mg/day divided into 3 or 4 doses.

Maximum dose: 60 mg/day.

Maintenance dosage: When satisfactory improvement has been reached, dosage should be reduced to the smallest amount that will maintain relief of symptoms.

Dosage adjustment: May be increased to 60 mg/day. Increases should be made in the morning dose.

➤*Children:*

Depression –

Adolescents: In general, lower dosages are recommended for these patients.

- *Initial dosage* – 5 mg 3 times/day, and increased gradually if necessary.
- *Maintenance dosage* – When satisfactory improvement has been reached, dosage should be reduced to the smallest amount that will maintain relief of symptoms.

➤*Elderly:* In general, lower dosages are recommended for these patients. The cardiovascular system must be monitored closely if the daily dose exceeds 20 mg.

Initial dosage – 5 mg 3 times/day and increased gradually if necessary.

Maintenance dosage – When satisfactory improvement has been reached, dosage should be reduced to the smallest amount that will maintain relief of symptoms.

➤*Storage/Stability:* Store at 20° to 25°C (68° to 77°F).in a tightly closed container.

TRIMIPRAMINE MALEATE

Rx	**Surmontil** (Duramed)	**Capsules:** 25 mg	Lactose. (Wyeth 4132). Opaque blue/yellow. In 100s.
		50 mg	Lactose. (Wyeth 4133). Opaque blue/orange. In 100s and UD 100s.
		100 mg	Lactose. (Wyeth 4158). Opaque blue/white. In 100s.

TRIMIPRAMINE MALEATE — ORAL

For complete and comparative prescribing information, refer to the Tricyclic Compounds group monograph.

WARNING

Suicidality in children and adolescents – Antidepressants increased the risk of suicidal thinking and behavior (suicidality) in short-term studies in children and adolescents with major depressive disorder (MDD) and other psychiatric disorders. Anyone considering the use of trimipramine or any other antidepressant in a child or adolescent must balance this risk with the clinical need. Patients who are started on therapy should be observed closely for clinical worsening, suicidality, or unusual changes in behavior. Families and caregivers should be advised of the need for close observation and communication with the prescriber. Trimipramine is not approved for use in pediatric patients.

Pooled analyses of short-term (4 to 16 weeks) placebo-controlled trials of 9 antidepressant drugs (SSRIs and others) in children and adolescents with MDD, obsessive-compulsive disorder (OCD), or other psychiatric disorders (a total of 24 trials involving over 4,400 patients) have revealed a greater risk of adverse reactions representing suicidal thinking or behavior (suicidality) during the first few months of treatment in those receiving antidepressants. The average risk of such reactions in patients receiving antidepressants was 4%, twice the placebo risk of 2%. No suicides occurred in these trials.

Indications

➤*Depression:* Trimipramine maleate is indicated for the relief of symptoms of depression. Endogenous depression is more likely to be alleviated than other depressive states. In studies with neurotic outpatients, the drug appeared to be equivalent to amitriptyline in the less-depressed patients but somewhat less effective than amitriptyline in the more severely depressed patients. In hospitalized depressed patients, trimipramine and imipramine were equally effective in relieving depression.

Administration and Dosage

➤*Adults:*

Depression –

Hospitalized patients:

- *Maximum dose* – 300 mg/day.
- *Initial dosage* – 100 mg/day in divided doses.
- *Dosage titration* – Increase gradually in a few days to 200 mg/day depending upon individual response and tolerance. If improvement does not occur in 2 to 3 weeks, increase to a maximum dose of 250 to 300 mg/day.
- *Maintenance dosage* – Maintenance medication may be required at the lowest dose that will maintain remission (range, 50 to 150 mg/day). Administer as a single bedtime dose. To minimize relapse, continue maintenance therapy for approximately 3 months.

Outpatients:

- *Maximum dose* – 200 mg/day.
- *Initial dosage* – 75 mg/day in divided doses; increase to 150 mg/day. The total dosage requirement may be given at bedtime.
- *Maintenance dosage* – Maintenance medication may be required at the lowest dose that will maintain remission (range, 50 to 150 mg/day). To minimize relapse, continue maintenance therapy for approximately 3 months. Administer as a single bedtime dose.

➤*Children:*

Depression –

Adolescents: Initially, 50 mg/day, with gradual increments up to 100 mg/day.

➤*Elderly:* Initially, 50 mg/day, with gradual increments up to 100 mg/day.

➤*Storage/Stability:* Store at 20° to 25°C (68° to 77°F). Keep bottles tightly closed. Dispense in a tight container.

Refer to the Antidepressants introduction.

WARNING

Suicidality and antidepressant drugs – Antidepressants increased the risk, compared with placebo, of suicidal thinking and behavior (suicidality) in children, adolescents, and young adults in short-term studies of major depressive disorder (MDD) and other psychiatric disorders. Anyone considering the use of maprotiline, mirtazapine, or any other antidepressant in a child, adolescent, or young adult must balance this risk with the clinical need. Short-term studies did not show an increase in the risk of suicidality with antidepressants compared with placebo in adults older than 24 years of age; there was a reduction in risk with antidepressants compared with placebo in adults 65 years of age and older. Depression and certain other psychiatric disorders are themselves associated with increases in the risk of suicide. Appropriately monitor patients of all ages who are started on antidepressant therapy and closely observe for clinical worsening, suicidality, or unusual changes in behavior. Advise families and caregivers of the need for close observation and communication with the prescriber. Maprotiline and mirtazapine are not approved for use in children.

Indications

➤*Depression:* **Maprotiline** is indicated for the treatment of depressive illness in patients with depressive neurosis (dysthymic disorder) and manic-depressive illness, depressed-type.

Mirtazapine is indicated for the treatment of MDD.

➤*Anxiety:* **Maprotiline** is effective for the relief of anxiety associated with depression.

➤*Off-label uses:* Refer to individual monographs for further information.

Chronic urticaria –

Mirtazapine: [3] = Safety concerns.

Hot flashes –

Mirtazapine: [4] = Insufficient documentation.

Hyperhidrosis (drug-induced) –

Mirtazapine: [4] = Insufficient documentation.

Postherpetic neuralgia –

Maprotiline: [1] = Good documentation.

Prevention of migraine (adults) –

Mirtazapine: [4] = Insufficient documentation.

Pruritus –

Mirtazapine: [3] = Safety concerns.

Actions

➤*Pharmacology:* The mechanism of action of tetracyclic antidepressants is not precisely known. **Maprotiline** and **mirtazapine** are both considered tetracyclic antidepressants (because of their chemical structures), but they each affect different neurotransmitters and, thus, have different adverse reaction profiles.

Maprotiline primarily acts by potentiation of central adrenergic synapses by blocking reuptake of norepinephrine at nerve endings. This pharmacologic action is thought to be responsible for its antidepressant and anxiolytic effects.

Evidence suggests that mirtazapine enhances central noradrenergic and serotonergic activity. It also acts as an antagonist at central presynaptic alpha-2 adrenergic inhibitory autoreceptors and heteroreceptors, an action that is postulated to result in an increase in central noradrenergic and serotonergic activity. Mirtazapine is a potent antagonist of 5-HT_2 and 5-HT_3 receptors. It does not have significant affinity for the 5-HT_{1A} and 5-HT_{1B} receptors. It is a potent antagonist of histamine (H_1) receptors, a property that may explain its prominent sedative effects. It also is a moderate antagonist at muscarinic receptors, a property that may explain the relatively low incidence of anticholinergic adverse reactions. Mirtazapine is a moderate peripheral alpha-1 adrenergic antagonist, a property that may explain the occasional orthostatic hypotension associated with its use.

➤*Pharmacokinetics:*

Summary of Pharmacokinetics of Tetracyclic Antidepressants

Parameter	Maprotiline	Mirtazapine
Bioavailability	66% to 75%	≈ 50%
T_{max}[a]	12 hours	2 hours
Protein binding	88%	≈ 85%
Metabolism	Metabolized to desmethyl-maprotiline (active)	Demethylation and hydroxylation followed by glucuronide conjugation. CYP2D6, 1A2, and 3A are also involved with formation of metabolites.
Routes of elimination	Urine (≈ 66%), feces (≈ 33%)	Urine (75%), feces (15%)
Half-life	51 hours	20 to 40 hours
Therapeutic plasma concentration	200 to 300 ng/mL	No data

[a] T_{max} = time to maximal concentration.

Absorption/Distribution – **Maprotiline** is slowly and completely absorbed after oral administration, and steady state is achieved after 1 week of therapy.

Mirtazapine tablets are rapidly and completely absorbed following oral administration. The presence of food in the stomach has a minimal effect on the rate and extent of absorption and does not require a dosage adjustment. Steady-state plasma levels of mirtazapine are attained within 5 days. Plasma levels are linearly related to dose over a dose range of 15 to 80 mg.

Metabolism/Excretion – **Maprotiline** is slowly eliminated, primarily as metabolites (most of which are glucuronides).

Mirtazapine is extensively metabolized after oral administration. Major pathways of biotransformation are demethylation and hydroxylation followed by glucuronide conjugation. In vitro, CYP2D6 and 1A2 are involved in the formation of the 8-hydroxy metabolite of mirtazapine, whereas CYP3A is considered to be responsible for the formation of the N-desmethyl and N-oxide metabolite. Several unconjugated metabolites possess pharmacologic activity but are present in the plasma at very low levels. The (−) enantiomer has an elimination half-life that is approximately twice as long as the (+) enantiomer and, therefore, achieves plasma levels that are approximately 3 times as high.

Special populations –

Renal function impairment: The disposition of **mirtazapine** was studied in patients with varying degrees of renal function. Elimination of mirtazapine is correlated with creatinine clearance (CrCl). Total body clearance of mirtazapine was reduced approximately 30% in patients with moderate (CrCl 11 to 39 mL/min per 1.73 m^2) renal function impairment and approximately 50% in patients with severe (CrCl less than 10 mL/min per 1.73 m^2) renal function impairment compared with healthy subjects. Caution is indicated when administering mirtazapine to patients with compromised renal function.

Hepatic function impairment: Following a single oral dose of **mirtazapine** 15 mg, the oral clearance of mirtazapine was decreased by approximately 30% in patients with hepatic function impairment, compared with subjects with healthy hepatic function. Caution is indicated when administering mirtazapine to patients with compromised hepatic function.

Elderly: Following oral administration of **mirtazapine** 20 mg/day for 7 days to subjects of varying ages (range, 25 to 74 years), oral clearance of mirtazapine was reduced in elderly patients compared with younger subjects. The differences were most striking in men, with a 40% lower clearance in elderly men compared with younger men, while the clearance in elderly women was only 10% lower compared with younger women. Caution is indicated when administering mirtazapine to elderly patients.

Gender: Women of all ages exhibited significantly longer elimination half-lives than men (mean half-life, 37 hours for women vs 26 hours for men) with use of **mirtazapine**.

Contraindications

Hypersensitivity to **maprotiline** or **mirtazapine**.

➤*Maprotiline:* Known or suspected seizure disorder; use during acute phase of myocardial infarction (MI); coadministration with monoamine oxidase inhibitors (MAOIs). (See also Warnings/Precautions and Drug Interactions.)

Warnings/Precautions

➤*Clinical worsening and suicide risk:* Adults and children with MDD may experience worsening of their depression and/or the emergence of suicidal ideation and behavior (suicidality) or unusual changes in behavior, whether or not they are taking antidepressant medications, and this risk may persist until significant remission occurs. Suicide is a known risk of depression and certain other psychiatric disorders, and these disorders themselves are the strongest predictors of suicide. There has been a long-standing concern, however, that antidepressants may have a role in inducing worsening of depression and the emergence of suicidality in certain patients during the early phases of treatment. Pooled analyses of short-term, placebo-controlled trials of antidepressant drugs (SSRIs and others) showed that these drugs increase the risk of suicidal thinking and behavior (suicidality) in children, adolescents, and young adults (18 to 24 years of age) with MDD and other psychiatric disorders. Short-term studies did not show an increase in the risk of suicidality with antidepressants compared with placebo in adults older than 24 years of age; there was a reduction in risk with antidepressants compared with placebo in adults 65 years of age and older.

The pooled analyses of placebo-controlled trials in children and adolescents with MDD, obsessive-compulsive disorder, or other psychiatric disorders included a total of 24 short-term trials of 9 antidepressant drugs in more than 4,400 patients. The pooled analyses of placebo-controlled trials in adults with MDD or other psychiatric disorders included a total of 295 short-term trials (median duration of 2 months) of 11 antidepressant drugs in more than 77,000 patients. There was considerable variation in risk of suicidality among drugs, but there was a tendency toward an increase in younger patients for almost all drugs studied. There were differences in absolute risk of suicidality across different indications, with the highest incidence in MDD. However, the risk differences (drug vs placebo) were relatively stable within age strata and across indications.

No suicides occurred in any of the pediatric trials. There were suicides in the adult trials, but the number was not sufficient to reach any conclusion about drug effect on suicide.

It is unknown whether the suicidality risk extends to longer-term use (ie, beyond several months). However, there is substantial evidence from placebo-controlled, maintenance trials in adults with depression that the use of antidepressants can delay the recurrence of depression.

Monitor all patients being treated with antidepressants for any indication and closely observe for clinical worsening, suicidality, and unusual changes in behavior, especially during the initial few months of a course of drug therapy, or at times of dose changes, either increases or decreases.

The following symptoms have been reported in adults and children being treated with antidepressants for MDD as well as for other indications, both psychiatric and nonpsychiatric: anxiety, agitation, panic attacks, insomnia, irritability, hostility, aggressiveness, impulsivity, akathisia (psychomotor restlessness), hypomania, and mania. Although a causal link between the emergence of such symptoms and the worsening of depression and/or the emergence of suicidal impulses has not been established, there is concern that such symptoms may represent precursors to emerging suicidality.

Consider changing the therapeutic regimen, including possibly discontinuing the medication, in patients whose depression is persistently worse or who are experiencing emergent suicidality or symptoms that might be precursors to worsening depression or suicidality, especially if these symptoms are severe, abrupt in onset, or were not part of the patient's presenting symptoms.

Alert families and caregivers of patients being treated with antidepressants for MDD or other indications, both psychiatric and nonpsychiatric, about the need to monitor patients for the emergence of agitation, irritability, unusual changes in behavior, and other symptoms previously described, as well as the emergence of suicidality, and to report such symptoms immediately to the health care provider. Such monitoring should include daily observation by family and caregivers. Prescribe the smallest quantity of tablets consistent with good patient management in order to reduce the risk of overdose.

➤*Screening for bipolar disorder:* A major depressive episode may be the initial presentation of bipolar disorder. It is generally believed (although not established in controlled trials) that treating such an episode with an antidepressant alone may increase the likelihood of precipitation of a mixed/manic episode in patients at risk for bipolar disorder. Whether any of the symptoms described represent such a conversion is unknown. However, prior to initiating treatment with an antidepressant, adequately screen patients with depressive symptoms to determine whether they are at risk for bipolar disorder; such screening should include a detailed psychiatric history, including a family history of suicide, bipolar disorder, and depression. Note that **maprotiline** and **mirtazapine** are not approved for treating bipolar disorder.

➤*Seizures:* Seizures have been associated with the use of **maprotiline**. Most of the seizures have occurred in patients without a known history of seizures. However, in some of these cases, other confounding factors were present, including concomitant medications known to lower the seizure threshold, rapid escalation of the dosage of maprotiline, and dosage that exceeded the recommended therapeutic range. The incidence of direct reports is less than 0.1%. The risk of seizures may be increased when maprotiline is taken concomitantly with phenothiazines, when the dosage of benzodiazepines is rapidly tapered in patients receiving maprotiline, or when the recommended dosage of maprotiline is exceeded. While a cause-and-effect relationship has not been established, the risk of seizures in patients treated with maprotiline may be reduced by initiating therapy at a low dosage; maintaining the initial dosage for 2 weeks before raising it gradually in small increments as necessitated by the long half-life of maprotiline (average, 51 hours); and keeping the dosage at the minimally effective level during maintenance therapy.

In premarketing clinical trials, only 1 seizure was reported among 2,796 patients treated with **mirtazapine**.

➤*Agranulocytosis:* In premarketing clinical trials, 2 (one with Sjögren syndrome) of 2,796 patients treated with **mirtazapine** developed agranulocytosis (absolute neutrophil count [ANC] less than 500/mm^3 with associated signs and symptoms [eg, fever, infection]), and a third patient developed severe neutropenia (ANC less than 500/mm^3 without any associated symptoms). For these 3 patients, onset of severe neutropenia was detected on days 61, 9, and 14 of treatment, respectively. All 3 patients recovered after mirtazapine was stopped. These 3 cases yield a crude incidence of severe neutropenia (with or without associated infection) of approximately 1.1 per 1,000 patients exposed, with a very wide 95% confidence interval (ie, 2.2 cases per 10,000 to 3.1 cases per 1,000). If a patient develops a sore throat, fever, stomatitis, or other signs of infection, along with a low white blood cell count (WBC), discontinue treatment with mirtazapine and closely monitor the patient.

➤*MAOIs:* In patients receiving other drugs for MDD in combination with an MAOI and in patients who have recently discontinued a drug for MDD and then are started on an MAOI, there have been reports of serious and sometimes fatal reactions, including autonomic instability with rapid fluctuations of vital signs, diaphoresis, dizziness, flushing, hyperthermia, mental status changes ranging from agitation to coma, myoclonus, nausea, rigidity, seizures, tremor, and vomiting. Although there are no human data pertinent to such an interaction with **mirtazapine**, it is recommended that mirtazapine not be used in combination with an MAOI or within 14 days of initiating or discontinuing therapy with an MAOI. Concomitant use of **maprotiline** with an MAOI is contraindicated. Allow a minimum of 14 days after discontinuing an MAOI before initiating maprotiline.

➤*Somnolence:* In US controlled studies, somnolence was reported in 54% of patients treated with **mirtazapine**, compared with 18% for placebo and 60% for amitriptyline. In these studies, somnolence resulted in discontinuation of treatment for 10.4% of mirtazapine-treated patients, compared with 2.2% of patients for placebo. It is unclear whether tolerance develops to the somnolent effects of mirtazapine.

➤*Dizziness:* Dizziness was reported in 7% of patients treated with **mirtazapine** compared with 3% for placebo and 14% for amitriptyline. It is unclear whether tolerance to the dizziness develops.

➤*Increased appetite/weight gain:* In US controlled studies, appetite increase was reported in 17% of patients treated with **mirtazapine**, compared with 2% for placebo and 6% for amitriptyline. In these trials, weight gain of at least 7% of body weight was reported in 7.5% of patients treated with mirtazapine, compared with 0% for placebo and 5.9% for amitriptyline. In a pool of premarketing US studies, including many patients for long-term, open-label treatment, 8% of patients receiving mirtazapine discontinued because of weight gain. In an 8-week, pediatric clinical trial of doses between 15 and 45 mg/day, 49% of mirtazapine-treated patients had a weight gain of at least 7%, compared with 5.7% of placebo-treated patients.

➤*Cholesterol/Triglycerides:* In US controlled studies, nonfasting cholesterol increases to at least 20% above the upper limits of normal (ULN) were observed in 15% of patients treated with **mirtazapine**, compared with 7% for placebo and 8% for amitriptyline. In these studies, nonfasting triglyceride increases to 500 mg/dL or more were observed in 6% of patients treated with mirtazapine, compared with 3% for placebo and 3% for amitriptyline.

➤*Transaminase levels:* Clinically significant ALT elevations (at least 3 times the ULN range) were observed in 2% of patients exposed to **mirtazapine** in a pool of US, short-term, controlled trials, compared with 0.3% of placebo-treated patients and 2% of amitriptyline-treated patients. Most of these patients with ALT increases did not develop signs or symptoms associated with compromised liver function. While some patients were discontinued for the ALT increases, in other cases, the enzyme levels returned to normal despite continued mirtazapine treatment. Use mirtazapine with caution in patients with hepatic function impairment.

➤*Mania/Hypomania:* Mania/hypomania occurred in approximately 0.2% of patients receiving **mirtazapine**. Hypomanic or manic episodes have occurred in some patients taking tricyclic antidepressant drugs, particularly in patients with cyclic disorders. Such occurrences also have been noted rarely with **maprotiline**. Although the incidence of mania/hypomania was very low during treatment with tetracyclics, use carefully in patients with a history of mania/hypomania.

➤*Elective surgery:* Prior to elective surgery, discontinue **maprotiline** for as long as possible, because little is known about the interaction between maprotiline and general anesthetics.

➤*Electroshock therapy:* Avoid coadministration of **maprotiline** and electroshock therapy because of the lack of experience in this area.

➤*Orthostatic hypotension:* **Mirtazapine** was associated with significant orthostatic hypotension in clinical trials with healthy volunteers. Orthostatic hypotension was infrequently observed in clinical trials with depressed patients. Use with caution in patients with known cardiovascular or cerebrovascular disease that could be exacerbated by hypotension (eg, angina, history of MI, ischemic stroke) and conditions that would predispose patients to hypotension (eg, dehydration, hypovolemia, treatment with antihypertensive medication).

➤*Renal/Hepatic function impairment:* **Mirtazapine** clearance is decreased in patients with moderate (glomerular filtration rate [GFR] 11 to 39 mL/min per 1.73 m^2) and severe (GFR less than 10 mL/min per 1.73 m^2) renal function impairment, and also in patients with hepatic function impairment. Caution is indicated when administering mirtazapine to such patients.

➤*Special risk:* Administer **maprotiline** with caution in patients with increased intraocular pressure, history of urinary retention, or history of narrow-angle glaucoma because of the drug's anticholinergic properties. Exercise caution when administering maprotiline to hyperthyroid patients because of enhanced potential for cardiovascular toxicity of maprotiline. Exercise extreme caution when administering maprotiline to patients with a history of MI and with a history or presence of cardiovascular disease because of the possibility of conduction defects, arrhythmia, MI, stroke, and tachycardia.

Clinical experience with **mirtazapine** in patients with concomitant systemic illness is limited. Accordingly, care is advisable in prescribing mirtazapine for patients with diseases or conditions that affect metabolism or hemodynamic responses.

Mirtazapine has not been systematically evaluated or used to any appreciable extent in patients with a recent history of MI or other significant heart disease. Mirtazapine was associated with significant orthostatic hypotension in early clinical pharmacology trials with healthy volunteers. Orthostatic hypotension was infrequently observed in clinical trials in patients with depression. Use mirtazapine with caution in patients with known cardiovascular or cerebrovascular disease that could be exacerbated by hypotension (eg, angina, history of MI, ischemic stroke) and conditions that would predispose patients to hypotension (eg, dehydration, hypovolemia, treatment with antihypertensive medication).

➤*Hazardous tasks:* Caution patients about engaging in hazardous activities until they are reasonably certain that tetracyclics do not adversely affect their ability to engage in such activities; because of their prominent sedative effects, tetracyclics may impair judgment, thinking, and, particularly, motor skills.

➤*Pregnancy: Category B* (**maprotiline**); *Category C* (**mirtazapine**). There are no adequate and well-controlled studies in pregnant women. However, there have been no published reports found that link maprotiline use with the development of congenital defects. Anticipate the transfer of mirtazapine to the fetus because of the drug's low molecular weight. Use these drugs during pregnancy only if clearly needed.

In rats, there was an increase in postimplantation losses in dams treated with mirtazapine at doses up to 100 mg/kg. There was an increase in pup deaths during the first 3 days of lactation and a decrease in pup birth weights. The cause of these deaths is not known. The effects occurred at doses that were 20 times the maximum recommended human dose (MRHD), but not at 3 times the MRHD, on a mg/m² basis.

Labor and delivery – As with any drug with CNS-depressant action, exercise caution during labor and delivery.

➤*Lactation:* **Maprotiline** is excreted in breast milk. At steady state, the concentration in milk corresponds closely to the concentrations in whole blood. Exercise caution when maprotiline is administered to a breast-feeding woman.

It is not known if **mirtazapine** is excreted in breast milk. However, expect passage into the breast milk because of mirtazapine's low molecular weight. Use caution when mirtazapine is administered to a breast-feeding woman.

➤*Children:* Safety and efficacy in children have not been established. Anyone considering the use of a tetracyclic antidepressant in a child or adolescent must balance the potential risks with the clinical need.

Two placebo-controlled trials in 258 children with MDD have been conducted with **mirtazapine**, and the data were not sufficient to support a claim for use in children.

➤*Elderly:* **Mirtazapine** is known to be substantially excreted by the kidney (75%), and the risk of decreased clearance of this drug is greater in patients with renal function impairment. Because elderly patients are more likely to have decreased renal function, take care in dose selection. Sedating drugs may cause confusion and oversedation in elderly patients. Caution is indicated when administering mirtazapine to elderly patients.

➤*Monitoring:* Appropriately monitor and closely observe all patients being treated with antidepressants for any indication for clinical worsening, suicidality, and unusual changes in behavior, especially during the initial few months of a course of drug therapy or at times of dose changes, either increases or decreases.

Discontinue **maprotiline** if there is evidence of pathological neutrophil depression. Perform leukocyte and differential counts in patients who develop fever and sore throat during therapy.

If a patient develops a sore throat, fever, stomatitis, or other signs of infection, along with a low WBC, discontinue treatment with **mirtazapine** and closely monitor the patient.

Drug Interactions

➤*QT prolongation:* An additive effect of **maprotiline** with other drugs that prolong the QT interval cannot be excluded. The following drugs may prolong the QT interval and increase the risk of life-threatening cardiac arrhythmia, including torsades de pointes: antiarrhythmic agents (eg, amiodarone, bretylium, disopyramide, dofetilide, procainamide, quinidine, sotalol), arsenic trioxide, chlorpromazine, cisapride, dolasetron, droperidol, mefloquine, mesoridazine, moxifloxacin, pentamidine, pimozide, tacrolimus, thioridazine, and ziprasidone. For a more complete list of drugs that may prolong the QT interval, see the appendix "Drug-Induced Prolongation of the QT Interval and Torsades de Pointes."

➤*CYP-450:* Because of the pharmacologic similarity of **maprotiline** to the tricyclic antidepressants, the plasma concentration of maprotiline may be increased when the drug is given concomitantly with hepatic enzyme inhibitors (eg, cimetidine, fluoxetine) and decreased by coadministration with hepatic enzyme inducers (eg, barbiturates, phenytoin), as has occurred with tricyclic antidepressants. Adjustment of the dosage of maprotiline may therefore be necessary in such cases.

In vitro, **mirtazapine** is a substrate for several of CYP-450 enzymes, including 2D6, 1A2, and 3A4. While in vitro studies have shown that mirtazapine is not a potent inhibitor of any of these enzymes, an indication that mirtazapine is not likely to have a clinically significant inhibitory effect on the metabolism of other drugs that are substrates for these CYP-450 enzymes, the concomitant use of mirtazapine with most other drugs metabolized by these enzymes has not been formally studied. Consequently, it is not possible to make any definitive statements about the risks of coadministration of mirtazapine with such drugs.

Tetracyclic Antidepressants Drug Interactions

Precipitant drug	Object drug[a]		Description
Alcohol	Tetracyclic antidepressants	↑	The impairment of cognitive and motor skills may be additive with those produced by alcohol. Advise patients to avoid alcohol while taking mirtazapine.
Tetracyclic antidepressants	Alcohol		
Anticholinergics (eg, hyoscyamine, scopolamine)	Tetracyclic antidepressants Maprotiline	↑	Additive atropine-like effects may occur. Closely supervise and carefully adjust dosage when coadministering.
Tetracyclic antidepressants Maprotiline	Anticholinergics (eg, hyoscyamine, scopolamine)		

Tetracyclic Antidepressants Drug Interactions

Precipitant drug	Object drug[a]		Description
Benzodiazepines (eg, diazepam)	Tetracyclic antidepressants	↑	The impairment of motor skills from mirtazapine has been shown to be additive with impairment caused by diazepam. Advise patients to avoid diazepam and other similar drugs while taking mirtazapine. The risk of seizures may be increased when the dosage of benzodiazepines is rapidly tapered in patients receiving maprotiline.
Tetracyclic antidepressants	Benzodiazepines (eg, diazepam)		
Cisapride[b]	Tetracyclic antidepressants Maprotiline	↑	The risk of life-threatening cardiac arrhythmia, including torsades de pointes, may be increased because of possible additive prolongation of the QT interval. Coadministration is contraindicated.
Tetracyclic antidepressants Maprotiline	Cisapride[b]		
CYP inducers (eg, barbiturates, phenytoin)	Tetracyclic antidepressants	↓	Because of the pharmacologic similarity of maprotiline to the tricyclic antidepressants, the plasma concentration of maprotiline may be decreased when given with hepatic enzyme inducers. In vitro, mirtazapine is a substrate for several CYP-450 enzymes (eg, 2D6, 1A2, 3A4) and theoretically may be affected by CYP inducers. In one study, coadministration of phenytoin with mirtazapine decreased both the mirtazapine AUC[c] (by 47%) and C_{max}[d].
CYP inhibitors (eg, cimetidine, fluoxetine)	Tetracyclic antidepressants	↑	Because of the pharmacologic similarity of maprotiline to the tricyclic antidepressants, the plasma concentration of maprotiline may be increased when given with hepatic enzyme inhibitors. In vitro, mirtazapine is a substrate for several CYP-450 enzymes (eg, 2D6, 1A2, 3A4) and theoretically may be affected by CYP inhibitors.
MAOIs (eg, phenelzine, selegiline)	Tetracyclic antidepressants	↑	Concomitant use of maprotiline with an MAOI is contraindicated. Allow a minimum of 14 days after discontinuing an MAOI before initiating maprotiline. Although there are no human data pertinent to such an interaction with mirtazapine, it is recommended that mirtazapine not be used in combination with an MAOI or within 14 days of initiating or discontinuing therapy with an MAOI.
Tetracyclic antidepressants	MAOIs (eg, phenelzine)		
Phenothiazines (eg, chlorpromazine, thioridazine)	Tetracyclic antidepressants Maprotiline	↑	The risk of seizures may be increased with concomitant use.
SSRIs (eg, fluoxetine, fluvoxamine)	Tetracyclic antidepressants Mirtazapine	↑	A 3- to 4-fold increase in mirtazapine serum levels was reported in 2 patients after fluvoxamine was added to their treatment regimens. Adjust the mirtazapine dose as needed.
Sympathomimetics (eg, epinephrine)	Tetracyclic antidepressants Maprotiline	↑	Additive atropine-like effects may occur. Closely supervise and carefully adjust dosage when coadministering.
Tetracyclic antidepressants Maprotiline	Sympathomimetics (eg, epinephrine)		
Tetracyclic antidepressants Maprotiline	Guanethidine[e]	↓	Maprotiline may block the pharmacologic effects of guanethidine[e] or similar drugs.

Tetracyclic Antidepressants Drug Interactions			
Precipitant drug	Object drug[a]		Description
Tetracyclic antidepressants Maprotiline	Thyroid hormones (eg, levothyroxine)	↑	Use caution when administering maprotiline to hyperthyroid patients or those on thyroid medication because of the possibility of enhanced potential for cardiovascular toxicity of maprotiline.

[a] ↑ = object drug increased; ↓ = object drug decreased.
[b] Available from the manufacturer on a limited-access protocol.
[c] AUC = area under the curve.
[d] C_{max} = maximum plasma concentration.
[e] No longer marketed in the United States.

Adverse Reactions

Tetracyclic Antidepressants Adverse Reactions[a]		
Adverse reactions	Maprotiline	Mirtazapine
Cardiovascular		
Hypertension	rare	≥ 1%
Hypotension	rare	0.1% to 1%
CNS		
Abnormal dreams	—	4%
Agitation	2%	≥ 1%
Anxiety	3%	≥ 1%
Asthenia	—	8%
Ataxia	rare	0.1% to 1%
Confusion	rare	2%
Dizziness	8%	7%
Drowsiness	16%	—
Extrapyramidal symptoms	rare	0.1% to 1%
Hallucinations	rare	0.1% to 1%
Headache	4%	—
Insomnia	2%	—
Mania/Manic reaction	rare	0.1% to 1%
Nervousness	6%	—
Somnolence	—	54%
Thinking abnormal	—	3%
Tremor	3%	2%
Weakness and fatigue	4%	—
Dermatologic		
Alopecia	rare	0.1% to 1%
Pruritus	—	≥ 1%
Rash	rare	≥ 1%
GI		
Constipation	6%	13%
Dry mouth	22%	25%
Increased appetite	—	17%
Nausea	2%	—
Nausea and vomiting		0.1% to 1%
Vomiting	rare	≥ 1%
Metabolic/Nutritional		
Edema	rare	1%
Peripheral edema	—	2%
Weight gain	rare	12%
Weight loss	rare	0.1% to 1%
Miscellaneous		
Altered liver function	rare	0.1% to 1%
Back pain	—	2%
Blurred vision	4%	
Dyspnea	—	1%
Flu syndrome	—	5%
Myalgia	—	2%
Urinary frequency	rare	2%

[a] Data are pooled from different studies and are not necessarily comparable.

➤*Maprotiline:*

Cardiovascular – Arrhythmia, heart block, palpitation, syncope, tachycardia (rare).

CNS – Akathisia, decrease in memory, delusions, disorientation, dysarthria, electroencephalogram alterations, exacerbation of psychosis, feelings of unreality, hypomania, motor hyperactivity, nightmares, numbness, restlessness, seizures, tingling (rare).

Dermatologic – Excessive perspiration, flushing (rare).

Endocrine – Elevation or depression of blood sugar levels, increased or decreased libido (rare).

GI – Abdominal cramps, bitter taste, diarrhea, dysphagia, epigastric distress, increased salivation (rare).

GU – Delayed micturition, impotence, urinary retention (rare).

Hypersensitivity – Drug fever, edema, itching, petechiae, photosensitization, skin rash (rare).

Special senses – Accommodation disturbances, mydriasis, tinnitus (rare).

Miscellaneous – Jaundice, nasal congestion (rare).

Because of maprotiline's pharmacologic similarity to tricyclic antidepressants and isolated reports of the following adverse reactions, consider each reaction when administering maprotiline: black tongue, bone marrow depression (including agranulocytosis, eosinophilia, purpura, and thrombocytopenia), breast enlargement and galactorrhea in women, gynecomastia in men, MI, paralytic ileus, peripheral neuropathy, stomatitis, stroke, sublingual adenitis, and testicular swelling.

➤*Mirtazapine:*

Cardiovascular – Vasodilatation (1% or more); angina pectoris, bradycardia, MI, migraine, syncope, ventricular extrasystoles (0.1% to 1%); atrial arrhythmia, bigeminy, cardiomegaly, cerebral ischemia, left-sided heart failure, phlebitis, pulmonary embolus, vascular headache (less than 0.1%).

CNS – Amnesia, apathy, depression, hyperkinesia, hypesthesia, hypokinesia, paresthesia, twitching, vertigo (1% or more); abnormal coordination, delirium, delusions, depersonalization, dysarthria, dyskinesia, dystonia, emotional lability, euphoria, hostility, increased libido, increased reflexes, neurosis, paranoid reaction (0.1% to 1%); akathisia, aphasia, dementia, diplopia, drug dependence, hypotonia, myoclonus, nystagmus, paralysis, psychotic depression, stupor, tonic-clonic seizures, withdrawal syndrome (less than 0.1%).

Dermatologic – Acne, dry skin, exfoliative dermatitis, herpes simplex (0.1% to 1%); herpes zoster, seborrhea, skin hypertrophy, skin ulcer, urticaria (less than 0.1%).

Endocrine – Goiter, hypothyroidism (less than 0.1%).

GI – Abdominal pain, acute abdominal syndrome, anorexia (1% or more); cholecystitis, colitis, enlarged abdomen, eructation, glossitis, gum hemorrhage, stomatitis, ulcer (0.1% to 1%); aphthous stomatitis, cirrhosis of the liver, gastritis, gastroenteritis, increased salivation, intestinal obstruction, oral moniliasis, pancreatitis, salivary gland enlargement, tongue discoloration, tongue edema, ulcerative stomatitis (less than 0.1%).

GU – Urinary tract infection (1% or more); amenorrhea, breast pain, cystitis, dysmenorrhea, dysuria, hematuria, impotence, kidney calculus, leukorrhea, urinary incontinence, urinary retention, vaginitis (0.1% to 1%); abnormal ejaculation, breast engorgement, breast enlargement, menorrhagia, metrorrhagia, polyuria, urethritis, urinary urgency (less than 0.1%).

Hematologic/Lymphatic – Anemia, leukopenia, lymphadenopathy, lymphocytosis, pancytopenia, petechiae, thrombocytopenia (less than 0.1%).

Metabolic/Nutritional – Thirst (1% or more); dehydration (0.1% to 1%); acid phosphatase increased, ALT increased, AST increased, diabetes mellitus, gout (less than 0.1%).

Musculoskeletal – Arthralgia, myasthenia (1% or more); arthritis, tenosynovitis (0.1% to 1%); arthrosis, bone pain, bursitis, myositis, osteoporosis fracture, pathological fracture, tendon rupture (less than 0.1%).

Respiratory – Cough increased, sinusitis (1% or more); asthma, bronchitis, epistaxis, pneumonia (0.1% to 1%); asphyxia, hiccough, laryngitis, pneumothorax (less than 0.1%).

Special senses – Abnormality of accommodation, conjunctivitis, deafness, ear pain, eye pain, glaucoma, hyperacusis, keratoconjunctivitis, lacrimation disorder (0.1% to 1%); blepharitis, otitis media, parosmia, partial transitory deafness, taste loss (less than 0.1%).

Miscellaneous – Malaise (1% or more); chills, face edema, fever, neck pain, neck rigidity, photosensitivity reaction (0.1% to 1%); cellulitis, healing abnormal, substernal chest pain (less than 0.1%).

➤*Postmarketing:*

Maprotiline – Interstitial pneumonitis, which in some cases was associated with eosinophilia and increased liver enzymes; Stevens-Johnson syndrome; toxic epidermal necrolysis.

Mirtazapine – Four cases of the ventricular arrhythmia torsades de pointes. In 3 of the 4 cases, however, concomitant drugs were implicated. All patients recovered.

Overdosage

➤*Symptoms:*

Maprotiline – Deaths may occur from overdosage with this class of drugs. Signs and symptoms of maprotiline overdose are similar to those seen with tricyclic antidepressant overdose. Critical manifestations of overdose include cardiac dysrhythmias, convulsions, CNS depression, including coma and severe hypotension. Changes in the electrocardiogram (ECG), particularly in QRS axis or width, are clinically significant indicators of toxicity. Other clinical manifestations include drowsiness, tachycardia, ataxia, vomiting, cyanosis, shock, restlessness, agitation, hyperpyrexia, muscle rigidity, athetoid movements, and mydriasis. Because congestive heart failure (CHF) has been seen with overdosage of tricyclic antidepressants, consider CHF with maprotiline overdosage as well.

Mirtazapine – Signs and symptoms reported in association with overdose included disorientation, drowsiness, impaired memory, and tachycardia. There were no reports of ECG abnormalities, coma, or convulsions following overdose with mirtazapine alone.

➤*Treatment:*

Maprotiline – Obtain an ECG and immediately initiate cardiac monitoring. Protect the patient's airway, establish an intravenous (IV) line, and initiate gastric decontamination. A minimum of 6 hours of observation with cardiac monitoring and observation for signs of CNS or respiratory depression, hypotension, cardiac dysrhythmia and/or conduction blocks, and seizures is necessary. If signs of toxicity occur at any time during this period, extended monitoring is required. There are case reports of patients succumbing to fatal dysrhythmias late after tricyclic overdose; these patients had clinical evidence of significant poisoning prior to death and most received inadequate GI decontamination. Do not guide management of the patient through monitoring of plasma drug levels.

GI decontamination: All patients suspected of overdose should receive GI decontamination. This should include large-volume gastric lavage followed by activated charcoal. Emesis is contraindicated.

Cardiovascular: A maximal limb-lead QRS duration of 0.1 seconds or more may be the best indication of the severity of the overdose. Use IV sodium bicarbonate to maintain the serum pH of 7.45 to 7.55. If the pH response is inadequate, hyperventilation may also be used. Concomitant use of hyperventilation and sodium bicarbonate should be done with extreme caution, with frequent pH monitoring. A pH higher than 7.6 or a carbon dioxide partial pressure (PCO_2) less than 20 mm Hg is undesirable. Dysrhythmias unresponsive to sodium bicarbonate therapy/hyperventilation may respond to lidocaine, bretylium, or phenytoin. Type 1A and 1C antiarrhythmics (eg, disopyramide, procainamide, quinidine) are generally contraindicated.

In rare instances, hemoperfusion may be beneficial in acute refractory cardiovascular instability in patients with acute toxicity. However, hemodialysis, peritoneal dialysis, exchange transfusions, and forced diuresis generally have been ineffective.

CNS: In patients with CNS depression, early intubation is advised because of the potential for abrupt deterioration. Control seizures with benzodiazepines, or, if these are ineffective, other anticonvulsants (eg, phenobarbital, phenytoin). Physostigmine is not recommended except to treat life-threatening symptoms that have been unresponsive to other therapies, and then only in consultation with a poison control center.

Mirtazapine – Treatment should consist of those general measures employed in the management of overdose with any drug effective in the treatment of major depressive disorder. Ensure an adequate airway, oxygenation, and ventilation. Monitor cardiac rhythm and vital signs. General supportive and symptomatic measures are also recommended. Induction of emesis is not recommended. Gastric lavage with a large-bore orogastric tube with appropriate airway protection, if needed, may be indicated if performed soon after ingestion or in symptomatic patients. Because of the rapid disintegration of mirtazapine orally disintegrating tablets, pill fragments may not appear in gastric contents obtained with lavage. Administer activated charcoal. There is no experience with the use of forced diuresis, dialysis, hemoperfusion, or exchange transfusion in the treatment of mirtazapine overdosage. No specific antidotes for mirtazapine are known. In managing overdosage, consider the possibility of multiple-drug involvement. Consider contacting a poison control center for additional information on the treatment of any overdose. The American Association of Poison Control Centers' phone number is 1-800-222-1222.

Patient Information

➤*Clinical worsening and suicide risk:* Encourage patients, their families, and their caregivers to be alert to the emergence of aggressiveness, akathisia (psychomotor restlessness), anxiety, agitation, hostility, hypomania, impulsivity, insomnia, irritability, mania, other unusual changes in behavior, panic attacks, suicidal ideation, and worsening of depression, especially early during antidepressant treatment and when the dose is adjusted up or down. Advise families and caregivers to observe for the emergence of such symptoms on a day-to-day basis, because changes may be abrupt. Advise patients and caregivers to report such symptoms to a health care provider, especially if they are severe, abrupt in onset, or were not part of a patient's presenting symptoms. Symptoms such as these may be associated with an increased risk for suicidal thinking and behavior and indicate a need for very close monitoring and, possibly, changes in the medication.

➤*Hazardous tasks:* Caution patients about engaging in hazardous activities until they are reasonably certain that tetracyclics do not adversely affect their ability to engage in such activities; because of their prominent sedative effects, tetracyclics may impair judgment, thinking, and, particularly, motor skills.

➤*Alcohol:* Advise patients to avoid alcohol while taking tetracyclic antidepressants because of the additive impairment of cognitive and motor skills.

➤*Pregnancy and breast-feeding:* Advise patients to notify their health care provider if they become pregnant, intend to become pregnant, or are breast-feeding during tetracyclic therapy.

➤*Maprotiline:*

Seizures – Warn patients of the association between seizures and maprotiline use. Inform patients that this association is enhanced in patients with a history of seizures and in those taking certain other drugs.

➤*Mirtazapine:*

Agranulocystosis – Warn patients who are to receive mirtazapine about the risk of developing agranulocytosis. Instruct patients to contact their health care provider if they experience any indication of infection such as fever, chills, sore throat, mucous membrane ulceration, or other possible signs of infection. Pay particular attention to any flu-like complaints or other symptoms that might suggest infection.

Phenylketonuria – Inform phenylketonuric patients that mirtazapine orally disintegrating tablets contain phenylalanine 2.6 mg per 15 mg tablet, 5.2 mg per 30 mg tablet, and 7.8 mg per 45 mg tablet.

Therapy – While patients may notice improvement with therapy in 1 to 4 weeks, advise them to continue therapy as directed.

MAPROTILINE HYDROCHLORIDE

Rx	**Maprotiline Hydrochloride** (Mylan)	**Tablets; oral:** 25 mg	PEG, polydextrose. (6 0 M). Scored. Film-coated. In 100s.
		50 mg	PEG, polydextrose. (8 7 M). Lt. blue, scored. Film-coated. In 100s.
		75 mg	PEG, polydextrose. (9 2 M). Scored. Film-coated. In 100s.

MAPROTILINE HYDROCHLORIDE — ORAL

For complete and comparative prescribing information, refer to the Tetracyclic Compounds group monograph.

WARNING

Suicidality and antidepressant drugs – Antidepressants increased the risk compared with placebo of suicidal thinking and behavior (suicidality) in children, adolescents, and young adults in short-term studies of major depressive disorder (MDD) and other psychiatric disorders. Anyone considering the use of maprotiline or any other antidepressant in a child, adolescent, or young adult must balance this risk with the clinical need. Short-term studies did not show an increase in the risk of suicidality with antidepressants compared with placebo in adults older than 24 years of age; there was a reduction in risk with antidepressants compared with placebo in adults 65 years of age and older. Depression and certain other psychiatric disorders are associated with increases in suicide risk. Appropriately monitor and closely observe patients of all ages who are started on antidepressant therapy for clinical worsening, suicidality, or unusual changes in behavior. Advise families and caregivers of the need for close observation and communication with the prescriber. Maprotiline is not approved for use in children.

Indications

➤*Anxiety:* For the relief of anxiety associated with depression.

➤*Depression:* For the treatment of depressive illness in patients with depressive neurosis (dysthymic disorder) and manic-depressive illness, depressed type (MDD).

➤*Off-label uses:*

Postherpetic neuralgia – [1] = Good documentation. Evidence from a controlled trial showed maprotiline was effective for the treatment of postherpetic neuralgia (PHN). American Academy of Neurology clinical practice guidelines consider maprotiline to be effective for the treatment of PHN and state that it should be used (level A, class I and II). (See Administration and Dosage.)

Administration and Dosage

➤*General dosing considerations:* May be given as a single daily dose or in divided doses. Therapeutic effects are sometimes seen within 3 to 7 days, although 2 to 3 weeks are usually necessary.

➤*Adults:*

Mild to moderate depression –

Maximum dose: 150 mg/day.

Initial dosage: 75 mg/day. In some patients, an initial dosage of 25 mg/day may be used. Because of the long half-life of maprotiline, maintain the initial dosage for 2 weeks.

Dosage titration: The dose may be increased gradually in 25 mg increments, as required and tolerated. A maximum daily dose of 150 mg/day will result in therapeutic efficacy in most outpatients.

Maintenance dosage: Keep dosage during prolonged maintenance therapy at the lowest effective level. The dose may be reduced to 75 to 150 mg/day, with adjustment depending on therapeutic response.

Severe depression (hospitalized patients) –

Maximum dose: 225 mg/day.

Initial dosage: 100 to 150 mg/day.

MAPROTILINE HYDROCHLORIDE — ORAL

Dosage titration: Gradually increase the dose as required and tolerated. Most hospitalized patients respond to a dose of 150 mg/day, although doses as high as 225 mg/day may be required.

Maintenance dosage: Keep dosage during prolonged maintenance therapy at the lowest effective level. The dose may be reduced to 75 to 150 mg/day with adjustment depending on therapeutic response.

Off-label dosing –

Postherpetic neuralgia: [1] = Good documentation. Oral maprotiline (mean dose, 100 mg) daily for 5 weeks.

➤*Elderly:* Lower doses are recommended for patients older than 60 years of age.

Initial dosage – 25 mg/day.

Maintenance dosage – 50 to 75 mg/day is usually satisfactory as maintenance therapy for elderly patients who do not tolerate higher amounts.

➤*Storage/Stability:* Store at 20° to 25°C (68° to 77°F). Dispense in a tight, light-resistant container.

MIRTAZAPINE

Rx	**Mirtazapine** (Caraco)	**Tablets; oral:** 7.5 mg	May contain lactose. In 30s, 500s, and 1,000s.
Rx	**Mirtazapine** (Various, eg, Mylan, Teva, Watson)	**Tablets; oral:** 15 mg	May contain lactose. In 30s, 90s, 100s, 500s, and 1,000s.
Rx	**Remeron** (Organon)		Lactose. (Organon T3Z). Yellow, oval, scored. Film-coated. In 30s.
Rx	**Mirtazapine** (Various, eg, Aurobindo, Caraco, Teva)	**Tablets; oral:** 30 mg	May contain lactose. In 30s, 60s, 90s, 100s, 500s, and 1,000s.
Rx	**Remeron** (Organon)		Lactose. (Organon T5Z). Red-brown, oval, scored. Film-coated. In 30s.
Rx	**Mirtazapine** (Various, eg, Aurobindo, Teva, Watson)	**Tablets; oral:** 45 mg	May contain lactose. In 30s, 90s, 100s, 500s, and 1,000s.
Rx	**Remeron** (Organon)		Lactose. (Organon T7Z). Oval, white. Film-coated. In 30s.
Rx	**Mirtazapine** (Various, eg, Actavis Totowa, Barr, Teva)	**Tablets, disintegrating; oral:** 15 mg	May contain aspartame, corn syrup, mannitol, phenylalanine, xylitol. In UD 30s.
Rx	**Remeron SolTab** (Organon)		Aspartame, mannitol, phenylalanine 2.6 mg, sucrose. (T1Z). Orange flavor. In UD 30s.
Rx	**Mirtazapine** (Various, eg, Actavis Totowa, Barr, Teva)	**Tablets, disintegrating; oral:** 30 mg	May contain aspartame, corn syrup, mannitol, phenylalanine, xylitol. In UD 30s.
Rx	**Remeron SolTab** (Organon)		Aspartame, mannitol, phenylalanine 5.2 mg, sucrose. (T2Z). Orange flavor. In UD 30s.
Rx	**Mirtazapine** (Various, eg, Actavis Totowa, Barr, Teva)	**Tablets, disintegrating; oral:** 45 mg	May contain aspartame, corn syrup, mannitol, phenylalanine, xylitol. In UD 30s.
Rx	**Remeron SolTab** (Organon)		Aspartame, mannitol, phenylalanine 7.8 mg, sucrose. (T4Z). Orange flavor. In UD 30s.

MIRTAZAPINE — ORAL

For complete and comparative prescribing information, refer to the Tetracyclic Compounds group monograph.

WARNING

Suicidality and antidepressant drugs – Antidepressants increased the risk compared with placebo of suicidal thinking and behavior (suicidality) in children, adolescents, and young adults in short-term studies of major depressive disorder (MDD) and other psychiatric disorders. Anyone considering the use of mirtazapine or any other antidepressant in a child, adolescent, or young adult must balance this risk with the clinical need. Short-term studies did not show an increase in the risk of suicidality with antidepressants compared with placebo in adults older than 24 years of age; there was a reduction in risk with antidepressants compared with placebo in adults 65 years of age and older. Depression and certain other psychiatric disorders are associated with increases in suicide risk. Appropriately monitor and closely observe patients of all ages who are started on antidepressant therapy for clinical worsening, suicidality, or unusual changes in behavior. Advise families and caregivers of the need for close observation and communication with the prescriber. Mirtazapine is not approved for use in children. (See also Warnings/Precautions.)

Indications

➤*Major depressive disorder:* For the treatment of MDD.

➤*Off-label uses:*

Chronic urticaria – [3] = Safety concerns. Initial data from isolated case reports suggest that mirtazapine may be of benefit in some patients with severe chronic urticaria who have been unresponsive to previous therapy. These data are limited by a small population, and the urticaria has been of varied etiology. (See Administration and Dosage.)

Hot flashes – [4] = Insufficient documentation. Initial data note a partial benefit of mirtazapine in the treatment of hot flashes related to menopause. (See Administration and Dosage.)

Hyperhidrosis (drug-induced) – [4] = Insufficient documentation. There is limited information regarding the use of mirtazapine in the management of selective serotonin reuptake inhibitor (SSRI)–induced excessive sweating. (See Administration and Dosage.)

Prevention of migraine (adults) – [4] = Insufficient documentation. The use of mirtazapine for migraine prophylaxis in adults has been reported in only 2 patients. These cases provide some support for use with this indication, but clinical trials are needed. American Academy of Neurology practice guidelines consider mirtazapine to be clinically efficacious based on consensus and clinical experience, despite the lack of scientific evidence of efficacy. (See Administration and Dosage.)

Pruritus – [3] = Safety concerns. Initial data from isolated case reports suggest that mirtazapine may benefit some patients with cancer-related severe chronic pruritus unresponsive to previous therapy. However, these data are limited by a small population of patients with pruritus of varied etiology. (See Administration and Dosage.)

Administration and Dosage

➤*Adults:*

Major depressive disorder –

Initial dosage: 15 mg/day as a single dose, preferably in the evening prior to sleep. The effective dose range is generally 15 to 45 mg/day.

Maintenance dosage: It is generally agreed that acute episodes of depression require several months or longer of sustained pharmacological therapy beyond response to the acute episode. Systematic evaluation of mirtazapine has demonstrated that its efficacy in MDD is maintained for periods of up to 40 weeks following 8 to 12 weeks of initial treatment at a dosage of 15 to 45 mg/day. Based on these limited data, it is unknown whether the dose of mirtazapine needed for maintenance treatment is identical to the dose needed to achieve an initial response. Patients should be periodically reassessed to determine the need for maintenance treatment and the appropriate dose for such treatment.

Off-label dosing –

Chronic urticaria: [3] = Safety concerns. Initial dosages ranged from 15 to 30 mg daily.

Hot flashes: [4] = Insufficient documentation. 7.5 to 60 mg daily.

Hyperhidrosis (drug-induced): [4] = Insufficient documentation. Initial dosages of 15 mg daily. Maintenance dosages titrated up to 60 mg daily.

Prevention of migraine (adults): [4] = Insufficient documentation. 7.5 mg at bedtime or 15 mg daily for up to several months.

Pruritus: [3] = Safety concerns. Initial dosages ranged from 15 to 30 mg daily. Most patients were controlled with 15 mg nightly.

➤*Discontinuation of therapy:* Symptoms associated with the discontinuation or dose reduction of mirtazapine have been reported. Patients should be monitored for these and other symptoms when discontinuing treatment or during dosage reduction. A gradual reduction in the dose over several weeks, rather than abrupt cessation, is recommended whenever possible. If intolerable symptoms occur following a decrease in the dose or upon discontinuation of treatment, dose titration should be managed on the basis of the patient's clinical response.

➤*Administration:*

Orally disintegrating tablets – Patients should be instructed to open the tablet blister pack with dry hands and place the tablet on the tongue. The tablet should be used immediately after removal from its blister; once removed, it cannot be stored. Mirtazapine orally disintegrating tablets will disintegrate rapidly on the tongue and can be swallowed with saliva. No water is needed for taking the tablet. Patients should not attempt to split the tablet.

➤*Storage/Stability:* Store at 25°C (77°F); excursions are permitted to 15° to 30°C (59° to 86°F). Protect from light and moisture. Use orally disintegrating tablets immediately upon opening individual tablet blister.

TRAZODONE HYDROCHLORIDE

Rx	**Trazodone Hydrochloride** (Various, eg, Apotex, Mylan)	**Tablets; oral:** 50 mg	In 100s, 500s, 1,000s, and UD 100s.
		100 mg	In 100s, 500s, 1,000s, and UD 100s.
		150 mg	In 100s, 500s, and 1,000s.
		300 mg	In 100s and 500s.
Rx	**Oleptro** (Labopharm)	**Tablets, extended-release; oral:** 150 mg	PEG. (DDS 080). Yellowish-beige, capsule-shaped, scored. Film-coated. In 30s, 90s, 500s, and UD 30s.
		300 mg	PEG. (DDS 081). Beige-orange, capsule-shaped, scored. Film-coated. In 30s, 90s, 500s, and UD 30s.

TRAZODONE HYDROCHLORIDE — ORAL

WARNING

Suicidality and antidepressant drugs – Antidepressants increase the risk, compared with placebo, of suicidal thinking and behavior (suicidality) in children, adolescents, and young adults in short-term studies of major depressive disorder (MDD) and other psychiatric disorders. Anyone considering the use of trazodone or any other antidepressant in a child, adolescent, or young adult must balance the risk with the clinical need. Short-term studies did not show an increase in the risk of suicidality with antidepressants compared with placebo in adults older than 24 years of age; there was a reduction in risk with antidepressants compared with placebo in adults 65 years of age and older. Depression and certain other psychiatric disorders are themselves associated with increases in the risk of suicide. Appropriately monitor patients of all ages who are started on antidepressant therapy and observe them closely for clinical worsening, suicidality, or unusual changes in behavior. Advise families and caregivers of the need for close observation and communication with the prescriber. Trazodone is not approved for use in children.

Indications

➤*Depression:* For the treatment of depression (immediate release) and MDD in adults (extended release [ER]).

➤*Off-label uses:*

Aggressive behavior – [4] = Insufficient documentation. Case reports, case series, small, noncontrolled trials, and N-of-1 studies have described successful trazodone treatment in adults and children for aggressive behavior resulting from a variety of causes, including mental retardation and other developmental disorders, behavioral disorders, Alzheimer dementia, degenerative dementia, alcoholic dementia, and organic brain syndromes. Doses varied considerably and were often titrated up over several weeks based on tolerance and response. The potential for orthostatic hypotension and excessive drowsiness, especially in elderly patients with dementia, should be carefully weighed against the potential benefits of trazodone.

Alcohol withdrawal – [4] = Insufficient documentation. Trazodone may be useful in patients suffering from sleep disturbances following alcohol withdrawal; however, there is a lack of evidence demonstrating benefit for the treatment of alcohol withdrawal syndrome. Further studies assessing trazodone in the acute phase of alcohol withdrawal are needed.

Cocaine withdrawal – [4] = Insufficient documentation. Limited case reports suggest that trazodone may decrease compulsive searching behavior seen in patients who abuse cocaine; however, there have been no clinical trials evaluating the safety and efficacy of trazodone for treating cocaine withdrawal. Data from larger controlled trials are needed.

Insomnia – [2] = Fair documentation. Multiple trials confirm trazodone's effectiveness for the treatment of insomnia associated with antidepressant use, depression, and mood disorders. Although patients with primary insomnia experienced significant improvement with trazodone, results were similar to placebo as treatment duration lengthened. Clinical data evaluating the efficacy of trazodone in the treatment of primary insomnia are limited to one study. Additional evidence is needed before a determination of trazodone's treatment effects can be established.

Panic disorder with agoraphobia – [5] = Poor documentation. Canadian Psychiatric Association guidelines recommend against the use of trazodone for the treatment of agoraphobia with panic attacks. Numerous other drug therapies are indicated for use in this setting. Although 1 small, noncontrolled study reported beneficial effects with trazodone compared with baseline, a larger and controlled study found that positive outcomes from trazodone use were small, of minimal clinical significance, and inferior to those achieved with a tricyclic antidepressant or benzodiazepine. Dropout rates for lack of efficacy and poor tolerance were high in the limited clinical experiences reported. Considering the availability of numerous other therapies with proven efficacy and more favorable safety profiles, trazodone is not recommended as a therapeutic option for agoraphobia with panic attacks.

Prevention of migraine (adults) – [2] = Fair documentation. There are no controlled trials evaluating the efficacy of trazodone for the prevention of migraine in adult patients. However, American Academy of Neurology practice guidelines state that trazodone is clinically efficacious based on consensus and clinical experience, despite the lack of scientific evidence of efficacy.

Prevention of migraine (children/adolescents) – [5] = Poor documentation. Current practice guidelines state that recommendations regarding the use of trazodone for the prevention of migraine headache in children cannot be made because of conflicting evidence.

Administration and Dosage

➤*Adults:*

Depression –

Immediate-release tablets:

• *Maximum dose* –
Inpatients: 600 mg/day in divided doses.
Outpatients: 400 mg/day in divided doses.

• *Initial dosage* – 150 mg/day in divided doses.

• *Dosage titration* – Increase gradually by 50 mg/day every 3 to 4 days.

• *Maintenance dosage* – Keep the dosage at the lowest effective level during prolonged therapy. Once an adequate response has been achieved, the dosage may be gradually reduced, with subsequent adjustment depending on therapeutic response.

• *Duration of therapy* – Although there has been no systematic evaluation of the efficacy of trazodone beyond 6 weeks, it is generally recommended that a course of antidepressant drug treatment should be continued for several months.

Extended-release tablets:

• *Maximum dose* – 375 mg/day.

• *Initial dosage* – 150 mg once daily.

• *Dosage titration* – Increase by 75 mg/day every 3 days (ie, start 225 mg on day 4 of therapy).

• *Maintenance dosage* – Patients should be maintained on the lowest effective dose and periodically reassessed to determine the continued need for maintenance treatment.

• *Dosage adjustment* – Once an adequate response has been achieved, the dosage may be gradually reduced, with subsequent adjustment depending on therapeutic response.

• *Duration of therapy* – While there is no body of evidence available to answer the question of how long a patient treated with trazodone should continue the drug, it is generally recommended that treatment be continued for several months after an initial response.

• *Discontinuation of therapy* – Patients should be monitored for withdrawal symptoms when discontinuing treatment with trazodone. The dose should be gradually reduced whenever possible.

Off-label dosing –

Aggressive behavior: [4] = Insufficient documentation. 50 mg orally twice daily. The dose may then be titrated up over 1 to 6 weeks based on response and tolerability.

• *Maintenance dosage* – 75 to 400 mg/day, divided into 2 to 4 daily doses.

Alcohol withdrawal: [4] = Insufficient documentation. 100 to 600 mg/day orally.

Cocaine withdrawal: [4] = Insufficient documentation. 150 to 200 mg orally daily.

Insomnia: [2] = Fair documentation. Used as monotherapy at dosages ranging from 50 to 100 mg daily.

Prevention of migraine: [2] = Fair documentation. 100 mg daily.

➤*Children:*

Off-label dosing –

Depression:

• *6 years of age and older* –
Maximum dose: 6 mg/kg/day divided 3 times a day.
Initial dosage: 1.5 to 2 mg/kg/day divided 2 to 3 times a day.
Dosage titration: Gradually increase every 3 to 4 days.

Aggressive behavior: [4] = Insufficient documentation. Initial dosage is 50 mg orally once daily at bedtime, titrated up as tolerated and based on response over approximately 1 week.

• *Maintenance dosage* – 150 to 200 mg/day, divided into 3 daily doses. Higher doses may be appropriate in some patients based on tolerance and efficacy.

➤*Elderly:* Use with caution.

➤*Renal function impairment:* Use with caution.

➤*Hepatic function impairment:* Use with caution.

➤*Administration:*

Immediate-release tablets – Instruct patient to take shortly after a meal or light snack. Drowsiness may require a major portion of the trazodone immediate-release daily dose to be administered at bedtime or an overall reduction of dosage.

Extended-release tablets – Trazodone ER should be taken at the same time every day in the late evening, preferably at bedtime, on an empty stomach. Trazodone ER can be swallowed whole or administered as a half tablet

TRAZODONE HYDROCHLORIDE — ORAL

by breaking the tablet along the score line. Breaking the tablet in half does not affect the controlled-release properties of the tablet. In order to maintain its controlled-release properties, trazodone ER should not be chewed or crushed.

➤*Storage/Stability:* Store between 20° and 25°C (68° and 77°F); excursions are permitted to 15° to 30°C (59° to 86°F).

Actions

➤*Pharmacology:* The mechanism of trazodone's antidepressant action in humans is not fully understood, but it is thought to be related to its potentiation of serotonergic activity in the CNS. Preclinical studies have shown that trazodone selectively inhibits neuronal reuptake of serotonin and acts as an antagonist at 5-HT-2A/2C serotonin receptors.

Pharmacodynamics – Trazodone antagonizes alpha-1 adrenergic receptors, a property which may be associated with postural hypotension.

Trazodone is not a monoamine oxidase inhibitor (MAOI) and, unlike amphetamine-type drugs, does not stimulate the CNS.

➤*Pharmacokinetics:* Trazodone ER tablets are dose proportional following single-dose administration of doses ranging from 75 to 375 mg as intact or bisected tablets.

Absorption – Trazodone is well absorbed after oral administration, without selective localization in any tissue.

Peak plasma levels of trazodone immediate-release tablets occur approximately 1 hour after dosing when taken on an empty stomach. Following single-dose administration of trazodone 300 mg ER tablets under fasting conditions, a mean peak trazodone plasma concentration (C_{max}) of 1188 ± 362 ng/mL was reported at a median time to peak plasma concentration (T_{max}) of 9 hours postdose.

Steady-state area under the curve (AUC) of trazodone is equivalent after administration of trazodone 100 mg immediate-release tablets 3 times a day (mean ± standard deviation [SD] AUC_{ss} = 33,058 ± 8,006 ng•h/mL) and trazodone 300 mg ER tablets once daily (mean ± SD AUC_{ss} = 29,131 ± 9,931 ng•h/mL) for 1 week. Steady-state C_{max} and minimum plasma concentration (C_{min}) of trazodone were not equivalent after administration of trazodone 100 mg immediate-release tablets 3 times a day (mean ± SD $C_{max,ss}$ = 3,118 ± 758 ng/mL, $C_{min,ss}$ = 843 ± 274 ng/mL) and trazodone 300 mg ER tablets once daily (mean ± SD $C_{max,ss}$ = 1,812 ± 621 ng/mL, $C_{min,ss}$ = 674 ± 355 ng/mL) for 1 week.

Effect of food: When trazodone immediate-release tablets are taken shortly after ingestion of food, there may be an increase in the amount of drug absorbed, a decrease in C_{max}, and a lengthening in the T_{max}. Peak plasma levels occur approximately 2 hours after dosing when taken with food.

When trazodone 300 mg ER tablets are taken shortly after ingestion of a high-fat meal, C_{max} increases by approximately 86%, compared with taking it under fasting conditions.

Distribution – Trazodone is 89% to 95% protein bound in vitro at concentrations attained with therapeutic doses in humans.

Metabolism – In vitro studies in human liver microsomes show that trazodone is metabolized via oxidative cleavage to an active metabolite, m-chlorophenylpiperazine by cytochrome P450 3A4 (CYP3A4). Trazodone is extensively metabolized; less than 1% of an oral dose is excreted unchanged in the urine.

Excretion – In some patients, trazodone may accumulate in the plasma. Elimination is predominantly renal, with 70% to 75% of an oral dose being recovered in the urine within the first 72 hours of ingestion. Following single-dose administration of trazodone 300 mg ER tablets, a mean apparent terminal half-life of 10 hours was reported.

Contraindications

Hypersensitivity to trazodone.

Warnings/Precautions

➤*Clinical worsening and suicide risk:* Patients with MDD, both adults and children, may experience worsening of their depression and/or the emergence of suicidal ideation and behavior (suicidality) or unusual changes in behavior, whether or not they are taking antidepressant medications, and this risk may persist until significant remission occurs. Suicide is a known risk of depression and certain other psychiatric disorders and these disorders themselves are the strongest predictors of suicide. There has been a long standing concern, however, that antidepressants may have a role in inducing worsening of depression and the emergence of suicidality in certain patients during the early phases of treatment. Pooled analyses of short-term, placebo-controlled trials of antidepressant drugs (selective serotonin reuptake inhibitors [SSRIs] and others) showed that these drugs increase the risk of suicidal thinking and behavior (suicidality) in children, adolescents, and young adults (18 to 24 years of age) with MDD and other psychiatric disorders. Short-term studies did not show an increase in the risk of suicidality with antidepressants compared with placebo in adults older than 24 years of age; there was a reduction with antidepressants compared with placebo in adults 65 years of age and older.

No suicides occurred in any of the pediatric trials. There were suicides in the adult trials, but the number was not sufficient to reach any conclusion about drug effect on suicide.

It is unknown whether the suicidality risk extends to longer-term use (beyond several months). However, there is substantial evidence from placebo-controlled maintenance trials in adults with depression that the use of antidepressants can delay the recurrence of depression.

Appropriately monitor all patients being treated with antidepressants for any indication and closely observe for clinical worsening, suicidality, and unusual changes in behavior, especially during the initial few months of a course of drug therapy or at times of dosage changes, either increases or decreases.

The following symptoms, including anxiety, agitation, panic attacks, insomnia, irritability, hostility, aggressiveness, impulsivity, akathisia (psychomotor restlessness), hypomania, and mania, have been reported in adults and children being treated with antidepressants for MDD as well as for other indications, both psychiatric and nonpsychiatric. Although a causal link between the emergence of such symptoms and either the worsening of depression and/or the emergence of suicidal impulses has not been established, there is concern that such symptoms may represent precursors to emerging suicidality.

Give consideration to changing the therapeutic regimen, including possibly discontinuing the medication, in patients whose depression is persistently worse or those who are experiencing emergent suicidality or symptoms that might be precursors to worsening depression or suicidality, especially if these symptoms are severe, abrupt in onset, or were not part of the patient's presenting symptoms.

Alert families and caregivers of patients being treated with antidepressants for MDD or other indications, both psychiatric and nonpsychiatric, about the need to monitor patients for the emergence of agitation, irritability, unusual changes in behavior, and the other symptoms described previously, as well as the emergence of suicidality, and to report such symptoms immediately to health care providers. Such monitoring should include daily observation by families and caregivers. Write prescriptions for trazodone for the smallest quantity of tablets consistent with good patient management in order to reduce the risk of overdose.

➤*Serotonin syndrome/neuroleptic malignant syndrome–like reactions:* The development of potentially life-threatening serotonin syndrome or neuroleptic malignant syndrome (NMS)–like reactions have been reported with antidepressants alone and may occur with trazodone treatment, but particularly with concomitant use of other serotonergic drugs (including SSRIs, serotonin-norepinephrine reuptake inhibitors (SNRIs), and triptans) and with drugs that impair metabolism of serotonin (including MAOIs), or with antipsychotics or other dopamine antagonists. Serotonin syndrome symptoms may include mental status changes (eg, agitation, hallucinations, coma), autonomic instability (eg, tachycardia, labile blood pressure, hyperthermia), neuromuscular aberrations (eg, hyperreflexia, incoordination), and/or GI symptoms (eg, nausea, vomiting, diarrhea). Serotonin syndrome, in its most severe form, can resemble NMS, which includes hyperthermia, muscle rigidity, autonomic instability with possible rapid fluctuation of vital signs, and mental status changes.

Immediately discontinue treatment with trazodone and any concomitant serotonergic or antidopaminergic agents, including antipsychotics, if the reactions mentioned previously occur and initiate supportive symptomatic treatment.

➤*Bipolar disorder:* A major depressive episode may be the initial presentation of bipolar disorder. It is generally believed (though not established in controlled trials) that treating such an episode with an antidepressant alone may increase the likelihood of precipitation of a mixed/manic episode in patients at risk for bipolar disorder. Whether any of the symptoms described previously represent such a conversion is unknown. However, prior to initiating treatment with an antidepressant, adequately screen patients with depressive symptoms to determine if they are at risk of bipolar disorder; such screening should include a detailed psychiatric history, including a family history of suicide, bipolar disorder, and depression. Note that trazodone is not approved for use in treating bipolar depression.

➤*Cardiovascular effects:*

QT prolongation and risk of sudden death – Trazodone is known to prolong the QT/QTc interval. Some drugs that prolong the QT/QTc interval can cause torsades de pointes with sudden, unexplained death. The relationship of QT prolongation is clearest for larger increases (20 msec and greater), but it is possible that smaller QT/QTc prolongations may also increase the risk, especially in susceptible individuals, such as those with hypokalemia, hypomagnesemia, or a genetic predisposition to prolonged QT/QTc.

Although torsades de pointes has not been observed with the use of trazodone ER at recommended doses in premarketing trials, experience is too limited to rule out an increased risk. However, there have been postmarketing reports of torsades de pointes with the immediate-release form of trazodone (in the presence of multiple confounding factors), even at dosages of 100 mg/day or less.

Preexisting cardiac disease – Trazodone is not recommended for use during the initial recovery phase of myocardial infarction (MI).

Use caution when administering trazodone to patients with cardiac disease and closely monitor such patients, because antidepressant drugs (including trazodone) have been associated with the occurrence of cardiac arrhythmias.

Clinical studies in patients with preexisting cardiac disease indicate that trazodone may be arrhythmogenic in some patients in that population. Arrhythmias identified included isolated premature ventricular contractions, ventricular couplets, and tachycardia with syncope and torsades de pointes. In 2 patients, short episodes (3 to 4 beats) of ventricular tachycardia occurred.

Hypotension – Hypotension, including orthostatic hypotension and syncope, has been reported in patients receiving trazodone. Coadministration of antihypertensive therapy with trazodone may require a reduction in the dose of the antihypertensive drug.

TRAZODONE HYDROCHLORIDE — ORAL

➤*Abnormal bleeding:* Postmarketing data have shown an association between the use of drugs that interfere with serotonin reuptake and the occurrence of GI bleeding. While no association between trazodone and bleeding events, in particular GI bleeding, was shown, caution patients about the potential risk of bleeding associated with the concomitant use of trazodone and nonsteroidal anti-inflammatory drugs (NSAIDs), aspirin, or other drugs that affect coagulation or bleeding. Other bleeding events related to SSRIs and SNRIs have ranged from ecchymosis, hematoma, epistaxis, and petechiae to life-threatening hemorrhages.

➤*Priapism:* Rare cases of priapism (painful erections more than 6 hours in duration) were reported in men receiving trazodone. Priapism, if not treated promptly, can result in irreversible damage to the erectile tissue. In many of the cases reported, surgical intervention was required and, in a portion of these cases, permanent impairment of erectile function or impotence resulted. Men who have an erection lasting more than 6 hours, whether painful or not, should immediately discontinue the drug and seek emergency medical attention.

The detumescence of priapism and drug-induced penile erections has been accomplished by pharmacologic (eg, the intracavernosal injection of alpha-adrenergic stimulants, such as epinephrine and norepinephrine) and surgical procedures. Perform any pharmacologic or surgical procedure utilized in the treatment of priapism under the supervision of a urologist or a health care provider familiar with the procedure and do not initiate without urologic consultation if the priapism has persisted for more than 24 hours.

Trazodone should be used with caution in men who have conditions that might predispose them to priapism (eg, sickle cell anemia, multiple myeloma, leukemia) or in men with anatomical deformation of the penis (eg, angulation, cavernosal fibrosis, Peyronie disease).

➤*Hyponatremia:* Hyponatremia may occur as a result of treatment with antidepressants. In many cases, this hyponatremia appears to be the result of the syndrome of inappropriate secretion of antidiuretic hormone (SIADH). Cases with serum sodium lower than 110 mmol/L have been reported. Elderly patients may be at greater risk of developing hyponatremia with antidepressants. Also, patients taking diuretics or who are otherwise volume-depleted can be at greater risk. Consider discontinuation of trazodone in patients with symptomatic hyponatremia and institute appropriate medical intervention.

➤*Elective surgery:* Little is known about the interaction between trazodone and general anesthetics; therefore, prior to elective surgery, discontinue trazodone for as long as clinically feasible.

➤*Electroconvulsive therapy:* Avoid coadministration with electroshock therapy because of the absence of experience in this area.

➤*Discontinuation:* See Administration and Dosage for more information.

➤*Hematologic effects:* Occasional low white blood cell (WBC) and neutrophil counts have been noted in patients receiving trazodone. These were not considered clinically significant and did not necessitate discontinuation of the drug; however, discontinue the drug in any patient whose WBC count or absolute neutrophil count falls below normal levels.

➤*Renal function impairment:* Use trazodone with caution in this population.

➤*Hepatic function impairment:* Use trazodone with caution in this population.

➤*Hazardous tasks:* Trazodone may cause somnolence or sedation and may impair the mental and/or physical ability required for the performance of potentially hazardous tasks. Caution patients about operating hazardous machinery, including automobiles, until they are reasonably certain that the drug treatment does not affect them adversely.

➤*Pregnancy: Category C.* There are no adequate and well-controlled studies in pregnant women. Trazodone has been shown to cause increased fetal resorption and other adverse effects on the fetus in 2 studies using the rat when given at dose levels of approximately 30 to 50 times the proposed maximum human dose. There was also an increase in congenital anomalies in 1 of 3 rabbit studies at approximately 15 to 50 times the maximum human dose. Use trazodone during pregnancy only if the potential benefit justifies the potential risk to the fetus.

➤*Lactation:* In a study of 6 healthy lactating women, trazodone was excreted into breast milk, with a mean milk:plasma ratio of 0.142. Trazodone and/or its metabolites have been found in the milk of lactating rats. Exercise caution when trazodone is administered to a breast-feeding woman.

Although the amount of trazodone in milk is very small, the American Academy of Pediatrics classifies trazodone as a drug for which the effect on breast-fed infants is unknown, but may be of concern.

➤*Children:* Safety and efficacy in children have not been established.

Anyone considering the use of trazodone immediate-release tablets in a child or adolescent must balance the potential risks with the clinical need. Trazodone ER tablets should not be used in children or adolescents.

➤*Elderly:* Antidepressants have been associated with cases of clinically significant hyponatremia in elderly patients who may be at greater risk for this adverse reaction.

➤*Monitoring:* Appropriately monitor all patients being treated with antidepressants for any indication and closely observe for clinical worsening, suicidality, and unusual changes in behavior, especially during the initial few months of a course of drug therapy or at times of dosage changes, either increases or decreases.

WBC and differential counts are recommended for patients who develop fever and sore throat (or other signs of infection) during therapy. Closely monitor patients with preexisting cardiac disease.

Drug Interactions

➤*QT prolongation:* An additive effect of trazodone with other drugs that prolong the QT interval cannot be excluded. The following drugs may prolong the QT interval and increase the risk of life-threatening cardiac arrhythmias, including torsades de pointes: antiarrhythmic agents (eg, amiodarone, bretylium, disopyramide, dofetilide, procainamide, quinidine, sotalol), arsenic trioxide, chlorpromazine, cisapride, dolasetron, droperidol, mefloquine, mesoridazine, moxifloxacin, pentamidine, pimozide, tacrolimus, thioridazine, and ziprasidone. For a more complete list of drugs that may prolong the QT interval, see the appendix, Drug-Induced Prolongation of the QT Interval and Torsades de Pointes.

Trazodone Drug Interactions

Precipitant drug	Object drug[a]		Description
Alcohol, barbiturates, CNS depressants	Trazodone	↑	Effects may be additive, enhancing the CNS depressant response to these agents. Avoid coadministration.
Trazodone	Alcohol, barbiturates, CNS depressants		
Antihypertensives (eg, propranolol)	Trazodone	↑	May cause additive hypotensive effects. Monitor blood pressure and be prepared to adjust the antihypertensive agent dose as needed.
Trazodone	Antihypertensives (eg, propranolol)		
Azole antifungals (eg, itraconazole, ketoconazole)	Trazodone	↑	Coadministration may lead to substantial increases in trazodone plasma concentrations, with the potential for adverse reactions. Monitor patient response and adjust dose of trazodone as needed. Caution the patient about the increased risk of sedation when an azole antifungal agent is started.
Carbamazepine	Trazodone	↑↓	Plasma concentrations of trazodone and its active metabolite may be decreased. Coadministration may increase carbamazepine levels. Monitor patient when starting or stopping either agent and adjust the trazodone or carbamazepine dose as needed.
Trazodone	Carbamazepine		
Delavirdine	Trazodone	↑	Plasma concentrations of trazodone may be elevated, increasing the pharmacologic effects and risk of adverse reactions. Coadminister with caution. Consider a lower dose of trazodone.
Ginkgo biloba	Trazodone	↑	Trazodone plasma concentrations may be elevated, increasing the pharmacologic effects and risk of adverse reactions (eg, sedation). If coadministration cannot be avoided, monitor the response of the patient when *Ginkgo biloba* is started or stopped. Adjust the trazodone dose as needed. Caution the patient about the increased risk of sedation when *Ginkgo biloba* is started.
Macrolide antibiotics (eg, clarithromycin)	Trazodone	↑	Plasma concentrations of trazodone may be elevated. Coadminister with caution. Monitor the response of the patient when a macrolide or related antibiotic is started or stopped. Adjust the trazodone dose as needed.
MAOIs (eg, phenelzine)	Trazodone	↑	In patients receiving serotonergic drugs in combination with MAOIs, serious, sometimes fatal reactions have been reported. It is recommended that trazodone not be coadministered with an MAOI or within 14 days of discontinuing an MAOI. Similarly, an MAOI should not be given within 14 days of stopping trazodone.
Trazodone	MAOIs (eg, phenelzine)		

TRAZODONE HYDROCHLORIDE — ORAL

Trazodone Drug Interactions

Precipitant drug	Object drug[a]		Description
Phenothiazines (eg, chlorpromazine)	Trazodone	↑	Elevated trazodone serum concentrations have occurred. Monitor the patient and adjust the dose of trazodone as needed. Caution the patient about the increased risk of sedation when a phenothiazine is started.
Protease inhibitors (eg, indinavir, ritonavir)	Trazodone	↑	Trazodone plasma concentrations may be elevated, increasing the pharmacologic and adverse reactions. Monitor patient and adjust the dose of trazodone as needed. Caution the patient about the increased risk of sedation when a protease inhibitor is started.
Serotonergic drugs (eg, dopamine antagonists [eg, metoclopramide], SNRIs [eg, nefazodone], SSRIs [eg, fluoxetine], triptans [eg, sumatriptan], tryptophan)	Trazodone	↑	A serotonin syndrome, including irritability, increased muscle tone, shivering, myoclonus, and altered consciousness, may occur. If coadministration cannot be avoided, start with a low dose of trazodone and closely monitor the patient. Serotonin syndrome requires immediate medical attention, including supportive care and withdrawal of the serotonergic agent. Concomitant use with tryptophan is not recommended.
Trazodone	Serotonergic drugs (eg, dopamine antagonists [eg, metoclopramide], SNRIs [eg, nefazodone], SSRIs [eg, fluoxetine], triptans [eg, sumatriptan], tryptophan)		
Sodium oxybate	Trazodone	↑	Concurrent use of sodium oxybate and trazodone may result in an increase in sleep duration and CNS depression. Sodium oxybate is contraindicated in patients receiving other sedative hypnotics.
Trazodone	Sodium oxybate		
Trazodone	Digoxin	↑	Increased serum digoxin levels have been reported to occur in patients receiving concurrent trazodone. Monitor digoxin levels regularly and adjust the digoxin dose as needed.
Trazodone	NSAIDs (eg, ibuprofen)	↑	The risk of bleeding may be increased. Use with caution. Monitor for bleeding and caution patients about the potential risk of bleeding.
Trazodone	Phenytoin	↑	Phenytoin serum levels were increased with concurrent trazodone therapy. Monitor phenytoin plasma levels regularly and adjust the phenytoin dose as needed.
Trazodone	Salicylates (eg, aspirin)	↑	The risk of bleeding may be increased. Use with caution. Monitor for bleeding and caution patients about the potential risk of bleeding.
Trazodone	Warfarin	↑↓	There have been reports of increased and decreased prothrombin time occurring in patients taking warfarin and trazodone concurrently. Monitor anticoagulant parameters frequently when starting or stopping trazodone. Adjust the warfarin dose as needed.

[a] ↑ = object drug increased; ↑↓ = object drug both increased and decreased.

➤*Drug/Food interactions:*

Immediate-release tablets – See Actions for more information.

Extended-release tablets – See Actions for more information.

Adverse Reactions

➤*Immediate-release tablets:*

Trazodone Immediate-Release Tablets Adverse Reactions

	Inpatients		Outpatients	
Adverse reactions	Trazodone (n = 142)	Placebo (n = 95)	Trazodone (n = 157)	Placebo (n = 158)
Cardiovascular				
Hypertension	2.1%	1.1%	1.3%	< 1%
Hypotension	7%	1.1%	3.8%	0%
Syncope	2.8%	2.1%	4.5%	1.3%
Tachycardia/Palpitations	0%	0%	7%	7%
CNS				
Anger/Hostility	3.5%	6.3%	1.3%	2.5%
Confusion	4.9%	0%	5.7%	7.6%
Decreased concentration	2.8%	2.1%	1.3%	0%
Disorientation	2.1%	0%	< 1%	0%
Dizziness/Light-headedness	19.7%	5.3%	28%	15.2%
Drowsiness	23.9%	6.3%	40.8%	19.6%
Excitement	1.4%	1.1%	5.1%	5.7%
Fatigue	11.3%	4.2%	5.7%	2.5%
Head full (heavy)	2.8%	0%	0%	0%
Headache	9.9%	5.3%	19.8%	15.8%
Impaired memory	1.4%	0%	< 1%	< 1%
Incoordination	4.9%	0%	1.9%	0%
Insomnia	9.9%	10.5%	6.4%	12%
Malaise	2.8%	0%	0%	0%
Nervousness	14.8%	10.5%	6.4%	8.2%
Nightmares/Vivid dreams	< 1%	1.1%	5.1%	5.7%
Paresthesia	1.4%	0%	0%	< 1%
Tremors	2.8%	1.1%	5.1%	3.8%
Dermatologic				
Skin condition/Edema	2.8%	1.1%	7%	1.3%
Sweating/Clamminess	1.4%	1.1%	< 1%	< 1%
GI				
Abdominal/Gastric disorder	3.5%	4.2%	5.7%	4.4%
Bad taste in mouth	1.4%	0%	0%	0%
Constipation	7%	4.2%	7.6%	5.7%
Decreased appetite	3.5%	5.3%	0%	< 1%
Diarrhea	0%	1.1%	4.5%	1.9%
Dry mouth	14.8%	8.4%	33.8%	20.3%
Nausea/Vomiting	9.9%	1.1%	12.7%	9.5%
Respiratory				
Nasal/Sinus congestion	2.8%	0%	5.7%	3.2%
Shortness of breath	< 1%	1.1%	1.3%	0%
Special senses				
Blurred vision	6.3%	4.2%	14.7%	3.8%
Eyes red/tired/itching	2.8%	0%	0%	0%
Tinnitus	1.4%	0%	0%	< 1%
Miscellaneous				
Decreased libido	< 1%	1.1%	1.3%	< 1%
Musculoskeletal aches/pains	5.6%	3.2%	5.1%	2.5%
Weight gain	1.4%	0%	4.5%	1.9%
Weight loss	< 1%	3.2%	5.7%	2.5%

Sinus bradycardia – Occasional sinus bradycardia has occurred in long-term studies.

Other adverse reactions – In addition to the relatively common (greater than 1%) adverse reactions enumerated previously, the following adverse reactions have been reported to occur in association with the use of trazodone in the controlled clinical studies.

TRAZODONE HYDROCHLORIDE — ORAL

CNS – Akathisia, hallucinations/delusions, hypomania, impaired speech, increased libido, numbness.

GI – Flatulence, hypersalivation, increased appetite.

GU – Delayed urine flow, early menses, hematuria, impotence, increased urinary frequency, missed periods, retrograde ejaculation.

Miscellaneous – Allergic reaction, anemia, chest pain, muscle twitches.

➤*Extended-release tablets:*

Most common adverse reactions – The most common adverse reactions (reported in at least 5% of patients and at twice the rate of placebo) are constipation, dizziness, somnolence/sedation, and vision blurred.

Adverse reactions (at least 5%) –

Trazodone Extended Release Adverse Reactions (≥ 5%)

Adverse reactions	Trazodone ER (n = 202)	Placebo (n = 204)
CNS		
Dizziness	25%	12%
Fatigue	15%	8%
Headache	33%	27%
Somnolence/Sedation	46%	19%
GI		
Constipation	8%	2%
Diarrhea	9%	11%
Dry mouth	25%	13%
Nausea	21%	13%
Miscellaneous		
Back pain	5%	3%
Vision blurred	5%	0%

Sexual dysfunction – Adverse reactions related to sexual dysfunction (regardless of causality) were reported by 4.9% and 1.5% of patients treated with trazodone ER and placebo, respectively. In the trazodone ER group, ejaculation disorders occurred in 1.5% of patients, decreased libido occurred in 1.5% of patients, and erectile dysfunction and abnormal orgasm in less than 1% of patients.

Other adverse reactions – The following is a list of treatment-emergent adverse reactions with an incidence of at least 1% to less than 5%.

CNS – Agitation, confusional state, coordination abnormal, disorientation, dysgeusia, memory impairment, migraine, paraesthesia, tremor (at least 1%); amnesia, aphasia, hypesthesia, speech disorder (less than 1%).

Dermatologic – Night sweats (at least 1%); acne, flushing, hyperhidrosis (less than 1%).

GI – Abdominal pain, vomiting (at least 1%); reflux esophagitis (less than 1%).

GU – Micturition urgency (at least 1%); bladder pain, urinary incontinence (less than 1%).

Musculoskeletal – Musculoskeletal complaints, myalgia (at least 1%); muscle twitching (less than 1%).

Special senses – Visual disturbance (at least 1%); dry eye, eye pain, hypoacusis, photophobia, tinnitus, vertigo (less than 1%).

Miscellaneous – Dyspnea, edema (at least 1%); gait disturbance, hypersensitivity, photosensitivity reaction (less than 1%).

➤*Postmarketing:*

Cardiovascular – Arrhythmia, atrial fibrillation, bradycardia, cardiac arrest, cardiospasm, cerebrovascular accident, conduction block, congestive heart failure, MI, orthostatic hypotension and syncope, palpitations, torsades de pointes, vasodilation, ventricular ectopic activity, including ventricular tachycardia and QT prolongation.

CNS – Abnormal dreams, agitation, anxiety, aphasia, ataxia, extrapyramidal symptoms, generalized tonic-clonic seizures, hallucinations, insomnia, paranoid reaction, paresthesia, psychosis, stupor, tardive dyskinesia, vertigo, weakness.

Dermatologic – Alopecia, hirsutism, leukonychia, pruritus, psoriasis, rash, urticaria.

GI – Cholestasis, increased salivation, nausea/vomiting.

GU – Breast enlargement or engorgement, clitorism, lactation, priapism (some patients have required surgical intervention), urinary incontinence, urinary retention.

Hematologic / Lymphatic – Hemolytic anemia, leukocytosis, methemoglobinemia.

Hepatic – Hyperbilirubinemia, jaundice, liver enzyme alterations.

Metabolic / Nutritional – Edema, increased amylase.

Miscellaneous – Apnea, chills, diplopia, SIADH, unexplained death.

Overdosage

➤*Symptoms:* Death from overdosage has occurred in patients ingesting trazodone and other CNS depressant drugs concurrently (namely, alcohol; alcohol, chloral hydrate, and diazepam; amobarbital; chlordiazepoxide; or meprobamate).

The most severe reactions reported to have occurred with overdosage of trazodone alone have been priapism, respiratory arrest, seizures, and electrocardiogram changes, including QT prolongation. The reactions reported most frequently have been drowsiness and vomiting. Overdosage may cause an increase in incidence or severity of any of the reported adverse reactions.

➤*Treatment:* Ensure an adequate airway, oxygenation, and ventilation. Monitor cardiac rhythm and vital signs. General supportive and symptomatic measures are also recommended (eg, for hypotension or excessive sedation). Induction of emesis is not recommended. Gastric lavage with a large bore orogastric tube with appropriate airway protection, if needed, may be indicated if performed soon after ingestion or in symptomatic patients. Activated charcoal should be administered. Forced diuresis may be useful in facilitating elimination of the drug.

In managing overdosage, consider the possibility of multiple drug involvement. Consider contacting a poison control center for additional information on the treatment of any overdose.

Patient Information

Encourage patients, their families, and their caregivers to be alert to the emergence of anxiety, agitation, panic attacks, insomnia, irritability, hostility, aggressiveness, impulsivity, akathisia (psychomotor restlessness), hypomania, mania, other unusual changes in behavior, worsening of depression, and suicidal ideation, especially early during antidepressant treatment and when the dose is adjusted up or down. Advise families and caregivers of patients to observe for the emergence of such symptoms on a day to day basis because changes may be abrupt. Advise them to report such symptoms to the patient's health care provider, especially if they are severe, abrupt in onset, or were not part of the patient's presenting symptoms. Symptoms such as these may be associated with an increased risk of suicidal thinking and behavior and indicate a need for very close monitoring and possibly changes in the medication.

Advise patients to inform their health care provider if they have a history of bipolar disorder, cardiac disease, or MI.

Inform patients that serotonin syndrome could occur and symptoms may include changes in mental status (eg, agitation, hallucinations, coma), autonomic instability (eg, tachycardia, labile blood pressure, hyperthermia), neuromuscular aberrations (eg, hyperreflexia, incoordination) and/or GI symptoms (eg, nausea, vomiting, diarrhea).

Advise patients with prolonged or inappropriate penile erection to immediately discontinue the drug and consult with their health care provider.

Inform patients of the potential for hypotension, including orthostatic hypotension and syncope.

Inform patients of the potential risk of bleeding (including life-threatening hemorrhages) and bleeding related events (including ecchymosis, hematoma, epistaxis, and petechiae) with the concomitant use of trazodone and NSAIDs, aspirin, or other drugs that affect coagulation or bleeding.

Advise patients that withdrawal symptoms, including anxiety, agitation and sleep disturbances, have been reported. Inform patients not to discontinue trazodone abruptly without contacting their health care provider.

Advise patients that trazodone may cause somnolence or sedation and may impair the mental and/or physical ability required for the performance of potentially hazardous tasks. Caution patients about operating hazardous machinery, including automobiles, until they are reasonably certain that the drug treatment does not affect them adversely.

Inform patients that trazodone may enhance the response to alcohol, barbiturates, and other CNS depressants.

Advise women who intend to become pregnant or who are breast-feeding to discuss with their health care provider whether to continue to use trazodone because use in pregnant and breast-feeding women is not recommended.

Instruct patients to take trazodone immediate-release tablets shortly after a meal or light snack. Tell patients that the total drug absorption may be up to 20% higher when the drug is taken with food, rather than on an empty stomach, and the risk of dizziness/light-headedness may increase under fasting conditions.

Instruct patients to take trazodone ER at the same time every day in the late evening, preferably at bedtime, and on an empty stomach. ER tablets are to be swallowed whole or broken in half along the score line. Instruct patients not to chew or crush the tablets.

BUPROPION

	Product	Dosage form	How supplied
Rx	**Bupropion Hydrochloride** (Various, eg, Sandoz, Teva)	**Tablets; oral:** 75 mg	In 30s, 100s, 500s, and 1,000s.
Rx	**Wellbutrin** (GlaxoSmithKline)		As bupropion hydrochloride. (Wellbutrin 75). Yellow-gold. Film-coated. In 100s.
Rx	**Bupropion Hydrochloride** (Various, eg, Sandoz, Teva)	**Tablets; oral:** 100 mg	In 30s, 100s, 500s, and 1,000s.
Rx	**Wellbutrin** (GlaxoSmithKline)		As bupropion hydrochloride. (Wellbutrin 100). Red. Film-coated. In 100s.
Rx	**Bupropion Hydrochloride** (Various, eg, Sandoz, Watson)	**Tablets, extended-release (12-hour); oral:** 100 mg	In 60s, 100s, and 500s.
Rx	**Budeprion SR**[a] (Teva)		As bupropion hydrochloride. Tartrazine. (G 2442). Yellow. Film-coated. In 60s and 100s.
Rx	**Wellbutrin SR**[a] (GlaxoSmithKline)		As bupropion hydrochloride. (Wellbutrin SR 100). Blue. Film-coated. In 60s.
Rx	**Bupropion Hydrochloride** (Various, eg, Sandoz, Watson)	**Tablets, extended-release (12-hour); oral:** 150 mg	In 60s, 100s, 250s, and 500s.
Rx	**Budeprion SR**[a] (Teva)		As bupropion hydrochloride. (G 2444). Lt. yellow. Film-coated. In 60s and 100s.
Rx	**Wellbutrin SR**[a] (GlaxoSmithKline)		As bupropion hydrochloride. (Wellbutrin SR 150). Purple. Film-coated. In 60s.
Rx	**Zyban** (GlaxoSmithKline)	**Tablets, extended-release; oral:** 150 mg	As bupropion hydrochloride. (ZYBAN 150). Purple. Film-coated. In 60s.
Rx	**Bupropion Hydrochloride** (Various, eg, Global, Sandoz, Watson)	**Tablets, extended-release (12-hour); oral:** 200 mg	In 60s, 100s, 180s, 500s, and 1,000s.
Rx	**Wellbutrin SR**[a] (GlaxoSmithKline)		As bupropion hydrochloride. (Wellbutrin SR 200). Lt. pink. Film-coated. In 60s.
Rx	**Bupropion Hydrochloride** (Anchen)	**Tablets, extended-release (24-hour); oral:** 150 mg	(A101). White to off-white. In 30s, 60s, 90s, and 500s.
Rx	**Budeprion XL** (Teva)		As bupropion hydrochloride. (A101). White to off-white, round. In 30s and 500s.
Rx	**Wellbutrin XL**[a] (BTA Pharmaceuticals)		As bupropion hydrochloride. Polyvinyl alcohol. (Wellbutrin XL 150). Creamy white to pale yellow. In 30s and 90s.
Rx	**Bupropion Hydrochloride** (Various, eg, Anchen, Watson)	**Tablets, extended-release (24-hour); oral:** 300 mg	In 30s, 60s, 90s, and 500s.
Rx	**Budeprion XL**[a] (Teva)		As bupropion hydrochloride. Lactose, tartrazine. (682). Yellow, oval. Film-coated. In 30s and 500s.
Rx	**Wellbutrin XL**[a] (BTA Pharmaceuticals)		As bupropion hydrochloride. Polyvinyl alcohol. (Wellbutrin XL 300). Creamy white to pale yellow. In 30s.
Rx	**Aplenzin** (Sanofi-Aventis)	**Tablets, extended-release; oral:** 174 mg	As bupropion hydrobromide. Polyethylene glycol. (BR 174). White to off-white, round. In 30s.
		348 mg	As bupropion hydrobromide. Polyethylene glycol. (BR 348) White to off-white, round. In 30s.
		522 mg	As bupropion hydrobromide. Polyethylene glycol. (BR 522). White to off-white, round. In 30s.

[a] Please note that "SR" refers to the 12-hour tablets and "XL" refers to the 24-hour tablets.

BUPROPION HYDROCHLORIDE — ORAL

For additional information, refer to the Antidepressants introduction.

WARNING

Suicidality and antidepressant drugs – Antidepressants increased the risk of suicidal thinking and behavior (suicidality) in children, adolescents, and young adults in short-term studies of major depressive disorder (MDD) and other psychiatric disorders compared with placebo. Anyone considering the use of bupropion or any other antidepressant in a child, adolescent, or young adult must balance this risk with the clinical need. Short-term studies did not show an increase in the risk of suicidality with antidepressants compared with placebo in adults older than 24 years of age; there was a reduction in risk with antidepressants compared with placebo in adults 65 years of age and older. Depression and certain other psychiatric disorders are themselves associated with increases in suicide risk. Appropriately monitor patients of all ages who are started on antidepressant therapy and closely observe them for clinical worsening, suicidality, or unusual changes in behavior. Advise families and caregivers of the need for close observation and communication with the prescriber. Bupropion is not approved for use in children.

Zyban: Although *Zyban* is not indicated for treatment of depression, it contains the same active ingredient as the antidepressant bupropion medications *Wellbutrin*, *Wellbutrin SR*, and *Wellbutrin XL*.

Indications

➤*Major depressive disorder (MDD):* Immediate-release and extended-release bupropion are indicated for the treatment of MDD.

➤*Seasonal affective disorder (Wellbutrin XL* only): For the prevention of seasonal major depressive episodes in patients with a diagnosis of seasonal affective disorder.

➤*Smoking cessation (Zyban* only): Indicated as an aid to smoking-cessation treatment.

➤*Off-label uses:*

Aphthous ulcers – [4] = Insufficient documentation. The use of bupropion has been limited to one case report that suggests a beneficial effect in the treatment of aphthous ulcers.

Attention deficit hyperactivity disorder (adults) – [2] = Fair documentation. Initial data suggest that bupropion offers an alternative drug therapy option for patients who have an inadequate response to or do not tolerate standard therapy for ADHD with stimulant medications. Larger, controlled trials are needed to fully define the efficacy of bupropion in the treatment of adult ADHD.

Attention deficit hyperactivity disorder (children and adolescents) – [1] = Good documentation. Evidence-based guidelines confirm the efficacy of bupropion for the second-line treatment of attention deficit hyperactivity disorder (ADHD).

Neuropathic pain – [3] = Safety concerns. Several medications and medication classes are recommended as first-line treatment for neuropathic pain by the International Association for the Study of Pain (IASP). The IASP recommends bupropion as a third-line agent for neuropathic pain in patients requiring antidepressant and analgesic effects who have not responded to therapy with preferred antidepressants.

Premenstrual dysphoric disorder – [4] = Insufficient documentation. Selective serotonin reuptake inhibitors (SSRIs) and other antidepressants have shown benefit for the treatment of premenstrual syndrome (PMS)/ premenstrual dysphoric disorder (PMDD). A single trial comparing bupropion with fluoxetine found that fluoxetine was superior to placebo and bupropion for the treatment of PMDD. In addition, bupropion was not statistically different from placebo.

Prevention of migraine (adults) – [4] = Insufficient documentation. Bupropion has not been formally studied for the prevention of migraine. However, American Academy of Neurology practice guidelines state that bupropion is clinically efficacious based on consensus and clinical experience, despite a lack of scientific evidence of efficacy. No dosage was reported.

BUPROPION HYDROCHLORIDE — ORAL

Promotion of weight loss – [2] = Fair documentation. Initial data suggest that bupropion, especially in women, may have some benefit in promoting weight loss when used in combination with lifestyle changes. Additional long-term controlled trials with larger sample sizes including both genders are needed to confirm these preliminary results and to assess the effect on body weight after bupropion is discontinued.

Other possible off-label uses – Sustained-release bupropion has been effective in the treatment of neuropathic pain.

Administration and Dosage

➤*General dosing considerations:* It is particularly important to administer immediate-release bupropion and extended-release (XL and SR) bupropion in a manner most likely to minimize the risk of seizure. Gradual escalation in dosage is also important if agitation, insomnia, and motor restlessness, often seen during the initial days of treatment, are to be minimized. If necessary, these effects may be managed by temporary reduction of the dose or the short-term administration of an intermediate- to long-acting sedative hypnotic. A sedative hypnotic usually is not required beyond the first week of treatment. Insomnia also may be minimized by avoiding bedtime doses. If distressing, untoward effects supervene, dose escalation should be stopped.

➤*Adults:*

Major Depressive Disorder –

Immediate release:

• *Usual dosage* – 300 mg/day given as 100 mg 3 times daily.

• *Maximum dose* – 450 mg/day. No single dose should exceed 150 mg.

• *Initial dosage* – 200 mg/day, given as 100 mg twice daily.

• *Maintenance dosage* – The lowest dose that maintains remission is recommended.

• *Dosage adjustment* – Based on clinical response, this dose may be increased to 300 mg/day, given as 100 mg 3 times daily, no sooner than 3 days after beginning therapy. Increases in dose should not exceed 100 mg/day in a 3-day period.

As with other antidepressants, the full antidepressant effect of immediate-release bupropion may not be evident until 4 weeks of treatment or longer. An increase in dose, up to a maximum of 450 mg/day, given in divided doses of not more than 150 mg each, may be considered for patients in whom no clinical improvement is noted after several weeks of treatment at 300 mg/day.

• *Duration of therapy* – Although it is not known how long a patient should remain on immediate-release bupropion, it is generally recognized that acute episodes of depression require several months or longer of antidepressant drug treatment.

• *Discontinuation of therapy* – Immediate-release bupropion should be discontinued in patients who do not demonstrate an adequate response after an appropriate period of treatment at 450 mg/day.

Extended-release:

• *Usual dosage* – 300 mg/day, given once daily in the morning (*Wellbutrin XL*) or given as 150 mg twice daily (*Wellbutrin SR*).

• *Maximum dose* – 450 mg/day administered as a single dose (*Wellbutrin XL*) or 400 mg/day given as 200 mg twice daily (*Wellbutrin SR*).

• *Initial dosage* – 150 mg/day (*Wellbutrin XL* and *Wellbutrin SR*), given as a single daily dose in the morning.

• *Maintenance dosage* – It is unknown if the dosage of extended-release bupropion needed for maintenance treatment is identical to the dosage needed to achieve an initial response. Patients should be periodically reassessed to determine appropriate dosage for such treatment.

• *Dosage adjustment* – If the 150 mg initial dose is adequately tolerated, an increase to the 300 mg/day target dose, given once daily (*Wellbutrin XL*) or given as 150 mg twice daily (*Wellbutrin SR*), may be made as early as day 4 of dosing.

As with other antidepressants, the full antidepressant effect of extended-release bupropion may not be evident until 4 weeks of treatment or longer. An increase in dose to the maximum of 450 mg/day administered as a single dose (*Wellbutrin XL*) or 400 mg/day given as 200 mg twice daily (*Wellbutrin SR*), may be considered for patients in whom no clinical improvement is noted after several weeks of treatment at 300 mg/day.

• *Duration of therapy* – It is generally agreed that acute episodes of depression require several months or longer of sustained pharmacological therapy beyond response to the acute episode. Patients should be periodically reassessed to determine the need for maintenance treatment.

Longer-term efficacy was demonstrated in a study in which patients with recurrent type MDD who had responded during 8 weeks of acute treatment with *Wellbutrin SR* were assigned randomly to placebo or to the same dose of *Wellbutrin SR* (150 mg twice daily) during 44 weeks of maintenance treatment as they had received during the acute stabilization phase.

• *Conversion* – When switching patients from immediate-release bupropion to *Wellbutrin XL* or from *Wellbutrin SR* to *Wellbutrin XL*, administer the same total daily dosage when possible. Patients who are currently being treated with immediate-release bupropion 300 mg/day (eg, 100 mg 3 times/day) may be switched to *Wellbutrin XL* 300 mg once daily. Patients who are currently being treated with *Wellbutrin SR* 300 mg/day (eg, 150 mg twice daily) may be switched to *Wellbutrin XL* 300 mg once daily.

Seasonal affective disorder (Wellbutrin XL only) – The timing of initiation and duration of treatment should be individualized based on the patient's historical pattern of seasonal major depressive episodes. Patients whose seasonal depressive episodes are infrequent or not associated with significant impairment should not generally be treated prophylactically.

Usual dosage: 300 mg/day, given once daily in the morning.

Doses above 300 mg/day have not been studied for the prevention of seasonal major depressive episodes.

Initial dosage: 150 mg/day given as a single daily dose in the morning, generally initiated in the autumn prior to the onset of depressive symptoms.

Dosage adjustment: If the 150 mg initial dose is adequately tolerated, the dose should be increased to the 300 mg/day dose after 1 week. If the 300 mg dose is not adequately tolerated, the dose can be reduced to 150 mg/day.

Duration of therapy: Treatment should continue through the winter season and should be tapered and discontinued in early spring.

Discontinuation of therapy: For patients taking 300 mg/day during the autumn-winter season, the dose should be tapered to 150 mg/day for 2 weeks prior to discontinuation.

Smoking cessation (Zyban only) – It is important that patients continue to receive counseling and support throughout treatment and for a period of time thereafter.

Usual dosage: 300 mg/day, given as 150 mg twice daily.

Maximum dose: 300 mg/day.

Initial dosage: 150 mg/day given every day for the first 3 days, followed by a dosage increase for most patients to the recommended dose of 300 mg/day.

Treatment should be initiated while the patient is still smoking because approximately 1 week of treatment is required to achieve steady-state blood levels of bupropion. Patients should set a target quit date within the first 2 weeks of treatment with *Zyban*, generally in the second week.

Maintenance dosage: Systematic evaluation of 300 mg/day for maintenance therapy demonstrated that treatment for up to 6 months was efficacious. Whether to continue treatment for periods longer than 12 weeks for smoking cessation must be determined for individual patients.

Duration of therapy: Treatment should be continued for 7 to 12 weeks; longer treatment should be guided by the relative benefits and risks for individual patients. If a patient has not made significant progress towards abstinence by the seventh week of therapy with *Zyban*, it is unlikely that he or she will quit during that attempt, and treatment should probably be discontinued. Conversely, a patient who successfully quits after 7 to 12 weeks of treatment should be considered for ongoing therapy.

Nicotine dependence is a chronic condition. Some patients may need continuous treatment.

Concomitant therapy: Combination treatment with *Zyban* and nicotine transdermal system may be prescribed for smoking cessation. Monitoring for treatment-emergent hypertension in patients treated with this combination is recommended.

Discontinuation of therapy: Dose tapering is not required when discontinuing treatment.

Individualization of therapy: Patients are more likely to quit smoking and remain abstinent if they are seen frequently and receive support from their health care provider. It is important to ensure that patients read the instructions provided to them and have their questions answered. Health care providers should review the patient's overall smoking-cessation program that includes treatment with *Zyban*. Patients should be advised of the importance of participating in the behavioral interventions, counseling, and/or support services to be used in conjunction with *Zyban*.

The goal of therapy is complete abstinence. If a patient has not made significant progress towards abstinence by the seventh week of therapy, it is unlikely that he or she will quit during that attempt, and treatment should probably be discontinued.

Patients who fail to quit smoking during an attempt may benefit from interventions to improve their chances for success on subsequent attempts. Patients who are unsuccessful should be evaluated to determine why they failed. A new quit attempt should be encouraged when factors that contributed to failure can be eliminated or reduced and conditions are more favorable.

Off-label dosing –

Aphthous ulcers: [4] = Insufficient documentation. Titrate up to 300 mg. Duration not provided.

Attention deficit hyperactivity disorder (adults): [2] = Fair documentation. Dosages ranged from 150 to 450 mg/day. Initiate therapy with 150 mg/day and titrate based on tolerability and efficacy. Doses can be given as divided doses or in extended- or sustained-release formulations.

Neuropathic pain: [3] = Safety concerns. Bupropion sustained-release formulation titrated to 150 mg twice daily for 6 weeks.

Premenstrual dysphoric disorder: [4] = Insufficient documentation. 100 mg 3 times daily.

Promotion of weight loss: [2] = Fair documentation. Initial dosage of 100 to 150 mg daily, then titrated to 300 to 400 mg daily for 24 to 48 weeks.

➤*Children:*

Off-label dosing –

Attention deficit hyperactivity disorder (children and adolescents): [1] = Good documentation.

• *Immediate-release* – Up to 3 mg/kg/day or 150 mg/day orally initially, titrated to a maximum dosage of up to 6 mg/kg/day or 300 mg/day; single dose should not exceed 150 mg. Usually given as divided doses for safety and effectiveness: twice daily for children and 3 times daily for adolescents.

• *Extended-release* – Up to 3 mg/kg/day or 150 mg/day orally initially, titrated to a maximum dosage of up to 6 mg/kg/day or 300 mg/day; single dose should not exceed 150 mg. Usually given as divided doses for safety and effectiveness: twice daily for children and 3 times daily for adolescents.

• *Sustained-release* – Up to 3 mg/kg/day or 150 mg/day orally initially, titrated to a maximum dosage of up to 6 mg/kg/day or 300 mg/day; single dose should not exceed 150 mg. Usually given as divided doses for safety and effectiveness: twice daily for children and 3 times daily for adolescents.

➤*Elderly:* Because elderly patients are more likely to have decreased renal function, take care in dose selection; it may be useful to monitor renal function.

BUPROPION HYDROCHLORIDE — ORAL

➤*Renal function impairment:* Bupropion should be used with caution in patients with renal function impairment, and a reduced frequency and/or dosage should be considered.

➤*Hepatic function impairment:* Bupropion should be used with caution in patients with hepatic function impairment (including mild to moderate hepatic cirrhosis), and a reduced frequency and/or dosage should be considered in patients with mild to moderate hepatic cirrhosis.

Bupropion should be used with extreme caution in patients with severe hepatic cirrhosis. In these patients, the dosage should not exceed 75 mg once daily for immediate-release bupropion; 100 mg every day or 150 mg every other day for *Wellbutrin SR*; and 150 mg every other day for *Wellbutrin XL* and *Zyban*).

➤*Administration:*

Immediate-release – Administered 3 times daily, preferably with at least 6 hours between successive doses.

Dosing above 300 mg/day may be accomplished using the 75 or 100 mg tablets. The 100 mg tablet must be administered 4 times/day with at least 4 hours between successive doses in order not to exceed the limit of 150 mg in a single dose.

Extended-release – Should be swallowed whole, not crushed, divided, or chewed, and may be taken without regard to meals. There should be an interval of at least 24 hours (*Wellbutrin XL*) or at least 8 hours (*Wellbutrin SR*) between successive doses.

Zyban – Tablets should be swallowed whole, not crushed, divided, or chewed. There should be an interval of at least 8 hours between successive doses.

➤*Storage/Stability:*

Immediate-release – Store at 15° to 25°C (59° to 77°F). Protect from light and moisture.

Wellbutrin XL – Store at 25°C (77°F); excursions are permitted to 15° to 30°C (59° to 86°F).

Wellbutrin SR and *Zyban* – Store at 20° to 25°C (68° to 77°F). Dispense in a tight, light-resistant container.

Actions

➤*Pharmacology:* Bupropion, an antidepressant of the aminoketone class or a nonnicotine aid to smoking cessation, is chemically unrelated to other known antidepressants. Bupropion is a relatively weak inhibitor of the neuronal uptake of norepinephrine, serotonin, and dopamine, and does not inhibit monoamine oxidase (MAO). While the mechanism of action of bupropion as an antidepressant or as a smoking deterrent is unknown, it is presumed that this action is mediated by noradrenergic and/or dopaminergic mechanisms.

Bupropion produces dose-related CNS-stimulant effects in animals, as evidenced by increased locomotor activity, increased rates of responding in various schedule-controlled operant behavior tasks, and, at high doses, the induction of mild stereotyped behavior.

Bupropion causes convulsions in rodents and dogs at doses approximately 10-fold the dose recommended as the human antidepressant dose.

➤*Pharmacokinetics:*

Absorption – Bupropion is a racemic mixture. The pharmacologic activity and pharmacokinetics of the individual enantiomers have not been studied. Bupropion follows biphasic pharmacokinetics best described by a 2-compartment model. The steady-state plasma concentrations of bupropion are reached within 8 days.

Plasma bupropion concentrations are dose proportional following single doses of 100 to 250 mg; however, it is not known if the proportionality between dose and plasma level are maintained in chronic use.

Bupropion has not been administered intravenously (IV) to humans; therefore, the absolute bioavailability of bupropion tablets in humans has not been determined. However, it appears likely that only a small proportion of any orally administered dose reaches the systemic circulation intact. In rat and dog studies, the bioavailability of bupropion ranged from 5% to 20%.

Immediate-release: In humans, following oral administration of immediate-release bupropion, peak plasma concentrations are usually achieved within 2 hours, followed by a biphasic decline.

Zyban and *Wellbutrin SR*: Following oral administration of *Zyban* or *Wellbutrin SR* to healthy volunteers, peak plasma concentrations of bupropion are achieved within 3 hours. The mean maximum drug concentration (C_{max}) values for *Zyban* were 91 and 143 ng/mL from 2 single-dose (150 mg) studies. At steady state, the mean C_{max} following a 150 mg dose every 12 hours is 136 ng/mL.

Wellbutrin XL: Following oral administration of *Wellbutrin XL* to healthy volunteers, time to reach C_{max} (T_{max}) for bupropion was approximately 5 hours, and food did not affect the C_{max} or area under the curve (AUC) of bupropion.

Effect of food:

Bioequivalency: In a study comparing chronic dosing with *Wellbutrin SR* 150 mg twice daily to immediate-release bupropion 100 mg 3 times daily, peak plasma concentrations of bupropion at steady state for *Wellbutrin SR* tablets were approximately 85% of those achieved with the immediate-release formulation. There was equivalence for bupropion AUCs and equivalence for both peak plasma concentration and AUCs for all 3 of the detectable bupropion metabolites. Thus, at steady state, *Wellbutrin SR* given twice daily and immediate-release bupropion given 3 times daily are essentially bioequivalent for bupropion and the 3 quantitatively important metabolites.

In a study comparing 14-day dosing with *Wellbutrin XL* 300 mg once daily to immediate-release bupropion at 100 mg 3 times daily, equivalence was demonstrated for peak plasma concentration and AUC for bupropion and the 3 metabolites (hydroxybupropion, threohydrobupropion, and erythrohydrobupropion).

Additionally, in a study comparing 14-day dosing with *Wellbutrin XL* 300 mg once daily to *Wellbutrin SR* 150 mg 2 times daily, equivalence was demonstrated for peak plasma concentration and AUC for bupropion and the 3 metabolites.

Distribution – In vitro tests show that bupropion is 84% bound to human plasma protein at concentrations up to 200 mcg/mL. The extent of protein binding of the hydroxybupropion metabolite is similar to that of bupropion, whereas the extent of protein binding of the threohydrobupropion metabolite is about half that seen with bupropion.

The distribution phase has a mean half-life of 3 to 4 hours.

Zyban: The volume of distribution estimated from a single 150 mg dose given to 17 subjects is 1,950 L (20% coefficient of variation [CV]).

Metabolism/Excretion – Bupropion is extensively metabolized in humans. The following 3 metabolites have been shown to be active: hydroxybupropion, which is formed via hydroxylation of the tert-butyl group of bupropion, and the amino-alcohol isomers threohydrobupropion and erythrohydrobupropion, which are formed via reduction of the carbonyl group. In vitro findings suggest that CYP-450 2B6 (CYP2B6) is the principal isoenzyme involved in the formation of hydroxybupropion, while CYP-450 isoenzymes are not involved in the formation of threohydrobupropion. Oxidation of the bupropion side chain results in the formation of a glycine conjugate of metachlorobenzoic acid, which then is excreted as the major urinary metabolite. The potency and toxicity of the metabolites relative to bupropion have not been fully characterized. However, it has been demonstrated in an antidepressant screening test in mice that hydroxybupropion is one-half as potent as bupropion, while threohydrobupropion and erythrohydrobupropion are 5-fold less potent than bupropion. This may be of clinical importance because the plasma concentrations of the metabolites are as high or higher than those of bupropion.

Bupropion and its metabolites exhibit linear kinetics following chronic administration of 300 to 450 mg/day.

Following a single dose in humans, peak plasma concentrations of hydroxybupropion occur approximately 3 hours after administration of immediate-release bupropion, approximately 6 hours after *Wellbutrin SR* and *Zyban* tablets, and approximately 7 hours after administration of *Wellbutrin XL*. For the immediate-release tablets, *Wellbutrin SR*, and *Zyban*, peak plasma concentrations of hydroxybupropion are approximately 10 times the peak level of the parent drug at steady state. Following administration of extended-release bupropion, peak plasma concentrations of hydroxybupropion are approximately 7 times the peak level of the parent drug at steady state. The elimination half-life of hydroxybupropion is approximately 20 (± 5) hours, and its AUC at steady state is about 17 times that of bupropion for the immediate-release tablets, *Wellbutrin SR*, and *Zyban*, and about 13 times that of bupropion for *Wellbutrin XL*. The times to peak concentrations for the erythrohydrobupropion and threohydrobupropion metabolites are similar to that of the hydroxybupropion metabolite. However, their elimination half-lives are longer, approximately 33 (± 10) and 37 (± 13) hours, respectively, and steady-state AUCs are 1.5 (1.4 for *Wellbutrin XL*) and 7 times that of bupropion, respectively.

Following oral administration of ^{14}C-bupropion 200 mg in humans, 87% and 10% of the radioactive dose were recovered in the urine and feces, respectively. However, the fraction of the oral dose of bupropion excreted unchanged was only 0.5%, a finding consistent with the extensive metabolism of bupropion.

The mean elimination half-life (± standard deviation [SD]) of bupropion after chronic dosing is 21 (± 9) hours.

Immediate-release: The terminal phase has a mean half-life of 14 hours, with a range of 8 to 24 hours.

Zyban: The terminal phase has a mean half-life (± % CV) of 21 hours (± 20%). The mean (± % CV) apparent clearance (Cl/F) estimated from 2 single-dose (150 mg) studies are 135 (± 20%) and 209 L/h (± 21%). Following chronic dosing of 150 mg of *Zyban* every 12 hours for 14 days (n = 34), the mean Cl/F at steady state was 160 L/h (± 23%). The mean elimination half-life of *Zyban*, estimated from a series of studies, is approximately 21 hours. Estimates of the half-lives of the metabolites determined from a multiple-dose study were 20 hours (± 25%) for hydroxybupropion, 37 hours (± 35%) for threohydrobupropion, and 33 hours (± 30%) for erythrohydrobupropion. Steady-state plasma concentrations of bupropion and its metabolites are reached within 5 and 8 days, respectively.

Special populations –

Renal function impairment: There is limited information on the pharmacokinetics of bupropion in patients with renal function impairment. An interstudy comparison between healthy subjects and patients with end-stage renal failure demonstrated that the parent drug C_{max} and AUC values were comparable in the 2 groups, whereas the hydroxybupropion and threohydrobupropion metabolites had a 2.3- and 2.8-fold increase, respectively, in AUC for patients with end-stage renal failure. The elimination of the major metabolites of bupropion may be reduced by renal function impairment.

Hepatic function impairment: The effect of hepatic function impairment on the pharmacokinetics of bupropion was characterized in 2 single-dose studies, one in patients with alcoholic liver disease and one in patients with mild to severe cirrhosis. The first study showed that the half-life of hydroxybupropion was significantly longer in 8 patients with alcoholic liver disease than in 8 healthy volunteers (32 ± 14 hours versus 21 ± 5 hours, respectively). Although not statistically significant, the AUCs for bupropion and hydroxybupropion were more variable and tended to be greater (by 53% to

BUPROPION HYDROCHLORIDE — ORAL

57%) in patients with alcoholic liver disease. The differences in half-life for bupropion and the other metabolites in the 2 patient groups were minimal.

The second study showed that there were no statistically significant differences in the pharmacokinetics of bupropion and its active metabolites in 9 patients with mild to moderate hepatic cirrhosis, compared with 8 healthy volunteers. However, more variability was observed in some of the pharmacokinetic parameters for bupropion (AUC, C_{max}, and T_{max}) and its active metabolites ($t_{½}$) in patients with mild to moderate hepatic cirrhosis. In addition, in patients with severe hepatic cirrhosis, the bupropion C_{max} and AUC were substantially increased (mean difference, approximately 70% and 3-fold, respectively) and more variable when compared with values in healthy volunteers; the mean bupropion half-life also was longer (29 hours in patients with severe hepatic cirrhosis versus 19 hours in healthy subjects). For the metabolite hydroxybupropion, the mean C_{max} was approximately 69% lower.

For the combined amino-alcohol isomers threohydrobupropion and erythrohydrobupropion, the mean C_{max} was approximately 31% lower.

The mean AUC increased about 1.5-fold (28% for *Zyban*) for hydroxybupropion and about 2.5-fold (50% for *Zyban*) for threo/erythrohydrobupropion.

The median T_{max} was observed 19 hours later for hydroxybupropion and 31 hours later (21 hours later for *Zyban*) for threo/erythrohydrobupropion. The mean half-lives for hydroxybupropion and threo/erythrohydrobupropion were increased 5- and 2-fold (2- and 4-fold, respectively, with *Zyban*), respectively, in patients with severe hepatic cirrhosis, compared with healthy volunteers.

Elderly: A pharmacokinetic study, single and multiple dose, has suggested that elderly individuals are at increased risk for accumulation of bupropion and its metabolites.

Contraindications

Seizure disorder; in patients treated with other bupropion products because the incidence of seizure is dose dependent; current or prior diagnosis of bulimia or anorexia nervosa because of a higher incidence of seizures noted in patients treated for bulimia with immediate-release bupropion; in patients undergoing abrupt discontinuation of alcohol or sedatives (including benzodiazepines); coadministration of an MAO inhibitor (MAOI); hypersensitivity to bupropion or the other ingredients.

Warnings/Precautions

➤*Clinical worsening and suicide risk:* Patients with MDD, both adults and children, may experience worsening of their depression and/or the emergence of suicidal ideation and behavior (suicidality) or unusual changes in behavior, whether or not they are taking antidepressant medications; this risk may persist until significant remission occurs. Suicide is a known risk of depression and certain other psychiatric disorders, and these disorders themselves are the strongest predictors of suicide. There has been a longstanding concern, however, that antidepressants may have a role in inducing worsening of depression and the emergence of suicidality in certain patients during the early phases of treatment.

Pooled analyses of short-term, placebo-controlled trials of antidepressant drugs (selective serotonin reuptake inhibitors [SSRIs] and others) showed that these drugs increase the risk of suicidal thinking and behavior (suicidality) in children, adolescents, and young adults (18 to 24 years of age) with MDD and other psychiatric disorders. Short-term studies did not show an increase in the risk of suicidality with antidepressants compared with placebo in adults older than 24 years of age; there was a reduction with antidepressants compared with placebo in adults 65 years of age and older.

The pooled analyses of placebo-controlled trials in children and adolescents with MDD, obsessive-compulsive disorder (OCD), or other psychiatric disorders included a total of 24 short-term trials of 9 antidepressant drugs in more than 4,400 patients. The pooled analyses of placebo-controlled trials in adults with MDD or other psychiatric disorders included a total of 295 short-term trials (median duration, 2 months) of 11 antidepressant drugs in more than 77,000 patients. There was considerable variation in the risk of suicidality among drugs but a tendency toward an increase in the younger patients for almost all drugs studied. There were differences in absolute risk of suicidality across the different indications, with the highest incidence in MDD. However, the risk differences (drug vs placebo) were relatively stable within age strata and across indications. These risk differences (drug-placebo difference in the number of cases of suicidality per 1,000 patients treated) are provided in the following table.

Suicidality per 1,000 Patients Treated: Antidepressants vs. Placebo

Age range	Number of cases
Increases compared with placebo	
< 18 years of age	14 additional cases
18 to 24 years of age	5 additional cases
Decreases compared with placebo	
25 to 64 years of age	1 fewer case
≥ 65 years of age	6 fewer cases

No suicides occurred in any of the pediatric trials. There were suicides in the adult trials, but the number was not sufficient to reach any conclusion about drug effect on suicide.

It is unknown whether the suicidality risk extends to longer-term use (ie, beyond several months). However, there is substantial evidence from placebo-controlled maintenance trials in adults with depression that the use of antidepressants can delay the recurrence of depression.

Appropriately monitor all patients being treated with antidepressants for any indication and closely observe them for clinical worsening, suicidality, and unusual changes in behavior, especially during the initial few months of a course of drug therapy, or at times of dose change, either increases or decreases.

Anxiety, agitation, panic attacks, insomnia, irritability, hostility, aggressiveness, impulsivity, akathisia (psychomotor restlessness), hypomania, and mania have been reported in adults and children being treated with antidepressants for MDD and other indications, both psychiatric and nonpsychiatric. Although a causal link between the emergence of such symptoms and either the worsening of depression and/or emergence of suicidal impulses has not been established, there is concern that such symptoms may represent precursors to emerging suicidality.

Consider changing the therapeutic regimen, including possibly discontinuing the medication, in patients whose depression is persistently worse or who are experiencing emergent suicidality or symptoms that might be precursors to worsening depression or suicidality, especially if these symptoms are severe, abrupt in onset, or were not part of the patient's presenting symptoms.

See the Patient Information section for more information.

➤*Screening patients for bipolar disorder:* A major depressive episode may be the initial presentation of bipolar disorder. It generally is believed (although not established in controlled trials) that treating such an episode with an antidepressant alone may increase the likelihood of precipitation of a mixed/manic episode in patients at risk for bipolar disorder. Whether any of the symptoms described above represent such a conversion is unknown. However, prior to initiating treatment with an antidepressant, adequately screen patients with depressive symptoms to determine if they are at risk for bipolar disorder; such screening should include a detailed psychiatric history, including a family history of suicide, bipolar disorder, and depression. Note that bupropion is not approved for use in treating bipolar depression.

➤*Other bupropion medications:* Bupropion immediate-release, *Wellbutrin SR*, and *Wellbutrin XL* contain the same active ingredient found in *Zyban*, used as an aid to smoking cessation treatment. Do not use bupropion in combination with *Zyban* or any other medications that contain bupropion.

➤*Seizures:* Bupropion is associated with a dose-related risk of seizures. Discontinue bupropion and do not restart in patients who experience a seizure while on treatment. The risk of seizures is also related to patient factors, clinical situations, and concomitant medications, which must be considered in selection of patients for therapy with bupropion.

Immediate-release – Bupropion is associated with seizures in approximately 0.4% (4/1,000) of patients treated at doses of up to 450 mg/day. This incidence of seizures may exceed that of other marketed antidepressants by as much as 4-fold. This relative risk is only an approximate estimate because no direct comparative studies have been conducted. The estimated seizure incidence for immediate-release bupropion increases almost 10-fold between 450 and 600 mg/day, which is twice the usually required daily dose (300 mg) and one and one-third the maximum recommended daily dose (450 mg). Given the wide variability among individuals and their capacity to metabolize and eliminate drugs, this disproportionate increase in seizure incidence with dose escalation calls for caution in dosing.

During the initial development, 25 of approximately 2,400 patients treated with immediate-release bupropion experienced seizures. At the time of seizure, 7 patients were receiving daily doses of 450 mg or below for an incidence of 0.33% (3/1,000) within the recommended dosage range. Twelve patients experienced seizures at 600 mg/day (2.3% incidence); 6 additional patients had seizures at daily doses between 600 and 900 mg (2.8% incidence).

A separate, prospective study was conducted to determine the incidence of seizure during an 8-week treatment exposure in approximately 3,200 additional patients who received daily doses of up to 450 mg. Patients were permitted to continue treatment beyond 8 weeks if clinically indicated. Eight seizures occurred during the initial 8-week treatment period, and 5 seizures were reported in patients continuing treatment beyond 8 weeks, resulting in a total seizure incidence of 0.4%.

The risk of seizure appears to be strongly associated with dose. Sudden and large increments in dose may contribute to increased risk. While many seizures occurred early in the course of treatment, some seizures did occur after several weeks at a fixed dosage.

Wellbutrin SR – At doses of *Wellbutrin SR* up to a dose of 300 mg/day, the incidence of seizure is approximately 0.1% and increases to approximately 0.4% at the maximum recommended dose of 400 mg/day.

Zyban – For smoking cessation, do not use doses higher than 300 mg/day. The seizure rate associated with doses of *Wellbutrin SR* up to 300 mg/day is approximately 0.1%. This incidence was prospectively determined during an 8-week treatment exposure in approximately 3,100 depressed patients.

Patient factors – Predisposing factors that may increase the risk of seizure with bupropion use include history of head trauma or seizure, CNS tumor, the presence of severe hepatic cirrhosis, and concomitant medications that lower seizure threshold.

Clinical situations – Circumstances associated with an increased seizure risk include, among others, excessive use of alcohol or sedatives (including benzodiazepines); addiction to opiates, cocaine, or stimulants; use of nonprescription stimulants and anorectics; and diabetes treated with oral hypoglycemics or insulin.

Concomitant medications – Many medications (eg, antidepressants, antipsychotics, systemic steroids, theophylline) are known to lower seizure threshold.

BUPROPION HYDROCHLORIDE — ORAL

Recommendations for reducing the risk of seizure – Use extreme caution when bupropion is administered to patients with a history of seizure, cranial trauma, or other predisposition(s) toward seizure, or is prescribed with other agents (eg, antipsychotics, other antidepressants, systemic steroids, theophylline) that lower seizure threshold.

Retrospective analysis of clinical experience gained during the development of bupropion suggests that the risk of seizure may be minimized if 1) the total daily dose does not exceed immediate-release bupropion 450 mg (400 mg for *Wellbutrin SR*; 450 mg for *Wellbutrin XL*; 300 mg for *Zyban*), 2) the daily dose of immediate-release bupropion is administered 3 times/day with each single dose not to exceed 150 mg to avoid high peak concentrations of bupropion and/or its metabolites (twice daily for *Wellbutrin SR* tablets with each single dose not to exceed 200 mg; twice daily for *Zyban* with each single dose not to exceed 150 mg), and 3) the rate of incrementation of the dosage is very gradual.

➤*Hepatotoxicity:* In rats receiving large doses of bupropion chronically, there was an increase in incidence of hepatic hyperplastic nodules and hepatocellular hypertrophy. In dogs receiving large doses of bupropion chronically, various histologic changes were seen in the liver, and laboratory tests suggesting mild hepatocellular injury were noted.

➤*Altered appetite and weight:*

Immediate-release – A weight loss of more than 5 lbs (2.3 kg) occurred in 28% of patients receiving immediate-release bupropion. This incidence is approximately double that seen in comparable patients treated with tricyclics or placebo. Furthermore, while 35% of patients receiving tricyclic antidepressants gained weight, only 9.4% of patients treated with immediate-release bupropion did. Consequently, if weight loss is a major presenting sign of a patient's depressive illness, consider the anorectic and/or weight-reducing potential of immediate-release bupropion.

Wellbutrin SR – In placebo-controlled studies using *Wellbutrin SR*, patients experienced weight gain or weight loss as shown in the following table.

Incidence of Weight Gain and Weight Loss of *Wellbutrin SR*

Weight change	*Wellbutrin SR* 300 mg/day (n = 339)	*Wellbutrin SR* 400 mg/day (n = 112)	Placebo (n = 347)
Gained > 5 lbs	3%	2%	4%
Lost > 5 lbs	14%	19%	6%

Wellbutrin XL – In 3 placebo-controlled clinical trials of seasonal affective disorder with *Wellbutrin XL*, the percentage of patients with weight gain or weight loss are shown in the following table.

Incidence of Weight Gain and Weight Loss of *Wellbutrin XL*

Weight change	*Wellbutrin XL* 150 to 300 mg/day (n = 537)	Placebo (n = 511)
Gained > 5 lbs	11%	21%
Lost > 5 lbs	23%	11%

➤*Cardiovascular effects:* In clinical practice, hypertension (in some cases, severe) requiring acute treatment, has been reported in patients receiving bupropion alone and in combination with nicotine-replacement therapy. These events have been observed in patients with and without evidence of preexisting hypertension.

There is no clinical experience establishing the safety of bupropion in patients with a recent history of myocardial infarction (MI) or unstable heart disease. Therefore, exercise care if it is used in these groups. Bupropion was well tolerated in depressed patients who had previously developed orthostatic hypotension while receiving tricyclic antidepressants, and also was generally well tolerated in a group of 36 depressed inpatients with stable congestive heart failure (CHF). However, bupropion was associated with a rise in supine blood pressure in the study of patients with CHF, resulting in discontinuation of treatment in 2 patients for exacerbation of baseline hypertension.

➤*CNS effects:*

Agitation/Insomnia –

Immediate-release: A substantial proportion of patients treated with immediate-release bupropion experiences some degree of agitation, anxiety, increased restlessness, and insomnia, especially shortly after initiation of treatment. In clinical studies, these symptoms were sometimes of sufficient magnitude to require treatment with sedative/hypnotic drugs. In approximately 2% of patients, symptoms were sufficiently severe to require discontinuation of treatment with immediate-release bupropion.

Wellbutrin SR: Patients in placebo-controlled trials with *Wellbutrin SR* experienced agitation, anxiety, and insomnia as shown in the following table.

Incidence of Agitation, Anxiety, and Insomnia With *Wellbutrin SR*

Adverse reaction	*Wellbutrin SR* 300 mg/day (n = 376)	*Wellbutrin SR* 400 mg/day (n = 114)	Placebo (n = 385)
Agitation[a]	3%	9%	2%
Anxiety[a]	5%	6%	3%
Insomnia[a]	11%	16%	6%

[a] In clinical studies, these symptoms were sometimes of sufficient magnitude to require treatment with sedative/hypnotic drugs.

Symptoms were sufficiently severe to require discontinuation of treatment in 1% and 2.6% of patients treated with 300 and 400 mg/day, respectively, of *Wellbutrin SR* and 0.8% of patients treated with placebo.

Wellbutrin XL: In 3 placebo-controlled clinical trials of seasonal affective disorder with *Wellbutrin XL*, the incidence of agitation, anxiety, and insomnia are shown in the following table.

Incidence of Agitation, Anxiety, and Insomnia With *Wellbutrin XL* for Seasonal Affective Disorder

Adverse reaction	*Wellbutrin XL* 150 to 300 mg/day (n = 537)	Placebo (n = 511)
Agitation	2%	< 1%
Anxiety	7%	5%
Insomnia	20%	13%

Zyban: In the dose-response smoking-cessation trial, 29% of patients treated with *Zyban* 150 mg/day and 35% of patients treated with *Zyban* 300 mg/day experienced insomnia, compared with 21% of placebo-treated patients. Symptoms were sufficiently severe to require discontinuation of treatment in 0.6% of patients treated with *Zyban* and none of the patients treated with placebo.

In the comparative trial, 40% of the patients treated with *Zyban* 300 mg/day, 28% of the patients treated with 21 mg/day of nicotine transdermal system, and 45% of the patients treated with the combination of *Zyban* and nicotine transdermal system experienced insomnia, compared with 18% of placebo-treated patients. Symptoms were sufficiently severe to require discontinuation of treatment in 0.8% of patients treated with *Zyban* and none of the patients in the other 3 treatment groups.

Insomnia may be minimized by avoiding bedtime doses and, if necessary, by reduction in dosage.

Depression and nicotine withdrawal – Depressed mood may be a symptom of nicotine withdrawal. Depression, rarely including suicidal ideation, has been reported in patients undergoing a smoking cessation attempt.

Neuropsychiatric phenomena – Depressed patients treated with bupropion have been reported to show a variety of neuropsychiatric signs and symptoms, including concentration disturbance, confusion, delusions, hallucinations, paranoia, and psychosis. Because of the uncontrolled nature of many studies, it is impossible to provide a precise estimate of the extent of risk imposed by treatment with bupropion. In some cases, these symptoms abated upon dose reduction and/or withdrawal of treatment. In clinical trials with *Zyban* conducted in nondepressed smokers, the incidence of neuropsychiatric adverse reactions was generally comparable with placebo.

Psychosis or mania – Antidepressants can precipitate manic episodes in bipolar disorder patients during the depressed phases of their illnesses and may activate latent psychosis in other susceptible patients. Bupropion is expected to pose similar risks. There were no reports of activation of psychosis or mania in clinical trials with *Zyban* conducted in nondepressed smokers.

➤*Hypersensitivity reactions:* Anaphylactoid/anaphylactic reactions characterized by symptoms such as angioedema, dyspnea, pruritus, and urticaria requiring medical treatment have been reported in clinical trials with bupropion. In clinical trials with *Zyban*, the reported rate was about 1 to 3 per 1,000. In addition, there have been rare, spontaneous postmarketing reports of anaphylactic shock, erythema multiforme, and Stevens-Johnson syndrome associated with bupropion. A patient experiencing allergic or anaphylactoid/anaphylactic reactions (eg, skin rash, pruritus, hives, chest pain, edema, shortness of breath) during treatment should stop taking bupropion and consult a health care provider.

Arthralgia, myalgia, and fever with rash and other symptoms suggestive of delayed hypersensitivity have been reported in association with bupropion. These symptoms may resemble serum sickness.

➤*Tartrazine sensitivity:* Some of these products contain tartrazine, which may cause allergic-type reactions (including bronchial asthma) in susceptible individuals. Although the incidence of tartrazine sensitivity in the general population is low, it is frequently seen in patients who also have aspirin sensitivity.

➤*Renal function impairment:* Use bupropion with caution in patients with renal function impairment, and consider a reduced frequency and/or dose (reduced frequency of dosing with *Zyban*) because bupropion and the metabolites of bupropion may accumulate in such patients to a greater extent than usual. Closely monitor the patient for possible adverse reactions that could indicate high drug or metabolite levels.

➤*Hepatic function impairment:* See Administration and Dosage for more information.

Closely monitor all patients with hepatic function impairment for possible adverse reactions that could indicate high drug and metabolite levels.

➤*Drug abuse and dependence:*

Controlled substance class – Bupropion is not a controlled substance. Controlled clinical studies of immediate-release bupropion conducted in healthy volunteers, in subjects with a history of multiple-drug abuse, and in depressed patients showed some increase in motor activity and agitation/excitement.

There have been few reported cases of drug dependence and withdrawal symptoms associated with immediate-release bupropion.

In human studies of abuse liability, individuals experienced with drugs of abuse reported that bupropion produced a feeling of euphoria and desirabil-

BUPROPION HYDROCHLORIDE — ORAL

ity. In these subjects, a single dose of bupropion 400 mg (1.33 times the recommended daily dose) produced mild amphetamine-like effects compared with placebo on the Morphine-Benzedrine Subscale of the Addiction Research Center Inventories (ARCI), which is indicative of euphorigenic properties, and a score intermediate between placebo and amphetamine on the Drug Liking scale of the ARCI. These scales measure general feelings of euphoria and drug desirability.

Zyban – Zyban is likely to have a low abuse potential. When evaluating the desirability of including the drug in smoking cessation programs of individual patients, keep in mind the possibility that bupropion may induce dependence.

➤*Hazardous tasks:* Any CNS-active drug like bupropion may impair the ability to perform tasks requiring judgment or motor and cognitive skills. Consequently, until patients are reasonably certain that bupropion does not adversely affect their performance, they should refrain from driving an automobile or operating complex, hazardous machinery.

➤*Photosensitivity:* Photosensitization may occur; therefore, caution patients to take protective measures (eg, use sunscreens, wear protective clothing) against exposure to ultraviolet light or sunlight until tolerance is determined.

➤*Pregnancy:* Category C (per manufacturer prescribing information). *Category B* (per Briggs' *Drugs in Pregnancy and Lactation*). Use bupropion during pregnancy only if the potential benefit justifies the potential risk to the fetus.

In studies conducted in rats and rabbits, bupropion was administered orally at doses of up to 450 and 150 mg/kg/day, respectively (approximately 11 and 7 times the MRHD, respectively, for immediate- and extended-release bupropion, and approximately 14 and 10 times the MRHD for *Zyban*, respectively, on a mg/m^2 basis), during the period of organogenesis. No clear evidence of teratogenic activity was found in either species; however, in rabbits, slightly increased incidences of fetal malformations and skeletal variations were observed at the lowest dose tested (25 mg/kg/day, approximately equal to the MRHD for immediate- and extended-release bupropion and approximately 2 times greater the MRHD for *Zyban* on a mg/m^2 basis) and greater. Decreased fetal weights were seen at 50 mg/kg and greater.

Pregnancy registry – To monitor fetal outcomes of pregnant women exposed to bupropion, the manufacturer maintains a bupropion pregnancy registry. Health care providers are encouraged to register patients by calling 1-800-336-2176.

➤*Lactation:* Like many other drugs, bupropion and its metabolites are secreted in human milk. Because of the potential for serious adverse reactions in breast-feeding infants from bupropion, decide whether to discontinue breast-feeding or the drug, taking into account the importance of the drug to the mother.

➤*Children:* The safety and effectiveness of bupropion in children have not been established. Anyone considering the use of bupropion in a child or adolescent must balance the potential risks with clinical need.

See the Warning box for more information.

➤*Elderly:* A single-dose pharmacokinetic study demonstrated that the disposition of bupropion and its metabolites in elderly subjects was similar to that of younger subjects; however, another pharmacokinetic study, single and multiple dose, has suggested that elderly individuals are at increased risk for accumulation of bupropion and its metabolites.

Bupropion is extensively metabolized in the liver to active metabolites, which are further metabolized and excreted by the kidneys. The risk of toxic reaction to this drug may be greater in patients with renal function impairment. Because elderly patients are more likely to have decreased renal function, take care in dose selection; it may be useful to monitor renal function.

➤*Monitoring:* Closely monitor all patients with hepatic or renal function impairment for possible adverse reactions that could indicate high drug and metabolite levels. Monitoring of blood pressure is recommended in patients who receive the combination of bupropion and nicotine replacement. Monitor patients closely for clinical worsening, suicidality, and unusual changes in behavior, especially during the initial few months of a course of drug therapy or at times of dosage increases or decreases.

Drug Interactions

➤*CYP-450 system:* In vitro studies indicate that bupropion is primarily metabolized to hydroxybupropion by the CYP2B6 isoenzyme. Therefore, the potential exists for a drug interaction between bupropion and drugs that are substrates or inhibitors of the CYP2B6 isoenzyme (eg, cyclophosphamide, orphenadrine, thiotepa). While not systematically studied, certain drugs may induce the metabolism of bupropion (eg, carbamazepine, phenobarbital, phenytoin).

Bupropion and hydroxybupropion are inhibitors of the CYP2D6 isoenzyme in vitro. Cautiously approach the coadministration of bupropion with drugs that are metabolized by the CYP2D6 isoenzyme, including certain antiarrhythmics, antidepressants (SSRIs, many tricyclics), antipsychotics, and beta-blockers, and initiate coadministration at the lower end of the dosage range of the concomitant medication. If bupropion is added to the treatment regimen of a patient already receiving a drug metabolized by CYP2D6, consider the need to decrease the dose of the original medication, particularly for those concomitant medications with a narrow therapeutic index.

➤*Drugs that lower the seizure threshold:* Use caution during coadministration of bupropion and agents (eg, antipsychotics, other antidepressants, systemic steroids, theophylline) or treatment regimens (eg, abrupt discontinuation of benzodiazepines) that lower the seizure threshold. Use low initial dosing and small, gradual dose increases.

Bupropion Drug Interactions

Precipitant drug	Object drug[a]		Description
Amantadine, Levodopa	Bupropion	↑	There is a higher incidence of adverse reactions (eg, neurotoxicity) with concurrent use of bupropion with either levodopa or amantadine. Use small initial dosages and small, gradual dosage increases of bupropion.
Carbamazepine	Bupropion	↓	Serum concentrations of bupropion may be decreased, reducing the pharmacologic effects.
Clopidogrel	Bupropion	↑	Bupropion plasma concentrations may be elevated, increasing the pharmacologic and adverse effects. The bupropion dosage may need to be adjusted when clopidogrel is started or stopped.
CYP2B6 inducers (eg, phenobarbital, phenytoin)	Bupropion	↓	Inducers of CYP2B6 may decrease serum levels and efficacy of bupropion.
CYP2B6 inhibitors (eg, cimetidine)	Bupropion	↑	Inhibitors of CYP2B6 may increase serum levels, increasing the pharmacologic and adverse effects.
Drugs that lower the seizure threshold (eg, antidepressants, antipsychotics, systemic steroids, theophylline)	Bupropion	↑	Bupropion is associated with a dose-dependent risk of seizures. Undertake the coadministration of bupropion and agents that lower the seizure threshold only with extreme caution.
Bupropion	Drugs that lower the seizure threshold (eg, antidepressants, antipsychotics, systemic steroids, theophylline)		
Guanfacine	Bupropion	↑	The risk of bupropion toxicity may be increased. Closely monitor patients. If an interaction is suspected, adjust therapy as needed.
Linezolid	Bupropion	↑	The risk of hypertensive crisis may be increased. Because coadministration of bupropion and traditional MAOIs is contraindicated, avoid concurrent use of bupropion and linezolid until more clinical information is available.
MAOIs	Bupropion	↑	Coadministration is contraindicated. Risk of acute bupropion toxicity may be increased. Allow at least 14 days to elapse between discontinuing an MAOI and starting bupropion.
Nicotine replacement therapy (ie, nicotine transdermal system)	Bupropion	↑	Hypertension (sometimes severe) requiring acute treatment has been reported in patients receiving bupropion alone and in combination with nicotine replacement therapy. These events have been observed in patients with and without evidence of preexisting hypertension.
Bupropion	Nicotine replacement therapy (ie, nicotine transdermal system)		
Rifampin	Bupropion	↓	Bupropion plasma concentrations may be reduced, decreasing the therapeutic effect.
Ritonavir	Bupropion	↓	Bupropion levels may be reduced, decreasing therapeutic effects.

BUPROPION HYDROCHLORIDE — ORAL

Bupropion Drug Interactions			
Precipitant drug	Object drug[a]		Description
Ticlopidine	Bupropion	↑	Bupropion plasma concentrations may be elevated, increasing the pharmacologic and adverse effects. Adjust bupropion dosage when ticlopidine is started or stopped.
Bupropion	Alcohol	↑	There have been rare reports of adverse neuropsychiatric events or reduced alcohol tolerance in patients who were drinking alcohol during treatment with bupropion. Advise patients to minimize or avoid alcohol consumption while taking bupropion.
Bupropion	Antiarrhythmics, type 1C (eg, flecainide, propafenone)	↑	Bupropion is an inhibitor of the CYP2D6 isoenzyme. If bupropion is added to the treatment regimen of a patient receiving a drug metabolized by CYP2D6, consider a dosage reduction in the medication.
	Antipsychotics (eg, haloperidol, risperidone, thioridazine)		
	Beta-blockers (eg, metoprolol)		
Bupropion	Cyclosporine	↓	Cyclosporine concentrations may be reduced, decreasing the pharmacologic effects.
Bupropion	SSRIs (eg, fluoxetine, paroxetine, sertraline)	↑	Bupropion is an inhibitor of the CYP2D6 isoenzyme. If bupropion is added to the treatment regimen of a patient receiving a drug metabolized by CYP2D6, consider a dosage reduction in the medication.
	Tricyclic antidepressants (eg, desipramine, imipramine, nortriptyline)		

[a] ↑ = object drug increased; ↓ = object drug decreased.

Adverse Reactions

➤*Immediate-release:* Adverse reactions commonly encountered in patients treated with immediate-release bupropion are agitation, constipation, dry mouth, headache/migraine, insomnia, nausea/vomiting, and tremor.

Discontinuation of treatment – Adverse reactions were sufficiently troublesome to cause discontinuation of treatment with immediate-release bupropion in approximately 10% of the 2,400 patients and volunteers who participated in clinical trials during the product's initial development. The more common reactions causing discontinuation include neuropsychiatric disturbances (3%), primarily agitation and abnormalities in mental status; GI disturbances (2.1%), primarily nausea and vomiting; neurological disturbances (1.7%), primarily headache, seizures, and sleep disturbances; and dermatological problems (1.4%), primarily rashes. It is important to note, however, that many of these reactions occurred at doses that exceed the recommended daily dosage.

Adverse reactions (1% or more) –

Immediate-Release Bupropion Adverse Reactions (≥ 1%)[a]		
Adverse reaction	Immediate-release bupropion (n = 323)	Placebo (n = 185)
Cardiovascular		
Cardiac arrhythmias	5.3%	4.3%
Hypertension	4.3%	1.6%
Hypotension	2.5%	2.2%
Palpitations	3.7%	2.2%
Syncope	1.2%	0.5%
Tachycardia	10.8%	8.6%
CNS		
Agitation	31.9%	22.2%
Akathisia	1.5%	1.1%
Akinesia/Bradykinesia	8%	8.6%
Anxiety	3.1%	1.1%
Confusion	8.4%	4.9%
Cutaneous temperature disturbance	1.9%	1.6%
Decreased libido	3.1%	1.6%
Delusions	1.2%	1.1%
Disturbed concentration	3.1%	3.8%
Dizziness	22.3%	16.2%
Euphoria	1.2%	0.5%
Fatigue	5%	8.6%
Headache/Migraine	25.7%	22.2%
Hostility	5.6%	3.8%
Impaired sleep quality	4%	1.6%
Insomnia	18.6%	15.7%
Pseudoparkinsonism	1.5%	1.6%
Sedation	19.8%	19.5%
Sensory disturbance	4%	3.2%
Tremor	21.1%	7.6%
Dermatologic		
Excessive sweating	22.3%	14.6%
Pruritus	2.2%	0%
Rash	8%	6.5%
GI		
Anorexia	18.3%	18.4%
Appetite increase	3.7%	2.2%
Constipation	26%	17.3%
Diarrhea	6.8%	8.6%
Dry mouth	27.6%	18.4%
Dyspepsia	3.1%	2.2%
Increased salivary flow	3.4%	3.8%
Nausea/Vomiting	22.9%	18.9%
Weight gain	13.6%	22.7%
Weight loss	23.2%	23.2%
GU		
Impotence	3.4%	3.1%
Menstrual complaints	4.7%	1.1%
Urinary frequency	2.5%	2.2%
Urinary retention	1.9%	2.2%
Musculoskeletal		
Arthritis	3.1%	2.7%
Muscle spasms	1.9%	3.2%
Respiratory		
Upper respiratory tract complaints	5%	11.4%
Special senses		
Auditory disturbance	5.3%	3.2%
Blurred vision	14.6%	10.3%
Gustatory disturbance	3.1%	1.1%
Miscellaneous		
Fever/Chills	1.2%	0.5%

[a] Reactions reported by at least 1% of patients receiving immediate-release bupropion are included.

Other adverse reactions

Cardiovascular: Chest pain, electrocardiogram (ECG) abnormalities (premature beats and nonspecific ST-T changes), and shortness of breath/dyspnea (0.1% to 1%); electroencephalogram (EEG) abnormality, flushing, pallor, phlebitis, and MI (less than 0.1%).

CNS: Ataxia/incoordination, decrease in sexual function, depression, dyskinesia, dystonia, hallucinations, increased libido, mania/hypomania, myoclonus, seizure (at least 1%); depersonalization, dysarthria, dysphoria, formal thought disorder, frigidity, memory impairment, mood instability, mydriasis, paranoia, psychosis, vertigo (0.1% to 1%); abnormal neurological exam, aphasia, impaired attention, sciatica, suicidal ideation (less than 0.1%).

Dermatologic: Nonspecific rashes (at least 1%); alopecia, dry skin (0.1% to 1%); acne, change in hair color, hirsutism (less than 0.1%).

Endocrine: Gynecomastia (0.1% to 1%); glycosuria, hormone level change (less than 0.1%).

GI: Stomatitis (at least 1%); bruxism, dysphagia, gum irritation, oral edema, thirst disturbance, toothache (0.1% to 1%); colitis, GI bleeding, glossitis, intestinal perforation, rectal complaints, stomach ulcer (less than 0.1%).

BUPROPION HYDROCHLORIDE — ORAL

GU: Nocturia (at least 1%); painful erection, retarded ejaculation, testicular swelling, urinary tract infection, vaginal irritation, (0.1% to 1%); cystitis, dyspareunia, dysuria, enuresis, menopause, ovarian disorder, painful ejaculation, pelvic infection, urinary incontinence (less than 0.1%).

Hematologic/Lymphatic: Anemia, lymphadenopathy, pancytopenia (less than 0.1%).

Hepatic: Liver damage/jaundice (0.1% to 1%).

Hypersensitivity: See Warnings/Precautions for more information.

Musculoskeletal: Musculoskeletal chest pain (less than 0.1%).

Respiratory: Bronchitis, shortness of breath/dyspnea (0.1% to 1%); epistaxis, pneumonia, pulmonary embolism, rate or rhythm disorder (less than 0.1%).

Special senses: Visual disturbance (0.1% to 1%); diplopia (less than 0.1%).

Miscellaneous: Edema, flu-type symptoms (at least 1%); nonspecific pain (0.1% to 1%); body odor, infection, medication reaction, overdose, surgically related pain (less than 0.1%).

➤*Extended-release (Wellbutrin XL):*

Seasonal affective disorder –

Discontinuation of treatment: In placebo-controlled clinical trials, 9% of patients treated with extended-release bupropion and 5% of patients treated with placebo discontinued treatment because of adverse reactions. The adverse reactions in these trials that led to discontinuation in at least 1% of patients treated with extended-release bupropion and at a rate numerically greater than the placebo rate were insomnia (2% vs less than 1%) and headache (1% vs less than 1%).

Adverse reactions (2% or more):

Adverse Reactions for *Wellbutrin XL* in Seasonal Affective Disorder (≥ 2%)		
Adverse reaction	*Wellbutrin XL* (n = 537)	Placebo (n = 511)
Cardiovascular		
Hypertension	2%	0%
CNS		
Abnormal dreams	3%	2%
Agitation	2%	< 1%
Anxiety	7%	5%
Dizziness	6%	5%
Feeling jittery	3%	2%
Headache	34%	26%
Insomnia	20%	13%
Tremor	3%	< 1%
Dermatologic		
Rash	3%	2%
GI		
Abdominal pain	2%	< 1%
Appetite decreased	4%	1%
Constipation	9%	2%
Dry mouth	26%	15%
Flatulence	6%	3%
Nausea	13%	8%
GU		
Dysmenorrhea	2%	< 1%
Musculoskeletal		
Myalgia	3%	2%
Pain in extremity	3%	2%
Respiratory		
Cough	4%	3%
Nasopharyngitis	13%	12%
Sinusitis	5%	4%
Upper respiratory tract infection	9%	8%
Miscellaneous		
Tinnitus	3%	< 1%

Adverse reactions that occurred in at least 2% of patients treated with *Wellbutrin XL* but equally or more frequently in the placebo group were arthralgia, back pain, diarrhea, dyspepsia, fatigue, hyperhidrosis, influenza, irritability, migraine, nasal congestion, neck pain, palpitations, pharyngolaryngeal pain, sinus congestion, upper abdominal pain, and viral gastroenteritis.

Common adverse reactions: Adverse reactions from the previous table occurring in at least 5% of patients treated with *Wellbutrin XL* and at a rate at least twice the placebo rate were constipation and flatulence.

Adverse reactions during taper or following discontinuation: Adverse reactions with onset during the 2 weeks following down titration of *Wellbutrin XL* from 300 mg/day to 150 mg/day were reported by 14% of patients compared with 18% of patients who continued on placebo.

Adverse reactions with onset during the 2 weeks following discontinuation of *Wellbutrin XL* were reported by 9% of patients compared with 12% of patients following discontinuation of placebo.

➤*Extended-release (Wellbutrin SR):*

Discontinuation of treatment – In placebo-controlled clinical trials, 9% and 11% of patients treated with 300 and 400 mg/day, respectively, of *Wellbutrin SR* and 4% of patients treated with placebo discontinued treatment because of adverse reactions. The specific adverse reactions in these trials that led to discontinuation in at least 1% of patients treated with *Wellbutrin SR* 300 or 400 mg/day and at a rate at least twice the placebo rate are listed in the following table.

Discontinuation of Treatment With *Wellbutrin SR*			
Adverse reaction	*Wellbutrin SR* 300 mg/day (n = 376)	*Wellbutrin SR* 400 mg/day (n = 114)	Placebo (n = 385)
Agitation	0.3%	1.8%	0.3%
Migraine	0%	1.8%	0.3%
Nausea	0.8%	1.8%	0.3%
Rash	2.4%	0.9%	0%

Adverse reactions (1% or more) –

Wellbutrin SR Adverse Reactions (≥ 1%)[a]			
Adverse reaction	*Wellbutrin SR* 300 mg/day (n = 376)	*Wellbutrin SR* 400 mg/day (n = 114)	Placebo (n = 385)
Cardiovascular			
Flushing	1%	4%	—[b]
Hot flashes	1%	3%	1%
Palpitation	2%	6%	2%
CNS			
Agitation	3%	9%	2%
Anxiety	5%	6%	3%
Asthenia	2%	4%	2%
CNS stimulation	2%	1%	1%
Dizziness	7%	11%	5%
Headache	26%	25%	23%
Insomnia	11%	16%	6%
Irritability	3%	2%	2%
Memory decreased	—	3%	1%
Migraine	1%	4%	1%
Nervousness	5%	3%	3%
Paresthesia	1%	2%	1%
Somnolence	2%	3%	2%
Tremor	6%	3%	1%
Dermatologic			
Pruritus	2%	4%	2%
Rash	5%	4%	1%
Sweating	6%	5%	2%
Urticaria	2%	1%	0%
GI			
Abdominal pain	3%	9%	2%
Anorexia	5%	3%	2%
Constipation	10%	5%	7%
Diarrhea	5%	7%	6%
Dry mouth	17%	24%	7%
Dysphagia	0%	2%	0%
Nausea	13%	18%	8%
Vomiting	4%	2%	2%
GU			
Urinary frequency	2%	5%	2%
Urinary tract infection	1%	0%	—
Urinary urgency	—	2%	0%
Vaginal hemorrhage[c]	0%	2%	—
Musculoskeletal			
Arthralgia	1%	4%	1%
Arthritis	0%	2%	0%
Myalgia	2%	6%	3%
Twitch	1%	2%	—

BUPROPION HYDROCHLORIDE — ORAL

Wellbutrin SR Adverse Reactions (≥ 1%)[a]			
Adverse reaction	*Wellbutrin SR* 300 mg/day (n = 376)	*Wellbutrin SR* 400 mg/day (n = 114)	Placebo (n = 385)
Respiratory			
Increased cough	1%	2%	1%
Pharyngitis	3%	11%	2%
Sinusitis	3%	1%	2%
Special senses			
Amblyopia	3%	2%	2%
Taste perversion	2%	4%	2%
Tinnitus	6%	6%	2%
Miscellaneous			
Chest pain	3%	4%	1%
Fever	1%	2%	—
Infection	8%	9%	6%
Pain	2%	3%	2%

[a] Adverse reactions that occurred in at least 1% of patients treated with *Wellbutrin SR* 300 or 400 mg/day, but equally or more frequently in the placebo group, were abnormal dreams, accidental injury, acne, back pain, bronchitis, dysmenorrhea, dyspepsia, flatulence, flu syndrome, hypertension, increased appetite, neck pain, respiratory disorder, rhinitis, and tooth disorder.
[b] Denotes adverse reactions occurring in more than 0% but less than 0.5% of patients.
[c] Incidence based on the number of women.

Common adverse reactions – The following adverse reactions from the previous table occurring in at least 5% of patients treated with *Wellbutrin SR* and at a rate at least twice the placebo rate are listed for the 300 and 400 mg/day dose groups.

Wellbutrin SR 300 mg/day: Anorexia, dry mouth, rash, sweating, tinnitus, and tremor.

Wellbutrin SR 400 mg/day: Abdominal pain, agitation, anxiety, dizziness, dry mouth, insomnia, myalgia, nausea, palpitation, pharyngitis, sweating, tinnitus, and urinary frequency.

Other adverse reactions –

Cardiovascular: Flushing, postural hypotension, stroke, tachycardia, vasodilation (0.1% to 1%); syncope (less than 0.1%). Also observed were complete atrioventricular block, extrasystoles, hypertension (in some cases severe), hypotension, MI, phlebitis, and pulmonary embolism.

CNS: Abnormal coordination, CNS stimulation, confusion, decreased libido, decreased memory, depersonalization, dysphoria, emotional lability, hostility, hyperkinesia, hypertonia, hypesthesia, migraine, paresthesia, suicidal ideation, vertigo (0.1% to 1%); amnesia, ataxia, derealization, hypomania (less than 0.1%). Also observed were abnormal EEG, aggression, akinesia, aphasia, coma, delirium, delusions, dysarthria, dyskinesia, dystonia, euphoria, extrapyramidal syndrome, hallucinations, hypokinesia, increased libido, manic reaction, neuralgia, neuropathy, paranoid ideation, restlessness, unmasking tardive dyskinesia.

Dermatologic: Photosensitivity (0.1% to 1%); maculopapular rash (less than 0.1%). Also observed were alopecia, angioedema, exfoliative dermatitis, hirsutism.

Endocrine: Hyperglycemia, hypoglycemia, syndrome of inappropriate antidiuretic hormone were observed.

GI: Bruxism, gastric reflux, gingivitis, glossitis, increased salivation, mouth ulcers, stomatitis, thirst (0.1% to 1%); edema of the tongue (less than 0.1%). Also observed were colitis, esophagitis, GI hemorrhage, gum hemorrhage, intestinal perforation, pancreatitis, stomach ulcer, stool abnormality.

GU: Impotence, polyuria, prostate disorder (0.1% to 1%). Also observed were abnormal ejaculation, cystitis, dyspareunia, dysuria, gynecomastia, menopause, painful erection, prostate disorder, salpingitis, urinary incontinence, urinary retention, urinary tract disorder, vaginitis.

Hematologic/Lymphatic: Ecchymosis (0.1% to 1%). Also observed were anemia, leukocytosis, leukopenia, lymphadenopathy, pancytopenia, thrombocytopenia.

Altered prothrombin time (PT) and/or international normalized ratio (INR), infrequently associated with hemorrhagic or thrombotic complications, were observed when bupropion was coadministered with warfarin.

Hepatic: Abnormal liver function, jaundice (0.1% to 1%). Also observed were hepatitis and liver damage.

Hypersensitivity: See Warnings/Precautions for more information.

Metabolic/Nutritional: Edema, increased weight, peripheral edema (0.1% to 1%). Also observed was glycosuria.

Musculoskeletal: Leg cramps (0.1% to 1%). Also observed were arthritis, muscle rigidity/fever/rhabdomyolysis, muscle weakness.

Respiratory: Bronchospasm (less than 0.1%). Also observed was pneumonia.

Special senses: Accommodation abnormality, dry eye (0.1% to 1%). Also observed were deafness, diplopia, increased intraocular pressure, mydriasis.

Miscellaneous: Chills, facial edema, musculoskeletal chest pain (0.1% to 1%); malaise (less than 0.1%). Also observed were arthralgia, fever with rash and other symptoms suggestive of delayed hypersensitivity, myalgia. These symptoms may resemble serum sickness.

➤*Extended-release (Zyban):*

Discontinuation of treatment – Adverse reactions were sufficiently troublesome to cause discontinuation of treatment in 8% of the 706 patients treated with *Zyban* and 5% of the 313 patients treated with placebo. The more common reactions leading to discontinuation of treatment with *Zyban* included nervous system disturbances (3.4%), primarily tremors, and skin disorders (2.4%), primarily rashes.

Common adverse reactions – The most commonly observed adverse reactions consistently associated with the use of *Zyban* were dry mouth and insomnia. The most commonly observed adverse reactions were those that consistently occurred at a rate of 5 percentage points higher than that for placebo across clinical studies.

Dose dependency adverse reactions – The incidence of dry mouth and insomnia may be related to the dose of *Zyban*. The occurrence of these adverse reactions may be minimized by reducing the dose of *Zyban*. In addition, insomnia may be minimized by avoiding bedtime doses.

Adverse reactions (1% or more) –

Zyban Adverse Reactions in the Dose-Response Trial (≥ 1%)[a]		
Adverse reaction	*Zyban* 100 to 300 mg/day (n = 461)	Placebo (n = 150)
Cardiovascular		
Hot flashes	1%	0%
Hypertension	1%	< 1%
CNS		
Abnormal thinking	1%	0%
Dizziness	8%	7%
Insomnia	31%	21%
Somnolence	2%	1%
Tremor	2%	1%
Dermatologic		
Dry skin	2%	0%
Pruritus	3%	< 1%
Rash	3%	< 1%
Urticaria	1%	0%
GI		
Anorexia	1%	< 1%
Dry mouth	11%	5%
Increased appetite	2%	< 1%
Taste perversion	2%	< 1%
Musculoskeletal		
Arthralgia	4%	3%
Myalgia	2%	1%
Respiratory		
Bronchitis	2%	0%
Miscellaneous		
Allergic reaction	1%	0%
Neck pain	2%	< 1%

[a] Selected adverse reactions with an incidence of at least 1% of patients treated with *Zyban* and more frequent than in the placebo group.

Zyban Adverse Reactions in the Comparative Trial (≥ 1%)[a]				
Adverse reaction	*Zyban* 300 mg/day (n = 243)	Nicotine 21 mg/day transdermal system (n = 243)	*Zyban* and nicotine transdermal system (n = 244)	Placebo (n = 159)
Cardiovascular				
Hypertension	1%	< 1%	2%	0%
Palpitations	2%	0%	1%	0%
CNS				
Anxiety	8%	6%	9%	6%
Disturbed concentration	9%	3%	9%	4%
Dizziness	10%	2%	8%	6%
Dream abnormality	5%	18%	13%	3%
Dysphoria	< 1%	1%	2%	1%
Insomnia	40%	28%	45%	18%
Nervousness	4%	< 1%	2%	2%
Tremor	1%	< 1%	2%	0%
Dermatologic				
Application-site reaction[b]	11%	17%	15%	7%
Pruritus	3%	1%	5%	1%
Rash	4%	3%	3%	2%

BUPROPION HYDROCHLORIDE — ORAL

Zyban Adverse Reactions in the Comparative Trial (≥ 1%)[a]				
Adverse reaction	*Zyban* 300 mg/day (n = 243)	Nicotine 21 mg/day transdermal system (n = 243)	*Zyban* and nicotine transdermal system (n = 244)	Placebo (n = 159)[b]
Urticaria	2%	0%	2%	0%
GI				
Abdominal pain	3%	4%	1%	1%
Anorexia	3%	1%	5%	1%
Constipation	8%	4%	9%	3%
Diarrhea	4%	4%	3%	1%
Dry mouth	10%	4%	9%	4%
Mouth ulcer	2%	1%	1%	1%
Nausea	9%	7%	11%	4%
Thirst	< 1%	< 1%	2%	0%
Musculoskeletal				
Arthralgia	5%	3%	3%	2%
Myalgia	4%	3%	5%	3%
Respiratory				
Dyspnea	1%	0%	2%	1%
Epistaxis	2%	1%	1%	0%
Increased cough	3%	5%	< 1%	1%
Pharyngitis	3%	2%	3%	0%
Rhinitis	12%	11%	9%	8%
Sinusitis	2%	2%	2%	1%
Special senses				
Taste perversion	3%	1%	3%	2%
Tinnitus	1%	0%	< 1%	0%
Miscellaneous				
Accidental injury	2%	2%	1%	1%
Chest pain	< 1%	1%	3%	1%
Facial edema	< 1%	0%	1%	0%
Neck pain	2%	1%	< 1%	0%

[a] Selected adverse reactions with an incidence of at least 1% of patients treated with *Zyban,* nicotine transdermal system, or the combination of *Zyban* and nicotine transdermal system, and more frequent than in the placebo group.
[b] Patients randomized to *Zyban* or placebo received placebo patches.

➤*Postmarketing:*

Cardiovascular – Hypertension (in some cases severe), orthostatic hypotension, third-degree heart block.

CNS – Aggression, coma, delirium, dream abnormalities, myalgia, paranoid ideation, paresthesia, restlessness, unmasking of tardive dyskinesia.

Dermatologic – Exfoliative dermatitis, Stevens-Johnson syndrome, urticaria.

Endocrine – Hyperglycemia, hypoglycemia, syndrome of inappropriate antidiuretic hormone secretion.

GI – Esophagitis.

Hematologic / Lymphatic – Ecchymosis, leukocytosis, leukopenia, thrombocytopenia.

Altered PT and/or INR, infrequently associated with hemorrhagic or thrombotic complications, were observed when bupropion was coadministered with warfarin.

Hepatic – Hepatitis, liver damage.

Musculoskeletal – Arthralgia, muscle rigidity/fever/rhabdomyolysis, muscle weakness, myalgia.

Special senses – Increased intraocular pressure, tinnitus.

Miscellaneous – Angioedema; fever with rash and other symptoms suggestive of delayed hypersensitivity that may resemble serum sickness.

Overdosage

➤*Symptoms:* Overdoses of 30 g or more of bupropion have been reported. Seizure was reported in approximately one-third of all cases. Other serious reactions reported with overdoses of bupropion alone included ECG changes (eg, conduction disturbances, arrhythmia), hallucinations, loss of consciousness, and sinus tachycardia. Coma, fever, hypotension, muscle rigidity, rhabdomyolysis, respiratory failure, and stupor have been reported, mainly when bupropion was part of multiple-drug overdoses.

Although most patients recovered without sequelae, deaths associated with overdoses of bupropion alone have been reported rarely in patients ingesting large doses of the drug. Multiple uncontrolled seizures, bradycardia, cardiac failure, and cardiac arrest prior to death were reported in these patients.

➤*Treatment:* Ensure an adequate airway, oxygenation, and ventilation. Monitor cardiac rhythm and vital signs. EEG monitoring also is recommended for the first 48 hours postingestion. General supportive and symptomatic measures also are recommended. Induction of emesis is not recommended. Gastric lavage with a large-bore orogastric tube with appropriate airway protection, if needed, may be indicated if performed soon after ingestion or in symptomatic patients.

Administer activated charcoal. There is no experience with the use of forced diuresis, dialysis, hemoperfusion, or exchange transfusion in the management of bupropion overdoses. No specific antidotes for bupropion are known.

Consider hospitalization following suspected overdose because of the dose-related risk of seizures with bupropion. Based on studies in animals, it is recommended that seizures be treated with benzodiazepine IV and other supportive measures, as appropriate.

Consider the possibility of multiple drug involvement in managing overdosage. Consider contacting a poison control center for additional information on the treatment of any overdose.

Patient Information

Inform patients, their families, and their caregivers about the benefits and risks associated with treatment with bupropion and counsel them in its appropriate use. A patient Medication Guide about using antidepressants in depression and other serious mental illnesses is available for bupropion. Instruct patients, their families, and their caregivers to read the Medication Guide and assist them in understanding its contents. Give patients the opportunity to discuss the contents of the Medication Guide and obtain answers to any questions they may have.

Inform patients that immediate-release bupropion, *Wellbutrin SR*, and *Wellbutrin XL*, used to treat depression, contain the same active ingredient found in *Zyban*, used as an aid in smoking cessation, and that immediate-release bupropion, *Wellbutrin SR*, and *Wellbutrin XL* should not be used in combination with *Zyban* or any other medications that contain bupropion.

Advise patients to discontinue bupropion and not to restart it if they experience a seizure while on treatment.

Any CNS-active drug like bupropion may impair the ability to perform tasks requiring judgment or motor and cognitive skills. Consequently, until patients are reasonably certain that bupropion does not adversely affect their performance, they should refrain from driving an automobile or operating complex, hazardous machinery.

Inform patients that excessive use or abrupt discontinuation of alcohol or sedatives (including benzodiazepines) may alter the seizure threshold. Some patients have reported lower alcohol tolerance during treatment with bupropion. Advise patients that the consumption of alcohol should be minimized or avoided.

Advise patients to inform their health care provider if they are taking or planning to take any prescription or nonprescription drugs. Concern is warranted because bupropion and other drugs may affect each other's metabolism.

Advise patients to notify their health care provider if they become pregnant or intend to become pregnant during therapy.

➤*Clinical worsening and suicide risk:* Encourage patients, their families, and their caregivers to be alert to the emergence of anxiety, agitation, panic attacks, insomnia, irritability, hostility, aggressiveness, impulsivity, akathisia (psychomotor restlessness), hypomania, mania, other unusual changes in behavior, worsening of depression, and suicidal ideation, especially early during antidepressant treatment and when the dose is adjusted up or down. Advise families and caregivers of patients to watch for the emergence of such symptoms on a day-to-day basis because changes may be abrupt. Advise patients to report such symptoms to a health care provider, especially if they are severe, abrupt in onset, or were not part of the patient's presenting symptoms. Symptoms such as these may be associated with an increased risk for suicidal thinking and behavior and indicate a need for very close monitoring and possibly changes in the medication.

➤*Immediate-release:* Instruct patients to take immediate-release bupropion in equally divided doses 3 or 4 times a day to minimize the risk of seizure.

➤*Extended-release:* Advise patients to swallow *Wellbutrin SR* and *Wellbutrin XL* tablets whole so that the release rate is not altered. Patients should not chew, divide, or crush tablets.

Advise patients that they may notice in their stool something that looks like a tablet. This is normal. The medication in *Wellbutrin XL* is contained in a nonabsorbable shell that has been specially designed to slowly release the drug in the body. When this process is completed, the empty shell is eliminated from the body.

As dosage is increased during initial titration to doses above 150 mg/day, instruct patients to take *Wellbutrin SR* in 2 divides doses, preferably with at least 8 hours between successive doses, to minimize the risk of seizures.

BUPROPION HYDROBROMIDE — ORAL

WARNING

Suicidality and antidepressant drugs – Antidepressants increased the risk of suicidal thinking and behavior (suicidality) in children, adolescents, and young adults in short-term studies of major depressive disorder (MDD) and other psychiatric disorders compared with placebo. Anyone considering the use of bupropion or any other antidepressant in a child, adolescent, or young adult must balance this risk with the clinical need. Short-term studies did not show an increase in the risk of suicidality with antidepressants compared with placebo in adults older than 24 years of age; there was a reduction in risk with antidepressants compared with placebo in adults 65 years of age and older. Depression and certain other psychiatric disorders are associated with increases in suicide risk. Appropriately monitor patients of all ages who are started on antidepressant therapy, and closely observe them for clinical worsening, suicidality, or unusual changes in behavior. Advise families and caregivers of the need for close observation and communication with the prescriber. Bupropion is not approved for use in children.

Indications

➤*Major depressive disorder:* For the treatment of MDD.

Administration and Dosage

➤*General dosing considerations:* It is particularly important to administer bupropion in a manner most likely to minimize the risk of seizure. Gradual escalation in dosage is also important if agitation, motor restlessness, and insomnia, often seen during the initial days of treatment, are to be minimized. If necessary, these effects may be managed by temporary reduction of dose or the short-term administration of an intermediate to long-acting sedative hypnotic. A sedative hypnotic usually is not required beyond the first week of treatment. Insomnia may also be minimized by avoiding bedtime doses. If distressing, untoward effects supervene, dose escalation should be stopped.

The full antidepressant effect of bupropion may not be evident until 4 weeks of treatment or longer.

➤*Adults:*

Major depressive disorder –

Usual dosage: 348 mg/day (equivalent to bupropion hydrochloride 300 mg/day) given once daily in the morning.

Maximum dose: 522 mg/day.

Initial dosage: 174 mg/day (equivalent to bupropion hydrochloride 150 mg/day) given as a single daily dose in the morning. The 174 mg tablet is currently not marketed. It is expected to launch in mid-2009.

Dosage titration: If the 174 mg initial dose is adequately tolerated, an increase to the 348 mg/day target dosage, given once daily, may be made as early as day 4 of dosing. There should be an interval of at least 24 hours between successive doses. An increase in dosage to the maximum of 522 mg/day, given as a single dose, may be considered for patients in whom no clinical improvement is noted after several weeks of treatment at 348 mg/day.

Maintenance dosage: It is generally agreed that acute episodes of depression require several months or longer of sustained pharmacological therapy beyond response to the acute episode. It is unknown whether or not the dose of bupropion needed for maintenance treatment is identical to the dose needed to achieve an initial response. Patients should be periodically reassessed to determine the need for maintenance treatment and the appropriate dose for such treatment.

Conversion: When switching patients from bupropion hydrochloride to bupropion hydrobromide, give the equivalent total daily dose when possible (bupropion hydrobromide 522 mg is equivalent to bupropion hydrochloride 450 mg; bupropion hydrobromide 348 mg is equivalent to bupropion hydrochloride 300 mg; bupropion hydrobromide 174 mg is equivalent to bupropion hydrochloride 150 mg). Patients who are currently being treated with bupropion hydrochloride tablets at 300 mg/day (eg, 100 mg 3 times a day) may be switched to bupropion hydrobromide 348 mg once daily. Patients who are currently being treated with bupropion hydrochloride tablets at 300 mg/day (eg, 150 mg twice daily) may be switched to bupropion hydrobromide 348 mg once daily.

➤*Elderly:* Care should be taken in dose selection, and it may be useful to monitor renal function.

➤*Renal function impairment:* Use with caution in patients with renal impairment and a reduced frequency and/or dose should be considered.

➤*Hepatic function impairment:* Use with extreme caution in patients with severe hepatic cirrhosis. The dose should not exceed 174 mg every other day in these patients. Bupropion should be used with caution in patients with hepatic impairment (including mild to moderate hepatic cirrhosis) and a reduced frequency and/or dose should be considered in patients with mild to moderate hepatic cirrhosis.

➤*Administration:* Swallow whole and do not crush, divide, or chew tablets. May be taken without regard to meals.

➤*Storage/Stability:* Store at 25°C (77°F); excursions are permitted to 15° to 30°C (59° to 86°F).

Actions

➤*Pharmacology:* The mechanism of action of bupropion an antidepressant of the aminoketone class, is unknown, as is the case with other antidepressants. However, it is presumed that this action is mediated by noradrenergic and/or dopaminergic mechanisms.

➤*Pharmacokinetics:*

Absorption – Following chronic dosing of bupropion 348 mg tablets, the mean peak steady-state plasma concentration and AUC of bupropion were 134.3 (± 38.2) ng/mL and 1,409 (± 346) ng•h/mL, respectively. Steady-state plasma concentrations of bupropion were reached within 8 days.

Following single oral administration of bupropion to healthy volunteers, the median time to peak plasma concentrations for bupropion was approximately 5 hours.

Effect of food: The presence of food did not affect the peak concentration and time to peak plasma concentration of bupropion; AUC was increased by 19%.

Distribution – In vitro tests show that bupropion is 84% bound to human plasma proteins at concentrations up to 200 mcg/mL. The extent of protein binding of the hydroxybupropion metabolite is similar to that for bupropion, whereas the extent of protein binding of the threohydrobupropion metabolite is about half that seen with bupropion.

Metabolism – Bupropion is extensively metabolized in humans. Three metabolites have been shown to be active: hydroxybupropion, which is formed via hydroxylation of the tert-butyl group of bupropion, and the amino-alcohol isomers threohydrobupropion and erythrohydrobupropion, which are formed via reduction of the carbonyl group. In vitro findings suggest that cytochrome P450IIB6 (CYP2B6) is the principal isoenzyme involved in the formation of hydroxybupropion, while cytochrome P450 isoenzymes are not involved in the formation of threohydrobupropion. Oxidation of the bupropion side chain results in the formation of a glycine conjugate of metachlorobenzoic acid, which is then excreted as the major urinary metabolite. The potency and toxicity of the metabolites relative to bupropion have not been fully characterized. However, it has been demonstrated in an antidepressant screening test in mice that hydroxybupropion is one half as potent as bupropion, while threohydrobupropion and erythrohydrobupropion are 5-fold less potent than bupropion. This may be of clinical importance because the plasma concentrations of the metabolites are as high or higher than those of bupropion.

Following chronic administration in healthy volunteers, peak plasma concentration of hydroxybupropion occurred approximately 6 hours after administration of bupropion. The peak plasma concentrations of hydroxybupropion were approximately 9 times the peak level of the parent drug at steady state. The elimination half-life of hydroxybupropion is approximately 24.3 (± 4.9) hours, and its area under the curve (AUC) at steady state is about 15.6 times that of bupropion. The times to peak concentrations for the erythrohydrobupropion and threohydrobupropion metabolites are similar to that of hydroxybupropion. However, the elimination half-lives of erythrohydrobupropion and threohydrobupropion are longer, approximately 31.1 (± 7.8) and 50.8 (± 8.5) hours, respectively, and steady-state AUCs were 1.5 and 6.8 times that of bupropion, respectively.

Bupropion and its metabolites exhibit linear kinetics following chronic administration of bupropion hydrochloride 300 to 450 mg/day (equivalent to bupropion hydrobromide 348 and 522 mg, respectively).

Excretion – The elimination half-life (± standard deviation [SD]) of bupropion after a single dose is 21.3 (± 6.7) hours.

Following oral administration of 200 mg of ^{14}C-bupropion in humans, 87% and 10% of the radioactive dose were recovered in the urine and feces, respectively. However, the fraction of the oral dose of bupropion excreted unchanged was only 0.5%, a finding consistent with the extensive metabolism of bupropion.

Special populations –

Renal function impairment: There is limited information on the pharmacokinetics of bupropion in patients with renal impairment. An inter-study comparison between normal subjects and patients with end-stage renal failure demonstrated that the parent drug maximum plasma concentration (C_{max}) and AUC values were comparable in the 2 groups, whereas the hydroxybupropion and threohydrobupropion metabolites had a 2.3- and 2.8-fold increase, respectively, in AUC for patients with end-stage renal failure. The elimination of the major metabolites of bupropion may be reduced by impaired renal function.

Hepatic function impairment: The effect of hepatic impairment on the pharmacokinetics of bupropion was characterized in 2 single-dose studies, one in patients with alcoholic liver disease and one in patients with mild to severe cirrhosis. The first study showed that the half-life of hydroxybupropion was significantly longer in 8 patients with alcoholic liver disease than in 8 healthy volunteers (32 ± 14 hours vs 21 ± 5 hours, respectively). Although not statistically significant, the AUCs for bupropion and hydroxybupropion were more variable and tended to be greater (by 53% to 57%) in patients with alcoholic liver disease. The differences in half-life for bupropion and the other metabolites in the 2 patient groups were minimal.

The second study showed no statistically significant differences in the pharmacokinetics of bupropion and its active metabolites in 9 patients with mild to moderate hepatic cirrhosis compared with 8 healthy volunteers. However, more variability was observed in some of the pharmacokinetic parameters for bupropion (AUC, C_{max}, and time of maximal concentration [T_{max}]) and its active metabolites (half-life) in patients with mild to moderate hepatic cirrhosis. In addition, in patients with severe hepatic cirrhosis, the bupropion C_{max} and AUC were substantially increased (mean difference: by approximately 70% and 3-fold, respectively) and more variable when compared with values in healthy volunteers; the mean bupropion half-life was also longer (29 hours in patients with severe hepatic cirrhosis versus 19 hours in healthy subjects). For the metabolite hydroxybupropion, the mean C_{max} was approximately 69% lower. For the combined amino-alcohol isomers threohydrobupropion and erythrohydrobupropion, the mean C_{max} was approximately 31% lower. The mean AUC increased by about 1½-fold

BUPROPION HYDROBROMIDE — ORAL

for hydroxybupropion and about 2½-fold for threo/erythrohydrobupropion. The median T_{max} was observed 19 hours later for hydroxybupropion and 31 hours later for threo/erythrohydrobupropion. The mean half-lives for hydroxybupropion and threo/erythrohydrobupropion were increased 5- and 2-fold, respectively, in patients with severe hepatic cirrhosis compared with healthy volunteers.

Elderly: A pharmacokinetic study, single and multiple dose, suggested that elderly subjects are at an increased risk for accumulation of bupropion and its metabolites.

Gender: The mean systemic exposure (AUC) was approximately 13% higher in men compared with women. The clinical significance of this finding is unknown.

Special risk patients: Factors or conditions altering metabolic capacity (eg, congestive heart failure [CHF], concomitant medications) or elimination may be expected to influence the degree and extent of accumulation of the active metabolites of bupropion.

Contraindications

Seizure disorder; patients treated with *Zyban*, *Wellbutrin*, *Wellbutrin SR*, *Wellbutrin XL*, or any other medications that contain bupropion because the incidence of seizure is dose dependent; patients with a current or prior diagnosis of bulimia or anorexia nervosa because of a higher incidence of seizures noted in patients treated for bulimia with the bupropion immediate-release formulation; patients undergoing abrupt discontinuation of alcohol or sedatives (including benzodiazepines); coadministration with a monoamine oxidase inhibitor (MAOI); patients who have shown an allergic response to bupropion or the other ingredients that make up bupropion tablets.

Warnings/Precautions

➤*Clinical worsening and suicide risk:* Patients with MDD, adults and children, may experience worsening of their depression and/or the emergence of suicidal ideation and behavior (suicidality) or unusual changes in behavior, whether or not they are taking antidepressant medications, and this risk may persist until significant remission occurs. Suicide is a known risk of depression and certain other psychiatric disorders, and these disorders themselves are the strongest predictors of suicide. There has been a long-standing concern that antidepressants may have a role in inducing worsening of depression and the emergence of suicidality in certain patients during the early phases of treatment. Pooled analyses of short-term, placebo-controlled trials of antidepressant drugs (selective serotonin reuptake inhibitors [SSRIs] and others) show that these drugs increase the risk of suicidal thinking and behavior (suicidality) in children, adolescents, and young adults (18 to 24 years of age) with MDD and other psychiatric disorders. Short-term studies did not show an increase in the risk of suicidality with antidepressants compared with placebo in adults older than 24 years of age; there was a reduction with antidepressants compared with placebo in adults 65 years of age and older.

The pooled analyses of placebo-controlled trials in children and adolescents with MDD, obsessive compulsive disorder, or other psychiatric disorders included a total of 24 short-term trials of 9 antidepressant drugs in over 4,400 patients. The pooled analyses of placebo-controlled trials in adults with MDD or other psychiatric disorders included a total of 295 short-term trials (median duration, 2 months) of 11 antidepressant drugs in over 77,000 patients. There was considerable variation in risk of suicidality among drugs, but a tendency toward an increase in the younger patients for almost all drugs studied. There were differences in absolute risk of suicidality across the different indications, with the highest incidence in MDD. The risk differences (drug versus placebo), however, were relatively stable within age strata and across indications.

Suicidality per 1,000 Patients Treated: Antidepressants vs. Placebo	
Age range	Number of cases
	Increases/Decreases compared with placebo
	Increases compared with placebo
< 18 years of age	14 additional cases
18 to 24 years of age	5 additional cases
	Decreases compared with placebo
25 to 64 years of age	1 fewer case
≥ 65 years of age	6 fewer cases

No suicides occurred in any of the pediatric trials. There were suicides in the adult trials, but the number was not sufficient to reach any conclusion about drug effect on suicide.

It is unknown whether the suicidality risk extends to longer-term use (ie, beyond several months). However, there is substantial evidence from placebo-controlled maintenance trials in adults with depression that the use of antidepressants can delay the recurrence of depression.

All patients being treated with antidepressants for any indication should be monitored appropriately and observed closely for clinical worsening, suicidality, and unusual changes in behavior, especially during the initial few months of a course of drug therapy, or at times of dose changes, either increases or decreases.

The following symptoms, anxiety, agitation, panic attacks, insomnia, irritability, hostility, aggressiveness, impulsivity, akathisia (psychomotor restlessness), hypomania, and mania, have been reported in adults and children being treated with antidepressants for MDD as well as for other indications, both psychiatric and nonpsychiatric. Although a causal link between the emergence of such symptoms and either the worsening of depression and/or the emergence of suicidal impulses has not been established, there is concern that such symptoms may represent precursors to emerging suicidality.

Consider changing the therapeutic regimen, including possibly discontinuing the medication, in patients whose depression is persistently worse, or who are experiencing emergent suicidality or symptoms that might be precursors to worsening depression or suicidality, especially if these symptoms are severe, abrupt in onset, or were not part of the patients presenting symptoms.

Alert families and caregivers of patients being treated with antidepressants for MDD or other indications, both psychiatric and nonpsychiatric, about the need to monitor patients for the emergence of agitation, irritability, unusual changes in behavior, and the other symptoms described previously, as well as the emergence of suicidality, and to report such symptoms immediately to health care providers. Such monitoring should include daily observation by families and caregivers.

Write prescriptions for bupropion for the smallest quantity of tablets consistent with good patient management, in order to reduce the risk of overdose. Advise families and caregivers of adults being treated for depression similarly.

➤*Activation of psychosis and/or mania:* Antidepressants can precipitate manic episodes in bipolar disorder patients during the depressed phase of their illness and may activate latent psychosis in other susceptible patients. Bupropion is expected to pose similar risks.

➤*Screening patients for bipolar disorder:* An MDD may be the initial presentation of bipolar disorder. It is generally believed (though not established in controlled trials) that treating such an episode with an antidepressant alone may increase the likelihood of precipitation of a mixed/manic episode in patients at risk for bipolar disorder. Whether any of the symptoms described above represent such a conversion is unknown. However, prior to initiating treatment with an antidepressant, adequately screen patients with depressive symptoms to determine if they are at risk for bipolar disorder; include in the screening a detailed psychiatric history, including a family history of suicide, bipolar disorder, and depression. Note that bupropion is not approved for use in treating bipolar depression.

➤*Other bupropion medications:* Inform patients that bupropion is the same active ingredient found in *Zyban*, used as an aid to smoking cessation treatment, and that bupropion should not be used in combination with *Zyban*, or any other medications that contain bupropion, such as *Wellbutrin XL*, *Wellbutrin SR*, or *Wellbutrin*.

➤*Seizures:* Bupropion is associated with a dose-related risk of seizures. The risk of seizures is also related to patient factors, clinical situations, and concomitant medications, which must be considered in selection of patients for therapy with bupropion. Discontinue bupropion and do not restart bupropion in patients who experience a seizure while on treatment.

The seizure incidence with bupropion has not been formally evaluated in clinical trials. Studies in mice suggest the potential for a significant reduction in the risk of seizure with bupropion hydrobromide as compared with bupropion hydrochloride. The seizure incidence is not expected to be worse than for comparable doses of the immediate-release and sustained release formulations of bupropion hydrochloride.

Dose – At dosages up to 300 mg/day (equivalent to bupropion hydrobromide 348 mg/day) of the *Wellbutrin SR*, the incidence of seizure is approximately 0.1% (1/1,000).

Data for the *Wellbutrin* revealed a seizure incidence of approximately 0.4% (ie, 13 of 3,200 patients followed prospectively) in patients treated at dosages in a range of 300 to 450 mg/day (equivalent to a range of 348 to 522 mg/day of bupropion hydrobromide). This seizure incidence (0.4%) may exceed that of some other marketed antidepressants.

Additional data accumulated for *Wellbutrin* suggested that the estimated seizure incidence increases almost 10-fold between 450 and 600 mg/day (equivalent to bupropion hydrobromide 522 and 696 mg/day). The 600 mg dose is twice the usual adult dose and one and one-third the maximum recommended daily dose (450 mg) of *Wellbutrin XL* (equivalent to bupropion hydrobromide 522 mg) tablets. This disproportionate increase in seizure incidence with dose incrementation calls for caution in dosing.

Patient factors – Predisposing factors that may increase the risk of seizure with bupropion use include history of head trauma or prior seizure, CNS tumor, the presence of severe hepatic cirrhosis, and concomitant medications that lower seizure threshold.

Clinical situations – Circumstances associated with an increased seizure risk include, among others, excessive use of alcohol or sedatives (including benzodiazepines); addiction to opiates, cocaine, or stimulants; use of over-the-counter stimulants and anorectics; and diabetes treated with oral hypoglycemics or insulin.

Recommendations for reducing the risk of seizure – Retrospective analysis of clinical experience gained during the development of bupropion suggests that the risk of seizure may be minimized if the total daily dose of bupropion does not exceed 522 mg and the rate of incrementation of dose is gradual.

Administer bupropion with extreme caution to patients with a history of seizure, cranial trauma, or other predisposition(s) toward seizure, or patients treated with other agents (eg, antipsychotics, other antidepressants, theophylline, systemic steroids) that lower seizure threshold.

➤*Hepatotoxicity:* In rats receiving large doses of bupropion chronically, there was an increase in incidence of hepatic hyperplastic nodules and hepatocellular hypertrophy. In dogs receiving large doses of bupropion chronically, various histologic changes were seen in the liver, and laboratory tests suggesting mild hepatocellular injury were noted.

BUPROPION HYDROBROMIDE — ORAL

➤*CNS effects:*

Agitation/Insomnia – Increased restlessness, agitation, anxiety, and insomnia, especially shortly after initiation of treatment, have been associated with treatment with bupropion.

Patients in placebo-controlled trials of MDD with *Wellbutrin SR* experienced agitation, anxiety, and insomnia as shown in the following table.

Incidence of Agitation, Anxiety, and Insomnia in Trials of *Wellbutrin SR*			
Adverse reactions	*Wellbutrin SR* 300 mg/day[a] (n = 376)	*Wellbutrin SR* 400 mg/day[b] (n = 114)	Placebo (n = 385)
Agitation	3%	9%	2%
Anxiety	5%	6%	3%
Insomnia	11%	16%	6%

[a] Equivalent to bupropion hydrobromide 348 mg/day.
[b] Equivalent to bupropion hydrobromide 464 mg/day.

In clinical studies of MDD, these symptoms were sometimes of sufficient magnitude to require treatment with sedative/hypnotic drugs.

Symptoms in these studies were sufficiently severe to require discontinuation of treatment in 1% and 2.6% of patients treated with *Wellbutrin SR* 300 and 400 mg/day, respectively, and 0.8% of patients treated with placebo.

Psychosis, confusion, and other neuropsychiatric phenomena – Depressed patients treated with bupropion have been reported to show a variety of neuropsychiatric signs and symptoms, including delusions, hallucinations, psychosis, concentration disturbance, paranoia, and confusion. In some cases, these symptoms abated upon dose reduction and/or withdrawal of treatment.

➤*Altered appetite and weight:* In placebo-controlled studies of MDD using *Wellbutrin SR*, patients experienced weight gain or weight loss.

Weight Gain/Loss in Trials of *Wellbutrin SR*			
Weight change	*Wellbutrin SR* 300 mg/day[a] (n = 339)	*Wellbutrin SR* 400 mg/day[b] (n = 112)	Placebo (n = 347)
Gained > 5 lbs	3%	2%	4%
Lost > 5 lbs	14%	19%	6%

[a] Equivalent to bupropion hydrobromide 348 mg/day.
[b] Equivalent to bupropion hydrobromide 464 mg/day.

In studies conducted with the *Wellbutrin*, 35% of patients receiving tricyclic antidepressants gained weight, compared with 9% of patients treated with the *Wellbutrin*. If weight loss is a major presenting sign of a patient's depressive illness, consider the anorectic and/or weight-reducing potential of bupropion tablets.

➤*Cardiovascular effects:* In clinical practice, hypertension, in some cases severe, requiring acute treatment, has been reported in patients receiving bupropion alone and in combination with nicotine replacement therapy. These reactions have been observed in both patients with and without evidence of preexisting hypertension.

There is no clinical experience establishing the safety of bupropion in patients with a recent history of myocardial infarction or unstable heart disease. Therefore, exercise caution if it is used in these groups. Bupropion was well tolerated in depressed patients who had previously developed orthostatic hypotension while receiving tricyclic antidepressants, and was also generally well tolerated in a group of 36 depressed inpatients with stable CHF. However, bupropion was associated with a rise in supine blood pressure in the study of patients with CHF, resulting in discontinuation of treatment in 2 patients for exacerbation of baseline hypertension.

➤*Hypersensitivity reactions:* Anaphylactoid/anaphylactic reactions characterized by symptoms such as pruritus, urticaria, angioedema, and dyspnea requiring medical treatment have been reported in clinical trials with bupropion. In addition, there have been rare spontaneous postmarketing reports of erythema multiforme, Stevens-Johnson syndrome, and anaphylactic shock associated with bupropion. A patient should stop taking bupropion and consult a health care provider if experiencing allergic or anaphylactoid/anaphylactic reactions (eg, chest pain, edema, hives, pruritus, shortness of breath, skin rash) during treatment.

Arthralgia, myalgia, and fever with rash and other symptoms suggestive of delayed hypersensitivity have been reported in association with bupropion. These symptoms may resemble serum sickness.

➤*Renal function impairment:* There is limited information on the pharmacokinetics of bupropion in patients with renal impairment. An interstudy comparison between normal subjects and patients with end-stage renal failure demonstrated that the parent drug C_{max} and AUC values were comparable in the 2 groups, whereas the hydroxybupropion and threohydrobupropion metabolites had a 2.3- and 2.8-fold increase, respectively, in AUC for patients with end-stage renal failure. Bupropion is extensively metabolized in the liver to active metabolites, which are further metabolized and subsequently excreted by the kidneys. Use bupropion with caution in patients with renal impairment and consider a reduced frequency and/or dose as bupropion and the metabolites of bupropion may accumulate in such patients to a greater extent than usual. Closely monitor the patient for possible adverse effects that could indicate high drug or metabolite levels.

➤*Hepatic function impairment:* Use bupropion with extreme caution in patients with severe hepatic cirrhosis. In these patients a reduced frequency and/or dose is required, as peak bupropion, as well as AUC, levels are substantially increased and accumulation is likely to occur in such patients to a greater extent than usual. The dose should not exceed 174 mg every other day in these patients.

Use bupropion with caution in patients with hepatic impairment (including mild to moderate hepatic cirrhosis) and consider reduced frequency and/or dose in patients with mild to moderate hepatic cirrhosis.

Monitor all patients with hepatic impairment for possible adverse effects that could indicate high drug and metabolite levels.

➤*Drug abuse and dependence:*

Controlled substance – Bupropion is not a controlled substance.

Abuse –

Humans: Controlled clinical studies of bupropion hydrochloride (immediate-release formulation) conducted in normal volunteers, in subjects with a history of multiple drug abuse, and in depressed patients showed some increase in motor activity and agitation/excitement.

In a population of individuals experienced with drugs of abuse, a single dose of bupropion hydrochloride 400 mg produced mild amphetamine-like activity as compared with placebo on the Morphine-Benzedrine Subscale of the Addiction Research Center Inventories (ARCI), and a score intermediate between placebo and amphetamine on the Liking Scale of the ARCI. These scales measure general feelings of euphoria and drug desirability.

Findings in clinical trials, however, are not known to reliably predict the abuse potential of drugs. Nonetheless, evidence from single-dose studies does suggest that the recommended daily dosage of bupropion when administered in divided doses is not likely to be especially reinforcing to amphetamine or stimulant abusers. However, higher doses that could not be tested because of the risk of seizure might be modestly attractive to those who abuse stimulant drugs.

Animals: Studies in rodents and primates have shown that bupropion exhibits some pharmacologic actions common to psychostimulants. In rodents, it has been shown to increase locomotor activity, elicit a mild stereotyped behavioral response, and increase rates of responding in several schedule controlled behavior paradigms. In primate models to assess the positive reinforcing effects of psychoactive drugs, bupropion was self-administered intravenously. In rats, bupropion produced amphetamine-like and cocaine-like discriminative stimulus effects in drug discrimination paradigms used to characterize the subjective effects of psychoactive drugs.

➤*Pregnancy: Category C* (per manufacturer's prescribing information; *Category B* (per Briggs' *Drugs in Pregnancy and Lactation*). Use bupropion during pregnancy only if the potential benefit justifies the potential risk to the fetus.

In studies conducted in rats and rabbits, bupropion hydrochloride was administered orally at dosages up to 450 and 150 mg/kg/day, respectively (approximately 11 and 7 times the MRHD, respectively, on a mg/m^2 basis), during the period of organogenesis. No clear evidence of teratogenic activity was found in either species; however, in rabbits, slightly increased incidences of fetal malformations and skeletal variations were observed at the lowest dosage tested (25 mg/kg/day, approximately equal to the MRHD on a mg/m^2 basis) and greater. Decreased fetal weights were seen at 50 mg/kg and greater.

When rats were administered bupropion hydrochloride at oral dosages of up to 300 mg/kg/day (approximately 7 times the MRHD on a mg/m^2 basis) prior to mating and throughout pregnancy and lactation, there were no apparent adverse effects on offspring development.

One study has been conducted in pregnant women. This retrospective, managed-care database study assessed the risk of congenital malformations overall, and cardiovascular malformations specifically, following exposure to bupropion in the first trimester compared with the risk of these malformations following exposure to other antidepressants in the first trimester and bupropion outside of the first trimester. This study included 7,005 infants with antidepressant exposure during pregnancy, 1,213 of whom were exposed to bupropion in the first trimester. The study showed no greater risk for congenital malformations overall, or cardiovascular malformations specifically, following first trimester bupropion exposure compared with exposure to all other antidepressants in the first trimester, or bupropion outside of the first trimester. The results of this study have not been corroborated.

Labor and delivery – The effect of bupropion on labor and delivery in humans is unknown.

➤*Lactation:* Like many other drugs, bupropion and its metabolites are secreted in human milk. Because of the potential for serious adverse reactions in nursing infants from bupropion tablets, make a decision whether to discontinue breast-feeding or to discontinue the drug, taking into account the importance of the drug to the mother. The American Academy of Pediatrics classifies bupropion as a drug whose effect on the breast-feeding infant is unknown, but may be of concern.

➤*Children:* Safety and effectiveness in children have not been established. Anyone considering the use of bupropion in a child or adolescent must balance the potential risks with the clinical need.

➤*Elderly:* A single-dose pharmacokinetic study demonstrated that the disposition of bupropion and its metabolites in elderly subjects was similar to that of younger subjects; however, another pharmacokinetic study, single and multiple dose, has suggested that elderly patients are at increased risk for accumulation of bupropion and its metabolites.

Bupropion is extensively metabolized in the liver to active metabolites, which are further metabolized and excreted by the kidneys. The risk of toxic reaction to this drug may be greater in patients with impaired renal function. Because elderly patients are more likely to have decreased renal function, care should be taken in dose selection, and it may be useful to monitor renal function.

➤*Monitoring:* Closely monitor all patients with hepatic or renal impairment for possible adverse reactions that could indicate high drug and metabolite levels. Monitoring of blood pressure is recommended in patients who receive the combination of bupropion and nicotine replacement. Monitor patients closely for clinical worsening, suicidality, and unusual changes in behavior, especially during the initial few months of a course of drug therapy or at times of dosage increases or decreases.

Drug Interactions

Bupropion Drug Interactions

Precipitant drug	Object drug[a]		Description
Amantadine, Levodopa	Bupropion	↑	There is a higher incidence of adverse reactions (eg, neurotoxicity) with concurrent use of bupropion with either levodopa or amantadine. Use small initial dosages and small, gradual dosage increases of bupropion.
Carbamazepine	Bupropion	↓	Serum concentrations of bupropion may be decreased, reducing the pharmacologic effects.
Clopidogrel	Bupropion	↑	Bupropion plasma concentrations may be elevated, increasing the pharmacologic and adverse effects. The bupropion dosage may need to be adjusted when clopidogrel is started or stopped.
CYP2B6 inducers (eg, phenobarbital, phenytoin)	Bupropion	↓	Inducers of CYP2B6 may decrease serum levels and efficacy of bupropion.
CYP2B6 inhibitors (eg, cimetidine)	Bupropion	↑	Inhibitors of CYP2B6 may increase serum levels, increasing the pharmacologic and adverse effects.
Drugs that lower the seizure threshold (eg, antidepressants, antipsychotics, systemic steroids, theophylline)	Bupropion	↑	Bupropion is associated with a dose-dependent risk of seizures. Undertake the coadministration of bupropion and agents that lower the seizure threshold only with extreme caution.
Bupropion	Drugs that lower the seizure threshold (eg, antidepressants, antipsychotics, systemic steroids, theophylline)		
Guanfacine	Bupropion	↑	The risk of bupropion toxicity may be increased. Closely monitor patients. If an interaction is suspected, adjust therapy as needed.
Linezolid	Bupropion	↑	The risk of hypertensive crisis may be increased. Because coadministration of bupropion and traditional MAOIs is contraindicated, avoid concurrent use of bupropion and linezolid until more clinical information is available.
MAOIs (eg, phenelzine)	Bupropion	↑	Coadministration is contraindicated. Risk of acute bupropion toxicity may be increased. Allow at least 14 days to elapse between discontinuing an MAOI and starting bupropion.
Bupropion	MAOIs (eg, phenelzine)		

Bupropion Drug Interactions

Precipitant drug	Object drug[a]		Description
Nicotine replacement therapy (ie, nicotine transdermal system)	Bupropion	↑	Hypertension (sometimes severe) requiring acute treatment has been reported in patients receiving bupropion alone and in combination with nicotine replacement therapy. These events have been observed in patients with and without evidence of preexisting hypertension. Monitor blood pressure in patients receiving this combination.
Bupropion	Nicotine replacement therapy (ie, nicotine transdermal system)		
Rifampin	Bupropion	↓	Bupropion plasma concentrations may be reduced, decreasing the therapeutic effect.
Ritonavir	Bupropion	↓	Bupropion levels may be reduced, decreasing therapeutic effects.
Ticlopidine	Bupropion	↑	Bupropion plasma concentrations may be elevated, increasing the pharmacologic and adverse effects. Adjust bupropion dosage when ticlopidine is started or stopped.
Bupropion	Alcohol	↑	There have been rare reports of adverse neuropsychiatric events or reduced alcohol tolerance in patients who were drinking alcohol during treatment with bupropion. Advise patients to minimize or avoid alcohol consumption while taking bupropion.
Bupropion	Anticoagulants, (eg, warfarin)	↑	Altered prothrombin time and/or international normalized ratio infrequently associated with hemorrhagic or thrombotic complications were observed when bupropion was administered with warfarin.
Bupropion	Antiarrhythmics, type 1C (eg, flecainide, propafenone)	↑	Bupropion is an inhibitor of the CYP2D6 isoenzyme. If bupropion is added to the treatment regimen of a patient receiving a drug metabolized by CYP2D6, consider a dosage reduction in the medication.
	Antipsychotics (eg, haloperidol, risperidone, thioridazine)		
	Beta-blockers (eg, metoprolol)		
Bupropion	Cyclosporine	↓	Cyclosporine concentrations may be reduced, decreasing the pharmacologic effects.
Bupropion	SSRIs (eg, fluoxetine, paroxetine, sertraline)	↑	Bupropion is an inhibitor of the CYP2D6 isoenzyme. If bupropion is added to the treatment regimen of a patient receiving a drug metabolized by CYP2D6, consider a dosage reduction in the medication.
	Tricyclic antidepressants (eg, desipramine, imipramine, nortriptyline)		

[a] ↑ = object drug increased; ↓ = object drug decreased.

➤*Drug/Food interactions:* See Actions for more information.

Adverse Reactions

➤*Common adverse reactions:*

Wellbutrin SR 300 mg/day (equivalent to bupropion hydrobromide 348 mg/day) – Anorexia, dry mouth, rash, sweating, tinnitus, tremor (at least 5%).

Wellbutrin SR 400 mg/day (equivalent to bupropion hydrobromide 464 mg/day) – Abdominal pain, agitation, anxiety, dizziness, dry mouth, insomnia, myalgia, nausea, palpitation, pharyngitis, sweating, tinnitus, urinary frequency (at least 5%).

Discontinuation – In placebo-controlled clinical trials, 9% and 11% of patients treated with 300 and 400 mg/day, respectively, of *Wellbutrin SR* and 4% of patients treated with placebo discontinued treatment due to adverse reactions.

BUPROPION HYDROBROMIDE — ORAL

Treatment Discontinuations Due to Bupropion Adverse Reactions			
Adverse reactions	*Wellbutrin SR* 300 mg/day[a] (n = 376)	*Wellbutrin SR* 400 mg/day[b] (n = 114)	Placebo (n = 385)
CNS			
Agitation	0.3%	1.8%	0.3%
Migraine	0%	1.8%	0.3%
Miscellaneous			
Nausea	0.8%	1.8%	0.3%
Rash	2.4%	0.9%	0%

[a] Equivalent to bupropion hydrobromide 348 mg/day.
[b] Equivalent to bupropion hydrobromide 464 mg/day.

In clinical trials with the immediate-release formulation of bupropion, 10% of patients and volunteers discontinued because of an adverse reaction. Reactions resulting in discontinuation, in addition to those listed previously for the sustained-release formulation of bupropion hydrochloride, include vomiting, seizures, and sleep disturbances.

Adverse reactions (1% or more) –

Bupropion Adverse Reactions (≥ 1%)[a]			
Adverse reactions	*Wellbutrin SR* 300 mg/day[b] (n = 376)	*Wellbutrin SR* 400 mg/day[c] (n = 114)	Placebo (n = 385)
Cardiovascular			
Chest pain	3%	4%	1%
Flushing	1%	4%	–
Hot flashes	1%	3%	1%
Palpitation	2%	6%	2%
CNS			
Agitation	3%	9%	2%
Anxiety	5%	6%	3%
Asthenia	2%	4%	2%
CNS stimulation	2%	1%	1%
Dizziness	7%	11%	5%
Headache	26%	25%	23%
Insomnia	11%	16%	6%
Irritability	3%	2%	2%
Memory decreased	–	3%	1%
Migraine	1%	4%	1%
Nervousness	5%	3%	3%
Paresthesia	1%	2%	1%
Somnolence	2%	3%	2%
Tremor	6%	3%	1%
Dermatology			
Pruritus	2%	4%	2%
Rash	5%	4%	1%
Sweating	6%	5%	2%
Urticaria	2%	1%	0%
GI			
Abdominal pain	3%	9%	2%
Anorexia	5%	3%	2%
Constipation	10%	5%	7%
Diarrhea	5%	7%	6%
Dry mouth	17%	24%	7%
Dysphagia	0%	2%	0%
Nausea	13%	18%	8%
Vomiting	4%	2%	2%
GU			
Urinary frequency	2%	5%	2%
Urinary tract infection	1%	0%	–
Urinary urgency	–	2%	0%
Vaginal hemorrhage[d]	0%	2%	–
Musculoskeletal			
Arthralgia	1%	4%	1%
Arthritis	0%	2%	0%
Myalgia	2%	6%	3%

Bupropion Adverse Reactions (≥ 1%)[a]			
Adverse reactions	*Wellbutrin SR* 300 mg/day[b] (n = 376)	*Wellbutrin SR* 400 mg/day[c] (n = 114)	Placebo (n = 385)
Twitch	1%	2%	–
Respiratory			
Cough increased	1%	2%	1%
Pharyngitis	3%	11%	2%
Sinusitis	3%	1%	2%
Special senses			
Blurred vision or diplopia	3%	2%	2%
Taste perversion	2%	4%	–
Tinnitus	6%	6%	2%
Miscellaneous			
Fever	1%	2%	–[e]
Infection	8%	9%	6%
Pain	2%	3%	2%

[a] Adverse reactions that occurred in ≥ 1% of patients treated with *Wellbutrin SR* 300 or 400 mg/day, but equally or more frequently in the placebo group, were as follows: abnormal dreams, accidental injury, acne, appetite increased, back pain, bronchitis, dysmenorrhea, dyspepsia, flatulence, flu syndrome, hypertension, neck pain, respiratory disorder, rhinitis, and tooth disorder.
[b] Equivalent to bupropion hydrobromide 348 mg/day.
[c] Equivalent to bupropion hydrobromide 464 mg/day.
[d] Incidence based on the number of women.
[e] Hyphen denotes adverse reactions occurring in > 0% but

Additional reactions to those listed that occurred at an incidence of at least 1% in controlled clinical trials of the immediate-release formulation of bupropion hydrochloride (300 to 600 mg/day) and that were numerically more frequent than placebo were: cardiac arrhythmias (5% vs 4%), hypertension (4% vs 2%), hypotension (3% vs 2%), tachycardia (11% vs 9%), appetite increase (4% vs 2%), dyspepsia (3% vs 2%), menstrual complaints (5% vs 1%), akathisia (2% vs 1%), impaired sleep quality (4% vs 2%), sensory disturbance (4% vs 3%), confusion (8% vs 5%), decreased libido (3% vs 2%), hostility (6% vs 4%), auditory disturbance (5% vs 3%), and gustatory disturbance (3% vs 1%).

Cardiovascular – Postural hypotension, stroke, tachycardia, vasodilation (0.1% to 1%); syncope (less than 0.1%); complete atrioventricular block, extrasystoles, hypertension (in some cases severe), hypotension, myocardial infarction, phlebitis, pulmonary embolism.

CNS – Abnormal coordination, decreased libido, depersonalization, dysphoria, emotional lability, hostility, hyperkinesia, hypertonia, hypesthesia, suicidal ideation, vertigo (0.1% to 1%); amnesia, ataxia, derealization, hypomania (less than 0.1%); abnormal electroencephalogram, aggression, akinesia, aphasia, coma, delirium, delusions, dysarthria, dyskinesia, dystonia, euphoria, extrapyramidal syndrome, hallucinations, hypokinesia, increased libido, manic reaction, neuralgia, neuropathy, paranoid ideation, restlessness, unmasking tardive dyskinesia.

Dermatologic – Maculopapular rash (less than 0.1%); alopecia, angioedema, exfoliative dermatitis, hirsutism.

Endocrine – Hyperglycemia, hypoglycemia, syndrome of inappropriate antidiuretic hormone.

GI – Abnormal liver function, bruxism, gastric reflux, gingivitis, glossitis, increased salivation, jaundice, mouth ulcers, stomatitis, and thirst (0.1% to 1%); edema of tongue (less than 0.1%); colitis, esophagitis, GI hemorrhage, gum hemorrhage, hepatitis, intestinal perforation, liver damage, pancreatitis, stomach ulcer.

GU – Impotence, polyuria, prostate disorder (0.1% to 1%); abnormal ejaculation, cystitis, dyspareunia, dysuria, gynecomastia, menopause, painful erection, salpingitis, urinary incontinence, urinary retention, vaginitis.

Hematologic/Lymphatic – Ecchymosis (0.1% to 1%). Also observed were anemia, leukocytosis, leukopenia, lymphadenopathy, pancytopenia, and thrombocytopenia. Altered prothrombin time and/or international normalized ratio, infrequently associated with hemorrhagic or thrombotic complications, were observed when bupropion was coadministered with warfarin.

Metabolic/Nutritional – Edema, peripheral edema (0.1% to 1%); glycosuria.

Musculoskeletal – Leg cramps (0.1% to 1%); muscle rigidity/fever/rhabdomyolysis, muscle weakness.

Respiratory – Bronchospasm (less than 0.1%); pneumonia.

Special senses – Accommodation abnormality, dry eye (0.1% to 1%); deafness, diplopia, increased intraocular pressure, mydriasis.

Miscellaneous – Chills, facial edema, musculoskeletal chest pain, photosensitivity (0.1% to 1%); malaise (less than 0.1%); arthralgia, myalgia, and fever with rash and other symptoms suggestive of delayed hypersensitivity. These symptoms may resemble serum sickness.

BUPROPION HYDROBROMIDE — ORAL

Overdosage

➤*Symptoms:* Overdoses of up to 30 g or more of bupropion have been reported. Seizure was reported in approximately one third of all cases. Other serious reactions reported with overdoses of bupropion alone included hallucinations, loss of consciousness, sinus tachycardia, and electrocardiogram changes, such as conduction disturbances or arrhythmias. Fever, muscle rigidity, rhabdomyolysis, hypotension, stupor, coma, and respiratory failure have been reported mainly when bupropion was part of multiple drug overdoses.

Although most patients recovered without sequelae, deaths associated with overdoses of bupropion alone have been reported in patients ingesting large doses of the drug. Multiple uncontrolled seizures, bradycardia, cardiac failure, and cardiac arrest prior to death were reported in these patients.

➤*Treatment:* Ensure an adequate airway, oxygenation, and ventilation. Monitor cardiac rhythm and vital signs. Electroencephalograph monitoring is also recommended for the first 48 hours postingestion. General supportive and symptomatic measures are also recommended. Induction of emesis is not recommended. Gastric lavage with a large-bore orogastric tube with appropriate airway protection, if needed, may be indicated if performed soon after ingestion or in symptomatic patients.

Activated charcoal should be administered. There is no experience with the use of forced diuresis, dialysis, hemoperfusion, or exchange transfusion in the management of bupropion overdoses. No specific antidotes for bupropion are known.

Because of the dose-related risk of seizures with bupropion, hospitalization following suspected overdose should be considered. Based on studies in animals, it is recommended that seizures be treated with IV benzodiazepine administration and other supportive measures, as appropriate.

In managing overdosage, consider the possibility of multiple drug involvement. The health care provider should consider contacting a poison control center for additional information on the treatment of any overdose.

Patient Information

Inform patients, their families, and their caregivers about the benefits and risks associated with treatment with bupropion and counsel them in its appropriate use. A patient Medication Guide with important information about bupropion is available. Instruct patients, their families, and their caregivers to read the Medication Guide and assist them in understanding its contents. Give patients the opportunity to discuss the contents of the Medication Guide and to obtain answers to any questions they may have.

Advise patients of the following issues and ask them to alert their health care provider if these occur while taking bupropion:

➤*Clinical worsening and suicide:* Encourage patients, their families, and their caregivers to be alert to the emergence of anxiety, agitation, panic attacks, insomnia, irritability, hostility, aggressiveness, impulsivity, akathisia (psychomotor restlessness), hypomania, mania, other unusual changes in behavior, worsening of depression, and suicidal ideation, especially early during antidepressant treatment and when the dose is adjusted up or down. Advise families and caregivers of patients to observe for the emergence of such symptoms on a day-to-day basis, because changes may be abrupt. Instruct them to report such symptoms to their health care provider, especially if they are severe, abrupt in onset, or were not part of the patient's presenting symptoms. Symptoms such as these may be associated with an increased risk for suicidal thinking and behavior and indicate a need for very close monitoring and possibly changes in the medication.

Inform patients that *Aplenzin* contains the same active ingredient (bupropion) found in *Zyban*, which is used as an aid to smoking cessation treatment, and that *Aplenzin* should not be used in combination with *Zyban* or any other medications that contain bupropion hydrochloride (such as *Wellbutrin XL*, the ER formulation, *Wellbutrin SR*, the sustained-release formulation, and *Wellbutrin*, the immediate-release formulation).

Tell patients that bupropion should be discontinued and not restarted if they experience a seizure while on treatment.

Inform patients that any CNS-active drug like bupropion may impair their ability to perform tasks requiring judgment or motor and cognitive skills. Consequently, until they are reasonably certain that bupropion does not adversely affect their performance, they should refrain from driving an automobile or operating complex, hazardous machinery.

Tell patients that the excessive use or abrupt discontinuation of alcohol or sedatives (including benzodiazepines) may alter the seizure threshold. Some patients have reported lower alcohol tolerance during treatment with bupropion. Advise patients that the consumption of alcohol should be minimized or avoided.

Advise patients to notify their health care provider if they are taking or plan to take any prescription or over-the-counter drugs. Concern is warranted because bupropion and other drugs may affect each other's metabolism.

Advise patients to notify their health care provider if they become pregnant or intend to become pregnant during therapy.

Tell patients to swallow bupropion tablets whole so that the release rate is not altered, and not to chew, divide, or crush the tablets.

Advise patients that they may notice something that looks like a tablet in their stool. This is normal. The medication in bupropion is contained in a nonabsorbable shell that has been specially designed to slowly release the drug in the body. When this process is completed, the empty shell is eliminated from the body.

NEFAZODONE HYDROCHLORIDE

Rx	**Nefazodone HCl** (Various, eg, Eon, Par, Teva)	**Tablets:** 50 mg	In 60s and 100s.
		100 mg	In 60s.
		150 mg	In 60s.
		200 mg	In 60s.
		250 mg	In 60s.

NEFAZODONE HYDROCHLORIDE — ORAL

For additional information, refer to the Antidepressants introduction.

WARNING

Cases of life-threatening hepatic failure have been reported in patients treated with nefazodone.

The reported rate in the US is approximately 1 case of liver failure resulting in death or transplant per 250,000 to 300,000 patient-years of nefazodone treatment. The total patient-years is a summation of each patient's duration of exposure expressed in years. For example, 1 patient-year is equal to 2 patients each treated for 6 months, 3 patients each treated for 4 months, etc. This represents a rate of about 3 to 4 times the estimated background rate of liver failure. This rate is an underestimate because of underreporting, and the true risk could be considerably greater than this. A large cohort study of antidepressant users found no cases of liver failure leading to death or transplant among nefazodone users in approximately 30,000 patient-years of exposure. The spontaneous report data and the cohort study results provide estimates of the upper and lower limits of the risk of liver failure in nefazodone-treated patients, but are not capable of providing a precise risk estimate.

Ordinarily, treatment with nefazodone should not be initiated in individuals with active liver disease or with elevated baseline serum transaminases. There is no evidence that preexisting liver disease increases the likelihood of developing liver failure; however, baseline abnormalities can complicate patient monitoring.

Advise patients to be alert for signs and symptoms of liver dysfunction (eg, jaundice, anorexia, GI complaints, malaise) and to report them to their health care provider immediately if they occur.

Discontinue nefazodone if clinical signs or symptoms suggest liver failure. If nefazodone-treated patients develop evidence of hepatocellular injury such as increased serum AST or serum ALT levels greater than or equal to 3 times the upper limit of normal, withdraw the drug. These patients should be presumed to be at increased risk for liver injury if nefazodone is reintroduced. Accordingly, do not consider such patients for retreatment.

Indications

➤*Depression:* For the treatment of depression.

Administration and Dosage

➤*Adults:*

Depression –

Initial dosage: 100 mg twice daily.

Dosage titration: Dosage increases should occur in increments of 100 to 200 mg/day, again on a twice-daily schedule, at intervals of no less than 1 week.

Most patients, depending on tolerability and the need for further clinical effect, should have their dose increased. As with all antidepressants, several weeks on treatment may be required to obtain a full antidepressant response.

Maintenance dosage: 300 to 600 mg/day.

➤*Elderly:*

Initial dosage – 50 mg twice daily.

➤*Hepatic function impairment:* Patients with active liver disease should not be treated with nefazodone.

➤*Debilitated patients:*

Initial dosage – 50 mg twice daily.

➤*Switching patients to or from a monoamine oxidase inhibitor:* At least 14 days should elapse between discontinuation of an monoamine oxidase inhibitor (MAOI) and initiation of therapy with nefazodone. In addition, allow at least 7 days after stopping nefazodone before starting an MAOI.

➤*Duration of therapy:* There is no body of evidence available from controlled trials to indicate how long the depressed patient should be treated with nefazodone. It is generally agreed, however, that pharmacological treatment for acute episodes of depression should continue for up to 6 months or longer. Whether the dose of antidepressant needed to induce

NEFAZODONE HYDROCHLORIDE — ORAL

remission is identical to the dose needed to maintain euthymia is unknown. Systematic evaluation of the efficacy of nefazodone has shown that efficacy is maintained for periods of up to 36 weeks following 16 weeks of open-label acute treatment (treated for 52 weeks total) at dosages that averaged 438 mg/day. For most patients, their maintenance dose was that associated with response during acute treatment. The safety of nefazodone in long-term use is supported by data from both double-blind and open-label trials involving more than 250 patients treated for at least 1 year.

➤*Administration:* Take with or without food.

➤*Storage/Stability:* Store at 15° to 30°C (59° to 86°F) and dispense in a tight, light-resistant container using a child-resistant closure.

Actions

➤*Pharmacology:* The mechanism of action of nefazodone, as with other antidepressants, is unknown.

Preclinical studies have shown that nefazodone inhibits neuronal uptake of serotonin and norepinephrine.

Nefazodone occupies central 5-HT_2 receptors at nanomolar concentrations, and acts as an antagonist at this receptor. Nefazodone was shown to antagonize alpha-1-adrenergic receptors, a property which may be associated with postural hypotension. In vitro binding studies showed that nefazodone had not significant affinity for the following receptors: alpha-2 and beta-adrenergic, 5-HT_{1A}, cholinergic, dopaminergic, or benzodiazepine.

➤*Pharmacokinetics:*

Absorption – Nefazodone is rapidly and completely absorbed but is subject to extensive metabolism, so that its absolute bioavailability is low (about 20%) and variable. Peak plasma concentrations occur at about 1 hour and the half-life of nefazodone is 2 to 4 hours.

Both nefazodone and its pharmacologically similar metabolite, hydroxynefazodone, exhibit nonlinear kinetics for both dose and time, with AUC and C_{max} increasing more than proportionally with dose increases and more than expected upon multiple dosing over time, compared with single dosing. For example, in a multiple-dose study involving twice-daily dosing with 50, 100, and 200 mg, the AUC for nefazodone and hydroxynefazodone increased by about 4-fold with an increase in dosage from 200 to 400 mg/day; C_{max} increased by about 3-fold with the same dose increase. In a multiple-dose study involving twice-daily dosing with 25, 50, 100, and 150 mg, the accumulation ratios for nefazodone and hydroxynefazodone AUC, after 5 days of twice-daily dosing relative to the first dose, ranged from approximately 3 to 4 at the lower dosages (50 to 100 mg/day) and from 5 to 7 at the higher dosages (200 to 300 mg/day); there were also approximately 2- to 4-fold increases in C_{max} after 5 days of twice-daily dosing relative to the first dose, suggesting extensive and greater than predicted accumulation of nefazodone and its hydroxy metabolite with multiple dosing. Steady-state plasma nefazodone and metabolite concentrations are attained within 4 to 5 days of initiation of twice-daily dosing or upon dose increase or decrease.

Effect of food: Food delays the absorption of nefazodone and decreases the bioavailability of nefazodone by approximately 20%.

Distribution – Nefazodone is widely distributed in body tissues, including the CNS. In humans the volume of distribution of nefazodone ranges from 0.22 to 0.87 L/kg.

At concentrations of 25 to 2,500 ng/mL, nefazodone is extensively (greater than 99%) bound to human plasma proteins in vitro.

Metabolism – Nefazodone is extensively metabolized after oral administration by n-dealkylation and aliphatic and aromatic hydroxylation, and less than 1% of administered nefazodone is excreted unchanged in urine. Attempts to characterize 3 metabolites identified in plasma, hydroxynefazodone (HO-NEF), meta-chlorophenylpiperazine (mCPP), and a triazoledione metabolite, have been carried out. The AUC (expressed as a multiple of the AUC for nefazodone dosed at 100 mg twice daily) and elimination half-lives for these 3 metabolites were as follows:

AUC Multiples and t ½ for 3 Metabolites of Nefazodone (100 mg twice a day)		
Metabolite	AUC multiple	t ½
HO-NEF	0.4	1.5 to 4 hours
mCPP	0.07	4 to 8 hours
Triazole-dionemetabolite	4	18 hours

HO-NEF possesses a pharmacological profile qualitatively and quantitatively similar to that of nefazodone. mCPP has some similarities to nefazodone, but also has agonist activity at some serotonergic receptor subtypes. The pharmacological profile of the triazole-dione metabolite has not yet been well characterized. In addition to the above compounds, several other metabolites were present in plasma but have not been tested for pharmacological activity.

Excretion – After oral administration of radiolabeled nefazodone, the mean half-life of total label ranged between 11 and 24 hours. Approximately 55% of the administered radioactivity was detected in urine and about 20% to 30% in feces.

Special populations –

Renal function impairment: In studies involving 29 renally impaired patients, renal impairment (creatinine clearances ranging from 7 to 60 mL/min/1.73 m^2) had no effect on steady-state nefazodone plasma concentrations.

Liver function impairment: In a multidose study of patients with liver cirrhosis, the AUC values for nefazodone and HO-NEF at steady state were approximately 25% greater than those observed in healthy volunteers.

Age/gender effects: After single doses of 300 mg to younger (18 to 45 years of age) and older patients (older than 65 years of age), C_{max} and AUC for nefazodone and hydroxynefazodone were up to twice as high in the older patients. With multiple doses, however, differences were much smaller, 10% to 20%. A similar result was seen for gender, with a higher C_{max} and AUC in women after single doses but no difference after multiple doses.

Initiate treatment with nefazodone initiated at half the usual dose in elderly patients, especially women; however, the therapeutic dose range is similar in younger and older patients.

Contraindications

Coadministration of terfenadine, astemizole, cisapride, pimozide, or carbamazepine with nefazodone is contraindicated.

Nefazodone tablets are contraindicated in patients withdrawn from nefazodone because of evidence of liver injury. Nefazodone tablets are also contraindicated in patients who have demonstrated hypersensitivity to nefazodone, its inactive ingredients, or other phenylpiperazine antidepressants.

The coadministration of triazolam and nefazodone causes a significant increase in the plasma level of triazolam; a 75% reduction in the initial triazolam dosage is recommended if the 2 drugs are to be given together. Because not all commercially available dosage forms of triazolam permit a sufficient dosage reduction, the coadministration of triazolam and nefazodone should be avoided for most patients, including the elderly.

Warnings/Precautions

➤*Hepatotoxicity:* See the Warning box for more information.

The time to liver injury for the reported liver failure cases resulting in death or transplant generally ranged from 2 weeks to 6 months on nefazodone therapy. Although some reports described dark urine and nonspecific prodromal symptoms (eg, anorexia, malaise, GI symptoms), other reports did not describe the onset of clear prodromal symptoms prior to the onset of jaundice.

Consider the value of liver function testing. Periodic serum transaminase testing has not been proven to prevent serious injury, but it is generally believed that early detection of drug-induced hepatic injury along with immediate withdrawal of the suspect drug enhances the likelihood for recovery.

Advise patients to be alert for signs and symptoms of liver dysfunction (jaundice, anorexia, GI complaints, malaise) and to report them to their health care provider immediately if they occur. Ongoing clinical assessment of patients should govern physician interventions, including diagnostic evaluations and treatment.

➤*Potential for interaction with MAOIs:* In patients receiving antidepressants with pharmacological properties similar to nefazodone in combination with a MAOI, there have been reports of serious, sometimes fatal, reactions. For an SSRI, these reactions have included hyperthermia, rigidity, myoclonus, autonomic instability with possible rapid fluctuations of vital signs, and mental status changes that include extreme agitation progressing to delirium and coma. These reactions have also been reported in patients who have recently discontinued that drug and have been started on an MAOI. Some cases presented with features resembling neuroleptic malignant syndrome. Severe hyperthermia and seizures, sometimes fatal, have been reported in association with the combined use of tricyclic antidepressants and MAOIs. These reactions have also been reported in patients who have recently discontinued these drugs and have been started on an MAOI.

Although the effects of combined use of nefazodone and MAOIs have not been evaluated in humans or animals, because nefazodone is an inhibitor of both serotonin and norepinephrine reuptake, do not use nefazodone in combination with an MAOI, or within 14 days of discontinuing treatment with an MAOI. Allow at least 1 week after stopping nefazodone before starting an MAOI.

➤*Interaction with triazolobenzodiazepines:* Interaction studies of nefazodone with 2 triazolobenzodiazepines (ie, triazolam and alprazolam) metabolized by cytochrome P450 3A4, have revealed substantial and clinically important increases in plasma concentrations of these compounds when administered concomitantly with nefazodone.

Triazolam – See Drug Interactions for more information.

Alprazolam – See Drug Interactions for more information.

➤*Electroconvulsive therapy (ECT):* There are no clinical studies of the combined use of ECT and nefazodone.

➤*Postural hypotension:* A pooled analysis of the vital signs monitored during placebo-controlled premarketing studies revealed that 5.1% of nefazodone patients compared with 2.5% of placebo patients ($P \le 0.01$) met criteria for a potentially important decrease in blood pressure at some time during treatment (systolic blood pressure less than or equal to 90 mm Hg and a change from baseline of greater than or equal to 20 mm Hg). While there was no difference in the proportion of nefazodone and placebo patients having adverse reactions characterized as "syncope" (nefazodone, 0.2%; placebo, 0.3%), the rates for adverse reactions characterized as "postural hypotension" were as follows: nefazodone (2.8%), tricyclic antidepressants (10.9%), SSRIs (1.1%), and placebo (0.8%). Thus, the prescriber should be aware that there is some risk of postural hypotension in association with nefazodone use. Use nefazodone with caution in patients with known cardiovascular or cerebrovascular disease that could be exacerbated by hypotension (history of myocardial infarction [MI], angina, or ischemic stroke) and conditions that would predispose patients to hypotension (dehydration, hypovolemia, and treatment with antihypertensive medication).

➤*Activation of mania/hypomania:* During premarketing testing, hypomania or mania occurred in 0.3% of nefazodone-treated unipolar patients, compared with 0.3% of tricyclic- and 0.4% of placebo-treated patients. In

NEFAZODONE HYDROCHLORIDE — ORAL

patients classified as bipolar the rate of manic episodes was 1.6% for nefazodone, 5.1% for the combined tricyclic-treated groups, and 0% for placebo-treated patients. Activation of mania/hypomania is a known risk in a small proportion of patients with major affective disorder treated with other marketed antidepressants. As with all antidepressants, use nefazodone cautiously in patients with a history of mania.

➤*Suicide:* The possibility of a suicide attempt is inherent in depression and may persist until significant remission occurs. Closely supervise high-risk patients during initial drug therapy. Write prescriptions for nefazodone for the smallest quantity of tablets consistent with good patient management in order to reduce the risk of overdose.

➤*Seizures:* During premarketing testing, a recurrence of a petit mal seizure was observed in a patient receiving nefazodone who had a history of such seizures. One nonstudy participant took 2,000 to 3,000 mg nefazodone with methocarbamol and alcohol; this person reportedly experienced a convulsion (type not documented). Neither of these patients died. Rare occurrences of convulsions (including grand mal seizures) following nefazodone administration have been reported since market introduction. A causal relationship to nefazodone has not been established.

➤*Priapism:* While priapism did not occur during premarketing experience with nefazodone, rare reports of priapism have been received since market introduction. A causal relationship to nefazodone has not been established. If patients present with prolonged or inappropriate erections, they should discontinue therapy immediately and consult their health care providers. If the condition persists for more than 24 hours, consult a urologist to determine appropriate management.

➤*Use in patients with concomitant illness:* Nefazodone has not been evaluated or used to any appreciable extent in patients with a history of MI or unstable heart disease. Patients with these diagnoses were systematically excluded from clinical studies during the product's premarketing testing. Evaluation of electrocardiograms of 1,153 patients who received nefazodone in 6- to 8-week, double-blind, placebo-controlled trials did not indicate that nefazodone is associated with the development of clinically important ECG abnormalities. However, sinus bradycardia, defined as heart rate less than or equal to 50 bpm and a decrease of at least 15 bpm from baseline, was observed in 1.5% of nefazodone-treated patients compared with 0.4% of placebo-treated patients ($P \le 0.05$). Because patients with a history of MI or unstable heart disease were excluded from clinical trials, treat such patients with caution.

In patients with cirrhosis of the liver, the AUC values of nefazodone and HO-NEF were increased by approximately 25%.

➤*Hazardous tasks:* Since any psychoactive drug may impair judgment, thinking, or motor skills, caution patients about operating hazardous machinery, including automobiles, until they are reasonably certain that nefazodone therapy does not adversely affect their ability to engage in such activities.

➤*Pregnancy: Category C.*

Teratogenic – Reproduction studies have been performed in pregnant rabbits and rats at daily doses up to 200 and 300 mg/kg, respectively (approximately 6 and 5 times, respectively, the maximum human daily dose on a mg/m^2 basis). No malformations were observed in the offspring as a result of nefazodone treatment. However, increased early pup mortality was seen in rats at a dose approximately 5 times the maximum human dose, and decreased pup weights were seen at this and lower doses, when dosing began during pregnancy and continued until weaning. The cause of these deaths is not known. The no-effect dose for rat pup mortality was 1.3 times the human dose on a mg/m^2 basis. There are no adequate and well-controlled studies in pregnant women. Use nefazodone during pregnancy only if the potential benefit justifies the potential risk to the fetus.

Labor and delivery – The effect of nefazodone on labor and delivery in humans is unknown.

➤*Lactation:* It is not known whether nefazodone or its metabolites are excreted in human milk. Because many drugs are excreted in human milk, exercise caution when nefazodone is administered to a nursing woman.

➤*Children:* Safety and efficacy in individuals younger than 18 years of age have not been established.

➤*Elderly:* Of the approximately 7,000 patients in clinical studies who received nefazodone for the treatment of depression, 18% were 65 years of age or older, while 5% were 75 years of age or older. Based on monitoring of adverse reactions, vital signs, electrocardiograms, and results of laboratory tests, no overall differences in safety between elderly and younger patients were observed in clinical studies. Efficacy in the elderly has not been demonstrated in placebo-controlled trials. Other reported clinical experience has not identified differences in responses between elderly and younger patients, but greater sensitivity of some older individuals cannot be ruled out.

Due to the increased systemic exposure to nefazodone seen in single-dose studies in elderly patients, initiate treatment at half the usual dose; titration upward should take place over the same range as in younger patients. Observe the usual precautions in elderly patients who have concomitant medical illnesses or who are receiving concomitant drugs.

Drug Interactions

➤*CYP450 system:* Terfenadine, astemizole, cisapride, and pimozide are all metabolized by the cytochrome P450 3A4 (CYP3A4) isozyme, and it has been demonstrated that ketoconazole, erythromycin, and other inhibitors of CYP3A4 can block the metabolism of these drugs, which can result in increased plasma concentrations of parent drug. Increased plasma concentrations of terfenadine, astemizole, cisapride, and pimozide are associated with QT prolongation and with rare cases of serious cardiovascular adverse reactions, including death, principally caused by ventricular tachycardia of the torsades de pointes type. Nefazodone has been shown in vitro to be an inhibitor of CYP3A4. Consequently, do not use nefazodone not be used in combination with either terfenadine, astemizole, cisapride, or pimozide.

➤*Drugs highly bound to plasma protein:* Because nefazodone is highly bound to plasma protein, administration of nefazodone to a patient taking another drug that is highly protein bound may cause increased free concentrations of the other drug, potentially resulting in adverse reactions. Conversely, adverse reactions could result from displacement of nefazodone by other highly bound drugs.

➤*CNS-active drugs:*

MAOIs –

Potential for interaction with MAOIs: In patients receiving antidepressants with pharmacological properties similar to nefazodone in combination with an MAOI, there have been reports of serious, sometimes fatal, reactions. For an SSRI, these reactions have included hyperthermia, rigidity, myoclonus, autonomic instability with possible rapid fluctuations of vital signs, and mental status changes that include extreme agitation progressing to delirium and coma. These reactions have also been reported in patients who have recently discontinued that drug and have been started on an MAOI. Some cases presented with features resembling neuroleptic malignant syndrome. Severe hyperthermia and seizures, sometimes fatal, have been reported in association with the combined use of tricyclic antidepressants and MAOIs. These reactions have also been reported in patients who have recently discontinued these drugs and have been started on an MAOI.

Although the effects of combined use of nefazodone and MAOI have not been evaluated in humans or animals, because nefazodone is an inhibitor of both serotonin and norepinephrine reuptake, do not use nefazodone in combination with an MAOI, or within 14 days of discontinuing treatment with an MAOI. Allow at least 1 week after stopping nefazodone before starting an MAOI.

Haloperidol – When a single oral dose of 5 mg haloperidol was coadministered with twice daily 200 mg nefazodone at steady state, haloperidol apparent clearance decreased by 35% with no significant increase in peak haloperidol plasma concentrations or time of peak. This change is of unknown clinical significance. Pharmacodynamic effects of haloperidol were generally not altered significantly. There were no changes in the pharmacokinetic parameters for nefazodone. Dosage adjustment of haloperidol may be necessary when coadministered with nefazodone.

Triazolam/alprazolam –

Triazolam: When a single oral dose of 0.25 mg triazolam was coadministered with twice daily 200 mg nefazodone at steady state, triazolam half-life and AUC increased 4-fold and peak concentrations increased 1.7-fold. Nefazodone plasma concentrations were unaffected by triazolam. Coadministration of nefazodone potentiated the effects of triazolam on psychomotor performance tests. If triazolam is coadministered with nefazodone, a 75% reduction in the initial triazolam dosage is recommended. Because not all commercially available dosage forms of triazolam permit sufficient dosage reduction, avoid coadministration of triazolam with nefazodone for most patients, including the elderly. In the exceptional case where coadministration of triazolam with nefazodone may be considered appropriate, use only the lowest possible dose of triazolam.

Alprazolam: When 1 mg alprazolam and 200 mg nefazodone were coadministered twice daily, steady-state peak concentrations, AUC and half-life values for alprazolam increased by approximately 2-fold. Nefazodone plasma concentrations were unaffected by alprazolam. If alprazolam is coadministered with nefazodone, reduce the initial alprazolam dosage by 50%. No dosage adjustment is required for nefazodone.

Alcohol – Although nefazodone did not potentiate the cognitive and psychomotor effects of alcohol in experiments with healthy subjects, the concomitant use of nefazodone and alcohol in depressed patients is not advised.

Buspirone – In a study of steady-state pharmacokinetics in healthy volunteers, twice daily coadministration of 2.5 or 5 mg buspirone with 250 mg nefazodone resulted in marked increases in plasma buspirone concentrations (increases up to 20-fold in C_{max} and up to 50-fold in AUC) and statistically significant decreases (about 50%) in plasma concentrations of the buspirone metabolite 1-pyrimidinylpiperazine. With twice-daily doses of 5 mg buspirone, slight increases in AUC were observed for nefazodone (23%) and its metabolites hydroxynefazodone (17%) and mCPP (9%). Subjects receiving 250 mg nefazodone twice daily and 5 mg buspirone twice daily experienced light-headedness, asthenia, dizziness, and somnolence, adverse reactions also observed with either drug alone. If the 2 drugs are to be used in combination, a low dose of buspirone (eg, 2.5 mg daily) is recommended. Base subsequent dose adjustment of either drug clinical assessment.

Fluoxetine – When 20 mg fluoxetine once daily and 200 mg nefazodone twice daily were administered at steady state, there were no changes in the pharmacokinetic parameters for fluoxetine or its metabolite, norfluoxetine. Similarly, there were no changes in the pharmacokinetic parameters of nefazodone or HO-NEF; however, the mean AUC levels of the nefazodone metabolites mCPP and triazole-dione increased by 3- to 6-fold and 1.3-fold, respectively. When a 200 mg nefazodone dose was administered to subjects who had been receiving fluoxetine for 1 week, there was an increased incidence of transient adverse events such as headache, light-headedness, nausea, or paresthesia, possibly due to the elevated mCPP levels. Patients who are switched from fluoxetine to nefazodone without an adequate washout period may experience similar transient adverse events. The possibility of this happening can be minimized by allowing a washout period before initiating nefazodone therapy and by reducing the initial dose of nefazodone. Because of the long half-life of fluoxetine and its metabolites, this washout period may range from 1 to several weeks depending on the dose of fluoxetine and other individual patient variables.

NEFAZODONE HYDROCHLORIDE — ORAL

Desipramine – When 150 mg nefazodone twice daily and 75 mg desipramine once daily were administered together, there were no changes in the pharmacokinetics of desipramine or its metabolite, 2-hydroxy desipramine. There were also no changes in the pharmacokinetics of nefazodone or its triazole-dione metabolite, but the AUC and C_{max} of mCPP increased by 44% and 48%, respectively, while the AUC of HO-NEF decreased by 19%. No changes in doses of either nefazodone or desipramine are necessary when the 2 drugs are given concomitantly. Subsequent dose adjustments should be made on the basis of clinical response.

Carbamazepine – The coadministration of 200 mg nefazodone twice daily for 5 days to 12 healthy subjects on carbamazepine who had achieved steady state (200 mg twice daily) was found to be well-tolerated. Steady-state conditions for carbamazepine, nefazodone, and several of their metabolites were achieved by day 5 of coadministration. With coadministration of the 2 drugs there were significant increases in the steady-state C_{max} and AUC of carbamazepine (23% and 23%, respectively), while the steady-state C_{max} and the AUC of the carbamazepine metabolite, 10,11 epoxycarbamazepine, decreased by 21% and 20%, respectively. The coadministration of the 2 drugs significantly reduced the steady-state C_{max} and AUC of nefazodone by 86% and 93%, respectively. Similar reductions in the C_{max} and AUC of HO-NEF were also observed (85% and 94%), while the reductions in C_{max} and AUC of mCPP and triazole-dione were more modest (13% and 44% for the former and 28% and 57% for the latter). Due to the potential for coadministration of carbamazepine to result in insufficient plasma nefazodone and hydroxynefazodone concentrations for achieving an antidepressant effect for nefazodone, it is recommended that nefazodone not be used in combination with carbamazepine.

General anesthetics – Little is known about the potential for interaction between nefazodone and general anesthetics; therefore, prior to elective surgery, discontinue nefazodone for as long as clinically feasible.

➤*Cardiovascularly active drugs:*

Digoxin – When 200 mg nefazodone twice daily and 0.2 mg digoxin once daily were coadministered for 9 days to healthy male volunteers (n = 18) who were phenotyped as CYP2D6 extensive metabolizers, C_{max}, C_{min}, and AUC of digoxin were increased by 29%, 27%, and 15%, respectively. Digoxin had no effects on the pharmacokinetics of nefazodone and its active metabolites. Because of the narrow therapeutic index of digoxin, exercise caution when nefazodone and digoxin are coadministered; plasma level monitoring for digoxin is recommended.

Propranolol – The coadministration of 200 mg nefazodone twice daily and 40 mg propranolol twice daily for 5.5 days to healthy male volunteers (n = 18), including 3 poor and 15 extensive CYP2D6 metabolizers, resulted in 30% and 14% reductions in C_{max} and AUC of propranolol, respectively, and a 14% reduction in C_{max} for the metabolite, 4-hydroxypropranolol. The kinetics of nefazodone, hydroxynefazodone, and triazole-dione were not affected by coadministration of propranolol. However, C_{max}, C_{min}, and AUC of m-chlorophenylpiperazine were increased by 23%, 54%, and 28%, respectively. No change in initial dose of either drug is necessary; make dose adjustments on the basis of clinical response.

HMG-CoA reductase inhibitors – When single 40 mg doses of simvastatin or atorvastatin, both substrates of CYP3A4, were given to healthy adult volunteers who had received 200 mg nefazodone twice daily for 6 days, approximately 20-fold increases in plasma concentrations of simvastatin and simvastatin acid and 3- to 4-fold increases in plasma concentrations of atorvastatin and atorvastatin lactone were seen. These effects appear to be due to the inhibition of CYP3A4 by nefazodone because, in the same study, nefazodone had no significant effect on the plasma concentrations of pravastatin, which is not metabolized by CYP3A4 to a clinically significant extent.

There have been rare reports of rhabdomyolysis involving patients receiving the combination of nefazodone and either simvastatin or lovastatin, also a substrate of CYP3A4. Rhabdomyolysis has been observed in patients receiving HMG-CoA reductase inhibitors administered alone (at recommended dosages) and in particular, for certain drugs in this class, when given in combination with inhibitors of the CYP3A4 isozyme.

Use caution if nefazodone is administered in combination with HMG-CoA reductase inhibitors that are metabolized by CYP3A4, such as simvastatin, atorvastatin, and lovastatin, and dosage adjustments of these HMG-CoA reductase inhibitors are recommended. Since metabolic interactions are unlikely between nefazodone and HMG-CoA reductase inhibitors that undergo little or no metabolism by the CYP3A4 isozyme, such as pravastatin or fluvastatin, dosage adjustments should not be necessary.

➤*Immunosuppressive agents:* There have been reports of increased blood concentrations of cyclosporine and tacrolimus into toxic ranges when patients received these drugs concomitantly with nefazodone. Both cyclosporine and tacrolimus are substrates of CYP3A4, and nefazodone is known to inhibit this enzyme. If either cyclosporine or tacrolimus is administered with nefazodone, blood concentrations of the immunosuppressive agent should be monitored and dosage adjusted accordingly.

➤*Pharmacokinetics of nefazodone in "poor metabolizers" and potential interaction with drugs that inhibit or are metabolized by cytochrome P450 isozymes:*

CYP3A4 isozyme – Nefazodone has been shown in vitro to be an inhibitor of CYP3A4. This is consistent with the interactions observed between nefazodone and triazolam, alprazolam, buspirone, atorvastatin, and simvastatin, drugs metabolized by this isozyme. Consequently, caution is indicated in the combined use of nefazodone with any drugs known to be metabolized by CYP3A4. In particular, avoid the combined use of nefazodone with triazolam for most patients, including the elderly. The combined use of nefazodone with terfenadine, astemizole, cisapride, or pimozide is contraindicated.

CYP2D6 isozyme – A subset (3% to 10%) of the population has reduced activity of the drug-metabolizing enzyme CYP2D6. Such individuals are referred to commonly as "poor metabolizers" of drugs such as debrisoquin, dextromethorphan, and the tricyclic antidepressants. The pharmacokinetics of nefazodone and its major metabolites are not altered in these "poor metabolizers." Plasma concentrations of 1 minor metabolite (mCPP) are increased in this population; the adjustment of nefazodone dosage is not required when administered to "poor metabolizers." Nefazodone and its metabolites have been shown in vitro to be extremely weak inhibitors of CYP2D6. Thus, it is not likely that nefazodone will decrease the metabolic clearance of drugs metabolized by this isozyme.

CYP1A2 isozyme – Nefazodone and its metabolites have been shown in vitro not to inhibit CYP1A2. Thus, metabolic interactions between nefazodone and drugs metabolized by this isozyme are unlikely.

Adverse Reactions

➤*Associated with discontinuation of treatment:* Approximately 16% of the 3,496 patients who received nefazodone in worldwide premarketing clinical trials discontinued treatment due to an adverse reaction. The more common (greater than or equal to 1%) reactions in clinical trials associated with discontinuation and considered to be drug related (ie, those reactions associated with dropout at a rate approximately twice or greater for nefazodone compared with placebo) included the following: nausea (3.5%), dizziness (1.9%), insomnia (1.5%), asthenia (1.3%), and agitation (1.2%).

➤*Commonly observed adverse reactions in controlled clinical trials:* The most commonly observed adverse reactions associated with the use of nefazodone (incidence of greater than or equal to 5%) and not seen at an equivalent incidence among placebo-treated patients (ie, significantly higher incidence for nefazodone compared with placebo, $P \le 0.05$), derived from the following table, were the following: somnolence, dry mouth, nausea, dizziness, constipation, asthenia, light-headedness, blurred vision, confusion, and abnormal vision.

Adverse reactions occurring at an incidence of 1% or more among nefazodone-treated patients – The table that follows enumerates adverse reactions that occurred at an incidence of greater than or equal to 1%, and were more frequent than in the placebo group, among nefazodone-treated patients who participated in short-term (6- to 8-week) placebo-controlled trials in which patients were dosed with nefazodone to ranges of 300 to 600 mg/day. This table shows the percentage of patients in each group who had at least 1 episode of a reaction at some time during their treatment. Reported adverse reactions were classified using standard Coding Symbols for a Thesaurus of Adverse Reaction Terms (COSTART)-based dictionary terminology.

Nefazodone Adverse Reactions[a]

Body system	Preferred term	Nefazodone (n = 393)	Placebo (n = 394)
Cardiovascular	Hypotension	2%	1%
	Postural hypotension	4%	1%
CNS	Abnormal dreams	3%	2%
	Ataxia	2%	0%
	Concentration decreased	3%	1%
	Confusion	7%	2%
	Dizziness	17%	5%
	Hypertonia	1%	0%
	Incoordination	2%	1%
	Insomnia	11%	9%
	Libido decreased	1%	< 1%
	Light-headedness	10%	3%
	Memory impairment	4%	2%
	Paresthesia	4%	2%
	Psychomotor retardation	2%	1%
	Somnolence	25%	14%
	Tremor	2%	1%
	Vasodilatation[b]	4%	2%
Dermatologic	Pruritus	2%	1%
	Rash	2%	1%
GI	Constipation	14%	8%
	Diarrhea	8%	7%
	Dry mouth	25%	13%
	Dyspepsia	9%	7%
	Increased appetite	5%	3%
	Nausea	22%	12%
	Nausea/vomiting	2%	1%

NEFAZODONE HYDROCHLORIDE — ORAL

Nefazodone Adverse Reactions[a]

Body system	Preferred term	Nefazodone (n = 393)	Placebo (n = 394)
GU	Breast pain[d]	1%	< 1%
	Urinary frequency	2%	1%
	Urinary retention	2%	1%
	Urinary tract infection	2%	1%
	Vaginitis[d]	2%	1%
Metabolic	Peripheral edema	3%	2%
	Thirst	1%	< 1%
Musculoskeletal	Arthralgia	1%	< 1%
Respiratory	Cough increased	3%	1%
	Pharyngitis	6%	5%
Special senses	Abnormal vision[c]	7%	1%
	Blurred vision	9%	3%
	Taste perversion	2%	1%
	Tinnitus	2%	1%
	Visual field defect	2%	0%
Miscellaneous	Asthenia	11%	5%
	Chills	2%	1%
	Fever	2%	1%
	Flu syndrome	3%	2%
	Headache	36%	33%
	Infection	8%	6%
	Neck rigidity	1%	0%

[a] Reactions reported by at least 1% of patients treated with nefazodone and more frequent than the placebo group are included; incidence is rounded to the nearest 1% (< 1% indicates an incidence less than 0.5%). Reactions for which the nefazodone incidence was equal to or less than placebo are not listed in the table, but included the following: abdominal pain, pain, back pain, accidental injury, chest pain, neck pain, palpitation, migraine, sweating, flatulence, vomiting, anorexia, tooth disorder, weight gain, edema, myalgia, cramp, agitation, anxiety, depression, hypesthesia, CNS stimulation, dysphoria, emotional lability, sinusitis, rhinitis, dysmenorrhea, dysuria.

[b] Vasodilatation (flushing, feeling warm).

[c] Abnormal vision (scotoma, visual trails).

[d] Incidence adjusted for gender.

➤*Dose dependency of adverse reactions:* The table that follows enumerates adverse reactions that were more frequent in the nefazodone dosage range of 300 to 600 mg/day than in the nefazodone dosage range of up to 300 mg/day. This table shows only those adverse reactions for which there was a statistically significant difference ($P \le 0.05$) in incidence between the nefazodone dose ranges as well as a difference between the high dose range and placebo.

Nefazodone Dose Dependency of Adverse Reactions in Placebo-Controlled Trials[a]

Body system	Preferred term	Nefazodone 300 to 600 mg/day (n = 209)	Nefazodone ≤ 300 mg/day (n = 211)	Placebo (n = 212)
CNS	Confusion	8%	2%	1%
	Dizziness	22%	11%	4%
	Somnolence	28%	16%	13%
GI	Constipation	17%	10%	9%
	Nausea	23%	14%	12%
Special senses	Abnormal vision	10%	0%	2%
	Blurred vision	9%	3%	2%
	Tinnitus	3%	0%	1%

[a] Reactions for which there was a statistically significant difference ($P \le 0.05$) between the nefazodone dose groups.

➤*Visual disturbances:* In controlled clinical trials, blurred vision occurred in 9% of nefazodone-treated patients compared with 3% of placebo-treated patients. In these same trials, abnormal vision, including scotomata and visual trails, occurred in 7% of nefazodone-treated patients compared with 1% of placebo-treated (see the preceding table). Dose dependency was observed for these reactions in these trials, with none of the scotomata and visual trails at doses below 300 mg/day. However, scotomata and visual trails observed at dosages less than 300 mg/day have been reported in postmarketing experience with nefazodone.

➤*Vital sign changes:*

Postural hypotension – See Warnings/Precautions for more information.

➤*Weight changes:* In a pooled analysis of placebo-controlled premarketing studies, there were no differences between nefazodone and placebo groups in the proportions of patients meeting criteria for potentially important increases or decreases in body weight (a change of greater than or equal to 7%).

➤*Laboratory changes:* Of the serum chemistry, serum hematology, and urinalysis parameters monitored during placebo-controlled premarketing studies with nefazodone, a pooled analysis revealed a statistical trend between nefazodone and placebo for hematocrit (ie, 2.8% of nefazodone patients met criteria for a potentially important decrease in hematocrit [less than or equal to 37% in men or less than or equal to 32% in women]) compared with 1.5% of placebo patients (0.05 less than $P \le 0.1$). Decreases in hematocrit, presumably dilutional, have been reported with many other drugs that block alpha-1-adrenergic receptors. There was no apparent clinical significance of the observed changes in the few patients meeting these criteria.

➤*ECG changes:* Of the ECG parameters monitored during placebo-controlled premarketing studies with nefazodone, a pooled analysis revealed a statistically significant difference between nefazodone and placebo for sinus bradycardia (ie, 1.5% of nefazodone patients met criteria for a potentially important decrease in heart rate [less than or equal to 50 bpm and a decrease of greater than or equal to 15 bpm]) compared with 0.4% of placebo patients (*P*

➤*Other reactions observed during the premarketing evaluation of nefazodone:* During its premarketing assessment, multiple doses of nefazodone were administered to 3,496 patients in clinical studies, including more than 250 patients treated for at least 1 year. The conditions and duration of exposure to nefazodone varied greatly, and included (in overlapping categories) open and double-blind studies, uncontrolled and controlled studies, inpatient and outpatient studies, fixed-dose and titration studies. Untoward reactions associated with this exposure were recorded by clinical investigators using terminology of their own choosing. Consequently, it is not possible to provide a meaningful estimate of the proportion of individuals experiencing adverse reactions without first grouping similar types of untoward reactions into a smaller number of standardized reaction categories.

Reactions are further categorized by body system and listed in order of decreasing frequency according to the following definitions: frequent adverse reactions are those occurring on 1 or more occasions in at least 1 of 100 patients (only those not already listed in the tabulated results from placebo-controlled trials appear in this listing); infrequent adverse reactions are those occurring in 1 of 100 to 1 of 1,000 patients; rare reactions are those occurring in less than 1 of 1,000 patients.

Cardiovascular –

Infrequent: Tachycardia, hypertension, syncope, ventricular extrasystoles, and angina pectoris.

Rare: AV block, congestive heart failure, hemorrhage, pallor, and varicose vein.

CNS –

Infrequent: Vertigo, twitching, depersonalization, hallucinations, suicide attempt, apathy, euphoria, hostility, suicidal thoughts, abnormal gait, thinking abnormal, attention decreased, derealization, neuralgia, paranoid reaction, dysarthria, increased libido, suicide, and myoclonus.

Rare: Hyperkinesia, increased salivation, cerebrovascular accident, hyperesthesia, hypotonia, ptosis, and neuroleptic malignant syndrome.

Dermatologic –

Infrequent: Dry skin, acne, alopecia, urticaria, maculopapular rash, vesiculobullous rash, and eczema.

GI –

Frequent: Gastroenteritis.

Infrequent: Eructation, periodontal abscess, abnormal liver function tests, gingivitis, colitis, gastritis, mouth ulceration, stomatitis, esophagitis, peptic ulcer, and rectal hemorrhage.

Rare: Glossitis, hepatitis, dysphagia, GI hemorrhage, oral moniliasis, and ulcerative colitis.

GU –

Frequent: Impotence.

Infrequent: Cystitis, urinary urgency, metrorrhagia, amenorrhea, polyuria, vaginal hemorrhage, breast enlargement, menorrhagia, urinary incontinence, abnormal ejaculation, hematuria, nocturia, and kidney calculus.

Rare: Uterine fibroids enlarged, uterine hemorrhage, anorgasmia, and oliguria.

Hematologic/Lymphatic –

Infrequent: Ecchymosis, anemia, leukopenia, and lymphadenopathy.

Metabolic/Nutritional –

Infrequent: Weight loss, gout, dehydration, lactic dehydrogenase increased, AST increased, and ALT increased.

Rare: Hypercholesteremia and hypoglycemia.

Musculoskeletal –

Infrequent: Arthritis, tenosynovitis, muscle stiffness, and bursitis.

Rare: Tendinous contracture.

Respiratory –

Frequent: Dyspnea and bronchitis.

Infrequent: Asthma, pneumonia, laryngitis, voice alteration, epistaxis, hiccup.

Rare: Hyperventilation and yawn.

Special senses –

Frequent: Eye pain.

Infrequent: Dry eye, ear pain, abnormality of accommodation, diplopia, conjunctivitis, mydriasis, keratoconjunctivitis, hyperacusis, and photophobia.

Rare: Deafness, glaucoma, night blindness, and taste loss.

NEFAZODONE HYDROCHLORIDE — ORAL

Miscellaneous –

Infrequent: Allergic reaction, malaise, photosensitivity reaction, face edema, hangover effect, abdomen enlarged, hernia, pelvic pain, and halitosis.

Rare: Cellulitis.

➤*Postmarketing:* Postmarketing experience with nefazodone has shown an adverse reaction profile similar to that seen during the premarketing evaluation of nefazodone. Voluntary reports of adverse reactions temporally associated with nefazodone have been received since market introduction that are not listed above and for which a causal relationship has not been established. These include the following:

Hypersensitivity – Anaphylactic reactions; angioedema; convulsions (including grand mal seizures); galactorrhea; gynecomastia (men); hyponatremia; liver necrosis and liver failure, in some cases leading to liver transplantation or death; priapism; prolactin increased; rhabdomyolysis involving patients receiving the combination of nefazodone and lovastatin or simvastatin; serotonin syndrome; Stevens-Johnson syndrome; and thrombocytopenia.

Overdosage

➤*Symptoms:*

Human experience – In premarketing clinical studies, there were 7 reports of nefazodone overdose alone or in combination with other pharmacological agents. The amount of nefazodone ingested ranged from 1,000 mg to 11,200 mg. Commonly reported symptoms from overdose of nefazodone included nausea, vomiting, and somnolence. One nonstudy participant took 2,000 to 3,000 mg nefazodone with methocarbamol and alcohol; this person reportedly experienced a convulsion (type not documented). None of these patients died. In postmarketing experience, overdose with nefazodone alone and in combination with alcohol or other substances has been reported. Commonly reported symptoms were similar to those reported from overdose in premarketing experience. While there have been rare reports of fatalities in patients taking overdoses of nefazodone, predominantly in combination with alcohol or other substances, no causal relationship to nefazodone has been established.

➤*Treatment:* Treatment should consist of those general measures employed in the management of overdosage with any antidepressant.

Ensure an adequate airway, oxygenation, and ventilation. Monitor cardiac rhythm and vital signs. General supportive and symptomatic measures are also recommended. Induction of emesis is not recommended. Gastric lavage with a large-bore orogastric tube with appropriate airway protection, if needed, may be indicated if performed soon after ingestion, or in symptomatic patients.

Administer activated charcoal. Due to the wide distribution of nefazodone in body tissues, forced diuresis, dialysis, hemoperfusion, and exchange transfusion are unlikely to be of benefit. No specific antidotes for nefazodone are known.

In managing overdosage, consider the possibility of multiple drug involvement. Consider contacting a poison control center for additional information on the treatment of any overdose.

Patient Information

Discuss the following issues with nefazodone-treated patients:

➤*Hepatotoxicity:* Patients should be informed that nefazodone therapy has been associated with liver abnormalities ranging from asymptomatic reversible serum transaminase increases to cases of liver failure resulting in transplant or death. At present, there is no way to predict who is likely to develop liver failure. Ordinarily, patients with active liver disease should not be treated with nefazodone. Advise patients to be alert for signs of liver dysfunction (eg, jaundice, anorexia, GI complaints, malaise) and to report them to their health care provider immediately if they occur.

➤*Time to response/continuation:* As with all antidepressants, several weeks on treatment may be required to obtain the full antidepressant effect. Once improvement is noted, it is important for patients to continue drug treatment as directed by their health care provider.

➤*Interference with cognitive and motor performance:* Since any psychoactive drug may impair judgment, thinking, or motor skills, caution patients about operating hazardous machinery, including automobiles, until they are reasonably certain that nefazodone therapy does not adversely affect their ability to engage in such activities.

➤*Pregnancy:* Advise patients to notify their health care provider if they become pregnant or intend to become pregnant during therapy. Reproduction studies have been performed in pregnant rabbits and rats at daily doses up to 200 and 300 mg/kg, respectively (approximately 6 and 5 times, respectively, the maximum human daily dose on a mg/m^2 basis). No malformations were observed in the offspring as a result of nefazodone treatment. However, increased early pup mortality was seen in rats at a dose approximately 5 times the maximum human dose, and decreased pup weights were seen at this and lower doses, when dosing began during pregnancy and continued until weaning. The cause of these deaths is not known. The no-effect dose for rat pup mortality was 1.3 times the human dose on a mg/m^2 basis. There are no adequate and well-controlled studies in pregnant women. Use nefazodone during pregnancy only if the potential benefit justifies the potential risk to the fetus.

➤*Nursing:* Advise patients to notify their health care provider if they are breastfeeding an infant. It is not known whether nefazodone or its metabolites are excreted in human milk. Because many drugs are excreted in human milk, exercise caution when nefazodone is administered to a nursing woman.

➤*Concomitant medication:* Advise patients to inform their health care providers if they are taking, or plan to take, any prescription or over-the-counter drugs, since there is a potential for interactions. Significant caution is indicated if nefazodone is to be used in combination with alprazolam; concomitant use with triazolam should be avoided for most patients, including the elderly; and concomitant use with terfenadine (not available in the US), astemizole (not available in the US), cisapride, pimozide, or carbamazepine is contraindicated.

➤*Alcohol:* Advise patients to avoid alcohol while taking nefazodone.

➤*Allergic reactions:* Advise patients to notify their health care provider if they develop a rash, hives, or a related allergic phenomenon.

➤*Visual disturbances:* There have been reports of visual disturbances associated with the use of nefazodone, including blurred vision, scotoma, and visual trails. Advise patients to notify their healthcare provider if they develop visual disturbances. In controlled clinical trials, blurred vision occurred in 9% of nefazodone-treated patients compared to 3% of placebo-treated patients. In these same trials, abnormal vision, including scotomata and visual trails, occurred in 7% of nefazodone-treated patients compared with 1% of placebo-treated patients. Dose dependency was observed for these reactions in these trials, with none of the scotomata and visual trails at dosages below 300 mg/day. However, scotomata and visual trails observed at dosages below 300 mg/day have been reported in postmarketing experience with nefazodone.

Serotonin and Norepinephrine Reuptake Inhibitors

DULOXETINE

Rx	**Cymbalta** (Eli Lilly)	**Capsules, delayed-release**[a]**; oral:** 20 mg	Equiv. to duloxetine hydrochloride 22.4 mg. Sucrose, sugar spheres. (Lilly 3235 20 mg). Opaque green. In 60s.
		30 mg	Equiv. to duloxetine hydrochloride 33.7 mg. Sucrose, sugar spheres. (Lilly 3240 30 mg). Opaque white and blue. In 30s, 90s, 1,000s, and UD 100s.
		60 mg	Equiv. to duloxetine hydrochloride 67.3 mg. Sucrose, sugar spheres. (Lilly 3270 60 mg). Opaque green and blue. In 30s, 1,000s, and UD 100s.

[a] Contains enteric-coated pellets.

DULOXETINE HYDROCHLORIDE — ORAL

For complete and comparative prescribing information, refer to the Antidepressants class monograph.

WARNING

Suicidality and antidepressant drugs – Antidepressants increased the risk compared with placebo of suicidal thinking and behavior (suicidality) in children, adolescents, and young adults in short-term studies of major depressive disorder (MDD) and other psychiatric disorders. Anyone considering the use of duloxetine or any other antidepressant in a child, adolescent, or young adult must balance this risk with the clinical need. Short-term studies did not show an increase in the risk of suicidality with antidepressants compared with placebo in adults older than 24 years of age; there was a reduction in risk with antidepressants compared with placebo in adults 65 years of age and older. Depression and certain other psychiatric disorders are themselves associated with increases in the risk of suicide. Appropriately monitor patients of all ages who are started on antidepressant therapy and closely observe patients for clinical worsening, suicidality, or unusual changes in behavior. Advise families and caregivers of the need for close observation and communication with the prescribing health care provider. Duloxetine is not approved for use in children.

Indications

➤*Chronic musculoskeletal pain:* For the management of chronic musculoskeletal pain.

This has been established in studies in patients with chronic low back pain and chronic pain caused by osteoarthritis.

➤*Diabetic peripheral neuropathic pain:* For the management of neuropathic pain associated with diabetic peripheral neuropathy.

➤*Fibromyalgia:* For the management of fibromyalgia.

➤*Generalized anxiety disorder:* For the treatment of generalized anxiety disorder (GAD).

➤*Major depressive disorder:* For the treatment of MDD.

➤*Off-label uses:*

Stress urinary incontinence – [2] = Fair documentation. Duloxetine appeared to be safe and had some modest benefit in the majority of patients with stress urinary incontinence. It was approved in August 2004 by the European Medicines Agency for the treatment of women with moderate to severe stress urinary incontinence and is presently approved in 42 countries. No other oral drug therapies for stress urinary incontinence are more widely accepted. However, no definitive recommendation can be made at this time because of the lack of long-term follow-up safety and efficacy studies, studies with more objectively measurable outcomes, and studies that included more men.

Administration and Dosage

➤*Adults:*

Chronic musculoskeletal pain –

Usual dosage: 60 mg once daily.

Initial dosage: 30 mg daily for 1 week to allow patients to adjust to the medication before increasing to 60 mg once daily.

Diabetic peripheral neuropathic pain –

Usual dosage: 60 mg administered once daily.

Fibromyalgia –

Usual dosage: 60 mg once daily.

Initial dosage: 30 mg once daily for 1 week to allow patient to adjust to the medication before increasing to 60 mg once daily. Some patients may respond to the starting dose.

Generalized anxiety disorder –

Usual dosage: 60 to 120 mg once daily.

Initial dosage: 60 mg once daily. For some patients, it may be desirable to start at 30 mg once daily for 1 week to allow patients to adjust to the medication before increasing to 60 mg once daily.

Dosage adjustment: While a 120 mg once-daily dosage was shown to be effective, there is no evidence that dosages of more than 60 mg once daily confer additional benefit. Nevertheless, if a decision is made to increase the dosage beyond 60 mg once daily, dosage increases should be made in increments of 30 mg once daily.

Major depressive disorder –

Initial dosage: 40 mg/day (given as 20 mg twice daily) to 60 mg/day (given once a day or as 30 mg twice daily). For some patients, it may be desirable to start at 30 mg once daily for 1 week to allow patients to adjust to the medication before increasing to 60 mg once daily.

Maintenance dosage: Total daily dosage of 60 mg once daily. While a 120 mg/day dosage was shown to be effective, there is no evidence that dosages of more than 60 mg/day confer any additional benefits.

Duration of therapy: It is generally agreed that acute episodes of major depression require several months or longer of sustained pharmacologic therapy. Patients should be periodically reassessed to determine the need for maintenance treatment and the appropriate dose for such treatment.

Off-label dosing –

Stress urinary incontinence: [2] = Fair documentation. 80 mg orally once daily or in 2 divided doses (range, 20 to 120 mg) for 12 weeks. Study duration ranged from 3 to 36 weeks.

➤*Renal function impairment:* A lower starting dosage and gradual increase in dosage should be considered for patients with renal impairment. Duloxetine is not recommended for patients with end-stage renal disease (ESRD) or severe renal impairment (estimated creatinine clearance [CrCl] less than 30 mL/min).

➤*Hepatic function impairment:* It is recommended that duloxetine should ordinarily not be administered to patients with any hepatic impairment.

➤*Switching patients to or from a monoamine oxidase inhibitor:* At least 14 days should elapse between discontinuation of an monoamine oxidase inhibitor (MAOI) and initiation of therapy with duloxetine. In addition, at least 5 days should be allowed after stopping duloxetine before starting an MAOI.

➤*Discontinuation of therapy:* Symptoms associated with discontinuation of duloxetine and other selective serotonin reuptake inhibitors (SSRIs) and serotonin-norepinephrine reuptake inhibitors (SNRIs) have been reported. A gradual reduction in the dose, rather than abrupt cessation, is recommended whenever possible. If intolerable symptoms occur following a decrease in the dose or upon discontinuation of treatment, consider resuming the previously prescribed dose. Subsequently, the dose may continue to be decreased, but at a more gradual rate. (See Warnings/Precautions.)

➤*Administration:* Duloxetine should be swallowed whole, and should not be chewed, crushed, or opened sprinkled on food or mixed with liquids. All of these might affect the enteric coating. Duloxetine should be given without regard to meals.

➤*Storage/Stability:* Store at 25°C (77°F); excursions are permitted between 15° and 30°C (59° and 86°F).

Actions

➤*Pharmacology:* Preclinical studies have shown that duloxetine is a potent inhibitor of neuronal serotonin and norepinephrine reuptake and a less potent inhibitor of dopamine reuptake. Although the exact mechanisms of the antidepressant and central pain inhibitory and anxiolytic actions of duloxetine in humans are unknown, these actions are believed to be related to its potentiation of serotonergic and noradrenergic activity in the CNS.

➤*Pharmacokinetics:*

Absorption/Distribution – Orally administered duloxetine is well absorbed. There is a median 2-hour lag until absorption begins, with maximal plasma concentrations (C_{max}) of duloxetine occurring 6 hours postdose. There is a 3-hour delay in absorption and a one-third increase in apparent clearance of duloxetine after an evening dose compared with a morning dose. Steady-state plasma concentrations are typically achieved after 3 days of dosing.

The apparent volume of distribution averages approximately 1,640 L. Duloxetine is highly bound (more than 90%) to proteins in human plasma, binding primarily to albumin and alpha-1 acid glycoprotein.

Food effects: Food does not affect the C_{max} of duloxetine, but delays the time to reach C_{max} from 6 to 10 hours and marginally decreases the extent of absorption (area under the curve [AUC]) by approximately 10%.

Metabolism/Excretion – Duloxetine undergoes extensive metabolism, but the major circulating metabolites have not been shown to contribute significantly to the pharmacologic activity of duloxetine. Duloxetine has an elimination half-life of approximately 12 hours (range, 8 to 17 hours). Elimination of duloxetine is mainly through hepatic metabolism involving 2 cytochrome P450 (CYP-450) isozymes, CYP2D6 and CYP1A2.

Biotransformation and disposition of duloxetine in humans have been determined following oral administration of ^{14}C-labeled duloxetine. Duloxetine comprises approximately 3% of the total radiolabeled material in the plasma, indicating that it undergoes extensive metabolism to numerous metabolites. The major biotransformation pathways for duloxetine involve oxidation of the naphthyl ring, followed by conjugation and further oxidation. Both CYP2D6 and CYP1A2 catalyze the oxidation of the naphthyl ring in vitro. Metabolites found in plasma include 4-hydroxy duloxetine glucuronide and 5-hydroxy, 6-methoxy duloxetine sulfate. Many additional metabolites have been identified in urine, some representing only minor pathways of elimination. Only trace (less than 1% of the dose) amounts of unchanged duloxetine are present in the urine. Most (approximately 70%) of the duloxetine dose appears in the urine as metabolites of duloxetine; approximately 20% is excreted in the feces.

Special populations –

Renal function impairment: After a single dose of duloxetine 60 mg, C_{max} and AUC values were approximately 100% greater in patients with ESRD receiving long-term intermittent hemodialysis than in subjects with healthy renal function. The elimination half-life, however, was similar in both groups. The AUCs of the major circulating metabolites, 4-hydroxy duloxetine glucuronide and 5-hydroxy, 6-methoxy duloxetine sulfate, largely excreted in urine, were approximately 7- to 9-fold higher and would be expected to increase further with multiple dosing.

Hepatic function impairment: Patients with clinically evident hepatic impairment have decreased duloxetine metabolism and elimination. After a single dose of duloxetine 20 mg, 6 cirrhotic patients with moderate hepatic impairment (Child-Pugh class B) had a mean plasma duloxetine clearance of approximately 15% that of age- and gender-matched healthy subjects, with a 5-fold increase in mean exposure (AUC). Although C_{max} was similar to healthy subjects in the cirrhotic patients, the half-life was approximately 3 times longer.

Elderly: The pharmacokinetics of duloxetine after a single dose of 40 mg were compared in healthy elderly women (65 to 77 years of age) and healthy middle-age women (32 to 50 years of age). There was no difference in the C_{max}, but the AUC of duloxetine was somewhat (approximately 25%) higher, and the half-life was approximately 4 hours longer in elderly women. Popu-

DULOXETINE HYDROCHLORIDE — ORAL

lation pharmacokinetic analyses suggest that the typical values for clearance decrease by approximately 1% each year between 25 and 75 years of age, but age as a predictive factor only accounts for a small percentage of between-patient variability. Dosage adjustment based on the age of the patient is not necessary.

Lactation: Lactation did not influence duloxetine pharmacokinetics. The disposition of duloxetine was studied in 6 breast-feeding women who were at least 12 weeks postpartum. Duloxetine 40 mg twice daily was given for 3.5 days. Like many other drugs, duloxetine is detected in breast milk, and steady-state concentrations in breast milk are about one-fourth those in plasma. The amount of duloxetine in breast milk is approximately 7 mcg/day while on 40 mg twice-daily dosing. The excretion of duloxetine metabolites into breast milk was not examined.

Smoking: Duloxetine bioavailability (AUC) appears to be reduced approximately one-third in smokers. Dosage modifications are not recommended for smokers.

Contraindications

Concomitant use in patients taking MAOIs (see Drug Interactions); use in patients with uncontrolled narrow-angle glaucoma.

Warnings/Precautions

➤*Clinical worsening and suicide risk:* Patients with MDD, both adults and children, may experience worsening of their depression and/or the emergence of suicidal ideation and behavior (suicidality) or unusual changes in behavior, whether or not they are taking antidepressant medications. This risk may persist until significant remission occurs. Suicide is a known risk of depression and certain other psychiatric disorders, and these disorders themselves are the strongest predictors of suicide. There has been a longstanding concern that antidepressants may have a role in inducing worsening of depression and the emergence of suicidality in certain patients during the early phases of treatment.

Pooled analyses of short-term, placebo-controlled trials of antidepressant drugs (SSRIs and others) showed that these drugs increase the risk of suicidal thinking and behavior (suicidality) in children, adolescents, and young adults (18 to 24 years of age) with MDD and other psychiatric disorders. Short-term studies did not show an increase in the risk of suicidality with antidepressants compared with placebo in adults older than 24 years of age; there was a reduction with antidepressants compared with placebo in adults 65 years of age and older.

No suicides occurred in any of the pediatric trials. There were suicides in the adult trials, but the number was not sufficient to reach any conclusion about drug effect on suicide.

It is unknown whether the suicidality risk extends to longer-term use (ie, beyond several months). However, there is substantial evidence from placebo-controlled maintenance trials in adults with depression that the use of antidepressants can delay the recurrence of depression.

Appropriately monitor all patients being treated with antidepressants for any indication, and observe them closely for clinical worsening, suicidality, and unusual changes in behavior, especially during the initial few months of a course of drug therapy, or at times of dose changes, either increases or decreases.

The following symptoms have been reported in adults and children treated with antidepressants for MDD, as well as for other indications, both psychiatric and nonpsychiatric, including agitation, akathisia (psychomotor restlessness), anxiety, hostility, aggressiveness, hypomania, impulsivity, insomnia, irritability, mania, and panic attacks. Although a causal link between the emergence of such symptoms and either the worsening of depression and/or the emergence of suicidal impulses has not been established, there is concern that such symptoms may represent precursors to emerging suicidality.

Consider changing the therapeutic regimen, including possibly discontinuing the medication, in patients whose depression is persistently worse or in patients who are experiencing emergent suicidality or symptoms that might be precursors to worsening depression or suicidality, especially if these symptoms are severe, abrupt in onset, or were not part of the patient's presenting symptoms.

If the decision has been made to discontinue treatment, taper medication as rapidly as feasible but with recognition that abrupt discontinuation can be associated with certain symptoms (eg, dizziness, headache, irritability, nausea, nightmares, paresthesia, vomiting).

Alert families and caregivers of patients being treated with antidepressants for MDD or other indications, both psychiatric and nonpsychiatric, about the need to monitor patients for the emergence of agitation, irritability, suicidality, unusual changes in behavior, and the other symptoms previously described, and to immediately report such symptoms to the health care provider. Such monitoring includes daily observation by families and caregivers. In order to reduce the risk of overdose, write prescriptions for duloxetine for the smallest quantity of capsules consistent with good patient management, in order to reduce the risk of overdose.

➤*Screening patients for bipolar disorder:* A major depressive episode may be the initial presentation of bipolar disorder. It is generally believed (although not established in controlled trials) that treating such an episode with an antidepressant alone may increase the likelihood of precipitation of a mixed/manic episode in patients at risk for bipolar disorder. It is unknown whether any of the symptoms previously described represent such a conversion. However, prior to initiating treatment with an antidepressant, adequately screen patients with depressive symptoms to determine if they are at risk for bipolar disorder; include in such screening a detailed psychiatric history, including a family history of suicide, bipolar disorder, and depression. Duloxetine is not approved for use in treating bipolar depression.

➤*Hepatotoxicity:* There have been reports of hepatic failure, sometimes fatal, in patients treated with duloxetine. These cases have presented as hepatitis with abdominal pain, hepatomegaly, and elevation of transaminase levels to more than 20 times the upper limits of normal (ULN), with or without jaundice, reflecting a mixed or hepatocellular pattern of liver injury. Discontinue duloxetine in patients who develop jaundice or other evidence of clinically significant liver dysfunction and do not resume unless another cause can be established.

Cases of cholestatic jaundice with minimal elevation of transaminase levels also have been reported. Other postmarketing reports indicate that elevated transaminases, bilirubin, and alkaline phosphatase have occurred in patients with chronic liver disease or cirrhosis.

Duloxetine increased the risk of elevation of serum transaminase levels in development program clinical trials. Liver transaminase elevations resulted in the discontinuation of 0.3% of duloxetine-treated patients. In most patients, the median time to detection of the transaminase elevation was approximately 2 months. In placebo-controlled trials in any indication, for patients with normal and abnormal baseline ALT values, elevation of ALT more than 3 times the ULN occurred in 1.37% of duloxetine-treated patients compared with 0.49% of placebo-treated patients. In placebo-controlled studies using a fixed-dose design, there was evidence of a dose-response relationship for ALT and AST elevation of more than 3 times the ULN and more than 5 times the ULN, respectively.

Because it is possible that duloxetine and alcohol may interact to cause liver injury or that duloxetine may aggravate preexisting liver disease, ordinarily do not prescribe duloxetine to patients with substantial alcohol use or evidence of chronic liver disease.

➤*Orthostatic hypotension and syncope:* Orthostatic hypotension and syncope have been reported with therapeutic doses of duloxetine. Syncope and orthostatic hypotension tend to occur within the first week of therapy but can occur at any time during duloxetine treatment, particularly after dose increases. The risk of blood pressure decreases may be greater in patients taking concomitant medications that induce orthostatic hypotension (eg, antihypertensives) or are potent CYP1A2 inhibitors, and in patients taking duloxetine at dosages higher than 60 mg/day. Consider discontinuing duloxetine in patients who experience symptomatic orthostatic hypotension and/or syncope during duloxetine therapy.

➤*Serotonin syndrome or neuroleptic malignant syndrome–like reactions:* The development of a potentially life-threatening serotonin syndrome or neuroleptic malignant syndrome (NMS)–like reactions have been reported with SNRIs and SSRIs alone, including duloxetine treatment, but particularly with concomitant use of serotonergic drugs (including triptans) with drugs that impair metabolism of serotonin (including MAOIs), or with antipsychotics or other dopamine antagonists. Serotonin syndrome symptoms may include mental status changes (eg, agitation, coma, hallucinations), autonomic instability (eg, hyperthermia, labile blood pressure, tachycardia), neuromuscular aberrations (eg, hyperreflexia, incoordination), and/or GI symptoms (eg, diarrhea, nausea, vomiting). (See also Drug Interactions.) Serotonin syndrome, in its most severe form, can resemble NMS, which includes hyperthermia, muscle rigidity, autonomic instability with possible rapid fluctuation of vital signs, and mental status changes. Monitor patients for the emergence of serotonin syndrome or NMS-like signs and symptoms.

Immediately discontinue treatment with duloxetine and any concomitant serotonergic or antidopaminergic agents, including antipsychotics, if the previously listed events occur; initiate supportive symptomatic treatment.

➤*Abnormal bleeding:* SSRIs and SNRIs, including duloxetine, may increase the risk of bleeding events. Concomitant use of aspirin, nonsteroidal anti-inflammatory drugs (NSAIDs), warfarin, and other anticoagulants may add to this risk. Case reports and epidemiological studies (case-control and cohort design) have demonstrated an association between use of drugs that interfere with serotonin reuptake and the occurrence of GI bleeding. Bleeding events related to SSRI and SNRI use have ranged from ecchymoses, hematomas, epistaxis, and petechiae to life-threatening hemorrhages.

Caution patients about the risk of bleeding associated with the concomitant use of duloxetine and NSAIDs, aspirin, or other drugs that affect coagulation.

➤*Discontinuation of treatment:* Discontinuation symptoms have been systematically evaluated in patients taking duloxetine. Following abrupt or tapered discontinuation in placebo-controlled clinical trials, the following symptoms occurred at a rate of 1% or more and at a significantly higher rate in duloxetine-treated patients compared with those discontinuing from placebo: anxiety, diarrhea, dizziness, fatigue, headache, hyperhidrosis, insomnia, irritability, nausea, nightmares, paresthesia, vertigo, and vomiting.

During marketing of other SSRIs and SNRIs, there have been spontaneous reports of adverse reactions occurring upon discontinuation of these drugs, particularly when abruptly discontinued. These adverse reactions included the following: agitation, anxiety, confusion, dizziness, dysphoric mood, emotional lability, headache, hypomania, insomnia, irritability, lethargy, seizures, sensory disturbances (eg, paresthesias such as electric shock sensations), and tinnitus. Although these reactions are generally self-limiting, some have been reported to be severe.

See Administration and Dosage for more information.

➤*Mania/Hypomania activation:* In placebo-controlled trials in patients with MDD, activation of mania or hypomania was reported in 0.1% of duloxetine-treated patients and 0.1% of placebo-treated patients. No activation of mania or hypomania was reported in diabetic peripheral neuropathic pain, fibromyalgia, or GAD placebo-controlled trials. Activation of mania or

DULOXETINE HYDROCHLORIDE — ORAL

hypomania has been reported in a small proportion of patients with mood disorders who were treated with other marketed drugs effective in the treatment of MDD. As with these other agents, use duloxetine cautiously in patients with a history of mania.

➤*Seizures:* Duloxetine has not been systematically evaluated in patients with a seizure disorder, and such patients were excluded from clinical studies. In placebo-controlled clinical trials, seizures/convulsions occurred in 0.03% of patients treated with duloxetine and 0.01% of patients treated with placebo. Prescribe duloxetine with care in patients with a history of a seizure disorder.

➤*Blood pressure effects:* In placebo-controlled clinical trials across indications from baseline to end point, duloxetine treatment was associated with mean increases of 0.5 mm Hg in systolic blood pressure and 0.8 mm Hg in diastolic blood pressure compared with mean decreases of 0.6 mm Hg systolic and 0.4 mm Hg diastolic in placebo-treated patients. There was no significant difference in the frequency of sustained (3 consecutive visits) elevated blood pressure. In a clinical pharmacology study designed to evaluate the effects of duloxetine on various parameters, including blood pressure at supratherapeutic doses with an accelerated dose titration, there was evidence of increases in supine blood pressure at dosages of up to 200 mg twice daily. At the highest 200 mg twice-daily dosage, the increase in mean pulse rate was 5 to 6.8 beats and increases in mean blood pressure were 4.7 to 6.8 mm Hg (systolic) and 4.5 to 7 mm Hg (diastolic) up to 12 hours after dosing. Measure blood pressure prior to initiating treatment and periodically throughout treatment.

➤*Hyponatremia:* Hyponatremia may occur as a result of treatment with SSRIs and SNRIs, including duloxetine. In many cases, hyponatremia appears to be the result of the syndrome of inappropriate antidiuretic hormone secretion. Cases with serum sodium lower than 110 mmol/L have been reported and appeared to be reversible when duloxetine was discontinued. Elderly patients may be at greater risk of developing hyponatremia with SSRIs and SNRIs. Also, patients taking diuretics or who are otherwise volume depleted may be at greater risk. Consider discontinuing duloxetine in patients with symptomatic hyponatremia and institute appropriate medical intervention.

Signs and symptoms of hyponatremia include headache, difficulty concentrating, memory impairment, confusion, weakness, and unsteadiness, which may lead to falls. More severe and/or acute cases have been associated with hallucination, syncope, seizure, coma, respiratory arrest, and death.

➤*Gastric motility alteration:* Clinical experience with duloxetine in patients with concomitant systemic illnesses is limited. There is no information on the effect that alterations in gastric motility may have on the stability of duloxetine's enteric coating. In extremely acidic conditions, duloxetine, unprotected by the enteric coating, may undergo hydrolysis to form naphthol. Caution is advised when using duloxetine in patients with conditions that may slow gastric emptying (eg, some patients with diabetes).

➤*Narrow-angle glaucoma:* In clinical trials, duloxetine was associated with an increased risk of mydriasis; therefore, avoid use in patients with uncontrolled narrow-angle glaucoma and use cautiously in patients with controlled narrow-angle glaucoma.

➤*Diabetes:* As observed in diabetic peripheral neuropathic pain trials, duloxetine treatment worsens glycemic control in some patients with diabetes. In 3 clinical trials of duloxetine for the management of neuropathic pain associated with diabetic peripheral neuropathy, the mean duration of diabetes was approximately 12 years, the mean baseline fasting blood glucose was 176 mg/dL, and the mean baseline glycosylated hemoglobin (HbA_{1c}) was 7.8%. In the 12-week, acute treatment phase of these studies, duloxetine was associated with a small increase in mean fasting blood glucose compared with placebo. In the extension phase of these studies, which lasted up to 52 weeks, mean fasting blood glucose increased by 12 mg/dL in the duloxetine group and decreased by 11.5 mg/dL in the routine care group. HbA_{1c} increased 0.5% in the duloxetine group and 0.2% in the routine care groups.

➤*Urinary effects:* Duloxetine is in a class of drugs known to affect urethral resistance. If symptoms of urinary hesitation develop during treatment with duloxetine, consider the possibility that they might be drug-related.

In postmarketing experience, cases of urinary retention have been observed. In some instances of urinary retention associated with duloxetine use, hospitalization and/or catheterization have been needed.

➤*Renal function impairment:* See Administration and Dosage for more information. See Actions for more information.

➤*Hepatic function impairment:* See Administration and Dosage for more information. See Actions for more information.

➤*Pregnancy: Category C; Category D* if taken in the second half of pregnancy (per *Drugs in Pregnancy and Lactation*). There are no adequate and well-controlled studies in pregnant women; therefore, use duloxetine during pregnancy only if the potential benefit justifies the potential risk to the fetus.

Based on a case report, duloxetine crosses the placenta at term. The drug's relatively low molecular weight and long half-life suggest that it would cross the placenta. However, duloxetine is highly protein bound and undergoes extensive metabolism, which lessens embryo/fetal exposure. When treating a pregnant woman with duloxetine during the third trimester, carefully consider the potential risks and benefits of treatment. Consider tapering duloxetine in the third trimester.

Teratogenic – In animal reproduction studies, duloxetine had adverse effects on embryofetal and postnatal development. When duloxetine was administered orally to pregnant rats and rabbits during the period of organogenesis, there was no evidence of teratogenicity at dosages of up to 45 mg/kg/day (7 times the MRHD of 60 mg/day and 4 times the human dosage of 120 mg/day on a mg/m^2 basis in rats; 15 times the MRHD and 7 times the human dosage of 120 mg/day on a mg/m^2 basis in rabbits). However, fetal weights were decreased at this dose, with a no-effect dosage of 10 mg/kg/day (2 times the MRHD and approximately 1 times the human dosage of 120 mg/day on a mg/m^2 basis in rats; 3 times the MRHD and 2 times the human dosage of 120 mg/day on a mg/m^2 basis in rabbits).

When duloxetine was administered orally to pregnant rats throughout gestation and lactation, the survival of pups to 1 day postpartum and pup body weights at birth and during the lactation period were decreased at a dosage of 30 mg/kg/day (5 times the MRHD and 2 times the human dosage of 120 mg/day on a mg/m^2 basis); the no-effect dosage was 10 mg/kg/day. Furthermore, behaviors consistent with increased reactivity, such as increased startle response to noise and decreased habituation of locomotor activity, were observed in pups following maternal exposure to 30 mg/kg/day. Postweaning growth and reproductive performance of the progeny were not adversely affected by maternal duloxetine treatment.

Nonteratogenic – Neonates exposed to SSRIs or SNRIs late in the third trimester have developed complications requiring prolonged hospitalization, respiratory support, and tube feeding. Such complications can arise immediately upon delivery. Reported clinical findings included apnea, constant crying, cyanosis, feeding difficulty, hyperreflexia, hypertonia, hypoglycemia, hypotonia, irritability, jitteriness, respiratory distress, seizures, temperature instability, tremor, and vomiting. These features are consistent with a direct toxic effect of SSRIs and SNRIs or, possibly, a drug discontinuation syndrome. In some cases, the clinical picture is consistent with serotonin syndrome.

Based on a case report of an infant exposed to duloxetine in utero during the second half of gestation and during breast-feeding, there were no developmental toxicities or other signs of toxicity noted. However, the possibility of the development of functional/neurobehavioral deficits later in life cannot be excluded.

➤*Lactation:* Duloxetine is excreted in the milk of breast-feeding women. The estimated daily infant dose on a mg/kg basis is approximately 0.14% of the maternal dose. Because the safety of duloxetine in infants is not known, breast-feeding while taking duloxetine is not recommended. However, if the health care provider determines that the benefit of duloxetine therapy for the mother outweighs any potential risk to the infant, no dosage adjustment is required. According to the American Academy of Pediatrics, antidepressants are classified as drugs for which the effect on breast-fed infants is unknown but may be of concern.

Case report – In one case report, a woman 29 years of age was treated with duloxetine 60 mg extended release daily for depression during the second half of an uncomplicated pregnancy and during breast-feeding. No developmental toxicity or other signs for toxicity were observed in the infant exposed to duloxetine during the second half of gestation and during breast-feeding in the first 32 days after birth. However, the possibility of functional/neurobehavioral deficits appearing later in life cannot be excluded.

➤*Children:* Safety and effectiveness in children have not been established. Anyone considering the use of duloxetine in a child or adolescent must balance the potential risks with the clinical need. Duloxetine is not approved for use in children.

➤*Monitoring:* Measure blood pressure prior to initiating treatment and periodically during treatment. Monitor all patients for the emergence of agitation, irritability, suicidality, unusual changes in behavior, and clinical worsening, especially during the initial few months of a course of drug therapy or at times of dose changes. When discontinuing therapy, monitor patients for symptoms, such as agitation, anxiety, confusion, dizziness, dysphoric mood, emotional lability, headache, hypomania, irritability, insomnia, lethargy, seizures, sensory disturbances, and tinnitus.

Monitor for possible sexual adverse reactions.

Carefully evaluate patients for a history of drug abuse and follow such patients closely, observing them for signs of misuse or abuse of duloxetine (eg, development of tolerance, incrementation of dose, drug-seeking behavior).

Monitor patients for the emergence of serotonin syndrome or NMS-like signs and symptoms.

Drug Interactions

➤*Drugs that affect gastric acidity:* Duloxetine has an enteric coating that resists dissolution until reaching a segment of the GI tract where the pH exceeds 5.5. In extremely acidic conditions, duloxetine, unprotected by the enteric coating, may undergo hydrolysis to form naphthol. Caution is advised when using duloxetine in patients with conditions that may slow gastric emptying (eg, some patients with diabetes). Drugs that raise the GI pH may lead to an earlier release of duloxetine.

Duloxetine Drug Interactions

Precipitant drug	Object drug[a]		Description
Alcohol	Duloxetine	↑	Liver injury manifested by ALT and total bilirubin elevations with evidence of obstruction occurred from heavy alcohol use and duloxetine. Ordinarily, do not prescribe duloxetine to patients with substantial alcohol use.
Duloxetine	Alcohol		

DULOXETINE HYDROCHLORIDE — ORAL

Duloxetine Drug Interactions

Precipitant drug	Object drug[a]		Description
CNS-acting drugs (eg, narcotic analgesics)	Duloxetine	↑	Given the primary CNS effects of duloxetine, use with caution when taken in combination with, or substituted for, other centrally acting drugs, including those with a similar mechanism of action.
Duloxetine	CNS-acting drugs (eg, narcotic analgesics)		
CYP1A2 inhibitors (eg, cimetidine, ciprofloxacin, fluvoxamine)	Duloxetine	↑	Avoid coadministration of duloxetine with potent CYP1A2 inhibitors. Concomitant use of duloxetine with fluvoxamine resulted in an approximate 6-fold increase in AUC, an approximate 2.5-fold increase in C_{max}, and a 3-fold increase in the half-life of duloxetine.
CYP2D6 inhibitors (eg, fluoxetine, paroxetine, quinidine, terbinafine)	Duloxetine	↑	Concomitant use of duloxetine with potent inhibitors of CYP2D6 may result in higher concentrations of duloxetine. Paroxetine (20 mg daily) increased the concentration of duloxetine (40 mg daily) AUC by approximately 60%. Monitor the clinical response. Adjust the duloxetine dose as needed.
Linezolid	Duloxetine	↑	Coadministration of linezolid and duloxetine may result in serotonin syndrome (eg, agitation, altered consciousness, ataxia, myoclonus, overactive reflexes, shivering). Because linezolid has MAOI activity, allow at least 2 weeks between stopping linezolid and starting duloxetine.
Duloxetine	Linezolid		
MAOIs (eg, phenelzine, rasagiline, selegiline)	Duloxetine	↑	Coadministration is contraindicated. Serious, sometimes fatal, reactions may occur, including hyperthermia, rigidity, myoclonus, autonomic instability with possible rapid fluctuations of vital signs, and mental status changes that include extreme agitation progressing to delirium and coma. It is recommended that duloxetine not be used in combination with an MAOI or within at least 14 days of discontinuing treatment with an MAOI. Allow at least 5 days after stopping duloxetine before starting an MAOI.
Duloxetine	MAOIs (eg, phenelzine, rasagiline, selegiline)		
Methylene blue	Duloxetine		Neurologic adverse reactions, including symptoms of serotonin syndrome, may occur. Avoid concurrent use.
Duloxetine	Methylene blue		
Serotonergic drugs (eg, cyclobenzaprine, lithium, other SNRIs, SSRIs, tramadol, tryptophan)	Duloxetine	↑	A serotonin syndrome (eg, agitation, altered consciousness, ataxia, myoclonus, overactive reflexes, shivering) may occur. Coadministration is not recommended.
Duloxetine	Serotonergic drugs (eg, cyclobenzaprine, lithium, other SNRIs, SSRIs, tramadol, tryptophan)		
St. John's wort	Duloxetine	↑	Coadministration may result in increased sedative-hypnotic effects. Coadministration may also result in serotonin syndrome. Avoid concurrent use.
Duloxetine	St. John's wort		
Triptans (eg, almotriptan, eletriptan, naratriptan, sumatriptan)	Duloxetine	↑	Concomitant use may result in serotonin syndrome, including agitation, overactive reflexes, ataxia, shivering, myoclonus, and altered consciousness. Careful observation of the patient is advised, particularly during treatment initiation and dose increases. Serotonin syndrome requires immediate medical attention, including supportive care and withdrawal of the serotonergic agent. Administration of an antiserotonergic agent (eg, cyproheptadine) may be helpful.
Duloxetine	Triptans (eg, almotriptan, eletriptan, naratriptan, sumatriptan)		
Duloxetine	Antiarrhythmics, type 1C (eg, flecainide, propafenone)	↑	Duloxetine may inhibit the metabolism (CYP2D6) of propafenone and flecainide, increasing plasma levels. Coadminister with caution.
Duloxetine	Aspirin, NSAIDs (eg, naproxen)	↑	Concomitant use may increase the risk of bleeding. Use with caution and warn patients of the risk of increased bleeding.
Duloxetine	Beta-blockers (eg, carvedilol, metoprolol, propranolol)	↑	Excessive beta-blockade (bradycardia) may occur. Duloxetine may inhibit the metabolism (CYP2D6) of certain beta-blockers. Monitor cardiac function.
Duloxetine	Phenothiazines (eg, thioridazine)	↑	Thioridazine plasma concentrations may be elevated, increasing the risk of life-threatening ventricular arrhythmias and sudden death. Do not coadminister.
Duloxetine	Sympathomimetics (eg, amphetamine, dextroamphetamine, phentermine)	↑	Increased sensitivity to sympathomimetic effects and increased risk of serotonin syndrome may occur. If coadministration cannot be avoided, monitor for increased CNS effects. Adjust therapy as needed.
Duloxetine	TCAs[b] (eg, amitriptyline, desipramine, imipramine, nortriptyline)	↑	Plasma TCA levels may be increased; coadminister with caution. Monitor TCA levels; TCA dose may need to be reduced.
Duloxetine	Theophylline	↑	Theophylline AUC was increased by as much as 20% when coadministered with duloxetine. This increase would not be expected to be clinically important. Monitor the clinical response and if an interaction is suspected, adjust the theophylline dose as needed.
Duloxetine	Warfarin	↑	Altered anticoagulant effects, including increased bleeding, have been reported. Carefully monitor warfarin therapy when duloxetine is initiated or discontinued.

[a] ↑ = object drug increased.
[b] TCAs = tricyclic antidepressants.

➤*Drug/Food interactions:* See Actions for more information.

Adverse Reactions

For more information concerning suicide risk, worsening of depression, hepatotoxicity, orthostatic hypotension and syncope, hyponatremia, gastric motility, narrow-angle glaucoma, urinary effects, serotonin syndrome, NMS-like reactions, abnormal bleeding, seizures, and blood pressure effects, refer to Warnings/Precautions.

➤*Discontinuation of treatment:*

Chronic pain caused by osteoarthritis – Approximately 16.3% of the patients who received duloxetine in 13-week, placebo-controlled trials for chronic pain caused by osteoarthritis discontinued treatment because of an adverse reaction compared with 5.6% for placebo. Common adverse reactions reported as a reason for discontinuation and considered to be drug-related (as previously defined) included nausea (duloxetine 2.9%, placebo 0.8%) and asthenia (duloxetine 1.3%, placebo 0%).

Chronic low back pain – Approximately 16.5% of the patients who received duloxetine in 13-week, placebo-controlled trials for chronic low back

DULOXETINE HYDROCHLORIDE — ORAL

pain discontinued treatment because of an adverse reaction, compared with 6.3% for placebo. Common adverse reactions reported as a reason for discontinuation and considered to be drug-related (as previously defined) included nausea (duloxetine 3%, placebo 0.7%) and somnolence (duloxetine 1%, placebo 0%).

Diabetic peripheral neuropathic pain – Approximately 12.9% of patients who received duloxetine in the diabetic peripheral neuropathic pain placebo-controlled trials discontinued treatment because of an adverse reaction compared with 5.1% for placebo. Nausea (duloxetine 3.5%, placebo 0.7%), dizziness (duloxetine 1.2%, placebo 0.4%), and somnolence (duloxetine 1.1%, placebo 0%) were the common adverse reactions reported as reasons for discontinuation and considered to be drug-related (ie, discontinuation occurring in at least 1% of duloxetine-treated patients and at a rate of at least twice that of placebo).

Fibromyalgia – Approximately 19.6% of the patients who received duloxetine in 3- to 6-month, placebo-controlled trials for fibromyalgia discontinued treatment because of an adverse reaction compared with 11.8% for placebo. Common adverse reactions reported as a reason for discontinuation and considered to be drug-related (as previously defined) included nausea (duloxetine 1.9%, placebo 0.7%), somnolence (duloxetine 1.5%, placebo 0%), and fatigue (duloxetine 1.3%, placebo 0.2%).

Generalized anxiety disorder – Approximately 15.3% of patients who received duloxetine in the GAD placebo-controlled trials discontinued treatment because of an adverse reaction compared with 4% for placebo. Nausea (duloxetine 3.7%, placebo 0.2%), vomiting (duloxetine 1.3%, placebo 0%), and dizziness (duloxetine 1%, placebo 0.2%) were the common adverse reactions reported as reasons for discontinuation and considered to be drug-related.

Major depressive disorder – Approximately 9% of patients who received duloxetine in the MDD placebo-controlled trials discontinued treatment because of an adverse reaction compared with 4.7% of patients receiving placebo. Nausea (duloxetine 1.3%, placebo 0.5%) was the only common adverse reaction reported as reason for discontinuation and considered to be drug-related.

➤*Most common adverse reactions:*

Pooled trials for all indications – The most commonly observed adverse reactions in duloxetine-treated patients (incidence of at least 5% and at least twice the incidence in placebo patients) were constipation, decreased appetite, dry mouth, fatigue, hyperhidrosis, nausea, and somnolence.

Chronic pain caused by osteoarthritis – The most commonly observed adverse reactions in duloxetine-treated patients (as defined previously) were constipation, fatigue, and nausea.

Chronic low back pain – The most commonly observed adverse reactions in duloxetine-treated patients (as defined previously) were constipation, dizziness, dry mouth, fatigue, insomnia, nausea, and somnolence.

Diabetic peripheral neuropathic pain – The most commonly observed adverse reactions in duloxetine-treated patients (as defined previously) were constipation, decreased appetite, dry mouth, hyperhidrosis, nausea, and somnolence.

Fibromyalgia – The most commonly observed adverse reactions in duloxetine-treated patients (as defined previously) were agitation, constipation, decreased appetite, dry mouth, hyperhidrosis, nausea, and somnolence.

➤*Adverse reactions for all indications:*

Duloxetine Adverse Reactions for All Indications in Clinical Trials (≥ 5%)

Adverse reactions	Duloxetine (n = 6,020)	Placebo (n = 3,962)
CNS		
Dizziness	10%	5%
Fatigue[a]	10%	5%
Headache	14%	13%
Insomnia[b,c]	10%	6%
Somnolence[b,d]	10%	3%
Dermatologic		
Hyperhidrosis	7%	2%
GI		
Appetite decreased[b,e]	8%	2%
Constipation[b]	10%	4%
Diarrhea	9%	6%
Dry mouth	13%	5%
Nausea	24%	8%

[a] Also includes asthenia.
[b] Events for which there was a significant dose-dependent relationship in fixed-dose studies, excluding 3 MDD studies that did not have a placebo lead-in period or dose titration.
[c] Also includes early morning awakening, initial insomnia, and middle insomnia.
[d] Also includes hypersomnia and sedation.
[e] Also includes anorexia.

➤*Diabetic peripheral neuropathic pain, fibromyalgia, osteoarthritis, and chronic low back pain:*

Duloxetine Adverse Reactions in Diabetic Peripheral Neuropathic Pain, Fibromyalgia, Osteoarthritis, and Chronic Low Back Pain Trials (≥ 2%)

Adverse reactions	Duloxetine (n = 2,621)	Placebo (n = 1,672)
CNS		
Agitation[a]	3%	< 1%
Dizziness	10%	5%
Fatigue[b]	11%	5%
Headache	13%	9%
Insomnia[c,d]	10%	6%
Paraesthesia[e]	2%	2%
Somnolence[c,f]	12%	3%
Tremor[c]	2%	< 1%
GI		
Abdominal pain[g]	6%	5%
Appetite decreased[c,h]	9%	1%
Constipation[c]	10%	3%
Diarrhea	9%	6%
Dry mouth[c]	11%	3%
Dyspepsia[i]	2%	1%
Nausea	23%	7%
Vomiting	3%	2%
GU		
Ejaculation disorder[j]	2%	< 1%
Erectile dysfunction[c,k]	4%	< 1%
Musculoskeletal		
Muscle spasms	3%	2%
Musculoskeletal pain[c,l]	4%	4%
Respiratory		
Cough	3%	2%
Influenza	3%	2%
Nasopharyngitis	5%	4%
Oropharyngeal pain[c]	2%	2%
Upper respiratory tract infection	4%	4%
Miscellaneous		
Flushing[m]	3%	1%
Hyperhidrosis	6%	1%

[a] Also includes feeling jittery, nervousness, restlessness, tension and psychomotor hyperactivity.
[b] Also includes asthenia.
[c] Incidence of 120 mg/day is significantly greater than the incidence for 60 mg/day.
[d] Also includes middle insomnia, early morning awakening, and initial insomnia.
[e] Also includes hypoaesthesia, hypoaesthesia facial, and paraesthesia oral.
[f] Also includes hypersomnia and sedation.
[g] Also includes abdominal discomfort, abdominal pain lower, abdominal pain upper, abdominal tenderness, and GI pain.
[h] Also includes anorexia.
[i] Also includes stomach discomfort.
[j] Men only (885 for duloxetine, 494 for placebo); also includes ejaculation failure.
[k] Men only (885 for duloxetine, 494 for placebo).
[l] Also includes myalgia and neck pain.
[m] Also includes hot flush.

➤*Generalized anxiety disorder/major depressive disorder:*

Duloxetine Adverse Reactions in Generalized Anxiety Disorder/ Major Depressive Disorder Trials (≥ 2%)

Adverse reactions	Duloxetine (n = 2,995)	Placebo (n = 1,955)
Cardiovascular		
Hot flush	2%	< 1%
Palpitations	2%	2%
CNS		
Abnormal dreams[a]	2%	1%
Agitation[b]	5%	3%
Anxiety	3%	2%
Dizziness	10%	6%
Fatigue[c]	10%	6%
Insomnia[d]	10%	6%
Somnolence[e]	10%	4%

DULOXETINE HYDROCHLORIDE — ORAL

Duloxetine Adverse Reactions in Generalized Anxiety Disorder/ Major Depressive Disorder Trials (≥ 2%)		
Adverse reactions	Duloxetine (n = 2,995)	Placebo (n = 1,955)
Tremor	3%	< 1%
GI		
Abdominal pain[f]	4%	4%
Appetite decreased[g]	7%	2%
Constipation[h]	10%	4%
Diarrhea	10%	7%
Dry mouth	15%	6%
Nausea	25%	9%
Vomiting	5%	2%
Weight decreased[h]	2%	< 1%
GU		
Ejaculation delayed[h,i]	3%	< 1%
Ejaculation disorder[i,j]	2%	< 1%
Erectile dysfunction[i]	5%	1%
Libido decreased[k]	4%	1%
Orgasm abnormal[l]	3%	< 1%
Miscellaneous		
Hyperhidrosis	6%	2%
Vision blurred	3%	2%
Yawning	2%	< 1%

[a] Also includes nightmare.
[b] Also includes feeling jittery, nervousness, restlessness, tension, and psychomotor agitation.
[c] Also includes asthenia.
[d] Also includes early morning awakening, initial insomnia, and middle insomnia.
[e] Also includes hypersomnia and sedation.
[f] Term includes abdominal discomfort, abdominal pain lower, abdominal pain upper, abdominal tenderness, and GI pain.
[g] Term includes anorexia.
[h] Reactions for which there was a significant dose-dependent relationship in fixed-dose studies, excluding 3 MDD studies that did not have a placebo lead-in period or dose titration.
[i] Men only.
[j] Also includes ejaculation dysfunction and ejaculation failure.
[k] Also includes loss of libido.
[l] Also includes anorgasmia.

➤*Effects on sexual function in men and women:* Changes in sexual desire, sexual performance, and sexual satisfaction often occur as manifestations of a psychiatric disorder or diabetes; they may also be a consequence of pharmacologic treatment.

Duloxetine Mean Change in ASEX Scores by Gender in Major Depressive Disorder Trials					
		Men[a]		Women[a]	
		Duloxetine (n = 175)	Placebo (n = 83)	Duloxetine (n = 241)	Placebo (n = 126)
ASEX total (items 1 to 5)		0.56[b]	−1.07	−1.15	−1.07
Item 1	Sex drive	−0.07	−0.12	−0.32	−0.24
Item 2	Arousal	0.01	−0.26	−0.21	−0.18
Item 3	Ability to achieve erection (men); lubrication (women)	0.03	−0.25	−0.17	−0.18
Item 4	Ease of reaching orgasm	0.4[c]	−0.24	−0.09	−0.13
Item 5	Orgasm satisfaction	0.09	−0.13	−0.11	−0.17

[a] n = number of patients with non-missing change score for ASEX total.
[b] $P = 0.013$ vs placebo.
[c] $P < 0.001$ vs placebo.

➤*Other adverse reactions:*

Cardiovascular – Hot flush, palpitations (at least 1%); flushing, myocardial infarction, orthostatic hypotension, peripheral coldness, tachycardia (0.1% to 1%).

In placebo-controlled clinical trials across approved indications for change from baseline to end point, duloxetine treatment was associated with mean increases in systolic blood pressure of 0.07 mm Hg and in diastolic blood pressure of 0.62 mm Hg compared with mean decreases of 1.31 mm Hg systolic and 0.73 mm Hg diastolic in placebo-treated patients. There was no significant difference in the frequency of sustained (3 consecutive visits) elevated blood pressure.

Duloxetine treatment for up to 26 weeks in placebo-controlled trials typically caused a small increase in heart rate compared with placebo of up to 1.4 beats per minute.

CNS – Abnormal dreams, chills/rigors, dysgeusia, lethargy, paresthesia/hypesthesia, sleep disorder (at least 1%); apathy, bruxism, disorientation/confusional state, disturbance in attention, dyskinesia, feeling abnormal, irritability, malaise, mood swings, myoclonus, poor quality sleep, suicide attempt (0.1% to 1%); completed suicide, dysarthria, gait disturbance (less than 0.1%).

Dermatologic – Cold sweat, dermatitis contact, erythema, increased tendency to bruise, night sweats, photosensitivity reaction (0.1% to 1%); ecchymosis (less than 0.1%).

GI – Flatulence (at least 1%); eructation, gastritis, gastroenteritis, halitosis, stomatitis (0.1% to 1%); gastric ulcer, hematochezia, melena (less than 0.1%).

GU – Abnormal orgasm/anorgasmia (at least 1%); dysuria, menopausal symptoms, micturition urgency, nocturia, polyuria, sexual dysfunction, urine odor abnormal (0.1% to 1%).

Lab test abnormalities – Duloxetine treatment in placebo-controlled clinical trials was associated with small mean increases from baseline to end point in ALT, AST, creatine phosphokinase, and alkaline phosphatase; infrequent, modest, transient, abnormal values were observed for these analyses in duloxetine-treated patients when compared with placebo-treated patients.

Metabolic/Nutritional – Weight increased (at least 1%); blood cholesterol increased, dehydration, hyperlipidemia, hypothyroidism, thirst (0.1% to 1%); dyslipidemia (less than 0.1%).

In MDD and GAD placebo-controlled clinical trials, patients treated with duloxetine for up to 10 weeks experienced a mean weight loss of approximately 0.5 kg, compared with a mean weight gain of approximately 0.2 kg in placebo-treated patients. In studies of diabetic peripheral neuropathic pain, fibromyalgia, osteoarthritis, and chronic low back pain, patients treated with duloxetine for up to 26 weeks experienced a mean weight loss of approximately 0.6 kg compared with a mean weight gain of approximately 0.2 kg in placebo-treated patients. In one long-term fibromyalgia 60-week uncontrolled study, duloxetine patients had a mean weight increase of 0.7 kg. In one long-term, chronic low back pain, 54-week study (13-week placebo-controlled acute phase and 41-week uncontrolled extension phase), duloxetine patients had a mean weight decrease of 0.6 kg in 13 weeks of acute phase compared with study entry, then a mean weight increase of 1.4 kg in 41 weeks of extension phase compared with end of acute phase.

Musculoskeletal – Musculoskeletal pain (at least 1%); muscle tightness, muscle twitching (0.1% to 1%).

Respiratory – Yawning (at least 1%); laryngitis, throat tightness (0.1% to 1%).

Special senses – Vertigo, vision blurred (at least 1%); diplopia, ear pain, tinnitus, visual disturbance (0.1% to 1%).

Miscellaneous – Feeling hot and/or cold (0.1% to 1%).

➤*Postmarketing:*

Cardiovascular – Hypertensive crisis, supraventricular arrhythmia.

CNS – Aggression and anger (particularly early in treatment or after treatment discontinuation), extrapyramidal disorder, hallucinations, restless legs syndrome, seizures upon treatment discontinuation, trismus.

Dermatologic – Erythema multiforme, rash, urticaria; serious skin reactions, including Stevens-Johnson syndrome, that have required drug discontinuation and/or hospitalization.

Special senses – Glaucoma, tinnitus (upon treatment discontinuation).

Miscellaneous – Anaphylactic reaction, angioneurotic edema, gynecological bleeding, hyperglycemia, hypersensitivity, muscle spasm.

Overdosage

➤*Symptoms:* In postmarketing experience, fatal outcomes have been reported for acute overdoses (primarily with mixed overdoses, but also with duloxetine only) at doses as low as 1,000 mg. Signs and symptoms of overdose (duloxetine alone or with mixed drugs) included coma, hypertension, hypotension, seizures, serotonin syndrome, somnolence, syncope, tachycardia, and vomiting.

➤*Treatment:* There is no specific antidote to duloxetine overdose, but if serotonin syndrome ensues, consider specific treatment (eg, with cyproheptadine and/or temperature control). In case of acute overdose, treatment should consist of those general measures employed in the management of overdose with any drug.

Ensure an adequate airway, oxygenation, and ventilation, and monitor cardiac rhythm and vital signs. Induction of emesis is not recommended. Gastric lavage with a large-bore orogastric tube with appropriate airway protection, if needed, may be indicated if performed soon after ingestion or in symptomatic patients.

Activated charcoal may be useful in limiting absorption of duloxetine from the GI tract. Administration of activated charcoal has been shown to decrease AUC and C_{max} by an average of one-third, although some subjects had a limited effect of activated charcoal. Because of the large volume of distribution of this drug, forced diuresis, dialysis, hemoperfusion, and exchange transfusion are unlikely to be beneficial.

In managing overdose, consider the possibility of multiple drug involvement. A specific caution involves patients who are taking or have recently taken duloxetine and might ingest excessive quantities of a TCA. In such a case, decreased clearance of the parent tricyclic and/or its active metabolite may increase the possibility of clinically significant sequelae and extend the time

DULOXETINE HYDROCHLORIDE — ORAL

needed for close medical observation. Consider contacting a poison control center (1-800-222-1222) for additional information on the treatment of any overdose.

Patient Information

Encourage patients, their families, and their caregivers to be alert to the emergence of aggressiveness, agitation, akathisia (psychomotor restlessness), anxiety, hostility, hypomania, impulsivity, insomnia, irritability, mania, panic attacks, or other unusual changes in behavior; worsening of depression; and suicidal ideation, especially early during antidepressant treatment and when the dose is adjusted up or down. Advise families and caregivers of patients to observe for the emergence of such symptoms on a day-to-day basis because changes may be abrupt. Report such symptoms to the patient's prescribing health care provider, especially if they are severe, abrupt in onset, or were not part of the patient's presenting symptoms. Symptoms such as these may be associated with an increased risk for suicidal thinking and behavior and indicate a need for very close monitoring and possible changes in the medication.

Instruct patients to swallow duloxetine whole and not to chew, crush, or open the capsules and sprinkle the contents on food or mix with liquids. All of these may affect the enteric coating.

Any psychoactive drug may impair judgment, thinking, or motor skills. Although in controlled studies duloxetine has not been shown to impair psychomotor performance, cognitive function, or memory, it may be associated with sedation and dizziness. Therefore, caution patients about operating hazardous machinery, including automobiles, until they are reasonably certain that duloxetine therapy does not affect their ability to engage in such activities.

Advise patients to inform their health care provider if they are taking or planning to take any prescription or nonprescription medications because there is a potential for interactions.

Although duloxetine does not increase the impairment of mental and motor skills caused by alcohol, concomitant use with heavy alcohol intake may be associated with severe liver injury. For this reason, do not generally prescribe duloxetine for patients with substantial alcohol use.

Caution patients about the risk of serotonin syndrome with the concomitant use of duloxetine and triptans, tramadol, or other serotonergic agents.

Advise patients of the risk of orthostatic hypotension and syncope, especially during the period of initial use and subsequent dose escalation, and in association with the use of concomitant drugs that might potentiate the orthostatic effect of duloxetine.

Advise patients to notify their health care provider if they become pregnant or intend to become pregnant during therapy.

Advise patients to notify their health care provider if they are breastfeeding.

While patients may notice improvement with duloxetine therapy in 1 to 4 weeks, advise them to continue therapy as directed.

Caution patients about the concomitant use of duloxetine and NSAIDs, aspirin, warfarin, or other drugs that affect coagulation because combined use of psychotropic drugs that interfere with serotonin reuptake and these agents has been associated with an increased risk of bleeding.

VENLAFAXINE

Rx	**Venlafaxine** (Various, eg, Dr. Reddy's, Mylan, Zydus)	**Tablets; oral:** 25 mg	As venlafaxine hydrochloride. May contain lactose. In 30s, 60s, 90s, 100s, 500s, 1,000s, and UD 100s.
		37.5 mg	As venlafaxine hydrochloride. May contain lactose. In 30s, 60s, 90s, 100s, 500s, 1,000s, and UD 100s.
		50 mg	As venlafaxine hydrochloride. May contain lactose. In 30s, 60s, 90s, 100s, 500s, 1,000s, and UD 100s.
		75 mg	As venlafaxine hydrochloride. May contain lactose. In 30s, 60s, 90s, 100s, 500s, 1,000s, and UD 100s.
		100 mg	As venlafaxine hydrochloride. May contain lactose. In 30s, 60s, 90s, 100s, 500s, 1,000s, and UD 100s.
Rx	**Venlafaxine** (Teva Pharmaceuticals USA)	**Capsules, extended-release; oral:** 37.5 mg	As venlafaxine hydrochloride. May contain sugar spheres. In 30s and 90s.
Rx	**Effexor XR** (Wyeth)		As venlafaxine hydrochloride. (W Effexor XR 37.5). Gray/Peach. In 15s, 30s, 90s, and *Redipak* 100s.
Rx	**Venlafaxine** (Teva Pharmaceuticals USA)	**Capsules, extended-release; oral:** 75 mg	As venlafaxine hydrochloride. May contain sugar spheres. In 30s and 90s.
Rx	**Effexor XR** (Wyeth)		As venlafaxine hydrochloride. (W Effexor XR 75). Peach. In 15s, 30s, 90s, and *Redipak* 100s.
Rx	**Venlafaxine** (Teva Pharmaceuticals USA)	**Capsules, extended-release; oral:** 150 mg	As venlafaxine hydrochloride. May contain sugar spheres. In 30s and 90s.
Rx	**Effexor XR** (Wyeth)		As venlafaxine hydrochloride. (W Effexor XR 150). Dark orange. In 15s, 30s, 90s, and *Redipak* 100s.
Rx	**Venlafaxine** (Upstate Pharma)	**Tablets, extended-release; oral:** 37.5 mg	As venlafaxine hydrochloride. May contain lactose and mannitol. In 30s and 90s.
		75 mg	As venlafaxine hydrochloride. May contain lactose and mannitol. In 30s and 90s.
		150 mg	As venlafaxine hydrochloride. May contain lactose and mannitol. In 30s and 90s.
		225 mg	As venlafaxine hydrochloride. May contain lactose and mannitol. In 30s and 90s.

VENLAFAXINE HYDROCHLORIDE — ORAL

For additional information, refer to the Antidepressants introduction.

WARNING

Suicidality and antidepressant drugs – Antidepressants increased the risk of suicidal thinking and behavior (suicidality) compared with placebo in short-term studies in children, adolescents, and young adults with major depressive disorder (MDD) and other psychiatric disorders. Anyone considering the use of venlafaxine or any other antidepressant in a child, adolescent, or young adult must balance this risk with the clinical need. Short-term studies did not show an increase in the risk of suicidality with antidepressants compared with placebo in adults older than 24 years of age; there was a reduction in risk with antidepressants compared with placebo in adults 65 years of age and older. Depression and certain other psychiatric disorders are themselves associated with increases in the risk of suicide. Closely observe and appropriately monitor patients of all ages who are started on antidepressant therapy for clinical worsening, suicidality, or unusual changes in behavior. Advise families and caregivers of the need for close observation and communication with the health care provider. Venlafaxine is not approved for use in children.

Indications

➤*Generalized anxiety disorder (extended-release capsules only):* For the treatment of generalized anxiety disorder (GAD) as defined in the *Diagnostic and Statistical Manual of Mental Disorders* (Fourth Edition) (*DSM-IV*). Anxiety or tension associated with the stress of everyday life usually does not require treatment with an anxiolytic.

➤*Major depressive disorder:* For the treatment of MDD.

➤*Panic disorder (extended-release capsules only):* For the treatment of panic disorder, with or without agoraphobia, as defined in *DSM-IV*. Panic disorder is characterized by the occurrence of unexpected panic attacks and associated concern about having additional attacks, worry about the implications or consequences of the attacks, and/or a significant change in behavior related to the attacks.

➤*Social anxiety disorder (extended-release capsules and tablets only):* For the treatment of social anxiety disorder, also known as social phobia, as defined in *DSM-IV*.

➤*Off-label uses:*

Autism – [4] = Insufficient documentation. The safety and efficacy of venlafaxine in the treatment of autism disorders have been suggested by a very small retrospective study of 10 children, adolescents, and young adults.

Binge eating disorder – [4] = Insufficient documentation. Preliminary data on the use of venlafaxine in the treatment of binge eating disorders suggest a beneficial effect.

Hot flashes – [2] = Fair documentation. Initial data note venlafaxine's benefit in the treatment of hot flashes in women (postmenopausal or history of breast cancer) and in men (prostate cancer).

VENLAFAXINE HYDROCHLORIDE — ORAL

Pain – [4] = Insufficient documentation. Venlafaxine has been studied in a variety of pain syndromes; however, data are from a limited number of patients with short-term use and noncontrolled settings. In case series data from fewer than 20 patients, venlafaxine was effective in the treatment of painful peripheral diabetic neuropathy. Various chronic pain syndromes in a very limited number of patients (fewer than 20) have also responded to short-term venlafaxine use (4 weeks to 3 months). In an open trial, 15 adult patients with fibromyalgia for 6 months or longer received a mean dose of 167 mg daily. At 8 weeks, there was a significant improvement from baseline. In a retrospective review of 170 adult patients with migraine or chronic tension-type headache, venlafaxine significantly decreased the monthly frequency of headaches, particularly moderate to severe headaches.

Premenstrual dysphoric disorder – [2] = Fair documentation. Venlafaxine was well tolerated and decreased the severity of premenstrual dysphoric symptoms in small studies.

Prevention of migraine (adults) – [4] = Insufficient documentation. American Academy of Neurology practice guidelines consider venlafaxine to be clinically effective based on consensus and clinical experience. The majority of the data evaluating venlafaxine were published after the practice guidelines. The results from these trials are favorable; however, additional data are needed to determine the optimal dosing regimen and the patient population that would most benefit from therapy.

Other possible off-label uses – Posttraumatic stress disorder (not recommended for use after no response with a selective serotonin reuptake inhibitor SSRI] for 8 weeks).

Administration and Dosage

➤*General dosing considerations:* Dosage adjustment required for patients with renal impairment (see Renal Function Impairment).

Dosage adjustment required for patients with hepatic impairment (see Hepatic Function Impairment).

Bioequivalency – Equal doses of venlafaxine extended-release tablets are bioequivalent (but not AB rated) to *Effexor XR* capsules when administered under fed conditions.

➤*Adults:*

Immediate-release tablets –

Major depressive disorder:

- *Usual dosage* – 75 to 225 mg/day.
- *Maximum dose* – 375 mg/day in 3 divided doses.
- *Initial dosage* – 75 mg/day administered in 2 or 3 divided doses and taken with food.
- *Maintenance dosage* – In outpatient settings, there was no evidence of usefulness of dosages higher than 225 mg/day for moderately depressed patients. More severely depressed inpatients respond to a mean dosage of 350 mg/day. Certain patients, including more severely depressed patients, may respond to higher dosages of up to a maximum of 375 mg/day, generally in 3 divided doses.
- *Dosage adjustment* – Depending on tolerability and the need for further clinical effect, the dosage may be increased to 150 mg/day. If needed, the dosage should be further increased up to 225 mg/day. When increasing the dose, make dosage increases in increments of up to 75 mg/day as needed and at intervals of no less than 4 days.

Extended-release capsules –

Generalized anxiety disorder:

- *Maximum dose* – 225 mg/day.
- *Initial dosage* – 75 mg/day as a single dose. For some patients, it may be desirable to start at 37.5 mg/day for 4 to 7 days to allow new patients to adjust to the medication before increasing to 75 mg/day.
- *Maintenance dosage* – 75 to 225 mg/day.
- *Dosage adjustment* – Make dosage increases in increments of up to 75 mg/day as needed and at intervals of no less than 4 days.

Major depressive disorder:

- *Maximum dose* – 225 mg/day.
- *Initial dosage* – 75 mg/day in a single dose. For some patients, it may be desirable to start at 37.5 mg/day for 4 to 7 days to allow new patients to adjust to the medication before increasing to 75 mg/day.
- *Maintenance dosage* – 75 to 225 mg/day.
- *Dosage adjustment* – Make dosage increases in increments of up to 75 mg/day as needed at intervals of no less than 4 days.
- *Conversion* – Depressed patients who are currently being treated at a therapeutic dose with venlafaxine may be switched to venlafaxine ER at the nearest equivalent dose (mg/day) (ie, venlafaxine 37.5 mg 2 times daily to venlafaxine ER 75 mg once daily). However, individual dosage adjustments may be necessary.

Panic disorder:

- *Maximum dose* – 225 mg/day.
- *Initial dosage* – 37.5 mg/day for 7 days.
- *Maintenance dosage* – 75 to 225 mg/day.
- *Dosage adjustment* – Make dosage increases in increments of up to 75 mg/day as needed at intervals of no less than 7 days.

Social anxiety disorder: 75 mg/day as a single dose.

Extended-release tablets –

Major depressive disorder: See ER capsules for dosing.

Social anxiety disorder: See ER capsules for dosing.

Off-label dosing –

Autism: [4] = Insufficient documentation. 12.5 to 50 mg daily (mean dosage, 24.37 mg daily) for a range of 1.75 to 10 months.

Binge eating disorder: [4] = Insufficient documentation. Initial dosage of 35 mg/day administered in the morning. Doses were titrated by 37.5 to 75 mg weekly to the target or maximum dosage of 300 mg/day. Median duration of 120 days (range, 28 to 300 days).

Hot flashes: [2] = Fair documentation.

- *Immediate-release formulation* – 12.5 mg twice a day for 4 weeks.
- *Extended-release formulation* – 37.5 to 150 mg once daily for up to 3 months. Doses were titrated.

Pain: [4] = Insufficient documentation. 37.5 to 375 mg daily in divided doses for up to 6 months. The most common initial dosage was 37.5 mg twice daily.

Premenstrual dysphoric disorder: [2] = Fair documentation. 37.5 to 200 mg/day, starting with either 37.5 mg once daily or 25 mg twice daily during the first menstrual cycle, then decreasing the dose as necessary at the start of subsequent menstrual cycles. Alternatively, intermittent dosing has been used, including starting 14 days prior to the start of menses with either 37.5 or 75 mg daily for 2 days, then increasing to either 75 or 112.5 mg daily for 12 days or until the start of menses, followed by 37.5 or 75 mg daily for 2 days.

Prevention of migraine (adults): [4] = Insufficient documentation. Venlafaxine doses ranged from 37.5 to 225 mg daily using the ER formulation. The 150 mg dose was most commonly studied.

➤*Children:*

Off-label dosing –

Anxiety:

- *Adolescent* –
  Initial dosage: 37.5 to 75 mg/day orally.
  Maintenance dosage: 150 to 300 mg/day orally.
- *Children* –
  Initial dosage: 37.5 mg/day orally.
  Maintenance dosage: 75 to 150 mg/day orally.

Autism (3.66 years of age and older): [4] = Insufficient documentation. 12.5 to 50 mg daily (mean dosage, 24.37 mg daily) for a range of 1.75 to 10 months.

Depression:

- *Adolescent* –
  Initial dosage: 37.5 to 75 mg/day orally.
  Maintenance dosage: 150 to 300 mg/day orally.
- *Children* –
  Initial dosage: 37.5 mg/day orally.
  Maintenance dosage: 75 to 150 mg/day orally.

➤*Elderly:* No dose adjustment is recommended for elderly patients solely on the basis of age. As with any drug for the treatment of MDD, GAD, social anxiety disorder, or panic disorder, exercise caution in elderly patients. When individualizing the dosage, take extra care when increasing the dose.

➤*Renal function impairment:* Reduce the total daily dose by 25% to 50% in patients taking ER formulations with mild to moderate renal impairment. Reduce the total daily dose by 25% in patients taking immediate release formulations. Withhold the dose until dialysis treatment is completed (4 hours) in patients undergoing hemodialysis. Because there was much individual variability in clearance between patients with renal impairment, individualization of dosing may be desirable in some patients.

➤*Hepatic function impairment:* Reduce the total daily dose by 50% in patients with mild to moderate hepatic impairment. In patients with cirrhosis, it may be necessary to reduce the dose more than 50%, and individualization of dosing may be desirable in some patients.

➤*Pregnant women during the third trimester:* Neonates exposed to venlafaxine, other serotonin-norepinephrine reuptake inhibitors (SNRIs), or SSRIs late in the third trimester have developed complications requiring prolonged hospitalization, respiratory support, and tube feeding. When treating pregnant women with venlafaxine during the third trimester, carefully consider the potential risk and benefits of treatment. Consider tapering venlafaxine in the third trimester.

➤*Switching patients to or from a monoamine oxidase inhibitor:* At least 14 days should elapse between discontinuation of a monoamine oxidase inhibitor (MAOI) and initiation of therapy with venlafaxine. In addition, allow at least 7 days after stopping venlafaxine before starting an MAOI.

➤*Discontinuation of therapy:* Symptoms associated with discontinuation of venlafaxine, other SNRIs, and SSRIs have been reported. Patients should be monitored for these symptoms when discontinuing treatment. A gradual reduction in the dose rather than abrupt cessation is recommended whenever possible. If intolerable symptoms occur following a decrease in the dose or upon discontinuation of treatment, then resuming the previously prescribed dose may be considered. Subsequently, the health care provider may continue decreasing the dose but at a more gradual rate.

➤*Administration:*

Immediate-release tablets – Administer with food.

Extended-release capsules – Administer in a single dose with food either in the morning or in the evening at approximately the same time each day. Each capsule should be swallowed whole with fluid, and not divided, crushed, chewed, or placed in water. It also may be administered by carefully opening the capsule and sprinkling the entire contents on a spoonful of applesauce. This drug/food mixture should be swallowed immediately without chewing and followed with a glass of water to ensure complete swallowing of the pellets.

VENLAFAXINE HYDROCHLORIDE — ORAL

Extended-release tablets – Administer in a single dose with food either in the morning or in the evening at approximately the same time each day. Each tablet should be swallowed whole with fluid, and not divided, crushed, chewed, or placed in water.

➤*Storage/Stability:* Store immediate-release tablets and ER capsules at 20° to 25°C (68° to 77°F) in a dry place. Store ER tablets at 25°C (77°F); excursions are permitted to between 15° and 30°C (59° and 86°F).

Actions

➤*Pharmacology:* The mechanism of the antidepressant action of venlafaxine in humans is believed to be associated with its potentiation of neurotransmitter activity in the CNS. Preclinical studies have shown that venlafaxine and its active metabolite, O-desmethylvenlafaxine, are potent inhibitors of neuronal serotonin and norepinephrine reuptake and weak inhibitors of dopamine reuptake. Venlafaxine and O-desmethylvenlafaxine have no significant affinity for muscarinic cholinergic, H_1-histaminergic, or $alpha_1$-adrenergic receptors in vitro. Pharmacologic activity at these receptors is hypothesized to be associated with the various anticholinergic, sedative, and cardiovascular effects seen with other psychotropic drugs. Venlafaxine and O-desmethylvenlafaxine do not possess MAOI activity.

➤*Pharmacokinetics:*

Absorption/Distribution – Venlafaxine is well absorbed. On the basis of mass balance studies, at least 92% of a single oral dose of venlafaxine is absorbed. The absolute bioavailability of venlafaxine is approximately 45%.

Steady-state concentrations of venlafaxine and O-desmethylvenlafaxine in plasma are attained within 3 days of oral multiple-dose therapy. Venlafaxine and O-desmethylvenlafaxine exhibited linear kinetics over the dosage range of 75 to 450 mg/day (for immediate-release tablets, administered on a schedule every 8 hours). Apparent (steady-state) volume of distribution is 7.5 ± 3.7 and 5.7 ± 1.8 L/kg, of venlafaxine and O-desmethylvenlafaxine, respectively. Venlafaxine and O-desmethylvenlafaxine are minimally bound at therapeutic concentrations to plasma proteins (27% and 30%, respectively). When equal daily doses of venlafaxine immediate-release were administered as either twice-daily or 3-times-daily regimens, the drug exposure (area under the curve AUC]) and fluctuation in plasma levels of venlafaxine and O-desmethylvenlafaxine were comparable following both regimens. Steady-state volume of distribution was unaltered for venlafaxine and O-desmethylvenlafaxine after multiple dosing.

Immediate-release: The relative bioavailability of venlafaxine from a tablet was 100% when compared with an oral solution.

Extended-release capsules: Administration of venlafaxine ER (150 mg every 24 hours) generally resulted in a lower maximum plasma concentration (C_{max}) (150 ng/mL for venlafaxine and 260 ng/mL for O-desmethylvenlafaxine) and later time to maximum plasma concentration (T_{max}) (5.5 hours for venlafaxine and 9 hours for O-desmethylvenlafaxine) than for immediate-release venlafaxine tablets (C_{max} for immediate-release 75 mg every 12 hours was 225 ng/mL for venlafaxine and 290 ng/mL for O-desmethylvenlafaxine; T_{max} was 2 hours for venlafaxine and 3 hours for O-desmethylvenlafaxine). When equal daily doses of venlafaxine were administered as either an immediate-release tablet or an ER capsule, the exposure to venlafaxine and O-desmethylvenlafaxine was similar for the 2 treatments, and the fluctuation in plasma concentrations was slightly lower with the venlafaxine ER capsule. Therefore, venlafaxine ER provides a slower rate of absorption but the same extent of absorption compared with the immediate-release tablet.

Time of administration (AM vs PM) did not affect the pharmacokinetics of venlafaxine and O-desmethylvenlafaxine from the venlafaxine ER 75 mg capsule.

Extended-release tablets: Administration of venlafaxine ER tablets 75 mg under fed conditions resulted in mean ± standard deviation (SD) venlafaxine C_{max} of 26.9 ± 13.4 ng/mL and AUC of 1,536.3 ± 496.8 ng•h/mL. T_{max} was 6.3 ± 2.3 hours. O-desmethylvenlafaxine mean ± SD C_{max}, AUC, and T_{max} after administration of venlafaxine ER tablets 75 mg were 97.9 ± 29.4 ng/mL, 2,926 ± 746.1 ng•h/mL, and 11.6 ± 2.9 hours, respectively.

- *Bioequivalency* – See Administration and Dosage for more information.
- *Effect of food* – Food did not affect the bioavailability of venlafaxine or its active metabolite, O-desmethylvenlafaxine. Food did not affect the pharmacokinetic parameters AUC, C_{max}, and T_{max} of venlafaxine or O-desmethylvenlafaxine after administration of venlafaxine ER tablets.

Metabolism/Excretion – Following absorption, venlafaxine undergoes extensive presystemic metabolism in the liver, primarily to O-desmethylvenlafaxine, but also to N-desmethylvenlafaxine, N,O-didesmethylvenlafaxine, and other minor metabolites. In vitro studies indicate that the formation of O-desmethylvenlafaxine is catalyzed by CYP2D6; this has been confirmed in a clinical study showing that patients with low CYP2D6 levels ("poor metabolizers") had increased levels of venlafaxine and reduced levels of O-desmethylvenlafaxine compared with people with normal CYP2D6 ("extensive metabolizers"). The differences between the CYP2D6 poor and extensive metabolizers are not expected to be clinically important because the sum of venlafaxine and O-desmethylvenlafaxine is similar in the 2 groups, and venlafaxine and O-desmethylvenlafaxine are pharmacologically approximately equiactive and equipotent.

Approximately 87% of a venlafaxine dose is recovered in the urine within 48 hours as unchanged venlafaxine (5%), unconjugated O-desmethylvenlafaxine (29%), conjugated O-desmethylvenlafaxine (26%), or other minor inactive metabolites (27%). Renal elimination is the primary route of excretion for venlafaxine and its metabolite. Plasma clearance and elimination half-life were unaltered for venlafaxine and O-desmethylvenlafaxine after multiple dosing. Mean ± SD steady-state plasma clearance of venlafaxine and O-desmethylvenlafaxine is 1.3 ± 0.6 and 0.4 ± 0.2 L/h/kg, respectively; apparent elimination half-life is 5 ± 2 and 11 ± 2 hours, respectively.

Special populations –

Renal function impairment: In a renal impairment study, venlafaxine elimination half-life after oral administration was prolonged approximately 50%, and clearance was reduced approximately 24% in renally impaired patients (glomerular filtration rate GFR], 10 to 70 mL/min), compared with healthy subjects. In dialysis patients, venlafaxine elimination half-life was prolonged approximately 180%, and clearance was reduced approximately 57% compared with healthy subjects. Similarly, O-desmethylvenlafaxine elimination half-life was prolonged approximately 40%, although clearance was unchanged in patients with renal impairment (GFR, 10 to 70 mL/min) compared with healthy subjects. In dialysis patients, O-desmethylvenlafaxine elimination half-life was prolonged approximately 142% and clearance was reduced approximately 56% compared with healthy subjects. A large degree of intersubject variability was noted. Dosage adjustment is necessary in these patients.

Hepatic function impairment: In 9 patients with hepatic cirrhosis, the pharmacokinetic disposition of venlafaxine and O-desmethylvenlafaxine was significantly altered after oral administration of venlafaxine. Venlafaxine elimination half-life was prolonged approximately 30%, and clearance decreased approximately 50% in cirrhotic patients compared with healthy subjects. O-desmethylvenlafaxine elimination half-life was prolonged approximately 60%, and clearance decreased approximately 30% in cirrhotic patients compared with healthy subjects. A large degree of intersubject variability was noted. Three patients with more severe cirrhosis had a more substantial decrease in venlafaxine clearance (approximately 90%) compared with healthy subjects. In a second study, venlafaxine was administered orally and intravenously in healthy (n = 21) subjects, and in Child-Pugh class A (n = 8) and Child-Pugh class B (n = 11) subjects (mildly and moderately impaired, respectively). Compared with healthy subjects, venlafaxine oral bioavailability was increased 2- to 3-fold, oral elimination half-life was approximately twice as long, and oral clearance was reduced by more than half. In hepatically impaired subjects, O-desmethylvenlafaxine oral elimination half-life was prolonged by about 40%, while oral clearance for O-desmethylvenlafaxine was similar to that for healthy subjects. A large degree of intersubject variability was noted. Dosage adjustment is necessary in these patients.

Poor/Extensive metabolizers: Plasma concentrations of venlafaxine were higher in CYP2D6 poor metabolizers than extensive metabolizers. However, because the total exposure (AUC) of venlafaxine and O-desmethylvenlafaxine was similar in poor and extensive metabolizer groups, there is no need for different venlafaxine dosing regimens for these 2 groups.

Contraindications

Hypersensitivity to venlafaxine or to any excipients in the formulation; concomitant use in patients taking MAOIs or in patients who have taken MAOIs within the preceding 14 days.

Warnings/Precautions

➤*Clinical worsening and suicide risk:* Adults and children with MDD may experience worsening of their depression and/or the emergence of suicidal ideation and behavior (suicidality) or unusual changes in behavior, whether or not they are taking antidepressant medications, and this risk may persist until significant remission occurs. Suicide is a known risk of depression and certain other psychiatric disorders, and these disorders themselves are the strongest predictors of suicide. There has been a longstanding concern that antidepressants may have a role in inducing worsening of depression and the emergence of suicidality in certain patients during the early phases of treatment.

See the Warning box for more information.

Suicidality per 1,000 Patients Treated: Antidepressants vs. Placebo	
Age range (years)	Cases
Increases compared with placebo	
< 18	14 additional cases
18 to 24	5 additional cases
Decreases compared with placebo	
25 to 64	1 fewer case
≥ 65	6 fewer cases

No suicides occurred in any of the children's trials. There were suicides in the adult trials, but the number was not sufficient to reach any conclusion about drug effect on suicide.

It is unknown whether the suicidality risk extends to longer-term use (ie, beyond several months). However, there is substantial evidence from placebo-controlled maintenance trials in adults with depression that the use of antidepressants can delay the recurrence of depression.

Closely monitor and observe all patients being treated with antidepressants for any indication of clinical worsening, suicidality, and unusual changes in behavior, especially during the initial few months of a course of drug therapy or at times of dose changes, either increases or decreases.

Consider changing the therapeutic regimen, including possibly discontinuing the medication, in patients whose depression is persistently worse or who are experiencing emergent suicidality or symptoms that might be precursors to worsening depression or suicidality, especially if these symptoms are severe, abrupt in onset, or were not part of the patient's presenting symptoms.

VENLAFAXINE HYDROCHLORIDE — ORAL

If the decision has been made to discontinue treatment, taper the medication as rapidly as is feasible but with recognition that abrupt discontinuation can be associated with certain symptoms.

➤*Bipolar disorder:* A major depressive episode may be the initial presentation of bipolar disorder. It is generally believed (though not established in controlled trials) that treating such an episode with an antidepressant alone may increase the likelihood of precipitation of a mixed/manic episode in patients at risk for bipolar disorder. Whether any of the symptoms previously described represent such a conversion is unknown. However, prior to initiating treatment with an antidepressant, adequately screen patients with depressive symptoms to determine if they are at risk for bipolar disorder; such screening should include a detailed psychiatric history, including a family history of suicide, bipolar disorder, and depression. Venlafaxine is not approved for use in treating bipolar depression.

➤*Serotonin syndrome or neuroleptic malignant syndrome–like reactions:* The development of a potentially life-threatening serotonin syndrome or neuroleptic malignant syndrome (NMS)–like reactions have been reported with SNRI and SSRIs alone, including venlafaxine treatment, but particularly with concomitant use of serotonergic drugs (including triptans) with drugs that impair metabolism of serotonin (including MAOIs), or with antipsychotics or other dopamine antagonists. Serotonin syndrome symptoms may include mental status changes (eg, agitation, coma, hallucinations), autonomic instability (eg, hyperthermia, labile blood pressure, tachycardia), neuromuscular aberrations (eg, hyperreflexia, incoordination), and/or GI symptoms (eg, diarrhea, nausea, vomiting). Serotonin syndrome in its most severe form can resemble NMS, which includes hyperthermia, muscle rigidity, autonomic instability with possible rapid fluctuations of vital signs, and mental status changes. Monitor patients for the emergence of serotonin syndrome or NMS-like signs and symptoms.

The concomitant use of venlafaxine with MAOIs intended to treat depression is contraindicated.

If concomitant use of venlafaxine with a 5-hydroxytryptamine receptor agonist (triptan) is clinically warranted, careful observation of the patient is advised, particularly during treatment initiation and dose increases.

The concomitant use of venlafaxine with serotonin precursors (eg, tryptophan) is not recommended.

Immediately discontinue treatment with venlafaxine and any concomitant serotonergic or antidopaminergic agents, including antipsychotics, if the previously described reactions occur, and initiate supportive symptomatic treatment.

➤*Blood pressure effects:*

Sustained hypertension – Venlafaxine treatment is associated with sustained hypertension (defined as treatment-emergent supine diastolic blood pressure SDBP]) 90 mm Hg or higher and 10 mm Hg or higher above baseline for 3 consecutive on-therapy visits.

Sustained increases of SDBP could have adverse consequences. Cases of elevated blood pressure requiring immediate treatment have been reported in postmarketing experience. Control preexisting hypertension before treatment with venlafaxine. It is recommended that patients receiving venlafaxine have regular monitoring of blood pressure. For patients who experience a sustained increase in blood pressure while receiving venlafaxine, consider dose reduction or discontinuation.

Immediate-release: An analysis for patients meeting the criteria for sustained hypertension revealed a dose-dependent increase in the incidence of sustained hypertension for venlafaxine.

An analysis of the patients with sustained hypertension and the 19 venlafaxine patients who were discontinued from treatment because of hypertension (less than 1% of total venlafaxine-treated group) revealed that most of the blood pressure increases were in a modest range (SDBP 10 to 15 mm Hg). Nevertheless, sustained increases of this magnitude could have adverse consequences (see Adverse Reactions).

Elevations in systolic and diastolic blood pressure –

Extended-release: In placebo-controlled premarketing studies, there were changes in mean blood pressure. Across most indications, a dose-related increase in supine systolic and diastolic blood pressure was evident in venlafaxine ER–treated patients (see Adverse Reactions).

➤*Mydriasis:* Mydriasis has been reported in association with venlafaxine; therefore, monitor patients with increased intraocular pressure or those at risk of acute narrow-angle glaucoma (angle-closure glaucoma).

➤*Discontinuation of treatment:* Discontinuation symptoms have been systematically evaluated in patients taking venlafaxine to include prospective analyses of clinical trials and retrospective surveys of trials in MDD and social anxiety disorder. Abrupt discontinuation or dose reduction of venlafaxine at various doses has been associated with the appearance of new symptoms, the frequency of which increased with increased dose level and with longer duration of treatment. Reported symptoms include agitation, anorexia, anxiety, confusion, impaired coordination and balance, diarrhea, dizziness, dry mouth, dysphoric mood, fasciculation, fatigue, flu-like symptoms, headaches, hypomania, insomnia, nausea, nervousness, nightmares, sensory disturbances (including shock-like electrical sensations), somnolence, sweating, tremor, vertigo, and vomiting.

During marketing of venlafaxine, other SNRIs, and SSRIs, there have been spontaneous reports of adverse reactions occurring with the discontinuation of these drugs, particularly when abrupt, including the following: agitation, anxiety, confusion, dizziness, dysphoric mood, emotional lability, headache, hypomania, insomnia, irritability, lethargy, seizures, sensory disturbances (ie, paresthesias such as electric shock sensations), and tinnitus. While these reactions are generally self-limiting, there have been reports of serious discontinuation symptoms.

Monitor patients for these symptoms when discontinuing treatment with venlafaxine. A gradual reduction in the dose rather than abrupt cessation is recommended whenever possible. If intolerable symptoms occur following a decrease in the dose or upon discontinuation of treatment, consider resuming the previously prescribed dose. Subsequently, the health care provider may continue decreasing the dose but at a more gradual rate.

➤*CNS effects:*

Immediate-release – Treatment-emergent anxiety, nervousness, and insomnia were more commonly reported for patients treated with venlafaxine than with placebo in a pooled analysis of short-term, double-blind, placebo-controlled depression studies.

Extended-release – Treatment-emergent insomnia and nervousness were more commonly reported for patients treated with venlafaxine ER than with placebo in pooled analyses of short-term MDD, GAD, social anxiety disorder, and panic disorder studies (see Adverse Reactions).

➤*Changes in weight:*

Immediate-release –

Adults: Dose-dependent weight loss was noted in adult patients treated with venlafaxine for several weeks. A loss of 5% or more of body weight occurred in 6% of patients treated with venlafaxine compared with 1% of patients treated with placebo and 3% of patients treated with another antidepressant. However, discontinuation of venlafaxine for weight loss was uncommon (0.1% of patients treated with venlafaxine in phase 2 and 3 depression trials).

Extended-release –

Adults: A loss of 5% or more of body weight occurred in 7% of venlafaxine ER–treated patients and 2% of patients treated with placebo in the short-term, placebo-controlled MDD trials. The discontinuation rate for weight loss associated with venlafaxine ER was 0.1% in MDD studies. In placebo-controlled GAD studies, a loss of 7% or more of body weight occurred in 3% of venlafaxine ER patients and 1% of placebo patients who received treatment for up to 6 months. The discontinuation rate for weight loss was 0.3% for patients receiving venlafaxine ER in GAD studies for up to 8 weeks. In placebo-controlled social anxiety disorder trials, 4% of venlafaxine ER–treated and 1% of treated with placebo sustained a loss of 7% or more of body weight with up to 6 months of treatment. None of the patients receiving venlafaxine ER in social anxiety disorder studies discontinued for weight loss. In placebo-controlled panic disorder trials, 3% of the venlafaxine ER–treated and 2% of the patients treated with placebo sustained a loss of 7% or more of body weight with up to 12 weeks of treatment. None of the patients receiving venlafaxine ER in panic disorder studies discontinued for weight loss.

Children: Weight loss has been observed in children 6 to 17 years of age receiving venlafaxine ER. In a pooled analysis of four 8-week, double-blind, placebo-controlled, flexible-dose outpatient trials for MDD and GAD, venlafaxine ER–treated patients lost an average of 0.45 kg (n = 333), while patients treated with placebo gained an average of 0.77 kg (n = 333). More patients treated with venlafaxine ER than with placebo experienced a weight loss of at least 3.5% in the MDD and the GAD studies (18% of venlafaxine ER–treated patients vs 3.6% of patients treated with placebo; $P < 0.001$). In a 16-week double-blind, placebo-controlled, flexible-dose outpatient trial for social anxiety disorder, venlafaxine ER–treated patients lost an average of 0.75 kg (n = 137), while patients treated with placebo gained an average of 0.76 kg (n = 148). More patients treated with venlafaxine ER than with placebo experienced a weight loss of at least 3.5% in the social anxiety disorder study (47% of venlafaxine ER–treated patients vs 14% of patients treated with placebo; $P < 0.001$). Weight loss was not limited to patients with treatment-emergent anorexia.

The risks associated with longer-term venlafaxine ER use were assessed in an open-label MDD study of children and adolescents who received venlafaxine ER for up to 6 months. The children and adolescents in the study had increases in weight that were less than expected based on data from age- and sex-matched peers. The difference between observed weight gain and expected weight gain was larger for children (younger than 12 years of age) than for adolescents (12 years of age and older).

Coadministration with weight-loss agents – The safety and efficacy of venlafaxine therapy in combination with weight-loss agents, including phentermine, have not been established. Coadministration of venlafaxine and weight-loss agents is not recommended. Venlafaxine is not indicated for weight loss alone or in combination with other products.

➤*Changes in height:* During the 8-week, placebo-controlled GAD studies, patients (6 to 17 years of age) treated with venlafaxine ER grew an average of 0.3 cm (n = 122), while patients treated with placebo grew an average of 1 cm (n = 132; $P = 0.041$). This difference in height increase was most notable in patients younger than 12 years of age. During the 8-week placebo-controlled MDD studies, patients treated with venlafaxine ER grew an average of 0.8 cm (n = 146), while patients treated with placebo grew an average of 0.7 cm (n = 147). During the 16-week placebo-controlled social anxiety disorder study, the patients treated with venlafaxine ER (n = 109) and the patients treated with placebo (n = 112) each grew an average of 1 cm. In the 6-month, open-label MDD study, children and adolescents had height increases that were less than expected based on data from age- and sex-matched peers. The difference between observed growth rates and expected growth rates was larger for children (younger than 12 years of age) than for adolescents (12 years of age and older).

VENLAFAXINE HYDROCHLORIDE — ORAL

➤*Changes in appetite:*

Immediate-release – Treatment-emergent anorexia was more commonly reported for venlafaxine-treated (11%) than adult patients treated with placebo (2%) in the pool of short-term, double-blind, placebo-controlled depression studies.

Extended-release –

Adults: Treatment-emergent anorexia was more commonly reported for venlafaxine ER–treated (8%) than patients treated with placebo (4%) in the pool of short-term, double-blind, placebo-controlled MDD studies. The discontinuation rate for anorexia associated with venlafaxine ER was 1% in MDD studies. Treatment-emergent anorexia was more commonly reported for venlafaxine ER–treated (8%) than patients treated with placebo (2%) in the pool of short-term, double-blind, placebo-controlled GAD studies. The discontinuation rate for anorexia was 0.9% for patients receiving venlafaxine ER for up to 8 weeks in GAD studies. Treatment-emergent anorexia was more commonly reported for venlafaxine ER–treated (17%) than patients treated with placebo (2%) in the pool of short-term, double-blind, placebo-controlled social anxiety disorder studies. The discontinuation rate for anorexia was 0.6% for patients receiving venlafaxine for up to 12 weeks in social anxiety disorder studies; no patients discontinued because of anorexia between week 12 and month 6. Treatment-emergent anorexia was more commonly reported for venlafaxine ER–treated (8%) than patients treated with placebo (3%) in the pool of short-term, double-blind, placebo-controlled panic disorder studies. The discontinuation rate for anorexia was 0.4% for patients receiving venlafaxine ER for up to 12 weeks in panic disorder studies.

Children: Decreased appetite has been observed in children receiving venlafaxine ER. In the placebo-controlled trials for GAD and MDD, 10% of patients 6 to 17 years of age treated with venlafaxine ER for up to 8 weeks and 3% of patients treated with placebo reported treatment-emergent anorexia. None of the patients receiving venlafaxine ER discontinued for anorexia or weight loss. In the placebo-controlled trial for social anxiety disorder, 22% and 3% of patients 8 to 17 years of age treated for up to 16 weeks with venlafaxine ER and placebo, respectively, reported treatment-emergent anorexia. The discontinuation rates for anorexia were 0.7% and 0% for patients receiving venlafaxine ER and placebo, respectively; the discontinuation rates for weight loss were 0.7% for patients receiving either venlafaxine ER or placebo.

➤*Activation of mania/hypomania:* Activation of mania/hypomania has also been reported in a small proportion of patients with major affective disorder who were treated with other marketed antidepressants. As with all antidepressants, use venlafaxine cautiously in patients with a history of mania.

Immediate-release – During phase 2 and 3 trials, hypomania or mania occurred in 0.5% of patients treated with venlafaxine.

Extended-release – During premarketing MDD studies, mania or hypomania occurred in 0.3% of venlafaxine ER–treated patients and no placebo patients. In premarketing GAD studies, no venlafaxine ER–treated patients and 0.2% of patients treated with placebo experienced mania or hypomania. In premarketing social anxiety disorder studies, 0.2% venlafaxine ER–treated patients and no patients treated with placebo experienced mania or hypomania. In premarketing panic disorder studies, 0.1% of venlafaxine ER–treated patients and no patients treated with placebo experienced mania or hypomania.

➤*Hyponatremia:* Hyponatremia may occur as a result of treatment with SSRIs and SNRIs, including venlafaxine. In many cases, this hyponatremia appears to be the result of the syndrome of inappropriate antidiuretic hormone secretion. Cases with serum sodium lower than 110 mmol/L have been reported. Elderly patients may be at a greater risk of developing hyponatremia with SSRIs and SNRIs. Also, patients taking diuretics or who are otherwise volume depleted may be at greater risk. Consider discontinuation of venlafaxine in patients with symptomatic hyponatremia and institute appropriate medical intervention.

Signs and symptoms of hyponatremia include headache, difficulty concentrating, memory impairment, confusion, weakness, and unsteadiness, which may lead to falls. Signs and symptoms associated with more severe and/or acute cases have included hallucination, syncope, seizure, coma, respiration arrest, and death.

➤*Seizures:* Use venlafaxine cautiously in patients with a history of seizures. Discontinue the drug in any patient who develops seizures.

Immediate-release – During premarketing testing, seizures were reported in 0.26% of patients treated with venlafaxine. Most seizures (5/8) occurred in patients receiving dosages of 150 mg/day or less.

Extended-release – During premarketing experience, no seizures occurred among 705 venlafaxine ER–treated patients in the MDD studies, among 1,381 patients treated with venlafaxine ER in GAD studies, or among 819 patients treated with venlafaxine ER patients in social anxiety disorder studies. In panic disorder studies, 1 seizure occurred among 1,001 patients treated with venlafaxine ER.

➤*Abnormal bleeding:* SSRIs and SNRIs, including venlafaxine, may increase the risk of bleeding reactions. Concomitant use of aspirin, nonsteroidal anti-inflammatory drugs (NSAIDs), warfarin, and other anticoagulants may add to this risk. Case reports and epidemiological studies (case-control and cohort design) have demonstrated an association between use of drugs that interfere with serotonin reuptake and the occurrence of GI bleeding. Bleeding reactions related to SSRI and SNRI use have ranged from ecchymoses, hematomas, epistaxis, and petechiae to life-threatening hemorrhages.

➤*Serum cholesterol elevation:* Clinically relevant increases in serum cholesterol were recorded in 5.3% of patients treated with venlafaxine and 0% of patients treated with placebo treated for at least 3 months in placebo-controlled trials. Consider measurement of serum cholesterol levels during long-term treatment.

➤*Interstitial lung disease and eosinophilic pneumonia:* Interstitial lung disease and eosinophilic pneumonia associated with venlafaxine therapy have been rarely reported. Consider the possibility of these adverse reactions in patients treated with venlafaxine who present with progressive dyspnea, cough, or chest discomfort. Such patients should undergo a prompt medical evaluation. Consider discontinuation of venlafaxine therapy.

➤*Cardiac effects:* Venlafaxine has not been evaluated or used to any appreciable extent in patients with a recent history of myocardial infarction or unstable heart disease. Patients with these diagnoses were systematically excluded from many clinical studies during venlafaxine's premarketing testing.

Exercise caution in patients whose underlying medical conditions might be compromised by increases in heart rate (ie, patients with hyperthyroidism, heart failure, or recent myocardial infarction), particularly when using dosages of venlafaxine of more than 200 mg/day (see Adverse Reactions for more information).

➤*Electroconvulsive therapy:* There are no clinical data establishing the benefit of electroconvulsive therapy combined with venlafaxine treatment.

➤*Renal/Hepatic function impairment:* In patients with renal impairment (GFR, 10 to 70 mL/min) or cirrhosis of the liver, the clearances of venlafaxine and its active metabolites were decreased, thus prolonging the elimination half-lives of these substances. A lower dose may be necessary. Like all antidepressants, use venlafaxine with caution in such patients.

➤*Pregnancy: Category C* (per manufacturer's prescribing information); *Category C/Category D* in second half of pregnancy (per Briggs *Drugs in Pregnancy and Lactation*). There are no adequate and well-controlled studies in pregnant women. Because animal reproduction studies are not always predictive of human response, use this drug during pregnancy only if clearly needed.

Teratogenic – Venlafaxine did not cause malformations in offspring of rats or rabbits given doses of up to 11 times (rat) or 12 times (rabbit) the maximum recommended human daily dose on a mg/kg basis, or 2.5 times (rat) and 4 times (rabbit) the human daily dose on a mg/m^2 basis. However, in rats, there was a decrease in pup weight, an increase in stillborn pups, and an increase in pup deaths during the first 5 days of lactation, when dosing began during pregnancy and continued until weaning. The cause of these deaths is not known. These effects occurred at 10 times (mg/kg) or 2.5 times (mg/m^2) the maximum human daily dose. The no-effect dose for rat pup mortality was 1.4 times the human dose on a mg/kg basis or 0.25 times the human dose on a mg/m^2 basis.

Nonteratogenic – Neonates exposed to venlafaxine, other SNRIs, or SSRIs late in the third trimester have developed complications requiring prolonged hospitalization, respiratory support, and tube feeding. Such complications can arise immediately upon delivery. Reported clinical findings have included respiratory distress, cyanosis, apnea, seizures, temperature instability, feeding difficulty, vomiting, hypoglycemia, hypotonia, hypertonia, hyperreflexia, tremor, jitteriness, irritability, and constant crying. These features are consistent with either a direct toxic effect of SSRIs and SNRIs or, possibly, a drug discontinuation syndrome. It should be noted that, in some cases, the clinical picture is consistent with serotonin syndrome. When treating a pregnant woman with venlafaxine during the third trimester, carefully consider the potential risks and benefits of treatment.

SSRIs and venlafaxine have been associated with developmental toxicities, including spontaneous abortions, low birth weight, prematurity, neonatal serotonin syndrome, neonatal behavioral syndrome (withdrawal, including seizures), possibly sustained abnormal neuro-behavior beyond the neonatal period, and respiratory distress. Persistent pulmonary hypertension of the newborn is an additional potential risk, but confirmation is needed.

➤*Lactation:* Venlafaxine and O-desmethylvenlafaxine have been reported to be excreted in human milk. Because of the potential for serious adverse reactions in breast-feeding infants from venlafaxine, decide whether to discontinue breast-feeding or the drug, taking into account the importance of the drug to the mother.

The American Academy of Pediatrics classifies other antidepressants as drugs for which the effect on breast-feeding infants is unknown but may be of concern. Monitor breast-fed infants for excessive sedation and adequate weight gain if venlafaxine is used during lactation, possibly including O-desmethylvenlafaxine serum levels to rule out toxicity if there is concern.

➤*Children:* Safety and effectiveness in children have not been established. Two placebo-controlled trials in 766 children with MDD and 2 placebo-controlled trials in 793 children with GAD have been conducted with venlafaxine ER, and the data were not sufficient to support a claim for use in children.

Anyone considering the use of venlafaxine in a child or adolescent must balance the potential risks with the clinical need.

Although no studies have been designed to primarily assess the impact of venlafaxine ER on the growth, development, and maturation of children and adolescents, studies suggest that venlafaxine ER may adversely affect weight and height. Should the decision be made to treat a child with venlafaxine, regular monitoring of weight and height is recommended during treatment, particularly if it is continued long term. The safety of venlafaxine ER treatment for children has not been systematically assessed for treatment longer than 6 months.

VENLAFAXINE HYDROCHLORIDE — ORAL

In the studies conducted in children 6 to 17 years of age, the occurrence of blood pressure and cholesterol increases considered to be clinically relevant in children was similar to that observed in adult patients. Consequently, the precautions for adults apply to children.

➤*Monitoring:* Monitor all patients for clinical worsening, suicidality, and unusual changes in behavior. Monitor patients for adverse reactions during discontinuation of therapy. Monitor sodium levels periodically during venlafaxine therapy. Consider measurement of serum cholesterol levels during long-term treatment. Monitor blood pressure and heart rate regularly during venlafaxine treatment. Monitor patients with raised intraocular pressure or who are at risk of acute narrow-angle glaucoma (angle-closure glaucoma).

Drug Interactions

➤*QT prolongation:* An additive effect of venlafaxine with other drugs that prolong the QT interval cannot be excluded. The following drugs may prolong the QT interval and increase the risk of life-threatening cardiac arrhythmias, including torsades de pointes: antiarrhythmic agents (eg, amiodarone, bretylium, disopyramide, dofetilide, procainamide, quinidine, sotalol), arsenic trioxide, chlorpromazine, cisapride, dolasetron, droperidol, mefloquine, mesoridazine, moxifloxacin, pentamidine, pimozide, tacrolimus, thioridazine, and ziprasidone. For a more complete list of drugs that may prolong the QT interval, see the appendix, Drug-Induced Prolongation of the QT Interval and Torsades de Pointes.

Venlafaxine Drug Interactions

Precipitant drug	Object drug[a]		Description
Aspirin, NSAIDs (eg, ibuprofen, naproxen)	Venlafaxine	↑	Concurrent use of NSAIDs or aspirin may increase the risk of upper GI bleeding. Caution patients about the increased risk of bleeding.
Azole antifungals (eg, itraconazole, ketoconazole)	Venlafaxine	↑	Ketoconazole increased venlafaxine C_{max} 26% in EMs[b] and 48% in PMs and AUC 21% in EMs and 70% in PMs. O-desmethylvenlafaxine C_{max} was increased 14% in EMs and 29% in PMs; AUC was increased 23% and 141% in EMs and PMs, respectively. Closely monitor the clinical response when starting or stopping an azole antifungal agent. Adjust the venlafaxine dose as needed.
Cimetidine	Venlafaxine	↑	Concomitant use reduced oral clearance by ≈ 43%, and AUC and C_{max} increased by ≈ 60%. However, cimetidine had no apparent effect on O-desmethylvenlafaxine. Consequently, the overall pharmacologic activity is expected to increase only slightly in healthy subjects. Use with caution in patients with hypertension and hepatic impairment, and in elderly patients.
Cyproheptadine	Venlafaxine	↓	Decreased pharmacologic effects of venlafaxine may occur. If coadministration cannot be avoided, closely monitor the clinical response. If an interaction is suspected, consider discontinuing cyproheptadine.
Fenfluramine	Venlafaxine	↑	Serotonin syndrome may occur because of additive serotonergic effects. Concurrent use is not recommended.
Venlafaxine	Fenfluramine		
Lithium	Venlafaxine	↑	Elevated lithium levels and neurotoxicity may occur. Serotonin syndrome, including irritability, increased muscle tone, shivering, myoclonus, and altered consciousness, may occur. Closely monitor the patient for adverse reactions, including signs and symptoms of serotonin syndrome. Serotonin syndrome requires immediate medical attention, including withdrawal of the serotonergic agent and supportive care.
Venlafaxine	Lithium		

Venlafaxine Drug Interactions

Precipitant drug	Object drug[a]		Description
MAOIs (eg, phenelzine)	Venlafaxine	↑	Serious and sometimes fatal reactions may occur, including hyperthermia, rigidity, myoclonus, autonomic instability with possible rapid fluctuation of vital signs, and mental status changes that include extreme agitation progressing to delirium and coma (see Warnings/Precautions). Concomitant use as well as use in patients who have taken MAOIs within the preceding 14 days is contraindicated.
Methylene blue	Venlafaxine	↑	The risk of CNS toxicity, including serotonin syndrome, may be increased. Use an alternative agent for methylene blue.
Methylphenidate	Venlafaxine	↑	Serotonin syndrome may occur because of additive effects. Closely monitor the patient for adverse reactions. Serotonin syndrome requires immediate medical attention, including withdrawal of the serotonergic agent and supportive care.
Venlafaxine	Methylphenidate		
Nefazodone	Venlafaxine	↑	Serotonin syndrome may occur because of additive serotonergic effects. Closely monitor the patient for adverse reactions. Serotonin syndrome requires immediate medical attention, including withdrawal of the serotonergic agent and supportive care.
Venlafaxine	Nefazodone		
Opioid analgesics (eg, meperidine)	Venlafaxine	↑	Serotonin syndrome may occur because of additive serotonergic effects. Closely monitor the patient for adverse reactions. Serotonin syndrome requires immediate medical attention, including withdrawal of the serotonergic agent and supportive care.
Venlafaxine	Opioid analgesics (eg, meperidine)		
Propafenone	Venlafaxine	↑	Propafenone and venlafaxine plasma concentrations may be increased. Closely monitor for increased pharmacologic and toxic effects of propafenone and venlafaxine. Adjust treatment as needed.
Venlafaxine	Propafenone		
Rasagiline	Venlafaxine	↑	Serotonin syndrome may occur because of additive or synergistic serotonergic effects. Closely monitor the patient for adverse reactions. Serotonin syndrome requires immediate medical attention, including withdrawal of the serotonergic agent and supportive care.
Venlafaxine	Rasagiline		
Sour date nut	Venlafaxine	↑	The risk of serotonin syndrome may be increased. Closely monitor the patient for adverse reactions. Patients taking venlafaxine should avoid sour date nut.
Terbinafine	Venlafaxine	↑	Venlafaxine plasma concentrations may be elevated, increasing the pharmacologic and adverse reactions. Monitor the clinical response and observe the patient for adverse reactions. Adjust the venlafaxine dose as needed.
L-tryptophan	Venlafaxine	↑	Serotonin syndrome may occur because of additive or synergistic serotonergic effects. Concurrent use is not recommended.
Venlafaxine	L-tryptophan		

VENLAFAXINE HYDROCHLORIDE — ORAL

Venlafaxine Drug Interactions

Precipitant drug	Object drug[a]		Description
Venlafaxine	Bupropion	↑	Unexpected adverse reactions, including serotonin syndrome, may occur. Closely monitor the patient. If an interaction is suspected, stop one or both drugs. Serotonin syndrome requires immediate medical attention, including withdrawal of the serotonergic agent and supportive care.
Bupropion	Venlafaxine		Paradoxical worsening of obsessive compulsive disorder or serotonin syndrome has been reported. If coadministration cannot be avoided, closely monitor the patient for worsening clinical status, as well as serotonin syndrome. Serotonin syndrome requires immediate medical attention, including withdrawal of the serotonergic agent and supportive care.
Venlafaxine	Clozapine	↑	There have been reports of elevated clozapine levels resulting in adverse reactions, including seizures, following the addition of venlafaxine. Monitor the clinical response and adjust the clozapine dose as needed when venlafaxine is started or stopped.
Venlafaxine	Dextromethorphan	↑	Dextromethorphan plasma concentrations and risk of toxicity may be increased. If coadministration cannot be avoided, closely monitor the clinical response and adjust the dextromethorphan dose as needed.
Venlafaxine	Haloperidol	↑	Venlafaxine decreased total oral-dose clearance of a single dose of haloperidol 42%, which resulted in a 70% increase in haloperidol AUC. In addition, the haloperidol C_{max} increased 88%. Monitor haloperidol concentrations and the clinical response. Adjust the haloperidol dose as needed.
Venlafaxine	Indinavir	↓	Venlafaxine resulted in a 28% decrease in the AUC of a single oral dose of indinavir and a 36% decrease in indinavir C_{max}. The clinical significance of this is unknown. Use with caution and monitor the clinical response.
Venlafaxine	Metoprolol	↓	Venlafaxine reduced the blood pressure–lowering effect of metoprolol. The clinical relevance of this finding is unknown; however, exercise caution with coadministration. Closely monitor blood pressure.
Venlafaxine	Serotonergic drugs (eg, linezolid, metoclopramide); sibutramine, tramadol, trazodone	↑	Serotonin syndrome, including irritability, increased muscle tone, shivering, myoclonus, and altered consciousness, may occur. If coadministration cannot be avoided, closely monitor the patient for adverse reactions, including signs and symptoms of serotonin syndrome. Serotonin syndrome requires immediate medical attention, including withdrawal of the serotonergic agent and supportive care.
Venlafaxine	SSRIs or SNRIs (eg, fluoxetine, paroxetine)	↑	Serotonin syndrome, including irritability, increased muscle tone, shivering, myoclonus, and altered consciousness, may occur. Closely monitor the patient for adverse reactions, including signs and symptoms of serotonin syndrome. Serotonin syndrome requires immediate medical attention, including withdrawal of the serotonergic agent and supportive care.
Venlafaxine	St. John's wort	↑	Serotonin syndrome, including irritability, increased muscle tone, shivering, myoclonus, and altered consciousness, may occur. Closely monitor the patient for adverse reactions, including signs and symptoms of serotonin syndrome. Serotonin syndrome requires immediate medical attention, including withdrawal of the serotonergic agent and supportive care.
Venlafaxine	Sympathomimetics (eg, amphetamine)	↑	Serotonin syndrome, including irritability, increased muscle tone, shivering, myoclonus, and altered consciousness, may occur. Closely monitor the patient for adverse reactions, including signs and symptoms of serotonin syndrome. Serotonin syndrome requires immediate medical attention, including withdrawal of the serotonergic agent and supportive care.
Venlafaxine	Tricyclic antidepressants (eg, desipramine)	↑	TCA levels may be elevated, increasing the pharmacologic and adverse effects. Desipramine AUC, C_{max}, and C_{min} increased approximately 35% in the presence of venlafaxine. The 2-OH-desipramine AUC increased at least 2.5- to 4.5-fold. Monitor the clinical response and plasma concentrations when starting or stopping venlafaxine. Adjust the TCA dose as needed.
Venlafaxine	Triptans (eg, sumatriptan, zolmitriptan)	↑	Serotonin syndrome, including irritability, increased muscle tone, shivering, myoclonus, and altered consciousness, may occur. Closely monitor the patient for adverse reactions, including signs and symptoms of serotonin syndrome. Serotonin syndrome requires immediate medical attention, including withdrawal of the serotonergic agent and supportive care.
Venlafaxine	Warfarin	↑	There have been reports of increases in prothrombin time, partial thromboplastin time, or international normalized ratio when venlafaxine was administered to patients also receiving warfarin. Monitor coagulation parameters when starting or stopping venlafaxine and adjust the warfarin dose as needed. Caution patients about the increased risk of bleeding.

[a] ↑ = object drug increased; ↓ = object drug decreased.
[b] EM = extensive metabolizer; PM = poor metabolizer; TCA = tricyclic antidepressant; C_{min} = minimum plasma concentration.

➤*Drug/Lab test interactions:* Venlafaxine may reduce uptake and diagnostic efficacy of lobenguane. False-negative lobenguane imaging test may result.

VENLAFAXINE HYDROCHLORIDE — ORAL

Adverse Reactions

➤*Immediate-release tablets:*

Discontinuation of treatment – Nineteen percent of venlafaxine patients in phase 2 and 3 depression studies discontinued treatment because of an adverse reaction.

Venlafaxine Adverse Reactions Associated With Discontinuation		
	Venlafaxine	Placebo
CNS		
Anxiety	2%	1%
Asthenia	2%	< 1%
Dizziness	3%	< 1%
Dry mouth	2%	< 1%
Headache	3%	1%
Insomnia	3%	1%
Nervousness	2%	< 1%
Somnolence	3%	1%
Miscellaneous		
Abnormal ejaculation[a]	3%	< 1%
Nausea	6%	1%
Sweating	2%	< 1%

[a] Percentages based on the number of males.

Common adverse reactions – The most commonly observed adverse reactions associated with the use of venlafaxine (incidence of 5% or more) and not seen at an equivalent incidence among patients treated with placebo (ie, incidence for venlafaxine at least twice that for placebo), derived from the 1% incidence, were anorexia, anxiety, asthenia, blurred vision, constipation, dizziness, dry mouth, nausea, nervousness, somnolence, sweating, tremor, and vomiting, as well as abnormal ejaculation/orgasm and impotence in men.

Dose-dependent adverse reactions: A comparison of adverse reaction rates in a fixed-dosage study comparing venlafaxine 75, 225, and 375 mg/day with placebo revealed a dosage dependency for some of the more common adverse reactions associated with venlafaxine use. The rule for including reactions was to enumerate those that occurred at an incidence of 5% or more for at least 1 of the venlafaxine groups and for which the incidence was at least twice the placebo incidence for at least 1 venlafaxine group. Tests for potential dosage relationships for these reactions (Cochran-Armitage test, with a criterion of exact 2-sided $P \leq 0.05$) suggested a dosage-dependency for several adverse reactions in this list, including abnormal ejaculation, agitation, anorexia, chills, dizziness, hypertension, nausea, somnolence, sweating, tremor, and yawning.

Venlafaxine Adverse Reactions in a Dosage-Comparison Trial				
Adverse reactions	Venlafaxine 75 mg/day (n = 89)	Venlafaxine 225 mg/day (n = 89)	Venlafaxine 375 mg/day (n = 88)	Placebo (n = 92)
Cardiovascular				
Hypertension	1.1%	2.2%	4.5%	1.1%
Vasodilation	4.5%	5.6%	2.3%	0%
CNS				
Agitation	1.1%	2.2%	4.5%	0%
Anxiety	11.2%	4.5%	2.3%	4.3%
Asthenia	16.9%	14.6%	14.8%	3.3%
Decreased libido	2.2%	1.1%	5.7%	1.1%
Dizziness	19.1%	22.5%	23.9%	4.3%
Insomnia	22.5%	20.2%	13.6%	9.8%
Nervousness	21.3%	13.5%	12.5%	4.3%
Somnolence	16.9%	18%	26.1%	4.3%
Tremor	1.1%	2.2%	10.2%	0%
GI				
Abdominal pain	3.4%	2.2%	8%	3.3%
Anorexia	14.6%	13.5%	17%	2.2%
Dyspepsia	6.7%	6.7%	4.5%	2.2%
Nausea	32.6%	38.2%	58%	14.1%
Vomiting	7.9%	3.4%	6.8%	1.1%
GU				
Abnormal ejaculation/orgasm	4.5%	2.2%	12.5%	0%
Impotence (number of men)	5.8%	2.1%	3.6%	0%
Miscellaneous				
Abnormality of accommodation	9.1%	7.9%	5.6%	0%
Chills	2.2%	5.6%	6.8%	1.1%
Infection	2.2%	5.6%	2.3%	2.2%
Sweating	6.7%	12.4%	19.3%	5.4%
Yawning	4.5%	5.6%	8%	0%

Adaptation to adverse reactions: Over a 6-week period, there was evidence of adaptation to some adverse reactions with continued therapy (eg, dizziness, nausea) but less to other reactions (eg, abnormal ejaculation, dry mouth).

➤*Extended-release:*

Discontinuation of treatment – Approximately 11% of the 357 patients who received venlafaxine ER in placebo-controlled clinical trials for MDD discontinued treatment because of an adverse reaction, compared with 6% of the 285 patients treated with placebo in those studies. Approximately 18% of the 1,381 patients who received venlafaxine ER in placebo-controlled clinical trials for GAD discontinued treatment because of an adverse reaction, compared with 12% of the 555 patients treated with placebo in those studies. Approximately 15% of the 819 patients who received venlafaxine ER capsules in placebo-controlled clinical trials for social anxiety disorder discontinued treatment because of an adverse reaction, compared with 5% of the 695 patients treated with placebo in those studies. Approximately 7% of the 1,001 patients who received venlafaxine ER in placebo-controlled clinical trials for panic disorder discontinued treatment because of an adverse reaction, compared with 6% of the 662 patients treated with placebo in those studies. The most common reactions leading to discontinuation and considered to be drug-related (ie, leading to discontinuation in at least 1% of the patients treated with venlafaxine ER at a rate at least twice that of placebo for any indication) are provided.

Venlafaxine ER Adverse Reactions Leading to Discontinuation[a]								
	MDD[b]		GAD[c,d]		Social anxiety disorder[e]		Panic disorder	
Adverse reactions	Venlafaxine ER (n = 357)	Placebo (n = 285)	Venlafaxine ER (n = 1,381)	Placebo (n = 555)	Venlafaxine ER (n = 819)	Placebo (n = 695)	Venlafaxine ER (n = 1,001)	Placebo (n = 662)
CNS								
Asthenia	—	—	3%	< 1%	2%	< 1%	1%	0%
Dizziness	2%	1%	—	—	2%	< 1%	—	—
Headache	—	—	—	—	1%	< 1%	—	—
Insomnia	1%	< 1%	3%	< 1%	2%	< 1%	1%	< 1%
Nervousness	—	—	2%	< 1%	—	—	—	—
Somnolence	2%	< 1%	3%	< 1%	2%	< 1%	—	—
Tremor	—	—	1%	0%	—	—	—	—
GI								
Anorexia	1%	< 1%	—	—	—	—	—	—
Dry mouth	1%	0%	2%	< 1%	—	—	—	—
Nausea	4%	< 1%	8%	< 1%	3%	< 1%	2%	< 1%
Vomiting	—	—	1%	< 1%	—	—	—	—

VENLAFAXINE HYDROCHLORIDE — ORAL

Venlafaxine ER Adverse Reactions Leading to Discontinuation[a]

Adverse reactions	MDD[b]		GAD[c,d]		Social anxiety disorder[e]		Panic disorder	
	Venlafaxine ER (n = 357)	Placebo (n = 285)	Venlafaxine ER (n = 1,381)	Placebo (n = 555)	Venlafaxine ER (n = 819)	Placebo (n = 695)	Venlafaxine ER (n = 1,001)	Placebo (n = 662)
Miscellaneous								
Impotence[f]	—	—	—	—	2%	0%	—	—
Sweating	—	—	2%	< 1%	—	—	—	—

[a] Two of the MDD studies were flexible dose and 1 was fixed dose. Four of the GAD studies were fixed dose and 1 was flexible dose. Four of the social anxiety disorder studies were flexible dose and 1 was fixed/flexible dose. Two of the panic disorder studies were flexible dose and 2 were fixed dose.
[b] In US placebo-controlled trials for MDD, the following were also common reactions leading to discontinuation and were considered to be drug-related for patients treated with venlafaxine ER (percent venlafaxine ER, n = 192, percent placebo, n = 202): hypertension (1%, < 1%); diarrhea (1%, 0%); paresthesia (1%, 0%); tremor (1%, 0%); abnormal vision, mostly blurred vision (1%, 0%); abnormal, mostly delayed, ejaculation (1%, 0%).
[c] In 2 short-term, US, placebo-controlled trials for GAD, the following were also common reactions leading to discontinuation and were considered to be drug-related for patients treated with venlafaxine ER (percent venlafaxine ER, n = 476, percent placebo, n = 201): headache (4%, < 1%); vasodilation (1%, 0%); anorexia (2%, < 1%); dizziness (4%, 1%); abnormal thinking (1%, 0%); abnormal vision (1%, 0%).
[d] In long-term, placebo-controlled trials for GAD, the following was also a common reaction leading to discontinuation and was considered to be drug-related for patients treated with venlafaxine ER (percent venlafaxine ER, n = 535, percent placebo, n = 257): decreased libido (1%, 0%).
[e] In a 6-month placebo-controlled trial for social anxiety disorder, the following was also a common reaction leading to discontinuation and was considered to be drug-related for venlafaxine ER–treated patients (percent venlafaxine ER, n = 257, percent placebo, n = 129: depression (5%, 0%); libido decrease (1%, 0%); nervousness (3%, 0%).
[f] Incidence is based on the number of men (venlafaxine ER = 454, placebo = 357).

Major depressive disorder –

Common adverse reactions: The following adverse reactions occurred in at least 5% of the patients treated with venlafaxine and at a rate of at least twice that of the placebo group for all placebo-controlled trials for MDD: abnormal ejaculation, CNS complaints (dizziness, somnolence, and abnormal dreams), GI complaints (nausea, dry mouth, and anorexia), and sweating. In the 2 US, placebo-controlled trials, the following additional reactions occurred in at least 5% of patients treated with venlafaxine ER (n = 192) and at a rate at least twice that of the placebo group: abnormalities of sexual function (anorgasmia in women, impotence in men, and decreased libido), cardiovascular effects (hypertension and vasodilation), CNS complaints (insomnia, nervousness, and tremor), GI complaints (constipation and flatulence), problems of special senses (abnormal vision), and yawning.

Venlafaxine ER Adverse Reactions (≥ 2%) in Major Depressive Disorder[a,b]

Adverse reactions	Venlafaxine ER (n = 357)	Placebo (n = 285)
Cardiovascular		
Hypertension	4%	1%
Vasodilation[c]	4%	2%
CNS		
Abnormal dreams[d]	7%	2%
Agitation	3%	1%
Asthenia	8%	7%
Decreased libido	3%	< 1%
Depression	3%	< 1%
Dizziness	20%	9%
Insomnia	17%	11%
Nervousness	10%	5%
Paresthesia	3%	1%
Somnolence	17%	8%
Tremor	5%	2%
GI		
Anorexia	8%	4%
Constipation	8%	5%
Dry mouth	12%	6%
Flatulence	4%	3%
Nausea	31%	12%
Vomiting	4%	2%
GU		
Abnormal ejaculation (male)[e,f]	16%	< 1%
Anorgasmia (female)[g,h]	3%	< 1%
Impotence[f]	4%	< 1%
Respiratory		
Pharyngitis	7%	6%
Yawning	3%	0%
Miscellaneous		
Abnormal vision[i]	4%	< 1%
Sweating	14%	3%
Weight loss	3%	0%

[a] Incidence, rounded to the nearest percent, for reactions reported by ≥ 2% of patients treated with venlafaxine ER, except the following reactions that had an incidence less than or equal to placebo: abdominal pain, accidental injury, anxiety, back pain, bronchitis, diarrhea, dysmenorrhea, dyspepsia, flu syndrome, headache, infection, pain, palpitation, rhinitis, and sinusitis.
[b] < 1% indicates an incidence > 0% but < 1%.
[c] Mostly hot flashes.
[d] Mostly vivid dreams, nightmares, and increased dreaming.
[e] Mostly delayed ejaculation.
[f] Incidence is based on the number of men.
[g] Mostly delayed orgasm or anorgasmia.
[h] Incidence is based on the number of women.
[i] Mostly blurred vision and difficulty focusing eyes.

Generalized anxiety disorder –

Most common adverse reactions: The following adverse reactions occurred in at least 5% of the venlafaxine ER patients and at a rate at least twice that of the placebo group for all placebo-controlled trials for the GAD indication: abnormalities of sexual function (abnormal ejaculation and impotence), GI complaints (anorexia, constipation, dry mouth, and nausea), problems of special senses (abnormal vision), and sweating.

Venlafaxine ER Adverse Reactions (≥ 2%) in Generalized Anxiety Disorder[a,b]

Adverse reactions	Venlafaxine ER (n = 1,381)	Placebo (n = 555)
CNS		
Abnormal dreams[c]	3%	2%
Asthenia	12%	8%
Decreased libido	4%	2%
Dizziness	16%	11%
Hypertonia	3%	2%
Insomnia	15%	10%
Nervousness	6%	4%
Paresthesia	2%	1%
Somnolence	14%	8%
Tremor	4%	< 1%
GI		
Anorexia	8%	2%
Constipation	10%	4%
Dry mouth	16%	6%
Nausea	35%	12%
Vomiting	5%	3%
GU		
Abnormal ejaculation[d,e]	11%	< 1%
Impotence[e]	5%	< 1%
Orgasmic dysfunction (women)[f,g]	2%	0%
Miscellaneous		
Abnormal vision[h]	5%	< 1%
Sweating	10%	3%
Vasodilation[i]	4%	2%
Yawning	3%	< 1%

[a] Adverse reactions for which the venlafaxine ER reporting rate was less than or equal to the placebo rate are not included. These reactions are abdominal pain, accidental injury, anxiety, back pain, diarrhea, dysmenorrhea, dyspepsia, flu syndrome, headache, infection, myalgia, pain, palpitation, pharyngitis, rhinitis, tinnitus, and urinary frequency.
[b] < 1% means > 0% but < 1%.
[c] Mostly vivid dreams, nightmares, and increased dreaming.
[d] Includes delayed ejaculation and anorgasmia.
[e] Percentages based on the number of men (venlafaxine ER = 525, placebo = 220).
[f] Includes delayed orgasm, abnormal orgasm, and anorgasmia.
[g] Percentages based on the number of women (venlafaxine ER = 856, placebo = 335).
[h] Mostly blurred vision and difficulty focusing eyes.
[i] Mostly hot flashes.

VENLAFAXINE HYDROCHLORIDE — ORAL

Social anxiety disorder –

Most common adverse reactions: The following adverse reactions occurred in at least 5% of the venlafaxine ER patients and at a rate of at least twice that of the placebo group for the 5 placebo-controlled trials for social anxiety disorder: abnormalities of sexual function (abnormal ejaculation, impotence), asthenia, CNS complaints (decreased libido, insomnia, nervousness, somnolence, tremor), GI complaints (anorexia, constipation, dry mouth, nausea), yawning, and sweating.

In the 6-month trial, the following adverse reactions occurred twice as often in the venlafaxine ER 150 to 225 mg/day group compared with the venlafaxine ER 75 mg/day group and placebo: abnormal vision, decreased libido, impotence, tremor, vasodilation, yawning.

Venlafaxine ER Adverse Reactions (≥ 2%) in Social Anxiety Disorder[a,b]

Adverse reactions	Venlafaxine ER (n = 819)	Placebo (n = 695)
Cardiovascular		
Hypertension	5%	3%
Palpitation	3%	1%
Vasodilation[c]	3%	2%
CNS		
Abnormal dreams[d]	3%	< 1%
Agitation	3%	1%
Anxiety	5%	4%
Asthenia	19%	9%
Decreased libido	8%	2%
Dizziness	16%	8%
Headache	38%	34%
Insomnia	24%	8%
Nervousness	10%	5%
Somnolence	20%	8%
Tremor	5%	2%
Twitching	3%	< 1%
GI		
Abdominal pain	6%	4%
Anorexia[e]	17%	2%
Constipation	9%	3%
Diarrhea	8%	6%
Dry mouth	17%	4%
Dyspepsia	7%	6%
Nausea	31%	9%
Vomiting	3%	2%
GU		
Abnormal ejaculation[f,g]	19%	< 1%
Impotence[g]	6%	< 1%
Orgasmic dysfunction[h,i]	5%	< 1%
Miscellaneous		
Abnormal vision[j]	4%	2%
Accidental injury	4%	3%
Sweating	13%	4%
Weight loss	2%	< 1%
Yawning	5%	< 1%

[a] Adverse reactions for which the venlafaxine ER reporting rate was less than or equal to the placebo rate are not included. These reactions are arthralgia, back pain, dysmenorrhea, flu syndrome, infection, pain, pharyngitis, rhinitis, and upper respiratory tract infection.
[b] < 1% means > 0% but < 1%.
[c] Mostly hot flashes.
[d] Mostly vivid dreams, nightmares, and increased dreaming.
[e] Mostly decreased appetite and loss of appetite.
[f] Includes delayed ejaculation and anorgasmia.
[g] Percentages based on the number of men (venlafaxine ER = 454, placebo = 357).
[h] Includes abnormal orgasm and anorgasmia.
[i] Percentages based on the number of women (venlafaxine ER = 365, placebo = 338).
[j] Mostly blurred vision.

Panic disorder –

Most common adverse reactions: The following adverse reactions occurred in at least 5% of the venlafaxine ER patients and at a rate at least twice that of the placebo group for 4 placebo-controlled trials for panic disorder: abnormalities of sexual function (abnormal ejaculation), CNS complaints (somnolence, tremor), GI complaints (anorexia, constipation, dry mouth), and sweating.

Venlafaxine ER Adverse Reactions (≥ 2%) in Panic Disorder[a,b]

Adverse reactions	Venlafaxine ER (n = 1,001)	Placebo (n = 662)
Cardiovascular		
Hypertension	4%	3%
Vasodilation[c]	3%	2%
CNS		
Asthenia	10%	8%
Decreased libido	4%	2%
Dizziness	11%	10%
Insomnia	17%	9%
Somnolence	12%	6%
Tremor	5%	2%
GI		
Anorexia[d]	8%	3%
Constipation	9%	3%
Dry mouth	12%	6%
Nausea	21%	14%
GU		
Abnormal ejaculation[e,f]	8%	< 1%
Impotence[f]	4%	< 1%
Orgasmic dysfunction[g,h]	2%	< 1%
Miscellaneous		
Sweating	10%	2%

[a] Adverse reactions for which the venlafaxine ER reporting rate was less than or equal to the placebo rate are not included. These reactions are abdominal pain, abnormal vision, accidental injury, anxiety, back pain, diarrhea, dysmenorrhea, dyspepsia, flu syndrome, headache, infection, nervousness, pain, paresthesia, pharyngitis, rash, rhinitis, and vomiting.
[b] < 1% means > 0% but < 1%.
[c] Mostly hot flushes.
[d] Mostly decreased appetite and loss of appetite.
[e] Includes delayed or retarded ejaculation and anorgasmia.
[f] Percentage based on the number of men (venlafaxine ER = 335, placebo = 238).
[g] Includes anorgasmia and delayed orgasm.
[h] Percentage based on the number of women (venlafaxine ER = 666, placebo = 424).

CNS

Venlafaxine Treatment-Emergent Anxiety, Insomnia, and Nervousness

Symptoms	Venlafaxine (n = 1,033)	Placebo (n = 609)
Anxiety	6%	3%
Insomnia	18%	10%
Nervousness	13%	6%

Anxiety, nervousness, and insomnia led to drug discontinuation in 2%, 2%, and 3%, respectively, of the patients treated with venlafaxine in the phase 2 and 3 depression studies.

Venlafaxine ER Treatment-Emergent Insomnia and Nervousness

	MDD		GAD		Social anxiety disorder		Panic disorder	
Symptoms	Venlafaxine ER (n = 357)	Placebo (n = 285)	Venlafaxine ER (n = 1,381)	Placebo (n = 555)	Venlafaxine ER (n = 819)	Placebo (n = 695)	Venlafaxine ER (n = 1,001)	Placebo (n = 662)
Insomnia	17%	11%	15%	10%	24%	8%	17%	9%
Nervousness	10%	5%	6%	4%	10%	5%	4%	6%

Insomnia and nervousness each led to drug discontinuation in 0.9% of the patients treated with venlafaxine ER in MDD studies.

In GAD trials, insomnia and nervousness led to drug discontinuation in 3% and 2%, respectively, of the patients treated with venlafaxine ER for up to 8 weeks and 2% and 0.7%, respectively, of the patients treated with venlafaxine ER for up to 6 months.

In social anxiety disorder trials, insomnia and nervousness led to drug discontinuation in 2% and 1%, respectively, of the patients treated with venlafaxine ER for up to 12 weeks and 2% and 3%, respectively, of the patients treated with venlafaxine ER for up to 6 months.

In panic disorder trials, insomnia and nervousness led to drug discontinuation in 1% and 0.1%, respectively, of the patients treated with venlafaxine ER for up to 12 weeks.

➤*Vital sign changes:*

Immediate-release – Venlafaxine treatment (averaged over all dose groups) in clinical trials was associated with a mean increase in pulse rate of approximately 3 beats per minute, compared with no change for placebo. In

VENLAFAXINE HYDROCHLORIDE — ORAL

a flexible-dose study, with dosages in the range of 200 to 375 mg/day and mean dosage of more than 300 mg/day, the mean pulse was increased by about 2 beats per minute compared with a decrease of about 1 beat per minute for placebo.

In controlled clinical trials, venlafaxine was associated with mean increases in diastolic blood pressure ranging from 0.7 to 2.5 mm Hg averaged over all dose groups, compared with mean decreases ranging from 0.9 to 3.8 mm Hg for placebo. However, there is a dose dependency for blood pressure increase.

In a premarketing study comparing 3 fixed dosages of venlafaxine (75, 225, and 375 mg/day) and placebo, a mean increase in SDBP of 7.2 mm Hg was seen in the 375 mg/day group at week 6 compared with essentially no changes in the 75 and 225 mg/day groups and a mean decrease in SDBP of 2.2 mm Hg in the placebo group (see Warnings/Precautions).

Venlafaxine Probability of Sustained Elevation in Supine Diastolic Blood Pressure

Treatment group	Incidence of sustained elevation in SDBP
Venlafaxine	
< 100 mg/day	3%
101 to 200 mg/day	5%
201 to 300 mg/day	7%
> 300 mg/day	13%
Placebo	2%

Extended-release – Venlafaxine ER treatment for up to 12 weeks in premarketing placebo-controlled MDD trials was associated with a mean final on-therapy increase in pulse rate of approximately 2 beats per minute, compared with 1 beat per minute for placebo. Venlafaxine ER treatment for up to 8 weeks in premarketing placebo-controlled GAD trials was associated with a mean final on-therapy increase in pulse rate of approximately 2 beats per minute, compared with less than 1 beat per minute for placebo. Venlafaxine ER treatment for up to 12 weeks in the premarketing placebo-controlled social anxiety disorder trials was associated with mean final on-therapy increase in pulse rate of approximately 3 beats per minute, compared with an increase of about 1 beat per minute for placebo. Venlafaxine ER treatment for up to 12 weeks in premarketing placebo-controlled panic disorder trials was associated with a mean final on-therapy increase in pulse rate of approximately 1 beat per minute, compared with a decrease of less than 1 beat per minute for placebo.

An insufficient number of patients received mean dosages of venlafaxine more than 300 mg/day to fully evaluate the incidence of sustained increases in blood pressure at these higher doses.

Venlafaxine ER Sustained Elevations in Supine Diastolic Blood Pressure by Indication

MDD (75 to 375 mg/day)	GAD (37.5 to 225 mg/day)	Social anxiety disorder (75 to 225 mg/day)	Panic disorder (75 to 225 mg/day)
3%	0.5%	0.6%	0.9%

In premarketing MDD studies, 0.7% of the patients treated with venlafaxine ER discontinued treatment because of elevated blood pressure. Among these patients, most of the blood pressure increases were in a modest range (SDBP, 12 to 16 mm Hg). In premarketing GAD studies for up to 8 weeks and for up to 6 months, 0.7% and 1.3% of the patients treated with venlafaxine ER, respectively, discontinued treatment because of elevated blood pressure. Among these patients, most of the blood pressure increases were in a modest range (SDBP, 12 to 25 mm Hg in up to 8 weeks; 8 to 28 mm Hg up to 6 months). In premarketing social anxiety disorder studies for up to 6 months, 0.6% of the patients treated with venlafaxine ER discontinued treatment because of elevated blood pressure. In these patients, the blood pressure increases were modest (SDBP, 1 to 24 mm Hg). In premarketing panic disorder studies for up to 12 weeks, 0.5% of the patients treated with venlafaxine ER discontinued treatment because of elevated blood pressure. In these patients, the blood pressure increases were in a modest range (SDBP, 7 to 19 mm Hg).

Across all clinical trials in MDD, GAD, social anxiety disorder, and panic disorder, 1.4% of patients in the venlafaxine ER–treated groups experienced a 15 mm Hg or more increase in supine diastolic blood pressure with blood pressure 105 mm Hg or more, compared with 0.9% of patients in the placebo groups. Similarly, 1% of patients in the venlafaxine ER–treated groups experienced a 20 mm Hg or more increase in supine systolic blood pressure with blood pressure 180 mm Hg or more, compared with 0.3% of patients in the placebo groups.

Venlafaxine ER Mean Changes from Baseline in Supine Systolic and Diastolic Blood Pressure (mm Hg)

	Venlafaxine ER				Placebo	
	≤ 75 mg/day		> 75 mg/day			
	SSBP[a]	SDBP	SSBP	SDBP	SSBP	SDBP
MDD						
8 to 12 weeks	−0.28	0.37	2.93	3.56	−1.08	−0.1
GAD						
8 weeks	−0.28	0.02	2.4	1.68	−1.26	−0.92
6 months	1.27	−0.69	2.06	1.28	−1.29	−0.74
Social anxiety disorder						
12 weeks	−0.29	−1.26	1.18	1.34	−1.96	−1.22
6 months	−0.98	−0.49	2.51	1.96	−1.84	−0.65
Panic disorder						
10 to 12 weeks	−1.15	0.97	−0.36	0.16	−1.29	−0.99

[a] SSBP = supine systolic blood pressure.

➤*Lab test abnormalities:*

Immediate-release – Of the serum chemistry and hematology parameters monitored during clinical trials with venlafaxine, a statistically significant difference with placebo was seen only for serum cholesterol. In premarketing trials, treatment with venlafaxine tablets was associated with a mean final on-therapy increase in total cholesterol of 3 mg/dL.

Patients treated with venlafaxine tablets for at least 3 months in placebo-controlled, 12-month extension trials had a mean final on-therapy increase in total cholesterol of 9.1 mg/dL compared with a decrease of 7.1 mg/dL among patients treated with placebo. This increase was duration-dependent over the study period and tended to be greater with higher doses. Clinically relevant increases in serum cholesterol, defined as

1.) a final on-therapy increase in serum cholesterol of 50 mg/dL or more from baseline and to a value of 261 mg/dL or more
2.) an average on-therapy increase in serum cholesterol of 50 mg/dL or more from baseline and to a value of 261 mg/dL or more were recorded in 5.3% of patients treated with venlafaxine and 0% of patients treated with placebo.

Extended-release –

Serum cholesterol: Venlafaxine ER treatment for up to 12 weeks in premarketing placebo-controlled MDD trials was associated with a mean final on-therapy increase in serum cholesterol concentration of approximately 1.5 mg/dL compared with a mean final decrease of 7.4 mg/dL for placebo. Venlafaxine ER treatment for up to 8 weeks and for up to 6 months in premarketing placebo-controlled GAD trials was associated with mean final on-therapy increases in serum cholesterol concentration of approximately 1 and 2.3 mg/dL, respectively, while placebo subjects experienced mean final decreases of 4.9 and 7.7 mg/dL, respectively. Venlafaxine ER treatment for up to 12 weeks and for up to 6 months in premarketing placebo-controlled social anxiety disorder trials was associated with mean final on-therapy increases in serum cholesterol concentration of approximately 7.9 and 5.6 mg/dL, respectively, compared with a mean final decrease of 2.9 and 4.2 mg/dL, respectively, for placebo. Venlafaxine ER treatment for up to 12 weeks in premarketing placebo-controlled panic disorder trials was associated with mean final on-therapy increases in serum cholesterol concentration of approximately 5.8 mg/dL, compared with a mean final decrease of 3.7 mg/dL for placebo.

Serum triglycerides: Venlafaxine ER treatment for up to 12 weeks in pooled premarketing social anxiety disorder trials was associated with a mean final on-therapy increase in fasting serum triglyceride concentration of approximately 8.2 mg/dL, compared with a mean final increase of 0.4 mg/dL for placebo. Venlafaxine ER treatment for up to 6 months in a premarketing social anxiety disorder trial was associated with a mean final on-therapy increase in fasting serum triglyceride concentration of approximately 11.8 mg/dL, compared with a mean final on-therapy increase of 1.8 mg/dL for placebo.

Venlafaxine ER treatment for up to 12 weeks in pooled premarketing panic disorder trials was associated with a mean final on-therapy increase in fasting serum triglyceride concentration of approximately 5.9 mg/dL, compared with a mean final increase of 0.9 mg/dL for placebo. Venlafaxine ER treatment for up to 6 months in a premarketing panic disorder trial was associated with a mean final on-therapy increase in fasting serum triglyceride concentration of approximately 9.3 mg/dL, compared with a mean final on-therapy decrease of 0.3 mg/dL for placebo.

➤*Electrocardiogram changes:*

Immediate-release – In an analysis of electrocardiograms (ECGs) obtained in 769 patients treated with venlafaxine and 450 patients treated with placebo in controlled clinical trials, the only statistically significant difference observed was for heart rate (ie, a mean increase from baseline of 4 beats per minute for venlafaxine). In a flexible-dosage study, with dosages in the range of 200 to 375 mg/day and mean dosage of more than 300 mg/day, the mean change in heart rate was 8.5 beats per minute with venlafaxine compared with 1.7 beats per minute for placebo.

Extended-release – ECGs were analyzed for 275 patients who received venlafaxine ER and 220 patients who received placebo in 8- to 12-week, double-blind, placebo-controlled trials in MDD; for 610 patients who received venlafaxine ER and 298 patients who received placebo in 8-week, double-blind, placebo-controlled trials in GAD; for 593 patients who received venlafaxine ER and 534 patients who received placebo in 12-week, double-blind, placebo-controlled trials in social anxiety disorder; and for 661 patients who received venlafaxine ER and 395 patients who received placebo in three 10- to 12-week, double-blind, placebo-controlled trials in panic disorder. The mean change from baseline in QTc for patients treated with venlafaxine ER in MDD studies was increased relative to that for patients treated with placebo (an increase of 4.7 msec for venlafaxine ER and a decrease of 1.9 msec for placebo). The mean change from baseline in

VENLAFAXINE HYDROCHLORIDE — ORAL

QTc for patients treated with venlafaxine ER in the GAD studies did not differ significantly from that with placebo. The mean change from baseline in QTc for patients treated with venlafaxine ER in the social anxiety disorder studies was increased relative to that for patients treated with placebo (an increase of 3.4 msec for venlafaxine ER and a decrease of 1.6 msec for placebo). The mean change from baseline in QTc for patients treated with venlafaxine ER in the panic disorder studies was increased relative to that for patients treated with placebo (an increase of 1.5 msec for venlafaxine ER and a decrease of 0.7 msec for placebo).

In these same trials, the mean change from baseline in heart rate for patients treated with venlafaxine ER in the MDD studies was significantly higher than that for placebo (a mean increase of 4 beats per minute for venlafaxine ER and 1 beat per minute for placebo). The mean change from baseline in heart rate for patients treated with venlafaxine ER in the GAD studies was significantly higher than that for placebo (a mean increase of 3 beats per minute for venlafaxine ER and no change for placebo). The mean change from baseline in heart rate for patients treated with venlafaxine ER in the social anxiety disorder studies was significantly higher than that for placebo (a mean increase of 5 beats per minute for venlafaxine ER and no change for placebo). The mean change from baseline in heart rate for venlafaxine ER–treated patients in the panic disorder studies was significantly higher than that for placebo (a mean increase of 3 beats per minute for venlafaxine ER and a mean decrease of less than 1 beat per minute for placebo).

➤*Other adverse reactions:* Reactions are further categorized by body system and listed using the following definitions: frequent adverse reactions are defined as those occurring on 1 or more occasions in at least 1 of 100 (1%) patients; infrequent adverse reactions are those occurring in 1 of 100 to 1 of 1,000 (0.1% to 1%) patients; and rare reactions are those occurring in fewer than 1 of 1,000 (less than 0.1%) patients.

Cardiovascular – Tachycardia (at least 1%); angina pectoris, arrhythmia, bradycardia, extrasystoles, hypotension, peripheral vascular disorder (mainly cold feet or cold hands), postural hypotension, syncope, thrombophlebitis (0.1% to 1%); aortic aneurysm, arteritis, bigeminy, bundle branch block, capillary fragility, cardiovascular disorder (mitral valve disorder and circulatory disturbance), cerebral ischemia, congestive heart failure, coronary artery disease, first-degree atrioventricular block, heart arrest, hematoma, mucocutaneous hemorrhage, myocardial infarct, pallor, sinus arrythmia (less than 0.1%).

CNS – Abnormal thinking, amnesia, confusion, depersonalization, hypesthesia, migraine, trismus, vertigo (at least 1%); abnormal speech, akathisia, apathy, ataxia, circumoral paresthesia, CNS stimulation, emotional lability, euphoria, hallucinations, hostility, hyperesthesia, hyperkinesia, hypotonia, incoordination, increased libido, malaise, manic reaction, myoclonus, neuralgia, neuropathy, psychosis, seizure, stupor, suicidal ideation, suicide attempt (0.1% to 1%); abnormal/changed behavior, abnormal gait, adjustment disorder, akinesia, alcohol abuse, aphasia, bradykinesia, buccoglossal syndrome, cerebrovascular accident, delusions, dementia, dystonia, energy increased, facial paralysis, feeling drunk, Guillain-Barré syndrome, homicidal ideation, hyperchlorhydria, hypokinesia, hysteria, impulse control difficulties, loss of consciousness, motion sickness, neuritis, nystagmus, paranoid reaction, paresis, psychotic depression, reflexes decreased, reflexes increased, torticollis (less than 0.1%).

Dermatologic – Pruritus (at least 1%); acne, alopecia, brittle nails, contact dermatitis, dry skin, eczema, maculopapular rash, psoriasis, skin hypertrophy, urticaria (0.1% to 1%); erythema nodosum, exfoliative dermatitis, furunculosis, hair discoloration, hirsutism, leukoderma, lichenoid dermatitis, miliaria, petechial rash, pruritic rash, pustular rash, seborrhea, skin atrophy, skin discoloration, skin striae, sweating decreased, vesiculobullous rash (less than 0.1%).

Endocrine – Galactorrhea, goiter, hyperthyroidism, hypothyroidism, thyroid nodule, thyroiditis (less than 0.1%).

GI – Eructation, increased appetite (at least 1%); bruxism, colitis, dysphagia, esophagitis, gastritis, gastroenteritis, GI ulcer, gingivitis, glossitis, hemorrhoids, melena, mouth ulceration, oral moniliasis, rectal hemorrhage, stomatitis, tongue edema (0.1% to 1%); abdominal distension, appendicitis, biliary pain, cellulitis, cheilitis, cholecystitis, cholelithiasis, duodenitis, esophageal spasms, gastroesophageal reflux disease, GI hemorrhage, gum hemorrhage, hematemesis, hepatitis, ileitis, increased salivation, intestinal obstruction, jaundice, liver tenderness, parotitis, periodontitis, proctitis, rectal disorder, salivary gland enlargement, soft stools, tongue discoloration (less than 0.1%).

GU – Based on the number of men and women as appropriate.

Albuminuria, metrorrhagia, prostatic disorder (prostatitis, enlarged prostate, and prostate irritability), urination impaired, vaginitis (at least 1%); amenorrhea, breast pain, cystitis, dysuria, hematuria, kidney calculus, kidney pain, leukorrhea, menorrhagia, nocturia, pelvic pain, polyuria, pyuria, urinary incontinence, urinary retention, urinary urgency, vaginal hemorrhage (0.1% to 1%); abortion, anuria, balanitis, bladder pain, breast discharge, breast engorgement, breast enlargement, calcium crystalluria, cervicitis, endometriosis, female lactation, fibrocystic breast, gynecomastia (male), hypomenorrhea, kidney function abnormal, mastitis, menopause, oliguria, orchitis, ovarian cyst, prolonged erection, pyelonephritis, salpingitis, urolithiasis, uterine hemorrhage, uterine spasm, vaginal dryness (less than 0.1%).

Hematologic/Lymphatic – Ecchymosis (at least 1%); anemia, leukocytosis, leukopenia, lymphadenopathy, thrombocythemia, thrombocytopenia (0.1% to 1%); basophilia, bleeding time increased, cyanosis, eosinophilia, lymphocytosis, multiple myeloma, purpura (less than 0.1%).

Metabolic/Nutritional – Edema, weight gain (at least 1%); alkaline phosphatase increased, dehydration, hypercholesteremia, hyperglycemia, hyperlipidemia, hypokalemia, ALT increased, AST increased, thirst (0.1% to 1%); alcohol intolerance, bilirubinemia, creatinine increased, diabetes mellitus, glycosuria, gout, healing abnormal, hemochromatosis, hypercalcinuria, hyperkalemia, hyperphosphatemia, hyperuricemia, hypocholesteremia, hypoglycemia, hyponatremia, hypophosphatemia, hypoproteinemia, serum urea nitrogen increased, uremia (less than 0.1%).

Musculoskeletal – Neck pain (at least 1%); arthritis, arthrosis, bone pain, bone spurs, bursitis, leg cramps, myasthenia, neck rigidity, tenosynovitis (0.1% to 1%); muscle cramp, muscle spasms, musculoskeletal stiffness, myopathy, osteoporosis, osteosclerosis, pathological fracture, plantar fasciitis, rheumatoid arthritis, tendon rupture (less than 0.1%).

Respiratory – Bronchitis, cough increased, dyspnea (at least 1%); asthma, chest congestion, epistaxis, hyperventilation, laryngismus, laryngitis, pneumonia, voice alteration (0.1% to 1%); atelectasis, hemoptysis, hypoventilation, hypoxia, larynx edema, pleurisy, pulmonary embolus, sleep apnea (less than 0.1%).

Special senses – Abnormal vision, abnormality of accommodation, mydriasis, taste perversion (at least 1%); cataract, conjunctivitis, corneal lesion, diplopia, dry eyes, eye pain, hyperacusis, otitis media, parosmia, photophobia, taste loss, visual field defect (0.1% to 1%); blepharitis, chromatopsia, conjunctival edema, deafness, decreased pupillary reflex, exophthalmos, eye hemorrhage, glaucoma, retinal hemorrhage, subconjunctival hemorrhage, keratitis, labyrinthitis, miosis, papilledema, otitis externa, scleritis, uveitis (less than 0.1%).

Miscellaneous – Accidental injury, chest pain substernal, chills, fever (at least 1%); face edema, intentional injury, moniliasis, photosensitivity reaction, withdrawal syndrome (0.1% to 1%); bacteremia, carcinoma, granuloma (less than 0.1%).

➤*Postmarketing:* Voluntary reports of other adverse reactions temporarily associated with the use of venlafaxine that have been received since market introduction and that may have no causal relationship with the use of venlafaxine include the following: agranulocytosis; anaphylaxis; angioedema; angle-closure glaucoma; aplastic anemia; catatonia; congenital anomalies; creatine phosphokinase increased; deep vein thrombophlebitis; delirium, ECG abnormalities such as QT prolongation; impaired coordination and balance; cardiac arrhythmias, including atrial fibrillation, supraventricular tachycardia, ventricular extrasystoles, and rare reports of ventricular fibrillation and ventricular tachycardia, including torsades de pointes; toxic epidermal necrosis/Stevens-Johnson syndrome; erythema multiforme; extrapyramidal symptoms (including dyskinesia and tardive dyskinesia); hemorrhage (including eye and GI bleeding); hepatic reactions (including gamma glutamyltransferase elevation; abnormalities of unspecified liver function tests; liver damage, necrosis, or failure; and fatty liver); interstitial lung disease; involuntary movements; lactate dehydrogenase increased; neutropenia; night sweats; pancreatitis; pancytopenia; panic; prolactin increased; renal failure; rhabdomyolysis; serotonin syndrome; shock-like electrical sensations or tinnitus (in some cases, subsequent to the discontinuation of venlafaxine or tapering of dose); and syndrome of inappropriate antidiuretic hormone secretion (usually in elderly patients).

Overdosage

➤*Symptoms:*

Immediate-release – There were 14 reports of acute overdose with venlafaxine, either alone or in combination with other drugs and/or alcohol, among the patients included in the premarketing evaluation. The majority of the reports involved ingestions in which the total dose of venlafaxine taken was estimated to be no more than several-fold higher than the usual therapeutic dose. The 3 patients who took the highest doses were estimated to have ingested approximately 6.75, 2.75, and 2.5 g. The resulting peak plasma levels of venlafaxine for the latter 2 patients were 6.24 and 2.35 mcg/mL, respectively, and the peak plasma levels of O-desmethylvenlafaxine were 3.37 and 1.3 mcg/mL, respectively. Plasma venlafaxine levels were not obtained for the patient who ingested venlafaxine 6.75 g. All 14 patients recovered without sequelae. Most patients reported no symptoms. Among the remaining patients, somnolence was the most commonly reported symptom. The patient who ingested venlafaxine 2.75 g was observed to have 2 generalized convulsions and a prolongation of QTc to 500 msec, compared with 405 msec at baseline. Mild sinus tachycardia was reported in 2 of the other patients.

Extended-release – Among the patients included in the premarketing evaluation of venlafaxine ER, there were 2 reports of acute overdosage with venlafaxine ER in MDD trials, either alone or in combination with other drugs. One patient took a combination of venlafaxine ER 6 g and lorazepam 2.5 mg. This patient was hospitalized, treated symptomatically, and recovered without any untoward effects. The other patient took venlafaxine ER 2.85 g. This patient reported paresthesia of all 4 limbs but recovered without sequelae.

There were 2 reports of acute overdose with venlafaxine ER in GAD trials. One patient took a combination of venlafaxine ER 0.75 g, paroxetine 200 mg, and zolpidem 50 mg. This patient was described as being alert, able to communicate, and a little sleepy. This patient was hospitalized, treated with activated charcoal, and recovered without any untoward effects. The other patient took venlafaxine ER 1.2 g. This patient recovered, and no other specific problems were found. The patient had moderate dizziness, nausea, numb hands and feet, and hot-cold spells 5 days after the overdose. These symptoms resolved over the next week.

There were 2 reports of acute overdose with venlafaxine ER in panic disorder trials. One patient took venlafaxine ER 0.675 g once, and the other patient took venlafaxine ER 0.45 g for 2 days. No signs or symptoms were

VENLAFAXINE HYDROCHLORIDE — ORAL

associated with either overdose, and no actions were taken to treat them. In postmarketing experience, overdose with venlafaxine has occurred predominantly in combination with alcohol or other drugs. The most commonly reported reactions in overdosage include tachycardia, changes in level of consciousness (ranging from somnolence to coma), mydriasis, seizures, and vomiting. ECG changes (eg, prolongation of QT interval, bundle branch block, QRS prolongation), ventricular tachycardia, bradycardia, hypotension, liver necrosis, rhabdomyolysis, serotonin syndrome, vertigo, and death have also been reported.

Published retrospective studies report that venlafaxine overdosage may be associated with an increased risk of fatal outcomes compared with that observed with SSRI antidepressant products, but lower than that for tricyclic antidepressants. Epidemiological studies have shown that patients treated with venlafaxine have a higher preexisting burden of suicide risk factors than patients treated with SSRIs. The extent to which the finding of an increased risk of fatal outcomes can be attributed to the toxicity of venlafaxine in overdosage as opposed to some characteristics of patients treated with venlafaxine is not clear. Prescriptions for venlafaxine should be written for the smallest quantity consistent with good patient management, in order to reduce the risk of overdose.

➤*Treatment:* Treatment should consist of general measures employed in the management of overdosage with any antidepressant.

Ensure an adequate airway, oxygenation, and ventilation. Monitor cardiac rhythm and vital signs. General supportive and symptomatic measures are also recommended. Induction of emesis is not recommended. Gastric lavage with a large bore orogastric tube with appropriate airway protection, if needed, may be indicated if performed soon after ingestion or in symptomatic patients.

Administer activated charcoal. Because of the large volume of distribution of this drug, forced diuresis, dialysis, hemoperfusion, and exchange transfusion are unlikely to be of benefit. No specific antidotes for venlafaxine are known.

In managing overdosage, consider the possibility of multiple drug involvement. Consider contacting a poison control center for additional information on the treatment of any overdose.

Patient Information

Inform patients, their families, and their caregivers about the benefits and risks associated with treatment with venlafaxine and counsel them in its appropriate use. A patient Medication Guide called "Antidepressant Medicines, Depression and Other Serious Mental Illness, and Suicidal Thoughts or Actions" is available for venlafaxine. Instruct patients, their families, and their caregivers to read the Medication Guide, and assist them in understanding its contents. Give patients the opportunity to discuss the contents of the Medication Guide and to obtain answers to any questions they may have.

Encourage patients, their families, and their caregivers to be alert to the emergence of anxiety, agitation, panic attacks, insomnia, irritability, hostility, aggressiveness, impulsivity, akathisia (psychomotor restlessness), hypomania, mania, other unusual changes in behavior, worsening of depression, and suicidal ideation, especially early during antidepressant treatment and when the dose is adjusted up or down. Advise families and caregivers of patients to observe for the emergence of such symptoms on a day-to-day basis, because changes may be abrupt. Report such symptoms to the patient's health care provider, especially if they are severe, abrupt in onset, or were not part of the patients presenting symptoms. Symptoms such as these may be associated with an increased risk for suicidal thinking and behavior and indicate a need for very close monitoring and possibly changes in the medication.

Caution patients about operating hazardous machinery, including automobiles, until they are reasonably certain that venlafaxine therapy does not adversely affect their ability to engage in such activities.

Inform patients who are taking venlafaxine ER tablets that the inert components of the tablet remain intact during GI transit and are eliminated in the feces as an insoluble shell.

Advise patients to inform their health care provider if they are taking or planning to take any prescription or nonprescription drugs, because there is a potential for interactions.

Caution patients about the risk of serotonin syndrome with the concomitant use of venlafaxine and triptans, tramadol, tryptophan supplements, or other serotonergic agents.

Caution patients about the concomitant use of venlafaxine and NSAIDs, aspirin, warfarin, or other drugs that affect coagulation because combined use of psychotropic drugs that interfere with serotonin reuptake and these agents has been associated with an increased risk of bleeding.

Although venlafaxine has not been shown to increase the impairment of mental and motor skills caused by alcohol, advise patients to avoid alcohol while taking venlafaxine.

Advise patients to notify their health care provider if they develop a rash, hives, or a related allergic phenomenon.

Advise patients to notify their health care provider if they become pregnant or intend to become pregnant during therapy.

Advise patients to notify their health care provider if they are breast-feeding an infant.

Mydriasis (prolonged dilation of the pupils of the eye) has been reported with venlafaxine. Advise patients to notify their health care provider if they have a history of glaucoma or a history of increased intraocular pressure.

DESVENLAFAXINE

Rx	**Pristiq** (Wyeth)	**Tablets, extended-release; oral:** 50 mg	Equiv. to desvenlafaxine succinate 76 mg. (W 50). Light pink, square pyramid. Film-coated. In 14s, 30s, 90s, and UD 100s.
		100 mg	Equiv. to desvenlafaxine succinate 152 mg. (W 100). Red-orange, square pyramid. Film-coated. In 14s, 30s, 90s, and UD 100s.

DESVENLAFAXINE SUCCINATE — ORAL

WARNING

Suicidality and antidepressant drugs – Antidepressants increased the risk compared with placebo of suicidal thinking and behavior (suicidality) in children, adolescents, and young adults in short-term studies of major depressive disorder (MDD) and other psychiatric disorders. Anyone considering the use of desvenlafaxine or any other antidepressant in a child, adolescent, or young adult must balance this risk with the clinical need. Short-term studies did not show an increase in the risk of suicidality with antidepressants compared with placebo in adults older than 24 years of age; there was a reduction in risk with antidepressants compared with placebo in adults 65 years of age and older. Depression and certain other psychiatric disorders are associated with increases in the risk of suicide. Monitor patients of all ages who are started on antidepressant therapy appropriately and observe closely for clinical worsening, suicidality, or unusual changes in behavior. Advise families and caregivers of the need for close observation and communication with the prescriber. Desvenlafaxine is not approved for use in children.

Indications

➤*Major depressive disorder:* For the treatment of MDD.

Administration and Dosage

➤*General dosing considerations:* A gradual reduction in the dose rather than abrupt cessation is recommended. (See Discontinuation of therapy.)

Consider tapering desvenlafaxine in the third trimester of pregnancy. (See Pregnancy.)

➤*Adults:*

Major depressive disorder – 50 mg once daily.

➤*Renal function impairment:*

Moderate renal impairment (24-hour creatinine clearance [CrCl] 30 to 50 mL/min) – 50 mg/day.

Severe renal impairment (24-hour CrCl less than 30 mL/min) or end-stage renal disease – 50 mg every other day.

Dialysis – Supplemental doses should not be given to patients after dialysis.

➤*Hepatic function impairment:* Dose escalation above 100 mg/day is not recommended.

➤*Pregnancy:* Neonates exposed to serotonin-norepinephrine reuptake inhibitor (SNRIs) or selective serotonin uptake inhibitors (SSRIs) late in the third trimester have developed complications requiring prolonged hospitalization, respiratory support, and tube feeding. When treating pregnant women with desvenlafaxine during the third trimester, carefully consider the potential risks and benefits of treatment. Consider tapering desvenlafaxine in the third trimester.

➤*Concomitant monoamine oxidase inhibitor therapy:* At least 14 days must elapse between discontinuation of an monoamine oxidase inhibitor (MAOI) and initiation of therapy with desvenlafaxine. In addition, at least 7 days must be allowed after stopping desvenlafaxine before starting an MAOI.

➤*Duration of therapy:* It is generally agreed that acute episodes of MDD require at least several months of sustained pharmacologic therapy. Patients should be periodically reassessed to determine the need for continued treatment.

➤*Discontinuation of therapy:* A gradual reduction in the dose (by giving desvenlafaxine 50 mg less frequently) rather than abrupt cessation is recommended whenever possible. If intolerable symptoms occur following a decrease in the dose or upon discontinuation of treatment, resuming the previously prescribed dose may be considered. Subsequently, continue decreasing the dose, but at a more gradual rate.

➤*Administration:* Desvenlafaxine should be taken at approximately the same time each day with or without food. Tablets must be swallowed whole with fluid and not divided, crushed, chewed, or dissolved.

➤*Storage/Stability:* Store at 20° to 25°C (68° to 77°F); excursions are permitted between 15° and 30°C (59° and 86°F).

DESVENLAFAXINE SUCCINATE — ORAL

Actions

➤*Pharmacology:* Desvenlafaxine is a structurally novel SNRI for the treatment of MDD.

Nonclinical studies have shown that desvenlafaxine is a potent SNRI. The clinical efficacy of desvenlafaxine is thought to be related to the potentiation of these neurotransmitters in the CNS.

➤*Pharmacokinetics:*

Absorption/Distribution – The absolute oral bioavailability of desvenlafaxine after oral administration is approximately 80%. Mean time to peak plasma concentrations (T_{max}) is approximately 7.5 hours after oral administration. With once-daily dosing, steady-state plasma concentrations are achieved within approximately 4 to 5 days.

The plasma protein binding of desvenlafaxine is low (30%) and is independent of drug concentration. The desvenlafaxine volume of distribution at steady state following intravenous (IV) administration is 3.4 L/kg, indicating distribution into nonvascular compartments.

Metabolism/Excretion – Desvenlafaxine is primarily metabolized by conjugation (mediated by UDP-glucuronosyltransferase isoforms) and, to a minor extent, through oxidative metabolism. CYP3A4 is the cytochrome P450 isozyme mediating the oxidative metabolism (N-demethylation) of desvenlafaxine. The CYP2D6 metabolic pathway is not involved, and after administration of 100 mg, the pharmacokinetics of desvenlafaxine were similar in subjects with CYP2D6 poor- and extensive-metabolizer phenotype. Approximately 45% of desvenlafaxine is excreted unchanged in urine 72 hours after oral administration. Approximately 19% of the administered dose is excreted as the glucuronide metabolite and less than 5% as the oxidative metabolite (N,O-didesmethylvenlafaxine) in urine. The mean terminal half-life is approximately 11 hours.

Special populations –

Renal function impairment: Elimination was significantly correlated with CrCl. Increases in areas under the curve (AUC) of approximately 42% in mild renal impairment (24-hour CrCl 50 to 80 mL/min), approximately 46% in moderate renal impairment (24-hour CrCl 30 to 50 mL/min), approximately 108% in severe renal impairment (24-hour CrCl 30 mL/min or less), and approximately 116% in end-stage renal disease (ESRD) subjects were observed, compared with healthy, age-matched, control subjects.

The mean terminal half-life was prolonged from 11.1 hours in the control subjects to approximately 13.5, 15.5, 17.6, and 22.8 hours in mild, moderate, and severe renal impairment, and ESRD subjects, respectively. Less than 5% of the drug in the body was cleared during a standard 4-hour hemodialysis procedure.

Dosage adjustment (every-other-day dosing) is recommended in patients with significant renal impairment.

Hepatic function impairment: Average AUC was increased approximately 31% and 35% in patients with moderate and severe hepatic impairment, respectively, as compared with healthy subjects. Average AUC values were similar in subjects with mild hepatic impairment and healthy subjects (less than 5% difference).

Systemic clearance (Cl/F) was decreased approximately 20% and 36% in patients with moderate and severe hepatic impairment, respectively, compared with healthy subjects. Cl/F values were comparable in mild hepatic impairment and healthy subjects (less than 5% difference).

The mean half-life changed from approximately 10 hours in healthy subjects and subjects with mild hepatic impairment to 13 and 14 hours in subjects with moderate and severe hepatic impairment, respectively. No adjustment in starting dosage is necessary for patients with hepatic impairment.

Elderly: In a study of healthy subjects administered doses of up to of 300 mg, there was an approximate 32% increase in maximal drug concentration (C_{max}) and a 55% increase in AUC in subjects older than 75 years of age (n = 17), compared with subjects 18 to 45 years of age (n = 16). Subjects 65 to 75 years of age (n = 15) had no change in C_{max} and an approximately 32% increase in AUC, compared with subjects 18 to 45 years of age.

Gender: In a study of healthy subjects administered doses of up to of 300 mg, women had an approximately 25% higher C_{max} and an approximately 10% higher AUC than age-matched men. No adjustment of dosage on the basis of gender is needed.

Contraindications

Hypersensitivity to desvenlafaxine, venlafaxine, or to any excipients in the desvenlafaxine formulation; concomitant use in patients taking MAOIs.

Warnings/Precautions

➤*Clinical worsening and suicide risk:* Adults and children with MDD may experience worsening of their depression and/or the emergence of suicidal ideation and behavior (suicidality) or unusual changes in behavior, whether or not they are taking antidepressant medications. This risk may persist until significant remission occurs. Suicide is a known risk of depression and certain other psychiatric disorders, and these disorders themselves are the strongest predictors of suicide. There has been a long-standing concern, however, that antidepressants may have a role in inducing worsening of depression and the emergence of suicidality in certain patients during the early phases of treatment. Pooled analyses of short-term, placebo-controlled studies of antidepressant drugs (SSRIs and others) showed that these drugs increase the risk of suicidal thinking and behavior (suicidality) in children, adolescents, and young adults (18 to 24 years of age) with MDD and other psychiatric disorders. Short-term studies did not show an increase in the risk of suicidality with antidepressants compared with placebo in adults older than 24 years of age. There was a reduction with antidepressants compared with placebo in adults 65 years of age and older.

The pooled analyses of placebo-controlled studies in children and adolescents with MDD, obsessive-compulsive disorder, or other psychiatric disorders included a total of 24 short-term studies of 9 antidepressant drugs in more than 4,400 patients. The pooled analyses of placebo-controlled studies in adults with MDD or other psychiatric disorders included a total of 295 short-term studies (median duration, 2 months) of 11 antidepressant drugs in more than 77,000 patients. There was considerable variation in risk of suicidality between drugs, but a tendency toward an increase in the younger patients for almost all drugs studied. There were differences in absolute risk of suicidality across the different indications, with the highest incidence in MDD. The risk differences (drug vs placebo), however, were relatively stable within age strata and across indications.

No suicides occurred in any of the pediatric studies. There were suicides in the adult studies, but the number was not sufficient to reach any conclusion about drug effect on suicide.

It is unknown whether the suicidality risk extends to longer-term use (beyond several months). However, there is substantial evidence from placebo-controlled maintenance studies in adults with depression that the use of antidepressants can delay the recurrence of depression.

Appropriately monitor all patients being treated with antidepressants for any indication and observe closely for clinical worsening, suicidality, and unusual changes in behavior, especially during the initial few months of a course of drug therapy, or at times of dose changes, either increases or decreases.

The following symptoms have been reported in adults and children being treated with antidepressants for MDD as well as for other indications (psychiatric and nonpsychiatric): aggressiveness, agitation, akathisia (psychomotor restlessness), anxiety, hostility, hypomania, impulsivity, insomnia, irritability, mania, and panic attacks. Although a causal link between the emergence of such symptoms and either the worsening of depression and/or the emergence of suicidal impulses has not been established, there is concern that such symptoms may represent precursors to emerging suicidality.

Consider changing the therapeutic regimen, including possibly discontinuing the medication, in patients whose depression is persistently worse, or who are experiencing emergent suicidality or symptoms that might be precursors to worsening depression or suicidality, especially if these symptoms are severe, abrupt in onset, or were not part of the patient's presenting symptoms.

If the decision has been made to discontinue treatment, taper the medication as rapidly as feasible, but with recognition that abrupt discontinuation can be associated with certain symptoms.

Alert families and caregivers of patients being treated with antidepressants for MDD or other indications (psychiatric and nonpsychiatric) about the need to monitor patients for the emergence of agitation, irritability, unusual changes in behavior, and the other symptoms described previously, as well as the emergence of suicidality, and to report such symptoms immediately to their health care provider. Include in such monitoring daily observation by families and caregivers. Write prescriptions for desvenlafaxine for the smallest quantity of tablets consistent with good patient management in order to reduce the risk of overdose.

➤*Screening patients for bipolar disorder:* A major depressive episode may be the initial presentation of bipolar disorder. It is generally believed (though not established in controlled studies) that treating such an episode with an antidepressant alone may increase the likelihood of precipitation of a mixed/manic episode in patients at risk for bipolar disorder. Whether any of the symptoms described previously represent such a conversion is unknown. However, prior to initiating treatment with an antidepressant, adequately screen patients with depressive symptoms to determine if they are at risk for bipolar disorder; in the screening include a detailed psychiatric history, including a family history of suicide, bipolar disorder, and depression. Note that desvenlafaxine is not approved for use in treating bipolar depression.

➤*Serotonin syndrome or neuroleptic malignant syndrome–like reactions:* The development of a potentially life-threatening serotonin syndrome or neuroleptic malignant syndrome (NMS)–like reactions have been reported with SNRIs and SSRIs alone, including desvenlafaxine treatment, but particularly with concomitant use of serotonergic drugs (including triptans) with drugs that impair metabolism of serotonin (including MAOIs), or with antipsychotics or other dopamine antagonists. Serotonin syndrome may include mental status changes (eg, agitation, coma, hallucinations), autonomic instability (eg, hyperthermia, labile blood pressure, tachycardia), neuromuscular aberrations (eg, hyperreflexia, incoordination), and/or GI symptoms (eg, diarrhea, nausea, vomiting). Serotonin syndrome in its most severe form can resemble NMS, which includes hyperthermia, muscle rigidity, autonomic instability with possible rapid fluctuation of vital signs, and mental status changes. Monitor patients for the emergence of serotonin syndrome or NMS-like signs and symptoms.

➤*Elevated blood pressure:* Regularly monitor blood pressure of patients receiving desvenlafaxine because sustained increases in blood pressure were observed in clinical studies. Control preexisting hypertension before initiating treatment with desvenlafaxine. Exercise caution in treating patients with preexisting hypertension or other underlying conditions that might be compromised by increases in blood pressure. Cases of elevated blood pressure requiring immediate treatment have been reported with desvenlafaxine.

Sustained hypertension – Sustained blood pressure increases could have adverse consequences. For patients who experience a sustained increase in blood pressure while receiving desvenlafaxine, consider dose reduction or discontinuation. Treatment with desvenlafaxine at all dosages from 50 to 400 mg/day in controlled studies was associated with sustained hypertension, defined as treatment-emergent supine diastolic blood pressure 90 mm Hg or more and 10 mm Hg or more above baseline for 3 consecutive on-therapy visits. Analy-

DESVENLAFAXINE SUCCINATE — ORAL

ses of patients in desvenlafaxine controlled studies who met criteria for sustained hypertension revealed a consistent increase in the proportion of subjects who developed sustained hypertension. This was seen at all doses with a suggestion of a higher rate at 400 mg/day.

➤*Abnormal bleeding:* SSRIs and SNRIs, including desvenlafaxine, may increase the risk of bleeding events. Concomitant use of aspirin, nonsteroidal anti-inflammatory drugs (NSAIDs), warfarin, and other anticoagulants may add to this risk. Case reports and epidemiological studies (case-control and cohort design) have demonstrated an association between the use of drugs that interfere with serotonin reuptake and the occurrence of GI bleeding. Bleeding events related to SSRIs and SNRIs have ranged from ecchymosis, hematoma, epistaxis, and petechiae to life-threatening hemorrhages. Caution patients about the risk of bleeding associated with the concomitant use of desvenlafaxine and NSAIDs, aspirin, or other drugs that affect coagulation or bleeding.

➤*Narrow-angle glaucoma:* Mydriasis has been reported in association with desvenlafaxine; therefore, monitor patients with raised intraocular pressure or those at risk of acute narrow-angle glaucoma (angle-closure glaucoma).

➤*Mania / Hypomania activation:* During all MDD and vasomotor symptoms phase 2 and 3 studies, mania was reported for approximately 0.1% of patients treated with desvenlafaxine. Activation of mania/hypomania has also been reported in a small proportion of patients with major affective disorder who were treated with other marketed antidepressants. As with all antidepressants, use desvenlafaxine cautiously in patients with a history or family history of mania or hypomania.

➤*Cardiac effects:* Caution is advised in administering desvenlafaxine to patients with cardiovascular or cerebrovascular disorders. Increases in blood pressure and small increases in heart rate were observed in clinical studies with desvenlafaxine. Desvenlafaxine has not been evaluated systematically in patients with a recent history of myocardial infarction, unstable heart disease, uncontrolled hypertension, or cerebrovascular disease. Patients with these diagnoses, except for cerebrovascular disease, were excluded from clinical studies.

➤*Lipid effects:* Caution is advised in administering desvenlafaxine to patients with lipid metabolism disorders. Dose-related elevations in fasting serum total cholesterol, low-density lipoprotein (LDL) cholesterol, and triglycerides were observed in the controlled studies. Consider measurement of serum lipids during treatment with desvenlafaxine.

➤*Discontinuation of treatment:* Discontinuation symptoms have been systematically and prospectively evaluated in patients treated with desvenlafaxine during clinical studies in MDD. Abrupt discontinuation or dose reduction has been associated with the appearance of new symptoms that include abnormal dreams, anxiety, diarrhea, dizziness, fatigue, headache, hyperhidrosis, insomnia, irritability, and nausea. In general, discontinuation events occurred more frequently with longer duration of therapy.

During marketing of SNRIs and SSRIs, there have been spontaneous reports of adverse reactions occurring upon discontinuation of these drugs, particularly when abrupt, including the following: agitation, anxiety, confusion, dizziness, dysphoric mood, emotional lability, headache, hypomania, insomnia, irritability, lethargy, seizures, sensory disturbances (eg, paresthesia, such as electric shock sensations), and tinnitus. While these reactions are generally self-limiting, there have been reports of serious discontinuation symptoms.

Monitor patients for these symptoms when discontinuing treatment with desvenlafaxine. A gradual reduction in the dose rather than abrupt cessation is recommended whenever possible. If intolerable symptoms occur following a decrease in the dose or upon discontinuation of treatment, then resuming the previously prescribed dose may be considered. Subsequently, continue decreasing the dose, but at a more gradual rate.

➤*Seizure:* Cases of seizure have been reported in premarketing clinical studies with desvenlafaxine. Desvenlafaxine has not been systematically evaluated in patients with a seizure disorder. Patients with a history of seizures were excluded from premarketing clinical studies. Prescribe desvenlafaxine with caution in patients with a seizure disorder.

➤*Hyponatremia:* Hyponatremia may occur as a result of treatment with SSRIs and SNRIs, including desvenlafaxine. In many cases, this hyponatremia appears to be the result of the syndrome of inappropriate antidiuretic hormone secretion. Cases with serum sodium lower than 110 mmol/L have been reported. Elderly patients may be at greater risk of developing hyponatremia with SSRIs and SNRIs. Also, patients taking diuretics or who are otherwise volume depleted can be at greater risk. Consider discontinuing desvenlafaxine in patients with symptomatic hyponatremia and institute appropriate medical intervention.

Signs and symptoms of hyponatremia include headache, difficulty concentrating, memory impairment, confusion, weakness, and unsteadiness, which can lead to falls. Signs and symptoms associated with more severe and/or acute cases have included coma, death, hallucination, respiratory arrest, seizure, and syncope.

➤*Interstitial lung disease and eosinophilic pneumonia:* Interstitial lung disease and eosinophilic pneumonia associated with venlafaxine (the parent drug of desvenlafaxine) therapy have been rarely reported. Consider the possibility of these adverse reactions in patients treated with desvenlafaxine who present with progressive dyspnea, cough, or chest discomfort. Ensure that such patients undergo a prompt medical evaluation, and consider discontinuation of desvenlafaxine.

➤*Renal function impairment:* In patients with moderate or severe renal impairment or ESRD, the clearance of desvenlafaxine was decreased, thus prolonging the elimination half-life of the drug. As a result, there were potentially clinically significant increases in exposures to desvenlafaxine. Dosage adjustment (50 mg every other day) is necessary in patients with severe renal impairment or ESRD. Do not escalate the doses in patients with moderate or severe renal impairment or ESRD.

In subjects with renal impairment, the clearance of desvenlafaxine was decreased. In subjects with severe renal function impairment (24-hour CrCl less than 30 mL/min) and ESRD, elimination half-lives were significantly prolonged, increasing exposures to desvenlafaxine; therefore, dosage adjustment is recommended in these patients.

➤*Hepatic function impairment:* The mean half-life changed from approximately 10 hours in healthy subjects and subjects with mild hepatic impairment to 13 and 14 hours in subjects with moderate and severe hepatic impairment, respectively. No adjustment in starting dosage is necessary for patients with hepatic impairment.

➤*Pregnancy:* *Category C.* Advise patients to notify their health care provider if they become pregnant or intend to become pregnant during therapy.

Teratogenic –

Fetal weights were decreased in rats, with a no-effect dose 10 times a human dosage of 100 mg/day (on a mg/m^2 basis).

When desvenlafaxine was administered orally to pregnant rats throughout gestation and lactation, there was a decrease in pup weights and an increase in pup deaths during the first 4 days of lactation. The cause of these deaths is not known. The no-effect dose for rat pup mortality was 10 times a human dosage of 100 mg/day (on a mg/m^2 basis). Postweaning growth and reproductive performance of the progeny were not affected by maternal treatment with desvenlafaxine at a dose 29 times a human dosage of 100 mg/day (on a mg/m^2 basis).

There are no adequate and well-controlled studies of desvenlafaxine in pregnant women. It is not known if venlafaxine or O-desmethylvenlafaxine (ODV) cross the human placenta. The molecular weight of venlafaxine (approximately 314) and the minimal protein binding and moderately long elimination half-lives of venlafaxine and ODV suggest that both will cross to the embryo and/or fetus. Therefore, use desvenlafaxine during pregnancy only if the potential benefits justify the potential risks.

Nonteratogenic – Neonates exposed to SNRIs or SSRIs late in the third trimester have developed complications requiring prolonged hospitalization, respiratory support, and tube feeding. Such complications can arise immediately upon delivery. Reported clinical findings have included respiratory distress, cyanosis, apnea, seizures, temperature instability, feeding difficulty, vomiting, hypoglycemia, hypotonia, hypertonia, hyperreflexia, tremor, jitteriness, irritability, and constant crying. These features are consistent with either a direct toxic effect of SSRIs and SNRIs or, possibly, a drug discontinuation syndrome. Note that, in some cases, the clinical picture is consistent with serotonin syndrome. When treating a pregnant woman with desvenlafaxine during the third trimester, carefully consider the potential risks and benefits of treatment.

➤*Lactation:* Desvenlafaxine (ODV) is excreted in human milk. Because of the potential for serious adverse reactions in breast-feeding infants from desvenlafaxine, decide whether to discontinue breast-feeding or the drug, taking into account the importance of the drug to the mother. Only administer desvenlafaxine to breast-feeding women if the expected benefits outweigh any possible risk. The American Academy of Pediatrics classifies other antidepressants as drugs for which the effect on breast-feeding infants is unknown but may be of concern.

➤*Children:* Safety and effectiveness in children have not been established. Anyone considering the use of desvenlafaxine in a child or adolescent must balance the potential risks with the clinical need. Desvenlafaxine is not approved for use in children.

➤*Elderly:* Of the 3,292 patients in clinical studies with desvenlafaxine, 5% were 65 years of age and older. No overall differences in safety or efficacy were observed between these patients and younger patients; however, in the short-term, placebo-controlled studies, there was a higher incidence of systolic orthostatic hypotension in patients 65 years of age or older compared with patients younger than 65 years of age treated with desvenlafaxine. For elderly patients, consider possible reduced renal clearance of desvenlafaxine when determining dose. If desvenlafaxine is poorly tolerated, every other day dosing can be considered.

SSRIs and SNRIs, including desvenlafaxine, have been associated with cases of clinically significant hyponatremia in elderly patients, who may be at greater risk for this adverse reaction.

Greater sensitivity of some older patients cannot be ruled out.

➤*Monitoring:* Measure serum lipids during desvenlafaxine treatment. Appropriately monitor all patients being treated with antidepressants for any indication and observe closely for clinical worsening, suicidality, and unusual changes in behavior, especially during the initial few months of a course of drug therapy, or at times of dose changes, either increases or decreases. Regularly monitor blood pressure. Monitor patients with raised intraocular pressure or those at risk of acute narrow-angle glaucoma (angle-closure glaucoma). Carefully evaluate patients for a history of drug abuse and follow such patients closely, observing them for signs of misuse or abuse of desvenlafaxine (eg, development of tolerance, incrementation of dose, drug-seeking behavior). Monitor patients for the emergence of serotonin-syndrome or NMS-like signs and symptoms.

Monitor patients for symptoms (eg, agitation, anxiety, confusion, headache, hypomania, insomnia, lethargy, seizures) when discontinuing desvenlafaxine treatment.

DESVENLAFAXINE SUCCINATE — ORAL

Drug Interactions

➤*Venlafaxine:* Desvenlafaxine is the major active metabolite of venlafaxine. Do not use products containing desvenlafaxine and venlafaxine concomitantly.

Desvenlafaxine Drug Interactions

Precipitant drug	Object drug[a]		Description
CNS-acting drugs (eg, alcohol)	Desvenlafaxine	↑	Given the primary CNS effects of desvenlafaxine, use with caution when taken in combination with, or substituted for, other centrally acting drugs, including those with a similar mechanism. Avoid alcohol consumption while taking desvenlafaxine.
Desvenlafaxine	CNS-acting drugs (eg, alcohol)		
CYP3A4 inhibitors (eg, ketoconazole)	Desvenlafaxine	↑	Concomitant use of desvenlafaxine with potent inhibitors of CYP3A4 may result in higher concentrations of desvenlafaxine. Ketoconazole 200 mg twice daily increased the AUC and C_{max} of desvenlafaxine 400 mg by approximately 43% and 8%, respectively.
MAOIs (eg, phenelzine, selegiline)	Desvenlafaxine	↑	Concomitant use is contraindicated. Desvenlafaxine must not be used in patients who have taken MAOIs within the preceding 14 days because serious, sometimes fatal, reactions may occur, including hyperthermia, rigidity, myoclonus, autonomic instability with possible rapid fluctuation of vital signs, and mental status changes that include extreme agitation progressing to delirium and coma. Allow at least 7 days after stopping desvenlafaxine before starting an MAOI.
Desvenlafaxine	MAOIs (eg, phenelzine, selegiline)		
Serotonergic drugs (eg, linezolid, metoclopramide, sibutramine, SNRIs, SSRIs, tramadol, trazodone, triptans)	Desvenlafaxine	↑	The development of a potentially life-threatening serotonin syndrome (eg, agitation, hallucinations, tachycardia, hyperthermia, hyperreflexia, nausea, vomiting) may occur with desvenlafaxine treatment, particularly with concomitant use of other serotonergic drugs.
Desvenlafaxine	Serotonergic drugs (eg, linezolid, metoclopramide, sibutramine, SNRIs, SSRIs, tramadol, trazodone, triptans)		
Desvenlafaxine	Aspirin, NSAIDs	↑	Concurrent use of aspirin or NSAIDs may increase the risk of GI bleeding.
Desvenlafaxine	Lithium	↑	Serotonin syndrome may occur.
Desvenlafaxine	Midazolam	↓	Coadministration of desvenlafaxine 400 mg daily with midazolam 4 mg, a CYP3A4 substrate, decreased midazolam AUC and C_{max} approximately 31% and 16%, respectively.
Desvenlafaxine	St. John's wort	↑	Serotonin syndrome may occur.
Desvenlafaxine	Tricyclic antidepressants (eg, desipramine)	↑	Tricyclic antidepressant levels may be elevated. Desvenlafaxine 100 mg daily administered with desipramine 50 mg, a CYP2D6 substrate, increased the C_{max} and AUC of desipramine approximately 25% and 17%, respectively.
Desvenlafaxine	Tryptophan	↑	Concurrent use is not recommended.
Desvenlafaxine	Warfarin	↑	Altered anticoagulant effects, including increased bleeding, have been reported when SSRIs and SNRIs are coadministered with warfarin. Monitor patients receiving warfarin therapy when desvenlafaxine is initiated or discontinued.

[a] ↑ = object drug increased; ↓ = object drug decreased.

Adverse Reactions

➤*Most common:* The most commonly observed adverse reactions in desvenlafaxine-treated MDD patients in short-term, fixed-dose studies (incidence of 5% or more and at least twice the rate of placebo in the 50 or 100 mg dose groups) were anxiety, constipation, decreased appetite, dizziness, hyperhidrosis, insomnia, nausea, somnolence, and specific male sexual function disorders.

➤*Discontinuation:* The most common adverse reactions leading to discontinuation in at least 2% of the desvenlafaxine-treated patients in the short-term studies, up to 8 weeks, were nausea (4%), and dizziness, headache, and vomiting (2% each). In the long-term study (up to 9 months' duration), the most common adverse reaction leading to discontinuation was vomiting (2%).

➤*Common adverse reactions:*

Desvenlafaxine Adverse Reactions (≥ 2%)[a]

Adverse reaction	Desvenlafaxine				
	50 mg	100 mg	200 mg	400 mg	Placebo
Cardiovascular					
Blood pressure increased	1%	1%	2%	2%	1%
Hot flush	1%	1%	2%	2%	< 1%
Palpitations	1%	3%	2%	3%	2%
Tachycardia	1%	< 1%	1%	2%	1%
CNS					
Abnormal dreams	2%	3%	2%	4%	1%
Anxiety	3%	5%	4%	4%	2%
Asthenia	1%	2%	1%	1%	1%
Disturbance in attention	< 1%	1%	2%	1%	< 1%
Dizziness	13%	10%	15%	16%	5%
Fatigue	7%	7%	10%	11%	4%
Feeling jittery	1%	2%	3%	3%	1%
Headache	20%	22%	29%	25%	23%
Insomnia	9%	12%	14%	15%	6%
Irritability	2%	2%	2%	2%	1%
Nervousness	< 1%	1%	2%	2%	1%
Paraesthesia	2%	2%	1%	3%	1%
Somnolence	4%	9%	12%	12%	4%
Tremor	2%	3%	9%	9%	2%
Dermatologic					
Hyperhidrosis	10%	11%	18%	21%	4%
Rash	1%	1%	2%	< 1%	< 1%
GI					
Constipation	9%	9%	10%	14%	4%
Diarrhea	11%	9%	7%	5%	9%
Dry mouth	11%	17%	21%	25%	9%
Dysgeusia	1%	1%	1%	2%	1%
Nausea	22%	26%	36%	41%	10%
Vomiting	3%	4%	6%	9%	3%
Metabolic and nutritional					
Decreased appetite	5%	8%	10%	10%	2%
Weight decreased	2%	1%	1%	2%	1%
Special senses					
Mydriasis	2%	2%	6%	6%	< 1%
Tinnitus	2%	1%	1%	2%	1%
Vision blurred	3%	4%	4%	4%	1%

DESVENLAFAXINE SUCCINATE — ORAL

Desvenlafaxine Adverse Reactions (≥ 2%)[a]					
	Desvenlafaxine				
Adverse reaction	50 mg	100 mg	200 mg	400 mg	Placebo
Miscellaneous					
Chills	1%	< 1%	3%	4%	1%
Urinary hesitation	< 1%	1%	2%	2%	0%
Yawning	1%	1%	4%	3%	< 1%

[a] Percentage based on the number of patients (placebo, n = 636; desvenlafaxine 50 mg, n = 317; desvenlafaxine 100 mg, n = 424; desvenlafaxine 200 mg, n = 307; desvenlafaxine 400 mg, n = 317). In general, the adverse reactions were most frequent in the first week of treatment.

➤*Sexual function adverse reactions:*

Desvenlafaxine Sexual Function: Adverse Reactions (≥ 2%) in Men[a] or Women[b]					
	Desvenlafaxine				
Adverse reaction	50 mg	100 mg	200 mg	400 mg	Placebo
Men only					
Anorgasmia	0%	3%	5%	8%	0%
Ejaculation delayed	1%	5%	7%	6%	≤1%
Ejaculation disorder	0%	1%	2%	5%	0%
Ejaculation failure	1%	0%	2%	2%	0%
Erectile dysfunction	3%	6%	8%	11%	1%
Libido decreased	4%	5%	6%	3%	1%
Orgasm abnormal	0%	1%	2%	3%	0%
Sexual dysfunction	1%	0%	0%	2%	0%
Women only					
Anorgasmia	1%	1%	0%	3%	0%

[a] Percentage based on the number of men (placebo, n = 239; desvenlafaxine 50 mg, n = 108; desvenlafaxine 100 mg, n = 157; desvenlafaxine 200 mg, n = 131; desvenlafaxine 400 mg, n = 154).
[b] Percentage based on the number of women (placebo, n = 397; desvenlafaxine 50 mg, n = 209; desvenlafaxine 100 mg, n = 267; desvenlafaxine 200 mg, n = 176; desvenlafaxine 400 mg, n = 163).

➤*Other adverse reactions:*

Cardiovascular – Orthostatic hypotension, syncope (less than 2%).

In clinical studies, there were uncommon reports of ischemic cardiac adverse reactions, including coronary occlusion requiring revascularization, myocardial infarction, and myocardial ischemia; these patients had multiple underlying cardiac risk factors. More patients experienced these reactions during desvenlafaxine treatment compared with placebo.

CNS – Convulsion, depersonalization, extrapyramidal disorder, hypomania (less than 2%).

Miscellaneous – Blood prolactin increased, epistaxis, hypersensitivity, liver function test abnormal (less than 2%).

➤*Abrupt discontinuation adverse reactions:* Adverse reactions reported in association with abrupt discontinuation, dose reduction, or tapering of treatment in MDD clinical studies at a rate of 5% or more include abnormal dreams, anxiety, diarrhea, dizziness, fatigue, headache, hyperhidrosis, insomnia, irritability, and nausea. In general, discontinuation reactions occurred more frequently with longer duration of therapy.

➤*Lab test abnormalities:*

Lipids –

Desvenlafaxine Patients With Lipid Abnormalities					
	Desvenlafaxine				
	50 mg	100 mg	200 mg	400 mg	Placebo
Total cholesterol (increase of ≥ 50 mg/dL and an absolute value of ≥ 261 mg/dL)	3%	4%	4%	10%	2%
LDL cholesterol (increase of ≥ 50 mg/dL and an absolute value of ≥ 190 mg/dL)	1%	0%	1%	2%	0%
Triglycerides, fasting (fasting: ≥ 327 mg/dL)	2%	1%	4%	6%	3%

Proteinuria –

Desvenlafaxine Patients With Proteinuria					
	Desvenlafaxine				
	50 mg	100 mg	200 mg	400 mg	Placebo
Proteinuria	6%	8%	5%	7%	4%

➤*Vital sign changes:*

Desvenlafaxine Mean Changes in Vital Signs					
	Desvenlafaxine				
	50 mg	100 mg	200 mg	400 mg	Placebo
Supine systolic blood pressure (mm Hg)	1.2	2	2.5	2.1	−1.4
Supine diastolic blood pressure (mm Hg)	0.7	0.8	1.8	2.3	−0.6
Supine pulse (bpm)	1.3	1.3	0.9	4.1	−0.3
Weight (kg)	−0.4	−0.6	−0.9	−1.1	0

➤*Orthostatic hypotension:* In the short-term, placebo-controlled clinical studies with doses of 50 to 400 mg, systolic orthostatic hypotension (decrease of 30 mm Hg or more from supine to standing position) occurred more frequently in patients 65 years of age and older receiving desvenlafaxine (8%) versus placebo (2.5%), compared with patients younger than 65 years of age receiving desvenlafaxine (0.9%) versus placebo (0.7%).

Overdosage

➤*Symptoms:* There is limited clinical experience with desvenlafaxine overdosage in humans. In premarketing clinical studies, no cases of fatal acute overdose of desvenlafaxine were reported.

Among the patients included in the MDD premarketing studies of desvenlafaxine, there were 4 adults who ingested desvenlafaxine (4,000 mg [desvenlafaxine alone], 900, 1,800, and 5,200 mg [in combination with other drugs]); all patients recovered. In addition, one patient's 11-month-old child accidentally ingested desvenlafaxine 600 mg, was treated, and recovered. The adverse reactions reported within 5 days of an overdose of more than 600 mg that were possibly related to desvenlafaxine included agitation, constipation, diarrhea, dizziness, dry mouth, headache, nausea, paresthesia, tachycardia, and vomiting.

Desvenlafaxine is the major active metabolite of venlafaxine. Overdose experience reported with venlafaxine (the parent drug of desvenlafaxine) is presented as follows.

In postmarketing experience, overdose with venlafaxine (the parent drug of desvenlafaxine) has occurred predominantly in combination with alcohol and/or other drugs. The most commonly reported reactions in overdosage include changes in level of consciousness (ranging from somnolence to coma), mydriasis, seizures, tachycardia, and vomiting. Electrocardiogram changes (eg, prolongation of QT interval, bundle branch block, QRS prolongation), sinus and ventricular tachycardia, bradycardia, hypotension, rhabdomyolysis, vertigo, liver necrosis, serotonin syndrome, and death have been reported.

Published retrospective studies report that venlafaxine overdosage may be associated with an increased risk of fatal outcomes compared with that observed with SSRI antidepressant products, but lower than that for tricyclic antidepressants. Epidemiological studies have shown that venlafaxine-treated patients have a higher preexisting burden of suicide risk factors than SSRI-treated patients. The extent to which the finding of an increased risk of fatal outcomes can be attributed to the toxicity of venlafaxine in overdosage, as opposed to some characteristic(s) of venlafaxine-treated patients, is not clear.

Write prescriptions for desvenlafaxine for the smallest quantity of tablets consistent with good patient management in order to reduce the risk of overdose.

➤*Treatment:* Employ general measures used in the management of overdosage with any SSRI or SNRI.

Ensure an adequate airway, oxygenation, and ventilation. Monitor cardiac rhythm and vital signs. General supportive and symptomatic measures are also recommended. Gastric lavage with a large-bore orogastric tube with appropriate airway protection, if needed, may be indicated if performed soon after ingestion or in symptomatic patients. Administer activated charcoal.

Induction of emesis is not recommended. Because of the moderate volume of distribution of this drug, forced diuresis, dialysis, hemoperfusion, and exchange transfusion are unlikely to be of benefit. No specific antidotes for desvenlafaxine are known.

In managing an overdose, consider the possibility of multiple drug involvement. Consider contacting a poison control center for additional information on the treatment of any overdose.

Patient Information

Advise patients and their families and caregivers about the benefits and risks associated with treatment with desvenlafaxine and counsel them in its appropriate use.

Advise patients and their families and caregivers to read the Medication Guide and assist them in understanding its contents.

Advise patients and their families and caregivers to look for the emergence of suicidality, especially early during treatment and when the dose is adjusted up or down.

DESVENLAFAXINE SUCCINATE — ORAL

Advise patients taking desvenlafaxine not to use it concomitantly with other products containing desvenlafaxine or venlafaxine. Instruct patients not to take desvenlafaxine with an MAOI or within 14 days of stopping an MAOI and to allow 7 days after stopping desvenlafaxine before starting an MAOI.

Caution patients about the risk of serotonin syndrome or NMS-like reactions, particularly with the concomitant use of desvenlafaxine and triptans, tramadol, tryptophan supplements, or other serotonergic agents or antipsychotic drugs.

Advise patients that their blood pressure will be regularly monitored while they are taking desvenlafaxine.

Caution patients about the concomitant use of desvenlafaxine and NSAIDs, aspirin, warfarin, or other drugs that affect coagulation because combined use of these agents and psychotropic drugs that interfere with serotonin reuptake has been associated with an increased risk of bleeding.

Advise patients with raised intraocular pressure or those at risk of acute narrow-angle glaucoma (angle-closure glaucoma) that mydriasis has been reported and they should be monitored.

Advise patients, their families, and caregivers to watch for signs of activation of mania/hypomania.

Caution is advised in administering desvenlafaxine to patients with cardiovascular, cerebrovascular, or lipid metabolism disorders.

Advise patients that elevations in total cholesterol, LDL, and triglycerides may occur and that measurement of serum lipids may be considered.

Advise patients not to stop taking desvenlafaxine without first talking with their health care provider. Make patients aware that discontinuation effects may occur when stopping desvenlafaxine.

Caution patients about operating hazardous machinery, including automobiles, until they are reasonably certain that desvenlafaxine therapy does not adversely affect their ability to engage in such activities.

Advise patients to avoid alcohol while taking desvenlafaxine.

Advise patients to notify their health care provider if they develop allergic phenomena such as rash, hives, swelling, or difficulty breathing.

Advise patients to notify their health care provider if they become pregnant or intend to become pregnant during therapy.

Advise patients to notify their health care provider if they are breast-feeding an infant.

Patients receiving desvenlafaxine may notice an inert matrix tablet passing in the stool or via colostomy. Inform patients that the active medication has already been absorbed by the time the patient sees the inert matrix tablet.

MILNACIPRAN HYDROCHLORIDE

Rx	**Savella** (Forest)	**Tablets; oral:** 12.5 mg	(F L). Blue, round. Film-coated. In 60s, UD titration pack 5s, and UD 100s.
		25 mg	(FL 25). White, round. Film-coated. In 60s, 180s, UD titration pack 8s, and UD 100s.
		50 mg	(FL 50). White, oval. Film-coated. In 60s, 180s, UD titration pack 42s, and UD 100s.
		100 mg	(FL 100). Pink, oval. Film-coated. In 60s, 180s, and UD 100s.

MILNACIPRAN HYDROCHLORIDE — ORAL

WARNING

Suicidality and antidepressant drugs – Milnacipran is a selective serotonin-norepinephrine reuptake inhibitor (SNRI), similar to some drugs used for the treatment of depression and other psychiatric disorders. Antidepressants increased the risk, compared with placebo, of suicidal thinking and behavior (suicidality) in children, adolescents, and young adults in short-term studies of major depressive disorder (MDD) and other psychiatric disorders. Anyone considering the use of such drugs in a child, adolescent, or young adult must balance this risk with the clinical need. Short-term studies did not show an increase in the risk of suicidality with antidepressants compared with placebo in adults older than 24 years of age; there was a reduction in risk with antidepressants compared with placebo in adults 65 years of age and older. Depression and certain other psychiatric disorders are themselves associated with increases in the risk of suicide. Appropriately monitor patients of all ages who are started on milnacipran and observe closely for clinical worsening, suicidality, or unusual changes in behavior. Advise families and caregivers of the need for close observation and communication with their health care provider. Milnacipran is not approved for use in the treatment of MDD. Milnacipran is not approved for use in children.

Indications

➤*Fibromyalgia:* For the management of fibromyalgia.

Administration and Dosage

➤*General dosing considerations:* Dosing adjustment required for patients with severe renal impairment (see Renal Function Impairment).

Milnacipran should be tapered and not abruptly discontinued after extended use (see Discontinuation of Therapy).

➤*Adults:*

Fibromyalgia –

Usual dosage: 50 mg twice daily.

Initial dosage: 12.5 mg once on day 1.

Dosage titration: 12.5 mg twice daily on days 2 and 3, 25 mg twice daily on days 4 to 7, and 50 mg twice daily after day 7.

Dosage adjustment: May increase to 100 mg twice daily based on individual response.

Concomitant therapy: At least 14 days should elapse between discontinuation of a monoamine oxidase inhibitor (MAOI) and initiation of therapy with milnacipran. In addition, at least 5 days should be allowed after stopping milnacipran before starting an MAOI.

Discontinuation of therapy: Milnacipran should be tapered and not abruptly discontinued after extended use. If intolerable symptoms occur following a decrease in the dose or upon discontinuation of treatment, then consider resuming the previously prescribed dose. Subsequently, continue decreasing the dose, but at a more gradual rate.

➤*Administration:* Should be taken orally with or without food. Taking milnacipran with food may improve the tolerability of the drug.

➤*Storage/Stability:* Store at 25°C (77°F); excursions are permitted between 15° and 30°C (59° and 86°F).

Actions

➤*Pharmacology:* The exact mechanism of the central pain inhibitory action of milnacipran and its ability to improve the symptoms of fibromyalgia in humans are unknown. Preclinical studies have shown that milnacipran is a potent inhibitor of neuronal norepinephrine and serotonin reuptake; milnacipran inhibits norepinephrine uptake with an approximately 3-fold higher potency in vitro than serotonin without directly affecting the uptake of dopamine or other neurotransmitters.

➤*Pharmacokinetics:*

Absorption/Distribution – Milnacipran is absorbed following oral administration with maximum concentrations (C_{max}) reached within 2 to 4 hours postdose. The absolute bioavailability is approximately 85% to 90%. The exposure to milnacipran increased proportionally within the therapeutic dose range. Steady-state levels are reached within 36 to 48 hours and can be predicted from single-dose data. The mean volume of distribution of milnacipran following a single intravenous (IV) dose to healthy subjects is approximately 400 L. Plasma protein binding is 13%.

Metabolism/Excretion – Milnacipran and its metabolites are eliminated primarily by renal excretion. Following oral administration of ^{14}C-milnacipran, approximately 55% of the dose was excreted in urine as unchanged milnacipran (24% as *l*-milnacipran and 31% as *d*-milnacipran). The *l*-milnacipran carbamoyl-O-glucuronide was the major metabolite excreted in urine and accounted for approximately 17% of the dose; approximately 2% of the dose was excreted in urine as *d*-milnacipran carbamoyl-O-glucuronide. Approximately 8% of the dose was excreted in urine as the N-desethyl milnacipran metabolite. The active enantiomer, *d*-milnacipran, has a longer elimination half-life (8 to 10 hours) than the *l*-enantiomer (4 to 6 hours). There is no interconversion between the enantiomers. Milnacipran has a terminal elimination half-life of about 6 to 8 hours.

Special populations –

Renal function impairment: The mean area under the curve ($AUC_{0-\infty}$) increased by 16%, 52%, and 199%, and terminal elimination half-life increased by 38%, 41%, and 122% in patients with mild, moderate, and severe renal impairment, respectively, compared with healthy patients.

See Administration and Dosage for more information.

Hepatic function impairment: Patients with severe hepatic impairment had a 31% higher $AUC_{0-\infty}$ and a 55% higher half-life than healthy patients. Exercise caution in patients with severe hepatic impairment.

Elderly: C_{max} and AUC parameters of milnacipran were approximately 30% higher in elderly (older than 65 years of age) patients compared with younger patients because of age-related decreases in renal function.

Gender: C_{max} and AUC parameters of milnacipran were approximately 20% higher in women compared with men.

Contraindications

Concomitant use with MAOIs or within 14 days of discontinuing treatment with an MAOI; uncontrolled narrow-angle glaucoma.

Warnings/Precautions

➤*Suicide risk:* Milnacipran is an SNRI, similar to some drugs used for the treatment of depression and other psychiatric disorders.

Patients, both adults and children, with depression or other psychiatric disorders may experience worsening of their depression and/or the emergence of suicidal ideation and behavior (suicidality) or unusual changes in behav-

MILNACIPRAN HYDROCHLORIDE — ORAL

ior, whether or not they are taking these medications, and this risk may persist until significant remission occurs. Suicide is a known risk of depression and certain other psychiatric disorders, and these disorders themselves are the strongest predictors of suicide. There has been a long-standing concern, however, that antidepressants, including drugs that inhibit the reuptake of norepinephrine and/or serotonin, may have a role in inducing worsening of depression and the emergence of suicidality in certain patients during the early phases of treatment.

In the placebo-controlled clinical trials of adults with fibromyalgia, among the patients who had a history of depression at treatment initiation, the incidence of suicidal ideation was 0.5% in patients treated with placebo, 0% in patients treated with milnacipran 100 mg/day, and 1.3% in patients treated with milnacipran 200 mg/day. No suicides occurred in the short-term or longer-term (up to 1 year) fibromyalgia trials.

See the Warning box for more information.

Appropriately monitor all patients being treated with drugs inhibiting the reuptake of norepinephrine and/or serotonin for any indication and observe them closely for clinical worsening, suicidality, and unusual changes in behavior, especially during the initial few months of a course of drug therapy or at times of dose changes, either increases or decreases.

Aggressiveness, agitation, akathisia (psychomotor restlessness), anxiety, hostility, hypomania, impulsivity, insomnia, irritability, mania, and panic attacks have been reported in adults and children being treated with drugs inhibiting the reuptake of norepinephrine and/or serotonin for MDD as well as for other indications, both psychiatric and nonpsychiatric. Although a causal link between the emergence of such symptoms and either the worsening of depression and/or the emergence of suicidal impulses has not been established, there is concern that such symptoms may represent precursors to emerging suicidality.

Consider changing the therapeutic regimen, including possibly discontinuing the medication, in patients who may experience worsening depressive symptoms or who are experiencing emergent suicidality or symptoms that might be precursors to worsening depression or suicidality, especially if these symptoms are severe or abrupt in onset, or were not part of the patient's presenting symptoms.

If the decision has been made to discontinue treatment because of worsening depressive symptoms or emergent suicidality, taper the medication as rapidly as is feasible, but with recognition that abrupt discontinuation can produce withdrawal symptoms.

Alert families and caregivers of patients being treated with drugs inhibiting the reuptake of norepinephrine and/or serotonin for MDD or other indications, both psychiatric and nonpsychiatric, about the need to monitor patients for the emergence of agitation, irritability, unusual changes in behavior, and the other symptoms described previously, as well as the emergence of suicidality, and to report such symptoms immediately to health care providers. Include in such monitoring daily observation by families and caregivers. Write prescriptions for milnacipran for the smallest quantity of tablets consistent with good patient management in order to reduce the risk of overdose.

➤*Serotonin syndrome or neuroleptic malignant syndrome–like reactions:* The development of a potentially life-threatening serotonin syndrome or neuroleptic malignant syndrome (NMS)–like reactions have been reported with SNRIs and selective serotonin reuptake inhibitors (SSRIs) alone, including milnacipran, particularly with concomitant use of serotonergic drugs (including triptans), with drugs that impair metabolism of serotonin (including MAOIs) or with antipsychotics or other dopamine antagonists. Serotonin syndrome symptoms may include mental status changes (eg, agitation, coma, hallucinations), autonomic instability (eg, hyperthermia, labile blood pressure, tachycardia), neuromuscular aberrations (eg, hyperreflexia, incoordination), and/or GI symptoms (eg, diarrhea, nausea, vomiting). Serotonin syndrome, in its most severe form, can resemble NMS, which includes hyperthermia, muscle rigidity, autonomic instability with possible rapid fluctuation of vital signs, and mental status changes. Monitor patients for the emergence of serotonin syndrome or NMS-like signs and symptoms.

Immediately discontinue treatment with milnacipran and any concomitant serotonergic or antidopaminergic agents, including antipsychotics, if the previously discussed events occur, and initiate supportive symptomatic treatment.

See Drug Interactions for more information.

➤*Cardiovascular effects:*

Blood pressure – Inhibition of the reuptake of norepinephrine and serotonin (5-HT) can lead to cardiovascular effects. SNRIs, including milnacipran, have been associated with reports of increase in blood pressure.

Sustained increases in blood pressure could have adverse consequences. Cases of elevated blood pressure requiring immediate treatment have been reported.

Concomitant use of milnacipran with drugs that increase blood pressure and pulse has not been evaluated; use such combinations with caution.

Effects of milnacipran on blood pressure in patients with significant hypertension or cardiac disease have not been systematically evaluated. Use milnacipran with caution in these patients.

Measure blood pressure prior to initiating treatment and periodically throughout milnacipran treatment. Treat preexisting hypertension and other cardiovascular disease before starting therapy with milnacipran. For patients who experience a sustained increase in blood pressure while receiving milnacipran, consider dose reduction or discontinuation. (See Adverse Reactions for more information.)

Heart rate – SNRIs have been associated with reports of increase in heart rate.

Measure heart rate prior to initiating treatment and periodically throughout milnacipran treatment. Treat preexisting tachyarrhythmias and other cardiac disease before starting therapy with milnacipran. For patients who experience a sustained increase in heart rate while receiving milnacipran, consider dose reduction or discontinuation. (See Adverse Reactions for more information.)

➤*Seizures:* Milnacipran has not been systematically evaluated in patients with a seizure disorder. In clinical trials evaluating milnacipran in patients with fibromyalgia, seizures/convulsions have not been reported. However, seizures have been reported infrequently in patients treated with milnacipran for disorders other than fibromyalgia. Prescribe milnacipran with care in patients with a history of a seizure disorder.

➤*Hepatotoxicity:* In the placebo-controlled fibromyalgia trials, increases in the number of patients treated with milnacipran with mild elevations of ALT or AST (1 to 3 times the upper limit of normal [ULN]) were observed. Increases in ALT were more frequently observed in the patients treated with milnacipran 100 mg/day (6%) and milnacipran 200 mg/day (7%) compared with the patients treated with placebo (3%). One (0.2%) patient receiving milnacipran 100 mg/day had an increase in ALT of more than 5 times the ULN, but did not exceed 10 times the ULN. Increases in AST were more frequently observed in patients treated with milnacipran 100 mg/day (3%) and milnacipran 200 mg/day (5%) compared with patients treated with placebo (2%).

There have been cases of increased liver enzymes and reports of severe liver injury, including fulminant hepatitis, with milnacipran from foreign postmarketing experience. In the cases of severe liver injury, there were significant underlying clinical conditions and/or the use of multiple concomitant medications. Because of underreporting, it is impossible to provide an accurate estimate of the true incidence of these reactions.

Discontinue milnacipran in patients who develop jaundice or other evidence of liver dysfunction. Do not resume treatment with milnacipran unless another cause can be established.

Ordinarily, do not prescribe milnacipran to patients with substantial alcohol use or evidence of chronic liver disease.

➤*Discontinuation of treatment:* Withdrawal symptoms have been observed in clinical trials following discontinuation of milnacipran, as with other SNRIs and SSRIs.

During marketing of milnacipran and other SNRIs and SSRIs, there have been spontaneous reports of adverse reactions indicative of withdrawal and physical dependence occurring upon discontinuation of these drugs, particularly when discontinuation is abrupt. The adverse reactions included agitation, anxiety, confusion, dizziness, dysphoric mood, emotional lability, headache, hypomania, insomnia, irritability, lethargy, sensory disturbances (eg, paresthesias such as electric shock sensations), seizures, and tinnitus. Although these reactions are generally self-limiting, some have been reported to be severe. Monitor patients for these symptoms when discontinuing treatment with milnacipran.

See Administration and Dosage for more information.

➤*Hyponatremia:* Hyponatremia may occur as a result of treatment with SSRIs and SNRIs, including milnacipran. In many cases, this hyponatremia appears to be the result of the syndrome of inappropriate antidiuretic hormone secretion. Cases with serum sodium lower than 110 mmol/L have been reported. Elderly patients may be at greater risk of developing hyponatremia with SNRIs, SSRIs, or milnacipran. Also, patients taking diuretics or who are otherwise volume-depleted may be at a greater risk. Consider discontinuation of milnacipran in patients with symptomatic hyponatremia.

➤*Abnormal bleeding:* SSRIs and SNRIs, including milnacipran, may increase the risk of bleeding events. Concomitant use of aspirin, nonsteroidal anti-inflammatory drugs (NSAIDs), warfarin, and other anticoagulants may add to this risk. Case reports and epidemiological studies (case-control and cohort design) have demonstrated an association between use of drugs that interfere with serotonin reuptake and the occurrence of GI bleeding. Bleeding events related to SSRI and SNRI use have ranged from ecchymoses, epistaxis, hematomas, and petechiae to life-threatening hemorrhages.

➤*Mania/Hypomania activation:* No activation of mania or hypomania was reported in the clinical trials evaluating effects of milnacipran in patients with fibromyalgia. However, those clinical trials excluded patients with a current major depressive episode. Activation of mania and hypomania have been reported in patients with mood disorders who were treated with other similar drugs for MDD. As with these other agents, use milnacipran cautiously in patients with a history of mania.

➤*GU effects:* Because of their noradrenergic effect, SNRIs, including milnacipran, can affect urethral resistance and micturition. In the controlled fibromyalgia trials, dysuria occurred more frequently in patients treated with milnacipran (1%) than in placebo-treated patients (0.5%). Caution is advised in use of milnacipran in patients with a history of dysuria, notably in men with prostatic hypertrophy, prostatitis, and other lower urinary tract obstructive disorders. Men are more prone to GU adverse reactions, such as dysuria or urinary retention, and may experience testicular pain or ejaculation disorders.

➤*Glaucoma:* Mydriasis has been reported in association with SNRIs and milnacipran; therefore, use milnacipran cautiously in patients with controlled narrow-angle glaucoma. Use of milnacipran in patients with uncontrolled narrow-angle glaucoma is contraindicated.

MILNACIPRAN HYDROCHLORIDE — ORAL

➤*Drug abuse and dependence:*

Dependence – Milnacipran produces physical dependence, as evidenced by the emergence of withdrawal symptoms following drug discontinuation, similar to other SNRIs and SSRIs. These withdrawal symptoms can be severe; therefore, taper milnacipran and do not abruptly discontinue after extended use.

➤*Hazardous tasks:* Milnacipran might diminish mental and physical capacities necessary to perform certain tasks such as operating machinery, including motor vehicles. Caution patients about operating machinery or driving motor vehicles until they are reasonably certain that milnacipran treatment does not affect their ability to engage in such activities.

➤*Pregnancy: Category C.* There are no adequate and well-controlled studies in pregnant women. Use milnacipran during pregnancy only if the potential benefit justifies the potential risk to the fetus.

Milnacipran increased the incidence of dead fetuses in utero in rats at dosages of 5 mg/kg/day (0.25 times the maximum recommended human dosage [MRHD] on a mg/m^2 basis). In rabbits, the incidence of the skeletal variation extra single rib was increased following administration of milnacipran at 15 mg/kg/day during the period of organogenesis.

Pregnancy registry – To provide information regarding the exposure to milnacipran during pregnancy, health care providers are advised to recommend that pregnant patients taking milnacipran enroll in the milnacipran pregnancy registry. Enrollment is voluntary and may be initiated by pregnant patients or their health care providers by contacting the registry at 1-877-643-3010 or by email at registrieskendle.com. Data forms may also be downloaded from the registry Web site at http://www.savellapregnancyregistry.com.

Nonteratogenic – Neonates exposed to dual reuptake inhibitors of serotonin and norepinephrine or to SSRIs late in the third trimester have developed complications requiring prolonged hospitalization, respiratory support, and tube feeding. Such complications can arise immediately upon delivery. Reported clinical findings have included apnea, constant crying, cyanosis, feeding difficulty, hyperreflexia, hypertonia, hypoglycemia, hypotonia, irritability, jitteriness, respiratory distress, seizures, temperature instability, tremor, and vomiting. These features are consistent with a direct toxic effect of these classes of drugs or, possibly, a drug discontinuation syndrome. Note that, in some cases, the clinical picture is consistent with serotonin syndrome.

A decrease in pup body weight and viability on postpartum day 4 were observed when milnacipran, at a dosage of 5 mg/kg/day (approximately 0.2 times the MRHD on a mg/m^2 basis), was administered orally to rats during late gestation. The no-effect dosage for maternal and offspring toxicity was 2.5 mg/kg/day (approximately 0.1 times the MRHD on a mg/m^2 basis).

➤*Lactation:* There are no adequate and well-controlled studies in breastfeeding women. It is not known if milnacipran is excreted in human breast milk. Studies in animals have shown that milnacipran or its metabolites are excreted in breast milk. Because many drugs are excreted in human breast milk and because of the potential for serious adverse reactions in breastfeeding infants from milnacipran, decide whether to discontinue breastfeeding or the drug, taking into account the importance of the drug to the mother. Because the safety of milnacipran in infants is not known, breastfeeding while on milnacipran is not recommended.

➤*Children:* Safety and effectiveness of milnacipran in children younger than 17 years of age with fibromyalgia have not been established. The use of milnacipran is not recommended in children.

➤*Elderly:* In view of the predominant excretion of unchanged milnacipran via the kidneys and the expected decrease in renal function with age, consider renal function prior to use of milnacipran in elderly patients.

SNRIs, SSRIs, and milnacipran have been associated with cases of clinically significant hyponatremia in elderly patients, who may be at greater risk for this adverse reaction.

➤*Monitoring:* Measure heart rate and blood pressure prior to initiating treatment and periodically throughout milnacipran treatment. Monitor patients for withdrawal symptoms when discontinuing treatment with milnacipran. Advise family and caregivers to monitor patients of all ages for the emergence of agitation, irritability, unusual changes in behavior, and the other symptoms described previously, as well as the emergence of suicidality, and to report such symptoms immediately to health care providers. Include in such monitoring daily observation by families and caregivers. Monitor patients for the emergence of serotonin syndrome or NMS-like signs and symptoms.

Drug Interactions

Milnacipran Drug Interactions

Precipitant drug	Object drug[a]		Description
Alcohol	Milnacipran	↑	Milnacipran may aggravate preexisting liver disease; therefore, do not administer to patients with substantial alcohol use or chronic liver disease.
Antipsychotic agents (eg, risperidone)	Milnacipran	↑	Serotonin syndrome may occur when an antipsychotic agent is coadministered with milnacipran. If coadministration cannot be avoided, closely monitor patients for signs and symptoms of serotonin syndrome or NMS-like reactions. Serotonin syndrome requires immediate medical attention, including withdrawal of the serotonergic agent and supportive care.
Clomipramine	Milnacipran	↑	An increase in euphoria and postural hypotension was observed in patients who switched from clomipramine to milnacipran. Use with caution. Closely monitor the patient during treatment switch.
CNS drugs (eg, amphetamine)	Milnacipran	↑	Given the primary CNS effects of milnacipran, use caution when taken in combination with other centrally acting drugs. Adjust therapy as needed.
Milnacipran	CNS drugs (eg, amphetamine)		
Cyclobenzaprine	Milnacipran	↑	Serotonergic effects of these agents may be additive. Serotonin syndrome may occur when a cyclobenzaprine is coadministered with milnacipran. If coadministration cannot be avoided, closely monitor patients for signs and symptoms of serotonin syndrome. Serotonin syndrome requires immediate medical attention, including withdrawal of the serotonergic agent and supportive care.
Milnacipran	Cyclobenzaprine		
Dopamine antagonists (eg, metaclopramide)	Milnacipran	↑	Serotonin syndrome may occur when a dopamine antagonist is coadministered with milnacipran. If coadministration cannot be avoided, closely monitor patients for signs and symptoms of serotonin syndrome or NMS-like reactions. Serotonin syndrome requires immediate medical attention, including withdrawal of the serotonergic agent and supportive care.
Lithium	Milnacipran	↑	Serotonin syndrome may occur when lithium is coadministered with milnacipran. If coadministration cannot be avoided, closely monitor patients for signs and symptoms of serotonin syndrome or NMS-like reactions. Serotonin syndrome requires immediate medical attention, including withdrawal of the serotonergic agent and supportive care.
MAOIs (eg, phenelzine, rasagiline)	Milnacipran	↑	Cocomitant use is contraindicated. Serotonin syndrome may occur. Do not start milnacipran within 14 days of discontinuation of an MAOI. Similarly, allow at least 5 days after stopping milnacipran before starting an MAOI.
Milnacipran	MAOIs (eg, phenelzine, rasagiline)		
Methylene blue	Milnacipran	↑	Coadministration of milnacipran and methylene blue may increase the risk of CNS toxicity, including serotonin syndrome. Avoid coadministration.

MILNACIPRAN HYDROCHLORIDE — ORAL

Milnacipran Drug Interactions			
Precipitant drug	Object drug[a]		Description
Serotonergic drugs (eg, SNRIs [eg, duloxetine], SSRIs [eg, fluoxetine], tramadol, triptans [eg, sumatriptan])	Milnacipran	↑	Coadministration of milnacipran with other inhibitors of serotonin reuptake may result in hypertension and coronary artery vasoconstriction through additive serotonergic effects. Coadministration is not recommended.
Milnacipran	Serotonergic drugs (eg, SNRIs [eg, duloxetine], SSRIs [eg, fluoxetine], tramadol, triptans [eg, sumatriptan])		
L-tryptophan	Milnacipran	↑	Coadministration may produce symptoms associated with serotonin syndrome (eg, dizziness, headache, nausea, sweating, vomiting). Coadministration is not recommended.
Milnacipran	Clonidine	↓	Milnacipran inhibits norepinephrine reuptake; coadministration with clonidine may inhibit clonidine's antihypertensive effect. Use with caution. Closely monitor blood pressure.
Milnacipran	Digoxin	↑	Use of milnacipran concomitantly with digoxin may be associated with potentiation of adverse hemodynamic effects. Postural hypotension and tachycardia have been reported in combination therapy with digoxin (1 mg) administered IV. Avoid coadministration.
Milnacipran	Drugs that interfere with hemostasis (eg, aspirin, NSAIDs, warfarin)	↑	Milnacipran may increase the bleeding effects of NSAIDs, aspirin, and/or warfarin. Caution patients about the risk of bleeding associated with the use of these drugs concurrently with milnacipran.
Milnacipran	Epinephrine Norepinephrine	↓	Milnacipran inhibits the reuptake of norepinephrine. Therefore, concomitant use of milnacipran with epinephrine and norepinephrine may be associated with paroxysmal hypertension and possible arrhythmia. Use with caution. Closely monitor blood pressure and pulse.

[a] ↑ = object drug increased; ↓ = object drug decreased.

Adverse Reactions

➤*Discontinuation of therapy:* In placebo-controlled trials in patients with fibromyalgia, 23% of patients treated with milnacipran 100 mg/day and 26% of patients treated with milnacipran 200 mg/day discontinued prematurely because of adverse reactions, compared with 12% of patients treated with placebo. The adverse reactions that led to withdrawal in 1% or more of patients in the milnacipran treatment group and with an incidence rate higher than that in the placebo treatment group were nausea (milnacipran, 6%; placebo, 1%), palpitations (milnacipran, 3%; placebo, 1%), headache (milnacipran, 2%; placebo, 0%), constipation (milnacipran, 1%; placebo, 0%), heart rate increased (milnacipran, 1%; placebo, 0%), hyperhidrosis (milnacipran, 1%; placebo, 0%), vomiting (milnacipran, 1%; placebo, 0%), and dizziness (milnacipran, 1%; placebo, 0.5%). Discontinuation because of adverse reactions was generally more common among patients treated with milnacipran 200 mg/day compared with milnacipran 100 mg/day.

➤*Most common adverse reactions:* In the placebo-controlled fibromyalgia trials, the most frequently occurring adverse reaction in clinical trials was nausea. The most common adverse reactions (incidence at least 5% and twice placebo) in patients treated with milnacipran were constipation, dry mouth, heart rate increased, hot flush, hyperhidrosis, hypertension palpitations, and vomiting.

➤*Adverse reactions (at least 2%):*

Milnacipran Adverse Reactions (≥ 2%)				
Adverse reactions	Milnacipran 100 mg/day (n = 623)	Milnacipran 200 mg/day (n = 934)	All milnacipran (n = 1,557)	Placebo (n = 652)
Cardiovascular				
Blood pressure increased	3%	3%	3%	1%
Flushing	2%	3%	3%	1%
Heart rate increased	5%	6%	6%	1%
Hot flush	11%	12%	12%	2%
Hypertension	7%	4%	5%	2%
Palpitations	8%	7%	7%	2%
Tachycardia	3%	2%	2%	1%
CNS				
Anxiety	5%	3%	4%	4%
Dizziness	11%	10%	10%	6%
Headache	19%	17%	18%	14%
Hypesthesia	1%	2%	1%	1%
Insomnia	12%	12%	12%	10%
Migraine	6%	4%	5%	3%
Paresthesia	2%	3%	2%	2%
Tension headache	2%	1%	1%	1%
Tremor	2%	2%	2%	1%
Dermatologic				
Hyperhidrosis	8%	9%	9%	2%
Pruritus	3%	2%	2%	2%
Rash	3%	4%	3%	2%
GI				
Abdominal pain	3%	3%	3%	2%
Constipation	16%	15%	16%	4%
Decreased appetite	1%	2%	2%	0%
Dry mouth	5%	5%	5%	2%
Nausea	35%	39%	37%	20%
Vomiting	6%	7%	7%	2%
Respiratory				
Dyspnea	2%	2%	2%	1%
Upper respiratory tract infection	7%	6%	6%	6%
Miscellaneous				
Chest discomfort	2%	1%	1%	1%
Chest pain	3%	2%	2%	2%
Chills	1%	2%	2%	0%
Vision blurred	1%	2%	2%	1%

➤*Weight changes:* In placebo-controlled fibromyalgia clinical trials, patients treated with milnacipran for up to 3 months experienced a mean weight loss of approximately 0.8 kg in both the milnacipran 100 mg/day and the milnacipran 200 mg/day treatment groups compared with a mean weight loss of approximately 0.2 kg in placebo-treated patients.

➤*GU:* In the placebo-controlled fibromyalgia studies, the following treatment-emergent adverse reactions related to the GU system were observed in at least 2% of men treated with milnacipran and occurred at a rate higher than in placebo-treated men: dysuria, ejaculation disorder, ejaculation failure, erectile dysfunction, libido decreased, prostatitis, scrotal pain, testicular pain, testicular swelling, urethral pain, urinary hesitation, urinary retention, and urine flow decreased.

➤*Blood pressure effects:* In a double-blind, placebo-controlled clinical pharmacology study in healthy patients designed to evaluate the effects of milnacipran on various parameters, including blood pressure at supratherapeutic doses, there was evidence of mean increases in supine blood pressure at dosages of up to 300 mg twice daily (600 mg/day). At the highest 300 mg twice-daily dosage, the mean increase in systolic blood pressure was up to 8.1 mm Hg for the placebo group and up to 10 mm Hg for the milnacipran-treated group over the 12-hour steady-state dosing interval. The corresponding mean increase in diastolic blood pressure over this interval was up to 4.6 mm Hg for placebo and up to 11.5 mm Hg for the milnacipran-treated group.

In the 3-month, placebo-controlled fibromyalgia clinical trials, milnacipran treatment was associated with mean increases of up to 3.1 mm Hg in systolic blood pressure and diastolic blood pressure.

In the placebo-controlled trials, among fibromyalgia patients who were non-hypertensive at baseline, approximately twice as many patients in the milnacipran treatment arms became hypertensive at the end of the study

MILNACIPRAN HYDROCHLORIDE — ORAL

(systolic blood pressure at least 140 mm Hg or diastolic blood pressure at least 90 mm Hg) compared with the placebo patients: 7.2% of patients in the placebo arm versus 19.5% of patients treated with milnacipran 100 mg/day and 16.6% of patients treated with milnacipran 200 mg/day. Among patients who met systolic criteria for prehypertension at baseline (systolic blood pressure 120 to 139 mm Hg), more patients became hypertensive at the end of the study in the milnacipran treatment arms than placebo: 9% of patients in the placebo arm versus 14% in both the milnacipran 100 and 200 mg/day treatment arms.

Among fibromyalgia patients who were hypertensive at baseline, more patients in the milnacipran treatment arms had a more than 15 mm Hg increase in systolic blood pressure than in the placebo arm at the end of the study: 1% of patients in the placebo arm versus 7% in the milnacipran 100 mg/day and 2% in the milnacipran 200 mg/day treatment arms. Similarly, more patients who were hypertensive at baseline and were treated with milnacipran had diastolic blood pressure increases more than 10 mm Hg than those who received placebo at the end of study: 3% of patients in the placebo arm versus 8% in the milnacipran 100 mg/day and 6% in the milnacipran 200 mg/day treatment arms.

Sustained increases in systolic blood pressure (increase of 15 mm Hg or more on 3 consecutive postbaseline visits) occurred in 2% of placebo patients versus 9% of patients receiving milnacipran 100 mg/day and 6% of patients receiving milnacipran 200 mg/day. Sustained increases in diastolic blood pressure (increase of at least 10 mm Hg on 3 consecutive postbaseline visits) occurred in 4% of patients receiving placebo versus 13% of patients receiving milnacipran 100 mg/day and 10% of patients receiving milnacipran 200 mg/day.

➤*Heart rate effects:* In clinical trials, relative to placebo, milnacipran treatment was associated with mean increases in pulse rate of approximately 7 to 8 beats per minute (bpm).

Increases in pulse of 20 bpm or more occurred more frequently in milnacipran-treated patients when compared with placebo: 0.3% in the placebo arm versus 8% in both the milnacipran 100 and 200 mg/day treatment arms. The effect of milnacipran on heart rate did not appear to increase with increasing dose.

➤*Other adverse reactions (at least 1%):*

CNS – Depression, fatigue, irritability, somnolence, stress.

GI – Abdominal distension, diarrhea, dysgeusia, dyspepsia, flatulence, gastroesophageal reflux disease.

GU – Cystitis, urinary tract infection.

Metabolic/Nutritional – Hypercholesterolemia, peripheral edema, weight decreased or increased.

Miscellaneous – Contusion, fall, night sweats, pyrexia.

➤*Postmarketing:*

Cardiovascular – Hypertensive crisis, supraventricular tachycardia.

CNS – Convulsions (including tonic-clonic), delirium, hallucination, loss of consciousness, parkinsonism, serotonin syndrome.

Dermatologic – Erythema multiforme, Stevens-Johnson syndrome.

GU – Acute renal failure, galactorrhea.

Hematologic/Lymphatic – Leukopenia, neutropenia, thrombocytopenia.

Metabolic/Nutritional – Anorexia, hyponatremia.

Miscellaneous – Accommodation disorder, hepatitis, hyperprolactinemia, rhabdomyolysis.

Overdosage

➤*Symptoms:* In postmarketing experience, fatal outcomes have been reported for acute overdoses primarily involving multiple drugs, but also with milnacipran only. The most common signs and symptoms included increased blood pressure, cardiorespiratory arrest, changes in the level of consciousness (ranging from somnolence to coma), confusional state, dizziness, and increased hepatic enzymes.

➤*Treatment:* There is no specific antidote to milnacipran, but if serotonin syndrome ensues, specific treatment (such as with cyproheptadine and/or temperature control) may be considered. In case of acute overdose, treatment consists of those general measures employed in the management of overdose with any drug.

Ensure an adequate airway, oxygenation, and ventilation, and monitor cardiac rhythm and vital signs. Gastric lavage with a large-bore orogastric tube with appropriate airway protection, if needed, may be indicated if performed soon after ingestion or in symptomatic patients. Because there is no specific antidote for milnacipran, consider symptomatic care and treatment with gastric lavage and activated charcoal as soon as possible for patients who experience a milnacipran overdose.

Patient Information

Inform patients, families, and caregivers about the benefits and risks associated with treatment with milnacipran, and counsel them in its appropriate use. A patient Medication Guide is available for milnacipran. Instruct patients, their families, and caregivers to read the Medication Guide and assist them in understanding its contents. Give patients the opportunity to discuss the contents of the Medication Guide and to obtain answers to any questions they may have.

Advise patients, families, and caregivers that milnacipran is a selective norepinephrine and serotonin reuptake inhibitor and, therefore, belongs to the same class of drugs as antidepressants. Advise patients, families, and caregivers that patients with depression may be at an increased risk for clinical worsening and/or suicidal ideation if they stop taking antidepressant medication, change the dose, or start a new medication.

Encourage patients, families, and caregivers to be alert to the emergence of aggressiveness, agitation, akathisia (psychomotor restlessness), anxiety, hostility, hypomania, impulsivity, insomnia, irritability, panic attacks, or other unusual changes in behavior, worsening of depression, and suicidal ideation, especially early during treatment with milnacipran or other drugs that inhibit the reuptake of norepinephrine and/or serotonin, and when the dose is adjusted up or down. Advise families and caregivers to monitor patients for the emergence of such symptoms on a day-to-day basis because changes may be abrupt. Advise families and caregivers to report such symptoms to the patient's health care provider, especially if they are severe or abrupt in onset, or were not part of the patient's presenting symptoms.

Caution patients about the risk of serotonin syndrome with concomitant use of milnacipran and triptans, tramadol, or other serotonergic agents.

Advise patients to monitor their blood pressure and pulse at regular intervals when receiving treatment with milnacipran.

Caution patients about the concomitant use of milnacipran and NSAIDs, aspirin, or other drugs that affect coagulation because the combined use of agents that interfere with serotonin reuptake and these agents has been associated with an increased risk of abnormal bleeding.

Milnacipran may diminish mental and physical capacities necessary to perform certain tasks such as operating machinery, including motor vehicles. Caution patients about operating machinery or driving motor vehicles until they are reasonably certain that milnacipran treatment does not affect their ability to engage in such activities.

Advise patients to avoid consumption of alcohol while taking milnacipran.

Advise patients that withdrawal symptoms can occur when discontinuing treatment with milnacipran, particularly when discontinuation is abrupt.

Advise patients to notify their health care provider if they become pregnant or intend to become pregnant during milnacipran therapy. Encourage patients to enroll in the milnacipran pregnancy registry if they become pregnant, preferably before any prenatal testing is done. This registry is collecting information about the safety of milnacipran during pregnancy. To enroll, patients or their health care providers may call the toll-free number 1-877-643-3010, download data forms from http://www.savellapregnancyregistry.com, or email the registry for further information at registrieskendle.com.

Advise patients to notify their health care provider if they are breast-feeding.

Selective Serotonin Reuptake Inhibitors

Refer to the Antidepressants introduction.

Indications

Refer to individual monographs for further information.

SSRIs — Summary of Indications

Indication ✓ - FDA approved X - Off-label	Citalopram	Escitalopram	Fluoxetine	Fluvoxamine	Paroxetine	Sertraline
Alcoholism	X[g]		X[f]			
Binge-eating disorder	X[f]					
Borderline personality disorder			X[d]			
Bulimia nervosa			✓	X[e]		
Depression	✓	✓	✓	X[h]	✓	✓
Diabetic neuropathy	X[g]				X[e]	
Fibromyalgia			X[g]			
GAD[i]	X[f]	✓	X[h]		✓[a]	
Hot flashes (men)					X[g]	X[g]

SSRIs — Summary of Indications

Indication ✓ - FDA approved X - Off-label	Citalopram	Escitalopram	Fluoxetine	Fluvoxamine	Paroxetine	Sertraline
Hot flashes (women)			X[g]		X[e]	
Irritable bowel syndrome (IBS)	X[g]					
Nocturnal enuresis			X[f]	X[f]	X[f]	X[f]
Obsessive-compulsive disorder (OCD)	X[d]		✓	✓	✓[a]	✓
Panic disorder	X[h]	X[h]	✓	X[d]	✓	✓
Pathological gambling	X[g]					
Postherpetic neuralgia			X[g]			
Posttraumatic stress disorder (PTSD)	X[h]	X[d] (adults only)	X[d]	X[d]	✓[a]	✓
Premenstrual disorders	X[e]				X[e]	
Premenstrual dysphoric disorder (PMDD)	X[h]		✓[b]		✓[c]	✓
Prevention of migraine (adults)			X[g]	X[e]	X[g]	X[g]
Pruritus					X[g]	
Pruritus (cholestatic)						X[e]
Raynaud phenomenon			X[e]			
Social anxiety disorder				✓[k]	✓	✓
Stuttering	X[g]				X[g]	
TBI[j]					X[f]	

[a] Immediate-release only.
[b] *Sarafem* only.
[c] Controlled-release only.
[d] Good documentation.
[e] Fair documentation.
[f] Safety concerns.
[g] Insufficient documentation.
[h] Not rated.
[i] GAD = generalized anxiety disorder.
[j] TBI = traumatic brain injury.
[k] Capsules only.

➤*Off-label uses:* Refer to individual monographs for further information.

Alcoholism –
Citalopram: [4] = Insufficient documentation.
Fluoxetine: [3] = Safety concerns.

Binge-eating disorder –
Citalopram: [3] = Safety concerns.

Borderline personality disorder –
Fluoxetine: [1] = Good documentation.

Bulimia nervosa –
Fluvoxamine: [2] = Fair documentation.

Diabetic neuropathy –
Citalopram: [4] = Insufficient documentation.
Fluoxetine: [5] = Poor documentation.
Paroxetine: [2] = Fair documentation.

Fibromyalgia –
Citalopram: [5] = Poor documentation.
Fluoxetine: [4] = Insufficient documentation.

Generalized anxiety disorder –
Citalopram: [3] = Safety concerns.

Hot flashes (men) –
Paroxetine: [4] = Insufficient documentation.
Sertraline: [4] = Insufficient documentation.

Hot flashes (women) –
Citalopram: [5] = Poor documentation.
Fluoxetine: [4] = Insufficient documentation.
Paroxetine: [2] = Fair documentation.
Sertraline: [5] = Poor documentation.

Impulsive aggressive behavior (adults) –
Citalopram: [4] = Insufficient documentation.

Impulsive aggressive behavior (children/adolescents) –
Citalopram: [4] = Insufficient documentation.

Irritable bowel syndrome –
Citalopram: [4] = Insufficient documentation.

Nocturnal enuresis –
Fluoxetine: [3] = Safety concerns.
Fluvoxamine: [3] = Safety concerns.
Paroxetine: [3] = Safety concerns.
Sertraline: [3] = Safety concerns.

Obsessive-compulsive disorder –
Citalopram: [1] = Good documentation.

Panic disorder –
Fluvoxamine: [1] = Good documentation.

Pathological gambling –
Citalopram: [4] = Insufficient documentation.

Postherpetic neuralgia –
Fluoxetine: [4] = Insufficient documentation.

Posttraumatic stress disorder (adults) –
Escitalopram: [1] = Good documentation.
Fluoxetine: [1] = Good documentation.
Fluvoxamine: [1] = Good documentation.

Posttraumatic stress disorder (children/adolescents) –
Fluoxetine: [1] = Good documentation.
Fluvoxamine: [1] = Good documentation.

Premenstrual disorders –
Citalopram: [2] = Fair documentation.
Paroxetine: [2] = Fair documentation.

Prevention of migraine (adults) –
Fluoxetine: [4] = Insufficient documentation.
Fluvoxamine: [2] = Fair documentation.
Paroxetine: [4] = Insufficient documentation.
Sertraline: [4] = Insufficient documentation.

Pruritus –
Paroxetine: [4] = Insufficient documentation.

Pruritus (cholestatic) –
Sertraline: [2] = Fair documentation.

Raynaud phenomenon –
Fluoxetine: [2] = Fair documentation.

Smoking cessation –
Fluoxetine: [5] = Poor documentation.
Paroxetine: [5] = Poor documentation.
Sertraline: [5] = Poor documentation.

Stuttering –
Citalopram: [4] = Insufficient documentation.
Paroxetine: [4] = Insufficient documentation.

Traumatic brain injury –
Paroxetine: [3] = Safety concerns.
Sertraline: [3] = Safety concerns.

Trichotillomania –
Fluoxetine: [5] = Poor documentation.

Other possible off-label uses –
Citalopram: Panic disorder; premenstrual dysphoric syndrome; posttraumatic stress disorder.

Escitalopram: Panic disorder.
Fluoxetine: GAD.
Fluvoxamine: Depression.

Actions

➤*Pharmacology:* Selective serotonin reuptake inhibitors (SSRIs) are oral antidepressant agents chemically unrelated to the tricyclic, tetracyclic, or other available antidepressants. The antidepressant action of the SSRIs is presumed to be linked to their inhibition of CNS neuronal uptake of serotonin (5HT). Human and in vitro studies have demonstrated that **fluoxetine** (and its active metabolite S-norfluoxetine), **fluvoxamine**, **paroxetine**, **sertraline**, **escitalopram**, and **citalopram** are potent and selective inhibitors of neuronal serotonin reuptake, and they also have a weak effect on norepinephrine and dopamine neuronal reuptake. SSRIs have little affinity for muscarinic, gamma aminobutyric acid (GABA), benzodiazepine, $alpha_1$, $alpha_2$, beta-adrenergic, dopamine (D_2), $5\text{-}HT_1$, $5\text{-}HT_2$, and histamine (H_1) receptors; antagonism of muscarinic, histaminergic, and $alpha_1$-adrenergic receptors has been associated with various anticholinergic, sedative, and cardiovascular effects for other psychotropic drugs. The chronic administration of sertraline in animals was found to down-regulate brain norepinephrine receptors, as has been observed with other clinically effective antidepressants.

➤*Pharmacokinetics:*

SSRI Pharmacokinetics							
SSRIs	Time to peak plasma concentration (h)	Peak plasma concentration (ng/mL)	Half-life (h)	Protein binding (%)	Time to reach steady state (days)	Primary route of elimination	Bioavailability (%)
Citalopram	≈ 4	nd[a]	≈ 35	≈ 80	≈ 7	20% renal, fecal	≈ 80
Escitalopram	5	nd[a]	27 - 32	≈ 56	≈ 7	7% renal	80[c]
Fluoxetine	6 - 8	15 - 55	24 - 384[b]	≈ 94.5	≈ 28	hepatic	nd[a]
Fluvoxamine	3 - 8	88 - 546	13.6 - 15.6	≈ 80	≈ 7	≈ 94% renal	53
Paroxetine	5.2	61.7	21	≈ 93-95	≈10	64% renal, 36% fecal	100
Paroxetine CR	6 - 10	30	15 - 20		14		
Sertraline	4.5 - 8.4	nd[a]	26 - 104[b]	98	≈ 7	40% - 45% renal, 40% - 45% fecal	nd[a]

[a] nd = No data.
[b] t½ includes the active metabolite.
[c] Based on citalopram data.

Special populations –
Elderly:
• *Citalopram* – In a single-dose study, citalopram AUC and half-life were increased in the elderly by 30% and 50%, respectively, whereas in a multiple-dose study they were increased by 23% and 30%, respectively.
• *Escitalopram* – Half-life was increased by approximately 50% in elderly subjects, and C_{max} was unchanged.
• *Fluvoxamine* – Mean C_{max} was 40% higher in elderly subjects, and the elimination half-life also increased. The clearance also was reduced by approximately 50%.
• *Paroxetine* – C_{min} concentrations were approximately 70% to 80% higher in elderly patients.
• *Sertraline* – Plasma clearance was approximately 40% lower in elderly patients. Therefore, steady state should be achieved after 2 to 3 weeks in older patients.
Hepatic function impairment:
• *Citalopram* – Oral clearance was reduced by 37% and half-life was doubled in patients with reduced hepatic function.
• *Fluoxetine* – Elimination half-life was prolonged in a study of cirrhotic patients, with a mean of 7.6 days; norfluoxetine elimination also was delayed, with a mean duration of 12 days for cirrhotic patients.
• *Fluvoxamine* – Clearance decreased 30% in patients with hepatic dysfunction.
• *Paroxetine* – Patients with hepatic function impairment had about a 2-fold increase in plasma concentrations (AUC, C_{max}).
• *Sertraline* – In patients with mild liver impairment, clearance was reduced, resulting in approximately 3-fold greater exposure.
Renal function impairment:
• *Citalopram* – In patients with mild to moderate renal function impairment, oral clearance was reduced by 17%.
• *Fluoxetine* – In depressed patients on dialysis (N = 12), fluoxetine administered as 20 mg once daily for 2 months produced steady-state fluoxetine and norfluoxetine plasma concentrations comparable with those seen in patients with normal renal function. The possibility exists that renally excreted metabolites of fluoxetine may accumulate to higher levels in patients with severe renal dysfunction.
• *Paroxetine* – The mean plasma concentrations in patients with Ccr less than 30 mL/min were approximately 4 times greater than normal subjects. Patients with Ccr of 30 to 60 mL/min had about a 2-fold increase in plasma concentrations (AUC, C_{max}).

Contraindications

Hypersensitivity to SSRIs or any inactive ingredients; in combination with a monoamine oxidase inhibitor (MAOI), or within 14 days of discontinuing an MAOI (see Drug Interactions);administration of thioridazine with **fluoxetine** or within a minimum of 5 weeks after fluoxetine has been discontinued; coadministration of **fluvoxamine** with cisapride, thioridazine or pimozide (see Drug Interactions); concomitant use of thioridazine with **paroxetine**; concomitant use of pimozide with **sertraline**; coadministration of sertraline oral concentrate and disulfiram.

Warnings/Precautions

➤*Long-term use:* The effectiveness of long-term use of SSRIs for OCD, panic disorder, social anxiety disorder, PMDD, PTSD, GAD, and bulimia has not been systematically evaluated. However, the long-term use of SSRIs for depression has been evaluated and demonstrated to maintain antidepressant response for up to 1 year. Periodically reevaluate the SSRI used for extended periods to determine long-term usefulness of the drug for the individual patient.

➤*MAOIs:* In patients receiving an SSRI in combination with an MAOI, serious, sometimes fatal reactions have occurred, including hyperthermia, rigidity, myoclonus, autonomic instability with possible rapid fluctuations of vital signs, and mental status changes that include confusion, irritability, extreme agitation progressing to delirium, and coma. These reactions also have occurred in patients who have recently discontinued an SSRI and have been started on an MAOI. Some cases presented with features resembling neuroleptic malignant syndrome. While no human data show such an interaction with **paroxetine**, limited animal data suggest that the drugs may act synergistically to elevate blood pressure and evoke behavioral excitation. Therefore, it is recommended that SSRIs not be used in combination with an MAOI or within 14 days of discontinuing treatment with an MAOI. Allow at least 2 weeks after stopping the SSRIs before starting an MAOI; allow at least 5 weeks after stopping **fluoxetine** before starting an MAOI (see Drug Interactions).

➤*Suicide risk:* Patients with major depressive disorder, both adult and pediatric, may experience worsening of their depression and/or the emergence of suicidal ideation and behavior (suicidality), whether or not they are taking antidepressant medications, and this risk may persist until significant remission occurs. Although there has been a long-standing concern that antidepressants may have a role in inducing worsening of depression and the emergence of suicidality in certain patients, a causal role for antidepressants in inducing such behaviors has not been established. Nevertheless, closely observe patients being treated with antidepressants for clinical worsening and suicidality, especially at the beginning of a course of drug therapy or at the time of dose changes, either increases or decreases. Consider changing the therapeutic regimen, including possibly discontinuing the medication, in patients whose depression is persistently worse or whose emergent suicidality is severe, abrupt in onset, or was not part of the patient's presenting symptoms. Write prescriptions for the smallest quantity of tablets or capsules in order to reduce the risk of overdose.

➤*Rash and accompanying events:* Seven percent of patients taking **fluoxetine** have developed a rash and/or urticaria; almost one third were withdrawn from treatment. Clinical findings reported in association with rash include: arthralgias, edema, carpal tunnel syndrome, fever, leukocytosis, lymphadenopathy, mild transaminase elevation, proteinuria, and respiratory distress. Most patients improved promptly with discontinuation of fluoxetine and/or adjunctive treatment with antihistamines or steroids; all patients recovered completely. Two patients treated with fluoxetine developed a serious cutaneous systemic illness. Neither had an unequivocal diagnosis, but one had a leukocytoclastic vasculitis; the other had a severe desquamating syndrome that was considered to be vasculitis or erythema multiforme. Other patients have had systemic syndromes suggestive of serum sickness.

Systemic events, possibly related to vasculitis and including lupus-like syndrome, have developed in patients with rash. Although rare, these events may be serious, involving the lung, kidney, or liver. Death has been associated with the events. Anaphylactoid events, including bronchospasm, angioedema, and urticaria, alone and in combination, have occurred with fluoxetine. Pulmonary events, including inflammatory processes of varying histopathology and/or fibrosis, have occurred rarely. These events have occurred with dyspnea as the only preceding symptom. Whether these systemic events and rash have a common underlying cause or are caused by different etiologies or pathogenic processes is not known. Furthermore, a specific underlying immunologic basis for these events has not been identified. Upon the appearance of rash or of other possibly allergic phenomena for which an alternative etiology cannot be identified, discontinue the SSRI.

➤*Abnormal bleeding:* Altered platelet function and/or abnormal results from laboratory studies in patients taking **fluoxetine**, **paroxetine**, or **ser-**

traline have occurred. There have been reports of abnormal bleeding or purpura in several patients; it is unclear whether the SSRIs had a causative role.

Published case reports have documented the occurrence of bleeding episodes in patients treated with psychotropic drugs that interfere with serotonin reuptake. Subsequent epidemiological studies, both of the case-control and cohort design, have demonstrated an association between the use of psychotropic drugs that interfere with serotonin reuptake and the occurrence of upper GI bleeding. In 2 studies, concurrent use of a nonsteroidal anti-inflammatory drug (NSAID) or aspirin potentiated the risk of bleeding. Although these studies focused on upper GI bleeding, there is reason to believe that bleeding at other sites may be similarly potentiated. Caution patients regarding the risk of bleeding associated with the concomitant use of SSRIs with NSAIDs, aspirin, or other drugs that affect coagulation.

➤*Anxiety, nervousness, and insomnia:* Anxiety, nervousness, and insomnia occurred in 2% to 22% of patients treated with an SSRI. In clinical trials for bulimia nervosa, insomnia occurred in 33% of patients treated with **fluoxetine**.

➤*Altered appetite and weight:* Significant weight loss, especially in underweight depressed or bulimic patients, has occurred. Approximately 3% to 17% of patients treated with an SSRI initially experienced anorexia. Significant weight loss may be an undesirable result of treatment for some patients but on average, patients in controlled trials treated with **paroxetine**, **citalopram**, or **sertraline** had a minimal 1- to 2-pound weight loss vs smaller changes with placebo. Only rarely have the SSRIs been discontinued because of weight loss or anorexia (see Adverse Reactions); however, after prolonged treatments, patients tend to gain weight. Monitor weight change during therapy.

➤*Activation of mania/hypomania:* Activation of mania/hypomania occurred infrequently in approximately 0.1% to 2.6% of patients taking SSRIs. Activation of mania/hypomania also has occurred in a small proportion of patients with major affective disorder treated with other antidepressants. Use cautiously in patients with a history of mania.

➤*Seizures:* Seizures have occurred with **fluoxetine** (0.1%), **fluvoxamine** (0.2%), **paroxetine** (0.1%), **sertraline** (0.2%), and **citalopram** (0.3%). Sertraline, citalopram, and **escitalopram** have not been evaluated in patients with a seizure disorder. These percentages appear similar to the rate associated with other antidepressants and placebo treatment. Use with care in patients with history of seizures; discontinue therapy if seizures occur.

➤*Cardiac effects:* SSRIs have not been systematically evaluated in patients with a recent history of MI or unstable heart disease. Patients with these diagnoses were generally excluded from clinical studies during the product's premarketing testing. However, the ECGs of patients who received SSRIs in clinical trials were evaluated and the data indicate that they are not associated with the development of clinically significant ECG abnormalities.

➤*Fluoxetine dose changes:* The long elimination half-life of **fluoxetine** and norfluoxetine means that changes in dose will not be fully reflected in plasma for several weeks, affecting titration to final dose and withdrawal from treatment.

➤*Concomitant illness:* Clinical experience is limited. Use caution in patients with diseases or conditions that could affect metabolism or hemodynamic responses.

➤*Glaucoma:* Mydriasis has been reported infrequently in premarketing studies with SSRIs. A few cases of acute angle-closure glaucoma associated with **paroxetine** therapy have been reported in the literature. As mydriasis can cause acute angle closure in patients with narrow-angle glaucoma, use caution when SSRIs are prescribed for patients with narrow-angle glaucoma.

➤*Effects of smoking:* Smokers had a 25% increase in the metabolism of **fluvoxamine** compared with nonsmokers.

➤*Electroconvulsive therapy (ECT):* There are no clinical studies establishing the benefit of the combined use of ECT and SSRIs. Rare prolonged seizure in patients on **fluoxetine** has occurred.

➤*Hyponatremia:* Several cases of **fluoxetine**, **fluvoxamine**, **sertraline**, **paroxetine**, **escitalopram**, and **citalopram**-induced hyponatremia (some with serum sodium less than 110 mmol/L) have occurred. The hyponatremia appeared to be reversible when fluoxetine, sertraline, paroxetine, citalopram, escitalopram, and fluvoxamine were discontinued. Although these cases were complex with varying possible etiologies, some were possibly because of the syndrome of inappropriate antidiuretic hormone secretion (SIADH). The majority have been in older patients and in patients taking diuretics or who were otherwise volume-depleted.

➤*Diabetes:* **Fluoxetine** may alter glycemic control. Hypoglycemia has occurred during therapy, and hyperglycemia has developed following discontinuation of the drug. The dosage of insulin and/or oral hypoglycemic agents may need to be adjusted when fluoxetine is started or discontinued.

➤*Uricosuric effect:* **Sertraline** is associated with a mean decrease in serum uric acid of approximately 7%. The clinical significance of this weak uricosuric effect is unknown.

➤*Discontinuation of SSRIs:* During marketing of SSRIs and SNRIs, there have been spontaneous reports of adverse events occurring upon discontinuation of these drugs, particularly when abrupt, including the following: agitation, anxiety, confusion, dizziness, dysphoric mood, emotional lability, headache, hypomania, insomnia, irritability, lethargy, and sensory disturbances (eg, paresthesias such as electric shock sensations). While these events are generally self-limiting, there have been reports of serious discontinuation symptoms.

Monitor patients for these symptoms when discontinuing treatment with SSRIs. A gradual reduction in the dose rather than abrupt cessation is recommended whenever possible. If intolerable symptoms occur following a decrease in the dose or upon discontinuation of treatment, then resuming the previously prescribed dose may be considered. Subsequently, the physician may continue decreasing the dose but at a more gradual rate.

➤*Renal function impairment:* In depressed patients on dialysis (N = 12), **fluoxetine** administered as 20 mg once daily for 2 months produced steady-state fluoxetine and norfluoxetine plasma concentrations comparable with those seen in patients with normal renal function. The possibility exists that renally excreted metabolites of fluoxetine may accumulate to higher levels in patients with severe renal dysfunction. Use of a lower or less-frequent dose for renally impaired patients is not routinely necessary (see Administration and Dosage).

Increased plasma concentrations of **paroxetine** occur in subjects with severe renal (Ccr less than 30 mL/min). Reduce the initial dosage of paroxetine in patients with severe renal impairment; if necessary, increase upward titration intervals (see Administration and Dosage).

Because **sertraline** and **escitalopram** are extensively metabolized by the liver, excretion of unchanged drug in the urine is a minor route of elimination. However, use with caution in patients with severe renal impairment.

In patients with mild to moderate renal function impairment, oral clearance of **citalopram** was reduced by 17% compared with healthy subjects. No adjustment of dosage for such patients is recommended. No information is available about pharmacokinetics of citalopram in patients with severely reduced renal function (Ccr less than 20 mL/min). Because citalopram is extensively metabolized, excretion of unchanged drug in urine is a minor route of elimination. Until an adequate number of patients with severe renal impairment have been evaluated during chronic treatment with citalopram, use with caution in such patients.

The mean minimum plasma concentrations in renally impaired patients (Ccr 5 to 45 mL/min) after 4 and 6 weeks of treatment (50 mg twice daily, n = 13) were comparable to each other, suggesting no accumulation of **fluvoxamine** in these patients.

➤*Hepatic function impairment:* SSRIs are extensively metabolized by the liver. Use with caution in patients with severe liver impairment. The elimination half-life of **fluoxetine** was prolonged in a study of cirrhotic patients, with a mean of 7.6 days; norfluoxetine elimination also was delayed, with a mean duration of 12 days. **Fluvoxamine** clearance was decreased by 30%; slowly titrate fluvoxamine during initiation of treatment. Increased plasma concentrations of **paroxetine** occur in patients with severe hepatic impairment. Initial dose should be reduced and upward titration, if necessary, should be at increased intervals. The clearance of **sertraline** is decreased in mild, chronic liver impairment. Give a lower or less-frequent dose in patients with liver impairment; if necessary, increase upward titration intervals.

Citalopram oral clearance was reduced by 37% and half-life was doubled in patients with reduced hepatic function compared with healthy subjects. The recommended dose for most hepatically impaired patients is 20 mg.

In subjects with hepatic impairment, clearance of racemic citalopram was decreased and plasma concentrations were increased. The recommended dose of **escitalopram** in hepatically impaired patients is 10 mg/day.

➤*Drug abuse and dependence:* Premarketing clinical experience did not reveal any tendency for a withdrawal syndrome or any drug-seeking behavior. It is not possible to predict on the basis of this limited experience the extent to which a CNS-active drug will be misused, diverted, or abused once marketed. Consequently, before starting an SSRI, carefully evaluate patients for history of drug abuse and follow such patients closely, observing them for signs of misuse or abuse.

➤*Hazardous tasks:* Any psychoactive drug may impair judgment, thinking, or motor skills; caution patients about operating hazardous machinery, including automobiles, until they are reasonably certain that the drug treatment does not affect them adversely.

➤*Photosensitivity:* Photosensitization may occur; therefore, caution patients to take protective measures (eg, sunscreens, protective clothing) against exposure to ultraviolet light or sunlight until tolerance is determined.

➤*Pregnancy: Category C.* There are no adequate and well-controlled studies in pregnant women. Use during pregnancy only if clearly needed. In a study involving 228 women who had received **fluoxetine** during pregnancy, 5.5% of the women who took fluoxetine in the first trimester delivered infants with major structural anomalies. At doses 0.5 to 4 times the MRHD mg/kg, **sertraline** was associated with delayed ossification in fetuses of rats and rabbits, respectively. The decrease in pup survival was most probably caused by in utero exposure to sertraline. In rats, **fluvoxamine** increased pup mortality at birth and decreased postnatal pup weight and survival. **Paroxetine** reproduction studies in rats revealed no evidence of teratogenic effects. However, in rats, there was an increase in pup deaths during the first 4 days of lactation when dosing occurred during the last trimester of gestation and continued throughout lactation. In 2 rat embryo/fetal development studies, oral administration of **citalopram** (32, 56, or 112 mg/kg/day) to pregnant animals during the period of organogenesis resulted in decreased embryo/fetal growth and survival and an increased incidence of fetal abnormalities (including cardiovascular and skeletal defects) at the high dose, which is approximately 18 times the MRHD. Female rats treated with citalopram from late gestation through weaning increased offspring mortality during the first 4 days after birth, and persistent offspring growth retardation was observed at the highest dose (32 mg/kg/day).

Oral administration of **escitalopram** to pregnant animals during the period of organogenesis resulted in decreased fetal body weight and associated delays in ossification. Maternal toxicity (clinical signs and decreased body weight gain and food consumption) was present at all dose levels. When female rats were treated with escitalopram during pregnancy and through weaning, slightly increased offspring mortality and growth retardation were noted at 48 mg/kg/day. Slight maternal toxicity (clinical signs and decreased body weight gain and food consumption) were seen at this dose.

Neonates exposed to SSRIs or serotonin-norepinephrine reuptake inhibitors (SNRIs) late in the third trimester have developed complications requiring prolonged hospitalization, respiratory support, and tube feeding. Such complications can arise immediately upon delivery. Reported clinical findings have included apnea, constant crying; cyanosis, feeding difficulty, hyperreflexia, hypertonia, hypoglycemia, hypotonia, irritability, jitteriness, respiratory distress, seizures, temperature instability, tremor, vomiting. These features are consistent with either a direct toxic effect of SSRIs and SNRIs or, possibly, a drug discontinuation syndrome. It should be noted that, in some cases, the clinical picture is consistent with serotonin syndrome. When treating a pregnant woman with SSRIs during the third trimester, the physician should carefully consider the potential risks and benefits of treatment.

➤*Lactation:* **Fluoxetine**, **fluvoxamine**, **paroxetine**, **citalopram**, and **escitalopram** are excreted in breast milk. It is not known whether **sertraline** or its metabolites are excreted in breast milk. In one breast milk sample, the concentration of fluoxetine plus norfluoxetine was 70.4 ng/mL; the mother's plasma concentration was 295 ng/mL. No adverse effects were noted in the infant. In another case, an infant nursed by a mother on fluoxetine developed crying, sleep disturbance, vomiting, and watery stools. The infant's plasma drug levels were 340 ng/mL of fluoxetine and 208 ng/mL of norfluoxetine on the second day of feeding. There have been 2 reports of infants experiencing excessive somnolence, decreased feeding, and weight loss in association with breastfeeding from a citalopram-treated mother; in one case, the infant was reported to recover completely upon discontinuation of citalopram by its mother. Exercise caution when SSRIs are administered to a nursing woman. Decide whether to discontinue nursing or discontinue the drug taking into account the importance of the drug to the mother.

➤*Children:* Safety and efficacy in children have not been established.

Regular monitoring of weight and growth is recommended if treatment of a child with an SSRI is to be continued long-term.

The safety and efficacy in pediatric patients younger than 8 years of age in major depressive disorder and younger than 7 years of age in OCD have not been established.

The efficacy of **sertraline** for the treatment of OCD was demonstrated in a 12-week, multicenter, placebo-controlled study with 187 outpatients 6 to 17 years of age. The efficacy of sertraline in pediatric patients with depression, panic disorder, PTSD, PMDD, or social anxiety disorder has not been established.

The efficacy of **fluvoxamine** for the treatment of OCD was demonstrated in a 10-week, multicenter, placebo-controlled study with 120 outpatients 8 to 17 years of age. The adverse event profile was similar to that observed in adult studies. The risks, if any, that may be associated with fluvoxamine's extended use in children and adolescents with OCD have not been systematically assessed. Have the prescriber be mindful that the evidence supporting fluvoxamine use in children and adolescents derives from relatively short-term clinical studies and from extrapolation of experience gained with adult patients.

➤*Elderly:* The disposition of single doses of **fluoxetine** in healthy elderly subjects (older than 65 years of age) did not differ significantly from that in younger healthy subjects. However, data are insufficient to rule out possible age-related differences during chronic use. Clearance of **fluvoxamine** is decreased by approximately 50% in elderly patients, and greater sensitivity of some older individuals cannot be ruled out. Consequently, slowly titrate fluvoxamine during initiation of therapy. **Paroxetine** pharmacokinetic studies revealed a decreased clearance in the elderly, and a lower starting dose is recommended; there was, however, no overall difference in the adverse event profile between elderly and younger patients, and efficacy was similar. For **sertraline**, the pattern of adverse reactions in the elderly was similar to that in younger patients. However, sertraline plasma clearance may be lower (see Pharmacokinetics). In 2 pharmacokinetic studies, **citalopram** AUC was increased by 23% and 30%, respectively, in elderly subjects as compared with younger subjects, and its half-life was increased by 30% and 50%, respectively. In 2 pharmacokinetic studies, **escitalopram** half-life was increased by approximately 50% in elderly subjects as compared with young subjects and C_{max} was unchanged.

Per the Beers list, fluoxetine has a long half-life and risk of producing excessive CNS stimulation, sleep disturbances, and increasing agitation. Safer alternatives exist.

➤*Monitoring:* In patients receiving SSRIs and suffering from SIADH, displacement syndromes, edematous states, adrenal disease, or conditions of fluid loss, it is recommended that serum electrolytes, especially sodium, as well as BUN and plasma creatinine be monitored regularly. Monitor patients for the emergence of agitation, irritability, and other symptoms, as well as emergence of suicidality, especially at the beginning of drug therapy or at the time of dose changes. Regular monitoring of weight and growth is recommended, especially if treatment of a child with an SSRI is to be continued long-term.

Drug Interactions

➤*Drugs highly bound to plasma protein:* Because SSRIs are highly bound to plasma protein, administration to a patient taking another drug that is highly protein-bound (eg, warfarin, digoxin) may cause increased free concentrations of the other drug, potentially resulting in adverse events. Conversely, adverse effects could result from displacement of SSRIs by other highly bound drugs.

➤*CYP450 system:* Concomitant use of SSRIs with drugs metabolized by cytochrome P450 2D6 may require lower doses than usually prescribed for either SSRIs or the other drug because SSRIs may significantly inhibit the activity of this isozyme. In most patients (more than 90%), this isozyme is saturated early during dosing. Therefore, coadministration of **paroxetine** with other drugs that are metabolized by this isozyme (eg, certain antidepressants, phenothiazines, risperidone, type IC antiarrhythmics) or drugs that inhibit this enzyme (eg, quinidine) should be approached with caution. **Fluvoxamine** is a relatively weak inhibitor of this isozyme. However, in vitro the drug inhibits the 1A2, 2C9, and 3A4 isozymes, which are involved in the metabolism of warfarin, theophylline, propranolol, and alprazolam. Therapy with medications that are predominantly metabolized by the CYP2D6 system and that have a relatively narrow therapeutic index (eg, flecainide, vinblastine, TCAs) should be initiated at the low end of the dose range if a patient is receiving **fluoxetine** concurrently or has taken it in the previous 5 weeks.

In vitro studies indicate that cytochrome P450 3A4 and 2C19 are the primary enzymes involved in metabolism of **citalopram** and **escitalopram**. Inhibitors of 3A4 (eg, azole antifungals, macrolide antibiotics) and 2C19 (eg, omeprazole) would be expected to increase plasma citalopram levels. Inducers of 3A4 (eg, carbamazepine) would be expected to decrease citalopram and escitalopram levels.

➤*Serotonin syndrome:* The serotonin syndrome is a complication of therapy with serotonergic drugs. It is most commonly observed when 2 drugs that potentiate serotonergic neurotransmission are used concurrently. When this problem occurs with SSRIs, it is most commonly in the setting of other concurrent medications, such as MAOIs, which increase serotonin by different mechanisms. Other such drugs include tryptophan, amphetamines, or other psychostimulants, other antidepressants that increase 5-HT levels, buspirone, lithium, or dopamine agonists (eg, amantadine, bromocriptine). Serotonin syndrome has been reported in 2 patients who were concomitantly receiving linezolid, an antibiotic that is a reversible non-selective MAOI.

➤*Drugs that interfere with hemostasis (eg, NSAIDs, aspirin, warfarin):* Serotonin release by platelets plays an important role in hemostasis. Epidemiological studies of the case-control and cohort design that have demonstrated an association between use of psychotropic drugs that interfere with serotonin reuptake and the occurrence of upper GI bleeding also have shown that concurrent use of an NSAID or aspirin potentiated the risk of bleeding. Thus, caution patients about the use of such drugs concurrently with an SSRI.

SSRI Drug Interactions

Precipitant drug	Object drug[a]		Description
Barbiturates	SSRIs Paroxetine	⬇	Phenobarbital decreased the AUC and half-life of paroxetine by 25% and 38%, respectively.
Cimetidine	SSRIs	⬆	Cimetidine increased steady-state paroxetine concentrations by ≈ 50%. Cimetidine increased sertraline AUC (50%), C_{max} (24%), and half-life (26%). Citalopram and escitalopram AUC (43%) and C_{max} (39%) also increased. Adjust paroxetine dosage as needed.
Cyproheptadine	SSRIs Fluoxetine Paroxetine	⬇	The pharmacologic effects of SSRIs may be decreased or reversed.
Linezolid	SSRIs		A serotonin syndrome has been reported to occur after coadministration of linezolid and paroxetine. It may be prudent to allow at least 2 weeks after stopping linezolid before giving an SSRI.
MAO inhibitors	SSRIs	⬆	Serious, sometimes fatal, reactions have occurred in patients receiving SSRIs in combination with a MAOI or who have recently discontinued the SSRI and are then started on an MAOI (see Warnings).
Metoclopramide Sibutramine Tramadol	SSRIs	⬆	A serotonin syndrome (eg, CNS irritability, shivering, myoclonus, altered consciousness) may occur.

SSRI Drug Interactions

Precipitant drug	Object drug[a]		Description
Phenytoin	SSRIs Paroxetine	↓	Phenytoin reduced the AUC and half-life of paroxetine by 50% and 35%, respectively. Also, paroxetine reduced the AUC of phenytoin by 12%, and sertraline, fluoxetine, and fluvoxamine may increase hydantoin levels.
SSRIs Fluoxetine Fluvoxamine Sertraline	Hydantoins	↑↓	
Smoking	SSRIs Fluvoxamine	↓	Smokers had a 25% increase in the metabolism of fluvoxamine.
L-tryptophan	SSRIs	↑	Concurrent use with fluoxetine or paroxetine may produce symptoms related to both central toxicity (eg, headache, sweating, dizziness, agitation, restlessness) and peripheral toxicity (eg, GI distress, nausea, vomiting). Concomitant use is not recommended. Tryptophan may enhance the serotonergic effects of fluvoxamine; use the combination with caution. Severe vomiting has been reported with the coadministration of fluvoxamine and tryptophan.
St. John's wort	SSRIs Paroxetine Sertraline	↑	Increased sedative-hypnotic effects may occur. Avoid concurrent use.
SSRIs	Alcohol	↔	Although potentiation of impairment of mental and motor skills caused by alcohol has not occurred, concurrent use is not recommended in patients.
SSRIs	Antidepressants, tricyclic	↑	Plasma TCA levels may be increased; use caution when coadministering. Monitor TCA levels; may need to reduce TCA dose.
SSRIs Fluoxetine Fluvoxamine Sertraline	Benzodiazepines	↑	Clearance of benzodiazepines metabolized by hepatic oxidation may be decreased; those metabolized by glucuronidation are unlikely to be affected. Coadministration of alprazolam and fluoxetine or fluvoxamine has resulted in increased alprazolam levels and decreased psychomotor performance. Halve the initial alprazolam dose, and titrate to the lowest effective dose. Avoid coadministration of fluvoxamine and diazepam.
SSRIs	Beta blockers	↑	Certain SSRIs may inhibit the metabolism of certain beta blockers. Concurrent use of citalopram or escitalopram and metoprolol produced an increase in metoprolol levels. Fluvoxamine administered with propranolol produced a 5-fold increase in propranolol C_{min}. If propranolol or metoprolol is given with fluvoxamine, reduce the initial beta blocker dose.
SSRIs Fluoxetine Fluvoxamine	Buspirone	↓	Effects of buspirone may be decreased; plasma concentrations may be increased with fluvoxamine but clinical response may be decreased. Paradoxical worsening of OCD or serotonin syndrome has occurred.
SSRIs Fluoxetine Fluvoxamine	Carbamazepine	↑	Serum carbamazepine levels may be increased with fluoxetine or fluvoxamine, possibly resulting in toxicity. The clearance of citalopram and escitalopram may be increased. The therapeutic effect of sertraline may be decreased.
Carbamazepine	SSRIs Citalopram Escitalopram Sertraline	↓	
SSRIs Fluvoxamine Sertraline	Cisapride	↓	Concurrent use of sertraline and cisapride reduced cisapride AUC and C_{max}. Use with fluvoxamine is contraindicated.
SSRIs Citalopram Fluoxetine Fluvoxamine Sertraline	Clozapine	↑	Elevated serum clozapine levels have occurred. Closely monitor patients on concomitant administration.
SSRIs Fluoxetine Fluvoxamine	Cyclosporine	↑	Elevated cyclosporine concentrations were reported in case reports during concomitant administration.
SSRIs Paroxetine	Digoxin	↓	Paroxetine decreased the AUC of digoxin by 15%. The coadministration of paroxetine and digoxin should be undertaken with caution.
SSRIs Fluvoxamine	Diltiazem	↑	Bradycardia has occurred with concurrent use.
SSRIs Fluoxetine Fluvoxamine	Haloperidol	↑	Serum concentrations of haloperidol may be increased. Closely monitor patients on concomitant therapy.
SSRIs Citalopram	Ketoconazole	↓	Coadministration decreased ketoconazole C_{max} (21%) and AUC (10%).
SSRIs Citalopram Escitalopram Fluoxetine Fluvoxamine Sertraline	Lithium	↑↓	Lithium levels may be increased or decreased by fluoxetine with possible neurotoxicity and increased serotonergic effects. In healthy volunteers, sertraline did not affect lithium levels. It is recommended that plasma lithium levels be monitored following initiation of sertraline, fluoxetine, citalopram, and escitalopram with appropriate adjustments to lithium dose. Concurrent use may enhance serotonergic effects of SSRIs. Use caution when coadministering. Lithium may enhance the serotonergic effects of fluvoxamine. Use with caution in combination; seizures have been reported.
Lithium	SSRIs	↑	
SSRIs Fluvoxamine	Methadone	↑	Significantly increased methadone concentrations have occurred. One patient developed opioid intoxication; another had opioid withdrawal symptoms with fluvoxamine discontinuation.
SSRIs Fluvoxamine	Mexiletine	↑	Mexiletine serum levels may be elevated, increasing the risk of side effects.
SSRIs	NSAIDs	↑	The risk of GI adverse effects may be increased. If possible, avoid concurrent use.
SSRIs Fluoxetine Fluvoxamine	Olanzapine	↑	Olanzapine plasma concentrations may be elevated. Observe the patient closely.

Selective Serotonin Reuptake Inhibitors

SSRI Drug Interactions			
Precipitant drug	Object drug[a]		Description
SSRIs Fluoxetine Fluvoxamine Paroxetine	Phenothiazines	↑	Plasma phenothiazine concentrations may be elevated, increasing the pharmacologic and adverse effects, including life-threatening cardiac arrhythmias. Thioridazine is contraindicated with fluvoxamine, fluoxetine, and paroxetine (see Contraindications).
SSRIs Fluvoxamine Sertraline	Pimozide	↑	Concurrent use of sertraline and pimozide 2 mg produced a mean increase in pimozide AUC and C_{max} of ≈ 40%, increasing the risk of life-threatening cardiac arrhythmias. Because of pimozide's narrow therapeutic index, administration with sertraline or fluvoxamine is contraindicated.
SSRIs Paroxetine	Procyclidine	↑	Paroxetine increased the AUC, C_{max}, and C_{min} of procyclidine by 35%, 37%, and 67%, respectively. Reduce procyclidine dose if anticholinergic effects occur.
SSRIs Fluoxetine	Propafenone	↑	Coadministration of fluoxetine and propafenone produced elevated propafenone plasma levels. Certain SSRIs may inhibit the metabolism (CYP2D6) of propafenone.
SSRIs Paroxetine	Risperidone	↑	Coadministration may increase risperidone concentrations, increasing the risk of side effects. Serotonin syndrome may occur.
SSRIs Fluoxetine	Ritonavir	↑	The AUC of ritonavir may be increased. Serotonin syndrome may occur.
SSRIs Fluvoxamine	Ropivacaine	↑	Ropivacaine plasma concentrations may be elevated; the pharmacologic effects may be prolonged, increasing the risk of toxicity.
SSRIs Fluvoxamine Sertraline	Sulfonylureas Glimepiride Tolbutamide	↑	Fluvoxamine and sertraline have been shown to decrease the clearance of tolbutamide. Fluvoxamine also has been shown to increase the peak plasma concentration of glimepiride.
SSRIs	Sumatriptan	↑	Weakness, hyperreflexia, and incoordination have occurred with coadministration. Observe patient closely.
SSRIs	Sympathomimetics	↑	Increased sensitivity to the effect of sympathomimetics and increased risk of serotonin syndrome may occur.
SSRIs Fluvoxamine	Tacrine	↑	Plasma tacrine concentrations may be elevated, increasing the pharmacologic and cholinergic adverse effects.
SSRIs Fluvoxamine Paroxetine	Theophylline	↑	Clearance of theophylline may be decreased by 3-fold when coadministered with fluvoxamine; reduce dosage. Elevated theophylline levels have occurred with paroxetine. It is recommended that theophylline levels be monitored when these drugs are concurrently administered.
SSRIs Fluoxetine Paroxetine	Trazodone	↑	Plasma trazodone levels may be elevated, resulting in increased pharmacologic and toxic effects. If coadministration cannot be avoided, start with a low dose of the SSRI or trazodone.
SSRIs	Warfarin	↑	A pharmacodynamic interaction of altered anticoagulant effects including increased bleeding diathesis with unaltered prothrombin time (PT) may occur with paroxetine or fluoxetine. Coadministration of sertraline and warfarin and citalopram and warfarin has resulted in an 8% and 5% increase in PT, respectively, and delayed PT normalization. Fluvoxamine increased warfarin plasma levels by 98%; PT was prolonged. Monitor PT. Use caution with coadministration and monitor patient.
SSRIs Sertraline	Zolpidem	↑	Coadministration of sertraline and zolpidem produced a shortened onset of action of zolpidem and an increased effect.

[a] ↑ = object drug increased; ↓ = object drug decreased; ↔ = undetermined clinical effect.

➤*Drug/Food interactions:* In one study following a single dose of **sertraline** with and without food, sertraline AUC was slightly increased with food and C_{max} was 25% greater. Time to reach peak plasma level decreased from 8 hours post dosing to 5.5 hours. For **paroxetine**, AUC was only slightly increased (6%) when drug was administered with food but the C_{max} was 29% greater, while the time to reach peak plasma concentration decreased from 6.4 hours postdosing to 4.9 hours.

Food does not appear to affect systemic bioavailability of **fluoxetine**, although it may delay absorption by 1 to 2 hours. **Fluvoxamine** and paroxetine CR bioavailability are not affected by food. **Citalopram** and **escitalopram** absorption is not affected by food. Thus, all SSRIs may be given with or without food.

Adverse Reactions

Discontinuation of treatment – In clinical trials, 9.4% to 20% of **paroxetine** patients, 3% to 13% of paroxetine CR patients, 10% to 15% of **sertraline** patients, 22% of **fluvoxamine** patients, 16% of **citalopram** patients, and 6% to 8% of **escitalopram** patients discontinued treatment because of an adverse event.

SSRIs Adverse Reactions (%)[a]							
Adverse reaction	Citalopram	Escitalopram	Fluoxetine	Fluvoxamine	Paroxetine IR/CR		Sertraline
Cardiovascular							
Chest pain	—	≥ 1	≥ 1	—	3	1	≥ 1
Hot flushes	0.1 - 1	≥ 1	—	—	—	—	0.1 - 1
Hypertension	0.1 - 1	≥ 1	≥ 1	≥ 1	≥ 1	2	0.1 - 1
Hypotension (postural)	≥ 1	—	0.1 - 1	≥ 1	—	0.1 - 1	0.1 - 1
Palpitations	—	≥ 1	1 - 3	3	2 - 3	0.1 - 1	≥ 1
Syncope	0.1 - 1	0.1 - 1	0.1 - 1	≥ 1	≥ 1	—	0.1 - 1
Tachycardia	≥ 1	0.1 - 1	0.1 - 1	≥ 1	≥ 1	1 - 2	0.1 - 1
Vasodilation	—	—	2 - 3	3	2 - 4	2 - 3	
CNS							
Abnormal dreams	—	3	3	—	3 - 4	1	0.1 - 1
Abnormal thinking	—	—	2 - 6	—	0.1 - 1	0.1 - 1	—
Agitation	3	0.1 - 1	≥ 1	2	3 - 6	2 - 3	1 - 6
Amnesia	≥ 1	0.1 - 1	≥ 1	≥ 1	2	0.1 - 1	0.1 - 1
Anxiety	4	—	12 - 13	1 - 5	2 - 6	2 - 5	4
Apathy	≥ 1	0.1 - 1		≥ 1	—	—	0.1 - 1
CNS stimulation	—	—	0.1 - 1	2	—	—	—
Concentration, decreased/impaired	≥ 1	≥ 1	—	—	3 - 4	1 - 3	—
Confusion	≥ 1	0.1 - 1	≥ 1	—	1	1	0.1 - 1
Depersonalization	0.1 - 1	0.1 - 1	0.1 - 1	0.1 - 1	3	0.1 - 1	—

SSRIs Adverse Reactions (%)[a]

Adverse reaction	Citalopram	Escitalopram	Fluoxetine	Fluvoxamine	Paroxetine IR/CR		Sertraline
Depression	≥ 1	0.1 - 1	—	2	—	2	0.1 - 1
Dizziness	—	4 - 7	2 - 11	2 - 11	6 - 14	6 - 14	6 - 17
Drugged feeling	—	—	—	—	2	—	—
Emotional lability	0.1 - 1	0.1 - 1	≥ 1	0.1 - 1	≥ 1	0.1 - 1	0.1 - 1
Fatigue	5	2-8	—	—	—	—	10 - 16
Headache	—	24	13 - 24	3 - 22	17 - 18	15 - 27	25
Hypertonia	0.1 - 1	—	0.1 - 1	2	0.1 - 1	2 - 3	≥ 1
Hypoesthesia	0.1 - 1	—	0.1 - 1	—	0.1 - 1	0.1 - 1	≥ 1
Hypo-/Hyperkinesia	0.1 - 1	—	—	≥ 1	0.1 - 1	0.1 - 1	0.1 - 1
Insomnia	15	7 - 14	9 - 24	4 - 21	11 - 24	7 - 20	12 - 28
Libido decreased	1 - 4	3 - 7	3 - 9	2	3 - 12	7 - 12	1 - 11
Manic reaction	—	—	—	≥ 1		—	—
Myoclonus/twitching	—	0.1 - 1	0.1 - 1	≥ 1	2 - 3	1 - 2	0.1 - 1
Nervousness	—	0.1 - 1	3 - 14	2 - 12	3 - 9	2 - 8	5
Paresthesia	≥ 1	2	—	—	4	1 - 3	2
Psychotic reaction	—	—	—	≥ 1	—	—	—
Sleep disorder	—	—	≥ 1	0.1-1	—	—	—
Somnolence	18	4 - 13	12 - 13	4 - 22	13 - 24	3 - 22	2 - 15
Tremor	8	0.1 - 1	9 - 12	5	4 - 15	4 - 8	< 1 - 11
Vertigo	0.1 - 1	0.1 - 1	—	0.1 - 1	≥ 1	2	0.1 - 1
Dermatologic							
Acne	0.1 - 1	0.1 - 1	0.1 - 1	0.1 - 1	0.1 - 1	0.1 - 1	0.1 - 1
Pruritus	≥ 1	0.1 - 1	3	—	≥ 1	0.1 - 1	0.1 - 1
Rash	≥ 1	≥ 1	4 - 5	—	2 - 3	≥ 1	3
Sweating, excessive/increased	11	3 - 8	7 - 8	7	1 - 14	6 - 14	3 - 11
GI							
Abdominal pain	3	2	6	1	4	3-7	2-7
Anorexia	4	—	10 - 11	1 - 6	—	—	3-11
Constipation	—	3 - 6	5	10	5 - 16	2 - 13	1 - 8
Decreased appetite	—	3	—	—	2 - 9	1 - 12	—
Diarrhea/loose stools	8	6 - 14	2 - 11	1 - 11	9 - 19	6 - 18	13 - 24
Dry mouth	20	4 - 9	9 - 11	1 - 14	9 - 21	2 - 18	6 - 16
Dyspepsia	5	2 - 6	7 - 8	1 - 10	2 - 5	2 - 13	6 - 13
Dysphagia	0.1 - 1	—	0.1 - 1	2	0.1 - 1	—	0.1 - 1
Flatulence	≥ 1	2	3	4	4	6 - 8	—
Gastroenteritis	0.1 - 1	≥ 1	0.1 - 1	0.1 - 1	0.1 - 1	0.1 - 1	0.1 - 1
Increased appetite	≥ 1	≥ 1	≥ 1	—	2 - 4	—	≥ 1
Melena	—	—	0.1 - 1	—	—	—	
Nausea	21	15 - 18	9 - 27	9 - 40	15 - 36	17 - 23	13 - 30
Oropharynx disorder	—	—	—	—	2	—	—
Tooth disorder/caries	—	2	—	3	< 0.1	0.1 - 1	0.1 - 1
Vomiting	4	3	1 - 3	2 - 5	2 - 3	2	4
GU							
Abnormal ejaculation	6	9 - 14	—	8	6 - 28	15 - 27	7 - 19
Female genital disorders	—	—	—	—	2 - 9	2 - 10	—
Male genital disorders, others	—	—	—	—	4 - 10	—	—
Menstrual disorder	—	2	—	—	—	1 - 2	0.1 - 1
Sexual dysfunction/impotence/ anorgasmia	1 - 3	2 - 6	0.1 - 1	2	2 - 13	5 - 10	≥ 1
Urinary frequency	—	≥ 1	2	3	2 - 3	2	0.1 - 1
Urinary tract infection	—	≥ 1	—	0.1 - 1	2	3	—
Urination disorder/retention	0.1 - 1	—	0.1- 1	1	3	2	0.1 - 1
Musculoskeletal							
Arthralgia	2	≥ 1	—	0.1 - 1	≥ 1	2	0.1 - 1
Myalgia	2	≥ 1	—	—	2 - 4	5	≥ 1
Myasthenia		—	< 0.1	0.1 - 1	1	< 0.1	—
Myopathy		—			2		—
Respiratory							
Bronchitis	0.1 - 1	≥ 1		0.1 - 1	0.1 - 1	1 - 2	< 0.1
Cough (increased)	≥ 1	≥ 1	—	≥ 1	≥ 1	1 - 2	0.1 - 1
Dyspnea	0.1 - 1	—	—	2	0.1 - 1	—	0.1 - 1
Pharyngitis	—	—	6 - 10		4	8	—
Respiratory disorder	—	—		—	7		
Rhinitis	5	5	16 - 23	—	3	4	≥ 1
Sinusitis	3	3	—	≥ 1	4	4 - 8	0.1 - 1
Upper respiratory tract infection	5	—		9		—	0.1 - 1
Yawn	2	2	3 - 5	2	2 - 5	2 - 5	≥ 1
Special senses							
Amblyopia	—	—		3		—	—
Taste perversion/change	≥ 1	0.1 - 1	≥ 1	3	2	2	—
Tinnitus	0.1 - 1	≥ 1	≥ 1		≥ 1	0.1 - 1	≥ 1
Vision disturbances/blurred vision/ abnormal vision	≥ 1	≥ 1	2 - 3	—	2 - 8	1 - 5	3
Miscellaneous							
Accidental injury/trauma	—		1 - 8	≥ 1	3 - 6	3 - 8	—
Allergy/allergic reaction	—	≥ 1		0.1 - 1	0.1 - 1	2	< 0.1

SSRIs Adverse Reactions (%)[a]							
Adverse reaction	Citalopram	Escitalopram	Fluoxetine	Fluvoxamine	Paroxetine IR/CR		Sertraline
Asthenia	—	0.1 - 1	8 - 14	2 - 14	3 - 22	14 - 18	≥ 1
Back pain	—	—	—	—	3	4 - 5	≥ 1
Chills	—	0.1 - 1	≥ 1	2	2	0.1 - 1	
Edema	0.1 - 1	—	—	≥ 1	0.1 - 1	0.1 - 1	0.1 - 1
Fever	2	≥ 1	2 - 5	—	—	0.1 - 1	0.1 - 1
Flu syndrome	0.1 - 1	5	3 - 12	3	5 - 6	6 - 8	—
Malaise	—	0.1 - 1	0.1 - 1	≥ 1	0.1 - 1	0.1 - 1	< 1 - 10
Pain	—	—	3 - 9			3	1 - 6
Weight gain	≥ 1	≥ 1	≥ 1	≥ 1	≥ 1	1 - 3	≥ 1
Weight loss	≥ 1	0.1 - 1	2 - 3	≥ 1	0.1 - 1	1	0.1 - 1

[a] Data are pooled from different studies and are not necessarily comparable.

Dose dependency of adverse reactions – A comparison of adverse event rates in a fixed-dose study comparing **paroxetine** 10, 20, 30, and 40 mg/day with placebo revealed a clear dose dependency for some of the more common adverse events associated with paroxetine use.

Fluoxetine Adverse Reactions (≥ 5%) by Indications								
	Depression		OCD		Bulimia		Panic disorder	
Adverse reaction	Fluoxetine (n = 1728)	Placebo (n = 975)	Fluoxetine (n = 266)	Placebo (n = 89)	Fluoxetine (n = 450)	Placebo (n = 267)	Fluoxetine (n = 425)	Placebo (n = 342)
CNS								
Abnormal dreams	1	1	5	2	5	3	1	1
Anxiety	12	7	14	7	15	9	6	2
Insomnia	16	9	28	22	33	13	10	7
Libido decreased	3	< 1	11	2	5	1	1	2
Nervousness	14	9	14	15	11	5	8	6
Somnolence	13	6	17	7	13	5	5	2
Tremor	10	3	9	1	13	1	3	1
Dermatologic								
Rash	4	3	6	3	4	4	2	2
Sweating	8	3	7	< 1	8	3	2	2
GI								
Anorexia	11	2	17	10	8	4	4	1
Diarrhea	12	8	18	13	8	6	9	4
Dry mouth	10	7	12	3	9	6	4	4
Dyspepsia	7	5	10	4	10	6	6	2
Nausea	21	9	26	13	29	11	12	7
GU								
Abnormal ejaculation			7		7		2	1
Impotence	2	< 1	< 1	< 1	7	< 1	1	< 1
Respiratory								
Pharyngitis	3	3	11	9	10	5	3	3
Sinusitis	1	4	5	2	6	4	2	3
Yawn	< 1	< 1	7	< 1	11	< 1	1	< 1
Miscellaneous								
Asthenia	9	5	15	11	21	9	7	7
Flu syndrome	3	4	10	7	8	3	5	5
Vasodilation	3	2	5	< 1	2	1	1	< 1

Adaptation to certain adverse events – Over a 4- to 6-week period, there was evidence of adaptation to some adverse events with continued therapy (eg, nausea, dizziness), but less to other effects (eg, dry mouth, somnolence, asthenia).

➤*Cardiovascular:*

Citalopram – Angina pectoris, bradycardia, cardiac failure, cerebrovascular accident, extrasystoles, MI, myocardial ischemia (0.1% to 1%); atrial fibrillation, bundle branch block, cardiac arrest, phlebitis, pulmonary embolism, transient ischemic attack (less than 0.1%); chest pain, torsade de pointes, ventricular arrhythmia, QT prolonged (postmarketing).

Escitalopram – Bradycardia, ECG abnormal, varicose vein (0.1% to 1%); atrial fibrillation, hypotension, MI, orthostatic hypotension, pulmonary embolism, QT prolongation, torsade de pointes, ventricular tachycardia (postmarketing).

Fluoxetine – Hemorrhage (at least 1%); angina pectoris, arrhythmia, CHF, hypotension, migraine, myocardial infarct, vascular headache (0.1% to 1%); atrial fibrillation, bradycardia, cerebral embolism, cerebral ischemia, cerebrovascular accident, extrasystoles, heart arrest, heart block, pallor, peripheral vascular disorder, phlebitis, shock, thrombophlebitis, thrombosis, vasospasm, ventricular arrhythmia, ventricular extrasystoles, ventricular fibrillation (less than 0.1%); atrial fibrillation, cerebrovascular accident, heart arrest, pulmonary embolism, pulmonary hypertension, QT prolongation, ventricular tachycardia (including torsade de pointes) (postmarketing).

Fluvoxamine – Angina pectoris, bradycardia, cardiomyopathy, cardiovascular disease, cold extremities, conduction delay, heart failure, MI, pallor, pulse irregular, ST segment changes (0.1% to 1%); AV block, cerebrovascular accident, coronary artery disease, embolus, pericarditis, phlebitis, pulmonary infarction, supraventricular extrasystoles (less than 0.1%); ventricular tachycardia (including torsade de pointes) (postmarketing).

Paroxetine and paroxetine CR – Bradycardia, hematoma, hypotension, supraventricular tachycardia, syncope (0.1% to 1%); angina pectoris, arrhythmia nodal, atrial fibrillation, bundle branch block, cardiospasm, cerebral ischemia, cerebrovascular accident, CHF, heart block, low cardiac output, MI, myocardial ischemia, pallor, phlebitis, pulmonary embolus, supraventricular/ventricular extrasystoles, thrombophlebitis, thrombosis, vascular headache (less than 0.1%); pulmonary hypertension, ventricular fibrillation, ventricular tachycardia (including torsade de pointes) (postmarketing).

Sertraline – Edema (dependent, general, periorbital, peripheral), hypotension, peripheral ischemia, postural dizziness (0.1% to 1%); aggravated hypertension, cerebrovascular disorder, MI, precordial/substernal chest pain (less than 0.1%); atrial arrhythmias, AV block, bradycardia, pulmonary hypertension, QT prolongation, ventricular tachycardia (including torsade de pointes-type arrhythmias) (postmarketing).

➤*CNS:*

Citalopram – Aggravated depression, increased appetite, migraine, suicide attempt (at least 1%); abnormal gait, aggressive reaction, alcohol intolerance, ataxia, delusion, drug dependence, dystonia, euphoria, extrapyramidal disorder, hallucinations, increased libido, involuntary muscle contractions, leg cramps, neuralgia, panic reaction, paranoia, paranoid reaction, psychosis, psychotic depression, rigors (0.1% to 1%); abnormal coordination, catatonic reaction, hyperesthesia, melancholia, ptosis, stupor (less than 0.1%); choreoathetosis; delirium; dyskinesia; neuroleptic malignant syndrome; serotonin syndrome; withdrawal syndrome; grand mal convulsions (postmarketing).

Escitalopram – Irritability, lethargy, lightheaded feeling, migraine (at least 1%); aggravated depression, aggravated restlessness, anxiety attack, auditory hallucination, bruxism, carbohydrate craving, carpal tunnel syndrome, coordination abnormal, crying abnormal, disorientation, dysequilibrium, excitability, faintness, feeling unreal, forgetfulness, hyperreflexia, jitteriness, panic reaction, restless legs, shaking, sluggishness, suicidal tendency, suicide attempt, tics, tremulousness nervous (0.1% to 1%); abnormal gait, aggression, dystonia, extrapyramidal disorders, grand mal seizures (or convulsions), neuroleptic malignant syndrome, seizures, serotonin syndrome, visual hallucinations (postmarketing).

Fluoxetine – Abnormal gait, acute brain syndrome, akathisia, apathy, ataxia, buccoglossal syndrome, CNS depression, euphoria, hallucinations, hostility, hyperkinesia, incoordination, increased libido, neuralgia, neuropathy, neurosis, paranoid reaction, personality disorder, psychosis, vertigo (0.1% to 1%); abnormal EEG, antisocial reaction, circumoral paresthesia, coma, delusions, dysarthria, dystonia, extrapyramidal syndrome, foot drop, hyperesthesia, neuritis, paralysis, reflexes decreased/increased, stupor, (less than 0.1%); confusion, dyskinesia, movement disorders, neuroleptic malignant syndrome-like events, suicidal ideation, violent behaviors, serotonin syndrome (postmarketing).

Fluvoxamine – Agoraphobia, akathisia, ataxia, CNS depression, convulsion, delirium, delusion, drug dependence, dyskinesia, dystonia, euphoria, extrapyramidal syndrome, gait unsteady, hallucinations, hemiplegia, hostility, hypersomnia, hypochondriasis, hypotonia, hysteria, incoordination, increased salivation, increased libido, neuralgia, paralysis, paranoid reaction, phobia, psychosis, stupor, twitching (0.1% to 1%); akinesia, coma, fibrillations, mutism, obsessions, reflexes decreased, slurred speech, tardive dyskinesia, torticollis, trismus, withdrawal syndrome (less than 0.1%); neuropathy, serotonin syndrome (postmarketing).

Paroxetine and paroxetine CR – Alcohol abuse, ataxia, dyskinesia, dystonia, euphoria, hallucinations, hostility, incoordination, increased libido, lack of emotion, manic reaction, migraine, neuralgia, neurosis, neuropathy, paralysis, paranoid reaction (0.1% to 1%); abnormal gait, akinesia, antisocial reaction, aphasia, choreoathetosis, circumoral paresthesias, coma, convulsion, delirium, delusions, diplopia, drug dependence, dysarthria, extrapyramidal syndrome, fasciculations, grand mal convulsion, hostility, hyperalgesia, hysteria, manic-depressive reaction, meningitis, myelitis, nystagmus, peripheral neuritis, psychosis, psychotic depression, reflexes decreased/increased, stupor, torticollis, trismus, withdrawal syndrome (less than 0.1%); akathisia; irritability; meningitis; myelitis; peripheral neuritis; psychosis; psychotic depression; reflexes decreased; reflexes increased; stupor; extrapyramidal symptoms (which have included akathisia, bradykinesia, cogwheel rigidity, dystonia, and hypertonia), Guillain-Barre syndrome, neuroleptic malignant syndrome-like events, serotonin syndrome associated in some cases with concomitant use of serotonergic drugs and with drugs that may have impaired paroxetine metabolism (symptoms included agitation, confusion, diaphoresis, hallucinations, hyperreflexia, myoclonus, shivering, tachycardia, and tremor), status epilepticus, tremor (postmarketing).

Sertraline – Abnormal coordination, abnormal gait, aggravated depression, aggressive reaction, ataxia, delusion, euphoria, hallucination, hyperesthesia, leg cramps, migraine, nystagmus, paranoid reaction, paroniria (0.1% to 1%); choreoathetosis, coma, dyskinesia, dysphonia, hyporeflexia, hypotonia, illusion, libido increased, ptosis, somnambulism, suicidal ideation, withdrawal syndrome (less than 0.1%); extrapyramidal symptoms, neuroleptic malignant syndrome-like events, psychosis, serotonin syndrome (postmarketing).

➤*Dermatologic:*

Citalopram – Alopecia, dermatitis, dry skin, eczema, photosensitivity reaction, psoriasis, skin discoloration, urticaria (0.1% to 1%); cellulitis, decreased sweating, hypertrichosis, keratitis, melanosis, pruritus ani (less than 0.1%); angioedema, epidermal necrolysis, erythema multiforme (postmarketing).

Escitalopram – Alopecia, dermatitis, dry lips, dry skin, eczema, folliculitis, furunculosis, lipoma, skin nodule (0.1% to 1%); toxic epidermal necrolysis (postmarketing).

Fluoxetine – Alopecia, contact dermatitis, eczema, maculopapular rash, skin discoloration, skin ulcer, vesiculobullous rash (0.1% to 1%); furunculosis, herpes zoster, hirsutism, petechial rash, photosensitivity, psoriasis, purpuric rash, pustular rash, seborrhea (less than 0.1%); epidermal necrolysis, erythema nodosum, exfoliative dermatitis, Stevens-Johnson syndrome (postmarketing).

Fluvoxamine – Alopecia, dry skin, eczema, exfoliative dermatitis, furunculosis, photosensitivity, seborrhea, skin discoloration, urticaria (0.1% to 1%); bullous eruption, Henoch-Schöenlein purpura, Stevens-Johnson syndrome, toxic epidermal necrolysis, porphyria (postmarketing).

Paroxetine and paroxetine CR – Acne, alopecia, contact dermatitis, dry skin, ecchymosis, eczema, herpes simplex, photosensitivity, urticaria (0.1% to 1%); angioedema, erythema multiforme, erythema nodosum, exfoliative dermatitis, fungal dermatitis, furunculosis, herpes zoster, hirsutism, maculopapular rash, pustular rash, seborrhea, skin discoloration, skin hypertrophy, skin ulcer, vesiculobullous rash, ecchymosis, skin hypertrophy, sweating decreased (less than 0.1%); toxic epidermal necrolysis (postmarketing).

Sertraline – Alopecia, cold clammy skin, dry skin, erythematous rash, maculopapular rash, photosensitivity, urticaria (0.1% to 1%); bullous eruption, contact dermatitis, dermatitis, eczema, hypertrichosis, follicular rash, pustular rash, skin discoloration (less than 0.1%); severe skin reactions that potentially can be fatal, such as Stevens-Johnson syndrome, vasculitis, photosensitivity, and other severe cutaneous disorders (postmarketing).

➤*GI:*

Citalopram – Increased saliva (at least 1%); eructation, esophagitis, gastritis, gingivitis, hemorrhoids, stomatitis, teeth grinding, thirst (0.1% to 1%); cholecystitis, cholelithiasis, colitis, diverticulitis, duodenal ulcer, gastric ulcer, gastroesophageal reflux, glossitis, hiccoughs, jaundice, rectal hemorrhage (less than 0.1%); GI hemorrhage, pancreatitis (postmarketing).

Escitalopram – Abdominal cramp, heartburn (at least 1%); abdominal discomfort, belching, bloating, gagging, gastritis, gastroesophageal reflux, hemorrhoids, increased stool frequency, polyposis gastric, swallowing difficulty (0.1% to 1%); GI hemorrhage, pancreatitis (postmarketing).

Fluoxetine – Abnormal liver function tests, aphthous stomatitis, cholelithiasis, colitis, eructation, esophagitis, gastritis, glossitis, gum hemorrhage, hyperchlorhydria, increased salivation, melena, mouth ulceration, stomach ulcer/hemorrhage, stomatitis, thirst (0.1% to 1%); biliary pain, bloody diarrhea, cholecystitis, duodenal ulcer, enteritis, esophageal ulcer, fecal incontinence, GI hemorrhage, hematemesis, hemorrhage of colon, hepatitis, intestinal obstruction, liver fatty deposit, pancreatitis, peptic ulcer, rectal hemorrhage, salivary gland enlargement, tongue edema (less than 0.1%).

Fluvoxamine – Colitis, eructation, esophagitis, gastritis, GI hemorrhage, GI ulcer, gingivitis, glossitis, hemorrhoids, melena, rectal hemorrhage, stomatitis (0.1% to 1%); biliary pain, cholecystitis, cholelithiasis, fecal incontinence, hematemesis, intestinal obstruction, jaundice (less than 0.1%).

Paroxetine and paroxetine CR – Abnormal liver function tests, bruxism, colitis, dysphagia, eructation, gastritis, gastroesophageal reflux, gingivitis, glossitis, hemorrhoids, increased salivation, pancreatitis, rectal hemorrhage, ulcerative stomatitis (0.1% to 1%); aphthous stomatitis, bloody diarrhea, bulimia, cholelithiasis, duodenitis, enteritis, esophagitis, fecal impaction/incontinence, gum hemorrhage/hyperplasia, hematemesis, hepatitis, hepatosplenomegaly, ileitis, ileus, intestinal obstruction, jaundice, melena, mouth ulceration, peptic ulcer, salivary gland enlargement, stomach ulcer, stomatitis, throat tightness, tongue discoloration, tongue edema, sialadenitis (less than 0.1%).

Sertraline – Eructation, esophagitis, increased saliva, teeth grinding, (0.1% to 1%); aphthous stomatitis, colitis, diverticulitis, fecal incontinence, gastritis, glossitis, gum hyperplasia, hemorrhagic peptic ulcer, hiccough, melena, proctitis, rectal hemorrhage, stomatitis, tenesmus, tongue edema/ulceration, ulcerative stomatitis (less than 0.1%).

➤*GU:*

Citalopram – Dysmenorrhea (3%); amenorrhea, polyuria (at least 1%); breast enlargement, breast pain, dysuria, galactorrhea, micturition frequency, urinary incontinence, vaginal hemorrhage (0.1% to 1%); facial edema, hematuria, oliguria, pyelonephritis, renal calculus, renal pain (less than 0.1%); priapism, spontaneous abortion, acute renal failure (postmarketing).

Escitalopram – Menstrual cramps (at least 1%); blood in urine, breast neoplasm, dysuria, kidney stone, menorrhagia, pelvic inflammation, premenstrual syndrome, spotting between menses, urinary urgency (0.1% to 1%); acute renal failure (postmarketing).

Fluoxetine – Abortion, albuminuria, amenorrhea, breast enlargement, breast pain, cystitis, dysuria, female lactation, fibrocystic breast, hematuria, leukorrhea, menorrhagia, metrorrhagia, nocturia, polyuria, urinary incontinence/urgency, vaginal hemorrhage (0.1% to 1%); breast engorgement, hypomenorrhea, glycosuria, kidney pain, oliguria, priapism, uterine fibroids enlarged, uterine hemorrhage (less than 0.1%); gynecomastia, kidney failure, priapism, vaginal bleeding after drug withdrawal (postmarketing).

Fluvoxamine – Anuria, breast pain, cystitis, delayed menstruation, dysuria, female lactation, hematuria, menopause, menorrhagia, metrorrhagia, nocturia, polyuria, premenstrual syndrome, urinary incontinence/urgency, urination impaired, vaginal hemorrhage, vaginitis (0.1% to 1%); hematospermia, kidney calculus, oliguria (less than 0.1%); priapism (postmarketing).

Paroxetine and paroxetine CR – Dysmenorrhea (at least 1%); albuminuria, amenorrhea, breast pain, cystitis, dysuria, hematuria, menorrhagia, nocturia, polyuria, prostate disorder, prostatitis, pyuria, urinary incontinence/retention/urgency, vaginitis (0.1% to 1%); abortion, breast atrophy/enlargement/neoplasm, ejaculatory disturbance, endometrial disorder; epididymitis, female lactation, fibrocystic breast, kidney calculus, kidney pain, leukorrhea, mastitis, metrorrhagia, nephritis, oliguria, pregnancy and puerperal disorders, salpingitis, urethritis, urinary casts, urolith, uterine fibroids enlarged, uterine spasm, urethritis, vaginal hemorrhage, vaginal moniliasis (less than 0.1%); acute renal failure, priapism (postmarketing).

Sertraline – Amenorrhea, dysmenorrhea, dysuria, intermenstrual bleeding, leukorrhea, nocturia, polyuria, urinary incontinence, vaginal hemorrhage (0.1% to 1%); acute female mastitis, atrophic vaginitis, balanoposthitis, breast enlargement, cystitis, female breast pain, gynecomastia, hematuria, libido increased, menorrhagia, oliguria, priapism, pyelonephritis, renal pain, strangury (less than 0.1%); acute renal failure (postmarketing).

➤*Musculoskeletal:*

Citalopram – Arthritis, muscle weakness, skeletal pain (0.1% to 1%); bursitis, osteoporosis (less than 0.1%).

Escitalopram – Neck/Shoulder pain (3%); arthritis, arthropathy, back discomfort, jaw pain, jaw stiffness, joint stiffness, muscle contractions involuntary, muscle cramp, muscle stiffness, muscle weakness, muscular tone increased (0.1% to 1%).

Fluoxetine – Arthritis, bone pain, bursitis, leg cramps, tenosynovitis (0.1% to 1%); arthrosis, chondrodystrophy, myositis, osteomyelitis, osteoporosis, rheumatoid arthritis (less than 0.1%).

Fluvoxamine – Arthritis, bursitis, generalized muscle spasm, tendinous contracture, tenosynovitis (0.1% to 1%); arthrosis, pathological fracture (less than 0.1%).

Paroxetine and paroxetine CR – Arthritis, arthrosis, tendonitis (0.1% to 1%); bursitis, generalized spasm, myositis, osteoporosis, tenosynovitis, tetany (less than 0.1%).

Sertraline – Arthrosis, dystonia, muscle cramps/weakness (0.1% to 1%).

➤*Respiratory:*

Citalopram – Pneumonia (0.1% to 1%); asthma, bronchospasm, laryngitis, pneumonitis, sputum increased (less than 0.1%).

Escitalopram – Nasal congestion, sinus congestion, sinus headache (at least 1%); asthma, breath shortness, laryngitis, pneumonia, tracheitis (0.1% to 1%).

Fluoxetine – Asthma, epistaxis, hiccoughs, hyperventilation (0.1% to 1%); apnea, atelectasis, cough decreased, emphysema, hemoptysis, hypoventilation, hypoxia, laryngeal edema, lung edema, pneumothorax, stridor (less than 0.1%); eosinophilic pneumonia (postmarketing).

Fluvoxamine – Asthma, epistaxis, hoarseness, hyperventilation (0.1% to 1%); apnea, congestion of upper airway, hemoptysis, hiccoughs, laryngismus, obstructive pulmonary disease, pneumonia (less than 0.1%).

Paroxetine and paroxetine CR – Asthma, epistaxis, hyperventilation, laryngitis, pneumonia, respiratory flu (0.1% to 1%); dysphonia; emphysema, hemoptysis, hiccoughs, lung fibrosis, pulmonary edema, sputum increased, stridor, voice alterations (less than 0.1%).

Sertraline – Bronchospasm, epistaxis (0.1% to 1%); apnea, bradypnea, hemoptysis, hyperventilation, hypoventilation, laryngismus, laryngitis, stridor (less than 0.1%).

➤*Special senses:*

Citalopram – Conjunctivitis, dry eyes, eye pain (0.1% to 1%); abnormal lacrimation, cataract, diplopia, mydriasis, photophobia, taste loss (less than 0.1%); nystagmus (postmarketing).

Escitalopram – Conjunctivitis, dry eyes, earache, eye infection, eye irritation, metallic taste, pupils dilated, vision abnormal, visual disturbance (0.1% to 1%); diplopia (postmarketing).

Fluoxetine – Ear pain (at least 1%); conjunctivitis, dry eyes, mydriasis, photophobia (0.1% to 1%); blepharitis, deafness, diplopia, exophthalmos, eye hemorrhage, glaucoma, hyperacusis, iritis, parosmia, scleritis, strabismus, taste loss, visual field defect (less than 0.1%); cataract, optic neuritis (postmarketing).

Fluvoxamine – Abnormal accommodation, conjunctivitis, deafness, diplopia, dry eyes, ear pain, eye pain, mydriasis, otitis media, parosmia, photophobia, taste loss, visual field defect (0.1% to 1%); corneal ulcer, retinal detachment (less than 0.1%).

Paroxetine and paroxetine CR – Abnormal accommodation, conjunctivitis, ear ache/pain, eye pain, keratoconjunctivitis, mydriasis, otitis media, (0.1% to 1%); amblyopia, anisocoria, blepharitis, cataract, conjunctival edema, corneal ulcer, deafness, exophthalmos, eye hemorrhage, glaucoma, hyperacusis, night blindness, otitis externa, parosmia, photophobia, ptosis, retinal hemorrhage, taste loss, visual field defect (less than 0.1%).

Sertraline – Abnormal accommodation, conjunctivitis, earache, eye pain, mydriasis (0.1% to 1%); abnormal lacrimation, diplopia, exophthalmos, glaucoma, hyperacusis, labyrinthine disorder, photophobia, scotoma, visual field defect, xerophthalmia (less than 0.1%) blindness, optic neuritis, cataract (postmarketing).

➤*Miscellaneous:*

Citalopram – Abnormal glucose tolerance, anemia, epistaxis, increased alkaline phosphatase, increased hepatic enzymes, leukocytosis, leukopenia, lymphadenopathy, purpura (0.1% to 1%); bilirubinemia, coagulation disorder, dehydration, gingival bleeding, goiter, granulocytopenia, gynecomastia, hayfever; hepatitis, hypochromic anemia, hypoglycemia, hypokalemia, hypothyroidism, lymphocytosis, lymphopenia, obesity (less than 0.1%);akathisia, allergic reaction, anaphylaxis, ecchymosis, hemolytic anemia, hepatic necrosis, myoclonus, prolactinemia, prothrombin decreased, rhabdomyolysis, thrombocytopenia, thrombosis (postmarketing).

Escitalopram – Lethargy (3%); pain in limb (at least 1%); anaphylaxis, anemia, bilirubin increased, bruise, edema of extremities, fall, gout, hematoma, hepatic enzymes increased, hypercholesterolemia, hyperglycemia, leg pain, lymphadenopathy cervical, nosebleed, thirst, tightness of chest (0.1% to 1%); angioedema, hepatitis, rhabdomyolysis, SIADH, thrombocytopenia (postmarketing).

Fluoxetine – Anemia, dehydration, ecchymosis, facial edema, generalized edema, gout, hypercholesterolemia, hyperlipemia, hypokalemia, hypothyroidism, intentional overdose, pelvic pain, peripheral edema; suicide attempt (0.1% to 1%); abdominal syndrome acute, alcohol intolerance, alkaline phosphatase increased, ALT increased, blood dyscrasia, BUN increased, creatine phosphokinase increased, diabetic acidosis, diabetes mellitus, hyperkalemia, hyperuricemia, hypocalcemia, hypochromic anemia, hypothermia, intentional injury, iron deficiency anemia, leukopenia, lymphedema, lymphocytosis, neuroleptic malignant syndrome, petechiae, purpura, thrombocythemia, thrombocytopenia (less than 0.1%); aplastic anemia, cholestatic jaundice, hepatic failure/necrosis, hyperprolactinemia, immune-related hemolytic anemia, misuse/abuse, pancreatitis, pancytopenia, sudden unexpected death, thrombocytopenic purpura, hypoglycemia (postmarketing).

Fluvoxamine – Increased liver transaminase (at least 1%); anemia, dehydration, ecchymosis, hypercholesterolemia, hypothyroidism, leukocytosis, lymphadenopathy, neck pain/rigidity, overdose, suicide attempt, thrombocytopenia (0.1% to 1%); cyst, diabetes mellitus, goiter, hyperglycemia, hyperlipidemia, hypoglycemia, hypokalemia, lactate dehydrogenase increased, leukopenia, pelvic pain, purpura, sudden death (less than 0.1%); acute renal failure, agranulocytosis, anaphylactic reaction, aplastic anemia, hepatitis, hyponatremia, ileus, laryngismus, pancreatitis, vasculitis, angioedema (postmarketing).

Paroxetine and paroxetine CR – Trauma (6%); infection (5% to 6%); pain (at least 1%); anemia, AST/ALT increased, facial edema, flu syndrome, leukopenia, lymphadenopathy, moniliasis, neck pain, purpura, peripheral edema, thirst (0.1% to 1%); abnormal erythrocytes, abnormal lymphocytes, abscess, adrenergic syndrome, anisocytosis, anticholinergic syndrome, basophilia, bilirubinemia, bleeding time increased, BUN increased, cellulitis, creatine phosphokinase increased, dehydration, diabetes mellitus, eosinophilia, goiter, gout, hypercalcemia, hypercholesterolemia, hyperglycemia, hyperkalemia, hyperphosphatemia, hyperthyroidism, hypocalcemia, hypochromic anemia, hypoglycemia, hypokalemia, hyponatremia, hypothermia, hypothyroidism, increased alkaline phosphatase, increased lactic dehydrogenase, increased gamma globulins, iron deficiency anemia, ketosis, leukocytosis, lymphedema, lymphocytosis, lymphopenia, microcytic/normocytic anemia, monocytosis, neck rigidity, non-protein nitrogen increased, obesity, pelvic pain, peritonitis, sepsis, thrombocythemia, thrombocytopenia, thyroiditis, ulcer, varicose vein (less than 0.1%); acute pancreatitis, allergic alveolitis, anaphylaxis, elevated liver function tests (the most severe cases were deaths because of liver necrosis and grossly elevated transaminases associated with severe liver dysfunction), events related to impaired hematopoiesis (including aplastic anemia, pancytopenia, bone marrow aplasia, and agranulocytosis), hemolytic anemia, laryngismus, myopathy, oculogyric crisis which has been associated with concomitant use of pimozide, optic neuritis, porphyria, symptoms suggestive of prolactinemia and galactorrhea, syndrome of inappropriate ADH secretion, vasculitis syndromes (such as Henoch-Schönlein purpura) (postmarketing).

Sertraline – Thirst (0.1% to 1%); abnormal hepatic function, anemia, anterior chamber eye hemorrhage, facial edema, hypoglycemia, pallor, rigors (less than 0.1%); anaphylactoid reaction, angioedema, agranulocytosis, aplastic anemia, galactorrhea, hyperglycemia, hyperprolactinemia, hypothyroidism, increased coagulation time, leukopenia; lupus-like syndrome, oculogyric crisis, pancreatitis, pancytopenia, serum sickness, thrombocytopenia, liver events including elevated enzymes, increased bilirubin, hepatomegaly, hepatitis, jaundice, abdominal pain, vomiting, liver failure, and death (postmarketing).

➤*Lab test abnormalities:*

Sertraline – Asymptomatic elevations in serum transaminases (AST or ALT) have occurred infrequently (approximately 0.8%) in association with sertraline administration. These hepatic enzyme elevations usually occurred within the first 1 to 9 weeks of drug treatment and promptly diminished upon drug discontinuation.

Sertraline therapy was associated with small mean increases in total cholesterol (approximately 3%) and triglycerides (approximately 5%) and a small mean decrease in serum uric acid (approximately 7%) of no apparent clinical importance.

Overdosage

➤*Symptoms:*

Citalopram – Although there were no reports of fatal citalopram overdose in clinical trials involving overdoses of up to 2,000 mg, postmarketing reports of drug overdoses involving citalopram have included 12 fatalities, 10 in combination with other drugs and/or alcohol, and 2 with citalopram alone (2,800 and 3,920 mg), as well as nonfatal overdoses of up to 6,000 mg. Symptoms most often accompanying citalopram overdose, alone or in combination with other drugs or alcohol, included dizziness, nausea, sinus tachycardia, somnolence, sweating, tremor, and vomiting. In more rare cases, observed symptoms included amnesia, coma, confusion, convulsions, cyanosis, hyperventilation, rhabdomyolysis, and ECG changes (including nodal rhythm, QT_c prolongation, ventricular arrhythmia, and 1 possible case of torsade de pointes).

Escitalopram – There have been reports of escitalopram overdose involving doses of up to 600 mg. All patients recovered and no symptoms associated with the overdoses were reported.

Fluoxetine – Of the 1578 cases of overdose involving fluoxetine, alone or with other drugs, there were 195 deaths. Among 633 adult patients who overdosed on fluoxetine alone, 34 resulted in a fatal outcome, 378 completely recovered, and 15 patients experienced sequelae after overdosage, including abnormal accommodation, abnormal gait, confusion, unresponsiveness, nervousness, pulmonary dysfunction, vertigo, tremor, elevated blood pressure, impotence, movement disorder, and hypomania. The remaining 206 patients had an unknown outcome. The most common signs and symptoms associated with nonfatal overdosage were seizures, somnolence, nausea, tachycardia, and vomiting. The largest known ingestion of fluoxetine in adult patients was 8 g in a patient who took fluoxetine alone and who subsequently recovered. However, in an adult patient who took fluoxetine alone, an ingestion as low as 520 mg has been associated with lethal outcome, but causality has not been established.

Among pediatric patients (3 months to 17 years of age), there were 156 cases of overdose involving fluoxetine alone or in combination with other drugs. Six patients died, 127 patients completely recovered, 1 patient experienced renal failure, and 22 patients had an unknown outcome. One of the 6 fatalities was a boy 9 years of age who had a history of OCD, Tourette syndrome with tics, attention deficit disorder, and fetal alcohol syndrome. He had been receiving 100 mg fluoxetine daily for 6 months in addition to clonidine, methylphenidate, and promethazine. Mixed-drug ingestion or other methods of suicide complicated all 6 overdoses in children that resulted in fatalities. The largest ingestion in a pediatric patient was 3 g, which was nonlethal.

Other important adverse events reported with fluoxetine overdose (single or multiple drugs) include coma, delirium, ECG abnormalities (such as QT interval prolongation and ventricular tachycardia, including torsade de pointes-type arrhythmias), hypotension, mania, neuroleptic malignant syndrome-like events, pyrexia, stupor, and syncope.

Fluvoxamine – Of the 462 cases of deliberate or accidental overdose involving fluvoxamine, there were 44 deaths. Of these, 6 were in patients taking fluvoxamine alone and the remaining 38 were in patients taking fluvoxamine along with other drugs. Among nonfatal overdose cases, 373 patients had complete recovery; 4 patients experienced adverse sequelae of overdosage, including persistent mydriasis, unsteady gait, kidney complications (from trauma associated with overdose), and bowel infarction requiring a hemicolectomy. In the remaining 41 patients, the outcome was unknown. The largest known ingestion of fluvoxamine involved 12,000 mg (equivalent of 2 to 3 months' dosage). The patient fully recovered. However, ingestion as low as 1,400 mg have been associated with lethal outcome, indicating considerable prognostic variability.

Commonly (at least 5%) observed adverse events associated with fluvoxamine overdose include coma, hypokalemia, hypotension, nausea, respiratory difficulties, somnolence, tachycardia, and vomiting. Other notable signs and symptoms seen with fluvoxamine overdose (single or multiple drugs) included bradycardia, ECG abnormalities (such as heart arrest, QT interval prolongation, first-degree atrioventricular block, bundle branch block, and junctional rhythm), convulsions, tremor, diarrhea, and increased reflexes.

Paroxetine – Since the introduction of paroxetine in the United States, 342 spontaneous cases of deliberate or accidental overdosage during paroxetine treatment have been reported worldwide. These include overdoses with paroxetine alone and in combination with other substances. Of these, 48 cases were fatal and of the fatalities, 17 appeared to involve paroxetine alone. Eight fatal cases that documented the amount of paroxetine ingested were generally confounded by the ingestion of other drugs or alcohol or the presence of significant comorbid conditions. Of 145 nonfatal cases with known outcome, most recovered without sequelae. The largest known ingestion involved 2,000 mg paroxetine (33 times the maximum recommended daily dose) in a patient who recovered. Commonly reported adverse events associated with paroxetine overdosage include coma, confusion, dizziness, nausea, somnolence, tachycardia, tremor, and vomiting. Other notable signs and symptoms observed with overdoses involving paroxetine (alone or with other substances) include acute renal failure, aggressive reactions, bradycardia, convulsions (including status epilepticus), dystonia, hypertension, hypotension, manic reactions, mydriasis, myoclonus, rhabdomyolysis, serotonin syndrome, stupor, symptoms of hepatic dysfunction (including hepatic failure, hepatic necrosis, jaundice, hepatitis, and hepatic steatosis), syncope, urinary retention, and ventricular dysrhythmias (including torsade de pointes).

Sertraline – Of 1027 cases of overdose involving sertraline worldwide, alone or with other drugs, there were 72 deaths.

Among 634 overdoses in which sertraline was the only drug ingested, 8 resulted in fatal outcome, 75 completely recovered, and 27 patients experienced sequelae after overdosage to include alopecia, decreased libido, diarrhea, ejaculation disorder, fatigue, insomnia, serotonin syndrome, and somnolence. The remaining 524 cases had an unknown outcome. The most common signs and symptoms associated with nonfatal sertraline overdosage were agitation, dizziness, nausea, somnolence, tachycardia, tremor, and vomiting.

The largest known ingestion was 13.5 g in a patient who took sertraline alone and subsequently recovered. However, another patient who took 2.5 g sertraline alone experienced a fatal outcome.

Other important adverse events reported with sertraline overdose (single or multiple drugs) include bradycardia, bundle branch block, coma, convulsions, delirium, hallucinations, hypertension, hypotension, manic reactions, pancreatitis, QT interval prolongation, serotonin syndrome, stupor, and syncope.

➤*Treatment:* There are no specific antidotes. Establish and maintain an airway; ensure adequate oxygenation and ventilation. Activated charcoal, which may be used with sorbitol, may be as or more effective than emesis or lavage.

Monitor cardiac and vital signs along with general symptomatic and supportive measures. SSRI-induced seizures that fail to respond spontaneously may respond to diazepam.

Because of the large volume of distribution of SSRIs, forced diuresis, dialysis, hemoperfusion, and exchange transfusion are unlikely to be of benefit.

Treatment includes usual supportive measures. Refer to General Management of Acute Overdosage.

During overdose management, consider the possibility that multiple medications were ingested. Consider contacting a poison control center for advice.

Patient Information

➤*Hazardous tasks:* Any psychoactive drug may impair judgment, thinking, or motor skills; caution patients about operating hazardous machinery, including automobiles, until they are reasonably certain that the drug treatment does not affect them adversely.

➤*Alcohol:* Although SSRIs have not been shown to increase the impairment of mental and motor skills caused by alcohol, advise patients to avoid alcohol during therapy.

➤*Concomitant medication:* Advise patients to consult their physician or pharmacist before taking concomitant OTC, prescription, or alternative medicinal drugs (see Drug Interactions). Instruct patients to avoid alcohol or other depressant medications.

Caution patients about the concomitant use of SSRIs and NSAIDs, aspirin, or other drugs that affect coagulation because the combined use of psychotropic drugs that interfere with serotonin reuptake and these agents has been associated with an increased risk of bleeding.

➤*Pregnancy or lactation:* Women should notify their physician if they are pregnant, intend to become pregnant, or are breastfeeding.

➤*Rash:* Advise patients to notify their physician if rash, hives, or a related allergic phenomenon develops.

➤*Completing course of therapy:* While patients may notice improvement in 1 to 4 weeks, advise patients to continue therapy as directed.

➤*Photosensitivity:* May cause photosensitivity (sensitivity to sunlight). Instruct patients to avoid prolonged exposure to the sun and other ultraviolet light and to use sunscreens and wear protective clothing until tolerance is determined.

➤*Emergence of adverse reactions:* Encourage patients and their families to be alert to the emergence of akathisia, anxiety, agitation, hostility, hypomania, impulsivity, insomnia, irritability, mania, panic attacks, suicidal ideation, and worsening of depression, especially early during antidepressant treatment. Such symptoms should be reported to the patient's physician, especially if they are severe, abrupt in onset, or were not part of the patient's presenting symptoms.

➤*Controlled-release tablet:* Instruct patients to swallow **paroxetine** CR whole and not to chew or crush.

➤*Citalopram/escitalopram:* Advise patients that **escitalopram** is the active isomer of **citalopram** and that the 2 medications should not be taken concomitantly.

➤*Disulfiram:* Advise patients taking disulfiram not to take concomitant paroxetine oral concentrate because of the alcohol content of the concentrate.

CITALOPRAM HYDROBROMIDE

Rx	**Citalopram Hydrobromide** (Various, eg, Caraco, Eon, Ivax, Watson)	**Tablets**: 10 mg (as base)	May contain lactose. In 30s, 100s, 500s, 1,000s, and 5,000s.
Rx	**Celexa** (Forest)		Lactose. (FP 10 mg). Beige, oval. Film-coated. In 100s.
Rx	**Citalopram Hydrobromide** (Various, eg, Caraco, Eon, Ivax, Watson)	**Tablets**: 20 mg (as base)	May contain lactose. In 30s, 100s, 500s, 1,000s, 5,000s, and UD 100s.
Rx	**Celexa** (Forest)		Lactose. (F P 20 mg). Pink, oval, scored. Film-coated. In 100s and UD 100s.
Rx	**Citalopram Hydrobromide** (Various, eg, Caraco, Eon, Ivax, Watson)	**Tablets**: 40 mg (as base)	May contain lactose. In 30s, 100s, 500s, 1,000s, 5,000s, and UD 100s.
Rx	**Celexa** (Forest)		Lactose. (F P 40 mg). White, oval, scored. Film-coated. In 100s and UD 100s.
Rx	**Citalopram Hydrobromide** (Roxane)	**Solution, oral**: 10 mg (as base) per 5 mL	Sorbitol, parabens. Peppermint flavor. In 240 mL.
Rx	**Celexa** (Forest)		Sorbitol, parabens. Peppermint flavor. In 240 mL.

CITALOPRAM HYDROBROMIDE — ORAL

WARNING

Suicidality in children and adolescents – Antidepressants increased the risk of suicidal thinking and behavior (suicidality) in short-term studies in children and adolescents with major depressive disorder (MDD) and other psychiatric disorders. Anyone considering the use of citalopram or any other antidepressant in a child or adolescent must balance this risk with the clinical need. Closely observe patients who are started on therapy for clinical worsening, suicidality, or unusual changes in behavior. Advise families and caregivers of the need for close observation and communication with the health care provider. Citalopram is not approved for use in pediatric patients.

Pooled analyses of short-term (4- to 16-week), placebo-controlled trials of 9 antidepressant drugs (selective serotonin reuptake inhibitors [SSRIs] and others) in children and adolescents with MDD, obsessive-compulsive disorder (OCD), or other psychiatric disorders (a total of 24 trials involving over 4,400 patients) have revealed a greater risk of adverse reactions representing suicidal thinking or behavior (suicidality) during the first few months of treatment in those receiving antidepressants. The average risk of such reactions in patients receiving antidepressants was 4%, twice the placebo risk of 2%. No suicides occurred in these trials.

Indications

➤*Depression:* For the treatment of depression.

➤*Off-label uses:*

Alcoholism – [4] = Insufficient documentation. Literature suggests that citalopram may be useful in the treatment of alcoholism, particularly on a short-term basis. However, data supporting a lasting effect on alcohol reduction are lacking. It appears that men may respond more favorably to this treatment than women, although these data are preliminary.

Binge-eating disorder – [3] = Safety concerns. Data regarding the use of citalopram in binge-eating disorder are very limited. A randomized, controlled trial showed benefit in reducing frequency of binging. The American Psychiatric Association published a practice guideline for the treatment of patients with eating disorders in 2006. The guideline reports SSRIs and tricyclic antidepressants have been associated with significant benefit in binge-eating disorder.

Diabetic neuropathy – [4] = Insufficient documentation. According to published, evidence-based recommendations, citalopram should generally be used as a third-line treatment rather than a first-line treatment. Initial data from a controlled study showed that citalopram caused relief of the symptoms of chronic diabetic neuropathy.

Fibromyalgia – [5] = Poor documentation. Preliminary data from a limited number of patients (less than 100) indicate that citalopram is not effective for the treatment of fibromyalgia.

Generalized anxiety disorder – [3] = Safety concerns. Initial data suggest that citalopram may be an effective option for the treatment of generalized anxiety disorder. The controlled trial demonstrated efficacy and safety; however, the study was on a narrow geriatric study population with a small number of patients. Larger, controlled trials are needed to confirm these data and identify appropriate candidates for therapy and optimal dosing.

Hot flashes – [5] = Poor documentation. Initial data are conflicting regarding the use of citalopram in the management of hot flashes in menopausal women. A large controlled trial showed no benefit of citalopram when compared with placebo or fluoxetine. A smaller open trial demonstrated some improvement in women unresponsive to venlafaxine. Based on this information, this drug is not recommended for use in the management of menopausal symptoms.

Impulsive aggressive behavior – Data suggest that citalopram may have some benefit in treating impulsive aggressive behavior in adults and children. Double-blind, placebo-controlled studies with a larger patient population are needed to further assess safety and efficacy.

Impulsive aggressive behavior (adults): [4] = Insufficient documentation.

Impulsive aggressive behavior (children/adolescents): [4] = Insufficient documentation.

Irritable bowel syndrome – [4] = Insufficient documentation. Initial data from a limited number of patients in controlled trials on citalopram's effectiveness in the treatment of irritable bowel syndrome (IBS) are conflicting, demonstrating comparable or superior activity when compared with placebo in improving symptoms. Larger trials are needed before this drug can be routinely recommended as established therapy in patients with IBS.

Obsessive-compulsive disorder – [1] = Good documentation. In controlled trials, citalopram was effective in the treatment of OCD. American Psychiatric Association practice guidelines support SSRI therapy for first-line treatment of OCD. Although several SSRIs are indicated for treatment of OCD, practice guidelines suggest all medications in this drug class, including citalopram, are equally effective for treatment of this condition. Choice of individual drug should be based on patient-specific parameters.

Pathological gambling – [4] = Insufficient documentation. Data regarding the use of citalopram for the treatment of pathological gambling are limited to 1 small, controlled trial (15 patients). These initial data are positive, suggesting beneficial effects of the drug in patients with or without depressive disorders. Larger placebo-controlled trials are needed before the clear benefits of this treatment can be determined.

Premenstrual disorders – [2] = Fair documentation. There are limited data available regarding the use of citalopram for the treatment of premenstrual disorders. Although intermittent citalopram dosing appeared to be effective in reducing irritability via self-reports, there is no information regarding its efficacy in the reduction of other symptoms (eg, breast tenderness, bloating). Patients should be counseled that reduction of libido may affect up to 39% of patients in the first treatment cycle. Further trials are required.

Stuttering – [4] = Insufficient documentation. Published information regarding the use of citalopram in the treatment of stuttering is limited. Because benefits appear to be dramatic, this agent may be considered when treating comorbidities (eg, anxiety, depression) in patients with stuttering. Larger controlled studies are needed to validate these initial results.

Other possible off-label uses – Panic disorder; premenstrual dysphoric syndrome; posttraumatic stress disorder; treatment of depression in children.

Administration and Dosage

➤*General dosing considerations:* May take with or without food.

Dose increases should usually occur in increments of 20 mg at intervals of no less than 1 week.

➤*Adults:*

Depression –

Initial dosage: 20 mg once daily, in the morning or evening, with or without food, generally with an increase to a dosage of 40 mg/day.

Dosage titration: Dose increases should usually occur in increments of 20 mg at intervals of no less than 1 week. Although certain patients may require a dosage of 60 mg/day, the only study pertinent to dose response for efficacy did not demonstrate an advantage for the 60 mg/day dosage over the 40 mg/day dosage; doses above 40 mg are therefore not ordinarily recommended.

Maintenance dosage: 20 to 60 mg/day. Acute episodes of depression require several months or longer of sustained pharmacologic therapy.

Concomitant therapy: At least 14 days should elapse between discontinuation of a monoamine oxidase inhibitor (MAOI) and initiation of citalopram therapy. Similarly, allow at least 14 days after stopping citalopram before starting an MAOI.

Off-label dosing –

Alcoholism: [4] = Insufficient documentation. 20 to 40 mg/day.

Binge eating disorder: [3] = Safety concerns. 20 to 60 mg/day.

Diabetic neuropathy: [4] = Insufficient documentation. 40 mg/day.

Generalized anxiety disorder: [3] = Safety concerns. Starting dosage 10 mg/day, titrated up to 40 mg/day.

Impulsive aggressive behavior (adults): [4] = Insufficient documentation. 20 mg orally daily, titrated to 60 mg daily as tolerated.

Irritable bowel syndrome: [4] = Insufficient documentation. Oral dosages of 20 mg daily for the first 2 to 3 weeks, followed by 40 mg daily for up to 10 additional weeks.

Obsessive-compulsive disorder: [1] = Good documentation.

- *Maximum dose* – The typical maximum dosage is 80 mg/day.
- *Initial dosage* – The recommended starting dosage is 20 mg daily orally, titrated to a target dosage of 40 to 60 mg/day. Generally, significant improvement is seen 4 to 6 weeks after starting therapy.

Pathological gambling: [4] = Insufficient documentation. Initiate at 10 mg/day and titrate up to 60 mg/day for 12 weeks.

Premenstrual disorders: [2] = Fair documentation. Intermittent dosing consisted of initiation of treatment on the estimated day of ovulation at 5 mg. Each day the dose was increased 5 mg to the maximum dose of 30 mg, which was continued until menstruation began. On the first day of menstruation, the dose was decreased to 20 mg and halved to 10 mg the next day. No drug was provided from menstruation day 3 until estimated ovulation began. The regimen then repeated itself.

Stuttering: [4] = Insufficient documentation. 10 to 20 mg at bedtime.

➤*Elderly:* 20 mg/day, with titration to 40 mg/day only for nonresponsive patients.

➤*Hepatic function impairment:* 20 mg/day, with titration to 40 mg/day only for nonresponsive patients.

➤*Discontinuation of therapy:* A gradual reduction in the dose rather than abrupt cessation is recommended whenever possible. If intolerable symptoms occur following a decrease in the dose or upon discontinuation of treatment, then resuming the previously prescribed dose may be considered. Subsequently, the health care provider may continue decreasing the dose but at a more gradual rate.

➤*Storage/Stability:* Store at 25°C (77°F); excursions are permitted to 15° to 30°C (59° to 86°F).

ESCITALOPRAM

Rx	**Lexapro** (Forest)	**Tablets; oral:** 5 mg	As escitalopram oxalate. (FL 5). White to off-white, round. Film-coated. In 100s.
		10 mg	As escitalopram oxalate. (F L 10). White to off-white, round, scored. Film-coated. In 100s and UD 100s.
		20 mg	As escitalopram oxalate. (F L 20). White to off-white, round, scored. Film-coated. In 100s and UD 100s.
		Solution; oral: 1 mg/mL	As escitalopram oxalate. Sorbitol, parabens. Peppermint flavor. In 240 mL.

ESCITALOPRAM OXALATE — ORAL

For complete prescribing information, refer to the Selective Serotonin Reuptake Inhibitors class monograph.

WARNING

Suicidality and antidepressant drugs – Antidepressants increased the risk compared with placebo of suicidal thinking and behavior (suicidality) in children, adolescents, and young adults in short-term studies of major depressive disorder (MDD) and other psychiatric disorders. Anyone considering the use of escitalopram or any other antidepressant in a child, adolescent, or young adult must balance this risk with the clinical need. Short-term studies did not show an increase in the risk of suicidality with antidepressants compared with placebo in adults older than 24 years of age; there was a reduction in risk with antidepressants compared with placebo in adults 65 years of age and older. Depression and certain other psychiatric disorders are themselves associated with increases in the risk of suicide. Appropriately monitor patients of all ages who are started on antidepressant therapy and closely observe for clinical worsening, suicidality, or unusual changes in behavior. Advise families and caregivers of the need for close observation and communication with the prescriber. Escitalopram is not approved for use in children younger than 12 years of age.

Indications

➤*Generalized anxiety disorder:* For the acute treatment of generalized anxiety disorder (GAD) in adults.

➤*Major depressive disorder:* For the acute and maintenance treatment of MDD in adults and in adolescents 12 to 17 years of age.

➤*Off-label uses:*

Posttraumatic stress disorder – [1] = Good documentation. Although few studies have specifically evaluated the use of escitalopram for the treatment of posttraumatic stress disorder (PTSD), national guidelines consider all drugs in the selective serotonin reuptake inhibitor (SSRI) class to have similar efficacy for treating PTSD. Escitalopram may be an appropriate choice based on its pharmacokinetic drug interaction or adverse effect profile compared with other drugs in the SSRI class. (See Administration and Dosage.)

Other possible off-label uses – Panic disorder.

Administration and Dosage

➤*General dosing considerations:* Patients should be periodically reassessed to determine the need for maintenance treatment.

Consider tapering escitalopram in the third trimester of pregnancy.

➤*Adults:*

Generalized anxiety disorder –

Initial dosage: 10 mg once daily.

Dosage adjustment: If the dose is increased to 20 mg, this should occur after a minimum of 1 week.

Duration of therapy: GAD is recognized as a chronic condition. The efficacy of escitalopram in the treatment of GAD beyond 8 weeks has not been systematically studied. The health care provider who elects to use escitalopram for extended periods should periodically reevaluate the long-term usefulness of the drug for the individual patient.

Major depressive disorder –

Initial dosage: 10 mg once daily.

Maintenance dosage: It is generally agreed that acute episodes of MDD require several months or longer of sustained pharmacological therapy beyond response to the acute episode. Systematic evaluation of continuing escitalopram 10 or 20 mg/day in adult patients with MDD who responded while taking escitalopram during an 8-week, acute-treatment phase demonstrated a benefit of such maintenance treatment. Nevertheless, the health care provider who elects to use escitalopram for extended periods should periodically reevaluate the long-term usefulness of the drug for the individual patient. Patients should be periodically reassessed to determine the need for maintenance treatment.

Dosage adjustment: If the dose is increased to 20 mg, this should occur after a minimum of 1 week.

Off-label dosing –

Posttraumatic stress disorder: [1] = Good documentation. 10 mg by mouth once daily, increased to 20 mg once daily after 4 weeks. Because PTSD is a chronic disorder, responders may need to continue therapy indefinitely. Tapering may be considered after 6 to 12 months in patients with acute PTSD, after 12 to 24 months in patients with chronic PTSD who have had an excellent response to therapy, and after at least 24 months or longer in patients with chronic PTSD and residual symptoms. Tapering should occur gradually over 2 weeks to 1 month to avoid withdrawal symptoms. In patients at risk of relapse, tapering should take place over 4 to 12 weeks.

➤*Children:*

Major depressive disorder –

12 to 17 years of age:

- *Initial dosage* – 10 mg once daily. A flexible-dose trial of escitalopram (10 to 20 mg/day) demonstrated the effectiveness of escitalopram.
- *Maintenance dosage* – See Adults for dosing.
- *Dosage adjustment* – If the dose is increased to 20 mg, this should occur over a minimum of 3 weeks.

➤*Elderly:* 10 mg/day.

➤*Hepatic function impairment:* 10 mg/day.

➤*Pregnancy:* Consider tapering escitalopram in the third trimester.

➤*Concomitant therapy:* At least 14 days should elapse between discontinuation of a monoamine oxidase inhibitor (MAOI) and initiation of escitalopram therapy. Similarly, at least 14 days should be allowed after stopping escitalopram before starting an MAOI.

➤*Discontinuation of therapy:* Symptoms associated with discontinuation of escitalopram and other SSRIs and selective-norepinephrine reuptake inhibitors (SNRIs) have been reported. Patients should be monitored for these symptoms (eg, agitation, anxiety, confusion, dizziness, dysphoric mood, emotional lability, headache, hypomania, insomnia, irritability, lethargy, sensory disturbances) when discontinuing treatment. A gradual reduction in the dose rather than abrupt cessation is recommended whenever possible. If intolerable symptoms occur following a decrease in the dose or upon discontinuation of treatment, then resuming the previously prescribed dose may be considered. Subsequently, the health care provider may continue decreasing the dose at a more gradual rate.

➤*Administration:* Administer once daily, in the morning or evening, with or without food.

➤*Storage/Stability:* Store at 25°C (77°F); excursions are permitted between 15° and 30°C (59° and 86°F).

FLUOXETINE

Rx	**Fluoxetine** (Various, eg, Teva)	**Tablets; oral:** 10 mg	As fluoxetine hydrochloride. May contain lactose or PEG. In 30s, 100s, and 1,000s.
Rx	**Sarafem** (Warner Chilcott)		As fluoxetine hydrochloride. (S10). Cream. In UD 28s.
Rx	**Sarafem** (Warner Chilcott)	**Tablets; oral:** 15 mg	As fluoxetine hydrochloride. (S15). White. In UD 28s.
Rx	**Sarafem** (Warner Chilcott)	**Tablets; oral:** 20 mg	As fluoxetine hydrochloride. (S20). Yellow. In UD 28s.
Rx	**Fluoxetine** (Various, eg, Aurobindo, Ivax, Mylan)	**Capsules; oral:** 10 mg	As fluoxetine hydrochloride. In 28s, 30s, 84s, 100s, 500s, 1,000s, and UD 100s.
Rx	**Prozac** (Eli Lilly/Dista)		As fluoxetine hydrochloride. (DISTA 3104 Prozac 10 mg). Green/Green. In 100s.
Rx	**Selfemra** (Teva)		As fluoxetine hydrochloride. (93 7225). Purple. In UD 28s.
Rx	**Fluoxetine** (Various, eg, Ivax, Mylan, Sandoz)	**Capsules; oral:** 20 mg	As fluoxetine hydrochloride. In 28s, 30s, 84s, 100s, 500s, 1,000s, and UD 100s.
Rx	**Prozac** (Eli Lilly/Dista)		As fluoxetine hydrochloride. (DISTA 3105 Prozac 20 mg). Green/Yellow. In 30s, 100s, 2,000s.
Rx	**Selfemra** (Teva)		As fluoxetine hydrochloride. (93 7226). Purple/Flesh. In UD 28s.

FLUOXETINE

Rx	**Fluoxetine** (Various, eg, Aurobindo, Ivax, Par)	**Capsules; oral**: 40 mg	As fluoxetine hydrochloride. In 30s, 100s, 500s, 1,000s, and UD 100s.
Rx	**Prozac** (Eli Lilly/Dista)		As fluoxetine hydrochloride. (DISTA 3107 Prozac 40 mg). Green/Orange. In 30s.
Rx	**Fluoxetine** (Various, eg, Dr. Reddy's, Teva)	**Capsules, delayed-release; oral**: 90 mg	As fluoxetine hydrochloride. May contain isopropyl alcohol, PEG, sugar. In UD 4s.
Rx	**Prozac Weekly** (Eli Lilly/Dista)		As fluoxetine hydrochloride. Sucrose, sugar. (Lilly 3004 90 mg). Green/Clear. Enteric-coated pellets. In UD 4s.
Rx	**Fluoxetine** (Various, eg, Teva)	**Solution; oral**: 20 mg per 5 mL	As fluoxetine hydrochloride. May contain alcohol, sucrose. In 120 mL.
Rx	**Prozac** (Eli Lilly/Dista)		As fluoxetine hydrochloride. Alcohol 0.23%, sucrose. Mint flavor. In 120 mL.

FLUOXETINE HYDROCHLORIDE — ORAL

For complete and comparative prescribing information, refer to theSelective Serotonin Reuptake Inhibitors group monograph.

WARNING

Suicidality and antidepressant drugs – Antidepressants increased the risk compared with placebo of suicidal thinking and behavior (suicidality) in short-term studies in children, adolescents, and young adults with major depressive disorder (MDD) and other psychiatric disorders. Anyone considering the use of fluoxetine or any other antidepressant in a child, adolescent, or young adult must balance this risk with the clinical need. Short-term studies did not show an increase in the risk of suicidality with antidepressants compared with placebo in adults older than 24 years of age; there was a reduction in risk with antidepressants compared with placebo in adults 65 years of age and older. Depression and certain other psychiatric disorders are themselves associated with increases in the risk of suicide. Appropriately monitor and closely observe patients of all ages who are started on antidepressant therapy for clinical worsening, suicidality, or unusual changes in behavior. Advise families and caregivers of the need for close observation and communication with the prescribing health care provider.

Fluoxetine is approved for use in children with MDD and obsessive-compulsive disorder (OCD). *Sarafem* and *Selfemra* are not approved for use in children.

Indications

➤*Bulimia nervosa (excluding Sarafem* and *Selfemra)*: For the acute and maintenance treatment of binge eating and vomiting behaviors in adult patients with moderate to severe bulimia nervosa.

➤*Depressive episodes associated with bipolar I disorder (fluoxetine and olanzapine in combination):* For the acute treatment of depressive episodes associated with bipolar I disorder in adult patients.

Fluoxetine monotherapy is not indicated for the treatment of depressive episodes associated with bipolar I disorder.

➤*Major depressive disorder (excluding Sarafem* and *Selfemra)*: For the acute and maintenance treatment of MDD in adults and children 8 to 18 years of age.

➤*Obsessive-compulsive disorder (excluding Sarafem* and *Selfemra)*: For the acute and maintenance treatment of obsessions and compulsions in adults and children 7 to 17 years of age with OCD.

➤*Panic disorder (excluding Sarafem* and *Selfemra)*: For the acute treatment of panic disorder, with or without agoraphobia, in adult patients.

➤*Premenstrual dysphoric disorder (Sarafem* and *Selfemra* only): For the treatment of premenstrual dysphoric disorder (PMDD).

➤*Treatment-resistant depression (fluoxetine and olanzapine in combination):* For the acute treatment of treatment-resistant depression (MDD in adults who do not respond to 2 separate trials of different antidepressants of adequate dose and duration in the current episode).

Fluoxetine monotherapy is not indicated for treatment of treatment-resistant depression.

➤*Off-label uses:*

Alcoholism – [3] = Safety concerns. Evidence-based guidelines suggest that fluoxetine may be used to treat alcoholism in adults who have failed treatment with a Food and Drug Administration (FDA)–approved medication. Fluoxetine may decrease depressive symptoms, as well as alcohol consumption, in adults and adolescents with alcoholism and comorbid depression. The use of fluoxetine is controversial in nondepressed alcoholic patients, and may increase their alcohol consumption. More studies are needed to determine the benefit of fluoxetine in nondepressed alcoholic patients. Selective serotonin reuptake inhibitors (SSRIs) are generally well tolerated; evaluate the patient to differentiate between medication adverse effects and effects of alcohol consumption or withdrawal.

Borderline personality disorder – [1] = Good documentation. The mainstay of treatment for borderline personality disorder is psychotherapy, but medications may be appropriate for acute exacerbations of disease or long-term management of selected symptoms. For affective dysregulation symptoms, SSRIs such as fluoxetine are considered the drugs of first choice because of their relative safety in overdose, favorable safety profile, and literature support in clinical trials. Published experience suggests that nonresponse to one SSRI is not predictive of lack of efficacy with other SSRIs. Impulsive behavior often responds rapidly to SSRI treatment, with improvements noted within the first week of treatment; however, it can also recur rapidly with treatment nonadherence or discontinuation.

Diabetic neuropathy – [5] = Poor documentation. There are not sufficient published data to support the use of fluoxetine in the management of diabetic neuropathy.

Fibromyalgia – [4] = Insufficient documentation. Preliminary data from a limited number of patients (less than 40) indicate that conflicting results may need to be clarified via larger controlled trials. To date, trials have utilized low doses of fluoxetine in combination with low-dose tricyclic antidepressants (TCAs). It should be noted that increased serum concentrations of TCAs have occurred during combination fluoxetine/TCA therapy, most likely as a result of fluoxetine cytochrome P450 (CYP-450) inhibition.

Hot flashes – [4] = Insufficient documentation. An initial controlled trial in women suggests that fluoxetine may have some benefit in the reduction of hot flash severity and frequency. However, the lack of a washout period in this trial makes it difficult to assess the validity of the results.

Nocturnal enuresis – [3] = Safety concerns. Uncontrolled evaluation of a very small number of children suggests some benefit with SSRI use for the treatment of nocturnal enuresis. In some cases, such as with fluvoxamine, the data are conflicting. Information from a health care provider survey suggests that SSRIs may be prescribed for enuresis despite the lack of controlled data. However, newer warnings regarding the possible association between suicidality and the use of antidepressants, including SSRIs, may limit the utility of these drugs for this indication. More data from larger controlled trials are needed.

Postherpetic neuralgia – [4] = Insufficient documentation. One study has shown positive results with the use of fluoxetine for the management of pain associated with postherpetic neuralgia (PHN). American Academy of Neurology clinical practice guidelines do not make a statement on the use of fluoxetine.

Posttraumatic stress disorder (adults) – [1] = Good documentation. National guidelines consider all drugs in the SSRI class to have similar efficacy for the treatment of posttraumatic stress disorder (PTSD). Fluoxetine may be an appropriate choice based on its pharmacokinetic, drug interaction, or adverse effect profile compared with other drugs in the SSRI class.

Posttraumatic stress disorder (children/adolescents) – [1] = Good documentation. Most national guidelines consider all drugs in the SSRI class to have similar efficacy in the treatment of PTSD. Fluoxetine may be an appropriate choice based on its pharmacokinetic, drug interaction, or adverse effect profile compared with other drugs in the SSRI class.

Prevention of migraine (adults) – [4] = Insufficient documentation. Early trials studying fluoxetine for the prevention of migraine headaches in adult patients show favorable results, but they are limited by the small number of subjects. Practice guidelines from the American Academy of Neurology consider fluoxetine to be somewhat effective for the prevention of migraines. Additional data are needed to determine the optimal dosing regimen and patient population who would most benefit from therapy.

Raynaud phenomenon – [2] = Fair documentation. Data from limited studies and cases in a small number of patients (approximately 60) suggest that fluoxetine may have some benefit in the reduction of the severity and frequency of attacks of Raynaud phenomenon.

Smoking cessation – [5] = Poor documentation. Studies evaluating fluoxetine as an aid in smoking cessation have produced inconsistent data. No randomized, placebo-controlled trials have shown a long-term benefit in using fluoxetine to improve cessation rates or evidence that fluoxetine is superior to FDA-approved first-line smoking cessation agents such as bupropion and varenicline. Guidelines from the Veterans Administration specify that treatment with antidepressants other than bupropion or nortriptyline is not recommended.

Trichotillomania – [5] = Poor documentation. Studies of fluoxetine treatment for trichotillomania have not been favorable. In a meta-analysis of trichotillomania interventions, the largest treatment effect was observed with habit-reversal therapy. Clomipramine was associated with a modest treatment effect, and fluoxetine was associated with no treatment effect. Nevertheless, a survey of 1,697 patients with trichotillomania found that the most commonly used intervention was drug therapy, that SSRIs were the most commonly prescribed class, and that fluoxetine was the most commonly prescribed agent. In keeping with the findings of the meta-analysis and controlled studies, 53.7% of survey patients rated the interventions as having no effect or making them feel worse, and another 20.8% reported experiencing minimal improvement. Given these results, clinicians considering fluoxetine treatment for trichotillomania should consider behavioral therapies instead.

Administration and Dosage

➤*Maximum dose:* 80 mg/day, but may vary by indication.

➤*General dosing considerations:* Individualize dosing.

FLUOXETINE HYDROCHLORIDE — ORAL

A gradual reduction in the dose rather than abrupt cessation is recommended with fluoxetine. (See Discontinuation of Therapy.)

Consider tapering fluoxetine in the third trimester. (See Pregnancy.)

➤*Adults:*

Bulimia nervosa –

Usual dosage: 60 mg/day, administered in the morning. For some patients, it may be advisable to titrate up to this target dosage over several days.

Maintenance dosage: Systematic evaluation of continuing fluoxetine 60 mg/day for periods of up to 52 weeks in patients with bulimia who have responded while taking fluoxetine 60 mg/day during an 8-week, short-term treatment phase has demonstrated a benefit of such maintenance treatment.

Duration of therapy: Continuing fluoxetine for periods of up to 52 weeks in patients with bulimia has demonstrated benefit. Nevertheless, periodically reassess patients to determine the need for maintenance treatment.

Depressive episodes associated with bipolar I disorder (fluoxetine and olanzapine in combination) –

Usual dosage: Fluoxetine should be administered in combination with oral olanzapine once daily in the evening without regard to meals, generally beginning with oral olanzapine 5 mg and fluoxetine 20 mg. Dosage adjustments, if indicated, should be made with the individual components according to efficacy and tolerability.

Safety of coadministration of doses above olanzapine 18 mg with fluoxetine 75 mg has not been evaluated in clinical studies.

Fluoxetine monotherapy is not indicated for the treatment of depressive episodes associated with bipolar I disorder.

Dosage adjustment: Dosage adjustments, if indicated, can be made according to efficacy and tolerability within dose ranges of fluoxetine 20 to 50 mg and oral olanzapine 5 to 12.5 mg.

Approximate Dose Correspondence Between *Symbyax*[a] and the Combination of Fluoxetine and Olanzapine

	Use in combination	
For *Symbyax* (mg/day)	Olanzapine (mg/day)	Fluoxetine (mg/day)
Olanzapine 3 mg/ Fluoxetine 25 mg	2.5	20
Olanzapine 6 mg/ Fluoxetine 25 mg	5	20
Olanzapine 12 mg/ Fluoxetine 25 mg	10 + 2.5	20
Olanzapine 6 mg/ Fluoxetine 50 mg	5	40 + 10
Olanzapine 12 mg/ Fluoxetine 50 mg	10 + 2.5	40 + 10

[a] *Symbyax* (olanzapine/fluoxetine) is a fixed-dose combination of fluoxetine and olanzapine.

Duration of therapy: While there is no body of evidence to answer the question of how long a patient treated with fluoxetine and olanzapine in combination should remain on it, it is generally accepted that bipolar I disorder, including the depressive episodes associated with bipolar I disorder, is a chronic illness requiring maintenance treatment. Periodically reexamine the need for continued pharmacotherapy.

Major depressive disorder –

Usual dosage: 20 to 80 mg/day.

Maximum dose: 80 mg/day.

Initial dosage: 20 mg/day, administered in the morning.

Maintenance dosage: It is generally agreed that acute episodes of MDD require several months or longer of sustained pharmacologic therapy. Whether the dose needed to induce remission is identical to the dose needed to maintain and/or sustain euthymia is unknown.

Dosage adjustment: A dosage increase may be considered after several weeks if insufficient clinical improvement is observed.

As with other drugs effective in the treatment of MDD, the full effect may be delayed until 4 weeks of treatment or longer.

Alternative dosage: Systemic evaluation of *Prozac Weekly* in adult patients has shown that its efficacy in MDD is maintained for periods of up to 25 weeks with once-weekly dosing following 13 weeks of open-label treatment with fluoxetine 20 mg once daily. However, therapeutic equivalence of *Prozac Weekly* given on a once-weekly basis with fluoxetine 20 mg given daily for delaying time to relapse has not been established.

Weekly dosing with *Prozac Weekly* capsules is recommended to be initiated 7 days after the last daily dose of fluoxetine 20 mg.

If satisfactory response is not maintained with *Prozac Weekly*, consider reestablishing a daily dosing regimen.

Duration of therapy: Systemic evaluation of fluoxetine in adult patients has shown that its efficacy in MDD is maintained for periods of up to 38 weeks following 12 weeks of open-label acute treatment (50 weeks total) at a dosage of 20 mg/day.

Concomitant therapy: The dose of a TCA may need to be reduced, and plasma TCA concentrations may need to be monitored temporarily when fluoxetine is coadministered or has been recently discontinued.

Obsessive-compulsive disorder –

Usual dosage: 20 to 60 mg/day is recommended; however, dosages of up to 80 mg/day have been well tolerated in open studies of OCD.

Maximum dose: 80 mg/day.

Initial dosage: 20 mg/day, administered in the morning.

Dosage adjustment: In controlled clinical trials of fluoxetine supporting its effectiveness in the treatment of OCD, patients were administered fixed daily doses of fluoxetine 20, 40, or 60 mg or placebo. In one of these studies, no dose-response relationship for effectiveness was demonstrated. Because there was a suggestion of a possible dose-response relationship for efficacy in the second study, a dose increase may be considered after several weeks if insufficient clinical improvement is observed. The full therapeutic effect may be delayed until 5 weeks of treatment or longer.

Duration of therapy: While there are no systematic studies that answer the question of how long to continue fluoxetine, OCD is a chronic condition, and it is reasonable to consider continuation for a responding patient. Although the efficacy of fluoxetine after 13 weeks has not been documented in controlled trials, adult patients have continued in therapy under double-blind conditions for up to an additional 6 months without loss of benefit. However, make dosage adjustments to maintain the patient on the lowest effective dose, and periodically reassess patients to determine the need for treatment.

Panic disorder –

Usual dosage: 20 mg/day was the most frequently administered dosage in the 2 flexible-dosage clinical trials.

In controlled clinical trials of fluoxetine supporting its effectiveness in the treatment of panic disorder, patients were administered fluoxetine dosages in the range of 10 to 60 mg/day.

Initial dosage: 10 mg/day. After 1 week, increase the dosage to 20 mg/day.

Dosage adjustment: A dosage increase may be considered after several weeks if no clinical improvement is observed. Fluoxetine dosages above 60 mg/day have not been systematically evaluated in patients with panic disorder.

Duration of therapy: While there are no systematic studies that answer the question of how long to continue fluoxetine, panic disorder is a chronic condition, and it is reasonable to consider continuation for a responding patient. Nevertheless, periodically reassess patients to determine the need for continued treatment.

*Premenstrual dysphoric disorder (*Sarafem *and* Selfemra *only) –*

Usual dosage: 20 mg/day given continuously (every day of the menstrual cycle) or intermittently (defined as starting a daily dose 14 days prior to the anticipated onset of menstruation through the first full day of menses and repeating with each new cycle).

In a study comparing continuous dosing of fluoxetine 20 and 60 mg/day with placebo, both dosages were proven to be effective, but there was no statistically significant added benefit for the 60 mg/day dosage compared with the 20 mg/day dosage. Fluoxetine dosages above 60 mg/day have not been systematically studied in patients with PMDD.

Maximum dose: 80 mg/day.

Duration of therapy: Systematic evaluation has shown that the efficacy of fluoxetine is maintained for periods of up to 6 months at a dosage of 20 mg/day given continuously and up to 3 months at a dosage of 20 mg/day given intermittently. Reassess patients periodically to determine the need for continued treatment.

Treatment-resistant depression (fluoxetine and olanzapine in combination) –

Usual dosage: Fluoxetine should be administered in combination with oral olanzapine once daily in the evening without regard to meals, generally beginning with oral olanzapine 5 mg and fluoxetine 20 mg.

Safety of coadministration of doses above 18 mg of olanzapine with 75 mg of fluoxetine has not been evaluated in clinical studies.

Fluoxetine monotherapy is not indicated for the treatment of treatment-resistant depression (MDD in patients who do not respond to 2 antidepressants of adequate dose and duration in the current episode).

Dosage adjustment: Dosage adjustments, if indicated, can be made according to efficacy and tolerability within dose ranges of fluoxetine 20 to 50 mg and oral olanzapine 5 to 20 mg.

Dosage adjustments, if indicated, should be made with the individual components according to efficacy and tolerability.

Duration of therapy: While there is no body of evidence to answer the question of how long a patient treated with fluoxetine and olanzapine in combination should remain on it, it is generally accepted that treatment-resistant depression (MDD in adult patients who do not respond to 2 separate trials of different antidepressants of adequate dose and duration in the current episode) is a chronic illness requiring maintenance treatment. Periodically reexamine the need for continued pharmacotherapy.

Off-label dosing –

Alcoholism: [3] = Safety concerns. Initially, 20 mg daily orally, titrated to 40 mg daily after 2 weeks if needed.

Borderline personality disorder: [1] = Good documentation. 20 to 80 mg/day orally. A reasonable trial period for treatment of borderline personality disorder is at least 12 weeks.

Fibromyalgia: [4] = Insufficient documentation. 20 mg/day (in the morning) for up to 6 weeks.

Hot flashes: [4] = Insufficient documentation. 20 mg/day for 4 weeks.

Nocturnal enuresis: [3] = Safety concerns. 20 to 40 mg daily (11 to 15 years of age).

Postherpetic neuralgia: [4] = Insufficient documentation. 52 mg daily (peak dose) for at least 6 weeks.

Posttraumatic stress disorder (adults): [1] = Good documentation. Initially, 10 to 20 mg/day orally. Evaluate for response every 1 to 2 weeks and increase the dose as needed for at least an 8-week treatment trial. The average target daily dose is 20 to 50 mg in adults and 20 mg in older adults. The highest target dosage is 80 mg/day. The recommended duration of therapy is 6 to 12 months for acute PTSD, 12 to 24 months for chronic PTSD with excellent response, and at least 24 months for chronic PTSD with residual symptoms. Discontinuation may be attempted after 6 to 24 months,

FLUOXETINE HYDROCHLORIDE — ORAL

depending on the type of PTSD and the patient's response. To avoid withdrawal syndrome, dose tapering over 2 weeks to 1 month is recommended.

Prevention of migraine (adults): [4] = Insufficient documentation. 20 mg every other day to 40 mg daily for 8 weeks. S-fluoxetine was dosed at 40 mg daily (equivalent to 80 mg of the racemic fluoxetine).

Raynaud phenomenon: [2] = Fair documentation. 20 to 60 mg daily.

➤*Children:*

Major depressive disorder –

8 years of age and older:

- *Usual dosage* – 10 to 20 mg/day.
- *Initial dosage* – 10 or 20 mg/day. After 1 week at 10 mg/day, the dosage should be increased to 20 mg/day.

Because of higher plasma levels in lower weight children, the starting and target dosage in this group may be 10 mg/day. A dosage increase to 20 mg/day may be considered after several weeks if sufficient clinical improvement is observed.

Obsessive-compulsive disorder –

Adolescents and higher-weight children:

- *7 years of age and older –*

  Usual dosage: 20 to 60 mg/day is recommended.

  Initial dosage: 10 mg/day. After 2 weeks, the dosage should be increased to 20 mg/day.

  Dosage adjustment: Additional dosage increases may be considered after several more weeks if insufficient clinical improvement is observed.

- *Lower-weight children –*

  Usual dosage: 20 to 30 mg/day is recommended. Experience with daily doses of more than 20 mg is very minimal, and there is no experience with doses of more than 60 mg.

  Initial dosage: 10 mg/day.

  Dosage adjustment: Additional dosage increases may be considered after several more weeks if insufficient clinical improvement is observed.

Off-label dosing –

Major depressive disorder:

- *Younger than 12 years of age –*

  Initial dosage: 5 to 10 mg/day.

  Maintenance dosage: 10 to 30 mg/day.

Posttraumatic stress disorder (children / adolescents): [1] = Good documentation. The average target daily dose is 10 to 20 mg in children. Evaluate for response every 1 to 2 weeks and increase the dose as needed for at least an 8-week treatment trial. The recommended duration of therapy is 6 to 12 months for acute PTSD, 12 to 24 months for chronic PTSD with excellent response, and at least 24 months for chronic PTSD with residual symptoms. Discontinuation may be attempted after 6 to 24 months, depending on the type of PTSD and the patient's response. To avoid withdrawal syndrome, dose tapering over 2 weeks to 1 month is recommended.

➤*Elderly:* Consider lower or less frequent dosing for elderly patients (does not apply to *Sarafem* and *Selfemra*).

➤*Hepatic function impairment:* Use lower or less frequent dosing.

➤*Concomitant illness:* Patients with concurrent disease or on multiple concomitant medications may require dosage adjustments.

➤*Fluoxetine and olanzapine in combination:* The starting dose of oral olanzapine 2.5 to 5 mg with fluoxetine 20 mg should be used for patients with a predisposition to hypotensive reactions, patients with hepatic impairment, or patients who exhibit a combination of factors that may slow the metabolism of olanzapine or fluoxetine in combination (women, elderly patients, nonsmokers), or those patients who may be pharmacodynamically sensitive to olanzapine. Dosing modifications may be necessary in patients who exhibit a combination of factors that may slow metabolism. When indicated, dose escalation should be performed with caution in these patients. Fluoxetine and olanzapine in combination have not been systematically studied in patients older than 65 years of age or in patients younger than 18 years of age.

➤*Pregnancy:* Neonates exposed to fluoxetine and other SSRIs or serotonin and norepinephrine reuptake inhibitors (SNRIs) late in the third trimester have developed complications requiring prolonged hospitalization, respiratory support, and tube feeding. When treating pregnant women with fluoxetine during the third trimester, carefully consider the potential risks and benefits of treatment. The health care provider may consider tapering fluoxetine in the third trimester.

➤*Switching patients to or from a monoamine oxidase inhibitor:* At least 14 days should elapse between the discontinuation of a monoamine oxidase inhibitor (MAOI) and initiation of therapy with fluoxetine. In addition, allow at least 5 weeks, perhaps longer, after stopping fluoxetine before starting an MAOI.

➤*Discontinuation of therapy:* Symptoms associated with discontinuation of fluoxetine and other SSRIs and SNRIs have been reported. Monitor patients for these symptoms when discontinuing treatment. A gradual reduction in dose rather than abrupt cessation is recommended whenever possible. If intolerable symptoms occur following a decrease in the dose or upon discontinuation of treatment, resuming the previously prescribed dose may be considered. Subsequently, the health care provider may continue decreasing the dose but at a more gradual rate. Plasma fluoxetine and norfluoxetine concentration decrease gradually at the conclusion of therapy, which may minimize the risk of discontinuation symptoms with this drug.

➤*Administration:* Dosages above 20 mg/day may be administered on a once-daily (ie, morning) or twice-daily schedule (ie, morning and noon).

When given in combination with olanzapine, administer once daily in the evening.

➤*Storage / Stability:* Store fluoxetine and *Sarafem*at 15° to 30°C (59° to 86°F). Store *Selfemra* at 20° to 25°C (68° to 77°F). Protect *Sarafem* and *Selfemra* from light.

FLUVOXAMINE MALEATE

Rx	**Fluvoxamine Maleate** (Various, eg, Apotex, Barr, Sandoz)	**Tablets; oral:** 25 mg	In 100s and 500s.
Rx	**Luvox** (Jazz Pharmaceuticals)		Mannitol, PEG. (LT25). White. Film-coated. In 100s.
Rx	**Fluvoxamine Maleate** (Various, eg, Apotex, Barr, Sandoz)	**Tablets; oral:** 50 mg	In 100s and 500s.
Rx	**Luvox** (Jazz Pharmaceuticals)		Mannitol, PEG. (LT50). Yellow, scored. Film-coated. In 100s.
Rx	**Fluvoxamine Maleate** (Various, eg, Apotex, Barr, Sandoz)	**Tablets; oral:** 100 mg	In 100s and 500s.
Rx	**Luvox** (Jazz Pharmaceuticals)		Mannitol, PEG. (LT100). Beige, scored. Film-coated. In 100s.
Rx	**Luvox CR** (Jazz Pharmaceuticals)	**Capsules, extended-release; oral:** 100 mg	Sugar spheres. Gluten-free. (LCR 100). Dark blue opaque/white opaque. In 30s.
		150 mg	Sugar spheres. Gluten-free. (LCR 150). Dark blue opaque/powder blue opaque. In 30s.

FLUVOXAMINE MALEATE — ORAL

For complete and comparative prescribing information, refer to the Selective Serotonin Reuptake Inhibitors (SSRIs) group monograph.

WARNING

Suicidality in children and adolescents – Antidepressants increased the risk of suicidal thinking and behavior (suicidality) in short-term studies in children, adolescents, and young adults with major depressive disorder (MDD) and other psychiatric disorders. Anyone considering the use of fluvoxamine or any other antidepressant in a child, adolescent, or young adult must balance this risk with the clinical need. Short-term studies did not show an increase in the risk of suicidality with antidepressants compared with placebo in adults older than 24 years of age; there was a reduction in risk with antidepressants compared with placebo in adults 65 years of age and older. Depression and certain other psychiatric disorders are associated with increases in the risk of suicide. Closely observe patients of all ages who are started on therapy for clinical worsening, suicidality, or unusual changes in behavior. Advise families and caregivers of the need for close observation and communication with the prescriber. Fluvoxamine tablets are not approved for use in children, except for patients with obsessive-compulsive disorder (OCD). Fluvoxamine extended-release capsules are not approved for use in children.

Indications

➤*Obsessive compulsive disorder (capsules and tablets):* For the treatment of obsessions and compulsions in patients with OCD as defined in the *Diagnostic and Statistical Manual of Mental Disorders* (*DSM-IV*, capsules; *DSM-III-R*, tablets). The obsessions or compulsions cause marked distress, are time-consuming, or significantly interfere with social or occupational functioning.

The efficacy of fluvoxamine was demonstrated in one 12-week trial (capsules) or three 10-week trials (tablets) with obsessive-compulsive outpatients with the diagnosis of OCD as defined in *DSM-IV* (capsules) or *DSM-III-R* (tablets).

OCD is characterized by recurrent and persistent ideas, thoughts, impulses, or images (obsessions) that are ego-dystonic and/or repetitive, purposeful, and intentional behaviors (compulsions) recognized by the person as excessive or unreasonable.

The effectiveness of fluvoxamine for long-term use (ie, more than 12 weeks for capsules or 10 weeks for tablets) has not been systemically evaluated in placebo-controlled trials. Therefore, the health care provider who elects to prescribe fluvoxamine for extended periods should periodically reevaluate the long-term usefulness of the drug for the individual patient.

➤*Social anxiety disorder (capsules only):* For the treatment of social anxiety disorder, also known as social phobia, as defined in *DSM-IV*.

FLUVOXAMINE MALEATE — ORAL

The efficacy of fluvoxamine was demonstrated in two 12-week trials in adult patients with social anxiety disorder (*DSM-IV*). Fluvoxamine capsules have not been studied in children or adolescents with social anxiety disorder.

➤*Off-label uses:*

Bulimia nervosa – [2] = Fair documentation. Limited clinical trials have shown modest benefit with fluvoxamine for the treatment of bulimia nervosa. According to American Psychiatric Association guidelines, SSRIs are the preferred class of antidepressants for the initial treatment of bulimia nervosa. Although fluoxetine is the only FDA-approved product for this indication, other SSRIs, including sertraline and fluvoxamine, may be beneficial in some patients.

Nocturnal enuresis – [3] = Safety concerns. Uncontrolled evaluation of a very small number of children suggests some benefit with SSRI use for the treatment of nocturnal enuresis. In some cases, such as with fluvoxamine, the data are conflicting. Information from a health care provider survey suggests that SSRIs may be prescribed for enuresis, despite the lack of controlled data. However, newer warnings regarding the possible association between suicidality and the use of antidepressants, including SSRIs, may limit the utility of these drugs for this indication. More data from larger controlled trials are needed.

Panic disorder – [1] = Good documentation. In several controlled trials, fluvoxamine demonstrated superiority over placebo in controlling panic. American Psychiatric Association guidelines state that SSRIs, tricyclic antidepressants (TCAs), benzodiazepines, and monoamine oxidase inhibitors (MAOIs) all have roughly comparable efficacy in the treatment of panic disorder but that SSRIs, such as fluvoxamine, are likely to have the most favorable balance of efficacy and adverse effects for most patients.

Posttraumatic stress disorder (adults) – [1] = Good documentation. Although few studies have specifically evaluated the use of fluvoxamine for the treatment of posttraumatic stress disorder (PTSD), national guidelines consider all drugs in the SSRI class to have similar efficacy for this disorder. Fluvoxamine may be an appropriate choice based on its pharmacokinetic, drug interaction, or adverse effect profile compared with other drugs in the SSRI class.

Posttraumatic stress disorder (children/adolescents) – [1] = Good documentation. Few studies have specifically evaluated the use of fluvoxamine in the treatment of PTSD. Guidelines suggest this drug may be an appropriate choice, but medication should be selected based on the prominent comorbid condition.

Prevention of migraine (adults) – [2] = Fair documentation. American Academy of Neurology practice guidelines consider fluvoxamine to be clinically efficacious based on consensus and clinical experience, despite the lack of scientific evidence of efficacy. One controlled trial showed favorable results, but it was limited by a small sample size. Additional data are needed to determine the optimal dosing regimen and patient population who would most benefit from therapy.

Other possible off-label uses – Depression.

Fluvoxamine has also been used in children for the treatment of depression and anxiety disorder (See Off-label dosing).

Administration and Dosage

➤*General dosing considerations:* A gradual reduction in the dose rather than abrupt cessation is recommended for fluvoxamine. (See Discontinuation of therapy.)

Consider tapering fluvoxamine in the third trimester of pregnancy. (See Pregnancy.)

➤*Adults:*

Obsessive-compulsive disorder –

Extended-release capsules:

- *Maximum dose* – 300 mg/day.
- *Initial dosage* – 100 mg once per day, administered with or without food, as a single daily dose at bedtime.
- *Dosage titration* – The dose should be increased in 50 mg increments every week, as tolerated, until maximum therapeutic benefit is achieved, not to exceed 300 mg/day.

Tablets:

- *Maximum dose* – 300 mg/day.
- *Initial dosage* – 50 mg as a single daily dose at bedtime.
- *Dosage titration* – Increase dose in 50 mg increments every 4 to 7 days, as tolerated, until maximum therapeutic benefit is achieved (not to exceed 300 mg/day). It is advisable to give total daily doses greater than 100 mg in 2 divided doses; if the doses are not equal, give the larger dose at bedtime.

In trials, patients were titrated within a range of 100 to 300 mg/day.

Social anxiety disorder –

Extended-release capsules:

- *Maximum dose* – 300 mg/day.
- *Initial dosage* – 100 mg once per day, administered with or without food as a single daily dose at bedtime.
- *Dosage titration* – The dose should be increased in 50 mg increments every week, as tolerated, until maximum therapeutic benefit is achieved.

Off-label dosing –

Bulimia nervosa: [2] = Fair documentation. 50 mg daily, titrated up based on therapeutic response to 200 mg/day for up to 12 weeks.

Panic disorder: [1] = Good documentation. The recommended starting dosage is 50 mg/day; maintain for several days and then gradually increase to 150 mg/day. Further dosage increases of up to 300 mg/day may be considered for patients who fail to respond after several weeks of treatment. Therapy should continue for 1 to 2 years after a response, after which discontinuation may be attempted with close supervision. When discontinuing therapy, a slow taper over 2 to 6 months is recommended.

Posttraumatic stress disorder (adults): [1] = Good documentation. Initially 50 mg/day orally. The average daily target dose is 100 to 250 mg in adults and 100 mg in older adults. The maximum recommended dosage is 300 mg/day. Because PTSD can be a chronic disorder, responders may need to continue therapy indefinitely. Tapering may be considered after 6 to 12 months in patients with acute PTSD, after 12 to 24 months in patients with chronic PTSD who have had an excellent response to therapy, and after at least 24 months or longer in patients with chronic PTSD and residual symptoms. Tapering should occur gradually over 2 weeks to 1 month to avoid withdrawal symptoms. In patients at risk of relapse, tapering should take place over 4 to 12 weeks.

Prevention of migraine (adults): [2] = Fair documentation. 50 mg at bedtime for 12 weeks.

➤*Children:*

Obsessive-compulsive disorder –

8 to 17 years of age:

- *Tablets* –
  - *Maximum dose:* 200 mg/day in children younger than 11 years of age; up to 300 mg/day in adolescents.
  - *Initial dosage:* 25 mg as a single daily dose at bedtime.
  - *Dosage titration:* Increase the dose in 25 mg increments every 4 to 7 days, as tolerated, until maximum therapeutic benefit is achieved. In trials, patients were titrated within a dose range of 50 to 200 mg/day. Dose adjustment in adolescents (up to the adult maximum dose of 300 mg) may be indicated to achieve therapeutic benefit. Health care providers should consider age and gender differences when dosing pediatric patients. Therapeutic effect in female children may be achieved with lower doses. Divide total daily doses of more than 50 mg into 2 doses. If the 2 divided doses are not equal, give the larger dose at bedtime.

Off-label dosing –

Anxiety disorder:

- *12 years of age and older* –
  - *Initial dosage:* 25 to 50 mg at bedtime.
  - *Maintenance dosage:* 150 to 300 mg/day.
- *Younger than 12 years of age* –
  - *Initial dosage:* 25 mg at bedtime.
  - *Maintenance dosage:* 100 to 200 mg/day.

Depression:

- *12 years of age and older* –
  - *Initial dosage:* 25 to 50 mg at bedtime.
  - *Maintenance dosage:* 150 to 300 mg/day.
- *Younger than 12 years of age* –
  - *Initial dosage:* 25 mg at bedtime.
  - *Maintenance dosage:* 100 to 200 mg/day.

Nocturnal enuresis: [3] = Safety concerns. 25 to 75 mg at bedtime; 25 mg twice daily; or 25 mg in the morning and 50 mg at bedtime (7 to 15 years of age).

Posttraumatic stress disorder (children/adolescents): [1] = Good documentation. The average daily target dose is 50 mg in children and younger adolescents. Because PTSD can be a chronic disorder, responders may need to continue therapy indefinitely. Tapering may be considered after 6 to 12 months in patients with acute PTSD, after 12 to 24 months in patients with chronic PTSD who have had an excellent response to therapy, and after at least 24 months in patients with chronic PTSD and residual symptoms. Tapering should occur gradually over 2 weeks to 1 month to avoid withdrawal symptoms. In patients at risk of relapse, tapering should take place over 4 to 12 weeks.

➤*Elderly:* Elderly patients have been observed to have a decreased clearance of fluvoxamine. In these patients, it may be appropriate to titrate slowly following the initial dose of 100 mg (capsules) and subsequent dose titration.

➤*Hepatic function impairment:* Patients with hepatic function impairment have been observed to have a decreased clearance of fluvoxamine. In these patients, it may be appropriate to titrate slowly following the initial dose of 100 mg (capsules) and subsequent dose titration.

➤*Pregnancy:* No neonates have been exposed to fluvoxamine capsules. Neonates exposed to fluvoxamine tablets and other SSRIs or serotonin-norepinephrine reuptake inhibitors (SNRIs) late in the third trimester have developed complications requiring prolonged hospitalization, respiratory support, and tube feeding.

When treating pregnant women with fluvoxamine during the third trimester, the health care provider should carefully consider the potential risks and benefits of treatment. The health care provider may consider tapering fluvoxamine in the third trimester.

➤*Switching patients to or from an MAOI:* At least 14 days should elapse between discontinuation of an MAOI and initiation of therapy with fluvoxamine. Similarly, at least 14 days should be allowed after stopping fluvoxamine before starting an MAOI.

➤*Duration of therapy:* Although the efficacy of fluvoxamine extended-release capsules beyond 12 weeks of dosing for social anxiety disorder and OCD, and for tablets beyond 10 weeks of dosing for OCD, has not been documented in controlled trials, social anxiety disorder and OCD are chronic conditions. It is reasonable to consider continuation for a responding patient. Dosage adjustments should be made to maintain the patient on the lowest

FLUVOXAMINE MALEATE — ORAL

effective dosage, and patients should be periodically reassessed to determine the need for continued treatment.

➤*Discontinuation of therapy:* Symptoms associated with discontinuation of other SSRIs or SNRIs have been reported. Patients should be monitored for these symptoms when discontinuing treatment. A gradual reduction in the dose rather than abrupt cessation is recommended whenever possible. If intolerable symptoms occur following a decrease in the dose or upon discontinuation of treatment, then resuming the previously prescribed dose may be considered. Subsequently, the health care provider may continue decreasing the dose, but at a more gradual rate.

➤*Administration:* Capsules should not be crushed or chewed; administer capsules with or without food. Oral bioavailability of fluvoxamine tablets is not significantly affected by food.

For adults, it is advisable to give total daily doses greater than 100 mg in 2 divided doses; if the doses are not equal, give the larger dose at bedtime.

For children, divide total daily doses of more than 50 mg into 2 doses. If the 2 divided doses are not equal, give the larger dose at bedtime.

➤*Storage/Stability:*

Capsules – Protect from high humidity and store at 25°C (77°F); excursions are permitted to 15° to 30°C (59° to 86°F). Avoid exposure to temperatures above 30°C.

Tablets – Store at 20° to 25°C (68° to 77°F). Protect from high humidity and dispense in tight, light-resistant containers.

PAROXETINE

Rx	**Paroxetine** (Various, eg, Apotex USA, Par, Sandoz)	**Tablets; oral:** 10 mg	As paroxetine hydrochloride. In 30s, 100s, 1,000s, and UD 100s.
Rx	**Paxil** (GlaxoSmithKline)		As paroxetine hydrochloride. (PAXIL 10). Yellow, oval, scored. Film-coated. In 30s.
Rx	**Paroxetine** (Various, eg, Apotex USA, Par, Sandoz)	**Tablets; oral:** 20 mg	As paroxetine hydrochloride. In 30s, 100s, 1,000s, and UD 100s.
Rx	**Paxil** (GlaxoSmithKline)		As paroxetine hydrochloride. (PAXIL 20). Pink, oval, scored. Film-coated. In 30s, 90s, and SUP[a] 100s.
Rx	**Paroxetine** (Various, eg, Apotex USA, Par, Sandoz)	**Tablets; oral:** 30 mg	As paroxetine hydrochloride. In 30s, 100s, 1,000s, and UD 100s.
Rx	**Paxil** (GlaxoSmithKline)		As paroxetine hydrochloride. (PAXIL 30). Blue, oval. Film-coated. In 30s.
Rx	**Paroxetine** (Various, eg, Apotex USA, Par, Sandoz)	**Tablets; oral:** 40 mg	As paroxetine hydrochloride. In 30s, 100s, 1,000s, and UD 100s.
Rx	**Paxil** (GlaxoSmithKline)		As paroxetine hydrochloride. (PAXIL 40). Green, oval. Film-coated. In 30s.
Rx	**Pexeva** (Synthon)	**Tablets; oral:** 10 mg	As paroxetine mesylate. (POT 10). White, oval. In 30s.
		20 mg	As paroxetine mesylate. (POT 20). Dark orange, oval, scored. In 30s, 100s, and 500s.
		30 mg	As paroxetine mesylate. (POT 30). Yellow, oval. In 30s.
		40 mg	As paroxetine mesylate. (POT 40). Rose, oval. In 30s.
Rx	**Paroxetine Hydrochloride** (Mylan)	**Tablets, controlled-release; oral:** 12.5 mg	As paroxetine hydrochloride. Lactose, PEG. (M P3). Enteric-coated. In 30s, 100s, and 500s.
Rx	**Paxil CR** (Apotex)		As paroxetine hydrochloride. Lactose. (Paxil CR 12.5). Yellow. Enteric-coated. In 30s.
Rx	**Paroxetine Hydrochloride** (Mylan)	**Tablets, controlled-release; oral:** 25 mg	As paroxetine hydrochloride. Lactose, PEG. (M P4). Lavender. Enteric-coated. In 30s, 100s, and 500s.
Rx	**Paxil CR** (Apotex)		As paroxetine hydrochloride. Lactose. (Paxil CR 25). Pink. Enteric-coated. In 30s.
Rx	**Paroxetine Hydrochloride** (Mylan)	**Tablets, controlled-release; oral:** 37.5 mg	As paroxetine hydrochloride. Lactose, PEG. (PL PCR 37.5). Blue. Enteric-coated. In 30s.
Rx	**Paxil CR** (Apotex)		As paroxetine hydrochloride. Lactose. (Paxil CR 37.5). Blue. Enteric-coated. In 30s.
Rx	**Paroxetine Hydrochloride** (Apotex USA)	**Suspension; oral:** 10 mg per 5 mL	As paroxetine hydrochloride. In 250 mL.
Rx	**Paxil** (GlaxoSmithKline)		As paroxetine hydrochloride. Parabens, saccharin, sorbitol. Orange flavor. In 250 mL.

[a] SUP = single unit packages. Intended for institutional use only.

PAROXETINE HYDROCHLORIDE — ORAL

For complete prescribing information, refer to the SSRIs group monograph.

WARNING

Suicidality in children and adolescents – Antidepressants increased the risk of suicidal thinking and behavior (suicidality) in short-term studies in children and adolescents with major depressive disorder (MDD) and other psychiatric disorders. Anyone considering the use of paroxetine or any other antidepressant in a child or adolescent must balance this risk with the clinical need. Closely observe patients who are started on therapy for clinical worsening, suicidality, or unusual changes in behavior. Advise families and caregivers of the need for close observation and communication with the health care provider. Paroxetine is not approved for use in children.

Pooled analyses of short-term (4- to 16-weeks) placebo-controlled trials of 9 antidepressant drugs (selective serotonin reuptake inhibitors [SSRIs] and others) in children and adolescents with MDD, obsessive-compulsive disorder (OCD), or other psychiatric disorders (a total of 24 trials involving more than 4,400 patients) have revealed a greater risk of adverse reactions representing suicidal thinking or behavior (suicidality) during the first few months of treatment in those receiving antidepressants. The average risk of such reactions in patients receiving antidepressants was 4%, twice the placebo risk of 2%. No suicides occurred in these trials.

Indications

➤*Generalized anxiety disorder (GAD) (immediate-release):* For the treatment of GAD, as defined in *Diagnostic and Statistical Manual of Mental Disorders* (Fourth Edition) (*DSM-IV*). Anxiety or tension associated with the stress of everyday life usually does not require treatment with an anxiolytic.

➤*Major Depressive Disorder (MDD) (immediate- and controlled-release):* For the treatment of MDD.

➤*Obsessive-compulsive disorder (OCD) (immediate-release):* For the treatment of obsessions and compulsions in patients with OCD as defined in the *DSM-IV*. The obsessions or compulsions cause marked distress, are time-consuming, or significantly interfere with social or occupational functioning.

➤*Panic disorder (immediate- and controlled-release):* For the treatment of panic disorder, with or without agoraphobia, as defined in *DSM-IV*.

➤*Posttraumatic stress disorder (PTSD) (immediate-release):* For the treatment of PTSD.

➤*Premenstrual dysphoric disorder (PMDD) (controlled-release):* For the treatment of PMDD.

➤*Social anxiety disorder (immediate- and controlled-release):* For the treatment of social anxiety disorder, also known as social phobia, as defined in *DSM-IV*.

➤*Off-label uses:*

Diabetic neuropathy – [2] = Fair documentation. In small trials, paroxetine was not as effective as imipramine at relieving symptoms associated with neuropathic pain, although it appears to be more effective than gabapentin. In addition, paroxetine was better tolerated than imipramine and gabapentin. Larger controlled trials are needed to define the role of paroxe-

PAROXETINE HYDROCHLORIDE — ORAL

tine in the treatment of diabetic neuropathy. Future studies comparing paroxetine with newer agents are also needed.

Hot flashes – [2] = Fair documentation. Initial data suggest that paroxetine may have some benefit in the reduction of hot flash severity and frequency. This drug may be useful in treating hot flashes and depression in menopausal women or in those who are breast cancer survivors.

Hot flashes (men) – [4] = Insufficient documentation. Initial data suggest that paroxetine may have some benefit in the reduction of hot flash severity and frequency in men who have a history of prostate cancer and are receiving androgen ablation therapy. Limited data to date (18 patients) make it difficult to recommend an optimal dose because a wide range was used in the published study.

Nocturnal enuresis – [3] = Safety concerns. Noncontrolled evaluation of a very small number of children suggests some benefit with SSRI use for the treatment of nocturnal enuresis. In some cases, such as with the use of fluvoxamine, data are conflicting. Information from a physician survey suggests that SSRIs may be prescribed for enuresis despite the lack of controlled data. However, newer warnings regarding the possible association between suicidality and the use of antidepressants, including SSRIs, may limit the utility of these drugs for this indication. More data from larger controlled trials are needed.

Premenstrual disorders – [2] = Fair documentation. Data from a limited number of studies suggest that paroxetine may be beneficial in the treatment of premenstrual disorders. However, further study is required to determine if intermittent use or other dosing regimens would be beneficial.

Prevention of migraine (adults) – [4] = Insufficient documentation. Information from 4 case reports provides some support for the use of paroxetine; however, clinical trials are needed to determine efficacy, optimal dosing, and the patient population who would most benefit from therapy. American Academy of Neurology practice guidelines consider paroxetine to be clinically efficacious for the prevention of migraines based on consensus and clinical experience, despite the lack of scientific evidence of efficacy.

Pruritus – [4] = Insufficient documentation. The role, if any, of paroxetine in the treatment of pruritus has not been established. Available data are limited by noncontrolled study designs and the small number of patients.

Smoking cessation – [5] = Poor documentation. Studies evaluating paroxetine as an aid in smoking cessation have produced inconsistent data for its efficacy in this setting. To date, no randomized, placebo-controlled trials have shown a long-term benefit in using paroxetine to improve cessation rates or evidence that paroxetine is superior to FDA-approved first-line smoking cessation agents such as bupropion and varenicline. Guidelines from the VA specify that treatment with antidepressants other than bupropion or nortriptyline is not recommended. As evidenced by the black box warning for paroxetine, this drug is not without risk. With no evidence of benefit in this setting, the risk of using paroxetine cannot be justified.

Stuttering – [4] = Insufficient documentation. Published information regarding the use of paroxetine in the treatment of stuttering is limited to a small number of experiences. Because benefits appear to be dramatic, this agent may be considered when treating comorbidities (eg, depression, anxiety) in patients with stuttering.

Traumatic brain injury – [3] = Safety concerns. Given that paroxetine was classified as an option, the lowest level of recommendation, rather than a standard or guideline, patients started on therapy should be closely monitored for response, and therapy should be continued only in those patients with sufficient benefit to outweigh the risks of therapy.

Other off-label uses – Paroxetine has also been used in children to treat obsessive-compulsive disorder and social anxiety disorder. (See also Administration and Dosage).

Administration and Dosage

➤*General dosing considerations:* A gradual reduction in the dose rather than abrupt cessation is recommended with paroxetine. (See Discontinuation of therapy.)

Pregnancy – Consider tapering paroxetine in the third trimester. (See Pregnancy.)

➤*Adults:*

Immediate-release –

General anxiety disorder:

• *Usual dosage* – The recommended starting dose and the established effective dose is 20 mg/day. In clinical trials, the efficacy of paroxetine was demonstrated in patients dosed within a range of 20 to 50 mg/day. There is not sufficient evidence to suggest a greater benefit to doses higher than 20 mg/day.

• *Dosage titration* – Dose changes should occur in 10 mg/day increments and at intervals of at least 1 week.

• *Duration of therapy* – Systematic evaluation of continuing paroxetine for periods of up to 24 weeks in patients with GAD who had responded while taking paroxetine during an 8-week, acute-treatment phase has demonstrated a benefit of such maintenance.

Major depressive disorder:

• *Maximum dose* – 50 mg/day.

• *Initial dosage* – 20 mg/day.

• *Dosage titration* – Some patients not responding to a 20 mg dose may benefit from dose increases in 10 mg/day increments. Dose changes should occur at intervals of at least 1 week.

• *Maintenance dosage* – It is generally agreed that acute episodes of MDD require at least several months of sustained pharmacologic therapy. Whether the dose needed to induce remission is identical to the dose needed to maintain and/or sustain euthymia is unknown.

Obsessive-compulsive disorder:

• *Maximum dose* – 60 mg/day.

• *Initial dosage* – 20 mg/day.

• *Dosage titration* – The dose can be increased in 10 mg/day increments. Dose changes should occur at intervals of at least 1 week.

• *Maintenance dosage* – 40 mg/day.

• *Duration of therapy* – Long-term maintenance of efficacy was demonstrated in a 6-month relapse prevention trial. In this trial, patients with OCD assigned to paroxetine demonstrated a lower relapse rate compared with patients on placebo. OCD is a chronic condition, and it is reasonable to consider continuation for a responding patient.

Panic disorder:

• *Maximum dose* – 60 mg/day.

• *Initial dosage* – 10 mg/day.

• *Dosage titration* – Dose changes should occur in 10 mg/day increments and at intervals of at least 1 week.

• *Maintenance dosage* – 40 mg/day.

• *Duration of therapy* – Long-term maintenance of efficacy was demonstrated with immediate-release paroxetine in a 3-month relapse prevention trial. In this trial, patients with panic disorder assigned to paroxetine demonstrated a lower relapse rate compared with patients on placebo. Panic disorder is a chronic condition, and it is reasonable to consider continuation for a responding patient.

Posttraumatic stress disorder:

• *Usual dosage* – The recommended starting dose and the established effective dose is 20 mg/day. In a fixed-dose study, there was not sufficient evidence to suggest a greater benefit for a dose of 40 mg/day compared with 20 mg/day.

• *Dosage titration* – Dose changes, if indicated, should occur in 10 mg/day increments and at intervals of at least 1 week.

• *Duration of therapy* – Although the efficacy of paroxetine beyond 12 weeks of dosing has not been demonstrated in controlled clinical trials, PTSD is recognized as a chronic condition, and it is reasonable to consider continuation of treatment for a responding patient.

Social anxiety disorder:

• *Usual dosage* – The recommended and initial dose is 20 mg/day. While the safety of paroxetine has been evaluated in patients with social anxiety disorder at doses up to 60 mg/day, available information does not suggest any additional benefit for doses above 20 mg/day.

• *Duration of therapy* – Although the efficacy of paroxetine beyond 12 weeks of dosing has not been demonstrated in controlled clinical trials, social anxiety disorder is recognized as a chronic condition, and it is reasonable to consider continuation of treatment for a responding patient.

Controlled-release –

Major depressive disorder:

• *Maximum dose* – 62.5 mg/day.

• *Initial dosage* – 25 mg/day.

• *Dosage titration* – Some patients not responding to a 25 mg dose may benefit from dose increases in 12.5 mg/day increments. Dose changes should occur at intervals of at least 1 week.

• *Maintenance dosage* – It is generally agreed that acute episodes of MDD require at least several months of sustained pharmacologic therapy. Whether the dose needed to induce remission is identical to the dose needed to maintain and/or sustain euthymia is unknown.

Panic disorder:

• *Maximum dose* – 75 mg/day.

• *Initial dosage* – 12.5 mg/day.

• *Dosage titration* – Dose changes should occur in 12.5 mg/day increments and at intervals of at least 1 week.

• *Duration of therapy* – Long-term maintenance of efficacy was demonstrated with immediate-release paroxetine in a 3-month relapse prevention trial. In this trial, patients with panic disorder assigned to paroxetine demonstrated a lower relapse rate compared with patients on placebo. Panic disorder is a chronic condition, and it is reasonable to consider continuation for a responding patient.

Premenstrual dysphoric disorder:

• *Initial dosage* – 12.5 mg/day. Paroxetine controlled-release tablets may be administered either daily throughout the menstrual cycle or limited to the luteal phase of the menstrual cycle, depending on health care provider assessment. In clinical trials, both 12.5 and 25 mg/day were shown to be effective.

• *Dosage titration* – Dose changes should occur at intervals of at least 1 week.

• *Duration of therapy* – The efficacy of paroxetine controlled-release tablets for a period exceeding 3 menstrual cycles has not been systematically evaluated in controlled trials. However, women commonly report that symptoms worsen with age until relieved by the onset of menopause. Therefore, it is reasonable to consider continuation of a responding patient.

Social anxiety disorder:

• *Maximum dose* – 37.5 mg/day.

• *Initial dosage* – 12.5 mg/day.

• *Dosage titration* – If the dose is increased, this should occur at intervals of at least 1 week, in increments of 12.5 mg/day.

• *Duration of therapy* – Although the efficacy of paroxetine beyond 12 weeks of dosing has not been demonstrated in controlled clinical trials, social anxiety disorder is recognized as a chronic condition, and it is reasonable to consider continuation of treatment for a responding patient.

Off-label dosing –

Diabetic neuropathy: [2] = Fair documentation. 10 mg/day initially, titrated to 20 to 60 mg/day.

Hot flashes: [2] = Fair documentation.

• *Breast cancer patients* – 20 mg daily or nightly.

PAROXETINE HYDROCHLORIDE — ORAL

• *Menopausal patients* – 12.5 or 25 mg daily (controlled-release formulation) or 10 or 20 mg daily (immediate-release formulation).

Hot flashes (men): [4] = Insufficient documentation. 12.5 mg daily titrated weekly over a 4-week period to 37.5 mg daily.

Premenstrual disorders: [2] = Fair documentation. 10 to 30 mg daily, taken continuously throughout cycles.

Prevention of migraine (adults): [4] = Insufficient documentation. The dose used in a case study was 20 mg daily. The doses used in a case series were standard doses for the treatment of depression (specific doses were not reported).

Pruritus: [4] = Insufficient documentation. Initial dosages have ranged from 10 to 20 mg once daily. Effective dosages ranged from 5 to 30 mg once daily.

Stuttering: [4] = Insufficient documentation. Initial dosage of 20 mg daily.

Traumatic brain injury: [3] = Safety concerns. 20 mg/day orally. The optimal duration of therapy has not been established; however, long-term administration may be required to maintain symptom control.

➤*Children:*

Off-label dosing –

Nocturnal enuresis: [3] = Safety concerns. 40 mg daily (in a patient 16 years of age).

Obsessive-compulsive disorder:

• *7 to 17 years of age –*
Maximum dose: 50 mg/day.
Initial dosage: 10 mg/day.
Dosage titration: Increase dose by 10 mg/day no more frequently than every 7 days, if needed.

Pruritus: [4] = Insufficient documentation. 5 mg once daily was used in 1 patient.

Social anxiety disorder:

• *8 to 17 years of age –*
Maximum dose: 50 mg/day.
Initial dosage: 10 mg/day
Dosage titration: Increase dose by 10 mg/day no more frequently than every 7 days, if needed.

➤*Elderly:*

Immediate-release –
Maximum dose: 40 mg/day.
Initial dosage: 10 mg/day. Increases may be made if indicated.

Controlled-release –
Maximum dose: 50 mg/day.
Initial dosage: 12.5 mg/day. Increases may be made if indicated

➤*Renal function impairment:* Dosing for patients with severe renal function impairment (CrCl less than 30 mL/min) is the same for elderly patients.

➤*Hepatic function impairment:* Dosing for patients with severe hepatic impairment is the same for elderly patients.

➤*Pregnancy:* Neonates exposed to paroxetine and other SSRIs or selective norepinephrine reuptake inhibitors (SNRIs) late in the third trimester have developed complications requiring prolonged hospitalization, respiratory support, and tube feeding. When treating pregnant women with paroxetine during the third trimester, the health care provider should carefully consider the potential risks and benefits of treatment. Consider tapering paroxetine in the third trimester.

➤*Switching patients to or from a monoamine oxidase inhibitor:* At least 14 days should elapse between discontinuation of an monoamine oxidase inhibitor (MAOI) and initiation of therapy with paroxetine. Similarly, at least 14 days should be allowed after stopping paroxetine before starting an MAOI.

➤*Duration of therapy:* There is no body of evidence available to answer the question of how long the patient treated with paroxetine should remain on it. Patients should be periodically reassessed to determine the need for continued therapy. Dosage adjustments should be made to maintain the patient on the lowest effective dose.

➤*Discontinuation of therapy:* Symptoms associated with discontinuation of paroxetine have been reported. Patients should be monitored for these symptoms when discontinuing treatment, regardless of the indication for which paroxetine is being prescribed. A gradual reduction in the dose rather than abrupt cessation is recommended whenever possible. If intolerable symptoms occur following a decrease in the dose or upon discontinuation of treatment, then resuming the previously prescribed dose may be considered. Subsequently, the health care provider may continue decreasing the dose but at a more gradual rate.

➤*Administration:* Paroxetine immediate- and controlled-release tablets should be administered as a single daily dose with or without food, usually in the morning. Paroxetine controlled-release tablets should not be chewed or crushed and should be swallowed whole. Shake suspension well before using.

➤*Storage / Stability:*

Tablets – Store immediate-release tablets between 15° and 30°C (59° and 86°F) and controlled-release tablets at or below 25°C (77°F).

Suspension – Store at or below 25°C (77°F).

PAROXETINE MESYLATE — ORAL

WARNING

Suicidality in children and adolescents – Antidepressants increased the risk of suicidal thinking and behavior (suicidality) in short-term studies in children and adolescents with major depressive disorder (MDD) and other psychiatric disorders. Anyone considering the use of paroxetine or any other antidepressant in a child or adolescent must balance this risk with the clinical need. Closely observe patients who are started on therapy for clinical worsening, suicidality, or unusual changes in behavior. Advise families and caregivers of the need for close observation and communication with the health care provider. Paroxetine is not approved for use in children.

Pooled analyses of short-term (4- to 16-week) placebo-controlled trials of 9 antidepressant drugs (selective serotonin reuptake inhibitors [SSRIs] and others) in children and adolescents with MDD, obsessive compulsive disorder (OCD), or other psychiatric disorders (a total of 24 trials involving more than 4,400 patients) have revealed a greater risk of adverse reactions representing suicidal thinking or behavior (suicidality) during the first few months of treatment in those receiving antidepressants. The average risk of such reactions in patients receiving antidepressants was 4%, twice the placebo risk of 2%. No suicides occurred in these trials.

Indications

➤*Major depressive disorder (MDD):* For the treatment of MDD.

The efficacy of paroxetine in the treatment of a major depressive episode was established in 6-week controlled trials of outpatients whose diagnoses corresponded most closely to the *Diagnostic and Statistical Manual of Mental Disorders* (Third Edition) (*DSM-III*) category of MDD. A major depressive episode implies a prominent and relatively persistent depressed or dysphoric mood that usually interferes with daily functioning (nearly every day for at least 2 weeks); it should include at least 4 of the following 8 symptoms: change in appetite, change in sleep, psychomotor agitation or retardation, loss of interest in usual activities or decrease in sexual drive, increased fatigue, feelings of guilt or worthlessness, slowed thinking or impaired concentration, and a suicide attempt or suicidal ideation.

The effects of paroxetine in hospitalized depressed patients have not been adequately studied.

The efficacy of paroxetine in maintaining a response in MDD for up to 1 year was demonstrated in a placebo-controlled trial.

Nevertheless, if electing to prescribe paroxetine for extended periods, periodically reevaluate the long-term usefulness of the drug for the individual patient.

➤*Obsessive compulsive disorder (OCD):* For the treatment of obsessions and compulsions in patients with OCD as defined in the *DSM* (Fourth Edition) (*DSM-IV*). The obsessions or compulsions cause marked distress, are time consuming, or significantly interfere with social or occupational functioning.

The efficacy of paroxetine was established in two 12-week trials with obsessive-compulsive outpatients whose diagnoses corresponded most closely to the *DSM* (Third Edition Revised) (*DSM-III-R*) category of OCD.

OCD is characterized by recurrent and persistent ideas, thoughts, impulses, or images (obsessions) that are ego-dystonic or repetitive, purposeful and intentional behaviors (compulsions) that are recognized by the person as excessive or unreasonable.

Long-term maintenance of efficacy was demonstrated in a 6-month relapse prevention trial. In this trial, patients assigned to paroxetine showed a lower relapse rate compared with patients on placebo. Nevertheless, if electing to prescribe paroxetine for extended periods, periodically reevaluate the long-term usefulness of the drug for the individual patient.

➤*Panic disorder:* For the treatment of panic disorder, with or without agoraphobia, as defined in *DSM-IV*. Panic disorder is characterized by the occurrence of unexpected panic attacks and associated concern about having additional attacks, worry about the implications or consequences of the attacks, or a significant change in behavior related to the attacks.

The efficacy of paroxetine was established in three 10- to 12-week trials in panic disorder patients whose diagnoses corresponded to the *DSM-III-R* category of panic disorder.

Panic disorder (*DSM-IV*) is characterized by recurrent unexpected panic attacks (ie, a discrete period of intense fear or discomfort in which 4 [or more] of the following symptoms develop abruptly and reach a peak within 10 minutes):

1.) palpitations, pounding heart, or accelerated heart rate
2.) sweating
3.) trembling or shaking
4.) sensations of shortness of breath or smothering
5.) feeling of choking
6.) chest pain or discomfort
7.) nausea or abdominal distress
8.) feeling dizzy, unsteady, light-headed, or faint
9.) derealization (feelings of unreality) or depersonalization (being detached from oneself)
10.) fear of losing control
11.) fear of dying
12.) paresthesias (numbness or tingling sensations), or
13.) chills or hot flushes.

PAROXETINE MESYLATE — ORAL

Long-term maintenance of efficacy was demonstrated in a 3-month relapse prevention trial. In this trial, patients with panic disorder assigned to paroxetine demonstrated a lower relapse rate compared with patients on placebo. Nevertheless, if electing to prescribe paroxetine mesylate for extended periods, periodically reevaluate the long-term usefulness of the drug for the individual patient.

➤*Off-label uses:*

Diabetic neuropathy – [2] = Fair documentation. In small trials, paroxetine was not as effective as imipramine at relieving symptoms associated with neuropathic pain, although it appears to be more effective than gabapentin. In addition, paroxetine was better tolerated than imipramine and gabapentin. Larger controlled trials are needed to define the role of paroxetine in the treatment of diabetic neuropathy. Future studies comparing paroxetine with newer agents are also needed.

Hot flashes – [2] = Fair documentation. Initial data suggest that paroxetine may have some benefit in the reduction of hot flash severity and frequency. This drug may be useful in treating hot flashes and depression in menopausal women or in those who are breast cancer survivors.

Hot flashes (men) – [4] = Insufficient documentation. Initial data suggest that paroxetine may have some benefit in the reduction of hot flash severity and frequency in men who have a history of prostate cancer and are receiving androgen ablation therapy. The limited data to date (18 patients) make it difficult to recommend an optimal dose because a wide range was used in the published study.

Nocturnal enuresis – [3] = Safety concerns. Noncontrolled evaluation of a very small number of children suggests some benefit with SSRI use for the treatment of nocturnal enuresis. In some cases, such as with the use of fluvoxamine, data are conflicting. Information from a physician survey suggests that SSRIs may be prescribed for enuresis despite the lack of controlled data. However, newer warnings regarding the possible association between suicidality and the use of antidepressants, including SSRIs, may limit the utility of these drugs for this indication. More data from larger controlled trials are needed.

Premenstrual disorders – [2] = Fair documentation. Data from a limited number of studies suggest that paroxetine may be beneficial in the treatment of premenstrual disorders. However, further study is required to determine if intermittent use or other dosing regimens would be beneficial.

Prevention of migraine (adults) – [4] = Insufficient documentation. Information from 4 case reports provides some support for the use of paroxetine; however, clinical trials are needed to determine efficacy, optimal dosing, and the patient population who would most benefit from therapy. American Academy of Neurology practice guidelines consider paroxetine to be clinically efficacious for the prevention of migraines based on consensus and clinical experience, despite the lack of scientific evidence of efficacy.

Pruritus – [4] = Insufficient documentation. The role, if any, of paroxetine in the treatment of pruritus has not been established. Available data are limited by noncontrolled study designs and the small number of patients.

Smoking cessation – [5] = Poor documentation. Studies evaluating paroxetine as an aid in smoking cessation have produced inconsistent data for its efficacy in this setting. To date, no randomized, placebo-controlled trials have shown a long-term benefit in using paroxetine to improve cessation rates or evidence that paroxetine is superior to FDA-approved first-line smoking cessation agents such as bupropion and varenicline. Guidelines from the VA specify that treatment with antidepressants other than bupropion or nortriptyline is not recommended. As evidenced by the black box warning for paroxetine, this drug is not without risk. With no evidence of benefit in this setting, the risk of using paroxetine cannot be justified.

Stuttering – [4] = Insufficient documentation. Published information regarding the use of paroxetine in the treatment of stuttering is limited to a small number of experiences. Because benefits appear to be dramatic, this agent may be considered when treating comorbidities (eg, depression, anxiety) in patients with stuttering.

Traumatic brain injury – [3] = Safety concerns. Given that paroxetine was classified as an option, the lowest level of recommendation, rather than a standard or guideline, patients started on therapy should be closely monitored for response, and therapy should be continued only in those patients with sufficient benefit to outweigh the risks of therapy.

Other off-label uses – Paroxetine has also been used in children to treat obsessive-compulsive disorder and social anxiety disorder. (See also Administration and Dosage).

Administration and Dosage

➤*General dosing considerations:* A gradual reduction in the dose rather than abrupt cessation is recommended with paroxetine. (See Discontinuation of therapy.)

➤*Adults:*

Major depressive disorder –

Maximum dose: 50 mg/day.

Initial dosage: 20 mg/day.

Dosage titration: Some patients not responding to a 20 mg dose may benefit from dosage increases, in 10 mg/day increments, up to a maximum of 50 mg/day. Dosage changes should occur at intervals of at least 1 week.

Maintenance dosage: It is generally agreed that acute episodes of MDD require several months or longer of sustained pharmacologic therapy. Whether the dose needed to induce remission is identical to the dose needed to maintain euthymia is unknown.

Obsessive-compulsive disorder –

Maximum dose: 60 mg/day.

Initial dosage: 20 mg/day.

Dosage titration: The dosage can be increased in 10 mg/day increments. Dosage changes should occur at intervals of at least 1 week.

Maintenance dosage: 40 mg/day.

Duration of therapy: Long-term maintenance of efficacy was demonstrated in a 6-month relapse prevention trial. In this trial, patients with OCD assigned to paroxetine demonstrated a lower relapse rate compared with patients on placebo. OCD is a chronic condition, and it is reasonable to consider continuation for a responding patient.

Panic disorder –

Maximum dose: 60 mg/day.

Initial dosage: 10 mg/day.

Dosage titration: Dosage changes should occur in 10 mg/day increments and at intervals of at least 1 week.

Maintenance dosage: 40 mg/day.

Duration of therapy: Long-term maintenance of efficacy was demonstrated with immediate-release paroxetine in a 3-month relapse prevention trial. In this trial, patients with panic disorder assigned to paroxetine demonstrated a lower relapse rate compared with patients on placebo. Panic disorder is a chronic condition, and it is reasonable to consider continuation for a responding patient.

Off-label dosing –

Diabetic neuropathy: [2] = Fair documentation. 10 mg/day initially, titrated to 20 to 60 mg/day.

Hot flashes: [2] = Fair documentation.

- *Breast cancer patients* – 20 mg daily or nightly.
- *Menopausal patients* – 12.5 or 25 mg daily (controlled-release formulation [as paroxetine hydrochloride]) or 10 or 20 mg daily (immediate-release formulation)

Hot flashes (men): [4] = Insufficient documentation. 12.5 mg daily titrated weekly over a 4-week period to 37.5 mg daily.

Premenstrual disorders: [2] = Fair documentation. 10 to 30 mg daily, taken continuously throughout cycles.

Prevention of migraine (adults): [4] = Insufficient documentation. The dose used in a case study was 20 mg daily. The doses used in a case series were standard doses for the treatment of depression (specific doses were not reported).

Pruritus: [4] = Insufficient documentation. Initial dosages have ranged from 10 to 20 mg once daily. Effective dosages ranged from 5 to 30 mg once daily.

Stuttering: [4] = Insufficient documentation. Initial dosage of 20 mg daily.

Traumatic brain injury: [3] = Safety concerns. 20 mg/day orally. The optimal duration of therapy has not been established; however, long-term administration may be required to maintain symptom control.

➤*Children:*

Off-label dosing –

Nocturnal enuresis: [3] = Safety concerns. 40 mg daily (in a patient 16 years of age).

Obsessive-compulsive disorder:

- *7 to 17 years of age* –
  Maximum dose: 50 mg/day.
  Initial dosage: 10 mg/day.
  Dosage titration: Increase dose by 10 mg/day no more frequently than every 7 days, if needed.

Pruritus: [4] = Insufficient documentation. 5 mg once daily was used in 1 patient.

Social anxiety disorder:

- *8 to 17 years of age* –
  Maximum dose: 50 mg/day.
  Initial dosage: 10 mg/day
  Dosage titration: Increase dose by 10 mg/day no more frequently than every 7 days, if needed.

➤*Elderly:*

Maximum dose – 40 mg/day.

Initial dosage – 10 mg/day. Increases may be made if indicated.

➤*Renal function impairment:* The following dosing is for patients with severe renal function impairment.

Maximum dose – 40 mg/day.

Initial dosage – 10 mg/day; upward titration, if necessary, should be at increased intervals.

➤*Hepatic function impairment:* The following dosing is for patients with severe hepatic function impairment.

Maximum dose – 40 mg/day.

Initial dosage – 10 mg/day; upward titration, if necessary, should be at increased intervals.

➤*Debilitated patients:*

Maximum dose – 40 mg/day.

Initial dosage – 10 mg/day. Increases may be made if indicated.

➤*Switching patients to or from a monoamine oxidase inhibitor:* At least 14 days should elapse between discontinuation of an monoamine oxidase inhibitor (MAOI) and initiation of therapy with paroxetine. Similarly, at least 14 days should be allowed after stopping paroxetine before starting an MAOI.

➤*Discontinuation of therapy:* Symptoms associated with discontinuation of paroxetine have been reported. During paroxetine marketing there

PAROXETINE MESYLATE — ORAL

have been spontaneous reports of similar adverse reactions, which may have no causal relationship to the drug, upon discontinuation of paroxetine (particularly when abrupt), including the following: dizziness, sensory disturbances (eg, paresthesias, such as electric shock sensations), agitation, anxiety, nausea, and sweating. These reactions are generally self-limiting. Similar reactions have been reported for other SSRIs. Monitor patients for these symptoms when discontinuing treatment, regardless of the indication for which paroxetine is being prescribed. A gradual reduction in the dose rather than abrupt cessation is recommended whenever possible. If intolerable symptoms occur following a decrease in the dose or upon discontinuation of treatment, then resuming the previously prescribed dose may be considered. Subsequently, the health care provider may continue decreasing the dose but at a more gradual rate.

➤*Administration:* Administer as a single daily dose with or without food, usually in the morning.

➤*Storage/Stability:* Protect from humidity. Store at 25°C (77°F); excursions are permitted to 15° to 30°C (59° to 86°F).

SERTRALINE

Rx	**Sertraline Hydrochloride** (Various, eg, Actavis Elizabeth, Greenstone, Ivax, Roxane, Teva)	**Tablets; oral:** 25 mg	As sertraline hydrochloride. May contain lactose, polydextrose. In 30s, 50s, 90s, 100s, 180s, 500s, 1,000s, and 5,000s.
Rx	**Zoloft** (Pfizer)		As sertraline hydrochloride. (ZOLOFT 25 mg). Lt. green, capsule shape, scored. Film-coated. In 30s and 50s.
Rx	**Sertraline Hydrochloride** (Various, eg, Greenstone, Roxane, Teva, UDL Labs, Watson)	**Tablets; oral:** 50 mg	As sertraline hydrochloride. May contain lactose, polydextrose. In 30s, 50s, 90s, 100s, 180s, 500s, 1,000s, 5,000s, and UD 100s.
Rx	**Zoloft** (Pfizer)		As sertraline hydrochloride. (ZOLOFT 50 mg). Lt. blue, capsule shape, scored. Film-coated. In 30s, 100s, 500s, 5,000s, and UD 100s.
Rx	**Sertraline Hydrochloride** (Various, eg, Pliva, Roxane, Teva, UDL Labs, Watson)	**Tablets; oral:** 100 mg	As sertraline hydrochloride. May contain lactose, polydextrose. In 30s, 50s, 90s, 100s, 180s, 500s, 1,000s, 5,000s, and UD 100s.
Rx	**Zoloft** (Pfizer)		As sertraline hydrochloride. (ZOLOFT 100 mg). Lt. yellow, capsule shape, scored. Film-coated. In 30s, 100s, 500s, 5,000s, and UD 100s.
Rx	**Sertraline Hydrochloride** (Various, eg, Greenstone, Ranbaxy Pharmaceuticals, Roxane)	**Solution, concentrate; oral:** 20 mg/mL	As sertraline hydrochloride. May contain alcohol, menthol. In 60 mL bottle with calibrated dropper.
Rx	**Zoloft** (Pfizer)		As sertraline hydrochloride. Alcohol 12%, menthol. In 60 mL.[a]

[a] Dropper dispenser contains dry natural rubber.

SERTRALINE HYDROCHLORIDE — ORAL

For complete and comparative prescribing information, refer to the Selective Serotonin Reuptake Inhibitors class monograph.

WARNING

Suicidality and antidepressant drugs – Antidepressants increased the risk compared with placebo of suicidal thinking and behavior (suicidality) in children, adolescents, and young adults in short-term studies of major depressive disorder (MDD) and other psychiatric disorders. Anyone considering the use of sertraline or any other antidepressant in a child, adolescent, or young adult must balance this risk with the clinical need. Short-term studies did not show an increase in the risk of suicidality with antidepressants compared with placebo in adults older than 24 years of age; there was a reduction in risk with antidepressants compared with placebo in adults 65 years of age and older. Depression and certain other psychiatric disorders are themselves associated with increases in the risk of suicide. Monitor patients of all ages who are started on antidepressant therapy appropriately and observe them closely for clinical worsening, suicidality, or unusual changes in behavior. Families and caregivers should be advised of the need for close observation and communication with the prescriber. Sertraline is not approved for use in children except for patients with obsessive compulsive disorder (OCD).

Indications

➤*Major depressive disorder:* For the treatment of MDD as defined in the *Diagnostic and Statistical Manual of Mental Disorders*, (Third Edition) (*DSM*-III).

➤*Obsessive-compulsive disorder:* For the treatment of obsessions and compulsions in patients with OCD, as defined in the *DSM*-III-*R*.

➤*Panic disorder:* For the treatment of panic disorder with or without agoraphobia, as defined in the *DSM*-IV.

➤*Posttraumatic stress disorder:* For the treatment of posttraumatic stress disorder (PTSD), as defined in the *DSM*-III-*R*/*DSM*-IV.

➤*Premenstrual dysphoric disorder:* For the treatment of premenstrual dysphoric disorder (PMDD), as defined in the *DSM*-III-*R*/*DSM*-IV.

➤*Social anxiety disorder:* For the treatment of social anxiety disorder (social phobia), as defined by *DSM*-IV.

➤*Off-label uses:*

Extended-interval dosing – [2] = Fair documentation. Currently there are very little clinical data regarding the clinical and safety effects of converting patients from once-daily to 3-times-weekly sertraline dosing. If effective, this regimen may reduce daily doses and cost.

Hot flashes (men) – [4] = Insufficient documentation. Initial uncontrolled case reports suggest that sertraline may have beneficial effects in reducing the frequency and severity of hot flashes in prostate cancer patients. Other serotonin reuptake inhibitors have demonstrated similar effects in hot flashes caused by varied etiology.

Hot flashes (women) – [5] = Poor documentation. Initial data suggest varied response to the use of sertraline in the management of hot flashes related to tamoxifen use in breast cancer patients or to menopausal changes. At this time, several other drugs in this class have demonstrated better efficacy for this use.

Nocturnal enuresis – [3] = Safety concerns. Noncontrolled evaluation of a very small number of children suggests some benefit with selective serotonin reuptake inhibitor (SSRI) use for the treatment of nocturnal enuresis. In some cases, such as with the use of fluvoxamine, data are conflicting. Information from a physician survey suggests that SSRIs may be prescribed for enuresis despite the lack of controlled data. However, newer warnings regarding the possible association between suicidality and the use of antidepressants, including SSRIs, may limit the utility of these drugs for this indication.

Prevention of migraine (adults) – [4] = Insufficient documentation. American Academy of Neurology practice guidelines consider sertraline to be clinically efficacious based on consensus and clinical experience, despite the lack of scientific evidence of efficacy. Results from a small, controlled trial did not show efficacy. Additional data are needed to determine efficacy, the optimal dosing regimen, and the patient population that would most benefit from therapy.

Pruritus (cholestatic) – [2] = Fair documentation. Data from published trials suggest that sertraline is effective in the management of cholestatic-related pruritus. Despite limited published data, guidelines recommend the use of this agent in patients who fail cholestyramine, rifampicin, or naltrexone.

Smoking cessation – [5] = Poor documentation. Studies evaluating sertraline as an aid in smoking cessation have produced inconsistent data for its efficacy in this setting. No randomized, placebo-controlled trials have shown a long-term benefit in using sertraline to improve cessation rates or evidence that sertraline is superior to Food and Drug Administration (FDA)–approved first-line smoking cessation agents, such as bupropion and varenicline. Guidelines from the Veterans Administration specify that treatment with antidepressants other than bupropion or nortriptyline is not recommended. As evidenced by the black box warning for sertraline, this drug is not without risk. With no evidence of benefit in this setting, the risk of using sertraline cannot be justified.

Traumatic brain injury – [3] = Safety concerns. SSRIs were recommended by the Neurobehavioral Guidelines Working Group at the option level (the lowest level of recommendation) for the management of aggression after traumatic brain injury (TBI). Among the SSRIs, sertraline has the most published experience in post-TBI aggression. Sertraline was also recommended at the option level by the guideline authors for the treatment of post-TBI depression. Sertraline therapy may be particularly useful for patients with concurrent depression and aggression after TBI.

Administration and Dosage

➤*General dosing considerations:* A gradual reduction in the dose rather than abrupt cessation is recommended whenever possible. (See Discontinuation of therapy.)

Oral concentrate – The oral concentrate is contraindicated with disulfiram because of the alcohol content of the concentrate. Use caution for patients with latex sensitivity, as the dropper dispenser may contain dry natural rubber. Sertraline oral concentrate must be diluted before use. (See Preparation for administration.)

SERTRALINE HYDROCHLORIDE — ORAL

Pregnancy – Consider tapering sertraline in the third trimester. (See Pregnancy.)

➤*Adults:* Given the 24-hour elimination half-life of sertraline, dose changes should not occur at intervals of less than 1 week. Periodically reassess patients to determine the need for maintenance treatment.

Major depressive disorder –

Initial dosage: 50 mg once daily.

Maintenance dosage: 50 to 200 mg/day. Dose changes should not occur at intervals of less than 1 week.

Obsessive-compulsive disorder –

Initial dosage: 50 mg once daily.

Maintenance dosage: 50 to 200 mg/day. Dose changes should not occur at intervals of less than 1 week.

Panic disorder –

Initial dosage: 25 mg once daily. After 1 week, increase the dosage to 50 mg once daily.

Maintenance dosage: 50 to 200 mg/day. Dose changes should not occur at intervals of less than 1 week.

Posttraumatic stress disorder –

Initial dosage: 25 mg once daily. After 1 week, increase the dosage to 50 mg once daily.

Maintenance dosage: 50 to 200 mg/day. Dose changes should not occur at intervals of less than 1 week.

Premenstrual dysphoric disorder –

Initial dosage: 50 mg/day, either daily throughout the menstrual cycle or limited to the luteal phase of the menstrual cycle, depending on the health care provider's assessment.

Dosage titration: Patients not responding to a 50 mg/day dosage may benefit from dose increases (at 50 mg increments per menstrual cycle) of up to 150 mg/day when dosing daily throughout the menstrual cycle, or 100 mg/day when dosing during the luteal phase of the menstrual cycle. If a 100 mg/day dosage has been established with luteal phase dosing, utilize a 50 mg/day titration step for 3 days at the beginning of each luteal phase dosing period.

Maintenance dosage: 50 to 150 mg/day. While a relationship between dose and effect has not been established for PMDD, patients were dosed in the range of 50 to 150 mg/day, with dose increases at the onset of each new menstrual cycle.

Dosage adjustment: Dosage adjustments, which may include changes between dosage regimens (eg, daily throughout the menstrual cycle vs during the luteal phase of the menstrual cycle), may be needed to maintain the patient on the lowest effective dosage.

Social anxiety disorder –

Initial dosage: 25 mg once daily. After 1 week, increase the dosage to 50 mg once daily.

Maintenance dosage: 50 to 200 mg/day. Dose changes should not occur at intervals of less than 1 week.

Off-label dosing –

Extended-interval dosing: [2] = Fair documentation. Daily dosing converted to equivalent dosing 3 times a week (50 mg daily switched to 100 mg 3 times weekly).

Hot flashes (men): [4] = Insufficient documentation. 25 mg daily (initial) titrated to 75 to 150 mg daily.

Prevention of migraine (adults): [4] = Insufficient documentation. Sertraline dosages ranged from 50 to 100 mg/day orally in a controlled trial.

Pruritus (cholestatic): [2] = Fair documentation. 25 to 100 mg daily for up to 5 years. The most effective dosages ranged from 75 to 100 mg daily.

Traumatic brain injury: [3] = Safety concerns. 25 to 200 mg/day.

➤*Children:* To avoid excess dosing in children with OCD, take into account their generally lower body weights compared with adults when increasing the dose.

Obsessive compulsive disorder –

Maximum dose: 200 mg/day.

13 to 17 years of age – Initiate dosage with 50 mg once daily. Patients not responding to an initial dosage of 50 mg/day may benefit from dose increases of up to a maximum of 200 mg/day. Dose changes should not occur at intervals of less than 1 week.

6 to 12 years of age – Initiate dosage with 25 mg once daily. Patients not responding to an initial dosage of 25 mg/day may benefit from dose increases of up to a maximum of 200 mg/day. Dose changes should not occur at intervals of less than 1 week.

Off-label dosing –

Depression:

- *13 years of age and older* –
  Maximum dose: 200 mg daily.
  Initial dosage: 50 mg orally daily.
  Dosage titration: May increase dosage by 50 mg at 1-week intervals.
- *6 to 12 years of age* –
  Maximum dose: 200 mg daily.
  Initial dosage: 12.5 to 25 mg orally daily.
  Dosage titration: May increase dosage by 25 mg at 1-week intervals.

Nocturnal enuresis: [3] = Safety concerns. 50 mg daily (in a patient 13 years of age).

➤*Hepatic function impairment:* Give a lower or less frequent dosage in patients with hepatic impairment. Use with caution in these patients.

➤*Pregnancy:* Consider tapering sertraline in the third trimester. Neonates exposed to sertraline and other SSRIs or serotonin and norepinephrine reuptake inhibitors (SNRIs) late in the third trimester have developed complications requiring prolonged hospitalization, respiratory support, and tube feeding. When treating pregnant women with sertraline during the third trimester, carefully consider the potential risks and benefits of treatment.

➤*Switching patients to or from a monoamine oxidase inhibitor (MAOI):* At least 14 days should elapse between discontinuation of a MAOI and initiation of therapy with sertraline. In addition, allow at least 14 days after stopping sertraline before starting an MAOI.

➤*Discontinuation of therapy:* A gradual reduction in the dose rather than abrupt cessation is recommended whenever possible. Symptoms associated with discontinuation of sertraline and other SSRIs and SNRIs have been reported. Monitor patients for these symptoms (eg, dysphoric mood, irritability, agitation, dizziness, sensory disturbances, anxiety, confusion, headache, lethargy, emotional lability, insomnia, hypomania) when discontinuing treatment. If intolerable symptoms occur following a decrease in the dose or upon discontinuation of treatment, resuming the previously prescribed dose may be considered. Subsequently, the health care provider may continue decreasing the dose, but at a more gradual rate.

➤*Preparation for administration:* Sertraline oral concentrate contains 20 mg/mL of sertraline (as the hydrochloride) as the active ingredient and 12% of alcohol. Sertraline oral concentrate must be diluted before use. Just before taking, use the dropper provided to remove the required amount of sertraline oral concentrate and mix with 4 oz (½ cup) of water, ginger ale, lemon/lime soda, lemonade, or orange juice only. Do not mix sertraline oral concentrate with anything other than the liquids listed. The dose should be taken immediately after mixing. Do not mix in advance. At times, a slight haze may appear after mixing; this is normal. Note that caution should be exercised for patients with latex sensitivity, as the dropper dispenser may contain dry natural rubber.

➤*Administration:* Administer sertraline once daily in the morning or evening.

➤*Storage/Stability:* Store at 25°C (77°F); excursions are permitted to 15° to 30°C (59° to 86°F).

5HT^{1a} Receptor Agonists

VILAZODONE HYDROCHLORIDE

Rx	**Viibryd** (Trovis Pharmaceuticals)	**Tablets; oral:** 10 mg	Lactose, PEG. (10). Pink, oval. In 30s, 90s, 500s, and UD 100s.
		20 mg	Lactose, PEG. (20). Orange, oval. In 30s, 90s, 500s, and UD 100s.
		40 mg	Lactose, PEG. (40). Blue, oval. In 30s, 90s, 500s, and UD 100s.
Rx	**Viibryd** Patient Starter Kit (Trovis Pharmaceuticals)	**Tablets; oral:** 10 mg	Lactose, PEG. (10). Pink, oval. In UD 30s (7 tablets).[a]
		20 mg	Lactose, PEG. (20). Orange, oval. In UD 30s (7 tablets).[a]
		40 mg	Lactose, PEG. (40). Blue, oval. In UD 30s (16 tablets).[a]

[a] Starter kit is a 30-tablet blister card containing seven 10 mg tablets, seven 20 mg tablets, and sixteen 40 mg tablets.

VILAZODONE HYDROCHLORIDE — ORAL

WARNING

Suicidality in children and adolescents – Antidepressants increased the risk compared with placebo of suicidal thinking and behavior (suicidality) in children, adolescents, and young adults in short-term studies of major depressive disorder (MDD) and other psychiatric disorders. Anyone considering the use of vilazodone or any other antidepressant in a child, adolescent, or young adult must balance this risk with the clinical need. Short-term studies did not show an increase in the risk of suicidality with antidepressants compared with placebo in adults older than 24 years of age; there was a reduction in risk with antidepressants compared with placebo in adults 65 years of age and older. Depression and certain other psychiatric disorders are themselves associated with increases in the risk of suicide. Patients of all ages who are started on antidepressant therapy should be monitored appropriately and observed closely for clinical worsening, suicidality, or unusual changes in behavior. Families and caregivers should be advised of the need for close observation and communication with the prescriber. Vilazodone is not approved for use in children.

Indications

➤*Major depressive disorder:* For the treatment of MDD.

Administration and Dosage

➤*Adults:*

Major depressive disorder –

Usual dosage: 40 mg once daily.

Dosage titration: Titrate, starting with an initial dose of 10 mg once daily for 7 days, followed by 20 mg once daily for an additional 7 days, and then an increase to 40 mg once daily.

Duration of therapy:

Periodically reassess patients to determine the need for maintenance treatment and the appropriate dose for treatment.

Concomitant therapy: At least 14 days must elapse between discontinuation of a monoamine oxidase inhibitor (MAOI) and initiation of therapy with vilazodone. In addition, at least 14 days must be allowed after stopping vilazodone before starting an MAOI.

➤*Discontinuation of therapy:* Discontinuation symptoms have been reported with discontinuation of serotonergic drugs such as vilazodone. Gradual dose reduction is recommended, instead of abrupt discontinuation, whenever possible. Monitor patients for these symptoms when discontinuing vilazodone. If intolerable symptoms occur following a dose decrease or upon discontinuation of treatment, consider resuming the previously prescribed dose and decreasing the dose at a more gradual rate.

➤*Administration:* Administer with food. Vilazodone blood concentrations (area under the curve [AUC]) in the fasted state can be decreased by approximately 50% compared with the fed state, and may result in diminished effectiveness in some patients.

➤*Storage/Stability:* Store at 25°C (77°F) with excursions permitted between 15° and 30°C (59° and 86°F).

Indications

➤*Depression:* In general, the MAOIs are indicated in patients with atypical (exogenous) depression and in some patients unresponsive to other antidepressive therapy. They are rarely a drug of first choice.

➤*Off-label uses:* Refer to individual monographs for further information.

Prevention of migraine (adults) –

Phenelzine: [5] = Poor documentation.

Other possible off-label uses – MAOIs have shown promise in the treatment of bulimia (having characteristics of atypical depression). Phenelzine has been investigated in the treatment of cocaine addiction; careful supervision is required. Anecdotal cases and small studies indicate beneficial effects of phenelzine in patients with night terrors (30 mg twice daily); posttraumatic stress disorder (60 to 75 mg/day); some migraines resistant to other therapies (15 mg 3 times/day); likewise, with tranylcypromine in Binswanger's encephalopathy (40 mg/day), seasonal affective disorder (≈ 30 mg/day), and subjective symptoms in multiple sclerosis patients (10 to 120 mg/day). MAOIs have also been used in the treatment of panic disorder with associated agoraphobia and globus hystericus syndrome.

Actions

➤*Pharmacology:* Monoamine oxidase is a complex enzyme system, widely distributed throughout the body, which is responsible for the metabolic decomposition of biogenic amines (eg, norepinephrine, epinephrine, dopamine, serotonin). Monoamine oxidase inhibitors (MAOIs) inhibit this enzyme system, causing an increase in the concentration of these endogenous amines.

Two types of MAO enzymes have been identified, MAO-A and MAO-B, which exhibit different preferences for substrates and different sensitivities to inhibitors. MAO-A preferentially de-aminates epinephrine, norepinephrine, and serotonin, while MAO-B metabolizes benzylamine and phenylethylamine. Dopamine and tyramine are metabolized by both isozymes. In neural tissues, this enzyme system regulates the metabolic decomposition of catecholamines and serotonin. Hepatic MAO inactivates circulating monoamines or those that are introduced via the GI tract into portal circulation (eg, tyramine).

Except for selegiline, MAOIs currently in use in the US are nonselective. Selegiline, an MAO-B selective agent, is used therapeutically for the treatment of Parkinson's disease. The nonselective agents are used for their antidepressant effects. All of these agents are irreversible inhibitors of MAO, and therefore, may require up to 2 weeks for normal amine metabolism to be restored following drug discontinuation. Studies have also indicated that chronic therapy with MAOIs causes down-regulation in adrenergic and serotonergic receptors.

Drugs that have MAOI activity cause a wide range of clinical effects and have the potential for serious interactions with other substances. Clinicians and patients should be fully aware of the potential hazards associated with their use.

➤*Pharmacokinetics:*

Absorption/Distribution – Limited information is available on MAOI pharmacokinetics. They appear to be well absorbed following oral administration. Peak levels of tranylcypromine and phenelzine are reached in ≈ 2 and 3 hours, respectively. However, maximal inhibition of MAO occurs within 5 to 10 days.

Metabolism/Excretion – The hydrazine MAOIs (phenelzine, isocarboxazid) are thought to be metabolized with the release of active metabolites. Inactivation is primarily by acetylation. The clinical effects of phenelzine may continue for up to 2 weeks after discontinuation of therapy. Upon withdrawal of tranylcypromine, MAO activity is recovered in 3 to 5 days (possibly up to 10 days). Phenelzine and isocarboxazid are excreted in the urine mostly as metabolites.

Special populations –

"Slow acetylators": Slow acetylation of hydrazine MAOIs may yield exaggerated effects after standard dosing.

Contraindications

Hypersensitivity to these agents; pheochromocytoma; CHF; history of liver disease or abnormal liver function tests; severe impairment of renal function; confirmed or suspected cerebrovascular disorders; cardiovascular disease; hypertension; history of headache; coadministration with other MAOIs; dibenzazepine-related agents including tricyclic antidepressants, carbamazepine, and cyclobenzaprine; buproprion; SSRIs; buspirone; sympathomimetics; meperidine; dextromethorphan; anesthetic agents; CNS depressants; antihypertensives; caffeine; cheese or other foods with high tyramine content (see Warnings and Drug Interactions).

Warnings/Precautions

➤*Hypertensive crises:* The most serious reactions involve changes in blood pressure; it is inadvisable to use these drugs in elderly or debilitated patients or in the presence of hypertension, cardiovascular or cerebrovascular disease, or coadministered with certain drugs or foods (see Warnings and Drug Interactions).

Hypertensive crises have sometimes been fatal. These crises usually occur within several hours after ingestion of a contraindicated substance and are characterized by some or all of the following symptoms: Occipital headache that may radiate frontally; palpitation; neck stiffness/soreness; nausea; vomiting; sweating (sometimes with fever or cold, clammy skin); dilated pupils; photophobia. Either tachycardia or bradycardia may be present and can be associated with constricting chest pain.

Note – Intracranial bleeding (sometimes fatal) has been reported in association with the paradoxical increase in blood pressure. Monitor blood pressure frequently to detect evidence of any pressor response. Do not rely completely on blood pressure readings, but observe patient frequently.

Discontinue therapy immediately if palpitations or frequent headaches occur. These signs may be prodromal of a hypertensive crisis.

Treatment – If a hypertensive crisis occurs, discontinue these drugs immediately and institute therapy to lower blood pressure. Do not use parenteral reserpine. Headaches tend to abate as blood pressure is lowered. Administer alpha-adrenergic blocking agents such as phentolamine 5 mg IV slowly to avoid producing an excessive hypotensive effect. Manage fever by means of external cooling.

Warning to the patient – Warn all patients against eating foods with high tyramine, dopamine, or tryptophan content (see table) during treatment and for 2 weeks after discontinuing MAOIs. Any high-protein food that is aged or undergoes breakdown by putrefaction process to improve flavor is suspect of being able to produce a hypertensive crisis in patients taking MAOIs. Also warn patients against drinking alcoholic beverages and against self-medication with certain proprietary agents such as cold, hay fever, or weight reduction preparations containing sympathomimetic amines while undergoing therapy. Instruct patients not to consume excessive amounts of caffeine in any form and to report promptly the occurrence of headache or other unusual symptoms.

Monoamine Oxidase Inhibitors

Tyramine-Containing Foods[a]		
Cheese/Dairy Products		
American Blue[b] Boursault[b] Brie	Camembert[b] Cheddar[b] Emmenthaler[b] Gruyere Mozzarella Parmesan	Romano Roquefort Sour cream Stilton[b] Swiss[b] Yogurt
Meat/Fish		
Anchovies Beef or chicken liver,[b] other meats, fish (unrefrigerated, fermented, spoiled, smoked, pickled) Caviar	Fermented sausages (bologna, pepperoni, salami, summer sausage)[b] Dried fish (salted herring) Dry sausage Game meat[b]	Meat extracts Meats prepared with tenderizer Herring, pickled, spoiled[b] Shrimp paste
Alcoholic Beverages (Undistilled)		
Beer (imports, some nonalcoholic)	Red wine (especially Chianti)[b]	Sherry[b] Distilled spirits Liqueurs
Fruit/Vegetables		
Bananas Bean curd Dried fruits (eg, raisins, prunes)	Fruit (eg, avocados, especially overripe) Figs, canned (overripe) Miso soup Raspberries	Sauerkraut[b] Soy sauce Yeast extracts (eg, Marmite)[b]
Foods Containing Other Vasopressors		
Broad beans (eg, fava beans, overripe) – dopa[b]	Caffeine (eg, coffee, tea, colas)	Chocolate – phenylethylamine Ginseng

[a] Tyramine contents are not predictable and may vary. The amounts of tyramine are estimated from low to very high.
[b] Contains high to very high amounts of tyramine.

➤*Suicidal risks:* In patients who may be suicidal, no single form of treatment, such as MAOIs, electroconvulsive, or other therapy, should be relied upon as a sole therapeutic measure. Strict supervision and, preferably, hospitalization are advised.

➤*Concomitant antidepressants:* In patients receiving a selective serotonin reuptake inhibitor (SSRI) in combination with an MAOI, there have been reports of serious, sometimes fatal, reactions including hyperthermia, rigidity, myoclonus, autonomic instability with possible rapid fluctuations of vital signs, and mental status changes that include extreme agitation progressing to delirium and coma. These reactions have also occurred in patients who have recently discontinued an SSRI and have been started on a MAOI. Some cases presented with features resembling neuroleptic malignant syndrome. It is recommended that SSRIs not be used in combination with a MAOI, or within 14 days of a MAOI. Allow at least 2 weeks after stopping the SSRI before starting a MAOI (see Drug Interactions). Allow at least 5 weeks after stopping fluoxetine before starting a MAOI.

Do not administer MAOIs with or immediately following tricyclic antidepressants (TCAs). Such combinations can produce seizures, sweating, coma, hyperexcitability, hyperthermia, tachycardia, tachypnea, headache, mydriasis, flushing, confusion, disseminated intravascular coagulation, and death. Allow at least 14 days to elapse between the discontinuation of the MAOIs and the institution of a TCA. Some TCAs have been used safely and successfully in combination with MAOIs.

➤*Withdrawal:* Withdrawal may be associated with nausea, vomiting, and malaise. An uncommon withdrawal syndrome following abrupt withdrawal of MAOIs has been infrequently reported. Signs and symptoms of this syndrome generally commence 24 to 72 hours after drug discontinuation and may range from vivid nightmares with agitation to frank psychosis and convulsions. This syndrome generally responds to reinstitution of low-dose MAOI therapy followed by cautious downward titration and discontinuation.

➤*Coexisting symptoms:* **Tranylcypromine** and **isocarboxazid** may aggravate coexisting symptoms in depression, such as anxiety and agitation.

➤*Hypotension:* Observe all patients for symptoms of postural hypotension. Hypotensive side effects have occurred in hypertensive as well as healthy and hypotensive patients. Blood pressure usually returns to pretreatment levels rapidly when the drug is discontinued or the dosage is reduced.

At doses > 30 mg/day, postural hypotension is a major side effect and may result in syncope. Make dosage increases more gradually in patients showing a tendency toward hypotension at the beginning of therapy. Postural hypotension may be relieved by the patient lying down until blood pressure returns to normal.

➤*Hypomania:* Hypomania has been the most common severe psychiatric side effect reported. This has been largely limited to patients in whom disorders characterized by hyperkinetic symptoms coexist with, but are obscured by, depressive affect; hypomania usually appeared as depression improved. If agitation is present, it may be increased with MAOIs. Hypomania and agitation have also occurred at higher than recommended doses or following long-term therapy.

These drugs may cause excessive stimulation in agitated or schizophrenic patients; in manic-depressive states, it may result in a swing from a depressive to a manic phase.

➤*Diabetes:* There is conflicting evidence as to whether MAOIs affect glucose metabolism or potentiate hypoglycemic agents. Consider this if used in diabetics.

➤*Epilepsy:* The effect of MAOIs on the convulsive threshold may vary. Do not use with metrizamide; discontinue MAOI ≥ 48 hours prior to myelography and resume ≥ 24 hours postprocedure.

➤*Hepatotoxicity:* There is a low incidence of altered liver function or jaundice in patients treated with **isocarboxazid**. In the past, it was difficult to differentiate most cases of drug-induced hepatocellular jaundice from viral hepatitis although this is no longer true. Perform periodic liver chemistry tests during therapy. Discontinue the drug at the first sign of hepatic dysfunction or jaundice.

➤*Myocardial ischemia:* MAOIs may suppress anginal pain that would otherwise serve as a warning of myocardial ischemia.

➤*Hyperthyroid patients:* Use **tranylcypromine** and **isocarboxazid** cautiously because of increased sensitivity to pressor amines.

➤*Switching MAOIs:* In several case reports, hypertensive crisis, cerebral hemorrhage, and death have possibly resulted from switching from one MAOI to another without a waiting period. However, in other patients no adverse reactions occurred. Nevertheless, a waiting period of 10 to 14 days is recommended when switching from one MAOI to another or from a dibenzazepine-related agent (eg, amitriptyline, perphenazine).

➤*Renal function impairment:* Observe caution in patients with impaired renal function because there is a possibility of cumulative effects in such patients.

➤*Drug abuse and dependence:* There have been reports of drug dependency in patients using doses of **tranylcypromine** and **isocarboxazid** significantly in excess of the therapeutic range. Some of these patients had a history of previous substance abuse. The following withdrawal symptoms have been reported: Restlessness; anxiety; depression; confusion; hallucinations; headaches; weakness; diarrhea.

➤*Pregnancy:* *Category C.* Safety for use during pregnancy has not been established. Use during pregnancy or in women of childbearing age only when clearly needed and when the potential benefits outweigh the potential hazards to the fetus.

Doses of **phenelzine** in pregnant mice well exceeding the maximum recommended human dose have caused a significant decrease in the number of viable offspring per mouse. The growth of dogs and rats has been retarded by doses exceeding the maximum human dose. **Tranylcypromine** passes through the placental barrier of animals into the fetus.

➤*Lactation:* Safety for use during lactation has not been established. **Tranylcypromine** is excreted in breast milk. Because of the potential for serious adverse effects in the nursing infant, decide whether to discontinue nursing or the drug, taking into account the importance of the drug to the mother.

➤*Children:* Not recommended for patients < 16 years of age.

➤*Elderly:* Older patients may suffer more morbidity than younger patients during and following an episode of hypertension or malignant hyperthermia with MAOI use. Older patients have less compensatory reserve to cope with any serious adverse reactions. Therefore, use **tranylcypromine** with caution in the elderly.

Drug Interactions

MAOI Drug Interactions

Precipitant drug	Object drug[a]		Description
Methylphenidate	MAOIs	↑	Coadministration may cause a hypertensive crisis.
Metrizamide	MAOIs	↑	Discontinue MAOIs at least 48 hours before myelography and do not resume for at least 24 hours postprocedure because of the decrease of the seizure threshold.
MAOIs	Anesthetics	↑	Patients taking MAOIs should not undergo elective surgery requiring general anesthesia. Do not give cocaine or local anesthesia containing sympathomimetic vasoconstrictors. Keep in mind the possible combined hypotensive effects of MAOIs and spinal anesthesia. Discontinue the MAOI at least 10 days before elective surgery.

Monoamine Oxidase Inhibitors

MAOI Drug Interactions			
Precipitant drug	Object drug[a]		Description
MAOIs	Antidepressants	↑	Do not administer MAOIs together with or immediately following these agents (see Warnings). There have been reports of serious, sometimes fatal, reactions (including hyperthermia, rigidity, myoclonus, autonomic instability with possible fluctuations of vital signs, and mental status changes that include extreme agitation and confusion progressing to delirium and coma). Do not administer MAOIs together or in rapid succession with other MAOIs.
MAOIs	Antidiabetic agents	↑	MAOIs may potentiate the hypoglycemic response to insulin or sulfonylureas and delay recovery from hypoglycemia.
MAOIs	Barbiturates	↑	Give barbiturates at a reduced dose with MAOIs.
MAOIs	Beta blockers	↑	Bradycardia may develop during concurrent use of certain MAOIs and beta blockers.
MAOIs	Bupropion	↑	The concurrent use of an MAOI and bupropion HCl is contraindicated. Allow at least 14 days between discontinuation of an MAOI and initiation of bupropion HCl treatment.
MAOIs	Buspirone	↑	Do not take isocarboxazid in combination with buspirone. Several cases of elevated blood pressure have occurred. Allow at least 10 days between discontinuation of isocarboxazid and institution of buspirone.
MAOIs	Carbamazepine	↑	Hypertensive crises, severe convulsive seizures, coma, or circulatory collapse may occur in patients receiving such combinations.
MAOIs	Cyclobenzaprine	↑	Because cyclobenzaprine is structurally related to the tricyclic antidepressants, use with caution with MAOIs (see MAOIs/Antidepressants).
MAOIs	Dextromethorphan	↑	Hyperpyrexia, abnormal muscle movement, psychosis, bizarre behavior, hypotension, coma, and death have been associated with this combination.
MAOIs	Guanethidine	↓	MAOIs may inhibit the hypotensive effects of guanethidine.
MAOIs	Levodopa	↑	Hypertensive reactions occur if levodopa is given to patients receiving MAOIs.
MAOIs	Meperidine	↑	Coadministration or use within 2 to 3 weeks of one another may result in agitation, seizures, diaphoresis, and fever, and progress to coma, apnea, and death. Adverse reactions are possible weeks after MAOI withdrawal. Avoid this combination; administer other narcotic analgesics with caution.
MAOIs	Methyldopa	↑	Coadministration may cause loss of blood pressure control or signs of central stimulation (eg, excitation, hallucinations).
MAOIs	Rauwolfia alkaloids	↑	MAOIs inhibit the destruction of serotonin and norepinephrine, which are believed to be released from tissue stores by rauwolfia alkaloids. Exercise caution when rauwolfia is used concomitantly with MAOIs.
MAOIs	Sulfonamide	↑	Coadministration may cause sulfonamide or MAOI toxicity.
Sulfonamide	MAOIs		
MAOIs	Sumatriptan	↑	Systemic exposure to sumatriptan may be increased, producing toxicity.
MAOIs	Sympathomimetics	↑	The MAOIs' potentiation of indirect- or mixed-acting sympathomimetic substances, including anorexiants, may result in severe headache, hypertension, high fever, and hyperpyrexia, possibly resulting in hypertensive crisis; avoid coadministration.
MAOIs	Thiazide diuretics	↑	Exaggerated hypotensive effects may result from concurrent use.
MAOIs	L-Tryptophan	↑	Coadministration may result in hyperreflexia, confusion, disorientation, shivering, myoclonic jerks, agitation, amnesia, delirium, hypomanic signs, ataxia, ocular oscillations, Babinski signs.

[a] ↑ = object drug increased; ↓ = object drug decreased.

➤*Drug/Food interactions:* Warn all patients against eating foods with a high **tyramine** content. Hypertensive crisis may result (see Warnings).

Adverse Reactions

➤*Common:*

Cardiovascular – Orthostatic and postural hypotension; syncope; palpitations; tachycardia.

CNS – Dizziness; headache; hyperreflexia; tremors; muscle twitching; mania; hypomania (see Precautions); confusion; memory impairment; sleep disturbances including hypersomnia and insomnia; weakness; myoclonic movements; fatigue; drowsiness; restlessness; overstimulation including increased anxiety, agitation, and manic symptoms.

GI – Constipation; GI disturbances; nausea; diarrhea; abdominal pain.

Miscellaneous – Edema; dry mouth; elevated serum transaminases; weight gain; sexual disturbances; anorexia; blurred vision; impotence; chills.

➤*Less common:*

CNS – Jitteriness; euphoria; palilalia; paresthesia; chills; myoclonic jerks; anxiety; hyperactivity; lethargy; sedation.

GU – Urinary retention/frequency; impotence.

Hematologic – Hematologic changes including anemia, agranulocytosis and thrombocytopenia; leukopenia.

Ophthalmic – Glaucoma; nystagmus; blurred vision.

Miscellaneous – Sweating; skin rash; hypernatremia; syncope; heavy feeling; palpitations.

➤*Rare:*

CNS – Convulsions; ataxia; shock-like coma; acute anxiety reaction; precipitation of schizophrenia; toxic delirium; manic reaction; headaches without blood pressure elevation; muscle spasm; myoclonic jerks; numbness; confusion; memory loss.

GU – Impaired water excretion compatible with the syndrome of inappropriate secretion of antidiuretic hormone (SIADH).

Hepatic – Reversible jaundice; hepatitis; fatal progressive necrotizing hepatocellular damage.

Metabolic – Hypermetabolic syndrome that may include, but is not limited to, hyperpyrexia, tachycardia, tachypnea, muscular rigidity, elevated CK levels, metabolic acidosis, hypoxia, and coma and may resemble an overdose.

Miscellaneous – Edema of the glottis; transient respiratory and cardiovascular depression following ECT; leukopenia; lupus-like syndrome; fever associated with increased muscle tone; tinnitus; localized scleroderma, cystic acne flare-up, ataxia, akinesia, disorientation, urinary frequency or incontinence, urticaria, fissuring in corner of mouth (tranylcypromine); skin rash; ejaculation problems; tremors.

Overdosage

➤*Symptoms:* Depending on the amount of overdosage, a mixed clinical picture may develop involving signs and symptoms of the CNS, cardiovascular stimulation or depression. Signs and symptoms may be absent or minimal during the initial 12–hour period following ingestion and may develop slowly thereafter, reaching a maximum in 24 to 48 hours. Some symptoms may persist for 8 to 14 days. Immediate hospitalization, with continuous patient monitoring throughout this period, is essential.

Early symptoms of MAOI toxicity include: Irritability; hyperactivity; anxiety; hypotension; vascular collapse; insomnia; restlessness; dizziness; faintness; weakness; drowsiness; hallucinations; trismus; flushing; sweating; tachypnea; tachycardia; movement disorders including grimacing, opisthotonus, rigidity, clonic movements and muscular fasciculation; severe headache. In serious cases, coma, convulsions, hypertension with severe headache, precordial pain, respiratory depression and failure, pyrexia, hyperpyrexia, diaphoresis, cool and clammy skin, cardiorespiratory arrest, incoherence, agitation, mental confusion, extreme dizziness, shock, and death may occur. Rare instances have been reported in which hypertension was accompanied by twitching or myoclonic fibrillation of skeletal muscles with hyperpyrexia, sometimes progressing to generalized rigidity and coma.

➤*Treatment:* Induce emesis or gastric lavage with instillation of charcoal slurry in early poisoning; protect the airway against aspiration. Support respiration by appropriate measures, including management of the airway, use of supplemental oxygen, and mechanical ventilatory assistance, as required. Refer to General Management of Acute Overdosage.

Cardiovascular – Cardiovascular complications include hypertension and hypotension; hence, any cardiovascular agent must be administered cautiously and blood pressure monitored frequently. Severe hypertension may be treated with an alpha-adrenergic blocker (eg, phentolamine, phenoxybenzamine). Beta blocking agents are not necessarily contraindicated and may be useful for tachycardia, tachypnea, and hyperpyrexia; however, more data are needed. Treat hypotension and vascular collapse with IV fluids and, if necessary, titrate blood pressure with an IV infusion of a dilute pressor agent. Administration of pressor amines such as norepinephrine may be of limited value; their effects may be potentiated. Plasma may be of value, as well. Adrenergic agents may produce a markedly increased pressor response.

CNS – CNS stimulation, including convulsions, may be treated with IV diazepam given slowly. Avoid phenothiazine derivatives and CNS stimulants. Monitor body temperature closely. Intensive management of hyperpyrexia may be required. Maintenance of fluid and electrolyte balance is essential.

Hemodialysis, peritoneal dialysis, and charcoal hemoperfusion may be of value in massive overdosage, but sufficient data are not available to recommend their routine use. External cooling is recommended if hyperpyrexia occurs. Barbiturates have been reported to help relieve myoclonic reactions.

The pathophysiologic effects of massive overdosage may persist for several days; recovery from mild overdosage may be expected within 3 to 4 days. Continue treatment for several days until homeostasis is restored. Liver function studies are recommended during the 4 to 6 weeks after recovery. It is not known if tranylcypromine is dialyzable.

Patient Information

Do not discontinue this medication or adjust dosage except on the advice of a physician. Consult physician before taking any other medication, including *otc* items.

Avoid tyramine-containing foods and certain *otc* drug products (see Warnings).

May cause drowsiness or blurred vision; use with caution when driving or performing other tasks requiring alertness, coordination, or physical dexterity.

Dizziness, weakness, or fainting may occur when arising from a sitting position.

Effects may be delayed a few weeks. Take as directed. Avoid alcohol and tryptophan.

Notify physician if severe headache, palpitation, or tachycardia, a sense of constriction in the throat or chest, sweating, dizziness, neck stiffness, nausea or vomiting, or other unusual symptoms occur.

Inform physician and dentist about the use of MAOIs.

PHENELZINE

Rx	**Phenelzine** (Gavis Pharmaceuticals)	**Tablets; oral:** 15 mg	As phenelzine sulfate. Edetate disodium, mannitol, PEG. (NL 360). Orange. Film-coated. In 60s.
Rx	**Nardil** (Parke-Davis)		As phenelzine sulfate. Mannitol. (P-D 270). Orange. Biconvex. Film-coated. In 60s.

PHENELZINE SULFATE — ORAL

WARNING

Suicidality in children and adolescents – Antidepressants increased the risk of suicidal thinking and behavior (suicidality) in short-term studies in children and adolescents with major depressive disorder (MDD) and other psychiatric disorders. Anyone considering the use of phenelzine or any other antidepressant in a child or adolescent must balance this risk with the clinical need. Closely observe patients who are started on therapy for clinical worsening, suicidality, or unusual changes in behavior. Advise families and caregivers of the need for close observation and communication with the prescriber. Phenelzine is not approved for use in children.

Pooled analyses of short-term (4- to 16-week) placebo-controlled trials of 9 antidepressant drugs (selective serotonin reuptake inhibitors [SSRIs] and others) in children and adolescents with MDD, obsessive compulsive disorder (OCD), or other psychiatric disorders (a total of 24 trials involving over 4,400 patients) have revealed a greater risk of adverse reactions representing suicidality during the first few months of treatment in those receiving antidepressants. The average risk of such reactions in patients receiving antidepressants was 4%, twice the placebo risk of 2%. No suicides occurred in these trials.

Indications

➤*Depression:* For depressed patients clinically characterized as "atypical," "nonendogenous," or "neurotic." These patients often have mixed anxiety and depression and phobic or hypochondriacal features. There is less conclusive evidence of its usefulness with severely depressed patients with endogenous features.

Phenelzine should rarely be the first antidepressant drug administered. Rather, it is more suitable for use with patients who have failed to respond to the drugs more commonly used for these conditions.

➤*Off-label uses:*

Prevention of migraine (adults) – [5] = Poor documentation. Evidence from noncontrolled trials evaluating the use of phenelzine for the prevention of migraine headaches in adults showed favorable results; however, the trials were limited by small sample size and lack of a control group. American Academy of Neurology practice guidelines consider phenelzine to be clinically efficacious based on consensus and clinical experience, despite the lack of scientific evidence of efficacy, but note that there are safety concerns. Given the numerous alternative therapies available for the prevention of migraine and the safety concerns that exist with monoamine oxidase inhibitors, routine use of phenelzine is not recommended.

Other possible off-label uses – Bulimia; chronic migraine not responsive to standard agents; panic disorder; posttraumatic stress disorder; and social anxiety disorder.

Administration and Dosage

➤*General dosing considerations:* Phenelzine should rarely be the first antidepressant drug administered. Rather, it is more suitable for use with patients who have failed to respond to the drugs more commonly used for these conditions.

➤*Adults:*

Depression –

Initial dosage: 15 mg 3 times per day.

Dosage titration: Dosage should be increased to at least 60 mg per day at a fairly rapid pace consistent with patient tolerance. It may be necessary to increase dosage to 90 mg per day to obtain sufficient monoamine oxidase (MAO) inhibition. Many patients do not show a clinical response until treatment at 60 mg has been continued for at least 4 weeks.

Maintenance dosage: After maximum benefit from phenelzine is achieved, dosage should be reduced slowly over several weeks. Maintenance dosage may be as low as 15 mg every day or every other day, and should be continued for as long as is required.

➤*Renal function impairment:* Contraindicated in patients with severe renal impairment or renal disease.

➤*Hepatic function impairment:* Contraindicated in patients with a history of liver disease or abnormal liver function tests.

➤*Storage/Stability:* Store between 15° and 30°C (59° and 86°F).

TRANYLCYPROMINE

Rx	**Tranylcypromine** (Par)	**Tablets; oral:** 10 mg	As tranylcypromine sulfate (250 K). Dark pink. Film-coated. In 100s.
Rx	**Parnate** (GlaxoSmithKline)		As tranylcypromine sulfate. Lactose. (PARNATE SB). Rose-red. Film-coated. In 100s.

Monoamine Oxidase Inhibitors

TRANYLCYPROMINE SULFATE — ORAL

WARNING

Suicidality in children and adolescents – Antidepressants increased the risk compared with placebo of suicidal thinking and behavior (suicidality) in children, adolescents, and young adults in short-term studies in children and adolescents with major depressive disorder (MDD) and other psychiatric disorders. Anyone considering the use of tranylcypromine or any other antidepressant in a child or adolescent must balance the risk with the clinical need. Short-term studies did not show an increase in the risk of suicidality with antidepressants compared with placebo in adults older than 24 years of age; there was a reduction in risk with antidepressants compared with placebo in adults 65 years of age and older. Depression and certain other psychiatric disorders are associated with increases in the risk of suicide. Closely observe and appropriately monitor patients of all ages who are started on antidepressant therapy for clinical worsening, suicidality, or unusual changes in behavior. Advise families and caregivers of the need for close observation and communication with the health care provider. Tranylcypromine is not approved for use in children.

Indications

➤*Major depression:* For the treatment of a major depressive episode without melancholia.

Use tranylcypromine in adult patients who can be closely supervised. It should rarely be the first antidepressant drug given. Rather, the drug is suited for patients who have failed to respond to the drugs more commonly administered for depression.

➤*Off-label uses:* For migraine prevention; social anxiety disorder; panic disorder; bipolar depression; Alzheimer and Parkinson disease (only in individuals who are unresponsive or unable to take other agents).

Administration and Dosage

➤*Adults:*

Major depression –

Usual dosage: 30 mg/day, usually given in divided doses.

Dosage adjustment: Dosage should be adjusted to the requirements of the individual patient. Improvement should be seen within 48 hours to 3 weeks after starting therapy.

If there are no signs of improvement after a reasonable period (up to 2 weeks), the dose may be increased in 10 mg/day increments at intervals of 1 to 3 weeks; the dose range may be extended to a maximum of 60 mg/day from the usual 30 mg/day.

➤*Renal function impairment:* Observe the usual precautions in patients with renal function impairment because there is a possibility of cumulative effects in such patients.

➤*Hepatic function impairment:* Do not use tranylcypromine in patients with a history of liver disease or in those with abnormal liver function tests.

➤*Storage/Stability:* Store between 15° and 30°C (59° and 86°F).

ISOCARBOXAZID

Rx	**Marplan** (Validus)[a]	**Tablets; oral:** 10 mg	Lactose. Peach, scored. In 100s.

[a] Validus Pharmaceuticals, Inc, 2001 Route 46 East, Suite 310, Parsippany, NJ 07054; 1-866-952-4387; http://www.validuspharma.com.

ISOCARBOXAZID — ORAL

WARNING

Suicidality in children and adolescents – Antidepressants increased the risk of suicidal thinking and behavior (suicidality) in short-term studies in children and adolescents with major depressive disorder (MDD) and other psychiatric disorders. Anyone considering the use of isocarboxazid or any other antidepressant in a child or adolescent must balance this risk with the clinical need. Closely observe patients who are started on therapy for clinical worsening, suicidality, or unusual changes in behavior. Advise families and caregivers of the need for close observation and communication with the prescriber. Isocarboxazid is not approved for use in children.

Pooled analyses of short-term (4- to 16-week), placebo-controlled trials of 9 antidepressant drugs (selective serotonin reuptake inhibitors [SSRIs] and others) in children and adolescents with MDD, obsessive-compulsive disorder (OCD), or other psychiatric disorders (a total of 24 trials involving more than 4,400 patients) have revealed a greater risk of adverse reactions representing suicidal thinking or behavior (suicidality) during the first few months of treatment in those receiving antidepressants. The average risk of such reactions in patients receiving antidepressants was 4%, twice the placebo risk of 2%. No suicides occurred in these trials.

Indications

➤*Depression:* For the treatment of depression. Because of its potentially serious adverse reactions, isocarboxazid is not an antidepressant of first choice in the treatment of newly diagnosed depressed patients.

➤*Off-label uses:* Isocarboxazid has shown promise in the treatment of bulimia (having characteristics of atypical depression).

Administration and Dosage

➤*Adults:*

Depression –

Maximum dose: 60 mg/day.

Initial dosage: 10 mg twice daily.

Dosage titration: If tolerated, the dose may be increased by increments of 10 mg every 2 to 4 days to achieve a dose of 40 mg daily by the end of the first week of treatment. The dose can then be increased by increments of up to 20 mg/week, if needed and tolerated, to a maximum dose of 60 mg/day. The daily dose should be divided into 2 to 4 doses.

Maintenance dosage: After maximum clinical response is achieved, an attempt should be made to slowly reduce the dosage over a period of several weeks without jeopardizing the therapeutic response. Beneficial effect may not be seen in some patients for 3 to 6 weeks. If no response is obtained by then, continued administration is unlikely to help.

Because of the limited experience with systematically monitored patients receiving isocarboxazid at the higher end of the currently recommended dose range (up to 60 mg/day), caution is indicated in patients for whom a dose of 40 mg/day is exceeded.

➤*Renal function impairment:* In patients with renal function impairment, use isocarboxazid cautiously to prevent accumulation. Isocarboxazid is contraindicated in patients with severe renal function impairment.

➤*Hepatic function impairment:* Do not use isocarboxazid in patients with a history of liver disease or abnormal liver function tests.

➤*Duration of therapy:* The efficacy of isocarboxazid in long-term use, that is, for more than 6 weeks, has not been systematically evaluated in controlled trials. Therefore, if electing to use isocarboxazid for extended periods, periodically evaluate the long-term usefulness of the drug for the individual patient.

ANTIPSYCHOTIC AGENTS

WARNING

Atypical antipsychotics –

Increased mortality in elderly patients with dementia-related psychosis: Elderly patients with dementia-related psychosis treated with atypical antipsychotic drugs are at an increased risk of death compared with placebo. Analyses of 17 placebo-controlled trials (modal duration of 10 weeks) in these patients revealed a risk of death in the drug-treated patients of between 1.6 to 1.7 times that seen in placebo-treated patients. Over the course of a typical 10-week controlled trial, the rate of death in drug-treated patients was about 4.5%, compared with a rate of about 2.6% in the placebo group. Although the causes of death were varied, most of the deaths appeared to be either cardiovascular (eg, heart failure, sudden death) or infectious (eg, pneumonia) in nature. Atypical antipsychotics are not approved for the treatment of patients with dementia-related psychosis.

WARNING (cont.)

Clozapine –

Agranulocytosis: Because of a significant risk of agranulocytosis, a potentially life-threatening adverse event, reserve **clozapine** use in 1) the treatment of severely ill patients with schizophrenia who fail to show an acceptable response to adequate courses of standard antipsychotic drug treatment, or 2) for reducing the risk of recurrent suicidal behavior in patients with schizophrenia or schizoaffective disorder who are judged to be at risk of re-experiencing suicidal behavior. Patients being treated with clozapine must have a baseline white blood cell (WBC) and differential count before initiation of treatment, as well as regular WBC counts during treatment and for 4 weeks after discontinuation of treatment. Clozapine is available only through a distribution system that ensures monitoring of WBC counts according to the following schedule, prior to delivery of the next supply of medication (see Warnings/Precautions).

Seizures: Seizures have been associated with the use of **clozapine**. Dose appears to be an important seizure predictor, with a greater likelihood at higher clozapine doses. Use caution when administering clozapine to patients with a history of seizures or other predisposing factors. Advise patients not to engage in any activity where sudden loss of consciousness could cause serious risk to themselves or others (see Warnings/Precautions).

WARNING (cont.)

Myocarditis: Analyses of postmarketing safety databases suggest **clozapine** is associated with an increased risk of fatal myocarditis, especially during, but not limited to, the first month of therapy. In patients in whom myocarditis is suspected, discontinue clozapine treatment promptly (see Warnings/Precautions).

Other adverse cardiovascular and respiratory effects: Orthostatic hypotension, with or without syncope, can occur with **clozapine** treatment. Rarely, collapse can be profound and accompanied by respiratory and/or cardiac arrest. Orthostatic hypotension is more likely to occur during initial titration in association with rapid dose escalation. In patients who have had even a brief interval without clozapine (2 or more days since the last dose), start treatment with 12.5 mg once or twice daily (see Warnings/Precautions). Because collapse, respiratory arrest, and cardiac arrest during initial treatment have occurred in patients receiving benzodiazepines or other psychotropic drugs, caution is advised when clozapine is initiated in patients taking a benzodiazepine or any other psychotropic drug (see Warnings/Precautions).

Mesoridazine, thioridazine – Some antipsychotics have been shown to prolong the QTc interval in a dose-related manner, and drugs with this potential, including **mesoridazine** and **thioridazine**, have been associated with torsades de pointes–type arrhythmias and sudden death. Because of their potential for significant, possibly life-threatening, proarrhythmic effects, reserve use of mesoridazine and thioridazine for the treatment of schizophrenic patients who fail to show an acceptable response to adequate courses of treatment with other antipsychotic drugs, either because of insufficient effectiveness or the inability to achieve an effective dose because of intolerable adverse effects from those drugs.

WARNING (cont.)

Olanzapine –

Postinjection delirium/sedation syndrome: Adverse events with signs and symptoms consistent with olanzapine overdose, in particular, sedation (including coma) and/or delirium, have been reported following injections of olanzapine extended-release (ER) injection. Olanzapine ER injection must be administered in a registered health care facility with ready access to emergency response services. After each injection, patients must be observed at the health care facility by a health care provider for at least 3 hours. Because of this risk, olanzapine ER injection is available only through a restricted distribution program and requires prescriber, health care facility, patient, and pharmacy enrollment.

Indications

Antipsychotics — Summary of Indications[a]

Indications ✓ = FDA-approved X = Off-label	Aripiprazole	Asenapine	Chlorpromazine	Clozapine	Fluphenazine	Haloperidol	Iloperidone	Loxapine	Lurasidone	Molindone	Olanzapine	Paliperidone	Perphenazine	Pimozide	Prochlorperazine	Quetiapine	Risperidone	Thioridazine	Thiothixene	Trifluoperazine	Ziprasidone
Acute agitation associated with bipolar I mania	✓ (IM[b])										✓ (IM)										
Acute agitation in schizophrenia	✓ (IM)										✓ (IM)										✓ (IM)
Acute intermittent porphyria			✓																		
Acute manic and/or mixed episodes associated with bipolar disorder	✓	✓[k]	✓	X[c]							✓					✓[d]	✓				✓
Depressive episodes associated with bipolar disorder											✓[i]										
Hyperactivity (children)			✓			✓															
Intractable hiccups			✓			X[e]															
Nausea/Vomiting			✓		X[c]	X[c]							✓		✓						
Nonpsychotic anxiety															✓					✓	
Presurgical apprehension/restlessness			✓																		
Prevention of chemotherapy-induced nausea and vomiting						X[e]															
Psychotic disorders					✓	✓							✓								
Recurrent suicidal behavior				✓																	
Schizophrenia	✓	✓	✓	✓	✓	✓	✓	✓	✓	✓	✓	✓	✓	X[c]	✓	✓	✓	✓	✓	✓	✓
Severe behavioral problems (children)			✓														X[c]				
Tetanus			✓ (IM)	✓																	
Tourette disorder						✓					X[f] (adults); X[g] (children)			✓		X[g] (children)	X[f]				X[g]
Treatment-resistant depression											✓[i]										
Off-label uses																					
Alcohol dependence																X[h]					
Autism																					X[h]
Behavioral problems associated with autism																	X[c]				
Cocaine dependence	X[g]																				
Migraines (acute treatment)			X (IV[b,h])												X[e]						
OCD[b] (refractory to SSRIs[b])						X[h]					X[e]					X[e]	X[e]				
Phencyclidine-induced psychosis						X[c]															
Parasitosis (delusional)											X[g]			X[h]							
Psychosis/Agitation in dementia or Alzheimer disease				X[c]		X[c]					X[c]					X[c]	X[c]	X[c]			X[c]
Psychosis in Parkinson disease				X[c]												X[c]	X[c]				
RLS[b]	X[g]																				

Antipsychotics — Summary of Indications[a]

Indications ✓ = FDA-approved X = Off-label	Aripiprazole	Asenapine	Chlorpromazine	Clozapine	Fluphenazine	Haloperidol	Iloperidone	Loxapine	Lurasidone	Molindone	Olanzapine	Paliperidone	Perphenazine	Pimozide	Prochlorperazine	Quetiapine	Risperidone	Thioridazine	Thiothixene	Trifluoperazine	Ziprasidone
Stuttering											X[g]						X[g]				
Tourette syndrome (adults)											X[f]					X[i]	X[f]				X[g]
Tourette syndrome (children and adolescents)	X[h]										X[g]					X[g]					

[a] For more detailed information, see the information below and individual drug monographs.
[b] IM = intramuscular; IV = intravenous; OCD = obsessive-compulsive disorder; SSRIs = selective serotonin reuptake inhibitors; RLS = restless legs syndrome.
[c] Not rated.
[d] Immediate release only.
[e] Good documentation.
[f] Fair documentation.
[g] Insufficient documentation.
[h] Safety concerns.
[i] Poor documentation.
[j] In combination with fluoxetine.
[k] May also be used as adjunctive therapy with lithium or valproate.

➤*Acute agitation associated with bipolar I mania:* **Olanzapine** IM, **aripiprazole** IM.

➤*Acute agitation in schizophrenia:* **Ziprasidone** IM, **aripiprazole** IM, **olanzapine** IM.

➤*Acute intermittent porphyria:* **Chlorpromazine**.

➤*Acute manic and/or mixed episodes associated with bipolar disorder:* **Chlorpromazine** is indicated to control the manifestations of the manic type of manic-depressive illness. **Olanzapine** is indicated as monotherapy for the acute mixed or manic episodes associated with bipolar I disorder and for the maintenance monotherapy of bipolar disorder or in combination with lithium or valproate for the short-term treatment of acute manic episodes associated with bipolar I disorder. **Quetiapine** is indicated for the short-term treatment of acute manic episodes associated with bipolar I disorder as monotherapy or adjunct therapy to lithium or divalproex. **Ziprasidone** IM is indicated for the treatment of acute manic or mixed episodes associated with bipolar disorder, with or without psychotic features. **Aripiprazole** is indicated for the treatment of acute manic and mixed episodes associated with bipolar disorder. **Risperidone** is indicated for the short-term treatment of acute manic or mixed episodes associated with bipolar I disorder. **Asenapine** is indicated for the acute treatment of manic or mixed episodes associated with bipolar I disorder, as monotherapy or adjuvant therapy with lithium or valproate.

➤*Behavioral problems (children):* **Chlorpromazine** and **haloperidol**. For the treatment of severe behavioral problems in children marked by combativeness and/or explosive hyperexcitable behavior (out of proportion to immediate provocations).

➤*Hyperactivity (children):* **Chlorpromazine** and **haloperidol**. For the short-term treatment of hyperactive children who show excessive motor activity with accompanying conduct disorders consisting of some or all of the following symptoms: aggressiveness, difficulty sustaining attention, impulsiveness, mood lability, poor frustration tolerance.

➤*Intractable hiccups:* **Chlorpromazine**.

➤*Nausea/Vomiting:* **Chlorpromazine**, **perphenazine**, and **prochlorperazine**. To control severe nausea and vomiting.

➤*Nonpsychotic anxiety:* **Prochlorperazine** and **trifluoperazine**. For the short-term treatment of generalized nonpsychotic anxiety; however, they are not the first drugs to be used.

➤*Presurgical apprehension/restlessness:* **Chlorpromazine** is indicated for relief of restlessness and apprehension before surgery.

➤*Psychotic disorders:* **Fluphenazine**, **haloperidol**, and **perphenazine**. For use in the management of the manifestations of psychotic disorders.

➤*Recurrent suicidal behavior:* **Clozapine** is indicated for reducing the risk of recurrent suicidal behavior in patients with schizophrenia or schizoaffective disorder who are judged to be at long-term risk of re-experiencing suicidal behavior.

➤*Schizophrenia:* **Aripiprazole**, **asenapine**, **chlorpromazine**, **clozapine**, **fluphenazine**, **iloperidone**, **loxapine**, **lurasidone**, **molindone**, **olanzapine**, **paliperidone**, **perphenazine**, **prochlorperazine**, **quetiapine**, **risperidone**, **haloperidol**, **thioridazine**, **thiothixene**, **trifluoperazine**, and **ziprasidone**. Clozapine, mesoridazine, and thioridazine should only be used in patients who have failed to respond adequately to other antipsychotic drugs.

➤*Tetanus:* **Chlorpromazine** is indicated as an adjunct in the treatment of tetanus.

➤*Tourette disorder:* **Haloperidol** is indicated for the control of tics and vocal utterances of Tourette disorder in children and adults. **Pimozide** is indicated for the suppression of motor and phonic tics in patients with Tourette disorder who have failed to respond satisfactorily to standard treatment.

➤*Off-label uses:* Refer to individual monographs for further information.

Alcohol dependence –
Quetiapine: [3] = Safety concerns.

Autism –
Ziprasidone: [3] = Safety concerns.

Cocaine dependence –
Aripiprazole: [4] = Insufficient documentation.

Hiccups (singultus) –
Haloperidol: [1] = Good documentation.

Obsessive-compulsive disorder –
Haloperidol: [3] = Safety concerns.
Olanzapine: [1] = Good documentation.
Quetiapine: [1] = Good documentation.
Risperidone: [1] = Good documentation.

Parasitosis (delusional) –
Olanzapine: [4] = Insufficient documentation.
Pimozide: [3] = Safety concerns.

Postherpetic neuralgia –
Fluphenazine: [5] = Poor documentation.

Prevention of chemotherapy-induced nausea and vomiting –
Haloperidol: [1] = Good documentation.

Restless legs syndrome –
Aripiprazole: [4] = Insufficient documentation.

Stuttering –
Olanzapine: [4] = Insufficient documentation.
Risperidone: [4] = Insufficient documentation.

Tardive dyskinesia –
Clozapine: [5] = Poor documentation.

Tourette syndrome –
Risperidone: [2] = Fair documentation.
Ziprasidone: [4] = Insufficient documentation.

Tourette syndrome (adults) –
Olanzapine: [2] = Fair documentation.
Quetiapine: [5] = Poor documentation.

Tourette syndrome (children and adolescents) –
Aripiprazole: [3] = Safety concerns. Initial data from noncontrolled trials and case reports suggest that aripiprazole may have some benefit in the treatment of Tourette syndrome and other tic disorders in children, adolescents, and adults.
Olanzapine: [4] = Insufficient documentation.
Quetiapine: [4] = Insufficient documentation.

Treatment of migraine (adults) –
Chlorpromazine, IM: [5] = Poor documentation.
Chlorpromazine, IV: [3] = Safety concerns.

Other possible off-label uses –
Acute manic episodes associated with bipolar disorder: **Clozapine** also may be an option in the treatment of refractory bipolar mania.

Behavioral problems associated with autism: **Risperidone** was shown to be effective for the treatment of tantrums, aggression, or self-injurious behavior in autistic children.

Behavioral problems (children): **Risperidone** has demonstrated efficacy in reducing aggression in children with a variety of comorbid disorders. Risperidone has also improved severely disruptive behavior in children with subaverage intelligence.

Migraines: **Chlorpromazine** IM and **prochlorperazine** IM have been used as abortive treatments of acute migraine attacks in adults.

Nausea/Vomiting: **Haloperidol** and **fluphenazine** also have been used as antiemetics.

Obsessive-compulsive disorder (refractory to SSRIs): Patients with OCD refractory to SSRIs may respond to the addition of **risperidone** or **olanzapine**.

Phencyclidine psychosis: **Haloperidol** has shown to be effective in improving phencyclidine-induced aggression, combativeness, and schizophreniform symptoms (eg, hallucinations, delusions, disorganized thinking.)

Psychosis/Agitation in dementia or Alzheimer disease: **Clozapine**, **haloperidol**, **olanzapine**, **quetiapine**, **risperidone**, **thioridazine**, and **ziprasidone** may be useful in the management of agitation and psychotic events in patients with dementia and Alzheimer disease.

Psychosis in Parkinson disease: In the treatment of psychosis in patients with Parkinson disease, **clozapine** has been shown to be beneficial in alleviating psychosis without compromising motor function. Other alternatives include **quetiapine** and **risperidone**.

Tourette disorder: **Risperidone** has shown efficacy in the treatment of tics in patients with Tourette disorder.

Administration and Dosage

See individual product listings for specific dosing.

Individualize dosage. The milligram-for-milligram potency relationship among all dosage forms has not been precisely established. Increase dosage until symptoms are controlled. Increase dosage gradually in elderly, debilitated, or emaciated patients. In continued therapy, gradually reduce dosage to the lowest effective maintenance level after symptoms have been controlled.

Actions

➤*Pharmacology:* The exact mechanism of action of the antipsychotic agents is unknown; however, it is thought to be caused by their antagonistic actions on the receptors of several neurotransmitters. The following table provides information on antipsychotic receptor affinity. All produce antagonist effects on the receptors unless otherwise specified.

Antipsychotic Receptor Affinity

Antipsychotic agent	Receptor affinity
	Conventional agents
Chlorpromazine	**High** — adrenergic **Weak** — peripheral anticholinergic, histaminergic, serotonergic
Fluphenazine	Dopamine D_2, histamine H_1, alpha-adrenergic, serotonin 5-HT$_2$
Haloperidol	Dopamine D_2, alpha-adrenergic, serotonin 5-HT$_2$
Loxapine	Dopamine D_2, histamine H_1, alpha-adrenergic, muscarinic M_1
Molindone	**Low** — dopamine D_2, alpha-adrenergic, serotonin 5-HT$_2$
Perphenazine	Dopamine D_2, histamine H_1, alpha-adrenergic
Pimozide	Dopamine D_2, alpha-adrenergic, serotonin 5-HT$_2$
Prochlorperazine	Dopamine D_2, histamine H_1, alpha-D_2adrenergic, serotonin 5-HT$_2$
Promethazine[a]	Histamine H_1, muscarinic, some serotonin
Thioridazine	Dopamine D_2, histamine H_1, alpha adrenergic, muscarinic M_1, serotonin 5-HT$_2$
Thiothixene	**High** — dopamine D_2 **Low** — histamine H_1, alpha-adrenergic
Trifluoperazine	Dopamine D_2, histamine H_1, alpha-adrenergic, muscarinic M_1, serotonin 5-HT$_2$
	Atypical agents
Aripiprazole	**High** — dopamine D_2[b], D_3, serotonin 5-HT$_{1A}$[b], 5-HT$_{2A}$ **Moderate** — dopamine D_4, 5-HT$_{2C}$, 5-HT$_7$, alpha-1 adrenergic, histamine H_1
Asenapine	**High** — dopamine D_1, D_2, D_3, D_4, alpha-1 and -2 adrenergic, histamine H_1, serotonin 5-HT$_{1A}$, 5-HT$_{1B}$, 5-HT$_{2A}$, 5-HT$_{2B}$, 5-HT$_{2C}$, 5-HT$_5$, 5-HT$_6$, 5-HT$_7$ *Moderate* — Histamine H_2
Clozapine	**High** — dopamine D_4 Other receptors — dopamine D_1, D_2, D_3, D_5, adrenergic, cholinergic, histaminergic, serotonergic
Iloperidone	**High** — serotonin 5-HT$_{2A}$, dopamine D_2 and D_3, **Moderate** — dopamine D_4, serotonin 5-HT$_6$, 5-HT$_7$, norepinephrine $NE_{alpha\text{-}1}$ **Low** — serotonin 5-HT$_{1A}$, dopamine D_1, histamine H_1
Lurasidone	**High** — serotonin 5-HT$_{2A}$, 5-HT$_7$, dopamine D_2 **Moderate** — alpha-2a and -2c adrenergic, serotonin 5-HT$_{1A}$
Olanzapine	**High** — serotonin 5-HT$_{2A}$, 5-HT$_{2C}$, dopamine D_1, D_2, D_3, D_4, muscarinic M_1, M_2, M_3, M_4, M_5, histamine H_1, alpha-1 adrenergic **Weak** — GABA$_A$, benzodiazepine receptor, beta-adrenergic
Paliperidone	**High** — dopamine D_2, serotonin 5-HT$_{2A}$ **Low to moderate** — alpha-adrenergic, histamine H_1
Quetiapine	Serotonin 5-HT$_{1A}$, 5-HT$_2$, dopamine D_1, D_2, alpha-1 and -2 adrenergic, histamine H_1
Risperidone	**High** — dopamine D_2, serotonin 5-HT$_2$ **Low to moderate** — 5-HT$_{1C}$, 5-HT$_{1D}$, 5-HT$_{1A}$, histamine H_1, alpha-adrenergic **Weak** — dopamine D_1, haloperidol-sensitive sigma site
Ziprasidone	**High** — dopamine D_2, D_3, 5-HT$_{2A}$, 5-HT$_{2C}$, 5-HT$_{1A}$[1], 5-HT$_{1D}$, alpha-1 adrenergic **Moderate** — histamine H_1

[a] Promethazine is classified as a phenothiazine but not indicated as an antipsychotic.
[b] Partial agonist activity.

Conventional (typical) antipsychotics can be grouped into several classes; the phenothiazines, structurally related thioxanthenes, butyrophenones (phenylbutylpiperadines), diphenylbutylpiperadines, and the indolones. As a group, these agents are dopamine receptor antagonists with a higher affinity for D_2 over D_1 receptors. They exhibit varying degrees of selectivity among the cortical dopamine tracts: nigrostriatal (movement disorders), mesolimbic (relief of hallucinations and delusions), mesocortical (relief of psychosis, worsening of negative symptoms) or tuberoinfundibular (prolactin release). They also bind with varying affinities to nondopaminergic sites, such as cholinergic, alpha-1 adrenergic and histaminic receptors, which can partially explain the varied side effect profiles for each agent. Typical antipsychotics are likely to induce extrapyramidal side effects (EPS) and have similar efficacies when used in equipotent doses. Lower-potency agents tend to be more sedating and high-potency agents usually have a higher incidence of acute EPS.

Novel (atypical) antipsychotics were introduced with the development of **clozapine** and can be structurally classified as dibenzepines, benzisoxazoles, benzoisothiazol, or quinolinone. As a group, they have diverse pharmacodynamic profiles differing considerably from the typical antipsychotics, but in general have an increased affinity for serotonin 5-HT$_2$ receptors compared with D_2 receptors. They act on several neurotransmitter systems, including antagonism at 1 or more types of dopamine receptors (eg, D_1, D_2, D_4, D_5); selectivity for limbic dopamine receptors; antagonism at 1 or more types of serotonin receptors (eg, 5-HT$_1$, 5-HT$_2$); antagonism at alpha-1 adrenergic receptors; and activity at muscarinic or histamine H_1 receptors. They are considered atypical because of their decreased ability or inability to induce EPS; newer agents also have a decreased propensity to induce agranulocytosis compared with clozapine. Studies indicate that some atypical agents are effective in patients resistant to conventional antipsychotic therapy and may be more effective in relieving negative symptoms than conventional agents.

Pharmacological Parameters of Antipsychotics

Antipsychotic agent	Approx. equiv. dose (mg)	Usual oral adult daily dose range (mg)	Sedation	EPS	Anticholinergic effects	Orthostatic hypotension	Weight gain
Phenothiazines							
Aliphatic							
Chlorpromazine	100	30 to 800	+++	++	++	+++	
Piperazine							
Fluphenazine	2	1 to 40	+	++++	+	+	
Perphenazine	10	12 to 64	++	++	+	+	
Prochlorperazine		15 to 150					
Trifluoperazine	5	2 to 15	+	+++	+	+	
Piperidines							
Thioridazine	100	150 to 800	+++	+	+++	+++	
Thioxanthenes							
Thiothixene	4	6 to 60	+	+++	+	+	
Phenylbutylpiperadines							
Butyrophenone							
Haloperidol	2	1 to 100	+	++++	+	+	
Diphenylbutylpiperadine							
Pimozide		1 to 10	+	+++	++	+	
Dibenzepines							
Dibenzoxazepines							
Asenapine		10 to 20	++	+	0 to +	++	+
Loxapine	10	20 to 250	+	++	+	+	
Dibenzodiazepine							
Clozapine	50	300 to 900	+++	0	+++	+++	++++
Thienbenzodiazepine							
Olanzapine		5 to 20	++	+	++	++	++++
Dibenzothiazepine							
Quetiapine		50 to 800	++	0	0 to +	++	+++
Benzisoxazole							
Iloperidone		12 to 24	++	+	+	++	+
Ziprasidone		40-200	++	++	+	++	+
Paliperidone		3 to 12	+		0 to +		

Pharmacological Parameters of Antipsychotics							
Antipsychotic agent	Approx. equiv. dose (mg)	Usual oral adult daily dose range (mg)	Sedation	EPS	Anticholinergic effects	Orthostatic hypotension	Weight gain
Risperidone		4 to 16	+	++	0 to +	++	+++
Benzoisothazol							
Lurasidone		40 to 80	+	+++	0	+	++
Quinolinone							
Aripiprazole		10 to 30	+	0	0 to +	+	+

++++ = Very high incidence of side effects, +++ = High incidence of side effects, ++ = Moderate incidence of side effects, + = Low incidence of side effects

➤*Pharmacokinetics:*

Metabolism – CYP2D6 is the enzyme responsible for metabolism of many antipsychotics. CYP2D6 is subject to genetic polymorphism and to inhibition by a variety of substrates and some nonsubstrates. Extensive CYP2D6 metabolizers convert drugs rapidly, whereas poor metabolizers convert the drugs much more slowly.

Special populations –

Renal function impairment:

• *Aripiprazole* – In patients with severe renal impairment (creatinine clearance [CrCl] less than 30 mL/min), **aripiprazole** and dehydro-aripiprazole maximum plasma concentration (C_{max}) increased 36% and 53%, respectively. Area under the curve (AUC) decreased 15% for aripiprazole and increased 7% for dehydro-aripiprazole.

• *Iloperidone* – $AUC_{0-\infty}$ was increased by 24%, decreased by 6%, and increased by 52% for iloperidone, P88, and P95, respectively, in patients with renal impairment.

• *Lurasidone* – After administration of a single dose of **lurasidone** 40 mg to patients with mild, moderate, and severe renal impairment, mean C_{max} increased by 40%, 92%, and 54%, respectively, and mean $AUC_{(0-\infty)}$ increased by 53%, 91%, and 2 times, respectively, compared with healthy matched subjects.

• *Quetiapine* – Patients with severe renal failure (CrCl 10 to 30 mL/min/1.73 m^2) had a 25% lower mean oral clearance than healthy subjects (CrCl greater than 80 mL/min/1.73m^2); however, plasma concentrations were within the same range.

• *Paliperidone* – In patients with moderate to severe renal function impairment, clearance was reduced 64% and 71%, respectively. The mean terminal elimination half-life was 40 and 51 hours, respectively. Reduce dose in moderate or severe renal function impairment patients.

• *Ziprasidone* – IM **ziprasidone** has not been fully evaluated in renal impairment; however, the cyclodextrin excipient is cleared renally. Therefore, administer IM formulation with caution in these patients.

• *Risperidone* – In patients with moderate to severe renal disease, clearance of the sum of **risperidone** and its active metabolite decreased 60%. Reduce dose in renal function impairment.

Hepatic function impairment:

• *Aripiprazole* – AUC increased 31% in mild, 8% in moderate, and decreased 20% in severe hepatic function impairment.

• *Asenapine* – Severe hepatic impairment exposure was 7 times higher than in healthy patients.

• *Lurasidone* – In a single-dose study of **lurasidone** 20 mg, mean $AUC_{(0-last)}$ was 1.5 times higher in subjects with mild hepatic impairment (Child-Pugh class A), 1.7 times higher in subjects with moderate hepatic impairment (Child-Pugh class B), and 3 times higher in subjects with severe hepatic impairment (Child-Pugh class C) compared with the values for healthy matched subjects. Mean C_{max} was 1.3, 1.2, and 1.3 times higher for mild, moderate, and severe hepatically impaired patients respectively, compared with the values for healthy matched subjects.

• *Quetiapine* – Mean oral clearance decreased 30% in patients with hepatic impairment and AUC and C_{max} increased by 3 times. Dosage adjustment may be needed.

• *Ziprasidone* – In patients with clinically significant cirrhosis (Child-Pugh class A and B), an increase in AUC of 13% and 34% occurred, respectively, and half-life was 7.1 hours compared with 4.8 hours in healthy subjects.

• *Risperidone* – The mean free fraction in plasma was increased by about 35% because of the diminished concentration of albumin and alpha-acid glycoprotein. Reduce dose in hepatic impairment.

Elderly:

• *Aripiprazole* – Clearance decreased 20% after a single 15 mg dose in patients 65 years of age or older.

• *Asenapine* – Clearance decreased, increasing exposure by 30% in elderly patients.

• *Quetiapine* – Oral clearance decreased 40% in patients 65 years of age or older. A dosage adjustment may be necessary.

• *Risperidone* – Renal clearance of **risperidone** and its active metabolite were decreased. Modify dose accordingly.

• *Olanzapine* – Mean elimination half-life was about 1.5 times greater in patients 65 years of age or older.

Gender:

• *Aripiprazole* – C_{max} and AUC of **aripiprazole** and dehydro-aripiprazole are 30% to 40% higher in women, and correspondingly, the oral clearance is lower in women. These differences are largely explained by differences in body weight.

• *Lurasidone* – Mean AUC of **lurasidone** was 18% higher in women than in men, and correspondingly, the apparent oral clearance was lower in women.

• *Olanzapine* – Clearance is approximately 30% lower in women.

Race:

• *Olanzapine* – Comparisons between study data collected in Japan versus the United States suggest exposure to **olanzapine** could be about 2-fold greater in Japanese patients when equivalent doses are administered.

Smoking:

• *Olanzapine* – Clearance is about 40% higher in smokers.

Antipsychotic Pharmacokinetics[a]

Drug	Bioavailability	Mean C_{max}	T_{max}	Mean Vd	Protein bound (%)	Routes of metabolism	Active metabolite	t½	Routes of excretion
Conventional agents									
Chlorpromazine	20% to 40%	25 to 150 ng/mL	1 to 4 h	≈ 21 L/kg	92% to 97%			24 h	
Fluphenazine	2.7% (oral); 3.4% (SC/IM)	≈ 2.3 ng/mL (oral); 1.3 ng/mL (SC/IM)	≈ 2.8 h (oral); 24 to 48 h (SC/IM)	20 L/kg				18 h (oral)	
Haloperidol	60% to 65% (oral)	≈ 9.2 ng/mL (oral): ≈ 22 ng/mL (IM)	6 days (decanoate)	≈ 18 L/kg	≈ 92%			≈ 18 h (oral); ≈ 3 wk (decanoate)	Feces, urine (≈ 1%)
Loxapine	≈ 100%							8 h	Urine, feces
Molindone			1.5 h					12 h	Urine, feces
Perphenazine	20%	984 pg/mL	1 to 3 h	10 to 34 L/kg		Sulfoxidation, hydroxylation, dealkylation, and glucuronidation by CYP2D6		9 to 12 h	
Pimozide	> 50%	≈ 10 ng/mL	4 to 12 h	≈ 28 L/kg[b]	99%	N-dealkylation by CYP3A and CYP1A2 to a lesser extent		≈ 55 h	Urine (main route)
Prochlorperazine				20 L/kg				3 to 5 h (oral); 6.9 h (IV)	
Promethazine[c]			2 to 3 h	13 L/kg	76% to 80%	N-demethylation and sulfoxidation		5 to 14 h	Urine, bile
Thioridazine				18 L/kg	99%		Mesoridazine	24 h	
Thiothixene								34 h	
Trifluoperazine								18 h	

Antipsychotic Pharmacokinetics[a]									
Drug	Bioavailability	Mean C_{max}	T_{max}	Mean Vd	Protein bound (%)	Routes of metabolism	Active metabolite	t½	Routes of excretion
Atypical agents									
Aripiprazole	87%	3 to 5 h		4.9 L/kg[b]	> 99%[d]	Dehydrogenation, hydroxylation, and N-dealkylation by CYP3A4 and CYP2D6	Dehydro-aripiprazole	75[e] to 146[f] h	Feces (≈ 55%), urine (≈ 25%)
Asenapine	35%	≈ 4 ng/mL	0.5 to 1.5 h	20 to 25 L/kg	95%	Glucuronidation by UGT1A4 and oxidation by CYP1A2	N+ glucuronide	≈ 24 h	Urine (≈ 50%), feces (≈ 40%)
Clozapine	27% to 47%	319 ng/mL[b]	2.5 h	≈ 5.4 L/kg	≈ 97%	Demethylation, hydroxylation, and N-oxidation	Desmethyl metabolite has limited activity	8 h[g], 12 h[b]	Urine (≈ 50%), feces (≈ 30%)
Iloperidone	96%		2 to 4 h	1,340 to 2,800 L	≈ 95%	Carbonyl reduction, hydroxylation, and o-demethylation by CYP2D6 and CYP3A4	P 95 and P 88	≈ 18 h[e] ≈ 33 h[f]	Urine (58.2%[e]) (45.1%[f]), feces (19.9%[e]) (22.1%[f])
Lurasidone	9% to 19%		1 to 3 h	6,173 L	99%	Oxidative N-dealkylation, hydroxylation, S-oxidation by CYP3A4	ID-14283 and ID-14326	18 h	Feces (80%), urine (9%)
Olanzapine	≈ 60%	≈ 12.9 ng/mL	≈ 6 h	≈ 1,000 L	93% over a concentration range of 7-1100 ng/mL	Glucuronidation and oxidation by CYP1A2 and CYP2D6		21 to 54 h (oral); 30 days (ER injection)	Urine (≈ 57%), feces (≈ 30%)
Paliperidone	28%		24 h 13 days (IM)	487 L	74%	Dealkylation, hydroxylation, dehydrogenation, benzisoxazole scission		23 h 25 to 49 days (IM)	Urine ≈ 80%, feces ≈11%
Quetiapine	≥ 73%	778 to 1,080 mcg/L	1.5 h	≈ 10 L/kg	83%[c]	Sulfoxidation and oxidation by CYP3A4	None	≈ 6 h	Urine (≈ 73%), feces (≈20%)
Risperidone	70%	10 ng/mL	≈ 1 h	1 to 2 L/kg	90%	Hydroxylation by CYP2D6 and N-dealkylation	9-hydroxy-risperidone	3[e] to 20[f] h	Urine (≈ 70%), feces (≈ 14%)
Ziprasidone	≈ 60% (oral); 100% (IM)	44.6 to 139.4 mcg/L	6 to 8 h (oral); ≈ 60 min (IM)	1.5 L/kg	> 99%	Reduction by aldehyde oxidase, methylation, and oxidation by CYP3A4 and CYP1A2 to a lesser extent		≈ 7 h (oral); 2-5 h (IM)	Feces (≈ 66%), urine (≈ 20%)

[a] T_{max} = time to reach maximum concentration; t½ = half-life; SC = subcutaneous.
[b] At steady-state.
[c] Promethazine is classified as a phenothiazine but not indicated as an antipsychotic.
[d] At therapeutic concentrations.
[e] Extensive metabolizers.
[f] Poor metabolizers.
[g] Single dose.

Contraindications

Hypersensitivity to drug or any other component of the product (cross-sensitivity between phenothiazines may occur); comatose or greatly depressed states because of CNS depressants or from any other cause (phenothiazines, **clozapine**, **loxapine**, **molindone**, **pimozide**, **haloperidol**); coadministration with other drugs that prolong the QT interval and in patients with congenital long QT syndrome or history of cardiac arrhythmias (**thioridazine**, **pimozide**, **ziprasidone**; see Drug Interactions).

➤*Phenothiazines:* Suspected or established subcortical brain damage (**fluphenazine**); blood dyscrasias (**perphenazine**, **trifluoperazine**, **fluphenazine**); bone marrow depression (**perphenazine**, **trifluoperazine**, **fluphenazine**); preexisting liver damage (**perphenazine**, **trifluoperazine**, **fluphenazine**); pediatric surgery (**prochlorperazine**); hypertensive or hypotensive heart disease of extreme degree (**thioridazine**).

➤*Thiothixene:* Circulatory collapse; blood dyscrasias.

➤*Haloperidol:* Parkinson disease.

➤*Lurasidone:* Coadministration with strong CYP3A4 inhibitors (eg, ketoconazole) and strong CYP3A4 inducers (eg, rifampin).

➤*Pimozide:* Treatment of simple tics or tics other than those associated with Tourette disorder; in combination with drugs (eg, pemoline, methylphenidate, amphetamines) that may themselves cause motor or phonic tics until it is determined whether or not the drugs, rather than Tourette disorder, are responsible for the tics. (See also Drug Interactions.)

➤*Paliperidone:* Hypersensitivity to **risperidone**.

➤*Clozapine:* Myeloproliferative disorders; uncontrolled epilepsy; history of **clozapine**-induced agranulocytosis or severe granulocytopenia; should not be used with other agents having a well-known potential to cause agranulocytosis or suppress bone marrow function.

➤*Ziprasidone:* Recent acute myocardial infarction (MI); uncompensated heart failure.

Warnings/Precautions

➤*Increased mortality in elderly patients with dementia-related psychosis:* See boxed warning for more information.

➤*Postinjection delirium/sedation syndrome:* See boxed warning for more information.

➤*Tardive dyskinesia:* Tardive dyskinesia (TD), a syndrome consisting of potentially irreversible, involuntary dyskinetic movements, may develop in patients treated with antipsychotic drugs. Although prevalence of TD appears highest among elderly patients, especially women, it is impossible to rely on prevalence estimates to predict, at the inception of antipsychotic treatment, which patients are likely to develop the syndrome. Whether antipsychotic drugs differ in their potential to cause TD is unknown. However, atypical antipsychotics appear to have a lower risk of TD. Both the risk of developing TD and the likelihood that it will become irreversible are increased as duration of treatment and total cumulative dose administered increase. However, the syndrome can develop, although much less commonly, after relatively brief treatment periods at low doses.

There is no known treatment for established cases of TD, although it may remit, partially or completely, if antipsychotics are withdrawn. Antipsychotic treatment itself, however, may suppress (or partially suppress) signs and symptoms of TD, possibly masking the underlying disease process. The effect of symptomatic suppression on the long-term course of the syndrome is unknown.

Given these considerations, prescribe antipsychotics in a manner most likely to minimize the occurrence of TD. In general, reserve chronic antipsychotic treatment for patients who suffer from a chronic illness that responds to antipsychotic drugs and for whom alternative, equally effective, but potentially less harmful treatments are not available or appropriate. In patients who require chronic treatment, use the smallest dose and the shortest duration of treatment producing a satisfactory clinical response. Periodically reassess the need for continued treatment.

If signs and symptoms of TD appear, consider drug discontinuation. However, some patients may require treatment despite the presence of the syndrome.

➤*Extrapyramidal symptoms:* Dystonic reactions develop primarily with the use of traditional antipsychotics. EPS has occurred during the administration of **haloperidol** and **pimozide** frequently, often during the first few days of treatment. EPS during the administration of haloperidol have been reported frequently, often during the first few days of treatment. EPS can be categorized generally as Parkinson symptoms, akathisia, or dystonia (including opisthotonos and oculogyric crisis). While all can occur at relatively low doses, they occur more frequently and with greater severity at higher doses. The symptoms may be controlled with dose reductions or administration of antiparkinson drugs such as benztropine mesylate or trihexyphenidyl HCl. It should be noted that persistent EPS has been reported; the drug may have to be discontinued in such cases.

➤*Neuroleptic malignant syndrome:* A potentially fatal symptom complex sometimes referred to as neuroleptic malignant syndrome (NMS) has been reported in association with administration of antipsychotic drugs. NMS has been reported with **asenapine** use and 2 possible cases (0.1%) have been reported in clinical trials with **quetiapine**. Clinical manifestations of NMS are hyperpyrexia, muscle rigidity, altered mental status, and evidence of autonomic instability (irregular pulse or blood pressure [BP], tachycardia, diaphoresis, cardiac dysrhythmia). Additional signs may include elevated creatine phosphokinase, myoglobinuria (rhabdomyolysis), and acute renal failure. The onset may be after hours to months of treatment or may occur after discontinuation of therapy. Once started, NMS proceeds rapidly over 24 to 72 hours.

The risk of NMS is higher in patients receiving high-potency, injectable, or depot antipsychotics. NMS may occur with atypical antipsychotics, but the risk is lower. There have been several reported cases of NMS in patients receiving **clozapine** alone or in combination with lithium or other CNS-active agents. The diagnostic evaluation of patients with this syndrome is complicated. In arriving at a diagnosis, it is important to exclude cases where the clinical presentation includes both serious medical illness (eg, pneumonia, systemic infection) and untreated or inadequately treated EPS. Other important considerations in the differential diagnosis include central anticholinergic toxicity, heat stroke, drug fever, and primary CNS pathology.

Include the following in the management of NMS: 1) immediate discontinuation of antipsychotic drugs and other drugs not essential to concurrent therapy; 2) intensive symptomatic treatment and medical monitoring; and 3) treatment of any concomitant serious medical problems for which specific treatments are available. There is no general agreement about specific pharmacological treatment regimens for NMS.

If a patient requires antipsychotic drug treatment after recovery from NMS, carefully consider the potential reintroduction of drug therapy. Carefully monitor the patient because recurrences of NMS have been reported.

➤*CNS effects:* Use cautiously in depressed patients. Use with caution in agitated states with depression (particularly if a suicidal tendency is recognized). When **haloperidol** is used for mania in cyclic disorders, a rapid mood swing to depression may occur.

Encephalopathic syndrome – An encephalopathic syndrome (characterized by weakness, lethargy, fever, tremulousness and confusion, extrapyramidal symptoms, leukocytosis, elevated serum enzymes, serum urea nitrogen [BUN], fasting blood sugar) has occurred in a few patients treated with lithium plus an antipsychotic (**haloperidol**). In some instances, the syndrome was followed by irreversible brain damage. Because of a possible causal relationship between these events and the coadministration of lithium and antipsychotics, closely monitor patients receiving such combined therapy for early evidence of neurologic toxicity and promptly discontinue treatment if such signs appear. This encephalopathic syndrome may be similar to or the same as NMS.

➤*Cardiovascular effects:* Use with caution in patients with cardiovascular disease (history of MI or ischemic heart disease, heart failure, or conduction abnormalities), cerebrovascular disease, conditions that would predispose patients to hypotension (dehydration, hypovolemia, and treatment with antihypertensive medications), or mitral insufficiency. Increased pulse rates occur in most patients. Large doses and parenteral administration should be avoided in patients with impaired cardiovascular systems. To minimize the occurrence of hypotension after injection, keep patient lying down and observe for at least 30 minutes. One result of therapy may be an increase in mental and physical activity. For example, a few patients with angina pectoris have complained of increased pain while taking **trifluoperazine**. Therefore, withdraw the drug from patients with angina if an unfavorable response is noted.

Electrocardiogram changes – A minority of **clozapine** patients experience electrocardiogram (ECG) repolarization changes similar to those seen with other antipsychotic drugs, including S-T segment depression and flattening or inversion of T waves, all of which normalize after discontinuation of clozapine. The clinical significance is unclear. However, several patients have experienced significant cardiac events, including ischemic changes, MI, arrhythmias, and sudden death. In addition, there have been postmarketing reports of congestive heart failure (CHF), pericarditis, and pericardial effusions. Causality assessment was difficult in many of these cases because of serious preexisting cardiac disease and plausible alternative causes. Rare instances of sudden death have been reported in psychiatric patients, with or without associated antipsychotic drug treatment, and the relationship of these events to antipsychotic drug use is unknown.

Paliperidone, **iloperidone**, **asenapine**, **ziprasidone**, **pimozide**, and **thioridazine** have been shown to prolong the QT interval, and drugs with this potential have been associated with torsades de pointes–type arrhythmias and sudden death. Certain circumstances may increase the risk of torsades de pointes and/or sudden death in association with the use of drugs that prolong the QT interval, including the following: 1) bradycardia; 2) hypokalemia or hypomagnesemia; 3) concomitant use of other drugs that prolong the QT interval; and 4) presence of congenital prolongation of the QT interval. Perform a baseline ECG and measure serum potassium and magnesium before initiation of treatment and periodically during treatment, especially during a period of dose adjustment. Patients with QT interval over 450 msec should not receive **thioridazine**. **Paliperidone** should be avoided in patients with congenital long QT syndrome and in patients with a history of cardiac arrhythmias. **Ziprasidone** should be avoided in patients with histories of significant cardiovascular illness (eg, QT prolongation, recent acute MI, uncompensated heart failure, cardiac arrhythmia). Low serum potassium and/or magnesium should be replaced with those electrolytes in patients before proceeding with treatment. Discontinue treatment if the QT interval is longer than 500 msec. Patients who experience symptoms that may be associated with the occurrence of torsades de pointes (eg, dizziness, palpitations, syncope) may warrant further cardiac evaluation; in particular, consider Holter monitoring. (See Black Box Warning, Contraindications, and Drug Interactions).

Nonspecific ECG changes, usually reversible Q- and T-wave distortions, have been observed in some patients receiving phenothiazines. Nonspecific ECG changes have been observed in some patients receiving **thiothixene**. These changes are usually reversible and frequently disappear on continued thiothixene therapy. The incidence of these changes is lower than that observed with some phenothiazines. The clinical significance of these changes is not known.

Haloperidol has been associated with ECG changes, including QT interval prolongation and ECG pattern changes compatible with the polymorphous configuration of torsades de pointes.

Rare, transient, nonspecific T-wave changes have been reported on ECG in patients taking **molindone**.

Prolongation of the QT interval and torsades de pointes have been reported with risperidone overdoses.

Other drugs that prolong the QT interval have been associated with the occurrence of torsades de pointes. Bradycardia, electrolyte imbalance, concomitant use with other drugs that prolong QT, or the presence of congenital prolongation in QT can increase the risk.

Myocarditis – Postmarketing **clozapine** surveillance data from 4 countries revealed cases of myocarditis, some fatal. The rate of myocarditis in clozapine-treated patients appears to be 17 to 322 times greater than the general population and is associated with an increased risk of fatal myocarditis that is 14 to 161 times greater than the general population. Therefore, consider the possibility of myocarditis in patients receiving clozapine who present with unexplained fatigue, dyspnea, tachypnea, fever, chest pain, palpitations, other signs or symptoms of heart failure, or ECG findings such as ST-T wave abnormalities or arrhythmias. It is not known whether eosinophilia is a reliable predictor of myocarditis. Tachycardia, which has been associated with clozapine treatment, also has been noted as a presenting sign in patients with myocarditis. Therefore, tachycardia during the first month of therapy warrants close monitoring for other signs of myocarditis. Prompt discontinuation of clozapine treatment is warranted upon suspicion of myocarditis. Patients with clozapine-related myocarditis should not be rechallenged with clozapine.

Cardiomyopathy – Cases of cardiomyopathy have been reported in patients treated with **clozapine**. Approximately 80% of clozapine-treated patients in whom cardiomyopathy was reported were younger than 50 years of age; the duration of treatment with clozapine prior to cardiomyopathy diagnosis varied, but was more than 6 months in 65% of the reports. Dilated cardiomyopathy was most frequently reported. Signs and symptoms suggestive of cardiomyopathy, particularly exertional dyspnea, fatigue, orthopnea, paroxysmal nocturnal dyspnea, and peripheral edema should alert the clinician to perform further investigations. If the diagnosis of cardiomyopathy is confirmed, discontinue clozapine unless the benefit to the patient clearly outweighs the risk.

Pulmonary embolism – Consider the possibility of pulmonary embolism in patients receiving **clozapine** who present with deep vein thrombosis (DVT), acute dyspnea, chest pain, or with other respiratory signs and symptoms. DVT also has been observed in association with clozapine therapy. Whether pulmonary embolus can be attributed to clozapine or some characteristics of its users is not clear, but the occurrence of DVT or respiratory symptomatology should suggest its presence.

Hypotension – Orthostatic hypotension with or without syncope can occur, especially during initial titration in association with rapid dose escalation, and may represent a continuing risk in some patients. In 1 report, initial **clozapine** doses as low as 12.5 mg were associated with collapse and respiratory arrest.

Patients taking **asenapine** may experience orthostatic hypotension and syncope early in treatment because of its alpha-1 adrenergic antagonist activity.

Severe, acute hypotension has occurred with the use of phenothiazines and is particularly likely to occur in patients with mitral insufficiency or pheochromocytoma. Rebound hypertension may occur in pheochromocytoma patients.

Carefully watch patients who are undergoing surgery and patients who are on large doses of phenothiazines, for hypotensive phenomena. It may be necessary to reduce amounts of anesthetics or CNS depressants. The hypotensive effects may occur after the first injection of the antipsychotic, occasionally after subsequent injections, and rarely after the first oral dose.

Recovery is usually spontaneous and symptoms disappear within 0.5 to 2 hours. If hypotension occurs, place the patient in a recumbent position. Women have a greater tendency to experience orthostatic hypotension. Patients with hypovolemia have increased sensitivity to the hypotensive effects of these agents. Volume replacement, when needed, should precede use of vasopressors. If a vasopressor is indicated, use phenylephrine or norepinephrine. Avoid using epinephrine in drug-induced hypotension (see Drug Interactions).

Tachycardia – Tachycardia, which may be sustained, also has been observed in approximately 25% of patients taking **clozapine**, with an average increase in pulse rate of 10 to 15 bpm. The sustained tachycardia is not simply a reflex response to hypotension, and is present in all positions monitored. Either tachycardia or hypotension may pose a serious risk for an individual with compromised cardiovascular function. Pulse rates have increased in most patients receiving antipsychotics.

➤*Cerebrovascular effects:* Cerebrovascular adverse events (eg, stroke, transient ischemic attack), including fatalities, were reported in elderly patients with dementia-related psychosis (mean, 85 years of age; range, 73 to 97 years of age) enrolled in trials of **risperidone**, **aripiprazole**, **asenapine**, and **olanzapine**. In placebo-controlled trials, there was a significantly higher incidence of cerebrovascular adverse events in patients treated with **risperidone**, **aripiprazole**, and **olanzapine** compared with patients treated with placebo. See Black box warning for more information.

➤*Sudden death:* Sudden, unexpected, and unexplained deaths have been reported in psychotic patients receiving phenothiazines. Previous brain damage or seizures may be predisposing factors; avoid high doses in known seizure patients. Several patients have shown sudden flare-ups of psychotic behavior patterns shortly before death. In some cases, death was apparently caused by cardiac arrest; in others, asphyxia was caused by failure of the cough reflex. Autopsy findings usually reveal acute fulminating pneumonia or pneumonitis, aspiration of gastric contents, or intramyocardial lesions. In some patients, cause could not be determined.

Sudden, unexpected deaths have occurred in experimental studies of **pimozide** in conditions other than Tourette disorder. These deaths occurred while patients were receiving pimozide dosages in the range of 1 mg/kg. One possible mechanism for such deaths is prolongation of the QT interval predisposing patients to ventricular arrhythmia.

➤*Priapism:* Rare cases of priapism have been associated with **risperidone**, **ziprasidone**, **quetiapine**, **aripiprazole**, and **olanzapine**. While the relationship of the event to these antipsychotics has not been established, other drugs with alpha-adrenergic blocking effects have been reported to induce priapism. Severe priapism may require surgical intervention.

➤*Hyperprolactinemia:* Antipsychotic drugs elevate prolactin levels; the elevation persists during chronic administration. However, in contrast to more typical antipsychotic drugs, **clozapine** therapy produces little or no prolactin elevation. Drugs that antagonize dopamine D_2 receptors elevate prolactin levels. Experiments indicate that approximately 33% of human breast cancers are prolactin-dependent in vitro, a factor of potential importance if the prescription of these drugs is contemplated in a patient with previously detected breast cancer.

Disturbances such as galactorrhea, amenorrhea, gynecomastia, and impotence have been reported with prolactin-elevating compounds. Longstanding hyperprolactinemia when associated with hypogonadism may lead to decreased bone density in both female and male patients.

Risperidone, **ziprasidone**, **asenapine**, **lurasidone**, **paliperidone**, and **olanzapine** elevate prolactin levels. As is common with compounds that increase prolactin release, an increase in pituitary gland, mammary gland, and pancreatic islet cell hyperplasia or neoplasia was observed in risperidone carcinogenicity studies conducted in mice and rats. An increase in mammary gland neoplasia was observed in the olanzapine and ziprasidone carcinogenicity studies conducted in mice and in the olanzapine studies in rats.

Elevated prolactin levels were not demonstrated in clinical trials with **quetiapine**. However, increased prolactin levels were observed in rats studied with this compound.

➤*Hyperglycemia and diabetes mellitus:* Hyperglycemia, in some cases extreme and associated with ketoacidosis or hyperosmolar coma or death, has been reported in patients treated with atypical antipsychotics. Assessment of the relationship between atypical antipsychotic use and glucose abnormalities is complicated by the possibility of an increased background risk of diabetes mellitus in patients with schizophrenia and the increasing incidence of diabetes mellitus in the general population. Given these confounders, the relationship between atypical antipsychotic use and hyperglycemia-related adverse events is not completely understood. However, epidemiological studies suggest an increased risk of treatment-emergent hyperglycemia-related adverse events in patients treated with atypical antipsychotics. Precise risk estimates for hyperglycemia-related adverse events in patients treated with atypical antipsychotics are not available.

Regularly monitor for worsening of glucose control in patients with an established diagnosis of diabetes mellitus who are started on atypical antipsychotics. Ensure that patients with risk factors for diabetes mellitus (eg, obesity, family history of diabetes) who are starting treatment with atypical antipsychotics undergo fasting blood glucose testing at baseline and periodically during treatment. Monitor any patient treated with atypical antipsychotics for symptoms of hyperglycemia, including polydipsia, polyuria, polyphagia, and weakness. Ensure that patients who develop symptoms of hyperglycemia during treatment with atypical antipsychotics undergo fasting blood glucose testing. In some cases, hyperglycemia resolved when the atypical antipsychotic was discontinued; however, some patients required continuation of antidiabetic treatment despite discontinuation of the suspect drug.

➤*Antiemetic effects:* Drugs with an antiemetic effect can obscure signs of toxicity of other drugs (eg, cancer chemotherapeutic drugs) or mask symptoms of disease (eg, brain tumor, intestinal obstruction, Reye syndrome). They can suppress the cough reflex; aspiration of vomitus is possible.

Paliperidone, **risperidone**, **thiothixene**, **loxapine**, and **molindone** have an antiemetic effect in animals that may also occur in humans.

➤*Pulmonary:* Cases of bronchopneumonia (some fatal) have followed the use of antipsychotic agents. Lethargy and decreased sensation of thirst caused by central inhibition may lead to dehydration, hemoconcentration, and reduced pulmonary ventilation. If these signs appear, especially in elderly patients, institute remedial therapy promptly.

Use with caution in respiratory impairment caused by acute pulmonary infections or chronic respiratory disorders, such as severe asthma or emphysema. "Silent pneumonias" may develop in patients treated with **phenothiazines**.

➤*GI effects:* Because the **paliperidone** tablet is nondeformable and does not appreciably change in shape in the GI tract, **paliperidone** should not be ordinarily administered to patients with preexisting severe GI narrowing (pathologic or iatrogenic). There have been rare reports of obstructive symptoms in patients with known strictures in association with the ingestion of drugs nondeformable controlled-release formulations. Because of the controlled-release design of the tablet, only use **paliperidone** in patients who are able to swallow the tablet whole.

➤*Agranulocytosis:* Agranulocytosis, defined as an absolute neutrophil count of less than 500/mm^3, occurs in association with **clozapine** use at a cumulative incidence at 1 year of approximately 1.3%, based on 15 cases out of 1,743 patients exposed to clozapine during clinical testing. All of these cases occurred when the need for close monitoring of WBC counts was already recognized. This reaction could prove fatal if not detected early and therapy interrupted. Of the 149 cases of agranulocytosis reported worldwide in association with clozapine use as of December 31, 1989, 32% were fatal. However, few of these deaths occurred since 1977, when knowledge of clozapine-induced agranulocytosis became more widespread, and close monitoring of WBC counts more widely practiced. In the United States, under a weekly WBC monitoring system with clozapine, there have been 585 cases of agranulocytosis as of August 21, 1997; 19 were fatal. During this period 150,409 patients received clozapine. The incidence rates of agranulocytosis based on a weekly monitoring schedule, rose steeply during the first 2 months of therapy, peaking in the third month. Among clozapine patients who continued the drug beyond the third month, the weekly incidence of agranulocytosis fell to a substantial degree, so that by the sixth month, the weekly incidence of agranulocytosis was reduced to 3 per 1,000 person-years. After 6 months, the weekly incidence of agranulocytosis declined still further, however, never reaching zero.

Patients must have a blood sample drawn for a WBC count before initiation of treatment with **clozapine**, and must have subsequent WBC counts done at least weekly for the first 6 months of treatment, as well as for 4 weeks after discontinuation. The distribution of clozapine is contingent on performance of the required blood tests (see Administration and Dosage of individual monograph).

Except for evidence of significant bone marrow suppression during initial **clozapine** therapy, there are no established risk factors for the development of agranulocytosis. However, a disproportionate number of the US cases of agranulocytosis occurred in patients of Jewish background compared with the overall proportion of such patients exposed during clozapine's domestic development. Most of the US cases occurred within 4 to 10 weeks of exposure, but neither dose nor duration is a reliable predictor. No patient characteristics have been clearly linked to the development of agranulocytosis in association with clozapine use, but agranulocytosis associated with other antipsychotic drugs occurred with a greater frequency in women, elderly patients, and in patients who are cachetic or have serious underlying medical illness; such patients may also be at particular risk with clozapine.

In clinical trials, leukopenia/neutropenia have been reported temporally related to **asenapine** use.

To reduce the risk of agranulocytosis developing undetected, **clozapine** will be dispensed only within the clozapine Patient Management System. For more information, call 1-800-448-5938.

➤*Ophthalmic effects:* As with all drugs that exert anticholinergic effect and/or cause mydriasis, use with caution in patients with a history of glaucoma. During prolonged therapy, ocular changes may occur; these include particle deposition in the cornea and lens, progressing in more severe cases to star-shaped lenticular opacities.

Pigmentary retinopathy – Carefully observe for pigmentary retinopathy and lenticular pigmentation (fine lenticular pigmentation has been noted in a small number of patients treated for prolonged periods). Pigmentary retinopathy, which has been observed primarily in patients taking larger than recommended thioridazine doses, is characterized by diminution of visual acuity, brownish coloring of vision, and impairment of night vision; examination of the fundus discloses deposits of pigment.

Cataracts – In dogs receiving **quetiapine** for 6 or 12 months, focal triangular cataracts occurred at the junction of the posterior sutures in the outer cortex of the lens at a dose of 4 times the maximum recommended human dose. The finding may be because of inhibition of cholesterol biosynthesis by quetiapine.

Lens changes have also been observed in patients during long-term treatment, but a causal relationship has not been established. Examination of the lens by methods adequate to detect cataract formation, such as slit-lamp exam, is recommended at initiation of treatment or shortly thereafter, and at 6-month intervals.

➤*Seizure disorders:* Some antipsychotics can lower the convulsive threshold and may precipitate seizures. Grand mal seizures have occurred, particularly in patients with electroencephalogram (EEG) abnormalities or a history of such disorders. Use cautiously in patients with a history of epilepsy, those in a state of alcohol withdrawal, or those with conditions that lower the seizure threshold (eg, Alzheimer dementia). These drugs may be used concomitantly with anticonvulsants; maintain an adequate anticonvulsant dosage (see Drug Interactions).

Seizure has been estimated to occur in association with **clozapine** use at a cumulative incidence at 1 year of approximately 5%, based on the occurrence of 1 or more seizures during its clinical testing prior to domestic marketing. Dose appears to be an important predictor of seizure, with a greater likelihood of seizure at the higher clozapine doses used. Exercise caution in administering clozapine to patients having a history of seizures or other predisposing factors. Because of the substantial risk of seizure associated with clozapine use, advise patients not to engage in any activity in which sudden loss of consciousness could cause serious risk to themselves or others. Caution should also be advised in patients with a history of seizures taking **asenapine**.

➤*GI dysmotility:* Esophageal dysmotility and aspiration have been associated with antipsychotic drug use. Aspiration pneumonia is a common cause of morbidity and mortality in elderly patients, in particular those with advanced Alzheimer dementia. Use **quetiapine**, **paliperidone**, **asenapine**, **ziprasidone**, **risperidone**, **olanzapine**, **aripiprazole**, and others cautiously in patients at risk of aspiration pneumonia. Do not use **lurasidone** in patients at risk of aspiration pneumonia.

➤*Anticholinergic effects:* Use caution in patients with clinically significant prostatic hypertrophy, narrow-angle glaucoma, or a history of paralytic ileus. Anticholinergic effects of **clozapine** are very potent. **Clozapine** use has been associated with varying degrees of impairment of intestinal peristalsis, ranging from constipation to intestinal obstruction, fecal impaction, and paralytic ileus. On rare occasions, these cases have been fatal. Treat constipation initially by ensuring adequate hydration, and use of ancillary therapy such as bulk laxatives. **Olanzapine** exhibits in vitro muscarinic receptor affinity and was associated with constipation, dry mouth, and tachycardia. **Thiothixene** and **chlorpromazine** exhibit rather weak anticholinergic properties. **Risperidone**, **aripiprazole**, **lurasidone**, **paliperidone**, **ziprasidone**, and **quetiapine** have no affinity for cholinergic muscarinic receptors.

➤*Cholesterol:* **Quetiapine**-treated patients had increases from baseline in cholesterol and triglyceride of 11% and 17%, respectively. **Lurasidone** was associated with a mean change in total cholesterol and triglycerides of −4.2 and −13.6 mg/dL at week 24, −1.9 and −3.5 mg/dL at week 36, and −3.6 and −6.5 mg/dL at week 52, respectively.

➤*Concomitant conditions:* Use with caution in patients exposed to extreme heat or phosphorus insecticides, taking atropine or related drugs because of additive anticholinergic effects, in a state of alcohol withdrawal, with dermatoses or other allergic reactions to phenothiazine derivatives because of the possibility of cross-sensitivity, and those who have exhibited idiosyncrasy to other centrally acting drugs.

➤*Hematologic:* Various blood dyscrasias have occurred (see Adverse Reactions). In clinical trials, 1% of **clozapine** patients developed eosinophilia, which, in rare cases, can be substantial. If a differential count reveals a total eosinophil count above 4,000/mm^3, clozapine therapy should be interrupted until eosinophil count falls below 3,000/mm^3. If sore throat or other sign of infection occurs, or if WBC and differential counts indicate cellular depression, stop treatment and institute an antibiotic and other suitable therapy. A single case of transient granulocytopenia has been associated with **mesoridazine**. Patients with bone marrow depression with a phenothiazine should not receive any phenothiazines, unless the potential benefits outweigh the possible hazard.

Ensure that patients with a history of leukopenia, neutropenia, and/or agranulocytosis have a complete blood cell count drawn frequently during the first few months of therapy with **asenapine**. Discontinue **asenapine** if WBC count decreases without other underlying factors.

Routine blood counts are advisable during therapy because blood dyscrasias, including leukopenia, agranulocytosis, thrombocytopenic or nonthrombocytopenic purpura, eosinophilia, and pancytopenia, have been observed with phenothiazine derivatives.

➤*Myelography:* Discontinue phenothiazines at least 48 hours before myelography because of the possibility of seizures; do not resume therapy for at least 24 hours postprocedure. Do not use phenothiazines to control nausea and vomiting occurring before or after myelography.

➤*Thrombotic thrombocytopenic purpura:* A single case of thrombotic thrombocytopenic purpura (TTP) was reported in a 28-year-old woman receiving **risperidone**. She experienced jaundice, fever, and bruising, but eventually recovered after receiving plasmapheresis. The relationship to therapy is unknown.

➤*Parkinson disease/dementia:* Patients with Parkinson disease or dementia with Lewy bodies are reported to have an increased sensitivity to antipsychotic medication. Manifestations of this increased sensitivity include confusion, obtundation, postural instability with frequent falls, EPS, and clinical features consistent with the NMS.

➤*Thyroid:* Severe neurotoxicity (rigidity, inability to walk or talk) may occur in patients with thyrotoxicosis who also are receiving antipsychotics.

Hypothyroidism – **Quetiapine** demonstrated a dose-related decrease in total and free thyroxine (T_4) of approximately 20% at the higher end of the therapeutic dose range that was maximal in the first 2 to 4 weeks of treatment and maintained without adaptation or progression during more chronic therapy. Generally, these changes were of no clinical significance and thyroid-stimulating hormone (TSH) and thyroxine-binding globulin were unchanged in most patients, but approximately 0.4% of quetiapine patients did experience TSH increases. Six of the patients with TSH increases needed replacement thyroid treatment.

➤*Hyperpyrexia:* A significant, not otherwise explained rise in body temperature may indicate intolerance to antipsychotics. Discontinue in this case. Disruption of the body's ability to reduce core body temperature has been attributed to antipsychotic agents. Appropriate care is advised for patients who will be experiencing conditions that may contribute to an elevation in core body temperature (eg, exercising strenuously, exposure to extreme heat, receiving concomitant medication with anticholinergic activity, being subject to dehydration). Heat stroke has been reported with **haloperidol** use.

During **clozapine** therapy, patients may experience transient temperature elevations above 100.4°F (38°C), with the peak incidence within the first 3 weeks of treatment. While this fever is generally benign and self-limiting, it may necessitate discontinuing patients from treatment. On occasion, there may be an associated increase or decrease in WBC count. Carefully evaluate patients with fever to rule out the possibility of an underlying infectious process or the development of agranulocytosis. In the presence of high fever, the possibility of NMS must be considered.

➤*Abrupt withdrawal:* These drugs are not known to cause psychic dependence. However, following abrupt withdrawal of high-dose therapy, symptoms such as gastritis, nausea, vomiting, dizziness, headache, restlessness, sweating, increased salivation, and insomnia have occurred. To lessen the likelihood of adverse reactions related to cumulative drug effects, periodically determine whether the maintenance dosage could be lowered or drug therapy discontinued. These symptoms can be reduced by gradual reduction of the dosage or by continuing antiparkinson agents for several weeks after the antipsychotic is withdrawn.

Some patients on **pimozide** or **haloperidol** maintenance treatment experience transient dyskinetic signs after abrupt withdrawal. This may be indistinguishable from the syndrome of persistent TD except for duration. It is not known whether gradual withdrawal of antipsychotic drugs will reduce the rate of occurrence, but it seems reasonable to gradually withdraw use of the drug.

➤*Suicide:* Suicide remains a possibility in psychotic illnesses and bipolar disorder and close supervision of high-risk patients should accompany drug therapy. Do not allow these patients to have access to large quantities of the drug.

➤*Weight gain:* Weight gain has been observed with atypical antipsychotic use.

➤*Cutaneous pigmentation changes:* Rare instances of skin pigmentation have occurred, primarily in women on long-term, high-dose phenothiazine therapy. These changes, restricted to exposed areas of the skin, range from almost imperceptible darkening to a slate gray color, sometimes with a violet hue. Pigmentation may fade following drug discontinuation.

➤*Phenylketonurics:* Inform phenylketonuric patients that some of these products contain phenylalanine.

➤*Benzyl alcohol:* Some of these products contain benzyl alcohol, which has been associated with a fatal "gasping syndrome" in premature infants.

➤*Hypersensitivity reactions:* Patients who have demonstrated a hypersensitivity reaction (eg, blood dyscrasias, jaundice) with a phenothiazine should not be re-exposed to any phenothiazine unless the potential benefits of treatment outweigh the possible hazards. Angioedema has been observed with **lurasidone**.

➤*Sulfite sensitivity:* Some of these products contain sulfites that may cause allergic-type reactions, including anaphylactic symptoms and life-threatening or less severe asthmatic episodes in certain susceptible persons. The overall prevalence of sulfite sensitivity in the general population is unknown and probably low. It is seen more frequently in asthmatic or atopic nonasthmatic persons.

➤*Renal function impairment:* Administer cautiously to those with diminished renal function. Monitor renal function in long-term therapy; lower the dose or discontinue if BUN becomes abnormal.

➤*Hepatic function impairment:* Jaundice usually occurs between the second and fourth weeks of **phenothiazine** treatment and is regarded as a hypersensitivity reaction. The clinical picture resembles infectious hepatitis with laboratory features of obstructive jaundice. It is usually reversible; however, long-term jaundice has occurred. If fever with flu-like symptoms occurs, perform liver function tests. If tests are abnormal, discontinue treatment. Withhold exploratory laparotomy until extrahepatic obstruction is confirmed. Because of the possibility of liver damage, periodically monitor hepatic function. There is no conclusive evidence that preexisting liver disease makes patients more susceptible to jaundice. Alcoholic patients with cirrhosis have been successfully treated with **chlorpromazine** without complications. Nevertheless, use cautiously in patients with liver disease. Do not re-expose patients who have experienced jaundice to a **phenothiazine**.

Use with caution in patients with impaired hepatic function. Patients with a history of hepatic encephalopathy caused by cirrhosis have increased sensitivity to the CNS effects of antipsychotic drugs (eg, impaired cerebration and abnormal slowing of the EEG).

Iloperidone is not recommended for patients with hepatic impairment. **Asenapine** is not recommended in patients with severe hepatic impairment (Child-Pugh class C).

Elevations of serum transaminase and alkaline phosphatase, usually transient, have been infrequently observed in some patients. No clinically confirmed cases of jaundice attributable to **thiothixene** have been reported.

Caution is advised in patients using **clozapine** who have concurrent hepatic disease. Hepatitis has been reported in patients with healthy liver function and those with preexisting liver function abnormalities. Immediately perform liver function tests in patients who develop nausea, vomiting, and/or anorexia during clozapine treatment. If the elevation of these values is clinically relevant or if symptoms of jaundice occur, discontinue clozapine treatment.

Patients with impaired hepatic function may have increases in the free fraction of **risperidone**, possibly resulting in an enhanced effect.

Six percent of **quetiapine** and 2% of **olanzapine** patients had transaminase elevations more than 3 times the upper limit of normal. Hepatic enzyme elevations usually occurred within the first 3 weeks of quetiapine treatment and promptly returned to prestudy levels with ongoing treatment. Because quetiapine is extensively metabolized by the liver, higher plasma levels are expected in patients with hepatic impairment and dosage adjustment may be needed.

➤*Drug abuse and dependence:* Evaluate patients for history of drug abuse, and observe such patients closely for signs of misuse or abuse (eg, development of tolerance, increases in dose, drug-seeking behavior).

➤*Hazardous tasks:* These agents may impair mental or physical abilities, especially during the first few days. Drowsiness may occur during the first or second week, after which it generally disappears. If troublesome, lower the dosage. Caution patients about performing activities requiring mental alertness until they are reasonably certain that antipsychotic therapy does not adversely affect them.

➤*Photosensitivity:* Because photosensitivity has been reported (rarely with **thioridazine**), advise patients to avoid undue exposure to the sun during phenothiazine treatment.

➤*Pregnancy: Category C; Category B* (**clozapine**, **lurasidone**). Safety for use during pregnancy has not been established. Use only when clearly needed and when potential benefits outweigh potential hazards to the fetus.

There are reported instances of prolonged jaundice, EPS, hyperreflexia or hyporeflexia in newborn infants whose mothers received **phenothiazines**. **Prochlorperazine** is not recommended for use in pregnant patients except in cases of severe nausea and vomiting that are so serious and intractable that drug intervention is required and potential benefits outweigh possible hazards.

Reproductive studies of **chlorpromazine** in rodents have demonstrated potential for embryotoxicity and increased neonatal mortality. Tests in the offspring of the rodent demonstrate decreased performance. The possibility of permanent neurological damage cannot be excluded. It is not recommended that chlorpromazine be given to pregnant patients except when it is essential.

There are reports of cases of limb malformations observed following maternal use of **haloperidol**. Causal relationships were not established in these cases.

Perinatal studies have shown renal papillary abnormalities in offspring of rats treated from mid-pregnancy with **loxapine** doses of 0.6 to 1.8 mg/kg.

In the rat, doses of **pimozide** up to 8 times the maximum human dose resulted in decreased pregnancies and in the retarded development of fetuses. In the rabbit, maternal toxicity, mortality, decreased weight gain, and embryotoxicity including increased resorption were dose-related.

In animal studies, **ziprasidone** and **aripiprazole** demonstrated developmental toxicity, including possible teratogenic effects.

Animal studies of **iloperidone** showed increased early intrauterine deaths, decreased fetal weight and length, decreased fetal skeletal ossification, and an increased incidence of minor fetal skeletal anomalies.

In the rat, dosages of **asenapine** of up to 1.5 mg/kg/day showed increases in postimplantation loss, early pup deaths, and decreases in subsequent pup survival and weight gain.

Placental transfer of **risperidone** occurs in rat pups and studies showed a decrease in the number of live pups and an increase in the number of dead pups at birth, and decrease in birth weight in pups. There was 1 report of a case of agenesis of the corpus callosum in an infant exposed to risperidone in utero. The causal relationship is unknown.

Placental transfer of **olanzapine** occurs in rat pups and studies showed early resorptions and increased numbers of nonviable fetuses.

Animal studies of **quetiapine** showed evidence of embryofetal toxicity, including delays in skeletal ossification, reduced fetal body weights, increased incidence of a minor soft tissue anomaly, increases in fetal and pup death, and decreases in mean litter weight. Evidence of maternal toxicity was also observed at high doses.

Reproductive studies in animals and clinical experience to date have failed to show a teratogenic effect with **thioridazine**, **thiothixene**, **clozapine**, **lurasidone**, and **molindone**.

➤*Lactation:* There is evidence that **phenothiazines** are excreted in the breast milk of breast-feeding mothers. Decide whether to discontinue breast-feeding or the drug, taking into account the importance of the drug to the mother.

Animal studies suggest that **loxapine** (and its metabolites), **paliperidone**, **clozapine**, **lurasidone**, **olanzapine**, **quetiapine**, and **aripiprazole** may be excreted in breast milk. **Risperidone** is excreted in human breast milk. Avoid breast-feeding during **loxapine** therapy if possible. Instruct women receiving **risperidone**, **paliperidone**, **iloperidone**, **asenapine**, **clozapine**, **olanzapine**, **quetiapine**, or **aripiprazole** not to breast-feed.

Infants should not be breast-fed during **haloperidol** or **ziprasidone** treatment.

Because of the tumorigenicity and unknown cardiovascular effects in the infant, decide whether to discontinue breast-feeding or discontinue **pimozide**, taking into account the importance of the drug to the mother.

➤*Children:* Children with acute illnesses (eg, chickenpox, CNS infections, measles, gastroenteritis) or dehydration are much more susceptible to neuromuscular reactions, particularly dystonias, than adults. Children seem more prone to develop extrapyramidal reactions, even at moderate doses. Therefore, use the lowest effective dosage.

EPS can occur and be confused with CNS signs of an undiagnosed primary disease responsible for the vomiting (eg, Reye syndrome or other encephalopathy). Avoid antipsychotics and other potential hepatotoxins in children and adolescents whose signs and symptoms suggest Reye syndrome.

Safety and effectiveness of **fluphenazine**, **asenapine**, **clozapine**, **haloperidol** (decanoate), **loxapine**, **iloperidone**, **lurasidone**, **paliperidone**, **risperidone**, **aripiprazole**, **quetiapine**, and **ziprasidone** in children have not been established.

Olanzapine is not recommended for treatment of bipolar disorder or schizophrenia in children younger than 13 years of age; safety and efficacy not established for use in combination with fluoxetine or for the injection formulations in patients younger than 18 years of age. **Thiothixene**, **perphenazine**, and **molindone** are not recommended in children younger than 12 years of age. Information on the use and efficacy of **pimozide** in patients younger than 12 years of age is limited. **Trifluoperazine** is indicated for the treatment of schizophrenia in children 6 to 12 years of age. When treating children for severe nausea and vomiting, do not use **prochlorperazine** in children weighing less than 9 kg (20 lb) or younger than 2 years of age. **Chlorpromazine** should not be used in children younger than 6 months of age, except where potentially life-saving. Oral **haloperidol** is not intended for children younger than 3 years of age.

➤*Elderly:* Dosages in the lower range are sufficient for most elderly patients. Because these patients appear more susceptible to various cardiovascular, neuromuscular, and anticholinergic reactions, observe patients closely. The prevalence of TD appears to be highest among elderly patients, especially elderly women. Monitor response and adjust dosage accordingly. Increase dosage gradually in elderly patients.

Per the Beers list, **thioridazine** has greater potential for CNS and extrapyramidal adverse effects. Thioridazine is also considered a high-risk medication for elderly patients according to the Centers of Medicare and Medicaid Services.

Drug Interactions

➤*QT prolongation:* An additive effect of **iloperidone** with other drugs that prolong the QT interval cannot be excluded. The following drugs may prolong the QT interval and increase the risk of life-threatening cardiac arrhythmias, including torsades de pointes: antiarrhythmic agents (eg, amiodarone, bretylium, disopyramide, dofetilide, procainamide, quinidine, and sotalol), arsenic trioxide, chlorpromazine, cisapride, dolasetron, droperidol, mefloquine, mesoridazine, moxifloxacin, pentamidine, pimozide, tacrolimus, thioridazine, and ziprasidone. For a more complete list of drugs that may prolong the QT interval, see the appendix, Drug-Induced Prolongation of the QT Interval and Torsades de Pointes.

➤*Cytochrome P450:* Several antipsychotics are metabolized by the cytochrome P450 (CYP-450) enzyme system. Therefore, several drug interactions may be possible involving drugs that are potent inhibitors or inducers of this enzyme system. Monitor and adjust therapy as needed when these antipsychotics are coadministered with potent inhibitors or inducers of the following isoenzymes.

Antipsychotics and Enzymes Involved with Metabolism

Antipsychotic agent	Enzyme(s)
Aripiprazole	CYP3A4, 2D6
Asenapine	CYP1A2, 3A4, 2D6
Clozapine	CYP1A2, 2D6, 3A4
Iloperidone	CYP3A4, 2D6
Lurasidone	CYP3A4
Olanzapine	CYP1A2, 2D6
Perphenazine	CYP2D6
Pimozide	CYP3A, 1A2
Quetiapine	CYP3A4
Risperidone	CYP2D6
Thioridazine	CYP2D6
Ziprasidone	Aldehyde oxidase, CYP3A4, 1A2

Antipsychotic Contraindications

Antipsychotic	Contraindicated with
Clozapine	Drugs having a well-known potential to cause agranulocytosis or suppress bone marrow function.
Phenothiazines	Cisapride, sparfloxacin (because of possible additive QT interval prolongation.
Ziprasidone	Drugs that prolong the QT interval.[a]

Antipsychotic Contraindications

Antipsychotic	Contraindicated with
Pimozide	Drugs that prolong the QT interval;[a] CYP3A inhibitors (eg, clarithromycin, dirithromycin, erythromycin, itraconazole, ketoconazole, nefazodone, protease inhibitors, sertraline, telithromycin, troleandomycin, voriconazole).
Thioridazine	Drugs that prolong the QT interval;[a] CYP2D6 inhibitors (eg, fluoxetine, fluvoxamine, paroxetine, pindolol, propranolol).
Lurasidone	Strong CYP3A4 inhibitors (eg, ketoconazole); strong CYP3A4 inducers (eg, rifampin).

[a] The following drugs may prolong the QT interval and increase the risk of life-threatening cardiac arrhythmias, including torsades de pointes: antiarrhythmic agents (eg, amiodarone, bretylium, disopyramide, dofetilide, procainamide, quinidine, sotalol), arsenic trioxide, chlorpromazine, cisapride, dolasetron mesylate, droperidol, gatifloxacin, halofantrine, levomethadyl acetate, mefloquine, mesoridazine, moxifloxacin, pentamidine, pimozide, probucol, sparfloxacin, tacrolimus, thioridazine, ziprasidone.

Antipsychotic Drug Interactions

Precipitant drug	Object drug[a]		Description
Anticholinergic agents	Haloperidol	↓	Decreased serum concentrations of haloperidol, worsening schizophrenic symptoms, and tardive dyskinesia have been reported with coadministration. Coadminister with caution.
Anticholinergic agents Phenothiazines	Phenothiazines Anticholinergic agents	↑↓	Therapeutic effects of phenothiazines may be decreased by centrally acting anticholinergics. Coadministration may lead to an increase in anticholinergic effects. Coadminister with caution.
Antipsychotic agents	Alcohol CNS depressants	↑	Coadministration may lead to enhanced CNS depression, especially impairment of motor skills. Dystonic reactions may be precipitated by alcohol. Avoid concurrent use or use with caution.
Antipsychotic agents	Antihypertensive agents	↑	May enhance the effects of antihypertensive agents. Antipsychotics produce alpha-adrenergic blockage and may potentiate orthostatic hypotension.
Antipsychotic agents	Dopamine Epinephrine	↓	For the treatment of antipsychotic-induced hypotension, do not use epinephrine, dopamine, or other sympathomimetics with beta-agonist activity because beta stimulation may worsen the hypotension caused by the antipsychotic-induced alpha blockade.
Azole antifungal agents	Haloperidol	↑	Haloperidol plasma concentrations may be elevated, increasing risk of side effects with coadministration. Adjust dose of haloperidol as needed.
Beta-blockers (eg, pindolol, propranolol) Phenothiazines (eg, thioridazine, chlorpromazine)	Phenothiazines (eg, thioridazine, chlorpromazine) Beta-blockers (eg, pindolol, propranolol)	↑	Coadministration may lead to increased effects from either or both drugs, including increased risk of life-threatening arrhythmias with thioridazine. Thioridazine is contraindicated in patients taking pindolol or propranolol.
Caffeine	Clozapine	↑	Plasma levels of clozapine may be increased, resulting in increased adverse effects. Avoid caffeine if interaction is suspected.
Carbamazepine	Aripiprazole Olanzapine Risperidone Ziprasidone	↓	The antipsychotic plasma concentrations may be decreased, resulting in decreased therapeutic effect. Adjust antipsychotic dose as needed. When carbamazepine is added to aripiprazole therapy, double the aripiprazole dose.
Carbamazepine Haloperidol	Haloperidol Carbamazepine	↓ ↑	Therapeutic effects of haloperidol may be decreased. Adjust dose of therapy as needed.
Charcoal	Antipsychotics	↓	Charcoal can decrease the absorption of antipsychotics, reducing their effectiveness or toxicity.
Cimetidine	Quetiapine	↑	Cimetidine decreased quetiapine oral clearance 20%.
Citalopram Fluoxetine Fluvoxamine Sertraline	Clozapine	↑	Plasma levels of clozapine may be increased, resulting in increased pharmacologic and toxic effects. Adjust clozapine dose as needed when starting or stopping certain SSRIs.
Clozapine Loxapine	Benzodiazepines	↑	Cases of orthostatic hypotension, collapse, respiratory arrest, and cardiac arrest have been reported with concomitant use of certain benzodiazepines. Coadminister with caution.
Clozapine	Risperidone	↑	Chronic administration of clozapine with risperidone may decrease risperidone clearance.
CYP1A2 inducers (eg, carbamazepine, omeprazole, rifampin)	Clozapine Olanzapine	↓	May decrease clozapine or olanzapine serum concentrations. May need dosage increase for olanzapine. Carbamazepine increased olanzapine clearance 50%.
CYP1A2 inhibitors (eg, fluvoxamine)	Clozapine Olanzapine	↑	May increase clozapine or olanzapine serum concentrations. Dose reduction may be needed. Fluvoxamine decreased olanzapine clearance, resulting in a mean increase in C_{max} of 54% in nonsmoking women and 77% in smoking men; AUC increased 52% and 108%, respectively.
CYP3A4 inducers (eg, carbamazepine, dexamethasone, phenobarbital, phenytoin, rifampin)	Lurasidone	↓	Coadministration is contraindicated.
CYP3A4 inhibitors (eg, ketoconazole)	Aripiprazole Clozapine Iloperidone Lurasidone Quetiapine Ziprasidone	↑	The plasma concentrations of the antipsychotic may be increased. Reduce aripiprazole and iloperidone dose 50% with coadministration of ketoconazole, then increase the aripiprazole and iloperidone dose when the CYP3A4 inhibitor is withdrawn. Lurasidone and strong CYP3A4 inhibitor coadministration is contraindicated. Do not exceed lurasidone 40 mg/day when coadministered with a moderate CYP3A4 inhibitor.

Antipsychotic Drug Interactions			
Precipitant drug	Object drug[a]		Description
CYP2D6 inhibitors (eg, fluoxetine, paroxetine)	Iloperidone	↑	Iloperidone plasma concentrations may be elevated, increasing the pharmacologic effects and adverse reactions. During coadministration, reduce the iloperidone dose to 50% of the normal dose. When the CYP2D6 inhibitor is discontinued, increase the dose of iloperidone.
Famotidine	Aripiprazole	↓	Coadministration of a single dose of aripiprazole and famotidine resulted in decreased aripiprazole solubility and, therefore, decreased its rate of absorption, C_{max}, and AUC.
Fluoxetine	Haloperidol	↑	Coadministration has been associated with an increase in haloperidol concentrations. Severe extrapyramidal reactions also have been reported.
Fluoxetine	Olanzapine	↑	Coadministration resulted in a small (approximately 16%) increase in C_{max} and decrease in olanzapine clearance.
Fluoxetine Paroxetine	Risperidone	↑	Risperidone concentrations may be elevated, increasing the risk of adverse effects. Fluoxetine increased risperidone plasma levels 2.5- to 2.8-fold. Adjust risperidone dose as needed.
Fluvoxamine	Asenapine	↑	Fluvoxamine may increase asenapine plasma concentrations. Coadminister with caution.
Lurasidone	Digoxin	↑	Coadministration of lurasidone 120 mg daily at steady state with a single dose of digoxin 0.25 mg increased the digoxin C_{max} and AUC approximately 9% and 13%, respectively. No adjustment in the digoxin dosage is needed.
Haloperidol	Lithium	↑	Alterations in consciousness, encephalopathy, extrapyramidal effects, fever, leukocytosis, and increased serum enzymes have occurred with coadministration with haloperidol. Monitor coadministration closely and discontinue either drug if interaction is suspected.
Lithium	Haloperidol Lurasidone		
Meperidine	Phenothiazines	↑	Excessive sedation and hypotension may occur with coadministration. Coadministration not recommended.
Phenothiazines	Meperidine		
Lurasidone	Midazolam	↑	Coadministration of lurasidone 120 mg daily at steady state with a single dose of midazolam 5 mg increased the midazolam C_{max} and AUC approximately 21% and 44%, respectively. No adjustment in the midazolam dosage is needed.
Olanzapine Quetiapine Risperidone Ziprasidone Paliperidone	Levodopa and dopamine agonists	↓	May antagonize the effects of levodopa and dopamine agonists.
Paroxetine	Phenothiazines	↑	Phenothiazine plasma levels may be increased, increasing the pharmacologic and adverse effects of these agents. Thioridazine is contraindicated. Adjust other phenothiazine doses as needed.
Phenobarbital	Clozapine	↓	Plasma levels of clozapine may be decreased, resulting in decreased pharmacologic effects.
Phenothiazines	Guanethidine	↓	Hypotensive effect of guanethidine is inhibited. Use alternate antihypertensive therapy if blood pressure is uncontrolled.
Phenothiazines	Oral anticoagulants	↓	Phenothiazines may diminish oral anticoagulant effects.
Phenothiazines	Phenytoin	↑↓	Phenothiazines have been reported to increase or decrease phenytoin levels. Monitor phenytoin levels.
Phenothiazines	Thiazide diuretics	↑	Coadministration may potentiate orthostatic hypotension.
Thiazide diuretics	Phenothiazines		
Prochlorperazine	Dofetilide	↑	Elevated dofetilide concentrations may occur with increased risk of ventricular arrhythmia, including torsades de pointes. It is not recommended to use prochlorperazine in patients receiving dofetilide.
Quetiapine	Lorazepam	↑	Lorazepam mean oral clearance was reduced 20% with coadministration.
Quinidine	Aripiprazole	↑	Coadministration increased aripiprazole AUC 112% and decreased the AUC of the active metabolite 35%. Reduce aripiprazole dose 50% with coadministration.
Rifamycins	Haloperidol	↓	Rifamycins may decrease the plasma concentration and therapeutic effects of haloperidol. Adjust haloperidol as needed.
Phenytoin	Quetiapine	↓	Quetiapine plasma levels may be decreased, resulting in decreased pharmacologic effects. Adjust quetiapine dose as needed.
Risperidone	Clozapine	↑	Pharmacologic and adverse effects of clozapine may be increased. Adjust dose as needed.
Risperidone	Valproate	↑	Coadministration resulted in a 20% increase in valproate C_{max}. Adjust therapy as needed.
Ritonavir	Clozapine Perphenazine Risperidone Thioridazine	↑	Increases in serum antipsychotic concentrations may occur, increasing risk of toxicity.
Thioridazine	Quetiapine	↓	Thioridazine increased quetiapine oral clearance 65%.
Valproate	Aripiprazole	↓	Aripiprazole C_{max} and AUC were decreased 25% with coadministration.

[a] ↑ = object drug increased; ↓ = object drug decreased; ↑↓ = object drug both increased and decreased.

➤*Drug/Lab test interactions:* Phenothiazines may produce false-positive phenylketonuria test results. Phenothiazines may cause false-positive pregnancy test results.

➤*Drug/Food interactions:* Grapefruit juice may inhibit the metabolism of **pimozide** via CYP3A. Food slows the absorption of oral **prochlorperazine** and decreases C_{max} by 23% and AUC by 13%. The **lurasidone** dose should not exceed 40 mg/day when coadministered with a moderate CYP3A4 inhibitor such as grapefruit juice or grapefruit-containing products. Administration of **lurasidone** with food increased the **lurasidone** mean C_{max} and AUC 3-fold and 2-fold, respectively, compared with administration under fasting conditions. Advise patients to take **lurasidone** with at least 350 calories of food.

Adverse Reactions

Antipsychotic Adverse Reactions[a] (%)

		Conventional Antipsychotics											Atypical Antipsychotics									
	Adverse reactions	Chlorpromazine	Fluphenazine	Haloperidol	Loxapine	Molindone	Perphenazine	Pimozide	Prochlorperazine	Thioridazine	Thiothixene	Trifluoperazine	Aripiprazole	Asenapine	Clozapine	Lurasidone	Iloperidone	Olanzapine	Paliperidone	Quetiapine	Risperidone	Ziprasidone, oral (IM)
Cardiovascular	Angina pectoris												0.1-1		1	0.1-1				< 0.1	< 0.1	0.1-1
	Atrial contractions, premature/atrial fibrillation/flutter												0.1-1		✓			< 0.1		< 0.1	< 0.1	0.1-1
	AV block												0.1-1			0.1-1			2	< 0.1	0.1-1	< 0.1
	Bradycardia						✓						> 1		✓	0.1-1	0.5-0.6	0.1-1	0.1-1	0.1-1		0.1-1 (≤ 2)
	Cardiac arrest	✓					✓		✓	Rare	✓	✓	0.1-1					0.1-1				
	Cerebral vascular accident												0.1-1			0.1-1		0.1-1		0.1-1	✓	< 0.1
	CHF												0.1-1		✓			0.1-1		< 0.1		
	ECG changes	✓	✓	✓	✓	✓	✓	✓	✓	✓	✓	✓			1							✓
	Hypertension		✓	✓	✓		✓	✓					2	3	4	0.1-1		2	2	✓	0.1-1	> 1 (≤ 2)
	Hypotension	✓	Rare	✓	✓[b]	Rare	✓	✓[b]	✓[c]	✓	✓	✓[c]	> 1		9		< 1 to 3	3-5[b]		7[b]	0.1-1	1[b] (≤ 5)
	MI												0.1-1		✓						0.1-1	
	Orthostatic hypotension															0.1-1	3- 5					
	Palpitation							✓					0.1-1				≥ 1	0.1-1	> 1	> 1	0.1-1	
	Phlebitis												0.1-1		✓						< 0.1	< 0.1
	Pulmonary embolus												< 0.1		✓			< 0.1	< 0.1		✓	< 0.1
	Q- and T-wave distortions	✓							✓			✓										
	QTc interval prolongation			✓				✓		✓			0.1-1						5	0.1-1		✓
	T-wave flattening							✓		✓					✓					0.1-1		
	T-wave inversion							✓		✓					✓					0.1-1	< 0.1	
	Tachycardia	✓	✓	✓	✓	✓[d]	✓	✓			✓		> 1		25	≥ 1	3-12	3	14	7	3-5	2
	Thrombophlebitis, including deep												< 0.1		✓					0.1-1		< 0.1
	Twitch												0.1-1		✓					0.1-1		
	Vasodilation												0.1-1					0.1-1		0.1-1		(≤ 1)
CNS	Accommodation abnormality																	0.1-1		< 0.1	0.1-1	
	Agitation	✓		✓	✓				✓	✓	✓	✓	25		4	6					22-26	> 1 (≤ 2)
	Akathisia		✓	✓	Freq	✓	✓	40	✓	✓	✓	✓	15-17	11	3	15	≈ 2	3	10	< 5		8 (≤ 2)
	Akinesia				✓	✓		40		✓			0.1-1		4			< 0.1				> 1
	Amnesia												0.1-1		✓		0.1-1	0.1-1		0.1-1	0.1-1	> 1
	Anxiety			✓									20	4	1	6			9		12-20	(≤ 2)
	Apathy												0.1-1							0.1-1	0.1-1	
	Asthenia							45					8					10-15	2	4		5 (≤ 2)
	Ataxia						✓						0.1-1		1			0.1-1		0.1-1		> 1
	Bradykinesia																0.5-0.6					
	Catatonic-like states	Rare	✓	✓			✓		✓			✓					0.1-1			0.1-1	0.1-1	
	Confusion			✓	✓		✓[e]			Rare[e]			> 1		3		0.1-1		0.1-1	0.1-1	0.1-1	> 1
	Convulsions[f]	✓		✓	✓		✓	✓	✓		Infreq	✓			3	< 0.1						
	Delirium												0.1-1		✓		0.1-1	0.1-1		< 0.1	< 0.1	> 1
	Depression			✓		✓		10					> 1	2	1		0.1-1				0.1-1	
	Dizziness	✓			✓		✓	✓	✓			✓		11	19	5	10-20	11-18	6	10	4-7	8 (3-10)
	Dreams, abnormal/ bizarre/increased		✓				✓	3		✓			≥ 1		✓	0.1-1		> 1		0.1-1	≥ 1	
	Drowsiness/sedation/ somnolence	✓	✓	✓	✓	✓	✓	25-70	✓	✓	✓	✓	7.5-15.3		39-46	22		29-35	11	18	3-8	14 (8-20)
	Dysarthria												0.1-1		✓	0.1-1		0.1-1		> 1	0.1-1	> 1
	Dyskinesia		✓				✓	✓	✓			✓	0.1-1				≈ 2	≤ 2		0.1-1		> 1
	Dystonia	✓	✓	✓		✓	✓	✓	✓	✓	✓	✓	0.1-1			5	≈ 1	2-3	5	< 5		4
	EPS	✓	✓	Freq	Freq	✓	✓	Freq	✓	Infreq	✓	✓	6	12		26	4-5		7	✓	17-34	5 (≤ 2)
	Euphoria			✓		✓							< 0.1					> 1		< 0.1	0.1-1	
	Excitement		✓				✓	✓		✓												
	Fainting/Faintness	✓			✓		✓	✓														
	Fatigue											✓		4	2	4	4-6		2		> 1	
	Gait, abnormal												> 1					6		0.1-1		> 1
	Gait, staggering/shuffling	✓			✓				✓			✓										

Antipsychotic Adverse Reactions[a] (%)

		Conventional Antipsychotics											Atypical Antipsychotics									
	Adverse reactions	Chlorpromazine	Fluphenazine	Haloperidol	Loxapine	Molindone	Perphenazine	Pimozide	Prochlorperazine	Thioridazine	Thiothixene	Trifluoperazine	Aripiprazole	Asenapine	Clozapine	Lurasidone	Iloperidone	Olanzapine	Paliperidone	Quetiapine	Risperidone	Ziprasidone, oral (IM)
CNS	Hallucinations			✓									≥ 1		✓					0.1-1		
	Headache		✓	✓	✓		✓	5-22	✓	Rare		✓	31	12	7				14	19	12-14	(3-13)
	Hostility												> 1				0.1-1			✓		> 1
	Hyperactivity					✓	✓			Rare			0.1-1				0.1-1					
	Hyperkinesia							6					0.1-1		1					0.1-1		> 1
	Hyperreflexia		✓				✓	✓	✓		✓	✓	0.1-1								< 0.1	< 0.1
	Hypesthesia												0.1-1					0.1-1			< 0.1	> 1
	Hypokinesia												0.1-1		4			0.1-1				> 1
	Incoordination												< 0.1					0.1-1	< 0.1	0.1-1		> 1
	Insomnia	✓		✓	✓		✓	10	✓		✓	✓	20	16	2	8		12		✓	23-26	< 3
	Jitteriness	✓							✓			✓										
	Lethargy		✓	✓			✓			Rare					1		1-3					
	Libido, increased		✓[g]	✓		✓							0.1-1		✓			0.1-1		0.1-1	0.1-1	
	Libido, decreased/loss of						✓	✓					0.1-1		✓		0.1-1			< 0.1	≥ 5	
	Lightheadedness				✓						✓		11									
	Malaise												0.1-1					0.1-1		0.1-1	0.1-1	
	Migraine												0.1-1					0.1-1		0.1-1	< 0.1	
	Motor restlessness (EPS)	✓				✓	✓	✓	✓	✓		✓										
	Nervousness												> 1							✓	≥ 1	
	NMS	✓	✓	✓	Freq		✓	✓	✓	✓	✓	✓				< 0.1		✓				
	Neuropathy												0.1-1					< 0.1				> 1
	Paresthesia				✓								0.1-1				0.1-1	> 1		✓	0.1-1	> 1 (≤ 2)
	Pseudoparkinsonism	✓	✓	✓	✓	✓	✓	✓	✓	Infreq	✓	✓			< 1		≈ 0.3	✓	2		✓	
	Psychosis	Rare	✓	✓			✓		✓	Rare	Infreq	✓	✓		✓					0.1-1		(≤ 1)
	Restlessness		✓	✓			✓			Rare	✓				4	3	≥ 1					
	Somnolence													24		22	9-15					
	Speech slurred				✓		✓								1							
	Suicide attempt/thought												0.1-1/ 1			< 0.1		> 1		0.1-1		
	Stupor												0.1-1							0.1-1	0.1-1	
	Syncope				✓						✓				6	0.1-1				< 5		
	Tardive dyskinesia	✓	✓	✓	✓	✓	✓	✓	✓	✓	✓	✓	0.1-1			0.1-1		0.1-1		0.1-1		> 1
	Tardive dystonia	✓		✓					✓				4-9									
	Tremor	✓			✓	✓		1	✓	✓		✓			6		3	4-6		✓		> 1
	Trismus	✓					✓		✓	✓		✓										< 0.1
	Vertigo			✓									0.1-1		19	0.1-1	< 0.1	0.1-1		0.1-1	0.1-1	> 1
	Weakness				✓						✓	✓			1							
Dermatologic	Acne			✓									0.1-1					0.1-1		0.1-1	0.1-1	
	Alopecia			✓	✓								0.1-1					0.1-1			0.1-1	0.1-1
	Dermatitis	✓[h,i]	✓[h]		✓		✓[h,i]		✓[h]	Infreq[h,i]		✓	< 0.1[h]		✓			0.1-1		0.1-1	0.1-1	0.1-2[h,i,j]
	Ecchymosis												> 1		✓			5		0.1-1		0.1-1
	Eczema		✓				✓		✓			✓	0.1-1		✓			0.1-1		0.1-1	2-4	0.1-1
	Erythema		✓				✓		✓	✓		✓			✓							
	Maculopapular skin reactions			✓									< 0.1					0.1-1		✓		0.1-1
	Pallor						✓			✓			0.1-1					0.1-1			< 0.1	
	Photosensitivity	✓	✓	✓			✓		✓	Rare	✓	✓	0.1-1		✓			0.1-1		0.1-1	> 1	> 1
	Pruritus		✓		✓		✓		✓		✓	✓	0.1-1			≥ 1		0.1-1		0.1-1	0.1-1	
	Psoriasis												0.1-1							< 0.1	< 0.1	
	Purpura, thrombocytopenic	✓	✓				✓		✓			✓										
	Rash				✓	✓		8			✓	✓	✓		2	≥ 1	2-3			< 5	2-5	4
	Rash, vesiculobullous												0.1-1					0.1-1				0.1-1
	Seborrhea		✓		✓								0.1-1					0.1-1		0.1-1	≤ 1	
	Skin pigmentation changes	✓	✓				✓		✓	✓		✓										
	Urticaria		✓				✓		✓	Infreq	✓	✓	< 0.1		✓			< 0.1			< 0.1	0.1-1

Antipsychotic Adverse Reactions[a] (%)

		Conventional Antipsychotics											Atypical Antipsychotics									
	Adverse reactions	Chlorpromazine	Fluphenazine	Haloperidol	Loxapine	Molindone	Perphenazine	Pimozide	Prochlorperazine	Thioridazine	Thiothixene	Trifluoperazine	Aripiprazole	Asenapine	Clozapine	Lurasidone	Iloperidone	Olanzapine	Paliperidone	Quetiapine	Risperidone	Ziprasidone, oral (IM)
GI	Abdominal discomfort/ pain												✓		4	≥ 1	1-3		3	3	1-4	> 1 (≤ 2)
	Abdominal distention/ enlargement												0.1-1					0.1-1		< 0.1	< 0.1	
	Adynamic ileus	✓					✓		✓		✓	✓										
	Anorexia		✓	✓			✓	✓		✓	✓	✓	✓		1					> 1	> 1	2 (≤ 2)
	Appetite increased	✓					✓	5	✓		✓	✓	0.1-1	4	✓		0.1-1	3-6		0.1-1	0.1-1	
	Atonic colon	✓							✓			✓										
	Constipation	✓	✓	✓	✓	✓	✓	20	✓	✓	Infreq	✓	13	7	14			9-11		9	7-13	9 (≤ 2)
	Diarrhea			✓			✓	5		✓	✓		✓		2	≥ 1	5-7			✓	≥ 5	5 (≤ 3)
	Diverticulitis																				< 0.1	
	Drooling	✓							✓			✓										
	Dry mouth	✓	✓	✓	✓	✓	✓	25	✓	✓	Infreq	✓	✓	3	6		8-10	9-22	3	12	≥ 5	4 (≤ 1)
	Dyspepsia			✓									15	4	14	8		7-11	5	6	5-10	8 (1-3)
	Dysphagia	✓					✓	3	✓			✓	0.1-1		✓	0.1-1		0.1-1		< 5	0.1-1	0.1-1
	Eructation												0.1-1		✓			0.1-1			< 0.1	
	Esophageal ulcer/ esophagitis												< 0.1				< 0.1	< 0.1			< 0.1	
	Fecal impaction		✓				✓						0.1-1		✓			0.1-1				< 0.1
	Flatulence												0.1-1					0.1-1		0.1-1	0.1-1	
	Gastritis												0.1-1			0.1-1	0.1-1	0.1-1		0.1-1	0.1-1	
	Gastroenteritis												0.1-1		✓			0.1-1		0.1-1	< 0.1	
	Gastroesophageal reflux												0.1-1		4		< 0.1			0.1-1	< 0.1	
	Gingivitis												0.1-1					0.1-1		0.1-1	< 0.1	
	Glossitis												< 0.1					< 0.1		< 0.1		
	Gum hemorrhage												< 0.1							0.1-1		< 0.1
	Hematemesis												< 0.1		✓					< 0.1	< 0.1	< 0.1
	Hemorrhoids												0.1-1							0.1-1	0.1-1	
	Incontinence, fecal												0.1-1					0.1-1		0.1-1	< 0.1	
	Intestinal obstruction												0.1-1		✓			< 0.1		< 0.1	✓	
	Melena												< 0.1					0.1-1		0.1-1	0.1-1	< 0.1
	Mouth ulceration												0.1-1				0.1-1	0.1-1		0.1-1		
	Nausea	✓	✓	✓	✓	✓	✓	✓	✓	✓	✓	✓	16		5	12	7-10	0.1-1	6	✓	4-6	10 (4-12)
	Obstipation	✓					✓		✓	✓		✓										
	Paralytic ileus		✓		✓					✓								< 0.1				
	Polydipsia				✓			5			✓	✓	0.1-1					> 1		0.1-1	> 1	0.1-1 (≤ 2)
	Rectal hemorrhage												0.1-1		✓			0.1-1		0.1-1		< 2
	Salivation		✓	✓	✓	✓	✓	14			Infreq		3	4	31	2	0.1-1	> 1	4	0.1-1	≤ 2	✓
	Stomatitis												0.1-1				< 0.1	0.1-1		0.1-1	0.1-1	0.1-1
	Taste altered							5					0.1-1							0.1-1		
	Tongue discoloration																	< 0.1			< 0.1	
	Tongue protrusion	✓	✓				✓		✓			✓										
	Tooth caries												0.1-1					0.1-1		0.1-1		
	Vomiting			✓	✓		✓	✓		✓	✓	✓	11	7	3	8		4		✓	5-7	> 1 (< 3)
	Weight gain	✓			✓	✓	✓	✓	✓	✓	✓	✓	3-8[k]	5	4		1-9	5-6	9	2	18	10[k]
	Weight loss				✓	✓		✓					> 1		✓		≥ 1			0.1-1	0.1-1	

Antipsychotic Adverse Reactions[a] (%)

		Conventional Antipsychotics											Atypical Antipsychotics									
	Adverse reactions	Chlorpromazine	Fluphenazine	Haloperidol	Loxapine	Molindone	Perphenazine	Pimozide	Prochlorperazine	Thioridazine	Thiothixene	Trifluoperazine	Aripiprazole	Asenapine	Clozapine	Lurasidone	Iloperidone	Olanzapine	Paliperidone	Quetiapine	Risperidone	Ziprasidone, oral (IM)
GU	Albuminuria												0.1-1					< 0.1				0.1-1
	Amenorrhea	✓			Rare	Infreq	✓		✓	✓	✓	✓	0.1-1			0.1-1	0.1-1	> 1		0.1-1	0.1-1	0.1-1
	Breast engorgement	✓		✓			✓			✓						0.1-1						
	Dysmenorrhea												✓		✓	0.1-1				0.1-1	0.1-1	(≤ 2)
	Ejaculation disorders	✓					✓		✓	✓		✓	0.1-1		1		2	0.1-1		0.1-1	≥ 5	0.1-1
	Galactorrhea	✓	✓	✓	Rare	Infreq	✓		✓	✓	✓	✓				< 0.1		0.1-1		0.1-1	0.1-1	0.1-1
	Glycosuria	✓					✓		✓		✓	✓	< 0.1					0.1-1		< 0.1		0.1-1
	Gynecomastia	✓	✓	✓	Rare	Infreq	✓		✓	✓	✓	✓	0.1-1				< 0.1	< 0.1		< 0.1	< 0.1	< 0.1
	Hematuria												0.1-1					> 1			0.1-1	0.1-1
	Impotence	✓	✓	✓				15	✓		Infreq	✓	0.1-1		✓			0.1-1		0.1-1	≥ 5	0.1-1
	Incontinence, urinary						✓			✓			> 1				≥ 1	2		0.1-1	0.1-1	
	Mastalgia			✓									0.1-1		✓			0.1-1			0.1-1	
	Menorrhagia					✓							< 0.1				< 0.1	0.1-1			≥ 5	0.1-1
	Menstrual irregularities		✓	✓	Rare		✓		✓	✓		✓					< 0.1					
	Metrorrhagia																< 0.1	> 1		0.1-1		0.1-1
	Nocturia							✓					< 0.1							< 0.1		< 0.1
	Polyuria		✓				✓						< 0.1					0.1-1		< 0.1	> 1	0.1-1
	Priapism	✓		✓		✓	✓		✓	✓		✓	< 0.1		✓			0.1-1				(≤ 1)
	Renal failure, acute		✓										0.1-1			< 0.1	< 0.1			< 0.1		
	Urinary frequency/ urgency increased						✓	✓					0.1-1		1			0.1-1		0.1-1		
	Urinary retention	✓		✓	✓	✓	✓		✓	✓		✓	0.1-1		1		< 0.1	0.1-1		0.1-1	> 1	0.1-1
	Vaginal hemorrhage												0.1-1					0.1-1		0.1-1	0.1-1	< 0.1
Hematologic/Lymphatic	Agranulocytosis	✓	✓	Rare	Rare		✓		✓	✓		✓			1							
	Anemia			✓						✓			> 1		✓	0.1-1	0.1 to 1	0.1-1		0.1-1	0.1-1	0.1-1
	Anemia, aplastic	✓							✓	✓		✓										
	Anemia, hemolytic	✓					✓	✓	✓			✓										
	Anemia, hypochromic												0.1-1							0.1-1	0.1-1	< 0.1
	Blood dyscrasias		✓				✓		✓			✓										
	Eosinophilia	✓	✓				✓		✓	✓		✓	< 0.1		1					0.1-1		0.1-1
	Hemorrhage												0.1-1					0.1-1			< 0.1	
	Hypercholesterolemia												0.1-1					0.1-1		✓		0.1-1
	Hyperglycemia	✓		✓					✓		✓	✓	0.1-1		✓			0.1-1		0.1-1	✓	0.1-1
	Hyperkalemia												0.1-1					< 0.1				< 0.1
	Hyperlipemia												0.1-1					0.1-1		0.1-1		< 0.1
	Hyperuricemia												0.1-1		✓							< 0.1
	Hypoglycemia	✓		✓			✓		✓		✓	✓	0.1-1					0.1-1		0.1-1	< 0.1	< 0.1
	Hypokalemia												0.1-1					0.1-1		< 0.1	< 0.1	0.1-1
	Hyponatremia			✓				✓					0.1-1		✓			0.1-1			0.1-1	< 0.1
	Hypoproteinemia																	< 0.1			< 0.1	< 0.1
	Leukocytosis		✓	✓		Rare					✓		0.1-1		✓			0.1-1		0.1-1	< 0.1	0.1-1
	Leukopenia	✓	✓	✓	Rare	Rare	✓		✓	✓	✓	✓	0.1-1		3	< 0.1	< 0.1	> 1		> 1	< 0.1	0.1-1
	Lymphadenopathy												0.1-1					0.1-1		0.1-1		0.1-1
	Pancytopenia	✓	✓				✓		✓			✓										< 0.1
	Thrombocythemia												< 0.1		✓			0.1-1				< 0.1
	Thrombocytopenia				Rare					✓			< 0.1		✓		< 0.1	0.1-1	< 0.1	< 0.1		< 0.1
Hepatic	ALT/AST elevation				✓						Infreq		0.1-1			1				✓	0.1-1	0.1-1
	Biliary stasis						✓		✓	✓		✓										
	Cholecystitis												0.1-1								< 0.1	
	Cholelithiasis												0.1-1		✓		0.1-1				< 0.1	
	Hepatitis				Rare								< 0.1		✓			0.1-1			< 0.1	< 0.1
	Jaundice	✓	✓[l]	✓	Rare		✓		✓[l]	✓		✓			✓						✓	< 0.1[l]
	Liver function impaired		✓	✓		Rare	✓					✓			1							
Hypersensitivity	Allergic reaction	✓							✓			✓	✓		✓			✓			< 0.1	
	Anaphylactoid reactions	✓	✓				✓		✓		Rare	✓						✓	< 0.1	✓	✓	

Antipsychotic Adverse Reactions[a] (%)

		Conventional Antipsychotics											Atypical Antipsychotics									
	Adverse reactions	Chlorpromazine	Fluphenazine	Haloperidol	Loxapine	Molindone	Perphenazine	Pimozide	Prochlorperazine	Thioridazine	Thiothixene	Trifluoperazine	Aripiprazole	Asenapine	Clozapine	Lurasidone	Iloperidone	Olanzapine	Paliperidone	Quetiapine	Risperidone	Ziprasidone, oral (IM)
Lab Test Abn.	Alkaline phosphatase increased										Infreq		0.1-1					0.1-1		0.1-1		0.1-1
	Cerebrospinal fluid proteins abnormality	✓	✓				✓		✓		✓	✓										
	Creatine phosphokinase elevated		✓										> 1		✓	≥ 1						0.1-1
	Creatinine increased												0.1-1			3				0.1-1	0.1-1	< 0.1
Metabolic/Nutritional	Cyanosis												0.1-1		✓			0.1-1		0.1-1		
	Edema									✓			0.1-1		✓		0.1-1		0.1-1		0.1-1	
	Edema, angioneurotic	✓	✓				✓		✓	✓		✓										
	Edema, cerebral	✓	✓				Rare		✓		✓	✓										
	Edema, facial				✓								0.1-1					0.1-1		0.1-1		> 1
	Edema, laryngeal	✓	✓				✓		✓	✓		✓										
	Edema, peripheral	✓	✓				✓		✓	✓	✓	✓	2	3				3		> 1		0.1-1
	Edema, tongue												0.1-1					0.1-1		0.1-1	< 0.1	0.1-1
Musculoskeletal	Arthralgia/Joint pain												0.1-1	3	✓		3	5		0.1-1	2-3	✓
	Arthritis												0.1-1					0.1-1		0.1-1	< 0.1	
	Bone pain												0.1-1					< 0.1		0.1-1		
	Bursitis												0.1-1					0.1-1			< 0.1	
	Muscle rigidity		✓			✓		15	✓	✓					✓							
	Muscle weakness						✓					✓	0.1-1		1					0.1-1		
	Musculoskeletal stiffness																1-3					
	Myalgia							3					4		1		≥ 1			✓	0.1-1	1
	Myoclonus				✓								0.1-1		1					0.1-1		< 0.1
	Myopathy												0.1-1					< 0.1				< 0.1
	Opisthotonos	✓	✓	✓			✓	✓	✓	✓		✓										< 0.1
	Rigidity							10							5						0.1-1	
	Spasm, carpopedal	✓							✓	✓		✓										
	Spasm of neck muscles	✓			✓				✓	✓		✓										
	Torticollis	✓					✓	3	✓	✓		✓					< 0.1				< 0.1	< 0.1
Respiratory	Apnea												< 0.1					0.1-1			✓	
	Asphyxia	✓					✓		✓		✓	✓										
	Aspiration														✓						< 0.1	
	Asthma	✓	✓				✓		✓	✓		✓	≥ 1				0.1-1	0.1-1		0.1-1	< 0.1	
	Cough, increased												3		✓			6	3	> 1	3	3
	Cough reflex failure	✓					✓		✓		✓	✓										
	Dyspnea				✓								> 1		1		2	> 1	> 1	> 1	≤ 1	> 1
	Epistaxis												0.1-1		✓		0.1-1	0.1-1		0.1-1	0.1-1	0.1-1
	Hemoptysis												< 0.1					0.1-1				< 0.1
	Hyperventilation														✓					< 0.1	0.1-1	
	Nasal congestion	✓	✓		✓		✓		✓	✓	Infreq	✓			1		5- 8					
	Nasopharyngitis																3-4					
	Pharyngitis												4					4		> 1	2-3	
	Pneumonia												> 1		✓			0.1-1		0.1-1	0.1-1	0.1-1
	Rhinitis												4					7		3	8-10	4 (≤ 1)
	Upper respiratory tract infection																2-3					

Antipsychotic Adverse Reactions[a] (%)

		Conventional Antipsychotics											Atypical Antipsychotics									
	Adverse reactions	Chlorpromazine	Fluphenazine	Haloperidol	Loxapine	Molindone	Perphenazine	Pimozide	Prochlorperazine	Thioridazine	Thiothixene	Trifluoperazine	Aripiprazole	Asenapine	Clozapine	Lurasidone	Iloperidone	Olanzapine	Paliperidone	Quetiapine	Risperidone	Ziprasidone, oral (IM)
Special senses	Blepharitis												0.1-1				0.1-1	0.1-1		0.1-1	< 0.1	0.1-1
	Cataracts			✓				✓					0.1-1				0.1-1	0.1-1				0.1-1
	Conjunctivitis												> 1		✓		≥ 1	> 1		0.1-1		0.1-1
	Diplopia												< 0.1					0.1-1			< 0.1	> 1
	Dry eyes												0.1-1				0.1-1	0.1-1		0.1-1		0.1-1
	Epithelial keratopathy	✓					✓		✓			✓										
	Eye hemorrhage												0.1-1					0.1-1				< 0.1
	Glaucoma	✓					✓		✓						✓[m]			< 0.1		< 0.1		
	Lenticular/Corneal opacities	✓	✓				✓		✓	✓	✓	✓					0.1-1					
	Miosis	✓					✓		✓		✓	✓						< 0.1				
	Mydriasis	✓					✓		✓		✓	✓						< 0.1				
	Oculogyric crisis	✓	✓	✓			✓		✓	✓	✓	✓	< 0.1									> 1
	Parotid swelling						Rare			Rare					✓							
	Photophobia	✓											< 0.1								< 0.1	0.1-1
	Pigmentary retinopathy	✓					✓		✓	✓		✓										
	Tinnitus												0.1-1				< 0.1	0.1-1		0.1-1		0.1-1
	Vision, abnormal																			0.1-1	1-2	3
	Vision, blurred	✓	✓	✓	✓	✓	✓	✓	✓	✓	Infreq	✓	3		≥ 1		1-3		2	< 5		
	Visual disturbances			✓											5							
Miscellaneous	Accidental injury												6					12		✓		4
	Back pain												✓		1	4		5	2	2	≤ 2	(≤ 1)
	Chest pain												> 1		1			3		✓	2-3	
	Chills												0.1-1		✓			0.1-1		0.1-1		> 1
	Choreoathetosis																	< 0.1		< 0.1		> 1
	Cogwheel rigidity	✓										✓	0.1-1					0.1-1				> 1 (≤ 1)
	Dehydration												≥ 1				0.1-1	0.1-1		0.1-1	< 0.1	0.1-1
	Diaphoresis		✓	✓			✓	✓			Infreq		> 1		6			> 1		> 1	0.1-1	(≤ 2)
	Fever						✓		✓	✓		✓	≥ 1		5			6	2	< 5	2-3	> 1
	Flu syndrome												> 1					> 1		> 1	0.1-1	> 1 (≤ 1)
	Gout												< 0.1					< 0.1		< 0.1		< 0.1
	Hyperpyrexia/ Hyperthermia	✓	✓	✓	✓		✓	✓	✓	✓	✓	✓					< 0.1					
	Hyperthyroidism												< 0.1							< 0.1		< 0.1
	Hypertonia												✓					3	4	> 1		3
	Hypothyroidism												0.1-1				0.1-1			0.1-1		< 0.1
	Hypotonia												< 0.1					0.1-1			< 0.1	> 1
	Mask-like faces	✓							✓			✓										
	Moniliasis																	0.1-1		0.1-1		
	Neck pain/rigidity												> 1		1			0.1-1		0.1-1		
	Pain, pelvic												≥ 1					0.1-1		0.1-1		
	Pillrolling motion	✓							✓			✓										
	Ptosis				✓																	
	Sudden death	✓	✓	✓			Rare	✓	✓	✓	✓	✓			✓	< 0.1		< 0.1			< 0.1	
	Systemic lupus erythematosus–like syndrome	✓	✓				✓		✓	✓		✓										
	Thyroiditis																	0.1-1			< 0.1	< 0.1
	Withdrawal syndrome			✓				✓	✓									1			< 0.1	> 1

[a] ✓ = occurs; incidence unknown. Data are pooled from separate trials and are not necessarily comparable; AV = atrioventricular.
[b] Includes orthostatic.
[c] Sometimes fatal.
[d] Especially with sudden marked increase in dosage.
[e] Nocturnal confusion.
[f] Includes petit and grand mal seizures.
[g] In women.
[h] Exfoliative dermatitis included.
[i] Contact dermatitis included.
[j] Fungal dermatitis.
[k] Gained at least 7% body weight.
[l] Includes cholestatic.
[m] Narrow-angle glaucoma.

➤*Other adverse reactions:*

Chlorpromazine – Ocular changes; back muscle rigidity; shock-like reaction.

Fluphenazine – Altered EEG tracings; nonthrombocytopenic purpura; appetite decreased; weight change; local tissue reactions (rare).

Loxapine – Flushed face; numbness; tension.

Molindone – Menses resumption; blood glucose alteration; BUN alteration; red blood cell (RBC) count alteration; thyroid function alteration.

Perphenazine – Pulse-rate change; paranoid reaction; polyphagia; throat tight; ocular changes; inappropriate antidiuretic hormone secretion; limb ache/numbness; shock-like reaction; hypnotic effects; tongue ache; tongue rounding; circulatory collapse (rare).

Pimozide – Adverse behavior effect (5% to 10%); sensitivity of eyes to light (5%); accommodation decrease (4%); speech disorder, stooped posture (2%); gingival hyperplasia, handwriting change (1%); skin irritation; GI distress; tonic spasm; transient dyskinetic signs; periorbital edema; T-wave notching; U-wave appearance.

Thioridazine – Arrhythmias; torsades de pointes–type arrhythmias; autonomic instability; blood glucose alteration; conjunctiva pigmentation; cornea discoloration; altered mental status; paradoxical reaction; irregular pulse; sclera discoloration; altered libido; U-wave appearance; skin eruption (infrequent).

Trifluoperazine – Skin reaction; back muscle rigidity; heat prolongation/ intensification.

Haloperidol – BP fluctuations; torsades de pointes–type arrhythmias; hyperammonemia (postmarketing); lymphomonocytosis; RBC count decreased; bronchospasm; laryngospasm; respiration depth increased; retinopathy; heat stroke; local tissue reactions; transient dyskinetic signs.

Atypicals –

Aripiprazole: Ear pain (0.1% to 1%), manic reaction, muscle cramp, dry skin, skin ulcer (at least 1%); DVT, concentration impaired, bloating, periodontal abscess, cystitis, uterine hemorrhage (less than 0.1%), bilirubinemia, increased BUN, increased lactic dehydrogenase (less than 0.1%), jaw pain/tightness, depersonalization, diabetes mellitus, iron deficiency anemia, bradykinesia, chest tightness, colitis, dysphoria, dysuria, extrasystoles, eye pain, hiccough, hypersomnia, GI hemorrhage, kidney calculus, laryngitis, leukorrhea, impaired memory, myocardial ischemia, obesity, otitis media, panic attack, peptic ulcer (less than 0.1%), restless leg, spasm, thinking slowed, vaginal moniliasis; hyperesthesia, arthrosis (0.1% to 1); cardiomegaly, throat tight, anorgasmia, hepatomegaly, amblyopia, increased lacrimation, tenosynovitis, heat stroke, increased sputum, cerebral ischemia, deafness, macrocytic anemia (0.1% to 1%), aspiration pneumonia (0.1% to 1%), increased blinking, blunted affect, cervicitis, cheilitis, decreased consciousness, duodenal ulcer, pulmonary edema, goiter, head heaviness, intracranial hemorrhage, hypernatremia, hypoxia, Mendelson syndrome, dry nasal passages, obsessive thought, otitis externa, pancreatitis, decreased reflexes, respiratory failure, rhabdomyolysis, rheumatoid arthritis, tendonitis, throat pain (0.1% to 1%), urinary burning (0.1% to 1%), urolithiasis, vasovagal reaction buccoglossal syndrome (less than 0.1%); oral moniliasis (0.1% to 1%); upper respiratory infection; dental pain; QT interval shortened; vaginitis.

Asenapine: Elevated triglycerides (15%); elevated creatinine kinase (11%); elevated total cholesterol (9%); elevated fasting glucose (7%); elevated prolactin levels, elevated transaminases, dysgeusia, stomach discomfort, toothache (3%); irritability, pain in extremity (2%); tachycardia, temporary bundle branch block, glossodynia, oral paresthesia, swollen tongue, anemia, accommodation disorder, hyponatremia, dysarthria (0.1% to less than 1%); thrombocytopenia, idiosyncratic drug reaction (less than 0.1%).

Clozapine: Arrhythmias, cardiomyopathy, DVT, ST-depression, aphasia, altered EEG tracings, GI distress, hypothermia, periorbital edema, delusions, amentia, bitter taste, bronchitis, mild cataplexy, chills with fever, cholestasis, poor coordination, ear disorder, epileptiform movements, erythema multiforme, increased erythrocyte sedimentation rate, eyelid disorder, bloodshot eyes, gastric ulcer, granulocytopenia, elevated hematocrit, elevated hemoglobin, histrionic movements, hot flashes, acute interstitial nephritis, involuntary movements, irritability, ischemic changes, laryngitis, impaired memory, numbness, overdose, acute pancreatitis, pericardial effusions, pericarditis, petechiae, pleural effusion, pneumonia-like symptoms, premature ventricular contraction, rhabdomyolysis, rhinorrhea, sepsis, shakiness, sneezing, status epilepticus, Stevens-Johnson syndrome, stuttering, abnormal stools, dry throat, throat pain/discomfort, tics, tongue numb/ sore, vaginal infections/itch, vasculitis, ventricular fibrillation, wheezing, nightmares, sleep disturbance (4%); neutropenia, WBC count decreased (3%); urinary abnormalities (2%); incontinence, cardiac abnormality, leg pain (1%).

Iloperidone: Aggression, delusion, erectile dysfunction, muscle spasms (at least 1%); anorgasmia, breast pain, bulimia nervosa, difficulty in walking, dysuria, enuresis, eyelid edema, eye swelling, fecal incontinence, fluid retention, hematocrit decreased, hemoglobin decreased, hyperemia (including conjunctival), hypokalemia, impulse-control disorder, iron deficiency anemia, mania, mood swings, nasal dryness, nephrolithiasis, neutrophil count increased, nystagmus, OCD, panic attack, paranoia, pollakiuria, polydipsia psychogenic, rhinorrhea, sinus congestion, testicular pain, thirst (0.1% to 1%); arrhythmia, AV block first degree, cardiac failure (including congestive and acute), dry throat, duodenal ulcer, dyspnea exertional, hiatus hernia, hyperchlorhydria, hyperthermia, lip ulceration, postmenopausal hemorrhage, prostatitis, restless legs syndrome, sleep apnea syndrome (less than 0.1%).

Lurasidone: Parkinsonism (11%); dysuria, panic attack, sleep disorder (0.1% to 1%); angioedema, breast pain, erectile dysfunction, neutropenia, rhabdomyolysis (less than 0.1%).

Olanzapine: Personality disorder (8%); extremity pain (not joint) (5%); amblyopia (3%); articulation impaired, urinary tract infection (UTI) (2%); angioedema, dental pain, intentional injury (at least 1%); antisocial reaction, CNS stimulation, arthrosis, voice alteration, laryngitis, obsessive compulsive symptoms, phobias, tobacco misuse (0.1% to 1%); normocytic anemia, arteritis, fatty liver deposits, keratoconjunctivitis, nystagmus, ketosis, hangover effect, encephalopathy, hiccough, hyperventilation, hypoxia, lung edema, stridor, breast pain, cystitis, uterine fibroids (less than 0.1%); aphthous stomatitis, enteritis, periodontal abscess, acidosis, bilirubinemia, atelectasis, alcohol misuse, coma (rare).

Paliperidone: Injection-site reactions (0% to 10%); tremor, orthostatic hypotension (4%); bundle branch block (3%); sinus arrhythmia, blood insulin increased, abnormal ECG T-wave, pain in extremity (2%); swollen tongue (0.1% to 1%); ischemia, venous thrombosis (< 0.1%);hyperprolactinemia.

Quetiapine: UTI, infection, pain, ear pain, dry skin, increased triglycerides (1%); bundle branch block, paranoid reaction, cystitis, vulvovaginitis, leg cramps, increased gamma glutamyl transferase (GGT), alcohol intolerance, bruxism, cerebral ischemia, delusions, depersonalization, diabetes mellitus, dysuria, eye pain, hemiplegia, involuntary movements, leukorrhea, manic reaction, orchitis, pathological fracture, irregular pulse, increased QRS duration, skin ulcer, abnormal thinking, vaginitis (0.1% to 1%); aphasia, emotional lability, deafness, hand edema, hemolysis, hiccough, neuralgia, neutropenia, skin discoloration, ST abnormality, ST elevated, stuttering, subdural hematoma, T-wave abnormality, water intoxication (less than 0.1%).

Risperidone: Lymphedema (8%); upper respiratory infection (3%); angioedema, cerebral vascular disorder, aggressive reaction (1% to 3%); toothache, sinusitis (2% or less); hyperpigmentation (at least 1%); concentration impaired, hyperkeratosis, nonthrombocytopenic purpura, skin exfoliation, bronchospasm, stridor, xerophthalmia (0.1% to 1%); myocarditis, ST-depression, cholinergic syndrome, emotional lability, nightmares, bullous eruption, furunculosis, hypertrichosis, skin ulceration, verruca, feces discoloration, GI hemorrhage, tongue paralysis, genital pruritus, normocytic anemia, ascites, yawning, eye pain, abnormal lacrimation, photopsia, arthrosis, leg cramps, cachexia, coma, increased sputum, sarcoidosis (less than 0.1%).

Ziprasidone: Injection-site pain (7% to 9%); respiratory disorder (8%); personality disorder, speech disorder, furunculosis (2% or less); hypotonia, buccoglossal syndrome, accidental fall, hypothermia, motor vehicle accident, flank pain, hypertonia (at least 1%); tooth disorder (less than 1%); cerebral infarct, polycythemia, anorgasmia, male sex dysfunction, tenosynovitis, increased lactic dehydrogenase (0.1% to 1%); bundle branch block, cardiomegaly, myocarditis, keratitis, leukoplakia of the mouth, female sex dysfunction, uterine hemorrhage, basophilia, hypocalcemia, hypochloremia, hypocholesterolemia, lymphedema, lymphocytosis, monocytosis, fatty liver deposits, hepatomegaly, laryngismus, respiratory alkalosis, keratoconjunctivitis, nystagmus, visual field defect, increased BUN, increased GGT, decreased glucose tolerance, ketosis, cerebral infarct, hyperchloremia, oliguria (less than 0.1%).

Overdosage

➤*Symptoms:* CNS depression to the point of somnolence, deep sleep from which patient cannot be aroused, or coma. Hypotension and EPS may occur. Other manifestations include agitation, autonomic reactions, cardiac arrest, cardiac arrhythmias, coma, convulsions, confusion, death, delirium, dilated or constricted pupils, dry mouth, ECG changes, fever, hyperpyrexia, hypertension, hyperthermia, hypothermia, ileus, NMS, renal failure (**loxapine**), respiratory depression or failure, restlessness, salivation, seizures, slurred speech, tachycardia, and vomiting.

Other symptoms temporally related to risperidone and paliperidone overdose include torsades de pointes, prolonged QT interval, and cardiopulmonary arrest.

➤*Treatment:* Includes usual supportive measures. Refer to General Management of Acute Overdosage. In case of acute overdosage, establish and maintain an airway and ensure adequate oxygenation and ventilation. Establish IV access and consider gastric lavage (after intubation, if patient is unconscious) and administration of activated charcoal. The possibility of obtundation, seizure, or dystonic reaction of the head and neck following overdose may create a risk of aspiration with induced emesis. Cardiovascular monitoring should commence immediately and include continuous ECG monitoring to detect possible arrhythmias. Treat EPS with anticholinergic drugs or diphenhydramine (see Adverse Reactions).

If hypotension occurs, initiate the standard measures for managing circulatory shock, including volume replacement. If a vasoconstrictor is desired, use norepinephrine or phenylephrine. Do not administer epinephrine, dopamine, or other sympathomimetics with beta-agonist activity, because beta stimulation may worsen hypotension of drug-induced alpha blockade (eg, **asenapine**, **lurasidone**, **olanzapine**, **paliperidone**, **quetiapine**, **risperidone**, **ziprasidone**) (see Drug Interactions).

Disopyramide, procainamide, and quinidine carry a theoretical hazard of QT-prolonging effects when administered in patients with acute overdosing. Similarly, it is reasonable to expect that the alpha-adrenergic blocking properties of bretylium might be additive, resulting in problematic hypertension.

Limited experience indicates antipsychotic drugs are not dialyzable.

Because of the long half-life of **pimozide**, observe patients for at least 4 days. Continue additional surveillance after overdosage of **clozapine** and **thioridazine** for several days because of the risk of delayed effects.

Patient Information

Because some patients exposed chronically to antipsychotics will develop TD, inform all patients in whom chronic use is contemplated, if possible, about this risk. The decision to inform patients or their guardians must obviously take into account the clinical circumstances and the patient's competence to understand the information (see Warnings/Precautions).

Counsel patients and caregivers that a potentially fatal symptom complex referred to as NMS has been reported in association with administration of antipsychotic drugs. Signs and symptoms of NMS include hyperpyrexia, muscle rigidity, altered mental status, and evidence of autonomic instability (irregular pulse or blood pressure, tachycardia, diaphoresis, and cardiac dysrhythmia).

May cause impaired judgment, thinking, or motor skills; use caution while driving or performing other tasks requiring alertness. Avoid alcohol and other CNS depressants because of possible additive effects and hypotension.

Avoid skin contact with injection and oral concentrates (contact dermatitis may occur). Oral concentrates are most conveniently used when diluted in fruit juices or other liquids. Use immediately after dilution. See individual products for specific guidelines.

Photosensitivity may occur with some antipsychotics. Avoid exposure to ultraviolet light or sunlight. Use sunscreen and protective clothing until tolerance is determined.

Advise patients of the risk of orthostatic hypotension, especially during the period of initial dose titration.

Use caution in hot weather. These drugs may increase susceptibility to heat stroke. Avoid overheating and dehydration.

Notify health care provider if sore throat, fever, skin rash, impaired vision, tremors, involuntary muscle twitching, muscle stiffness, or jaundice occurs.

Instruct patients to notify their health care provider if they become pregnant or intend to become pregnant during therapy.

Instruct patients to notify their health care provider if they are taking, or plan to take, any prescription or over-the-counter drugs.

Advise patients not to breast-feed if they are taking **clozapine, olanzapine, loxapine, iloperidone, risperidone, aripiprazole, ziprasidone, haloperidol, quetiapine,** or **paliperidone**. Safety of the typical antipsychotics in the breast-feeding mother has not been established.

False-positive pregnancy tests have occurred with some **phenothiazines** but are less likely to occur when a serum test is used.

Warn patients receiving **clozapine** about the significant risk of developing agranulocytosis and advise them that frequent blood tests are required. Instruct patients to report immediately the appearance of lethargy, weakness, fever, sore throat, malaise, mucous membrane ulceration, or other possible signs of infection. Inform patients of the significant risk of seizures during clozapine treatment. Inform patients that if they stop taking clozapine for more than 2 days, not to restart their medication at the same dosage, but to contact their health care provider for dosing instructions.

Advise patients of the risk of postinjection delirium/sedation syndrome each time they receive an olanzapine ER injection. Advise patients that after each injection, they must be observed at the health care facility for at least 3 hours and must be accompanied to their destination upon leaving the facility.

Advise patients taking **asenapine** to not remove the tablet until ready to administer, to place the tablet under the tongue, and to let it dissolve completely. Do not crush, chew, or swallow the tablet whole; do not eat or drink for 10 minutes following administration of the tablet.

Phenothiazine Derivatives

CHLORPROMAZINE HYDROCHLORIDE

Rx	**Chlorpromazine HCl** (Various, eg, Geneva, Major)	**Tablets:** 10 mg	In 100s, 1000s, and UD 100s.
Rx	**Chlorpromazine HCl** (Various, eg, Geneva, Major)	**Tablets:** 25 mg	In 100s, 1000s, and UD 100s.
Rx	**Chlorpromazine HCl** (Various, eg, Geneva, Major)	**Tablets:** 50 mg	In 100s, 1000s, and UD 100s.
Rx	**Chlorpromazine HCl** (Various, eg, Geneva, Major)	**Tablets:** 100 mg	In 100s, 1000s, and UD 100s.
Rx	**Chlorpromazine HCl** (Various, eg, Geneva, Major)	**Tablets:** 200 mg	In 100s, 1000s, and UD 100s.
Rx	**Chlorpromazine HCl** (Various)	**Injection:** 25 mg/mL	In 1 and 2 mL amps.[a]

[a] With sodium metabisulfite and sodium sulfite.

CHLORPROMAZINE — ORAL

Complete and comparative prescribing information begins in the Antipsychotic Agents group monograph. Also see the Antiemetic/Antivertigo Agents monograph.

Indications

➤*Emesis/Hiccoughs:* For the control of nausea and vomiting and relief of intractable hiccoughs (see Antiemetic/Antivertigo Agents).

➤*Manic-depressive illness:* For the control of manifestations of the manic type of manic-depressive illness.

➤*Porphyria, acute intermittent:* For the treatment of acute intermittent porphyria.

➤*Schizophrenia:* For the treatment of schizophrenia.

➤*Surgery:* For the relief of restlessness and apprehension prior to surgery.

➤*Behavioral problems:* For the treatment of severe behavioral problems in children 1 to 12 years of age marked by combativeness and/or explosive hyperexcitable behavior (out of proportion to immediate provocations).

➤*Hyperactivity:* For the short-term treatment of hyperactive children who show excessive motor activity with accompanying conduct disorders consisting of some or all of the following symptoms: Impulsivity, difficulty sustaining attention, aggressiveness, mood lability, and poor frustration tolerance.

Administration and Dosage

➤*General dosing considerations:* Individualize dosage based on condition severity. Increase dosage until symptoms are controlled, then gradually reduce dosage to the lowest effective maintenance level.

➤*Adults:*

Acute intermittent porphyria – 25 to 50 mg 3 or 4 times/day.

Intractable hiccoughs – 25 to 50 mg 3 or 4 times daily. If symptoms persist for 2 to 3 days, give parenteral therapy. (See the Chlorpromazine Injection monograph for more information.)

Nausea and vomiting – 10 to 25 mg every 4 to 6 hours, as needed; increase if necessary.

Preoperative apprehension – 25 to 50 mg 2 to 3 hours before surgery.

Psychotic disorders – Maximum improvement may not be seen for weeks or even months. Continue optimum dosage for 2 weeks, then gradually reduce to lowest effective maintenance level. A dosage of 200 mg/day is not unusual. Some patients require higher dosages (eg, 800 mg/day is not uncommon in discharged mental patients).

Hospitalized patients:

• *Acute schizophrenic or manic states* –

Usual dosage: 500 mg a day is generally sufficient.

Initial dosage: Initial treatment should be with chlorpromazine injection until patient is controlled. Usually patient becomes quiet and co-operative within 24 to 48 hours and oral doses may be substituted and increased until the patient is calm.

Dosage titration: While gradual increases to 2,000 mg a day or more may be necessary, there is usually little therapeutic gain to be achieved by exceeding 1,000 mg a day for extended periods.

• *Less acutely disturbed* – 25 mg 3 times/day. Increase gradually until effective dose is reached, usually 400 mg/day.

Outpatients:

• *Usual dosage* – 10 mg 3 or 4 times/day, or 25 mg 2 or 3 times/day.

• *More severe cases* – 25 mg 3 times/day. After 1 or 2 days, daily dosage may be increased by 20 to 50 mg at semiweekly intervals until patient becomes calm and cooperative.

➤*Children:*

Older than 12 years of age – See Adults for dosing for children older than 12 years of age.

6 months to 12 years of age –

Behavioral disorders/Hyperactivity:

• *Hospitalized patients* – Start with low doses and increase gradually. In severe behavior disorders, 50 to 100 mg/day, or in older children, 200 mg/day or more may be necessary. There is little evidence that improvement in severely disturbed mentally retarded patients is enhanced by doses beyond 500 mg/day.

• *Outpatients* – 0.55 mg/kg (0.25 mg/lb) every 4 to 6 hours, as needed.

Nausea and vomiting: 0.55 mg/kg (0.25 mg/lb) every 4 to 6 hours, as needed.

Preoperative apprehension: 0.55 mg/kg (0.25 mg/lb) 2 to 3 hours before surgery.

➤*Elderly:* Lower initial doses and more gradual adjustments are recommended.

➤*Debilitated/Emaciated patients:* Lower initial doses and more gradual adjustments are recommended.

➤*Storage/Stability:* Store between 15° and 30°C (59° and 86°F).

CHLORPROMAZINE — INJECTION

Complete and comparative prescribing information begins in the Antipsychotic Agents group monograph. Also see the Antiemetic/Antivertigo Agents monograph.

Indications

➤*Emesis/Hiccoughs:* For the control of nausea and vomiting and relief of intractable hiccoughs.

➤*Manic-depressive illness:* For the control of manifestations of the manic type of manic-depressive illness.

➤*Porphyria, acute intermittent:* For the treatment of acute intermittent porphyria.

➤*Schizophrenia:* For the treatment of schizophrenia.

➤*Surgery:* For the relief of restlessness and apprehension prior to surgery.

➤*Tetanus:* An adjunct in treatment of tetanus.

➤*Behavioral problems:* For the treatment of severe behavioral problems in children 1 to 12 years of age marked by combativeness and/or explosive hyperexcitable behavior (out of proportion to immediate provocations).

➤*Hyperactivity:* For the short-term treatment of hyperactive children who show excessive motor activity with accompanying conduct disorders consisting of some or all of the following symptoms: Impulsivity, difficulty sustaining attention, aggressiveness, mood lability, and poor frustration tolerance.

➤*Off-label uses:*

Treatment of migraine (intramuscular) (adults) – [5] = Poor documentation. The data evaluating the efficacy of intramuscular (IM) chlorpromazine for the treatment of an acute migraine attack are limited and show conflicting results. American Academy of Neurology clinical practice guidelines for the pharmacologic treatment of migraine headache in adults consider IM chlorpromazine to be ineffective.

CHLORPROMAZINE — INJECTION

Treatment of migraine (intravenous) (adults) – [3] = Safety concerns. Data evaluating the efficacy of intravenous (IV) chlorpromazine for the treatment of an acute migraine attack consistently show favorable results. American Academy of Neurology clinical practice guidelines for the pharmacologic treatment of migraine headache in adults consider IV chlorpromazine to be a choice for migraine in the appropriate setting (grade B evidence). However, because of significant safety concerns, including hypotension and akathisias, avoid routine use. (See Administration and Dosage.)

Administration and Dosage

➤*General dosing considerations:* Because of possible hypotensive effects, reserve for bedfast patients or for acute ambulatory cases and keep patient recumbent for at least 30 minutes after injection.

Individualize dosage based on condition severity. Increase dosage until symptoms are controlled, then gradually reduce dosage to the lowest effective maintenance level. Increase parenteral dosage only if hypotension has not occurred.

➤*Adults:*

Acute intermittent porphyria – 25 mg intramuscularly (IM) 3 or 4 times/day until patient can take oral therapy.

Intractable hiccoughs – 25 to 50 mg orally 3 or 4 times daily. If symptoms persist for 2 to 3 days, give 25 to 50 mg IM. If symptoms persist, use slow intravenous (IV) infusion with patient flat in bed. Administer 25 to 50 mg in 500 to 1,000 mL of saline. Monitor blood pressure.

Nausea and vomiting –

Usual dosage: 25 mg IM. If no hypotension occurs, give 25 to 50 mg every 3 to 4 hours, as needed, until vomiting stops. Then switch to oral dosage.

Intraoperative (to control acute nausea/vomiting): For IM use, give 12.5 mg IM; repeat in 30 minutes if necessary and if no hypotension occurs. For IV use, give 2 mg per fractional injection at 2-minute intervals. Do not exceed 25 mg (dilute 1 mg/mL with saline).

Preoperative apprehension – 12.5 to 25 mg IM 1 to 2 hours before surgery.

Psychotic disorders – Maximum improvement may not be seen for weeks or even months. Continue optimum dosage for 2 weeks, then gradually reduce to lowest effective maintenance level. A dosage of 200 mg/day is not unusual. Some patients require higher dosages (eg, 800 mg/day is not uncommon in discharged mental patients).

Hospitalized patients:

• *Acute schizophrenic or manic states* –

Maximum dose: 400 mg every 4 to 6 hours.

Initial dosage: 25 mg IM. If necessary, give an additional 25 to 50 mg injection in 1 hour.

Dosage titration: Increase gradually over several days (up to 400 mg every 4 to 6 hours in exceptionally severe cases) until patient is controlled. Patient usually becomes quiet and cooperative within 24 to 48 hours. Substitute oral dosage and increase until the patient is calm. (See the Chlorpromazine oral monograph for more information.)

Prompt control of severe symptoms: 25 mg IM; if necessary, repeat in 1 hour. Give subsequent doses orally, 25 to 50 mg 3 times/day.

Tetanus –

IM: 25 to 50 mg IM 3 or 4 times/day, usually with barbiturates.

IV: 25 to 50 mg diluted to at least 1 mg/mL and administered at a rate of 1 mg/min.

Off-label dosing –

Treatment of migraine (IV): [3] = Safety concerns. 5 to 50 mg (total dose) IV as a single dose. Some trials allowed for repeat dosing in nonresponders. One trial used weight-based dosing at 0.1 mg/kg.

➤*Children:*

Older than 12 years of age – See Adults for dosing for children older than 12 years of age.

6 months to 12 years of age –

Behavioral disorders/Hyperactivity:

• *Hospitalized patients* –

Usual dosage: Start with low doses and increase gradually. In severe behavior disorders, 50 to 100 mg/day, or in older children, 200 mg/day or more may be necessary. There is little evidence that improvement in severely disturbed mentally retarded patients is enhanced by doses beyond 500 mg/day.

Maximum dose: 40 mg/day IM for children up to 5 years of age (or 50 lbs); 75 mg/day IM for children 5 to 12 years of age (or 50 to 100 lbs), except in unmanageable cases.

• *Outpatients* – 0.55 mg/kg (0.25 mg/lb) IM every 6 to 8 hours, as needed.

Nausea and vomiting: The activity following IM use may last 12 hours.

• *Usual dosage* – 0.55 mg/kg (0.25 mg/lb) IM every 6 to 8 hours, as needed.

• *Maximum dose* – 40 mg/day IM for children up to 5 years (or 50 lbs); 75 mg/day IM for children 5 to 12 years of age (or 50 to 100 lbs), except in severe cases.

• *Intraoperative (to control acute nausea/vomiting)* – For IM use, give 0.275 mg/kg (0.125 mg/lb) IM; repeat in 30 minutes if needed and if no hypotension occurs.

For IV use, give 1 mg per fractional injection at 2-minute intervals; do not exceed IM dosage. Always dilute to 1 mg/mL with saline.

Preoperative apprehension: 0.55 mg/kg (0.25 mg/lb) IM 1 to 2 hours before surgery.

Tetanus:

• *Usual dosage* – 0.55 mg/kg (0.25 mg/lb) IM or IV every 6 to 8 hours. When given IV, dilute to at least 1 mg/mL and administer at a rate of 1 mg per 2 minutes.

• *Maximum dose* – 40 mg/day for children up to 23 kg (50 lbs); 75 mg/day for children 23 to 45 kg (50 to 100 lbs), except in severe cases.

➤*Elderly:* Lower initial doses and more gradual adjustments are recommended.

➤*Debilitated/Emaciated patients:* Lower initial doses and more gradual adjustments are recommended.

➤*Administration:* Subcutaneous administration is not advised. Inject IM slowly, deep into upper outer quadrant of buttock. If irritation is a problem, dilute injection with saline or procaine 2%; do not mix with other agents in the syringe. Avoid injecting undiluted into vein. Use the IV route only for severe hiccoughs, surgery, and tetanus.

Because of the possibility of contact dermatitis, avoid getting solution on hands or clothing.

➤*Storage/Stability:* Store between 15° and 30°C (59° and 86°F). Protect the injection solution from light, or discoloration may occur. Slight yellowing will not alter potency. Discard if markedly discolored.

FLUPHENAZINE

Rx	**Fluphenazine HCl** (Various, eg, Geneva)	**Tablets**: 1 mg	In 50s, 100s, 500s, 1000s, and UD 100s.
Rx	**Fluphenazine HCl** (Various, eg, Geneva)	**Tablets**: 2.5 mg	In 50s, 100s, 500s, 1000s, and UD 100s.
Rx	**Fluphenazine HCl** (Various, eg, Geneva)	**Tablets**: 5 mg	In 50s, 100s, 500s, 1000s, and UD 100s.
Rx	**Fluphenazine HCl** (Various, eg, Geneva, Par)	**Tablets**: 10 mg	In 50s, 100s, 500s, 1000s, and UD 100s.
Rx	**Fluphenazine HCl** (Various, eg, Pharmaceuticals Associates)	**Elixir**: 2.5 mg/5 mL	May contain 14% alcohol and sucrose. In 60 and 473 mL.
Rx	**Fluphenazine HCl** (Pharmaceuticals Associates)	**Oral solution, concentrate**: 5 mg/mL	14% alcohol. In 120 mL with safety-cap dropper calibrated at 0.1 mL and in 0.2 mL increments.
Rx	**Fluphenazine HCl** (American Pharmaceutical Partners)	**Injection**: 2.5 mg/mL	Parabens. In 10 mL vials.
Rx	**Fluphenazine Decanoate** (Various, eg, Bedford Labs, Geneva)	**Injection**: 25 mg/mL	May contain sesame oil and benzyl alcohol. In 5 mL multidose vials.

FLUPHENAZINE HYDROCHLORIDE — ORAL

Complete and comparative prescribing information begins in the Antipsychotic Agents group monograph.

Indications

➤*Psychotic disorders:* For the management of manifestations of psychotic disorders.

➤*Off-label uses:*

Postherpetic neuralgia – [5] = Poor documentation. The efficacy of fluphenazine for postherpetic neuralgia (PHN) has been evaluated in one trial in which it failed to show benefit either alone or in combination with amitriptyline. While American Academy of Neurology clinical practice guidelines do not make a statement regarding fluphenazine, they consider the efficacy of chlorprothixine (another neuroleptic) to be unproven. Given the documented lack of efficacy and possibility of significant adverse effects, fluphenazine should not be used for the treatment of PHN.

Administration and Dosage

➤*General dosing considerations:* The oral dose is approximately 2 to 3 times the parenteral dose.

Individualize dosage. Institute treatment with a low initial dosage; increase as necessary. Therapeutic effect is often achieved with doses under 20 mg/day. However, daily doses up to 40 mg may be needed.

➤*Adults:*

Psychotic disorders –

Initial dosage: 2.5 to 10 mg/day in divided doses at 6 to 8 hour intervals.

Maintenance dosage: When symptoms are controlled, reduce dosage gradually to daily maintenance doses of 1 or 5 mg, often given as a single daily dose. Continued treatment is needed to achieve maximum therapeutic benefits; further adjustments in dosage may be necessary during the course of therapy to meet the patient's requirements.

FLUPHENAZINE HYDROCHLORIDE — ORAL

Conversion: For psychotic patients stabilized on a fixed daily dosage of orally administered fluphenazine, conversion from oral therapy to the long-acting injectable fluphenazine decanoate may be indicated.

➤*Elderly:* Initially, 1 to 2.5 mg/day, adjusted according to response.

➤*Hepatic function impairment:* Contraindicated in patients with liver damage.

➤*Administration:*

Oral concentrate – When the oral concentrate dosage form is to be used, the desired dose (measured by a calibrated device only) should be added to at least 60 mL (2 fluid ounces) of a suitable diluent just prior to administration to ensure palatability and stability. Suggested diluents include tomato or fruit juice, milk, and uncaffeinated soft drinks. The oral concentrate should not be mixed with beverages containing caffeine (coffee, cola), tannics (tea), or pectinates (apple juice) because of the potential incompatibility.

➤*Storage/Stability:* Store at 15° to 30°C (59° to 86°F); avoid excessive heat. Protect from light and keep tightly closed. Do not freeze elixir or oral concentrate.

FLUPHENAZINE HYDROCHLORIDE — INJECTION

Complete and comparative prescribing information begins in the Antipsychotic Agents group monograph.

Indications

➤*Psychotic disorders:* For the management of manifestations of psychotic disorders.

➤*Off-label uses:*

Postherpetic neuralgia – [5] = Poor documentation. The efficacy of fluphenazine for postherpetic neuralgia (PHN) has been evaluated in one trial in which it failed to show benefit either alone or in combination with amitriptyline. While American Academy of Neurology clinical practice guidelines do not make a statement regarding fluphenazine, they consider the efficacy of chlorprothixine (another neuroleptic) to be unproven. Given the documented lack of efficacy and possibility of significant adverse effects, fluphenazine should not be used for the treatment of PHN.

Administration and Dosage

➤*General dosing considerations:* The oral dose is approximately 2 to 3 times the parenteral dose.

Administer intramuscularly (IM). Individualize dosage. Institute treatment with a low initial dosage; increase as necessary. Therapeutic effect is often achieved with doses under 20 mg/day. However, daily doses up to 40 mg may be needed.

➤*Adults:*

Psychotic disorders –

Initial dosage: 1.25 mg (0.5 mL) IM. Initial total daily dose may range from 2.5 to 10 mg and should be divided and given at 6- to 8-hour intervals. Use dosages exceeding 10 mg per day with caution.

Maintenance dosage: When symptoms are controlled, oral maintenance therapy can generally be instituted, often with single daily doses.

➤*Hepatic function impairment:* Contraindicated in patients with liver damage.

➤*Administration:* Administer IM.

➤*Storage/Stability:* Store at 15° to 30°C (59° to 86°F); avoid excessive heat. Protect from light. Do not freeze. Parenteral solutions may vary in color from essentially colorless to light amber. If a solution has become any darker than light amber or is discolored in any other way, it should not be used.

FLUPHENAZINE DECANOATE — INJECTION

Complete and comparative prescribing information begins in the Antipsychotic Agents group monograph.

Indications

➤*Psychotic disorders:* For patients requiring prolonged and parenteral neuroleptic therapy (eg, chronic schizophrenic patients).

Administration and Dosage

➤*General dosing considerations:* The oral dose is approximately 2 to 3 times the parenteral dose.

Initially, treat patients who have never taken phenothiazines with a shorter-acting form of the drug before administering the decanoate. This helps to determine the response to fluphenazine and to establish appropriate dosage.

Individualize dosage. Institute treatment with a low initial dosage; increase as necessary. Therapeutic effect is often achieved with doses less than 20 mg/day. However, daily doses up to 40 mg may be needed. The optimal amount of the drug and the frequency of administration must be determined for each patient because dosage requirements have been found to vary with clinical circumstances as well as with individual response to the drug.

➤*Adults:*

Psychotic disorders –

Maximum dose: 100 mg.

Initial dosage: 12.5 to 25 mg (0.5 to 1 mL) intramuscularly (IM) or subcutaneously. The onset of action generally appears between 24 and 72 hours after injection, and the effects of the drug on psychotic symptoms become significant within 48 to 96 hours.

Dosage titration: Determine subsequent injections and dosage interval in accordance with patient response. If doses greater than 50 mg are needed, increase succeeding doses cautiously in 12.5 mg increments.

Maintenance dosage: A single injection may be effective in controlling schizophrenic symptoms up to 4 weeks or longer. The response to a single dose has been found to last as long as 6 weeks in a few patients on maintenance therapy.

Conversion: For psychotic patients stabilized on a fixed daily dosage of orally administered fluphenazine, conversion from oral therapy to the long-acting injectable fluphenazine decanoate may be indicated.

No precise formula can be given to convert to fluphenazine decanoate use. However, in a controlled multicenter study, 20 mg/day of oral fluphenazine hydrochloride was equivalent to fluphenazine decanoate 25 mg every 3 weeks. This is an approximate conversion ratio of 12.5 mg (0.5 mL) decanoate every 3 weeks for every fluphenazine hydrochloride 10 mg daily. Do not exceed 100 mg. Once conversion to fluphenazine decanoate is made, careful clinical monitoring of the patient and appropriate dosage adjustment should be made at the time of each injection.

Severely agitated patients: Initially treat with a rapid-acting phenothiazine. When acute symptoms subside, administer 25 mg of the fluphenazine decanoate; adjust subsequent dosage as necessary.

Poor risk patients: In poor risk patients (known phenothiazine hypersensitivity or with disorders predisposing to undue reactions), cautiously initiate oral or parenteral fluphenazine. When appropriate dosage is established, give equivalent dose of fluphenazine decanoate.

➤*Hepatic function impairment:* Contraindicated in patients with liver damage.

➤*Administration:* Administer IM or subcutaneously. Use a dry syringe and needle of at least 21 gauge. A wet needle or syringe may cause the solution to become cloudy.

➤*Storage/Stability:* Store at 15° to 30°C (59° to 86°F); avoid excessive heat. Do not freeze. Protect from light. Retain vial in carton until ready for use.

PERPHENAZINE

Rx	**Perphenazine** (Various, eg, Geneva, Ivax)	**Tablets:** 2 mg	In 100s, 1000s, and UD 100s.
Rx	**Perphenazine** (Various, eg, Geneva, Ivax)	**Tablets:** 4 mg	In 100s, 500s, 1000s, and UD 100s.
Rx	**Perphenazine** (Various, eg, Geneva, Ivax)	**Tablets:** 8 mg	In 100s, 500s, 1000s, and UD 100s.
Rx	**Perphenazine** (Various, eg, Geneva, Ivax)	**Tablets:** 16 mg	In 100s, 1000s, and UD 100s.

PERPHENAZINE — ORAL

For complete and comparative prescribing information refer to the Antipsychotic Agents group monograph.

Indications

➤*Psychotic disorders:* For the treatment of schizophrenia (tablets).

➤*Emesis:* To control severe nausea and vomiting in adults.

Administration and Dosage

➤*General dosing considerations:* Individualize the dosage and adjust according to the severity of the condition and the response obtained.

➤*Adults:*

Intractable hiccoughs – 8 to 16 mg daily in divided doses; occasionally, 24 mg may be necessary. Early dosage reduction is desirable.

Nausea/Vomiting – 8 to 16 mg daily in divided doses; occasionally, 24 mg may be necessary. Early dosage reduction is desirable.

Schizophrenia –

Hospitalized patients: 8 to 16 mg 2 to 4 times/day; avoid dosages greater than 64 mg/day.

Reserve prolonged administration of doses exceeding 24 mg/day for hospitalized patients or patients under continued observation for early detection and management of adverse reactions. An antiparkinsonian agent, such as trihexyphenidyl or benztropine, is valuable in controlling drug-induced extrapyramidal symptoms.

Outpatients: 4 to 8 mg 3 times/day initially; reduce as soon as possible to minimum effective dosage.

➤*Children:*

12 years of age and older – See Adults for dosing for children 12 years of age and older. Perphenazine is not indicated for the treatment of severe nausea and vomiting in children.

PERPHENAZINE — ORAL

➤*Hepatic function impairment:* Contraindicated in patients with liver damage.

➤*Storage / Stability:*
Tablets – Store at 15° to 30°C (59° to 86°F). Dispense in a tight, light-resistant container.

PROCHLORPERAZINE

Rx	**Prochlorperazine** (Various, eg, Barr, Geneva, Par, UDL, Ivax)	**Tablets:** 5 mg (as maleate)	In 100s, 500s, 1000s, blister pack 25s, and UD 100s.
Rx	**Prochlorperazine** (Various, eg, Barr, Geneva, Par, UDL, Ivax)	**Tablets:** 10 mg (as maleate)	In 100s, 500s, 1000s, blister pack 25s, and UD 100s.
Rx	**Prochlorperazine** (Various, eg, Abbott)	**Injection:** 5 mg/mL (as edisylate)	In 2 mL vials.
Rx	**Prochlorperazine** (Various, eg, G & W Labs)	**Suppositories:** 25 mg	In 12s.
Rx	**Compro** (Paddock)		Glycerin and coconut oil. In 12s.

[a] With sodium saccharin, benzyl alcohol, sodium biphosphate, and sodium tartrate.

PROCHLORPERAZINE — ORAL

For complete and comparative prescribing information refer to the Antipsychotic Agents class monograph. See also the Antiemetic/Antivertigo Agents monograph.

Indications

➤*Schizophrenia:* For the treatment of schizophrenia.

➤*Nonpsychotic anxiety:* For the short-term treatment of generalized nonpsychotic anxiety; however, prochlorperazine is not the first drug of choice for this indication.

➤*Emesis:* To control severe nausea and vomiting.

Administration and Dosage

➤*Adults:*

Nausea and vomiting –
Tablets: 5 to 10 mg, 3 or 4 times daily.
Spansule capsule: Initially, 15 mg upon arising or 10 mg every 12 hours.

Nonpsychotic anxiety –
Usual dosage:
• *Tablets* – 5 mg 3 to 4 times/day.
• *Spansule capsule* – 15 mg upon arising, or 10 mg every 12 hours.
Maximum dose: 20 mg/day or for longer than 12 weeks.

Schizophrenia – Adjust dosage to the response of the individual and according to the severity of the condition. Begin with the lowest recommended dose. Although response is ordinarily seen within a day or 2, longer treatment is usually required before maximal improvement is seen.
Mild conditions: 5 or 10 mg 3 or 4 times/day.
Moderate to severe conditions:
• *Initial dosage* – 10 mg 3 or 4 times/day.
• *Dosage titration* – Gradually increase dosage until symptoms are controlled or adverse reactions become bothersome. When dosage is increased by small increments every 2 or 3 days, adverse reactions either do not occur or are easily controlled. Some patients respond satisfactorily on 50 to 75 mg/day.
Severe conditions: 100 to 150 mg/day.

➤*Children:* Children seem more prone to develop extrapyramidal reactions, even on moderate doses. Use the lowest effective dose. Occasionally the patients may react to the drug with signs of restlessness and excitement. Do not administer additional doses if this occurs. Take particular precaution in administering the drug to children with acute illnesses or dehydration.

Adjust dosage and frequency of administration according to the severity of the symptoms and the response of the patient.

Do not use in pediatric surgery.

Nausea and vomiting –
2 years of age and older and at least 9.1 kg (20 lbs): More than 1 days' therapy is seldom necessary.

Prochlorperazine Oral Dosing in Children 2 Years of age and older		
Weight	Usual dosage	Not to exceed
Under 20 lbs: Use is not recommended		
9.1 to 13.2 kg (20 to 29 lbs)	2.5 mg 1 or 2 times/day	7.5 mg/day
13.6 to 17.7 kg (30 to 39 lbs)	2.5 mg 2 or 3 times/day	10 mg/day
18.2 to 38.6 kg (40 to 85 lbs)	2.5 mg 3 times/day or 5 mg 2 times /day	15 mg/day

Schizophrenia –
2 to 12 years of age:
• *Maximum dose* – 20 mg/day (2 to 5 years of age); 25 mg/day (6 to 12 years of age).
• *Initial dosage* – 2.5 mg 2 or 3 times/day. Do not give more than 10 mg on the first day.
• *Dosage titration* – Increase dosage according to the patient's response.

➤*Elderly:* Dosages in the lower range are sufficient for most elderly patients. Because they appear to be more susceptible to hypotension and neuromuscular reactions, observe such patients closely. Tailor dosage to the individual, carefully monitor response, and adjust dose accordingly. Increase dosage more gradually in elderly patients.

➤*Debilitated / emaciated patients:* Increase dosage more gradually in debilitated or emaciated patients.

➤*Storage / Stability:* Store between 15° and 30°C (59° and 86°F). Protect from light.

PROCHLORPERAZINE — INJECTION

For complete and comparative prescribing information refer to the Antipsychotic Agents group monograph. See also the Antiemetic/Antivertigo Agents monograph.

Indications

➤*Schizophrenia:* For the treatment of schizophrenia.

➤*Nonpsychotic anxiety:* For the short-term treatment of generalized nonpsychotic anxiety; however, prochlorperazine is not the first drug of choice for this indication.

➤*Emesis:* To control severe nausea and vomiting.

Administration and Dosage

➤*General dosing considerations:* Hypotension may occur if the drug is given by intravenous (IV) injection or by infusion. Do not give by bolus injection. (See Administration).

➤*Adults:*

Nausea and vomiting –
Intramuscular (IM) use:
• *Usual dosage* – 5 to 10 mg given by deep IM injection. If necessary, repeat every 3 or 4 hours.
• *Maximum dose* – 40 mg/day.
IV use:
• *Usual dosage* – 2.5 to 10 mg by slow IV injection or infusion at a rate not to exceed 5 mg/min.
• *Maximum dose* – 10 mg (single dose); 40 mg/day (total daily dose).

Surgery-related nausea and vomiting –
IM use:
• *Usual dosage* – 5 to 10 mg given by deep IM injection, 1 to 2 hours before induction of anesthesia (may repeat once in 30 minutes), or to control acute symptoms during and after surgery (may repeat once).
• *Maximum dose* – 40 mg/day.
IV use:
• *Usual dosage* – 5 to 10 mg by slow IV injection or infusion (at a rate not to exceed 5 mg/min) 15 to 30 minutes before induction of anesthesia or to control acute symptoms during and after surgery. Repeat once if necessary.
• *Maximum dose* – 10 mg (single dose); 40 mg/day (total daily dose).

Schizophrenia (severe symptoms) – Adjust dosage to the response of the individual and according to the severity of the condition. Begin with the lowest recommended dose. Although response is ordinarily seen within 1 or 2 days, longer treatment is usually required before maximal improvement is seen.
Initial dosage: 10 to 20 mg given by deep IM injection. Many patients respond shortly after the first injection. If necessary, repeat the initial dose every 2 to 4 hours (or, in resistant cases, every hour) to gain control of the patient, if necessary. More than 3 or 4 doses are seldom necessary.
Maintenance dosage: If, in rare cases, parenteral therapy is needed for a prolonged period, give 10 to 20 mg IM every 4 to 6 hours.
Conversion: After control is achieved, switch patient to an oral form of the drug at the same dosage levels or higher.

➤*Children:* Children seem more prone to develop extrapyramidal reactions, even on moderate doses. Use the lowest effective dose. Occasionally the patients may react to the drug with signs of restlessness and excitement. Do not administer additional doses if this occurs. Take particular precaution in administering the drug to children with acute illnesses or dehydration.

Adjust dosage and frequency of administration according to the severity of the symptoms and the response of the patient. The duration of activity following IM administration may last up to 12 hours. Subsequent doses may be given by the same route if necessary.

Do not use in pediatric surgery.

Nausea and vomiting –
2 years of age and older and at least 9.1 kg (20 lbs): 0.132 mg/kg (0.06 mg/lb) given by deep IM injection. Control is usually obtained with one dose. Duration of action may be 12 hours. Subsequent doses may be given if necessary.

PROCHLORPERAZINE — INJECTION

Schizophrenia –

Younger than 12 years of age:

• *Initial dosage* – 0.132 mg/kg (0.06 mg/lb) given by deep IM injection. Control is usually obtained with 1 dose.

• *Conversion* – After control is achieved, switch the patient to an oral form of the drug at the same dosage level or higher.

➤*Elderly:* Dosages in the lower range are sufficient for most elderly patients. Because they appear to be more susceptible to hypotension and neuromuscular reactions, observe such patients closely. Tailor dosage to the individual, carefully monitor response, and adjust dose accordingly. Increase dosage more gradually in elderly patients.

➤*Debilitated/emaciated patients:* Increase dosage more gradually in debilitated or emaciated patients.

➤*Administration:* Subcutaneous administration is not advisable because of local irritation. Hypotension may occur if the drug is given by IV injection or by infusion. Do not give by bolus injection. When administering by IV injection or infusion, administer at a rate not to exceed 5 mg/min.

Administer IM injections deeply into the upper outer quadrant of the buttock.

➤*Admixture compatibility:* Do not mix prochlorperazine injection with other agents in the syringe.

➤*Storage/Stability:* Store at 15° to 30°C (59° to 86°F). Do not freeze. Protect from light.

PROCHLORPERAZINE — RECTAL

For complete and comparative prescribing information refer to the Antipsychotic Agents group monograph. See also the Antiemetic/Antivertigo Agents monograph.

Indications

➤*Schizophrenia:* For the treatment of schizophrenia.

➤*Nonpsychotic anxiety:* For the short-term treatment of generalized nonpsychotic anxiety; however, prochlorperazine is not the first drug of choice for this indication.

➤*Emesis:* To control severe nausea and vomiting. (*Compro* is only indicated for severe nausea and vomiting in adults.)

Administration and Dosage

➤*General dosing considerations:* Adjust dosage to the response of the individual. Begin with the lowest recommended dosage.

➤*Adults:*

Nausea and vomiting – 25 mg twice daily administered rectally.

➤*Children:* No pediatric prochlorperazine rectal strength is commercially available. For pediatric dosing information, see the Prochlorperazine Oral monograph.

Do not use in pediatric surgery. Do not use prochlorperazine in children younger than 2 years of age or under 9.1 kg (20 lbs).

➤*Elderly:* In general, dosages in the lower range are sufficient for most elderly patients. Because they appear to be more susceptible to hypotension and neuromuscular reactions, such patients should be observed closely. Dosage should be tailored to the individual, response carefully monitored and dosage adjusted accordingly. Dosage should be increased more gradually in elderly patients.

➤*Debilitated/emaciated patients:* Dosage should be increased more gradually in debilitated or emaciated patients.

➤*Storage/Stability:* Store between 15° and 30°C (59° and 86°F). Protect from light.

TRIFLUOPERAZINE HYDROCHLORIDE

Rx	**Trifluoperazine** (Various, eg, Sandoz, UDL)	**Tablets:** 1 mg	In 100s, 500s, 1000s, and UD 100s.
		2 mg	In 100s, 500s, 1000s, and UD 100s.
		5 mg	In 100s, 500s, 1000s, and UD 100s.
		10 mg	In 100s, 500s, 1000s, and UD 100s.

TRIFLUOPERAZINE HYDROCHLORIDE — ORAL

For complete and comparative prescribing information refer to the Antipsychotic Agents group monograph.

Indications

➤*Schizophrenia:* For the management of schizophrenia.

➤*Nonpsychotic anxiety:* For the short-term treatment of nonpsychotic anxiety (not the first drug of choice in most patients).

Administration and Dosage

➤*General dosing considerations:* Individualize dosage. Increase dosage more gradually in debilitated or emaciated patients. When maximum response is achieved, reduce dosage gradually to a maintenance level. Use the lowest effective dosage. Patients may be controlled with once- or twice-daily administration.

➤*Adults:*

Nonpsychotic anxiety –

Usual dosage: 1 or 2 mg twice daily.

Maximum dose: 6 mg/day or for longer than 12 weeks because trifluoperazine use at higher doses or for longer intervals may cause persistent tardive dyskinesia that may prove irreversible.

Schizophrenia –

Initial dosage: 2 to 5 mg twice daily. Start small or emaciated patients on the lower dosage.

Maintenance dosage: Optimum therapeutic dosage levels should be reached within 2 or 3 weeks. Most patients will show optimum response with 15 or 20 mg/day, although a few may require 40 mg/day or more.

➤*Children:*

Schizophrenia –

Older than 12 years of age: See Adults for dosing for children older than 12 years of age.

6 to 12 years of age: Adjust dosage to the weight of the child and severity of the symptoms. These dosages are for children 6 to 12 years of age who are hospitalized or under close supervision.

• *Initial dosage* – 1 mg administered once or twice daily.

• *Dosage titration* – Dosage may be increased gradually until symptoms are controlled or until adverse reactions become troublesome. While it is usually not necessary to exceed 15 mg/day, older children with severe symptoms may require higher doses.

➤*Elderly:* Usually, lower dosages are sufficient. Elderly patients appear more susceptible to hypotension and neuromuscular reactions; observe closely and increase dosage more gradually.

➤*Hepatic function impairment:* Contraindicated in patients with preexisting liver damage.

➤*Storage/Stability:* Store between 15° and 30°C (59° and 86°F).

THIORIDAZINE HYDROCHLORIDE

Rx	**Thioridazine HCl** (Various, eg, Geneva, Mylan, URL/Mutual)	**Tablets:** 10 mg	In 60s, 100s, 1000s, and UD 100s.
Rx	**Thioridazine HCl** (Various, eg, Geneva)	**Tablets:** 15 mg	In 100s, 1000s, and UD 100s.
Rx	**Thioridazine HCl** (Various, eg, Geneva, Mylan, URL/Mutual)	**Tablets:** 25 mg	In 60s, 100s, 1000s, and UD 100s.
Rx	**Thioridazine HCl** (Various, eg, Geneva, Mylan, URL/Mutual)	**Tablets:** 50 mg	In 60s, 100s, 1000s, and UD 100s.
Rx	**Thioridazine HCl** (Various, eg, Geneva, Mylan, URL/Mutual)	**Tablets:** 100 mg	In 60s, 100s, 1000s, and UD 100s.
Rx	**Thioridazine HCl** (Various, eg, Geneva)	**Tablets:** 150 mg	In 100s and 1000s.
Rx	**Thioridazine HCl** (Various, eg, Geneva)	**Tablets:** 200 mg	In 100s and 1000s.

Phenothiazine Derivatives

THIORIDAZINE HYDROCHLORIDE — ORAL

For complete and comparative prescribing information refer to the Antipsychotic Agents group monograph.

WARNING

Thioridazine has been shown to prolong the QTc interval in a dose-related manner. Drugs with this potential, including thioridazine, have been associated with torsade de pointes-type arrhythmias and sudden death. Because of its potential for significant, possibly life-threatening, proarrhythmic effects, reserve thioridazine use in the treatment of schizophrenic patients who fail to show an acceptable response to adequate courses of treatment with other antipsychotic drugs, either because of insufficient effectiveness or the inability to achieve an effective dose because of intolerable adverse effects from those drugs.

Indications

➤*Schizophrenia:* For the management of schizophrenic patients who fail to respond adequately to treatment with other antipsychotic drugs. Before initiating treatment with thioridazine, it is strongly recommended that a patient be given at least 2 trials, each with a different antipsychotic drug product, at an adequate dose and for an adequate duration.

Administration and Dosage

➤*General dosing considerations:* Dosage must be individualized and the smallest effective dosage should be determined for each patient.

➤*Adults:*

Schizophrenia –

Maximum dose: 800 mg/day.

Initial dosage: 50 to 100 mg 3 times/day.

Dosage titration: Gradually increase dose to a maximum of 800 mg/day, if necessary. Once effective control of symptoms has been achieved, the dosage may be reduced gradually to determine the minimum maintenance dose.

Maintenance dosage: 200 to 800 mg/day, divided into 2 to 4 doses.

➤*Children:* For patients unresponsive to other agents.

Schizophrenia –

Maximum dose: 3 mg/kg/day.

Initial dosage: 0.5 mg/kg/day given in divided doses.

Dosage titration: Dosage may be increased gradually until optimum therapeutic effect is obtained or the maximum dose of 3 mg/kg/day has been reached.

➤*Storage/Stability:* Store at 15° to 30°C (59° to 86°F); dispense in a tight, light-resistant container.

Thioxanthene Derivatives

THIOTHIXENE

Rx	**Thiothixene** (Various, eg, Sandoz)	**Capsules; oral:** 1 mg	May contain lactose. In 100s and 1,000s.
Rx	**Navane** (Pfizer)		Lactose. In 100s.
Rx	**Thiothixene** (Various, eg, Sandoz)	**Capsules; oral:** 2 mg	May contain lactose. In 100s, 1,000s, and UD 100s.
Rx	**Navane** (Pfizer)		Lactose. In 100s.
Rx	**Thiothixene** (Various, eg, Sandoz)	**Capsules; oral:** 5 mg	May contain lactose. In 100s, 1,000s, and UD 100s.
Rx	**Navane** (Pfizer)		Lactose. In 100s.
Rx	**Thiothixene** (Various, eg, Sandoz)	**Capsules; oral:** 10 mg	May contain lactose. In 100s, 1,000s, and UD 100s.
Rx	**Navane** (Pfizer)		Lactose. In 100s.
Rx	**Navane** (Pfizer)	**Capsules; oral:** 20 mg	Lactose. In 100s.

THIOTHIXENE — ORAL

For complete and comparative prescribing information refer to the class monograph.Antipsychotic Agents

WARNING

Increased mortality in elderly patients with dementia-related psychosis –

Elderly patients with dementia-related psychosis treated with antipsychotic drugs are at an increased risk of death. Analyses of 17 placebo-controlled trials (modal duration of 10 weeks), largely in patients taking atypical antipsychotic drugs, revealed a risk of death in drug-treated patients of between 1.6 and 1.7 times the risk of death in placebo-treated patients. Over the course of a typical 10-week controlled trial, the rate of death in drug-treated patients was about 4.5%, compared with a rate of about 2.6% in the placebo group. Although the causes of death were varied, most of the deaths appeared to be either cardiovascular (eg, heart failure, sudden death) or infectious (eg, pneumonia) in nature. Observational studies suggest that, similar to atypical antipsychotic drugs, treatment with conventional antipsychotic drugs may increase mortality. The extent to which the findings of increased mortality in observational studies may be attributed to the antipsychotic drug as opposed to some characteristic(s) of the patients is not clear. Thiothixene is not approved for the treatment of patients with dementia-related psychosis.

Indications

➤*Schizophrenia:* For the management of schizophrenia.

Administration and Dosage

➤*General dosing considerations:* Individualize dose depending on the chronicity and severity of the symptoms of schizophrenia.

In general, use small doses initially and gradually increase to the optimal effective level based on patient response.

Some patients have been successfully maintained on once-a-day therapy.

➤*Adults:*

Schizophrenia –

Mild conditions: Initially, 2 mg 3 times/day is recommended. If indicated, a subsequent increase to 15 mg/day is often effective.

Severe conditions:

• *Usual dosage* – The optimum dosage is 20 to 30 mg/day. If indicated, an increase to 60 mg/day total daily dosage is often effective. Exceeding a total daily dosage of 60 mg/day rarely increases the beneficial response.

• *Initial dosage* – Initially, 5 mg twice daily is recommended.

➤*Children:* See Adults for dosing in children 12 years of age and older.

➤*Storage/Stability:* Store at controlled room temperature of up to 30°C (86°F).

Phenylbutylpiperadine Derivatives

HALOPERIDOL

Rx	**Haloperidol** (Various, eg, Mallinckrodt, Sandoz, UDL)	**Tablets; oral:** 0.5 mg	May contain lactose. In 100s and UD 100s.
		1 mg	May contain lactose. In 100s, 1,000s, and UD 100s.
		2 mg	May contain lactose. In 100s, 1,000s, and UD 100s.
		5 mg	May contain lactose. In 100s, 1,000s, UD 100s, and UD 300s.
		10 mg	May contain lactose. In 100s, 1,000s, and UD 100s.
		20 mg	May contain lactose. In 100s.
Rx	**Haloperidol** (Various, eg, PAI, Qualitest, Teva)	**Solution, concentrate; oral:** 2 mg/mL	As haloperidol lactate. In 15 and 120 mL, and 5 mL UD 100s.
Rx	**Haloperidol** (Various, eg, APP, Teva)	**Injection, solution:** 5 mg/mL	As haloperidol lactate. May contain parabens. In 1, 2, and 10 mL vials.
Rx	**Haldol** (Ortho-McNeil)		As haloperidol lactate. In 1 mL ampuls.

Phenylbutylpiperadine Derivatives

HALOPERIDOL

Rx	**Haloperidol Decanoate** (Various, eg, Bedford, Teva)	**Injection, oil, extended-release:** 50 mg/mL	Equiv. to decanoate 70.5 mg/mL. May contain sesame oil and benzyl alcohol 1.2%. In 1 mL single-dose vials and 5 mL multidose vials.
Rx	**Haldol Decanoate 50** (Janssen)		In 1 mL ampuls.[a]
Rx	**Haloperidol Decanoate** (Various, eg, Bedford, Teva)	**Injection, oil, extended-release:** 100 mg/mL	Equiv. to decanoate 141.04 mg/mL. May contain sesame oil and benzyl alcohol 1.2%. In 1 mL single-dose vials and 5 mL multidose vials.
Rx	**Haldol Decanoate 100** (Janssen)		In 1 mL ampuls.[a]

[a] In sesame oil with benzyl alcohol 1.2%.

HALOPERIDOL — ORAL

For complete and comparative prescribing information, refer to the Antipsychotic Agents class monograph.

WARNING

Increased mortality in elderly patients with dementia-related psychosis – Elderly patients with dementia-related psychosis treated with antipsychotic drugs are at an increased risk of death. Analyses of 17 placebo-controlled trials (modal duration, 10 weeks), largely in patients taking atypical antipsychotic drugs, revealed a risk of death in drug-treated patients of between 1.6 to 1.7 times the risk of death in placebo-treated patients. Over the course of a typical 10-week controlled trial, the rate of death in drug-treated patients was about 4.5% compared with a rate of about 2.6% in the placebo group. Although the causes of death were varied, most of the deaths appeared to be cardiovascular (eg, heart failure, sudden death) or infectious (eg, pneumonia) in nature. Observational studies suggest that, similar to atypical antipsychotic drugs, treatment with conventional antipsychotic drugs may increase mortality. The extent to which the findings of increased mortality in observational studies may be attributed to the antipsychotic drug as opposed to some characteristic(s) of the patients is not clear. Haloperidol is not approved for the treatment of patients with dementia-related psychosis.

Indications

➤*Behavioral disorders:* For the treatment of severe behavioral problems in children with combative, explosive hyperexcitability that cannot be accounted for by immediate provocation. Reserve for use in these children only after failure to respond to psychotherapy or medications other than antipsychotics.

➤*Hyperactivity:* For short-term treatment of hyperactive children who show excessive motor activity with accompanying conduct disorders consisting of some or all of the following symptoms: impulsivity, difficulty sustaining attention, aggression, mood lability, or poor frustration tolerance. Reserve for use in these children only after failure to respond to psychotherapy or medications other than antipsychotics.

➤*Psychotic disorders:* For use in the management of manifestations of psychotic disorders.

➤*Tourette disorder:* For the control of tics and vocal utterances in Tourette disorder in adults and children.

➤*Off-label uses:*

Hiccups (singultus) – [1] = Good documentation. Haloperidol may be a useful alternative in patients with intractable hiccups from various causes that have been unresponsive to other therapies.

Obsessive-compulsive disorder – [3] = Safety concerns. According to American Psychiatric Association guidelines, the addition of haloperidol or another first-generation antipsychotic agent may be appropriate as part of a step-wise approach for patients with obsessive-compulsive disorder (OCD) who fail to respond to initial therapy with a selective serotonin reuptake inhibitor or cognitive-behavioral therapy; however, avoid indiscriminate use of haloperidol for the treatment of OCD because of the potential for tardive dyskinesia.

Prevention of chemotherapy-induced nausea and vomiting – [1] = Good documentation. More recent medications are preferable to haloperidol because of a lower risk of adverse effects. In general, the National Comprehensive Cancer Network guidelines provide an outline that includes the use of haloperidol in a limited role for the prevention and treatment of breakthrough chemotherapy-induced nausea and vomiting.

Administration and Dosage

➤*General dosing considerations:* There is considerable variation from patient to patient in the amount of medication required for treatment. Individualize dosage. Children, debilitated or elderly patients, and those with a history of adverse reactions to neuroleptic drugs may require less haloperidol; optimal response is usually obtained with more gradual dosage adjustments and at lower dosage levels. Dosage adjustments, either upward or downward, should be carried out as rapidly as practicable to achieve optimum therapeutic control.

➤*Adults:*

Psychotic disorders –

Initial dosage:

- *Moderate symptoms* – 0.5 to 2 mg given 2 or 3 times daily.
- *Severe symptoms or chronic or resistant patients* – 3 to 5 mg given 2 or 3 times daily. To achieve prompt control, higher doses may be required.

Dosage titration: Patients who remain severely disturbed or inadequately controlled may require dosage adjustment. Daily doses of up to 100 mg may be necessary. Infrequently, doses greater than 100 mg have been used for severely resistant patients; however, safety of prolonged administration of such doses has not been demonstrated.

Tourette disorder – See Psychotic Disorders for dosing.

Off-label dosing –

Hiccups (singultus): [1] = Good documentation. Per guidelines, the recommended dosage is 0.5 to 2 mg administered 1 to 3 times daily. Dosages from published reports vary. After a single intramuscular (IM) dose of 2 mg, oral dosing for 2 days ranged from 1 mg 2 to 4 times daily.

Obsessive-compulsive disorder: [3] = Safety concerns. Initial dosing is suggested as 2 mg/day orally, titrated up to 10 mg/day based on response and tolerance. A mean dosage of 6 mg/day was effective in a meta-analysis. Once successful management is achieved, therapy should continue for 1 to 2 years before tapering is attempted. During tapering, dosages may be reduced by 10% to 25% every 1 to 2 months while monitoring for symptom exacerbation or return.

Prevention of chemotherapy-induced nausea and vomiting: [1] = Good documentation. 1 to 2 mg orally every 4 to 6 hours as needed for the treatment and prevention of breakthrough emesis. When used for preventative means, haloperidol should be given on a set schedule and not used on an as-needed basis.

➤*Children:*

Behavioral disorders/hyperactivity –

3 to 12 years of age (15 to 40 kg):

- *Initial dosage* – Start at the lowest dosage possible (0.5 mg/day).
- *Dosage titration* – If required, increase dose in 0.5 mg increments at 5- to 7-day intervals until therapeutic effect is obtained.
- *Maintenance dosage* – 0.05 to 0.075 mg/kg/day given in 2 to 3 divided doses. Upon achieving a satisfactory therapeutic response, dosage should then be gradually reduced to the lowest effective maintenance level.

In severely disturbed, nonpsychotic children or in hyperactive children with conduct disorders, short-term administration may suffice. There is little evidence that behavior improvement is further enhanced by dosages greater than 6 mg/day.

Psychotic disorders –

3 to 12 years of age (15 to 40 kg):

- *Initial dosage* – Start at the lowest dosage possible (0.5 mg/day).
- *Dosage titration* – If required, increase dose in 0.5 mg increments at 5- to 7-day intervals until therapeutic effect is obtained. Severely disturbed psychotic children may require higher doses.
- *Maintenance dosage* – 0.05 to 0.15 mg/kg/day given in 2 to 3 divided doses. Upon achieving a satisfactory therapeutic response, dosage should then be gradually reduced to the lowest effective maintenance level.

Tourette disorder – See Behavioral Disorders/Hyperactivity for dosing.

Off-label dosing –

Older than 12 years of age:

- *Acute agitation* – 1 to 15 mg/dose; repeat in 1 hour as needed.
- *Psychosis* – 1 to 15 mg/day, given in 2 to 3 divided doses.
- *Tourette disorder* – 0.5 to 2 mg/dose given 2 to 3 times daily.

➤*Elderly:* Lower initial doses and more gradual adjustments are recommended. Initial dosage is 0.5 to 2 mg given 2 or 3 times daily.

➤*Debilitated patients:* Lower initial doses and more gradual adjustments are recommended. Initial dosage is 0.5 to 2 mg given 2 or 3 times daily.

➤*Conversion:* Replace the injectable with the oral form as soon as feasible. For an approximation of the total daily dose required, use the parenteral dose administered in the preceding 24 hours; carefully monitor the patient for the first several days. Give the first oral dose within 12 to 24 hours following the last parenteral dose.

➤*Discontinuation of therapy:* It is not known whether gradual withdrawal of antipsychotic drugs will reduce the rate of occurrence of withdrawal emergent neurological signs, but until further evidence becomes available, it would be reasonable to gradually withdraw use of haloperidol.

➤*Storage/Stability:* Store at 20° to 25°C (68° to 77°F). Protect from light. Dispense in a tight, light-resistant container.

HALOPERIDOL LACTATE — ORAL

For complete and comparative prescribing information, refer to the Antipsychotic Agentsclass monograph.

WARNING

Increased mortality in elderly patients with dementia-related psychosis – Elderly patients with dementia-related psychosis treated with antipsychotic drugs are at an increased risk of death. Analyses of 17 placebo-controlled trials (modal duration, 10 weeks), largely in patients taking atypical antipsychotic drugs, revealed a risk of death in drug-treated patients of between 1.6 to 1.7 times the risk of death in placebo-treated patients. Over the course of a typical 10-week controlled trial, the rate of death in drug-treated patients was about 4.5%, compared with a rate of about 2.6% in the placebo group. Although the causes of death were varied, most of the deaths appeared to be cardiovascular (eg, heart failure, sudden death) or infectious (eg, pneumonia) in nature. Observational studies suggest that, similar to atypical antipsychotic drugs, treatment with conventional antipsychotic drugs may increase mortality. The extent to which the findings of increased mortality in observational studies may be attributed to the antipsychotic drug as opposed to some characteristic(s) of the patients is not clear. Haloperidol is not approved for the treatment of patients with dementia-related psychosis.

Indications

➤*Behavioral disorders:* For the treatment of severe behavioral problems in children with combative, explosive hyperexcitability that cannot be accounted for by immediate provocation. Reserve for use in these children only after failure to respond to psychotherapy or medications other than antipsychotics.

➤*Hyperactivity:* For short-term treatment of hyperactive children who show excessive motor activity with accompanying conduct disorders consisting of some or all of the following symptoms: impulsivity, difficulty sustaining attention, aggression, mood lability, or poor frustration tolerance. Reserve for use in these children only after failure to respond to psychotherapy or medications other than antipsychotics.

➤*Psychotic disorders:* For use in the management of manifestations of psychotic disorders.

➤*Tourette disorder:* For the control of tics and vocal utterances in Tourette disorder in adults and children.

➤*Off-label uses:*

Hiccups (singultus) – [1] = Good documentation. Haloperidol may be a useful alternative in patients with intractable hiccups from various causes that have been unresponsive to other therapies.

Obsessive-compulsive disorder – [3] = Safety concerns. According to American Psychiatric Association guidelines, the addition of haloperidol or another first-generation antipsychotic agent may be appropriate as part of a step-wise approach for patients with obsessive-compulsive disorder (OCD) who fail to respond to initial therapy with a selective serotonin reuptake inhibitor or cognitive-behavioral therapy; however, avoid indiscriminate use of haloperidol for the treatment of OCD because of the potential for tardive dyskinesia.

Prevention of chemotherapy-induced nausea and vomiting – [1] = Good documentation. More recent medications are preferable to haloperidol because of a lower risk of adverse effects. In general, the National Comprehensive Cancer Network guidelines provide an outline that includes the use of haloperidol in a limited role for the prevention and treatment of breakthrough chemotherapy-induced nausea and vomiting.

Administration and Dosage

➤*General dosing considerations:* Individualize dosage. Children, debilitated or elderly patients, and those with a history of adverse reactions to neuroleptic drugs may require less haloperidol; optimal response is usually obtained with more gradual dosage adjustments and at lower dosage levels.

➤*Adults:*

Psychotic Disorders –

Initial dosage:

- *Moderate symptoms* – 0.5 to 2 mg given 2 or 3 times daily.
- *Severe symptoms or chronic or resistant patients* – 3 to 5 mg 2 or 3 times daily. To achieve prompt control, higher doses may be required.

Dosage titration: Patients who remain severely disturbed or inadequately controlled may require dosage adjustment. Daily doses up to 100 mg may be necessary. Infrequently, doses greater than 100 mg have been used for severely resistant patients; however, safety of prolonged administration of such doses has not been demonstrated.

Tourette disorder – See Psychotic Disorders for dosing.

Off-label dosing –

Hiccups (singultus): [1] = Good documentation. Per guidelines, the recommended dosage is 0.5 to 2 mg administered 1 to 3 times daily. Doses from published reports vary. After a single intramuscular (IM) dose of 2 mg, the oral dosing for 2 days ranged from 1 mg 2 to 4 times daily.

Obsessive-compulsive disorder: [3] = Safety concerns. Initial dosing is suggested as 2 mg/day orally, titrated up to 10 mg/day based on response and tolerance. A mean dosage of 6 mg/day was effective in a meta-analysis. Once successful management is achieved, therapy should continue for 1 to 2 years before taper is attempted. During tapering, doses may be reduced by 10% to 25% every 1 to 2 months while monitoring for symptom exacerbation or return.

Prevention of chemotherapy-induced nausea and vomiting: [1] = Good documentation. 1 to 2 mg orally every 4 to 6 hours as needed for the treatment and prevention of breakthrough emesis. When used for preventative means, haloperidol should be given on a set schedule and not used on an as-needed basis.

➤*Children:*

Behavioral disorders/hyperactivity –

3 to 12 years of age (15 to 40 kg):

- *Initial dosage* – Start at the lowest dosage possible (0.5 mg/day).
- *Dosage titration* – If required, increase dose in 0.5 mg increments at 5- to 7-day intervals until therapeutic effect is obtained.
- *Maintenance dosage* – 0.05 to 0.075 mg/kg/day given in 2 to 3 divided doses. Upon achieving a satisfactory therapeutic response, dosage should then be gradually reduced to the lowest effective maintenance level.

In severely disturbed, nonpsychotic children or in hyperactive children with conduct disorders, short-term administration may suffice. There is little evidence that behavior improvement is further enhanced by dosages greater than 6 mg/day.

Psychotic disorders –

3 to 12 years of age (15 to 40 kg):

- *Initial dosage* – Start at the lowest dosage possible (0.5 mg/day).
- *Dosage titration* – If required, increase dose in 0.5 mg increments at 5- to 7-day intervals until therapeutic effect is obtained. Severely disturbed psychotic children may require higher doses.
- *Maintenance dosage* – 0.05 to 0.15 mg/kg/day given in 2 to 3 divided doses. Upon achieving a satisfactory therapeutic response, dosage should then be gradually reduced to the lowest effective maintenance level.

Tourette disorder – See Behavioral Disorders/Hyperactivity for dosing.

Off-label dosing –

Older than 12 years of age:

- *Acute agitation* – 1 to 15 mg/dose; repeat in 1 hour as needed.
- *Psychosis* – 1 to 15 mg/day given in 2 to 3 divided doses.
- *Tourette disorder* – 0.5 to 2 mg/dose given 2 to 3 times daily.

➤*Elderly:* Lower initial doses and more gradual adjustments are recommended. Initial dosage is 0.5 to 2 mg given 2 or 3 times daily.

➤*Debilitated patients:* Lower initial doses and more gradual adjustments are recommended. Initial dosage is 0.5 to 2 mg given 2 or 3 times daily.

➤*Conversion:* Replace the injectable with the oral form as soon as feasible. For an approximation of the total daily dose required, use the parenteral dose administered in the preceding 24 hours; carefully monitor the patient for the first several days. Give the first oral dose within 12 to 24 hours following the last parenteral dose.

➤*Discontinuation of therapy:* It is not known whether gradual withdrawal of antipsychotic drugs will reduce the rate of occurrence of withdrawal emergent neurological signs but until further evidence becomes available, it would be reasonable to gradually withdraw use of haloperidol.

➤*Administration:* Measure prescribed dose of oral concentrate using the calibrated dropper or dosing syringe.

➤*Storage/Stability:* Store at 20° to 25°C (68° to 77°F). Protect from light. Do not freeze. Dispense in a tight, light-resistant container.

HALOPERIDOL LACTATE — INJECTION

For complete and comparative prescribing information, refer to the Antipsychotic Agents class monograph.

WARNING

Increased mortality in elderly patients with dementia-related psychosis – Elderly patients with dementia-related psychosis treated with antipsychotic drugs are at an increased risk of death. Analyses of 17 placebo-controlled trials (modal duration, 10 weeks), largely in patients taking atypical antipsychotic drugs, revealed a risk of death in drug-treated patients of between 1.6 to 1.7 times the risk of death in placebo-treated patients. Over the course of a typical 10-week controlled trial, the rate of death in drug-treated patients was approximately 4.5%, compared with a rate of approximately 2.6% in the placebo group. Although the causes of death were varied, most of the deaths appeared to be cardiovascular (eg, heart failure, sudden death) or infectious (eg, pneumonia) in nature. Observational studies suggest that, similar to atypical antipsychotic drugs, treatment with conventional antipsychotic drugs may increase mortality. The extent to which the findings of increased mortality in observational studies may be attributed to the antipsychotic drug as opposed to some characteristic(s) of the patients is not clear. Haloperidol is not approved for the treatment of patients with dementia-related psychosis.

Indications

➤*Schizophrenia:* For use in the treatment of schizophrenia.

➤*Tourette disorder:* For the control of tics and vocal utterances in Tourette disorder.

➤*Off-label uses:*

Hiccups (singultus) – [1] = Good documentation. Haloperidol may be a useful alternative in patients with intractable hiccups from various causes that have been unresponsive to other therapies.

Other possible off-label uses – Prevention and treatment of chemotherapy-induced nausea or vomiting.

Administration and Dosage

➤*General dosing considerations:* There is considerable variation from patient to patient in the amount of medication required for treatment.

Individualize dosage. Patients with a history of adverse reactions to antipsychotic drugs may require less haloperidol.

➤*Adults:*

Schizophrenia –

Usual dosage: 2 to 5 mg intramuscularly (IM). To determine the initial dosage, consideration should be given to the patient's age, severity of illness, previous response to other antipsychotic drugs, and any concomitant medication or disease state.

Administer subsequent doses as often as every 60 minutes, although 4- to 8-hour intervals may be satisfactory.

Dosage adjustment: Dosage adjustments, either upward or downward, should be carried out as rapidly as practicable to achieve optimum therapeutic control. Optimal response is usually obtained with more gradual dosage adjustments and at lower dosage levels.

Conversion: An oral form should supplant the injectable as soon as practicable. For an initial approximation of the total daily dose required, the parenteral dose administered in the preceding 24 hours may be used. Because this dose is only an initial estimate, it is recommended that careful monitoring of clinical signs and symptoms, including clinical efficacy, sedation, and adverse effects, be carried out periodically for the first several days following the initiation of switchover. In this way, dosage adjustments, either upward or downward, can be quickly accomplished. Depending on the patient's clinical status, the first oral dose should be given within 12 to 24 hours following the last parenteral dose.

Off-label dosing –

Hiccups (singultus): [1] = Good documentation. Per guidelines, the recommended dosage is 2.5 to 5 mg administered IM 1 to 3 times, or 5 to 10 mg/day administered by subcutaneous/intravenous (IV) infusion. Doses from published reports vary. IV infusion of 5 mg every 6 hours has been used.

➤*Children:*

Off-label dosing –

Older than 12 years of age:

- *Acute agitation* – 2 to 5 mg/dose IM; repeat in 1 hour as needed.
- *Psychosis* – 2 to 5 mg IM every 4 to 8 hours as needed.

6 to 12 years of age:

- *Psychosis* –
  Usual dosage: 1 to 3 mg every 4 to 8 hours.
  Maximum dose: 0.15 mg/kg per 24 hours.

➤*Elderly:* Lower initial doses and more gradual dosage adjustments are recommended.

➤*Debilitated patients:* Lower initial doses and more dosage gradual adjustments are recommended.

➤*Discontinuation of therapy:* It is not known whether gradual withdrawal of antipsychotic drugs will reduce the rate of occurrence of withdrawal-emergent neurological signs, but until further evidence becomes available, it would be reasonable to gradually withdraw use of haloperidol.

➤*Administration:* Administer by IM injection. Haloperidol injection is not approved for IV administration. If administered IV, the electrocardiogram (ECG) should be monitored for QT prolongation and arrhythmias.

➤*Storage/Stability:* Store at 15° to 30°C (59° to 86°F). Protect from light; do not freeze.

HALOPERIDOL DECANOATE — INJECTION

For complete and comparative prescribing information, refer to the Antipsychotic Agents class monograph.

WARNING

Increased mortality in elderly patients with dementia-related psychosis – Elderly patients with dementia-related psychosis treated with antipsychotic drugs are at an increased risk of death. Analyses of 17 placebo-controlled trials (modal duration, 10 weeks), largely in patients taking atypical antipsychotic drugs, revealed a risk of death in drug-treated patients of between 1.6 to 1.7 times the risk of death in placebo-treated patients. Over the course of a typical 10-week controlled trial, the rate of death in drug-treated patients was approximately 4.5%, compared with a rate of approximately 2.6% in the placebo group. Although the causes of death were varied, most of the deaths appeared to be cardiovascular (eg, heart failure, sudden death) or infectious (eg, pneumonia) in nature. Observational studies suggest that, similar to atypical antipsychotic drugs, treatment with conventional antipsychotic drugs may increase mortality. The extent to which the findings of increased mortality in observational studies may be attributed to the antipsychotic drug as opposed to some characteristic(s) of the patients is not clear. Haloperidol is not approved for the treatment of patients with dementia-related psychosis.

Indications

➤*Schizophrenia:* For the treatment of patient with schizophrenia who require prolonged parenteral antipsychotic therapy.

Administration and Dosage

➤*General dosing considerations:* Individualize dosage. Debilitated or elderly patients and those with a history of adverse reactions to neuroleptic drugs may require less haloperidol; optimal response is usually obtained with more gradual dosage adjustments and at lower dosage levels.

Provide close clinical supervision during initiation and stabilization of therapy. The recommended interval between doses is monthly or every 4 weeks. However, variation in patient response may dictate a need for adjustment of the dosing interval as well as the dose. To determine the minimum effective dose, begin with lower initial doses and adjust the dose upward as needed.

Intended for use in chronic psychotic patients who require prolonged parenteral antipsychotic therapy. These patients should be previously stabilized on antipsychotic medication and should have been treated with, and tolerated well, short-acting haloperidol to exclude the possibility of an unexpected adverse sensitivity to haloperidol. Close clinical supervision is required during the initial period of dose adjustment to minimize the risk of overdosage or reappearance of psychotic symptoms before the next injection.

During dose adjustment or episodes of exacerbation of psychotic symptoms, haloperidol decanoate therapy can be supplemented with short-acting forms of haloperidol.

➤*Adults:*

Schizophrenia –

Maximum dose: 100 mg (as the initial dose).

Initial dosage: See the following table for the conversion from oral haloperidol to haloperidol decanoate injection. The initial dose should not exceed 100 mg regardless of previous antipsychotic dose requirements. If the conversion requires more than 100 mg of haloperidol decanoate as an initial dose, administer that dose in 2 injections (maximum of 100 mg initially, followed by the balance in 3 to 7 days).

Haloperidol Decanoate Dosing Recommendations[a]

Patients	First month[b]	Monthly maintenance
Stabilized on low daily oral dosages (≤ 10 mg/day)	10 to 15 × daily oral dosage	10 to 15 × previous daily oral dosage
Stabilized on higher dosages; risk of relapse	20 × daily oral dosage	10 to 15 × previous daily oral dosage
Tolerant to oral haloperidol		

[a] Clinical experience with dosages greater than 450 mg/month has been limited.
[b] Initial dose should not exceed 100 mg. See the previous paragraph for more information.

Maintenance dosage: See the previous table for monthly maintenance dose information. The recommended interval between doses is monthly or every 4 weeks. However, variation in patient response may dictate a need for adjustment of the dosing interval as well as the dose.

Upon achieving a satisfactory therapeutic response, gradually reduce dosage to the lowest effective maintenance level.

Dosage adjustment: To determine the minimum effective dose, begin with lower initial doses and adjust the dose upward as needed. Individualize with

Phenylbutylpiperadine Derivatives

HALOPERIDOL DECANOATE — INJECTION

titration upward or downward based on therapeutic response. Variation in patient response may dictate a need for adjustment of the dosing interval as well as the dose.

Conversion: Conversion from oral haloperidol to haloperidol decanoate can be achieved by using an initial dose of haloperidol decanoate that is 10 to 20 times the previous daily dose in oral haloperidol equivalent.

➤*Elderly:* Lower initial doses and more gradual adjustments are recommended. The recommended initial and maintenance dosage is 10 to 15 times daily oral dose administered intramuscularly (IM) monthly or every 4 weeks.

➤*Debilitated patients:* See Elderly for dosing.

➤*Administration:* Administer by deep IM injection. A 21-gauge needle is recommended. The maximum volume per injection site should not exceed 3 mL. The recommended interval between doses is monthly or every 4 weeks. Do not administer intravenously (IV).

➤*Storage/Stability:* Store at 15° to 30°C (59° to 86°F). Do not refrigerate or freeze. Protect from light. Retain vial in carton until contents are used.

PIMOZIDE

Rx	**Orap** (Gate)	**Tablets; oral:** 1 mg	Lactose. (ORAP 1). White, oval, scored. In 100s.
		2 mg	Lactose. (LEMMON ORAP 2). White, oval, scored. In 100s.

PIMOZIDE — ORAL

For complete and comparative prescribing information, refer to the Antipsychotic Agents class monograph.

Indications

➤*Tourette syndrome:* For suppression of motor and phonic tics in patients with Tourette syndrome who have failed to respond satisfactorily to standard treatment.

➤*Off-label uses:*

Parasitosis (delusional) – [3] = Safety concerns. Despite a significant adverse reaction profile, pimozide remains an effective choice in patients with chronic delusional parasitosis refractory to other treatment. A treatment paradigm for the management of psychogenic parasitosis has recently been published, with neuroleptics haloperidol or pimozide recommended as first-line therapy in patients with psychogenic parasitosis without depression. (See Administration and Dosage.)

Administration and Dosage

➤*General dosing considerations:* The suppression of tics by pimozide requires a slow and gradual introduction of the drug. Carefully adjust the patient's dose to a point where the suppression of tics and the relief afforded is balanced against the adverse effects of the drug.

An electrocardiogram (ECG) should be performed at baseline and periodically thereafter, especially during the period of dose adjustment.

➤*Adults:*

Tourette syndrome –

Maximum dose: 0.2 mg/kg/day or 10 mg/day, whichever is less.

Initial dosage: 1 to 2 mg/day in divided doses.

Dosage titration: Increase dose every other day.

Maintenance dosage: Most patients are maintained at less than 0.2 mg/kg/day or 10 mg/day, whichever is less.

Tapering: Periodically attempt to reduce dosage to see if tics persist at the level and extent first identified. In attempts to reduce the dosage of pimozide, give consideration to the possibility that increases of tic intensity and frequency may represent a transient, withdrawal-related phenomenon rather than a return of disease symptoms. Allow 1 to 2 weeks to elapse before concluding that an increase in tic manifestations is caused by the underlying disease rather than drug withdrawal. A gradual withdrawal is recommended in any case.

Off-label dosing –

Parasitosis (delusional): [3] = Safety concerns. Initial dosages of 1 to 2 mg daily and titrated slowly (1 mg every 5 to 7 days) to the effective dose that is best tolerated. Typical maintenance dosages have been between 2 and 4 mg daily. The lowest possible dose of pimozide should be used for the shortest duration.

➤*Children:*

Tourette syndrome –

12 years of age and older:

- *Maximum dose* – 0.2 mg/kg, not to exceed 10 mg/day.
- *Initial dosage* – 0.05 mg/kg, preferably taken once at bedtime.
- *Dosage titration* – Dose may be increased every third day to a maximum of 0.2 mg/kg, not to exceed 10 mg/day.

➤*Storage/Stability:* Store at 25°C (77°F); excursions are permitted between 15° and 30°C (59° and 86°F). Dispense in a tight, light-resistant container.

Dibenzapine Derivatives

CLOZAPINE

Rx	**Clozapine** (Various, eg, IVAX)	**Tablets; oral:** 12.5 mg	In 100s.
Rx	**Clozapine** (Various, eg, IVAX, Mylan, UDL)	**Tablets; oral:** 25 mg	In 100s, 500s, and UD 100s.
Rx	**Clozaril** (Novartis)		Lactose, talc. (CLOZARIL 25). Pale yellow, round, scored. In 100s, 500s, and UD 100s.
Rx	**Clozapine** (Various, eg, Teva)	**Tablets; oral:** 50 mg	In 100s, 500s, and UD 100s.
Rx	**Clozapine** (Various, eg, IVAX, Mylan, UDL)	**Tablets; oral:** 100 mg	In 100s, 500s, and UD 100s.
Rx	**Clozaril** (Novartis)		Lactose, talc. (CLOZARIL 100). Pale yellow, round, scored. In 100s, 500s, and UD 100s.
Rx	**Clozapine** (Teva)	**Tablets; oral:** 200 mg	In 100s, 500s, and UD 100s.
Rx	**FazaClo** (Azur Pharma)	**Tablets, disintegrating; oral:** 12.5 mg	Aspartame, mannitol, phenylalanine 0.87 mg. (A05). Yellow, round, mint flavor. In 100s.
		25 mg	Aspartame, mannitol, phenylalanine 1.74 mg. (A06). Yellow, round, mint flavor. In 100s and UD 48s.
		100 mg	Aspartame, mannitol, phenylalanine 6.96 mg. (A08). Yellow, round, mint flavor. In 100s and UD 48s.
		150 mg	Aspartame, mannitol, phenylalanine 10.44 mg. (A09). Yellow, round, mint flavor. In 100s and UD 48s.
		200 mg	Aspartame, mannitol, phenylalanine 13.92 mg. (A10). Yellow, round, mint flavor. In 100s and UD 48s.

CLOZAPINE — ORAL

For complete and comparative prescribing information refer to the Antipsychotic Agents class monograph.

WARNING

Agranulocytosis – Because of a significant risk of agranulocytosis, a potentially life-threatening adverse reaction, reserve clozapine for use in the treatment of severely ill patients with schizophrenia who fail to show an acceptable response to adequate courses of standard antipsychotic drug treatment or for use in reducing the risk of recurrent suicidal behavior in patients with schizophrenia or schizoaffective disorder who are judged to be at risk of reexperiencing suicidal behavior.

Patients being treated with clozapine must have a baseline white blood cell (WBC) count and absolute neutrophil count (ANC) before initiation of treatment, as well as regular WBC counts and ANCs during treatment and for at least 4 weeks after discontinuation of treatment.

Clozapine is available only through a distribution system that ensures monitoring of WBC counts and ANCs according to the following schedule prior to delivery of the next supply of medication.

Seizures – Seizures have been associated with the use of clozapine. Dose appears to be an important predictor of seizure, with a greater likelihood at higher clozapine doses. Use caution when administering clozapine to patients who have a history of seizures or other predisposing factors. Advise patients not to engage in any activity in which sudden loss of consciousness could cause serious risk to themselves or others.

Myocarditis – Analyses of postmarketing safety databases suggest that clozapine is associated with an increased risk of fatal myocarditis, especially during, but not limited to, the first month of therapy. In patients in whom myocarditis is suspected, promptly discontinue clozapine treatment.

Other adverse cardiovascular and respiratory reactions – Orthostatic hypotension, with or without syncope, can occur with clozapine treatment. Rarely, collapse can be profound and be accompanied by respiratory and/or cardiac arrest. Orthostatic hypotension is more likely to occur during initial titration in association with rapid dose escalation. In patients who have had even a brief interval off clozapine (2 or more days since the last dose), start treatment with 12.5 mg once or twice daily.

Because collapse, respiratory arrest, and cardiac arrest during initial treatment have occurred in patients who were being administered benzodiazepines or other psychotropic drugs, caution is advised when clozapine is initiated in patients taking a benzodiazepine or any other psychotropic drug. (See group monograph.) Antipsychotic Agents.

Elderly patients with dementia-related psychosis – Elderly patients with dementia-related psychosis treated with antipsychotic drugs are at an increased risk of death. Analyses of 17 placebo-controlled trials (modal duration of 10 weeks), largely in patients taking atypical antipsychotic drugs, revealed a risk of death in the drug-treated patients between 1.6 and 1.7 times that seen in placebo-treated patients. Over the course of a typical 10-week controlled trial, the rate of death in drug-treated patients was about 4.5%, compared with a rate of about 2.6% in the placebo group. Although the causes of death were varied, most of the deaths appeared to be either cardiovascular (eg, heart failure, sudden death) or infectious (eg, pneumonia) in nature. Observational studies suggest that, similar to atypical antipsychotic drugs, treatment with conventional antipsychotic drugs may increase mortality. The extent to which the findings of increased mortality in observational studies may be attributed to the antipsychotic drug as opposed to some characteristic(s) of the patients is not clear. Clozapine is not approved for the treatment of patients with dementia-related psychosis.

Indications

➤*Recurrent suicidal behavior:* For reducing the risk of recurrent suicidal behavior in patients with schizophrenia or schizoaffective disorder who are judged to be at chronic risk for reexperiencing suicidal behavior, based on history and recent clinical state. Suicidal behavior refers to actions by a patient that put himself or herself at risk for death.

➤*Treatment-resistent schizophrenia:* For the management of severely ill schizophrenic patients who fail to respond adequately to standard drug treatment for schizophrenia. Because of the significant risk of agranulocytosis and seizure associated with its use, use clozapine only in patients who have failed to respond adequately to treatment with appropriate courses of standard drug treatments for schizophrenia, either because of insufficient effectiveness or the inability to achieve an effective dose because of intolerable adverse reactions from those drugs.

➤*Off-label uses:*

Tardive dyskinesia – [5] = Poor documentation. Limited evidence from noncontrolled data suggests that clozapine may be effective in the treatment of tardive dyskinesia; however, clozapine has been associated with causing or exacerbating tardive dyskinesia symptoms. Clozapine has several black box warnings, and safety was not assessed in the reviewed studies. Based on limited data and safety considerations, this drug is not recommended for treatment of tardive dyskinesia.

Administration and Dosage

➤*General dosing considerations:* Drug dispensing should not ordinarily exceed a weekly supply. Upon initiation of clozapine therapy, up to a 1-week supply of additional clozapine may be provided to the patient to be held for emergencies (eg, weather, holidays).

If a patient is eligible for WBC count and ANC testing every 2 weeks, then a 2-week supply of clozapine can be dispensed. If a patient is eligible for WBC count and ANC testing every 4 weeks, then a 4-week supply of clozapine can be dispensed. Dispensing is contingent upon the WBC count and ANC test results.

Because of the significant risk of agranulocytosis and seizure, the extended treatment of patients failing to show an acceptable level of clinical response should ordinarily be avoided.

Patients discontinued for WBC counts below 2,000/mm^3 or an ANC below 1,000/mm^3 must not be restarted on clozapine.

Patients previously treated with other antipsychotics were cross-titrated to clozapine over a 1-month interval; the dose of the previous antipsychotic was gradually decreased simultaneously with a gradual increase in clozapine dose over the first month of the study. Patients on depot antipsychotic medication began clozapine after 1 full dosing interval since the last injection.

➤*Adults:*

Recurrent suicidal behavior –

Usual dosage: 300 to 450 mg/day. The InterSePT study demonstrated the efficacy of clozapine in treatment of patients with schizophrenia or schizoaffective disorder at risk for recurrent suicidal behavior where the mean daily dose was about 300 mg (range, 12.5 to 900 mg).

Maximum dose: 900 mg/day.

Initial dosage: 12.5 mg dose once or twice daily. The dosing should be continued with daily dose increments of 25 to 50 mg/day, if well tolerated, to achieve a target dosage of 300 to 450 mg/day by the end of 2 weeks.

Dosage titration: Subsequent dose increments should be made no more than once or twice weekly, in increments not to exceed 100 mg. Cautious titration and a divided dosage schedule are necessary to minimize the risks of hypotension, seizure, and sedation.

Maintenance dosage: It is recommended that responding patients be continued on clozapine, but at the lowest level needed to maintain remission. Because of the significant risk associated with the use of clozapine, patients should be periodically reassessed to determine the need for maintenance treatment.

Dosage adjustment: While many patients may respond adequately at dosages between 300 and 600 mg/day, it may be necessary to raise the dosage to the 600 to 900 mg/day range to obtain an acceptable response.

Because of the possibility of increased adverse reactions at higher doses, particularly seizures, patients should ordinarily be given adequate time to respond to a given dose level before escalation to a higher dose is contemplated. Clozapine can cause electroencephalographic (EEG) changes, including the occurrence of spike and wave complexes. It lowers the seizures threshold in a dose-dependent manner and may induce myoclonic jerks or generalized seizures. These symptoms may be likely to occur with rapid dose increase and in patients with preexisting epilepsy. In this case, the dose should be reduced and, if necessary, anticonvulsant treatment initiated.

Discontinuation of therapy: Gradual reduction in dose is recommended over a 1- to 2-week period. However, if a patient's medical condition requires abrupt discontinuation (eg, leukopenia), the patient should be carefully observed for the recurrence of psychotic symptoms and symptoms related to cholinergic rebound, such as headache, nausea, vomiting, and diarrhea.

Reinitiation of treatment: When restarting patients who have had even a brief interval off clozapine (ie, 2 days or more since the last dose), it is recommended that treatment be reinitiated with a 12.5 mg dose once or twice daily. If that dose is well tolerated, it may be feasible to titrate patients back to a therapeutic dose more quickly than is recommended for initial treatment. However, for any patient who has previously experienced respiratory or cardiac arrest with initial dosing but was then able to be successfully titrated to a therapeutic dose, retitrate with extreme caution, even after 24 hours of discontinuation.

Certain additional precautions seem prudent when reinitiating treatment. The mechanisms underlying clozapine-induced adverse reactions are unknown. It is conceivable, however, that reexposure of a patient might enhance the risk of an untoward event's occurrence and increase its severity. Such phenomena, for example, occur when immune-mediated mechanisms are responsible. Consequently, during the reinitiation of treatment, additional caution is advised.

Patients discontinued for WBC counts below 2,000/mm^3 or an ANC below 1,000/mm^3 must not be restarted on clozapine.

Treatment-resistant schizophrenia – See Recurrent suicidal behavior.

Off-label dosing –

➤*Elderly:* Dose selection for an elderly patient should be cautious, reflecting the greater frequency of decreased hepatic, renal, or cardiac function, and of concomitant disease or other drug therapy. Other reported clinical experience does suggest that the prevalence of tardive dyskinesia appears to be highest among the elderly, especially elderly women.

➤*Hepatic function impairment:* Caution is advised in patients using clozapine who have concurrent hepatic disease. Hepatitis has been reported in patients with healthy liver function and those with preexisting liver function abnormalities. In patients who develop nausea, vomiting, and/or anorexia during clozapine treatment, perform liver function tests immediately. If the elevation of these values is clinically relevant or if symptoms of jaundice occur, discontinue treatment with clozapine.

➤*Duration of therapy:* The results of the InterSePT study demonstrated that, for a 2-year treatment period, the probability of a suicide attempt or a hospitalization because of imminent suicide risk is stable at approximately 24% after 1 year of treatment with clozapine. A course of treatment with clozapine of at least 2 years is, therefore, recommended in order to maintain the reduction of risk for suicidal behavior. After 2 years, it is recommended that the patient's risk of suicidal behavior be assessed. If the health care

CLOZAPINE — ORAL

provider's assessment indicates that a significant risk for suicidal behavior is still present, treatment with clozapine should be continued. Thereafter, the decision to continue treatment with clozapine should be revisited at regular intervals, based on thorough assessments of the patient's risk for suicidal behavior during treatment. If the health care provider determines that the patient is no longer at risk for suicidal behavior, treatment with clozapine may be discontinued and treatment of the underlying disorder with an antipsychotic medication to which the patient has previously responded may be resumed.

➤*Administration:* Clozapine orally disintegrating tablets rapidly disintegrate after placement in the mouth. The clozapine orally disintegrating tablet should be left in the unopened blister until time of use. The orally disintegrating tablet should not be pushed through the foil. Just prior to use, peel the foil from the blister and gently remove the tablet. Immediately place the tablet in the mouth, allow it to disintegrate, and swallow with saliva. No water is needed to take clozapine orally disintegrating tablets.

➤*Storage/Stability:* Storage of tablets should not exceed 30°C (86°F). Store orally disintegrating tablets at 25°C (77°F); excursions are permitted between 15° and 30°C (59° and 86°F). Protect from moisture.

LOXAPINE

Rx	**Loxapine Succinate** (Various, eg, Dixon-Shane, UDL, Watson)	**Capsules:** 5 mg (6.8 mg as loxapine succinate)	In 100s and 1,000s.
Rx	**Loxitane** (Watson)		Lactose. (WATSON LOXITANE 5 mg). Dark green. In 100s and 1,000s.
Rx	**Loxapine Succinate** (Various, eg, Dixon-Shane, UDL, Watson)	**Capsules:** 10 mg (13.6 mg as loxapine succinate)	In 100s.
Rx	**Loxitane** (Watson)		Lactose. (WATSON LOXITANE 10 mg). Dark green/yellow. In 100s and 1,000s.
Rx	**Loxapine Succinate** (Various, eg, Dixon-Shane, UDL, Watson)	**Capsules:** 25 mg (34 mg as loxapine succinate)	In 100s.
Rx	**Loxitane** (Watson)		Lactose. (WATSON LOXITANE 25 mg). Two-tone green. In 100s and 1,000s.
Rx	**Loxapine Succinate** (Various, eg, Dixon-Shane, UDL, Watson)	**Capsules:** 50 mg (68.1 mg loxapine succinate)	In 100s.
Rx	**Loxitane** (Watson)		Lactose. (WATSON LOXITANE 50 mg). Dark green/blue. In 100s and 1,000s.

LOXAPINE — ORAL

For complete and comparative prescribing information, refer to the Antipsychotic Agents group monograph.

Indications

➤*Schizophrenia:* For the treatment of schizophrenia.

Administration and Dosage

➤*General dosing considerations:* Individualize dosage. Administer in divided doses, 2 to 4 times/day.

➤*Adults:*

Schizophrenia –

Maximum dose: 250 mg/day.

Initial dosage: 10 mg twice daily. In severely disturbed patients, up to 50 mg/day may be desirable.

Dosage titration: Increase dosage fairly rapidly over the first 7 to 10 days until symptoms are controlled.

Maintenance dosage: Reduce dosage to the lowest level compatible with control of symptoms. Usual therapeutic and maintenance range is 60 to 100 mg/day. Many patients have been maintained satisfactorily at dosages in the range of 20 to 60 mg/day.

➤*Storage/Stability:* Store at 15° to 30°C (59° to 86°F). Dispense capsules in a tight, child-resistant container.

OLANZAPINE

Rx	**Zyprexa** (Eli Lilly)	**Tablets; oral:** 2.5 mg	Lactose. (LILLY 4112). White, round. In 30s, 1,000s, and UD 100s.
		5 mg	Lactose. (LILLY 4115). White, round. In 30s, 1,000s, and UD 100s.
		7.5 mg	Lactose. (LILLY 4116). White, round. In 30s, 1,000s, and UD 100s.
		10 mg	Lactose. (LILLY 4117). White, round. In 30s, 1,000s, and UD 100s.
		15 mg	Lactose. (LILLY 4415). Blue, elliptical. In 30s, 1,000s, and UD 100s.
		20 mg	Lactose. (LILLY 4420). Pink, elliptical. In 30s, 1,000s, and UD 100s.
Rx	**Zyprexa Zydis** (Eli Lilly)	**Tablets, disintegrating; oral:** 5 mg	Aspartame, mannitol, parabens, phenylalanine 0.34 mg. (5). Yellow, round. In UD 30s.
		10 mg	Aspartame, mannitol, parabens, phenylalanine 0.45 mg. (10). Yellow, round. In UD 30s.
		15 mg	Aspartame, mannitol, parabens, phenylalanine 0.67 mg. (15). Yellow, round. In UD 30s.
		20 mg	Aspartame, mannitol, parabens, phenylalanine 0.9 mg. (20). Yellow, round. In UD 30s.
Rx	**Zyprexa IntraMuscular** (Eli Lilly)	**Injection, powder for solution:** 10 mg	Lactose 50 mg. In 10 mg vials.
Rx	**Zyprexa Relprevv** (Eli Lilly)	**Injection, powder for suspension, extended-release:** 210 mg	Mannitol, polysorbate 80. As olanzapine pamoate 483 mg. In single-use vials with diluent.
		300 mg	Mannitol, polysorbate 80. As olanzapine pamoate 690 mg. In single-use vials with diluent.
		405 mg	Mannitol, polysorbate 80. As olanzapine pamoate 931 mg. In single-use vials with diluent.

OLANZAPINE — ORAL

For complete and comparative prescribing information, refer to the Antipsychotic Agents class monograph. When using olanzapine and fluoxetine in combination, also refer to the olanzapine/fluoxetine monograph.

WARNING

Increased mortality in elderly patients with dementia-related psychosis –

Elderly patients with dementia-related psychosis treated with antipsychotic drugs are at an increased risk of death. Analyses of 17 placebo-controlled trials (modal duration, 10 weeks), largely in patients taking atypical antipsychotic drugs, revealed a risk of death in drug-treated patients between 1.6 and 1.7 times the risk of death in placebo-treated patients. Over the course of a typical 10-week controlled trial, the rate of death in drug-treated patients was approximately 4.5%, compared with a rate of about 2.6% in the placebo group. Although the causes of death were varied, most of the deaths appeared to be either cardiovascular (eg, heart failure, sudden death) or infectious (eg, pneumonia) in nature. Observational studies suggest that, similar to atypical antipsychotic drugs, treatment with conventional antipsychotic drugs may increase mortality. The extent to which the findings of increased mortality in observational studies may be attributed to the antipsychotic drug as opposed to some characteristic(s) of the patient is not clear. Olanzapine is not approved for treatment of patients with dementia-related psychosis.

Indications

➤*Bipolar disorder:*

Monotherapy – For the treatment of acute mixed or manic episodes associated with bipolar I disorder and for the maintenance monotherapy of bipolar disorder.

Adjunctive therapy with lithium or valproate – As an adjunct to lithium or valproate for the treatment of mixed or manic episodes associated with bipolar I disorder.

Depressive episodes associated with bipolar I disorder – In combination with fluoxetine for the treatment of depressive episodes associated with bipolar I disorder, based on clinical studies in adult patients.

➤*Treatment-resistant depression:* In combination with fluoxetine for the treatment of treatment-resistant depression (major depressive disorder in patients who do not respond to 2 separate trials of different antidepressants of adequate dose and duration in the current episode), based on clinical studies in adult patients.

➤*Schizophrenia:* For the treatment of schizophrenia.

➤*Children:* Pediatric schizophrenia and bipolar I disorder are serious mental disorders; however, diagnosis can be challenging. For pediatric schizophrenia, symptom profiles can be variable. For bipolar I disorder, children may have variable patterns of periodicity of manic or mixed symptoms. It is recommended that medication therapy for pediatric schizophrenia and bipolar I disorder be initiated only after a thorough diagnostic evaluation has been performed and careful consideration given to the risks associated with medication treatment. Medication treatment for both pediatric schizophrenia and bipolar I disorder should be part of a total treatment program that often includes psychological, educational, and social interventions.

When deciding among the alternative treatments available for adolescents, health care providers should consider the increased potential (in adolescents as compared with adults) for weight gain and hyperlipidemia. Health care providers should consider the potential long-term risks when prescribing to adolescents, and in many cases this may lead them to consider prescribing other drugs first in adolescents.

➤*Off-label uses:*

Obsessive-compulsive disorder – [1] = Good documentation. According to American Psychiatric Association guidelines, the addition of olanzapine or another second-generation antipsychotic agent may be appropriate as part of a step-wise approach to patients with obsessive-compulsive disorder who fail to respond to initial therapy with a selective serotonin reuptake inhibitor or cognitive-behavioral therapy.

Parasitosis (delusional) – [4] = Insufficient documentation. Published information regarding the use of olanzapine in the treatment of delusional parasitosis is limited to 3 case reports. Although olanzapine offers a better safety profile than pimozide, which is considered a first-line agent in the management of delusional parasitosis, sufficient evidence is not available at this time.

Stuttering – [4] = Insufficient documentation. Although published information regarding the use of olanzapine in the treatment of stuttering is limited to a small number of patients, initial controlled data suggest a benefit, particularly in adults with developmental stuttering. Little information is available regarding the use of this agent in children and adolescents (3 cases). This drug may be a therapeutic option in the management of stuttering but requires further evaluation in larger, controlled trials.

Tourette syndrome – Initial data suggest that olanzapine may be beneficial in the treatment of patients with Tourette syndrome. However, study limitations included a largely male population and small sample size. Larger, controlled studies with a more gender-equal population are needed to validate the promising initial figures.

Tourette syndrome (adults): [2] = Fair documentation.

Tourette syndrome (children/adolescents): [4] = Insufficient documentation.

Administration and Dosage

➤*Maximum dose:*

Adults and children 13 years of age and older – 20 mg/day for the treatment of schizophrenia according to the prescribing information. There is no well-established maximum dose for the other approved indication according to the prescribing information.

➤*Adults:*

Bipolar disorder –

Monotherapy:

- *Initial dosage* – 10 to 15 mg orally once daily without regard to meals.
- *Maintenance dosage* – 5 to 20 mg/day, after achieving a responder status for an average duration of 2 weeks.
- *Dosage adjustment* – Adjust dosage, if indicated, at 5 mg/day increments or decrements in intervals of not less than 24 hours.

Adjunctive therapy:

- *Usual dosage* – 5 to 20 mg/day.
- *Initial dosage* – 10 mg orally once daily without regard to meals when coadministered with lithium or valproate.

Treatment-resistant depression – Refer to Depressive episodes associated with bipolar I disorder for dosing.

Schizophrenia –

Usual dosage: 10 mg/day within several days of initiation.

Efficacy was demonstrated in a dosage range of 10 to 15 mg/day in clinical trials. However, dosages above 10 mg/day were not demonstrated to be more efficacious than the 10 mg/day dosage. Dosages larger than 10 mg/day (ie, to a dosage of 15 mg/day or more) are recommended only after clinical assessment.

Maximum dose: Olanzapine is not indicated for use in dosages above 20 mg/day.

Initial dosage: 5 to 10 mg orally once daily without regard to meals.

Maintenance dosage: 10 to 20 mg/day.

Dosage adjustment: Adjust dosage, if indicated, at 5 mg/day increments or decrements in intervals of not less than 1 week because steady state for olanzapine is not achieved for approximately 1 week in the typical patient.

Depressive episodes associated with bipolar I disorder –

Initial dosage: Olanzapine 5 mg and fluoxetine 20 mg once daily in the evening, without regard to meals.

Dosage adjustment: Dosage adjustments, if indicated, can be made according to efficacy and tolerability within dose ranges of oral olanzapine 5 to 12.5 mg and fluoxetine 20 to 50 mg.

Duration of therapy: While there is no body of evidence to answer the question of how long a patient treated with the combination of olanzapine and fluoxetine should remain on it, it is generally accepted that this disorder is a chronic illness requiring long-term treatment. The health care provider should periodically reexamine the need for continued pharmacotherapy.

Conversion from fixed-dose combination olanzapine/fluoxetine: Safety and efficacy of olanzapine and fluoxetine in combination were determined in clinical trials supporting approval of olanzapine/fluoxetine (fixed-dose combination of olanzapine and fluoxetine). Olanzapine/fluoxetine is dosed between 3 mg/25 mg per day (olanzapine/fluoxetine) and 12 mg/50 mg per day (olanzapine/fluoxetine). The following table demonstrates the appropriate individual component dosages of olanzapine and fluoxetine versus olanzapine/fluoxetine. Dosage adjustments, if indicated, should be made with the individual components according to efficacy and tolerability

Approximate Oral Dosage Correspondence Between Olanzapine/Fluoxetine and the Combination of Olanzapine and Fluoxetine

	Use in combination	
Olanzapine/Fluoxetine	Olanzapine	Fluoxetine
3 mg/25 mg per day	2.5 mg/day	20 mg/day
6 mg/25 mg per day	5 mg/day	20 mg/day
12 mg/25 mg per day	10 + 2.5 mg/day	20 mg/day
6 mg/50 mg per day	5 mg/day	40 + 10 mg/day
12 mg/50 mg per day	10 + 2.5 mg/day	40 + 10 mg/day

Off-label dosing –

Obsessive-compulsive disorder: [1] = Good documentation. Initial dose is 5 mg/day and increased based on therapeutic effect and tolerance. The mean final daily dose in trials was 6 or 11 mg (range, 5 to 20 mg/day). Once successful management is achieved, therapy should continue for 1 to 2 years before a taper is attempted. During tapering, doses may be reduced by 10% to 25% every 1 to 2 months while monitoring for symptom exacerbation or return.

Parasitosis (delusional): [4] = Insufficient documentation. Initial dosages of 5 mg daily.

Stuttering: [4] = Insufficient documentation. Initial dosage of 2.5 mg daily for 4 weeks, then increased to 5 mg daily for another 12 weeks.

Tourette syndrome (adults): [2] = Fair documentation. 5 mg orally daily (initial) titrated to a maximum of 20 mg daily for 6 to 8 weeks (maximum studied, 16 weeks).

➤*Children:*

13 years of age and older –

Bipolar I disorder:

- *Initial dosage* – 2.5 or 5 mg once daily without regard to meals.

OLANZAPINE — ORAL

• *Maintenance dosage* – 10 mg/day. It is generally recommended that responding patients be continued beyond the acute response, but at the lowest dose needed to maintain remission. Patients should be periodically reassessed to determine the need for maintenance treatment.

• *Dosage adjustment* – When dosage adjustments are necessary, dose increments/decrements of 2.5 or 5 mg are recommended.

Schizophrenia:

• *Initial dosage* – 2.5 or 5 mg once daily without regard to meals.

• *Maintenance dosage* – 10 mg/day. It is generally recommended that responding patients be continued beyond the acute response, but at the lowest dose needed to maintain remission. Patients should be periodically reassessed to determine the need for maintenance treatment.

• *Dosage adjustment* – When dosage adjustments are necessary, dose increments/decrements of 2.5 or 5 mg are recommended.

Off-label dosing –

Stuttering: [4] = Insufficient documentation.

• *Children* – Initial dosage of 1.25 mg at bedtime for 1 month, then increased to 2.5 mg at bedtime.

• *Adolescents* – Initial dose of 5 mg at bedtime was not well tolerated, requiring dosage reduction.

Tourette syndrome (children/adolescents): [4] = Insufficient documentation. 2.5 mg orally daily (initial) titrated to a maximum of 20 mg for 8 weeks.

➤*Elderly:* Consider a lower starting dose for any elderly patient if factors are present that might decrease pharmacokinetic clearance or increase the pharmacodynamic response to olanzapine.

➤*Special risk patients:*

Schizophrenia – 5 mg is the recommended starting dose in patients who are debilitated, who have a predisposition to hypotensive reactions, who otherwise exhibit a combination of factors that may result in slower metabolism of olanzapine (eg, nonsmoking women 65 years of age and older), or who may be more pharmacodynamically sensitive to olanzapine. When indicated, dose escalation should be performed with caution in these patients.

Olanzapine/Fluoxetine – The starting dose of oral olanzapine 2.5 to 5 mg with fluoxetine 20 mg should be used for patients with a predisposition to hypotensive reactions or patients who exhibit a combination of factors that may slow the metabolism of olanzapine or fluoxetine in combination (women, elderly, nonsmoking status), or those patients who may be pharmacodynamically sensitive to olanzapine. Dosing modification may be necessary in patients who exhibit a combination of factors that may slow metabolism. When indicated, dose escalation should be performed with caution in these patients.

➤*Administration:* May be taken without regard to meals.

Orally disintegrating tablets – Peel back the foil on the blister; do not push the tablet through the foil. Using dry hands, remove and immediately place the entire tablet in the mouth. The tablet disintegration occurs rapidly in saliva so it can be easily swallowed with or without liquid.

➤*Storage/Stability:* Store at controlled room temperature, 20° to 25°C (68° to 77°F). Protect from light and moisture.

OLANZAPINE — INJECTION

For complete and comparative prescribing information, refer to the Antipsychotic Agents class monograph.

WARNING

Increased mortality in elderly patients with dementia-related psychosis – Elderly patients with dementia-related psychosis treated with antipsychotic drugs are at an increased risk of death. Analyses of 17 placebo-controlled trials (modal duration, 10 weeks), largely in patients taking atypical antipsychotic drugs, revealed a risk of death in drug-treated patients between 1.6 and 1.7 times the risk of death in placebo-treated patients. Over the course of a typical 10-week controlled trial, the rate of death in drug-treated patients was approximately 4.5%, compared with a rate of about 2.6% in the placebo group. Although the causes of death were varied, most of the deaths appeared to be cardiovascular (eg, heart failure, sudden death) or infectious (eg, pneumonia) in nature. Observational studies suggest that, similar to atypical antipsychotic drugs, treatment with conventional antipsychotic drugs may increase mortality. The extent to which the findings of increased mortality in observational studies may be attributed to the antipsychotic drug as opposed to some characteristic(s) of the patients is not clear. Olanzapine is not approved for the treatment of patients with dementia-related psychosis.

Indications

➤*Agitation associated with schizophrenia and bipolar I mania:* For the treatment of acute agitation associated with schizophrenia and bipolar I mania.

Administration and Dosage

➤*General dosing considerations:* Be aware that there are 2 olanzapine intramuscular (IM) formulations with different dosing schedules. Olanzapine short-acting (10 mg/vial) formulation should not be confused with olanzapine ER.

Maximal dosing of olanzapine short-acting injection (eg, 3 doses of 10 mg administered 2 to 4 hours apart) may be associated with a substantial occurrence of significant orthostatic hypotension. It is recommended that patients requiring subsequent short-acting injections be assessed for orthostatic hypotension prior to the administration of any subsequent doses of olanzapine short-acting injection. The administration of an additional dose to a patient with a clinically significant postural change in systolic blood pressure is not recommended.

The efficacy of repeated doses of olanzapine injection in agitated patients has not been systematically evaluated in controlled clinical trials.

Olanzapine injection is intended for IM use only.

Dosage adjustments are required for elderly patients. (See Elderly.)

Dosage adjustments are required for debilitated patients. (See Special-Risk Patients.)

➤*Adults:*

Agitation associated with schizophrenia and bipolar I mania –

Usual dosage: 10 mg IM. If agitation warranting additional IM doses persists following the initial dose, subsequent doses of up to 10 mg IM may be given.

Maximum dose: 30 mg/day IM.

Dosage adjustment: A lower dose of 5 to 7.5 mg IM may be considered when clinical factors warrant.

Conversion: If ongoing olanzapine therapy is clinically indicated, oral olanzapine may be initiated in a range of 5 to 20 mg/day as soon as clinically appropriate.

➤*Elderly:* A dose of 5 mg per injection should be considered for elderly patients or when other clinical factors warrant.

➤*Special-risk patients:* A lower dose of 2.5 mg per injection should be considered for patients who otherwise might be debilitated, predisposed to hypotensive reactions, or more pharmacodynamically sensitive to olanzapine.

➤*Administration:* Olanzapine is intended for IM use only. Inject slowly, deep into the muscle mass. Do not administer intravenously or subcutaneously.

➤*Admixture compatibility:* Olanzapine injection should be reconstituted only with sterile water for injection. Olanzapine injection should not be combined in a syringe with diazepam injection because precipitation occurs when these products are mixed. Lorazepam injection should not be used to reconstitute olanzapine injection because this combination results in a delayed reconstitution time. Olanzapine injection should not be combined in a syringe with haloperidol injection because the resulting low pH has been shown to degrade olanzapine over time.

➤*Storage/Stability:* Store vials at 20° to 25°C (68° to 77°F). Reconstituted olanzapine may be stored at 20° to 25°C (68° to 77°F) for up to 1 hour if necessary. Discard any unused portion of reconstituted olanzapine. Protect from light. Do not freeze.

OLANZAPINE PAMOATE — INJECTION

For complete and comparative prescribing information, refer to the Antipsychotic Agents class monograph.

WARNING

Increased mortality in elderly patients with dementia-related psychosis – Elderly patients with dementia-related psychosis treated with antipsychotic drugs are at an increased risk of death. Analyses of 17 placebo-controlled trials (modal duration, 10 weeks), largely in patients taking atypical antipsychotic drugs, revealed a risk of death in drug-treated patients between 1.6 and 1.7 times the risk of death in placebo-treated patients. Over the course of a typical 10-week controlled trial, the rate of death in drug-treated patients was approximately 4.5%, compared with a rate of about 2.6% in the placebo group. Although the causes of death were varied, most of the deaths appeared to be cardiovascular (eg, heart failure, sudden death) or infectious (eg, pneumonia) in nature. Observational studies suggest that, similar to atypical antipsychotic drugs, treatment with conventional antipsychotic drugs may increase mortality. The extent to which the findings of increased mortality in observational studies may be attributed to the antipsychotic drug as opposed to some characteristic(s) of the patients is not clear. Olanzapine is not approved for the treatment of patients with dementia-related psychosis.

WARNING (cont.)

Postinjection delirium/sedation syndrome – Adverse reactions with signs and symptoms consistent with olanzapine overdose, in particular, sedation (including coma) and/or delirium, have been reported following injections of olanzapine extended release (ER). Olanzapine ER must be administered in a registered health care facility with ready access to emergency response services. After each injection, patients must be observed at the health care facility by a health care provider for at least 3 hours. Because of this risk, olanzapine ER is available only through a restricted distribution program called *Zyprexa Relprevv* Patient Care Program, and requires health care provider, health care facility, patient, and pharmacy enrollment.

Indications

➤*Schizophrenia:* For the treatment of schizophrenia.

OLANZAPINE PAMOATE — INJECTION

Administration and Dosage

➤*General dosing considerations:* Be aware that there are 2 olanzapine intramuscular (IM) formulations with different dosing schedules. Olanzapine short-acting (10 mg/vial) formulation should not be confused with olanzapine ER.

Establish tolerability with oral olanzapine prior to initiating treatment with olanzapine ER.

Olanzapine injection is intended for IM use only.

Dosage adjustments are required for debilitated patients. (See Special-Risk Patients.)

➤*Adults:*

Schizophrenia –

Usual dosage: 150 to 300 mg every 2 weeks or 405 mg every 4 weeks.

Maintenance dosage: Although no controlled studies have been conducted to determine how long patients should be treated, efficacy has been demonstrated over a period of 24 weeks in patients with stabilized schizophrenia. Patients should be periodically reassessed to determine the need for continued treatment.

Conversion:

Recommended Dosing for Extended-Release Olanzapine Injection Based on Correspondence to Oral Olanzapine Doses

Target oral olanzapine dosage	Dosing of olanzapine ER during the first 8 weeks	Maintenance dose after 8 weeks of olanzapine ER treatment
10 mg/day	210 mg per 2 weeks or 405 mg per 4 weeks	150 mg per 2 weeks or 300 mg per 4 weeks
15 mg/day	300 mg per 2 weeks	210 mg per 2 weeks or 405 mg per 4 weeks
20 mg/day	300 mg per 2 weeks	300 mg per 2 weeks

➤*Special-risk patients:* The recommended starting dose is 150 mg per 4 weeks in patients who are debilitated, who have a predisposition to hypotensive reactions, who otherwise exhibit a combination of factors that may result in slower metabolism of olanzapine (eg, nonsmoking women 65 years of age and older), or who may be more pharmacodynamically sensitive to olanzapine. When indicated, dose escalation should be undertaken with caution in these patients.

➤*Preparation for administration:* Olanzapine ER must be suspended using only the diluent supplied in the convenience kit. It is recommended that gloves are used when reconstituting because olanzapine ER may be irritating to the skin. Flush with water if contact is made with skin. It is important to note that there is more diluent in the vial than is needed to reconstitute.

Step 1: determine reconstitution volume –

Directions for Reconstituting Olanzapine Extended Release Injection

Olanzapine ER dose	Vial strength	Diluent to add
150 mg	210 mg	1.3 mL
210 mg	210 mg	1.3 mL
300 mg	300 mg	1.8 mL
405 mg	405 mg	2.3 mL

Step 2: reconstituting olanzapine extended release – Read the *Hypodermic Needle-Pro* instructions for use before proceeding with step 2. Failure to follow these instructions may result in a needlestick injury.

Loosen the powder by lightly tapping the vial. Open the prepackaged *Hypodermic Needle-Pro* syringe and needle with needle protection device. Withdraw the predetermined diluent volume (step 1) into the syringe. Inject the diluent into the powder vial. Withdraw air to equalize the pressure in the vial by pulling back slightly on the plunger in the syringe. Remove the needle from the vial, holding the vial upright to prevent any loss of material. Engage the needle safety device (refer to complete *Hypodermic Needle-Pro* instructions for use). Pad a hard surface to cushion the impact. Tap the vial firmly and repeatedly on the surface until no powder is visible. Visually check the vial for clumps. Unsuspended powder appears as yellow, dry clumps clinging to the vial. Additional tapping may be required if large clumps remain. Shake the vial vigorously until the suspension appears smooth and is consistent in color and texture. The suspended product will be yellow and opaque. If foam forms, let vial stand to allow foam to dissipate. If the product is not used right away, it should be shaken vigorously to resuspend. Reconstituted olanzapine ER remains stable for up to 24 hours in the vial.

Step 3: determine final volume to inject – Suspension concentration is olanzapine ER 150 mg/mL.

Olanzapine Extended Release Injection Volume

Olanzapine ER dose	Final volume to inject
150 mg	1 mL
210 mg	1.4 mL
300 mg	2 mL
405 mg	2.7 mL

Attach a new safety needle to the syringe. Slowly withdraw the desired amount into the syringe. Some excess product will remain in the vial. Engage the needle safety device and remove needle from syringe. Once the suspension has been removed from the vial, it should be injected immediately.

➤*Administration:* Olanzapine ER injection is intended for deep IM gluteal injection only. Do not administer either formulations intravenously or subcutaneously.

Before administering the injection, confirm there will be someone to accompany the patient after the 3-hour observation period. If this cannot be confirmed, do not give the injection. For administration, select the 19-gauge, 1.5-inch (38 mm) *Hypodermic Needle-Pro* needle with needle protection device. For obese patients, a 2-inch (50 mm), 19-gauge or larger needle (not included in convenience kit) may be used. To help prevent clogging, a 19-gauge or larger needle must be used. Attach the new safety needle to the syringe prior to injection.

Select and prepare a site for injection in the gluteal area. After insertion of the needle into the muscle, aspirate for several seconds to ensure that no blood appears. If any blood is drawn into the syringe, discard the syringe and the dose and begin with a new convenience kit. The injection should be performed with steady, continuous pressure. Engage the needle safety device. Do not massage the injection site. Dispose of the vials, needles, and syringe appropriately after injection.

Postinjection delirium/sedation syndrome – See the Warning box for more information.

After each injection, a health care provider must continuously observe the patient at the health care facility for at least 3 hours for symptoms consistent with olanzapine overdose, including sedation (ranging from mild in severity to coma) and/or delirium (including confusion, disorientation, agitation, anxiety, and other cognitive impairment). Other symptoms noted include extrapyramidal symptoms, dysarthria, ataxia, aggression, dizziness, weakness, hypertension, and convulsion. The potential for onset of a reaction is greatest within the first hour. The majority of cases have occurred within the first 3 hours after injection; however, the reaction has occurred after 3 hours. Following the 3-hour observation period, health care providers must confirm that the patient is alert, oriented, and absent of any signs and symptoms of postinjection delirium/sedation syndrome prior to being released. All patients must be accompanied to their destination upon leaving the facility. For the remainder of the day of each injection, patients should not drive or operate heavy machinery, and should be advised to be vigilant for symptoms of postinjection delirium/sedation syndrome and be able to obtain medical assistance if needed. If postinjection delirium/sedation syndrome is suspected, close medical supervision and monitoring should be instituted in a facility capable of resuscitation.

➤*Admixture compatibility:* Olanzapine ER must be suspended using only the diluent provided in the convenience kit.

➤*Storage/Stability:* Store vials at room temperature, not to exceed 30°C (86°F). When the drug product is suspended in the solution, it may be held at room temperature for 24 hours. The vial should be agitated immediately prior to product withdrawal. Once the suspension is withdrawn into the syringe, it should be used immediately.

QUETIAPINE

Rx	**Seroquel** (AstraZeneca)	**Tablets; oral:** 25 mg	As quetiapine fumarate. Lactose, PEG. (SEROQUEL 25). Peach, round. Film-coated. In 100s, 1,000s, and UD 100s.
		50 mg	As quetiapine fumarate. Lactose, PEG. (SEROQUEL 50). White, round. Film-coated. In 100s, 1,000s, and UD 100s.
		100 mg	As quetiapine fumarate. Lactose, PEG. (SEROQUEL 100). Yellow, round. Film-coated. In 100s and UD 100s.
		200 mg	As quetiapine fumarate. Lactose, PEG. (SEROQUEL 200). White, round. Film-coated. In 100s and UD 100s.
		300 mg	As quetiapine fumarate. Lactose, PEG. (SEROQUEL 300). White, capsule shape. Film-coated. In 60s and UD 100s.
		400 mg	As quetiapine fumarate. Lactose, PEG. (SEROQUEL 400). Yellow, capsule shape. Film-coated. In 100s and UD 100s.

Dibenzapine Derivatives

QUETIAPINE

Rx	**Seroquel XR** (AstraZeneca)	**Tablets, extended-release; oral:** 50 mg	Equiv. to quetiapine fumarate 58 mg. Lactose. (XR 50). Peach, capsule shape. Film-coated. In 60s, 500s, and UD 100s.
		150 mg	Equiv. to quetiapine fumarate 173 mg. Lactose. (XR 150). White, capsule shape. Film-coated. In 60s, 500s, and UD 100s.
		200 mg	Equiv. to quetiapine fumarate 230 mg. Lactose. (XR 200). Yellow, capsule shape. Film-coated. In 60s, 500s, and UD 100s.
		300 mg	Equiv. to quetiapine fumarate 345 mg. Lactose. (XR 300). Pale yellow, capsule shape. Film-coated. In 60s, 500s, and UD 100s.
		400 mg	Equiv. to quetiapine fumarate 461 mg. Lactose. (XR 400). White, capsule shape. Film-coated. In 60s, 500s, and UD 100s.

QUETIAPINE FUMARATE — ORAL

For complete and comparative prescribing information, refer to the Antipsychotic Agents class monograph.

WARNING

Increased mortality in elderly patients with dementia-related psychosis –

Elderly patients with dementia-related psychosis treated with atypical antipsychotic drugs are at an increased risk of death. Analyses of 17 placebo-controlled trials (modal duration of 10 weeks), largely in patients taking atypical antipsychotic drugs, revealed a risk of death in the drug-treated patients between 1.6 and 1.7 times that seen in placebo-treated patients. Over the course of a typical 10-week controlled trial, the rate of death in drug-treated patients was about 4.5%, compared with a rate of about 2.6% in the placebo group. Although the causes of death were varied, most of the deaths appeared to be either cardiovascular (eg, heart failure, sudden death) or infectious (eg, pneumonia) in nature. Observational studies suggest that, similar to atypical antipsychotic drugs, treatment with conventional antipsychotic drugs may increase mortality. The extent to which the findings of increased mortality in observational studies may be attributed to the antipsychotic drug as opposed to some characteristic(s) of the patients is not clear. Quetiapine is not approved for the treatment of patients with dementia-related psychosis.

Suicidality and antidepressant drugs – Antidepressants increased the risk compared with placebo of suicidal thinking and behavior (suicidality) in children, adolescents, and young adults in short-term studies of major depressive disorder and other psychiatric disorders. Anyone considering the use of quetiapine or any other antidepressant in a child, adolescent, or young adult must balance this risk with the clinical need. Short-term studies did not show an increase in the risk of suicidality with antidepressants compared with placebo in adults older than 24 years of age; there was a reduction in risk with antidepressants compared with placebo in adults 65 years of age and older. Depression and certain other psychiatric disorders are themselves associated with increases in the risk of suicide. Monitor patients of all ages who are started on antidepressant therapy appropriately and observe these patients closely for clinical worsening, suicidality, or unusual changes in behavior. Advise families and caregivers of the need for close observation and communication with the prescriber. Quetiapine is not approved for use in children younger than 10 years of age (immediate release) or younger than 18 years of age (extended release [ER]).

Indications

➤*Bipolar disorder:* For the acute treatment of manic (immediate release and ER) or mixed (ER) episodes associated with bipolar I disorder, both as monotherapy and as an adjunct to lithium or divalproex.

Quetiapine immediate release and quetiapine ER are indicated for the acute treatment of depressive episodes associated with bipolar disorder.

Quetiapine immediate release and quetiapine ER are indicated for the maintenance treatment of bipolar I disorder, as an adjunct to lithium or divalproex.

➤*Major depressive disorder, adjunct therapy (ER only):* For use as adjunctive therapy to antidepressants for the treatment of major depressive disorder.

➤*Schizophrenia:* For the treatment of schizophrenia.

➤*Off-label uses:*

Alcohol dependence – [3] = Safety concerns. Initial data with quetiapine from noncontrolled trials suggest that this agent may have beneficial effects on reduction of alcohol consumption and/or cravings.

Obsessive-compulsive disorder – [1] = Good documentation. According to American Psychiatric Association guidelines, the addition of quetiapine or another second-generation antipsychotic agent may be appropriate as part of a stepwise approach to patients with obsessive-compulsive disorder who fail to respond to initial therapy with a selective serotonin reuptake inhibitor (SSRI) or cognitive-behavioral therapy.

Tourette syndrome (adults) – [5] = Poor documentation. Initial data suggest that quetiapine may not be an effective treatment option for Tourette syndrome in adults. Larger, controlled trials with long-term studies are needed to further expand upon the efficacy and tolerability of this therapy.

Tourette syndrome (children / adolescents) – [4] = Insufficient documentation. Initial data suggest that quetiapine may be an effective treatment option for Tourette syndrome. Larger, controlled trials with long-term studies are needed to further expand upon the efficacy and tolerability of this therapy.

Administration and Dosage

➤*Adults:*

Bipolar disorder –

Acute manic episodes:

• *Extended release –*

Initial dosage: 300 mg on day 1 and 600 mg on day 2, once daily in the evening. Use as monotherapy or adjunct therapy (with lithium or divalproex).

Dosage adjustment: Dose may be adjusted between 400 and 800 mg beginning on day 3, depending on the response and tolerance of the individual patient.

• *Immediate release –*

Usual dosage: 400 and 800 mg/day.

Initial dosage: When used as monotherapy or adjunct therapy (with lithium or divalproex), initiate in twice-daily doses totaling 100 mg/day on day 1 and increased to 400 mg/day on day 4 in increments of up to 100 mg/day in twice-daily divided doses.

Dosage adjustment: Further dosage adjustments of up to 800 mg/day by day 6 should be in increments of no more than 200 mg/day.

Depressive episodes:

• *Extended release* – 50 mg on day 1; 100 mg on day 2; 200 mg on day 3; 300 mg on day 4 given once daily in the evening.

• *Immediate release –*

Usual dosage: Antidepressant efficacy was demonstrated at both 300 and 600 mg; however, no additional benefit was seen in the 600 mg group.

Initial dosage: Initiate with 50 mg on day 1, increase to 100 mg on day 2, 200 mg on day 3, and 300 mg on day 4 given once daily at bedtime.

In these clinical trials supporting effectiveness, the dosing schedule was 50, 100, 200, and 300 mg/day for days 1 through 4, respectively. Patients receiving 600 mg increased to 400 mg on day 5 and to 600 mg on day 8 (week 1).

Maintenance of bipolar I disorder:

• *Extended release* – Generally, in the maintenance phase, patients continued on the same dose on which they were stabilized during the stabilization phase. Patients should be periodically reassessed to determine the need for maintenance treatment and the appropriate dose for such treatment.

• *Immediate release* – Administer twice daily (totaling 400 to 800 mg/day) as adjunct therapy to lithium or divalproex. Generally, in the maintenance phase, patients continued on the same dose on which they were stabilized during the stabilization phase.

Major depressive disorder, adjunctive therapy –

Extended release:

• *Usual dosage* – 150 to 300 mg/day.

• *Initial dosage* – 50 mg once daily in the evening. On day 3, the dose can be increased to 150 mg once daily in the evening.

Schizophrenia –

Extended release:

• *Initial dosage* – 300 mg/day once daily, preferably in the evening.

• *Dosage titration* – Dose increases can be made at intervals as short as 1 day and in increments of 300 mg/day. Patients should be titrated within a dosage range of 400 to 800 mg/day, depending on the response and tolerance of the individual patient.

• *Maintenance dosage* – A maintenance trial in adult patients with schizophrenia treated with quetiapine ER has shown this drug to be effective in delaying time to relapse in patients who were stabilized on quetiapine ER at dosages of 400 to 800 mg/day for 16 weeks. Patients should be periodically reassessed to determine the need for maintenance treatment and the appropriate dose for such treatment.

Immediate release:

• *Usual dosage* – 150 to 750 mg/day.

• *Initial dosage* – 25 mg twice daily, with increases in total daily dose of 25 to 50 mg divided in 2 or 3 doses on the second and third day, as tolerated, to a target dosage range of 300 to 400 mg/day by the fourth day.

• *Maintenance dosage* – While there is no body of evidence available to answer the question of how long the patient treated with quetiapine should be maintained, it is generally recommended that responding patients be continued beyond the acute response, but at the lowest dose needed to maintain remission. Patients should be periodically reassessed to determine the need for maintenance treatment.

QUETIAPINE FUMARATE — ORAL

• *Dosage adjustment* – Further dosage adjustments, if indicated, should generally occur at intervals of no less than 2 days because steady state for quetiapine would not be achieved for approximately 1 to 2 days in the typical patient. When dosage adjustments are necessary, increments/decrements of 25 to 50 mg divided twice daily are recommended.

• *Duration of therapy* – The effectiveness of quetiapine for longer than 6 weeks has not been evaluated in controlled clinical trials.

Off-label dosing –

Alcohol dependence: [3] = Safety concerns. Initial dosage ranged from 25 to 50 mg nightly and was titrated to a maximum of 300 mg nightly based on tolerance and efficacy.

Obsessive-compulsive disorder: [1] = Good documentation. Initial dosage is 50 mg daily orally and increased based on therapeutic effect and tolerance. The mean daily doses in trials were 169 or 215 mg (range, 25 to 400 mg/day). Once successful management is achieved, therapy should continue for 1 to 2 years before attempting to taper the dose. During tapering, doses may be reduced by 10% to 25% every 1 to 2 months while monitoring for symptom exacerbation or return.

➤*Children:*

Bipolar I disorder, acute manic episodes –

10 to 17 years of age:

• *Immediate release –*

Usual dosage: Efficacy was demonstrated at 400 and 600 mg; however, no additional benefit was seen in the 600 mg group.

Initial dosage: The total daily dose for the initial 5 days of therapy is 50 (day 1), 100 (day 2), 200 (day 3), 300 (day 4), and 400 mg (day 5).

Maintenance dosage: While there is no body of evidence available to answer the question of how long the patient treated with quetiapine should be maintained, it is generally recommended that responding patients be continued beyond the acute response but at the lowest dose needed to maintain remission. Patients should be periodically reassessed to determine the need for maintenance treatment.

Dosage adjustment: After day 5, the dose should be adjusted within the recommended dosage range of 400 to 600 mg/day, based on response and tolerability. Dosage adjustments should be in increments of no greater than 100 mg/day.

Duration of therapy: The effectiveness of quetiapine for longer than 3 weeks has not been evaluated in controlled clinical trials of children and adolescents.

Schizophrenia –

13 to 17 years of age:

• *Immediate release –*

Usual dosage: 400 to 800 mg/day.

Initial dosage: The total daily dose for the initial 5 days of therapy is 50 (day 1), 100 (day 2), 200 (day 3), 300 (day 4), and 400 mg (day 5).

Maintenance dosage: While there is no body of evidence available to answer the question of how long the patient treated with quetiapine should be maintained, it is generally recommended that responding patients be continued beyond the acute responses but at the lowest dose needed to maintain remission. Patients should be periodically reassessed to determine the need for maintenance treatment.

Dosage adjustment: After day 5, the dose should be adjusted within the recommended dosage range of 400 to 800 mg/day based on response and tolerability. Dosage adjustments should be in increments of no greater than 100 mg/day.

Duration of therapy: The effectiveness of quetiapine for longer than 6 weeks has not been evaluated in controlled clinical trials.

Off-label dosing –

Schizophrenia (children): 12.5 to 750 mg/day orally.

Tourette syndrome (children/adolescents): [4] = Insufficient documentation. Dosing ranged from 25 to 175 mg/day for 8 weeks based on treatment evaluations and tolerability. Initiate dose at the low end of the range and titrate based on tolerability and efficacy.

➤*Elderly:* Consider a slower rate of dose titration and a lower target dose. When indicated, dose escalation should be performed with caution in these patients.

Extended release – Start elderly patients on quetiapine ER 50 mg/day; the dosage can be increased in increments of 50 mg/day, depending on the response and tolerance of the individual patient.

➤*Hepatic function impairment:*

Immediate release – Patients should be started on quetiapine immediate release 25 mg/day. The dosage should be increased daily in increments of 25 to 50 mg/day to an effective dosage, depending on the clinical response and tolerability of the patient.

Extended release – Patients should be started on quetiapine ER 50 mg/day. The dosage can be increased daily in increments of 50 mg/day to an effective dosage, depending on the clinical response and tolerance of the patient.

➤*Debilitated patients:* Consider a slower rate of dose titration and a lower target dose. When indicated, dose escalation should be performed with caution in these patients.

➤*Patients with predisposition to hypotensive reactions:* See Debilitated patients.

➤*Reinitiation of treatment in patients previously discontinued:* Although there are no data to specifically address reinitiation of treatment, it is recommended that, when restarting patients who have discontinued quetiapine ER for an interval of more than 1 week, the initial dosing schedule should be followed. When restarting patients who have been off quetiapine ER for less than 1 week, gradual dose escalation may not be required and the maintenance dose may be reinitiated. When restarting patients who have had an interval of less than 1 week off quetiapine immediate release, titration of quetiapine immediate release is not required and the maintenance dose may be reinitiated. When restarting therapy for patients who have discontinued quetiapine immediate release for longer than 1 week, the initial titration schedule should be followed.

➤*Conversion:* Schizophrenic patients who are currently being treated with divided doses of quetiapine immediate release (eg, 2 to 3 times per day) may be switched to quetiapine ER at the equivalent total daily dose taken once daily. Individual dosage adjustments may be necessary.

➤*Switching from other antipsychotics:* While immediate discontinuation of the previous antipsychotic treatment may be acceptable for some patients with schizophrenia, more gradual discontinuation may be most appropriate for others. In all cases, the period of overlapping antipsychotic administration should be minimized. When switching patients with schizophrenia from depot antipsychotics, if medically appropriate, initiate quetiapine therapy in place of the next scheduled injection. The need for continuing existing extrapyramidal syndrome medication should be periodically reevaluated.

➤*Concomitant therapy:* The elimination of quetiapine was enhanced in the presence of phenytoin. Higher maintenance doses of quetiapine may be required when it is coadministered with phenytoin and other enzyme inducers, such as carbamazepine and phenobarbital.

➤*Duration of therapy:* Patients should be periodically reassessed to determine the need for maintenance treatment and the appropriate dose for such treatment.

➤*Discontinuation of therapy:* Acute withdrawal symptoms, such as insomnia, nausea, and vomiting, have very rarely been described after abrupt cessation of atypical antipsychotic drugs, including quetiapine. Gradual withdrawal is advised.

➤*Administration:*

Immediate release – Quetiapine can be taken with or without food.

Quetiapine should be administered twice daily. However, based on response and tolerability, quetiapine may be administered 3 times daily where needed.

Extended release – Quetiapine ER tablets should be swallowed whole and not split, chewed, or crushed. It is recommended that quetiapine ER be taken without food or with a light meal (approximately 300 calories).

Quetiapine ER should be administered once daily, preferably in the evening.

➤*Storage/Stability:* Store at 25°C (77°F); excursions are permitted between 15° and 30°C (59° and 86°F).

ASENAPINE

Rx	**Saphris** (Organon)	**Tablets; sublingual:** 5 mg	Mannitol, sucralose (black cherry flavor only). (5). Round, white to off-white. Unflavored or black cherry flavor. In UD 60s and 100s.
		10 mg	Mannitol, sucralose (black cherry flavor only). (10). Round, white to off-white. Unflavored or black cherry flavor. In UD 60s and 100s.

For complete and comparative prescribing information, refer to the Antipsychotic Agents class monograph.

Dibenzapine Derivatives

ASENAPINE — ORAL

WARNING

Increased mortality in elderly patients with dementia-related psychosis –

Elderly patients with dementia-related psychosis treated with antipsychotic drugs are at an increased risk of death. Analyses of 17 placebo-controlled trials (modal duration of 10 weeks), largely in patients taking atypical antipsychotic drugs, revealed a risk of death in the drug-treated patients of between 1.6 and 1.7 times that seen in placebo-treated patients. Over the course of a typical 10-week controlled trial, the rate of death in drug-treated patients was about 4.5%, compared with a rate of about 2.6% in the placebo group. Although the causes of death were varied, most of the deaths appeared to be cardiovascular (eg, heart failure, sudden death) or infectious (eg, pneumonia) in nature. Observational studies suggest that similar to atypical antipsychotic drugs, treatment with conventional antipsychotic drugs may increase mortality. The extent to which the findings of increased mortality in observational studies may be attributed to the antipsychotic drug as opposed to some characteristic(s) of the patient is not clear. Asenapine is not approved for the treatment of patients with dementia-related psychosis.

Indications

➤*Bipolar disorder:*

Monotherapy – For the acute treatment of manic or mixed episodes associated with bipolar I disorder.

Adjunctive therapy – As adjunctive therapy with lithium or valproate for the acute treatment of manic or mixed episodes associated with bipolar I disorder.

➤*Schizophrenia:* For the treatment of schizophrenia in adults.

Administration and Dosage

➤*Adults:*

Bipolar disorder –

Monotherapy:

- *Maximum dose* – 10 mg twice daily.
- *Initial dosage* – 10 mg twice daily.
- *Dosage adjustment* – Decrease to 5 mg twice daily if there are adverse effects or based on individual tolerability.

Adjunctive therapy:

- *Maximum dose* – 10 mg twice daily.
- *Initial dosage* – 5 mg twice daily.
- *Dosage adjustment* – Increase to 10 mg twice daily depending on the clinical response and tolerability.
- *Concomitant therapy* – Administer with lithium or valproate.

Schizophrenia –

Usual dosage: 5 mg twice daily.
Maximum dose: 10 mg twice daily.
Dosage adjustment: Increase up to 10 mg twice daily after 1 week based on tolerability.

➤*Hepatic function impairment:* Not recommended in patients with severe hepatic impairment (Child-Pugh class C).

➤*Switching from other antipsychotics:* There are no systematically collected data to specifically address switching patients with schizophrenia or bipolar mania from other antipsychotics to asenapine or concerning coadministration with other antipsychotics. While immediate discontinuation of the previous antipsychotic treatment may be acceptable for some patients with schizophrenia, more gradual discontinuation may be most appropriate for others. In all cases, the period of overlapping antipsychotic administration should be minimized.

➤*Maintenance dosage:* Patients should be periodically reassessed to determine the need for maintenance treatment. While there is no body of evidence available to answer the question of how long a patient should remain on asenapine, it is generally recommended that responding bipolar patients be continued beyond the acute response.

➤*Duration of therapy:* If asenapine is used for extended periods, periodically reevaluate the long-term risks and benefits of the drug for the individual patient.

➤*Administration:* For sublingual use only. Place the tablet under the tongue and allow it to dissolve completely. The tablet will dissolve in saliva within seconds. The tablets should not be crushed, chewed, or swallowed. Do not eat or drink for 10 minutes after administration. Use dry hands when handling the tablets.

➤*Storage/Stability:* Store at 15° to 30°C (59° to 86°F). Do not remove the tablet from packaging until ready to administer.

Benzisoxazole Derivatives

PALIPERIDONE

Rx	**Invega** (Janssen)	**Tablets, extended-release; oral:** 1.5 mg	PEG. (PAL 1.5). Orange-brown, capsule shape. In 30s.
		3 mg	Lactose, PEG. (PAL 3). White, capsule shape. In 30s and UD 100s.
		6 mg	PEG. (PAL 6). Beige, capsule shape. In 30s and UD 100s.
		9 mg	PEG. (PAL 9). Pink, capsule shape. In 30s and UD 100s.
Rx	**Invega Sustenna** (Janssen)	**Injection, suspension, extended-release:** 39 mg	As paliperidone palmitate. PEG 4000. In single-use prefilled syringes.[a]
		78 mg	As paliperidone palmitate. PEG 4000. In single-use prefilled syringes.[a]
		117 mg	As paliperidone palmitate. PEG 4000. In single-use prefilled syringes.[a]
		156 mg	As paliperidone palmitate. PEG 4000. In single-use prefilled syringes.[a]
		234 mg	As paliperidone palmitate. PEG 4000. In single-use prefilled syringes.[a]

[a] Each kit contains a single-use syringe and 2 safety needles (a 1½-inch, 22-gauge safety needle and a 1-inch, 23-gauge safety needle).

PALIPERIDONE — ORAL

For complete and comparative prescribing information, refer to the Antipsychotic Agents class monograph.

WARNING

Increased mortality in elderly patients with dementia-related psychosis –

Elderly patients with dementia-related psychosis treated with antipsychotic drugs are at an increased risk of death. Analyses of 17 placebo-controlled trials (modal duration of 10 weeks), largely in patients taking atypical antipsychotic drugs, revealed a risk of death in the drug-treated subjects between 1.6 and 1.7 times that seen in placebo-treated subjects. Over the course of a typical 10-week controlled trial, the rate of death in drug-treated subjects was approximately 4.5%, compared with a rate of approximately 2.6% in the placebo group. Although the causes of death were varied, most of the deaths appeared to be cardiovascular (eg, heart failure, sudden death) or infectious (eg, pneumonia) in nature. Observational studies suggest that, similar to atypical drugs, treatment with conventional antipsychotic drugs may increase mortality. The extent to which the findings of increased mortality in observational studies may be attributed to the antipsychotic drug as opposed to some characteristic(s) of the patients is not clear. Paliperidone is not approved for the treatment of patients with dementia-related psychosis.

Indications

➤*Schizoaffective disorder:* For the treatment of schizoaffective disorder as monotherapy and as an adjunct to mood stabilizers and/or antidepressants.

The efficacy of paliperidone in schizoaffective disorder was established in two 6-week trials in adults.

➤*Schizophrenia:* For the treatment of schizophrenia.

The efficacy of paliperidone in schizophrenia was established in three 6-week trials in adults and one 6-week trial in adolescents, as well as 1 maintenance trial in adults.

Administration and Dosage

➤*Adults:*

Schizoaffective disorder –

Usual dosage: 6 mg once daily. Initial dose titration is not required.
Maximum dose: 12 mg/day.
Dosage adjustment: Some patients may benefit from lower or higher doses within the recommended dosage range of 3 to 12 mg once daily. Dosage increases, if indicated, should occur only at intervals of more than 4 days in increments of 3 mg/day. Dosage adjustment, if indicated, should occur only after clinical reassessment.

Schizophrenia –

Usual dosage: 6 mg once daily. Initial dose titration is not required.
Maximum dose: 12 mg/day.
Dosage adjustment: Some patients may benefit from higher dosages of up to 12 mg/day, and for some patients, a lower dosage of 3 mg/day may be sufficient. Dosage increases above 6 mg/day should be made only after clinical reassessment and generally should occur at intervals of more than 5 days. When dosage increases are indicated, increments of 3 mg/day are recommended.
Duration of therapy: Paliperidone should be prescribed at the lowest effective dose for maintaining clinical stability, and periodic reevaluation of the long-term usefulness of the drug in individual patients should be made.

PALIPERIDONE — ORAL

➤*Children:*

Schizophrenia –

12 to 17 years of age:

• *Usual dosage* – 3 mg once daily. Initial dose titration is not required.

• *Dosage adjustment* – Dose increases, if considered necessary, should be made only after clinical reassessment and should occur at increments of 3 mg/day at intervals of more than 5 days.

➤*Elderly:* Dose adjustments may be required according to their renal function status. (See Renal Function Impairment.)

➤*Renal function impairment:*

Mild renal impairment (creatinine clearance 50 to less than 80 mL/min) –

Maximum dose: 6 mg daily.

Initial dosage: 3 mg daily.

Moderate to severe renal impairment (creatinine clearance 10 to less than 50 mL/min) –

Maximum dose: 3 mg once daily.

Initial dosage: 1.5 mg once daily.

Creatinine clearance less than 10 mL/min –

Use is not recommended in such patients.

➤*Concomitant therapy:* Because paliperidone is the major active metabolite of risperidone, consideration should be given to the additive paliperidone exposure if risperidone is coadministered with paliperidone.

➤*Administration:* Paliperidone can be taken with our without food.

Paliperidone must be swallowed whole with the aid of liquids. Tablets should not be chewed, divided, or crushed. The medication is contained within a nonabsorbable shell designed to release the drug at a controlled rate. The tablet shell, along with insoluble core components, is eliminated from the body; patients should not be concerned if they occasionally notice something that looks like a tablet in their stool.

➤*Storage/Stability:* Store up to 25°C (77°F); excursions are permitted between 15° and 30°C (59° and 86°F). Protect from moisture.

PALIPERIDONE PALMITATE — INJECTION

For complete and comparative prescribing information, refer to the Antipsychotic Agents class monograph.

WARNING

Increased mortality in elderly patients with dementia-related psychosis – Elderly patients with dementia-related psychosis treated with antipsychotic drugs are at an increased risk of death. Analyses of 17 placebo-controlled trials (modal duration of 10 weeks), largely in patients taking atypical antipsychotic drugs, revealed a risk of death in drug-treated patients of between 1.6 and 1.7 times the risk of death in placebo-treated patients. Over the course of a typical 10-week controlled trial, the rate of death in drug-treated patients was approximately 4.5%, compared with a rate of approximately 2.6% in the placebo group. Although the causes of death varied, most of the deaths appeared to be either cardiovascular (eg, heart failure, sudden death) or infectious (eg, pneumonia) in nature. Observational studies suggest that, similar to atypical antipsychotic drugs, treatment with conventional antipsychotic drugs may increase mortality. The extent to which the findings of increased mortality in observational studies may be attributed to the antipsychotic drug as opposed to some characteristic(s) of the patients is not clear. Paliperidone is not approved for the treatment of patients with dementia-related psychosis.

Indications

➤*Schizophrenia:* For the acute and maintenance treatment of schizophrenia in adults.

Administration and Dosage

➤*General dosing considerations:* For patients who have never taken oral paliperidone or oral or injectable risperidone, it is recommended that tolerability with oral paliperidone or oral risperidone be established prior to initiating treatment with paliperidone injection.

➤*Adults:*

Schizophrenia –

Initial dosage: 234 mg intramuscularly (IM) on treatment day 1 and 156 mg 1 week later, both administered in the deltoid muscle.

Maintenance dosage: The recommended monthly maintenance dose is 117 mg; some patients may benefit from lower or higher maintenance doses within the recommended range of 39 to 234 mg based on individual patient tolerability and/or efficacy. Following the second dose, monthly maintenance doses can be administered in the deltoid or gluteal muscle.

Dosage adjustment: Adjustment of the maintenance dose may be made monthly. When making dose adjustments, the prolonged-release characteristics of paliperidone injection should be considered, as the full effect of the dose adjustment may not be evident for several months.

Duration of therapy: Paliperidone has been shown to be effective in delaying time to relapse of symptoms of schizophrenia in long-term use. It is recommended that responding patients be continued on treatment at the lowest dose needed. Patients should be periodically reassessed to determine the need for continued treatment.

Concomitant therapy: Concomitant use of paliperidone injection with oral paliperidone or oral or injectable risperidone has not been studied. Because paliperidone is the major active metabolite of risperidone, consideration should be given to the additive paliperidone exposure if any of these medications are coadministered with paliperidone injection.

Discontinuation of therapy: If paliperidone injection is discontinued, its prolonged-release characteristics must be considered. As recommended with other antipsychotic medications, the need for continuing existing extrapyramidal symptoms medication should be reevaluated periodically.

Switching from other antipsychotics: There are no systematically collected data that specifically address switching patients with schizophrenia from other antipsychotics to paliperidone injection, or concerning coadministration with other antipsychotics.

For patients who have never taken oral paliperidone or oral or injectable risperidone, tolerability should be established with oral paliperidone or oral risperidone prior to initiating treatment with paliperidone injection.

• *Switching from oral antipsychotics* – Previous oral antipsychotics can be discontinued at the time of initiation of treatment with paliperidone injection. Patients previously stabilized on different doses of paliperidone extended-release (ER) tablets can attain similar paliperidone steady-state exposure during maintenance treatment with paliperidone injection monthly doses.

Doses of Oral Paliperidone and IM Paliperidone Needed to Attain Similar Paliperidone Exposure at Steady State

Formulation	Paliperidone ER tablet	Paliperidone injection
Dosing frequency	Once daily	Once every 4 weeks
Dose	12 mg	234 mg
	6 mg	117 mg
	3 mg	39 to 78 mg

• *Switching from long-acting injectable antipsychotics* – When switching patients from previous long-acting injectable antipsychotics, initiate paliperidone injection in place of the next scheduled injection. Paliperidone should then be continued at monthly intervals. The 1-week initiation dosing regimen is not required.

Missed doses:

• *Avoiding missed doses –*

To avoid a missed dose, patients may be given the second dose 2 days before or after the 1-week time point. To avoid a missed monthly dose, patients may be given the injection up to 7 days before or after the monthly time point.

• *Missed dose (1 month to 6 weeks) –*

If less than 6 weeks have elapsed since the last injection, the previously stabilized dose should be administered as soon as possible, followed by injections at monthly intervals.

• *Missed dose (more than 6 weeks to 6 months)* – If more than 6 weeks have elapsed since the last injection of paliperidone, resume the same dose the patient was previously stabilized on (unless the patient was stabilized on a dose of 234 mg, then the first 2 injections should each be 156 mg) in the following manner: 1) a deltoid injection as soon as practically possible, followed by 2) another deltoid injection (same dose) 1 week later, and 3) resumption of either deltoid or gluteal dosing at monthly intervals.

• *Missed dose (more than 6 months)* – If more than 6 months have elapsed since the last injection of paliperidone, initiate dosing as described in Initial Dosage.

➤*Renal function impairment:*

Mild renal impairment (creatinine clearance of 50 mL/min to less than 80 mL/min) –

Initial dosage: 156 mg IM on treatment day 1 and 117 mg 1 week later, both administered in the deltoid muscle.

Maintenance dosage: Monthly injections of 78 mg IM in the deltoid or gluteal muscle.

Moderate or severe renal impairment (creatinine clearance less than 50 mL/min) – Paliperidone is not recommended.

➤*Administration:* Paliperidone injection is intended for IM use only. Inject slowly, deep into the muscle. Care should be taken to avoid inadvertent injection into a blood vessel.

Administration should be in a single injection. Do not administer the dose in divided injections. Do not administer intravascularly or subcutaneously.

The recommended needle size for administration of paliperidone into the deltoid muscle is determined by the patient's weight. For those weighing 90 kg or more (200 lb or more), the 1½-inch, 22-gauge needle is recommended. For those weighing less than 90 kg (less than 200 lb), the 1-inch, 23-gauge needle is recommended. Deltoid injections should be alternated between the 2 deltoid muscles.

The recommended needle size for administration of paliperidone into the gluteal muscle is the 1½-inch, 22-gauge needle. Administration should be made into the upper-outer quadrant of the gluteal area. Gluteal injections should be alternated between the 2 gluteal muscles.

➤*Storage/Stability:* Store at room temperature, 25°C (77°F); excursions are permitted between 15° and 30°C (59° and 86°F). Paliperidone injection is for single use only.

RISPERIDONE

Rx	**Risperidone** (Teva)	**Tablets; oral:** 0.25 mg	Lactose, PEG. (93 221). Dark yellow. Film-coated. In 60s and 500s.
Rx	**Risperdal** (Janssen)		Lactose. (JANSSEN Ris 0.25). Dark yellow, capsule shape. In 60s, 500s, and UD 100s.
Rx	**Risperidone** (Teva)	**Tablets; oral:** 0.5 mg	Lactose, PEG. (93 225). Red-brown. Film-coated. In 60s and 500s.
Rx	**Risperdal** (Janssen)		Lactose. (JANSSEN Ris 0.5). Red-brown, capsule shape. In 60s, 500s, and UD 100s.
Rx	**Risperidone** (Teva)	**Tablets; oral:** 1 mg	Lactose, PEG. (93 7240). White. Film-coated. In 60s and 500s.
Rx	**Risperdal** (Janssen)		Lactose. (JANSSEN R 1). White, capsule shape. In 60s, 500s, and UD 100s.
Rx	**Risperidone** (Teva)	**Tablets; oral:** 2 mg	Lactose, PEG. (93 7241). Orange. Film-coated. In 60s and 500s.
Rx	**Risperdal** (Janssen)		Lactose. (JANSSEN R 2). Orange, capsule shape. In 60s, 500s, and UD 100s.
Rx	**Risperidone** (Teva)	**Tablets; oral:** 3 mg	Lactose, PEG. (93 7242). Yellow. Film-coated. In 60s and 500s.
Rx	**Risperdal** (Janssen)		Lactose. (JANSSEN R 3). Yellow, capsule shape. In 60s, 500s, and UD 100s.
Rx	**Risperidone** (Teva)	**Tablets; oral:** 4 mg	Lactose, PEG. (93 7243). Green. Film-coated. In 60s.
Rx	**Risperdal** (Janssen)		Lactose. (JANSSEN R 4). Green, capsule shape. In 60s and UD 100s.
Rx	**Risperidone** (Dr. Reddy's Labs)	**Tablets, disintegrating; oral:** 0.5 mg	Aspartame, mannitol, phenylalanine. (R-207). White to off-white, capsule shape. In UD 30s and 100s.
Rx	**Risperdal M-TAB** (Janssen)		Phenylalanine 0.14 mg, mannitol, aspartame, peppermint oil. (R0.5). Light coral, round. In UD 28s and 30s.
Rx	**Risperidone** (Dr. Reddy's Labs)	**Tablets, disintegrating; oral:** 1 mg	Aspartame, mannitol, phenylalanine. (R-208). White to off-white, capsule shape. In UD 30s and 100s.
Rx	**Risperdal M-TAB** (Janssen)		Phenylalanine 0.28 mg, mannitol, aspartame, peppermint oil. (R1). Light coral, square. In UD 28s and 30s
Rs	**Risperidone** (Dr. Reddy's Labs)	**Tablets, disintegrating; oral:** 2 mg	Aspartame, mannitol, phenylalanine. (R-209). White to off-white, capsule shape. In UD 30s and 100s.
Rx	**Risperdal M-TAB** (Janssen)		Phenylalanine 0.42 mg, mannitol, aspartame, peppermint oil. (R2). Coral, square. In UD 28s.
Rx	**Risperidone** (Dr. Reddy's Labs)	**Tablets, disintegrating; oral:** 3 mg	Aspartame, mannitol, phenylalanine. (R470). White to off-white, round. In UD 30s and 100s.
Rx	**Risperdal M-TAB** (Janssen)		Phenylalanine 0.63 mg, mannitol, aspartame, peppermint oil. (R3). Coral, round. In UD 28s.
Rx	**Risperidone** (Dr. Reddy's Labs)	**Tablets, disintegrating; oral:** 4 mg	Aspartame, mannitol, phenylalanine. (R471). White to off-white, square. In UD 30s and 100s.
Rx	**Risperdal M-TAB** (Janssen)		Phenylalanine 0.84 mg, mannitol, aspartame, peppermint oil. (R4). Coral, round. In UD 28s.
Rx	**Risperidone** (Various, eg, Apotex, Roxane Laboratories, Teva)	**Solution; oral:** 1 mg/mL	May contain sorbitol. In 30 mL with calibrated pipette.
Rx	**Risperdal** (Janssen)		In 30 mL with calibrated pipette.
Rx	**Risperdal Consta** (Janssen)	**Injection, powder for suspension, extended-release:** 12.5 mg	In vials/kits with 2 mL of diluent.
		25 mg	In vials/kits with 2 mL of diluent.
		37.5 mg	In vials/kits with 2 mL of diluent.
		50 mg	In vials/kits with 2 mL of diluent.

RISPERIDONE — ORAL

Complete and comparative prescribing information begins in the Antipsychotic Agents class monograph.

WARNING

Increased mortality in elderly patients with dementia-related psychosis –

Elderly patients with dementia-related psychosis treated with antipsychotic drugs are at an increased risk of death. Analyses of 17 placebo-controlled trials (modal duration of 10 weeks), largely in patients taking atypical antipsychotic drugs, revealed a risk of death in the drug-treated patients of between 1.6 and 1.7 times that seen in placebo-treated patients. Over the course of a typical 10-week controlled trial, the rate of death in drug-treated patients was approximately 4.5%, compared with a rate of approximately 2.6% in the placebo group. Although the causes of death were varied, most of the deaths appeared to be either cardiovascular (eg, heart failure, sudden death) or infectious (eg, pneumonia) in nature. Observational studies suggest that, similar to atypical antipsychotic drugs, treatment with conventional antipsychotic drugs may increase mortality. The extent to which the findings of increased mortality in observational studies may be attributed to the antipsychotic drug as opposed to some characteristic(s) of the patients is not clear. Risperidone is not approved for the treatment of patients with dementia-related psychosis.

Indications

➤ *Bipolar mania:*

Monotherapy (adults and children) – For the short-term treatment of acute manic or mixed episodes associated with bipolar I disorder in adults and in children and adolescents 10 to 17 years of age.

Combination therapy (adults) – The combination of risperidone with lithium or valproate is indicated for the short-term treatment of adults with acute manic or mixed episodes associated with bipolar I disorder.

➤ *Irritability associated with autistic disorder (children):* For the treatment of irritability associated with autistic disorder in children and adolescents 5 to 16 years of age, including symptoms of aggression towards others, deliberate self-injuriousness, temper tantrums, and quickly changing moods.

➤ *Schizophrenia:*

Adults – For the acute and maintenance treatment of schizophrenia.

Adolescents – For the treatment of schizophrenia in adolescents 13 to 17 years of age.

➤ *Off-label uses:*

Obsessive-compulsive disorder – [1] = Good documentation. No evidence supports the use of risperidone monotherapy for the treatment of obsessive-compulsive disorder (OCD). According to American Psychiatric Association guidelines, the addition of risperidone or another second-generation antipsychotic agent may be appropriate as part of a step-wise approach for patients with OCD who fail to respond to initial therapy with a selective serotonin reuptake inhibitor (SSRI) or cognitive-behavioral therapy.

Stuttering – [4] = Insufficient documentation. Although published information regarding the use of risperidone in the treatment of stuttering is limited to a small number of patients, initial controlled data suggest a benefit, particularly in adult patients with developmental stuttering. Little information is available regarding the use of this agent in children or adolescents (1 case). This drug may be a therapeutic option in the management of stuttering in adults, but it requires further evaluation in larger controlled trials.

Tourette syndrome – [2] = Fair documentation. The use of risperidone to treat Tourette syndrome or chronic tic disorder has been studied in both controlled and noncontrolled studies with some success. Various titration schedules and dosing regimens have been utilized. While initial data suggest that risperidone may be a useful alternative in patients with refractory tic disorders, further controlled trials are needed to determine the optimal dosage schedule and its role in current therapy options.

RISPERIDONE — ORAL

Administration and Dosage

➤*General dosing considerations:* Periodically reevaluate the long-term risks and benefits of the drug for the individual patient.

➤*Adults:*

Bipolar mania –

Usual dosage: 1 to 6 mg/day.

Initial dosage: 2 to 3 mg/day, administered once daily.

Dosage adjustment: Dosage adjustments, if indicated, should occur at intervals of no less than 24 hours and in increments/decrements of 1 mg/day. In trials, short-term (3-week) antimanic efficacy was demonstrated in a flexible dosage range of 1 to 6 mg/day. Risperidone dosages higher than 6 mg/day were not studied.

Duration of therapy: There is no body of evidence available from controlled trials to guide in the longer-term management of a patient who improves during treatment of an acute manic episode with risperidone. While it is generally agreed that pharmacological treatment beyond an acute response in mania is desirable, both for maintenance of the initial response and for prevention of new manic episodes, there are no systematically obtained data to support the use of risperidone in such longer-term treatment (ie, beyond 3 weeks).

Schizophrenia –

Usual dosage: 4 to 8 mg/day.

Initial dosage: 2 mg/day, administered once daily or half the total daily dose administered twice daily.

Dosage titration: Dosage increases should occur at intervals of no less than 24 hours, in increments of 1 to 2 mg/day, as tolerated, to a recommended dosage of 4 to 8 mg/day. In some patients, slower titration may be appropriate. Efficacy has been demonstrated in a range of 4 to 16 mg/day. However, dosages above 6 mg/day for twice-daily dosing were not demonstrated to be more efficacious than lower doses, were associated with more extrapyramidal symptoms and other adverse reactions, and are generally not recommended. In a single study supporting once-daily dosing, the efficacy results were generally stronger for 8 mg than for 4 mg. The safety of dosages above 16 mg/day has not been evaluated in clinical trials.

Duration of therapy: While it is unknown how long a patient with schizophrenia should remain on risperidone, the effectiveness of risperidone 2 to 8 mg/day at delaying relapse was demonstrated in a controlled trial in patients who had been clinically stable for at least 4 weeks and were then followed for a period of 1 to 2 years.

Conversion:

While immediate discontinuation of the previous antipsychotic treatment may be acceptable for some patients with schizophrenia, more gradual discontinuation may be most appropriate for other patients. In all cases, minimize the period of overlapping antipsychotic administration. When switching patients with schizophrenia from depot antipsychotic agents, if medically appropriate, initiate risperidone therapy in place of the next scheduled injection. Reevaluate the need for continuing existing extrapyramidal symptom medication periodically.

Reinitiation of therapy – Although there are no data to specifically address reinitiation of treatment, it is recommended that, after an interval off risperidone, the initial titration schedule should be followed.

Off-label dosing –

Obsessive-compulsive disorder: [1] = Good documentation. Initial dosage is 0.5 or 1 mg daily and increased by 0.5 or 1 mg weekly based on therapeutic effect and tolerance. The mean daily dose in trials was 0.5 or 2.2 mg (range, 0.5 to 4 mg/day). Once successful management is achieved, therapy should continue for 1 to 2 years before a taper is attempted. During tapering, doses may be reduced by 10% to 25% every 1 to 2 months, while monitoring for symptom exacerbation or return.

Stuttering: [4] = Insufficient documentation. Initial dosing was 0.5 mg nightly, increased by 0.5 mg daily every 4 days or more as tolerated to a maximum of 2 mg daily.

Tourette syndrome: [2] = Fair documentation. Initial dosing in trials was 0.5 to 1 mg/day with various titration schedules. Doses were titrated by 0.5 or 1 mg every 5 days. In 2 studies enrolling children and adults, the mean dosages were less than 4 mg/day (2.7 and 3.9 mg), but dosages reached as high as 6 to 9 mg/day.

➤*Children:*

Bipolar mania (10 to 17 years of age) –

Usual dosage: 2.5 mg/day. Patients experiencing persistent somnolence may benefit from administering half the daily dose twice daily.

Initial dosage: 0.5 mg/day, administered as a single daily dose in either the morning or evening.

Dosage titration: Dosage adjustments, if indicated, should occur at intervals of no less than 24 hours in increments of 0.5 or 1 mg/day, as tolerated, to a recommended dosage of 2.5 mg/day. Although efficacy has been demonstrated in studies of children with bipolar mania at dosages between 0.5 and 6 mg/day, no additional benefit was seen above 2.5 mg/day, and higher dosages were associated with more adverse reactions. Dosages higher than 6 mg/day have not been studied.

Duration of therapy: There is no body of evidence available from controlled trials to guide in the longer-term management of a patient who improves during treatment of an acute manic episode with risperidone. While it is generally agreed that pharmacologic treatment beyond an acute response in mania is desirable, both for maintenance of the initial response and for prevention of new manic episodes, there are no systematically obtained data to support the use of risperidone in such longer-term treatment (ie, beyond 3 weeks).

Irritability associated with autistic disorder (5 to 16 years of age) –

Usual dosage: 0.5 mg/day for patients weighing less than 20 kg and 1 mg/day for patients weighing 20 kg or more. Patients experiencing persistent somnolence may benefit from a once-daily dose administered at bedtime, administering half the daily dose twice daily, or a reduction of the dose.

Initial dosage: 0.25 mg/day for patients weighing less than 20 kg and 0.5 mg/day for patients weighing 20 kg or more. The dose may be administered once daily or half the total daily dose may be administered twice daily.

Dosage titration: After a minimum of 4 days from treatment initiation, the dosage may be increased to the recommended dosage of 0.5 mg/day for patients weighing less than 20 kg and 1 mg/day for patients weighing 20 kg or more. This dose should be maintained for a minimum of 14 days. In patients not achieving sufficient clinical response, dose increases may be considered at intervals of at least 2 weeks in increments of 0.25 mg/day for patients weighing less than 20 kg or 0.5 mg/day for patients weighing 20 kg or more. Caution should be exercised with dosage for smaller children who weigh less than 15 kg.

Maintenance dosage: Once sufficient clinical response has been achieved and maintained, consider gradually lowering the dose to achieve the optimal balance of efficacy and safety.

Schizophrenia (13 to 17 years of age) –

Usual dosage: 3 mg/day. Patients experiencing persistent somnolence may benefit from administering half the daily dose twice daily.

Initial dosage: 0.5 mg/day, administered as a single daily dose in either the morning or evening.

Dosage titration: Dosage adjustments, if indicated, should occur at intervals of no less than 24 hours in increments of 0.5 or 1 mg/day, as tolerated, to a recommended dosage of 3 mg/day. Although efficacy has been demonstrated in studies of adolescent patients with schizophrenia at dosages between 1 and 6 mg/day, no additional benefit was seen above 3 mg/day, and higher doses were associated with more adverse reactions. Dosages higher than 6 mg/day have not been studied.

Duration of therapy: There are no controlled data to support the longer term use of risperidone beyond 8 weeks in adolescents with schizophrenia.

Conversion:

While immediate discontinuation of the previous antipsychotic treatment may be acceptable for some patients with schizophrenia, more gradual discontinuation may be most appropriate for other patients. In all cases, the period of overlapping antipsychotic administration should be minimized. When switching schizophrenic patients from depot antipsychotic agents, if medically appropriate, initiate risperidone therapy in place of the next scheduled injection. The need for continuing existing extrapyramidal symptom medication should be reevaluated periodically.

Reinitiation of therapy – Although there are no data to specifically address reinitiation of treatment, it is recommended that, after an interval off risperidone, the initial titration schedule should be followed.

Off-label dosing –

Stuttering: [4] = Insufficient documentation. 0.25 mg daily.

Tourette syndrome: [2] = Fair documentation. Initial dosing in trials was 0.5 to 1 mg/day with various titration schedules. Doses were titrated by 0.5 or 1 mg every 5 days. In 2 studies enrolling children and adults, the mean dosages were less than 4 mg/day (2.7 and 3.9 mg), but dosages reached as high as 6 to 9 mg/day. One study enrolling only children titrated doses to a maximum of 2.5 mg/day (in divided doses).

➤*Elderly:* Initial dosage is 0.5 mg twice daily. Dosage increases should be in increments of no more than 0.5 mg twice daily. Increases to dosages greater than 1.5 mg twice daily should generally occur at intervals of at least 1 week. In some patients, slower titration may be medically appropriate. If a once-daily dosing regimen is being considered, it is recommended that the patient be titrated on a twice-a-day regimen for 2 to 3 days at the target dose. Subsequent switches to a once-a-day dosing regimen can be done thereafter.

➤*Renal function impairment:* For patients with severe renal impairment, the initial dosage is 0.5 mg twice daily. Dosage increases should be in increments of no more than 0.5 mg twice daily. Increases to dosages greater than 1.5 mg twice daily should generally occur at intervals of at least 1 week. In some patients, slower titration may be medically appropriate.

➤*Administration:* May be given with or without food.

Oral solution – Risperidone oral solution can be administered directly from the calibrated pipette or can be mixed with a beverage prior to administration. Risperidone oral solution is compatible in the following beverages: water, coffee, orange juice, and low-fat milk; it is not compatible with cola or tea.

Orally disintegrating tablets –

Using dry hands, remove the tablet from the blister unit and immediately place the entire orally disintegrating tablet on the tongue. The orally disintegrating tablet should be consumed immediately, because the tablet cannot be stored once removed from the blister unit. Risperidone orally disintegrating tablets disintegrate in the mouth within seconds and can be swallowed subsequently with or without liquid. Patients should not attempt to split or chew the tablet.

➤*Storage/Stability:* Store at 15° to 25°C (59° to 77°F). Protect from light and moisture. Protect oral solution from freezing.

RISPERIDONE — INJECTION

For complete and comparative prescribing information refer to the Antipsychotic Agents group monograph.

WARNING

Increased mortality in elderly patients with dementia-related psychosis – Elderly patients with dementia-related psychosis treated with antipsychotic drugs are at an increased risk of death. Analyses of 17 placebo-controlled trials (modal duration of 10 weeks), largely in patients taking atypical antipsychotic drugs, revealed a risk of death in the drug-treated patients of between 1.6 and 1.7 times that seen in placebo-treated patients. Over the course of a typical 10-week controlled trial, the rate of death in drug-treated patients was approximately 4.5%, compared with a rate of approximately 2.6% in the placebo group. Although the causes of death were varied, most of the deaths appeared to be either cardiovascular (eg, heart failure, sudden death) or infectious (eg, pneumonia) in nature. Observational studies suggest that, similar to atypical antipsychotic drugs, treatment with conventional antipsychotic drugs may increase mortality. The extent to which the findings of increased mortality in observational studies may be attributed to the antipsychotic drug as opposed to some characteristic(s) of the patients is not clear. Risperidone is not approved for the treatment of patients with dementia-related psychosis.

Indications

➤*Bipolar disorder:* As monotherapy or as adjunctive therapy to lithium or valproate for the maintenance treatment of bipolar I disorder.

➤*Schizophrenia:* For the treatment of schizophrenia.

Administration and Dosage

➤*General dosing considerations:* For patients who have never taken oral risperidone, it is recommended to establish tolerability with oral risperidone prior to initiating treatment with risperidone injection. (See Concomitant therapy.)

➤*Adults:*

Bipolar disorder – The recommended dosage for monotherapy or adjunctive therapy to lithium or valproate for the maintenance treatment of bipolar I disorder is 25 mg IM every 2 weeks. Some patients may benefit from a higher dose of 37.5 or 50 mg. Doses above 50 mg have not been studied in this population. The health care provider who elects to use risperidone for extended periods should periodically reevaluate the long-term risks and benefits of the drug for the individual patient.

Schizophrenia –

Usual dosage: 25 mg IM every 2 weeks.

Maximum dose: 50 mg IM every 2 weeks.

Dosage titration: Although dose response for efficacy has not been established for risperidone, some patients not responding to 25 mg may benefit from a higher dose of 37.5 or 50 mg. Upward dosage adjustment should not be made more frequently than every 4 weeks. The clinical effects of this dose adjustment should not be anticipated earlier than 3 weeks after the first injection with the higher dose. No additional benefit was observed with doses greater than 50 mg; however, a higher incidence of adverse reactions was observed.

Duration of therapy:

It is recommended that responding patients continue on treatment with risperidone injection at the lowest dose needed. Patients should be periodically reassessed to determine the need for continued treatment.

Reinitiation of treatment: There are no data to specifically address reinitiation of treatment. When restarting patients who have had an interval off treatment with risperidone injection, supplementation with oral risperidone (or another antipsychotic medication) should be administered.

➤*Elderly:*

For elderly patients treated with risperidone injection, the recommended dosage is 25 mg IM every 2 weeks. Oral risperidone (or another antipsychotic medication) should be given with the first injection of risperidone and should be continued for 3 weeks to ensure that adequate therapeutic plasma concentrations are maintained prior to the main release phase of risperidone from the injection site.

➤*Renal function impairment:*

Usual dosage – Patients with renal impairment should be treated with titrated doses of oral risperidone prior to initiating treatment with risperidone injection. The recommended starting dosage is oral risperidone 0.5 mg twice daily during the first week, which can be increased to 1 mg twice daily or 2 mg once daily during the second week. If a total daily dose of at least 2 mg of oral risperidone is well tolerated, an IM injection of risperidone 25 mg can be administered every 2 weeks. Oral supplementation should be continued for 3 weeks after the first injection until the main release of risperidone from the injection site has begun. In some patients, slower titration may be medically appropriate.

Alternatively, a starting dose of 12.5 mg IM may be appropriate.

Dosage adjustment – Upward dosage adjustment should not be made more frequently than every 4 weeks. The clinical effects of this dose adjustment should not be anticipated earlier than 3 weeks after the first injection with the higher dose. Dose reduction as low as 12.5 mg may be appropriate.

➤*Hepatic function impairment:* See Renal Function Impairment for dosing.

Usual dosage –

➤*Patients who have a history of poor tolerability to psychotropic medications:*

Initial dosage – A lower initial dose of 12.5 mg IM may be appropriate.

Dosage adjustment – Upward dosage adjustment should not be made more frequently than every 4 weeks. The clinical effects of this dose adjustment should not be anticipated earlier than 3 weeks after the first injection with the higher dose.

➤*Switching from other antipsychotics:* There are no systematically collected data to specifically address switching patients from other antipsychotics to risperidone injection or concerning coadministration with other antipsychotics. Previous antipsychotics should be continued for 3 weeks after the first injection of risperidone to ensure that therapeutic concentrations are maintained until the main release phase of risperidone from the injection site has begun. For patients who have never taken oral risperidone, it is recommended to establish tolerability with oral risperidone prior to initiating treatment with risperidone injection. As recommended with other antipsychotic medications, the need for continuing existing extrapyramidal symptom medication should be reevaluated periodically.

Concomitant therapy –

Oral risperidone or another antipsychotic: Oral risperidone (or another antipsychotic medication) should be given with the first injection of risperidone and continued for 3 weeks (and then discontinued) to ensure that adequate therapeutic plasma concentrations are maintained prior to the main release phase of risperidone from the injection site.

CYP3A4 inducers (eg, carbamazepine, phenobarbital, phenytoin, rifampin): Coadministration of carbamazepine and other CYP3A4 enzyme inducers (eg, phenytoin, rifampin, phenobarbital) with risperidone would be expected to cause decreases in the plasma concentrations of the sum of risperidone and 9-hydroxyrisperidone, which could lead to decreased efficacy of risperidone treatment.

The dose of risperidone needs to be titrated accordingly for patients receiving these enzyme inducers, especially during initiation or discontinuation of therapy with these inducers. At the initiation of therapy with CYP3A4 inducers, patients should be closely monitored during the first 4 to 8 weeks, because the dose of risperidone may need to be adjusted. A dose increase, or additional oral risperidone, may need to be considered. On discontinuation of CYP3A4 inducers, the dosage of risperidone should be reevaluated and, if necessary, decreased. Patients may be placed on a lower dose of risperidone between 2 and 4 weeks before the planned discontinuation of CYP3A4 inducers to adjust for the expected increase in plasma concentrations of risperidone plus 9-hydroxyrisperidone.

For patients treated with the recommended dose of risperidone 25 mg injection and discontinuing from CYP3A4 inducers, it is recommended to continue treatment with the 25 mg dose unless clinical judgment necessitates lowering the risperidone injection dose to 12.5 mg or necessitates interruption of risperidone treatment. The efficacy of the 12.5 mg dose has not been investigated in clinical trials.

CYP2D6 inhibitors (eg, fluoxetine, paroxetine): Fluoxetine and paroxetine, CYP2D6 inhibitors, have been shown to increase the plasma concentration of risperidone 2.5- to 2.8-fold and 3- to 9-fold, respectively. Fluoxetine did not affect the plasma concentration of 9-hydroxyrisperidone. Paroxetine lowered the concentration of 9-hydroxyrisperidone by about 10%.

The dose of risperidone needs to be titrated accordingly when fluoxetine or paroxetine is coadministered. When either fluoxetine or paroxetine is initiated or discontinued, reevaluate the dose of risperidone injection. When initiation of fluoxetine or paroxetine is considered, patients may be placed on a lower dose of risperidone injection between 2 and 4 weeks before the planned start of fluoxetine or paroxetine therapy to adjust for the expected increase in plasma concentrations of risperidone.

When fluoxetine or paroxetine is initiated in patients receiving the recommended dose of risperidone 25 mg injection, it is recommended to continue treatment with the 25 mg dose unless clinical judgment necessitates lowering the risperidone dose to 12.5 mg or necessitates interruption of risperidone treatment. When risperidone injection is initiated in patients already receiving fluoxetine or paroxetine, a starting dose of 12.5 mg can be considered. The efficacy of the 12.5 mg dose has not been investigated in clinical trials. The effects of discontinuation of concomitant fluoxetine or paroxetine therapy on the pharmacokinetics of risperidone and 9-hydroxyrisperidone have not been studied.

➤*Predisposition to hypotension:* Elderly patients and patients with a predisposition to hypotensive reactions or for whom such reactions would pose a particular risk should be instructed in nonpharmacologic interventions that help to reduce the occurrence of orthostatic hypotension (eg, sitting on the edge of the bed for several minutes before attempting to stand in the morning and slowly rising from a seated position). These patients should avoid sodium depletion or dehydration, and circumstances that accentuate hypotension (eg, alcohol intake, high ambient temperature). Monitoring of orthostatic vital signs should be considered.

➤*Preparation for administration:* Risperidone must be reconstituted only in the diluent supplied in the dose pack, and must be administered with the needle supplied in the dose pack. All components are required for administration. Do not substitute any components of the dose pack. To ensure that the intended dose of risperidone is delivered, the full contents from the vial must be administered. Administration of partial contents may not deliver the intended dose of risperidone.

Remove the dose pack of risperidone from the refrigerator and allow it to come to room temperature prior to reconstitution.

Upon suspension in the diluent, it is recommended to use risperidone injection immediately. Risperidone must be used within 6 hours of suspension. If

Benzisoxazole Derivatives

RISPERIDONE — INJECTION

risperidone is not administered within 2 minutes of reconstitution, settling of the microspheres will occur and resuspension by shaking will be necessary prior to administration. Keeping the vial upright, shake vigorously back and forth for as long as it takes to resuspend the microspheres.

➤*Administration:* Risperidone should be administered every 2 weeks by deep IM deltoid or gluteal injection. Each injection should be administered by a health care provider using the enclosed safety needle. For deltoid administration, use the 1-inch needle, alternating injections between the 2 arms. For gluteal administration, use the 2-inch needle, alternating between the 2 buttocks. Do not administer IV.

Do not combine 2 different dosage strengths of risperidone in a single administration.

➤*Storage/Stability:* The entire dose pack should be stored in the refrigerator (2° to 8°C; 36° to 46°F) and protected from light. If refrigeration is unavailable, risperidone can be stored at temperatures not exceeding 25°C (77°F) for no more than 7 days prior to administration. Do not expose unrefrigerated product to temperatures above 25°C (77°F). Once in suspension, the product should not be exposed to temperatures above 25°C (77°F). Risperidone must be used within 6 hours of suspension.

ILOPERIDONE

Rx	**Fanapt** (Novartis)	**Tablets; oral:** 1 mg	Lactose. (1). White, round. In 60s and a titration pack.[a]
		2 mg	Lactose. (2). White, round. In 60s and a titration pack.[a]
		4 mg	Lactose. (4). White, round. In 60s and a titration pack.[a]
		6 mg	Lactose. (6). White, round. In 60s and a titration pack.[a]
		8 mg	Lactose. (8). White, round. In 60s.
		10 mg	Lactose. (10). White, round. In 60s.
		12 mg	Lactose. (12). White, round. In 60s.

[a] Titration pack contains two 1 mg tablets, two 2 mg tablets, two 4 mg tablets, and two 6 mg tablets (total of 8 tablets).

ILOPERIDONE — ORAL

For complete and comparative product information, refer to the Antipsychotic Agents class monograph.

WARNING

Increased mortality in elderly patients with dementia-related psychosis – Elderly patients with dementia-related psychosis treated with antipsychotic drugs are at an increased risk of death. Analysis of 17 placebo-controlled trials (modal duration, 10 weeks), largely in patients taking atypical antipsychotic drugs, revealed a risk of death in the drug-treated patients of between 1.6 and 1.7 times the risk of death in placebo-treated patients. Over the course of a typical 10-week controlled trial, the rate of death in drug-treated patients was about 4.5%, compared with a rate of about 2.6% in the placebo group. Although the causes of death were varied, most of the deaths appeared to be either cardiovascular (eg, heart failure, sudden death) or infectious (eg, pneumonia) in nature.

Observational studies suggest that, similar to atypical antipsychotic drugs, treatment with conventional antipsychotic drugs may increase mortality. The extent to which the findings of increased mortality in observational studies may be attributed to the antipsychotic drug as opposed to some characteristic(s) of the patients is not clear. Iloperidone is not approved for the treatment of patients with dementia-related psychosis.

Indications

➤*Schizophrenia:* For the acute treatment of adults with schizophrenia.

Administration and Dosage

➤*General dosing considerations:* Iloperidone must be titrated slowly from a low starting dose to avoid orthostatic hypotension because of its alpha-adrenergic blocking properties.

Be aware that some adverse effects associated with iloperidone use are dose related.

➤*Adults:*

Schizophrenia –

Maximum dose: 12 mg twice daily (24 mg/day).

Initial dosage: 1 mg twice daily on day 1.

Dosage titration: 2, 4, 6, 8, 10, and 12 mg twice daily on days 2, 3, 4, 5, 6, and 7, respectively.

Be mindful of the fact that patients need to be titrated to an effective dose of iloperidone. Thus, control of symptoms may be delayed during the first 1 to 2 weeks of treatment compared with some other antipsychotic drugs that do not require similar titration.

Maintenance dosage: 6 to 12 mg twice daily is the target dose range.

Although there is no body of evidence available to answer the question of how long the patient treated with iloperidone should be maintained, it is generally recommended that responding patients be continued beyond the acute response. Patients should be periodically reassessed to determine the need for maintenance treatment.

Duration of therapy: The effectiveness of iloperidone in long-term use, that is, for more than 6 weeks, has not been systematically evaluated in controlled trials. Therefore, the health care provider who elects to use iloperidone for extended periods should periodically re-evaluate the long-term usefulness of the drug for the individual patient.

Concomitant therapy:

• *CYP2D6 inhibitors* – Iloperidone dose should be reduced by one-half when coadministered with strong CYP2D6 inhibitors such as fluoxetine or paroxetine. When the CYP2D6 inhibitor is withdrawn from the combination therapy, the iloperidone dose should then be increased to where it was before.

• *CYP3A4 inhibitors* – Iloperidone dose should be reduced by one-half when coadministered with strong CYP3A4 inhibitors such as ketoconazole or clarithromycin. When the CYP3A4 inhibitor is withdrawn from the combination therapy, the iloperidone dose should be increased to where it was before.

➤*Elderly:* See Adults for dosing. Studies suggest that there may be a different tolerability profile (ie, increased risk in mortality and cerebrovascular events, including stroke) in this population compared with younger patients with schizophrenia. Exercise vigilance when electing to treat such patients.

➤*Hepatic function impairment:* Iloperidone is not recommended for patients with hepatic impairment.

➤*Reinitiation of treatment in patients previously discontinued:* Although there are no data to specifically address reinitiation of treatment, it is recommended that the initiation titration schedule be followed whenever patients have had an interval of more than 3 days off iloperidone.

➤*Switching from other antipsychotics:* There are no specific data to address how patients with schizophrenia can be switched from other antipsychotics to iloperidone or how iloperidone can be used concomitantly with other antipsychotics. Although immediate discontinuation of the previous antipsychotic treatment may be acceptable for some patients with schizophrenia, more gradual discontinuation may be most appropriate for others. In all cases, the period of overlapping antipsychotic administration should be minimized.

➤*Poor metabolizers of CYP2D6:* Poor metabolizers of CYP2D6 have higher exposure to iloperidone compared with extensive metabolizers. Laboratory tests are available to identify CYP2D6 poor metabolizers and dosing adjustments should be considered in this group of patients.

➤*Administration:* Iloperidone can be administered without regard to meals.

➤*Storage/Stability:* Store at 25°C (77°F); excursions are permitted between 15° and 30°C (59° and 86°F). Protect from exposure to light and moisture.

ZIPRASIDONE

Rx	**Geodon** (Pfizer)	**Capsules; oral:** 20 mg	As ziprasidone hydrochloride. Lactose. (Pfizer 396). Blue/White. In 60s and UD 80s.
		40 mg	As ziprasidone hydrochloride. Lactose. (Pfizer 397). Blue/Blue. In 60s and UD 80s.
		60 mg	As ziprasidone hydrochloride. Lactose. (Pfizer 398). White. In 60s and UD 80s.
		80 mg	As ziprasidone hydrochloride. Lactose. (Pfizer 399). Blue/White. In 60s and UD 80s.
		Injection, lyophilized powder for solution: 20 mg/mL	As ziprasidone mesylate. In single-use vials.

ZIPRASIDONE HYDROCHLORIDE — ORAL

For complete and comparative prescribing information, refer to the Antipsychotic Agents group monograph.

WARNING

Increased mortality in elderly patients with dementia-related psychosis – Elderly patients with dementia-related psychosis treated with antipsychotic drugs are at an increased risk of death. Analyses of 17 placebo-controlled trials (modal duration of 10 weeks), largely in patients taking atypical antipsychotic drugs, revealed a risk of death in the drug-treated patients between 1.6 and 1.7 times that seen in placebo-treated patients. Over the course of a typical 10-week controlled trial, the rate of death in drug-treated patients was approximately 4.5%, compared with a rate of approximately 2.6% in the placebo group. Although the causes of death were varied, most of the deaths appeared to be either cardiovascular (eg, heart failure, sudden death) or infectious (eg, pneumonia) in nature. Observational studies suggest that, similar to atypical antipsychotic drugs, treatment with conventional antipsychotic drugs may increase mortality. The extent to which the findings of increased mortality in observational studies may be attributed to the antipsychotic drug as opposed to some characteristic(s) of the patients is not clear. Ziprasidone is not approved for the treatment of patients with dementia-related psychosis.

Indications

➤*Bipolar I disorder:* For the treatment of acute manic or mixed episodes associated with bipolar disorder, with or without psychotic features.

For the maintenance treatment of bipolar I disorder as an adjunct to lithium or valproate.

➤*Schizophrenia:* For the treatment of schizophrenia.

➤*Off-label uses:*

Autism – [3] = Safety concerns. The safety and efficacy of ziprasidone in the treatment of autism in children and adolescents have not been clearly established. Strongly consider safety issues, most notably potential for QT prolongation and CYP3A4 drug interactions. (See Administration and Dosage.)

Tourette syndrome – [4] = Insufficient documentation. The use of ziprasidone to treat Tourette syndrome or chronic tic disorder has been primarily studied in a controlled trial enrolling a small number of children and adolescents. Although initial data suggest that this drug may be a useful alternative in patients with refractory tic disorders, larger controlled trials are needed to determine the optimal dosage schedule and to verify results observed in this small trial. (See Administration and Dosage.)

Administration and Dosage

➤*Adults:*

Bipolar I disorder –

Usual dosage: 40 to 80 mg twice daily. In the flexible-dose clinical trials, the daily dose administered was approximately 120 mg.

Initial dosage: 40 mg twice daily. The dose should be increased to 60 or 80 mg twice daily on the second day of treatment and subsequently adjusted on the basis of toleration and efficacy, within the range of 40 to 80 mg twice daily.

Maintenance dosage: Continue treatment at the same dose on which the patient was initially stabilized, within the range of 40 to 80 mg twice daily with food. Periodically reassess patients to determine the need for maintenance treatment.

Schizophrenia –

Usual dosage: 20 to 100 mg twice daily. Generally, an increase to a dosage of more than 80 mg twice daily is not recommended. The safety of dosages above 100 mg twice daily has not been systematically evaluated in clinical trials.

Initial dosage: 20 mg twice daily. In some patients, daily dosage subsequently may be adjusted on the basis of individual clinical status, up to 80 mg twice daily. Dosage adjustments generally should occur at intervals of 2 days or more because steady state is achieved within 1 to 3 days. To ensure use of the lowest effective dose, ordinarily patients should be observed for improvement for several weeks before upward dosage adjustment.

Maintenance dosage: While there is no body of evidence available to answer the question of how long to treat a patient with ziprasidone, a maintenance study in patients who had been symptomatically stable and then randomized to continue ziprasidone or switch to placebo demonstrated a delay in time to relapse for patients receiving ziprasidone. No additional benefit was demonstrated for dosages above 20 mg twice daily. Periodically reassess patients to determine the need for maintenance treatment.

Off-label dosing –

Autism:

• *Initial dosage* – Initial dose of 20 mg nightly, increased by 10 to 20 mg weekly in a twice-daily regimen. Mean final dose was 59.23 mg (range, 20 to 120 mg daily) for a mean of 14.15 weeks (range, 6 to 30 weeks).

Tourette syndrome:

• *Initial dosage* – Initial dosage was 10 mg twice daily, titrated to 30 mg 3 times daily over an 8-week period.

➤*Elderly:* Consider a lower starting dose, slower titration, and careful monitoring during the initial dosing period for some elderly patients.

➤*Administration:* Take with food.

➤*Storage/Stability:* Store at 25°C (77°F); excursions are permitted to 15° to 30°C (59°F to 86°F).

ZIPRASIDONE MESYLATE — INJECTION

For complete and comparative prescribing information, refer to the Antipsychotic Agents group monograph.

WARNING

Increased mortality in elderly patients with dementia-related psychosis – Elderly patients with dementia-related psychosis treated with antipsychotic drugs are at an increased risk of death. Analyses of 17 placebo-controlled trials (modal duration of 10 weeks), largely in patients taking atypical antipsychotic drugs, revealed a risk of death in the drug-treated patients between 1.6 and 1.7 times that seen in placebo-treated patients. Over the course of a typical 10-week controlled trial, the rate of death in drug-treated patients was approximately 4.5%, compared with a rate of approximately 2.6% in the placebo group. Although the causes of death were varied, most of the deaths appeared to be cardiovascular (eg, heart failure, sudden death) or infectious (eg, pneumonia) in nature. Observational studies suggest that, similar to atypical antipsychotic drugs, treatment with conventional antipsychotic drugs may increase mortality. The extent to which the findings of increased mortality in observational studies may be attributed to the antipsychotic drug as opposed to some characteristic(s) of the patients is not clear. Ziprasidone is not approved for the treatment of patients with dementia-related psychosis.

Indications

➤*Acute agitation:* For the treatment of acute agitation in patients with schizophrenia for whom treatment with ziprasidone is appropriate and who need intramuscular (IM) antipsychotic medication for rapid control of the agitation.

Administration and Dosage

➤*General dosing considerations:* If long-term therapy is indicated, ziprasidone oral should replace the IM administration as soon as possible. Because there is no experience regarding the safety of administering ziprasidone IM to patients with schizophrenia who already take oral ziprasidone, coadministration is not recommended.

➤*Adults:*

Acute agitation –

Usual dosage: 10 to 20 mg IM as required. Doses of 10 mg may be administered every 2 hours; doses of 20 mg may be administered every 4 hours, up to a maximum of 40 mg/day.

Maximum dose: 40 mg/day.

Duration of therapy – IM administration of ziprasidone for more than 3 consecutive days has not been studied.

➤*Elderly:* Consider a lower starting dose, slower titration, and careful monitoring during the initial dosing period for some elderly patients.

➤*Renal function impairment:* Because the cyclodextrin excipient is cleared by renal filtration, ziprasidone IM should be administered with caution to patients with renal impairment.

➤*Preparation for administration:* Ziprasidone injection should only be administered IM. Single-dose vials require reconstitution prior to administration; any unused portion should be discarded.

Add sterile water for injection 1.2 mL to the vial and shake vigorously until all of the drug is dissolved. Each mL of reconstituted solution contains ziprasidone 20 mg. To administer a 10 mg dose, draw up 0.5 mL of the reconstituted solution. To administer a 20 mg dose, draw up 1 mL of the reconstituted solution. Because no preservative or bacteriostatic agent is present in this product, aseptic technique must be used in preparation of the final solution.

➤*Admixture compatibility:* This product must not be mixed with other medicinal products or solvents other than sterile water for injection.

➤*Storage/Stability:* Store at 25°C (77°F); excursions are permitted between 15° and 30°C (59° and 86°F) in dry form. Protect from light. Following reconstitution, ziprasidone can be stored, when protected from light, for up to 24 hours at 15° to 30°C (59° to 86°F), or up to 7 days refrigerated (2° to 8°C [36° to 46°F]).

Quinolinone Derivatives

ARIPIPRAZOLE

Rx	Abilify (Otsuka America)	Tablets; oral: 2 mg	Lactose. (A-006 2). Green, rectangular. In 30s.
		5 mg	Lactose. (A-007 5). Blue, rectangular. In 30s and UD 100s.
		10 mg	Lactose. (A-008 10). Pink, rectangular. In 30s and UD 100s.
		15 mg	Lactose. (A-009 15). Yellow, round. In 30s and UD 100s.
		20 mg	Lactose. (A-010 20). White, round. In 30s and UD 100s.
		30 mg	Lactose. (A-011 30). Pink, round. In 30s and UD 100s.
Rx	Abilify Discmelt (Otsuka America)	Tablets, disintegrating; oral: 10 mg	Acesulfame K, aspartame, phenylalanine 1.12 mg, xylitol. (A 640 10). Pink (with scattered specks), round. Vanilla cream flavor. In UD 30s.
		15 mg	Acesulfame K, aspartame, phenylalanine 1.68 mg, xylitol. (A 641 15). Yellow (with scattered specks), round. Vanilla cream flavor. In UD 30s.
Rx	Abilify (Otsuka America)	Solution; oral: 1 mg/mL	Disodium edetate, fructose, glycerin, parabens, propylene glycol, sucrose. Orange cream flavor. In 150 mL bottle.
Rx	Abilify (Otsuka America)	Injection, solution: 7.5 mg/mL	In single-dose vials.

ARIPIPRAZOLE — ORAL

For complete and comparative prescribing information, refer to the Antipsychotic Agents class monograph.

WARNING

Increased mortality in elderly patients with dementia-related psychosis – Elderly patients with dementia-related psychosis treated with antipsychotic drugs are at an increased risk of death. Analyses of 17 placebo-controlled trials (modal duration of 10 weeks), largely in patients taking atypical antipsychotic drugs, revealed a risk of death in drug-treated patients of between 1.6 and 1.7 times the risk of death in placebo-treated patients. Over the course of a typical 10-week controlled trial, the rate of death in drug-treated patients was approximately 4.5%, compared with a rate of approximately 2.6% in the placebo group. Although the causes of death were varied, most of the deaths appeared to be either cardiovascular (eg, heart failure, sudden death) or infectious (eg, pneumonia) in nature. Observational studies suggest that, similar to atypical antipsychotic drugs, treatment with conventional antipsychotic drugs may increase mortality. The extent to which the findings of increased mortality in observational studies may be attributed to the antipsychotic drug as opposed to some characteristic(s) of the patients is not clear. Aripiprazole is not approved for the treatment of patients with dementia-related psychosis.

Suicidality and antidepressant drugs – Antidepressants increased the risk compared with placebo of suicidal thinking and behavior (suicidality) in children, adolescents, and young adults in short-term studies of major depressive disorder and other psychiatric disorders. Anyone considering the use of adjunctive aripiprazole or any other antidepressant in a child, adolescent, or young adult must balance this risk with the clinical need. Short-term studies did not show an increase in the risk of suicidality with antidepressants compared with placebo in adults older than 24 years of age; there was a reduction in risk with antidepressants compared with placebo in adults 65 years of age and older. Depression and certain other psychiatric disorders are themselves associated with increases in the risk of suicide. Appropriately monitor patients of all ages who are started on antidepressant therapy and closely observe them for clinical worsening, suicidality, or unusual changes in behavior. Advise families and caregivers of the need for close observation and communication with the prescriber. Aripiprazole is not approved for use in children with depression.

Indications

➤*Bipolar I disorder:*

Monotherapy – For acute treatment of manic and mixed episodes associated with bipolar I disorder, both as monotherapy and as an adjunct to lithium or valproate.

Maintenance treatment – For the maintenance treatment of bipolar I disorder, both as monotherapy and as an adjunct to either lithium or valproate.

➤*Irritability associated with autistic disorder:* For the treatment of irritability associated with autistic disorder in children.

➤*Major depressive disorder:* For use as an adjunctive treatment to antidepressants for the treatment of major depressive disorder in adults.

➤*Schizophrenia:* For the treatment of schizophrenia.

➤*Off-label uses:*

Cocaine dependence – [4] = Insufficient documentation. Although statistical improvement was demonstrated for some end points related to cocaine dependence, the trials were open-label and conducted in a small number of patients (mostly men), who had concomitant psychiatric illnesses. However, considering the serious nature of cocaine use in this population and the lack of other treatments, aripiprazole may be a reasonable option. Larger, controlled trials are needed to fully evaluate the effectiveness and potential for extrapolation to other patients.

Restless legs syndrome – [4] = Insufficient documentation. Limited available evidence suggests that aripiprazole may be a reasonable alternative in patients with restless legs syndrome.

Tourette syndrome (children/adolescents) – [3] = Safety concerns. Initial data from noncontrolled trials and case reports suggest that aripiprazole may have some benefit in the treatment of Tourette syndrome and other tic disorders in children, adolescents, and adults.

Administration and Dosage

➤*General dosing considerations:* The oral solution can be substituted for tablets on a mg-per-mg basis up to the 25 mg dose level. Patients receiving 30 mg tablets should receive 25 mg of the solution.

The dosing for aripiprazole orally disintegrating tablets is the same as for the oral tablets.

➤*Adults:*

Bipolar disorder –

Initial dosage: 15 mg as monotherapy or 10 to 15 mg as adjunctive therapy with lithium or valproate given once a day. The safety of dosages above 30 mg/day has not been evaluated in clinical trials. The recommended target dosage is 15 mg/day, as monotherapy or as adjunctive therapy with lithium or valproate.

Dosage adjustment: The dosage can be increased to 30 mg/day based on clinical response.

Major depressive disorder –

Initial dosage: 2 to 5 mg/day as adjunctive treatment for patients already taking an antidepressant.

Maintenance dosage: 2 to 15 mg/day.

Dosage adjustment: Dosage adjustments of up to 5 mg/day should occur gradually, at intervals of no less than 1 week.

Schizophrenia –

Initial dosage: 10 or 15 mg/day once daily.

Dosage titration: Dosage increases should not be made before 2 weeks, the time needed to achieve steady state.

Maintenance dosage: 10 to 30 mg/day (tablets); however, dosages higher than 10 or 15 mg/day were not more effective.

Off-label dosing –

Cocaine dependence: [4] = Insufficient documentation. 10 mg once daily orally (initial), titrated to 15 mg once daily for 8 weeks or 15 mg once daily (initial), titrated to 30 mg once daily for 12 weeks. Most patients were maintained at the higher dosages in both studies.

Restless legs syndrome: [4] = Insufficient documentation. Oral doses included 3 to 5 mg daily administered in the morning. In 1 case report, the patient was started on 5 mg every morning and increased to 15 mg/day. No titration schedule was provided.

➤*Children:*

Bipolar disorder –

10 to 17 years of age:

- *Usual dosage* – 10 mg/day as monotherapy, or as adjunctive therapy with lithium or valproate.
- *Initial dosage* – 2 mg/day.
- *Dosage titration* – Titrate to 5 mg/day after 2 days and to the target dosage of 10 mg/day after 2 additional days. Subsequent dosage increases should be administered in 5 mg/day increments.
- *Maintenance dosage* – 10 or 30 mg/day.

It is generally recommended that responding patients be continued beyond the acute response but at the lowest dose needed to maintain remission.

The recommended dose for maintenance treatment, whether as monotherapy or as adjunctive therapy, is the same dose needed to stabilize patients during acute treatment.

Irritability associated with autistic disorder –

6 to 17 years of age:

- *Usual dosage* – 5 to 15 mg/day.
- *Initial dosage* – 2 mg/day.
- *Dosage titration* – The dosage should be increased to 5 mg/day, with subsequent increases to 10 or 15 mg/day if needed.

Dosage adjustments of up to 5 mg/day should occur gradually, at intervals of no less than 1 week.

Quinolinone Derivatives

ARIPIPRAZOLE — ORAL

Schizophrenia –

13 to 17 years of age:

- *Usual dosage* – 10 mg/day.
- *Initial dosage* – 2 mg/day.
- *Dosage titration* – Titrate to 5 mg after 2 days and to the target dose of 10 mg after 2 additional days. Subsequent dose increases should be administered in 5 mg increments.
- *Maintenance dosage* – 10 to 30 mg/day. The 30 mg/day dosage was not shown to be more efficacious than the 10 mg/day dosage.

It is generally recommended that responding patients be continued beyond the acute response but at the lowest dose needed to maintain remission.

Off-label dosing –

Tourette syndrome (children/adolescents): [3] = Safety concerns. Initially, 2.5 to 5 mg daily and titrated based on tolerability (mean, 8 to 10 mg; range, 2.5 to 20 mg).

➤*Concomitant medications:*

Strong CYP3A4 inhibitors – When coadministration of aripiprazole with strong CYP3A4 inhibitors, such as ketoconazole or clarithromycin, is indicated, the aripiprazole dose should be reduced to one-half the usual dose. When the CYP3A4 inhibitor is withdrawn from combination therapy, the aripiprazole dose should then be increased.

Potential CYP2D6 inhibitors – When coadministration of aripiprazole with potential CYP2D6 inhibitors, such as quinidine, fluoxetine, or paroxetine, occurs, the aripiprazole dose should be reduced to at least one-half of the normal dose. When the CYP2D6 inhibitor is withdrawn from combination therapy, the aripiprazole dose should then be increased.

When adjunctive aripiprazole is administered to patients with major depressive disorder, aripiprazole should be administered without dosage adjustment.

Potential CYP3A4 inducers – When a potential CYP3A4 inducer, such as carbamazepine, is added to aripiprazole therapy, the aripiprazole dose should be doubled. Additional dose increases should be based on clinical evaluation. When the CYP3A4 inducer is withdrawn from combination therapy, the aripiprazole dose should be reduced to 10 to 15 mg.

➤*Switching from other antipsychotics:* There are no systematically collected data to specifically address switching patients with schizophrenia from other antipsychotics to aripiprazole or concerning coadministration with other antipsychotics. While immediate discontinuation of the previous antipsychotic treatment may be acceptable for some patients with schizophrenia, more gradual discontinuation may be most appropriate for others. In all cases, the period of overlapping antipsychotic administration should be minimized.

➤*Duration of therapy:* Patients should be periodically reassessed to determine the need for maintenance therapy.

➤*Administration:* Aripiprazole may be administered with or without food.

Orally disintegrating tablets – Do not open the blister until ready to administer. For single tablet removal, open the package and peel back the foil on the blister to expose the tablet. Do not push the tablet through the foil because this could damage the tablet. Immediately upon opening the blister, remove the tablet using dry hands and place the entire orally disintegrating tablet on the tongue. Tablet disintegration occurs rapidly in saliva. It is recommended that the orally disintegrating tablet be taken without liquid; however, if needed, it can be taken with liquid. Do not attempt to split the tablet.

➤*Storage/Stability:* Store at 25°C (77°F); excursions are permitted between 15° and 30°C (59° and 86°F). Open bottles of oral solution can be used for up to 6 months after opening.

ARIPIPRAZOLE — INJECTION

For complete and comparative prescribing information, refer to the Antipsychotic Agents class monograph.

WARNING

Increased mortality in elderly patients with dementia-related psychosis – Elderly patients with dementia-related psychosis treated with antipsychotic drugs are at an increased risk of death. Analyses of 17 placebo-controlled trials (modal duration of 10 weeks), largely in patients taking atypical antipsychotic drugs, revealed a risk of death in drug-treated patients of between 1.6 and 1.7 times the risk of death in placebo-treated patients. Over the course of a typical 10-week controlled trial, the rate of death in drug-treated patients was approximately 4.5%, compared with a rate of approximately 2.6% in the placebo group. Although the causes of death were varied, most of the deaths appeared to be either cardiovascular (eg, heart failure, sudden death) or infectious (eg, pneumonia) in nature. Observational studies suggest that, similar to atypical antipsychotic drugs, treatment with conventional antipsychotic drugs may increase mortality. The extent to which the findings of increased mortality in observational studies may be attributed to the antipsychotic drug as opposed to some characteristic(s) of the patients is not clear. Aripiprazole is not approved for the treatment of patients with dementia-related psychosis.

Suicidality and antidepressant drugs – Antidepressants increased the risk compared with placebo of suicidal thinking and behavior (suicidality) in children, adolescents, and young adults in short-term studies of major depressive disorder and other psychiatric disorders. Anyone considering the use of adjunctive aripiprazole or any other antidepressant in a child, adolescent, or young adult must balance this risk with the clinical need. Short-term studies did not show an increase in the risk of suicidality with antidepressants compared with placebo in adults older than 24 years of age; there was a reduction in risk with antidepressants compared with placebo in adults 65 years of age and older. Depression and certain other psychiatric disorders are themselves associated with increases in the risk of suicide. Appropriately monitor patients of all ages who are started on antidepressant therapy and closely observe them for clinical worsening, suicidality, or unusual changes in behavior. Families and caregivers should be advised of the need for close observation and communication with the prescriber. Aripiprazole is not approved for use in children with depression.

Indications

➤*Agitation associated with schizophrenia or bipolar mania:* For the acute treatment of agitation associated with schizophrenia or bipolar disorder, manic or mixed in adults.

Administration and Dosage

➤*Adults:*

Agitation associated with schizophrenia or bipolar mania –

Usual dosage: 9.75 mg intramuscularly (IM). A lower dose of 5.25 mg IM may be considered when clinical factors warrant. If agitation warranting a second dose persists following the initial dose, cumulative doses up to a total of 30 mg/day may be given.

Maximum dose: 30 mg IM per day.

Concomitant therapy:

- *Strong CYP3A4 inhibitors* – When coadministration of aripiprazole with strong CYP3A4 inhibitors such as ketoconazole or clarithromycin is indicated, the aripiprazole dose should be reduced to one-half of the usual dose. When the CYP3A4 inhibitor is withdrawn from combination therapy, the aripiprazole dose should then be increased.
- *Potential CYP2D6 inhibitors* – When coadministration of potential CYP2D6 inhibitors such as quinidine, fluoxetine, or paroxetine with aripiprazole occurs, the aripiprazole dose should be reduced to at least one-half of its normal dose. When the CYP2D6 inhibitor is withdrawn from combination therapy, the aripiprazole dose should then be increased.

When adjunctive aripiprazole is administered to patients with major depressive disorder, aripiprazole should be administered without dosage adjustment.

- *Potential CYP3A4 inducers* – When a potential CYP3A4 inducer such as carbamazepine is added to aripiprazole therapy, the aripiprazole dose should be doubled. Additional dose increases should be based on clinical evaluation. When the CYP3A4 inducer is withdrawn from combination therapy, the aripiprazole dose should be reduced to 10 to 15 mg.

Conversion: If ongoing aripiprazole therapy is clinically indicated, oral aripiprazole in a range of 10 to 30 mg/day should replace aripiprazole injection as soon as possible.

➤*Preparation for administration:* To administer aripiprazole, draw up the required volume of solution into the syringe (5.25 mg = 0.7 mL, 9.75 mg = 1.3 mL, 15 mg = 2 mL).

➤*Administration:* For IM use only. Do not administer intravenously (IV) or subcutaneously. Inject slowly, deep into the muscle mass.

➤*Storage/Stability:* Store at 25°C (77°F); excursions are permitted to between 15° and 30°C (59° and 86°F). Protect from light. Retain in carton until time of use. Discard any unused portion.

Benzoisothiazol Derivatives

LURASIDONE HYDROCHLORIDE

Rx	**Latuda** (Sunovion)	**Tablets; oral:** 40 mg	Mannitol. (L40). White to off-white, round. In 30s, 90s, 500s, and UD 70s and 100s.
		80 mg	Mannitol. (L80). Pale green, oval. In 30s, 90s, 500s, and UD 70s and 100s.

Benzoisothiazol Derivatives

LURASIDONE HYDROCHLORIDE — ORAL

For complete and comparative prescribing information, refer to the Antipsychotic Agents class monograph.

WARNING

Increased mortality in elderly patients with dementia-related psychosis – Elderly patients with dementia-related psychosis treated with antipsychotic drugs are at an increased risk of death. Analyses of 17 placebo-controlled trials (modal duration of 10 weeks), largely in patients taking atypical antipsychotic drugs, revealed a risk of death in drug-treated patients of between 1.6 to 1.7 times the risk of death in placebo-treated patients. Over the course of a typical 10-week controlled trial, the rate of death in drug-treated patients was approximately 4.5%, compared with a rate of approximately 2.6% in the placebo group. Although the causes of death were varied, most of the deaths appeared to be either cardiovascular (eg, heart failure, sudden death) or infectious (eg, pneumonia) in nature. Observational studies suggest that, similar to atypical antipsychotic drugs, treatment with conventional antipsychotic drugs may increase mortality. The extent to which the findings of increased mortality in observational studies may be attributed to the antipsychotic drug as opposed to some characteristic(s) of the patients is not clear. Lurasidone is not approved for the treatment of patients with dementia-related psychosis.

Indications

➤*Schizophrenia:* For the treatment of patients with schizophrenia.

Administration and Dosage

➤*Adults:*

Schizophrenia –

Usual dosage: 40 to 80 mg/day.

Maximum dose: 80 mg/day.

Initial dosage: 40 mg once daily.

Concomitant therapy:

• *Cytochrome P450 3A4 inhibitors* – When coadministration with a moderate cytochrome P450 3A4 (CYP3A4) inhibitor such as diltiazem is considered, the dosage should not exceed 40 mg/day. Do not use in combination with a strong CYP3A4 inhibitor (eg, ketoconazole).

• *CYP3A4 inducers* – Do not use in combination with a strong CYP3A4 inducer (eg, rifampin).

➤*Renal function impairment:*

Moderate to severe renal impairment – Do not exceed 40 mg/day.

➤*Hepatic function impairment:*

Moderate to severe hepatic impairment – Do not exceed 40 mg/day.

➤*Administration:* Take with food (at least 350 calories).

➤*Storage/Stability:* Store at 25°C (77°F); excursions are permitted between 15° and 30°C (59° and 86°F).

ANTIPSYCHOTIC AGENTS

LITHIUM

Rx	**Lithium Carbonate** (Various, eg, Harber, International Labs, Roxane)	**Tablets; oral:** 300 mg lithium carbonate (8.12 mEq lithium)	In 100s, 1,000s, and UD 100s.
Rx	**Lithium Carbonate** (Various, eg, Roxane)	**Tablets, extended-release; oral:** 300 mg lithium carbonate (8.12 mEq lithium)	In 100s and 500s.
Rx	**Lithobid** (Noven Therapeutics)		(Lithobid 300). Peach. Film coated. In 100s.
Rx	**Lithium Carbonate** (Roxane)	**Tablets, extended-release; oral:** 450 mg lithium carbonate	In 100s.
Rx	**Lithium Carbonate** (Roxane)	**Capsules; oral:** 150 mg lithium carbonate (4.06 mEq lithium)	(54 213). White. In 100s, 1,000s, and UD 100s.
Rx	**Lithium Carbonate** (Various, eg, Dixon-Shane, Geneva, Goldline, Moore, Roxane)	**Capsules; oral:** 300 mg lithium carbonate (8.12 mEq lithium)	In 100s, 500s, 1,000s, and UD 100s.
Rx	**Lithium Carbonate** (Roxane)	**Capsules; oral:** 600 mg lithium carbonate (16.24 mEq lithium)	(54 702). White and flesh. In 100s, 1,000s, and UD 100s.
Rx	**Lithium Citrate** (Various, eg, Geneva, Major, PBI, Roxane)	**Syrup; oral:** 8 mEq lithium (as citrate equivalent to 300 mg lithium carbonate) per 5 mL	In 480 and 500 mL and UD 5 and 10 mL.

LITHIUM CARBONATE — ORAL

Complete prescribing information begins in the Antipsychotic Agents group monograph.

WARNING

Lithium toxicity is closely related to serum lithium levels, and can occur at doses close to therapeutic levels. Facilities for prompt and accurate serum lithium determinations should be available before initiating therapy.

Indications

➤*Bipolar disorder:* Lithium is indicated in the treatment of manic episodes of manic-depressive illness.

Typical symptoms of mania include pressure of speech, motor hyperactivity, reduced need for sleep, flight of ideas, grandiosity, elation, poor judgment, aggressiveness, and possibly hostility. When given to a patient experiencing a manic episode, lithium may produce a normalization of symptomatology within 1 to 3 weeks.

➤*Off-label uses:*

Borderline personality disorder – [1] = Good documentation. Lithium has a narrow margin of safety overdose, requires blood level monitoring, and poses a risk of hypothyroidism with long-term use. Nevertheless, it is recommended in national guidelines as a second-line or adjunctive treatment of borderline personality disorder associated with symptoms of either affective dysregulation or impulsive-behavioral control. The mainstay of treatment is psychotherapy, but medications may be appropriate for either acute exacerbations of disease or long-term management of selected symptoms.

Traumatic brain injury – [3] = Safety concerns. Lithium is approved by the Food and Drug Administration for the management of manic episodes of bipolar disorder. Patients with traumatic brain injury (TBI), however, are more likely to be refractory to standard therapies for psychiatric indications. The Neurobehavioral Guidelines Working Group concluded that there was insufficient experience specifically in patients with TBI to support or refute use of lithium for bipolar disorder or mania following TBI. Nevertheless, standard treatments such as lithium were recommended for a trial first in patients with TBI-associated mania or bipolar disorder. Thus, lithium therapy may be useful for patients with concurrent mania or bipolar disorder and aggression after TBI.

Given that lithium was assigned the lowest level of recommendation, classification as an option rather than a standard or guideline, patients started on therapy should be closely monitored for response, and therapy should be continued only in those patients with sufficient benefit to outweigh the risks of therapy.

Other possible off-label uses – Lithium carbonate (300 to 1000 mg/day) has improved the neutrophil count in patients with cancer chemotherapy-induced neutropenia, in children with chronic neutropenia, and in AIDS patients receiving zidovudine.

Lithium has also been used successfully in the prophylaxis of cluster headache; premenstrual tension; bulimia; alcoholism (especially if patient has a concomitant affective disorder such as depression); syndrome of inappropriate secretion of antidiuretic hormone (ADH); tardive dyskinesia; hyperthyroidism; postpartum affective psychosis; corticosteroid-induced psychosis.

A topical lithium succinate preparation has been studied in the treatment of seborrheic dermatitis and genital herpes.

Administration and Dosage

➤*General dosing considerations:* Individualize dosage according to both serum levels and clinical response. Do not rely on serum levels alone.

➤*Adults:*

Bipolar disorder –

Usual dosage: Optimal patient response for acute mania is usually established and maintained with 600 mg 3 times daily or 900 mg twice/day for the slow-release form. Such doses normally produce an effective serum lithium level ranging between 1 and 1.5 mEq/L.

Maintenance dosage: For long-term control, the dosage will vary, but 900 to 1,200 mg daily in divided doses will usually maintain desired serum levels between 0.6 to 1.2 mEq/L.

Maintenance therapy reduces the frequency of manic episodes and diminishes the intensity of those episodes which may occur.

Off-label dosing –

Borderline personality disorder: [1] = Good documentation. 900 to 2,400 mg/day in 3 to 4 divided doses or 900 to 1,800 mg/day (sustained-release) in 2 divided doses, titrated to maintain serum levels of 0.8 to 1 mEq/L. Pharmacotherapy may be limited to short-term treatment during periods of acute decompensation or may continue indefinitely for long-term treatment of trait vulnerabilities.

Traumatic brain injury: [3] = Safety concerns. 900 mg per day orally, titrated to achieve therapeutic serum levels. The optimal duration of

LITHIUM CARBONATE — ORAL

therapy has not been established; however, long-term administration may be required for symptom control.

A behavioral response to lithium was observed at serum levels of 0.48 to 1.4 mEq/L. Careful monitoring of cognitive status was recommended during lithium use for management of post-TBI aggression.

➤*Children:* See Adults for dosing in children 12 years of age and older.

Off-label dosing –

Bipolar disorder:

• *Adolescents –*

Usual dosage: 600 to 1,800 mg/day orally administered in 3 to 4 divided doses. Administer extended-release formulations in 2 divided doses.

• *Children –*

Initial dosage: 15 to 60 mg/kg/day orally administered in 3 to 4 divided doses.

Dosage adjustment: Adjust weekly as needed to achieve therapeutic levels.

➤*Therapeutic drug monitoring:*

Serum lithium levels – Draw blood samples immediately prior to the next dose (8 to 12 hours after the previous dose) when lithium concentrations are relatively stable. Do not rely on serum levels alone.

Usual dosage: Determine serum levels twice weekly during the acute phase and until the serum level and clinical condition of the patient have been stabilized.

Maintenance dosage: Monitor serum levels in uncomplicated cases on maintenance therapy during remission at least every 2 months.

➤*Administration:* Immediate-release products are usually given 3 or 4 times daily. Extended-release products are usually given twice daily (12-hour intervals).

Swallow extended/controlled-release tablets whole; do not chew or crush.

➤*Storage/Stability:* Store at 25°C (77°F); excursions permitted between 15° to 30°C (59° to 86°F). Protect from moisture.

Actions

➤*Pharmacology:* Preclinical studies have shown that lithium alters sodium transport in nerve and muscle cells and effects a shift toward intraneuronal metabolism of catecholamines, but the specific biochemical mechanism of lithium action in mania is unknown.

➤*Pharmacokinetics:* The distribution space of lithium approximates that of total body water. Lithium is primarily excreted in urine with insignificant excretion in feces. Renal excretion of lithium is proportional to its plasma concentration. The half-life of elimination of lithium is approximately 24 hours. Lithium decreases sodium reabsorption by the renal tubules which could lead to sodium depletion. Therefore, it is essential for the patient to maintain a normal diet, including salt, and an adequate fluid intake (2500 to 3000 mL) at least during the initial stabilization period. Decreased tolerance to lithium has been reported to ensue from protracted sweating or diarrhea and, if such occur, supplemental fluid and salt should be administered under careful medical supervision and lithium intake reduced or suspended until the condition is resolved.

Contraindications

Lithium should generally not be given to patients with significant renal or cardiovascular disease, severe debilitation or dehydration, or sodium depletion, and to patients receiving diuretics or angiotensin-converting enzyme (ACE) inhibitors, since the risk of lithium toxicity is very high in such patients. If the psychiatric indication is life-threatening, and if such a patient fails to respond to other measures, lithium treatment may be undertaken with extreme caution, including daily serum lithium determinations and adjustment to the usually low doses ordinarily tolerated by these individuals. In such instances, hospitalization is a necessity.

Warnings/Precautions

➤*Toxicity:* Lithium toxicity is closely related to serum lithium levels, and can occur at doses close to therapeutic levels. The desirable serum lithium levels are 0.6 to 1.2 mEq/L. Patients abnormally sensitive to lithium may exhibit toxic signs at serum levels of 1 to 1.5 mEq/L.

Outpatients and their families should be warned that the patient must discontinue lithium therapy and contact his physician if such clinical signs of lithium toxicity as diarrhea, vomiting, tremor, mild ataxia, drowsiness, or muscular weakness occur.

➤*Renal function impairment:* Chronic lithium therapy may be associated with diminution of renal concentrating ability, occasionally presenting as nephrogenic diabetes insipidus, with polyuria and polydipsia. Such patients should be carefully managed to avoid dehydration with resulting lithium retention and toxicity. This condition is usually reversible when lithium is discontinued.

Morphologic changes with glomerular and interstitial fibrosis and nephron-atrophy have been reported in patients on chronic lithium therapy. Morphologic changes have also been seen in bipolar patients never exposed to lithium. The relationship between renal functional and morphologic changes and their association with lithium therapy has not been established. To date, lithium in therapeutic doses has not been reported to cause end-stage renal disease.

When kidney function is assessed, for baseline data prior to starting lithium therapy or thereafter, routine urinalysis and other tests may be used to evaluate tubular function (eg, urine specific gravity or osmolality following a period of water deprivation, or 24-hour urine volume) and glomerular function (eg, serum creatinine or creatinine clearance). During lithium therapy, progressive or sudden changes in renal function, even within the normal range, indicate the need for reevaluation of treatment.

➤*Special risk:* Lithium should generally not be given to patients with significant renal or cardiovascular disease, severe debilitation, dehydration, sodium depletion, and to patients receiving diuretics, or ACE inhibitors, since the risk of lithium toxicity is very high in such patients. If the psychiatric indication is life threatening, and if such a patient fails to respond to other measures, lithium treatment may be undertaken with extreme caution, including daily serum lithium determinations and adjustment to the usually low doses ordinarily tolerated by these individuals. In such instances, hospitalization is a necessity.

In addition to sweating and diarrhea, concomitant infection with elevated temperatures may also necessitate a temporary reduction or cessation of medication.

The ability to tolerate lithium is greater during the acute manic phase and decreases when manic symptoms subside.

➤*Hazardous tasks:* Lithium may impair mental or physical abilities. Caution patients about activities requiring alertness (eg, operating vehicles or machinery).

➤*Pregnancy:* *Category D.* In humans, lithium may cause fetal harm when administered to a pregnant woman. There have been reports of lithium having adverse effects on nidations in rats, embryo viability in mice, and metabolism in vitro of rat testis and human spermatozoa have been attributed to lithium, as have teratogenicity in submammalian species, and cleft palate in mice. Studies in rats, rabbits and monkeys have shown no evidence of lithium-induced teratology. Data from lithium birth registries suggest an increase in cardiac and other anomalies, especially Ebstein's anomaly. If the patient becomes pregnant while taking lithium, she should be apprised of the potential risk to the fetus. If possible, lithium should be withdrawn for at least the first trimester unless it is determined that this would seriously endanger the mother.

➤*Lactation:* Lithium is excreted in human milk. Nursing should not be undertaken during lithium therapy except in rare and unusual circumstances where, in the view of the physician, the potential benefits to the mother outweigh possible hazards to the child. Signs and symptoms of lithium toxicity such as hypertonia, hypothermia, cyanosis and ECG changes have been reported in some infants and neonates.

➤*Children:* Since information regarding the safety and effectiveness of lithium in children under 12 years of age is not available, its use in such patients is not recommended at this time.

There has been a report of a transient syndrome of acute dystonia and hyperreflexia occurring in a 15 kg child who ingested 300 mg of lithium carbonate.

➤*Elderly:* Elderly patients often require lower lithium dosages to achieve therapeutic serum levels. They may also exhibit adverse reactions at serum levels ordinarily tolerated by younger patients.

In general, dose selection for an elderly patient should be cautious, usually starting at the low end of the dosing range, reflecting the greater frequency of decreased hepatic, renal, or cardiac function, and of concomitant disease or other therapy.

➤*Monitoring:* Previously existing underlying thyroid disorders do not necessarily constitute a contraindication to lithium treatment; where hypothyroidism exists, careful monitoring of thyroid function during lithium stabilization and maintenance allows for correction of changing thyroid parameters, if any. Where hypothyroidism occurs during lithium stabilization and maintenance, supplemental thyroid treatment may be used.

Lithium levels should be closely monitored when patients initiate or discontinue NSAID use. In some cases, lithium toxicity has resulted from interactions between an NSAID and lithium.

Kidney function should be assessed prior to and during lithium therapy. Routine urinalysis and other tests may be used to evaluate tubular function (eg, urine specific gravity or osmolality following a period of water deprivation, or 24-hour urine volume) and glomerular function (eg, serum creatinine or creatinine clearance). During lithium therapy, progressive or sudden changes in renal function, even within the normal range, indicate the need for reevaluation of treatment.

Drug Interactions

➤*QT prolongation:* An additive effect of lithium with other drugs that prolong the QT interval cannot be excluded. The following drugs may prolong the QT interval and increase the risk of life-threatening cardiac arrhythmias, including torsades de pointes: Antiarrhythmic agents (eg, amiodarone, bretylium, disopyramide, dofetilide, procainamide, quinidine, and sotalol), arsenic trioxide, chlorpromazine, cisapride, dolasetron, droperidol, mefloquine, mesoridazine, moxifloxacin, pentamidine, pimozide, tacrolimus, thioridazine, and ziprasidone. For a more complete list of drugs that may prolong the QT interval, see the appendix, Drug-Induced Prolongation of the QT Interval and Torsades de Pointes.

LITHIUM CARBONATE — ORAL

Lithium Drug Interactions			
Precipitant drug	Object drug[a]		Description
Acetazolamide	Lithium	↓	Increased renal excretion of lithium.
Carbamazepine	Lithium	↑	Increased neurotoxic effects despite therapeutic serum levels and normal dosage range.
Fluoxetine	Lithium	↓↑	Increased lithium serum levels; mechanism unknown.
Haloperidol	Lithium	↑	Increased or decreased neurotoxic effects despite therapeutic serum levels and normal dosage range.
Loop diuretics	Lithium	↑	Increased lithium serum levels; mechanism unknown.
Methyldopa	Lithium	↑	Increased neurotoxic effects with or without increased lithium serum levels.
NSAIDs	Lithium	↑	Decreased renal clearance of lithium possibly caused by inhibition of renal prostaglandin synthesis.
Osmotic diuretics (urea)	Lithium	↓	Increased renal excretion of lithium.
Theophyllines	Lithium	↓	Increased renal excretion of lithium.
Thiazide diuretics	Lithium	↑	Increased lithium serum levels caused by decreased renal lithium clearance.
Urinary alkalinizers	Lithium	↓	Enhanced renal lithium clearance.
Verapamil	Lithium	↔	Both a reduction in lithium levels and lithium toxicity have occurred.
Lithium	Iodide salts	↑	Synergistic action to more readily produce hypothyroidism.
Lithium	Neuromuscular blocking agents	↑	Neuromuscular blocking effects may be increased; profound and severe respiratory depression may occur.
Lithium	Phenothiazines	↔	Neurotoxicity, decreased phenothiazine concentrations or increased lithium concentrations may occur.
Lithium	Sympathomimetics	↓	The pressor sensitivity of the sympathomimetic may be decreased.
Lithium	Tricyclic antidepressants	↑	Pharmacologic effects of the tricyclic may be increased.

[a] ↑ = Object drug increased. ↓ = Object drug decreased. ↔ = Undetermined clinical effect.

The following drugs can lower serum lithium concentrations by increasing urinary lithium excretion: Acetazolamide, urea, xanthine preparations and alkalinizing agents such as sodium bicarbonate.

The following have also been shown to interact with lithium: Methyldopa and phenytoin.

➤*Antipsychotic medication:* The possibility of similar adverse interactions with other antipsychotic medication exists.

➤*Calcium channel blocking agents:* Concurrent use of calcium channel blocking agents with lithium may increase the risk of neurotoxicity in the form of ataxia, tremors, nausea, vomiting, diarrhea or tinnitus. Caution is recommended.

➤*Diuretics or angiotensin-converting enzyme (ACE) inhibitors:* In general, the concomitant use of diuretics or angiotensin-converting enzyme (ACE) inhibitors with lithium carbonate should be avoided. In those cases where concomitant use is necessary, extreme caution is advised since sodium loss from these drugs may reduce the renal clearance of lithium resulting in increased serum lithium concentrations with the risk of lithium toxicity.

There is evidence that ACE inhibitors, such as enalapril and captopril, and angiotensin II receptor antagonists, such as losartan, may substantially increase steady-state plasma lithium levels, sometimes resulting in lithium toxicity. When such combinations are used, the lithium dosage may need to be decreased, and more frequent monitoring of lithium serum concentrations is recommended.

➤*Neuroleptics:* An encephalopathic syndrome (characterized by weakness, lethargy, fever, tremulousness and confusion, extrapyramidal symptoms, leucocytosis, elevated serum enzymes, BUN and FBS) followed by irreversible brain damage has occurred in a few patients treated with lithium plus a neuroleptic, most notably haloperidol. Because of a possible causal relationship between these events and the concomitant administration of lithium and neuroleptic drugs, patients receiving such combined therapy or patients with organic brain syndrome or other CNS impairment should be monitored closely for early evidence of neurological toxicity and treatment discontinued promptly if such signs appear. This encephalopathic syndrome may be similar to or the same as neuroleptic malignant syndrome (NMS).

➤*Metronidazole:* Concurrent use of metronidazole with lithium may provoke lithium toxicity due to reduced renal clearance. Patients receiving such combined therapy should be monitored closely.

➤*Selective serotonin reuptake inhibitors:* The concomitant administration of lithium with selective serotonin reuptake inhibitors (SSRIs) should be undertaken with caution as this combination has been reported to result in symptoms such as diarrhea, confusion, tremor, dizziness, and agitation.

Adverse Reactions

➤*Lithium toxicity:* The likelihood of toxicity increases with increasing serum lithium levels. Serum lithium levels greater than 1.5 mEq/L carry a greater risk than lower levels. However, patients sensitive to lithium may exhibit toxic signs at serum levels below 1.5 mEq/L.

Diarrhea, vomiting, drowsiness, muscular weakness and lack of coordination may be early signs of lithium toxicity, and can occur at lithium levels below 2 mEq/L. At higher levels, giddiness, ataxia, blurred vision, tinnitus and a large output of dilute urine may be seen. Serum lithium levels above 3 mEq/L may produce a complex clinical picture involving multiple organs and organ systems. Serum lithium levels should not be permitted to exceed 2 mEq/L during the acute treatment phase.

Fine hand tremor, polyuria and mild thirst may occur during initial therapy for the acute manic phase, and may persist throughout treatment. Transient and mild nausea and general discomfort may also appear during the first few days of lithium administration.

These side effects are an inconvenience rather than a disabling condition, and usually subside with continued treatment or a temporary reduction or cessation of dosage. If persistent, a cessation of dosage is indicated.

➤*Adverse reactions directly related to serum lithium levels:* The following adverse reactions have been reported and appear to be directly related to serum lithium levels, including concentrations within the therapeutic range.

Cardiovascular – Cardiac arrhythmia, hypotension, peripheral circulatory collapse, bradycardia, sinus node dysfunction with severe bradycardia (which may result in syncope).

EKG changes: Reversible flattening, isoelectricity or inversion of T-waves.

CNS – Blackout spells, epileptiform seizures, slurred speech, dizziness, vertigo, incontinence of urine or feces, somnolence, psychomotor retardation, restlessness, confusion, stupor, coma, acute dystonia, downbeat nystagmus, tongue movements, tics, tinnitus, hallucinations, poor memory, slowed intellectual functioning, startled response, worsening of organic brain syndromes, myasthenia gravis (rarely).

Cases of pseudotumor cerebri (increased intracranial pressure and papilledema) have been reported with lithium use. If undetected, this condition may result in enlargement of the blind spot, constriction of visual fields and eventual blindness due to optic atrophy. Lithium should be discontinued, if clinically possible, if this syndrome occurs.

Autonomic nervous system: Blurred vision, dry mouth, impotence/sexual dysfunction.

EEG changes: Diffuse slowing, widening of frequency spectrum, potentiation and disorganization of background rhythm.

Dermatologic – Drying and thinning of hair, anesthesia of skin, acne, chronic folliculitis, xerosis cutis, alopecia and exacerbation of psoriasis, generalized pruritus with or without rash, angioedema, cutaneous ulcers.

Endocrine – Euthyroid goiter or hypothyroidism (including myxedema) accompanied by lower T_3 and T_4. ^{131}Iodine uptake may be elevated. Paradoxically, rare cases of hyperthyroidism have been reported.

GI – Anorexia, nausea, vomiting, diarrhea, gastritis, salivary gland swelling, abdominal pain, excessive salivation, flatulence, indigestion.

GU – Albuminuria, oliguria, polyuria, glycosuria, decreased creatinine clearance, symptoms of nephrogenic diabetes insipidus including polyuria, thirst and polydipsia.

Musculoskeletal – Tremor, muscle hyperirritability (fasciculations, twitching, clonic movements of whole limbs), ataxia, hypertonicity, choreoathetotic movements, hyperactive deep tendon reflexes, extrapyramidal symptoms including acute dystonia, cogwheel rigidity.

Miscellaneous – Fatigue, lethargy, transient scotomata, dehydration, weight loss, tendency to sleep.

Miscellaneous reactions unrelated to dosage are: Transient electroencephalographic and electrocardiographic changes, leucocytosis, headache, diffuse nontoxic goiter with or without hypothyroidism, transient hyperglycemia, excessive weight gain, edematous swelling of ankles or wrists, and metallic taste.

Exophthalmos, hypercalcemia, hyperparathyroidism, dysgeusia/taste distortion, salty taste, swollen lips, tightness in chest, swollen or painful joints, fever, polyarthralgia, dental caries.

A few reports have been received of the development of painful discoloration of fingers and toes and coldness of the extremities within 1 day of the starting of treatment of lithium. The mechanism through which these symptoms (resembling Raynaud's syndrome) developed is not known. Recovery followed discontinuance.

LITHIUM CARBONATE — ORAL

Some reports of nephrogenic diabetes insipidus, hyperparathyroidism, and hypothyroidism which persist after lithium discontinuation have been received.

Overdosage

➤*Symptoms:* The toxic concentrations for lithium (greater than or equal to 1.5 mEq/L) are close to the therapeutic concentrations (0.6 to 1.2 mEq/L). It is therefore important that patients and their families be cautioned to watch for early symptoms and to discontinue the drug and inform the physician should they occur. Diarrhea, vomiting, drowsiness, muscular weakness, and lack of coordination may be early signs of lithium toxicity, and can occur at lithium levels below 2 mEq/L. At higher levels, giddiness, ataxia, blurred vision, tinnitus, and a large output of dilute urine may be seen. Serum lithium levels above 3 mEq/L may produce a complex clinical picture involving multiple organs and organ systems. Serum lithium levels should not be permitted to exceed 2 mEq/L during the acute treatment phase.

➤*Treatment:* No specific antidote for lithium poisoning is known. Treatment is supportive. Early symptoms of lithium toxicity can usually be treated by reduction of cessation of dosage of the drug and resumption of the treatment at a lower dose after 24 to 48 hours. In severe cases of lithium poisoning, the first and foremost goal of treatment consists of elimination of this ion from the patient.

Treatment is essentially the same as that used in barbiturate poisoning:

1.) Gastric lavage.
2.) Correction of fluid and electrolyte imbalance.
3.) Regulation of kidney functioning.

Urea, mannitol, and aminophylline all produce significant increases in lithium excretion. Hemodialysis is an effective and rapid means of removing the ion from the severely toxic patient. However, patient recovery may be slow. Infection prophylaxis, regular chest x-rays, and preservation of adequate respiration are essential.

Patient Information

Outpatients and their families should be warned that the patient must discontinue lithium therapy and contact his physician if such clinical signs of lithium toxicity as diarrhea, vomiting, tremor, mild ataxia, drowsiness, or muscular weakness occur.

Lithium may impair mental or physical abilities. Caution patients about activities requiring alertness (eg, operating vehicles or machinery).

Take immediately after meals or with food or milk to avoid stomach upset.

Drink 8 to 12 glasses of water or other liquid every day while on this drug. Prolonged exposure to the sun can lead to dehydration. Maintain a regular diet (including salt). Contact a physician if fever or diarrhea develops.

LITHIUM CITRATE — ORAL

Complete prescribing information begins in the Antipsychotic Agents group monograph.

WARNING

Lithium toxicity is closely related to serum lithium levels, and can occur at doses close to therapeutic levels. Facilities for prompt and accurate serum lithium determinations should be available before initiating therapy.

Indications

➤*Bipolar disorder:* Lithium is indicated in the treatment of manic episodes of bipolar disorder.

Maintenance therapy reduces the frequency of manic episodes and diminishes the intensity of those episodes which may occur.

Typical symptoms of mania include pressure of speech, motor hyperactivity, reduced need for sleep, flight of ideas, grandiosity, elation, poor judgment, aggressiveness, and possibly hostility. When given to a patient experiencing a manic episode, lithium may produce a normalization of symptomatology within 1 to 3 weeks.

➤*Off-label uses:*

Borderline personality disorder – [1] = Good documentation. Lithium has a narrow margin of safety overdose, requires blood level monitoring, and poses a risk of hypothyroidism with long-term use. Nevertheless, it is recommended in national guidelines as a second-line or adjunctive treatment of borderline personality disorder associated with symptoms of either affective dysregulation or impulsive-behavioral control. The mainstay of treatment is psychotherapy, but medications may be appropriate for either acute exacerbations of disease or long-term management of selected symptoms.

Traumatic brain injury – [3] = Safety concerns. Lithium is approved by the Food and Drug Administration for the management of manic episodes of bipolar disorder. Patients with traumatic brain injury (TBI), however, are more likely to be refractory to standard therapies for psychiatric indications. The Neurobehavioral Guidelines Working Group concluded that there was insufficient experience specifically in patients with TBI to support or refute use of lithium for bipolar disorder or mania following TBI. Nevertheless, standard treatments such as lithium were recommended for a trial first in patients with TBI-associated mania or bipolar disorder. Thus, lithium therapy may be useful for patients with concurrent mania or bipolar disorder and aggression after TBI.

Given that lithium was assigned the lowest level of recommendation, classification as an option rather than a standard or guideline, patients started on therapy should be closely monitored for response, and therapy should be continued only in those patients with sufficient benefit to outweigh the risks of therapy.

Administration and Dosage

➤*General dosing considerations:* Dosage must be individualized according to serum levels and clinical response. Regular monitoring of the patient's clinical state and of serum lithium levels is necessary.

Patients abnormally sensitive to lithium may exhibit toxic signs at serum levels of 1 to 1.5 mEq/L.

Each lithium citrate 5 mL syrup contains lithium ion 8 mEq, equivalent to the amount of lithium in lithium carbonate 300 mg.

➤*Adults:*

Bipolar disorder –

Initial dosage: 10 mL (lithium 16 mEq) 3 times daily for the treatment of acute mania. Such doses will normally produce an effective serum lithium level ranging between 1 and 1.5 mEq/L. Dosage must be individualized according to serum levels and clinical response. (See Therapeutic Drug Monitoring).

Maintenance dosage: The desirable serum lithium levels are 0.6 to 1.2 mEq/L. Dosage will vary from one individual to another, but usually 5 mL (lithium 8 mEq) 3 or 4 times daily will maintain this level. (See Therapeutic Drug Monitoring).

Off-label dosing –

Borderline personality disorder: [1] = Good documentation. The following dosages are based on lithium carbonate: 900 to 2,400 mg/day in 3 to 4 divided doses or 900 to 1,800 mg/day (sustained-release) in 2 divided doses, titrated to maintain serum levels of 0.8 to 1 mEq/L. Pharmacotherapy may be limited to short-term treatment during periods of acute decompensation or may continue indefinitely for long-term treatment of trait vulnerabilities.

Traumatic brain injury: [3] = Safety concerns. 900 mg per day orally, titrated to achieve therapeutic serum levels. The optimal duration of therapy has not been established; however, long-term administration may be required for symptom control.

A behavioral response to lithium was observed at serum levels of 0.48 to 1.4 mEq/L. Careful monitoring of cognitive status was recommended during lithium use for management of post-TBI aggression.

➤*Children:*

Bipolar disorder – See Adults for dosing for children 12 years of age and older.

Younger than 12 years of age: See Off-Label Dosing.

Off-label dosing –

Bipolar disorder:

• *Adolescents* –

Usual dosage: 600 to 1,800 mg/day orally administered in 3 to 4 divided doses.

• *Children* –

Initial dosage: 15 to 60 mg/kg/day orally administered in 3 to 4 divided doses.

Dosage adjustment: Adjust weekly as needed to achieve therapeutic levels.

➤*Elderly:* Elderly patients often require lower lithium dosages to achieve therapeutic serum concentrations. They may also exhibit adverse reactions at serum concentrations ordinarily tolerated by younger patients.

➤*Renal function impairment:* Patients with renal impairment may require lower lithium doses.

➤*Therapeutic drug monitoring:* Regular monitoring of the patient's clinical state and of serum lithium levels is necessary. Serum levels should be determined twice per week during the acute phase, and until the serum level and clinical condition of the patient has been stabilized.

Serum lithium levels in uncomplicated cases receiving maintenance therapy during remission should be monitored at least every 2 months.

Blood samples for serum lithium determination should be drawn immediately prior to the next dose when lithium concentrations are relatively stable (ie, 8 to 12 hours after the previous dose). Total reliance must not be placed on serum levels alone. Accurate patient evaluation requires both clinical and laboratory analysis.

➤*Administration:* Take immediately after meals or with food or milk to avoid stomach upset.

Drink 8 to 12 glasses of water or other liquid every day while on this drug. Maintain a regular diet (including salt).

➤*Storage/Stability:* Store at 25°C (77°F); excursions are permitted to 15° to 30°C (59° to 86°F). Dispense in a tight container.

Actions

➤*Pharmacology:* Preclinical studies have shown that lithium alters sodium transport in nerve and muscle cells and effects a shift toward intraneuronal metabolism of catecholamines, but the specific biochemical mechanism of lithium action in mania is unknown.

➤*Pharmacokinetics:* The distribution space of lithium approximates that of total body water. Lithium is primarily excreted in urine with insignificant excretion in feces. Renal excretion of lithium is proportional to its plasma concentration. The half-life of elimination of lithium is approximately 24 hours. Lithium decreases sodium reabsorption by the renal tubules which could lead to sodium depletion. Therefore, it is essential for the patient to maintain a normal diet, including salt, and an adequate fluid

LITHIUM CITRATE — ORAL

intake (2500 to 3000 mL) at least during the initial stabilization period. Decreased tolerance to lithium has been reported to ensue from protracted sweating or diarrhea and, if such occur, supplemental fluid and salt should be administered.

Contraindications

Lithium should generally not be given to patients with significant renal or cardiovascular disease, severe debilitation or dehydration, or sodium depletion, and to patients receiving diuretics, since the risk of lithium toxicity is very high in such patients. If the psychiatric indication is life-threatening, and if such a patient fails to respond to other measures, lithium treatment may be undertaken with extreme caution, including daily serum lithium determinations and adjustment to the usually low doses ordinarily tolerated by these individuals. In such instances, hospitalization is a necessity.

Warnings/Precautions

➤*Toxicity:* Lithium toxicity is closely related to serum lithium levels, and can occur at doses close to therapeutic levels. The desirable serum lithium levels are 0.6 to 1.2 mEq/L. Patients abnormally sensitive to lithium may exhibit toxic signs at serum levels of 1 to 1.5 mEq/L.

➤*Renal effects:* Chronic lithium therapy may be associated with diminution of renal concentrating ability, occasionally presenting as nephrogenic diabetes insipidus, with polyuria and polydipsia. Such patients should be carefully managed to avoid dehydration with resulting lithium retention and toxicity. This condition is usually reversible when lithium is discontinued.

Morphologic changes with glomerular and interstitial fibrosis and nephron atrophy have been reported in patients on chronic lithium therapy. Morphologic changes have also been seen in bipolar patients never exposed to lithium. The relationship between renal functional and morphologic changes and their association with lithium therapy has not been established. To date, lithium in therapeutic doses has not been reported to cause end-stage renal disease.

When kidney function is assessed, for baseline data prior to starting lithium therapy or thereafter, routine urinalysis and other tests may be used to evaluate tubular function (eg, urine specific gravity or osmolality following a period of water deprivation, or 24-hour urine volume) and glomerular function (eg, serum creatinine or creatinine clearance). During lithium therapy, progressive or sudden changes in renal function, even within the normal range, indicate the need for reevaluation of treatment.

➤*Special risk:* In addition to sweating and diarrhea, concomitant infection with elevated temperatures may also necessitate a temporary reduction or cessation of medication.

The ability to tolerate lithium is greater during the acute manic phase and decreases when manic symptoms subside.

➤*Hazardous tasks:* Lithium may impair mental or physical abilities. Caution patients about activities requiring alertness (eg, operating vehicles or machinery).

➤*Pregnancy: Category D.* Lithium may cause fetal harm when administered to a pregnant woman. There have been reports of lithium having adverse effects on nidations in rats, embryo viability in mice, and metabolism in vitro of rat testis and human spermatozoa have been attributed to lithium, as have teratogenicity in submammalian species, and cleft palates in mice. Studies in rats, rabbits and monkeys have shown no evidence of lithium-induced teratology. Data from lithium birth registries suggest an increase in cardiac and other anomalies, especially Ebstein's anomaly. If the patient becomes pregnant while taking lithium, she should be apprised of the potential risk to the fetus. If possible, lithium should be withdrawn for at least the first trimester unless it is determined that this would seriously endanger the mother.

➤*Lactation:* Lithium is excreted in human milk. Nursing should not be undertaken during lithium therapy except in rare and unusual circumstances where, in the view of the physician, the potential benefits to the mother outweigh possible hazards to the child.

➤*Children:* Since information regarding the safety and effectiveness of lithium in children under 12 years of age is not available, its use in such patients is not recommended at this time. There has been a report of a transient syndrome of acute dystonia and hyperreflexia occurring in a 15 kg child who ingested 300 mg of lithium carbonate.

➤*Elderly:* Elderly patients often require lower lithium dosages to achieve therapeutic serum concentrations. They may also exhibit adverse reactions at serum concentrations ordinarily tolerated by younger patients. Additionally, patients with renal impairment may also require lower lithium doses.

➤*Monitoring:* Previously existing underlying thyroid disorders do not necessarily constitute a contraindication to lithium treatment; where hypothyroidism exists, careful monitoring of thyroid function during lithium stabilization and maintenance allows for correction of changing thyroid parameters, if any. Where hypothyroidism occurs during lithium stabilization and maintenance, supplemental thyroid treatment may be used.

Drug Interactions

➤*QT prolongation:* An additive effect of lithium with other drugs that prolong the QT interval cannot be excluded. The following drugs may prolong the QT interval and increase the risk of life-threatening cardiac arrhythmias, including torsades de pointes: Antiarrhythmic agents (eg, amiodarone, bretylium, disopyramide, dofetilide, procainamide, quinidine, and sotalol), arsenic trioxide, chlorpromazine, cisapride, dolasetron, droperidol, mefloquine, mesoridazine, moxifloxacin, pentamidine, pimozide, tacrolimus, thioridazine, and ziprasidone. For a more complete list of drugs that may prolong the QT interval, see the appendix, Drug-Induced Prolongation of the QT Interval and Torsades de Pointes.

The following drugs can lower serum lithium concentrations by increasing urinary lithium excretion: Acetazolamide, urea, xanthine preparations and alkalinizing agents such as sodium bicarbonate.

The following have also been shown to interact with lithium: Methyldopa and phenytoin.

➤*Antipsychotic medication:* The possibility of similar adverse interactions with other antipsychotic medication exists (see Haloperidol).

➤*Calcium channel blocking agents:* Concurrent use of calcium channel blocking agents with lithium may increase the risk of neurotoxicity in the form of ataxia, tremors, nausea, vomiting, diarrhea or tinnitus.

➤*Carbamazepine:* Concomitant administration of carbamazepine and lithium may increase the risk of neurotoxic side effects.

➤*Diuretics or angiotensin-converting enzyme (ACE) inhibitors:* Caution should be used when lithium and diuretics or angiotensin-converting enzyme (ACE) inhibitors are used concomitantly because sodium loss may reduce the renal clearance of lithium and increase serum lithium levels with risk of lithium toxicity. When such combinations are used, the lithium dosage may need to be decreased, and more frequent monitoring of lithium plasma levels is recommended.

There is evidence that angiotensin-converting enzyme inhibitors (eg, enalapril and captopril) may substantially increase steady-state plasma lithium levels, sometimes resulting in lithium toxicity.

➤*Fluoxetine:* Concurrent use of fluoxetine with lithium has resulted in both increased and decreased serum lithium concentrations. Patients receiving such combined therapy should be monitored closely.

➤*Haloperidol:* An encephalopathic syndrome (characterized by weakness, lethargy, fever, tremulousness and confusion, extrapyramidal symptoms, leucocytosis, elevated serum enzymes, BUN and fasting blood sugar [FBS]) followed by irreversible brain damage has occurred in a few patients treated with lithium plus haloperidol. A causal relationship between these events and the concomitant administration of lithium and haloperidol has not been established; however, patients receiving such combined therapy should be monitored closely for early evidence of neurological toxicity and treatment discontinued promptly if such signs appear.

➤*NSAIDs:* Indomethacin and piroxicam have been reported to increase significantly, steady state plasma lithium levels. In some cases lithium toxicity has resulted from such interactions. There is also evidence that other nonsteroidal, anti-inflammatory agents may have a similar effect. When such combinations are used, increased plasma lithium level monitoring is recommended. Lithium levels should be closely monitored when patients initiate or discontinue NSAID use.

➤*Iodide preparations:* Concomitant extended use of iodide preparations, especially potassium iodide, with lithium may produce hypothyroidism.

➤*Metronidazole:* Concurrent use of metronidazole with lithium may provoke lithium toxicity due to reduced renal clearance. Patients receiving such combined therapy should be monitored closely.

➤*Neuromuscular blocking agents:* Lithium may prolong the effects of neuromuscular blocking agents. Therefore, neuromuscular blocking agents should be given with caution to patients receiving lithium.

➤*Selective serotonin reuptake inhibitors:* The concomitant administration of lithium with selective serotonin reuptake inhibitors should be undertaken with caution as this combination has been reported to result in symptoms such as diarrhea, confusion, tremor, dizziness and agitation.

Adverse Reactions

➤*Lithium toxicity:* The likelihood of toxicity increases with increasing serum lithium levels. Serum lithium levels greater than 1.5 mEq/L carry a greater risk than lower levels. However, patients sensitive to lithium may exhibit toxic signs at serum levels below 1.5 mEq/L.

Diarrhea, vomiting, drowsiness, muscular weakness and lack of coordination may be early signs of lithium toxicity, and can occur at lithium levels below 2 mEq/L. At higher levels, giddiness, ataxia, blurred vision, tinnitus and a large output of dilute urine may be seen. Serum lithium levels above 3 mEq/L may produce a complex clinical picture involving multiple organs and organ systems. Serum lithium levels should not be permitted to exceed 2 mEq/L during the acute treatment phase.

Fine hand tremor, polyuria and mild thirst may occur during initial therapy for the acute manic phase, and may persist throughout treatment. Transient and mild nausea and general discomfort may also appear during the first few days of lithium administration.

These side effects are an inconvenience rather than a disabling condition, and usually subside with continued treatment or a temporary reduction or cessation of dosage. If persistent, a cessation of dosage is indicated.

➤*Adverse reactions not directly related to serum lithium levels:* The following adverse reactions have been reported and do not appear to be directly related to serum lithium levels.

Cardiovascular – Cardiac arrhythmia, hypotension, peripheral circulatory collapse, sinus node dysfunction with severe bradycardia (which may result in syncope).

EKG changes: Reversible flattening, isoelectricity or inversion of T-waves.

LITHIUM CITRATE — ORAL

CNS – Blackout spells, epileptiform seizures, slurred speech, dizziness, vertigo, incontinence of urine or feces, somnolence, psychomotor retardation, restlessness, confusion, stupor, coma, acute dystonia, downbeat nystagmus.

Autonomic nervous system: Blurred vision, dry mouth.

EEG changes: Diffuse slowing, widening of frequency spectrum, potentiation and disorganization of background rhythm.

Neurological: Cases of pseudotumor cerebri (increased intracranial pressure and papilledema) have been reported with lithium use. If undetected, this condition may result in enlargement of the blind spot, constriction of visual fields and eventual blindness due to optic atrophy. Lithium should be discontinued, if clinically possible, if this syndrome occurs.

Dermatologic – Drying and thinning of hair, anesthesia of skin, chronic folliculitis, xerosis cutis, alopecia and exacerbation of psoriasis.

GI – Anorexia, nausea, vomiting, diarrhea.

GU – Albuminuria, oliguria, polyuria, glycosuria.

Musculoskeletal – Tremor, muscle hyperirritability (fasciculations, twitching, clonic movements of whole limbs), ataxia, choreoathetotic movements, hyperactive deep tendon reflexes.

Endocrine – Euthyroid goiter or hypothyroidism (including myxedema) accompanied by lower T_3 and T_4. ^{131}Iodine uptake may be elevated. Paradoxically, rare cases of hyperthyroidism have been reported.

Miscellaneous – Fatigue, lethargy, transient scotomata, dehydration, weight loss, tendency to sleep.

Miscellaneous reactions unrelated to dosage are the following: Transient electroencephalographic and electrocardiographic changes, leucocytosis, headache, diffuse nontoxic goiter with or without hypothyroidism, transient hyperglycemia, generalized pruritus with or without rash, cutaneous ulcers, albuminuria, worsening of organic brain syndromes, excessive weight gain, edematous swelling of ankles or wrists, and thirst or polyuria, sometimes resembling diabetes insipidus, and metallic taste.

A single report has been received of the development of painful discoloration of fingers and toes and coldness of the extremities within 1 day of the starting of treatment of lithium. The mechanism through which these symptoms (resembling Raynaud's syndrome) developed is not known. Recovery followed discontinuance.

Overdosage

➤*Symptoms:* The toxic levels for lithium are close to the therapeutic levels. It is therefore important that patients and their families be cautioned to watch for early symptoms and to discontinue the drug and inform the physician should they occur. Toxic symptoms include the following: Giddiness; ataxia; blurred vision; tinnitus; vertigo; increasing confusion; slurred speech; blackouts; fasciculations; myoclonic twitching or movement of entire limbs; choreoathetoid movements; urinary or fecal incontinence; agitation or manic-like behavior; hyperreflexia; hypertonia; dysarthria; seizures (generalized and focal); arrhythmias; hypotension; peripheral vascular collapse; stupor; muscle group twitching; spasticity; coma.

➤*Treatment:* No specific antidote for lithium poisoning is known. Early symptoms of lithium toxicity can usually be treated by reduction of cessation of dosage of the drug and resumption of the treatment at a lower dose after 24 to 48 hours. In severe cases of lithium poisoning, the first and foremost goal of treatment consists of elimination of this ion from the patient.

Treatment is essentially the same as that used in barbiturate poisoning:

1.) Gastric lavage.
2.) Correction of fluid and electrolyte imbalance.
3.) Regulation of kidney functioning. Urea, mannitol, and aminophylline all produce significant increases in lithium excretion. Hemodialysis is an effective and rapid means of removing the ion from the severely toxic patient. Infection prophylaxis, regular chest x-rays, and preservation of adequate respiration are essential.

Patient Information

Outpatients and their families should be warned that the patient must discontinue lithium therapy and contact his physician if such clinical signs of lithium toxicity as diarrhea, vomiting, tremor, mild ataxia, drowsiness, or muscular weakness occur.

Lithium may impair mental or physical abilities. Caution patients about activities requiring alertness (eg, operating vehicles or machinery).

Take immediately after meals or with food or milk to avoid stomach upset.

Drink 8 to 12 glasses of water or other liquid every day while on this drug. Prolonged exposure to the sun can lead to dehydration. Maintain a regular diet (including salt). Contact a physician if fever or diarrhea develops.

NMDA RECEPTOR ANTAGONISTS

MEMANTINE HYDROCHLORIDE

Rx	**Namenda** (Forest Laboratories)	**Tablets; oral:** 5 mg	(5 FL). Tan, capsule shape. Film-coated. In 60s, UD 100s, and titration paks.[a]
		10 mg	(10 FL). Gray, capsule shape. Film-coated. In 60s, UD 100s, and titration paks.[a]
Rx	**Namenda XR** (Forest Laboratories)	**Capsules, extended-release; oral:** 7 mg	PEG, sugar. (FLI 7 mg). Yellow, opaque. In 30s and titration paks.[b]
		14 mg	PEG, sugar. (FLI 14 mg). Yellow/dark green, opaque. In 30s, 90s, UD 100s, and titration paks.[b]
		21 mg	PEG, sugar. (FLI 21 mg). White to off-white/dark green, opaque. In 30s and titration paks.[b]
		28 mg	PEG, sugar. (FLI 28 mg). Dark green, opaque. In 30s, 90s, UD 100s, and titration paks.[b]
Rx	**Namenda** (Forest Laboratories)	**Solution; oral:** 2 mg/mL	Glycerin, parabens, sorbitol. Alcohol free, sugar free. Peppermint flavor. In 360 mL

[a] Titration paks are blister packages containing 49 tablets (28 × 5 mg and 21 × 10 mg).

[b] Titration paks are blister packages containing 28 capsules (7 × 7 mg, 7 × 14 mg, 7 × 21 mg, 7 × 28 mg).

MEMANTINE HYDROCHLORIDE — ORAL

Indications

➤*Alzheimer disease:* For the treatment of moderate to severe dementia of the Alzheimer type.

➤*Off-label uses:*

Attention deficit hyperactivity disorder – [4] = Insufficient documentation. Initial data from a noncontrolled study suggest that memantine may have some benefit as adjunctive therapy in the management of attention deficit hyperactivity disorder (ADHD) as demonstrated by improved ADHD scores after 8 weeks. Larger, controlled trials are needed to verify and expand on these results. (See Administration and Dosage.)

Postherpetic neuralgia – [5] = Poor documentation. Use is not recommended. Memantine has been studied in patients with postherpetic neuralgia (PHN) in 2 controlled trials, neither of which showed any benefit. The American Academy of Neurology clinical practice guidelines do not make a statement on the efficacy of memantine for the treatment of PHN. However, they state that 2 other N-methyl-D-aspartate (NMDA) antagonists, dextromethorphan and ketamine, are of limited to no value.

Prevention of migraine (adults) – [4] = Insufficient documentation. Results from a retrospective trial evaluating the use of memantine for the prevention of migraine headaches in adults showed favorable results but was limited by small sample size and lack of a control group. (See Administration and Dosage.)

Other possible off-label uses – Treatment of vascular dementia.

Administration and Dosage

➤*Adults:*

Alzheimer disease –

Immediate release:

- *Usual dosage* – 20 mg/day.
- *Initial dosage* – 5 mg once daily.
- *Dosage titration* – Increase in 5 mg increments to 10 mg/day (5 mg twice a day), 15 mg/day (5 and 10 mg as separate doses), and 20 mg/day (10 mg twice a day). The minimum recommended interval between dose increases is 1 week.

Extended release:

- *Usual dosage* – 28 mg once daily.
- *Maximum dose* – 28 mg once daily.
- *Initial dosage* – 7 mg once daily.
- *Dosage titration* – Increased in 7 mg increments to 28 mg once daily. The minimum recommended interval between dose increases is 1 week, and only if the previous dose has been well tolerated.
- *Conversion* – Patients taking 10 mg immediate-release tablets twice daily may switch to 28 mg extended-release (ER) capsules once daily the day following the last dose of an immediate-release 10 mg tablet.

Off-label dosing –

Prevention of migraine: [4] = Insufficient documentation. Rational use cannot be established as evidenced by data in limited patient populations (less than 30 patients) or inconsistent results. Assessment of appropriate patient population, dose, or efficacy cannot be adequately determined. In addition, significant safety data have been identified by the Food and Drug Administration (FDA) or manufacturer safety notifications (eg, black box warnings).
5 to 20 mg daily for at least 2 months.

MEMANTINE HYDROCHLORIDE — ORAL

➤*Children:*

Off-label dosing –

Attention deficit hyperactivity disorder: [4] = Insufficient documentation. Rational use cannot be established as evidenced by data in limited patient populations (less than 30 patients) or inconsistent results. Assessment of appropriate patient population, dose, or efficacy cannot be adequately determined. In addition, significant safety data have been identified by the FDA or manufacturer safety notifications (eg, black box warnings).

20 mg/day, titrated up over 4 weeks from a starting dosage of 4.8 mg/day. The one study to date had a duration of only 8 weeks, but ADHD pharmacotherapy is usually long term.

➤*Renal function impairment:*

Immediate release –

Severe renal impairment (creatinine clearance [CrCl] 5 to 29 mL/min):

- *Usual dose* – A target dosage of 5 mg twice daily is recommended.
- *Conversion* – Patients taking the 5 mg tablet twice daily may switch to the 14 mg ER capsule once daily the day following the last dose of an immediate-release 5 mg tablet.

Extended release –

Severe renal impairment (CrCl 5 to 29 mL/min): A target dosage of 14 mg/day is recommended.

➤*Administration:* May be taken with or without food.

Extended release – Capsules can be taken intact or may be opened, sprinkled on applesauce, and thereby swallowed. The entire contents of each capsule should be consumed; the dose should not be divided. The capsules should be swallowed whole and not be divided, chewed, or crushed.

➤*Storage/Stability:* Store at 25°C (77°F); excursions are permitted from 15° to 30°C (59° to 86°F).

Actions

➤*Pharmacology:* Persistent activation of CNS NMDA receptors by the excitatory amino acid glutamate has been hypothesized to contribute to the symptomatology of Alzheimer disease. Memantine is postulated to exert its therapeutic effect through its action as a low to moderate affinity uncompetitive (open-channel) NMDA receptor antagonist, that binds preferentially to the NMDA receptor-operated cation channels. There is no evidence that memantine prevents or slows neurodegeneration in patients with Alzheimer disease.

➤*Pharmacokinetics:*

Absorption/Distribution – Memantine is well-absorbed after oral administration and has linear pharmacokinetics over the therapeutic dose range. Following oral administration, memantine is highly absorbed with peak concentrations reached in about 3 to 7 hours. The mean volume of distribution of memantine is 9 to 11 L/kg, and the plasma protein binding is low (45%).

In a study comparing memantine 28 mg once daily ER to memantine immediate-release 10 mg twice daily, maximum drug concentration (C_{max}) and area under the curve ($AUC_{0\text{-}24}$) values were 48% and 33% higher for the ER dosage regimen, respectively.

After multiple dose administration of memantine ER, memantine peak concentrations occur around 9 to 12 hours postdose.

Effect of food: There is no difference in memantine exposure, based on C_{max} or AUC, for memantine ER whether administered with food or on an empty stomach. However, peak plasma concentrations are achieved about 18 hours after administration with food versus approximately 25 hours after administration on an empty stomach.

Metabolism/Excretion – Memantine undergoes partial hepatic metabolism; about 48% of administered drug is excreted unchanged in urine. The remainder is converted primarily to 3 polar metabolites, which posses minimal NMDA receptor antagonists activity: N-glucuronide conjugate, 6-hydroxy memantine, and 1-nitroso-deaminated memantine. A total of 74% of the administered dose is excreted as the sum of the parent drug and the N-glucuonide conjugate. The hepatic microsomal cytochrome P450 (CYP-450) enzyme system does not play a significant role in the metabolism of memantine. Renal clearance involves active tubular secretion moderated by pH-dependent tubular reabsorption. Memantine has a terminal elimination half-life of about 60 to 80 hours.

Special populations –

Renal function impairment: Mean AUC $_{0-\infty}$ increased 4%, 60%, and 115% in subjects with mild, moderate, and severe renal impairment, respectively, compared with healthy subjects. The terminal elimination half-life increased 18%, 41%, and 95% in subjects with mild, moderate, and severe renal impairment, respectively, compared with healthy subjects.

Hepatic function impairment: Terminal elimination half-life increased by approximately 16% in subjects with moderate hepatic impairment when compared with healthy subjects. The pharmacokinetics of memantine have not been evaluated in patients with severe hepatic impairment.

Gender: Following multiple-dose administration of memantine 20 mg twice daily, women had an approximately 45% higher exposure than men, but there was no difference in exposure when body weight was taken into account.

Contraindications

Hypersensitivity to memantine or to any excipients used in the formulation.

Warnings/Precautions

➤*Seizures:* Memantine has not been systematically evaluated in patients with a seizure disorder. In clinical trials of memantine immediate-release and ER, seizures occurred in 0.2% and 0.3% of patients treated with memantine and 0.5% and 0.6% of patients treated with placebo, respectively.

➤*Genitourinary conditions:* Conditions that raise urine pH may decrease the urinary elimination of memantine, resulting in increased plasma levels of memantine.

➤*Renal function impairment:* See Administration and Dosage for more information.

➤*Hepatic function impairment:* See Administration and Dosage for more information.

➤*Pregnancy:* Category B. There are no adequate and well-controlled studies of memantine in pregnant women. Use memantine during pregnancy only if the potential benefit justifies the potential risk to the fetus.

Slight maternal toxicity, decreased pup weights, and an increased incidence of nonossified cervical vertebrae were seen at an oral dosage of 18 mg/kg/day in a study in which rats were given oral memantine beginning premating and continuing through the postpartum period. Slight maternal toxicity and decreased pup weights also were seen at this dosage in a study in which rats were treated from day 15 of gestation through the postpartum period. The no-effect dose for these effects was 6 mg/kg, which is 3 times (immediate release) and 2 times (ER) the MRHD on a mg/m^2 basis.

➤*Lactation:* It is not known whether memantine is excreted in human breast milk. Due to the large volume of distribution, it is unlikely that memantine would transfer to any measurable extent. Because many drugs are excreted in human milk, exercise caution when memantine is administered to a breast-feeding woman.

➤*Children:* There are no adequate and well-controlled trials documenting the safety and efficacy of memantine in any illness occurring in children.

Drug Interactions

Memantine Drug Interactions

Precipitant drug	Object drug[a]		Description
NMDA antagonists (eg, amantadine, ketamine, dextromethorphan)	Memantine	↔	Concurrent use of memantine with other NMDA antagonists has not been evaluated. Use with caution.
Urinary alkalinizers (eg, carbonic anhydrase inhibitors, sodium bicarbonate)	Memantine	↑	Memantine plasma concentrations may be elevated, increasing the risk of adverse reactions. Use with caution. Monitor the clinical response of the patient. Adjust the memantine dose as needed.
Memantine	Thiazide diuretics (eg, hydrochlorothiazide)	↓	Coadministration of memantine and hydrochlorothiazide/triamterene did not affect the bioavailability of triamterene; however, the bioavailability of hydrochlorothiazide decreased 20%. Monitor the clinical response of the patient. If an interaction is suspected, adjust the thiazide dose as needed.

[a] ↑ = object drug increased; ↓ = object drug decreased; ↔ = undetermined clinical effect.

➤*Drug/Food interactions:* There is no difference in memantine exposure whether the drug is taken with food or on an empty stomach. However, C_{max} is achieved about 18 hours after administration with food compared with 25 hours after administration on an empty stomach. Memantine may be taken without regard to food.

Adverse Reactions

➤*Immediate release:*

Adverse reactions (2% or more) and higher frequency than placebo) –

Memantine Immediate Release Adverse Reactions (≥ 2% and Higher Frequency Than Placebo)

Adverse reactions	Memantine (n = 940)	Placebo (n = 922)
CNS		
Confusion	6%	5%
Dizziness	7%	5%
Fatigue	2%	1%
Hallucination	3%	2%
Headache	6%	3%
Somnolence	3%	2%

MEMANTINE HYDROCHLORIDE — ORAL

Memantine Immediate Release Adverse Reactions (≥ 2% and Higher Frequency Than Placebo)		
Adverse reactions	Memantine (n = 940)	Placebo (n = 922)
GI		
Constipation	5%	3%
Vomiting	3%	2%
Respiratory		
Coughing	4%	3%
Dyspnea	2%	1%
Miscellaneous		
Back pain	3%	2%
Hypertension	4%	2%
Pain	3%	1%

Adverse reactions (2% or more) and at a greater or equal rate as placebo –

CNS: Agitation, anxiety, depression, gait abnormal, insomnia.

GI: Diarrhea, nausea.

GU: Urinary incontinence, urinary tract infection.

Respiratory: Bronchitis, upper respiratory tract infection.

Miscellaneous: Anorexia, arthralgia, fall, inflicted injury, influenza-like symptoms, peripheral edema.

Other adverse reactions –

Cardiovascular: Cardiac failure, cerebrovascular accident, syncope transient ischemic attack (at least 1%); angina pectoris, atrial fibrillation, bradycardia, cardiac arrest, hypotension, myocardial infarction, postural hypotension, pulmonary edema, pulmonary embolism, thrombophlebitis (0.1% to 1%).

CNS: Aggressive reaction, ataxia, hypokinesia, vertigo (at least 1%); abnormal coordination, abnormal crying, abnormal thinking, amnesia, apathy, aphasia, cerebral hemorrhage, convulsions, delirium, delusion, depersonalization, emotional lability, extrapyramidal disorder, hemiplegia, hyperkinesia, hypertonia, hypesthesia, increased appetite, increased libido, involuntary muscle contractions, nervousness, neuralgia, neuropathy, neurosis, paranoid reaction, paresthesia, paroniria, personality disorder, psychosis, ptosis, sleep disorder, stupor, suicide attempt, tremor (0.1% to 1%).

Dermatologic: Rash (at least 1%); alopecia, cellulitis, dermatitis, eczema, erythematous rash, pruritus, skin ulceration, urticaria (0.1% to 1%).

GI: Diverticulitis, esophageal ulceration, gastroenteritis, GI hemorrhage, melena (0.1% to 1%).

GU: Frequent micturition (at least 1%); dysuria, hematuria, urinary retention (0.1% to 1%).

Hematologic / lymphatic: Anemia (at least 1%); leukopenia (0.1% to 1%).

Metabolic / nutritional: Decreased weight, increased alkaline phosphatase (at least 1%); aggravated diabetes mellitus, dehydration, hyponatremia (0.1% to 1%).

Respiratory: Pneumonia (at least 1%); apnea, asthma, hemoptysis (0.1% to 1%).

Special senses: Cataract, conjunctivitis (at least 1%); abnormal lacrimation, blepharitis, blurred vision, conjunctival hemorrhage, corneal opacity, decreased hearing, decreased visual acuity, diplopia, eye pain, glaucoma, macula lutea degeneration, myopia, retinal detachment, retinal hemorrhage, tinnitus, xerophthalmia (0.1% to 1%).

Miscellaneous: Allergic reaction, hypothermia (0.1% to 1%).

➤*Extended release:*

Discontinuation of therapy – In the placebo-controlled clinical trial of memantine ER, which treated a total of 676 patients, the proportion of patients in the memantine ER 28 mg/day dosage and placebo groups who discontinued treatment due to adverse reactions were 10% and 6.3%, respectively. The most common adverse reaction in the memantine ER treated group that led to treatment discontinuation in this study was dizziness at a rate of 1.5%.

Adverse reactions (2% or more) –

Memantine Extended-Release Adverse Reactions (≥ 2%)		
Adverse reactions	Memantine ER 28 mg (n = 341)	Placebo (n = 335)
Cardiovascular		
Hypertension	4%	2%
Hypotension	2%	1%
CNS		
Aggression	2%	1%
Anxiety	4%	3%
Depression	3%	1%
Dizziness	5%	1%
Headache	6%	5%
Somnolence	3%	1%
GI		
Abdominal pain	2%	1%
Constipation	3%	1%
Diarrhea	5%	4%
Vomiting	2%	1%
Miscellaneous		
Back pain	3%	1%
Influenza	4%	3%
Urinary incontinence	2%	1%
Weight increased	3%	1%

Other adverse reactions –

Cardiovascular: Bradycardia, myocardial infarction, syncope.

CNS: Agitation, asthenia, confusional state, convulsion, delirium, delusion, dementia of the Alzheimer type, disorientation, fall, fatigue, gait disturbance, hallucinations (both visual and auditory), insomnia, irritability, malaise, restlessness, suicidal ideation, tremor.

GI: Fecal incontinence, nausea.

Metabolic / nutritional: Anorexia, decreased appetite, dehydration, hyperglycemia, peripheral edema, weight decreased.

Musculoskeletal: Arthralgia, pain in extremity.

Respiratory: Bronchitis, cough, dyspnea, nasopharyngitis, pneumonia, upper respiratory tract infection.

Miscellaneous: Anemia, pyrexia, urinary tract infection.

➤*Postmarketing:*

Cardiovascular – Atrial fibrillation, atrioventricular block (including 2nd and 3rd degree block), cardiac failure, cerebral infarction, cerebrovascular accident, deep venous thrombosis, electrocardiogram QT prolonged, international normalized ratio increased, orthostatic hypotension, pulmonary embolism, supraventricular tachycardia, tachycardia, thrombophlebitis, torsades de pointes, transient ischemic attack.

CNS – Claudication, convulsions (including tonic clonic), depressed levels of consciousness (including rare reports of coma), dyskinesia, encephalopathy, extrapyramidal disorder, hallucinations (both visual and auditory), hypertonia, intracranial hemorrhage, lethargy, loss of consciousness, malaise, neuroleptic malignant syndrome, parkinsonism, restlessness, suicidal ideation, tardive dyskinesia.

Dermatologic – Rash, Stevens-Johnson syndrome.

GI – Colitis, dysphagia, gastritis, gastroesophageal reflux, ileus, pancreatitis.

GU – Acute renal failure (including abnormal renal function test), impotence, urinary retention.

Hematologic / Lymphatic – Agranulocytosis, leukopenia (including neutropenia), pancytopenia, thrombocytopenia, thrombotic thrombocytopenic purpura.

Hepatic – Cholelithiasis, hepatic failure, hepatitis (including abnormal hepatic function test, cytolytic and cholestatic hepatitis).

Metabolic / Nutritional – Hyperglycemia, hyperlipidemia, hypoglycemia, hyponatremia.

Musculoskeletal – Bone fracture, carpal tunnel syndrome, myoclonus.

Miscellaneous – Aspiration pneumonia, chest pain, inappropriate antidiuretic hormone secretion, sepsis, sudden death.

Overdosage

➤*Symptoms:* Signs and symptoms associated with memantine overdosage in clinical trials and from worldwide marketing experience alone or in combination with other drugs and/or alcohol include agitation, asthenia, bradycardia, coma, confusion, dizziness, electrocardiogram (ECG) changes, increased blood pressure, lethargy, loss of consciousness, psychosis, restlessness, slowed movement, somnolence, stupor, unsteady gait, visual hallucinations, vertigo, vomiting, and weakness. The largest known ingestion of memantine worldwide was 2 g in a patient who took memantine in conjunction with unspecified antidiabetic medications. The patient experienced agitation, coma, and diplopia but subsequently recovered.

One patient participating in a memantine ER clinical trial unintentionally took memantine ER 112 mg daily for 31 days and experienced an elevated serum uric acid, elevated serum alkaline phosphatase, and low platelet count.

➤*Treatment:* Utilize general supportive measures and symptomatic treatment. Elimination of memantine can be enhanced by acidification of urine.

Patient Information

Instruct caregivers of the recommended administration.

Instruct patients and caregivers that memantine ER capsules should be swallowed whole. Alternatively, memantine ER capsules may be opened, sprinkled on applesauce, and thereby swallowed. The entire contents of each capsule should be consumed. Do not divide, chew, or crush capsules.

Advise patients and caregivers that memantine may cause headache, diarrhea, and dizziness.

TACRINE HYDROCHLORIDE (Tetrahydroacridinamine; THA)

Rx	Cognex[a] (Parke-Davis)	Capsules: 10 mg	Lactose. (Cognex 10). Yellow/dark green. In 120s and UD 100s.
		20 mg	Lactose. (Cognex 20). Yellow/light blue. In 120s and UD 100s.
		30 mg	Lactose. (Cognex 30). Yellow/orange. In 120s and UD 100s.
		40 mg	Lactose. (Cognex 40). Yellow/lavender. In 120s and UD 100s.

[a] This product is no longer being manufactured.

TACRINE HYDROCHLORIDE — ORAL

Indications

➤*Alzheimer disease:* For the treatment of mild-to-moderate dementia of the Alzheimer type.

Administration and Dosage

➤*General dosing considerations:* The rate of dose escalation may be slowed if a patient is intolerant to the titration schedule recommended below. However, it is not advisable to accelerate the dose incrementation plan.

Following initiation of therapy, or any dosage increase, patients should be observed carefully for adverse effects.

➤*Adults:*

Alzheimer disease –

Initial dosage: 40 mg/day (10 mg 4 times daily). This dose should be maintained for a minimum of 4 weeks with every other week monitoring of transaminase levels beginning 4 weeks after initiation of treatment. It is important that the dose is not increased during this period because of the potential for delayed onset of transaminase elevations.

Dosage titration: Following 4 weeks of treatment at 40 mg/day (10 mg 4 times daily), the dose of tacrine should then be increased to 80 mg/day (20 mg 4 times daily), providing there are no significant transaminase elevations and the patient is tolerating treatment. Titrate patients to higher doses (120 and 160 mg/day, in divided doses on a 4 times daily schedule) at 4-week intervals on the basis of tolerance.

Dosage adjustment: Monitor serum ALT every other week from at least week 4 to week 16 following initiation of treatment, after which monitoring may be decreased to every 3 months. For patients who develop ALT elevations greater than 2 times the upper limit of normal, the dose and monitoring regimen should be modified as described.

A full monitoring and dose titration sequence must be repeated in the event that a patient suspends treatment with tacrine for more than 4 weeks.

Tacrine Dose and Monitoring Regimen Modification in Response to ALT Elevations

ALT level	Treatment and monitoring regimen
≤ 2 × ULN	Continue treatment according to recommended titration and monitoring schedule.
> 2 to ≤ 3 × ULN	Continue treatment according to recommended titration. Monitor ALT levels weekly until levels return to normal limits.
> 3 to ≤ 5 × ULN	Reduce the daily dose of tacrine by 40 mg/day. Monitor ALT levels weekly. Resume dose titration and every other week monitoring when the levels of the ALT return to normal limits.
> 5 × ULN	Stop tacrine treatment. Monitor the patient closely for signs and symptoms associated with hepatitis and follow ALT levels until within normal limits. See Rechallenge section.
	Experience is limited in patients with ALT > 10 × ULN. The risk of rechallenge must be considered against demonstrated clinical benefit.
	Patients with clinical jaundice confirmed by a significant elevation in total bilirubin (> 3 mg/dL) or those exhibiting clinical signs or symptoms of hypersensitivity (eg, rash, fever) in association with ALT elevations should immediately and permanently discontinue tacrine and not be rechallenged.

Rechallenge: Patients who are required to discontinue tacrine treatment because of ALT elevations may be rechallenged once ALT levels return to healthy limits.

Rechallenge of patients with ALT elevations less than 10 times ULN has not resulted in serious liver injury. However, because experience in the rechallenge of patients who had elevations greater than 10 times ULN is limited, the risks associated with the rechallenge of these patients are not well characterized. Careful, frequent (weekly) monitoring of serum ALT should be undertaken when rechallenging such patients.

If rechallenged, patients should be given an initial dose of 40 mg/day (10 mg 4 times daily) and ALT levels monitored weekly. If, after 6 weeks on 40 mg/day, the patient is tolerating the dosage with no unacceptable elevations in ALT, the recommended dose-titration may be resumed. Weekly monitoring of the ALT levels should continue for a total of 16 weeks after which monitoring may be decreased to monthly for 2 months and every 3 months thereafter.

➤*Hepatic function impairment:* Tacrine should be prescribed with care in patients with current evidence or history of abnormal liver function.

➤*Monitoring:* Serum ALT should be monitored every other week from at least week 4 to week 16 following initiation of treatment, after which monitoring may be decreased to every 3 months.

➤*Administration:* Tacrine should be taken between meals whenever possible; however, if minor GI upset occurs, tacrine may be taken with meals to improve tolerability. Taking tacrine with meals can be expected to reduce plasma levels approximately 30% to 40%.

➤*Storage / Stability:* Store at 15° to 30°C (59° to 86°F) away from moisture.

Actions

➤*Pharmacology:* Although widespread degeneration of multiple CNS neuronal systems eventually occurs, early pathological changes in Alzheimer disease involve, in a relatively selective manner, cholinergic neuronal pathways that project from the basal forebrain to the cerebral cortex and hippocampus. The resulting deficiency of cortical acetylcholine is believed to account for some of the clinical manifestations of mild-to-moderate dementia. Tacrine HCl, an orally bioavailable, centrally active, reversible cholinesterase inhibitor, presumably acts by elevating acetylcholine concentrations in the cerebral cortex by slowing the degradation of acetylcholine released by still intact cholinergic neurons. If this theoretical mechanism of action is correct, tacrine HCl's effects may lessen as the disease process advances and fewer cholinergic neurons remain functionally intact. There is no evidence that tacrine HCl alters the course of the underlying dementing process.

➤*Pharmacokinetics:*

Absorption – Tacrine HCl is rapidly absorbed after oral administration; maximal plasma concentrations occur within 1 to 2 hours. The rate and extent of tacrine HCl absorption following administration of tacrine HCl capsules and solution are virtually indistinguishable. Absolute bioavailability of tacrine HCl is ≈ 17 (SD ± 13)%. Food reduces tacrine HCl bioavailability by ≈ 30% to 40%; however, there is no food effect if tacrine HCl is administered at least 1 hour before meals. The effect of achlorhydria on the absorption of tacrine HCl is unknown.

Distribution – Mean volume of distribution of tacrine HCl is ≈ 349 (SD ± 193) L. Tacrine HCl is ≈ 55% bound to plasma proteins. The extent and degree of tacrine HCl's distribution within various body compartments has not been systematically studied. However, 336 hours after the administration of a single radiolabeled dose, ≈ 25% of the radiolabel was not recovered in a mass balance study, suggesting the possibility that tacrine HCl or one or more of its metabolites may be retained.

Metabolism – Tacrine HCl is extensively metabolized by the cytochrome P450 system to multiple metabolites, not all of which have been identified. The vast majority of radiolabeled species present in the plasma following a single dose of ^{14}C radiolabeled tacrine HCl are unidentified (ie, only 5% of radioactivity in plasma has been identified [tacrine HCl and 3-hydroxylated metabolites; 1-, 2-, and 4-hydroxytacrine]).

Studies utilizing human liver preparations demonstrated that cytochrome P450 1A2 is the principal isozyme involved in tacrine HCl metabolism. These findings are consistent with the observation that tacrine HCl or one of its metabolites inhibits the metabolism of theophylline in humans (see Drug Interactions). Results from a study utilizing quinidine to inhibit cytochrome P450 2D6 indicate that tacrine HCl is not metabolized extensively by this enzyme system.

Following aromatic ring hydroxylation, tacrine HCl's metabolites undergo glucuronidation. Whether tacrine HCl or its metabolites undergo biliary excretion or enterohepatic circulation is unknown.

Excretion – Tacrine HCl undergoes presystemic clearance (ie, first-pass metabolism). The extent of this first-pass metabolism depends upon the dose of tacrine HCl administered. Because the enzyme system involved can be saturated at relatively low doses, a larger fraction of a high dose of tacrine HCl will escape first-pass elimination than of a smaller dose. Thus, when a 40 mg daily dose is increased by 40 mg, the average plasma concentration will be increased by ≈ 6 ng/mL. However, when a daily dose of 80 or 120 mg is increased by 40 mg, the increment in average plasma concentration is ≈ 10 ng/mL.

Elimination of tacrine HCl from the plasma, however, is not dose dependent (ie, the half-life is independent of dose or plasma concentration). The elimination half-life is ≈ 2 to 4 hours. Following initiation of therapy or a change in daily dose, steady-state tacrine HCl plasma concentration should be attained within 24 to 36 hours.

Special populations –

Gender: Average tacrine HCl plasma concentrations are ≈ 50% higher in females than in males. This is not explained by differences in body surface

TACRINE HYDROCHLORIDE — ORAL

area or elimination half-life. The difference is probably due to higher systemic availability after oral dosing and may reflect the known lower activity of cytochrome P450 1A2 in women.

Smoking: Mean plasma tacrine HCl concentrations in current smokers are approximately one-third the concentrations in nonsmokers. Cigarette smoking is known to induce cytochrome P450 1A2.

Contraindications

Hypersensitivity to tacrine HCl or acridine derivatives; in patients previously treated with tacrine HCl who developed treatment-associated jaundice; a serum bilirubin ≥ 3 mg/dL; or those exhibiting clinical signs or symptoms of hypersensitivity (eg, rash or fever) in association with ALT elevations.

Warnings/Precautions

➤*Anesthesia:* Tacrine, as a cholinesterase inhibitor, is likely to exaggerate succinylcholine-type muscle relaxation during anesthesia.

➤*Cardiovascular conditions:* Because of its cholinomimetic action, tacrine HCl may have vagotonic effects on the heart rate (eg, bradycardia). This action may be particularly important to patients with conduction abnormalities, bradyarrhythmia, or a sick sinus syndrome.

➤*GI effects:* Tacrine HCl is an inhibitor of cholinesterase and may be expected to increase gastric acid secretion due to increased cholinergic activity. Therefore, patients are at increased risk for developing ulcers. Those with a history of ulcer disease or those receiving concurrent nonsteroidal anti-inflammatory drugs (NSAIDs) should be monitored closely for symptoms of active or occult GI disease.

Tacrine HCl also as a predictable consequence of its pharmacological properties, can cause nausea, vomiting, and loose stools at recommended doses.

➤*Genitourinary effects:* Cholinomimetics may cause bladder outflow obstruction.

➤*Neurological conditions:*

Seizures – Cholinomimetics are believed to have some potential to cause generalized convulsions; seizure activity may, however, also be a manifestation of Alzheimer disease.

Sudden worsening of the degree of cognitive impairment – Worsening of cognitive function has been reported following abrupt discontinuation of tacrine HCl or after a large reduction in total daily dose (≥ 80 mg/day).

➤*Pulmonary conditions:* Because of its cholinomimetic action, tacrine HCl should be prescribed with care to patients with a history of asthma.

➤*Hepatic effects:* The use of tacrine HCl in patients without a history of liver disease is commonly associated with serum aminotransferase elevations, some to levels ordinarily considered to indicate clinically important hepatic injury (see above information).

Experience gained in more than 12,000 patients who received tacrine HCl in clinical studies and the treatment IND program indicates that if tacrine HCl is promptly withdrawn following detection of these elevations, clinically evident signs and symptoms of liver injury are rare.

Long-term follow-up of patients who experience transaminase elevations, however, is limited and it is impossible, therefore, to exclude, with certainty, the possibility of chronic sequelae.

➤*Hepatic function impairment:* Tacrine HCl should be prescribed with care in patients with current evidence or history of abnormal liver function indicated by significant abnormalities in serum transaminase (ALT; AST), bilirubin, and gamma-glutamyl transpeptidase (GGT) levels.

Clinically evident liver toxicity – One of more than 12,000 patients exposed to tacrine HCl in clinical studies and the treatment IND program had documented elevated bilirubin (5.3 times upper limit of normal, [ULN]) and jaundice with transaminase levels (AST) nearly 20 times the ULN.

Rare cases of liver toxicity associated with jaundice, raised serum bilirubin, pyrexia, hepatitis and liver failure have been reported in postmarketing experience. Most of these cases have been reversible but some deaths have occurred. Since there was multiple pathology including infection, gallstones and carcinoma it was not possible to clearly establish the relationship to tacrine HCl treatment.

Blood chemistry signs of liver injury – Experience from the 30-week clinical study (described earlier) provides a representative estimate of the frequency of ALT elevations expected for patients whose transaminase levels are monitored weekly and who receive tacrine HCl according to the recommended regimen for dose introduction and titration (see below). A dosing regimen employing a more rapid escalation of the daily dose of tacrine HCl may be associated with more serious clinical events (see below).

Tacrine Cumulative Incidence of ALT Elevations Based on Maximum Values with Weekly Monitoring (Number and (%) of Patients)

Maximum ALT	Males (n = 229)	Females (n = 250)	Total (n = 479)
Within normal limits	121 (53%)	100 (40%)	221 (46%)
> ULN	108 (47%)	150 (60%)	258 (54%)
> 2 times ULN	77 (34%)	104 (42%)	181 (38%)
> 3 times ULN	58 (25%)	81 (32%)	139 (29%)
> 10 times ULN	12 (5%)	19 (8%)	31 (6%)
> 20 times ULN	3 (1%)	6 (2%)	9 (2%)

Experience in 2446 patients who participated in all clinical trials, including the 30-week study, indicates ≈ 50% of patients treated with tacrine HCl can be expected to have at least 1 ALT level above ULN; ≈ 25% of patients are likely to develop elevations > 3 times ULN, and ≈ 7% of patients may develop elevations > 10 times ULN. Data collected from the treatment IND program were consistent with those obtained during clinical studies, and showed 3% of 5665 patients experiencing an ALT elevation > 10 times ULN.

In clinical trials where transaminases were monitored weekly, the median time to onset of the first ALT elevation above ULN was ≈ 6 weeks, with maximum ALT occurring 1 week later, even in instances when tacrine HCl treatment was stopped. Under the conditions of forced slow upwards dose titration (increases of 40 mg/day every 6 weeks) employed in clinical studies, 95% of transaminase elevations > 3 times ULN occurred within the first 18 weeks of tacrine HCl therapy, and 99% of the 10-fold elevations occurred by the 12th week and on not more than 80 mg; note, however, that for most patients ALT was monitored weekly and tacrine HCl was stopped when liver enzymes exceeded 3 times ULN. A total of 276 patients were monitored for ALT levels every other week in 2 double-blind clinical studies, an open-label study, and amended treatment IND. The incidence, severity, time to onset, peak and recovery of ALT levels were similar to weekly monitoring. With less frequent monitoring than every other week or the less stringent discontinuation criteria recommended below, it is possible that marked elevations might be more common. It must also be appreciated that experience with prolonged exposure to the high dose (160 mg/day) is limited. In all cases, transaminase levels returned to within normal limits upon discontinuation of tacrine HCl treatment or following dosage reduction, usually within 4 to 6 weeks.

This relatively benign experience may be the consequence of careful laboratory monitoring that facilitated the discontinuation of patients early on after the onset of their transaminase elevations. Consequently, frequent monitoring of serum transaminase levels is recommended.

Liver biopsy experience – Liver biopsy results in 7 patients who received tacrine HCl (1 in a Parke-Davis sponsored study and 6 in studies reported in the literature) revealed hepatocellular necrosis in 6 patients, and granulomatous changes in the seventh. In all cases, liver function tests returned to normal with no evidence of persisting hepatic dysfunction.

Experience with the rechallenge of patients with transaminase elevations following recovery – Two hundred and twelve patients among the 866 patients assigned to tacrine HCl in the 12- and 30-week studies were withdrawn because they developed transaminase elevations > 3 times ULN. One hundred and forty-five of these patients were subsequently rechallenged with weekly monitoring of ALT. During their initial exposure to tacrine, 20 of these 145 had experienced initial elevations > 10 times ULN, while the remainder had experienced elevations between 3 and 10 times ULN.

Upon rechallenge with an initial dose of 40 mg/day, only 48 (33%) of the 145 patients developed transaminase elevations > 3 times ULN. Of these patients, 44 had elevations that were between 3 and 10 times ULN and 4 had elevations that were > 10 times ULN.

The mean time to onset of elevations occurred earlier on rechallenge than on initial exposure (22 vs 48 days). Of the 145 patients rechallenged, 127 (88%) were able to continue tacrine HCl treatment, and 91 of these 127 patients titrated to doses higher than those associated with the initial transaminase elevation.

Predictors of the risk of transaminase elevations – The incidence of transaminase elevations is higher among females. There are no other known predictors of the risk of hepatocellular injury.

Monitoring of liver function and the management of the patient who develops transaminase elevations –

Blood chemistries: Serum transaminase levels (specifically ALT) should be monitored every other week from at least week 4 to week 16 following initiation of treatment, after which monitoring may be decreased to every 3 months. For patients who develop ALT elevations > 2 times the ULN, the dose and monitoring regimen should be modified.

A full monitoring sequence should be repeated in the event that a patient suspends treatment with tacrine HCl for > 4 weeks.

If ALT elevations occur, the frequency of monitoring and the dose of tacrine HCl should be modified.

Rechallenge: Patients with clinical jaundice confirmed by a significant elevation in total bilirubin (> 3 mg/dL) or those exhibiting clinical signs or symptoms of hypersensitivity (eg, rash, fever) in association with ALT elevations should immediately and permanently discontinue tacrine HCl and not be rechallenged. Other patients who are required to discontinue tacrine HCl treatment because of ALT elevations may be rechallenged once ALT levels return to within healthy limits.

See Administration and Dosage for more information.

Liver biopsy: Liver biopsy is not indicated in cases of uncomplicated transaminase elevation.

➤*Pregnancy: Category C.* Animal reproduction studies have not been conducted with tacrine HCl. It is also not known whether tacrine HCl can cause fetal harm when administered to a pregnant woman or can affect reproductive capacity.

➤*Lactation:* It is not known whether this drug is excreted in human milk.

➤*Children:* There are no adequate and well-controlled trials to document the safety and efficacy of tacrine HCl in any dementing illness occurring in pediatric patients.

➤*Lab test abnormalities:* An absolute neutrophil count (ANC) < 500/mcL occurred in 4 patients who received tacrine HCl during the course of clinical trials. Three of the 4 patients had concurrent medical conditions commonly associated with a low ANC; 2 of these patients remained on tacrine. The fourth patient, who had a history of hypersensitivity (penicillin allergy), withdrew from the study as a result of a rash and also developed an ANC < 500/mcL, which returned to normal; this patient was not rechallenged and, therefore, the role played by tacrine HCl in this reaction is unknown.

Six patients had an absolute neutrophil count ≤ 1500/mcL, associated with an elevation of ALT.

The total clinical experience in > 12,000 patients does not indicate a clear association between tacrine HCl treatment and serious white blood cell abnormalities.

➤*Monitoring:* See Warnings/Precautions for more information.

Drug Interactions

➤*CYP450 system:* Tacrine HCl is primarily eliminated by hepatic metabolism via cytochrome P450 drug metabolizing enzymes. Drug interactions may occur when tacrine HCl is given concurrently with agents such as theophylline that undergo extensive metabolism via cytochrome P450 1A2.

Tacrine Drug Interactions

Precipitant drug	Object drug[a]		Description
Cimetidine	Tacrine	↑	Cimetidine increased the C_{max} and AUC of tacrine by ≈ 54% and 64%, respectively.
Tacrine	Anticholinergics	↓	Because of its mechanism of action, tacrine has the potential to interfere with the activity of anticholinergic medications.
Tacrine	Cholinomimetics/ Cholinesterase inhibitors	↑	A synergistic effect is expected when tacrine is given concurrently with succinylcholine, cholinesterase inhibitors or cholinergic agonists (eg, bethanechol).
Tacrine	Theophylline	↑	Coadministration increased theophylline elimination half-life and average plasma levels by ≈ 2-fold; monitor plasma theophylline concentrations and reduce theophylline dose as appropriate.

[a] ↑ = object drug increased; ↓ = object drug decreased.

➤*Fluvoxamine:* In a study of 13 healthy, male volunteers, a single 40 mg dose of tacrine HCl added to fluvoxamine 100 mg/day administered at steady-state was associated with 5- and 8-fold increases in tacrine HCl C_{max} and AUC, respectively, compared to the administration of tacrine HCl alone. Five subjects experienced nausea, vomiting, sweating, and diarrhea following coadministration, consistent with the cholinergic effects of tacrine.

Adverse Reactions

➤*Common adverse events leading to discontinuation:* In clinical trials, ≈ 17% of the 2706 patients who received tacrine and 5% of the 1886 patients who received placebo withdrew permanently because of adverse events. It should be noted that some of the placebo-treated patients were exposed to tacrine HCl prior to receiving placebo due to the variety of study designs used, including crossover studies. Apart from withdrawals due to transaminase elevations, 244 patients (9%) withdrew for adverse events while receiving tacrine HCl.

Hepatic – Transaminase elevations were the most common reason for withdrawals during tacrine treatment (8% of all tacrine-treated patients, or 212 of 456 patients withdrawn). The controlled clinical trial protocols required that any patient with an ALT elevation > 3 times ULN be withdrawn, because of concern about potential hepatotoxicity.

Miscellaneous – Other adverse events that most frequently led to the withdrawal of tacrine-treated patients in clinical trials were nausea or vomiting (1.5%), agitation (0.9%), rash (0.7%), anorexia (0.7%), and confusion (0.5%). These adverse events also most frequently led to the withdrawal of placebo-treated patients, although at lower frequencies (0.1% to 0.2%).

➤*Most frequent:* The events identified here are those that occurred at an absolute incidence of at least 5% of patients treated with tacrine HCl, and at a rate at least 2-fold higher in patients treated with tacrine HCl than placebo. The most common adverse events associated with the use of tacrine HCl were elevated transaminases, nausea or vomiting, diarrhea, dyspepsia, myalgia, anorexia, and ataxia. Of these events, nausea or vomiting, diarrhea, dyspepsia, and anorexia appeared to be dose dependent.

➤*Adverse events reported in controlled trials:*

Tacrine HCl Adverse Events (≥ 2%) (Number [%] of Patients)[a]

Body system/adverse events	Tacrine HCl (n = 634)	Placebo (n = 342)
Laboratory abnormalities		
Elevated transaminase[b]	184 (29%)	5 (2%)
Miscellaneous		
Headache	67 (11%)	52 (15%)
Fatigue	26 (4%)	9 (3%)
Chest pain	24 (4%)	18 (5%)
Weight decrease	21 (3%)	4 (1%)
Back pain	15 (2%)	14 (4%)
Asthenia	15 (2%)	7 (2%)
GI		
Nausea or vomiting	178 (28%)	29 (9%)
Diarrhea	99 (16%)	18 (5%)
Dyspepsia	57 (9%)	22 (6%)
Anorexia	54 (9%)	11 (3%)
Abdominal pain	48 (8%)	24 (7%)
Flatulence	22 (4%)	5 (2%)
Constipation	24 (4%)	8 (2%)
Hematologic-lymphatic system		
Purpura	15 (2%)	8 (2%)
Musculoskeletal system		
Myalgia	54 (9%)	18 (5%)
CNS		
Dizziness	73 (12%)	39 (11%)
Confusion	42 (7%)	24 (7%)
Ataxia	36 (6%)	12 (4%)
Insomnia	37 (6%)	18 (5%)
Somnolence	22 (4%)	11 (3%)
Tremor	14 (2%)	2 (< 1%)
Psychiatric		
Agitation	43 (7%)	30 (9%)
Depression	22 (4%)	14 (4%)
Thinking abnormal	17 (3%)	14 (4%)
Anxiety	16 (3%)	7 (2%)
Hallucination	15 (2%)	12 (4%)
Hostility	15 (2%)	5 (2%)
Respiratory system		
Rhinitis	51 (8%)	22 (6%)
Upper respiratory tract infection	18 (3%)	11 (3%)
Coughing	17 (3%)	18 (5%)
Dermatologic		
Rash[c]	46 (7%)	18 (5%)
Facial flushing, skin flushing	16 (3%)	3 (< 1%)
GU		
Urination frequency	21 (3%)	12 (4%)
Urinary tract infection	21 (3%)	20 (6%)
Urinary incontinence	16 (3%)	9 (3%)

[a] Adverse events occurring in at least 2% of patients receiving tacrine hydrochloride at a starting dose of 40 mg/day with titration in 40 mg/day increments every 6 weeks in controlled clinical trials

[b] ALT or AST value of ≈ 3 × ULN or greater or that resulted in a change in patient management. Patients were monitored weekly.

[c] Includes COSTART terms: rash, rash-erythematous, rash-maculopapular, urticaria, petechial rash, rash-vesiculobullous, and pruritus.

➤*Other adverse events observed during all clinical trials:* Tacrine HCl has been administered to 2,706 individuals during clinical trials. A total of 1,471 patients were treated for at least 3 months, 1,137 for at least 6 months, and 773 for at least 1 year. Any untoward reactions that occurred during these trials were recorded as adverse events by the clinical investigators using terminology of their own choosing. To provide a meaningful estimate of the proportion of individuals having similar types of events, the events were grouped into a smaller number of standardized categories using a modified dictionary. These categories are used in the listing below. The frequencies represent the proportion of the 2,706 individuals exposed to tacrine HCl who experienced that event while receiving tacrine HCl. All adverse events are included except those already listed in the previous paragraphs and those terms too general to be informative. Events are further classified by body system categories and listed using the following definitions: Frequent adverse events are defined as those occurring in at least 1/100 patients; infrequent adverse events are those occurring in 1/100 to 1/1,000 patients; and rare adverse events are those occurring in < 1/1,000 patients. These adverse events are not necessarily related to tacrine HCl treatment. Only rare adverse events deemed to be potentially important are included.

Cardiovascular –

Frequent: Hypotension, hypertension.

Infrequent: Heart failure, MI, angina pectoris, cerebrovascular accident, transient ischemic attack, phlebitis, venous insufficiency, abdominal aortic

TACRINE HYDROCHLORIDE — ORAL

aneurysm, atrial fibrillation or flutter, palpitation, tachycardia, bradycardia, pulmonary embolus, migraine, hypercholesterolemia.

Rare: Heart arrest, premature atrial contractions, AV block, bundle branch block.

CNS –

Frequent: Convulsions, vertigo, syncope, hyperkinesia, paresthesia.

Infrequent: Dreaming abnormal, dysarthria, aphasia, amnesia, wandering, twitching, hypesthesia, delirium, paralysis, bradykinesia, movement disorder, cogwheel rigidity, paresis, neuritis, hemiplegia, Parkinson's disease, neuropathy, extrapyramidal syndrome, reflexes decreased/absent.

Rare: Tardive dyskinesia, dysesthesia, dystonia, encephalitis, coma, apraxia, oculogyric crisis, akathisia, oral facial dyskinesia, Bell's palsy, exacerbation of Parkinson's disease.

Dermatologic –

Frequent: Sweating increased.

Infrequent: Acne, alopecia, dermatitis, eczema, skin dry, herpes zoster, psoriasis, cellulitis, cyst, furunculosis, herpes simplex, hyperkeratosis, basal cell carcinoma, skin cancer.

Rare: Desquamation, seborrhea, squamous cell carcinoma, ulcer (skin), skin necrosis, melanoma.

Endocrine –

Infrequent: Diabetes.

Rare: Hyperthyroid, hypothyroid.

GI –

Infrequent: Glossitis, gingivitis, mouth or throat dry, stomatitis, increased salivation, dysphagia, esophagitis, gastritis, gastroenteritis, GI hemorrhage, stomach ulcer, hiatal hernia, hemorrhoids, stools bloody, diverticulitis, fecal impaction, fecal incontinence, hemorrhage (rectum), cholelithiasis, cholecystitis, increased appetite.

Rare: Duodenal ulcer, bowel obstruction.

GU –

Infrequent: Hematuria, renal stone, kidney infection, glycosuria, dysuria, polyuria, nocturia, pyuria, cystitis, urinary retention, urination urgency, vaginal hemorrhage, pruritus (genital), breast pain, impotence, prostate cancer.

Rare: Bladder tumor, renal tumor, renal failure, urinary obstruction, breast cancer, epididymitis, carcinoma (ovary).

Hematologic / Lymphatic –

Infrequent: Anemia, lymphadenopathy.

Rare: Leukopenia, thrombocytopenia, hemolysis, pancytopenia.

Musculoskeletal –

Frequent: Fracture, arthralgia, arthritis, hypertonia.

Infrequent: Osteoporosis, tendinitis, bursitis, gout.

Rare: Myopathy.

Psychiatric –

Frequent: Nervousness.

Infrequent: Apathy, increased libido, paranoia, neurosis.

Rare: Suicidal ideation, psychosis, hysteria.

Respiratory –

Frequent: Pharyngitis, sinusitis, bronchitis, pneumonia, dyspnea.

Infrequent: Epistaxis, chest congestion, asthma, hyperventilation, lower respiratory tract infection.

Rare: Hemoptysis, lung edema, lung cancer, acute epiglottitis.

Special senses –

Frequent: Conjunctivitis.

Infrequent: Cataract, eyes dry, eye pain, visual field defect, diplopia, amblyopia, glaucoma, hordeolum, deafness, earache, tinnitus, inner ear infection, otitis media, unusual taste.

Rare: Vision loss, ptosis, blepharitis, labyrinthitis, inner ear disturbance.

Miscellaneous –

Frequent: Chill, fever, malaise, peripheral edema.

Infrequent: Face edema, dehydration, weight increase, cachexia, edema (generalized), lipoma.

Rare: Heat exhaustion, sepsis, cholinergic crisis, death.

➤*Postmarketing:* Voluntary reports of adverse events temporally associated with tacrine HCl that have been received since market introduction, that are not listed above, and that may have no causal relationship with the drug include the following: Pancreatitis, perforated peptic ulcer, and falling.

Overdosage

➤*Symptoms:* Overdosage with cholinesterase inhibitors can cause a cholinergic crisis characterized by severe nausea/vomiting, salivation, sweating, bradycardia, hypotension, collapse, and convulsions. Increasing muscle weakness is a possibility and may result in death if respiratory muscles are involved.

➤*Treatment:* As in any case of overdose, general supportive measures should be used. Tertiary anticholinergics such as atropine may be used as an antidote for tacrine HCl overdosage. IV atropine sulfate titrated to effect is recommended.

It is not known whether tacrine HCl or its metabolites can be eliminated by dialysis (hemodialysis, peritoneal dialysis, or hemofiltration).

Patient Information

Patients and caregivers should be advised that the effect of tacrine HCl therapy is thought to depend upon its administration at regular intervals, as directed.

The caregiver should be advised about the possibility of adverse effects. Two types should be distinguished: Those occurring in close temporal association with the initiation of treatment or an increase in dose (eg, nausea, vomiting, loose stools, diarrhea), and those with a delayed onset (eg, rash, jaundice, changes in the color of stool—black, very dark or light [ie, acholic]).

Patients and caregivers should be encouraged to inform the physician about the emergence of new events or any increase in the severity of existing adverse clinical events.

Caregivers should be advised that abrupt discontinuation of tacrine HCl or a large reduction in total daily dose (≥ 80 mg/day) may cause a decline in cognitive function and behavioral disturbances. Unsupervised increases in the dose of tacrine HCl may also have serious consequences. Consequently, changes in dose should not be undertaken in the absence of direct instruction of a physician.

DONEPEZIL HYDROCHLORIDE

Rx	**Donepezil** (UDL)	**Tablets; oral:** 5 mg	Lactose. (5 G). White, round. Film-coated. In UD blister pack 300s.
Rx	**Aricept** (Eisai)		Lactose. (ARICEPT 5). White, round. Film-coated. In 30s, 90s, 1,000s, and UD 100s.
Rx	**Donepezil** (UDL)	**Tablets; oral:** 10 mg	Lactose. (10 G). Yellow, round. Film-coated. In UD blister pack 300s.
Rx	**Aricept** (Eisai)		Lactose. (ARICEPT 10). Yellow, round. Film-coated. In 30s, 90s, 1,000s, and UD blister pack 100s.
Rx	**Aricept** (Eisai)	**Tablets; oral:** 23 mg	Lactose. (ARICEPT 23). Red, round. Film-coated. In 30s, 90s.
Rx	**Donepezil** (Teva)	**Tablets, disintegrating; oral:** 5 mg	Aspartame, mannitol, phenylalanine, strawberry flavoring, xylitol. (b 151). White to off-white, round. In UD 30s.
Rx	**Aricept ODT** (Eisai)		Mannitol, polyvinyl alcohol. (ARICEPT 5). White, round. In UD 30s.
Rx	**Donepezil** (Teva)	**Tablets, disintegrating; oral:** 10 mg	Aspartame, mannitol, phenylalanine, strawberry flavoring, xylitol. (b 152). White to off-white, round. In UD 30s.
Rx	**Aricept ODT** (Eisai)		Mannitol, polyvinyl alcohol. (ARICEPT 10). Yellow, round. In UD 30s.

DONEPEZIL HYDROCHLORIDE — ORAL

Indications

➤*Alzheimer disease:* For the treatment of dementia of the Alzheimer type.

➤*Off-label uses:*

Autism – [4] = Insufficient documentation. Only 1 small retrospective trial has examined the utility of donepezil in the management of patients with autistic disorders. Larger controlled trials are required before this agent may be recommended for the treatment of this condition.

Traumatic brain injury – [1] = Good documentation. The Neurobehavioral Guidelines Working Group assigned different levels to their recommendations for drug therapy of neurobehavioral sequelae of traumatic brain injury (TBI). They ranged from options to guidelines to the highest level, standards, based on the quality of available evidence and the extent of observed efficacy. Donepezil was recommended at the guideline level for use in patients with TBI and deficits in attention, processing speed, or memory.

Other possible off-label uses – Possible treatment for vascular dementia and poststroke aphasia, and improvement of memory in multiple sclerosis patients.

Administration and Dosage

➤*Adults:*

Alzheimer disease –

Usual dosage:

- *Mild to moderate Alzheimer disease* – 5 or 10 mg once daily.
- *Moderate to severe Alzheimer disease* – 10 or 23 mg once daily.

Initial dosage: 5 mg once daily.

Dosage titration: Evidence from the controlled trials in mild to moderate Alzheimer disease indicates that the 10 mg dose, with a 1-week titration, is likely to be associated with a higher incidence of cholinergic adverse reactions than the 5 mg dose. In open-label trials using 6-week titration, the type and frequency of these same adverse reactions were similar between the 5 and 10 mg dose groups. Therefore, because steady state is achieved approximately 15 days after it is started and the incidence of untoward reac-

DONEPEZIL HYDROCHLORIDE — ORAL

tions may be influenced by the rate of dose escalation, a dose of 10 mg should not be administered until patients have been on a daily dose of 5 mg for 4 to 6 weeks. A dosage of donepezil 23 mg once daily can be administered once patients have been on a dosage of donepezil 10 mg once daily for at least 3 months.

Off-label dosing –

Traumatic brain injury: [1] = Good documentation. 5 to 10 mg/day orally, continued through subacute or chronic periods of recovery if response is adequate.

➤*Children:*

Off-label dosing –

Autism: [4] = Insufficient documentation. 2.5 mg/day for 1 week, then increased by 2.5 mg/wk until a maximal tolerated dose or 10 mg/day is reached.

➤*Administration:* Instruct patients to take in the evening, just prior to retiring, with or without food. Tablets should be swallowed whole with water. Do not split or crush the tablets. The 23 mg tablet should not be crushed or chewed because this may increase its rate of absorption. Allow donepezil orally disintegrating tablets to dissolve on the tongue and follow with water.

➤*Storage/Stability:* Store at 15° to 30°C (59° to 86°F).

Actions

➤*Pharmacology:* Donepezil, a reversible inhibitor of the enzyme acetylcholinesterase, is postulated to exert its therapeutic effect by enhancing cholinergic function. This is accomplished by increasing the concentration of acetylcholine through reversible inhibition of its hydrolysis by acetylcholinesterase.

➤*Pharmacokinetics:*

Absorption – Based on population pharmacokinetic analysis of plasma donepezil concentrations measured in patients with Alzheimer disease, following oral dosing, maximal drug concentration (C_{max}) is achieved for donepezil 23 mg tablets in approximately 8 hours, compared with 3 hours for donepezil 10 mg tablets. C_{max} was almost 2-fold higher for donepezil 23 mg tablets than donepezil 10 mg tablets.

Distribution – Following multiple-dose administration, donepezil accumulates in plasma by 4- to 7-fold, and steady state is reached within 15 days. The steady-state volume of distribution is 12 to 16 L/kg. Donepezil is approximately 96% bound to human plasma proteins, mainly to albumins (approximately 75%) and alpha-1 acid glycoprotein (approximately 21%) over the concentration range of 2 to 1,000 ng/mL.

Metabolism – Donepezil is extensively metabolized to 4 major metabolites (2 of which are known to be active) and a number of minor metabolites, not all of which have been identified. Donepezil is metabolized by the cytochrome P450 (CYP-450) isoenzymes 2D6 and 3A4, and undergoes glucuronidation. Following administration of ^{14}C-labeled donepezil, plasma radioactivity, expressed as a percent of the administered dose, was present primarily as intact donepezil (53%) and as 6-O-desmethyl donepezil (11%). 6-O-desmethyl donepezil has been reported to inhibit acetylcholinesterase to the same extent as donepezil in vitro and was found in plasma at concentrations equal to approximately 20% of donepezil.

Excretion – The elimination half-life of donepezil is approximately 70 hours and the mean apparent plasma clearance is 0.13 to 0.19 L/h/kg. Donepezil is excreted in the urine intact. Approximately 57% and 15% of the total radioactivity was recovered in urine and feces, respectively, over a period of 10 days, while 28% remained unrecovered. Approximately 17% of the donepezil dose was recovered in the urine as unchanged drug. Examination of the effect of CYP2D6 genotype in patients with Alzheimer disease showed differences in clearance values among CYP2D6 genotype subgroups. When compared with the extensive metabolizers, poor metabolizers had a 31.5% slower clearance, and ultra-rapid metabolizers had a 24% faster clearance. These results suggest CYP2D6 has a minor role in the metabolism of donepezil.

Special populations –

Hepatic function impairment: In a study of 10 patients with stable alcoholic cirrhosis, the clearance of donepezil was decreased 20% relative to 10 age- and sex-matched healthy subjects.

Body weight: There was a relationship noted between body weight and clearance. Over the range of body weight from 50 to 110 kg, clearance increased from 7.77 to 14.04 L/h, with a value of 10 L/h for 70 kg individuals.

Contraindications

Hypersensitivity to donepezil or to piperidine derivatives.

Warnings/Precautions

➤*Cardiovascular effects:* Because of their pharmacological action, cholinesterase inhibitors may have vagotonic effects on the sinoatrial and atrioventricular nodes. This effect may manifest as bradycardia or heart block in patients with and without known underlying cardiac conduction abnormalities. Syncopal episodes have been reported in association with the use of donepezil.

➤*GI effects:*

Peptic ulcer/GI bleeding – Through their primary action, cholinesterase inhibitors may be expected to increase gastric acid secretion because of increased cholinergic activity. Therefore, monitor patients closely for symptoms of active or occult GI bleeding, especially those at increased risk for developing ulcers (eg, those with a history of ulcer disease or those receiving concurrent nonsteroidal anti-inflammatory drugs [NSAIDs]). Clinical studies of donepezil 5 to 10 mg/day have shown no increase relative to placebo in the incidence of peptic ulcer disease or GI bleeding. Results of a controlled clinical study with donepezil 23 mg/day showed an increase, relative to a dosage of 10 mg/day, in the incidence of peptic ulcer disease (0.4% vs 0.2%) and GI bleeding from any site (1.1% vs 0.6%).

Nausea/Vomiting – Donepezil, as a predictable consequence of its pharmacological properties, produced diarrhea, nausea, and vomiting. These effects, when they occur, appear more frequently with the 10 mg/day dosage than with the 5 mg/day dosage and more frequently with the 23 mg dose than with the 10 mg dose. Specifically, in a controlled trial that compared a dose of 23 mg/day to 10 mg/day in patients who had been treated with donepezil 10 mg/day for at least 3 months, the incidence of nausea in the 23 mg group was markedly greater than in the patients who continued on 10 mg/day (11.8% vs 3.4%, respectively), and the incidence of vomiting in the 23 mg group was markedly greater than in the 10 mg group (9.2% vs 2.5%, respectively). The percent of patients who discontinued treatment because of vomiting in the 23 mg group was markedly higher than in the 10 mg group (2.9% vs 0.4%, respectively). Although in most cases, these effects were mild and transient, sometimes lasting 1 to 3 weeks, and resolved during continued use of donepezil, closely observe patients at the initiation of treatment and after dose increases.

➤*Weight loss:* Weight loss was reported as an adverse reaction in 4.7% of patients assigned to donepezil in a dosage of 23 mg/day compared with 2.5% of patients assigned to 10 mg/day. Compared with their baseline weights, 8.4% of patients taking 23 mg/day had a weight decrease of 7% or more by the end of the study, while 4.9% of patients taking 10 mg/day experienced a weight loss of 7% or more at the end of the study.

➤*Genitourinary effects:* Although not observed in clinical trials, cholinomimetics may cause bladder outflow obstruction.

➤*Seizures:* Cholinomimetics are believed to have some potential to cause generalized convulsions. However, seizure activity also may be a manifestation of Alzheimer disease.

➤*Pulmonary effects:* Because of their cholinomimetic actions, prescribe cholinesterase inhibitors with care to patients with a history of asthma or obstructive pulmonary disease.

➤*Lower-weight individuals:* In the controlled clinical trial, among patients in the donepezil 23 mg treatment group, patients weighing less than 55 kg reported more nausea, vomiting, and decreased weight than patients weighing 55 kg or more. There were also more withdrawals due to adverse reactions. This finding may be related to higher plasma exposure associated with lower weight.

➤*Lactation:* It is not known whether donepezil is excreted in breast milk. The molecular weight of the parent compound (approximately 416) and its long plasma elimination half-life (about 70 hours) suggest that donepezil, and possibly the active metabolites, will be excreted into breast milk. The extensive protein binding (approximately 96%), however, should limit this excretion. The effects of this exposure on a breast-feeding infant are unknown.Exercise caution when donepezil is administered to a breast-feeding woman.

➤*Children:* The safety and effectiveness of donepezil in children have not been established.

➤*Monitoring:* Monitor patients closely for symptoms of active or occult GI bleeding, especially those at increased risk for developing ulcers (eg, those with a history of ulcer disease or those receiving NSAIDs). Evaluate patients' mental status, cognitive function, and activities of daily living prior to initiation of therapy and periodically thereafter during prolonged treatment.

Drug Interactions

Donepezil Drug Interactions

Precipitant drug	Object drug[a]		Description
Cholinomimetics/ Cholinesterase inhibitors (eg, bethanechol, succinylcholine)	Donepezil	⬆	A synergistic effect may be expected when cholinesterase inhibitors are given concurrently with succinylcholine, similar neuromuscular-blocking agents, or cholinergic agonists, such as bethanechol. Monitor the clinical response and adjust treatment as needed.
Donepezil	Cholinomimetics/ Cholinesterase inhibitors (eg, bethanechol succinylcholine)		
CYP-450 3A4 and 2D6 inducers (eg, carbamazepine, dexamethasone, phenobarbital, phenytoin, rifampin)	Donepezil	⬇	Inducers of CYP3A4 and CYP2D6 could increase the rate of elimination of donepezil. Monitor the clinical response and adjust the donepezil dose as needed.

DONEPEZIL HYDROCHLORIDE — ORAL

Donepezil Drug Interactions			
Precipitant drug	Object drug[a]		Description
CYP-450 3A4 and 2D6 inhibitors (eg, ketoconazole, quinidine)	Donepezil	⬆	Ketoconazole 200 mg daily increased mean donepezil 5 mg daily concentrations (AUC_{0-24}[b] and C_{max}) 36%. The clinical relevance of this increase in concentration is unknown. Monitor the clinical response and adjust the donepezil dose as needed.
Donepezil	Anticholinergics (eg, atropine)	⬇	Because of their mechanism of action, cholinesterase inhibitors have the potential to interfere with the activity of anticholinergic medications. Monitor the clinical response and adjust treatment as needed.
Donepezil	Aspirin, NSAIDs (eg, ibuprofen, naproxen)	⬆	Donepezil increases gastric acid secretions caused by increased cholinergic activity. The risk of stomach ulcers may be increased. Therefore, monitor for active or occult GI bleeding.

[a] ⬆ = object drug increased; ⬇ = object drug decreased.
[b] AUC = area under the curve.

Adverse Reactions

➤*Mild to moderate Alzheimer disease:*
Discontinuation –

Donepezil Common Adverse Reactions Leading to Withdrawal in Mild to Moderate Patients (≥ 2%)			
Adverse reactions	Donepezil 5 mg/day (n = 350)	Donepezil 10 mg/day (n = 315)	Placebo (n = 355)
GI			
Diarrhea	< 1%	3%	0%
Nausea	1%	3%	1%
Vomiting	< 1%	2%	< 1%

Common adverse reactions (at least 5%) –

Donepezil Common Adverse Reactions in Mild to Moderate Patients (≥ 5%)				
	No titration		1-week titration	6-week titration
Adverse reactions	Donepezil 5 mg/day (n = 311)	Placebo (n = 315)	Donepezil 10 mg/day (n = 315)	Donepezil 10 mg/day (n = 269)
CNS				
Fatigue	4%	3%	8%	3%
Insomnia	6%	6%	14%	6%
GI				
Anorexia	3%	2%	7%	3%
Diarrhea	8%	5%	15%	9%
Nausea	5%	6%	19%	6%
Vomiting	3%	3%	8%	5%
Musculoskeletal				
Muscle cramps	6%	2%	8%	3%

Adverse reactions (at least 2%) –

Donepezil Adverse Reactions in Mild to Moderate Patients (≥ 2%)		
Adverse reactions	Donepezil (n = 747)	Placebo (n = 355)
Any adverse reaction	74%	72%
CNS		
Abnormal dreams	3%	0%
Depression	3%	< 1%
Dizziness	8%	6%
Fatigue	5%	3%
Headache	10%	9%
Insomnia	9%	6%
Somnolence	2%	< 1%
GI		
Anorexia	4%	2%
Diarrhea	10%	5%
Nausea	11%	6%
Vomiting	5%	3%
Musculoskeletal		
Arthritis	2%	1%
Muscle cramps	6%	2%
Miscellaneous		
Accident	7%	6%
Ecchymosis	4%	3%
Frequent urination	2%	1%
Pain, various locations	9%	8%
Syncope	2%	1%
Weight decrease	3%	1%

➤*Other adverse reactions:*

Cardiovascular – Atrial fibrillation, hot flashes, hypertension, hypotension, vasodilation (at least 1%); angina pectoris, arteritis, atrioventricular block (first degree), bradycardia, congestive heart failure, deep vein thrombosis, myocardial infarction, peripheral vascular disease, postural hypotension, supraventricular tachycardia, transient ischemic attack (0.1% to 1%).

CNS – Abnormal crying, aggression, aphasia, ataxia, delusions, increased libido, irritability, nervousness, paresthesia, restlessness, tremor, vertigo (at least 1%); cerebrovascular accident, coldness (localized), decreased libido, dysarthria, dysphasia, dysphoria, emotional lability, emotional withdrawal, gait abnormality, generalized coldness, head fullness, hostility, hypertonia, hypokinesia, intracranial hemorrhage, listlessness, melancholia, neuralgia, neurodermatitis, numbness (localized), pacing, paranoia (0.1% to 1%).

Dermatologic – Diaphoresis, pruritus, urticaria (at least 1%); alopecia, dermatitis, erythema, fungal dermatitis, herpes zoster, hirsutism, hyperkeratosis, night sweats, skin discoloration, skin striae, skin ulcer (0.1% to 1%).

Endocrine – Diabetes mellitus, goiter (0.1% to 1%).

GI – Bloating, epigastric pain, fecal incontinence, GI bleeding, toothache (at least 1%); cholelithiasis, diverticulitis, drooling, dry mouth, duodenal ulcer, epigastric distress, eructation, fever sore, flatulence, gastritis, gastroenteritis, gingivitis, hemorrhoids, ileus, increased appetite, increased thirst, increased transaminases, irritable colon, jaundice, melena, periodontal abscess, polydipsia, stomach ulcer, tongue edema (0.1% to 1%).

GU – Nocturia, urinary incontinence (at least 1%); breast fibroadenosis, cystitis, dysuria, enuresis, fibrocystic breast, hematuria, inability to empty bladder, mastitis, metrorrhagia, prostate hypertrophy, pyelonephritis, pyuria, renal failure, urinary urgency, vaginitis (0.1% to 1%).

Hematologic/Lymphatic – Anemia, eosinophilia, erythrocytopenia, thrombocythemia, thrombocytopenia (0.1% to 1%).

Metabolic/Nutritional – Dehydration (at least 1%); gout, hyperglycemia, hypokalemia, increased creatine kinase, increased lactate dehydrogenase, weight increase (0.1% to 1%).

Musculoskeletal – Bone fracture (at least 1%); muscle fasciculation, muscle spasm, muscle weakness (0.1% to 1%).

Respiratory – Bronchitis, dyspnea, sore throat (at least 1%); epistaxis, hyperventilation, hypoxia, pharyngitis, pleurisy, pneumonia, postnasal drip, pulmonary collapse, pulmonary congestion, sleep apnea, snoring, wheezing (0.1% to 1%).

Special senses – Cataract, eye irritation, vision blurred (at least 1%); bad taste, blepharitis, conjunctival hemorrhage, decreased hearing, dry eyes, ear buzzing, earache, glaucoma, motion sickness, nystagmus, otitis externa, otitis media, periorbital edema, retinal hemorrhage, spots before eyes, tinnitus (0.1% to 1%).

Miscellaneous – Chest pain, influenza (at least 1%); abscess, cellulitis, chills, face edema, fever, hiatal hernia (0.1% to 1%).

➤*Severe Alzheimer disease:*

Discontinuation – The rates of discontinuation from controlled clinical trials of donepezil because of adverse reactions in the donepezil patients were approximately 12% compared with 7% for placebo patients.

The most common adverse reactions leading to discontinuation, defined as those occurring in at least 2% of donepezil patients and at twice or more the incidence seen in placebo patients, were anorexia, urinary tract infection (2% vs 1% placebo), nausea (2% vs less than 1% placebo), diarrhea (2% vs 0% placebo).

Adverse reactions (at least 2%) –

Donepezil Adverse Reactions (≥ 2%)		
Adverse reactions	Donepezil (n = 501)	Placebo (n = 392)
Any adverse reaction	81%	73%
Cardiovascular		
Hemorrhage	2%	1%
Hypertension	3%	2%

DONEPEZIL HYDROCHLORIDE — ORAL

Donepezil Adverse Reactions (≥ 2%)		
Adverse reactions	Donepezil (n = 501)	Placebo (n = 392)
Syncope	2%	1%
CNS		
Confusion	2%	1%
Depression	2%	1%
Dizziness	2%	1%
Emotional lability	2%	1%
Hallucinations	3%	1%
Headache	4%	3%
Hostility	3%	2%
Insomnia	5%	4%
Nervousness	3%	2%
Personality disorder	2%	1%
Somnolence	2%	1%
GI		
Anorexia	8%	4%
Diarrhea	10%	4%
Nausea	6%	2%
Vomiting	8%	4%
Metabolic/Nutritional		
Creatine phosphokinase increased	3%	1%
Dehydration	2%	1%
Hyperlipemia	2%	< 1%
Miscellaneous		
Accident	13%	12%
Back pain	3%	2%
Chest pain	2%	< 1%
Ecchymosis	5%	2%
Eczema	3%	2%
Fever	2%	1%
Infection	11%	9%
Pain	3%	2%
Urinary incontinence	2%	1%

Other adverse reactions –

Cardiovascular: Bradycardia, electrocardiogram abnormal, heart failure, hypotension (at least 1%); angina pectoris, atrial fibrillation, cardiomegaly, congestive heart failure, myocardial infarction, peripheral vascular disorder, supraventricular extrasystoles, vasodilatation, ventricular extrasystoles (0.1% to 1%).

CNS: Abnormal gait, agitation, anxiety, asthenia, convulsion, tremor, wandering (at least 1%); abnormal dreams, apathy, ataxia, cerebral hemorrhage, cerebral infarction, cerebral ischemia, cerebrovascular accident, delusions, dementia, euphoria, extrapyramidal syndrome, grand mal convulsion, hemiplegia, hypertonia, hypokinesia, malaise, vertigo (0.1% to 1%).

Dermatologic: Pruritus, rash, skin ulcer (at least 1%); dry skin, herpes zoster, psoriasis, skin discoloration, sweating, urticaria, vesiculobullous rash (0.1% to 1%).

GI: Abdominal pain, ALT increased, AST increased, constipation, dyspepsia, fecal incontinence, gastroenteritis (at least 1%); dysphagia, eructation, esophagitis, flatulence, gamma-glutamyl transpeptidase increase, gastritis, increased salivation, liver function tests abnormal, periodontal abscess, periodontitis, rectal hemorrhage, stomach ulcer (0.1% to 1%).

GU: Cystitis, glycosuria, hematuria, urinary tract infection (at least 1%); albuminuria, dysuria, urinary frequency, vaginitis (0.1% to 1%).

Hematologic-Lymphatic: Anemia (at least 1%); B_{12}-deficiency anemia, iron-deficiency anemia, leukocytosis (0.1% to 1%).

Metabolic/Nutritional: Alkaline phosphatase increased, edema, lactic dehydrogenase increased, peripheral edema, weight loss (at least 1%); bilirubinemia, cachexia, creatinine increased, gout, hypercholesteremia, hypoglycemia, hypokalemia, hyponatremia, hypoproteinemia, serum urea nitrogen increased, weight gain (0.1% to 1%).

Musculoskeletal: Arthritis (at least 1%); arthralgia, arthrosis, bone fracture, leg cramps, myalgia, osteoporosis (0.1% to 1%).

Respiratory: Bronchitis, cough increased, pharyngitis, pneumonia (at least 0.1%); asthma, dyspnea, rhinitis (0.1% to 1%).

Special Senses: Abnormal vision, conjunctivitis, ear pain, glaucoma, lacrimation disorder (0.1% to 1%).

Miscellaneous: Flu syndrome, fungal infection (at least 1%); allergic reaction, cellulitis, diabetes mellitus, face edema, hernia, sepsis (0.1% to 1%).

➤*Donepezil 23 mg/day:*

Discontinuation – The rate of discontinuation from a controlled trial of donepezil 23 mg/day due to adverse reactions was higher (18.6%) than for the 10 mg/day treatment group (7.9%). The majority of discontinuations due to adverse reactions in the 23 mg group occurred during the first month of treatment.

Donepezil Adverse Reactions Leading to Discontinuation (≥ 1%)		
Adverse reactions	Donepezil 23 mg/day (n = 963)	Donepezil 10 mg/day (n = 471)
CNS		
Dizziness	1%	0
GI		
Diarrhea	2%	0
Nausea	2%	0
Vomiting	3%	0

Adverse reactions (≥ 2%) –

Donepezil Adverse Reactions Reported (≥ 2%)		
Adverse reactions	Donepezil 23 mg/day (n = 963)	Donepezil 10 mg/day (n = 471)
Any adverse reaction	74%	64%
CNS		
Asthenia	2%	1%
Dizziness	5%	3%
Fatigue	2%	1%
Headache	4%	3%
Insomnia	3%	2%
Somnolence	2%	1%
GI		
Diarrhea	8%	5%
Nausea	12%	3%
Vomiting	9%	3%
Metabolic/Nutritional		
Anorexia	5%	2%
Weight decreased	5%	3%
Miscellaneous		
Contusion	2%	0%
Urinary incontinence	3%	1%

➤*Postmarketing:*

CNS – Agitation, confusion, convulsions, hallucinations neuroleptic malignant syndrome.

GI – Abdominal pain, cholecystitis, hepatitis, pancreatitis.

Miscellaneous – Heart block (all types), hemolytic anemia, hyponatremia, rash.

Overdosage

➤*Symptoms:* Overdosage with cholinesterase inhibitors can result in cholinergic crisis characterized by severe nausea, vomiting, salivation, sweating, bradycardia, hypotension, respiratory depression, collapse, and convulsions. Increasing muscle weakness is a possibility and may result in death if respiratory muscles are involved.

➤*Treatment:* As in any case of overdose, use general supportive measures. Tertiary anticholinergics such as atropine may be used as an antidote for donepezil overdosage. Intravenous (IV) atropine titrated to effect is recommended as follows: an initial dose of 1 to 2 mg IV with subsequent doses based upon clinical response. Atypical responses in blood pressure and heart rate have been reported with other cholinomimetics when coadministered with quarternary anticholinergics such as glycopyrrolate. It is not known whether donepezil and/or its metabolites can be removed by dialysis (eg, hemodialysis, peritoneal dialysis, hemofiltration).

Patient Information

Inform patients to take donepezil in the evening, just prior to retiring.

Donepezil may be taken with or without food.

Advise patients not to swallow the orally disintegrating tablets whole but to allow the tablets to dissolve on the tongue and follow by drinking water.

Inform patients to swallow the tablets whole, and not to split or crush the tablets.

Inform patients that donepezil may cause nausea, diarrhea, insomnia, vomiting, muscle cramps, fatigue, and decreased appetite.

RIVASTIGMINE

Rx	**Rivastigmine** (Dr. Reddy's Laboratories)	**Capsules; oral:** 1.5 mg	As rivastigmine tartrate. (RDY 352). Tan. In 30s, 60s, 100s, and 500s.
Rx	**Exelon** (Novartis)		As rivastigmine tartrate. (Exelon 1, 5 mg). Yellow. In 60s, 500s, UD 30s, and UD 100s.
Rx	**Rivastigmine** (Dr. Reddy's Laboratories)	**Capsules; oral:** 3 mg	As rivastigmine tartrate. (RDY 353). Brown. In 30s, 60s, 100s, and 500s.
Rx	**Exelon** (Novartis)		As rivastigmine tartrate. (Exelon 3 mg). Orange. In 60s, 500s, UD 30s, and UD 100s.
Rx	**Rivastigmine** (Dr. Reddy's Laboratories)	**Capsules; oral:** 4.5 mg	As rivastigmine tartrate. (RDY 354). Brick red. In 30s, 60s, 100s, and 500s.
Rx	**Exelon** (Novartis)		As rivastigmine tartrate. (Exelon 4, 5 mg). Red. In 60s, 500s, UD 30s, and UD 100s.
Rx	**Rivastigmine** (Dr. Reddy's Laboratories)	**Capsules; oral:** 6 mg	As rivastigmine tartrate. (RDY 355). Brick red/brown. In 30s, 60s, 100s, and 500s.
Rx	**Exelon** (Novartis)		As rivastigmine tartrate. (Exelon 6 mg). Orange/red. In 60s, 500s, UD 30s, and UD 100s.
Rx	**Exelon** (Novartis)	**Solution; oral:** 2 mg/mL	As rivastigmine tartrate. In 120 mL bottles.
Rx	**Exelon** (Novartis)	**Patch; transdermal:** 4.6 mg/24 h	9 mg total rivastigmine per transdermal system. 5 cm^2. (4.6 mg/24/AMCX). In 30s.
		9.5 mg/24 h	18 mg total rivastigmine per transdermal system. 10 cm^2. (9.5 mg/24/BHDI). In 30s.

RIVASTIGMINE TARTRATE — ORAL

Indications

➤*Alzheimer dementia:* For the treatment of mild to moderate dementia of the Alzheimer type.

➤*Dementia associated with Parkinson disease:* For the treatment of mild to moderate dementia associated with Parkinson disease.

➤*Off-label uses:*

Diffuse Lewy body disease – [1] = Good documentation. Therapeutic options for the management of behavioral symptoms associated with Lewy body dementia are limited. Cholinesterase inhibitors are recommended for treatment of neuropsychiatric symptoms associated with Lewy body dementia by the Dementia with Lewy Bodies Consortium; however, rivastigmine is the only cholinesterase inhibitor with placebo-controlled data supporting its use. Although limited to fewer than 200 patients, initial data indicate rivastigmine provides statistically significant early improvement in clinical and cognitive assessments in patients with dementia with Lewy bodies and no deterioration with long-term therapy. In patients who do not respond to cholinesterase inhibitors, a cautious trial of an atypical antipsychotic agent may be warranted after warning the patient and caregiver about the potential for severe sensitivity reactions.

Administration and Dosage

➤*General dosing considerations:* Rivastigmine oral solution and capsules may be interchanged at equal doses.

➤*Adults:*

Alzheimer dementia –

Maximum dose: 12 mg/day (6 mg twice daily).

Initial dosage: 1.5 mg twice a day.

Dosage titration: If the initial dose is well-tolerated after a minimum of 2 weeks of treatment, it may be increased to 3 mg twice daily. Subsequent increases to 4.5 mg twice daily and 6 mg twice daily should be attempted after a minimum of 2 weeks at the previous dose.

Maintenance dosage: 3 to 6 mg twice daily (6 to 12 mg/day). There is evidence from the clinical trials that doses at the higher end of this range may be more beneficial.

Dosage adjustment: If adverse reactions (eg, nausea, vomiting, abdominal pain, loss of appetite) cause intolerance during treatment, the patient should be instructed to discontinue treatment for several doses and then restart at the same or next lower dose level. If treatment is interrupted for longer than several days, treatment should be reinitiated with the lowest daily dose and titrated as previously described.

Dementia associated with Parkinson disease –

Initial dosage: 1.5 mg twice daily.

Dosage titration: The dose may be increased to 3 mg twice daily and further to 4.5 mg twice daily and 6 mg twice daily, based on tolerability, with a minimum of 4 weeks at each dose.

Maintenance dosage: 1.5 to 6 mg twice daily (3 to 12 mg/day).

Off-label dosing –

Diffuse Lewy body disease: [1] = Good documentation. 1.5 mg orally twice daily initially, increased as tolerated by 1.5 mg twice daily every 2 weeks to a maximum of 6 mg twice daily. Ongoing therapy is required; rivastigmine has been studied for up to 96 weeks in patients with dementia with Lewy bodies.

➤*Administration:* Rivastigmine should be taken with food in divided doses in the morning and evening.

Administration of oral solution –

Each dose of rivastigmine oral solution may be swallowed directly from the syringe or first mixed with a small glass of water, cold fruit juice, or soda. Patients should be instructed to stir and drink the mixture.

➤*Storage/Stability:* Store at 25°C (77°F); excursions are permitted between 15° and 30°C (59° and 86°F). Store capsules in a tight container. Store oral solution in an upright position and protect from freezing. When rivastigmine oral solution is combined with cold fruit juice or soda, the mixture is stable at room temperature for up to 4 hours.

Actions

➤*Pharmacology:* Pathological changes in dementia of the Alzheimer type and dementia associated with Parkinson disease involve cholinergic neuronal pathways that project from the basal forebrain to the cerebral cortex and hippocampus. These pathways are thought to be intricately involved in memory, attention, learning, and other cognitive processes. While the precise mechanism of rivastigmine's action is unknown, it is postulated to exert its therapeutic effect by enhancing cholinergic function. This is accomplished by increasing the concentration of acetylcholine through reversible inhibition of its hydrolysis by cholinesterase. If this proposed mechanism is correct, rivastigmine's effect may lessen as the disease process advances and fewer cholinergic neurons remain functionally intact. There is no evidence that rivastigmine alters the course of the underlying dementing process. After a dose of rivastigmine 6 mg, anticholinesterase activity is present in cerebrospinal fluid (CSF) for about 10 hours, with a maximum inhibition of about 60% five hours after dosing.

➤*Pharmacokinetics:*

Absorption – Rivastigmine is rapidly and completely absorbed, with absolute bioavailability of about 40% (3 mg dose). It shows linear pharmacokinetics at doses up to 3 mg twice daily but is nonlinear at higher dosages. Doubling the dose from 3 to 6 mg twice daily results in a 3-fold increase in the AUC. Peak plasma concentrations are reached in approximately 1 hour. Absolute bioavailability after a 3 mg dose is about 36%.

Food effects: Administration of rivastigmine with food delays absorption (time to maximum concentration [T_{max}]) by 90 minutes, lowers maximal drug concentration (C_{max}) approximately 30%, and increases area under the curve (AUC) approximately 30%.

Distribution – Rivastigmine is widely distributed throughout the body, with a volume of distribution in the range of 1.8 to 2.7 L/kg. Rivastigmine penetrates the blood-brain barrier, reaching CSF peak concentrations in 1.4 to 2.6 hours. The mean $AUC_{1\text{-}12\ h}$ ratio of CSF/plasma averaged 40 ± 0.5% following 1 to 6 mg twice-daily doses.

Rivastigmine is about 40% bound to plasma proteins at concentrations of 1 to 400 ng/mL, which cover the therapeutic concentration range. Rivastigmine distributes equally between blood and plasma, with a blood-to-plasma partition ratio of 0.9 at concentrations ranging from 1 to 400 ng/mL.

Metabolism – Rivastigmine is rapidly and extensively metabolized, primarily via cholinesterase-mediated hydrolysis to the decarbamylated metabolite. Based on evidence from in vitro and animal studies, the major CYP-450 isozymes are minimally involved in rivastigmine metabolism. Consistent with these observations is the finding that no drug interactions related to CYP-450 have been observed in humans.

Excretion – The elimination half-life is about 1.5 hours, with most elimination as metabolites via the urine. The major pathway of elimination is the kidneys. Following administration of ^{14}C-rivastigmine to 6 healthy volunteers, total recovery of radioactivity over 120 hours was 97% in urine and 0.4% in feces. No parent drug was detected in urine. The sulfate conjugate of the decarbamylated metabolite is the major component excreted in urine and represents 40% of the dose. Mean oral clearance of rivastigmine is 1.8 ± 0.6 L/min after 6 mg twice daily.

Special populations –

Renal function impairment: Following a single 3 mg dose, mean oral clearance of rivastigmine is 64% lower in moderately impaired renal patients (n = 8, glomerular filtration rate [GFR] 10 to 50 mL/min) than in healthy subjects (n = 10, GFR 60 mL/min); plasma clearance (Cl/F) was 1.7 L/min (coefficient of variation [CV] 45%) and 4.8 L/min (CV 80%), respectively. In

RIVASTIGMINE TARTRATE — ORAL

severely impaired renal patients (n = 8, GFR less than 10 mL/min), mean oral clearance of rivastigmine is 43% higher than in healthy subjects (n = 10, GFR equal to 60 mL/min); Cl/F was 6.9 and 4.8 L/min, respectively. For unexplained reasons, the severely impaired renal patients had a higher clearance of rivastigmine than moderately impaired patients. However, dosage adjustment may not be necessary in renally impaired patients because the dose of the drug is individually titrated to tolerability.

Hepatic function impairment: Following a single 3 mg dose, mean oral clearance of rivastigmine was 60% lower in hepatically impaired patients (n = 10, biopsy proven) than in healthy subjects (n = 10). After multiple 6 mg twice-daily oral doses, the mean clearance of rivastigmine was 65% lower in mild (n = 7, Child-Pugh score 5 to 6) and moderate (n = 3, Child-Pugh score 7 to 9) hepatically impaired patients (biopsy proven, liver cirrhosis) than in healthy subjects (n = 10). Dosage adjustment is not necessary in hepatically impaired patients because the dose of drug is individually titrated to tolerability.

Age: Following a single 2.5 mg oral dose to elderly volunteers (older than 60 years of age, n = 24) and younger volunteers (n = 24), mean oral clearance of rivastigmine was 30% lower in elderly (7 L/min) than in younger subjects (10 L/min).

Nicotine use: Population pharmacokinetic analysis showed that nicotine use increases the oral clearance of rivastigmine 23% (75 smokers, 549 nonsmokers).

Contraindications

Known hypersensitivity to rivastigmine, other carbamate derivatives, or other components of the formulation.

Warnings/Precautions

➤*GI adverse reactions:* Rivastigmine use is associated with significant GI adverse reactions, including nausea and vomiting, anorexia, and weight loss. For this reason, always start patients at a dose of 1.5 mg twice daily and titrate to their maintenance dose. If treatment is interrupted for longer than several days, reinitiate treatment with the lowest daily dose to reduce the possibility of severe vomiting and its potentially serious sequelae (eg, there has been 1 postmarketing report of severe vomiting with esophageal rupture following inappropriate reinitiation of treatment with a 4.5 mg dose after 8 weeks of treatment interruption).

Nausea and vomiting – In the controlled clinical trials, 47% of the patients treated with a rivastigmine dose in the therapeutic range of 6 to 12 mg/day (n = 1,189) developed nausea (compared with 12% in placebo). A total of 31% of rivastigmine-treated patients developed at least 1 episode of vomiting (compared with 6% for placebo). The rate of vomiting was higher during the titration phase (24% vs 3% for placebo) than in the maintenance phase (14% vs 3% for placebo). The rates were higher in women than men. Five percent of patients discontinued for vomiting, compared with less than 1% for patients on placebo. Vomiting was severe in 2% of rivastigmine-treated patients and was rated as mild or moderate in 14% of patients. The rate of nausea was higher during the titration phase (43% vs 9% for placebo) than in the maintenance phase (17% vs 4% for placebo).

Weight loss – In the controlled trials, approximately 26% of women on high dosages of rivastigmine (greater than 9 mg/day) had weight loss of greater than or equal to 7% of their baseline weight, compared with 6% in the placebo-treated patients. About 18% of the men in the high-dosage group experienced a similar degree of weight loss, compared with 4% in placebo-treated patients. It is not clear how much of the weight loss was caused by anorexia, nausea, vomiting, and diarrhea associated with the drug.

Anorexia – In the controlled trials, of the patients treated with a dosage of rivastigmine 6 to 12 mg/day, 17% developed anorexia, compared with 3% of the placebo patients. Neither the time course or the severity of the anorexia is known.

Peptic ulcers/GI bleeding – Because of their pharmacological action, cholinesterase inhibitors may be expected to increase gastric acid secretion as a result of increased cholinergic activity. Therefore, monitor patients closely for symptoms of active or occult GI bleeding, especially those at increased risk for developing ulcers (eg, those with a history of ulcer disease, those receiving concurrent nonsteroidal anti-inflammatory drugs [NSAIDs]). Clinical studies of rivastigmine have shown no significant increase, relative to placebo, in the incidence of peptic ulcer disease or GI bleeding.

➤*Anesthesia:* Rivastigmine, as a cholinesterase inhibitor, is likely to exaggerate succinylcholine-type muscle relaxation during anesthesia.

➤*Cardiovascular effects:* Drugs that increase cholinergic activity may have vagotonic effects on heart rate (eg, bradycardia). The potential for this action may be particularly important to patients with sick sinus syndrome or other supraventricular cardiac conduction conditions. In clinical trials, rivastigmine was not associated with any increased incidence of cardiovascular adverse reactions, heart rate or blood pressure changes, or electrocardiogram abnormalities. Syncopal episodes have been reported in 3% of patients receiving rivastigmine 6 to 12 mg/day, compared with 2% of placebo patients.

➤*Urinary obstruction:* Although this was not observed in clinical trials of rivastigmine, drugs that increase cholinergic activity may cause urinary obstruction.

➤*Seizures:* Drugs that increase cholinergic activity are believed to have some potential for causing seizures. However, seizure activity also may be a manifestation of Alzheimer disease.

➤*Pulmonary effects:* Like other drugs that increase cholinergic activity, use rivastigmine with care in patients with a history of asthma or obstructive pulmonary disease.

➤*Pregnancy:* Category B. Reproduction studies conducted in pregnant rats at doses up to 2.3 mg base/kg/day (approximately 2 times the MRHD on a mg/m² basis) and in pregnant rabbits at doses up to 2.3 mg base/kg/day (approximately 4 times the MRHD on a mg/m² basis) revealed no evidence of teratogenicity.

Studies in rats showed slightly decreased fetal/pup weights, usually at doses causing some maternal toxicity; decreased weights were seen at doses that were several fold lower than the MRHD on a mg/m² basis. There are no adequate or well-controlled studies in pregnant women. Because animal reproduction studies are not always predictive of human response, use rivastigmine during pregnancy only if the potential benefit justifies the potential risk to the fetus.

➤*Lactation:* It is not known whether rivastigmine is excreted in breast milk. Rivastigmine has no indication for use in breast-feeding mothers.

➤*Children:* There are no adequate and well-controlled trials documenting the safety and efficacy of rivastigmine in any illness occurring in children.

Drug Interactions

➤*Anticholinergics:* Because of their mechanism of action, cholinesterase inhibitors have the potential to interfere with the activity of anticholinergic medications.

➤*Cholinomimetics and other cholinesterase inhibitors:* A synergistic effect may be expected when cholinesterase inhibitors are given concurrently with succinylcholine, similar neuromuscular blocking agents, or cholinergic agonists such as bethanechol. Rivastigmine is likely to exaggerate succinylcholine-type muscle relaxation during anesthesia.

➤*Drug/Food interactions:* Administration of rivastigmine with food delays absorption (T_{max}) by 90 minutes, lowers C_{max} approximately 30%, and increases AUC approximately 30%.

Adverse Reactions

➤*Alzheimer-type dementia:* The rate of discontinuation because of adverse reactions in controlled clinical trials of rivastigmine was 15% for patients receiving 6 to 12 mg/day, compared with 5% for patients on placebo, during forced, weekly dose titration. While on a maintenance dose, the rates were 6% for patients on rivastigmine, compared with 4% for those on placebo.

The most common adverse reactions leading to discontinuation, defined as those occurring in at least 2% of patients and at twice the incidence seen in placebo patients, are shown in the following table.

Rivastigmine Oral Adverse Reactions (% Discontinuing)

Adverse reaction	Titration		Maintenance		Overall	
	Placebo (n = 868)	Rivastigmine ≥ 6 to 12 mg/day (n = 1,189)	Placebo (n = 788)	Rivastigmine ≥ 6 to 12 mg/day (n = 987)	Placebo (n = 868)	Rivastigmine ≥ 6 to 12 mg/day (n = 1,189)
CNS						
Dizziness	< 1%	2%	< 1%	1%	< 1%	2%
GI						
Anorexia	0%	2%	< 1%	1%	< 1%	3%
Nausea	< 1%	8%	< 1%	1%	1%	8%
Vomiting	< 1%	4%	< 1%	1%	< 1%	5%

Most common adverse reactions – The most common adverse reactions, defined as those occurring at a frequency of at least 5% and twice the placebo rate, are largely predicted by rivastigmine's cholinergic effects. These include anorexia, asthenia, dyspepsia, nausea, and vomiting.

GI – Rivastigmine use is associated with significant nausea, vomiting, and weight loss.

Nausea and vomiting: In the controlled clinical trials, 47% of the patients treated with a rivastigmine dose in the therapeutic range of 6 to 12 mg/day (n = 1,189) developed nausea (compared with 12% in placebo). A total of 31% of rivastigmine-treated patients developed at least 1 episode of vomiting (compared with 6% for placebo). The rate of vomiting was higher during the titration phase (24% vs 3% for placebo) than in the maintenance phase (14% vs 3% for placebo). The rates were higher in women than men. Five percent of patients discontinued for vomiting, compared with less than 1% for patients on placebo. Vomiting was severe in 2% of rivastigmine-treated patients and was rated as mild or moderate in 14% of patients. The rate of nausea was higher during the titration phase (43% vs 9% for placebo) than in the maintenance phase (17% vs 4% for placebo).

Weight loss: In the controlled trials, approximately 26% of women on high doses of rivastigmine (greater than 9 mg/day) had weight loss of greater than or equal to 7% of their baseline weight, compared with 6% in the placebo-treated patients. About 18% of the men in the high-dose group experienced a similar degree of weight loss, compared with 4% in placebo-treated patients. It is not clear how much of the weight loss was due to anorexia, nausea, vomiting, and diarrhea associated with the drug.

Adverse reactions reported in controlled trials – The following are treatment-emergent signs and symptoms that were reported in at least 2% of patients in placebo-controlled trials and for which the rate of occurrence was greater for patients treated with rivastigmine doses of 6 to 12 mg/day than for those treated with placebo (see the following table). Be aware that these figures cannot be used to predict the frequency of adverse reactions in the course of usual medical practice, when patient characteristics and other factors may differ from those prevailing during clinical studies. Similarly, the cited frequencies cannot be directly compared with figures obtained from other clinical investigations involving different treatments, uses, or investigators. An inspection of these frequencies, however, does provide 1 basis by which to estimate the relative contribution of drug and nondrug factors to the adverse reaction incidences in the population studied.

RIVASTIGMINE TARTRATE — ORAL

In general, adverse reactions were less frequent later in the course of treatment.

No systematic effect of race or age could be determined on the incidence of adverse reactions in the controlled studies. Nausea, vomiting, and weight loss were more frequent in women than men.

Rivastigmine Oral 6 to 12 mg/day Adverse Reactions (≥ 2%)		
Adverse reaction	Placebo (n = 868)	Rivastigmine (6 to 12 mg/day) (n = 1,189)
Patients with any adverse reaction	79%	92%
Cardiovascular		
Hypertension	2%	3%
CNS		
Aggressive reaction	2%	3%
Anxiety	3%	5%
Confusion	7%	8%
Depression	4%	6%
Dizziness	11%	21%
Fatigue	5%	9%
Hallucination	3%	4%
Headache	12%	17%
Insomnia	7%	9%
Somnolence	3%	5%
Syncope	2%	3%
Tremor	1%	4%
GI		
Abdominal pain	6%	13%
Anorexia	3%	17%
Constipation	4%	5%
Diarrhea	11%	19%
Dyspepsia	4%	9%
Eructation	1%	2%
Flatulence	2%	4%
Nausea	12%	47%
Vomiting	6%	31%
Respiratory		
Rhinitis	3%	4%
Miscellaneous		
Accidental trauma	9%	10%
Asthenia	2%	6%
Influenza-like symptoms	2%	3%
Malaise	2%	5%
Sweating increased	1%	4%
Urinary tract infection	6%	7%
Weight decrease	< 1%	3%

➤*Other adverse reactions (2% or more):* Other adverse reactions observed at a rate of 2% or more on rivastigmine 6 to 12 mg/day but at a greater or equal rate on placebo were as follows:

CNS – Agitation, delusion, nervousness, paranoid reaction, vertigo.

Dermatologic – Rash (general).

GU – Urinary incontinence.

Musculoskeletal – Arthralgia, back pain, bone fracture.

Respiratory – Bronchitis, coughing, pharyngitis, upper respiratory tract infections.

Miscellaneous – Chest pain, infection (general), pain, peripheral edema.

➤*Parkinson-associated dementia:*

Adverse reactions leading to discontinuation – The rate of discontinuation due to adverse reactions in the single controlled trial of rivastigmine was 18.2% for patients receiving 3 to 12 mg/day, compared with 11.2% for patients on placebo during the 24-week study.

The most frequent adverse reactions that led to discontinuation from this study, defined as those occurring in at least 1% of patients receiving rivastigmine and more frequently than in those receiving placebo, were nausea (3.6% rivastigmine vs 0.6% placebo), vomiting (1.9% rivastigmine vs 0.6% placebo), and tremor (1.7% rivastigmine vs 0% placebo).

Most frequent adverse reactions – The most common adverse reactions, defined as those occurring at a frequency of at least 5% and twice the placebo rate, are largely predicted by rivastigmine's cholinergic effects. These include anorexia, dizziness, nausea, tremor, and vomiting.

Adverse reactions reported in controlled trials – The following table lists treatment-emergent signs and symptoms that were reported in at least 2% of patients in placebo-controlled trials and for which the rate of occurrence was greater for patients treated with rivastigmine doses of 3 to 12 mg/day than for those treated with placebo. Be aware that these figures cannot be used to predict the frequency of adverse reactions in the course of usual medical practice, when patient characteristics and other factors may differ from those prevailing during clinical studies. Similarly, the cited frequencies cannot be directly compared with figures obtained from other clinical investigations involving different treatments, uses, or investigators. An inspection of these frequencies, however, provides one basis by which to estimate the relative contribution of drug and nondrug factors to the adverse reaction incidences in the population studied.

In general, adverse reactions were less frequent later in the course of treatment.

Rivastigmine Oral 3 to 12 mg/day Adverse Reactions (≥ 2%)		
Adverse reaction	Placebo (n = 179)	Rivastigmine (3 to 12 mg/day) (n = 362)
Patients with any adverse reaction	71%	84%
CNS		
Anxiety	1%	4%
Dizziness	1%	6%
Fatigue	3%	4%
Headache	3%	4%
Insomnia	2%	3%
Parkinson disease (worsening)	1%	3%
Parkinsonism	1%	2%
Somnolence	3%	4%
Tremor	4%	10%
GI		
Anorexia	3%	6%
Diarrhea	4%	7%
Nausea	11%	29%
Upper abdominal pain	1%	4%
Vomiting	2%	17%
Miscellaneous		
Asthenia	1%	2%
Dehydration	1%	2%

➤*Other adverse reactions observed during clinical trials:*

Alzheimer-type dementia – Rivastigmine has been administered to over 5,297 patients during clinical trials worldwide. Of these, 4,326 patients have been treated for at least 3 months, 3,407 patients have been treated for at least 6 months, 2,150 patients have been treated for 1 year, 1,250 have been treated for 2 years, and 168 have been treated for over 3 years. With regard to exposure to the highest dose, 2,809 patients were exposed to doses of 10 to 12 mg, 2,615 patients have been treated for 3 months, 2,328 patients have been treated for 6 months, 1,378 patients have been treated for 1 year, 917 patients have been treated for 2 years, and 129 have been treated for over 3 years.

Treatment-emergent signs and symptoms that occurred during 8 controlled clinical trials and 9 open-label trials in North America, Western Europe, Australia, South Africa, and Japan were recorded as adverse reactions by the clinical investigators using terminology of their own choosing. To provide an overall estimate of the proportion of individuals having similar types of reactions, the reactions were grouped into a smaller number of standardized categories using a modified World Health Organization (WHO) dictionary, and reaction frequencies were calculated across all studies. These categories are used in the following listing. The frequencies represent the proportion of 5,297 patients from these trials who experienced that reaction while receiving rivastigmine. All adverse reactions occurring in at least 6 patients (approximately 0.1%) are included, except for those already listed elsewhere in labeling, WHO terms too general to be informative, relatively minor reactions, or reactions unlikely to be drug-caused. Reactions are classified by body system and listed using the following definitions: frequent adverse reactions, those occurring in at least 1 of 100 patients; and infrequent adverse reactions, those occurring in 1 of 100 to 1 of 1,000 patients. These adverse reactions are not necessarily related to rivastigmine treatment and, in most cases, were observed at a similar frequency in placebo-treated patients in the controlled studies.

Cardiovascular – Angina pectoris, atrial fibrillation, bradycardia, cardiac failure, hypotension, myocardial infarction, palpitation, postural hypotension (1% or more).

Aneurysm, atrioventricular block, bundle-branch block, cardiac arrest, deep thrombophlebitis, extrasystoles, intracranial hemorrhage, peripheral ischemia, pulmonary embolism, sick sinus syndrome, supraventricular tachycardia, tachycardia, thrombosis (0.1% to 1%).

CNS – Abnormal gait, ataxia, confusion, convulsions, paranoid reaction, paresthesia (1% or more).

RIVASTIGMINE TARTRATE — ORAL

Abnormal dreaming, amnesia, apathy, aphasia, apraxia, decreased libido, delirium, dementia, depersonalization, dysphonia, emotional lability, hyperkinesia, hyperreflexia, hypertonia, hypesthesia, hypokinesia, impaired concentration, increased libido, migraine, neuralgia, neurosis, nystagmus, paresis, peripheral neuropathy, personality disorder, psychosis, suicidal ideation, suicide attempt (0.1% to 1%).

Dermatologic – Rashes of various kinds (bullous, eczema, erythematous, exfoliative, maculopapular, psoriaform) (1% or more).

Alopecia, cold clammy skin, contact dermatitis, flushing, skin ulceration, urticaria (0.1% to 1%).

Endocrine – Goiter, hypothyroidism (0.1% to 1%).

GI – Fecal incontinence, gastritis (1% or more).

Colitis, dry mouth, duodenal ulcer, dysphagia, esophagitis, gastric ulcer, gastroenteritis, gastroesophageal reflux, GI hemorrhage, gingivitis, glossitis, hematemesis, hernia, increased saliva, intestinal obstruction, melena, pancreatitis, rectal hemorrhage, tenesmus, ulcerative stomatitis (0.1% to 1%).

GU – Hematuria (1% or more).

Acute renal failure, albuminuria, atrophic vaginitis, breast pain, dysuria, impotence, micturition urgency, nocturia, oliguria, polyuria, renal calculus, urinary retention (0.1% to 1%).

Hematologic/Lymphatic – Anemia, epistaxis (1% or more).

Hematoma, hypochromic anemia, leukocytosis, purpura, thrombocytopenia (0.1% to 1%).

Hepatic – Abnormal hepatic function, cholecystitis (0.1% to 1%).

Metabolic/Nutritional – Dehydration, hypokalemia (1% or more).

Cachexia, diabetes mellitus, gout, hypercholesterolemia, hyperglycemia, hyperlipemia, hypoglycemia, hyponatremia, thirst (0.1% to 1%).

Musculoskeletal – Arthritis, leg cramps, myalgia, rigors (1% or more).

Cramps, hernia, muscle weakness (0.1% to 1%).

Ophthalmic – Cataract (1% or more).

Blepharitis, conjunctival hemorrhage, diplopia, eye pain, glaucoma (0.1% to 1%).

Respiratory – Apnea, bronchospasm, laryngitis (0.1% to 1%).

Special senses – Tinnitus (1% or more).

Loss of taste, perversion of taste (0.1% to 1%).

Miscellaneous – Accidental trauma, allergy, edema, fever, hot flushes (1% or more).

Cellulitis, cystitis, feeling cold, halitosis, hemorrhoids, herpes simplex, hypothermia, otitis media, periorbital or facial edema (0.1% to 1%).

Parkinson-associated dementia – Rivastigmine has been administered to 485 individuals during clinical trials worldwide. Of these, 413 patients have been treated for at least 3 months, 253 patients have been treated for at least 6 months, and 113 patients have been treated for 1 year.

Additional treatment-emergent adverse reactions in patients with Parkinson disease dementia occurring in at least 1 patient (approximately 0.3%) follow, excluding reactions that are already listed previously for the dementia of the Alzheimer type or elsewhere in labeling, WHO terms too general to be informative, relatively minor reactions, or reactions unlikely to be drug-caused. Reactions are classified by body system and listed using the following definitions: frequent adverse reactions, those occurring in at least 1 of 100 patients; infrequent adverse reactions, those occurring in 1 of 100 to 1 of 1,000 patients. These adverse reactions are not necessarily related to rivastigmine treatment and in most cases were observed at a similar frequency in placebo-treated patients in the controlled studies.

Cardiovascular – Chest pain (1% or more).

Adam-Stokes syndrome, sudden cardiac death, vasculitis, vasovagal syncope (0.1% to 1%).

CNS – Agitation, bradykinesia, depression, dyskinesia, restlessness, transient ischemic attack, vertigo (1% or more).

Delusion, dystonia, epilepsy, hemiparesis, insomnia, restless leg syndrome (0.1% to 1%).

Endocrine – Elevated prolactin level (0.1% to 1%).

GI – Dyspepsia (1% or more).

Diverticulitis, dysphagia, fecaloma, peritonitis (0.1% to 1%).

GU – Endometrial hypertrophy, mastitis, neurogenic bladder, prostatic adenoma, urinary incontinence (0.1% to 1%).

Hepatic – Elevated alkaline phosphatase level, elevated gamma-glutamyltransferase level (0.1% to 1%).

Musculoskeletal – Back pain (1% or more).

Freezing phenomenon, muscle stiffness, myoclonus (0.1% to 1%).

Ophthalmic – Blepharospasm, blurred vision, conjunctivitis, retinopathy (0.1% to 1%).

Respiratory – Dyspnea (1% or more).

Cough (0.1% to 1%).

Miscellaneous –

Meniere disease (0.1% to 1%).

➤*Postmarketing:* Voluntary reports of adverse reactions temporally associated with rivastigmine that have been received since market introduction and are not listed above, and that may or may not be causally related to the drug include the following: Stevens-Johnson syndrome.

Overdosage

➤*Symptoms:* Overdosage with cholinesterase inhibitors can result in cholinergic crisis, characterized by severe nausea, vomiting, salivation, sweating, bradycardia, hypotension, respiratory depression, collapse, and convulsions. Increasing muscle weakness is a possibility and may result in death if respiratory muscles are involved. Atypical responses in blood pressure and heart rate have been reported with other drugs that increase cholinergic activity when coadministered with quaternary anticholinergics such as glycopyrrolate.

➤*Treatment:* Because strategies for the management of overdose are continually evolving, it is advisable to contact a poison control center to determine the latest recommendations for the management of an overdose of any drug.

As rivastigmine has a short plasma half-life of about 1 hour and a moderate duration of acetylcholinesterase inhibition of 8 to 10 hours, it is recommended that a further dose of rivastigmine not be administered for the next 24 hours in cases of asymptomatic overdoses.

As in any case of overdose, utilize general supportive measures.

Because of the short half-life of rivastigmine, dialysis (hemodialysis, peritoneal dialysis, or hemofiltration) would not be clinically indicated in the event of an overdose.

In overdoses accompanied by severe nausea and vomiting, consider using antiemetics. In a documented case of a rivastigmine 46 mg overdose, the patient experienced vomiting, incontinence, hypertension, psychomotor retardation, and loss of consciousness. The patient fully recovered within 24 hours and conservative management was all that was required for treatment.

Patient Information

Advise caregivers of the high incidence of nausea and vomiting associated with the use of the drug, along with the possibility of anorexia and weight loss. Encourage caregivers to monitor for these adverse reactions and inform the patient's health care provider if they occur. It is critical to inform caregivers that if therapy has been interrupted for more than several days, not to administer the next dose until they have discussed with this with the health care provider.

Instruct caregivers in the correct procedure for administering rivastigmine oral solution. In addition, inform caregivers of the existence of an instruction sheet (included with the product) describing how the solution is to be administered. Urge caregivers to read this sheet prior to administering rivastigmine oral solution. Tell caregivers to direct questions about the administration of the solution to the patient's doctor or pharmacist.

Advise caregivers and patients that, like other cholinomimetics, rivastigmine may exacerbate or induce extrapyramidal symptoms. Worsening in patients with Parkinson disease, including an increased incidence or intensity of tremor, has been observed.

RIVASTIGMINE — TRANSDERMAL

Indications

➤*Alzheimer disease:* For the treatment of mild to moderate dementia of the Alzheimer type.

➤*Parkinson disease dementia:* For the treatment of mild to moderate dementia associated with Parkinson disease.

Administration and Dosage

➤*General dosing considerations:* Patients with a body weight below 50 kg may experience more adverse reactions and may be more likely to discontinue treatment because of adverse reactions. Particular caution should be exercised in titrating these patients above the recommended maintenance dose of the rivastigmine 9.5 mg/24 h transdermal patch.

➤*Adults:*

Alzheimer dementia –

Maximum dose: 9.5 mg/24 h.

Initial dosage: 4.6 mg/24 h.

Dosage titration: After a minimum of 4 weeks of treatment and if well tolerated, the dose should be increased to the rivastigmine 9.5 mg/24 h transdermal patch.

Maintenance dosage: 9.5 mg/24 h. Higher doses confer no appreciable additional benefit and are associated with a significant increase in the incidence of adverse reactions.

Dosage adjustment: If adverse reactions (eg, diarrhea, loss of appetite, nausea, vomiting) cause intolerance during treatment, the patient should be instructed to discontinue treatment for several days and then restart at the same or next lower dose level. If treatment is interrupted for longer than several days, treatment should be reinitiated with the lowest daily dose and titrated as previously described.

Conversion: Patients treated with rivastigmine capsules or oral solution may be switched to rivastigmine transdermal according to the following:

A patient who is on a total daily dose of oral rivastigmine less than 6 mg can be switched to the rivastigmine 4.6 mg/24 h transdermal patch.

A patient who is on a total daily dose of oral rivastigmine 6 to 12 mg may be directly switched to the rivastigmine 9.5 mg/24 h transdermal patch.

It is recommended to apply the first transdermal patch on the day following the last oral dose.

RIVASTIGMINE — TRANSDERMAL

Dementia associated with Parkinson disease – See Alzheimer Dementia for dosing.

➤*Administration:* Rivastigmine transdermal should be applied once a day to clean, dry, hairless, intact, healthy skin in a place that will not be rubbed by tight clothing. The upper or lower back is recommended as the site of application because the transdermal patch is less likely to be removed by the patient; however, when sites on the back are not accessible, the transdermal patch can be applied to the upper arm or chest. The transdermal patch should not be applied to skin that is red, irritated, or cut. It is recommended that the transdermal patch application site be changed daily to avoid potential irritation, although consecutive transdermal patches can be applied to the same anatomic site (eg, another spot on the upper back). The same site should not be used within 14 days. The transdermal patch should be replaced with a new one every 24 hours.

The transdermal patch should be pressed down firmly until the edges stick well. The transdermal patch can be used in situations that include bathing and hot weather. To prevent interference with the adhesive properties of the transdermal patch, it should not be applied to a skin area where cream, lotion, or powder has been recently applied.

If the patch falls off, apply a new patch for the rest of the day, then replace the patch the next day at the same time as usual.

➤*Storage / Stability:* Store at 25°C (77°F); excursions are permitted to 15° to 30°C (59° to 86°F). Keep rivastigmine transdermal system in the individually sealed pouches until ready to use. Used systems should be folded, with the adhesive surfaces pressed together, and discarded safely.

Actions

➤*Pharmacology:* Pathological changes in dementia of the Alzheimer type and dementia associated with Parkinson disease involve cholinergic neuronal pathways that project from the basal forebrain to the cerebral cortex and hippocampus. These pathways are thought to be intricately involved in memory, attention, learning, and other cognitive processes. While the precise mechanism of rivastigmine's action is unknown, it is postulated to exert its therapeutic effect by enhancing cholinergic function. This is accomplished by increasing the concentration of acetylcholine through reversible inhibition of its hydrolysis by cholinesterase. If this proposed mechanism is correct, rivastigmine's effect may lessen as the disease process advances and fewer cholinergic neurons remain functionally intact. There is no evidence that rivastigmine alters the course of the underlying dementing process.

Pharmacodynamics – After a 6 mg oral dose of rivastigmine in humans, anticholinesterase activity is present in cerebrospinal fluid (CSF) for about 10 hours, with a maximum inhibition of about 60% 5 hours after dosing.

In vitro and in vivo studies demonstrate that the inhibition of cholinesterase by rivastigmine is not affected by the concomitant administration of memantine, an N-methyl-D-aspartate receptor antagonist.

➤*Pharmacokinetics:*

Absorption – After the first dose, there is a lag time of 0.5 to 1 hours in the absorption of rivastigmine from the rivastigmine transdermal patch. Concentrations then rise slowly, typically reaching a maximum after 8 hours, although maximum values (C_{max}) are often reached at later times as well (10 to 16 h). After the peak, plasma concentrations slowly decrease over the remainder of the 24-hour period of application. At steady-state, trough levels are approximately 60% to 80% of peak levels. Fluctuation (between C_{max} and minimum concentration [C_{min}]) is lower for the rivastigmine transdermal than for the oral formulation. Rivastigmine 9.5 mg/24 h transdermal patch exhibited exposure approximately the same as that provided by an oral dose of 6 mg twice daily (ie, 12 mg/day).

Intersubject variability in exposure was lower (43% to 49%) for the rivastigmine transdermal formulation as compared with the oral formulations (73% to 103%).

A relationship between drug exposure at steady state (rivastigmine and metabolite NAP226-90) and body weight was observed in patients with Alzheimer dementia. Compared with a patient with a body weight of 65 kg, the rivastigmine steady-state concentrations in a patient with a body weight of 35 kg are approximately doubled, while for a patient with a body weight of 100 kg, the concentrations are approximately halved. The effect of body weight on drug exposure suggests special attention to patients with very low body weight during up-titration.

Over a 24-hour dermal application, approximately 50% of the drug load is released from the system.

Exposure (area under the curve [AUC_∞]) to rivastigmine (and metabolite NAP266-90) was highest when the transdermal patch was applied to the upper back, chest, or upper arm. Two other sites (abdomen and thigh) could be used if none of the 3 other sites is available, but keep in mind that the rivastigmine plasma exposure associated with these sites was approximately 20% to 30% lower.

There was no relevant accumulation of rivastigmine or the metabolite NAP226-90 in plasma in patients with Alzheimer disease upon multiple dosing.

Distribution – Rivastigmine is weakly bound to plasma proteins (approximately 40%) over therapeutic range. It readily crosses the blood-brain barrier, reaching CSF peak concentrations in 1.4 to 2.6 hours. It has an apparent volume of distribution in the range of 1.8 to 2.7 L/kg.

Metabolism – Rivastigmine is extensively metabolized primarily via cholinesterase-mediated hydrolysis to the decarbamylated metabolite NAP226-90. In vitro, this metabolite shows minimal inhibition of acetylcholinesterase (less than 10%). Based on evidence from in-vitro and animal studies, the major CYP-450 isoenzymes are minimally involved in rivastigmine metabolism.

The metabolite-to-parent AUC_∞ ratio was approximately 0.7 after rivastigmine transdermal application versus 3.5 after oral administration, indicating that much less metabolism occurred after dermal treatment. Less NAP226-90 is formed following transdermal application, presumably because of the lack of presystemic (hepatic first pass) metabolism. Based on in vitro studies, no unique metabolic routes were detected in human skin.

Excretion – Renal excretion of the metabolites is the major route of elimination. Unchanged rivastigmine is found in trace amounts in the urine. Following administration of ^{14}C-rivastigmine, renal elimination was rapid and essentially complete (greater than 90%) within 24 hours. Less than 1% of the administered dose is excreted in the feces. The apparent elimination half-life in plasma is approximately 3 hours after transdermal removal. Renal clearance was approximately 2.1 to 2.8 L/h.

Special populations –

Renal function impairment: No study was conducted with rivastigmine transdermal in subjects with renal function impairment. Following a single 3 mg dose, mean oral clearance of rivastigmine is 64% lower in patients with moderate renal function impairment (n = 8, glomular filtration rate [GFR] = 10 to 50 mL/min) than in healthy subjects (n = 10, GFR 60 mL/min or more); apparent total clearance (Cl/F) = 1.7 L/min (covariance [cv] = 45%) and 4.8 L/min (cv = 80%), respectively. In patients with severe renal function impairment (n = 8, GFR less than 10 mL/min), mean oral clearance of rivastigmine is 43% higher than in healthy subjects (n = 10, GFR 60 mL/min or more); Cl/F = 6.9 L/min and 4.8 L/min, respectively. For unexplained reasons, patients with severe renal function impairment had a higher clearance of rivastigmine than moderately impaired patients. However, dosage adjustment may not be necessary in patients with renal function impairment, as the dose of the drug is individually titrated to tolerability.

Hepatic function impairment: No pharmacokinetic study was conducted with rivastigmine transdermal in subjects with hepatic function impairment. Following a single 3 mg dose, mean oral clearance of rivastigmine was 60% lower in patients with hepatic function impairment (n = 10, biopsy proven) than in healthy subjects (n = 10). After multiple 6 mg twice-daily oral dosing, the mean clearance of rivastigmine was 65% lower in mild (n = 7, Child-Pugh score 5 to 6) and moderate (n = 3, Child-Pugh score 7 to 9) patients with hepatic function impairment (biopsy proven, liver cirrhosis) than in healthy subjects (n = 10). Dosage adjustment is not necessary in patients with hepatic function impairment, as the dose of the drug is individually titrated to tolerability.

Gender and race: No specific pharmacokinetic study was conducted to investigate the effect of gender and race on the disposition of rivastigmine, but a population pharmacokinetic analysis indicates that gender (277 men and 348 women) and race (575 white, 34 black, 4 Asian, and 12 other) did not affect the clearance of rivastigmine administered orally. Similar results were seen with analyses of pharmacokinetic data obtained after the administration of rivastigmine transdermal.

Nicotine: Population pharmacokinetic analysis showed that nicotine use increases the oral clearance of rivastigmine by 23% (75 smokers and 549 nonsmokers). No dose adjustment is necessary, as the dose of the drug is individually titrated to tolerability.

Contraindications

Known hypersensitivity to rivastigmine, other carbamate derivatives, or other components of the formulation.

Warnings/Precautions

➤*GI effects:* At higher than recommended doses, rivastigmine transdermal system use is associated with significant GI adverse reactions, including anorexia/decreased appetite, diarrhea, nausea, vomiting, and weight loss. For this reason, patients administered rivastigmine transdermal should always be started at a dose of 4.6 mg/24 h and titrated to the maintenance dose of 9.5 mg/24 h. If treatment is interrupted for longer than several days, reinitiate treatment with the lowest daily dose to reduce the possibility of severe vomiting and its potentially serious sequelae (eg, there has been 1 postmarketing report of severe vomiting with esophageal rupture following inappropriate reinitiation of treatment with a 4.5 mg dose of an oral formulation after 8 weeks of treatment interruption).

At higher than recommended doses, advise caregivers of the high incidence of nausea and vomiting associated with the use of rivastigmine transdermal along with the possibility of anorexia and weight loss. Encourage caregivers to monitor for these adverse reactions and inform the health care provider if they occur. It is critical to inform caregivers that if therapy has been interrupted for more than several days, the next dose should not be administered until they have discussed this with the health care provider.

Nausea and vomiting – In the controlled clinical trial, 7% of patients treated with rivastigmine 9.5 mg/24 h transdermal developed nausea, as compared with 23% of patients who received the rivastigmine capsule at doses up to 6 mg twice daily and 5% of those who received placebo. In the same clinical trial, 6% of patients treated with rivastigmine 9.5 mg/24 h transdermal developed vomiting, as compared with 17% of patients who received the rivastigmine capsule at doses up to 6 mg twice daily and 3% of those who received placebo. The proportion of patients who discontinued treatment due to vomiting was 0% of the patients who received rivastigmine 9.5 mg/24 h transdermal and 2% of patients who received rivastigmine capsules at doses up to 6 mg twice daily and 0% of those who received placebo. Vomiting was severe in 0% of patients who received rivastigmine 9.5 mg/24 h transdermal and 1% of patients who received rivastigmine capsules at doses up to 6 mg twice daily and 0% of those who received placebo.

In the same clinical trial, 21% of the patients treated with the higher dose of rivastigmine 17.4 mg/24 h transdermal developed nausea, 19% developed vomiting, and the proportion of these patients who discontinued treatment due to vomiting was 2%. Vomiting was severe in 1% of the patients treated with rivastigmine 17.4 mg/24 h transdermal.

RIVASTIGMINE — TRANSDERMAL

Weight loss – In the controlled clinical trial, the proportion of patients who had weight loss of 7% or more of their baseline weight was 8% of those treated with rivastigmine 9.5 mg/24 h transdermal, 11% of patients who received rivastigmine capsules at doses up to 6 mg twice daily, and 6% of those who received placebo.

In the same clinical trial, 12% of those treated with rivastigmine 17.4 mg/24 h transdermal had weight loss of 7% or more of their baseline weight. It is not clear how much of the weight loss was associated with the anorexia, diarrhea, nausea, and vomiting associated with the drug.

Diarrhea – In the controlled clinical trial, 6% of the patients treated with rivastigmine 9.5 mg/24 h transdermal developed diarrhea, as compared with 5% of patients who received rivastigmine capsules at doses up to 6 mg twice daily, 10% of those treated with rivastigmine 17.4 mg/24 h transdermal, and 3% of those who received placebo.

Anorexia/Decreased appetite – In the controlled clinical trial, 3% of the patients treated with rivastigmine 9.5 mg/24 h transdermal were recorded as developing decreased appetite or anorexia, as compared with 9% of patients who received rivastigmine capsules at doses up to 6 mg twice daily, 9% of those treated with rivastigmine transdermal 17.4 mg/24 h, and 2% of those who received placebo.

Peptic ulcers/GI bleeding – Because of their pharmacological action, cholinesterase inhibitors may be expected to increase gastric acid secretion due to increased cholinergic activity. Therefore, monitor patients closely for symptoms of active or occult GI bleeding, especially those at increased risk for developing ulcers (eg, those with a history of ulcer disease, those receiving concurrent nonsteroidal anti-inflammatory drugs [NSAIDs]). Clinical studies of rivastigmine have shown no significant increase, relative to placebo, in the incidence of either peptic ulcer disease or GI bleeding.

➤*Anesthesia:* Rivastigmine, as a cholinesterase inhibitor, is likely to exaggerate succinylcholine-type muscle relaxation during anesthesia.

➤*Cardiovascular effects:* Drugs that increase cholinergic activity may have vagotonic effects on heart rate (eg, bradycardia). The potential for this action may be particularly important to patients with sick sinus syndrome or other supraventricular cardiac conduction conditions. In clinical trials, rivastigmine was not associated with any increased incidence of cardiovascular adverse reactions, heart rate or blood pressure changes, or electrocardiogram (ECG) abnormalities.

➤*Urinary obstruction:* Although this was not observed in clinical trials of rivastigmine, drugs that increase cholinergic activity may cause urinary obstruction.

➤*CNS effects:*

Seizures – Drugs that increase cholinergic activity are believed to have some potential for causing seizures. However, seizure activity also may be a manifestation of Alzheimer disease.

Extrapyramidal symptoms – Like other cholinomimetics, rivastigmine may exacerbate or induce extrapyramidal symptoms. Worsening of parkinsonian symptoms, particularly tremor, has been observed in patients with dementia associated with Parkinson disease who were treated with rivastigmine capsules.

➤*Pulmonary effects:* Like other drugs that increase cholinergic activity, use rivastigmine with care in patients with a history of asthma or obstructive pulmonary disease.

➤*Low body weight:* Rivastigmine exposure is higher in subjects with low body weight. Compared with a patient with a body weight of 65 kg, the rivastigmine steady-state concentrations in a patient with a body weight of 35 kg would be approximately doubled, while for a patient with a body weight of 100 kg, the concentrations would be approximately halved. This suggests special attention should be given to patients with very low body weight during up-titration.

➤*Hazardous tasks:* Dementia may cause gradual impairment of driving performance or compromise the ability to use machinery. The administration of rivastigmine may also result in adverse reactions that are detrimental to these functions. Thus, routinely evaluate the patient's ability to continue driving or operate machinery.

➤*Pregnancy: Category B.* There are no adequate or well-controlled studies in pregnant women. Because animal reproduction studies are not always predictive of human response, use rivastigmine transdermal during pregnancy only if the potential benefit outweighs the potential risk to the fetus.

No dermal reproduction studies in animals have been conducted. Oral reproduction studies conducted in pregnant rats at doses of up to 2.3 mg base/kg/day and in pregnant rabbits at doses of up to 2.3 mg base/kg/day revealed no evidence of teratogenicity. Studies in rats showed slightly decreased fetal/pup weights, usually at doses causing some maternal toxicity.

➤*Lactation:* Milk transfer studies in animals have not been conducted with dermal rivastigmine. In rats given rivastigmine orally, concentrations of rivastigmine plus metabolites were approximately 2 times higher in milk than plasma. It is not known whether rivastigmine is excreted in human breast milk. The rivastigmine transdermal system has no indication for use in breast-feeding mothers.

➤*Children:* There are no adequate and well-controlled trials documenting the safety and efficacy of rivastigmine in any illness occurring in children.

➤*Elderly:* Age had no impact on the exposure to rivastigmine in patients with Alzheimer disease treated with the rivastigmine transdermal.

➤*Monitoring:* Monitor patients closely for symptoms of active or occult GI bleeding, especially those at increased risk for developing ulcers (eg, history of ulcer disease, concurrent NSAID use). Monitor patients for loss of appetite and/or weight loss.

Drug Interactions

Rivastigmine Drug Interactions

Precipitant drug	Object drug[a]		Description
Rivastigmine	Anesthesia	↑	Rivastigmine, as a cholinesterase inhibitor, is likely to exaggerate succinylcholine-type muscle relaxation during anesthesia.
Rivastigmine	Anticholinergics	↓	Because of their mechanism of action, cholinesterase inhibitors have the potential to interfere with the activity of anticholinergic medications.
Rivastigmine	Cholinomimetics/ Cholinesterase inhibitors	↑	A synergistic effect may be expected when cholinesterase inhibitors are given concurrently with succinylcholine, similar neuromuscular blocking agents, or cholinergic agonists, such as bethanechol.
Rivastigmine	NSAIDs	↑	Rivastigmine increases gastric acid secretions caused by increased cholinergic activity. Therefore, monitor for active or occult GI bleeding (see Warnings/Precautions).

[a] ↑ = object drug increased; ↓ = object drug decreased.

Adverse Reactions

Significant GI adverse reactions, including anorexia, nausea, vomiting, and weight loss, have been reported with rivastigmine transdermal at higher than recommended doses.

➤*Discontinuation of treatment:* In the single controlled clinical trial of rivastigmine transdermal, which randomized a total of 1,195 patients, the proportions of patients in the rivastigmine 9.5 mg/24 h transdermal, rivastigmine 17.4 mg/24 h transdermal, rivastigmine 6 mg capsules twice daily, and placebo groups who discontinued treatment because of adverse reactions were 9.6%, 8.6%, 8.1%, and 5%, respectively.

The most common adverse reactions in the rivastigmine transdermal–treated groups that led to treatment discontinuation in this study were nausea and vomiting. The proportions of patients who discontinued treatment because of nausea were 0.7%, 1.7%, 1.7%, and 1.3% in the rivastigmine 9.5 mg/24 h transdermal, rivastigmine 17.4 mg/24 h transdermal, rivastigmine 6 mg capsules twice daily, and placebo groups, respectively. The proportions of patients who discontinued treatment because of vomiting were 0%, 1.7%, 2%, and 0.3% in the rivastigmine 9.5 mg/24 h transdermal, rivastigmine 17.4 mg/24 h transdermal, rivastigmine 6 mg capsules twice daily, and placebo groups, respectively.

Most common reactions – The most commonly observed adverse reactions seen in patients administered the rivastigmine transdermal in the controlled clinical trial, defined as those occurring at a frequency of at least 5% in the 9.5 mg/24 h group and at a frequency at least as high as in the placebo group, are largely predicted by rivastigmine's cholinergic effects. These are diarrhea, nausea, and vomiting. All these reactions were more common at the higher rivastigmine transdermal dose of 17.4 mg/24 h than at a dose of 9.5 mg/24 h.

Adverse reactions (≥ 2%) –

Rivastigmine Adverse Reactions (≥ 2%)

	Rivastigmine 9.5 mg/24 h transdermal (n = 291)	Rivastigmine 17.4 mg/24 h transdermal (n = 303)	Rivastigmine 6 mg capsule twice daily (n = 294)	Placebo (n = 302)
Percentage of patients with adverse reactions	51%	66%	63%	46%
CNS				
Anxiety	3%	3%	2%	1%
Asthenia	2%	3%	6%	1%
Depression	4%	4%	4%	1%
Dizziness	2%	7%	7%	2%
Fatigue	2%	2%	1%	1%
Headache	3%	4%	6%	2%
Insomnia	1%	4%	2%	2%
Vertigo	0%	2%	1%	1%
GI				
Abdominal pain	2%	4%	1%	1%
Anorexia/ Decreased appetite	3%	9%	9%	2%
Diarrhea	6%	10%	5%	3%
Nausea	7%	21%	23%	5%

RIVASTIGMINE — TRANSDERMAL

Rivastigmine Adverse Reactions (≥ 2%)				
	Rivastigmine 9.5 mg/24 h transdermal (n = 291)	Rivastigmine 17.4 mg/24 h transdermal (n = 303)	Rivastigmine 6 mg capsule twice daily (n = 294)	Placebo (n = 302)
Upper abdominal pain	1%	3%	2%	2%
Vomiting	6%	19%	17%	3%
Weight decreased	3%	8%	5%	1%
Miscellaneous				
Urinary tract infection	2%	2%	1%	1%

Application-site reactions – The vast majority of patients participating in the controlled clinical trial had either no observed skin irritation or mild to moderate skin reactions. The incidence of severe reactions was very low, regardless of the administered dosage.

➤*Other adverse reactions:* Reactions are classified by system organ class and listed using the following definitions: Frequent adverse reactions are those occurring in at least 1/100 patients (at least 1%); and infrequent adverse reactions are those occurring in 1/100 to 1/1,000 patients (0.1% to 1%). These adverse reactions are not necessarily related to the rivastigmine transdermal treatment and in most cases were observed at a similar frequency in placebo-treated patients in the controlled studies.

Cardiovascular – Angina pectoris, arrhythmia, atrial fibrillation, atrioventricular block, bradycardia, cardiac failure, ECG QT prolonged, hypotension, myocardial infarction, supraventricular extrasystoles, tachycardia (0.1% to 1%).

CNS – Tremor (at least 1%); delusion, epilepsy, migraine, parkinsonism (0.1% to 1%).

Dermatologic – Pruritus (at least 1%); application-site dermatitis, application-site eczema, application-site irritation, dermatitis, eczema, erythema, erythematous rash, skin ulcer (0.1% to 1%).

GI – Constipation, gastritis (at least 1%); diverticulitis, gastroesophageal reflux disease, hematemesis, hematochezia, pancreatitis, peptic ulcer, salivary hypersecretion (0.1% to 1%).

GU – Urinary incontinence (at least 1%); benign prostatic hyperplasia, hematuria, nocturia, pollakiuria, renal failure (0.1% to 1%).

Metabolic/Nutritional – Dehydration (at least 1%); blood amylase increased, blood creatine phosphokinase increased, hyperlipidemia, hypokalemia, hyponatremia, lipase increased, peripheral edema (0.1% to 1%).

Musculoskeletal – Arthralgia, muscle spasms, myalgia (0.1% to 1%).

Respiratory – Nasopharyngitis, pneumonia (at least 1%); bronchospasm, chronic obstructive pulmonary disease, dyspnea (0.1% to 1%).

Special senses – Cataract, glaucoma, tinnitus, vision blurred (0.1% to 1%).

Miscellaneous – Anemia, fall (at least 1%); chest pain, cholecystitis, hip fracture, hyperpyrexia, subdural hematoma (0.1% to 1%).

Overdosage

➤*Symptoms:* Overdosage with cholinesterase inhibitors can result in cholinergic crisis characterized by bradycardia, collapse, convulsions, hypotension, respiratory depression, salivation, severe nausea, sweating, and vomiting. Increasing muscle weakness is a possibility and may result in death if respiratory muscles are involved. Atypical responses in blood pressure and heart rate have been reported with other drugs that increase cholinergic activity when coadministered with quaternary anticholinergics such as glycopyrrolate.

➤*Treatment:* Because rivastigmine has a plasma half-life of about 3.4 hours after transdermal administration and a duration of acetylcholinesterase inhibition of about 9 hours, it is recommended that in cases of asymptomatic overdose, the transdermal patch be immediately removed and no transdermal patch applied for the next 24 hours.

Due to the short plasma elimination half-life of rivastigmine after transdermal administration, dialysis (hemodialysis, hemofiltration, or peritoneal dialysis) would not be clinically indicated in the event of an overdose.

In overdose accompanied by severe nausea and vomiting, consider the use of antiemetics. In a documented case of an oral 46 mg overdose with rivastigmine, the patient experienced hypertension, incontinence, loss of consciousness, psychomotor retardation, and vomiting. The patient fully recovered within 24 hours and conservative management was all that was required for treatment.

Because strategies for the management of overdose are continually evolving, it is advisable to contact a poison control center to determine the latest recommendations for the management of an overdose of any drug. As in any case of overdose, utilize general supportive measures.

There are currently no data on overdose with the rivastigmine transdermal system.

Patient Information

To assure safe and effective use of rivastigmine transdermal, discuss this information and instructions provided in the patient information section with patients.

Inform patients or caregivers of the importance of applying the correct dose on the correct part of their body. Also instruct them to rotate the application site in order to minimize skin irritation. The same site should not be used within 14 days. Instruct the patient to replace the transdermal patch every 24 hours at the same time every day. It may be helpful for this to be part of a daily routine, such as the daily bath or shower.

Tell patients or caregivers to avoid exposure of the transdermal patch to external heat sources (excess sunlight, saunas, solarium) for long periods of time.

Instruct patients or caregivers to fold the transdermal patch in half after use and discard it in a place out of the reach and sight of children and pets. Also inform them that drug still remains in the transdermal patch after 24-hour use. Instruct them to avoid eye contact and to wash their hands after handling the transdermal patch.

Tell patients or caregivers that while wearing the rivastigmine transdermal patch, the patient should not take rivastigmine capsules, rivastigmine oral solution, or other drugs with cholinergic effects.

Inform patients or caregivers of potential GI adverse reactions, such as diarrhea, nausea, and vomiting. Instruct patients and caregivers to observe for these adverse reactions at all times, and in particular when treatment is initiated or the dose is increased. Instruct patients and caregivers to inform their health care provider if these adverse reactions persist, as a dose adjustment/reduction may be required.

Inform patients or caregivers that rivastigmine transdermal may affect the patient's appetite and/or the patient's weight. Any loss of appetite or weight reduction needs to be monitored.

If patients miss a dose, instruct them to apply a new transdermal immediately. They may apply the next transdermal patch at the usual time the next day. Advise patients not to apply 2 rivastigmine transdermal patches to make up for the one missed.

If treatment has been missed for several days, inform patients or caregivers to restart treatment with the starting transdermal dose of 4.6 mg/24 h. Titration to the next transdermal dose should proceed after 4 weeks.

GALANTAMINE

Rx	**Galantamine Hydrobromide** (Various, eg, Patriot, Mylan)	**Tablets; oral:** 4 mg	As galantamine hydrobromide. May contain lactose. In 60s and 1,000s.
Rx	**Razadyne** (Janssen)		As galantamine hydrobromide. Lactose. (JANSSEN G 4). Off-white. Film-coated. In 60s.
Rx	**Galantamine Hydrobromide** (Various, eg, Patriot, Mylan)	**Tablets; oral:** 8 mg	As galantamine hydrobromide. May contain lactose. In 60s and 1,000s.
Rx	**Razadyne** (Janssen)		As galantamine hydrobromide. Lactose. (JANSSEN G 8). Pink. Film-coated. In 60s.
Rx	**Galantamine Hydrobromide** (Various, eg, Patriot, Mylan)	**Tablets; oral:** 12 mg	As galantamine hydrobromide. May contain lactose. In 60s and 1,000s.
Rx	**Razadyne** (Janssen)		As galantamine hydrobromide. Lactose. (JANSSEN G 12). Orange-brown. Film-coated. In 60s.
Rx	**Galantamine Hydrobromide** (Various, eg, Barr Labs, Patriot)	**Capsules, extended-release; oral:** 8 mg	As galantamine hydrobromide. May contain sugar spheres. In 30s, 500s, and unit-use 30s.
Rx	**Razadyne ER** (Janssen)		As galantamine hydrobromide. Sucrose. (GAL 8). White opaque. Pellet-filled. In 30s.
Rx	**Galantamine Hydrobromide** (Various, eg, Barr Labs, Patriot)	**Capsules, extended-release; oral:** 16 mg	As galantamine hydrobromide. May contain sugar spheres. In 30s, 500s, and unit-use 30s.
Rx	**Razadyne ER** (Janssen)		As galantamine hydrobromide. Sucrose. (GAL 16). Pink opaque. Pellet-filled. In 30s.

GALANTAMINE

Rx	**Galantamine Hydrobromide** (Various, eg, Barr Labs, Patriot)	**Capsules, extended-release; oral:** 24 mg	As galantamine hydrobromide. May contain sugar spheres. In 30s, 500s, and unit-use 30s.
Rx	**Razadyne ER** (Janssen)		As galantamine hydrobromide. Sucrose. (GAL 24). Caramel opaque. Pellet-filled. In 30s.
Rx	**Razadyne** (Janssen)	**Solution, oral:** 4 mg/mL	As galantamine hydrobromide. Saccharin. In 100 mL w/calibrated pipette.

GALANTAMINE HYDROBROMIDE — ORAL

Indications

➤*Alzheimer disease:* For the treatment of mild to moderate dementia of the Alzheimer type.

Administration and Dosage

➤*General dosing considerations:* Patients and caregivers of patients should be advised to ensure adequate fluid intake during treatment. Inform patients and caregivers that if therapy has been interrupted for several days or longer, the patient should be restarted at the lowest dose and titrated to the current dose.

➤*Adults:*

Alzheimer disease –

Extended-Release:

- *Initial dosage* – 8 mg once daily.
- *Dosage titration* – Increase to 16 mg once daily after a minimum of 4 weeks. A further increase to 24 mg once daily should be attempted after a minimum of 4 weeks of 16 mg/day. Base dose increases on assessment of clinical benefit and tolerability of the previous dose.
- *Maintenance dosage* – 16 to 24 mg once daily.

Immediate-release:

- *Initial dosage* – 4 mg twice daily (8 mg/day).
- *Dosage titration* – After a minimum of 4 weeks of treatment, if well-tolerated, increase the dosage to 8 mg twice daily (16 mg/day). Attempt a further increase to 12 mg twice daily (24 mg/day) only after a minimum of 4 weeks at the 8 mg twice-daily dose. Dose increases should be based upon assessment of clinical benefit and tolerability of the previous dose.
- *Maintenance dosage* – 8 to 12 mg twice daily (16 to 24 mg/day). The 24 mg/day dose did not provide a statistically significant greater clinical benefit than the 16 mg/day dose. However, it is possible that 24 mg/day might provide additional benefit for some patients.

➤*Renal function impairment:* For patients with moderate renal function impairment, the dose generally should not exceed 16 mg/day. In patients with severe renal function impairment (CrCl less than 9 mL/min), the use of galantamine is not recommended.

➤*Hepatic function impairment:* Galantamine plasma concentrations may be increased in patients with moderate to severe hepatic function impairment. In patients with moderately impaired hepatic function (Child-Pugh class 7 to 9), the dose generally should not exceed 16 mg/day. The use of galantamine in patients with severe hepatic function impairment (Child-Pugh class 10 to 15) is not recommended.

➤*Discontinuation of therapy:* The abrupt withdrawal of galantamine in those patients who had been receiving doses in the effective range was not associated with an increased frequency of adverse reactions in comparison with those continuing to receive the same doses of that drug. However, the beneficial effects of galantamine are lost when the drug is discontinued.

➤*Administration:*

Extended-release – Administer once daily in the morning, preferably with food (but not required).

Immediate-release – Administer twice daily, preferably with morning and evening meals.

➤*Storage/Stability:* Store at 25°C (77°F); excursions are permitted between 15° and 30°C (59° and 86°F). Do not freeze the oral solution.

Actions

➤*Pharmacology:* Although the etiology of cognitive impairment in Alzheimer disease is not fully understood, it has been reported that acetylcholine-producing neurons degenerate in the brains of patients with Alzheimer disease. The degree of this cholinergic loss has been correlated with degree of cognitive impairment and density of amyloid plaques (a neuropathological hallmark of Alzheimer disease).

Galantamine, a tertiary alkaloid, is a competitive and reversible inhibitor of acetylcholinesterase. While the precise mechanism of galantamine's action is unknown, it is postulated to exert its therapeutic effect by enhancing cholinergic function. This is accomplished by increasing the concentration of acetylcholine through reversible inhibition of its hydrolysis by cholinesterase. If this mechanism is correct, galantamine's effect may lessen as the disease process advances and fewer cholinergic neurons remain functionally intact. There is no evidence that galantamine alters the course of the underlying dementing process.

➤*Pharmacokinetics:*

Absorption/Distribution – Galantamine is well absorbed with absolute oral bioavailability of approximately 90%.

The maximum inhibition of anticholinesterase activity, approximately 40%, was achieved approximately 1 hour after a single oral dose of galantamine 8 mg in healthy men.

Galantamine is rapidly and completely absorbed with time to peak concentration (T_{max}) approximately 1 hour. Bioavailability of the tablet was the same as the bioavailability of an oral solution. Food did not affect the area under the curve (AUC) of galantamine but maximal drug concentrations (C_{max}) decreased 25% and T_{max} was delayed by 1.5 hours.

Galantamine 24 mg ER capsules administered once daily under fasting conditions are bioequivalent to galantamine 12 mg tablets twice daily with respect to AUC_{24h} and minimum drug concentrations (C_{min}). The C_{max} and T_{max} of the ER capsules were lower and occurred later, respectively, compared with the IR tablets, with C_{max} about 25% lower and median T_{max} occurring about 4.5 to 5 hours after dosing. Dose-proportionality is observed for galantamine ER capsules over the dose range of 8 to 24 mg daily and steady state is achieved within a week.

There are no appreciable differences in pharmacokinetic parameters when galantamine ER capsules are given with food, compared with when they are given in the fasted state.

The mean volume of distribution of galantamine is 175 L. The plasma protein binding of galantamine is 18% at therapeutically relevant concentrations. In whole blood, galantamine is mainly distributed to blood cells (52.7%). The blood to plasma concentration ratio of galantamine is 1.2.

Metabolism/Excretion – Galantamine has a terminal elimination half-life of approximately 7 hours and pharmacokinetics are linear over the range of 8 to 32 mg/day.

Galantamine is metabolized by hepatic CYP-450 enzymes, glucuronidated, and excreted unchanged in the urine. In vitro studies indicate that CYP2D6 and CYP3A4 were the major CYP-450 isoenzymes involved in the metabolism of galantamine, and inhibitors of both pathways increase oral bioavailability of galantamine modestly. O-demethylation, mediated by CYP2D6, was greater in extensive metabolizers of CYP2D6 than in poor metabolizers. In plasma from both poor and extensive metabolizers, however, unchanged galantamine and its glucuronide accounted for most of the sample radioactivity.

In studies of oral ^{3}H-galantamine, unchanged galantamine and its glucuronide accounted for most plasma radioactivity in poor and extensive CYP2D6 metabolizers. Up to 8 hours postdose, unchanged galantamine accounted for 39% to 77% of the total radioactivity in the plasma, and galantamine glucuronide for 14% to 24%. By 7 days, 93% to 99% of the radioactivity had been recovered, with approximately 95% in urine and 5% in the feces. Total urinary recovery of unchanged galantamine accounted for, on average, 32% of the dose; urinary recovery of galantamine glucuronide accounted for another 12%, on average.

Within 24 hours after intravenous (IV) or oral administration, approximately 20% of the dose was excreted in the urine as unchanged galantamine, representing a renal clearance of approximately 65 mL/min, approximately 20% to 25% of the total plasma clearance of approximately 300 mL/min.

Special populations –

Renal function impairment: Following a single dose of galantamine 8 mg, AUC increased 37% and 67% in moderate and severe renal function impairment patients compared with healthy volunteers.

Hepatic function impairment: Following a single dose of galantamine 4 mg IR tablets, the pharmacokinetics of galantamine in subjects with mild hepatic function impairment (n = 8; Child-Pugh class 5 to 6) were similar to those in healthy subjects. In patients with moderate hepatic function impairment (n = 8; Child-Pugh class 7 to 9), galantamine clearance was decreased approximately 25% compared with healthy volunteers. Exposure would be expected to increase further with increasing degree of hepatic function impairment.

Elderly: Data from clinical trials in patients with Alzheimer disease indicate that galantamine concentrations are 30% to 40% higher than in younger healthy subjects. There was no effect of age on the pharmacokinetics of galantamine ER capsules.

Gender and race: No specific pharmacokinetic study was conducted to investigate the effect of gender and race on the disposition of galantamine, but a population pharmacokinetic analysis indicates (n = 539 male and 550 female patients) that galantamine clearance is approximately 20% lower in female than in male patients (explained by lower body weight in female patients), and race (n = 1,029 white, 24 black, 13 Asian, and 23 other) did not affect the clearance of galantamine.

CYP2D6 poor metabolizers: Approximately 7% of the healthy population has a genetic variation that leads to reduced levels of activity of CYP2D6 isozyme. Such individuals have been referred to as poor metabolizers. After a single oral dose of galantamine 4 or 8 mg, CYP2D6 poor metabolizers demonstrated a similar C_{max} and approximately 35% AUC_{∞} increase of unchanged galantamine compared with extensive metabolizers.

CYP2D6 poor metabolizers had drug exposures that were approximately 50% higher than extensive metabolizers.

A total of 356 patients with Alzheimer disease enrolled in 2 phase 3 studies were genotyped with respect to CYP2D6 (n = 210 heteroextensive metabolizers, 126 homoextensive metabolizers, and 20 poor metabolizers). Population pharmacokinetic analysis indicated that there was a 25% decrease in median clearance in poor metabolizers compared with extensive metaboliz-

GALANTAMINE HYDROBROMIDE — ORAL

ers. Dosage adjustment is not necessary in patients identified as poor metabolizers as the dose of drug is individually titrated to tolerability.

Contraindications

Known hypersensitivity to galantamine or to any excipients used in the formulation.

Warnings/Precautions

➤*Anesthesia:* Galantamine, as a cholinesterase inhibitor, is likely to exaggerate the neuromuscular blockade effects of succinylcholine-type and similar neuromuscular-blocking agents during anesthesia.

➤*Cardiovascular conditions:* Because of their pharmacological action, cholinesterase inhibitors have vagotonic effects on the sinoatrial and atrioventricular (AV) nodes, leading to bradycardia and AV block. These actions may be particularly important to patients with supraventricular cardiac conduction disorders or to patients taking other drugs concomitantly that significantly slow heart rate. Postmarketing surveillance of marketed anticholinesterase inhibitors has shown, however, that bradycardia and all types of heart block have been reported in patients both with and without known underlying cardiac conduction abnormalities. Therefore, consider all patients at risk for adverse reactions on cardiac conduction.

➤*GI conditions:* Through their primary action, cholinomimetics may be expected to increase gastric acid secretion because of increased cholinergic activity. Therefore, closely monitor patients for symptoms of active or occult GI bleeding, especially those with an increased risk for developing ulcers (eg, those with a history of ulcer disease, patients using concurrent nonsteroidal anti-inflammatory drugs [NSAIDs]). Clinical studies of galantamine have shown no increase, relative to placebo, in the incidence of either peptic ulcer disease or GI bleeding.

Galantamine, as a predictable consequence of its pharmacological properties, has been shown to produce nausea, vomiting, diarrhea, anorexia, and weight loss.

➤*Genitourinary:* Although this was not observed in clinical trials with galantamine, cholinomimetics may cause bladder outflow obstruction.

➤*Pulmonary conditions:* Because of its cholinomimetic action, prescribe galantamine with care to patients with a history of severe asthma or obstructive pulmonary disease.

➤*Seizures:* Cholinesterase inhibitors are believed to have some potential to cause generalized seizures. However, seizure activity may also be a manifestation of Alzheimer disease. In clinical trials, there was no increase in the incidence of seizures with galantamine compared with placebo.

➤*Renal function impairment:* In patients with moderate renal function impairment, cautiously proceed with dose titration. Do not exceed a dose of 16 mg/day. In patients with severe renal function impairment (creatinine clearance [Ccr] less than 9 mL/min), the use of galantamine is not recommended.

➤*Hepatic function impairment:* In patients with moderate hepatic function impairment, cautiously proceed dose titration. Do not exceed a dosage of 16 mg/day. The use of galantamine in patients with severe hepatic function impairment (Child-Pugh class 10 to 15) is not recommended.

➤*Pregnancy: Category B.* In a study in which rats were dosed from day 14 (females) or day 60 (males) prior to mating through the period of organogenesis, a slightly increased incidence of skeletal variations was observed at doses of 8 mg/kg/day (3 times the MRHD on a mg/m^2 basis) and 16 mg/kg/day. In a study in which pregnant rats were dosed from the beginning of organogenesis through day 21 postpartum, pup weights were decreased at doses of 8 and 16 mg/kg/day, but no adverse reactions on other postnatal developmental parameters were seen. The doses causing the previously listed reactions in rats produced slight maternal toxicity.

There are no adequate and well-controlled studies of galantamine in pregnant women. Use galantamine during pregnancy only if the potential benefit justifies the potential risk to the fetus.

➤*Lactation:* It is not known whether galantamine is excreted in human breast milk. Galantamine has no indication for use in breast-feeding mothers.

➤*Children:* There are no adequate and well-controlled trials documenting the safety and efficacy of galantamine in any illness occurring in children. Therefore, use of galantamine in children is not recommended.

➤*Monitoring:* Monitor patients for symptoms of active or occult GI bleeding, especially those with increased risk of developing ulcers (eg, history of ulcer disease).

Drug Interactions

Galantamine Drug Interactions

Precipitant drug	Object drug[a]		Description
Cimetidine	Galantamine	↑	Cimetidine increased the bioavailability of galantamine approximately 16%.
CYP2D6 or CYP3A4 inhibitors	Galantamine	↑	Drugs that are potent inhibitors of CYP2D6 or CYP3A4 may increase the AUC of galantamine.
Erythromycin	Galantamine	↑	Erythromycin increased the AUC of galantamine 10%.
Ketoconazole	Galantamine	↑	Ketoconazole increased the AUC of galantamine approximately 30%.
Paroxetine	Galantamine	↑	Paroxetine increased the oral bioavailability of galantamine approximately 40%.
Galantamine	Anticholinergics	↓	Galantamine has the potential to interfere with the activity of anticholinergic medications.
Galantamine	Neuromuscular-blocking agents	↑	Galantamine may exaggerate the neuromuscular blockade effects of succinylcholine-type and similar neuromuscular-blocking agents during anesthesia.
Galantamine	NSAIDs	↑	Galantamine may increase gastric acid secretion because of increased cholinergic activity. Monitor patients for symptoms of active or occult GI bleeding.
Galantamine	Succinylcholine, cholinergic agonists (eg, bethanechol), other cholinesterase inhibitors	↑	A synergistic effect is expected when combined.
Succinylcholine, cholinergic agonists (eg, bethanechol), other cholinesterase inhibitors	Galantamine		

[a] ↑ = object drug increased; ↓ = object drug decreased.

➤*Drug/Food interactions:* Food did not affect the AUC of galantamine but C_{max} decreased 25% and T_{max} was delayed 1.5 hours.

Adverse Reactions

➤*Premarketing clinical trial experience:* The specific adverse reaction data described in this section are based on studies of the IR tablet formulation. In clinical trials, once-daily treatment with galantamine ER capsules was well tolerated and adverse reactions were similar with those seen with galantamine IR tablets.

Discontinuation of treatment – In 2 large-scale, placebo-controlled trials of 6 months' duration, in which patients were titrated weekly from 8 to 16 to 24, and to 32 mg/day, the risk of discontinuation because of an adverse reaction in the galantamine group exceeded that in the placebo group by about 3-fold. In contrast, in a 5-month trial with escalation of the dose by 8 mg/day every 4 weeks, the overall risk of discontinuation because of an adverse reaction was 7%, 7%, and 10% for the placebo, galantamine 16 mg/day, and galantamine 24 mg/day groups, respectively, with GI adverse reactions the principle reason for discontinuing galantamine. The following table shows the most frequent adverse reactions leading to discontinuation in this study.

Most Frequent Galantamine Adverse Reactions Leading to Discontinuation

	4-week escalation		
Adverse reaction	Placebo (n = 286)	16 mg/day (n = 279)	24 mg/day (n = 273)
CNS			
Dizziness	< 1%	2%	1%
Syncope	0%	0%	1%
GI			
Anorexia	< 1%	1%	< 1%
Nausea	< 1%	2%	4%
Vomiting	0%	1%	3%

➤*Adverse reactions reported in controlled trials:* The reported adverse reactions in galantamine IR tablet trials reflect experience gained under closely monitored conditions in a highly selected patient population. In actual practice or in other clinical trials, these frequency estimates may not apply, as the conditions of use, reporting behavior, and the types of patients treated may differ.

The majority of these adverse reactions occurred during the dose-escalation period. In those patients who experienced the most frequent adverse reaction, nausea, the median duration was 5 to 7 days.

Administration of galantamine with food, the use of antiemetic medication, and ensuring adequate fluid intake may reduce the impact of these reactions.

The most frequent adverse reactions, defined as those occurring at a frequency of at least 5% and at least twice the rate on placebo with the recommended maintenance dose of either 16 or 24 mg/day of galantamine under

GALANTAMINE HYDROBROMIDE — ORAL

conditions of every 4-week dose-escalation for each dose increment of 8 mg/day, are shown in the following table. These reactions were primarily GI and tended to be less frequent with the 16 mg/day recommended initial maintenance dose.

Galantamine IR Adverse Reactions (≥ 5%)			
Adverse reaction	Placebo (n = 286)	Galantamine 16 mg/day (n = 279)	Galantamine 24 mg/day (n = 273)
GI			
Anorexia	3%	7%	9%
Diarrhea	6%	12%	6%
Nausea	5%	13%	17%
Vomiting	1%	6%	10%
Miscellaneous			
Weight decrease	1%	5%	5%

The most common adverse reactions (adverse reactions occurring with an incidence of at least 2% with galantamine IR tablets and in which the incidence was greater than with placebo treatment) are listed in the following table for 4 placebo-controlled trials for patients treated with galantamine 16 or 24 mg/day.

Galantamine IR Adverse Reactions (≥ 2%)		
Adverse reaction	Placebo (n = 801)	Galantamine[a] (n = 1,040)
CNS		
Depression	5%	7%
Dizziness	6%	9%
Headache	5%	8%
Insomnia	4%	5%
Somnolence	3%	4%
Tremor	2%	3%
GI		
Abdominal pain	4%	5%
Anorexia	3%	9%
Diarrhea	7%	9%
Dyspepsia	2%	5%
Nausea	9%	24%
Vomiting	4%	13%
GU		
Hematuria	2%	3%
Urinary tract infection	7%	8%
Miscellaneous		
Anemia	2%	3%
Bradycardia	1%	2%
Fatigue	3%	5%
Rhinitis	3%	4%
Syncope	1%	2%
Weight decrease	2%	7%

[a] Adverse reactions in patients treated with galantamine 16 or 24 mg/day in 4 placebo-controlled trials are included.

Adverse reactions occurring with an incidence of at least 2% in placebo-treated patients that were either equal to or greater than adverse reactions in galantamine-treated patients were agitation, anxiety, asthenia, back pain, bronchitis, chest pain, confusion, constipation, coughing, fall, hallucination, hypertension, injury, peripheral edema, purpura, upper respiratory tract infection, and urinary incontinence.

There were no important differences in adverse reaction rate related to dose or sex. There were too few nonwhite patients to assess the effects of race on adverse reaction rates.

No clinically relevant abnormalities in laboratory values were observed.

➤*Other observed adverse reactions:* Galantamine IR tablets were administered to 3,055 patients with Alzheimer disease. A total of 2,357 patients received galantamine in placebo-controlled trials and 761 patients with Alzheimer disease received galantamine 24 mg/day, the maximum recommended maintenance dose. About 1,000 patients received galantamine for at least 1 year, and approximately 200 patients received galantamine for 2 years.

To establish the rate of adverse reactions, data from all patients receiving any dose of galantamine in 8 placebo-controlled trials and 6 open-label extension trials were pooled. The methodology to gather and codify these adverse reactions was standardized across trials, using World Health Organization (WHO) terminology. All adverse reactions occurring in approximately 0.1% are included, except for those already listed elsewhere in labeling, WHO terms too general to be informative, or events unlikely to be drug caused. Reactions are classified by body system and listed using the following definitions: frequent adverse reactions (those occurring in at least 1/100 patients), infrequent adverse reactions (those occurring in 1/100 to 1/1,000 patients), rare adverse reactions (those occurring in less than 1/1,000 to 1/10,000 patients), very rare adverse reactions (those occurring in fewer than 1/10,000 patients). These adverse reactions are not necessarily related to galantamine treatment and in most cases were observed at a similar frequency in placebo-treated patients in the controlled studies.

Cardiovascular – Atrial arrhythmias including atrial fibrillation and supraventricular tachycardia, AV block, bundle branch block, cardiac failure, dependent edema, hypotension, myocardial ischemia or infarction, palpitation, postural hypotension, QT prolonged, T-wave inversion, ventricular tachycardia (infrequent); severe bradycardia (rare).

CNS – Apathy, aphasia, apraxia, ataxia, delirium, hyperkinesia, hypertonia, hypokinesia, involuntary muscle contractions, leg cramps, libido increased, paranoid reaction, paresthesia, paroniria, seizures, tinnitus, transient ischemic attack or cerebrovascular accident, vertigo (infrequent); suicidal ideation (rare); suicide (very rare).

GI – Flatulence (frequent); diverticulitis, dry mouth, dysphagia, gastritis, gastroenteritis, hiccup, melena, rectal hemorrhage, saliva increased (infrequent); esophageal perforation (rare).

GU – Incontinence (frequent); cystitis, hematuria, micturition frequency, nocturia, renal calculi, urinary retention (infrequent).

Hematologic – Epistaxis, purpura, thrombocytopenia (infrequent).

Metabolic – Alkaline phosphatase increased, hyperglycemia (infrequent).

Miscellaneous – Asthenia, chest pain, fever, malaise (frequent).

➤*Postmarketing:* Other adverse reactions from post-approval controlled and uncontrolled clinical trials and postmarketing experience observed in patients treated with galantamine IR tablets are listed in the following sections. These adverse reactions may or may not be causally related to the drug.

CNS – Aggression.

GI – Upper and lower GI bleeding.

Metabolic/Nutritional – Hypokalemia.

Miscellaneous – Dehydration (including rare, severe cases leading to renal function impairment and renal failure).

Overdosage

➤*Symptoms:* Signs and symptoms of significant overdosing of galantamine are predicted to be similar with those of overdosing of other cholinomimetics. These effects generally involve the CNS, the parasympathetic nervous system, and the neuromuscular junction. In addition to muscle weakness or fasciculations, some or all of the following signs of cholinergic crisis may develop: severe nausea, vomiting, GI cramping, salivation, lacrimation, urination, defecation, sweating, bradycardia, hypotension, respiratory depression, collapse, and convulsions. Increasing muscle weakness is a possibility and may result in death if respiratory muscles are involved.

In a postmarketing report, 1 patient who had been taking galantamine 4 mg daily for a week inadvertently ingested eight 4 mg tablets (32 mg total) on a single day. Subsequently, she developed bradycardia, QT prolongation, ventricular tachycardia, and torsades de pointes, accompanied by a brief loss of consciousness for which she required hospital treatment. Two additional cases of accidental ingestion of 32 mg (nausea, vomiting, and dry mouth; nausea, vomiting, and substernal chest pain) and one of 40 mg (vomiting) resulted in brief hospitalizations for observation with full recovery. One patient, who was prescribed 24 mg/day and had a history of hallucinations over the previous 2 years, mistakenly received 24 mg twice daily for 34 days and developed hallucinations requiring hospitalization. Another patient, who was prescribed 16 mg/day of oral solution, inadvertently ingested 160 mg (40 mL) and experienced sweating, vomiting, bradycardia, and near-syncope 1 hour later, which necessitated hospital treatment. His symptoms resolved within 24 hours.

➤*Treatment:* As in any case of overdose, use general supportive measures. Tertiary anticholinergics, such as atropine, may be used as an antidote for galantamine overdosage. IV atropine sulfate titrated to effect is recommended at an initial dose of 0.5 to 1 mg IV with subsequent doses based upon clinical response. Atypical responses in blood pressure and heart rate have been reported with other cholinomimetics when coadministered with quaternary anticholinergics. It is not known whether galantamine and/or its metabolites can be removed by dialysis (hemodialysis, peritoneal dialysis, or hemofiltration). Dose-related signs of toxicity in animals included chromodacryorrhea, clonic seizures, dyspnea, hypoactivity, lacrimation, mucoid feces, salivation, and tremors.

Because strategies for the management of overdose are continually evolving, it is advisable to contact a poison control center to determine the latest recommendations for the management of an overdose of any drug.

Patient Information

Instruct caregivers about the recommended dosage and administration of galantamine. Administer galantamine ER capsules once daily in the morning, preferably with food (although not required). Administer galantamine IR tablets and oral solution twice per day, preferably with morning and evening meals. Dose escalation (dose increase) should follow a minimum of 4 weeks at prior dose.

Advise patients and caregivers that the most frequent adverse reactions associated with use of the drug can be minimized by following the recommended dosage and administration.

Advise patients and caregivers to ensure adequate fluid intake during treatment. If therapy has been interrupted for several days or longer, restart the patient at the lowest dose and escalate the dose to the current dose.

Instruct caregivers in the correct procedure for administering galantamine oral solution. In addition, inform caregivers of the existence of an instruction

GALANTAMINE HYDROBROMIDE — ORAL

sheet describing how the solution is to be administered. Urge caregivers to read this sheet prior to administering galantamine oral solution. Caregivers should direct questions about the administration of the solution to either their health care provider or pharmacist.

MISCELLANEOUS PSYCHOTHERAPEUTIC AGENTS

ATOMOXETINE

Rx	Strattera (Eli Lilly)	Capsules; oral: 10 mg	As atomoxetine hydrochloride. (LILLY 3227 10 mg). Opaque white. In 30s.
		18 mg	As atomoxetine hydrochloride. (LILLY 3238 18 mg). Gold/opaque white. In 30s.
		25 mg	As atomoxetine hydrochloride. (LILLY 3228 25 mg). Opaque blue/opaque white. In 30s.
		40 mg	As atomoxetine hydrochloride. (LILLY 3229 40 mg). Opaque blue. In 30s.
		60 mg	As atomoxetine hydrochloride. (LILLY 3239 60 mg). Opaque blue/gold. In 30s.
		80 mg	As atomoxetine hydrochloride. (LILLY 3250 80 mg). Opaque brown/opaque white. In 30s.
		100 mg	As atomoxetine hydrochloride. (LILLY 3251 100 mg). Opaque brown. In 30s.

ATOMOXETINE HYDROCHLORIDE — ORAL

WARNING

Suicidal ideation in children and adolescents – Atomoxetine increased the risk of suicidal ideation in short-term studies in children or adolescents with attention deficit hyperactivity disorder (ADHD). Anyone considering the use of atomoxetine in a child or adolescent must balance this risk with the clinical need. Comorbidities occurring with ADHD may be associated with an increase in the risk of suicidal ideation and/or behavior. Closely monitor patients who are started on therapy for suicidality (suicidal thinking and behavior), clinical worsening, or unusual changes in behavior. Advise families and caregivers of the need for close observation and communication with the prescribing health care provider. Atomoxetine is approved for ADHD in children and adults. Atomoxetine is not approved for major depressive disorder (MDD).

Pooled analyses of short-term (6- to 18-week), placebo-controlled trials of atomoxetine in children and adolescents (12 trials involving more than 2,200 patients, including 11 trials in ADHD and 1 trial in enuresis) have revealed a greater risk of suicidal ideation early during treatment in those receiving atomoxetine compared with placebo. The average risk of suicidal ideation in patients receiving atomoxetine was 0.4% compared with none in placebo-treated patients. No suicides occurred in these trials.

Indications

➤*Attention deficit hyperactivity disorder:* For the treatment of ADHD.

For the inattentive type, at least 6 of the following symptoms must have persisted for at least 6 months: lack of attention to details/careless mistakes, lack of sustained attention, poor listening, failure to follow through on tasks, poor organization, avoidance of tasks requiring sustained mental effort, losing things, tendency to be easily distracted, forgetfulness.

For the hyperactive-impulsive type, at least 6 of the following symptoms must have persisted for at least 6 months: fidgeting/squirming, leaving his or her seat, inappropriate running/climbing, difficulty with quiet activities, being "on the go," excessive talking, blurting answers, inability to wait his or her turn, intrusiveness.

For a combined-type diagnosis, both inattentive and hyperactive-impulsive criteria must be met.

➤*Off-label uses:*

Binge eating disorder – [4] = Insufficient documentation. Initial data suggest that atomoxetine may be beneficial for overweight adults with binge eating disorder. However, the patient population studied was largely female. Further studies are needed to determine efficacy in other patient populations, including those with psychiatric disorders. In addition, larger, longer-term studies and studies comparing atomoxetine with cognitive-behavioral and interpersonal therapies and selective serotonin reuptake inhibitors are needed.

Nocturnal enuresis – [2] = Fair documentation. Initial data suggest that atomoxetine may be beneficial for children with nocturnal enuresis, including patients with concomitant ADHD.

Obesity – [4] = Insufficient documentation. Based on limited data, the use of atomoxetine for weight reduction in women with obesity has shown benefits in one trial. However, the number of patients completing the trial was small (N = 21), and larger controlled trials are needed before this agent can be recommended for the management of obesity.

Administration and Dosage

➤*Adults:*

Attention deficit hyperactivity disorder –

Maximum dose: 100 mg/day.

Initial dosage: 40 mg/day.

Dosage adjustment: Increase after a minimum of 3 days to a target total daily dose of approximately 80 mg. After 2 to 4 additional weeks, the dose may be increased to a maximum of 100 mg in patients who have not achieved optimal response.

Concomitant therapy with strong CYP2D6 inhibitors (eg, fluoxetine, paroxetine, quinidine) or in patients who are known to be CYP2D6 poor metabolizers: Initiate at 40 mg/day and only increase to the usual target dosage of 80 mg/day if symptoms fail to improve after 4 weeks and the initial dose is well tolerated.

Off-label dosing –

Binge eating disorder: [4] = Insufficient documentation. 40 mg orally daily, titrated to 120 mg daily for 10 weeks (mean, 106 mg daily).

Obesity: [4] = Insufficient documentation. Initial dosing was 25 mg daily for the first 3 days, followed by 50 mg for days 4 through 7, then 100 mg daily for the remaining 12 weeks.

➤*Children:*

Attention deficit hyperactivity disorder –

6 years and older:

- *Children more than 70 kg body weight* – See Adults for dosing.
- *Children up to 70 kg body weight* –

Maximum dose: Should not exceed 1.4 mg/kg/day or 100 mg/day, whichever is less.

Initial dosage: 0.5 mg/kg/day.

Dosage adjustment: Increase after a minimum of 3 days to a target total daily dose of approximately 1.2 mg/kg. No additional benefit has been demonstrated for dosages higher than 1.2 mg/kg/day.

Concomitant therapy with strong CYP2D6 inhibitors (eg, fluoxetine, paroxetine, quinidine) or in patients who are known to be CYP2D6 poor metabolizers: Initiate at 0.5 mg/kg/day and only increase to the usual target dosage of 1.2 mg/kg/day if symptoms fail to improve after 4 weeks and the initial dose is well tolerated.

Off-label dosing –

Nocturnal enuresis: [2] = Fair documentation. In a randomized trial, 1.5 mg/kg/day given orally in 2 divided doses was given for 12 weeks; 1 to 1.6 mg/kg/day orally for up to 4 months was used in a case series.

➤*Hepatic function impairment:* For patients with moderate hepatic impairment (Child-Pugh class B), the initial and target doses should be reduced to 50% of the usual dose (for patients without hepatic impairment). For patients with severe hepatic impairment (Child-Pugh class C), initial dose and target doses should be reduced to 25% of the usual dose.

➤*Duration of therapy:* Pharmacological treatment of ADHD may be needed for extended periods. The health care provider who elects to use atomoxetine for extended periods should periodically reevaluate the long-term usefulness of the drug for the individual patient.

➤*Discontinuation of therapy:* Atomoxetine can be discontinued without being tapered.

➤*Administration:* Administer as a single daily dose in the morning or as evenly divided doses in the morning and late afternoon/early evening. May be taken with or without food. Atomoxetine capsules are not intended to be opened; they should be taken whole.

➤*Storage/Stability:* Store at 25°C (77°F); excursions are permitted between 15° and 30°C (59° and 86°F).

Actions

➤*Pharmacology:* Atomoxetine is a selective norepinephrine reuptake inhibitor. The precise mechanism by which atomoxetine produces its therapeutic effects in ADHD is unknown, but is thought to be related to selective inhibition of the presynaptic norepinephrine transporter, as determined in ex vivo uptake and neurotransmitter depletion studies.

➤*Pharmacokinetics:*

Absorption/Distribution – Atomoxetine is rapidly absorbed after oral administration and is minimally affected by food, with an absolute bioavailability of approximately 63% in extensive metabolizers and 94% in poor metabolizers. Maximal plasma concentrations (C_{max}) are reached approximately 1 to 2 hours after dosing.

The steady-state volume of distribution after intravenous administration is 0.85 L/kg, indicating that atomoxetine distributes primarily into total body water. Volume of distribution is similar across the patient weight range after normalizing for body weight. At therapeutic concentrations, 98% of atomoxetine in plasma is bound to protein, primarily albumin.

Effect of food: Atomoxetine may be administered with or without food. Administration of atomoxetine with a standard high-fat meal in adults did not affect the extent of oral absorption of atomoxetine (area under the curve [AUC]), but did decrease the rate of absorption, resulting in a 37% lower C_{max} and delayed time of maximal concentration (T_{max}) by 3 hours. In clini-

ATOMOXETINE HYDROCHLORIDE — ORAL

cal trials with children and adolescents, administration of atomoxetine with food resulted in a 9% lower C_{max}.

Metabolism/Excretion – Atomoxetine is metabolized primarily by oxidative metabolism through the cytochrome P450 (CYP) 2D6 enzymatic pathway and subsequent glucuronidation. People with reduced activity in this pathway (poor metabolizers) have higher plasma concentrations of atomoxetine compared with people with normal activity (extensive metabolizers). A fraction of the population (approximately 7% of white patients and 2% of black patients) are poor metabolizers of CYP2D6-metabolized drugs. For poor metabolizers, the AUC of atomoxetine is approximately 10-fold, and $C_{ss\ max}$ is about 5-fold greater than extensive metabolizers. Laboratory tests are available to identify CYP2D6 poor metabolizers. Atomoxetine did not inhibit or induce the CYP2D6 pathway.

The major oxidative metabolite formed, regardless of CYP2D6 status, is 4-hydroxyatomoxetine, which is glucuronidated. Four-hydroxyatomoxetine is equipotent to atomoxetine as an inhibitor of the norepinephrine transporter, but circulates in plasma at much lower concentrations (1% of atomoxetine concentration in extensive metabolizers and 0.1% of atomoxetine concentration in poor metabolizers). Four-hydroxyatomoxetine is primarily formed by CYP2D6, but in poor metabolizers, 4-hydroxyatomoxetine is formed at a slower rate by several other cytochrome CYP-450 enzymes. N-desmethylatomoxetine is formed by CYP2C19 and other CYP-450 enzymes but has substantially less pharmacological activity compared with atomoxetine and circulates in plasma at lower concentrations (5% of atomoxetine concentration in extensive metabolizers and 45% of atomoxetine concentration in poor metabolizers).

Mean apparent plasma clearance of atomoxetine after oral administration in adult extensive metabolizers was 0.35 L/h/kg, and the mean half-life was 5.2 hours. Following oral administration of atomoxetine to poor metabolizers, mean apparent plasma clearance was 0.03 L/h/kg, and mean half-life was 21.6 hours. For poor metabolizers, AUC of atomoxetine was approximately 10-fold and $C_{ss\ max}$ was approximately 5-fold greater than extensive metabolizers. The elimination half-life of 4-hydroxyatomoxetine was similar to that of N-desmethylatomoxetine (6 to 8 hours) in extensive metabolizers, whereas the half-life of N-desmethylatomoxetine was much longer in poor metabolizers (34 to 40 hours).

Atomoxetine was excreted primarily as 4-hydroxyatomoxetine-*O*-glucuronide, mainly in the urine (more than 80% of the dose) and, to a lesser extent, in the feces (less than 17% of the dose). Only a small fraction of the atomoxetine dose was excreted as unchanged atomoxetine (less than 3% of the dose), indicating extensive biotransformation.

Special populations –

Hepatic function impairment: Atomoxetine exposure (AUC) was increased, compared with healthy subjects, in extensive metabolizers with moderate (Child-Pugh class B) (2-fold increase) and severe (Child-Pugh class C) (4-fold increase) hepatic insufficiency. Dosage adjustment is recommended for patients with moderate or severe hepatic insufficiency.

Poor metabolizers of CYP2D6: Poor metabolizers of CYP2D6 have a 10-fold higher AUC and a 5-fold higher peak concentration and slower elimination (plasma half-life of about 24 hours) to a given dose of atomoxetine compared with extensive metabolizers. Approximately 7% of a white population and 2% of a black population are poor metabolizers. Laboratory tests are available to identify CYP2D6 poor metabolizers. The blood levels in poor metabolizers are similar to those attained by taking strong inhibitors of CYP2D6. The higher blood levels in poor metabolizers lead to a higher rate of some adverse reactions of atomoxetine.

Contraindications

Hypersensitivity to atomoxetine or other constituents of the product; narrow-angle glaucoma; use with a monoamine oxidase inhibitor (MAOI) or within 2 weeks of discontinuing an MAOI.

Warnings/Precautions

➤*Suicidal ideation:* Atomoxetine increased the risk of suicidal ideation in short-term studies in children and adolescents with ADHD. Pooled analyses of short-term (6- to 18-weeks), placebo-controlled trials of atomoxetine in children and adolescents have revealed a greater risk of suicidal ideation early during treatment in those receiving atomoxetine. There were 12 trials (11 in ADHD; 1 in enuresis) involving more than 2,200 patients (including 1,357 patients receiving atomoxetine and 851 receiving placebo). The average risk of suicidal ideation in patients receiving atomoxetine was 0.4% compared with none in the placebo-treated patients. There was 1 suicide attempt (among approximately 2,200 patients) occurring in a patient treated with atomoxetine. No suicides occurred in these trials. All reactions occurred in children 12 years of age and younger. All reactions occurred during the first month of treatment. It is unknown whether the risk of suicidal ideation in children extends to longer-term use. A similar analysis in adult patients treated with atomoxetine for ADHD or MDD did not reveal an increased risk of suicidal ideation or behavior in association with the use of atomoxetine.

Monitor all children being treated with atomoxetine appropriately and observe closely for clinical worsening, suicidality, and unusual changes in behavior, especially during the initial few months of a course of drug therapy or at times of dose changes, either increases or decreases.

The following symptoms have been reported with atomoxetine: aggressiveness, agitation, akathisia (psychomotor restlessness), anxiety, hostility, hypomania, impulsivity, insomnia, irritability, mania, and panic attacks. Although a causal link between the emergence of such symptoms and the emergence of suicidal impulses has not been established, there is a concern that such symptoms may represent precursors to emerging suicidality. Thus, observe for the emergence of such symptoms in patients being treated with atomoxetine.

Consider changing the therapeutic regimen, including possibly discontinuing the medication, in patients who experience emerging suicidality or symptoms that might be precursors to emerging suicidality, especially if these symptoms are severe or abrupt in onset or were not part of the patient's presenting symptoms.

Alert families and caregivers of children being treated with atomoxetine about the need to monitor patients for the emergence of agitation, irritability, unusual changes in behavior, and the other symptoms described previously, as well as the emergence of suicidality, and to report such symptoms immediately to a health care provider. Include daily observation by families and caregivers in this monitoring.

➤*Hepatic effects:* Postmarketing reports indicate that atomoxetine can cause severe liver injury. Although no evidence of liver injury was detected in clinical trials of approximately 6,000 patients, there have been rare cases of clinically significant liver injury that were considered probably or possibly related to atomoxetine use in postmarketing experience. Because of probable underreporting, it is impossible to provide an accurate estimate of the true incidence of these reactions. Reported cases of liver injury occurred within 120 days of initiation of atomoxetine in the majority of cases and some patients presented with markedly elevated liver enzymes (greater than 20 times the upper limit of normal [ULN]), and jaundice with significantly elevated bilirubin levels (greater than 2 times the ULN), followed by recovery upon atomoxetine discontinuation. In 1 patient, liver injury, manifested by elevated hepatic enzymes (up to 40 times the ULN) and jaundice (bilirubin up to 12 times the ULN), recurred upon rechallenge and was followed by recovery upon drug discontinuation, providing evidence that atomoxetine caused the liver injury. Such reactions may occur several months after therapy is started, but laboratory abnormalities may continue to worsen for several weeks after the drug is stopped. The patient described previously recovered from his liver injury and did not require a liver transplant. However, severe liver injury caused by any drug may potentially progress to acute liver failure, resulting in death or the need for a liver transplant.

Discontinue atomoxetine in patients with jaundice or laboratory evidence of liver injury, and do not restart therapy. Conduct laboratory testing to determine liver enzyme levels upon the first symptom or sign of liver dysfunction (eg, dark urine, jaundice, pruritus, right upper quadrant tenderness, unexplained "flu-like" symptoms).

➤*Cardiovascular effects:*

Sudden death and other serious heart problems –

Children and adolescents: Sudden death has been reported in association with atomoxetine treatment at usual doses in children and adolescents with structural cardiac abnormalities or other serious heart problems. Although some serious heart problems alone carry an increased risk of sudden death, generally, do not use atomoxetine in children or adolescents with known serious structural cardiac abnormalities, cardiomyopathy, serious heart rhythm abnormalities, or other serious cardiac problems that may place them at increased vulnerability to the noradrenergic effects of atomoxetine.

Adults: Sudden death, stroke, and myocardial infarction have been reported in adults taking atomoxetine at usual doses for ADHD. Although the role of atomoxetine in these adult cases is also unknown, adults have a greater likelihood than children of having serious structural cardiac abnormalities, cardiomyopathy, serious heart rhythm abnormalities, coronary artery disease, or other serious cardiac problems. Consider not treating adults with clinically significant cardiac abnormalities.

Assessing cardiovascular status – Children, adolescents, or adults who are being considered for treatment with atomoxetine should have a careful history (including assessment for a family history of sudden death or ventricular arrhythmia) and physical exam to assess for the presence of cardiac disease, and should receive further cardiac evaluation if findings suggest such disease (eg, echocardiogram, electrocardiogram). Conduct a prompt cardiac evaluation for patients who develop symptoms such as exertional chest pain, unexplained syncope, or other symptoms suggestive of cardiac disease during atomoxetine treatment.

Blood pressure and heart rate effects – Use atomoxetine with caution in patients with hypertension, tachycardia, or cardiovascular or cerebrovascular disease because it can increase blood pressure and heart rate. Measure pulse and blood pressure at baseline, following atomoxetine dose increases, and periodically while on therapy.

Children: In placebo-controlled trials, atomoxetine-treated subjects experienced a mean increase in heart rate of about 6 beats per min (bpm) compared with placebo-treated subjects. At the final study visit before drug discontinuation, 2.5% of atomoxetine-treated subjects had heart rate increases of at least 25 bpm and a heart rate of at least 110 bpm, compared with 0.2% of placebo subjects. There were 1.1% atomoxetine-treated children with a heart rate increase of at least 25 bpm and a heart rate of at least 110 bpm on more than 1 occasion. Tachycardia was identified as an adverse reaction for 0.3% of these children compared with 0% of placebo subjects. The mean heart rate increase in extensive metabolizer patients was 5 bpm and 9.4 bpm in poor metabolizer patients.

Atomoxetine-treated children experienced mean increases of about 1.6 and 2.4 mm Hg in systolic and diastolic blood pressures, respectively, compared with placebo. At the final study visit before drug discontinuation, 4.8% of atomoxetine-treated children had high systolic blood pressure measurements compared with 3.5% of placebo subjects. High diastolic blood pressures were measured on 2 or more occasions in 4.4% of atomoxetine-treated subjects and 1.9% of placebo subjects. At the final study visit before drug discontinuation, 4% of atomoxetine-treated children had high diastolic blood pressure measurements compared with 1.1% of placebo subjects. High systolic blood pressures were measured on 2 or more occasions in 3.5% of atomoxetine-treated subjects and 0.5% of placebo subjects. High systolic and diastolic blood pressure measurements were defined as those exceeding the 95th percentile, stratified by age, gender, and height percentile, according to

ATOMOXETINE HYDROCHLORIDE — ORAL

the National High Blood Pressure Education Working Group on Hypertension Control in Children and Adolescents)

Orthostatic hypotension and syncope have been reported in patients taking atomoxetine. In child and adolescent trials, 0.2% of atomoxetine-treated patients experienced orthostatic hypotension and 0.8% experienced syncope. In short-term child and adolescent controlled trials, 1.8% of atomoxetine-treated patients experienced orthostatic hypotension compared with 0.5% of placebo-treated patients. Syncope was not reported during short-term child and adolescent placebo-controlled ADHD trials. Use atomoxetine with caution in any condition that may predispose patients to hypotension, or conditions associated with abrupt heart rate or blood pressure changes.

Adults: In adult placebo-controlled trials, atomoxetine-treated subjects experienced a mean increase in heart rate of 5 bpm compared with placebo-treated subjects. Tachycardia was identified as an adverse reaction for 1.5% of these adult atomoxetine-treated subjects compared with 0.5% of placebo-treated subjects.

Atomoxetine-treated adult subjects experienced mean increases in systolic (approximately 2 mm Hg) and diastolic (approximately 1 mm Hg) blood pressures compared with placebo. At the final study visit before drug discontinuation, 2.2% of atomoxetine-treated adult subjects had systolic blood pressure measurements of 150 mm Hg or more compared with 1% of placebo subjects. At the final study visit before drug discontinuation, 0.4% of atomoxetine-treated adult subjects had diastolic blood pressure measurements of 100 mm Hg or more compared with 0.5% of placebo subjects. No adult subject had a high systolic or diastolic blood pressure detected on more than 1 occasion.

Peripheral vascular effects – There have been spontaneous postmarketing reports of Raynaud phenomenon (new-onset and exacerbation of preexisting condition).

➤*Emergence of new psychotic or manic symptoms:* Treatment-emergent psychotic or manic symptoms (eg, delusional thinking, hallucinations, mania) in children and adolescents without a prior history of psychotic illness or mania can be caused by atomoxetine at usual doses. If such symptoms occur, consider a possible causal role of atomoxetine and consider discontinuation of treatment. In a pooled analysis of multiple short-term, placebo-controlled studies, such symptoms occurred in about 0.2% (4 of 1,939 patients exposed to atomoxetine for several weeks at usual doses) of atomoxetine-treated patients compared with 0 of 1,056 placebo-treated patients.

➤*Screening patients for bipolar disorder:* In general, take particular care in treating ADHD in patients with comorbid bipolar disorder because of the concern of possible induction of a mixed/manic episode in patients at risk of bipolar disorder. Whether any of the symptoms described previously represent such a conversion is unknown. However, prior to initiating treatment with atomoxetine, adequately screen patients with comorbid depressive symptoms to determine if they are at risk of bipolar disorder; include a detailed psychiatric history in the screening, as well as family history of bipolar disorder, depression, and suicide.

➤*Aggressive behavior or hostility:* Monitor patients beginning treatment for ADHD for the appearance or worsening of aggressive behavior or hostility. Aggressive behavior or hostility is often observed in children and adolescents with ADHD. In short-term, controlled clinical trials, 1.6% of atomoxetine-treated patients versus 1.1% of placebo-treated patients spontaneously reported treatment-emergent, hostility-related adverse events. Although this is not conclusive evidence that atomoxetine causes aggressive behavior or hostility, these behaviors were more frequently observed in clinical trials in children and adolescents treated with atomoxetine compared with placebo (overall risk ratio of 1.33 [95% confidence interval, 0.67 to 2.64; not statistically significant]).

➤*Urinary effects:* In adult ADHD controlled trials, the rates of urinary retention (1.7%) and urinary hesitation (5.6%) were increased among atomoxetine-treated subjects compared with placebo-treated subjects (0% [0/402]; 0.5%, respectively). Two adult atomoxetine-treated subjects and no placebo-treated subjects discontinued from controlled clinical trials because of urinary retention. Consider a complaint of urinary retention or urinary hesitancy to be potentially related to atomoxetine.

➤*Priapism:* Rare postmarketing cases of priapism, defined as painful and nonpainful penile erection lasting more than 4 hours, have been reported for children and adults treated with atomoxetine. The erections resolved in cases in which follow-up information was available, some following discontinuation of atomoxetine. Prompt medical attention is required in the event of suspected priapism.

➤*Effects on growth:* Data on the long-term effects of atomoxetine on growth come from open-label studies, and weight and height changes are compared with normative population data. In general, the weight and height gain of children treated with atomoxetine lags behind that predicated by normative population data for about the first 9 to 12 months of treatment. Subsequently, weight gain rebounds and, at about 3 years of treatment, patients treated with atomoxetine have gained 17.9 kg on average, 0.5 kg more than predicted by their baseline data. After about 12 months, gain in height stabilizes and, at 3 years, patients treated with atomoxetine have gained 19.4 cm on average, 0.4 cm less than predicted by their baseline data.

This growth pattern was generally similar regardless of pubertal status at the time of treatment initiation. Patients who were prepubertal at the start of treatment (girls 8 years and younger, boys 9 years and younger) gained an average of 2.1 kg and 1.2 cm less than predicted after 3 years. Patients who were pubertal (girls older than 8 to 13 years, boys older than 9 to 14 years) or late pubertal (girls older than 13 years, boys older than 14 years) had average weight and height gains that were close to or exceeded those predicted after 3 years of treatment.

Growth followed a similar pattern in extensive metabolizers and poor metabolizers. Poor metabolizers treated for at least 2 years gained an average of 2.4 kg and 1.1 cm less than predicted, while extensive metabolizers gained an average of 0.2 kg and 0.4 cm less than predicted.

In short-term (up to 9-week) control studies, atomoxetine-treated patients lost an average of 0.4 kg and gained an average of 0.9 cm, compared with a gain of 1.5 kg and 1.1 cm in the placebo-treated patients. In a fixed-dose controlled trial, 1.3%, 7.1%, 19.3%, and 29.1% of patients lost at least 3.5% of their body weight in the placebo, 0.5, 1.2, and 1.8 mg/kg/day dosage groups, respectively. Monitor growth during treatment with atomoxetine.

➤*Narrow-angle glaucoma:* In clinical trials, atomoxetine use was associated with an increased risk of mydriasis; therefore, its use is contraindicated in patients with narrow-angle glaucoma.

➤*Hypersensitivity reactions:* Although uncommon, allergic reactions, including angioneurotic edema, rash, and urticaria, have been reported in patients taking atomoxetine.

➤*Hazardous tasks:* Advise patients to use caution when driving a car or operating hazardous machinery until they are reasonably certain that their performance is not affected by atomoxetine.

➤*Pregnancy:* *Category C.* No adequate and well-controlled studies have been conducted in pregnant women.

It is not known if atomoxetine or its active metabolites cross the human placenta. The molecular weight for the parent drug (about 256 for the free base) and the elimination half-life suggest that atomoxetine will cross to the embryo and/or fetus. The extensive protein binding, however, will limit the amount available for transfer.

Do not use atomoxetine during pregnancy unless the potential benefit justifies the potential risk to the fetus.

Pregnant rabbits were treated with up to 100 mg/kg/day of atomoxetine given by gavage throughout the period of organogenesis. At this dosage, in 1 of 3 studies, a decrease in live fetuses and an increase in early resorption were observed. Slight increases in the incidences of atypical origin of carotid artery and absent subclavian artery were observed. These findings were observed at dosages that caused slight maternal toxicity. The no-effect dosage for these findings was 30 mg/kg/day. The 100 mg/kg dose is approximately 23 times the maximum human dose on a mg/m^2 basis. Plasma levels (AUC) of atomoxetine at this dose in rabbits are estimated to be 3.3 (extensive metabolizers) or 0.4 (poor metabolizers) times those in humans receiving the maximum human dose.

Rats were treated with up to approximately 50 mg/kg/day of atomoxetine (approximately 6 times the maximum human dose on a mg/m^2 basis) given in the diet from 2 weeks (females) or 10 weeks (males) prior to mating through the periods of organogenesis and lactation. In 1 of 2 studies, decreases in pup weight and pup survival were observed. The decreased pup survival was also seen at 25 mg/kg (but not at 13 mg/kg). In a study in which rats were treated with atomoxetine given in the diet from 2 weeks (females) or 10 weeks (males) prior to mating throughout the period of organogenesis, a decrease in fetal weight (female only) and an increase in the incidence of incomplete ossification of the vertebral arch in fetuses were observed at 40 mg/kg/day (approximately 5 times the maximum human dose on a mg/m^2 basis), but not at 20 mg/kg/day.

➤*Lactation:* Atomoxetine and/or its metabolites were excreted in the milk of rats. It is not known if atomoxetine is excreted in human milk.

The molecular weight of the parent drug (about 256 for the free base) and the relatively long elimination half-life (5 hours for normal metabolizers; 24 hours for poor metabolizers) suggest that atomoxetine and/or its metabolites will be excreted into breast milk. The effects of this exposure on a breast-feeding infant are unknown.

Exercise caution if atomoxetine is administered to a breast-feeding woman.

If a mother chooses to breast-feed while taking atomoxetine, monitor the infant for potential toxicity (eg, constipation, dyspepsia, upper abdominal pain).

➤*Children:* The safety and efficacy of atomoxetine in children younger than 6 years have not been evaluated. Anyone considering the use of atomoxetine in a child or adolescent must balance the potential risks with the clinical need.

➤*Monitoring:* Closely monitor patients being treated with atomoxetine for suicidality, clinical worsening, and unusual changes in behavior, especially during the initial few months of a course of drug therapy or at times of dose changes.

Monitor growth, pulse, and blood pressure at baseline, at dose increases, and periodically during atomoxetine therapy. Monitor patients beginning treatment for the appearance or worsening of aggressive behavior or hostility.

Drug Interactions

➤*QT prolongation:* An additive effect of atomoxetine with other drugs that prolong the QT interval cannot be excluded. The following drugs may prolong the QT interval and increase the risk of life-threatening cardiac arrhythmias, including torsade de pointes: antiarrhythmic agents (eg, amiodarone, bretylium, disopyramide, dofetilide, procainamide, quinidine, sotalol), arsenic trioxide, chlorpromazine, cisapride, dolasetron, droperidol, gatifloxacin, halofantrine, levomethadyl, mefloquine, mesoridazine, moxifloxacin, pentamidine, pimozide, probucol, sparfloxacin, thioridazine, ziprasidone. (See Drug-Induced Prolongation of the QT Interval and Torsades de Pointes.)

ATOMOXETINE HYDROCHLORIDE — ORAL

Atomoxetine Drug Interactions			
Precipitant drug	Object drug[a]		Description
CYP2D6 inhibitors (eg, fluoxetine, paroxetine, quinidine)	Atomoxetine	↑	Coadministration causes an increase in AUC and C_{max} at steady state. Dosage adjustment may be necessary.
MAOIs (eg, phenelzine)	Atomoxetine	↑	There have been reports of serious, sometimes fatal reactions (including hyperthermia, rigidity, myoclonus, autonomic instability with possible rapid fluctuations of vital signs, and mental status changes that include extreme agitation progressing to delirium and coma) when taken in combination with an MAOI. Some cases presented with features resembling neuroleptic malignant syndrome. Such reactions may occur when these drugs are given concurrently or in close proximity. Coadministration is contraindicated. Do not administer atomoxetine within 2 weeks after discontinuing an MAOI and do not initiate treatment with an MAOI within 2 weeks after discontinuing atomoxetine.
Atomoxetine	MAOIs (eg, phenelzine)		
Pressor agents (eg, dobutamine, dopamine)	Atomoxetine	↑	Administer with caution because of possible effects on blood pressure.
Atomoxetine	Pressor agents (eg, dobutamine, dopamine)		
Atomoxetine	Albuterol	↑	Administer with caution because the cardiovascular action of albuterol can be potentiated (eg, increased heart rate and blood pressure).
Atomoxetine	CYP3A substrates (eg, midazolam)	↑	Coadministration resulted in a 15% increase in midazolam AUC. No dosage adjustment is needed.
Atomoxetine	Iobenguane	↓	Atomoxetine may reduce uptake and diagnostic efficacy of iobenguane. False-negative iobenguane imaging tests may result. Discontinue atomoxetine for at least 5 biological half- lives (approximately 24 hours) prior to iobenguane administration.

[a] ↑ = object drug increased; ↓ = object drug decreased.

➤*Minimally or non-interacting drugs:* Coadministration of methylphenidate with atomoxetine did not increase cardiovascular effects compared with giving methylphenidate alone. Consumption of alcohol with atomoxetine did not change the intoxicating effects of alcohol. Drugs that elevate gastric pH (eg, magnesium hydroxide/aluminum hydroxide) did not affect atomoxetine bioavailability.

In vitro drug-displacement studies with atomoxetine and other highly-bound drugs at therapeutic concentrations, atomoxetine did not affect binding of acetylsalicylic acid, diazepam, phenytoin, or warfarin to human albumin. Likewise, these agents did not affect the binding of atomoxetine to human albumin.

➤*Drug/Food interactions:* See Actions for more information.

Adverse Reactions

➤*Children and adolescents:*

Discontinuation – In acute placebo-controlled trials in children and adolescents, 3% of atomoxetine-treated subjects and 1.4% of placebo-treated subjects discontinued because of adverse reactions. For all studies, (including open-label and long-term studies), 6.3% of extensive metabolizers and 11.2% of poor metabolizers discontinued because of an adverse reaction. Among atomoxetine-treated patients, constipation, fatigue, feeling abnormal, and headache (0.1%); abdominal pain, aggression, nausea, and vomiting (0.2%); and irritability and somnolence (0.3%) were the reasons for discontinuation reported by more than 1 patient.

Seizures – Atomoxetine has not been systematically evaluated in children with seizure disorder because these patients were excluded from clinical studies during the product's premarket testing. In the clinical development program, seizures were reported in 0.2% of children whose average age was 10 years (range, 6 to 16 years of age). In these clinical trials, the seizure risk among poor metabolizers was 0.3% compared with 0.2% for extensive metabolizers.

Common adverse reactions –

Atomoxetine Adverse Reactions in Acute (Up to 18 Weeks) Child and Adolescent Trials (≥ 2%)[a]		
Adverse reactions	Atomoxetine (n = 1,597)	Placebo (n = 934)
CNS		
Dizziness	5%	2%
Fatigue	8%	3%
Headache	19%	15%
Irritability	6%	3%
Somnolence[b]	11%	4%
GI		
Abdominal pain[c]	18%	10%
Anorexia	3%	1%
Nausea	10%	5%
Vomiting	11%	6%
Metabolic/Nutritional		
Appetite decreased	16%	4%
Weight decreased	3%	0%
Miscellaneous		
Rash	2%	1%
Therapeutic response unexpected	2%	1%

[a] Reactions reported by ≥ 2% of patients treated with atomoxetine and more than with placebo. The following reactions did not meet this criterion, but were reported by more atomoxetine-treated patients than placebo-treated patients and are possibly related to atomoxetine treatment: asthenia, blood pressure increased, constipation, early morning awakening, flushing, mood swings, mydriasis, palpitations, and sinus tachycardia. The following reactions were reported by ≥ 2% of patients treated with atomoxetine and less than or equal to placebo: insomnia (insomnia includes the terms initial insomnia, insomnia, and middle insomnia) and pharyngolaryngeal pain. The following reaction did not meet this criterion, but shows a statistically significant dose relationship: pruritus.
[b] Somnolence includes the terms sedation and somnolence.
[c] Abdominal pain includes the terms abdominal discomfort, abdominal pain, abdominal pain upper, epigastric discomfort, and stomach discomfort.

Atomoxetine Adverse Reactions in Acute (Up to 18 Weeks) Child and Adolescent Twice Daily and Once Daily Trials				
	Twice-daily trials		Once-daily trials	
Adverse reactions	Atomoxetine (n = 715)	Placebo (n =434)	Atomoxetine (n = 882)	Placebo (n = 500)
CNS				
Fatigue	6%	4%	9%	2%
Mood swings[a]	2%	0%	1%	1%
GI				
Abdominal pain[b]	17%	13%	18%	7%
Constipation[c]	2%	1%	1%	0%
Nausea	7%	6%	13%	4%
Vomiting	11%	8%	11%	4%

[a] Mood swings did not meet the statistical significance on Breslow-Day test at 0.05 level, but *P* value was < 0.1 (trend).
[b] Abdominal pain includes the terms abdominal discomfort, abdominal pain, abdominal pain upper, epigastric discomfort, and stomach discomfort.
[c] Constipation did not meet the statistical significance on Breslow-Day test, but is included in the table because of pharmacologic plausibility.

Other adverse reactions (at least 2%) – The following adverse reactions occurred in at least 2% of poor metabolizers and were twice as frequent or statistically significantly more frequent in poor metabolizers compared with extensive metabolizers:

CNS: Depression (includes depressed mood, depression, depressive symptoms, dysphoria, major depression) (7% of poor metabolizers, 4% of extensive metabolizers), insomnia (15% of poor metabolizers, 10% of extensive metabolizers), tremor (5% of poor metabolizers, 1% of extensive metabolizers).

GI: Constipation (7% of poor metabolizers, 4% of extensive metabolizers), weight decreased (7% of poor metabolizers, 4% of extensive metabolizers).

Special senses: Conjunctivitis (3% of poor metabolizers, 1% of extensive metabolizers), mydriasis (2% of poor metabolizers, 1% of extensive metabolizers).

Miscellaneous: Early morning awakening (2% of poor metabolizers, 1% of extensive metabolizers), excoriation (4% of poor metabolizers, 2% of extensive metabolizers), syncope(3% of poor metabolizers, 1% of extensive metabolizers).

➤*Adults:*

Discontinuation – In acute adult placebo-controlled trials, 11.3% of atomoxetine patients and 3% of placebo patients discontinued for adverse reactions. Among atomoxetine-treated patients, anxiety, erectile dysfunction, mood swings, nervousness, palpitations, and urinary retention (0.4%); chest pain and fatigue (0.6%); insomnia and nausea (0.9%), were the reasons for discontinuation reported by more than 1 patient.

ATOMOXETINE HYDROCHLORIDE — ORAL

Seizures – Atomoxetine has not been systematically evaluated in adult patients with seizure disorder because these patients were excluded from clinical studies during the product's premarket testing. In the clinical development program, seizures were reported in 0.1% of adult patients. In these clinical trials, no poor metabolizers reported seizures compared with 0.1% of extensive metabolizers.

Common adverse reactions –

Atomoxetine Adverse Reactions in Acute (Up to 25 Weeks) Adult Trials (≥ 2%)[a]

Adverse reactions	Atomoxetine (n = 540)	Placebo (n = 402)
Cardiovascular		
Hot flush	8%	1%
Palpitations	3%	1%
CNS		
Chills	3%	1%
Dizziness	6%	4%
Fatigue	9%	4%
Feeling jittery	2%	0%
Insomnia[b]	15%	7%
Libido decreased	4%	2%
Paraesthesia	3%	1%
Sinus headache	3%	1%
Sleep disorder	3%	1%
Somnolence[c]	4%	3%
Tremor	2%	0%
Dermatologic		
Hyperhidrosis	4%	1%
Rash	2%	1%
GI		
Abdominal pain[d]	7%	5%
Constipation	9%	3%
Dry mouth	21%	7%
Dyspepsia	4%	2%
Nausea	21%	5%
Vomiting	3%	2%
GU		
Dysmenorrhea[e]	6%	2%
Dysuria	3%	0%
Ejaculation delayed[f] and/or ejaculation disorder[f]	3%	1%
Erectile dysfunction[f]	9%	1%
Menstruation irregular[e]	2%	0%
Urinary hesitation and/or urinary retention	7%	1%
Metabolic/Nutritional		
Appetite decreased	11%	2%
Weight decreased	2%	1%
Miscellaneous		
Therapeutic response unexpected	3%	1%

[a] Reactions reported by ≥ 2% of patients treated with atomoxetine and more than with placebo. The following reactions did not meet this criterion, but were reported by more atomoxetine-treated patients than placebo-treated patients and are possibly related to atomoxetine treatment: early morning awakening, orgasm abnormal, peripheral coldness, prostatitis, tachycardia, and testicular pain. The following reactions were reported by ≥ 2% of patients treated with atomoxetine and less than or equal to placebo: headache, irritability, and pharyngolaryngeal pain.
[b] Insomnia includes the terms initial insomnia, insomnia, and middle insomnia.
[c] Somnolence includes the terms sedation and somnolence.
[d] Abdominal pain includes the terms abdominal discomfort, abdominal pain, abdominal pain upper, epigastric discomfort, and stomach discomfort.
[e] Based on total number of women (atomoxetine, n = 214; placebo, n = 142).
[f] Based on total number of men (atomoxetine, n = 326; placebo, n = 260).

➤*Sexual dysfunction:* Atomoxetine appears to impair sexual function in some patients. Changes in sexual desire, performance, and satisfaction are not well assessed in most clinical trials because they need special attention and patients and health care providers may be reluctant to discuss them. Accordingly, estimates of the incidence of untoward sexual experience and performance are likely to underestimate the actual incidence. The previous table displays the incidence of sexual adverse reactions reported by at least 2% of adult patients taking atomoxetine in placebo-controlled trials.

➤*Postmarketing:*

Cardiovascular – QT prolongation, syncope.

CNS – Anxiety, depressed mood, depression, hypoasthesia, lethargy, paraesthesia in children and adolescents, sensory disturbances, tics.Seizures have been reported in the postmarketing period. Postmarketing seizure cases include patients with preexisting seizure disorders and those with identified risk factors of seizures, as well as patients with neither a history of nor identified risk factors of seizures. The exact relationship between atomoxetine and seizures is difficult to evaluate because of uncertainty about the background risk of seizures in patients with ADHD.

Dermatologic – Hyperhidrosis.

GU – Pelvic pain (men only), urinary hesitation in children and adolescents, urinary retention in children and adolescents.

Overdosage

➤*Symptoms:* In some cases of overdose involving atomoxetine, seizures have been reported. The most commonly reported symptoms accompanying acute and chronic overdoses of atomoxetine were abnormal behavior, agitation, dizziness, GI symptoms, hyperactivity, somnolence, tremor. Signs and symptoms consistent with mild to moderate sympathetic nervous system activation (eg, blood pressure increased, dry mouth, mydriasis, tachycardia) have also been observed. Most events were mild to moderate. Less commonly, there have been reports of QT prolongation and mental changes, including disorientation and hallucinations.

➤*Treatment:* Consult with a certified Poison Control Center for up-to-date guidance and advice. Because atomoxetine is highly protein-bound, dialysis is not likely to be useful in the treatment of overdose.

Patient Information

Encourage patients, their families, and their caregivers to be alert to the emergence of agitation, aggressiveness, akathisia (psychomotor restlessness), anxiety, depression, hostility, hypomania, impulsivity, insomnia, irritability, mania, panic attacks, other unusual changes in behavior, and suicidal ideation, especially during early atomoxetine treatment and when the dose is adjusted. Advise families and caregivers of patients to observe for the emergence of such symptoms on a day-to-day basis, because changes may be abrupt. Instruct families and caregivers to report such symptoms to the patient's health care provider, especially if they are severe, abrupt in onset, or were not part of the patient's presenting symptoms. Symptoms such as these may be associated with an increased risk of suicidal thinking and behavior and indicate a need for very close monitoring and possible changes in the medication.

Caution patients initiating atomoxetine therapy that severe liver injury may develop. Instruct patients to contact their health care provider immediately if they develop dark urine, jaundice, pruritus, right upper quadrant tenderness, or unexpected flu-like symptoms.

Instruct patients to call their health care provider as soon as possible if they notice an increase in aggression or hostility.

Rare postmarketing cases of priapism, defined as painful and nonpainful penile erection lasting more than 4 hours, have been reported for children and adults treated with atomoxetine. Instruct the parents or guardians of children taking atomoxetine and adults taking atomoxetine that priapism requires prompt medical attention.

Inform patients that atomoxetine is an ocular irritant. Atomoxetine capsules are not intended to be opened. In the event that capsule contents come in contact with the eye, instruct the patient to immediately flush the affected eye with water and obtain medical advice. Instruct the patient to wash hands and any potentially contaminated surfaces as soon as possible.

Instruct patients to consult their health care provider if they are taking or planning to take any prescription or nonprescription medicines, dietary supplements, or herbal remedies.

Instruct patients to consult their health care provider if they are breast-feeding, pregnant, or thinking of becoming pregnant while taking atomoxetine.

Advise patients that atomoxetine may be taken with or without food.

Tell patients that if they miss a dose, they should take it as soon as possible. However, they should not take more than the prescribed total daily amount of atomoxetine in any 24-hour period.

Instruct patients to use caution when driving a car or operating hazardous machinery until they are reasonably certain that their performance is not affected by atomoxetine.

SODIUM OXYBATE

c-iii	**Xyrem**[a] (Jazz Pharmaceuticals)	**Solution; oral:** 500 mg/mL[b]	In 180 mL with syringe and dosing cups.

[a] Available only through the *Xyrem* Success Program. Call 1-866-997-3688 for more information.

[b] With sodium 91 mg/mL.

SODIUM OXYBATE — ORAL

WARNING

Sodium oxybate is a gamma hydroxybutyrate (GHB), a known drug of abuse. Abuse has been associated with some important CNS adverse reactions, including death. Even at recommended doses, use has been associated with confusion, depression, and other neuropsychiatric reactions. Reports of respiratory depression occurred in clinical trials. Almost all of the patients who received sodium oxybate during clinical trials were receiving CNS stimulants.

Important CNS adverse reactions associated with abuse of sodium oxybate include respiratory depression, seizure, and profound decreases in level of consciousness, with instances of coma and death. For reactions that occurred outside of clinical trials, in people taking sodium oxybate for recreational purposes, the circumstances surrounding the reactions often are unclear (eg, dose of sodium oxybate taken, the nature and amount of alcohol or any concomitant drugs).

Sodium oxybate is available through the *Xyrem* Success Program, using a centralized pharmacy (1-866-997-3688). The Success Program provides educational materials to the prescriber and the patient explaining the risks and proper use of sodium oxybate and the required prescription form. Once it is documented that the patient has read and/or understands the materials, the drug will be shipped to the patient. The *Xyrem* Success Program also recommends patient follow-up every 3 months. Health care providers are expected to report all serious adverse reactions to the manufacturer.

Indications

➤*Excessive daytime sleepiness/cataplexy:* For the treatment of excessive daytime sleepiness and cataplexy in patients with narcolepsy.

➤*Off-label uses:*

Fibromyalgia – [3] = Safety concerns. Initial data from 2 trials indicate that sodium oxybate may be beneficial in reducing pain and fatigue in patients with fibromyalgia. However, there was a relatively high drop out rate in one trial, and both trials were conducted by the same study group. Studies of sodium oxybate in the treatment of narcolepsy have shown that longer use (3 months) is required for maximal effectiveness, and the same may be true for this indication. Larger, controlled trials are needed.

Other possible off-label uses – Fatigue.

Administration and Dosage

➤*Adults:*

Excessive daytime sleepiness/cataplexy –

Usual dosage: 6 to 9 g/night.

Maximum dose: 9 g/night.

Initial dosage: 4.5 g/night divided into 2 equal doses of 2.25 g. The first dose is taken while in bed, and the second dose is taken 2.5 to 4 hours later. (See Administration.)

Dosage titration: The starting dose can be increased to a maximum of 9 g/night in increments of 1.5 g/night (0.75 g/dose). One to 2 weeks are recommended between dosage increases to evaluate clinical response and minimize adverse reactions.

Off-label dosing –

Fibromyalgia: [3] = Safety concerns. 2.25 to 3 g orally at bedtime and 4 hours later for 1 month.

➤*Elderly:* Closely monitor elderly patients for impaired motor and/or cognitive function.

➤*Hepatic function impairment:* Patients with compromised liver function will have increased elimination half-life and systemic exposure along with reduced clearance. As a result, the starting dose should be decreased by one-half, and dose increments should be titrated to effect while closely monitoring potential adverse reactions.

➤*Preparation for administration:* Prepare both doses of sodium oxybate prior to bedtime. Each dose of sodium oxybate must be diluted with 2 ounces (ie, 60 mL, one-fourth cup, 4 tablespoons) of water in the child-resistant dosing cups provided prior to ingestion. The second dose must be prepared prior to ingesting the first dose and should be placed in close proximity to the patient's bed.

➤*Administration:* The first dose should be taken at bedtime while in bed, and the second dose should be taken 2.5 to 4 hours later; both doses should be taken while seated in bed. Patients probably will need to set an alarm to awaken for the second dose. After ingesting each dose, patients should lie down and remain in bed.

Because food significantly reduces the bioavailability of sodium oxybate, the patient should allow at least 2 hours after eating before taking the first dose of sodium oxybate. Patients should try to minimize variability in time of dosing in relation to meals.

➤*Storage/Stability:* Store at 25°C (77°F); excursions are permitted up to 15° to 30°C (59° to 86°F). Solutions prepared following dilution should be consumed within 24 hours to minimize bacterial growth and contamination.

Actions

➤*Pharmacology:* The precise mechanism by which sodium oxybate produces an effect on cataplexy is unknown.

➤*Pharmacokinetics:*

Absorption – Sodium oxybate is absorbed rapidly following oral administration, with an absolute bioavailability of about 25%. The average peak plasma concentrations (C_{max}); 1st and 2nd peak following administration of a 9 g daily dose divided into 2 equivalent doses given 4 hours apart were 78 and 142 mcg/mL, respectively. The average time to peak plasma concentration (T_{max}) ranged from 0.5 to 1.25 hours in 8 pharmacokinetic studies. Following oral administration, the plasma levels of sodium oxybate increase more than proportionally with increasing dose. Single doses greater than 4.5 g have not been studied.

Sodium oxybate is rapidly but incompletely absorbed after oral administration; absorption is delayed and decreased by a high-fat meal. Pharmacokinetics are nonlinear, with blood levels increasing 3.7-fold as the dose is doubled from 4.5 to 9 g. The pharmacokinetics are not altered with repeat dosing.

Food effects: Administration of sodium oxybate immediately after a high-fat meal resulted in delayed absorption (average T_{max} increased from 0.75 to 2 hours) and a reduction in C_{max} by a mean of 58% and systemic exposure (area under the curve [AUC]) by 37%.

Distribution – Sodium oxybate is a hydrophilic compound with an apparent volume of distribution averaging 190 to 384 mL/kg. At sodium oxybate concentrations ranging from 3 to 300 mcg/mL, less than 1% is bound to plasma proteins.

Metabolism – Animal studies indicate that metabolism is the major elimination pathway for sodium oxybate, producing carbon dioxide and water via the tricarboxylic acid (Krebs) cycle and secondarily by beta-oxidation. The primary pathway involves a cytosolic nicotineamide adenine dinucleotide phosphate positive-linked enzyme, sodium oxybate dehydrogenase, that catalyses the conversion of sodium oxybate to succinic semialdehyde, which then is biotransformed to succinic acid by the enzyme succinic semialdehyde dehydrogenase. Succinic acid enters the Krebs cycle, where it is metabolized to carbon dioxide and water. A second mitochondrial oxidoreductase enzyme, a transhydrogenase, also catalyses the conversion to succinic semialdehyde in the presence of α-ketoglutarate. An alternate pathway of biotransformation involves β-oxidation via 3,4-dihydroxybutyrate to carbon dioxide and water. No active metabolites have been identified.

Excretion – The clearance of sodium oxybate is almost entirely by biotransformation to carbon dioxide, which then is eliminated by expiration. On average, less than 5% of unchanged drug appears in human urine within 6 to 8 hours after dosing. Fecal excretion is negligible. Sodium oxybate is eliminated mainly by metabolism with a half-life of 0.5 to 1 hour.

Special populations –

Hepatic function impairment: Sodium oxybate undergoes significant presystemic (hepatic first-pass) metabolism. The kinetics of sodium oxybate in 16 patients with cirrhosis, half without ascites (Child-Pugh class A) and half with ascites (Child-Pugh class C), were compared with the kinetics in 8 healthy adults after a single oral dose of 25 mg/kg. AUC values were double in the patients with cirrhosis, with apparent oral clearance reduced from 9.1 in healthy adults to 4.5 and 4.1 mL/min/kg in class A and Child-Pugh class C patients, respectively. Elimination half-life was significantly longer in Child-Pugh class C and class A patients than in control subjects (mean $t_{1/2}$ of 59; 32 versus 22 minutes). It is prudent to reduce the starting dose of sodium oxybate by half in patients with liver dysfunction.

Contraindications

Patients being treated with sedative hypnotic agents; succinic semialdehyde dehydrogenase deficiency.

Warnings/Precautions

➤*Respiratory effects:* Sodium oxybate is a CNS depressant with the potential to impair respiratory drive, especially in patients with already compromised respiratory function. In overdoses, life-threatening respiratory depression has been reported. In clinical trials, 2 subjects had profound CNS depression. A healthy 39-year-old woman received a single dose of sodium oxybate 4.5 g after fasting for 10 hours. An hour later, while asleep, she developed decreased respiration and was treated with an oxygen mask. An hour later, this event recurred. She also vomited and had fecal incontinence. In another case, a 64-year-old man with narcolepsy was found unresponsive on the floor on day 170 of treatment with sodium oxybate at a total daily dose of 4.5 g/night. He was taken to an emergency room where he was intubated. He improved and was able to return home later the same day. Two other patients discontinued sodium oxybate because of severe difficulty breathing and an increase in obstructive sleep apnea.

The respiratory depressant effects of sodium oxybate, at recommended doses, were assessed in 21 patients with narcolepsy, and no dose-related changes in oxygen saturation were demonstrated in the group as a whole. One of these patients had significant concomitant pulmonary illness, and 4 of the 21 had moderate to severe sleep apnea. One of the 4 patients with sleep apnea had significant worsening of the apnea/hypopnea index during treatment, but worsening did not increase at higher doses. Another patient discontinued treatment because of a perceived increase in clinical apnea events. In the randomized, controlled trials 3 and 4, a total of 40 narcolepsy

SODIUM OXYBATE — ORAL

patients were included with a baseline apnea/hypopnea index of 16 to 67 events/hour, indicative of mild to severe sleep disordered breathing. None of the 40 patients had a clinically significant worsening of their respiratory function as measured by apnea/hypopnea index and pulse oximetry while receiving sodium oxybate at dosages of 4.5 to 9 g/night in divided dosages. Observe caution if sodium oxybate is prescribed to patients with compromised respiratory function. Be aware that sleep apnea has been reported with a high incidence (even 50%) in some cohorts of patients with narcolepsy.

➤*CNS effects:* During clinical trials, 2.6% of patients treated with sodium oxybate experienced confusion. Fewer than 1% of patients discontinued the drug because of confusion. Confusion was reported at all recommended dosages from 6 to 9 g/night. In a controlled trial in which patients were randomized to fixed total daily doses of 3, 6, and 9 g/night or placebo, a dose-response relationship for confusion was demonstrated, with 17% of patients at 9 g/night experiencing confusion. In all cases in that controlled trial, the confusion resolved soon after termination of treatment. In trial 3, in which sodium oxybate was titrated from an initial 4.5 g/night dose, there was a single event of confusion in 1 patient at the 9 g/night dose. In the majority of cases in all clinical trials, confusion resolved either soon after termination of dosing or with continued treatment. However, fully evaluate patients treated with sodium oxybate who become confused, and consider appropriate intervention on an individual basis.

Other neuropsychiatric events included agitation, hallucinations, paranoia, and psychosis. The emergence of thought disorders and/or behavior abnormalities when patients are treated with sodium oxybate requires careful and immediate evaluation.

➤*Depression:* In clinical trials, 3.2% of patients treated with sodium oxybate reported depressive symptoms. In the majority of cases, no change in sodium oxybate treatment was required. Four (less than 1%) patients discontinued because of depressive symptoms. In the controlled clinical trial in which patients were randomized to fixed dosages of 3, 6, and 9 g/night or placebo, there was a single event of depression at the 3 g/night dosage. In trial 3, in which patients were titrated from an initial 4.5 g/night starting dose, the incidence of depression was 1 (1.7%), 1 (1.5%), 2 (3.2%), and 2 (3.6%) for the placebo, 4.5, 6, and 9 g/night doses, respectively.

In the 717 patient dataset, there were 2 suicides and 1 attempted suicide recorded in patients with a previous history of depressive psychiatric disorder. Of the 2 suicides, 1 patient used sodium oxybate in conjunction with other drugs. Sodium oxybate was not involved in the second suicide. Sodium oxybate was the only drug involved in the attempted suicide. A fourth patient without a history of depression attempted suicide by taking an overdose of a drug other than sodium oxybate.

The emergence of depression when patients are treated with sodium oxybate requires careful and immediate evaluation. Monitor patients with a history of a depressive illness and/or suicide attempt especially carefully for the emergence of depressive symptoms while they are taking sodium oxybate.

➤*Incontinence:* During clinical trials, 7% of patients with narcolepsy treated with sodium oxybate experienced either a single or sporadic episode of nocturnal urinary incontinence, and less than 1% experienced a single episode of nocturnal fecal incontinence. Less than 1% of patients discontinued as a result of incontinence. Incontinence has been reported at all doses tested.

In a controlled trial in which patients were randomized to fixed total daily doses of 3, 6, and 9 g/night, or placebo, a dose-response relationship for urinary incontinence was demonstrated, with 14% of patients at 9 g/night experiencing urinary incontinence. In the same trial, 1 patient experienced fecal incontinence at a dosage of 9 g/night and discontinued treatment as a result.

If a patient experiences urinary or fecal incontinence during sodium oxybate therapy, consider pursuing investigations to rule out underlying etiologies, including worsening sleep apnea or nocturnal seizures, although there is no evidence to suggest that incontinence has been associated with seizures in patients being treated with sodium oxybate.

➤*Sleepwalking:* The term "sleepwalking" in this section refers to confused behavior occurring at night and, at times, associated with wandering. It is unclear if some or all of these episodes correspond to true somnambulism, which is a parasomnia occurring during nonrapid eye movement sleep, or to any other specific medical disorder. Sleepwalking was reported in 4% of 717 patients treated in clinical trials with sodium oxybate. In sodium oxybate–treated patients, less than 1% discontinued because of sleepwalking. In controlled trials of up to 4 weeks' duration, the incidence of sleepwalking was 1% in both placebo- and sodium oxybate–treated patients. Sleepwalking was reported by 32% of patients treated with sodium oxybate for periods up to 16 years in 1 independent, uncontrolled trial. Fewer than 1% of the patients discontinued because of sleepwalking. Five instances of significant injury or potential injury were associated with sleepwalking during a clinical trial of sodium oxybate, including a fall, clothing set on fire while attempting to smoke, attempted ingestion of nail polish remover, and overdose of sodium oxybate. Therefore, fully evaluate episodes of sleepwalking and consider appropriate interventions.

➤*Sodium intake:* Daily sodium intake in patients taking sodium oxybate is provided in the following table. Consider this in patients with compromised renal function, heart failure, or hypertension.

Sodium Content per Total Nightly Dose in Sodium Oxybate		
Sodium oxybate (g)	Sodium oxybate (mL)	Sodium content/dose
3 g	6 mL	546 mg
4.5 g	9 mL	819 mg
6 g	12 mL	1,092 mg
7.5 g	15 mL	1,365 mg
9 g	18 mL	1,638 mg

➤*Renal function impairment:* Consider the sodium load associated with administration of sodium oxybate in patients with renal function impairment.

➤*Hepatic function impairment:* Patients with compromised liver function will have an increased elimination half-life and systemic exposure to sodium oxybate. Decrease the starting dose by half in such patients and closely monitor response to dose increments.

➤*Drug abuse and dependence:*

Controlled substance class – Sodium oxybate is classified as a Schedule III controlled substance by federal law. The active ingredient, sodium oxybate or gamma hydroxybutyrate, is listed in the most restrictive schedule of the Controlled Substances Act (Schedule I). Thus, nonmedical uses of sodium oxybate are classified under Schedule I.

Abuse, dependence, and tolerance –

Abuse: Although sodium oxybate has not been systematically studied in clinical trials for its potential for abuse, illicit use and abuse have been reported. Sodium oxybate is a psychoactive drug that produces a wide range of pharmacological effects. It is a sedative-hypnotic that produces dose- and concentration-dependent CNS effects in humans. The onset of effect is rapid, enhancing its desirability as a drug of abuse or misuse.

The rapid onset of sedation, coupled with the amnestic features of sodium oxybate, particularly when combined with alcohol, has proven to be dangerous for the voluntary and involuntary (assault victim) user.

Sodium oxybate is abused in social settings primarily by young adults. Sodium oxybate has some commonalties with ethanol over a limited dose range and some cross-tolerance with ethanol has been reported as well. Cases of severe dependence and craving for sodium oxybate have been reported. Dependence is indicated by the use of increasingly large doses, increased frequency of use, and continued use despite adverse consequences. Some of the doses reported abused in the "rave" setting have been similar to the dose range studied for therapeutic treatment of cataplexy.

Hospital emergency department (ED) reports increased 100-fold from 1992 to 1999 (source: Substance Abuse Mental Health Services Administration, Drug Abuse Warning Network [DAWN]). Sixty percent of the ED reports involved individuals 25 years of age and younger. Numerous deaths have been reported over that period of time, typically involving sodium oxybate in combination with alcohol and other drugs, including 5 in the DAWN system in which sodium oxybate was the only drug that could be identified. However, the incidence of hospital ED reports of reactions involving sodium oxybate and sodium oxybate–related analogs has decreased by about 33% since 2000, and reports to the American Association of Poison Control Centers of sodium oxybate exposures has decreased from 1,916 (involving 6 deaths) in 2001 to 800 (without any deaths) in 2003.

Dependence: There have been case reports of dependence after illicit use of sodium oxybate at frequent repeated dosages (18 to 250 g/day), in excess of the therapeutic dosage range. In these cases, the signs and symptoms of abrupt discontinuation included an abstinence syndrome consisting of anxiety, insomnia, lethargy, muscle cramps, nausea, psychosis, restlessness, sweating, tachycardia, and tremor. These symptoms generally abated in 3 to 14 days. The discontinuation effects of sodium oxybate have not been systematically evaluated in controlled clinical trials. An abstinence syndrome has not been reported in clinical investigations. Although the clinical trial experience with sodium oxybate in patients with narcolepsy/cataplexy at therapeutic doses does not show clear evidence of a withdrawal syndrome, 2 patients reported anxiety and 1 reported insomnia following abrupt discontinuation at the termination of the clinical trial; in the 2 patients with anxiety, the frequency of cataplexy had increased markedly at the same time.

Tolerance: Tolerance to sodium oxybate has not been systematically studied in controlled clinical trials. Open-label, long-term (greater than or equal to 6 months) clinical trials did not demonstrate development of tolerance. There have been some case reports of symptoms of tolerance developing after illicit use at dosages far in excess of the recommended sodium oxybate dosage regimen. Clinical studies of sodium oxybate in the treatment of alcohol withdrawal suggest a potential cross-tolerance with alcohol. Because illicit use and abuse of sodium oxybate have been reported, carefully evaluate patients for a history of drug abuse and follow such patients closely, observing them for signs of misuse or abuse of sodium oxybate (eg, increase in size or frequency of dosing, drug-seeking behavior). Document the diagnosis and indication for sodium oxybate, being alert to drug-seeking behavior and/or feigned cataplexy.

➤*Hazardous tasks:* Because of the rapid onset of its CNS-depressant effects, sodium oxybate should only be ingested at bedtime, and while in bed. For at least 6 hours after ingesting sodium oxybate, patients must not engage in hazardous occupations or activities requiring complete mental alertness or motor coordination, such as operating machinery, driving a motor vehicle, or flying an airplane. When patients first start taking sodium oxybate or any other sleep medicine, until they know whether the medicine will still have some carryover effect on them the next day, they should use extreme care while driving a car, operating heavy machinery, or performing any other task that could be dangerous or requires full mental alertness.

➤*Pregnancy: Category B.* In a study in which rats were given sodium oxybate from day 6 of gestation through day 21 postpartum, slight decreases in pup and maternal weight gains were seen at 1,000 mg/kg; there were no drug effects on other developmental parameters. There are, however, no adequate and well-controlled studies in pregnant women. Because animal

SODIUM OXYBATE — ORAL

reproduction studies are not always predictive of human response, use this drug during pregnancy only if clearly needed.

Labor and delivery – Sodium oxybate has not been studied in labor or delivery. In obstetric anesthesia using an injectable formulation of sodium oxybate, newborns had stable cardiovascular and respiratory measures but were very sleepy, causing a slight decrease in Apgar scores. There was a fall in the rate of uterine contractions 20 minutes after injection. Placental transfer is rapid, but umbilical vein levels of sodium oxybate were no more than 25% of the maternal concentration. No sodium oxybate was detected in the infant's blood 30 minutes after delivery. Elimination curves of sodium oxybate between a 2-day-old infant and a 15-year-old patient were similar.

➤*Lactation:* It is not known whether sodium oxybate is excreted in human milk. The molecular weight of the acid form (about 104) and the minimal plasma protein binding (< 1%) suggest that it will be excreted into breast milk, but the extensive, rapid metabolism and short half-life (0.5 to 1 hour) should limit the amount excreted. Because many drugs are excreted in human milk, exercise caution when sodium oxybate is administered to a breast-feeding woman. Because the drug is taken immediately before bedtime, nursing no sooner than 5 hours after a dose to just before the next dose should prevent clinically significant exposure of an infant.

➤*Children:* Safety and efficacy in patients younger than 16 years of age have not been established.

➤*Elderly:* There is very limited experience with sodium oxybate in elderly patients. Therefore, closely monitor elderly patients taking sodium oxybate for impaired motor and/or cognitive function.

➤*Lab test abnormalities:* In an open-label trial of long-term exposure to sodium oxybate, which extended as long as 16 years for some patients, 30% (26/87) of patients tested had at least 1 positive antinuclear antibody (ANA) test. Of the 26, 17 patients had multiple positive ANA tests over time. The clinical course of these patients was not always clearly recorded, but 1 patient was clearly diagnosed with rheumatoid arthritis at the time of the first recorded positive ANA test. No instances of systemic lupus erythematosus have been reported in patients taking sodium oxybate.

➤*Monitoring:* Monitor patients with a history of a depressive illness and/or suicide attempt especially carefully for the emergence of depressive symptoms while they are taking sodium oxybate. Monitor elderly patients taking sodium oxybate closely for impaired motor and/or cognitive function. Monitor patients for signs of abuse, dependence, or tolerance.

Drug Interactions

➤*Alcohol:* The combined use of alcohol (ethanol) with sodium oxybate may result in potentiation of the CNS-depressant effects of sodium oxybate and alcohol. Therefore, warn patients strongly against the use of any alcoholic beverages in conjunction with sodium oxybate.

➤*CNS depressants/sedative hypnotics:* Interactions between sodium oxybate and 3 drugs commonly used in patients with narcolepsy (modafinil, protriptyline, and zolpidem) have been evaluated in formal studies. Sodium oxybate, in combination with these drugs, produced no significant pharmacokinetic changes for either drug. However, pharmacodynamic interactions cannot be ruled out. Nonetheless, do not use sodium oxybate in combination with sedative hypnotics or other CNS depressants.

➤*Drug/Food interactions:* Administration of sodium oxybate immediately after a high-fat meal resulted in delayed absorption (average T_{max} increased from 0.75 to 2 hours) and a reduction in C_{max} by a mean of 58% and of systemic exposure (AUC) by 37%.

Adverse Reactions

A total of 717 patients with narcolepsy were exposed to sodium oxybate in clinical trials. The most commonly observed adverse reactions associated with the use of sodium oxybate were as follows: headache (22%); nausea (21%); dizziness (17%); nasopharyngitis, somnolence, vomiting (8%); urinary incontinence (7%).

Two deaths occurred in these clinical trials, both from drug overdoses. Both of these deaths resulted from ingestion of multiple drugs, including sodium oxybate in 1 patient.

➤*Discontinuation of treatment:* In these clinical trials, 10% of patients discontinued because of adverse reactions. The most frequent (greater than 1%) reasons for discontinuation were dizziness, nausea (2%); and vomiting (1%).

Approximately 9% of patients receiving sodium oxybate in 5 placebo-controlled clinical trials (n = 443) withdrew because of an adverse reaction, compared with 1% receiving placebo (n = 79). The reasons for discontinuation that occurred more frequently in sodium oxybate–treated patients than placebo-treated patients were as follows: dizziness, nausea (2%); vomiting (1%); blurred vision, confusional state, dyspnea, hypesthesia, paresthesia, somnolence, tremor, urinary incontinence, vertigo (less than 1%).

➤*Adverse reactions (≥ 5%):* The most commonly reported adverse reactions (at least 5%) in placebo-controlled clinical trials associated with the use of sodium oxybate and occurring more frequently than in placebo-treated patients were as follows: nausea (19%); dizziness, headache (18%); vomiting (8%); nasopharyngitis, somnolence, urinary incontinence (6%).

These incidences are based on combined data from trials 1, 2, and 3, and 2 smaller, randomized, double-blind, placebo-controlled, crossover trials (n = 655).

Because clinical trials are conducted under widely varying conditions, adverse reaction rates observed in the clinical trials of a drug cannot be directly compared with rates in the clinical trials of another drug and may not reflect the rates observed in practice. The adverse reaction information from clinical trials does, however, provide a basis for identifying the adverse reactions that appear to be related to drug use and for approximating incidence rates.

The data presented in the following tables come from 2 placebo-controlled, clinical trials, trial 1 and 3.

Sodium Oxybate Adverse Reactions from Trial 1

Adverse reaction	Placebo (n = 34)	Sodium oxybate dose at onset: 3 g/night (n = 34)	6 g/night (n = 33)	9 g/night (n = 35)
CNS				
Cataplexy	0%	0%	0%	9%
Confusion	0%	6%	3%	6%
Depression	0%	6%	0%	0%
Disorientation	3%	3%	0%	9%
Disturbance in attention	0%	3%	0%	9%
Dizziness	6%	24%	30%	37%
Feeling drunk	0%	0%	0%	9%
Headache	24%	9%	21%	37%
Hypesthesia	0%	6%	0%	0%
Lethargy	0%	6%	0%	0%
Nightmare	0%	3%	6%	0%
Sleep disorder	0%	0%	6%	3%
Sleep paralysis	3%	3%	6%	14%
Sleep walking	0%	0%	0%	6%
Somnolence	9%	12%	12%	14%
GI				
Abdominal pain, upper	0%	0%	3%	11%
Diarrhea	0%	0%	6%	9%
Dyspepsia	6%	3%	9%	9%
Gastroenteritis, viral	0%	0%	6%	0%
Nausea	6%	9%	24%	40%
Vomiting	0%	0%	9%	23%
Musculoskeletal				
Back pain	6%	0%	6%	6%
Muscular weakness	0%	6%	3%	0%
Respiratory				
Nasopharyngitis	3%	3%	6%	6%
Pharyngolaryngeal pain	6%	0%	9%	3%
Upper respiratory tract infection	3%	3%	6%	0%
Special senses				
Tinnitus	0%	6%	0%	0%
Vision blurred	3%	6%	0%	0%
Miscellaneous				
Blood pressure increase	3%	0%	6%	0%
Enuresis	0%	0%	3%	17%
Hyperhidrosis	0%	3%	3%	6%
Pain	3%	3%	3%	6%
Postprocedural pain	0%	0%	0%	6%

Sodium Oxybate Adverse Reactions in Trial 3[a]

Adverse reaction	Placebo (n = 60)	Sodium oxybate dose at onset: 4.5 g/night (n = 185)	6 g/night (n = 114)	9 g/night (n = 46)
CNS				
Disturbance in attention	0%	1%	0%	7%
Dizziness	2%	9%	8%	9%
Somnolence	0%	1%	0%	11%
GI				
Nausea	3%	8%	11%	20%
Vomiting	2%	2%	4%	9%
GU				
Enuresis	2%	3%	4%	13%

[a] Dose titration from 4.5 to 9 g occurred in weekly intervals.

➤*Dose response adverse reactions:* Discontinuations of treatment because of adverse reactions were most common at the highest dose of sodium oxybate. A dose-response relationship was observed for disorientation, disturbance in attention, enuresis, feeling drunk, irritability, nausea,

SODIUM OXYBATE — ORAL

paresthesia, sleepwalking, and vomiting. The incidence of all these reactions was notably higher at 9 g/day. Dizziness was most common at 3 and 9 g/night.

➤*Other adverse reactions:*

Cardiovascular – Hypertension (at least 1%); heart rate increased, hypotension, syncope, tachycardia (0.1% to 1%).

CNS – Abnormal dreams, asthenia, balance disorder, confusional state, depression, fatigue, headache, hypesthesia, insomnia, malaise, memory impairment, nervousness, nightmare, sleep disorder, vertigo (at least 1%); abnormal coordination, abnormal feeling, abnormal gait, affect lability, crying, depressed level of consciousness, dysarthria, dysgeusia, dyskinesia, dysstasia, emotional disorder, euphoric mood, fear, feeling jittery, hallucination auditory, hangover, head discomfort, hyperaesthesia, hypnagogic hallucination, initial insomnia, lethargy, libido increased, mental impairment, middle insomnia, migraine, mood altered, myoclonus, panic disorder, paralysis, paranoia, postural dizziness, psychomotor hyperactivity, restless leg syndrome, restlessness, sedation, sinus headache, sleep attacks, sleep talking, sluggishness, stress symptoms, sudden onset of sleep, tension headache (0.1% to 1%).

Dermatologic – Pruritus (at least 1%); acne, alopecia, cold sweat, contact dermatitis, night sweats, rosacea, skin irritation, urticaria (0.1% to 1%).

GI – Anorexia, constipation, dyspepsia, toothache, viral gastroenteritis (at least 1%); abdominal distension, dysphagia, eructation, fecal incontinence, flatulence, gastroenteritis, gastroesophageal reflux disease, oral pain, retching, salivary hypersecretion, stomach discomfort (0.1% to 1%).

GU – Urinary tract infection (at least 1%); bladder infection, chromaturia, hematuria, incontinence, micturition urgency, nocturia, ovarian cyst, pollakiuria, proteinuria, urinary incontinence, vaginal hemorrhage, vaginal infection, vaginal mycosis (0.1% to 1%).

Hematologic/Lymphatic – Leukopenia, lymphadenopathy (0.1% to 1%).

Hypersensitivity – Hypersensitivity, multiple allergies (0.1% to 1%).

Lab test abnormalities – Abnormal electrocardiogram, abnormal urine analysis, ALT increased, blood alkaline phosphatase increased, blood calcium decreased, blood cholesterol increased, blood glucose increased, blood uric acid increased, blood urine, liver function test abnormal, protein urine (0.1% to 1%).

Metabolic/Nutritional – Weight decreased (at least 1%); decreased appetite, edema, hypernatremia, hypocalcemia, increased appetite (0.1% to 1%).

Musculoskeletal – Arthralgia, back pain, myalgia, neck pain (at least 1%); arthritis, chest wall pain, joint stiffness, joint swelling, muscle tightness, muscle twitching, muscular weakness, musculoskeletal discomfort, musculoskeletal stiffness, polyarthritis, sensation of heaviness, tendonitis (0.1% to 1%).

Ophthalmic – Vision blurred (at least 1%); conjunctivitis, eye irritation, eye pain, eye redness, eye swelling, keratoconjunctivitis sicca, miosis (0.1% to 1%).

Respiratory – Bronchitis, cough, dyspnea, nasal congestion, nasopharyngitis, pharyngolaryngeal pain, sinus congestion, sinusitis, upper respiratory tract infection (at least 1%); allergic rhinitis, allergic sinusitis, apnea, asthma, bronchial infection, dry throat, hiccups, hyperventilation, increased throat secretion, laryngitis, nocturnal dyspnea, oropharyngeal swelling, pharyngitis, pneumonia, respiratory disorder, respiratory rate increased, rhinitis, sinus disorder, snoring, upper respiratory tract congestion (0.1% to 1%).

Special senses – Ear pain (at least 1%); ear discomfort, ear infection, otitis externa, tinnitus (0.1% to 1%).

Miscellaneous – Ankle fracture, back injury, chest pain, concussion, contusion, fall, head injury, influenza, influenza-like illness, pyrexia, trauma pain activated (at least 1%); cellulitis, chest discomfort, cyst, dental caries, discomfort, endodontic procedure, feeling cold, feeling hot, feeling hot and cold, fungal infection, herpes simplex, herpes zoster, joint sprain, limb injury, localized infection, muscle strain, peripheral coldness, postprocedural pain, road traffic accident, sensation of foreign body, skin laceration, tinea pedis, tooth abscess, tooth infection, tooth injury (0.1% to 1%).

Overdosage

➤*Symptoms:* Information regarding overdose with sodium oxybate is derived from reports in the medical literature that describe symptoms and signs in individuals who have ingested sodium oxybate illicitly. In these circumstances, the coingestion of other drugs and alcohol is common, and may influence the presentation and severity of clinical manifestations of overdose. In addition, overdose with sodium oxybate may be indistinguishable from overdose with other drugs, or from several other medical conditions that result in similar symptoms.

In clinical trials, 2 cases of overdose with sodium oxybate were reported. In the first case, an estimated dose of 150 g, more than 15 times the maximum recommended dose, caused a patient to be unresponsive with brief periods of apnea and to be incontinent of urine and feces. This individual recovered without sequelae. In the second case, death was reported following a multiple-drug overdose consisting of sodium oxybate and numerous other drugs.

Information about signs and symptoms associated with overdosage with sodium oxybate derives from reports of its illicit use. Patient presentation following overdose is influenced by the dose ingested, the time since ingestion, the coingestion of other drugs and alcohol, and the fed or fasted state. Patients have exhibited varying degrees of depressed consciousness that may fluctuate rapidly between a confusional, agitated combative state with ataxia and coma. Emesis (even when obtunded), diaphoresis, headache, and impaired psychomotor skills may be observed. No typical pupillary changes have been described to assist in diagnosis; pupillary reactivity to light is maintained. Blurred vision has been reported. An increasing depth of coma has been observed at higher doses. Myoclonus and tonic-clonic seizures have been reported. Respiration may be unaffected or compromised in rate and depth. Cheyne-Stokes respiration and apnea have been observed. Bradycardia and hypothermia may accompany unconsciousness, as well as muscular hypotonia, but tendon reflexes remain intact.

➤*Treatment:* Immediately institute general symptomatic and supportive care, and consider gastric decontamination if coingestants are suspected. Because emesis may occur in the presence of obtundation, appropriate posture (left lateral recumbent position) and protection of the airway by intubation may be warranted. Although the gag reflex may be absent in deeply comatose patients, even unconscious patients may become combative to intubation; consider rapid-sequence induction (without the use of sedative). Closely monitor vital signs and consciousness. The bradycardia reported with sodium oxybate overdose has been responsive to atropine intravenous administration. No reversal of the CNS-depressant effects of sodium oxybate can be expected from naloxone or flumazenil administration. The use of hemodialysis and other forms of extracorporeal drug removal have not been studied in sodium oxybate overdose. However, because of the rapid metabolism of sodium oxybate, these measures are not warranted.

As with the management of all cases of drug overdosage, consider the possibility of multiple drug ingestion. Collect urine and blood samples for routine toxicologic screening, and consult with a regional poison control center (1-800-222-1222) for current treatment recommendations.

Patient Information

The *Xyrem* Patient Success Program includes detailed information about the safe and proper use of sodium oxybate, as well as information to help the patient prevent accidental use or abuse of sodium oxybate by others. Patients must read and/or understand the materials before initiating therapy. Discuss dosing, including the procedure for preparing the dose to be administered, prior to the initiation of treatment. Inform patients that they must be seen by their health care providers frequently during the course of their treatment to review dose titration, symptom response, and adverse reactions. Food significantly decreases the bioavailability of sodium oxybate. Whether sodium oxybate is taken in the fed or fasted state may affect both the efficacy and safety of sodium oxybate for a given patient. Patients should be made aware of this and try to take the first dose several hours after a meal. Inform patients that sodium oxybate is associated with urinary and, less frequently, fecal incontinence. As a safety precaution, instruct patients to lie down and sleep after each dose of sodium oxybate, and not to take sodium oxybate at any time other than at night, immediately before bedtime and again 2.5 to 4 hours later. Instruct patients that they should not take alcohol or other sedative hypnotics with sodium oxybate.

OLANZAPINE/FLUOXETINE

Rx	**Symbyax** (Eli Lilly)	**Capsules; oral:** olanzapine 3 mg/ fluoxetine 25 mg	As fluoxetine hydrochloride. (Lilly 3230 3/25). Peach/Lt. yellow. In 30s.
		olanzapine 6 mg/fluoxetine 25 mg	As fluoxetine hydrochloride. (Lilly 3231 6/25). Mustard yellow/Lt. yellow. In 30s, 100s, 1,000s, and UD 100s.
		olanzapine 6 mg/fluoxetine 50 mg	As fluoxetine hydrochloride. (Lilly 3233 6/50). Mustard yellow/Lt. grey. In 30s, 100s, 1,000s, and UD 100s.
		olanzapine 12 mg/fluoxetine 25 mg	As fluoxetine hydrochloride. (Lilly 3232 12/25). Red/Lt. yellow. In 30s, 100s, 1,000s, and UD 100s.
		olanzapine 12 mg/fluoxetine 50 mg	As fluoxetine hydrochloride. (Lilly 3234 12/50). Red/Lt. grey. In 30s, 100s, 1,000s, and UD 100s.

OLANZAPINE/FLUOXETINE HYDROCHLORIDE — ORAL

For complete and comparative prescribing information, refer to the Selective Serotonin Reuptake Inhibitors and the Antipsychotic Agents class monographs.

WARNING

Suicidality and antidepressant drugs – Antidepressants increased the risk of suicidal thinking and behavior (suicidality) in children, adolescents, and young adults compared with placebo in short-term studies of major depressive disorder (MDD) and other psychiatric disorders. Anyone considering the use of olanzapine/fluoxetine or any other antidepressant in a child, adolescent, or young adult must balance this risk with the clinical need. Short-term studies did not show an increase in the risk of suicidality with antidepressants compared with placebo in adults older than 24 years of age; there was a reduction in risk with antidepressants compared with placebo in adults 65 years of age and older. Depression and certain other psychiatric disorders are themselves associated with increases in the risk of suicide. Appropriately monitor and closely observe patients of all ages who are started on antidepressant therapy for clinical worsening, suicidality, or unusual changes in behavior. Advise families and caregivers of the need for close observation and communication with the health care provider. Olanzapine/fluoxetine is not approved for use in children.

Increased mortality in elderly patients with dementia-related psychosis – Elderly patients with dementia-related psychosis treated with antipsychotic drugs are at an increased risk of death. Analyses of 17 placebo-controlled trials (modal duration of 10 weeks), largely in patients taking atypical antipsychotic drugs, revealed a risk of death in drug-treated patients of 1.6 to 1.7 times the risk of death in placebo-treated patients. Over the course of a typical 10-week controlled trial, the rate of death in drug-treated patients was approximately 4.5% compared with a rate of approximately 2.6% in the placebo group. Although the causes of death were varied, most of the deaths appeared to be either cardiovascular (CV) (eg, heart failure, sudden death) or infectious (eg, pneumonia) in nature. Observational studies suggest that, similar to atypical antipsychotic drugs, treatment with conventional antipsychotic drugs may increase mortality. The extent to which the findings of increased mortality in observational studies may be attributed to the antipsychotic drug, as opposed to some characteristic(s) of the patients, is not clear. Olanzapine/fluoxetine is not approved for the treatment of patients with dementia-related psychosis.

Indications

➤*Bipolar I disorder:* For the acute treatment of depressive episodes associated with bipolar I disorder in adults.

➤*Depression:* For the acute treatment of treatment-resistant depression (MDD in adults who do not respond to 2 separate trials of different antidepressants of adequate dose and duration in the current episode).

Administration and Dosage

➤*General dosing considerations:* Because of the long elimination half-lives of fluoxetine and its major active metabolite, changes in dose will not be fully reflected in plasma for several weeks, affecting strategies for titration to final dose and withdrawal from treatment. This is of potential consequence when drug discontinuation is required or when drugs are prescribed that might interact with fluoxetine and norfluoxetine following the discontinuation of fluoxetine.

➤*Adults:*

Bipolar I disorder –

Usual dosage: Antidepressant efficacy was demonstrated with olanzapine/fluoxetine in a dose range of olanzapine 6 to 12 mg and fluoxetine 25 to 50 mg. The safety of doses above olanzapine 18 mg/fluoxetine 75 mg has not been evaluated in clinical studies.

Initial dosage: Olanzapine 6 mg/fluoxetine 25 mg once daily in the evening.

Dosage adjustment: Dosage adjustments, if indicated, can be made according to efficacy and tolerability.

Depression –

Usual dosage: Antidepressant efficacy was demonstrated with olanzapine/fluoxetine in a dose range of olanzapine 6 to 18 mg and fluoxetine 25 to 50 mg. The safety of doses above olanzapine 18 mg/fluoxetine 75 mg has not been evaluated in clinical studies.

Initial dosage: Olanzapine 6 mg/fluoxetine 25 mg once daily in the evening.

Dosage adjustment: Dosage adjustments, if indicated, can be made according to efficacy and tolerability.

➤*Elderly:* Olanzapine/fluoxetine has not been systemically studied in patients older than 65 years of age.

Initial dosage – Olanzapine 3 mg/fluoxetine 25 mg to olanzapine 6 mg/fluoxetine 25 mg.

Dosage adjustments – Perform dose escalation with caution.

➤*Hepatic function impairment:*

Initial dosage – Olanzapine 3 mg/fluoxetine 25 mg to olanzapine 6 mg/fluoxetine 25 mg.

Dosage adjustments – Perform dose escalation with caution.

➤*Pregnant women during the third trimester:* Neonates exposed to serotonin-norepinephrine reuptake inhibitors (SNRIs) or selective serotonin reuptake inhibitors (SSRIs) late in the third trimester have developed complications requiring prolonged hospitalizations, respiratory support, and tube feeding. Consider using a lower dose of fluoxetine in the third trimester.

➤*Special risk patients:* Use a starting dose of olanzapine 3 mg/fluoxetine 25 mg to olanzapine 6 mg/fluoxetine 25 mg for patients with a predisposition to hypotensive reactions, patients who exhibit a combination of factors that may slow the metabolism of olanzapine/fluoxetine (eg, women, nonsmokers), or patients who may be pharmacodynamically sensitive to olanzapine. Dosing modification may be necessary in patients who exhibit a combination of factors that may slow metabolism. When indicated, perform dose escalation with caution.

➤*Duration of therapy:* While there is no body of evidence to answer the question of how long a patient treated with olanzapine/fluoxetine should remain on it, it is generally accepted that bipolar I disorder and treatment-resistant depression are chronic illnesses requiring long-term treatment. The health care provider should periodically reexamine the need for continued pharmacotherapy.

➤*Discontinuation of therapy:* Symptoms associated with discontinuation of fluoxetine have been reported.

A gradual reduction in the dose rather than abrupt cessation is recommended whenever possible.

➤*Administration:* Administer once daily in the evening.

➤*Storage/Stability:* Store at 25°C (77°F); excursions are permitted between 15° and 30°C (59° and 86°F). Keep the bottle tightly closed and protect from moisture.

CHLORDIAZEPOXIDE/AMITRIPTYLINE

c-iv	**Chlordiazepoxide and Amitriptyline** (Various, eg, Geneva, Lemmon, Par)	**Tablets:** 5 mg chlordiazepoxide and 12.5 mg amitriptyline	In 100s and 500s.
c-iv	**Limbitrol** (Valeant)		(V 3805). Blue. Film-coated. In 100s.
c-iv	**Chlordiazepoxide and Amitriptyline** (Various, eg, Goldline, Lemmon)	**Tablets:** 10 mg chlordiazepoxide and 25 mg amitriptyline	In 100s and 500s.
c-iv	**Limbitrol DS** (Valeant)		(V 3806). White. Film coated. In 100s.

CHLORDIAZEPOXIDE/AMITRIPTYLINE — ORAL

Consider the prescribing information for chlordiazepoxide in the Antianxiety Agents monograph and amitriptyline in the Antidepressants monograph.

WARNING

Suicidality in children and adolescents – Antidepressants increased the risk of suicidal thinking and behavior (suicidality) in short-term studies in children and adolescents with major depressive disorder (MDD) and other psychiatric disorders. Anyone considering the use of chlordiazepoxide/amitriptyline or any other antidepressant in a child or adolescent must balance this risk with the clinical need. Patients who are started on therapy should be observed closely for clinical worsening, suicidality, or unusual changes in behavior. Families and caregivers should be advised of the need for close observation and communication with the prescriber. Chlordiazepoxide/amitriptyline is not approved for use in pediatric patients.

Pooled analyses of short-term (4 to 16 weeks) placebo-controlled trials of 9 antidepressant drugs (SSRIs and others) in children and adolescents with MDD, obsessive-compulsive disorder (OCD), or other psychiatric disorders (a total of 24 trials involving over 4,400 patients) have revealed a greater risk of adverse reactions representing suicidal thinking or behavior (suicidality) during the first few months of treatment in those receiving antidepressants. The average risk of such reactions in patients receiving antidepressants was 4%, twice the placebo risk of 2%. No suicides occurred in these trials.

Indications

➤*Severe depression:* Treatment of moderate to severe depression associated with moderate to severe anxiety. The therapeutic response to this combination has occurred earlier and with fewer treatment failures than when either ingredient is used alone. Symptoms likely to respond in the first week of treatment include: Insomnia; feelings of guilt or worthlessness; agitation; psychic and somatic anxiety; suicidal ideation; anorexia.

Administration and Dosage

➤*Adults:*

Severe depression –

Initial dosage: 3 or 4 tablets daily of chlordiazepoxide 10 mg with amitriptyline 25 mg given in divided doses.

The chlordiazepoxide 5 mg with amitriptyline 12.5 mg in an initial dosage of 3 or 4 tablets daily in divided doses may be satisfactory in patients who do not tolerate higher doses.

Dosage titration: Increase to 6 tablets daily, as required. Some patients respond to smaller doses and can be maintained on 2 tablets daily.

Maintenance dosage: After a satisfactory response is obtained, reduce dosage to smallest amount needed. The larger portion of the total daily dose may be taken at bedtime. In some patients, a single dose at bedtime may be sufficient.

➤*Elderly:* Lower dosages are recommended for elderly patients.

➤*Storage/Stability:* Store at 25°C (77°F); excursions permitted to 15° to 30°C (59° to 86° F). Store in a dry place.

PERPHENAZINE/AMITRIPTYLINE HYDROCHLORIDE

Rx	**Perphenazine/Amitriptyline** (Various, eg, Bolar, Geneva, Goldline, Lemmon, Par, Zenith)	**Tablets:** 2 mg perphenazine and 10 mg amitriptyline	In 21s, 100s, 500s and 1000s.
Rx	**Perphenazine/Amitriptyline** (Various, eg, Bolar, Geneva, Goldline, Lemmon, Par, Zenith)	**Tablets:** 2 mg perphenazine and 25 mg amitriptyline	In 100s, 500s and 1000s.
Rx	**Perphenazine/Amitriptyline** (Various, eg, Bolar, Geneva, Goldline, Lemmon, Par, Zenith)	**Tablets:** 4 mg perphenazine and 10 mg amitriptyline	In 100s, 250s, 500s and 1000s.
Rx	**Perphenazine/Amitriptyline** (Various, eg, Bolar, Geneva, Goldline, Lemmon, Par, Zenith)	**Tablets:** 4 mg perphenazine and 25 mg amitriptyline	In 100s, 500s, 800s and 1000s.
Rx	**Perphenazine/Amitriptyline** (Various, eg, Bolar, Geneva, Goldline, Lemmon, Par, Zenith)	**Tablets:** 4 mg perphenazine and 50 mg amitriptyline	In 100s and 250s.

PERPHENAZINE/AMITRIPTYLINE HYDROCHLORIDE — ORAL

Consider the prescribing information for perphenazine in the Antipsychotic Agents monograph and amitriptyline in the Antidepressants monograph.

WARNING

Suicidality in children and adolescents – Antidepressants increased the risk of suicidal thinking and behavior (suicidality) in short-term studies in children and adolescents with major depressive disorder (MDD) and other psychiatric disorders. Anyone considering the use of perphenazine/amitriptyline or any other antidepressant in a child or adolescent must balance this risk with the clinical need. Patients who are started on therapy should be observed closely for clinical worsening, suicidality, or unusual changes in behavior. Families and caregivers should be advised of the need for close observation and communication with the prescriber. Perphenazine/amitriptyline is not approved for use in pediatric patients.

Pooled analyses of short-term (4 to 16 weeks) placebo-controlled trials of 9 antidepressant drugs (SSRIs and others) in children and adolescents with MDD, obsessive-compulsive disorder (OCD), or other psychiatric disorders (a total of 24 trials involving over 4,400 patients) have revealed a greater risk of adverse reactions representing suicidal thinking or behavior (suicidality) during the first few months of treatment in those receiving antidepressants. The average risk of such reactions in patients receiving antidepressants was 4%, twice the placebo risk of 2%. No suicides occurred in these trials.

Indications

➤*Anxiety/Agitation/Depression:* Treatment of moderate to severe anxiety or agitation and depressed mood; patients with depression in whom anxiety or agitation are moderate or severe; patients with anxiety and depression associated with chronic physical disease; patients in whom depression and anxiety cannot be clearly differentiated; schizophrenic patients who have associated symptoms of depression.

Many patients presenting symptoms such as agitation, anxiety, insomnia, psychomotor retardation, functional somatic complaints, tiredness, loss of interest and anorexia have responded well to this combination.

Administration and Dosage

➤*Adults:*

Anxiety/Agitation/Depression –

Initial dosage: 2 to 4 mg perphenazine with 10 to 25 mg amitriptyline given 3 or 4 times daily, or 4 mg perphenazine with 50 mg amitriptyline given twice daily.

In more severely ill patients with schizophrenia, 4 mg perphenazine with 25 mg amitriptyline is recommended in an initial dose of two tablets three times a day. If necessary, a fourth dose may be given at bedtime.

Dosage adjustment: After a satisfactory response is noted, reduce to smallest amount necessary to obtain relief.

➤*Storage/Stability:* Store at 20° to 25°C (68° to 77°F). Protect from light. Dispense in a tight, light-resistant container.

DEXTROMETHORPHAN HYDROBROMIDE/QUINIDINE SULFATE

Rx	**Nuedexta** (Avanir)	**Capsules; oral:** dextromethorphan hydrobromide 20 mg/ quinidine sulfate 10 mg	Lactose. (DMQ/20-10). Brick red. In 60s.

DEXTROMETHORPHAN HYDROBROMIDE/QUINIDINE SULFATE — ORAL

Indications

➤*Pseudobulbar affect:* For the treatment of pseudobulbar affect.

Administration and Dosage

➤*Adults:*

Pseudobulbar affect –

Initial dosage: 1 capsule daily for the initial 7 days of therapy.

Maintenance dosage: 2 capsules daily, given as 1 capsule every 12 hours.

Duration of therapy: The need for continued treatment should be reassessed periodically because spontaneous improvement of pseudobulbar affect occurs in some patients.

➤*Storage/Stability:* Store at 25°C (77°F); excursions are permitted between 15° and 30°C (59° and 86°F).

Actions

➤*Pharmacology:* Dextromethorphan is a sigma-1 receptor agonist and an uncompetitive N-methyl-D-aspartate (NMDA) receptor antagonist. Quinidine increases plasma levels of dextromethorphan by competitively inhibiting cytochrome P450 2D6 (CYP2D6), which catalyzes a major biotransformation pathway for dextromethorphan. The mechanism by which dextromethorphan exerts therapeutic effects in patients with pseudobulbar affect is unknown.

➤*Pharmacokinetics:*

Absorption – Following single and repeated combination doses of dextromethorphan 30 mg/quinidine 10 mg, dextromethorphan/quinidine-treated subjects had an approximately 20-fold increase in dextromethorphan exposure compared with dextromethorphan given without quinidine.

DEXTROMETHORPHAN HYDROBROMIDE/ QUINIDINE SULFATE — ORAL

Following repeated doses of dextromethorphan 30 mg/quinidine 10 mg and dextromethorphan 20 mg/quinidine 10 mg, maximal plasma concentrations (C_{max}) of dextromethorphan are reached approximately 3 to 4 hours after dosing and C_{max} of quinidine are reached approximately 1 to 2 hours after dosing.

In extensive metabolizers, mean C_{max} and area under the curve (AUC_{0-12}) values of dextromethorphan and dextrorphan increased as doses of dextromethorphan increased from 20 to 30 mg; mean C_{max} and AUC_{0-12} values of quinidine appeared similar.

The mean plasma C_{max} of quinidine following twice daily coadministration of dextromethorphan 30 mg/quinidine 10 mg in patients with pseudobulbar affect was within 1% to 3% of the concentrations required for antiarrhythmic efficacy (2 to 5 mcg/mL).

Distribution – After dextromethorphan/quinidine administration, protein binding remains essentially the same as that after administration of the individual components; dextromethorphan is approximately 60% to 70% protein bound and quinidine is approximately 80% to 89% protein bound.

Metabolism/Excretion – Dextromethorphan is metabolized by CYP2D6 and quinidine is metabolized by CYP3A4. After dextromethorphan 30 mg/quinidine 30 mg administration in extensive metabolizers, the elimination half-life of dextromethorphan was approximately 13 hours and the elimination half-life of quinidine was approximately 7 hours.

There are several hydroxylated metabolites of quinidine. The major metabolite of quinidine is 3-hydroxyquinidine. The 3-hydroxymetabolite is considered to be at least half as pharmacologically active as quinidine with respect to cardiac effects (eg, QT prolongation).

When the urine pH is less than 7, approximately 20% of administered quinidine appears unchanged in the urine, but this fraction drops to as little as 5% when the urine is more alkaline. Renal clearance involves glomerular filtration and active tubular secretion, moderated by (pH-dependent) tubular reabsorption.

Special populations –

Hepatic function impairment: Patients with moderate impairment showed an increased frequency of adverse reactions. Therefore, dosage adjustment is not required in patients with mild and moderate hepatic impairment, although additional monitoring for adverse reactions should be considered.

Poor metabolizers: The quinidine component of dextromethorphan/quinidine is intended to inhibit CYP2D6 so that higher exposure to dextromethorphan can be achieved compared with dextromethorphan alone. Approximately 7% to 10% of white patients and 3% to 8% of black patients generally lack the capacity to metabolize CYP2D6 substrates and are classified as poor metabolizers (PMs). The quinidine component of dextromethorphan/quinidine is not expected to contribute to the effectiveness of dextromethorphan/quinidine in PMs, but adverse reactions of the quinidine are still possible. In those patients who may be at risk of significant toxicity due to quinidine, consider genotyping to determine if they are PMs prior to making the decision to treat with dextromethorphan/quinidine.

Contraindications

Prolonged QT interval, congenital long QT syndrome, or a history suggestive of torsades de pointes; heart failure; concurrent use with drugs that both prolong QT interval and are metabolized by CYP2D6 (eg, thioridazine, pimozide); complete atrioventricular (AV) block without implanted pacemakers, or in patients who are at high risk of complete AV block; history of dextromethorphan/quinidine-, quinine-, mefloquine-, or quinidine-induced thrombocytopenia, hepatitis, bone marrow depression, or lupus-like syndrome; hypersensitivity to dextromethorphan (eg, rash, hives); concurrent monoamine oxidase inhibitor (MAOI) use or in patients who have taken MAOIs within the preceding 14 days; concurrent use with other drugs containing quinidine, quinine, or mefloquine.

Warnings/Precautions

➤*Thrombocytopenia:* Quinidine can cause immune-mediated thrombocytopenia that can be severe or fatal. Nonspecific symptoms, such as lightheadedness, chills, fever, nausea, and vomiting, can precede or occur with thrombocytopenia. Discontinue dextromethorphan/quinidine immediately if thrombocytopenia occurs, unless the thrombocytopenia is clearly not drug-related, because continued use increases the risk for fatal hemorrhage. Likewise, do not restart dextromethorphan/quinidine in sensitized patients because more rapid and more severe thrombocytopenia than the original episode can occur. Do not use dextromethorphan/quinidine if immune-mediated thrombocytopenia from structurally related drugs, including quinine and mefloquine, is suspected because cross-sensitivity can occur. Quinidine-associated thrombocytopenia usually, but not always, resolves within a few days of discontinuation of the sensitizing drug.

➤*Lupus-like syndrome:* Quinidine has also been associated with a lupus-like syndrome involving polyarthritis, sometimes with a positive antinuclear antibody test. Other associations include rash, bronchospasm, lymphadenopathy, hemolytic anemia, vasculitis, uveitis, angioedema, agranulocytosis, the sicca syndrome, myalgia, elevation in serum levels of skeletal-muscle enzymes, and pneumonitis.

➤*Hepatotoxicity:* Hepatitis, including granulomatous hepatitis, has been reported in patients receiving quinidine, generally during the first few weeks of therapy. Fever may be a presenting symptom, and thrombocytopenia or other signs of hypersensitivity may also occur. Most cases remit when quinidine is withdrawn.

➤*Cardiac effects:* Dextromethorphan/quinidine causes dose-dependent QTc prolongation. QT prolongation can cause torsades de pointes-type ventricular tachycardia, with the risk increasing as the degree of prolongation increases. When initiating dextromethorphan/quinidine in patients at risk of QT prolongation and torsades de pointes, conduct an electrocardiographic (ECG) evaluation of QT interval at baseline and 3 to 4 hours after the first dose. This includes patients concomitantly taking/initiating drugs that prolong the QT interval or that are strong or moderate CYP3A4 inhibitors, and patients with left ventricular hypertrophy (LVH) or left ventricular dysfunction (LVD). LVH and LVD are more likely to be present in patients with chronic hypertension, known coronary artery disease, or history of stroke. LVH and LVD can be diagnosed utilizing echocardiography or another suitable cardiac imaging modality.

Reevaluate ECG if risk factors for arrhythmia change during the course of treatment with dextromethorphan/quinidine. Risk factors include concomitant use of drugs associated with QT prolongation, electrolyte abnormality (hypokalemia, hypomagnesemia), bradycardia, and family history of QT abnormality. Correct for hypokalemia and hypomagnesemia prior to initiation of therapy with dextromethorphan/quinidine and monitor during treatment.

If patients taking dextromethorphan/quinidine experience symptoms that could indicate the occurrence of cardiac arrhythmias (eg, syncope, palpitations), discontinue dextromethorphan/quinidine and further evaluate the patient.

➤*Dizziness:* Dextromethorphan/quinidine may cause dizziness. Take precautions to reduce the risk of falls, particularly for patients with motor impairment affecting gait or a history of falls. In a controlled trial of dextromethorphan/quinidine, 10% of patients taking dextromethorphan/quinidine and 5% taking placebo experienced dizziness.

➤*Anticholinergic effects:* Monitor for worsening clinical condition in myasthenia gravis and other conditions that may be adversely affected by anticholinergic effects.

➤*CYP2D6 poor metabolizers:* Quinidine is intended to inhibit CYP2D6 so that higher exposure to dextromethorphan can be achieved compared with dextromethorphan alone. Approximately 7% to 10% of white patients and 3% to 8% of black patients lack the capacity to metabolize CYP2D6 substrates and are classified as PMs. The quinidine component of dextromethorphan/quinidine is not expected to contribute to the effectiveness of dextromethorphan/quinidine in PMs, but adverse reactions of quinidine are still possible. In those patients who may be at risk of significant toxicity due to quinidine, consider genotyping to determine if they are PMs prior to making the decision to treat with dextromethorphan/quinidine.

➤*Renal function impairment:* Increases in dextromethorphan and/or quinidine levels are likely to be observed in patients with severe renal impairment.

➤*Hepatic function impairment:* Increases in dextromethorphan and/or quinidine levels are likely to be observed in patients with severe hepatic impairment.

➤*Drug abuse and dependence:* Dextromethorphan/quinidine is a low-affinity uncompetitive NMDA antagonist and sigma-1 receptor agonist that has not been systematically studied in animals or humans for its potential for abuse, tolerance, or physical dependence. However, dextromethorphan/quinidine is a combination product containing dextromethorphan and quinidine, and cases of dextromethorphan abuse have been reported, predominantly in adolescents.

While clinical trials did not reveal drug-seeking behavior, these observations were not systematic and it is not possible to predict on the basis of this experience the extent to which dextromethorphan/quinidine will be misused, diverted, and/or abused once marketed. Therefore, closely observe patients with a history of drug abuse for signs of dextromethorphan/quinidine misuse or abuse (eg, development of tolerance, increases in dose, drug-seeking behavior).

➤*Pregnancy: Category C.* There are no adequate and well-controlled studies of dextromethorphan/quinidine in pregnant women. Quinidine crosses the placenta and achieves fetal serum levels similar to maternal levels. No information is available on the placental transfer of dextromethorphan. The molecular weight (approximately 271) is low enough that transfer to the fetus should be expected. In oral studies conducted in rats and rabbits, a combination of dextromethorphan/quinidine demonstrated developmental toxicity, including teratogenicity (rabbits) and embryolethality, when given to pregnant animals. Use dextromethorphan/quinidine during pregnancy only if the potential benefit justifies the potential risk to the fetus.

When dextromethorphan/quinidine was administered orally (dextromethorphan 0 mg/quinidine 0 mg/kg/day, dextromethorphan 5 mg/quinidine 100 mg/kg/day, dextromethorphan 15 mg/quinidine 100 mg, and dextromethorphan 50 mg/quinidine 100 mg/kg/day) to pregnant rats during the period of organogenesis, embryo-fetal deaths were observed at the highest dosage tested and reduced skeletal ossification was observed at all dosages. The lowest dosage tested (dextromethorphan 5 mg/quinidine 100 mg/kg/day) is approximately 1/50 times the recommended human dosage of dextromethorphan 40 mg/quinidine 20 mg/day on a mg/m^2 basis. Oral administration (dextromethorphan 0 mg/quinidine 0 mg/kg/day, dextromethorphan 5 mg/quinidine 60 mg/kg/day, dextromethorphan 15 mg/quinidine 60 mg/kg/day, and dextromethorphan 30 mg/quinidine 60 mg/kg/day) to pregnant rabbits during organogenesis resulted in an increased incidence of fetal malformations at all but the lowest dosage tested. The no-effect dosage (dextromethorphan 5 mg/quinidine 60 mg/kg/day) is approximately 2/60 times the recommended human dosage on a mg/m^2 basis.

When dextromethorphan/quinidine was orally administered (dextromethorphan 0 mg/quinidine 0 mg/kg/day, dextromethorphan 5 mg/quinidine 100 mg/kg/day, dextromethorphan 15 mg/quinidine 100 mg/kg/day, and dex-

DEXTROMETHORPHAN HYDROBROMIDE/ QUINIDINE SULFATE — ORAL

tromethorphan 30 mg/quinidine 100 mg/kg/day) to female rats during pregnancy and lactation, pup survival and pup weight were decreased at all dosages and developmental delay was seen in offspring at the mid- and high-dosages. The lowest dosage tested (dextromethorphan 5 mg/quinidine 100 mg/kg/day) is approximately 1/50 times the recommended human dosage on a mg/m^2 basis.

➤*Lactation:* Quinidine is excreted into breast milk for a milk:serum ratio of 0.71. It is not known whether dextromethorphan is excreted in human milk. The relatively low molecular weight of dextromethorphan (approximately 271) suggests that passage into milk probably occurs. Because many drugs are excreted in human milk, exercise caution when dextromethorphan/quinidine is administered to a breast-feeding mother.

➤*Children:* The safety and effectiveness in children younger than 18 years of age have not been established.

➤*Monitoring:* When initiating dextromethorphan/quinidine in patients at risk of QT prolongation and torsades de pointes, conduct ECG evaluation of QT interval at baseline and 3 to 4 hours after the first dose. This includes patients concomitantly taking/initiating drugs that prolong the QT interval or that are strong or moderate CYP3A4 inhibitors, and patients with LVH or LVD.

Reevaluate ECG if risk factors for arrhythmia change during the course of treatment with dextromethorphan/quinidine. Risk factors include concomitant use of drugs associated with QT prolongation, electrolyte abnormality (hypokalemia, hypomagnesemia), bradycardia, and family history of QT abnormality. Correct hypokalemia and hypomagnesemia prior to initiation of therapy with dextromethorphan/quinidine and monitor during treatment.

Monitor for worsening clinical condition in myasthenia gravis and other conditions that may be adversely affected by anticholinergic effects.

Closely observe patients with a history of drug abuse for signs of dextromethorphan/quinidine misuse or abuse (eg, development of tolerance, increases in dose, drug-seeking behavior).

Drug Interactions

➤*QT prolongation:* An additive effect of dextromethorphan/quinidine with other drugs that prolong the QT interval cannot be excluded. The following drugs may prolong the QT interval and increase the risk of life-threatening cardiac arrhythmias, including torsades de pointes: antiarrhythmic agents (eg, amiodarone, bretylium, disopyramide, dofetilide, procainamide, quinidine, sotalol), arsenic trioxide, chlorpromazine, cisapride, dolasetron, droperidol, gatifloxacin, halofantrine, levomethadyl, mefloquine, mesoridazine, moxifloxacin, pentamidine, pimozide, probucol, sparfloxacin, thioridazine, ziprasidone. (See Drug-Induced Prolongation of the QT Interval and Torsades De Pointes.)

Dextromethorphan/Quinidine Drug Interactions

Precipitant drug	Object drug[a]		Description
Alcohol	Dextromethorphan/ Quinidine	↑	CNS effectsmay be increased. Use with caution.
Dextromethorphan/ Quinidine	Alcohol		
Drugs that prolong the QT interval and are CYP2D6 substrates (eg, pimozide, thioridazine)	Dextromethorphan/ Quinidine	↑	The risk of QT prolongation may be increased, increasing the risk of torsades de pointes–type ventricular tachycardia. Concomitant use is contraindicated.
Drugs that prolong the QT interval	Dextromethorphan/ Quinidine	↑	The risk of QT prolongation may be increased, increasing the risk of torsades de pointes–type ventricular tachycardia. Conduct an ECG evaluation of the QT interval at baseline and 3 to 4 hours after the first dose of dextromethorphan/quinidine in patients taking drugs that prolong the QT interval. If patients experience symptoms of cardiac arrhythmias, discontinue dextromethorphan/quinidine.
Dextromethorphan/ Quinidine	Drugs that prolong the QT interval		
Mefloquine, quinidine, quinine	Dextromethorphan/ Quinidine	↑	Concomitant use is contraindicated. The risk of adverse reactions may be increased.
Dextromethorphan/ Quinidine	Mefloquine, quinidine, quinine		

Dextromethorphan/Quinidine Drug Interactions

Precipitant drug	Object drug[a]		Description
NMDA receptor antagonists (eg, memantine)	Dextromethorphan/ Quinidine	↑	Both memantine and dextromethorphan are NMDA antagonists and could theoretically result in an additive effect at NMDA receptors and potentially an increased incidence of adverse reactions.
Dextromethorphan/ Quinidine	NMDA receptor antagonists (eg, memantine)		
Selective serotonin reuptake inhibitors (eg, fluoxetine)	Dextromethorphan/ Quinidine	↑	The risk of serotonin syndrome may be increased. Closely monitor the patient. Serotonin syndrome requires immediate medical attention, including withdrawal of the sertonergic agent and supportive care.
Dextromethorphan/ Quinidine	Selective serotonin reuptake inhibitors (eg, fluoxetine)		
Strong (eg, atazanavir, clarithromycin, indinavir, itraconazole, ketoconazole, nefazodone, nelfinavir, ritonavir, saquinavir, telithromycin) or moderate (eg, aprepitant, diltiazem, erythromycin, fluconazole, fosamprenavir, verapamil) CYP3A inhibitors	Dextromethorphan/ Quinidine	↑	The risk of QT prolongation may be increased, increasing the risk of torsades de pointes–type ventricular tachycardia. Conduct an ECG evaluation of the QT interval at baseline and 3 to 4 hours after the first dose of dextromethorphan/quinidine in patients taking drugs that are strong or moderate CYP3A inhibitors. If patients experience symptoms of cardiac arrhythmias, discontinue dextromethorphan/ quinidine.
Tricyclic antidepressants (eg, clomipramine, imipramine)	Dextromethorphan/ Quinidine	↑	The risk of serotonin syndrome may be increased. Closely monitor the patient. Serotonin syndrome requires immediate medical attention, including withdrawal of the serotonergic agent and supportive care.
Dextromethorphan/ Quinidine	Tricyclic antidepressants (eg, clomipramine, imipramine)		
Dextromethorphan/ Quinidine	CYP2D6 substrates (eg, codeine, desipramine, hydrocodone, paroxetine)	↑↓	Quinidine may elevate plasma concentrations of the CYP2D6 substrate (eg, desipramine, paroxetine) and increase the risk for adverse reactions. In this instance, a lower dose of the substrate may be needed. A dosage greater than desipramine 40 mg/day or paroxetine 35 mg/day is not recommended. Monitor the clinical response. By inhibiting CYP2D6, quinidine may also reduce metabolism of a substrate (eg, codeine, hydrocodone) to its active metabolite (eg, morphine, hydromorphone, respectively), decreasing the pharmacologic effects (eg, analgesia, antitussive). In this instance, alternative treatment may be necessary.
Dextromethorphan/ Quinidine	Digoxin	↑	Digoxin levels may be increased. Closely monitor digoxin plasma concentrations and adjust the digoxin dose as needed.
Dextromethorphan/ Quinidine	MAOIs (eg, phenelzine)	↑	Concomitant use is contraindicated in patients taking MAOIs or who have taken MAOIs within the preceding 14 days. Allow at least 14 days after stopping dextromethorphan/quinidine before starting an MAOI.
MAOIs (eg, phenelzine)	Dextromethorphan/ Quinidine		

[a] ↑ = object drug increased. ↑↓ = object drug both increased and decreased.

DEXTROMETHORPHAN HYDROBROMIDE/ QUINIDINE SULFATE — ORAL

➤*Drug/Food interactions:* Grapefruit juice is a moderate CYP3A inhibitor. Concurrent use may increase the risk of QT prolongation, increasing the risk of torsades de pointes–type ventricular tachycardia.

Adverse Reactions

➤*Mortality:* Three ALS patients in each drug treatment arm and 1 ALS patient in the placebo arm died during the 12-week placebo-control period. All deaths were consistent with the natural progression of ALS.

➤*Discontinuation of therapy:* The most commonly reported adverse reactions (incidence greater than 2% and greater than placebo) that led to discontinuation with the dextromethorphan 20 mg/quinidine 10 mg twice daily dose were muscle spasticity (3%), respiratory failure (1%), abdominal pain (2%), asthenia (2%), dizziness (2%), fall (1%), and muscle spasms (2%).

➤*Most common adverse reactions (3% or more):*

Dextromethorphan/Quinidine Adverse Reactions (≥ 3%)		
Adverse reactions	Dextromethorphan/ Quinidine (n = 107)	Placebo (n = 109)
CNS		
Asthenia	5%	2%
Dizziness	10%	5%
GI		
Diarrhea	13%	6%
Flatulence	3%	1%
Vomiting	5%	1%
Miscellaneous		
Cough	5%	2%
Increased gamma-glutamyltransferase	3%	0%
Influenza	4%	1%
Peripheral edema	5%	1%
Urinary tract infection	4%	1%

➤*Postmarketing:*

Dextromethorphan – Dizziness, drowsiness, nausea, nervousness, restlessness, stomach pain, and vomiting.

Quinidine – Cinchonism is most often a sign of chronic quinidine toxicity, but it may appear in sensitive patients after a single moderate dose of several hundred milligrams. Cinchonism is characterized by blurred vision, confusion, delirium, diarrhea, diplopia, headache, hearing loss, nausea, photophobia, tinnitus, vertigo, and vomiting.

Apprehension, ataxia, and convulsions have been reported with quinidine therapy, but it is not clear that these were not simply the results of hypotension and consequent cerebral hypoperfusion in patients being treated for cardiovascular indications. Acute psychotic reactions have been reported to follow the first dose of quinidine, but these reactions appear to be extremely rare. Other adverse reactions occasionally reported with quinidine therapy include abnormalities of skin pigmentation, depression, disturbed color perception, keratopathy, mydriasis, night blindness, optic neuritis, photosensitivity, scotomata, and visual field loss.

Overdosage

➤*Symptoms:*

Dextromethorphan/Quinidine – During development of dextromethorphan/quinidine, dose combinations of dextromethorphan/quinidine containing up to 6-times higher dextromethorphan dose and 12-times higher quinidine dose were studied. The most common adverse reactions were mild to moderate nausea, dizziness, and headache.

Quinidine – The most important adverse effects of acute quinidine overdose are ventricular arrhythmias and hypotension. Other signs and symptoms of overdose may include vomiting, diarrhea, tinnitus, high-frequency hearing loss, vertigo, blurred vision, diplopia, photophobia, headache, confusion, and delirium.

While therapeutic doses of quinidine for treatment of cardiac arrhythmia or malaria are generally 10-fold or more higher than the dose of quinidine in dextromethorphan/quinidine, potentially fatal cardiac arrhythmia, including torsades de pointes, can occur at quinidine exposures that are possible from dextromethorphan/quinidine overdose.

Dextromethorphan – Adverse effects of dextromethorphan overdose include nausea, vomiting, stupor, coma, respiratory depression, seizures, tachycardia, hyperexcitability, and toxic psychosis. Other adverse effects include ataxia, nystagmus, dystonia, blurred vision, and changes in muscle reflexes. Dextromethorphan may cause serotonin syndrome, and this risk is increased by overdose, particularly if taken with other serotonergic agents, selective serotonin reuptake inhibitors, or tricyclic antidepressants.

➤*Treatment:* While serum quinidine levels can be measured, ECG monitoring of the QTc interval is a better predictor of quinidine-induced arrhythmia. Treatment of hemodynamically unstable polymorphic ventricular tachycardia (including torsades de pointes) is either immediate cardioversion or, if a cardiac pacemaker is in place or immediately available, immediate overdrive pacing. After pacing or cardioversion, further management must be guided by the length of the QTc interval. Identify and (if possible) aggressively correct factors contributing to QTc prolongation (especially hypokalemia and hypomagnesemia). Prevention of recurrent torsades de pointes may require sustained overdrive pacing or the cautious administration of isoproterenol (30 to 150 ng/kg/min).

Because of the theoretical possibility of QT-prolonging effects that might be additive to those of quinidine, avoid other antiarrhythmics with class I (procainamide) or class III activities whenever possible.

If the post-cardioversion QTc interval is prolonged, then the pre-cardioversion polymorphic ventricular tachyarrhythmia was (by definition) torsades de pointes. In this case, class Ib antiarrhythmics like lidocaine are unlikely to be of value, and other class I and class III antiarrhythmics are likely to exacerbate the situation.

Quinidine-induced hypotension that is not due to an arrhythmia is likely to be a consequence of quinidine-related alpha-blockade and vasorelaxation. Direct treatment of hypotension at symptomatic and supportive measures. Repletion of central volume (Trendelenburg positioning, saline infusion) may be sufficient therapy; other interventions reported to have been beneficial in this setting are those that increase peripheral vascular resistance, including alpha-agonist catecholamines (norepinephrine).

Quinidine – Adequate studies of orally administered activated charcoal in human overdoses of quinidine have not been reported, but there are animal data showing significant enhancement of systemic elimination following this intervention, and there is at least 1 human case report in which the elimination half-life of quinidine in the serum was apparently shortened by repeated gastric lavage. Avoid activated charcoal if an ileus is present; the conventional dose is 1 g/kg, administered every 2 to 6 hours as a slurry with 8 mL/kg of tap water. Although renal elimination of quinidine might theoretically be accelerated by maneuvers to acidify the urine, such maneuvers are potentially hazardous and of no demonstrated benefit. Quinidine is not usefully removed from the circulation by dialysis. Following quinidine overdose, discontinue drugs that delay elimination of quinidine (cimetidine, carbonic anhydrase inhibitors, thiazide diuretics) unless absolutely required.

Dextromethorphan – Direct treatment of dextromethorphan overdosage at symptomatic and supportive measures.

Patient Information

Advise patients that a hypersensitivity reaction to dextromethorphan/quinidine could occur. Instruct patients to seek medical attention immediately if they experience symptoms indicative of hypersensitivity after taking dextromethorphan/quinidine.

Advise patients to consult their health care provider immediately if they feel faint or lose consciousness. Counsel patients to inform their health care provider if they have any personal or family history of QTc prolongation.

Advise patients that dextromethorphan/quinidine may cause dizziness. Take precautions to reduce the risk of falls, particularly for patients with motor impairment affecting gait or a history of falls.

Inform patients that dextromethorphan/quinidine increases the risk of adverse drug interactions. Instruct patients to inform their health care provider about all the medications that they are taking before taking dextromethorphan/quinidine. Inform patients to tell their health care provider that they are taking dextromethorphan/quinidine before taking any new medicine.

Summarize for patients the risks of treatment with dextromethorphan/quinidine. Advise patients to tell their health care provider if they have adverse effects that bother them or do not go away.

Instruct patients to take dextromethorphan/quinidine exactly as prescribed. Instruct patients not to take more than 2 capsules in a 24-hour period and to make sure that there is an approximate 12-hour interval between doses, and not to take a double dose after they miss a dose.

Advise patients to contact their health care provider if their pseudobulbar affect symptoms persist or worsen.

ERGOLOID MESYLATES (Dihydrogenated Ergot Alkaloids, Dihydroergotoxine)

Rx	**Ergoloid Mesylates** (Various, eg, Ivax, Major, Mutual, URL)	**Tablets, sublingual:** 1 mg	In 100s, 500s, 1000s and UD 100s.
Rx	**Ergoloid Mesylates** (Various, eg, Ivax, Major, Mutual, URL)	**Tablets, oral:** 1 mg	In 60s, 100s, 500s, 1000s and UD 32s, 100s and 1000s.

ERGOLOID MESYLATES — ORAL

Indications

➤*Mental capacity decline:* A proportion of individuals older than 60 years of age who manifest signs and symptoms of an idiopathic decline in mental capacity (ie, cognitive and interpersonal skills, mood, self-care, apparent motivation) can experience some symptomatic relief upon treatment with ergoloid mesylates preparations. The identity of the specific trait(s) or condition(s), if any, which would usefully predict a response to ergoloid mesylates therapy is not known. It appears, however, that those individuals who do respond come from groups of patients who would be considered clinically to suffer from some ill-defined process related to aging or to have some underlying dementing condition (ie, primary progressive dementia, Alzheimer's dementia, senile onset, multi-infarct dementia).

Administration and Dosage

➤*General dosing considerations:* Alleviation of symptoms is usually gradual and results may not be observed for 3 to 4 weeks.

➤*Adults:*

Mental capacity decline – 1 mg 3 times daily.

➤*Storage/Stability:* Store in a tight, light-resistant container below 25°C (77°F).

Actions

➤*Pharmacology:* There is no specific evidence which clearly establishes the mechanism by which ergoloid mesylates preparations produce mental effects, nor is there conclusive evidence that the drug particularly affects cerebral arteriosclerosis or cerebrovascular insufficiency.

➤*Pharmacokinetics:* Pharmacokinetic studies have been performed in healthy volunteers with the help of radiolabeled drug as well as employing a specific radioimmunoassay technique. From the urinary excretion quotient of orally and intravenously administered tritium-labelled ergoloid mesylates the absorption of ergoloid was calculated to be 25%. Following oral administration, peak levels of 0.5 ng Eq/mL/mg were achieved within 1.5 to 3 hours. Bioavailability studies with the specific radioimmunoassay confirm that ergoloid is rapidly absorbed from the gastrointestinal tract, with mean peak levels of 0.05 to 0.13 ng/mL/mg (with extremes of 0.03 and 0.18 ng/mL/mg) achieved within 0.6 to 1.3 hours (with extremes of 0.4 and 2.8 hours). The finding of lower peak levels of ergoloid compared to the total drug-metabolite composite is consistent with a considerable first pass liver metabolism, with < 50% of the therapeutic moiety reaching the systemic circulation. The elimination of radioactivity, representing ergoloid plus metabolites bearing the radiolabel, was biphasic with half-lives of 4 and 13 hours. The mean half-life of unchanged ergoloid in plasma is about 2.6 to 5.1 hours; after 3 half-lives ergoloid plasma levels are < 10% of radioactivity levels, and by 24 hours no ergoloid is detectable.

Bioequivalence studies were performed comparing ergoloid mesylates oral tablets (administered orally) with ergoloid mesylates sublingual tablets (administered sublingually).

Contraindications

Individuals who have previously shown hypersensitivity to the drug; in patients who have psychosis, acute or chronic, regardless of etiology.

Warnings/Precautions

➤*Diagnosis:* Practitioners are advised that because the target symptoms are of unknown etiology, careful diagnosis should be attempted before prescribing ergoloid mesylates preparations.

➤*Pregnancy: Category: Undetermined*. Do not use this medication in pregnant women.

➤*Lactation:* Ergoloid is excreted in breast milk. Do not use this medication in breast-feeding women.

Adverse Reactions

Ergoloid mesylates preparations have not been found to produce serious side effects. Transient nausea and gastric disturbances have been reported. Ergoloid mesylates preparations do not possess the vasoconstrictor properties of the natural ergot alkaloids.

SEDATIVES AND HYPNOTICS, NONBARBITURATE

The following is a general discussion of nonbarbiturate sedative/hypnotics.

To facilitate comparison, the products are divided into two groups: The miscellaneous nonbarbiturates and the benzodiazepines. Although sedative doses can be given, these agents are primarily intended to be hypnotics (agents that produce drowsiness and facilitate sleep). Agents intended primarily for sedation or tranquilization are discussed in other parts of this chapter.

In the table below, some pharmacokinetic properties of the nonbarbiturate sedative/hypnotics are compared. Do not use this table to predict exact duration of effect, but use as a guide in drug selection.

Nonbarbiturate Sedative/Hypnotics Pharmacokinetic Parameters

Drug	Adult oral dose		Onset (min)	Duration of action (hrs)	Half-life (hrs)	Protein binding (%)	Urinary excretion, unchanged (%)
	Hypnotic	Sedative					
Imidazopyridines							
Zolpidem	10 mg	na[a]	nd[a]	nd[a]	≈ 2.5	92.5	0
Ureides							
Acetylcarbromal	nd[a]	250-500 mg bid or tid	nd[a]	nd[a]	nd[a]	nd[a]	nd[a]
Tertiary Acetylenic Alcohols							
Ethchlorvynol	500 mg	100-200 mg bid or tid	15-60	5	10-20[c]	nd[a]	40[d]
Piperidine Derivatives							
Glutethimide	250-500 mg	nd[a]	30	4-8	10-12	50	< 2
Benzodiazepines							
Estazolam	1-2 mg	na[a]	nd[a]	nd[a]	10-24	93	< 5
Flurazepam	15-30 mg	na[a]	17	7-8	50-100[c]	97	< 1[e]
Quazepam	15 mg	na[a]	nd[a]	nd[a]	25-41	> 95	trace
Temazepam	15-30 mg	na[a]	nd[a]	nd[a]	10-17	98	1.5
Triazolam	0.125-0.5 mg	na[a]	nd[a]	nd[a]	1.5-5.5	90	2
Miscellaneous nonbarbiturates							
Chloral hydrate	0.5-1 g	250 mg tid pc	30	nd[a]	7-10[b]	35-41	nd[a]
Paraldehyde	10-30 ml	5-10 ml	10-15	8-12	3.4-9.8	nd[a]	small
Propiomazine	nd[a]	10-20 mg	nd[a]	nd[a]	nd[a]	nd[a]	nd[a]

[a] na – Not applicable. nd = No data.
[b] Trichloroethanol, the principal metabolite.
[c] In acute use, half-life of the distribution phase (1 to 3 hours) is more appropriate.
[d] Free and conjugated forms of the major metabolite, secondary alcohol of ethchlorvynol.
[e] Active metabolite, desalkylflurazepam.

ZOLPIDEM TARTRATE

c-iv	**Zolpidem Tartrate** (Various, eg, Mylan, Sandoz, Teva)	**Tablets; oral:** 5 mg	May contain lactose. In 10s, 30s, 60s, 100s, 250s, 500s, 1,000s, and UD 30s and 100s.
c-iv	**Ambien** (Sanofi-Aventis)		Lactose, PEG. (AMB 5 5401). Pink, capsule shape. Film-coated. In 100s and 500s.
c-iv	**Zolpidem Tartrate** (Various, eg, Mylan, Sandoz, Teva)	**Tablets; oral:** 10 mg	May contain lactose. In 10s, 30s, 60s, 100s, 250s, 500s, 1,000s, and UD 30s and 100s.
c-iv	**Ambien** (Sanofi-Aventis)		Lactose, PEG. (AMB 10 5421). White, capsule shape. Film-coated. In 100s and 500s.
c-iv	**Zolpidem** (Winthrop US)	**Tablets, extended-release; oral:** 6.25 mg	Lactose, PEG. (ZCR). Pink, bilayered, round. In 100s.
c-iv	**Ambien CR** (Sanofi-Aventis)		Lactose, PEG. (A~). Pink, bilayered, round. In 100s, 500s, and UD 30s and 100s.
c-iv	**Zolpidem** (Winthrop US)	**Tablets, extended-release; oral:** 12.5 mg	Lactose, PEG. (ZCR). Blue, bilayered, round. In 100s.
c-iv	**Ambien CR** (Sanofi-Aventis)		Lactose, PEG. (A~). Blue, bilayered, round. In 100s, 500s, and UD 30s and 100s.
c-iv	**Edluar** (Meda Pharmaceuticals)	**Tablets; sublingual:** 5 mg	Mannitol, saccharin. (V). White, round. In UD 10s, UD 30s, and UD 100s.
		10 mg	Mannitol, saccharin. (X). White, round. In UD 10s, UD 30s, and UD 100s.
c-iv	**Zolpimist** (ECR[a])	**Spray, solution; lingual:** 5 mg per actuation	Neotame. Cherry flavor. In 60 metered actuations per container.

[a] 25 Minneakoning Road; Flemington, NJ 08822; phone: (908) 782-3431; fax: (908) 782-2445; http://www.novadel.com/index.html.

ZOLPIDEM TARTRATE — ORAL

Refer to the general discussion beginning in the Sedatives and Hypnotics, Nonbarbiturate introduction.

Indications

➤*Insomnia:*

Immediate-release tablets, sublingual tablets, and oral spray – For the short-term treatment of insomnia characterized by difficulties in sleep initiation.

Extended-release (ER) tablets – For the short-term treatment of insomnia, characterized by difficulties with sleep onset and/or sleep maintenance (as measured by wake time after sleep onset).

➤*Off-label uses:*

Parkinson disease – [4] = Insufficient documentation. Preliminary data suggest that zolpidem administration may be effective in promoting improvement in motor symptoms associated with Parkinson disease.

Restless legs syndrome – [4] = Insufficient documentation. Zolpidem has been studied for restless legs syndrome (RLS) in fewer than 10 patients. Despite evidence of probable efficacy with clonazepam, most guidelines either do not include sedative hypnotics or state that there is insufficient evidence to make a recommendation on the use of zolpidem in the management of RLS. Larger, controlled trials are needed to establish the use of zolpidem in the management of RLS.

Administration and Dosage

➤*Adults:*

Insomnia –

Immediate-release tablets, sublingual tablets, and oral spray:

- *Usual dosage* – 10 mg immediately before bedtime.
- *Maximum dose* – 10 mg/day.

ER tablets: 12.5 mg immediately before bedtime.

- *Maximum dose* – 12.5 mg/day.

Off-label dosing –

Parkinson disease: [4] = Insufficient documentation. Initial dosages typically have been 10 mg nightly with gradual titration to dosages as high as 40 mg/day or 10 mg every 2 hours.

Restless legs syndrome: [4] = Insufficient documentation. 10 mg nightly for up to 30 months has been documented.

➤*Elderly:* Elderly patients may be especially sensitive to the effects of zolpidem.

Immediate-release tablets, sublingual tablets, and oral spray – 5 mg once daily taken immediately before bedtime.

ER tablets – 6.25 mg taken immediately before bedtime.

➤*Hepatic function impairment:*

Immediate-release tablets, sublingual tablets, and oral spray – 5 mg taken immediately before bedtime.

ER tablets – 6.25 mg taken immediately before bedtime.

➤*Debilitated patients:* Debilitated patients may be especially sensitive to the effects of zolpidem.

See Elderly for dosing.

➤*Concomitant therapy:* Dosage adjustment may be necessary when zolpidem is administered with agents having known CNS-depressant effects because of the potentially additive effects.

➤*Administration:*

Immediate-release tablets, sublingual tablets, and oral spray – The effect of zolpidem may be slowed by ingestion with or immediately after a meal.

Sublingual tablets should not be given with or immediately after a meal. Sublingual tablets should be placed under the tongue, where it will disintegrate. The tablet should not be swallowed, and the tablets should not be taken with water.

Zolpidem oral spray is packaged in a child-resistant container. Zolpidem oral spray must be primed before it is used for the first time. To prime, patients should be told to point the black spray opening away from their face and other people and spray 5 times. For administration, the child-resistant container should be held upright with the black spray opening pointed directly into the mouth. The patient should fully press down on the pump to make sure a full dose (5 mg) of oral spray is sprayed directly into the mouth over the tongue. If a 10 mg dose is prescribed, a second spray should be administered.

If the patient does not use zolpidem oral spray for at least 14 days, it must be primed again with 1 spray. The patient should be referred to the Patient Instructions for Use included at the end of the Medication Guide.

ER tablets – ER tablets should be swallowed whole and not divided, crushed, or chewed. The effect of zolpidem ER tablets may be slowed by ingestion with or immediately after a meal.

➤*Storage/Stability:*

Immediate-release tablets and sublingual tablets – Store at 20° to 25°C (68° to 77°F).

Oral spray – Store upright at 25°C (77°F), with excursions permitted to 15° to 30°C (59° to 86°F). Do not freeze. Avoid prolonged product exposure to temperatures above 30°C (86°F). The child-resistant container should be discarded when the labeled number of actuations (60 sprays) have been used.

ER tablets – Store between 15° and 25°C (59° and 77°F). Limited excursions are permissible up to 30°C (86°F).

Actions

➤*Pharmacology:* Zolpidem is a nonbenzodiazepine hypnotic of the imidazopyridine class. Subunit modulation of the gamma-aminobutyric acid A ($GABA_A$) receptor chloride channel macromolecular complex is hypothesized to be responsible for sedative, anticonvulsant, anxiolytic, and myorelaxant drug properties. The major modulatory site of the $GABA_A$ receptor complex is located on its alpha subunit and is referred to as the benzodiazepine or omega receptor. At least 3 subtypes of the omega receptor have been identified.

Zolpidem, the active moiety of zolpidem tartrate, is a hypnotic agent with a chemical structure unrelated to benzodiazepines, barbiturates, pyrrolopyrazines, pyrazolopyrimidines, or other drugs with known hypnotic properties; it interacts with a GABA-benzodiazepine receptor complex and shares some of the pharmacological properties of the benzodiazepines. In contrast to the benzodiazepines, which nonselectively bind to and activate all benzodiazepine or omega receptor subtypes, zolpidem in vitro binds the benzodiazepine$_1$ receptor (omega-1 receptor) preferentially with a high-affinity ratio of the alpha$_1$/alpha$_5$ subunits. The benzodiazepine$_1$ receptor is found primarily on the lamina IV of the sensorimotor cortical regions, substantia nigra (pars reticulata), cerebellum molecular layer, olfactory bulb, ventral thalamic complex, pons, inferior colliculus, and globus pallidus. This selective binding of zolpidem on the benzodiazepine$_1$ receptor is not absolute, but it may explain the relative absence of myorelaxant and anticonvulsant effects in animal studies as well as the preservation of deep sleep (stages 3 and 4) in human studies of zolpidem at hypnotic doses.

➤*Pharmacokinetics:*

Absorption/Distribution – Total protein binding was found to be 92.5 ± 0.1% and remained constant, independent of concentration between 40 and 790 ng/mL.

Immediate-release tablets and oral spray: Zolpidem oral spray is bioequivalent to zolpidem immediate-release tablets. The pharmacokinetic profile of zolpidem is characterized by rapid absorption from the oral mucosa and GI tract and a short elimination half-life ($t_{½}$) in healthy subjects.

In a single-dose crossover study in 45 healthy subjects administered zolpidem 5 and 10 mg immediate-release tablets, the mean peak concentrations (C_{max}) were 59 ng/mL (range, 29 to 113 ng/mL) and 121 ng/mL (range, 58 to 272 ng/mL), respectively, occurring at a mean time (T_{max}) of 1.6 hours for both. Zolpidem demonstrated linear kinetics in the dose range of 5 to 20 mg.

ZOLPIDEM TARTRATE — ORAL

In a single-dose crossover study in 10 healthy young (18 to 40 years of age) men administered zolpidem 2.5, 5, and 10 mg oral spray, the results demonstrated a linear relationship to dose for mean C_{max} and area under the curve ($AUC_{0-\infty}$) over the range of doses administered in the study.

In a single-dose crossover study in 43 healthy young (18 to 45 years of age) subjects administered zolpidem 5 and 10 mg oral spray, the means for C_{max} were 114 ng/mL (range, 19 to 197 ng/mL) and 210 ng/mL (range, 77 to 401 ng/mL), respectively, occurring at a mean T_{max} of approximately 0.9 hours for both. In the same study, the means for C_{max} were 123 ng/mL (range, 53 to 221 ng/mL) and 219 ng/mL (range, 101 to 446 ng/mL) for 5 and 10 mg immediate-release tablets, respectively, occurring at a mean T_{max} of 0.9 and 1 hour, respectively. The mean zolpidem $t_{½}$ was 2.8 (range, 1.5 to 6) and 3.1 (range, 1.1 to 8.6) hours for the 5 and 10 mg immediate-release tablets, respectively.

• *Food effect* – A food-effect study in 30 healthy men compared the pharmacokinetics of zolpidem 10 mg immediate-release tablets when administered while fasting or 20 minutes after a meal. Results demonstrated that with food, mean area under the curve (AUC) and C_{max} were decreased by 15% and 25%, respectively, while mean T_{max} was prolonged by 60% (from 1.4 to 2.2 hours). The half-life remained unchanged. These results suggest that for faster sleep onset, do not administer zolpidem with or immediately after a meal.

A food-effect crossover study in 14 healthy young men (18 to 45 years of age) compared the pharmacokinetics of zolpidem 10 mg oral spray when administered while fasting at least 8 hours or 5 minutes after eating a standard high-fat meal. Results demonstrated that with food, mean $AUC_{0-\infty}$ and C_{max} were decreased by 27% and 58%, respectively, while mean T_{max} was prolonged by 225% (from 0.8 to 2.6 hours). These results suggest that for faster sleep onset, as with all zolpidem products, zolpidem oral spray should not be administered with or immediately after a meal.

ER tablets: Zolpidem ER exhibits biphasic absorption characteristics, which results in rapid initial absorption from the GI tract similar to zolpidem immediate release, then provides extended plasma concentrations more than 3 hours after administration. A study in 24 healthy men was conducted to compare mean zolpidem plasma concentration–time profiles obtained after single oral administration of zolpidem 12.5 mg ER and of an immediate-release formulation of zolpidem 10 mg.

Following administration of zolpidem ER administered as a single 12.5 mg dose in healthy men, the C_{max} of zolpidem was 134 ng/mL (range, 68.9 to 197 ng/mL), occurring at a median T_{max} of 1.5 hours. The mean AUC of zolpidem was 740 ng•h/mL (range, 295 to 1,359 ng•h/mL).

• *Food effect* – A food-effect study in 45 healthy volunteers compared the pharmacokinetics of zolpidem 12.5 mg ER when administered while fasting or within 30 minutes after a meal. Results demonstrated that with food, mean AUC and C_{max} were decreased by 23% and 30%, respectively, while median T_{max} was increased from 2 to 4 hours. The half-life was not changed. These results suggest that, for faster sleep onset, zolpidem ER should not be administered with or immediately after a meal.

Metabolism/Excretion – Zolpidem is converted to inactive metabolites that are eliminated primarily by renal excretion.

Immediate-release tablets: The mean zolpidem elimination half-life was 2.6 hours (range, 1.4 to 4.5 hours) and 2.5 hours (range, 1.4 to 3.8 hours) for the 5 and 10 mg tablets, respectively. Zolpidem did not accumulate in young adults following nightly dosing with zolpidem 20 mg tablets for 2 weeks.

Oral spray: The mean zolpidem elimination half-life was 2.7 hours (range, 1.7 to 5 hours) and 3 hours (range, 1.7 to 8.4 hours) for zolpidem 5 and 10 mg oral spray, respectively.

ER tablets: The terminal elimination half-life observed with zolpidem 12.5 mg ER was similar to that obtained with zolpidem 10 mg immediate release. When zolpidem ER was administered as a single 12.5 mg dose in healthy men, the mean zolpidem elimination half-life was 2.8 hours (range, 1.62 to 4.05 hours).

Special populations –

Hepatic function impairment:

• *Immediate-release tablets and oral spray* – The pharmacokinetics of zolpidem in 8 patients with chronic hepatic function impairment were compared with results in healthy subjects. Following a single oral zolpidem 20 mg dose, mean C_{max} and AUC were found to be 2 times (250 vs 499 ng/mL) and 5 times (788 vs 4,203 ng•h/mL) higher, respectively, in hepatically compromised patients. T_{max} did not change. The mean half-life in cirrhotic patients of 9.9 hours (range, 4.1 to 25.8 hours) was greater than that observed in healthy patients of 2.2 hours (range, 1.6 to 2.4 hours). Modify dosing accordingly in patients with hepatic function impairment.

• *ER tablets* – Zolpidem ER was not studied in patients with hepatic function impairment. Based on the pharmacokinetics of immediate-release zolpidem, modify doses in patients with hepatic function impairment.

Elderly:

• *Immediate-release tablets and oral spray* – In elderly patients, the dose for zolpidem should be 5 mg. This recommendation is based on several studies in which the mean C_{max}, half-life, and AUC were significantly increased when compared with results in young adults. In one study of 8 elderly subjects (older than 70 years of age), the means for C_{max}, half-life, and AUC significantly increased by 50% (255 vs 384 ng/mL), 32% (2.2 vs 2.9 hours), and 64% (955 vs 1,562 ng•h/mL), respectively, compared with younger adults (20 to 40 years of age) following a single oral zolpidem 20 mg dose. In a pharmacokinetic study of 24 elderly subjects (65 years of age and older) administered zolpidem 5 mg oral spray, the means for C_{max} and AUC were 134 ng/mL and 493 ng•h/mL, respectively, following administration of a single dose of zolpidem 5 mg oral spray. Zolpidem did not accumulate in elderly subjects following nightly oral dosing of 10 mg for 1 week.

• *ER tablets* – In 24 elderly (at least 65 years of age) healthy subjects administered a single dose of zolpidem 6.25 mg ER, the mean C_{max} of zolpidem was 70.6 ng/mL (range, 35 to 161 ng/mL), occurring at a T_{max} of 2 hours. The mean AUC of zolpidem was 413 ng•h/mL (range, 124 to 1,190 ng•h/mL) and the mean elimination half-life was 2.9 hours (range, 1.59 to 5.5 hours).

Contraindications

Known hypersensitivity to zolpidem or any of the inactive ingredients in the formulation. Observed reactions include anaphylaxis and angioedema.

Warnings/Precautions

➤*CNS effects:*

Psychiatric/Physical disorder – Because sleep disturbances may be the presenting manifestation of a physical and/or psychiatric disorder, initiate symptomatic treatment of insomnia only after a careful evaluation of the patient. The failure of insomnia to remit after 7 to 10 days of treatment may indicate the presence of a primary psychiatric and/or medical illness that should be evaluated. Worsening of insomnia or the emergence of new thinking or behavior abnormalities may be the consequence of an unrecognized psychiatric or physical disorder. Such findings have emerged during the course of treatment with sedative-hypnotic drugs, including zolpidem.

Abnormal thinking and behavior changes – A variety of abnormal thinking and behavior changes have been reported to occur in association with the use of sedative-hypnotics. Some of these changes may be characterized by decreased inhibition (eg, aggressiveness and extroversion that seem out of character), similar to effects produced by alcohol and other CNS depressants. Visual and auditory hallucinations have been reported, as well as behavioral changes such as agitation, bizarre behavior, and depersonalization. In controlled trials, less than 1% of adults with insomnia who received zolpidem reported hallucinations. In a clinical trial, 7.4% of children with insomnia associated with attention deficit hyperactivity disorder (ADHD) who received zolpidem reported hallucinations. Amnesia, anxiety, and other neuropsychiatric symptoms may occur unpredictably. In primarily depressed patients, worsening of depression (including suicidal thinking) and actions (including completed suicides) have been reported in association with the use of sedative-hypnotics.

Complex behaviors: Complex behaviors such as "sleep driving" (ie, driving while not fully awake after ingestion of a sedative-hypnotic, with amnesia for the event) have been reported with sedative-hypnotics, including zolpidem. These events can occur in sedative-hypnotic–naive as well as sedative-hypnotic–experienced people. Although behaviors such as "sleep driving" may occur with zolpidem alone at therapeutic doses, the use of alcohol and other CNS depressants with zolpidem appears to increase the risk of such behaviors, as does the use of zolpidem at doses exceeding the maximum recommended dose. Because of the risk to the patient and the community, strongly consider discontinuation of zolpidem for patients who report a "sleep driving" episode. Other complex behaviors (eg, preparing and eating food, making phone calls, having sex) have been reported in patients who are not fully awake after taking a sedative-hypnotic. As with "sleep driving," patients usually do not remember these events.

It can rarely be determined with certainty whether a particular instance of the abnormal behaviors previously listed are drug induced, spontaneous in origin, or a result of an underlying psychiatric or physical disorder. Nonetheless, the emergence of any new behavioral sign or symptom of concern requires careful and immediate evaluation.

Depression – As with other sedative-hypnotic drugs, administer zolpidem with caution to patients exhibiting signs or symptoms of depression. Suicidal tendencies may be present in such patients and protective measures may be required. Intentional overdosage is more common in this group of patients; therefore, prescribe the least amount of drug that is feasible for the patient at any one time.

➤*Abrupt discontinuation:* Following the rapid dose decrease or abrupt discontinuation of sedative-hypnotics, there have been reports of signs and symptoms similar to those associated with withdrawal from other CNS-depressant drugs.

➤*Concomitant illness:* Clinical experience with zolpidem in patients with concomitant systemic illness is limited. Caution is advisable in using zolpidem in patients with diseases or conditions that could affect metabolism or hemodynamic responses.

➤*Respiratory illness:* Although studies did not reveal respiratory-depressant effects at hypnotic doses of zolpidem in healthy patients or patients with mild to moderate chronic obstructive pulmonary disease, a reduction in the Total Arousal Index together with a reduction in lowest oxygen saturation and increase in the times of oxygen desaturation below 80% and 90% were observed in patients with mild to moderate sleep apnea when treated with a zolpidem immediate-release formulation (10 mg) compared with placebo. However, observe precautions if zolpidem is prescribed to patients with compromised respiratory function because sedative-hypnotics have the capacity to depress respiratory drive. Postmarketing reports of respiratory insufficiency, most of which involved patients with preexisting respiratory impairment, have been received. Use zolpidem with caution in patients with sleep apnea syndrome or myasthenia gravis.

➤*Hypersensitivity reactions:* Rare cases of angioedema involving the glottis, larynx, or tongue have been reported in patients after taking the first or subsequent doses of sedative-hypnotics, including zolpidem. Some patients have had additional symptoms, such as dyspnea, throat closing, or nausea and vomiting, which suggest anaphylaxis. Some patients have required medical therapy in the emergency department. If angioedema involves the throat, glottis, or larynx, airway obstruction may occur and be fatal. Patients who develop angioedema after treatment with zolpidem should not be rechallenged with the drug.

ZOLPIDEM TARTRATE — ORAL

➤*Renal function impairment:* No dosage adjustment in patients with renal function impairment is required; however, closely monitor these patients.

➤*Hepatic function impairment:* A study in subjects with hepatic function impairment did reveal prolonged elimination; therefore, initiate treatment with zolpidem 6.25 mg ER and zolpidem 5 mg immediate-release tablets and oral spray in patients with hepatic compromise, and closely monitor these patients.

➤*Drug abuse and dependence:* Sedative-hypnotics have produced withdrawal signs and symptoms following abrupt discontinuation. These reported symptoms range from mild dysphoria and insomnia to a withdrawal syndrome that may include abdominal and muscle cramps, convulsions, sweating, tremors, and vomiting. The following adverse reactions, which are considered to meet *Diagnostic and Statistical Manual of Mental Disorders* (Third Edition Revised) (*DSM-III-R*) criteria for uncomplicated sedative-hypnotic withdrawal, were reported during US clinical trials following placebo substitution occurring within 48 hours following the last zolpidem treatment: abdominal discomfort, emesis, fatigue, flushing, lightheadedness, nausea, nervousness, panic attack, stomach cramps, and uncontrolled crying. These reported adverse reactions occurred at an incidence of 1% or less. However, available data cannot provide a reliable estimate of the incidence, if any, of dependence during treatment at recommended doses. Postmarketing reports of abuse, dependence, and withdrawal have been received.

History of psychiatric disorders or addiction to drugs/alcohol – Because people with a history of addiction to or abuse of drugs or alcohol are at increased risk for misuse and abuse of and addiction to zolpidem, monitor these patients carefully when administering zolpidem or any other hypnotic.

➤*Hazardous tasks:* Zolpidem, like other sedative-hypnotic drugs, has CNS-depressant effects. Because of the rapid onset of action, zolpidem should only be ingested immediately prior to going to bed. Caution patients against engaging in hazardous occupations requiring complete mental alertness or motor coordination, such as operating machinery or driving a motor vehicle, after ingesting the drug. Also caution patients that potential impairment of the performance of such activities may occur the day following ingestion of zolpidem. Zolpidem showed additive effects when combined with alcohol and should not be taken with alcohol. Also caution patients about possible combined effects with other CNS-depressant drugs. Dosage adjustments may be necessary when zolpidem is administered with such agents because of the potentially additive effects.

➤*Pregnancy:* Category C There are no adequate and well-controlled studies in pregnant women. Use zolpidem during pregnancy only if the potential benefit justifies the potential risk to the fetus.

Studies to assess the effects on children whose mothers took zolpidem during pregnancy have not been conducted. There is a published case report documenting the presence of zolpidem in human umbilical cord blood. However, children born of mothers taking sedative-hypnotic drugs may be at some risk for withdrawal symptoms from the drug during the postnatal period. In addition, neonatal flaccidity has been reported in infants born to mothers who received sedative-hypnotic drugs during pregnancy.

Oral studies of zolpidem in pregnant rats and rabbits showed adverse effects on the development of offspring only at dosages greater than the MRHD of 10 mg/day for immediate-release tablets and oral spray and 12.5 mg/day for ER tablets. These doses were also maternally toxic in animals. A teratogenic effect was not observed in these studies. Administration to pregnant rats during the period of organogenesis produced dose-related maternal toxicity and decreases in fetal skull ossification at doses 25 to 125 times the MRHD for immediate-release tablets, 24 to 120 times the MRHD for oral spray, and 20 to 100 times the MRHD for ER tablets. The no-effect dose for embryofetal toxicity was between 4 and 5 times the MRHD for immediate-release tablets, 5 times the MRHD for oral spray, and 4 times the MRHD for ER tablets. Treatment of pregnant rabbits during organogenesis resulted in maternal toxicity at all doses studied and increased postimplantation embryofetal loss and under ossification of fetal sternebrae at the highest dose (more than 35 times the MRHD for immediate-release tablets, 40 times the MRHD for oral spray, and 30 times the MRHD for ER tablets). The no-effect level for embryofetal toxicity was between 9 and 10 times the MRHD for immediate-release tablets, 10 times the MRHD for oral spray, and 8 times the MRHD for ER tablets. Administration to rats during the latter part of pregnancy and throughout lactation produced maternal toxicity and decreased pup growth and survival at doses approximately 25 to 125 times the MRHD for immediate-release tablets, 24 to 120 times the MRHD for oral spray, and 20 to 100 times the MRHD for ER tablets. The no-effect dose for offspring toxicity was between 4 and 5 times the MRHD for immediate-release tablets, 5 times the MRHD for oral spray, and approximately 4 times the MRHD for ER tablets.

➤*Lactation:* Zolpidem is excreted into human milk. Studies in lactating mothers indicate that the half-life of zolpidem is similar to that in young healthy nonlactating volunteers (2.6 ± 0.3 hours). Between 0.004% and 0.019% of the total administered dose is excreted into milk, but the effect of zolpidem on the infant is unknown. Exercise caution when administering zolpidem to a breast-feeding mother.

Because of the low levels of zolpidem in breast milk and its short half-life, the amount ingested by the infants is small and would not be expected to cause any adverse effects in breast-fed infants.

In those instances in which the mother is taking zolpidem, she should observe the breast-feeding infant for increased sedation, lethargy, and changes in feeding habits.

The American Academy of Pediatrics classifies zolpidem as usually compatible with breast-feeding.

➤*Children:* Safety and effectiveness of zolpidem have not been established in pediatric patients.

In an 8-week controlled study, 201 pediatric patients (6 to 17 years of age) with insomnia associated with ADHD (90% of the patients were using psychoanaleptics) were treated with an oral solution of zolpidem (n = 136) or placebo (n = 65). Zolpidem did not significantly decrease latency to persistent sleep compared with placebo, as measured by PSG after 4 weeks of treatment. Psychiatric and nervous system disorders comprised the most frequent (greater than 5%) treatment-emergent adverse reactions observed with zolpidem tartrate versus placebo and included dizziness (23.5% vs 1.5%), headache (12.5% vs 9.2%), and hallucinations (7.4% vs 0%). Ten patients taking zolpidem (7.4%) discontinued treatment because of an adverse reaction.

➤*Elderly:* Impaired motor and/or cognitive performance after repeated exposure or unusual sensitivity to sedative-hypnotic drugs is a concern in the treatment of elderly and/or debilitated patients. Therefore, the recommended zolpidem ER dose is 6.25 mg and the recommended dose for zolpidem immediate-release tablets and oral spray is 5 mg in such patients to decrease the possibility of adverse reactions. Monitor these patients closely.

➤*Monitoring:* Monitor patients with a history of addiction to, or abuse of, drugs and alcohol when administering zolpidem. Monitor for abnormal thinking and behavior changes.

Monitor patients with hepatic function impairment and respiratory illness, and monitor elderly patients for increased adverse reactions.

Drug Interactions

Zolpidem Drug Interactions

Precipitant drug	Object drug[a]		Description
Azole antifungals (eg, fluconazole, itraconazole, ketoconazole)	Zolpidem	↑	Plasma concentrations and therapeutic effects of zolpidem may be increased. Monitor closely and adjust the zolpidem dose as needed.
Chlorpromazine	Zolpidem	↑	Coadministration produced an additive effect of decreased alertness and psychomotor performance.
Zolpidem	Chlorpromazine		
Flumazenil	Zolpidem	↓	Zolpidem's effect may be reversed by flumazenil.
Imipramine	Zolpidem	↑↓	Coadministration produced a 20% decrease in peak levels of imipramine; however, an additive effect of decreased alertness was seen.
Zolpidem	Imipramine		
Rifamycins (eg, rifampin)	Zolpidem	↓	Plasma concentrations and therapeutic effects of zolpidem may be decreased. Monitor closely and adjust the zolpidem dose as needed.
Ritonavir	Zolpidem	↑	Coadministration may cause severe sedation and respiratory depression. Concurrent use is contraindicated.
SSRIs[b] (eg, sertraline)	Zolpidem	↑	The onset of action of zolpidem may be shortened and the effect increased. Coadministration with sertraline produced an increase in zolpidem C_{max} (43%) and a decrease in T_{max} (53%). Observe patients closely.
Zolpidem	Amiodarone	↑	The risk of life-threatening cardiac arrhythmias, including torsades de pointes, may be increased. Coadminister with caution and careful monitoring of cardiac function.
Zolpidem	CNS depressants (eg, alcohol)	↑	May enhance the CNS depressant effects of zolpidem. An additive effect on psychomotor performance between alcohol and zolpidem has been demonstrated.
CNS depressants (eg, alcohol)	Zolpidem		

[a] ↑ = object drug increased; ↓ = object drug decreased; ↑↓ = object drug both increased and decreased.
[b] SSRIs = selective serotonin reuptake inhibitors.

➤*Drug/Lab test interactions:* Zolpidem is not known to interfere with commonly employed clinical laboratory tests. In addition, clinical data indicate that zolpidem does not cross-react with amphetamines, barbiturates, benzodiazepines, cannabinoids, cocaine, or opiates in 2 standard urine drug screens.

➤*Drug/Food interactions:* A study of 30 healthy men compared the pharmacokinetics of zolpidem 10 mg immediate release when administered

ZOLPIDEM TARTRATE — ORAL

while fasting or 20 minutes after a meal. With food, mean AUC and C_{max} were decreased by 15% and 25%, respectively, while mean T_{max} was prolonged by 60% (from 1.4 to 2.2 hours). The half-life remained unchanged. For faster sleep onset, do not administer with or immediately after a meal.

A food-effect study in 45 healthy volunteers compared the pharmacokinetics of zolpidem 12.5 mg ER when administered while fasting or within 30 minutes after a meal. Results demonstrated that with food, mean AUC and C_{max} were decreased by 23% and 30%, respectively, while median T_{max} was increased from 2 to 4 hours. The half-life was unchanged. These results suggest that for faster sleep onset, do not administer zolpidem ER with or immediately after meal.

Adverse Reactions

The following serious adverse reactions are discussed in greater detail in the Warnings/Precautions section of the labeling: serious anaphylactic and anaphylactoid reactions; abnormal thinking, behavior changes, and complex behaviors; withdrawal effects; CNS-depressant effects.

➤*Immediate-release tablets and oral spray:*

Discontinuation of treatment – Approximately 4% of 1,701 patients who received zolpidem at all doses (1.25 to 90 mg) in US premarketing clinical trials discontinued treatment because of an adverse reaction. Reactions most commonly associated with discontinuation from US trials were nausea (0.6%), daytime drowsiness (0.5%), headache (0.5%), vomiting (0.5%), and dizziness/vertigo (0.4%).

Approximately 4% of 1,959 patients who received zolpidem at all doses (1 to 50 mg) in similar foreign trials discontinued treatment because of an adverse reaction. Reactions most commonly associated with discontinuation from these trials were daytime drowsiness (1.1%), dizziness/vertigo (0.8%), amnesia (0.5%), nausea (0.5%), falls (0.4%), and headache (0.4%).

Data from a clinical study in which SSRI-treated patients were given zolpidem revealed that 4 of the 7 discontinuations during double-blind treatment with zolpidem (n = 95) were associated with impaired concentration, continuing or aggravated depression, and manic reaction; 1 patient treated with placebo (n = 97) was discontinued after an attempted suicide.

Most common adverse reactions – During short-term treatment (up to 10 nights) with zolpidem at doses of up to 10 mg, the most commonly observed adverse reactions associated with the use of zolpidem and seen at statistically significant differences from placebo-treated patients were drowsiness (reported by 2% of zolpidem patients), diarrhea (1%), and dizziness (1%). During longer-term treatment (28 to 35 nights) with zolpidem at doses of up to 10 mg, the most commonly observed adverse reactions associated with the use of zolpidem and seen at statistically significant differences from placebo-treated patients were dizziness (5%) and drugged feelings (3%).

Adverse reactions (1% or more) –

Short-term, placebo-controlled trials: The following table was derived from a pool of 11 placebo-controlled, short-term US efficacy trials involving zolpidem in doses ranging from 1.25 to 20 mg. The information is limited to data from doses up to and including 10 mg, the highest dose recommended for use.

Zolpidem Immediate-Release Tablets and Oral Spray Adverse Reactions in Short-Term, Placebo-Controlled Clinical Trials (≥ 1%)

Adverse reactions[a]	Zolpidem (≤ 10 mg) (n = 685)	Placebo (n = 473)
CNS		
Dizziness	1%	0%
Drowsiness	2%	0%
Headache	7%	6%
GI		
Diarrhea	1%	0%

[a] Reactions reported by ≥ 1% of zolpidem patients and at a greater frequency than placebo are included.

Long-term, placebo-controlled clinical trials: The following table was derived from a pool of 3 placebo-controlled, long-term efficacy trials involving zolpidem. These trials involved patients with chronic insomnia who were treated for 28 to 35 nights with zolpidem at doses of 5, 10, or 15 mg. The information is limited to data from doses up to and including 10 mg, the highest dose recommended for use. The table includes only adverse reactions occurring at an incidence of at least 1% for zolpidem patients.

Zolpidem Immediate-Release Tablets and Oral Spray Adverse Reactions in Long-Term, Placebo-Controlled Clinical Trials (≥ 1%)

Adverse reactions[a]	Zolpidem (≤ 10 mg) (n = 152)	Placebo (n = 161)
CNS		
Abnormal dreams	1%	0%
Amnesia	1%	0%
Depression	2%	1%
Dizziness	5%	1%
Drowsiness	8%	5%
Drugged feeling	3%	0%
Lethargy	3%	1%
Light-headedness	2%	1%
Sleep disorder	1%	0%
GI		
Abdominal pain	2%	2%
Constipation	2%	1%
Diarrhea	3%	2%
Dry mouth	3%	1%
Respiratory		
Pharyngitis	3%	1%
Sinusitis	4%	2%
Miscellaneous		
Allergy	4%	1%
Back pain	3%	2%
Chest pain	1%	0%
Influenza-like symptoms	2%	0%
Palpitation	2%	0%
Rash	2%	1%

[a] Reactions reported by ≥ 1% of patients treated with zolpidem and at a greater frequency than placebo.

• *Adverse reactions in elderly patients* –

Zolpidem Adverse Reactions in Elderly Patients (≥ 3% and at Least Twice the Placebo Incidence)

Adverse reactions	Zolpidem	Placebo
Diarrhea	3%	1%
Dizziness	3%	0%
Drowsiness	5%	2%

• *Oral tissue-related adverse reactions in zolpidem oral spray pharmacokinetics studies* – The effect of chronic daily administrations of zolpidem oral spray on oral tissue has not been evaluated. In pharmacokinetic studies conducted with zolpidem oral spray in healthy subjects, an oral soft tissue exam was performed and no signs of oral irritation were noted following administration of single doses of zolpidem oral spray.

Other adverse reactions – The frequencies presented represent the proportions of the 3,660 individuals exposed to zolpidem at all doses who experienced a reaction of the type cited on at least 1 occasion while receiving zolpidem immediate release. All reported treatment-emergent adverse reactions are included, except those already listed in the preceding table of adverse reactions in placebo-controlled studies, those coding terms that are so general as to be uninformative, and those reactions in which a drug cause was remote. It is important to emphasize that although the reactions reported did occur during treatment with zolpidem immediate release, they were not necessarily caused by it.

Cardiovascular – Cerebrovascular disorder, hypertension, postural hypotension, syncope, tachycardia (0.1% to 1%); aggravated hypertension, angina pectoris, arrhythmia, arteritis, circulatory failure, extrasystoles, hypotension, myocardial infarction, phlebitis, pulmonary edema, pulmonary embolism, varicose veins, ventricular tachycardia (less than 0.1%).

CNS – Asthenia, ataxia, confusion, drowsiness, drugged feeling, dry mouth, euphoria, headache, insomnia, lethargy, light-headedness, vertigo (greater than 1%); agitation, anxiety, decreased cognition, detached feeling, difficulty concentrating, dysarthria, emotional lability, hallucination, hypesthesia, illusion, leg cramps, migraine, nervousness, paresthesia, sleeping (after daytime dosing), speech disorder, stupor, tremor (0.1% to 1%); abnormal gait, abnormal thinking, aggressive reaction, apathy, appetite increased, decreased libido, delusion, dementia, depersonalization, dysphasia, feeling strange, hypokinesia, hypotonia, hysteria, intoxicated feeling, manic reaction, neuralgia, neuritis, neuropathy, neurosis, panic attacks, paresis, personality disorder, restless legs, rigors, somnambulism, suicide attempts, tenesmus, tetany, yawning (less than 0.1%).

Dermatologic – Increased sweating, pallor, pruritus (0.1% to 1%); acne, bullous eruption, dermatitis, flushing, furunculosis, injection-site inflammation, photosensitivity reaction, urticaria (less than 0.1%).

GI – Diarrhea, dyspepsia, hiccup, nausea (greater than 1%); anorexia, constipation, dysphagia, flatulence, gastroenteritis, vomiting (0.1% to 1%); altered saliva, enteritis, eructation, esophagospasm, gastritis, hemorrhoids, increased saliva, intestinal obstruction, rectal hemorrhage, tooth caries (less than 0.1%).

GU – Urinary tract infection (greater than 1%); cystitis, menstrual disorder, urinary incontinence, vaginitis (0.1% to 1%); acute renal failure, breast fibroadenosis, breast neoplasm, breast pain, dysuria, impotence, micturition frequency, nocturia, polyuria, pyelonephritis, renal pain, urinary retention (less than 0.1%).

ZOLPIDEM TARTRATE — ORAL

Hematologic/Lymphatic – Anemia, hyperhemoglobinemia, increased erythrocyte sedimentation rate, leukopenia, lymphadenopathy, macrocytic anemia, purpura, thrombosis (less than 0.1%).

Hepatic – Abnormal hepatic function, increased ALT (0.1% to 1%); bilirubinemia, increased AST (less than 0.1%).

Metabolic/Nutritional – Edema, hyperglycemia, thirst (0.1% to 1%); gout, hypercholesteremia, hyperlipidemia, increased alkaline phosphatase, increased serum urea nitrogen, periorbital edema, weight decrease (less than 0.1%).

Musculoskeletal – Arthralgia, back pain, myalgia (greater than 1%); arthritis (0.1% to 1%); arthrosis, muscle weakness, sciatica, tendinitis (less than 0.1%).

Respiratory – Sinusitis, upper respiratory tract infection (greater than 1%); bronchitis, coughing, dyspnea, rhinitis (0.1% to 1%); bronchospasm, epistaxis, hypoxia, laryngitis, pneumonia (less than 0.1%).

Special senses – Abnormal vision, diplopia (greater than 1%); eye irritation, eye pain, scleritis, taste perversion, tinnitus (0.1% to 1%); abnormal accommodation, conjunctivitis, corneal ulceration, glaucoma, lacrimation abnormal, otitis externa, otitis media, parosmia, photopsia (less than 0.1%).

Miscellaneous – Chest pain, falling, fatigue, fever, infection, malaise, trauma (0.1% to 1%); abscess, allergic reaction, allergy aggravated, anaphylactic shock, face edema, herpes simplex, herpes zoster, hot flashes, pain, tolerance increased (less than 0.1%).

➤*ER tablets:*

Discontinuation of treatment – In 3-week trials in adults and elderly patients (older than 65 years of age), 3.5% (7/201) of patients receiving zolpidem 6.25 or 12.5 mg ER discontinued treatment because of an adverse reaction compared with 0.9% (2/216) of patients on placebo. The reaction most commonly associated with discontinuation in patients treated with zolpidem ER was somnolence (1%).

In a 6-month study in adult patients (18 to 64 years of age), 8.5% (57/669) of patients receiving zolpidem 12.5 mg ER compared with 4.6% (16/349) on placebo discontinued treatment because of an adverse reaction. Reactions most commonly associated with discontinuation of zolpidem ER included anxiety (anxiety, restlessness, or agitation) reported in 1.5% (10/669) of patients compared with 0.3% (1/349) of patients on placebo, and depression (depression, major depression, or depressed mood) reported in 1.5% (10/669) of patients compared with 0.3% (1/349) of patients on placebo.

Most common adverse reactions – During treatment with zolpidem ER in adults and elderly patients at daily doses of 12.5 and 6.25 mg, respectively, each for 3 weeks, the most commonly observed adverse reactions associated with the use of zolpidem ER were dizziness, headache, and next-day somnolence.

In the 6-month trial evaluating zolpidem 12.5 mg, the adverse reaction profile was consistent with that reported in short-term trials, except for a higher incidence of anxiety (6.3% for zolpidem ER vs 2.6% for placebo).

Placebo-controlled clinical trials in healthy adults – The following tables were derived from results of 2 placebo-controlled efficacy trials involving zolpidem ER. These trials involved patients with primary insomnia who were treated for 3 weeks with zolpidem ER at doses of 12.5 or 6.25 mg, respectively. The tables include only adverse reactions occurring at an incidence of at least 1% for zolpidem ER patients and with an incidence greater than that seen in placebo patients. Events reported by investigators were classified using the *MedDRA* dictionary for establishing reaction frequencies.

Zolpidem ER Tablets Adverse Reactions (%)

Adverse reactions[a]	Zolpidem 12.5 mg ER (n = 102)	Placebo (n = 110)
CNS		
Anxiety	2%	0%
Asthenia	1%	0%
Ataxia	1%	0%
Balance disorder	2%	0%
Binge eating	1%	0%
Depersonalization	1%	0%
Depression	2%	0%
Disinhibition	1%	0%
Disorientation	3%	2%
Disturbance in attention	2%	0%
Dizziness	12%	5%
Euphoric mood	1%	0%
Fatigue	3%	2%
Hallucinations[b]	4%	0%
Headache	19%	16%
Hypesthesia	2%	1%
Memory disorders[c]	3%	0%
Mood swings	1%	0%
Paresthesia	1%	0%
Psychomotor retardation	2%	0%
Somnolence	15%	2%
Stress symptoms	1%	0%
Dermatologic		
Rash	1%	0%
Skin wrinkling	1%	0%
Urticaria	1%	0%
GI		
Abdominal discomfort	1%	0%
Abdominal tenderness	1%	0%
Constipation	2%	0%
Frequent bowel movements	1%	0%
Gastroenteritis	1%	0%
Gastroesophageal reflux disease	1%	0%
Nausea	7%	4%
Vomiting	1%	0%
Musculoskeletal		
Back pain	4%	3%
Myalgia	4%	0%
Neck pain	1%	0%
Special senses		
Altered visual depth perception	1%	0%
Asthenopia	1%	0%
Eye redness	2%	0%
Labyrinthitis	1%	0%
Tinnitus	1%	0%
Vertigo	2%	0%
Vision blurred	2%	1%
Visual disturbance	3%	0%
Miscellaneous		
Appetite disorder	1%	0%
Blood pressure increased	1%	0%
Body temperature increased	1%	0%
Chest discomfort	1%	0%
Contusion	1%	0%
Exposure to poisonous plant	1%	0%
Influenza	3%	0%
Menorrhagia	1%	0%
Throat irritation	1%	0%

[a] Reactions reported by ≥ 1% of patients treated with zolpidem ER and at a greater frequency than the placebo group.
[b] Hallucinations included hallucinations not otherwise specified, as well as visual and hypnogogic hallucinations.
[c] Memory disorders include the following: amnesia, anterograde amnesia, and memory impairment.

Adverse reactions in elderly patients –

Zolpidem ER Adverse Reactions in Elderly Patients (%)

Adverse reactions[a]	Zolpidem 6.25 mg ER (n = 99)	Placebo (n = 106)
CNS		
Anxiety	3%	2%
Apathy	1%	0%
Burning sensation	1%	0%
Depressed mood	1%	0%
Dizziness	8%	3%
Dizziness postural	1%	0%
Headache	14%	11%
Memory disorders[b]	1%	0%
Muscle contractions, involuntary	1%	0%
Paresthesia	1%	0%
Psychomotor retardation	2%	0%
Somnolence	6%	5%
Tremor	1%	0%

ZOLPIDEM TARTRATE – ORAL

Zolpidem ER Adverse Reactions in Elderly Patients (%)		
Adverse reactions[a]	Zolpidem 6.25 mg ER (n = 99)	Placebo (n = 106)
Dermatologic		
Rash	1%	0%
Urticaria	1%	0%
GI		
Flatulence	1%	0%
Vomiting	1%	0%
GU		
Dysuria	1%	0%
Vulvovaginal dryness	1%	0%
Musculoskeletal		
Arthralgia	2%	0%
Muscle cramp	2%	1%
Neck injury	1%	0%
Neck pain	2%	0%
Respiratory		
Dry throat	1%	0%
Lower respiratory tract infection	1%	0%
Nasopharyngitis	6%	4%
Otitis externa	1%	0%
Upper respiratory tract infection	1%	0%
Miscellaneous		
Influenza-like illness	1%	0%
Palpitations	2%	0%
Pyrexia	1%	0%

[a] Reactions reported by ≥ 1% of patients treated with zolpidem ER and at a greater frequency than the placebo group.
[b] Memory disorders include the following: amnesia, anterograde amnesia, and memory impairment.

Overdosage

➤*Symptoms:* In postmarketing experience of overdose with zolpidem alone or in combination with CNS-depressant agents, impairment of consciousness ranging from somnolence to coma, cardiovascular and/or respiratory compromise, and fatal outcomes have been reported.

➤*Treatment:* As with the management of all overdosage, consider the possibility of multiple-drug ingestion. Also consider contacting a poison control center for up-to-date information on the management of hypnotic drug product overdosage. Use general symptomatic and supportive measures along with immediate gastric lavage when appropriate. Administer intravenous fluids as needed. Zolpidem's sedative-hypnotic effect was shown to be reduced by flumazenil and therefore may be useful; however, flumazenil administration may contribute to the appearance of neurological symptoms (convulsions). As in all cases of drug overdose, monitor respiration, pulse, blood pressure, and other appropriate signs, and employ general supportive measures. Monitor hypotension and CNS depression and treat by appropriate medical intervention. Withhold sedating drugs following zolpidem overdosage, even if excitation occurs. The value of dialysis in the treatment of overdosage has not been determined, although hemodialysis studies in patients with renal failure receiving therapeutic doses have demonstrated that zolpidem is not dialyzable.

Patient Information

Inform patients, their families, and their caregivers about the benefits and risks associated with treatment with sedative-hypnotics, counsel them in its appropriate use, and instruct them to read the accompanying Medication Guide and Patient Instructions for Use.

Inform patients that severe anaphylactic and anaphylactoid reactions have occurred with zolpidem. Describe the signs/symptoms of these reactions and advise patients to seek medical attention immediately if any of them occur.

Inform patients that there have been reports of people getting out of bed after taking a sedative-hypnotic and driving their cars while not fully awake, often with no memory of the event. If a patient experiences such an episode, advise them to report it immediately to their doctor immediately because "sleep driving" can be dangerous. This behavior is more likely to occur when zolpidem is taken with alcohol or other CNS depressants. Other complex behaviors (eg, preparing and eating food, making phone calls, or having sex) have been reported in patients who are not fully awake after taking a sedative-hypnotic. As with "sleep driving," patients usually do not remember these events.

In addition, advise patients to report all concomitant medications to the prescriber. Instruct patients to report events such as "sleep driving" and other complex behaviors immediately to the prescriber.

Counsel patients to take zolpidem right before they get into bed and only when they are able to stay in bed a full night (7 to 8 hours) before being active again. Zolpidem tablets should not be crushed, divided, or chewed and should not be taken with or immediately after a meal. Advise patients not to take zolpidem when drinking alcohol.

➤*Oral spray:* See the Dosage and Administration section. Zolpidem oral spray is packaged in a child-resistant container. Refer patients to the Patient Instructions for Use (following the Medication Guide) for detailed instructions on how to use zolpidem oral spray.

ZALEPLON

c-iv	**Zaleplon** (Corepharma)	**Capsules; oral:** 5 mg	Lactose. (322). Green/pale green, opaque. In 100s.
c-iv	**Sonata** (King)		Lactose, tartrazine. (5 mg SONATA). Green/pale green. In 100s.
c-iv	**Zaleplon** (Corepharma)	**Capsules; oral:** 10 mg	Lactose. (323). Green/light green, opaque. In 100s.
c-iv	**Sonata** (King)		Lactose, tartrazine. (10 mg SONATA). Green/lt. green. In 100s.

ZALEPLON — ORAL

Indications

➤*Insomnia:* Zaleplon is indicated for the short-term treatment of insomnia. Zaleplon has been shown to decrease the time to sleep onset for up to 30 days in controlled clinical studies. It has not been shown to increase total sleep time or decrease the number of awakenings.

Hypnotics should generally be limited to 7 to 10 days of use, and reevaluation of the patient is recommended if they are to be taken for > 2 to 3 weeks. Zaleplon should not be prescribed in quantities exceeding a 1-month supply.

Administration and Dosage

➤*Adults:*

Insomnia –

Usual dosage: 10 mg at bedtime. For certain low weight individuals, 5 mg may be a sufficient dose.

Maximum dose: 20 mg/day.

Dosage adjustment: Although the risk of certain adverse events associated with the use of zaleplon appears to be dose dependent, the 20 mg dose has been shown to be adequately tolerated and may be considered for the occasional patient who does not benefit from a trial of a lower dose.

➤*Elderly:*

Maximum dose – 10 mg/day.

Usual dosage – 5 mg/day. Elderly patients appear to be more sensitive to the effects of hypnotics, and respond to 5 mg of zaleplon.

➤*Hepatic function impairment:*

Mild to moderate hepatic impairment – 5 mg/day. Zaleplon clearance is reduced in this population.

Severe hepatic impairment – Use is not recommended.

➤*Debilitated patients:* See Elderly for dosing.

➤*Concomitant therapy:* An initial dose of 5 mg should be given to patients concomitantly taking cimetidine because zaleplon clearance is reduced in this population (see Drug interactions).

➤*Administration:* Zaleplon should be taken immediately before bedtime or after the patient has gone to bed and has experienced difficulty falling asleep. Taking zaleplon with or immediately after a heavy, high-fat meal results in slower absorption and would be expected to reduce the effect of zaleplon on sleep latency.

➤*Storage/Stability:* Store at 20° to 25°C (68° to 77°F). Dispense in a light-resistant container.

Actions

➤*Pharmacology:* While zaleplon is a hypnotic agent with a chemical structure unrelated to benzodiazepines, barbiturates, or other drugs with known hypnotic properties, it interacts with the gamma-aminobutyric acid-benzodiazepine (GABA-BZ) receptor complex. Subunit modulation of the GABA-BZ receptor chloride channel macromolecular complex is hypothesized to be responsible for some of the pharmacological properties of benzodiazepines, which include sedative, anxiolytic, muscle relaxant, and anticonvulsive effects in animal models.

Other nonclinical studies have also shown that zaleplon binds selectively to the brain omega-1 receptor situated on the alpha subunit of the $GABA_A$/chloride ion channel receptor complex and potentiates t-butyl-bicyclophosphorothionate (TBPS) binding. Studies of binding of zaleplon to recombinant $GABA_A$ receptors ($\alpha_1\beta_1\gamma_2$ "omega-1" and $\alpha_2\beta_1\gamma_2$ "omega-2")

ZALEPLON — ORAL

have shown that zaleplon has a low affinity for these receptors, with preferential binding to the omega-1 receptor.

➤*Pharmacokinetics:*

Absorption – The pharmacokinetics of zaleplon have been investigated in more than 500 healthy subjects (young and elderly), nursing mothers, and patients with hepatic disease or renal disease. In healthy subjects, the pharmacokinetic profile has been examined after single doses of up to 60 mg and once-daily administration at 15 mg and 30 mg for 10 days. Zaleplon was rapidly absorbed with a time to peak concentration (t_{max}) of ≈ 1 hour and a terminal-phase elimination half-life ($t_{½}$) of ≈ 1 hour. Zaleplon does not accumulate with once-daily administration and its pharmacokinetics are dose proportional in the therapeutic range.

Zaleplon is rapidly and almost completely absorbed following oral administration. Peak plasma concentrations are attained within ≈ 1 hour after oral administration. Although zaleplon is well absorbed, its absolute bioavailability is ≈ 30% because it undergoes significant presystemic metabolism.

Effect of food: In healthy adults a high-fat/heavy meal prolonged the absorption of zaleplon compared to the fasted state, delaying t_{max} by ≈ 2 hours and reducing C_{max} by ≈ 35%. Zaleplon AUC and elimination half-life were not significantly affected. These results suggest that the effects of zaleplon on sleep onset may be reduced if it is taken with or immediately after a high-fat/heavy meal.

Distribution – Zaleplon is a lipophilic compound with a volume of distribution of ≈ 1.4 L/kg following intravenous (IV) administration, indicating substantial distribution into extravascular tissues. The in vitro plasma protein binding is ≈ 60% ± 15% and is independent of zaleplon concentration over the range of 10 ng/mL to 1000 ng/mL. This suggests that zaleplon disposition should not be sensitive to alterations in protein binding. The blood to plasma ratio for zaleplon is ≈ 1, indicating that zaleplon is uniformly distributed throughout the blood with no extensive distribution into red blood cells.

Metabolism – After oral administration, zaleplon is extensively metabolized, with

Excretion – After either oral or IV administration, zaleplon is rapidly eliminated with a mean $t_{½}$ of ≈ 1 hour. The oral-dose plasma clearance of zaleplon is about 3 L/hr/kg and the IV zaleplon plasma clearance is ≈ 1 L/hr/kg. Assuming normal hepatic blood flow and negligible renal clearance of zaleplon, the estimated hepatic extraction ratio of zaleplon is ≈ 0.7, indicating that zaleplon is subject to high first-pass metabolism.

After administration of a radiolabeled dose of zaleplon, 70% of the administered dose is recovered in urine within 48 hours (71% recovered within 6 days), almost all as zaleplon metabolites and their glucuronides. An additional 17% is recovered in feces within 6 days, most as 5-oxo-zaleplon.

Special populations –

Hepatic function impairment: Zaleplon is metabolized primarily by the liver and undergoes significant presystemic metabolism. Consequently, the oral clearance of zaleplon was reduced by 70% and 87% in compensated and decompensated cirrhotic patients, respectively, leading to marked increases in mean C_{max} and AUC (up to 4-fold and 7-fold in compensated and decompensated patients, respectively), in comparison with healthy subjects. The dose of zaleplon should therefore be reduced in patients with mild to moderate hepatic impairment (see Administration and Dosage). Zaleplon is not recommended for use in patients with severe hepatic impairment.

Race: The pharmacokinetics of zaleplon have been studied in Japanese subjects as representative of Asian populations. For this group, C_{max} and AUC were increased 37% and 64%, respectively. This finding can likely be attributed to differences in body weight, or alternatively, may represent differences in enzyme activities resulting from differences in diet, environment, or other factors. The effects of race on pharmacokinetic characteristics in other ethnic groups have not been well characterized.

Contraindications

None known.

Warnings/Precautions

➤*Psychiatric / Physical disorder:* Because sleep disturbances may be the presenting manifestation of a physical or psychiatric disorder, symptomatic treatment of insomnia should be initiated only after a careful evaluation of the patient. The failure of insomnia to remit after 7 to 10 days of treatment may indicate the presence of a primary psychiatric or medical illness that should be evaluated. Worsening of insomnia or the emergence of new thinking or behavior abnormalities may be the consequence of an unrecognized psychiatric or physical disorder. Such findings have emerged during the course of treatment with sedative/hypnotic drugs, including zaleplon. Because some of the important adverse effects of zaleplon appear to be dose-related, it is important to use the lowest possible effective dose, especially in the elderly (see Administration and Dosage).

A variety of abnormal thinking and behavior changes have been reported to occur in association with the use of sedative/hypnotics. Some of these changes may be characterized by decreased inhibition (eg, aggressiveness and extroversion that seem out of character), similar to effects produced by alcohol and other CNS depressants. Other reported behavioral changes have included bizarre behavior, agitation, hallucinations, and depersonalization. Amnesia and other neuropsychiatric symptoms may occur unpredictably. In primarily depressed patients, worsening of depression, including suicidal thinking, has been reported in association with the use of sedative/hypnotics.

It can rarely be determined with certainty whether a particular instance of the abnormal behaviors listed above are drug induced, spontaneous in origin, or a result of an underlying psychiatric or physical disorder. Nonetheless, the emergence of any new behavioral sign or symptom of concern requires careful and immediate evaluation.

Following rapid dose decrease or abrupt discontinuation of the use of sedative/hypnotics, there have been reports of signs and symptoms similar to those associated with withdrawal from other CNS-depressant drugs (see Precautions, Drug abuse and dependence).

➤*Timing of drug administration:* Zaleplon should be taken immediately before bedtime or after the patient has gone to bed and has experienced difficulty falling asleep. As with all sedative/hypnotics, taking zaleplon while still up and about may result in short-term memory impairment, hallucinations, impaired coordination, dizziness, and lightheadedness.

➤*Tartrazine sensitivity:* This product contains FD&C Yellow No. 5 (tartrazine) which may cause allergic-type reactions (including bronchial asthma) in certain susceptible persons. Although the overall incidence of FD&C Yellow No. 5 (tartrazine) sensitivity in the general population is low, it is frequently seen in patients who also have aspirin hypersensitivity.

➤*Hepatic function impairment:* The dose of zaleplon should be reduced to 5 mg in patients with mild to moderate hepatic impairment. It is not recommended for use in patients with severe hepatic impairment.

➤*Special risk:*

Use in the elderly or debilitated patients – Impaired motor or cognitive performance after repeated exposure or unusual sensitivity to sedative/hypnotic drugs is a concern in the treatment of elderly or debilitated patients. A dose of 5 mg is recommended for elderly patients to decrease the possibility of side effects (see Administration and Dosage). Elderly or debilitated patients should be monitored closely.

Use in patients with concomitant illness – Clinical experience with zaleplon in patients with concomitant systemic illness is limited. Zaleplon should be used with caution in patients with diseases or conditions that could affect metabolism or hemodynamic responses.

Although preliminary studies did not reveal respiratory depressant effects at hypnotic doses of zaleplon in healthy subjects, caution should be observed if zaleplon is prescribed to patients with compromised respiratory function, because sedative/hypnotics have the capacity to depress respiratory drive. Controlled trials of acute administration of zaleplon 10 mg in patients with chronic obstructive pulmonary disease or moderate obstructive sleep apnea showed no evidence of alterations in blood gases or apnea/hypopnea index, respectively. However, patients with compromised respiration due to preexisting illness should be monitored carefully.

Use in patients with depression – As with other sedative/hypnotic drugs, zaleplon should be administered with caution to patients exhibiting signs or symptoms of depression. Suicidal tendencies may be present in such patients and protective measures may be required. Intentional overdosage is more common in this group of patients (see Overdosage); therefore, the least amount of drug that is feasible should be prescribed for the patient at any one time.

➤*Drug abuse and dependence:*

Abuse – Two studies assessed the abuse liability of zaleplon at doses of 25 mg, 50 mg, and 75 mg in subjects with known histories of sedative drug abuse. The results of these studies indicate that zaleplon has an abuse potential similar to benzodiazepine and benzodiazepine-like hypnotics.

Dependence – The potential for developing physical dependence on zaleplon and a subsequent withdrawal syndrome was assessed in controlled studies of 14-, 28-, and 35-night durations and in open-label studies of 6- and 12-month durations by examining for the emergence of rebound insomnia following drug discontinuation. Some patients (mostly those treated with 20 mg) experienced a mild rebound insomnia on the first night following withdrawal that appeared to be resolved by the second night. The use of the Benzodiazepine Withdrawal Symptom Questionnaire and examination of any other withdrawal emergent events did not detect any other evidence for a withdrawal syndrome following abrupt discontinuation of zaleplon therapy in premarketing studies.

However, available data cannot provide a reliable estimate of the incidence of dependence during treatment at recommended doses of zaleplon. Other sedative/hypnotics have been associated with various signs and symptoms following abrupt discontinuation, ranging from mild dysphoria and insomnia to a withdrawal syndrome that may include abdominal and muscle cramps, vomiting, sweating, tremors, and convulsions. Seizures have been observed in 2 patients, one of which had a prior seizure, in clinical trials with zaleplon. Seizures and death have been seen following the withdrawal of zaleplon from animals at doses many times higher than those proposed for human use. Because individuals with a history of addiction to, or abuse of, drugs or alcohol are at risk of habituation and dependence, they should be under careful surveillance when receiving zaleplon or any other hypnotic.

➤*Hazardous tasks:* Zaleplon, like other hypnotics, has CNS-depressant effects. Because of the rapid onset of action, zaleplon should only be ingested immediately prior to going to bed or after the patient has gone to bed and has experienced difficulty falling asleep. Patients receiving zaleplon should be cautioned against engaging in hazardous occupations requiring complete mental alertness or motor coordination (eg, operating machinery or driving a motor vehicle) after ingesting the drug, including potential impairment of the performance of such activities that may occur the day following ingestion of zaleplon. Zaleplon, as well as other hypnotics, may produce additive CNS depressant effects when coadministered with other psychotropic medications, anticonvulsants, antihistamines, ethanol, and other drugs that themselves produce CNS depression. Zaleplon should not be taken with alcohol. Dosage adjustment may be necessary when zaleplon is administered with other CNS-depressant agents because of the potentially additive effects.

ZALEPLON — ORAL

➤*Pregnancy: Category C.* In embryofetal development studies in rats and rabbits, oral administration of up to 100 mg/kg/day and 50 mg/kg/day, respectively, to pregnant animals throughout organogenesis produced no evidence of teratogenicity. These doses are equivalent to 49 (rat) and 48 (rabbit) times the MRHD of 20 mg on a mg/m^2 basis. In rats, pre- and postnatal growth was reduced in the offspring of dams receiving 100 mg/kg/day. This dose was also maternally toxic, as evidenced by clinical signs and decreased maternal body weight gain during gestation. The no-effect dose for rat offspring growth reduction was 10 mg/kg (a dose equivalent to 5 times the MRHD of 20 mg on a mg/m^2 basis). No adverse effects on embryofetal development were observed in rabbits at the doses examined.

In a pre- and postnatal development study in rats, increased stillbirth and postnatal mortality, and decreased growth and physical development, were observed in the offspring of females treated with doses of 7 mg/kg/day or greater during the latter part of gestation and throughout lactation. There was no evidence of maternal toxicity at this dose. The no-effect dose for offspring development was 1 mg/kg/day (a dose equivalent to 0.5 times the MRHD of 20 mg on a mg/m^2 basis). When the adverse effects on offspring viability and growth were examined in a cross-fostering study, they appeared to result from both in utero and lactational exposure to the drug.

There are no studies of zaleplon in pregnant women; therefore, zaleplon is not recommended for use in women during pregnancy.

Labor and delivery – Zaleplon has no established use in labor and delivery.

➤*Lactation:* A study in lactating mothers indicated that the clearance and half-life of zaleplon is similar to that in young healthy subjects. A small amount of zaleplon is excreted in breast milk, with the highest excreted amount occurring during a feeding at ≈ 1 hour after zaleplon administration. Since the small amount of the drug from breast milk may result in potentially important concentrations in infants, and because the effects of zaleplon on a nursing infant are not known, it is recommended that nursing mothers not take zaleplon.

➤*Children:* The safety and effectiveness of zaleplon in pediatric patients have not been established.

➤*Elderly:* A total of 628 patients in double-blind, placebo-controlled, parallel-group clinical trials who received zaleplon were at least 65 years of age; of these, 311 received 5 mg and 317 received 10 mg. In both sleep laboratory and outpatient studies, elderly patients with insomnia responded to a 5 mg dose with a reduced sleep latency, and thus 5 mg is the recommended dose in this population. During short-term treatment (14 night studies) of elderly patients with zaleplon, no adverse event with a frequency of at least 1% occurred at a significantly higher rate with either 5 mg or 10 mg zaleplon than with placebo.

Drug Interactions

➤*CNS-active drugs:*

Ethanol – Zaleplon 10 mg potentiated the CNS-impairing effects of ethanol 0.75 g/kg on balance testing and reaction time for 1 hour after ethanol administration and on the digit symbol substitution test (DSST), symbol copying test, and the variability component of the divided attention test for 2.5 hours after ethanol administration. The potentiation resulted from a CNS pharmacodynamic interaction; zaleplon did not affect the pharmacokinetics of ethanol.

Imipramine – Coadministration of single doses of zaleplon 20 mg and imipramine 75 mg produced additive effects on decreased alertness and impaired psychomotor performance for 2 to 4 hours after administration. The interaction was pharmacodynamic with no alteration of the pharmacokinetics of either drug.

Thioridazine – Coadministration of single doses of zaleplon 20 mg and thioridazine 50 mg produced additive effects on decreased alertness and impaired psychomotor performance for 2 to 4 hours after administration. The interaction was phamacodynamic with no alteration of the pharmacokinetics of either drug.

➤*Drugs that induce CYP3A4:*

Rifampin – CYP3A4 is ordinarily a minor metabolizing enzyme of zaleplon. Multiple-dose administration of the potent CYP3A4 inducer rifampin (600 mg every 24 hours for 14 days), however, reduced zaleplon C_{max} and AUC by ≈ 80%. The coadministration of a potent CYP3A4 enzyme inducer, although not posing a safety concern, thus could lead to ineffectiveness of zaleplon. An alternative non-CYP3A4 substrate hypnotic agent may be considered in patients taking CYP3A4 inducers such as rifampin, phenytoin, carbamazepine, and phenobarbital.

➤*Drugs that inhibit both aldehyde oxidase and CYP3A4:*

Cimetidine – Cimetidine inhibits both aldehyde oxidase (in vitro) and CYP3A4 (in vitro and in vivo), the primary and secondary enzymes, respectively, responsible for zaleplon metabolism. Concomitant administration of zaleplon (10 mg) and cimetidine (800 mg) produced an 85% increase in the mean C_{max} and AUC of zaleplon. An initial dose of 5 mg should be given to patients who are concomitantly being treated with cimetidine.

Adverse Reactions

➤*Adverse findings observed in short-term, placebo-controlled trials:*

Adverse events occurring at an incidence of 1% or more among zaleplon 20 mg-treated patients – The table below enumerates the incidence of treatment-emergent adverse events for a pool of three 28-night and one 35-night placebo-controlled studies of zaleplon at doses of 5 mg or 10 mg and 20 mg. The table includes only those events that occurred in 1% or more of patients treated with zaleplon 20 mg and that had a higher incidence in patients treated with zaleplon 20 mg than in placebo-treated patients.

Zaleplon Adverse Events (%)[a]			
Body system/preferred term	Placebo (n = 344)	Zaleplon 5 mg or 10 mg (n = 569)	Zaleplon 20 mg (n = 297)
Miscellaneous			
Abdominal pain	3%	6%	6%
Asthenia	5%	5%	7%
Headache	35%	30%	42%
Malaise	< 1%	< 1%	2%
Photosensitivity reaction	< 1%	< 1%	1%
GI			
Anorexia	< 1%	< 1%	2%
Colitis	0%	0%	1%
Nausea	7%	6%	8%
Metabolic and nutritional			
Peripheral edema	< 1%	< 1%	1%
CNS			
Amnesia	1%	2%	4%
Confusion	< 1%	< 1%	1%
Depersonalization	< 1%	< 1%	2%
Dizziness	7%	7%	9%
Hallucinations	< 1%	< 1%	1%
Hypertonia	< 1%	1%	1%
Hypesthesia	< 1%	< 1%	2%
Paresthesia	1%	3%	3%
Somnolence	4%	5%	6%
Tremor	1%	2%	2%
Vertigo	< 1%	< 1%	1%
Respiratory			
Epistaxis	< 1%	< 1%	1%
Special senses			
Abnormal vision	< 1%	< 1%	2%
Ear pain	0%	< 1%	1%
Eye pain	2%	4%	3%
Hyperacusis	< 1%	1%	2%
Parosmia	< 1%	< 1%	2%
GU			
Dysmenorrhea	2%	3%	4%

[a] Events for which the incidence for zaleplon 20 mg-treated patients was at least 1% and greater than the incidence among placebo-treated patients. Incidence greater than 1% has been rounded to the nearest whole number.

➤*Other adverse events observed during the premarketing evaluation of zaleplon:* Events are further categorized by body system and listed in order of decreasing frequency according to the following definitions: Frequent adverse events are those occurring on one or more occasions in at least 1/100 patients; infrequent adverse events are those occurring in < 1/100 patients but at least 1/1000 patients; rare events are those occurring in < 1/1000 patients.

Cardiovascular –

Frequent: Migraine.

Infrequent: Angina pectoris, bundle branch block, hypertension, hypotension, palpitation, syncope, tachycardia, vasodilatation, ventricular extrasystoles.

Rare: Bigeminy, cerebral ischemia, cyanosis, pericardial effusion, postural hypotension, pulmonary embolus, sinus bradycardia, thrombophlebitis, ventricular tachycardia.

CNS –

Frequent: Anxiety, depression, nervousness, thinking abnormal (mainly difficulty concentrating).

Infrequent: Abnormal gait, agitation, apathy, ataxia, circumoral paresthesia, emotional lability, euphoria, hyperesthesia, hyperkinesia, hypotonia, incoordination, insomnia, libido decreased, neuralgia, nystagmus.

Rare: CNS stimulation, delusions, dysarthria, dystonia, facial paralysis, hostility, hypokinesia, myoclonus, neuropathy, psychomotor retardation, ptosis, reflexes decreased, reflexes increased, sleep talking, sleep walking, slurred speech, stupor, trismus.

Dermatologic –

Frequent: Pruritus, rash.

Infrequent: Acne, alopecia, contact dermatitis, dry skin, eczema, maculopapular rash, skin hypertrophy, sweating, urticaria, vesiculobullous rash.

Rare: Melanosis, psoriasis, pustular rash, skin discoloration.

Pyrazolopyrimidine

ZALEPLON — ORAL

Endocrine –

Rare: Diabetes mellitus, goiter, hypothyroidism.

GI –

Frequent: Constipation, dry mouth, dyspepsia.

Infrequent: Eructation, esophagitis, flatulence, gastritis, gastroenteritis, gingivitis, glossitis, increased appetite, melena, mouth ulceration, rectal hemorrhage, stomatitis.

Rare: Aphthous stomatitis, biliary pain, bruxism, cardiospasm, cheilitis, cholelithiasis, duodenal ulcer, dysphagia, enteritis, gum hemorrhage, increased salivation, intestinal obstruction, abnormal liver function tests, peptic ulcer, tongue discoloration, tongue edema, ulcerative stomatitis.

GU –

Infrequent: Bladder pain, breast pain, cystitis, decreased urine stream, dysuria, hematuria, impotence, kidney calculus, kidney pain, menorrhagia, metrorrhagia, urinary frequency, urinary incontinence, urinary urgency, vaginitis.

Rare: Albuminuria, delayed menstrual period, leukorrhea, menopause, urethritis, urinary retention, vaginal hemorrhage.

Hematologic / Lymphatic –

Infrequent: Anemia, ecchymosis, lymphadenopathy.

Rare: Eosinophilia, leukocytosis, lymphocytosis, purpura.

Metabolic / Nutritional –

Infrequent: Edema, gout, hypercholesteremia, thirst, weight gain.

Rare: Bilirubinemia, hyperglycemia, hyperuricemia, hypoglycemia, hypoglycemic reaction, ketosis, lactose intolerance, AST increased, ALT increased, weight loss.

Musculoskeletal –

Frequent: Arthralgia, arthritis, myalgia.

Infrequent: Arthrosis, bursitis, joint disorder (mainly swelling, stiffness, and pain), myasthenia, tenosynovitis.

Rare: Myositis, osteoporosis.

Special senses –

Frequent: Conjunctivitis, taste perversion.

Infrequent: Diplopia, dry eyes, photophobia, tinnitus, watery eyes.

Rare: Abnormality of accommodation, blepharitis, cataract specified, corneal erosion, deafness, eye hemorrhage, glaucoma, labyrinthitis, retinal detachment, taste loss, visual field defect.

Miscellaneous –

Frequent: Back pain, chest pain, fever.

Infrequent: Chest pain substernal, chills, face edema, generalized edema, hangover effect, neck rigidity.

Overdosage

➤*Symptoms:* Signs and symptoms of overdose effects of CNS depressants can be expected to present as exaggerations of the pharmacological effects noted in preclinical testing. Overdose is usually manifested by degrees of central nervous system depression ranging from drowsiness to coma. In mild cases, symptoms include drowsiness, mental confusion, and lethargy; in more serious cases, symptoms may include ataxia, hypotonia, hypotension, respiratory depression, rarely coma, and very rarely death.

There is limited premarketing clinical experience with the effects of an overdosage of zaleplon. Two cases of overdose were reported. One was the accidental ingestion by a 2½-year-old boy of 20 mg to 40 mg of zaleplon. The second was a 20-year-old man who took 100 mg zaleplon plus 2.25 mg of triazolam. Both were treated and recovered uneventfully.

➤*Treatment:* General symptomatic and supportive measures should be used along with immediate gastric lavage where appropriate. Intravenous fluids should be administered as needed. Animal studies suggest that flumazenil is an antagonist to zaleplon. However, there is no premarketing clinical experience with the use of flumazenil as an antidote to a zaleplon overdose. As in all cases of drug overdose, respiration, pulse, blood pressure, and other appropriate signs should be monitored and general supportive measures employed. Hypotension and CNS depression should be monitored and treated by appropriate medical intervention.

Melatonin Receptor Agonist

RAMELTEON

Rx	**Rozerem** (Takeda Pharmaceuticals America)	**Tablets; oral:** 8 mg	Lactose, PEG 8000. (TAK RAM-8). Pale orange-yellow, round. Film coated. In 30s, 100s, and 500s.

RAMELTEON — ORAL

Indications

➤*Insomnia:* For the treatment of insomnia characterized by difficulty with sleep onset.

Administration and Dosage

➤*Adults:*

Insomnia –

Usual dosage: 8 mg taken within 30 minutes of going to bed.

Maximum dose: 8 mg/day.

Concomitant therapy: Do not use in combination with fluvoxamine; use caution in patients taking other CYP1A2-inhibiting drugs.

➤*Hepatic function impairment:* Ramelteon should be used with caution in patients with moderate hepatic impairment. Ramelteon should not be used in patients with severe hepatic impairment.

➤*Administration:* It is recommended that ramelteon not be taken with or immediately after a high-fat meal. After taking ramelteon, patients should confine their activities to those necessary to prepare for bed.

➤*Storage / Stability:* Store at 25°C (77°F); excursions are permitted between 15° and 30°C (59° and 86°F). Protect from moisture and humidity.

Actions

➤*Pharmacology:* Ramelteon is a melatonin receptor agonist with high affinity for melatonin MT_1 and MT_2 receptors and selectivity over the MT_3 receptor. Ramelteon demonstrates full agonist activity in vitro in cells expressing human MT_1 or MT_2 receptors.

The activity of ramelteon at the MT_1 and MT_2 receptors is believed to contribute to its sleep-promoting properties because these receptors, acted upon by endogenous melatonin, are thought to be involved in the maintenance of the circadian rhythm underlying the normal sleep-wake cycle.

The major metabolite of ramelteon, M-II, is active and has approximately one-tenth and one-fifth the binding affinity of the parent molecule for the human MT_1 and MT_2 receptors, respectively, and is 17- to 25-fold less potent than ramelteon in in vitro functional assays. Although the potency of M-II at MT_1 and MT_2 receptors is lower than the parent drug, M-II circulates at higher concentrations than the parent, producing 20- to 100-fold greater mean systemic exposure compared with ramelteon.

➤*Pharmacokinetics:*

Absorption – Ramelteon is absorbed rapidly, with median peak concentrations occurring at approximately 0.75 hours (range, 0.5 to 1.5 hours) after fasted oral administration. Although the total absorption of ramelteon is at least 84%, the absolute oral bioavailability is only 1.8% because of extensive first-pass metabolism.

Effect of food: When administered with a high-fat meal, the area under the curve ($AUC_{0\text{-}inf}$) for a single 16 mg dose of ramelteon was 31% higher, and the maximum serum concentration (C_{max}) was 22% lower than when given in a fasted state. Median time to C_{max} (T_{max}) was delayed by approximately 45 minutes when ramelteon was administered with food. Effects of food on the AUC values for M-II were similar. Therefore, it is recommended that ramelteon not be taken with or immediately after a high-fat meal.

Distribution – Ramelteon has a mean volume of distribution after intravenous (IV) administration of 73.6 L, suggesting substantial tissue distribution. In vitro protein binding of ramelteon is approximately 82% in human serum, independent of concentration. Binding to albumin accounts for most of that binding because 70% of the drug is bound in human serum albumin.

Metabolism – When administered orally to humans in doses ranging from 4 to 64 mg, ramelteon undergoes rapid, high first-pass metabolism and exhibits linear pharmacokinetics. C_{max} and AUC data show substantial intersubject variability, consistent with the high first-pass effect; the coefficient of variation for these values is approximately 100%. Several metabolites have been identified in human serum and urine.

Metabolism of ramelteon consists primarily of oxidation to hydroxyl and carbonyl derivatives, with secondary metabolism producing glucuronide conjugates. CYP1A2 is the major isozyme involved in the hepatic metabolism of ramelteon; the CYP2C subfamily and CYP3A4 isozymes also are involved to a minor degree.

The rank order of the principal metabolites by prevalence in human serum is M-II, M-IV, M-I, and M-III. These metabolites are formed rapidly and exhibit a monophasic decline and rapid elimination. The overall mean systemic exposure of M-II is approximately 20- to 100-fold higher than the parent drug.

Excretion – Following oral administration of radio-labeled ramelteon, 84% of total radioactivity was excreted in urine and approximately 4% in feces, resulting in a mean recovery of 88%. Less than 0.1% of the dose was excreted in urine and feces as the parent compound. Elimination was essentially complete by 96 hours postdose.

Repeated once-daily dosing with ramelteon does not result in significant accumulation because of the short elimination half-life of ramelteon (on average, approximately 1 to 2.6 hours).

The half-life of M-II is 2 to 5 hours and is independent of dose. Serum concentrations of the parent drug and its metabolites in humans are at or below the lower limits of quantitation within 24 hours.

Special populations –

Hepatic function impairment: Exposure to ramelteon was increased almost 4-fold in subjects with mild hepatic impairment after 7 days of dosing with 16 mg/day; exposure was further increased (more than 10-fold) in subjects with moderate hepatic impairment. Exposure to M-II was only marginally increased in mildly and moderately impaired subjects relative to healthy matched controls. The pharmacokinetics of ramelteon have not been evaluated in subjects with severe hepatic impairment (Child-Pugh class C). Ramelteon is not recommended for use in patients with severe hepatic impairment. Use ramelteon with caution in patients with moderate hepatic impairment.

Elderly: In a group of 24 elderly subjects 63 to 79 years of age who were administered a single ramelteon 16 mg dose, the mean C_{max} and $AUC_{0\text{-}inf}$

RAMELTEON — ORAL

values were 11.6 ng/mL (standard deviation "SD", 13.8) and 18.7 ng•h/mL (SD, 19.4), respectively. The elimination half-life was 2.6 hours (SD, 1.1). Compared with younger adults, the total exposure ($AUC_{0\text{-inf}}$) and C_{max} of ramelteon were 97% and 86% higher, respectively, in elderly subjects. The $AUC_{0\text{-inf}}$ and C_{max} of M-II were increased by 30% and 13%, respectively, in elderly subjects.

Contraindications

Patients who develop angioedema after treatment with ramelteon; concomitant use with fluvoxamine.

Warnings/Precautions

➤*Psychiatric/Physical disorder:* Because sleep disturbances may be the presenting manifestation of a physical and/or psychiatric disorder, initiate symptomatic treatment of insomnia only after a careful evaluation of the patient. The failure of insomnia to remit after 7 to 10 days of treatment may indicate the presence of a primary psychiatric and/or medical illness that should be evaluated. Worsening of insomnia or the emergence of new cognitive or behavioral abnormalities may be the result of an unrecognized underlying psychiatric or physical disorder and requires further evaluation of the patient. Exacerbation of insomnia and emergence of cognitive and behavioral abnormalities were seen with ramelteon during the clinical development program.

➤*CNS effects:* A variety of cognitive and behavior changes have been reported to occur in association with the use of hypnotics. In primarily depressed patients, worsening of depression (including suicidal ideation and completed suicides) has been reported in association with the use of hypnotics.

Hallucinations, as well as behavioral changes, such as bizarre behavior, agitation, and mania, have been reported with ramelteon use. Amnesia, anxiety, and other neuropsychiatric symptoms may also occur unpredictably.

Complex behaviors, such as "sleep driving" (ie, driving while not fully awake after ingestion of a hypnotic) and other complex behaviors (eg, preparing and eating food, making phone calls, having sex) with amnesia for the event, have been reported in association with hypnotic use. The use of alcohol and other CNS depressants may increase the risk of such behaviors. These reactions can occur in hypnotic-naive as well as hypnotic-experienced persons. Complex behaviors have been reported with the use of ramelteon. Strongly consider discontinuation of ramelteon for patients who report any complex sleep behavior.

➤*Sleep apnea:* Ramelteon has not been studied in subjects with severe sleep apnea and is not recommended for use in those populations.

➤*Chronic obstructive pulmonary disease:* Treatment with a single dose of ramelteon has no demonstrated respiratory depressant effects in subjects with mild to severe COPD, as measured by arterial oxygen saturation. There is no available information on the respiratory effects of multiple doses of ramelteon in patients with COPD. The respiratory depressant effects in patients with COPD cannot be definitively known from this study.

➤*Hypersensitivity reactions:* Rare cases of angioedema involving the tongue, glottis, or larynx have been reported in patients after taking the first or subsequent doses of ramelteon. Some patients have had additional symptoms, such as dyspnea, throat closing, or nausea and vomiting, that suggest anaphylaxis. Some patients have required medical therapy in the emergency department. If angioedema involves the tongue, glottis, or larynx, airway obstruction may occur and be fatal. Do not rechallenge patients who develop angioedema after treatment with ramelteon.

➤*Hepatic function impairment:* See Actions for more information.

➤*Hazardous tasks:* Advise patients to avoid engaging in hazardous activities that require concentration (eg, operating a motor vehicle or heavy machinery) after taking ramelteon.

➤*Pregnancy: Category C.* In animal studies, ramelteon produced evidence of developmental toxicity, including teratogenic effects in rats at doses much greater than the recommended human dose of 8 mg/day. There are no adequate and well-controlled studies in pregnant women. It is not known if ramelteon or its active metabolite crosses the placenta. The molecular weight of ramelteon (about 259) and the elimination half-lives of ramelteon and its metabolite suggest that exposure of the embryo and/or fetus to both will probably occur. Use ramelteon during pregnancy only if the potential benefit justifies the potential risk to the fetus. Infrequent or inadvertent exposure during gestation does not appear to represent a significant risk to the embryo or fetus. However, long-term exposure in rodents was associated with cardinogenic effects; consider this if ramelteon is used frequently in pregnancy.

Oral administration of ramelteon 10, 40, 150, or 600 mg/kg/day to pregnant rats during the period of organogenesis was associated with increased incidences of fetal structural abnormalities (malformations and variations) at dosages of more than 40 mg/kg/day. The no-effect dose is approximately 50 times the recommended human dose on a body surface area (mg/m^2) basis. Treatment of pregnant rabbits during the period of organogenesis produced no evidence of embryofetal toxicity at oral dosages of up to 300 mg/kg/day (or up to 720 times the recommended human dose on a mg/m^2 basis).

When rats were orally administered ramelteon 30, 100, or 300 mg/kg/day throughout gestation and lactation, growth retardation, developmental delay, and behavioral changes were observed in the offspring at dosages of more than 30 mg/kg/day. The no-effect dose is 36 times the recommended human dose on a mg/m^2 basis. Increased incidences of malformation and death among offspring were seen at the highest dose.

➤*Lactation:* It is not known whether this drug is excreted in human milk; however, ramelteon is secreted into the milk of lactating rats. The molecular weight of ramelteon (about 259) and the elimination half-lives of ramelteon and its active metabolite suggest that both will be excreted into breast milk. Because many drugs are excreted into human milk, exercise caution when administering ramelteon to a breast-feeding woman. Moreover, if a breast-feeding mother uses this drug frequently, consider the fact that it is carcinogenic in rodents with long-term exposure.

➤*Children:* Safety and effectiveness of ramelteon in children have not been established. Further study is needed prior to determining that this product may be used safely in prepubescent and pubescent patients. Ramelteon has been associated with an effect on reproductive hormones in adults (eg, decreased testosterone levels, increased prolactin levels). It is not known what effect chronic or even chronic, intermittent use of ramelteon may have on the reproductive axis in developing humans.

➤*Monitoring:* For patients presenting with unexplained amenorrhea, galactorrhea, decreased libido, or problems with fertility, consider assessment of prolactin levels and testosterone levels as appropriate.

Drug Interactions

➤*CYP450 enzymes:* Ramelteon has a highly variable intersubject pharmacokinetic profile (approximately 100% coefficient of variation in C_{max} and AUC). CYP1A2 is the major isozyme involved in the metabolism of ramelteon; the CYP2C subfamily and CYP3A4 isozymes also are involved to a minor degree. Ramelteon is contraindicated for use with fluvoxamine; use with caution in patients taking less strong CYP1A2 inhibitors. Administer with caution to patients taking strong CYP3A4 or 2C9 inhibitors.

Ramelteon Drug Interactions

Precipitant drug	Object drug[a]		Description
Alcohol	Ramelteon	⬆	Concomitant use may produce additive CNS effects. Advise patients taking ramelteon not to consume alcohol.
Ramelteon	Alcohol		
Azole antifungals (eg, fluconazole, ketoconazole)	Ramelteon	⬆	When administered with ketoconazole, the AUC and C_{max} of ramelteon increased by ≈ 84% and 36%, respectively. The AUC and C_{max} of ramelteon also were increased by ≈ 150% when administered with fluconazole. Similar increases also were seen in M-II exposure. Use with caution. Closely monitor the clinical response of the patient and adjust the ramelteon dose as needed.
Fluvoxamine	Ramelteon	⬆	Ramelteon AUC increased ≈ 190-fold, and the C_{max} increased ≈ 70-fold. Do not use ramelteon in combination with fluvoxamine.
Rifampin	Ramelteon	⬇	Ramelteon and metabolite M-II had a decrease in both AUC and C_{max} by ≈ 80% when administered with rifampin. Ramelteon efficacy may be reduced when used with a strong CYP enzyme inducer, such as rifampin. Closely monitor the clinical response of the patient when rifampin is started or stopped. Adjust the ramelteon dose as needed.

[a] ⬆ = object drug increased; ⬇ = object drug decreased.

➤*Drug/Food interactions:* See Actions for more information.

Adverse Reactions

➤*Discontinuation:* Six percent of the 5,373 individual subjects exposed to ramelteon in clinical trials discontinued treatment because of an adverse reaction compared with 2% of the 2,279 subjects receiving placebo. The most frequent adverse reactions leading to discontinuation in subjects receiving ramelteon were dizziness, fatigue, headache, insomnia, nausea, and somnolence, all of which occurred in 1% or less of patients.

Most common adverse reactions –

Ramelteon Adverse Reactions

Adverse reactions	Ramelteon 8 mg (n = 1,405)	Placebo (n = 1,456)
CNS		
Dizziness	4%	3%
Fatigue	3%	2%
Insomnia exacerbated	3%	2%
Somnolence	3%	2%
GI		
Nausea	3%	2%

Melatonin Receptor Agonist

RAMELTEON — ORAL

Overdosage

➤*Treatment:* Use general symptomatic and supportive measures, along with immediate gastric lavage when appropriate. Administer IV fluids as needed. As in all cases of drug overdose, monitor respiration, pulse, blood pressure, and other appropriate vital signs and employ general supportive measures.

Patient Information

Inform patients, their families, and their caregivers about the benefits and risks associated with treatment with hypnotics, counsel them in their appropriate use, and instruct them to read the accompanying Medication Guide.

Inform patients that severe anaphylactic and anaphylactoid reactions have occurred with ramelteon. Describe the relevant signs/symptoms and advise them to seek immediate medical attention if they occur.

There have been reports of people getting out of bed after taking a sleep medication and driving their cars while not fully awake, often with no memory of the event. If a patient experiences such an episode, advise them to report it to their health care provider immediately because "sleep driving" can be dangerous. This behavior is more likely to occur when sleep medications are taken with alcohol or other CNS depressants. Other complex behaviors (eg, preparing and eating food, making phone calls, having sex) have been reported in patients who are not fully awake after taking a sleep medication. As with sleep driving, patients usually do not remember these events.

Advise patients to take ramelteon within 30 minutes prior to going to bed and to confine their activities to those necessary to prepare for bed.

Advise patients to avoid engaging in hazardous activities (eg, operating a motor vehicle or heavy machinery) after taking ramelteon.

Advise patients not to take ramelteon with or immediately after a high-fat meal.

Advise patients to consult their health care provider if they experience worsening of insomnia or any new behavioral signs or symptoms of concern.

Advise patients to consult their health care provider if they experience 1 of the following: cessation of menses or galactorrhea in women, decreased libido, or problems with fertility.

Advise patients to avoid alcohol in combination with ramelteon.

Tell patients not to break the tablet, but to swallow it whole.

Benzodiazepines

Refer to the general discussion beginning in the Sedative and Hypnotic, Nonbarbiturate introduction. For information on benzodiazepines used as antianxiety agents, refer to the group monograph in the Antianxiety Agents section.

Indications

➤*Insomnia:* Insomnia characterized by difficulty in falling asleep, frequent nocturnal awakenings or early morning awakening. Can be used for recurring insomnia or poor sleeping habits and in acute or chronic medical situations requiring restful sleep.

Insomnia is often transient and intermittent; therefore, prolonged administration is generally not recommended. Because insomnia may be a symptom of other disorders, consider the possibility that the complaint may be related to a condition for which there is more specific treatment.

Actions

➤*Pharmacology:* Estazolam, flurazepam, quazepam, temazepam and triazolam are benzodiazepine derivatives useful as hypnotics. Benzodiazepines are believed to potentiate gamma aminobutyric acid (GABA) neuronal inhibition. The sedative and anticonvulsant actions involve GABA receptors located in the limbic, neocortical and mesencephalic reticular systems.

At least two benzodiazepine receptor subtypes have been identified in the brain, BZ_1 and BZ_2. BZ_1 is thought to be associated with sleep mechanisms; BZ_2 with memory, motor, sensory and cognitive functions. Quazepam and its active metabolite 2-oxoquazepam have a high affinity for BZ_1 receptors; this selectivity is not seen with estazolam, flurazepam, temazepam and triazolam. It is possible this selectivity of quazepam facilitates GABA transmission; however, further study is needed to determine the clinical significance of this receptor sensitivity.

Benzodiazepines generally decrease sleep latency, the number of awakenings and the time spent in stage 0 (awake stage). Flurazepam, quazepam and temazepam decrease stage 1 (descending drowsiness). Stage 2 (unequivocal sleep) is increased by all benzodiazepines, and most benzodiazepines shorten stages 3 and 4 (slow wave sleep). Temazepam has prolonged stage 3 and shortened stage 4 in neurotic patients or patients with depression. All but flurazepam prolong REM latency. REM sleep is usually shortened, but with temazepam or low-dose flurazepam, this may not be the case. The result of benzodiazepine administration is an increase in total sleep time.

If benzodiazepines are discontinued after 3 or 4 weeks of continued use, the patient may experience REM rebound; however, REM rebound with flurazepam, quazepam and possibly estazolam is slight.

➤*Pharmacokinetics:*

Absorption – These agents are rapidly and completely absorbed within 1 to 3 hours of oral administration. All have high lipid:water distribution coefficients in the non-ionized form. Times to peak plasma concentration range from 0.5 to 2 hours for parent compounds. The major active metabolite of flurazepam reaches peak plasma levels in ≈ 10 hours.

Distribution – Plasma protein binding ranges from 70% to 99% with free-drug concentrations closely approximating CSF levels. IV and rapidly absorbed oral benzodiazepines are rapidly taken into the brain and other highly perfused organs. Redistribution, favoring lipophilic compounds, follows and can greatly influence the duration of CNS effects. They also cross the placenta and are secreted into breast milk.

Metabolism – Benzodiazepines are extensively metabolized in the liver. Biotransformation to active metabolites is an important factor in product selection especially in the elderly or patients with severe liver disease. Flurazepam is biotransformed to an active metabolite, N-desalkylflurazepam, which has a half-life ranging from 47 to 100 hours. Quazepam is extensively metabolized to 2-oxoquazepam, an active metabolite; 2-oxoquazepam is further biotransformed to N-desalkyl-2-oxoquazepam, which is identical to N-desalkylflurazepam and is therefore also active. Temazepam, estazolam and triazolam do not form active long-acting metabolites.

Select Benzodiazepine (Hypnotic) Pharmacokinetic Parameters

Drug	Usual adult oral dose (mg)	Time to peak plasma levels (hrs)	Half-life (hrs)	Protein binding (%)	Urinary excretion, unchanged (%)
Estazolam	1-2	2	8-28	93	< 5
Flurazepam	15-30	0.5-1 (7.6-13.6)[a]	2-3 (47-100)[a]	97	< 1
Quazepam	7.5-15	2 (1-2)	41 (47-100)[a]	> 95	trace
Temazepam	15-30	1.2-1.6	3.5-18.4 (9-15)	96	0.2
Triazolam	0.125-0.5	1-2	1.5-5.5	78-89	2

[a] N-desalkylflurazepam, active metabolite.

Contraindications

Hypersensitivity to other benzodiazepines; pregnancy (see Warnings); established or suspected sleep apnea (quazepam).

Concurrent use with ketoconazole, itraconazole and nefazodone, medications that significantly impair the oxidative metabolism of **triazolam** mediated by cytochrome P450 3A (CYP3A).

Warnings/Precautions

➤*Anterograde amnesia:* Anterograde amnesia of varying severity and paradoxical reactions have occurred following therapeutic doses of **triazolam**. Although these effects generally occurred with a 0.5 mg dose, they have also been reported with 0.125 and 0.25 mg doses. These effect may occur with some other benzodiazepines, but data suggest that they may occur at a higher rate with triazolam.

Cases of "traveler's amnesia" have been reported by individuals who have taken **triazolam** to induce sleep while traveling. In some of these cases, insufficient time was allowed for the sleep period prior to awakening and before beginning activity. Also, the concomitant use of alcohol may have been a factor in some cases.

➤*Depression:* Administer with caution in severely depressed patients or in those in whom there is evidence of latent depression or suicidal tendencies. Signs or symptoms of depression may be intensified by hypnotic drugs. Protective measures may be required. Intentional overdosage is more common in these patients, and the least amount of drug that is feasible should be available to the patient at any one time.

➤*Rebound sleep disorder:* Rebound sleep disorder, which is characterized by recurrence of insomnia to levels worse than before treatment began, may occur following abrupt withdrawal of triazolam, usually during the first 1 to 3 nights. Gradual rather than abrupt discontinuation of the drug may help avoid this syndrome. Rebound insomnia appears to be less likely after withdrawal of agents with intermediate or long half-lives (eg, estazolam, flurazepam, quazepam).

➤*Disturbed nocturnal sleep:* Disturbed nocturnal sleep may occur for the first or second night after discontinuing use.

➤*Early morning insomnia:* Early morning insomnia, or early morning awakenings, appears to be more common with the use of short half-life agents (temazepam, triazolam) than agents with intermediate or long half-lives (estazolam, flurazepam, quazepam). However, daytime sleepiness appears to be more prevalent with the long half-life agents.

➤*Respiratory depression and sleep apnea:* Observe caution. In patients with compromised respiratory function, respiratory depression and sleep apnea have occurred. Estazolam may cause dose-related respiratory depression that is ordinarily not clinically relevant at recommended doses in patients with normal respiratory function. However, patients with compromised respiratory function may be at risk; therefore, monitor appropriately. Benzodiazepines have the capacity to depress respiratory drive, although there are insufficient data to characterize the relative potency of these agents in depressing respiratory drive at clinically recommended doses.

➤*Renal/Hepatic function impairment:* Observe usual precautions under these conditions; the potential for excessive sedation or impaired coordination exists.

Abnormal liver function tests as well as blood dyscrasias have been reported with benzodiazepines.

➤*Drug abuse and dependence:* Withdrawal symptoms following abrupt discontinuation of benzodiazepines have occurred in patients receiving excessive doses over extended periods of time. Symptoms are similar to those noted with barbiturates and alcohol following abrupt discontinuance and range from mild dysphoria to abdominal and muscle cramps, vomiting, sweating, tremor and convulsions.

Milder withdrawal symptoms infrequently occur following abrupt discontinuance of higher therapeutic levels of benzodiazepines taken continuously for several months. Exercise caution in administering to individuals known to be addiction-prone or those who may increase the dosage on their own initiative. Limit repeated prescriptions without adequate medical supervision.

Gradual withdrawal is the preferred course for any patient taking benzodiazepines for a prolonged period. Patients with a history of seizures, regardless of their concomitant anti-seizure therapy, should not be withdrawn abruptly from benzodiazepines.

➤*Hazardous tasks:* Observe caution while driving or performing tasks requiring alertness. Be aware of potential impairment of the performance of such activities the day following ingestion.

Amnesia, paradoxical reactions (eg, excitement, agitation) and other adverse behavioral effects may occur unpredictably.

➤*Pregnancy: Category X* (estazolam, quazepam, temazepam, triazolam). Flurazepam is contraindicated in pregnancy.

A neonate whose mother received 30 mg **flurazepam** nightly for insomnia during the 10 days prior to delivery appeared hypotonic and inactive during the first 4 days of life. Serum levels of N–desalkylflurazepam in the infant indicated transplacental circulation.

Teratogenic – Benzodiazepines may cause fetal damage when administered during pregnancy. An increased risk of congenital malformations associated with the use of diazepam and chlordiazepoxide during the first trimester of pregnancy has been suggested. Transplacental distribution results in neonatal CNS depression following ingestion of therapeutic doses of a benzodiazepine hypnotic during the last weeks of pregnancy.

Reproduction studies with **temazepam** in animals demonstrated an increased nursling mortality, increased fetal resorptions and increased occurrence of rudimentary ribs. Exencephaly and fusion or asymmetry of the ribs occurred without dose relationship.

Warn the patient of the potential risk to the fetus if there is a likelihood of the patient becoming pregnant while receiving benzodiazepines. Instruct patients to discontinue the drug prior to becoming pregnant. Consider the possibility that a woman of childbearing potential may be pregnant at the time of therapy institution.

Nonteratogenic – A child born to a mother taking benzodiazepines may be at some risk of withdrawal symptoms during the postnatal period. Neonatal flaccidity has occurred in an infant whose mother had been receiving benzodiazepines.

➤*Lactation:* Safety for use in the nursing mother has not been established. Benzodiazepines are excreted in breast milk. One study showed only 0.11% of quazepam and its metabolites were excreted in breast milk 48 hours after administration. Animal studies indicate that **triazolam, estazolam** and their metabolites are secreted in milk. Therefore, administration to nursing mothers is not recommended.

➤*Children:*

Flurazepam – Not for use in children < 15 years of age.

Estazolam, quazepam, temazepam, triazolam – Not for use in children < 18 years of age.

➤*Elderly:* The risk of developing oversedation, dizziness, confusion or ataxia increases substantially with larger doses of benzodiazepines in elderly and debilitated patients. Initiate with lowest effective dose.

Per the Beers list, **flurazepam** and **quazepam** have an extremely long half-life in elderly patients (often days), producing prolonged sedation and increasing the incidence of falls and fracture. Medium or short acting benzodiazepines are preferable to flurazepam. Short and intermediate acting benzodiazepines are preferable to quazepam. Flurazepam is also considered a high risk medication for the elderly according to the Centers of Medicare and Medicaid Services.

Per the Beers list, **temazepam** doses greater than 15 mg, and **triazolam** doses greater than 0.25 mg should not be used because of increased sensitivity to benzodiazepines in elderly patients. Smaller doses may be effective as well as safer. Total daily doses should rarely exceed the suggested maximums.

➤*Monitoring:* When triazolam or estazolam treatment is protracted, obtain periodic blood counts, urinalysis and blood chemistry analyses. Minor EEG changes, usually low-voltage fast activity, are of no known significance.

Drug Interactions

Benzodiazepine (Hypnotic) Drug Interactions			
Precipitant drug	Object drug[a]		Description
Alcohol/CNS depressants	Benzodiazepines	⬆	Additive CNS depressant effects. Potential for this interaction continues for several days following flurazepam withdrawal.
Azole antifungals (itraconazole, ketoconazole, voriconazole)	Benzodiazepines	⬆	Azole antifungals decrease the metabolism of benzodiazepines, leading to increased sedation and prolonged CNS depression. Triazolam is contraindicated with itraconazole and ketoconazole; midazolam is contraindicated with itraconazole.
Carbamazepine	Benzodiazepines	⬇	May increase hepatic metabolism, resulting in decreased pharmacologic effects. Consider increased benzodiazepine dose.
Cimetidine Contraceptives, oral Disulfiram Isoniazid	Benzodiazepines (metabolized by oxidation)	⬆	The hepatic metabolism of the benzodiazepines may be inhibited, their half-life prolonged and their clearance decreased, possibly resulting in increased pharmacologic and CNS depressant effects. Temazepam, metabolized by glucuronidation, would probably not interact; however, its half-life may be decreased by oral contraceptive agents.
Clozapine	Benzodiazepines	⬆	Delirium, sedation, sialorrhea, and ataxia may occur. Do not start simultaneously; it may be better to add clozapine to established clonazepam therapy than vice versa. Carefully monitor.
Probenecid	Benzodiazepines	⬆	More rapid onset or more prolonged benzodiazepine effect.
Protease inhibitors (eg, ritonavir, nelfinavir)	Benzodiazepines	⬆	May decrease the oxidative metabolism of benzodiazepines, leading to severe sedation and respiratory depression. Midazolam and triazolam are contraindicated with atazanavir or darunavir.
Rifampin	Benzodiazepines (metabolized by oxidation)	⬇	Increased clearance and decreased half-life of benzodiazepines may occur. Temazepam would probably not interact.
St. John's Wort	Benzodiazepines	⬇	May increase hepatic metabolism, resulting in decreased pharmacologic effects. Adjust benzodiazepine dose as needed.
Smoking	Benzodiazepines	⬇	Benzodiazepine clearance is increased in cigarette smokers, probably due to enzyme induction.
Theophyllines	Benzodiazepines	⬇	Benzodiazepine pharmacologic effects may be antagonized.
Macrolides	Triazolam	⬆	Bioavailability of triazolam may be increased.
Benzodiazepines	Digoxin	⬆	Digoxin serum levels and toxicity may increase.
Benzodiazepines	Neuromuscular blocking agents (nondepolarizing)	⟷	Benzodiazepines may potentiate, counteract or have no effect on these agents.
Benzodiazepines	Phenytoin	⬆	Phenytoin serum levels may be increased, resulting in toxicity, but data are conflicting.

[a] ⬆ = object drug increased; ⬇ = object drug decreased; ⟷ = undetermined clinical effect.

Adverse Reactions

➤*Cardiovascular:* Palpitations; chest pains; tachycardia; hypotension (rare).

➤*CNS:* Headache; nervousness; talkativeness; apprehension; irritability; confusion; euphoria; relaxed feeling; weakness; tremor; lack of concentration; coordination disorders; confusional states/memory impairment; depression; dreaming/nightmares; insomnia; paresthesia; restlessness; tiredness; dysesthesia. Hallucinations, horizontal nystagmus and paradoxical reactions, including excitement, stimulation and hyperactivity were rare. Dizziness, drowsiness, lightheadedness, staggering, ataxia, falling, particularly in elderly or debilitated patients. Severe sedation, lethargy, disorientation and coma are probably indicative of drug intolerance or overdosage.

➤*Dermatologic:* Dermatitis/allergy; sweating, flushes, pruritus, skin rash (rare).

➤*GI:* Heartburn; nausea; vomiting; diarrhea; constipation; GI pain; anorexia; taste alterations; dry mouth; excessive salivation (rare); death from hepatic failure in a patient also receiving diuretics; jaundice; glossitis, stomatitis (triazolam).

➤*Lab test abnormalities:* Elevated AST, ALT, total and direct bilirubin and alkaline phosphatase with **flurazepam**.

➤*Miscellaneous:* Body/joint pain; tinnitus; GU complaints; cramps/pain; congestion. Leukopenia, granulocytopenia, blurred vision, burning eyes, faintness, difficulty in focusing, visual disturbances, shortness of breath, apnea, slurred speech (rare).

➤*Estazolam:* Other adverse reactions reported only for estazolam include the following:

Cardiovascular – Arrhythmia, syncope (< 0.1%).

CNS – Somnolence (42%); asthenia (11%); hypokinesia (8%); hangover (3%); abnormal thinking (2%); anxiety (1%); agitation, amnesia, apathy, emotional lability, hostility, seizure, sleep disorder, stupor, twitch (0.1% to 1%); ataxia, decreased libido, decreased reflexes, neuritis (< 0.1%).

Dermatologic – Urticaria (0.1% to 1%); acne, dry skin, photosensitivity (< 0.1%).

GI – Dyspepsia (2%); decreased/increased appetite, flatulence, gastritis (0.1% to 1%); enterocolitis, melena, mouth ulceration (< 0.1%).

GU – Frequent urination, menstrual cramps, urinary hesitancy/urgency, vaginal discharge/itching (0.1% to 1%); hematuria, nocturia, oliguria, penile discharge, urinary incontinence (< 0.1%).

Respiratory – Cold symptoms (3%); pharyngitis (1%); asthma, cough, dyspnea, rhinitis, sinusitis (0.1% to 1%); epistaxis, hyperventilation, laryngitis (< 0.1%).

Special senses – Ear pain, eye irritation/pain/swelling, photophobia (0.1% to 1%); decreased hearing, diplopia, nystagmus, scotomata (< 0.1%).

Miscellaneous – Lower extremity/back/abdominal pain (1% to 3%); stiffness (1%); allergic reaction, chills, fever, neck/upper extremity pain, thirst, arthritis, muscle spasm, myalgia (0.1% to 1%); edema, jaw pain, swollen breast, thyroid nodule, purpura, swollen lymph nodes, agranulocytosis, increased AST, weight gain/loss, arthralgia (< 0.1%).

Overdosage

➤*Symptoms:* Somnolence; confusion with reduced or absent reflexes; respiratory depression; apnea; hypotension; impaired coordination; slurred speech; seizures; ultimately, coma. Death has occurred with overdoses of benzodiazepines alone and with alcohol.

➤*Treatment:* If excitation occurs, do not use barbiturates. Consider the possibility that multiple agents may have been ingested. Monitor respiration, pulse and blood pressure. Employ general supportive measures. Administer IV fluids and maintain an adequate airway. Perform gastric lavage. Refer to General Management of Acute Overdosage. Hemodialysis and forced diuresis are of little value.

Use of IV pressor agents may be necessary to treat hypotension. Administer IV fluids to encourage diuresis.

Patient Information

Avoid alcohol and other CNS depressants. Do not exceed prescribed dosage.

Do not discontinue medication abruptly after prolonged therapy.

Advise patients that they may experience disturbed nocturnal sleep for the first or second night after discontinuing the drug.

May cause drowsiness or dizziness; observe caution while driving or performing other tasks requiring alertness.

Inform your physician if you are planning to become pregnant, if you are pregnant, or if you become pregnant while taking this medicine.

➤*Triazolam:* Advise patients not to take triazolam in circumstances where a full night's sleep and clearance of the drug from the body are not possible before they would again need to be active and functional.

ESTAZOLAM

c-iv	**Estazolam** (Zenith-Goldline)	**Tablets:** 1 mg	In 30s, 100s, 500s and 1000s.
c-iv	**Estazolam** (Zenith-Goldline)	2 mg	In 30s, 100s, 500s and 1000s.

ESTAZOLAM — ORAL

For complete and comparative prescribing information, refer to the Benzodiazepines group monograph.

Indications

➤*Insomnia:* Estazolam is indicated for the short-term management of insomnia characterized by difficulty in falling asleep, frequent nocturnal awakenings, and/or early morning awakenings. Both outpatient studies and a sleep laboratory study have shown that estazolam administered at bedtime improved sleep induction and sleep maintenance.

Administration and Dosage

➤*Adults:*

Insomnia –

Initial dosage: 1 mg at bedtime.

Dosage adjustment: Up to 2 mg at bedtime may be required by some patients.

➤*Elderly:* In healthy elderly patients, 1 mg is the appropriate starting dose, but increases should be initiated with particular care. In small or debilitated older patients, a starting dose of 0.5 mg, while only marginally effective in the overall elderly population, should be considered.

➤*Storage/Stability:* Store at 15° to 30°C (59° to 86°F).

FLURAZEPAM HYDROCHLORIDE

c-iv	**Flurazepam** (Various, eg, Goldline, Major, PBI, Warner Chilcott)	**Capsules; oral:** 15 mg	In 100s and 100s.
c-iv	**Flurazepam** (Various, eg, Goldline, Major, PBI, Warner Chilcott)	**Capsules; oral:** 30 mg	In 100s and 100s.

FLURAZEPAM HYDROCHLORIDE — ORAL

For complete and comparative prescribing information, refer to the Benzodiazepines group monograph.

Indications

➤*Insomnia:* Flurazepam hydrochloride is a hypnotic agent useful for the treatment of insomnia characterized by difficulty in falling asleep, frequent nocturnal awakenings, or early morning awakening. Flurazepam hydrochloride can be used effectively in patients with recurring insomnia or poor sleeping habits, and in acute or chronic medical situations requiring restful sleep. Sleep laboratory studies have objectively determined that flurazepam hydrochloride is effective for at least 28 consecutive nights of drug administration. Since insomnia is often transient and intermittent, short-term use is usually sufficient. Prolonged use of hypnotics is usually not indicated and should only be undertaken concomitantly with appropriate evaluation of the patient.

Administration and Dosage

➤*Adults:*

Insomnia – 30 mg before bedtime. In some patients, 15 mg may suffice.

➤*Elderly:* Initial dosage is 15 mg before bedtime.

➤*Debilitated patients:* Initial dosage is 15 mg before bedtime.

➤*Storage/Stability:* Store at 15° to 30°C (59° to 86°F). Protect from light. Dispense in a tight, light-resistant container using a child-resistant closure.

TEMAZEPAM

c-iv	**Temazepam** (Mallinckrodt)	**Capsules; oral:** 7.5 mg	Lactose. (FOR SLEEP M 7.5 mg). Blue/Pink. In 100s.
c-iv	**Restoril** (Mallinckrodt)		Lactose. In 100s.
c-iv	**Temazepam** (Various, eg, McKesson, Mylan, Sandoz, UDL)	**Capsules; oral:** 15 mg	In 100s and 500s.
c-iv	**Restoril** (Mallinckrodt)		Lactose. (FOR SLEEP M RESTORIL 15 mg). Maroon/Pink. In 100s.

TEMAZEPAM

c-iv	Temazepam (Mallinckrodt)	Capsules; oral: 22.5 mg	Lactose. In 30s.
c-iv	Restoril (Mallinckrodt)		Lactose. (FOR SLEEP M RESTORIL 22.5 mg). Opaque blue. In 30s.
c-iv	Temazepam (Various, eg, McKesson, Mylan, Sandoz, UDL)	Capsules; oral: 30 mg	In 100s and 500s.
c-iv	Restoril (Mallinckrodt)		Lactose. (FOR SLEEP M RESTORIL 30 mg). Maroon/Blue. In 100s.

TEMAZEPAM — ORAL

For complete and comparative prescribing information, refer to the Benzodiazepines group monograph.

Indications

➤*Insomnia:* For the short-term treatment of insomnia (generally 7 to 10 days).

Administration and Dosage

➤*Adults:*

Insomnia –

Usual dosage: 15 mg at bedtime.

Dosage adjustment: 7.5 mg may be sufficient for some patients, and others may need 30 mg. In transient insomnia, a 7.5 mg dose may be sufficient to improve sleep latency.

➤*Elderly:* Initiate therapy with 7.5 mg until individual responses are determined.

Per the Beers list, temazepam doses greater than 15 mg should not be used because of increased sensitivity to benzodiazepines in elderly patients. Smaller doses may be effective as well as safer. Total daily doses should rarely exceed the suggested maximums.

➤*Debilitated patients:* Initiate therapy with 7.5 mg until individual responses are determined.

➤*Storage/Stability:* Store at 20° to 25°C (68° to 77°F). Dispense in a tight, light-resistant container.

TRIAZOLAM

c-iv	Triazolam (Various, eg, Geneva, Goldline, Par, Roxane)	Tablets: 0.125 mg	In 10s, 100s, 500s and UD 100s.
c-iv	Triazolam (Various, eg, Geneva, Goldline, Par, Roxane)	Tablets: 0.25 mg	In 10s, 100s, 500s and UD 100s.
c-iv	Halcion (Upjohn)		(0.25 Halcion 17). Blue, scored. In 100s, UD 100s, and *Visipak* 100s.

TRIAZOLAM — ORAL

For complete and comparative prescribing information, refer to the Benzodiazepines group monograph.

Indications

➤*Insomnia:* Triazolam is indicated for the short-term treatment of insomnia (generally 7 to 10 days). Use for more than 2 to 3 weeks requires complete reevaluation of the patient.

Administration and Dosage

➤*Adults:*

Insomnia –

Usual dosage: 0.25 mg at bedtime.

Maximum dose: 0.5 mg/day.

Dosage adjustment: A dose of 0.125 mg may be sufficient for some patients (eg, low body weight). A dose of 0.5 mg should be used only for exceptional patients who do not respond adequately to a trial of a lower dose because the risk of several adverse reactions increases with the size of the dose administered.

➤*Elderly:*

Insomnia –

Usual dosage: 0.125 to 0.25 mg to decrease the possibility of development of oversedation, dizziness, or impaired coordination in elderly patients.

Maximum dose: 0.25 mg/day.

The Beers list also recommends a maximum dose of 0.25 mg in the elderly because of increased sensitivity to benzodiazepines in elderly patients. Smaller doses may be effective as well as safer. Total daily doses should rarely exceed the suggested maximums.

Initial dosage: 0.125 mg.

Dosage adjustment: The 0.25 mg dose should be used only for exceptional patients who do not respond to a trial of the lower dose.

➤*Debilitated patients:* See Elderly for dosing.

➤*Storage/Stability:* Store at 20° to 25°C (68° to 77°F).

QUAZEPAM

c-iv	Doral (Questcor)	Tablets; oral: 7.5 mg	(7.5 Doral). Light orange w/white speckles. Capsule shaped. In 100s, 500s, UD 100s.
		15 mg	(15 Doral). Light orange w/white speckles. Capsule shaped. In 100s, 500s, UD 100s.

QUAZEPAM — ORAL

For complete and comparative prescribing information, refer to the Benzodiazepines group monograph.

Indications

➤*Insomnia:* Quazepam tablets are indicated for the treatment of insomnia characterized by difficulty in falling asleep, frequent nocturnal awakenings, or early morning awakenings. The effectiveness of quazepam has been established in placebo-controlled clinical studies of 5 nights' duration in acute and chronic insomnia. The sustained effectiveness of quazepam has been established in chronic insomnia in a sleep lab (polysomnographic) study of 28 nights duration.

Administration and Dosage

➤*Adults:*

Insomnia –

Initial dosage: 15 mg until individual responses are determined.

Dosage adjustment: In some patients, the dose may then be reduced to 7.5 mg.

➤*Elderly:*

Insomnia –

Initial dosage: 7.5 mg.

Dosage adjustment: If the initial dosage is not effective after 1 to 2 nights, dosage may be increased to 15 mg. In some patients, the dose may then be reduced to 7.5 mg.

Because the elderly may be more sensitive to benzodiazepines, attempts to reduce the nightly dosage after the first 1 or 2 nights of therapy are suggested.

➤*Debilitated patients:* Because debilitated patients may be more sensitive to benzodiazepines, attempts to reduce the nightly dosage after the first 1 or 2 nights of therapy are suggested.

➤*Storage/Stability:* Store at c 20° to 25°C (68° to 77°F). Protect unit doses from excessive moisture.

CHLORAL HYDRATE

c-iv	**Chloral Hydrate** (Various, eg, URL)	**Capsules:** 500 mg	In 100s, 500s, 1,000s, and UD 100s.
c-iv	**Somnote** (Breckenridge		(B-080). In 50s and UD 50s.
c-iv	**Chloral Hydrate** (Various, eg, Pharmaceutical Assoc., Roxane)	**Syrup:** 250 mg per 5 mL	In UD 10 mL (40s and 100s).
c-iv	**Chloral Hydrate** (Various, eg, UDL, URL)	**Syrup:** 500 mg per 5 mL	In pt, gal, and UD 5 mL (100s) and 10 mL (40s and 100s).

CHLORAL HYDRATE — ORAL

Refer to the general discussion beginning in the Sedative and Hypnotic, Nonbarbiturate introduction.

Indications

➤*Nocturnal sedation:* For nocturnal sedation.

➤*Preoperative sedation:* For use in preoperative sedation to lessen anxiety and induce sleep without depressing respiration or cough reflex.

➤*Postoperative pain; adjunct:* In postoperative care and control of pain as an adjunct to opiates and analgesics.

➤*Off-label uses:* Chloral hydrate has been used in infants and children for procedural sedation (See also Administration and Dosage).

Administration and Dosage

➤*Adults:*

Hypnotic –

Usual dosage: 500 mg to 1 g 15 to 30 minutes before bedtime or 30 minutes before surgery.

Maximum dose: Single doses or daily dosage should not exceed 2 g.

Sedative –

Usual dosage: 250 mg 3 times daily after meals.

Maximum dose: Single doses or daily dosage should not exceed 2 g.

➤*Children:*

Hypnotic – 50 mg/kg/day, up to 1 g per single dose. May be given in divided doses. (See also Off-label Dosing.)

Sedative – 25 mg/kg/day, up to 500 mg per single dose. May be given in divided doses. (See also Off-label Dosing.)

Dental sedation – Higher doses than those suggested by the manufacturer are generally used. Doses of 75 mg/kg supplemented by nitrous oxide may provide better sedation than the lower dose with no change in the vital signs or adverse effects.

Off-label dosing –

Hypnotic:

- *Neonatal* – 25 to 75 mg/kg per dose orally. Dilute or administer after a feeding to reduce gastric irritation.

Procedural sedation:

- *Usual dose* – 50 to 75 mg/kg/dose orally 30 to 60 minutes before procedure. May repeat the dose in 30 minutes if needed.
- *Maximum dose* – 120 mg/kg or 1 g total for infants and 2 g total for children.

Sedative:

- *Children –*
  Usual dosage: 25 to 50 mg/kg/day orally administered in divided doses every 6 to 8 hours.
  Maximum dose: 500 mg per dose.
- *Neonatal* – 25 to 75 mg/kg per dose by mouth. Dilute or administer after a feeding to reduce gastric irritation.

➤*Duration of therapy:* Chloral hydrate is effective as a hypnotic only for short-term use; it loses much of its effectiveness for inducing and maintaining sleep after 2 weeks of use.

➤*Administration:* Take capsules with a full glass of liquid. Swallow capsules whole do not chew. Administer syrup in ½ glass of water, fruit juice, or ginger ale.

Actions

➤*Pharmacology:* The mechanism of action by which the CNS is affected is not known. Hypnotic dosage produces mild cerebral depression and quiet, deep sleep. In therapeutic doses, chloral hydrate has little effect on respiration, blood pressure and reflexes. "Hangover" is less common than with most barbiturates and some benzodiazepines. It has generally been replaced by safer and more effective agents.

➤*Pharmacokinetics:* Chloral hydrate is readily absorbed and metabolized to trichloroethanol, the principal active metabolite. Trichloroethanol has a plasma half-life of 7 to 10 hours; plasma protein binding is 35% to 41%. The drug is converted in the liver and kidney to trichloroacetic acid and excreted in the urine and bile. Although inactive, trichloroacetic acid is 71% to 88% protein bound and can displace other acidic drugs from plasma protein binding sites.

Contraindications

Marked hepatic or renal impairment; severe cardiac disease; gastritis; hypersensitivity or idiosyncrasy to chloral derivatives.

Warnings/Precautions

➤*Cardiac disease:* Continued use of therapeutic doses does not have a deleterious effect on the heart. However, do not use large doses in patients with severe cardiac disease.

➤*GI conditions:* Avoid use in patients with esophagitis, gastritis or gastric or duodenal ulcers.

➤*Acute intermittent porphyria:* Acute intermittent porphyria attacks may be precipitated by chloral hydrate; use with caution in susceptible patients.

➤*Skin/mucous membrane irritation:* Chloral derivatives irritate the skin and mucous membranes; gastric necrosis has occurred following intoxicating doses.

➤*Tartrazine sensitivity:* Some of these products contain tartrazine, which may cause allergic-type reactions (including bronchial asthma) in susceptible individuals. Although the incidence of tartrazine sensitivity in the general population is low, it is frequently seen in patients who also have aspirin hypersensitivity. Specific products containing tartrazine are identified in the product listings.

➤*Drug abuse and dependence:* May be habit forming. Exercise caution in administering to patients prone to addiction. Slurred speech, incoordination, tremulousness and nystagmus should arouse suspicion. Drowsiness, lethargy and hangover are frequently observed from excessive drug intake.

Prolonged use of large doses may result in psychic and physical dependence. Tolerance and psychologic dependence may develop by the second week of continued administration. Chloral hydrate addicts may take huge doses of the drug (up to 12 g nightly). Sudden withdrawal may result in CNS excitation with tremor, anxiety, hallucinations or even delirium, which may be fatal. Gastritis, skin eruptions and parenchymatous renal injury may also occur. Undertake withdrawal in a hospital using supportive therapy similar to that used for barbiturate withdrawal.

➤*Hazardous tasks:* May produce drowsiness; patients should observe caution while driving or performing other tasks requiring alertness.

➤*Pregnancy: Category C.* Safety for use during pregnancy has not been established. Chloral hydrate crosses the placenta; chronic use during pregnancy may cause withdrawal symptoms in the neonate. Congenital defects have not been reported. Use only when clearly needed and when potential benefits outweigh potential hazards to the fetus.

➤*Lactation:* Chloral hydrate is excreted in breast milk; use by nursing mothers may cause sedation in the infant.

Drug Interactions

Chloral Hydrate Drug Interactions

Precipitant drug	Object drug[a]		Description
Alcohol	Chloral hydrate	⬆	Alcohol may have synergistic effects with chloral hydrate. With alcohol, there is mutual inhibition of metabolism in addition to the combined depressant effect.
Chloral hydrate	Alcohol		Disulfiram-like reactions (eg, increased respiration and pulse rate, flushing), although rare, have occurred. Avoid concomitant use.
Chloral hydrate	Anticoagulants, oral	⬆	Hypoprothrombinemic effects may occur by displacement from protein binding sites. However, this effect is usually small and fleeting. Monitor prothrombin levels and adjust coumarin dose accordingly.
Chloral hydrate	CNS depressants	⬆	CNS depressants (eg, barbiturates, narcotics) may have additive CNS effects with chloral hydrate coadministration.
CNS depressants	Chloral hydrate		
Furosemide	Chloral hydrate	⬆	Administration of chloral hydrate followed by IV furosemide may result in sweating, hot flashes, tachycardia, hypertension, weakness and nausea.
Chloral hydrate	Hydantoins	⬇	The elimination of phenytoin may be increased by concurrent chloral hydrate, possibly reducing its effectiveness.

[a] ⬆ = object drug increased; ⬇ = object drug decreased.

➤*Drug/Lab test interactions:* Chloral hydrate may interfere with the **copper sulfate test** for glycosuria (confirm suspected glycosuria by a glucose oxidase test), **fluorometric tests** for urine catecholamines (do not administer medication for 48 hours preceding the test) or **urinary 17-hydroxycorticosteroid determinations** (when using the Reddy, Jenkins and Thorn procedure).

CHLORAL HYDRATE — ORAL

Adverse Reactions

➤*CNS:* Somnambulism, disorientation, incoherence, paranoid behavior (occasional); excitement, delirium, drowsiness, staggering gait, ataxia, lightheadedness, vertigo, dizziness, nightmares, malaise, mental confusion, headache, hallucinations (rare).

➤*Dermatologic:* Allergic skin rashes including hives, erythema, eczematoid dermatitis, urticaria, scarlatiniform exanthems (occasional).

➤*GI:* Gastric irritation; nausea and vomiting (occasional); flatulence; diarrhea; unpleasant taste in mouth.

➤*Hematologic:* Leukopenia, eosinophilia (occasional).

➤*Miscellaneous:* Hangover, idiosyncratic syndrome, ketonuria (rare).

Overdosage

➤*Symptoms:* Stupor; coma; pinpoint pupils; hypotension; slow or rapid and shallow respiration; hypothermia; areflexia; muscle flaccidity.

Corrosive action – Nausea; vomiting; esophagitis; gastritis; hemorrhagic gastritis; gastric necrosis; enteritis.

Organ damage – Hepatic damage (jaundice); renal damage (albuminuria); cardiac damage (ventricular and atrial arrhythmias).

Doses greater than 2 g may produce symptoms of toxicity. The toxic oral dose of chloral hydrate for adults is approximately 5 to 10 g; however, death has occurred following doses of 1.25 and 3 g; some patients have survived after taking 36 g.

➤*Treatment:* Perform gastric lavage or induce vomiting to empty the stomach. Activated charcoal may prevent drug absorption. Treatment includes usual supportive measures. Refer to General Management of Acute Overdosage. Hemoperfusion and hemodialysis are effective, but peritoneal dialysis is not useful. Hemodialysis is reported to promote the clearance of trichloroethanol.

Patient Information

May cause GI upset. Take capsules with a full glass of water or fruit juice; swallow capsules whole – do not chew. Dilute syrup in a half glass of water or fruit juice.

May cause drowsiness; use caution when performing tasks requiring alertness. Avoid alcohol and other CNS depressants.

May be habit forming; do not discontinue the drug abruptly.

DEXMEDETOMIDINE

Rx	**Precedex** (Hospira)	**Injection, solution, concentrate:** 100 mcg/mL	Equiv. to dexmedetomidine hydrochloride 118 mcg. Preservative free. Sodium chloride 9 mg. In single-use 2 mL vials.

DEXMEDETOMIDINE HYDROCHLORIDE — INJECTION

Indications

➤*Intensive care unit sedation:* For sedation of initially intubated and mechanically ventilated patients during treatment in an intensive care unit (ICU) setting.

➤*Procedural sedation:* For sedation of nonintubated patients prior to and/or during surgical and other procedures.

➤*Off-label uses:*

Adjunct to epidural or spinal anesthesia – [2] = Fair documentation. Dexmedetomidine has been used successfully as an adjunct to spinal and epidural anesthesia. Data from 3 randomized, controlled trials suggest that its use may increase the duration of anesthesia and decrease the need for additional analgesic medications in the perioperative and postoperative periods. More data are needed to determine the clinical significance of its use, optimal dosing regimen, adverse events, and place in therapy.

Benzodiazepine withdrawal (adults) – [4] = Insufficient documentation. Dexmedetomidine has been used successfully in 3 patients to eliminate symptoms of withdrawal from benzodiazepines. Larger, controlled studies are needed to confirm this use and to determine additional safety data for the drug.

Benzodiazepine withdrawal (children) – [4] = Insufficient documentation. Dexmedetomidine has been reported in 1 case study in a patient 8 months of age to eliminate symptoms of withdrawal from benzodiazepines. Larger, controlled studies are needed to confirm this use and to determine additional safety data for the drug.

Cyclic vomiting syndrome (children) – [4] = Insufficient documentation. Data from 3 case reports suggest dexmedetomidine may reduce nausea and vomiting in children with cyclic vomiting syndrome. Randomized, controlled trials are needed to determine the dose, duration, and effects in this patient population.

Postanesthetic shivering (adults) – [2] = Fair documentation. Dexmedetomidine has been used successfully to prevent and treat postanesthetic shivering in more than 200 adults. Adverse events included higher sedation scores and increased intraoperative bradycardia, as well as longer times to extubation, orientation, and awakening, which resolved with no permanent negative outcomes. More data are needed to determine the optimal dosing regimen, adverse events, and place in therapy.

Postanesthetic shivering (children/adolescents) – [4] = Insufficient documentation. Dexmedetomidine has been used successfully to prevent and treat postanesthetic shivering in a small sample of 24 children. No adverse effects were observed. More data are needed to validate these results and determine the optimal dosing regimen, adverse events, and place in therapy.

Sedation during awake craniotomy – [2] = Fair documentation. Data from 3 controlled studies and a case series enrolling more than 175 patients indicate that dexmedetomidine can be used successfully to provide sedation during awake craniotomy, and may help reduce length of stay, as well as the need for other perioperative pharmacological interventions. Additional prospective, placebo-controlled trials are needed to determine an optimal dose and dexmedetomidine's specific place in therapy.

Other possible off-label uses – To treat shivering; as an adjunct to regional or general anesthesia; as a bridge to ICU sedation and analgesia; as a supplement to regional block in patients undergoing carotid endarterectomy; in selected patients with congestive heart failure; to control agitation while receiving noninvasive ventilatory support, such as mask continuous or bilevel positive airway pressure.

Administration and Dosage

➤*General dosing considerations:* Dexmedetomidine is not indicated for infusions lasting longer than 24 hours.

Dexmedetomidine injection is a concentrated solution and must be diluted prior to administration (see Preparation for Administration).

➤*Adults:*

Intensive care unit sedation –

Loading dose: Up to 1 mcg/kg over 10 minutes. For patients being converted from alternate sedative therapy, a loading dose may not be required.

Maintenance dosage: 0.2 to 0.7 mcg/kg/h.

Procedural sedation –

Loading dose: 1 mcg/kg over 10 minutes, including awake fiberoptic intubation patients. For less invasive procedures, such as ophthalmic surgery, a loading infusion of 0.5 mcg/kg over 10 minutes may be suitable.

Maintenance dosage: Initiate at 0.6 mcg/kg/h and titrate to achieve desired clinical effect, with doses ranging from 0.2 to 1 mcg/kg/h. For awake fiberoptic intubation patients, 0.7 mcg/kg/h is recommended until the endotracheal tube is secured.

Off-label dosing –

Adjunct to epidural or spinal anesthesia: [2] = Fair documentation. Doses used in studies included 1 mcg/kg intravenously (IV) as a loading dose followed by 0.4 mcg/kg/h continuous IV infusion, 0.5 mcg/kg IV as a loading dose followed by 0.4 mcg/kg/h continuous IV infusion, or 3 mcg administered intrathecally as a 1-time dose.

Benzodiazepine withdrawal (adults): [4] = Insufficient documentation.

• *IV* – Loading dose of 1 mcg/kg over 10 to 20 minutes, followed by a continuous infusion at a rate of 0.2 to 0.7 mcg/kg/h.

Postanesthetic shivering (adults): [2] = Fair documentation. 0.1 mcg/kg as a single bolus dose administered over 3 to 5 minutes, or a loading dose of 0.1 mcg/kg over 10 minutes followed by a maintenance infusion of 0.4 mcg/kg/h.

Sedation during awake craniotomy: [2] = Fair documentation. Doses studied for use in awake craniotomy ranged from a loading dose of 0.5 to 1 mcg/kg, followed by a continuous infusion of 0.1 to 0.7 mcg/kg/h. Food and Drug Administration (FDA)–approved dosing for dexmedetomidine for sedation in other clinical scenarios consists of a loading dose of 1 mcg/kg over 10 minutes, followed by a maintenance infusion of 0.2 to 0.7 mcg/kg/h, not to exceed 24 hours.

➤*Elderly:*

Intensive care unit sedation – A dose reduction should be considered.

Procedural sedation –

Loading dose: 0.5 mcg/kg over 10 minutes.

Maintenance dosage: A dose reduction should be considered.

➤*Hepatic function impairment:* A dose reduction should be considered.

➤*Dosage adjustment:* Because of possible pharmacodynamic interactions, a reduction in dosage of dexmedetomidine or other concomitant anesthetics, sedatives, hypnotics, or opioids may be required when coadministered.

➤*Preparation for administration:* Dexmedetomidine must be diluted in sodium chloride 0.9% solution to achieve required concentration (4 mcg/mL) prior to administration. Preparation of solutions is the same, whether for the loading dose or maintenance infusion.

To prepare the infusion, withdraw 2 mL of dexmedetomidine and add to 48 mL of sodium chloride 0.9% injection to a total of 50 mL. Shake gently to mix well.

➤*Administration:* Administer dexmedetomidine by continuous IV infusion using a controlled infusion device, not to exceed 24 hours.

➤*Admixture compatibility:*

Incompatibility – Dexmedetomidine infusion should not be coadministered through the same IV catheter with blood or plasma because physical compatibility has not been established.

Dexmedetomidine has been shown to be incompatible when administered with amphotericin B and diazepam.

Compatibility – Dexmedetomidine has been shown to be compatible when administered with the following IV fluids and drugs: sodium chloride 0.9% in

DEXMEDETOMIDINE HYDROCHLORIDE — INJECTION

water, dextrose 5% in water, mannitol 20%, Ringer's lactate solution, magnesium sulfate 100 mg/mL solution, potassium chloride 0.3% solution.

Compatibility studies have demonstrated the potential for absorption of dexmedetomidine to some types of natural rubber. Although dexmedetomidine is dosed to effect, it is advisable to use administration components made with synthetic or coated natural rubber gaskets.

➤*Storage/Stability:* Store at 25°C (77°F); excursions are permitted between 15° and 30°C (59° and 86°F).

Actions

➤*Pharmacology:* Dexmedetomidine is a relatively selective alpha-2 adrenergic agonist with sedative properties. Alpha-2 selectivity was observed in animals following slow IV infusion of low and medium doses (10 to 300 mcg/kg).

Both alpha-1 and alpha-2 activity was observed following slow IV infusion of high doses (1,000 mcg/kg or more) or with rapid IV administration.

➤*Pharmacokinetics:*

Dexmedetomidine Mean ± SD[a,b] Pharmacokinetic Parameters

Parameter	Loading infusion (min)/total infusion duration (h)			
	10/12	10/24	10/24	35/24
	Target plasma concentration (ng/mL)/dose (mcg/kg/h)			
	0.3/0.17	0.3/0.17	0.6/0.33	1.25/0.7
Half-life[c], h	1.78 ± 0.3	2.22 ± 0.59	2.23 ± 0.21	2.5 ± 0.61
Cl, L/h	46.3 ± 8.3	43.1 ± 6.5	35.3 ± 6.8	36.5 ± 7.5
Vd_{ss}, L	88.7 ± 22.9	102.4 ± 20.3	93.6 ± 17	99.6 ± 17.8
Average C_{ss}[d], ng/mL	0.27 ± 0.05	0.27 ± 0.05	0.67 ± 0.1	1.37 ± 0.2

[a] SD = standard deviation; Cl = clearance; Vd_{ss} = apparent volume of distribution at steady state.
[b] The loading doses for each of the groups were 0.5, 0.5, 1, and 2.2 mcg/kg, respectively.
[c] Presented as a harmonic mean and pseudo standard deviation.
[d] C_{ss} = steady-state concentration of dexmedetomidine (2.5- to 9-hour postdose samples for 12-hour infusion and 2.5- to 18-hour postdose samples for 24-hour infusions).

Absorption/Distribution – Following IV administration, dexmedetomidine exhibits a rapid distribution phase with a distribution half-life of approximately 6 minutes.

Dexmedetomidine exhibits linear pharmacokinetics in the dosage range of 0.2 to 0.7 mg/kg/h when administered by IV infusion for up to 24 hours.

The steady-state volume of distribution (Vd_{ss}) of dexmedetomidine is approximately 118 L. Dexmedetomidine pharmacokinetic parameters after maintenance dosages of 0.2 to 1.4 mcg/kg/h for more than 24 hours were similar to the pharmacokinetic parameters after maintenance dosing for less than 24 hours in other studies. Vd_{ss} was 152 L. Dexmedetomidine protein binding was assessed in the plasma of healthy men and women. The average protein binding was 94% and was constant across the different concentrations tested. Protein binding was similar in men and women. The fraction of dexmedetomidine that was bound to plasma proteins was statistically significantly decreased in subjects with hepatic impairment compared with healthy subjects.

Metabolism – Dexmedetomidine undergoes almost complete biotransformation, with very little unchanged dexmedetomidine excreted in urine and feces. Biotransformation involves both direct glucuronidation as well as cytochrome P450–mediated metabolism. The major metabolic pathways of dexmedetomidine are as follows: direct N-glucuronidation to inactive metabolites; aliphatic hydroxylation (mediated primarily by CYP2A6) of dexmedetomidine to generate 3-hydroxy dexmedetomidine, the glucuronide of 3-hydroxy dexmedetomidine, and 3-carboxy dexmedetomidine; and N-methylation of dexmedetomidine to generate 3-hydroxy N-methyl dexmedetomidine, 3-carboxy N-methyl dexmedetomidine, and N-methyl O-glucuronide dexmedetomidine.

Excretion – The terminal elimination half-life of dexmedetomidine is approximately 2 hours, and clearance is estimated to be approximately 39 L/h. The mean body weight associated with this clearance estimate was 72 kg. Pharmacokinetic parameters after dexmedetomidine maintenance doses of 0.2 to 1.4 mcg/kg/h for more than 24 hours were similar to those after maintenance dosing for less than 24 hours in other studies. The values for clearance and half-life were 39.4 L/h and 2.67 hours, respectively. A mass-balance study demonstrated that after 9 days, an average of 95% of the radioactivity following IV administration of radiolabeled dexmedetomidine was recovered in the urine and 4% in the feces. No unchanged dexmedetomidine was detected in the urine. Approximately 85% of the radioactivity recovered in the urine was excreted within 24 hours after the infusion. Fractionation of the radioactivity excreted in urine demonstrated that products of N-glucuronidation accounted for approximately 34% of the cumulative urinary excretion. In addition, aliphatic hydroxylation of parent drug to form 3-hydroxy dexmedetomidine, the glucuronide of 3-hydroxy dexmedetomidine, and 3-carboxylic acid dexmedetomidine together represented approximately 14% of the dose in urine. N-methylation of dexmedetomidine to form 3-hydroxy N-methyl dexmedetomidine, 3-carboxy N-methyl dexmedetomidine, and N-methyl O-glucuronide dexmedetomidine accounted for approximately 18% of the dose in urine. The N-methyl metabolite itself was a minor circulating component and was undetected in urine. Approximately 28% of the urinary metabolites have not been identified.

Special populations –

Hepatic function impairment: In subjects with varying degrees of hepatic impairment (Child-Pugh class A, B, or C), clearance values for dexmedetomidine were lower than in healthy subjects. The mean clearance values for patients with mild, moderate, and severe hepatic impairment were 74%, 64%, and 53%, respectively, of those observed in healthy subjects. Mean clearances for free drug were 59%, 51%, and 32%, respectively, of those observed in healthy subjects.

Although dexmedetomidine is dosed to effect, it may be necessary to consider a dose reduction in subjects with hepatic impairment.

Contraindications

None well documented.

Warnings/Precautions

➤*Administration:* Only administer dexmedetomidine if skilled in the management of patients in the intensive care or operating room setting. Because of the known pharmacological effects of dexmedetomidine, continuously monitor patients while they are receiving dexmedetomidine.

➤*Cardiovascular effects:* Clinically significant episodes of bradycardia and sinus arrest have been reported with dexmedetomidine administration in young, healthy volunteers with high vagal tone or with different routes of administration, including rapid IV or bolus administration.

Reports of hypotension and bradycardia have been associated with dexmedetomidine infusion. If medical intervention is required, treatment may include decreasing or stopping the infusion of dexmedetomidine, increasing the rate of IV fluid administration, elevating the lower extremities, and using pressor agents. Because dexmedetomidine has the potential to augment bradycardia induced by vagal stimuli, be prepared to intervene. Consider the IV administration of anticholinergic agents (eg, atropine, glycopyrrolate) to modify vagal tone. In clinical trials, atropine and glycopyrrolate were effective in the treatment of most episodes of dexmedetomidine-induced bradycardia. However, in some patients with significant cardiovascular dysfunction, more advanced resuscitative measures were required.

Transient hypertension has been observed primarily during the loading dose in association with the initial peripheral vasoconstrictive effects of dexmedetomidine. Treatment of transient hypertension has generally not been necessary, although reduction of the loading infusion rate may be desirable.

Exercise caution when administering dexmedetomidine injection to patients with advanced heart block or severe ventricular dysfunction. Because dexmedetomidine decreases sympathetic nervous system activity, hypotension and/or bradycardia may be expected to be more pronounced in patients with hypovolemia, diabetes mellitus, or chronic hypertension, and in elderly patients.

In clinical trials where other vasodilators or negative chronotropic agents were coadministered with dexmedetomidine, an additive pharmacodynamic effect was not observed. Nonetheless, exercise caution when such agents are coadministered.

➤*Alertness:* Some patients receiving dexmedetomidine have been observed to be arousable and alert when stimulated. Do not consider this alone as evidence of lack of efficacy in the absence of other clinical signs and symptoms.

➤*Withdrawal:*

Intensive care unit sedation – With administration up to 7 days, regardless of dose, 5% of dexmedetomidine subjects experienced at least 1 event related to withdrawal within the first 24 hours after discontinuing study drug and 3% of dexmedetomidine subjects experienced at least 1 event 24 to 48 hours after the end of study drug. The most common events were nausea, vomiting, and agitation.

Tachycardia and hypertension requiring intervention in 48 hours following study drug discontinuation occurred at frequencies of less than 5%. If tachycardia and/or hypertension occurs after discontinuation of dexmedetomidine, supportive therapy is indicated.

Procedural sedation – Withdrawal symptoms were not seen after discontinuation of short-term infusions of dexmedetomidine (less than 6 hours).

➤*Tolerance and tachyphylaxis:* Use of dexmedetomidine beyond 24 hours has been associated with tolerance and tachyphylaxis and a dose-related increase in adverse reactions.

➤*Hepatic function impairment:* Because dexmedetomidine clearance decreases with severity of hepatic impairment, consider dose reduction in patients with impaired hepatic function.

➤*Drug abuse and dependence:* Dexmedetomidine is not a controlled substance. The dependence potential of dexmedetomidine has not been studied in humans. However, because studies in rodents and primates have demonstrated that dexmedetomidine exhibits pharmacologic actions similar to those of clonidine, it is possible that dexmedetomidine may produce a clonidine-like withdrawal syndrome upon abrupt discontinuation.

➤*Pregnancy:* *Category C.* There are no adequate and well-controlled studies in pregnant women. Use dexmedetomidine during pregnancy only if the potential benefits justify the potential risk to the fetus.

Teratogenic –

Fetal toxicity, as evidenced by increased postimplantation losses and reduced live pups, was observed in rats at a subcutaneous dose of 200 mcg/kg. The no-effect dose was 20 mcg/kg (less than the maximum recommended human IV dose on a body surface area [BSA] comparison). In another reproductive toxicity study where dexmedetomidine was administered subcutaneously to pregnant rats at doses of 8 and 32 mcg/kg (representing a dose less than the maximum recommended human IV dose based on a BSA comparison) from gestation day 16 through weaning, lower offspring weights were observed. In addition, when offspring of the 32 mcg/kg group were allowed to mate, elevated fetal and embryocidal toxicity and delayed motor development were observed in second-generation offspring.

DEXMEDETOMIDINE HYDROCHLORIDE — INJECTION

Placental transfer of dexmedetomidine was observed when radiolabeled dexmedetomidine was administered subcutaneously to pregnant rats. In an in vitro human placenta study, placental transfer of dexmedetomidine occurred. Fetal exposure should be expected in humans.

➤*Lactation:* It is not known whether dexmedetomidine is excreted in human milk. Radiolabeled dexmedetomidine administered subcutaneously to lactating female rats was excreted in milk. Because many drugs are excreted in human milk, exercise caution when dexmedetomidine is administered to a breast-feeding woman.

➤*Children:* The efficacy, safety, and pharmacokinetics of dexmedetomidine in children younger than 18 years of age have not been established. Therefore, do not use dexmedetomidine in this population.

➤*Elderly:* A total of 729 patients in the ICU sedation clinical studies were 65 years of age and older. A total of 200 patients were 75 years of age and older. In patients older than 65 years of age, a higher incidence of bradycardia and hypotension was observed following administration of dexmedetomidine. Therefore, a dose reduction may be considered in patients older than 65 years of age.

A total of 131 patients in the procedural sedation clinical studies were 65 years of age and older. A total of 47 patients were 75 years of age and older. Hypotension occurred at a higher incidence in dexmedetomidine-treated patients 65 years of age and older (72%) and 75 years of age and older (74%) compared with patients younger than 65 years of age (47%). A reduced loading dose of 0.5 mcg/kg given over 10 minutes is recommended; consider a reduction in the maintenance infusion for patients older than 65 years of age.

➤*Monitoring:* Because of the known pharmacological effects of dexmedetomidine, continuously monitor patients while they are receiving dexmedetomidine.

Drug Interactions

➤*Anesthetics, sedatives, hypnotics, and opioids:* Coadministration of dexmedetomidine with anesthetics, sedatives, hypnotics, and opioids is likely to lead to an enhancement of effects. Specific studies have confirmed these effects with sevoflurane, isoflurane, propofol, alfentanil, and midazolam. No pharmacokinetic interactions between dexmedetomidine and isoflurane, propofol, alfentanil, and midazolam have been demonstrated. However, because of possible pharmacodynamic interactions, when coadministered with dexmedetomidine, a reduction in dosage of dexmedetomidine or the concomitant anesthetic, sedative, hypnotic, or opioid may be required.

Adverse Reactions

➤*Serious adverse reactions:* Use of dexmedetomidine has been associated with the following serious adverse reactions: bradycardia, hypotension, sinus arrest, and transient hypertension.

➤*Common adverse reactions:* Most common treatment-emergent reactions, occurring in more than 2% of patients in both ICU and procedural sedation studies, include bradycardia, dry mouth, and hypotension.

➤*Intensive care unit sedation:*

Dexmedetomidine Adverse Reactions in Intensive Care Unit Sedation (> 2%)[a]

Adverse reactions	All dexmedetomidine (n = 1,007)	Randomized dexmedetomidine (n = 798)	Placebo (n = 400)	Propofol (n = 188)
Cardiovascular				
Atrial fibrillation	4%	5%	3%	7%
Bradycardia	5%	5%	3%	0%
Hypertension	12%	13%	19%	4%
Hypotension	25%	24%	12%	13%
Sinus tachycardia	1%	1%	1%	2%
Tachycardia	2%	2%	4%	1%
Ventricular tachycardia	< 1%	1%	1%	5%
GI				
Dry mouth	4%	3%	1%	1%
Nausea	9%	9%	9%	11%
Vomiting	3%	3%	5%	3%
Metabolic/Nutritional				
Acidosis	1%	1%	1%	2%
Edema, peripheral	< 1%	0%	1%	2%
Hyperglycemia	2%	2%	2%	3%
Hypocalcemia	1%	1%	0%	2%
Hypovolemia	3%	3%	2%	5%
Respiratory				
Atelectasis	3%	3%	3%	6%
Hypoxia	2%	2%	2%	3%
Pleural effusion	2%	2%	1%	6%
Pulmonary edema	1%	1%	1%	3%
Wheezing	< 1%	1%	0%	2%
Miscellaneous				
Agitation	2%	2%	3%	1%
Anemia	2%	2%	2%	2%
Chills	2%	2%	3%	2%
Hyperthermia	2%	2%	3%	0%
Postprocedural hemorrhage	2%	2%	3%	4%
Pyrexia	4%	4%	4%	4%
Urine output decreased	1%	1%	0%	2%

[a] Twenty-six subjects in the all-dexmedetomidine group and 10 subjects in the randomized dexmedetomidine group had exposure for longer than 24 hours.

Adverse Reactions in Dexmedetomidine-Treated Patients in the Infusion < 24 Hours Intensive Care Unit Sedation Studies (> 1%)

Adverse reactions	Randomized dexmedetomidine (n = 387)	Placebo (n = 379)
Cardiovascular		
Atrial fibrillation	4%	3%
Bradycardia	7%	3%
Hypertension	16%	18%
Hypotension	28%	13%
Tachycardia	3%	5%
GI		
Dry mouth	3%	1%
Nausea	11%	9%
Vomiting	4%	6%
Hematologic		
Anemia	3%	2%
Hemorrhage	3%	4%
Metabolic		
Acidosis	2%	2%
Hyperglycemia	2%	2%
Respiratory		
Hypoxia	4%	4%
Pleural effusion	2%	1%
Miscellaneous		
Agitation	2%	3%
Fever	5%	4%
Hyperpyrexia	2%	3%
Oliguria	2%	< 1%
Pain	2%	2%
Rigors	2%	3%
Thirst	2%	< 1%

Adverse Reactions in Dexmedetomidine- or Midazolam-Treated Patients in the Long-Term (> 24 h) Intensive Care Unit Sedation Study

Adverse reactions	Dexmedetomidine (n = 244)	Midazolam (n = 122)
Cardiovascular		
Bradycardia[b]	42%	19%
Bradycardia requiring intervention	5%	1%
Diastolic hypertension[c]	12%	15%
Hypertension[c]	11%	15%
Hypertension requiring intervention[e]	19%	30%
Hypotension[a]	56%	56%
Hypotension requiring intervention	28%	27%
Systolic hypertension[c]	28%	42%
Tachycardia[d]	25%	44%

DEXMEDETOMIDINE HYDROCHLORIDE — INJECTION

Adverse Reactions in Dexmedetomidine- or Midazolam-Treated Patients in the Long-Term (> 24 h) Intensive Care Unit Sedation Study		
Adverse reactions	Dexmedetomidine (n = 244)	Midazolam (n = 122)
Tachycardia requiring intervention	10%	10%
Metabolic		
Generalized edema	2%	6%
Hyperglycemia	7%	2%
Hypoglycemia	5%	6%
Hypokalemia	9%	13%
Hypomagnesemia	1%	7%
Respiratory		
Acute respiratory distress syndrome	2%	1%
Respiratory failure	5%	3%
Miscellaneous		
Acute renal failure	2%	1%
Agitation	7%	6%
Constipation	6%	6%
Pyrexia	7%	2%

[a] Hypotension was defined in absolute terms as systolic blood pressure < 80 mm Hg or diastolic blood pressure < 50 mm Hg, or in relative terms as ≤ 30% lower than pre–study drug infusion value.
[b] Bradycardia was defined in absolute terms as < 40 beats per minute (bpm), or in relative terms as ≤ 30% lower than pre–study drug infusion value.
[c] Hypertension was defined in absolute terms as systolic blood pressure> 180 mm Hg or diastolic blood pressure > 100 mm Hg, or in relative terms as ≥ 30% higher than pre–study drug infusion value.
[d] Tachycardia was defined in absolute terms as > 120 bpm, or in relative terms as ≥ 30% higher than pre–study drug infusion value.
[e] Includes any type of hypertension.

The following adverse reactions occurred between 2% and 5% for dexmedetomidine and midazolam, respectively: acute renal failure (2.5%, 0.8%), acute respiratory distress syndrome (2.5%, 0.8%), and respiratory failure (4.5%, 3.3%).

Dexmedetomidine Dose-Related Adverse Reactions			
Adverse events	Dexmedetomidine ≤ 0.7 mcg/kg/h[a] (n = 95)	Dexmedetomidine > 0.7 to ≤ 1.1 mcg/kg/h[a] (n = 78)	Dexmedetomidine > 1.1 mcg/kg/h[a] (n = 71)
CNS			
Agitation	5%	8%	14%
Anxiety	5%	5%	9%
Respiratory			
Acute respiratory distress syndrome	1%	3%	9%
Respiratory failure	2%	6%	10%
Miscellaneous			
Atrial fibrillation	2%	4%	9%
Constipation	6%	5%	14%
Peripheral edema	3%	5%	7%

[a] Average maintenance dosage over the entire study drug administration.

➤*Procedural sedation:* The most frequent adverse reactions were bradycardia, dry mouth, and hypotension. The decrease in respiratory rate and hypoxia were similar between dexmedetomidine and comparator groups in both studies.

Dexmedetomidine Adverse Reactions in Procedural Sedation (> 2%)		
Adverse reactions	Dexmedetomidine (n = 318)	Placebo (n = 113)
Cardiovascular		
Bradycardia[a]	14%	4%
Hypertension[b]	13%	24%
Hypotension[c]	54%	30%
Tachycardia[d]	5%	17%
GI		
Dry mouth	3%	1%
Nausea	3%	2%
Respiratory		
Bradypnea	2%	4%
Hypoxia[e]	2%	3%
Respiratory depression[f]	37%	32%

[a] Bradycardia was defined in absolute and relative terms as < 40 bpm or ≤ 30% lower than pre–study drug infusion value.
[b] Hypertension was defined in absolute and relative terms as systolic blood pressure > 180 mm Hg or ≥ 30% higher than pre–study drug infusion value or diastolic blood pressure > 100 mm Hg.
[c] Hypotension was defined in absolute and relative terms as systolic blood pressure < 80 mm Hg or ≤ 30% lower than pre–study drug infusion value, or diastolic blood pressure < 50 mm Hg.
[d] Tachycardia was defined in absolute and relative terms as > 120 bpm or ≥ 30% greater than pre–study drug infusion value.
[e] Hypoxia was defined in absolute and relative terms as SpO_2 < 90% or 10% decrease from baseline.
[f] Respiratory depression was defined in absolute and relative terms as respiratory rate < 8 breaths or > 25% decrease from baseline.

➤*Postmarketing:*

Cardiovascular – Hypotension and bradycardia were the most common adverse reactions associated with the use of dexmedetomidine during post-approval use of the drug.

Arrhythmia, atrial fibrillation, atrioventricular (AV) block, blood pressure fluctuation, cardiac arrest, extrasystoles, heart block, heart disorder, hypertension, myocardial infarction, supraventricular tachycardia, tachycardia, T wave inversion, ventricular arrhythmia, ventricular tachycardia.

CNS – Agitation, confusion, convulsion, delirium, dizziness, hallucination, headache, illusion, neuralgia, neuritis, speech disorder.

GI – Abdominal pain, diarrhea, nausea, vomiting.

Hepatic – ALT, AST, hepatic function abnormal, hyperbilirubinemia, increased gamma-glutamyl transpeptidase.

Metabolic/Nutritional – Acidosis, hyperkalemia, hypoglycemia, hypovolemia, increased alkaline phosphatase, respiratory acidosis, thirst.

Renal – Oliguria, serum urea nitrogen increased.

Respiratory – Apnea, bronchospasm, dyspnea, hypercapnia, hypoventilation, hypoxia, pulmonary congestion.

Special senses – Abnormal vision, photopsia.

Miscellaneous – Anemia, fever, hemorrhage, hyperpyrexia, increased sweating, light anesthesia, pain, rigors.

Overdosage

➤*Symptoms:* The tolerability of dexmedetomidine was noted in 1 study in which healthy subjects were administered doses at and above the recommended dose of 0.2 to 0.7 mcg/kg/h. The maximum blood concentration achieved in this study was approximately 13 times the upper boundary of the therapeutic range. The most notable effects observed in 2 subjects who achieved the highest doses were first-degree AV block and second-degree heart block. No hemodynamic compromise was noted with the AV block, and the heart block resolved spontaneously within 1 minute.

Five patients received an overdose of dexmedetomidine in the ICU sedation studies. Two of these patients had no symptoms reported; 1 patient received a 2 mcg/kg loading dose over 10 minutes (twice the recommended loading dose), and 1 patient received a maintenance infusion of 0.8 mcg/kg/h. Two other patients who received a 2 mcg/kg loading dose over 10 minutes experienced bradycardia and/or hypotension. One patient who received a loading bolus dose of undiluted dexmedetomidine (19.4 mcg/kg) had cardiac arrest, from which he was successfully resuscitated.

Patient Information

Inform patients that dexmedetomidine is indicated for short-term IV sedation. Dosage must be individualized and titrated to the desired clinical effect. Blood pressure, heart rate, and oxygen levels will be monitored continuously during the infusion of dexmedetomidine and as clinically appropriate after discontinuation.

When dexmedetomidine is infused for more than 6 hours, instruct patients to report nervousness, agitation, and headaches that may occur for up to 48 hours.

Advise patients to report symptoms that may occur within 48 hours after the administration of dexmedetomidine, such as weakness, confusion, excessive sweating, weight loss, abdominal pain, salt cravings, diarrhea, constipation, dizziness, or light-headedness.

ESZOPICLONE

c-iv	**Lunesta** (Sepracor)	**Tablets; oral:** 1 mg	Lactose, PEG. (S190). Lt. blue. Film-coated. In 100s.
		2 mg	Lactose, PEG. (S191). Film-coated. In 100s and cartons of 90.
		3 mg	Lactose, PEG. (S193). Dk. blue. Film-coated. In 100s and cartons of 90.

ESZOPICLONE — ORAL

Indications

➤*Insomnia:* For the treatment of insomnia.

Administration and Dosage

➤*Adults:*

Insomnia –

Initial dosage: 2 mg immediately before bedtime.

Dosage adjustment: Dosing can be initiated at or raised to 3 mg if clinically indicated because 3 mg is more effective for sleep maintenance.

➤*Elderly:* For elderly patients whose primary complaint is difficulty falling asleep, the starting dose is 1 mg immediately before bedtime. In these patients, the dose may be increased to 2 mg if clinically indicated.

For elderly patients whose primary complaint is difficulty staying asleep, the recommended dose is 2 mg immediately before bedtime.

➤*Hepatic function impairment:* The starting dose should be 1 mg in patients with severe hepatic function impairment. Use eszopiclone with caution in these patients.

➤*Coadministration with CYP-450 3A4 inhibitors:* The starting dose should not exceed 1 mg in patients coadministered eszopiclone with potent CYP3A4 inhibitors. If needed, the dose can be raised to 2 mg.

➤*Administration:* Swallow tablets whole. Avoid taking with meals. Taking eszopiclone with or immediately after a heavy, high-fat meal results in slower absorption and would be expected to reduce the effect of eszopiclone on sleep latency.

➤*Storage/Stability:* Store at 25°C (77°F); excursions are permitted between 15° and 30°C (59° and 86°F).

Actions

➤*Pharmacology:* The precise mechanism of action of eszopiclone as a hypnotic is unknown, but its effect is believed to result from its interaction with gamma-aminobutyric acid (GABA)–receptor complexes at binding domains located close to or allosterically coupled to benzodiazepine receptors. Eszopiclone is a nonbenzodiazepine hypnotic that is a pyrrolopyrazine derivative of the cyclopyrrolone class, with a chemical structure unrelated to barbiturates, benzodiazepines, imidazopyridines, pyrazolopyrimidines, or other drugs with known hypnotic properties.

➤*Pharmacokinetics:*

Absorption/Distribution –

Eszopiclone is rapidly absorbed following oral administration. Peak plasma concentrations are achieved within approximately 1 hour after oral administration. In healthy adults, eszopiclone does not accumulate with once-daily administration, and its exposure is dose-proportional over the range of 1 to 6 mg. Eszopiclone is weakly bound to plasma protein (52% to 59%). The large free fraction suggests that eszopiclone disposition should not be affected by drug-drug interactions caused by protein binding. The blood-to-plasma ratio for eszopiclone is less than 1, indicating no selective uptake by red blood cells.

Effect of food: In healthy adults, administration of eszopiclone 3 mg after a high-fat meal resulted in no change in the area under the curve (AUC), a reduction in mean maximal drug concentration (C_{max}) of 21%, and delayed time to peak concentration (T_{max}) by approximately 1 hour. The half-life remained unchanged, approximately 6 hours. The effects of eszopiclone on sleep onset may be reduced if it is taken with or immediately after a high-fat/heavy meal.

Metabolism – Following oral administration, eszopiclone is extensively metabolized by oxidation and demethylation. The primary plasma metabolites are (*S*)-zopiclone-N-oxide and (*S*)-N-desmethyl zopiclone; the latter compound binds to GABA receptors with substantially lower potency than eszopiclone, and the former compound shows no significant binding to this receptor. In vitro studies have shown that CYP3A4 and CYP2E1 enzymes are involved in the metabolism of eszopiclone. Eszopiclone did not show any inhibitory potential on CYP1A2, 2A6, 2C9, 2C19, 2D6, 2E1, and 3A4 in cryopreserved human hepatocytes.

Excretion – After oral administration, eszopiclone is eliminated with a mean half-life of approximately 6 hours. Up to 75% of an oral dose of racemic zopiclone is excreted in the urine, primarily as metabolites. A similar excretion profile would be expected for eszopiclone, the S-isomer of racemic zopiclone. Less than 10% of the oral eszopiclone dose is excreted in the urine as parent drug.

Special populations –

Hepatic function impairment: The pharmacokinetics of eszopiclone 2 mg were assessed in 16 healthy volunteers and 8 subjects with mild, moderate, and severe liver disease. Exposure was increased 2-fold in patients with severe impairment compared with healthy volunteers. C_{max} and T_{max} were unchanged. Do not increase the dose of eszopiclone above 2 mg in patients with severe hepatic function impairment. No dose adjustment is necessary for patients with mild to moderate hepatic function impairment. Use eszopiclone with caution in patients with hepatic function impairment.

Elderly: Compared with nonelderly adults, subjects 65 years of age and older had an increase of 41% in total exposure (AUC) and a slightly prolonged elimination of eszopiclone (half-life, approximately 9 hours). C_{max} was unchanged. Therefore, decrease the starting dose of eszopiclone to 1 mg in elderly patients. The dose should not exceed 2 mg.

Contraindications

None known.

Warnings/Precautions

➤*Psychiatric/Physical disorder:* Because sleep disturbances may be the presenting manifestation of a physical and/or psychiatric disorder, initiate symptomatic treatment of insomnia only after careful evaluation of the patient. The failure of insomnia to remit after 7 to 10 days of treatment may indicate the presence of a primary psychiatric and/or medical illness that should be evaluated. Worsening of insomnia or the emergence of new thinking or behavior abnormalities may be the consequence of an unrecognized psychiatric or physical disorder. Such findings have emerged during the course of treatment with sedative/hypnotic drugs, including eszopiclone. Because some of the important adverse reactions of eszopiclone appear to be dose related, use the lowest possible effective dose, especially in elderly patients.

➤*Abnormal thinking and behavioral changes:* A variety of abnormal thinking and behavioral changes have been reported to occur in association with the use of sedative/hypnotic drugs. Some of these changes may be characterized by decreased inhibition (ie, aggressiveness and extroversion that seem out of character) similar to effects produced by alcohol and other CNS depressants. Other reported behavioral changes have included agitation, bizarre behavior, depersonalization, and hallucinations. Complex behaviors such as sleep-driving (ie, driving while not fully awake after ingestion of a sedative/hypnotic, with amnesia for the reaction) have been reported. These reactions can occur in sedative/hypnotic-naive and sedative/hypnotic-experienced people. Although behaviors such as sleep-driving may occur with eszopiclone alone at therapeutic doses, the use of alcohol and other CNS depressants with eszopiclone appears to increase the risk of such behaviors, as does the use of eszopiclone at doses exceeding the maximum recommended dose. Because of the risk to the patients and the community, strongly consider discontinuation of eszopiclone for patients who report a sleep-driving episode. Other complex behaviors (eg, having sex, making phone calls, preparing and eating food) have been reported in patients who are not fully awake after taking a sedative/hypnotic. As with sleep-driving, patients usually do not remember these events. Amnesia and other neuropsychiatric symptoms may occur unpredictably. In primarily depressed patients, worsening of depression, including suicidal thoughts and actions (including completed suicides), have been reported in association with the use of sedative/hypnotic drugs.

It can rarely be determined with certainty whether a particular instance of the abnormal behaviors previously listed are drug induced, spontaneous in origin, or a result of an underlying psychiatric or physical disorder. Nonetheless, the emergence of any new behavioral sign or symptom of concern requires careful and immediate evaluation.

➤*Rapid dose decrease/discontinuation:* Following rapid dose decrease or abrupt discontinuation of the use of a sedative/hypnotic, there have been reports of signs and symptoms similar to those associated with withdrawal from other CNS-depressant drugs.

➤*CNS effects:* Eszopiclone, like other hypnotics, has CNS-depressant effects. Because of the rapid onset of action, the patient should ingest eszopiclone immediately prior to going to bed or after having gone to bed and experiencing difficulty falling asleep. Eszopiclone, like other hypnotic drugs, may produce additive CNS-depressant effects when coadministered with anticonvulsants, antihistamines, ethanol, psychotropic medications, and other drugs that produce CNS depression. Eszopiclone should not be taken with alcohol. Dose adjustment may be necessary when eszopiclone is administered with other CNS-depressant agents because of the potentially additive effects.

➤*Administration:* Take eszopiclone immediately before bedtime. Taking a sedative/hypnotic while still ambulatory may result in dizziness, hallucinations, impaired coordination, light-headedness, and short-term memory impairment.

➤*Elderly/Debilitated patients:* Impaired motor and/or cognitive performance after repeated exposure or unusual sensitivity to sedative/hypnotic drugs is a concern in the treatment of elderly and/or debilitated patients. The recommended starting dose of eszopiclone for these patients is 1 mg.

➤*Concomitant illness:* Clinical experience with eszopiclone in patients with concomitant illness is limited. Use eszopiclone with caution in patients with diseases or conditions that could affect metabolism or hemodynamic responses.

A study in healthy volunteers did not reveal respiratory-depressant effects at doses 2.5-fold higher (7 mg) than the recommended dose of eszopiclone. However, caution is advised if eszopiclone is prescribed to patients with compromised respiratory function.

➤*Depression:* Administer sedative/hypnotic drugs with caution to patients exhibiting signs and symptoms of depression. Suicidal tendencies may be present in such patients, and protective measures may be required. Intentional overdose is more common in this group of patients; therefore, prescribe the least amount of drug that is feasible for the patient at any one time.

➤*Hypersensitivity reactions:* Rare cases of angioedema involving the tongue, glottis, or larynx have been reported in patients after taking the first or subsequent doses of sedative/hypnotic drugs, including eszopiclone. Some patients have had additional symptoms such as dyspnea, nausea and vomiting, or throat closing that suggest anaphylaxis. Some patients have required medical therapy in the emergency department. If angioedema involves the tongue, glottis, or larynx, airway obstruction may occur and be fatal. Do not rechallenge patients who develop angioedema after treatment with eszopiclone.

ESZOPICLONE — ORAL

➤*Hepatic function impairment:* Reduce the dose of eszopiclone to 1 mg in patients with severe hepatic function impairment because systemic exposure is doubled in such subjects.

➤*Drug abuse and dependence:*

Abuse and dependence – In a study of abuse liability conducted in individuals with known histories of benzodiazepine abuse, doses of eszopiclone 6 and 12 mg produced euphoric effects similar to those of diazepam 20 mg. In this study, at doses 2-fold or greater than the maximum recommended doses, a dose-related increase in reports of amnesia and hallucinations was observed for eszopiclone and diazepam.

The clinical trial experience with eszopiclone revealed no evidence of a serious withdrawal syndrome. Nevertheless, the following adverse reactions included in *Diagnostic and Statistical Manual of Mental Disorders* (Fourth Edition) (*DSM-IV*) criteria for uncomplicated sedative/hypnotic withdrawal were reported during clinical trials following placebo substitution within 48 hours of the last eszopiclone treatment: abnormal dreams, anxiety, nausea, and upset stomach. These reported adverse reactions occurred at an incidence of 2% or less. Use of benzodiazepines and similar agents may lead to physical and psychological dependence. The risk of abuse and dependence increases with the dose and duration of treatment and concomitant use of other psychoactive drugs. The risk is also greater for patients who have a history of alcohol or drug abuse or a history of psychiatric disorders. Place these patients under careful surveillance when they are receiving eszopiclone or any other hypnotic.

➤*Hazardous tasks:* Caution patients receiving eszopiclone against engaging in hazardous occupations requiring complete mental alertness or motor coordination (eg, driving a motor vehicle, operating machinery) after ingesting the drug. Also, caution them about potential impairment of the performance of such activities on the day following ingestion of eszopiclone.

➤*Pregnancy: Category C.* In rats, slight reductions in fetal weight and evidence of developmental delay were seen at maternally toxic doses of 125 and 150 mg/kg/day, but not at 62.5 mg/kg/day (200 times the MRHD on a mg/m^2 basis).

Eszopiclone also was administered by oral gavage to pregnant rats throughout pregnancy and lactation at doses of up to 180 mg/kg/day. Increased postimplantation loss, decreased postnatal pup weights and survival, and increased pup startle response were seen at all doses; the lowest dose tested, 60 mg/kg/day, is 200 times the MRHD on a mg/m^2 basis. These doses did not produce significant maternal toxicity. Eszopiclone had no effects on other behavioral measures or reproductive function in the offspring.

There are no adequate and well-controlled studies of eszopiclone in pregnant women. Use eszopiclone during pregnancy only if the potential benefit justifies the potential risk to the fetus.

➤*Lactation:* It is not known whether eszopiclone is excreted in human milk. Because many drugs are excreted in human milk, exercise caution when eszopiclone is administered to a breast-feeding woman.

➤*Children:* Safety and efficacy of eszopiclone in children younger than 18 years of age have not been established.

➤*Elderly:* Eszopiclone 2 mg exhibited significant reduction in sleep latency and improvement in sleep maintenance in the elderly population.

Drug Interactions

Eszopiclone Drug Interactions

Precipitant drug	Object drug[a]		Description
CNS depressants (eg, ethanol)	Eszopiclone	↑	An additive effect on psychomotor performance was seen with coadministration of eszopiclone and ethanol 0.7 g/kg for up to 4 hours after ethanol administration.
Eszopiclone	CNS depressants (eg, ethanol)		
CYP3A4 inducers (eg, rifampin)	Eszopiclone	↓	Racemic zopiclone exposure was decreased 80% by concomitant use of rifampin. A similar effect would be expected with eszopiclone.
CYP3A4 inhibitors (eg, clarithromycin, itraconazole, ketoconazole, nefazodone, nelfinavir, ritonavir)	Eszopiclone	↑	The AUC, C_{max}, and half-life of eszopiclone may be increased when given with a strong CYP3A4 inhibitor. Do not exceed a starting dose of eszopiclone 1 mg when coadministered with potent CYP3A4 inhibitors.
Lorazepam	Eszopiclone	↓	Eszopiclone and lorazepam decreased each other's C_{max} by 22%.
Eszopiclone	Lorazepam		

[a] ↓ = object drug decreased; ↑ = object drug increased.

➤*Drug/Food interactions:* See Actions for more information.

Adverse Reactions

➤*Discontinuation:* In placebo-controlled, parallel-group clinical trials in elderly patients, 3.8% of 208 patients who received placebo, 2.3% of 215 patients who received eszopiclone 2 mg, and 1.4% of 72 patients who received eszopiclone 1 mg discontinued treatment because of an adverse reaction. In the 6-week, parallel-group study in adults, no patients in the 3 mg arm discontinued because of an adverse reaction. In the long-term, 6-month study in adult insomnia patients, 7.2% of 195 patients who received placebo and 12.8% of 593 patients who received eszopiclone 3 mg discontinued because of an adverse reaction. No reaction that resulted in discontinuation occurred at a rate of greater than 2%.

➤*Adverse reactions (≥ 2%):*

Eszopiclone Adverse Reactions in Nonelderly Adults (≥ 2%)[a]

Adverse reaction	Placebo (n = 99)	Eszopiclone 2 mg (n = 104)	Eszopiclone 3 mg (n = 105)
CNS			
Anxiety	0%	3%	1%
Confusion	0%	0%	3%
Depression	0%	4%	1%
Dizziness	4%	5%	7%
Hallucinations	0%	1%	3%
Headache	13%	21%	17%
Libido decreased	0%	0%	3%
Nervousness	3%	5%	0%
Somnolence	3%	10%	8%
Dermatologic			
Rash	1%	3%	4%
GI			
Dry mouth	3%	5%	7%
Dyspepsia	4%	4%	5%
Nausea	4%	5%	4%
Unpleasant taste	3%	17%	34%
Vomiting	1%	3%	0%
GU			
Dysmenorrhea[b]	0%	3%	0%
Gynecomastia[c]	0%	3%	0%
Miscellaneous			
Infection	3%	5%	10%
Viral infection	1%	3%	3%

[a] Reactions for which the eszopiclone incidence was equal to or less than placebo are not listed in the table, but included the following: abnormal dreams, accidental injury, back pain, diarrhea, flu syndrome, myalgia, pain, pharyngitis, and rhinitis.
[b] Gender-specific adverse reactions in women.
[c] Gender-specific adverse reactions in men.

Adverse reactions from the previous table that suggest a dose-response relationship in adults include dizziness, dry mouth, hallucinations, infection, rash, unpleasant taste, and viral infection, with this relationship most clear for unpleasant taste.

The following table shows the incidence of treatment-emergent adverse reactions from combined phase 3, placebo-controlled studies of eszopiclone at doses of 1 or 2 mg in elderly adults (65 to 86 years of age).

Treatment duration in these trials was 14 days. The table includes only reactions that occurred in 2% or more of patients treated with eszopiclone 1 or 2 mg in which the incidence in patients treated with eszopiclone was greater than the incidence in placebo-treated patients.

Eszopiclone Adverse Reactions in Elderly Adults (65 to 86 Years of Age) (≥ 2%)[a]

Adverse reaction	Placebo (n = 208)	Eszopiclone 1 mg (n = 72)	Eszopiclone 2 mg (n = 215)
CNS			
Abnormal dreams	0%	3%	1%
Dizziness	2%	1%	6%
Headache	14%	15%	13%
Nervousness	1%	0%	2%
Neuralgia	0%	3%	0%
Dermatologic			
Pruritus	1%	4%	1%
GI			
Diarrhea	2%	4%	2%
Dry mouth	2%	3%	7%
Dyspepsia	2%	6%	2%
Unpleasant taste	0%	8%	12%
GU			
Urinary tract infection	0%	3%	0%

ESZOPICLONE — ORAL

Eszopiclone Adverse Reactions in Elderly Adults (65 to 86 Years of Age) (≥ 2%)[a]			
Adverse reaction	Placebo (n = 208)	Eszopiclone 1 mg (n = 72)	Eszopiclone 2 mg (n = 215)
Miscellaneous			
Accidental injury	1%	0%	3%
Pain	2%	4%	5%

[a] Reactions for which the eszopiclone incidence was equal to or less than placebo are not listed in the table, but included the following: abdominal pain, asthenia, nausea, rash, and somnolence.

Adverse reactions from the previous table that suggest a dose-response relationship in elderly adults include dry mouth, pain, and unpleasant taste, with this relationship, again, clearest for unpleasant taste.

➤*Other adverse reactions:*

Cardiovascular – Hypertension (0.1% to less than 1%); thrombophlebitis (less than 0.1%).

CNS – Migraine (1% or more); agitation, apathy, ataxia, emotional lability, hostility, hypertonia, hypesthesia, incoordination, insomnia, memory impairment, neurosis, paresthesia, reflexes decreased, thinking abnormal (mainly difficulty concentrating), vertigo (0.1% to less than 1%); abnormal gait, euphoria, hyperesthesia, hypokinesia, neuritis, neuropathy, stupor, tremor (less than 0.1%).

Dermatologic – Acne, alopecia, contact dermatitis, dry skin, eczema, skin discoloration, sweating, urticaria (0.1% to less than 1%); erythema multiforme, furunculosis, herpes zoster, hirsutism, maculopapular rash, vesiculobullous rash (less than 0.1%).

GI – Anorexia, cholelithiasis, increased appetite, melena, mouth ulceration, thirst, ulcerative stomatitis (0.1% to less than 1%); colitis, dysphagia, gastritis, hepatitis, hepatomegaly, liver damage, rectal hemorrhage, stomach ulcer, stomatitis, tongue edema (less than 0.1%).

GU – Amenorrhea, breast engorgement, breast enlargement, breast neoplasm, breast pain, cystitis, dysuria, female lactation, hematuria, kidney calculus, kidney pain, mastitis, menorrhagia, metrorrhagia, urinary frequency, urinary incontinence, uterine hemorrhage, vaginal hemorrhage, vaginitis (0.1% to less than 1%); oliguria, pyelonephritis, urethritis (less than 0.1%).

Hematologic/Lymphatic – Anemia, lymphadenopathy (0.1% to less than 1%).

Metabolic/Nutritional – Peripheral edema (1% or more); hypercholesteremia, weight gain, weight loss (0.1% to less than 1%); dehydration, gout, hyperlipemia, hypokalemia (less than 0.1%).

Musculoskeletal – Arthritis, bursitis, joint disorder (mainly pain, stiffness, and swelling), leg cramps, myasthenia, twitching (0.1% to less than 1%); arthrosis, myopathy, ptosis (less than 0.1%).

Respiratory – Asthma, bronchitis, dyspnea, epistaxis, hiccup, laryngitis (0.1% to less than 1%).

Special senses – Conjunctivitis, dry eyes, ear pain, nystagmus, otitis externa, otitis media, tinnitus, vestibular disorder (0.1% to less than 1%); hyperacusis, iritis, mydriasis, photophobia (less than 0.1%).

Miscellaneous – Chest pain (1% or more); allergic reaction, cellulitis, face edema, fever, halitosis, heat stroke, hernia, malaise, neck rigidity, photosensitivity (0.1% to less than 1%).

Overdosage

➤*Symptoms:* Signs and symptoms of overdose of CNS depressants can be expected to present as exaggerations of the pharmacological effects noted in preclinical testing. Impairment of consciousness ranging from somnolence to coma has been described. Rare individual instances of fatal outcomes following overdose with racemic zopiclone have been reported in European postmarketing reports, most often associated with overdose of other CNS-depressant agents.

➤*Treatment:* Use general symptomatic and supportive measures along with immediate gastric lavage when appropriate. Administer intravenous fluids as needed. Flumazenil may be useful. As in all cases of drug overdose, monitor respiration, pulse, blood pressure, and other appropriate signs, and employ general supportive measures. Monitor hypotension and CNS depression and treat by appropriate medical intervention. The value of dialysis in the treatment of overdosage has not been determined.

As with the management of all overdosage, consider the possibility of multiple drug ingestion. The health care provider may wish to consider contacting a poison control center (1-800-221-2222) for up-to-date information on the management of hypnotic drug product overdosage.

Patient Information

There have been reports of people getting out of bed after taking a sedative/hypnotic drug and driving their cars while not fully awake, often with no memory of the event. If patients experience such an episode, advise them to report it to their health care provider immediately because sleep-driving can be dangerous. This behavior is more likely to occur when eszopiclone is taken with alcohol or CNS depressants. Other complex behaviors (eg, having sex, making phone calls, preparing and eating food) have been reported in patients who are not fully awake after taking a sedative-hypnotic drug. As with sleep-driving, patients usually do not remember these events.

Caution patients receiving eszopiclone against engaging in hazardous activities requiring complete mental alertness or motor coordination (eg, operating machinery, driving a motor vehicle) after ingesting the drug, and caution them about potential impairment of the performance of such activities on the day following ingestion of eszopiclone.

Instruct patients to take eszopiclone immediately prior to going to bed and only if they can dedicate 8 hours to sleep.

Instruct patients not to take eszopiclone with alcohol or with other sedating medications.

Advise patients to consult with their health care providers if they have a history of depression, mental illness, or suicidal thoughts, have a history of drug or alcohol abuse, or have liver disease.

Advise women to contact their health care provider if they become pregnant, plan to become pregnant, or if they are breast-feeding.

Advise patients that taking eszopiclone with or immediately after a heavy, high-fat meal results in slower absorption and would be expected to reduce the effect of eszopiclone on sleep latency.

SEDATIVES AND HYPNOTICS, BARBITURATES

The following general discussion of the barbiturates refers to their use as sedative-hypnotic agents and as anticonvulsants. In addition, barbiturates are discussed under General Anesthetics, Barbiturates.

Indications

The following indications apply to most barbiturates. For specific indications, refer to the individual monographs.

➤*Acute convulsive episodes:* Emergency control of certain acute convulsive episodes (eg, those associated with status epilepticus, cholera, eclampsia, meningitis, tetanus, and toxic reactions to strychnine or local anesthetics).

➤*Anticonvulsant (mephobarbital, phenobarbital):* Treatment of partial and generalized tonic-clonic and cortical focal seizures.

➤*Hypnotic:* Short-term treatment of insomnia, since barbiturates appear to lose their effectiveness in sleep induction and maintenance after 2 weeks. If insomnia persists, seek alternative therapy (including nondrug) for chronic insomnia.

➤*Preanesthetic:* Used as preanesthetic sedatives.

➤*Sedation:* Although traditionally used as nonspecific CNS depressants for daytime sedation, the barbiturates generally have been replaced by the benzodiazepines.

Administration and Dosage

Individualize dosage; consider patient's age, weight and condition. Use parenteral routes only when oral administration is impossible or impractical.

➤*Intramuscular (IM) injection:* IM injection of the sodium salts should be made deeply into a large muscle. Do not exceed 5 mL at any one site because of possible tissue irritation. Monitor patient's vital signs.

➤*Intravenous (IV):* Restrict to conditions in which other routes are not feasible, either because the patient is unconscious (as in cerebral hemorrhage, eclampsia or status epilepticus), or because the patient resists (as in delirium), or because prompt action is imperative. Slow IV injection is essential; observe patients carefully during administration. Maintain blood pressure, respiratory and cardiac function, monitor vital signs, and have equipment for resuscitation and artificial ventilation available.

➤*Rectal administration:* Rectally administered barbiturates are absorbed from the colon and are used occasionally in infants for prolonged convulsive states, or when oral or parenteral administration may be undesirable. If the rectal form is not available, the soluble sodium salt may be incorporated in a retention enema.

➤*Elderly/Debilitated:* Reduce dosage because these patients may be more sensitive to barbiturates.

➤*Hepatic/Renal function impairment:* Reduce dosage.

Actions

➤*Pharmacology:* Barbiturates can produce all levels of CNS mood alteration from excitation to mild sedation, hypnosis, and deep coma. In sufficiently high therapeutic doses, barbiturates induce anesthesia. Overdosage can produce death.

These agents depress the sensory cortex, decrease motor activity, alter cerebellar function, and produce drowsiness, sedation, and hypnosis.

Barbiturates have little analgesic action at subanesthetic doses and may increase the reaction to painful stimuli. All barbiturates exhibit anticonvulsant activity in anesthetic doses. However, only phenobarbital and mephobarbital are effective as oral anticonvulsants in subhypnotic doses.

Barbiturates are respiratory depressants; the degree of respiratory depression is dose-dependent. With hypnotic doses, respiratory depression is similar to that which occurs during physiologic sleep and is accompanied by a slight decrease in blood pressure and heart rate.

➤*Pharmacokinetics:*

Absorption – Barbiturates are absorbed in varying degrees following oral, rectal, or parenteral administration. The salts are more rapidly absorbed than the acids. The rate of absorption is increased if the sodium salt is ingested as a dilute solution or taken on an empty stomach.

Onset: Onset of action for oral or rectal administration varies from 20 to 60 minutes. For IM administration, onset is slightly faster than the oral route. Following IV administration, onset ranges from almost immediate for pentobarbital sodium and secobarbital to 5 minutes for phenobarbital sodium. Maximal CNS depression may not occur for at least 15 minutes after IV administration of phenobarbital sodium.

Duration: Duration of action varies and is related to dose and to the rate at which the barbiturates are redistributed throughout the body. In the following table, the barbiturates are classified according to their duration of action. Do not use this classification to predict the exact duration of effect, but use as a guide in drug selection.

Pharmacokinetics of Sedatives and Hypnotic Barbiturates

		Half-life (h)		Oral dosage range (mg)		Onset (min)	Duration (h)
	Barbiturate	Range	Mean	Sedative[a]	Hypnotic		
Long-Acting	Mephobarbital	11 to 67	34	32 to 200	—	30 to ≥ 60	10 to 16
	Phenobarbital	53 to 118	79	30 to 120	100 to 320		
Intermediate	Amobarbital[b]	16 to 40	25	—	—	45 to 60	6 to 8
	Butabarbital	66 to 140	100	45 to 120	50 to 100		
Short-Acting	Pentobarbital	15 to 50	†[c]	40 to 120	100	10 to 15	3 to 4
	Secobarbital	15 to 40	28	—	100		

[a] Total daily dose; administered in 2 to 4 divided doses.
[b] Available as injection only.
[c] May follow dose-dependent kinetics. Mean half-life is 50 hours for 50 mg and 22 hours for 100 mg.

Distribution – Barbiturates are weak acids that are rapidly distributed to all tissues and fluids with high concentrations in the brain, liver, and kidneys. Lipid solubility of the barbiturates is the dominant factor in their distribution. The more lipid soluble the barbiturate, the more rapidly it penetrates body tissue. Barbiturates are bound to plasma and tissue proteins; the degree of binding increases directly as a function of lipid solubility.

Phenobarbital has the lowest lipid solubility, plasma binding and brain protein binding, the longest delay in onset of activity, and the longest duration of action. Secobarbital has the highest lipid solubility, plasma protein binding and brain protein binding, the shortest delay in onset of activity, and the shortest duration of action.

Excretion – Barbiturates are metabolized primarily by the hepatic microsomal enzyme system, and the metabolic products are excreted in the urine, and less commonly, in the feces. Approximately 25% to 50% of a phenobarbital dose is eliminated unchanged in the urine, whereas the amount of other barbiturates excreted unchanged in the urine is negligible. The excretion of unmetabolized barbiturate is one feature that distinguishes the long-acting agents. The inactive metabolites of the barbiturates are excreted as conjugates of glucuronic acid.

Contraindications

Barbiturate sensitivity; manifest or latent porphyria; marked liver function impairment; nephritic patients; patients with respiratory disease where dyspnea or obstruction is present; intra-arterial administration (consequences vary from transient pain to gangrene); subcutaneous administration (produces tissue irritation ranging from tenderness and redness to necrosis); previous addiction to the sedative/hypnotic group (ordinary doses may be ineffective and may contribute to further addiction).

Warnings/Precautions

➤*Habit forming:* Tolerance or psychological and physical dependence may occur with continued use (see Drug abuse and dependence in the Precautions section). Administer with caution, if at all, to patients who are mentally depressed, have suicidal tendencies or a history of drug abuse (eg, alcoholics, opiate abusers, other sedative-hypnotic and amphetamine abusers). Limit prescribing and dispensing to the amount required for the interval until the next appointment.

➤*IV administration:* Too rapid administration may cause respiratory depression, apnea, laryngospasm, or vasodilation with fall in blood pressure. Parenteral solutions of barbiturates are highly alkaline. Therefore, use extreme care to avoid perivascular extravasation or intra-arterial injection. Extravascular injection may cause local tissue damage with subsequent necrosis; consequences of intra-arterial injection may vary from transient pain to gangrene of the limb. Any complaint of pain in the limb warrants stopping the injection.

Phenobarbital sodium may be administered IM or IV as an anticonvulsant for emergency use. When administered IV, it may require at least 15 minutes before reaching peak concentrations in the brain. Therefore, injecting phenobarbital sodium until the convulsions stop may cause the brain level to exceed that required to control the convulsions and may lead to severe barbiturate-induced depression.

➤*Pain:* Exercise caution when administering to patients with acute or chronic pain, because paradoxical excitement may be induced or important symptoms may be masked. However, the use of barbiturates as sedatives in postoperative surgery and as adjuncts to cancer chemotherapy is well established.

➤*Seizure disorders:* Status epilepticus may result from abrupt discontinuation, even when administered in small daily doses in the treatment of epilepsy.

➤*Effects on vitamin D:* Barbiturates may increase vitamin D requirements, possibly by increasing the metabolism of vitamin D via enzyme induction. Rickets and osteomalacia have been reported rarely following prolonged use of barbiturates.

➤*Tartrazine sensitivity:* Some of these products contain tartrazine, which may cause allergic-type reactions (including bronchial asthma) in susceptible individuals. Although the incidence of tartrazine sensitivity in the general population is low, it is frequently seen in patients who also have aspirin hypersensitivity. Specific products containing tartrazine are identified in the product listings.

➤*Renal function impairment:* Barbiturates are excreted either partially or completely unchanged in the urine and are contraindicated in patients with renal function impairment.

➤*Hepatic function impairment:* Barbiturates are metabolized primarily by hepatic microsomal enzymes. Administer with caution and initially in reduced doses to patients with hepatic function impairment. Do not use in patients showing premonitory signs of hepatic coma.

➤*Special risk:* Untoward reactions may occur in the presence of fever, hyperthyroidism, diabetes mellitus, and severe anemia. Use with caution.

Use **mephobarbital** with caution in patients with myasthenia gravis and myxedema.

➤*Drug abuse and dependence:* Barbiturates may be habit forming. Tolerance, psychological dependence, and physical dependence may occur, especially following prolonged use of high doses. Doses in excess of 400 mg/day **pentobarbital** or **secobarbital** for approximately 90 days are likely to produce some degree of physical dependence. A dose of 600 to 800 mg taken for at least 35 days is sufficient to produce withdrawal seizures. The average daily dose for the barbiturate addict is usually about 1.5 g. As tolerance develops, the amount needed to maintain the same level of intoxication increases; tolerance to a fatal dosage, however, does not increase more than 2-fold. As this occurs, the margin between an intoxicating dosage and fatal dosage becomes smaller.

Intoxication – Symptoms of acute intoxication include unsteady gait, slurred speech, and sustained nystagmus. Mental signs of chronic intoxication include confusion, poor judgment, irritability, insomnia, and somatic complaints. If an individual appears to be intoxicated with alcohol to a degree that is radically disproportionate to the amount of alcohol in his/her blood, suspect the use of barbiturates. The lethal dose of a barbiturate is less if accompanied with alcohol.

Dependence – Symptoms are similar to those of chronic alcoholism and include the following: a strong desire or need to continue taking the drug; tendency to increase the dose; psychological dependence on the effects of the drug related to subjective and individual appreciation of those effects; and physical dependence on the effects of the drug requiring its presence for maintenance of homeostasis resulting in a definite, characteristic, and self-limited abstinence syndrome when the drug is withdrawn.

Withdrawal symptoms – Withdrawal symptoms can be severe and may cause death.

Minor symptoms: These may appear 8 to 12 hours after the last dose of a barbiturate and usually appear in the following order: anxiety, muscle twitching, tremor of hands and fingers, progressive weakness, dizziness, distortion in visual perception, nausea, vomiting, insomnia, and orthostatic hypotension.

Major symptoms: Convulsions and delirium may occur within 16 hours and last up to 5 days after abrupt cessation of these drugs. Intensity of withdrawal symptoms gradually declines within about 15 days.

Treatment of dependence – Treatment of dependence consists of cautious and gradual withdrawal of the drug, which takes an extended period of time.

One method involves substituting 30 mg phenobarbital for each 100 to 200 mg barbiturate dose the patient is taking. The total daily amount of **phenobarbital** is administered in 3 to 4 divided doses, not to exceed 600 mg/day. Should signs of withdrawal occur on the first day of treatment, administer an IM loading dose of phenobarbital 100 to 200 mg in addition to the oral dose. After stabilization on phenobarbital, decrease the total daily dose by 30 mg/day as long as withdrawal is proceeding smoothly. A modification of this regimen involves initiating treatment at the patient's regular dosage level and decreasing the daily dosage by 10%, if tolerated. Severely dependent individuals generally may be withdrawn over 2 to 3 weeks.

Infants physically dependent on barbiturates may be given phenobarbital 3 to 10 mg/kg/day. After withdrawal symptoms (eg, hyperactivity, disturbed sleep, tremors, hyperreflexia) are relieved, gradually decrease the dosage of phenobarbital; completely withdraw over 2 weeks.

➤*Pregnancy: Category D.* Barbiturates may cause fetal damage when administered to a pregnant woman. Studies suggest a connection between maternal consumption of barbiturates and a higher incidence of fetal abnormalities. If this drug is used during pregnancy, or if the patient becomes pregnant while taking this drug, apprise her of the potential hazards to the fetus.

Barbiturates readily cross the placental barrier and are distributed throughout fetal tissues. Fetal blood levels approach maternal blood levels following parenteral use.

Withdrawal symptoms occur in infants born to mothers who receive barbiturates throughout the last trimester of pregnancy. Reports include the acute withdrawal syndrome of seizures and hyperirritability from birth to a delayed onset of up to 14 days.

Anticonvulsant use – Because of the strong possibility of precipitating status epilepticus with attendant hypoxia and the risk to the mother and unborn child, do not discontinue anticonvulsants when used to prevent major seizures. However, consider discontinuing anticonvulsants prior to and during pregnancy when the nature, frequency and severity of the seizures do not pose a serious threat to the patient. It is not known whether even minor seizures constitute some risk to the embryo or fetus.

Maternal ingestion of anticonvulsants, particularly barbiturates, may be associated with a neonatal coagulation defect that may cause bleeding, usually within 24 hours of birth. The defect is characterized by decreased levels of vitamin K-dependent clotting factors, and prolongation of prothrombin time, partial thromboplastin time or both. Give prophylactic vitamin K to the mother 1 month prior to and during delivery, and to the infant immediately after birth.

Labor and delivery – Hypnotic doses do not appear to significantly impair uterine activity during labor. Full anesthetic doses decrease the force and frequency of uterine contractions. Administration to the mother during labor may result in respiratory depression in the newborn; premature infants are particularly susceptible. If barbiturates are used during labor and delivery, have resuscitation equipment available.

➤*Lactation:* Exercise caution when administering to a breast-feeding mother, because small amounts of drug are excreted in breast milk. Drowsiness in the nursing infant has been reported.

➤*Children:* In some patients, especially children, barbiturates repeatedly produce excitement rather than depression. Barbiturates may produce irritability, excitability, inappropriate tearfulness, and aggression in children. Hyperkinetic states also may be induced and are primarily related to a specific drug sensitivity. Cognitive deficits have been associated with phenobarbital use for complicated febrile seizures in children. Safety and efficacy of amobarbital (children

➤*Elderly:* May produce marked excitement, depression, and confusion in elderly patients. In some people, barbiturates repeatedly produce excitement rather than depression.

Per the Beers list, all barbiturates (except **phenobarbital**) are highly addictive and cause more adverse effects than most sedative or hypnotic drugs in elderly patients except when used to control seizures.

➤*Monitoring:* During prolonged therapy, perform periodic laboratory evaluation of organ systems, including hematopoietic, renal, and hepatic systems.

Drug Interactions

Most reports of clinically significant drug interactions occurring with the barbiturates have involved phenobarbital.

Sedative/Hypnotic Barbiturate Drug Interactions

Precipitant drug	Object drug[a]		Description
Alcohol	Barbiturates	↑	Concomitant use may produce additive CNS effects and death.
Charcoal	Barbiturates	↓	Charcoal may reduce the absorption of barbiturates. Depending on the clinical situation, this will reduce their efficacy or toxicity.
Chloramphenicol	Barbiturates	↓	Chloramphenicol may inhibit phenobarbital metabolism. Barbiturates may enhance chloramphenicol metabolism.
Barbiturates	Chloramphenicol	↑	
Monoamine oxidase inhibitors	Barbiturates	↑	MAOIs may enhance the sedative effects of barbiturates.
Rifampin	Barbiturates	↓	Rifampin induces hepatic microsomal enzymes and may decrease the effectiveness of barbiturates.
Valproic acid	Barbiturates	↑	Valproic acid appears to decrease barbiturate metabolism, resulting in an increased effect.
Barbiturates	Anticoagulants	↓	Barbiturates may increase metabolism of anticoagulants, resulting in a decreased response. Patients stabilized on anticoagulants may require dosage adjustments if barbiturates are added to or withdrawn from their regimen.
Barbiturates	Beta blockers	↓	Pharmacokinetic parameters of certain beta-blockers (metoprolol and propranolol) may be altered by barbiturates. Timolol does not appear to be affected.
Barbiturates	Carbamazepine	↓	Decreased serum carbamazepine levels may occur.
Barbiturates	Clonazepam	↓	Increased clonazepam clearance may occur, which may lead to lower steady-state levels and loss of efficacy.
Barbiturates	Contraceptives, oral	↓	Decreased contraceptive effect may occur due to induction of microsomal enzymes. Menstrual irregularities (eg, spotting, breakthrough bleeding) or pregnancy may occur. An alternate form of birth control is suggested.
Barbiturates	Corticosteroids	↓	Barbiturates may enhance corticosteroid metabolism through the induction of hepatic microsomal enzymes.
Barbiturates	Digitoxin	↓	Barbiturates may increase digitoxin metabolism.
Barbiturates	Doxorubicin	↓	Total doxorubicin plasma clearance may be increased.
Barbiturates	Doxycycline	↓	Phenobarbital decreases doxycycline's half-life and serum levels, which may persist for 2 weeks after barbiturate therapy is discontinued.
Barbiturates	Felodipine	↓	Felodipine plasma levels and bioavailability may be reduced.
Barbiturates	Fenoprofen	↓	Fenoprofen bioavailability may be decreased.
Barbiturates	Griseofulvin	↓	Phenobarbital appears to interfere with the absorption of oral griseofulvin, thus decreasing its blood level; however, the effect on therapeutic response has not been established.
Barbiturates	Hydantoins	↔	The effect of barbiturates on metabolism is unpredictable; monitor hydantoin and barbiturate blood levels frequently if these drugs are given concurrently.
Barbiturates	Methoxyflurane	↑	Enhanced renal toxicity may occur.
Barbiturates	Metronidazole	↓	Barbiturates may decrease the antimicrobial effectiveness of metronidazole.
Barbiturates	Narcotics	↔	Methadone actions may be reduced. CNS depressant effects of meperidine may be prolonged.
Barbiturates	Phenylbutazone	↓	The elimination half-life of phenylbutazone may be reduced.
Barbiturates	Quinidine	↓	Phenobarbital may significantly reduce the serum levels and half-life of quinidine.
Barbiturates	Theophylline	↓	Barbiturates decrease theophylline levels, possibly resulting in decreased effects.
Barbiturates	Verapamil	↓	The clearance of verapamil may be increased and its bioavailability decreased.

[a] ↓ = object drug decreased; ↑ = object drug increased; ↔ = undetermined clinical effect.

Adverse Reactions

The following adverse reactions and their incidence were from observations of hospitalized patients. Because such patients may be less aware of milder adverse reactions of barbiturates, the incidence may be higher in fully ambulatory patients.

➤*Cardiovascular:* Bradycardia, hypotension, syncope (less than 1%).

➤*CNS:* Somnolence (1% to 3%); abnormal thinking, agitation, anxiety, ataxia, CNS depression, confusion, dizziness, fever (especially with chronic phenobarbital use), hallucinations, headache, hyperkinesia, insomnia, nervousness, nightmares, psychiatric disturbance (less than 1%); drowsiness; lethargy; residual sedation (hangover effect); vertigo.

Emotional disturbances and phobias may be accentuated with phenobarbital use. In some patients, barbiturates repeatedly produce excitement rather than depression; the patient may appear to be inebriated. Irritability and hyperactivity can occur in children.

Barbiturates, when given in the presence of pain, may cause restlessness, excitement, and even delirium. Rarely, the use of barbiturates results in localized or diffuse myalgic, neuralgic, or arthritic pain, especially in psychoneurotic patients with insomnia. The pain may appear in paroxysms, is most intense in the early morning hours, and is most frequently located in the region of the neck, shoulder girdle, and upper limbs. Symptoms may last for days after the drug is discontinued.

➤*GI:* Constipation, nausea, vomiting (less than 1%); liver damage, particularly with chronic **phenobarbital** use (less than 1%).

➤*Hematologic:* Megaloblastic anemia (rarely, following chronic **phenobarbital** use).

➤*Hypersensitivity:* Skin rashes, angioedema (particularly following chronic phenobarbital use) (less than 1%); exfoliative dermatitis (eg, Stevens-Johnson syndrome and toxic epidermal necrolysis) may be caused by phenobarbital and may be fatal (rare).

Acquired hypersensitivity to barbiturates consists chiefly in allergic reactions that occur especially in persons who tend to have asthma, urticaria, angioedema, and similar conditions. Hypersensitivity reactions in this category include localized swelling, particularly of the eyelids, cheeks or lips, and erythematous dermatitis. The skin eruption may be associated with fever, delirium, and marked degenerative changes in the liver and other parenchymatous organs.

➤*Local:* Inadvertent intra-arterial injection may produce arterial spasm with resultant thrombosis and gangrene of an extremity. Reactions range from transient pain to severe tissue necrosis and neurological deficit. Subcutaneous injection may produce tissue necrosis, pain, tenderness and redness. Injection into or near peripheral nerves may result in permanent neurological deficit. Thrombophlebitis after IV use and pain at IM injection site have been reported.

➤*Respiratory:* Apnea, hypoventilation (less than 1%); circulatory collapse; respiratory depression.

Overdosage

The toxic dose of barbiturates varies considerably. In general, an oral dose of 1 g produces serious poisoning in an adult. Death commonly occurs after 2 to 10 g of ingested barbiturate.

➤*Symptoms:* Onset of symptoms may not occur until several hours after ingestion. Acute barbiturate overdosage is manifested by CNS and respiratory depression which may progress to Cheyne-Stokes respiration, areflexia, constriction of the pupils to a slight degree (though in severe poisoning they may show paralytic dilation), nystagmus, ataxia, oliguria, tachycardia, hypotension, lowered body temperature, and coma. Typical shock syndrome (eg, apnea, circulatory collapse, respiratory arrest, death) may occur.

In extreme overdose, all electrical activity in the brain may cease, in which case a "flat" electroencephalogram normally equated with clinical death cannot be accepted. This effect is fully reversible unless hypoxic damage occurs. Consider the possibility of barbiturate intoxication even in situations that appear to involve trauma.

Complications such as pneumonia, pulmonary edema, cardiac arrhythmias, congestive heart failure and renal failure may occur. Uremia may increase CNS sensitivity to barbiturates if renal function is impaired. Differential diagnosis should include hypoglycemia, head trauma, cerebrovascular accidents, convulsive states and diabetic coma.

➤*Treatment:* Treatment is mainly supportive. Maintain an adequate airway, with assisted respiration and oxygen administration, as necessary. Monitor vital signs and fluid balance. Refer to General Management of Acute Overdosage.

Administer 30 g activated charcoal. Nasogastric administration of multiple doses of activated charcoal has been successful in accelerating the elimination of phenobarbital from the body. Consider gastric lavage with a cuffed endotracheal tube in place with the patient in the face-down position. Activated charcoal may be left in the emptied stomach and a saline cathartic administered.

Administer fluid and other standard treatments for shock, if needed. If renal function is normal, forced diuresis may aid in the elimination of the barbiturate. However, diuresis and peritoneal dialysis are of little value. Alkalinization of the urine increases renal excretion of some barbiturates, especially **phenobarbital** and **mephobarbital** (which is metabolized to phenobarbital).

Hemodialysis and hemoperfusion may be used in severe barbiturate intoxication or if the patient is anuric or in shock. The patient should be rolled from side to side every 30 minutes.

Patient Information

Instruct the patient not to increase the dose of the drug without consulting a health care provider.

Advise patients that barbiturates may impair mental or physical abilities required for the performance of potentially hazardous tasks (eg, driving, operating machinery).

Advise patients not to consume alcohol while taking barbiturates. Concurrent use of barbiturates with other CNS depressants (eg, alcohol, narcotics, tranquilizers, antihistamines) may result in additional CNS depressant effects.

Instruct patient to notify the health care provider if any of the following occur: fever; sore throat; mouth sores; easy bruising or bleeding; tiny broken blood vessels under the skin.

Patients may use these drugs on a limited basis as a sleep aid; advise patients not to use for longer than 2 weeks.

Long-Acting

PHENOBARBITAL

c-iv	**Phenobarbital** (Various, eg, Harber, Lilly, Major, Moore, PBI, Parmed, Roxane, Warner Chilcott)	**Tablets**: 15 mg	In 100s, 1000s, 5,000s, and UD 100s.
c-iv	**Solfoton** (ECR Pharm.)	**Tablets**: 16 mg	In 100s and 500s.
c-iv	**Phenobarbital** (Various, eg, Goldline, Harber, Lilly, Major, Moore, PBI, Parmed, Roxane)	**Tablets**: 30 mg	In 100s, 1,000s, 5,000s, and UD 100s.
c-iv	**Phenobarbital** (Various, eg, Century, Harber, Lilly, Moore, PBI, Parmed, Roxane)	**Tablets**: 60 mg	In 100s, 1,000s, and UD 100s.
c-iv	**Phenobarbital** (Various, eg, URL)	**Tablets**: 90 mg	In 1,000s.
c-iv	**Phenobarbital** (Various, eg, Century, Harber, Lilly, Roxane)	**Tablets**: 100 mg	In 100s and 1,000s.
c-iv	**Solfoton** (ECR Pharm.)	**Capsules**: 16 mg	In 100s and 500s.
c-iv	**Phenobarbital** (Pharmaceutical Associates)	**Elixir**: 15 mg per 5 mL	13.5% alcohol. Fruit flavor. In pt and UD 5, 10, and 20 mL.
c-iv	**Phenobarbital** (Various, eg, Barre-National, Century, Goldline, Harber, Lilly, Roxane)	**Elixir**: 20 mg per 5 mL	Alcohol. In pt, gal, UD 5 mL and UD 7.5 mL.
c-iv	**Phenobarbital Sodium** (Wyeth-Ayerst)	**Injection**: 30 mg/mL	In 1 mL *Tubex*.
c-iv	**Luminal Sodium** (Hospira)	**Injection**: 60 mg/mL	In 1 mL *Carpuject* with *Luer Lock*.[a]
c-iv	**Phenobarbital Sodium** (Wyeth-Ayerst)		In 1 mL *Tubex*.
c-iv	**Phenobarbital Sodium** (Wyeth-Ayerst)	**Injection**: 65 mg/mL	In 1 mL vials.
c-iv	**Phenobarbital Sodium** (Various)	**Injection**: 130 mg/mL	In 1 mL *Tubex* and 1 mL vials.
c-iv	**Luminal Sodium** (Hospira)		In 1 mL *Carpuject* with *Luer Lock*.[a]

[a] With 10% alcohol and 67.8% propylene glycol.

Long-Acting

PHENOBARBITAL — ORAL

For complete and comparative prescribing information, refer to the Barbiturates group monograph.

Indications

➤*Sedation:* For use as a sedative.

➤*Anticonvulsant:* For use as an anticonvulsant for the treatment of generalized and partial seizures.

Administration and Dosage

➤*Adults:*

Sedation –

Usual dosage: 30 to 120 mg daily in 2 to 3 divided doses.

Maximum dose: 400 mg/day.

Single dose: 30 to 120 mg repeated at intervals; frequency will be determined by the patient's response.

Hypnosis – 100 to 320 mg.

Anticonvulsant – 60 to 300 mg/day in divided doses.

➤*Children:*

Anticonvulsant – 3 to 6 mg/kg/day. 15 to 50 mg 2 or 3 times daily has also been used.

Sedation – 6 mg/kg/day in 3 divided doses.

Off-label dosing –

Hyperbilirubinemia:

• *Younger than 12 years of age –*

Usual dosage: 3 to 8 mg/kg/day divided 2 to 3 times daily.

Maximum dose: 12 mg/kg/day.

Preoperative sedation: 1 to 3 mg/kg once 60 to 90 minutes before procedure.

Status epilepticus maintenance:

• *Older than 12 years of age* – 1 to 3 mg/kg/day divided once to twice daily. Begin 12 to 24 hours after IV loading dose.

• *6 to 12 years of age* – 4 to 6 mg/kg/day divided once to twice daily. Begin 12 to 24 hours after IV loading dose.

• *1 to 5 years of age* – 6 to 8 mg/kg/day divided once to twice daily. Begin 12 to 24 hours after IV loading dose.

• *Infant* – 5 to 6 mg/kg/day divided once to twice daily. Begin 12 to 24 hours after IV loading dose.

• *Neonates* – 3 to 5 mg/kg/day divided once to twice daily. Begin 12 to 24 hours after IV loading dose.

➤*Elderly:* Dosage should be reduced in the elderly patient because these patients may be more sensitive to barbiturates.

See Warnings/Precautions.

➤*Renal function impairment:* Dosage should be reduced for patients with impaired renal function.

➤*Hepatic function impairment:* Dosage should be reduced for patients with hepatic disease.

See Warnings/Precautions.

➤*Therapeutic drug monitoring:* Clinical laboratory reference values should be used to determine the therapeutic anticonvulsant level of phenobarbital in the serum. To achieve the blood levels considered therapeutic in children, higher per-kilogram dosages are generally necessary for phenobarbital and most other anticonvulsants. In children and infants, phenobarbital at a loading dose of 15 to 20 mg/kg produces blood levels of about 20 mcg/mL shortly after administration.

➤*Storage/Stability:* Store at 20° to 25°C (68° to 77°F).

PHENOBARBITAL SODIUM — INJECTION

For complete and comparative prescribing information, refer to the Barbiturates groupmonograph.

Indications

➤*Hypnotic:* As a hypnotic, for the short-term management of insomnia.

➤*Sedative:* As a sedative, for the relief of anxiety, tension, and apprehension.

➤*Anticonvulsant:* As an anticonvulsant, for the treatment of epilepsy (generalized tonic-clonic and cortical focal seizures).

Administration and Dosage

➤*General dosing considerations:* Alkalis should be given and the bowels regulated during prolonged use.

In the emergency control of certain acute convulsive episodes (eg, those associated with status epilepticus, cholera, eclampsia, meningitis, tetanus, and toxic reactions to strychnine or local anesthetics); phenobarbital sodium may be administered IM or IV as an anticonvulsant for emergency use. When administered IV, it may require 15 or more minutes before reaching peak concentrations in the brain. Therefore, injecting phenobarbital sodium until the convulsions stop may cause the brain level to exceed that required to control the convulsions and lead to severe barbiturate-induced depression.

➤*Adults:*

Maximum dose – 600 mg/day.

Usual dosage – 100 to 320 mg. Larger doses may occasionally be necessary in people with status epilepticus, psychoses, and pronounced excitement, and in mental patients with insomnia. The effect of large doses must be closely watched.

➤*Children:*

Off-label dosing –

Preoperative sedation: 1 to 3 mg/kg intramuscularly (IM) or intravenously (IV) once 60 to 90 minutes before procedure.

Status epilepticus:

• *Loading dose* – 15 to 20 mg/kg IV in single or divided dose slowly over 10 to 15 minutes. May give additional 5 mg/kg doses every 15 to 30 minutes up to 30 to 40 mg/kg.

• *Maintenance dosage –*

Older than 12 years of age: 1 to 3 mg/kg/day IV divided once or twice daily. Begin 12 to 24 hours after the loading dose.

6 to 12 years of age: 4 to 6 mg/kg/day IV divided once or twice daily. Begin 12 to 24 hours after the loading dose.

1 to 5 years of age: 6 to 8 mg/kg/day IV divided once or twice daily. Begin 12 to 24 hours after the loading dose.

Infant: 5 to 6 mg/kg/day IV divided once or twice daily. Begin 12 to 24 hours after the loading dose.

Neonate: 3 to 5 mg/kg/day IV divided once or twice daily. Begin 12 to 24 hours after the loading dose.

➤*Hepatic function impairment:* In patients with hepatic damage, barbiturates should be administered with caution and initially in reduced doses. Barbiturates should not be administered to patients showing the premonitory signs of hepatic coma.

➤*Administration:* IV injection should be administered slowly.

➤*Storage/Stability:* Protect from light. Store at room temperature up to 30°C (86°F).

MEPHOBARBITAL

c-iv	**Mebaral** (Ovation)	**Tablets:** 32 mg	(M 31). In 250s.
		50 mg	(M 32). In 250s.
		100 mg	(M 33). In 250s.

MEPHOBARBITAL — ORAL

For complete and comparative prescribing information, refer to the Barbiturates group monograph.

Indications

➤*Sedative:* Mephobarbital is indicated for use as a sedative for the relief of anxiety, tension, and apprehension.

➤*Anticonvulsant:* For use as an anticonvulsant for the treatment of grand mal and petit mal epilepsy.

Administration and Dosage

➤*General dosing considerations:* Mephobarbital is best taken at bedtime if seizures generally occur at night, and during the day if attacks are diurnal.

➤*Adults:*

Epilepsy –

Usual dosage: 400 to 600 mg (6 to 9 grains) daily.

Dosage titration: Treatment should be started with a small dose that is gradually increased over 4 or 5 days until the optimum dosage is determined.

Maintenance dosage: When the dose is lowered to a maintenance level, the amount should be reduced gradually over 4 or 5 days.

Concomitant therapy: If the patient has been taking some other antiepileptic drug, it should be tapered off as the doses of mephobarbital are increased to guard against the temporary marked attacks that may occur when any treatment for epilepsy is changed abruptly.

Mephobarbital may be used in combination with phenobarbital, either in the form of alternating courses or concurrently. When the 2 drugs are used at the same time, the dose should be about one-half the amount of each used alone. The average daily dose for an adult is from 50 to 100 mg (¾ to 1½ grains) of phenobarbital and from 200 to 300 mg (3 to 4½ grains) of mephobarbital.

Mephobarbital may also be used with phenytoin; in some cases, combined therapy appears to give better results than either agent used alone because phenytoin is particularly effective for the psychomotor types of seizure but relatively ineffective for petit mal. When the drugs are employed concurrently, a reduced dose of phenytoin is advisable, but the full dose of mephobarbital may be given. Satisfactory results have been obtained with an average daily dose of 230 mg (3½ grains) of phenytoin plus approximately 600 mg (9 grains) of mephobarbital.

Long-Acting

MEPHOBARBITAL — ORAL

Discontinuation of therapy: When the dose is to be discontinued, the amount should be reduced gradually over 4 or 5 days.

Sedation – 32 to 100 mg (½ to 1½ grains) 3 to 4 times daily; optimum dose is 50 mg (¾ grain) 3 to 4 times daily.

➤*Children:*

Epilepsy – See Adults for more information.

5 years of age and older: 32 to 64 mg (½ to 1 grain) by mouth 3 or 4 times daily.

Younger than 5 years of age: 16 to 32 mg (¼ to ½ grain) by mouth 3 or 4 times daily.

Sedation – 16 to 32 mg (¼ to ½ grain) 3 to 4 times daily.

➤*Elderly:* Dosage should be reduced in elderly or debilitated patients because these patients may be more sensitive to barbiturates.

➤*Renal function impairment:* Dosage should be reduced for patients with impaired renal function.

➤*Hepatic function impairment:* Dosage should be reduced for patients with hepatic disease.

➤*Storage/Stability:* Store at room temperature up to 25°C (77°F).

Intermediate-Acting

AMOBARBITAL SODIUM

c-ii	**Amytal Sodium** (Marathon Pharmaceuticals)	**Injection, lyophilized powder for solution:** 500 mg	In vials.

AMOBARBITAL SODIUM — INJECTION

For complete prescribing information, refer to the Barbiturates group monograph.

Indications

➤*Sedative/Hypnotic:* For use as a sedative, hypnotic (short-term treatment of insomnia since it appears to lose its effectiveness after 2 weeks), or preanesthetic.

Administration and Dosage

➤*Adults:*

Hypnotic –

Usual dosage: 65 to 200 mg at bedtime.

Maximum dose: 1 g (as a single dose).

Sedative –

Usual dosage: 30 to 50 mg given 2 or 3 times daily.

Maximum dose: 1 g (as a single dose).

➤*Children:*

Sedative/Hypnotic –

6 years to 12 years of age: 65 to 500 mg IV.

➤*Elderly:* Dosage should be reduced in elderly or debilitated patients because these patients may be more sensitive to barbiturates.

➤*Renal function impairment:* Dosage should be reduced for patients with impaired renal function.

➤*Hepatic function impairment:* Dosage should be reduced for patients with hepatic disease.

➤*Preparation for administration:* Add sterile water for injection to the vial. The vial should be rotated to facilitate solution of the powder. Do not shake the vial.

Several minutes may be required for the drug to dissolve completely, but under no circumstances should a solution be injected if it has not become absolutely clear within 5 minutes. Also, a solution that forms a precipitate after clearing should not be used. Amobarbital hydrolyzes in solution or on exposure to air. No more than 30 minutes should elapse from the time the vial is opened until its contents are injected.

The following table will aid in preparing solutions of various concentrations. Ordinarily, a 10% solution is used.

Reconstitution of Amobarbital With Sterile Water[a]

Content in weight	1%	2.5%	5%	10%	20%
0.5 g	50 mL	20 mL	10 mL	5 mL	2.5 mL

[a] Quantity of sterile water for injection required to dilute the contents of a given vial of amobarbital sodium to obtain the percentages listed. Solutions derived will be in weight/volume.

➤*Administration:*

Intramuscular (IM) administration – IM injection of the sodium salts of barbiturates should be made deeply into a large muscle. The average IM dose ranges from 65 mg to 0.5 g. A volume of 5 mL (irrespective of concentration) should not be exceeded at any one site because of possible tissue irritation. Twenty percent solutions may be used so that a small volume can contain a large dose. After IM injection of a hypnotic dose, the patient's vital signs should be monitored. Superficial IM or subcutaneous injections may be painful and may produce sterile abscesses or sloughs.

IV administration – IV injection is restricted to conditions in which other routes are not feasible, either because the patient is unconscious (as in cerebral hemorrhage, eclampsia, or status epilepticus), the patient resists (as in delirium), or prompt action is imperative. Slow IV injection is essential, and patients should be carefully observed during administration. This requires that blood pressure, respiration, and cardiac function be maintained, vital signs be recorded, and equipment for resuscitation and artificial ventilation be available. The rate of IV injection for adults should not exceed 50 mg/min to prevent sleep or sudden respiratory depression. The final dosage is determined to a great extent by the patient's reaction to the slow administration of the drug.

➤*Storage/Stability:* Store at 59° to 86°F (15° to 30°C). Do not use a solution that is not absolutely clear after 5 minutes; amobarbital hydrolyzes in solution or upon exposure to air. No more than 30 minutes should elapse from the time the vial is opened until the contents are injected.

BUTABARBITAL SODIUM

c-iii	**Butisol Sodium** (MedPointe Healthcare)	**Tablets; oral:** 30 mg	Tartrazine. (Butisol Sodium 37 113). Green, scored. In 100s.
c-iii	**Butisol Sodium** (MedPointe Healthcare)	**Tablets; oral:** 50 mg	Tartrazine. (Butisol Sodium 37 114). Orange, scored. In 100s.
c-iii	**Butisol Sodium** (MedPointe Healthcare)	**Elixir; oral:** 30 mg/5 ml	7% alcohol, EDTA, tartrazine, saccharin. In 473 mL.

BUTABARBITAL SODIUM — ORAL

For complete prescribing information, refer to the Barbiturates class monograph.

Indications

➤*Sedative/Hypnotic. :* For use as a Sedative or hypnotic.

Administration and Dosage

➤*Adults:*

Hypnotic – 50 to 100 mg at bedtime.

Sedative –

Daytime sedation: 15 to 30 mg, 3 or 4 times daily.

Preoperative sedation: 50 to 100 mg, 60 to 90 minutes before surgery.

➤*Children:*

Preoperative sedation –

Usual dosage: 2 to 6 mg/kg.

Maximum dose: 100 mg.

➤*Elderly:* Reduce dosage; these patients may be more sensitive to the drug.

➤*Renal function impairment:* Reduce dosage.

➤*Hepatic function impairment:* Reduce dosage.

➤*Duration of therapy:* Barbiturates appear to lose their effectiveness for sleep induction and maintenance after 2 weeks.

➤*Storage/Stability:* Store 20° to 25°C (68° to 77°F). Dispense in a tight container.

Short-Acting

SECOBARBITAL SODIUM

c-ii	**Seconal Sodium Pulvules** (Marathon Pharm[a])	**Capsules; oral:** 100 mg	(RX679). Orange. In 100s.

[a] Marathon Pharmaceuticals, LLC, 1751 Lake Cook Road, Suite 400, Deerfield, IL 60015; 866-945-7860; http://www.marathonpharma.com

SECOBARBITAL SODIUM — ORAL

For complete and comparative prescribing information, refer to the Barbiturates group monograph.

Indications

➤*Hypnotic:* Hypnotic, for the short-term treatment of insomnia, since it appears to lose its effectiveness for sleep induction and sleep maintenance after 2 weeks.

➤*Preanesthetic:* For use as a preanesthetic.

Administration and Dosage

➤*Adults:*

Hypnotic – 100 mg at bedtime.

Preanesthetic – 200 to 300 mg 1 to 2 hours before surgery.

➤*Children:*

Preanesthetic –

Usual dosage: 2 to 6 mg/kg.
Maximum dose: 100 mg.

➤*Elderly:* Dosage should be reduced in elderly or debilitated patients because these patients may be more sensitive to barbiturates.

➤*Renal function impairment:* Dosage should be reduced for patients with impaired renal function.

➤*Hepatic function impairment:* Dosage should be reduced for patients with hepatic disease.

➤*Duration of therapy:* Secobarbital appears to lose its effectiveness for sleep induction and sleep maintenance after 2 weeks.

➤*Storage/Stability:* Store at 15° to 30°C (59° to 86°F). Dispense in a tight container.

PENTOBARBITAL SODIUM

c-ii	**Pentobarbital Sodium** (Wyeth-Ayerst)	**Injection:** 50 mg/mL	In 2 mL *Tubex*.[a]

[a] With propylene glycol and 10% alcohol.

PENTOBARBITAL SODIUM — INJECTION

For complete and comparative prescribing information, refer to the Barbiturates group monograph.

Indications

➤*Hypnotic:* Hypnotic, for the short-term treatment of insomnia, since barbiturates appear to lose their effectiveness for sleep induction and sleep maintenance after 2 weeks.

➤*Anticonvulsant:* For use as an anticonvulsant, in anesthetic doses, for the emergency control of certain acute convulsive episodes (eg, those associated with status epilepticus, eclampsia, meningitis, tetanus, and toxic reactions to strychnine or local anesthetics).

➤*Preanesthetic:* For use as a preanesthetic in pediatric patients.

Administration and Dosage

➤*General dosing considerations:* The clinical response is the basis for dosage determination, although the patient's weight and age may influence the total amount of the drug required. At least 1 minute is necessary to determine the full effect.

Anticonvulsant use – In status epilepticus, it is imperative to achieve therapeutic blood levels of a barbiturate (or other anticonvulsants) as rapidly as possible. Inject slowly with regard to the time needed for the drug to penetrate the blood-brain barrier.

A barbiturate-induced depression may occur along with a postictal depression once the seizures are controlled; therefore, it is important to use the minimal amount required and to wait for the anticonvulsant effect to develop before administering a second dose.

➤*Adults:*

Hypnotic –

Initial dosage: 100 mg intravenously (IV) initially (commonly used initial dose for a 70 kg adult) or 150 to 200 mg IM.

Dosage adjustment: At least 1 minute is necessary to determine the full effect. If needed, small increments of the drug may be given to a total of 200 to 500 mg for healthy adults.

➤*Children:*

Anticonvulsant use – To achieve the blood levels considered therapeutic in children, higher per-kilogram dosages are generally necessary for phenobarbital and most other anticonvulsants.

Hypnotic – The initial dose for a 70 kg adult is 100 mg; reduce dosage proportionally for children.

Preanesthetic sedation –

Usual dosage: 2 to 6 mg/kg IM.
Maximum dose: 100 mg IM.

➤*Elderly:* Dosage should be reduced in elderly or debilitated patients because these patients may be more sensitive to barbiturates.

➤*Renal function impairment:* Dosage should be reduced for patients with impaired renal function.

➤*Hepatic function impairment:* Dosage should be reduced for patients with hepatic disease.

➤*Treatment of adverse effects due to inadvertent error in administration:* Extravasation into subcutaneous tissues causes tissue irritation. This may vary from slight tenderness and redness to necrosis. Recommended treatment includes application of moist heat and injection of procaine 0.5% solution into the affected area.

Intra-arterial injection of any barbiturate must be avoided. The accidental intra-arterial injection of a small amount of the solution may cause spasm and severe pain along the course of the artery. The injection should be terminated if the patient complains of pain or if other indications of accidental intra-arterial injection occur, such as a white hand with cyanosed skin or patches of discolored skin and delayed onset of hypnosis.

The consequences of intra-arterial injection of pentobarbital can vary from transient pain to gangrene. It is not possible to formulate strict rules for management of such accidents. Although no specific treatment has proved entirely successful, the following procedures have been suggested:

1.) Release of the tourniquet or restrictive garments to permit dilution of injected drug,
2.) relief of arterial spasm by injecting 10 mL of procaine 1% solution into the artery and, if necessary, brachial plexus block,
3.) prevention of thrombosis by early anticoagulant therapy, and
4.) supportive treatment.

➤*Monitoring:* Closely monitor the physical signs to accurately obtain and maintain the desired degree of sedation. This requires maintaining blood pressure, respiration, and cardiac function; recording vital signs; and making available equipment for resuscitation and artificial ventilation.

➤*Administration:* IM injection of the sodium salts of barbiturates should be made deeply into a large muscle, and a volume of 5 mL should not be exceeded at any one site because of possible tissue irritation. After IM injection of a hypnotic dose, the patient's vital signs should be monitored.

IV injection is restricted to conditions in which other routes are not feasible because the patient is unconscious (as in cerebral hemorrhage, eclampsia, or status epilepticus), the patient resists (as in delirium), or prompt action is imperative. Slow IV injection is essential, and patients should be carefully observed during administration. The rate of IV injection should not exceed 50 mg/min. No average IV dose can be relied upon to produce similar effects in different patients. The possibility of overdose and respiratory depression is remote when the drug is injected slowly in fractional doses.

Any vein may be used, but preference should be given to a larger vein (to minimize the risk of irritation with the possibility of resultant thrombosis). Avoid administration into varicose veins because circulation there is retarded.

Inadvertent injection into or adjacent to an artery has resulted in gangrene requiring amputation of an extremity or a portion thereof. Careful technique, including aspiration, is necessary to avoid inadvertent intra-arterial injection.

➤*Storage/Stability:* Store at room temperature, approximately 25° C (77° F).

NONPRESCRIPTION SLEEP AID COMBINATIONS

otc	**Extra Strength Tylenol PM** (McNeil-CPC)	**Tablets; oral:** 25 mg diphenhydramine, 500 mg acetaminophen	**Tablets:** (Tylenol PM). In 24s, 50s. **Caplets:** (Tylenol PM). In 24s and 50s.
otc	**Extra Strength Pain Reliever PM Tablets** (Magno-Humphries)		Capsule shape. In 100s.
otc	**Bayer Select Maximum Strength Night Time Pain Relief** (Bayer)		In 24s and 50s.
otc	**Sominex Pain Relief** (SmithKline-Beecham)		In 16s and 32s.
otc	**Tycolene P.M.** (Pfeiffer Pharmaceuticals)		In 50s.
otc	**Doan's P.M. Extra Strength** (Novartis Consumer Health)	**Tablets; oral:** 25 mg diphenhydramine hydrochloride, 580 mg magnesium salicylate	PEG, methylparaben. Capsule shape. In 20s.
otc	**Unisom PM Pain** (Chattem)	**Tablets; oral:** 50 mg diphenhydramine hydrochloride, 325 mg acetaminophen	Mineral oil. Capsule shape. In 30s.
otc	**Legatrin PM** (Columbia)	**Tablets; oral:** 50 mg diphenhydramine hydrochloride, 500 mg acetaminophen	In 30s and 50s.
otc	**Unisom with Pain Relief** (Pfizer)	**Tablets; oral:** 50 mg diphenhydramine hydrochloride, 650 mg acetaminophen	In 16s.
otc	**Bayer PM Extra Strength Aspirin Plus Sleep Aid Caplet** (Pfizer)	**Tablets; oral:** 25 mg diphenhydramine hydrochloride, 500 mg aspirin	(BAYER PM). Capsule shape. In 24s.
otc	**Melagesic PM** (B.F. Ascher)	**Tablets; oral:** 500 mg acetaminophen, 1.5 mg melatonin.	In 32s.
otc	**Excedrin PM Tablets and Caplets** (Novartis Consumer Health)	**Tablets; oral:** 38 mg diphenhydramine citrate, 500 mg acetaminophen	Parabens, mineral oil. In 24s, 50s, 100s.
otc	**Unisom SleepMelts** (Chattem)	**Tablets, disintegrating; oral:** 25 mg diphenhydramine hydrochloride	Mannitol, sucralose, sucrose. Cherry flavor. In 24s.
otc	**Alka-Seltzer PM** (Bayer Consumer)	**Tablets, effervescent; oral:** 38 mg diphenhydramine citrate, 325 mg aspirin	Acesulfame K, aspartame, mannitol, 4 mg phenylalanine, 504 mg sodium. In 24s.
otc	**Extra Strength Tylenol PM Gelcaps** (McNeil-CPC)	**Capsules; oral:** 25 mg diphenhydramine hydrochloride, 500 mg acetaminophen	EDTA, propylparaben. In 20s and 40s.
otc	**Advil PM** (Wyeth Consumer Health)	**Capsules; oral:** 25 mg diphenhydramine hydrochloride, 200 mg ibuprofen	Sorbitol. In 32s.
otc	**Goody's PM** (Glaxo Consumer)	**Powder; oral:** 38 mg diphenhydramine citrate, 500 mg acetaminophen	Lactose. In 6 packets.
otc	**Nighttime Pamprin** (Chattem)	**Powder; oral:** 50 mg diphenhydramine hydrochloride, 650 mg acetaminophen	Sugar. Apple cinnamon and hot chocolate flavors. In 4s.
otc	**Excedrin P.M.** (B-M Squibb)	**Liquid; oral:** 167 mg acetaminophen, 8.3 mg diphenhydramine hydrochloride/5 mL	10% alcohol, sucrose. Wild berry flavor. In 180 mL.
		Liquid; oral: 1000 mg acetaminophen 50 mg diphenhydramine hydrochloride/30 mL.	10% alcohol, sucrose. Wild berry flavor. In 180 mL.
otc	**Advil PM** (Wyeth Consumer Health)	**Tablets; oral:** 38 mg diphenhydramine citrate, 200 mg ibuprofen	Lactose. Capsule shape. In 20s and UD 50s.

NONPRESCRIPTION SLEEP AIDS — ORAL

Certain doxylamine and diphenhydramine single-ingredient products may also be used to induce sleep. For complete prescribing information and a complete listing of these products, refer to the Doxylamine and Diphenhydramine monographs in the Respiratory Drugs section.

Indications

➤*Insomnia:* Aid in the relief of insomnia.

Traditionally, products containing analgesics have been used for relief of insomnia due to minor pain.

Administration and Dosage

➤*Adults:*

Insomnia –

Diphenhydramine citrate: 76 mg before bedtime.

Diphenhydramine hydrochloride: 50 mg before bedtime.

➤*Children:*

Insomnia – See Adults for dosing for children 12 years of age and older.

Actions

➤*Pharmacology:* These products contain antihistamines which act on the CNS, producing prominent sedative effects.

Contraindications

Asthma, glaucoma or prostate gland enlargement, except under a physician's advice.

Warnings/Precautions

➤*Prolonged insomnia:* Not for use more than 2 weeks. If insomnia persists for more than 2 weeks, consult a physician; it may be a symptom of a serious underlying illness.

➤*Hazardous tasks:* May cause drowsiness; observe caution while driving or performing other tasks requiring alertness, coordination or physical dexterity.

➤*Pregnancy: Category undetermined.* Consult a physician before using these products. **Doxylamine** should not be taken by pregnant women.

➤*Lactation:* **Doxylamine** should not be taken by a nursing woman.

➤*Children:* Do not use in children younger than 12 years of age.

Adverse Reactions

Occasional anticholinergic effects may occur with doxylamine.

Overdosage

Antihistamine overdosage reactions may vary from CNS depression to stimulation. See the Antihistamines monograph for a more complete description of reactions.

Patient Information

Avoid alcoholic beverages while taking this product. Do not take this product if you are taking sedatives or tranquilizers without first consulting the physician.

May cause drowsiness; observe caution while driving or performing other tasks requiring alertness, coordination or physical dexterity.

Do not use if you have asthma, glaucoma, emphysema, chronic pulmonary disease, shortness of breath, difficulty in breathing or difficulty in urination due to prostate enlargement unless directed by the physician.

Indications

➤*Anesthesia:* For the induction of anesthesia; supplementation of other anesthetic agents; IV anesthesia for short surgical procedures with minimal painful stimuli.

➤*Hypnotic:* For the induction of a hypnotic state.

➤*Thiopental (IV):* Control of convulsive states and in neurosurgical patients with increased intracranial pressure if adequate ventilation is provided.

➤*Thiopental (rectal suspension):* Used when preanesthetic sedation or basal narcosis by the rectal route is desired. It may be employed as the sole agent in selected brief, minor procedures where muscular relaxation and analgesia are not required.

Actions

➤*Pharmacology:* The ultrashort-acting barbiturates, thiopental and methohexital, depress the CNS to produce hypnosis and anesthesia without analgesia. Methohexital does not possess muscle relaxant properties. These drugs are frequently used to provide hypnosis during balanced anesthesia with other agents for muscle relaxation and analgesia.

Biotransformation products of thiopental are pharmacologically inactive and mostly excreted in the urine.

➤*Pharmacokinetics:* The rapid onset and brief duration of action of these drugs is a function of their high lipid solubility. They quickly cross the blood-brain barrier and are rapidly redistributed from the brain to other body tissues, first to highly perfused visceral organs (liver, kidneys, heart) and muscle, and later to fatty tissues.

Administered IV as the sodium salts, these agents produce anesthesia within 1 minute. Recovery after a small dose is rapid, with somnolence and retrograde amnesia. Muscle relaxation occurs at the onset of anesthesia. The duration of anesthetic activity following a single IV dose is 20 to 30 minutes for thiopental and somewhat shorter for methohexital. Thiopental is readily absorbed by the rectal route when administered as a suspension; onset of action usually occurs within 8 to 10 minutes. Thiopental IV produces hypnosis within 30 to 40 seconds following administration. Repeated doses or continuous infusion of these agents causes accumulation. Slow release of the drug from lipoidal storage sites results in prolonged anesthesia, somnolence, and respiratory and circulatory depression. The plasma half-life is 3 to 8 hours.

Contraindications

➤*Absolute:* Latent or manifest porphyria; hypersensitivity to barbiturates; absence of suitable veins for IV administration.

➤*Relative:* Severe cardiovascular disease; hypotension or shock; conditions in which hypnotic effects may be prolonged or potentiated (excessive premedication, Addison disease, hepatic or renal dysfunction, myxedema, increased blood urea, severe anemia); increased intracranial pressure; asthma; myasthenia gravis; status asthmaticus (thiopental).

If barbiturates are used in conditions involving relative contraindications, reduce dosage and administer slowly.

Warnings/Precautions

➤*Status asthmaticus:* Use **methohexital** with extreme caution in patients with status asthmaticus.

➤*Repeated or continuous infusion:* Repeated or continuous infusion may cause cumulative effects resulting in prolonged somnolence and respiratory and circulatory depression. Have resuscitative and endotracheal intubation equipment and oxygen immediately available. Maintain patency of the airway at all times.

➤*Extravascular injection:* Extravascular injection may cause pain, swelling, ulceration, and necrosis. Intra-arterial injection is dangerous and may produce gangrene on an extremity.

➤*Rectal dose:* If evacuation of the instilled rectal dose occurs, assess the effects of any retained portion before administering a repeat dose.

➤*Special risk:* Respiratory depression, apnea, or hypotension may occur due to individual variations in tolerance or to the physical status of the patient. Exercise caution in debilitated patients, or those with impaired function of respiratory, circulatory, cardiac, renal, hepatic, or endocrine systems.

➤*Drug abuse and dependence:* May be habit-forming.

➤*Pregnancy: Category C* (thiopental); *Category B* (methohexital). Safety for use during pregnancy has not been established. Use only when clearly needed and when the potential benefits outweigh the potential hazards to the fetus.

Thiopental – Thiopental readily crosses the placental barrier.

Methohexital – Methohexital has been used in cesarean section delivery, but because of its solubility and lack of protein binding, it readily and rapidly traverses the placenta.

➤*Lactation:* Small amounts of **thiopental** may appear in breast milk following administration of large doses. Exercise caution when administering barbiturates to a breast-feeding woman.

➤*Children:*

Methohexital – Safety and efficacy in children have not been established.

➤*Elderly:* Per the Beers list, all barbiturates (except **phenobarbital**) are highly addictive and cause more adverse effects than most sedative or hypnotic drugs in elderly patients except when used to control seizures.

Drug Interactions

Barbiturate Drug Interactions

Precipitant drug	Object drug[a]		Description
Narcotics	Barbiturate anesthetics	↑	The barbiturate dose required to induce anesthesia may be reduced. Apnea may be more common with this combination.
Phenothiazines	Barbiturate anesthetics	↑	Preanesthetic use of phenothiazines may raise the frequency and severity of neuromuscular excitation and hypotension in patients who receive barbiturate anesthesia.
Probenecid	Barbiturate anesthetics	↑	The anesthesia produced by the barbiturate may be extended or achieved at lower doses.
Sulfisoxazole	Barbiturate anesthetics	↑	Sulfisoxazole may enhance the anesthetic effects of the barbiturate.

[a] ↑ = object drug increased.

➤*Drug/Lab test interactions:* Body segment parameter and liver function studies may be influenced by administration of a single dose of barbiturates.

Adverse Reactions

➤*Cardiovascular:* Circulatory depression; thrombophlebitis; hypotension; peripheral vascular collapse; convulsions in association with cardiorespiratory arrest; myocardial depression; cardiac arrhythmias.

➤*CNS:* Emergence delirium; headache; restlessness; anxiety; seizures; prolonged somnolence and recovery.

➤*GI:* Nausea; emesis; abdominal pain. Rectal irritation; diarrhea; cramping; rectal bleeding (rectal administration).

➤*Hypersensitivity:*

Acute allergic reactions – Erythema; pruritus; urticaria; anaphylactic reaction.

➤*Respiratory:* Respiratory depression including apnea; dyspnea; rhinitis; laryngospasm; bronchospasm; sneezing; coughing.

➤*Miscellaneous:* Salivation; hiccups, skin rashes; skeletal muscle hyperactivity; shivering.

Rarely, immune hemolytic anemia with renal failure and radial nerve palsy have occurred.

Overdosage

➤*Symptoms:* Overdosage may occur from too rapid or repeated injections. Too rapid injection may be followed by an alarming fall in blood pressure, even to shock levels. Apnea, occasional laryngospasm, coughing, and other respiratory difficulties with excessive or too rapid injections may occur.

➤*Treatment:* In the event of suspected or apparent overdosage, discontinue the drug, maintain or establish a patent airway (intubate if necessary), and administer oxygen with assisted ventilation if necessary. The lethal dose of barbiturates varies and cannot be stated with certainty. Lethal blood levels may be as low as 1 mg/dL for short-acting barbiturates; less if other depressant drugs or alcohol are also present.

THIOPENTAL SODIUM

c-iii	**Thiopental Sodium** (IMS)	**Powder for Injection:** 2% (20 mg/ml)	In 400 mg *Min-I-Mix* vials with *Min-I-Mix* injector.
c-iii	**Pentothal** (Abbott)		In 1, 2.5 and 5 g kits, 400 mg *Ready-to-Mix* syringes and 400 mg *Ready-to-Mix LifeShield* syringes.
c-iii	**Thiopental Sodium** (Various, eg, Gensia, IMS)	**Powder for Injection:** 2.5% (25 mg/ml)	In 250 and 500 mg *Min-I-Mix* vials with *Min-I-Mix* and 500 mg, 1, 2.5, 5 and 10 g kits.
c-iii	**Pentothal** (Abbott)		In 1, 2.5, 5 g and 500 mg kits, 250 and 500 mg *Ready-to-Mix* syringes and 250 and 500 mg *Ready-to-Mix LifeShield* syringes.

THIOPENTAL SODIUM — INJECTION

For complete and comparative prescribing information refer to the Barbiturate Anesthetics group monograph.

Indications

➤*Anesthesia:* As the sole anesthetic agent for brief (15 minute) procedures; induction of anesthesia prior to administration of other anesthetic agents; to supplement regional anesthesia; to provide hypnosis during balanced anesthesia with other agents for analgesia or muscle relaxation.

➤*Convulsive states:* For the control of convulsive states during or following inhalation anesthesia, local anesthesia or other causes.

➤*Neurosurgical patients with increased intracranial pressure:* For use in neurosurgical patients with increased intracranial pressure, if adequate ventilation is provided.

➤*Narcoanalysis/Narcosynthesis:* For narcoanalysis and narcosynthesis in psychiatric disorders.

Administration and Dosage

➤*General dosing considerations:* Thiopental should be administered only by IV injection and by individuals experienced in the conduct of IV anesthesia.

Individual response to the drug is so varied that there can be no fixed dosage. The drug should be titrated against patient requirements as governed by age, sex, and body weight. Prepuberty requirements are the same for both sexes, but adult women require less than adult men. Dose is usually proportional to body weight, and obese patients require a larger dose than relatively lean persons of the same weight.

A test dose is advisable. See Test dose.

➤*Adults:*

Anesthesia – Moderately slow induction can usually be accomplished in the "average" adult by injection of 50 to 75 mg (2 to 3 mL of a 2.5% solution) at intervals of 20 to 40 seconds, depending on the reaction of the patient. Once anesthesia is established, additional injections of 25 to 50 mg can be given whenever the patient moves.

Slow injection is recommended to minimize respiratory depression and the possibility of overdosage. The smallest dose consistent with attaining the surgical objective is the desired goal. Momentary apnea following each injection is typical, and progressive decrease in the amplitude of respiration appears with increasing dosage. Pulse remains normal or increases slightly and returns to normal. Blood pressure usually falls slightly, but returns toward normal. Muscles usually relax about 30 seconds after unconsciousness is attained, but this may be masked if a skeletal muscle relaxant is used. The tone of jaw muscles is a fairly reliable index. The pupils may dilate, but later contract; sensitivity to light is not usually lost until a level of anesthesia deep enough to permit surgery is attained. Nystagmus and divergent strabismus are characteristic during early stages, but at the level of surgical anesthesia the eyes are central and fixed. Corneal and conjunctival reflexes disappear during surgical anesthesia.

Balanced anesthesia: When thiopental is used for induction in balanced anesthesia with a skeletal muscle relaxant and an inhalation agent, the total dose of thiopental can be estimated and then injected in 2 to 4 fractional doses. With this technique, brief periods of apnea may occur, which may require assisted or controlled pulmonary ventilation. As an initial dose, 210 to 280 mg (3 to 4 mg/kg) of thiopental is usually required for rapid induction in the average adult (70 kg).

Sole anesthetic agent: When thiopental is used as the sole anesthetic agent, the desired level of anesthesia can be maintained by injection of small repeated doses as needed, or by using a continuous IV drip in a 0.2% or 0.4% concentration. (Sterile water should not be used as the diluent in these concentrations, since hemolysis will occur.) With continuous drip, the depth of anesthesia is controlled by adjusting the rate of infusion.

Convulsive states – 75 to 125 mg (3 to 5 mL of a 2.5% solution) should be given as soon as possible after the convulsion begins. Convulsions following the use of a local anesthetic may require thiopental 125 to 250 mg given over a 10-minute period. If the convulsion is caused by a local anesthetic, the required dose of thiopental will depend upon the amount of local anesthetic given and its convulsant properties.

Narcoanalysis/narcosynthesis – Premedication with an anticholinergic agent may precede administration of thiopental. After a test dose (see Test dose), thiopental is injected at a slow rate of 100 mg/min (4 mL/min of a 2.5% solution) with the patient counting backwards from 100. Shortly after counting becomes confused, but before actual sleep is produced, the injection is discontinued. Allow the patient to return to a semidrowsy state where conversation is coherent. Alternatively, thiopental may be administered by rapid IV drip using 0.2% concentration in 5% dextrose and water. At this concentration, the rate of administration should not exceed 50 mL/min.

Neurosurgical patients with increased intracranial pressure – Intermittent bolus injections of 1.5 to 3.5 mg/kg may be given to reduce intraoperative elevations of intracranial pressure, if adequate ventilation is provided.

➤*Children:* Younger patients require relatively larger doses than middle-aged and elderly patients.

➤*Test dose:* It is advisable to inject a small "test" dose of 25 to 75 mg (1 to 3 mL of a 2.5% solution) of thiopental to assess tolerance or unusual sensitivity to thiopental and pausing to observe patient reaction for at least 60 seconds. If unexpectedly deep anesthesia develops or if respiratory depression occurs consider these possibilities:

1.) the patient may be unusually sensitive to thiopental,
2.) the solution may be more concentrated than had been assumed, or
3.) the patient may have received too much premedication.

➤*Premedication:* Premedication usually consists of atropine or scopolamine to suppress vagal reflexes and inhibit secretions. In addition, a barbiturate or an opiate is often given. Sodium pentobarbital injection is suggested because it provides a preliminary indication of how the patient will react to barbiturate anesthesia. Ideally, the peak effect of these medications should be reached shortly before the time of induction.

➤*Preparation for administration:* The volume and choice of diluent for preparing thiopental depends on the concentration and vehicle desired. Thiopental kits provide only sterile water for injection as the diluent for individual or multipatient use, or sodium chloride 0.9% injection as the diluent for individual patient use.

Thiopental is supplied as a yellowish, hygroscopic powder in a variety of different containers. Solutions should be prepared aseptically with one of the 3 following diluents: sterile water for injection, sodium chloride 0.9% injection or dextrose 5% injection. Clinical concentrations used for intermittent IV administration vary between 2% and 5%. A 2% or 2.5% solution is most commonly used. A 3.4% concentration in sterile water for injection is isotonic; concentrations less than 2% in this diluent are not used because they cause hemolysis. For continuous IV drip administration, concentrations of 0.2% or 0.4% are used. Solutions may be prepared by adding thiopental to dextrose 5% injection, sodium chloride 0.9% injection or a combined electrolyte solution (pH 7.4).

Because thiopental contains no added bacteriostatic agent, extreme care in preparation and handling should be exercised at all times to prevent the introduction of microbial contaminants. Solutions should be freshly prepared and used promptly; when reconstituted for administration to several patients, unused portions should be discarded after 24 hours. Sterilization by heating should not be attempted.

Warning – The 2.5 g and larger sizes contain adequate medication for several patients.

Calculations for Various Concentrations of Thiopental

Concentration desired		Thiopental	Diluent
Percent	mg/mL	g	mL
0.2	2	1	500
0.4	4	1	250
		2	500
2	20	5	250
		10	500
2.5	25	1	40
		5	200
5	50	1	20
		5	100

➤*Administration:* Thiopental is administered by the IV route only.

➤*Admixture compatibility:* Any solution of thiopental with a visible precipitate should not be administered. The stability of thiopental solutions depends on several factors, including the diluent, temperature of storage, and the amount of carbon dioxide from room air that gains access to the solution. Any factor or condition that tends to lower pH (increase acidity) of thiopental solutions will increase the likelihood of precipitation of thiopental acid. Such factors include the use of diluents that are too acidic and the absorption of carbon dioxide, which can combine with water to form carbonic acid.

Solutions of succinylcholine, tubocurarine, or other drugs that have an acid pH should not be mixed with thiopental solutions. The most stable solutions are those reconstituted in water or isotonic saline, kept under refrigeration, and tightly stoppered. The presence or absence of a visible precipitate offers

THIOPENTAL SODIUM — INJECTION

a practical guide to the physical compatibility of prepared solutions of thiopental.

➤*Storage/Stability:* Store product prior to reconstitution at 15° to 30°C (59° to 86°F). Store reconstituted solution in a cool place and use within 24 hours of mixing. Administer only clear solution.

METHOHEXITAL SODIUM

c-iv	**Brevital Sodium** (JHP Pharm)	**Powder for Injection**[a]: 500 mg	30 mg anhydrous sodium carbonate. In 50 mL multiple dose vials.
		2.5 g	150 mg anhydrous sodium carbonate. In 50 mL multiple dose vials.

[a] May be administered IV, IM, or rectally.

METHOHEXITAL SODIUM — INJECTION

For complete and comparative prescribing information, refer to the Barbiturate Anesthetics group monograph.

WARNING

Use methohexital only in hospital or ambulatory care settings that provide for continuous monitoring of respiratory (eg, pulse oximetry) and cardiac function. Ensure immediate availability of resuscitative drugs and age- and size-appropriate equipment for bag/valve/mask ventilation and intubation and personnel trained in their use and skilled in airway management. For deeply sedated patients, a designated individual other than the practitioner performing the procedure should be present to continuously monitor the patient.

Indications

➤*Adult usage:* Methohexital can be used in adults as follows:

- For intravenous (IV) induction of anesthesia prior to the use of other general anesthetic agents.
- For IV induction of anesthesia and as an adjunct to subpotent inhalational anesthetic agents (such as nitrous oxide in oxygen) for short surgical procedures; give methohexital by infusion or intermittent injection.
- For use along with other parenteral agents, usually narcotic analgesics, to supplement subpotent inhalational anesthetic agents (such as nitrous oxide in oxygen) for longer surgical procedures.
- As IV anesthesia for short surgical, diagnostic, or therapeutic procedures associated with minimal painful stimuli.
- As an agent for inducing a hypnotic state.

➤*Child usage:* Methohexital can be used in children older than 1 month as follows:

- For intramuscular (IM) induction of anesthesia prior to the use of other general anesthetic agents.
- For IM induction of anesthesia and as an adjunct to subpotent inhalational anesthetic agents for short surgical procedures.
- As IM anesthesia for short surgical, diagnostic, or therapeutic procedures associated with minimal painful stimuli.

Administration and Dosage

➤*General dosing considerations:* Dosage is highly individualized; the drug should be administered only by those completely familiar with its quantitative differences from other barbiturate anesthetics.

Facilities for assisting ventilation and administering oxygen are necessary adjuncts for all routes of administration of anesthesia. Because cardiorespiratory arrest may occur, carefully observe patients during and after use of methohexital. Age- and size-appropriate resuscitative equipment (ie, intubation and cardioversion equipment, oxygen, suction, and a secure IV line) and personnel qualified in its use must be immediately available.

Preanesthetic medication is generally advisable. Methohexital may be used with any of the recognized preanesthetic medications.

➤*Adults:*

Induction of anesthesia –

Usual dosage: 50 to 120 mg or more, but averages approximately 70 mg. The usual dose in adults ranges from 1 to 1.5 mg/kg. The induction dose usually provides anesthesia for 5 to 7 minutes. A 1% solution is administered at a rate of approximately 1 mL per 5 seconds.

Concomitant therapy: Gaseous anesthetics and/or skeletal muscle relaxants may be administered concomitantly.

Maintenance of anesthesia –

Usual dosage: Intermittent injections of the 1% solution or, more easily, by continuous IV drip of a 0.2% solution. Give intermittent injections of approximately 20 to 40 mg (2 to 4 mL of a 1% solution) as required, usually every 4 to 7 minutes. For continuous drip, the average rate of administration of a 0.2% solution is approximately 3 mL/min (1 drop/second). Individualize the rate of flow for each patient. For longer surgical procedures, gradual reduction in the rate of administration is recommended.

Prolonged administration may result in cumulative effects, including extended somnolence, protracted unconsciousness, and respiratory and cardiovascular depression. Respiratory depression in the presence of an impaired airway may lead to hypoxia, cardiac arrest, and death.

Concomitant therapy: Other parenteral agents, usually narcotic analgesics, are ordinarily employed along with methohexital during longer procedures.

➤*Children:*

Induction of anesthesia –

One month of age and older: 6.6 to 10 mg/kg IM of the 5% concentration.

➤*Renal function impairment:* Exercise caution in patients with impaired renal function.

➤*Hepatic function impairment:* Exercise caution in patients with impaired hepatic function.

➤*Preparation for administration:* Follow diluting instructions exactly. Freshly prepare and promptly use solutions of methohexital. Reconstituted solutions of methohexital are chemically stable at room temperature for 24 hours.

Do not use a bacteriostatic-containing diluent. The preferred diluent is sterile water for injection. Acceptable diluents are dextrose 5% injection and sodium chloride 0.9% injection. Ringer's lactate injection is an incompatible diluent.

IV administration – 1% solutions (10 mg/mL) should be prepared for IV use. Contents of vials should be diluted according to the following.

Methohexital Dilution for IV Administration		
Strength	Amount of diluent to be added to the contents of the vial	For 1% solution
500 mg	50 mL	No further dilution needed
2.5 g	15 mL	Added to 235 mL for 250 mL total volume

When the first dilution is made with 2.5 g, the solution in the vial will be yellow. When further diluted to make a 1% solution, the solution must be clear and colorless or it should not be used.

For continuous drip anesthesia, prepare a 0.2% solution by adding methohexital 500 mg to 250 mL of diluent. For this dilution, either glucose 5% solution or isotonic (0.9%) sodium chloride solution is recommended instead of distilled water to avoid extreme hypotonicity.

IM administration – Contents of the vials should be diluted according to the following.

Methohexital Dilution for IM Administration		
Strength	Amount of diluent to be added to the contents of the vial	Concentration after dilution
500 mg vial	10 mL	5% solution (50 mg/mL)
2.5 g vial	50 mL	5% solution (50 mg/mL)

➤*Administration:* Methohexital may be administered by direct IV injection, continuous IV drip, or IM routes.

For adults, a 1% solution is administered at a rate of approximately 1 mL per 5 seconds. Administer methohexital IV at a concentration no higher than 1%. Higher concentrations markedly increase the incidence of muscular movements and irregularities in respiration and blood pressure.

For children, administer methohexital IM in a 5% concentration.

➤*Admixture compatibility:* Do not use a bacteriostatic-containing diluent. Ringer's lactate injection is an incompatible diluent. Do not mix solutions of methohexital in the same syringe or administer simultaneously during IV infusion through the same needle with acid solutions such as atropine sulfate, metocurine iodide, and succinylcholine chloride. Alteration of pH may cause free barbituric acid to be precipitated. Solubility of the soluble sodium salts of barbiturates, including methohexital, is maintained only at a relatively high (basic) pH.

Because of numerous requests from anesthesiologists for information regarding the chemical compatibility of these mixtures, the following chart contains information obtained from compatibility studies in which a methohexital 1% solution was mixed with therapeutic amounts of agents whose solutions have a low (acidic) pH.

Methohexital Compatibility						
Active ingredient	Potency/ mL	Volume used	Physical change			
			Immediate	15 min	30 min	1 h
Methohexital	10 mg	10 mL			control	
Atropine sulfate	1/150 g	1 mL	none	haze		
Atropine sulfate	1/100 g	1 mL	none	precipitate	precipitate	

Barbiturates

METHOHEXITAL SODIUM — INJECTION

Methohexital Compatibility							
Active ingredient	Potency/ mL	Volume used	Physical change				
			Immediate	15 min	30 min	1 h	
Succinyl-choline chloride	0.5 mg	4 mL	none	none	haze		
Succinyl-choline chloride	1 mg	4 mL	none	none	haze		
Metocurine iodide	0.5 mg	4 mL	none	none	precipitate		
Metocurine iodide	1 mg	4 mL	none	none	precipitate		
Scopol-amine hydrobro-mide	1/120 gr	1 mL	none	none	none	haze	
Tubocura-rine chloride	3 mg	4 mL	none	haze			

➤*Storage/Stability:* Store at 20° to 25°C (68° to 77°F). Reconstituted solutions of methohexital are chemically stable at room temperature for 24 hours.

METHOHEXITAL SODIUM — RECTAL

For complete and comparative prescribing information, refer to the Barbiturate Anesthetics group monograph.

WARNING

Methohexital sodium should be used only in hospital or ambulatory care settings that provide for continuous monitoring of respiratory (eg, pulse oximetry) and cardiac function. Immediate availability of resuscitative drugs and age- and size-appropriate equipment for bag/valve/mask ventilation and intubation and personnel trained in their use and skilled in airway management should be assured. For deeply sedated patients, a designated individual other than the practitioner performing the procedure should be present to continuously monitor the patient.

Indications

➤*Child usage:* Methohexital sodium can be used in children older than 1 month as follows:
- For rectal induction of anesthesia prior to the use of other general anesthetic agents.
- For rectal induction of anesthesia and as an adjunct to subpotent inhalational anesthetic agents for short surgical procedures.
- As rectal anesthesia for short surgical, diagnostic, or therapeutic procedures associated with minimal painful stimuli.

Administration and Dosage

➤*General dosing considerations:* Dosage is highly individualized; the drug should be administered only by those completely familiar with its quantitative differences from other barbiturate anesthetics.

Facilities for assisting ventilation and administering oxygen are necessary adjuncts for all routes of administration of anesthesia. Because cardiorespiratory arrest may occur, patients should be observed carefully during and after use of methohexital sodium. Age- and size-appropriate resuscitative equipment (ie, intubation and cardioversion equipment, oxygen, suction, and a secure IV line) and personnel qualified in its use must be immediately available.

Preanesthetic medication is generally advisable. Methohexital sodium may be used with any of the recognized preanesthetic medications.

➤*Children:*

Induction of anesthesia –

1 month of age and older: 25 mg/kg administered rectally using the 1% solution.

➤*Preparation for administration:* Freshly prepare and use promptly solutions of methohexital.

Do not use diluents containing bacteriostatics. The preferred diluent is sterile water for injection. Acceptable diluents are dextrose 5% injection and sodium chloride 0.9% injection. Lactated Ringer's injection is an incompatible diluent.

Methohexital Dilution for Rectal Administration		
Strength	Amount of diluent to be added to the contents of the vial	Concentration after dilution
500 mg vial	50 mL	1% solution (10 mg/mL)
2.5 g vial (larger vial needed)	250 mL	1% solution (10 mg/mL)

➤*Admixture compatibility:* Do not use diluents containing bacteriostatics. Lactated Ringer's injection is an incompatible diluent.

➤*Storage/Stability:* Store at 20° to 25°C (68° to 77°F). Reconstituted solutions of methohexital are chemically stable at room temperature for 24 hours.

Benzodiazepines

MIDAZOLAM HYDROCHLORIDE

c-iv	Midazolam Hydrochloride (Roxane)	Syrup: 2 mg/mL	EDTA, saccharin, sorbitol. Cherry flavor. In 118 mL.
c-iv	Midazolam Hydrochloride (Various, eg, Bedford, Hospira)	Injection: 1 mg (as HCl)/mL	In 2 and 5 mL vials and *Carpuject* vials and 10 mL vials.
		5 mg (as HCl)/mL	In 1, 2, and 5 mL vials and *Carpuject* vials, 10 mL vials, and 2 mL syringes.

For complete and comparative prescribing information, refer to the Benzodiazepines monograph in the Antianxiety Agents section.

MIDAZOLAM HYDROCHLORIDE — ORAL

WARNING

Midazolam syrup has been associated with respiratory depression and respiratory arrest, especially when used for sedation in noncritical care settings. Midazolam syrup has been associated with reports of respiratory depression, airway obstruction, desaturation, hypoxia, and apnea, most often when used concomitantly with other CNS depressants (eg, opioids). Midazolam syrup should be used only in hospital or ambulatory care settings, including physicians' and dentists' offices, that can provide for continuous monitoring of respiratory and cardiac function. Immediate availability of resuscitative drugs and age- and size-appropriate equipment for ventilation and intubation, and personnel trained in their use and skilled in airway management should be ensured (see Warnings). For deeply sedated patients, a dedicated individual, other than the practitioner performing the procedure, should monitor the patient throughout the procedure.

Indications

➤*Sedation/Anxiolysis/Amnesia:* For use in children for sedation, anxiolysis, and amnesia prior to diagnostic, therapeutic or endoscopic procedures or before induction of anesthesia.

Administration and Dosage

➤*General dosing considerations:* Children undergoing procedures involving the upper airway, such as upper endoscopy or dental care, are particularly vulnerable to episodes of desaturation and hypoventilation due to partial airway obstruction.

Patients must be monitored for signs of cardiorespiratory depression after receiving midazolam.

In obese children, the dose should be calculated based on ideal body weight.

Midazolam has not been studied, nor is it intended for chronic use.

➤*Children:*

Amnesia –

6 to 16 years of age or cooperative patients:
- *Maximum dose* – 20 mg.
- *Single dose* – 0.25 to 0.5 mg/kg.

6 months to 6 years of age or less cooperative patients: Up to 1 mg/kg.

Cardiac or respiratory compromise, concurrent CNS depressive drug, or high-risk surgery: 0.25 mg/kg.

Concomitant therapy: When given in conjunction with opioids or other sedatives, the potential for respiratory depression, airway obstruction, or hypoventilation is increased.

Anxiolysis – See Amnesia for dosing.

Sedation – See Amnesia for dosing.

➤*Hepatic function impairment:* Titrate in patients with chronic hepatic disease.

MIDAZOLAM HYDROCHLORIDE — ORAL

➤*Preparation for administration:* Insertion of press-in bottle adapter (PIBA):

1.) Remove the cap and push bottle adapter into neck of bottle.
2.) Close the bottle tightly with cap. This will ensure the proper seating of the bottle adapter in the bottle.

Use of oral dispensers and PIBA:

1.) Remove the cap.
2.) Before inserting the tip of the oral dispenser into bottle adapter, push the plunger completely down toward the tip of the oral dispenser. Insert tip firmly into opening of the bottle adapter.
3.) The tip of the dispenser may be covered with a tip cap until time of use.
4.) Close bottle with cap after each use.

➤*Administration:* Dispense directly into mouth. Do not mix with any liquid (such as grapefruit juice) prior to dispensing.

➤*Storage/Stability:* Store at 25°C (77°F); excursions are permitted to 15° to 30°C (59° to 86°F).

Actions

➤*Pharmacology:* Midazolam is a short-acting benzodiazepine CNS depressant.

Pharmacodynamic properties of midazolam and its metabolites, which are similar to those of other benzodiazepines, include sedative, anxiolytic, amnesic and hypnotic activities. Benzodiazepine pharmacologic effects appear to result from reversible interactions with the gamma-amino butyric acid (GABA) benzodiazepine receptor, the major inhibitory neurotransmitter in the CNS. The action of midazolam is readily reversed by the benzodiazepine receptor antagonist, flumazenil.

See Warnings/Precautions for more information.

See Drug Interactions for more information.

Pharmacodynamics – The relationship between plasma concentration and sedation and anxiolysis scores of oral midazolam syrup (single oral doses of 0.25, 0.5, or 1 mg/kg) was investigated in 3 age groups of pediatric patients (6 months to < 2 years, 2 to < 12 years, and 12 to < 16 years old). In this study, the patient's sedation scores were recorded at baseline and at 10-minute intervals up to 30 minutes after oral dosing until satisfactory sedation ("drowsy" or "asleep but responsive to mild shaking" or "asleep and not responsive to mild shaking") was achieved. Anxiolysis scores were measured at the time when the patient was separated from his/her parents and at mask induction. The results of the analyses showed that the mean midazolam plasma concentration as well as the mean of midazolam plus alpha-hydroxymidazolam for those patients with a sedation score of 4 (asleep but responsive to mild shaking) is significantly different than the mean concentrations for those patients with a sedation score of 3 (drowsy), which is significantly different than the mean concentrations for patients with a sedation score of 2 (awake/calm). The statistical analysis indicates that the greater the midazolam, or midazolam plus alpha-hydroxymidazolam concentration, the greater the maximum sedation score for pediatric patients. No such trend was observed between anxiolysis scores and the mean midazolam concentration or mean of midazolam plus alpha-hydroxymidazolam concentration; however, anxiolysis is a more variable surrogate measurement of clinical response.

➤*Pharmacokinetics:*

Midazolam Syrup Pharmacokinetics

Number of subjects	Dose (mg/kg)	t_{max} (hr)	C_{max} (ng/mL)	t½ (hr)	$AUC_{0-\infty}$ (ng•hr/mL)
6 months to < 2 years old					
1	0.25	0.17	28	5.82	67.6
1	0.5	0.35	66	2.22	152
1	1	0.17	61.2	2.97	224
2 to < 12 years old					
18	0.25	0.72 ± 0.44	63 ± 30	3.16 ± 1.5	138 ± 89.5
18	0.5	0.95 ± 0.53	126 ± 75.8	2.71 ± 1.09	306 ± 196
18	1	0.88 ± 0.99	201 ± 101	2.37 ± 0.96	743 ± 642
12 to < 16 years old					
4	0.25	2.09 ± 1.35	29.1 ± 8.2	6.83 ± 3.84	155 ± 84.6
4	0.5	2.65 ± 1.58	118 ± 81.2	4.35 ± 3.31	821 ± 568
2	1	0.55 ± 0.28	191 ± 47.4	2.51 ± 0.18	566 ± 15.7

Absorption – Midazolam is rapidly absorbed after oral administration and is subject to substantial intestinal and hepatic first-pass metabolism. The pharmacokinetics of midazolam and its major metabolite, alpha-hydroxymidazolam, and the absolute bioavailability of midazolam hydrochloride syrup were studied in pediatric patients of different ages (6 months to < 16 years old) over a 0.25 to 1 mg/kg dose range. Pharmacokinetic parameters from this study are presented in the following paragraphs. The mean t_{max} values across dose groups (0.25, 0.5, and 1 mg/kg) range from 0.17 to 2.65 hours. Midazolam exhibits linear pharmacokinetics between oral doses of 0.25 to 1 mg/kg (up to a maximum dose of 40 mg) across the age groups ranging from 6 months to < 16 years. Linearity was also demonstrated across the doses within the age group of 2 years to < 12 years having 18 patients at each of the 3 doses. The absolute bioavailability of the midazolam syrup in pediatric patients is about 36%, which is not affected by pediatric age or weight. The $AUC_{0-\infty}$ ratio of alpha-hydroxymidazolam to midazolam for the oral dose in pediatric patients is higher than for an IV dose (0.38 to 0.75 vs 0.21 to 0.39 across the age group of 6 months to < 16 years), and the AUC $_{0-\infty}$ ratio of alpha-hydroxymidazolam to midazolam for the oral dose is higher in pediatric patients than in adults (0.38 to 0.75 vs 0.4 to 0.56).

Distribution – The extent of plasma protein binding of midazolam is moderately high and concentration-independent. In adults and pediatric patients > 1 year of age, midazolam is ≈ 97% bound to plasma protein, principally albumin. In healthy volunteers, alpha-hydroxymidazolam is bound to the extent of 89%. In pediatric patients (6 months to < 16 years) receiving 0.15 mg/kg IV midazolam, the mean steady-state volume of distribution ranged from 1.24 to 2.02 L/kg.

Metabolism – Midazolam is primarily metabolized in the liver and gut by human cytochrome P450 3A4 (CYP3A4) to its pharmacologic active metabolite, alpha-hydroxymidazolam, followed by glucuronidation of the alpha-hydroxyl metabolite which is present in unconjugated and conjugated forms in human plasma. The alpha-hydroxymidazolam glucuronide is then excreted in urine. In a study in which adult volunteers were administered IV midazolam (0.1 mg/kg) and alpha-hydroxymidazolam (0.15 mg/kg), the pharmacodynamic parameter values of the maximum effect (E_{max}) and concentration eliciting half-maximal effect (EC_{50}) were similar for both compounds. The effects studied were reaction time and errors in tracing tests. The results indicate that alpha-hydroxymidazolam is equipotent and equally effective as unchanged midazolam on a total plasma concentration basis. After oral or IV administration, 63% to 80% of midazolam is recovered in urine as alpha-hydroxymidazolam glucuronide. No significant amount of parent drug or metabolites is extractable from urine before beta-glucuronidase and sulfatase deconjugation, indicating that the urinary metabolites are excreted mainly as conjugates.

Midazolam is also metabolized to 2 other minor metabolites: 4-hydroxy metabolite (about 3% of the dose) and 1,4-dihydroxy metabolite (about 1% of the dose) are excreted in small amounts in the urine as conjugates.

Excretion – The mean elimination half-life of midazolam ranged from 2.2 to 6.8 hours following single oral doses of 0.25, 0.5, and 1 mg/kg of midazolam (midazolam hydrochloride syrup). Similar results (ranged from 2.9 to 4.5 hours) for the mean elimination half-life were observed following IV administration of 0.15 mg/kg of midazolam to pediatric patients (6 months to < 16 years old). In the same group of patients receiving the 0.15 mg/kg IV dose, the mean total clearance ranged from 9.3 to 11 mL/min/kg.

Special populations –

Hepatic function impairment: Chronic hepatic disease alters the pharmacokinetics of midazolam. Following oral administration of 15 mg of midazolam, C_{max} and bioavailability values were 43% and 100% higher, respectively, in adult patients with hepatic cirrhosis than adult subjects with healthy liver function. In the same patients with hepatic cirrhosis, following IV administration of 7.5 mg of midazolam, the clearance of midazolam was reduced by about 40% and the elimination half-life was increased by about 90% compared with subjects with healthy liver function. Midazolam should be titrated for the desired effect in patients with chronic hepatic disease.

Congestive heart failure: Following oral administration of 7.5 mg of midazolam, elimination half-life values were 43% higher in adult patients with congestive heart failure than in control subjects.

Contraindications

Hypersensitivity to the drug or allergies to cherries or formulation excipients; acute narrow-angle glaucoma. Benzodiazepines may be used in patients with open-angle glaucoma only if they are receiving appropriate therapy. Measurements of intraocular pressure in patients without eye disease show a moderate lowering following induction of general anesthesia with injectable midazolam hydrochloride; patients with glaucoma have not been studied.

Warnings/Precautions

➤*Respiratory effects:* Serious respiratory adverse reactions have occurred after administration of oral midazolam hydrochloride, most often when midazolam hydrochloride was used in combination with other CNS depressants. These adverse reactions have included respiratory depression, airway obstruction, oxygen desaturation, apnea, and rarely, respiratory or cardiac arrest. When oral midazolam is administered as the sole agent at recommended doses respiratory depression, airway obstruction, oxygen desaturation, and apnea occur infrequently.

Patients should be continuously monitored for early signs of hypoventilation, airway obstruction, or apnea with means for detection readily available (eg, pulse oximetry). Hypoventilation, airway obstruction, and apnea can lead to hypoxia or cardiac arrest unless effective countermeasures are taken immediately. The immediate availability of specific reversal agents (flumazenil) is highly recommended. Vital signs should continue to be monitored during the recovery period. Because midazolam hydrochloride can depress respiration (see Pharmacology), especially when used concomitantly with opioid agonists and other sedatives (see Administration and Dosage), it should be used for sedation/anxiolysis/amnesia only in the presence of personnel skilled in early detection of hypoventilation, maintaining a patent airway, and supporting ventilation.

Episodes of oxygen desaturation, respiratory depression, apnea, and airway obstruction have been occasionally reported following premedication (sedation prior to induction of anesthesia) with oral midazolam; such events are markedly increased when oral midazolam is combined with other CNS-depressing agents and in patients with abnormal airway anatomy, patients with cyanotic congenital heart disease, or patients with sepsis or severe pulmonary disease.

➤*Monitoring:* Prior to the administration of midazolam hydrochloride in any dose, the immediate availability of oxygen, resuscitative drugs, age- and

MIDAZOLAM HYDROCHLORIDE — ORAL

size-appropriate equipment for bag/valve/mask ventilation and intubation, and skilled personnel for the maintenance of a patent airway and support of ventilation should be ensured. Midazolam hydrochloride syrup must never be used without individualization of dosage, particularly when used with other medications capable of producing CNS depression.

Midazolam hydrochloride syrup should be used only in hospital or ambulatory care settings, including physicians' and dentists' offices, that are equipped to provide continuous monitoring of respiratory and cardiac function. Midazolam hydrochloride syrup must only be administered to patients if they will be monitored by direct visual observation by a healthcare professional. If midazolam hydrochloride syrup will be administered in combination with other anesthetic drugs or drugs which depress the CNS, patients must be monitored by persons specifically trained in the use of these drugs and, in particular, in the management of respiratory effects of these drugs, including respiratory and cardiac resuscitation of patients in the age group being treated.

➤*Improper dosing:* Reactions such as agitation, involuntary movements (including tonic/clonic movements and muscle tremor), hyperactivity and combativeness have been reported in both adult and pediatric patients. Consideration should be given to the possibility of paradoxical reaction. Should such reactions occur, the response to each dose of midazolam hydrochloride and all other drugs, including local anesthetics, should be evaluated before proceeding. Reversal of such responses with flumazenil has been reported in pediatric and adult patients.

➤*Special risk:* Higher-risk pediatric surgical patients may require lower doses, whether or not concomitant, sedating medications have been administered. Pediatric patients with cardiac or respiratory compromise may be unusually sensitive to the respiratory-depressant effect of midazolam hydrochloride. Pediatric patients undergoing procedures involving the upper airway such as upper endoscopy or dental care, are particularly vulnerable to episodes of desaturation and hypoventilation due to partial airway obstruction. Patients with chronic renal failure and patients with congestive heart failure eliminate midazolam more slowly.

➤*Use with other CNS depressants:* The efficacy and safety of midazolam hydrochloride in clinical use are functions of the dose administered, the clinical status of the individual patient, and the use of concomitant medications capable of depressing the CNS. Anticipated effects may range from mild sedation to deep levels of sedation with a potential loss of protective reflexes, particularly when coadministered with anesthetic agents or other CNS depressants. Care must be taken to individualize the dose of midazolam hydrochloride based on the patient's age, underlying medical/surgical conditions, concomitant medications, and to have the personnel, age- and size-appropriate equipment and facilities available for monitoring and intervention. Practitioners administering midazolam hydrochloride must have the skills necessary to manage reasonably foreseeable adverse effects, particularly skills in airway management.

➤*Special risk:* Following oral administration of 7.5 mg of midazolam to adult patients with congestive heart failure, the half-life of midazolam was 43% higher than in control subjects. One study suggests that hypercarbia or hypoxia following premedication with oral midazolam might pose a risk to children with congenital heart disease and pulmonary hypertension, although there are no known reports of pulmonary hypertensive crises that had been triggered by premedication. In the study, 22 children were premedicated with oral midazolam (0.75 mg/kg) or IM morphine plus scopolamine prior to elective repair of congenital cardiac defects. Both premedication regimens increased $PtcCO_2$ and decreased SpO_2 and respiratory rates preferentially in patients with pulmonary hypertension.

➤*Drug abuse and dependence:* Midazolam hydrochloride syrup is a benzodiazepine and is a schedule IV controlled substance that can produce drug dependence of the diazepam-type. Therefore, midazolam hydrochloride syrup may be subject to misuse, abuse and addiction. Benzodiazepines can cause physical dependence. Physical dependence results in withdrawal symptoms in patients who abruptly discontinue the drug. Withdrawal symptoms (ie, convulsions, hallucinations, tremors, abdominal and muscle cramps, vomiting and sweating), similar in characteristics to those noted with barbiturates and alcohol have occurred following abrupt discontinuation of midazolam following chronic administration. Abdominal distention, nausea, vomiting, and tachycardia are prominent symptoms of withdrawal in infants. The handling of midazolam hydrochloride syrup should be managed to minimize the risk of diversion, including restriction of access and accounting procedures as appropriate to the clinical setting and as required by law.

➤*Hazardous tasks:* The decision as to when patients who have received midazolam hydrochloride syrup, particularly on an outpatient basis, may again engage in activities requiring complete mental alertness, operate hazardous machinery or drive a motor vehicle must be individualized. Gross tests of recovery from the effects of midazolam hydrochloride syrup (see Pharmacology) cannot be relied upon to predict reaction time under stress. It is recommended that no patient operate hazardous machinery or a motor vehicle until the effects of the drug, such as drowsiness, have subsided or until one full day after anesthesia and surgery, whichever is longer. Particular care should be taken to assure safe ambulation.

➤*Pregnancy: Category D.* Although midazolam hydrochloride syrup has not been studied in pregnant patients, an increased risk of congenital malformations associated with the use of benzodiazepine drugs (diazepam and chlordiazepoxide) have been suggested in several studies. If this drug is used during pregnancy, the patient should be apprised of the potential hazard to the fetus.

Labor and delivery – In humans, measurable levels of midazolam were found in maternal venous serum, umbilical venous and arterial serum and amniotic fluid, indicating placental transfer of the drug. The use of midazolam hydrochloride syrup in obstetrics has not been evaluated in clinical trials. Because midazolam is transferred transplacentally and because other benzodiazepines given in the last weeks of pregnancy have resulted in neonatal CNS depression, midazolam hydrochloride syrup is not recommended for obstetrical use.

➤*Lactation:* Midazolam is excreted in human milk. Caution should be exercised when midazolam hydrochloride syrup is administered to a nursing woman.

➤*Children:* Midazolam hydrochloride syrup has not been studied in patients

Drug Interactions

➤*CNS agents:* Concomitant use of barbiturates, alcohol or other CNS depressants may increase the risk of hypoventilation, airway obstruction, desaturation, or apnea and may contribute to profound or prolonged drug effect. Narcotic premedication also depresses the ventilatory response to carbon dioxide stimulation.

➤*Inhibitors of CYP3A4 isozymes:*

Oral Midazolam Interactions with Inhibitors of CYP3A4 Isozymes

Interacting drug	Adult doses studied	% Increase in C_{max} of oral midazolam	% Increase in AUC of oral midazolam
Cimetidine	800 to 1200 mg up to 4 times daily in divided doses	6 to 138	10 to 102
Diltiazem	60 mg 3 times daily	105	275
Erythromycin	500 mg 3 times daily	170 to 171	281 to 341
Fluconazole	200 mg once daily	150	250
Grapefruit juice	200 mL	56	52
Itraconazole	100 to 200 mg once daily	80 to 240	240 to 980
Ketoconazole	400 mg once daily	309	1490
Ranitidine	150 mg twice daily or 3 times daily; 300 mg once daily	15 to 67	9 to 66
Roxithromycin	300 mg once daily	37	47
Saquinavir	120 mg 3 times daily	235	514
Verapamil	80 mg 3 times daily	97	192

Other drugs known to inhibit the effects of CYP3A4 would be expected to have similar effects on these midazolam pharmacokinetic parameters.

➤*Inducers of CYP3A4 isozymes:*

Oral Midazolam Interactions with Inducers of CYP3A4 Isozymes

Interacting drug	Adult doses studied	% Decrease in C_{max} of oral midazolam	% Decrease in AUC of oral midazolam
Carbamazepine	Therapeutic doses	93	94
Phenytoin	Therapeutic doses	93	94
Rifampin	600 mg/day	94	96

Although not tested, phenobarbital, rifabutin and other drugs known to induce the effects of CYP3A4 would be expected to have similar effects on these midazolam pharmacokinetic parameters.

➤*CNS depressants:* One case was reported of inadequate sedation with chloral hydrate and later with oral midazolam due to a possible interaction with methylphenidate administered chronically in a 2-year-old boy with a history of Williams syndrome. The difficulty in achieving adequate sedation may have been the result of decreased absorption of the sedatives due to both the GI effects and stimulant effects of methylphenidate.

The sedative effect of midazolam hydrochloride syrup is accentuated by any concomitantly administered medication which depresses the CNS, particularly narcotics (eg, morphine, meperidine, fentanyl), propofol, ketamine, nitrous oxide, secobarbital and droperidol. Consequently, the dose of midazolam hydrochloride syrup should be adjusted according to the type and amount of concomitant medications administered and the desired clinical response.

Adverse Reactions

The distribution of adverse reactions occurring in patients evaluated in a randomized, double-blind, parallel-group trial are presented below by body system in order of decreasing frequency. For the premedication period (eg, sedation period prior to induction of anesthesia) alone, see the first table below. For over the entire monitoring period including premedication, anesthesia and recovery, see the second table below.

The distribution of adverse events occurring during the premedication period, before induction of anesthesia, is presented in the first table below. Emesis, which occurred in 31/397 (8%) patients over the entire monitoring period (premedication, anesthesia and recovery), occurred in 3/397 (0.8%) of

MIDAZOLAM HYDROCHLORIDE — ORAL

patients during the premedication period (from midazolam administration to mask induction). Nausea, which occurred in $^{14}/_{397}$ (4%) patients over the entire monitoring period, occurred in $^{2}/_{397}$ (0.5%) patients during the premedication period.

For the entire monitoring period (premedication, anesthesia and recovery), adverse reactions were reported by $^{82}/_{397}$ (21%) patients who received midazolam overall. The most frequently reported adverse reactions were emesis occurring in $^{31}/_{397}$ (8%) patients and nausea occurring in $^{14}/_{397}$ (4%) patients. Most of these GI events occurred after the administration of other anesthetic agents.

For the respiratory system overall, adverse events (hypoxia, laryngospasm, rhonchi, coughing, respiratory depression, airway obstruction, upper-airway congestion, shallow respirations), occurred during the entire monitoring period in $^{31}/_{397}$ (8%) patients and increased in frequency as dosage was increased: $^{7}/_{132}$ (5%) patients in the 0.25 mg/kg dose group, $^{9}/_{132}$ (7%) patients in the 0.5 mg/kg dose group, and $^{15}/_{133}$ (11%) patients in the 1 mg/kg dose group.

Most of the respiratory adverse events occurred during induction, general anesthesia or recovery. One patient (0.25%) experienced a respiratory system adverse event (laryngospasm) during the premedication period. This adverse event occurred precisely at the time of induction. Although many of the respiratory complications occurred in settings of upper airway procedures or concurrently administered opioids, a number of these events occurred outside of these settings as well. In this study, administration of midazolam hydrochloride syrup was generally accompanied by a slight decrease in both systolic and diastolic blood pressures, as well as a slight increase in heart rate.

Midazolam Oral Adverse Reactions (Premedication Period Alone)

Adverse reaction	0.25 mg/kg (n = 132)	0.5 mg/kg (n = 132)	1 mg/kg (n = 133)	(n = 397)
GI				
Emesis	1 (0.76%)	1 (0.76%)	1 (0.75%)	3 (0.76%)
Nausea			2 (1.5%)	2 (0.5%)
Respiratory				
Laryngospasm			1[a] (0.75%)	1 (0.25%)
Sneezing/rhinorrhea			1 (0.75%)	1 (0.25%)
All body systems	1 (0.76%)	1 (0.76%)	5 (3.8%)	1 (1.8%)

[a] This adverse reaction occurred precisely at the time of induction.

Midazolam Oral Adverse Reactions (≥ 1%) (Entire Monitoring Period)

Adverse reaction	0.25 mg/kg (n = 132)	0.5 mg/kg (n = 132)	1 mg/kg (n = 133)	(n = 397)
GI				
Emesis	11 (8%)	5 (4%)	15 (11%)	31 (8%)
Nausea	6 (5%)	2 (2%)	6 (5%)	14 (4%)
Overall	16 (12%)	8 (6%)	16 (12%)	40 (10%)
Respiratory				
Hypoxia	0	5 (4%)	4 (3%)	9 (2%)
Laryngospasm	0	1 (< 1%)	5 (4%)	6 (2%)
Respiratory depression	2 (2%)	1 (< 1%)	2 (2%)	5 (1%)
Rhonchi	2 (2%)	1 (< 1%)	2 (2%)	5 (1%)
Airway obstruction	2 (2%)	2 (2%)	0	4 (1%)
Upper airway congestion	2 (2%)	0	2 (2%)	4 (1%)
Overall	7 (5%)	9 (7%)	15 (11%)	31 (8%)
Psychiatric				
Agitated	1 (< 1%)	2 (2%)	3 (2%)	6 (2%)
Overall	1 (< 1%)	3 (2%)	4 (3%)	8 (2%)
Heart rate, rhythm disorders				
Bradycardia	1 (< 1%)	3 (2%)	0	4 (1%)
Bigeminy	2 (2%)	0	0	2 (< 1%)
Overall	3 (2%)	3 (2%)	1 (< 1%)	7 (2%)
Central/peripheral nervous system				
Prolonged sedation	0	0	2 (2%)	2 (< 1%)
Overall	2 (2%)	0	3 (2%)	5 (1%)
Dermatologic				
Rash	2 (2%)	0	0	2 (< 1%)
Overall	2 (2%)	2 (2%)	0	4 (1%)

Midazolam Oral Adverse Reactions (≥ 1%) (Entire Monitoring Period)

Adverse reaction	0.25 mg/kg (n = 132)	0.5 mg/kg (n = 132)	1 mg/kg (n = 133)	(n = 397)
All body systems	26 (20%)	23 (17%)	33 (25%)	82 (21%)

There were no deaths during the study, and no patient withdrew from the study due to adverse events. Serious adverse events (both respiratory disorders) were experienced postoperatively by 2 patients: 1 case of airway obstruction and desaturation (SpO_2 of 33%) in a patient given midazolam hydrochloride syrup 0.25 mg/kg, and 1 case of upper airway obstruction and respiratory depression following 0.5 mg/kg. Both patients had received IV morphine sulfate (1.5 mg total for both patients).

Other adverse reactions that have been reported in the literature with the oral administration of midazolam (not necessarily midazolam hydrochloride syrup), are listed below. The incidence rate for these events was generally < 1%.

➤*Cardiovascular:* Decreased systolic and diastolic blood pressure, increased heart rate.

➤*CNS:* Dysphoria, disinhibition, excitation, aggression, mood swings, hallucinations, adverse behavior, agitation, dizziness, confusion, ataxia, vertigo, dysarthria.

➤*GI:* Nausea, vomiting, hiccoughs, gagging, salivation, drooling.

➤*Respiratory:* Apnea, hypercarbia, desaturation, stridor.

➤*Special senses:* Diplopia, strabismus, loss of balance, blurred vision.

Overdosage

➤*Symptoms:* The manifestations of midazolam hydrochloride overdosage reported are similar to those observed with other benzodiazepines, including sedation, somnolence, confusion, impaired coordination, diminished reflexes, coma, and deleterious effects on vital signs. No evidence of specific organ toxicity from midazolam hydrochloride overdosage has been reported.

➤*Treatment:* Treatment of midazolam hydrochloride overdosage is the same as that followed for overdosage with other benzodiazepines. Respiration, pulse rate and blood pressure should be monitored and general supportive measures should be employed. Attention should be given to the maintenance of a patent airway and support of ventilation, including administration of oxygen. Should hypotension develop, treatment may include IV fluid therapy, repositioning, judicious use of vasopressors appropriate to the clinical situation, if indicated, and other appropriate countermeasures. There is no information as to whether peritoneal dialysis, forced diuresis or hemodialysis are of any value in the treatment of midazolam overdosage.

GI decontamination with lavage or activated charcoal once the patient's airway is secure is also recommended.

Flumazenil, a specific benzodiazepine-receptor antagonist, is indicated for the complete or partial reversal of the sedative effects of midazolam hydrochloride and may be used in situations when an overdose with a benzodiazepine is known or suspected. There are anecdotal reports of adverse hemodynamic responses associated with midazolam hydrochloride following administration of flumazenil to pediatric patients. Prior to the administration of flumazenil, necessary measures should be instituted to secure the airway, ensure adequate ventilation, and establish adequate IV access. Flumazenil is intended as an adjunct to, not as a substitute for, proper management of benzodiazepine overdose. Patients treated with flumazenil should be monitored for resedation, respiratory depression and other residual benzodiazepine effects for an appropriate period after treatment. The prescriber should be aware of a risk of seizure in association with flumazenil treatment, particularly in long-term benzodiazepine users and in cyclic antidepressant overdose. The complete flumazenil package insert, including Contraindications, Warnings and Precautions, should be consulted prior to use.

Patient Information

Inform your physician about any alcohol consumption and medicine you are now taking, especially blood pressure medication and antibiotics, including drugs you buy without a prescription. Alcohol has an increased effect when consumed with benzodiazepines; therefore, caution should be exercised regarding simultaneous ingestion of alcohol during benzodiazepine treatment.

Inform your physician if you are pregnant or are planning to become pregnant.

Inform your physician if you are nursing.

Patients should be informed of the pharmacological effects of midazolam hydrochloride syrup, such as sedation and amnesia, which in some patients may be profound. The decision as to when patients who have received midazolam hydrochloride syrup, particularly on an outpatient basis, may again engage in activities requiring complete mental alertness, operate hazardous machinery or drive a motor vehicle must be individualized.

Midazolam hydrochloride syrup should not be taken in conjunction with grapefruit juice.

For pediatric patients, particular care should be taken to ensure safe ambulation.

MIDAZOLAM HYDROCHLORIDE — INJECTION

Benzodiazepine compounds used as antianxiety agents appear under the Antianxiety Agents monograph.

WARNING

Adults and pediatrics – IV midazolam hydrochloride has been associated with respiratory depression and respiratory arrest, especially when used for sedation in noncritical care settings. In some cases, where this was not recognized promptly and treated effectively, death or hypoxic encephalopathy has resulted. IV midazolam hydrochloride should be used only in hospital or ambulatory care settings, including physicians' and dental offices, that provide for continuous monitoring of respiratory and cardiac function (ie, pulse oximetry). Immediate availability of resuscitative drugs and age- and size-appropriate equipment for bag/valve/mask ventilation and intubation, and personnel trained in their use and skilled in airway management should be ensured. Patients should be continuously monitored with some means of detection for early signs of hypoventilation, airway obstruction, or apnea (ie, pulse oximetry). Hypoventilation, airway obstruction, and apnea can lead to hypoxia or cardiac arrest unless effective countermeasures are taken immediately. The immediate availability of specific reversal agents (flumazenil) is highly recommended. Vital signs should continue to be monitored during the recovery period. For deeply sedated pediatric patients, a dedicated individual, other than the practitioner performing the procedure, should monitor the patient throughout the procedure.

The initial dose for sedation in adult patients may be as little as 1 mg, but should not exceed 2.5 mg in a healthy adult. Lower doses are necessary for older (over 60 years) or debilitated patients and in patients receiving concomitant narcotics or other CNS depressants. The initial dose and all subsequent doses should always be titrated slowly; administer over at least 2 minutes and allow an additional 2 or more minutes to fully evaluate the sedative effect. The use of the 1 mg/mL formulation or dilution of the 1 mg/mL or 5 mg/mL formulation is recommended to facilitate slower injection. Doses of sedative medications in pediatric patients must be calculated on a mg/kg basis, and initial doses and all subsequent doses should always be titrated slowly. The initial pediatric dose of midazolam hydrochloride for sedation/anxiolysis/amnesia is age, procedure, and route dependent.

Neonates – Midazolam hydrochloride should not be administered by rapid injection in the neonatal population. Rapid injection should be avoided in the neonatal population. Midazolam hydrochloride administered rapidly as an IV injection (less than 2 minutes) has been associated with severe hypotension in neonates, particularly when the patient has also received fentanyl. Likewise, severe hypotension has been observed in neonates receiving a continuous infusion of midazolam who then receive a rapid IV injection of fentanyl. Seizures have been reported in several neonates following rapid IV administration.

Indications

➤*Preoperative sedation/Anxiolysis/Amnesia:* IM or IV for preoperative sedation/anxiolysis/amnesia.

➤*Procedural sedation:* IV as an agent for sedation/anxiolysis/amnesia prior to or during diagnostic, therapeutic, or endoscopic procedures, such as bronchoscopy, gastroscopy, cystoscopy, coronary angiography, cardiac catheterization, oncology procedures, radiologic procedures, suture of lacerations, and other procedures either alone or in combination with other CNS depressants.

➤*Anesthesia:* IV for induction of general anesthesia, before administration of other anesthetic agents. With the use of narcotic premedication, induction of anesthesia can be attained within a relatively narrow dose range and in a short period of time. IV midazolam hydrochloride can also be used as a component of IV supplementation of nitrous oxide and oxygen (balanced anesthesia).

➤*Sedation for mechanically ventilated patients:* For continuous IV infusion for sedation of intubated and mechanically ventilated patients as a component of anesthesia or during treatment in a critical care setting.

➤*Off-label uses:*

Buccal administration – [4] = Insufficient documentation. In an open trial, 42 young patients (age range, 5 to 19 years) with severe epilepsy were randomized to receive treatment with rectal diazepam or buccal midazolam for treatment of seizures longer than 5 minutes. Buccal midazolam was used to treat 40 seizures in 14 patients and rectal diazepam was used to treat 39 seizures in 14 patients. There was no significant difference between the 2 groups in stopping seizure activity (75% vs 59%), or time after drug administration to the end of seizure (17 vs 15 minutes). It should be noted that 2 patients had a total of 39 seizures during the study period, which could have affected results. (See Administration and Dosage.)

Administration and Dosage

➤*General dosing considerations:* Midazolam is a potent sedative agent that requires slow administration and individualization of dosage. Because serious and life-threatening cardiorespiratory adverse reactions have been reported, provision for monitoring, detection, and correction of these reactions must be made for every patient to whom midazolam is administered, regardless of age or health status. Excessive single doses or rapid IV administration may result in respiratory depression, airway obstruction, or arrest. The potential for these latter effects is increased in debilitated patients, those receiving concomitant medications capable of depressing the CNS, and patients without an endotracheal tube but undergoing a procedure involving the upper airway, such as endoscopy or dental.

Titration to effect with multiple small doses is essential for safe administration. It should be noted that adequate time to achieve peak CNS effect (3 to 5 minutes) for midazolam should be allowed between doses to minimize the potential for oversedation. Sufficient time must elapse between doses of concomitant sedative medications to allow the effect of each dose to be assessed before subsequent drug administration. This is an important consideration for all patients who receive IV midazolam. Immediate availability of resuscitative drugs and age- and size-appropriate equipment and personnel trained in their use and skilled in airway management should be ensured.

Injectable midazolam should not be administered to patients in shock or coma, or in acute alcohol intoxication with depression of vital signs. Particular care should be exercised in the use of IV midazolam patients with uncompensated acute illnesses, such as severe fluid or electrolyte disturbances.

The dose must be individualized and reduced when IM midazolam is administered to patients with chronic obstructive pulmonary disease, other higher-risk surgical patients, patients 60 years of age and older, and patients who have received concomitant narcotics or other CNS depressants. Higher-risk or debilitated patients may require lower dosages whether or not concomitant sedating medications have been administered. Patients undergoing procedures involving the upper airway, such as upper endoscopy or dental care, are particularly vulnerable to episodes of desaturation and hypoventilation due to partial airway obstruction. Administration of IM midazolam to elderly or higher-risk surgical patients has been associated with rare reports of death under circumstances compatible with cardiorespiratory depression. In most of these cases, the patients also received other CNS depressants capable of depressing respiration, especially narcotics. As with any potential respiratory depressant, these patients require observation for signs of cardiorespiratory depression after receiving IM midazolam.

➤*Adults:*

Premedication –

IM: 0.07 to 0.08 mg/kg IM (approximately 5 mg IM) administered up to 1 hour before surgery.

IV: Dosage must be individualized and titrated. Some patients may respond to as little as 1 mg. No more than 2.5 mg should be given over a period of at least 2 minutes. Wait an additional 2 or more minutes to fully evaluate the sedative effect. If further titration is necessary, continue to titrate, using small increments, to the appropriate level of sedation. Wait an additional 2 or more minutes after each increment to fully evaluate the sedative effect. A total dose greater than 5 mg is not usually necessary to reach the desired end point. If narcotic premedication or other CNS depressants are used, patients will require approximately 30% less midazolam than unpremedicated patients.

• *Maintenance dosage* – Additional doses to maintain the desired level of sedation may be given in increments of 25% of the dose used to first reach the sedative end point, but again only by slow titration, especially in elderly and chronically ill or debilitated patients. These additional doses should be given only after a thorough clinical evaluation clearly indicates the need for additional sedation.

Concomitant therapy: Narcotic premedication results in less variability in patient response and a reduction in dosage of midazolam. For preoral procedures, the use of an appropriate topical anesthetic is recommended. For bronchoscopic procedures, the use of narcotic premedication is recommended.

Induction of anesthesia – Individual response to the drug is variable, particularly when a narcotic premedication is not used. The dosage should be titrated to the desired effect according to the patient's age and clinical status. When midazolam is used before other IV agents for induction of anesthesia, the initial dose of each agent may be significantly reduced, at times to as low as 25% of the usual initial dose of the individual agents.

Continuous infusion: If a loading dose is necessary to rapidly initiate sedation, 0.01 to 0.05 mg/kg (approximately 0.5 to 4 mg for a typical adult) may be given slowly or infused over several minutes. This dose may be repeated at 10- to 15-minute intervals until adequate sedation is achieved. For maintenance of sedation, the usual initial infusion rate is 0.02 to 0.1 mg/kg/hr (1 to 7 mg/hr). Higher loading or maintenance infusion rates may occasionally be required in some patients. The lowest recommended doses should be used in patients with residual effects from anesthetic drugs or in those concurrently receiving other sedatives or opioids. Individual response to midazolam is variable. The infusion rate should be titrated to the desired level of sedation, taking into account the patient's age, clinical status, and current medications. In general, midazolam should be infused at the lowest rate that produces the desired level of sedation. Assessment of sedation should be performed at regular intervals and the midazolam infusion rate adjusted up or down by 25% to 50% of the initial infusion rate to ensure adequate titration of sedation level. Larger adjustments or even a small incremental dose may be necessary if rapid changes in the level of sedation are indicated. In addition, the infusion rate should be decreased by 10% to 25% every few hours to find the minimum effective infusion rate. Finding the minimum effective infusion rate decreases the potential accumulation of midazolam and provides for the most rapid recovery once the infusion is terminated. Patients who exhibit agitation, hypertension, or tachycardia in response to noxious stimulation, but who are otherwise adequately sedated, may benefit from coadministration of an opioid analgesic. Addition of an opioid will generally reduce the minimum effective midazolam infusion rate.

IV infusion:

• *Unpremedicated patients* – Initial dose of 0.3 to 0.35 mg/kg for induction, administered over 20 to 30 seconds and allowing 2 minutes for effect. If needed to complete induction, increments approximately 25% of the patient's initial dose may be used; induction may instead be completed with inhalational anesthetics. In resistant cases, up to 0.6 mg/kg total dose may be used for induction, but such larger doses may prolong recovery. Unpre-

MIDAZOLAM HYDROCHLORIDE — INJECTION

medicated patients older than 55 years of age usually require less midazolam for induction; an initial dose of 0.3 mg/kg is recommended. Unpremedicated patients with severe systemic disease or other debilitation usually require less midazolam for induction. An initial dose of 0.2 to 0.25 mg/kg will usually suffice; in some cases, as little as 0.15 mg/kg may suffice.

• *Premedicated patients* – 0.15 to 0.35 mg/kg. 0.25 mg/kg, administered over 20 to 30 seconds and allowing 2 minutes for effect, will usually suffice. The initial dose of 0.2 mg/kg is recommended for good-risk (ASA I & II) surgical patients. In some patients with severe systemic disease or debilitation, as little as 0.15 mg/kg may suffice. Narcotic premedication frequently used during clinical trials included fentanyl (1.5 to 2 mcg/kg IV administered 5 minutes before induction), morphine (dosage individualized, up to 0.15 mg/kg IM), and meperidine (dosage individualized, up to 1 mg/kg IM). Sedative premedications were hydroxyzine pamoate (100 mg orally) and sodium secobarbital (200 mg orally). Except for IV fentanyl, administered 5 minutes before induction, all other premedications should be administered approximately 1 hour prior to the time anticipated for midazolam induction.

Maintenance of anesthesia – Effective narcotic premedication is especially recommended in such cases. Incremental injections of approximately 25% of the induction dose should be given in response to signs of lightening of anesthesia and repeated as necessary.

Off-label dosing –

Buccal administration: [4] = Insufficient documentation. 10 mg per 2 mL of the injectable product squirted around the patient's buccal mucosa.

➤*Children:*

Premedication –

IM: Sedation after IM midazolam is age and dose dependent; higher doses may result in deeper and more prolonged sedation. Doses of 0.1 to 0.15 mg/kg are usually effective and do not prolong emergence from general anesthesia. For more anxious patients, doses of up to 0.5 mg/kg have been used. Although not systematically studied, the total dose usually does not exceed 10 mg. If midazolam is given with an opioid, the initial dose of each must be reduced.

IV by intermittent injection: It should be recognized that the depth of sedation/anxiolysis needed for children depends on the type of procedure to be performed. For example, simple light sedation/anxiolysis in the preoperative period is quite different from the deep sedation and analgesia required for an endoscopic procedure in a child. For this reason, there is a broad range of dosage. For all children, regardless of the indication for sedation/anxiolysis, it is vital to titrate midazolam and other concomitant medications slowly to the desired clinical effect. The initial dose of midazolam should be administered over 2 to 3 minutes. Because midazolam is water soluble, it takes approximately 3 times longer than diazepam to achieve peak EEG effects; therefore, one must wait an additional 2 to 3 minutes to fully evaluate the sedative effect before initiating a procedure or repeating a dose. If further sedation is necessary, continue to titrate with small increments until the appropriate level of sedation is achieved. If other medications capable of depressing the CNS are coadministered, the peak effect of those concomitant medications must be considered and the dose of midazolam adjusted. The importance of drug titration to effect is vital to the safe sedation/anxiolysis of the pediatric patient. The total dose of midazolam will depend on patient response, the type and duration of the procedure, as well as the type and dose of concomitant medications.

• *Children 12 to 16 years of age* – Should be dosed as adults. Prolonged sedation may be associated with higher doses; some patients in this age range will require higher than recommended adult doses, but the total dose usually does not exceed 10 mg.

• *Children 6 to 12 years of age* – Initial dose of 0.025 to 0.05 mg/kg; a total dose of up to 0.4 mg/kg may be needed to reach the desired end point but usually does not exceed 10 mg. Prolonged sedation and risk of hypoventilation may be associated with the higher doses.

• *Children 6 months to 5 years of age* – Initial dose of 0.05 to 0.1 mg/kg; a total dose of up to 0.6 mg/kg may be necessary to reach the desired end point but usually does not exceed 6 mg. Prolonged sedation and risk of hypoventilation may be associated with the higher doses.

• *Children younger than 6 months of age* – Children younger than 6 months of age are particularly vulnerable to airway obstruction and hypoventilation; therefore, titration with small increments to clinical effect and careful monitoring are essential.

Continuous IV infusion –

Non-neonatal: To initiate sedation, an IV loading dose of 0.05 to 0.2 mg/kg administered over at least 2 to 3 minutes can be used to establish the desired clinical effect in patients whose trachea is intubated. (Midazolam should not be administered as a rapid IV dose.) This loading dose may be followed by a continuous IV infusion to maintain the effect. An infusion of midazolam has been used in patients whose trachea was intubated but who were allowed to breathe spontaneously. Assisted ventilation is recommended for pediatric patients who are receiving other CNS-depressant medications such as opioids. Based on pharmacokinetic parameters and reported clinical experience, continuous IV infusions of midazolam should be initiated at a rate of 0.06 to 0.12 mg/kg/hr (1 to 2 mcg/kg/min). The rate of infusion can be increased or decreased (generally by 25% of the initial or subsequent infusion rate) as required, or supplemental IV doses of midazolam can be administered to increase or maintain the desired effect. Frequent assessment at regular intervals using standard pain/sedation scales is recommended. Drug elimination may be delayed in patients receiving erythromycin or other P450 3A4 enzyme inhibitors and in patients with liver dysfunction, low cardiac output (especially those requiring inotropic support), and in neonates. Hypotension may be observed in patients who are critically ill, particularly those receiving opioids or when midazolam is rapidly administered.

When initiating an infusion with midazolam in hemodynamically compromised patients, the usual loading dose of midazolam should be titrated in small increments and the patient monitored for hemodynamic instability (eg, hypotension). These patients are also vulnerable to the respiratory depressant effects of midazolam and require careful monitoring of respiratory rate and oxygen saturation.

Neonatal: Initiate at a rate of 0.03 mg/kg/hr (0.5 mcg/kg/min) in neonates younger than 32 weeks and 0.06 mg/kg/hr (0.5 mcg/kg/min) in neonates older than 32 weeks. IV loading doses should not be used in neonates. Rather the infusion may be run more rapidly for the first several hours to establish therapeutic plasma levels. The rate of infusion should be carefully and frequently reassessed, particularly after the first 24 hours, to administer the lowest possible effective dose and reduce the potential for drug accumulation.

Off-label dosing –

Intranasal: 0.2 to 0.3 mg/kg/dose using 5 mg/mL.

Refractory status epilepticus:

• *Two months of age and older* – 0.15 to 0.38 mg/kg IV loading dose, followed by a continuous infusion of 0.06 to 2 mg/kg/h, and titrate dose upward every 15 minutes with 0.06 mg/kg/h (mean range of maintenance infusion is 0.14 to 0.84 mg/kg/h).

Sublingual: 0.2 mg/kg/dose. The 5 mg/mL formulation can be mixed with a small amount of flavored syrup.

➤*Elderly:* In a study of patients 60 years of age and older who did not receive coadministration of narcotics, 2 to 3 mg (0.02 to 0.05 mg/kg) of midazolam produced adequate sedation during the preoperative period. The dose of 1 mg IM midazolam may suffice for some older patients if the anticipated intensity and duration of sedation are less critical. Because the danger of hypoventilation, airway obstruction, or apnea is greater in elderly patients and those with chronic disease states or decreased pulmonary reserve, and because the peak effect may take longer in these patients, increments should be smaller and the rate of injection slower. Titrate slowly to the desired effect (eg, the initiation of slurred speech). Some patients may respond to as little as 1 mg. No more than 1.5 mg should be given over a period of no less than 2 minutes. Wait an additional 2 or more minutes to fully evaluate the sedative effect. If additional titration is necessary, it should be given at a rate of no more than 1 mg over a period of 2 minutes, waiting an additional 2 or more minutes each time to fully evaluate the sedative effect. Total doses greater than 3.5 mg are not usually necessary. If concomitant CNS-depressant premedications are used in these patients, they will require at least 50% less midazolam than healthy, young, unpremedicated patients.

➤*Renal function impairment:* Patients with renal impairment may have longer elimination half-lives for midazolam and its metabolites, which may result in slower recovery.

➤*Monitoring:* Patient response to sedative agents and resultant respiratory status is variable. Regardless of the intended level of sedation or route of administration, sedation is a continuum; a patient may move easily from light to deep sedation, with potential loss of protective reflexes. This is especially true in children. Sedative doses should be individually titrated, taking into account patient age, clinical status, and concomitant use of other CNS depressants. Continuous monitoring of respiratory and cardiac function is required (ie, pulse oximetry). Hypoventilation, airway obstruction, and apnea can lead to hypoxia or cardiac arrest unless effective countermeasures are taken immediately. Vital signs should continue to be monitored during the recovery period.

For deeply sedated children, a dedicated individual (other than the practitioner performing the procedure) should monitor the patient throughout the procedure.

➤*Preparation for administration:*

Continuous infusion – Midazolam 5 mg/mL formulation is recommended diluted to a concentration of 0.5 mg/mL with 0.9% sodium chloride or 5% dextrose in water.

➤*Administration:* Midazolam should only be administered IM or IV. Care should be taken to avoid intra-arterial injection or extravasation. For IM use, midazolam should be injected deep in a large muscle mass.

Titrate IV doses slowly; administer over at least 2 minutes and allow an additional 2 or more minutes to fully evaluate the sedative effect.

Rapid injection should be avoided in the neonatal population. Midazolam administered rapidly as an IV injection (less than 2 minutes) has been associated with severe hypotension in neonates, particularly when the patient has also received fentanyl. Likewise, severe hypotension has been observed in neonates receiving a continuous infusion of midazolam who then receive a rapid IV injection of fentanyl. Seizures have been reported in several neonates following rapid IV administration. Neonates also have reduced and immature organ function and are also vulnerable to profound or prolonged respiratory effects of midazolam.

Midazolam 1 mg/mL formulation is recommended for sedation/anxiolysis/amnesia for procedures to facilitate slower injection.

➤*Admixture compatibility:* Midazolam may be mixed in the same syringe with the following frequently used premedications: morphine, meperidine, atropine, or scopolamine. Midazolam, at a concentration of 0.5 mg/mL, is compatible with 5% dextrose in water and 0.9% sodium chloride for up to 24 hours and with lactated Ringer's solution for up to 4 hours. Midazolam may be diluted with 0.9% sodium chloride or 5% dextrose in water. It can be administered concomitantly with atropine or scopolamine and reduced doses of narcotics.

➤*Storage/Stability:* Store at 15° to 30°C (59° to 86°F).

MIDAZOLAM HYDROCHLORIDE — INJECTION

Actions

➤*Pharmacology:* Midazolam hydrochloride is a short-acting benzodiazepine CNS depressant.

The effects of midazolam hydrochloride on the CNS are dependent on the dose administered, the route of administration, and the presence or absence of other medications. Onset time of sedative effects after IM administration in adults is 15 minutes, with peak sedation occurring 30 to 60 minutes following injection. In 1 adult study, when tested the following day, 73% of the patients who received midazolam hydrochloride IM had no recall of memory cards shown 30 minutes following drug administration; 40% had no recall of the memory cards shown 60 minutes following drug administration. Onset time of sedative effects in the pediatric population begins within 5 minutes and peaks at 15 to 30 minutes depending upon the dose administered. In pediatric patients, up to 85% had no recall of pictures shown after receiving IM midazolam hydrochloride compared with 5% of the placebo controls.

Sedation in adult and pediatric patients is achieved within 3 to 5 minutes after IV injection; the time of onset is affected by total dose administered and the concurrent administration of narcotic premedication. Seventy-one percent (71%) of the adult patients in endoscopy studies had no recall of introduction of the endoscope; 82% of the patients had no recall of withdrawal of the endoscope. In 1 study of pediatric patients undergoing lumbar puncture or bone marrow aspiration, 88% of patients had impaired recall vs 9% of the placebo controls. In another pediatric oncology study, 91% of midazolam hydrochloride treated patients were amnestic compared with 35% of patients who had received fentanyl alone.

When midazolam hydrochloride is given IV as an anesthetic induction agent, induction of anesthesia occurs in approximately 1.5 minutes when narcotic premedication has been administered and in 2 to 2.5 minutes without narcotic premedication or other sedative premedication. Some impairment in a test of memory was noted in 90% of the patients studied. A dose-response study of pediatric patients premedicated with 1 mg/kg IM meperidine found that only 4 out of 6 pediatric patients who received 600 mcg/kg IV midazolam hydrochloride lost consciousness, with eye closing at 108 ± 140 seconds. This group was compared with pediatric patients who were given thiopental 5 mg/kg IV; 6 out of 6 closed their eyes at 20 ± 3.2 seconds. Midazolam hydrochloride did not dependably induce anesthesia at this dose despite concomitant opioid administration in pediatric patients.

Midazolam hydrochloride, used as directed, does not delay awakening from general anesthesia in adults. Gross tests of recovery after awakening (orientation, ability to stand and walk, suitability for discharge from the recovery room, return to baseline Trieger competency) usually indicate recovery within 2 hours, but recovery may take up to 6 hours in some cases. When compared with patients who received thiopental, patients who received midazolam generally recovered at a slightly slower rate. Recovery from anesthesia or sedation for procedures in pediatric patients depends on the dose of midazolam hydrochloride administered, coadministration of other medications causing CNS depression and duration of the procedure.

The usual recommended IM premedicating doses of midazolam hydrochloride do not depress the ventilatory response to carbon dioxide stimulation to a clinically significant extent in adults. IV induction doses of midazolam hydrochloride depress the ventilatory response to carbon dioxide stimulation for 15 minutes or more beyond the duration of ventilatory depression following administration of thiopental in adults. Impairment of ventilatory response to carbon dioxide is more marked in adult patients with chronic obstructive pulmonary disease (COPD). Sedation with IV midazolam hydrochloride does not adversely affect the mechanics of respiration (resistance, static recoil, most lung volume measurements); total lung capacity and peak expiratory flow decrease significantly, but static compliance and maximum expiratory flow at 50% of awake total lung capacity (V_{max}) increase. In 1 study of pediatric patients under general anesthesia, IM midazolam hydrochloride (100 or 200 mcg/kg) was shown to depress the response to carbon dioxide in a dose-related manner.

In cardiac hemodynamic studies in adults, IV induction of general anesthesia with midazolam hydrochloride was associated with a slight-to-moderate decrease in mean arterial pressure, cardiac output, stroke volume and systemic vascular resistance. Slow heart rates (less than 65/minute), particularly in patients taking propranolol for angina, tended to rise slightly; faster heart rates (eg, 85/minute) tended to slow slightly. In pediatric patients, a comparison of IV midazolam hydrochloride (500 mcg/kg) with propofol (2.5 mg/kg) revealed a mean 15% decrease in systolic blood pressure in patients who had received IV midazolam hydrochloride vs a mean 25% decrease in systolic blood pressure following propofol.

Pharmacodynamics –

➤*Pharmacokinetics:*

Continuous infusion – The pharmacokinetic profile of midazolam following continuous infusion, based on 282 adult subjects, has been shown to be similar to that following single-dose administration for subjects of comparable age, gender, body habits and health status. However, midazolam can accumulate in peripheral tissues with continuous infusion. The effects of accumulation are greater after long-term infusions than after short-term infusions. The effects of accumulation can be reduced by maintaining the lowest midazolam infusion rate that produces satisfactory sedation.

Infrequent hypotensive episodes have occurred during continuous infusion; however, neither the time to onset nor the duration of the episode appeared to be related to plasma concentrations of midazolam or alpha-hydroxy-midazolam. Furthermore, there does not appear to be an increased chance of occurrence of a hypotensive episode with increased loading doses.

Absorption – The absolute bioavailability of the IM route was greater than 90% in a crossover study in which healthy subjects (n = 17) were administered a 7.5 mg IV or IM dose. The mean peak concentration (C_{max}) and time to peak (t_{max}) following the IM dose was 90 ng/mL (20% CV) and 0.5 hour (50% CV). C_{max} for the 1–hydroxy metabolite following the IM dose was 8 ng/mL (t_{max} = 1 hour).

Following IM administration, C_{max} for midazolam and its 1–hydroxy metabolite were approximately one-half of those achieved after IV injection.

Distribution – The volume of distribution (Vd), determined from 6 single-dose pharmacokinetic studies involving healthy adults, ranged from 1 to 3.1 L/kg. Female gender, old age, and obesity are associated with increased values of midazolam Vd. In humans, midazolam has been shown to cross the placenta and enter into fetal circulation and has been detected in human milk and CSF.

In adults and pediatric patients greater than 1 year of age, midazolam is approximately 97% bound to plasma protein, principally albumin.

Metabolism – In vitro studies with human liver microsomes indicate that the biotransformation of midazolam is mediated by cytochrome P450 3A4. This cytochrome also appears to be present in GI tract mucosa as well as liver. Sixty to seventy percent (60% to 70%) of the biotransformation products is 1-hydroxy-midazolam (also termed alpha-hydroxy-midazolam), while 4-hydroxy-midazolam constitutes less than or equal to 5%. Small amounts of dihydroxy derivative have also been detected but not quantified. The principal urinary excretion products are glucuronide conjugates of the hydroxylated derivatives.

Drugs that inhibit the activity of cytochrome P450 3A4 may inhibit midazolam clearance and elevate steady-state midazolam concentrations.

Studies of the IV administration of 1-hydroxy-midazolam in humans suggest that 1-hydroxy-midazolam is at least as potent as the parent compound and may contribute to the net pharmacologic activity of midazolam. In vitro studies have demonstrated that the affinities of 1- and 4-hydroxy-midazolam for the benzodiazepine receptor are approximately 20% and 7%, respectively, relative to midazolam.

Excretion – Clearance of midazolam is reduced in association with old age, congestive heart failure, liver disease (cirrhosis) or conditions which diminish cardiac output and hepatic blood flow.

The principal urinary excretion product is 1-hydroxy-midazolam in the form of a glucuronide conjugate; smaller amounts of the glucuronide conjugates of 4-hydroxy- and dihydroxy-midazolam are detected as well. The amount of midazolam excreted unchanged in the urine after a single IV dose is less than 0.5% (n = 5). Following a single IV infusion in 5 healthy volunteers, 45% to 57% of the dose was excreted in the urine as 1-hydroxymethyl midazolam conjugate.

Midazolam's activity is primarily due to the parent drug. Elimination of the parent drug takes place via hepatic metabolism of midazolam to hydroxylated metabolites that are conjugated and excreted in the urine. Six (6) single-dose pharmacokinetic studies involving healthy adults yield pharmacokinetic parameters for midazolam in the following ranges: Volume distribution (Vd), 1 to 3.1 L/kg; elimination half-life, 1.8 to 6.4 hours (mean approximately 3 hours); total clearance (Cl), 0.25 to 0.54 L/hr/kg. In a parallel-group study, there was no difference in the clearance, in subjects administered 0.15 mg/kg (n = 4) and 0.3 mg/kg (n = 4) IV doses indicating linear kinetics. The clearance was successively reduced by approximately 30% at doses of 0.45 mg/kg (n = 4) and 0.6 mg/kg (n = 5) indicating nonlinear kinetics in this dose range.

Special populations –

Renal function impairment: Patients with renal impairment may have longer elimination half-lives for midazolam and its metabolites, which may result in slower recovery.

Hepatic function impairment: Midazolam pharmacokinetics were studied after an IV single dose (0.075 mg/kg) was administered to 7 patients with biopsy-proven alcoholic cirrhosis and 8 control patients. The mean half-life of midazolam increased 2.5-fold in the alcoholic patients. Clearance was reduced by 50% and the Vd increased by 20%. In another study in 21 male patients with cirrhosis, without ascites and with healthy kidney function as determined by creatinine clearance, no changes in the pharmacokinetics of midazolam or 1-hydroxy-midazolam were observed when compared to healthy individuals.

Elderly: In 3 parallel-group studies, the pharmacokinetics of midazolam administered IV or IM were compared in young (mean age 29, n = 52) and healthy elderly subjects (mean age 73, n = 53). Plasma half-life was approximately 2-fold higher in the elderly. The mean Vd based on total body weight increased consistently between 15% to 100% in the elderly. The mean Cl decreased approximately 25% in the elderly in 2 studies and was similar to that of the younger patients in the other.

Children: In seriously ill neonates, the terminal elimination half-life of midazolam is substantially prolonged (6.5 to 12 hours) and the clearance reduced (0.07 to 0.12 L/hr/kg) compared to healthy adults or other groups of pediatric patients. It cannot be determined if these differences are due to age, immature organ function or metabolic pathways, underlying illness or debility.

Obese patients: In a study comparing healthy patients (n = 20) and obese patients (n = 20), the mean half-life was greater in the obese group (5.9 vs 2.3 hours). This was due to an increase of approximately 50% in the Vd corrected for total body weight. The clearance was not significantly different between groups.

Congestive heart failure: In patients suffering from congestive heart failure, there appeared to be a 2-fold increase in the elimination half-life, a 25% decrease in the plasma clearance and a 40% increase in the volume of distribution of midazolam.

MIDAZOLAM HYDROCHLORIDE — INJECTION

Contraindications

Hypersensitivity to the drug; acute narrow-angle glaucoma. Benzodiazepines may be used in patients with open-angle glaucoma only if they are receiving appropriate therapy. Measurements of intraocular pressure in patients without eye disease show a moderate lowering following induction with midazolam hydrochloride; patients with glaucoma have not been studied.

Midazolam hydrochloride is not intended for intrathecal or epidural administration due to the presence of the preservative benzyl alcohol in the dosage form.

Warnings/Precautions

➤*Administration:* See the Warning box for more information.

➤*Respiratory depression effects:* Hypoventilation, airway obstruction, and apnea can lead to hypoxia or cardiac arrest unless effective countermeasures are taken immediately. The immediate availability of specific reversal agents (flumazenil) is highly recommended. Vital signs should continue to be monitored during the recovery period. Because IV midazolam hydrochloride depresses respiration, and because opioid agonists and other sedatives can add to this depression, midazolam hydrochloride should be administered as an induction agent only by a person trained in general anesthesia and should be used for sedation/anxiolysis/amnesia only in the presence of personnel skilled in early detection of hypoventilation, maintaining a patent airway and supporting ventilation. When used for sedation/anxiolysis/amnesia, midazolam hydrochloride should always be titrated slowly in adult or pediatric patients. Adverse hemodynamic events have been reported in pediatric patients with cardiovascular instability; rapid IV administration should also be avoided in this population.

➤*Cardiorespiratory effects:* Serious cardiorespiratory adverse reactions have occurred after administration of midazolam hydrochloride. These have included respiratory depression, airway obstruction, oxygen desaturation, apnea, respiratory arrest or cardiac arrest, sometimes resulting in death or permanent neurologic injury. There have also been rare reports of hypotensive episodes requiring treatment during or after diagnostic or surgical manipulations particularly in adult or pediatric patients with hemodynamic instability. Hypotension occurred more frequently in the sedation studies in patients premedicated with a narcotic.

➤*Improper dosing:* Reactions such as agitation, involuntary movements (including tonic/clonic movements and muscle tremor), hyperactivity and combativeness have been reported in both adult and pediatric patients. These reactions may be due to inadequate or excessive dosing or improper administration of midazolam hydrochloride; however, consideration should be given to the possibility of cerebral hypoxia or true paradoxical reactions. Should such reactions occur, the response to each dose of midazolam hydrochloride and all other drugs, including local anesthetics, should be evaluated before proceeding. Reversal of such responses with flumazenil has been reported in pediatric patients.

➤*Special risk:* Higher risk adult and pediatric surgical patients, elderly patients and debilitated adult and pediatric patients require lower dosages, whether or not concomitant sedating medications have been administered. Adult or pediatric patients with chronic obstructive pulmonary disease (COPD) are unusually sensitive to the respiratory-depressant effect of midazolam hydrochloride. Pediatric and adult patients undergoing procedures involving the upper airway such as upper endoscopy or dental care, are particularly vulnerable to episodes of desaturation and hypoventilation due to partial airway obstruction. Adult and pediatric patients with chronic renal failure and patients with congestive heart failure eliminate midazolam more slowly. Because elderly patients frequently have inefficient function of 1 or more organ systems, and because dosage requirements have been shown to decrease with age, reduced initial dosage of midazolam hydrochloride is recommended, and the possibility of profound or prolonged effect should be considered.

Injectable midazolam hydrochloride should not be administered to adult or pediatric patients in shock or coma, or in acute alcohol intoxication with depression of vital signs. Particular care should be exercised in the use of IV midazolam hydrochloride in adult or pediatric patients with uncompensated acute illnesses, such as severe fluid or electrolyte disturbances.

➤*Intra-arterial injection:* There have been limited reports of intra-arterial injection of midazolam hydrochloride. Adverse events have included local reactions, as well as isolated reports of seizure activity in which no clear causal relationship was established. Precautions against unintended intra-arterial injection should be taken. Extravasation should also be avoided.

➤*Benzyl alcohol:* Exposure to excessive amounts of benzyl alcohol has been associated with toxicity (hypotension, metabolic acidosis), particularly in neonates, and an increased incidence of kernicterus, particularly in small preterm infants. There have been rare reports of deaths, primarily in preterm infants, associated with exposure to excessive amounts of benzyl alcohol. The amount of benzyl alcohol from medications is usually considered negligible compared to that received in flush solutions containing benzyl alcohol. Administration of high dosages of medications (including midazolam hydrochloride) containing this preservative must take into account the total amount of benzyl alcohol administered. The recommended dosage range of midazolam hydrochloride for preterm and term infants includes amounts of benzyl alcohol well below that associated with toxicity; however, the amount of benzyl alcohol at which toxicity may occur is not known. If the patient requires more than the recommended dosages or other medications containing this preservative, the practitioner must consider the daily metabolic load of benzyl alcohol from these combined sources.

➤*Intracranial pressure/cardiac effects:* Midazolam hydrochloride does not protect against the increase in intracranial pressure or against the heart rate rise and blood pressure rise associated with endotracheal intubation under light general anesthesia.

➤*Use with other CNS depressants:* The efficacy and safety of midazolam hydrochloride in clinical use are functions of the dose administered, the clinical status of the individual patient, and the use of concomitant medications capable of depressing the CNS. Anticipated effects range from mild sedation to deep levels of sedation virtually equivalent to a state of general anesthesia where the patient may require external support of vital functions. Care must be taken to individualize and carefully titrate the dose of midazolam hydrochloride to the patient's underlying medical/surgical conditions; administer to the desired effect, being certain to wait an adequate time for peak CNS effects of both midazolam hydrochloride and concomitant medications, and have the personnel and size-appropriate equipment and facilities available for monitoring and intervention. IV midazolam hydrochloride should be used only in hospital or ambulatory care settings, including physicians' and dental offices, that provide for continuous monitoring of respiratory and cardiac function (ie, pulse oximetry). For deeply sedated pediatric patients, a dedicated individual, other than the practitioner performing the procedure, should monitor the patient throughout the procedure. Practitioners administering midazolam hydrochloride must have the skills necessary to manage reasonably foreseeable adverse reactions, particularly skills in airway management.

➤*Drug abuse and dependence:* Midazolam produced physical dependence of a mild-to-moderate intensity in cynomolgus monkeys after 5 to 10 weeks of administration. Available data concerning the drug abuse and dependence potential of midazolam suggest that its abuse potential is at least equivalent to that of diazepam.

Withdrawal symptoms, similar in character to those noted with barbiturates and alcohol (convulsions, hallucinations, tremor, abdominal and muscle cramps, vomiting and sweating), have occurred following abrupt discontinuation of benzodiazepines, including midazolam. Abdominal distention, nausea, vomiting, and tachycardia are prominent symptoms of withdrawal in infants. The more severe withdrawal symptoms have usually been limited to those patients who had received excessive doses over an extended period of time. Generally milder withdrawal symptoms (eg, dysphoria, insomnia) have been reported following abrupt discontinuance of benzodiazepines taken continuously at therapeutic levels for several months. Consequently, after extended therapy, abrupt discontinuation should generally be avoided and a gradual dosage tapering schedule followed. There is no consensus in the medical literature regarding tapering schedules; therefore, practitioners are advised to individualize therapy to meet patient's needs. In some case reports, patients who have had severe withdrawal reactions due to abrupt discontinuation of high-dose, long-term midazolam, have been successfully weaned off of midazolam over a period of several days.

➤*Hazardous tasks:* The decision as to when patients who have received injectable midazolam hydrochloride, particularly on an outpatient basis, may again engage in activities requiring complete mental alertness, operate hazardous machinery or drive a motor vehicle must be individualized. Gross tests of recovery from the effects of midazolam hydrochloride cannot be relied upon to predict reaction time under stress. Gross tests of recovery after awakening (orientation, ability to stand and walk, suitability for discharge from the recovery room, return to baseline Trieger competency) usually indicate recovery within 2 hours, but recovery may take up to 6 hours in some cases. It is recommended that no patient operate hazardous machinery or a motor vehicle until the effects of the drug, such as drowsiness, have subsided, or until 1 full day after anesthesia and surgery, whichever is longer. For pediatric patients, particular care should be taken to ensure safe ambulation.

➤*Pregnancy: Category D.* An increased risk of congenital malformations associated with the use of benzodiazepine drugs (diazepam and chlordiazepoxide) has been suggested in several studies. If this drug is used during pregnancy, the patient should be apprised of the potential hazard to the fetus.

Labor and delivery – The use of injectable midazolam hydrochloride in obstetrics has not been evaluated in clinical studies. Because midazolam is transferred transplacentally and because other benzodiazepines given in the last weeks of pregnancy have resulted in neonatal CNS depression, midazolam hydrochloride is not recommended for obstetrical use.

➤*Lactation:* Midazolam is excreted in human milk. Caution should be exercised when midazolam hydrochloride is administered to a nursing woman.

➤*Children:* The safety and efficacy of midazolam hydrochloride for sedation/anxiolysis/amnesia following single-dose IM administration, IV by intermittent injections and continuous infusion have been established in pediatric and neonatal patients. Onset time of sedative effects in the pediatric population begins within 5 minutes and peaks at 15 to 30 minutes depending upon the dose administered. The following adverse reactions related to the use of IV midazolam hydrochloride in pediatric patients were reported in the medical literature: Desaturation (4.6%), apnea (2.8%), hypotension (2.7%), paradoxical reactions (2%), hiccups (1.2%), seizure-like activity (1.1%) and nystagmus (1.1%). The majority of airway-related events occurred in patients receiving other CNS depressing medications and in patients where midazolam hydrochloride was not used as a single sedating agent. Midazolam hydrochloride is a potent sedative agent that requires slow administration and individualization of dosage. Clinical experience has shown midazolam hydrochloride to be 3 to 4 times as potent per mg as diazepam. Because serious and life-threatening cardiorespiratory adverse events have been reported, provision for monitoring, detection and correction of these reactions must be made for every patient to whom midazolam hydro-

MIDAZOLAM HYDROCHLORIDE — INJECTION

chloride injection is administered, regardless of age or health status. Unlike adult patients, pediatric patients generally receive increments of midazolam hydrochloride on a mg/kg basis. As a group, pediatric patients generally require higher dosages of midazolam hydrochloride (mg/kg) than do adults. Younger (less than 6 years of age) pediatric patients may require higher dosages (mg/kg) than older pediatric patients, and may require closer monitoring. In obese pediatric patients, the dose should be calculated based on ideal body weight. When midazolam hydrochloride is given in conjunction with opioids or other sedatives, the potential for respiratory depression, airway obstruction, or hypoventilation is increased. The healthcare practitioner who uses this medication in pediatric patients should be aware of and follow accepted professional guidelines for pediatric sedation appropriate to their situation.

Preterm infants and neonates – Rapid injection should be avoided in the neonatal population. Midazolam hydrochloride administered rapidly as an IV injection (less than 2 minutes) has been associated with severe hypotension in neonates, particularly when the patient has also received fentanyl. Likewise, severe hypotension has been observed in neonates receiving a continuous infusion of midazolam who then receive a rapid IV injection of fentanyl. Seizures have been reported in several neonates following rapid IV administration.

The neonate also has reduced and immature organ function and is also vulnerable to profound or prolonged respiratory effects of midazolam hydrochloride.

➤*Elderly:* Because geriatric patients may have altered drug distribution and diminished hepatic or renal function, reduced doses of midazolam hydrochloride are recommended; IV and IM doses of midazolam hydrochloride should be decreased for elderly and for debilitated patients, whether or not concomitant sedating medications have been administered, and subjects over 70 years of age may be particularly sensitive. These patients will also probably take longer to recover completely after midazolam hydrochloride administration for the induction of anesthesia. Administration of IM and IV midazolam hydrochloride to elderly or high-risk surgical patients has been associated with rare reports of death under circumstances compatible with cardiorespiratory depression. In most of these cases, the patients also received other CNS depressants capable of depressing respiration, especially narcotics.

Drug Interactions

➤*CNS agents:* Concomitant use of barbiturates, alcohol or other CNS depressants may increase the risk of hypoventilation, airway obstruction, desaturation, or apnea and may contribute to profound or prolonged drug effect. Narcotic premedication also depresses the ventilatory response to carbon dioxide stimulation.

The sedative effect of IV midazolam is accentuated by any concomitantly administered medication which depresses the CNS, particularly narcotics (eg, morphine, meperidine, fentanyl) and also secobarbital and droperidol. Consequently, the dosage of midazolam should be adjusted according to the type and amount of concomitant medications administered and the desired clinical response.

➤*CYP450 system:* Caution is advised when midazolam is administered concomitantly with drugs that are known to inhibit the P450 3A4 enzyme system such as cimetidine (not ranitidine), erythromycin, diltiazem, verapamil, ketoconazole and itraconazole. These drug interactions may result in prolonged sedation due to a decrease in plasma clearance of midazolam.

➤*H_2 blockers:* The effect of single oral doses of 800 mg cimetidine and 300 mg ranitidine on steady-state concentrations of midazolam was examined in a randomized crossover study (n = 8). Cimetidine increased the mean steady-state concentration from 57 to 71 ng/mL. Ranitidine increased the mean steady-state concentration to 62 ng/mL. No change in choice reaction time or sedation index was detected after dosing with the H_2 receptor antagonists.

➤*Erythromycin:* In a placebo-controlled study, erythromycin administered as a 500 mg dose 3 times daily for 1 week (n = 6) reduced the clearance of midazolam following a single 0.5 mg/kg IV dose. The half-life was approximately doubled. Caution is advised when midazolam is administered to patients receiving erythromycin since this may result in a decrease in the plasma clearance of midazolam.

➤*Calcium channel blockers:* The effects of diltiazem (60 mg 3 times daily) and verapamil (80 mg 3 times daily) on the pharmacokinetics and pharmacodynamics of midazolam were investigated in a 3-way crossover study (n = 9). The half-life of midazolam increased from 5 to 7 hours when midazolam was taken in conjunction with verapamil or diltiazem. No interaction was observed in healthy subjects between midazolam and nifedipine.

➤*Thiopental:* A moderate reduction in induction dosage requirements of thiopental (about 15%) has been noted following use of IM midazolam hydrochloride for premedication in adults.

➤*Halothane:* The IV administration of midazolam hydrochloride decreases the minimum alveolar concentration (MAC) of halothane required for general anesthesia. This decrease correlates with the dose of midazolam hydrochloride administered; no similar studies have been carried out in pediatric patients, but there is no scientific reason to expect that pediatric patients would respond differently than adults.

➤*Other agents:* In neonates, severe hypotension has been reported with concomitant administration of fentanyl. This effect has been observed in neonates on an infusion of midazolam who received a rapid injection of fentanyl and in patients on an infusion of fentanyl who have received a rapid injection of midazolam.

Adverse Reactions

Fluctuations in vital signs were the most frequently seen findings following parenteral administration of midazolam hydrochloride in adults and included decreased tidal volume or respiratory rate decrease (23.3% of patients following IV and 10.8% of patients following IM administration) and apnea (15.4% of patients following IV administration), as well as variations in blood pressure and pulse rate. The majority of serious adverse reactions, particularly those associated with oxygenation and ventilation, have been reported when midazolam hydrochloride is administered with other medications capable of depressing the CNS. The incidence of such events is higher in patients undergoing procedures involving the airway without the protective effect of an endotracheal tube (eg, upper endoscopy, dental procedures).

➤*Cardiorespiratory effects:* See Warnings/Precautions for more information.

➤*Improper dosing:* See Warnings/Precautions for more information.

Adults – The following additional adverse reactions were reported after IM administration: Headache (1.3%) was reported as an adverse reaction. Local adverse effects at the IM injection site reported included pain (3.7%), induration (0.5%), redness (0.5%), and muscle stiffness (0.3%).

Administration of IM midazolam hydrochloride to elderly or higher risk surgical patients has been associated with rare reports of death under circumstances compatible with cardiorespiratory depression. In most of these cases, the patients also received other CNS depressants capable of depressing respiration, especially narcotics.

The following additional adverse reactions were reported subsequent to IV administration as a single sedative/anxiolytic/amnestic agent in adult patients: Hiccups (3.9%), nausea (2.8%), vomiting (2.6%), coughing (1.3%), "oversedation" (1.6%), headache (1.5%), and drowsiness (1.2%). Local adverse effects at the IV site reported included the following: Tenderness (5.6%), pain during injection (5%), redness (2.6%), induration (1.7%), and phlebitis (0.4%).

Children – The following adverse reactions related to the use of IV midazolam hydrochloride in pediatric patients were reported in the medical literature: Desaturation (4.6%), apnea (2.8%), hypotension (2.7%), paradoxical reactions (2%), hiccups (1.2%), seizure-like activity (1.1%) and nystagmus (1.1%). The majority of airway-related events occurred in patients receiving other CNS depressing medications and in patients where midazolam hydrochloride was not used as a single sedating agent.

Neonates – See Warnings/Precautions for more information.

➤*Occurrence less than 1% in adults and children:* Other adverse reactions, observed mainly following IV injection as a single sedative/anxiolytic/amnesia agent and occurring at an incidence of less than 1% in adult and pediatric patients, are as follows:

Cardiovascular – Bigeminy, premature ventricular contractions, vasovagal episode, bradycardia, tachycardia, nodal rhythm.

CNS – Retrograde amnesia, euphoria, hallucination, confusion, argumentativeness, nervousness, anxiety, grogginess, restlessness, emergence delirium or agitation, prolonged emergence from anesthesia, dreaming during emergence, sleep disturbance, insomnia, nightmares, athetoid movements, seizure-like activity, ataxia, dizziness, dysphoria, slurred speech, dysphonia, paresthesia.

GI – Acid taste, excessive salivation, retching.

Hypersensitivity – Allergic reactions including anaphylactoid reactions, hives, rash, pruritus.

Local – Hive-like elevation at injection site, swelling or feeling of burning, warmth or coldness at injection site.

Respiratory – Laryngospasm, bronchospasm, dyspnea, hyperventilation, wheezing, shallow respirations, airway obstruction, tachypnea.

Special senses – Blurred vision, diplopia, nystagmus, pinpoint pupils, cyclic movements of eyelids, visual disturbance, difficulty focusing eyes, ears blocked, loss of balance, lightheadedness.

Miscellaneous – Yawning, lethargy, chills, weakness, toothache, faint feeling, hematoma.

Overdosage

➤*Symptoms:* The manifestations of midazolam hydrochloride overdosage reported are similar to those observed with other benzodiazepines, including sedation, somnolence, confusion, impaired coordination, diminished reflexes, coma and untoward effects on vital signs. No evidence of specific organ toxicity from midazolam hydrochloride overdosage has been reported.

➤*Treatment:* Treatment of injectable midazolam hydrochloride overdosage is the same as that followed for overdosage with other benzodiazepines. Respiration, pulse rate and blood pressure should be monitored and general supportive measures should be employed. Attention should be given to the maintenance of a patent airway and support of ventilation, including administration of oxygen. An IV infusion should be started. Should hypotension develop, treatment may include IV fluid therapy, repositioning, judicious use of vasopressors appropriate to the clinical situation, if indicated, and other appropriate countermeasures. There is no information as to whether peritoneal dialysis, forced diuresis or hemodialysis are of any value in the treatment of midazolam overdosage.

Flumazenil, a specific benzodiazepine-receptor antagonist, is indicated for the complete or partial reversal of the sedative effects of benzodiazepines and may be used in situations when an overdose with a benzodiazepine is known or suspected. There are anecdotal reports of reversal of adverse

MIDAZOLAM HYDROCHLORIDE — INJECTION

hemodynamic responses associated with midazolam hydrochloride following administration of flumazenil to pediatric patients. Prior to the administration of flumazenil, necessary measures should be instituted to secure the airway, ensure adequate ventilation, and establish adequate IV access. Flumazenil is intended as an adjunct to, not as a substitute for, proper management of benzodiazepine overdose. Patients treated with flumazenil should be monitored for resedation, respiratory depression and other residual benzodiazepine effects for an appropriate period after treatment. Flumazenil will only reverse benzodiazepine-induced effects but will not reverse the effects of other concomitant medications. The reversal of benzodiazepine effects may be associated with the onset of seizures in certain high-risk patients. The prescriber should be aware of a risk of seizure in association with flumazenil treatment, particularly in long-term benzodiazepine users and in cyclic antidepressant overdose. The complete flumazenil monograph, including Contraindications, Warnings and Precautions, should be consulted prior to use.

Patient Information

Inform your physician about any alcohol consumption and medicine you are now taking, especially blood pressure medication and antibiotics, including drugs you buy without a prescription. Alcohol has an increased effect when consumed with benzodiazepines; therefore, caution should be exercised regarding simultaneous ingestion of alcohol during benzodiazepine treatment.

Inform your physician if you are pregnant or are planning to become pregnant.

Inform your physician if you are breastfeeding.

Patients should be informed of the pharmacological effects of midazolam hydrochloride, such as sedation and amnesia, which in some patients may be profound. The decision as to when patients who have received injectable midazolam hydrochloride, particularly on an outpatient basis, may again engage in activities requiring complete mental alertness, operate hazardous machinery or drive a motor vehicle must be individualized.

Patients receiving continuous infusion of midazolam in critical care settings over an extended period of time, may experience symptoms of withdrawal following abrupt discontinuation.

GENERAL ANESTHETICS

KETAMINE HYDROCHLORIDE

c-iii	**Ketamine HCl** (Various, eg, Bedford)	**Injection:** 10 mg/ml	In 20 ml vials.[a]
		50 mg/ml	In 10 ml vials.[a]
		100 mg/ml	In 5 ml vials.[a]
c-iii	**Ketalar** (JHP Pharmaceuticals)	**Injection; solution:** 10 mg/ml	In 20 ml vials (10s).[a]
		50 mg/ml	In 10 ml vials (10s).[a]
		100 mg/ml	In 5 ml vials (10s).[a]

[a] With benzethonium chloride.

KETAMINE HYDROCHLORIDE — INJECTION

Indications

➤*Procedural sedation:* As the sole anesthetic agent for diagnostic and surgical procedures that do not require skeletal muscle relaxation. Ketamine hydrochloride is best suited for short procedures, but it can be used, with additional doses, for longer procedures.

➤*Anesthesia:* For the induction of anesthesia prior to the administration of other general anesthetic agents; to supplement low-potency agents, such as nitrous oxide.

➤*Off-label uses:*

Postanesthetic shivering – [4] = Insufficient documentation. Initial data regarding the use of single-dose ketamine indicate that this agent is more effective than granisetron and comparable with meperidine in the prevention of anesthesia-induced shivering. (See Administration and Dosage.)

Postherpetic neuralgia – [5] = Poor documentation. Use is not recommended. The results from the 3 trials evaluating the efficacy of topical ketamine for the treatment of postherpetic neuralgia (PHN) are conflicting. American Academy of Neurology clinical practice guidelines state that the efficacy of ketamine for the treatment of PHN is unproven. Routine use of topical ketamine for PHN is not recommended until additional data defining the optimum dose and patient population are available.

Administration and Dosage

➤*General dosing considerations:* While vomiting has been reported following ketamine administration, some airway protection may be afforded because of active laryngeal-pharyngeal reflexes. However, because aspiration may occur with ketamine, and because protective reflexes may also be diminished by supplementary anesthetics and muscle relaxants, the possibility of aspiration must be considered. Ketamine is recommended for use in the patient whose stomach is not empty when, in the judgment of the practitioner, the benefits of the drug outweigh the possible risks.

Atropine, scopolamine, or another drying agent should be given at an appropriate interval prior to induction.

Because of rapid induction following the initial IV injection, the patient should be in a supported position during administration.

The onset of action of ketamine is rapid; an IV dose of 2 mg/kg (1 mg/lb) usually produces surgical anesthesia within 30 seconds after injection, with the anesthetic effect usually lasting 5 to 10 minutes. If a longer effect is desired, additional increments can be administered IV or IM to maintain anesthesia without producing significant cumulative effects.

IM doses, from experience primarily in children, in a range of 9 to 13 mg/kg (4 to 6 mg/lb) usually produce surgical anesthesia within 3 to 4 minutes following injection, with the anesthetic effect usually lasting 12 to 25 minutes.

As with other general anesthetic agents, the individual response to ketamine is somewhat varied depending on the dose, route of administration, and age of patient, so that dosage recommendation cannot be absolutely fixed. The drug should be titrated against the patient's requirements.

➤*Adults:*

Induction of Anesthesia –

IV use:

• *Initial dosage* – 1 to 4.5 mg/kg (0.5 to 2 mg/lb) given slowly IV. The average amount required to produce 5 to 10 minutes of surgical anesthesia has been 2 mg/kg (1 mg/lb).

• *Alternative dosage* – 1 to 2 mg/kg IV at a rate of 0.5 mg/kg/min may be used for induction of anesthesia. In addition, diazepam in 2 to 5 mg doses, administered in a separate syringe over 60 seconds, may be used. In most cases, IV diazepam 15 mg or less will suffice. The incidence of psychological manifestations during emergence, particularly dreamlike observations and emergence delirium, may be reduced by this induction dosage program.

IM use: The initial dose may range from 6.5 to 13 mg/kg (3 to 6 mg/lb). A dose of 10 mg/kg (5 mg/lb) will usually produce 12 to 25 minutes of surgical anesthesia.

Maintenance of anesthesia – The maintenance dose should be adjusted according to the patient's anesthetic needs and whether an additional anesthetic agent is employed.

It should be recognized that the larger the total dose of ketamine administered, the longer will be the time to complete recovery.

Usual dosage: Increments of one-half to the full induction dose may be repeated as needed for maintenance of anesthesia. However, it should be noted that purposeless and tonic-clonic movements of extremities may occur during the course of anesthesia. These movements do not imply a light plane and are not indicative of the need for additional doses of the anesthetic.

Alternative dosage: Adult patients induced with ketamine augmented with IV diazepam may be maintained on ketamine given by slow microdrip infusion technique at a dose of 0.1 to 0.5 mg/min, augmented with diazepam 2 to 5 mg administered IV as needed.

In many cases, IV diazepam 20 mg or less total for combined induction and maintenance will suffice. However, slightly more diazepam may be required depending on the nature and duration of the operation, physical status of the patient, and other factors. The incidence of psychological manifestations during emergence, particularly dreamlike observations and emergence delirium, may be reduced by this maintenance dosage program.

Off-label dosing –

Postanesthetic shivering: [4] = Insufficient documentation. Single 0.5 mg/kg IV bolus injection.

➤*Children:* As with other general anesthetic agents, the individual response to ketamine is somewhat varied depending on the dose, route of administration, and age of patient, so that dosage recommendation cannot be absolutely fixed. The drug should be titrated against the patient's requirements.

➤*Concomitant therapy:* Atropine, scopolamine, or another drying agent should be given at an appropriate interval prior to induction.

Ketamine is clinically compatible with the commonly used general and local anesthetic agents when an adequate respiratory exchange is maintained.

The regimen of a reduced dose of ketamine supplemented with diazepam can be used to produce balanced anesthesia by combination with other agents such as nitrous oxide and oxygen.

➤*Preparation for administration:* To prepare a dilute solution containing ketamine 1 mg/mL, aseptically transfer 10 mL (50 mg/mL *Steri-Vial*) or

KETAMINE HYDROCHLORIDE — INJECTION

5 mL (100 mg/mL *Steri-Vial*) to 500 mL of dextrose 5% injection or sodium chloride 0.9% injection and mix well. The resultant solution will contain ketamine 1 mg/mL.

The fluid requirements of the patient and duration of anesthesia must be considered when selecting the appropriate dilution of ketamine. If fluid restriction is required, ketamine can be added to a 250 mL infusion as described above to provide a ketamine concentration of 2 mg/mL.

Ketamine *Steri-Vials* 10 mg/mL are not recommended for dilution.

Note: The 100 mg/mL concentration of ketamine should not be injected IV without proper dilution. It is recommended the drug be diluted with an equal volume of either sterile water for injection, normal saline, or dextrose 5% in water.

➤*Administration:* May be given IV or IM. It is recommended that ketamine be administered slowly IV (over a period of 60 seconds). More rapid administration may result in respiratory depression and enhanced pressor response.

➤*Admixture compatibility:* Barbiturates and ketamine, being chemically incompatible because of precipitate formation, should not be injected from the same syringe.

If the ketamine dose is augmented with diazepam, the 2 drugs must be given separately. Do not mix ketamine and diazepam in syringe or infusion flask.

➤*Storage/Stability:* Store between 15° and 30°C (59° and 86°F). Protect from light.

Actions

➤*Pharmacology:* Ketamine hydrochloride is a rapidly acting general anesthetic producing an anesthetic state characterized by profound analgesia, normal pharyngeal-laryngeal reflexes, normal or slightly enhanced skeletal muscle tone, cardiovascular and respiratory stimulation, and occasionally a transient and minimal respiratory depression.

A patent airway is maintained partly by virtue of unimpaired pharyngeal and laryngeal reflexes.

The anesthetic state produced by ketamine hydrochloride has been termed "dissociative anesthesia" in that it appears to selectively interrupt association pathways of the brain before producing somatesthetic sensory blockade. It may selectively depress the thalamoneocortical system before significantly obtunding the more ancient cerebral centers and pathways (reticular-activating and limbic systems).

Elevation of blood pressure begins shortly after injection, reaches a maximum within a few minutes, and usually returns to preanesthetic values within 15 minutes after injection. In the majority of cases, the systolic and diastolic blood pressure peaks from 10% to 50% above preanesthetic levels shortly after induction of anesthesia, but the elevation can be higher or longer in individual cases (see Contraindications).

Ketamine has a wide margin of safety; several instances of unintentional administration of overdoses of ketamine hydrochloride (up to 10 times that usually required) have been followed by prolonged but complete recovery.

➤*Pharmacokinetics:*

Absorption/Distribution – Following IV administration, the ketamine concentration has an initial slope (alpha phase) lasting about 45 minutes with a half-life of 10 to 15 minutes. This first phase corresponds clinically to the anesthetic effect of the drug. The anesthetic action is terminated by a combination of redistribution from the CNS to slower equilibrating peripheral tissues and by hepatic biotransformation to metabolite I. This metabolite is about ⅓ as active as ketamine in reducing halothane requirements (MAC) of the rat.

Metabolism/Excretion – The later half-life of ketamine (beta phase) is 2.5 hours.

The biotransformation of ketamine hydrochloride includes N-dealkylation (metabolite 1), hydroxylation of the cyclohexone ring (metabolites 3 and 4), conjugation with glucuronic acid and dehydration of the hydroxylated metabolites to form the cyclohexene derivative (metabolite 2).

Contraindications

Those in whom a significant elevation of blood pressure would constitute a serious hazard; hypersensitivity to the drug.

Warnings/Precautions

➤*Emergence reaction:* Emergence reactions have occurred in approximately 12% of patients.

The psychological manifestations vary in severity between pleasant dream-like states, vivid imagery, hallucinations, and emergence delirium. In some cases, these states have been accompanied by confusion, excitement, and irrational behavior which a few patients recall as an unpleasant experience. The duration ordinarily is no more than a few hours; in a few cases, however, recurrences have taken place up to 24 hours postoperatively. No residual psychological effects are known to have resulted from use of ketamine hydrochloride.

The incidence of these emergence phenomena is least in the elderly (older than 65 years of age) patient. Also, they are less frequent when the drug is given IM, and the incidence is reduced as experience with the drug is gained.

The incidence of psychological manifestations during emergence, particularly dreamlike observations and emergence delirium, may be reduced by using lower recommended dosages of ketamine hydrochloride in conjunction with IV diazepam during induction and maintenance of anesthesia (see Administration and Dosage). Also, these reactions may be reduced if verbal, tactile, and visual stimulation of the patient is minimized during the recovery period. This does not preclude the monitoring of vital signs.

In order to terminate a severe emergence reaction, the use of a small hypnotic dose of a short-acting or ultra, short-acting barbiturate may be required.

➤*Confusional states:* Postoperative confusional states may occur during the recovery period.

➤*Respiratory depression:* Respiratory depression may occur with overdosage or too rapid a rate of administration of ketamine hydrochloride, in which case supportive ventilation should be employed. Mechanical support of respiration is preferred to administration of analeptics.

➤*Administration:* Ketamine hydrochloride should be used by or under the direction of physicians experienced in administering general anesthetics and in maintenance of an airway and in the control of respiration.

Because pharyngeal and laryngeal reflexes are usually active, ketamine hydrochloride should not be used alone in surgery or diagnostic procedures of the pharynx, larynx, or bronchial tree. Mechanical stimulation of the pharynx should be avoided, whenever possible, if ketamine hydrochloride is used alone. Muscle relaxants, with proper attention to respiration, may be required in both of these instances.

Resuscitative equipment should be ready for use.

The incidence of emergence reactions may be reduced if verbal and tactile stimulation of the patient is minimized during the recovery period. This does not preclude the monitoring of vital signs.

The IV dose should be administered over a period of 60 seconds. More rapid administration may result in respiratory depression or apnea and enhanced pressor response.

In surgical procedures involving visceral pain pathways, ketamine hydrochloride should be supplemented with an agent which obtunds visceral pain.

➤*Special risk:* Use with caution in the chronic alcoholic and the acutely alcohol-intoxicated patient.

An increase in CSF pressure has been reported following administration of ketamine hydrochloride. Use with extreme caution in patients with preanesthetic elevated cerebrospinal fluid pressure.

➤*Drug abuse and dependence:* Ketamine has been reported being used as a drug of abuse. Reports suggest that ketamine produces a variety of symptoms including, but not limited to, flashbacks, hallucinations, dysphoria, anxiety, insomnia, or disorientation. Ketamine dependence and tolerance may develop in individuals with a history of drug abuse or dependence. Therefore, ketamine should be prescribed and administered with caution.

➤*Hazardous tasks:* The patients should be cautioned that driving an automobile, operating hazardous machinery or engaging in hazardous activities should not be undertaken for 24 hours or more (depending upon the dosage of ketamine hydrochloride and consideration of other drugs employed) after anesthesia.

When ketamine is used on an outpatient basis, the patient should not be released until recovery from anesthesia is complete and then should be accompanied by a responsible adult.

➤*Pregnancy:* Category B (per Briggs' *Drugs in Pregnancy and Lactation*). Since the safe use in pregnancy, including obstetrics (either vaginal or abdominal delivery), has not been established, such use is not recommended.

Animal reproduction –

To determine the effect of ketamine hydrochloride on the perinatal and postnatal period, pregnant rats were given twice the average human IM dose during days 18 to 21 of pregnancy. Litter characteristics at birth and through the weaning period were equivalent to those of the control animals. There was a slight increase in incidence of delayed parturition by 1 day in treated dams of this group. Three groups each of mated beagle bitches were given 2.5 times the average human IM dose twice weekly for the 3 weeks of the first, second, and third trimesters of pregnancy, respectively, without the development of adverse reactions in the pups.

➤*Lactation:* The elimination half-life of ketamine is 2.17 hours; therefore, the drug should be undetectable in the mother's plasma approximately 11 hours after a dose. Breast-feeding after this time should not expose the infant to pharmacologically significant amounts of ketamine.

➤*Children:* As with other general anesthetic agents, the individual response to ketamine hydrochloride is somewhat varied depending on the dose, route of administration, and age of patient, so that dosage recommendation cannot be absolutely fixed. The drug should be titrated against the patient's requirements.

➤*Monitoring:* Cardiac function should be continually monitored during the procedure in patients found to have hypertension or cardiac decompensation.

Drug Interactions

Ketamine Drug Interactions

Precipitant drug	Object drug[a]		Description
Ketamine	Nondepolarizing muscle relaxants	⬆	Ketamine may increase the neuromuscular effects resulting in prolonged respiratory depression.
Ketamine	Thiopental	⬇	The hypnotic effect of thiopental may be antagonized.

KETAMINE HYDROCHLORIDE — INJECTION

Ketamine Drug Interactions			
Precipitant drug	Object drug[a]		Description
Barbiturates/ Narcotics	Ketamine	↑	Prolonged recovery time may occur if used with ketamine.
Halothane	Ketamine	↓	Cardiac output, blood pressure and pulse rate may be decreased. Halothane blocks the cardiovascular stimulatory effects of ketamine. Closely monitor cardiac function if ketamine and halothane are used together.
Theophyllines	Ketamine	↔	Unpredictable extensor-type seizures have been reported with coadministration.
Thyroid hormones	Ketamine	↑	Concurrent use may produce hypertension and tachycardia.

[a] ↑ = object drug increased; ↓ = object drug decreased; ↔ = undetermined effect.

Adverse Reactions

➤*Cardiovascular:* Blood pressure and pulse rate are frequently elevated following administration of ketamine hydrochloride alone. However, hypotension and bradycardia have been observed. Arrhythmia has also occurred.

➤*CNS:* In some patients, enhanced skeletal muscle tone may be manifested by tonic and clonic movements sometimes resembling seizures (see Administration and Dosage).

➤*Dermatologic:* Transient erythema or morbilliform rash have also been reported.

➤*GI:* Anorexia, nausea and vomiting have been observed; however, this is not usually severe and allows the great majority of patients to take liquids by mouth shortly after regaining consciousness (see Administration and Dosage).

➤*Hypersensitivity:* Anaphylaxis.

➤*Local:* Local pain and exanthema at the injection site have infrequently been reported.

➤*Ophthalmic:* Diplopia and nystagmus have been noted following ketamine hydrochloride administration. It also may cause a slight elevation in intraocular pressure measurement.

➤*Psychiatric:* See Warnings.

➤*Respiratory:* Although respiration is frequently stimulated, severe depression of respiration or apnea may occur following rapid IV administration of high doses of ketamine hydrochloride. Laryngospasms and other forms of airway obstruction have occurred during ketamine hydrochloride anesthesia.

Overdosage

➤*Symptoms:* Respiratory depression may occur with overdosage or too rapid a rate of administration of ketamine hydrochloride.

➤*Treatment:* In case of respiratory depression, supportive ventilation should be employed. Mechanical support of respiration is preferred to administration of analeptics.

Patient Information

As appropriate, especially in cases where early discharge is possible, the duration of ketamine hydrochloride and other drugs employed during the conduct of anesthesia should be considered. The patients should be cautioned that driving an automobile, operating hazardous machinery or engaging in hazardous activities should not be undertaken for 24 hours or more (depending upon the dosage of ketamine hydrochloride and consideration of other drugs employed) after anesthesia.

ETOMIDATE

Rx	**Etomidate** (Parenta)	**Injection, solution:** 2 mg/mL	In 10 and 20 mL single-dose vials.
Rx	**Amidate** (Hospira)		In 10 and 20 mL single-dose vials, 20 mL and in 10 and 20 mL amps, 20 mL *Abboject*.

ETOMIDATE — INJECTION

Indications

➤*Anesthesia:* For the induction of general anesthesia. When considering use of etomidate, the usefulness of its hemodynamic properties should be weighed against the high frequency of transient skeletal muscle movements.

➤*Supplementation of subpotent anesthetic agents:* For the supplementation of subpotent anesthetic agents, such as nitrous oxide in oxygen, during maintenance of anesthesia for short operative procedures, such as dilation and curettage or cervical conization.

Administration and Dosage

➤*Adults:*

Induction of anesthesia – 0.3 mg/kg injected IV over a period of 30 to 60 seconds. The dose will vary between 0.2 and 0.6 mg/kg, and it must be individualized in each case.

Supplementation of subpotent anesthetic agents – Smaller increments of IV etomidate may be administered to adult patients during short operative procedures to supplement subpotent anesthetic agents, such as nitrous oxide. Although usually smaller than the original induction dose, the dosage employed under these circumstances must be individualized. There are insufficient data to support the use of etomidate for longer adult procedures.

➤*Children:*

Induction of anesthesia – See Adults for dosing children 10 years of age and older.

➤*Elderly:* Elderly patients may require reduced doses of etomidate.

➤*Concomitant therapy:* The use of IV fentanyl and other neuroactive drugs employed during the conduct of anesthesia may alter the etomidate dosage requirements. Consult the prescribing information for all other such drugs before using.

Etomidate hypnosis does not significantly alter the usual dosage requirements of neuromuscular-blocking agents employed for endotracheal intubation or other purposes shortly after induction of anesthesia.

➤*Administration:* Etomidate injection is intended for administration only by the IV route.

➤*Admixture compatibility:* Etomidate injection is compatible with commonly administered preanesthetic medications, which may be employed as indicated.

➤*Storage/Stability:* Store at 15° to 30°C (59° to 86°F). Do not administer unless solution is clear and container is undamaged. Discard unused portion.

Actions

➤*Pharmacology:* Etomidate is a hypnotic drug without analgesic activity. IV etomidate produces hypnosis characterized by a rapid onset of action, usually within 1 minute. Duration of hypnosis is dose dependent but relatively brief, usually 3 to 5 minutes when an average dose of 0.3 mg/kg is employed. Immediate recovery from anesthesia (as assessed by awakening time, time needed to follow simple commands, and time to perform simple tests after anesthesia as well as they were performed before anesthesia), based upon data derived from short operative procedures where IV etomidate was used for induction and maintenance of anesthesia, is about as rapid as, or slightly faster than, immediate recovery after similar use of thiopental. These same data revealed that the immediate recovery period will usually be shortened in adult patients by the administration of approximately 0.1 mg of IV fentanyl, 1 or 2 minutes before induction of anesthesia, probably because less etomidate is generally required under these circumstances (consult the package insert for fentanyl before using).

The most characteristic effect of IV etomidate on the respiratory system is a slight elevation in arterial carbon dioxide tension.

Reduced plasma cortisol and aldosterone levels have been reported following induction doses of etomidate. These results persist for approximately 6 to 8 hours and appear to be unresponsive to adrenocorticotropic hormone stimulation.

The administration of up to 0.6 mg/kg of etomidate to patients with severe cardiovascular disease has little or no effect on myocardial metabolism, cardiac output, peripheral circulation, or pulmonary circulation. The hemodynamic effects of etomidate have, in most cases, been qualitatively similar to those of thiopental sodium, except that the heart rate tended to increase by a moderate amount following administration of thiopental under conditions where there was little or no change in heart rate following administration of etomidate. However, clinical data indicate that etomidate administration in elderly patients, particularly those with hypertension, may result in decreases in heart rate, cardiac index, and mean arterial blood pressure.There are insufficient data concerning use of etomidate in patients with recent severe trauma or hypovolemia to predict cardiovascular response under such circumstances.

Etomidate induction is associated with a transient 20% to 30% decrease in cerebral blood flow. This reduction in blood flow appears to be uniform in the absence of intracranial space–occupying lesions. As with other IV induction agents, reduction in cerebral oxygen utilization is roughly proportional to the reduction in cerebral blood flow. In patients with and without intracranial space–occupying lesions, etomidate induction is usually followed by a moderate lowering of intracranial pressure lasting several minutes. All of these studies provided for avoidance of hypercapnia. Information concerning regional cerebral perfusion in patients with intracranial space–occupying lesions is too limited to permit definitive conclusions.

Preliminary data suggest that etomidate will usually lower intraocular pressure moderately.

➤*Pharmacokinetics:*

Metabolism/Excretion – Etomidate is rapidly metabolized in the liver. Minimal hypnotic plasma levels of unchanged drug are 0.23 mcg/mL or more; they decrease rapidly up to 30 minutes following injection and thereafter more slowly with a half-life value of about 75 minutes. Approximately 75% of the administered dose is excreted in the urine during the first day after injection. The chief metabolite is R-(+)-1-(1-phenylethyl)-1H-imidazole-

ETOMIDATE — INJECTION

5-carboxylic acid, resulting from hydrolysis of etomidate, and accounts for about 80% of the urinary excretion.

Special populations –

Hepatic function impairment: Limited pharmacokinetic data in patients with cirrhosis and esophageal varices suggest that the volume of distribution and elimination half-life of etomidate are approximately double those seen in healthy subjects.

Elderly: In clinical studies, elderly patients demonstrated decreased initial distribution volumes and total clearance of etomidate. Protein binding of etomidate to serum albumin was also significantly decreased in these individuals.

Contraindications

Hypersensitivity to etomidate.

Warnings/Precautions

➤*Administration:* IV etomidate should be administered only by persons trained in the administration of general anesthetics and in the management of complications encountered during the conduct of general anesthesia.

Because of the hazards of prolonged suppression of endogenous cortisol and aldosterone production, this formulation is not intended for administration by prolonged infusion.

➤*Plasma cortisol levels:* Induction doses of etomidate have been associated with reduction in plasma cortisol and aldosterone concentrations. These have not been associated with changes in vital signs or evidence of increased mortality; however, consider exogenous replacement when concern exists for patients undergoing severe stress.

➤*Pregnancy: Category C.* Etomidate has been shown to have an embryocidal effect in rats when given in doses 1 and 4 times the human dose. There are no adequate and well-controlled studies in pregnant women. Use etomidate during pregnancy only if the potential benefit justifies the potential risks to the fetus. Etomidate has not been shown to be teratogenic in animals. Reproduction studies with etomidate have been shown to:

1.) decrease pup survival at 0.3 and 5 mg/kg in rats (approximately 1 and 16 times the human dosage, respectively) and at 1.5 and 4.5 mg/kg in rabbits (approximately 5 and 15 times the human dosage, respectively). No clear dose-related pattern was observed.
2.) increase slightly the number of stillborn fetuses in rats at 0.3 and 1.25 mg/kg (approximately 1 and 4 times the human dosage, respectively).
3.) cause maternal toxicity with deaths of 6 of 20 rats at 5 mg/kg (approximately 16 times the human dosage) and 6 of 20 rabbits at 4.5 mg/kg (approximately 15 times the human dosage).

Labor and delivery – There are insufficient data to support use of IV etomidate in obstetrics, including cesarean section deliveries. Therefore, such use is not recommended.

➤*Lactation:* It is not known whether this drug is excreted in human milk. Because many drugs are excreted in human milk, exercise caution when etomidate is administered to a breast-feeding mother.

➤*Children:* There are inadequate data to make dosage recommendations for induction of anesthesia in patients younger than 10 years of age; therefore, such use is not recommended.

➤*Elderly:* Clinical data indicates that etomidate may induce cardiac depression in elderly patients, particularly those with hypertension.

Elderly patients may require lower doses of etomidate than younger patients. Age-related differences in pharmacokinetic parameters have been observed in clinical studies.

This drug is known to be substantially excreted by the kidney, and the risk of toxic reactions to this drug may be greater in patients with renal function impairment. Because elderly patients are more likely to have decreased renal function, take care in dose selection; it may be useful to monitor renal function.

Drug Interactions

None known.

Adverse Reactions

The most frequent adverse reactions associated with use of IV etomidate are transient venous pain on injection and transient skeletal muscle movements, including myoclonus.

➤*Local:* Transient venous pain was observed immediately following IV injection of etomidate in about 20% of patients, with considerable difference in the reported incidence (1.2% to 42%). This pain is usually described as mild to moderate in severity, but it is occasionally judged disturbing. The observation of venous pain is not associated with a more than usual incidence of thrombosis or thrombophlebitis at the injection site. Pain also appears to be less frequently noted when larger, more proximal arm veins are employed, and it appears to be more frequently noted when smaller, more distal hand or wrist veins are employed.

➤*Musculoskeletal:* Transient skeletal muscle movements were noted following use of IV etomidate in about 32% of the patients, with considerable difference in the reported incidence (22.7% to 63%). Most of these observations were judged mild to moderate in severity, but some were judged disturbing. The incidence of disturbing movements was less when fentanyl 0.1 mg was given immediately before induction. These movements have been classified as myoclonic in the majority of cases (74%), but averting movements (7%), tonic movements (10%), and eye movements (9%) have also been reported. No exact classification is available, but these movements may also be placed into 3 groups by location.

Most movements are bilateral. The arms, legs, shoulders, neck, chest wall, trunk, and all 4 extremities have been described in some cases, with 1 or more of these muscle groups predominating in each individual case. Results of electroencephalographic studies suggest that these muscle movements are a manifestation of disinhibition of cortical activity; cortical electroencephalograms, taken during periods when these muscle movements were observed, have failed to reveal seizure activity.

Other movements are described as either unilateral or having a predominance of activity of 1 side over the other. These movements sometimes resemble a localized response to some stimuli, such as venous pain on injection, in the lightly anesthetized patient (averting movements). Any muscle group or groups may be involved, but a predominance of movement of the arm in which the IV infusion is started is frequently noted.

Still other movements probably represent a mixture of the first 2 types.

Skeletal muscle movements appear to be more frequent in patients who also manifest venous pain on injection.

➤*Other adverse reactions:*

Cardiovascular – Hypertension, hypotension, tachycardia, bradycardia and other arrhythmias have occasionally been observed during induction and maintenance of anesthesia. One case of severe hypotension and tachycardia, judged to be anaphylactoid in character, has been reported.

Elderly patients, particularly those with hypertension, may be at increased risk for the development of cardiac depression following etomidate administration.

GI – Postoperative nausea and/or vomiting following induction of anesthesia with etomidate is probably no more frequent than the general incidence. When etomidate was used for induction and maintenance of anesthesia in short procedures, such as dilation and curettage, or when insufficient analgesia was provided, the incidence of postoperative nausea and/or vomiting was higher than that noted in control patients who received thiopental.

Respiratory – Apnea of short duration (5 to 90 seconds with spontaneous recovery), hiccup, and snoring suggestive of partial upper airway obstruction have been observed in some patients. These conditions were managed by conventional countermeasures. Hyperventilation, hypoventilation, laryngospasm.

Overdosage

➤*Symptoms:* Overdosage may occur from too rapid or repeated injections. Too rapid injection may be followed by a fall in blood pressure. No adverse cardiovascular or respiratory reactions attributable to etomidate overdose have been reported.

➤*Treatment:* In the event of suspected or apparent overdosage, discontinue the drug, establish or maintain a patent airway (intubate, if necessary), and administer oxygen with assisted ventilation, if necessary.

PROPOFOL

Rx	**Propofol** (Baxter)	**Injectable, emulsion:** 10 mg/mL	In 20 mL single-use vials and 50 and 100 mL single-use infusion vials.[a]
Rx	**Diprivan** (AstraZeneca)		In 20 mL single-use amps, 50 and 100 mL single-use infusion vials, and 50 mL prefilled single-use syringes.[b]
Rx	**Fresenius Propoven** (APP Pharmaceutical)		In 20 mL single-use ampules and 20, 50, and 100 mL single-use vials.[c]

[a] With 100 mg/mL soybean oil, 22.5 mg/mL glycerol, 12 mg/mL egg yolk phospholipid, and 0.25 mg/mL sodium metabisulfite. pH = 4.5 to 6.4.
[b] With 100 mg/mL soybean oil, 22.5 mg/mL glycerol, 12 mg/mL egg lecithin, and 0.005% EDTA. pH = 7 to 8.5.
[c] With glycerol, oleic acid, purified egg phosphatides, soybean oil, triglycerides medium chain.

PROPOFOL — INJECTION

Indications

➤*Anesthesia:* Induction or maintenance of anesthesia as part of a balanced anesthetic technique for inpatient and outpatient surgery in adults and children at least 3 years of age. Can also be used for maintenance of anesthesia as part of a balanced anesthetic technique for inpatient and outpatient surgery in adult patients and children older than 2 months of age.

Propofol is not recommended for induction of anesthesia in patients younger than 3 years of age or for maintenance of anesthesia in patients younger than 2 months of age because safety and efficacy have not been established in those populations.

➤*Monitored anesthesia care (MAC) sedation:* To initiate and maintain MAC sedation during diagnostic procedures in adults, and it may also be

PROPOFOL — INJECTION

used for MAC sedation in conjunction with local/regional anesthesia in patients undergoing surgical procedures.

➤*Intensive care unit (ICU) sedation:* Continuous sedation and control of stress responses in intubated or respiratory-controlled adults in ICUs. Not indicated in pediatric ICU sedation because safety and efficacy have not been established.

Administration and Dosage

➤*General dosing considerations:* Individualize dosage and rate of administration and titrate to the desired effect according to clinically relevant factors, including preinduction and concomitant medications, age, American Society of Anesthesiologists (ASA) physical classification, and the patient's level of debilitation.

Steady-state propofol blood concentrations are generally proportional to infusion rates, especially within an individual patient. Undesirable effects such as cardiorespiratory depression are likely to occur at higher blood levels, which result from bolus dosing or rapid increase in the infusion rate.

An adequate interval (3 to 5 minutes) must be allowed between clinical dosage adjustments in order to assess drug effects.

Changes in vital signs (increases in pulse rate, blood pressure, sweating, and/or tearing) that indicate a response to surgical stimulation or lightening of anesthesia may be controlled by the administration of 25 to 50 mg (2.5 to 5 mL) incremental boluses and/or by increasing the infusion rate.

Always titrate infusion rates downward in the absence of clinical signs of light anesthesia until a mild response to surgical stimulation can be perceived in order to avoid the administration of propofol at rates higher than clinically necessary. Generally, achieve infusion rates of 50 to 100 mcg/kg/min in adults during maintenance therapy in order to optimize recovery times.

➤*Adults:*

Anesthesia –

Induction of general anesthesia: Most adult patients younger than 55 years of age and ASA physical classification I/II require 2 to 2.5 mg/kg IV for induction when not premedicated or when premedicated with oral benzodiazepines or intramuscular (IM) opioids. For induction, titrate propofol (approximately 40 mg every 10 seconds) against the patient response until the clinical signs show the onset of anesthesia.

For more information on neurosurgical patients or cardiac anesthesia, see Neurosurgical Patients or Cardiac Anesthesia.

Maintenance of general anesthesia: In adults, anesthesia can be maintained by administering propofol by infusion or intermittent IV bolus injection. The patient's clinical response will determine the infusion rate or the amount and frequency of incremental injections.

• *Continuous infusion* – 100 to 200 mcg/kg/min administered in a variable rate infusion with nitrous oxide 60% to 70% and oxygen provides anesthesia for patients undergoing general surgery. Maintenance by infusion should immediately follow the induction dose in order to provide satisfactory or continuous anesthesia during the induction phase. During this initial period following the induction dose, higher rates of infusion are generally required (150 to 200 mcg/kg/min) for the first 10 to 15 minutes. Subsequently decrease infusion rates 30% to 50% during the first half hour of maintenance. Generally, rates of 50 to 100 mcg/kg/min in adults should be achieved during maintenance in order to optimize recovery times.

• *Intermittent bolus* – Increments of 25 to 50 mg (2.5 to 5 mL) may be administered with nitrous oxide in adults undergoing general surgery. The incremental boluses should be administered when changes in vital signs indicate a response to surgical stimulation or light anesthesia.

MAC sedation –

Initiation of MAC sedation: Either a slow infusion or a slow injection method may be used while closely monitoring cardiorespiratory function. With the infusion method, sedation may be initiated by infusing propofol at 100 to 150 mcg/kg/min (6 to 9 mg/kg/h) for a period of 3 to 5 minutes and titrating to the desired clinical effect while closely monitoring respiratory function.

With the slow injection method for initiation, patients will require approximately 0.5 mg/kg administered over 3 to 5 minutes and titrated to clinical responses. When propofol is slowly administered over 3 to 5 minutes, most patients will be adequately sedated, and the peak drug effect can be achieved while minimizing undesirable cardiorespiratory effects occurring at high plasma levels.

Maintenance of MAC sedation: Propofol can be administered as the sole agent for maintenance as MAC sedation during surgical/diagnostic procedures.

A variable rate infusion method is preferable over an intermittent bolus dose method. With the variable rate infusion method, patients will generally require maintenance rates of 25 to 75 mcg/kg/min (1.5 to 4.5 mg/kg/h) during the first 10 to 15 minutes of sedation maintenance. Subsequently decrease infusion rates over time to 25 to 50 mcg/kg/min and adjust to clinical response. In titrating to clinical effect, allow approximately 2 minutes for onset of peak drug effect.

Always titrate downward in the absence of clinical signs of light sedation until mild responses to stimulation are obtained in order to avoid sedative administration at rates higher than are clinically necessary.

If intermittent bolus method is used, 10 or 20 mg (1 or 2 mL) increments can be given and titrated to desired level of sedation. With the intermittent bolus method of sedation maintenance, there is increased potential for respiratory depression, transient increases in sedation depth, and prolongation of recovery.

ICU sedation –

Initial dosage: For intubated, mechanically ventilated adults, slowly initiate with a continuous infusion of 5 mcg/kg/min (0.3 mg/kg/h) for at least 5 minutes to titrate to desired clinical effect and minimize hypotension.

Dosage titration: Subsequent increments of 5 to 10 mcg/kg/min (0.3 to 0.6 mg/kg/h) over 5- to 10-minute intervals may be used until desired sedation level is achieved. A minimum of 5 minutes between adjustments should be allowed for onset of peak drug effect.

Maintenance dosage: Most ICU adults recovering from the effects of general anesthesia or deep sedation will require maintenance rates of 5 to 50 mcg/kg/min (0.3 to 3 mg/kg/h) individualized and titrated to clinical response. With medical ICU patients or patients who have recovered from the effect of general anesthesia or deep sedation, the rate of administration of 50 mcg/kg/min or more may be required to achieve adequate sedation. These higher rates may increase the likelihood of hypotension.

In clinical studies, the mean infusion maintenance rate for all patients was approximately 27 mcg/kg/min. The maintenance infusion rates required to maintain adequate sedation ranged from 2.8 to 130 mcg/kg/min. The infusion rate was lower in patients older than 55 years of age (approximately 20 mcg/kg/min) compared with patients younger than 55 years of age (approximately 38 mcg/kg/min). In these studies, morphine or fentanyl was used as needed for analgesia.

Concomitant therapy: Although there are reports of reduced analgesic requirements, most patients received opioids for analgesia during maintenance of ICU sedation. Some patients also received benzodiazepines or neuromuscular-blocking agents. During long-term maintenance of sedation, some ICU patients were awakened once or twice every 24 hours for assessment of neurologic or respiratory function.

Discontinuation of therapy: Avoid discontinuation prior to weaning or for daily evaluation of sedation levels. This may result in rapid awakening with associated anxiety, agitation, and resistance to mechanical ventilation. Adjust infusions to maintain light sedation through these processes.

➤*Children:*

Anesthesia –

Induction of general anesthesia:

• *3 to 16 years of age* – Most patients 3 through 16 years of age and ASA physical class I/II require 2.5 to 3.5 mg/kg for induction when not premedicated or when lightly premedicated with oral benzodiazepines or intramuscular opioids. Within this dosage range, younger children may require higher induction doses than older children. A lower dosage is recommended for children ASA physical class III/IV.

Maintenance of general anesthesia:

• *3 to 16 years of age* – Propofol administered as a variable rate infusion supplemented with nitrous oxide 60% to 70% provides satisfactory anesthesia for most children 2 months of age or older, ASA physical class I or II, undergoing general anesthesia.

In general, for children, maintenance by infusion of propofol at a rate of 200 to 300 mcg/kg/min should immediately follow the induction dose. Following the first half-hour of maintenance, infusion rates of 125 to 150 mcg/kg/min are typically needed. Titrate propofol to achieve the desired clinical effect. Younger children may require higher maintenance infusion rates than older children.

➤*Elderly:* Use a lower induction dose and a slower maintenance rate of administration.

Induction of general anesthesia – Because of the reduced clearance and higher blood concentrations, most elderly patients require approximately 1 to 1.5 mg/kg (approximately 20 mg every 10 seconds) for induction of anesthesia according to their condition and responses. Do not use a rapid bolus because this will increase the likelihood of undesirable cardiorespiratory depression, including hypotension, apnea, airway obstruction, and/or oxygen desaturation.

Maintenance of general anesthesia – The maintenance infusion dose is 50 to 100 mcg/kg/min (3 to 6 mg/kg/h).

Initiation of MAC sedation – Do not use rapid (single or repeated) bolus dose administration for MAC sedation. The rate of administration should be over 3 to 5 minutes and the dosage of propofol should be reduced to approximately 80% of the usual adult dosage in these patients according to their condition, responses, and changes in vital signs.

Maintenance of MAC sedation – Do not use rapid (single or repeated) bolus dose administration for MAC sedation. Reduce the rate of administration and the dosage to approximately 80% of the usual adult dosage in these patients according to their condition, responses, and changes in vital signs.

Propofol can be the sole agent for maintenance of MAC sedation during surgical/diagnostic procedures, supplemented with opioids or benzodiazepines, which increase sedative and respiratory effects and may also result in a slower recovery profile.

➤*Debilitated or ASA physical class III/IV patients:* See Elderly for dosing information.

➤*Neurosurgical patients:*

Induction of general anesthesia – For induction of general anesthesia, slower induction is recommended using boluses of 20 mg every 10 seconds. Slower boluses or infusions of propofol for induction of anesthesia, titrated to clinical responses, will generally result in reduced induction dosage requirements (1 to 2 mg/kg).

Maintenance of general anesthesia – For maintenance of general anesthesia, the infusion dose is 100 to 200 mcg/kg/min (6 to 12 mg/kg/h).

➤*Cardiac anesthesia:*

Induction of general anesthesia – For induction of general anesthesia, morphine premedication (0.15 mg/kg) with nitrous oxide 67% in oxygen has been shown to decrease the necessary propofol maintenance infusion rates and therapeutic blood concentrations when compared with nonnarcotic premedication (eg, lorazepam). Determine the rate of propofol administration based on the patient's premedication and adjust according to clinical responses.

PROPOFOL — INJECTION

Avoid rapid bolus injection. Use a slow rate of approximately 20 mg every 10 seconds until induction onset (0.5 to 1.5 mg/kg). In order to ensure adequate anesthesia, when propofol is used as the primary agent, maintenance infusion rates should not be less than 100 mcg/kg/min and should be supplemented with analgesic levels of continuous opioid administration. When an opioid is used as the primary agent, propofol maintenance rates should be less than 50 mcg/kg/min and care should be taken to ensure amnesia with concomitant benzodiazepines. Higher doses of propofol will reduce the opioid requirements (see the following table). When propofol is used as the primary anesthetic, it should not be administered with the high-dose opioid technique because this may increase the likelihood of hypotension.

Maintenance of general anesthesia – For maintenance of general anesthesia, most patients require an infusion rate of 100 to 150 mcg/kg/min (6 to 9 mg/kg/h) when propofol is given with a secondary opioid. When low-dose propofol is used with a primary opioid, the infusion rate is 50 to 100 mcg/kg/min (see the following table).

In postcoronary artery bypass graft patients, the maintenance rate of propofol administration was usually low (median, 11 mcg/kg/min) because of the intraoperative administration of high opioid doses.

Propofol in Cardiac Anesthesia

Primary agent	Rate	Secondary agent/rate (following induction with primary agent)
Propofol		Opioid[a] 0.05 to 0.075 mcg/kg/min (no bolus)
Preinduction anxiolysis	25 mcg/kg/min	
Induction	0.5 to 1.5 mg/kg over 60 sec	
Maintenance (titrated to clinical response)	100 to 150 mcg/kg/min	
Opioid[b]		Propofol 50 to 100 mcg/kg/min (no bolus)
Induction	25 to 50 mcg/kg	
Maintenance	0.2 to 0.3 mcg/kg/min	

[a] Opioid is defined in terms of fentanyl equivalents (ie, fentanyl 1 mcg = alfentanil 5 mcg (for bolus), alfentanil 10 mcg (for maintenance), or sufentanil 0.1 mcg).
[b] Take care to ensure amnesia with concomitant benzodiazepine therapy.

➤*Concomitant therapy:* Nitrous oxide 60% to 70% can be combined with a variable rate of infusion to provide satisfactory anesthesia for minor surgical procedures (eg, body surface). With more stimulating surgical procedures (eg, intraabdominal), or if supplementation with nitrous oxide is not provided, increase administration rate(s) of propofol and/or opioids in order to provide adequate anesthesia.

Other drugs that cause CNS depression (eg, hypnotics/sedatives, inhalational anesthetics, opioids) can increase CNS depression induced by propofol. Morphine premedication (0.15 mg/kg) with nitrous oxide 67% in oxygen decreases the necessary propofol injection maintenance infusion rate and therapeutic blood concentrations when compared with nonnarcotic premedication (eg, lorazepam).

Transient local pain may occur during IV injection, which may be reduced if the larger veins of the forearm or antecubital fossa are used or by prior injection of IV lidocaine (1 mL of a 1% solution).

➤*Preparation for administration:* Propofol is provided as a ready-to-use formulation. However, should dilution be necessary, only dilute with dextrose 5% injection and do not dilute to a concentration of less than 2 mg/mL because it is an emulsion. In diluted form, it is more stable when in contact with glass than with plastic (95% potency after 2 hours of running infusion in plastic).

➤*Administration:* When administering propofol by infusion, syringe pumps or volumetric pumps are recommended to provide controlled infusion rates. When infusing propofol to patients undergoing magnetic resonance imaging, metered control devices may be used if mechanical pumps are impractical.

Elderly, debilitated, or ASA classification III/IV patients – Do not use rapid (single or repeated) bolus dose administration for general anesthesia or MAC sedation because this will increase the likelihood of undesirable cardiorespiratory depression, including hypotension, apnea, airway obstruction, and/or oxygen desaturation.

Children – Attempt to minimize pain on injection when administering propofol to children. Boluses of propofol may be administered via small veins if pretreated with lidocaine or via antecubital or larger veins.

➤*Admixture compatibility:* Although propofol appears to be compatible with other therapeutic agents for a very limited amount of time, the manufacturers do not recommend mixing it with other agents prior to administration.

Administration with other fluids – Compatibility of propofol with the coadministration of blood/serum/plasma has not been established (see Warnings/Precautions). Propofol is compatible with the following IV fluids when administered using a y-type infusion set: dextrose 5% injection; Ringer's lactate injection; Ringer's lactate and dextrose 5% injection; dextrose 5% and sodium chloride injection 0.45%; dextrose 5% and sodium chloride 0.2% injection.

➤*Storage/Stability:* Do not use if there is evidence of separation of the emulsion phases. Discard any unused portions of propofol or solutions containing propofol at the end of the anesthetic procedure or at 6 hours, whichever occurs sooner; for ICU sedation, discard after 12 hours (if administered directly from the vial or prefilled syringe) or 6 hours (if transferred to a syringe or other container).

Store at 4° to 22°C (40° to 72°F). Do not freeze. Protect from light. Shake well before use. Propofol undergoes oxidative degradation in the presence of oxygen, and is therefore packaged under nitrogen to eliminate this degradation path.

Always maintain strict aseptic technique during handling. Propofol injectable emulsion is a single-use, parenteral product that contains sodium metabisulfite (0.25 mg/mL) or 0.005% EDTA to retard the rate of growth of microorganisms in the event of accidental extrinsic contamination. However, propofol injectable emulsion can still support the growth of microorganisms because it is not an antimicrobially preserved product under USP standards. Do not use if contamination is suspected.

Actions

➤*Pharmacology:* Propofol is an IV hypnotic/sedative agent for induction and maintenance of anesthesia or sedation. IV injection of a therapeutic dose produces hypnosis rapidly and smoothly with minimal excitation, usually within 40 seconds from the start of an injection. As with other rapidly acting IV anesthetic agents, the half-time of blood-brain equilibration is ≈ 1 to 3 minutes, and this accounts for the rapid induction of anesthesia.

Pharmacodynamic properties of propofol depend on the therapeutic blood propofol concentrations. Steady-state concentrations are generally proportional to infusion rates, especially within an individual patient. Undesirable side effects such as cardiorespiratory depression are likely to occur at higher blood levels that result from bolus dosing or rapid increase in infusion rate. Allow an adequate interval (3 to 5 minutes) between clinical dosage adjustments in order to assess drug effects.

The hemodynamic effects of propofol injection during induction of anesthesia vary. If spontaneous ventilation is maintained, major cardiovascular effects are arterial hypotension (sometimes > 30% decrease) with little or no change in heart rate and no appreciable decrease in cardiac output. If ventilation is assisted or controlled (positive pressure ventilation), degree and incidence of decrease in cardiac output are accentuated. Addition of a potent opioid (eg, fentanyl) as a premedication further decreases cardiac output and respiratory drive.

If anesthesia is continued by infusion of propofol, endotracheal intubation and surgical stimulation may return arterial pressure towards normal. However, cardiac output may remain depressed. In comparative clinical studies, hemodynamic effects of propofol during induction are generally more pronounced than with traditional IV induction agents.

Induction of anesthesia with propofol is frequently associated with apnea. In 1573 adult patients given propofol (2 to 2.5 mg/kg), apnea lasted 0 to 30 sec in 7%, 30 to 60 seconds in 24%, and > 60 seconds in 12% of patients. In 218 children from birth to 16 years of age assessable for apnea who received bolus doses of propofol 1 to 3.6 mg/kg, the values were 12%, 10%, and 5%, respectively. During maintenance, propofol causes a decrease in ventilation usually associated with an increase in carbon dioxide tension which may be marked depending on the rate of administration and other concurrent agents (eg, opioids, sedatives).

In humans and animals, propofol does not suppress the adrenal response to ACTH. Preliminary findings in patients with normal intraocular pressure indicate that propofol anesthesia produces a decrease in intraocular pressure, which may be associated with a concomitant decrease in systemic vascular resistance. Animal studies and limited experience in susceptible patients have not indicated any propensity of propofol to induce malignant hyperthermia. Propofol is rarely associated with elevation of plasma histamine levels and does not cause signs of histamine release.

➤*Pharmacokinetics:*

Distribution – Following an IV bolus dose, plasma levels initially decline rapidly due to both high metabolic clearance and rapid drug distribution into tissues. Distribution accounts for about half of this decline following a bolus of propofol.

However, distribution is not constant over time, but decreases as body tissues equilibrate with plasma and become saturated. The rate at which equilibration occurs is a function of the rate and duration of the infusion. When equilibration occurs, there is no longer a net transfer of propofol between tissues and plasma.

Discontinuation of the recommended doses of propofol after the maintenance of anesthesia for ≈ 1 hour, or for sedation in the ICU for 1 day, results in a prompt decrease in blood propofol concentrations and rapid awakening. Longer infusions (10 days of ICU sedation) result in accumulation of significant tissue stores of propofol, such that the reduction in circulating propofol is slowed and the time to awakening is increased.

By daily titration of propofol dosage to achieve only the minimum effective therapeutic concentration, rapid awakening within 10 to 15 minutes will occur even after long-term administration. However, if higher than necessary infusion levels have been maintained for a long time, propofol will be redistributed from fat and muscle to the plasma, and this return of propofol from peripheral tissues will slow recovery.

The large contribution of distribution (≈ 50%) to the fall of propofol plasma levels following brief infusions means that after very long infusions (at steady state), about half the initial rate will maintain the same plasma levels. Thus, titration to clinical response and daily evaluation of sedation levels are important during use of propofol infusion for ICU sedation, especially infusions of long duration.

PROPOFOL — INJECTION

Clearance ranges from 23 to 50 mL/kg/min. It is chiefly eliminated by hepatic conjugation to inactive metabolites that are excreted by the kidneys. A glucuronide conjugate accounts for ≈ 50% of dose. Steady-state volume of distribution approaches 60 L/kg. Terminal half-life after a 10-day infusion is 1 to 3 days.

Special populations –

Elderly: With increasing age, the dose needed to achieve a defined anesthetic endpoint (dose requirement) decreases. This does not appear to be an age-related change. With increasing age, higher peak plasma levels occur, which can explain the decreased dose requirement. These higher levels can predispose patients to cardiorespiratory effects, including hypotension, apnea, airway obstruction, or oxygen desaturation. Lower doses are, therefore, recommended in the elderly.

Contraindications

When general anesthesia or sedation are contraindicated; hypersensitivity to propofol or components of the product.

Warnings/Precautions

➤*Administration:* Only people trained in the administration of general anesthesia and not involved in the conduct of the surgical/diagnostic procedure should administer propofol. Continuously monitor patients. Facilities for maintenance of a patent airway, artificial ventilation, and oxygen enrichment and circulatory resuscitation must be immediately available. For sedation of intubated, mechanically ventilated patients in the ICU, administer only by people skilled in the management of critically ill patients and trained in cardiovascular resuscitation and airway management.

See Administration and Dosage for more information.

➤*Blood/Plasma coadministration:* Do not coadminister through the same IV catheter with blood or plasma because compatibility has not been established. In vitro, aggregates of the globular component of the emulsion vehicle have occurred with blood/plasma/serum from humans and animals.

➤*Aseptic technique:* See Administration and Dosage for more information.

➤*Anaphylaxis:* Rarely, features of anaphylaxis, which may include angioedema, bronchospasm, erythema, and hypotension, have occurred after the administration of propofol, although the use of other drugs in most instances makes the relationship to propofol unclear.

➤*Special risk patients:* Use a lower induction dose and a slower maintenance rate of administration in elderly, debilitated, and ASA physical class III/IV patients. Continuously monitor patients for early signs of significant hypotension or bradycardia. Treatment may include increasing the rate of IV fluid administration, elevation of lower extremities, use of pressor agents, or administration of atropine. Apnea often occurs during induction and may persist for > 60 seconds. Ventilatory support may be required. Because propofol is an emulsion, use caution in patients with lipid metabolism disorders (eg, primary hyperlipoproteinemia, diabetic hyperlipidemia, pancreatitis).

➤*Epilepsy:* When administered to an epileptic patient, there may be a risk of seizure during the recovery phase.

➤*Transient local pain:* Transient local pain may occur during IV injection, which may be reduced if the larger veins of the forearm or antecubital fossa are used or by prior injection of IV lidocaine (1 mL of a 1% solution). Venous sequelae (phlebitis or thrombosis) have occurred rarely (< 1%). In 2 well-controlled clinical studies using dedicated IV catheters, no instances of venous sequelae were reported up to 14 days following induction. Intentional injection into SC or perivascular tissues of animals caused minimal tissue reaction. Intra-arterial injection in animals did not induce local tissue effects. Accidental intra-arterial injections have been reported in patients, and other than pain, there were no major sequelae.

➤*Perioperative myoclonia:* Perioperative myoclonia, rarely including convulsions and opisthotonus, has occurred.

➤*Pulmonary edema:* Pulmonary edema has been reported rarely with propofol use, although a causal relationship is not known.

➤*Cardiovascular effects:* Propofol has no vagolytic activity and has been associated with reports of bradycardia, asystole, and, rarely, cardiac arrest. Consider the IV administration of anticholinergic agents (eg, atropine, glycopyrrolate) to modify potential increases in vagal tone caused by concomitant agents (eg, succinylcholine) or surgical stimuli. There have been rare reports of cardiac arrest. Monitor patients for early signs of significant hypotension or cardiovascular depression, which may be profound. These effects are responsive to discontinuation of propofol, IV fluid administration, or vasopressor therapy.

➤*Hyperlipidemia:* Because propofol is formulated in an oil-in-water emulsion, elevations in serum triglycerides may occur when it is administered for extended periods of time. Monitor patients at risk of hyperlipidemia for increases in serum triglycerides or serum turbidity. Adjust if fat is being inadequately cleared from the body. A reduction in the quantity of concurrently administered lipids is indicated to compensate for the amount of lipid infused as part of the formulation; 1 mL of propofol contains ≈ 0.1 g of fat (1.1 kcal).

➤*Neurosurgical anesthesia:* When propofol is used in patients with increased intracranial pressure (ICP) or impaired cerebral circulation, avoid significant decreases in mean arterial pressure because of the resultant decreases in cerebral perfusion pressure. To avoid significant hypotension and decreases in cerebral perfusion pressure, use an infusion or slow bolus of ≈ 20 mg every 10 seconds instead of rapid, more frequent, and larger boluses. Slower induction titrated to clinical responses generally will result in reduced induction dosage requirements (1 to 2 mg/kg). When increased ICP is suspected, hyperventilation and hypocarbia should accompany use of propofol.

➤*Cardiac anesthesia:* Use slower rates of administration in premedicated patients, geriatric patients, patients with recent fluid shifts, or patients who are hemodynamically unstable. Correct any fluid deficits prior to administration. In those patients where additional fluid therapy may be contraindicated, other measures (eg, elevation of lower extremities, use of pressor agents) may be useful to offset the hypotension that is associated with the induction of anesthesia with propofol.

➤*Additives:*

Sodium metabisulfite – Propofol formulations that contain sodium metabisulfite, a sulfite, may cause allergic-type reactions including anaphylactic symptoms and life-threatening or less severe asthmatic episodes in certain susceptible people. The overall prevalence of sulfite sensitivity in the general population is unknown and probably low. Sulfite sensitivity is seen more frequently in asthmatic than nonasthmatic people.

EDTA – EDTA is a strong chelator of trace metals, including zinc. Although with propofol there are no reports of decreased zinc levels or zinc deficiency-related adverse events, do not infuse propofol for > 5 days without providing a drug holiday to safely replace estimated or measured urine zinc losses.

In clinical trials, mean urinary zinc loss was ≈ 2.5 to 3 mg/day in adult patients and 1.5 to 2 mg/day in pediatric patients. In patients who are predisposed to zinc deficiency, such as those with burns, diarrhea, or major sepsis, consider the need for supplemental zinc during prolonged therapy.

At high doses (2 to 3 g/day) EDTA has been reported, on rare occasions, to be toxic to the renal tubules. Studies to date in patients with normal or impaired renal function, have not shown any alterations in renal function with propofol injectable emulsion containing 0.005% EDTA. In patients at risk for renal impairment, check urinalysis and urine sediment before initiation of sedation and then monitor on alternate days during sedation.

➤*Pregnancy: Category B.* Reproduction studies have been performed in rats and rabbits at IV doses of 15 mg/kg/day (approximately equivalent to the recommended human induction dose on a mg/m^2 basis) and have revealed no evidence of impaired fertility or harm to the fetus caused by propofol. However, propofol has been shown to cause maternal deaths in rats and rabbits and decreased pup survival during the lactating period in dams treated with 15 mg/kg/day. The pharmacological activity (anesthesia) of the drug on the mother is probably responsible for the adverse effects seen in the offspring. However, there are no adequate and well-controlled studies in pregnant women. Use during pregnancy only if clearly needed.

Labor and delivery – Not recommended for obstetrics, including cesarean section deliveries. Propofol crosses the placenta and may be associated with neonatal depression.

➤*Lactation:* Not recommended for use in nursing mothers because propofol is excreted in breast milk and the effects of oral absorption of small amounts of propofol are not known.

➤*Children:* Safety and efficacy of propofol have been established for induction of anesthesia in children ≥ 3 years of age and for the maintenance of anesthesia in children ≥ 2 months of age. Not recommended for the induction of anesthesia in children < 3 years of age, in the maintenance of anesthesia in children < 2 months of age, or for ICU or MAC sedation in children because safety and efficacy have not been established. In pediatric patients, administration of fentanyl concomitantly with propofol may result in serious bradycardia. Although no causal relationship has been established, serious adverse events (including fatalities) have been reported in children with respiratory tract infections given propofol for ICU sedation. In pediatric patients, abrupt discontinuation following prolonged infusion may result in flushing of the hands and feet, agitation, tremulousness, and hyperirritability. Increased incidences of bradycardia (5%), agitation (4%), and jitteriness (9%) also have been reported.

➤*Elderly:* See Actions for more information.

➤*Monitoring:* MAC sedation patients should be continuously monitored by people not involved in the conduct of the surgical or diagnostic procedure; oxygen supplementation should be immediately available and provided where clinically indicated. Monitor oxygen saturation in all patients. Continuously monitor patients for early signs of hypotension, apnea, airway obstruction, or oxygen desaturation. These cardiorespiratory effects are more likely to occur following rapid initiation (loading) boluses or during supplemental maintenance boluses, especially in the elderly, debilitated, or ASA physical class III/IV patients.

Drug Interactions

➤*CNS depressants:* CNS depressants (eg, hypnotics/sedatives, inhalational anesthetics, opioids) can increase the CNS depression induced by propofol. Morphine premedication with nitrous oxide decreases the necessary propofol maintenance infusion rate and therapeutic blood concentrations when compared to nonnarcotic (eg, lorazepam) premedication (see Administration and Dosage). In addition, the induction dose requirements of propofol may be reduced in patients with IM or IV premedication, particularly with narcotics alone or in combination with sedatives. These agents may increase the anesthetic or sedative effects of propofol and may also result in more pronounced decreases in systolic, diastolic, and mean arterial pressures and cardiac output.

Adverse Reactions

➤*Anesthesia/MAC sedation:*

Cardiovascular – Hypotension (3% to 10%); arrhythmia, tachycardia, bradycardia (1% to 3%); hemorrhage/bleeding, premature atrial contractions, syncope, atrial fibrillation, atrial arrhythmia, AV heartblock,

PROPOFOL — INJECTION

bigeminy, bundle branch block, cardiac arrest, abnormal ECG, edema, extrasystole, heart block, hypertension, MI, myocardial ischemia, PVCs, ST segment depression, supraventricular tachycardia, ventricular fibrillation (< 1%).

CNS – Movement (3% to 10%); hypertonia/dystonia, paresthesia, abnormal dreams, agitation, anxiety, bucking/jerking/thrashing, chills/shivering, clonic/myoclonic movement, combativeness, confusion, delirium, depression, dizziness, emotional lability, euphoria, fatigue, headache, hysteria, insomnia, moaning, rigidity, seizures, somnolence, tremor, twitching, amorous behavior, hypotonia, hallucinations, neuropathy, opisthotonos (< 1%).

Dermatologic – Rash, pruritus (1% to 3%); flushing, diaphoresis, urticaria (< 1%).

GI – Hypersalivation, cramping, diarrhea, dry mouth, enlarged parotid, nausea, swallowing, vomiting (

GU – Cloudy urine, oliguria, urine retention (< 1%).

Local – Burning/stinging or pain (17.6%); hives/itching, phlebitis, redness/discoloration (< 1%).

Respiratory – Apnea (1% to 3%); bronchospasm, burning in throat, wheezing, cough, dyspnea, hiccough, hypoventilation, hyperventilation, hypoxia, laryngospasm, pharyngitis, sneezing, tachypnea, upper airway obstruction, decreased lung function (< 1%).

Special senses – Amblyopia, diplopia, ear pain, eye pain, taste perversion, tinnitus, conjunctival hyperemia, nystagmus, abnormal vision (< 1%).

Miscellaneous – Awareness, extremity pain, fever, increased drug effect, neck rigidity/stiffness, chest/trunk pain, myalgia, coagulation disorder, leukocytosis, hyperkalemia, asthenia, hyperlipidemia, anaphylaxis/anaphylactoid reaction, perinatal disorder, anticholinergic syndrome, hypomagnesemia (< 1%).

➤*ICU sedation:*

Cardiovascular – Hypotension (26%); bradycardia, decreased cardiac output (1% to 3%); arrhythmia, atrial fibrillation, bigeminy, cardiac arrest, extrasystole, ventricular tachycardia, right heart failure (< 1%).

CNS – Agitation, chills/shivering, intracranial hypertension, seizures, somnolence, abnormal thinking (< 1%).

Metabolic/Nutritional – Hyperlipidemia (3% to 10%); increased BUN, creatinine, and osmolality, dehydration, hyperglycemia, metabolic acidosis (< 1%).

Respiratory – Respiratory acidosis during weaning (3% to 10%); hypoxia (< 1%).

Miscellaneous – Fever, sepsis, trunk pain, weakness, rash, ileus, abnormal liver function, green urine, kidney failure (< 1%).

➤*Children:* Generally, the adverse reaction profile in children 6 days to 16 years of age is similar to adults. The following reactions have occurred: Hypotension, movement (17%); burning/stinging or pain (10%); hypertension (8%); rash (5%); pruritus (2%); nodal tachycardia (1.6%); arrhythmia (1.2%); apnea.

Overdosage

If accidental overdosage occurs, discontinue propofol immediately. Overdosage is likely to cause cardiorespiratory depression. Treat respiratory depression by artificial ventilation with oxygen. Cardiovascular depression may require raising the patient's legs, increasing the flow rate of IV fluids, and administering pressor agents or anticholinergic agents. Refer to General Management of Acute Overdosage.

Patient Information

Performance of activities requiring mental alertness, coordination, or physical dexterity may be impaired for some time after general anesthesia or sedation.

FOSPROPOFOL DISODIUM

c-iv	**Lusedra** (Eisai)	**Injection, solution:** 35 mg/mL	Preservative free. Single-use 30 mL vials.

FOSPROPOFOL DISODIUM — INJECTION

Indications

➤*Monitored anesthesia care:* For monitored anesthesia care sedation in adult patients undergoing diagnostic or therapeutic procedures.

Administration and Dosage

➤*General dosing considerations:* Use supplemental oxygen for all patients undergoing sedation with fospropofol.

Individualize the dosage of fospropofol and titrate to the level of sedation required for the procedure. Administer supplemental doses of fospropofol based on the patient's level of sedation and the level of sedation required for the procedure. Give supplemental doses only when patients can demonstrate purposeful movement in response to verbal or light tactile stimulation and no more frequently than every 4 minutes. Use only the minimum dosage required to facilitate the procedure.

➤*Adults:*

Monitored anesthesia care –

Standard dosing regimen: In adults who are healthy or have mild systemic disease as categorized by the American Society of Anesthesiology (ASA P1 or P2), the standard dosing regimen of fospropofol should be followed.

- *Maximum dose* – No initial dose should exceed 16.5 mL; no supplemental dose should exceed 4 mL.
- *Initial dosage* – Intravenous (IV) bolus of 6.5 mg/kg.

Supplemental doses: 1.6 mg/kg IV (25% of initial dosage) as needed to achieve the desired level of sedation.

Fospropofol Standard Dosing Regimen in Adults

Weight (kg)	Initial dose[a] mg	Initial dose[a] mL	Supplemental dose[a] No more frequently than every 4 min mg	Supplemental dose[a] No more frequently than every 4 min mL
≤ 60	385	11	105	3
61 to 63	402.5	11.5	105	3
64 to 65	420	12	105	3
66 to 68	437.5	12.5	105	3
69 to 71	455	13	105	3
72 to 74	472.5	13.5	122.5	3.5
75 to 76	490	14	122.5	3.5
77 to 79	507.5	14.5	122.5	3.5
80 to 82	525	15	140	4
83 to 84	542.5	15.5	140	4
85 to 87	560	16	140	4
88 to 89	577.5	16.5	140	4
≥ 90	577.5	16.5	140	4

[a] Doses in this table are rounded to the nearest half-milliliter volume to facilitate practical measurement, hence may differ slightly from the dose recommended on the basis of mg/kg.

Modified dosing regimen: Adults with severe systemic disease (ASA P3 or P4) should receive initial and supplemental IV dosages of 75% of the standard dosing regimen.

Fospropofol Modified Dosing Regimen in Adults

Weight (kg)	Initial dose[a] mg	Initial dose[a] mL	Supplemental dose[a] No more frequently than every 4 min mg	Supplemental dose[a] No more frequently than every 4 min mL
≤ 60	297.5	8.5	70	2
61 to 62	297.5	8.5	70	2
63 to 64	315	9	87.5	2.5
65 to 66	315	9	87.5	2.5
67 to 69	332.5	9.5	87.5	2.5
70 to 73	350	10	87.5	2.5
74 to 77	367.5	10.5	87.5	2.5
78 to 80	385	11	105	3
81 to 84	402.5	11.5	105	3
85 to 87	420	12	105	3
88 to 89	437.5	12.5	105	3
≥ 90	437.5	12.5	105	3

[a] Doses in this table are rounded to the nearest half-milliliter volume to facilitate practical measurement, hence may differ slightly from the dose recommended on the basis of mg/kg.

➤*Elderly:* See Adults modified dosing regimen.

➤*Concomitant therapy:* In clinical studies, an opioid premedication (fentanyl citrate 50 mcg IV) was administered 5 minutes prior to the initial dose of fospropofol.

Consider the potential for worsened cardio-respiratory depression prior to using fospropofol concomitantly with other drugs that have the same potential (eg, sedative-hypnotics or narcotic analgesics).

➤*Preparation for administration:* Fospropofol is provided as a ready to use formulation. Draw fospropofol into sterile syringes immediately after vials are opened. Discard any unused portion at the end of the procedure.

➤*Administration:* Administer fospropofol IV as a bolus injection. Administer fospropofol through a secure, freely flowing, peripheral IV line using commonly available IV administration sets. Flush the infusion line with normal saline before and after administration of fospropofol. Fospropofol is not light sensitive. Fospropofol does not need to be filtered before use.

➤*Admixture compatibility:* Fospropofol has been shown to be compatible with the following fluids: dextrose 5% injection, dextrose 5% and sodium chloride 0.2%, dextrose 5% and sodium chloride 0.45% injection, sodium chloride 0.9% injection, Ringer's lactate injection, Ringer's lactate and dextrose 5% injection, sodium chloride 0.45% injection, dextrose 5%, sodium chloride 0.45%, and potassium chloride 20 mEq.

FOSPROPOFOL DISODIUM — INJECTION

Do not mix fospropofol with other drugs or fluids prior to administration. Fospropofol is not physically compatible with midazolam or meperidine, and compatibility with other agents has not been adequately evaluated.

➤*Storage/Stability:* Store at controlled room temperature 25°C (77°F). Excursions are permitted between 15° and 30°C (59° and 86°F).

Actions

➤*Pharmacology:* Fospropofol is a sedative-hypnotic agent. Fospropofol is a prodrug of propofol. Following IV injection, fospropofol is metabolized by alkaline phosphatases. For every millimole of fospropofol administered, one millimole of propofol is produced (1.86 mg of fospropofol is the molar equivalent of 1 mg of propofol).

➤*Pharmacokinetics:*

Absorption – The maximum plasma concentration (C_{max}) and area under the curve ($AUC_{0-\infty}$) values of fospropofol were dose proportional. The intersubject variability in C_{max} and $AUC_{0-\infty}$ was low. Propofol was rapidly liberated reaching plasma C_{max} at a median time to C_{max}(T_{max}) of 12 minutes for fospropofol 6 mg/kg and 8 minutes for fospropofol 18 mg/kg. Concentration-time profiles showed a biexponential decline. The increase in C_{max} and $AUC_{0-\infty}$ of propofol was dose proportional.

Fospropofol Pharmacokinetics Parameters (Mean ± Standard Deviation [SD])

Pharmacokinetic parameter	Fospropofol			Propofol from fospropofol		
	Healthy (6 mg/kg) (n = 68)	Healthy (18 mg/kg) (n = 68)	Patient (6.5 mg/kg) (n = 667)	Healthy (6 mg/kg) (n = 68)	Healthy (18 mg/kg) (n = 68)	Patient (6.5 mg/kg) (n = 400)
C_{max} (mcg/mL)	78.7 ± 15.4	211 ± 48.6	–	1.08 ± 0.33	3.9 ± 0.822	–
T_{max} (min)	4	2	–	12	8	–
$AUC_{0-\infty}$ (mcg•h/mL)	19.2 ± 3.59	50.3 ± 8.4	19.0 ± 7.2	1.70 ± 0.29	5.67 ± 1.28	1.2 ± 0.39
Plasma clearance (CLp) (L/h/kg)	0.28 ± 0.053	0.32 ± 0.058	0.36 ± 0.16	1.95 ± 0.34	1.79 ± 0.39	3.2 ± 0.92
t½ (h)	0.81 ± 0.08	0.81 ± 0.09	0.88 ± 0.08	2.06 ± 0.77	1.76 ± 0.54	1.13 ± 0.28

Distribution – Fospropofol has a low volume of distribution (0.33 ± 0.069 L/kg), and the liberated propofol has a large volume of distribution (5.8 L/kg).

Both fospropofol and its active metabolite propofol are highly protein bound (approximately 98%), primarily to albumin. Fospropofol does not affect the binding of propofol to albumin.

Metabolism – Fospropofol is completely metabolized by alkaline phosphatases to propofol, formaldehyde, and phosphate. Formaldehyde and phosphate plasma concentrations are comparable to endogenous levels when fospropofol is administered as recommended. Formaldehyde is further metabolized to formate by several enzyme systems, including formaldehyde dehydrogenase, present in various tissues. Propofol liberated from fospropofol is further metabolized to major metabolites propofol glucuronide (34.8%), quinol-4-sulfate (4.6%), quinol-1- glucuronide (11.1%), and quinol-4-glucuronide (5.1%). Oxidation to CO_2 is the primary means of eliminating excess formate.

Excretion – After a single 400 mg IV dose of [^{14}C]-fospropofol in humans, approximately 71% of radioactivity was recovered in the urine within 192 hours. Total body clearance (CLp) of fospropofol was 0.28 ± 0.053 L/h/kg, and renal elimination of fospropofol was insignificant (less than 0.02% of dose). The terminal phase elimination half-life of fospropofol was 0.81 ± 0.08 and 0.88 ± 0.08 hours in healthy subjects and patients, respectively. In healthy subjects, the apparent total body clearance of liberated propofol (CLp/F) was 1.95 ± 0.345 L/h/kg and terminal elimination half-life was 2.06 ± 0.77 hours. In patients, the CLp of fospropofol was 0.31 ± 0.14 L/h/kg, and CLp/F for propofol was 2.74 ± 0.80 L/h/kg and is similar to that observed in healthy subjects.

Contraindications

None known.

Warnings/Precautions

➤*Respiratory depression:* Fospropofol may cause loss of spontaneous respiration. Apnea was reported in 1 of 455 (less than 1%) patients treated with fospropofol using the standard or modified dosing regimen. In patients treated with more than the recommended fospropofol dose, apnea was reported in 14 of 556 (3%).

Supplemental oxygen is recommended for all patients receiving fospropofol. Dosages of fospropofol must be individualized for each patient and titrated to effect. Use lower doses of fospropofol in patients who are 65 years of age or older or who have severe systemic disease. Consider the additive cardio-respiratory effects of narcotic analgesics and sedative-hypnotic agents when administered concomitantly with fospropofol.

Assess patients for their ability to demonstrate purposeful response while sedated with fospropofol as patients who are unable to do so may lose protective reflexes. Airway assistance maneuvers may be required in the management of respiratory depression.

➤*Hypoxemia:* Fospropofol may cause hypoxemia detectable by pulse oximetry. Hypoxemia was reported in 20 of 455 (4%) patients treated with fospropofol using the standard or modified dosing regimen. Hypoxemia was reported among patients who retained the ability to respond purposefully to their health care provider following administration of fospropofol. Therefore, retention of purposeful responsiveness did not prevent patients from becoming hypoxemic following administration of fospropofol. In patients treated with more than the recommended fospropofol dose, hypoxemia was reported in 151 of 556 (27%).

The risk of hypoxemia is reduced by appropriate positioning of the patient, and the use of supplemental oxygen in all patients receiving fospropofol. Airway assistance maneuvers may be required in the management of hypoxemia. The additive cardio-respiratory effects of narcotic analgesics and other sedative-hypnotic agents should be considered when administered concomitantly with fospropofol.

➤*Unresponsiveness:* Fospropofol has not been studied for use in general anesthesia. However, administration of fospropofol may inadvertently cause patients to become unresponsive or minimally responsive to vigorous tactile or painful stimulation. The incidence of patients sedated for colonoscopy who became minimally responsive or unresponsive to vigorous tactile or painful stimulation was 7 of 183 (4%). The duration of minimal or complete unresponsiveness in colonoscopy patients ranged from 2 to 16 minutes. Among patients sedated for bronchoscopy, the incidence of patients who became minimally or completely unresponsive to vigorous tactile or painful stimulation was 24 of 149 (16%). The duration of minimal to complete unresponsiveness in bronchoscopy patients ranged from 2 to 20 minutes.

➤*Hypotension:* Hypotension following the use of fospropofol may occur. Hypotension was reported in 18 of 455 (4%) patients treated with fospropofol using the standard or modified dosing regimen. In patients treated with more than the recommended fospropofol dose, hypotension was reported in 31 of 556 (6%).

Patients with compromised myocardial function, reduced vascular tone, or who have reduced intravascular volume may be at an increased risk for hypotension. A secure IV access catheter and supplemental volume replacement fluids should be readily available during the procedure. Additional pharmacological management may be necessary.

➤*Hepatic function impairment:* Fospropofol has not been adequately studied in patients with hepatic function impairment. Caution should be exercised when using fospropofol in patients with hepatic function impairment.

➤*Pregnancy: Category B.* There are no adequate and well-controlled studies in pregnant women. Because animal reproduction studies are not always predictive of human response, this drug should be used during pregnancy only if clearly needed.

Teratogenic –

Pregnant rats were treated with fospropofol (5, 20, or 45 mg/kg/day IV) from gestation day 7 through 17 (the highest dose is 0.6 times the anticipated human dose for a procedure of 16 minutes based on a comparison of doses expressed as mg/m^2). Doses of 20 and 45 mg/kg/day produced significant maternal toxicity. No drug-related adverse reactions on embryo-fetal development were noted.

Pregnant rabbits were treated with fospropofol (14, 28, 56, or 70 mg/kg/day IV) from gestation day 6 through 18 (the highest dose is 1.7 times the anticipated human dose for a procedure of 16 minutes based on a comparison of doses expressed as mg/m^2). Significant maternal toxicity was noted at all doses. No drug-related adverse reactions on embryo-fetal development were noted.

Labor and delivery – Fospropofol is not recommended for use in labor and delivery, including Cesarean section deliveries. It is not known if fospropofol crosses the placenta; however, propofol is known to cross the placenta, and as with other sedative-hypnotic agents, the administration of fospropofol may be associated with neonatal respiratory and cardiovascular depression.

➤*Lactation:* It is not known whether fospropofol is excreted in human milk; however, propofol has been reported to be excreted in human milk and the effects of oral absorption of fospropofol or propofol are not known. Fospropofol is not recommended for use in breast-feeding mothers.

➤*Children:* Safety and efficacy in children have not been established because fospropofol has not been studied in patients younger than 18 years of age. Fospropofol is not recommended for use in this population.

➤*Elderly:* Patients 65 years of age and older should receive the modified dosing regimen. Hypoxemia was reported more frequently among patients 75 years of age and older than among patients 65 years of age to younger than 75 years of age and less frequently among younger patients 18 years of age to younger than 65 years of age.

➤*Monitoring:* Fospropofol should be administered only by persons trained in the administration of general anesthesia and not involved in the conduct of the diagnostic or therapeutic procedure. Continuously monitor sedated patients and facilities for maintenance of a patent airway, providing artificial ventilation, administering supplemental oxygen, and instituting cardiovascular resuscitation must be immediately available. Continuously monitor patients during sedation and through the recovery process for early signs of hypotension, apnea, airway obstruction, and/or oxygen desaturation.

Drug Interactions

➤*Cardio-respiratory depressants:* Fospropofol may produce additive cardio-respiratory effects when administered with other cardio-respiratory depressants such as sedative-hypnotics and narcotic analgesics.

Adverse Reactions

For more information on respiratory depression, hypoxemia, loss of purposeful responsiveness or hypotension, refer to the Warnings/Precautions section.

➤*Most common adverse reactions:* The most common adverse reactions (reported in more than 20%) are paresthesia and pruritus. Paresthesias (including burning, tingling, stinging) and/or pruritus, usually manifested in the perineal region, were the most frequently recorded adverse reactions in clinical trials. Paresthesias and pruritus generally occurred within 5 min-

FOSPROPOFOL DISODIUM — INJECTION

utes after administration of the initial dose of fospropofol and were generally transient and mild to moderate in intensity. The pharmacologic basis of these sensory phenomena is unknown. No pretreatments, including the use of nonsteroidal anti-inflammatory drugs, opioids, or lidocaine, are known to have an effect on, or to reduce the incidence of these sensations.

➤*Discontinuation:* The most commonly reported reasons for discontinuation are paresthesia and cough.

➤*Clinical trials experience:*

Fospropofol Common Adverse Reactions (≥ 2%)			
Adverse reactions	Colonoscopy (n = 183)	Minor procedures (n = 123)	Bronchoscopy (n = 149)
CNS			
Headache	1%	2%	1%
Paresthesia[a]	74%	63%	52%
GI			
Nausea	0%	4%	1%
Vomiting	0%	3%	0%
Miscellaneous			
Hypotension	2%	3%	7%
Hypoxemia	2%	1%	11%
Procedural pain	0%	0%	2%
Pruritus[b]	16%	28%	16%

[a] Paresthesia includes the following terms: paresthesia genital male; burning sensation; genital burning sensation; vaginal burning sensation; skin burning sensation; genital pain (reported as burning); perineal pain (reported as burning); anal discomfort (reported as burning); chest pain (reported as burning); ear discomfort (reported as burning); nasal discomfort (reported as burning); buttock pain (reported as stinging); groin pain (reported as stinging); pain (reported as stinging); sensory disturbance (reported as nonspecific sensation in pubic area).

[b] Pruritus includes the following terms: genital pruritus female; genital pruritus male; pruritus genital; pruritus ani; pruritus generalized

Sedation-related adverse reactions – Sedation-related adverse reactions were experienced at the following rates for subjects receiving the standard or modified fospropofol dosing regimen: 20 of 455 (4%) hypoxemia, 18 of 455 (4%) hypotension, 1 of 455 (less than 1%) apnea. A higher rate of sedation-related adverse reactions necessitating intervention was observed in patients undergoing bronchoscopy compared with colonoscopy and minor surgical procedures. In the colonoscopy studies, 5 of 183 (3%) patients were ASA P3. In the minor surgical procedures study, 23 of 123 (19%) patients were ASA P3 or P4. In the flexible bronchoscopy study, 68 of 150 (46%) patients were ASA P3 or P4.

➤*Continuous sedation:* The safety of fospropofol for continuous sedation has not been established and therefore its use is not recommended. Fospropofol was administered to 38 intubated and mechanically ventilated patients in postoperative and intensive care settings. An occurrence of nonsustained ventricular tachycardia was observed as a serious adverse reaction in 1 patient in the study. Another patient with acute myeloid leukemia with renal and hepatic insufficiency experienced a further increase in plasma formate concentration from a baseline of 66 mcg/mL to a postdose level of 212 mcg/mL after a 12-hour infusion. The clinical significance of these findings is unknown.

Overdosage

➤*Symptoms:* Overdosage with fospropofol can cause cardiorespiratory depression.

Formate and phosphate are metabolites of fospropofol and may contribute to signs of toxicity following overdosage. Signs of formate toxicity are similar to those of methanol toxicity and are associated with anion-gap metabolic acidosis. IV exposure to a large amount of phosphate could potentially cause hypocalcemia with paresthesia, muscle spasms, and seizures.

➤*Treatment:* If overdosage occurs, discontinue fospropofol administration immediately. Respiratory depression may require manual or mechanical ventilation. Cardiovascular depression may require elevation of lower extremities, intravascular volume replacement, and/or pharmacological management.

Patient Information

Paresthesias (including burning, tingling, stinging) and/or pruritus, usually manifested in the perineal region are frequently experienced upon injection of the initial dose of fospropofol. Inform the patient that these sensations are typically mild to moderate in intensity, last a short time, and require no treatment.

Consider the requirement for a patient escort. The decision as to when patients who have received fospropofol, particularly on an outpatient basis, may again engage in activities requiring complete mental alertness, coordination and/or physical dexterity (eg, operate hazardous machinery, sign legal documents, drive a motor vehicle) must be individualized.

DROPERIDOL

Rx	**Droperidol** (Various, eg, Hospira, American Regent)	**Injection:** 2.5 mg/mL	In 2 mL vials.

DROPERIDOL — INJECTION

WARNING

Cases of QT prolongation and/or torsade de pointes have been reported in patients receiving droperidol at doses at or below recommended doses. Some cases have occurred in patients with no known risk factors for QT prolongation, and some cases have been fatal.

Due to its potential for serious proarrhythmic effects and death, reserve droperidol for use in the treatment of patients who fail to show an acceptable response to other adequate treatments, either because of insufficient effectiveness or the inability to achieve an effective dose due to intolerable adverse effects from those drugs.

Cases of QT prolongation and serious arrhythmias (eg, torsade de pointes) have been reported in patients treated with droperidol. Based on these reports, all patients should undergo a 12-lead ECG prior to administration of droperidol to determine if a prolonged QT interval (ie, QTc greater than 440 msec for males or 450 msec for females) is present. If there is a prolonged QT interval, do not administer droperidol. For patients in whom the potential benefit of droperidol treatment is felt to outweigh the risks of potentially serious arrhythmias, perform ECG monitoring prior to treatment and continue for 2 to 3 hours after completing treatment to monitor for arrhythmias.

Droperidol is contraindicated in patients with known or suspected QT prolongation, including patients with congenital long QT syndrome.

Administer droperidol with extreme caution to patients who may be at risk for development of prolonged QT syndrome (eg, congestive heart failure, bradycardia, use of a diuretic, cardiac hypertrophy, hypokalemia, hypomagnesemia, or administration of other drugs known to increase the QT interval). Other risk factors may include age greater than 65 years, alcohol abuse, and use of agents such as benzodiazepines, volatile anesthetics, and IV opiates. Initiate droperidol at a low dose and adjust upward, with caution, as needed to achieve the desired effect.

Indications

➤*Antiemetic:* To reduce the incidence of nausea and vomiting associated with surgical and diagnostic procedures.

➤*Off-label uses:* Treatment of breakthrough chemotherapy-induced nausea and vomiting; acute treatment of chemotherapy-induced nausea and vomiting. Prevention of nausea or vomiting associated with chemotherapy.

Administration and Dosage

➤*General dosing considerations:* Individualize dosage. Some of the factors to be considered in determining the dose include age, body weight, physical status, underlying pathological condition, use of other drugs, type of anesthesia to be used, and the surgical procedure involved.

Monitor vital signs and ECG routinely.

➤*Adults:*

Antiemetic –

Maximum dose: 2.5 mg (initial dose).

Initial dosage: 2.5 mg IM or slow IV.

Dosage adjustment: Additional 1.25 mg doses may be administered to achieve the desired effect. However, administer additional doses with caution and only if the potential benefit outweighs the potential risk.

➤*Children:*

Antiemetic –

Older than 12 years of age: See Adults for dosing for children older than 12 years of age.

2 to 12 years of age:

- *Maximum dose* – 0.1 mg/kg (initial dose).
- *Initial dosage* – 0.1 mg/kg IM or slow IV taking into account the patient's age and other clinical factors. Administer additional doses with caution and only if the potential benefit outweighs the potential risk.

➤*Elderly:* Reduce the initial dose of droperidol appropriately in elderly, debilitated, and other poor-risk patients.

➤*Concomitant therapy:* Other CNS depressant drugs (eg, barbiturates, tranquilizers, opioids, general anesthetics) have additive or potentiating effects with droperidol. When patients have received such drugs, the dose of droperidol required will be less than usual. Following the administration of droperidol, reduce the dose of other CNS depressant drugs.

➤*Storage/Stability:* Protect from light. Store at room temperature, between 15° and 30°C (59° and 86°F).

Actions

➤*Pharmacology:* Droperidol produces marked tranquilization and sedation. It allays apprehension and provides a state of mental detachment and indifference while maintaining a state of reflex alertness.

Droperidol produces an antiemetic effect as evidenced by the antagonism of apomorphine in dogs. It lowers the incidence of nausea and vomiting during surgical procedures and provides antiemetic protection in the postoperative period.

Droperidol potentiates other CNS depressants. It produces mild alpha-adrenergic blockade, peripheral vascular dilatation, and reduction of the pressor effect of epinephrine. It can produce hypotension and decreased peripheral vascular resistance and may decrease pulmonary arterial pres-

DROPERIDOL — INJECTION

sure (particularly if it is abnormally high). It may reduce the incidence of epinephrine-induced arrhythmias, but it does not prevent other cardiac arrhythmias.

The onset of action of single IM and IV doses is from 3 to 10 minutes following administration, although the peak effect may not be apparent for up to 30 minutes. The duration of the tranquilizing and sedative effects generally is 2 to 4 hours, although alteration of alertness may persist for as long as 12 hours.

Contraindications

Known or suspected QT prolongation (ie, QTc interval greater than 440 msec for males or 450 msec for females). This would include patients with congenital long QT syndrome.

Hypersensitivity to the drug.

Warnings/Precautions

➤*Risks for prolonged QT syndrome:* Administer droperidol with extreme caution in the presence of risk factors for development of prolonged QT syndrome, such as:

1.) clinically significant bradycardia (less than 50 bpm),
2.) any clinically significant cardiac disease,
3.) treatment with Class I and Class III antiarrhythmics,
4.) treatment with monoamine oxidase inhibitors (MAOIs),
5.) concomitant treatment with other drug products known to prolong the QT interval,
6.) electrolyte imbalance, in particular hypokalemia and hypomagnesemia, or concomitant treatment with drugs (eg, diuretics) that may cause electrolyte imbalance.

➤*Effects on cardiac conduction:* See the Warning box for more information.

Hypotension – Keep fluids and other countermeasures to manage hypotension readily available.

Opioids – When required, initially use opioids in reduced doses.

Neuroleptic malignant syndrome – As with other neuroleptic agents, very rare reports of neuroleptic malignant syndrome (altered consciousness, muscle rigidity and autonomic instability) have occurred in patients who have received droperidol.

Since it may be difficult to distinguish neuroleptic malignant syndrome from malignant hyperpyrexia in the perioperative period, consider prompt treatment with dantrolene if increases in temperature, heart rate, or carbon dioxide production occur.

➤*Special risk:* Reduce the initial dose of droperidol appropriately in elderly, debilitated and other poor-risk patients. Consider the effect of the initial dose in determining incremental doses.

➤*Conduction anesthesia:* Certain forms of conduction anesthesia, such as spinal anesthesia and some peridural anesthetics, can alter respiration by blocking intercostal nerves and can cause peripheral vasodilatation and hypotension because of sympathetic blockade. Through other mechanisms, droperidol can also alter circulation. Therefore, when droperidol is used to supplement these forms of anesthesia, the anesthetist should be familiar with the physiological alterations involved, and be prepared to manage them in the patients elected for these forms of anesthesia.

➤*Hypotension:* If hypotension occurs, consider the possibility of hypovolemia and manage with appropriate parenteral fluid therapy. Consider repositioning the patient to improve venous return to the heart when operative conditions permit. It should be noted that in spinal and peridural anesthesia, tilting the patient into a head-down position may result in a higher level of anesthesia than is desirable, as well as impair venous return to the heart. Exercise care in moving and positioning of patients because of a possibility of orthostatic hypotension. If volume expansion with fluids plus these other countermeasures do not correct the hypotension, then consider the administration of pressor agents other than epinephrine. Epinephrine may paradoxically decrease the blood pressure in patients treated with droperidol due to the alpha-adrenergic blocking action of droperidol.

➤*Pulmonary arterial pressure:* Since droperidol may decrease pulmonary arterial pressure, those who conduct diagnostic or surgical procedures where interpretation of pulmonary arterial pressure measurements might determine final management of the patient should consider this fact.

➤*Pheochromocytoma:* In patients with diagnosed/suspected pheochromocytoma, severe hypertension and tachycardia have been observed after the administration of droperidol.

➤*Renal/Hepatic function impairment:* Administer droperidol with caution to patients with liver and kidney dysfunction because of the importance of these organs in the metabolism and excretion of drugs.

➤*Pregnancy: Category C.* Droperidol administered intravenously has been shown to cause a slight increase in mortality of the newborn rat at 4.4 times the upper human dose. At 44 times the upper human dose, mortality rate was comparable to that for control animals. Following IM administration, increased mortality of the offspring at 1.8 times the upper human dose is attributed to CNS depression in the dams who neglected to remove placentae from their offspring. Droperidol has not been shown to be teratogenic in animals. There are no adequate and well-controlled studies in pregnant women. Use during pregnancy only if the potential benefit justifies the potential risk to the fetus.

Labor and delivery – There are insufficient data to support the use of droperidol in labor and delivery. Therefore, such use is not recommended.

➤*Lactation:* It is not known whether droperidol is excreted in human milk. Because many drugs are excreted in human milk, exercise caution when droperidol is administered to a nursing mother.

➤*Children:* The safety of droperidol in children less than 2 years of age has not been established.

➤*Monitoring:* Monitor vital signs and ECG routinely. When the EEG is used for postoperative monitoring, it may be found that the EEG pattern returns to normal slowly.

As with other CNS depressant drugs, patients who have received droperidol should have appropriate surveillance.

Drug Interactions

➤*QT prolongation:* An additive effect of droperidol with other drugs that prolong the QT interval cannot be excluded. The following drugs may prolong the QT interval and increase the risk of life-threatening cardiac arrhythmias, including torsade de pointes: Antiarrhythmic agents (eg, amiodarone, bretylium, disopyramide, dofetilide, procainamide, quinidine, and sotalol), arsenic trioxide, chlorpromazine, cisapride, dolasetron, mefloquine, mesoridazine, moxifloxacin, pentamidine, pimozide, tacrolimus, thioridazine, and ziprasidone. For a more complete list of drugs that may prolong the QT interval, see the appendix, Drug-Induced Prolongation of the QT Interval and Torsade de Pointes.

Use caution when patients are taking concomitant drugs known to induce hypokalemia or hypomagnesemia as they may precipitate QT prolongation and interact with droperidol. These would include diuretics, laxatives, and supraphysiological use of steroid hormones with mineralocorticoid potential.

Droperidol Drug Interactions

Precipitant drug	Object drug[a]		Description
Droperidol	Anesthesia	⬆	Certain forms of conduction anesthesia (eg, spinal anesthesia, some peridural anesthetics) can cause peripheral vasodilation and hypotension because of sympathetic blockade. Droperidol can alter circulation through other mechanisms.
CNS depressants (eg, barbiturates, tranquilizers, opioids, general anesthetics)	Droperidol	⬆	CNS depressants have additive or potentiating CNS effects with droperidol; thus, droperidol dose will be less than usual. Likewise, following the droperidol, reduce the dose of other CNS depressants.
Droperidol	CNS depressants (eg, barbiturates, tranquilizers, opioids, general anesthetics)		
Epinephrine	Droperidol	⬆	Epinephrine may paradoxically enhance droperidol-induced hypotension because of the alpha-adrenergic blocking action of droperidol. Epinephrine is not recommended as treatment of droperidol-induced hypotension.
Parenteral analgesics (eg, fentanyl)	Droperidol	⬆	Hypertension has been reported following coadministration of droperidol and fentanyl or other parenteral analgesics and may be due to unexplained alterations in sympathetic activity following large doses.

[a] ⬆ = object drug increased.

Adverse Reactions

See the Warning box for more information.

Be alert to palpitations, syncope, or other symptoms suggestive of episodes of irregular cardiac rhythm in patients taking droperidol and promptly evaluate such cases.

The most common somatic adverse reactions reported to occur with droperidol are mild to moderate hypotension and tachycardia, but these effects usually subside without treatment. If hypotension occurs and is severe or persists, consider the possibility of hypovolemia, and manage with appropriate parenteral fluid therapy.

The most common behavioral adverse effects of droperidol include dysphoria, postoperative drowsiness, restlessness, hyperactivity, and anxiety, which can either be the result of an inadequate dosage (lack of adequate treatment effect) or of an adverse drug reaction (part of the symptom complex of akathisia).

Take care to search for extrapyramidal signs and symptoms (dystonia, akathisia, oculogyric crisis) to differentiate these different clinical conditions. When extrapyramidal symptoms are the cause, they can usually be controlled with anticholinergic agents.

Postoperative hallucinatory episodes (sometimes associated with transient periods of mental depression) have also been reported.

DROPERIDOL — INJECTION

Other less common reported adverse reactions include anaphylaxis, dizziness, chills or shivering, laryngospasm, and bronchospasm.

Elevated blood pressure, with or without preexisting hypertension, has been reported following administration of droperidol combined with fentanyl citrate or other parenteral analgesics. This might be due to unexplained alterations in sympathetic activity following large doses; however, it is also frequently attributed to anesthetic or surgical stimulation during light anesthesia.

Overdosage

➤*Symptoms:* The manifestations of droperidol overdosage are an extension of its pharmacologic actions and may include QT prolongation and serious arrhythmias (eg, torsade de pointes).

➤*Treatment:* In the presence of hypoventilation or apnea, administer oxygen, and assist or control respiration as indicated. Maintain a patent airway; an oropharyngeal airway or endotracheal tube might be indicated. Carefully observe the patient for 24 hours; maintain body warmth and adequate fluid intake. If hypotension occurs and is severe or persists, consider the possibility of hypovolemia and manage with appropriate parenteral fluid therapy.

If significant extrapyramidal reactions occur in the context of an overdose, administer an anticholinergic.

Gases

NITROUS OXIDE

Nitrous Oxide (Airgas)	**Gas; inhalation:** 100%[a]	In cylinders.

[a] Provided as a liquefied compressed gas.

NITROUS OXIDE — INHALATION

Indications

➤*Anesthesia:* Nitrous oxide is primarily used as an adjuvant to opioids or other anesthetics to induce general anesthesia.

Administration and Dosage

➤*Adults:*

Anesthesia –

Usual dosage: The concentration and administration rate of nitrous oxide (given with oxygen) are patient- and usage-specific. Concentrations as low as 20% will usually produce analgesia, and concentrations between 30% and 80% will usually produce sedation. In outpatient dentistry, concentrations of approximately 50% are frequently used to produce analgesia and sedation. Higher concentrations of nitrous oxide will allow for lower concentrations of other anesthetics (eg, halothane), and therefore decrease the degree of adverse reactions. Do not give concentrations above 80% because nitrous oxide will limit the delivery of an adequate amount of oxygen.

Maximum dose: Do not give concentrations above 80% because nitrous oxide will limit the delivery of an adequate amount of oxygen.

➤*Children:*

Anesthesia – See Adults for more information.

➤*Handling:* Never allow any unprotected part of the body to touch uninsulated pipes or vessels that contain cryogenic liquids.

➤*Storage/Stability:* Avoid contact with combustible materials. Do not puncture or incinerate container. Cylinder temperatures should not exceed 52°C (125°F). Keep container in a cool, well-ventilated area. Keep container tightly closed. Store upright, with valve protection cap in place and firmly secured to prevent falling or being knocked over. Protect cylinders from physical damage; do not drag, roll, slide, or drop.

Actions

➤*Pharmacology:* Nitrous oxide is a sweet-smelling anesthetic gas with a low blood-gas partition coefficient (0.47) and low potency (minimum alveolar concentration [MAC] is 104%). Although the exact mechanism of action is not known, nitrous oxide produces general anesthesia through interaction with cellular membranes in the CNS.

Nitrous oxide also produces analgesia and may produce amnesia at concentrations of more than 60%. It may also act as a mild myocardial depressant and mild sympathetic nervous system stimulant. In adults, it does not usually affect heart rate or blood pressure, but it may increase pulmonary artery pressure and pulmonary vascular resistance when given in a 40% concentration. In sedated infants, nitrous oxide has not been shown to significantly increase pulmonary artery pressure or pulmonary vascular resistance. It also acts as a mild respiratory depressant and has powerful cerebral vasodilating properties. Nitrous oxide is not a skeletal muscle relaxant, but may cause skeletal muscle rigidity in doses greater than 1 MAC.

Nitrous oxide is 30 times more soluble than nitrogen in blood. Therefore, nitrous oxide diffuses into gas-containing body cavities from the bloodstream faster than the nitrogen in those cavities can diffuse out into circulation. This can contribute to excessive distension of gas-containing bowels, possible bowel ischemia, and increased difficulty with surgical exposure (see Warnings/Precautions).

Nitrous oxide also inhibits methionine synthesis and folate metabolism (see Warnings/Precautions).

➤*Pharmacokinetics:*

Absorption/Distribution – The uptake and elimination of nitrous oxide is relatively rapid, primarily because of the low blood-gas partition coefficient (0.47).

Metabolism/Excretion – Nitrous oxide is eliminated via exhalation and does not undergo significant biotransformation.

Contraindications

Nitrous oxide is relatively contraindicated during tympanoplasty because increased pressure caused by nitrous oxide can dislodge a tympanic graft.

Do not use immediately before, during, or after bypass.

Do not use in the presence of an existing pneumocephalus because it may elevate intracranial pressure (ICP) and precipitate a life-threatening tension pneumocephalus. Nitrous oxide may also be contraindicated in other settings involving air accumulation (eg, pneumothorax; pneumocephalus; pneumopericardium; bowel obstruction; any procedure associated with intracorporeal air enclosure, including middle ear surgery and ophthalmic surgery; all cases with an increased risk of air embolism).

Warnings/Precautions

➤*Bowel distension and/or ischemia:* Nitrous oxide is best avoided in situations in which the bowel is distended. However, the use of low concentrations of nitrous oxide during elective abdominal operations in which no significant amount of gas is present in the bowels is reasonable.

➤*Cardiovascular reactions:* Nitrous oxide may increase pulmonary vascular resistance, especially in patients with preexisting pulmonary hypertension. It is also a mild myocardial depressant, and therefore elicits a compensatory, sympathetically induced increase in systemic vascular resistance. In patients with mild cardiovascular reserve, these reactions may not be well-tolerated.

➤*Cerebrovascular reactions:* Nitrous oxide may increase ICP; however, the changes in ICP are reduced or eliminated by various concomitant anesthetics and also by hypocapnia. Consider avoiding or discontinuing the use of nitrous oxide in patients with a high likelihood of elevated ICP or significant cerebral ischemia.

➤*Hypoxia/Hypoxemia:* When nitrous oxide is discontinued, it rapidly diffuses from the blood into the lungs, causing a low partial pressure of oxygen in the alveoli. Therefore, supplemental oxygen is required to prevent hypoxia and hypoxemia when nitrous oxide is discontinued.

➤*Expansion of closed gas spaces:* Gas-containing spaces (eg, pneumothorax, occluded middle ear, bowel lumen, pneumocephalus) may excessively expand when nitrous oxide is administered. Nitrous oxide may also cause increased pressure within the cuff of an endotracheal tube and pulmonary artery catheters, possibly causing damage via increased pressure in the pulmonary trachea or artery, respectively. Assess this pressure intermittently and adjust the pressure as indicated.

➤*Hematologic reactions:* Megaloblastic changes have been seen in patients exposed to nitrous oxide for 24 hours, and agranulocytosis has been reported in patients exposed to nitrous oxide for 4 days.

➤*Malignant hyperthermia:* Unlike volatile anesthetic liquids, nitrous oxide is only a weak trigger for malignant hyperthermia.

➤*Special risk:* Use with caution in patients with vitamin B_{12} deficiency.

➤*Drug abuse and dependence:* There are reports in the literature of nitrous oxide intoxication, dependence, and abuse. Symptoms of intoxication have been described as feeling drunk, dreamy, coasting or spaced out, and pleasant bodily sensations. Chronic abuse has produced diffuse polyneuropathy and myelinopathy with extensive (sometimes reversible) neurological symptoms replicating those of pernicious anemia caused by vitamin B_{12} deficiency. Nitrous oxide abuse does not appear to cause clinically significant withdrawal symptoms because of the short duration of action and the intermittent inhalation patterns of the users.

➤*Pregnancy:* *Category C* per Briggs' *Drugs in Pregnancy and Lactation.* Nitrous oxide rapidly crosses the placenta to the fetus, producing nearly equivalent amounts of nitrous oxide in fetal circulation as in the mother. There have been retrospective reports of spontaneous abortion, infertility, and decreased birth weight; however, much of the data was based on voluntary self-reported outcomes. Chronic exposure to nitrous oxide has been associated with an increased incidence of spontaneous abortions and infertility. Exposure to general anesthesia during the first or second trimesters has been associated with reduced birth weight; however, the exact causative agent has not yet been identified. With regards to congenital anomalies, currently available data do not suggest that nitrous oxide exposure (acute or chronic) at any time during pregnancy is a significant risk for congenital malformations. However, it would be safest to postpone elective surgeries until after the pregnancy, or at least until after the organogenesis period.

In animals, nitrous oxide (usually in higher doses and for longer exposure than in humans) has caused abortions and growth retardation. Other effects have included structural anomalies (usually involving the skeleton) and neurotoxicities; therefore, nitrous oxide is considered to be an embryo and fetal toxin.

Gases

NITROUS OXIDE — INHALATION

➤*Lactation:* Although there are no published reports describing the use of nitrous oxide during breast-feeding, nitrous oxide is considered to be compatible with breast-feeding. This is because it is unlikely that a breastfeeding infant would be exposed to nitrous oxide in the milk because of the agent's low solubility and short half-life.

➤*Children:* Nitrous oxide appears to be a reasonable drug for use in neonates as long as there is no concern for expanding gas spaces (eg, intestinal obstruction, pneumocephalus, pneumothorax) and no need for a high fraction of inspired oxygen (FiO_2) to maintain oxygen saturation.

Adverse Reactions

➤*CNS:* Amnesia (concentration-dependent).

➤*Hematologic:* Agranulocytosis, megaloblastic changes (see Warnings/Precautions).

➤*Respiratory:* Mild respiratory depression.

➤*Miscellaneous:* Cases of subacute combined degeneration of the spinal cord precipitated by nitrous oxide have been reported.

Overdosage

➤*Symptoms:* Acute symptoms of toxicity initially include inebriation, euphoria, tachypnea, and tachycardia, followed by bradycardia, respiratory depression, and hypotension. Hypoxia along with diaphoresis and cyanosis may develop abruptly after increased exposure. Respiratory depression, lethargy, and coma may also develop as hypoxia worsens. Chronic abuse may cause sensory and motor neuropathy (see Warnings/Precautions).

➤*Treatment:* Oxygen therapy and general supportive care, including airway management, as appropriate.

Volatile Liquids

ENFLURANE

Rx	**Enflurane** (Abbott)	**Liquid; inhalation**	In 125 and 250 mL.
Rx	**Ethrane** (Baxter Healthcare)		In 125 and 250 mL.
Rx	**Compound 347** (Minrad)		In 250 mL.

ENFLURANE — INHALATION

Indications

➤*Anesthesia:* For induction and maintenance of general anesthesia. Enflurane may be used to provide analgesia for vaginal delivery. Low concentrations of enflurane may also be used to supplement other general anesthetic agents during delivery by Cesarean section. Higher concentrations of enflurane may produce uterine relaxation and an increase in uterine bleeding.

Administration and Dosage

➤*General dosing considerations:* Consult detailed literature before using. Enflurane should be administered only by those with appropriate training and experience.

The concentration of enflurane being delivered from a vaporizer during anesthesia should be known. This may be accomplished by using vaporizers calibrated specifically for enflurane or vaporizers from which delivered flows can easily and readily be calculated.

➤*Adults:*

Anesthesia –

Preanesthetic medication: Preanesthetic medication should be selected according to the need of the individual patient, taking into account that secretions are weakly stimulated by enflurane and that enflurane does not alter heart rate. The use of anticholinergic drugs is a matter of choice.

Surgical anesthesia:

• *Initial dosage* – In general, inspired concentrations of 2% to 4.5% enflurane produce surgical anesthesia in 7 to 10 minutes.

Induction may be achieved using enflurane alone with oxygen or in combination with oxygen-nitrous oxide mixtures. Under these conditions some excitement may be encountered. If excitement is to be avoided, a hypnotic dose of a short-acting barbiturate should be used to induce unconsciousness, followed by the enflurane mixture.

• *Maintenance dosage* – Surgical levels of anesthesia may be maintained with 0.5% to 3% enflurane. Maintenance concentrations should not exceed 3%. If added relaxation is required, supplemental doses of muscle relaxants may be used. Ventilation to maintain the tension of carbon dioxide in arterial blood in the 35 to 45 mmHg range is preferred. Hyperventilation should be avoided in order to minimize possible CNS excitation.

The level of blood pressure during maintenance is an inverse function of enflurane concentration in the absence of other complicating problems. Excessive decreases (unless related to hypovolemia) may be due to depth of anesthesia and in such instances should be corrected by lightening the level of anesthesia.

• *Cesarean section* – Enflurane should ordinarily be administered in the concentration range of 0.5% to 1% to supplement other general anesthetics.

Analgesia – Enflurane 0.25% to 1% provides analgesia for vaginal delivery equal to that produced by 30% to 60% nitrous oxide. These concentrations normally do not produce amnesia.

➤*Storage/Stability:* Store at 15° to 30°C (59° to 86°F). Enflurane contains no additives and has been demonstrated to be stable at room temperature for periods in excess of 5 years.

Actions

➤*Pharmacology:* The MAC (minimum alveolar concentration) in man is 1.68% in pure oxygen, 0.57 in 70% nitrous oxide, 30% oxygen, and 1.17 in 30% nitrous oxide, 70% oxygen.

Induction of and recovery from anesthesia with enflurane are rapid. Enflurane has a mild, sweet odor. Enflurane may provide a mild stimulus to salivation or tracheobronchial secretions. Pharyngeal and laryngeal reflexes are readily obtunded. The level of anesthesia can be changed rapidly by changing the inspired enflurane concentration. Enflurane reduces ventilation as depth of anesthesia increases. High $PaCO_2$ levels can be obtained at deeper levels of anesthesia if ventilation is not supported. Enflurane provokes a sigh response reminiscent of that seen with diethyl ether.

There is a decrease in blood pressure with induction of anesthesia, followed by a return to near normal with surgical stimulation. Progressive increases in depth of anesthesia produce corresponding increases in hypotension. Heart rate remains relatively constant without significant bradycardia. Electrocardiographic monitoring or recordings indicate that cardiac rhythm remains stable. Elevation of the carbon dioxide level in arterial blood does not alter cardiac rhythm.

Muscle relaxation may be adequate for intra-abdominal operations at normal levels of anesthesia. Muscle relaxants may be used to achieve greater relaxation and all commonly used muscle relaxants are compatible with enflurane. The nondepolarizing muscle relaxants are potentiated. In the healthy 70 kg adult, 6 to 9 mg of d-tubocurarine or 1 to 1.5 mg of pancuronium will produce a 90% or greater depression of twitch height. Neostigmine does not reverse the direct effect of enflurane.

➤*Pharmacokinetics:* Biotransformation of enflurane in man results in low peak levels of serum fluoride averaging 15 mcmol/L. These levels are well below the 50 mcmol/L threshold level which can produce minimal renal damage in healthy subjects. However, patients chronically ingesting isoniazid or other hydrazine-containing compounds may metabolize greater amounts of enflurane. Although no significant renal dysfunction has been found thus far in such patients, peak serum fluoride levels can exceed 50 mcmol/L, particularly when anesthesia goes beyond 2 MAC hours. Depression of lymphocyte transformation does not follow prolonged enflurane anesthesia in man in the absence of surgery. Thus enflurane does not depress this aspect of the immune response.

Contraindications

Seizure disorders; sensitivity to enflurane or other halogenated anesthetics; known or suspected genetic susceptibility to malignant hyperthermia.

Warnings/Precautions

➤*EEG changes:* Increasing depth of anesthesia with enflurane may produce a change in the electroencephalogram characterized by high voltage, fast frequency, progressing through spike-dome complexes alternating with periods of electrical silence to frank seizure activity. The latter may or may not be associated with motor movement. Motor activity, when encountered, generally consists of twitching or "jerks" of various muscle groups; it is self-limiting and can be terminated by lowering the anesthetic concentration. This electroencephalographic pattern associated with deep anesthesia is exacerbated by low arterial carbon dioxide tension. A reduction in ventilation and anesthetic concentrations usually suffices to eliminate seizure activity. Cerebral blood flow and metabolism studies in healthy volunteers immediately following seizure activity show no evidence of cerebral hypoxia. Mental function testing does not reveal any impairment of performance following prolonged enflurane anesthesia associated with or not associated with seizure activity.

➤*Depth of anesthesia:* Since levels of anesthesia may be altered easily and rapidly, only vaporizers producing predictable concentrations should be used. Hypotension and respiratory exchange can serve as a guide to depth of anesthesia. Deep levels of anesthesia may produce marked hypotension and respiratory depression.

➤*Hepatic effects:* When previous exposure to a halogenated anesthetic is known to have been followed by evidence of unexplained hepatic dysfunction, consideration should be given to use of an agent other than enflurane.

➤*Malignant hyperthermia:* In susceptible individuals, enflurane anesthesia may trigger a skeletal muscle hypermetabolic state leading to high oxygen demand and the clinical syndrome known as malignant hyperthermia. The syndrome includes nonspecific features such as muscle rigidity, tachycardia, tachypnea, cyanosis, arrhythmias, and unstable blood pressure. (It should also be noted that many of these nonspecific signs may appear with light anesthesia, acute hypoxia, etc. The syndrome of malignant hyperthermia secondary to enflurane appears to be rare; by March 1980, 35 cases had been reported in North America for an approximate incidence of 1:725,000 enflurane anesthetics.) An increase in overall metabolism may be reflected in an elevated temperature (which may rise rapidly early or late in the case, but usually is not the first sign of augmented metabolism) and an increased usage of CO_2 absorption system (hot cannister). PaO_2 and pH

ENFLURANE — INHALATION

may decrease, and hyperkalemia and a base deficit may appear. Treatment includes discontinuance of triggering agents (eg, enflurane), administration of intravenous dantrolene sodium, and application of supportive therapy. Such therapy includes vigorous efforts to restore body temperature to normal, respiratory and circulatory support as indicated, and management of electrolyte-fluid-acid-base derangement. (Consult prescribing information for dantrolene sodium intravenous for additional information on patient management.) Renal failure may appear later or damage may occur in already impaired kidneys due to release of fluoride ion; urine flow should be sustained if possible.

➤*Special risk:* Enflurane should be used with caution in patients who by virtue of medical or drug history could be considered more susceptible to cortical stimulation produced by the drug. Enflurane, like some other inhalational anesthetics, can react with desiccated carbon dioxide (CO_2) absorbents to produce carbon monoxide which may result in elevated levels of carboxyhemoglobin in some patients. Case reports suggest that barium hydroxide lime and soda lime become desiccated when fresh gases are passed through the CO_2 absorber cannister at high flow rates over many hours or days. When a clinician suspects that CO_2 absorbent may be desiccated, it should be replaced before the administration of enflurane.

➤*Pregnancy: Category B.* There are no adequate and well-controlled studies in pregnant women. Because animal reproduction studies are not always predictive of human response, this drug should be used during pregnancy only if clearly needed.

➤*Lactation:* It is not known whether this drug is excreted in human milk. Because many drugs are excreted in human milk, caution should be exercised when enflurane is administered to a nursing woman.

➤*Monitoring:* Bromsulfalein (BSP) retention is mildly elevated postoperatively in some cases. This may relate to the effect of surgery since prolonged anesthesia (5 to 7 hours) in human volunteers does not result in BSP elevation. There is some elevation of glucose and white blood count intraoperatively. Glucose elevation should be considered in diabetic patients.

Drug Interactions

➤*QT prolongation:* An additive effect of enflurane with other drugs that prolong the QT interval cannot be excluded. The following drugs may prolong the QT interval and increase the risk of life-threatening cardiac arrhythmias, including torsade de pointes: Antiarrhythmic agents (eg, amiodarone, bretylium, disopyramide, dofetilide, procainamide, quinidine, and sotalol), arsenic trioxide, chlorpromazine, cisapride, dolasetron, droperidol, mefloquine, mesoridazine, moxifloxacin, pentamidine, pimozide, tacrolimus, thioridazine, and ziprasidone. For a more complete list of drugs that may prolong the QT interval, see the appendix, Drug-Induced Prolongation of the QT Interval and Torsade de Pointes.

➤*Nondepolarizing relaxants:* The action of nondepolarizing relaxants is augmented by enflurane. Less than the usual amounts of these drugs should be used. If the usual amounts of nondepolarizing relaxants are given, the time for recovery from neuromuscular blockade will be longer in the presence of enflurane than when halothane or nitrous oxide with a balanced technique are used.

Adverse Reactions

➤*Cardiovascular:* Hypotension, arrhythmias.

➤*CNS:* Shivering motor activity exemplified by movements of various muscle groups or seizures may be encountered with deep levels of enflurane, USP, anesthesia, or light levels with hypocapnia.

➤*GI:* Nausea and vomiting have been reported.

➤*Hematologic:* Elevation of the white blood count has been observed.

➤*Hepatic:* Unexplained mild, moderate, and severe liver injury may rarely follow anesthesia with enflurane. Serum transaminases may be increased and histologic evidence of injury may be found. The histologic changes are neither unique nor consistent. In several of these cases, it has not been possible to exclude enflurane as the cause or as a contributing cause to liver injury. The incidence of unexplained hepatotoxicity following the administration of enflurane is unknown, but it appears to be rare and not dose related.

➤*Respiratory:* Respiratory depression has been reported.

➤*Miscellaneous:* Malignant hyperthermia (see Warnings).

Overdosage

In the event of overdosage, or what may appear to be overdosage, the following action should be taken: Stop drug administration, establish a clear airway, and initiate assisted or controlled ventilation with pure oxygen.

Patient Information

Enflurane, as well as other general anesthetics, may cause a slight decrease in intellectual function for 2 to 3 days following anesthesia. As with other anesthetics, small changes in moods and symptoms may persist for several days following administration.

ISOFLURANE

Rx	**Isoflurane** (Abbott)	**Liquid; inhalation**	In 100 mL.
Rx	**Forane** (Baxter Healthcare)		In 100 mL.
Rx	**Terrell** (Minrad)		In 100 and 250 mL.

ISOFLURANE — INHALATION

Indications

➤*Anesthesia:* For induction and maintenance of general anesthesia. Adequate data have not been developed to establish its application in obstetrical anesthesia.

Administration and Dosage

➤*General dosing considerations:* The concentration of isoflurane being delivered from a vaporizer during anesthesia should be known. This may be accomplished by using:

1.) Vaporizers calibrated specifically for isoflurane.
2.) Vaporizers from which delivered flows can be calculated, such as vaporizers delivering a saturated vapor which is then diluted. The delivered concentration from such a vaporizer may be calculated using the formula:

% isoflurane = 100 P_VF_V/F_T ($P_A - P_V$) where: P_A = Pressure of atmosphere P_V = Vapor pressure of isoflurane F_V = Flow of gas through vaporizer (mL/min) F_T = Total gas flow (mL/min)

Isoflurane contains no stabilizer. Nothing in the agent alters calibration or operation of these vaporizers.

The level of blood pressure during maintenance is an inverse function of isoflurane concentration in the absence of other complicating problems. Excessive decreases may be due to depth of anesthesia and in such instances may be corrected by lightening anesthesia.

➤*Adults:*

Anesthesia –

Preanesthetic medication: Premedication should be selected according to the need of the individual patient, taking into account that secretions are weakly stimulated by isoflurane, and the heart rate tends to be increased. The use of anticholinergic drugs is a matter of choice.

Induction: Inspired concentrations of 1.5% to 3% isoflurane usually produce surgical anesthesia in 7 to 10 minutes.

Induction with isoflurane in oxygen or in combination with oxygen-nitrous oxide mixtures may produce coughing, breathholding, or laryngospasm. These difficulties may be avoided by the use of a hypnotic dose of an ultrashort-acting barbiturate.

Maintenance: Surgical levels of anesthesia may be sustained with a 1% to 2.5% concentration when nitrous oxide is used concomitantly. An additional 0.5% to 1% may be required when isoflurane is given using oxygen alone. If added relaxation is required, supplemental doses of muscle relaxants may be used.

➤*Storage/Stability:* Store at 15° to 30°C (59° to 86°F). Isoflurane contains no additives and has been demonstrated to be stable at room temperature for periods in excess of 5 years.

Actions

➤*Pharmacology:* Isoflurane is an inhalation anesthetic. The MAC (minimum alveolar concentration) in humans is as follows:

Isoflurane MAC		
Age	100% oxygen	70% N_2O
26 ± 4	1.28	0.56
44 ± 7	1.15	0.5
64 ± 5	1.05	0.37

Induction of and recovery from isoflurane anesthesia are rapid. Isoflurane has a mild pungency which limits the rate of induction, although excessive salivation or tracheobronchial secretions do not appear to be stimulated. Pharyngeal and laryngeal reflexes are readily obtunded. The level of anesthesia may be changed rapidly with isoflurane. Isoflurane is a profound respiratory depressant. Respiration must be monitored closely and supported when necessary. As anesthetic dose is increased, tidal volume decreases and respiratory rate is unchanged. This depression is partially reversed by surgical stimulation, even at deeper levels of anesthesia. Isoflurane evokes a sigh response reminiscent of that seen with diethyl ether and enflurane, although the frequency is less than with enflurane.

Blood pressure decreases with induction of anesthesia but returns toward normal with surgical stimulation. Progressive increases in depth of anesthesia produce corresponding decreases in blood pressure. Nitrous oxide diminishes the inspiratory concentration of isoflurane required to reach a desired level of anesthesia and may reduce the arterial hypotension seen with isoflurane alone. Heart rhythm is remarkably stable. With controlled ventilation and normal $PaCO_2$, cardiac output is maintained despite increasing depth of anesthesia, primarily through an increase in heart rate which compensates for a reduction in stroke volume. The hypercapnia which attends spontaneous ventilation during isoflurane anesthesia further increases heart rate and raises cardiac output above awake levels. Isoflurane does not sensitize the myocardium to exogenously administered epinephrine in the

ISOFLURANE — INHALATION

dog. Limited data indicate that subcutaneous injection of 0.25 mg of epinephrine (50 mL of 1:200,000 solution) does not produce an increase in ventricular arrhythmias in patients anesthetized with isoflurane.

Muscle relaxation is often adequate for intra-abdominal operations at normal levels of anesthesia. Complete muscle paralysis can be attained with small doses of muscle relaxants. All commonly used muscle relaxants are markedly potentiated with isoflurane, the effect being most profound with the nondepolarizing type. Neostigmine reverses the effect of nondepolarizing muscle relaxants in the presence of isoflurane. All commonly used muscle relaxants are compatible with isoflurane.

Isoflurane can produce coronary vasodilation at the arteriolar level in selected animal models; the drug is probably also a coronary dilator in humans. Isoflurane, like some other coronary arteriolar dilators, has been shown to divert blood from collateral dependent myocardium to normally perfused areas in an animal model ("coronary steal"). Clinical studies to date evaluating myocardial ischemia, infarction and death as outcome parameters have not established that the coronary arteriolar dilation property of isoflurane is associated with coronary steal or myocardial ischemia in patients with coronary artery disease.

➤*Pharmacokinetics:* Isoflurane undergoes minimal biotransformation in man. In the postanesthesia period, only 0.17% of the isoflurane taken up can be recovered as urinary metabolites.

Contraindications

Known sensitivity to isoflurane or to other halogenated agents. Known or suspected genetic susceptibility to malignant hyperthermia.

Warnings/Precautions

➤*Depth of anesthesia:* Since levels of anesthesia may be altered easily and rapidly, only vaporizers producing predictable concentrations should be used. Hypotension and respiratory depression increase as anesthesia is deepened.

➤*Blood loss:* Increased blood loss comparable to that seen with halothane has been observed in patients undergoing abortions.

➤*Cerebral spinal fluid pressure:* Isoflurane markedly increased cerebral blood flow at deeper levels of anesthesia. There may be a transit rise in cerebral spinal fluid pressure which is fully reversible with hyperventilation.

➤*Maintenance of normal hemodynamics:* Regardless of the anesthetics employed, maintenance of normal hemodynamics is important to the avoidance of myocardial ischemia in patients with coronary artery disease.

➤*Desiccated carbon dioxide:* Isoflurane, like some other inhalational anesthetics, can react with desiccated carbon dioxide (CO_2) absorbents to produce carbon monoxide which may result in elevated levels of carboxyhemoglobin in some patients. Case reports suggest that barium hydroxide lime and soda have become desiccated when fresh gases are passed through the CO_2 absorber cannister at high flow rates over many hours or days. When a clinician suspects that CO_2 absorbent may be desiccated, it should be replaced before the administration of isoflurane.

➤*Hepatic effects:* As with other halogenated anesthetic agents, isoflurane may cause sensitivity hepatitis in patients who have been sensitized by previous exposure to halogenated anesthetics. Known sensitivity to isoflurane or other halogenated agents is a contraindication to the use of this drug.

➤*Malignant hyperthermia:* In susceptible individuals, isoflurane anesthesia may trigger a skeletal muscle hypermetabolic state leading to high oxygen demand and the clinical syndrome known as malignant hyperthermia. The syndrome includes nonspecific features such as muscle rigidity, tachycardia, tachypnea, cyanosis, arrhythmias, and unstable blood pressure. (It should also be noted that many of these nonspecific signs may appear with light anesthesia, acute hypoxia, etc.) An increase in overall metabolism may be reflected in an elevated temperature, (which may rise rapidly early or late in the case, but usually is not the first sign of augmented metabolism) and an increased usage of the CO_2 absorption system (hot cannister). PaO_2 and pH may decrease, and hyperkalemia and a base deficit may appear. Treatment includes discontinuance of triggering agents (eg, isoflurane), administration of IV dantrolene sodium, and application of supportive therapy. Such therapy includes vigorous efforts to restore body temperature to normal, respiratory and circulatory support as indicated, and management of electrolyte-fluid-acid-base derangements. Renal failure may appear later, and urine flow should be sustained if possible.

If patients judged malignant hyperthermia susceptible are administered IV or oral dantrolene sodium preoperatively, anesthetic preparation must still follow a standard malignant hyperthermia susceptible regimen, including the avoidance of known triggering agents. Monitoring for early clinical and metabolic signs of malignant hyperthermia is indicated because attenuation of malignant hyperthermia, rather than prevention, is possible. These signs usually call for the administration of additional IV dantrolene sodium.

➤*Pregnancy: Category C* per manufacturer's prescribing information. *Category B* per Briggs' *Drugs in Pregnancy and Lactation*. Isoflurane has been shown to have a possible anesthetic-related fetotoxic effect in mice when given in doses 6 times the human dose. There are no adequate and well-controlled studies in pregnant women. Isoflurane should be used during pregnancy only if the potential benefit justifies the potential risk to the fetus.

➤*Lactation:* It is not known whether this drug is excreted in human milk. Because many drugs are excreted in human milk, caution should be exercised when isoflurane is administered to a nursing woman.

➤*Lab test abnormalities:* Transient increases in BSP retention, blood glucose and serum creatinine with decrease in BUN, serum cholesterol and alkaline phosphatase have been observed.

Drug Interactions

Isoflurane potentiates the muscle relaxant effect of all muscle relaxants, most notably nondepolarizing muscle relaxants, and MAC (minimum alveolar concentration) is reduced by concomitant administration of N_2O. Nitrous oxide diminishes the inspiratory concentration of isoflurane required to reach a desired level of anesthesia and may reduce the arterial hypotension seen with isoflurane alone.

➤*QT prolongation:* An additive effect of isoflurane with other drugs that prolong the QT interval cannot be excluded. The following drugs may prolong the QT interval and increase the risk of life-threatening cardiac arrhythmias, including torsade de pointes: Antiarrhythmic agents (eg, amiodarone, bretylium, disopyramide, dofetilide, procainamide, quinidine, and sotalol), arsenic trioxide, chlorpromazine, cisapride, dolasetron, droperidol, mefloquine, mesoridazine, moxifloxacin, pentamidine, pimozide, tacrolimus, thioridazine, and ziprasidone. For a more complete list of drugs that may prolong the QT interval, see the appendix, Drug-Induced Prolongation of the QT Interval and Torsade de Pointes.

Adverse Reactions

Adverse reactions encountered in the administration of isoflurane are in general dose dependent extensions of pharmacophysiologic effects and include respiratory depression, hypotension and arrhythmias. Shivering, nausea, vomiting and ileus have been observed in the postoperative period.

As with all other general anesthetics, transient elevations in white blood count have been observed even in the absence of surgical stress. See Precautions for information regarding malignant hyperthermia. In susceptible individuals, isoflurane anesthesia may trigger a skeletal muscle hypermetabolic state leading to high oxygen demand and the clinical syndrome known as malignant hyperthermia. The syndrome includes nonspecific features such as muscle rigidity, tachycardia, tachypnea, cyanosis, arrhythmias, and unstable blood pressure. (It should also be noted that many of these nonspecific signs may appear with light anesthesia, acute hypoxia, etc.) An increase in overall metabolism may be reflected in an elevated temperature (which may rise rapidly early or late in the case, but usually is not the first sign of augmented metabolism) and an increased usage of the CO_2 absorption system (hot cannister). PaO_2 and pH may decrease, and hyperkalemia and a base deficit may appear.

During marketing, there have been rare reports of mild, moderate and severe (some fatal) postoperative hepatic dysfunction and hepatitis.

Overdosage

In the event of overdosage, or what may appear to be overdosage, the following action should be taken.

Stop drug administration, establish a clear airway, and initiate assisted or controlled ventilation with pure oxygen.

Patient Information

Isoflurane, as well as other general anesthetics, may cause a slight decrease in intellectual function for 2 or 3 days following anesthesia. As with other anesthetics, small changes in moods and symptoms may persist for up to 6 days after administration.

DESFLURANE

Rx	**Suprane** (Baxter)	**Inhalation; oral:**	In 240 mL.

DESFLURANE — INHALATION

Indications

➤*Anesthesia:* For induction or maintenance of anesthesia for inpatient and outpatient surgery in adults.

Desflurane is not recommended for induction of anesthesia in pediatric patients because of a high incidence of moderate-to-severe upper airway adverse events. After induction of anesthesia with agents other than desflurane, and tracheal intubation, desflurane is indicated for maintenance of anesthesia in infants and children.

Administration and Dosage

➤*General dosing considerations:* Deliver desflurane from a vaporizer specifically designed and designated for use with desflurane.

The administration of general anesthesia must be individualized based on the patient's response. The following table provides mean relative potency based upon age and drug interaction studies in predominantly ASA physical status I or II patients.

DESFLURANE — INHALATION

Effect of Age on MAC of Desflurane Mean ± SD (% Atmospheres)[a]				
Age	n[b]	O_2 100%	n	N_2O 60%
2 weeks	6	9.2 ± 0	-	-
10 weeks	5	9.4 ± 0.4	-	-
9 months	4	10 ± 0.7	5	7.5 ± 0.8
2 years	3	9.1 ± 0.6	-	-
3 years	-	-	5	6.4 ± 0.4
4 years	4	8.6 ± 0.6	-	-
7 years	5	8.1 ± 0.6.	-	-
25 years	4	7.3 ± 0	4	4 ± 0.3
45 years	4	6 ± 0.3	6	2.8 ± 0.6
70 years	6	5.2 ± 0.6	6	1.7 ± 0.4

[a] MAC = minimum alveolar concentration; SD = standard deviation.
[b] n = number of crossover pairs (using up-and-down method of quantal response).

➤*Adults:*

Anesthesia –

Preanesthetic medication: Issues such as whether or not to premedicate and the choice of premedicant(s) must be individualized. In clinical studies, patients scheduled to be anesthetized with desflurane frequently received intravenous (IV) preanesthetic medication, such as opioid and/or benzodiazepine.

Induction of anesthesia: In adults, some premedicated with opioid, a frequent starting concentration was desflurane 3%, increased in 0.5% to 1% increments every 2 to 3 breaths. End-tidal concentrations of desflurane 4% to 11%, with and without N_2O, produced anesthesia within 2 to 4 minutes. When desflurane was tested as the primary anesthetic induction agent, the incidence of upper airway irritation (apnea, breathholding, laryngospasm, coughing, and secretions) was high (see Adverse Reactions). During induction in adults, the overall incidence of oxyhemoglobin desaturation (arterial oxyhemoglobin saturation [SpO_2] less than 90%) was 6%.

After induction in adults with an IV drug such as thiopental or propofol, desflurane can be started at approximately 0.5 to 1 MAC, whether the carrier gas is O_2 or N_2O/O_2.

Maintenance of anesthesia: Surgical levels of anesthesia in adults may be maintained with concentrations of desflurane 2.5% to 8.5%, with or without the concomitant use of nitrous oxide.

During the maintenance of anesthesia, increasing concentrations of desflurane produce dose-dependent decreases in blood pressure. Excessive decreases in blood pressure may be because of depth of anesthesia and, in such instances, may be corrected by decreasing the inspired concentration of desflurane.

Concentrations of desflurane exceeding 1 MAC may increase heart rate. Thus, with this drug, an increased heart rate may not serve reliably as a sign of inadequate anesthesia. Desflurane decreases the doses of neuromuscular-blocking agents required.

During the maintenance of anesthesia with inflow rates of 2 L/min or more, the alveolar concentration of desflurane will usually be within 10% of the inspired concentration. (F_A/F_I).

Concomitant therapy: Opioids or benzodiazepines decrease the amounts of desflurane required to produce anesthesia. The following table is based on studies of drug interaction (MAC reduction).

Desflurane MAC with Fentanyl or Midazolam Mean ± SD (% reduction)		
Dose	18 to 30 years of age	31 to 65 years of age
No fentanyl	6.4 ± 0	6.3 ± 0.4
fentanyl 3 mcg/kg	3.5 ± 1.9 (46%)	3.1 ± 0.6 (51%)
fentanyl 6 mcg/kg	3 ± 1.2 (53%)	2.3 ± 1 (64%)
No midazolam	6.9 ± 0.1	5.9 ± 0.6
midazolam 25 mcg/kg	-	4.9 ± 0.9 (16%)
midazolam 50 mcg/kg	-	4.9 ± 0.5 (17%)

Desflurane decreases the doses of neuromuscular-blocking agents required (see Drug Interactions).

➤*Children:*

Induction – Desflurane is not recommended for induction of general anesthesia in infants or children because of a high incidence of moderate to severe laryngospasm, coughing, breathholding, and increased secretions. The occurrence of oxyhemoglobin desaturation was 26%. See also Adverse Reactions.

Maintenance of anesthesia – See Adults for more information.

In children, surgical levels of anesthesia may be maintained with concentrations of desflurane 5.2% to 10% with or without the concomitant use of nitrous oxide.

➤*Storage/Stability:* Store at 15° to 30°C (59° to 86°F).

Actions

➤*Pharmacology:* Desflurane is a volatile liquid inhalation anesthetic minimally biotransformed in the liver in humans. Less than 0.02% of the desflurane absorbed can be recovered as urinary metabolites (compared to 0.2% for isoflurane).

Minimum alveolar concentration (MAC) of desflurane in oxygen for a 25-year-old adult is 7.3%. The MAC of desflurane decreases with increasing age and with addition of depressants such as opioids or benzodiazepines (see Administration and Dosage).

➤*Pharmacokinetics:* Due to the volatile nature of desflurane in plasma samples, the washin-washout profile of desflurane was used as a surrogate of plasma pharmacokinetics. Eight healthy male volunteers first breathed 70% N_2O/30% O_2 for 30 minutes and then a mixture of desflurane 2%, isoflurane 0.4%, and halothane 0.2% for another 30 minutes. During this time, inspired and end-tidal concentrations (F_I and F_A) were measured. The F_A/F_I (washin) value at 30 minutes for desflurane was 0.91, compared to 1 for N_2O, 0.74 for isoflurane, and 0.58 for halothane. The washin rates for halothane and isoflurane were similar to literature values. The washin was faster for desflurane than for isoflurane and halothane at all time points. The F_A/F_{AO} (washout) value at 5 minutes was 0.12 for desflurane, 0.22 for isoflurane, and 0.25 for halothane. The washout for desflurane was more rapid than that for isoflurane and halothane at all elimination time points. By 5 days, the F_A/F_{AO} for desflurane is one-twentieth of that for halothane or isoflurane.

Contraindications

Known or suspected genetic susceptibility to malignant hyperthermia; sensitivity to desflurane or to other halogenated agents.

Warnings/Precautions

➤*Administration:* Desflurane should be administered only by persons trained in the administration of general anesthesia, using a vaporizer specifically designed and designated for use with desflurane. Facilities for maintenance of a patent airway, artificial ventilation, oxygen enrichment, and circulatory resuscitation must be immediately available. Hypotension and respiratory depression increase as anesthesia is deepened.

➤*Cardiovascular effects:* During the maintenance of anesthesia, increasing concentrations of desflurane produce dose-dependent decreases in blood pressure. Excessive decreases in blood pressure may be related to depth of anesthesia and in such instances may be corrected by decreasing the inspired concentration of desflurane.

Concentrations of desflurane exceeding 1 MAC may increase heart rate. Thus an increased heart rate may not be a sign of inadequate anesthesia.

➤*Intracranial space occupying lesions:* In patients with intracranial space occupying lesions, desflurane should be administered at 0.8 MAC or less, in conjunction with a barbiturate induction and hyperventilation (hypocapnia). Appropriate measures should be taken to maintain cerebral perfusion pressure.

➤*Coronary artery disease:* In patients with coronary artery disease, maintenance of normal hemodynamics is important to the avoidance of myocardial ischemia. Desflurane should not be used as the sole agent for anesthetic induction in patients with coronary artery disease or patients where increases in heart rate or blood pressure are undesirable. It should be used with other medications, preferably IV opioids and hypnotics (see Clinical trials).

➤*Concentrations greater than 12%:* Inspired concentrations of desflurane more than 12% have been safely administered to patients, particularly during induction of anesthesia. Such concentrations will proportionately dilute the concentration of oxygen; therefore, maintenance of an adequate concentration of oxygen may require a reduction of nitrous oxide or air if these gases are used concurrently.

➤*Desiccated carbon dioxide:* Desflurane, like some other inhalational anesthetics, can react with desiccated carbon dioxide (CO_2) absorbents to produce carbon monoxide which may result in elevated levels of carboxyhemoglobin in some patients. Case reports suggest that barium hydroxide lime and soda lime become desiccated when fresh gases are passed through the CO_2 absorber cannister at high flow rates over many hours or days. When a clinician suspects that CO_2 absorbent may be desiccated, it should be replaced before the administration of desflurane.

➤*Hepatic effects:* As with other halogenated anesthetic agents, desflurane may cause sensitivity hepatitis in patients who have been sensitized by previous exposure to halogenated anesthetics.

➤*Malignant hyperthermia:* In susceptible individuals, potent inhalation anesthetic agents may trigger a skeletal muscle hypermetabolic state leading to high oxygen demand and the clinical syndrome known as malignant hyperthermia. In genetically susceptible pigs, desflurane-induced malignant hyperthermia. The clinical syndrome is signalled by hypercapnia, and may include muscle rigidity, tachycardia, tachypnea, cyanosis, arrhythmias, or unstable blood pressure. Some of these nonspecific signs may also appear during light anesthesia: Acute hypoxia, hypercapnia, and hypovolemia.

Treatment of malignant hyperthermia includes discontinuation of triggering agents, administration of IV dantrolene sodium, and application of supportive therapy. (Consult prescribing information for dantrolene sodium IV for additional information on patient management.) Renal failure may appear later, and urine flow should be monitored and sustained if possible.

➤*Neurosurgical use:* Desflurane may produce a dose-dependent increase in cerebrospinal fluid pressure (CSFP) when administered to patients with intracranial space occupying lesions. Desflurane should be administered at 0.8 MAC or less, and in conjunction with a barbiturate induction and hyper-

DESFLURANE — INHALATION

ventilation (hypocapnia) until cerebral decompression in patients with known or suspected increases in CSFP. Appropriate attention must be paid to maintain cerebral perfusion pressure.

➤*Pregnancy: Category B.* There are no adequate and well-controlled studies in pregnant women. Desflurane should be used during pregnancy only if the potential benefit justifies the potential risk to the fetus.

No teratogenic effect was observed at ≈ 10 and 13 cumulative MAC-hour exposures at 1 MAC-hour/day during organogenesis in rats or rabbits. At higher doses increased incidences of post-implantation loss and maternal toxicity were observed. However, at 10 MAC-hours cumulative exposure in rats, about 6% decrease in the weight of male pups was observed at preterm caesarean delivery.

➤*Lactation:* The concentrations of desflurane in milk are probably of no clinical importance 24 hours after anesthesia. Because of rapid washout, desflurane concentrations in milk are predicted to be below those found with other volatile potent anesthetics.

➤*Children:* Desflurane is not recommended for induction of general anesthesia via mask in infants or children because of the high incidence of moderate to severe laryngospasm in 50% of patients, coughing 72%, breathholding 68%, increase in secretions 21% and oxyhemoglobin desaturation 26%.

➤*Elderly:* The average MAC for desflurane in a 70–year-old patient is two-thirds the MAC for a 20–year-old patient.

➤*Lab test abnormalities:* Transient elevations in glucose and white blood cell count may occur as with use of other anesthetic agents.

Drug Interactions

➤*Benzodiazepines and opioids (MAC reduction):* See Administration and Dosage for more information.

➤*Neuromuscular-blocking agents:* Anesthetic concentrations of desflurane at equilibrium (administered for 15 or more minutes before testing) reduced the ED_{95} of succinylcholine by ≈ 30% and that of atracurium and pancuronium by ≈ 50% compared to N_2O/opioid anesthesia. The effect of desflurane on duration of nondepolarizing neuromuscular blockade has not been studied.

Dosage of Muscle Relaxant Causing 95% Depression in Neuromuscular Blockade

Desflurane concentration	Mean ED_{95} (mcg/kg)		
	Pancuronium	Atracurium	Succinylcholine
0.65 MAC 60% N_2O/O_2	26	123	—
1.25 MAC 60% N_2O/O_2	18	91	
1.25 MAC O_2	22	120	362

Dosage reduction of neuromuscular-blocking agents during induction of anesthesia may result in delayed onset of conditions suitable for endotracheal intubation or inadequate muscle relaxation, because potentiation of neuromuscular blocking agents requires equilibration of muscle with the delivered partial pressure of desflurane.

Among nondepolarizing drugs, only pancuronium and atracurium interactions have been studied. In the absence of specific guidelines:

For endotracheal intubation, do not reduce the dose of nondepolarizing muscle relaxants or succinylcholine.

During maintenance of anesthesia, the dose of nondepolarizing muscle relaxants is likely to be reduced compared to that during N_2O/opioid anesthesia. Administration of supplemental doses of muscle relaxants should be guided by the response to nerve stimulation.

Adverse Reactions

➤*Probably causally related:*
Incidence greater than 1% –

Desflurane Induction (Use as a Mask Inhalation Agent)		
Adult patients (n = 370)		
Coughing		34%
Breath holding		30%
Apnea		15%
Increased secretions		[a]
Laryngospasm		[a]
Oxyhemoglobin desaturation (SpO_2		[a]
Pharyngitis		[a]
Pediatric patients (n = 152)		
Coughing		72%
Breath holding		68%
Laryngospasm		50%
Oxyhemoglobin desaturation (SpO_2		26%
Increased secretions		21%
Bronchospasm		[a]

[a] Incidence of events: 3% to 10%.

➤*Maintenance and recovery (probably causally related):* The following adverse events occurred in greater than 1% of patients during maintenance and recovery in adult and pediatric patients (n = 687) and are probably causally related:

Cardiovascular – Bradycardia, hypertension, nodal arrhythmia, tachycardia.

CNS – Increased salivation.

GI – Nausea (27%) and vomiting (16%).

Respiratory – Apnea (incidence 3% to 10%), breath holding, increased cough (incidence 3% to 10%), laryngospasm (incidence 3% to 10%), pharyngitis.

Special senses – Conjunctivitis (conjunctival hyperemia).

Miscellaneous – Headache.

➤*Probably causally related (incidence < 1%):* Other adverse events that were probably causally related and that were reported in < 1% of patients (3 or more patients, n = 1843) are as follows:

Cardiovascular – Arrhythmia, bigeminy, abnormal electrocardiogram, myocardial ischemia, vasodilation.

CNS – Agitation, dizziness.

Hepatic – Hepatitis was not seen in clinical trials, but has been reported in postmarketing experience or in the literature, and is considered rare.

Respiratory – Asthma, dyspnea, and hypoxia.

➤*Causal relationship unknown (incidence < 1%):* See Warnings for information regarding pediatric use and malignant hyperthermia.

For the following adverse events, which were reported in < 1% of patients, a causal relationship could not be established:

Cardiovascular – Hemorrhage, myocardial infarction (MI).

Dermatologic – Pruritus.

Metabolic/Nutritional – Increased creatine phosphokinase.

Musculoskeletal – Myalgia.

Miscellaneous – Fever.

Overdosage

➤*Treatment:* In the event of overdosage, or suspected overdosage take the following actions: Discontinue administration of desflurane, maintain a patent airway, initiate assisted or controlled ventilation with oxygen, and maintain adequate cardiovascular function.

SEVOFLURANE

Rx	**Sojourn** (Minrad)	In 250 mL.
Rx	**Ultane** (Abbott)	In 250 mL.

SEVOFLURANE — INHALATION

Indications

➤*Anesthesia:* Induction and maintenance of general anesthesia in adults and children for inpatient and outpatient surgery.

Administration and Dosage

➤*General dosing considerations:* Consult detailed literature before using. Sevoflurane should be administered only by those with appropriate training and experience.

The concentration of sevoflurane being delivered from a vaporizer should be known. This may be accomplished by using a vaporizer calibrated specifically for sevoflurane. Administration of general anesthesia must be individualized based on patient response.

➤*Adults:*
Anesthesia –

Preanesthetic medication: No specific premedication is either indicated or contraindicated. The decision as to whether or not to premedicate and choice of premedication is left to the discretion of the anesthesiologist.

Induction: Sevoflurane has a nonpungent odor and does not cause respiratory irritability; it is suitable for mask induction in children and adults.

SEVOFLURANE — INHALATION

Maintenance: Surgical levels of anesthesia can usually be obtained with concentrations of 0.5% to 3% with or without the concomitant use of nitrous oxide. Sevoflurane can be administered with any type of anesthesia circuit.

➤*Children:*

Anesthesia – See Adults for information.

➤*Preparation for administration:* Before administration of sevoflurane, replace the CO_2 absorbent if it is desiccated. The exothermic reaction that occurs with sevoflurane and CO_2 absorbents is increased when the CO_2 absorbent becomes desiccated, such as after an extended period of dry gas flow through the CO_2 absorbent canisters. Extremely rare cases of spontaneous fire in the respiratory circuit of the anesthesia machine have been reported during sevoflurane use in conjunction with the use of a desiccated CO_2 absorbent. Rapid changes in the color of some CO_2 absorbents or an unusually delayed rise in the delivered (inspired) gas concentration of sevoflurane compared with the vaporizer setting may indicate excessive heating of the CO_2 absorbent canister and chemical breakdown of sevoflurane.

➤*Storage/Stability:* Store at 15° to 30°C (59° to 86°F).

Actions

➤*Pharmacology:* Sevoflurane is an inhalational anesthetic. Minimum alveolar concentration (MAC) of sevoflurane in oxygen for an adult 40 years of age is 2.1%. The MAC of sevoflurane decreases with age.

Alveolar concentration/inspired concentration (F_A/F_I) of sevoflurane was compared with F_A/F_I data of other halogenated anesthetics in healthy volunteers. When all data were normalized to isoflurane, the uptake and distribution of sevoflurane was faster than isoflurane and halothane but slower than desflurane. Sevoflurane is a dose-related cardiac depressant. It does not produce increases in heart rate at doses less than 2 MAC.

➤*Pharmacokinetics:*

Metabolism/Excretion – Sevoflurane is metabolized by cytochrome P450 2E1 to hexafluoroisopropanol (HFIP) with release of inorganic fluoride and CO_2. Once formed HFIP is rapidly conjugated with glucuronic acid and eliminated as a urinary metabolite. No other metabolic pathways for sevoflurane have been identified. In vivo metabolism studies suggest that approximately 5% of the sevoflurane dose may be metabolized.

The low solubility of sevoflurane facilitates rapid elimination via the lungs. In healthy volunteers, rate of elimination was similar compared with desflurane, but faster compared with halothane or isoflurane. Up to 3.5% of the sevoflurane dose appears in the urine as inorganic fluoride. Studies on fluoride indicate that up to 50% of fluoride clearance is nonrenal (via fluoride being taken up into bone).

Contraindications

Known sensitivity to sevoflurane or to other halogenated agents or in patients with known or suspected susceptibility to malignant hyperthermia.

Warnings/Precautions

➤*Malignant hyperthermia:* Malignant hyperthermia may be triggered by most of the potent inhalational anesthetics. Treatment of malignant hyperthermia includes discontinuation of triggering agents, administration of IV dantrolene sodium and supportive therapy. Sevoflurane may present an increased risk in patients with known sensitivity to volatile halogenated anesthetic agents (see Contraindications).

➤*Pregnancy:* *Category C* per Briggs' *Drugs in Pregnancy and Lactation. Category B* per manufacturer's prescribing information. Sevoflurane is teratogenic in mice, but no reports of its use in early human gestation have been located.

➤*Lactation:* Sevoflurane is probably excreted into colostrum and milk as suggested by its presence in the maternal blood and its low molecular weight (about 200), but the toxic potential of this exposure for the infant is unknown. However, the risk to a breast-feeding infant from exposure to sevoflurane via milk is probably very low. Per the American Academy of Pediatrics, halothane, a related inhalational anesthetic, is classified as usually compatible with breast-feeding.

INJECTABLE LOCAL ANESTHETICS

This information on local anesthetics is not intended to be comprehensive. Consult standard textbooks for further discussion of techniques and applications.

WARNING

Have resuscitative equipment and drugs immediately available when any local anesthetic is used.

Do not use preparations containing preservatives for caudal epidural anesthesia. When using preparations without preservatives, discard any unused drug remaining in vial.

Obstetrical anesthesia – The 0.75% concentration of **bupivacaine** is not recommended for obstetrical anesthesia. Cardiac arrest with difficult resuscitation or death has occurred during use for epidural anesthesia in obstetrical patients. Resuscitation has been difficult or impossible despite adequate preparation and appropriate management. Cardiac arrest has occurred after convulsions resulting from systemic toxicity, presumably following unintentional intravascular injection. Reserve the 0.75% concentration for surgical procedures where a high degree of muscle relaxation and prolonged effect are necessary.

Historically, pregnant patients were reported to have a high risk for cardiac arrhythmias, cardiac/circulatory arrest, and death when bupivacaine was inadvertently rapidly injected intravenously (IV). Avoid levobupivacaine 0.75% in obstetrical patients. The concentration is indicated only for nonobstetrical surgery requiring profound muscle relaxation and long duration. For Cesarean section, the levobupivacaine 5 mg/mL (0.5%) solution in doses up to 150 mg is recommended.

Indications

Refer to individual product listings.

➤*Off-label uses:* Refer to individual monographs for further information.

Hiccups (singultus) –

Lidocaine: [3] = Safety concerns.

Administration and Dosage

The dose of local anesthetic administered varies with the procedure, vascularity of the tissues, depth of anesthesia, degree of required muscle relaxation, duration of anesthesia desired, and the physical condition of the patient. Reduce dosages for children, elderly patients, debilitated patients, and patients with cardiac or liver disease.

➤*Infiltration or regional block anesthesia:* Always inject slowly, with frequent aspirations, to prevent intravascular injection.

For detailed Administration and Dosage, refer to individual product listings and specific manufacturers' labeling.

Actions

➤*Pharmacology:* These agents prevent generation and conduction of nerve impulses by inhibiting ionic fluxes, increasing electrical excitation threshold, slowing nerve impulse propagation, and reducing rate of rise of action potential. Progression of anesthesia is related to the diameter, myelination, and conduction velocity of affected nerve fibers. The order of loss of nerve function is the following: pain, temperature, touch, proprioception, and skeletal muscle tone.

Systemic absorption of local anesthetics affects the cardiovascular system and CNS. At blood concentrations achieved with normal therapeutic doses, changes in cardiac conduction, excitability, refractoriness, contractility, and peripheral vascular resistance are minimal. However, toxic blood concentrations depress cardiac conduction and excitability, which may lead to atrioventricular block and ultimately to cardiac arrest. In addition, with toxic blood concentrations, myocardial contractility may be depressed and peripheral vasodilation may occur, leading to decreased cardiac output and arterial blood pressure.

Following systemic absorption, toxic blood concentrations can produce CNS stimulation, depression, or both. Apparent central stimulation may manifest as restlessness, tremors, and shivering, which may progress to convulsions. Depression and coma may occur, possibly progressing ultimately to respiratory arrest. Local anesthetics have a primary depressant effect on the medulla and on higher centers. The depressed stage may occur without a prior stage of CNS stimulation.

The use of vasoconstrictors (eg, epinephrine) with local anesthetics promotes local hemostasis, decreases systemic absorption, and prolongs duration of action.

➤*Pharmacokinetics:* Various pharmacokinetic parameters can be significantly altered by the presence of hepatic or renal disease, addition of epinephrine, factors affecting urinary pH, renal blood flow, administration route and age of patient, and the presence or absence of epinephrine in the anesthetic solution.

Injectable Local Anesthetics Pharmacokinetics

Anesthetic	Onset (minutes)	Duration (hours)	Equivalent anesthetic concentration (%)	pKa	Partition coefficient	Systemic protein binding (%)
Esters						
Procaine[a]	2 to 5	0.25 to 1	2	9.1	0.02[c]	5.8[d]
(w/epinephrine)	nd	0.5 to 1.5				
(Epidural)[b]	15 to 25	0.5 to 1.5				
Chloroprocaine[a]	6 to 12	0.5	2	9	0.14[c]	nd
(w/epinephrine)	nd	0.5 to 1.5				
(Epidural)[b]	5 to 15	0.5 to 1.5				
Tetracaine[a]	≤ 15	2 to 3	0.25	8.5	4.1[c]	75.6[e]
(Epidural)[b]	20 to 30	3 to 5				
(Spinal)	nd	1.25 to 3				
Amides						
Lidocaine[a]	< 2	0.5 to 1	1	7.9	2.9[c]	64.3
(w/epinephrine)	< 2	2 to 6				
(Epidural)[b]	5 to 15	1 to 3				
(Spinal)	nd	0.5 to 1.5				
Prilocaine[a]	< 2	≥ 1	1	7.9	0.9[c]	55
(w/epinephrine)	< 2	2.25				
(Epidural)[b]	5 to 15	1 to 3				
Mepivacaine[a]	3 to 5	0.75 to 1.5	1	7.8	0.8[c]	77.5[e]
(w/epinephrine)	nd	2 to 6				
(Epidural)[b]	5 to 15	1 to 3				
(Spinal)	nd	0.5 to 1.5				

Injectable Local Anesthetics Pharmacokinetics						
Anesthetic	Onset (minutes)	Duration (hours)	Equivalent anesthetic concentration (%)	pKa	Partition coefficient	Systemic protein binding (%)
Bupivacaine[a]	5	2 to 4	0.25	8.2	27.5[c]/ 1,565[f]	95.6[e]
(w/epinephrine)	nd	3 to 7				
(Epidural)[b]	10 to 20	3 to 5				
(Spinal)	nd	1.25 to 2.5				
Levobupivacaine	—	—	—	8.09	1,624[f]	> 97[e]
(Epidural)[g]	≈ 10	≈ 8	nd			
Ropivacaine	—	—	nd	8.07	2.9[h]	94
(Epidural)	10 to 30	0.5 to 6				

[a] Values in this line are for infiltrative anesthesia. nd – No data.
[b] With epinephrine 1:200,000.
[c] n-Heptane/Buffer, pH 7.4.
[d] Nerve homogenate binding.
[e] Plasma protein binding.
[f] Oleyl alcohol/water buffer.
[g] Administration in Cesarean section.
[h] n-heptane buffer.

Rate of systemic absorption depends on total dose and concentration of drug, vascularity of administration site, and presence of vasoconstrictors. Depending on route, local anesthetics are distributed to some extent to all body tissues. High concentrations are found in highly perfused organs (eg, liver, lungs, heart, brain). Rate and extent of placental diffusion are determined by plasma protein binding, ionization, and lipid solubility. Fetal/maternal ratios are inversely related to degree of protein binding. Only free, unbound drug is available for placental transfer. Drugs with the highest protein binding capacity may have the lowest fetal/maternal ratios. Lipid soluble, nonionized drugs readily enter fetal blood from maternal circulation.

The onset of local anesthesia is dependent on the dissociation constant (pKa), lipid solubility, pH at the injection site, protein binding and molecular size. In general, local anesthetics with high lipid solubility or low pKa have a faster onset.

Local anesthetics are divided into 2 groups: Esters, which are derivatives of para-aminobenzoic acid, and amides, which are derivatives of aniline. The "ester" local anesthetics are metabolized by hydrolysis of the ester linkage by plasma esterase, probably plasma cholinesterase. The "amide" local anesthetics are metabolized primarily in the liver, then excreted primarily in the urine as metabolites, with a small fraction of unchanged drug.

Contraindications

Hypersensitivity to local anesthetics or any components of the products, para-aminobenzoic acid (esters only) or parabens; congenital or idiopathic methemoglobinemia (**prilocaine**); spinal and caudal anesthesia in septicemia, existing neurologic disease, spinal deformities, and severe hypertension, hemorrhage, shock, or heart block; subarachnoid administration (**chloroprocaine**).

➤*Bupivacaine / Levobupivacaine:* Obstetrical paracervical block anesthesia (such use has resulted in fetal bradycardia and death); IV regional anesthesia (Bier block; cardiac arrest and death have occurred) (see Warnings).

Warnings/Precautions

➤*Head and neck area:* Small doses of local anesthetics injected into the head and neck area, including retrobulbar, dental, and stellate ganglion blocks, may produce adverse reactions similar to systemic toxicity seen with unintentional intravascular injections of larger doses. The injection procedures require the utmost care. Confusion, convulsions, respiratory depression or arrest, and cardiovascular stimulation or depression have been reported. These reactions may be caused by intra-arterial injection of the local anesthetic with retrograde flow to cerebral circulation. They also may be caused by puncture of the dural sheath of the optic nerve during retrobulbar block with diffusion of any local anesthetic along the subdural space to the midbrain. Observe patient carefully. Monitor respiration and circulation. Do not exceed dosage recommendations.

Ophthalmic surgery – When local anesthetic solutions are used for retrobulbar block, complete corneal anesthesia usually precedes onset of clinically acceptable external ocular muscle akinesia. Therefore, presence of akinesia rather than anesthesia alone should determine readiness of the patient for surgery. Clinicians who perform retrobulbar blocks should be aware that there have been reports of respiratory arrest following local anesthetic injection. The use of ropivacaine in retrobulbar blocks for ophthalmic surgery has not been studied. The use of ropivacaine in retrobulbar blocks for ophthalmic surgery has not been studied. The use of ropivacaine in retrobulbar blocks for ophthalmic surgery has not been studied.

Dentistry – Because of the long duration of anesthesia of **bupivacaine with epinephrine**, caution patients about the possibility of inadvertent trauma to tongue, lips, and buccal mucosa and advise against chewing solid foods or testing anesthetized area by biting or probing.

Cardiovascular effects – Cardiovascular reactions are depressant. They may be the result of direct drug effect, the result of vasovagal reaction, particularly if the patient is in the sitting position. Failure to recognize premonitory signs such as sweating, feeling of faintness, changes in pulse, or sensorium may result in progressive cerebral hypoxia and seizure, or serious cardiovascular catastrophe. Place patient in recumbent position and administer oxygen.

➤*Intravascular or subarachnoid administration:* It is essential that aspiration for blood or cerebrospinal fluid (where applicable) be done prior to injecting any local anesthetic, both the original dose and all subsequent doses, to avoid intravascular or subarachnoid injection. However, a negative aspiration does not ensure against an intravascular or subarachnoid injection.

In performing **ropivacaine** blocks, unintended intravascular injection is possible and may result in cardiac arrhythmia or cardiac arrest. The potential for successful resuscitation has not been studied in humans. Administer ropivacaine in incremental doses. It is not recommended for emergency situations in which a fast onset of surgical anesthesia is necessary. Historically, pregnant patients were reported to have a high risk for cardiac arrhythmias, cardiac/circulatory arrest, and death when **bupivacaine** 0.75% was inadvertently rapidly injected IV.

➤*Spinal anesthesia:* The following conditions may preclude the use of spinal anesthesia, depending on the physician's evaluation of the situation and ability to deal with the following complications or complaints that may occur:

- Preexisting diseases of the CNS, such as those attributable to pernicious anemia, poliomyelitis, syphilis, or tumor.
- Hematological disorders predisposing to coagulopathies or patients on anticoagulant therapy. Trauma to a blood vessel during the conduct of spinal anesthesia may, in some instances, result in uncontrollable CNS hemorrhage or soft tissue hemorrhage.
- Chronic backache and preoperative headache.
- Hypotension and hypertension.
- Technical problems (persistent paresthesias, persistent bloody tap).
- Arthritis or spinal deformity.
- Extremes of age.
- Psychosis or other causes of poor cooperation by the patient.

➤*Administration:* Use the lowest dosage that results in effective anesthesia to avoid high plasma levels and serious adverse effects. Inject slowly, with frequent aspirations before and during the injection, to avoid intravascular injection. Perform syringe aspirations before and during each supplemental injection in continuous (intermittent) catheter techniques. During the administration of epidural anesthesia, it is recommended that a test dose be administered initially and that the patient be monitored for CNS toxicity and cardiovascular toxicity, as well as for signs of unintended intrathecal administration, before proceeding.

➤*Inflammation or sepsis:* Use local anesthetic procedures with caution when there is inflammation or sepsis in the region of proposed injection.

➤*CNS toxicity:* Monitor cardiovascular and respiratory vital signs and state of consciousness after each injection. Restlessness, anxiety, incoherent speech, lightheadedness, numbness, and tingling of the mouth and lips, metallic taste, tinnitus, dizziness, blurred vision, tremors, twitching, depression, or drowsiness may be early signs of CNS toxicity.

➤*Malignant hyperthermia:* Many drugs used during anesthesia are considered potential triggering agents for familial malignant hyperthermia. It is not known whether local anesthetics may trigger this reaction and the need for supplemental general anesthesia cannot be predicted in advance; therefore, have a standard protocol for management available.

➤*Chondrolysis:* Intra-articular infusions of local anesthetics following arthroscopic and other surgical procedures is an unapproved use, and there have been postmarketing reports in patients receiving such infusions.

➤*Peripheral nerve block:* Major peripheral nerve blocks may result in the administration of a large volume of local anesthetics in highly vascularized areas, often close to large vessels where there is an increased risk of intravascular injection and/or rapid systemic absorption, which can lead to high plasma concentrations.

➤*Vasoconstrictors:* Use solutions containing a vasoconstrictor with caution and in carefully circumscribed quantities in areas of the body supplied by end arteries or having otherwise compromised blood supply (eg, digits, nose, external ear, penis). Use with extreme caution in patients whose medical history and physical evaluation suggest the existence of hypertension, peripheral vascular disease, arteriosclerotic heart disease, cerebral vascular insufficiency, or heart block; these individuals may exhibit exaggerated vasoconstrictor response.

Serious dose-related cardiac arrhythmias may occur if preparations containing a vasoconstrictor such as epinephrine are employed in patients during or following the administration of potent inhalation agents.

➤*IV regional anesthesia:* Cardiac arrest and death are reported with the use of **bupivacaine** for IV regional anesthesia (Bier block). Bupivacaine is not recommended for this technique.

➤*Hypersensitivity reactions:* These include anaphylaxis and may occur in a small segment of the population allergic to para-aminobenzoic acid derivatives (eg, procaine, tetracaine, benzocaine). The amide-type local anesthetics have not shown cross-sensitivity with the esters.

Reactions resulting in fatality have occurred on rare occasions with the use of local anesthetics, even in the absence of a history of hypersensitivity.

Administer ester-type local anesthetics cautiously to patients with abnormal or reduced levels of plasma esterases.

➤*Sulfite sensitivity:* Some of these products contain sulfites. Sulfites may cause allergic-type reactions (eg, hives, itching, wheezing, anaphylaxis) in certain susceptible people. Although the overall prevalence of sulfite sensitivity in the general population is probably low, it is seen more frequently in asthmatics or in atopic nonasthmatic people.

➤*Renal function impairment:* Use **mepivacaine** with caution in patients with renal disease.

➤*Hepatic function impairment:* Because amide-type local anesthetics are metabolized primarily in the liver and ester-type local anesthetics are hydrolyzed by plasma cholinesterase produced by the liver, patients with hepatic disease, especially severe hepatic disease, may be more susceptible to potential toxicity. Use cautiously in such patients.

➤*Special risk:*

Debilitated patients/acutely ill patients/elderly patients/children – Repeated doses may cause accumulation of the drug or its metabolites or slow metabolic degradation. Give reduced doses. Use anesthetics with caution in patients with severe disturbances of cardiac rhythm, hypotension, shock, or heart block. Also use local anesthetics with caution in patients with impaired cardiovascular function because they may be less able to compensate for functional changes associated with the prolongation of A-V conduction produced by these drugs.

➤*Pregnancy:* *Category B* (**levobupivacaine**, **lidocaine**, **prilocaine**, **ropivacaine**). *Category C* (**bupivacaine**, **chloroprocaine**, **mepivacaine**, **procaine**, **tetracaine**). Safety for use in pregnant women, other than those in labor, has not been established. Local anesthetics rapidly cross the placenta. When used for epidural, caudal, paracervical, or pudendal block, they can cause varying degrees of maternal, fetal, and neonatal toxicity involving alterations of the CNS, peripheral vascular tone, and cardiac function. The incidence and degree of toxicity depend upon the procedure, type and amount of drug used, and technique of administration.

Labor, delivery, and abortion – Fetal bradycardia and fetal acidosis may occur in patients receiving anesthetics for paracervical block. Always monitor fetal heart rate prior to and during paracervical anesthesia. Added risk appears to be present in prematurity, toxemia of pregnancy, and fetal distress. Weigh the possible advantages against dangers when considering paracervical block in these conditions. The use of some local anesthetics during labor and delivery may be followed by diminished muscle strength and tone for the infant's first day or 2 of life.

Careful adherence to recommended dosage is extremely important. Failure to achieve adequate analgesia via intended paracervical or pudendal block or both with these doses may indicate intravascular or fetal intracranial injection. Babies so affected present with unexplained neonatal depression at birth and usually manifest seizures within 6 hours. Prompt use of supportive measures and forced urinary excretion of the local anesthetic have been used successfully.

Maternal hypotension – Maternal hypotension has resulted from regional anesthesia. Local anesthetics produce vasodilation by blocking sympathetic nerves. Elevating the patient's legs and positioning her on her left side will help prevent decreases in blood pressure. Continuously monitor fetal heart rate; electronic monitoring is advisable. It is extremely important to avoid aortacaval compression by the gravid uterus during administration of regional block.

Epidural, caudal, paracervical, or pudendal anesthesia – These may alter the forces of parturition through changes in uterine contractility or maternal expulsive efforts. Epidural anesthesia has been reported to prolong the second stage of labor by removing the parturient's reflex urge to bear down or by interfering with motor function. The use of obstetrical anesthesia may increase the need for forceps assistance.

Rapid absorption – Maternal convulsions and cardiovascular collapse following use of some local anesthetics for paracervical block in early pregnancy (as anesthesia for elective abortion) suggest that systemic absorption may be rapid. Therefore, do not exceed the recommended maximum dose. Inject slowly, with frequent aspirations. Allow a 5-minute interval between sides.

➤*Lactation:* Safety for use in the nursing mother has not been established. **Bupivacaine** has been reported to be excreted in breast milk. However, it is not known whether local anesthetic drugs are excreted in breast milk.

➤*Children:* Because of lack of clinical experience, the administration of **bupivacaine** to children younger than 12 years of age and bupivacaine 0.75% in dextrose to children younger than 18 years of age is not recommended.

Safety and efficacy of **tetracaine**, **levobupivacaine**, and **ropivacaine** in children have not been established.

Lidocaine 0.5% to 2% with or without epinephrine (except for dentistry indications) is not indicated in children 3 years of age and younger. Lidocaine 5% in dextrose is not indicated in children younger than 16 years of age. Lidocaine 1.5% in dextrose is not indicated in children.

Chloroprocaine is not indicated in children younger than 3 years of age.

Reduce dosages in children, commensurate with age, body weight, and physical condition.

➤*Elderly:* Repeated doses may cause accumulation of the drug or its metabolites or slow metabolic degradation; give reduced doses. Take care in dose selection, starting at the low end of the dosage range; it may be useful to monitor renal function.

Drug Interactions

Some preparations contain vasoconstrictors. Keep this in mind when using concurrently with other drugs that may interact with vasoconstrictors (refer to the Vasopressors Used in Shock) monographs.

➤*Intercurrent use:* Mixtures of local anesthetics are sometimes employed to compensate for the slower onset of one drug and the shorter duration of action of the second drug. Toxicity is probably additive with mixtures of local anesthetics, but some experiments suggest synergisms. Exercise caution regarding toxic equivalence when mixtures of local anesthetics are employed.

➤*CYP450:* The metabolism of **levobupivacaine** may be affected by the known CYP3A4 inducers (eg, phenytoin, phenobarbital, rifampin), CYP3A4 inhibitors (azole antimycotics [eg, ketoconazole]; certain protease inhibitors [eg, ritonavir]; macrolide antibiotics [eg, erythromycin]; and calcium channel antagonists [eg, verapamil]), CYP1A2 inducers (omeprazole), and CYP1A2 inhibitors (furafylline and clarithromycin). Dosage adjustment may be warranted when levobupivacaine is concurrently administered with CYP3A4 inhibitors and CYP1A2 inhibitors, as systemic levobupivacaine levels may rise, resulting in toxicity.

The plasma concentration of **ropivacaine** was reduced 70% during coadministration of fluvoxamine (25 mg twice daily for 2 days), a selective and potent CYP1A2 inhibitor. Thus strong inhibitors of cytochrome P4501A2 such as fluvoxamine, given concomitantly during administration of ropivacaine, can interact with ropivacaine, leading to increased ropivacaine plasma levels. Exercise caution when CYP1A2 inhibitors are coadministered. Possible interactions with drugs known to be metabolized by CYP1A2 via competitive inhibition (eg, theophylline, imipramine) may also occur. Coadministration of a selective and potent inhibitor of CYP3A4, ketoconazole (100 mg twice daily for 2 days with ropivacaine infusion administered 1 hour after ketoconazole) caused a 15% reduction in in vivo plasma clearance of ropivacaine.

Injectable Local Anesthetic Drug Interactions

Precipitant drug	Object drug[a]		Description
Local anesthetics	Sedatives	↑	If employed to reduce patient apprehension during dental procedures, use reduced doses, since local anesthetics used in combination with CNS depressants may have additive effects. Give young children minimal doses of each agent.
Local anesthetics	Sulfonamides	↓	The para-aminobenzoic acid metabolite of procaine, chloroprocaine, and tetracaine inhibits the action of sulfonamides. Therefore, do not use procaine, chloroprocaine, or tetracaine in any condition in which a sulfonamide drug is employed.

[a] ↑ = object drug increased; ↓ = object drug decreased.

Adverse Reactions

The most common acute adverse reactions are related to the CNS and cardiovascular systems. These are generally dose-related and may result from overdosage, rapid absorption from the injection site, diminished tolerance, or unintentional intravascular injection.

➤*Cardiovascular:* Bradycardia, cardiac arrest, decreased cardiac output, fetal bradycardia (see Warnings), heart block, hypertension, hypotension (with spinal anesthesia caused by vasomotor paralysis and pooling of blood in the venous bed), myocardial depression, ventricular arrhythmias (including tachycardia and fibrillation).

➤*CNS:* Anxiety, blurred vision, chills, dizziness, pupil constriction, restlessness, tinnitus, or tremors may occur, possibly proceeding to convulsions (approximately 0.1% of local anesthetic epidural administrations). Excitement may be transient or absent, with depression being the first manifestation. This may quickly be followed by drowsiness merging into unconsciousness and respiratory arrest.

Apprehension, arachnoiditis, cold, double vision, euphoria, meningismus, numbness, palsies, postspinal headache, sensation of heat, and spinal nerve paralysis (spinal anesthesia) have also occurred.

➤*GI:* Nausea, vomiting.

➤*Hypersensitivity:* Anaphylactoid symptoms (including severe hypotension), angioneurotic edema (including laryngeal edema), elevated temperature, excessive sweating, cutaneous lesions, erythema, pruritus, urticaria, sneezing, syncope. Skin testing is of limited value.

➤*Respiratory:* Respiratory impairment or paralysis caused by level of anesthesia (spinal) extending to upper thoracic and cervical segments (see Warnings).

➤*Miscellaneous:* Occasional unintentional penetration of the subarachnoid space by the catheter may occur. Subsequent adverse effects may depend partially on amount of drug administered intrathecally. These may include the following: arachnoiditis; cranial nerve palsies caused by traction on nerves from loss of cerebrospinal fluid; fecal or urinary incontinence; headache and backache; high or total spinal block; hypotension secondary to spinal block; loss of perineal sensation and sexual function; meningismus; paresthesia, weakness, and paralysis of the lower extremities and loss of sphincter control; persistent anesthesia; persistent motor, sensory, or autonomic deficit of some lower spinal segments with slow (several months), incomplete, or no recovery; septic meningitis; slowing of labor and increased incidence of forceps delivery; urinary retention.

Methemoglobinemia – **Prilocaine** may produce dose-dependent methemoglobinemia. While methemoglobin values of less than 20% do not generally produce any clinical symptoms, evaluate the appearance of cyanosis at 2 to 4 hours following administration in terms of the patient's status.

➤*Levobupivacaine:*

Levobupivacaine Adverse Reactions (≥ 1%)	
Adverse reaction	Levobupivacaine (n = 509)
Cardiovascular	
Bradycardia	2.2%
ECG abnormal	3.1%
Hypertension	1%
Hypotension	19.6%
Tachycardia	1.8%
CNS	
Anxiety	1%
Delivery delayed	6.3%
Dizziness	5.1%
Fetal distress	9.6%
Headache	4.5%
Hypoesthesia	2.6%
Paresthesia	1.8%
Somnolence	1.2%
Dermatologic	
Pruritus	3.7%
Purpura	1.4%
GI	
Abdomen enlarged	2.9%
Abdominal pain	2.2%
Constipation	2.8%
Diarrhea	1%
Dyspepsia	2%
Flatulence	2.4%
Nausea	11.6%
Vomiting	8.3%
GU	
Albuminuria	2.9%
Breast pain (female)	1%
Hematuria	2%
Urinary incontinence	1.2%
Urinary tract infection	1%
Urine abnormal	1.8%
Urine flow decreased	1%
Miscellaneous	
Anemia	9.6%
Anesthesia, local	1%
Back pain	5.7%
Coughing	1.2%
Diplopia	2.6%
Fever	6.5%
Hemorrhage in pregnancy	1.8%
Hypothermia	2.2%
Leukocytosis	1.2%
Pain	3.5%
Postoperative pain	7.3%
Rigors	2.9%
Wound drainage increased	1.4%

The following adverse events were reported at an overall rate of less than 1% and were considered clinically relevant.

Cardiovascular – Arrhythmia, atrial fibrillation, cardiac arrest, extrasystoles, postural hypotension.

CNS – Confusion, hypokinesia, involuntary muscle contraction, spasm (generalized), syncope, tremor.

Dermatologic – Increased sweating, skin discoloration.

Respiratory – Apnea, bronchospasm, dyspnea, pulmonary edema, respiratory insufficiency.

Miscellaneous – Asthenia, edema, elevated bilirubin, ileus.

➤*Ropivacaine:* For the indications of epidural administration in surgery, Cesarean section, postoperative pain management, peripheral nerve block, and local infiltration, the following treatment-emergent adverse events were reported with an incidence of 5% or greater in all clinical studies (n = 3988): hypotension (37%); nausea (24.8%); vomiting (11.6%); bradycardia (9.3%); fever (9.2%); pain (8%); postoperative complications (7.1%); anemia (6.1%); paresthesia (5.6%); headache, pruritus (5.1%); back pain (5%).

Anxiety, chest pain, cramps, dizziness, dyspnea, hypertension, hypesthesia, hypokalemia, oliguria, rigors, tachycardia, urinary retention, and urinary tract infection occurred with an incidence of 1% to 5%.

Ropivacaine Adverse Events (≥ 1%) in Adult Patients Receiving Regional or Local Anesthesia[a]		
Adverse reaction	Ropivacaine (n = 1661)	Bupivacaine (n =1433)
Cardiovascular		
Bradycardia	5.8%	5.1%
Hypotension	32.3%	28.5%
CNS		
Anxiety	1.3%	0.8%
Dizziness	2.5%	1.6%
Headache	5.1%	4.7%
Paresthesia	4.9%	4%
GI		
Nausea	17%	14.4%
Vomiting	7%	6.1%
GU		
Breast disorder, breast feeding	1.3%	0.8%
Urinary retention	1.4%	1.4%
Miscellaneous		
Back pain	4.4%	5.2%
Fever	3.7%	2.6%
Hypesthesia	1.6%	1.7%
Pain	4.3%	5%
Postoperative complications	2.5%	3.1%
Progression of labor poor/failed	1.4%	1.5%
Pruritus	3.8%	2.8%
Rhinitis	1.1%	0.9%
Rigors (chills)	2.5%	1.7%

[a] Surgery, labor, Cesarean section, postoperative pain management, peripheral nerve block, local infiltration.

The following adverse events were reported during the clinical program in more than 1 patient (n = 3988), occurred at an overall incidence of less than 1%, and were considered relevant.

Cardiovascular – Atrial fibrillation, deep vein thrombosis, extrasystoles, nonspecific arrhythmias, nonspecific ECG abnormalities, MI, phlebitis, postural hypotension, pulmonary embolism, ST segment changes, syncope, vasovagal reaction.

CNS – Agitation, amnesia, coma, confusion, convulsion, dyskinesia, emotional lability, hallucination, Horner's syndrome, hypokinesia, hypotonia, insomnia, nervousness, neuropathy, nightmares, paresis, ptosis, somnolence, stupor, tremor, vertigo.

Dermatologic – Rash; urticaria.

GI – Fecal incontinence, neonatal vomiting, tenesmus.

GU – Micturition disorder, poor progression of labor, urinary incontinence, uterine atony.

Special senses – Hearing abnormalities, tinnitus, vision abnormalities.

Respiratory – Bronchospasm, coughing.

Miscellaneous – Accident or injury, asthenia, hypomagnesemia, hypothermia, injection-site pain, jaundice, malaise, myalgia.

For the indication of epidural anesthesia for surgery, the 15 most common adverse events were compared between different concentrations of **ropivacaine** and **bupivacaine**. The following table is based on data from trials in the US and other countries where ropivacaine was administered as an epidural anesthetic for surgery.

Ropivacaine vs Bupivacaine Adverse Reactions in Epidural Administration					
	Ropivacaine			Bupivacaine	
Adverse reaction	5 mg/mL (n = 256)	7.5 mg/mL (n = 297)	10 mg/mL (n = 207)	5 mg/mL (n = 236)	7.5 mg/mL (n = 174)
Cardiovascular					
Bradycardia	11.3%	19.5%	19.3%	13.6%	14.4%
Hypotension	38.7%	49.2%	54.6%	38.6%	51.1%
CNS					
Chills	2.3%	2.4%	2.9%	1.7%	1.7%
Headache	4.7%	6.7%	7.7%	5.5%	5.2%
Paresthesia	2%	3.4%	2.4%	3%	—

Ropivacaine vs Bupivacaine Adverse Reactions in Epidural Administration					
	Ropivacaine			Bupivacaine	
Adverse reaction	5 mg/mL (n = 256)	7.5 mg/mL (n = 297)	10 mg/mL (n = 207)	5 mg/mL (n = 236)	7.5 mg/mL (n = 174)
GI					
Nausea	13.3%	22.9%	—	17.4%	20.7%
Vomiting	7%	11.1%	11.1%	8.1%	8%
Miscellaneous					
Back pain	7%	7.7%	16.4%	8.9%	13.2%
Fever	3.1%	1.7%	8.7%	4.7%	—
Pruritus	—	4.7%	1.4%	—	4%
Urinary retention	2%	2.7%	4.8%	4.2%	—

Overdosage

Acute emergencies from local anesthetics are generally related to high plasma levels encountered during therapeutic use or to unintended subarachnoid injection.

➤*Management:* The first consideration is prevention.

Convulsions – Convulsions, as well as underventilation or apnea, are caused by unintentional subarachnoid injection; maintain patent airway and assist or control ventilation with oxygen and a delivery system capable of permitting immediate positive airway pressure by mask. Evaluate circulation. If convulsions persist despite respiratory support, and if the status of the circulation permits, give small increments of an ultra short-acting barbiturate (eg, thiopental) or a benzodiazepine (eg, diazepam) IV. Circulatory depression may require administration of IV fluids and a vasopressor.

If not treated immediately, convulsions and cardiovascular depression can result in hypoxia, acidosis, bradycardia, arrhythmias, and cardiac arrest. Underventilation or apnea may produce these same signs and also lead to cardiac arrest if ventilatory support is not instituted. If cardiac arrest occurs, institute standard cardiopulmonary resuscitative measures.

Endotracheal intubation may be indicated.

The supine position is dangerous in pregnant women at term because of aortacaval compression by the gravid uterus. Therefore, during treatment of systemic toxicity, maternal hypotension or fetal bradycardia following regional block, maintain the parturient in the left lateral decubitus position if possible, or accomplish manual displacement of the uterus off the great vessels. Resuscitation of obstetrical patients may take longer than resuscitation of nonpregnant patients and closed-chest cardiac compression may be ineffective. Rapid delivery of the fetus may improve the response to resuscitation efforts.

Patient Information

When appropriate, inform patients in advance that they may experience temporary loss of sensation and motor activity, usually in the lower half of the body, following proper administration of caudal or epidural anesthesia.

Advise the patient to exert caution to avoid inadvertent trauma to the lips, tongue, cheek, mucosae, or soft palate when these structures are anesthetized. The ingestion of food should therefore be postponed until normal function returns.

Advise the patient to consult the dentist if anesthesia persists or a rash develops.

Amide Local Anesthetics

BUPIVACAINE HYDROCHLORIDE

Rx	**Bupivacaine HCl** (Hospira)	**Injection, solution:** 0.25%	In 20, 30, and 50 mL amps, 10 and 30 mL vials, 50 mL multidose vials,[a] and 50 mL *Abboject*.
Rx	**Marcaine** (Hospira)		In 50 mL single-dose amps, 10 and 30 mL single-dose vials, 50 mL multidose vials.[a]
Rx	**Sensorcaine** (APP Pharmaceutical)		In 50[a] mL multidose vials.
Rx	**Sensorcaine MPF** (APP Pharmaceutical)		In 30 mL single-dose amps and 10 and 30 mL single-dose vials.
Rx	**Bupivacaine HCl** (Hospira)	**Injection, solution:** 0.5%	In 10 and 30 mL vials, 20 and 30 mL amps, 30 mL *Abboject*, and 50 mL multidose vials.[a]
Rx	**Marcaine** (Hospira)		In 10 and 30 mL single-dose vials, 30 mL single-dose amps, and 50 mL multidose vials.[a]
Rx	**Sensorcaine** (APP Pharmaceutical)		In 50[a] mL multidose vials.
Rx	**Sensorcaine MPF** (APP Pharmaceutical)		In 10 and 30 mL single-dose vials.
Rx	**Bupivacaine HCl** (Hospira)	**Injection, solution:** 0.75%	In 20 and 30 mL amps and 10 and 30 mL vials.
Rx	**Marcaine** (Hospira)		In 30 mL single-dose amps and 10 and 30 mL single-dose vials.
Rx	**Sensorcaine MPF** (APP Pharmaceutical)		In 30 mL single-dose amps and 10 and 30 mL single-dose vials.
Rx	**Bupivacaine HCl with Epinephrine 1:200,000** (Hospira)	**Injection, solution:** 0.25% with 1:200,000 epinephrine	In 50 mL amps, 10 and 30 mL vials, and 50 mL flip-top multidose vials.[a]
Rx	**Marcaine** (Hospira)		In 50 mL amps[b] and 10,[b] 30,[b] and 50[a,b] mL vials.
Rx	**Sensorcaine** (APP Pharmaceutical)		In 50 mL multidose vials.[a]
Rx	**Sensorcaine MPF** (APP Pharmaceutical)		In 10 and 30 mL single-dose vials.[c]
Rx	**Bupivacaine HCl with Epinephrine 1:200,000** (Hospira)	**Injection, solution:** 0.5% with 1:200,000 epinephrine	In 30 mL amps, 10 and 30 mL vials, and 50 mL flip-top multidose vials.[a]
Rx	**Marcaine** (Hospira)		In 3 and 30 mL single-dose amps[b] and 10 and 30 mL single-dose vials.[b]
Rx	**Sensorcaine** (APP Pharmaceutical)		In 50 mL multidose vials.[a]
Rx	**Sensorcaine MPF** (APP Pharmaceutical)		In 5 mL single-dose amps and 10 and 30 mL single-dose vials.[c]
Rx	**Marcaine** (Eastman-Kodak)		In 1.8 mL dental cartridges.[b]
Rx	**Bupivacaine HCl with Epinephrine 1:200,000** (Hospira)	**Injection, solution:** 0.75% with 1:200,000 epinephrine	In 30 mL amps.
Rx	**Marcaine** (Hospira)		In 30 mL amps.[b]
Rx	**Sensorcaine MPF** (APP Pharmaceutical)		In 30 mL single-dose vials.[c]
Rx	**Bupivacaine Spinal** (Abbott)	**Injection, solution:** 0.75% in 8.25% dextrose	Preservative-free. In 2 mL amps.
Rx	**Sensorcaine-MPF Spinal** (APP Pharmaceutical)		In 2 mL amps.

[a] With 1 mg methylparaben per mL.
[b] With 0.5 mg sodium metabisulfite and 0.1 mg EDTA per mL.
[c] With 0.5 mg sodium metabisulfite per mL.

BUPIVACAINE HYDROCHLORIDE — INJECTION

For complete and comparative prescribing information, refer to the Injectable Local Anesthetics group monograph.

WARNING

Injection – The 0.75% concentration of bupivacaine is not recommended for obstetrical anesthesia. There have been reports of cardiac arrest with difficult resuscitation or death during use of bupivacaine for epidural anesthesia in obstetrical patients. In most cases, this has followed use of the 0.75% concentration. Resuscitation has been difficult or impossible despite apparently adequate preparation and appropriate management. Cardiac arrest has occurred after convulsions resulting from systemic toxicity, presumably following unintentional intravascular injection. The 0.75% concentration should be reserved for surgical procedures where a high degree of muscle relaxation and prolonged effect are necessary.

Indications

➤*Injection:* For the production of local or regional anesthesia or analgesic for surgery, dental and oral surgery procedures, diagnostic and therapeutic procedures, and for obstetrical procedures. Only the 0.25% and 0.5% concentrations are indicated for obstetrical anesthesia.

Experience with nonobstetrical surgical procedures in pregnant patients is not sufficient to recommend use of 0.75% concentration of bupivacaine hydrochloride in these patients.

Bupivacaine hydrochloride is not recommended for IV regional anesthesia (Bier Block).

The routes of administration and indicated bupivacaine hydrochloride concentrations are local infiltration (0.25%); peripheral nerve block (0.25% and 0.5%); retrobulbar block (0.75%); sympathetic block (0.25%); lumbar epidural (0.25%, 0.5%, and 0.75%) (0.75% not for obstetrical anesthesia); caudal (0.25% and 0.5%); epidural test dose (0.5% with epinephrine 1:200,000); dental blocks (0.5% with epinephrine 1:200,000).

➤*Dextrose injection for spinal anesthesia:* Bupivacaine hydrochloride spinal is indicated for the production of subarachnoid block (spinal anesthesia). Standard textbooks should be consulted to determine the accepted procedures and techniques for the administration of spinal anesthesia.

Administration and Dosage

➤*General dosing considerations:* In recommended doses, bupivacaine produces complete sensory block, but the effect on motor function differs among the 3 concentrations.

0.25% – When used for caudal, epidural, or peripheral nerve block, produces incomplete motor block. Should be used for operations in which muscle relaxation is not important, or when another means of providing muscle relaxation is used concurrently. Onset of action may be slower than with the 0.5% or 0.75% solutions.

0.5% – Provides motor blockade for caudal, epidural, or nerve block, but muscle relaxation may be inadequate for operations in which complete muscle relaxation is essential.

0.75% – Produces complete motor block. Most useful for epidural block in abdominal operations requiring complete muscle relaxation, and for retrobulbar anesthesia. Not for obstetrical anesthesia.

A test dose may be needed for caudal and epidural blocks. (See Test Dose.)

➤*Adults:*

Anesthesia –

Usual dosage:

These doses may be repeated up to once every 3 hours. The duration of anesthetic effect may be prolonged by the addition of epinephrine. The duration of anesthesia with bupivacaine is such that for most indications, a single dose is sufficient.

Bupivacaine Recommended Concentrations and Doses

Type of block	Concentration	Each dose (mL)	Each dose (mg)	Motor block[a]
Local infiltration	0.25%[b]	up to maximum	up to maximum	-
Epidural	0.75%[b,c]	10 to 20	75 to 150	complete
	0.5%[b]	10 to 20	50 to 100	moderate to complete
	0.25%[b]	10 to 20	25 to 50	partial to moderate
Caudal	0.5%[b]	15 to 30	75 to 150	moderate to complete
	0.25%[b]	15 to 30	37.5 to 75	moderate
Peripheral nerves	0.5%[b]	5 to max	25 to max	moderate to complete
	0.25%[b]	5 to max	12.5 to max	moderate to complete
Retrobulbar	0.75%[b]	2 to 4	15 to 30	complete
Sympathetic	0.25%	20 to 50	50 to 125	-
Dental	0.5% w/epinephrine	1.8 to 3.6 per site	9 to 18 per site	-
Epidural test dose	0.5% w/epinephrine	2 to 3	10 to 15 (10 to 15 mcg epinephrine)	-

[a] With continuous (intermittent) techniques, repeat doses increase the degree of motor block. The first repeat dose of 0.5% may produce complete motor block. Intercostal nerve block with 0.25% may also produce complete motor block for intra-abdominal surgery.

[b] Solutions with or without epinephrine.

[c] For single-dose use, not for intermittent epidural technique. Not for obstetrical anesthesia.

Maximum dose: 400 mg total in 24 hours

Dentistry –

Usual dosage: The 0.5% concentration with epinephrine is recommended for infiltration and block injection in the maxillary and mandibular area when a longer duration of local anesthetic action is desired, such as for oral surgical procedures generally associated with significant postoperative pain. The average dose of 1.8 mL (9 mg) per injection site will usually suffice; an occasional second dose of 1.8 mL (9 mg) may be used if necessary to produce adequate anesthesia after making allowance for 2 to 10 minutes onset time (see Pharmacokinetics). The lowest effective dose should be employed and time should be allowed between injections.

Maximum dose: Total dose for all injection sites over a single dental sitting should not exceed 90 mg (ten 1.8 mL injections of bupivacaine 0.5% with epinephrine).

Epidural anesthesia (preservative-free) – Use only the single-dose ampules and single-dose vials for epidural anesthesia; the multiple-dose vials contain a preservative and, therefore, should not be used for these procedures.

Usual dosage: 3 to 5 mL increments of 0.5% and 0.75% solutions with sufficient time between doses to detect toxic manifestations of unintentional intravascular or intrathecal injection. Repeat doses should be preceded by a test dose containing epinephrine if not contraindicated.

Obstetrics: Use only the 0.5% and 0.25% concentrations; incremental doses of 3 mL to 5 mL of the 0.5% solution not exceeding 50 to 100 mg at any dosing interval are recommended.

Spinal anesthesia (with dextrose) –

Usual dosage: 7.5 mg (1 mL) bupivacaine spinal has generally proven satisfactory for spinal anesthesia for lower extremity and perineal procedures including TURP and vaginal hysterectomy. 12 mg (1.6 mL) has been used for lower abdominal procedures such as abdominal hysterectomy, tubal ligation, and appendectomy.

- *Vaginal delivery* – Doses as low as 6 mg.
- *Cesarean section* – 7.5 to 10.5 mg (1 to 1.4 mL).

➤*Children:*

Anesthesia –

12 years of age and older: See Adults for dosing.

Dentistry –

12 years of age and older: See Adults for dosing.

Epidural anesthesia (preservative-free) –

12 years of age and older: See Adults for dosing.

➤*Elderly:* Dosages should be reduced for the elderly.

➤*Hepatic function impairment:* Dosages should be reduced for patients with liver disease.

➤*Special risk patients:* Dosages should be reduced for debilitated or acutely ill patients and patients with cardiac disease.

➤*Test dose:* The test dose of bupivacaine (bupivacaine 0.5% with 1:200,000 epinephrine in a 3 mL ampul) is recommended for use as a test dose when clinical conditions permit prior to caudal and lumbar epidural blocks. This may serve as a warning of unintended intravascular or subarachnoid injection. The pulse rate and other signs should be monitored carefully immediately following each test dose administration to detect possible intravascular injection, and adequate time for onset of spinal block should be allotted to detect possible intrathecal injection. An intravascular or subarachnoid injection is still possible even if results of the test dose are negative. The test dose itself may produce a systemic toxic reaction, high spinal or cardiovascular effects from the epinephrine (see Warnings/Precautions and Overdosage).

➤*Administration:* The rapid injection of a large volume of local anesthetic solution should be avoided and fractional (incremental) doses should be used when feasible.

Dentistry – Injections should be made slowly and with frequent aspirations.

➤*Admixture compatibility:* Mixing or the prior or intercurrent use of any other local anesthetic with bupivacaine cannot be recommended because of insufficient data on the clinical use of such mixtures.

➤*Storage/Stability:* Store between 15° and 30°C (59° and 86°F). Unused portions of solution not containing preservatives (ie, single-dose ampuls and single-dose vials) and spinal solutions should be discarded following initial use. Bupivacaine spinal solution may be autoclaved once at 15 pound pressure, 121°C (250°F) for 15 minutes.

Amide Local Anesthetics

LIDOCAINE HYDROCHLORIDE

Rx	**Lidocaine HCl** (Various, eg, Hospira)	**Injection:** 0.5%	In 50 mL single-dose vials and 50 mL multidose vials.[a]
Rx	**Xylocaine** (APP Pharmaceutical)		In 50 mL multidose vials.[b]
Rx	**Xylocaine MPF** (APP Pharmaceutical)		In 50 mL single-dose vials.
Rx	**Lidocaine HCl** (Various, eg, Hospira, American Regent)	**Injection:** 1%	In 2 and 5 mL amps, 5 mL vials,[c] 30 mL single-dose vials, 20,[a] 30,[a] and 50 mL[a] multidose vials, 5 mL syringes, and cartridges.
Rx	**Xylocaine** (APP Pharmaceutical)		In 10, 20, and 50 mL multidose vials.[b]
Rx	**Xylocaine MPF** (APP Pharmaceutical)		In 2, 5 and 30 mL amps, 10 and 20 mL *PolyAmp DuoFit*, and 2, 5, 10, and 30 mL single-dose vials.
Rx	**Lidocaine HCl** (Various, eg, Hospira)	**Injection:** 1.5%	In 20 mL amps.
Rx	**Xylocaine MPF** (APP Pharmaceutical)		In 20 mL amps, 10 and 20 mL *PolyAmp DuoFit*, and 5 and 10 mL single-dose vials.
Rx	**Lidocaine HCl** (Various, eg, Hospira, American Regent)	**Injection:** 2%	In 2 and 10 mL amps, 5 mL vials,[c] 10 mL single-dose vials, 20[a] and 50 mL[a] multidose vials, and 5 mL syringes.
Rx	**Xylocaine** (APP Pharmaceutical)		In 10, 20, and 50 mL multidose vials[b] and 1.8 mL cartridges.
Rx	**Xylocaine MPF** (APP Pharmaceutical)		In 2 and 10 mL amps, 10 mL *PolyAmp DuoFit*, and 2, 5, and 10 mL single-dose vials.
Rx	**Lidocaine HCl** (Hospira)	**Injection:** 4%	In 5 mL single-dose amps.
Rx	**Xylocaine MPF** (APP Pharmaceutical)		In 5 mL amps and 5 mL syringe with laryngotracheal cannula.
Rx	**Lidocaine and Epinephrine** (Abbott)	**Injection:** 0.5% with 1:200,000 epinephrine	In 50 mL multidose vials.[d]
Rx	**Xylocaine** (APP Pharmaceutical)		In 50 mL multidose vials.[b]
Rx	**Lidocaine and Epinephrine** (Abbott)	**Injection:** 1% with 1:100,000 epinephrine	In 20, 30, and 50 mL multidose vials.[d]
Rx	**Xylocaine** (APP Pharmaceutical)		In 10, 20, and 50 mL multidose vials.[b]
Rx	**Lidocaine and Epinephrine** (Abbott)	**Injection:** 1% with 1:200,000 epinephrine	In 30 mL single-dose amps.[e]
Rx	**Xylocaine MPF** (APP Pharmaceutical)		In 30 mL amps and 5, 10, and 30 mL single-dose vials.[e]
Rx	**Lidocaine HCl** (Abbott)	**Injection:** 1.5% with 1:200,000 epinephrine	In 5 and 30 mL amps and 30 mL single-dose vials.[e]
Rx	**Lidocaine and Epinephrine** (Abbott)		In 5 and 30 mL single-dose amps and 30 mL single-dose vials.[e]
Rx	**Xylocaine MPF** (APP Pharmaceutical)		In 5 and 30 mL amps and 5, 10, and 30 mL single-dose vials.[e]
Rx	**Lidocaine HCl and Epinephrine** (Eastman Kodak)	**Injection:** 2% with 1:50,000 epinephrine	In 1.8 mL dental cartridges.[e]
Rx	**Octocaine** (Septodont)		In 1.8 mL cartridges.[f]
Rx	**Xylocaine** (APP Pharmaceutical)		In 1.8 mL dental cartridges.[e]
Rx	**Lidocaine and Epinephrine** (Various, eg, Abbott, Eastman Kodak)	**Injection:** 2% with 1:100,000 epinephrine	In 1.8 mL cartridges and 20, 30, and 50 mL multidose vials.[g]
Rx	**Xylocaine** (APP Pharmaceutical)		In 10[e], 20[e] and 50 mL[e] multidose vials and 1.8 mL cartridges.[f]
Rx	**Lidocaine and Epinephrine** (Abbott)	**Injection:** 2% with 1:200,000 epinephrine	In 20 mL single-dose vials.[e]
Rx	**Xylocaine MPF** (APP Pharmaceutical)		In 20 mL amps and 5, 10, and 20 mL single-dose vials.[e]
Rx	**Lidocaine HCl** (Abbott)	**Injection:** 1.5% with 7.5% dextrose	In 2 mL amps.
Rx	**Xylocaine** (APP Pharmaceutical)		In 2 mL amps.
Rx	**Xylocaine-MPF** (APP Pharmaceutical)		In 2 mL amps.
Rx	**Lidocaine HCl** (Abbott)	**Injection:** 5% with 7.5% dextrose	In 2 mL single-dose amps.
Rx	**Xylocaine MPF** (APP Pharmaceutical)		In 2 mL amps.

[a] May contain methylparaben.
[b] With methylparaben.
[c] Preservative-free.
[d] With methylparaben and sodium metabisulfite.
[e] With sodium metabisulfite.
[f] With sodium bisulfite.
[g] May contain sodium metabisulfite and methylparaben.

LIDOCAINE HYDROCHLORIDE — INJECTION

For complete and comparative prescribing information, refer to the Injectable Local Anesthetics group monograph.

Indications

➤*For infiltration and nerve block:* For production of local or regional anesthesia by infiltration techniques such as percutaneous injection and intravenous (IV) regional anesthesia by peripheral nerve block techniques such as brachial plexus and intercostal and by central neural techniques such as lumbar and caudal epidural blocks, when the accepted procedures for these techniques as described in standard textbooks are observed.

➤*For cardiac arrhythmias:*

IV – In the acute management of:

1.) Ventricular arrhythmias occurring during cardiac manipulation, such as cardiac surgery.
2.) Life-threatening arrhythmias, particularly those which are ventricular in origin, such as those which occur during acute MI.

IM – Single doses are justified in the following exceptional circumstances: When ECG equipment is not available to verify the diagnosis but the potential benefits outweigh the possible risks; when facilities for IV administration are not readily available; by the patient in the prehospital phase of suspected acute MI, directed by qualified medical personnel viewing the transmitted ECG.

➤*Off-label uses:*

Cough (fentanyl induced) – [3] = Safety concerns. Initial data from 3 large controlled trials suggest that lidocaine, in varying doses, is effective in reducing fentanyl-induced cough. The lowest effective dose studied to date was 0.5 mg/kg administered 1 minute prior to fentanyl administration. Some clinicians have raised concerns regarding the need for another drug during the induction of anesthesia that might carry an increased risk of adverse reactions.

Cough suppression (inhaled lidocaine) – [4] = Insufficient documentation. Evidence from a limited number of controlled and noncontrolled studies evaluating the use of nebulized lidocaine in the treatment of cough suggests that this agent may be of use in refractory cases.

Hiccups (singultus) – [3] = Safety concerns. IV lidocaine may be an useful alternative in patients with intractable hiccups from various causes that

LIDOCAINE HYDROCHLORIDE — INJECTION

have been unresponsive to other therapies. However, because current information is limited to isolated case reports, more information is needed before this agent can be recommended routinely.

Other possible off-label uses – In pediatric patients with cardiac arrest, less than 10% develop ventricular fibrillation, and others develop ventricular tachycardia; the hemodynamically compromised child may develop ventricular couplets or frequent premature ventricular beats. In these cases, lidocaine 1 mg/kg should be administered by the IV, intraosseous, or endotracheal route. A second 1 mg/kg dose may be given in 10 to 15 minutes. Start a lidocaine infusion if the second dose is required; a third bolus may be needed in 10 to 15 minutes to maintain therapeutic levels.

Administration and Dosage

➤*Maximum dose:*

Adults – The following maximum doses are according to the prescribing information.

Cardiac arrhythmias: 200 to 300 mg, administered during a 1-hour period.
IV regional anesthesia: 4 mg/kg.
Paracervical block: 200 mg total per 90-minute period in obstetric and nonobstetric patients.

There are no well-established maximum doses for the other approved indications according to the prescribing information.

Children – Total dosages not to exceed 3 mg/kg (1.4 mg/lb) for induction of IV regional anesthesia according to the prescribing information. There is no well-established maximum dose for the other approved indication according to the prescribing information.

➤*General dosing considerations:*

Infiltration and nerve block – These recommended doses serve only as a guide to the amount of anesthetic required for most routine procedures. The actual volumes and concentrations to be used depend on a number of factors, such as type and extent of surgical procedure, depth of anesthesia, degree of muscular relaxation required, duration of anesthesia required, and the physical condition of the patient. In all cases, the lowest concentration and smallest dose that will produce the desired result should be given.

Dosages should be reduced for debilitated patients and for patients with cardiac disease.

The onset of anesthesia, the duration of anesthesia, and the degree of muscular relaxation are proportional to the volume and concentration (ie, total dose) of local anesthetic used. Thus, an increase in volume and concentration of lidocaine hydrochloride injection will decrease the onset of anesthesia, prolong the duration of anesthesia, provide a greater degree of muscular relaxation, and increase the segmental spread of anesthesia. However, increasing the volume and concentration of lidocaine hydrochloride injection may result in a more profound fall in blood pressure when used in epidural anesthesia. Although the incidence of adverse effects with lidocaine hydrochloride is quite low, caution should be exercised when employing large volumes and concentrations because the incidence of adverse effects is directly proportional to the total dose of local anesthetic agent injected.

IV regional anesthesia – For IV regional anesthesia, only the 50 mL, single-dose vial containing lidocaine hydrochloride 0.5% injection should be used.

Epidural anesthesia – For epidural anesthesia, only the following dosage forms of lidocaine hydrochloride injection are recommended:

Lidocaine Epidural Anesthesia Dosage Forms	
1% without epinephrine	10 mL *Polyamp DuoFit*
1% without epinephrine	20 mL *Polyamp DuoFit*
1% without epinephrine	30 mL single-dose solutions
1.5% without epinephrine	10 mL *Polyamp DuoFit*
1.5% without epinephrine	20 mL *Polyamp DuoFit*
1.5% without epinephrine	20 mL ampules, 20 mL single-dose solutions
2% without epinephrine	10 mL *Polyamp DuoFit*
2% without epinephrine	10 mL ampules, 10 mL single-dose solutions

Although these solutions are intended specifically for epidural anesthesia, they may also be used for infiltration and peripheral nerve block, provided they are employed as single-dose units. These solutions contain no bacteriostatic agent.

Lidocaine hydrochloride injection for cardiac arrhythmias – This product is for direct infusion only. For continuous infusion protocol, see information for lidocaine hydrochloride for infusion solution.

Dosage forms listed as lidocaine methylparaben free (MPF) indicate single-dose solutions that are MPF.

➤*Adults:*

Cardiac arrhythmias –

Usual dosage: 50 to 100 mg, administered intravenously (IV) at a rate of approximately 25 to 50 mg/min. Administer under ECG monitoring. Allow a sufficient time to enable a slow circulation to carry the drug to the site of action. If the initial injection of 50 to 100 mg does not produce a desired response, a second dose may be repeated after 5 minutes.

Maximum dose: 200 to 300 mg, administered during a 1-hour period.

Alternative dosage: 300 mg intramuscularly (IM). The deltoid muscle is preferred. Avoid intravascular injection. Use only the 10% solution for IM injection. As soon as possible, change the patient to IV lidocaine or to an oral antiarrhythmic preparation for maintenance therapy. However, if necessary, an additional IM injection may be administered after 60 to 90 minutes.

Caudal and lumbar epidural block –

Usual dosage: See the following table.

Maximum dose: For continuous epidural or caudal anesthesia, the maximum recommended dosage should not be administered at intervals of less than 90 minutes. When continuous lumbar or caudal epidural anesthesia is used for nonobstetric procedures, more drug may be administered if required to produce adequate anesthesia.

Test dose: As a precaution against the adverse reaction sometimes observed following unintentional penetration of the subarachnoid space, a test dose such as 2 to 3 mL of lidocaine hydrochloride 1.5% should be administered at least 5 minutes prior to injecting the total volume required for a lumbar or caudal epidural block. The test dose should be repeated if the patient is moved in a manner that may have displaced the catheter. Epinephrine, if contained in the test dose (10 to 15 mcg has been suggested), may serve as a warning of unintentional intravascular injection. If injected into a blood vessel, this amount of epinephrine is likely to produce a transient "epinephrine response" within 45 seconds, consisting of an increase in heart rate and systolic blood pressure, circumoral pallor, palpitations, and nervousness in the unsedated patient. The sedated patient may exhibit only a pulse rate increase of 20 or more beats/minute for 15 or more seconds. Patients on beta-blockers may not manifest changes in heart rate, but blood pressure monitoring can detect an evanescent rise in systolic blood pressure. Adequate time should be allowed for onset of anesthesia after administration of each test dose. The rapid injection of a large volume of lidocaine hydrochloride injection through the catheter should be avoided, and, when feasible, fractional doses should be administered.

In the event of the known injection of a large volume of local anesthetic solution into the subarachnoid space, after suitable resuscitation and if the catheter is in place, consider attempting the recovery of drug by draining a moderate amount of cerebrospinal fluid (such as 10 mL) through the epidural catheter.

Epidural anesthesia – See the following table.

Dosage varies with the number of dermatomes to be anesthetized (generally 2 to 3 mL of the indicated concentration per dermatome).

IV regional anesthesia –

Usual dosage: See the following table.

Maximum dose: For IV regional anesthesia, the dose administered should not exceed 4 mg/kg in adults.

Paracervical block –

Usual dosage: See the following table.

Maximum dose: 200 mg total per 90-minute period in obstetric and nonobstetric patients. One-half of the total dose is usually administered to each side. Inject slowly, with 5 minutes between sides.

Infiltration and nerve block – The following table summarizes the recommended volumes and concentrations of lidocaine hydrochloride injection for various types of anesthetic procedures. The dosages suggested in this information are for healthy adults and refer to the use of epinephrine-free solutions. When larger volumes are required, only solutions containing epinephrine should be used, except in those cases where vasopressor drugs may be contraindicated.

Lidocaine Recommended Dosages			
	Lidocaine hydrochloride injection (without epinephrine)		
Procedure	Concentration (%)	Volume (mL)	Total dose (mg)
Infiltration			
Percutaneous	0.5 or 1	1 to 60	5 to 300
Intravenous regional	0.5	10 to 60	50 to 300
Peripheral nerve blocks			
Brachial	1.5	15 to 20	225 to 300
Dental	2	1 to 5	20 to 100
Intercostal	1	3	30
Paravertebral	1	3 to 5	30 to 50
Pudendal (each side)	1	10	100
Paracervical			
Obstetrical analgesia (each side)	1	10	100
Sympathetic nerve blocks			
Cervical (stellate ganglion)	1	5	50
Lumbar	1	5 to 10	50 to 100
Central neural blocks[a]			
Thoracic epidural	1	20 to 30	200 to 300
Lumbar epidural (analgesia)	1	25 to 30	250 to 300
Lumbar epidural (anesthesia)	1.5	15 to 20	225 to 300
	2	10 to 15	200 to 300

LIDOCAINE HYDROCHLORIDE — INJECTION

Lidocaine Recommended Dosages			
	Lidocaine hydrochloride injection (without epinephrine)		
Procedure	Concentration (%)	Volume (mL)	Total dose (mg)
Caudal			
Obstetrical analgesia	1	20 to 30	200 to 300
Surgical anesthesia	1.5	15 to 20	225 to 300

[a] Dose determined by number of dermatomes to be anesthetized (2 to 3 mL/dermatome).

The above suggested concentrations and volumes serve only as a guide. Other volumes and concentrations may be used provided the total maximum recommended dose is not exceeded.

Off-label dosing –

Cough (fentanyl induced): [3] = Safety concerns. Lidocaine IV 0.5 to 2 mg/kg, administered 1 minute prior to the administration of fentanyl.

Cough suppression (inhaled lidocaine): [4] = Insufficient documentation. Administered as inhalation/nebulization as a 1 mg/kg dose diluted in isotonic sodium chloride solution (normal saline) to a total volume of 4 mL and administered over a 15- to 25-minute period. Also administered as a 0.25% solution (4 mL) with oxygen 4 to 6 L/min until nebulization is complete and repeated every 4 to 6 hours as needed with concentrated solutions of 1% to 4%.

Hiccups (singultus): [3] = Safety concerns. 1 mg/kg (50 mg) or 1.5 mg/kg (100 mg) IV over 5 minutes or loading dose of 1 mg/kg followed by continuous infusion at 2 to 4 mg/min. Bolus doses of 0.5 mg/kg may be used.

➤*Children:*

Cardiac arrhythmias – Although controlled clinical studies to establish pediatric dosing schedules have not been conducted, the American Heart Associations Standards and Guidelines recommends a bolus dose of 1 mg/kg followed by an infusion rate of 30 mcg/kg/min. Administer under ECG monitoring.

IV regional anesthesia –

Usual dosage: Dosages in children should be reduced, commensurate with age, body weight and physical condition. In order to guard against systemic toxicity, the lowest effective concentration and lowest effective dose should be used at all times. In some cases, it will be necessary to dilute available concentrations with sodium chloride 0.9% injection in order to obtain the required final concentration.

Maximum dose: It is difficult to recommend a maximum dose of any drug for children because this varies as a function of age and weight. For children older than 3 years of age who have a normal lean body mass and normal body development, the maximum dose is determined by the child's age and weight. For example, in a child of 5 years of age weighing 50 lbs, the dose of lidocaine hydrochloride should not exceed 75 to 100 mg (1.5 to 2 mg/lb). The use of even more dilute solutions (ie, 0.25% to 0.5%) and total dosages not to exceed 3 mg/kg (1.4 mg/lb) are recommended for induction of IV regional anesthesia in children.

Off-label dosing –

Hiccups (singultus): [3] = Safety concerns. 1 mg/kg IV.

➤*Elderly:* Elderly patients should be given reduced doses commensurate with their age and physical condition.

➤*Renal function impairment:* Use caution with repeated or prolonged use in renal disease; possible toxic accumulation of lidocaine or its metabolites may occur.

➤*Hepatic function impairment:* Dosages should be reduced for patients with liver disease.

➤*Preparation for administration:*

Sterilization and technical procedures – Disinfecting agents containing heavy metals, which cause release of respective ions (eg, copper, mercury, zinc), should not be used for skin or mucous membrane disinfection because they have been related to incidents of swelling and edema. When chemical disinfection of multidose vials is desired, either isopropyl alcohol (91%) or ethyl alcohol (70%) is recommended. Many commercially available brands of rubbing alcohol, as well as solutions of ethyl alcohol not of USP grade, contain denaturants that are injurious to rubber and therefore are not to be used.

➤*Administration:*

Cardiac arrhythmias –

Adults: Administer lidocaine injection IV at a rate of approximately 25 to 50 mg/min. Administer under ECG monitoring.

Children: Administer a bolus dose, followed by an infusion rate of 30 mcg/kg/min. Administer under ECG monitoring.

Paracervical block – One-half of the total dose is usually administered to each side. Inject slowly, with 5 minutes between sides.

➤*Storage / Stability:* All solutions should be stored at room temperature, approximately 25°C (77°F). Protect from light.

Stable for 24 hours after dilution in 5% dextrose in water.

MEPIVACAINE HYDROCHLORIDE

Rx	**Carbocaine** (Hospira)	**Injection**: 1%	In 30 mL single-dose vials and 50 mL[a] multidose vials.
Rx	**Polocaine** (APP Pharmaceuticals)		In 50 mL multidose vials.[a]
Rx	**Polocaine MPF** (APP Pharmaceutical)		In 30 mL single-dose vials.[a]
Rx	**Carbocaine** (Hospira)	**Injection**: 1.5%	In 30 mL single-dose vials.
Rx	**Polocaine MPF** (APP Pharmaceutical)		In 30 mL single-dose vials.
Rx	**Carbocaine** (Hospira)	**Injection**: 2%	In 20 mL single-dose vials and 50 mL[a] multidose vials.
Rx	**Polocaine** (APP Pharmaceutical)		In 50 mL multidose vials.[a]
Rx	**Polocaine MPF** (APP Pharmaceutical)		In 20 mL single-dose vials.
Rx	**Mepivacaine HCl** (Septodont)	**Injection**: 3%	In 1.8 mL dental cartridge.
Rx	**Carbocaine** (Eastman-Kodak)		In 1.8 mL dental cartridge.[b]
Rx	**Polocaine** (AstraZeneca)		In 1.8 mL dental cartridge.[c]
Rx	**Carbocaine with Neo-Cobefrin** (Eastman-Kodak)	**Injection**: 2% with 1:20,000 levonordefrin	In 1.8 mL dental cartridge.[b]
Rx	**Polocaine with Levonordefrin** (AstraZeneca)		In 1.8 mL dental cartridge.[d]

[a] With methylparaben.
[b] With acetone sodium bisulfite.
[c] With sodium bisulfite.
[d] With sodium metabisulfite.

MEPIVACAINE HYDROCHLORIDE — INJECTION

For complete and comparative prescribing information, refer to the Injectable Local Anesthetics group monograph.

Indications

➤*Peripheral nerve block (eg, cervical, brachial, intercostal, pudendal):* 1% or 2% solution.

➤*Transvaginal block (paracervical plus pudendal):* 1% solution.

➤*Paracervical block in obstetrics:* 1% solution.

➤*Caudal and epidural block:* 1%, 1.5%, or 2% solution.

➤*Infiltration:* 0.5% (via dilution) or 1% solution.

➤*Therapeutic block (pain management):* 1% or 2% solution.

➤*Dental procedures (infiltration or nerve block):* 3% solution or 2% solution with levonordefrin.

Administration and Dosage

➤*General dosing considerations:* A test dose is recommended prior to administration (see Test dose).

➤*Adults:*

Local anesthesia –

Maximum dose: 400 mg/single dose or the total of a series of doses given in 1 procedure; 1,000 mg per 24 hours.

Dental procedures (infiltration or nerve block): In the upper or lower jaw, the average dose of 1 cartridge usually will suffice. Five cartridges (180 mg of the 2% solution or 270 mg of the 3% solution) usually are adequate to effect anesthesia of the entire oral cavity.

Mepivacaine Recommended Concentrations and Doses				
Procedure	Concentration	Total dose		Comments
Cervical, brachial, intercostal, pudendal nerve block	1%	5 to 40 mL	50 to 400 mg	Pudendal block: one-half of total dose injected on each side.
	2%	5 to 20 mL	100 to 400 mg	
Transvaginal block (paracervical plus pudendal)	1%	up to 30 mL (both sides)	up to 300 mg (both sides)	One-half of total dose injected on each side.

MEPIVACAINE HYDROCHLORIDE — INJECTION

Mepivacaine Recommended Concentrations and Doses				
Procedure	Concentration	Total dose		Comments
Paracervical block	1%	up to 20 mL (both sides)	up to 200 mg (both sides)	One-half of total dose injected on each side. This is the maximum recommended dose per 90-minute period in obstetrical and nonobstetrical patients. Inject slowly, 5 minutes between sides.
Caudal and epidural block	1%	15 to 30 mL	150 to 300 mg	Use only single-dose vials that do not contain a preservative.
	1.5%	10 to 25 mL	150 to 375 mg	
	2%	10 to 20 mL	200 to 400 mg	
Infiltration	1%	up to 40 mL	up to 400 mg	An equivalent amount of a 0.5% solution (prepared by diluting the 1% solution with Sodium Chloride Injection) may be used for large areas.
Therapeutic block (pain management)	1%	1 to 5 mL	10 to 50 mg	—
	2%	1 to 5 mL	20 to 100 mg	

➤*Children:*

Local anesthesia – Carefully measure the pediatric dose as a percentage of the total adult dose based on weight. In children younger than 3 years of age or weighing less than 13.6 kg, use concentrations less than 2% (eg, 0.5% to 1.5%).

Maximum dose: 5 to 6 mg/kg, especially in those weighing less than 13.6 kg.

See Adults for dosing in children.

➤*Elderly:* Clinical studies and other reported clinical experience indicates that use of the drug in elderly patients requires a decreased dosage.

➤*Debilitated and acutely ill patients:* Debilitated and acutely ill patients should be given reduced doses commensurate with their age and physical status.

➤*Test dose:* During the administration of epidural anesthesia, it is recommended that a test dose be administered initially and the effects monitored before the full dose is given. When using a "continuous" catheter technique, test doses should be given prior to both the original and all reinforcing doses because plastic tubing in the epidural space can migrate into a blood vessel or through the dura. When clinical conditions permit, an effective test dose should contain epinephrine (10 to 15 mcg have been suggested) to serve as a warning of unintended intravascular injection. If injected into a blood vessel, this amount of epinephrine is likely to produce an "epinephrine response" within 45 seconds, consisting of an increase of pulse and blood pressure, circumoral pallor, palpitations, and nervousness in the unsedated patient. The sedated patient may exhibit only a pulse rate increase of 20 or more beats per minute for 15 or more seconds. Therefore, following the test dose, the heart rate should be monitored for a heart rate increase. The test dose should also contain mepivacaine 45 to 50 mg to detect an unintended intrathecal administration. This will be evidenced within a few minutes by signs of spinal block (eg, decreased sensation of the buttocks, paresis of the leg, or, in the sedated patient, absent knee jerk).

➤*Administration:* Avoid the rapid injection of a large volume of a local anesthetic solution and use fractional (incremental) doses. Injections should be made slowly, with frequent aspirations before and during the injection to avoid intravascular injection. Current opinion favors fractional administration with constant attention to the patient rather than rapid bolus injection. Syringe aspirations should also be performed before and during each supplemental injection in continuous (intermittent) catheter techniques. An intravascular injection is still possible even if aspirations for blood are negative.

➤*Admixture compatibility:* Mixing or the prior or intercurrent use of any local anesthetic with mepivacaine cannot be recommended because of insufficient data on the clinical use of such mixtures.

➤*Storage/Stability:* Store at 15° to 30°C (59° to 86°F).

PRILOCAINE HYDROCHLORIDE

Rx	**Citanest Plain** (Dentsply Pharm)	**Injection, solution:** 4%	In 1.8 mL cartridge.
Rx	**Citanest Forte** (Dentsply Pharm)		Epinephrine 0.005 mg/mL, sodium metabisulfite 0.5 mg. In 1.8 mL cartridge.

PRILOCAINE HYDROCHLORIDE — INJECTION

For complete and comparative prescribing information, refer to the Injectable Local Anesthetics group monograph.

Indications

➤*Local anesthesia:* For the production of local anesthesia in dentistry by nerve block or infiltration techniques.

Administration and Dosage

➤*General dosing considerations:* Repeated doses of prilocaine may cause significant increases in blood levels with each repeated dose because of slow accumulation of the drug or its metabolites.

➤*Adults:*

Local anesthesia –

Maximum dose: The maximum recommended dose that should ever be administered within a 2-hour period in healthy adults should be calculated based on the patient's weight.

Prilocaine Maximum Dosing	
Weight	Max dose
< 70 kg	8 mg/kg
≥ 70 kg	600 mg (15 mL) or 8 cartridges

Inferior alveolar block: There are no practical clinical differences between prilocaine with and without epinephrine when used for inferior alveolar blocks.

Maxillary infiltration: Prilocaine plain is recommended for use in maxillary infiltration anesthesia for procedures in which the painful aspects can be completed within 15 minutes after the injection. Prilocaine plain is therefore especially suited to short procedures in the maxillary anterior teeth. For long procedures, or those involving maxillary posterior teeth where soft tissue numbness is not troublesome to the patient, prilocaine with epinephrine is recommended.

• *Initial dosage* – For most routine procedures, 1 to 2 mL of prilocaine plain or prilocaine with epinephrine will usually provide adequate infiltration or major nerve block anesthesia.

➤*Children:*

Local anesthesia – Reduce dosages in children, commensurate with age, body weight, and physical condition.

11 years of age and older: See Adults for dosing.

10 years of age and younger: It is rarely necessary to administer more than one-half of a cartridge (40 mg) of prilocaine plain or prilocaine with epinephrine per procedure to achieve local anesthesia for a procedure involving a single tooth. In maxillary infiltration, this amount will often suffice for the treatment of 2 or even 3 teeth. However, in the mandibular block, satisfactory anesthesia achieved with this amount of drug will allow treatment of the teeth in an entire quadrant.

• *Maximum dose* – In children who have a healthy lean body mass and healthy body development, the maximum dose may be determined by the application of one of the standard pediatric drug formulas (eg, Clark's rule).

➤*Elderly:* Give elderly patients reduced doses commensurate with their age and physical status.

➤*Special risk patients:* Give debilitated, acutely ill patients reduced doses commensurate with their age and physical status.

➤*Preparation for administration:* Cartridges of prilocaine plain and prilocaine with epinephrine should not be autoclaved because solutions of epinephrine and the closures employed in cartridges cannot withstand autoclaving temperatures and pressures.

If chemical disinfection of anesthetic cartridges is desired, either isopropyl alcohol 91% or ethyl alcohol 70% is recommended. Many commercially available brands of rubbing alcohol, as well as solutions of ethyl alcohol not of USP grade, contain denaturants that are injurious to rubber; therefore, they are not to be used. It is recommended that chemical disinfection be accomplished by wiping the cartridge cap thoroughly with a pledget of cotton that has been moistened with the recommended alcohol just prior to use. Immersion is not recommended.

To avoid leakage of solutions during injection, be sure to penetrate the center of the rubber diaphragm when loading the syringe. An off-center penetration produces an oval shaped puncture that allows leakage around the needle. Other causes of leakage and breakage include badly worn syringes, aspirating syringes with bent harpoons, the use of syringes not designed to take 1.8 mL cartridges, and inadvertent freezing.

Cracking of glass cartridges is most often the result of an attempt to use a cartridge with an extruded plunger. An extruded plunger loses its lubrication and only can be forced back into the cartridge with difficulty. Cartridges with extruded plungers should be discarded.

➤*Administration:* Aspiration prior to injection is recommended because it reduces the possibility of intravascular injection, thereby keeping the incidence of adverse reactions and anesthetic failure to a minimum. If blood is aspirated, the needle must be repositioned until no return of blood can be elicited by aspiration. However, note that the absence of blood in the syringe does not ensure that intravascular injection will be avoided.

➤*Admixture compatibility:* Certain metallic ions (mercury, zinc, copper) have been related to swelling and edema after local anesthesia in dentistry. Therefore, chemical disinfectants containing or releasing these ions are not recommended. Antirust tablets usually contain metal ions. Accordingly, aluminum-sealed cartridges should not be kept in such solutions.

Amide Local Anesthetics

PRILOCAINE HYDROCHLORIDE — INJECTION

Quaternary ammonium salts, such as benzalkonium chloride, are electrolytically incompatible with aluminum. Cartridges of prilocaine injection and prilocaine with epinephrine injection are sealed with aluminum caps; therefore, they should not be immersed in any solution containing these salts.

➤*Storage/Stability:* Store at approximately 25°C (77°F). Solutions containing epinephrine should be protected from light. Any unused portion of a cartridge of prilocaine plain or prilocaine with epinephrine should be discarded.

ROPIVACAINE HYDROCHLORIDE

Rx	**Naropin** (APP Pharmaceuticals)	**Injection; solution:** 2 mg/mL (0.2%)	Preservative free. In 10 and 20 mL *Polyamp DuoFit Sterile Paks* and 100 and 200 mL single-dose infusion bottles.
		5 mg/mL (0.5%)	Preservative free. In 20 mL *Polyamp DuoFit Sterile Paks* and 30 mL single-dose vials.
		7.5 mg/mL (0.75%)	Preservative free. In 20 mL *Polyamp DuoFit Sterile Paks.*
		10 mg/mL (1%)	Preservative free. In 10 and 20 mL *Polyamp DuoFit Sterile Paks.*

ROPIVACAINE HYDROCHLORIDE — INJECTION

For complete and comparative prescribing information, refer to the Injectable Local Anesthetics class monograph.

Indications

➤*Acute pain management:* For acute pain management administered as an epidural continuous infusion, intermittent bolus (eg, postoperative or labor), or local infiltration.

➤*Surgical anesthesia:* For the production of local or regional anesthesia for surgery administered as an epidural block, including cesarean section, major nerve block, or local infiltration.

Administration and Dosage

➤*General dosing considerations:* Exercise caution when administering for prolonged periods of time (eg, more than 70 hours in debilitated patients). (See Prolonged Exposure.)

A test dose is recommended prior to administration during epidural anesthesia. (See Administration.)

➤*Adults:*

Acute pain management –

Labor pain management:

Ropivacaine Dosage Recommendations for Labor Pain Management

Procedure	Concentration	Volume	Dose	Onset	Duration
Lumbar epidural administration					
Initial dose	2 mg/mL (0.2%)	10 to 20 mL	20 to 40 mg	10 to 15 min	0.5 to 1.5 h
Continuous infusion[a]	2 mg/mL (0.2%)	6 to 14 mL/h	12 to 28 mg/h	NA[b]	NA
Incremental injections (top-up)[a]	2 mg/mL (0.2%)	10 to 15 mL/h	20 to 30 mg/h	NA	NA

[a] Median dosage of 21 mg/h was administered by continuous infusion or incremental injections (top-ups) over a median delivery time of 5.5 hours.

[b] NA = not applicable.

Postoperative pain management: If regional anesthesia was not used intraoperatively, then an initial epidural block with ropivacaine 5 to 7 mL is induced via an epidural catheter. Analgesia is maintained with an infusion of 2 mg/mL (0.2%). Clinical studies have demonstrated that infusion rates of 6 to 14 mL (12 to 28 mg) per hour provide adequate analgesia with nonprogressive motor block. With this technique, a significant reduction in the need for opioids was demonstrated. Clinical experience supports the use of epidural infusions for up to 72 hours.

Ropivacaine Dosage Recommendations for Postoperative Pain Management

Procedure	Concentration	Volume	Dose	Onset	Duration
Lumbar epidural administration					
Continuous infusion[a]	2 mg/mL (0.2%)	6 to 14 mL/h	12 to 28 mg/h	NA	NA
Thoracic epidural administration					
Continuous infusion[a]	2 mg/mL (0.2%)	6 to 14 mL/h	12 to 28 mg/h	NA	NA
Infiltration (eg, minor nerve block)	2 mg/mL (0.2%)	1 to 100 mL	2 to 200 mg	1 to 5 min	2 to 6 h
	5 mg/mL (0.5%)	1 to 40 mL	5 to 200 mg	1 to 5 min	2 to 6 h

[a] Cumulative doses up to ropivacaine 770 mg over 24 hours (intraoperative block plus postoperative infusion); continuous epidural infusion at rates up to 28 mg/h for 72 hours have been well tolerated in adults (ie, 2,016 mg plus surgical dose of approximately 100 to 150 mg as top-up).

Surgical anesthesia:

Ropivacaine Dosage Recommendations for Surgical Anesthesia

Procedure	Concentration	Volume	Dose	Onset	Duration
Lumbar epidural administration for surgery	5 mg/mL (0.5%)	15 to 30 mL	75 to 150 mg	15 to 30 min	2 to 4 h
	7.5 mg/mL (0.75%)	15 to 25 mL	113 to 188 mg	10 to 20 min	3 to 5 h
	10 mg/mL (1%)	15 to 20 mL	150 to 200 mg	10 to 20 min	4 to 6 h
Lumbar epidural administration for cesarean section	5 mg/mL (0.5%)	20 to 30 mL	100 to 150 mg	15 to 25 min	2 to 4 h
	7.5 mg/mL (0.75%)	15 to 20 mL	113 to 150 mg	10 to 20 min	3 to 5 h
Thoracic epidural administration for surgery	5 mg/mL (0.5%)	5 to 15 mL	25 to 75 mg	10 to 20 min	NA
	7.5 mg/mL (0.75%)	5 to 15 mL	38 to 113 mg	10 to 20 min	NA
Major nerve block (eg, brachial plexus block)[a]	5 mg/mL (0.5%)	35 to 50 mL	175 to 250 mg	15 to 30 min	5 to 8 h
	7.5 mg/mL (0.75%)	10 to 40 mL	75 to 300 mg	10 to 25 min	6 to 10 h
Field block (eg, minor nerve blocks and infiltration)	5 mg/mL (0.5%)	1 to 40 mL	5 to 200 mg	1 to 15 min	2 to 6 h

[a] The dose for a major nerve block must be adjusted according to site of administration and patient status. Supraclavicular brachial plexus blocks may be associated with a higher frequency of serious adverse reactions, regardless of the local anesthetic used.

Amide Local Anesthetics

ROPIVACAINE HYDROCHLORIDE — INJECTION

➤*Children:*

Off-label dosing –

Caudal epidural block: 1.25 to 6.5 mg/kg or 1 mL/kg of the 0.2% strength.

Epidural continuous infusion:

- *7 to 12 years of age –*
  Loading dose: 3.6 mg.
  Additional doses: 3.2 mg/h continuous infusion; may be titrated up to 27.2 mg/h as needed.
- *4 months to 7 years of age –*
  Loading dose: 1 mg/kg.
  Additional doses: 0.2 to 0.4 mg/kg/h for 48 hours.

➤*Debilitated and acutely ill patients:* Give reduced doses commensurate with their age and physical condition.

➤*Prolonged exposure:* When prolonged blocks are used, either through continuous infusion or through repeated bolus administration, the risks of reaching a toxic plasma concentration or inducing local neural injury must be considered.

➤*Preparation for administration:* Disinfecting agents containing heavy metals, which cause release of respective ions (eg, mercury, zinc, copper), should not be used for skin or mucous membrane disinfection because they have been related to incidents of swelling and edema.

➤*Administration:* Avoid the rapid administration of a large volume of local anesthetic solution and use fractional (incremental) doses. Administer the smallest dose and concentration required to produce the desired result.

Inject the drug slowly and incrementally, with frequent aspirations before and during the injection to avoid intravascular injection. When a continuous catheter technique is used, also perform syringe aspirations before and during each supplemental injection.

It is essential that aspiration for blood or cerebrospinal fluid (where applicable) be done prior to injecting any local anesthetic (both the original dose and all subsequent doses) to avoid intravascular or subarachnoid injection. However, a negative aspiration does not ensure against an intravascular or subarachnoid injection.

Test dose – Use an adequate test dose (3 to 5 mL of a short-acting local anesthetic containing epinephrine) prior to induction of complete block. Repeat this test dose if patient movement potentiates epidural catheter displacement. Allow adequate time for onset of anesthesia following administration of each test dose.

During the administration of epidural anesthesia, it is recommended that a test dose of a local anesthetic with a fast onset be administered initially and that the patient be monitored for CNS and cardiovascular toxicity, as well as for signs of unintended intrathecal administration before proceeding. When clinical conditions permit, consider employing local anesthetic solutions, which contain epinephrine, for the test dose, because circulatory changes compatible with epinephrine may also serve as a warning sign of unintended intravascular injection. If injected into a blood vessel, this amount of epinephrine is likely to produce a transient "epinephrine response" within 45 seconds, consisting of an increase in heart rate and systolic blood pressure, circumoral pallor, palpitations, and nervousness in the unsedated patient. The sedated patient may exhibit only a pulse rate increase of 20 or more beats per minute for 15 or more seconds. Therefore, following the test dose, monitor the heart continuously for a heart rate increase. Patients receiving beta-blockers may not manifest changes in heart rate, but blood pressure monitoring can detect a rise in systolic blood pressure. A test dose of a short-acting amide anesthetic such as lidocaine is recommended to detect an unintentional intrathecal administration. This will be manifested within a few minutes by signs of spinal block (eg, decreased sensation of the buttocks, paresis of the legs, or, in the sedated patient, absent knee jerk). An intravascular injection is still possible even if aspirations for blood are negative. Administration of higher than recommended doses of ropivacaine to achieve greater motor blockade or increased duration of sensory blockade may result in cardiovascular depression, particularly in the event of inadvertent intravascular injection. The test dose itself may produce a systemic toxic reaction, or high spinal or epinephrine-induced cardiovascular effects.

➤*Admixture compatibility:* Solubility is limited at pH above 6. Thus, care must be taken because precipitation may occur if ropivacaine is mixed with alkaline solutions.

To screen for specific compatibilities, see *Trissel's IV-Chek*.

➤*Storage/Stability:* Store at 20° to 25°C (68° to 77°F). Any solution remaining from an opened container should be discarded promptly. Continuous infusion bottles should not be left in place for more than 24 hours.

ARTICAINE HYDROCHLORIDE

Rx	**Orabloc** (Pierrel)	**Injection; solution:** 4% with epinephrine 1:100,000	Sodium metabisulfite. In 1.8 mL single-use cartridges.
		Injection; solution: 4% with epinephrine 1:200,000	Sodium metabisulfite. In 1.8 mL single-use cartridges.

ARTICAINE HYDROCHLORIDE — INJECTION

Indications

➤*Dental procedure anesthesia:* For local, infiltrative, or conductive anesthesia in both simple and complex dental procedures.

Administration and Dosage

➤*General dosing considerations:* The onset of anesthesia and the duration of anesthesia are proportional to the volume and concentration (ie, total dose) of local anesthetic used. Caution should be exercised when employing large volumes because the incidence of side effects may be dose-related.

For most routine dental procedures, articaine containing epinephrine 1:200,000 is preferred. However, when more pronounced hemostasis or improved visualization of the surgical field is required, articaine containing epinephrine 1:100,000 may be used.

➤*Adults:* The following table summarizes the recommended volumes and concentrations of articaine for various types of anesthetic procedures. The dosages suggested in this table are for healthy adults, administered by submucosal infiltration or nerve block.

Articaine Recommended Dosages for Both Strengths

	Articaine injection	
Procedure	Volume	Total dose of articaine
Infiltration	0.5 to 2.5 mL	20 to 100 mg
Nerve block	0.5 to 3.4 mL	20 to 136 mg
Oral surgery	1 to 5.1 mL	40 to 204 mg

The recommended doses serve only as a guide to the amount of anesthetic required for most routine procedures. The actual volumes to be used depend on a number of factors such as type and extent of surgical procedure, depth of anesthesia, degree of muscular relaxation, and condition of the patient. In all cases, the smallest dose that will produce the desired result should be given.

➤*Children:*

4 to 16 years of age –

Usual dosage: The quantity of articaine in children ages 4 to 16 years of age to be injected should be determined by the age and weight of the child and the magnitude of the operation.

Maximum dose: The maximum dose of articaine should not exceed 7 mg/kg (0.175 mL/kg) of articaine.

Younger than 4 years of age – Safety and effectiveness of articaine in patients younger than 4 years of age have not been established.

➤*Dosing in special populations:* Dose reduction may be required in debilitated patients, acutely ill patients, elderly patients, and children commensurate with their age and physical condition. No studies have been performed in patients with renal or liver dysfunction. Caution should be used in patients with severe liver disease.

➤*Preparation for administration:* For chemical disinfection of the carpule, either isopropyl alcohol (91%) or ethyl alcohol (70%) is recommended. Many commercially available brands of isopropyl (rubbing) alcohol, as well as solutions of ethyl alcohol not of USP grade, contain denaturants that are injurious to rubber and therefore are not to be used.

Parenteral drug products should be inspected visually for particulate matter and discoloration prior to administration, whenever solution and container permit.

➤*Storage/Stability:* Store at 25°C (77°F), with brief excursions permitted between 15° and 30°C (59° and 86°F). Protect from light. Do not freeze.

Ester Local Anesthetics

CHLOROPROCAINE HYDROCHLORIDE

Rx	**Nesacaine** (APP Pharmaceuticals)	**Injection, solution:** 1% (10 mg/mL)	In 30 mL multidose vials.[a]
Rx	**Chloroprocaine Hydrochloride** (Various, eg, Bedford, Hospira)	**Injection, solution:** 2% (20 mg/mL)	Preservative free. May contain sodium chloride. In 20 and 30 mL single-dose vials.
Rx	**Nesacaine** (APP Pharmaceuticals)		In 30 mL multidose vials.[a]
Rx	**Nesacaine-MPF** (APP Pharmaceuticals)		Preservative free. In 20 mL single-dose vials.
Rx	**Chloroprocaine Hydrochloride** (Various, eg, Bedford, Hospira)	**Injection, solution:** 3% (30 mg/mL)	Preservative free. May contain sodium chloride. In 20 and 30 mL single-dose vials.
Rx	**Nesacaine-MPF** (APP Pharmaceuticals)		Preservative free. In 20 mL vials.

[a] Contains sodium chloride, methylparaben, and disodium EDTA.

CHLOROPROCAINE HYDROCHLORIDE — INJECTION

For complete prescribing information, refer to the Injectable Local Anesthetics class monograph.

Indications

➤*Local anesthesia:* Chloroprocaine 1% and 2% injections in multidose vials with methylparaben as preservative are indicated for the production of local anesthesia by infiltration and peripheral nerve block. Do not use for lumbar or caudal epidural anesthesia.

Chloroprocaine 2% and 3% injections in single-dose vials without preservative and without EDTA are indicated for the production of local anesthesia by infiltration and peripheral and central nerve block, including lumbar and caudal epidural blocks.

Administration and Dosage

➤*General dosing considerations:* Injection of repeated doses of local anesthetics may cause significant increases in plasma levels with each repeated dose because of slow accumulation of the drug or its metabolite. Tolerance to elevated blood levels varies with the physical condition of the patient.

In order to guard against adverse reactions sometimes noted following unintended penetration of the subarachnoid space, administer a test dose for caudal and lumbar epidural block (see Test dose).

➤*Adults:*

Local anesthesia –

Caudal block:

• *Usual dosage* – 15 to 25 mL of chloroprocaine 2% or 3% without preservatives. Repeated doses may be given at 40- to 60-minute intervals.

• *Maximum dose –*

Single dose (without epinephrine): 11 mg/kg, not to exceed a maximum total dose of 800 mg.

Single dose (with epinephrine): 14 mg/kg, not to exceed a maximum total dose of 1,000 mg.

Infiltration and peripheral nerve block –

Maximum dose:

• *Single dose (without epinephrine)* – 11 mg/kg, not to exceed a maximum total dose of 800 mg.

• *Single dose (with epinephrine)* – 14 mg/kg, not to exceed a maximum total dose of 1,000 mg.

Brachial plexus: 30 to 40 mL (600 to 800 mg) as a chloroprocaine 2% solution with or without preservatives.

Digital: 3 to 4 mL (30 to 40 mg) as a chloroprocaine 1% solution with or without preservatives (without epinephrine).

Infraorbital: 0.5 to 1 mL (10 to 20 mg) as a chloroprocaine 2% solution with or without preservatives.

Mandibular: 2 to 3 mL (40 to 60 mg) as a chloroprocaine 2% solution with or without preservatives.

Paracervical: 3 mL per each of 4 sites as a chloroprocaine 1% solution with or without preservatives; total dose of up to 120 mg.

Pudendal: 10 mL on each side as a chloroprocaine 2% solution with or without preservatives; total dose of 400 mg.

Lumbar epidural block –

Usual dosage: 2 to 2.5 mL per segment of a chloroprocaine 2% or 3% solution with or without preservatives can be used. The usual total volume is 15 to 25 mL. Repeated doses of 2 to 6 mL less than the original dose may be given at 40- to 50-minute intervals.

Maximum dose:

• *Single dose (without epinephrine)* – 11 mg/kg, not to exceed a maximum total dose of 800 mg.

• *Single dose (with epinephrine)* – 14 mg/kg, not to exceed a maximum total dose of 1,000 mg.

➤*Children:*

Older than 3 years of age –

Infiltration:

• *Usual dosage* – Use concentrations of 0.5% to 1%.

• *Maximum dose* – 11 mg/kg (5 mg/lb) (without epinephrine) determined by the child's age and weight. This maximum dose is for children who have a healthy lean body mass and healthy body weight.

Nerve block:

• *Usual dosage* – Use concentrations of 1% to 1.5%.

3 years of age and younger – Safety and efficacy have not been established.

➤*Elderly:* Reduce dosage for elderly patients.

➤*Hepatic function impairment:* Reduce dosage for patients with liver disease.

➤*Special risk patients:* Reduce dosage in cardiac, debilitated, and acutely ill patients.

➤*Test dose:* Use an adequate test dose (3 mL of chloroprocaine 3% injection without preservatives or 5 mL of chloroprocaine 2% injection without preservatives) prior to induction of complete block. Repeat this test dose if the patient is moved in such a fashion as to have displaced the epidural catheter. Allow adequate time for onset of anesthesia following administration of each test dose.

➤*Preparation for administration:*

Epinephrine injections – To prepare a 1:200,000 epinephrine:chloroprocaine injection, add 0.1 mL of a 1:1,000 epinephrine injection to 20 mL of chloroprocaine injection without preservatives.

Children – Some of the lower concentrations for use in infants and smaller children are not available in prepackaged containers; it will be necessary to dilute available concentrations with the amount of sodium chloride 0.9% injection necessary to obtain the required final concentration of chloroprocaine.

➤*Administration:* Administer as a single injection or continuously through an indwelling catheter. Avoid rapid injection of a large volume of local anesthetic injection through the catheter. Consider fractional doses when feasible.

Chloroprocaine with preservatives contains methylparaben and should not be used for lumbar or caudal epidural anesthesia because safety of this antimicrobial preservative has not been established with regard to intrathecal injection, intentional or unintentional.

To avoid intravascular injection, aspiration should be performed before the anesthetic solution is injected. The needle must be repositioned until no blood return can be elicited. However, the absence of blood in the syringe does not guarantee that intravascular injection has been avoided.

In the event of the known injection of a large volume of local anesthetic injection into the subarachnoid space, after suitable resuscitation and if the catheter is in place, consider attempting the recovery of drug by draining a moderate amount of cerebrospinal fluid (eg, 10 mL) through the epidural catheter.

➤*Admixture compatibility:* Chloroprocaine is incompatible with caustic alkalis and their carbonates, soaps, silver salts, iodine, and iodides.

➤*Storage/Stability:* Store at 20° to 25°C (68° to 77°F). Protect from freezing. Protect from light. Discard unused chloroprocaine injection without preservatives remaining in the vial after use because it contains no preservatives.

Chloroprocaine injection is slightly photosensitive and may become discolored after prolonged exposure to light. Store these vials in the original outer containers, protected from direct sunlight. Do not administer discolored injection. If exposed to low temperatures, chloroprocaine injection may deposit crystals of chloroprocaine, which will redissolve with shaking when returned to room temperature. Do not use the product if it contains undissolved (eg, particulate) material.

Actions

➤*Pharmacology:* Like other local anesthetics, chloroprocaine blocks the generation and conduction of nerve impulses, presumably by increasing the threshold for electrical excitation in the nerve, by slowing the propagation of the nerve impulse, and by reducing the rate of rise of the action potential. In general, the progression of anesthesia is related to the diameter, myelination, and conduction velocity of affected nerve fibers. Clinically, the order of loss of nerve function is as follows: pain, temperature, touch, proprioception, and skeletal muscle tone.

Systemic absorption of local anesthetics produces effects on the cardiovascular system and the CNS. At blood concentrations achieved with normal therapeutic doses, changes in cardiac conduction, excitability, refractoriness, contractility, and peripheral vascular resistance are minimal. However, toxic blood concentrations depress cardiac conduction and excitability, which may lead to atrioventricular block and ultimately to cardiac arrest. In addition, with toxic blood concentrations, myocardial contractility may be depressed and peripheral vasodilation may occur, leading to decreased cardiac output and arterial blood pressure.

Following systemic absorption, toxic blood concentrations of local anesthetics can produce CNS stimulation, depression, or both. Apparent central stimulation may be manifested as restlessness, tremors, and shivering, which may progress to convulsions. Depression and coma may occur, possibly progressing ultimately to respiratory arrest.

However, the local anesthetics have a primary depressant effect on the medulla and on higher centers. The depressed stage may occur without a prior stage of CNS stimulation

➤*Pharmacokinetics:*

Absorption/Distribution – The onset of action with chloroprocaine is rapid (usually within 6 to 12 minutes), and the duration of anesthesia, depending upon the amount used and the route of administration, may be up to 60 minutes.

Local anesthetics appear to cross the placenta by passive diffusion. However, the rate and degree of diffusion vary considerably among the different drugs, as governed by the degree of plasma protein binding, of ionization, and of lipid solubility. Fetal/maternal ratios of local anesthetics appear to be inversely related to the degree of plasma protein binding because only the free, unbound drug is available for placental transfer. Thus, drugs with the highest protein-binding capacity may have the lowest fetal/maternal ratios. The extent of placental transfer is also determined by the degree of ionization and lipid solubility of the drug. Lipid-soluble, nonionized drugs readily enter the fetal blood from the maternal circulation.

Depending upon the route of administration, local anesthetics are distributed to some extent to all body tissues, with high concentrations found in highly perfused organs, such as the liver, lungs, heart, and brain.

Metabolism/Excretion – Chloroprocaine is rapidly metabolized in plasma by hydrolysis of the ester linkage by pseudocholinesterase. The hydrolysis of chloroprocaine results in the production of beta-diethylaminoethanol and 2-chloro-4-aminobenzoic acid, which inhibits the action of the sulfonamides.

CHLOROPROCAINE HYDROCHLORIDE — INJECTION

The kidney is the main excretory organ for most local anesthetics and their metabolites. Urinary excretion is affected by urinary perfusion and factors affecting urinary pH.

Special populations –

Renal function impairment: Various pharmacokinetic parameters of the local anesthetics can be significantly altered by the presence of renal impairment and/or renal blood flow.

Hepatic function impairment: Various pharmacokinetic parameters of the local anesthetics can be significantly altered by the presence of hepatic impairment.

Elderly: Various pharmacokinetic parameters of local anesthetics can be significantly altered by the presence of advanced age.

Children: The in vitro plasma half-life in neonates is 43 ± 2 seconds.

Gender: The in vitro plasma half-life of chloroprocaine in adults is 21 ± 2 seconds for men and 25 ± 1 seconds for women.

Epinephrine, urinary pH, and route of administration: Various pharmacokinetic parameters of the local anesthetics can be significantly altered by the addition of epinephrine, by factors affecting urinary pH, and by the route of administration.

Contraindications

Hypersensitivity to drugs of the para-aminobenzoic acid (PABA) ester group.

Warnings/Precautions

➤*Administration:* Ensure that local anesthetics are employed by health care providers well versed in diagnosis and management of dose-related toxicity and other acute emergencies that might arise from the block to be employed, and then only after ensuring the immediate availability of oxygen, other resuscitative drugs, cardiopulmonary resuscitative equipment, and the personnel resources needed for proper management of toxic reactions and related emergencies. Delay in proper management of dose-related toxicity, underventilation from any cause, and/or altered sensitivity may lead to the development of acidosis, cardiac arrest, and, possibly, death.

The safety and effective use of chloroprocaine depend on proper dosage, correct technique, adequate precautions, and readiness for emergencies. Ensure that resuscitative equipment, oxygen, and other resuscitative drugs are available for immediate use. Use the lowest dosage that results in effective anesthesia to avoid high plasma levels and serious adverse effects. Make injections slowly, with frequent aspirations before and during the injection to avoid intravascular injection. Also, perform syringe aspirations before and during each supplemental injection in continuous (intermittent) catheter techniques. During the administration of epidural anesthesia, it is recommended that a test dose be administered (3 mL of chloroprocaine 3% or 5 mL of 2% without preservatives) initially and that the patient be monitored for CNS toxicity and cardiovascular toxicity, as well as for signs of unintended intrathecal administration, before proceeding. When clinical conditions permit, consider employing a chloroprocaine solution that contains epinephrine for the test dose because circulatory changes characteristic of epinephrine may also serve as a warning sign of unintended intravascular injection. An intravascular injection is still possible, even if aspirations for blood are negative. With the use of continuous catheter techniques, it is recommended that a fraction of each supplemental dose be administered as a test dose in order to verify proper location of the catheter.

➤*Mixtures of local anesthetics:* Mixtures of local anesthetics are sometimes employed to compensate for the slower onset of one drug and the shorter duration of action of the second drug. Experiments in primates suggest that toxicity is probably additive when mixtures of local anesthetics are employed, but some experiments in rodents suggest synergism. Exercise caution regarding toxic equivalence when mixtures of local anesthetics are employed.

➤*Vasoconstrictors:* Use local anesthetic injections containing a vasoconstrictor cautiously and in carefully circumscribed quantities in areas of the body supplied by end arteries or having otherwise compromised blood supply. Patients with peripheral vascular disease and those with hypertensive vascular disease may exhibit exaggerated vasoconstrictor response. Ischemic injury or necrosis may result.

➤*Ophthalmic surgery:* When local anesthetic injections are employed for retrobulbar block, do not rely upon lack of corneal sensation to determine whether or not the patient is ready for surgery. This is because complete lack of corneal sensation usually precedes clinically acceptable external ocular muscle akinesia.

➤*Hepatic function impairment:* Because ester-type local anesthetics are hydrolyzed by plasma cholinesterase produced by the liver, use chloroprocaine cautiously in patients with hepatic disease.

➤*Special risk:* Use lumbar and caudal epidural anesthesia with extreme caution in patients with existing neurological disease, spinal deformities, septicemia, and severe hypertension. Use local anesthetics with caution in patients with impaired cardiovascular function because they may be less able to compensate for functional changes associated with the prolongation of atrioventricular conduction produced by these drugs. Use local anesthetics with caution in patients with hypotension or heart block.

➤*Pregnancy: Category C.* Animal reproduction studies have not been conducted with chloroprocaine. It is also not known whether chloroprocaine can cause fetal harm when administered to a pregnant woman or can affect reproduction capacity. Give chloroprocaine to a pregnant woman only if clearly needed. This does not preclude the use of chloroprocaine at term for the production of obstetrical anesthesia.

Labor and delivery – Local anesthetics rapidly cross the placenta, and, when used for epidural, paracervical, pudendal, or caudal block anesthesia, can cause varying degrees of maternal, fetal, and neonatal toxicity.

The incidence and degree of toxicity depend upon the procedure performed, the type and amount of drug used, and the technique of drug administration. Adverse reactions in the parturient, fetus, and neonate involve alterations of the CNS, peripheral vascular tone, and cardiac function.

Maternal hypotension has resulted from regional anesthesia. Local anesthetics produce vasodilation by blocking sympathetic nerves. Elevating the patient's legs and positioning her on her left side will help prevent decreases in blood pressure. Monitor the fetal heart rate continuously, and electronic fetal monitoring is highly advisable.

Epidural, paracervical, or pudendal anesthesia may alter the forces of parturition through changes in uterine contractility or maternal expulsive efforts. In one study, paracervical block anesthesia was associated with a decrease in the mean duration of first-stage labor and facilitation of cervical dilation. However, epidural anesthesia has also been reported to prolong the second stage of labor by removing the parturient's reflex to bear down or by interfering with motor function. The use of obstetrical anesthesia may increase the need for forceps assistance.

The use of some local anesthetic drug products during labor and delivery may be followed by diminished muscle strength and tone for the first day or two of life. The long-term significance of these observations is unknown.

Careful adherence to recommended dosage is of the utmost importance in obstetrical paracervical block. Failure to achieve adequate analgesia with recommended doses should arouse suspicion of intravascular or fetal intracranial injection. Cases compatible with unintended fetal intracranial injection of local anesthetic injection have been reported following intended paracervical or pudendal block or both. Babies so affected present with unexplained neonatal depression at birth, which correlates with high local anesthetic serum levels and usually manifest seizures within 6 hours. Prompt use of supportive measures combined with forced urinary excretion of the local anesthetic has been used successfully to manage this complication.

Case reports of maternal convulsions and cardiovascular collapse following the use of some local anesthetics for paracervical block in early pregnancy (as anesthesia for elective abortion) suggest that systemic absorption under these circumstances may be rapid. Do not exceed the recommended maximum dose of each drug. Make the injection slowly and with frequent aspiration. Allow a 5-minute interval between sides.

There are no data concerning use of chloroprocaine for obstetrical paracervical block when toxemia of pregnancy is present or when fetal distress or prematurity is anticipated in advance of the block; therefore, such use is not recommended.

➤*Lactation:* It is not known whether this drug is excreted in human milk. Because many drugs are excreted in human milk, exercise caution when chloroprocaine is administered to a breast-feeding woman.

➤*Elderly:* In general, exercise caution in dose selection for an elderly patient, usually starting at the low end of the dosing range, reflecting the greater frequency of decreased hepatic, renal, or cardiac function, and of concomitant disease or other drug therapy.

This drug and its metabolites are known to be substantially excreted by the kidney, and the risk of toxic reactions to this drug may be greater in patients with impaired renal function. Because elderly patients are more likely to have decreased renal function, take care in dose selection; it may be useful to monitor renal function.

➤*Monitoring:* Careful and constant monitoring of cardiovascular and respiratory (adequacy of ventilation) vital signs and the patient's state of consciousness should be accomplished after each local anesthetic injection. Keep in mind at such times that restlessness, anxiety, tinnitus, dizziness, blurred vision, tremors, depression, or drowsiness may be early warning signs of CNS toxicity.

Drug Interactions

➤*Ergot-type oxytocic drugs:* Do not use vasopressors in the presence of ergot-type oxytocic drugs because severe, persistent hypertension or cerebrovascular accidents may occur.

➤*Sulfonamides:* The PABA metabolite of chloroprocaine inhibits the action of sulfonamides; do not coadminister.

➤*Epinephrine/Norepinephrine:* The administration of local anesthetic solutions containing epinephrine or norepinephrine to patients receiving monoamine oxidase inhibitors, tricyclic antidepressants, or phenothiazines may produce severe, prolonged hypotension or hypertension. Generally avoid concurrent use of these agents. In situations when concurrent therapy is necessary, careful patient monitoring is essential.

Adverse Reactions

➤*Allergic:* Allergic-type reactions are rare and may occur as a result of sensitivity to the local anesthetic or to other formulation ingredients, such as the antimicrobial preservative methylparaben, contained in multiple-dose vials. These reactions are characterized by signs such as urticaria, pruritus, erythema, angioneurotic edema (including laryngeal edema), tachycardia, sneezing, nausea, vomiting, dizziness, syncope, excessive sweating, elevated temperature, and, possibly, anaphylactoid-type symptomatology (including severe hypotension). Cross-sensitivity among members of the ester-type local anesthetic group has been reported. The usefulness of screening for sensitivity has not been definitely established.

CHLOROPROCAINE HYDROCHLORIDE — INJECTION

➤*Cardiovascular:* High doses, or unintended intravascular injection, may lead to high plasma levels and related depression of the myocardium, hypotension, bradycardia, ventricular arrhythmias, and, possibly, cardiac arrest.

➤*CNS:* CNS reactions are characterized by excitation and/or depression. Restlessness, anxiety, dizziness, tinnitus, blurred vision, or tremors may occur, possibly proceeding to convulsions. However, excitement may be transient or absent, with depression being the first manifestation of an adverse reaction. This may quickly be followed by drowsiness merging into unconsciousness and respiratory arrest.

The incidence of convulsions associated with the use of local anesthetics varies with the procedure used and the total dose administered. In a survey of studies of epidural anesthesia, overt toxicity progressing to convulsions occurred in approximately 0.1% of local anesthetic administrations.

In the practice of caudal or lumbar epidural block, occasional unintentional penetration of the subarachnoid space by the catheter may occur. Subsequent adverse observations may depend partially on the amount of drug administered intrathecally. These observations may include spinal block of varying magnitude (including total spinal block), hypotension secondary to spinal block, loss of bladder and bowel control, and loss of perineal sensation and sexual function. Arachnoiditis; persistent motor, sensory and/or autonomic (sphincter control) deficit of some lower spinal segments with slow recovery (several months); or incomplete recovery have been reported in rare instances. Backache and headache have also been noted following lumbar epidural or caudal block.

➤*Systemic:* The most commonly encountered acute adverse experiences that demand immediate countermeasures are related to the CNS and the cardiovascular system. These adverse experiences are generally dose related and may result from rapid absorption from the injection site, diminished tolerance, or unintentional intravascular injection of the local anesthetic solution. In addition to systemic dose-related toxicity, unintentional subarachnoid injection of drug during the intended performance of caudal or lumbar epidural block or nerve blocks near the vertebral column (especially in the head and neck region) may result in underventilation or apnea (total spinal). Factors influencing plasma protein binding, such as acidosis, systemic diseases that alter protein production, or competition of other drugs for protein binding sites, may diminish individual tolerance. Plasma cholinesterase deficiency may also account for diminished tolerance to ester-type local anesthetics.

Overdosage

➤*Animal toxicology:* In mice, the intravenous (IV) median lethal dose (LD_{50}) of chloroprocaine is 97 mg/kg and the subcutaneous LD_{50} of chloroprocaine is 950 mg/kg.

➤*Symptoms:* Acute emergencies from local anesthetics are generally related to high plasma levels encountered during therapeutic use of local anesthetics or to unintended subarachnoid injection of local anesthetic solution.

➤*Treatment:* The first consideration is prevention, best accomplished by careful and constant monitoring of cardiovascular and respiratory vital signs and the patient's state of consciousness after each local anesthetic injection. At the first sign of change, administer oxygen.

The first step in the management of convulsions, as well as underventilation or apnea caused by unintentional subarachnoid injection of drug solution, consists of immediate attention to the maintenance of a patent airway and assisted or controlled ventilation with oxygen and a delivery system capable of permitting immediate positive airway pressure by mask. Immediately after the institution of these ventilatory measures, evaluate the adequacy of the circulation, keeping in mind that drugs used to treat convulsions sometimes depress the circulation when administered IV. Should convulsions persist despite adequate respiratory support, and if the status of the circulation permits, small increments of an ultra–short-acting barbiturate (such as thiopental or thiamylal) or a benzodiazepine (such as diazepam) may be administered IV; prior to the use of anesthetics, be familiar with these anticonvulsant drugs. Supportive treatment of circulatory depression may require administration of IV fluids and, when appropriate, a vasopressor dictated by the clinical situation (such as ephedrine to enhance myocardial contractile force).

If not treated immediately, both convulsions and cardiovascular depression can result in hypoxia, acidosis, bradycardia, arrhythmias, and cardiac arrest. Underventilation or apnea caused by unintentional subarachnoid injection of local anesthetic solution may produce these same signs and can also lead to cardiac arrest if ventilatory support is not instituted. If cardiac arrest should occur, institute standard cardiopulmonary resuscitative measures. Recovery has been reported after prolonged resuscitative efforts.

Endotracheal intubation, employing drugs and techniques familiar to the health care provider, may be indicated after the initial administration of oxygen by mask if difficulty is encountered in the maintenance of a patent airway or if prolonged ventilatory support (assisted or controlled) is indicated.

Patient Information

When appropriate, inform patients in advance that they may experience temporary loss of sensation and motor activity, usually in the lower half of the body, following proper administration of epidural anesthesia.

PROCAINE HYDROCHLORIDE

Rx	**Novocain** (Abbott)	**Injection:** 1%	In 2 mL *Uni-Amps*, 6 mL single-dose amps,[a] and 30 mL multidose vials.[b]
Rx	**Procaine HCl** (Various, eg, IDE)	**Injection:** 2%	In 30 mL multidose vials.[c]
Rx	**Novocain** (Abbott)		In 30 mL multidose vials.[b]
Rx	**Novocain** (Abbott)	**Injection:** 10%	In 2 mL *Uni-Amps*.[a]

[a] With acetone sodium bisulfite.
[b] With acetone sodium bisulfite and chlorobutanol.
[c] May contain sodium metabisulfite.

PROCAINE HYDROCHLORIDE — INJECTION

For complete and comparative prescribing information, refer to the Injectable Local Anesthetics group monograph.

Indications

➤*Procaine hydrochloride injection 10%:* For spinal anesthesia.

➤*Procaine hydrochloride injection 1% and 2%:* For the production of local or regional analgesia and anesthesia by local infiltration and peripheral nerve block techniques.

The routes of administration and concentrations are: for local infiltration use 0.25% to 0.5% (via dilution) and for peripheral nerve blocks use 0.5% (via dilution), 1%, and 2% (see Administration and Dosage for additional information).

Administration and Dosage

➤*Adults:*

0.25% and 0.5% –

Infiltration anesthesia:

• *Usual dosage* – 350 to 600 mg is generally considered to be a single safe total dose.

• *Maximum dose* – 1,000 mg during one treatment.

0.5%, 1%, and 2% –

Peripheral nerve block:

• *Usual dosage* – 0.5% solution (up to 200 mL), 1% solution (up to 100 mL), or 2% solution (up to 50 mL). The use of the 2% solution should usually be limited to cases requiring a small volume of anesthetic solution (10 to 25 mL).

• *Maximum dose* – 1,000 mg during one treatment.

10% –

Spinal anesthesia:

Recommended Dosage of Procaine 10% for Spinal Anesthesia

Extent of anesthesia	Procaine 10% Volume of 10% solution	Volume of diluent	Total dose	Site of injection (lumbar interspace)
Perineum	0.5 mL	0.5 mL	50 mg	4th
Perineum and lower extremities	1 mL	1 mL	100 mg	3rd or 4th
Up to costal margin	2 mL	1 mL	200 mg	2nd, 3rd, or 4th

➤*Children:*

0.25% and 0.5% –

Infiltration anesthesia:

• *Usual dosage* – See Adults for dosing.

• *Maximum dose* – 15 mg/kg of a 0.5% solution for local infiltration.

0.5%, 1%, and 2% –

Peripheral nerve block: See Adults for dosing.

10% –

Spinal anesthesia: See Adults for dosing.

➤*Elderly:* Elderly patients should be given reduced doses commensurate with their age and physical status.

➤*Hepatic function impairment:* Dosages of procaine should be reduced for patients with liver disease.

PROCAINE HYDROCHLORIDE — INJECTION

➤*Special risk patients:* Dosages should be reduced for patients with cardiac disease, obstetric delivery, and patients with increased intra-abdominal pressure. Debilitated and acutely ill patients should be given reduced doses commensurate with their age and physical status.

➤*Preparation for administration:*

0.5% solution – To prepare 60 mL of a 0.5% solution (5 mg/mL), dilute 30 mL of the 1% solution with 30 mL sodium chloride 0.9%. An anesthetic solution of 0.5 mL to 1 mL of epinephrine 1:1,000 per 100 mL may be added for vasoconstrictive effect (1:200,000 to 1:100,000).

0.25% solution – To prepare 60 mL of a 0.25% solution (2.5 mg/mL), dilute 15 mL of the 1% solution with 45 mL sodium chloride 0.9%. An anesthetic solution of 0.5 mL to 1 mL of epinephrine 1:1,000 per 100 mL may be added for vasoconstrictive effect (1:200,000 to 1:100,000).

Sterilization – The drug in intact ampuls is sterile. The preferred method of destroying bacteria on the exterior of ampuls before opening is heat sterilization (autoclaving). Immersion in antiseptic solution is not recommended.

Single-dose containers and multiple-dose containers of procaine may be sterilized by autoclaving at 15-pound pressure, 121°C (250°F) for 15 minutes. The diluent dextrose may show some brown discoloration because of caramelization. Do not use solutions if crystals, cloudiness, or discoloration is observed. Examine solution carefully before use. Reautoclaving increases likelihood of crystal formation. Do not administer solutions that are discolored or that contain particulate matter.

➤*Administration:* The usual rate of injection is 1 mL per 5 seconds for the 10% solution. Full anesthesia and fixation usually occur in 5 minutes. The rapid injection of a large volume of local anesthetic solution should be avoided, and fractional doses should be used when feasible.

➤*Admixture compatibility:*

10% solution – The diluent may be sterile normal saline, sterile distilled water, spinal fluid; for hyperbaric technique, sterile dextrose solution.

➤*Storage/Stability:* Store at 15° to 30°C (59° to 86°F). Protect solutions from light. Unused portions of solutions not containing preservatives (ie, those supplied in ampuls) should be discarded following initial use.

TETRACAINE HYDROCHLORIDE

Rx	**Tetracaine** (Akorn)	**Injection, solution:** 1%	Preservative free. Sodium chloride 7.5 mg. In 2 mL amps.
Rx	**Pontocaine Hydrochloride** (Hospira)		In 2 mL amps.[a]
Rx	**Pontocaine Hydrochloride** (Hospira)	**Injection:** 0.2% in 6% dextrose	In 2 mL amps.
		0.3% in 6% dextrose	In 5 mL amps.
		Powder for reconstitution: 20 mg	In *Niphanoid* (instantly soluble) amps.

[a] With acetone sodium bisulfite.

TETRACAINE HYDROCHLORIDE — INJECTION

For complete and comparative prescribing information, refer to the Injectable Local Anesthetics class monograph.

Indications

➤*Spinal anesthesia:* For the production of spinal anesthesia for procedures requiring 2 to 3 hours.

Administration and Dosage

➤*General dosing considerations:* The dosage varies and depends upon the area to be anesthetized, the number of neuronal segments to be blocked, individual tolerance, and the technique of anesthesia. The lowest dosage needed to provide effective anesthesia should be administered. For specific techniques and procedures, refer to standard textbooks.

The extent and degree of spinal anesthesia depend upon dosage, specific gravity of the anesthetic solution, volume of solution used, force of the injection, level of puncture, position of the patient during and immediately after injection.

➤*Adults:*

Spinal anesthesia –

Tetracaine Suggested Dosage

	Using *Niphanoid*		Using 1% solution		
Extent of anesthesia	Dose of *Niphanoid* (mg)	Volume of spinal fluid (mL)	Dose of solution (mL)	Volume of spinal fluid (mL)	Site of injection (lumbar interspace)
Perineum	5[a]	1	0.5 (≈ 5 mg)[a]	0.5	4th
Perineum and lower extremities	10	2	1 (≈ 10 mg)	1	3rd or 4th
Up to coastal margin	15 to 20[b]	3	1.5 to 2 (≈ 15 to 20 mg)[b]	1.5 to 2	2nd, 3rd, or 4th

[a] For vaginal delivery (saddle block), from 2 to 5 mg in dextrose.
[b] Doses exceeding 15 mg are rarely required and should be used only in exceptional cases. Inject solution at rate of about 1 mL per 5 seconds.

➤*Preparation for administration:* When spinal fluid is added to either the *Niphanoid* or solution, some turbidity results, the degree depending on the pH of the spinal fluid, the temperature of the solution during mixing, as well as the amount of drug and diluent employed. This cloudiness is caused by the release of the base from the hydrochloride. Liberation of base (which is completed within the spinal canal) is held to be essential for satisfactory results with any spinal anesthetic.

The specific gravity of spinal fluid at 25°C/25°C (77°F/77°F) varies under normal conditions from 1.0063 to 1.0075. A solution of the instantly soluble form (*Niphanoid*) in spinal fluid has only a slightly greater specific gravity. The 1% concentration in saline solution has a specific gravity of 1.006 to 1.0074 at 25°C/25°C (77°F/77°F).

Hyperbaric solution – A hyperbaric solution may be prepared by mixing equal volumes of the 1% solution and dextrose 10%.

Hypobaric solution – A hypobaric solution may be prepared by dissolving the *Niphanoid* in sterile water for injection (1 mg per mL). The specific gravity of this solution is essentially the same as that of water, 1, at 25°C/25°C (77°F/77°F).

Niphanoid – If the *Niphanoid* form is preferred, it is first dissolved in dextrose 10% in a ratio of 1 mL dextrose to 10 mg of the anesthetic. Further dilution is made with an equal volume of spinal fluid. The resulting solution now contains dextrose 5% with 5 mg of anesthetic agent per mL.

Sterilization of ampuls – The drug in intact ampuls is sterile. The preferred method of destroying bacteria on the exterior of ampuls before opening is heat sterilization (autoclaving). Immersion in antiseptic solution is not recommended.

Autoclave at 15-pound pressure, at 121°C (250°F), for 15 minutes. The *Niphanoid* form may also be autoclaved in the same way but may lose its snowlike appearance and tend to adhere to the sides of the ampul. This may slightly decrease the rate at which the drug dissolves but does not interfere with its anesthetic potency.

Autoclaving increases likelihood of crystal formation. Unused autoclaved ampuls should be discarded. Under no circumstance should unused ampuls which have been autoclaved be returned to stock.

➤*Storage/Stability:* Store solution under refrigeration. Protect ampuls from light. These formulations do not contain preservatives; therefore, unused portions should be discarded and the reconstituted *Niphanoid* should be used immediately.

COMBINATION LOCAL ANESTHETICS

Rx	**Duocaine** (Amphastar)	**Injection, solution:** 10 mg/mL lidocaine HCl/3.75 mg/mL bupivacaine HCl	Preservative-free. In 10 mL single-dose vials. In cartons of 25.

For complete prescribing information, refer to the Injectable Local Anesthetics class monograph.

COMBINATION LOCAL ANESTHETICS — INJECTION

Indications

➤*Surgical anesthesia:* For the production of local or regional anesthesia for ophthalmologic surgery by peripheral nerve block techniques such as parabulbar, retrobulbar, and facial blocks. May be used with or without epinephrine and/or hyaluronidase.

Administration and Dosage

➤*Adults:*

Ophthalmic anesthesia –

Usual dosage:

- *Peribulbar nerve block* – 6 to 12 mL (lidocaine 60 to 120 mg and bupivacaine 22 to 45 mg).
- *Retrobulbar and facial nerve block* – 2 to 5 mL (lidocaine 20 to 50 mg and bupivacaine 7 to 18 mg). A portion of the dose is injected retrobulbarly, and the remainder may be used to block the facial nerve.

COMBINATION LOCAL ANESTHETICS — INJECTION

Maximum dose:

- *Without epinephrine* – 0.18 mL/kg or total dose of 12 mL (lidocaine 120 mg and bupivacaine 45 mg).
- *With epinephrine* – 0.28 mL/kg or total dose of 20 mL (lidocaine 200 mg and bupivacaine 75 mg).

➤*Children:*

Ophthalmic anesthesia –

12 years of age and older: See Adults for dosing.

➤*Elderly:* Elderly patients should be given reduced doses commensurate with their age and physical condition.

➤*Hepatic function impairment:* Because of their inability to metabolize local anesthetics normally, patients with severe hepatic disease are at greater risk of developing toxic plasma concentrations.

➤*Special risk patients:* Debilitated and acutely ill patients should be given reduced doses commensurate with their age and physical condition.

➤*Storage/Stability:* Store at 15° to 25°C (59° to 77°F). Discard unused portion after initial use.

ANTICONVULSANTS

Anticonvulsant drugs include a variety of agents, all possessing the ability to depress abnormal neuronal discharges in the CNS, thus inhibiting seizure activity. Because of differences in pharmacology, therapeutic use, and adverse reaction potential, these agents are discussed in groups as follows:

- Barbiturates
- Hydantoins
- Succinimides
- Oxazolidinediones
- Benzodiazepines
- Adjuvants to anticonvulsants

➤*Warnings:*

Pregnancy – Reports suggest an association between use of anticonvulsant drugs by women with epilepsy and an elevated incidence of birth defects in children born to these women. Data are more extensive with respect to phenytoin and phenobarbital; other reports indicate a possible similar association with other anticonvulsants. Other factors (eg, genetics or the seizure disorder per se) may also contribute to the higher incidence of birth defects. The great majority of mothers receiving anticonvulsant medication deliver healthy infants.

Do not discontinue anticonvulsant drugs in patients in whom the drug is administered to prevent major seizures because of the strong possibility of precipitating status epilepticus with attendant hypoxia and risk to both the mother and the unborn child. Consider discontinuation of anticonvulsants prior to and during pregnancy when the nature, frequency, and severity of the seizures do not pose a serious threat to the patient. It is not known whether even minor seizures constitute some risk to the developing embryo or fetus.

An increase in seizure frequency during pregnancy occurs in a high proportion of patients because of altered phenytoin absorption or metabolism. Periodic measurement of serum phenytoin levels is particularly valuable in the management of pregnant epileptic patients as a guide to an appropriate adjustment of dosage. However, postpartum restoration of the original dosage will probably be indicated.

Reports suggest that maternal ingestion of anticonvulsant drugs, particularly barbiturates and hydantoins, is associated with a neonatal coagulation defect that may cause bleeding during the early (usually within 24 hours of birth) neonatal period. The defect is characterized by decreased levels of vitamin K-dependent clotting factors, and prolongation of either the prothrombin time or the partial thromboplastin time, or both. It has been suggested that prophylactic vitamin K be given to the mother 1 month prior to and during delivery, and to the infant immediately after birth.

In addition to the reports of increased incidence of congenital malformations, such as cleft lip/palate and heart malformations in children of women receiving phenytoin and other antiepileptic drugs, there have been more recent reports of a fetal hydantoin syndrome. This consists of prenatal growth deficiency, microcephaly, and mental deficiency in children born to mothers who have received phenytoin, barbiturates, alcohol, or trimethadione. However, these features are all interrelated and are frequently associated with intrauterine growth retardation from other causes.

There have been isolated reports of malignancies, including neuroblastoma, in children whose mothers received phenytoin during pregnancy.

Seizures – Seizures may be classified based on their clinical form. The following is based on the International Classification of Epileptic Seizures (Commission on Classification and Terminology of the International League Against Epilepsy. *Epilepsia*. 1981;22:489-501 and 1989;30:389-99.):

1.) Partial seizures (generally involve 1 hemisphere of the brain at onset)
   a.) Simple (consciousness not impaired)
   b.) With motor symptoms (Jacksonian, adversive)
   c.) With somatosensory or other special sensory symptoms
   d.) With autonomic symptoms
   e.) With psychic symptoms
   f.) Complex (consciousness impaired)
   g.) Simple partial onset followed by impaired consciousness
   h.) Impaired consciousness at onset
   i.) Secondarily generalized
   j.) Simple partial seizures evolving to generalized tonic-clonic seizures
   k.) Complex partial seizures evolving to generalized tonic-clonic seizures
   l.) Simple partial seizures evolving to complex partial seizures, then to generalized tonic-clonic seizures.

2.) Generalized seizures (involve both hemispheres of the brain at onset, consciousness usually impaired)
   a.) Absence
   b.) Typical
   c.) Atypical
   d.) Myoclonic
   e.) Clonic
   f.) Tonic
   g.) Tonic-clonic
   h.) Atonic

3.) Localization-related (focal)
   a.) Idiopathic
   b.) Benign focal epilepsy of childhood
   c.) Symptomatic
   d.) Chronic progressive epilepsia partialis continua
   e.) Temporal-lobe
   f.) Extratemporal

4.) Generalized epilepsy
   a.) Idiopathic
   b.) Benign neonatal convulsions
   c.) Childhood absence
   d.) Juvenile myoclonic
   e.) Other
   f.) Cryptogenic or symptomatic
   g.) West syndrome (infantile spasms)
   h.) Early myoclonic encephalopathy
   i.) Lennox-Gastaut syndrome
   j.) Progressive myoclonic epilepsy

5.) Special syndromes
   a.) Febrile seizures

6.) Unclassified

Withdrawal of anticonvulsants – A long-term prospective study suggests that epileptic adults may remain seizure-free if their anticonvulsant is withdrawn following at least 2 years of a single therapy regimen. Approximately one-third of patients relapsed following withdrawal of the anticonvulsants.

Predictors of relapse include the following: Seizure type (highest relapse rates occurred with complex partial seizures with secondary generalization and generalized seizures).

Number of seizures (higher risk with > 100 seizures before control).

Number of drugs (highest rate with patients taking 2 or 3 drugs).

Treatment duration (longer duration of drug treatment resulted in higher relapse rate).

EEG classification (lower relapse rate with less severe EEG abnormalities).

Type of drug (higher relapse rate following withdrawal of valproic acid).

Anticonvulsants: Indications and Pharmacokinetics

	Drug	Labeled indications	Protein binding (%)	Metabolism/ Excretion	t½ (hrs)	Therapeutic serum levels (mcg/mL)
Barbiturates	Phenobarbital[a] (PB)	Status epilepticus Cortical focal Tonic-clonic	40-60	Liver; 25% eliminated unchanged in urine	53-140	20-40
Hydantoins	Ethotoin	Tonic-clonic Psychomotor	nd	Liver; renal excretion of metabolites	3-9[b]	15-50
	Mephenytoin	Tonic-clonic Psychomotor Focal Jacksonian	nd	Liver	95 (active metabolite)	nd
	Phenytoin	Tonic-clonic Psychomotor Status epilepticus	≈ 90	Liver; renal excretion. < 5% excreted unchanged	Dose-dependent[c]	10-20
Succinimides	Ethosuximide	Absence	0	Liver; 25% excreted unchanged in urine	30 (children 7-9 yrs) 40-60 (adults)	40-100
	Methsuximide	Absence	nd	Liver; < 1% excreted unchanged in urine	< 2 (40, active metabolite)	nd
	Phensuximide	Absence	nd	Urine, bile	8 (active metabolite)	nd
Oxazolidinediones	Trimethadione	Absence	0	Demethylated to dimethadione; 3% excreted unchanged	6-13 days (dimethadione)	≥ 700 (dimethadione)
Benzodiazepines	Clonazepam	Absence Myoclonic Akinetic	50-85	5 metabolites identified; urine is major excretion route	18-60	20-80 ng/ml
	Clorazepate	Partial[d]	97	Hydrolyzed in stomach to desmethyldiazepam (active); metabolized in liver, renally excreted	30-100	nd
	Diazepam	Status epilepticus[d] Convulsive disorders, all forms[d]	97-99	Liver, active metabolites	20-50	nd
Adjuncts to anticonvulsants	Lamotrigine	Partial (adults)	≈ 55	Glucuronic acid conjugation to inactive metabolites; 94% excreted in urine, 2% in feces.	≈ 33[e]	nd
	Carbamazepine	Tonic-clonic Mixed Psychomotor	≈ 75	Liver to active 10, 11–epoxide. 72% excreted in urine, 28% in feces	18-54 (initial) 10-20[e] ≈ 6 (10, 11- epoxide)	4-12
	Felbamate[f]	Partial (adults) Partial/generalized assoc. with Lennox-Gastaut syndrome (children)	22-25	40% to 50% unchanged in urine, 40% as unidentified metabolites and conjugates	20-23	nd[g]
	Gabapentin	Partial (adults) with and without secondary generalization	< 3	Not appreciably metabolized; excreted in urine unchanged	5-7	nd
	Lacosamide	Partial (adults)	< 15	Liver; 95% excreted in the urine (40% as unchanged drug, 30% as inactive metabolite)	13	nd
	Primidone	Tonic-clonic Psychomotor Focal	20-25	Metabolized to PB and PEMA, both active	5-15 (primidone) 10-18 (PEMA) 53-140 (PB)	5-12 (primidone) 15-40 (PB)
	Valproic acid	Absence	80-94	Liver; excreted in urine	5-20	50-150

[a] Other barbiturates are also used as anticonvulsants. See Sedatives/Hypnotics section.
[c] Exhibits dose-dependent, nonlinear pharmacokinetics.
[b] Below 8 mcg/ml; > 8 mcg/ml, t½ not defined due to dose-dependent, nonlinear pharmacokinetics.
[d] Recommended for adjunctive use.
[e] Following multiple administrations (150 mg twice daily) to normal volunteers taking no other medications, lamotrigine induced its own metabolism, resulting in a 25% decrease in half-life compared to values obtained in the same volunteers following a single dose. Evidence gathered from other sources suggests that self-induction may not occur when lamotrigine is given as adjunctive therapy in patients receiving enzyme-inducing antiepileptic drugs (EIAEDs).
[f] Because of cases of aplastic anemia, it has been recommended that the use of this drug be discontinued unless, in the judgment of the physician, continued therapy is warranted. Refer to the specific monograph.
[g] Value of monitoring blood levels not established.

Hydantoins

Refer to the general discussion beginning in the Anticonvulsants introduction.

Indications

Refer to individual product monographs for specific indications.

Hydantoins: Summary of Indications

FDA-approved indication	Ethotoin	Fosphenytoin[a]	Phenytoin Chewable tablets	Phenytoin ER[b] capsules	Phenytoin Oral suspension	Phenytoin Injection
Complex partial seizures[c]	✓	✓				
Generalized tonic-clonic seizures	✓	✓	✓	✓	✓	
Prevent/Treat seizures during or following neurosurgery		✓	✓	✓		✓
Status epilepticus		✓				✓ (IV)

[a] May be substituted short-term for oral phenytoin when other means of phenytoin administration are unavailable, inappropriate, or deemed less advantageous.
[b] ER = extended-release.
[c] Also called psychomotor or temporal lobe seizures.

➤*Off-label uses:* Phenytoin is useful as an antiarrhythmic agent, particularly in cardiac glycoside-induced arrhythmias. (Oral loading dose = 14 mg/kg; oral maintenance = 200 to 400 mg/day. Intravenous (IV) loading dose = 50 mg every 5 minutes to a total dose of 1 g; IV maintenance dose = 200 to 400 mg/day.) Pharmacokinetic, electrophysiologic, and electrocardiogram (ECG) effects of phenytoin are summarized in the Antiarrhythmic Agents monograph.

Phenytoin has been used as an alternative to magnesium sulfate for severe preeclampsia (15 mg/kg IV, given as 10 mg/kg initially and 5 mg/kg 2 hours later).

Phenytoin has been used in the treatment of trigeminal neuralgia (tic douloureux), recessive dystrophic epidermolysis bullosa, and junctional epidermolysis bullosa.

Actions

➤*Pharmacology:* Based on phenytoin, the primary site of action of the hydantoins appears to be the motor cortex, where the spread of seizure activity is inhibited. Possibly by promoting sodium efflux from neurons, hydantoins tend to stabilize the threshold against hyperexcitability caused by excessive stimulation or environmental changes capable of reducing membrane sodium gradient. This includes the reduction of posttetanic potentiation at synapses. Loss of posttetanic potentiation prevents cortical seizure foci from detonating adjacent cortical areas. Hydantoins reduce the maximal activity of brain stem centers responsible for the tonic phase of tonic-clonic seizures.

Phenytoin is available as phenytoin acid (ie, chewable tablets, oral suspension) or phenytoin sodium (ie, capsules, injection). There is approximately an 8% increase in drug content with the free acid form over that of the sodium salt.

Fosphenytoin is a prodrug of phenytoin and is converted to phenytoin following parenteral administration. For every millimole of fosphenytoin administered, phenytoin 1 mmol is produced. Each vial of fosphenytoin contains fosphenytoin 75 mg/mL, which is equivalent to phenytoin sodium 50 mg/mL after administration.

➤*Pharmacokinetics:*

Hydantoins: Summary of Pharmacokinetics

Pharmacokinetic parameter	Ethotoin	Fosphenytoin[a]	Phenytoin Chewable tablets	Phenytoin ER capsules	Phenytoin Oral suspension	Phenytoin Injection
T_{max}[b]	2 to 4 hours	IV: End of infusion (phenytoin plasma concentrations peak in 30 to 60 minutes). IM: 30 minutes postdose (phenytoin plasma concentrations peak in approximately 3 hours).	1.5 to 3 hours	4 to 12 hours	1.5 to 3 hours	24 hours (IM)
Protein binding	46%	95% to 99%	Approximately 90% (range, 69% to 96%)	Approximately 90% (range, 69% to 96%)	Approximately 90% (range, 69% to 96%)	Approximately 90% (range, 69% to 96%)
Plasma half-life		Approximately 15 minutes[a]	14 hours (range, 7 to 29 hours)	22 hours (range, 7 to 42 hours)	22 hours (range, 7 to 42 hours)	10 to 15 hours (IV)
Elimination half-life	3 to 12 hours (single dose)					24 hours (for concentration of 10 mcg/mL)
Excretion		Renal (0% to 4%)[c]	Urine and feces (as inactive metabolites)	Urine and feces (as inactive metabolites)	Urine and feces (as inactive metabolites)	Urine and feces (as inactive metabolites)
Therapeutic plasma concentration	15 to 50 mcg/mL	10 to 20 mcg/mL (as phenytoin)	10 to 20 mcg/mL[d]	10 to 20 mcg/mL[d]	10 to 20 mcg/mL[d]	10 to 20 mcg/mL

[a] Conversion half-life of fosphenytoin to phenytoin.
[b] T_{max} = time to maximal concentration.
[c] Phenytoin derived from fosphenytoin is excreted in the same way as injectable phenytoin.
[d] Steady state achieved at least 7 to 10 days (5 to 7 half-lives) after initiation of therapy with doses of 300 mg/day.

Absorption/Distribution –

Phenytoin: Phenytoin is highly protein bound; free phenytoin levels may be altered in patients whose protein-binding characteristics differ from normal.

Fosphenytoin: Fosphenytoin is completely bioavailable following intramuscular (IM) administration. It is extensively bound (95% to 99%) to human plasma proteins, primarily albumin. Binding to plasma proteins is saturable, with the result that the percent bound decreases as total fosphenytoin concentrations increase. Fosphenytoin displaces phenytoin from protein-binding sites. The volume of distribution of fosphenytoin increases with fosphenytoin dose and rate and ranges from 4.3 to 10.8 L.

Ethotoin: Ethotoin is fairly rapidly absorbed; the extent of oral absorption is not known.

Bioequivalency: Chewed and unchewed phenytoin chewable tablets are bioequivalent, yield approximately equivalent plasma levels, and are more rapidly absorbed than phenytoin 100 mg ER capsules.

Metabolism/Excretion –

Phenytoin: Phenytoin exhibits nonlinear (dose-dependent) pharmacokinetics. Most of phenytoin is excreted in the bile as inactive metabolites that are then reabsorbed from the intestinal tract and excreted in the urine. Urinary excretion of phenytoin and its metabolites occurs partly with glomerular filtration but, more importantly, by tubular excretion. Because phenytoin is hydroxylated in the liver by an enzyme system that is saturable at high plasma levels, small incremental doses may increase the half-life and produce very substantial increases in serum levels when they are in the upper range. The steady-state level may be disproportionately increased, with resultant intoxication, from an increase in dosage of 10% or more.

Fosphenytoin: The hydrolysis of fosphenytoin to phenytoin yields 2 metabolites, phosphate and formaldehyde. Formaldehyde is subsequently converted to formate, which is in turn metabolized via a folate-dependent mechanism. The mechanism of fosphenytoin conversion has not been determined, but phosphatases probably play a major role. Each millimole of fosphenytoin is metabolized to 1 mmol of phenytoin, phosphate, and formate.

Ethotoin: Ethotoin exhibits saturable metabolism with respect to the formation of 2 major metabolites. Ethotoin and, to a lesser extent, a major metabolite exhibit substantial nonlinear kinetics.

Special populations –

Renal/Hepatic function impairment: After IV administration to patients with renal and/or hepatic disease, or those with hypoalbuminemia, fosphenytoin clearance to phenytoin may be increased without a similar increase in phenytoin clearance. This has the potential to increase the frequency and severity of adverse reactions.

The liver is the primary site of biotransformation of phenytoin; patients with liver function impairment, elderly patients, or those who are gravely ill may show early signs of toxicity.

Contraindications

Hypersensitivity to hydantoinsor any component of the product; hepatic abnormalities or hematologic disorders (ethotoin only).

Because of the effect of parenteral phenytoin on ventricular automaticity, parenteral phenytoin and fosphenytoin are contraindicated in patients with sinus bradycardia, sinoatrial block, or second- or third-degree atrioventricular (AV) block, and patients with Adams-Stokes syndrome.

Warnings/Precautions

➤*Suicidal behavior and ideations:* Antiepileptic drugs (AEDs) increase the risk of suicidal thoughts or behavior in patients taking these drugs for any indication. Monitor patients treated with any AED for any indication for the emergence or worsening of depression, suicidal thoughts or behavior, and/or any unusual changes in mood or behavior.

When considering prescribing an AED, balance the risk of suicidal thoughts or behavior with the risk of untreated illness. Epilepsy and many other illnesses for which AEDs are prescribed are themselves associated with morbidity and mortality and an increased risk of suicidal thoughts and behavior. If suicidal thoughts and behavior emerge during treatment, consider whether the emergence of these symptoms in any given patient may be related to the illness being treated.

Inform patients, their caregivers, and families that AEDs increase the risk of suicidal thoughts and behavior and to be alert for the emergence or worsening of the signs and symptoms of depression, any unusual changes in mood or behavior, or the emergence of suicidal thoughts, behavior, or thoughts about self-harm. Advise them to report behaviors of concern immediately to health care providers.

➤*Administration:* The IM route is not recommended for the treatment of status epilepticus because blood levels of phenytoin in the therapeutic range cannot be readily achieved with doses and methods of administration ordinarily employed.

Phenytoin – Phenytoin chewable tablets can either be chewed thoroughly before being swallowed or can be swallowed whole.

IV administration of phenytoin should not exceed 50 mg/min in adults or 1 to 3 mg/kg/min in neonates. Inject phenytoin injection slowly (not exceeding 50 mg/min in adults) directly into a large vein through a large-gauge needle or IV catheter. Follow each injection of IV phenytoin by an injection of sterile saline through the same needle or IV catheter to avoid local venous irritation caused by the alkalinity of the solution.

Avoid continuous infusion because of the likelihood of precipitation when parenteral phenytoin is added to IV infusion fluids.

Fosphenytoin – The dose, concentration in dosing solutions, and infusion rate of fosphenytoin is expressed as phenytoin equivalents. Always prescribe and dispense fosphenytoin in phenytoin equivalent units. Because of the risk of hypotension, administer fosphenytoin no faster than 150 mg phenytoin equivalent/min.

Ethotoin – Take ethotoin after food, and space doses as evenly as practicable.

➤*Local effects:* Soft tissue irritation and inflammation have occurred at the site of injection with and without extravasation of IV phenytoin. Soft tissue irritation may vary from slight tenderness to extensive necrosis or sloughing and, in rare instances, has led to amputation. Avoid improper administration, including subcutaneous or perivascular injection, to help prevent the possibility of the previously listed reactions.

➤*Abrupt withdrawal:* Do not abruptly discontinue antiepileptic drugs because of the possibility of increased seizure frequency, including status epilepticus. When, in the judgement of the health care provider, the need for dosage reduction, discontinuation, or substitution of alternative antiepileptic medication arises, this should be done gradually. However, in the event of an allergic or hypersensitivity reaction, rapid substitution of alternative therapy may be necessary. In this case, alternative therapy should be an antiepileptic drug not belonging to the hydantoin chemical class.

➤*Cardiovascular effects:* Hypotension may occur, especially after IV administration of phenytoin and fosphenytoin at high doses and high rates of administration. Following administration of phenytoin, severe cardiovascular reactions and fatalities have been reported with atrial and ventricular conduction depression and ventricular fibrillation. Severe complications are most commonly encountered in elderly or gravely ill patients. Therefore, careful cardiac monitoring is needed. Reduction in rate of administration or discontinuation of dosing may be needed.

Use IV phenytoin and fosphenytoin with caution in patients with hypotension and severe myocardial insufficiency.

➤*Lymphadenopathy:* There have been a number of reports that have suggested a relationship between hydantoins and the development of lymphadenopathy (local or generalized), including benign lymph node hyperplasia, Hodgkin disease, lymphoma, and pseudolymphoma. Although a cause-and-effect relationship has not been established, the occurrence of lymphadenopathy indicates the need to differentiate such a condition from other types of lymph node pathology. Lymph node involvement may occur with or without symptoms and signs resembling serum sickness (eg, fever, liver involvement, rash). In all cases of lymphadenopathy, follow-up observation for an extended period is indicated; make every effort to achieve seizure control using alternative antiepileptic drugs.

➤*Alcohol use:* Acute alcohol intake may increase plasma phenytoin concentrations, while chronic alcohol use may decrease plasma concentrations.

➤*Dermatologic effects:* Discontinue fosphenytoin and phenytoin if a skin rash appears. If the rash is exfoliative, purpuric, or bullous, or if lupus erythematosus, Stevens-Johnson syndrome, or toxic epidermal necrolysis is suspected, do not resume use of the drug and consider alternative therapy. If the rash is of a milder type (measles-like or scarlatiniform), therapy may be resumed after the rash has completely disappeared. If the rash recurs upon reinstitution of therapy, further drug administration is contraindicated.

*HLA-B*1502* – Limited evidence suggests that HLA-B*1502 may be a risk factor for the development of Stevens-Johnson syndrome/toxic epidermal necrolysis in patients of Asian ancestry taking drugs associated with Stevens-Johnson syndrome/toxic epidermal necrolysis, including phenytoin. Consider avoiding the use of drugs associated with Stevens-Johnson syndrome/toxic epidermal necrolysis, including phenytoin, in HLA-B*1502-positive patients when alternative therapies are otherwise equally available.

➤*Hepatic effects:* Cases of acute hepatotoxicity, including infrequent cases of acute hepatic failure, have been reported with phenytoin. These incidents have been associated with a hypersensitivity syndrome characterized by fever, skin eruptions, and lymphadenopathy, and usually occur within the first 2 months of treatment. Other common manifestations include elevated serum transaminase levels, eosinophilia, hepatomegaly, jaundice, and leukocytosis. The clinical course of acute phenytoin hepatotoxicity ranges from prompt recovery to fatal outcomes. In these patients with acute hepatotoxicity, immediately discontinue and do not readminister the hydantoin.

➤*Hematologic effects:* Hemopoietic complications, some fatal, have occasionally been reported in association with administration of phenytoin. These have included agranulocytosis, granulocytopenia, leukopenia, pancytopenia with or without bone marrow suppression, and thrombocytopenia.

Blood dyscrasias have been reported in patients receiving ethotoin. Although the etiologic role of ethotoin has not been definitely established, be alert for general malaise, sore throat, and other symptoms indicative of possible blood dyscrasia. Ethotoin is contraindicated in patients with hematologic disorders.

➤*Sensory disturbances:* Severe burning, itching, and/or paresthesia were reported by 7 of 16 healthy volunteers administered IV fosphenytoin at a dose of 1,200 mg phenytoin equivalent at the maximum rate of administration (150 mg phenytoin equivalent/min). The severe sensory disturbance lasted from 3 to 50 minutes in 6 of these subjects and for 14 hours in the seventh subject. In some cases, milder sensory disturbances persisted for as long as 24 hours. The location of the discomfort varied among subjects, with the groin mentioned most frequently as an area of discomfort. In a separate cohort of 16 healthy volunteers (taken from 2 other studies) who were administered IV fosphenytoin at a dose of 1,200 mg phenytoin equivalent at the maximum rate of administration (150 mg phenytoin equivalent/min), none experienced severe disturbances, but most experienced mild to moderate itching or tingling.

Patients administered fosphenytoin at doses of 20 mg phenytoin equivalent/kg at 150 mg phenytoin equivalent/min are expected to experience discomfort of some degree. The occurrence and intensity of the discomfort can be lessened by slowing or temporarily stopping the infusion.

The effect of continuing infusion unaltered in the presence of these sensations is unknown. No permanent sequelae have been reported thus far. The pharmacologic basis for these positive sensory phenomena is unknown, but other phosphate ester drugs, which deliver smaller phosphate loads, have been associated with burning, itching, or tingling, predominantly in the groin area.

➤*Phosphate load:* Consider the phosphate load provided by fosphenytoin (0.0037 mmol of phosphate/mg phenytoin equivalent) when treating patients who require phosphate restriction, such as those with severe renal function impairment.

➤*Slow metabolism:* A small percentage of individuals treated with phenytoin have been shown to metabolize the drug slowly. Slow metabolism may be caused by limited enzyme availability and lack of induction; it appears to be genetically determined.

➤*Exacerbation of porphyria:* Phenytoin has been infrequently associated with the exacerbation of porphyria. Exercise caution when fosphenytoin or phenytoin is used in patients with this disease.

➤*Hyperglycemia:* Hyperglycemia, resulting from phenytoin's inhibitory effect on insulin release, has been reported. Phenytoin may also raise the serum glucose concentrations in patients with diabetes.

➤*Acute toxicity:* Plasma concentrations of phenytoin sustained above the optimal range may produce confusional states, referred to as "delirium," "psychosis," or "encephalopathy," or, rarely, irreversible cerebellar dysfunction. Accordingly, at the first sign of acute toxicity, determination of plasma phenytoin concentrations is recommended. Dose reduction is indicated if phenytoin concentrations are excessive; if symptoms persist, discontinue drug administration.

➤*Other seizures:* Hydantoins are not indicated for seizures caused by hypoglycemic or other metabolic causes. Perform appropriate diagnostic procedures as indicated. Hydantoins are not indicated for the treatment of absence seizures. If tonic-clonic and absence seizures are present, combined drug therapy is needed.

➤*Folate levels:* Phenytoin has the potential to lower serum folate levels. Evidence suggests that hydantoin-like compounds may interfere with folic acid metabolism, precipitating a megaloblastic anemia. If this occurs during gestation, consider folic acid therapy.

➤*Osteomalacia:* Osteomalacia has been associated with phenytoin therapy and is considered to be due to phenytoin's interference with vitamin D metabolism.

➤*Enteral feeding:* Literature reports suggest that patients who received enteral feeding preparations and/or related nutritional supplements had lower than expected phenytoin plasma levels. It is therefore suggested that phenytoin not be coadministered with an enteral feeding preparation. More frequent monitoring of serum phenytoin levels may be necessary in these patients.

➤*Hypersensitivity reactions:* Hydantoins are contraindicated in patients who have experienced phenytoin hypersensitivity. Additionally, exercise caution if using structurally similar drugs (eg, barbiturates, oxazolidinediones, succinimides, and other related compounds) in these same patients.

Published literature has suggested that there may be an increased, although still rare, risk of hypersensitivity reactions, including skin rashes, Stevens-Johnson syndrome, toxic epidermal necrolysis, hepatotoxicity, and anticonvulsant hypersensitivity syndrome in black patients.

Anticonvulsant hypersensitivity syndrome – Anticonvulsant hypersensitivity syndrome is a rare, drug-induced, multiorgan syndrome that is potentially fatal and occurs in some patients taking anticonvulsant medication. It is characterized by fever, rash, lymphadenopathy, and other multiorgan pathologies, often hepatic. The mechanism is unknown. The interval between first drug exposure and symptoms is usually 2 to 4 weeks but has been reported in individuals receiving anticonvulsants for 3 or more months. Although up to 1 in 5 patients on phenytoin may develop cutaneous eruptions, only a small proportion will progress to anticonvulsant hypersensitivity syndrome.

Patients at higher risk for developing anticonvulsant hypersensitivity syndrome include black patients, patients who have a family history of or who have experienced this syndrome in the past, and immunosuppressed patients. The syndrome is more severe in previously sensitized individuals. If a patient is diagnosed with anticonvulsant hypersensitivity syndrome, discontinue phenytoin and provide appropriate supportive measures.

➤*Renal/Hepatic function impairment:* After IV administration to patients with renal and/or hepatic disease, or those with hypoalbuminemia, fosphenytoin clearance to phenytoin may be increased without a similar increase in phenytoin clearance. This has the potential to increase the frequency and severity of adverse reactions.

The liver is the primary site of biotransformation of phenytoin; patients with hepatic function impairment, elderly patients, or patients who are gravely ill may show early signs of toxicity.

Ethotoin is contraindicated in patients with hepatic abnormalities.

➤*Pregnancy: Category D.* Hydantoins may cause fetal harm when administered to a pregnant woman. If a hydantoin is used during pregnancy, or if the patient becomes pregnant while taking a hydantoin, apprise the patient of the potential harm to the fetus.

A potentially life-threatening bleeding disorder related to decreased levels of vitamin K–dependent clotting factors may occur in newborns exposed to hydantoins (or other anticonvulsants) in utero. This drug-induced condition can be prevented with vitamin K administration to the mother before delivery and to the neonate after birth.

Phenytoin – Prenatal exposure to phenytoin may increase the risks for congenital malformations and other adverse developmental outcomes. Increased frequencies of major malformations (eg, cardiac defects, orofacial clefts), minor anomalies (dysmorphic facial features, nail and digit hypoplasia), growth abnormalities (eg, microcephaly), and mental deficiency have been reported among children born to epileptic women who took phenytoin alone or in combination with other antiepileptic drugs during pregnancy. There have also been several reported cases of malignancies, including neuroblastoma, in children whose mothers received phenytoin during pregnancy. The overall incidence of malformations for children of epileptic women treated with antiepileptic drugs (phenytoin and/or others) during pregnancy is about 10%, or 2- to 3-fold that in the general population. However, the relative contributions of antiepileptic drugs and other factors associated with epilepsy to this increased risk are uncertain and, in most cases, it has not been possible to attribute specific developmental abnormalities to particular antiepileptic drugs.

An increase in seizure frequency during pregnancy may occur during pregnancy because of altered phenytoin pharmacokinetics. Periodic measurement of serum phenytoin levels may be valuable in the management of pregnant women as a guide to appropriate dosage adjustment. However, postpartum restoration of the original dosage will probably be indicated.

Fosphenytoin – Increased frequencies of death, growth retardation, functional impairment (eg, chromodacryorrhea, circling, hyperactivity), and malformations (brain, cardiovascular, digit, and skeletal anomalies) were observed among the offspring of rats receiving fosphenytoin during pregnancy. Most of the adverse effects on embryo-fetal development occurred at doses of 33 mg phenytoin equivalent/kg or higher (approximately 30% of the maximum human loading dose or higher on a mg/m^2 basis), which produced peak maternal plasma phenytoin concentrations of approximately 20 mcg/mL or greater. Maternal toxicity was often associated with these doses and plasma concentrations; however, there is no evidence to suggest that the developmental effects were secondary to the maternal effects. The single occurrence of a rare brain malformation at a nonmaternotoxic dose of 17 mg phenytoin equivalent/kg (approximately 10% of the maximum human loading dose on a mg/m^2 basis) was also considered drug induced. The developmental effects of fosphenytoin in rats were similar to those reported following administration of phenytoin to pregnant rats.

➤*Lactation:* Following administration of phenytoin, the drug appears to be excreted in low concentrations in human milk. Therefore, according to manufacturers, breast-feeding is not recommended for women receiving phenytoin or fosphenytoin. However, the American Academy of Pediatrics considers phenytoin to be compatible with breast-feeding.

Ethotoin is excreted in breast milk. Because of the potential for serious adverse reactions in breast-feeding infants from ethotoin, decide whether to discontinue breast-feeding or the drug, taking into account the importance of the drug to the mother.

➤*Children:* Phenytoin and ethotoin are approved for use in children. The safety of fosphenytoin in children has not been established.

➤*Elderly:* Phenytoin clearance tends to decrease with increasing age. The liver is the primary site of biotransformation of phenytoin; patients with hepatic function impairment, elderly patients, or patients who are gravely ill may show early signs of toxicity.

Clinical studies of ethotoin did not include sufficient numbers of subjects 65 years of age and older to determine whether they respond differently from younger subjects. In general, dose selection for an elderly patient should be cautious, usually starting at the low end of the dosing range, reflecting the greater frequency of decreased hepatic, renal, or cardiac function, and of concomitant disease or other drug therapy.

➤*Lab test abnormalities:* Phenytoin may cause increased serum concentrations of alkaline phosphatase, gamma glutamyl transpeptidase (GGT), and glucose.

➤*Monitoring:* Perform liver function tests if clinical evidence suggests the possibility of hepatic function impairment.

Closely monitor all patients for the emergence of worsening of depression, suicidal thoughts or behaviors, and/or any unusual changes in mood or behavior.

Phenytoin – Phenytoin doses are usually selected to attain therapeutic plasma total phenytoin concentrations of 10 to 20 mcg/mL (unbound phenytoin concentrations of 1 to 2 mcg/mL). With recommended dosage, a period of 7 to 10 days may be required to achieve steady-state blood levels with phenytoin; changes in dosage (increase or decrease) should not be carried out at intervals shorter than 7 to 10 days.

Monitor serum concentrations when changing from the phenytoin sodium salt (ie, ER capsules, injection) to the free acid form (ie, chewable tablets, oral suspension).

During administration of phenytoin injection, continuous monitoring of ECG and blood pressure is essential. Also observe for signs of respiratory depression.

Fosphenytoin – Following fosphenytoin administration, it is recommended that phenytoin concentrations not be monitored until conversion to phenytoin is essentially complete. This occurs within approximately 2 hours after the end of IV infusion and 4 hours after IM injection.

Continuous monitoring of the ECG, blood pressure, and respiratory function is essential; observe the patient throughout the period during which maximal serum phenytoin concentrations occur, approximately 10 to 20 minutes after the end of the fosphenytoin infusion.

Ethotoin – It is recommended that blood cell counts and urinalyses be performed when therapy is begun and at monthly intervals for several months thereafter. As in patients receiving other hydantoin compounds and other antiepileptic drugs, blood dyscrasias have been reported in patients receiving ethotoin. Marked depression of the blood cell count is indication for withdrawal of the drug.

Drug Interactions

Hydantoins Drug Interactions

Precipitant drug	Object drug[a]		Description
Alcohol	Hydantoins Fosphenytoin Phenytoin	↑↓	Acute alcohol intake may increase phenytoin serum levels, while chronic alcoholic use may decrease serum levels.
Amiodarone	Hydantoins	↑	Increased serum hydantoin concentrations with symptoms of toxicity. Hydantoins may decrease amiodarone serum levels. Monitor drug concentrations and observe the patient for toxicity or loss of therapeutic effect when this combination is used.
Hydantoins	Amiodarone	↓	
Antacids (ie, calcium-containing)	Hydantoins Phenytoin (oral)	↓	Stagger ingestion times of phenytoin and antacid preparations containing calcium in patients with low serum phenytoin levels to prevent absorption problems.
Anticoagulants (eg, dicumarol,[b] warfarin)	Hydantoins	↑	Increased hydantoin serum concentrations with possible toxicity. Increased and decreased PT/INR[c] responses have been reported. May increase or decrease the anticoagulant effect of warfarin; the mechanism is unknown.
Hydantoins	Anticoagulants (eg, dicumarol,[b] warfarin)		
Antineoplastic agents (eg, bleomycin, carboplatin, carmustine, cisplatin, methotrexate, vinblastine)	Hydantoins	↓	Serum concentrations of hydantoins may be decreased, resulting in a loss of therapeutic effect. Monitor hydantoin serum levels and adjust dose appropriately.
Azole antifungals (eg, fluconazole, itraconazole, voriconazole)	Hydantoins	↑	Hydantoin plasma levels may be elevated, increasing the risk of toxicity, while itraconazole and voriconazole plasma levels may be reduced, resulting in decreased efficacy.
Hydantoins	Azole antifungals (ie, itraconazole, voriconazole)	↓	
Barbiturates (eg, phenobarbital)	Hydantoins	↔	The effect of barbiturates on hydantoins is unpredictable. Addition of hydantoins may increase barbiturate serum concentrations. Monitor serum concentrations of both drugs, seizure activity, and clinical symptoms when initiating or discontinuing either drug.
Hydantoins	Barbiturates (eg, phenobarbital)	↑	
Benzodiazepines (eg, alprazolam, chlordiazepoxide, diazepam)	Hydantoins	↑	Serum hydantoin concentrations may be increased, resulting in toxicity, but data is conflicting. Monitor serum hydantoin levels and effects when benzodiazepines are started or stopped. Clearance of midazolam and oxazepam may be increased.
Hydantoins	Benzodiazepines (ie, midazolam, oxazepam)	↓	
Carbamazepine	Hydantoins	↑↓	The effect of carbamazepine on hydantoins is variable. Hydantoins decrease serum carbamazepine levels. Monitor serum concentrations of both drugs, particularly when starting or stopping one drug.
Hydantoins	Carbamazepine	↓	
Chloral hydrate	Hydantoins Fosphenytoin Phenytoin	↓	The elimination of phenytoin is increased, possibly reducing therapeutic effects.

Hydantoins Drug Interactions

Precipitant drug	Object drug[a]		Description
Chloramphenicol	Hydantoins	↑	Increased serum hydantoin concentrations with potential toxicity. Chloramphenicol concentrations may be increased or decreased. Monitor serum concentrations of both drugs closely and adjust dose as needed.
Hydantoins	Chloramphenicol	↑↓	
Cimetidine	Hydantoins	↑	Serum hydantoin levels may be elevated, increasing the pharmacologic effects.
Colesevelam	Hydantoins Ethotoin Phenytoin (oral)	↓	Ethotoin plasma concentrations may be reduced, decreasing efficacy. Administer ethotoin 4 hours prior to colesevelam.
Contraceptives, hormonal	Hydantoins	↑	Hydantoin levels may be increased. Pharmacologic effects of hormonal contraceptives may be decreased. Alternative or nonhormonal contraception is recommended during hydantoin therapy.
Hydantoins	Contraceptives, hormonal	↓	
Corticosteroids	Hydantoins	↓	Hydantoin plasma concentrations may be reduced, decreasing the pharmacologic effect. Decreased steroid effects may occur within days of hydantoin initiation and persist for 3 weeks after discontinuation. A 2-fold or more increase in steroid dose may be needed. Measure hydantoin concentrations and adjust the dose as needed.
Hydantoins	Corticosteroids		
Diazoxide	Hydantoins	↓	Serum hydantoin levels may be decreased, resulting in a possible decrease in the anticonvulsant actions of hydantoin.
Disulfiram	Hydantoins	↑	Serum hydantoin levels may be increased, resulting in an increase in the pharmacologic and toxic effects of hydantoins.
Efavirenz	Hydantoins Phenytoin	↑	Phenytoin concentrations may be elevated. Efavirenz concentrations may be reduced. Monitor concentrations of both drugs and observe patient response. Adjust the dose as needed.
Hydantoins Phenytoin	Efavirenz	↓	
Estrogens (eg, conjugated estrogens, estradiol, ethinyl estradiol)	Hydantoins	↑	Protein binding of phenytoin may be affected. Monitor patients for loss of seizure control. Hydantoins may induce hepatic metabolism of estrogen compounds. This may result in breakthrough bleeding, spotting, and loss of efficacy of hormonal contraceptives. Consider alternate methods of contraception.
Hydantoins	Estrogens (eg, conjugated estrogens, estradiol, ethinyl estradiol)	↓	
Erlotinib	Hydantoins Phenytoin	↑	Phenytoin concentrations may be elevated. Measure phenytoin concentrations and monitor the patient response when starting, stopping, or changing the erlotinib dose. Erlotinib concentrations may be reduced. If alternative treatment lacking CYP3A4 activity is not available, consider increasing the erlotinib dose at 2-week intervals. If the dose is adjusted upward, reduce the erlotinib dose to the indicated starting dose immediately after stopping phenytoin.
Hydantoins Phenytoin	Erlotinib	↓	

Hydantoins Drug Interactions			
Precipitant drug	Object drug[a]		Description
Felbamate	Hydantoins	↑	Serum hydantoin concentrations may be increased, possibly resulting in an increase in the pharmacologic and toxic effects of hydantoins. Phenytoin may also decrease felbamate concentrations. Monitor hydantoin and felbamate concentrations and observe for changes in seizure control.
Hydantoins Phenytoin	Felbamate	↓	
Fluorouracil	Hydantoins	↑	Hydantoin plasma concentrations may be elevated, increasing the pharmacologic effect and risk of toxicity. Closely monitor hydantoin concentrations and adjust the dose as needed.
Folic acid	Hydantoins	↓	Serum hydantoin concentrations may be decreased, resulting in a possible decrease of pharmacologic effects. Monitor serum hydantoin concentrations and observe for decreased hydantoin activity or increased toxicity if folic acid is started or stopped.
Halothane	Hydantoins Fosphenytoin Phenytoin	↑	Serum phenytoin concentrations may be increased.
Isoniazid	Hydantoins	↑	Serum hydantoin concentrations may be increased, producing an increase in the pharmacologic and toxic effects of hydantoins.
Methylphenidate	Hydantoins Fosphenytoin Phenytoin	↑	Serum phenytoin concentrations may be increased.
Metronidazole	Hydantoins	↑	The pharmacologic effects of hydantoins may be increased. Monitor hydantoin plasma levels and adjust the dose accordingly.
Molindone	Hydantoins Phenytoin (oral)	↓	Serum phenytoin concentrations may be decreased. The commercial molindone product contains calcium ions that interfere with the absorption of oral phenytoin.
Omeprazole	Hydantoins	↑	Serum hydantoin levels may be increased, resulting in an increase in the pharmacologic and toxic effects.
Phenacemide[b]	Hydantoins	↑	Serum hydantoin levels may be increased, producing increased pharmacologic and toxic effects of hydantoins.
Phenothiazines (eg, fluphenazine, prochlorperazine, thioridazine)	Hydantoins Fosphenytoin Phenytoin	↑	An increase in pharmacologic effects of phenytoin and a decrease in thioridazine effectiveness may be observed.
Hydantoins Fosphenytoin Phenytoin	Phenothiazines (ie, thioridazine)	↓	
Phenylbutazone[b]	Hydantoins Fosphenytoin Phenytoin	↑	Serum phenytoin levels may be increased.
Protease inhibitors (eg, fosamprenavir, lopinavir/ritonavir)	Hydantoins Fosphenytoin Phenytoin	↓	Certain protease inhibitors and phenytoin plasma concentrations may be reduced during coadministration, decreasing the therapeutic effects of both drugs.
Hydantoins Fosphenytoin Phenytoin	Protease inhibitors (eg, fosamprenavir, lopinavir/ritonavir)		
Quinolones (eg, ciprofloxacin)	Hydantoins Fosphenytoin Phenytoin	↓	Serum levels of phenytoin may be decreased. Measure phenytoin levels and monitor the response of the patient; adjust the dose as needed.

Hydantoins Drug Interactions			
Precipitant drug	Object drug[a]		Description
Reserpine	Hydantoins Fosphenytoin Phenytoin	↓	Serum levels of phenytoin may be decreased.
Rifamycins (eg, rifabutin, rifampin)	Hydantoins	↓	Serum hydantoin levels may be decreased, resulting in a possible decrease in pharmacologic effects of hydantoins. Phenytoin may impair efficacy of rifampin.
Hydantoins Fosphenytoin Phenytoin	Rifamycins (ie, rifampin)		
Salicylates (eg, aspirin, bismuth subsalicylate)	Hydantoins	↑	Serum hydantoin levels may be increased.
SSRIs[c] (eg, fluoxetine, fluvoxamine, sertraline)	Hydantoins	↑	Serum hydantoin concentrations may be elevated, producing an increase in the pharmacologic and toxic effects. Efficacy of paroxetine and sertraline may be impaired by hydantoins.
Hydantoins	SSRIs (ie, paroxetine, sertraline)	↓	
Succinimides (eg, ethosuximide, methsuximide)	Hydantoins	↑	Serum hydantoin levels may be increased, resulting in increased pharmacologic and toxic effects of hydantoin.
Sucralfate	Hydantoins Phenytoin (oral)	↓	The absorption of oral phenytoin may be reduced by coadministration with sucralfate.
Sulfonamides (eg, sulfadiazine, sulfamethizole[b])	Hydantoins	↑	Serum hydantoin levels may be increased, resulting in an increase in the pharmacologic and toxic effects of hydantoins.
Tacrolimus	Hydantoins Fosphenytoin Phenytoin	↑	Phenytoin serum concentrations may be increased by tacrolimus, and tacrolimus serum concentrations may be decreased by phenytoin. Monitor serum concentrations of both tacrolimus and phenytoin.
Hydantoins Fosphenytoin Phenytoin	Tacrolimus	↓	
TCAs[c] (eg, imipramine)	Hydantoins Fosphenytoin Phenytoin	↑	TCAs may precipitate seizures in patients receiving hydantoins. Serum concentrations of phenytoin may be elevated, increasing the pharmacologic effects and risk of toxicity. Measure phenytoin concentrations and observe the response of the patient when a TCA is started or stopped. Adjust the hydantoin dose as needed.
Ticlopidine	Hydantoins	↑	Plasma hydantoin concentrations may be increased, resulting in an increase in adverse effects.
Theophylline	Hydantoins Fosphenytoin Phenytoin	↓	Decrease or loss of pharmacologic effects of theophyllines or phenytoin may occur. When either medication is added to or deleted from a patient's regimen, monitor plasma levels of each drug.
Hydantoins Fosphenytoin Phenytoin	Theophylline		
Tolbutamide	Hydantoins Fosphenytoin Phenytoin	↑	Serum hydantoin levels may be increased. Phenytoin may cause an increase in blood glucose levels, necessitating a higher dose of sulfonylurea for control of hyperglycemia.
Hydantoins Fosphenytoin Phenytoin	Tolbutamide	↓	
Topiramate	Hydantoins	↑	Topiramate may increase the effects of hydantoins, while hydantoins may decrease the pharmacologic effects of topiramate.
Hydantoins	Topiramate	↓	
Trazodone	Hydantoins Phenytoin	↑	The pharmacologic effects of phenytoin may be increased by trazodone. Limited evidence suggests that elevated phenytoin plasma levels, resulting in toxicity, could occur.

Hydantoins Drug Interactions			
Precipitant drug	Object drug[a]		Description
Trimethoprim	Hydantoins	↑	Serum hydantoin concentrations may be increased, producing an increase in the pharmacologic and toxic effects of hydantoins.
Valproic acid Sodium valproate Divalproex sodium	Hydantoins	↑	Hydantoin effects may be enhanced, while those of valproic acid may be decreased. Hydantoin toxicity may occur at therapeutic total plasma concentrations. Monitor the levels of free concentrations of hydantoin and serum valproic acid levels.
Hydantoins	Valproic acid Sodium valproate Divalproex sodium	↓	
Vigabatrin	Hydantoins Fosphenytoin Phenytoin	↓	Phenytoin plasma concentrations may be reduced, decreasing the pharmacologic effects. Measure phenytoin concentrations when vigabatrin is started or stopped. Adjust the hydantoin dose as needed.
Hydantoins	Acetaminophen	↑↓	The potential hepatotoxicity of acetaminophen may be increased when chronic doses of hydantoins are coadministered. The therapeutic effects of acetaminophen may be reduced with simultaneous hydantoin therapy.
Hydantoins	Cyclosporine	↓	Cyclosporine concentrations are decreased by hydantoins, resulting in a decrease in the immunosuppressive activity of cyclosporine, which may predispose patients to transplant rejection. Closely monitor cyclosporine concentrations.
Hydantoins Phenytoin	Deferasirox	↓	Plasma concentrations of deferasirox may be reduced. Avoid concurrent use.
Hydantoins Fosphenytoin Phenytoin	Digoxin	↓	Serum levels of digoxin may be decreased. Monitor for loss of therapeutic effect; increase digoxin dosage as needed.
Hydantoins	Disopyramide	↑↓	Coadministration decreased serum levels, half-life, and bioavailability of disopyramide. At the same time, plasma levels and AUC[d] of the disopyramide major metabolite increased.
Hydantoins Fosphenytoin Phenytoin	Dopamine	↓	The administration of phenytoin during a dopamine infusion may result in profound hypotension and possibly cardiac arrest. Use phenytoin with extreme caution in patients receiving a dopamine infusion.
Hydantoins Fosphenytoin Phenytoin	Doxycycline	↓	The half-life of doxycycline is significantly decreased by coadministration of phenytoin. Consider doubling the dose of doxycycline to maintain adequate serum levels.
Hydantoins	Dronedarone	↓	Dronedarone plasma concentrations may be reduced, decreasing the pharmacologic effects. Avoid coadministration.
Hydantoins Fosphenytoin Phenytoin	Exemestane	↓	Exemestane plasma concentrations may be reduced, decreasing the pharmacologic effects. The recommended dose of exemestane is 50 mg once daily after a meal if fosphenytoin or phenytoin is coadministered. If the hydantoin is discontinued, reduce the exemestane dose to 25 mg once daily with a meal.

Hydantoins Drug Interactions			
Precipitant drug	Object drug[a]		Description
Hydantoins	Felodipine	↓	The pharmacologic effects of felodipine may be decreased. Patients receiving long-term treatment with hydantoins and felodipine may require higher doses of felodipine.
Hydantoins	Gefitinib	↓	Gefitinib plasma concentrations may be reduced, decreasing the pharmacologic effect. Closely monitor for reduced gefitinib effects. Consider increasing the dose of gefitinib when coadministered with hydantoins.
Hydantoins	Haloperidol	↓	Hydantoins may decrease the serum concentration of haloperidol. Monitor patients taking haloperidol for loss of control of psychiatric symptoms or for haloperidol adverse reactions when a hydantoin is added or discontinued.
Hydantoins Fosphenytoin Phenytoin	HMG-CoA reductase inhibitors (eg, atorvastatin, simvastatin)	↓	HMG-CoA reductase inhibitor concentrations may be reduced, decreasing the pharmacologic effect. Monitor the clinical response of the patient. If an interaction is suspected, consider administering alternative therapy. Pravastatin may be less likely to interact.
Hydantoins Fosphenytoin Phenytoin	Imatinib	↓	Imatinib plasma concentrations may be reduced, decreasing the pharmacologic effect. Closely monitor for reduced imatinib effects. Consider increasing the dose of imatinib when fosphenytoin or phenytoin is coadministered.
Hydantoins Fosphenytoin Phenytoin	Irinotecan	↓	Irinotecan plasma concentrations may be reduced, decreasing the efficacy. Irinotecan dosage adjustments may be needed when the hydantoin is started or stopped.
Hydantoins Fosphenytoin Phenytoin	Ixabepilone	↓	Ixabepilone plasma concentrations may be reduced, decreasing the therapeutic effects. Use of therapeutic agents with low CYP3A4 induction potential should be considered for coadministration with ixabepilone.
Hydantoins	Levodopa	↓	Levodopa efficacy may be reduced. Use this combination with caution.
Hydantoins Fosphenytoin Phenytoin	Loop diuretics (ie, furosemide)	↓	Phenytoin may reduce the diuretic effects of furosemide.
Hydantoins Fosphenytoin Phenytoin	Maraviroc	↓	Maraviroc plasma concentrations may be reduced, decreasing the pharmacologic effects. Monitor the response of the patient and adjust the maraviroc dose as needed.
Hydantoins	Methadone	↓	The actions of methadone may be reduced. A higher dose of methadone may be required during coadministration of hydantoins.
Hydantoins	Metyrapone	↓	Coadministration resulted in subnormal pituitary-adrenal responses to oral metyrapone caused by hydantoin induction of metyrapone first-pass hepatic extraction. Consider using oral metyrapone doses as much as twice the usual amount.

Hydantoins

Hydantoins Drug Interactions			
Precipitant drug	Object drug[a]		Description
Hydantoins	Mexiletine	↓	Increased mexiletine clearance during coadministration of hydantoins, leading to lower steady-state plasma mexiletine concentrations and possibly loss of effectiveness.
Hydantoins	Mirtazapine	↓	Mirtazapine plasma concentrations may be reduced, decreasing the pharmacologic effects.
Hydantoins Fosphenytoin Phenytoin	mTOR[e] inhibitors (eg, everolimus, temsirolimus)	↓	Pharmacologic effects of mTOR inhibitors may be decreased. Avoid coadministration. If coadministration cannot be avoided, mTOR inhibitor dosage adjustment is needed.
Hydantoins	Nisoldipine	↓	The pharmacologic effects of nisoldipine may be decreased. Monitor the cardiovascular status of patients receiving this combination therapy.
Hydantoins	NNRT[f] inhibitors (eg, etravirine)	↓	The pharmacologic effects of the NNRT inhibitor may be reduced, decreasing the efficacy. Avoid coadministration.
Hydantoins Fosphenytoin Phenytoin	Nondepolarizing muscle relaxants (eg, cisatracurium, pancuronium, vecuronium)	↓	Nondepolarizing muscle relaxants may have a shorter than expected duration or be less effective. Nondepolarizing muscle relaxant dosage may need to be increased. Monitor for reduced effectiveness.
Hydantoins Fosphenytoin Phenytoin	Posaconazole	↓	The pharmacologic effects of posaconazole may be reduced, decreasing the efficacy. Avoid coadministration.
Hydantoins	Praziquantel	↓	Serum praziquantel concentrations may be reduced, possibly leading to treatment failures.
Hydantoins	Primidone	↑	Hydantoins may increase the serum primidone concentrations and its metabolites. Monitor primidone and primidone metabolites closely following any alteration in hydantoin therapy.
Hydantoins	Progestins (eg, levonorgestrel, norgestrel)	↓	Phenytoin may decrease the efficacy of contraceptive steroids, resulting in increased risk of contraceptive failure. Alternative or nonhormonal contraception is recommended during hydantoin therapy.
Hydantoins	Quetiapine	↓	Quetiapine plasma concentrations and pharmacologic effects may be decreased.
Hydantoins	Quinidine	↓	A decrease in the therapeutic effect of quinidine may occur. Frequent monitoring of serum quinidine concentrations is recommended.
Hydantoins Phenytoin	Ranolazine	↓	Serum levels of ranolazine may be reduced. Avoid coadministration.
Hydantoins Fosphenytoin Phenytoin	Teniposide	↓	Teniposide plasma concentrations may be reduced, decreasing the efficacy. Closely monitor the patient response to teniposide when starting, stopping, or changing the hydantoin dose. Adjust the teniposide dose as needed.
Hydantoins Fosphenytoin Phenytoin	Tolvaptan	↓	Tolvaptan plasma concentrations may be reduced, decreasing the efficacy. Avoid coadministration.
Hydantoins	Tyrosine kinase inhibitors (eg, dasatinib, lapatinib, nilotinib)	↓	Tyrosine kinase inhibitor plasma concentrations may be reduced, decreasing the efficacy. Avoid coadministration.
Hydantoins Fosphenytoin Phenytoin	Vitamin D	↓	Phenytoin may decrease the efficacy of vitamin D.

[a] ↑ = object drug increased; ↓ = object drug decreased; ↑↓ = object drug both increased and decreased; ↔ = undetermined clinical effect.
[b] No longer marketed in the United States.
[c] TCAs = tricyclic antidepressants.
[d] PT/INR = prothrombin time/international normalized ratio; SSRIs = selective serotonin reuptake inhibitors; AUC = area under the curve.
[e] mTOR = Mammalian target of rapamycin.
[f] NNRT = Non-nucleoside reverse transcriptase.

➤*Drug/Lab test interactions:* Phenytoin may cause decreased serum levels of protein-bound iodine. It may also produce artificially low results in dexamethasone or metyrapone tests.

Take care when using immunoanalytical methods to measure plasma phenytoin concentrations following fosphenytoin administration.

➤*Drug/Food interactions:* The anticonvulsant effects of phenytoin may be altered by food. Administer phenytoin consistently with respect to meals to avoid fluctuations in the amount of phenytoin absorbed. Literature reports suggest that patients who have received enteral feeding preparations and/or related nutritional supplements have lower than expected phenytoin plasma levels. It is therefore suggested that phenytoin not be coadministered with an enteral feeding preparation. More frequent phenytoin level monitoring may be necessary in these patients.

Adverse Reactions

Hydantoins: Summary of Adverse Reactions[a]

Adverse reaction	Ethotoin	Fosphenytoin	Phenytoin	
			Oral	Injection
Cardiovascular				
Atrial/Ventricular conduction depression				✓[b,c]
Cardiovascular collapse		✓		✓[b]
Hypotension		7.7% (IV)		✓[b]
Periarteritis nodosa			✓	✓
Tachycardia		2.2% (IV)		
Vasodilation		5.6% (IV)		
Ventricular fibrillation				✓
CNS				
Agitation		3.3% (IV)		
Ataxia	Rare	11.1% (IV); 8.4% (IM)[d]	✓	✓
Brain edema		2.2% (IV)		
CNS depression		0.1% to 1%		✓
Coordination, decreased			✓	✓
Dizziness	✓	31.1% (IV); 5% (IM)[d]	✓	✓
Dysarthria		2.2% (IV)		
Dyskinesias (chorea, dystonia, tremor, asterixis)			Rare	Rare
Extrapyramidal syndrome		4.4% (IV)		
Headache	✓	2.2% (IV); 8.9% (IM)[d]	✓	✓
Hypesthesia		2.2% (IV)		
Incoordination		4.4% (IV); 7.8% (IM)[d]		
Insomnia	✓	0.1% to 1%	✓	✓
Mental confusion		0.1% to 1%	✓	✓
Motor twitchings		0.1% to 1%	✓	✓
Nervousness		> 1%	✓	✓
Numbness	✓			
Nystagmus	✓	44.4% (IV); 15.1% (IM)[d]	✓	✓
Paresthesia		4.4% (IV)[b]; 3.9% (IM)[b,d]		
Peripheralpolyneuropathy			✓[e]	✓[e]
Reflexes decreased		2.8% (IM)[d]		
Slurred speech			✓	✓
Somnolence		20% (IV); 6.7% (IM)[d]		
Stupor		7.7% (IV)		

Hydantoins: Summary of Adverse Reactions[a]

Adverse reaction	Ethotoin	Fosphenytoin	Phenytoin	
			Oral	Injection
Tremor		3.3% (IV); 9.5% (IM)[d]		
Vertigo		2.2% (IV)		
Dermatologic				
Bullous, exfoliative or purpuric dermatitis			✓[b]	✓[b]
Dermatitis			✓	✓
Hypertrichosis			✓	✓
Morbilliform rash			✓	✓
Pruritus		48.9% (IV)[b]; 2.8% (IM)[b,d]		
Scarlatiniform rash			✓[b]	✓[b]
Skin rash	✓	> 1%	✓[b]	✓[b]
Toxic epidermal necrolysis			✓[b]	✓[b]
GI				
Constipation		> 1%	✓	✓
Diarrhea	✓	0.1% to 1%		
Dry mouth		4.4% (IV)		
Ecchymosis		7.3% (IM)[d]		
Gum/Gingival hypertrophy	Rare		✓	✓
Liver damage			✓[b]	✓[b]
Nausea	✓	8.9% (IV); 4.5% (IM)[d]	✓	✓
Tongue disorder		4.4% (IV)		
Toxic hepatitis			✓	✓
Vomiting	✓	2.2% (IV); 2.8% (IM)[d]	✓	✓
Hematologic/Lymphatic				
Agranulocytosis			✓[b]	✓[b]
Benign lymph node hyperplasia			✓[b]	✓[b]
Blood dyscrasias	✓[b]			
Granulocytopenia			✓[b]	✓[b]
Hodgkin disease			✓[b]	✓[b]
Leukopenia		0.1% to 1%	✓[b]	✓[b]
Lymphadenopathy	✓	0.1% to 1%	✓[b]	✓[b]
Lymphoma			✓[b]	✓[b]
Macrocytosis			✓[f]	✓[f]
Megaloblastic anemia			✓[f]	✓[f]
Pancytopenia (with or without bone marrow suppression)			✓[b]	✓[b]
Pseudolymphoma			✓[b]	✓[b]
Thrombocytopenia		0.1% to 1%	✓[b]	✓[b]
Hypersensitivity				
Hypersensitivity syndrome[g]			✓	
Stevens-Johnson syndrome	✓		✓[b]	✓[b]
Local				
Inflammation		0.1% to 1%		✓[b]
Local irritation				✓[b]
Necrosis				✓[b]
Sloughing				✓[b]
Tenderness/Pain		0.1% to 1%		✓[b]
Special senses				
Amblyopia		2.2% (IV)		
Deafness		2.2% (IV)		
Diplopia	✓	3.3% (IV)		
Taste perversion		3.3% (IV)		
Tinnitus		8.9% (IV)		
Miscellaneous				
Accidental injury		3.4% (IM)[d]		
Asthenia		2.2% (IV); 3.9% (IM)[d]		
Back pain		2.2% (IV)		
Chest pain	✓			
Coarsening of facial features			✓	✓
Enlargement of lips			✓	✓
Fatigue	✓			
Fever	✓	> 1%		
Hyperglycemia		✓[b]	✓[b]	✓[b]
Immunoglobulin abnormalities			✓	✓
Lupus erythematosus			✓[b]	✓[b]
Pelvic pain		4.4% (IV)		
Peyronie disease			✓	✓
Systemic lupus erythematosus	✓		✓	✓

[a] Data are pooled from separate studies and are not necessarily comparable.
[b] See Warnings/Precautions for more information.
[c] ✓ = reported; no incidence given.
[d] Adverse reaction following substitution of fosphenytoin IM for oral phenytoin.
[e] With long-term phenytoin therapy.
[f] Usually responds to folic acid therapy.
[g] May include, but is not limited to, symptoms such as arthralgias, eosinophilia, fever, liver dysfunction, lymphadenopathy, or rash.

➤*Fosphenytoin:*

Cardiovascular – Hypertension (greater than 1%); atrial flutter, bundle branch block, cardiac arrest, cardiomegaly, cerebral hemorrhage, cerebral infarct, congestive heart failure, migraine, palpitation, postural hypotension, pulmonary embolus, QT interval prolongation, sinus bradycardia, syncope, thrombophlebitis, ventricular extrasystoles (0.1% to 1%).

CNS – Dysarthria, intracranial hypertension, reflexes increased, speech disorder, thinking abnormal (greater than 1%); acute brain syndrome, akathisia, amnesia, aphasia, Babinski sign positive, brain edema, circumoral paresthesia, coma, convulsion, depersonalization, depression, emotional lability, encephalitis, encephalopathy, hematoma, hemiplegia, hyperesthesia, hyperkinesia, hypokinesia, hypotonia, meningitis, myoclonus, neurosis, paralysis, personality disorder, psychosis, subdural hostility (0.1% to 1%).

Dermatologic – Contact dermatitis, maculopapular rash, pustular rash, skin discoloration, skin nodule, sweating, urticaria (0.1% to 1%).

Endocrine – Diabetes insipidus (0.1% to 1%).

GI – Anorexia, dyspepsia, dysphagia, flatulence, gastritis, GI hemorrhage, ileus, increased salivation, liver function tests abnormal, tenesmus, tongue edema (0.1% to 1%).

GU – Albuminuria, dysuria, genital edema, kidney failure, oliguria, polyuria, urethral pain, urinary incontinence, urinary retention, vaginitis, vaginal moniliasis (0.1% to 1%).

Hematologic / Lymphatic – Anemia, cyanosis, hypochromic anemia, leukocytosis, petechia (0.1% to 1%).

Local – Injection-site reaction (greater than 1%); injection-site edema, injection-site hemorrhage (0.1% to 1%).

Metabolic / Nutritional – Face edema, hypokalemia (greater than 1%); acidosis, alkalosis, dehydration, generalized edema, hyperglycemia, hyperkalemia, hypophosphatemia, ketosis (0.1% to 1%).

Musculoskeletal – Myasthenia (greater than 1%); arthralgia, leg cramps, myalgia, myopathy (0.1% to 1%).

Respiratory – Pneumonia (greater than 1%); apnea, aspiration pneumonia, asthma, atelectasis, bronchitis, cough increased, dyspnea, epistaxis, hemoptysis, hyperventilation, hypoxia, pharyngitis, pneumothorax, rhinitis, sinusitis, sputum increased (0.1% to 1%).

Special senses – Conjunctivitis, ear pain, eye pain, hyperacusis, mydriasis, parosmia, photophobia, taste loss, visual field defect (0.1% to 1%).

Miscellaneous – Chills, infection, (greater than 1%); cachexia, cryptococcosis, flu syndrome, malaise, photosensitivity reaction, sepsis, shock (0.1% to 1%).

Overdosage

➤*Symptoms:*

Phenytoin – The lethal dose of phenytoin in children is not known. The lethal dose in adults is estimated to be 2 to 5 g. The initial symptoms are ataxia, dysarthria, and nystagmus. Other signs are hyperreflexia, lethargy, nausea, slurred speech, tremor, and vomiting. The patient may become comatose and hypotensive. Death is due to respiratory and circulatory depression.

There are marked variations among individuals with respect to phenytoin plasma levels in whom toxicity may occur. Nystagmus, on lateral gaze, usually appears at 20 mcg/mL, ataxia at 30 mcg/mL; dysarthria and lethargy appear when the plasma concentration is more than 40 mcg/mL, but as high a concentration as 50 mcg/mL has been reported without evidence of toxicity. As much as 25 times the therapeutic dose has been taken to result in a serum concentration of more than 100 mcg/mL with complete recovery.

Fosphenytoin – Asystole, bradycardia, cardiac arrest, death, hypocalcemia, hypotension, lethargy, metabolic acidosis, nausea, syncope, tachycardia, and vomiting have been reported in cases of overdosage with fosphenytoin.

Formate and phosphate are metabolites of fosphenytoin and therefore may contribute to signs of toxicity following overdosage. Signs of formate toxicity are similar to those of methanol toxicity and are associated with severe anion-gap metabolic acidosis. Large amounts of phosphate, delivered rapidly, could potentially cause hypocalcemia with paresthesia, muscle spasms, and seizures. Ionized free calcium levels can be measured and, if low, used to guide treatment.

The median lethal dose of fosphenytoin given IV in mice and rats was 156 mg phenytoin equivalent/kg and approximately 250 mg phenytoin equivalent/kg, or about 0.6 and 2 times, respectively, the maximum human loading dose on a mg/m^2 basis. Signs of acute toxicity in animals included ataxia, labored breathing, hypoactivity, and ptosis.

Ethotoin – Symptoms of acute overdosage include ataxia, drowsiness, nausea, and visual disturbance. Coma is possible at very high dosages.

➤*Treatment:* Treatment is nonspecific because there is no known antidote. Carefully observe the adequacy of the respiratory and circulatory systems and employ appropriate supportive measures. Total exchange transfusion has been used in the treatment of severe intoxication in children.

In acute overdosage, keep in mind the possibility of other CNS depressants, including alcohol.

Ethotoin – Carefully evaluate blood-forming organs following recovery.

Patient Information

Advise patients taking hydantoins of the importance of adhering strictly to the prescribed dosage regimen. Tell patients to inform their health care provider of any clinical condition in which it is not possible to take the drug orally as prescribed (eg, surgery).

Caution patients on the use of other drugs or alcoholic beverages without first seeking the health care provider's advice.

Instruct patients to call their health care provider if skin rash develops.

Stress the importance of good dental hygiene in order to minimize the development of gingival hyperplasia and its complications.

Counsel patients, their caregivers, and families that AEDs, including hydantoins, may increase the risk of suicidal thoughts and behavior. Advise them of the need to be alert for the emergence or worsening of symptoms of depression, any unusual changes in mood or behavior, or the emergence of suicidal thoughts, behavior, or thoughts of self-harm. Tell them to report behaviors of concern immediately to health care providers.

➤*Phenytoin oral suspension:* Instruct patients to use an accurately calibrated measuring device when using this medication to ensure accurate dosing. Shake well prior to use.

➤*Phenytoin chewable tablets:* Tablets can be either chewed thoroughly before being swallowed or can be swallowed whole.

➤*Ethotoin:* Take after food, and space doses as evenly as practicable. Advise patients to report immediately any signs and symptoms, such as easy bruising, epistaxis, fever, malaise, petechiae, or sore throat that may be indicative of an infection or bleeding tendency.

ETHOTOIN

Rx	**Peganone** (Lundbeck)	**Tablets; oral:** 250 mg	Lactose. (OV 61). White. In 100s.

ETHOTOIN — ORAL

For complete and comparative prescribing information, refer to the Hydantoins class monograph.

Indications

➤*Seizures:* For the control of tonic-clonic and complex partial (psychomotor) seizures.

Administration and Dosage

➤*General dosing considerations:* Drug may need to be tapered prior to discontinuation. (See Tapering.)

➤*Adults:*

Seizures –

Initial dosage: 1 g or less daily in 4 to 6 divided doses, with subsequent gradual dosage increases over a period of several days. The optimum dosage must be determined on an individual-response basis.

Maintenance dosage: 2 to 3 g daily in 4 to 6 divided doses. Less than 2 g daily was ineffective in most adults.

➤*Children:*

Seizures –

Children 1 year of age and older:

- *Initial dosage* – Do not exceed 750 mg daily in 4 to 6 divided doses.
- *Maintenance dosage* – 500 mg to 1 g daily in 4 to 6 divided doses, although occasionally, 2 or (rarely) 3 g daily in 4 to 6 divided doses may be necessary.

➤*Hepatic function impairment:* Contraindicated in patients with hepatic abnormalities.

➤*Tapering:* If a patient is receiving another antiepileptic drug (AED), it should not be discontinued when ethotoin therapy is begun. The dosage of the other drug should be gradually reduced as that of ethotoin is increased. Ethotoin may eventually replace the other drug or the optimal dosage of both antiepileptics may be established.

Concomitant therapy – In tonic-clonic seizures, use of the drug with phenobarbital may be beneficial.

➤*Administration:* Should be taken after food; doses should be spaced as evenly as possible.

Administer orally in 4 to 6 divided doses daily.

➤*Storage/Stability:* Store below 25°C (77°F). Protect from light.

FOSPHENYTOIN SODIUM

Rx	**Fosphenytoin Sodium** (Various, eg, Akorn, APP, Bedford, Hospira, Wockhard)	**Injection, solution, concentrate:** 75 mg/mL (equiv. to phenytoin sodium 50 mg/mL)	In 2 and 10 mL vials.
Rx	**Cerebyx** (Parke-Davis)		In 2 mL vials.

FOSPHENYTOIN SODIUM — INJECTION

For complete and comparative prescribing information, refer to the Hydantoins class monograph.

Indications

➤*Seizures:* For the control of generalized convulsive status epilepticus and the prevention and treatment of seizures occurring during neurosurgery. It can also be substituted, short term, for oral phenytoin.

Administration and Dosage

➤*General dosing considerations:* The dose, concentration in dosing solutions, and infusion rate of intravenous (IV) fosphenytoin is expressed as phenytoin sodium equivalent to avoid the need to perform molecular weight–based adjustments when converting between fosphenytoin and phenytoin doses.

Fosphenytoin should always be prescribed and dispensed in phenytoin sodium equivalent units.

Monitor patients for approximately 10 to 20 minutes after the end of fosphenytoin infusions.

Renal and hepatic impairment may alter total phenytoin plasma concentrations (see Therapeutic Drug Monitoring).

If rapid phenytoin loading is a primary goal, IV administration of fosphenytoin is preferred because the time to achieve therapeutic plasma phenytoin concentrations is greater following intramuscular (IM) administration than IV administration.

➤*Adults:*

Seizures –

Loading dose: Phenytoin sodium equivalent 15 to 20 mg/kg administered IV at phenytoin sodium equivalent 100 to 150 mg/min.

Maintenance dosage: The initial daily maintenance dosage is phenytoin sodium equivalent 4 to 6 mg/kg/day. The loading dose should be followed by maintenance doses of fosphenytoin or phenytoin orally or parenterally.

Concomitant therapy: Because the full antiepileptic effect of phenytoin, whether given as fosphenytoin or parenteral phenytoin, is not immediate, other measures, including coadministration of an IV benzodiazepine, will usually be necessary for the control of status epilepticus.

If administration of fosphenytoin does not terminate seizures, the use of other anticonvulsants and other appropriate measures should be considered.

Prevention of seizures occurring during neurosurgery –

Loading dose: Phenytoin sodium equivalent 10 to 20 mg/kg given IV or IM.

Maintenance dosage: Initial daily maintenance dosage is phenytoin sodium equivalent 4 to 6 mg/kg/day IM or IV.

➤*Children:*

Off-label dosing –

Status epilepticus:

- *Loading dose* –

  Neonates: Phenytoin sodium equivalent 15 to 24 mg/kg. Phenobarbital or a benzodiazepine may be preferable to fosphenytoin in this age group.

  Infants and children: Phenytoin sodium equivalent 15 to 20 mg/kg administered IV.

FOSPHENYTOIN SODIUM — INJECTION

Maintenance for seizure disorder:

• *Usual dose* –

Neonates (30 days of age and younger): Phenytoin sodium equivalent 4 to 8 mg/kg IV or IM divided 2 to 3 times daily.

6 months to 3 years of age: Phenytoin sodium equivalent 8 to 10 mg/kg IV or IM divided 2 to 3 times daily.

4 to 6 years of age: Phenytoin sodium equivalent 7.5 to 9 mg/kg IV or IM divided 2 to 3 times daily.

7 to 9 years of age: Phenytoin sodium equivalent 7 to 8 mg/kg IV or IM divided 2 to 3 times daily.

10 to 16 years of age: Phenytoin sodium equivalent 6 to 7 mg/kg IV or IM divided 2 to 3 times daily.

• *Initial dosage* –

Infants and children: Phenytoin sodium equivalent 5 mg/kg IV or IM divided 2 to 3 times daily. Follow with usual dose within 24 hours.

➤*Elderly:* Phenytoin clearance is decreased slightly in elderly patients; lower or less frequent dosing may be required.

➤*Substitution for oral phenytoin:* Fosphenytoin IM or IV can be substituted for oral phenytoin therapy at the same total daily dose.

Plasma phenytoin concentrations may increase modestly when IM or IV fosphenytoin is substituted for oral phenytoin therapy due to increased bioavailability.

➤*Therapeutic drug monitoring:* Typical therapeutic plasma total phenytoin concentrations are 10 to 20 mcg/mL (unbound phenytoin concentrations of 1 to 2 mcg/mL). It is recommended that phenytoin concentrations be monitored only after conversion to phenytoin is essentially complete approximately 2 hours after the end of IV infusion and 4 hours after IM injection.

Because of an increased fraction of unbound phenytoin in patients with renal or hepatic disease, or in those with hypoalbuminemia, the interpretation of total phenytoin plasma concentrations should be made with caution. Unbound phenytoin concentrations may be more useful in these patient populations.

➤*Discontinuation of therapy:* Fosphenytoin should not be abruptly discontinued because of the possibility of increased seizure frequency, including status epilepticus. If there is a need for dosage reduction, discontinuation, or substitution of alternative antiepileptic medication, this should be done gradually. In the event of an allergic or hypersensitivity reaction, rapid substitution of alternative therapy not belonging to the hydantoin chemical class is permissible.

➤*Preparation for administration:* Dilute fosphenytoin in dextrose 5% or saline 0.9% solution for injection to a concentration ranging from phenytoin sodium equivalent 1.5 to 25 mg/mL.

➤*Administration:* Because of the risk of hypotension, fosphenytoin should be administered no faster than phenytoin sodium equivalent 150 mg/min.

IM fosphenytoin should not be used in the treatment of status epilepticus because therapeutic phenytoin concentrations may not be reached as quickly as with IV administration. If IV access is impossible, loading doses of fosphenytoin have been given by the IM route for other indications.

In controlled trials, IM fosphenytoin was administered as a single daily dose utilizing either 1 or 2 injection sites. Some patients may require more frequent dosing.

The typical fosphenytoin infusion administered to a 50 kg patient would take between 5 and 7 minutes. Note that the delivery of an identical molar dose of phenytoin using parenteral phenytoin cannot be accomplished in less than 15 to 20 minutes because of the untoward cardiovascular effects that accompany the direct IV administration of phenytoin at rates more than 50 mg/min.

➤*Storage/Stability:* Store under refrigeration at 2° to 8°C (36° to 46°F). The product should not be stored at room temperature for more than 48 hours.

PHENYTOIN

Rx	**Dilantin Infatab** (Parke-Davis)	**Tablets, chewable; oral:** 50 mg	Saccharin, sucrose. Yellow, triangular, scored. In 100s and UD 100s.
Rx	**Dilantin** (Parke-Davis)	**Capsules, extended-release; oral:** 30 mg	As phenytoin sodium. Lactose, sugar. (PD Dilantin 30 mg). White opaque/pale pink opaque. In 100s.
Rx	**Phenytoin Sodium** (Wockhardt USA[a])	**Capsules, extended-release; oral:** 30 mg	As phenytoin sodium. In 100s and 1,000s.
Rx	**Dilantin** (Parke-Davis)	**Capsules, extended-release; oral:** 100 mg	As phenytoin sodium. Lactose, sugar. (PD Dilantin 100 mg). Orange/White opaque. In 100s, 1,000s, and UD 100s.
Rx	**Phenytoin Sodium** (Various, eg, Amneal, Taro)	**Capsules, extended-release; oral:** 100 mg	As phenytoin sodium. May contain lactose, mannitol, sugar. In 30s, 100s, 500s, 1,000s, and UD 100s.
Rx	**Phenytek** (Mylan)	**Capsules, extended-release; oral:** 200 mg	As phenytoin sodium. (BERTEK 670). Dark blue opaque/blue opaque. In 30s and 100s.
Rx	**Phenytoin Sodium** (Caraco)	**Capsules, extended-release; oral:** 200 mg	As phenytoin sodium. In 30s, 100s, and 500s.
Rx	**Phenytek** (Mylan)	**Capsules, extended-release; oral:** 300 mg	As phenytoin sodium. (BERTEK 750). Blue opaque. In 30s and 100s.
Rx	**Phenytoin Sodium** (Caraco)	**Capsules, extended-release; oral:** 300 mg	As phenytoin sodium. In 30s, 100s, and 500s.
Rx	**Phenytoin** (Various, eg, Actavis Mid Atlantic[b], Taro)	**Suspension; oral:** 125 mg per 5 mL	May contain alcohol, sucrose, sodium benzoate, glycerin. In 240 mL.
Rx	**Dilantin-125** (Pfizer)		0.6% or less alcohol, sucrose, sodium benzoate, glycerin. Orange-vanilla flavor. In 240 mL.
Rx	**Phenytoin Sodium** (Various, eg, Baxter, Hospira, West-Ward)	**Injection, solution:** 50 mg/mL	May contain alcohol. In 2 and 5 mL.

[a] Wockhardt USA, 135 Route 202–206, Bedminster, NJ 07921; 908-719-4350; http://www.wockhardtusa.com.

[b] Actavis Mid Atlantic, 7125 Columbia Gateway Dr., Columbia, MD 21046–2552; 410-277-1630.

PHENYTOIN — ORAL

For complete and comparative prescribing information, refer to the Hydantoins class monograph.

Indications

➤*Seizures:* For the control of generalized tonic-clonic and complex partial (psychomotor, temporal lobe) seizures; prevention and treatment of seizures occurring during or following neurosurgery(tablets only).

➤*Off-label uses:*

Rectal administration – [4] = Insufficient documentation. There are limited clinical and kinetic data available regarding the rectal administration of phenytoin.

Administration and Dosage

➤*General dosing considerations:* The dosage should be individualized to provide maximum benefit. Serum blood level determinations may be necessary for optimal dosage adjustments. (See Therapeutic drug monitoring.)

Tablets are not for once-daily dosing.

➤*Adults:*

Seizures –

Initial dosage: 2 tablets (100 mg) or 5 mL of suspension (125 mg) 3 times daily in patients who have received no previous treatment.

Maintenance dosage: 6 to 8 tablets (300 to 400 mg) daily; an increase to 12 tablets (600 mg) or 25 mL of suspension (625 mg) daily may be made if necessary.

Dosage adjustment: Adjust dose to suit individual requirements.

Off-label dosing –

Rectal administration: [4] = Insufficient documentation. 300 to 1,200 mg daily (as suppositories) for 10 days. Formulation information was not provided.

➤*Children:*

Seizures –

Usual dosage: 4 to 8 mg/kg/day in 2 or 3 equally divided doses. Children older than 6 years of age and adolescents may require the minimum adult dose (300 mg/day).

Maximum dose: 300 mg daily.

Initial dosage: 5 mg/kg/day in 2 or 3 equally divided doses, with subsequent dosage individualized.

Off-label dosing –

Seizures:

• *Usual dose* –

10 to 16 years of age: 6 to 7 mg/kg/day in 2 or 3 divided doses.

7 to 9 years of age: 7 to 8 mg/kg/day in 2 or 3 divided doses.

4 to 6 years of age: 7.5 to 9 mg/kg/day in 2 or 3 divided doses.

6 months to 3 years of age: 8 to 10 mg/kg/day in 2 or 3 divided doses.

Neonates: 5 to 8 mg/kg/day in 2 or 3 divided doses.

• *Initial dosage* –

6 months to 16 years of age: 5 mg/kg/day in 2 or 3 divided doses.

Neonates: 5 mg/kg/day in 2 divided doses.

PHENYTOIN — ORAL

➤*Conversion:* When given in equal doses, phenytoin yields higher plasma levels than phenytoin sodium. Because there is approximately an 8% increase in drug content with the free acid form over that of the sodium salt, dosage adjustments and serum level monitoring may be necessary when switching from a product formulated with the free acid to a product formulated with the sodium salt and vice versa.

➤*Therapeutic drug monitoring:* In some cases, serum blood level determinations may be necessary for optimal dosage adjustments; the clinically effective serum level is usually 10 to 20 mcg/mL. With recommended dosage, a period of 7 to 10 days may be required to achieve steady-state blood levels with phenytoin, and changes in dosage (increase or decrease) should not be carried out at intervals shorter than 7 to 10 days.

For patients with low albumin levels (hypoalbuminemia), renal impairment, hepatic impairment, or a critical illness, monitoring free phenytoin levels should be considered.

Alternatively, equations taking into account the patient's serum albumin and renal function may be used to estimate the serum phenytoin level that would have been observed if serum albumin and renal function were normal.

Total phenytoin level adjusted for hypoalbuminemia:

$$\text{Total } C_{normalized} = \text{Total } C_{measured} / [(0.2 \times \text{serum albumin [g/dL]}) + 0.1]$$

Total phenytoin level adjusted for hypoalbuminemia and end-stage renal disease requiring hemodialysis:

$$\text{Total } C_{normalized} = \text{Total } C_{measured} / [(0.1 \times \text{serum albumin [g/dL]}) + 0.1]$$

Total phenytoin – The therapeutic range is 10 to 20 mcg/mL. Levels less than 5 mcg/mL are rarely effective; levels more than 20 mcg/mL produce dose-related adverse effects.

Free phenytoin – The therapeutic range is 1 to 2 mcg/mL.

➤*Administration:* Tablets can be chewed thoroughly before swallowing or swallowed whole. Shake suspension well before preparing dose.

Children – If the daily dosage cannot be divided equally, the larger dose should be given before retiring.

➤*Storage/Stability:* Store tablets at room temperature, below 30°C (86°F). Store unit dose tablets at 15° to 30°C (59° to 86°F). Protect from moisture. Store suspension at 20° to 25°C (68° to 77°F). Protect from freezing and light.

PHENYTOIN SODIUM — ORAL

For complete and comparative prescribing information, refer to the Hydantoins class monograph.

Indications

➤*Seizures:* For the control of generalized tonic-clonic and complex partial (psychomotor, temporal lobe) seizures, and the prevention and treatment of seizures occurring during or following neurosurgery.

➤*Off-label uses:*

Rectal administration – [4] = Insufficient documentation. There are limited clinical and kinetic data available regarding the rectal administration of phenytoin.

Administration and Dosage

➤*General dosing considerations:* The dosage should be individualized to provide maximum benefit. Serum blood level determinations may be necessary for optimal dosage adjustments (see Therapeutic drug monitoring).

➤*Adults:*

Seizures –

Divided daily dosage:

• *Usual dosage* – 100 mg 3 to 4 times a day. An increase of up to 200 mg 3 times a day may be made if necessary.

• *Initial dosage* – 100 mg 3 times daily; the dosage should then be adjusted to suit individual requirements.

• *Loading dose* – Some authorities have advocated the use of an oral loading dose of phenytoin in adults who require rapid steady-state serum levels and in whom intravenous administration is not desirable. This dosing regimen should be reserved for patients in a clinical or hospital setting, where phenytoin serum levels can be closely monitored. Patients with a history of renal or liver disease should not receive the oral loading regimen.

Initial dosage: 1 g divided into 3 doses (400, 300, and 300 mg) and administered at 2-hour intervals.

Maintenance dosage: Normal maintenance dosage is then instituted 24 hours after the loading dose, with frequent serum level determinations.

Once-daily dosage: If seizure control is established with 100 mg 3 times daily, once-daily dosage with phenytoin 300 mg extended release (ER) may be considered.

➤*Children:*

Seizures –

Usual dosage: 4 to 8 mg/kg/day in 2 or 3 equally divided doses. Children older than 6 years of age and adolescents may require the minimum adult dose (300 mg/day).

Maximum dose: 300 mg daily.

Initial dosage: 5 mg/kg/day in 2 or 3 equally divided doses, with subsequent dosage individualized.

Off-label dosing –

Seizures:

• *Usual dose* –

10 to 16 years of age: 6 to 7 mg/kg/day in 2 or 3 divided doses.

7 to 9 years of age: 7 to 8 mg/kg/day in 2 or 3 divided doses.

4 to 6 years of age: 7.5 to 9 mg/kg/day in 2 or 3 divided doses.

6 months to 3 years of age: 8 to 10 mg/kg/day in 2 or 3 divided doses.

Neonates: 5 to 8 mg/kg/day in 2 or 3 divided doses.

• *Initial dosage* –

6 months to 16 years of age: 5 mg/kg/day in 2 or 3 divided doses.

Neonates: 5 mg/kg/day in 2 divided doses.

➤*Conversion:* Only phenytoin sodium ER capsules are recommended for once-daily dosing. Inherent differences in dissolution characteristics and resulting absorption rates of phenytoin due to different manufacturing procedures and/or dosage forms preclude such recommendations for other phenytoin products. When a change in dosage form or brand is prescribed, careful monitoring of phenytoin serum levels should be carried out.

Phenytoin sodium ER capsules are formulated with the sodium salt of phenytoin. The free acid form of phenytoin is used in phenytoin suspensions and tablets. Because there is an approximate 8% increase in drug content with the free acid form compared with the sodium salt, dosage adjustments and serum level monitoring may be necessary when switching from a product formulated with the free acid to a product formulated with the sodium salt and vice versa.

➤*Therapeutic drug monitoring:* In some cases, serum blood level determinations may be necessary for optimal dosage adjustments; the clinically effective serum level is usually 10 to 20 mcg/mL. With the recommended dosage, a period of 7 to 10 days may be required to achieve steady-state blood levels with phenytoin, and changes in dosage (increase or decrease) should not be carried out at intervals shorter than 7 to 10 days.

For patients with low albumin levels (hypoalbuminemia), renal impairment, hepatic impairment, or a critical illness, monitoring free phenytoin levels should be considered.

Alternatively, equations taking into account the patient's serum albumin and renal function may be used to estimate the serum phenytoin level that would have been observed if serum albumin and renal function were normal.

Total phenytoin level adjusted for hypoalbuminemia:

$$\text{Total } C_{normalized} = \text{Total } C_{measured} / [(0.2 \times \text{Serum albumin [g/dL]}) + 0.1]$$

Total phenytoin levels adjusted for hypoalbuminemia and end-stage renal disease requiring hemodialysis:

$$\text{Total } C_{normalized} = \text{Total } C_{measured} / [(0.1 \times \text{Serum albumin [g/dL]}) + 0.1]$$

Total phenytoin – The therapeutic range is 10 to 20 mcg/mL. Levels less than 5 mcg/mL are rarely effective; levels higher than 20 mcg/mL produce dose-related adverse effects.

Free phenytoin – The therapeutic range is 1 to 2 mcg/mL.

➤*Storage/Stability:* Store at 20° to 25°C (68° to 77°F). Protect from light and moisture.

PHENYTOIN SODIUM — INJECTION

For complete prescribing information, refer to the Hydantoins class monograph.

WARNING

This drug must be administered slowly. In adults, do not exceed 50 mg/min intravenously (IV). In neonates, administer the drug at a rate not exceeding 1 to 3 mg/kg/min.

Indications

➤*Seizures:* For the control of status epilepticus of the tonic-clonic type, and prevention and treatment of seizures occurring during neurosurgery.

➤*Off-label uses:*

Rectal administration – [4] = Insufficient documentation. There are limited clinical and kinetic data available regarding the rectal administration of phenytoin (see Administration and Dosage).

Administration and Dosage

➤*General dosing considerations:* If administration of phenytoin does not terminate seizures, the use of other anticonvulsants, IV barbiturates, general anesthesia, and other appropriate measures should be considered.

Continuous monitoring of the electrocardiogram and blood pressure is essential. Observe the patient for signs of respiratory depression.

PHENYTOIN SODIUM — INJECTION

The loading dose for obese patients may be calculated using an adjusted body weight based on the following formula:

Dosing weight (kg) = ideal body weight (IBW) + 1.33 × (measured weight − IBW).

➤*Adults:*

Status epilepticus –

Loading dose: 10 to 15 mg/kg.

Maintenance dosage: 100 mg orally or IV every 6 to 8 hours.

Concomitant therapy: Other measures, including coadministration of an IV benzodiazepine, such as diazepam, or an IV short-acting barbiturate, will usually be necessary for rapid control of seizures because of the required slow rate of administration of phenytoin.

Prevention of seizures during neurosurgery –

Usual dosage: 100 to 200 mg (2 to 4 mL) intramuscularly (IM) at approximately 4-hour intervals during surgery and continued during the postoperative period.

Conversion: When IM administration is required for a patient previously stabilized orally, compensating dosage adjustments are necessary to maintain therapeutic plasma levels. An IM dose of 50% more than the oral dose is necessary to maintain these levels. When returned to oral administration, the dose should be reduced by 50% of the original oral dose for 1 week to prevent excessive plasma levels caused by sustained release from IM tissue sites.

If the patient requires more than a week of IM phenytoin, alternative routes should be explored, such as gastric intubation. For time periods of less than 1 week, a patient shifted back from IM administration should receive 50% the original dose for the same period of time the patient received IM phenytoin. Monitoring plasma levels would help prevent a fall into the subtherapeutic range.

Off-label dosing –

Rectal administration: Single dose of 7 mg/kg (parenteral solution given rectally).

➤*Children:*

Status epilepticus –

Loading dose: 15 to 20 mg/kg.

Concomitant therapy: Other measures, including coadministration of an IV benzodiazepine, such as diazepam, or an IV short-acting barbiturate, will usually be necessary for rapid control of seizures because of the required slow rate of administration of phenytoin.

Off-label dosing –

Status epilepticus:

• *Infants and children –*

Maximum dose: 1 g (loading dose).

Loading dose: 10 to 20 mg/kg.

Maintenance dosage:

12 years of age and older: 4 to 8 mg/kg/day divided every 8 to 12 hours.

1 to 12 years of age: 8 to 10 mg/kg/day divided every 8 hours.

4 weeks to less than 1 year of age: 4 to 8 mg/kg day.

• *Neonates –*

Loading dose: 8 to 20 mg/kg.

Maintenance dosage: 4 to 8 mg/kg/day divided every 12 to 24 hours.

➤*Product interchangeability:* Phenytoin injection is formulated with the sodium salt of phenytoin. Because there is an approximate 8% increase in drug content with the free acid form over that of the sodium salt, dosage adjustments and serum level monitoring may be necessary when switching from a product formulated with the free acid to a product formulated with the sodium salt and vice versa.

➤*Therapeutic drug monitoring:* Determination of phenytoin plasma levels is advised when using phenytoin in the management of status epilepticus and in the subsequent establishment of maintenance dosage. Serum blood level determinations are especially helpful when possible drug interactions are suspected.

For patients with low albumin levels (hypoalbuminemia), renal impairment, hepatic impairment, or a critical illness, monitoring free phenytoin levels should be considered.

Alternatively, equations taking into account the patient's serum albumin and renal function may be used to estimate the serum phenytoin level that would have been observed if serum albumin and renal function were normal.

Total phenytoin levels is adjusted for hypoalbuminemia:

$$\text{Total } C_{normalized} = \text{Total } C_{measured} / [(0.2 \times \text{Serum albumin [g/dL]}) + 0.1].$$

Total phenytoin level adjusted for hypoalbuminemia and end-stage renal disease requiring hemodialysis:

$$\text{Total } C_{normalized} = \text{Total } C_{measured} / [(0.1 \times \text{Serum albumin [g/dL]}) + 0.1].$$

Total phenytoin – The therapeutic range is 10 to 20 mcg/mL. Levels less than 5 mcg/mL is rarely effective; levels more than 20 mcg/mL produce dose-related adverse effects.

Free phenytoin – The therapeutic range is 1 to 2 mcg/mL.

➤*Preparation for administration:* The injection solution is suitable for use as long as it remains free of haziness and precipitate. Upon refrigeration or freezing, a precipitate might form; this will dissolve again after the solution is allowed to stand at room temperature. The product is still suitable for use. Only a clear solution should be used. A faint yellow coloration may develop; however, this has no effect on the potency of the solution.

➤*Administration:* Do not exceed 50 mg/min IV in adults or 1 to 3 mg/kg/min in neonates. There is a relatively small margin between full therapeutic effect and minimally toxic doses of this drug.

Inject phenytoin slowly and directly into a large vein through a large-gauge needle or IV catheter. Each injection of IV phenytoin should be followed by an injection of sterile saline through the same needle or catheter to avoid local venous irritation due to the alkalinity of the solution. Continuous infusion should be avoided.

The manufacturer recommends IM administration for prevention of seizures during neurosurgery; however, most health care providers avoid IM administration of phenytoin because of severe pain and the potential for tissue necrosis and crystallization at the injection site.

IM administration should not be used in the treatment of status epilepticus because the attainment of peak plasma levels may require up to 24 hours.

➤*Admixture compatibility:* The addition of phenytoin to IV fluids is not recommended because of the lack of solubility and likelihood of precipitation.

➤*Storage/Stability:* Store at 15° to 30°C (59° to 86°F). Do not freeze.

Refer to the general discussion beginning in the Anticonvulsants introduction.

Indications

➤*Ethosuximide:* Control of absence (petit mal) seizures.

➤*Methsuximide:* For petit mal seizures when refractory to other drugs.

Actions

➤*Pharmacology:* Succinimides suppress the paroxysmal three cycle per second spike and wave activity associated with lapses of consciousness common in absence (petit mal) seizures. The frequency of epileptiform attacks is reduced, apparently by motor cortex depression and elevation of the threshold of the CNS to convulsive stimuli.

➤*Pharmacokinetics:*

Absorption/Distribution – These agents are readily absorbed from the GI tract. Peak serum levels of ethosuximide are achieved in 3 to 7 hours; peak levels of methsuximide and phensuximide are reached in 1 to 4 hours. Therapeutic serum concentrations of ethosuximide range from 40 to 100 mcg/ml.

Metabolism/Excretion – Ethosuximide is extensively metabolized to inactive metabolites; ≈ 20% is excreted unchanged via the kidneys. The plasma half-life is 30 hours in children and 60 hours in adults. Less than 1% of a dose of methsuximide is recovered unchanged in urine; plasma half-lives range from 2.6 to 4 hours. Phensuximide is excreted in urine and in bile; half-life is ≈ 4 hours.

Contraindications

Hypersensitivity to succinimides.

Warnings/Precautions

➤*Hematologic effects:* Blood dyscrasias, some fatal, have occurred; therefore, perform periodic blood counts. Should signs or symptoms of infection (eg, sore throat, fever) develop, consider blood counts at that point.

➤*Lupus:* Cases of systemic lupus erythematosus have occurred.

➤*Grand mal seizures:* Succinimides, when used alone in mixed types of epilepsy, may increase the frequency of grand mal seizures in some patients.

➤*Dosage changes/other medication:* It is important to proceed slowly when increasing or decreasing dosage, and when adding or eliminating other medication. Abrupt withdrawal of anticonvulsant medication may precipitate absence (petit mal) status.

➤*Acute intermittent porphyria:* Use phensuximide with caution.

➤*Renal/Hepatic function impairment:* Succinimides have produced morphological and functional changes in animal liver. Abnormal liver and renal function have been reported in humans. For this reason, administer with extreme caution to patients with known liver or renal disease. Perform periodic urinalyses and liver function studies for all patients receiving these drugs.

➤*Pregnancy:* Refer to information for use during pregnancy in the Anticonvulsant introduction.

Drug Interactions

Succinimide Drug Interactions

Precipitant drug	Object drug[a]		Description
Succinimides	Hydantoins	↑	Serum hydantoin levels may be increased.
Succinimides	Primidone	↓	Lower primidone and phenobarbital levels may occur.
Valproic acid	Succinimides	↔	Both increases and decreases in succinimide levels have occurred.

[a] ↑ = object drug increased; ↓ = object drug decreased; ↔ = undetermined clinical effect.

Adverse Reactions

The following have been reported with one or more of the succinimides:

➤*CNS:* Drowsiness; ataxia; dizziness; irritability; nervousness; headache; blurred vision; myopia; photophobia; hiccoughs; euphoria; dream-like state; lethargy; hyperactivity; fatigue; insomnia. Drowsiness, ataxia and dizziness are the most frequent **methsuximide** side effects.

➤*Dermatologic:* Pruritus; urticaria; Stevens-Johnson syndrome; pruritic erythematous rashes; skin eruptions; erythema multiforme; systemic lupus erythematosus; alopecia; hirsutism.

➤*GI:* (frequent): Nausea; vomiting; vague gastric upset; cramps; anorexia; diarrhea; weight loss; epigastric and abdominal pain; constipation.

➤*GU:* Urinary frequency, renal damage, hematuria (**phensuximide**); vaginal bleeding; microscopic hematuria.

➤*Hematologic:* Eosinophilia; granulocytopenia; leukopenia; agranulocytosis; monocytosis; pancytopenia, with or without bone marrow suppression.

➤*Psychiatric:* Confusion; instability; mental slowness; depression; hypochondriacal behavior; sleep disturbances; night terrors; aggressiveness; inability to concentrate. These effects may be noted particularly in patients who have previously exhibited psychological abnormalities. There have been rare reports of paranoid psychosis, suicidal behavior, auditory hallucinations, increased libido and increased state of depression.

➤*Miscellaneous:* Periorbital edema; hyperemia; muscle weakness; swelling of the tongue; gum hypertrophy.

Overdosage

The therapeutic range of ethosuximide serum levels is 40 to 100 mcg/ml, although levels as high as 150 mcg/ml have occurred without signs of toxicity. Methsuximide levels > 40 mcg/ml have caused toxicity; coma has been seen at levels of 150 mcg/ml.

➤*Symptoms:*

Acute overdosage – Confusion; sleepiness; unsteadiness; flaccid muscles; coma with slow, shallow respiration; hypotension; cyanosis; hypo- or hyperthermia; absent reflexes; nausea; vomiting; CNS depression including coma with respiratory depression.

Chronic overdosage – Skin rash; confusion; ataxia; dizziness; drowsiness; hangover; depression; irritability; poor judgment; periorbital edema; proteinuria; hepatic dysfunction; fatal bone marrow aplasia; delayed onset of coma; nausea; vomiting; muscular weakness; hematuria; casts; nephrosis.

➤*Treatment:* Treatment includes usual supportive measures. Refer to General Management of Acute Overdosage. Charcoal hemoperfusion may be indicated. Hemodialysis may be useful for ethosuximide. Forced diuresis and exchange transfusions are ineffective.

Patient Information

If GI upset occurs, take with food or milk.

Do not discontinue medication abruptly or change dosage, except on advice of physician.

Patients should carry identification (Medic Alert) indicating medication usage and epilepsy.

May cause drowsiness, dizziness or blurred vision; alcohol may exacerbate these effects. Use caution while driving or performing other tasks requiring alertness, coordination or physical dexterity.

Notify physician if any of the following occurs: Skin rash, joint pain, unexplained fever, sore throat, unusual bleeding or bruising, drowsiness, dizziness, blurred vision or pregnancy.

➤*Phensuximide:* Phensuximide may discolor the urine pink, red or red-brown. This is not harmful.

ETHOSUXIMIDE

Rx	**Ethosuximide** (Sidmak)	**Capsules:** 250 mg	In 100s.
Rx	**Zarontin** (Parke-Davis)		Sorbitol. (PD 237). In 100s.
Rx	**Ethosuximide** (Copley)	**Syrup:** 250 mg/5 ml	Saccharin, sucrose. Raspberry flavor. In 483 mL.
Rx	**Zarontin** (Parke-Davis)		Raspberry flavor. Saccharin, sucrose. In pt.

ETHOSUXIMIDE — ORAL

For complete and comparative prescribing information, refer to the Succinimides group monograph.

Indications

➤*Epilepsy:* For the control of absence (petit mal) epilepsy.

Administration and Dosage

➤*General dosing considerations:* Abrupt withdrawal of anticonvulsant medication may precipitate absence (petit mal) status.

➤*Adults:*

Epilepsy –

Initial dosage: 500 mg per day. The dose thereafter must be individualized according to the patient's response.

Dosage titration: Dosage should be increased by small increments. One useful method is to increase the daily dose by 250 mg every 4 to 7 days until control is achieved with minimal adverse reactions. Dosages exceeding 1.5 g daily, in divided doses, should be administered only under the strictest supervision of the health care provider. Subsequent dose schedules can be based upon effectiveness and plasma level determinations.

➤*Children:*

Epilepsy –

6 years of age and older: See Adults for dosing in children 6 years of age and older.

• *Maintenance dosage* – The optimal dose for most children is 20 mg/kg/day. This dose has given average plasma levels within the accepted therapeutic range of 40 to 100 mcg/mL. (See also Off-Label Dosing).

3 to 6 years of age:

• *Initial dosage* – 250 mg per day. Dosage should be increased by small increments every 4 to 7 days until control is achieved with minimal adverse reactions. (See also Off-Label Dosing).

• *Maintenance dosage* – The optimal dose for most children is 20 mg/kg/day. This dose has given average plasma levels within the accepted therapeutic range of 40 to 100 mcg/mL. Subsequent dose schedules can be based on effectiveness and plasma level determinations. (See also Off-Label Dosing).

Off-label dosing –

Epilepsy:

• *Older than 6 years of age* –
Maximum dose: 1,500 mg daily.
Initial dosage: 250 mg twice daily.
Maintenance dosage: 20 to 40 mg/kg/day, administered in 2 divided doses.

• *6 years of age and younger* –
Maximum dose: 500 mg daily.
Initial dosage: 15 mg/kg/day administered in 2 divided doses.
Dosage titration: Increase dose every 4 to 7 days as needed.
Maintenance dosage: 15 to 40 mg/kg/day administered in 2 divided doses.

➤*Concomitant therapy:* May be administered in combination with other anticonvulsants when other forms of epilepsy coexist with absence (petit mal).

➤*Administration:* May be given with or without food.

➤*Storage/Stability:*

Capsule – Store at 25°C (77°F); excursions are permitted to 15° to 30°C (59° to 86°F).

Syrup – Store below 30°C (86°F). Protect from freezing and light.

Succinimides

METHSUXIMIDE

Rx	Celontin (Pfizer U.S.)	**Capsules; oral:** 300 mg	In 100s.

METHSUXIMIDE — ORAL

For complete and comparative prescribing information, refer to the Succinimides class monograph.

Indications

➤*Seizures:* For the control of absence (petit mal) seizures that are refractory to other drugs.

Administration and Dosage

➤*Adults:*

Seizure –

Initial dosage: 300 mg per day for the first week.

Dosage titration: If required, dosage may be increased thereafter at weekly intervals by 300 mg per day for 3 weeks, following to a daily dosage of 1,200 mg.

Concomitant therapy: May be administered in combination with other anticonvulsants when other forms of epilepsy coexist with absence (petit mal) seizures.

➤*Children:*

Seizure – See Adults for dosing.

➤*Discontinuation of therapy:* Withdraw slowly; abrupt withdrawal may precipitate absence (petit mal) status.

➤*Administration:* The smaller capsule (150 mg) facilitates administration to small children. Do not use capsules that are not full or in which contents have melted. Effectiveness may be reduced.

➤*Storage/Stability:* Store at 25°C (77°F); excursions are permitted between 15° and 30°C (59° and 86°F).

Protect from light and moisture. Protect from excessive heat (40°C; 104°F). Avoid storage conditions that may promote high temperatures (eg, closed cars, delivery vans, storage near steam pipes).

Sulfonamides

ZONISAMIDE

Rx	Zonisamide (Various, eg, Barr, Mutual)	**Capsules:** 25 mg	In 30s, 60s, 100s, 250s, 500s, and 1,000s.
Rx	Zonegran (Eisai)		(ZONEGRAN 25). White. In 100s.
Rx	Zonisamide (Various, eg, Barr, Mutual)	**Capsules:** 50 mg	In 30s, 60s, 100s, 250s, 500s, and 1,000s.
Rx	Zonegran (Eisai)		(ZONEGRAN 50). White/Gray. In 100s.
Rx	Zonisamide (Various, eg, Barr, Dr. Reddy's, Mutual, UDL, Wockhardt)	**Capsules:** 100 mg	May contain lactose. In 30s, 60s, 100s, 250s, 500s, 1,000s, and UD 100s.
Rx	Zonegran (Eisai)		(ZONEGRAN 100). White/Red. In 100s.

ZONISAMIDE — ORAL

Indications

➤*Seizures:* As adjunctive therapy in the treatment of partial seizures in adults with epilepsy.

➤*Off-label uses:*

Binge eating disorder – [4] = Insufficient documentation. There are very limited data available regarding the use of zonisamide for binge eating disorders. This information is limited by a high withdrawal rate and adverse reaction profile.

Migraine prevention (children/adolescents) – [5] = Poor documentation. Published data on the use of zonisamide for the prevention of migraine headaches in children and adolescents are limited, and the number of patients studied is small. Current practice guidelines do not include a review or recommendation for zonisamide.

Weight gain or obesity – [4] = Insufficient documentation. Preliminary data with zonisamide for promoting weight loss are limited to 1 controlled trial. Although initial data suggest that this drug may be effective and well tolerated, additional studies are needed to compare it with more traditional therapies and determine its role in the management of obesity.

Other possible off-label uses – Zonisamide has also been used in children to treat infantile spasms and partial and generalized seizures.

Administration and Dosage

➤*General dosing considerations:* Because of the long half-life of zonisamide, up to 2 weeks may be required to achieve steady-state levels upon reaching a stable dose or following dosage adjustment.

➤*Adults:*

Seizures –

Initial dosage: 100 mg daily.

Maintenance dosage: Evidence from controlled trials suggests that zonisamide doses of 100 to 600 mg/day are effective, but there is no suggestion of increasing response above 400 mg/day. There is little experience with doses greater than 600 mg/day.

Dosage adjustment: After 2 weeks, the dose may be increased to 200 mg/day for at least 2 weeks. It can be increased to 300 and 400 mg/day, with the dose stable for at least 2 weeks to achieve steady state at each level.

Although the regimen described has been shown to be tolerated, the prescriber may wish to prolong the duration of treatment at the lower doses in order to fully assess the effects of zonisamide at steady state, noting that many of the adverse reactions of zonisamide are more frequent at doses of 300 mg/day and above. Although there is some evidence of greater response at doses above 100 to 200 mg/day, the increase appears small, and formal dose-response studies have not been conducted.

Off-label dosing –

Binge eating disorder: [4] = Insufficient documentation. Initial dose was 100 mg/day for the first week. Doses were titrated by 100 mg/wk initially to a maximum dose of 600 mg/day. The dose could be reduced to a minimum of 100 mg/day because of intolerance.

Weight gain or obesity: [4] = Insufficient documentation. Initial oral dose of 100 mg/day for 2 weeks, titrated by 100 mg increments every 2 weeks until week 12, when the dose could be increased to 600 mg/day in patients who had not lost at least 5% of initial body weight.

➤*Children:*

Seizures –

16 years of age and older: See Adults.

➤*Elderly:* Dose selection for an elderly patient should be cautious, usually starting at the low end of the dosing range, reflecting the greater frequency of decreased hepatic, renal, or cardiac function and of concomitant disease or other drug therapy.

➤*Renal function impairment:* Zonisamide should be discontinued in patients who develop acute renal failure or a clinically significant sustained increase in the creatinine/serum urea nitrogen (BUN) concentration. Zonisamide should not be used in patients with renal failure (estimated glomerular filtration rate [GFR] of less than 50 mL/min) because there has been insufficient experience concerning drug dosing and toxicity. Patients with renal disease should be treated with caution and might require slower titration and more frequent monitoring.

➤*Hepatic function impairment:* Patients with hepatic disease should be treated with caution and might require slower titration and more frequent monitoring.

➤*Administration:* Administer once or twice daily with or without food. Capsules should be swallowed whole.

➤*Storage/Stability:* Store at 25°C (77°F); excursions are permitted to 15° to 30°C (59° to 86°F). Store in a dry place, protected from light.

Actions

➤*Pharmacology:* The precise mechanism(s) by which zonisamide exerts its antiseizure effect is unknown. Zonisamide demonstrated anticonvulsant activity in several experimental models. In animals, zonisamide was effective against tonic extension seizures induced by maximal electroshock but ineffective against clonic seizures induced by subcutaneous pentylenetetrazol. Zonisamide raised the threshold for generalized seizures in the kindled rat model and reduced the duration of cortical focal seizures induced by electrical stimulation of the visual cortex in cats. Furthermore, zonisamide suppressed both interictal spikes and the secondarily generalized seizures produced by cortical application of tungstic acid gel in rats or by cortical freezing in cats. The relevance of these models to human epilepsy is unknown.

Zonisamide may produce these effects through action at sodium and calcium channels. In vitro pharmacological studies suggest that zonisamide blocks sodium channels and reduces voltage-dependent, transient inward currents (T-type Ca^{2+} currents), consequently stabilizing neuronal membranes and suppressing neuronal hypersynchronization. In vitro binding studies have demonstrated that zonisamide binds to the GABA/benzodiazepine receptor ionophore complex in an allosteric fashion which does not produce changes in chloride flux. Other in vitro studies have demonstrated that zonisamide (10 to 30 mcg/mL) suppresses synaptically driven electrical activity without

ZONISAMIDE — ORAL

affecting postsynaptic GABA or glutamate responses (cultured mouse spinal cord neurons) or neuronal or glial uptake of [^{3}H]-GABA (rat hippocampal slices). Thus, zonisamide does not appear to potentiate the synaptic activity of GABA. In vivo microdialysis studies demonstrated that zonisamide facilitates both dopaminergic and serotonergic neurotransmission. Zonisamide also has weak carbonic anhydrase inhibiting activity, but this pharmacologic effect is not thought to be a major contributing factor in the antiseizure activity of zonisamide.

➤*Pharmacokinetics:*

Absorption – Following a 200 to 400 mg oral zonisamide dose, peak plasma concentrations (range, 2 to 5 mcg/mL) in healthy volunteers occur within 2 to 6 hours. In the presence of food, the time to maximum concentration is delayed, occurring at 4 to 6 hours, but food has no effect on the bioavailability of zonisamide. Zonisamide extensively binds to erythrocytes, resulting in an 8-fold higher concentration of zonisamide in red blood cells (RBC) than in plasma. The pharmacokinetics of zonisamide are dose proportional in the range of 200 to 400 mg, but the C_{max} and AUC increase disproportionately at 800 mg, perhaps due to saturable binding of zonisamide to RBC. Once a stable dose is reached, steady state is achieved within 14 days. The elimination half-life of zonisamide in plasma is about 63 hours. The elimination half-life of zonisamide in RBC is approximately 105 hours.

Distribution – The apparent volume of distribution (V/F) of zonisamide is about 1.45 L/kg following a 400 mg oral dose. Zonisamide, at concentrations of 1 to 7 mcg/mL, is approximately 40% bound to human plasma proteins. Protein binding of zonisamide is unaffected in the presence of therapeutic concentrations of phenytoin, phenobarbital or carbamazepine.

Metabolism / Excretion – Following oral administration of ^{14}C-zonisamide to healthy volunteers, only zonisamide was detected in plasma. Zonisamide is excreted primarily in urine as parent drug and as the glucuronide of a metabolite. Following multiple dosing, 62% of the ^{14}C dose was recovered in the urine, with 3% in the feces by day 10. Zonisamide undergoes acetylation to form N-acetyl zonisamide and reduction to form the open ring metabolite, 2-sulfamoylacetyl phenol (SMAP). Of the excreted dose, 35% was recovered as zonisamide, 15% as N-acetyl zonisamide, and 50% as the glucuronide of SMAP. Reduction of zonisamide to SMAP is mediated by cytochrome P450 isozyme 3A4 (CYP3A4). Zonisamide does not induce its own metabolism. Plasma clearance of zonisamide is approximately 0.3 to 0.35 mL/min/kg in patients not receiving enzyme-inducing antiepilepsy drugs (AEDs). The clearance of zonisamide is increased to 0.5 mL/min/kg in patients concurrently on enzyme-inducing AEDs.

Renal clearance is about 3.5 mL/min. The clearance of an oral dose of zonisamide from RBC is 2 mL/min.

Special populations –
Renal function impairment: See Warnings/Precautions for more information.
Hepatic function impairment: See Warnings/Precautions for more information.

Contraindications

Zonisamide is contraindicated in patients who have demonstrated hypersensitivity to sulfonamides or zonisamide.

Warnings/Precautions

➤*Potentially fatal reactions to sulfonamides:* Fatalities have occurred, although rarely, as a result of severe reactions to sulfonamides (zonisamide is a sulfonamide) including Stevens-Johnson syndrome, toxic epidermal necrolysis, fulminant hepatic necrosis, agranulocytosis, aplastic anemia, and other blood dyscrasias. Such reactions may occur when a sulfonamide is readministered irrespective of the route of administration. If signs of hypersensitivity or other serious reactions occur, discontinue zonisamide immediately. Specific experience with sulfonamide-type adverse reaction to zonisamide is described below.

➤*Serious skin reactions:* Consideration should be given to discontinuing zonisamide in patients who develop an otherwise unexplained rash. If the drug is not discontinued, patients should be observed frequently. Seven deaths from severe rash (ie, Stevens-Johnson syndrome [SJS] and toxic epidermal necrolysis [TEN]) were reported in the first 11 years of marketing in Japan. All of the patients were receiving other drugs in addition to zonisamide. In postmarketing experience from Japan, a total of 49 cases of SJS or TEN have been reported, a reporting rate of 46 per million patient-years of exposure. Although this rate is greater than background, it is probably an underestimate of the true incidence because of under-reporting. There were no confirmed cases of SJS or TEN in the US, European, or Japanese development programs.

In the US and European randomized controlled trials, 6 of 269 (2.2%) zonisamide patients discontinued treatment because of rash compared to none on placebo. Across all trials during the US and European development, rash that led to discontinuation of zonisamide was reported in 1.4% of patients (12 events per 1000 patient-years of exposure). During Japanese development, serious rash or rash that led to study drug discontinuation was reported in 2% of patients (27.8 events per 1000 patient years). Rash usually occurred early in treatment, with 85% reported within 16 weeks in the US and European studies and 90% reported within 2 weeks in the Japanese studies. There was no apparent relationship of dose to the occurrence of rash.

➤*Serious hematologic events:* Two confirmed cases of aplastic anemia and 1 confirmed case of agranulocytosis were reported in the first 11 years of marketing in Japan, rates greater than generally accepted background rates. There were no cases of aplastic anemia and 2 confirmed cases of agranulocytosis in the US, European, or Japanese development programs. There is inadequate information to assess the relationship, if any, between dose and duration of treatment and these events.

➤*Seizures on withdrawal:* As with other AEDs, abrupt withdrawal of zonisamide in patients with epilepsy may precipitate increased seizure frequency or status epilepticus. Dose reduction or discontinuation of zonisamide should be done gradually.

➤*Cognitive / neuropsychiatric adverse reactions:* Use of zonisamide was frequently associated with central nervous system-related adverse reactions. The most significant of these can be classified into 3 general categories:

1.) Psychiatric symptoms, including depression and psychosis.
2.) Psychomotor slowing, difficulty with concentration, and speech or language problems, in particular, word-finding difficulties.
3.) Somnolence or fatigue.

In placebo-controlled trials, 2.2% of patients discontinued zonisamide or were hospitalized for depression compared to 0.4% of placebo patients, while 1.1% of zonisamide and 0.4% of placebo patients attempted suicide. Among all epilepsy patients treated with zonisamide, 1.4% were discontinued and 1% were hospitalized because of reported depression or suicide attempts. In placebo-controlled trials, 2.2% of patients discontinued zonisamide or were hospitalized due to psychosis or psychosis-related symptoms compared to none of the placebo patients. Among all epilepsy patients treated with zonisamide, 0.9% were discontinued and 1.4% were hospitalized because of reported psychosis or related symptoms.

Psychomotor slowing and difficulty with concentration occurred in the first month of treatment and were associated with doses above 300 mg/day. Speech and language problems tended to occur after 6 to 10 weeks of treatment and at doses above 300 mg/day. Although in most cases these reactions were of mild to moderate severity, they at times led to withdrawal from treatment.

Somnolence and fatigue were frequently reported CNS adverse reactions during clinical trials with zonisamide. Although in most cases these events were of mild to moderate severity, they led to withdrawal from treatment in 0.2% of the patients enrolled in controlled trials. Somnolence and fatigue tended to occur within the first month of treatment. Somnolence and fatigue occurred most frequently at doses of 300 to 500 mg/day. Patients should be cautioned about this possibility and special care should be taken by patients if they drive, operate machinery, or perform any hazardous task.

➤*Creatine phosphokinase (CPK) elevation and pancreatitis:* In the postmarketing setting, the following rare adverse events have been observed (less than 1:1000):

If patients taking zonisamide develop severe muscle pain and/or weakness, either in the presence or absence of a fever, markers of muscle damage should be assessed, including serum CPK and aldolase levels. If elevated, in the absence of another obvious cause (eg, trauma, grand mal seizures), tapering and/or discontinuance of zonisamide should be considered and appropriate treatment initiated.

Patients taking zonisamide that manifest clinical signs and symptoms of pancreatitis should have pancreatic lipase and amylase levels monitored. If pancreatitis is evident, in the absence of another obvious cause, tapering and/or discontinuation of zonisamide should be considered and appropriate treatment initiated.

➤*Kidney stones:* Among the 991 patients treated during the development of zonisamide, 40 patients (4%) with epilepsy receiving zonisamide developed clinically possible or confirmed kidney stones (eg, clinical symptomatology, sonography), a rate of 34 per 1000 patient-years of exposure (40 patients with 1168 years of exposure). Of these, 12 were symptomatic, and 28 were described as possible kidney stones based on sonographic detection. In 9 patients, the diagnosis was confirmed by a passage of a stone or by a definitive sonographic finding. The rate of occurrence of kidney stones was 28.7 per 1000 patient-years of exposure in the first 6 months, 62.6% per 1000 patient-years of exposure between 6 and 12 months, and 24.3% per 1000 patient-years of exposure after 12 months of use. There are no normative sonographic data available for either the general population or patients with epilepsy. The clinical significance of the sonographic finding is unknown. The analyzed stones were composed of calcium or urate salts. In general, increasing fluid intake and urine output can help reduce the risk of stone formation, particularly in those with predisposing risk factors. It is unknown, however, whether these measures will reduce the risk of stone formation in patients treated with zonisamide.

➤*Effect on renal function:* In several clinical studies, zonisamide was associated with a statistically significant 8% mean increase from baseline of serum creatinine and blood urea nitrogen (BUN) compared to essentially no change in the placebo patients. The increase appeared to persist over time but was not progressive; this has been interpreted as an effect on glomerular filtration rate (GFR). There were no episodes of unexplained acute renal failure in clinical development in the US, Europe, or Japan. The decrease in GFR appeared within the first 4 weeks of treatment. In a 30-day study, the GFR returned to baseline within 2 to 3 weeks of drug discontinuation. There is no information about reversibility, after drug discontinuation, of the effects on GFR after long-term use. Zonisamide should be discontinued in patients who develop acute renal failure or a clinically significant sustained increase in the creatinine/BUN concentration. Zonisamide should not be used in patients with renal failure (estimated GFR less than 50 mL/min) as there has been insufficient experience concerning drug dosing and toxicity.

➤*Sudden unexplained death in epilepsy:* During the development of zonisamide, 9 sudden unexplained deaths occurred among 991 patients with epilepsy receiving zonisamide for whom accurate exposure data are available. This represents an incidence of 7.7 deaths per 1000 patient years. Although this rate exceeds that expected in a healthy population, it is within

ZONISAMIDE — ORAL

the range of estimates for the incidence of sudden unexplained deaths in patients with refractory epilepsy not receiving zonisamide (ranging from 0.5 per 1000 patient-years for the general population of patients with epilepsy, to 2 to 5 per 1000 patient-years for patients with refractory epilepsy. Higher incidences range from 9 to 15 per 1000 patient-years among surgical candidates and surgical failures). Some of the deaths could represent seizure-related deaths in which the seizure was not observed.

➤*Status epilepticus:* Estimates of the incidence of treatment emergent status epilepticus in zonisamide treated patients are difficult because a standard definition was not employed. Nonetheless, in controlled trials, 1.1% of patients treated with zonisamide had an event labeled as status epilepticus compared to none of the patients treated with placebo. Among patients treated with zonisamide across all epilepsy studies (controlled and uncontrolled), 1% of patients had an event reported as status epilepticus.

➤*Renal/Hepatic function impairment:* Single 300 mg zonisamide doses were administered to 3 groups of volunteers. Group 1 was a healthy group with a creatinine clearance ranging from 70 to 152 mL/min. Group 2 and group 3 had creatinine clearances ranging from 14.5 to 59 mL/min and 10 to 20 mL/min, respectively. Zonisamide renal clearance decreased with decreasing renal function (3.42, 2.5, 2.23 mL/min, respectively). Marked renal impairment (creatinine clearance less than 20 mL/min) was associated with an increase in zonisamide AUC of 35%. The pharmacokinetics of zonisamide in patients with impaired liver function have not been studied. Somnolence is commonly reported, especially at higher doses of zonisamide. Zonisamide is metabolized by the liver and eliminated by the kidneys; caution should therefore be exercised when administering zonisamide to patients with hepatic and renal dysfunction.

➤*Hazardous tasks:* Patients should be cautioned about the possibility of drowsiness and fatigue, and special care should be taken by patients if they drive, operate machinery, or perform any hazardous task.

➤*Pregnancy: Category C.* Zonisamide was teratogenic in mice, rats, and dogs and embryolethal in monkeys when administered during the period of organogenesis. Fetal abnormalities or embryo-fetal deaths occurred in these species at zonisamide dosage and maternal plasma levels similar to or lower than therapeutic levels in humans, indicating that use of this drug in pregnancy entails a significant risk to the fetus. A variety of external, visceral, and skeletal malformations was produced in animals by prenatal exposure to zonisamide. Cardiovascular defects were prominent in both rats and dogs.

There are no adequate and well-controlled studies in pregnant women. Zonisamide should be used during pregnancy only if the potential benefit justifies the potential risk to the fetus.

Teratogenic – Women of childbearing potential who are given zonisamide should be advised to use effective contraception. Zonisamide was teratogenic in mice, rats, and dogs and embryolethal in monkeys when administered during the period of organogenesis. A variety of fetal abnormalities, including cardiovascular defects, and embryo-fetal deaths occurred at maternal plasma levels similar to or lower than therapeutic levels in humans. These findings suggest that the use of zonisamide during pregnancy in humans may present a significant risk to the fetus. It cannot be said with any confidence, however, that even mild seizures do not pose some hazards to the developing fetus. Zonisamide should be used during pregnancy only if the potential benefit justifies the potential risk to the fetus.

Labor and delivery – The effect of zonisamide on labor and delivery in humans is not known.

➤*Lactation:* It is not known whether zonisamide is excreted in human milk. Because many drugs are excreted in human milk and because of the potential for serious adverse reactions in nursing infants from zonisamide, a decision should be made whether to discontinue nursing or to discontinue the drug, taking into account the importance of the drug to the mother. Zonisamide should be used in nursing mothers only if the benefits outweigh the risks.

➤*Children:* The safety and effectiveness of zonisamide in children younger than 16 years of age have not been established. Cases of oligohidrosis and hyperpyrexia have been reported.

Oligohidrosis and hyperthermia in pediatric patients – Oligohidrosis, sometimes resulting in heat stroke and hospitalization, is seen in association with zonisamide in pediatric patients.

During the preapproval development program in Japan, 1 case of oligohidrosis was reported in 403 pediatric patients, an incidence of 1 case per 285 patient-years of exposure. While there were no cases reported in the US or European development programs, less than 100 pediatric patients participated in these trials.

In the first 11 years of marketing in Japan, 38 cases were reported, an estimated reporting rate of about 1 case per 10,000 patient-years of exposure. In the first year of marketing in the US, 2 cases were reported, an estimated reporting rate of about 12 cases per 10,000 patient-years of exposure. These rates are underestimates of the true incidence because of underreporting. There has been 1 report of heat stroke in an 18-year-old patient in the US.

Decreased sweating and an elevation in body temperature above normal characterized these cases. Many cases were reported after exposure to elevated environmental temperatures. Heat stroke, requiring hospitalization, was diagnosed in some cases. There have been no reported deaths.

Pediatric patients appear to be at an increased risk for zonisamide-associated oligohidrosis and hyperthermia. Patients, especially pediatric patients, treated with zonisamide should be monitored closely for evidence of decreased sweating and increased body temperature, especially in warm or hot weather. Caution should be used when zonisamide is prescribed with other drugs that predispose patients to heat-related disorders; these drugs include, but are not limited to, carbonic anhydrase inhibitors and drugs with anticholinergic activity.

➤*Elderly:* Single dose pharmacokinetic parameters are similar in elderly and young healthy volunteers. Clinical studies of zonisamide did not include sufficient numbers of subjects aged 65 years and over to determine whether they respond differently from younger subjects. Other reported clinical experience has not identified differences in responses between the elderly and younger patients. In general, dose selection for an elderly patient should be cautious, usually starting at the low end of the dosing range, reflecting the greater frequency of decreased hepatic, renal, or cardiac function, and of concomitant disease or other drug therapy.

➤*Lab test abnormalities:* In several clinical studies, zonisamide was associated with a mean increase in the concentration of serum creatinine and blood urea nitrogen (BUN) of approximately 8% over the baseline measurement. Consideration should be given to monitoring renal function periodically. Zonisamide was associated with an increase in serum alkaline phosphatase. In the randomized, controlled trials, a mean increase of approximately 7% over baseline was associated with zonisamide compared to a 3% mean increase in placebo-treated patients. These changes were not statistically significant. The clinical relevance of these changes is unknown.

Drug Interactions

➤*Effects of other drugs on zonisamide pharmacokinetics:* Drugs that induce liver enzymes increase the metabolism and clearance of zonisamide and decrease its half-life. The half-life of zonisamide following a 400 mg dose in patients concurrently on enzyme-inducing AEDs such as phenytoin, carbamazepine, or phenobarbital was between 27 to 38 hours; the half-life of zonisamide in patients concurrently on the non-enzyme-inducing AED, valproate, was 46 hours. Concurrent medication with drugs that either induce or inhibit CYP3A4 would be expected to alter serum concentrations of zonisamide.

Adverse Reactions

The most commonly observed adverse reactions associated with the use of zonisamide in controlled clinical trials that were not seen at an equivalent frequency among placebo-treated patients were somnolence, anorexia, dizziness, headache, nausea, and agitation/irritability.

In controlled clinical trials, 12% of patients receiving zonisamide as adjunctive therapy discontinued due to an adverse reaction compared to 6% receiving placebo. Approximately 21% of the 1336 patients with epilepsy who received zonisamide in clinical studies discontinued treatment because of an adverse reaction. The adverse reactions most commonly associated with discontinuation were somnolence, fatigue or ataxia (6%), anorexia (3%), difficulty concentrating (2%), difficulty with memory, mental slowing, nausea/vomiting (2%), and weight loss (1%). Many of these adverse reactions were dose-related.

➤*Adverse reaction incidence in controlled clinical trials:* The table below lists treatment-emergent adverse reaction that occurred in at least 2% of patients treated with zonisamide in controlled clinical trials that were numerically more common in the zonisamide group. In these studies, either zonisamide or placebo was added to the patient's current AED therapy. Adverse reactions were usually mild or moderate in intensity.

Zonisamide Adverse Reactions (≥ 2%)

Adverse reaction	Zonisamide (n = 269)	Placebo (n = 230)
CNS		
Agitation/irritability	9%	4%
Anxiety	3%	2%
Ataxia	6%	1%
Confusion	6%	3%
Depression	6%	3%
Difficulty concentrating	6%	2%
Difficulty in verbal expression	2%	< 1%
Difficulty with memory	6%	2%
Dizziness	13%	7%
Fatigue	8%	6%
Insomnia	6%	3%
Mental slowing	4%	2%
Nervousness	2%	1%
Nystagmus	4%	2%
Paresthesia	4%	1%
Schizophrenic/schizophreniform behavior	2%	0%
Somnolence	17%	7%
Speech abnormalities	5%	2%
Tiredness	7%	5%
Dermatologic		
Rash	3%	2%
GI		
Anorexia	13%	6%

Sulfonamides

ZONISAMIDE — ORAL

Zonisamide Adverse Reactions (≥ 2%)		
Adverse reaction	Zonisamide (n = 269)	Placebo (n = 230)
Constipation	2%	1%
Diarrhea	5%	2%
Dry mouth	2%	1%
Dyspepsia	3%	1%
Nausea	9%	6%
Hematologic/lymphatic		
Ecchymosis	2%	1%
Metabolic/Nutritional		
Weight loss	3%	2%
Respiratory		
Rhinitis	2%	1%
Special senses		
Diplopia	6%	3%
Taste perversion	2%	0%
Miscellaneous		
Abdominal pain	6%	3%
Flu syndrome	4%	3%
Headache	10%	8%

➤*Other adverse reactions observed during clinical trials:* Reactions are further classified within each category and listed in order of decreasing frequency as follows: Frequent occurring in at least 1:100 patient; infrequent occurring in 1:100 to 1:1000 patients; rare occurring in fewer than 1:1000 patients.

Cardiovascular –
Infrequent: Palpitation, tachycardia, vascular insufficiency, hypotension, hypertension, thrombophlebitis, syncope, bradycardia.
Rare: Atrial fibrillation, heart failure, pulmonary embolus, ventricular extrasystoles.

CNS –
Frequent: Tremor, convulsion, abnormal gait, hyperesthesia, incoordination.
Infrequent: Hypertonia, twitching, abnormal dreams, vertigo, libido decreased, neuropathy, hyperkinesia, movement disorder, dysarthria, cerebrovascular accident, hypotonia, peripheral neuritis, paraesthesia, reflexes increased.
Rare: Circumoral paresthesia, dyskinesia, dystonia, encephalopathy, facial paralysis, hypokinesia, hyperesthesia, myoclonus, oculogyric crisis.

Dermatologic –
Frequent: Pruritus.
Infrequent: Maculopapular rash, acne, alopecia, dry skin, sweating, eczema, urticaria, hirsutism, pustular rash, vesiculobullous rash.

GI –
Frequent: Vomiting.
Infrequent: Flatulence, gingivitis, gum hyperplasia, gastritis, gastroenteritis, stomatitis, cholelithiasis, glossitis, melena, rectal hemorrhage, ulcerative stomatitis, gastro-duodenal ulcer, dysphagia, gum hemorrhage.
Rare: Cholangitis, hematemesis, cholecystitis, cholestatic jaundice, colitis, duodenitis, esophagitis, fecal incontinence, mouth ulceration.

GU –
Infrequent: Urinary frequency, dysuria, urinary incontinence, hematuria, impotence, urinary retention, urinary urgency, amenorrhea, polyuria, nocturia.
Rare: Albuminuria, enuresis, bladder pain, bladder calculus, gynecomastia, mastitis, menorrhagia.

Hematologic / Lymphatic –
Infrequent: Leukopenia, anemia, immunodeficiency, lymphadenopathy.
Rare: Thrombocytopenia, microcytic anemia, petechia.

Metabolic / Nutritional –
Infrequent: Peripheral edema, weight gain, edema, thirst, dehydration.
Rare: Hypoglycemia, hyponatremia, increased lactic dehydrogenase, increased AST, increased ALT.

Musculoskeletal –
Infrequent: Leg cramps, myalgia, myasthenia, arthralgia, arthritis.

Psychiatric –
Infrequent: Euphoria.

Respiratory –
Frequent: Pharyngitis, cough increased.
Infrequent: Dyspnea.
Rare: Apnea, hemoptysis.

Special senses –
Frequent: Amblyopia, tinnitus.
Infrequent: Conjunctivitis, parosmia, deafness, visual field defect, glaucoma.
Rare: Photophobia, iritis.

Miscellaneous –
Frequent: Accidental injury, asthenia.
Infrequent: Chest pain, flank pain, malaise, allergic reaction, face edema, neck rigidity.
Rare: Lupus erythematosus.

Overdosage

➤*Symptoms:* Experience with zonisamide daily doses over 800 mg/day is limited. During zonisamide clinical development, 3 patients ingested unknown amounts of zonisamide as suicide attempts, and all 3 were hospitalized with CNS symptoms. One patient became comatose and developed bradycardia, hypotension, and respiratory depression; the zonisamide plasma level was 100.1 mcg/mL measured 31 hours post-ingestion. Zonisamide plasma levels fell with a half-life of 57 hours, and the patient became alert 5 days later.

➤*Treatment:* No specific antidotes for zonisamide overdosage are available. Following a suspected recent overdose, emesis should be induced or gastric lavage performed with the usual precautions to protect the airway. General supportive care is indicated, including frequent monitoring of vital signs and close observation. Zonisamide has a long half-life (approximately 105 hours). Due to the low protein binding of zonisamide (40%), renal dialysis may not be effective. A poison control center should be contacted for information on the management of zonisamide overdosage.

Patient Information

Patients should be advised as follows:

1.) Zonisamide may produce drowsiness, especially at higher doses. Patients should be advised not to drive a car or operate other complex machinery until they have gained experience on zonisamide sufficient to determine whether it affects their performance.
2.) Patients should contact their physicians immediately if a skin rash develops or seizures worsen.
3.) Patients should contact their physicians immediately if they develop signs or symptoms, such as sudden back pain, abdominal pain, or blood in the urine, that could indicate a kidney stone. Increasing fluid intake and urine output may reduce the risk of stone formation, particularly in those with predisposing risk factors for stones.
4.) Patients should contact their physicians immediately if a child has been taking zonisamide and is not sweating as usual with or without a fever.
5.) Because zonisamide can cause hematological complications, patients should contact their physicians immediately if they develop a fever, sore throat, oral ulcers, or easy bruising.
6.) As with other AEDs, patients should contact their physicians if they intend to become pregnant or are pregnant during zonisamide therapy. Patients should notify their physicians if they intend to breastfeed or are breastfeeding infants.
7.) Patients should contact their physicians if they develop severe muscle pain and/or weakness.

Benzodiazepines

CLONAZEPAM

Refer to the general discussion beginning in the Anticonvulsants introduction. For prescribing information, refer to the Clonazepam monograph in the Antianxiety Agents section.

CLORAZEPATE DIPOTASSIUM

For complete prescribing information, refer to the Clorazepate Dipotassium monograph in the Antianxiety Agents section.

DIAZEPAM

Refer to the general discussion beginning in the Anticonvulsants introduction. For prescribing information, refer to the Diazepam monographs in the Antianxiety Agents section.

LORAZEPAM

Refer to the general discussion beginning in the Anticonvulsants introduction. For prescribing information, refer to the lorazepam monograph in the Antianxiety Agents section.

CARBAMAZEPINE

Rx	**Carbamazepine** (Various, eg, Caraco, Taro, Teva, UDL)	**Tablets; oral:** 200 mg	May contain lactose. In 100s, 500s, 1,000s, and UD 25s, 50s, and 100s.
Rx	**Epitol** (Teva)		Lactose. (Epitol 93-93). Scored. In 100s.
Rx	**Tegretol** (Novartis)		(Tegretol 27 27). Pink, scored. Capsule shape. In 100s.
Rx	**Carbamazepine** (Various, eg, Caraco, Taro, Teva, UDL)	**Tablets, chewable; oral:** 100 mg	May contain lactose, sorbitol, sucrose. In 100s, 500s, and UD 50s and 100s.
Rx	**Tegretol** (Novartis)		Sucrose. (Tegretol 52 52). Pink, red-speckled, scored. In 100s and UD 100s.
Rx	**Carbamazepine** (Taro)	**Tablets, chewable; oral:** 200 mg	Sorbitol. (T27). White, oval, scored. Cherry flavor. In 100s and 400s.
Rx	**Carbamazepine** (Taro)	**Tablets, extended-release; oral:** 100 mg	Lactose. (T91). White to off-white, round. In 30s, 100s, and 1,000s.
Rx	**Tegretol-XR** (Novartis)		Mannitol. (T 100 mg). Yellow. Film-coated. In 100s.
Rx	**Carbamazepine** (Taro)	**Tablets, extended-release; oral:** 200 mg	Lactose. (T26). White to off-white, round. In 30s, 100s, and 1,000s.
Rx	**Tegretol-XR** (Novartis)		Mannitol. (T 200 mg). Pink. Film-coated. In 100s.
Rx	**Carbamazepine** (Taro)	**Tablets, extended-release; oral:** 400 mg	Lactose. (T29). White to off-white, capsule shape. In 30s, 100s, and 1,000s.
Rx	**Tegretol-XR** (Novartis)		Mannitol. (T 400 mg). Brown. Film-coated. In 100s.
Rx	**Carbatrol** (Shire)	**Capsules, extended-release; oral:** 100 mg	Lactose. (Shire logo). Bluish green. In 120s.
Rx	**Equetro** (Shire)		Lactose. (SPD417 100 mg). Yellow/bluish green. In 120s.
Rx	**Carbatrol** (Shire)	**Capsules, extended-release; oral:** 200 mg	Lactose. (Shire logo). Lt. gray/bluish green. In 120s.
Rx	**Equetro** (Shire)		Lactose. (SPD417 200 mg). Yellow/blue. In 120s.
Rx	**Carbatrol** (Shire)	**Capsules, extended-release; oral:** 300 mg	Lactose. (Shire logo). Black/bluish green. In 120s.
Rx	**Equetro** (Shire)		Lactose. (SPD417 300 mg). Yellow/blue. In 120s.
Rx	**Carbamazepine** (Various, eg, Morton, Taro)	**Suspension; oral:** 100 mg per 5 mL	May contain sorbitol, sucrose. In 450 mL and UD 5 mL and 10 mL.
Rx	**Tegretol** (Novartis)		Sorbitol, sucrose. Citrus/vanilla flavor. In 450 mL.

CARBAMAZEPINE — ORAL

Refer to the general discussion beginning in the Anticonvulsants introduction.

WARNING

Aplastic anemia and agranulocytosis have been reported in association with the use of carbamazepine. Data from a population-based case-control study demonstrate that the risk of developing these reactions is 5 to 8 times greater than in the general population. However, the overall risk of these reactions in the untreated general population is low, approximately 6 patients per 1 million population per year for agranulocytosis and 2 patients per 1 million population per year for aplastic anemia.

Although reports of transient or persistent decreased platelet or white blood cell counts are not uncommon in association with the use of carbamazepine, data are not available to accurately estimate their incidence or outcome. However, the vast majority of the cases of leukopenia have not progressed to the more serious conditions of aplastic anemia or agranulocytosis.

Because of the very low incidence of agranulocytosis and aplastic anemia, the vast majority of minor hematological changes observed while monitoring patients on carbamazepine are unlikely to signal the occurrence of either abnormality. Nonetheless, obtain complete pretreatment hematological testing as a baseline. If a patient in the course of treatment exhibits low or decreased white blood cell or platelet counts, monitor the patient closely. Consider discontinuation of the drug if any evidence of significant bone marrow depression develops.

Indications

➤*Bipolar I disorder (Equetro only)*: For the treatment of acute manic and mixed episodes associated with bipolar I disorder.

➤*Epilepsy (except Equetro)*: For use as an anticonvulsant drug. Evidence supporting the efficacy of carbamazepine as an anticonvulsant was derived from active, drug-controlled studies that enrolled patients with the following seizure types:

- Partial seizures with complex symptomatology (ie, psychomotor, temporal lobe). Patients with these seizures appear to show greater improvement than those with other types.
- Generalized tonic-clonic seizures (grand mal).
- Mixed seizure patterns that include those previously described or other partial or generalized seizures. Note: Absence seizures (petit mal) do not appear to be controlled by carbamazepine.

➤*Trigeminal neuralgia (except Equetro)*: For the treatment of pain associated with true trigeminal neuralgia. Beneficial results have also been reported in glossopharyngeal neuralgia. This drug is not a simple analgesic; do not use for the relief of trivial aches or pains.

➤*Off-label uses:*

Alcohol withdrawal – [2] = Fair documentation. Carbamazepine appears to be a promising alternative to other medications in the setting of alcohol withdrawal, but the doses used in clinical trials have varied considerably. Interpretation of some study results is confounded by use of carbamazepine in combination with agents that are not available in the United States.

Borderline personality disorder – [1] = Good documentation. Clinical trial data on the use of carbamazepine for the treatment of borderline personality disorder are limited, and carbamazepine may cause serious hematologic adverse effects. Nevertheless, carbamazepine is recommended in national guidelines as a second-line or adjunctive pharmacologic treatment of borderline personality disorder associated with symptoms of either affective dysregulation or impulsive-behavioral control. The mainstay of treatment is psychotherapy, but medications may be appropriate for acute exacerbations of disease or long-term management of selected symptoms.

Idiopathic muscle cramps – [4] = Insufficient documentation. Carbamazepine is frequently used for the management of idiopathic muscle cramps in clinical practice, but there are no published clinical trials evaluating its efficacy for this use. Guidelines did not recommend carbamazepine as a pharmacologic treatment for muscle cramps.

Postherpetic neuralgia – [4] = Insufficient documentation. There is insufficient evidence to make any recommendations regarding the use of carbamazepine for the treatment of postherpetic neuralgia.

Prevention of migraine (adults) – [5] = Poor documentation. Results from controlled and noncontrolled studies evaluating the use of carbamazepine for the prevention of migraine headaches in adults have been favorable, but the significance of the data is unclear. American Academy of Neurology practice guidelines consider carbamazepine to be no more effective than placebo for the prevention of migraines and note that, while the data show a statistically significant benefit, clinical experience has shown that most patients have no improvement.

Rectal administration – [2] = Fair documentation. Carbamazepine is too slowly absorbed rectally to be of clinical utility in status epilepticus but may be useful in maintaining current dosing if oral dosing is interrupted for short periods of time. Because there is variable rectal absorption between individuals, it has been recommended to monitor serum concentrations if prolonged rectal administration is planned.

Restless legs syndrome – [4] = Insufficient documentation. Although carbamazepine was the first anticonvulsant studied for treatment of restless legs syndrome (RLS), gabapentin is more frequently used because it has a more favorable adverse effect profile. In guideline statements, carbamazepine is rated as probably effective.

Schizophrenia – [4] = Insufficient documentation. Only 1 study has evaluated carbamazepine monotherapy for treatment of schizophrenia, and treatment was not proven to be more efficacious in preventing relapse than placebo. Most trials have focused on adjunctive use of carbamazepine with antipsychotics. None of the currently available data show consistently superior efficacy to warrant recommendation of carbamazepine therapy for schizophrenia. Sample sizes of the individual studies were often too small to detect statistically significant differences, and study designs varied greatly.

Traumatic brain injury – [4] = Insufficient documentation. Although carbamazepine was not recommended by the Neurobehavioral Guidelines Working Group for the management of aggression after traumatic brain injury, carbamazepine may be an appropriate therapy for patients who experience seizures as a result of traumatic brain injury.

CARBAMAZEPINE — ORAL

Administration and Dosage

➤*General dosing considerations:* Before prescribing carbamazepine, be thoroughly familiar with the details of this prescribing information, particularly regarding use with other drugs, especially those that accentuate toxicity potential.

Dosage should be adjusted to the needs of the individual patient. A low initial daily dosage with a gradual increase is advised. As soon as adequate control is achieved, the dosage may be reduced very gradually to the minimum effective level.

➤*Adults:*

Bipolar I disorder (Equetro only) –

Maximum dose: Doses higher than 1,600 mg/day have not been studied.

Initial dosage: 400 mg/day, given in divided doses twice daily.

Dosage adjustment: Adjusted in 200 mg daily increments to achieve optimal clinical response. Doses higher than 1,600 mg/day have not been studied.

Epilepsy (except Equetro) –

Usual dosage: Adjust dosage to the minimum effective level, usually 800 to 1,200 mg daily.

Maximum dose: Doses of up to 1,600 mg daily have been used in adults in rare instances.

Initial dosage: Either 200 mg twice daily for tablets and extended-release (ER) tablets/capsules or 5 mL 4 times daily for suspension (400 mg/day).

Dosage titration: Increase at weekly intervals by adding up to 200 mg/day using a twice-daily regimen of carbamazepine ER tablets/capsules or a 3- or 4-times-daily regimen of the other formulations until the optimal response is obtained. Doses of up to 1,600 mg daily have been used in adults in rare instances.

Trigeminal neuralgia (except Equetro) –

Usual dosage: Control of pain can be maintained in most patients with 400 to 800 mg daily. However, some patients may be maintained on as little as 200 mg daily, while others may require as much as 1,200 mg daily. At least once every 3 months throughout the treatment period, attempts should be made to reduce the dose to the minimum effective level or even discontinue the drug.

Maximum dose: Do not exceed 1,200 mg/day.

Initial dosage:

- *Epitol/Tegretol/Tegretol-XR* – On the first day, either 100 mg twice daily for tablets or ER tablets, or 2.5 mL 4 times daily for suspension, for a total daily dose of 200 mg.
- *Carbatrol* (only) – On the first day, start with one 200 mg capsule.

Dosage titration:

- *Epitol/Tegretol/Tegretol-XR* – The daily dose may be increased by up to 200 mg/day using increments of 100 mg every 12 hours for tablets or ER tablets, or 50 mg (2.5 mL) 4 times daily for suspension, only as needed to achieve freedom from pain. Do not exceed 1,200 mg daily.
- *Carbatrol* (only) – The daily dose may be increased by up to 200 mg/day every 12 hours, only as needed to achieve freedom from pain. Do not exceed 1,200 mg daily.

Off-label dosing –

Alcohol withdrawal: [2] = Fair documentation. 600 to 1,200 mg on day 1, tapered to 0 mg over 5 to 10 days.

Borderline personality disorder: [1] = Good documentation. Initial dose is 400 mg/day in 2 divided doses (tablets, ER tablets, or ER capsules) or 4 divided doses (oral suspension). May increase dose in increments of 200 mg/day depending on response, tolerability, and plasma concentrations (therapeutic plasma concentration is 4 to 12 mcg/mL). Maximum dosage is 1,600 mg/day.

Idiopathic muscle cramps: [4] = Insufficient documentation. An optimal dose has not been identified. For cramp fasciculation syndrome, the dosage of carbamazepine is increased to maximal clinical effect, not to exceed 1,600 mg/day. In this setting, carbamazepine was studied for 4 months.

Postherpetic neuralgia: [4] = Insufficient documentation. 100 to 200 mg daily, slowly increased to a maximum of 1,200 mg daily.

Rectal administration: [2] = Fair documentation. Dosage formulations varied between studies and, thus, optimal dosing recommendations are not established. In a clinical efficacy trial for pain relief and seizure control, a commercially available suppository was administered as 400 mg twice daily to 600 mg 3 times/day in adult cancer patients. In bioavailability studies, oral suspension was administered rectally as 200 mg per 10 mL or 6 mg/kg (single dose). Because the oral suspension contained a high sorbitol content, several patients expelled the product shortly after administration. One study suggested that dosing be repeated if defecation occurs within 2 hours after rectal dosing.

Restless legs syndrome: [4] = Insufficient documentation. 100 to 600 mg daily for up to 5 weeks. Guidelines state 100 to 300 mg at bedtime reduced RLS attacks.

Schizophrenia: [4] = Insufficient documentation. Doses used in clinical trials have varied considerably. Most studies adjusted dose to therapeutic plasma levels used for seizure treatment. Carbamazepine was used as monotherapy or adjunctive therapy in oral dosages ranging from 200 to 1,374 mg/day for 2.5 to 28 weeks.

Traumatic brain injury: [4] = Insufficient documentation. 200 mg daily, increased in increments of 200 mg at intervals of 4 days, up to a maximum of 600 to 1,200 mg daily, based on tolerance and effectiveness. In the one published study to date, the final dose range was 400 to 800 mg/day and the duration of the trial was 8 weeks.

➤*Children:*

Epilepsy –

Epitol/Tegretol/Tegretol-XR:

- *Older than 12 years of age –*

  Maximum dose: Dosage generally should not exceed 1,000 mg daily in children 12 to 15 years of age or 1,200 mg daily in patients older than 15 years of age.

  Initial dosage: Either 200 mg twice daily for tablets and extended-release (ER) tablets or 5 mL 4 times daily for suspension (400 mg/day).

  Dosage titration: Increase at weekly intervals by adding up to 200 mg/day using a twice-daily regimen of carbamazepine ER tablets or a 3- or 4-times-daily regimen of the other formulations until the optimal response is obtained.

  Maintenance dosage: Adjust dosage to the minimum effective level, usually 800 to 1,200 mg daily.

- *6 to 12 years of age –*

  Maximum dose: Dosage generally should not exceed 1,000 mg daily.

  Initial dosage: Either 100 mg twice daily for tablets and ER tablets or 2.5 mL 4 times daily for suspension (200 mg/day). See also Off-label dosing.

  Dosage titration: Increase at weekly intervals by adding up to 100 mg/day using a twice-daily regimen of carbamazepine ER tablets or a 3- or 4-times-daily regimen of the other formulations until the optimal response is obtained.

  Maintenance dosage: Adjust dosage to the minimum effective level, usually 400 to 800 mg daily. See also Off-label dosing.

- *Younger than 6 years of age –*

  Maximum dose: No recommendation regarding the safety of carbamazepine for use at doses of more than 35 mg/kg per 24 hours can be made.

  Initial dosage: 10 to 20 mg/kg/day twice daily or 3 times daily as tablets, or 4 times daily as suspension.

  Dosage titration: Increase the dosage weekly to achieve optimal clinical response, administered 3 or 4 times daily.

  Maintenance dosage: Ordinarily, optimal clinical response is achieved at daily doses of less than 35 mg/kg. If satisfactory clinical response has not been achieved, plasma levels should be measured to determine whether or not they are in the therapeutic range.

Carbatrol (only):

- *Older than 12 years of age –*

  Usual dosage: Adjust dosage to the minimum effective level, usually 800 to 1,200 mg/day.

  Maximum dose: Dosage generally should not exceed 1,000 mg/day in children 12 to 15 years of age and 1,200 mg daily in patients older than 15 years of age.

  Initial dosage: 200 mg twice daily.

  Dosage titration: Increase at weekly intervals by adding up to 200 mg/day until the optimal response is obtained.

- *12 years of age and younger –*

  Usual dosage: Ordinarily, optimal clinical response is achieved at daily doses of less than 35 mg/kg. If satisfactory clinical response has not been achieved, plasma levels should be measured to determine whether they are in the therapeutic range.

  Maximum dose: No recommendation regarding the safety of carbamazepine for use at doses of more than 35 mg/kg per 24 hours can be made.

  Conversion: Total daily doses of immediate-release carbamazepine 400 mg or more may be converted to the same total daily dose of carbamazepine ER capsules using a twice-daily regimen.

Off-label dosing –

Epilepsy:

- *6 to 12 years of age –*

  Initial dosage: 10 mg/kg per day in 2 divided doses up to a single maximum dosage of 100 mg per dose twice daily.

  Maintenance dosage: 20 to 30 mg/kg per day given in 2 to 4 divided doses per day up to a maximum dosage of 1,000 mg per day.

➤*Concomitant therapy:* Carbamazepine may be used alone or with other anticonvulsants. When added to existing anticonvulsant therapy, the drug should be added gradually while the other anticonvulsants are maintained or gradually decreased, except phenytoin, which may have to be increased.

Suspension – Carbamazepine suspension in combination with liquid chlorpromazine or thioridazine results in precipitate formation, and, in the case of chlorpromazine, there has been a report of a patient passing an orange rubbery precipitate in the stool following coadministration of the 2 drugs. Because the extent to which this occurs with other liquid medications is not known, carbamazepine suspension should not be administered simultaneously with other liquid medications or diluents.

➤*Conversion:*

Tablets to suspension – Patients should be converted by administering the same number of milligrams per day in smaller, more frequent doses (ie, twice-daily tablets to 3-times-daily suspension).

Conventional tablets to ER tablets/capsules – When converting patients from carbamazepine conventional tablets to ER tablets/capsules, the same total daily milligram dose of carbamazepine ER tablets/capsules should be administered.

➤*Administration:*

Tablets – This medication should be taken with meals.

Suspension – Shake suspension well before using.

CARBAMAZEPINE — ORAL

Because a given dose of carbamazepine suspension will produce higher peak levels than the same dose given as a tablet, it is recommended to start with low doses (children 6 to 12 years of age, 2.5 mL 4 times daily) and increase slowly to avoid unwanted adverse reactions.

ER tablets – Carbamazepine ER tablets must be swallowed whole and never crushed or chewed. Carbamazepine ER tablets should be inspected for chips or cracks. Damaged tablets or tablets without a release portal should not be consumed. Carbamazepine ER tablet coating is not absorbed and is excreted in the feces; these coatings may be noticeable in the stool.

ER capsules – Carbamazepine capsules may be opened and the beads sprinkled over food, such as a teaspoon of applesauce or other similar food products, if this method of administration is preferred. Carbamazepine capsules and their contents should not be crushed or chewed. Carbamazepine capsules can be taken with or without meals.

➤*Storage/Stability:*

Chewable tablets, tablets, and suspension – Do not store above 30°C (86°F). Protect from light and moisture.

ER tablets – Store at controlled room temperature, 15° to 30°C (59° to 86°F). Protect from moisture.

ER capsules – Store at 25°C (77°F); excursions are permitted from 15° to 30°C (59° to 86°F). Protect from light and moisture.

Actions

➤*Pharmacology:* The mechanism(s) of action of carbamazepine in the treatment of bipolar disorder has not been elucidated. Although numerous pharmacological effects of carbamazepine have been described in the published literature (eg, modulation of ion channels [sodium and calcium], receptor-mediated neurotransmission [gamma-aminobutyric acid (GABA)ergic, glutamatergic, and monoaminergic], and intracellular signaling pathways in experimental preparations), the contribution of these effects to the efficacy of carbamazepine in bipolar disorder is unknown.

Carbamazepine has demonstrated anticonvulsant properties in rats and mice with electrically and chemically induced seizures. It appears to act by reducing polysynaptic responses and blocking the posttetanic potentiation. Carbamazepine greatly reduces or abolishes pain induced by stimulation of the infraorbital nerve in cats and rats. It depresses thalamic potential and bulbar and polysynaptic reflexes, including the linguomandibular reflex in cats. Carbamazepine is chemically unrelated to other anticonvulsants or other drugs used to control the pain of trigeminal neuralgia. The mechanism of action remains unknown.

➤*Pharmacokinetics:*

Absorption – In clinical studies, carbamazepine suspension, conventional tablets, and ER tablets delivered equivalent amounts of drug to the systemic circulation. However, the suspension was absorbed somewhat faster, and ER tablets slightly slower, than conventional tablets. The bioavailability of ER tablets was 89% compared with suspension. Following a twice-daily dosage regimen, the suspension provides higher peak levels and lower trough levels than those obtained from the conventional tablet for the same dosage regimen.

On the other hand, following a 3-times-daily dosage regimen, carbamazepine suspension affords steady-state plasma levels comparable with carbamazepine tablets given twice daily when administered at the same total milligram daily dose. Following a twice-daily dosage regimen, ER carbamazepine tablets afford steady-state plasma levels comparable with conventional carbamazepine tablets given 4 times daily when administered at the same total milligram daily dose.

ER capsules: Taken every 12 hours, carbamazepine ER capsules provide steady-state plasma levels comparable with immediate-release carbamazepine tablets given every 6 hours when administered at the same total milligram daily dose. Following a single 200 mg oral ER dose of carbamazepine, peak plasma concentration was 1.9 ± 0.3 mcg/mL and the time to reach the peak was 19 ± 7 hours. Following chronic administration (800 mg every 12 hours), the peak levels were 11 ± 2.5 mcg/mL, and the time to reach the peak was 5.9 ± 1.8 hours. The pharmacokinetics of carbamazepine ER capsules are linear over the single-dose range of 200 to 800 mg.

• *Food effect* – A high-fat meal diet increased the rate of absorption of a single 400 mg dose (mean time to maximum concentration [T_{max}] was reduced from 24 hours in the fasting state to 14 hours, and maximum drug concentration [C_{max}] increased from 3.2 to 4.3 mcg/mL) but not the extent (area under the curve [AUC]) of absorption. The elimination half-life remains unchanged between fed and fasting states. The multiple-dose study conducted in the fed state showed that the steady-state C_{max} values were within the therapeutic concentration range. The pharmacokinetic profile of ER carbamazepine was similar when given by sprinkling the beads over applesauce, compared with the intact capsule administered in the fasted state.

Distribution – Carbamazepine in blood is 76% bound to plasma proteins. Plasma levels of carbamazepine are variable and may range from 0.5 to 25 mcg/mL, with no apparent relationship to the daily intake of the drug. Usual adult therapeutic levels are between 4 and 12 mcg/mL. In polytherapy, the concentration of carbamazepine and concomitant drugs may be increased or decreased during therapy, and drug effects may be altered.

Following chronic oral administration of suspension, plasma levels peak at approximately 1.5 hours, compared with 4 to 5 hours after administration of conventional carbamazepine tablets and 3 to 12 hours after administration of ER carbamazepine tablets. The cerebrospinal fluid/serum ratio is 0.22, similar to the 24% unbound carbamazepine in serum.

Metabolism/Excretion – Because carbamazepine induces its own metabolism, the half-life is also variable. Autoinduction is completed after 3 to 5 weeks of a fixed dosing regimen. Initial half-life values range from 25 to 65 hours, decreasing to 12 to 17 hours on repeated doses. Carbamazepine is primarily metabolized in the liver. CYP-450 3A4 was identified as the major isoform responsible for the formation of carbamazepine-10,11-epoxide from carbamazepine.

After oral administration of ^{14}C-carbamazepine, 72% of the administered radioactivity was found in the urine and 28% in the feces. This urinary radioactivity was composed largely of hydroxylated and conjugated metabolites, with only 3% of unchanged carbamazepine.

ER capsules: Following a single ER dose of carbamazepine, the average half-life ranged from 35 to 40 hours and 12 to 17 hours on repeated dosing. The apparent oral clearance following a single dose was 25 ± 5 mL/min and following multiple dosing, 80 ± 30 mL/min.

Carbamazepine-10,11-epoxide: Carbamazepine-10,11-epoxide is considered an active metabolite of carbamazepine. Following a single 200 mg oral ER dose of carbamazepine, the peak plasma concentration of carbamazepine-10,11-epoxide was 0.11 ± 0.012 mcg/mL, and the time to reach the peak was 36 ± 6 hours. Following chronic administration of an ER dose of carbamazepine (800 mg every 12 hours), the peak levels of carbamazepine-10,11-epoxide were 2.2 ± 0.9 mcg/mL, and the time to reach the peak was 14 ± 8 hours. The plasma half-life of carbamazepine-10,11-epoxide following administration of carbamazepine is 34 ± 9 hours. Following a single oral dose of ER carbamazepine (200 to 800 mg), the AUC and C_{max} of carbamazepine-10,11-epoxide were less than 10% of carbamazepine. Following multiple dosing of ER carbamazepine (800 to 1,600 mg daily for 14 days), the AUC and C_{max} of carbamazepine-10,11-epoxide were dose related, ranging from 15.7 mcg•h/mL and 1.5 mcg/mL at 800 mg/day to 32.6 mcg•h/mL and 3.2 mcg/mL at 1,600 mg/day, respectively, and were less than 30% of carbamazepine. Carbamazepine-10,11-epoxide is 50% bound to plasma proteins.

Special populations –

Hepatic function impairment: See Warnings/Precautions for more information.

Children: The pharmacokinetic parameters of carbamazepine disposition are similar in children and adults. However, there is a poor correlation between plasma concentrations of carbamazepine and the carbamazepine dose in children. Carbamazepine is more rapidly metabolized to carbamazepine-10,11-epoxide (a metabolite shown to be equipotent to carbamazepine as an anticonvulsant in animal screens) in younger age groups than in adults. In children younger than 15 years of age, there is an inverse relationship between carbamazepine-10,11-epoxide/carbamazepine ratio and increasing age (in 1 report, from 0.44 in children younger than 1 year of age to 0.18 in children between 10 and 15 years of age).

Contraindications

History of previous bone marrow depression, coadministration with nefazodone, hypersensitivity to the drug, or known sensitivity to any of the tricyclic compounds (eg, amitriptyline, desipramine, imipramine, nortriptyline, protriptyline). Likewise, on theoretical grounds, its use with monoamine oxidase inhibitors (MAOIs) is not recommended. Before administration of carbamazepine, discontinue MAOIs for a minimum of 14 days or longer, if the clinical situation permits.

Warnings/Precautions

➤*Hematologic:* Patients with a history of adverse hematologic reaction to any drug may be particularly at risk.

➤*Dermatologic:* Severe dermatologic reactions, including toxic epidermal necrolysis (Lyell syndrome) and Stevens-Johnson syndrome, have been reported with carbamazepine. These reactions have been extremely rare. However, a few fatalities have been reported.

➤*Discontinuation:* In patients with seizure disorder, do not discontinue carbamazepine abruptly because of the strong possibility of precipitating status epilepticus with attendant hypoxia and threat to life.

➤*Anticholinergic effects:* Carbamazepine has shown mild anticholinergic activity; therefore, closely observe patients with increased intraocular pressure during therapy.

➤*CNS effects:* Because of the relationship of the drug to other tricyclic compounds, keep in mind the possibility of activation of a latent psychosis and, in elderly patients, confusion or agitation.

➤*Hepatic effects:* Hepatic effects, ranging from slight elevations in liver enzymes to rare cases of hepatic failure, have been reported. In some cases, hepatic effects may progress despite discontinuation of the drug. Given that carbamazepine is primarily metabolized in the liver, it is prudent to proceed with caution in patients with hepatic function impairment.

Hepatic porphyria (Tegretol only) – Avoid the use of *Tegretol* in patients with a history of hepatic porphyria (eg, acute intermittent porphyria, porphyria cutanea tarda, variegate porphyria). Acute attacks have been reported in such patients receiving *Tegretol* therapy. Carbamazepine administration has also been demonstrated to increase porphyrin precursors in rodents, a presumed mechanism for the induction of acute attacks of porphyria.

➤*Hyponatremia:* Hyponatremia has been reported in association with carbamazepine use, alone or in combination with other drugs.

➤*Suicide (Equetro only):* The possibility of suicide attempt is inherent in bipolar disorder; accompany drug therapy with close supervision of high-risk patients. Write prescriptions for carbamazepine for the smallest quantity consistent with good patient management in order to reduce the risk of overdosage.

➤*Absence seizures:* Use carbamazepine with caution in patients with a mixed seizure disorder that includes atypical absence seizures because in these patients, carbamazepine has been associated with increased frequency of generalized convulsions.

CARBAMAZEPINE — ORAL

➤*Hypersensitivity reactions:* Multiorgan hypersensitivity reactions occurring days to weeks or months after initiating treatment have been reported in rare cases. Consider discontinuation of carbamazepine if any evidence of hypersensitivity develops.

Hypersensitivity reactions to carbamazepine have been reported in patients who previously experienced such reactions to anticonvulsants, including phenytoin and phenobarbital. Obtain a history of hypersensitivity reactions for the patient and immediate family members. If positive, use caution in prescribing carbamazepine.

➤*Special risk:* Prescribe therapy only after a critical benefit-to-risk appraisal in patients with a history of cardiac conduction disturbance, including second- and third-degree atrioventricular (AV) heart block; cardiac, hepatic, or renal damage; adverse hematologic or hypersensitivity reaction to other drugs, including reactions to other anticonvulsants or interrupted courses of therapy with carbamazepine.

AV heart block, including second- and third-degree block, have been reported following carbamazepine treatment. This occurred generally, but not solely, in patients with underlying electrocardiogram abnormalities or risk factors for conduction disturbances.

➤*Hazardous tasks:* Because dizziness and drowsiness may occur, caution patients about the hazards of operating machinery or automobiles or engaging in other potentially dangerous tasks requiring alertness, coordination, or physical dexterity.

➤*Pregnancy: Category D.* Carbamazepine can cause fetal harm when administered to a pregnant woman.

According to the American Academy of Neurology and the American Epilepsy Society, avoidance of carbamazepine during pregnancy should be considered in order to reduce the risk of major congenital malformations such as posterior cleft palate.

Epidemiological data suggest that there may be an association between the use of carbamazepine during pregnancy and congenital malformations, including spina bifida. There have also been reports that associate carbamazepine with congenital anomalies (eg, cardiovascular malformations and anomalies involving various body systems, craniofacial defects) and developmental disorders. Developmental delays based on neurobehavioral assessments have been reported. Weigh the benefits of therapy against the risks when treating or counseling women of childbearing potential. If this drug is used during pregnancy or if the patient becomes pregnant while taking this drug, apprise the patient of the potential hazard to the fetus.

Retrospective case reviews suggest that, compared with monotherapy, there may be a higher prevalence of teratogenic effects associated with the use of anticonvulsants in combination therapy. Therefore, if therapy is to be continued, monotherapy may be preferable for pregnant women.

In humans, transplacental passage of carbamazepine is rapid (30 to 60 minutes), and the drug is accumulated in the fetal tissues, with higher levels found in the liver and kidneys than in the brain and lungs.

Carbamazepine has been shown to have adverse reactions in reproduction studies in rats when given orally in doses 10 to 25 times the maximum human daily dose of 1,200 mg on a mg/kg basis or 1.5 to 4 times the maximum human daily dose on a mg/m^2 basis. In rat teratology studies, 2 of 135 offspring showed kinked ribs at 250 mg/kg, and 4 of 119 offspring at 650 mg/kg showed other anomalies (cleft palate, 1; talipes, 1; anophthalmos, 2). In reproduction studies in rats, nursing offspring demonstrated a lack of weight gain and an unkempt appearance at a maternal dosage level of 200 mg/kg.

Do not discontinue antiepileptic drugs abruptly in patients in whom the drug is administered to prevent major seizures because of the strong possibility of precipitating status epilepticus with attendant hypoxia and threat to life. In individual cases in which the severity and frequency of the seizure disorder are such that removal of medication does not pose a serious threat to the patient, discontinuation of the drug may be considered prior to and during pregnancy, although it cannot be said with any confidence that even minor seizures do not pose some hazard to the developing embryo or fetus.

Consider tests to detect defects using currently accepted procedures as part of routine prenatal care in pregnant women receiving carbamazepine.

There have been a few cases of neonatal seizures and/or respiratory depression associated with maternal carbamazepine and other concomitant anticonvulsant drug use. A few cases of neonatal vomiting, diarrhea, and/or decreased feeding have also been reported in association with maternal carbamazepine use. These symptoms may represent a neonatal withdrawal syndrome.

➤*Lactation:* Carbamazepine and its epoxide metabolite are transferred to breast milk. The ratio of the concentration in breast milk to that in maternal plasma is about 0.4 for carbamazepine and about 0.5 for the epoxide. The estimated doses given to the newborn during breast-feeding are in the range of 2 to 5 mg daily for carbamazepine and 1 to 2 mg daily for the epoxide. The concentrations of carbamazepine and its epoxide metabolite are approximately 50% of the maternal plasma concentration.

Because of the potential for serious adverse reactions in breast-feeding infants from carbamazepine, decide whether to discontinue breast-feeding or the drug, taking into account the importance of the drug to the mother.

➤*Elderly:* Because of the relationship of the drug to other tricyclic compounds, keep in mind the possibility of activation of a latent psychosis and, in elderly patients, confusion or agitation.

➤*Monitoring:* Obtain complete pretreatment blood counts, including platelets and possibly reticulocytes and serum iron, as a baseline. Monitoring of blood levels has increased the efficacy and safety of anticonvulsants. Monitoring of blood levels may be useful in cases of dramatic increase in seizure frequency for verification of drug compliance, assessment of safety, and determination of the cause of toxicity, including when more than 1 medication is being used. If a patient in the course of treatment exhibits low or decreased white blood cell or platelet counts, monitor the patient closely. Consider discontinuation of the drug if any evidence of significant bone marrow depression develops.

Baseline and periodic evaluations of liver function, particularly in patients with a history of liver disease, must be performed during treatment with this drug because liver damage may occur. Discontinue carbamazepine, based on clinical judgment, if indicated by newly occurring or worsening clinical or laboratory evidence of liver function impairment or hepatic damage, or in the case of active liver disease.

Baseline and periodic eye examinations, including slit-lamp, funduscopy, and tonometry, are recommended because many phenothiazines and related drugs have been shown to cause eye changes.

Baseline and periodic complete urinalysis and serum urea nitrogen (BUN) determinations are recommended for patients treated with this agent because of observed renal function impairment.

Increases in total cholesterol, low-density lipoprotein (LDL), and high-density lipoprotein (HDL) have been observed is some patients taking anticonvulsants. Therefore, periodic evaluation of these parameters is also recommended.

Drug Interactions

➤*Drugs highly bound to plasma protein:* Carbamazepine is not highly bound to plasma proteins; therefore, administration of carbamazepine to a patient taking another drug that is highly protein-bound should not cause increased free concentrations of the other drug.

➤*CYP-450 system:* Carbamazepine is metabolized mainly by CYP-450 3A4 to the active carbamazepine 10,11-epoxide, which is further metabolized to the trans-diol by epoxide hydrolase. Therefore, the potential exists for interaction between carbamazepine and any agent that inhibits or induces CYP3A4 and/or epoxide hydrolase.

Agents that are CYP3A4 inhibitors that have been found or are expected to increase plasma levels of carbamazepine are the following: acetazolamide, azole antifungals, cimetidine, clarithromycin, dalfopristin, danazol, delavirdine, diltiazem, erythromycin, fluoxetine, fluvoxamine, grapefruit juice, isoniazid, itraconazole, ketoconazole, loratadine, macrolides, nefazodone, niacinamide, nicotinamide, protease inhibitors, propoxyphene, quinine, quinupristin, terfenadine, troleandomycin, valproate, verapamil, and zileuton. Clarithromycin, erythromycin, and valproate also inhibit epoxide hydrolase, resulting in increased levels of the active metabolite carbamazepine 10,11-epoxide. Coadministration of carbamazepine and delavirdine may lead to loss of virologic response and possible resistance to delavirdine or to the class of nonnucleoside reverse transcriptase inhibitors (NNRTIs). Thus, if a patient has been titrated to a stable dosage of carbamazepine, and then begins a course of treatment with one of these CYP3A4 or epoxide hydrolase inhibitors, it is reasonable to expect that a dose reduction of carbamazepine may be necessary.

Agents that are CYP inducers that have been found or are expected to decrease plasma levels of carbamazepine are the following: cisplatin, doxorubicin, felbamate, methsuximide, phenobarbital, phenytoin, primidone, rifampin, and theophylline. Phenytoin plasma levels have also been reported to increase and decrease in the presence of carbamazepine. Thus, if a patient has been titrated to a stable dosage on carbamazepine and then begins a course of treatment with one of these CYP3A4 inducers, it is reasonable to expect that a dose increase for carbamazepine may be necessary.

Carbamazepine Drug Interactions

Precipitant drug	Object drug[a]		Description
Acetazolamide	Carbamazepine	⬆	Carbamazepine plasma levels may be increased. Adjust the dose of carbamazepine as needed.
Antimalarials (eg, chloroquine, mefloquine)	Carbamazepine	⬇	Chloroquine and mefloquine may antagonize the activity of carbamazepine. Adjust the dose of carbamazepine as needed.
Antipsychotics (eg, haloperidol, quetiapine)	Carbamazepine	⬆	The therapeutic effects of carbamazepine may be increased when coadministered with haloperidol or quetiapine. Consider adjusting the dose of carbamazepine as indicated. Coadministration may reduce the plasma levels of the antipsychotics.
Carbamazepine	Antipsychotics (eg, aripiprazole, clozapine, haloperidol, olanzapine, quetiapine, risperidone, ziprasidone)	⬇	
Azole antifungals (eg, itraconazole, ketoconazole)	Carbamazepine	⬆	Carbamazepine plasma levels may be increased. Closely monitor carbamazepine levels when an azole antifungal is started or stopped. Serum itraconazole or voriconazole levels may be decreased in the presence of carbamazepine.
Carbamazepine	Azole antifungals (eg, itraconazole, voriconazole)	⬇	

CARBAMAZEPINE — ORAL

Carbamazepine Drug Interactions

Precipitant drug	Object drug[a]		Description
Barbiturates (eg, phenobarbital)	Carbamazepine	↓	Carbamazepine plasma levels may be decreased. Monitor serum concentrations of both drugs regularly and adjust their doses appropriately.
Carbamazepine	Barbiturates (eg, phenobarbital)	↔	
Cimetidine	Carbamazepine	↑	Carbamazepine plasma levels may be increased; toxicity may result.
Cisplatin	Carbamazepine	↓	Carbamazepine plasma levels may be decreased. Monitor carbamazepine levels closely.
Dalfopristin	Carbamazepine	↑	Carbamazepine plasma levels may be increased resulting in possible toxicity.
Danazol	Carbamazepine	↑	Carbamazepine plasma levels may be increased, resulting in an increase in pharmacologic and toxic effects. Avoid coadministration if possible.
Delavirdine	Carbamazepine	↑	Carbamazepine plasma levels may be increased. Monitor carbamazepine levels closely. Coadministration may lead to loss of virologic response and possible resistance to delavirdine or to the class of NNRTIs.
Carbamazepine	Delavirdine	↓	
Diltiazem	Carbamazepine	↑	Carbamazepine plasma levels may be increased; toxicity may result. Monitor serum carbamazepine levels and observe the patient.
Doxorubicin	Carbamazepine	↓	Carbamazepine plasma levels may be decreased. Monitor carbamazepine levels.
Felbamate	Carbamazepine	↓	Carbamazepine plasma levels may be decreased. An average decrease of 25% in carbamazepine levels has been reported. Felbamate levels may be decreased, possibly resulting in loss of effectiveness.
Carbamazepine	Felbamate		
Isoniazid	Carbamazepine	↑	Isoniazid is suspected to inhibit carbamazepine metabolism. Carbamazepine toxicity may result. Carbamazepine may increase isoniazid degradation to hepatic metabolites, isoniazid toxicity may result.
Carbamazepine	Isoniazid	↑	
Macrolides (eg, clarithromycin, erythromycin, troleandomycin)	Carbamazepine	↑	Carbamazepine plasma levels may be increased. Avoid combination if possible.
MAOIs (eg, isocarboxazid, phenelzine)	Carbamazepine	↑	Coadministration is contraindicated. Discontinue MAOI at least 14 days prior to administration of carbamazepine.
Carbamazepine	MAOIs (eg, isocarboxazid, phenelzine)		
Nefazodone	Carbamazepine	↑	Carbamazepine plasma levels may be increased. Lower nefazodone levels may result. Coadministration is contraindicated.
Carbamazepine	Nefazodone	↓	
Niacin (eg, niacinamide, nicotinamide)	Carbamazepine	↑	Carbamazepine plasma levels may be increased. Monitor carbamazepine levels and adjust the dose accordingly.
Nonsedating antihistamines (eg, loratadine, terfenadine)	Carbamazepine	↑	Carbamazepine plasma levels may be increased. Closely monitor carbamazepine levels.

Carbamazepine Drug Interactions

Precipitant drug	Object drug[a]		Description
Phenytoin	Carbamazepine	↓	Carbamazepine plasma levels may be decreased. Monitor serum concentrations of both drugs regularly and adjust their dosages appropriately. Phenytoin plasma levels may increase or decrease in the presence of carbamazepine.
Carbamazepine	Phenytoin	↔	
Primidone	Carbamazepine	↓	Carbamazepine levels may be decreased. Primidone plasma levels may be increased or decreased. Monitor serum levels of both drugs regularly and adjust doses appropriately.
Carbamazepine	Primidone	↔	
Protease inhibitors (eg, amprenavir, indinavir)	Carbamazepine	↑	Carbamazepine plasma levels may be increased, increasing the risk of toxicity. Monitor serum carbamazepine levels. Antiretroviral treatment failure may occur.
Carbamazepine	Protease inhibitors (eg, amprenavir, indinavir)	↓	
Propoxyphene	Carbamazepine	↑	Increases in carbamazepine levels between 45% and 77% have been reported. Avoid coadministration if possible.
Quinine	Carbamazepine	↑	Carbamazepine plasma levels may be increased. Monitor carbamazepine levels and adjust the dose as needed.
Quinupristin	Carbamazepine	↑	Carbamazepine plasma levels may be increased. Monitor carbamazepine levels closely.
Rifampin	Carbamazepine	↓	Carbamazepine plasma levels may be decreased. Monitor serum carbamazepine levels and observe the patient.
SSRIs[b] (eg, fluoxetine, fluvoxamine)	Carbamazepine	↑	Carbamazepine plasma levels may be increased, producing possible toxicity. Monitor carbamazepine serum concentrations closely. Plasma levels of the SSRIs may be decreased. Closely monitor the response of the patient and be prepared to adjust the dose of the SSRI.
Carbamazepine	SSRIs (eg, citalopram, sertraline)	↓	
Succinimides (eg, methsuximide)	Carbamazepine	↓	Carbamazepine plasma level may be decreased. Succinimide levels may be decreased.
Carbamazepine	Succinimides (eg, ethosuximide, methsuximide, phensuximide)	↓	
Theophylline	Carbamazepine	↓	Carbamazepine plasma levels may be decreased. Theophylline levels may be decreased or increased. Monitor carbamazepine and theophylline levels. Adjust doses accordingly.
Carbamazepine	Theophylline	↔	
Tricyclic antidepressants (eg, amitriptyline, desipramine, nortriptyline)	Carbamazepine	↑	Carbamazepine serum levels may be elevated, increasing pharmacologic and toxic effects, while tricyclic antidepressant levels may be decreased. Monitor carbamazepine and tricyclic antidepressant levels and adjust dose as needed.
Carbamazepine	Tricyclic antidepressants (eg, amitriptyline, desipramine, imipramine, nortriptyline)	↓	
Valproate	Carbamazepine	↑	Carbamazepine plasma levels may be increased. Decreased valproate levels with possible loss of seizure control. Observe the patient for seizure activity and toxicity for at least 1 month after starting or stopping either drug.
Carbamazepine	Valproate	↓	

CARBAMAZEPINE — ORAL

Carbamazepine Drug Interactions

Precipitant drug	Object drug[a]		Description
Verapamil	Carbamazepine	↑	Carbamazepine plasma levels may be increased. Carbamazepine dose may need to be decreased 40% to 50% with coadministration.
Zileuton	Carbamazepine	↑	Carbamazepine plasma levels may be increased.
Carbamazepine	Acetaminophen	↓	Carbamazepine may increase the metabolism of acetaminophen, increasing the risk of acetaminophen-induced hepatotoxicity and/or decreasing its effectiveness.
Carbamazepine	Anticoagulants (eg, dicumarol, warfarin)	↓	The anticoagulant effect may be reduced during coadministration. Monitor prothrombin times when starting or stopping carbamazepine therapy.
Carbamazepine	Benzodiazepines (eg, alprazolam, clonazepam, clobazam, diazepam, lorazepam, midazolam, triazolam)	↓	The pharmacological effects of benzodiazepines may be reduced. Monitor patient response.
Carbamazepine	Bupropion	↓	Carbamazepine increased the hepatic P-450 metabolism of bupropion and has been reported to decrease bupropion peaks 87% and AUC 90%.
Carbamazepine	Buspirone	↓	Plasma levels of buspirone may be decreased. Monitor patient response.
Carbamazepine	Calcium channel blockers (eg, felodipine)	↓	Pharmacologic effects of felodipine may be decreased.
Carbamazepine	Clomipramine	↑	Carbamazepine increases the plasma levels of clomipramine.
Carbamazepine	Cyclosporine	↓	Plasma level of cyclosporine may be decreased, resulting in a reduction of pharmacologic effects. Monitor cyclosporine levels and observe the patient for signs of rejection or toxicity.
Carbamazepine	Doxycycline	↓	Carbamazepine may decrease the half-life and serum levels of doxycycline, possibly reducing its therapeutic efficacy.
Carbamazepine	Glucocorticoids (eg, dexamethasone, hydrocortisone)	↓	Plasma levels of glucocorticoids may be reduced.
Carbamazepine	HMG-CoA reductase inhibitors (eg, atorvastatin, simvastatin)	↓	Plasma concentration of certain HMG-CoA reductase inhibitors may be reduced, decreasing the therapeutic effect (resulting in hypercholesterolemia). Closely monitor clinical response of the patient.
Carbamazepine	Lamotrigine	↓	Serum lamotrigine levels may be decreased 40%.
Carbamazepine	Levothyroxine	↓	Plasma levels of levothyroxine may be decreased. Monitor thyroid-stimulating hormone.
Carbamazepine	Lithium	↑	Increased CNS toxicity may occur during concomitant therapy. Monitor serum lithium levels and adjust dose accordingly.
Carbamazepine	Methadone	↓	Pharmacologic effects of methadone may be decreased. A higher dose of methadone may be required.
Carbamazepine	Mirtazapine	↓	Plasma levels of mirtazapine may be decreased. Monitor patient response.
Carbamazepine	Nondepolarizing muscle relaxants (eg, atracurium, tubocurarine)	↓	Nondepolarizing muscle relaxants may have shorter than expected duration or be less effective. Monitor patient for reduced muscle relaxant effectiveness and increase the dose of the nondepolarizing muscle relaxant accordingly.
Carbamazepine	Oral and other hormonal contraceptives (eg, levonorgestrel subdermal implant, *Ortho-Novum*)	↓	Breakthrough bleeding and unintended pregnancies have been reported with coadministration; the reliability of the oral contraceptive may be adversely affected.
Carbamazepine	Oxcarbazepine	↓	Plasma levels of oxcarbazepine may be decreased.
Carbamazepine	Praziquantel	↓	Serum praziquantel may be decreased, possibly leading to treatment failures. It may be necessary to increase the dose of praziquantel during coadministration.
Carbamazepine	Tiagabine	↓	Plasma levels of tiagabine may be decreased.
Carbamazepine	Topiramate	↓	Carbamazepine may decrease the pharmacologic effects of topiramate.
Carbamazepine	Tramadol	↓	Plasma levels of tramadol may be decreased.
Carbamazepine	Trazodone	↓	Plasma levels of trazodone may be reduced.
Carbamazepine	Triazole antifungals (itraconazole)	↓	Plasma levels of itraconazole may be reduced.
Carbamazepine	Zonisamide	↓	Plasma levels of zonisamide may be reduced.

[a] ↑ = object drug increased; ↓ = object drug decreased; ↔ = undetermined clinical effect.
[b] SSRIs = selective serotonin reuptake inhibitors.

➤*Drug/Lab test interactions:* Thyroid function tests have been reported to show decreased values when carbamazepine is administered alone. Interference with some pregnancy tests has been reported.

➤*Drug/Food interactions:* See Actions for more information.

Grapefruit juice – Serum carbamazepine levels may be elevated. Avoid coadministration of carbamazepine and grapefruit products.

Adverse Reactions

If adverse reactions are of such severity that the drug must be discontinued, be aware that abrupt discontinuation of any anticonvulsant drug in a responsive epileptic patient may lead to seizures or even status epilepticus with life-threatening hazards.

The most severe adverse reactions have been observed in the cardiovascular system, hemopoietic system, skin, and liver.

The most frequently observed adverse reactions, particularly during the initial phases of therapy, are dizziness, drowsiness, nausea, unsteadiness, and vomiting. To minimize the possibility of such reactions, initiate therapy at the lowest dosage recommended.

Carbamazepine ER Adverse Reactions Reported in Bipolar I Disorder Trials (≥ 5%)

Adverse reaction	Carbamazepine (n = 251)	Placebo (n = 248)
CNS		
Ataxia	15%	0%
Dizziness	44%	12%
Somnolence	32%	13%
Dermatologic		
Pruritus	8%	2%
GI		
Dry mouth	8%	3%
Nausea	29%	10%
Vomiting	18%	3%
Special senses		
Amblyopia[a]	6%	2%
Speech disorder	6%	0%

[a] Reported as blurred vision.

CARBAMAZEPINE — ORAL

Carbamazepine ER Adverse Reactions (*Equetro* Only) (≥ 5%)	
Adverse reaction	
CNS	
Amnesia[a]	8%
Anxiety	7%
Asthenia	8%
Ataxia	5%
Depression[b]	7%
Dizziness	16%
Headache	22%
Manic depressive reaction	7%
Somnolence	12%
Dermatologic	
Pruritus	5%
Rash	13%
GI	
Constipation	5%
Diarrhea	10%
Dyspepsia	10%
Nausea	10%
Miscellaneous	
Accidental injury	7%
Back pain	5%
Chest pain	5%
Infection	12%
Pain	12%

[a] Amnesia includes forgetfulness, memory disturbance, and poor memory.
[b] Depression includes suicidal ideation.

Other significant adverse reactions seen in less than 5% of patients from bipolar I disorder trials include the following: abnormal liver function tests, allergic reaction, alopecia, bronchitis, depersonalization and extrapyramidal symptoms, diplopia, ear pain, edema, infections (eg, bacterial, fungal, viral), insomnia, leukopenia, lymphadenopathy, manic reaction, nervousness, peripheral edema, pharyngitis, photosensitivity reaction, rhinitis, sinusitis, suicide attempt, and urinary tract infection.

The following additional adverse reactions have been reported:

➤*Cardiovascular:* Adenopathy or lymphadenopathy, aggravation of coronary artery disease, aggravation of hypertension, arrhythmias and AV block, congestive heart failure, edema, hypotension, syncope and collapse, thromboembolism, thrombophlebitis. Some of these cardiovascular complications have resulted in fatalities. Myocardial infarction has been associated with other tricyclic compounds.

➤*CNS:* Abnormal involuntary movements, blurred vision, confusion, depression with agitation, disturbances of coordination, dizziness, drowsiness, fatigue, headache, hyperacusis, nystagmus, oculomotor disturbances, peripheral neuritis and paresthesias, speech disturbances, talkativeness, tinnitus, transient diplopia, visual hallucinations. There have been reports of associated paralysis and other symptoms of cerebral arterial insufficiency, but the exact relationship of these reactions to the drug has not been established. Isolated cases of neuroleptic malignant syndrome have been reported with concomitant use of psychotropic drugs.

➤*Dermatologic:* Aggravation of disseminated lupus erythematosus, alopecia, alterations in skin pigmentation, diaphoresis, erythema multiforme and nodosum, exfoliative dermatitis, photosensitivity reactions, pruritic and erythematous rashes, purpura, Stevens-Johnson syndrome, toxic epidermal necrolysis (Lyell syndrome), urticaria. In certain cases, discontinuation of therapy may be necessary. Isolated cases of hirsutism have been reported, but a causal relationship is not clear.

➤*GI:* Anorexia, constipation, diarrhea, dryness of the mouth and pharynx including glossitis and stomatitis, gastric distress and abdominal pain, nausea, pancreatitis, vomiting.

➤*GU:* Acute urinary retention, azotemia, impotence, oliguria with elevated blood pressure, renal failure, urinary frequency. Albuminuria, elevated BUN, glycosuria, and microscopic deposits in the urine have also been reported.

➤*Hematologic:* Acute intermittent porphyria, agranulocytosis, aplastic anemia, bone marrow depression, eosinophilia, leukocytosis, leukopenia, pancytopenia, thrombocytopenia.

➤*Hepatic:* Abnormalities in liver function tests, cholestatic and hepatocellular jaundice, hepatitis, very rare cases of hepatic failure.

➤*Hypersensitivity:* Multiorgan hypersensitivity reactions occurring days to weeks or months after initiating treatment have been reported in rare cases. Signs or symptoms may include, but are not limited to, abnormal liver function tests, arthralgia, disorders mimicking lymphoma, eosinophilia, fever, hepatosplenomegaly, leukopenia, lymphadenopathy, skin rashes, and vasculitis. These signs and symptoms may occur in various combinations and not necessarily concurrently. Signs and symptoms may initially be mild. Various organs, including but not limited to, the colon, liver, skin, immune system, lungs, kidneys, myocardium, and pancreas may be affected.

➤*Metabolic:* Inappropriate antidiuretic hormone secretion syndrome has been reported. Cases of frank water intoxication, with decreased serum sodium (hyponatremia) and confusion, have been reported in association with carbamazepine use. Decreased levels of plasma calcium have been reported.

➤*Musculoskeletal:* Aching joints and muscles, leg cramps.

➤*Ophthalmic:* Scattered punctate cortical lens opacities, as well as conjunctivitis, have been reported. Although a direct causal relationship has not been established, many phenothiazines and related drugs have been shown to cause eye changes.

➤*Respiratory:* Pulmonary hypersensitivity characterized by dyspnea, fever, pneumonia, or pneumonitis.

➤*Miscellaneous:* Chills, fever. Isolated cases of a lupus erythematosus-like syndrome have been reported. There have been occasional reports of elevated levels of cholesterol, HDL cholesterol, and triglycerides in patients taking anticonvulsants.

A case of aseptic meningitis accompanied by myoclonus and peripheral eosinophilia has been reported in a patient taking carbamazepine in combination with other medications. The patient was successfully dechallenged, and the meningitis reappeared upon rechallenge with carbamazepine.

Overdosage

➤*Symptoms:* Conduction disorders, hypotension or hypertension, impairment of consciousness ranging in severity to deep coma, irregular breathing, respiratory depression, tachycardia, and shock. Convulsions, especially in small children. Adiadochokinesia, ataxia, athetoid movements, ballism, dizziness, drowsiness, dysmetria, motor restlessness, muscular twitching, mydriasis, nystagmus, opisthotonos, psychomotor disturbances, and tremor. Initial hyperreflexia, followed by anuria or oliguria, hyporeflexia, nausea and vomiting, and urinary retention. Isolated instances of overdosage have included acetonuria, glycosuria, leukocytosis, and reduced leukocyte count. Electroencephalogram (EEG) may show dysrhythmias.

The first signs and symptoms appear after 1 to 3 hours. Neuromuscular disturbances are the most prominent. Cardiovascular disorders are generally milder, and severe cardiac complications occur only when very high doses (more than 60 g) have been ingested.

When alcohol, barbiturates, hydantoins, or tricyclic antidepressants are taken at the same time, the signs and symptoms of acute poisoning with carbamazepine may be aggravated or modified.

➤*Treatment:* There is no specific antidote. Successful management of large or intentional carbamazepine exposures requires implementation of supportive care, frequent monitoring of serum drug concentrations, as well as aggressive but appropriate gastric decontamination.

Elimination of the drug – For substantial recent ingestions, gastric lavage may be considered. Even when more than 4 hours have elapsed following ingestion of the drug, repeatedly irrigate the stomach, especially if the patient has also consumed alcohol.

Measures to reduce absorption –

Activated charcoal, laxatives: The primary method for gastric decontamination of carbamazepine overdose is use of activated charcoal. Administration of activated charcoal prior to hospital assessment has the potential to significantly reduce drug absorption. There is no specific antidote. In overdose, absorption of carbamazepine may be prolonged and delayed. More than 1 dose of activated charcoal may be beneficial in patients who have evidence of continued absorption (eg, rising serum carbamazepine levels).

Measures to accelerate elimination – Forced diuresis. Dialysis is indicated only in severe poisoning associated with renal failure. The data on use of dialysis to enhance elimination in carbamazepine are scarce. Dialysis, particularly high-flux or high-efficiency hemodialysis, may be considered in patients with severe carbamazepine poisoning associated with renal failure or in cases of status epilepticus, or where there are rising serum drug levels and worsening clinical status despite appropriate supportive care and gastric decontamination. For severe cases of carbamazepine overdose unresponsive to other measures, charcoal hemoperfusion may be used to enhance drug clearance. Replacement transfusion is indicated in severe poisoning in small children.

Respiratory depression – Keep the airways free; resort, if necessary, to endotracheal intubation, artificial respiration, and administration of oxygen.

Hypotension, shock – Keep the patient's legs raised and administer a plasma expander. If blood pressure fails to rise despite measures taken to increase plasma volume, consider use of vasoactive substances.

Convulsions –

Diazepam/Barbiturates: Diazepam or barbiturates may aggravate respiratory depression (especially in children), hypotension, and coma. However, do not use barbiturates if drugs that inhibit monoamine oxidase have also been taken by the patient in overdosage or recent therapy (within 1 week).

Monitoring – Monitor blood pressure, body temperature, cardiac function (ECG monitoring), pupillary reflexes, respiration, and kidney and bladder function for several days.

Hematologic abnormalities – If evidence of significant bone marrow depression develops, the following recommendations are suggested: Stop the drug. Perform daily complete blood cell count (CBC), platelet, and reticulocyte counts. Do a bone marrow aspiration and trephine biopsy immediately and repeat with sufficient frequency to monitor recovery.

CARBAMAZEPINE — ORAL

Special periodic studies might be helpful as follows: White cell and platelet antibodies. ^{59}Fe-ferrokinetic studies. Peripheral blood cell typing. Cytogenetic studies on marrow and peripheral blood. Bone marrow culture studies for colony-forming units. Hemoglobin electrophoresis for A_2 and F hemoglobin. Serum folic acid and B_{12} levels.

A fully developed aplastic anemia will require appropriate, intensive monitoring and therapy, for which specialized consultation should be sought.

Patient Information

Apprise patients of the early toxic signs and symptoms of a potential hematologic problem, as well as dermatologic, hypersensitivity, or hepatic reactions. These symptoms may include, but are not limited to, fever, sore throat, rash, ulcers in the mouth, easy bruising, lymphadenopathy, petechial or purpuric hemorrhage, and in the case of liver reactions, anorexia, nausea/vomiting, or jaundice. Advise the patient that, because these signs and symptoms may signal a serious reaction, they must report any occurrence immediately to a health care provider. In addition, advise the patient to report these signs and symptoms even if they are mild or occur after extended use.

Because dizziness and drowsiness may occur, caution patients about the hazards of operating machinery or automobiles or engaging in other potentially dangerous tasks.

If necessary, carbamazepine ER capsules can be opened and the contents sprinkled over food, such as a teaspoon of applesauce or other similar food products. Instruct patients not to crush or chew carbamazepine ER capsules or their contents.

Advise patients to use caution if alcohol is taken in combination with carbamazepine therapy because of possible additive sedative effect.

Carbamazepine may interact with some drugs. Therefore, advise patients to report to their doctors the use of any other prescription or nonprescription medication or herbal product.

Advise patients that carbamazepine may produce drowsiness, dizziness, or blurred vision; advise patients to observe caution while driving or performing other tasks requiring alertness, coordination, or physical dexterity.

Advise patients to notify their health care providers if any of the following occurs: unusual bleeding or bruising, fever, sore throat, rash or ulcers in the mouth, lymphadenopathy, and petechial or purpuric hemorrhage, and, in the case of liver reactions, anorexia, nausea/vomiting, or jaundice.

Advise patients to take the medication with food; however, the ER capsules can be taken with or without food.

Inform patients that the ER tablet coating is not absorbed and is excreted in the feces; these coatings may be noticeable in the stool.

Inform patients not to administer carbamazepine suspension simultaneously with other liquid medications.

Advise patients that if they are taking the suspension to shake it well before administering.

Inform patients that the capsule formulation may be opened and the beads sprinkled over food, such as applesauce or other similar foods. Instruct patients not to crush or chew the capsule.

Inform patients not to use carbamazepine in combination with any other medications containing carbamazepine.

MAGNESIUM SULFATE

For Magnesium Sulfate prescribing information, refer to the IV Nutritional, Minerals section.

ACETAZOLAMIDE

Refer to the general discussion beginning in the Anticonvulsants introduction. For complete prescribing information, refer to the Acetazolamide monograph in the Renal and Genitourinary Agents.

OXCARBAZEPINE

Rx	**Oxcarbazepine** (Various, eg, Caraco, Glenmark, Roxane)	**Tablets; oral:** 150 mg	Film-coated. In 30s, 100s, 500s, 1,000s, and UD 100s.
Rx	**Trileptal** (Novartis)		(T/D C/G). Pale gray-green, oval, scored. Film-coated. In 100s and UD 100s.
Rx	**Oxcarbazepine** (Various, eg, Caraco, Glenmark, Roxane)	**Tablets; oral:** 300 mg	Film-coated. In 30s, 100s, 500s, 1,000s, and UD 100s.
Rx	**Trileptal** (Novartis)		(TE/TE CG/CG). Yellow, oval, scored. Film-coated. In 100s and UD 100s.
Rx	**Oxcarbazepine** (Various, eg, Caraco, Glenmark, Roxane)	**Tablets; oral:** 600 mg	Film-coated. In 30s, 100s, 500s, 1,000s, and UD 100s.
Rx	**Trileptal** (Novartis)		(TF/TF CG/CG). Light pink, oval, scored. Film-coated. In 100s and UD 100s.
Rx	**Oxcarbazepine** (Sandoz)	**Suspension; oral:** 60 mg/mL	Ethanol, saccharin, sorbitol. In 250 mL with dosing syringe and adapter.
Rx	**Trileptal** (Novartis)		Ethanol, saccharin, sorbitol. In 250 mL with dosing syringe and adapter.

OXCARBAZEPINE — ORAL

Indications

➤*Epilepsy:* For use as monotherapy or adjunctive therapy in the treatment of partial seizures in adults and as monotherapy in the treatment of partial seizures in children 4 years of age and older with epilepsy, and as adjunctive therapy in children 2 years of age and older with epilepsy.

➤*Off-label uses:*

Alcohol withdrawal – [1] = Good documentation. Evidence-based guidelines suggest that oxcarbazepine may be an alternative or adjunctive option for patients with alcohol withdrawal syndrome who do not tolerate first-line treatment with benzodiazepines.

Bipolar disorder – [4] = Insufficient documentation. Although oxcarbazepine appears to be a useful and potentially effective alternative for the treatment of refractory bipolar disorder, it is unclear if this drug has a role as monotherapy or is most useful as adjunctive therapy to lithium.

Diabetic neuropathy – [4] = Insufficient documentation. Mixed data from randomized, controlled trials suggest that oxcarbazepine may be useful in the treatment of painful diabetic neuropathy. Additional open-label trials report similar mixed results. Given inconsistent study outcomes, along with potential confounding from placebo impact in this population, additional controlled trials are necessary to clarify the role of oxcarbazepine in treating pain associated with diabetic neuropathy.

Idiopathic muscle cramps – [4] = Insufficient documentation. Evidence-based pharmacologic treatments for idiopathic muscle cramps are limited. Although quinine derivatives are likely effective for the condition, the American Academy of Neurology (AAN) recommends they be considered only in cases in which cramps are disabling, no other agents provide relief, and adverse effects can be carefully monitored. Although oxcarbazepine is frequently used, there are no clinical trials evaluating its efficacy for the management of idiopathic muscle cramps. Further research is needed to establish appropriate therapy for idiopathic muscle cramps that offers an acceptable balance of efficacy and safety.

Neuralgia/Neuropathy – [4] = Insufficient documentation. Preliminary data suggest that oxcarbazepine, like other anticonvulsants, may be a useful alternative in the treatment of painful neuralgias and neuropathies. However, long-term study in a limited number of patients suggests that initial benefits may postpone eventual surgery in patients with severe neuropathies.

Administration and Dosage

➤*Adults:*

Adjunctive therapy in epilepsy –

Initial dosage: 600 mg/day as a twice-daily regimen.

Dosage adjustment: If clinically indicated, the dose may be increased by a maximum of 600 mg/day at approximately weekly intervals. The recommended daily dose is 1,200 mg. Daily doses above 1,200 mg show somewhat greater efficacy in controlled trials, but most patients were not able to tolerate the 2,400 mg/day dose, primarily because of CNS adverse reactions.

Conversion to monotherapy in epilepsy –

Initial dosage: 600 mg/day as a twice-daily regimen while simultaneously initiating the reduction of the dosage of the concomitant antiepileptic drugs (AEDs).

Dosage adjustment: The concomitant AEDs should be completely withdrawn over 3 to 6 weeks, while the maximum dose of oxcarbazepine should be reached in approximately 2 to 4 weeks. Increase as clinically indicated by a maximum increment of 600 mg/day at approximately weekly intervals to achieve the recommended daily dose of 2,400 mg. A daily dose of 1,200 mg was shown in 1 study to be effective in patients in whom monotherapy had been initiated with oxcarbazepine. Observe patients closely during this transition phase.

Initiation of monotherapy in epilepsy –

Initial dosage: 600 mg/day as a twice-daily regimen.

Dosage adjustment: Increase by 300 mg/day every third day to a dose of 1,200 mg/day. Controlled trials in these patients examined the efficacy of a 1,200 mg/day dose; a dose of 2,400 mg/day has been shown to be effective in patients converted from other AEDs to oxcarbazepine monotherapy.

Off-label dosing –

Alcohol withdrawal: [1] = Good documentation. 600 to 1,800 mg orally in divided doses for 6 weeks to 6 months.

Bipolar disorder: [4] = Insufficient documentation. Most studies employed a titration schedule starting with a dose of 300 mg daily and increasing to a maximum of 900 to 2,400 mg daily (adult doses).

OXCARBAZEPINE — ORAL

• *Adults* –

Maximum dose: 1,800 to 2,400 mg daily.

Diabetic neuropathy: [4] = Insufficient documentation. 900 to 1,200 mg/day is the general recommendation, typically titrated from an initial dose of 150 to 300 mg/day. Maximum dose of 1,800 mg/day has been studied with positive results. Studied treatment durations ranged from 8 weeks to 6 months.

Idiopathic muscle cramps: [4] = Insufficient documentation. No information is available on the appropriate dose and duration of oxcarbazepine for the treatment of idiopathic muscle cramps. When used for its approved indication (partial seizures), oxcarbazepine is initiated at a dosage of 300 mg orally twice daily. The dosage may then be increased gradually.

Neuralgia/Neuropathy: [4] = Insufficient documentation. 400 to 2,000 mg (or maximum tolerable dose) in 2 to 4 divided doses. Initial doses ranged from 300 mg 2 to 3 times/day and were titrated to the effective or maximum tolerable dose.

➤*Children:*

Adjunctive therapy in epilepsy –

4 to 16 years of age:

• *Initial dosage* – Initiate at a daily dose of 8 to 10 mg/kg, generally not to exceed 600 mg/day, given as a twice-daily regimen.

• *Maintenance dosage* – The target maintenance dose of oxcarbazepine should be achieved over 2 weeks and is dependent upon patient weight: for children weighing 20 to 29 kg, the dose is 900 mg/day; for children weighing 29.1 to 39 kg, the dose is 1,200 mg/day; and for children weighing more than 39 kg, the dose is 1,800 mg/day.

2 to 4 years of age:

• *Maximum dose* – 60 mg/kg/day as a twice daily regimen.

• *Initial dosage* – Initiated at a daily dose of 8 to 10 mg/kg, generally not to exceed 600 mg/day, given as a twice-daily regimen. For patients weighing less than 20 kg, a starting dose of 16 to 20 mg/kg may be considered.

• *Maintenance dosage* – The maximum maintenance dose of oxcarbazepine should be achieved over 2 to 4 weeks and should not exceed 60 mg/kg/day as a twice-daily regimen.

Conversion to monotherapy in epilepsy –

4 to 16 years of age:

• *Initial dosage* – 8 to 10 mg/kg/day given as a twice-daily regimen, while simultaneously initiating the reduction of the dose of the concomitant AEDs.

• *Dosage adjustment* – The concomitant AEDs can be completely withdrawn over 3 to 6 weeks, while oxcarbazepine may be increased as clinically indicated by a maximum increment of 10 mg/kg/day at approximately weekly intervals to achieve the recommended daily dose. Observe patients closely during this transition phase.

See table in Initiation of monotherapy in epilepsy.

Initiation of monotherapy in epilepsy –

4 to 16 years of age:

• *Initial dosage* – 8 to 10 mg/kg/day given as a twice-daily regimen.

• *Dosage adjustment* – The dose should be increased 5 mg/kg/day every third day to the recommended daily dose.

Range of Maintenance Dosages of Oxcarbazepine for Children by Weight During Monotherapy

Weight (kg)	From	To
20	600 mg/day	900 mg/day
25	900 mg/day	1,200 mg/day
30	900 mg/day	1,200 mg/day
35	900 mg/day	1,500 mg/day
40	900 mg/day	1,500 mg/day
45	1,200 mg/day	1,500 mg/day
50	1,200 mg/day	1,800 mg/day
55	1,200 mg/day	1,800 mg/day
60	1,200 mg/day	2,100 mg/day
65	1,200 mg/day	2,100 mg/day
70	1,500 mg/day	2,100 mg/day

Off-label dosing –

Bipolar disorder: [4] = Insufficient documentation. Most studies employed a titration schedule starting with a dose of 300 mg daily and increasing to a maximum of 900 to 2,400 mg daily (adult doses).

• *Adolescents* – 450 to 900 mg daily.

• *Children* – 150 mg twice daily.

➤*Renal function impairment:* In patients with impaired renal function (CrCl less than 30 mL/min), initiate oxcarbazepine therapy at one-half the usual starting dose (300 mg/day) and increase slowly to achieve the desired clinical response.

➤*Administration:* Oxcarbazepine can be taken with or without food. Give as a twice-daily regimen.

Before using oxcarbazepine oral suspension, shake the bottle well and prepare the dose immediately afterward. Withdraw the prescribed amount of oral suspension from the bottle using the supplied oral dosing syringe. Oxcarbazepine oral suspension can be mixed in a small glass of water just prior to administration or swallowed directly from the syringe. After each use, close the bottle and rinse the syringe with warm water and allow it to dry thoroughly.

➤*Storage/Stability:* Store at 25°C (77°F); excursions are permitted to 15° to 30°C (59° to 86°F). Store suspension in the original container. Use within 7 weeks of first opening the bottle.

Actions

➤*Pharmacology:* The pharmacological activity of oxcarbazepine is primarily exerted through the 10-monohydroxy metabolite (MHD) of oxcarbazepine. The precise mechanism by which oxcarbazepine and MHD exert their antiseizure effect is unknown; however, in vitro electrophysiological studies indicate that they produce a blockade of voltage-sensitive sodium channels, resulting in stabilization of hyperexcited neural membranes, inhibition of repetitive neuronal firing, and diminution of propagation of synaptic impulses. These actions are thought to be important in the prevention of seizure spread in the intact brain. In addition, increased potassium conductance and modulation of high-voltage activated calcium channels may contribute to the anticonvulsant effects of the drug. No significant interactions of oxcarbazepine or MHD with brain neurotransmitter or modulator receptor sites have been demonstrated.

➤*Pharmacokinetics:*

Absorption – Following oral administration of oxcarbazepine tablets, oxcarbazepine is completely absorbed and extensively metabolized to its pharmacologically active MHD. Based on MHD concentrations, oxcarbazepine tablets and suspension were shown to have similar bioavailability. After single-dose administration of oxcarbazepine tablets to healthy male volunteers under fasted conditions, the median time to maximum concentration (T_{max}) was 4.5 hours (range, 3 to 13 hours). After single-dose administration of oxcarbazepine oral suspension to healthy male volunteers under fasted conditions, the median T_{max} was 6 hours. In a mass balance study in humans, only 2% of total radioactivity in plasma was because of unchanged oxcarbazepine, with approximately 70% present as MHD, and the remainder attributable to minor metabolites.

Steady-state plasma concentrations of MHD are reached within 2 to 3 days in patients when oxcarbazepine is given twice daily. At steady state, the pharmacokinetics of MHD are linear and show dose proportionality over the dose range of 300 to 2,400 mg/day.

Distribution – The apparent volume of distribution of MHD is 49 L. Approximately 40% of MHD is bound to serum proteins, predominantly to albumin. Binding is independent of the serum concentration within the therapeutically relevant range. Oxcarbazepine and MHD do not bind to alpha-1-acid glycoprotein.

Metabolism/Excretion – Oxcarbazepine is rapidly reduced to MHD by cytosolic enzymes in the liver primarily responsible for the pharmacological effect of oxcarbazepine. MHD is metabolized further by conjugation with glucuronic acid. Minor amounts (4% of the dose) are oxidized to the pharmacologically inactive 10,11-dihydroxy metabolite (DHD).

Oxcarbazepine is cleared from the body mostly in the form of metabolites, which are predominantly excreted by the kidneys. More than 95% of the dose appears in the urine, with less than 1% as unchanged oxcarbazepine. Fecal excretion accounts for less than 4% of the administered dose. Approximately 80% of the dose is excreted in the urine either as glucuronides of MHD (49%) or as unchanged MHD (27%); the inactive DHD accounts for approximately 3% and conjugates of MHD and oxcarbazepine account for 13% of the dose. The half-life of the parent is approximately 2 hours, while the half-life of MHD is approximately 9 hours so that MHD is responsible for most antiepileptic activity.

Special populations –

Renal function impairment: There is a linear correlation between Ccr and the renal clearance of MHD. When oxcarbazepine 300 mg is administered as a single dose in renally impaired patients (Ccr less than 30 mL/min), the elimination half-life of MHD is prolonged to 19 hours, with a 2-fold increase in area under the curve (AUC). Dose adjustment for oxcarbazepine is recommended in these patients.

Hepatic function impairment: Exercise caution when dosing severely impaired patients.

Elderly: Following administration of single (300 mg) and multiple (600 mg/day) doses of oxcarbazepine to elderly volunteers (60 to 82 years of age), the maximum plasma concentrations (C_{max}) and AUC values of MHD were 30% to 60% higher than in younger volunteers (18 to 32 years of age). Comparisons of Ccr in younger and elderly volunteers indicate that the difference was because of age-related reductions in Ccr.

Children: Weight-adjusted MHD clearance decreases as age and weight increase, approaching that of adults. The mean weight-adjusted clearance in children 2 to younger than 4 years of age is approximately 80% higher on average than that of adults. Therefore, MHD exposure in these children is expected to be about one half that of adults when treated with a similar weight-adjusted dose. The mean weight-adjusted clearance in children 4 to 12 years of age is approximately 40% higher on average than that of adults. Therefore, MHD exposure in these children is expected to be about three quarters that of adults when treated with a similar weight-adjusted dose. As weight increases, for patients 13 years of age and older, the weight-adjusted MHD clearance is expected to reach that of adults.

Contraindications

Known hypersensitivity to oxcarbazepine or to any of its components.

Warnings/Precautions

➤*Hyponatremia:* Clinically significant hyponatremia (sodium less than 125 mmol/L) can develop during oxcarbazepine use. In the 14 controlled epilepsy studies, 2.5% of oxcarbazepine-treated patients (38/1,524) had a sodium of less than 125 mmol/L at some point during treatment, compared with no such patients assigned placebo or active control (carbamazepine and phenobarbital for adjunctive and monotherapy substitution studies and phenytoin and valproate for the monotherapy initiation studies). Clinically significant hyponatremia generally occurred during the first 3 months of treatment with oxcarbazepine, although there were patients who first developed a serum sodium less than 125 mmol/L more than 1 year after initiation of therapy. Most patients who developed hyponatremia were asymptomatic, but patients in the clinical trials were frequently monitored; some had their oxcarbazepine dose reduced or discontinued or had their fluid intake restricted for hyponatremia. Whether these maneuvers prevented the occurrence of more severe reactions is unknown. Cases of symptomatic hyponatremia have been reported during postmarketing use. In clinical trials, patients whose treatment with oxcarbazepine was discontinued because of hyponatremia generally experienced normalization of serum sodium within a few days without additional treatment.

➤*Serious dermatological reactions:* Serious dermatological reactions, including Stevens-Johnson syndrome and toxic epidermal necrolysis, have been reported in children and adults in association with oxcarbazepine use. The median time of onset for reported cases was 19 days. Such serious skin reactions may be life-threatening, and some patients have required hospitalization with very rare reports of fatal outcome. Recurrence of serious skin reactions following rechallenge with oxcarbazepine has also been reported.

The reporting rate of toxic epidermal necrolysis and Stevens-Johnson syndrome associated with oxcarbazepine use, which is generally accepted to be an underestimate because of underreporting, exceeds the background incidence rate estimates by a factor of 3- to 10-fold. Estimates of the background incidence rate for these serious skin reactions in the general population range between 0.5 and 6 cases per million person-years. Therefore, if a patient develops a skin reaction while taking oxcarbazepine, consider discontinuing oxcarbazepine use and prescribing another AED.

➤*Withdrawal of AEDs:* As with all AEDs, gradually withdraw oxcarbazepine to minimize the potential of increased seizure frequency.

➤*CNS effects:* Use of oxcarbazepine has been associated with CNS-related adverse reactions. The most significant of these can be classified into 3 general categories: cognitive symptoms, including difficulty with concentration, psychomotor slowing, and speech or language problems; somnolence or fatigue; and coordination abnormalities, including ataxia and gait disturbances.

➤*Multiorgan hypersensitivity:* Multiorgan hypersensitivity reactions have occurred in close temporal association (median time to detection, 13 days; range, 4 to 60) to the initiation of oxcarbazepine therapy in adults and children. Although there have been a limited number of reports, many of these cases resulted in hospitalization and some were considered life-threatening. Signs and symptoms of this disorder were diverse; however, patients typically, although not exclusively, presented with fever and rash associated with other organ system involvement. Other associated manifestations included arthralgia, asthenia, hematological abnormalities (eg, eosinophilia, neutropenia, thrombocytopenia), hepatitis, hepatorenal syndrome, liver function test abnormalities, lymphadenopathy, nephritis, oliguria, and pruritus. Because the disorder is variable in its expression, other organ system symptoms and signs not noted here may occur. If this reaction is suspected, discontinue oxcarbazepine and start an alternative treatment. Although there are no case reports to indicate cross-sensitivity with other drugs that produce this syndrome, the experience among drugs associated with multiorgan hypersensitivity would indicate this to be a possibility.

➤*Hypersensitivity reactions:* See Patient Information for more information.

➤*Renal function impairment:* In renally impaired patients (Ccr less than 30 mL/min), the elimination half-life of MHD is prolonged with a corresponding 2-fold increase in AUC. Initiate oxcarbazepine therapy at one half the usual starting dose and increase, if necessary, at a slower than usual rate until the desired clinical response is achieved.

➤*Hazardous tasks:* See Patient Information for more information.

➤*Pregnancy: Category C.* Increased incidences of fetal structural abnormalities and other manifestations of developmental toxicity (embryolethality, growth retardation) were observed in the offspring of animals treated with either oxcarbazepine or MHD during pregnancy at doses similar to the MRHD.

When pregnant rats were given oxcarbazepine (30, 300, or 1,000 mg/kg) orally throughout the period of organogenesis, increased incidences of fetal malformations (craniofacial, cardiovascular, and skeletal) and variations were observed at intermediate and high doses (approximately 1.2 and 4 times, respectively, the MRHD on a mg/m^2 basis). Increased embryofetal death and decreased fetal body weights were seen at the high dose. Doses at least 300 mg/kg were also maternally toxic (decreased body weight gain, clinical signs), but there is no evidence to suggest that teratogenicity was secondary to the maternal effects.

In a study in which pregnant rabbits were orally administered MHD (20, 100, or 200 mg/kg) during organogenesis, embryofetal mortality was increased at the highest dose (1.5 times the MRHD on a mg/m^2 basis). This dose produced only minimal maternal toxicity.

In a study in which female rats were dosed orally with oxcarbazepine (25, 50, or 150 mg/kg) during the latter part of gestation and throughout the lactation period, a persistent reduction in body weight and altered behavior (decreased activity) were observed in offspring exposed to the highest dose (0.6 times the MRHD on a mg/m^2 basis). Oral administration of MHD (25, 75, or 250 mg/kg) to rats during gestation and lactation resulted in a persistent reduction in offspring weights at the highest dose (equivalent to the MRHD on a mg/m^2 basis).

There are no adequate and well-controlled clinical studies of oxcarbazepine in pregnant women; however, oxcarbazepine is closely related structurally to carbamazepine, which is considered to be teratogenic in humans. Given this fact, and the results of the animal studies described, it is likely that oxcarbazepine is a human teratogen. Use oxcarbazepine during pregnancy only if the potential benefit justifies the potential risk to the fetus.

➤*Lactation:* Oxcarbazepine and MHD are excreted in human breast milk. A milk-to-plasma concentration ratio of 0.5 was found for both. Because of the potential for serious adverse reactions to oxcarbazepine in breast-feeding infants, decide whether to discontinue breast-feeding or the drug, taking into account the importance of the drug to the mother.

➤*Children:* Oxcarbazepine is indicated for use as adjunctive therapy for partial seizures in patients 2 to 16 years of age. Oxcarbazepine is also indicated as monotherapy for partial seizures in patients 4 to 16 years of age. Oxcarbazepine has been given to 898 patients between 1 month and 17 years of age in controlled clinical trials (332 treated as monotherapy) and about 677 patients between the 1 month and 17 years of age in other trials.

➤*Elderly:* There were 52 patients older than 65 years of age in controlled clinical trials and 565 patients older than 65 years of age in other trials. Following administration of single (300 mg) and multiple (600 mg/day) doses of oxcarbazepine in elderly volunteers (60 to 82 years of age), the C_{max} and AUC values of MHD were 30% to 60% higher than in younger volunteers (18 to 32 years of age). Comparisons of Ccr in younger and elderly volunteers indicate that the difference was because of age-related reductions in Ccr.

➤*Lab test abnormalities:* Serum sodium levels less than 125 mmol/L have been observed in patients treated with oxcarbazepine. Experience from clinical trials indicates that serum sodium levels return toward normal when the oxcarbazepine dosage is reduced or discontinued, or when the patient was treated conservatively (eg, fluid restriction).

Laboratory data from clinical trials suggest that oxcarbazepine use was associated with decreases in thyroxine (T_4), without changes in triiodothyronine (T_3) or thyroid-stimulating hormone.

➤*Monitoring:* It is recommended that the patient be closely observed and plasma levels of the concomitant AEDs be monitored during the period of oxcarbazepine titration, as these plasma levels may be altered, especially at oxcarbazepine doses above 1,200 mg/day.

Consider measurement of serum sodium levels for patients during maintenance treatment with oxcarbazepine, particularly if the patient is receiving other medications known to decrease serum sodium levels (eg, drugs associated with inappropriate antidiuretic hormone secretion) or if symptoms possibly indicating hyponatremia develop (eg, confusion, headache, increase in seizure frequency or severity, lethargy, malaise, nausea, obtundation).

Drug Interactions

Oxcarbazepine Drug Interactions

Precipitant drug	Object drug[a]		Description
Carbamazepine	Oxcarbazepine	↓	Concurrent use of carbamazepine and oxcarbazepine decreased MHD concentration ≈ 40%.
Phenobarbital	Oxcarbazepine	↓	Administration of phenobarbital with oxcarbazepine decreased MHD concentrations ≈ 25%, while phenobarbital concentrations increased ≈ 14%.
Oxcarbazepine	Phenobarbital	↑	
Phenytoin	Oxcarbazepine	↓	Coadministration of phenytoin with oxcarbazepine (600 to 1,800 mg/day) caused a 30% decrease in MHD AUC. Higher doses of oxcarbazepine (> 1,200 to 2,400 mg/day) increased phenytoin concentrations up to 40%. A decrease in phenytoin dose may be required when given with oxcarbazepine in doses > 1,200 mg/day.
Oxcarbazepine	Phenytoin	↑	
Valproic acid	Oxcarbazepine	↓	Concurrent use of valproic acid and oxcarbazepine decreased MHD concentrations ≈ 18%.
Verapamil	Oxcarbazepine	↓	Verapamil administration resulted in a 20% decrease of oxcarbazepine (MHD) plasma levels.
Oxcarbazepine	Contraceptives, oral	↓	The mean AUC of ethinyl estradiol decreased 48% to 52% and the mean AUC of levonorgestrel decreased 32% to 52% when coadministered with oxcarbazepine.
Oxcarbazepine	Felodipine	↓	The AUC of felodipine decreased 28% when repeatedly coadministered with oxcarbazepine.
Oxcarbazepine	Lamotrigine	↓	Oxcarbazepine administration reduced serum concentrations of lamotrigine 29%. Adjust the dose of lamotrigine as needed.

[a] ↑ = object drug increased; ↓ = object drug decreased.

Adverse Reactions

Be aware that the following figures cannot be used to predict the frequency of adverse reactions in the course of usual medical practice where patient characteristics and other factors may differ from those prevailing during clinical studies. Similarly, the cited frequencies cannot be directly compared

OXCARBAZEPINE — ORAL

with figures obtained from other clinical investigations involving different treatments, uses, or investigators. An inspection of these frequencies, however, provides a basis to estimate the relative contribution of drug and nondrug factors to the adverse reaction incidences in the population studied.

➤*Adjunctive therapy/monotherapy in adults previously treated with other AEDs:* The most commonly observed (at least 5%) adverse reactions seen in association with oxcarbazepine and substantially more frequent than in placebo-treated patients were as follows: abdominal pain, abnormal gait, abnormal vision, ataxia, diplopia, dizziness, dyspepsia, fatigue, nausea, somnolence, tremor, and vomiting.

Approximately 23% of 1,537 adult patients discontinued treatment because of an adverse reaction. The adverse reactions most commonly associated with discontinuation were as follows: abnormal gait (1.7%), abnormal vision (2.1%), ataxia (5.2%), diplopia (5.9%), dizziness (6.4%), fatigue (2.1%), headache (2.9%), hyponatremia (1%), nausea (4.9%), rash (1.4%), somnolence (3.8%), tremor (1.8%), and vomiting (5.1%).

The following table lists treatment-emergent signs and symptoms that occurred in at least 2% of adult patients with epilepsy treated with oxcarbazepine or placebo as adjunctive treatment and were numerically more common in the patients treated with any dose of oxcarbazepine. Treatment-emergent signs and symptoms in patients converted from other AEDs to either high-dose oxcarbazepine or low-dose (300 mg) oxcarbazepine are also listed. Note that in some of these monotherapy studies patients who dropped out during a preliminary tolerability phase are not included in the tables.

Oxcarbazepine (OXC) Adverse Reactions in Adults (%)								
	Patients on adjunctive therapy treated with oxcarbazepine (mg/day)				Patients on monotherapy previously treated with other AEDs (mg/day)		Patients on monotherapy not previously treated with other AEDs (mg/day)	
Adverse reactions	OXC 600 (n = 163)	OXC 1,200 (n = 171)	OXC 2,400 (n = 126)	Placebo (n = 166)	OXC 2,400 (n = 86)	OXC 300 (n = 86)	OXC (n = 55)	Placebo (n = 49)
Cardiovascular								
Abnormal EEG	0%	0%	2%	0%	—	—	—	—
Hypotension	0%	1%	2%	0%	—	—	—	—
CNS								
Abnormal coordination	1%	3%	2%	1%	2%	1%	4%	2%
Abnormal gait	5%	10%	17%	1%	—	—	—	—
Abnormal thinking	0%	2%	4%	0%	—	—	—	—
Agitation	1%	1%	2%	1%	—	—	—	—
Amnesia	—	—	—	—	5%	1%	4%	2%
Anxiety	—	—	—	—	7%	5%	—	—
Ataxia	9%	17%	31%	5%	7%	1%	5%	0%
Confusion	1%	1%	2%	1%	7%	0%	—	—
Convulsions aggravated	—	—	—	—	5%	2%	—	—
Cranial injury NOS[a]	1%	0%	2%	1%	—	—	—	—
Dizziness	26%	32%	49%	13%	28%	8%	22%	6%
Dysmetria	1%	2%	3%	0%	—	—	—	—
Emotional lability	—	—	—	—	3%	2%	—	—
Headache	32%	28%	26%	23%	31%	15%	13%	10%
Hypesthesia	—	—	—	—	3%	1%	—	—
Insomnia	4%	2%	3%	1%	6%	3%	—	—
Nervousness	2%	4%	2%	1%	7%	0%	5%	2%
Somnolence	20%	28%	36%	12%	19%	5%	—	—
Speech disorder	1%	1%	3%	0%	2%	0%	—	—
Tremor	3%	8%	16%	5%	6%	3%	4%	0%
Vertigo	6%	12%	15%	2%	3%	0%	—	—
Dermatologic								
Acne	1%	2%	2%	0%	—	—	—	—
Hot flushes	—	—	—	—	2%	1%	—	—
Purpura	—	—	—	—	2%	0%	—	—
Rash	—	—	—	—	—	—	4%	2%
GI								
Abdominal pain	10%	13%	11%	5%	5%	3%	—	—
Anorexia	—	—	—	—	5%	3%	—	—
Constipation	2%	2%	6%	4%	—	—	5%	0%
Diarrhea	5%	6%	7%	6%	7%	5%	7%	2%
Dry mouth	—	—	—	—	3%	0%	—	—
Dyspepsia	5%	5%	6%	2%	6%	1%	5%	4%
Gastritis	2%	1%	2%	1%	—	—	—	—
Nausea	15%	25%	29%	10%	22%	7%	16%	12%
Rectum hemorrhage	—	—	—	—	2%	0%	—	—
Toothache	—	—	—	—	2%	1%	—	—
Vomiting	13%	25%	36%	5%	15%	5%	7%	6%
GU								
Micturition frequency	—	—	—	—	2%	1%	—	—
Urinary tract infection	—	—	—	—	5%	1%	—	—
Vaginitis	—	—	—	—	2%	0%	—	—
Metabolic/Nutritional								
Hyponatremia	3%	1%	2%	1%	5%	0%	—	—
Thirst	—	—	—	—	2%	0%	—	—
Musculoskeletal								
Back pain	—	—	—	—	—	—	4%	2%
Muscle weakness	1%	2%	2%	0%	—	—	—	—

OXCARBAZEPINE — ORAL

Oxcarbazepine (OXC) Adverse Reactions in Adults (%)								
	Patients on adjunctive therapy treated with oxcarbazepine (mg/day)				Patients on monotherapy previously treated with other AEDs (mg/day)		Patients on monotherapy not previously treated with other AEDs (mg/day)	
Adverse reactions	OXC 600 (n = 163)	OXC 1,200 (n = 171)	OXC 2,400 (n = 126)	Placebo (n = 166)	OXC 2,400 (n = 86)	OXC 300 (n = 86)	OXC (n = 55)	Placebo (n = 49)
Sprains/Strains	0%	2%	2%	1%	—	—	—	—
Respiratory								
Bronchitis	—	—	—	—	3%	0%	—	—
Chest infection	—	—	—	—	—	—	4%	0%
Coughing	—	—	—	—	5%	0%	—	—
Epistaxis	—	—	—	—	—	—	4%	0%
Pharyngitis	—	—	—	—	3%	0%	—	—
Rhinitis	2%	4%	5%	4%	—	—	—	—
Sinusitis	—	—	—	—	—	—	4%	2%
Upper respiratory tract infection	—	—	—	—	10%	5%	7%	0%
Special senses								
Abnormal accommodation	0%	0%	2%	0%	—	—	—	—
Abnormal vision	6%	14%	13%	4%	14%	2%	4%	0%
Diplopia	14%	30%	40%	5%	12%	1%	—	—
Earache	—	—	—	—	2%	1%	—	—
Ear infection NOS[a]	—	—	—	—	2%	0%	—	—
Nystagmus	7%	20%	26%	5%	2%	0%	—	—
Taste perversion	—	—	—	—	5%	0%	—	—
Miscellaneous								
Abnormal feeling	0%	1%	2%	0%	—	—	—	—
Allergy	—	—	—	—	2%	0%	—	—
Asthenia	6%	3%	6%	5%	—	—	—	—
Chest pain	—	—	—	—	2%	0%	—	—
Edema, legs	2%	1%	2%	1%	—	—	—	—
Falling down NOS[a]	—	—	—	—	—	—	4%	0%
Fatigue	15%	12%	15%	7%	21%	5%	—	—
Fever	—	—	—	—	3%	0%	—	—
Generalized edema	—	—	—	—	2%	1%	—	—
Infection	—	—	—	—	2%	0%	—	—
Infection viral	—	—	—	—	7%	5%	—	—
Lymphadenopathy	—	—	—	—	2%	0%	—	—
Weight increase	1%	2%	2%	1%	—	—	—	—

[a] NOS = not otherwise specified.

➤*Monotherapy in adults not previously treated with other AEDs:* The most commonly observed (at least 5%) adverse reactions seen in association with oxcarbazepine in these patients were similar to those in previously treated patients.

Approximately 9% of 295 adult patients discontinued treatment because of an adverse reaction. The adverse reactions most commonly associated with discontinuation were the following: dizziness (1.7%), headache (1.4%), nausea (1.7%), and rash (1.7%).

➤*Adjunctive therapy/monotherapy in children 4 years of age and older previously treated with other AEDs:* The most commonly observed (at least 5%) adverse reactions seen in association with oxcarbazepine in these patients were similar to those seen in adults.

Approximately 11% of 456 children discontinued treatment because of an adverse reaction. The adverse reactions most commonly associated with discontinuation were ataxia (1.8%), diplopia (1.3%), dizziness (1.3%), fatigue (1.1%), nystagmus (1.1%), somnolence (2.4%), and vomiting (2%).

The following table lists treatment-emergent signs and symptoms that occurred in at least 2% of children with epilepsy treated with oxcarbazepine or placebo as adjunctive treatment and were numerically more common in the patients treated with oxcarbazepine.

Adverse Reactions of Oxcarbazepine Adjunctive Therapy/Monotherapy in Children Previously Treated With Other AEDs (≥ 2%)		
Adverse reaction	Oxcarbazepine (n = 171)	Placebo (n = 139)
CNS		
Abnormal gait	8%	3%
Ataxia	13%	4%
Convulsions	2%	1%
Dizziness	28%	8%
Emotional lability	8%	4%
Fatigue	13%	9%
Headache	31%	19%
Impaired concentration	2%	1%
Involuntary muscle contractions	2%	1%
Somnolence	31%	13%
Speech disorder	3%	1%
Tremor	6%	4%
Vertigo	2%	0%
Dermatologic		
Bruising	4%	2%
Increased sweating	3%	0%
GI		
Constipation	4%	1%
Dyspepsia	2%	0%
Nausea	19%	5%
Vomiting	33%	14%
Respiratory		
Pneumonia	2%	1%
Rhinitis	10%	9%
Special senses		
Abnormal vision	13%	1%

OXCARBAZEPINE — ORAL

Adverse Reactions of Oxcarbazepine Adjunctive Therapy/Monotherapy in Children Previously Treated With Other AEDs (≥ 2%)		
Adverse reaction	Oxcarbazepine (n = 171)	Placebo (n = 139)
Diplopia	17%	1%
Nystagmus	9%	1%
Miscellaneous		
Allergy	2%	0%
Asthenia	2%	1%

➤*Monotherapy in children 4 years of age and older not previously treated with other AEDs:* The most commonly observed (at least 5%) adverse reactions seen in association with oxcarbazepine in these patients were similar to those in adults. Approximately 9.2% of 152 children discontinued treatment because of an adverse reaction. The adverse reactions most commonly associated (at least 1%) with discontinuation were maculopapular rash (1.3%) and rash (5.3%).

➤*Adjunctive therapy / monotherapy in children 1 month to younger than 4 years of age previously treated or not previously treated with other AEDs:* The most commonly observed (at least 5%) adverse reactions seen in association with oxcarbazepine in these patients were similar to those seen in older children and adults except for infections and infestations, which were more frequently seen in these younger children.

Approximately 11% of these 241 children discontinued treatment because of an adverse reaction. The adverse reactions most commonly associated with discontinuation were convulsions (3.7%), ataxia (1.2%), and status epilepticus (1.2%).

➤*Other adverse reactions:* In the paragraphs that follow, the adverse reactions, other than those in the preceding tables or text, that occurred in a total of 565 children and 1,574 adults exposed to oxcarbazepine and that are reasonably likely to be related to drug use are presented. Reactions common in the population, reactions reflecting chronic illness, and reactions likely to reflect concomitant illness are omitted, particularly if minor. Because the reports cite reactions observed in open-label and uncontrolled trials, the role of oxcarbazepine in their causation cannot be reliably determined.

Cardiovascular – Bradycardia, cardiac failure, cerebral hemorrhage, hypertension, palpitation, postural hypotension, syncope, tachycardia.

CNS – Aggravated seizures, aggressive reaction, amnesia, anguish, anxiety, apathy, aphasia, aura, delirium, delusion, depressed level of consciousness, dysphonia, dystonia, emotional lability, euphoria, extrapyramidal disorder, feeling drunk, hemiplegia, hyperkinesia, hyperreflexia, hypesthesia, hypokinesia, hyporeflexia, hypotonia, hysteria, involuntary muscle contractions, libido decreased, libido increased, manic reaction, migraine, nervousness, neuralgia, oculogyric crisis, panic disorder, paralysis, paroniria, personality disorder, psychosis, ptosis, stupor, tetany.

Dermatologic – Acne, alopecia, angioedema, bruising, contact dermatitis, eczema, erythematous rash, facial rash, flushing, folliculitis, genital pruritus, heat rash, hot flushes, maculopapular rash, photosensitivity reaction, psoriasis, purpura, urticaria, vitiligo.

GI – Appetite increased, biliary pain, blood in stool, cholelithiasis, colitis, dry mouth, duodenal ulcer, dysphagia, enteritis, eructation, esophagitis, flatulence, gastric ulcer, gingival bleeding, gum hyperplasia, hematemesis, hemorrhoids, hiccup, rectum hemorrhage, retching, right hypochondrium pain, sialoadenitis, stomatitis, ulcerative stomatitis.

GU – Dysuria, hematuria, intermenstrual bleeding, leukorrhea, menorrhagia, micturition frequency, polyuria, priapism, renal calculus, renal pain, urinary tract pain.

Hematologic / Lymphatic – Leukopenia, thrombocytopenia.

Lab test abnormalities – Gamma-glutamyltransferase (GGT) increased, liver enzymes elevated, serum transaminase increased.

Metabolic – Hyperglycemia, hypocalcemia, hypoglycemia, hypokalemia, weight decrease.

Musculoskeletal – Muscle hypertonia.

Respiratory – Asthma, dyspnea, epistaxis, laryngismus, pleurisy.

Special senses – Accommodation abnormal, cataract, conjunctival hemorrhage, eye edema, hemianopia, mydriasis, otitis externa, photophobia, scotoma, taste perversion, tinnitus, xerophthalmia.

Miscellaneous – Dental oral procedure, female reproductive procedure, fever, malaise, musculoskeletal procedure, precordial chest pain, rigors, skin procedure, systemic lupus erythematosus.

➤*Postmarketing:* The following adverse reactions not seen in controlled clinical trials have been observed in named patient programs or postmarketing experience:

Dermatologic – Erythema multiforme, Stevens-Johnson syndrome, toxic epidermal necrolysis.

Hypersensitivity – Multiorgan hypersensitivity disorders characterized by features such as abnormal liver function tests, arthralgia, eosinophilia, fever, lymphadenopathy, and rash.

Overdosage

Isolated cases of overdose with oxcarbazepine have been reported. The maximum dose taken was approximately 24,000 mg. All patients recovered with symptomatic treatment.

➤*Treatment:* There is no specific antidote. Administer symptomatic and supportive treatment as appropriate. Consider removal of the drug by gastric lavage and/or inactivation by administering activated charcoal.

Patient Information

Inform patients who have exhibited hypersensitivity reactions to carbamazepine that approximately 25% to 30% of these patients may experience hypersensitivity reactions with oxcarbazepine. Advise patients to consult their health care provider immediately if they experience a hypersensitivity reaction while taking oxcarbazepine.

Advise patients that serious skin reactions have been reported in association with oxcarbazepine. In the event a skin reaction should occur while taking oxcarbazepine, instruct patients to consult their health care provider immediately.

Instruct patients that a fever associated with other organ system involvement (eg, lymphadenopathy, rash) may be drug-related and should be reported to their health care provider immediately.

Warn female patients of childbearing age that the concurrent use of oxcarbazepine with hormonal contraceptives may render this method of contraception less effective. Recommend additional nonhormonal forms of contraception when oxcarbazepine is used.

Advise patients to exercise caution if alcohol is taken in combination with oxcarbazepine therapy because of a possible additive sedative effect.

Advise patients that oxcarbazepine may cause dizziness and somnolence. Accordingly, advise patients not to drive or operate machinery until they have gained sufficient experience on oxcarbazepine to gauge whether it adversely affects their ability to drive or operate machinery.

LACOSAMIDE

c-v	**Vimpat** (UCB)	**Tablets; oral:** 50 mg	Alcohol, PEG. (SP 50). Pink, oval. Film-coated. In 60s.
		100 mg	Alcohol, PEG. (SP 100). Dark yellow, oval. Film-coated. In 60s.
		150 mg	Alcohol, PEG. (SP 150). Salmon, oval. Film-coated. In 60s.
		200 mg	Alcohol, PEG. (SP 200). Blue, oval. Film-coated. In 60s.
		Solution; oral: 10 mg/mL	Acesulfame potassium, aspartame, glycerin, parabens, PEG, phenylalanine 0.016 mg/mL, propylene glycol, sorbitol. Strawberry flavored. In 465 mL.
		Injection, solution: 10 mg/mL	Sodium chloride. In 20 mL single-use glass vials.

LACOSAMIDE — ORAL

Refer to the general discussion beginning in the Anticonvulsants Introduction.

Indications

➤*Partial-onset seizures:* As adjunctive therapy in the treatment of partial-onset seizures in patients 17 years of age and older with epilepsy.

➤*Off-label uses:*

Diabetic neuropathy – [4] = Insufficient documentation. Lacosamide in the management of diabetic neuropathy has been evaluated in controlled trials, demonstrating both a benefit and a lack of therapeutic benefit compared with placebo. Lacosamide is either not included in guidelines or is rated level A/B for inefficacy or discrepant results.

Administration and Dosage

➤*Adults:*

Partial-onset seizures –

Initial dosage: 50 mg twice daily (100 mg/day).

Dosage titration: Increase at weekly intervals by 100 mg/day given in 2 divided doses, up to the recommended maintenance dosage of 200 to 400 mg/day, based on individual patient response and tolerability. In clinical trials, the 600 mg daily dose was not more effective than the 400 mg daily dose and was associated with a substantially higher rate of adverse reactions.

Maintenance dosage: 200 to 400 mg/day.

Conversion:

• *Switching from oral to intravenous dosing* – When switching from oral to intravenous (IV) lacosamide, the initial total daily dosage of IV lacosamide should be equivalent to the total daily dosage and frequency of

LACOSAMIDE — ORAL

oral lacosamide and should be infused IV over a period of 30 to 60 minutes. There is experience with twice-daily IV infusion for up to 5 days.

• *Switching from IV to oral dosing* – At the end of the IV treatment period, the patient may be switched to oral lacosamide at the equivalent daily dosage and frequency of the IV administration.

Off-label dosing –

Diabetic neuropathy: [4] = Insufficient documentation. 200, 400, or 600 mg daily. Titration schedules have started at 50 mg twice daily for 1 to 3 weeks, with increases of 100 mg weekly to the target dose. Based on efficacy data and a high withdrawal rate during the titration phase, the optimal dose appears to be 400 mg daily. In published trials, treatment duration was 12 weeks after target dose was reached.

➤*Renal function impairment:*

Severe renal impairment/end-stage renal disease –

Maximum dose: A maximum dosage of 300 mg/day is recommended for patients with severe renal impairment (creatinine clearance [CrCl] 30 mL/min or less) and in patients with end-stage renal disease.

Dosage titration: Dose titration should be performed with caution in all renally impaired patients.

Hemodialysis – Lacosamide is effectively removed from plasma by hemodialysis. Following a 4-hour hemodialysis treatment, dosage supplementation of up to 50% should be considered.

➤*Hepatic function impairment:*

Mild or moderate hepatic impairment –

Maximum dose: A maximum dosage of 300 mg/day is recommended for patients with mild or moderate hepatic impairment.

Dosage titration: Dose titration should be performed with caution.

Severe hepatic impairment – Use is not recommended in patients with severe hepatic impairment.

➤*Discontinuation of therapy:* As with all antiepileptic drugs (AEDs), gradually withdraw lacosamide over a minimum of 1 week to minimize the potential of increased seizure frequency in patients with seizure disorders.

➤*Administration:* Lacosamide may be taken with or without food.

Lacosamide can be initiated orally or IV.

Oral solution – When using lacosamide oral solution, it is recommended that a calibrated measuring device be obtained and used. A household teaspoon or tablespoon is not an adequate measuring device.

➤*Storage/Stability:* Store at 20° to 25°C (68° to 77°F); excursions are permitted between 15° and 30°C (59° and 86°F).

Do not freeze lacosamide oral solution. Discard any unused lacosamide oral solution remaining after 7 weeks of first opening the bottle.

Actions

➤*Pharmacology:* The precise mechanism by which lacosamide exerts its antiepileptic effects in humans remains to be fully elucidated. In vitro electrophysiological studies have shown that lacosamide selectively enhances slow inactivation of voltage-gated sodium channels, resulting in stabilization of hyperexcitable neuronal membranes and inhibition of repetitive neuronal firing.

Lacosamide binds to collapsin response mediator protein-2, a phosphoprotein that is mainly expressed in the nervous system and is involved in neuronal differentiation and control of axonal outgrowth. The role of collapsin response mediator protein-2 binding in seizure control is unknown.

Pharmacodynamics –

Cardiac electrophysiology: Lacosamide produced a small, dose-related increase in mean PR interval. At steady state, the time of the maximum observed mean PR interval corresponded with time to maximal concentration (T_{max}). The placebo-subtracted maximum increase in PR interval (at T_{max}) was 7.3 ms for the 400 mg/day group and 11.9 ms for the 800 mg/day group. For patients who participated in the controlled trials, the placebo-subtracted mean maximum increase in PR interval for a lacosamide 400 mg/day dosage was 3.1 ms in patients with partial-onset seizures and 9.4 ms for patients with diabetic neuropathy.

➤*Pharmacokinetics:* Pharmacokinetics of lacosamide are dose proportional (100 to 800 mg) and time invariant, with low inter- and intrasubject variability.

Absorption – Lacosamide is completely absorbed after oral administration with negligible first-pass effect, with a high absolute bioavailability of approximately 100%. The maximum lacosamide plasma concentrations (C_{max}) occur approximately 1 to 4 hours postdose after oral dosing. Steady-state plasma concentrations are achieved after 3 days of twice-daily repeated administration.

In a trial comparing the oral tablet with an oral solution containing lacosamide 10 mg/mL, bioequivalence between both formulations was shown.

Distribution – The volume of distribution is approximately 0.6 L/kg and is close to the volume of total body water. Lacosamide is less than 15% bound to plasma proteins.

Metabolism/Excretion – Lacosamide is primarily eliminated from the systemic circulation by renal excretion and biotransformation.

After oral administration of 100 mg of [14C]-lacosamide, approximately 95% of radioactivity administered was recovered in the urine and less than 0.5% in the feces. The major compounds excreted were unchanged lacosamide (approximately 40% of the dose), its O-desmethyl metabolite (approximately 30%), and a structurally unknown polar fraction (approximately 20%). The plasma exposure of the major human metabolite, O-desmethyl-lacosamide, is approximately 10% of that of lacosamide. Compared with lacosamide, O-desmethyl metabolite has a longer T_{max} (0.5 to 12 hours) and elimination half-life (15 to 23 hours). This metabolite has no known pharmacological activity.

Lacosamide is a CYP2C19 substrate. The relative contribution of other CYP isoforms or non-CYP enzymes in the metabolism of lacosamide is not clear. The elimination half-life of the unchanged drug is approximately 13 hours and is not altered by different doses, multiple dosing, or IV administration.

Special populations –

Renal function impairment: Lacosamide and its major metabolite are eliminated from the systemic circulation primarily by renal excretion.

The area under the curve (AUC) of lacosamide was increased approximately 25% in mildly (CrCl 50 to 80 mL/min) and moderately (CrCl 30 to 50 mL/min) and 60% in severely (CrCl 30 mL/min or less) renally impaired patients compared with subjects with healthy renal function (CrCl greater than 80 mL/min), whereas C_{max} was unaffected. No dose adjustment is considered necessary in mildly and moderately renally impaired subjects. A maximum dosage of 300 mg/day is recommended for patients with severe renal impairment (CrCl 30 mL/min or less) and in patients with end-stage renal disease. Lacosamide is effectively removed from plasma by hemodialysis. Following a 4-hour hemodialysis treatment, the AUC of lacosamide is reduced by approximately 50%. Therefore, consider dosage supplementation of up to 50% following hemodialysis. In all renally impaired patients, perform dosage titration with caution.

Hepatic function impairment: Lacosamide undergoes metabolism. Subjects with moderate hepatic impairment (Child-Pugh B) showed higher plasma concentrations of lacosamide (approximately 50% to 60% higher AUC compared with healthy subjects). Perform dosage titration with caution in patients with hepatic impairment. A maximum dosage of 300 mg/day is recommended for patients with mild or moderate hepatic impairment.

The pharmacokinetics of lacosamide have not been evaluated in severe hepatic impairment; use is not recommended in patients with severe hepatic impairment. Closely monitor patients with coexisting hepatic and renal impairment during dose titration.

Elderly: In elderly patients (older than 65 years of age), dose and body weight–normalized AUC and C_{max} is approximately 20% increased compared with younger subjects (18 to 64 years of age). This may be related to body weight and decreased renal function in elderly subjects. Dose reduction is not considered to be necessary.

CYP2C19 polymorphism: There are no clinically relevant differences in the pharmacokinetics of lacosamide between CYP2C19 poor and extensive metabolizers. Results from a trial in poor metabolizers (n = 4) and extensive metabolizers (n = 8) of CYP2C19 showed that lacosamide plasma concentrations were similar in poor metabolizers and extensive metabolizers, but plasma concentrations and amount excreted into urine of the O-desmethyl metabolite were approximately 70% reduced in poor metabolizers compared with extensive metabolizers.

Contraindications

None well documented.

Warnings/Precautions

➤*Suicidal behavior and ideation:* AEDs, including lacosamide, increase the risk of suicidal thoughts or behavior in patients taking these drugs for any indication. Monitor patients treated with any AED for any indication for the emergence or worsening of depression, suicidal thoughts or behavior, and/or any unusual changes in mood or behavior.

Pooled analyses of 199 placebo-controlled clinical trials (monotherapy and adjunctive therapy) of 11 different AEDs showed that patients randomized to one of the AEDs had approximately twice the risk (adjusted relative risk, 1.8; 95% confidence interval, 1.2 to 2.7) of suicidal thinking or behavior compared with patients randomized to placebo. In these trials, which had a median treatment duration of 12 weeks, the estimated incidence of suicidal behavior or ideation among 27,863 AED-treated patients was 0.43%, compared with 0.24% among 16,029 placebo-treated patients, representing an increase of approximately 1 case of suicidal thinking or behavior for every 530 patients treated. There were 4 suicides in drug-treated patients in the trials and none in placebo-treated patients, but the number of events is too small to allow any conclusion about drug effect on suicide.

The increased risk of suicidal thoughts or behavior with AEDs was observed as early as 1 week after starting treatment with AEDs and persisted for the duration of treatment assessed. Because most trials included in the analysis did not extend beyond 24 weeks, the risk of suicidal thoughts or behavior beyond 24 weeks could not be assessed.

The risk of suicidal thoughts or behavior was generally consistent among drugs in the data analyzed. The finding of increased risk with AEDs of varying mechanisms of action and across a range of indications suggests that the risk applies to all AEDs used for any indication. The risk did not vary substantially by age (5 to 100 years of age) in the clinical trials analyzed.

The relative risk for suicidal thoughts or behavior was higher in clinical trials for epilepsy than in clinical trials for psychiatric or other conditions, but the absolute risk differences were similar.

Anyone considering prescribing lacosamide or any other AED must balance this risk with the risk of untreated illness. Epilepsy and many other illnesses for which antiepileptics are prescribed are themselves associated with morbidity and mortality and an increased risk of suicidal thoughts and behavior. If suicidal thoughts and behavior emerge during treatment, the health care provider needs to consider whether the emergence of these symptoms in any given patient may be related to the illness being treated.

Inform patients, their caregivers, and families that AEDs increase the risk of suicidal thoughts and behavior and advise them of the need to be alert for the emergence or worsening of the signs and symptoms of depression, any unusual changes in mood or behavior, or the emergence of suicidal thoughts

LACOSAMIDE — ORAL

or behavior, or thoughts about self-harm. Advise patients to report behaviors of concern immediately to their health care provider.

➤*CNS effects:* In patients with partial-onset seizures taking 1 to 3 concomitant AEDs, dizziness was experienced by 25% of patients randomized to the recommended dosages of lacosamide (200 to 400 mg/day), compared with 8% of placebo patients, and was the adverse reaction most frequently leading to discontinuation (3%). Ataxia was experienced by 6% of patients randomized to the recommended dosages of lacosamide (200 to 400 mg/day) compared with 2% of placebo patients. The onset of dizziness and ataxia was most commonly observed during titration. There was a substantial increase in these adverse reactions at dosages higher than 400 mg/day.

➤*Cardiovascular effects:*

PR interval prolongation – Dose-dependent prolongations in PR interval with lacosamide have been observed in clinical studies in patients and in healthy volunteers. In clinical trials in patients with partial-onset epilepsy, asymptomatic first-degree atrioventricular (AV) block was observed as an adverse reaction in 0.4% of patients randomized to receive lacosamide and 0% of patients randomized to receive placebo. In clinical trials in patients with diabetic neuropathy, asymptomatic first-degree AV block was observed as an adverse reaction in 0.5% of patients receiving lacosamide and 0% of patients receiving placebo. When lacosamide is given with other drugs that prolong the PR interval, further PR prolongation is possible.

Use lacosamide with caution in patients with known conduction problems (eg, marked first-degree AV block, second-degree or higher AV block, sick sinus syndrome without pacemaker) or with severe cardiac disease, such as myocardial ischemia or heart failure. In such patients, obtaining an electrocardiogram before beginning lacosamide, and after lacosamide is titrated to steady state, is recommended.

Atrial fibrillation/flutter – In the short-term investigational trials of lacosamide in epilepsy patients, there were no cases of atrial fibrillation or flutter. In patients with diabetic neuropathy, 0.5% of patients treated with lacosamide experienced an adverse reaction of atrial fibrillation or atrial flutter, compared with 0% of placebo-treated patients. Lacosamide administration may predispose to atrial arrhythmias (atrial fibrillation or flutter), especially in patients with diabetic neuropathy and/or cardiovascular disease. Inform patients of the symptoms of atrial fibrillation and flutter (eg, palpitations, rapid pulse, shortness of breath) and advise them to contact their health care provider if any of these symptoms occur.

Syncope – In the short-term controlled trials of lacosamide in epilepsy patients with no significant system illnesses, there was no increase in syncope compared with placebo. In the short-term controlled trials of lacosamide in patients with diabetic neuropathy, 1.2% of patients who were treated with lacosamide reported an adverse reaction of syncope or loss of consciousness compared with 0% of placebo-treated patients with diabetic neuropathy. Most of the cases of syncope were observed in patients receiving dosages higher than 400 mg/day. The cause of syncope was not determined in most cases. However, several were associated with changes in orthostatic blood pressure, atrial flutter/fibrillation (and associated tachycardia), or bradycardia.

➤*Discontinuation of therapy:* As with all AEDs, gradually withdraw lacosamide over a minimum of 1 week to minimize the potential of increased seizure frequency in patients with seizure disorders.

➤*Phenylketonurics:* Lacosamide oral solution contains aspartame, a source of phenylalanine. A dose of lacosamide 200 mg oral solution (equivalent to 20 mL) contains phenylalanine 0.32 mg.

➤*Hypersensitivity reactions:* One case of symptomatic hepatitis and nephritis was observed among 4,011 subjects exposed to lacosamide during clinical development. The event occurred in a healthy volunteer 10 days after stopping lacosamide treatment. The subject was not taking any concomitant medication, and potential known viral causes for hepatitis were ruled out. The subject fully recovered within a month without specific treatment. The case is consistent with a delayed multiorgan hypersensitivity reaction. Additional potential cases included 2 with rash and elevated liver enzymes and 1 with myocarditis and hepatitis of uncertain cause.

Multiorgan hypersensitivity reactions (also known as drug reaction with eosinophilia and systemic symptoms) have been reported with other anticonvulsants and typically, although not exclusively, present with fever and rash associated with other organ system involvement that may or may not include eosinophilia, hepatitis, nephritis, lymphadenopathy, and/or myocarditis. Because this disorder is variable in its expression, other organ system signs and symptoms not noted here may occur. If this reaction is suspected, discontinue lacosamide and start alternative treatment.

➤*Renal function impairment:* A maximum dosage of 300 mg/day is recommended for patients with severe renal impairment (CrCl 30 mL/min or less) and in patients with end-stage renal disease. Lacosamide is effectively removed from plasma by hemodialysis. Following a 4-hour hemodialysis treatment, AUC of lacosamide is reduced by approximately 50%. Therefore, consider dosage supplementation of up to 50% following hemodialysis. In all renally impaired patients, perform dosage titration with caution.

➤*Hepatic function impairment:* Closely observe patients with mild to moderate hepatic impairment during dose titration. A maximum dosage of 300 mg/day is recommended for patients with mild to moderate hepatic impairment. The pharmacokinetics of lacosamide have not been evaluated in severe hepatic impairment. Lacosamide use is not recommended in patients with severe hepatic impairment. Closely monitor patients with coexisting hepatic and renal impairment during dose titration.

➤*Drug abuse and dependence:* Lacosamide is a schedule V controlled substance. In a human abuse potential study, single doses of lacosamide 200 and 800 mg produced euphoria-type subjective responses that differentiated statistically from placebo; at 800 mg, these euphoria-type responses were statistically indistinguishable from those produced by alprazolam, a schedule IV drug. The duration of the euphoria-type responses following lacosamide was less than that following alprazolam. A high rate of euphoria was also reported as an adverse reaction in the human abuse potential study following single doses of lacosamide 800 mg (15%) compared with placebo (0%) and in 2 pharmacokinetic studies following single and multiple doses of lacosamide 300 to 800 mg (ranging from 6% to 25%) compared with placebo (0%). However, the rate of euphoria reported as an adverse reaction in the lacosamide development program at therapeutic doses was less than 1%.

Abrupt termination of lacosamide in clinical trials with diabetic neuropathic pain patients produced no signs or symptoms that are associated with a withdrawal syndrome indicative of physical dependence. However, psychological dependence cannot be excluded because of the ability of lacosamide to produce euphoria-type adverse reactions in humans.

➤*Hazardous tasks:* Advise patients that lacosamide may cause dizziness and ataxia. Accordingly, advise them not to drive a car or operate other complex machinery until they are familiar with the effects of lacosamide on their ability to perform such activities.

➤*Pregnancy: Category C.* There are no adequate and well-controlled studies in pregnant women. Use lacosamide during pregnancy only if the potential benefit justifies the potential risk to the fetus.

Lacosamide produced developmental toxicity (increased embryofetal and perinatal mortality, growth deficit) in rats following administration during pregnancy. Developmental neurotoxicity was observed in rats following administration during a period of postnatal development corresponding to the third trimester of human pregnancy. These effects were observed at doses associated with clinically relevant plasma exposures.

Lacosamide has been shown in vitro to interfere with the activity of collapsin response mediator protein-2, a protein involved in neuronal differentiation and control of axonal outgrowth. Potential adverse effects on CNS development cannot be ruled out.

Oral administration of lacosamide to pregnant rats (20, 75, or 200 mg/kg/day) and rabbits (6.25, 12.5, or 25 mg/kg/day) during the period of organogenesis did not produce any teratogenic effects. However, the maximum doses evaluated were limited by maternal toxicity in both species and embryofetal death in rats. These doses were associated with maternal plasma lacosamide exposures (AUC) approximately 2 and 1 times (rat and rabbit, respectively) that in humans at the maximum recommended human dose (MRHD) of 400 mg/day.

When lacosamide (25, 70, or 200 mg/kg/day) was orally administered to rats throughout gestation, parturition, and lactation, increased perinatal mortality and decreased body weights were observed in the offspring at the highest dose. The no-effect dosage for pre- and postnatal developmental toxicity in rats (70 mg/kg/day) was associated with a maternal plasma lacosamide AUC approximately equal to that in humans at the MRHD.

Oral administration of lacosamide (30, 90, or 180 mg/kg/day) to rats during the neonatal and juvenile periods of postnatal development resulted in decreased brain weights and long-term neurobehavioral changes (eg, altered open-field performance, deficits in learning and memory). The early postnatal period in rats is generally thought to correspond to late pregnancy in humans in terms of brain development. The no-effect dose for developmental neurotoxicity in rats was associated with a plasma lacosamide AUC approximately 0.5 times that in humans at the MRHD.

Pregnancy registry – The manufacturer has established the UCB AED Pregnancy Registry to advance scientific knowledge about safety and outcomes in pregnant women being treated with lacosamide. To ensure broad program access and reach, a health care provider or the patient can initiate enrollment in the UCB AED Pregnancy Registry by calling 1-888-537-7734.

Health care providers are also advised to recommend that pregnant patients taking lacosamide enroll in the North American Antiepileptic Drug Pregnancy Registry. This can be done by calling 1-888-233-2334, and must be done by patients themselves. Information on the registry can also be found at the Web site http://www.aedpregnancyregistry.org.

➤*Lactation:* Studies in lactating rats have shown that lacosamide and/or its metabolites are excreted in milk. The molecular weight (about 250), low plasma protein binding (about 15%), and long elimination half-life (about 13 hours) suggest that the drug will be excreted into breast milk. It is not known whether lacosamide is excreted in human milk. Because many drugs are excreted into human milk, decide whether to discontinue breast-feeding or lacosamide, taking into account the importance of the drug to the mother.

➤*Children:* The safety and effectiveness of lacosamide in children younger than 17 years of age have not been established.

Lacosamide has been shown in vitro to interfere with the activity of collapsin response mediator protein-2, a protein involved in neuronal differentiation and control of axonal outgrowth. Potential adverse effects on CNS development cannot be ruled out. Administration of lacosamide to rats during the neonatal and juvenile periods of postnatal development resulted in decreased brain weights and long-term neurobehavioral changes (eg, altered open-field performance, deficits in learning and memory). The no-effect dose for developmental neurotoxicity in rats was associated with a plasma lacosamide exposure (AUC) approximately 0.5 times the human plasma AUC at the MRHD of 400 mg/day.

➤*Elderly:* In healthy subjects, the dose and body weight–normalized pharmacokinetic parameters AUC and C_{max} were approximately 20% higher in elderly subjects compared with younger subjects. The slightly higher lacosamide plasma concentrations in elderly subjects are possibly caused by differences in total body water (lean body weight) and age-associated decreased renal clearance. No lacosamide dose adjustment based on age is considered necessary. Exercise caution for dose titration in elderly patients.

LACOSAMIDE — ORAL

➤*Monitoring:* Monitor patients treated with any AED for any indication of the emergence or worsening of depression, suicidal thoughts or behavior, and/or any unusual changes in mood or behavior.

Obtain an electrocardiogram before beginning therapy and after lacosamide is titrated to steady state in patients with known conduction problems or severe cardiac disease.

Closely monitor patients with coexisting hepatic and renal impairment during dose titration.

Drug Interactions

Lacosamide Drug Interactions			
Precipitant drug	Object drug[a]		Description
AEDs (eg, carbamazepine, phenobarbital, phenytoin)	Lacosamide	↓	Small reductions (15% to 20%) in lacosamide plasma concentrations resulted with coadministration. A clinically important pharmacokinetic interaction is unlikely.
Omeprazole	Lacosamide	↓	Plasma levels of the O-desmethyl-lacosamide metabolite were reduced approximately 60% in the presence of omeprazole. A clinically important pharmacokinetic interaction is unlikely.
Lacosamide	Contraceptives, hormonal	↑	A 20% increase in ethinyl estradiol C_{max} has been observed. A clinically important pharmacokinetic interaction is unlikely.

[a] ↑ = object drug increased; ↓ = object drug decreased.

Adverse Reactions

➤*Discontinuation:* In controlled clinical trials, the rate of discontinuation as a result of an adverse reaction was 8% and 17% in patients randomized to receive lacosamide at the recommended dosages of 200 and 400 mg/day, respectively, 29% at 600 mg/day, and 5% in patients randomized to receive placebo. The adverse reactions most commonly (more than 1% in the lacosamide total group and greater than placebo) leading to discontinuation were ataxia, diplopia, dizziness, nausea, vertigo, vision blurred, and vomiting.

➤*Most common adverse reactions:* The majority of adverse reactions in the lacosamide patients were reported with a maximum intensity of mild or moderate.

Lacosamide Adverse Reactions (≥ 2%)					
Adverse reactions	Lacosamide 200 mg/day (n = 270)	Lacosamide 400 mg/day (n = 471)	Lacosamide 600 mg/day (n = 203)	Lacosamide total (n = 944)	Placebo (n = 364)
CNS					
Asthenia	2%	2%	4%	2%	1%
Ataxia	4%	7%	15%	8%	2%
Balance disorder	1%	5%	6%	4%	0%
Depression	2%	2%	2%	2%	1%
Dizziness	16%	30%	53%	31%	8%
Fatigue	7%	7%	15%	9%	6%
Gait disturbance	< 1%	2%	4%	2%	< 1%
Headache	11%	14%	12%	13%	9%
Memory impairment	1%	2%	6%	2%	2%
Somnolence	5%	8%	8%	7%	5%
Tremor	4%	6%	12%	7%	4%
Dermatologic					
Contusion	3%	4%	2%	3%	3%
Pruritus	3%	2%	3%	2%	1%
Skin laceration	2%	3%	3%	3%	2%
GI					
Diarrhea	3%	5%	4%	4%	3%
Nausea	7%	11%	17%	11%	4%
Vomiting	6%	9%	16%	9%	3%
Special senses					
Diplopia	6%	10%	16%	11%	2%
Nystagmus	2%	5%	10%	5%	4%
Vertigo	5%	3%	4%	4%	1%
Vision blurred	2%	9%	16%	8%	3%

➤*Other adverse reactions:*

CNS – Cerebellar syndrome, cognitive disorder, confusional state, depressed mood, disturbance in attention, dysarthria, feeling drunk, hypoesthesia, irritability, mood altered, paresthesia.

GI – Constipation, dry mouth, dyspepsia, oral hypoesthesia.

Hematologic/Lymphatic – Anemia, neutropenia.

Miscellaneous – Fall, muscle spasms, palpitations, pyrexia, tinnitus.

➤*Lab test abnormalities:* Abnormalities in liver function tests have been observed in controlled trials with lacosamide in adult patients with partial-onset seizures who were taking 1 to 3 concomitant AEDs. Elevations of ALT to at least 3 × the upper limit of normal (ULN) occurred in 0.7% of lacosamide patients and 0% of placebo patients. One case of hepatitis with transaminases more than 20 × ULN was observed in 1 healthy subject 10 days after lacosamide treatment completion, along with nephritis (proteinuria and urine casts). Serologic studies were negative for viral hepatitis. Transaminases returned to normal within 1 month without specific treatment. At the time of this event, bilirubin was normal. The hepatitis/nephritis was interpreted as a delayed hypersensitivity reaction to lacosamide.

➤*Postmarketing:*

Cardiovascular – Bradycardia.

Dermatologic – Rash.

Overdosage

➤*Symptoms:* There is limited clinical experience with lacosamide overdose in humans. The highest reported accidental overdose of lacosamide during clinical development was 1,200 mg/day, which was nonfatal. The types of adverse reactions experienced by patients exposed to supratherapeutic doses during the trials were not clinically different from those of patients administered recommended doses of lacosamide.

There has been a single case of intentional overdose by a patient who self-administered lacosamide 12 g along with large doses of zonisamide, topiramate, and gabapentin. The patient presented in a coma and was hospitalized. An electroencephalograph revealed epileptic waveforms. The patient recovered 2 days later.

➤*Treatment:* There is no specific antidote for lacosamide overdose. Follow standard decontamination procedures. General supportive care of the patient is indicated, including monitoring of vital signs and observation of the clinical status of the patient. Contact a certified poison control center for up-to-date information on the management of overdose with lacosamide.

Standard hemodialysis procedures result in significant clearance of lacosamide (reduction of systemic exposure by 50% in 4 hours). Hemodialysis has not been performed in the few known cases of overdose, but may be indicated based on the patient's clinical state or in patients with significant renal impairment.

Patient Information

Recommend a device that can measure and deliver the prescribed dose of oral solution accurately, and provide instructions for measuring the dosage.

Counsel patients, their caregivers, and families that AEDs, including lacosamide, may increase the risk of suicidal thoughts and behavior and advise them of the need to be alert for the emergence or worsening of symptoms of depression, any unusual changes in mood or behavior, or the emergence of suicidal thoughts or behavior, or thoughts about self-harm. Advise them to report behaviors of concern immediately to a health care provider.

Counsel patients that lacosamide use may cause dizziness, double vision, abnormal coordination and balance, and somnolence. Advise patients taking lacosamide not to drive, operate complex machinery, or engage in other hazardous activities until they have become accustomed to any such effects associated with lacosamide.

Counsel patients that lacosamide is associated with electrocardiographic changes that may predispose to irregular beat and syncope, particularly in patients with underlying cardiovascular disease or heart conduction problems, or who are taking other medications that affect the heart. Advise patients who develop syncope to lie down with raised legs until recovered and contact their health care provider.

Inform patients that lacosamide may cause serious hypersensitivity reactions affecting multiple organs, such as the liver and kidney. Discontinue lacosamide if a serious hypersensitivity reaction is suspected. Instruct patients to report promptly to their health care provider any symptoms of liver toxicity (eg, fatigue, jaundice, dark urine).

The manufacturer has established the UCB AED Pregnancy Registry to advance scientific knowledge about safety and outcomes in pregnant women being treated with lacosamide. To ensure broad program access and reach, a health care provider or the patient can initiate enrollment in the UCB AED Pregnancy Registry by calling 1-888-537-7734.

Encourage patients to enroll in the North American Antiepileptic Drug Pregnancy Registry if they become pregnant. This registry is collecting information about the safety of AEDs during pregnancy. To enroll, patients can call 1-888-233-2334.

LACOSAMIDE — INJECTION

Refer to the general discussion beginning in the Anticonvulsants Introduction.

Indications

➤*Partial-onset seizures:* As adjunctive therapy in the treatment of partial-onset seizures in patients with epilepsy 17 years of age and older when oral administration is temporarily not feasible.

Administration and Dosage

➤*Adults:*

Partial-onset seizures –

Initial dosage: 50 mg intravenously (IV) twice daily (100 mg/day).

Dosage titration: Increase at weekly intervals by 100 mg/day IV given as 2 divided doses, up to the recommended maintenance dosage of 200 to 400 mg/day, based on individual patient response and tolerability. In clinical trials, the 600 mg daily dose was not more effective than the 400 mg daily dose and was associated with a substantially higher rate of adverse reactions.

Maintenance dosage: 200 to 400 mg/day I.

Conversion:

• *Switching from oral to IV dosing –* When switching from oral lacosamide, the initial total daily dosage of IV lacosamide should be equivalent to the total daily dosage and frequency of oral lacosamide and should be infused IV over a period of 30 to 60 minutes. There is experience with twice-daily IV infusion for up to 5 days.

• *Switching from IV to oral dosing –* At the end of the IV treatment period, the patient may be switched to lacosamide oral administration at the equivalent daily dosage and frequency of the IV administration.

➤*Elderly:* Caution should be exercised for dose titration in elderly patients (see Warnings/Precautions).

➤*Renal function impairment:*

Severe renal impairment / end-stage renal disease –

Maximum dose: 300 mg/day is recommended for patients with severe renal function impairment (creatinine clearance [CrCl] 30 mL/min or less) and in patients with end-stage renal disease.

Dosage titration: In all renally impaired patients, the dose titration should be performed with caution.

Hemodialysis – Lacosamide is effectively removed from plasma by hemodialysis. Following a 4-hour hemodialysis treatment, dosage supplementation of up to 50% should be considered.

➤*Hepatic function impairment:*

Mild or moderate hepatic impairment –

Maximum dose: 300 mg/day is recommended for patients with mild or moderate hepatic impairment.

Dosage titration: Dosage titration should be performed with caution.

Severe hepatic impairment – Lacosamide use is not recommended in patients with severe hepatic impairment.

➤*Discontinuation of therapy:* As with all antiepileptic drugs (AEDs), gradually withdraw lacosamide over a minimum of 1 week to minimize the potential of increased seizure frequency in patients with seizure disorders.

➤*Preparation for administration:* Lacosamide injection can be administered IV without further dilution or may be mixed with diluents.

➤*Admixture compatibility:* Lacosamide injection was found to be physically compatible and chemically stable when mixed with sodium chloride injection 0.9%, dextrose injection 5%, and Ringer's lactate injection for at least 24 hours and stored in glass or polyvinyl chloride (PVC) bags at ambient room temperature, 15° to 30°C (59° to 86°F).

The stability of lacosamide injection in other infusion solutions has not been evaluated.

➤*Storage / Stability:* Store at 20° to 25°C (68° to 77°F); excursions are permitted between 15° and 30°C (59° and 86°F). Do not freeze. Any unused portion of lacosamide injection should be discarded.

Actions

➤*Pharmacology:* The precise mechanism by which lacosamide exerts its antiepileptic effects in humans remains to be fully elucidated. In vitro electrophysiological studies have shown that lacosamide selectively enhances slow inactivation of voltage-gated sodium channels, resulting in stabilization of hyperexcitable neuronal membranes and inhibition of repetitive neuronal firing.

Lacosamide binds to collapsin response mediator protein-2, a phosphoprotein that is mainly expressed in the nervous system and is involved in neuronal differentiation and control of axonal outgrowth. The role of collapsin response mediator protein-2 binding in seizure control is unknown.

Pharmacodynamics –

Cardiac electrophysiology: Lacosamide produced a small, dose-related increase in mean PR interval. At steady state, the time of the maximum observed mean PR interval corresponded with time to maximal drug concentration (T_{max}). The placebo-subtracted maximum increase in PR interval (at T_{max}) was 7.3 ms for the 400 mg/day group and 11.9 ms for the 800 mg/day group. For patients who participated in the controlled trials, the placebo-subtracted mean maximum increase in PR interval for a lacosamide 400 mg/day dosage was 3.1 ms in patients with partial-onset seizures and 9.4 ms for patients with diabetic neuropathy.

➤*Pharmacokinetics:* There is no enantiomeric interconversion of lacosamide.

Absorption – After IV administration, maximal drug concentration (C_{max}) is reached at the end of infusion. The 30- and 60-minute IV infusions are bioequivalent to the oral tablet.

Distribution – The volume of distribution is approximately 0.6 L/kg and is close to the volume of total body water. Lacosamide is less than 15% bound to plasma proteins.

Metabolism / Excretion – Lacosamide is primarily eliminated from the systemic circulation by renal excretion and biotransformation.

After IV administration of 100 mg of [14C]-lacosamide, approximately 95% of radioactivity administered was recovered in the urine and less than 0.5% in the feces. The major compounds excreted were unchanged lacosamide (approximately 40% of the dose), its O-desmethyl metabolite (approximately 30%), and a structurally unknown polar fraction (approximately 20%). The plasma exposure of the major human metabolite, O-desmethyl-lacosamide, is approximately 10% of that of lacosamide. Compared with lacosamide, O-desmethyl metabolite has a longer T_{max} (0.5 to 12 hours) and elimination half-life (15 to 23 hours). This metabolite has no known pharmacological activity.

Lacosamide is a CYP2C19 substrate. The relative contribution of other CYP isoforms or non-CYP enzymes in the metabolism of lacosamide is not clear. The elimination half-life of the unchanged drug is approximately 13 hours and is not altered by different doses, multiple dosing, or IV administration.

Special populations –

Renal function impairment: The area under the curve (AUC) of lacosamide was increased approximately 25% in mildly (CrCl 50 to 80 mL/min) and moderately (CrCl 30 to 50 mL/min) and 60% in severely (CrCl 30 mL/min or less) renally impaired patients compared with subjects with healthy renal function (CrCl greater than 80 mL/min), whereas C_{max} was unaffected. No dose adjustment is considered necessary in mildly and moderately renally impaired subjects. A maximum dosage of 300 mg/day is recommended for patients with severe renal impairment (CrCl 30 mL/min or less) and in patients with end-stage renal disease. Lacosamide is effectively removed from plasma by hemodialysis. Following a 4-hour hemodialysis treatment, the AUC of lacosamide is reduced by approximately 50%. Therefore, consider dosage supplementation of up to 50% following hemodialysis. In all renally impaired patients, perform dosage titration with caution.

Hepatic function impairment: Lacosamide undergoes metabolism. Subjects with moderate hepatic impairment (Child-Pugh B) showed higher plasma concentrations of lacosamide (approximately 50% to 60% higher AUC compared with healthy subjects). Perform dosage titration with caution in patients with hepatic impairment. A maximum dosage of 300 mg/day is recommended for patients with mild or moderate hepatic impairment.

Closely observe patients with mild to moderate hepatic impairment during dose titration. A maximum dosage of 300 mg/day is recommended for patients with mild to moderate hepatic impairment. The pharmacokinetics of lacosamide have not been evaluated in severe hepatic impairment. Lacosamide use is not recommended in patients with severe hepatic impairment. Closely monitor patients with coexisting hepatic and renal impairment during dose titration.

Elderly: In elderly patients (older than 65 years of age), dose and body weight–normalized AUC and C_{max} is approximately 20% increased compared with younger subjects (18 to 64 years of age). This may be related to body weight and decreased renal function in elderly subjects. Dose reduction is not considered to be necessary.

CYP2C19 polymorphism: There are no clinically relevant differences in the pharmacokinetics of lacosamide between CYP2C19 poor metabolizers and extensive metabolizers. Results from a trial in poor (n = 4) and extensive metabolizers (n = 8) of CYP2C19 showed that lacosamide plasma concentrations were similar in poor metabolizers and extensive metabolizers, but plasma concentrations and the amount excreted into urine of the O-desmethyl metabolite were approximately 70% reduced in poor metabolizers compared with extensive metabolizers.

Contraindications

None well documented.

Warnings/Precautions

➤*Suicidal behavior and ideation:* AEDs, including lacosamide, increase the risk of suicidal thoughts or behavior in patients taking these drugs for any indication. Monitor patients treated with any AED for any indication of the emergence or worsening of depression, suicidal thoughts or behavior, and/or any unusual changes in mood or behavior.

Pooled analyses of 199 placebo-controlled clinical trials (monotherapy and adjunctive therapy) of 11 different AEDs showed that patients randomized to one of the AEDs had approximately twice the risk (adjusted relative risk, 1.8; 95% confidence interval, 1.2 to 2.7) of suicidal thinking or behavior compared with patients randomized to placebo. In these trials, which had a median treatment duration of 12 weeks, the estimated incidence of suicidal behavior or ideation among 27,863 AED-treated patients was 0.43% compared with 0.24% among 16,029 placebo-treated patients, representing an increase of approximately 1 case of suicidal thinking or behavior for every 530 patients treated. There were 4 suicides in drug-treated patients in the trials and none in placebo-treated patients, but the number of events is too small to allow any conclusion about drug effect on suicide.

The increased risk of suicidal thoughts or behavior with AEDs was observed as early as 1 week after starting treatment with AEDs and persisted for the duration of treatment assessed. Because most trials included in the analysis did not extend beyond 24 weeks, the risk of suicidal thoughts or behavior beyond 24 weeks could not be assessed.

The risk of suicidal thoughts or behavior was generally consistent among drugs in the data analyzed. The finding of increased risk with AEDs of varying mechanisms of action and across a range of indications suggests that the

LACOSAMIDE — INJECTION

risk applies to all AEDs used for any indication. The risk did not vary substantially by age (5 to 100 years of age) in the clinical trials analyzed.

The relative risk of suicidal thoughts or behavior was higher in clinical trials for epilepsy than in clinical trials for psychiatric or other conditions, but the absolute risk differences were similar.

Anyone considering prescribing lacosamide or any other AED must balance this risk with the risk of untreated illness. Epilepsy and many other illnesses for which antiepileptics are prescribed are associated with morbidity and mortality and an increased risk of suicidal thoughts and behavior. If suicidal thoughts and behavior emerge during treatment, the health care provider needs to consider whether the emergence of these symptoms in any given patient may be related to the illness being treated.

Inform patients, their caregivers, and families that AEDs increase the risk of suicidal thoughts and behavior and advise them of the need to be alert for the emergence or worsening of the signs and symptoms of depression, any unusual changes in mood or behavior, or the emergence of suicidal thoughts or behavior, or thoughts about self-harm. Advise patients to report behaviors of concern immediately to a health care provider.

➤*CNS effects:* In patients with partial-onset seizures taking 1 to 3 concomitant AEDs, dizziness was experienced by 25% of patients randomized to the recommended dosages of lacosamide (200 to 400 mg/day), compared with 8% of placebo patients, and was the adverse reaction most frequently leading to discontinuation (3%). Ataxia was experienced by 6% of patients randomized to the recommended dosages of lacosamide (200 to 400 mg/day) compared with 2% of placebo patients. The onset of dizziness and ataxia was most commonly observed during titration. There was a substantial increase in these adverse reactions at dosages higher than 400 mg/day.

➤*Cardiovascular effects:*

PR interval prolongation – Dose-dependent prolongations in PR interval with lacosamide have been observed in clinical studies in patients and healthy volunteers. In clinical trials in patients with partial-onset epilepsy, asymptomatic first-degree atrioventricular (AV) block was observed as an adverse reaction in 0.4% of patients randomized to receive lacosamide and 0% of patients randomized to receive placebo. In clinical trials in patients with diabetic neuropathy, asymptomatic first-degree AV block was observed as an adverse reaction in 0.5% of patients receiving lacosamide and 0% of patients receiving placebo. When lacosamide is given with other drugs that prolong the PR interval, further PR prolongation is possible.

Use lacosamide with caution in patients with known conduction problems (eg, marked first-degree AV block, second-degree or higher AV block, sick sinus syndrome without pacemaker) or with severe cardiac disease, such as myocardial ischemia or heart failure. In such patients, obtaining an electrocardiogram before beginning lacosamide, and after lacosamide is titrated to steady state, is recommended.

Atrial fibrillation/flutter – In the short-term investigational trials of lacosamide in epilepsy patients, there were no cases of atrial fibrillation or flutter. In patients with diabetic neuropathy, 0.5% of patients treated with lacosamide experienced an adverse reaction of atrial fibrillation or atrial flutter compared with 0% of placebo-treated patients. Lacosamide administration may predispose to atrial arrhythmias (atrial fibrillation or flutter), especially in patients with diabetic neuropathy and/or cardiovascular disease. Inform patients of the symptoms of atrial fibrillation and flutter (eg, palpitations, rapid pulse, shortness of breath) and tell patients to contact their health care provider if any of these symptoms occur.

Syncope – In the short-term controlled trials of lacosamide in epilepsy patients with no significant system illnesses, there was no increase in syncope compared with placebo. In the short-term controlled trials of lacosamide in patients with diabetic neuropathy, 1.2% of patients who were treated with lacosamide reported an adverse reaction of syncope or loss of consciousness compared with 0% of placebo-treated patients with diabetic neuropathy. Most of the cases of syncope were observed in patients receiving dosages above 400 mg/day. The cause of syncope was not determined in most cases. However, several were associated with changes in orthostatic blood pressure, atrial flutter/fibrillation (and associated tachycardia), or bradycardia.

➤*Discontinuation of therapy:* As with all AEDs, gradually withdraw lacosamide over a minimum of 1 week to minimize the potential of increased seizure frequency in patients with seizure disorders.

➤*Hypersensitivity reactions:* One case of symptomatic hepatitis and nephritis was observed among 4,011 subjects exposed to lacosamide during clinical development. The event occurred in a healthy volunteer 10 days after stopping lacosamide treatment. The subject was not taking any concomitant medication, and potential known viral causes for hepatitis were ruled out. The subject fully recovered within a month without specific treatment. The case is consistent with a delayed multiorgan hypersensitivity reaction. Additional potential cases included 2 with rash and elevated liver enzymes and 1 with myocarditis and hepatitis of uncertain cause.

Multiorgan hypersensitivity reactions (also known as drug reaction with eosinophilia and systemic symptoms) have been reported with other anticonvulsants and typically, although not exclusively, present with fever and rash associated with other organ system involvement that may or may not include eosinophilia, hepatitis, nephritis, lymphadenopathy, and/or myocarditis. Because this disorder is variable in its expression, other organ system signs and symptoms not noted here may occur. If this reaction is suspected, discontinue lacosamide and start alternative treatment.

➤*Renal function impairment:* A maximum dosage of 300 mg/day is recommended for patients with severe renal impairment (CrCl 30 mL/min or less) and in patients with end-stage renal disease. Lacosamide is effectively removed from plasma by hemodialysis. Following a 4-hour hemodialysis treatment, the AUC of lacosamide is reduced by approximately 50%. Therefore, consider dosage supplementation of up to 50% following hemodialysis. In all renally impaired patients, perform dose titration with caution.

➤*Hepatic function impairment:* Closely observe patients with mild to moderate hepatic impairment during dose titration. A maximum dosage of 300 mg/day is recommended for patients with mild to moderate hepatic function impairment. The pharmacokinetics of lacosamide have not been evaluated in severe hepatic impairment. Lacosamide use is not recommended in patients with severe hepatic function impairment. Closely monitor patients with coexisting hepatic and renal function impairment during dose titration.

➤*Drug abuse and dependence:* Lacosamide is a schedule V controlled substance. In a human abuse potential study, single doses of lacosamide 200 and 800 mg produced euphoria-type subjective responses that differentiated statistically from placebo; at 800 mg, these euphoria-type responses were statistically indistinguishable from those produced by alprazolam, a schedule IV drug. The duration of the euphoria-type responses following lacosamide was less than that following alprazolam. A high rate of euphoria was also reported as an adverse reaction in the human abuse potential study following single doses of lacosamide 800 mg (15%) compared with placebo (0%) and in 2 pharmacokinetic studies following single and multiple doses of lacosamide 300 to 800 mg (ranging from 6% to 25%) compared with placebo (0%). However, the rate of euphoria reported as an adverse reaction in the lacosamide development program at therapeutic doses was less than 1%.

Abrupt termination of lacosamide in clinical trials with diabetic neuropathic pain patients produced no signs or symptoms that are associated with a withdrawal syndrome indicative of physical dependence. However, psychological dependence cannot be excluded because of the ability of lacosamide to produce euphoria-type adverse events in humans.

➤*Hazardous tasks:* Advise patients that lacosamide may cause dizziness and ataxia. Accordingly, advise them not to drive a car or operate other complex machinery until they are familiar with the effects of lacosamide on their ability to perform such activities.

➤*Pregnancy: Category C.* There are no adequate and well-controlled studies in pregnant women. Use lacosamide during pregnancy only if the potential benefit justifies the potential risk to the fetus.

Lacosamide produced developmental toxicity (increased embryofetal and perinatal mortality, growth deficit) in rats following administration during pregnancy. Developmental neurotoxicity was observed in rats following administration during a period of postnatal development corresponding to the third trimester of human pregnancy. These effects were observed at doses associated with clinically relevant plasma exposures.

Lacosamide has been shown in vitro to interfere with the activity of collapsin response mediator protein-2, a protein involved in neuronal differentiation and control of axonal outgrowth. Potential adverse effects on CNS development cannot be ruled out.

Pregnancy registry – The manufacturer has established the UCB AED Pregnancy Registry to advance scientific knowledge about safety and outcomes in pregnant women being treated with lacosamide. To ensure broad program access and reach, a health care provider or patient can initiate enrollment in the UCB AED Pregnancy Registry by calling 1-888-537-7734.

Health care providers are also advised to recommend that pregnant patients taking lacosamide enroll in the North American Antiepileptic Drug Pregnancy Registry. This can be done by calling 1-888-233-2334, and must be done by patients themselves. Information on the registry can also be found at the Web site http://www.aedpregnancyregistry.org.

➤*Lactation:* Studies in lactating rats have shown that lacosamide and/or its metabolites are excreted in milk. It is not known whether lacosamide is excreted in human milk. The molecular weight (about 250), low plasma protein binding (about 15%), and long elimination half-life (about 13 hours) suggest that the drug will be excreted into breast milk. Because many drugs are excreted into human milk, decide whether to discontinue breast-feeding or lacosamide, taking into account the importance of the drug to the mother.

➤*Children:* The safety and effectiveness of lacosamide in children younger than 17 years of age have not been established.

Lacosamide has been shown in vitro to interfere with the activity of collapsin response mediator protein-2, a protein involved in neuronal differentiation and control of axonal outgrowth. Potential adverse effects on CNS development cannot be ruled out. Administration of lacosamide to rats during the neonatal and juvenile periods of postnatal development resulted in decreased brain weights and long-term neurobehavioral changes (eg, altered open-field performance, deficits in learning and memory). The no-effect dose for developmental neurotoxicity in rats was associated with a plasma lacosamide exposure (AUC) approximately 0.5 times the human plasma AUC at the maximum recommended human dose of 400 mg/day.

➤*Elderly:* In healthy subjects, the dose and body weight–normalized pharmacokinetic parameters of AUC and C_{max} were approximately 20% higher in elderly subjects compared with younger subjects. The slightly higher lacosamide plasma concentrations in elderly subjects are possibly caused by differences in total body water (lean body weight) and age-associated decreased renal clearance. No lacosamide dose adjustment based on age is considered necessary. Exercise caution for dose titration in elderly patients.

➤*Monitoring:* Monitor patients treated with any AED for any indication of the emergence or worsening of depression, suicidal thoughts or behavior, and/or any unusual changes in mood or behavior.

Obtain an electrocardiogram before beginning therapy and after lacosamide is titrated to steady state in patients with known conduction problems or severe cardiac disease.

Closely monitor patients with coexisting hepatic and renal impairment during dose titration.

LACOSAMIDE — INJECTION

Drug Interactions

Lacosamide Drug Interactions			
Precipitant drug	Object drug[a]		Description
AEDs (eg, carbamazepine, phenobarbital, phenytoin)	Lacosamide	⬇	Small reductions (15% to 20%) in lacosamide plasma concentrations resulted with coadministration. A clinically important pharmacokinetic interaction is unlikely.
Omeprazole	Lacosamide	⬇	Plasma levels of the O-desmethyl-lacosamide metabolite were reduced approximately 60% in the presence of omeprazole. A clinically important pharmacokinetic interaction is unlikely.
Lacosamide	Contraceptives, hormonal	⬆	A 20% increase in ethinyl estradiol C_{max} has been observed. A clinically important pharmacokinetic interaction is unlikely.

[a] ⬆ = object drug increased; ⬇ = object drug decreased.

Adverse Reactions

➤*Discontinuation:* In controlled clinical trials, the rate of discontinuation as a result of an adverse reaction was 8% and 17% in patients randomized to receive lacosamide at the recommended dosages of 200 and 400 mg/day, respectively, 29% at 600 mg/day, and 5% in patients randomized to receive placebo. The adverse reactions most commonly (more than 1% in the lacosamide total group and greater than placebo) leading to discontinuation were ataxia, diplopia, dizziness, nausea, vertigo, vision blurred, and vomiting.

➤*Most common adverse reactions:* The majority of adverse reactions in the lacosamide patients were reported with a maximum intensity of mild or moderate.

Lacosamide Adverse Reactions (≥ 2%)					
Adverse reaction	Lacosamide 200 mg/day (n = 270)	Lacosamide 400 mg/day (n = 471)	Lacosamide 600 mg/day (n = 203)	Lacosamide total (n = 944)	Placebo (n = 364)
CNS					
Ataxia	4%	7%	15%	8%	2%
Balance disorder	1%	5%	6%	4%	0%
Depression	2%	2%	2%	2%	1%
Dizziness	16%	30%	53%	31%	8%
Fatigue	7%	7%	15%	9%	6%
Gait disturbance	< 1%	2%	4%	2%	< 1%
Headache	11%	14%	12%	13%	9%
Memory impairment	1%	2%	6%	2%	2%
Somnolence	5%	8%	8%	7%	5%
Tremor	4%	6%	12%	7%	4%
Dermatologic					
Pruritus	3%	2%	3%	2%	1%
Skin laceration	2%	3%	3%	3%	2%
GI					
Diarrhea	3%	5%	4%	4%	3%
Nausea	7%	11%	17%	11%	4%
Vomiting	6%	9%	16%	9%	3%
Special senses					
Diplopia	6%	10%	16%	11%	2%
Nystagmus	2%	5%	10%	5%	4%
Vertigo	5%	3%	4%	4%	1%
Vision blurred	2%	9%	16%	8%	3%
Miscellaneous					
Asthenia	2%	2%	4%	2%	1%
Contusion	3%	4%	2%	3%	3%

➤*Other adverse reactions:*

CNS – Cerebellar syndrome, cognitive disorder, confusional state, depressed mood, disturbance in attention, dysarthria, feeling drunk, hypoesthesia, irritability, mood altered, paresthesia.

GI – Constipation, dry mouth, dyspepsia, oral hypoesthesia.

Hematologic/Lymphatic – Anemia, neutropenia.

Miscellaneous – Fall, muscle spasms, palpitations, pyrexia, tinnitus.

➤*Local adverse reactions:* IV administration was associated with local adverse reactions, such as injection-site pain or discomfort (2.5%), irritation (1%), and erythema (0.5%). One case of profound bradycardia (26 beats per minute, blood pressure 100/60 mm Hg) was observed in a patient during a 15-minute infusion of lacosamide 150 mg. This patient was on a beta-blocker. The infusion was discontinued and the patient experienced a rapid recovery.

➤*Lab test abnormalities:* Abnormalities in liver function tests have been observed in controlled trials with lacosamide in adult patients with partial-onset seizures who were taking 1 to 3 concomitant AEDs. Elevations of ALT× to at least 3 the upper limit of normal (ULN) occurred in 0.7% of lacosamide patients and 0% of placebo patients. One case of hepatitis with transaminases more than 20 × ULN was observed in 1 healthy subject 10 days after lacosamide treatment completion, along with nephritis (proteinuria and urine casts). Serologic studies were negative for viral hepatitis. Transaminases returned to normal within 1 month without specific treatment. At the time of this event, bilirubin was normal. The hepatitis/nephritis was interpreted as a delayed hypersensitivity reaction to lacosamide.

➤*Postmarketing:*

Cardiovascular – Bradycardia.

Dermatologic – Rash.

Overdosage

➤*Symptoms:* There is limited clinical experience with lacosamide overdose in humans. The highest reported accidental overdose of lacosamide during clinical development was 1,200 mg/day, which was nonfatal. The types of adverse reactions experienced by patients exposed to supratherapeutic doses during the trials were not clinically different from those of patients administered recommended doses of lacosamide.

There has been a single case of intentional overdose by a patient who self-administered lacosamide 12 g along with large doses of zonisamide, topiramate, and gabapentin. The patient presented in a coma and was hospitalized. An electroencephalograph revealed epileptic waveforms. The patient recovered 2 days later.

➤*Treatment:* There is no specific antidote for overdose with lacosamide. Follow standard decontamination procedures. General supportive care of the patient is indicated, including monitoring of vital signs and observation of the clinical status of the patient. Contact a certified poison control center for up-to-date information on the management of overdose with lacosamide.

Standard hemodialysis procedures result in significant clearance of lacosamide (reduction of systemic exposure by 50% in 4 hours). Hemodialysis has not been performed in the few known cases of overdose but may be indicated based on the patient's clinical state or in patients with significant renal function impairment.

Patient Information

Counsel patients, their caregivers, and families that AEDs, including lacosamide, may increase the risk of suicidal thoughts and behavior and advise them of the need to be alert for the emergence or worsening of symptoms of depression, any unusual changes in mood or behavior, or the emergence of suicidal thoughts or behavior, or thoughts about self-harm. Advise them to report behaviors of concern immediately to a health care provider.

Counsel patients that lacosamide use may cause dizziness, double vision, abnormal coordination and balance, and somnolence. Advise patients taking lacosamide not to drive, operate complex machinery, or engage in other hazardous activities until they have become accustomed to any such effects associated with lacosamide.

Counsel patients that lacosamide is associated with electrocardiographic changes that may predispose to irregular beat and syncope, particularly in patients with underlying cardiovascular disease or heart conduction problems, or who are taking other medications that affect the heart. Advise patients who develop syncope to lie down with raised legs until recovered and contact their health care provider.

Inform patients that lacosamide may cause serious hypersensitivity reactions affecting multiple organs, such as the liver and kidney. Discontinue lacosamide if a serious hypersensitivity reaction is suspected. Instruct patients to report promptly to their health care provider any symptoms of liver toxicity (eg, fatigue, jaundice, dark urine).

The manufacturer has established the UCB AED Pregnancy Registry to advance scientific knowledge about safety and outcomes in pregnant women being treated with lacosamide. To ensure broad program access and reach, a health care provider or the patient can initiate enrollment in the UCB AED Pregnancy Registry by calling 1-888-537-7734.

Encourage patients to enroll in the North American Antiepileptic Drug Pregnancy Registry if they become pregnant. This registry is collecting information about the safety of AEDs during pregnancy. To enroll, patients can call 1-888-233-2334.

FELBAMATE

Rx	**Felbatol**[a] (Wallace Labs)	**Tablets:** 400 mg	Lactose. (Wallace 0430). Yellow, scored. Capsule shape. In 100s and UD 100s.
		600 mg	Lactose. (Wallace 0431). Peach, scored. Capsule shape. In 100s.
		Suspension : 600 mg/5 ml	Sorbitol, parabens, saccharin. In 240 and 960 ml.

[a] It has been recommended that use of this drug be discontinued if aplastic anemia or hepatic failure occurs unless, in the judgment of the physician, continued therapy is warranted. See Warning box. For further information contact Wallace Labs at 800–526–3840.

FELBAMATE — ORAL

Refer to the general discussion beginning in the Anticonvulsants introduction.

WARNING

Felbamate should not be used by patients until there has been a complete discussion of the risks and the patient, parent, or guardian has provided written informed consent.

Aplastic anemia – The use of felbamate is associated with a marked increase in the incidence of aplastic anemia. Accordingly, felbamate should only be used in patients whose epilepsy is so severe that the risk of aplastic anemia is deemed acceptable in light of the benefits conferred by its use. Ordinarily, a patient should not be placed on or continued on felbamate without consideration of appropriate expert hematologic consultation.

Among felbamate treated patients, aplastic anemia (pancytopenia in the presence of a bone marrow largely depleted of hematopoietic precursors) occurs at an incidence that may be more than a 100-fold greater than that seen in the untreated population (ie, 2 to 5 per million persons per year). The risk of death in patients with aplastic anemia generally varies as a function of its severity and etiology; current estimates of the overall case fatality rate are in the range of 20% to 30%, but rates as high as 70% have been reported in the past.

There are too few felbamate associated cases, and too little known about them to provide a reliable estimate of the syndrome's incidence or its case fatality rate or to identify the factors, if any, that might conceivably be used to predict who is at greater or lesser risk.

In managing patients on felbamate, it should be borne in mind that the clinical manifestation of aplastic anemia may not be seen until after a patient has been on felbamate for several months (eg, onset of aplastic anemia among felbamate exposed patients for whom data are available has ranged from 5 to 30 weeks). However, the injury to bone marrow stem cells that is held to be ultimately responsible for the anemia may occur weeks to months earlier. Accordingly, patients who are discontinued from felbamate remain at risk for developing anemia for a variable, and unknown, period afterwards.

It is not known whether or not the risk of developing aplastic anemia changes with duration of exposure. Consequently, it is not safe to assume that a patient who has been on felbamate without signs of hematologic abnormality for long periods of time is without risk.

It is not known whether the dose of felbamate affects the incidence of aplastic anemia.

It is not known whether or not concomitant use of antiepileptic drugs or other drugs affects the incidence of aplastic anemia.

Aplastic anemia typically develops without premonitory clinical or laboratory signs, the full blown syndrome presenting with signs of infection, bleeding, or anemia. Accordingly, routine blood testing cannot be reliably used to reduce the incidence of aplastic anemia, but, it will, in some cases, allow the detection of the hematologic changes before the syndrome declares itself clinically. Felbamate should be discontinued if any evidence of bone marrow depression occurs.

Hepatic failure – Evaluation of postmarketing experience suggests that acute liver failure is associated with the use of felbamate. The reported rate in the US has been about 6 cases of liver failure leading to death or transplant per 75,000 patient years of use. This rate is an underestimate because of under reporting, and the true rate could be considerably greater than this. For example, if the reporting rate is 10%, the true rate would be 1 case per 1250 patient years of use.

Of the cases reported, about 67% resulted in death or liver transplantation, usually within 5 weeks of the onset of signs and symptoms of liver failure. The earliest onset of severe hepatic dysfunction followed subsequently by liver failure was 3 weeks after initiation of felbamate. Although some reports described dark urine and nonspecific prodromal symptoms (eg, anorexia, malaise, and gastrointestinal symptoms), in other reports it was not clear if any prodromal symptoms preceded the onset of jaundice.

It is not known whether or not the risk of developing hepatic failure changes with duration of exposure.

It is not known whether or not the dosage of felbamate affects the incidence of hepatic failure.

It is not known whether concomitant use of other antiepileptic drugs or other drugs affect the incidence of hepatic failure.

Felbamate should not be prescribed for anyone with a history of hepatic dysfunction.

WARNING (cont.)

Treatment with felbamate should be initiated only in individuals without active liver disease and with normal baseline serum transaminases. It has not been proved that periodic serum transaminase testing will prevent serious injury but it is generally believed that early detection of drug-induced hepatic injury along with immediate withdrawal of the suspect drug enhances the likelihood for recovery. There is no information available that documents how rapidly patients can progress from normal liver function to liver failure, but other drugs known to be hepatotoxins can cause liver failure rapidly (eg, from normal enzymes to liver failure in 2 to 4 weeks). Accordingly, monitoring of serum transaminase levels (AST and ALT) is recommended at baseline and periodically thereafter. While the more frequent the monitoring the greater the chances of early detection, the precise schedule for monitoring is a matter of clinical judgement.

Felbamate should be discontinued if either serum AST or serum ALT levels become increased greater than or equal to 2 times the upper limit of normal, or if clinical signs and symptoms suggest liver failure. Patients who develop evidence of hepatocellular injury while on felbamate and are withdrawn from the drug for any reason should be presumed to be at increased risk for liver injury if felbamate is reintroduced. Accordingly, such patients should not be considered for retreatment.

Indications

➤*Seizures:* Felbamate is not indicated as a first-line antiepileptic treatment. Felbamate is recommended for use only in those patients who respond inadequately to alternative treatments and whose epilepsy is so severe that a substantial risk of aplastic anemia or liver failure is deemed acceptable in light of the benefits conferred by its use.

If these criteria are met and the patient has been fully advised of the risk and has provided written, informed consent, felbamate can be considered for either monotherapy or adjunctive therapy in the treatment of partial seizures, with and without generalization, in adults with epilepsy and as adjunctive therapy in the treatment of partial and generalized seizures associated with Lennox-Gastaut syndrome in children.

➤*Off-label uses:*

Rectal administration – [5] = Poor documentation. Limited information is available regarding the rectal use of felbamate for seizure control. In 1 case report, rectal administration of felbamate for 4 days resulted in subtherapeutic serum concentrations. This use is not recommended based on current data.

Administration and Dosage

➤*Adults:*

Seizures –

Monotherapy:

• *Initial dosage* – 1,200 mg/day in divided doses 3 or 4 times daily.

• *Dosage titration* – Titrate previously untreated patients under close clinical supervision, increasing the dosage in 600 mg increments every 2 weeks to 2,400 mg/day based on clinical response and to 3,600 mg/day thereafter, if clinically indicated.

Conversion to monotherapy:

• *Initial dosage* – 1,200 mg/day in divided doses 3 or 4 times daily.

• *Dosage adjustment* – Reduce the dosage of concomitant AEDs by one-third at initiation of felbamate. At week 2, increase the felbamate dosage to 2,400 mg/day while reducing the dosage of other AEDs up to an additional one-third of their original dosage. At week 3, increase the felbamate dosage up to 3,600 mg/day and continue to reduce the dosage of other AEDs as clinically indicated. While the conversion guidelines may result in a felbamate 3,600 mg/day dose within 3 weeks, in some patients, titration to a felbamate 3,600 mg/day dose has been achieved in as little as 3 days with appropriate adjustment of other AEDs.

Adjunctive therapy:

• *Initial dosage* – 1,200 mg/day in divided doses 3 or 4 times daily.

• *Dosage titration* – Increase the dosage by 1,200 mg/day increments at weekly intervals to 3,600 mg/day. Most side effects seen resolve as the dosage of concomitant AEDs is decreased. While the conversion guidelines may result in a felbamate 3,600 mg/day dose within 3 weeks, in some patients, titration to a 3,600 mg/day felbamate dose has been achieved in as little as 3 days with appropriate adjustment of other AEDs.

• *Concomitant therapy* – Reduce present AEDs by 20% in order to control plasma concentrations of concurrent phenytoin, valproic acid, phenobarbital, and carbamazepine and its metabolites. Further reductions of the concomitant AEDs dosage may be necessary to minimize side effects due to drug interactions.

FELBAMATE — ORAL

➤*Children:*

Seizures –

14 years of age and older: See Adults for dosing for children 14 years of age and older.

Lennox-Gastaut syndrome –

2 to 14 years of age:

• *Adjunctive therapy –*

Initial dosage: 15 mg/kg/day in divided doses 3 or 4 times daily.

Dosage titration: Increase the dosage by 15 mg/kg/day increments at weekly intervals to 45 mg/kg/day. Most side effects seen resolve as the dosage of concomitant AEDs is decreased.

Concomitant therapy: Reduce present AEDs by 20% in order to control plasma levels of concurrent phenytoin, valproic acid, phenobarbital, and carbamazepine and its metabolites. Further reductions of the concomitant AEDs dosage may be necessary to minimize side effects due to drug interactions.

Off-label dosing –

➤*Renal function impairment:* Adjunctive therapy with medications that affect felbamate plasma concentrations, especially AEDs, may warrant further reductions in felbamate daily doses in patients with renal dysfunction.

➤*Hepatic function impairment:* Contraindicated in patients with a history of hepatic dysfunction.

➤*Administration:* Take the tablet whole with full glass of water; do not crush or chew. May administer tablet with food. Shake suspension well before using.

➤*Storage/Stability:* Store at 20° to 25°C (68° to 77°F).

Actions

➤*Pharmacology:* The mechanism by which felbamate exerts its anticonvulsant activity is unknown, but in animal test systems designed to detect anticonvulsant activity, felbamate has properties in common with other marketed anticonvulsants. Felbamate is effective in mice and rats in the maximal electroshock test, the subcutaneous pentylenetetrazol seizure test, and the subcutaneous picrotoxin seizure test. Felbamate also exhibits anticonvulsant activity against seizures induced by intracerebroventricular administration of glutamate in rats and N-methyl-D,L-aspartic acid in mice. Protection against maximal electroshock-induced seizures suggests that felbamate may reduce seizure spread, an effect possibly predictive of efficacy in generalized tonic-clonic or partial seizures. Protection against pentylenetetrazol-induced seizures suggests that felbamate may increase seizure threshold, an effect considered to be predictive of potential efficacy in absence seizures.

Receptor-binding studies in vitro indicate that felbamate has weak inhibitory effects on GABA-receptor binding, benzodiazepine receptor binding, and is devoid of activity at the MK-801 receptor binding site of the NMDA receptor-ionophore complex. However, felbamate does interact as an antagonist at the strychnine-insensitive glycine recognition site of the NMDA receptor-ionophore complex. Felbamate is not effective in protecting chick embryo retina tissue against the neurotoxic effects of the excitatory amino acid agonists NMDA, kainate, or quisqualate in vitro.

The monocarbamate, p-hydroxy, and 2-hydroxy metabolites were inactive in the maximal electroshock-induced seizure test in mice. The monocarbamate and p-hydroxy metabolites had only weak (0.2 to 0.6) activity compared with felbamate in the subcutaneous pentylenetetrazol seizure test. These metabolites did not contribute significantly to the anticonvulsant action of felbamate.

➤*Pharmacokinetics:*

Absorption – Felbamate is well-absorbed after oral administration. Over 90% of the radioactivity after a dose of 1000 mg ^{14}C felbamate was found in the urine. Absolute bioavailability (oral vs parenteral) has not been measured. The tablet and suspension were each shown to be bioequivalent to the capsule used in clinical trials, and pharmacokinetic parameters of the tablet and suspension are similar. There was no effect of food on absorption of the tablet; the effect of food on absorption of the suspension has not been evaluated.

Distribution – The apparent volume of distribution was 756 ± 82 mL/kg after a 1200 mg dose. Felbamate C_{max} and AUC are proportionate to dose after single and multiple doses over a range of 100 to 800 mg single doses and 1200 to 3600 mg daily doses. C_{min} (trough) blood levels are also dose proportional. Multiple-daily doses of 1200, 2400, and 3600 mg gave C_{min} values of 30 ± 5, 55 ± 8, and 83 ± 21 mcg/mL (n = 10 patients). Linear and dose proportional pharmacokinetics were also observed at doses above 3600 mg/day up to the maximum dose studied of 6000 mg/day. Felbamate gave dose proportional steady-state peak plasma concentrations in children age 4 to 12 over a range of 15, 30, and 45 mg/kg/day with peak concentrations of 17, 32, and 49 mcg/mL.

Binding of felbamate to human plasma protein was independent of felbamate concentrations between 10 and 310 mcg/mL. Binding ranged from 22% to 25%, mostly to albumin, and was dependent on the albumin concentration.

Metabolism – Following oral administration, felbamate is the predominant plasma species (about 90% of plasma radioactivity). About 40% to 50% of absorbed dose appears unchanged in urine, and an additional 40% is present as unidentified metabolites and conjugates. About 15% is present as parahydroxyfelbamate, 2-hydroxyfelbamate, and felbamate monocarbamate, none of which have significant anticonvulsant activity.

Excretion – Felbamate is excreted with a terminal half-life of 20 to 23 hours, which is unaltered after multiple doses. Clearance after a single 1200 mg dose is 26 ± 3 mL/hr/kg, and after multiple-daily doses of 3600 mg is 30 ± 8 mL/hr/kg.

Special populations –

Renal function impairment: Felbamate's single-dose monotherapy pharmacokinetic parameters were evaluated in 12 otherwise healthy individuals with renal impairment. Reduced felbamate clearance and a longer half-life were associated with diminishing renal function.

Contraindications

Hypersensitivity to felbamate, its ingredients, or other carbamates; history of any blood dyscrasia or hepatic dysfunction.

Warnings/Precautions

➤*Aplastic anemia:* The use of felbamate is associated with a marked increase in the incidence of aplastic anemia. Accordingly, felbamate should only be used in patients whose epilepsy is so severe that the risk of aplastic anemia is deemed acceptable in light of the benefits conferred by its use. Ordinarily, a patient should not be placed on or continued on felbamate without consideration of appropriate expert hematologic consultation.

See the Warning box for more information.

➤*Discontinuation:* Antiepileptic drugs should not be suddenly discontinued because of the possibility of increasing seizure frequency.

➤*Hepatic failure:* See the Warning box for more information.

➤*Renal function impairment:* A study in otherwise healthy individuals with renal dysfunction indicated that prolonged half-life and reduced clearance of felbamate are associated with diminishing renal function. Felbamate should be used with caution in patients with renal dysfunction. Adjunctive therapy with medications that affect felbamate plasma concentrations, especially AEDs, may warrant further reductions in felbamate daily doses in patients with renal dysfunction.

➤*Hepatic function impairment:* See the Warning box for more information.

➤*Pregnancy:* Category C. The incidence of malformations was not increased compared to control in offspring of rats or rabbits given doses up to 13.9 times (rat) and 4.2 times (rabbit) the human daily dose on a mg/kg basis, or 3 times (rat) and less than 2 times (rabbit) the human daily doses on a mg/m^2 basis. However, in rats, there was a decrease in pup weight and an increase in pup deaths during lactation. The cause for these deaths is not known. The no-effect dose for rat pup mortality was 6.9 times the human dose on a mg/kg basis or 1.5 times the human dose.

Placental transfer of felbamate occurs in rat pups. There are, however, no studies in pregnant women. Because animal reproduction studies are not always predictive of human response, this drug should be used during pregnancy only if clearly needed.

➤*Lactation:* Felbamate has been detected in human milk. The effect on the nursing infant is unknown. In rats, there was a decrease in pup weight and an increase in pup deaths during lactation. The cause for these deaths is not known.

➤*Children:* The safety and efficacy of felbamate in children other than those with Lennox-Gastaut syndrome have not been established.

➤*Elderly:* No systemic studies in geriatric patients have been conducted. Clinical studies of felbamate did not include sufficient numbers of patients aged 65 years and older to determine whether they respond differently from younger patients. Other reported clinical experience has not identified differences in responses between the elderly and younger patients. In general, dosage selection for an elderly patient should be cautious, usually starting at the low end of the dosing range, reflecting the greater frequency of hepatic, renal, or cardiac function, and of concomitant disease or other drug therapy.

➤*Monitoring:* Full hematologic evaluations should be performed before felbamate therapy, frequently during therapy, and for a significant period of time after discontinuation of felbamate therapy. While it might appear prudent to perform frequent CBCs in patients continuing on felbamate, there is no evidence that such monitoring will allow early detection of marrow suppression before aplastic anemia occurs. Complete pretreatment blood counts, including platelets and reticulocytes, should be obtained as a baseline. If any hematologic abnormalities are detected during the course of treatment, immediate consultation with a hematologist is advised. Felbamate should be discontinued if any evidence of bone marrow depression occurs.

Treatment with felbamate should be initiated only in individuals without active liver disease and with normal baseline serum transaminases. It has not been proved that periodic serum transaminase testing will prevent serious injury but it is generally believed that early detection of drug-induced hepatic injury along with immediate withdrawal of the suspect drug enhances the likelihood for recovery. There is no information available that documents how rapidly patients can progress from normal liver function to liver failure, but other drugs known to be hepatotoxins can cause liver failure rapidly (eg, from normal enzymes to liver failure in 2 to 4 weeks). Accordingly, monitoring of serum transaminase levels (AST and ALT) is recommended at baseline and periodically thereafter. While the more frequent the monitoring the greater the chances of early detection, the precise schedule for monitoring is a matter of clinical judgement. If significant, confirmed liver abnormalities are detected during the course of felbamate treatment, felbamate should be discontinued immediately with continued liver function monitoring until values return to normal.

Drug Interactions

➤*QT prolongation:* An additive effect of felbamate with other drugs that prolong the QT interval cannot be excluded. The following drugs may prolong the QT interval and increase the risk of life-threatening cardiac arrhythmias, including torsade de pointes: Antiarrhythmic agents (eg, amiodarone, bretylium, disopyramide, dofetilide, procainamide, quinidine, and

FELBAMATE — ORAL

sotalol), arsenic trioxide, chlorpromazine, cisapride, dolasetron, droperidol, mefloquine, mesoridazine, moxifloxacin, pentamidine, pimozide, tacrolimus, thioridazine, and ziprasidone. For a more complete list of drugs that may prolong the QT interval, see the appendix, Drug-Induced Prolongation of the QT Interval and Torsade de Pointes.

➤*Other antiepileptic drugs:* As felbamate is added to or substituted for existing antiepileptic drugs (AEDs), it is strongly recommended to reduce the dosage of those AEDs in the range of 20% to 33% to minimize side effects. Adjunctive therapy with medications that affect felbamate plasma concentrations, especially AEDs, may warrant further reductions in felbamate daily doses in patients with renal dysfunction. The net effect of these interactions is summarized in the following table:

Effects of Felbamate Interactions with Other Antiepileptic Drugs (AEDs)

AED coadministered	AED concentration	Felbamate concentration
Phenytoin	↑	↓
Valproate	↑	↔[a]
Carbamazepine (CBZ)	↓	↓
[b]CBZ epoxide	↑	
Phenobarbital	↑	↓

[a] No significant effect.
[b] Not administered, but an active metabolite of carbamazepine.

➤*Specific effects of felbamate on other antiepileptic drugs:*

Phenytoin – Felbamate causes an increase in steady-state phenytoin plasma concentrations. In 10 otherwise healthy subjects with epilepsy ingesting phenytoin, the steady-state trough (C_{min}) phenytoin plasma concentration was 17 ± 5 mcg/mL. The steady-state C_{min} increased to 21 ± 5 mcg/mL when 1200 mg/day of felbamate was coadministered. Increasing the felbamate dose to 1800 mg/day in 6 of these subjects increased the steady-state phenytoin C_{min} to 25 ± 7 mcg/mL. In order to maintain phenytoin levels, limit adverse experiences, and achieve the felbamate dose of 3600 mg/day, a phenytoin dose reduction of approximately 40% was necessary for 8 of these 10 subjects.

In a controlled clinical trial, a 20% reduction of the phenytoin dose at the initiation of felbamate therapy resulted in phenytoin levels comparable to those prior to felbamate administration.

Carbamazepine – Felbamate causes a decrease in the steady-state carbamazepine plasma concentrations and an increase in the steady-state carbamazepine epoxide plasma concentration. In 9 otherwise healthy subjects with epilepsy ingesting carbamazepine, the steady-state trough (C_{min}) carbamazepine concentration was 8 ± 2 mcg/mL. The carbamazepine steady-state C_{min} decreased 31% to 5 ± 1 mcg/mL when felbamate (3000 mg/day, divided into 3 doses) was coadministered. Carbamazepine epoxide steady-state C_{min} concentrations increased 57% from 1 ± 0.3 to 1.6 ± 0.4 mcg/mL with the addition of felbamate.

Valproate – Felbamate causes an increase in steady-state valproate concentrations. In 4 subjects with epilepsy ingesting valproate, the steady-state trough (C_{min}) valproate plasma concentration was 63 ± 16 mcg/mL. The steady-state C_{min} increased to 78 ± 14 mcg/mL when 1200 mg/day of felbamate was coadministered. Increasing the felbamate dose to 2400 mg/day increased the steady-state valproate C_{min} to 96 ± 25 mcg/mL. Corresponding values for free valproate C_{min} concentrations were 7 ± 3, 9 ± 4, and 11 ± 6 mcg/mL for 0, 1200, and 2400 mg/day felbamate, respectively. The ratios of the AUCs of unbound valproate to the AUCs of the total valproate were 11.1%, 13%, and 11.5%, with coadministration of 0, 1200, and 2400 mg/day of felbamate, respectively. This indicates that the protein binding of valproate did not change appreciably with increasing doses of felbamate.

Phenobarbital – Coadministration of felbamate with phenobarbital causes an increase in phenobarbital plasma concentrations. In 12 otherwise healthy male volunteers ingesting phenobarbital, the steady-state trough (C_{min}) phenobarbital concentration was 14.2 mcg/mL. The steady-state C_{min} concentration increased to 17.8 mcg/mL when 2400 mg/day of felbamate was coadministered for 1 week.

➤*Effects of other antiepileptic drugs on felbamate:*

Phenytoin – Phenytoin causes an approximate doubling of the clearance of felbamate at steady state and, therefore, the addition of phenytoin causes an approximately 45% decrease in the steady-state trough concentrations of felbamate as compared to the same dose of felbamate given as monotherapy.

Carbamazepine – Carbamazepine causes an approximately 50% increase in the clearance of felbamate at steady state and, therefore, the addition of carbamazepine results in an approximately 40% decrease in the steady-state trough concentrations of felbamate as compared to the same dose of felbamate given as monotherapy.

Phenobarbital – It appears that phenobarbital may reduce plasma felbamate concentrations. Steady-state plasma felbamate concentrations were found to be 29% lower than the mean concentrations of a group of newly diagnosed subjects with epilepsy also receiving 2400 mg of felbamate a day.

➤*Oral contraceptives:* A group of 24 nonsmoking, healthy white female volunteers established on an oral contraceptive regimen containing 30 mcg ethinyl estradiol and 75 mcg gestodene for at least 3 months received 2400 mg/day of felbamate from midcycle (day 15) to midcycle (day 14) of 2 consecutive oral contraceptive cycles. Felbamate treatment resulted in a 42% decrease in the gestodene $AUC_{(0-24)}$, but no clinically relevant effect was observed on the pharmacokinetic parameters of ethinyl estradiol. No volunteer showed hormonal evidence of ovulation, but 1 volunteer reported intermenstrual bleeding during felbamate treatment.

Adverse Reactions

➤*Most common adverse reactions in adults:* The most common adverse reactions seen in association with felbamate in adults during monotherapy are anorexia, vomiting, insomnia, nausea, and headache. The most common adverse reactions seen in association with felbamate in adults during adjunctive therapy are anorexia, vomiting, insomnia, nausea, dizziness, somnolence, and headache.

➤*Most common adverse reactions seen in children:* The most common adverse reactions seen in association with felbamate in children during adjunctive therapy are anorexia, vomiting, insomnia, headache, and somnolence.

➤*Dropout rate due to adverse reactions:* The dropout rate because of adverse reactions or intercurrent illnesses among adult felbamate patients was 12% (120/977). The dropout rate because of adverse reactions or intercurrent illnesses among pediatric felbamate patients was 6% (22/357). In adults, the body systems associated with causing these withdrawals in order of frequency were the following: Digestive (4.3%), psychological (2.2%), whole body (1.7%), neurological (1.5%), and dermatological (1.5%). In children, the body systems associated with causing these withdrawals in order of frequency were the following: Digestive (1.7%), neurological (1.4%), dermatological (1.4%), psychological (1.1%), and whole body (1%). In adults, specific reactions with an incidence of greater than or equal to 1% associated with causing these withdrawals, in order of frequency were the following: Anorexia (1.6%), nausea (1.4%), rash (1.2%), and weight decrease (1.1%). In children, specific reactions with an incidence of greater than or equal to 1% associated with causing these withdrawals, in order of frequency was rash (1.1%).

➤*Incidence in clinical trials:*

Adults: Incidence in controlled clinical trials (monotherapy studies in adults) – The table that follows enumerates adverse reactions that occurred at an incidence of greater than or equal to 2% among 58 adult patients who received felbamate monotherapy at dosages of 3600 mg/day in double-blind controlled trials. Reported adverse reactions were classified using standard WHO-based dictionary terminology.

Felbamate Adverse Reactions in Adults in Controlled Clinical Trials

Adverse reaction	Felbamate[a] (n = 58) %	Low dose valproate[b] (n = 50) %
Miscellaneous		
Fatigue	6.9%	4%
Weight decrease	3.4%	0%
Face edema	3.4%	0%
CNS		
Insomnia	8.6%	4%
Headache	6.9%	18%
Anxiety	5.2%	2%
Dermatological		
Acne	3.4%	0%
Rash	3.4%	0%
GI		
Dyspepsia	8.6%	2%
Vomiting	8.6 %	2%
Constipation	6.9%	2%
Diarrhea	5.2%	0%
ALT increased	5.2%	2%
Metabolic/Nutritional		
Hypophosphatemia	3.4%	0%
Respiratory		
Upper respiratory tract infection	8.6%	4%
Rhinitis	6.9%	0%
Special senses		
Diplopia	3.4%	4%
Otitis media	3.4%	0%
GU		
Intramenstrual bleeding	3.4%	0%
Urinary tract infection	3.4%	2%

[a] 3600 mg/day.
[b] 15 mg/kg/day.

Incidence in controlled add-on clinical studies in adults – The table that follows enumerates adverse reactions that occurred at an incidence of greater than or equal to 2% among 114 adult patients who received felbamate adjunctive therapy in add-on controlled trials at dosages up to 3600 mg/day. Reported adverse reactions were classified using standard WHO-based dictionary terminology.

Many adverse reactions that occurred during adjunctive therapy may be a result of drug interactions. Adverse reactions during adjunctive therapy typically resolved with conversion to monotherapy, or with adjustment of the dosage of other antiepileptic drugs.

FELBAMATE — ORAL

Felbamate Adverse Reactions in Adults in Controlled Add-On Clinical Trials		
Adverse reaction	Felbamate (n = 114) %	Placebo (n = 43) %
Miscellaneous		
Fatigue	16.8%	7%
Fever	2.6%	4.7%
Chest pain	2.6%	0%
CNS		
Headache	36.8%	9.3%
Somnolence	19.3%	7%
Dizziness	18.4%	14%
Insomnia	17.5%	7%
Nervousness	7%	2.3%
Tremor	6.1%	2.3%
Anxiety	5.3%	4.7%
Gait abnormal	5.3%	0%
Depression	5.3%	0%
Paraesthesia	3.5%	2.3%
Ataxia	3.5%	0%
Dry mouth	2.6%	0%
Stupor	2.6%	0%
Dermatological		
Rash	3.5%	4.7%
GI		
Nausea	34.2%	2.3%
Anorexia	19.3%	2.3%
Vomiting	16.7%	4.7%
Dyspepsia	12.3%	7%
Constipation	11.4%	2.3%
Diarrhea	5.3%	2.3%
Abdominal pain	5.3%	0%
ALT increased	3.5%	0%
Musculoskeletal		
Myalgia	2.6%	0%
Respiratory		
Upper respiratory tract infection	5.3%	7%
Sinusitis	3.5%	0%
Pharyngitis	2.6%	0%
Special senses		
Diplopia	6.1%	0%
Taste perversion	6.1%	0%
Vision abnormal	5.3%	2.3%

Children: Incidence in a controlled add-on trial in children with Lennox-Gastaut syndrome – The table that follows enumerates adverse reactions that occurred more than once among 31 pediatric patients who received felbamate up to 45 mg/kg/day or a maximum of 3600 mg/day. Reported adverse reactions were classified using standard WHO-based dictionary terminology.

Felbamate Adverse Reactions in Children		
Adverse reaction	Felbamate (n = 31) %	Placebo (n = 27) %
Miscellaneous		
Fever	22.6%	11.1%
Fatigue	9.7%	3.7%
Weight decrease	6.5%	0%
Pain	6.5%	0%
CNS		
Somnolence	48.4%	11.1%
Insomnia	16.1%	14.8%
Nervousness	16.1%	18.5%
Gait abnormal	9.7%	0%
Headache	6.5%	18.5%
Thinking abnormal	6.5%	3.7%
Ataxia	6.5%	3.7%
Urinary incontinence	6.5%	7.4%
Emotional lability	6.5%	0%
Miosis	6.5%	0%

Felbamate Adverse Reactions in Children		
Adverse reaction	Felbamate (n = 31) %	Placebo (n = 27) %
Dermatological		
Rash	9.7%	7.4%
GI		
Anorexia	54.8%	14.8%
Vomiting	38.7%	14.8%
Constipation	12.9%	0%
Hiccup	9.7%	3.7%
Nausea	6.5%	0%
Dyspepsia	6.5%	3.7%
Hematologic		
Purpura	12.9%	7.4%
Leukopenia	6.5%	0%
Respiratory		
Upper respiratory tract infection	45.2%	25.9%
Pharyngitis	9.7%	3.7%
Coughing	6.5%	0%
Special senses		
Otitis media	9.7%	0%

➤*Other reactions observed in association with the administration of felbamate:* In the paragraphs that follow, the adverse clinical reactions, other than those in the preceding tables, that occurred in a total of 977 adults and 357 children exposed to felbamate and that are reasonably associated with its use are presented. They are listed in order of decreasing frequency. Because the reports cite reactions observed in open-label and uncontrolled studies, the role of felbamate in their causation cannot be reliably determined.

Reactions are classified within body system categories and enumerated in order of decreasing frequency using the following definitions: Frequent adverse reactions are defined as those occurring on 1 or more occasions in at least 1/100 patients; infrequent adverse reactions are those occurring in 1/100 to 1/1000 patients; and rare reactions are those occurring in fewer than 1/1000 patients.

Reaction frequencies are calculated as the number of patients reporting an event divided by the total number of patients (n = 1334) exposed to felbamate.

Cardiovascular – Frequent: Palpitation, tachycardia. Rare: Supraventricular tachycardia.

CNS – Frequent: Agitation, psychological disturbance, aggressive reaction. Infrequent: Hallucination, euphoria, suicide attempt, migraine.

Dermatologic – Frequent: Pruritus. Infrequent: Urticaria, bullous eruption. Rare: Buccal mucous membrane swelling, Stevens-Johnson syndrome.

GI – Frequent: AST increased. Infrequent: Esophagitis, appetite increased. Rare: GGT elevated.

Hematologic – Infrequent: Lymphadenopathy, leukopenia, leukocytosis, thrombocytopenia, granulocytopenia. Rare: Antinuclear factor test positive, qualitative platelet disorder, agranulocytosis.

Metabolic/Nutritional – Infrequent: Hypokalemia, hyponatremia, LDH increased, alkaline phosphatase increased, hypophosphatemia. Rare: Creatine phosphokinase increased.

Musculoskeletal – Infrequent: Dystonia.

Special senses – Rare: Photosensitivityallergic reaction.

Miscellaneous – Frequent: Weight increase, asthenia, malaise, influenza-like symptoms. Rare: Anaphylactoid reaction, chest pain substernal.

➤*Postmarketing:*

Cardiovascular – Atrial fibrillation, atrial arrhythmia, cardiac arrest, torsade de pointes, cardiac failure, hypotension, hypertension, flushing, thrombophlebitis, ischemic necrosis, gangrene, peripheral ischemia, bradycardia, Henoch-Schönlein purpura (vasculitis).

CNS – Delusion, paralysis, mononeuritis, cerebrovascular disorder, cerebral edema, coma, manic reaction, encephalopathy, paranoid reaction, nystagmus, choreoathetosis, extrapyramidal disorder, confusion, psychosis, status epilepticus, dyskinesia, dysarthria, respiratory depression, apathy, concentration impaired.

Dermatologic – Abnormal body odor, sweating, lichen planus, livedo reticularis, alopecia, toxic epidermal necrolysis.

GI – Hepatitis, hepatic failure, GI hemorrhage, hyperammonemia, pancreatitis, hematemesis, gastritis, rectal hemorrhage, flatulence, gingival bleeding, acquired megacolon, ileus, intestinal obstruction, enteritis, ulcerative stomatitis, glossitis, dysphagia, jaundice, gastric ulcer, gastric dilatation, gastroesophageal reflux.

GU – Menstrual disorder, acute renal failure, hepatorenal syndrome, hematuria, urinary retention, nephrosis, vaginal hemorrhage, abnormal renal function, dysuria, placental disorder.

Hematologic – Increased and decreased prothrombin time, anemia, hypochromic anemia, aplastic anemia, pancytopenia, hemolytic uremic syn-

FELBAMATE — ORAL

drome, increased mean corpuscular volume (MCV) with and without anemia, coagulation disorder, embolism-limb, disseminated intravascular coagulation, eosinophilia, hemolytic anemia, leukemia, including myelogenous leukemia, and lymphoma, including T-cell and B-cell lymphoproliferative disorders.

Metabolic/Nutritional – Hypernatremia, hypoglycemia, SIADH, hypomagnesemia, dehydration, hyperglycemia, hypocalcemia.

Musculoskeletal – Arthralgia, muscle weakness, involuntary muscle contraction, rhabdomyolysis.

Respiratory – Dyspnea, pneumonia, pneumonitis, hypoxia, epistaxis, pleural effusion, respiratory insufficiency, pulmonary hemorrhage, asthma.

Special senses – Hemianopsia, decreased hearing, conjunctivitis.

Miscellaneous – Neoplasm, sepsis, LE syndrome, SIDS, sudden death, edema, hypothermia, rigors, hyperpyrexia.

Fetal disorders: Fetal death, microcephaly, genital malformation, anencephaly, encephalocele.

Overdosage

➤*Symptoms:* Four subjects inadvertently received felbamate as adjunctive therapy in dosages ranging from 5400 to 7200 mg/day for durations between 6 and 51 days. One subject who received 5400 mg/day as monotherapy for 1 week reported no adverse reactions. Another subject attempted suicide by ingesting 12,000 mg of felbamate in a 12-hour period. The only adverse reactions reported were mild gastric distress and a resting heart rate of 100 bpm. No serious adverse reactions have been reported.

➤*Treatment:* General supportive measures should be employed if overdosage occurs. It is not known whether felbamate is dialyzable.

Patient Information

Patients should be informed that the use of felbamate is associated with aplastic anemia and hepatic failure, potentially fatal conditions acutely or over a long term.

The physician should obtain written, informed consent prior to initiation of felbamate therapy.

➤*Aplastic anemia:* Aplastic anemia in the general population is relatively rare. The absolute risk for the individual patient is not known with any degree of reliability, but patients on felbamate may be at more than a 100-fold greater risk for developing the syndrome than the general population.

The long term outlook for patients with aplastic anemia is variable. Although many patients are apparently cured, others require repeated transfusions and other treatments for relapses, and some, although surviving for years, ultimately develop serious complications that sometimes prove fatal (eg, leukemia).

At present there is no way to predict who is likely to get aplastic anemia, nor is there a documented effective means to monitor the patient so as to avoid or reduce the risk. Patients with a history of any blood dyscrasia should not receive felbamate.

Patients should be advised to be alert for signs of infection, bleeding, easy bruising, or signs of anemia (eg, fatigue, weakness, lassitude) and should be advised to report to the physician immediately if any such signs or symptoms appear.

➤*Hepatic failure:* Hepatic failure in the general population is relatively rare. The absolute risk for an individual patient is not known with any degree of reliability but patients on felbamate are at a greater risk for developing hepatic failure than the general population.

At present, there is no way to predict who is likely to develop hepatic failure; however, patients with a history of hepatic dysfunction should not be started on felbamate.

Patients should be advised to follow their physician's directives for liver function testing both before starting felbamate and at frequent intervals while taking felbamate.

Patients should be advised to be alert for signs of liver dysfunction (eg, jaundice, anorexia, gastrointestinal complaints, malaise) and to report them to their doctor immediately if they should occur.

GABAPENTIN

Rx	**Gralise**[a] (Abbott Laboratories)	**Tablets; oral:** 300 mg	(SLV 300). White, oval shaped. In 30s, 90s, 300s, and UD 10s, starter pack.[b]
Rx	**Gabapentin** (Various, eg, Greenstone, Ivax, Teva)	**Tablets; oral:** 600 mg	May contain lactose. In 100s, 500s, 1,000s, and UD 100s.
Rx	**Gralise**[a] (Abbott Laboratories)		(SLV 600). Beige, oval-shaped. In 90s, 300s, and UD 10s, starter pack.[b]
Rx	**Neurontin** (Pfizer)		Talc. (NT 16). White, elliptical, scored. Film-coated. In 100s.
Rx	**Gabapentin** (Various, eg, Greenstone, Ivax, Teva)	**Tablets; oral:** 800 mg	May contain lactose. In 100s, 500s, 1,000s, and UD 100s.
Rx	**Neurontin** (Pfizer)		Talc. (NT 26). White, elliptical, scored. Film-coated. In 100s.
Rx	**Horizant** (GlaxoSmithKline)	**Tablets, extended-release; oral:** 600 mg	As gabapentin enacarbil. (GS LFG). White to off-white (may have black/grey spots), oval. In 30s.
Rx	**Gabapentin** (Various, eg, American Health, Greenstone, Ivax)	**Capsules; oral:** 100 mg	In 100s, 500s, and UD 50s.
Rx	**Neurontin** (Pfizer)		Lactose, talc. (PD Neurontin/100 mg). White. In 100s and UD 50s.
Rx	**Gabapentin** (Various, eg, American Health, Greenstone, Ivax)	**Capsules; oral:** 300 mg	In 100s, 500s, and UD 50s.
Rx	**Neurontin** (Pfizer)		Lactose, talc. (PD Neurontin/300 mg). Yellow. In 100s and UD 50s.
Rx	**Gabapentin** (Various, eg, American Health, Greenstone, Ivax)	**Capsules; oral:** 400 mg	In 100s, 500s, and UD 50s.
Rx	**Neurontin** (Pfizer)		Lactose, talc. (PD Neurontin/400 mg). Orange. In 100s and UD 50s.
Rx	**Gabapentin** (Hi-Tech Pharmacal)	**Solution; oral:** 250 mg per 5 mL	May contain xylitol, glycerin. In 470 mL.
Rx	**Neurontin** (Pfizer)		Xylitol. Cool strawberry anise flavor. In 470 mL.

[a] This product is not being marketed yet.

[b] 30 day starter pack is a blister package containing 78 tablets: 9 × 300 mg tablets and 69 × 600 mg tablets.

GABAPENTIN — ORAL

Refer to the general discussion beginning in the Anticonvulsants introduction.

Indications

➤*Epilepsy:* As adjunctive therapy in the treatment of partial seizures with and without secondary generalization in patients older than 12 years of age with epilepsy; as adjunctive therapy in the treatment of partial seizures in children 3 to 12 years of age.

➤*Postherpetic neuralgia:* For the management of postherpetic neuralgia in adults.

➤*Off-label uses:*

Agitation in dementia – [4] = Insufficient documentation. Initial data suggest that gabapentin may be a useful alternative for the treatment of agitation or behavioral disorders in patients with dementia.

Alcohol withdrawal – [4] = Insufficient documentation. Although initial data suggest that gabapentin may be effective in moderating the symptoms of alcohol withdrawal, there is a wide variance in the dosage schedule that has been studied. It appears that an established titration schedule and dosage range are needed before this product can be recommended on a routine basis.

Bipolar disorder – [5] = Poor documentation. Data from randomized, double-blind, controlled trials suggest that gabapentin is not effective alone or as adjunctive therapy in the treatment of bipolar disorders in adult patients. Open-label studies have shown moderate to marked improvement with gabapentin, but these results have not been reproduced in double-blind trials of large populations. Because of the lack of evidence, expert consensus-based guidelines do not recommend gabapentin monotherapy for any phase of bipolar disorder and recommend it as an adjunct only as third-line or later intervention. While gabapentin is not recommended for use in bipolar disorder, it may be reserved for patients with bipolar disorder who also have panic disorder as a comorbid condition, as gabapentin has shown strongest efficacy in this population. Because of the lack of evidence, further large, controlled trials are unlikely.

Cocaine withdrawal – [4] = Insufficient documentation. Currently, limited data from isolated case reports and 1 small open-label trial suggest that gabapentin may be used for cocaine withdrawal cravings.

Diabetic neuropathy – [1] = Good documentation. In guidelines for the management of diabetic neuropathy, gabapentin is among the medications recommended as first-line therapy and supported by level A evidence.

Fibromyalgia – [4] = Insufficient documentation. Preliminary data from a controlled trial suggest that gabapentin may be useful for the treatment of fibromyalgia.

Headaches – [4] = Insufficient documentation. To date, the study of gabapentin therapy for various migraine headaches has been limited to mostly case reports, inadequate controls, and small numbers of patients. The majority of these data demonstrate a favorable effect, particularly in refractory cases, and suggest that this drug may be a useful alternative in nonresponsive patients.

GABAPENTIN — ORAL

Hiccups (singultus) – [4] = Insufficient documentation. Gabapentin may be a useful alternative in patients with intractable hiccups from various causes that have been unresponsive to other therapies.

Hot flashes (cancer related) – [2] = Fair documentation. Gabapentin used to treat cancer-related hot flashes has been observed in both controlled and noncontrolled settings. Although these reports indicate beneficial results, they have been short term (8 weeks or less).

Hot flashes (postmenopausal) – [2] = Fair documentation. Gabapentin used to treat hot flashes in postmenopausal womenhas been observed in both controlled and noncontrolled settings. Although these reports indicate beneficial results, most controlled trials have been conducted for short periods (up to 12 weeks).

Hyperhidrosis – [4] = Insufficient documentation. A single case report suggests that gabapentin may be useful as an agent to treat hyperhidrosis associated with spinal cord injury.

Idiopathic muscle cramps – [5] = Poor documentation. Evidence-based pharmacologic treatments for idiopathic muscle cramps are limited. Although quinine derivatives are likely effective for the condition, the American Academy of Neurology recommends that they be considered only in cases in which cramps are disabling, no other agents provide relief, and adverse effects can be carefully monitored. Data on gabapentin suggest that it is probably not effective. Further research is needed to establish appropriate therapy for idiopathic muscle cramps that offers an acceptable balance of efficacy and safety.

Nausea (chemotherapy induced) – [4] = Insufficient documentation. Preliminary data from a very small open trial suggest that gabapentin may produce beneficial effects in reducing nausea associated with chemotherapy.

Neuralgia/Neuropathy/Chronic pain – [2] = Fair documentation. Preliminary data suggest that gabapentin, like other anticonvulsants, may be a useful alternative in the therapy of painful neuralgias and neuropathies due to various etiologies.

Prevention of migraine (adults) – [4] = Insufficient documentation. Trials evaluating gabapentin for the prevention of migraine headaches in adults have shown favorable results. American Academy of Neurology practice guidelines consider gabapentin to be clinically efficacious based on consensus and clinical experience, despite the lack of scientific evidence of efficacy. Additional data are needed to determine the optimal dosing regimen and the patient population who would most benefit from therapy.

Prevention of migraine (children/adolescents) – [5] = Poor documentation. Gabapentin was studied for the prevention of migraine headaches in children and adolescents in 1 small trial that exists only in abstract form. This trial was limited by the small number of patients studied and its retrospective study design. Current practice guidelines do not include a review or recommendation for gabapentin.

Prevention of spinal opioid–related pruritus – [4] = Insufficient documentation. Initial data based on a small clinical trial suggest that gabapentin may be beneficial in the prevention of spinal opioid–related pruritus.

Pruritus (brachioradial) – [4] = Insufficient documentation. Initial data from isolated case reports suggest that gabapentin may be beneficial in patients with brachioradial pruritus unresponsive to previous therapy. However, these data are limited by a small population, and further study is required in larger, controlled settings.

Pruritus (cholestatic) – [5] = Poor documentation. Although gabapentin may be of benefit in hemodialysis patients with uremic pruritus, initial data based on a small clinical trial suggest that it is of no benefit in the treatment of cholestatic pruritus.

Pruritus (uremic) – [2] = Fair documentation. Initial data suggest that gabapentin may be beneficial in hemodialysis patients with uremic pruritus unresponsive to previous therapy. However, these data are limited by a small population, and further study is needed in larger, controlled settings to identify optimal dosage recommendations.

Rectal administration – [5] = Poor documentation. Based on the limited data available, this route of administration is not currently recommended.

Restless legs syndrome – [2] = Fair documentation. Evidence suggests that gabapentin may be an alternative to dopamine agonists in patients with restless legs syndrome, particularly in hemodialysis patients. In patients with renal dysfunction, accumulation and CNS or GI adverse effects may occur. Guidelines recommend the use of gabapentin as an alternative when patients with restless leg syndrome do not respond to dopamine agonists.

Tremors in multiple sclerosis – [4] = Insufficient documentation. No large, controlled trials have evaluated the efficacy of gabapentin for tremors in patients with multiple sclerosis (MS). The majority of data on this indication come from patients who have tremor but not necessarily MS. Larger, controlled trials are needed.

Other possible off-label uses – For the treatment of neuropathic pain in children.

Administration and Dosage

➤*General dosing considerations:* Dosage adjustment required for patients with renal impairment. (See Renal Function Impairment.)

Gralise is not interchangeable with other gabapentin products because of differing pharmacokinetic profiles that affect the frequency of administration.

➤*Adults:*

Epilepsy –

Usual dosage: 900 to 1,800 mg/day given in divided doses (3 times a day) using 300 or 400 mg capsules or 600 or 800 mg tablets.

Dosages of up to 2,400 mg/day have been well tolerated in long-term clinical studies. Dosages of 3,600 mg/day have also been administered to a small number of patients for a relatively short duration, and have been well tolerated.

Initial dosage: 300 mg 3 times a day.

Dosage titration: If necessary, the dose may be increased using 300 or 400 mg capsules or 600 or 800 mg tablets 3 times a day up to 1,800 mg/day.

Postherpetic neuralgia –

Usual dosage: In clinical studies, efficacy was demonstrated over a range of doses from 1,800 mg/day to 3,600 mg/day with comparable effects across the dose range. Additional benefit of using doses greater than 1,800 mg/day was not demonstrated.

Initial dosage: 300 mg on day 1 (single dose), 600 mg/day on day 2 (divided twice daily), and 900 mg/day on day 3 (divided 3 times daily).

Dosage titration: The dose can subsequently be titrated up as needed for pain relief to a daily dose of 1,800 mg (divided 3 times daily).

Gralise only: Titrate to an 1,800 mg dose taken orally once daily with the evening meal. Tablets should be swallowed whole. Do not split, crush, or chew the tablets.

If dose is reduced, discontinued, or substituted with an alternative medication, this should be done gradually over a minimum of 1 week or longer (at the discretion of the prescriber).

In adults with postherpetic neuralgia, therapy should be initiated and titrated as follows:

***Gralise* Recommended Titration Schedule**

	Day 1	Day 2	Days 3 to 6	Days 7 to 10	Days 11 to 14	Day 15
Daily dose	300 mg	600 mg	900 mg	1,200 mg	1,500 mg	1,800 mg

Off-label dosing –

Agitation in dementia: [4] = Insufficient documentation. Initial dosage of 100 to 300 mg twice a day; titrated to 100 to 400 mg 3 times a day (maximum dose, 2,400 mg daily).

Alcohol withdrawal: [4] = Insufficient documentation. Various titration schedules have been utilized. In an open trial, 15 patients received an unspecified gabapentin titration schedule (mean dosage, 953 mg/day). In a case report, dosages included 300 mg twice daily during week 1 titrated to 600 mg twice daily by week 3 with final titration to 1,200 mg twice daily after 1-month follow-up. In a case series of 6 patients, 400 mg 3 times daily was tapered to 400 mg/day by day 5. In another case series, 400 mg every 6 hours was reduced by 400 mg/day.

Cocaine withdrawal: [4] = Insufficient documentation. 800 to 1,500 mg/day in divided doses for up to 9 months. In all cases, patients were titrated to final doses.

Diabetic neuropathy: [1] = Good documentation. 900 to 3,600 mg daily (or maximum tolerable dose) in 3 divided doses. All studies used a titration schedule with dosage increases every 3 days to weekly.

Fibromyalgia: [4] = Insufficient documentation. Dose was titrated from 300 mg nightly to a maximum of 1,200 mg daily (administered 3 times a day) over a 6-week period. The maintenance dose was continued for a total of 12 weeks. Tapering occurred at the end of the study, with decreases by 300 mg daily until the drug was discontinued.

Headaches: [4] = Insufficient documentation. Initial dosages have ranged from 300 to 400 mg once daily to 300 mg 3 times daily with various titration schedules of up to 2,400 mg daily (in divided doses).

Hiccups (singultus): [4] = Insufficient documentation. Initial dosages ranged from 100 mg 3 or 4 times daily or 300 to 400 mg 3 times a day for up to 3 days, followed by 400 mg 3 times a day for 3 additional days. Gabapentin has also been used in combination with baclofen or other agents (cisapride, omeprazole) as combination therapy. Some regimens have used short-term therapy (6 days) as needed and others have used continuous therapy.

Hot flashes (cancer related): [2] = Fair documentation. Doses have ranged from 200 to 1,600 mg given as various regimens (1 to 4 times per day). Therapy duration has ranged from 4 to 8 weeks.

Hot flashes (postmenopausal): [2] = Fair documentation. Doses have ranged from 200 to 2,700 mg given as various regimens (1 to 4 times per day). Therapy duration in controlled trials has continued for up to 12 weeks.

Hyperhidrosis: [4] = Insufficient documentation. Initial dosage of 300 mg twice daily and titrated for further response to 900 mg 3 times daily and, eventually, 1,200 mg 3 times daily.

Nausea (chemotherapy induced): [4] = Insufficient documentation. Five days prior to chemotherapy, gabapentin was started at 300 mg nightly for 2 days, followed by 300 mg twice daily for 2 days, followed by 300 mg 3 times daily for 6 days. Gabapentin was stopped at day 6 postchemotherapy administration. Patients also received adjunctive premedicants (eg, ondansetron, dexamethasone, with or without lorazepam) and rescue medications if needed (eg, ondansetron, dexamethasone, prochlorperazine).

Neuralgia/Neuropathy/Chronic pain: [2] = Fair documentation. 900 to 2,400 mg (or maximum tolerable dose) in 3 divided doses. Most studies initiated dosages as low as 150 mg every night or 100 mg 3 times a day, with dosage increases every 2 days or weekly to the effective or maximum tolerable dose.

Prevention of migraine (adults): [4] = Insufficient documentation. Doses ranged from 1,200 to 2,400 mg daily.

Prevention of spinal opioid–related pruritus: [4] = Insufficient documentation. 1,200 mg administered 2 hours prior to the operation.

Pruritus (brachioradial): [4] = Insufficient documentation. 100 to 300 mg daily initially, with titration up to 1,800 mg daily (300 mg 3 to 6 times daily; 600 mg 3 times daily; or 400 mg 3 times daily). Specific titration schedules were not provided.

GABAPENTIN — ORAL

Pruritus (uremic): [2] = Fair documentation. The most common dosage has ranged from 100 to 300 mg 3 times weekly, or 400 mg twice weekly, administered at the end of hemodialysis sessions for 4 weeks. In 1 study, some patients continued therapy for a median of 8 months (range, 7 to 10 months).

Because gabapentin is eliminated primarily through the kidneys and is removed by hemodialysis, it has a significantly longer half-life in patients on hemodialysis than in those with healthy renal function. Thus, these patients need lower doses at less frequent intervals.

Restless legs syndrome: [2] = Fair documentation. Initial dosages ranged from 100 to 300 mg nightly on the first day, with various titration schedules of up to 600 to 800 mg/day. Higher dosages than these were administered as divided doses 2 or 3 times daily. Maximum dosing was 2,400 mg in most trials. Guidelines for restless leg syndrome recommend doses ranging from 300 to 2,700 mg daily.

In trials enrolling hemodialysis patients, doses were administered at the end of hemodialysis sessions as 300 mg 3 times weekly for 6 weeks or 200 mg after each hemodialysis session for 4 weeks.

Tremors in multiple sclerosis: [4] = Insufficient documentation. Oral dosages of 1,200 to 1,800 mg daily as monotherapy for tremors.

➤*Children:*

Epilepsy –

13 years of age and older: See Adults for dosing.

3 to 12 years of age:

• *Usual dosage* – Dosages of up to 50 mg/kg/day have been well tolerated in a long-term clinical study.

5 to 12 years of age: 25 to 35 mg/kg/day given in divided doses (3 times a day).

3 and 4 years of age: 40 mg/kg/day given in divided doses (3 times a day).

• *Initial dosage* – 10 to 15 mg/kg/day in 3 divided doses, and the effective dose reached by upward titration over a period of approximately 3 days.

➤*Elderly:* Because elderly patients are more likely to have decreased renal function, care should be taken in dose selection, and dose should be adjusted based on creatinine clearance (CrCl) values in these patients.

➤*Renal function impairment:*

Adults –

Gabapentin Dosage for Adults Based on Renal Function

CrCl (mL/min)	Total daily dose range (mg/day)	Dose regimen				
≥ 60	900 to 3,600	300 mg 3 times daily	400 mg 3 times daily	600 mg 3 times daily	800 mg 3 times daily	1,200 mg 3 times daily
> 30 to 59	400 to 1,400	200 mg twice daily	300 mg twice daily	400 mg twice daily	500 mg twice daily	700 mg twice daily
> 15 to 29	200 to 700	200 mg every day	300 mg every day	400 mg every day	500 mg every day	700 mg every day
15[a]	100 to 300	100 mg once daily	125 mg once daily	150 mg once daily	200 mg once daily	300 mg once daily
		Posthemodialysis supplemental dose[b]				
Hemodialysis		125 mg[b]	150 mg[b]	200 mg[b]	250 mg[b]	350 mg[b]

[a] For patients with CrCl less than 15 mL/min, reduce daily dose in proportion to CrCl (eg, patients with a CrCl of 7.5 mL/min should receive one-half the daily dose that patients with a CrCl of 15 mL/min receive).

[b] For patients on hemodialysis, the maintenance dose should be based on the estimates of CrCl as indicated in the upper portion of the table and a supplemental posthemodialysis dose administered after each 4 hours of hemodialysis as indicated in the lower portion of the table.

Gralise only: Adjust the dose in patients with reduced renal function, according to the following table. Patients with reduced renal function must initiate *Gralise* at a daily dose of 300 mg. *Gralise* should be titrated following the schedule outlined in the *Gralise* recommended titration schedule. Daily dosing in patients with reduced renal function must be individualized based on tolerability and desired clinical benefit.

***Gralise* Dosage Based on Renal Function**

CrCl (mL/min)	Once-daily dosing: *Gralise* dose (once daily with evening meal)
≥ 60	1,800 mg
30 to 60	600 to 1,800 mg
< 30	Do not administer.
Patients receiving hemodialysis	Do not administer.

Children – The use of gabapentin in patients younger than 12 years of age with compromised renal function has not been studied.

➤*Discontinuation of therapy:* If gabapentin dose is reduced, discontinued, or substituted with alternative mediation, it should be done gradually over a minimum of 1 week (a longer period may be needed at the discretion of the health care provider).

➤*Administration:* Administer orally with or without food.

The maximum time between doses in the 3-times-a-day schedule should not exceed 12 hours.

Gabapentin may be administered as the oral solution, capsule, or tablet, or using combinations of these formulations.

To administer a half-tablet, break the scored 600 or 800 mg tablet; take the unused half-tablet as the next dose. Half-tablets not used within several days of breaking the scored tablet should be discarded.

➤*Storage/Stability:* Store tablets and capsules at 25°C (77°F); excursions are permitted between 15° and 30°C (59° and 86°F). Store oral solution between 2° and 8°C (36° and 46°F).

Actions

➤*Pharmacology:* Gabapentin is structurally related to the neurotransmitter gamma-aminobutyric acid (GABA), but it does not modify $GABA_A$ or $GABA_B$ radioligand binding, it is not converted metabolically into GABA or a GABA agonist, and it is not an inhibitor of GABA uptake or degradation. Gabapentin was tested in radioligand binding assays at concentrations up to 100 mcM and did not exhibit affinity for a number of other common receptor sites, including benzodiazepine, glutamate, N-methyl-D-aspartate (NMDA), quisqualate, kainate, strychnine-insensitive or strychnine-sensitive glycine, alpha-1, alpha-2, or beta adrenergic, $cannabinoid_1$, adenosine A_1 or A_2, cholinergic muscarinic or nicotinic, dopamine D_1 or D_2, histamine H_1, serotonin S_1 or S_2, opiate mu, delta or kappa, voltage-sensitive calcium channel sites labeled with nitrendipine or diltiazem, or at voltage-sensitive sodium channel sites with batrachotoxinin A 20-alpha-benzoate. Furthermore, gabapentin did not alter the cellular uptake of dopamine, norepinephrine, or serotonin.

Animal pharmacology – The mechanism by which gabapentin exerts its analgesic action is unknown, but in animal models of analgesia, gabapentin prevents allodynia (pain-related behavior in response to a normally innocuous stimulus) and hyperalgesia (exaggerated response to painful stimuli). In particular, gabapentin prevents pain-related responses in several models of neuropathic pain in rats or mice (eg, spinal nerve ligation models, streptozocin-induced diabetes model, spinal cord injury model, acute herpes zoster infection model). Gabapentin also decreases pain-related responses after peripheral inflammation (carrageenan footpad test, late phase of formalin test). Gabapentin did not alter immediate pain-related behaviors (rat tail flick test, formalin footpad acute phase, acetic acid abdominal constriction test, footpad heat irradiation test). The relevance of these models to human pain is not known.

The mechanism by which gabapentin exerts its anticonvulsant action is unknown, but in animal test systems designed to detect anticonvulsant activity, gabapentin prevents seizures as do other marketed anticonvulsants. Gabapentin exhibits antiseizure activity in mice and rats in both the maximal electroshock and pentylenetetrazole seizure models and other preclinical models (eg, strains with genetic epilepsy). The relevance of these models to human epilepsy is not known.

In vitro studies with radiolabeled gabapentin have revealed a gabapentin binding site in areas of rat brains, including the neocortex and hippocampus. A high-affinity binding protein in animal brain tissue has been identified as an auxiliary subunit of voltage-activated calcium channels. However, functional correlates of gabapentin binding, if any, remain to be elucidated.

➤*Pharmacokinetics:* All pharmacological actions following gabapentin administration are due to the activity of the parent compound.

Absorption – Gabapentin bioavailability is not dose-proportional (ie, as dose is increased, bioavailability decreases). Bioavailability of gabapentin is approximately 60%, 47%, 34%, 33%, and 27% following 900, 1,200, 2,400, 3,600, and 4,800 mg/day given in 3 divided doses, respectively.

Effect of food: Food has only a slight effect on the rate and extent of absorption of gabapentin (14% increase in area under the curve [AUC] and maximum plasma concentration [C_{max}]).

Distribution – Less than 3% of gabapentin circulates bound to plasma protein. The apparent volume of distribution of gabapentin after 150 mg intravenous administration is 58 ± 6 L (mean ± standard deviation [SD]). In patients with epilepsy, steady-state predose (minimum plasma concentration) concentrations of gabapentin in cerebrospinal fluid were approximately 20% of the corresponding plasma concentrations.

Excretion – Gabapentin is eliminated from the systemic circulation by renal excretion as unchanged drug.

Gabapentin elimination half-life is 5 to 7 hours and is unaltered by dose or following multiple dosing. Gabapentin elimination rate constant, plasma clearance, and renal clearance are directly proportional to CrCl. Gabapentin can be removed from plasma by hemodialysis.

Special populations –

Renal function impairment: Subjects (n = 60) with renal insufficiency (mean CrCl ranging from 13 to 114 mL/min) were administered single 400 mg oral doses of gabapentin. The mean gabapentin half-life ranged from approximately 6.5 hours (patients with CrCl greater than 60 mL/min) to 52 hours (CrCl less than 30 mL/min) and gabapentin renal clearance from approximately 90 mL/min (greater than 60 mL/min group) to approximately 10 mL/min (less than 30 mL/min). Mean plasma clearance (CL/F) decreased from approximately 190 to 20 mL/min. Children with renal insufficiency have not been studied. Dosage adjustment in patients with compromised renal function is necessary.

• *Hemodialysis* – In a study in anuric subjects (n = 11), the apparent elimination half-life of gabapentin on nondialysis days was approximately 132 hours; during dialysis, the apparent half-life of gabapentin was reduced

GABAPENTIN — ORAL

to 3.8 hours. Hemodialysis thus has a significant effect on gabapentin elimination in anuric subjects. Dosage adjustment in patients undergoing hemodialysis is necessary.

Elderly: The effect of age was studied in subjects 20 to 80 years of age. Apparent oral clearance (CL/F) of gabapentin decreased as age increased, from approximately 225 mL/min in those under 30 years of age to approximately 125 mL/min in those over 70 years of age. Renal clearance (CLr) and CLr adjusted for body surface area also declined with age; however, the decline in the renal clearance of gabapentin with age can largely be explained by the decline in renal function. Reduction of gabapentin dose may be required in patients who have age-related compromised renal function.

Children: Gabapentin pharmacokinetics were determined in 48 children between the ages of 1 month and 12 years following a dose of approximately 10 mg/kg. Peak plasma concentrations were similar across the entire age group and occurred 2 to 3 hours postdose. In general, children between 1 month and less than 5 years of age achieved approximately 30% lower exposure (AUC) than that observed in those 5 years of age and older. Accordingly, oral clearance normalized per body weight was higher in the younger children. Apparent oral clearance of gabapentin was directly proportional to CrCl. Gabapentin elimination half-life averaged 4.7 hours and was similar across the age groups studied.

A population pharmacokinetic analysis was performed in 253 children between 1 month and 13 years of age. Patients received 10 to 65 mg/kg/day given 3 times daily. Apparent oral clearance (CL/F) was directly proportional to CrCl and this relationship was similar following a single dose and at steady state. Higher oral clearance values were observed in children less than 5 years of age compared with those observed in children 5 years of age and older, when normalized per body weight. The clearance was highly variable in infants less than 1 year of age. The normalized CL/F values observed in children 5 years of age and older were consistent with values observed in adults after a single dose. The oral volume of distribution normalized per body weight was constant across the age range.

Contraindications

Hypersensitivity to the drug or its ingredients.

Warnings/Precautions

➤*Suicidal behavior and ideation:* Antiepileptic drugs (AEDs), including gabapentin, increase the risk of suicidal thoughts or behavior in patients taking these drugs for any indication. Patients treated with any AED for any indication should be monitored for the emergence or worsening of depression, suicidal thoughts or behavior, and/or any unusual changes in mood or behavior.

Pooled analysis of 199 placebo-controlled clinical trials (mono- and adjunctive therapy) of 11 different AEDs showed that patients randomized to 1 of the AEDs had approximately twice the risk (adjusted relative risk 1.8; 95% confidence interval, 2.1 to 2.7) of suicidal thinking or behavior compared with patients randomized to placebo. In these trials, which had a median treatment duration of 12 weeks, the estimated incidence rate of suicidal behavior or ideation among 27,863 AED-treated patients was 0.43%, compared with 0.24% among 16,029 placebo-treated patients, representing an increase of approximately 1 case of suicidal thinking or behavior for every 530 patients treated. There were 4 suicides in drug-treated patients in the trials and none in placebo-treated patients, but the number is too small to allow any conclusion about drug effect on suicide.

The increased risk of suicidal thoughts or behavior with AEDs was observed as early as 1 week after starting drug treatment with AEDs and persisted for the duration of treatment assessed. Because most trials included in the analysis did not extend beyond 24 weeks, the risk of suicidal thought or behavior beyond 24 weeks could not be assessed.

The risk of suicidal thoughts or behavior was generally consistent among drugs in the data analyzed. The finding of increased risk with AEDs of varying mechanisms of action and across a range of indications suggests that the risk applies to all AEDs used for any indication. The risk did not vary substantially by age (5 to 100 years of age) in the clinical trials analyzed.

Suicidal Thoughts or Behavior Risk By Indication for AED

Indication	Placebo patients with events per 1,000 patients	Drug patients with events per 1,000 patients	Relative risk: Incidence of events in drug patients/ incidence in placebo patients	Risk difference: Additional drug patients with events per 1,000 patients
Epilepsy	1	3.4	3.5	2.4
Psychiatric	5.7	8.5	1.5	2.9
Other	1	1.8	1.9	0.9
Total	2.4	4.3	1.8	1.9

The relative risk of suicidal thoughts or behavior was higher in clinical trials for epilepsy than in clinical trials for psychiatric or other conditions, but the absolute risk differences were similar for the epilepsy and psychiatric indications.

Anyone considering prescribing gabapentin or any other AED must balance the risk of suicidal thoughts or behavior with the risk of untreated illness. Epilepsy and many other illnesses for which AEDs are prescribed are themselves associated with morbidity and mortality and an increased risk of suicidal thoughts and behavior. Should suicidal thoughts and behavior emerge during treatment, the health care provider needs to consider whether the emergence of these symptoms in any given patient may be related to the illness being treated.

Inform patients, their caregivers, and families that AEDs increase the risk of suicidal thoughts and behavior and advise them to be alert for the emergence or worsening of the signs and symptoms of depression, any unusual changes in mood or behavior, or the emergence of suicidal thoughts, behavior, or thoughts about self-harm. Behaviors of concern should be reported immediately to healthcare providers.

➤*Neuropsychiatric effects:* Gabapentin use in children with epilepsy 3 to 12 years of age is associated with the occurrence of CNS-related adverse reactions. The most significant of these can be classified into the following categories: emotional lability (primarily behavioral problems); hostility, including aggressive behaviors; thought disorder, including concentration problems and change in school performance; hyperkinesia (primarily restlessness and hyperactivity). Among the gabapentin-treated patients, most of the reactions were mild to moderate in intensity.

In controlled trials in children 3 to 12 years of age, the incidence of these adverse reactions was: emotional lability 6% (gabapentin-treated patients) vs 1.3% (placebo-treated patients); hostility 5.2% vs 1.3%; hyperkinesia 4.7% vs 2.9%; and thought disorder 1.7% vs 0%. One of these reactions, a report of hostility, was considered serious. Discontinuation of gabapentin treatment occurred in 1.3% of patients reporting emotional lability and hyperkinesia and 0.9% of gabapentin-treated patients reporting hostility and thought disorder. One placebo-treated patient (0.4%) withdrew due to emotional lability.

➤*Withdrawal precipitated seizure:* AEDs should not be abruptly discontinued because of the possibility of increasing seizure frequency.

In the placebo-controlled studies in patients greater than 12 years of age, the incidence of status epilepticus in patients receiving gabapentin was 0.6% vs 0.5% in patients receiving placebo. Among the 2,074 patients greater than 12 years of age treated with gabapentin across all studies (controlled and uncontrolled) 1.5% had status epilepticus. Of these, 14 patients had no history of status epilepticus either before treatment or while on other medications. Because adequate historical data are not available, it is impossible to say whether or not treatment with gabapentin is associated with a higher or lower rate of status epilepticus than would be expected to occur in a similar population not treated with gabapentin.

➤*Tumorigenic potential:* In standard preclinical in vivo lifetime carcinogenicity studies, an unexpectedly high incidence of pancreatic acinar adenocarcinomas was identified in male, but not female, rats. The clinical significance of this finding is unknown. Clinical experience during gabapentin's premarketing development provides no direct means to assess its potential for inducing tumors in humans.

In clinical studies in adjunctive therapy in epilepsy comprising 2,085 patient-years of exposure in patients greater than 12 years of age, new tumors were reported in 10 patients (2 breast, 3 brain, 2 lung, 1 adrenal, 1 non-Hodgkin lymphoma, 1 endometrial carcinoma in situ), and preexisting tumors worsened in 11 patients (9 brain, 1 breast, 1 prostate) during or up to 2 years following discontinuation of gabapentin. Without knowledge of the background incidence and recurrence in a similar population not treated with gabapentin, it is impossible to know whether the incidence seen in this cohort is or is not affected by treatment.

➤*Sudden and unexplained deaths:* During the course of premarketing development of gabapentin, 8 sudden and unexplained deaths were recorded among a cohort of 2,203 patients treated (2,103 patient-years of exposure).

Some of these could represent seizure-related deaths in which the seizure was not observed (eg, at night). This represents an incidence of 0.0038 deaths per patient-year. Although this rate exceeds that expected in a healthy population matched for age and sex, it is within the range of estimates for the incidence of sudden unexplained deaths in patients with epilepsy not receiving gabapentin (ranging from 0.0005 for the general population of epileptics to 0.003 for a clinical trial population similar to that in the gabapentin program, to 0.005 for patients with refractory epilepsy). Consequently, whether these figures are reassuring or raise further concern depends on comparability of the populations reported on with the gabapentin cohort and the accuracy of the estimates provided.

➤*Renal function impairment:* See Administration and Dosage and/or Actions for more information.

➤*Hazardous tasks:* Patients should be advised that gabapentin may cause dizziness, somnolence and other symptoms and signs of CNS depression. Accordingly, they should be advised neither to drive a car nor to operate other complex machinery until they have gained sufficient experience on gabapentin to gauge whether or not it affects their mental and/or motor performance adversely.

➤*Pregnancy: Category C.* It is not known whether gabapentin crosses the human placenta to the fetus. Because of its lack of protein binding and low molecular weight (approximately 171), exposure of the embryo and fetus should be expected. There are no adequate and well-controlled studies in pregnant women. This drug should be used during pregnancy only if the potential benefit justifies the potential risk to the fetus.

Gabapentin has been shown to be fetotoxic in rodents, causing delayed ossification of several bones in the skull, vertebrae, forelimbs, and hindlimbs. These effects occurred when pregnant mice received oral doses of 1,000 or 3,000 mg/kg/day during the period of organogenesis, or approximately equal to 1 to 4 times the maximum dose of 3,600 mg/day given to epileptic patients on a mg/m^2 basis. The no-effect level was 500 mg/kg/day or approximately half of the human dose on a mg/m^2 basis.

When rats were dosed prior to and during mating, and throughout gestation, pups from all dosage groups (500, 1,000, and 2,000 mg/kg/day) were affected. These doses are equivalent to less than approximately 1 to 5 times the maximum human dose on a mg/m^2 basis. There was an increased inci-

GABAPENTIN — ORAL

dence of hydroureter and/or hydronephrosis in rats in a study of fertility and general reproductive performance at 2,000 mg/kg/day with no effect at 1,000 mg/kg/day, in a teratology study at 1,500 mg/kg/day with no effect at 300 mg/kg/day, and in a perinatal and postnatal study at all doses studied (500, 1,000, and 2,000 mg/kg/day). The doses at which the effects occurred are approximately 1 to 5 times the maximum human dose of 3,600 mg/day on a mg/m^2 basis; the no-effect doses were approximately 3 times (Fertility and General Reproductive Performance study) and approximately equal to (Teratogenicity study) the maximum human dose on a mg/m^2 basis. Other than hydroureter and hydronephrosis, the etiologies of which are unclear, the incidence of malformations was not increased compared with controls in offspring of mice, rats, or rabbits given doses up to 50 times (mice), 30 times (rats), and 25 times (rabbits) the human daily dose on a mg/kg basis, or 4 times (mice), 5 times (rats), or 8 times (rabbits) the human daily dose on a mg/m^2 basis.

In a teratology study in rabbits, an increased incidence of postimplantation fetal loss occurred in dams exposed to 60, 300, and 1,500 mg/kg/day, or less than approximately one-fourth to 8 times the maximum human dose on a mg/m^2 basis.

Pregnancy registry – To provide information regarding the effects of in utero exposure to gabapentin, physicians are advised to recommend that pregnant patients taking gabapentin enroll in the North American Antiepileptic Drug (NAAED) Pregnancy Registry if they become pregnant. This can be done by calling the toll-free number 1-888-233-2334, and must be done by patients themselves. Information on the registry can also be found at the Web site http://www.aedpregnancyregistry.org.

➤*Lactation:* Gabapentin is secreted into human milk following oral administration. A nursed infant could be exposed to a maximum dose of approximately 1 mg/kg/day of gabapentin. Because the effect on the nursing infant is unknown, gabapentin should be used in women who are nursing only if the benefits clearly outweigh the risks. Monitor the infant for drowsiness, adequate weight gain, and developmental milestones, especially in younger, exclusively breastfed infants and when using combinations of anticonvulsant or psychotropic drugs.

➤*Children:* Safety and effectiveness of gabapentin in the management of postherpetic neuralgia in children have not been established. Effectiveness as adjunctive therapy in the treatment of partial seizures in children younger than 3 years of age has not been established.

➤*Elderly:* Clinical studies of gabapentin in epilepsy did not include sufficient numbers of subjects aged 65 and over to determine whether they responded differently from younger subjects. Other reported clinical experience has not identified differences in responses between the elderly and younger patients. In general, dose selection for an elderly patient should be cautious, usually starting at the low end of the dosing range, reflecting the greater frequency of decreased hepatic, renal, or cardiac function, and of concomitant disease or other drug therapy.

This drug is known to be substantially excreted by the kidney, and the risk of toxic reactions to this drug may be greater in patients with impaired renal function. Because elderly patients are more likely to have decreased renal function, care should be taken in dose selection, and dose should be adjusted based on CrCl values in these patients.

➤*Monitoring:* Patients treated with any AED for any indication should be monitored for the emergence or worsening of depression, suicidal thoughts or behavior, and/or any unusual changes in mood or behavior.

Drug Interactions

Gabapentin Drug Interactions

Precipitant drug	Object drug[a]		Description
Antacids	Gabapentin	⬇	Antacids reduced the bioavailability of gabapentin by approximately 20%. This decrease in bioavailability was approximately 5% when gabapentin was given 2 hours after the antacid. Take gabapentin at least 2 hours following antacid administration.
Cimetidine	Gabapentin	⬆	The mean apparent oral clearance of gabapentin fell by 14% and CrCl fell by 10% with concurrent cimetidine. Thus, cimetidine seemed to alter the renal excretion of gabapentin and creatinine. This is not expected to be of clinical importance.
Hydrocodone	Gabapentin	⬆	Coadministration increases gabapentin AUC values by 14% and decreases hydrocodone C_{max} and AUC values in a dose-dependent manner. The mechanism for this interaction and the magnitude of interaction at other doses is unknown. Observe the clinical response of the patients when starting, stopping or changing the gabapentin dose. If an interaction is suspected, adjust the hydrocodone dose as needed.
Gabapentin	Hydrocodone	⬇	
Morphine	Gabapentin	⬆	Coadministration of controlled-release morphine 60 mg 2 hours prior to administration of gabapentin 600 mg resulted in an increase in gabapentin AUC by 44%. The magnitude of interaction at other doses is unknown. Observe the clinical response of the patients when starting, stopping or changing the gabapentin dose. If an interaction is suspected, adjust the gabapentin dose as needed.
Naproxen	Gabapentin	⬆	Coadministration (n = 18) of naproxen sodium capsules (250 mg) with gabapentin (125 mg) appears to increase the amount of gabapentin absorbed by 12% to 15%. The magnitude of interaction within the recommended dose ranges of either drug is not known. Observe the clinical response of the patients when starting, stopping or changing the dose of either drug. If an interaction is suspected, adjust the gabapentin dose as needed.
Gabapentin	Contraceptives, hormonal	⬆	The C_{max} of norethindrone was 13% higher when coadministered with gabapentin; this interaction is not expected to be clinically important.

[a] ⬆ = object drug increased; ⬇ = object drug decreased.

➤*Drug/Lab test interactions:* Because false positive readings were reported with the *Ames N-Multistix SG* dipstick test for urinary protein when gabapentin was added to other antiepileptic drugs, the more specific sulfosalicylic acid precipitation procedure is recommended to determine the presence of urine protein.

Adverse Reactions

➤*Postherpetic neuralgia:*

Common adverse reactions – The most commonly observed adverse reactions associated with the use of gabapentin in adults not seen at an equivalent frequency among placebo-treated patients were dizziness, somnolence, and peripheral edema.

Discontinuation – In the 2 controlled studies in postherpetic neuralgia, 16% of the 336 patients who received gabapentin and 9% of the 227 patients who received placebo discontinued treatment because of an adverse reaction. The adverse reactions that most frequently led to withdrawal in gabapentin-treated patients were dizziness, somnolence, and nausea.

Adverse reactions (at least 1%):

Gabapentin Adverse Reactions in Postherpetic Neuralgia Patients (≥ 1%)

Adverse reactions	Gabapentin (n = 336)	Placebo (n = 227)
CNS		
Abnormal gait	1.5%	0%
Abnormal thinking	2.7%	0%
Amnesia	1.2%	0.9%
Ataxia	3.3%	0%
Dizziness	28%	7.5%
Headache	3.3%	3.1%
Hypesthesia	1.2%	0.9%
Incoordination	1.5%	0%
Somnolence	21.4%	5.3%
GI		
Abdominal pain	2.7%	2.6%
Constipation	3.9%	1.8%
Diarrhea	5.7%	3.1%
Dry mouth	4.8%	1.3%
Flatulence	2.1%	1.8%
Nausea	3.9%	3.1%
Vomiting	3.3%	1.8%
Metabolic/Nutritional		
Hyperglycemia	1.2%	0.4%
Peripheral edema	8.3%	2.2%
Weight gain	1.8%	0%

GABAPENTIN — ORAL

Gabapentin Adverse Reactions in Postherpetic Neuralgia Patients (≥ 1%)		
Adverse reactions	Gabapentin (n = 336)	Placebo (n = 227)
Special senses		
Amblyopia[a]	2.7%	0.9%
Conjunctivitis	1.2%	0%
Diplopia	1.2%	0%
Otitis media	1.2%	0%
Miscellaneous		
Accidental injury	3.3%	1.3%
Asthenia	5.7%	4.8%
Infection	5.1%	3.5%
Pharyngitis	1.2%	0.4%
Rash	1.2%	0.9%

[a] Reported as blurred vision.

Other reactions in more than 1% of patients, but equally or more frequent in the placebo group included pain, tremor, neuralgia, back pain, dyspepsia, dyspnea, and flu syndrome.

Other adverse reactions –

Cardiovascular: Cardiovascular disorder, cerebrovascular accident, congestive heart failure, hypertension, hypotension, migraine, myocardial infarction, palpitation, peripheral vascular disorder, syncope, vasodilatation (0.1 to 1%); angina pectoris, heart failure, increased capillary fragility, phlebitis, thrombophlebitis, varicose vein (less than 0.1%).

CNS: Confusion, depression (at least 1%); abnormal dreams, anxiety, circumoral paresthesia, depersonalization, dysarthria, emotional lability, euphoria, insomnia, hyperesthesia, hypokinesia, libido decreased, nervousness, neuropathy, nystagmus, paresthesia, reflexes decreased, speech disorder, stupor, vertigo (0.1 to 1%); agitation, hypertonia, libido increased, movement disorder, myoclonus, vestibular disorder (less than 0.1%).

Dermatologic: Dry skin, fungal dermatitis, furunculosis, herpes simplex, herpes zoster, pruritus, psoriasis, skin disorder, skin ulcer, sweating, urticaria, vesiculobullous rash (0.1 to 1%); acne, hair disorder, maculopapular rash, nail disorder, skin carcinoma, skin discoloration, skin hypertrophy (less than 0.1%).

Endocrine: Diabetes mellitus (0.1 to 1%).

GI: Abnormal stools, anorexia, gastritis, gastroenteritis, GI disorder, increased appetite, liver function tests abnormal, oral moniliasis, periodontal abscess, thirst, tongue disorder, tooth disorder (0.1 to 1%); cholecystitis, cholelithiasis, duodenal ulcer, fecal incontinence, gamma glutamyl transpeptidase increased, gingivitis, intestinal obstruction, intestinal ulcer, melena, mouth ulceration, rectal disorder, rectal hemorrhage, stomatitis (less than 0.1%).

GU: Breast pain, dysuria, impotence, menstrual disorder, polyuria, urinary incontinence, urinary retention, urinary tract infection, vaginal moniliasis (0.1 to 1%); abnormal ejaculation, cystitis, gynecomastia, nocturia, pyelonephritis, swollen penis, swollen scrotum, urinary frequency, urinary urgency, urine abnormality (less than 0.1%).

Hematologic/Lymphatic: Anemia, ecchymosis (0.1 to 1%); lymphadenopathy, lymphoma-like reaction, prothrombin decreased (less than 0.1%).

Metabolic/Nutritional: Edema, gout, hypoglycemia, weight loss (0.1 to 1%); alkaline phosphatase increased, diabetic ketoacidosis, lactic dehydrogenase increased (less than 0.1%).

Musculoskeletal: Arthralgia, arthritis, arthrosis, leg cramps, myalgia, myasthenia (0.1 to 1%); joint disorder, shin bone pain, tendon disorder (less than 0.1%).

Respiratory: Asthma, bronchitis, cough increased, epistaxis, lung disorder, pneumonia, rhinitis, sinusitis (0.1 to 1%); hemoptysis, voice alteration (less than 0.1%).

Special senses: Abnormal vision, deafness, ear pain, eye disorder, taste perversion (0.1 to 1%); conjunctival hyperemia, diabetic retinopathy, eye pain, fundi with microhemorrhage, retinal vein thrombosis, taste loss (less than 0.1%).

Miscellaneous: Abscess, allergic reaction, cellulitis, chest pain, chills, chills and fever, face edema, malaise, mucous membrane disorder, neck pain (0.1 to 1%); abnormal serum urea nitrogen value, body odor, cyst, fever, hernia, lump in neck, pelvic pain, sepsis, viral infection (less than 0.1%).

➤*Epilepsy:*

Common adverse reactions – The most commonly observed adverse reactions associated with the use of gabapentin in combination with other AEDs in patients greater than 12 years of age, not seen at an equivalent frequency among placebo-treated patients, were somnolence, dizziness, ataxia, fatigue, and nystagmus. The most commonly observed adverse reactions reported with the use of gabapentin in combination with other AEDs in children 3 to 12 years of age, not seen at an equal frequency among placebo-treated patients, were viral infection, fever, nausea and/or vomiting, somnolence, and hostility.

Discontinuation – Approximately 7% of the 2,074 patients older than 12 years of age and approximately 7% of the 449 children 3 to 12 years of age who received gabapentin in premarketing clinical trials discontinued treatment because of an adverse reaction. The adverse reactions most commonly associated with withdrawal in patients older than 12 years of age were somnolence (1.2%), ataxia (0.8%), fatigue (0.6%), nausea and/or vomiting (0.6%), and dizziness (0.6%). The adverse reactions most commonly associated with withdrawal in children were emotional lability (1.6%), hostility (1.3%), and hyperkinesia (1.1%).

Adults and children 12 years of age and older –

Gabapentin Adverse Reactions in Add-On Epilepsy Trials in Patients Older than 12 Years of Age (≥ 1%)		
Adverse reaction	Gabapentin[a] (n = 543)	Placebo[a] (n = 378)
CNS		
Abnormal coordination	1.1%	0.3%
Abnormal thinking	1.7%	1.3%
Amnesia	2.2%	0%
Ataxia	12.5%	5.6%
Depression	1.8%	1.1%
Dizziness	17.1%	6.9%
Dysarthria	2.4%	0.5%
Fatigue	11%	5%
Nervousness	2.4%	1.9%
Nystagmus	8.3%	4%
Somnolence	19.3%	8.7%
Tremor	6.8%	3.2%
Twitching	1.3%	0.5%
Dermatologic		
Abrasion	1.3%	0%
Pruritus	1.3%	0.5%
GI		
Constipation	1.5%	0.8%
Dental abnormalities	1.5%	0.3%
Dyspepsia	2.2%	0.5%
Increased appetite	1.1%	0.8%
Mouth or throat dry	1.7%	0.5%
Musculoskeletal		
Back pain	1.8%	0.5%
Fracture	1.1%	0.8%
Myalgia	2%	1.9%
Respiratory		
Coughing	1.8%	1.3%
Pharyngitis	2.8%	1.6%
Rhinitis	4.1%	3.7%
Special senses		
Amblyopia[b]	4.2%	1.1%
Diplopia	5.9%	1.9%
Miscellaneous		
Impotence	1.5%	1.1%
Leukopenia	1.1%	0.5%
Peripheral edema	1.7%	0.5%
Vasodilatation	1.1%	0.3%
WBC[c] count decreased	1.1%	0.5%
Weight increase	2.9%	1.6%

[a] Plus background AED therapy.
[b] Amblyopia was often described as blurred vision.
[c] WBC = white blood cell.

Other adverse reactions: Other reactions in greater than 1% of patients older than 12 years of age but equally or more frequent in the placebo group included the following: headache, viral infection, fever, nausea and/or vomiting, abdominal pain, diarrhea, convulsions, confusion, insomnia, emotional lability, rash, and acne.

Among the treatment-emergent adverse events occurring at an incidence of at least 10% of gabapentin-treated patients, somnolence and ataxia appeared to exhibit a positive dose-response relationship.

Children 3 to 12 years of age –

Gabapentin Adverse Reactions in Add-On Epilepsy Trials in Children 3 to 12 Years of Age (≥2%)		
Adverse reaction	Gabapentin[a] (n = 119)	Placebo[a] (n = 128)
CNS		
Dizziness	2.5%	1.6%
Emotional lability	4.2%	1.6%
Fatigue	3.4%	1.6%
Hostility	7.6%	2.3%
Hyperkinesia	2.5%	0.8%
Somnolence	8.4%	4.7%

GABAPENTIN — ORAL

Gabapentin Adverse Reactions in Add-On Epilepsy Trials in Children 3 to 12 Years of Age (≥2%)		
Adverse reaction	Gabapentin[a] (n = 119)	Placebo[a] (n = 128)
Respiratory		
Bronchitis	3.4%	0.8%
Respiratory tract infection	2.5%	0.8%
Miscellaneous		
Fever	10.1%	3.1%
Nausea/Vomiting	8.4%	7%
Viral infection	10.9%	3.1%
Weight increase	3.4%	0.8%

[a] Plus background AED therapy.

Other adverse reactions: Other reactions in more than 2% of children 3 to 12 years of age but equally or more frequent in the placebo group included the following: pharyngitis, upper respiratory tract infection, headache, rhinitis, convulsions, diarrhea, anorexia, coughing, and otitis media. Adverse reactions during epilepsy clinical trials in 449 children 3 to 12 years of age treated with gabapentin that were not reported in adjunctive trials in adults are: aura disappeared, coagulation defect, dehydration, hepatitis, hoarseness, infectious mononucleosis, occipital neuralgia, pseudocroup, and sleep walking.

Additional adverse reactions in epilepsy trials –

Cardiovascular: Hypertension (at least 1%); angina pectoris, hypotension, migraine, murmur, palpitation, peripheral vascular disorder, tachycardia (0.1 to 1%); atrial fibrillation, bradycardia, cerebrovascular accident, deep thrombophlebitis, heart block, heart failure, hypercholesterolemia, hyperlipidemia, myocardial infarction, pericardial effusion, pericardial rub, pericarditis, premature atrial contraction, pulmonary embolus, pulmonary thrombosis, thrombophlebitis, ventricular extrasystoles (less than 0.1%).

CNS: Anxiety, decreased or absent reflexes, hostility, hyperkinesia, increased reflexes, paresthesia, vertigo (at least 1%); agitation, apathy, aphasia, cerebellar dysfunction, CNS tumors, decreased position sense, decrease or loss of libido, depersonalization, doped-up sensation, dreaming abnormal, dysesthesia, dystonia, euphoria, facial paralysis, feeling high, hallucination, hemiplegia, hypesthesia, hypotonia, intracranial hemorrhage, paresis, positive Babinski sign, paranoia, psychosis, subdural hematoma, stupor, syncope (0.1 to 1%); antisocial reaction, apraxia, choreoathetosis, encephalopathy, fine motor control disorder, hyperesthesia, hypokinesia, hysteria, increased libido, local myoclonus, mania, meningismus, nerve palsy, neurosis, orofacial dyskinesia, personality disorder, subdued temperament (less than 0.1%).

Dermatologic: Alopecia, cyst, dry skin, eczema, herpes simplex, hirsutism, increased sweating, seborrhea, urticaria (0.1 to 1%); desquamation, herpes zoster, leg ulcer, local swelling, maceration, melanosis, photosensitivity reaction, psoriasis, scalp seborrhea, skin discolor, skin nodules, skin papules, subcutaneous nodule, skin necrosis (less than 0.1%).

Endocrine: Cushingoid appearance, epididymitis, goiter, hyperthyroid, hypoestrogen, hypothyroid, ovarian failure, swollen testicle (less than 0.1%).

GI: Anorexia, flatulence, gingivitis (at least 1%); glossitis, gum hemorrhage, thirst, stomatitis, increased salivation, gastroenteritis, hemorrhoids, bloody stools, fecal incontinence, hepatomegaly (0.1 to 1%); dysphagia, eructation, pancreatitis, peptic ulcer, colitis, blisters in mouth, tooth discolor, perleche, salivary gland enlarged, lip hemorrhage, esophagitis, hiatal hernia, hematemesis, proctitis, irritable bowel syndrome, rectal hemorrhage, esophageal spasm (less than 0.1%).

GU: Amenorrhea, breast cancer, cystitis, dysmenorrhea, dysuria, ejaculation abnormal, hematuria, inability to climax, menorrhagia, urination frequency, urinary incontinence, urinary retention, vaginal hemorrhage (0.1 to 1%); acute renal failure, anuria, breast pain, glycosuria, kidney pain, leukorrhea, nephrosis, nocturia, pyuria, pruritus genital, renal stone, testicle pain, urination urgency, vaginal pain (less than 0.1%).

Hematologic/Lymphatic: Purpura most often described as bruises resulting from physical trauma (at least 1%); anemia, lymphadenopathy, thrombocytopenia (0.1 to 1%); bleeding time increased, lymphocytosis, non-Hodgkin lymphoma, WBC count increased (less than 0.1%).

Musculoskeletal: Arthralgia (at least 1%); arthritis, joint stiffness, joint swelling, positive Romberg test, tendinitis (0.1 to 1%); bursitis, contracture, costochondritis, osteoporosis (less than 0.1%).

Respiratory: Pneumonia (at least 1%); epistaxis, dyspnea, apnea (0.1 to 1%); aspiration pneumonia, bronchospasm, hiccup, hyperventilation, hypoventilation, laryngitis, lung edema, mucositis, nasal obstruction, snoring (less than 0.1%).

Special senses: Abnormal vision (at least 1%); bilateral or unilateral ptosis, cataract, conjunctivitis, earache, ear fullness, eyes dry, eye hemorrhage, eye pain, eye twitching, hearing loss, hordeolum, inner ear infection, photophobia, otitis, taste loss, tinnitus, unusual taste, visual field defect (0.1 to 1%); abnormal accommodation, blindness, chorioretinitis, corneal disorders, degenerative eye changes, eustachian tube dysfunction, eye focusing problem, eye itching, glaucoma, iritis, labyrinthitis, lacrimal dysfunction, miosis, perforated ear drum, retinal degeneration, retinopathy, sensitivity to noise, strabismus, otitis externa, odd smell, watery eyes (less than 0.1%).

Miscellaneous: Asthenia, face edema, malaise (at least 1%); allergy, chill, generalized edema, weight decrease (0.1 to 1%); alcohol intolerance, hangover effect, lassitude, strange feelings (less than 0.1%).

➤*Postmarketing:*

Dermatologic – Erythema multiforme, Stevens-Johnson syndrome.

Hepatic – Elevated liver function tests, jaundice.

Miscellaneous – Angioedema, blood glucose fluctuation, breast hypertrophy, fever, hyponatremia, movement disorder.

Adverse reactions following the abrupt discontinuation of gabapentin have also been reported. The most frequently reported reactions were anxiety, insomnia, nausea, pain, and sweating.

Overdosage

➤*Symptoms:* Acute oral overdoses of gabapentin of up to 49 g have been reported. In these cases, double vision, slurred speech, drowsiness, lethargy, and diarrhea were observed. All patients recovered with supportive care.

➤*Treatment:* Gabapentin can be removed by hemodialysis. Although hemodialysis has not been performed in the few overdose cases reported, it may be indicated by the patient's clinical state or in patients with significant renal impairment.

Patient Information

Instruct patients to take gabapentin only as prescribed.

Counsel patients, their caregivers, and families that AEDs, including gabapentin, may increase the risk of suicidal thoughts and behavior, and advise them of the need to be alert for the emergence or worsening of symptoms of depression, any unusual changes in mood or behavior, or the emergence of suicidal thoughts, behavior, or thoughts about self-harm. Behaviors of concern should be reported immediately to health care providers.

Advise patients that gabapentin may cause dizziness, somnolence and other symptoms and signs of CNS depression. Accordingly, advise them not to drive a car or operate other complex machinery until they have gained sufficient experience on gabapentin to gauge whether or not it affects their mental and/or motor performance adversely.

Patients who require concomitant treatment with morphine may experience increases in gabapentin concentrations. Observe patients carefully for signs of CNS depression, such as somnolence, and reduce the dose of gabapentin or morphine appropriately.

Encourage patients to enroll in the North American Antiepileptic Drug (NAAED) Pregnancy Registry if they become pregnant. This registry is collecting information about the safety of AEDs during pregnancy. To enroll, patients can call the toll-free number 1-888-233-2334.

GABAPENTIN ENACARBIL — ORAL

Refer to the general discussion beginning in the Anticonvulsants introduction.

Indications

➤*Restless legs syndrome:* For the treatment of moderate-to-severe primary restless legs syndrome (RLS) in adults.

Gabapentin is not recommended for patients who are required to sleep during the daytime and remain awake at night.

Administration and Dosage

➤*Adults:*

Restless legs syndrome –

Usual dosage: 600 mg once daily taken with food at approximately 5 PM.

Missed dose: If the dose is not taken at the recommended time, the next dose should be taken the following day as prescribed.

➤*Elderly:* Because elderly patients are more likely to have decreased renal function, the frequency of dosing may need to be adjusted based on calculated creatinine clearance in these patients.

➤*Renal function impairment:* In patients with compromised renal function (creatinine clearance [CrCl] 30 to 59 mL/min), 600 mg should be administered on day 1, day 3, and every day thereafter.

Gabapentin is not recommended for use in patients with a CrCl less than 30 mL/min or on hemodialysis because the dose cannot be reduced below 600 mg.

➤*Administration:* Gabapentin should be swallowed whole and should not be cut, crushed, or chewed.

➤*Storage/Stability:* Store at 25°C (77°F); excursions are permitted from 15° to 30°C (59° to 86°F). Protect from moisture. Do not remove desiccants. Dispense in original bottle.

PREGABALIN

c-v	Lyrica (Pfizer)	Capsules; oral: 25 mg	Lactose. (Pfizer PGN 25). White. In 90s.
		50 mg	Lactose. (Pfizer PGN 50). White. In 90s and UD 100s.
		75 mg	Lactose. (Pfizer PGN 75). White/Orange. In 90s and UD 100s.
		100 mg	Lactose. (Pfizer PGN 100). Orange. In 90s and UD 100s.
		150 mg	Lactose. (Pfizer PGN 150). White. In 90s and UD 100s.
		200 mg	Lactose. (Pfizer PGN 200). Lt. orange. In 90s.
		225 mg	Lactose. (Pfizer PGN 225). White/Lt. orange. In 90s.
		300 mg	Lactose. (Pfizer PGN 300). White/Orange. In 90s.
		Solution; oral: 20 mg/mL	Parabens, sucralose. Strawberry flavor. In 473 mL.

PREGABALIN — ORAL

Indications

➤*Fibromyalgia:* For the management of fibromyalgia.

➤*Neuropathic pain associated with diabetic peripheral neuropathy:* For the management of neuropathic pain associated with diabetic peripheral neuropathy.

➤*Partial-onset seizures:* Adjunctive therapy for adult patients with partial-onset seizures.

➤*Postherpetic neuralgia:* For the management of postherpetic neuralgia.

➤*Off-label uses:* Treatment of generalized anxiety disorder.

Administration and Dosage

➤*Adults:*

Fibromyalgia –

Maximum dose: 450 mg/day.

Initial dosage: 75 mg twice daily.

Maintenance dosage: 300 to 450 mg/day divided twice daily.

Dosage adjustment: Dosage may be increased to 150 mg twice daily within 1 week, based on efficacy and tolerability. Patients who do not experience sufficient benefit with 300 mg/day may be further increased to 225 mg twice daily.

Neuropathic pain associated with diabetic peripheral neuropathy –

Maximum dose: 300 mg/day.

Initial dosage: 50 mg 3 times a day.

Dosage adjustment: Dosage may be increased to 100 mg 3 times a day within 1 week, based on efficacy and tolerability.

Partial-onset seizures –

Maximum dose: 600 mg/day.

Initial dosage: 75 mg 2 times a day or 50 mg 3 times a day.

Maintenance dosage: 150 to 600 mg/day divided and given 2 or 3 times daily.

Dosage adjustment: Based on individual patient response and tolerability, the dose may be increased to a maximum dosage of 600 mg/day.

Postherpetic neuralgia –

Initial dosage: 75 mg twice daily or 50 mg 3 times a day.

Maintenance dosage: 75 to 150 mg twice daily or 50 to 100 mg 3 times a day.

In view of the dose-dependent adverse reactions and the higher rate of treatment discontinuation caused by adverse reactions, dosing higher than 300 mg/day should be reserved only for those patients who have ongoing pain and tolerate 300 mg daily.

Dosage adjustment: Dosage may be increased to 300 mg/day within 1 week, based on efficacy and tolerability.

Patients who do not experience sufficient pain relief following 2 to 4 weeks of treatment with 300 mg/day and are able to tolerate pregabalin may be treated with up to 300 mg 2 times a day or 200 mg 3 times a day.

➤*Elderly:* Dosage reduction required in elderly patients with renal impairment. (See Renal Function Impairment.)

➤*Renal function impairment:*

Pregabalin Dosage Adjustment Based on Renal Function

CrCl[a] (mL/min)	Total pregabalin daily dose[b]				Dose regimen
≥ 60	150 mg/day	300 mg/day	450 mg/day	600 mg/day	2 or 3 times daily
30 to 60	75 mg/day	150 mg/day	225 mg/day	300 mg/day	2 or 3 times daily
15 to 30	25 to 50 mg/day	75 mg/day	100 to 150 mg/day	150 mg/day	Single daily dose or 2 times daily
< 15	25 mg/day	25 to 50 mg/day	50 to 75 mg/day	75 mg/day	Single daily dose
Supplementary dosage following hemodialysis (mg)[c]					
Patients on the 25 mg single daily dose regimen (see < 15 CrCl): Take 1 supplemental dose of 25 or 50 mg.					
Patients on the 25 to 50 mg single daily dose regimen (see < 15 CrCl): Take 1 supplemental dose of 50 or 75 mg.					
Patients on the 50 to 75 mg single daily dose regimen (see < 15 CrCl): Take 1 supplemental dose of 75 or 100 mg.					
Patients on the 75 mg single daily dose regimen (see < 15 CrCl): Take 1 supplemental dose of 100 or 150 mg.					

[a] CrCl = creatinine clearance.
[b] Total daily dose (mg/day) should be divided as indicated by dose regimen to provide mg/dose.
[c] Supplementary dose is a single additional dose.

Hemodialysis – Adjust the pregabalin daily dosage based on renal function. In addition to the daily dosage adjustment, administer a supplemental dosage immediately following every 4-hour hemodialysis treatment.

➤*Discontinuation of therapy:* Taper gradually over a minimum of 1 week.

➤*Administration:* Give orally, with or without food, in 2 or 3 divided doses.

➤*Storage/Stability:* Store at 25°C (77°F); excursions are permitted to 15° to 30°C (59° to 86°F). For the oral solution, use within 45 days of first opening the bottle.

Actions

➤*Pharmacology:* Pregabalin binds with high affinity to the alpha-2 delta site (an auxiliary subunit of voltage-gated calcium channels) in CNS tissues. The mechanism of action of pregabalin is unknown. In vitro, pregabalin reduces the calcium-dependent release of several neurotransmitters, possibly by modulation of calcium channel function.

While pregabalin is a structural derivative of the inhibitory neurotransmitter gamma-aminobutyric acid (GABA), it does not bind directly to $GABA_A$, $GABA_B$, or benzodiazepine receptors; does not augment $GABA_A$ responses in cultured neurons; does not alter rat brain GABA concentration; or have acute effects on GABA uptake or degradation. However, in cultured neurons, prolonged application of pregabalin increases the density of GABA transporter protein and increases the rate of functional GABA transport. Pregabalin does not block sodium channels, is not active at opiate receptors, and does not alter cyclooxygenase enzyme activity. It is inactive at serotonin and dopamine receptors and does not inhibit dopamine, serotonin, or norepinephrine reuptake.

➤*Pharmacokinetics:*

Absorption/Distribution – Pregabalin is well absorbed after oral administration. Following oral administration of pregabalin capsules under fasting conditions, peak plasma concentrations occur within 1.5 hours. Pregabalin oral bioavailability is 90% or more and is independent of dose. Following single-dose (25 to 300 mg) and multiple-dose (75 to 900 mg/day) administration, maximum plasma concentrations (C_{max}) and area under the curve (AUC) values increase linearly. Following repeated administration, steady state is achieved within 24 to 48 hours. Multiple-dose pharmacokinetics can be predicted from single-dose data.

Pregabalin does not bind to plasma proteins. The apparent volume of distribution of pregabalin following oral administration is approximately 0.5 L/kg. Pregabalin is a substrate for system L transporter, which is responsible for the transport of large amino acids across the blood brain barrier. Although there are no data in humans, pregabalin crossed the blood brain barrier in mice, rats, and monkeys. In addition, pregabalin crossed the placenta in rats and was present in the milk of lactating rats.

Effect of food: The rate of pregabalin absorption is decreased when given with food, resulting in a decrease in C_{max} of approximately 25% to 30% and an increase in time of maximal concentration (T_{max}) to approximately 3 hours. However, administration of pregabalin with food has no clinically relevant effect on the total absorption of pregabalin. Therefore, pregabalin can be taken with or without food.

Metabolism/Excretion – Pregabalin undergoes negligible metabolism in humans. Following a dose of radiolabeled pregabalin, approximately 90% of the administered dose was recovered in the urine as unchanged pregabalin. The N-methylated derivative of pregabalin, the major metabolite of pregabalin found in urine, accounted for 0.9% of the dose. In preclinical studies, pregabalin (S-enantiomer) did not undergo racemization to the R-enantiomer in mice, rats, rabbits, or monkeys.

Pregabalin is eliminated from the systemic circulation primarily by renal excretion as unchanged drug, with a mean elimination half-life of 6.3 hours in subjects with healthy renal function. Mean renal clearance was estimated

PREGABALIN — ORAL

to be 67 to 80.9 mL/min in young, healthy subjects. Because pregabalin is not bound to plasma proteins, this clearance rate indicates that renal tubular reabsorption is involved. Pregabalin elimination is nearly proportional to CrCl.

Special populations –

Renal function impairment: Pregabalin clearance is nearly proportional to CrCl. Dosage reduction in patients with renal impairment is necessary. Pregabalin is effectively removed from plasma by hemodialysis. Following a 4-hour hemodialysis treatment, plasma pregabalin concentrations are reduced approximately 50%. For patients on hemodialysis, dosing must be modified.

Elderly: Pregabalin oral clearance tended to decrease with increasing age. This decrease in pregabalin oral clearance is consistent with age-related decreases in CrCl. Reduction of the pregabalin dose may be required in patients who have age-related compromised renal function.

Contraindications

Hypersensitivity to pregabalin or any of its components.

Warnings/Precautions

➤*Angioedema:* There have been postmarketing reports of angioedema in patients during initial and long-term treatment with pregabalin. Specific symptoms included swelling of the face, mouth (gums, lips, and tongue), and neck (larynx and throat). There were reports of life-threatening angioedema with respiratory compromise requiring emergency treatment. Discontinue pregabalin immediately in patients with these symptoms.

Exercise caution when prescribing pregabalin to patients who have had a previous episode of angioedema. In addition, patients who are taking other drugs associated with angioedema (eg, angiotensin-converting enzyme inhibitors) may be at increased risk of developing angioedema.

➤*Discontinuation of therapy:* As with all antiepileptic drugs (AEDs), withdraw pregabalin gradually to minimize the potential of increased seizure frequency in patients with seizure disorders. Following abrupt or rapid discontinuation of pregabalin, some patients reported symptoms, including diarrhea, headache, insomnia, and nausea. Taper pregabalin gradually over a minimum of 1 week rather than discontinuing abruptly.

➤*Suicidal behavior and ideation:* AEDs, including pregabalin, increase the risk of suicidal thoughts or behavior in patients taking these drugs for any indication. Monitor patients treated with any AED for any indication for the emergence of worsening of depression, suicidal thoughts or behavior, and/or any unusual changes in mood or behavior.

The increased risk of suicidal thoughts or behavior with AEDs was observed as early as 1 week after starting drug treatment with AEDs and persisted for the duration of treatment assessed. Because most trials included in the analysis did not extend beyond 24 weeks, the risk of suicidal thoughts or behavior beyond 24 weeks could not be assessed.

The relative risk (RR) for suicidal thoughts or behavior was higher in clinical trials for epilepsy than in clinical trials for psychiatric or other conditions, but the absolute risk differences were similar for the epilepsy and psychiatric indications.

Anyone considering prescribing pregabalin or any other AED must balance the risk of suicidal thoughts or behaviors with the risk of the untreated illness. Epilepsy and many other illnesses for which AEDs are prescribed are themselves associated with morbidity and mortality and an increased risk of suicidal thoughts and behavior. Should suicidal thoughts and behavior emerge during treatment, consider whether the emergence of these symptoms in any given patient may be related to the illness being treated.

Inform patients, their caregivers, and families that pregabalin and other AEDs increase the risk of suicidal thoughts and behavior and advise them of the need to be alert for the emergence or worsening of the signs and symptoms of depression, any unusual changes in mood or behavior, or the emergence of suicidal thoughts, behavior, or thoughts about self-harm. Immediately report any behaviors of concern to health care providers.

➤*Peripheral edema:* Pregabalin treatment may cause peripheral edema. In short-term trials of patients without clinically significant heart or peripheral vascular disease, there was no apparent association between peripheral edema and cardiovascular complications such as hypertension or congestive heart failure (CHF). Peripheral edema was not associated with laboratory changes suggestive of deterioration in renal or hepatic function.

In controlled clinical trials, the incidence of peripheral edema was 6% in the pregabalin group compared with 2% in the placebo group. In controlled clinical trials, 0.5% of pregabalin patients and 0.2% of placebo patients withdrew because of peripheral edema.

Higher frequencies of weight gain and peripheral edema were observed in patients taking both pregabalin and a thiazolidinedione antidiabetic agent compared with patients taking either drug alone. The majority of patients using thiazolidinedione antidiabetic agents in the overall safety database were participants in studies of pain associated with diabetic peripheral neuropathy. In this population, peripheral edema was reported in 3% of patients who were using thiazolidinedione antidiabetic agents only, 8% of patients who were treated with pregabalin only, and 19% of patients who were taking both pregabalin and thiazolidinedione antidiabetic agents. Similarly, weight gain was reported in 0% of patients taking thiazolidinediones only, 4% of patients taking pregabalin only, and 7.5% of patients taking both drugs.

Because the thiazolidinedione class of antidiabetic drugs can cause weight gain and/or fluid retention, possibly exacerbating or leading to heart failure, exercise caution when coadministering pregabalin and these agents.

Congestive heart failure – Because there are limited data on CHF patients with New York Heart Association class III or IV cardiac status, use pregabalin with caution in these patients.

➤*CNS effects:* Pregabalin may cause dizziness and somnolence. In the pregabalin controlled trials, dizziness was experienced by 31% of pregabalin-treated patients compared with 9% of placebo-treated patients; somnolence was experienced by 22% of pregabalin-treated patients compared with 7% of placebo-treated patients. Dizziness and somnolence generally began shortly after the initiation of pregabalin therapy and occurred more frequently at higher doses. Dizziness and somnolence were the adverse reactions most frequently leading to withdrawal (4% each) from controlled studies. In pregabalin-treated patients reporting these adverse reactions in short-term, controlled studies, dizziness persisted until the last dose in 30% of patients, and somnolence persisted until the last dose in 42% of patients.

➤*Weight gain:* Pregabalin treatment may cause weight gain. In pregabalin controlled clinical trials of up to 14 weeks, a gain of 7% or more over baseline weight was observed in 9% of pregabalin-treated patients and 2% of placebo-treated patients. Few patients treated with pregabalin (0.3%) withdrew from controlled trials because of weight gain. Pregabalin-associated weight gain was related to dose and duration of exposure but did not appear to be associated with baseline body mass index, gender, or age. Weight gain was not limited to patients with edema.

Among diabetic patients, pregabalin-treated patients gained an average of 1.6 kg (range, −16 to 16 kg), compared with an average 0.3 kg (range, −10 to 9 kg) weight gain in placebo-treated patients. In a cohort of 333 patients with diabetes who received pregabalin for at least 2 years, the average weight gain was 5.2 kg.

➤*Ophthalmic effects:* In controlled studies, a higher proportion of patients treated with pregabalin reported blurred vision (7%) than patients treated with placebo (2%), which resolved in the majority of cases with continued dosing. Less than 1% of patients discontinued pregabalin treatment because of vision-related reactions (primarily blurred vision).

Although the clinical significance of the ophthalmologic findings is unknown, inform patients to notify their health care provider if changes in vision occur. If visual disturbance persists, consider further assessment. Consider more frequent assessment for patients who are already routinely monitored for ocular conditions.

➤*Creatine kinase elevations:* Pregabalin treatment was associated with creatine kinase (CK) elevations. Mean changes in CK from baseline to the maximum value were 60 units/L for pregabalin-treated patients and 28 units/L for placebo-treated patients. In all controlled trials across multiple patient populations, 1.5% of patients on pregabalin and 0.7% of placebo-treated patients had a value of CK at least 3 times the upper limit of normal. Three pregabalin-treated subjects reported rhabdomyolysis in premarketing clinical trials. The relationship between these myopathy events and pregabalin is not completely understood because the cases had documented factors that may have caused or contributed to these events. Instruct patients to promptly report unexplained muscle pain, tenderness, or weakness, particularly if these muscle symptoms are accompanied by malaise or fever. Discontinue pregabalin treatment if myopathy is diagnosed or suspected or if markedly elevated CK levels occur.

➤*Decreased platelet count:* Pregabalin treatment was associated with a decrease in platelet count. Pregabalin-treated subjects experienced a mean maximal decrease in platelet count of 20×10^3/mcL, compared with 11×10^3/mcL in placebo-treated patients. In the overall database of controlled trials, 2% of placebo-treated patients and 3% of pregabalin-treated patients experienced a potentially clinically significant decrease in platelets, defined as 20% below baseline value and less than 150×10^3/mcL. A single pregabalin-treated subject developed severe thrombocytopenia with a platelet count of less than 20×10^3/mcL. In randomized, controlled trials, pregabalin was not associated with an increase in bleeding-related adverse reactions.

➤*PR interval prolongation:* Pregabalin treatment was associated with PR interval prolongation. In analyses of clinical trial electrocardiogram data, the mean PR interval increase was 3 to 6 msec at pregabalin dosages of 300 mg/day or more. This mean change difference was not associated with an increased risk of PR increase of 25% or more from baseline, an increased percentage of subjects with on-treatment PR of more than 200 msec, or an increased risk of adverse reactions of second- or third-degree atrioventricular block.

➤*Hypersensitivity reactions:* There have been postmarketing reports of hypersensitivity in patients shortly after initiation of treatment with pregabalin. Adverse reactions included blisters, dyspnea, hives, rash, skin redness, and wheezing. Discontinue pregabalin immediately in patients with these symptoms.

➤*Renal function impairment:* See Actions for more information.

➤*Hazardous tasks:* Pregabalin may cause dizziness and somnolence. Pregabalin-related dizziness and somnolence may impair abilities to perform tasks such as driving or operating machinery.

➤*Pregnancy: Category C.* Increased incidences of fetal structural abnormalities and other manifestations of developmental toxicity, including lethality, growth retardation, and nervous and reproductive system functional impairment, were observed in the offspring of rats and rabbits given pregabalin during pregnancy at doses that produced plasma pregabalin exposures (AUC) at least 5 times human exposure at the maximum recommended human dose of 600 mg/day.

There are no adequate and well-controlled studies in pregnant women. It is not known if pregabalin crosses the human placenta. The low molecular weight (approximately 159), minimal metabolism, lack of plasma protein binding, and the moderately long elimination half-life suggest that the drug will reach the embryo and fetus. Use pregabalin during pregnancy only if the potential benefit justifies the potential risk to the fetus.

Pregnancy registry – To provide information regarding the effects of in utero exposure to pregabalin, health care providers are advised to recom-

PREGABALIN — ORAL

mend that pregnant patients taking pregabalin enroll in the North American Antiepileptic Drug (NAAED) Pregnancy Registry. This can be done by calling the toll-free number 1-888-233-2334 and must be done by patients themselves. Information on the registry can also be found at the Web site http://www.aedpregnancyregistry.org.

Labor and delivery – The effects of pregabalin on labor and delivery in pregnant women are unknown. In the prenatal-postnatal study in rats, pregabalin prolonged gestation and induced dystocia at exposures of 50 times or more the mean human exposure ($AUC_{(0-24)}$ of 123 mcg•h/mL) at the maximum recommended clinical dosage of 600 mg/day.

➤*Lactation:* It is not known if pregabalin is excreted in human milk; it is, however, present in the milk of rats. The low molecular weight (approximately 159), minimal metabolism, lack of plasma protein binding, and the moderately long elimination half-life (6 hours) suggest that the drug will also be excreted into breast milk. Because it is freely soluble in water, the highest concentrations of the drug are found in foremilk. Because many drugs are excreted in human milk and because of the potential for tumorigenicity shown for pregabalin in animal studies, decide whether to discontinue breast-feeding or the drug, taking into account the importance of the drug to the mother.

➤*Children:* The safety and efficacy of pregabalin in children have not been established.

➤*Elderly:* In controlled clinical studies of pregabalin in fibromyalgia, 106 patients were 65 years of age and older. Although the adverse reaction profile was similar between the 2 age groups, the following neurological adverse reactions were more frequent in patients 65 years of age and older: abnormal coordination, balance disorder, blurred vision, confusional state, dizziness, lethargy, and tremor.

Pregabalin is known to be substantially excreted by the kidneys, and the risk of toxic reactions to pregabalin may be greater in patients with renal function impairment. Because pregabalin is eliminated primarily by renal excretion, adjust the dose for elderly patients with renal function impairment.

➤*Monitoring:* Monitor patients being treated with pregabalin for any indication of the emergence or worsening of depression, suicidal thoughts or behavior, and any unusual changes in behavior. Monitor patients for weight gain and/or fluid retention, possibly exacerbating or leading to heart failure. Carefully evaluate patients for a history of drug abuse and observe them for signs of pregabalin misuse or abuse (eg, development of tolerance, dose escalation, drug-seeking behavior).

Drug Interactions

Pregabalin Drug Interactions

Precipitant drug	Object drug[a]		Description
ACE[b] inhibitors (eg, captopril)	Pregabalin	↑	Coadministration of these agents may increase the risk of swelling and hives. Instruct patient to contact health care provider immediately if these signs occur.
Pregabalin	ACE inhibitors (eg, captopril)		
CNS depressants (eg, ethanol, lorazepam, oxycodone)	Pregabalin	↑	Multiple oral doses of pregabalin were coadministered with ethanol, lorazepam, or oxycodone. Although no pharmacokinetic interactions were seen, additive effects on cognitive and gross motor functioning occurred. No clinically important effects on respiration were seen. Instruct patients to avoid alcohol.
Pregabalin	CNS depressants (eg, ethanol, lorazepam, oxycodone)		
Thiazolidinedione (ie, pioglitazone, rosiglitazone)	Pregabalin	↑	Coadministration of pregabalin and a thiazolidinedione may lead to an additive effect on edema and weight gain and/or fluid retention, possibly exacerbating or leading to heart failure. Use with caution. Monitor the patient. If an interaction is suspected, it may be necessary to adjust the dose of one or both agents.
Pregabalin	Thiazolidinedione (ie, pioglitazone, rosiglitazone)		

[a] ↑ = object drug increased.
[b] ACE = angiotensin-converting enzyme.

➤*Drug/Food interactions:* The rate of pregabalin absorption is decreased when given with food, resulting in a decrease in C_{max} of approximately 25% to 30% and an increase in T_{max} to approximately 3 hours. However, administration of pregabalin with food has no clinically relevant effect on the total absorption of pregabalin. Therefore, pregabalin can be taken with or without food.

Adverse Reactions

➤*Discontinuation of therapy:* In premarketing controlled trials of all populations combined, 14% of patients treated with pregabalin and 7% of patients treated with placebo discontinued prematurely because of adverse reactions. In the pregabalin treatment group, the adverse reactions most frequently leading to discontinuation were dizziness (4%) and somnolence (3%). In the placebo group, 1% of patients withdrew because of dizziness and less than 1% withdrew because of somnolence. Other adverse reactions that led to discontinuation from controlled trials more frequently in the pregabalin group compared with the placebo group were abnormal thinking, asthenia, ataxia, blurred vision, confusion, incoordination, and peripheral edema (1% each).

➤*Most common adverse reactions:* In premarketing controlled trials of all patient populations combined, abnormal thinking (primarily difficulty with concentration/attention), blurred vision, dizziness, dry mouth, edema, somnolence, and weight gain were more commonly reported by subjects treated with pregabalin than by subjects treated with placebo (at least 5% and twice the rate of that seen in placebo).

➤*Neuropathic pain associated with diabetic peripheral neuropathy:*

Discontinuation of therapy – In clinical trials in patients with neuropathic pain associated with diabetic peripheral neuropathy, 9% of patients treated with pregabalin and 4% of patients treated with placebo discontinued prematurely because of adverse reactions. In the pregabalin treatment group, the most common reasons for discontinuation because of adverse reactions were dizziness (3%) and somnolence (2%). In comparison, less than 1% of placebo patients withdrew because of dizziness and somnolence. Other reasons for discontinuation from trials, occurring with greater frequency in the pregabalin group than the placebo group, were asthenia, confusion, and peripheral edema. Each of these reactions led to withdrawal in approximately 1% of patients.

Most common adverse reactions –

Pregabalin Adverse Reactions in Neuropathic Pain Associated With Diabetic Peripheral Neuropathy (≥ 1%)

Adverse reactions	75 mg/day (n = 77)	150 mg/day (n = 212)	300 mg/day (n = 321)	600 mg/day (n = 369)	All pregabalin (n = 979)	Placebo (n = 459)
CNS						
Abnormal gait	1%	0%	1%	3%	1%	0%
Abnormal thinking[a]	1%	0%	1%	3%	2%	0%
Amnesia	3%	1%	0%	2%	1%	0%
Asthenia	4%	2%	4%	7%	5%	2%
Ataxia	6%	1%	2%	4%	3%	1%
Confusion	0%	1%	2%	3%	2%	1%
Dizziness	8%	9%	23%	29%	21%	5%
Euphoria	0%	0%	3%	2%	2%	0%
Incoordination	1%	0%	2%	2%	2%	0%
Nervousness	0%	1%	1%	1%	1%	0%
Neuropathy	9%	2%	2%	5%	4%	3%
Somnolence	4%	6%	13%	16%	12%	3%
Tremor	1%	1%	1%	2%	1%	0%
Vertigo	1%	2%	2%	4%	3%	1%

PREGABALIN — ORAL

Adverse reactions	75 mg/day (n = 77)	150 mg/day (n = 212)	300 mg/day (n = 321)	600 mg/day (n = 369)	All pregabalin (n = 979)	Placebo (n = 459)
Pregabalin Adverse Reactions in Neuropathic Pain Associated With Diabetic Peripheral Neuropathy (≥ 1%)						
GI						
Constipation	0%	2%	4%	6%	4%	2%
Dry mouth	3%	2%	5%	7%	5%	1%
Flatulence	3%	0%	2%	3%	2%	1%
Metabolic/Nutritional						
Edema	0%	2%	4%	2%	2%	0%
Face edema	0%	1%	1%	2%	1%	0%
Hypoglycemia	1%	3%	2%	1%	2%	1%
Peripheral edema	4%	6%	9%	12%	9%	2%
Weight gain	0%	4%	4%	6%	4%	0%
Special senses						
Abnormal vision	1%	0%	1%	1%	1%	0%
Blurry vision[b]	3%	1%	3%	6%	4%	2%
Miscellaneous						
Accidental injury	5%	2%	2%	6%	4%	3%
Back pain	0%	2%	1%	2%	2%	0%
Chest pain	4%	1%	1%	2%	2%	1%
Dyspnea	3%	0%	2%	2%	2%	1%

[a] Abnormal thinking primarily consists of reactions related to difficulty with concentration/attention but also includes reactions related to cognition and language problems and slowed thinking.

[b] Investigator term; summary level term is amblyopia.

➤*Postherpetic neuralgia:*

Discontinuation of therapy – In clinical trials in patients with postherpetic neuralgia, 14% of patients treated with pregabalin and 7% of patients treated with placebo discontinued prematurely because of adverse reactions. In the pregabalin treatment group, the most common reasons for discontinuation because of adverse reactions were dizziness (4%) and somnolence (3%). In comparison, less than 1% of placebo patients withdrew because of dizziness and somnolence. Other reasons for discontinuation from the trials, occurring with greater frequency in the pregabalin group than the placebo group, were confusion (2%), as well as abnormal gait, asthenia, ataxia, and peripheral edema (1% each).

Most common adverse reactions –

Adverse reactions	75 mg/day (n = 84)	150 mg/day (n = 302)	300 mg/day (n = 312)	600 mg/day (n = 154)	All pregabalin (n = 852)	Placebo (n = 398)
Pregabalin Adverse Reactions in Neuropathic Pain Associated With Postherpetic Neuralgia (≥ 1%)						
CNS						
Abnormal gait	0%	2%	4%	8%	4%	1%
Abnormal thinking[a]	0%	2%	1%	6%	2%	2%
Amnesia	0%	1%	1%	4%	2%	0%
Ataxia	1%	2%	5%	9%	5%	1%
Confusion	1%	2%	3%	7%	3%	0%
Dizziness	11%	18%	31%	37%	26%	9%
Headache	5%	9%	5%	8%	7%	5%
Incoordination	2%	2%	1%	3%	2%	0%
Myasthenia	1%	1%	1%	1%	1%	0%
Somnolence	8%	12%	18%	25%	16%	5%
Speech disorder	0%	0%	1%	3%	1%	0%
GI						
Constipation	4%	5%	5%	5%	5%	2%
Dry mouth	7%	7%	6%	15%	8%	3%
Flatulence	2%	1%	2%	3%	2%	1%
Vomiting	1%	1%	3%	3%	2%	1%
Metabolic/Nutritional						
Edema	0%	1%	2%	6%	2%	1%
Face edema	0%	2%	1%	3%	2%	1%
Peripheral edema	0%	8%	16%	16%	12%	4%
Weight gain	1%	2%	5%	7%	4%	0%
Special senses						
Abnormal vision	0%	1%	2%	5%	2%	0%
Blurry vision[b]	1%	5%	5%	9%	5%	3%
Diplopia	0%	2%	2%	4%	2%	0%
Eye disorder	0%	1%	1%	2%	1%	0%
Miscellaneous						
Accidental injury	4%	3%	3%	5%	3%	2%
Bronchitis	0%	1%	1%	3%	1%	1%
Flu syndrome	1%	2%	2%	1%	2%	1%

PREGABALIN — ORAL

Pregabalin Adverse Reactions in Neuropathic Pain Associated With Postherpetic Neuralgia (≥ 1%)						
Adverse reactions	75 mg/day (n = 84)	150 mg/day (n = 302)	300 mg/day (n = 312)	600 mg/day (n = 154)	All pregabalin (n = 852)	Placebo (n = 398)
Infection	14%	8%	6%	3%	7%	4%
Pain	5%	4%	5%	5%	5%	4%
Urinary incontinence	0%	1%	1%	2%	1%	0%

[a] Abnormal thinking primarily consists of reactions related to difficulty with concentration/attention but also includes reactions related to cognition and language problems and slowed thinking.

[b] Investigator term; summary level term is amblyopia.

➤*Partial-onset seizures:*

Discontinuation of therapy – Approximately 15% of patients receiving pregabalin and 6% of patients receiving placebo in add-on epilepsy trials discontinued prematurely because of adverse reactions. In the pregabalin treatment group, the adverse reactions most frequently leading to discontinuation were dizziness (6%), ataxia (4%), and somnolence (3%). In comparison, less than 1% of patients in the placebo group withdrew because of each of these reactions. Other adverse reactions that led to discontinuation of at least 1% of patients in the pregabalin group and occurred at least twice as frequently compared with the placebo group were abnormal thinking, asthenia, blurred vision, confusion, diplopia, headache, nausea, tremor, and vertigo (each reaction led to withdrawal in 2% or less of patients).

Most common adverse reactions –

Pregabalin Adverse Reactions in Adjunctive Therapy for Adult Patients With Partial-Onset Seizures (≥ 2%)					
Adverse reactions	150 mg/day (n = 185)	300 mg/day (n = 90)	600 mg/day (n = 395)	All pregabalin (n = 670[a])	Placebo (n = 294)
CNS					
Abnormal gait	1%	3%	5%	4%	0%
Abnormal thinking[b]	4%	8%	9%	8%	2%
Amnesia	3%	2%	6%	5%	2%
Ataxia	6%	10%	20%	15%	4%
Confusion	1%	2%	5%	4%	2%
Dizziness	18%	31%	38%	32%	11%
Incoordination	1%	3%	6%	4%	1%
Myoclonus	1%	0%	4%	2%	0%
Somnolence	11%	18%	28%	22%	11%
Speech disorder	1%	2%	7%	5%	1%
Tremor	3%	7%	11%	8%	4%
Twitching	0%	4%	5%	4%	1%
GI					
Constipation	1%	1%	7%	4%	2%
Dry mouth	1%	2%	6%	4%	1%

Pregabalin Adverse Reactions in Adjunctive Therapy for Adult Patients With Partial-Onset Seizures (≥ 2%)					
Adverse reactions	150 mg/day (n = 185)	300 mg/day (n = 90)	600 mg/day (n = 395)	All pregabalin (n = 670[a])	Placebo (n = 294)
Metabolic/Nutritional					
Increased appetite	2%	3%	6%	5%	1%
Peripheral edema	3%	3%	6%	5%	2%
Weight gain	5%	7%	16%	12%	1%
Special senses					
Abnormal vision	3%	1%	5%	4%	1%
Blurred vision[c]	5%	8%	12%	10%	4%
Diplopia	5%	7%	12%	9%	4%
Miscellaneous					
Accidental injury	7%	11%	10%	9%	5%
Pain	3%	2%	5%	4%	3%

[a] Excludes patients who received the 50 mg dose in study E1.

[b] Abnormal thinking primarily consists of reactions related to difficulty with concentration/attention but also includes reactions related to cognition and language problems and slowed thinking.

[c] Investigator term; summary level term is amblyopia.

➤*Fibromyalgia:*

Discontinuation of therapy – In clinical trials of patients with fibromyalgia, 19% of patients treated with pregabalin 150 to 600 mg/day and 10% of patients treated with placebo discontinued prematurely because of adverse reactions. In the pregabalin treatment group, the most common reasons for discontinuation because of adverse reactions were dizziness (6%) and somnolence (3%). In comparison, less than 1% of placebo-treated patients withdrew because of dizziness and somnolence. Other reasons for discontinuation from trials, occurring with greater frequency in the pregabalin treatment group than the placebo treatment group, were balance disorder, fatigue, headache, and increased weight. Each of these adverse reactions led to withdrawal in approximately 1% of patients.

Most common adverse reactions –

Pregabalin Adverse Reactions in Fibromyalgia (≥ 2%)						
Adverse reactions	150 mg/day (n = 132)	300 mg/day (n = 502)	450 mg/day (n = 505)	600 mg/day (n = 378)	All pregabalin (n = 1,517)	Placebo (n = 505)
CNS						
Abnormal coordination	2%	1%	2%	2%	2%	1%
Anxiety	2%	2%	2%	2%	2%	1%
Attention disturbance	4%	4%	6%	6%	5%	1%
Balance disorder	2%	3%	6%	9%	5%	0%
Confusional state	0%	2%	3%	4%	3%	0%
Depression	2%	2%	2%	2%	2%	2%
Disorientation	1%	0%	2%	1%	2%	0%
Dizziness	23%	31%	43%	45%	38%	9%
Euphoric mood	2%	5%	6%	7%	6%	1%
Fatigue	5%	7%	6%	8%	7%	4%
Feeling abnormal	1%	3%	2%	2%	2%	0%
Feeling drunk	1%	2%	1%	2%	2%	0%
Headache	11%	12%	14%	10%	12%	12%
Hypesthesia	2%	2%	3%	2%	2%	1%
Lethargy	2%	2%	1%	2%	2%	0%
Memory impairment	1%	3%	4%	4%	3%	0%
Somnolence	13%	18%	22%	22%	20%	4%
Tremor	0%	1%	3%	2%	2%	0%

PREGABALIN — ORAL

Adverse reactions	Pregabalin Adverse Reactions in Fibromyalgia (≥ 2%) 150 mg/day (n = 132)	300 mg/day (n = 502)	450 mg/day (n = 505)	600 mg/day (n = 378)	All pregabalin (n = 1,517)	Placebo (n = 505)
Vertigo	2%	2%	2%	1%	2%	0%
GI						
Abdominal distention	2%	2%	2%	2%	2%	1%
Constipation	4%	4%	7%	10%	7%	2%
Dry mouth	7%	6%	9%	9%	8%	2%
Flatulence	1%	1%	2%	2%	2%	1%
Vomiting	2%	3%	3%	2%	3%	2%
Metabolic/Nutritional						
Edema	1%	2%	1%	2%	2%	1%
Fluid retention	2%	3%	3%	2%	2%	1%
Increased appetite	4%	3%	5%	7%	5%	1%
Increased weight	8%	10%	10%	14%	11%	2%
Peripheral edema	5%	5%	6%	9%	6%	2%
Musculoskeletal						
Arthralgia	4%	3%	3%	6%	4%	2%
Back pain	2%	3%	4%	3%	3%	3%
Muscle spasms	2%	4%	4%	4%	4%	2%
Respiratory						
Pharyngolaryngeal pain	2%	1%	3%	3%	2%	2%
Sinusitis	4%	5%	7%	5%	5%	4%
Miscellaneous						
Blurred vision	8%	7%	7%	12%	8%	1%
Chest pain	2%	1%	1%	2%	2%	1%

➤*Other adverse reactions:*

Cardiovascular – Deep thrombophlebitis, heart failure, hypotension, postural hypotension, retinal vascular disorder, syncope (0.1% to 1%); ST depressed, ventricular fibrillation (less than 0.1%).

CNS – Anxiety, depersonalization, hypertonia, hypesthesia, libido decreased, paresthesia, stupor, twitching (1% or more); abnormal dreams, agitation, apathy, aphasia, circumoral paresthesia, dysarthria, hallucinations, hostility, hyperalgesia, hyperesthesia, hyperkinesia, hypokinesia, hypotonia, increased libido, malaise, myoclonus, neuralgia (0.1% to 1%); addiction, cerebellar syndrome, cogwheel rigidity, coma, delirium, delusions, dysautonomia, dyskinesia, dystonia, encephalopathy, extrapyramidal syndrome, Guillain-Barré syndrome, hangover effect, hypalgesia, intracranial hypertension, manic reaction, paranoid reaction, peripheral neuritis, personality disorder, psychotic depression, schizophrenic reaction, sleep disorder, torticollis, trismus (less than 0.1%).

Dermatologic – Pruritus (1% or more); alopecia, dry skin, eczema, hirsutism, photosensitivity reaction, skin ulcer, urticaria, vesiculobullous rash (0.1% to 1%); angioedema, exfoliative dermatitis, lichenoid dermatitis, melanosis, nail disorder, petechial rash, purpuric rash, pustular rash, skin atrophy, skin necrosis, skin nodule, Stevens-Johnson syndrome, subcutaneous nodule (less than 0.1%).

GI – Abdominal pain, gastroenteritis (1% or more); cholecystitis, cholelithiasis, colitis, dysphagia, esophagitis, gastritis, GI hemorrhage, melena, mouth ulceration, pancreatitis, rectal hemorrhage, tongue edema (0.1% to 1%); aphthous stomatitis, esophageal ulcer, periodontal abscess (less than 0.1%).

GU – Anorgasmia, impotence, libido decreased, urinary frequency, urinary incontinence (1% or more); abnormal ejaculation, albuminuria, amenorrhea, dysmenorrhea, dysuria, hematuria, kidney calculus, leukorrhea, menorrhagia, metrorrhagia, nephritis, oliguria, pelvic pain, urinary retention, urine abnormality (0.1% to 1%); acute kidney failure, balanitis, bladder neoplasm, cervicitis, dyspareunia, epididymitis, female lactation, glomerulitis, ovarian disorder, pyelonephritis (less than 0.1%).

Hematologic/Lymphatic – Ecchymosis (1% or more); anemia, eosinophilia, hypochromic anemia, leukocytosis, leukopenia, lymphadenopathy, thrombocytopenia (0.1% to 1%); myelofibrosis, polycythemia, prothrombin decreased, purpura, thrombocythemia (less than 0.1%).

Metabolic/Nutritional – Increased appetite (1% or more); decreased glucose tolerance, urate crystalluria (less than 0.1%).

Musculoskeletal – Arthralgia, leg cramps, myalgia, myasthenia (1% or more); arthrosis, neck rigidity (0.1% to 1%); chondrodystrophy, generalized spasm (less than 0.1%).

Respiratory – Apnea, atelectasis, bronchiolitis, hiccup, laryngismus, lung edema, lung fibrosis, yawn (less than 0.1%).

Special senses – Conjunctivitis, diplopia, nystagmus, otitis media, tinnitus (1% or more); abnormality of accommodation, blepharitis, dry eyes, eye hemorrhage, hyperacusis, photophobia, retinal edema, taste loss, taste perversion (0.1% to 1%); anisocoria, blindness, corneal ulcer, exophthalmos, extraocular palsy, iritis, keratitis, keratoconjunctivitis, miosis, mydriasis, night blindness, ophthalmoplegia, optic atrophy, papilledema, parosmia, ptosis, uveitis (less than 0.1%).

Miscellaneous – Allergic reaction, fever (1% or more); abscess, cellulitis, chills, overdose (0.1% to 1%); anaphylactoid reaction, ascites, granuloma, intentional injury, retroperitoneal fibrosis, shock (less than 0.1%).

➤*Postmarketing:*

CNS – Headache.

GI – Diarrhea, nausea.

Overdosage

➤*Symptoms:* There is limited experience with overdose of pregabalin. The highest reported accidental overdose of pregabalin during the clinical development program was 8,000 mg, and there were no notable clinical consequences.

➤*Treatment:* There is no specific antidote for overdose with pregabalin. If indicated, elimination of unabsorbed drug may be attempted by gastric lavage; observe usual precautions to maintain the airway. General supportive care of the patient is indicated, including monitoring of vital signs and observation of the clinical status of the patient. Contact a certified poison control center for up-to-date information on the management of overdose with pregabalin.

Although hemodialysis has not been performed in the few known cases of overdose, it may be indicated by the patient's clinical state or in patients with significant renal function impairment. Standard hemodialysis procedures result in significant clearance of pregabalin (approximately 50% in 4 hours).

Patient Information

Advise patients that pregabalin may cause angioedema, with swelling of the face, mouth (lip, gum, and tongue), and neck (larynx and pharynx) that can lead to life-threatening respiratory compromise. Instruct patients to discontinue pregabalin and immediately seek medical care if they experience these symptoms.

Advise patients that pregabalin has been associated with hypersensitivity reactions such as blisters, dyspnea, hives, rash, and wheezing. Instruct patients to discontinue pregabalin and seek medical care immediately if they experience these symptoms.

Counsel patients, their caregivers, and families that AEDs, including pregabalin, may increase the risk of suicidal thoughts and behavior and advise them of the need to be alert for the emergence or worsening of symptoms of depression; any unusual changes in mood or behavior; or the emergence of suicidal thoughts, behavior, or thoughts about self-harm. Immediately report behaviors of concern to health care providers.

Counsel patients that pregabalin may cause blurred vision, dizziness, somnolence, and other CNS signs and symptoms. Accordingly, advise patients not to drive, operate complex machinery, or engage in other hazardous activities until they have gained sufficient experience on pregabalin to gauge whether it adversely affects their mental, visual, and/or motor performance.

Counsel patients that pregabalin may cause visual disturbances. Inform patients to notify their health care provider if changes in vision occur.

Advise patients to take pregabalin as prescribed. Abrupt or rapid discontinuation may result in diarrhea, headache, insomnia, or nausea.

Counsel patients that pregabalin may cause edema and weight gain.

PREGABALIN — ORAL

Advise patients that concomitant treatment with pregabalin and a thiazolidinedione antidiabetic agent may lead to an additive effect on edema and weight gain. For patients with preexisting cardiac conditions, this may increase the risk of heart failure.

Instruct patients to promptly report unexplained muscle pain, tenderness, or weakness, particularly if accompanied by malaise or fever.

Inform patients who require concomitant treatment with CNS depressants, such as opiates or benzodiazepines, that they may experience additive CNS adverse reactions, such as somnolence.

Tell patients to avoid consuming alcohol while taking pregabalin because it may potentiate the impairment of motor skills and cause sedation.

Instruct patients to notify their health care provider if they become pregnant or intend to become pregnant during therapy and to notify their health care provider if they are breast-feeding or intend to breast-feed during therapy.

Encourage patients to enroll in the NAAED Pregnancy Registry if they become pregnant. This registry is collecting information about the safety of antiepileptic drugs during pregnancy. To enroll, patients can call the toll-free number 1-888-233-2334.

Inform men being treated with pregabalin who plan to father a child of the potential risk of male-mediated teratogenicity. In preclinical studies in rats, pregabalin was associated with an increased risk of male-mediated teratogenicity. The clinical significance of this finding is uncertain.

Instruct diabetic patients to pay particular attention to skin integrity while being treated with pregabalin. Some animals treated with pregabalin developed skin ulcerations, although no increased incidence of skin lesions associated with pregabalin was observed in clinical trials.

LAMOTRIGINE

Rx	**Lamotrigine** (Various, eg, Taro, Teva)	**Tablets; oral**: 25 mg	May contain lactose. In 25s, 30s, 60s, 90s, 100s, 500s, 1,000s, and UD 100s.
Rx	**Lamictal** (GlaxoSmithKline)		Lactose. (Lamictal 25). White, shield-shaped, scored. In 100s.
Rx	**Lamotrigine Starter Kit** (Various, eg, Taro, Teva)	**Tablets; oral**: 25 mg	May contain lactose. In "Blue Kit."[a]
Rx	**Lamictal Starter Kit** (GlaxoSmith-Kline)		Lactose. (Lamictal 25). White, shield-shaped, scored. In "Blue Kit."[a]
Rx	**Lamotrigine** (ZyGenerics)	**Tablets; oral**: 50 mg	May contain lactose. In 90s, 100s, 500s, and 1,000s.
Rx	**Lamotrigine** (Various, eg, Taro, Teva)	**Tablets; oral**: 100 mg	May contain lactose. In 30s, 60s, 90s, 100s, 500s, 1,000s, 3,000s, and UD 100s.
Rx	**Lamictal** (GlaxoSmithKline)		Lactose. (Lamictal 100). Peach, shield-shaped, scored. In 100s.
Rx	**Lamotrigine** (Various, eg, Taro, Teva)	**Tablets; oral**: 150 mg	May contain lactose. In 30s, 60s, 90s, 100s, 500s, 1,000s, 2,000s, and UD 100s.
Rx	**Lamictal** (GlaxoSmithKline)		Lactose. (Lamictal 150). Cream, shield-shaped, scored. In 60s.
Rx	**Lamotrigine** (Various, eg, Taro, Teva)	**Tablets; oral**: 200 mg	May contain lactose. In 30s, 60s, 90s, 100s, 500s, 1,000s, 1,500s, and UD 100s.
Rx	**Lamictal** (GlaxoSmithKline)		Lactose. (Lamictal 200). Blue, shield-shaped, scored. In 60s.
Rx	**Lamotrigine** (ZyGenerics)	**Tablets; oral**: 250 mg	May contain lactose. In 60s, 90s, and 500s.
Rx	**Lamotrigine Starter Kit** (Various, eg, Taro, Teva	**Tablets; oral**: 25 mg	May contain lactose. In "Green Kit"[b] and "Orange Kit."[c]
		100 mg	May contain lactose. In "Green Kit"[b] and "Orange Kit."[c]
Rx	**Lamictal Starter Kit** (GlaxoSmith-Kline)	**Tablets; oral**: 25 mg	Lactose. (Lamictal 25). White, shield-shaped, scored. In "Green Kit"[b] and "Orange Kit."[c]
		100 mg	Lactose. (Lamictal 100). Peach, shield-shaped, scored. In "Green Kit"[b] and "Orange Kit."[c]
Rx	**Lamictal** (GlaxoSmithKline)	**Tablets, chewable, dispersible; oral**: 2 mg	Saccharin. (LTG 2). White to off-white, round. Black currant flavor. In 30s.
Rx	**Lamotrigine** (Various, eg, Greenstone, Taro, Teva)	**Tablets, chewable, dispersible; oral**: 5 mg	May contain mannitol, saccharin, and/or sucralose. In 30s, 90s, 100s, 500s, 1,000s, and UD 100s.
Rx	**Lamictal** (GlaxoSmithKline)		Saccharin. (GX CL2). White to off-white, capsule shaped. Black currant flavor. In 100s.
Rx	**Lamotrigine** (Various, eg, Greenstone, Taro, Teva)	**Tablets, chewable, dispersible; oral**: 25 mg	May contain mannitol, saccharin, and/or sucralose. In 30s, 90s, 100s, 500s, 1,000s, and UD 100s.
Rx	**Lamictal** (GlaxoSmithKline)		Saccharin. (GX CL5). White, elliptical-shaped. Black currant flavor. In 100s.
Rx	**Lamictal ODT** (GlaxoSmithKline)	**Tablets, orally disintegrating; oral**: 25 mg	Mannitol, sucralose. (LMT 25). White to off-white, round. Cherry flavor. In 30s.
		50 mg	Mannitol, sucralose. (LMT 50). White to off-white, round. Cherry flavor. In 30s.
		100 mg	Mannitol, sucralose. (LAMICTAL 100). White to off-white, round. Cherry flavor. In 30s.
		200 mg	Mannitol, sucralose. (LAMICTAL 200). White to off-white, round. Cherry flavor. In 30s.
Rx	**Lamictal ODT Patient Titration Kit** (GlaxoSmithKline)	**Tablets, orally disintegrating; oral**: 25 mg	Mannitol, sucralose. (LMT 25). White to off-white, round. Cherry flavor. In "Blue ODT Kit."[d]
		50 mg	Mannitol, sucralose. (LMT 50). White to off-white, round. Cherry flavor. In "Blue ODT Kit."[d]
Rx	**Lamictal ODT Patient Titration Kit** (GlaxoSmithKline)	**Tablets, orally disintegrating; oral**: 50 mg	Mannitol, sucralose. (LMT 50). White to off-white, round. Cherry flavor. In "Green ODT Kit."[e]
		100 mg	Mannitol, sucralose. (LMT 100). White to off-white, round. Cherry flavor. In "Green ODT Kit."[e]
Rx	**Lamictal ODT Patient Titration Kit** (GlaxoSmithKline)	**Tablets, orally disintegrating; oral**: 25 mg	Mannitol, sucralose. (LMT 25). White to off-white, round. Cherry flavor. In "Orange ODT Kit."[f]
		50 mg	Mannitol, sucralose. (LMT 50). White to off-white, round. Cherry flavor. In "Orange ODT Kit."[f]
		100 mg	Mannitol, sucralose. (LMT 100). White to off-white, round. Cherry flavor. In "Orange ODT Kit."[f]
Rx	**Lamictal XR** (GlaxoSmithKline)	**Tablets, extended-release; oral**: 25 mg	Lactose. (LAMICTAL XR 25). Yellow with white center, round. Film-coated. In 30s.
		50 mg	Lactose. (LAMICTAL XR 50). Green with white center, round. Film-coated. In 30s.
		100 mg	Lactose. (LAMICTAL XR 100). Orange with white center, round. Film-coated. In 30s.
		200 mg	Lactose. (LAMICTAL XR 200). Blue with white center, round. Film-coated. In 30s.

LAMOTRIGINE

Rx	**Lamictal XR Patient Titration Kit** (GlaxoSmithKline)	**Tablets, extended-release; oral:** 25 mg	Lactose. (LAMICTAL XR 25). Yellow with white center, round. Film-coated. In "Blue XR" Titration Kit.[g]
		50 mg	Lactose. (LAMICTAL XR 50). Green with white center, round. Film-coated. In "Blue XR" Titration Kit.[g]
Rx	**Lamictal XR Patient Titration Kit** (GlaxoSmithKline)	**Tablets, extended-release; oral:** 25 mg	Lactose. (LAMICTAL XR 25). Yellow with white center, round. Film-coated. In "Orange XR" Titration Kit.[h]
		50 mg	Lactose. (LAMICTAL XR 50). Green with white center, round. Film-coated. In "Orange XR" Titration Kit.[h]
		100 mg	Lactose. (LAMICTAL XR 100). Orange with white center, round. Film-coated. In "Orange XR" Titration Kit.[h]
Rx	**Lamictal XR Patient Titration Kit** (GlaxoSmithKline)	**Tablets, extended-release; oral:** 50 mg	Lactose. (LAMICTAL XR 50). Green with white center, round. Film-coated. In "Green XR" Titration Kit.[i]
		100 mg	Lactose. (LAMICTAL XR 100). Orange with white center, round. Film-coated. In "Green XR" Titration Kit.[i]
		200 mg	Lactose. (LAMICTAL XR 200). Blue with white center, round. Film-coated. In "Green XR" Titration Kit.[i]

[a] For patients already taking valproate. Starter kit (Blue Kit) contains 35 of the 25 mg tablets.
[b] For patients taking carbamazepine, phenobarbital, phenytoin, or primidone, and not taking valproate. Starter kit (Green Kit) contains 84 of the 25 mg tablets and 14 of the 100 mg tablets.
[c] For patients not taking carbamazepine, phenobarbital, phenytoin, primidone, or valproate. Starter kit (Orange Kit) contains 42 of the 25 mg tablets and 7 of the 100 mg tablets.
[d] For patients already taking valproate. Titration kits (Blue ODT Kit) contain 21 of the 25 mg orally disintegrating tablet (ODT) tablets and 7 of the 50 mg ODT tablets.
[e] For patients already taking carbamazepine, phenobarbital, phenytoin, or primidone, and not taking valproate. Titration kits (Green ODT Kit) contain 42 of the 50 mg ODT tablets and 14 of the 100 mg ODT tablets.
[f] For patients not taking carbamazepine, phenobarbital, phenytoin, primidone, or valproate. Titration kits (Orange ODT Kit) contain 14 of the 25 mg ODT tablets, 14 of the 50 mg ODT tablets, and 7 of the 100 mg ODT tablets.
[g] For patients already taking valproate. Titration kits (Blue XR Kit) contain 21 of the 25 mg extended-release (ER) tablets and 7 of the 50 mg ER tablets.
[h] For patients not taking carbamazepine, phenobarbital, phenytoin, primidone, or valproate. Titration kits (Orange XR Kit) contain 14 of the 25 mg ER tablets, 14 of the 50 mg ER tablets, and 7 of the 100 mg ER tablets.
[i] For patients already taking carbamazepine, phenobarbital, phenytoin, or primidone, and not taking valproate. Titration kits (Green XR Kit) contain 14 of the 50 mg ER tablets, 14 of the 100 mg ER tablets, and 7 of the 200 mg ER tablets.

LAMOTRIGINE — ORAL

For complete and comparative prescribing information, refer to the Anticonvulsants class monograph.

WARNING

Skin reactions – Lamotrigine can cause serious rashes requiring hospitalization and discontinuation of treatment. The incidence of these rashes, which have included Stevens-Johnson syndrome, is approximately 0.8% (8/1,000) in children (2 to 16 years of age) receiving lamotrigine immediate release as adjunctive therapy for epilepsy and 0.3% (3/1,000) in adults receiving adjunctive therapy for epilepsy. In clinical trials of bipolar and other mood disorders, the rate of serious rash was 0.08% (0.8/1,000) in adult patients receiving lamotrigine as initial monotherapy and 0.13% (1.3/1,000) in adult patients receiving lamotrigine as adjunctive therapy. In a prospectively followed cohort of 1,983 children (2 to 16 years of age) with epilepsy taking adjunctive lamotrigine immediate release, there was 1 rash-related death. In worldwide postmarketing experience, rare cases of toxic epidermal necrolysis and/or rash-related death have been reported in adults and children, but those numbers are too few to permit a precise estimate of the rate.

The risk of serious rash caused by treatment with lamotrigine ER is not expected to differ from that with the immediate-release formulation of lamotrigine. However, the relatively limited treatment experience with lamotrigine ER makes it difficult to characterize the frequency and risk of serious rashes caused by treatment with lamotrigine ER. Lamotrigine ER is not approved for patients younger than 13 years of age.

Other than age, there are no known factors identified to predict the risk of occurrence or the severity of rash associated with lamotrigine. There are suggestions, yet to be proven, that the risk of rash may also be increased by coadministration of lamotrigine with valproate (includes valproic acid and divalproex sodium), exceeding the recommended initial dose of lamotrigine, or exceeding the recommended dose escalation for lamotrigine. However, cases have been reported in the absence of these factors.

Nearly all cases of life-threatening rashes associated with lamotrigine have occurred within 2 to 8 weeks of treatment initiation. However, isolated cases have been reported after prolonged treatment (eg, 6 months). Accordingly, duration of therapy cannot be relied upon as a means to predict the potential risk heralded by the first appearance of a rash.

Although benign rashes also occur with lamotrigine, it is not possible to reliably predict which rashes will prove to be serious or life-threatening. Accordingly, discontinue lamotrigine at the first sign of rash unless the rash is clearly not drug-related. Discontinuation of treatment may not prevent a rash from becoming life-threatening or permanently disabling or disfiguring.

Indications

➤*Bipolar disorder (immediate release only):* For the maintenance treatment of bipolar I disorder to delay the time to occurrence of mood episodes (depression, mania, hypomania, mixed episodes) in adults treated for acute mood episodes with standard therapy. The efficacy of lamotrigine in the acute treatment of mood episodes has not been established.

➤*Epilepsy:*

Adjunctive therapy – As adjunctive therapy for partial seizures, the generalized seizures of Lennox-Gastaut syndrome, and primary generalized tonic-clonic seizures in adults and children 2 years of age and older (immediate release); for primary generalized tonic-clonic seizures and partial-onset seizures with or without secondary generalization in patients 13 years of age and older (ER).

Monotherapy (immediate release only) – For conversion to monotherapy in adults (16 years of age and older) with partial seizures who are receiving treatment with carbamazepine, phenytoin, phenobarbital, primidone, or valproate as the single antiepileptic drug (AED).

➤*Off-label uses:*

Depression – [2] = Fair documentation. Data from double-blind, randomized studies with placebo or active comparator (valproate) and an open-label monotherapy study suggest that lamotrigine is safe and effective for the treatment of depression with comorbid epilepsy. However, long-term efficacy studies in patients with depression and no comorbid conditions, safety studies, and more active comparator studies are needed.

Obesity – [2] = Fair documentation. Results from a small preliminary study indicate that lamotrigine, given at a dosage of 200 mg/day for 26 weeks, does not significantly reduce mean body weight in healthy obese patients; however, a statistically significant reduction in mean body mass index was observed. Given the small number of subjects, larger trials are needed before lamotrigine is used routinely for obesity.

Postpoliomyelitis syndrome – [4] = Insufficient documentation. Evidence from a controlled study in a limited number of patients suggests that lamotrigine may be of therapeutic benefit in the treatment of postpoliomyelitis syndrome–related symptoms.

Prevention of migraine (adults) – [5] = Poor documentation. Noncontrolled pilot studies suggest that lamotrigine may be effective for the prevention of migraine headache in adults, but these positive results were not supported in larger, controlled trials. The American Academy of Neurology practice guidelines do not include a review of lamotrigine, and a recent review of the use of anticonvulsants for migraine preventionconsiders lamotrigine to be no more effective than placebo. Based on the available data and the safety concerns, routine use of lamotrigine for the prevention of migraine is not recommended.

Rectal administration – [4] = Insufficient documentation. Lamotrigine is absorbed too slowly to be of clinical utility in status epilepticus, but may be useful in maintaining current dosing if oral dosing is interrupted for short periods of time. Because there is variable absorption among individuals, it has been recommended that serum concentrations be monitored if prolonged administration is planned.

Restless legs syndrome – [5] = Poor documentation. Although anticonvulsants (eg, gabapentin, carbamazepine, valproic acid) have been used in the management of restless legs syndrome (RLS), published data regarding lamotrigine for this use are insufficient. Guidelines also note that there is little supportive evidence available. Because of the availability of other agents to treat RLS and the unfavorable benefit-risk ratio (eg, probability of serious dermatological reactions) associated with lamotrigine, it is recommended that this drug not be used for RLS until further favorable evidence is available.

Schizophrenia – [4] = Insufficient documentation. Data from randomized trials enrolling more than 500 patients are conflicting on whether or not adjuvant lamotrigine improves schizophrenia symptoms. Data from 3 small, controlled studies, each assessing approximately 30 to 50 treatment-resistant schizophrenic patients, indicated a significant effect of lamotrigine over placebo in reducing Positive and Negative Syndrome Scale (PANSS) positive symptom scores and general psychopathological symptoms, as well as all assessed symptoms and total Scale for the Assessment of Positive Symptoms and Scale for the Assessment of Negative Symptoms (SANS) scores. Two larger trials enrolling more than 400 stable schizophrenic

LAMOTRIGINE — ORAL

patients produced conflicting results regarding the effectiveness of lamotrigine over placebo in reducing Brief Assessment of Cognition in Schizophrenia or SANS scores. Neither of these larger studies showed lamotrigine to be more effective than placebo in reducing PANSS general psychopathological or total score, nor SANS scores. More data are needed to determine the role of lamotrigine in the treatment of schizophrenia before it can be recommended as routine add-on therapy.

Other possible off-label uses – Management of children with absence seizures, juvenile myoclonic epilepsy, and temporal lobe seizures.

Administration and Dosage

➤*General dosing considerations:* To avoid an increased risk of rash, the recommended initial dose and subsequent dose escalations of lamotrigine should not be exceeded. See Black Box Warning for more information.

Lamotrigine starter kits, lamotrigine orally disintegrating tablet titration kits, and lamotrigine ER titration kits provide lamotrigine at doses consistent with the recommended titration schedule for the first 5 weeks of treatment, based on concomitant medication, and are intended to help reduce the potential for rash. The use of these kits is recommended for appropriate patients who are starting or restarting lamotrigine.

It is recommended that lamotrigine not be restarted in patients who discontinued therapy because of rash associated with prior treatment with lamotrigine, unless the potential benefits clearly outweigh the risks. If the decision is made to restart a patient who has discontinued lamotrigine, the need to restart with the initial dosing recommendations should be assessed. The greater the interval of time since the previous dose, the greater the consideration should be given to restarting with the initial dosing recommendations. If a patient has discontinued lamotrigine for a period of more than 5 half-lives, it is recommended that initial dosing recommendations and guidelines be followed. The half-life of lamotrigine is affected by other concomitant medications.

For patients receiving lamotrigine in combination with other AEDs, a reevaluation of all AEDs in the regimen should be considered if a change in seizure control or an appearance or worsening of adverse reactions is observed.

➤*Adults:*

Bipolar disorder –

Usual dosage: Target dosage is 200 mg/day, but may vary depending on concurrent medications. (See the following table.)

Dosage titration: Treatment with lamotrigine is introduced, based on concurrent medications, according to the regimen outlined in the following table.

To avoid an increased risk of rash, the recommended initial dose and subsequent dose escalations of lamotrigine should not be exceeded.

Lamotrigine Immediate Release Escalation Regimen for Bipolar Disorder[a]

	Patients taking valproate[b]	Patients not taking carbamazepine, phenobarbital, phenytoin, primidone,[c] or valproate[b]	Patients taking carbamazepine, phenobarbital, phenytoin, or primidone,[c] and not taking valproate[b]
Weeks 1 and 2	25 mg every other day	25 mg/day	50 mg/day
Weeks 3 and 4	25 mg/day	50 mg/day	100 mg/day in divided doses
Week 5	50 mg/day	100 mg/day	200 mg/day in divided doses
Week 6	100 mg/day	200 mg/day	300 mg/day in divided doses
Week 7	100 mg/day	200 mg/day	Up to 400 mg/day in divided doses

[a] See Drug Interactions for a description of known drug interactions.
[b] Valproate has been shown to inhibit glucuronidation and decrease the apparent clearance of lamotrigine.
[c] These drugs induce lamotrigine glucuronidation and increase clearance. Other drugs that have similar effects include estrogen-containing oral contraceptives. Dosing recommendations for oral contraceptives can be found in Concomitant Therapy. Patients taking rifampin, or other drugs that induce lamotrigine glucuronidation and increase clearance, should follow the same dosing titration/maintenance regimen as that used with anticonvulsants that have this effect.

Dosage adjustment:

• *Discontinuation of concomitant psychotropics* –

Adjustments to Lamotrigine Dosing for Patients With Bipolar Disorder Following Discontinuation of Psychotropic Medications

	Discontinuation of psychotropic drugs (excluding carbamazepine, phenobarbital, phenytoin, primidone,[a] and valproate[b])	After discontinuation of valproate[b]	After discontinuation of carbamazepine, phenobarbital, phenytoin, or primidone[a]
		Current lamotrigine dosage 100 mg/day	Current lamotrigine dosage 400 mg/day
Week 1	Maintain current lamotrigine dose	150 mg/day	400 mg/day
Week 2	Maintain current lamotrigine dose	200 mg/day	300 mg/day
Week 3 onward	Maintain current lamotrigine dose	200 mg/day	200 mg/day

[a] These drugs induce lamotrigine glucuronidation and increase clearance. Other drugs that have similar effects include estrogen-containing oral contraceptives. Dosing recommendations for oral contraceptives can be found in Concomitant Therapy. Patients taking rifampin, or other drugs that induce lamotrigine glucuronidation and increase clearance, should follow the same dosing titration/maintenance regimen as that used with anticonvulsants that have this effect.
[b] Valproate has been shown to inhibit glucuronidation and decrease the apparent clearance of lamotrigine.

• *Introduction of concomitant psychotropics* – If other drugs are subsequently introduced, the dose of lamotrigine may need to be adjusted. In particular, the introduction of valproate requires reduction in the dose of lamotrigine.

Duration of therapy: Patients should be periodically reassessed to determine the need for maintenance treatment.

Epilepsy –

Adjunctive therapy:

• *Immediate release* –

Dosage titration:

Lamotrigine Immediate Release Escalation Regimen in Patients With Epilepsy

	Patients taking valproate[a]	Patients not taking carbamazepine, phenobarbital, phenytoin, primidone,[b] or valproate[a]	Patients taking carbamazepine, phenobarbital, phenytoin, or primidone,[b] and not taking valproate[a]
Weeks 1 and 2	25 mg every other day	25 mg/day	50 mg/day
Weeks 3 and 4	25 mg/day	50 mg/day	100 mg/day (in 2 divided doses)
Week 5 onward to maintenance	Increase by 25 to 50 mg/day every 1 to 2 weeks	Increase by 50 mg/day every 1 to 2 weeks	Increase by 100 mg/day every 1 to 2 weeks
Usual maintenance dose	100 to 400 mg/day with valproate and other drugs that induce glucuronidation 100 to 200 mg/day with valproate alone (1 or 2 divided doses)	225 to 375 mg/day (in 2 divided doses)	300 to 500 mg/day (in 2 divided doses)

[a] Valproate has been shown to inhibit glucuronidation and decrease the apparent clearance of lamotrigine.
[b] These drugs induce glucuronidation and increase clearance. Other drugs that have similar effects include estrogen-containing oral contraceptives. Dosing recommendations for oral contraceptives can be found in Concomitant Therapy. Patients taking rifampin, or other drugs that induce lamotrigine glucuronidation and increase clearance, should follow the same dosing titration/maintenance regimen as that used with anticonvulsants that have this effect.

Maintenance dosage: See the previous table for lamotrigine immediate release maintenance dosing.

LAMOTRIGINE — ORAL

• *ER* –

Dosage titration:

Lamotrigine ER Escalation Regimen			
	Patients taking valproate[a]	Patients not taking carbamazepine, phenobarbital, phenytoin, primidone,[b] or valproate[a]	Patients taking carbamazepine, phenobarbital, phenytoin, or primidone,[b] and not taking valproate[a]
Weeks 1 and 2	25 mg every other day	25 mg/day	50 mg/day
Weeks 3 and 4	25 mg/day	50 mg/day	100 mg/day
Week 5	50 mg/day	100 mg/day	200 mg/day
Week 6	100 mg/day	150 mg/day	300 mg/day
Week 7	150 mg/day	200 mg/day	400 mg/day
Maintenance range (week 8 and onward)	200 to 250 mg/day[c]	300 to 400 mg/day[c]	400 to 600 mg/day[c]

[a] Valproate has been shown to inhibit glucuronidation and decrease the apparent clearance of lamotrigine.

[b] These drugs induce glucuronidation and increase clearance. Other drugs that have similar effects include estrogen-containing oral contraceptives. Dosing recommendations for oral contraceptives can be found in Concomitant Therapy. Patients taking rifampin, or other drugs that induce glucuronidation and increase clearance, should follow the same dosing titration/maintenance regimen as that used with anticonvulsants that have this effect.

[c] Dose increases at week 8 or later should not exceed 100 mg daily at weekly intervals.

Maintenance dosage: See the previous table for lamotrigine ER maintenance dosing.

Monotherapy (conversion from adjunctive therapy): The goal of the transition regimen is to effect the conversion to monotherapy with lamotrigine immediate release under conditions that ensure adequate seizure control while mitigating the risk of serious rash associated with the rapid titration of lamotrigine immediate release.

• *Immediate release* –

Maintenance dosage: 500 mg/day in 2 divided doses.

Conversion from adjunctive therapy with carbamazepine, phenobarbital, phenytoin, or primidone to monotherapy with lamotrigine: After achieving a dosage of 500 mg/day of lamotrigine immediate release according to the escalation regimen, the concomitant AED should be withdrawn by 20% decrements each week over a 4-week period.

Conversion from adjunctive therapy with valproate to monotherapy with lamotrigine:

Conversion From Adjunctive Therapy With Valproate to Monotherapy With Lamotrigine Immediate Release in Patients ≥ 16 Years of Age With Epilepsy		
	Lamotrigine immediate release	Valproate
Step 1	Achieve a dosage of 200 mg/day (if not already on 200 mg/day) according to escalation regimen	Maintain previous stable dose
Step 2	Maintain at 200 mg/day	Decrease to 500 mg/day by decrements no greater than 500 mg/day per week, and then maintain the dosage of 500 mg/day for 1 week
Step 3	Increase to 300 mg/day and maintain for 1 week	Simultaneously decrease to 250 mg/day and maintain for 1 week
Step 4	Increase by 100 mg/day every week to achieve maintenance dosage of 500 mg/day	Discontinue

Off-label dosing –

Depression: [2] = Fair documentation. 100 to 500 mg daily. Lamotrigine dose varied when used adjunctively with other AEDs.

Obesity: [2] = Fair documentation. 25 mg/day orally for 2 weeks, titrated to a maximum of 200 mg/day for up to 26 weeks.

Postpoliomyelitis syndrome: [4] = Insufficient documentation. 50 to 100 mg daily for 4 weeks.

Rectal administration: [4] = Insufficient documentation. Two kinetic studies used single doses of lamotrigine 100 mg as a chewable dispersible tablet or as a compressed tablet. Prior to rectal administration, each subject self-administered a *Fleet* enema. A lamotrigine 100 mg tablet was crushed and mixed with 6 mL of room temperature tap water followed by two 2 mL syringe tubing rinses. The suspension was administered via a small catheter into the rectal vault while in the lateral decubitus position. The supine position was maintained for 60 minutes to minimize expulsion of the drug.

Schizophrenia: [4] = Insufficient documentation. 100 to 400 mg/day orally for up to 24 weeks.

➤*Children:*

Epilepsy –

Adjunctive therapy:

• *Immediate release* –

Older than 12 years of age: See Adults for dosing.

Lamotrigine Immediate Release Escalation Regimen in Patients > 12 Years of Age With Epilepsy			
	Patients taking valproate[a]	Patients not taking carbamazepine, phenobarbital, phenytoin, primidone,[b] or valproate[a]	Patients taking carbamazepine, phenobarbital, phenytoin, or primidone,[b] and not taking valproate[a]
Weeks 1 and 2	25 mg every other day	25 mg/day	50 mg/day
Weeks 3 and 4	25 mg/day	50 mg/day	100 mg/day (in 2 divided doses)
Week 5 onwards to maintenance	Increase by 25 to 50 mg/day every 1 to 2 weeks	Increase by 50 mg/day every 1 to 2 weeks	Increase by 100 mg/day every 1 to 2 weeks
Usual maintenance dose	100 to 400 mg/day with valproate and other drugs that induce glucuronidation 100 to 200 mg/day with valproate alone (1 or 2 divided doses)	225 to 375 mg/day (in 2 divided doses)	300 to 500 mg/day (in 2 divided doses)

[a] Valproate has been shown to inhibit glucuronidation and decrease the apparent clearance of lamotrigine.

[b] These drugs induce glucuronidation and increase clearance. Other drugs that have similar effects include estrogen-containing oral contraceptives. Dosing recommendations for oral contraceptives can be found in Concomitant Therapy. Patients taking rifampin, or other drugs that induce lamotrigine glucuronidation and increase clearance, should follow the same dosing titration/maintenance regimen as that used with anticonvulsants that have this effect. See the previous table for lamotrigine immediate release maintenance dosing.

In patients receiving multidrug regimens employing carbamazepine, phenytoin, phenobarbital, or primidone without valproate, maintenance dosages of adjunctive lamotrigine immediate release as high as 700 mg/day have been used.

In patients receiving valproate alone, maintenance dosages of adjunctive lamotrigine immediate release as high as 200 mg/day have been used.

The advantage of using doses greater than those recommended has not been established in controlled trials.

2 to 12 years of age: Smaller starting doses and lower dose escalations than those used in clinical trials are recommended because of the suggestion that the risk of rash may be decreased by smaller starting doses and slower dose escalations. Therefore, maintenance doses will take longer to reach in clinical practice than in clinical trials.

Lamotrigine Immediate Release Escalation Regimen in Patients 2 to 12 Years of Age With Epilepsy[a]			
	Patients taking valproate[b]	For patients not taking carbamazepine, phenobarbital, phenytoin, primidone,[c] or valproate[b]	For patients taking carbamazepine, phenobarbital, phenytoin, or primidone,[c] and not taking valproate[b]
Weeks 1 and 2	0.15 mg/kg/day in 1 or 2 divided doses, rounded down to the nearest whole tablet	0.3 mg/kg/day in 1 or 2 divided doses, rounded down to the nearest whole tablet	0.6 mg/kg/day in 2 divided doses, rounded down to the nearest whole tablet
Weeks 3 and 4	0.3 mg/kg/day in 1 or 2 divided doses, rounded down to the nearest whole tablet	0.6 mg/kg/day in 2 divided doses, rounded down to the nearest whole tablet	1.2 mg/kg/day in 2 divided doses, rounded down to the nearest whole tablet
Week 5 onward to maintenance	The dose should be increased every 1 to 2 weeks as follows: Calculate 0.3 mg/kg/day, round this amount down to the nearest whole tablet, and add this amount to the previously administered daily dose.	The dose should be increased every 1 to 2 weeks as follows: Calculate 0.6 mg/kg/day, round this amount down to the nearest whole tablet, and add this amount to the previously administered daily dose.	The dose should be increased every 1 to 2 weeks as follows: Calculate 1.2 mg/kg/day, round this amount down to the nearest whole tablet, and add this amount to the previously administered daily dose.

LAMOTRIGINE — ORAL

Lamotrigine Immediate Release Escalation Regimen in Patients 2 to 12 Years of Age With Epilepsy[a]			
	Patients taking valproate[b]	For patients not taking carbamazepine, phenobarbital, phenytoin, primidone,[c] or valproate[b]	For patients taking carbamazepine, phenobarbital, phenytoin, or primidone,[c] and not taking valproate[b]
Usual maintenance dose	1 to 5 mg/kg/day (maximum, 200 mg/day in 1 or 2 divided doses); 1 to 3 mg/kg/day with valproate alone	4.5 to 7.5 mg/kg/day (maximum, 300 mg/day in 2 divided doses)	5 to 15 mg/kg/day (maximum, 400 mg/day in 2 divided doses)
Maintenance doses in patients weighing less than 30 kg	May need to be increased by as much as 50%, based on clinical response	May need to be increased by as much as 50%, based on clinical response	May need to be increased by as much as 50%, based on clinical response

[a] Note: Only whole tablets should be used for dosing.
[b] Valproate has been shown to inhibit glucuronidation and decrease the apparent clearance of lamotrigine.
[c] These drugs induce glucuronidation and increase the clearance. Other drugs that have similar effects include estrogen-containing oral contraceptives. Dosing recommendations for oral contraceptives can be found in Concomitant Therapy. Patients taking rifampin, or other drugs that induce lamotrigine glucuronidation and increase clearance, should follow the same dosing titration/maintenance regimen as that used with anticonvulsants that have this effect.

Initial Lamotrigine Immediate Release Weight-Based Dosing Guide for Patients 2 to 12 Years of Age Taking Valproate			
If the patient's weight is		Give this daily dose, using the most appropriate combination of lamotrigine immediate-release 2 and 5 mg tablets	
>	<	Weeks 1 and 2	Weeks 3 and 4
6.7 kg	14 kg	2 mg every other day	2 mg/day
14.1 kg	27 kg	2 mg/day	4 mg/day
27.1 kg	34 kg	4 mg/day	8 mg/day
34.1 kg	40 kg	5 mg/day	10 mg/day

See previous tables for lamotrigine immediate release maintenance dosing.

Maintenance doses in patients weighing less than 30 kg, regardless of age or concomitant AED, may need to be increased by as much as 50%, based on clinical response.

• *ER –*

13 years of age and older: See Adults for dosing.

Lamotrigine ER Escalation Regimen in Patients ≥ 13 Years of Age			
	Patients taking valproate[a]	Patients not taking carbamazepine, phenobarbital, phenytoin,[b] primidone,[b] or valproate[a]	Patients taking carbamazepine, phenobarbital, phenytoin, or primidone,[b] and not taking valproate[a]
Weeks 1 and 2	25 mg every other day	25 mg/day	50 mg/day
Weeks 3 and 4	25 mg/day	50 mg/day	100 mg/day
Week 5	50 mg/day	100 mg/day	200 mg/day
Week 6	100 mg/day	150 mg/day	300 mg/day
Week 7	150 mg/day	200 mg/day	400 mg/day
Maintenance range (week 8 and onward)	200 to 250 mg/day[c]	300 to 400 mg/day[c]	400 to 600 mg/day[c]

[a] Valproate has been shown to inhibit glucuronidation and decrease the apparent clearance of lamotrigine.
[b] These drugs induce glucuronidation and increase clearance. Other drugs that have similar effects include estrogen-containing oral contraceptives. Dosing recommendations for oral contraceptives can be found in Concomitant Therapy. Patients on rifampin, or other drugs that induce glucuronidation and increase clearance, should follow the same dosing titration/maintenance regimen as that used with anticonvulsants that have this effect.
[c] Dose increases at week 8 or later should not exceed 100 mg daily at weekly intervals.

See the previous table for lamotrigine ER maintenance dosing.

The advantage of using doses higher than those recommended has not been established in controlled trials.

➤*Renal function impairment:* Initial doses of lamotrigine should be based on patients' concomitant medications; reduced maintenance doses may be effective for patients with significant renal impairment.

➤*Hepatic function impairment:* Escalation and maintenance doses should be adjusted according to clinical response.

Moderate and severe hepatic impairment (without ascites) – Reduce initial, escalation, and maintenance doses by approximately 25%.

Severe hepatic impairment – Reduce initial, escalation, and maintenance doses by 50%.

➤*Concomitant therapy:*

Estrogen-containing oral contraceptives –

Dosage adjustment:

In women, starting estrogen-containing oral contraceptives while taking a stable dose of lamotrigine and not taking carbamazepine, phenobarbital, phenytoin, primidone, or other drugs such as rifampin that induce lamotrigine glucuronidation, the maintenance dose will in most cases need to be increased by as much as 2-fold in order to maintain a consistent lamotrigine plasma level. The dose increases should begin at the same time that the oral contraceptive is introduced and continue, based on clinical response, no more rapidly than 50 to 100 mg/day every week. Dose increases should not exceed the recommended rate unless lamotrigine plasma levels or clinical response support larger increases.

Discontinuation of estrogen-containing contraceptive therapy: For women not taking carbamazepine, phenobarbital, phenytoin, primidone, or other drugs, such as rifampin, that induce lamotrigine glucuronidation, the maintenance dose of lamotrigine will in most cases need to be decreased by as much as 50% in order to maintain a consistent lamotrigine plasma level. The decrease in dose of lamotrigine should not exceed 25% of the total daily dose per week over a 2-week period, unless clinical response or lamotrigine plasma levels indicate otherwise.

➤*Conversion:* Patients may be converted directly from immediate-release to ER tablets. The initial dose of lamotrigine ER should match the total daily dose of lamotrigine immediate release; however, some subjects on concomitant enzyme-inducing agents may have lower plasma levels of lamotrigine on conversion and should be monitored.

Following conversion to lamotrigine ER, all patients (but especially those on drugs that induce lamotrigine glucuronidation) should be closely monitored for seizure control. Depending on the therapeutic response after conversion, the total daily dose may need to be adjusted within the recommended dosing instructions.

➤*Discontinuation of therapy:* Lamotrigine should not be abruptly discontinued. A step-wise reduction of dose over at least 2 weeks (approximately 50% per week) is recommended unless safety concerns require a more rapid withdrawal.

➤*Administration:*

Chewable dispersible tablets – Only whole tablets should be administered. If the calculated dose cannot be achieved using whole tablets, the dose should be rounded down to the nearest whole tablet.

Chewable dispersible tablets may be swallowed whole, chewed, or dispersed in water or diluted fruit juice. If the tablets are chewed, consume a small amount of water or diluted fruit juice to aid in swallowing.

To disperse chewable dispersible tablets, add the tablets to a small amount of liquid (5 mL, or enough to cover the medication). Approximately 1 minute later, when the tablets are completely dispersed, swirl the solution and administer the entire quantity immediately. No attempt should be made to administer partial quantities of the dispersed tablets.

Orally disintegrating tablets – Orally disintegrating tablets should be placed on the tongue and moved around in the mouth. The tablet will disintegrate rapidly, can be swallowed with or without water, and can be taken with or without food.

ER tablets – Should be taken once daily, with or without food. Tablets must be swallowed whole and must not be chewed, crushed, or divided.

➤*Storage/Stability:* Store at 25°C (77°F); excursions are permitted to 15° to 30°C (59° to 86°F). Store in a dry place and protect from light.

Orally disintegrating tablets – Store between 20° and 25°C (68° and 77°F); excursions are permitted between 15° and 30°C (59° and 86°F).

Actions

➤*Pharmacology:* The precise mechanism(s) by which lamotrigine exerts its anticonvulsant action is unknown. In animal models designed to detect anticonvulsant activity, lamotrigine was effective in preventing seizure spread in the maximal electroshock and pentylenetetrazol tests and prevented seizures in the visually and electrically evoked after-discharge tests for antiepileptic activity. Lamotrigine also displayed inhibitory properties in the kindling model in rats during kindling development and in the fully kindled state. The relevance of these models to human epilepsy, however, is not known.

One proposed mechanism of action of lamotrigine, the relevance of which remains to be established in humans, involves an effect on sodium channels. In vitro pharmacological studies suggest that lamotrigine inhibits voltage-sensitive sodium channels, thereby stabilizing neuronal membranes and consequently modulating presynaptic transmitter release of excitatory amino acids (eg, glutamate, aspartate).

LAMOTRIGINE — ORAL

➤*Pharmacokinetics:*

Mean Lamotrigine Immediate Release Pharmacokinetic Parameters in Healthy Volunteers and Adults With Epilepsy[a,b]

Adult study population	T_{max} (h)	t½ (h)	Cl/F (mL/min/kg)
Healthy volunteers taking no other medication			
Single-dose lamotrigine (n = 179)	2.2 (0.25 to 12)	32.8 (14 to 103)	0.44 (0.12 to 1.1)
Multiple-dose lamotrigine (n = 36)	1.7 (0.5 to 4)	25.4 (11.6 to 61.6)	0.58 (0.24 to 1.15)
Healthy volunteers taking valproate			
Single-dose lamotrigine (n = 6)	1.8 (1 to 4)	48.3 (31.5 to 88.6)	0.3 (0.14 to 0.42)
Multiple-dose lamotrigine (n = 18)	1.9 (0.5 to 3.5)	70.3 (41.9 to 113.5)	0.18 (0.12 to 0.33)
Patients with epilepsy taking valproate only			
Single-dose lamotrigine (n = 4)	4.8 (1.8 to 8.4)	58.8 (30.5 to 88.8)	0.28 (0.16 to 0.4)
Patients with epilepsy taking EIAEDs plus valproate			
Single-dose lamotrigine (n = 25)	3.8 (1 to 10)	27.2 (11.2 to 51.6)	0.53 (0.27 to 1.04)
Patients with epilepsy taking EIAEDs[c]			
Single-dose lamotrigine (n = 24)	2.3 (0.5 to 5)	14.4 (6.4 to 30.4)	1.1 (0.51 to 2.22)
Multiple-dose lamotrigine (n = 17)	2 (0.75 to 5.93)	12.6 (7.5 to 23.1)	1.21 (0.66 to 1.82)

[a] T_{max} = time of maximal plasma concentration; t½ = reaction half-time; Cl/F = apparent plasma clearance; EIAEDs = enzyme-inducing antiepileptic drugs.

[b] The majority of the parameter means determined in each study had coefficients of variation between 20% and 40% for t½ and Cl/F and between 30% and 70% for T_{max}. The overall mean values were calculated from individual study means that were weighted based on the number of volunteers/patients in each study. The number in parentheses after each parameter mean represent the range of individual volunteer/patient values across studies.

[c] Carbamazepine, phenobarbital, phenytoin, and primidone have been shown to increase the apparent clearance of lamotrigine. Estrogen-containing oral contraceptives and other drugs, such as rifampin, that induce lamotrigine glucuronidation have also been shown to increase the apparent clearance of lamotrigine.

Absorption – Lamotrigine is rapidly and completely absorbed after oral administration with negligible first-pass metabolism (absolute bioavailability, 98%). Peak plasma concentrations of the immediate-release formulation occur anywhere from 1.4 to 4.8 hours following drug administration. Lamotrigine chewable/dispersible tablets were equivalent, whether they were administered dispersed in water, chewed and swallowed, or swallowed as whole, to lamotrigine compressed tablets in terms of rate and extent of absorption. In terms of rate and extent of absorption, lamotrigine orally disintegrating tablets, whether disintegrated in the mouth or swallowed whole with water, were equivalent to the lamotrigine compressed tablets swallowed with water.

In comparison with lamotrigine immediate release, the plasma lamotrigine levels following administration of lamotrigine ER are not associated with any significant changes in trough plasma concentrations and are characterized by lower peaks, longer time to peaks, and lower peak-to-trough fluctuation, as described in detail in the following.

In an open-label, crossover study of 44 subjects with epilepsy receiving concomitant AEDs, the steady-state pharmacokinetics of lamotrigine were compared following administration of equivalent total doses of lamotrigine ER given once daily with those of lamotrigine immediate release given twice daily. In this study, the T_{max} following administration of lamotrigine ER was 4 to 6 hours in patients taking carbamazepine, phenobarbital, phenytoin, or primidone; 9 to 11 hours in patients taking valproic acid; and 6 to 10 hours in patients taking AEDs other than carbamazepine, phenobarbital, phenytoin, primidone, or valproic acid. In comparison, the median T_{max} following administration of lamotrigine immediate release was between 1 and 1.5 hours.

The steady-state trough concentrations for lamotrigine ER were similar to or higher than those of lamotrigine immediate release depending on concomitant AED. A mean reduction in the lamotrigine peak plasma concentrations (maximal drug concentration [C_{max}]) by 11% to 29% was observed for lamotrigine ER compared with lamotrigine immediate release, resulting in a decrease in the peak-to-trough fluctuation in serum lamotrigine concentrations. However, in some subjects receiving enzyme-inducing AEDs, a reduction in C_{max} of 44% to 77% was observed. The degree of fluctuation was reduced by 17% in patients taking enzyme-inducing AEDs, 34% in patients taking valproic acid, and 37% in patients taking AEDs other than carbamazepine, phenobarbital, phenytoin, primidone, or valproic acid. Lamotrigine ER and immediate-release regimens were similar with respect to area under the curve (AUC, a measure of the extent of bioavailability) for patients receiving AEDs other than those known to induce the metabolism of lamotrigine. The relative bioavailability of lamotrigine ER was approximately 21% lower than lamotrigine immediate release in subjects receiving enzyme-inducing AEDs. However, in some subjects in this group, a reduction in exposure of up to 70% was observed when switched to lamotrigine ER. Therefore, doses may need to be adjusted in some subjects based on therapeutic response.

Steady-State Bioavailability of Lamotrigine Extended Release Relative to Immediate Release at Equivalent Daily Doses (Ratio of Extended Release to Immediate Release 90% CI)[a]

Concomitant AED	$AUC_{(0-24ss)}$	C_{max}	C_{min}
EIAEDs[b]	0.79 (0.69 to 0.9)	0.71 (0.61 to 0.82)	0.99 (0.89 to 1.09)
Valproic acid	0.94 (0.81 to 1.08)	0.88 (0.75 to 1.03)	0.99 (0.88 to 1.1)
AEDs other than EIAEDs[b] or valproic acid	1 (0.88 to 1.14)	0.89 (0.78 to 1.03)	1.14 (1.03 to 1.25)

[a] CI = confidence interval; C_{min} = trough plasma concentration.

[b] EIAEDs include carbamazepine, phenobarbital, phenytoin, and primidone.

Distribution – Estimates of the mean apparent volume of distribution (Vd/F) of lamotrigine following oral administration ranged from 0.9 to 1.3 L/kg. Vd/F is independent of dose and is similar following single and multiple doses in patients with epilepsy and in healthy volunteers.

Data from in vitro studies indicate that lamotrigine is approximately 55% bound to human plasma proteins at plasma lamotrigine concentrations from 1 to 10 mcg/mL (10 mcg/mL is 4 to 6 times the C_{min} observed in the controlled efficacy trials). Because lamotrigine is not highly bound to plasma proteins, clinically significant interactions with other drugs through competition for protein binding sites are unlikely. The binding of lamotrigine to plasma proteins did not change in the presence of therapeutic concentrations of phenobarbital, phenytoin, or valproate. Lamotrigine did not displace other AEDs (carbamazepine, phenobarbital, phenytoin) from protein binding sites.

Metabolism – Lamotrigine is metabolized predominantly by glucuronic acid conjugation; the major metabolite is an inactive 2-N-glucuronide conjugate.

Enzyme induction: Following multiple administrations (150 mg twice daily) to healthy volunteers taking no other medications, lamotrigine induced its own metabolism, resulting in a 25% decrease in half-life and a 37% increase in Cl/F at steady state compared with values obtained in the same volunteers following a single dose. Evidence gathered from other sources suggests that self-induction by lamotrigine may not occur when lamotrigine is given as adjunctive therapy in patients receiving carbamazepine, phenobarbital, phenytoin, primidone, or other drugs, such as rifampin, that induce lamotrigine glucuronidation.

Excretion – After oral administration of ^{14}C-lamotrigine 240 mg (15 mcCi) to 6 healthy volunteers, 94% was recovered in the urine and 2% was recovered in the feces. The radioactivity in the urine consisted of unchanged lamotrigine (10%), the 2-N-glucuronide (76%), a 5-N-glucuronide (10%), a 2-N-methyl metabolite (0.14%), and other unidentified minor metabolites (4%).

The elimination half-life and apparent clearance of lamotrigine following administration of lamotrigine immediate release to adults with epilepsy and healthy volunteers is summarized in the following table. Half-life and apparent oral clearance vary depending on concomitant AEDs.

Because the half-life of lamotrigine following administration of single doses of lamotrigine immediate release is comparable with that observed following administration of lamotrigine ER, similar changes in the half-life of lamotrigine would be expected for lamotrigine ER.

Special populations –

Renal function impairment: Twelve volunteers with long-term renal failure (mean creatinine clearance [CrCl], 13 mL/min; range, 6 to 23) and another 6 individuals undergoing hemodialysis were each given a single lamotrigine 100 mg immediate-release dose. The mean plasma half-lives determined in the study were 42.9 hours (long-term renal failure), 13 hours (during hemodialysis), and 57.4 hours (between hemodialysis) compared with 26.2 hours in healthy volunteers. On average, approximately 20% (range, 5.6 to 35.1) of the amount of lamotrigine present in the body was eliminated by hemodialysis during a 4-hour session.

Hepatic function impairment: The mean apparent clearance of lamotrigine in patients with mild (n = 12), moderate (n = 5), severe without ascites (n = 2), and severe with ascites (n = 5) hepatic impairment was 0.3 ± 0.09, 0.24 ± 0.1, 0.21 ± 0.04, and 0.15 ± 0.09 mL/min/kg, respectively, compared with 0.37 ± 0.1 mL/min/kg in healthy controls. Mean half-life of lamotrigine in patients with mild, moderate, severe without ascites, and severe with ascites hepatic impairment was 46 ± 20, 72 ± 44, 67 ± 11, and 100 ± 48 hours, respectively, compared with 33 ± 7 hours in healthy controls.

Elderly: The pharmacokinetics of lamotrigine immediate release following a single 150 mg dose were evaluated in 12 elderly volunteers between 65 and 76 years of age (mean CrCl, 61 mL/min; range, 33 to 108 mL/min). The mean half-life of lamotrigine in these subjects was 31.2 hours (range, 24.5 to 43.4 hours), and the mean clearance was 0.4 mL/min/kg (range, 0.26 to 0.48 mL/min/kg).

Children: Population pharmacokinetic analyses involving patients 2 to 18 years of age demonstrated that lamotrigine clearance was influenced predominantly by total body weight and concurrent AED therapy. The oral clearance of lamotrigine was higher, on a body weight basis, in children than in adults. Weight-normalized lamotrigine clearance was higher in those subjects weighing less than 30 kg compared with those weighing more than 30 kg. Accordingly, patients weighing less than 30 kg may need an increase of as much as 50% in maintenance doses, based on clinical response, as compared with patients weighing more than 30 kg being administered the same AEDs.

LAMOTRIGINE — ORAL

Mean Lamotrigine Pharmacokinetic Parameters in Children With Epilepsy			
Pediatric study population	T_{max} (h)	t½ (h)	Cl/F (mL/min/kg)
10 months to 5.3 years of age			
Patients taking EIAEDs[a] (n = 10)	3 (1 to 5.9)	7.7 (5.7 to 11.4)	3.62 (2.44 to 5.28)
Patients taking AEDs with no known effect on the apparent clearance of lamotrigine (n = 7)	5.2 (2.9 to 6.1)	19 (12.9 to 27.1)	1.2 (0.75 to 2.42)
Patients taking valproate only (n = 8)	2.9 (1 to 6)	44.9 (29.5 to 52.5)	0.47 (0.23 to 0.77)
5 to 11 years of age			
Patients taking EIAEDs [a] (n = 7)	1.6 (1 to 3)	7 (3.8 to 9.8)	2.54 (1.35 to 5.58)
Patients taking EIAEDs[a] plus valproate (n = 8)	3.3 (1 to 6.4)	19.1 (7 to 31.2)	0.89 (0.39 to 1.93)
Patients taking valproate only[b] (n = 3)	4.5 (3 to 6)	65.8 (50.7 to 73.7)	0.24 (0.21 to 0.26)
13 to 18 years of age			
Patients taking EIAEDs[a] (n = 11)	—[c]	—[c]	1.3
Patients taking EIAEDs[a] plus valproate (n = 8)	—[c]	—[c]	0.5
Patients taking valproate only (n = 4)	[c]	[c]	0.3

[a] Carbamazepine, phenobarbital, phenytoin, and primidone have been shown to increase the apparent clearance of lamotrigine. Estrogen-containing oral contraceptives and rifampin have also been shown to increase the apparent clearance of lamotrigine.
[b] Two subjects were included in the calculation for mean T_{max}.
[c] Parameter not estimated.

Gender: The clearance of lamotrigine is not affected by gender. However, during dose escalation of lamotrigine immediate release in 1 clinical trial in patients with epilepsy on a stable dose of valproate (n = 77), mean trough lamotrigine concentrations, unadjusted for weight, were 24% to 45% higher (0.3 to 1.7 mcg/mL) in women than men.

Race: The apparent oral clearance of lamotrigine was 25% lower in non-white patients than white patients.

Contraindications

Hypersensitivity to the drug or its ingredients.

Warnings/Precautions

➤*Dermatological reactions:* Serious rashes associated with hospitalization and discontinuation of lamotrigine have been reported. See the Black Box Warning for more information on serious skin conditions.

Children – The incidence of serious rash associated with hospitalization and discontinuation of lamotrigine immediate release in a prospectively followed cohort of children 2 to 16 years of age with epilepsy receiving adjunctive therapy was approximately 0.8%. There was 1 rash-related death in this 1,983-patient cohort. Additionally, there have been rare cases of toxic epidermal necrolysis with and without permanent sequelae or death in the US and foreign postmarketing experience.

There is evidence that the inclusion of valproate in a multidrug regimen increases the risk of serious, potentially life-threatening rash in children. In children who used valproate concomitantly, 1.2% experienced a serious rash compared with 0.6% of patients not taking valproate.

Lamotrigine ER is not approved in patients younger than 13 years of age.

Adults – Serious rash associated with hospitalization and discontinuation of lamotrigine immediate release occurred in 0.3% of adults who received lamotrigine in premarketing clinical trials of epilepsy. In the bipolar and other mood disorders clinical trials, the rate of serious rash was 0.08% of adult patients who received lamotrigine immediate release as initial monotherapy and 0.13% of adult patients who received lamotrigine immediate release as adjunctive therapy. No fatalities occurred among these individuals. However, in worldwide postmarketing experience, rare cases of rash-related death have been reported, but their numbers are too few to permit a precise estimate of the rate.

Among the rashes leading to hospitalization were Stevens-Johnson syndrome, toxic epidermal necrolysis, angioedema, and a rash associated with a variable number of the following systemic manifestations: facial swelling, fever, hematologic and hepatologic abnormalities, and lymphadenopathy.

There is evidence that the inclusion of valproate in a multidrug regimen increases the risk of serious and potentially life-threatening rash in adults. Specifically, of 584 patients administered lamotrigine with valproate in clinical trials, 1% were hospitalized in association with rash; in contrast, 0.16% of 2,398 clinical trial patients and volunteers administered lamotrigine in the absence of valproate were hospitalized.

Nonserious rash – The risk of nonserious rash may be increased in patients with a history of allergy or rash to other AEDs and also when the recommended initial dose and/or the rate of dose escalation of lamotrigine is exceeded.

➤*Acute multiorgan failure:* Multiorgan failure, which in some cases has been fatal or irreversible, has been observed in patients receiving lamotrigine. Fatalities associated with multiorgan failure and various degrees of hepatic failure have been reported in 2 of 3,796 adults and 4 of 2,435 children who received lamotrigine in clinical trials. No such fatalities have been reported in bipolar patients in clinical trials. Rare fatalities from multiorgan failure have also been reported in compassionate plea and postmarketing use. The majority of these deaths occurred in association with other serious medical events, including status epilepticus, overwhelming sepsis, and hantavirus, making it difficult to identify the initial cause.

Additionally, 3 patients (a woman 45 years of age, a boy 3.5 years of age, and a girl 11 years of age) developed multiorgan dysfunction and disseminated intravascular coagulation 9 to 14 days after lamotrigine was added to their AED regimens. Rash and elevated transaminases were also present in all patients, and rhabdomyolysis was noted in 2 patients. Both children were receiving concomitant therapy with valproate, while the woman was being treated with carbamazepine and clonazepam. All patients subsequently recovered with supportive care after treatment with lamotrigine was discontinued.

➤*Hematologic effects:* There have been reports of blood dyscrasias that may or may not be associated with the hypersensitivity syndrome. These have included anemia, leukopenia, neutropenia, pancytopenia, thrombocytopenia, and rarely, aplastic anemia and pure red cell aplasia.

➤*Suicidal behavior and ideation:* AEDs, including lamotrigine, increase the risk of suicidal thoughts or behavior in patients taking these drugs for any indication. Monitor patients treated with any AED for any indication for the emergence or worsening of depression, suicidal thoughts or behavior, and/or any unusual changes in mood or behavior.

Pooled analysis of 199 placebo-controlled clinical trials (mono- and adjunctive therapy) of 11 different AEDs showed that patients randomized to one of the AEDs had approximately twice the risk (adjusted relative risk, 1.8; 95% CI, 1.2 to 2.7) of suicidal thinking or behavior compared with patients randomized to placebo. In these trials, which had a median treatment duration of 12 weeks, the estimated incidence of suicidal behavior or ideation among 27,863 AED-treated patients was 0.43%, compared with 0.24% among 16,029 placebo-treated patients, representing an increase of approximately 1 case of suicidal thinking or behavior for every 530 patients treated. There were 4 suicides in drug-treated patients in the trials and none in placebo-treated patients, but the number of events is too small to allow any conclusion about drug effect on suicide.

The increased risk of suicidal thoughts or behavior with AEDs was observed as early as 1 week after starting treatment with AEDs and persisted for the duration of treatment assessed. Because most trials included in the analysis did not extend beyond 24 weeks, the risk of suicidal thoughts or behavior beyond 24 weeks could not be assessed.

The relative risk for suicidal thoughts or behavior was higher in clinical trials for epilepsy than in clinical trials for psychiatric or other conditions, but the absolute risk differences were similar for the epilepsy and psychiatric indications.

Anyone considering prescribing lamotrigine or any other AED must balance the risk of suicidal thoughts or behavior with the risk of untreated illness. Epilepsy and many other illnesses for which AEDs are prescribed are themselves associated with morbidity and mortality and an increased risk of suicidal thoughts and behavior. If suicidal thoughts and behavior emerge during treatment, consider whether the emergence of these symptoms in any given patients may be related to the illness being treated.

Patients, their caregivers, and families should be informed that AEDs increase the risk of suicidal thoughts and behavior and should be advised of the need to be alert for the emergence or worsening of the signs and symptoms of depression, any unusual changes in mood or behavior, or the emergence of suicidal thoughts, behavior, or thoughts about self-harm. Behaviors of concerns should be reported immediately to health care providers.

Bipolar disorder – Patients with bipolar disorder may experience worsening of their depressive symptoms and/or the emergence of suicidal ideation and behaviors (suicidality) whether or not they are taking medications for bipolar disorder.

In addition, patients with a history of suicidal behavior or thoughts, patients exhibiting a significant degree of suicidal ideation prior to commencement of treatment, and young adults are at increased risk of suicidal thoughts or suicide attempts and should receive careful monitoring during treatment.

Consider changing the therapeutic regimen, including possibly discontinuing the medication, in patients who experience clinical worsening (including development of new symptoms) and/or the emergence of suicidality, especially if these symptoms are severe, abrupt in onset, or were not part of the patient's presenting symptoms.

Write prescriptions for lamotrigine for the smallest quantity of tablets consistent with good patient management in order to reduce the risk of overdose. Overdoses have been reported for lamotrigine, some of which have been fatal.

➤*Withdrawal seizures:* As with other AEDs, do not abruptly discontinue lamotrigine. In patients with epilepsy, there is a possibility of increasing seizure frequency. In clinical trials in patients with bipolar disorder, 2 patients experienced seizures shortly after abrupt withdrawal of lamotrigine. However, there were confounding factors that may have contributed to the occurrence of seizures in these bipolar patients. Unless safety concerns require a more rapid withdrawal, taper the dose of lamotrigine over a period of at least 2 weeks (approximately 50% reduction per week).

➤*Status epilepticus:* Valid estimates of the incidence of treatment-emergent status epilepticus among patients treated with lamotrigine are difficult to obtain because reporters participating in clinical trials did not all employ identical rules for identifying cases. At a minimum, 7 of 2,343 adult

LAMOTRIGINE — ORAL

patients had episodes that could unequivocally be described as status epilepticus. In addition, a number of reports of variably defined episodes of seizure exacerbation (eg, seizure clusters, seizure flurries) were made.

➤*Sudden unexplained death in epilepsy:* During the premarketing development of lamotrigine, 20 sudden and unexplained deaths were recorded among a cohort of 4,700 patients with epilepsy (5,747 patient-years of exposure).

➤*Melanin-containing tissues:* Because lamotrigine binds to melanin, it could accumulate in melanin-rich tissues over time. This raises the possibility that lamotrigine may cause toxicity in these tissues after extended use. Although ophthalmological testing was performed in 1 controlled clinical trial, the testing was inadequate to exclude subtle effects or injury occurring after long-term exposure. Moreover, the capacity of available tests to detect potentially adverse consequences, if any, of lamotrigine's binding to melanin is unknown.

Accordingly, although there are no specific recommendations for periodic ophthalmological monitoring, be aware of the possibility of long-term ophthalmologic effects.

➤*Hypersensitivity reactions:* Hypersensitivity reactions, some fatal or life-threatening, have also occurred. Some of these reactions have included clinical features of multiorgan failure/function impairment, including hepatic abnormalities and evidence of disseminated intravascular coagulation. It is important to note that early manifestations of hypersensitivity (eg, fever, lymphadenopathy) may be present even though a rash is not evident. If such signs or symptoms are present, evaluate the patient immediately. Discontinue lamotrigine if an alternative etiology for the signs or symptoms cannot be established.

Prior to initiation of treatment with lamotrigine, instruct the patient that a rash or other signs or symptoms of hypersensitivity (eg, fever, lymphadenopathy) may herald a serious medical event; instruct the patient to report any such occurrence to a health care provider immediately.

➤*Renal function impairment:* Lamotrigine is metabolized mainly by glucuronic acid conjugation, with the majority of the metabolites being recovered in the urine. In a small study comparing a single dose of lamotrigine in patients with varying degrees of renal impairment with healthy volunteers, plasma half-life of lamotrigine was significantly longer in the patients with renal impairment.

Initial doses of lamotrigine should be based on patients' AED regimen; reduced maintenance doses may be effective for patients with significant renal impairment. Few patients with severe renal impairment have been evaluated during long-term treatment with lamotrigine. Because there is inadequate experience in this population, use lamotrigine with caution in these patients.

➤*Hepatic function impairment:* Experience in patients with hepatic impairment is limited. Based on a clinical pharmacology study in 24 patients with mild, moderate, and severe liver impairment, the following general recommendations can be made. No dosage adjustment is needed in patients with mild liver impairment. Reduce initial, escalation, and maintenance doses by approximately 25% in patients with moderate and severe liver impairment without ascites and 50% in patients with severe liver impairment with ascites. Escalation and maintenance doses may be adjusted according to clinical response.

➤*Pregnancy: Category C.* As with other antiepileptic drugs, physiological changes during pregnancy may affect lamotrigine concentrations or therapeutic effect. There have been reports of decreased lamotrigine concentrations during pregnancy and restoration of prepartum concentrations after delivery. Check lamotrigine blood levels before, during, and after pregnancy. Dose adjustments may be necessary to maintain clinical response.

There are no adequate and well-controlled studies in pregnant women. Lamotrigine crosses the human placenta. Because animal reproduction studies are not always predictive of human response, use this drug during pregnancy only if the potential benefit justifies the potential risk to the fetus.

No evidence of teratogenicity was found in mice, rats, or rabbits when lamotrigine was orally administered to pregnant animals during the period of organogenesis at doses of up to 1.2, 0.5, and 1.1 times, respectively, on a mg/m^2 basis, the highest usual human maintenance dosage (ie, 500 mg/day). However, maternal toxicity and secondary fetal toxicity producing reduced fetal weight and/or delayed ossification were seen in mice and rats, but not in rabbits, at these doses. Teratology studies were also conducted using bolus intravenous administration of the isethionate salt of lamotrigine in rats and rabbits. In rat dams administered an IV dose at 0.6 times the highest usual human maintenance dose, the incidence of intrauterine death without signs of teratogenicity was increased.

A behavioral teratology study was conducted in rats dosed during the period of organogenesis. At day 21 postpartum, offspring of dams receiving 5 mg/kg/day or higher displayed a significantly longer latent period for open field exploration and a lower frequency of rearing. In a swimming maze test performed on days 39 to 44 postpartum, time to completion was increased in offspring of dams receiving 25 mg/kg/day. These doses represent 0.1 and 0.5 times the clinical dose on a mg/m^2 basis, respectively.

When pregnant rats were orally dosed at 0.1, 0.14, or 0.3 times the highest human maintenance dose (on a mg/m^2 basis) during the latter part of gestation (days 15 to 20), maternal toxicity and fetal death were seen. In dams, food consumption and weight gain were reduced, and the gestation period was slightly prolonged (22.6 vs 22 days in the control group). Stillborn pups were found in all 3 drug-treated groups, with the highest number in the high-dose group. Postnatal death was also seen, but only in the 2 highest doses, and occurred between day 1 and 20. Some of these deaths appear to be drug-related and not secondary to the maternal toxicity. A no-observed-effect level could not be determined for this study.

Although lamotrigine was not found to be teratogenic in the previous studies, lamotrigine decreases fetal folate concentrations in rats, an effect known to be associated with teratogenesis in animals and humans.

Pregnancy registry – To provide information regarding the effects of in utero exposure to lamotrigine, health care providers are advised to recommend that pregnant patients taking lamotrigine enroll in the North American Antiepileptic Drug Pregnancy Registry. This can be done by calling the toll free number 1-888-233-2334 and must be done by patients themselves. Information on the registry can also be found at http://www.aedpregnancyregistry.org.

Health care providers are also encouraged to register patients in the Lamotrigine Pregnancy Registry; enrollment in this registry must be done prior to any prenatal diagnostic tests and before fetal outcome is known. Health care providers can obtain information by calling the Lamotrigine Pregnancy Registry at 1-800-336-2176.

➤*Lactation:* Lamotrigine passes into human milk. Because the effects on the infant exposed to lamotrigine by this route are unknown, breast-feeding while taking lamotrigine is not recommended.

There is a published case report describing a 16-day-old infant who developed several mild episodes of apnea that culminated into a severe cyanotic episode requiring resuscitation. The infant's mother had been using lamotrigine throughout the pregnancy and was taking 850 mg/day at the time of the infant's apneic episodes. The infant had been exclusively breastfed, and on admission had a lamotrigine serum concentration of 4.87 mcg/mL. The mother ceased breast-feeding the infant and the infant fully recovered.

As with any drug, a mother who must take lamotrigine to control her disease and who chooses to breast-feed her infant should carefully monitor the infant for adverse reactions. Some anticonvulsants have produced adverse reactions in breast-feeding infants, whereas others are considered compatible with breast-feeding. Although no adverse reactions have been seen in breast-feeding infants of mothers taking lamotrigine, the number of known cases still is too small to assess the safety of this drug during lactation. Consider monitoring infant serum levels of lamotrigine.

Because of the potential for therapeutic serum concentrations in the infant, the American Academy of Pediatrics classifies lamotrigine as a drug for which the effect on a breast-feeding infant is not known but may be of concern.

➤*Children:* Lamotrigine ER is indicated as adjunctive therapy for primary generalized tonic-clonic seizures and partial onset seizures with or without secondary generalization in patients 13 years of age and older. Safety and effectiveness of lamotrigine ER for any use in patients younger than 13 years of age have not been established.

Lamotrigine immediate release is indicated for adjunctive therapy in patients 2 years of age and older for partial seizures, the generalized seizures of Lennox-Gastaut syndrome, and primary generalized tonic-clonic seizures. Safety and efficacy of lamotrigine immediate release used as adjunctive treatment for partial seizures were not demonstrated in a small, randomized, double-blind, placebo-controlled, withdrawal study in very young children (1 to 24 months of age). Lamotrigine immediate release was associated with an increased risk for infectious adverse reactions (lamotrigine 37%, placebo 5%) and respiratory adverse reactions (lamotrigine 26%, placebo 5%). Infectious adverse reactions included bronchiolitis, bronchitis, ear infection, eye infection, otitis externa, pharyngitis, urinary tract infection, and viral infection. Respiratory adverse reactions included apnea, cough, and nasal congestion.

Safety and effectiveness of lamotrigine immediate release in patients younger than 18 years of age with bipolar disorder have not been established.

➤*Elderly:* In general, use caution in dose selection for an elderly patient, usually starting at the low end of the dosing range, reflecting the greater frequency of hepatic, renal, or cardiac function impairment, and of concomitant disease or other drug therapy.

➤*Monitoring:* The value of monitoring plasma concentrations of lamotrigine has not been established. Because of the possible pharmacokinetic interactions between lamotrigine and other drugs, including AEDs, monitoring of the plasma levels of lamotrigine and concomitant drugs may be indicated, particularly during dose adjustments. In general, exercise clinical judgment regarding monitoring of plasma levels of lamotrigine and other drugs and whether or not dose adjustments are necessary.

Closely monitor patients for clinical worsening (including development of new symptoms) and suicidality, especially at the beginning of a course of treatment or at the time of dose changes.

Drug Interactions

➤*Inducers or inhibitors of glucuronidation:* Because lamotrigine is metabolized predominately by glucuronic acid conjugation, drugs that are known to induce or inhibit glucuronidation may affect the apparent clearance of lamotrigine, and doses of lamotrigine may require adjustment based on clinical response.

➤*Folate inhibitors:* Lamotrigine is a weak inhibitor of dihydrofolate reductase. Be aware of this action when administering other medications that inhibit folate metabolism.

LAMOTRIGINE — ORAL

Lamotrigine Drug Interactions			
Precipitant drug	Object drug[a]		Description
Acetaminophen	Lamotrigine	⬇	Serum lamotrigine concentrations may be reduced, producing a decrease in therapeutic effects. With long-term administration of acetaminophen, monitor the clinical response of the patient and, if an interaction is suspected, it may be necessary to adjust the dose of lamotrigine.
Carbamazepine	Lamotrigine	⬇	Lamotrigine concentration is decreased ≈ 40%. Carbamazepine epoxide metabolite levels may be increased, increasing carbamazepine toxicity. Observe the clinical response of the patient and adjust the lamotrigine dose as needed when starting, stopping, or changing the carbamazepine dose. When adding lamotrigine to regimens containing carbamazepine, monitor for carbamazepine toxicity and reduce the carbamazepine dose as needed.
Lamotrigine	Carbamazepine	⬆	
Contraceptives, hormonal replacement therapy	Lamotrigine	⬇	Lamotrigine levels decreased by 50%. Similar effects may be seen with hormone replacement therapy. Dose adjustment may be necessary. Observe the clinical response of the patient and adjust the lamotrigine dose as needed when starting or stopping hormonal contraceptives.
Lamotrigine	Contraceptives, hormonal replacement therapy	⬇	Levonorgestrel concentrations are decreased by 19%.
Orlistat	Lamotrigine	⬇	Plasma concentrations and pharmacologic effects of lamotrigine may be decreased by orlistat. Observe the clinical response of the patient and adjust the lamotrigine dose as needed when starting or stopping orlistat.
Oxcarbazepine	Lamotrigine	⬇	Data are conflicting. Lamotrigine plasma concentrations may be reduced, decreasing the therapeutic effects. Observe the clinical response of the patient and adjust the lamotrigine dose as needed when starting, stopping, or changing the oxcarbazepine dose.
Phenobarbital, Primidone	Lamotrigine	⬇	Lamotrigine concentration is decreased ≈ 40%, reducing the therapeutic response. Observe the clinical response of the patient and adjust the lamotrigine dose as needed when starting, stopping, or changing the phenobarbital or primidone dose.
Phenytoin	Lamotrigine	⬇	Lamotrigine concentration is decreased ≈ 40%, reducing the therapeutic response. Observe the clinical response of the patient and adjust the lamotrigine dose as needed when starting, stopping, or changing the phenytoin dose.
Protease inhibitors (eg, ritonavir)	Lamotrigine	⬇	Lamotrigine concentration may be reduced, decreasing the therapeutic response. Observe the clinical response of the patient and adjust the lamotrigine dose as needed when starting, stopping, or changing the protease inhibitor dose.
Rifamycins (eg, rifampin)	Lamotrigine	⬇	Rifampin increased the apparent clearance of lamotrigine ≈ 2-fold (AUC decreased ≈ 40%). Observe the clinical response of the patient and adjust the lamotrigine dose as needed when starting, stopping, or changing the rifamycin dose.
Sertraline	Lamotrigine	⬆	Sertraline may elevate lamotrigine plasma concentrations, increasing the pharmacologic effects and risk of adverse reactions. Monitor the clinical response of the patient. If an interaction is suspected, adjust the lamotrigine dose as needed when starting or stopping sertraline.
Succinimides (eg, ethosuximide)	Lamotrigine	⬇	Lamotrigine serum concentrations may be reduced, decreasing the therapeutic effects. Observe the clinical response of the patient and adjust the dose of lamotrigine as needed when starting, stopping, or changing the succinimide dose.
Valproic acid	Lamotrigine	⬆	The addition of valproic acid increased lamotrigine steady-state concentration more than 2-fold. Trough steady-state valproic acid concentration decreased ≈ 25% when lamotrigine was added in 1 study. Another study showed no change in valproic acid concentrations. Because valproate reduces lamotrigine clearance, the dosage of lamotrigine in the presence of valproate is < 50% of that required without valproate. Monitor the clinical response of the patient and adjust the dose of 1 or both drugs as needed.
Lamotrigine	Valproic acid	⬇	
Lamotrigine	Clozapine	⬆	Clozapine plasma concentrations may be elevated, increasing the pharmacologic effects and risk of adverse reactions. Monitor the clinical response of the patient when starting or stopping lamotrigine. Adjust the clozapine dose as needed.
Lamotrigine	Topiramate	⬆	Administration of lamotrigine resulted in a 15% increase in topiramate concentrations. This change is not likely to be clinically important; however, monitor the clinical response of the patient. If an interaction is suspected, adjust the topiramate dose as needed.

[a] ⬆ = object drug increased; ⬇ = object drug decreased.

Adverse Reactions

➤*Adjunctive therapy in adults with epilepsy (immediate release):*
Most common adverse reactions – The most commonly observed (at least 5%) adverse reactions seen in association with lamotrigine during adjunctive therapy in adults and not seen at an equivalent frequency among placebo-treated patients were ataxia, blurred vision, diplopia, dizziness, headache, nausea, rash, somnolence, and vomiting. Ataxia, blurred vision, diplopia, dizziness, nausea, and vomiting were dose related. Ataxia, blurred vision, diplopia, and dizziness occurred more commonly in patients receiving carbamazepine with lamotrigine than in patients receiving other AEDs with lamotrigine. Clinical data suggest a higher incidence of rash, including serious rash, in patients receiving concomitant valproate than in patients not receiving valproate.

Discontinuation – Approximately 11% of the 3,378 adult patients who received lamotrigine as adjunctive therapy in premarketing clinical trials discontinued treatment because of an adverse reaction. The adverse reactions most commonly associated with discontinuation were dizziness (2.8%), headache (2.5%), and rash (3%).

In a dose response study in adults, the rate of discontinuation of lamotrigine for ataxia, blurred vision, diplopia, dizziness, nausea, and vomiting was dose-related.

LAMOTRIGINE — ORAL

Adverse reactions (2% or more) –

Lamotrigine Immediate Release Adjunctive Therapy Adverse Reactions in Adults With Epilepsy (≥ 2%)[a]

Adverse reactions	Lamotrigine (n = 711)	Placebo (n = 419)
CNS		
Anxiety	4%	3%
Ataxia	22%	6%
Concentration disturbance	2%	1%
Depression	4%	3%
Dizziness	38%	13%
Headache	29%	19%
Incoordination	6%	2%
Insomnia	6%	2%
Irritability	3%	2%
Seizure	3%	1%
Somnolence	14%	7%
Speech disorder	3%	0%
Tremor	4%	1%
Dermatologic		
Pruritus	3%	2%
Rash	10%	5%
GI		
Abdominal pain	5%	4%
Anorexia	2%	1%
Constipation	4%	3%
Diarrhea	6%	4%
Dyspepsia	5%	2%
Nausea	19%	10%
Vomiting	9%	4%
GU		
Female patients only	(n = 365)	(n = 207)
Amenorrhea	2%	1%
Dysmenorrhea	7%	6%
Vaginitis	4%	1%
Musculoskeletal		
Arthralgia	2%	0%
Neck pain	2%	1%
Respiratory		
Increased cough	8%	6%
Pharyngitis	10%	9%
Rhinitis	14%	9%
Special senses		
Blurred vision	16%	5%
Diplopia	28%	7%
Vision abnormality	3%	1%
Miscellaneous		
Fever	6%	4%
Flu syndrome	7%	6%
Reaction aggravated (seizure exacerbation)	2%	1%

[a] Patients in these adjunctive studies were receiving 1 to 3 concomitant AEDs (carbamazepine, phenobarbital, phenytoin, or primidone) in addition to lamotrigine or placebo. Patients may have reported multiple adverse reactions during the study or at discontinuation; thus, patients may be included in more than 1 category.

In a randomized, parallel study comparing placebo and lamotrigine 300 and 500 mg/day, some of the more common drug-related adverse reactions were dose-related.

Lamotrigine Immediate Release Dose-Related Adverse Reactions

Adverse reactions	Lamotrigine 300 mg (n = 71)	Lamotrigine 500 mg (n = 72)	Placebo (n = 73)
CNS			
Ataxia	10%	28%[a,b]	10%
Dizziness	31%	54%[a,b]	27%
GI			
Nausea	18%	25%[a]	11%
Vomiting	11%	18%[a]	4%
Special senses			
Blurred vision	11%	25%[a,b]	10%
Diplopia	24%[a]	49%[a,b]	8%

[a] Significantly greater than placebo group (P
[b] Significantly greater than group receiving lamotrigine 300 mg ($P < 0.05$).

Gender/Race – Generally, women receiving lamotrigine as adjunctive therapy or placebo were more likely to report adverse reactions than men. The only adverse reaction for which the reports on lamotrigine were greater than 10% more frequent in women than men (without a corresponding difference by gender with placebo) was dizziness (difference, 16.5%). There was little difference between women and men in the rates of discontinuation of lamotrigine for individual adverse reactions.

➤*Adjunctive therapy in adults with epilepsy (ER):*

Most common adverse reactions – The most commonly observed adverse reactions (at least 4% for lamotrigine ER and more common on drug than placebo) in these 2 double-blind, placebo-controlled trials of adjunctive therapy with lamotrigine ER were, in order of decreasing treatment difference (lamotrigine ER % − Placebo %) incidence, dizziness, tremor/intention tremor, vomiting, and diplopia.

Discontinuation – In these 2 trials, adverse reactions led to withdrawal of 4 (2%) patients in the group receiving placebo and 10 (5%) patients in the group receiving lamotrigine ER. Dizziness was the most common reason for withdrawal in the group receiving lamotrigine ER (5 patients [3%]). The next most common adverse reactions leading to withdrawal in 2 patients each (1%) were headache, nausea, nystagmus, and rash.

Adverse reactions (2% or more) –

Lamotrigine Extended-Release Adverse Reactions in Patients With Epilepsy (≥ 2%)[a]

Adverse reactions	Lamotrigine ER (n = 190)	Placebo (n = 195)
CNS		
Anxiety	3%	0%
Asthenia and fatigue	6%	4%
Cerebellar coordination/balance disorder	3%	0%
Depression	3%	< 1%
Dizziness	14%	6%
Nystagmus	2%	< 1%
Somnolence	5%	3%
Tremor/intention tremor	6%	1%
GI		
Anorexia	3%	2%
Constipation	2%	< 1%
Diarrhea	5%	3%
Dry mouth	2%	1%
Nausea	7%	4%
Vomiting	6%	3%
Respiratory		
Pharyngolaryngeal pain	3%	2%
Sinusitis	2%	1%
Special senses		
Diplopia	5%	< 1%
Vertigo	3%	< 1%
Vision blurred	3%	2%
Miscellaneous		
Hot flush	2%	0%
Myalgia	2%	0%

[a] Note: In these trials, the incidence of nonserious rash was 2% for lamotrigine ER and 3% for placebo. In clinical trials evaluating lamotrigine immediate release, the rate of serious rash was 0.3% in adults on adjunctive therapy for epilepsy.

Titration and maintenance period – The incidence for many adverse reactions caused by lamotrigine ER treatment was increased relative to placebo (ie, lamotrigine % − placebo % = treatment difference of at least 2%) in either the titration or maintenance phases of the study. During the titration phase, an increased incidence (shown in descending order of percent treatment difference) was observed for diarrhea, nausea, vomiting, somnolence, vertigo, myalgia, hot flush, and anxiety. During the maintenance phase, an increased incidence was observed for dizziness, tremor, and diplopia. Some adverse reactions developing in the titration phase were notable for persisting (more than 7 days) into the maintenance phase. These "persistent" adverse reactions included somnolence and dizziness.

LAMOTRIGINE — ORAL

➤*Monotherapy in adults with epilepsy (immediate release):*

Most common adverse reactions – The most commonly observed (at least 5%) adverse reactions associated with the use of lamotrigine during the monotherapy phase of the controlled trial in adults that were not seen at an equivalent rate in the control group were anxiety, chest pain, coordination abnormality, dizziness, dysmenorrhea, dyspepsia, infection, insomnia, nausea, pain, rhinitis, vomiting, and weight decrease. The most commonly observed (at least 5%) adverse reactions associated with the use of lamotrigine during the conversion to monotherapy (add-on) period that were not seen at an equivalent frequency among low-dose valproate-treated patients were accidental injury, asthenia, ataxia, blurred vision, coordination abnormality, diarrhea, diplopia, dizziness, headache, insomnia, lymphadenopathy, nausea, nystagmus, pruritus, rash, sinusitis, somnolence, tremor, and vomiting.

Discontinuation – Approximately 10% of the 420 adult patients who received lamotrigine as monotherapy in premarketing clinical trials discontinued treatment because of an adverse reaction. The adverse reactions most commonly associated with discontinuation were rash (4.5%), headache (3.1%), and asthenia (2.4%).

Adverse reactions (5% or more) –

Lamotrigine Immediate Release Monotherapy Adverse Reactions in Adults With Partial Seizures (≥ 5%)[a]

Adverse reactions	Lamotrigine monotherapy[b] (n = 43)	Low-dose valproate[c] monotherapy (n = 44)
CNS		
Anxiety	5%	0%
Coordination abnormality	7%	0%
Dizziness	7%	0%
Insomnia	5%	2%
GI		
Dyspepsia	7%	2%
Nausea	7%	2%
Vomiting	9%	0%
GU		
Women only	(n = 21)	(n = 28)
Dysmenorrhea	5%	0%
Miscellaneous		
Chest pain	5%	2%
Infection	5%	2%
Pain	5%	0%
Rhinitis	7%	2%
Weight decrease	5%	2%

[a] Patients in these studies were converted to lamotrigine or valproate monotherapy from adjunctive therapy with carbamazepine or phenytoin. Patients may have reported multiple adverse reactions during the study; thus, patients may be included in more than 1 category.
[b] Up to 500 mg/day.
[c] 1,000 mg/day.

Other adverse reactions (less than 5% and greater than 2%) –

CNS: Amnesia, asthenia, ataxia, decreased reflexes, depression, hypesthesia, increased reflexes, irritability, libido increase, nystagmus, suicidal ideation.

Dermatologic: Contact dermatitis, dry skin, sweating.
GI: Anorexia, dry mouth, peptic ulcer, rectal hemorrhage.
Respiratory: Bronchitis, dyspnea, epistaxis.
Miscellaneous: Fever, peripheral edema, vision abnormality.

➤*Adjunctive therapy in children with epilepsy (immediate release):*

Most common adverse reactions – The most commonly observed (at least 5%) adverse reactions seen in association with the use of lamotrigine as adjunctive treatment in children 2 to 16 years of age and not seen at an equivalent rate in the control group were abdominal pain, accidental injury, asthenia, ataxia, bronchitis, diarrhea, diplopia, dizziness, fever, flu syndrome, infection, nausea, rash, somnolence, tremor, and vomiting.

Discontinuation – In 339 patients 2 to 16 years of age with partial seizures or generalized seizures from Lennox-Gastaut syndrome, 4.2% of patients on lamotrigine and 2.9% of patients on placebo discontinued because of adverse reactions. The most commonly reported adverse reaction that led to discontinuation of lamotrigine was rash.

Approximately 11.5% of the 1,081 children 2 to 16 years of age who received lamotrigine as adjunctive therapy in premarketing clinical trials discontinued treatment because of an adverse reaction. The adverse reactions most commonly associated with discontinuation were rash (4.4%), reaction aggravated (1.7%), and ataxia (0.6%).

Adverse reactions (2% or more) –

Lamotrigine Immediate Release Adverse Reactions in Children With Epilepsy (≥ 2%)

Adverse reactions	Lamotrigine (n = 168)	Placebo (n = 171)
CNS		
Asthenia	8%	4%
Ataxia	11%	3%
Dizziness	14%	4%
Emotional lability	4%	2%
Gait abnormality	4%	2%
Nervousness	2%	1%
Seizures	2%	1%
Somnolence	17%	15%
Thinking abnormality	3%	2%
Tremor	10%	1%
Vertigo	2%	1%
Dermatologic		
Eczema	2%	1%
Photosensitivity	2%	0%
Pruritus	2%	1%
Rash	14%	12%
GI		
Abdominal pain	10%	5%
Constipation	4%	2%
Diarrhea	11%	9%
Dyspepsia	2%	1%
Nausea	10%	2%
Vomiting	20%	16%
Metabolic		
Edema	2%	0%
Facial edema	2%	1%
Respiratory		
Bronchitis	7%	5%
Bronchospasm	2%	1%
Increased cough	7%	6%
Pharyngitis	14%	11%
Sinusitis	2%	1%
Special senses		
Blurred vision	4%	1%
Diplopia	5%	1%
Visual abnormality	2%	0%
Miscellaneous		
Accidental injury	14%	12%
Fever	15%	14%
Flu syndrome	7%	6%
Hemorrhage	2%	1%
Infection	20%	17%
Lymphadenopathy	2%	1%
Pain	5%	4%
Urinary tract infection	3%	0%

➤*Bipolar disorder (immediate release):*

Most common adverse reactions – The most commonly observed (at least 5%) treatment-emergent adverse reactions seen in association with the use of lamotrigine (100 to 400 mg/day) as monotherapy in adults with bipolar disorder in the 2 double-blind, placebo-controlled trials of 18 months' duration and numerically more frequent than in placebo-treated patients are included in the following table. Adverse reactions that occurred in at least 5% of patients and were numerically more common during the dose escalation phase of lamotrigine in these trials (when patients may have been receiving concomitant medications) compared with the monotherapy phase were headache (25%), rash (11%), dizziness (10%), diarrhea (8%), dream abnormality (6%), and pruritus (6%).

Discontinuation – During the monotherapy phase of the double-blind, placebo-controlled trials of 18 months' duration, 13% of 227 patients who received lamotrigine (100 to 400 mg/day), 16% of 190 patients who received placebo, and 23% of 166 patients who received lithium discontinued therapy because of an adverse reaction. The adverse reactions that most commonly led to discontinuation of lamotrigine were rash (3%) and mania/hypomania/mixed mood adverse reactions (2%). Approximately 16% of 2,401 patients who received lamotrigine (50 to 500 mg/day) for bipolar disorder in premar-

LAMOTRIGINE — ORAL

keting trials discontinued therapy because of an adverse reaction, most commonly because of rash (5%) and mania/hypomania/mixed mood adverse reactions (2%).

Adverse reactions (5% or more) –

Lamotrigine Immediate Release Adverse Reactions in Adults With Bipolar Disorder (≥ 5%)[a]		
Adverse reactions	Lamotrigine (n = 227)	Placebo (n = 190)
CNS		
Fatigue	8%	5%
Insomnia	10%	6%
Somnolence	9%	7%
GI		
Abdominal pain	6%	3%
Constipation	5%	2%
Nausea	14%	11%
Vomiting	5%	2%
Xerostomia (dry mouth)	6%	4%
Respiratory		
Exacerbation of cough	5%	3%
Pharyngitis	5%	4%
Rhinitis	7%	4%
Miscellaneous		
Back pain	8%	6%
Rash (nonserious)[b]	7%	5%

[a] Patients in these studies were converted to lamotrigine (100 to 400 mg/day) or placebo monotherapy from add-on therapy with other psychotropic medications. Patients may have reported multiple adverse reactions during the study; thus, patients may be included in more than 1 category.
[b] In the overall bipolar and other mood disorders clinical trials, the rate of serious rash was 0.08% of adult patients who received lamotrigine as initial monotherapy and 0.13% of adult patients who received lamotrigine as adjunctive therapy.

Other reactions that occurred in 5% or more patients, but equally or more frequently in the placebo group, included accidental injury, diarrhea, dizziness, dyspepsia, headache, infection, influenza, mania, and pain.

Other adverse reactions (less than 5% and greater than 1%) –

CNS: Abnormal thoughts, agitation, amnesia, depression, dream abnormality, dyspraxia, emotional lability, hypesthesia, migraine.
Metabolic/Nutritional: Edema, weight gain.
Musculoskeletal: Arthralgia, myalgia, neck pain.
Miscellaneous: Fever, flatulence, sinusitis, urinary frequency.

Abrupt discontinuation – In the 2 maintenance trials, there was no increase in the incidence, severity, or type of adverse reactions in bipolar disorder patients after abruptly terminating lamotrigine therapy. In clinical trials in patients with bipolar disorder, 2 patients experienced seizures shortly after abrupt withdrawal of lamotrigine. However, there were confounding factors that may have contributed to the occurrence of seizures in these bipolar patients.

Mania/Hypomania/Mixed episodes – During the double-blind, placebo-controlled clinical trials in bipolar I disorder in which patients were converted to lamotrigine (100 to 400 mg/day) monotherapy from other psychotropic medications and followed for durations of up to 18 months, the rate of manic, hypomanic, or mixed mood episodes reported as adverse reactions was 5% for patients treated with lamotrigine (n = 227), 4% for patients treated with lithium (n = 166), and 7% for patients treated with placebo (n = 190). In all bipolar controlled trials combined, adverse reactions of mania (including hypomania and mixed mood episodes) were reported in 5% of patients treated with lamotrigine (n = 956), 3% of patients treated with lithium (n = 280), and 4% of patients treated with placebo (n = 803).

➤*Other adverse reactions:*

Cardiovascular – Flushing, hot flashes, hypertension, palpitations, postural hypotension, syncope, tachycardia, vasodilation (0.1% to 1%).

CNS – Confusion, paresthesia (1% or more); akathisia, apathy, aphasia, CNS depression, depersonalization, dysarthria, dyskinesia, euphoria, hallucinations, hostility, hyperkinesia, hypertonia, libido decreased, memory decrease, mind racing, movement disorder, myoclonus, panic attack, paranoid reaction, personality disorder, psychosis, sleep disorder, stupor, suicide ideation (0.1% to 1%); abnormality of accommodation, choreoathetosis, delirium, delusions, dysphoria, dystonia, extrapyramidal syndrome, faintness, hemiplegia, hyperalgesia, hyperesthesia, hypokinesia, hypotonia, manic depression reaction, muscle spasm, neuralgia, neurosis, paralysis, peripheral neuritis, tonic-clonic seizures (less than 0.1%).

Dermatologic – Acne, alopecia, hirsutism, maculopapular rash, skin discoloration, urticaria (0.1% to 1%); angioedema, erythema, erythema multiforme, exfoliative dermatitis, fungal dermatitis, herpes zoster, leukoderma, petechial rash, pustular rash, Stevens-Johnson syndrome, vesiculobullous rash (less than 0.1%).

Endocrine – Goiter, hypothyroidism (less than 0.1%).

GI – Dysphagia, eructation, gastritis, gingivitis, increased appetite, increased salivation, mouth ulceration (0.1% to 1%); GI hemorrhage, glossitis, gum hemorrhage, gum hyperplasia, hematemesis, hemorrhagic colitis, hepatitis, melena, stomach ulcer, stomatitis, tongue edema (less than 0.1%).

GU – Abnormal ejaculation, hematuria, impotence, menorrhagia, polyuria, urinary incontinence (0.1% to 1%); acute kidney failure, anorgasmia, breast abscess, breast neoplasm, creatinine increase, cystitis, dysuria, epididymitis, female lactation, kidney failure, kidney pain, nocturia, urinary retention, urinary urgency (less than 0.1%).

Hematologic/Lymphatic – Ecchymosis, leukopenia (0.1% to 1%); anemia, eosinophilia, fibrin decrease, fibrinogen decrease, iron deficiency anemia, leukocytosis, lymphocytosis, macrocytic anemia, petechia, thrombocytopenia (less than 0.1%).

Hepatic – Abnormal liver function tests, AST increased (0.1% to 1%); ALT increased, bilirubinemia, gamma-glutamyl transpeptidase increase (less than 0.1%)

Metabolic/Nutritional – Alcohol intolerance, alkaline phosphatase increase, general edema, hyperglycemia (less than 0.1%).

Musculoskeletal – Arthritis, leg cramps, myasthenia, twitching (0.1% to 1%); bursitis, muscle atrophy, pathological fracture, tendinous contracture (less than 0.1%).

Respiratory – Yawn (0.1% to 1%); hiccup, hyperventilation (less than 0.1%).

Special senses – Amblyopia (1% or more); conjunctivitis, dry eyes, ear pain, photophobia, taste perversion, tinnitus (0.1% to 1%); deafness, lacrimation disorder, oscillopsia, parosmia, ptosis, strabismus, taste loss, uveitis, visual field defect (less than 0.1%).

Miscellaneous – Allergic reaction, chills, malaise (0.1% to 1%).

➤*Lab test abnormalities:* Treatment with lamotrigine ER caused an increased incidence of subnormal (below the reference range) values in some hematology analytes (eg, total white blood cells, monocytes). The treatment effect (lamotrigine ER % − placebo %) incidence of subnormal counts was 3% for total white blood cells and 4% for monocytes.

➤*Postmarketing:*

CNS – Aseptic meningitis, exacerbation of parkinsonian symptoms in patients with preexisting Parkinson disease, tics.

GI – Esophagitis, pancreatitis.

Hematologic/Lymphatic – Agranulocytosis, hemolytic anemia, lymphadenopathy not associated with hypersensitivity disorder.

Miscellaneous – Apnea, lupus-like reaction, progressive immunosuppression, rhabdomyolysis in patients experiencing hypersensitivity reactions, vasculitis.

Overdosage

➤*Symptoms:* Overdoses involving quantities of up to 15 g have been reported for lamotrigine, some of which have been fatal. Overdose has resulted in ataxia, coma, decreased level of consciousness, increased seizures, intraventricular conduction delay, and nystagmus.

➤*Treatment:* There are no specific antidotes for lamotrigine. Following a suspected overdose, hospitalization of the patient is advised. General supportive care is indicated, including frequent monitoring of vital signs and close observation of the patient. Lamotrigine is rapidly absorbed. It is uncertain whether hemodialysis is an effective means of removing lamotrigine from the blood. In 6 renal failure patients, about 20% of the amount of lamotrigine in the body was removed by hemodialysis during a 4-hour session. Contact a poison control center for information on the management of overdose of lamotrigine.

Patient Information

Prior to initiation of treatment with lamotrigine, inform patients that a rash or other signs or symptoms of hypersensitivity (eg, fever, lymphadenopathy) may herald a serious medical event and instruct patients to report any such occurrence to their health care provider immediately. In addition, instruct patients to notify their health care provider if worsening of seizure control occurs.

Advise patients that lamotrigine may cause dizziness, somnolence, and other symptoms and signs of CNS depression. Accordingly, advise patients not to drive a car or to operate other complex machinery until they have gained sufficient experience on lamotrigine to gauge whether or not it adversely affects their mental or motor performance.

Counsel patients, their caregivers, and families that AEDs, including lamotrigine, may increase the risk of suicidal thoughts and behavior and advise them of the need to be alert for the emergence or worsening of symptoms of depression, any unusual changes in mood or behavior, or the emergence of suicidal thoughts, behavior, or thoughts about self-harm. Report behaviors of concern immediately to health care providers.

Advise patients of the possibility of blood dyscrasias and/or acute multiorgan failure and to contact their health care provider immediately if they experience any signs or symptoms of these conditions.

Advise patients to notify their health care provider if they become pregnant or intend to become pregnant during therapy. Advise patients to notify their health care provider if they intend to breast-feed or are breast-feeding an infant.

Encourage patients to enroll in the NAAED Pregnancy Registry if they become pregnant. This registry is collecting information about the safety of antiepileptic drugs during pregnancy. To enroll, patients can call the toll-free number 1-888-233-2334.

To avoid a medication error of using the wrong drug or formulation, strongly advise patients to visually inspect their tablets to verify that they are lamotrigine as well as the correct formulation each time they fill their pre-

LAMOTRIGINE — ORAL

scription and to immediately talk to their health care provider/pharmacist if they feel they may have received the wrong medication.

Advise women to notify their health care provider if they plan to start or stop use of oral contraceptives or other female hormonal preparations. Inform women that starting estrogen-containing oral contraceptives may significantly decrease lamotrigine plasma levels and that stopping estrogen-containing oral contraceptives (including the "pill-free" week) may significantly increase lamotrigine plasma levels. Also advise women to promptly notify their health care provider if they experience adverse reactions or changes in menstrual pattern (eg, breakthrough bleeding) while receiving lamotrigine in combination with these medications.

Advise patients to notify their health care provider if they stop taking lamotrigine for any reason and not to resume lamotrigine without consulting their health care provider.

Instruct patients to swallow lamotrigine ER tablets whole and not to chew, crush, or divide the tablets.

Instruct patients to swallow lamotrigine tablets whole; chewing the tablets may leave a bitter taste.

Inform patients that lamotrigine chewable dispersible tablets may be swallowed whole, chewed, or mixed in water or diluted fruit juice. If the tablets are chewed, instruct patients to consume a small amount of water or diluted fruit juice to aid in swallowing.

To disperse lamotrigine chewable dispersible tablets, instruct patients to add the tablets to a small amount of liquid (5 mL, or enough to cover the medication) in a glass or spoon. Instruct patients to wait until the tablets are completely dispersed (approximately 1 minute later), mix the solution, and take the entire amount immediately.

RUFINAMIDE

Rx	**Banzel** (Novartis Pharma AG)	**Tablets; oral:** 200 mg	Lactose, PEG. (262). Pink, oblong, scored. Film-coated. In 30s.
		400 mg	Lactose, PEG. (263). Pink, oblong, scored. Film-coated. In 120s.
		Suspension; oral: 40 mg/mL	Parabens, potassium sorbate, propylene glycol. Orange-flavored. In bottles of 460 mL.

RUFINAMIDE — ORAL

Indications

➤*Seizures:* For adjunctive treatment of seizures associated with Lennox-Gastaut syndrome in adults and children 4 years and older.

Administration and Dosage

➤*General dosing considerations:* Tablets can be administered whole, as half tablets, or crushed for dosing flexibility. (See Administration.)

➤*Adults:*

Seizures –

Maximum dose: 3,200 mg/day, administered in 2 equally divided doses.

Initial dosage: 400 to 800 mg/day, administered in 2 equally divided doses.

Dosage titration: Increase the dosage by 400 to 800 mg/day every 2 days until a maximum daily dosage of 3,200 mg/day, administered in 2 equally divided doses, is reached.

Maintenance dosage: 3,200 mg/day.

➤*Children:*

Seizures –

4 years and older:

• *Initial dosage* – Approximately 10 mg/kg/day, administered in 2 equally divided doses.

• *Dosage titration* – Increase the dose by approximately 10 mg/kg increments every other day to a target dosage of 45 mg/kg/day or 3,200 mg/day (whichever is less), administered in 2 equally divided doses.

• *Maintenance dosage* – 45 mg/kg/day or 3,200 mg/day (whichever is less), administered in 2 equally divided doses.

➤*Renal function impairment:*

Hemodialysis – Hemodialysis may reduce exposure to a limited extent (approximately 30%). Accordingly, consider adjusting the rufinamide dose during the dialysis process.

➤*Hepatic function impairment:* Use of rufinamide in patients with hepatic impairment has not been studied. Therefore, use in patients with severe hepatic impairment is not recommended. Caution should be exercised in treating patients with mild to moderate hepatic impairment.

➤*Discontinuation of therapy:* Rufinamide should be withdrawn gradually to minimize the risk of precipitating seizures, seizure exacerbation, or status epilepticus. If abrupt discontinuation of the drug is medically necessary, the transition to another antiepileptic drug (AED) should be made under close medical supervision. In clinical trials, rufinamide discontinuation was achieved by reducing the dose by approximately 25% every 2 days.

➤*Administration:* Rufinamide tablets are scored on both sides and can be cut in half for dosing flexibility. Tablets can be administered whole, as half tablets, or crushed.

Rufinamide should be given with food.

Rufinamide oral suspension should be shaken well before every administration. The provided adapter and calibrated oral dosing syringe should be used to administer the oral suspension. The adapter that is supplied in the product carton should be inserted firmly into the neck of the bottle before use and remain in place for the duration of the usage of the bottle. The dosing syringe should be inserted into the adapter and the dose withdrawn from the inverted bottle. The cap should be replaced after each use. The cap fits properly when the adapter is in place.

➤*Storage/Stability:* Store the tablets at 25°C (77°F); excursions are permitted between 15° and 30°C (59° and 86°F). Protect from moisture. Replace cap securely after opening.

Store the oral suspension at 25°C (77°F); excursions are permitted between 15° and 30°C (59° and 86°F). Replace the cap securely after opening. The cap fits properly in place when the adapter is in place.

Actions

➤*Pharmacology:* The precise mechanism(s) by which rufinamide exerts its antiepileptic effect is unknown. The results of in vitro studies suggest that the principal mechanism of action of rufinamide is modulation of the activity of sodium channels and, in particular, prolongation of the inactive state of the channel. Rufinamide (1 mcM or more) significantly slowed sodium channel recovery from inactivation after a prolonged prepulse in cultured cortical neurons and limited sustained repetitive firing of sodium-dependent action potentials (EC_{50} of 3.8 mcM).

➤*Pharmacokinetics:*

Absorption/Distribution – Rufinamide is well absorbed after oral administration. However, the rate of absorption is relatively slow, and the extent of absorption is decreased as the dose is increased. The pharmacokinetics do not change with multiple dosing.

Following oral administration of rufinamide, peak plasma concentrations (C_{max}) occur between 4 and 6 hours both under fed and fasted conditions. Rufinamide displays decreasing bioavailability with increasing dose after single- and multiple-dose administration. Based on urinary excretion, the extent of absorption was at least 85% following oral administration of a single dose of rufinamide 600 mg under fed conditions.

Multiple-dose pharmacokinetics can be predicted from single-dose data for both rufinamide and its metabolite. Given the dosing frequency of every 12 hours and the half-life of 6 to 10 hours, an observed steady-state peak concentration of about 2 to 3 times the peak concentration after a single dose is expected.

Only a small fraction of rufinamide (34%) is bound to human serum proteins, predominantly to albumin (27%), giving little risk of displacement drug-drug interactions. Rufinamide was evenly distributed between erythrocytes and plasma. The apparent volume of distribution is dependent upon dose and varies with body surface area. The apparent volume of distribution was approximately 50 L at 3,200 mg/day.

Food effects: Food increased the extent of absorption of rufinamide in healthy volunteers by 34% and increased peak exposure by 56% after a single dose of 400 mg, although the time to C_{max} (T_{max}) was not elevated. Clinical trials were performed under fed conditions, and dosing is recommended with food.

Metabolism – Most elimination of rufinamide is via metabolism, with the primary metabolite resulting from enzymatic hydrolysis of the carboxamide moiety to form the carboxylic acid. This metabolic route is not cytochrome P450 (CYP-450) dependent. There are no known active metabolites.

Rufinamide is extensively metabolized but has no active metabolites. Following a radiolabeled dose of rufinamide, less than 2% of the dose was recovered unchanged in urine. The primary biotransformation pathway is carboxylesterase(s)-mediated hydrolysis of the carboxylamide group to the acid derivative CGP 47292. A few minor additional metabolites were detected in urine, which appeared to be acyl-glucuronides of CGP 47292. There is no involvement of oxidizing CYP-450 enzymes or glutathione in the biotransformation process.

Rufinamide is a weak inhibitor of CYP2E1. It did not show significant inhibition of other CYP-450 enzymes. Rufinamide is a weak inducer of CYP3A4 enzymes.

Excretion – Plasma half-life of rufinamide is approximately 6 to 10 hours. Renal excretion is the predominant route of elimination for drug-related material, accounting for 85% of the dose based on a radiolabeled study. Of the metabolites identified in urine, at least 66% of the rufinamide dose was excreted as the acid metabolite CGP 47292, with 2% of the dose excreted as rufinamide.

The plasma elimination half-life is approximately 6 to 10 hours in healthy subjects and patients with epilepsy.

Special populations –

Renal function impairment: Rufinamide pharmacokinetics in 9 patients with severe renal impairment (CrCl of less than 30 mL/min) was similar to that of healthy subjects. Patients undergoing dialysis 3 hours after rufinamide dosing showed a reduction in area under the curve (AUC) and C_{max} by 29% and 16%, respectively. Consider adjusting rufinamide dose for the loss of drug upon dialysis.

Hepatic function impairment: There have been no specific studies investigating the effect of hepatic impairment on the pharmacokinetics of rufinamide. Therefore, use in patients with severe hepatic impairment is not recommended. Exercise caution in treating patients with mild to moderate hepatic impairment.

RUFINAMIDE — ORAL

Contraindications

Patients with familial short QT syndrome.

Warnings/Precautions

➤*Suicidal behavior and ideation:* AEDs increase the risk of suicidal thoughts or behavior in patients taking these drugs for any indication. Monitor patients treated with any AED for any indication for the emergence or worsening of depression, suicidal thoughts or behavior, or any unusual changes in mood or behavior.

Pooled analyses of 199 placebo-controlled clinical trials (mono- and adjunctive therapy) of 11 different AEDs showed that patients randomized to one of the AEDs had approximately twice the risk (adjusted relative risk, 1.8; 95% confidence interval, 1.2% to 2.7%) of suicidal thinking or behavior compared with patients randomized to placebo. In these trials, (median treatment duration, 12 weeks), the estimated incidence rate of suicidal behavior or ideation among 27,863 AED-treated patients was 0.43% compared with 0.24% among 16,029 placebo-treated patients, representing an increase of approximately 1 case of suicidal thinking or behavior for every 530 patients treated. There were 4 suicides in drug-treated patients in the trials and none in placebo-treated patients, but the number of events is too small to allow any conclusion about drug effect on suicide.

The increased risk of suicidal thoughts or behavior was observed as early as 1 week after starting drug treatment and persisted for at least 24 weeks. Because most trials included in the analysis did not extend beyond 24 weeks, the risk of suicidal thoughts or behavior beyond 24 weeks could not be assessed.

The risk of suicidal thoughts or behavior was generally consistent among drugs in the data analyzed. The finding of increased risk with AEDs of varying mechanisms of action and across a range of indications suggests that the risk applies to all AEDs used for any indication. The risk did not vary substantially by age in the clinical trials analyzed.

The relative risk for suicidal thoughts or behavior was higher in clinical trials for epilepsy than in clinical trials for psychiatric or other conditions, but the absolute risk differences were similar.

Anyone considering prescribing rufinamide or any other AED must balance this risk with the risk of untreated illness. Epilepsy and many other illnesses for which AEDs are prescribed are themselves associated with morbidity and mortality and an increased risk of suicidal thoughts and behavior. Consider whether the emergence of these symptoms in any given patient may be related to the illness being treated if suicidal thoughts and behavior emerge during treatment.

Inform patients, their caregivers, and families that AEDs increase the risk of suicidal thoughts and behavior, and advise them of the need to be alert for the emergence or worsening of the signs and symptoms of depression; any unusual changes in mood or behavior; or the emergence of suicidal thoughts, behavior, or thoughts about self-harm. Report behaviors of concern immediately to health care providers.

➤*CNS reactions:* Use of rufinamide has been associated with CNS-related adverse reactions. The most significant of these can be classified into 2 general categories: somnolence or fatigue and coordination abnormalities, dizziness, gait disturbances, and ataxia.

➤*QT interval:* Formal cardiac electrocardiographic studies demonstrated shortening of the QT interval (up to 20 msec) with rufinamide treatment. In a placebo-controlled study of the QT interval, a higher percentage of rufinamide-treated subjects (46% at 2,400 mg, 46% at 3,200 mg, and 65% at 4,800 mg) had a QT shortening of more than 20 msec at T_{max} compared with placebo (5% to 10%).

Reductions of the QT interval below 300 msec were not observed in the formal QT studies with doses of up to 7,200 mg/day. Moreover, there was no signal for drug-induced sudden death or ventricular arrhythmias.

The degree of QT shortening induced by rufinamide is without any known clinical risk. Familial short QT syndrome is associated with an increased risk of sudden death and ventricular arrhythmias, particularly ventricular fibrillation. Such events in this syndrome are believed to occur primarily when the corrected QT interval falls below 300 msec. Nonclinical data also indicate that QT shortening is associated with ventricular fibrillation. Do not treat patients with familial short QT syndrome with rufinamide. Use caution when administering rufinamide with other drugs that shorten the QT interval.

➤*Withdrawal of AEDs:* See Administration and Dosage for more information.

➤*Status epilepticus:* Estimates of the incidence of treatment-emergent status epilepticus among patients treated with rufinamide are difficult because standard definitions were not employed. In a controlled Lennox-Gastaut syndrome trial, 3 of 74 (4.1%) rufinamide-treated patients had episodes that could be described as status epilepticus compared with none of the 64 placebo-treated patients. In all controlled trials that included patients with different epilepsies, 11 of 1,240 (0.9%) rufinamide-treated patients had episodes that could be described as status epilepticus compared with none of 635 placebo-treated patients.

➤*Hypersensitivity reactions:* Multiorgan hypersensitivity syndrome, a serious condition sometimes induced by AEDs, has occurred in association with rufinamide therapy in clinical trials. One patient experienced rash, urticaria, facial edema, fever, elevated eosinophils, stuporous state, and severe hepatitis beginning on day 29 of rufinamide therapy and extending over a course of 30 days of continued rufinamide therapy, with resolution 11 days after discontinuation. Additional possible cases presented with rash and one or more of the following: elevated liver function studies, fever, hematuria, and lymphadenopathy. These cases occurred in children younger than 12 years of age, within 4 weeks of treatment initiation, and were noted to resolve and/or improve upon rufinamide discontinuation. This syndrome has been reported with other anticonvulsants and typically, although not exclusively, presents with fever and rash associated with other organ system involvement. Because this disorder is variable in its expression, other organ system signs and symptoms not noted here may occur. If this reaction is suspected, discontinue rufinamide and start an alternative treatment.

All patients who develop a rash while taking rufinamide must be closely supervised.

➤*Pregnancy: Category C.* Rufinamide produced developmental toxicity when administered orally to pregnant animals at clinically relevant doses.

Rufinamide was administered orally to rats at doses of 20, 100, and 300 mg/kg/day and to rabbits at doses of 30, 200, and 1,000 mg/kg/day during the period of organogenesis (implantation to closure of the hard palate); the high doses are associated with plasma AUCs approximately 2 times the human plasma AUC at the MRHD (3,200 mg/day). Decreased fetal weights and increased incidences of fetal skeletal abnormalities were observed in rats at doses associated with maternal toxicity. In rabbits, embryofetal death, decreased fetal body weights, and increased incidences of fetal visceral and skeletal abnormalities occurred at all but the low dose. The highest dose tested in rabbits was associated with abortion. The no-effect doses for adverse effects on rat and rabbit embryofetal development (20 and 30 mg/kg/day, respectively) were associated with plasma AUCs approximately 0.2 times that in humans at the MRHD).

In a rat pre- and postnatal developmental study (dosing from implantation through weaning) conducted at oral doses of 5, 30, and 150 mg/kg/day (associated with plasma AUCs of up to approximately 1.5 times that in humans at the MRHD), decreased offspring growth and survival were observed at all doses tested. A no-effect dose for adverse effects on pre- and postnatal development was not established. The lowest dose tested was associated with plasma AUC of less than 0.1 times that in humans at the MRHD.

There are no adequate and well-controlled studies in pregnant women. Use rufinamide during pregnancy only if the potential benefit justifies the potential risk to the fetus.

➤*Lactation:* Rufinamide is likely to be excreted in breast milk. Because of the potential for serious adverse reactions in breast-feeding infants from rufinamide, decide whether to discontinue breast-feeding or the drug, taking into account the importance of the drug to the mother.

➤*Children:* The safety and effectiveness in patients with Lennox-Gastaut syndrome have not been established in children younger than 4 years of age.

➤*Elderly:* In general, use caution in dose selection for an elderly patient, usually starting at the low end of the dosing range, reflecting the greater frequency of decreased hepatic, renal, or cardiac function, and of concomitant disease or other drug therapy in elderly patients.

➤*Monitoring:* Monitor patients treated with any AED for any indication for the emergence or worsening of depression, suicidal thoughts or behavior, or any unusual changes in mood or behavior.

Drug Interactions

Based on in vitro studies, rufinamide shows little or no inhibition of most CYP-450 enzymes at clinically relevant concentrations, with weak inhibition of CYP2E1. Drugs that are substrates of CYP2E1 (eg, chlorzoxazone) may have increased plasma levels in the presence of rufinamide, but this has not been studied.

Based on in vivo drug interaction studies with triazolam and oral contraceptives, rufinamide is a weak inducer of CYP3A4 and can decrease exposure of drugs that are substrates of CYP3A4.

Rufinamide Drug Interactions

Precipitant drug	Object drug[a]		Description
Carbamazepine	Rufinamide	↓	Carbamazepine can decrease plasma levels of rufinamide by 19% to 26%, depending on the carbamazepine concentration. Rufinamide can decrease plasma levels of carbamazepine by 7% to 13% based on the maximum recommended dose of rufinamide.
Rufinamide	Carbamazepine		
Phenobarbital	Rufinamide	↓	Phenobarbital can decrease rufinamide plasma concentrations by 25% to 46%, with greater effects in children. Rufinamide can increase phenobarbital concentrations by 8% to 13% in a concentration-dependent manner, especially in children.
Rufinamide	Phenobarbital	↑	
Phenytoin	Rufinamide	↓	Phenytoin can decrease rufinamide plasma concentrations by 25% to 46%, with greater effects in children. Rufinamide can increase phenytoin concentrations by 7% to 21% in a concentration-dependent manner, especially in children.
Rufinamide	Phenytoin	↑	

RUFINAMIDE — ORAL

Rufinamide Drug Interactions			
Precipitant drug	Object drug[a]		Description
Primidone	Rufinamide	↓	Primidone can decrease rufinamide concentrations by 25% to 46%, with greater effects in children.
Valproate	Rufinamide	↑	Valproate can increase rufinamide concentrations by 16% to 70%, with greater effects in children.
Rufinamide	Contraceptive, hormonal	↓	Rufinamide decreased C_{max} and AUC of ethinyl estradiol/norethindrone. Additional nonhormonal forms of contraception are recommended.
Rufinamide	Lamotrigine	↓	Rufinamide can decrease lamotrigine concentrations by 7% to 13% in a concentration-dependent manner, especially in children.
Rufinamide	Triazolam	↓	Rufinamide decreases C_{max} and AUC by 23% and 37%, respectively.

[a] ↑ = object drug increased; ↓ = object drug decreased.

➤*Drug/Food interactions:* Food increased the extent of absorption of rufinamide in healthy volunteers by 34% and increased peak exposure by 56% after a single dose of 400 mg, although the T_{max} was not elevated.

Adverse Reactions

➤*Common CNS reactions:* Somnolence was reported in 24.3% of rufinamide-treated patients compared with 12.5% of placebo-treated patients and led to study discontinuation in 2.7% of rufinamide-treated patients compared with 0% of placebo-treated patients. Fatigue was reported in 9.5% of rufinamide-treated patients compared with 7.8% of placebo-treated patients. It led to study discontinuation in 1.4% of rufinamide-treated patients and 0% of placebo-treated patients.

Dizziness was reported in 2.7% of rufinamide-treated patients compared with 0% of placebo-treated patients, and did not lead to study discontinuation.

Ataxia and gait disturbance were reported in 5.4% and 1.4% of rufinamide-treated patients, respectively, and in no placebo patients. Balance disorder and abnormal coordination were each reported in 0% of rufinamide-treated patients and 1.6% of placebo patients. None of these reactions led to study discontinuation.

➤*Adverse reactions for all treated patients with epilepsy:* The most commonly observed (10% or more) adverse reactions in rufinamide-treated patients, when used as adjunctive therapy at all doses studied (200 to 3,200 mg/day) with a higher frequency than in placebo were dizziness, fatigue, headache, nausea, and somnolence.

At the target dose of 45 mg/kg/day in children, the most commonly observed (5% or more) adverse reactions in rufinamide-treated patients, given as adjunctive therapy, with a higher frequency than placebo were convulsion, dizziness, fatigue, headache, nausea, somnolence, and vomiting.

At doses of up to 3,200 mg/day in adults, the most commonly observed (5% or more) adverse reactions in rufinamide-treated patients, given as adjunctive therapy, at all doses studied, with a higher frequency than placebo were blurred vision, diplopia, dizziness, fatigue, headache, nasopharyngitis, nausea, nystagmus, somnolence, tremor, and vomiting.

Children – Treatment-emergent adverse reactions that occurred in at least 3% of children with epilepsy treated with rufinamide in controlled, adjunctive studies and were numerically more common in patients treated with rufinamide than placebo are presented in the following table.

Rufinamide Adverse Reactions in Children (≥ 3%)		
Adverse reactions	Rufinamide (n = 187)	Placebo (n = 182)
CNS		
Aggression	3%	2%
Ataxia	4%	1%
Disturbance in attention	3%	1%
Dizziness	8%	6%
Fatigue	9%	8%
Headache	16%	8%
Psychomotor hyperactivity	3%	1%
Somnolence	17%	9%
GI		
Abdominal pain upper	3%	2%
Decreased appetite	5%	2%
Nausea	7%	3%
Vomiting	17%	7%
Dermatologic		
Pruritus	3%	0%
Rash	4%	2%
Respiratory		
Bronchitis	3%	2%
Sinusitis	3%	2%
Special senses		
Diplopia	4%	1%
Ear infection	3%	1%
Nasopharyngitis	5%	3%
Miscellaneous		
Influenza	5%	3%

Adults – Treatment-emergent adverse reactions that occurred in at least 3% of adult patients with epilepsy treated with rufinamide (up to 3,200 mg/day) in adjunctive controlled studies and were numerically more common in patients treated with rufinamide than placebo are presented in the following table. In these studies, either rufinamide or placebo was added to current AED therapy.

Rufinamide Adverse Reactions in Adults (≥ 3%)		
Adverse reactions	Rufinamide (n = 823)	Placebo (n = 376)
CNS		
Anxiety	3%	2%
Ataxia	4%	0%
Dizziness	19%	12%
Fatigue	16%	10%
Gait disturbance	3%	1%
Headache	27%	26%
Somnolence	11%	9%
Tremor	6%	5%
Vertigo	3%	1%
GI		
Abdominal pain upper	3%	2%
Constipation	3%	2%
Dyspepsia	3%	2%
Nausea	12%	9%
Vomiting	5%	4%
Special senses		
Diplopia	9%	3%
Nystagmus	6%	5%
Vision blurred	6%	2%
Miscellaneous		
Back pain	3%	1%

➤*Discontinuation of therapy:* In controlled, double-blind, adjunctive clinical studies, 9% of patients receiving rufinamide as adjunctive therapy and 4.4% receiving placebo discontinued as a result of an adverse reaction. The adverse reactions most commonly leading to discontinuation of rufinamide (more than 1%) used as adjunctive therapy were generally similar in adults and children.

In pediatric double-blind, adjunctive clinical studies, 8% of patients receiving rufinamide as adjunctive therapy and 2.2% receiving placebo discontinued as a result of an adverse reaction.

Rufinamide Adverse Reactions Leading to Discontinuation In Children (> 1%)		
Adverse reactions	Rufinamide (n = 187)	Placebo (n = 182)
Convulsion	2%	1%
Fatigue	2%	0%
Rash	2%	1%
Vomiting	1%	0%

In adult double-blind, adjunctive clinical studies (up to 3,200 mg/day), 9.5% of patients receiving rufinamide as adjunctive therapy and 5.9% receiving placebo discontinued as a result of an adverse reaction.

Rufinamide Adverse Reactions Leading to Discontinuation In Adults (> 1%)		
Adverse reactions	Rufinamide (n = 823)	Placebo (n = 376)
Ataxia	1%	0%
Dizziness	3%	1%

RUFINAMIDE — ORAL

Rufinamide Adverse Reactions Leading to Discontinuation In Adults (> 1%)		
Adverse reactions	Rufinamide (n = 823)	Placebo (n = 376)
Fatigue	2%	1%
Headache	2%	1%
Nausea	1%	0%

➤*Other adverse reactions:*

Cardiovascular – First-degree atrioventricular block, right bundle branch block (0.1% to 1%).

GU – Pollakiuria (at least 1%); dysuria, enuresis, hematuria, incontinence, nephrolithiasis, nocturia, polyuria, urinary incontinence (0.1% to 1%).

Hematologic/Lymphatic – Anemia (at least 1%); iron deficiency anemia, leukopenia, lymphadenopathy, neutropenia, thrombocytopenia (0.1% to 1%).

Metabolic/Nutritional – Decreased appetite, increased appetite (at least 1%).

➤*Lab test abnormalities:* Leukopenia (white blood cell count of lower than 3×10^9 L) was more commonly observed in rufinamide-treated patients (43/1,171 [3.7%]) than placebo-treated patients (7/579 [1.2%]) in all controlled trials.

Overdosage

➤*Symptoms:* Because strategies for the management of overdose are continually evolving, it is advisable to contact a certified poison control center to determine the latest recommendations for the management of an overdose of any drug.

One overdose of 7,200 mg/day rufinamide was reported in an adult during the clinical trials. The overdose was associated with no major signs or symptoms, no medical intervention was required, and the patient continued in the study at the target dose.

➤*Treatment:* There is no specific antidote for overdose with rufinamide. If clinically indicated, attempt elimination of unabsorbed drug by induction of gastric lavage. Observe usual precautions to maintain the airway. General supportive care of the patient is indicated, including monitoring of vital signs and observation of the clinical status of the patient.

Hemodialysis – Standard hemodialysis procedures may result in limited clearance of rufinamide. Although there is no experience to date in treating overdose with hemodialysis, the procedure may be considered when indicated by the patient's clinical state.

Patient Information

Inform patients, their families, and their caregivers about the benefits and risks associated with treatment with rufinamide and counsel them in its appropriate use.

Inform patients, their caregivers, and families that AEDs increase the risk of suicidal thoughts and behavior and advise them of the need to be alert for the emergence or worsening of the signs and symptoms of depression, any unusual changes in mood or behavior, or the emergence of suicidal thoughts, behavior, or thoughts about self-harm. Report behaviors of concern immediately to health care providers.

Instruct patients to take rufinamide only as prescribed.

Instruct patients to take rufinamide with food.

Advise patients that, like with all centrally acting medications, alcohol in combination with rufinamide may cause additive CNS effects.

Advise patients about the potential for somnolence or dizziness and advise them not to drive or operate machinery until they have gained sufficient experience on rufinamide to gauge whether it adversely affects their mental and/or motor performance.

Warn women of childbearing age that the concurrent use of rufinamide with hormonal contraceptives may render this method of contraception less effective. Additional nonhormonal forms of contraception are recommended when using rufinamide.

Advise patients to notify their health care provider if they become pregnant or intend to become pregnant during therapy. Advise patients to notify their health care provider if they are breast-feeding or intend to breast-feed.

Advise patients to notify their health care provider if they experience a rash associated with fever.

LEVETIRACETAM

Rx	**Levetiracetam** (Mylan)	**Tablets; oral:** 250 mg	Polydextrose. (M 613). White, round, scored. Film-coated. In 120s and 500s.
Rx	**Keppra** (UCB)		Lactose free, gluten free. PEG, polyvinyl alcohol. (ucb 250). Blue, oblong, scored. Film-coated. In 120s.
Rx	**Levetiracetam** (Various, eg, Boca[a], Mylan)	**Tablets; oral:** 500 mg	May contain polydextrose. (M 615). In 120s and 500s.
Rx	**Keppra** (UCB)		Lactose free, gluten free. PEG, polyvinyl alcohol. (ucb 500). Yellow, oblong, scored. Film-coated. In 120s.
Rx	**Levetiracetam** (Mylan)	**Tablets; oral:** 750 mg	Polydextrose. (M 617). White, capsule shape, scored. Film-coated. In 120s and 500s.
Rx	**Keppra** (UCB)		Lactose free, gluten free. PEG, polyvinyl alcohol. (ucb 750). Orange, oblong, scored. Film-coated. In 120s.
Rx	**Levetiracetam** (Various, eg, Dr. Reddy's Labs, Roxane, Sandoz, Teva, Torrent)	**Tablets; oral:** 1,000 mg	May contain PEG. In 30s, 60s, 100s, 120s, 250s, 500s, and UD 10s.
Rx	**Keppra** (UCB)		Lactose free, gluten free. PEG, polyvinyl alcohol. (ucb 1000). White, oblong, scored. Film-coated. In 60s.
Rx	**Levetiracetam** (Various, eg, Actavis Mid Atlantic, Aurobindo, Roxane)	**Solution; oral:** 100 mg/mL	May contain acesulfame K, maltitol, parabens. In 473 and 500 mL.
Rx	**Keppra** (UCB)		Dye free. Acesulfame K, ammonium glycyrrhizinate, maltitol, parabens. Grape flavor. In 480 mL.
Rx	**Keppra XR** (UCB)	**Tablets, extended-release; oral:** 500 mg	Lactose free, gluten free. PEG 6000. (UCB 500 XR). White/red, oblong. Film-coated. In 60s.
		750 mg	PEG-6000. (UCB 750XR). White, oblong. Film-coated. In 60s.
Rx	**Levetiracetam** (Sun Pharmaceutical)	**Injection, solution, concentrate:** 100 mg/mL	In 5 mL single-use vials.
Rx	**Keppra** (UCB)		In 5 mL single-use vials.

[a] This manufacturer's tablets are gluten-free.

LEVETIRACETAM — ORAL

Refer to the general discussion beginning in the Anticonvulsants introduction.

Indications

➤*Myoclonic seizures:*

Immediate-release tablets/oral solution – Adjunctive therapy in the treatment of myoclonic seizures in adults and adolescents 12 years of age and older with juvenile myoclonic epilepsy.

➤*Partial-onset seizures:*

Immediate-release tablets/oral solution – Adjunctive therapy in the treatment of partial-onset seizures in adults and children 4 years of age and older with epilepsy.

Extended-release (ER) tablets – Adjunctive therapy in the treatment of partial-onset seizures in adults and adolescents 16 years of age and older with epilepsy.

➤*Primary generalized tonic-clonic seizures:*

Immediate-release tablets/oral solution – Adjunctive therapy in the treatment of primary generalized tonic-clonic seizures in adults and children 6 years of age and older with idiopathic generalized epilepsy.

➤*Off-label uses:*

Bipolar disorder (adolescents) – [4] = Insufficient documentation. There are several reports of the use of levetiracetam in adult patients with bipolar disease but the data in adolescents are limited to case reports and demonstrate that levetiracetam has some benefit.

Bipolar disorder – Depressive episodes (adults) – [4] = Insufficient documentation. Reports of levetiracetam use in adults with depressive episodes of bipolar disorder are limited to noncontrolled settings. Results from the largest open-label trial were inconsistent.

Bipolar disorder – Manic or mixed episodes (adults) – [4] = Insufficient documentation. There are several reports of levetiracetam use in adult patients with bipolar disorder presenting as acute mania or mixed episode, but data are limited to noncontrolled settings and results to date have been variable. The majority of the published reports show levetiracetam to have some benefit in these patients, most of whom had refractory disease. However, the results from the largest open-label trial were inconsistent.

Bipolar disorder – Rapid cycling (adults) – [4] = Insufficient documentation. There are several reports of levetiracetam use in adult patients with bipolar disorder, but data are limited to small, open-label trials and case reports. The majority of published reports show levetiracetam had some benefit in these patients, most of whom had refractory disease. However, results from the largest open-label trial were inconsistent.

Migraine prevention (adults) – [4] = Insufficient documentation. Levetiracetam for the prevention of migraine headaches in adults has shown favorable results with a tolerable safety profile; however, these data are limited by small population and noncontrolled study design.

Migraine prevention(children/adolescents) – [4] = Insufficient documentation. Preliminary results suggest that levetiracetam may be effective in preventing migraines in children and adolescents; however, the results are limited by small sample population and open-label study design. Current practice guidelines consider there to be insufficient evidence to make a recommendation for use.

Tardive dyskinesia (neuroleptic induced) – [4] = Insufficient documentation. Initial data suggest levetiracetam may have use in the management of tardive dyskinesia.

Other possible off-label uses – Levetiracetam oral has been used in the neonatal period as a second line of therapy for seizures that have proven refractory to phenobarbital and other anticonvulsants.

Administration and Dosage

➤*Adults:*

Immediate-release tablets/oral solution –

Myoclonic seizures:

• *Initial dosage* – 1,000 mg/day, given as twice-daily dosing (500 mg twice daily).

• *Dosage titration* – Increase dosage by 1,000 mg/day every 2 weeks to the recommended daily dose of 3,000 mg.

• *Maintenance dosage* – 3,000 mg/day. The efficacy of dosages lower than 3,000 mg/day has not been studied.

Partial-onset seizures:

• *Maximum dose* – 3,000 mg/day.

• *Initial dosage* – 1,000 mg/day, given as twice-daily dosing (500 mg twice daily).

• *Dosage titration* – Additional dosing increments may be given (additional 1,000 mg/day every 2 weeks) to a maximum recommended daily dose of 3,000 mg. Dosages greater than 3,000 mg/day have been used in open-label studies for periods of 6 months and longer. There is no evidence that dosages greater than 3,000 mg/day confer additional benefit.

Primary generalized tonic-clonic seizures:

• *Initial dosage* – 1,000 mg/day, given as twice-daily dosing (500 mg twice daily).

• *Dosage titration* – Increase dosage by 1,000 mg/day every 2 weeks to the recommended daily dose of 3,000 mg.

• *Maintenance dosage* – 3,000 mg/day. The efficacy of dosages lower than 3,000 mg/day has not been adequately studied.

ER tablets –

Partial-onset seizures:

• *Maximum dose* – 3,000 mg/day.

• *Initial dosage* – 1,000 mg once daily.

• *Dosage titration* – The daily dosage may be adjusted in increments of 1,000 mg every 2 weeks to a maximum recommended daily dose of 3,000 mg.

Off-label dosing –

Bipolar disorder – Depressive episodes: [4] = Insufficient documentation. Dosages were initiated at 500 mg once or twice daily and titrated to maintenance dosages of up to 3,000 mg daily for up to 8 weeks.

Bipolar disorder – Manic or mixed episodes: [4] = Insufficient documentation. Dosages were initiated at 500 mg daily and titrated to maintenance dosages of up to 4,000 mg daily for up to 6 months.

Bipolar disorder – Rapid cycling: [4] = Insufficient documentation. Dosages were initiated at 500 mg daily and titrated to maintenance dosages of up to 3,000 mg daily for 8 weeks to 6 months.

Prevention of migraine (adults): [4] = Insufficient documentation. 500 to 2,000 mg daily orally (mean, 1,125 mg daily). Levetiracetam 1,000 mg was administered for 6 months in an open-label trial.

Tardive dyskinesia (neuroleptic induced): [4] = Insufficient documentation. Dosages were initiated at 250 mg twice daily and titrated to response based on the Abnormal Involuntary Movement Scale.

➤*Children:*

Immediate-release tablets/oral solution –

Myoclonic seizures:

• *12 years of age and older* – See Adults for dosing.

Partial-onset seizures:

• *4 to younger than 16 years of age* –

Initial dosage: 20 mg/kg in 2 divided doses (10 mg/kg twice daily).

Dosage titration: Increase the daily dose every 2 weeks by increments of 20 mg/kg to the recommended daily dose of 60 mg/kg (30 mg/kg twice daily). If a patient cannot tolerate a daily dose of 60 mg/kg, the daily dose may be reduced. In the clinical trial, the mean daily dose was 52 mg/kg.

Maintenance dosage: 60 mg/kg/day (30 mg/kg twice daily).

Dosage adjustment: Dose patients with a body weight of 20 kg or less with oral solution. Patients with a body weight greater than 20 kg can be dosed with tablets or oral solution.

Levetiracetam Immediate-Release Tablets Weight-Based Dosing for Children

Patient weight	Immediate-release tablets daily dose		
	20 mg/kg/day (twice-daily dosing)	40 mg/kg/day (twice-daily dosing)	60 mg/kg/day (twice-daily dosing)
20.1 to 40 kg	500 mg/day (1 × 250 mg tablet twice daily)	1,000 mg/day (1 × 500 mg tablet twice daily)	1,500 mg/day (1 × 750 mg tablet twice daily)
> 40 kg	1,000 mg/day (1 × 500 mg tablet twice daily)	2,000 mg/day (2 × 500 mg tablets twice daily)	3,000 mg/day (2 × 750 mg tablets twice daily)

• *Oral solution* – Use the dosing calculation provided to determine the appropriate daily dose of oral solution for children based on a daily dosage of 20, 40, or 60 mg/kg/day:

Total daily dosage (mL/day) = (daily dosage [mg/kg/day] × patient weight [kg]) ÷ 100 mg/mL.

Primary generalized tonic-clonic seizures:

• *6 to younger than 16 years of age* –

Initial dosage: 20 mg/kg in 2 divided doses (10 mg/kg twice daily).

Dosage titration: Increase the daily dose every 2 weeks by increments of 20 mg/kg to the recommended daily dose of 60 mg/kg (30 mg/kg twice daily).

Maintenance dosage: 60 mg/kg/day (30 mg/kg twice daily). The efficacy of dosages lower than 60 mg/kg/day has not been adequately studied.

Dosage adjustment: Dose patients with a body weight of 20 kg or less with oral solution. Patients with a body weight greater than 20 kg can be dosed with tablets or oral solution.

Off-label dosing –

Bipolar disorder (adolescents): [4] = Insufficient documentation. As adjunctive therapy administered orally as 250 to 500 mg twice daily for at least 8 weeks. Total duration not specified.

Rational use cannot be established as evidenced by data in limited patient population (less than 30 patients) or inconsistent results. Assessment of appropriate patient population, dose, or efficacy cannot be adequately determined. In addition, significant safety data have been identified by FDA or manufacturer safety notifications (eg, black box warnings).

Epilepsy (neonatal):

• *Maximum dose* – 30 mg/kg/dose.

• *Initial dosage* – 10 mg/kg/dose orally. Administer every 24 hours in the neonatal period, then every 12 hours later in infancy.

• *Dosage titration* – May increase dose upward as needed every 1 to 2 weeks.

Migraine prevention (children/adolescents): [4] = Insufficient documentation. Rational use cannot be established as evidenced by data in limited patient population (less than 30 patients) or inconsistent results. Assessment of appropriate patient population, dose, or efficacy cannot be adequately determined. In addition, significant safety data have been identified by FDA or manufacturer safety notifications (eg, black box warnings).

Levetiracetam oral doses ranged from 250 to 1,500 mg daily, administered on a twice-daily schedule. In one trial, levetiracetam was dosed at 20 to 40 mg/kg/day orally for up to 3 months.

Refractory seizures (6 months to 4 years of age):

• *Maximum dose* – 60 mg/kg/day.

• *Initial dosage* – 5 to 10 mg/kg/day orally, administered in 2 or 3 divided doses.

• *Dosage titration* – Increase the dose if needed and tolerated by 10 mg/kg/day at weekly intervals.

➤*Renal function impairment:* Levetiracetam dosing must be individualized according to the patient's renal function status.

Immediate-release tablets/oral solution –

Levetiracetam Immediate-Release Tablets and Oral Solution Dosage for Adults With Renal Function Impairment[a]

Renal function status	CrCl (mL/min)	Dosage (mg)	Frequency
Healthy	> 80	500 to 1,500	Every 12 h
Mild	50 to 80	500 to 1,000	Every 12 h
Moderate	30 to 50	250 to 750	Every 12 h
Severe	< 30	250 to 500	Every 12 h
ESRD patients using dialysis	—	500 to 1,000	Every 24 h[b]

[a] CrCl = creatinine clearance; ESRD = end-stage renal disease.
[b] Following dialysis, a 250 to 500 mg supplemental dose is recommended.

LEVETIRACETAM — ORAL

ER tablets –

Levetiracetam ER Tablets Dosage for Adult With Renal Function Impairment			
Renal function status	CrCl (mL/min per 1.73 m²)	Dosage (mg)	Frequency
Healthy	> 80	1,000 to 3,000	Every 24 h
Mild	50 to 80	1,000 to 2,000	Every 24 h
Moderate	30 to 50	500 to 1,500	Every 24 h
Severe	< 30	500 to 1,000	Every 24 h

➤*Discontinuation of therapy:* Withdraw antiepileptic drugs (AEDs), including levetiracetam, gradually to minimize the potential of increased seizure frequency.

➤*Administration:* Levetiracetam is given orally, with or without food. Only whole tablets should be administered. Swallow the levetiracetam ER tablets whole; do not chew, break, or crush tablets. Take levetiracetam at the same time(s) each day.

➤*Storage/Stability:* Store at 25°C (77°F); excursions are permitted between 15° and 30°C (59° and 86°F).

Actions

➤*Pharmacology:* The precise mechanism by which levetiracetam exerts its antiepileptic effect is unknown. The antiepileptic activity of levetiracetam was assessed in a number of animal models of epileptic seizures. Levetiracetam did not inhibit single seizures induced by maximal stimulation with electrical current or different chemoconvulsants and showed only minimal activity in submaximal stimulation and in threshold tests. Protection was observed, however, against secondarily generalized activity from focal seizures induced by pilocarpine and kainic acid, 2 chemoconvulsants that induce seizures that mimic some features of human complex-partial seizures with secondary generalization. Levetiracetam also displayed inhibitory properties in the kindling model in rats, another model of human complex-partial seizures, both during kindling development and in the fully kindled state. The predictive value of these animal models for specific types of human epilepsy is uncertain.

In vitro and in vivo recordings of epileptiform activity from the hippocampus have shown that levetiracetam inhibits burst firing without affecting normal neuronal excitability, suggesting that levetiracetam may selectively prevent hypersynchronization of epileptiform burst firing and propagation of seizure activity.

➤*Pharmacokinetics:*

Absorption/Distribution –

Immediate-release tablets/oral solution: Absorption of levetiracetam is rapid, with peak plasma concentrations occurring in about 1 hour following oral administration in fasted subjects. The oral bioavailability of levetiracetam tablets is 100%, and the tablets and oral solution are bioequivalent in rate and extent of absorption. The pharmacokinetics of levetiracetam are linear over the dose range of 500 to 5,000 mg. Steady state is achieved after 2 days of multiple, twice-daily dosing. Levetiracetam and its major metabolite are less than 10% bound to plasma proteins; clinically significant interactions with other drugs through competition for protein-binding sites are therefore unlikely. Its volume of distribution is close to the volume of intracellular and extracellular water.

ER tablets: Levetiracetam ER peak plasma concentrations occur in about 4 hours. The time to peak plasma concentrations is about 3 hours longer with levetiracetam ER than with immediate-release tablets.

Bioequivalency: Single administration of 2 levetiracetam 500 mg ER tablets once daily produced comparable Maximal drug concentration (C_{max}) and area under the curve (AUC) as did the administration of one 500 mg immediate-release tablet twice daily in fasting conditions. After multiple-dose levetiracetam ER tablets intake, extent of exposure (AUC_{0-24}) was similar to extent of exposure after multiple-dose immediate-release tablets intake. C_{max} and minimal drug concentration were lower by 17% and 26%, respectively, after multiple-dose levetiracetam ER tablets intake in comparison with multiple-dose immediate-release tablets intake.

Food effects: Food does not affect the extent of absorption of levetiracetam, but it decreases C_{max} by 20% and delays time to C_{max} (T_{max}) by 1.5 hours. Intake of a high-fat, high-calorie breakfast before the administration of levetiracetam ER tablets resulted in a higher peak concentration and longer median time to peak. The median T_{max} was 2 hours longer in the fed state.

Metabolism – Levetiracetam is not extensively metabolized in humans. The major metabolic pathway is the enzymatic hydrolysis of the acetamide group, which produces the carboxylic acid metabolite ucb L057 (24% of the dose) and is not dependent on any liver CYP-450 isoenzymes. The major metabolite is inactive in animal seizure models. Two minor metabolites were identified as the product of hydroxylation of the 2-oxo-pyrrolidine ring (2% of the dose) and opening of the 2-oxo-pyrrolidine ring in position 5 (1% of the dose). There is no enantiomeric interconversion of levetiracetam or its major metabolite.

Excretion – Levetiracetam plasma half-life in adults is 7 ± 1 hour and is unaffected by dose or repeated administration. Levetiracetam is eliminated from the systemic circulation by renal excretion as unchanged drug, which represents 66% of the administered dose. The total body clearance is 0.96 mL/min/kg, and the renal clearance is 0.6 mL/min/kg. The mechanism of excretion is glomerular filtration with subsequent partial tubular reabsorption. The metabolite ucb L057 is excreted by glomerular filtration and active tubular secretion with a renal clearance of 4 mL/min/kg. Levetiracetam elimination is correlated to CrCl. Levetiracetam clearance is reduced in patients with renal function impairment. Plasma half-life of levetiracetam ER is approximately 7 hours.

Special populations –

Renal function impairment: The disposition of levetiracetam immediate-release was studied in subjects with varying degrees of renal function. Total body clearance of levetiracetam in patients with renal function impairment is reduced by 40% in the mild group (CrCl = 50 to 80 mL/min), 50% in the moderate group (CrCl = 30 to 50 mL/min), and 60% in the severe renal function impairment group (CrCl less than 30 mL/min). Clearance of levetiracetam is correlated with CrCl.

In anuric (ESRD) patients, the total body clearance decreased by 70% compared with healthy subjects (CrCl more than 80 mL/min). Approximately 50% of the pool of levetiracetam in the body is removed during a standard 4-hour hemodialysis procedure.

See Administration and Dosage for more information.

• *ER tablets* – The effect of levetiracetam ER on patients with renal impairment was not assessed in the well-controlled study. However, it is expected that the effect on levetiracetam ER–treated patients would be similar to that seen in well-controlled studies of levetiracetam immediate-release tablets. In patients with ESRD on dialysis, it is recommended that levetiracetam immediate-release be used instead of levetiracetam ER.

Elderly: Pharmacokinetics of levetiracetam immediate-release were evaluated in 16 elderly subjects (61 to 88 years of age) with CrCl ranging from 30 to 74 mL/min. Following oral administration of twice-daily dosing for 10 days, total body clearance decreased by 38%, and the half-life was 2.5 hours longer in elderly patients compared with healthy, younger adults. This is most likely because of the decrease in renal function in elderly patients.

Children:

• *Immediate-release tablets/oral solution* – Pharmacokinetics of levetiracetam immediate-release were evaluated in 24 children 6 to 12 years of age after a single dose (20 mg/kg). The body weight–adjusted apparent clearance of levetiracetam immediate-release was approximately 40% higher than in adults.

A repeat-dose pharmacokinetic study was conducted in children 4 to 12 years of age at doses of 20, 40, and 60 mg/kg/day. The evaluation of the pharmacokinetic profile of levetiracetam immediate release and its metabolite, ucb L057, in 14 children demonstrated rapid absorption of levetiracetam at all doses, with a T_{max} of approximately 1 hour and a half-life of 5 hours across the 3 dosing levels. The pharmacokinetics of levetiracetam immediate-release in children were linear between 20 and 60 mg/kg/day. Population pharmacokinetic analysis showed that body weight was significantly correlated to clearance of levetiracetam in children; clearance increased with an increase in body weight.

Contraindications

None known.

Warnings/Precautions

➤*CNS effects:*

Myoclonic seizures –

Somnolence: In the double-blind, controlled trial in adults and adolescents with juvenile myoclonic epilepsy who were experiencing myoclonic seizures, 11.7% of levetiracetam-treated patients experienced somnolence, compared with 1.7% of placebo patients. No patient discontinued treatment as a result of somnolence. In 1.7% of levetiracetam-treated patients and in 0% of placebo patients, the dose was reduced as a result of somnolence.

Behavioral disorders: A total of 13.3% of levetiracetam patients experienced other behavioral symptoms (eg, aggression, agitation, anger, anxiety, apathy, depersonalization, depression, emotional lability, hostility, irritability), compared with 6.2% of placebo patients. Approximately half of these patients reported these reactions within the first 4 weeks. A total of 1.7% of treated patients discontinued treatment because of these reactions, compared with 0.2% of placebo patients. The treatment dose was reduced in 0.8% of treated patients and in 0.5% of placebo patients. A total of 0.8% of treated patients experienced a serious behavioral reaction (compared with 0.2% of placebo patients) and were hospitalized.

Nonpsychotic behavioral disorders (reported as aggression and irritability) occurred in 5% of levetiracetam-treated patients, compared with 0% of placebo patients. Nonpsychotic mood disorders (reported as depressed mood, depression, and mood swings) occurred in 6.7% of levetiracetam-treated patients, compared with 3.3% of placebo patients. A total of 5% of levetiracetam-treated patients had a reduction in dose or discontinued treatment because of behavior or psychiatric reactions (reported as anxiety, depressed mood, depression, irritability, and nervousness), compared with 1.7% of placebo patients.

Partial-onset seizures – Somnolence, asthenia, and coordination difficulties occurred most frequently within the first 4 weeks of treatment.

Dizziness: Dizziness was reported in 5.2% of levetiracetam ER–treated patients compared with 2.5% of placebo-treated patients.

Somnolence: In controlled trials of adult patients with epilepsy experiencing partial-onset seizures, 14.8% of levetiracetam-treated patients reported somnolence, compared with 8.4% of placebo patients. There was no clear dose response up to 3,000 mg/day. In a study where there was no titration, about 45% of patients receiving 4,000 mg/day reported somnolence. The somnolence was considered serious in 0.3% of the treated patients, compared with 0% in the placebo group. About 3% of levetiracetam-treated patients discontinued treatment because of somnolence, compared with 0.7% of placebo patients. In 1.4% of levetiracetam-treated patients and 0.9% of placebo patients, the dose was reduced; 0.3% of the levetiracetam-treated patients were hospitalized because of somnolence.

• *ER tablets* – In the levetiracetam ER double-blind, controlled trial in patients experiencing partial-onset seizures, 7.8% of levetiracetam ER–treated patients experienced somnolence compared with 2.5% of placebo-treated patients.

LEVETIRACETAM — ORAL

• *Children* – In the double-blind, controlled trial in children with epilepsy experiencing partial-onset seizures, 22.8% of levetiracetam-treated patients experienced somnolence, compared with 11.3% of placebo patients. The design of the study prevented the accurate assessment of dose-response effects. No patient discontinued treatment because of somnolence. In approximately 3% of levetiracetam-treated patients and 3.1% of placebo patients, the dose was reduced as a result of somnolence.

Asthenia: In controlled trials of adult patients with epilepsy experiencing partial-onset seizures, 14.7% of levetiracetam-treated patients reported asthenia, compared with 9.1% of placebo patients. Treatment was discontinued in 0.8% of levetiracetam-treated patients, compared with 0.5% of placebo patients. In 0.5% of levetiracetam-treated patients and in 0.2% of placebo patients, the dose was reduced.

• *Children* – Asthenia was reported in 8.9% of levetiracetam-treated patients, compared with 3.1% of placebo patients. No patient discontinued treatment for asthenia, but asthenia led to a dose reduction in 3% of levetiracetam-treated patients, compared with 0% of placebo patients.

Coordination difficulties: A total of 3.4% of levetiracetam-treated patients experienced coordination difficulties (reported as ataxia, abnormal gait, or incoordination), compared with 1.6% of placebo patients. A total of 0.4% of patients in controlled trials discontinued levetiracetam treatment because of ataxia, compared with 0% of placebo patients. In 0.7% of levetiracetam-treated patients and 0.2% of placebo patients, the dose was reduced because of coordination difficulties; 1 of the levetiracetam-treated patients was hospitalized because of worsening of preexisting ataxia.

Psychotic symptoms: In controlled trials of patients with epilepsy experiencing partial-onset seizures, 5 (0.7%) levetiracetam-treated patients experienced psychotic symptoms, compared with 1 (0.2%) placebo-treated patient. Two (0.3%) levetiracetam-treated patients were hospitalized, and their treatment was discontinued. Both reactions, reported as psychosis, developed within the first week of treatment and resolved within 1 to 2 weeks following treatment discontinuation. Two other reactions, reported as hallucinations, occurred after 1 to 5 months and resolved within 2 to 7 days while the patients remained on treatment. In 1 patient experiencing psychotic depression occurring within a month, symptoms resolved within 45 days while the patient continued treatment.

Suicide attempts: In addition, 4 (0.5%) of the treated patients attempted suicide, compared with 0% of placebo patients. Of these patients, 1 successfully committed suicide. In the other 3 patients, the reactions did not lead to discontinuation or dose reduction. The reactions occurred between 4 weeks and 6 months of treatment. One levetiracetam-treated patient experienced suicidal ideation.

Behavioral symptoms: A total of 13.3% of levetiracetam patients experienced other behavioral symptoms (eg, aggression, agitation, anger, anxiety, apathy, depersonalization, depression, emotional lability, hostility, irritability), compared with 6.2% of placebo patients. Approximately half of these patients reported these reactions within the first 4 weeks. A total of 1.7% of treated patients discontinued treatment because of these reactions, compared with 0.2% of placebo patients. The treatment dose was reduced in 0.8% of treated patients and in 0.5% of placebo patients. A total of 0.8% of treated patients experienced a serious behavioral reaction (compared with 0.2% of placebo patients) and were hospitalized.

• *ER tablets* – A total of 6.5% of levetiracetam ER–treated patients experienced nonpsychotic behavioral disorders (reported as irritability and aggression) compared with 0% of placebo-treated patients. Irritability was reported in 6.5% of levetiracetam ER–treated patients. Aggression was reported in 1.3% of levetiracetam ER–treated patients. No patient discontinued treatment or had a dose reduction as a result of these adverse reactions.

• *Children* – A total of 37.6% of the levetiracetam-treated patients experienced behavioral symptoms (eg, agitation, anxiety, apathy, depersonalization, depression, emotional lability, hostility, hyperkinesia, nervousness, neurosis, personality disorder), compared with 18.6% of placebo patients. Hostility was reported in 11.9% of levetiracetam-treated patients, compared with 6.2% of placebo patients. Nervousness was reported in 9.9% of levetiracetam-treated patients, compared with 2.1% of placebo patients. Depression was reported in 3% of levetiracetam-treated patients, compared with 1% of placebo patients.

A total of 3% of levetiracetam-treated patients discontinued treatment because of psychotic and nonpsychotic adverse reactions, compared with 4.1% of placebo patients. Overall, 10.9% of levetiracetam-treated patients experienced behavioral symptoms associated with discontinuation or dose reduction, compared with 6.2% of placebo patients.

Primary generalized epilepsy – In a long-term, open-label study that examined patients with various forms of primary generalized epilepsy, along with the nonpsychotic behavioral disorders, 2 of 192 patients studied exhibited psychotic-like behavior. Behavior in one case was characterized by auditory hallucinations and suicidal thoughts, and led to levetiracetam discontinuation. The other case was described as worsening of preexistent schizophrenia and did not lead to drug discontinuation.

Primary generalized tonic-clonic seizures – In patients 6 years of age and older experiencing primary generalized tonic-clonic seizures, levetiracetam is associated with behavioral abnormalities.

In the double-blind, controlled trial in patients with idiopathic generalized epilepsy experiencing primary generalized tonic-clonic seizures, irritability was the most frequently reported psychiatric adverse reaction occurring in 6.3% of levetiracetam-treated patients, compared with 2.4% of placebo patients. Additionally, nonpsychotic behavioral disorders (reported as abnormal behavior, aggression, conduct disorder, and irritability) occurred in 11.4% of the levetiracetam-treated patients, compared with 3.6% of placebo patients. Of the levetiracetam-treated patients experiencing nonpsychotic behavioral disorders, 1 patient discontinued treatment because of aggression. Nonpsychotic mood disorders (reported as anger, apathy, depression, mood altered, mood swings, negativism, suicidal ideation, and tearfulness) occurred in 12.7% of levetiracetam-treated patients, compared with 8.3% of placebo patients. No levetiracetam-treated patients discontinued or had a dose reduction as a result of these reactions. One levetiracetam-treated patient experienced suicidal ideation. One patient experienced delusional behavior that required the lowering of the dose of levetiracetam.

➤*Withdrawal seizures:* Withdraw AEDs, including levetiracetam, gradually to minimize the potential of increased seizure frequency.

➤*Hematologic effects:*

Partial-onset seizures –

Immediate-release tablets/oral solution: Minor, but statistically significant, decreases compared with placebo in total mean red blood cell count ($0.03 \times 10^6/mm^3$), mean hemoglobin (0.09 g/dL), and mean hematocrit (0.38%) were seen in levetiracetam-treated patients in controlled trials.

A total of 3.2% of levetiracetam-treated and 1.8% of placebo patients had at least 1 possibly significant (2.8×10^9/L or less) decreased white blood cell count (WBC), and 2.4% of treated and 1.4% of placebo patients had at least 1 possibly significant (1×10^9/L or less) decreased neutrophil count. Of the treated patients with a low neutrophil count, all but 1 rose toward or to baseline with continued treatment. No patient was discontinued secondary to low neutrophil counts.

Children: Minor, but statistically significant, decreases in WBC and neutrophil counts were seen in levetiracetam-treated children compared with placebo. The mean decreases from baseline in the levetiracetam-treated group were -0.4×10^9/L and -0.3×10^9/L, respectively, whereas there were small increases in the placebo group. Mean relative lymphocyte counts increased by 1.7% in levetiracetam-treated patients, compared with a decrease of 4% in placebo patients (statistically significant).

Myoclonic seizures – Although there were no obvious hematologic abnormalities observed in patients with juvenile myoclonic epilepsy, the limited number of patients makes any conclusion tentative. Consider the data from the partial seizure patients to be relevant for juvenile myoclonic epilepsy patients.

➤*Hepatic effects:*

ER tablets – There were no meaningful changes in mean liver function tests in the levetiracetam ER controlled trial. No patients were discontinued from the controlled trial for liver function test abnormalities.

➤*Renal function impairment:*

Immediate-release tablets/oral solution – See Actions for more information.

ER tablets – The effect of levetiracetam ER on renally impaired patients was not assessed in the well-controlled study. However, it is expected that the effect on levetiracetam ER–treated patients would be similar to the effect seen in well-controlled studies of levetiracetam immediate-release tablets. Use caution in dosing patients with moderate and severe renal function impairment and in patients undergoing hemodialysis. Reduce the dosage in patients with impaired renal function receiving levetiracetam ER. (Also see Administration and Dosage.)

➤*Hazardous tasks:* Advise patients that levetiracetam may cause dizziness and somnolence. Accordingly, advise patients not to drive or operate machinery, or engage in other hazardous activities until they have gained sufficient experience on levetiracetam and can gauge whether it adversely affects their performance of these activities.

➤*Pregnancy: Category C.* There are no adequate and well-controlled studies in pregnant women. Use levetiracetam during pregnancy only if the potential benefit justifies the potential risk to the fetus. Although confirmation is needed, severe growth restriction has been observed in limited human pregnancy experience. Also, it is not known if levetiracetam crosses the placenta. However, exposure to the embryo and fetus is expected because of levetiracetam's low molecular weight and lack of protein binding.

In animal studies, levetiracetam produced evidence of developmental toxicity, including teratogenic effects, at doses similar to or more than human therapeutic doses.

Administration to female rats throughout pregnancy and lactation was associated with increased incidences of minor fetal skeletal abnormalities and retarded offspring growth prenatally and/or postnatally at dosages of 350 mg/kg/day or more (approximately equivalent to the maximum recommended human daily dose (MRHD) of 3,000 mg on a mg/m^2 basis) and with increased pup mortality and offspring behavioral alterations at a dosage of 1,800 mg/kg/day (6 times the MRHD on a mg/m^2 basis). The developmental, no-effect dosage was 70 mg/kg/day (0.2 times the MRHD on a mg/m^2 basis). There was no overt maternal toxicity at the doses used in this study.

Treatment of pregnant rabbits during the period of organogenesis resulted in increased embryofetal mortality and increased incidences of minor fetal skeletal abnormalities at dosages of 600 mg/kg/day or more (approximately 4 times MRHD on a mg/m^2 basis) and in decreased fetal weights and increased incidences of fetal malformations at a dosage of 1,800 mg/kg/day (12 times the MRHD on a mg/m^2 basis). The developmental, no-effect dosage was 200 mg/kg/day (1.3 times the MRHD on a mg/m^2 basis). Maternal toxicity was also observed at 1,800 mg/kg/day.

When pregnant rats were treated during the period of organogenesis, fetal weights were decreased and the incidence of fetal skeletal variations was increased at a dosage of 3,600 mg/kg/day (12 times the MRHD). The developmental, no-effect dosage was 1,200 mg/kg/day (4 times the MRHD). There was no evidence of maternal toxicity in this study.

Pregnancy registry – The manufacturer has established the levetiracetam pregnancy registry to advance scientific knowledge about safety and outcomes associated with pregnant women being treated with levetiracetam. To ensure broad program access and reach, either a health care provider or the patient can initiate enrollment in the levetiracetam preg-

LEVETIRACETAM — ORAL

nancy registry by calling 1-888-537-7734. Patients may also enroll in the North American Antiepileptic Drug Pregnancy Registry by calling 1-888-233-2334.

➤*Lactation:* Levetiracetam is excreted in low levels in breast milk, but would not be expected to cause any adverse effects in breast-fed infants, especially infants older than 2 months of age. Because of the potential for serious adverse reactions in breast-feeding infants from levetiracetam, decide whether to discontinue breast-feeding or the drug, taking into account the importance of the drug to the mother. Other anticonvulsants (eg, carbamazepine, phenytoin, valproic acid) are classified as compatible with breast-feeding by the American Academy of Pediatrics.

➤*Children:*

Immediate-release tablets/oral solution – Safety and effectiveness in patients younger than 4 years of age have not been established.

ER tablets – Safety and effectiveness of levetiracetam ER in patients younger than 16 years of age have not been established.

➤*Elderly:* Levetiracetam is known to be substantially excreted by the kidney, and the risk of adverse reactions to this drug may be greater in patients with renal function impairment. Because elderly patients are more likely to have decreased renal function, take care in dose selection; it may be useful to monitor renal function.

➤*Lab test abnormalities:* Although most laboratory tests are not systematically altered with levetiracetam immediate-release treatment, there have been relatively infrequent abnormalities seen in hematologic parameters and liver function tests.

Drug Interactions

➤*Probenecid:* The maximum plasma concentration at steady-state of the metabolite, ucb L057, was approximately doubled in the presence of probenecid while the fraction of drug excreted unchanged in the urine remained the same. Renal clearance of ucb L057 in the presence of probenecid decreased by 60%, probably related to competitive inhibition of tubular secretion of ucb L057.

➤*Drug/Food interactions:* See Actions for more information.

Adverse Reactions

For more information on dizziness, somnolence, asthenia, coordination difficulties, psychotic symptoms, suicide attempts, and behavioral disorders/symptoms, see the Warnings/Precautions section.

➤*Myoclonic seizures:* In the well-controlled clinical study that included both adolescent (12 to 16 years of age) and adult patients with myoclonic seizures, the most frequently reported adverse reactions associated with the use of levetiracetam in combination with other AEDs not seen at an equivalent frequency among placebo-treated patients were neck pain, pharyngitis, and somnolence.

Levetiracetam Adverse Reactions in Patients 12 Years of Age and Older With Myoclonic Seizures (≥ 5%)

Adverse reaction	Levetiracetam (n = 60)	Placebo (n = 60)
CNS		
Depression	5%	2%
Somnolence	12%	2%
Vertigo	5%	3%
Respiratory		
Influenza	5%	2%
Pharyngitis	7%	0%
Miscellaneous		
Neck pain	8%	2%

➤*Partial-onset seizures in adults:*

Immediate-release tablets/oral solution – In well-controlled clinical studies in adults with partial-onset seizures, the most frequently reported adverse reactions associated with the use of levetiracetam in combination with other AEDs not seen at an equivalent frequency among placebo-treated patients were asthenia, dizziness, infection, and somnolence.

Of the most frequently reported adverse reactions in adults experiencing partial-onset seizures, asthenia, dizziness, and somnolence appeared to occur predominantly during the first 4 weeks of treatment.

Levetiracetam Adverse Reactions in Adults With Partial-Onset Seizures (≥ 1%)

Adverse reaction	Levetiracetam (n = 769)	Placebo (n = 439)
CNS		
Amnesia	2%	1%
Anxiety	2%	1%
Asthenia	15%	9%
Ataxia	3%	1%
Depression	4%	2%
Dizziness	9%	4%
Emotional lability	2%	0%
Headache	14%	13%
Hostility	2%	1%
Nervousness	4%	2%
Paresthesia	2%	1%
Somnolence	15%	8%
Vertigo	3%	1%
Respiratory		
Increased cough	2%	1%
Pharyngitis	6%	4%
Rhinitis	4%	3%
Sinusitis	2%	1%
Miscellaneous		
Anorexia	3%	2%
Diplopia	2%	1%
Infection	13%	8%
Pain	7%	6%

Other reactions reported by at least 1% of patients treated with levetiracetam, but as often or more frequently in the placebo group, were the following.

CNS: Abnormal thinking, confusion, convulsion, generalized tonic-clonic seizure, insomnia, tremor.

GI: Abdominal pain, constipation, diarrhea, dyspepsia, gastroenteritis, gingivitis, nausea, vomiting, weight gain.

Musculoskeletal: Arthralgia, back pain.

Special senses: Amblyopia, otitis media.

Miscellaneous: Accidental injury, bronchitis, chest pain, drug level increased, ecchymosis, fever, flu syndrome, fungal infection, rash, urinary tract infection.

ER tablets – In the well-controlled clinical study using levetiracetam ER in patients with partial-onset seizures, the most frequently reported adverse reactions in patients receiving levetiracetam ER in combination with other AEDs, not seen at an equivalent frequency among placebo-treated patients, were irritability and somnolence.

Levetiracetam ER Tablets Adverse Reactions (≥ 5%)

Adverse reaction	Levetiracetam ER (n = 77)	Placebo (n = 79)
CNS		
Dizziness	5%	3%
Irritability	7%	0%
Somnolence	8%	3%
Miscellaneous		
Influenza	8%	4%
Nasopharyngitis	7%	5%
Nausea	5%	3%

➤*Partial-onset seizures in children:* In the well-controlled clinical study of children 4 to 16 years of age with partial-onset seizures, the adverse reactions most frequently reported with the use of levetiracetam in combination with other AEDs not seen at an equivalent frequency among placebo-treated patients were accidental injury, asthenia, hostility, nervousness, and somnolence.

Levetiracetam Adverse Reactions in Children (4 to 16 Years of Age) With Partial-Onset Seizures (≥ 2%)

Adverse reaction	Levetiracetam ER (n = 101)	Placebo (n = 97)
CNS		
Agitation	6%	1%
Asthenia	9%	3%
Confusion	2%	0%
Depression	3%	1%
Dizziness	7%	2%
Emotional lability	6%	4%
Hostility	12%	6%
Increased reflexes	2%	1%
Nervousness	10%	2%
Personality disorder	8%	7%
Somnolence	23%	11%
Vertigo	3%	1%

LEVETIRACETAM — ORAL

Levetiracetam Adverse Reactions in Children (4 to 16 Years of Age) With Partial-Onset Seizures (≥ 2%)		
Adverse reaction	Levetiracetam ER (n = 101)	Placebo (n = 97)
Dermatologic		
Pruritus	2%	0%
Skin discoloration	2%	0%
Vesiculobullous rash	2%	0%
GI		
Anorexia	13%	8%
Constipation	3%	1%
Diarrhea	8%	7%
Gastroenteritis	4%	2%
Vomiting	15%	13%
GU		
Albuminuria	4%	0%
Urine abnormality	2%	1%
Metabolic/Nutritional		
Dehydration	2%	1%
Facial edema	2%	1%
Respiratory		
Asthma	2%	1%
Increased cough	11%	7%
Pharyngitis	10%	8%
Rhinitis	13%	8%
Special senses		
Amblyopia	2%	0%
Conjunctivitis	3%	2%
Ear pain	2%	0%
Miscellaneous		
Accidental injury	17%	10%
Ecchymosis	4%	1%
Flu syndrome	3%	2%
Neck pain	2%	1%
Pain	6%	3%
Viral infection	2%	1%

➤*Primary generalized tonic-clonic seizures:* In the well-controlled clinical study that included patients 4 years of age and older with primary generalized tonic-clonic seizures, the most frequently reported adverse reaction associated with the use of levetiracetam in combination with other AEDs, not seen at an equivalent frequency among placebo-treated patients, was nasopharyngitis.

Levetiracetam Adverse Reactions in Patients 4 Years of Age and Older With Primary Generalized Tonic-Clonic Seizures (≥5%)		
Adverse reaction	Levetiracetam (n = 79)	Placebo (n = 84)
CNS		
Fatigue	10%	8%
Irritability	6%	2%
Mood swings	5%	1%
Miscellaneous		
Diarrhea	8%	7%
Nasopharyngitis	14%	5%

➤*Discontinuation or dose reduction:*

Myoclonic seizures – In the placebo-controlled study, 8.3% of patients receiving levetiracetam and 1.7% receiving placebo discontinued or had a dose reduction as a result of an adverse reaction.

Levetiracetam Adverse Reactions Resulting in Discontinuation or Dose Reduction in Juvenile Myoclonic Epilepsy		
Adverse reaction	Levetiracetam (n = 60)	Placebo (n = 60)
CNS		
Anxiety	3.3%	1.7%
Depressed mood	1.7%	0%
Depression	1.7%	0%
Hypersomnia	1.7%	0%
Insomnia	1.7%	0%
Irritability	1.7%	0%
Nervousness	1.7%	0%
Somnolence	1.7%	0%
Special senses		
Diplopia	1.7%	0%

Partial-onset seizures –

Immediate-release tablets/oral solution: In well-controlled, adult clinical studies, 15% of patients receiving levetiracetam and 11.6% receiving placebo discontinued or had a dose reduction as a result of an adverse reaction.

Levetiracetam Adverse Reactions Resulting in Discontinuation or Dose Reduction in Adults With Partial-Onset Seizures		
Adverse reaction	Levetiracetam (n = 769)	Placebo (n = 439)
CNS		
Asthenia	1.3%	0.7%
Convulsion	3%	3.4%
Dizziness	1.4%	0%
Somnolence	4.4%	1.6%
Dermatologic		
Rash	0%	1.1%

In the well-controlled clinical study in children, 16.8% of patients receiving levetiracetam and 20.6% receiving placebo discontinued or had a dose reduction as a result of an adverse reaction.

Levetiracetam Adverse Reactions Resulting in Discontinuation or Dose Reduction in Children (4 to 16 Years of Age) With Partial-Onset Seizures		
Adverse reaction	Levetiracetam (n = 101)	Placebo (n = 97)
CNS		
Asthenia	3%	0%
Hostility	6.9%	2.1%
Somnolence	3%	3.1%

ER tablets: In the well-controlled clinical study using levetiracetam ER, 5.2% of patients receiving levetiracetam ER and 2.5% receiving placebo discontinued as a result of an adverse reaction. The adverse reactions that resulted in discontinuation and that occurred more frequently in levetiracetam ER–treated patients than in placebo-treated patients were asthenia, epilepsy, mouth ulceration, rash, and respiratory failure. Each of these adverse reactions led to discontinuation in a levetiracetam-treated patient and no placebo-treated patients.

Primary generalized tonic-clonic seizures – In the placebo-controlled study, 5.1% of patients receiving levetiracetam and 8.3% receiving placebo discontinued or had a dose reduction during the treatment period as a result of a treatment-emergent adverse reaction.

➤*Postmarketing:*

CNS – Suicidal behavior (including completed suicide).

GI – Pancreatitis, weight loss.

Hematologic – Leukopenia, neutropenia, pancytopenia (with bone marrow suppression identified in some of these cases), thrombocytopenia.

Hepatic – Abnormal liver function test, hepatic failure, hepatitis.

Miscellaneous – Alopecia has been reported with levetiracetam immediate-release use; recovery was observed in a majority of cases in which levetiracetam was discontinued.

Overdosage

➤*Symptoms:* The highest known dosage of levetiracetam received in the clinical development program was 6,000 mg/day. Other than drowsiness, there were no adverse reactions in the few known cases of overdose in clinical trials. Cases of aggression, agitation, coma, depressed level of consciousness, respiratory depression, and somnolence were observed with levetiracetam immediate-release overdoses in postmarketing use.

➤*Treatment:* There is no specific antidote for overdose with levetiracetam. If indicated, attempt elimination of unabsorbed drug by gastric lavage; observe the usual precautions to maintain the airway. General supportive care of the patient is indicated, including monitoring of vital signs and observation of the patient's clinical status. Contact a certified poison control center (800-222-1222) for up-to-date information on the management of overdose with levetiracetam.

In cases of overdose, consider standard hemodialysis procedures, which result in significant clearance of levetiracetam (approximately 50% in 4 hours). Although hemodialysis has not been performed in the few known cases of overdose, it may be indicated by the patient's clinical state or in patients with significant renal function impairment.

LEVETIRACETAM — ORAL

Patient Information

Instruct patients to take levetiracetam only as prescribed. Instruct patients to swallow the ER tablets whole, and not to chew, break, or crush.

Advise patients to notify their health care provider if they become pregnant or intend to become pregnant during therapy.

Advise patients that levetiracetam may cause dizziness and somnolence. Advise patients not to drive or operate machinery, or engage in other hazardous activities until they have gained sufficient experience on levetiracetam and can gauge whether it adversely affects their performance of these activities.

Advise patients that levetiracetam may cause changes in behavior (eg, aggression, agitation, anger, anxiety, apathy, depression, hostility, irritability), and in rare cases, patients may experience psychotic symptoms.

Advise patients to immediately report any symptoms of depression and/or suicidal ideation to their prescribing health care provider, because suicide, suicide attempt, and suicidal ideation have been reported in patients treated with levetiracetam.

LEVETIRACETAM — INJECTION

Refer to the general discussion beginning in the Anticonvulsants introduction.

Indications

➤*Myoclonic seizures:* Adjunctive therapy in the treatment of myoclonic seizures in adults with juvenile myoclonic epilepsy.

➤*Partial-onset seizures:* Adjunctive therapy in the treatment of partial-onset seizures in adults with epilepsy.

➤*Primary generalized tonic-clonic seizures:* Adjunctive therapy in the treatment of primary generalized tonic-clonic seizures in adults with idiopathic generalized epilepsy.

➤*Off-label uses:*

Other possible off-label uses – May be used in the neonatal period as second-line therapy for seizures that have been refractory to phenobarbital and other anticonvulsants (See also Administration and Dosage).

Administration and Dosage

➤*General dosing considerations:* Treatment can be initiated with either intravenous (IV) or oral administration.

➤*Adults:*

Myoclonic seizures –

16 years of age and older:

• *Initial dosage* – 1,000 mg/day given IV as twice-daily dosing (500 mg IV twice daily).

• *Dosage titration* – Dosage should be increased by 1,000 mg/day every 2 weeks to the recommended daily dose of 3,000 mg.

• *Maintenance dosage* – 3,000 mg/day. The effectiveness of dosages lower than 3,000 mg/day has not been studied.

Partial-onset seizures –

16 years of age and older:

• *Maximum dose* – 3,000 mg/day.

• *Initial dosage* – 1,000 mg IV, given as twice-daily dosing (500 mg IV twice daily).

• *Dosage titration* – Additional dosing increments may be given (1,000 mg/day additional every 2 weeks) to a maximum recommended daily dose of 3,000 mg.

• *Maintenance dosage* – 3,000 mg/day. Dosages greater than 3,000 mg/day have been used in open-label studies with levetiracetam tablets for periods of 6 months and longer. There is no evidence that dosages greater than 3,000 mg/day confer additional benefit.

Primary generalized tonic-clonic seizures –

16 years of age and older:

• *Initial dosage* – 1,000 mg/day, given IV as twice-daily dosing (500 mg IV twice daily).

• *Dosage titration* – Dosage should be increased by 1,000 mg/day every 2 weeks to the recommended daily dose of 3,000 mg.

• *Maintenance dosage* – 3,000 mg/day. The effectiveness of dosages lower than 3,000 mg/day has not been adequately studied.

➤*Children:*

Off-label dosing –

Anticonvulsant:

• *Neonates* –

Maximum dose: 30 mg/kg/dose.

Initial dosage: 10 mg/kg/dose administered IV slowly over 15 minutes every 24 hours in the immediate neonatal period. Administer every 12 hours later in infancy.

Dilute to a concentration of 5 mg/ml with compatible diluent prior to administration.

Dosage adjustment: Adjust dosage upward as needed every 1 to 2 weeks to a maximum of 30 mg/kg/dose.

➤*Renal function impairment:* Levetiracetam dosing must be individualized according to the patient's renal function status.

Levetiracetam Injection Dosage Adjustment for Adults With Renal Function Impairment[a]

Renal function status	CrCl (mL/min)	Dosage (mg)	Frequency
Healthy	> 80	500 to 1,500	Every 12 h
Mild	50 to 80	500 to 1,000	Every 12 h
Moderate	30 to 50	250 to 750	Every 12 h
Severe	< 30	250 to 500	Every 12 h

Levetiracetam Injection Dosage Adjustment for Adults With Renal Function Impairment[a]

Renal function status	CrCl (mL/min)	Dosage (mg)	Frequency
ESRD patients using dialysis	—	500 to 1,000	Every 24 h[b]

[a] CrCl = creatinine clearance; ESRD = end-stage renal disease.
[b] Following dialysis, a 250 to 500 mg supplemental dose is recommended.

➤*Conversion:* When switching from oral levetiracetam, the initial total daily IV dosage of levetiracetam should be equivalent to the total daily dosage and frequency of oral levetiracetam, and should be administered as a 15-minute IV infusion following dilution in 100 mL of a compatible diluent. At the end of the IV treatment period, the patient may be switched to levetiracetam oral administration at the equivalent daily dosage and frequency of the IV administration.

➤*Discontinuation of therapy:* Gradually withdraw antiepileptic drugs (AEDs), including levetiracetam, in order to minimize the potential of increased seizure frequency.

➤*Preparation for administration:* Levetiracetam injection (500 mg per 5 mL) should be diluted in 100 mL of a compatible diluent and administered IV as a 15-minute IV infusion. Any unused portion of the vial contents should be discarded. A product with particulate matter or discoloration should not be used.

Preparation of Levetiracetam Injection

Dose	Withdraw volume	Volume of diluent
500 mg	5 mL (one 5 mL vial)	100 mL
1,000 mg	10 mL (two 5 mL vials)	100 mL
1,500 mg	15 mL (three 5 mL vials)	100 mL

➤*Administration:* Levetiracetam injection is for IV use only and must be diluted prior to administration. It should be administered as a 15-minute IV infusion.

➤*Admixture compatibility:* Levetiracetam is physically compatible and chemically stable with the following diluents: sodium chloride 0.9% injection, dextrose 5% injection, and Ringer's lactate injection. Levetiracetam is compatible with the following AEDs: lorazepam, diazepam, and valproate sodium. There are no data to support the physical compatibility of levetiracetam with AEDs that are not listed.

➤*Storage/Stability:* Store at 25°C (77°F); excursions are permitted between 15° and 30°C (59° and 86°F).

Levetiracetam was found to be physically compatible and chemically stable for at least 24 hours when mixed with compatible diluents and AEDs, and stored in polyvinyl chloride bags at controlled room temperature, 15° to 30°C (59° to 86°F).

Actions

➤*Pharmacology:* The precise mechanism by which levetiracetam exerts its antiepileptic effect is unknown. The antiepileptic activity of levetiracetam was assessed in a number of animal models of epileptic seizures. Levetiracetam did not inhibit single seizures induced by maximal stimulation with electrical current or different chemoconvulsants and showed only minimal activity in submaximal stimulation and in threshold tests. Protection was observed, however, against secondarily generalized activity from focal seizures induced by pilocarpine and kainic acid, 2 chemoconvulsants that induce seizures that mimic some features of human complex partial seizures with secondary generalization. Levetiracetam also displayed inhibitory properties in the kindling model in rats, another model of human complex partial seizures, both during kindling development and in the fully kindled state. The predictive value of these animal models for specific types of human epilepsy is uncertain.

In vitro and in vivo recordings of epileptiform activity from the hippocampus have shown that levetiracetam inhibits burst firing without affecting normal neuronal excitability, suggesting that levetiracetam may selectively prevent hypersynchronization of epileptiform burst firing and propagation of seizure activity.

➤*Pharmacokinetics:*

Absorption – Equivalent doses of IV levetiracetam and oral levetiracetam result in equivalent maximal drug concentration (C_{max}), minimal drug concentration, and total systemic exposure to levetiracetam when IV levetiracetam is administered as a 15-minute infusion.

Levetiracetam is rapidly and almost completely absorbed after oral administration. Levetiracetam injection and tablets are bioequivalent. The phar-

LEVETIRACETAM — INJECTION

macokinetics of levetiracetam are linear and time-invariant, with low intra- and intersubject variability.

Distribution – The equivalence of levetiracetam injection and the oral formulation was demonstrated in a bioavailability study of 17 healthy volunteers. In this study, levetiracetam 1,500 mg was diluted in 100 mL of sterile saline 0.9% solution and was infused over 15 minutes. The selected infusion rate provided plasma concentrations of levetiracetam at the end of the infusion period that were similar to those achieved at the time to maximum serum concentration after an equivalent oral dose. It was demonstrated that a levetiracetam 1,500 mg IV infusion is equivalent to levetiracetam 3 × 500 mg oral tablets. The time-independent pharmacokinetic profile of levetiracetam was demonstrated following 1,500 mg IV infusion twice daily for 4 days. The area under the curve ($AUC_{0\text{-}12\ h}$) at steady state was equivalent to AUC_{∞} following an equivalent single dose.

Levetiracetam and its major metabolite are less than 10% bound to plasma proteins; clinically significant interactions with other drugs through competition for protein-binding sites are therefore unlikely. The volume of distribution of levetiracetam is close to the volume of intracellular and extracellular water.

Metabolism – Levetiracetam is not extensively metabolized in humans. The major metabolic pathway is the enzymatic hydrolysis of the acetamide group, which produces the carboxylic acid metabolite, ucb L057 (24% of the dose), and is not dependent on any liver CYP-450 isoenzymes. The major metabolite is inactive in animal seizure models. Two minor metabolites were identified as the product of hydroxylation of the 2-oxo-pyrrolidine ring (2% of the dose) and as the opening of the 2-oxo-pyrrolidine ring in position 5 (1% of the dose). There is no enantiomeric interconversion of levetiracetam or its major metabolite.

Excretion – Levetiracetam plasma half-life in adults is 7 ± 1 hour and is unaffected by dose, route of administration, or repeated administration. Levetiracetam is eliminated from the systemic circulation as unchanged drug by renal excretion (66% of the dose). The total body clearance is 0.96 mL/min/kg, and the renal clearance is 0.6 mL/min/kg. The mechanism of excretion is glomerular filtration with subsequent partial tubular reabsorption. The metabolite ucb L057 is excreted by glomerular filtration and active tubular secretion, with a renal clearance of 4 mL/min/kg. Levetiracetam elimination is correlated to CrCl. Levetiracetam clearance is reduced in patients with renal function impairment.

Special populations –

Renal function impairment: The disposition of levetiracetam was studied in adult subjects with varying degrees of renal function. Total body clearance of levetiracetam is reduced in patients with renal function impairment by 40% in the mild group (CrCl = 50 to 80 mL/min), 50% in the moderate group (CrCl = 30 to 50 mL/min), and 60% in the severe renal function impairment group (CrCl = less than 30 mL/min). Clearance of levetiracetam is correlated with CrCl.

In anuric (ESRD) patients, the total body clearance decreased by 70% compared with healthy subjects (CrCl more than 80 mL/min). Approximately 50% of the pool of levetiracetam in the body is removed during a standard 4-hour hemodialysis procedure.

See Administration and Dosage for more information.

Elderly: Pharmacokinetics of levetiracetam were evaluated in 16 elderly subjects (61 to 88 years of age) with CrCl ranging from 30 to 74 mL/min. Following oral administration of twice-daily dosing for 10 days, total body clearance decreased by 38%, and the half-life was 2.5 hours longer in elderly subjects compared with healthy adults. This is most likely because of the decrease in renal function in these subjects.

Contraindications

None known.

Warnings/Precautions

➤*CNS effects:*

Myoclonic seizures – During clinical development, the number of patients with myoclonic seizures exposed to levetiracetam was considerably smaller than the number with partial seizures. Therefore, under-reporting of certain adverse reactions was more likely to occur in the myoclonic seizure population. In some patients experiencing myoclonic seizures, levetiracetam causes somnolence and behavioral abnormalities. It is expected that the events seen in partial seizure patients would occur in patients with juvenile myoclonic epilepsy.

Somnolence: In the double-blind, controlled trial in patients with juvenile myoclonic epilepsy experiencing myoclonic seizures, 11.7% of levetiracetam-treated patients experienced somnolence compared with 1.7% of placebo patients. No patient discontinued treatment as a result of somnolence. In 1.7% of levetiracetam patients and in 0% of placebo patients, the dose was reduced as a result of somnolence.

Other behavioral symptoms: Nonpsychotic behavioral disorders (reported as aggression and irritability) occurred in 5% of the levetiracetam patients compared with 0% of placebo patients. Nonpsychotic mood disorders (reported as depressed mood, depression, and mood swings) occurred in 6.7% of levetiracetam-treated patients compared with 3.3% of placebo patients. A total of 5% of levetiracetam-treated patients had a reduction in dose or discontinued treatment because of behavioral or psychiatric reactions (reported as anxiety, depressed mood, depression, irritability, and nervousness), compared with 1.7% of placebo patients.

Partial-onset seizures – Somnolence, asthenia, and coordination difficulties occurred most frequently within the first 4 weeks of treatment.

Somnolence: In controlled trials of adult patients with epilepsy experiencing partial-onset seizures, 14.8% of levetiracetam-treated patients reported somnolence, compared with 8.4% of placebo patients. There was no clear dosage response up to 3,000 mg/day. In a study in which there was no titration, approximately 45% of patients receiving 4,000 mg/day reported somnolence. The somnolence was considered serious in 0.3% of the treated patients, compared with 0% in the placebo group. Approximately 3% of levetiracetam-treated patients discontinued treatment because of somnolence, compared with 0.7% of placebo patients. In 1.4% of treated patients and in 0.9% of placebo patients, the dose was reduced; 0.3% of the treated patients were hospitalized because of somnolence.

Asthenia: In controlled trials of adult patients with epilepsy experiencing partial-onset seizures, 14.7% of treated patients reported asthenia, compared with 9.1% of placebo patients. Treatment was discontinued in 0.8% of treated patients compared with 0.5% of placebo patients. In 0.5% of treated patients and in 0.2% of placebo patients, the dose was reduced.

Coordination difficulties: A total of 3.4% of levetiracetam-treated patients reported coordination difficulties (eg, abnormal gait, ataxia, incoordination), compared with 1.6% of placebo patients. A total of 0.4% of patients in controlled trials discontinued levetiracetam treatment because of ataxia, compared with 0% of placebo patients. In 0.7% of levetiracetam-treated patients and in 0.2% of placebo patients, the dose was reduced because of coordination difficulties; 1 of the levetiracetam-treated patients was hospitalized because of worsening of preexisting ataxia.

Psychotic symptoms: In controlled trials of patients with epilepsy experiencing partial-onset seizures, 5 (0.7%) of levetiracetam-treated patients experienced psychotic symptoms, compared with 1 (0.2%) placebo-treated patient. Two (0.3%) levetiracetam-treated patients were hospitalized, and their treatment was discontinued. Both reactions, reported as psychosis, developed within the first week of treatment and resolved within 1 to 2 weeks of treatment discontinuation. Two other reactions, reported as hallucinations, occurred after 1 to 5 months and resolved within 2 to 7 days, while the patients remained on treatment. In 1 patient who experienced psychotic depression within a month, symptoms resolved within 45 days and the patient continued treatment. A total of 13.3% of levetiracetam patients experienced other behavioral symptoms (eg, aggression, agitation, anger, anxiety, apathy, depersonalization, depression, emotional lability, hostility, irritability), compared with 6.2% of placebo patients. Approximately half of the patients reported these reactions within the first 4 weeks. A total of 1.7% of treated patients discontinued treatment because of these reactions, compared with 0.2% of placebo patients. The treatment dose was reduced in 0.8% of treated patients and in 0.5% of placebo patients. A total of 0.8% of treated patients experienced a serious behavioral reaction and were hospitalized, compared with 0.2% of placebo patients.

Suicide attempts: In addition, 4 (0.5%) levetiracetam-treated patients attempted suicide, compared with 0% of placebo patients. One of these patients completed suicide. In the other 3 patients, the reactions did not lead to discontinuation or dose reduction. The reactions occurred after patients had been treated between 4 weeks and 6 months.

Primary generalized tonic-clonic seizures – During clinical development, the number of patients with primary generalized tonic-clonic epilepsy exposed to levetiracetam was considerably smaller than the number with partial epilepsy described previously. As in the partial seizure patients, behavioral symptoms appeared to be associated with levetiracetam treatment. Gait disorders and somnolence were also described in the study in the primary generalized seizures, but with no difference between placebo and levetiracetam treatment groups and no appreciable discontinuations. Although it may be expected that drug-related reactions seen in partial seizure patients would be seen in primary generalized epilepsy patients (eg, somnolence, gait disturbance), these reactions may not have been observed because of the smaller sample size.

In some patients experiencing primary generalized tonic-clonic seizures, levetiracetam causes behavioral abnormalities.

Nonpsychotic disorders: In the double-blind controlled trial in patients with idiopathic generalized epilepsy experiencing primary generalized tonic-clonic seizures, irritability was the most frequently reported psychiatric adverse reaction occurring in 6.3% of levetiracetam-treated patients compared with 2.4% of placebo patients. Additionally, nonpsychotic behavioral disorders (reported as abnormal behavior, aggression, conduct disorder, and irritability) occurred in 11.4% of the levetiracetam-treated patients compared with 3.6% of placebo patients. Of the levetiracetam-treated patients experiencing nonpsychotic behavioral disorders, 1 patient discontinued treatment because of aggression.

Nonpsychotic mood disorders (reported as anger, apathy, depression, mood altered, mood swings, negativism, suicidal ideation, and tearfulness) occurred in 12.7% of levetiracetam-treated patients compared with 8.3% of placebo patients. No levetiracetam-treated patients discontinued or had a dose reduction as a result of these reactions. One levetiracetam-treated patient experienced suicidal ideation. One patient experienced delusional behavior that required lowering of the dose of levetiracetam.

Psychotic-like disorders: In a long-term, open-label study that examined patients with various forms of primary generalized epilepsy, along with the nonpsychotic behavioral disorders, 2 of 192 patients studied exhibited psychotic-like behavior. Behavior in one case was characterized by auditory hallucinations and suicidal thoughts, and led to levetiracetam discontinuation. The other case was described as worsening of pre-existent schizophrenia and did not lead to drug discontinuation.

➤*Withdrawal seizures:* Gradually withdraw AEDs, including levetiracetam, to minimize the potential of increased seizure frequency.

➤*Hematologic effects:* Minor, but statistically significant, decreases compared with placebo in total mean red blood cell count ($0.03 \times 10^6/mm^3$), mean hemoglobin (0.09 g/dL), and mean hematocrit (0.38%) were observed in levetiracetam-treated patients in partial-onset seizures controlled trials.

A total of 3.2% of levetiracetam-treated and 1.8% of placebo patients had at least 1 possibly significant ($2.8 \times 10^9/L$ or less) decreased white blood cell count, and 2.4% of levetiracetam-treated and 1.4% of placebo patients had at least 1 possibly significant (less than or equal to $1 \times 10^9/L$) decreased neutrophil count. Of the treated patients with a low neutrophil count, all but 1

LEVETIRACETAM — INJECTION

rose toward or to baseline with continued treatment. No patient discontinued treatment because of low neutrophil counts.

➤*Renal function impairment:* Clearance of levetiracetam is decreased in patients with renal function impairment and is correlated with CrCl. Use caution during dose selection in patients with moderate and severe renal function impairment and in patients undergoing hemodialysis. Reduce the dosage in patients with renal function impairment who are receiving levetiracetam. Give supplemental doses to patients after dialysis. (Also see Administration and Dosage.)

➤*Hazardous tasks:* Advise patients that levetiracetam may cause dizziness and somnolence. Advise patients not to drive or operate machinery, or engage in other hazardous activities until they have gained sufficient experience on levetiracetam and can gauge whether it adversely affects their performance in these activities.

➤*Pregnancy: Category C.* There are no adequate and well-controlled studies in pregnant women. Use levetiracetam during pregnancy only if the potential benefit justifies the potential risk to the fetus. Although confirmation is needed, severe growth restriction has been observed in limited human pregnancy experience. Also, it is not known if levetiracetam crosses the placenta. However, exposure to the embryo and fetus should be expected because of levetiracetam's low molecular weight and lack of protein binding.

In animal studies, levetiracetam produced evidence of developmental toxicity, including teratogenic effects, at doses similar to or greater than human therapeutic doses.

Administration of levetiracetam to female rats throughout pregnancy and lactation was associated with increased incidences of minor fetal skeletal abnormalities and retarded offspring growth pre- and/or postnatally at dosages of 350 mg/kg/day or more (approximately equivalent to the maximum recommended human daily dose [MRHD] of 3,000 mg on a mg/m^2 basis), and was associated with increased pup mortality and offspring behavioral alterations at a dosage of 1,800 mg/kg/day (6 times the MRHD on a mg/m^2 basis). The developmental, no-effect dosage was 70 mg/kg/day (0.2 times the MRHD on a mg/m^2 basis). There was no overt maternal toxicity at the doses used in this study.

Treatment of pregnant rabbits during the period of organogenesis resulted in increased embryofetal mortality and increased incidences of minor fetal skeletal abnormalities at dosages of 600 mg/kg/day or more (approximately 4 times MRHD on a mg/m^2 basis). Treatment also resulted in decreased fetal weights and increased incidences of fetal malformations at a dosage of 1,800 mg/kg/day (12 times the MRHD on a mg/m^2 basis). The developmental, no-effect dosage was 200 mg/kg/day (1.3 times the MRHD on a mg/m^2 basis). Maternal toxicity was also observed at 1,800 mg/kg/day.

When pregnant rats were treated during the period of organogenesis, fetal weights were decreased and the incidence of fetal skeletal variations was increased at a dosage of 3,600 mg/kg/day (12 times the MRHD). The developmental, no-effect dosage was 1,200 mg/kg/day (4 times the MRHD). There was no evidence of maternal toxicity in this study.

Pregnancy registry – The manufacturer has established the levetiracetam pregnancy registry to advance scientific knowledge about safety and outcomes associated with pregnant women being treated with levetiracetam. To ensure broad program access and reach, a health care provider or the patient can initiate enrollment in the levetiracetam pregnancy registry by calling 1-888-537-7734. Patients may also enroll in the North American Antiepileptic Drug Pregnancy Registry by calling 1-888-233-2334.

➤*Lactation:* Levetiracetam is excreted in low levels in breast milk, but would not be expected to cause any adverse effects in breast-fed infants, especially infants older than 2 months of age. Because of the potential for serious adverse reactions in breast-feeding infants, decide whether to discontinue breast-feeding or levetiracetam, taking into account the importance of the drug to the mother. Other anticonvulsants are classified as compatible with breast-feeding by the American Academy of Pediatrics.

➤*Children:* Safety and effectiveness of levetiracetam injection in patients younger than 16 years of age have not been established.

➤*Elderly:* Levetiracetam is known to be substantially excreted by the kidney, and the risk of adverse reactions to this drug may be greater in patients with renal function impairment. Because elderly patients are more likely to have decreased renal function, take care in dose selection and monitor renal function.

➤*Lab test abnormalities:* Although most laboratory tests are not systematically altered with levetiracetam treatment, there have been relatively infrequent abnormalities observed in hematologic parameters and liver function tests.

Drug Interactions

➤*Probenecid:* The maximum plasma concentration at steady-state of the levetiracetam metabolite ucb L057 was approximately doubled in the presence of probenecid, while the fraction of drug excreted unchanged in the urine remained the same. Renal clearance of ucb L057 in the presence of probenecid decreased 60%; this decrease was probably related to competitive inhibition of tubular secretion of ucb L057.

Adverse Reactions

For more information on somnolence, asthenia, coordination difficulties, psychotic symptoms and other behavioral symptoms, see the Warnings/Precautions section.

➤*Myoclonic seizures:* The following tables lists adverse reactions that occurred in at least 5% of juvenile myoclonic epilepsy patients treated with levetiracetam tablets and that were numerically more common than in patients treated with placebo. In this study, either levetiracetam or placebo was added to concurrent AED therapy. Adverse reactions were usually mild to moderate in intensity.

Levetiracetam Adverse Reactions in Myoclonic Seizures (≥ 5%)		
Adverse reaction	Levetiracetam (n = 60)	Placebo (n = 60)
CNS		
Depression	5%	2%
Somnolence	12%	2%
Vertigo	5%	3%
Respiratory		
Pharyngitis	7%	0%
Influenza	5%	2%
Miscellaneous		
Neck pain	8%	2%

➤*Partial-onset seizures:*

Levetiracetam Adverse Reactions in Adults With Partial-Onset Seizures (≥ 1%)		
Adverse reaction	Levetiracetam (n = 769)	Placebo (n = 439)
CNS		
Amnesia	2%	1%
Anxiety	2%	1%
Asthenia	15%	9%
Ataxia	3%	1%
Depression	4%	2%
Dizziness	9%	4%
Emotional lability	2%	0%
Headache	14%	13%
Hostility	2%	1%
Nervousness	4%	2%
Paresthesia	2%	1%
Somnolence	15%	8%
Vertigo	3%	1%
Respiratory		
Increased cough	2%	1%
Pharyngitis	6%	4%
Rhinitis	4%	3%
Sinusitis	2%	1%
Miscellaneous		
Anorexia	3%	2%
Diplopia	2%	1%
Infection	13%	8%
Pain	7%	6%

➤*Primary generalized tonic-clonic seizures:* The following tables lists adverse reactions that occurred in at least 5% of idiopathic generalized epilepsy patients experiencing primary generalized tonic-clonic seizures treated with levetiracetam and were numerically more common than in patients treated with placebo. In this study, either levetiracetam or placebo was added to concurrent AED therapy. Adverse reactions were usually mild to moderate in intensity.

Levetiracetam Adverse Reactions in Patients 4 Years of Age and Older With Primary Generalized Tonic-Clonic Seizures (≥ 5%)		
Adverse reaction	Levetiracetam (n = 79)	Placebo (n = 84)
CNS		
Fatigue	10%	8%
Irritability	6%	2%
Mood swings	5%	1%
Miscellaneous		
Diarrhea	8%	7%
Nasopharyngitis	14%	5%

LEVETIRACETAM — INJECTION

➤*Discontinuation or dose reduction:*

Myoclonic seizures –

Levetiracetam Adverse Reactions Resulting in Discontinuation or Dose Reduction in Juvenile Myoclonic Epilepsy		
Adverse reaction	Levetiracetam (n = 60)	Placebo (n = 60)
CNS		
Anxiety	3.3%	1.7%
Depressed mood	1.7%	0%
Depression	1.7%	0%
Hypersomnia	1.7%	0%
Insomnia	1.7%	0%
Irritability	1.7%	0%
Nervousness	1.7%	0%
Somnolence	1.7%	0%
Special senses		
Diplopia	1.7%	0%

Partial-onset seizures –

Levetiracetam Adverse Reactions Resulting in Discontinuation or Dose Reduction in Adults With Partial-Onset Seizures		
Adverse reaction	Levetiracetam (n = 769)	Placebo (n = 439)
CNS		
Asthenia	1.3%	0.7%
Dizziness	1.4%	0%
Somnolence	4.4%	1.6%

➤*Postmarketing:*

CNS – Suicidal behavior (including completed suicide).

GI – Pancreatitis, weight loss.

Hematologic – Leukopenia, neutropenia, pancytopenia (with bone marrow suppression identified in some of these cases), thrombocytopenia.

Hepatic – Abnormal liver function test, hepatic failure, hepatitis.

Miscellaneous – Alopecia has been reported with levetiracetam use; recovery was observed in a majority of cases in which levetiracetam was discontinued.

Overdosage

➤*Symptoms:* The highest known dosage of oral levetiracetam received in the clinical development program was 6,000 mg/day. Other than drowsiness, there were no adverse reactions in the few known cases of overdose in clinical trials. Cases of aggression, agitation, coma, depressed level of consciousness, respiratory depression, and somnolence were observed with levetiracetam overdoses in postmarketing use.

➤*Treatment:* There is no specific antidote for overdose with levetiracetam. If indicated, attempt elimination of unabsorbed drug by gastric lavage; observe the usual precautions to maintain the airway. General supportive care of the patient is indicated, including monitoring of vital signs and observation of the patient's clinical status. Contact a certified poison control center (800-222-1222) for up-to-date information on the management of overdose with levetiracetam.

In cases of overdose, consider standard hemodialysis procedures, which results in significant clearance of levetiracetam (approximately 50% in 4 hours). Although hemodialysis has not been performed in the few known cases of overdose, it may be indicated by the patient's clinical state or in patients with significant renal function impairment.

Patient Information

Advise patients to notify their health care provider if they are pregnant prior to therapy.

Advise patients that levetiracetam may cause dizziness and somnolence. Advise patients not to drive or operate machinery, or engage in other hazardous activities until they have gained sufficient experience on levetiracetam to gauge whether it adversely affects their performance in these activities.

Advise patients that levetiracetam may cause changes in behavior (eg, aggression, agitation, anger, anxiety, apathy, depression, hostility, irritability), and in rare cases, patients may experience psychotic symptoms and/or suicidal ideation.

PRIMIDONE

Rx	**Primidone** (Various, eg, Global)	**Tablets:** 50 mg	In 100s, 500s, and 1000s.
Rx	**Mysoline** (Valeant)		Lactose. (Mysoline 50 M). White, scored. Square. In 100s.
Rx	**Primidone** (Various, eg, Danbury, Global, Major, Marlex)	**Tablets:** 250 mg	In 100s, 500s, and 1000s.
Rx	**Mysoline** (Valeant)		Lactose. (Mysoline 250 M). Yellow, scored. Square. In 100s.

PRIMIDONE — ORAL

Refer to the general discussion beginning in the Anticonvulsants introduction.

Indications

➤*Seizures:* Primidone, used alone or concomitantly with other anticonvulsants, is indicated in the control of grand mal, psychomotor, and focal epileptic seizures. It may control grand mal seizures refractory to other anticonvulsant therapy.

➤*Off-label uses:* Benign familial tremor (essential tremor, 750 mg/day).

Administration and Dosage

➤*General dosing considerations:* In some cases, serum blood level determinations of primidone may be necessary for optimal dosage adjustment. (See Therapeutic Drug Monitoring.)

➤*Adults:*

Seizures –

Maximum dose: 500 mg 4 times per day.

Initial dosage: 100 to 125 mg at bedtime on days 1 to 3.

Dosage titration:

- *Days 4 to 6* – 100 to 125 mg twice daily (morning and evening).
- *Days 7 to 9* – 100 to 125 mg 3 times daily (morning, noon, and evening).
- *Day 10 to maintenance* – 250 mg 3 times daily (morning, noon, and evening).

Maintenance dosage: 250 mg 3 to 4 times daily. If required, an increase to 250 mg 5 or 6 times daily may be made, but daily doses should not exceed 500 mg 4 times daily.

➤*Children:*

Seizures –

8 years of age and older: See Adults for dosing.

Younger than 8 years of age:

- *Initial dosage* – 50 mg at bedtime on days 1 to 3.
- *Dosage titration* –
  Days 4 to 6: 50 mg twice daily.
  Days 7 to 9: 100 mg twice daily.
  Day 10 to maintenance: 125 mg 3 times daily to 250 mg 3 times daily.
- *Maintenance dosage* – 125 to 250 mg 3 times daily, or 10 to 25 mg/kg/day in divided doses.

➤*Concomitant therapy with other anticonvulsants:* Primidone should be started at 100 to 125 mg at bedtime and gradually increased to maintenance level as the other drug is gradually decreased. This regimen should be continued until satisfactory dosage level is achieved for the combination or the other medication is completely withdrawn. When therapy with primidone alone is the objective, the transition from concomitant therapy should not be completed in less than 2 weeks.

➤*Therapeutic drug monitoring:* The clinically effective serum level is between 5 to 12 mcg/mL.

➤*Administration:* Administer without regard to meals.

➤*Storage/Stability:* Store at 15° to 30°C (59° to 86°F).

Actions

➤*Pharmacology:* Primidone raises electro- or chemoshock seizure thresholds or alters seizure patterns in experimental animals. The mechanism(s) of primidone's antiepileptic action is not known.

Primidone per se has anticonvulsant activity, as do its 2 metabolites, phenobarbital and phenylethylmalonamide (PEMA). In addition to its anticonvulsant activity, PEMA potentiates the anticonvulsant activity of phenobarbital in experimental animals.

Contraindications

Porphyria; hypersensitivity to phenobarbital, a metabolite of primidone.

Warnings/Precautions

➤*Withdrawal precipitated seizures:* The abrupt withdrawal of antiepileptic medication may precipitate status epilepticus.

➤*Therapeutic efficacy:* The therapeutic efficacy of a dosage regimen takes several weeks before it can be assessed.

➤*Pregnancy: Category D.* The effects of primidone in human pregnancy and nursing infants are unknown. Recent reports suggest an association between the use of anticonvulsant drugs by women with epilepsy and an elevated incidence of birth defects in children born to these women. Data are more extensive with respect to diphenylhydantoin and phenobarbital, but these are also the most commonly prescribed anticonvulsants; less systematic or anecdotal reports suggest a possible similar association with the use of all known anticonvulsant drugs.

The reports suggesting an elevated incidence of birth defects in children of drug-treated epileptic women cannot be regarded as adequate to prove a definite cause-and-effect relationship. There are intrinsic methodologic problems in obtaining adequate data on drug teratogenicity in humans; the possibility also exists that other factors leading to birth defects (eg, genetic factors, the epileptic condition itself), may be more important than drug

PRIMIDONE — ORAL

therapy. The majority of mothers on anticonvulsant medication deliver healthy infants. It is important to note that anticonvulsant drugs should not be discontinued in patients in whom the drug is administered to prevent major seizures because of the strong possibility of precipitating status epilepticus with attendant hypoxia and threat to life. In individual cases where the severity and frequency of the seizure disorders are such that the removal of medication does not pose a serious threat to the patient, discontinuation of the drug may be considered prior to and during pregnancy, although it cannot be said with any confidence that even minor seizures do not pose some hazard to the developing embryo or fetus.

The prescribing physician will wish to weigh these considerations in treating or counseling epileptic women of childbearing potential.

Neonatal hemorrhage, with a coagulation defect resembling vitamin K deficiency, has been described in newborns whose mothers were taking primidone and other anticonvulsants. Pregnant women under anticonvulsant therapy should receive prophylactic vitamin K_1 therapy for 1 month prior to, and during, delivery.

➤*Lactation:* There is evidence that in mothers treated with primidone, the drug appears in the milk in substantial quantities. Since tests for the presence of primidone in biological fluids are too complex to be carried out in the average clinical laboratory. It is suggested that the presence of undue somnolence and drowsiness in nursing newborns of primidone-treated mothers be taken as an indication that nursing should be discontinued.

➤*Monitoring:* Since primidone therapy generally extends over prolonged periods, a complete blood count and a sequential multiple analysis-12 (SMA-12) test should be made every 6 months.

Drug Interactions

Primidone Drug Interactions

Precipitant drug	Object drug[a]		Description
Carbamazepine	Primidone	↓	Concomitant primidone and carbamazepine may result in decreased primidone, its metabolite phenobarbital, and carbamazepine serum concentrations.
Primidone	Carbamazepine		
Hydantoins (eg, phenytoin)	Primidone	↑	Hydantoins may increase serum primidone and its metabolites. Patients on concomitant treatment with hydantoins and primidone should be monitored closely following any alteration in hydantoin therapy.
Succinimides (eg, ethosuximide, methsuximide)	Primidone	↓	Coadministration of primidone and a succinimide may result in lower primidone and phenobarbital serum concentrations.
Valproic Acid	Primidone	↑	Plasma primidone concentrations may be elevated, increasing the pharmacologic and adverse effects. Primidone dosage may need to be decreased in some patients.
Primidone	Anticoagulants (eg, warfarin sodium)	↓	Primidone reduces the effect of anticoagulants. Monitor anticoagulation dose and tailor doses as needed.
Primidone	Beta-blockers (eg, propranolol)	↓	Pharmacokinetic effects of certain beta-blockers may be reduced. Consider a higher beta-blocker dose during coadministration of primidone.
Primidone	Corticosteroids (eg, prednisone)	↓	Decreased effect of corticosteroid may be observed. If possible, avoid this combination.
Primidone	Doxycycline	↓	Coadministration may decrease doxycycline half-life and serum levels, possibly resulting in a decreased therapeutic effect. These effects may persist for weeks following primidone discontinuation. Consider an alternate tetracycline.
Primidone	Estrogens Oral contraceptives	↓	AUC of estrogen may be decreased. Contraceptive failure has been reported. Alternate contraception methods are recommended.
Primidone	Ethanol	↑	Impaired hand-eye coordination, additive CNS effects, and death have been noted upon acute ingestion. Chronic ethanol ingestion may manifest as drug tolerance. Avoid concomitant use.
Primidone	Felodipine	↓	Pharmacologic effects of felodipine may be decreased. Patients receiving long-term treatment with both drugs may require higher doses of felodipine.
Primidone	Methadone	↓	The actions of methadone may be reduced. Patients receiving chronic methadone treatment may experience opiate withdrawal symptoms. A higher dose of methadone may be required during coadministration with primidone.
Primidone	Metronidazole	↓	Therapeutic failure of metronidazole has been observed. May need to use higher initial metronidazole doses in patients also receiving primidone.
Primidone	Nifedipine	↓	Decreased serum nifedipine concentrations, possibly reducing efficacy have been observed. Titrate dose according to response. A larger nifedipine dose may be needed.
Primidone	Quinidine	↓	Primidone appears to produce decreased quinidine serum concentrations and a decreased quinidine elimination half-life.
Primidone	Theophyllines	↓	Decreased theophylline levels, possibly resulting in reduced therapeutic effects have been observed. Increased theophylline dosages may be required with use of primidone.

[a] ↑ = object drug increased; ↓ = object drug decreased.

Adverse Reactions

The most frequently occurring early side effects are ataxia and vertigo. These tend to disappear with continued therapy, or with reduction of initial dosage. Occasionally, the following have been reported: Nausea, anorexia, vomiting, fatigue, hyperirritability, emotional disturbances, sexual impotency, diplopia, nystagmus, drowsiness, and morbilliform skin eruptions. Granulocytopenia, agranulocytosis, and red-cell hypoplasia and aplasia, have been reported rarely. These and, occasionally, other persistent or severe side effects may necessitate withdrawal of the drug. Megaloblastic anemia may occur as a rare idiosyncrasy to primidone and to other anticonvulsants. The anemia responds to folic acid without necessity of discontinuing medication.

VIGABATRIN

Rx	**Sabril** (Lundbeck)	**Powder for solution; oral:** 500 mg	In packets (50s).
		Tablets; oral: 500 mg	White, oval, scored. Film-coated. (OV 111). In 100s.

VIGABATRIN — ORAL

Refer to the general discussion beginning in the Anticonvulsants introduction.

WARNING

Vision loss – Vigabatrin causes permanent vision loss in infants, children, and adults. Because assessing vision loss is difficult in children, the frequency and extent of vision loss in infants and children is poorly characterized. For this reason, the following data are primarily based on the adult experience.

In adults, vigabatrin causes permanent bilateral concentric visual field constriction in 30% or more of patients; it ranges in severity from mild to severe, including tunnel vision to within 10 degrees of visual fixation, and can result in disability. In some cases, vigabatrin also can damage the central retina and may decrease visual acuity.

The onset of vision loss from vigabatrin is unpredictable, and can occur within weeks of starting treatment or sooner, or at any time during treatment, even after months or years.

The risk of vision loss increases with increasing dose and cumulative exposure, but there is no dose or exposure known to be free of risk of vision loss.

Vision testing at baseline (no later than 4 weeks after starting vigabatrin) and at least every 3 months during therapy is required for adults on vigabatrin. In infants and children, vision loss may not be detected until it is severe. Nonetheless, assess vision to the extent possible at baseline (no later than 4 weeks after starting vigabatrin) and at least every 3 months during therapy. Vision testing is also required about 3 to 6 months after the discontinuation of vigabatrin therapy. Once detected, vision loss caused by vigabatrin is not reversible. It is expected that, even with frequent monitoring, some patients will develop severe vision loss.

It is possible that vision loss can worsen despite discontinuing vigabatrin.

Because of the risk of vision loss, withdraw vigabatrin from patients who fail to show substantial clinical benefit within 2 to 4 weeks of initiation when used in children or within 3 months when used in adults, or sooner if treatment failure becomes obvious. Periodically reassess patient response to and continued need for vigabatrin.

Symptoms of vision loss from vigabatrin are unlikely to be recognized by the parent or caregiver before vision loss is severe. Vision loss of milder severity, although unrecognized by the caregiver, may still adversely affect function.

Do not use vigabatrin in patients with, or at high risk of, other types of irreversible vision loss unless the benefits of treatment clearly outweigh the risks. The interaction of other types of irreversible vision damage with vision damage from vigabatrin has not been well characterized, but is likely adverse.

Do not use vigabatrin with other drugs associated with serious adverse ophthalmic effects such as retinopathy or glaucoma unless the benefits clearly outweigh the risks.

Use the lowest dose and shortest exposure to vigabatrin that is consistent with clinical objectives.

The possibility that vision loss from vigabatrin may be more common, more severe, or have more severe functional consequences in infants and children than in adults cannot be excluded.

Because of the risk of permanent vision loss, vigabatrin is available only through a special restricted distribution program called SHARE, by calling 1-888-457-4273. Only prescribers and pharmacies registered with SHARE may prescribe and distribute vigabatrin. In addition, vigabatrin may be dispensed only to patients who are enrolled in and meet all conditions of SHARE.

Indications

➤*Infantile spasms (1 month to 2 years of age):* As monotherapy for infants and children with infantile spasms for whom the potential benefits outweigh the potential risk of vision loss.

➤*Refractory complex partial seizures:* As adjunctive therapy for adults with refractory complex partial seizures who have inadequately responded to several alternative treatments and for whom the potential benefits outweigh the risk of vision loss.

Administration and Dosage

➤*General dosing considerations:* Monitoring of vigabatrin concentrations to optimize therapy is not helpful.

Vigabatrin must be tapered prior to discontinuation.

➤*Adults:*

Refractory complex partial seizures –
Usual dosage: 3 g/day (1.5 g twice daily).
Maximum dose: 6 g/day.
Initial dosage: 1 g/day (500 mg twice daily).
Dosage titration: Total daily dose may be increased in 500 mg increments at weekly intervals depending on response.

Tapering: Vigabatrin should be withdrawn gradually. In controlled clinical studies in adults with complex partial seizures, vigabatrin was tapered by decreasing the daily dose 1 g/day on a weekly basis until discontinued.

➤*Children:*

Infantile spasms –
1 month to 2 years of age:
• *Maximum dose* – 150 mg/kg/day.
• *Initial dosage* – 50 mg/kg/day given in 2 divided doses.

Vigabatrin Infant Dosing Table

Weight (kg)	Starting dose 50 mg/kg/day	Maximum dose 150 mg/kg/day
3	1.5 mL twice daily	4.5 mL twice daily
4	2 mL twice daily	6 mL twice daily
5	2.5 mL twice daily	7.5 mL twice daily
6	3 mL twice daily	9 mL twice daily
7	3.5 mL twice daily	10.5 mL twice daily
8	4 mL twice daily	12 mL twice daily
9	4.5 mL twice daily	13.5 mL twice daily
10	5 mL twice daily	15 mL twice daily
11	5.5 mL twice daily	16.5 mL twice daily
12	6 mL twice daily	18 mL twice daily
13	6.5 mL twice daily	19.5 mL twice daily
14	7 mL twice daily	21 mL twice daily
15	7.5 mL twice daily	22.5 mL twice daily
16	8 mL twice daily	24 mL twice daily

• *Dosage titration* – Titrate by 25 to 50 mg/kg/day increments every 3 days, up to a maximum of 150 mg/kg/day.
• *Tapering* – If a decision is made to discontinue vigabatrin, the dose should be gradually reduced. In a controlled clinical study in patients with infantile spasms, vigabatrin was tapered by decreasing the dose at a rate of 25 to 50 mg/kg every 3 to 4 days.

Refractory complex partial seizures –
16 years of age and older: See Adults for dosing.
Younger than 16 years of age: Safety and efficacy of vigabatrin in children younger than 16 years of age with complex partial seizures have not been established.

➤*Renal function impairment:* Information about how to adjust the dose in children with renal impairment is unavailable.

The following dose adjustments are pertinent to the use of the oral solution in adults with renal impairment.

Mild renal impairment (creatinine clearance greater than 50 to 80 mL/min) – Decrease the dose by 25%.

Moderate renal impairment (creatinine clearance greater than 30 to 50 mL/min) – Decrease the dose by 50%.

Severe renal impairment (creatinine clearance greater than 10 to less than 30 mL/min) – Decrease the dose by 75%.

➤*Preparation for administration:* The entire contents of the appropriate number of packets (500 mg/packet) of powder should be emptied into an empty cup, and should be dissolved in 10 mL of cold or room temperature water per packet using the 10 mL oral syringe supplied with the medication. The concentration of the final solution is 50 mg/mL. The following table describes how many packets and how many mL of water will be needed to prepare each individual dose. Each individual dose should be prepared immediately before use and administered cold or at room temperature.

Number of Packages of Vigabatrin and mL of Water Used for Each Individual Dose

Each individual dose (prepared and given twice daily)	Number of vigabatrin packets	Number of mL of water for dissolving
0 to 500 mg	1 packet	10 mL
501 to 1,000 mg	2 packets	20 mL
1,001 to 1,500 mg	3 packets	30 mL

➤*Administration:* Vigabatrin should be given as twice-daily oral administration with or without food.

Health care providers should confirm that caregiver(s) understand how to reconstitute vigabatrin and to administer the correct dose to their infants.

➤*Storage/Stability:* Store at 20° to 25°C (68° to 77°F).

Actions

➤*Pharmacology:* The precise mechanism of vigabatrin's antiseizure effect is unknown, but it is believed to be the result of its action as an irreversible inhibitor of gamma-aminobutyric acid transaminase (GABA-T), the enzyme

VIGABATRIN — ORAL

responsible for the metabolism of the inhibitory neurotransmitter GABA. This action results in increased levels of GABA in the CNS.

No direct correlation between plasma concentration and efficacy has been established. The duration of drug effect is presumed to be dependent on the rate of enzyme resynthesis, rather than on the rate of elimination of the drug from the systemic circulation.

➤*Pharmacokinetics:* Vigabatrin displayed linear pharmacokinetics after administration of single doses ranging from 0.5 to 4 g, and after administration of repeated dosages of 0.5 to 2 g twice daily.

Absorption – Following oral administration, vigabatrin is essentially completely absorbed.

Time to maximum concentration (T_{max}) is approximately 2.5 hours in infants and approximately 1 hour in children and adults following a single dose. There was little accumulation with multiple dosing.

Effect of food: A food effect study involving administration of vigabatrin to healthy adult volunteers under fasting and fed conditions indicated that the maximum plasma concentration (C_{max}) was decreased by 33%, T_{max} increased to 2 hours, and area under the curve (AUC) was unchanged under fed conditions.

Bioequivalence: Bioequivalence has been established between the oral solution and tablet formulations.

Distribution – Vigabatrin does not bind to plasma proteins. Vigabatrin is widely distributed throughout the body; mean steady-state volume of distribution is 1.1 L/Kg (coefficient of variation, 20%).

Metabolism/Excretion – Vigabatrin is not significantly metabolized; it is eliminated primarily through renal excretion. The half-life of vigabatrin in adults is approximately 7.5 hours and approximately 5.7 hours in infants. Following administration of ^{14}C-vigabatrin to healthy adult male volunteers, approximately 95% of total radioactivity was recovered in the urine over 72 hours, with the parent drug representing about 80% of this. Vigabatrin induces CYP2C9, but does not induce other hepatic cytochrome P450 enzyme systems.

Special populations –

Renal function impairment: In patients with mild renal impairment (creatinine clearance [CrCl] greater than 50 to 80 mL/min), mean AUC increased by 30% and the terminal half-life increased by 55% (8.1 vs 12.5 h) in comparison with healthy subjects. Mean AUC increased by 2-fold and the terminal half-life increased by 2-fold in patients with moderate renal impairment (CrCl greater than 30 to 50 mL/min) in comparison with healthy subjects. Mean AUC increased by 4.5-fold and the terminal half-life increased by 3.5-fold in patients with severe renal impairment (CrCl greater than 10 to 30 mL/min) in comparison with healthy subjects.

While dose adjustments are warranted in children with renal impairment, no data are available to guide dose adjustments in this patient population. Dosage adjustment, including starting at a lower dose, is recommended in adults with any degree of renal impairment.

Elderly: The renal clearance of vigabatrin in healthy elderly patients (65 years of age and older) was 36% less than those in healthy younger patients.

Children: The clearance of infants and children were 2.4 ± 0.8 and 5.7 ± 2.5 L/h, respectively compared with 7 L/h in adults.

Race: The mean renal clearance of white patients (5.2 L/h) was approximately 25% higher than the Japanese patients (4 L/h). Intersubject variability in renal clearance was 20% in white patients and 30% in Japanese patients.

Contraindications

None well documented.

Warnings/Precautions

➤*Vision loss:* Because of the risk of vision loss and because vigabatrin, when it is effective, provides an observable symptomatic benefit, withdraw the patient who fails to show substantial clinical benefit within 2 to 4 weeks of initiation of treatment for infants and children and within 3 months for adults from vigabatrin. If, in the clinical judgment of the health care provider, evidence of treatment failure becomes obvious earlier than 2 to 4 weeks (infants and children) or 3 months (adults), discontinue treatment with vigabatrin at that time. Periodically assess patient response to and continued need for treatment. Also see Warning Box for more information.

Monitoring of vision – Because vision testing in infants and children is difficult, vision loss may not be detected until it is severe. However, monitoring of vision by an ophthalmic professional with expertise in visual field interpretation and the ability to perform dilated indirect ophthalmoscopy of the retina must be performed at baseline (no later than 4 weeks after starting vigabatrin) and at least every 3 months while on therapy. Vision testing is also required about 3 to 6 months after the discontinuation of vigabatrin therapy. Ensure that this assessment includes visual acuity and visual field whenever possible.

Individualize the diagnostic approach for the patient and clinical situation, but, for all patients, attempts to monitor vision periodically must be documented under the SHARE program. Perimetry is recommended, preferably by automated threshold visual field testing. Additional testing may also include electrophysiology (eg, electroretinography), retinal imaging (eg, optical coherence tomography), and/or other methods appropriate for the patient. In patients in whom vision testing is not possible, treatment may continue according to clinical judgment, with appropriate patient and caregiver(s) counseling, and with documentation in the SHARE program of the inability to test vision. Because of variability, results from ophthalmic monitoring must be interpreted with caution, and repeat testing is recommended if results are abnormal or uninterpretable. Repeat testing in the first few weeks of treatment is recommended to establish if, and to what degree, reproducible results can be obtained, and to guide selection of appropriate ongoing monitoring for the patient.

The onset and progression of vision loss from vigabatrin are unpredictable, and may occur or worsen precipitously. Once detected, vision loss caused by vigabatrin is not reversible. It is expected that, even with frequent monitoring, some vigabatrin patients will develop severe vision loss.

➤*Distribution program:* Vigabatrin is available only under a special restricted distribution program called the SHARE program. Under the SHARE program, only prescribers and pharmacies registered with the program are able to prescribe and distribute vigabatrin. In addition, vigabatrin may be dispensed only to patients who are enrolled in and meet all conditions of SHARE. Contact the SHARE program at 1-888-457-4273. To enroll in SHARE, prescribers must understand the risks of vigabatrin and complete the SHARE Prescriber Enrollment and Agreement Form indicating agreement to:

- Enroll all patients in SHARE.
- Review the vigabatrin Medication Guide with every patient and/or caregiver.
- Educate caregiver(s) and patients on the risks of vigabatrin, including the risk of vision loss.
- Arrange for visual field and retinal exam by an expert examiner and review visual evaluation prior to initiation of vigabatrin treatment and every 3 months during therapy.
- Remove patients from vigabatrin therapy if the patients do not experience a meaningful reduction in seizures.
- Counsel caregiver(s) and patients who fail to comply with the program requirements.
- Remove patients who fail to comply, or whose caregiver(s) fail to comply, with the program requirements after appropriate counseling from vigabatrin therapy.

➤*Magnetic resonance imaging:* Abnormal magnetic resonance imaging (MRI) signal changes characterized by increased T2 signal and restricted diffusion in a symmetric pattern involving the thalamus, basal ganglia, brain stem, and cerebellum have been observed in some infants treated for infantile spasms with vigabatrin. In a retrospective epidemiologic study in infants with infantile spasms (N = 205), the prevalence of these changes was 21.5% in vigabatrin-treated patients versus 4.1% in patients treated with other therapies.

In the previously mentioned study, in postmarketing experience, and in published literature reports, these changes generally resolved with discontinuation of treatment. In a few patients, the lesion resolved despite continued use. It has been reported that some infants exhibited coincident motor abnormalities, but no causal relationship has been established and the potential for long-term clinical sequelae has not been adequately studied.

The specific pattern of signal changes observed in patients with infantile spasms was not observed in older children and adult patients treated with vigabatrin for refractory complex partial seizures. In a blinded review of MRI images obtained in prospective clinical trials in patients with refractory complex partial seizures 3 years of age and older (N = 656), no difference was observed in anatomic distribution or prevalence of MRI signal changes between vigabatrin-treated and placebo patients. For adults treated with vigabatrin, routine MRI surveillance is unnecessary because there is no evidence that vigabatrin causes MRI changes in this population.

➤*Neurotoxicity:* Vacuolization, characterized by fluid accumulation and separation of the outer layers of myelin, has been observed in brain white matter tracts in adult and juvenile rats and adult mice, dogs, and possibly monkeys following administration of vigabatrin. This lesion, referred to as intramyelinic edema, was seen in animals at doses within the human therapeutic range. A no-effect dose was not established in rodents or dogs. In the rat and dog, vacuolization was reversible following discontinuation of vigabatrin treatment, but, in the rat, pathologic changes consisting of swollen or degenerating axons, mineralization, and gliosis were seen in brain areas in which vacuolation had been previously observed. Vacuolization in adult animals was correlated with alterations in MRI and changes in visual and somatosensory evoked potentials.

Administration of vigabatrin to rats during the neonatal and juvenile periods of development produced vacuolar changes in the gray matter (areas including the thalamus, midbrain, deep cerebellar nuclei, substantia nigra, hippocampus, and forebrain), which are considered distinct from the intramyelinic edema observed in vigabatrin-treated adult animals. Decreased myelination, retinal dysplasia, and neurobehavioral abnormalities (convulsions, neuromotor impairment, learning deficits) were also observed following vigabatrin treatment of young rats. These effects occurred at doses associated with plasma vigabatrin levels substantially lower than those achieved clinically in infants and children.

In a published study, vigabatrin (200 and 400 mg/kg/day) induced apoptotic neurodegeneration in the brain of young rats when administered by intraperitoneal injection on postnatal days 5 to 7.

Administration of vigabatrin to female rats during pregnancy and lactation at doses below those used clinically resulted in hippocampal vacuolation and convulsions in the mature offspring.

Abnormal MRI signal changes characterized by increased T2 signal and restricted diffusion in a symmetric pattern involving the thalamus, basal ganglia, brain stem, and cerebellum have been observed in some infants treated for infantile spasms with vigabatrin. Studies of the effects of vigabatrin on MRI and evoked potentials in adult epilepsy patients have demonstrated no clear-cut abnormalities.

➤*Suicidal behavior and ideation:* Antiepileptic drugs (AEDs), including vigabatrin, increase the risk of suicidal thoughts or behavior in patients taking these drugs for any indication. Monitor patients treated with any AED

VIGABATRIN — ORAL

for any indication for the emergence or worsening of depression, suicidal thoughts or behavior, and/or any unusual changes in mood or behavior.

The increased risk of suicidal thoughts or behavior with AEDs was observed as early as 1 week after starting drug treatment with AEDs and persisted for the duration of treatment assessed. Because most trials included in the analysis did not extend beyond 24 weeks, the risk of suicidal thoughts or behavior beyond 24 weeks could not be assessed.

The risk of suicidal thoughts or behavior was generally consistent among drugs in the data analyzed. The finding of increased risk with AEDs of varying mechanisms of action and across a range of indications suggests that the risk applies to all AEDs used for any indication. The risk did not vary substantially by age (5 to 100 years) in the clinical trials analyzed.

The RR for suicidal thoughts or behavior was higher in clinical trials for epilepsy than in clinical trials for psychiatric or other conditions, but the absolute risk differences were similar for the epilepsy and psychiatric indications.

Anyone considering prescribing vigabatrin or any other AED must balance the risk of suicidal thoughts or behavior with the risk of untreated illness. Epilepsy and many other illnesses for which AEDs are prescribed are themselves associated with morbidity and mortality and an increased risk of suicidal thoughts and behavior. Should suicidal thoughts and behavior emerge during treatment, consider whether the emergence of these symptoms in any given patient may be related to the illness being treated.

Inform patients, caregiver(s), and families that AEDs increase the risk of suicidal thoughts and behavior and advise them of the need to be alert for the emergence or worsening of the signs and symptoms of depression, any unusual changes in mood or behavior, or the emergence of suicidal thoughts, behavior, or thoughts about self-harm. Instruct patients, caregiver(s), and families to report behaviors of concern immediately to health care providers.

➤*Withdrawal:* As with all AEDs, withdraw vigabatrin gradually.

Tell caregivers not to suddenly discontinue vigabatrin therapy. In a controlled clinical study in patients with infantile spasms, vigabatrin was tapered by decreasing the daily dose at a rate of 25 to 50 mg/kg every 3 to 4 days.

In controlled clinical studies in adults with complex partial seizures, vigabatrin was tapered by decreasing the daily dose 1 g/day on a weekly basis until discontinued.

➤*Anemia:* In North American controlled trials in adults, 5.7% of patients receiving vigabatrin and 1.6% of patients receiving placebo had adverse events of anemia and/or met criteria for potentially clinically important hematology changes involving hemoglobin, hematocrit, and/or red blood cell indices. Across US controlled trials, there were mean decreases in hemoglobin of approximately 3% and 0% in vigabatrin- and placebo-treated patients, respectively, and in hematocrit of approximately 1% in vigabatrin-treated patients compared with a gain of approximately 1% in patients treated with placebo.

In controlled and open-label epilepsy trials in adults and children, 3 (0.06%) vigabatrin patients discontinued for anemia and 2 vigabatrin patients experienced unexplained declines in hemoglobin to below 8 g/dL and/or hematocrit below 24%.

➤*Peripheral neuropathy:* Vigabatrin has been shown to cause symptoms of peripheral neuropathy in adults. The clinical trials in children were not adequately designed to assess whether or not these symptoms occur in children.

There is insufficient evidence to determine if development of these signs and symptoms were related to duration of vigabatrin treatment or cumulative dose, or if the findings of peripheral neuropathy were completely reversible upon discontinuation of vigabatrin.

➤*Weight gain:* Vigabatrin has been shown to cause weight gain in adults. The clinical trials in children were not adequately designed to assess whether or not weight gain occurs in children.

The long-term effects of vigabatrin related weight gain are not known. Weight gain was not related to the occurrence of edema.

➤*Edema:* Vigabatrin has been shown to cause edema in adults. The clinical trials in children were not adequately designed to assess whether or not edema occurs in children.

➤*Renal function impairment:* Information about how to adjust the dose in children with renal impairment is unavailable.

In adults, dose adjustment, including initiating treatment with a lower dose, is necessary in patients with mild (CrCl greater than 50 to 80 mL/min), moderate (CrCl greater than 30 to 50 mL/min), and severe (CrCl greater than 10 to 30 mL/min) renal impairment.

➤*Hazardous tasks:* Vigabatrin causes somnolence and fatigue. Advise patients not to drive a car or operate other complex machinery until they are familiar with the effects of vigabatrin on their ability to perform such activities.

➤*Pregnancy: Category C.* There are no adequate and well-controlled studies in pregnant women. Use vigabatrin during pregnancy only if the potential benefit justifies the potential risk to the fetus. Vigabatrin produced developmental toxicity, including teratogenic and neurohistopathological effects, when administered to pregnant animals at clinically relevant doses. In addition, developmental neurotoxicity was observed in rats treated with vigabatrin during a period of postnatal development corresponding to the third trimester of human pregnancy.

Administration of vigabatrin (oral doses of 50 to 200 mg/kg) to pregnant rabbits throughout the period of organogenesis was associated with an increased incidence of malformations (cleft palate) and embryofetal death; these findings were observed in 2 separate studies. The no-effect dose for teratogenicity and embryolethality in rabbits (100 mg/kg) is approximately one-half of the maximum recommended human dose (MRHD) of 3 g/day on a body surface area (mg/m^2) basis for adults treated for refractory complex partial seizures with vigabatrin. In rats, oral administration of vigabatrin (50, 100, or 150 mg/kg) throughout organogenesis resulted in decreased fetal body weights and increased incidences of fetal anatomic variations. The no-effect dose for embryofetal toxicity in rats (50 mg/kg) is approximately one-fifth of the MRHD in adults on a mg/m^2 basis. Oral administration of vigabatrin (50, 100, 150 mg/kg) to rats from the latter part of pregnancy through weaning produced long-term neurohistopathological (hippocampal vacuolation) and neurobehavioral (convulsions) abnormalities in the offspring. A no-effect dose for developmental neurotoxicity in rats was not established; the low-effect dose (50 mg/kg) is approximately one-fifth of the MRHD in adults on a mg/m^2 basis.

In a published study, vigabatrin (300 or 450 mg/kg) was administered by intraperitoneal injection to a mutant mouse strain on a single day during organogenesis (day 7, 8, 9, 10, 11, or 12). An increase in malformations (including cleft palate) was observed at both doses.

Oral administration of vigabatrin (5, 15, or 50 mg/kg) to young rats during the neonatal and juvenile periods of development (postnatal days 4 to 65) produced neurobehavioral (convulsions, neuromotor impairment, learning deficits) and neurohistopathological (brain vacuolation, decreased myelination, and retinal dysplasia) abnormalities in treated animals. The early postnatal period in rats is generally thought to correspond to late pregnancy in humans in terms of brain development. The no-effect dose for developmental neurotoxicity in juvenile rats (5 mg/kg) was associated with plasma vigabatrin exposures (AUC) less than one-thirtieth of those measured in children receiving an oral dose of 50 mg/kg.

Pregnancy registry – To provide information regarding the effects of in utero exposure to vigabatrin, recommend that pregnant patients taking vigabatrin enroll in the North American Antiepileptic Drug (NAAED) Pregnancy Registry. This can be done by calling the toll-free number 1-888-233-2334, and must be done by patients themselves. Information on the registry can also be found at the Web site http://www.aedpregnancyregistry.org/.

➤*Lactation:* Vigabatrin is excreted in human milk. Because of the potential for serious adverse reactions from vigabatrin in breast-feeding infants, decide whether to discontinue breast-feeding or the drug, taking into account the importance of the drug to the mother.

➤*Children:* Vigabatrin is indicated as monotherapy for infants and children with infantile spasms (1 month to 2 years of age) for whom the potential benefits outweigh the potential risk for developing permanent vision loss.

The safety and efficacy of vigabatrin in children younger than 16 years of age with complex partial seizures have not been established.

Abnormal MRI signal changes characterized by increased T2 signal and restricted diffusion in a symmetric pattern involving the thalamus, basal ganglia, brain stem, and cerebellum have been observed in some infants treated for infantile spasms with vigabatrin. In a retrospective epidemiologic study in infants with infantile spasms (N = 205), the prevalence of these changes was 21.5% in vigabatrin-treated patients versus 4.1% in patients treated with other therapies. A dose-dependent relationship may exist, because children with infantile spasms who were exposed to a higher vigabatrin dose (at least 125 mg/kg/day) had a prevalence of 29.5%, while those exposed to lower doses of vigabatrin had a prevalence of 12.5%; however, these differences were not statistically significant (P = 0.099).

In the previous study, in postmarketing experience, and in published literature reports, these changes generally resolved with discontinuation of treatment, although in a few patients, the lesion resolved despite continued use. It has been reported that some infants exhibited coincident motor abnormalities, but no causal relationship has been established and the potential for long-term clinical sequelae has not been adequately studied.

➤*Elderly:* Vigabatrin is known to be substantially excreted by the kidney, and the risk of toxic reactions to this drug may be greater in patients with impaired renal function. Because elderly patients are more likely to have decreased renal function, exercise care in dose selection; it may be useful to monitor renal function.

Oral administration of a single dose of vigabatrin 1.5 g to elderly (older than 65 years of age) patients with reduced CrCl (less than 50 mL/min) was associated with moderate to severe sedation and confusion in 4 of 5 patients, lasting up to 5 days. The renal clearance of vigabatrin was 36% lower in healthy elderly subjects (older than 65 years of age) than in young healthy men. Consider adjustment of dose or frequency of administration. Such patients may respond to a lower maintenance dose.

➤*Monitoring:* Monitoring of vision by an ophthalmic professional with expertise in visual field interpretation and the ability to perform dilated indirect ophthalmoscopy of the retina must be performed at baseline (no later than 4 weeks after starting vigabatrin) and at least every 3 months while on therapy. Vision testing is also required about 3 to 6 months after the discontinuation of vigabatrin therapy. Ensure that this assessment includes visual acuity and visual field whenever possible.

Monitor patients for the emergence or worsening of the signs and symptoms of depression, any unusual changes in mood or behavior, or the emergence of suicidal thoughts, behavior, or thoughts about self-harm.

VIGABATRIN — ORAL

Drug Interactions

Vigabatrin Drug Interactions			
Precipitant drug	Object drug[a]		Description
Drugs associated with serious adverse ophthalmic effects such as retinopathy (eg, hydroxychloroquine) or glaucoma (eg, corticosteroids [open-angle], tricyclic antidepressants [closed-angle])	Vigabatrin	↑	Risk of serious adverse ophthalmic effects may be increased. Avoid coadministration unless the benefits clearly outweigh the risks.
Vigabatrin	Clonazepam	↑	Clonazepam plasma concentrations may be increased while the T_{max} may be reduced, increasing the pharmacologic effects and risk of adverse reactions. Monitor the patient when starting or stopping vigabatrin. Adjust the clonazepam dose as needed.
Vigabatrin	Hydantoins (eg, phenytoin)	↓	Vigabatrin coadministration has been reported to decrease phenytoin plasma concentrations 16% to 20%. Monitor the patient when starting or stopping vigabatrin. Be prepared to adjust the hydantoin dose if an interaction is suspected.
Vigabatrin	Phenobarbital, primidone	↓	On average, phenobarbital plasma concentrations may be reduced 8% to 16%. This change is not likely to be clinically important.
Vigabatrin	Valproic acid	↓	On average, valproate plasma concentrations may be reduced 8%. This change is not likely to be clinically important.

[a] ↑ = object drug increased; ↓ = object drug decreased.

➤*Drug/Lab test interactions:* Vigabatrin suppresses ALT and AST enzyme activity in up to 90% of patients. In some patients, these enzymes become undetectable. The suppression of ALT and AST activity may preclude the use of these markers to detect early hepatic injury.

Vigabatrin may increase the amount of amino acids in the urine, possibly leading to a false-positive test for certain rare genetic metabolic diseases (eg, alpha-aminoadipic aciduria).

➤*Drug/Food interactions:* Under fed conditions, vigabatrin C_{max} was decreased 33%, the T_{max} was prolonged to 2 hours, and the AUC was unchanged. However, vigabatrin may be given without regard to food.

Adverse Reactions

➤*Common adverse reactions:* In US and primary non-US clinical studies of 4,079 patients treated with vigabatrin, the most commonly observed (at least 5%) adverse reactions associated with the use of vigabatrin in combination with other AEDs were headache (18%); somnolence (17%); fatigue (16%); dizziness (15%); convulsion (11%); nasopharyngitis, upper respiratory tract infection, weight increased (10%); visual field defect (9%); depression (8%); coordination abnormal, diarrhea, insomnia, irritability, memory impairment, nausea, nystagmus, tremor (7%); diplopia, influenza, pyrexia, rash, vision blurred, vomiting (6%).

➤*Discontinuation:* The adverse reactions most commonly associated with vigabatrin treatment discontinuation in at least 1% of infantile spasms patients were infections (1.5%); developmental coordination disorder, dystonia, hypertonia, hypotonia, insomnia, status epilepticus, weight increased (1.2%). The adverse reactions most commonly associated with vigabatrin treatment discontinuation in at least 1% of patients with complex partial seizures were convulsion (1.4%) and depression (1.5%).

➤*Infantile spasms:* In a randomized, placebo-controlled infantile spasms study with a 5-day double-blind treatment phase (n = 40), the adverse reactions reported by more than 5% of vigabatrin patients and that occurred more frequently than in placebo patients were somnolence (vigabatrin 45%, placebo 30%), bronchitis (vigabatrin 30%, placebo 15%), ear infection (vigabatrin 10%, placebo 5%), and otitis media acute(vigabatrin 10%, placebo 0%).

In a dose-response study of low-dose (18 to 36 mg/kg/day) versus high-dose (100 to 148 mg/kg/day) vigabatrin, no clear correlation between dose and incidence of adverse reactions was observed.

Vigabatrin Adverse Reactions in Children With Infantile Spasms (≥ 5%)		
Adverse reaction	Vigabatrin low dose (n = 114)	Vigabatrin high dose (n = 108)
CNS		
Convulsion	4%	7%
Hypotonia	4%	6%
Insomnia	10%	12%
Irritability	16%	23%
Lethargy	5%	7%
Sedation	19%	17%
Somnolence	17%	19%
Status epilepticus	6%	4%
GI		
Constipation	14%	12%
Decreased appetite	9%	7%
Diarrhea	13%	12%
Gastroenteritis viral	6%	5%
Vomiting	14%	20%
GU		
Urinary tract infection	5%	6%
Respiratory		
Cough	3%	8%
Nasal congestion	13%	4%
Pneumonia	13%	11%
Sinusitis	5%	9%
Upper respiratory tract infection	51%	46%
Special senses		
Conjunctivitis	5%	2%
Ear infection	7%	14%
Otitis media	44%	30%
Strabismus	5%	5%
Miscellaneous		
Candidiasis	8%	3%
Croup infectious	5%	1%
Fever	29%	19%
Influenza	5%	3%
Rash	8%	11%
Viral infection	20%	19%

➤*Refractory complex partial seizures:*

Vigabatrin Adverse Reactions in Adults With Refractory Complex Partial Seizures (≥ 2%)			
Adverse reaction	Vigabatrin 3 g/day (n = 134)	Vigabatrin 6 g/day (n = 43)	Placebo (n = 135)
CNS			
Abnormal behavior	3%	5%	1%
Abnormal dreams	1%	5%	1%
Anxiety	4%	0%	3%
Asthenia	5%	7%	1%
Confusional state	4%	14%	1%
Coordination abnormal	7%	16%	2%
Depressed mood	5%	0%	1%
Depression	6%	14%	3%
Disturbance in attention	9%	0%	1%
Dizziness	24%	26%	17%
Dysarthria	2%	2%	1%
Expressive language disorder	1%	7%	1%
Fatigue	23%	40%	16%
Gait disturbance	6%	12%	7%
Headache	33%	26%	31%
Hypesthesia	4%	5%	1%
Hyperreflexia	4%	2%	3%
Hyporeflexia	4%	5%	1%
Irritability	7%	23%	7%

VIGABATRIN — ORAL

Vigabatrin Adverse Reactions in Adults With Refractory Complex Partial Seizures (≥ 2%)			
Adverse reaction	Vigabatrin 3 g/day (n = 134)	Vigabatrin 6 g/day (n = 43)	Placebo (n = 135)
Lethargy	4%	7%	2%
Malaise	0%	5%	0%
Memory impairment	7%	16%	3%
Nervousness	2%	5%	2%
Paresthesia	7%	2%	1%
Postictal state	2%	0%	1%
Sedation	4%	0%	0%
Sensory disturbance	4%	7%	2%
Sensory loss	0%	5%	0%
Somnolence	22%	26%	13%
Status epilepticus	2%	5%	0%
Thinking abnormal	3%	7%	0%
Tremor	15%	16%	8%
GI			
Abdominal distension	2%	0%	1%
Abdominal pain	3%	2%	1%
Abdominal pain upper	5%	5%	1%
Constipation	8%	5%	3%
Diarrhea	10%	16%	7%
Dyspepsia	4%	5%	3%
Nausea	10%	2%	8%
Stomach discomfort	4%	2%	1%
Toothache	2%	5%	2%
Vomiting	7%	9%	6%
GU			
Dysmenorrhea	9%	5%	3%
Erectile dysfunction	0%	5%	0%
Urinary tract infection	4%	5%	0%
Metabolic/Nutritional			
Increased appetite	1%	5%	1%
Peripheral edema	5%	7%	1%
Weight increased	6%	14%	3%
Musculoskeletal			
Arthralgia	10%	5%	3%
Back pain	4%	7%	2%
Joint sprain	1%	2%	1%
Muscle spasms	3%	0%	1%
Muscle strain	1%	2%	1%
Muscle twitching	1%	9%	1%
Myalgia	3%	5%	1%
Pain in extremity	6%	2%	4%
Respiratory			
Bronchitis	0%	5%	1%
Cough	2%	14%	7%
Nasopharyngitis	14%	9%	10%
Pharyngolaryngeal pain	7%	14%	5%
Pulmonary congestion	0%	5%	1%
Upper respiratory tract infection	7%	9%	6%
Sinus headache	6%	2%	1%
Special senses			
Asthenopia	2%	2%	0%
Diplopia	7%	16%	3%
Eye pain	0%	5%	0%
Nystagmus	13%	19%	9%
Tinnitus	2%	0%	1%
Vertigo	2%	5%	1%
Vision blurred	13%	16%	5%
Miscellaneous			
Chest pain	1%	5%	1%
Contusion	3%	5%	2%
Fever	4%	7%	3%
Influenza	5%	7%	4%
Rash	4%	5%	4%
Thirst	2%	0%	0%
Wound secretion	0%	2%	0%

➤*Postmarketing:*

Birth defects – Congenital cardiac defects, congenital external ear anomaly, congenital hemangioma, congenital hydronephrosis, congenital male genital malformation, congenital oral malformation, congenital vesicoureteric reflux, dentofacial anomaly, dysmorphism, fetal anticonvulsant syndrome, hamartomas, hip dysplasia, limb malformation, limb reduction defect, low set ears, renal aplasia, retinitis pigmentosa, supernumerary nipple, talipes.

CNS – Acute psychosis, apathy, delirium, dystonia, encephalopathy, hypertonia, hypomania, hypotonia, malignant hyperthermia, muscle spasticity, myoclonus, neonatal agitation, psychotic disorder.

Dermatologic – Angioedema, maculopapular rash, pruritus.

GI – Esophagitis, GI hemorrhage.

Respiratory – Laryngeal edema, pulmonary embolism, respiratory failure, stridor.

Special senses – Deafness, optic neuritis.

Miscellaneous – Cholestasis, delayed puberty, developmental delay, facial edema, multiorgan failure.

Overdosage

➤*Symptoms:* Confirmed and/or suspected vigabatrin overdoses have been reported during clinical studies and in post marketing surveillance. No vigabatrin overdoses resulted in death. When reported, the vigabatrin dose ingested ranged from 3 to 90 g, but most were between 7.5 and 30 g. Nearly half the cases involved multiple drug ingestions, including carbamazepine, barbiturates, benzodiazepines, lamotrigine, valproic acid, acetaminophen, and/or chlorpheniramine.

Coma, unconsciousness, and/or drowsiness were described in the majority of cases of vigabatrin overdose. Other less commonly reported symptoms included vertigo, psychosis, apnea or respiratory depression, bradycardia, agitation, irritability, confusion, headache, hypotension, abnormal behavior, increased seizure activity, status epilepticus, and speech disorder. These symptoms resolved with supportive care.

➤*Treatment:* There is no specific antidote for vigabatrin overdose. Use standard measures to remove unabsorbed drug, including elimination by gastric lavage. Employ supportive measures, including monitoring of vital signs and observation of the clinical status of the patient.

In an in vitro study, activated charcoal did not significantly adsorb vigabatrin.

The effectiveness of hemodialysis in the treatment of vigabatrin overdose is unknown. In isolated case reports in patients with renal failure receiving therapeutic doses of vigabatrin, hemodialysis reduced vigabatrin plasma concentrations by 40% to 60%.

Patient Information

Instruct patients and caregivers on the appropriate procedure for reconstituting the powder for oral solution and administering the correct dose of vigabatrin.

Inform patients and caregivers of the risk of permanent vision loss, particularly loss of peripheral vision, from vigabatrin, and the need for monitoring vision.

Inform patients and caregiver(s) that monitoring of vision, including assessment of visual fields and visual acuity, is required for adults at baseline (no later than 4 weeks after starting vigabatrin) and at least every 3 months while on therapy unless after repeated attempts it is not possible. In those patients in whom vision testing is not possible, treatment may continue according to clinical judgment with appropriate patient counseling and with documentation in the SHARE program of the inability to test vision. Inform patients that if baseline or subsequent vision is not normal, only to use vigabatrin if the benefits of treatment clearly outweigh the risks of additional vision loss.

Ensure that patients and caregiver(s) understand that vision testing may be insensitive, especially in infants, and may not detect vision loss before it is severe. Also ensure that they understand that if vision loss is documented, such loss is irreversible.

Inform patients and caregivers that if changes in vision are suspected, they should notify their health care provider immediately.

Inform patients and caregivers of the possibility of developing abnormal MRI signal changes of unknown clinical significance.

Counsel patients, families, and caregivers that AEDs, including vigabatrin, may increase the risk of suicidal thoughts and behavior and should be advised of the need to be alert for the emergence or worsening of symptoms of depression, any unusual changes in mood or behavior, or the emergence of

VIGABATRIN — ORAL

suicidal thoughts, behavior, or thoughts of self-harm. Advise patients, families, and caregivers to immediately report behaviors of concern to health care providers.

Instruct patients to notify their health care provider if they become pregnant or intend to become pregnant during therapy, and to notify their health care provider if they are breast-feeding or intend to breast-feed during therapy.

Advise patients to enroll in the NAAED Pregnancy Registry if they become pregnant. This registry is collecting information about the safety of antiepileptic drugs during pregnancy. To enroll, patients can call the toll-free number, 1-888-233-2334. Information on the registry can also be found at the Web site http://www.aedpregnancyregistry.org/.

Advise patients and caregivers not to suddenly discontinue vigabatrin therapy. As with all AEDs, withdrawal should be gradual. In infants and children with infantile spasms, taper vigabatrin by decreasing the daily dose at a rate of 25 to 50 mg/kg every 3 to 4 days. In adults with complex partial seizures, taper vigabatrin by decreasing the daily dose 1 g/day on a weekly basis until discontinued.

TIAGABINE HYDROCHLORIDE

Rx	**Gabitril** (Cephalon)	**Tablets; oral:** 2 mg	Lactose. (C 402). Orange-peach. Round. In 30s.
		4 mg	Lactose. (C 404). Yellow. Round. In 30s.
		12 mg	Lactose. (C 412). Green. Ovaloid. In 30s.
		16 mg	Lactose. (C 416). Blue. Ovaloid. In 30s.

TIAGABINE HYDROCHLORIDE — ORAL

Indications

➤*Partial seizures:* Adjunctive therapy in adults and children 12 years of age and older in the treatment of partial seizures.

➤*Off-label uses:*

Bipolar disorders – [3] = Safety concerns. Conflicting data regarding efficacy and new information documenting an increased risk of significant adverse reactions (eg, seizures) with off-label use suggest that tiagabine is not beneficial in the treatment of bipolar disorders. In light of new safety data, this drug does not offer a clear benefit-risk ratio and is not recommended for use in the treatment of bipolar disorders. (See Administration and Dosage.)

Posttraumatic stress disorder (adults) – [4] = Insufficient documentation. The use of tiagabine in the management of posttraumatic stress disorder (PTSD) has produced conflicting results, demonstrating beneficial effects in noncontrolled settings and less favorable effects in controlled settings. (See Administration and Dosage.)

Other possible off-label uses – For the treatment of refractory seizures in children. (See Administration and Dosage.)

Administration and Dosage

➤*General dosing considerations:* Dosing should take the presence of concomitant medications into account.

Do not use a loading dose.

➤*Adults:*

Partial seizures –

Patients taking enzyme-inducing antiepilepsy drugs:

- *Maximum dose* – 56 mg/day.
- *Initial dosage* – 4 mg once daily.
- *Dosage titration* – Increase by 4 to 8 mg at weekly intervals until clinical response is achieved or up to 56 mg/day in 2 to 4 divided doses.
- *Maintenance dosage* – 32 to 56 mg/day in 2 to 4 divided doses.
- *Dosage adjustment* – Dosage adjustment should be considered whenever a change in patient's enzyme-inducing status occurs as a result of the addition, discontinuation, or dose change of the enzyme-inducing agent.
- *Concomitant therapy* – Modification of concomitant antiepilepsy drugs (AEDs) is not necessary unless clinically indicated.

Patients not taking an enzyme-inducing AED: Following a given dose of tiagabine, the estimated plasma concentration in the noninduced patients is more than twice that in patients receiving enzyme-inducing agents. Use in noninduced patients requires lower doses of tiagabine. These patients may also require a slower titration of tiagabine compared with that of induced patients.

Off-label dosing –

Bipolar disorders: [3] = Safety concerns.

- *Initial dosage* – 1 to 4 mg daily titrated by 1 to 4 mg weekly.
- *Maintenance dosage* – Doses as high as 40 mg have been documented but typically have been between 3 and 8 mg daily for up to several months.

Posttraumatic stress disorder (adults): [4] = Insufficient documentation.

- *Maximum dose* – 16 mg/day.
- *Initial dosage* – 4 mg daily (2 mg twice daily) for 1 week.
- *Dosage titration* – Titrate by increments of 4 mg/day weekly.
- *Alternative dosage* – 2 mg daily, with weekly increases by 2 mg increments every week or 2 to 3 days to a maximum of 8 mg daily.

➤*Children:*

Partial seizures –

12 to 18 years of age:

- *Patients taking enzyme-inducing AEDs* –
  Maximum dose: 32 mg/day.
  Initial dosage: 4 mg once daily.
  Dosage titration: Increase by 4 mg at the beginning of week 2. Thereafter, the total daily dose may be increased by 4 to 8 mg at weekly intervals until clinical response is achieved or up to 32 mg/day in 2 to 4 divided doses.
  Dosage adjustment: See Adults.
  Concomitant therapy: See Adults.
- *Patients not taking an enzyme-inducing AED* – See Adults.

Off-label dosing –

Refractory seizures:

- *2 years of age and older* –
  Maximum dose: 0.73 ± 0.44 mg/kg/day in patients receiving enzyme-inducing AED; 0.61 ± 0.32 mg/kg/day in patients receiving nonenzyme-inducing AED.
  Initial dosage: 0.25 mg/kg/day divided 3 times daily for 4 weeks.
  Dosage titration: Increase at 4-week intervals to 0.5, 1, and 1.5 mg/kg/day until effective dose is established.

➤*Hepatic function impairment:* Patients with impaired liver function may require reduced initial and maintenance doses and/or longer dosing intervals.

➤*Missed dose:* If a dose is not taken at the scheduled time, do not attempt to make up for the missed dose alone by increasing the next dose. If multiple doses have been missed, possible retitration may be required.

➤*Discontinuation of therapy:* Do not abruptly discontinue tiagabine. Withdraw gradually to minimize the potential for increased seizure frequency, unless safety concerns require a more rapid withdrawal.

➤*Therapeutic drug monitoring:* The blood level of tiagabine obtained after a given dose depends on whether the patient also is receiving a drug that induces the metabolism of tiagabine. The presence of an inducer means that the attained blood level will be substantially reduced.

➤*Administration:* Tiagabine should be taken with food.

➤*Storage/Stability:* Store between 20° and 25°C (68° and 77°F). Protect from light and moisture.

Actions

➤*Pharmacology:* The precise mechanism by which tiagabine exerts its antiseizure effect is unknown, although it is believed to be related to its ability, documented in in vitro experiments, to enhance the activity of gamma-aminobutyric acid (GABA), the major inhibitory neurotransmitter in the CNS. These experiments have shown that tiagabine binds to recognition sites associated with the GABA uptake carrier. It is thought that, by this action, tiagabine blocks GABA uptake into presynaptic neurons, permitting more GABA to be available for receptor binding on the surfaces of postsynaptic cells. Inhibition of GABA uptake has been shown for synaptosomes, neuronal cell cultures, and glial cell cultures. In rat-derived hippocampal slices, tiagabine has been shown to prolong GABA-mediated inhibitory postsynaptic potentials. Tiagabine increases the amount of GABA available in the extracellular space of the globus pallidus, ventral palladum, and substantia nigra in rats at the median effective dose (ED_{50}) and near maximal effective dose (ED_{85}) for inhibition of pentylenetetrazol-induced tonic seizures. This suggests that tiagabine prevents the propagation of neural impulses that contribute to seizures by a GABA-ergic action.

➤*Pharmacokinetics:*

Absorption/Distribution – Tiagabine is well absorbed. Absorption of tiagabine is rapid, with peak plasma concentrations (C_{max}) occurring at approximately 45 minutes after an oral dose in the fasting state. Tiagabine is nearly completely absorbed (more than 95%), with an absolute oral bioavailability of approximately 90%. Following multiple dosing, steady state is achieved within 2 days.

The pharmacokinetics of tiagabine are linear over the single dose range of 2 to 24 mg. Mean steady-state minimum plasma concentration (C_{min}) values were 40% lower in the evening than in the morning. Tiagabine steady-state area under the curve (AUC) values were also found to be 15% lower after the evening tiagabine dose compared with the AUC after the morning dose.

Tiagabine is 96% bound to human plasma proteins, mainly to serum albumin and alpha-1 acid glycoprotein over the concentration range of 10 to 10,000 ng/mL. While the relationship between tiagabine plasma concentrations and clinical response is not currently understood, trough plasma concentrations observed in controlled clinical trials at dosages from 30 to 56 mg/day ranged from less than 1 to 234 ng/mL.

Effect of food: Food slows the absorption rate of tiagabine but not the extent of absorption. A high-fat meal decreases the absorption rate (mean time of maximal drug concentration [T_{max}] prolonged to 2.5 hours, mean C_{max} reduced by approximately 40%) but not the extent (AUC) of tiagabine absorption. In all clinical trials, tiagabine was given with meals.

Metabolism/Excretion – Although the metabolism of tiagabine has not been fully elucidated, in vivo and in vitro studies suggest that at least 2 metabolic pathways for tiagabine have been identified in humans: 1) thiophene ring oxidation leading to the formation of 5-oxo-tiagabine, and 2) gluc-

TIAGABINE HYDROCHLORIDE — ORAL

uronidation. The 5-oxo-tiagabine metabolite does not contribute to the pharmacologic activity of tiagabine.

Based on in vitro data, tiagabine is likely to be metabolized primarily by the 3A isoform subfamily of hepatic cytochrome P450 (CYP3A), although contributions to the metabolism of tiagabine from CYP1A2, CYP2D6, or CYP2C19 have not been excluded.

Approximately 2% of an oral dose of tiagabine is excreted unchanged, with 25% and 63% of the remaining dose excreted into the urine and feces, respectively, primarily as metabolites, at least 2 of which have not been identified. The mean systemic plasma clearance is 109 mL/min (coefficient of variation, 23%) and the average elimination half-life for tiagabine in healthy subjects ranged from 7 to 9 hours. The elimination half-life decreased 50% to 65% in hepatic enzyme-induced patients with epilepsy compared with noninduced patients with epilepsy.

The systemic clearance of tiagabine in induced patients is approximately 60% greater, resulting in considerably lower plasma concentrations and an elimination half-life of 2 to 5 hours. Given this difference in clearance, the systemic exposure after a dosage of 32 mg/day in an induced population is expected to be comparable with the systemic exposure after a dosage of 12 mg/day in a noninduced population. Similarly, the systemic exposure after a dosage of 56 mg/day in an induced population is expected to be comparable with the systemic exposure after a dosage of 22 mg/day in a noninduced population.

Special populations –

Hepatic function impairment: In patients with moderate hepatic impairment (Child-Pugh class B), clearance of unbound tiagabine was reduced by approximately 60%.

See Administration and Dosage for more information.

Children: In children who were taking a noninducing AED (eg, valproate), the clearance of tiagabine based upon body weight and body surface area was 2- and 1.5-fold higher, respectively, than in noninduced adults with epilepsy.

Contraindications

Hypersensitivity to the drug or its ingredients.

Warnings/Precautions

➤*Seizures in patients without epilepsy:* Postmarketing reports have shown that tiagabine use has been associated with new-onset seizures and status epilepticus in patients without epilepsy. Dose may be an important predisposing factor in the development of seizures, although seizures have been reported in patients taking daily doses of tiagabine as low as 4 mg. In most cases, patients were using concomitant medications (eg, antidepressants, antipsychotics, stimulants, narcotics) that are thought to lower the seizure threshold. Some seizures occurred near the time of a dose increase, even after periods of prior stable dosing.

The tiagabine dosing recommendations in current labeling for treatment of epilepsy were based on use in patients 12 years of age and older with partial seizures, most of whom were taking enzyme-inducing AEDs (eg, carbamazepine, phenytoin, primidone, phenobarbital), which lower plasma levels of tiagabine by inducing its metabolism. Use of tiagabine without enzyme-inducing AEDs results in blood levels approximately twice those attained in the studies on which current dosing recommendations are based.

In nonepileptic patients who develop seizures while on tiagabine treatment, discontinue tiagabine and evaluate patients for an underlying seizure disorder.

➤*Suicidal behavior and ideation:* AEDs, including tiagabine, increase the risk of suicidal thoughts or behavior in patients taking these drugs for any indication. Monitor patients treated with any AED for any indication for the emergence of worsening of depression, suicidal thoughts or behavior, and/or any unusual changes in mood or behavior.

The increased risk of suicidal thoughts or behavior with AEDs was observed as early as 1 week after starting drug treatment with AEDs and persisted for the duration of treatment assessed. Because most trials included in the analysis did not extend beyond 24 weeks, the risk of suicidal thoughts or behavior beyond 24 weeks could not be assessed.

The RR for suicidal thoughts or behavior was higher in clinical trials for epilepsy than in clinical trials for psychiatric or other conditions, but the absolute risk differences were similar for the epilepsy and psychiatric indications.

When considering prescribing tiagabine or any other AED, balance the risk of suicidal thoughts or behavior with the risk of untreated illness. Epilepsy and many other illnesses for which AEDs are prescribed are associated with morbidity and mortality and an increased risk of suicidal thoughts and behavior. If suicidal thoughts and behavior emerge during treatment, consider whether the emergence of these symptoms in any given patient may be related to the illness being treated.

Inform patients, their caregivers, and their families that AEDs increase the risk of suicidal thoughts and behavior and advise them of the need to be alert for the emergence or worsening of the signs and symptoms of depression, any unusual changes in mood or behavior, or the emergence of suicidal thoughts, behavior, or thoughts about self-harm. Behaviors of concern should be reported immediately to health care providers.

➤*Withdrawal seizures:* As a rule, do not abruptly discontinue AEDs because of the possibility of increasing seizure frequency. In a placebo-controlled, double-blind, dose-response study designed in part to investigate the capacity of tiagabine to induce withdrawal seizures, study drug was tapered over a 4-week period after 16 weeks of treatment. Patients' seizure frequency during this 4-week withdrawal period was compared with their baseline seizure frequency (before study drug). For each partial seizure type, for all partial seizure types combined, and for secondarily generalized tonic-clonic seizures, more patients experienced increases in their seizure frequencies during the withdrawal period in the 3 tiagabine groups than in the placebo group. The increase in seizure frequency was not affected by dose. Withdraw tiagabine gradually to minimize the potential of increased seizure frequency, unless safety concerns require a more rapid withdrawal.

➤*CNS effects:* Adverse reactions most often associated with the use of tiagabine were related to the CNS. The most significant of these can be classified into the following 2 general categories: 1) impaired concentration, speech or language problems, and confusion (effects on thought processes) and 2) somnolence and fatigue (effects on level of consciousness). The majority of these reactions were mild to moderate. In controlled clinical trials, these reactions led to discontinuation of treatment with tiagabine in 6% of patients compared with 2% of the placebo-treated patients. A total of 1.6% of the tiagabine-treated patients in the controlled trials were hospitalized secondary to the occurrence of these reactions, compared with 0% of the placebo-treated patients. Some of these reactions were dose related and usually began during initial titration.

Patients with a history of spike and wave discharges on electroencephalogram (EEG) have been reported to have exacerbations of their EEG abnormalities associated with the cognitive/neuropsychiatric events. This raises the possibility that these clinical events may, in some cases, be a manifestation of underlying seizure activity. In the documented cases of spike and wave discharges on EEG with cognitive/neuropsychiatric events, patients usually continued tiagabine but required dosage adjustment.

Additionally, there have been postmarketing reports of patients who have experienced cognitive/neuropsychiatric symptoms, some accompanied by EEG abnormalities such as generalized spike and wave activity, that have been reported as nonconvulsant status epilepticus. Some reports describe recovery following reduction of dose or discontinuation of tiagabine.

➤*Status epilepticus:* In the 3 double-blind, placebo-controlled, parallel-group studies (studies 1, 2, and 3), the incidence of any type of status epilepticus (simple, complex, or generalized tonic-clonic) in patients receiving tiagabine was 0.8% versus 0.7% receiving placebo. Among the patients treated with tiagabine across all epilepsy studies (controlled and uncontrolled), 5% had some form of status epilepticus. Of the 5%, 57% of patients experienced complex partial status epilepticus. A critical risk factor for status epilepticus was the presence of a history of this condition; 33% of patients with a history of status epilepticus had recurrence during tiagabine treatment. Because adequate information about the incidence of status epilepticus in a similar population of patients with epilepsy who have not received treatment with tiagabine is not available, it is impossible to state whether treatment with tiagabine is associated with a higher or lower rate of status epilepticus than would be expected to occur in a similar population not treated with tiagabine.

➤*Sudden unexpected death:* There have been as many as 10 cases of sudden unexpected deaths during the clinical development of tiagabine among 2,531 patients with epilepsy (3,831 patient-years of exposure).

This represents an estimated incidence of 0.0026 deaths/patient-year. This rate is within the range of estimates for the incidence of sudden and unexpected deaths in patients with epilepsy not receiving tiagabine (0.0005 for the general population with epilepsy, 0.003 to 0.004 for clinical trial populations similar to that in the clinical development program for tiagabine, and 0.005 for patients with refractory epilepsy). The estimated sudden unexpected death in epilepsy rates in patients receiving tiagabine are also similar to those observed in patients receiving other AEDs, chemically unrelated to tiagabine, who underwent clinical testing in similar populations at about the same time. This evidence suggests that the sudden unexpected death in epilepsy rates reflect population rates, not a drug effect.

➤*Generalized weakness:* Moderately severe to incapacitating generalized weakness has been reported after administration of tiagabine in approximately 1% of patients with epilepsy. The weakness resolved in all cases after a reduction in dose or discontinuation of tiagabine.

➤*Ophthalmic effects:* When dogs received a single dose of radiolabeled tiagabine, there was evidence of residual binding in the retina and uvea after 3 weeks (the latest time point measured). Although not directly measured, melanin binding is suggested. The ability of available tests to detect potentially adverse consequences, if any, of the binding of tiagabine to melanin-containing tissue is unknown, and there was no systematic monitoring for relevant ophthalmological changes during the clinical development of tiagabine. However, long-term (up to 1 year) toxicological studies of tiagabine in dogs showed no treatment-related ophthalmoscopic changes and macro- and microscopic examinations of the eye were unremarkable. Accordingly, although there are no specific recommendations for periodic ophthalmologic monitoring, be aware of the possibility of long-term ophthalmologic effects.

➤*Serious rash:* Four patients treated with tiagabine during the product's premarketing clinical testing developed what were considered to be serious rashes. In 2 patients, the rash was described as maculopapular; in one it was described as vesiculobullous; and in the fourth case, a diagnosis of Stevens-Johnson syndrome was made. In none of the 4 cases is it certain that tiagabine was the primary, or even a contributory, cause of the rash. Nevertheless, drug-associated rash can, if extensive and serious, cause irreversible morbidity, even death.

➤*EEG abnormalities:* Patients with a history of spike and wave discharges on EEG have been reported to have exacerbations of their EEG abnormalities associated with cognitive/neuropsychiatric events. This raises the possibility that these clinical reactions may, in some cases, be a manifestation of underlying seizure activity. In the documented cases of spike and wave discharges on EEG with cognitive/neuropsychiatric reactions, patients usually continued tiagabine, but required dosage adjustment.

➤*Hepatic function impairment:* See Administration and Dosage for more information.

TIAGABINE HYDROCHLORIDE — ORAL

➤*Hazardous tasks:* Advise patients that tiagabine may cause dizziness, somnolence, and other symptoms and signs of CNS depression. Accordingly, advise patients not to drive or operate other complex machinery until they have gained sufficient experience on tiagabine to gauge whether it affects their mental or motor performance adversely. Because of the possible additive depressive effects, use caution when patients are taking other CNS depressants in combination with tiagabine.

➤*Pregnancy: Category C.* There are no adequate and well-controlled studies in pregnant women. It is not known if tiagabine crosses the human placenta. The molecular weight (376 for the free base) is low enough that exposure of the embryo and fetus should be expected. The moderately long elimination half-life will result in prolonged concentrations of the drug at the maternal blood-placenta interface, thus increasing the opportunity for embryofetal exposure. Use tiagabine during pregnancy only if clearly needed. Metabolism of tiagabine results in epoxide metabolites. These intermediate arene oxide metabolites from other anticonvulsants (eg, carbamazepine, phenytoin, valproic acid) have been associated with human teratogenicity. Therefore, the safest course is to avoid tiagabine during the first trimester, if possible. However, there is no evidence that exposure during organogenesis or at any other time during gestation will result in fetal harm. If tiagabine is required, monotherapy using the lowest effective dose is preferred, but because of its status as adjunctive therapy, this may not be possible. In addition, administer folic acid 4 mg/day with tiagabine.

Tiagabine has been shown to have adverse effects on embryofetal development, including teratogenic effects, when administered to pregnant rats and rabbits at doses higher than the human therapeutic dose.

An increased incidence of malformed fetuses (various craniofacial, appendicular, and visceral defects) and decreased fetal weights were observed following oral administration of 100 mg/kg/day to pregnant rats during the period of organogenesis. This dosage is approximately 16 times the MRHD of 56 mg/day, based on body surface area (mg/m^2). Maternal toxicity (transient weight loss/reduced maternal weight gain during gestation) was associated with this dosage, but there is no evidence to suggest that the teratogenic effects were secondary to the maternal effects. No adverse maternal or embryofetal effects were seen at a dosage of 20 mg/kg/day (3 times the MRHD on a mg/m^2 basis).

Decreased maternal weight gain, increased resorption of embryos, and increased incidences of fetal variations, but not malformations, were observed when pregnant rabbits were given 25 mg/kg/day (8 times the MRHD on a mg/m^2 basis) during organogenesis. The no effect level for maternal and embryofetal toxicity in rabbits was 5 mg/kg/day (equivalent to the MRHD on a mg/m^2 basis).

When female rats were given tiagabine 100 mg/kg/day during late gestation and throughout parturition and lactation, decreased maternal weight gain during gestation, an increase in stillbirths, and decreased postnatal offspring viability and growth were found.

Pregnancy registry – To provide additional information regarding the effects of in utero exposure to tiagabine, recommended that pregnant patients taking tiagabine enroll in the North American Antiepileptic Drug (NAAED) Pregnancy Registry. This can be done by calling the toll-free number 1-888-233-2334 and must be done by patients themselves. Information on the registry can also be found at the Web site http://www.aedpregnancyregistry.org.

➤*Lactation:* Studies in rats have shown that tiagabine and/or its metabolites are excreted in the milk of that species. Levels of excretion of tiagabine and/or its metabolites in human milk have not been determined and effects on the breast-feeding infant are unknown. The molecular weight (approximately 376 for the free base) and the moderately long elimination half-life (as long as 13 hours) suggest that excretion into breast milk should be expected. Use tiagabine in women who are breast-feeding only if the benefits clearly outweigh the risks.

➤*Children:* Safety and efficacy in children younger than 12 years of age have not been established.

➤*Monitoring:* Monitor patients treated with any AED for any indication for the emergence of worsening of depression, suicidal thoughts or behavior, and/or any unusual changes in mood or behavior.

A therapeutic range for tiagabine plasma concentrations has not been established. In controlled trials, trough plasma concentrations observed among patients randomized to doses of tiagabine that were statistically significantly more effective than placebo ranged from less than 1 to 234 ng/mL (median, 10th, and 90th percentiles are 23.7, 5.4, and 69.8 ng/mL, respectively). Because of the potential for pharmacokinetic interactions between tiagabine and drugs that induce or inhibit hepatic metabolizing enzymes, it may be useful to obtain plasma levels of tiagabine before and after changes are made in the therapeutic regimen.

Drug Interactions

In evaluating the potential for interactions among coadministered AEDs, whether an AED induces or does not induce metabolic enzymes is an important consideration. Carbamazepine, phenytoin, primidone, and phenobarbital are generally classified as enzyme-inducers; valproate and gabapentin are not. Tiagabine is considered to be a nonenzyme-inducing AED.

Tiagabine Drug Interactions

Precipitant drug	Object drug[a]		Description
Bupropion	Tiagabine	↑	The risk of seizures may be increased in patients receiving tiagabine with drugs, such as bupropion, that are known to lower the seizure threshold. Use with caution. Consider using alternate therapy for one of the agents.
Carbamazepine	Tiagabine	↓	Tiagabine had no effect on the steady-state plasma concentrations of carbamazepine or its epoxide metabolite in patients with epilepsy. However, tiagabine clearance is 60% greater in patients taking carbamazepine with or without other enzyme-inducing AEDs. Monitor the response of the patient. Adjust the tiagabine dose accordingly.
Gemfibrozil	Tiagabine	↑	Tiagabine plasma concentrations may be increased, resulting in increased toxicity (eg, confusion, seizures, coma). Closely monitor the patient and adjust the tiagabine dose as needed.
Highly protein-bound drugs	Tiagabine	↔	Tiagabine is 96% bound to plasma protein and, therefore, has the potential to interact with other highly protein-bound drugs. Such an interaction can potentially lead to higher free fractions of either drug. Monitor the response of the patient. If an interaction is suspected, adjust the dose of either drug as needed.
Tiagabine	Highly protein-bound drugs		
Phenobarbital Primidone	Tiagabine	↓	In a limited number of patients in 3 well-controlled studies, tiagabine caused no systematic changes in phenobarbital or primidone concentrations when compared with placebo. However, tiagabine clearance is 60% greater in patients taking phenobarbital or primidone with or without other enzyme-inducing AEDs. Monitor the response of the patient. Adjust the tiagabine dose accordingly.
Phenytoin	Tiagabine	↓	Tiagabine had no effect on the steady-state plasma concentrations of phenytoin in patients with epilepsy. However, tiagabine clearance is 60% greater in patients taking phenytoin with or without other enzyme-inducing AEDs. Monitor the response of the patient. Adjust the tiagabine dose accordingly.
Tramadol	Tiagabine	↑	The risk of seizures may be increased in patients receiving tiagabine with drugs such as tramadol that are known to lower the seizure threshold. Use with caution. Consider using alternate therapy for one of the agents.
Valproate	Tiagabine	↔	Tiagabine causes a slight decrease (approximately 10%) in steady-sate valproate concentrations. Valproate significantly decreased tiagabine binding in vitro from 96.3% to 94.8%, which resulted in an increase of approximately 40% in the free tiagabine. The clinical relevance is unknown.
Tiagabine	Valproate		

[a] ↑ = object drug increased; ↓ = object drug decreased; ↔ = undetermined clinical effect.

➤*Drug/Food interactions:* See Actions for more information.

Adverse Reactions

➤*Common adverse reactions:* The most commonly observed adverse reactions in placebo-controlled, parallel-group, add-on epilepsy trials associated with the use of tiagabine in combination with other AEDs not seen at

TIAGABINE HYDROCHLORIDE — ORAL

an equivalent frequency among placebo-treated patients were dizziness/light-headedness, asthenia/lack of energy, somnolence, nausea, nervousness/irritability, tremor, abdominal pain, and thinking abnormal/difficulty with concentration or attention.

➤*Discontinuation of treatment:* Approximately 21% of patients who received tiagabine in clinical trials of epilepsy discontinued treatment because of an adverse reaction. The adverse reactions most commonly associated with discontinuation were dizziness (1.7%), somnolence (1.6%), depression (1.3%), confusion (1.1%), and asthenia (1.1%).

➤*Adverse reactions (1% or more):*

Tiagabine Adverse Reactions (≥ 1%)[a]

Adverse reaction	Tiagabine (n = 494)	Placebo (n = 275)
CNS		
Abnormal gait	3%	2%
Agitation	1%	0%
Asthenia	20%	14%
Ataxia	5%	3%
Confusion	5%	3%
Depression	3%	1%
Difficulty with concentration/attention	6%	2%
Difficulty with memory	4%	3%
Dizziness	27%	15%
Emotional lability	3%	2%
Hostility	2%	1%
Insomnia	6%	4%
Language problems	2%	0%
Nervousness	10%	3%
Nystagmus	2%	1%
Paresthesia	4%	2%
Somnolence	18%	15%
Speech disorder	4%	2%
Tremor	9%	3%
Dermatologic		
Pruritus	2%	0%
Rash	5%	4%
GI		
Abdominal pain	7%	3%
Diarrhea	7%	3%
Increased appetite	2%	0%
Mouth ulceration	1%	0%
Nausea	11%	9%
Vomiting	7%	4%
Respiratory		
Cough increased	4%	3%
Pharyngitis	7%	4%
Miscellaneous		
Myasthenia	1%	0%
Pain (unspecified)	5%	3%
Vasodilation	2%	1%

[a] Patients in these add-on studies were receiving 1 to 3 concomitant enzyme-inducing AEDs in addition to tiagabine or placebo. Patients may have reported multiple adverse reactions; thus, patients may be included in more than 1 category.

Other adverse reactions – Other reactions reported by 1% or more of patients treated with tiagabine but equally or more frequent in the placebo group were as follows:

CNS: Anxiety, headache, incoordination, twitching.

GI: Anorexia, constipation, dry mouth, dyspepsia, flatulence, gastroenteritis, nausea, vomiting.

GU: Urinary frequency, urinary tract infection.

Musculoskeletal: Back pain, myalgia.

Special senses: Amblyopia, conjunctivitis, diplopia, rhinitis, sinusitis.

Miscellaneous: Accidental injury, acne, chest pain, ecchymosis, fever, flu syndrome, infection.

➤*Dose-response study:*

Tiagabine Adverse Reactions (≥ 5%) in Study 1[a]

Adverse reaction	Tiagabine 32 mg (n = 88)	Tiagabine 56 mg (n = 57)	Placebo (n = 91)
CNS			
Abnormal gait	5%	5%	3%
Asthenia	18%	23%	15%
Ataxia	6%	9%	6%
Depression	1%	7%	0%
Difficulty with concentration/attention	7%	14%	3%
Dizziness	31%	28%	12%
Hostility	5%	5%	2%
Insomnia	6%	5%	3%
Nervousness	11%	14%	6%
Somnolence	21%	19%	17%
Tremor	14%	21%	1%
GI			
Abdominal pain	7%	5%	4%
Diarrhea	10%	2%	6%
Miscellaneous			
Accidental injury	15%	21%	20%
Amblyopia	9%	4%	8%
Ecchymosis	6%	0%	1%
Flu syndrome	6%	9%	3%
Infection	10%	19%	12%
Myalgia	2%	5%	3%
Pain	2%	7%	3%
Pharyngitis	8%	7%	6%
Urinary tract infection	0%	5%	2%

[a] Patients in this study were receiving 1 to 3 concomitant enzyme-inducing AEDs in addition to tiagabine or placebo. Patients may have reported multiple adverse reactions; thus, patients may be included in more than 1 category.

➤*Other adverse reactions in all clinical trials:*

Cardiovascular – Hypertension, palpitation, syncope, tachycardia (at least 1%); angina pectoris, cerebral ischemia, ECG abnormal, hypotension, myocardial infarct, pallor, peripheral vascular disorder, phlebitis, postural hypotension, thrombophlebitis (0.1% to 1%).

CNS – Depersonalization, dysarthria, euphoria, hallucination, hyperkinesia, hypertonia, hypesthesia, hypokinesia, hypotonia, malaise, migraine, myoclonus, paranoid reaction, personality disorder, reflexes decreased, stupor, twitching, vertigo (at least 1%); abnormal dreams, apathy, choreoathetosis, circumoral paresthesia, CNS neoplasm, coma, delusions, dystonia, encephalopathy, hemiplegia, libido decreased, libido increased, movement disorder, neuritis, neurosis, paralysis, peripheral neuritis, psychosis, reflexes increased, suicide attempt (0.1% to 1%).

Dermatologic – Alopecia, dry skin, sweating (at least 1%); contact dermatitis, eczema, exfoliative dermatitis, furunculosis, herpes simplex, herpes zoster, hirsutism, maculopapular rash, photosensitivity reaction, psoriasis, skin benign neoplasm, skin carcinoma, skin discolorations, skin nodules, skin ulcer, subcutaneous nodule, urticaria, vesiculobullous rash (0.1% to 1%).

Endocrine – Goiter, hypothyroidism (0.1% to 1%).

GI – Gingivitis, stomatitis (at least 1%); abnormal stools, cholecystitis, cholelithiasis, dry mouth, dysphagia, eructation, esophagitis, fecal incontinence, gastritis, GI hemorrhage, glossitis, gum hyperplasia, hepatomegaly, increased salivation, liver function tests abnormal, melena, periodontal abscess, rectal hemorrhage, thirst, tooth caries, ulcerative stomatitis (0.1% to 1%).

GU – Dysmenorrhea, dysuria, metrorrhagia, urinary incontinence, vaginitis (at least 1%); abortion, amenorrhea, breast enlargement, breast pain, cystitis, fibrocystic breast, hematuria, impotence, kidney failure, menorrhagia, nocturia, pelvic pain, polyuria, pyelonephritis, salpingitis, suspicious Pap smear, urethritis, urinary retention, urinary urgency, vaginal hemorrhage (0.1% to 1%).

Hematologic/Lymphatic – Lymphadenopathy (at least 1%); anemia, erythrocytes abnormal, hemorrhage, leukopenia, petechia, thrombocytopenia (0.1% to 1%).

Metabolic/Nutritional – Edema, peripheral edema, weight gain, weight loss (at least 1%); dehydration, hypercholesteremia, hyperglycemia, hyperlipemia, hypoglycemia, hypokalemia, hyponatremia (0.1% to 1%).

Musculoskeletal – Arthralgia, neck pain (at least 1%); arthritis, arthrosis, bursitis, generalized spasm, leg cramps, neck rigidity, tendinous contracture (0.1% to 1%).

Respiratory – Bronchitis, dyspnea, epistaxis, pneumonia (at least 1%); apnea, asthma, hemoptysis, hiccups, hyperventilation, laryngitis, respiratory disorder, voice alteration (0.1% to 1%).

TIAGABINE HYDROCHLORIDE — ORAL

Special senses – Abnormal vision, ear pain, otitis media, tinnitus (at least 1%); blepharitis, blindness, deafness, eye pain, halitosis, hyperacusis, keratoconjunctivitis, otitis externa, parosmia, photophobia, taste loss, taste perversion, visual field defect (0.1% to 1%).

Miscellaneous – Allergic reaction, chest pain, chills, cyst (at least 1%); abscess, cellulitis, facial edema, hernia, neoplasm, sepsis, sudden death (0.1% to 1%).

Overdosage

➤*Symptoms:* The most common symptoms reported after overdose included agitation, confusion, depression, hostility, impaired consciousness, myoclonus, somnolence, speech difficulty, and weakness. One patient who ingested a single dose of 400 mg experienced generalized tonic-clonic status epilepticus, which responded to intravenous phenobarbital.

From postmarketing experience, there have been no reports of fatal overdoses involving tiagabine alone (doses up to 720 mg), although a number of patients required intubation and ventilatory support as part of the management of their status epilepticus. Overdoses involving multiple drugs, including tiagabine, have resulted in fatal outcomes. Symptoms most often accompanying tiagabine overdose, alone or with other drugs, have included seizures, including status epilepticus in patients with and without underlying seizure disorders; nonconvulsive status epilepticus; coma; ataxia; confusion; somnolence; drowsiness; impaired speech; agitation; lethargy; myoclonus; spike wave stupor; tremors, disorientation; vomiting; hostility; and temporary paralysis. Respiratory depression was seen in a number of patients, including children, in the context of seizures.

➤*Treatment:* There is no specific antidote for overdose with tiagabine. If indicated, elimination of unabsorbed drug should be achieved by gastric lavage; observe usual precautions to maintain the airway. General supportive care of the patient is indicated, including monitoring of vital signs and observation of clinical status of the patient. Because tiagabine is mostly metabolized by the liver and is highly protein bound, dialysis is unlikely to be beneficial. Consult a certified poison control center for up-to-date information on the management of overdose with tiagabine.

Patient Information

Counsel patients, their caregivers, and their families that AEDs, including tiagabine, may increase the risk of suicidal thoughts and behavior and advise them of the need to be alert for the emergence or worsening of symptoms of depression, any unusual changes in mood or behavior, or the emergence of suicidal thoughts, behavior, or thoughts about self-harm. Report behaviors of concern immediately to health care providers.

Advise patients that tiagabine may cause dizziness, somnolence, and other symptoms and signs of CNS depression. Accordingly, advise patients not to drive or operate other complex machinery until they have gained sufficient experience on tiagabine to gauge whether it affects their mental and/or motor performance adversely. Because of the possible additive depressive effects, advise patients to use caution when taking other CNS depressants in combination with tiagabine.

Because teratogenic effects were seen in the offspring of rats exposed to maternally toxic doses of tiagabine and because experience in humans is limited, advise patients to notify their health care providers if they become pregnant or intend to become pregnant during therapy.

Because of the possibility that tiagabine may be excreted in breast milk, advise patients to notify those providing care to themselves and their children if they intend to breast-feed or are breast-feeding an infant.

Encourage patients to enroll in the NAAED Pregnancy Registry if they become pregnant. This registry is collecting information about the safety of AEDs during pregnancy. To enroll, patients can call the toll-free number 1-888-233-2334.

If the patient forgets to take the prescribed dose of tiagabine at the scheduled time, advise the patient not to attempt to make up for the missed dose by increasing the next dose. If a patient has missed multiple doses, advise the patient to refer back to his or her health care provider for possible retitration as clinically indicated.

TOPIRAMATE

Rx	**Topiramate** (Various, eg, Apotex, Aurobindo, Zydus)	**Tablets; oral**: 25 mg	May contain lactose and PEG. In 30s, 60s, 90s, 100s, 500s, 1,000s, and UD 100s.
Rx	**Topamax** (Janssen)		Lactose. (TOP 25). In 60s.
Rx	**Topiragen** (Upsher-Smith)		Lactose, PEG. (USL 25). White, round. In 60s, 100s, 500s, 1,000s, and UD 100s.
Rx	**Topiramate** (Various, eg, Apotex, Aurobindo, Zydus)	**Tablets; oral**: 50 mg	May contain lactose and PEG. In 30s, 60s, 90s, 100s, 500s, 1,000s, and UD 100s.
Rx	**Topamax** (Janssen)		Lactose. (TOPAMAX 50). Lt. yellow. In 60s.
Rx	**Topiragen** (Upsher-Smith)		Lactose, PEG. (USL 50). Lt. yellow, round. In 60s, 100s, 500s, 1,000s, and UD 100s.
Rx	**Topiramate** (Various, eg, Apotex, Aurobindo, Zydus)	**Tablets; oral**: 100 mg	May contain lactose and PEG. In 30s, 60s, 90s, 100s, 500s, 1,000s, and UD 100s.
Rx	**Topamax** (Janssen)		Lactose. (TOPAMAX 100). Yellow. In 60s.
Rx	**Topiragen** (Upsher-Smith)		Lactose, PEG. (USL 100). Dk. yellow, round. In 60s, 100s, 500s, 1,000s, and UD 100s.
Rx	**Topiramate** (Various, eg, Apotex, Aurobindo, Zydus)	**Tablets; oral**: 200 mg	May contain lactose and PEG. In 30s, 60s, 90s, 100s, 500s, 1,000s, and UD 100s.
Rx	**Topamax** (Janssen)		Lactose. (TOPAMAX 200). Salmon. In 60s.
Rx	**Topiragen** (Upsher-Smith)		Lactose, PEG. (USL 200). Dk. red, round. In 60s, 100s, 500s, 1,000s, and UD 100s.
Rx	**Topiramate** (Teva)	**Capsules, sprinkle; oral**: 15 mg	PEG, sugar. (93 7335). White. In 60s.
Rx	**Topamax** (Janssen)		Sucrose. (TOP 15 mg). White/clear. In 60s.
Rx	**Topiramate** (Teva)	**Capsules, sprinkle; oral**: 25 mg	PEG, sugar. (93 7336). White. In 60s.
Rx	**Topamax** (Janssen)		Sucrose. (TOP 25 mg). White/clear. In 60s.

TOPIRAMATE — ORAL

Refer to the general discussion beginning in the Anticonvulsants introduction.

Indications

➤*Epilepsy:*

Monotherapy – As initial monotherapy in patients 10 years of age and older with partial-onset or primary generalized tonic-clonic seizures.

Adjunctive therapy – As adjunctive therapy for adults and children 2 to 16 years of age with partial-onset seizures or primary generalized tonic-clonic seizures and in patients 2 years of age and older with seizures associated with Lennox-Gastaut syndrome.

➤*Migraine:* For the prophylaxis of migraine headache in adults.

The use of topiramate in the acute treatment of migraine headache has not been studied.

➤*Off-label uses:*

Alcohol dependence – [4] = Insufficient documentation. Preliminary data from controlled trials suggest that topiramate may be effective in the management of alcohol dependence. It is important to note that all controlled trial studies have been investigated by the same group.

Binge eating disorder – [4] = Insufficient documentation. Preliminary data with topiramate in other disease states suggest a possible relationship with this drug and weight loss. However, limited data are available regarding the use of this agent for binge eating disorders.

Bipolar disorders – [2] = Fair documentation. Topiramate has been studied in a limited number of patients (fewer than 75) for the treatment of various bipolar disorders. Onset of clinical improvement was not provided in most reports and is an important factor when selecting drug regimens. In most cases, topiramate has been used with preexisting medication regimens. Thus, it is not clear if this drug is effective only as adjunctive therapy.

Bulimia nervosa – [1] = Good documentation. In a small, controlled trial, topiramate demonstrated efficacy for the treatment of bulimia nervosa; however, adverse reactions with topiramate are common. American Psychiatric Association guidelines state that topiramate is preferred over lithium and valproic acid because of its weight loss effects for patients who require a mood stabilizer. Larger, controlled studies are needed to compare the efficacy of topiramate with selective serotonin reuptake inhibitors.

Cluster headaches – [4] = Insufficient documentation. Limited published information suggests that topiramate may be useful as adjunctive therapy in patients with refractory episodic or chronic cluster headaches. However, the utility of this agent may be limited by intolerable CNS effects

TOPIRAMATE — ORAL

in some patients when used at higher doses. This drug should be considered in patients who have not responded to other therapies.

Essential tremor – [4] = Insufficient documentation. To date, the utility of topiramate in the management of patients with essential tremor has been evaluated in only a small patient sample (fewer than 40 patients). Initial data suggest a beneficial, but not curative, effect.

Hyperhidrosis (palmar, plantar, axillary) – [4] = Insufficient documentation. Information from a single case report suggests that topiramate should be studied further as an agent to treat hyperhidrosis. However, an exact mechanism of action is unclear at this time. Further controlled trials in larger patient numbers are needed before this drug can be recommended.

Infantile spasm – [2] = Fair documentation. Topiramate may be effective as adjunctive therapy or monotherapy for the treatment of infantile spasm. Data from noncontrolled studies in more than 100 patients indicated at least 50% of infants experienced a reduction in spasm frequency, while a smaller percentage became spasm free. Controlled trials are needed to determine optimal dosing and topiramate's specific place in the management of infantile spasm.

Migraine prevention(children/adolescents) – [4] = Insufficient documentation. Topiramate has been studied for the prevention of migraine headaches in children. While data from early studies showed reduction in headache frequency and severity, there was concern with the adverse reaction profile. More recent studies have been published that used lower doses of topiramate. The results appear to be promising, but the adverse reaction profile, although more tolerable, is still of concern. Published data are limited and the number of patients studied is small. Current practice guidelines consider the evidence insufficient to make a recommendation for use. Additional data are needed to determine the optimal dosing regimen and the patient population that would most benefit from therapy, particularly given the safety concerns when higher doses are used.

Neuralgias/Neuropathy/Pain – [4] = Insufficient documentation. Although there is limited published information, abstract citations indicate that topiramate is being extensively investigated for the management of various pain syndromes and neuropathies.

Restless legs syndrome – [5] = Poor documentation. Although anticonvulsants (eg, gabapentin, carbamazepine, valproic acid) have been used in the management of restless legs syndrome (RLS), published data are insufficient regarding the use of topiramate for this purpose. Guideline statements also note that little supportive evidence is available. In addition, there are case reports of topiramate-induced RLS. Because other agents are available, this drug is not recommended for treatment of RLS until there is further favorable evidence.

Smoking cessation – [4] = Insufficient documentation. Preliminary data from 2 controlled trials and 1 small, open-label study have shown conflicting results when topiramate was used as a smoking cessation agent. Recent trials suggest that topiramate may have gender-based advantage in men; however, additional controlled studies are needed to identify best candidates. Because of the availability of agents already approved to promote smoking cessation, it is unlikely that topiramate will be considered first- or second-line therapy.

Weight gain or obesity (antipsychotic-induced) – [4] = Insufficient documentation. Preliminary data with topiramate in other disease states suggest a possible relationship with this drug and weight loss. Limited data are available as evidence of weight reduction associated with antipsychotics that currently offer consistent results.

Administration and Dosage

➤*General dosing considerations:*

Bioequivalence – The sprinkle formulation is bioequivalent to the immediate-release tablet formulation and, therefore, may be substituted as a therapeutic equivalent.

➤*Adults:*

Epilepsy (monotherapy) –

Usual dosage: 400 mg/day in 2 divided doses.

Dosage titration:

Topiramate Titration Schedule for Epilepsy (Monotherapy)

	Morning dose	Evening dose
Week 1	25 mg	25 mg
Week 2	50 mg	50 mg
Week 3	75 mg	75 mg
Week 4	100 mg	100 mg
Week 5	150 mg	150 mg
Week 6	200 mg	200 mg

Epilepsy (adjunctive therapy) –

Partial-onset seizures:

• *Initial dosage* – 25 to 50 mg/day, followed by titration to an effective dose.

• *Dosage titration* – Titrate in increments of 25 to 50 mg/week. Titrating in increments of 25 mg/week may delay the time to reach an effective dose.

• *Maintenance dosage* – 200 to 400 mg/day in 2 divided doses.

Primary generalized tonic-clonic seizures:

• *Initial dosage* – 25 to 50 mg/day, followed by titration to an effective dose.

• *Dosage titration* – Titrate in increments of 25 to 50 mg/week. Titrating in increments of 25 mg/week may delay the time to reach an effective dose.

• *Maintenance dosage* – 400 mg/day in 2 divided doses.

Migraine prophylaxis –

Usual dosage: 100 mg/day, administered in 2 divided doses.

Dosage titration: The recommended titration rate to 100 mg/day is shown in the following table. Guide dose titration rate by clinical outcome. If required, longer intervals between dose adjustments can be used.

Topiramate Titration Rate for Migraine Prophylaxis

	Morning dose	Evening dose
Week 1	None	25 mg
Week 2	25 mg	25 mg
Week 3	25 mg	50 mg
Week 4	50 mg	50 mg

Off-label dosing –

Alcohol dependence: [4] = Insufficient documentation. In controlled trials, a weekly titration schedule was used. Topiramate was initiated at 25 mg daily at week 1 and increased to a maximum of 300 mg daily by weeks 5 to 14 or weeks 8 to 12. In one case report, 2 patients received 100 mg 3 times daily.

Binge eating disorder: [4] = Insufficient documentation. Initial doses of 25 to 50 mg/day. Doses were titrated by 25 to 50 mg/week initially. The target or maximum dose was varied with as low as 150 mg/day in one noncontrolled study to a maximum of 1,400 mg/day in another open study. In a controlled trial, initial titration occurred over a 2-week period (25 to 50 mg/week increments), with additional titration up to a maximum of 600 mg/day over an 8-week period. Mean doses in this controlled trial were 212 mg/day.

Bipolar disorders: [2] = Fair documentation. 50 to 200 mg/day (maximum daily dose: 400 mg/day).

Bulimia nervosa: [1] = Good documentation. 25 mg/day for the first week, then titrated by 25 to 50 mg/week to the minimal effective dosage or a maximum dosage of 400 mg/day.

Cluster headaches: [4] = Insufficient documentation. Initial dose has ranged from 25 to 50 mg/day, typically titrated by 25 to 50 mg/week to a maximum dose ranging from 200 to 600 mg/day. In clinical trials, mean doses have ranged from 87.5 to 310 mg/day.

Essential tremor: [4] = Insufficient documentation. Initial doses of 25 to 50 mg daily and titrated to a maximum of 400 mg/day or maximum tolerated dose for up to 21 months. Mean doses have ranged from 144 to 333 mg/day.

Neuralgias/Neuropathy/Pain: [4] = Insufficient documentation. 50 to 125 mg/day with a titration to maximum tolerable dose.

Smoking cessation: [4] = Insufficient documentation. A weekly titration schedule was employed in one controlled trial, starting at topiramate 25 mg daily at week 1 titrated to a maximum of 300 mg daily by week 12. The mean daily dose at week 12 was 279.2 mg.

Weight gain or obesity (antipsychotic-induced): [4] = Insufficient documentation. Initiate oral doses of 25 mg/day with various titration schedules to a maximum of 300 mg/day.

➤*Children:*

Epilepsy (monotherapy) –

10 years of age and older: See Adults for dosing for children 10 years of age and older.

Epilepsy (adjunctive therapy) – See Adults for dosing for children older than 16 years of age.

2 to 16 years of age:

• *Partial seizures, primary generalized tonic-clonic seizures, and seizures associated with Lennox-Gastaut syndrome* –

Initial dosage: 25 mg (or less, based on a range of 1 to 3 mg/kg/day) nightly for the first week.

Dosage titration: Increase the dose at 1- or 2-week intervals by increments of 1 to 3 mg/kg/day (administered in 2 divided doses) to achieve optimal clinical response. Guide dose titration by clinical outcome.

Maintenance dosage: 5 to 9 mg/kg/day in 2 divided doses.

Off-label dosing –

Hyperhidrosis (palmar, plantar, axillary): [4] = Insufficient documentation. Initial doses of 25 to 50 mg and titrated to 200 mg/day.

Infantile spasm: [2] = Fair documentation.

• *Initial dosages* – 1 to 3 mg/kg/day.

• *Maximum dosages* – 12 to 27 mg/kg/day. Therapy has been evaluated for up to 4 years. The optimal dose of topiramate has not been established. Doses should be tapered up every 2 to 5 days until a response is reached or patients cannot tolerate the medication.

Migraine prevention (children/adolescents): [4] = Insufficient documentation. Oral doses ranged from 12.5 to 200 mg daily in 2 of the trials. In another trial, topiramate was dosed at 1.8 to 6 mg/kg/day. Lower total daily doses (25 to 100 mg) were used in the most recent trials in an effort to minimize toxicities seen with higher doses.

➤*Renal function impairment:* In renally impaired patients (creatinine clearance [CrCl] less than 70 mL/min per 1.73 m^2), one-half of the usual adult dose is recommended. Such patients will require a longer time to reach steady state at each dose.

Hemodialysis – Topiramate is cleared by hemodialysis at a rate that is 4 to 6 times greater than a healthy individual. Accordingly, a prolonged period of dialysis may cause topiramate concentration to fall below that required to maintain an antiseizure effect. To avoid rapid drops in topiramate plasma concentration during hemodialysis, a supplemental dose of topiramate may be required. The actual adjustment should take into account the following:

TOPIRAMATE — ORAL

the duration of the dialysis period, the clearance rate of the dialysis system being used, and the effective renal clearance of topiramate in the patient being dialyzed.

➤*Concomitant therapy:* On occasion, the addition of topiramate to phenytoin may require an adjustment of the phenytoin dose to achieve optimal clinical outcome. Addition or withdrawal of phenytoin and/or carbamazepine during adjunctive therapy with topiramate may require adjustment of the topiramate dose.

➤*Administration:* Topiramate can be taken without regard to meals. Because of the bitter taste, tablets should not be broken.

Topiramate capsules may be swallowed whole or administered by carefully opening the capsule and sprinkling the entire contents on a small amount (teaspoon) of soft food. This drug/food mixture should be swallowed immediately and not chewed. Do not store for future use.

➤*Storage / Stability:* Protect from moisture. Store tablets in tightly closed containers at controlled room temperature, 15° to 30°C (59° to 86°F). Store capsules in tightly closed containers at or below 25°C (77°F).

Actions

➤*Pharmacology:* The precise mechanism by which topiramate exerts its anticonvulsant and migraine prophylaxis effects are unknown; however, preclinical studies have revealed 4 properties that may contribute to topiramate's efficacy for epilepsy and migraine prophylaxis. Electrophysiological and biochemical evidence suggests that topiramate, at pharmacologically relevant concentrations, blocks voltage-dependent sodium channels, augments the activity of the neurotransmitter gamma-aminobutyrate at some subtypes of the gamma-aminobutyric acid (GABA)-A receptor, antagonizes the alpha-amino-3–hydroxy-5–methylisoxazole-4–propionic acid/kainate subtype of the glutamate receptor, and inhibits the carbonic anhydrase enzyme, particularly isozymes II and IV.

➤*Pharmacokinetics:*

Absorption / Distribution – Absorption of topiramate is rapid, with peak plasma concentrations occurring at approximately 2 hours following a 400 mg oral dose. The relative bioavailability of topiramate from the tablet formulation is approximately 80% compared with a solution. The bioavailability of topiramate is not affected by food.

The pharmacokinetics of topiramate are linear, with dose-proportional increases in plasma concentration over the dosage range studied (200 to 800 mg/day). Steady state is reached in about 4 days in patients with healthy renal function. Topiramate is 15% to 41% bound to human plasma proteins over the blood concentration range of 0.5 to 250 mcg/mL. The fraction bound decreased as blood concentration increased.

Carbamazepine and phenytoin do not alter the binding of topiramate. Sodium valproate, at 500 mcg/mL (a concentration 5 to 10 times higher than considered therapeutic for valproate), decreased the protein binding of topiramate from 23% to 13%. Topiramate does not influence the binding of sodium valproate.

Metabolism / Excretion – Topiramate is not extensively metabolized and is primarily eliminated unchanged in the urine (approximately 70% of an administered dose). Six metabolites have been identified in humans, none of which constitute more than 5% of an administered dose. The metabolites are formed via hydroxylation, hydrolysis, and glucuronidation. There is evidence of renal tubular reabsorption of topiramate. In rats given probenecid to inhibit tubular reabsorption along with topiramate, a significant increase in renal clearance of topiramate was observed. This interaction has not been evaluated in humans. Overall, oral plasma clearance (CL/F) is approximately 20 to 30 mL/min in humans following oral administration.

The mean plasma elimination half-life is 21 hours after single or multiple doses.

Special populations –

Renal function impairment: The clearance of topiramate was reduced 42% in moderately renally impaired subjects (CrCl 30 to 69 mL/min per 1.73 m^2) and 54% in severely renally impaired subjects (CrCl less than 30 mL/min per 1.73 m^2) compared with subjects with healthy renal function (CrCl greater than 70 mL/min per 1.73 m^2). Because topiramate is presumed to undergo significant tubular reabsorption, it is uncertain whether this experience can be generalized to all situations of renal function impairment. It is conceivable that some forms of renal disease could differentially affect glomerular filtration rate and tubular reabsorption, resulting in a clearance of topiramate not predicted by CrCl. In general, however, one-half the usual starting and maintenance dose is recommended in patients with moderate or severe renal function impairment.

Topiramate is cleared by hemodialysis. Using a high-efficiency, counterflow, single-pass, dialysate hemodialysis procedure, topiramate dialysis clearance was 120 mL/min with blood flow through the dialyzer at 400 mL/min. This high clearance (compared with 20 to 30 mL/min total oral clearance in healthy adults) will remove a clinically significant amount of topiramate from the patient over the hemodialysis treatment period; therefore, a supplemental dose may be required.

Hepatic function impairment: In hepatically impaired subjects, the clearance of topiramate may be decreased; the mechanism underlying the decrease is not well understood.

Elderly: The pharmacokinetics of topiramate in elderly subjects (65 to 85 years of age; n = 16) were evaluated in a controlled clinical study. The elderly subject population had reduced renal function (CrCl 20% lower) compared with younger adults. Following a single dose of topiramate 100 mg oral, maximum plasma concentration for elderly and younger adults was achieved at approximately 1 to 2 hours. Reflecting the primary renal elimination of topiramate, topiramate plasma and renal clearance were reduced 21% and 19%, respectively, in elderly subjects, compared with younger adults. Similarly, topiramate half-life was longer (13%) in elderly subjects. Reduced topiramate clearance resulted in slightly higher maximum plasma concentration (23%) and area under the curve (AUC) (25%) in elderly subjects than observed in younger adults. Topiramate clearance is decreased in elderly patients only to the extent that renal function is reduced. As recommended for all patients, dosage adjustment may be indicated in elderly patients with renal function impairment (CrCl less than or equal to 70 mL/min per 1.73 m^2). It may be useful to monitor renal function in elderly patients.

Children: Pharmacokinetics of topiramate were evaluated in patients 4 to 17 years of age receiving 1 or 2 other antiepileptic drugs (AEDs). Pharmacokinetic profiles were obtained after 1 week at doses of 1, 3, and 9 mg/kg/day. Clearance was independent of dose.

Children have a 50% higher clearance and shorter elimination half-life than adults. Consequently, the plasma concentration for the same mg/kg dose may be lower in children compared with adults. Similar to adults, hepatic enzyme–inducing AEDs decrease the steady-state plasma concentrations of topiramate.

Contraindications

Hypersensitivity to any component of this product.

Warnings/Precautions

➤*Metabolic acidosis:* Hyperchloremic, nonanion gap, metabolic acidosis (ie, decreased serum bicarbonate below the normal reference range in the absence of chronic respiratory alkalosis) is associated with topiramate treatment. This metabolic acidosis is caused by renal bicarbonate loss because of the inhibitory effect of topiramate on carbonic anhydrase. Such electrolyte imbalance has been observed with the use of topiramate in placebo-controlled clinical trials and in the postmarketing period. Generally, topiramate-induced metabolic acidosis occurs early in treatment, although cases can occur at any time during treatment. Bicarbonate decrements are usually mild to moderate (average decrease of 4 mEq/L at daily doses of 400 mg in adults and at approximately 6 mg/kg/day in children); rarely, patients can experience severe decrements to values less than 10 mEq/L. Conditions or therapies that predispose to acidosis (eg, renal disease, severe respiratory disorders, status epilepticus, diarrhea, surgery, ketogenic diet, drugs) may be additive to the bicarbonate-lowering effects of topiramate.

Some manifestations of acute or chronic metabolic acidosis may include hyperventilation, nonspecific symptoms such as fatigue and anorexia, or more severe sequelae including cardiac arrhythmias or stupor. Chronic, untreated metabolic acidosis may increase the risk for nephrolithiasis or nephrocalcinosis, and also may result in osteomalacia (referred to as rickets in children) and/or osteoporosis with an increased risk for fractures. Chronic metabolic acidosis in children also may reduce growth rates. A reduction in growth rate may eventually decrease the maximal height achieved. The effect of topiramate on growth and bone-related sequelae has not been systematically investigated.

Measurement of baseline and periodic serum bicarbonate during topiramate treatment is recommended. If metabolic acidosis develops and persists, consider reducing the dose or discontinuing topiramate (using dose tapering). If the decision is made to continue patients on topiramate in the face of persistent acidosis, consider alkali treatment.

Adults – In adults, the incidence of persistent treatment-emergent decreases in serum bicarbonate (levels of less than 20 mEq/L at 2 consecutive visits or at the final visit) in controlled clinical trials for adjunctive treatment of epilepsy was 32% for 400 mg/day and 1% for placebo. Metabolic acidosis has been observed at dosages as low as 50 mg/day. The incidence of persistent treatment-emergent decreases in serum bicarbonate in adults in the epilepsy controlled clinical trial for monotherapy was 15% for 50 mg/day and 25% for 400 mg/day. The incidence of a markedly abnormally low serum bicarbonate (absolute value less than 17 mEq/L and more than 5 mEq/L decrease from pretreatment) in the adjunctive therapy trials was 3% for 400 mg/day and 0% for placebo, and in the monotherapy trial was 1% for 50 mg/day and 7% for 400 mg/day. Serum bicarbonate levels have not been systematically evaluated at daily doses greater than 400 mg/day.

The incidence of persistent treatment-emergent decreases in serum bicarbonate in adult placebo-controlled trials for prophylaxis of migraine was 44% for 200 mg/day, 39% for 100 mg/day, 23% for 50 mg/day, and 7% for placebo. The incidence of a markedly abnormally low serum bicarbonate (absolute value less than 17 mEq/L and more than 5 mEq/L decrease from pretreatment) in these trials was 11% for 200 mg/day, 9% for 100 mg/day, 2% for 50 mg/day, and less than 1% for placebo.

Children – In children younger than 16 years of age, the incidence of persistent treatment-emergent decreases in serum bicarbonate in placebo-controlled trials for adjunctive treatment of Lennox-Gastaut syndrome or refractory partial-onset seizures was 67% for topiramate (at approximately 6 mg/kg/day) and 10% for placebo. The incidence of a markedly abnormally low serum bicarbonate (absolute value less than 17 mEq/L and more than 5 mEq/L decrease from pretreatment) in these trials was 11% for topiramate and 0% for placebo. Cases of moderately severe metabolic acidosis have been reported in children as young as 5 months of age, especially at daily doses of more than 5 mg/kg/day.

In children 10 to 16 years of age, the incidence of persistent treatment-emergent decreases in serum bicarbonate in the epilepsy controlled clinical trial for monotherapy was 7% for 50 mg/day and 20% for 400 mg/day. The incidence of a abnormally low serum bicarbonate (absolute value less than 17 mEq/L and more than 5 mEq/L decreased from pretreatment) in this trial was 4% for 50 mg/day and 4% for 400 mg/day.

➤*Acute myopia and secondary angle-closure glaucoma:* A syndrome consisting of acute myopia associated with secondary angle-closure glaucoma has been reported in patients receiving topiramate. Symptoms include acute onset of decreased visual acuity and/or ocular pain. Ophthalmologic findings can include myopia, anterior chamber shallowing, ocular hyperemia (redness), and increased intraocular pressure; mydriasis may or may not be

TOPIRAMATE — ORAL

present. This syndrome may be associated with supracillary effusion resulting in anterior displacement of the lens and iris, with secondary angle-closure glaucoma. Symptoms typically occur within 1 month of initiating topiramate therapy. In contrast to primary narrow-angle glaucoma, which is rare in patients younger than 40 years of age, secondary angle-closure glaucoma associated with topiramate has been reported in children as well as adults. The primary treatment to reverse symptoms is discontinuation of topiramate as rapidly as possible, according to the judgement of the treating health care provider. Other measures in conjunction with discontinuation of topiramate may be helpful.

Elevated intraocular pressure of any etiology, if left untreated, can lead to serious sequelae, including permanent vision loss.

➤*Oligohidrosis and hyperthermia:* Oligohidrosis (decreased sweating), infrequently resulting in hospitalization, has been reported in association with topiramate use. Decreased sweating and an elevation in body temperature above normal characterized these cases. Some of the cases were reported after exposure to elevated environmental temperatures.

The majority of the reports have been in children. Closely monitor patients, especially children, treated with topiramate for evidence of decreased sweating and increased body temperature, especially in hot weather. Use caution when topiramate is prescribed with other drugs that predispose patients to heat-related disorders; these drugs include, but are not limited to, other carbonic anhydrase inhibitors and drugs with anticholinergic activity.

➤*Withdrawal of AEDs:* In patients with or without a history of seizures or epilepsy, gradually withdraw AEDs, including topiramate, to minimize the potential for seizures or increased seizure frequency. In situations in which rapid withdrawal of topiramate is medically required, monitor patients appropriately.

➤*CNS effects:*

Adults – Adverse reactions most often associated with the use of topiramate were related to the CNS and were observed in epilepsy and migraine populations. In adults, the most frequent of these can be classified into 3 general categories:

1.) cognitive-related dysfunction (eg, confusion, psychomotor slowing, difficulty with concentration/attention, difficulty with memory, speech or language problems, particularly word-finding difficulties)
2.) psychiatric/behavioral disturbances (eg, depression, mood problems)
3.) somnolence or fatigue.

Cognitive-related dysfunction – The majority of cognitive-related adverse reactions were mild to moderate in severity, and they frequently occurred in isolation. Rapid titration rate and higher initial dose were associated with higher incidences of these reactions. Many of these reactions contributed to withdrawal from treatment.

Psychiatric/Behavioral disturbances – Depression or mood problems were dose-related for the add-on epilepsy and migraine populations.

In the double-blind phases of clinical trials with topiramate in approved and investigational indications, suicide attempts occurred at a rate of 3 per 1,000 patient-years (13 reactions per 3,999 patient-years) on topiramate versus 0 (0 reactions per 1,430 patient-years) on placebo. One completed suicide was reported in a bipolar disorder trial in a patient taking topiramate.

Somnolence/Fatigue – Somnolence and fatigue were the adverse reactions most frequently reported during clinical trials of topiramate for adjunctive epilepsy. For the adjunctive epilepsy population, the incidence of somnolence did not differ substantially between 200 and 1,000 mg/day, but the incidence of fatigue was dose-related and increased at doses above 400 mg/day. For the monotherapy epilepsy population in the 50 and 400 mg/day groups, the incidence of somnolence was dose-related (9% for the 50 mg/day group and 15% for the 400 mg/day group), and the incidence of fatigue was comparable in both treatment groups (14% each). For the migraine population, fatigue and somnolence were dose-related and more common in the titration phase.

Additional nonspecific CNS reactions commonly observed with topiramate in the add-on epilepsy population include dizziness or ataxia.

Children – In double-blind adjunctive therapy and monotherapy epilepsy clinical studies, the incidences of cognitive/neuropsychiatric adverse reactions in children were generally lower than those previously observed in adults. These reactions included psychomotor slowing, difficulty with concentration/attention, speech disorders/related speech problems, and language problems. The most frequently reported neuropsychiatric reactions in children during adjunctive therapy double-blind studies were somnolence and fatigue. The most frequently reported neuropsychiatric events in children in the 50 and 400 mg/day groups during the monotherapy double-blind study were headache, dizziness, anorexia, and somnolence.

➤*Sudden unexplained death in epilepsy:* During the course of premarketing development of topiramate tablets, 10 sudden and unexplained deaths were recorded among a cohort of treated patients (2,796 subject-years of exposure). This represents an incidence of 0.0035 deaths per patient-year. Although this rate exceeds that expected in a healthy population matched for age and sex, it is within the range of estimates for the incidence of sudden unexplained deaths in patients with epilepsy who are not receiving topiramate (ranging from 0.0005 for the general population of patients with epilepsy to 0.003 for a clinical trial population similar to that in the topiramate program to 0.005 for patients with refractory epilepsy).

➤*Hyperammonemia and encephalopathy associated with concomitant valproic acid use:* Coadministration of topiramate and valproic acid has been associated with hyperammonemia with or without encephalopathy in patients who have tolerated either drug alone. Clinical symptoms of hyperammonemic encephalopathy often include acute alterations in level of consciousness and/or cognitive function with lethargy or vomiting. In most cases, symptoms and signs abated with discontinuation of either drug. This adverse reaction is not caused by a pharmacokinetic interaction.

It is not known if topiramate monotherapy is associated with hyperammonemia.

Patients with inborn errors of metabolism or reduced hepatic mitochondrial activity may be at an increased risk for hyperammonemia with or without encephalopathy. Although not studied, an interaction of topiramate and valproic acid may exacerbate existing defects or unmask deficiencies in susceptible people.

In patients who develop unexplained lethargy, vomiting, or changes in mental status, consider hyperammonemic encephalopathy and measure an ammonia level.

➤*Kidney stones:* A total of 32 out of 2,086 (1.5%) of adults exposed to topiramate during its adjunctive epilepsy therapy development reported the occurrence of kidney stones, an incidence about 2 to 4 times that expected in a similar, untreated population. In the double-blind monotherapy epilepsy study, a total of 4 of 319 (1.3%) adults exposed to topiramate reported the occurrence of kidney stones. As in the general population, the incidence of stone formation among topiramate-treated patients was higher in men. Kidney stones also have been reported in children.

An explanation for the association of topiramate and kidney stones may be that topiramate is a weak carbonic anhydrase inhibitor. Carbonic anhydrase inhibitors (eg, acetazolamide, dichlorphenamide) promote stone formation by reducing urinary citrate excretion and by increasing urinary pH. The concomitant use of topiramate with other carbonic anhydrase inhibitors or potentially in patients on a ketogenic diet may create a physiological environment that increases the risk of kidney stone formation; therefore, avoid concomitant use.

Increased fluid intake increases the urinary output, lowering the concentration of substances involved in stone formation. Hydration is recommended to reduce new stone formation.

➤*Paresthesia:* Paresthesia (usually tingling of the extremities), an effect associated with the use of other carbonic anhydrase inhibitors, also appears to be a common effect of topiramate. Paresthesia was more frequently reported in the monotherapy epilepsy trials and migraine prophylaxis trials versus the adjunctive therapy trials in epilepsy. In the majority of instances, paresthesia did not lead to treatment discontinuation.

➤*Renal function impairment:* The major route of elimination of unchanged topiramate and its metabolites is via the kidney. Dosage adjustment may be required in patients with reduced renal function.

➤*Hepatic function impairment:* In hepatically impaired patients, administer topiramate with caution because the clearance of topiramate may be decreased.

➤*Pregnancy: Category C.* Topiramate has demonstrated selective developmental toxicity, including teratogenicity, in experimental animal studies. When oral doses of 20, 100, or 500 mg/kg were administered to pregnant mice during the period of organogenesis, the incidence of fetal malformations (primarily craniofacial defects) was increased at all doses. The low dose is approximately 0.2 times the recommended human dose (400 mg/day) on a mg/m^2 basis. Fetal body weights and skeletal ossification were reduced at 500 mg/kg in conjunction with decreased maternal body weight gain.

In rat studies (oral doses of 20, 100, and 500 mg/kg or 0.2, 2.5, 30, and 400 mg/kg), the frequency of limb malformations (ectrodactyly, micromelia, and amelia) was increased among the offspring of dams treated with 400 mg/kg (10 times the recommended human dose on a mg/m^2 basis) or more during the organogenesis period of pregnancy. Embryotoxicity (reduced fetal body weights, increased incidence of structural variations) was observed at doses as low as 20 mg/kg (0.5 times the recommended human dose on a mg/m^2 basis). Clinical signs of maternal toxicity were seen at 400 mg/kg or more, and maternal body weight gain was reduced during treatment with 100 mg/kg or more.

In rabbit studies (20, 60, and 180 mg/kg or 10, 35, and 120 mg/kg orally during organogenesis), embryo/fetal mortality was increased at 35 mg/kg (2 times the recommended human dose on a mg/m^2 basis) or more, and teratogenic effects (primarily rib and vertebral malformations) were observed at 120 mg/kg (6 times the recommended human dose on a mg/m^2 basis). Evidence of maternal toxicity (decreased body weight gain, clinical signs, and/or mortality) was seen at 35 mg/kg or more.

When female rats were treated during the latter part of gestation and throughout lactation (0.2, 4, 20, and 100 mg/kg or 2, 20, and 200 mg/kg), offspring exhibited decreased viability and delayed physical development at 200 mg/kg (5 times the recommended human dose on a mg/m^2 basis) and reductions in preweaning and/or postweaning body weight gain at 2 mg/kg (0.05 times the recommended human dose on a mg/m^2 basis) and higher. Maternal toxicity (decreased body weight gain, clinical signs) was evident at 100 mg/kg or more.

In a rat embryo/fetal development study with a postnatal component (0.2, 2.5, 30, or 400 mg/kg during organogenesis; noted above), pups exhibited delayed physical development at 400 mg/kg (10 times the recommended human dose on a mg/m^2 basis) and persistent reductions in body weight gain at 30 mg/kg (1 times the recommended human dose on a mg/m^2 basis) and higher.

There are no studies using topiramate in pregnant women. Use topiramate during pregnancy only if the potential benefit outweighs the potential risk to the fetus.

In postmarketing experience, cases of hypospadias have been reported in male infants exposed in utero to topiramate, with or without other anticonvulsants; however, a causal relationship with topiramate has not been established.

TOPIRAMATE — ORAL

➤*Lactation:* Topiramate is excreted in the milk of lactating rats. The excretion of topiramate in human milk has not been evaluated in controlled studies. Limited observations in patients suggest an extensive secretion of topiramate into breast milk. Because many drugs are excreted in human milk and because the potential for serious adverse reactions in breast-feeding infants to topiramate is unknown, weigh the potential benefit to the mother against the potential risk to the infant when considering recommendations regarding breast-feeding.

➤*Children:* Safety and efficacy in children younger than 2 years of age have not been established for the adjunctive therapy treatment of partial-onset seizures, primary generalized tonic-clonic seizures, or seizures associated with Lennox-Gastaut syndrome. Safety and efficacy in children younger than 10 years of age have not been established for the monotherapy treatment of epilepsy.

Topiramate is associated with metabolic acidosis. Chronic untreated metabolic acidosis in children may cause osteomalacia (rickets) and may reduce growth rates. A reduction in growth rate may eventually decrease the maximal height achieved. The effect of topiramate on growth and bone-related sequelae has not been systematically investigated.

Safety and efficacy in children have not been established for the prophylaxis treatment of migraine headache.

➤*Elderly:* In clinical trials, 3% of patients were older than 60 years of age. No age-related differences in efficacy or adverse reactions were evident. However, clinical studies of topiramate did not include sufficient numbers of subjects 65 years of age and older to determine whether they respond differently than younger subjects. Dosage adjustment may be necessary for elderly patients with renal function impairment (CrCl 70 mL/min per 1.73 m^2 or less) because of reduced clearance of topiramate.

➤*Monitoring:* Measurement of baseline and periodic serum bicarbonate during topiramate treatment is recommended. Closely monitor patients, especially children, treated with topiramate for evidence of decreased sweating and increased body temperature, especially in hot weather.

In situations in which rapid withdrawal of topiramate is medically required, appropriate monitoring is recommended.

In patients who develop unexplained lethargy, vomiting, or changes in mental status, consider hyperammonemic encephalopathy and measure an ammonia level.

Drug Interactions

Topiramate Drug Interactions

Precipitant drug	Object drug[a]		Description
Carbamazepine	Topiramate	⬇	Carbamazepine may increase the metabolism of topiramate, causing a 40% decrease in serum concentrations. Adjust the dose if needed.
Carbonic anhydrase inhibitors (eg, acetazolamide)	Topiramate	⬆	Because topiramate is also a carbonic anhydrase inhibitor, concomitant use may increase the risk for renal stone formation. Avoid concurrent use.
Topiramate	Carbonic anhydrase inhibitors (eg, acetazolamide)		
Hydantoins (eg, phenytoin)	Topiramate	⬇	Hydantoins may increase the metabolism of topiramate, causing a 48% decrease in serum concentration. Topiramate may decrease the metabolism of phenytoin, causing a 25% increase in serum concentrations in some patients. Adjust the hydantoin dose if needed.
Topiramate	Hydantoins (eg, phenytoin)	⬆	
Hydrochlorothiazide	Topiramate	⬆	Coadministration increased topiramate C_{max}[b] 27% and AUC 29%. Adjust the topiramate dose accordingly.
Lamotrigine	Topiramate	⬇	Coadministration produced a 13% decrease in topiramate concentration.
Metformin	Topiramate	⬆	Coadministration caused metformin C_{max} and AUC to increase 18% and 25%, respectively, and clearance to decrease 20%. Oral plasma clearance of topiramate is reduced with coadministration. The clinical significance of these effects is not known.
Topiramate	Metformin		
Valproic acid	Topiramate	⬇	Coadministration caused a 14% decrease in topiramate serum concentrations and an 11% decrease in valproic acid serum concentrations. Administration has been associated with hyperammonemia with and without encephalopathy.
Topiramate	Valproic acid		
Topiramate	Alcohol, CNS depressants	⬆	Use topiramate with extreme caution because of its potential to cause CNS depression, as well as other cognitive and/or neuropsychiatric adverse reactions.
Topiramate	Amitriptyline	⬆	There was a 12% increase of amitriptyline AUC and C_{max}. Adjust amitriptyline dose according to patient response, not on the basis of plasma levels.
Topiramate	Digoxin	⬇	Serum digoxin AUC was decreased 12% when given with topiramate. The clinical relevance of this observation has not been established.
Topiramate	Lithium	⬇	Lithium AUC and C_{max} decreased 20%.
Topiramate	Oral contraceptives	⬇	Oral contraceptive efficacy may be reduced, even in the absence of breakthrough bleeding.
Topiramate	Pioglitazone	⬇	Pioglitazone AUC decreased 15%. Monitor patients for control of diabetic disease state.
Topiramate	Risperidone	⬇	Coadministration produced a 25% decrease in exposure to risperidone. Monitor closely.

[a] ⬆ = object drug increased; ⬇ = object drug decreased.
[b] C_{max} = maximum plasma concentration.

Adverse Reactions

The data described in the following sections were obtained using topiramate tablets.

➤*Epilepsy, monotherapy:*

Adults – In the controlled trial, the adverse reactions that occurred most frequently in adults in the 400 mg/day group and at a rate higher than the 50 mg/day group were anorexia, difficulty with memory not otherwise specified (NOS) (see the following table), dizziness, paresthesia, somnolence, and weight decrease.

Approximately 21% of the 159 adult patients in the 400 mg/day group who received topiramate as monotherapy in the controlled clinical trial discontinued therapy because of adverse reactions. Adverse reactions associated with discontinuing therapy (2% or more) included depression, difficulty with memory (NOS), dizziness, insomnia, nausea, paresthesia, psychomotor slowing, and somnolence.

Topiramate Adverse Reactions in the Monotherapy Epilepsy Trial in Adults[a] (≥ 2%)

Adverse reaction	Topiramate 50 mg/day (n = 160)	Topiramate 400 mg/day (n = 159)
CNS		
Anxiety	4%	6%
Asthenia	4%	6%
Ataxia	3%	4%
Cognitive problem NOS	1%	4%
Confusion	3%	4%
Depression	7%	9%
Difficulty with concentration/attention	7%	8%
Difficulty with memory NOS	5%	10%
Dizziness	13%	14%
Hypertonia	0%	3%
Hypesthesia	4%	5%
Insomnia	8%	9%
Libido decreased	0%	3%
Mood problems	2%	5%
Paresthesia	21%	40%
Psychomotor slowing	3%	5%
Somnolence	9%	15%

TOPIRAMATE — ORAL

Topiramate Adverse Reactions in the Monotherapy Epilepsy Trial in Adults[a] (≥ 2%)		
Adverse reaction	Topiramate 50 mg/day (n = 160)	Topiramate 400 mg/day (n = 159)
Dermatologic		
Acne	2%	3%
Pruritus	1%	4%
Rash	1%	4%
GI		
Anorexia	4%	14%
Constipation	1%	4%
Diarrhea	5%	6%
Dry mouth	1%	3%
Gastritis	0%	3%
Gastroesophageal reflux	1%	2%
Taste perversion	3%	5%
GU		
Cystitis	1%	3%
Dysuria	0%	2%
Micturition frequency	0%	2%
Renal calculus	0%	3%
Urinary tract infection	1%	2%
Vaginal hemorrhage	0%	3%
Respiratory		
Bronchitis	3%	4%
Dyspnea	1%	2%
Rhinitis	2%	4%
Miscellaneous		
Anemia	1%	2%
Chest pain	1%	2%
Gamma-glutamyl transferase increased	1%	3%
Infection	2%	3%
Infection viral	6%	8%
Leg pain	2%	3%
Weight decrease	6%	16%

[a] Patients may have reported more than 1 adverse reaction during the study and can be included in more than 1 adverse reaction category.

Children – In the controlled trial, the adverse reactions that occurred most frequently in children 10 to 16 years of age in the 400 mg/day group and at a rate higher than the 50 mg/day group were anorexia, diarrhea, mood problems paresthesia, upper respiratory tract infection, and weight decrease (see the following table).

Approximately 12% of the 57 children in the 400 mg/day group who received topiramate as monotherapy in the controlled clinical trial discontinued therapy because of adverse reactions. Adverse reactions associated with discontinuing therapy (5% or more) included difficulty with concentration/attention.

Topiramate Adverse Reactions in the Monotherapy Epilepsy Trial in Children[a] (≥ 5%)		
Adverse reaction	Topiramate 50 mg/day (n = 57)	Topiramate 400 mg/day (n = 57)
CNS		
Cognitive problems NOS	0%	7%
Difficulty with concentration/attention	4%	9%
Mood problems	2%	11%
Nervousness	4%	5%
Paresthesia	2%	16%
GI		
Anorexia	11%	14%
Diarrhea	5%	11%
Respiratory		
Bronchitis	2%	7%
Rhinitis	2%	7%
Sinusitis	2%	5%
Upper respiratory tract infection	16%	18%
Miscellaneous		
Alopecia	2%	5%
Fever	0%	9%
Infection	2%	7%
Infection viral	4%	9%
Weight decrease	7%	21%

[a] Patients may have reported more than 1 adverse reaction during the study and can be included in more than 1 adverse reaction category.

➤*Epilepsy, adjunctive therapy:*

Adults – The most frequently observed adverse reactions associated with the use of topiramate at doses of 200 to 400 mg/day in controlled trials in adults with partial-onset-seizures, primary generalized tonic-clonic seizures, or Lennox-Gastaut syndrome, which were seen at greater frequency in topiramate-treated patients and did not appear to be dose-related, were abnormal vision, ataxia, difficulty with memory, diplopia, dizziness, paresthesia, psychomotor slowing, somnolence, and speech disorders and related speech problems. The most common dose-related adverse reactions at doses of 200 to 1,000 mg/day were as follows: anorexia, anxiety, confusion, depression, difficulty with concentration/attention, fatigue, language problems, mood problems, nervousness, and weight decrease.

In controlled clinical trials in adults, 11% of patients receiving topiramate 200 to 400 mg/day as adjunctive therapy discontinued because of adverse reactions. This rate appeared to increase at doses of more than 400 mg/day. Adverse reactions associated with discontinuing therapy included somnolence, anxiety,difficulty with concentration/attention, dizziness, fatigue, and paresthesia, and increased at dosages of more than 400 mg/day.

Approximately 28% of the 1,757 adults with epilepsy who received topiramate at doses of 200 to 1,600 mg/day in clinical studies discontinued treatment because of adverse reactions; an individual patient could have reported more than 1 adverse reaction. These adverse reactions were psychomotor slowing (4%), difficulty with memory (3.2%), fatigue (3.2%), somnolence (3.2%), confusion (3.1%), difficulty with concentration/attention (2.9%), anorexia (2.7%), depression (2.6%), dizziness (2.5%), weight decrease (2.5%), nervousness (2.3%), ataxia (2.1%), and paresthesia (2%). Approximately 11% of the 310 children who received topiramate at doses of up to 30 mg/kg/day discontinued because of adverse reactions. Adverse reactions associated with discontinuing therapy included aggravated convulsions (2.3%), difficulty with concentration/attention (1.6%), language problems (1.3%), personality disorder (1.3%), and somnolence (1.3%).

Children – Adverse reactions associated with the use of topiramate at doses of 5 to 9 mg/kg/day in controlled trials in children with partial-onset seizures, primary generalized tonic-clonic seizures, or Lennox-Gastaut syndrome, which were seen at greater frequency in topiramate-treated patients, were aggressive reaction, anorexia, difficulty with concentration/attention, difficulty with memory, fatigue, nervousness, somnolence, and weight decrease. None of the children who received topiramate adjunctive therapy at 5 to 9 mg/kg/day in controlled clinical trials discontinued because of adverse reactions.

➤*Incidence in epilepsy controlled clinical trials (adjunctive therapy), including partial-onset seizures, primary generalized tonic-clonic seizures, and Lennox-Gastaut syndrome:*

Adults – The following table lists treatment-emergent adverse reactions that occurred in at least 1% of adults treated with topiramate 200 to 400 mg/day in controlled trials that were numerically more common at this dose than in the patients treated with placebo. In general, most patients who experienced adverse reactions during the first 8 weeks of these trials no longer experienced them by their last visit. Other events that occurred in more than 1% of adults treated with topiramate 200 to 400 mg in placebo-controlled epilepsy trials but with equal or greater frequency in the placebo group were anxiety, convulsions aggravated, coughing, diarrhea, dysmenorrhea, eye pain, fever, headache, injury, insomnia, muscle weakness, pain, personality disorder, rash, upper respiratory tract infection, and vomiting.

Topiramate Adverse Reactions in Add-on Epilepsy Trials in Adults[a,b] (≥ 1%)			
Adverse reaction[c]	Topiramate 200 to 400 mg/day (n = 183)	Topiramate 600 to 1,000 mg/day (n = 414)	Placebo (n = 291)
CNS			
Aggressive reaction	3%	3%	2%
Agitation	3%	3%	2%
Apathy	1%	3%	1%
Asthenia	6%	3%	1%
Ataxia	16%	14%	7%
Cognitive problems	3%	3%	1%
Confusion	11%	14%	5%
Coordination abnormal	4%	4%	2%
Depersonalization	1%	2%	1%
Depression	5%	13%	5%

TOPIRAMATE — ORAL

Topiramate Adverse Reactions in Add-on Epilepsy Trials in Adults[a,b] (≥ 1%)			
Adverse reaction[c]	Topiramate 200 to 400 mg/day (n = 183)	Topiramate 600 to 1,000 mg/day (n = 414)	Placebo (n = 291)
Difficulty with concentration/attention	6%	14%	2%
Difficulty with memory	12%	14%	3%
Dizziness	25%	32%	15%
Emotional lability	3%	3%	1%
Fatigue	15%	30%	13%
Gait abnormal	3%	2%	1%
Hypesthesia	2%	1%	1%
Language problems	6%	10%	1%
Libido decreased	2%	< 1%	1%
Mood problems	4%	9%	2%
Muscle contractions involuntary	2%	2%	1%
Nervousness	16%	19%	6%
Nystagmus	10%	11%	7%
Paresthesia	11%	19%	4%
Psychomotor slowing	13%	21%	2%
Rigors	1%	< 1%	0%
Somnolence	29%	28%	12%
Speech disorders/related speech problems	13%	11%	2%
Stupor	2%	1%	0%
Tremor	9%	9%	6%
Vertigo	1%	2%	1%
Dermatologic			
Rash erythematous	1%	< 1%	< 1%
Skin disorder	2%	1%	< 1%
Sweating increased	1%	< 1%	< 1%
GI			
Abdominal pain	6%	7%	4%
Anorexia	10%	12%	4%
Constipation	4%	3%	2%
Dry mouth	2%	4%	1%
Dyspepsia	7%	6%	6%
Epistaxis	2%	1%	1%
Gastroenteritis	2%	1%	1%
GI disorder	1%	0%	< 1%
Gingivitis	1%	1%	< 1%
Nausea	10%	12%	8%
GU			
Amenorrhea	2%	2%	1%
Breast pain	4%	0%	2%
Hematuria	2%	< 1%	1%
Menorrhagia	2%	1%	0%
Menstrual disorder	2%	1%	1%
Micturition frequency	1%	2%	1%
Prostatic disorder	2%	0%	< 1%
Urinary incontinence	2%	1%	< 1%
Urinary tract infection	2%	3%	1%
Urine abnormal	1%	< 1%	0%
Musculoskeletal			
Myalgia	2%	2%	1%
Skeletal pain	1%	0%	0%
Respiratory			
Dyspnea	1%	2%	1%
Pharyngitis	6%	3%	2%
Rhinitis	7%	6%	6%
Sinusitis	5%	6%	4%
Special senses			
Abnormal vision	13%	10%	2%
Diplopia	10%	10%	5%
Hearing decreased	2%	1%	1%
Taste perversion	2%	4%	0%
Miscellaneous			
Allergy	2%	3%	1%
Back pain	5%	3%	4%
Body odor	1%	0%	0%
Chest pain	4%	2%	3%
Edema	2%	1%	1%
Hot flushes	2%	1%	1%
Infection	2%	1%	1%
Influenza-like symptoms	3%	4%	2%
Leg pain	2%	4%	2%
Leukopenia	2%	1%	1%
Moniliasis	1%	0%	< 1%
Viral infection	2%	< 1%	1%
Weight decrease	9%	13%	3%

[a] Patients in these add-on trials were receiving 1 to 2 concomitant AEDs in addition to topiramate or placebo.
[b] Patients may have reported more than 1 adverse reaction during the study and can be included in more than 1 adverse reaction category.
[c] Adverse reactions reported by at least 1% of patients in the topiramate 200 to 400 mg/day group and more common than in the placebo group are listed in this table.

➤*Partial-onset seizures (add-on therapy):*

Adults – Study 119 was a randomized, double-blind, placebo-controlled, parallel-group study with 3 treatment arms: placebo; topiramate 200 mg/day with a 25 mg/day starting dosage, increased by 25 mg/day each week for 8 weeks until the 200 mg/day maintenance dosage was reached; and topiramate 200 mg/day with a 50 mg/day starting dosage, increased by 50 mg/day each week for 4 weeks until the 200 mg/day maintenance dosage was reached. All patients were maintained on concomitant carbamazepine with or without another concomitant AED.

The incidence of adverse reactions (see the following table) did not differ significantly between the 2 topiramate regimens. Because the frequencies of adverse reactions reported in this study were markedly lower than those reported in the previous epilepsy studies, they cannot be directly compared with data obtained in other studies.

Topiramate Treatment-Emergent Adverse Reactions in Add-On Therapy in Adults[a,b] with Partial-Onset Seizures (≥ 2%)		
Adverse reaction[c]	Placebo (n = 92)	Topiramate dosage 200 mg/day (n = 171)
CNS		
Aggressive reaction	0%	2%
Difficulty with concentration/attention	0%	5%
Difficulty with memory	1%	2%
Dizziness	4%	7%
Fatigue	4%	9%
Hypesthesia	0%	2%
Insomnia	3%	4%
Language problems	0%	2%
Nervousness	2%	9%
Paresthesia	2%	9%
Somnolence	9%	15%
Tremor	2%	3%
GI		
Abdominal pain	3%	5%
Anorexia	7%	9%
Constipation	0%	4%
Diarrhea	1%	2%
Dry mouth	0%	2%
Dyspepsia	0%	2%

TOPIRAMATE — ORAL

Topiramate Treatment-Emergent Adverse Reactions in Add-On Therapy in Adults[a,b] with Partial-Onset Seizures (≥ 2%)		
Adverse reaction[c]	Placebo (n = 92)	Topiramate dosage 200 mg/day (n = 171)
Special senses		
Diplopia	0%	2%
Tinnitus	0%	2%
Vision abnormal	0%	2%
Miscellaneous		
Chest pain	1%	2%
Cystitis	0%	2%
Hypertension	0%	2%
Leg cramps	0%	2%
Rhinitis	0%	4%
Weight decrease	4%	8%

[a] Patients in these add-on trials were receiving 1 to 2 concomitant AEDs in addition to topiramate or placebo.
[b] Patients may have reported more than 1 adverse reaction during the study and can be included in more than 1 adverse reaction category.
[c] Adverse reactions reported by 2% or more of patients in the topiramate 200 mg/day group and more common than in the placebo group are listed in this table.

Topiramate Dose-Related Adverse Reactions in Add-On Trials in Adults with Partial-Onset Seizures[a]				
Adverse reaction	Topiramate 200 mg/day (n = 45)	Topiramate 400 mg/day (n = 68)	Topiramate 600 to 1,000 mg/day (n = 414)	Placebo (n = 216)
CNS				
Anxiety	2%	3%	10%	6%
Confusion	9%	10%	14%	4%
Depression	9%	7%	13%	6%
Difficulty with concentration/ attention	7%	9%	14%	1%
Fatigue	11%	12%	30%	13%
Language problems	2%	9%	10%	< 1%
Mood problems	0%	6%	9%	2%
Nervousness	13%	18%	19%	7%
Miscellaneous				
Anorexia	4%	6%	12%	4%
Weight decrease	4%	9%	13%	3%

[a] Dose-response studies were not conducted for other adult indications or for child indications.

Children – The following table lists the percentage of incidence of treatment-emergent adverse reactions in placebo-controlled, add-on epilepsy trials in children 2 to 16 years of age (reactions that occurred in at least 1% of topiramate-treated patients and occurred more frequently in topiramate-treated than placebo-treated patients).

Topiramate Adverse Reactions in Add-On Epilepsy Trials in Children[a,b] (≥ 1%)		
Adverse reaction	Topiramate (n = 98)	Placebo (n = 101)
Cardiovascular		
Bradycardia	1%	0%
Hypertension	1%	0%
CNS		
Aggressive reaction	9%	4%
Ataxia	6%	2%
Confusion	4%	3%
Convulsions tonic-clonic	1%	0%
Difficulty with concentration/attention	10%	2%
Difficulty with memory NOS	5%	0%
Dizziness	4%	2%
Fatigue	16%	5%
Gait abnormal	8%	5%
Hyperkinesia	5%	4%
Hyporeflexia	2%	0%
Insomnia	8%	7%
Nervousness	14%	7%
Neurosis	1%	0%
Paresthesia	1%	0%
Personality disorder (behavior problems)	11%	9%
Psychomotor slowing	3%	2%
Somnolence	26%	16%
Speech disorders/ related speech problems	4%	2%
Dermatologic		
Alopecia	2%	1%
Dermatitis	2%	0%
Eczema	1%	0%
Hypertrichosis	2%	1%
Rash erythematous	2%	0%
Seborrhea	1%	0%
Skin discoloration	1%	0%
Skin disorder	3%	2%
GI		
Anorexia	24%	15%
Appetite increased	1%	0%
Constipation	5%	4%
Dysphagia	1%	0%
Epistaxis	4%	1%
Fecal incontinence	1%	0%
Flatulence	1%	0%
Gastroenteritis	3%	2%
Gastroesophageal reflux	1%	0%
Glossitis	1%	0%
Gum hyperplasia	1%	0%
Nausea	6%	5%
Saliva increased	6%	4%
GU		
Leukorrhea	2%	0%
Nocturia	1%	0%
Urinary incontinence	4%	2%
Hematologic/Lymphatic		
Hematoma	1%	0%
Leukopenia	2%	0%
Prothrombin increased	1%	0%
Purpura	8%	4%
Thrombocytopenia	1%	0%
Metabolic/Nutritional		
Hypoglycemia	1%	0%
Thirst	2%	1%
Weight decrease	9%	1%
Weight increase	1%	0%
Ophthalmic		
Abnormal vision	2%	1%
Diplopia	1%	0%
Eye abnormality	2%	1%
Lacrimation abnormal	1%	0%
Myopia	1%	0%
Respiratory		
Pneumonia	5%	1%
Respiratory disorder	1%	0%

TOPIRAMATE — ORAL

Topiramate Adverse Reactions in Add-On Epilepsy Trials in Children[a,b] (≥ 1%)		
Adverse reaction	Topiramate (n = 98)	Placebo (n = 101)
Miscellaneous		
Allergic reaction	2%	1%
Back pain	1%	0%
Injury	14%	13%
Pallor	1%	0%
Viral infection	7%	3%

[a] Patients in these add-on trials were receiving 1 to 2 concomitant AEDs in addition to topiramate or placebo.

[b] Patients may have reported more than 1 adverse reaction during the study and can be included in more than 1 adverse reaction category.

➤*Other adverse reactions observed during all epilepsy clinical trials:*

Cardiovascular – Angina pectoris, atrioventricular block, deep vein thrombosis, flushing, hypotension, phlebitis, postural hypotension, syncope, vasodilation (0.1% to 1%); pulmonary embolism, vasospasm (less than 0.1%).

CNS – Electroencephalogram abnormal, euphoria, hallucination, psychosis, suicide attempt (1% or more); abnormal dreaming, apraxia, delirium, delusion, dyskinesia, dysphonia, dystonia, encephalopathy, hyperesthesia, neuropathy, paranoia, paranoid reaction, ptosis, scotoma (0.1% to 1%); cerebellar syndrome, increased libido, manic reaction, tongue paralysis, upper motor neuron lesion (less than 0.1%).

Dermatologic – Abnormal hair texture, photosensitivity reaction, urticaria (0.1% to 1%); chloasma (less than 0.1%).

GI – Abdomen enlarged, esophagitis, gastritis, gingival bleeding, hemorrhoids, melena, stomatitis (0.1% to 1%); tongue edema (less than 0.1%).

GU – Impotence (1% or more); albuminuria, breast discharge, ejaculation disorder, oliguria, polyuria, renal pain, urinary retention (0.1% to 1%).

Hematologic/Lymphatic – Anemia, eosinophilia, granulocytopenia, lymphadenopathy, lymphopenia, thrombocythemia (0.1% to 1%); lymphocytosis, marrow depression , pancytopenia, polycythemia (less than 0.1%).

Hepatic – ALT, AST, and gamma-glutamyl transferase increased (0.1% to 1%).

Metabolic/Nutritional – Dehydration (1% or more); face edema, hyperglycemia, hyperlipidemia, hypocalcemia, hypokalemia, increased alkaline phosphatase, xerophthalmia (0.1% to 1%); diabetes mellitus, hyperchloremia, hypernatremia, hypocholesterolemia, hyponatremia, hypophosphatemia, increased creatinine (less than 0.1%).

Musculoskeletal – Arthralgia (1% or more); arthrosis (0.1% to 1%).

Ophthalmic – Conjunctivitis (1% or more); abnormal accommodation, photophobia, strabismus, visual field defect (0.1% to 1%); iritis, mydriasis (less than 0.1%).

Special senses – Parosmia, taste loss (0.1% to 1%).

Miscellaneous – Alcohol intolerance (less than 0.1%).

➤*Migraine:* The following table includes those adverse reactions reported for patients in the placebo-controlled trials in which the incidence rate in any topiramate treatment group was at least 2% and was more than that for placebo patients.

Topiramate Adverse Reactions in Migraine Trials (≥ 2%)[a]				
Adverse reaction	Topiramate 50 mg/day (n = 235)	Topiramate 100 mg/day (n = 386)	Topiramate 200 mg/day (n = 514)	Placebo (n = 445)
CNS				
Aggravated depression	1%	2%	2%	1%
Agitation	2%	2%	1%	1%
Anxiety	4%	5%	6%	3%
Asthenia	< 1%	2%	2%	1%
Ataxia	1%	2%	1%	< 1%
Cognitive problems NOS	< 1%	2%	2%	1%
Confusion	2%	3%	4%	2%
Depression	3%	4%	6%	4%
Difficulty with concentration/attention	3%	6%	10%	2%
Difficulty with memory NOS	7%	7%	11%	2%
Dizziness	8%	9%	12%	10%
Fatigue	14%	15%	19%	11%
Hypesthesia	6%	7%	8%	2%
Insomnia	6%	7%	6%	5%
Language problems	7%	6%	7%	2%
Mood problems	3%	6%	5%	2%
Nervousness	4%	4%	4%	2%
Paresthesia	35%	51%	49%	6%
Psychomotor slowing	3%	2%	4%	1%
Somnolence	8%	7%	10%	5%
Speech disorders/related speech problems	1%	< 1%	2%	< 1%
GI				
Abdominal pain	6%	6%	7%	5%
Anorexia	9%	15%	14%	6%
Diarrhea	9%	11%	11%	4%
Dry mouth	2%	3%	5%	2%
Dyspepsia	4%	5%	3%	3%
Gastroenteritis	3%	3%	2%	1%
Nausea	9%	13%	14%	8%
Vomiting	1%	2%	3%	2%
GU				
Ejaculation premature	3%	0%	0%	0%
Libido decreased	1%	1%	2%	1%
Menstrual disorder	3%	2%	2%	2%
Renal calculus	0%	1%	2%	0%
Urinary tract infection	4%	2%	4%	2%
Metabolic/Nutritional				
Thirst	2%	2%	1%	< 1%
Weight decrease	6%	9%	11%	1%
Musculoskeletal				
Arthralgia	7%	3%	1%	2%
Involuntary muscle contractions	2%	2%	4%	1%
Ophthalmic				
Abnormal vision	1%	2%	3%	< 1%
Blurred vision[b]	4%	2%	4%	2%
Conjunctivitis	1%	2%	1%	1%
Respiratory				
Bronchitis	3%	3%	3%	2%
Coughing	2%	4%	3%	2%
Dyspnea	1%	3%	2%	2%
Pharyngitis	5%	6%	2%	4%
Rhinitis	1%	2%	2%	1%
Sinusitis	10%	6%	8%	6%
Upper respiratory tract infection	13%	14%	12%	12%
Special senses				
Otitis media	2%	1%	1%	< 1%
Taste loss	1%	1%	2%	< 1%
Taste perversion	15%	8%	12%	1%
Tinnitus	< 1%	1%	2%	1%
Miscellaneous				
Allergy	2%	< 1%	< 1%	< 1%
Fever	1%	1%	2%	1%
Influenza-like symptoms	< 1%	< 1%	2%	< 1%
Injury	9%	6%	6%	7%
Neoplasm NOS	2%	< 1%	< 1%	< 1%
Pruritus	4%	2%	2%	2%
Viral infection	4%	4%	3%	3%

[a] Patients may have reported more than 1 adverse reaction during the study and can be included in more than 1 adverse reaction category.

[b] Blurred vision was the most common term considered as vision abnormal. Blurred vision was an included term that accounted for 50% or more of reactions coded as vision abnormal, a preferred term.

Of the 1,135 patients exposed to topiramate in the placebo-controlled studies, 25% discontinued because of adverse reactions, compared with 10% of the 445 placebo patients. The adverse reactions associated with discontinuation of therapy in the topiramate-treated patients included paresthesia (7%), fatigue (4%), nausea (4%), difficulty with concentration/attention (3%), insomnia (3%), anorexia (2%), and dizziness (2%).

TOPIRAMATE — ORAL

Patients treated with topiramate experienced dose-dependent mean percent reductions in body weight. This change was not seen in the placebo group. Mean changes of 0%, −2%, −3%, and −4% were seen for the placebo group, topiramate 50, 100, and 200 mg groups, respectively.

The following table shows adverse reactions that were dose-dependent. Several CNS adverse reactions, including some that represented cognitive dysfunction, were dose-related. The most common dose-related adverse reactions were anorexia, diarrhea, difficulty with concentration/attention, difficulty with memory, dizziness, fatigue, nausea, paresthesia, somnolence, and weight decrease.

Topiramate Dose-Related Adverse Reactions From Migraine Trials[a]

Adverse reaction	Topiramate 50 mg/day (n = 235)	Topiramate 100 mg/day (n = 386)	Topiramate 200 mg/day (n = 514)	Placebo (n = 445)
CNS				
Anxiety	4%	5%	6%	3%
Confusion	2%	3%	4%	2%
Depression	3%	4%	6%	4%
Difficulty with concentration/attention	3%	6%	10%	2%
Difficulty with memory NOS	7%	7%	11%	2%
Dizziness	8%	9%	12%	10%
Fatigue	14%	15%	19%	11%
Hypesthesia	6%	7%	8%	2%
Mood problems	3%	6%	5%	2%
Paresthesia	35%	51%	49%	6%
Somnolence	8%	7%	10%	5%
GI				
Anorexia	9%	15%	14%	6%
Diarrhea	9%	11%	11%	4%
Dry mouth	2%	3%	5%	2%
Nausea	9%	13%	14%	8%
Miscellaneous				
Abnormal vision	1%	2%	3%	< 1%
Involuntary muscle contractions	2%	2%	4%	1%
Renal calculus	0%	1%	2%	0%
Weight decrease	6%	9%	11%	1%

[a] The incidence rate of the adverse reaction in the 200 mg/day group was 2% or more than the rate in both the placebo group and the 50 mg/day group.

➤*Other adverse reactions observed during migraine clinical trials:* The following additional adverse reactions that were not described earlier were reported by more than 1% of the 1,367 topiramate-treated patients in the controlled clinical trials.

CNS – Headache, migraine aggravated, sensory disturbance, tremor, vertigo.

Dermatologic – Alopecia, rash.

GI – Constipation, epistaxis, gastroesophageal reflux, tooth disorder.

GU – Genital moniliasis, intermenstrual bleeding.

Ophthalmic – Abnormal accommodation, eye pain.

Respiratory – Asthma, pneumonia.

Miscellaneous – Allergic reaction, chest pain, infection, myalgia, pain.

➤*Postmarketing:* In addition to the adverse reactions reported during clinical testing of topiramate, the following adverse reactions have been reported worldwide in patients receiving topiramate postapproval. These adverse reactions have not been listed previously. Data are insufficient to support an estimate of their incidence or to establish causation. The listing is alphabetized as follows: bullous skin reactions (including erythema multiforme, Stevens-Johnson syndrome, toxic epidermal necrolysis), hepatic failure (including fatalities), hepatitis, pancreatitis, pemphigus, and renal tubular acidosis.

Overdosage

➤*Symptoms:* Overdoses of topiramate have been reported. Signs and symptoms included abdominal pain, abnormal coordination, agitation, blurred vision, convulsions, depression, diplopia, dizziness, drowsiness, hypotension, lethargy, mentation impaired, speech disturbance, and stupor. The clinical consequences were not severe in most cases, but deaths have been reported after polydrug overdoses involving topiramate.

Topiramate overdose has resulted in severe metabolic acidosis.

A patient who ingested a dose between 96 and 110 g was admitted to a hospital with a coma lasting 20 to 24 hours followed by full recovery after 3 to 4 days.

➤*Treatment:* In acute topiramate overdose, if the ingestion is recent, immediately empty the stomach by lavage. Activated charcoal adsorbs topiramate in vitro. Use supportive treatment. Hemodialysis is an effective means of removing topiramate from the body.

Patient Information

Instruct patients to read the patient information before starting treatment with topiramate and each time their prescription is renewed.

Tell patients taking topiramate to seek immediate medical attention if they experience blurred vision, visual disturbances, or periorbital pain.

Tell patients, especially children, treated with topiramate to watch for evidence of decreased sweating and increased body temperature, especially in hot weather.

Instruct patients, particularly those with predisposing factors, to maintain an adequate fluid intake in order to minimize the risk of renal stone formation.

Warn patients about the potential for somnolence, dizziness, confusion, and difficulty concentrating, and advise them not to drive or operate machinery until they have gained sufficient experience on topiramate to gauge whether it adversely affects their mental or motor performance.

Consider advising additional food intake if the patient is losing weight while on this medication.

Even when taking topiramate or other anticonvulsants, some patients with epilepsy will continue to have unpredictable seizures. Therefore, tell all patients taking topiramate for epilepsy to exercise appropriate caution when engaging in any activities where loss of consciousness could result in serious danger to themselves or those around them (eg, swimming, driving a car, climbing in high places). Some patients with refractory epilepsy will need to avoid such activities altogether. Discuss the appropriate level of caution before patients with epilepsy engage in such activities.

VALPROIC ACID

Rx	**Valproic Acid** (Various, eg, Ivax, Pliva, UDL)	**Capsules; oral:** 250 mg	In 10s, 30s, 31s, and 100s.
Rx	**Depakene** (Abbott)		Parabens, corn oil. (Depakene). Orange. In 100s.
Rx	**Divalproex Sodium** (Various, eg, Apotex, Lupin, Teva, Upsher-Smith, Wockhardt)	**Tablets, delayed-release; oral:** 125 mg	May contain lactose. In 30s, 100s, 500s, and 1,000s.
Rx	**Depakote** (Abbott)		As divalproex sodium. Talc. Salmon pink. In 100s and *Abbo-Pac* UD 100s.
Rx	**Divalproex Sodium** (Various, eg, Apotex, Lupin, Teva, Upsher-Smith, Wockhardt)	**Tablets, delayed-release; oral:** 250 mg	May contain lactose. In 30s, 100s, 500s, and 1,000s.
	Depakote (Abbott)		As divalproex sodium. Talc. Peach. In 100s, 500s, and *Abbo-Pac* UD 100s.
Rx	**Divalproex Sodium** (Various, eg, Apotex, Lupin, Teva, Upsher-Smith, Wockhardt)	**Tablets, delayed-release; oral:** 500 mg	May contain lactose. In 30s, 100s, 500s, and 1,000s.
	Depakote (Abbott)		As divalproex sodium. Talc. Lavender. In 100s, 500s, and *Abbo-Pac* UD 100s.
Rx	**Depakote ER** (Abbott)	**Tablets, extended-release; oral:** 250 mg	As divalproex sodium. Lactose. (a HF). White, oval. In 60s, 100s, 500s, and *Abbo-Pac* UD 100s.
		500 mg	As divalproex sodium. Lactose, polydextrose. (a HC). Gray, oval. In 100s, 500s, and *Abbo-Pac* UD 100s.
Rx	**Stavzor** (Noven Therapeutics)	**Capsules, delayed-release; oral:** 125 mg	As valproic acid. (NVN). Orange, oval. In 100s.
		250 mg	As valproic acid. (NVN1). Orange, oval. In 100s.
		500 mg	As valproic acid. (NVN2). Orange, oval. In 100s.

VALPROIC ACID

Rx	**Divalproex Sodium** (Various, eg, Dr. Reddy's Lab, ZyGenerics)	**Capsules, sprinkle; oral**[a]: 125 mg	May contain sugar. In 30s, 100s, 500s, 1,000s, and UD 100s.
Rx	**Depakote** (Abbott)		As divalproex sodium. White/Blue. In 100s and *Abbo-Pac* UD 100s.
Rx	**Valproic Acid** (Various, eg, Hi-Tech, Teva)	**Syrup; oral**: 250 mg per 5 mL	In 473 mL.
Rx	**Depakene** (Abbott)		Parabens, sorbitol, sucrose. In 473 mL.
Rx	**Valproate** (Various, eg, Abraxis, Bedford)	**Injection, concentrate**: 100 mg/mL	May be preservative free. In 5 mL single-dose vials.
Rx	**Depacon** (Abbott)		EDTA. Preservative free. In 5 mL single-dose vials.

[a] Sprinkle capsules contain coated particles.

VALPROIC ACID — ORAL

Refer to the general discussion beginning in the Anticonvulsants introduction.

WARNING

Hepatotoxicity – Hepatic failure resulting in fatalities has occurred in patients receiving valproic acid. Experience has indicated that children younger than 2 years of age are at a considerably increased risk of developing fatal hepatotoxicity, especially those on multiple anticonvulsants, those with congenital metabolic disorders, those with severe seizure disorders accompanied by mental retardation, and those with organic brain disease. When valproic acid products are used in this patient group, use them with extreme caution and as a sole agent. Weigh the benefits of therapy against the risks. Above this age group, experience in epilepsy has indicated that the incidence of fatal hepatotoxicity decreases considerably in progressively older patient groups.

These incidents usually have occurred during the first 6 months of treatment. Serious or fatal hepatotoxicity may be preceded by nonspecific symptoms such as anorexia, facial edema, lethargy, malaise, vomiting, and weakness. In patients with epilepsy, a loss of seizure control may also occur. Closely monitor patients for appearance of these symptoms. Perform liver function tests prior to therapy and at frequent intervals thereafter, especially during the first 6 months.

Teratogenicity – Valproate can produce teratogenic effects such as neural tube defects (eg, spina bifida). Accordingly, the use of valproate products in women of childbearing potential requires that the benefits of its use be weighed against the risk of injury to the fetus. This is especially important when the treatment of a spontaneously reversible condition not ordinarily associated with permanent injury or risk of death (eg, migraine) is contemplated.

An information sheet describing the teratogenic potential of valproate is available for patients.

Pancreatitis – Cases of life-threatening pancreatitis have been reported in both children and adults receiving valproate. Some of the cases have been described as hemorrhagic with a rapid progression from initial symptoms to death. Cases have been reported shortly after initial use as well as after several years of use. Warn patients and guardians that abdominal pain, nausea, vomiting, and/or anorexia can be symptoms of pancreatitis that require prompt medical evaluation. If pancreatitis is diagnosed, valproate should ordinarily be discontinued. Initiate alternative treatment for the underlying medical condition as clinically indicated.

Indications

➤*Complex partial seizures:* As monotherapy and adjunctive therapy in the treatment of patients with complex partial seizures in adults and children 10 years of age and older that occur either in isolation or in association with other types of seizures.

➤*Simple and complex absence seizures:* For use as sole and adjunctive therapy in the treatment of simple and complex absence seizures, and adjunctively in patients with multiple seizure types, including absence seizures.

➤*Stavzor*:

Mania – *Stavzor* is indicated for the treatment of the manic episodes associated with bipolar disorder. A manic episode is a distinct period of abnormally and persistently elevated, expansive, or irritable mood. Typical symptoms of mania include pressure of speech, motor hyperactivity, reduced need for sleep, flight of ideas, grandiosity, poor judgment, aggressiveness, and possible hostility.

Migraine – *Stavzor* is indicated for prophylaxis of migraine headaches. There is no evidence that *Stavzor* is useful in the acute treatment of migraine headaches. Because it may be a hazard to the fetus, *Stavzor* should be considered for women of childbearing potential only after this risk has been thoroughly discussed with the patient and weighed against the potential benefits of treatment.

➤*Off-label uses:*

Bipolar disorder – Current practice guidelines suggest that valproic acid is safe and effective for the treatment of bipolar I disorder, including acute mania, rapid cycling, and maintenance therapy. Further randomized, controlled trials are needed to determine its effectiveness in bipolar II disorder and bipolar depression. Valproic acid should be avoided in pregnant women, and hematologic and liver function tests should be conducted routinely to monitor for severe adverse events.

Bipolar disorder – Depressive episodes (adults): [4] = Insufficient documentation.

Bipolar disorder – Manic or mixed episodes (adults): [1] = Good documentation.

Bipolar disorder – Rapid cycling (adults): [1] = Good documentation.

Borderline personality disorder – [1] = Good documentation. The mainstay of treatment for borderline personality disorder is psychotherapy, but medications may be appropriate for acute exacerbations of disease or long-term management of selected symptoms. Although clinical trial data on the use of valproate for the treatment of borderline personality disorder are limited and it may cause serious adverse effects, it is recommended in national guidelines as a second-line or adjunctive pharmacotherapy for symptoms of either affective dysregulation or impulsive-behavioral control in patients with borderline personality disorder.

Rectal administration – [2] = Fair documentation. Various rectal formulations of valproic acid used in kinetic and clinical settings make it difficult to establish optimal dosing recommendations. This administration route may offer an alternative method of drug delivery in patients who are refractory to current treatment and who are not able to take anticonvulsants orally.

Restless legs syndrome – [3] = Safety concerns. Limited evidence is available regarding valproic acid for the treatment of primary restless legs syndrome. In guidelines, valproic acid has been rated as probably effective, but there is little evidence to support use.

Traumatic brain injury – [3] = Safety concerns. Given that valproic acid has a black box warning and was given the lowest guideline recommendation level (classification as an option rather than a standard or guideline), patients started on therapy should be monitored closely. Valproic acid should be continued only in those patients with sufficient benefit to outweigh the risks of therapy.

In addition to its possible role in managing aggression resulting from traumatic brain injury, valproic acid may also be an appropriate therapy for patients who experience seizures as a result of traumatic brain injury.

Administration and Dosage

➤*Maximum dose:*

Adults – 60 mg/kg/day for the treatment of simple and complex absence seizures and mania according to the prescribing information. There are no well-established maximum doses for the other approved indications according to the prescribing information.

Children – 60 mg/kg/day for the treatment of simple and complex absence seizures according to the prescribing information. There is no well-established maximum dose for the other approved indication according to the prescribing information.

➤*General dosing considerations:* If satisfactory clinical response has not been achieved, plasma levels should be measured to determine whether they are in the usually accepted therapeutic range (50 to 100 mcg/mL).

If the total daily dose exceeds 250 mg, it should be given in divided doses.

➤*Adults:*

Complex partial seizures –

Monotherapy (initial therapy):

• *Initial dosage* – 10 to 15 mg/kg/day.

• *Dosage titration* – The dose should be increased by 5 to 10 mg/kg/week to achieve optimal clinical response. Ordinarily, optimal clinical response is achieved at daily doses less than 60 mg/kg/day.

Conversion to monotherapy: See Monotherapy (initial therapy) for dosing.

• *Initial dosage* – 10 to 15 mg/kg/day.

• *Conversion* – Concomitant antiepilepsy drug (AED) dosage can ordinarily be reduced by approximately 25% every 2 weeks. This reduction may be started at initiation of valproic acid therapy or delayed by 1 to 2 weeks if there is a concern that seizures are likely to occur with a reduction. The speed and duration of withdrawal of the concomitant AED can be highly variable; patients should be monitored closely during this period for increased seizure frequency.

Adjunctive therapy:

• *Initial dosage* – May be added to the patient's regimen at a dose of 10 to 15 mg/kg/day.

• *Dosage titration* – The dose may be increased by 5 to 10 mg/kg/week to achieve optimal clinical response. Ordinarily, optimal clinical response is achieved at daily doses less than 60 mg/kg/day.

Simple and complex absence seizures –

Maximum dose: 60 mg/kg/day.

Initial dosage: 15 mg/kg/day.

VALPROIC ACID — ORAL

Valproic Acid Initial Dose (15 mg/kg/day)					
Weight		Total daily dose	Number of capsules or teaspoonfuls of syrup		
(kg)	(lb)	(mg)	Dose 1	Dose 2	Dose 3
10 to 24.9	22 to 54.9	250	0	0	1
25 to 39.9	55 to 87.9	500	1	0	1
40 to 59.9	88 to 131.9	750	1	1	1
60 to 74.9	132 to 164.9	1,000	1	1	2
75 to 89.9	165 to 197.9	1,250	2	1	2

Dosage titration: Increase at 1-week intervals by 5 to 10 mg/kg/day until seizures are controlled or adverse reactions preclude further increases. If the total daily dose exceeds 250 mg, it should be given in divided doses.

Mania (Stavzor only) – See also Off-label uses.

Maximum dose: 60 mg/kg/day.

Initial dosage: 750 mg daily in divided doses.

Dosage titration: The dose should be increased as rapidly as possible to achieve the lowest therapeutic dose which produces the desired clinical effect or the desired range of plasma concentrations. In placebo-controlled clinical trials of acute mania, patients were dosed to a clinical response with a trough plasma concentration between 50 and 125 mcg/mL. Maximum concentrations were generally achieved within 14 days.

Duration of therapy:

Although there are no efficacy data that specifically address longer-term antimanic treatment with *Stavzor*, the safety of *Stavzor* in long-term use is supported by data from record reviews involving approximately 360 patients treated with valproate for more than 3 months.

Migraine (Stavzor only) – Starting dosage is 250 mg twice daily. Some patients may benefit from doses of up to 1,000 mg/day.

Off-label dosing –

Bipolar disorder – Manic or mixed episodes: [1] = Good documentation. The starting dosage of valproic acid for adult outpatients was 250 mg 3 times daily, increased by 250 to 500 mg every few days or as tolerated. The target serum concentration was 50 to 125 mcg/mL. Some studies have shown efficacy and tolerability with a higher starting dosage of 20 to 30 mg/kg/day in adult inpatients. Doses should be titrated downward until the target serum concentration is reached.

Serum valproate levels should be measured at steady state (3 to 5 days after initiation and subsequent dose changes) approximately 12 hours after the last dose to determine the trough point. After 2 consecutive therapeutic levels, subsequent monitoring can take place every 3 to 6 months unless dosing changes are needed.

Bipolar disorder – Rapid cycling: [1] = Good documentation. See Bipolar disorder – Manic or mixed episodes for dosing information.

Borderline personality disorder: [1] = Good documentation. 750 mg/day orally in divided doses, titrated to maintain a therapeutic plasma level of 50 to 100 mcg/mL. Pharmacotherapy may be limited to short-term treatment during periods of acute decompensation or may be continued indefinitely for long-term treatment of trait vulnerabilities.

Rectal administration: [2] = Fair documentation. Valproic acid has been administered rectally as either a suppository or retention enema, 250 mg every 8 hours, increased to 500 mg every 6 hours over a 36-hour period (1 case report).

Restless legs syndrome: [3] = Safety concerns. Oral doses of slow-release valproic acid 300 to 600 mg administered 90 minutes before bedtime for 3 weeks. Guidelines recommend oral dosages of slow-release valproic acid 600 mg/day.

Traumatic brain injury: [3] = Safety concerns. 750 to 2,250 mg daily orally, titrated to achieve therapeutic serum levels.

➤*Children:*

Complex partial seizures – See Adults for dosing for children 10 years of age and older.

Simple and complex absence seizures – See Adults for dosing.

Off-label dosing –

Migraine prophylaxis: 15 to 30 mg/kg/day orally administered in divided doses twice daily.

Rectal administration: [2] = Fair documentation. Valproic acid has been administered rectally as either a suppository or retention enema.

Rectal valproic acid was dosed at 150 mg (children less than 10 kg) and 300 mg (children more than 10 kg) every 12 hours for febrile seizures with follow-up to 1 year. In pediatric intensive care unit patients, a rectal loading dose of 10 to 20 mg/kg was used, followed 8 hours later by 10 to 15 mg/kg every 8 hours for 1 to 8 days. In case reports, single doses were 12 and 20 mg/kg in a neonate 14 days of age and an infant 5 months of age, respectively.

➤*Elderly:* Because of a decrease in unbound clearance of valproate and possibly a greater sensitivity to somnolence in elderly patients, the starting dose should be reduced in these patients. Dosage should be increased more slowly and with regular monitoring for fluid and nutritional intake, dehydration, somnolence, and other adverse reactions. Dose reductions or discontinuation of valproate should be considered in patients with decreased food or fluid intake and in patients with excessive somnolence. The ultimate therapeutic dose should be achieved on the basis of both tolerability and clinical response.

➤*Dose-related adverse reactions:* The frequency of adverse reactions (particularly elevated liver enzymes and thrombocytopenia) may be dose related. The probability of thrombocytopenia increases significantly at total trough valproate plasma concentrations above 110 mcg/mL in women and 135 mcg/mL in men. The benefit of improved seizure control with higher doses should be weighed against the possibility of a greater incidence of adverse reactions.

➤*Therapeutic drug monitoring:* The therapeutic range is commonly considered to be 50 to 100 mcg/mL of total valproate, although some patients may be controlled with lower or higher plasma concentrations.

➤*Discontinuation of therapy:* AEDs should not be abruptly discontinued in patients in whom the drug is administered to prevent major seizures because of the strong possibility of precipitating status epilepticus with attendant hypoxia and threat to life.

➤*Administration:* The capsules should be swallowed without chewing to avoid local irritation of the mouth and throat. Patients who experience GI irritation may benefit from administration of the drug with food or by slowly building up the dose from an initial low level.

➤*Storage / Stability:* Store capsules at 15° to 25°C (59° to 77°F). Store oral solution below 30°C (86°F).

Stavzor – Store at 25°C (77°F). Excursions are permitted between 15° and 30°C (59° and 86° F).

Actions

➤*Pharmacology:* Valproic acid is a carboxylic acid antiepileptic. The mechanisms by which valproate exerts its antiepileptic effects have not been established. It has been suggested that its activity in epilepsy is related to increased brain concentrations of gamma-aminobutyric acid (GABA).

➤*Pharmacokinetics:*

Absorption – Valproic acid dissociates to the valproate ion in the GI tract. Equivalent oral doses of divalproex products and valproic acid products deliver equivalent quantities of valproate ion systemically. Although the rate of valproate ion absorption may vary with the formulation administered (liquid, solid, or sprinkle), conditions of use (eg, fasting, postprandial), and the method of administration (ie, whether the contents of the capsule are sprinkled on food or the capsule is taken intact), these differences should be of minor clinical importance under the steady-state conditions achieved in chronic use in the treatment of epilepsy.

However, it is possible that differences among the various valproate products in time to maximal concentration (T_{max}) and maximal drug concentration (C_{max}) could be important upon initiation of treatment. For example, in single-dose studies, the effect of feeding had a greater influence on the rate of absorption of the divalproex tablet (increase in T_{max} from 4 to 8 hours) than on the absorption of the divalproex sprinkle capsules (increase in T_{max} from 3.3 to 4.8 hours).

While the absorption rate from the GI tract and fluctuation in valproate plasma concentrations vary with dosing regimen and formulation, the efficacy of valproate as an anticonvulsant in chronic use is unlikely to be affected. Experience employing dosing regimens from once a day to 4 times a day, as well as studies in primate epilepsy models involving constant rate infusion, indicate that total daily systemic bioavailability (extent of absorption) is the primary determinant of seizure control and that differences in the ratios of plasma peak to trough concentrations between valproate formulations are inconsequential from a practical clinical standpoint.

Distribution – The plasma protein binding of valproate is concentration dependent, and the free fraction increases from approximately 10% at 40 mcg/mL to 18.5% at 130 mcg/mL. Protein binding of valproate is reduced in elderly patients, in patients with chronic hepatic diseases, in patients with renal function impairment, and in the presence of other drugs (eg, aspirin). Conversely, valproate may displace certain protein-bound drugs (eg, carbamazepine, phenytoin, tolbutamide, warfarin).

Valproate concentrations in cerebrospinal fluid (CSF) approximate unbound concentrations in plasma (about 10% of total concentration). Mean volume of distribution for total valproate is 11 L per 1.73 m^2. Mean volume of distribution for free valproic acid is 92 L per 1.73 m^2.

The relationship between plasma concentration and clinical response is not well documented. One contributing factor is the nonlinear, concentration dependent protein binding of valproate, which affects the clearance of the drug. Thus, monitoring of total serum valproate cannot provide a reliable index of the bioactive valproate species.

For example, because the plasma protein binding of valproate is concentration dependent, the free fraction increases from approximately 10% at 40 mcg/mL to 18.5% at 130 mcg/mL. Higher than expected free fractions occur in elderly patients, in hyperlipidemic patients, and in patients with hepatic and renal function impairment.

Metabolism – Valproate is metabolized almost entirely by the liver. In adult patients on monotherapy, 30% to 50% of an administered dose appears in urine as a glucuronide conjugate. Mitochondrial beta-oxidation is the other major metabolic pathway, typically accounting for more than 40% of the dose. Usually, less than 15% to 20% of the dose is eliminated by other oxidative mechanisms.

The relationship between dose and total valproate concentration is nonlinear; concentration does not increase proportionally with the dose but rather increases to a lesser extent because of saturable plasma protein binding. The kinetics of unbound drug are linear.

Excretion – Less than 3% of an administered dose is excreted unchanged in urine. Mean plasma clearance for total valproate is 0.56 L/h per 1.73 m^2. Mean plasma clearance for free valproate is 4.6 L/h per 1.73 m^2. Mean terminal half-life for valproate monotherapy ranged from 9 to 16 hours following oral dosing regimens of 250 to 1,000 mg.

VALPROIC ACID — ORAL

The estimates cited apply primarily to patients who are not taking drugs that affect hepatic metabolizing enzyme systems. For example, patients taking enzyme-inducing AEDs (eg, carbamazepine, phenobarbital, phenytoin) will clear valproate more rapidly. Because of these changes in valproate clearance, intensify monitoring of antiepileptic concentrations whenever concomitant antiepileptics are introduced or withdrawn.

Special populations –

Renal function impairment: A slight reduction (27%) in the unbound clearance of valproate has been reported in patients with renal failure (creatinine clearance [CrCl] less than 10 mL/min); however, hemodialysis typically reduces valproate concentrations by about 20%. Therefore, no dosage adjustment appears to be necessary in patients with renal failure. Protein binding in these patients is substantially reduced; thus, monitoring total concentrations may be misleading.

Hepatic function impairment: Liver disease impairs the capacity to eliminate valproate. In 1 study, the clearance of free valproate was decreased 50% in 7 patients with cirrhosis and 16% in 4 patients with acute hepatitis, compared with 6 healthy subjects. In that study, the half-life of valproate was increased from 12 to 18 hours. Liver disease is also associated with decreased albumin concentrations and larger unbound fractions (2- to 2.6-fold increase) of valproate. Accordingly, monitoring of total concentrations may be misleading because free concentrations may be substantially elevated in patients with hepatic disease, whereas total concentrations may appear to be normal.

Elderly: The capacity of elderly patients (range, 68 to 89 years of age) to eliminate valproate has been shown to be reduced, compared with younger adults (range, 22 to 26 years of age). Intrinsic clearance is reduced by 39%; the free fraction is increased by 44%. Accordingly, reduce the initial dosage in elderly patients.

Children: Children within the first 2 months of life have a markedly decreased ability to eliminate valproate, compared with older children and adults. This is a result of reduced clearance (perhaps due to a delay in development of glucuronosyltransferase and other enzyme systems involved in valproate elimination) as well as increased volume of distribution (in part due to decreased plasma protein binding). For example, in one study, the half-life in children younger than 10 days of age ranged from 10 to 67 hours, compared with a range of 7 to 13 hours in children older than 2 months of age.

Children (ie, between 3 months and 10 years of age) have 50% higher clearances expressed on weight (ie, mL/min/kg) than adults. Older than 10 years of age, children have pharmacokinetic parameters that approximate those of adults.

Contraindications

Hepatic disease or significant hepatic function impairment; hypersensitivity to the drug; known urea cycle disorders.

Warnings/Precautions

➤*Hepatotoxicity:* See the Warning box for more information.

Observe caution when administering valproic acid to patients with a history of hepatic disease. Patients of multiple anticonvulsants, children, those with congenital metabolic disorders, those with severe seizure disorders accompanied by mental retardation, and those with organic brain disease may be at particular risk. Experience has indicated that children younger than 2 years of age are at a considerably increased risk of developing fatal hepatotoxicity, especially those with the aforementioned conditions. When valproic acid products are used in this patient group, use them with extreme caution and as a sole agent. Weigh the benefits of therapy against the risks. Above this age group, experience has indicated that the incidence of fatal hepatotoxicity decreases considerably in progressively older patient groups. Immediately discontinue the drug in the presence of significant hepatic function impairment, suspected or apparent. In some cases, hepatic function impairment has progressed in spite of discontinuation of the drug.

➤*Pancreatitis:* See the Warning box for more information.

➤*Urea cycle disorders:* Valproic acid is contraindicated in patients with known urea cycle disorders.

Hyperammonemic encephalopathy, sometimes fatal, has been reported following initiation of valproate therapy in patients with urea cycle disorders, a group of uncommon genetic abnormalities, particularly ornithine transcarbamylase deficiency. Prior to the initiation of valproate therapy, consider evaluation for urea cycle disorders in the following patients: 1) those with a history of unexplained encephalopathy or coma, encephalopathy associated with a protein load, pregnancy-related or postpartum encephalopathy, unexplained mental retardation, or history of elevated plasma ammonia or glutamine; 2) those with ataxia, cyclical vomiting and lethargy, episodic extreme irritability, low blood urea nitrogen (BUN), or protein avoidance; 3) those with a family history of urea cycle disorders or a family history of unexplained infant deaths (particularly men); 4) those with other signs or symptoms of urea cycle disorders. Give prompt treatment to patients who develop symptoms of unexplained hyperammonemic encephalopathy while receiving valproate (including discontinuation of valproate therapy) and evaluate them for underlying urea cycle disorders.

Hyperammonemia – Hyperammonemia has been reported in association with valproate therapy and may be present despite healthy liver function tests. In patients who develop unexplained lethargy and vomiting or changes in mental status, consider hyperammonemic encephalopathy and measure an ammonia level. If ammonia is increased, discontinue valproate therapy. Initiate appropriate interventions for treatment of hyperammonemia; evaluate such patients for underlying urea cycle disorders.

Asymptomatic elevations of ammonia are more common, and, when present, require close monitoring of plasma ammonia levels. If the elevation persists, consider discontinuation of valproate therapy.

Hyperammonemia and encephalopathy associated with concomitant topiramate use – Coadministration of topiramate and valproic acid has been associated with hyperammonemia with or without encephalopathy in patients who have tolerated either drug alone. Clinical symptoms of hyperammonemic encephalopathy often include acute alterations in level of consciousness and/or cognitive function with lethargy or vomiting. In most cases, symptoms and signs abated with discontinuation of either drug. This adverse reaction is not due to a pharmacokinetic interaction. It is not known if topiramate monotherapy is associated with hyperammonemia. Patients with inborn errors of metabolism or reduced hepatic mitochondrial activity may be at an increased risk for hyperammonemia with or without encephalopathy. Although not studied, an interaction of topiramate and valproic acid may exacerbate existing defects or unmask deficiencies in susceptible persons. In patients who develop unexplained lethargy, vomiting, or changes in mental status, consider hyperammonemic encephalopathy and measure an ammonia level.

➤*Thrombocytopenia:* The frequency of adverse reactions (particularly elevated liver enzymes and thrombocytopenia) may be dose related. In a clinical trial of divalproex as monotherapy in patients with epilepsy, 34/126 (27%) patients receiving approximately 50 mg/kg/day on average had at least 1 value of platelets 75×10^9/L or less. Approximately half of these patients had treatment discontinued, with return of platelet counts to normal. In the remaining patients, platelet counts normalized with continued treatment. In this study, the probability of thrombocytopenia appeared to increase significantly at total valproate concentrations of 110 mcg/mL or more (women) or 135 mcg/mL or more (men). Weigh the therapeutic benefit, which may accompany the higher doses, against the possibility of a greater incidence of adverse reactions.

Because of reports of thrombocytopenia, inhibition of the secondary phase of platelet aggregation, and abnormal coagulation parameters (eg, low fibrinogen), platelet counts and coagulation tests are recommended before initiating therapy and at periodic intervals. It is recommended that patients receiving valproic acid be monitored for platelet count and coagulation parameters prior to planned surgery. Evidence of hemorrhage, bruising, or a disorder of hemostasis/coagulation is an indication for reduction of the dosage or withdrawal of therapy.

➤*Multiorgan hypersensitivity reaction:* Multiorgan hypersensitivity reactions have been rarely reported in close temporal association to the initiation of valproate therapy in adults and children (median time to detection, 21 days; range, 1 to 40 days). Although there have been a limited number of reports, many of these cases resulted in hospitalization and at least 1 death has been reported. Signs and symptoms of this disorder were diverse; however, patients typically, although not exclusively, presented with fever and rash associated with other organ system involvement. Other associated manifestations may include arthralgia, asthenia, hematological abnormalities (eg, eosinophilia, neutropenia, thrombocytopenia), hepatitis, hepatorenal syndrome, liver function test abnormalities, lymphadenopathy, nephritis, oliguria, or pruritus. Because the disorder is variable in its expression, other organ system symptoms and signs, not noted here, may occur. If this reaction is suspected, discontinue valproate and start an alternative treatment. Although the existence of cross-sensitivity with other drugs that produce this syndrome is unclear, the experience among drugs associated with multiorgan hypersensitivity would indicate this to be a possibility.

➤*HIV:* There are in vitro studies that suggest valproate stimulates the replication of the HIV and cytomegalovirus (CMV) under certain experimental conditions. The clinical consequence, if any, is not known. Additionally, the relevance of these in vitro findings is uncertain for patients receiving maximally suppressive antiretroviral therapy. Nevertheless, these data should be borne in mind when interpreting the results from regular monitoring of the viral load in HIV-infected patients receiving valproate, or when following CMV-infected patients clinically.

➤*Hepatic function impairment:* Observe caution when administering valproic acid to patients with a history of hepatic function impairment. Patients on multiple anticonvulsants, children, those with congenital metabolic disorders, those with severe disorders accompanied by mental retardation, and those with organic brain disease may be at particular risk.

Discontinue the drug immediately in the presence of significant hepatic function impairment, suspected or apparent. In some cases, hepatic function impairment has progressed in spite of discontinuation of drug.

➤*Hazardous tasks:* Because valproic acid products may produce CNS depression, especially when combined with another CNS depressant (eg, alcohol), advise patients not to engage in hazardous activities, such as driving an automobile or operating dangerous machinery, until it is known that they do not become drowsy from the drug.

➤*Pregnancy: Category D.* According to the American Academy of Neurology and the American Epilepsy Society, valproic acid should be avoided if possible during pregnancy, especially during the first trimester. Valproic acid has been associated with major congenital malformations (eg, neural tube defects, facial clefts) in the offspring of women with epilepsy taking valproic acid monotherapy or as part of polytherapy. Valproic acid has also been associated with an increased risk of impaired cognitive function in children at 3 years of age. If possible, switch patients from valproic acid to a less teratogenic antiepileptic drug well before pregnancy. If a patient is already several weeks into her pregnancy, switching to another AED will not avoid the risk of major congenital malformations, since these effects occur very early in the pregnancy. A patient should consult her physician before stopping valproic acid since stopping an antiepileptic drug could lead to seizures and other serious consequences.

Teratogenic – Valproate can produce teratogenic effects. Data suggest that there is an increased incidence of congenital malformations associated with the use of valproate by women with seizure disorders during pregnancy when compared with the incidence in women with seizure disorders who do

VALPROIC ACID — ORAL

not use AEDs during pregnancy, the incidence in women with seizure disorders who use other AEDs, and the background incidence for the general population. Therefore, consider valproate for women of childbearing potential only after the risks have been thoroughly discussed with the patient and weighed against the potential benefits of treatment.

There are multiple reports in the clinical literature that indicate that the use of AEDs during pregnancy results in an increased incidence of congenital malformations in the offspring. Therefore, administer AEDs, including valproate, to women of childbearing potential only if they are clearly shown to be essential in the management of their seizures.

Do not discontinue AEDs abruptly in patients in whom the drug is administered to prevent major seizures because of the strong possibility of precipitating status epilepticus with attendant hypoxia and threat to life. In individual cases in which the severity and frequency of the seizure disorder are such that the removal of medication does not pose a serious threat to the patient, discontinuation of the drug may be considered prior to and during pregnancy, although it cannot be said with any confidence that even minor seizures do not pose some hazard to the developing embryo or fetus.

Congenital malformations – The North American Antiepileptic Drug Pregnancy Registry reported 16 cases of congenital malformations among the offspring of 149 women with epilepsy who were exposed to valproic acid monotherapy during the first trimester of pregnancy at doses of approximately 1,000 mg/day, for a prevalence rate of 10.7% (95% confidence interval [CI], 6.3% to 16.9%). Three (2%) of the 149 offspring had neural tube defects and 6 (4%) of the 149 had less severe malformations. Among epileptic women who were exposed to other AED monotherapies during pregnancy (1,048 patients), the malformation rate was 2.9% (95% CI, 2% to 4.1%). There was a 4-fold increase in congenital malformations among infants with valproic acid–exposed mothers, compared with those treated with other antiepileptic monotherapies as a group (odds ratio, 4; 95% CI, 2.1% to 7.4%). This increased risk does not reflect a comparison versus any specific AED, but the risk versus the heterogeneous group of all other AED monotherapies combined. The increased teratogenic risk from valproic acid in women with epilepsy is expected to be reflected in an increased risk in other indications (eg, migraine, bipolar disorder).

The strongest association of maternal valproate usage with congenital malformations is with neural tube defects. However, other congenital anomalies (eg, anomalies involving various body systems, cardiovascular malformations, craniofacial defects), compatible and incompatible with life, have been reported. Sufficient data to determine the incidence of these congenital anomalies is not available.

Neural tube defects – The incidence of neural tube defects in the fetus is increased in mothers receiving valproate during the first trimester of pregnancy. The Centers for Disease Control (CDC) has estimated the risk of valproic acid–exposed women having children with spina bifida to be approximately 1% to 2%. The American College of Obstetricians and Gynecologists estimates the general population risk for congenital neural tube defects as 0.14% to 0.2%.

Consider tests to detect neural tube and other defects using current accepted procedures a part of routine prenatal care in childbearing women receiving valproate.

Evidence suggests that pregnant women who receive folic acid supplementation may be at a decreased risk for congenital neural tube defects in their offspring, compared with pregnant women not receiving folic acid. Whether the risk of neural tube defects in the offspring of women receiving valproate specifically is reduced by folic acid supplementation is unknown. Routinely recommend dietary folic acid supplementation prior to and during pregnancy to patients contemplating pregnancy.

Other adverse pregnancy reactions – Patients taking valproate may develop clotting abnormalities. A patient who had low fibrinogen when taking multiple anticonvulsants, including valproate, gave birth to an infant with afibrinogenemia who subsequently died of hemorrhage. If valproate is used in pregnancy, carefully monitor the clotting parameters.

Patients taking valproate may develop hepatic failure. Hepatic failure, resulting in the death of a newborn and of an infant, has been reported following the use of valproate during pregnancy.

➤*Lactation:* Valproate is excreted in breast milk. Concentrations in breast milk have been reported to be 1% to 10% of serum concentrations. It is not known what effect this would have on a breast-feeding infant. Consider discontinuing breast-feeding when valproic acid is administered to a breast-feeding woman.

➤*Children:* Experience has indicated that children younger than 2 years of age are at a considerably increased risk of developing fatal hepatotoxicity, especially those on multiple anticonvulsants, those with congenital metabolic disorders, those with severe seizure disorders accompanied by mental retardation, and those with organic brain disease. When valproic acid is used in this patient group, use it with extreme caution and as a sole agent. Weigh the benefits of therapy against the risks. Older than 2 years of age, experience in epilepsy has indicated that the incidence of fatal hepatotoxicity decreases considerably in progressively older patient groups.

Younger children, especially those receiving enzyme-inducing drugs, will require larger maintenance doses to attain targeted total and unbound valproic acid concentrations.

The variability in free fraction limits the clinical usefulness of monitoring total serum valproic acid concentrations. Interpretation of valproic acid concentrations in children should include consideration of factors that affect hepatic metabolism and protein binding.

➤*Elderly:* No patients older than 65 years of age were enrolled in double-blind prospective clinical trials of mania associated with bipolar illness. In a case-review study of 583 patients, 72 (12%) patients were older than 65 years of age. A higher percentage of patients older than 65 years of age reported accidental injury, infection, pain, somnolence, and tremor. Discontinuation of valproate was occasionally associated with the latter 2 reactions. It is not clear whether these reactions indicate additional risk or whether they result from preexisting medical illness and concomitant medication use among these patients.

In a double-blind, multicenter trial of valproate in elderly patients with dementia (mean age, 83 years), doses were increased by 125 mg/day to a target dose of 20 mg/kg/day. A significantly higher proportion of valproate patients had somnolence compared with placebo, and although not statistically significant, there was a higher proportion of patients with dehydration. Discontinuations for somnolence were also significantly higher than with placebo. In some patients with somnolence (approximately one-half), there was associated reduced nutritional intake and weight loss. There was a trend for the patients who experienced these reactions to have a lower baseline albumin concentration, lower valproate clearance, and a higher BUN. In elderly patients, increase dosage more slowly and with regular monitoring for fluid and nutritional intake, dehydration, somnolence, and other adverse reactions. Consider dose reductions or discontinuation of valproate in patients with decreased food or fluid intake and in patients with excessive somnolence.

➤*Monitoring:* Perform liver function tests prior to therapy and at frequent intervals thereafter, especially during the first 6 months. However, do not rely totally on serum biochemistry because these tests may not be abnormal in all instances; also consider the results of careful interim medical history and physical examination.

Because valproate may interact with coadministered drugs that are capable of enzyme induction, periodic plasma concentration determinations of valproate and concomitant drugs are recommended during the early course of therapy.

Platelet counts and coagulation tests are recommended before initiating therapy and at periodic intervals thereafter.

Any changes in dosage administration, or the addition or discontinuance of concomitant drugs should ordinarily be accompanied by close monitoring of clinical status and valproate plasma concentrations.

Asymptomatic elevations of ammonia are more common, and, when present, require close monitoring of plasma ammonia levels. If the elevation persists, consider discontinuation of valproate therapy.

In patients who develop unexplained lethargy, vomiting, or changes in mental status, consider hyperammonemic encephalopathy and measure an ammonia level.

Drug Interactions

Valproic Acid Drug Interactions

Precipitant drug	Object drug[a]		Description
Carbapenem antibiotics (eg, meropenem)	Valproic acid	↓	Subtherapeutic valproic acid levels have been reported with coadministration.
Chlorpromazine	Valproic acid	↑	Valproate elimination half-life and trough levels may increase; clearance may decrease.
Cholestyramine	Valproic acid	↓	Serum concentrations and bioavailability of valproic acid may be reduced, resulting in a decrease in therapeutic effects. Administer valproic acid at least 3 hours before, but not within 3 hours following cholestyramine.
Felbamate	Valproic acid	↑	Coadministration revealed a 35% increase in mean peak valproate levels.
Rifampin	Valproic acid	↓	In one study, rifampin increased the oral clearance of valproate by 40%.
Salicylates (eg, aspirin)	Valproic acid	↑	Salicylates may displace valproic acid from protein binding sites and may inhibit metabolism of valproate. Monitor serum concentrations.
Valproic acid	Barbiturates (eg, phenobarbital, primidone)	↑	Valproic acid may decrease hepatic metabolism of barbiturates. Barbiturate dosage may need to be decreased in some patients. Phenobarbital or primidone can double the clearance of valproate.
Barbiturates (eg, phenobarbital, primidone)	Valproic acid	↓	
Valproic acid	Benzodiazepines (eg, clonazepam, diazepam, lorazepam)	↑	Valproate displaces benzodiazepines from their plasma albumin binding sites and inhibits their metabolism, resulting in increased CNS depression. Concomitant use with clonazepam may induce absence status in patients with a history of absence seizures.

VALPROIC ACID — ORAL

Valproic Acid Drug Interactions			
Precipitant drug	Object drug[a]		Description
Valproic acid	Carbamazepine	↑	Variable changes in carbamazepine concentrations with increased levels of the active metabolite; carbamazepine may decrease valproic acid levels, and possible loss of seizure control may occur.
Carbamazepine	Valproic acid	↓	
Valproic acid	Ethosuximide	↑↓	Increases and decreases in ethosuximide blood levels and decreases in valproic acid levels have been reported. Valproic acid appears to inhibit the metabolism of ethosuximide.
Ethosuximide	Valproic acid	↓	
Valproic acid	Hydantoins (eg, phenytoin)	↑	Increased action of phenytoin, even at therapeutic levels; increased metabolism of valproic acid with decreased pharmacologic effects may occur. Monitor the levels of the free concentrations of hydantoin and serum valproic acid.
Hydantoins (eg, phenytoin)	Valproic acid	↓	
Valproic acid	Lamotrigine	↑	Serum valproic acid concentrations may be decreased while lamotrigine levels increase. In one study, coadministration increased the half-life of lamotrigine from 26 to 70 hours. Reduce lamotrigine dose.
Lamotrigine	Valproic acid	↓	
Valproic acid	Tolbutamide	↔	The unbound fraction of tolbutamide may be increased from 20% to 50%. The clinical relevance of this displacement is unknown.
Valproic acid	Topiramate	↓	Possible increased metabolism of both agents. Coadministration has been associated with hyperammonemia with and without encephalopathy.
Topiramate	Valproic acid		
Valproic acid	Tricyclic antidepressants (eg, amitriptyline, nortriptyline)	↑	Plasma concentrations and adverse reactions of the tricyclic antidepressant may be increased. Coadministration resulted in a 21% decrease in the plasma clearance of amitriptyline and a 34% decrease in the net clearance of nortriptyline.
Valproic acid	Warfarin	↑	The potential exists for valproate to displace warfarin from protein binding sites. Monitor coagulation tests.
Valproic acid	Zidovudine	↑	Zidovudine clearance was decreased by 38% in 6 HIV-seropositive patients.

[a] ↑ = object drug increased; ↓ = object drug decreased; ↔ = undetermined clinical effect.

➤*Drug/Lab test interactions:* Valproate is partially eliminated in the urine as a keto-metabolite, which may lead to a false interpretation of the urine ketone test.

There have been reports of altered thyroid function tests associated with valproate. The clinical significance of these is unknown.

Adverse Reactions

➤*Epilepsy:* The data described in the following section were obtained using divalproex tablets.

Adjunctive therapy for complex partial seizures – Based on a placebo-controlled trial of adjunctive therapy for treatment of complex partial seizures, divalproex was generally well tolerated with most adverse reactions rated as mild to moderate in severity. Intolerance was the primary reason for discontinuation in the divalproex-treated patients (6%), compared with 1% of placebo-treated patients.

The following table lists treatment-emergent adverse reactions that were reported by 5% or more of divalproex-treated patients and for which the incidence was greater than in the placebo group in a placebo-controlled trial of adjunctive therapy for the treatment of complex partial seizures. Because patients were also treated with other AEDs, it is not possible, in most cases, to determine whether the following adverse reactions can be ascribed to divalproex alone, or the combination of divalproex and other AEDs.

Divalproex Adverse Reactions (≥ 5%) in Adjunctive Therapy for Complex Partial Seizures		
Adverse reaction	Divalproex (n = 77)	Placebo (n = 70)
CNS		
Abnormal thinking	6%	0%
Amnesia	5%	1%
Asthenia	27%	7%
Ataxia	8%	1%
Dizziness	25%	13%
Emotional lability	6%	4%
Headache	31%	21%
Somnolence	27%	11%
Tremor	25%	6%
GI		
Abdominal pain	23%	6%
Anorexia	12%	0%
Constipation	5%	1%
Diarrhea	13%	6%
Dyspepsia	8%	4%
Nausea	48%	14%
Vomiting	27%	7%
Respiratory		
Bronchitis	5%	1%
Flu syndrome	12%	9%
Infection	12%	6%
Rhinitis	5%	4%
Special senses		
Amblyopia/Blurred vision	12%	9%
Diplopia	16%	9%
Nystagmus	8%	1%
Miscellaneous		
Alopecia	6%	1%
Fever	6%	4%
Weight loss	6%	0%

High-dose monotherapy for complex partial seizures – The following table lists treatment-emergent adverse reactions that were reported by 5% or more of patients in the high-dose divalproex group and for which the incidence was greater than in the low-dose group in a controlled trial of divalproex monotherapy treatment of complex partial seizures. Because patients were being titrated off another AED during the first portion of the trial, it is not possible, in many cases, to determine whether the following adverse reactions can be ascribed to divalproex alone, or the combination of divalproex and other AEDs.

Divalproex Adverse Reactions (≥ 5%) in the High-Dose Monotherapy for Complex Partial Seizures[a]		
Adverse reaction	High-dose (n = 131)	Low-dose (n = 134)
CNS		
Amnesia	7%	4%
Asthenia	21%	10%
Depression	5%	4%
Dizziness	18%	13%
Insomnia	15%	9%
Nervousness	11%	7%
Somnolence	30%	18%
Tremor	57%	19%
GI		
Abdominal pain	12%	9%
Anorexia	11%	4%
Diarrhea	23%	19%
Dyspepsia	11%	10%
Nausea	34%	26%
Vomiting	23%	15%
Hematologic/Lymphatic		
Ecchymosis	5%	4%
Thrombocytopenia	24%	1%

VALPROIC ACID — ORAL

Divalproex Adverse Reactions (≥ 5%) in the High-Dose Monotherapy for Complex Partial Seizures[a]		
Adverse reaction	High-dose (n = 131)	Low-dose (n = 134)
Metabolic/Nutritional		
Peripheral edema	8%	3%
Weight gain	9%	4%
Respiratory		
Dyspnea	5%	1%
Infection	20%	13%
Pharyngitis	8%	2%
Special senses		
Amblyopia/Blurred vision	8%	4%
Nystagmus	7%	1%
Tinnitus	7%	1%
Miscellaneous		
Alopecia	24%	13%

[a] Headache was the only adverse reaction that occurred in 5% or more of patients in the high-dose group and at an equal or greater incidence in the low-dose group.

➤*Complex partial seizures (more than 1% to less than 5%):*

Cardiovascular – Hypertension, palpitation, tachycardia.

CNS – Abnormal dreams, abnormal gait, anxiety, confusion, hypertonia, incoordination, paresthesia, personality disorder.

Dermatologic – Dry skin, pruritus, rash.

GI – Eructation, flatulence, hematemesis, increased appetite, pancreatitis, periodontal abscess.

GU – Amenorrhea, dysmenorrhea, urinary frequency, urinary incontinence, vaginitis.

Hematologic / Lymphatic – Petechia.

Hepatic – ALT increased, AST increased.

Musculoskeletal – Arthralgia, leg cramps, myalgia, myasthenia, twitching.

Respiratory – Cough increased, pneumonia, sinusitis.

Special senses – Abnormal vision, deafness, epistaxis, otitis media, taste perversion.

Miscellaneous – Back pain, chest pain, malaise.

➤*Mania:* Although valproic acid has not been evaluated for safety and efficacy in the treatment of manic episodes associated with bipolar disorder, the following adverse reactions not previously listed were reported by 1% or more of patients from 2 placebo-controlled clinical trials of divalproex tablets.

Cardiovascular – Hypotension, postural hypotension, vasodilation.

CNS – Agitation, catatonic reaction, hypokinesia, reflexes increased, tardive dyskinesia, vertigo.

Dermatologic – Furunculosis, maculopapular rash, seborrhea.

GI – Fecal incontinence, gastroenteritis, glossitis.

GU – Dysuria.

Musculoskeletal – Arthrosis, neck pain, neck rigidity.

Special senses – Conjunctivitis, dry eyes, eye pain.

Miscellaneous – Chills.

➤*Migraine:* Although valproic acid has not been evaluated for safety and efficacy in the treatment of prophylaxis of migraine headaches, the following adverse reactions not previously listed were reported by 1% or more of patients from 2 placebo-controlled clinical trials of divalproex tablets.

GI – Dry mouth, stomatitis.

GU – Cystitis, metrorrhagia, vaginal hemorrhage.

Miscellaneous – Facial edema.

➤*Other adverse reactions (all dosage forms):* Adverse reactions that have been reported with all dosage forms of valproate from epilepsy trials, spontaneous reports, and other sources are listed by body system.

CNS – Aggression, behavioral deterioration, depression, emotional upset, hostility, hyperactivity, psychosis.

Sedative effects have occurred in patients receiving valproate alone but occur most often in patients receiving combination therapy. Sedation usually abates upon reduction of other antiepileptic medication. Asterixis, ataxia, confusion, diplopia, dizziness, dysarthria, hallucinations, headache, hypesthesia, incoordination, nystagmus, parkinsonism, "spots before eyes," tremor (may be dose related), and vertigo have been reported with the use of valproate. Rare cases of coma have occurred in patients receiving valproic acid alone or in conjunction with phenobarbital. In rare instances, encephalopathy with or without fever has developed shortly after the introduction of valproate monotherapy without evidence of hepatic function impairment or inappropriately high plasma valproate levels. Although recovery has been described following drug withdrawal, there have been fatalities in patients with hyperammonemic encephalopathy, particularly in patients with underlying urea cycle disorders.

Several reports have noted reversible cerebral atrophy and dementia in association with valproate therapy.

Dermatologic – Erythema multiforme, generalized pruritus, photosensitivity, skin rash, Stevens-Johnson syndrome, transient hair loss. Rare cases of toxic epidermal necrolysis have been reported, including a fatal case in a 6-month-old infant taking valproate and several other concomitant medications. An additional case of toxic epidermal necrosis resulting in death was reported in a 35-year-old patient with AIDS taking several concomitant medications and with a history of multiple cutaneous drug reactions. Serious skin reactions have been reported with coadministration of lamotrigine and valproate.

Endocrine – Breast enlargement, galactorrhea, irregular menses, abnormal thyroid function tests, secondary amenorrhea, andparotid gland swelling.

There have been rare spontaneous reports of polycystic ovary disease. A cause-and-effect relationship has not been established.

GI – The most commonly reported adverse reactions at the initiation of therapy are indigestion, nausea, and vomiting. These reactions are usually transient and rarely require discontinuation of therapy. Abdominal cramps, constipation, and diarrhea have been reported. Both anorexia with some weight loss and increased appetite with weight gain have also been reported. The administration of delayed-release divalproex may result in reduction of GI adverse reactions in some patients.

Acute pancreatitis, including fatalities.

GU – Enuresis, urinary tract infection.

Hematologic – Thrombocytopenia and inhibition of the secondary phase of platelet aggregation may be reflected in altered bleeding time, bruising, epistaxis, frank hemorrhage, hematoma formation, and petechiae. Relative acute intermittent porphyria, anemia (including macrocytic, with or without folate deficiency), aplastic anemia, bone marrow suppression, eosinophilia, hypofibrinogenemia, leukopenia, lymphocytosis, macrocytosis, and pancytopenia.

Hepatic – Minor elevations of transaminases (eg, ALT, AST) and lactate dehydrogenase are frequent and appear to be dose related. Occasionally, laboratory test results include increases in serum bilirubin and abnormal changes in other liver function tests. These results may reflect potentially serious hepatotoxicity.

Metabolic – Hyperammonemia, hyponatremia, inappropriate antidiuretic hormone secretion. There have been rare reports of Fanconi syndrome occurring chiefly in children. Decreased carnitine concentrations have been reported, although the clinical relevance is undetermined. Hyperglycinemia has occurred and was associated with a fatal outcome in a patient with preexistent nonketotic hyperglycinemia.

Musculoskeletal – Weakness.

Special senses – Hearing loss, either reversible or irreversible, has been reported; however, a cause-and-effect relationship has not been established. Ear pain has also been reported.

Miscellaneous – Allergic reaction, anaphylaxis, bone pain, bradycardia, cough increased, cutaneous vasculitis, edema of the extremities, fever, hypothermia, lupus erythematosus, otitis media, pneumonia.

Overdosage

➤*Symptoms:* Overdosage with valproate may result in somnolence, heart block, and deep coma. Fatalities have been reported; however, patients have recovered from valproate levels as high as 2,120 mcg/mL.

➤*Treatment:* In overdose situations, the fraction of drug not bound to protein is high and hemodialysis or tandem hemodialysis plus hemoperfusion may result in significant removal of drug. The benefit of gastric lavage or emesis will vary with the time since ingestion. Apply general supportive measures with particular attention to the maintenance of adequate urinary output.

Naloxone has been reported to reverse the CNS-depressant effects of valproate overdosage. Because naloxone could theoretically also reverse the antiepileptic effects of valproate, use it with caution in patients with epilepsy.

Patient Information

Warn patients and guardians that abdominal pain, anorexia, nausea, and/or vomiting can be symptoms of pancreatitis and, therefore, require further medical evaluation promptly.

Inform patients of the signs and symptoms associated with hyperammonemic encephalopathy and tell them to inform the prescriber if any of these symptoms occur.

Because valproic acid products may produce CNS depression, especially when combined with another CNS depressant (eg, alcohol), advise patients not to engage in hazardous activities, such as driving an automobile or operating dangerous machinery, until it is known that they do not become drowsy from the drug.

Because valproic acid has been associated with certain types of birth defects, advise women of childbearing age considering the use of valproic acid of the risk and of alternative therapeutic options; tell them to read the patient information section, which appears as the last section of the labeling. This is especially important when the treatment of a spontaneously reversible condition not ordinarily associated with permanent injury or risk of death (eg, migraine) is considered.

Instruct patients that a fever associated with other organ system involvement (eg, lymphadenopathy, rash) may be drug related; instruct patients to report such reactions to their health care provider immediately.

DIVALPROEX SODIUM — ORAL

WARNING

Hepatotoxicity – Hepatic failure resulting in fatalities has occurred in patients receiving valproic acid and its derivatives. Experience has indicated that children younger than 2 years of age are at a considerably increased risk of developing fatal hepatotoxicity, especially those on multiple anticonvulsants, those with congenital metabolic disorders, those with severe seizure disorders accompanied by mental retardation, and those with organic brain disease. Use divalproex in this patient group with extreme caution and as a sole agent. Weigh the benefits of therapy against the risks. Above this age group, experience in epilepsy has indicated that the incidence of fatal hepatotoxicity decreases considerably in progressively older patient groups.

These incidents usually have occurred during the first 6 months of treatment. Serious or fatal hepatotoxicity may be preceded by nonspecific symptoms such as malaise, weakness, lethargy, facial edema, anorexia, and vomiting. In patients with epilepsy, a loss of seizure control may also occur. Closely monitor patients for appearance of these symptoms. Perform liver function tests prior to therapy and at frequent intervals thereafter, especially during the first 6 months.

Teratogenicity – Valproate can produce teratogenic effects, such as neural tube defects (eg, spina bifida). Accordingly, the use of valproate products in women of childbearing potential requires that the benefits of its use be weighed against the risk of injury to the fetus. This is especially important when the treatment of a spontaneously reversible condition not ordinarily associated with permanent injury or risk of death (eg, migraine) is contemplated.

An information sheet describing the teratogenic potential of valproate is available for patients.

Pancreatitis – Cases of life-threatening pancreatitis have been reported in both children and adults receiving valproate. Some of the cases have been described as hemorrhagic with a rapid progression from initial symptoms to death. Cases have been reported shortly after initial use and after several years of use. Warn patients and guardians that abdominal pain, anorexia, nausea, and/or vomiting can be symptoms of pancreatitis that require prompt medical evaluation. If pancreatitis is diagnosed, valproate should ordinarily be discontinued. Initiate alternative treatment for the underlying medical condition as clinically indicated.

Indications

➤*Epilepsy:*

Complex partial seizures – As monotherapy or adjunctive therapy in the treatment of adults and children 10 years of age and older with complex partial seizures that occur either in isolation or in association with other types of seizures.

Simple and complex absence seizures – For use as sole and adjunctive therapy in the treatment of simple and complex absence seizures, and adjunctively in patients with multiple seizure types that include absence seizures in adults and children 10 years of age or older.

➤*Mania (delayed-release and extended-release [ER]):* For the treatment of the manic episodes (delayed-release) and acute manic or mixed episodes, with or without psychotic features (ER), associated with bipolar disorder.

➤*Migraine (delayed-release and ER):* For prophylaxis of migraine headaches in adults. There is no evidence that divalproex is useful in the acute treatment of migraine headaches.

➤*Off-label uses:*

Bipolar disorder – Current practice guidelines suggest that valproic acid and its other formulations (ie, divalproex, sodium valproate) are safe and effective for the treatment of bipolar I disorder, including acute mania, rapid cycling, and maintenance therapy. Further randomized, controlled trials are needed to determine its effectiveness in bipolar II disorder and bipolar depression. Valproic acid should be avoided in pregnant women, and hematologic and liver function tests should be conducted routinely to monitor for severe adverse events.

Bipolar disorder – Depressive episodes (adults): [4] = Insufficient documentation. No dosing information was provided.

Bipolar disorder – Manic or mixed episodes (adults): [1] = Good documentation.

Bipolar disorder – Rapid cycling (adults): [1] = Good documentation.

Migraine prevention (children / adolescents) – [4] = Insufficient documentation. Published data on the use of divalproex sodium for the prevention of migraine headaches in children and adolescents are limited, and the number of patients studied is small. Current practice guidelines consider the evidence to be insufficient to make a recommendation for use.

Postherpetic neuralgia – [4] = Insufficient documentation. Evidence from a controlled trial evaluating divalproex for the treatment of postherpetic neuralgia (PHN) showed some benefit. American Academy of Neurology clinical practice guidelines do not make a statement on the efficacy of divalproex for PHN, likely because the available data are more recent than the guidelines.

Restless legs syndrome – [3] = Safety concerns. Limited evidence is available regarding valproic acid for the treatment of primary restless legs syndrome. In guidelines, valproic acid has been rated as probably effective, but there is little evidence to support use.

Administration and Dosage

➤*General dosing considerations:* In patients with epilepsy previously receiving valproic acid therapy, divalproex delayed-release tablets and divalproex sprinkle capsules should be initiated at the same daily dose and dosing schedule. After the patient is stabilized on divalproex delayed-release tablets or divalproex sprinkle capsules, a dosing schedule of 2 or 3 times a day may be elected in selected patients.

Antiepilepsy drugs should not be abruptly discontinued in patients whom the drug is administered to prevent major seizures. (See Discontinuation of therapy.)

➤*Adults:*

Epilepsy –

Complex partial seizures:

- *Monotherapy* –

Initial dosage: 10 to 15 mg/kg/day; may increase dosage by 5 to 10 mg/kg/week to achieve optimal clinical response. If satisfactory clinical response has not been achieved, plasma levels should be measured to determine whether or not they are in the usually accepted therapeutic range (50 to 100 mcg/mL). No recommendation regarding the safety of valproate for use at doses of more than 60 mg/kg/day can be made.

Dosage titration: The dosage should be increased by 5 to 10 mg/kg/week to achieve optimal clinical response. Ordinarily, optimal clinical response is achieved at daily doses of less than 60 mg/kg/day.

Conversion (to monotherapy): This reduction may be started at initiation of divalproex therapy or delayed by 1 to 2 weeks if there is a concern that seizures are likely to occur with a reduction. The speed and duration of withdrawal of the concomitant AED can be highly variable, and patients should be monitored closely during this period for increased seizure frequency.

- *Adjunctive therapy* –

Initial dosage: Divalproex may be added to the patient's regimen at a dose of 10 to 15 mg/kg/day. The dose may be increased by 5 to 10 mg/kg/week to achieve optimal clinical response. Ordinarily, optimal clinical response is achieved at daily doses of less than 60 mg/kg/day. If satisfactory clinical response has not been achieved, plasma levels should be measured to determine whether they are in the usually accepted therapeutic range (50 to 100 mcg/mL). No recommendation regarding the safety of valproate for use at doses of more than 60 mg/kg/day can be made. If the total daily dose exceeds 250 mg, it should be given in divided doses.

Dosage titration: The dose may be increased by 5 to 10 mg/kg/week to achieve optimal clinical response. Ordinarily, optimal clinical response is achieved at daily doses of less than 60 mg/kg/day.

Concomitant therapy: In a study of adjunctive therapy for complex partial seizures in which patients were receiving either carbamazepine or phenytoin in addition to divalproex, no adjustment of carbamazepine or phenytoin dosage was needed. However, because valproate may interact with these or other coadministered AEDs and other drugs, periodic plasma concentration determinations of concomitant AEDs are recommended during the early course of therapy.

Simple and complex absence seizures:

- *Usual dosage* – Initial dose is 15 mg/kg/day and may increase at 1-week intervals by 5 to 10 mg/kg/day until seizures are controlled.

A good correlation has not been established between daily dose, serum concentrations, and therapeutic effect. However, therapeutic valproate serum concentrations for most patients with absence seizures is considered to range from 50 to 100 mcg/mL. Some patients may be controlled with lower or higher serum concentrations.

- *Maximum dose* – 60 mg/kg/day.
- *Dosage titration* – Increase at 1-week intervals by 5 to 10 mg/kg/day until seizures are controlled or adverse reactions preclude further increases. If the total daily dose exceeds 250 mg, it should be given in divided doses.

As the divalproex dosage is titrated upward, blood concentrations of phenobarbital and phenytoin may be affected.

Mania –

Extended-release:

- *Maximum dose* – 60 mg/kg/day.
- *Initial dosage* – 25 mg/kg/day given once daily. The dose should be increased as rapidly as possible to achieve the lowest therapeutic dose that produces the desired clinical effect or the desired range of plasma concentrations. In placebo-controlled clinical trials of acute mania or mixed type, patients were dosed to a clinical response with a trough plasma concentration between 85 and 125 mcg/mL.
- *Duration of therapy* – While it is generally agreed that pharmacological treatment beyond an acute response in mania is desirable, both for maintenance of the initial response and for prevention of new manic episodes, there are no systemically obtained data to support the benefits of divalproex extended release (ER) in such long-term treatment (ie, beyond 3 weeks).

Delayed-release:

- *Maximum dose* – 60 mg/kg/day.
- *Initial dosage* – 750 mg daily, orally in divided doses. The dose should be increased as rapidly as possible to achieve the lowest therapeutic dose, which produces the desired clinical effect or the desired range of plasma concentrations. In placebo-controlled clinical trials of acute mania, patients

DIVALPROEX SODIUM — ORAL

were dosed to a clinical response with a trough plasma concentration between 50 and 125 mcg/mL. Maximum concentrations were generally achieved within 14 days.

• *Duration of therapy* – Although there are no efficacy data that specifically address longer-term antimanic treatment with divalproex, the safety of divalproex in long-term use is supported by data from record reviews involving approximately 360 patients treated with divalproex for more than 3 months.

Migraine –

Extended-release:

• *Initial dosage* – 500 mg once daily for 1 week, thereafter increasing to 1,000 mg once daily.

• *Maintenance dosage* – Although dosages other than 1,000 mg once daily have not been evaluated in patients with migraine, the effective dose range is 500 to 1,000 mg/day.

• *Dosage adjustment* – As with other valproate products, doses of divalproex ER should be individualized and dose adjustment may be necessary. If a patient requires smaller dose adjustments than that available with divalproex ER, divalproex delayed-release should be used instead.

Delayed-release: The recommended starting dosage is 250 mg orally, twice daily. Some patients may benefit from doses of up to 1,000 mg/day. In the clinical trials, there was no evidence that higher doses led to greater efficacy.

Off-label dosing –

Bipolar disorder – Manic or mixed episodes: [1] = Good documentation. Dosing was not provided for divalproex, but was provided for valproic acid. The starting dosage of valproic acid for adult outpatients was 250 mg 3 times daily, increased by 250 to 500 mg every few days or as tolerated. The target serum concentration was 50 to 125 mcg/mL. Some studies have shown efficacy and tolerability with a higher starting dosage of 20 to 30 mg/kg/day in adult inpatients. Doses should be titrated downward until the target serum concentration is reached.

Serum valproate levels should be measured at steady state (3 to 5 days after initiation and subsequent dose changes) approximately 12 hours after the last dose to determine the trough point. After 2 consecutive therapeutic levels, subsequent monitoring can take place every 3 to 6 months unless dosing changes are needed.

Bipolar disorder – Rapid cycling: [1] = Good documentation. See Bipolar disorder – Manic or mixed episodes for dosing information.

Postherpetic neuralgia: [4] = Insufficient documentation. 1,000 mg daily for 8 weeks.

Restless legs syndrome: [3] = Safety concerns. Dosing was not provided for divalproex, but was provided for valproic acid. Oral doses of slow-release valproic acid 300 to 600 mg administered 90 minutes before bedtime for 3 weeks. Guidelines recommend oral dosages of slow-release valproic acid 600 mg/day.

➤*Children:*

Epilepsy –

10 years of age and older: See Adults for dosing.

Off-label dosing –

Anticonvulsant:

• *Maintenance dosage* – A maintenance dose of 30 to 60 mg/kg/day orally has been suggested for children with epilepsy. Administer in 2 or 3 divided doses. Because of drug interactions, higher doses may be required in children on other anticonvulsants.

Migraine prevention (children/adolescents): [4] = Insufficient documentation. Doses ranged from 10 to 45 mg/kg daily.

➤*Elderly:* Because of a decrease in unbound clearance of valproate and possibly a sensitivity to somnolence in elderly patients, the starting dose of divalproex should be reduced in these patients. Starting doses in elderly patients lower than 250 mg can only be achieved by the use of divalproex delayed-release. Dosage should be increased more slowly and with regular monitoring for dehydration, fluid and nutritional intake, somnolence, and other adverse reactions. Dose reductions or discontinuation of valproate should be considered in patients with decreased food or fluid intake and in patients with excessive somnolence. The ultimate therapeutic dose should be achieved on the basis of both tolerability and clinical response.

➤*Hepatic function impairment:* Observe caution when administering divalproex to patients with a history of hepatic function impairment. Discontinue the drug immediately in the presence of hepatic function impairment, suspected, or apparent. In some cases, hepatic function impairment has progressed in spite of discontinuation of the drug.

➤*Conversion (divalproex delayed-release to divalproex extended-release):* In adult patients and children 10 years of age and older with epilepsy previously receiving divalproex delayed-release, divalproex ER should be administered once daily, using a dose 8% to 20% higher than the total daily dose of divalproex delayed-release (see the following table). For patients whose divalproex delayed-release total daily dose cannot be directly converted to divalproex ER, consideration may be given at the health care provider's discretion to increase the patient's divalproex delayed-release total daily dose to the next higher dosage before converting to the appropriate total daily dose of divalproex ER.

Divalproex Dose Conversion

Divalproex delayed-release	Divalproex ER
500[a] to 625 mg	750 mg
750[a] to 875 mg	1,000 mg
1,000[a] to 1,125 mg	1,250 mg
1,250 to 1,375 mg	1,500 mg
1,500 to 1,625 mg	1,750 mg
1,750 mg	2,000 mg
1,875 to 2,000 mg	2,250 mg
2,125 to 2,250 mg	2,500 mg
2,375 mg	2,750 mg
2,500 to 2,750 mg	3,000 mg
2,875 mg	3,250 mg
3,000 to 3,125 mg	3,500 mg

[a] Total daily doses of delayed-release divalproex 500, 750, and 1,000 mg cannot be directly converted to an 8% to 20% higher total daily dose of divalproex ER because the required dosing strengths of divalproex ER are not available. Consideration may be given at the health care provider's discretion to increase the patient's divalproex total daily dose to the next higher dosage before converting to the appropriate total daily dose of divalproex ER.

There are insufficient data to allow a conversion factor recommendation for patients with divalproex doses higher than 3,125 mg/day.

Plasma valproate minimum drug concentrations (C_{min}) for divalproex ER on average are equivalent to divalproex delayed-release, but may vary across patients after conversion. If satisfactory clinical response has not been achieved, plasma level should be measured to determine whether they are in the usually accepted therapeutic range (50 to 100 mcg/mL)

➤*Dose-related adverse reactions:* The frequency of adverse reactions (particularly elevated liver enzymes and thrombocytopenia) may be dose related. The probability of thrombocytopenia appears to increase significantly at total valproate concentrations of 110 mcg/mL or more (women) or 135 mcg/mL or more (men). The benefit of improved therapeutic effect with higher doses should be weighed against the possibility of a greater incidence of adverse reactions.

➤*Therapeutic drug monitoring:*

Therapeutic range – The therapeutic range in epilepsy is commonly considered to be 50 to 100 mcg/mL of total valproate, although some patients may be controlled with lower or higher plasma concentrations.

In placebo-controlled clinical trials of acute mania with delayed-release tablets, patients were dosed to clinical response with trough plasma concentrations between 50 and 125 mcg/mL. In a placebo-controlled clinical trial of acute mania with ER divalproex, patients were dosed to clinical response with trough plasma concentrations between 85 and 125 mcg/mL.

➤*Discontinuation of therapy:* Antiepilepsy drugs (AEDs) should not be abruptly discontinued in patients in whom the drug is administered to prevent major seizures because of the strong possibility of precipitating status epilepticus with attendant hypoxia and threat to life.

➤*Administration:*

Extended-release tablets – Divalproex ER is for once-a-day oral administration. Divalproex ER should be swallowed whole and should not be crushed or chewed.

Sprinkle capsules – Divalproex sprinkle capsules may be swallowed whole or may be administered by carefully opening the capsule and sprinkling the entire contents on a small amount (teaspoonful) of soft food such as applesauce or pudding. The drug/food mixture should be swallowed immediately (avoid chewing) and not stored for future use. Each capsule is oversized to allow ease of opening.

Patients who experience GI irritation may benefit from administration of the drug with food, by slowly building up the dose from an initial low level or by initiating therapy with a lower dose of divalproex delayed-release.

➤*Storage/Stability:*

Delayed-release – Store tablets below 30°C (86°F).

Extended-release – Store tablets at 25°C (77°F); excursions are permitted to 15° to 30°C (59° to 86°F).

Sprinkle capsules – Store capsules below 25°C (77°F).

Actions

➤*Pharmacology:* Divalproex dissociates to the valproate ion in the GI tract. The mechanisms by which valproate exerts its therapeutic effects have not been established. It has been suggested that its activity in epilepsy is related to increased brain concentrations of gamma-aminobutyric acid (GABA).

➤*Pharmacokinetics:*

Absorption –

Sprinkle capsules and delayed-release tablets: Equivalent oral doses of divalproex products and valproic acid capsules deliver equivalent quantities of valproate ion systemically. Although the rate of valproate ion absorption may vary with the formulation administered (ie, liquid, solid, sprinkle), conditions of use (eg, fasting, postprandial), and the method of administration (eg, whether the contents of the capsule are sprinkled on food or the capsule is taken intact), these differences should be of minor clinical importance under the steady-state conditions achieved in chronic use in the treatment of epilepsy.

However, it is possible that differences among the various valproate products in time to maximum plasma concentration (T_{max}) and maximum drug concentration (C_{max}) could be important upon initiation of treatment. For example, in single-dose studies, the effect of feeding had a greater influence

DIVALPROEX SODIUM — ORAL

on the rate of absorption of the tablet (increase in T_{max} from 4 to 8 hours) than on the absorption of the sprinkle capsules (increase in T_{max} from 3.3 to 4.8 hours).

While the absorption rate from the GI tract and fluctuation in valproate plasma concentrations vary with dosing regimen and formulation, the efficacy of valproate as an anticonvulsant in chronic use is unlikely to be affected. Experience employing dosing regimens from once a day to 4 times daily, as well as studies in primate epilepsy models involving constant rate infusion, indicate that total daily systemic bioavailability (extent of absorption) is the primary determinant of seizure control, and that differences in the ratios of plasma peak to trough concentrations between valproate formulations are inconsequential from a practical clinical standpoint. Whether or not rate of absorption influences the efficacy of valproate as an antimanic or antimigraine agent is unknown.

Coadministration of oral valproate products with food and substitution among the various divalproex and valproic acid formulations should cause no clinical problems in the management of patients with epilepsy. Nonetheless, accompany any changes in dosage administration or the addition or discontinuance of concomitant drugs with close monitoring of clinical status and valproate plasma concentrations.

ER: The absolute bioavailability of divalproex ER administered as a single dose after a meal was approximately 90% relative to intravenous (IV) infusion.

When given in equal total daily doses, the bioavailability of divalproex ER is less than that of divalproex delayed-release. In 5 multiple-dose studies in healthy subjects (n = 82) and in subjects with epilepsy (n = 86), when administered under fasting and nonfasting conditions, divalproex ER given once daily produced an average bioavailability of 89% relative to an equal total daily dose of divalproex delayed-release given twice daily, 3 times daily, or 4 times daily. The median time to maximum plasma valproate concentrations (C_{max}) after divalproex ER administration ranged from 4 to 17 hours. After multiple once-daily dosing of divalproex ER, the peak-to-trough fluctuation in plasma valproate concentrations was 10% to 20% lower than that of regular divalproex given twice daily, 3 times daily, or 4 times daily.

Distribution – The plasma protein binding of valproate is concentration dependent, and the free fraction increases from approximately 10% at 40 mcg/mL to 18.5% at 130 mcg/mL. Protein binding of valproate is reduced in elderly patients, in patients with chronic hepatic diseases, in patients with renal function impairment, and in the presence of other drugs (eg, aspirin). Conversely, valproate may displace certain protein-bound drugs (eg, carbamazepine, phenytoin, warfarin, tolbutamide).

Valproate concentrations in cerebrospinal fluid (CSF) approximate unbound concentrations in plasma (approximately 10% of total concentration).

Volume of distribution for total valproate is 11 L per 1.73 m^2 and 92 L per 1.73 m^2 for free valproate.

Metabolism – Valproate is metabolized almost entirely by the liver. In adult patients on monotherapy, 30% to 50% of an administered dose appears in urine as a glucuronide conjugate. Mitochondrial beta-oxidation is the other major metabolic pathway, typically accounting for more than 40% of the dose. Usually, less than 15% to 20% of the dose is eliminated by other oxidative mechanisms. Less than 3% of an administered dose is excreted unchanged in urine.

The relationship between dose and total valproate concentration is nonlinear; concentration does not increase proportionally with the dose but rather increases to a lesser extent because of saturable plasma protein binding. The kinetics of unbound drug are linear.

Excretion – Mean plasma clearance for total valproate is 0.56 L/h per 1.73 m^2. Mean plasma clearance for free valproate is 4.6 L/h per 1.73 m^2. Mean terminal half-life for valproate monotherapy ranged from 9 to 16 hours following oral dosing regimens of 250 to 1,000 mg.

The estimates cited apply primarily to patients who are not taking drugs that affect hepatic-metabolizing enzyme systems. For example, patients taking enzyme-inducing AEDs (carbamazepine, phenobarbital, and phenytoin) will clear valproate more rapidly. Because of these changes in valproate clearance, intensify monitoring of antiepileptic concentrations whenever concomitant antiepileptics are introduced or withdrawn.

Special populations –

Renal function impairment: A slight reduction (27%) in the unbound clearance of valproate has been reported in patients with renal failure (creatinine clearance [CrCl] less than 10 mL/min); however, hemodialysis typically reduces valproate concentrations by approximately 20%. Therefore, no dosage adjustment appears to be necessary in patients with renal failure. Protein binding in these patients is substantially reduced; thus, monitoring total concentrations may be misleading.

Hepatic function impairment: Liver disease impairs the capacity to eliminate valproate. In one study, the clearance of free valproate was decreased by 50% in 7 patients with cirrhosis and by 16% in 4 patients with acute hepatitis, compared with 6 healthy subjects. In that study, the half-life of valproate was increased from 12 to 18 hours. Liver disease is also associated with decreased albumin concentrations and larger unbound fractions (2- to 2.6-fold increase) of valproate. Accordingly, monitoring of total concentrations may be misleading because free concentrations may be substantially elevated in patients with hepatic disease, whereas total concentrations may appear to be normal.

Elderly: The capacity of elderly patients (range, 68 to 89 years of age) to eliminate valproate has been shown to be reduced, compared with younger adults (range, 22 to 26 years of age). Intrinsic clearance is reduced by 39%; the free fraction is increased by 44%. Accordingly, the initial dosage should be reduced in elderly patients.

Children: Children within the first 2 months of life have a markedly decreased ability to eliminate valproate, compared with older children and adults. This is a result of reduced clearance (perhaps due to a delay in development of glucuronosyltransferase and other enzyme systems involved in valproate elimination) as well as increased volume of distribution (in part due to decreased plasma protein binding). For example, in one study, the half-life in children younger than 10 days of age ranged from 10 to 67 hours, compared with a range of 7 to 13 hours in children older than 2 months of age.

Children (ie, between 3 months and 10 years of age) have 50% higher clearances expressed in weight (ie, mL/min/kg) than do adults. Older than 10 years of age, children have pharmacokinetic parameters that approximate those of adults.

Contraindications

Hepatic disease or significant hepatic function impairment; hypersensitivity to the drug; known urea cycle disorders.

Warnings/Precautions

➤*Hepatotoxicity:* See the Warning box for more information.

Observe caution when administering divalproex products to patients with a history of hepatic disease. Patients on multiple anticonvulsants, children, those with congenital metabolic disorders, those with severe seizure disorders accompanied by mental retardation, and those with organic brain disease may be at particular risk. Experience has indicated that children younger than 2 years of age are at a considerably increased risk of developing fatal hepatotoxicity, especially those with the aforementioned conditions. When divalproex is used in this patient group, use it with extreme caution and as a sole agent. Weigh the benefits of therapy against the risks. Above this age group, experience in epilepsy has indicated that the incidence of fatal hepatotoxicity decreases considerably in progressively older patient groups.

Discontinue the drug immediately in the presence of significant hepatic function impairment, suspected or apparent. In some cases, hepatic function impairment has progressed in spite of discontinuation of drug.

➤*Pancreatitis:* See the Warning box for more information.

➤*Urea cycle disorders:* Divalproex is contraindicated in patients with known urea cycle disorders.

Hyperammonemic encephalopathy, sometimes fatal, has been reported following initiation of valproate therapy in patients with urea cycle disorders, a group of uncommon genetic abnormalities, particularly ornithine transcarbamylase deficiency. Prior to the initiation of valproate therapy, consider evaluation for urea cycle disorders in the following patients: 1) those with a history of unexplained encephalopathy or coma, encephalopathy associated with a protein load, pregnancy-related or postpartum encephalopathy, unexplained mental retardation, or history of elevated plasma ammonia or glutamine; 2) those with cyclical vomiting and lethargy, episodic extreme irritability, ataxia, low blood urea nitrogen (BUN), or protein avoidance; 3) those with a family history of urea cycle disorders or a family history of unexplained infant deaths (particularly men); 4) those with other signs and symptoms of urea cycle disorders. Patients who develop symptoms of unexplained hyperammonemic encephalopathy while receiving valproate therapy should receive prompt treatment (including discontinuation of valproate therapy) and be evaluated for underlying urea cycle disorders.

Hyperammonemia – Hyperammonemia has been reported in association with valproate therapy and may be present despite normal liver function tests. In patients who develop unexplained lethargy and vomiting or changes in mental status, consider hyperammonemic encephalopathy and measure an ammonia level. If ammonia is increased, discontinue valproate therapy. Initiate appropriate interventions for treatment of hyperammonemia and evaluate patients for underlying urea cycle disorders. Asymptomatic elevations of ammonia are more common and when present, require close monitoring of ammonia levels. If the elevation persists, consider discontinuation of valproate therapy.

Hyperammonemia and encephalopathy associated with concomitant topiramate use – Coadministration of topiramate and valproic acid has been associated with hyperammonemia with or without encephalopathy in patients who have tolerated either drug alone. Clinical symptoms of hyperammonemic encephalopathy often include acute alterations in level of consciousness and/or cognitive function with lethargy or vomiting. In most cases, symptoms and signs abated with discontinuation of either drug. This adverse reaction is not due to a pharmacokinetic interaction. It is not known if topiramate monotherapy is associated with hyperammonemia. Patients with inborn errors of metabolism or reduced hepatic mitochondrial activity may be at an increased risk for hyperammonemia with or without encephalopathy. Although not studied, an interaction of topiramate and valproic acid may exacerbate existing defects or unmask deficiencies in susceptible persons. In patients who develop unexplained lethargy, vomiting, or changes in mental status, consider hyperammonemic encephalopathy and measure an ammonia level.

➤*Multiorgan hypersensitivity reaction:* Multiorgan hypersensitivity reactions have been rarely reported in close temporal association to the initiation of valproate therapy in adults and children (median time to detection, 21 days; range, 1 to 40 days). Although there have been a limited number of reports, many of these cases resulted in hospitalization and at least 1 death has been reported. Signs and symptoms of this disorder were diverse; however, patients typically, although not exclusively, presented with fever and rash associated with other organ system involvement. Other associated manifestations may include arthralgia, asthenia, hematological abnormalities (eg, eosinophilia, thrombocytopenia, neutropenia), hepatitis, hepatorenal syndrome, liver function test abnormalities, lymphadenopathy, nephritis, oliguria, and pruritis. Because the disorder is variable in its expression, other organ system symptoms and signs, not noted here, may occur. If this reaction is suspected, discontinue valproate and start an alternative treatment. Although the existence of cross-sensitivity with other

DIVALPROEX SODIUM — ORAL

drugs that produce this syndrome is unclear, the experience among drugs associated with multiorgan hypersensitivity would indicate this to be a possibility.

➤*Thrombocytopenia:* Because of reports of thrombocytopenia, inhibition of the secondary phase of platelet aggregation, and abnormal coagulation parameters (eg, low fibrinogen), platelet counts and coagulation tests are recommended before initiating therapy and at periodic intervals. It is recommended that patients receiving divalproex be monitored for platelet count and coagulation parameters prior to planned surgery. In a clinical trial of divalproex as monotherapy in patients with epilepsy, 34/126 (27%) patients receiving approximately 50 mg/kg/day on average, had at least 1 value of platelets of 75×10^9/L or less. Approximately half of these patients had treatment discontinued, with return of platelet counts to normal. In the remaining patients, platelet counts normalized with continued treatment. In this study, the probability of thrombocytopenia appeared to increase significantly at total valproate concentrations of 110 mcg/mL or more (women) or 135 mcg/mL or more (men). Therefore, weigh the therapeutic benefit that may accompany the higher doses against the possibility of a greater incidence of adverse reactions. Evidence of bruising, hemorrhage, or a disorder of hemostasis/coagulation is an indication for reduction of the dosage or withdrawal of therapy.

➤*Suicidal ideation:* Suicidal ideation may be a manifestation of certain psychiatric disorders and may persist until significant remission of symptoms occurs. Close supervision of high-risk patients should accompany initial drug therapy.

➤*HIV:* There are in vitro studies that suggest valproate stimulates the replication of the HIV and cytomegalovirus (CMV) under certain experimental conditions. The clinical consequence, if any, is not known. Additionally, the relevance of these in vitro findings is uncertain for patients receiving maximally suppressive antiretroviral therapy. Nevertheless, keep these data in mind when interpreting the results from regular monitoring of the viral load in HIV-infected patients receiving valproate or when following CMV-infected patients clinically.

➤*Hepatic function impairment:* Observe caution when administering divalproex to patients with a history of hepatic function impairment. Patients on multiple anticonvulsants, children, those with congenital metabolic disorders, those with severe disorders accompanied by mental retardation, and those with organic brain disease may be at particular risk. Discontinue the drug immediately in the presence of hepatic function impairment, suspected or apparent. In some cases, hepatic function impairment has progressed in spite of discontinuation of the drug.

➤*Hazardous tasks:* Because divalproex products may produce CNS depression, especially when combined with another CNS depressant (eg, alcohol), advise patients not to engage in hazardous activities, such as driving an automobile or operating dangerous machinery, until it is known that they do not become drowsy from the drug.

➤*Pregnancy: Category D.* According to the American Academy of Neurology and the American Epilepsy Society, valproic acid should be avoided if possible during pregnancy, especially during the first trimester. Valproic acid has been associated with major congenital malformations (eg, neural tube defects, facial clefts) in the offspring of women with epilepsy taking valproic acid monotherapy or as part of polytherapy. Valproic acid has also been associated with an increased risk of impaired cognitive function in children at 3 years of age. If possible, switch patients from valproic acid to a less teratogenic antiepileptic drug well before pregnancy. If a patient is already several weeks into her pregnancy, switching to another AED will not avoid the risk of major congenital malformations, since these effects occur very early in the pregnancy. A patient should consult her physician before stopping valproic acid since stopping an antiepileptic drug could lead to seizures and other serious consequences.

Teratogenic – Valproate can produce teratogenic effects. Data suggest that there is an increased incidence of congenital malformations associated with the use of valproate by women with seizure disorders during pregnancy when compared with the incidence in women with seizure disorders who do not use AEDs during pregnancy, the incidence in women with seizure disorders who use other AEDs, and the background incidence for the general population. Therefore, consider valproate for women of childbearing potential only after the risks have been thoroughly discussed with the patient and weighed against the potential benefits of treatment.

The following data were gained almost exclusively from women who received valproate to treat epilepsy. There are multiple reports in the clinical literature that indicate that the use of AEDs during pregnancy results in an increased incidence of congenital malformations in the offspring. Although data are more extensive with respect to paramethadione, phenobarbital, phenytoin, and trimethadione, reports indicate a possible similar association with the use of other AEDs. Therefore, administer AEDs, including valproate, to women of childbearing potential only if they are clearly shown to be essential in the management of their seizures.

Do not abruptly discontinue AEDs in patients in whom the drug is administered to prevent major seizures because of the strong possibility of precipitating status epilepticus with attendant hypoxia and threat to life. In individual cases in which the severity and frequency of the seizure disorder are such that the removal of medication does not pose a serious threat to the patient, consider discontinuation of the drug prior to and during pregnancy, although it cannot be said with any confidence that even minor seizures do not pose some hazard to the developing embryo or fetus.

Congenital malformations – The North American Antiepileptic Drug Pregnancy Registry reported 16 cases of congenital malformations among the offspring of 149 women with epilepsy who were exposed to valproic acid monotherapy during the first trimester of pregnancy at doses of approximately 1,000 mg per day, for a prevalence rate of 10.7% (95% confidence interval [CI], 6.3% to 16.9%). Three (2%) of the 149 offspring had neural tube defects and 6 (4%) of the 149 had less severe malformations. Among epileptic women who were exposed to other AED monotherapies during pregnancy (1,048 patients), the malformation rate was 2.9% (95% CI, 2% to 4.1%). There was a 4-fold increase in congenital malformations among infants with valproic acid-exposed mothers, compared with those treated with other antiepileptic monotherapies as a group (odds ratio, 4; 95% CI, 2.1% to 7.4%). This increased risk does not reflect a comparison versus any specific AED but the risk versus the heterogeneous group of all other AED monotherapies combined. The increased teratogenic risk from valproic acid in women with epilepsy is expected to be reflected in an increased risk in other indications (eg, bipolar disorder, migraine).

The strongest association of maternal valproate usage with congenital malformations is with neural tube defects. However, other congenital anomalies (eg, anomalies involving various body systems, cardiovascular malformations, craniofacial defects), compatible and incompatible with life, have been reported. Sufficient data to determine the incidence of these congenital anomalies are not available.

Neural tube defects – The incidence of neural tube defects in the fetus may be increased in mothers receiving valproate during the first trimester of pregnancy. The Centers for Disease Control and Prevention (CDC) has estimated the risk of valproic acid-exposed women having children with spina bifida to be approximately 1% to 2%. The American College of Obstetricians and Gynecologists (ACOG) estimates the general population risk for congenital neural tube defects as 0.14% to 0.2%.

Consider tests to detect neural tube and other defects using currently accepted procedures as a part of routine prenatal care in childbearing women receiving valproate.

Evidence suggests that pregnant women who receive folic acid supplementation may be at decreased risk for congenital neural tube defects in their offspring, compared with pregnant women not receiving folic acid. Whether the risk of neural tube defects in the offspring of women receiving valproate specifically is reduced by folic acid supplementation is unknown. Routinely recommend dietary folic acid supplementation prior to and during pregnancy to patients contemplating pregnancy.

Other adverse pregnancy reactions – Patients taking valproate may develop clotting abnormalities. A patient who had low fibrinogen when taking multiple anticonvulsants, including valproate, gave birth to an infant with afibrinogenemia who subsequently died of hemorrhage. If valproate is used in pregnancy, carefully monitor the clotting parameters.

Patients taking valproate may develop hepatic failure. Hepatic failure resulting in the death of a newborn and of an infant has been reported following the use of valproate during pregnancy.

➤*Lactation:* Valproate is excreted in breast milk. Concentrations in breast milk have been reported to be 1% to 10% of serum concentrations. It is not known what effect this would have on a breast-feeding infant. Consider discontinuing breast-feeding when divalproex is administered to a breast-feeding woman.

➤*Children:* Experience has indicated that children younger than 2 years of age are at a considerably increased risk of developing fatal hepatotoxicity, especially those on multiple anticonvulsants, those with congenital metabolic disorders, those with severe seizure disorders accompanied by mental retardation, and those with organic brain disease. Use divalproex in this patient group with extreme caution and as a sole agent. Weigh the benefits of therapy against the risks. Older than 2 years of age, experience in epilepsy has indicated that the incidence of fatal hepatotoxicity decreases considerably in progressively older patient groups.

Younger children, especially those receiving enzyme-inducing drugs, will require larger maintenance doses to attain targeted total and unbound valproic acid concentrations.

The variability in free fraction limits the clinical usefulness of monitoring total serum valproic acid concentrations. In interpretation of valproic acid concentrations in children, consider factors that affect hepatic metabolism and protein binding.

The safety and efficacy of divalproex delayed-release have not been studied for the treatment of acute mania in persons younger than 18 years of age and have not been studied for the prophylaxis of migraines in children younger than 16 years of age.

The safety and efficacy of divalproex ER for the prophylaxis of migraine headaches in children have not been established.

The safety and efficacy of divalproex for the treatment of complex partial seizures, simple and complex absence seizures, and multiple seizure types that include absence seizures have not been established in children younger than 10 years of age.

➤*Elderly:* In a double-blind, multicenter trial of valproate in elderly patients with dementia (mean age, 83 years), doses were increased by 125 mg/day to a target dose of 20 mg/kg/day. A significantly higher proportion of valproate patients had somnolence compared with placebo patients, and, although not statistically significant, there was a higher proportion of patients with dehydration. Discontinuations for somnolence were also significantly higher than with placebo. In some patients with somnolence (approximately one-half), there was associated reduced nutritional intake and weight loss. There was a trend for the patients who experienced these reactions to have a lower baseline albumin concentration, lower valproate clearance, and a higher BUN. In elderly patients, increase dosage more slowly and regularly monitor for dehydration, fluid and nutritional intake, somnolence, and other adverse reactions. Consider dose reductions or discontinuation of valproate in patients with decreased food or fluid intake and in patients with excessive somnolence.

A higher percentage of patients older than 65 years of age reported accidental injury, infection, pain, somnolence, and tremor. Discontinuation of val-

DIVALPROEX SODIUM — ORAL

proate was occasionally associated with the latter 2 events. It is not clear whether these events indicate additional risk or whether they result from preexisting medical illness and concomitant medication use among these patients.

➤*Monitoring:* Perform liver function tests prior to therapy and at frequent intervals thereafter, especially during the first 6 months. However, do not rely totally on serum biochemistry because these tests may not be abnormal in all instances; also consider the results of careful interim medical history and physical examination.

Platelet counts and coagulation tests are recommended before initiating therapy and at periodic intervals.

Because divalproex may interact with coadministered drugs that are capable of enzyme induction, periodic plasma concentration determinations of valproate and concomitant drugs are recommended during the early course of therapy.

Asymptomatic elevations of ammonia are more common and when present, require close monitoring of plasma ammonia levels. If the elevation persists, consider discontinuation of valproate therapy.

In patients who develop unexplained lethargy, vomiting, or changes in mental status, consider hyperammonemic encephalopathy and measure an ammonia level.

Drug Interactions

Divalproex Drug Interactions

Precipitant drug	Object drug[a]		Description
Carbapenem antibiotics (eg, meropenem)	Divalproex	↓	Subtherapeutic valproic acid levels have been reported with coadministration.
Chlorpromazine	Divalproex	↑	Valproate elimination half-life and trough levels may increase; clearance may decrease.
Cholestyramine	Divalproex	↓	Serum concentrations and bioavailability of valproic acid may be reduced, resulting in a decrease in therapeutic effects. Administer valproic acid at least 3 hours before, but not within 3 hours following, cholestyramine.
Felbamate	Divalproex	↑	Coadministration revealed a 35% increase in mean peak valproate levels.
Rifampin	Divalproex	↓	In one study, rifampin increased the oral clearance of valproate by 40%.
Salicylates (eg, aspirin)	Divalproex	↑	Salicylates may displace divalproex from protein binding sites and may inhibit metabolism of valproate. Monitor serum concentrations.
Divalproex	Barbiturates (eg, phenobarbital, primidone)	↑	Valproic acid may decrease hepatic metabolism of barbiturates. Barbiturate dosage may need to be decreased in some patients. Phenobarbital or primidone can double the clearance of valproate.
Barbiturates (eg, phenobarbital, primidone)	Divalproex	↓	
Divalproex	Benzodiazepines (eg, clonazepam, diazepam, lorazepam)	↑	Valproate displaces benzodiazepines from their plasma albumin binding sites and inhibits their metabolism, resulting in increased CNS depression. Concomitant use with clonazepam may induce absence status in patients with a history of absence seizures.
Divalproex	Carbamazepine	↑	Variable changes in carbamazepine concentrations with increased levels of the active metabolite; carbamazepine may decrease divalproex levels, and possible loss of seizure control may occur.
Carbamazepine	Divalproex	↓	
Divalproex	Ethosuximide	↑↓	Increases and decreases in ethosuximide blood levels and decreases in valproic acid levels have been reported. Valproic acid appears to inhibit the metabolism of ethosuximide.
Ethosuximide	Divalproex	↓	
Divalproex	Hydantoins (eg, phenytoin)	↑	Increased action of phenytoin, even at therapeutic levels; increased metabolism of valproic acid with decreased pharmacologic effects may occur. Monitor the levels of the free concentrations of hydantoin and serum valproic acid.
Hydantoins (eg, phenytoin)	Divalproex	↓	
Divalproex	Lamotrigine	↑	Serum valproic acid concentrations may be decreased while lamotrigine levels increase. In one study, coadministration increased the half-life of lamotrigine from 26 to 70 hours. Consider reducing lamotrigine dose.
Lamotrigine	Divalproex	↓	
Divalproex	Tolbutamide	↔	The unbound fraction of tolbutamide may be increased from 20% to 50%. The clinical relevance of this displacement is unknown.
Divalproex	Topiramate	↓	Possible increased metabolism of both agents. Coadministration has been associated with hyperammonemia with and without encephalopathy.
Topiramate	Divalproex		
Divalproex	Tricyclic antidepressants (eg, amitriptyline, nortriptyline)	↑	Plasma concentrations and adverse reactions of the tricyclic antidepressant may be increased. Coadministration resulted in a 21% decrease in the plasma clearance of amitriptyline and a 34% decrease in the net clearance of nortriptyline.
Divalproex	Warfarin	↑	The potential exists for valproate to displace warfarin from protein binding sites. Monitor coagulation tests.
Divalproex	Zidovudine	↑	Zidovudine clearance was decreased by 38% in 6 HIV-seropositive patients.

[a] ↑ = object drug increased; ↓ = object drug decreased; ↔ = undetermined clinical effect.

➤*Drug/Lab test interactions:* There have been reports of altered thyroid function tests associated with valproate. The clinical significance of these is unknown.

Valproate is partially eliminated in the urine as a ketometabolite, which may lead to a false interpretation of the urine ketone test.

Adverse Reactions

➤*Epilepsy:*

Adjunctive therapy for complex partial seizures – Based on a placebo-controlled trial of adjunctive therapy for the treatment of complex partial seizures, divalproex was generally well tolerated, with most adverse reactions rated as mild to moderate in severity. Intolerance was the primary reason for discontinuation in the divalproex-treated patients (6%), compared with 1% of placebo-treated patients.

The following table lists treatment-emergent adverse reactions that were reported by 5% or more of divalproex-treated patients and for which the incidence was greater than in the placebo group in the placebo-controlled trial of adjunctive therapy for treatment of complex partial seizures. Because patients were also treated with other AEDs, it is not possible, in most cases, to determine whether the following adverse reactions can be ascribed to divalproex alone or the combination of divalproex and other AEDs.

Divalproex Adverse Reactions (≥ 5%) in Adjunctive Therapy for Complex Partial Seizures

Adverse reaction	Divalproex (n = 77)	Placebo (n = 70)
CNS		
Abnormal thinking	6%	0%
Amnesia	5%	1%
Asthenia	27%	7%
Ataxia	8%	1%
Dizziness	25%	13%
Emotional lability	6%	4%
Headache	31%	21%
Somnolence	27%	11%
Tremor	25%	6%

DIVALPROEX SODIUM — ORAL

Divalproex Adverse Reactions (≥ 5%) in Adjunctive Therapy for Complex Partial Seizures		
Adverse reaction	Divalproex (n = 77)	Placebo (n = 70)
GI		
Abdominal pain	23%	6%
Anorexia	12%	0%
Constipation	5%	1%
Diarrhea	13%	6%
Dyspepsia	8%	4%
Nausea	48%	14%
Vomiting	27%	7%
Respiratory		
Bronchitis	5%	1%
Flu syndrome	12%	9%
Infection	12%	6%
Rhinitis	5%	4%
Special senses		
Amblyopia/ Blurred vision	12%	9%
Diplopia	16%	9%
Nystagmus	8%	1%
Miscellaneous		
Alopecia	6%	1%
Fever	6%	4%
Weight loss	6%	0%

High-dose monotherapy for complex partial seizures – The following table lists treatment-emergent adverse reactions that were reported by 5% or more of patients in the high-dose divalproex group, and for which the incidence was greater than in the low-dose group, in a controlled trial of divalproex monotherapy treatment of complex partial seizures. Because patients were being titrated off another AED during the first portion of the trial, it is not possible, in many cases, to determine whether the following adverse reactions can be ascribed to divalproex alone or the combination of divalproex and other AEDs.

Divalproex Adverse Reactions (≥ 5%) in the High-Dose Monotherapy for Complex Partial Seizures[a]		
Adverse reaction	High-dose (n = 131)	Low-dose (n = 134)
CNS		
Amnesia	7%	4%
Asthenia	21%	10%
Depression	5%	4%
Dizziness	18%	13%
Insomnia	15%	9%
Nervousness	11%	7%
Somnolence	30%	18%
Tremor	57%	19%
GI		
Abdominal pain	12%	9%
Anorexia	11%	4%
Diarrhea	23%	19%
Dyspepsia	11%	10%
Nausea	34%	26%
Vomiting	23%	15%
Hematologic/Lymphatic		
Ecchymosis	5%	4%
Thrombocytopenia	24%	1%
Metabolic/Nutritional		
Peripheral edema	8%	3%
Weight gain	9%	4%
Respiratory		
Dyspnea	5%	1%
Infection	20%	13%
Pharyngitis	8%	2%
Special senses		
Amblyopia/ Blurred vision	8%	4%
Nystagmus	7%	1%
Tinnitus	7%	1%
Miscellaneous		
Alopecia	24%	13%

[a] Headache was the only adverse reaction that occurred in 5% or more of patients in the high-dose group and at an equal or greater incidence in the low-dose group.

➤*Complex partial seizures (more than 1% to less than 5%):*
Cardiovascular – Hypertension, palpitation, tachycardia.
CNS – Abnormal dreams, abnormal gait, anxiety, confusion, hypertonia, incoordination, paresthesia, personality disorder.
Dermatologic – Dry skin, pruritus, rash.
GI – Eructation, flatulence, hematemesis, increased appetite, pancreatitis, periodontal abscess.
GU – Amenorrhea, dysmenorrhea, urinary frequency, urinary incontinence, vaginitis.
Hematologic / Lymphatic – Petechia.
Hepatic – ALT increased, AST increased.
Musculoskeletal – Arthralgia, leg cramps, myalgia, myasthenia, twitching.
Respiratory – Cough increased, epistaxis, pneumonia, sinusitis.
Special senses – Abnormal vision, deafness, otitis media, taste perversion.
Miscellaneous – Back pain, chest pain, malaise.

➤*Mania:*
Delayed-release –

Divalproex Delayed-Release Adverse Reactions (> 5%) in Acute Mania[a]		
Adverse reaction	Divalproex delayed-release (n = 89)	Placebo (n = 97)
CNS		
Asthenia	10%	7%
Dizziness	12%	4%
Somnolence	19%	12%
Dermatologic		
Rash	6%	3%
GI		
Abdominal pain	9%	8%
Dyspepsia	9%	8%
Nausea	22%	15%
Vomiting	12%	3%

[a] The following adverse reactions occurred at an equal or greater incidence for placebo than for divalproex: back pain, constipation, diarrhea, headache, pharyngitis, and tremor.

➤*Additional adverse reactions in the treatment of mania (delayed-release):* The following additional adverse reactions were reported by more than 1% but less than 5% of the 89 divalproex-treated patients in controlled clinical trials:
Cardiovascular – Hypertension, hypotension, palpitations, postural hypotension, tachycardia, vasodilation.
CNS – Abnormal dreams, abnormal gait, agitation, ataxia, catatonic reaction, chills, confusion, depression, diplopia, dysarthria, hallucinations, hypertonia, hypokinesia, insomnia, paresthesia, reflexes increased, tardive dyskinesia, thinking abnormalities, vertigo.
Dermatologic – Alopecia, discoid lupus erythematosis, dry skin, furunculosis, maculopapular rash, seborrhea.
GI – Anorexia, fecal incontinence, flatulence, gastroenteritis, glossitis, periodontal abscess.
GU – Dysmenorrhea, dysuria, urinary incontinence.
Hematologic / Lymphatic – Ecchymosis.
Metabolic / Nutritional – Edema, peripheral edema.
Musculoskeletal – Arthralgia, arthrosis, leg cramps, twitching.
Respiratory – Dyspnea, rhinitis.
Special senses – Amblyopia, conjunctivitis, deafness, dry eyes, ear pain, eye pain, tinnitus.
Miscellaneous – Chest pain, chills and fever, fever, neck pain, neck rigidity.

DIVALPROEX SODIUM — ORAL

➤*Mania:*

ER –

Divalproex ER Adverse Reactions (> 5%) in Acute Mania[a]		
Adverse reaction	Divalproex ER (n = 338)	Placebo (n = 263)
CNS		
Asthenia	6%	5%
Dizziness	12%	7%
Somnolence	26%	14%
GI		
Abdominal pain	10%	5%
Diarrhea	12%	8%
Dyspepsia	23%	11%
Nausea	19%	13%
Vomiting	13%	5%
Miscellaneous		
Accidental injury	6%	5%
Pain	11%	10%
Pharyngitis	6%	5%

[a] The following adverse reaction occurred at an equal to or greater incidence for placebo than for divalproex ER: headache.

➤*Additional adverse reactions in the treatment of mania (ER):* The following additional adverse reactions were reported by more than 1% but not more than 5% of the divalproex ER-treated patients in controlled clinical trials.

Cardiovascular – Hypertension.

CNS – Abnormal gait, hypertonia, tremor.

Dermatologic – Pruritus, rash.

GI – Constipation, dry mouth, flatulence.

GU – Urinary tract infection, vaginitis.

Hematologic/Lymphatic – Ecchymosis.

Metabolic/Nutritional – Peripheral edema.

Musculoskeletal – Myalgia.

Respiratory – Rhinitis.

Special senses – Conjunctivitis.

Miscellaneous – Back pain, flu syndrome, fungal infection, infection.

➤*Other adverse reactions in the treatment of mania (> 1%):*

Cardiovascular – Arrhythmia, hypotension, postural hypotension.

CNS – Agitation, catatonic reaction, chills, dysarthria, hallucinations, hypokinesia, increased reflexes, psychosis, sleep disorder, tardive dyskinesia.

Dermatologic – Discoid lupus erythematosis, erythema nodosum, furunculosis, maculopapular rash, seborrhea, sweating, vesiculobullous rash.

GI – Dysphagia, fecal incontinence, gastroenteritis, glossitis, gum hemorrhage, mouth ulceration.

GU – Cystitis, menstrual disorder.

Hematologic/Lymphatic – Anemia, increased bleeding time, leukopenia.

Metabolic/Nutritional – Hypoproteinemia.

Musculoskeletal – Arthrosis.

Respiratory – Hiccup.

Special senses – Conjunctivitis, dry eyes, eye disorder, eye pain, photophobia, taste perversion.

Miscellaneous – Chills and fever, increased drug level, neck rigidity.

➤*Migraine:*

Delayed-release –

Divalproex Delayed-Release Adverse Reactions (> 5%) in Migraine[a]		
Adverse reaction	Divalproex delayed-release (n = 202)	Placebo (n = 81)
CNS		
Asthenia	20%	9%
Dizziness	12%	6%
Somnolence	17%	5%
Tremor	9%	0%
GI		
Abdominal pain	9%	4%
Diarrhea	12%	7%
Dyspepsia	13%	9%
Increased appetite	6%	4%
Nausea	31%	10%
Vomiting	11%	1%
Miscellaneous		
Alopecia	7%	1%
Back pain	8%	6%
Weight gain	8%	2%

[a] The following adverse reactions occurred in at least 5% of divalproex delayed-release-treated patients and at an equal or greater incidence for placebo than for divalproex delayed-release: flu syndrome and pharyngitis.

➤*Additional adverse reactions in the treatment of migraine (delayed-release):* The following additional adverse reactions were reported by more than 1% but not more than 5% of the 202 divalproex-treated patients in the controlled clinical trials.

Cardiovascular – Vasodilatation.

CNS – Abnormal dreams, amnesia, chills, confusion, depression, emotional lability, insomnia, nervousness, paresthesia, speech disorder, thinking abnormalities, vertigo.

Dermatologic – Pruritus, rash.

GI – Anorexia, constipation, dry mouth, flatulence, GI disorder (unspecified), stomatitis.

GU – Cystitis, metrorrhagia, vaginal hemorrhage.

Hematologic/Lymphatic – Ecchymosis.

Metabolic/Nutritional – ALT increased, AST increased, peripheral edema.

Musculoskeletal – Leg cramps, myalgia.

Respiratory – Cough increased, dyspnea, rhinitis, sinusitis.

Special senses – Conjunctivitis, ear disorder, taste perversion, tinnitus.

Miscellaneous – Chest pain, face edema, malaise.

➤*Migraine:*

ER –

Divalproex ER Adverse Reactions (> 5%) in Migraine[a]		
Adverse reaction	Divalproex ER (n = 122)	Placebo (n = 115)
CNS		
Somnolence	7%	2%
GI		
Abdominal pain	7%	5%
Diarrhea	7%	3%
Dyspepsia	7%	4%
Nausea	15%	9%
Vomiting	7%	2%
Miscellaneous		
Infection	15%	14%

[a] The following adverse reactions occurred in more than 5% of divalproex ER-treated patients and at a greater incidence for placebo than for divalproex ER: asthenia and flu syndrome.

➤*Additional adverse reactions in the treatment of migraine (ER):* The following additional adverse reactions were reported by more than 1% but not more than 5% of divalproex ER-treated patients with a greater incidence than placebo in the placebo-controlled clinical trial for migraine prophylaxis:

Cardiovascular – Vasodilation.

CNS – Abnormal dreams, abnormal gait, abnormal thinking, confusion, dizziness, hypertonia, insomnia, nervousness, paresthesia, speech disorder, tremor, vertigo.

Dermatologic – Pruritus, rash.

GI – Constipation, dry mouth, flatulence, increased appetite, stomatitis, tooth disorder.

GU – Metrorrhagia.

Hematologic/Lymphatic – Ecchymosis.

Metabolic/Nutritional – Edema, peripheral edema, weight gain.

Musculoskeletal – Leg cramps.

Respiratory – Dyspnea, pharyngitis, rhinitis, sinusitis.

Special senses – Tinnitus.

DIVALPROEX SODIUM — ORAL

Miscellaneous – Accidental injury, chest pain, viral infection.

➤*Other adverse reactions (all dosage forms):* The following adverse reactions have been reported with all dosage forms of valproate from epilepsy trials, spontaneous reports, and other sources, and are listed by body system.

Cardiovascular – Bradycardia.

CNS – Aggression, behavioral deterioration, depression, emotional upset, hostility, hyperactivity, psychosis.

Sedative effects have occurred in patients receiving valproate alone but occur most often in patients receiving combination therapy. Sedation usually abates upon reduction of other antiepileptic medication. Asterixis, ataxia, confusion, diplopia, dizziness, dysarthria, hallucinations, headache, hypesthesia, incoordination, nystagmus, parkinsonism, "spots before eyes," tremor (may be dose related), and vertigo have been reported with the use of valproate. Rare cases of coma have occurred in patients receiving valproate alone or in conjunction with phenobarbital. In rare instances, encephalopathy with fever has developed shortly after the introduction of valproate monotherapy without evidence of hepatic function impairment or inappropriately high plasma levels. Although recovery has been described following drug withdrawal, there have been fatalities in patients with hyperammonemic encephalopathy, particularly in patients with underlying urea cycle disorders.

Several reports have noted reversible cerebral atrophy and dementia in association with valproate therapy.

Dermatologic – Erythema multiforme, generalized pruritus, photosensitivity, skin rash, Stevens-Johnson syndrome, transient hair loss. Rare cases of toxic epidermal necrolysis have been reported, including a fatal case in a 6-month-old infant taking valproate and several other concomitant medications. An additional case of toxic epidermal necrosis resulting in death was reported in a 35-year-old patient with AIDS taking several concomitant medications and a history of multiple cutaneous drug reactions. Serious skin reactions have been reported with coadministration of lamotrigine and valproate.

Endocrine – Abnormal thyroid function tests, breast enlargement, galactorrhea, irregular menses, parotid gland swelling, secondary amenorrhea.

There have been rare spontaneous reports of polycystic ovary disease. A cause-and-effect relationship has not been established.

GI – The most commonly reported reactions at the initiation of therapy are indigestion, nausea, and vomiting. These reactions are usually transient and rarely require discontinuation of therapy. Abdominal cramps, constipation, and diarrhea have been reported. Both anorexia with some weight loss and increased appetite with weight gain have also been reported. In some patients, many of whom have functional or anatomic (including ileostomy or colostomy) GI disorders with shortened GI transit times, there have been postmarketing reports of divalproex ER in the stool. The administration of delayed-release divalproex may result in reduction of GI reactions in some patients.

GU – Enuresis, urinary tract infection.

Hematologic – Thrombocytopenia and inhibition of the secondary phase of platelet aggregation may be reflected in acute intermittent porphyria, altered bleeding time, anemia (including macrocytic with or without folate deficiency), aplastic anemia, bone marrow suppression, bruising, eosinophilia, epistaxis, frank hemorrhage, hematoma formation, hypofibrinogenemia, leukopenia, macrocytosis, pancytopenia, petechiae, relative lymphocytosis.

Hepatic – Minor elevations of transaminases (eg, ALT, AST) and lactate dehydrogenase are frequent and appear to be dose related. Occasionally, laboratory test results include increases in serum bilirubin and abnormal changes in other liver function tests. These results may reflect potentially serious hepatotoxicity.

Metabolic – Hyperammonemia, hyponatremia, inappropriate antidiuretic hormone secretion.

There have been rare reports of Fanconi syndrome occurring chiefly in children.

Decreased carnitine concentrations have been reported, although the clinical relevance is undetermined.

Hyperglycinemia has occurred and was associated with a fatal outcome in a patient with preexistent nonketotic hyperglycinemia.

Musculoskeletal – Weakness.

Special senses – Hearing loss, either reversible or irreversible, has been reported; however, a cause-and-effect relationship has not been established. Ear pain and otitis media have also been reported.

Miscellaneous – Acute pancreatitis (including fatalities), allergic reaction, anaphylaxis, bone pain, cough increased, cutaneous vasculitis, edema of the extremities, fever, hypothermia, lupus erythematosus, pneumonia.

Overdosage

➤*Symptoms:* Overdosage with valproate may result in deep coma, heart block, and somnolence. Fatalities have been reported; however, patients have recovered from valproate levels as high as 2,120 mcg/mL.

➤*Treatment:* In overdose situations, the fraction of drug not bound to protein is high, and hemodialysis or tandem hemodialysis plus hemoperfusion may result in significant removal of drug. The benefit of gastric lavage or emesis will vary with the time since ingestion. Apply general supportive measures; pay particular attention to the maintenance of adequate urinary output.

Naloxone has been reported to reverse the CNS-depressant effects of valproate overdosage. Because naloxone could theoretically also reverse the antiepileptic effects of valproate, use it with caution in patients with epilepsy.

Patient Information

Warn patients and guardians that abdominal pain, anorexia, nausea, and/or vomiting can be symptoms of pancreatitis and, therefore, require further medical evaluation promptly.

Inform patients of the signs and symptoms associated with hyperammonemic encephalopathy and tell them to inform the prescriber if any of these symptoms occur. In patients who develop unexplained lethargy and vomiting or changes in mental status, consider hyperammonemic encephalopathy and measure an ammonia level. If ammonia is increased, discontinue valproate therapy.

Because divalproex products may produce CNS depression, especially when combined with another CNS depressant (eg, alcohol), advise patients not to engage in hazardous activities, such as driving an automobile or operating dangerous machinery, until it is known that they do not become drowsy from the drug.

The specially coated particles in divalproex sprinkle capsules have been observed in the stool, but this occurrence has not been associated with clinically significant effects.

Because divalproex has been associated with certain types of birth defects, advise female patients of childbearing age considering the use of divalproex for the prevention of migraine of the risk and of alternative therapeutic options. Tell patients to read the enclosed patient information labeling that comes with their medication. This is especially important when the treatment of a spontaneously reversible condition not ordinarily associated with permanent injury or risk of death (eg, migraine) is considered.

Inform patients that a fever associated with other organ system involvement (eg, lymphadenopathy, rash) may be drug related; tell them to report a fever to their health care provider immediately.

Instruct patients to take divalproex ER every day as prescribed. If a dose is missed, it should be taken as soon as possible, unless it is almost time for the next dose. If a dose is skipped, the patient should not double the next dose.

VALPROATE — INJECTION

Refer to the general discussion beginning in the Anticonvulsants introduction.

WARNING

Hepatotoxicity – Hepatic failure resulting in fatalities has occurred in patients receiving valproic acid and its derivatives. Experience has indicated that children younger than 2 years of age are at a considerably increased risk of developing fatal hepatotoxicity, especially those on multiple anticonvulsants, those with congenital metabolic disorders, those with severe seizure disorders accompanied by mental retardation, and those with organic brain disease. When using valproate sodium in this patient group, use it with extreme caution and as a sole agent. Weigh the benefits of therapy against the risks. Above this age group, experience in epilepsy has indicated that the incidence of fatal hepatotoxicity decreases considerably in progressively older patient groups.

These incidents usually have occurred during the first 6 months of treatment. Serious or fatal hepatotoxicity may be preceded by nonspecific symptoms, such as anorexia, facial edema, lethargy, malaise, vomiting, and weakness. In patients with epilepsy, a loss of seizure control may also occur. Closely monitor patients for appearance of these symptoms. Perform liver function tests prior to therapy and at frequent intervals thereafter, especially during the first 6 months.

WARNING (cont.)

Teratogenicity – Valproate can produce teratogenic effects such as neural tube defects (eg, spina bifida). Accordingly, the use of valproate products in women of childbearing potential requires that the benefits of its use be weighed against the risk of injury to the fetus. This is especially important when the treatment of a spontaneously reversible condition not ordinarily associated with permanent injury or risk of death (eg, migraine) is contemplated.

Pancreatitis – Cases of life-threatening pancreatitis have been reported in both children and adults receiving valproate. Some of the cases have been described as hemorrhagic, with a rapid progression from initial symptoms to death. Cases have been reported shortly after initial use as well as after several years of use. Warn patients and guardians that abdominal pain, anorexia, nausea, or vomiting can be symptoms of pancreatitis that require prompt medical evaluation. If pancreatitis is diagnosed, valproate should ordinarily be discontinued. Initiate alternative treatment for the underlying medical condition as clinically indicated.

Indications

➤*Complex partial seizures:* As monotherapy and adjunctive therapy in the treatment of patients with complex partial seizures that occur either in isolation or in association with other types of seizures.

VALPROATE — INJECTION

➤*Simple and complex absence seizures:* For use as sole and adjunctive therapy in the treatment of patients with simple and complex absence seizures, and adjunctively in patients with multiple seizure types that include absence seizures.

➤*Off-label uses:*

Other possible off-label uses – Headaches, treatment of status epilepticus in children.

Administration and Dosage

➤*Maximum dose:*

Adults and children 2 years of age and older – 60 mg/kg/day for the treatment of simple and complex absence seizures according to the prescribing information. There is no well-established maximum dose for the other approved indications according to the prescribing information.

➤*General dosing considerations:* Valproate injection may be used as an intravenous (IV) alternative in patients for whom oral administration of valproate products is temporarily not feasible.

Equivalent doses of valproate injection and divalproex sodium yield equivalent plasma levels of the valproate ion. (See Conversion from oral products to injection.)

If satisfactory clinical response has not been achieved, plasma levels should be measured to determine whether they are in the usually accepted therapeutic range (50 to 100 mcg/mL).

If the total daily dose exceeds 250 mg, it should be given in divided doses.

➤*Adults:*

Complex partial seizures –

Monotherapy (initial therapy):

• *Initial dosage* – 10 to 15 mg/kg/day given by IV infusion.

• *Dosage titration* – The dose should be increased by 5 to 10 mg/kg/week to achieve optimal clinical response. Ordinarily, optimal clinical response is achieved at daily doses below 60 mg/kg/day.

Conversion to monotherapy: See Monotherapy (initial therapy) for dosing.

• *Conversion* – Concomitant antiepilepsy drug (AED) dosage can ordinarily be reduced approximately 25% every 2 weeks. This reduction may be started at initiation of valproate injection therapy or delayed by 1 to 2 weeks if there is a concern that seizures are likely to occur with a reduction. The speed and duration of withdrawal of the concomitant AED can be highly variable, and patients should be monitored closely during this period for increased seizure frequency.

Adjunctive therapy:

• *Initial dosage* – May be added to the patient's regimen at a dose of 10 to 15 mg/kg/day.

• *Dosage titration* – The dose may be increased by 5 to 10 mg/kg/week to achieve optimal clinical response. Ordinarily, optimal clinical response is achieved at daily doses less than 60 mg/kg/day.

Simple and complex absence seizures –

Maximum dose: 60 mg/kg/day.

Initial dosage: 15 mg/kg/day.

Dosage titration: Increase at 1-week intervals by 5 to 10 mg/kg/day until seizures are controlled or reactions preclude further increases. If the total daily dose exceeds 250 mg, it should be given in divided doses.

➤*Children:* Younger children, especially those receiving enzyme-inducing drugs, will require larger maintenance doses to attain targeted total and unbound valproic acid concentrations.

Complex partial seizures – See Adults for dosing for children 10 years of age and older.

Simple and complex absence seizures – See Adults for dosing for children 2 years of age and older.

Off-label dosing –

Headache:

• *Adolescents* –

Usual dosage: 1,000 mg as an initial dose infused at 50 mg/min. A second dose of 500 mg/dose may be given if response is not sufficient.

Alternative dosage: 20 to 40 mg/kg IV as a loading dose followed by a continuous IV infusion of 1 to 1.5 mg/kg/hour.

Seizures (acute, nonstatus epilepticus):

• *2 years of age and older* –

Usual dosage: 10 to 15 mg/kg IV every 6 hours.

Dosage titration: Increase weekly by 5 to 10 mg/kg/day until seizures are controlled.

Maintenance dosage: 30 to 60 mg/kg/day administered in divided doses every 6 hours.

Alternative dosage: 20 to 40 mg/kg IV as a loading dose followed by a continuous IV infusion of 1 to 1.5 mg/kg/hour.

Seizures (generalized status epilepticus):

• *Neonates/infants* – 10 to 25 mg/kg IV. Use only if all other options have failed and give in combination with carnitine.

• *2 years of age and older* –

Usual dosage: 13.4 to 40 mg/kg or 500 mg IV given as a loading dose. Administer further loading doses based on clinical response and serum concentrations.

Maintenance dosage: 1 mg/kg/hour IV initially. For patients on concomitant CYP-450 inducers, use 2 mg/kg/hour IV; for patients on CYP-450 inducers and also in a pentobarbital coma, use 4 to 6 mg/kg/hour.

Seizures (nonconvulsive status epilepticus):

• *2 years of age and older* – 13.4 to 25 mg/kg administered as a loading dose followed by 4 mg/kg every 6 hours.

➤*Elderly:* Because of a decrease in unbound clearance of valproate and possibly a greater sensitivity to somnolence in elderly patients, the starting dose should be reduced in these patients. Dosage should be increased more slowly and regular monitoring for fluid and nutritional intake, dehydration, somnolence, and other adverse reactions should be performed. Dose reductions or discontinuation of valproate should be considered in patients with decreased food or fluid intake and in patients with excessive somnolence. The ultimate therapeutic dose should be achieved on the basis of both tolerability and clinical response.

➤*Conversion from oral products to injection:* When switching from oral valproate products, the total daily dose of valproate injection should be equivalent to the total daily dose of the oral valproate product, and should be administered as a 60-minute infusion (but not more than 20 mg/min) with the same frequency as the oral products, although plasma concentration monitoring and dosage adjustments may be necessary. Patients receiving doses near the maximum recommended human daily dose (MRHD) of 60 mg/kg/day, particularly those not receiving enzyme-inducing drugs, should be monitored more closely. If the total daily dose exceeds 250 mg, it should be given in a divided regimen. The equivalence shown between valproate injection and oral valproate products (divalproex) at steady state was only evaluated in an every 6-hour regimen. When valproate injection is given less frequently (ie, 2 or 3 times a day), it is unknown if trough levels fall below those that result from an oral dosage form given via the same regimen. For this reason, when valproate injection is given 2 or 3 times a day, close monitoring of trough plasma levels may be needed.

➤*Dose-related adverse reactions:* The frequency of adverse reactions (particularly elevated liver enzymes and thrombocytopenia) may be dose related. The probability of thrombocytopenia appears to increase significantly at total valproate concentrations of 110 mcg/mL or more (women) or 135 mcg/mL or more (men). The benefit of improved therapeutic effect with higher doses should be weighed against the possibility of a greater incidence of adverse reactions.

➤*Therapeutic drug monitoring:* The therapeutic range in epilepsy is commonly considered to be 50 to 100 mcg/mL of total valproate, although some patients may be controlled with lower or higher plasma concentrations.

➤*Duration of therapy:* Use of valproate injection for periods of more than 14 days has not been studied. Patients should be switched to oral valproate products as soon as it is clinically feasible.

➤*Discontinuation of therapy:* AEDs should not be abruptly discontinued in patients in whom the drug is administered to prevent major seizures because of the strong possibility of precipitating status epilepticus with attendant hypoxia and threat to life.

➤*Preparation for administration:* Valproate injection should be diluted with at least 50 mL of a compatible diluent. (See Admixture compatibility.) Any unused portion of the vial contents should be discarded.

➤*Administration:* Valproate injection is for IV use only. Valproate injection should be administered as a 60-minute infusion (but not more than 20 mg/min) with the same frequency as the oral products, although plasma concentration monitoring and dosage adjustments may be necessary. If the total daily dose exceeds 250 mg, it should be given in divided doses.

Rapid infusion of valproate injection has been associated with an increase in adverse reactions. There is limited experience with infusion times of less than 60 minutes or rates of infusion greater than 20 mg/min in patients with epilepsy.

In one clinical safety study, approximately 90 patients with epilepsy and with no measurable plasma levels of valproate were given single infusions of valproate (up to 15 mg/kg and mean dose of 1,184 mg) over 5 to 10 minutes (1.5 to 3 mg/kg/min). Patients generally tolerated the more rapid infusions well. This study was not designed to assess the efficacy of these regimens.

➤*Admixture compatibility:* Valproate injection was found to be physically compatible and chemically stable in the following parenteral solutions for at least 24 hours when stored in glass or polyvinyl chloride (PVC) bags at 15° to 30°C (59° to 86°F): dextrose (5%) injection, sodium chloride (0.9%) injection, Ringer's lactate injection.

➤*Storage/Stability:* Store vials at 15° to 30°C (59° to 86°F). No preservatives have been added. Any unused portion of the container should be discarded.

Actions

➤*Pharmacology:* Valproate exists as the valproate ion in the blood. The mechanisms by which valproate exerts its therapeutic effects have not been established. It has been suggested that its activity in epilepsy is related to increased brain concentrations of gamma-aminobutyric acid (GABA).

➤*Pharmacokinetics:*

Absorption – Equivalent doses of IV valproate, oral valproate products, and divalproex are expected to result in equivalent maximal drug concentration (C_{max}), minimum concentration (C_{min}), and total systemic exposure to the valproate ion when the IV valproate is administered as a 60-minute infusion. However, the rate of valproate ion absorption may vary with the formulation used. These differences should be of minor clinical importance under the steady-state conditions achieved in chronic use in the treatment of epilepsy.

Administration of divalproex tablets and IV valproate (given as a 1-hour infusion) 250 mg every 6 hours for 4 days to 18 healthy male volunteers resulted in equivalent area under the curve (AUC), C_{max}, and C_{min} at steady state, as well as after the first dose. The T_{max} after valproate IV injection occurs at the end of the 1-hour infusion, while the T_{max} after oral dosing with divalproex occurs at approximately 4 hours. Because the kinetics of unbound valproate are linear, bioequivalence between valproate injection

VALPROATE — INJECTION

and divalproex up to the maximum recommended dose of 60 mg/kg/day can be assumed. The AUC and C_{max} resulting from administration of valproate 500 mg IV as a single 1-hour infusion and a single 500 mg dose of valproic acid syrup to 17 healthy male volunteers were also equivalent.

Patients maintained on valproic acid doses of 750 to 4,250 mg daily (given in divided doses every 6 hours) as oral divalproex alone (n = 24) or with another stabilized AED (carbamazepine [n = 15], phenobarbital [n = 1], or phenytoin [n = 11]) showed comparable plasma levels for valproic acid when switching from oral divalproex to IV valproate (1-hour infusion).

Eleven healthy volunteers were given single infusions of valproate 1,000 mg IV over 5, 10, 30, and 60 minutes in a 4-period crossover study. Total valproate concentrations were measured; unbound concentrations were not measured. After the 5-minute infusions (mean rate of 2.8 mg/kg/min), mean C_{max} was 145 ± 32 mcg/mL, while after the 60-minute infusions, mean C_{max} was 115 ± 8 mcg/mL. Total valproate concentrations were similar for all 4 rates of infusion at 90 to 120 minutes after infusion initiation. Because protein binding is nonlinear at higher total valproate concentrations, the corresponding increase in unbound C_{max} at faster infusion rates will be greater.

Distribution – The plasma protein binding of valproate is concentration dependent and the free fraction increases from approximately 10% at 40 mcg/mL to 18.5% at 130 mcg/mL. Protein binding of valproate is reduced in elderly patients, in patients with chronic hepatic diseases, in patients with renal function impairment, and in the presence of other drugs (eg, aspirin). Conversely, valproate may displace certain protein-bound drugs (eg, carbamazepine, phenytoin, tolbutamide, warfarin).

Valproate concentrations in cerebrospinal fluid (CSF) approximate unbound concentrations in plasma (about 10% of total concentration). Mean volume of distribution for total valproate is 11 L per 1.73 m^2.

The relationship between plasma concentration and clinical response is not well documented. One contributing factor is the nonlinear, concentration dependent protein binding of valproate, which affects the clearance of the drug. Thus, monitoring of total serum valproate cannot provide a reliable index of the bioactive valproate species.

For example, because the plasma protein binding of valproate is concentration dependent, the free fraction increases from approximately 10% at 40 mcg/mL to 18.5% at 130 mcg/mL. Higher than expected free fractions occur in elderly patients, in hyperlipidemic patients, and in patients with hepatic and renal diseases.

Metabolism – Valproate is metabolized almost entirely by the liver. In adult patients on monotherapy, 30% to 50% of an administered dose appears in urine as a glucuronide conjugate. Mitochondrial beta-oxidation is the other major metabolic pathway, typically accounting for over 40% of the dose. Usually, less than 15% to 20% of the dose is eliminated by other oxidative mechanisms. Less than 3% of an administered dose is excreted unchanged in urine.

The relationship between dose and total valproate concentration is nonlinear; concentration does not increase proportionally with the dose, but, rather, increases to a lesser extent because of saturable plasma protein binding. The kinetics of unbound drug are linear.

Excretion – Mean plasma clearance for total valproate is 0.56 L/h per 1.73 m^2. Mean terminal half-life for valproate monotherapy after a 60-minute IV infusion of 1,000 mg was 16 ± 3 hours.

The estimates cited apply primarily to patients who are not taking drugs that affect hepatic-metabolizing enzyme systems. For example, patients taking enzyme-inducing AEDs (carbamazepine, phenobarbital, and phenytoin) will clear valproate more rapidly. Because of these changes in valproate clearance, intensify monitoring of antiepileptic concentrations whenever concomitant antiepileptics are introduced or withdrawn.

Special populations –

Renal function impairment: A slight reduction (27%) in the unbound clearance of valproate has been reported in patients with renal failure (creatinine clearance [CrCl] less than 10 mL/min); however, hemodialysis typically reduces valproate concentrations by about 20%. Therefore, no dosage adjustment appears to be necessary in patients with renal failure. Protein binding in these patients is substantially reduced; thus, monitoring total concentrations may be misleading.

Hepatic function impairment: Liver disease impairs the capacity to eliminate valproate. In one study, the clearance of free valproate was decreased by 50% in 7 patients with cirrhosis and by 16% in 4 patients with acute hepatitis, compared with 6 healthy subjects. In that study, the half-life of valproate was increased from 12 to 18 hours. Liver disease is also associated with decreased albumin concentrations and larger unbound fractions (2- to 2.6-fold increase) of valproate. Accordingly, monitoring of total concentrations may be misleading because free concentrations may be substantially elevated in patients with hepatic disease, whereas total concentrations may appear to be normal.

Elderly: The capacity of elderly patients (range, 68 to 89 years of age) to eliminate valproate has been shown to be reduced, compared with younger adults (range, 22 to 26 years of age). Intrinsic clearance is reduced by 39%; the free fraction is increased by 44%. Accordingly, reduce the initial dosage in elderly patients.

Children: Children within the first 2 months of life have a markedly decreased ability to eliminate valproate, compared with older children and adults. This is a result of reduced clearance (perhaps due to delay in development of glucuronosyltransferase and other enzyme systems involved in valproate elimination) as well as increased volume of distribution (in part due to decreased plasma protein binding). For example, in one study, the half-life in children younger than 10 days of age ranged from 10 to 67 hours, compared with a range of 7 to 13 hours in children older than 2 months of age. Children (ie, between 3 months and 10 years of age) have 50% higher clearances expressed on weight (ie, mL/min/kg) than do adults. Older than 10 years of age, children have pharmacokinetic parameters that approximate those of adults.

Contraindications

Hepatic disease or significant hepatic function impairment; hypersensitivity to the drug; known urea cycle disorders.

Warnings/Precautions

➤*Hepatotoxicity:* See the Warning box for more information.

Observe caution when administering valproate products to patients with a history of hepatic disease. Patients on multiple anticonvulsants, children, those with congenital metabolic disorders, those with severe seizure disorders accompanied by mental retardation, and those with organic brain disease may be at particular risk. Experience has indicated that children younger than 2 years of age are at a considerably increased risk of developing fatal hepatotoxicity, especially those with the aforementioned conditions. When valproate injection is used in this patient group, use it with extreme caution and as a sole agent. Weigh the benefits of therapy against the risks. Use of valproate injection has not been studied in children younger than 2 years of age. Above this age group, experience with valproate products in epilepsy has indicated that the incidence of fatal hepatotoxicity decreases considerably in progressively older patient groups.

Discontinue the drug immediately in the presence of significant hepatic function impairment, suspected or apparent. In some cases, hepatic function impairment has progressed in spite of discontinuation of the drug.

➤*Pancreatitis:* See the Warning box for more information.

➤*Urea cycle disorders:* Valproate is contraindicated in patients with known urea cycle disorders.

Hyperammonemic encephalopathy, sometimes fatal, has been reported following initiation of valproate therapy in patients with urea cycle disorders, a group of uncommon genetic abnormalities, particularly ornithine transcarbamylase deficiency. Prior to the initiation of valproate therapy, consider evaluation for urea cycle disorders in the following patients: 1) those with a history of unexplained encephalopathy or coma, encephalopathy associated with a protein load, pregnancy-related or postpartum encephalopathy, unexplained mental retardation, or history of elevated plasma ammonia or glutamine; 2) those with ataxia, cyclical vomiting and lethargy, episodic extreme irritability, low blood urea nitrogen (BUN), or protein avoidance; 3) those with a family history of urea cycle disorders or a family history of unexplained infant deaths (particularly men); 4) those with other signs or symptoms of urea cycle disorders. Give patients who develop symptoms of unexplained hyperammonemic encephalopathy while receiving valproate therapy prompt treatment (including discontinuation of valproate therapy) and evaluate for underlying urea cycle disorders.

Hyperammonemia – Hyperammonemia has been reported in association with valproate therapy and may be present despite normal liver function tests. In patients who develop unexplained lethargy and vomiting or changes in mental status, consider hyperammonemic encephalopathy and measure an ammonia level. If ammonia is increased, discontinue valproate therapy. Initiate appropriate interventions for treatment of hyperammonemia and evaluate such patients for underlying urea cycle disorders.

Asymptomatic elevations of ammonia are more common and, when present, require close monitoring of plasma ammonia levels. If the elevation persists, consider discontinuation of valproate therapy.

Hyperammonemia and encephalopathy associated with concomitant topiramate use – Coadministration of topiramate and valproic acid has been associated with hyperammonemia with or without encephalopathy in patients who have tolerated either drug alone. Clinical symptoms of hyperammonemic encephalopathy often include acute alterations in level of consciousness and/or cognitive function with lethargy or vomiting. In most cases, symptoms and signs abated with discontinuation of either drug. This adverse reaction is not due to a pharmacokinetic interaction. It is not known if topiramate monotherapy is associated with hyperammonemia. Patients with inborn errors of metabolism or reduced hepatic mitochondrial activity may be at an increased risk for hyperammonemia with or without encephalopathy. Although not studied, an interaction of topiramate and valproic acid may exacerbate existing defects or unmask deficiencies in susceptible persons. In patients who develop unexplained changes in mental status, lethargy, or vomiting, consider hyperammonemic encephalopathy and measure an ammonia level.

➤*Thrombocytopenia:* The frequency of adverse reactions (particularly elevated liver enzymes and thrombocytopenia) may be dose related. In a clinical trial of divalproex as monotherapy in patients with epilepsy, 34 of 126 (27%) patients receiving approximately 50 mg/kg/day on average had at least 1 value of platelets 75 × 10^9/L or less. Approximately half of these patients had treatment discontinued, with return of platelet counts to normal. In the remaining patients, platelet counts normalized with continued treatment. In this study, the probability of thrombocytopenia appeared to increase significantly at total valproate concentrations of 110 mcg/mL or more (women) or 135 mcg/mL or more (men). Weigh the therapeutic benefit that may accompany the higher doses against the possibility of a greater incidence of adverse reactions. Because of reports of thrombocytopenia, inhibition of the secondary phase of platelet aggregation and abnormal coagulation parameters (eg, low fibrinogen), platelet counts, and coagulation tests are recommended before initiating therapy and at periodic intervals. It is recommended that patients receiving valproate be monitored for platelet and coagulation parameters prior to planned surgery. Evidence of hemorrhage, bruising, or a disorder of hemostasis/coagulation is an indication for reduction of the dosage or withdrawal of therapy.

VALPROATE — INJECTION

➤*Post-traumatic seizures:* A study was conducted to evaluate the effect of IV valproate in the prevention of post-traumatic seizures in patients with acute head injuries. Patients were randomly assigned to receive either IV valproate given for 1 week (followed by oral valproate products for either 1 or 6 months per random treatment assignment) or IV phenytoin given for 1 week (followed by placebo). In this study, the incidence of death was found to be higher in the 2 groups assigned to valproate treatment compared with the rate in those assigned to the IV phenytoin treatment group (13% vs 8.5%, respectively). Many of these patients were critically ill with multiple or severe injuries, and evaluation of the causes of death did not suggest any specific drug-related causation. Further, in the absence of a concurrent placebo control during the initial week of IV therapy, it is impossible to determine if the mortality rate in the patients treated with valproate was greater or less than that expected in a similar group not treated with valproate, or whether the rate seen in the IV phenytoin–treated patients was lower than would be expected. Nonetheless, until further information is available, it seems prudent not to use valproate injection in patients with acute head trauma for the prophylaxis of post-traumatic seizures.

➤*Multiorgan hypersensitivity reaction:* Multiorgan hypersensitivity reactions have been rarely reported in close temporal association with the initiation of valproate therapy in adults and children (median time to detection, 21 days; range, 1 to 40 days). Although there have been a limited number of reports, many of these cases resulted in hospitalization, and at least 1 death has been reported. Signs and symptoms of this disorder were diverse; however, patients typically, although not exclusively, presented with fever and rash associated with other organ system involvement. Other associated manifestations may include arthralgia, asthenia, hematological abnormalities (eg, eosinophilia, neutropenia, thrombocytopenia), hepatitis, hepatorenal syndrome, liver function test abnormalities, lymphadenopathy, nephritis, oliguria, and pruritis. Because the disorder is variable in its expression, other organ system symptoms and signs, not noted here, may occur. If this reaction is suspected, discontinue valproate and start an alternative treatment. Although the existence of cross-sensitivity with other drugs that produce this syndrome is unclear, the experience among drugs associated with multiorgan hypersensitivity would indicate this to be a possibility.

➤*HIV:* There are in vitro studies that suggest valproate stimulates the replication of the HIV and cytomegalovirus (CMV) under certain experimental conditions. The clinical consequence, if any, is not known. Additionally, the relevance of these in vitro findings is uncertain for patients receiving maximally suppressive antiretroviral therapy. Nevertheless, keep these data in mind when interpreting the results from regular monitoring of the viral load in HIV-infected patients receiving valproate or when following CMV-infected patients clinically.

➤*Hepatic function impairment:* Observe caution when administering valproate products to patients with a history of hepatic disease. Patients on multiple anticonvulsants, children, those with congenital metabolic disorders, those with severe seizure disorders accompanied by mental retardation, and those with organic brain disease may be at particular risk.

Discontinue the drug immediately in the presence of significant hepatic function impairment, suspected or apparent. In some cases, hepatic function impairment has progressed in spite of discontinuation of the drug.

➤*Hazardous tasks:* Because valproate injection may produce CNS depression, especially when combined with another CNS depressant (eg, alcohol), advise patients not to engage in hazardous activities, such as driving an automobile or operating dangerous machinery, until it is known that they do not become drowsy from the drug.

➤*Pregnancy:* Category D. According to the American Academy of Neurology and the American Epilepsy Society, valproic acid should be avoided if possible during pregnancy, especially during the first trimester. Valproic acid has been associated with major congenital malformations (eg, neural tube defects, facial clefts) in the offspring of women with epilepsy taking valproic acid monotherapy or as part of polytherapy. Valproic acid has also been associated with an increased risk of impaired cognitive function in children at 3 years of age. If possible, switch patients from valproic acid to a less teratogenic antiepileptic drug well before pregnancy. If a patient is already several weeks into her pregnancy, switching to another AED will not avoid the risk of major congenital malformations, since these effects occur very early in the pregnancy. A patient should consult her physician before stopping valproic acid since stopping an antiepileptic drug could lead to seizures and other serious consequences.

Teratogenic – Valproate can produce teratogenic effects. Data suggest that there is an increased incidence of congenital malformations associated with the use of valproate by women with seizure disorders during pregnancy when compared with the incidence in women with seizure disorders who do not use AEDs during pregnancy, the incidence in women with seizure disorders who use other AEDs, and the background incidence for the general population. Therefore, consider valproate for women of childbearing potential only after the risks have been thoroughly discussed with the patient and weighed against the potential benefits of treatment.

There are multiple reports in the clinical literature that indicate that the use of AEDs during pregnancy results in an increased incidence of birth defects in the offspring. Therefore, administer AEDs, including valproate, to women of childbearing potential only if they are clearly shown to be essential in the management of their medical condition.

Do not abruptly discontinue AEDs in patients in whom the drug is administered to prevent major seizures because of the strong possibility of precipitating status epilepticus with attendant hypoxia and threat to life. In individual cases in which the severity and frequency of the seizure disorder are such that the removal of medication does not pose a serious threat to the patient, discontinuation of the drug may be considered prior to and during pregnancy, although it cannot be said with any confidence that even minor seizures do not pose some hazard to the developing embryo or fetus.

Congenital malformations – The North American Antiepileptic Drug Pregnancy Registry reported 16 cases of congenital malformations among the offspring of 149 women with epilepsy who were exposed to valproic acid monotherapy during the first trimester of pregnancy at doses of approximately 1,000 mg/day, for a prevalence rate of 10.7% (95% confidence interval [CI], 6.3% to 16.9%). Three (2%) of the 149 offspring had neural tube defects and 6 (4%) of the 149 offspring had less severe malformations. Among epileptic women who were exposed to other AED monotherapies during pregnancy (1,048 patients), the malformation rate was 2.9% (95% CI, 2% to 4.1%). There was a 4-fold increase in congenital malformations among infants with valproic acid–exposed mothers, compared with those treated with other antiepileptic monotherapies as a group (odds ratio, 4; 95% CI, 2.1% to 7.4%). This increased risk does not reflect a comparison versus any specific AED, but the risk versus the heterogeneous group of all other AED monotherapies combined. The increased teratogenic risk from valproic acid in women with epilepsy is expected to be reflected in an increased risk in other indications (eg, bipolar disorder, migraine).

The strongest association of maternal valproate usage with congenital malformations is with neural tube defects. Other congenital anomalies (eg, cardiovascular malformations and anomalies involving various body systems, craniofacial defects), compatible and incompatible with life, have been reported. Sufficient data to determine the incidence of these congenital anomalies is not available.

Neural tube defects – The incidence of neural tube defects in the fetus may be increased in mothers receiving valproate during the first trimester of pregnancy. The Centers for Disease Control (CDC) has estimated the risk of valproic acid–exposed women having children with spina bifida to be approximately 1% to 2%. The American College of Obstetricians and Gynecologists (ACOG) estimates the general population risk for congenital neural tube defects as 0.14% to 0.2%.

Consider tests to detect neural tube and other defects using currently accepted procedures as a part of routine prenatal care in childbearing women receiving valproate.

Evidence suggests that pregnant women who receive folic acid supplementation may be at a decreased risk for congenital neural tube defects in their offspring, compared with pregnant women not receiving folic acid. Whether the risk of neural tube defects in the offspring of women receiving valproate specifically is reduced by folic acid supplementation is unknown. Routinely recommend dietary folic acid supplementation prior to and during pregnancy to patients contemplating pregnancy.

Other adverse pregnancy reactions – Patients taking valproate may develop clotting abnormalities. A patient who had low fibrinogen when taking multiple anticonvulsants, including valproate, gave birth to an infant with afibrinogenemia who subsequently died of hemorrhage. If valproate is used in pregnancy, monitor the clotting parameters carefully.

Patients taking valproate may develop hepatic failure. Hepatic failure, resulting in the death of a newborn and of an infant, have been reported following the use of valproate during pregnancy.

➤*Lactation:* Valproate is excreted in breast milk. Concentrations in breast milk have been reported to be 1% to 10% of serum concentrations. It is not known what effect this would have on a breast-feeding infant. Consider discontinuing breast-feeding when valproate is administered to a breast-feeding woman.

➤*Children:* Experience with oral valproate has indicated that children younger than 2 years of age are at a considerably increased risk of developing fatal hepatotoxicity, especially those on multiple anticonvulsants, those with congenital metabolic disorders, those with severe seizure disorders accompanied by mental retardation, and those with organic brain disease. The safety of valproate injection has not been studied in children younger than 2 years of age. If a decision is made to use valproate injection in this age group, use it with extreme caution and as a sole agent. Weigh the benefits of therapy against the risks. Older than 2 years of age, experience in epilepsy has indicated that the incidence of fatal hepatotoxicity decreases considerably in progressively older patient groups.

Younger children, especially those receiving enzyme-inducing drugs, will require larger maintenance doses to attain targeted total and unbound valproic acid concentrations.

The variability in free fraction limits the clinical usefulness of monitoring total serum valproic acid concentrations. Interpretation of valproic acid concentrations in children should include consideration of factors that affect hepatic metabolism and protein binding.

➤*Elderly:* No patients older than 65 years of age were enrolled in double-blind, prospective clinical trials of mania associated with bipolar illness. In a case review study of 583 patients, 72 (12%) subjects were older than 65 years of age. A higher percentage of patients older than 65 years of age reported accidental injury, infection, pain, somnolence, and tremor. Discontinuation of valproate was occasionally associated with the latter 2 reactions. It is not clear whether these reactions indicate additional risk or whether they result from preexisting medical illness and concomitant medication use among these patients.

In a double-blind, multicenter trial of valproate in elderly patients with dementia (mean age, 83 years), doses were increased by 125 mg/day to a target dose of 20 mg/kg/day. A significantly higher proportion of valproate patients had somnolence compared with placebo patients, and although not statistically significant, there was a higher proportion of patients with dehydration. Discontinuations for somnolence were also significantly higher than with placebo. In some patients with somnolence (approximately 50%), there was associated reduced nutritional intake and weight loss. There was a trend for the patients who experienced these reactions to have a lower baseline albumin concentration, lower valproate clearance, and a higher BUN.

VALPROATE — INJECTION

In elderly patients, increase dosage more slowly and regularly monitor for dehydration, fluid and nutritional intake, somnolence, and other adverse reactions. Consider dose reductions or discontinuation of valproate in patients with decreased food or fluid intake and in patients with excessive somnolence.

➤*Monitoring:* Platelet counts and coagulation tests are recommended before initiating therapy and at periodic intervals. It is recommended that patients receiving valproate injection be monitored for platelet count and coagulation parameters prior to planned surgery.

Because valproate injection may interact with coadministered drugs that are capable of enzyme induction (eg, carbamazepine, phenobarbital, phenytoin), periodic plasma concentration determinations of valproate and concomitant drugs are recommended during the early course of therapy.

Perform liver function tests prior to therapy and at frequent intervals thereafter, especially during the first 6 months of valproate therapy. However, do not rely totally on serum biochemistry because these tests may not be abnormal in all instances; also consider the results of careful interim medical history and physical examination.

Asymptomatic elevations of ammonia are more common and, when present, require close monitoring of plasma ammonia levels. If the elevation persists, consider discontinuation of valproate therapy.

In patients who develop unexplained changes in mental status, lethargy, or vomiting, consider hyperammonemic encephalopathy and measure an ammonia level.

Drug Interactions

Valproate Injection Drug Interactions

Precipitant drug	Object drug[a]		Description
Carbapenem antibiotics (eg, meropenem)	Valproate	↓	Subtherapeutic valproate levels have been reported with coadministration.
Chlorpromazine	Valproate	↑	Valproate elimination half-life and trough levels may increase; clearance may decrease.
Felbamate	Valproate	↑	Coadministration revealed a 35% increase in mean peak valproate levels.
Rifampin	Valproate	↓	In one study, rifampin increased the oral clearance of valproate by 40%.
Salicylates (eg, aspirin)	Valproate	↑	Salicylates may displace valproate from protein binding sites and may inhibit metabolism of valproate. Monitor serum concentrations.
Valproate	Barbiturates (eg, phenobarbital, primidone)	↑	Valproate may decrease hepatic metabolism of barbiturates. Barbiturate dosage may need to be decreased in some patients. Phenobarbital or primidone can double the clearance of valproate.
Barbiturates (eg, phenobarbital, primidone)	Valproate	↓	
Valproate	Benzodiazepines (eg, clonazepam, diazepam, lorazepam)	↑	Valproate displaces benzodiazepines from their plasma albumin binding sites and inhibits their metabolism, resulting in increased CNS depression. Concomitant use with clonazepam may induce absence status in patients with a history of absence seizures.
Valproate	Carbamazepine	↑	Variable changes in carbamazepine concentrations with increased levels of the active metabolite; carbamazepine decreased valproate levels with possible loss of seizure control.
Carbamazepine	Valproate	↓	
Valproate	Ethosuximide	↑↓	Increases and decreases in ethosuximide blood levels and decreases in valproate levels have been reported. Valproate appears to inhibit the metabolism of ethosuximide.
Ethosuximide	Valproate	↓	
Valproate	Hydantoins (eg, phenytoin)	↑	Increased action of phenytoin, even at therapeutic levels; increased metabolism of valproate with decreased pharmacologic effects may occur. Monitor the levels of the free concentrations of hydantoin and serum valproate.
Hydantoins (eg, phenytoin)	Valproate	↓	
Valproate	Lamotrigine	↑	Serum valproate concentrations may be decreased while lamotrigine levels increase. In one study, coadministration increased the elimination half-life of lamotrigine from 26 to 70 hours. Reduce lamotrigine dose.
Lamotrigine	Valproate	↓	
Valproate	Tolbutamide	↔	The unbound fraction of tolbutamide may be increased from 20% to 50%. The clinical relevance of this displacement is unknown.
Valproate	Topiramate	↓	Possible increased metabolism of both agents. Coadministration has been associated with hyperammonemia with and without encephalopathy.
Topiramate	Valproate		
Valproate	Tricyclic antidepressants (eg, amitriptyline, nortriptyline)	↑	Plasma concentrations and adverse reactions of the tricyclic antidepressant may be increased. Coadministration resulted in a 21% decrease in the plasma clearance of amitriptyline and a 34% decrease in the net clearance of nortriptyline.
Valproate	Warfarin	↑	The potential exists for valproate to displace warfarin from protein binding sites. Monitor coagulation tests.
Valproate	Zidovudine	↑	Zidovudine clearance was decreased by 38% in 6 HIV-seropositive patients.

[a] ↑ = object drug increased; ↓ = object drug decreased; ↔ = undetermined clinical effect.

➤*Drug/Lab test interactions:* Valproate is partially eliminated in the urine as a keto-metabolite, which may lead to a false interpretation of the urine ketone test.

There have been reports of altered thyroid function tests associated with valproate. The clinical significance of these is unknown.

Adverse Reactions

The adverse reactions that can result from valproate injection use include all of those associated with oral forms of valproate. The following describes experience specifically with valproate injection. Valproate injection has been generally well tolerated in clinical trials involving 111 healthy adult male volunteers and 352 patients with epilepsy, given at doses of 125 to 6,000 mg (total daily dose). A total of 2% of patients discontinued treatment with valproate injection because of adverse reactions. The most common adverse reactions leading to discontinuation were 2 cases each of nausea/vomiting and elevated amylase. Other adverse reactions leading to discontinuation were abnormal gait, hallucinations, headache, injection-site reaction, and pneumonia. Dizziness and injection-site pain were observed more frequently at a 100 mg/min infusion rate than at rates of up to 33 mg/min. At a 200 mg/min rate, dizziness and taste perversion occurred more frequently than at a 100 mg/min rate. The maximum rate of infusion studied was 200 mg/min.

Adverse reactions reported by 0.5% or more of all subjects/patients in clinical trials of valproate are summarized in the following table.

Valproate Injection Adverse Reactions (≥ 0.5%)

Adverse reaction	(n = 463)
Cardiovascular	
Vasodilation	0.9%
CNS	
Dizziness	5.2%
Euphoria	0.9%
Headache	4.3%
Hypesthesia	0.6%
Nervousness	0.9%
Paresthesia	0.9%
Somnolence	1.7%
Tremor	0.6%
Dermatologic	
Sweating	0.9%
GI	
Abdominal pain	1.1%
Diarrhea	0.9%
Nausea	3.2%

VALPROATE — INJECTION

Valproate Injection Adverse Reactions (≥ 0.5%)	
Adverse reaction	(n = 463)
Vomiting	1.3%
Local	
Injection-site inflammation	0.6%
Injection-site pain	2.6%
Injection-site reaction	2.4%
Respiratory	
Pharyngitis	0.6%
Special senses	
Taste perversion	1.9%
Miscellaneous	
Chest pain	1.7%
Pain (unspecified)	1.3%

In a separate clinical safety trial, 112 patients with epilepsy were given infusions of valproate (up to 15 mg/kg) over 5 to 10 minutes (1.5 to 3 mg/kg/min). The common adverse reactions (greater than 2%) were asthenia (7.1%), dizziness (7.1%), headache (2.7%), nausea (6.3%), paresthesia (7.1%), and somnolence (10.7%). While the incidence of these adverse reactions was generally higher than in the table (experience encompassing the standard, much slower infusion rates) (eg, asthenia [0%], dizziness [5.2%], headache [4.3%], nausea [3.2%], paresthesia [0.9%], somnolence [1.7%]), a direct comparison between the incidence of adverse reactions in the 2 cohorts cannot be made because of differences in patient populations and study designs.

Ammonia levels have not been systematically studied after IV valproate, so an estimate of the incidence of hyperammonemia after IV valproate cannot be provided. Hyperammonemia with encephalopathy has been reported in 2 patients after infusions of valproate.

➤*Epilepsy:*

Adjunctive therapy for complex partial seizures – Based on a placebo-controlled trial of adjunctive therapy for treatment of complex partial seizures, divalproex was generally well tolerated, with most adverse reactions rated as mild to moderate in severity. Intolerance was the primary reason for discontinuation in the divalproex-treated patients (6%), compared with 1% of placebo-treated patients.

The following table lists treatment-emergent adverse reactions that were reported by 5% or more of divalproex-treated patients and for which the incidence was greater than in the placebo group, in the placebo-controlled trial of adjunctive therapy for treatment of complex partial seizures. Because patients were also treated with other AEDs, it is not possible, in most cases, to determine whether the following adverse reactions can be ascribed to divalproex alone or the combination of divalproex and other AEDs.

Divalproex Adverse Reactions (≥ 5%) in Adjunctive Therapy for Complex Partial Seizures		
Adverse reaction	Divalproex (n = 77)	Placebo (n = 70)
CNS		
Abnormal thinking	6%	0%
Amnesia	5%	1%
Asthenia	27%	7%
Ataxia	8%	1%
Dizziness	25%	13%
Emotional lability	6%	4%
Headache	31%	21%
Somnolence	27%	11%
Tremor	25%	6%
GI		
Abdominal pain	23%	6%
Anorexia	12%	0%
Constipation	5%	1%
Diarrhea	13%	6%
Dyspepsia	8%	4%
Nausea	48%	14%
Vomiting	27%	7%
Respiratory		
Bronchitis	5%	1%
Flu syndrome	12%	9%
Infection	12%	6%
Rhinitis	5%	4%
Special senses		
Amblyopia/ Blurred vision	12%	9%
Diplopia	16%	9%
Nystagmus	8%	1%
Miscellaneous		
Alopecia	6%	1%
Fever	6%	4%
Weight loss	6%	0%

High-dose monotherapy for complex partial seizures – The following table lists treatment-emergent adverse reactions that were reported by 5% or more of patients in the high-dose divalproex group, and for which the incidence was greater than in the low-dose group, in a controlled trial of divalproex monotherapy treatment of complex partial seizures. Because patients were being titrated off another AED during the first portion of the trial, it is not possible, in many cases, to determine whether the following adverse reactions can be ascribed to divalproex alone, or the combination of divalproex and other AEDs.

Divalproex Adverse Reactions (≥ 5%) in the High-Dose Monotherapy for Complex Partial Seizures[a]		
Adverse reaction	High-dose (n = 131)	Low-dose (n = 134)
CNS		
Amnesia	7%	4%
Asthenia	21%	10%
Depression	5%	4%
Dizziness	18%	13%
Insomnia	15%	9%
Nervousness	11%	7%
Somnolence	30%	18%
Tremor	57%	19%
Dermatologic		
Alopecia	24%	13%
GI		
Abdominal pain	12%	9%
Anorexia	11%	4%
Diarrhea	23%	19%
Dyspepsia	11%	10%
Nausea	34%	26%
Vomiting	23%	15%
Hematologic/Lymphatic		
Ecchymosis	5%	4%
Thrombocytopenia	24%	1%
Metabolic/Nutritional		
Peripheral edema	8%	3%
Weight gain	9%	4%
Respiratory		
Dyspnea	5%	1%
Infection	20%	13%
Pharyngitis	8%	2%
Special senses		
Amblyopia/ Blurred vision	8%	4%
Nystagmus	7%	1%
Tinnitus	7%	1%

[a] Headache was the only adverse reaction that occurred in 5% or more of patients in the high-dose group and at an equal or greater incidence in the low-dose group.

➤*Complex partial seizures:* The following additional adverse reactions were reported by more than 1% but less than 5% of the 358 patients treated with divalproex in the controlled trials of complex partial seizures:

Cardiovascular – Hypertension, palpitation, tachycardia.

CNS – Abnormal dreams, abnormal gait, anxiety, confusion, hypertonia, incoordination, malaise, paresthesia, personality disorder.

Dermatologic – Dry skin, pruritus, rash.

GI – Eructation, flatulence, hematemesis, increased appetite, pancreatitis, periodontal abscess.

GU – Amenorrhea, dysmenorrhea, urinary frequency, urinary incontinence, vaginitis.

Hematologic/Lymphatic – Petechia.

Hepatic – ALT increased, AST increased.

VALPROATE — INJECTION

Musculoskeletal – Arthralgia, leg cramps, myalgia, myasthenia, twitching.

Respiratory – Epistaxis, cough increased, pneumonia, sinusitis.

Special senses – Abnormal vision, deafness, otitis media, taste perversion.

Miscellaneous – Back pain, chest pain.

➤*Mania:* Although valproate injection has not been evaluated for safety and efficacy in the treatment of manic episodes associated with bipolar disorder, the following adverse reactions not previously listed were reported by 1% or more of patients from 2 placebo-controlled clinical trials of divalproex tablets.

Cardiovascular – Hypotension, postural hypotension, vasodilation.

CNS – Agitation, catatonic reaction, hypokinesia, reflexes increased, tardive dyskinesia, vertigo.

Dermatologic – Furunculosis, maculopapular rash, seborrhea.

GI – Fecal incontinence, gastroenteritis, glossitis.

GU – Dysuria.

Musculoskeletal – Arthrosis.

Special senses – Conjunctivitis, dry eyes, eye pain.

Miscellaneous – Chills, neck pain, neck rigidity.

➤*Migraine:* Although valproate injection has not been evaluated for safety and efficacy in the prophylactic treatment of migraine headaches, the following adverse reactions not previously listed were reported by 1% or more of patients from 2 placebo-controlled clinical trials of divalproex tablets.

GI – Dry mouth, stomatitis.

GU – Cystitis, metrorrhagia, vaginal hemorrhage.

Miscellaneous – Face edema.

➤*Other adverse reactions (all dosage forms):*

CNS – Aggression, behavioral deterioration, depression, emotional upset, hostility, hyperactivity, psychosis.

Sedative effects have occurred in patients receiving valproate alone but occur most often in patients receiving combination therapy. Sedation usually abates upon reduction of other antiepileptic medication. Asterixis, ataxia, confusion, diplopia, dizziness, dysarthria, hallucinations, headache, hypesthesia, incoordination, nystagmus, parkinsonism, "spots before eyes," tremor (may be dose related), and vertigo have been reported with the use of valproate. Rare cases of coma have occurred in patients receiving valproate alone or in conjunction with phenobarbital. In rare instances, encephalopathy with or without fever, has developed shortly after the introduction of valproate monotherapy without evidence of hepatic function impairment or inappropriately high plasma valproate levels. Although recovery has been described following drug withdrawal, there have been fatalities in patients with hyperammonemic encephalopathy, particularly in patients with underlying urea cycle disorders.

Several reports have noted reversible cerebral atrophy and dementia in association with valproate therapy.

Dermatologic – Erythema multiforme, generalized pruritus, photosensitivity, skin rash, Stevens-Johnson syndrome, and transient hair loss. Rare cases of toxic epidermal necrolysis have been reported including a fatal case in a 6-month-old infant taking valproate and several other concomitant medications. An additional case of toxic epidermal necrosis resulting in death was reported in a 35-year-old patient with AIDS taking several concomitant medications and with a history of multiple cutaneous drug reactions. Serious skin reactions have been reported with coadministration of lamotrigine and valproate.

Endocrine – Breast enlargement, galactorrhea, irregular menses, parotid gland swelling, and secondary amenorrhea; abnormal thyroid function tests.

There have been rare spontaneous reports of polycystic ovary disease. A cause-and-effect relationship has not been established.

GI – The most commonly reported adverse reactions at the initiation of therapy are nausea, indigestion, and vomiting. These effects are usually transient and rarely require discontinuation of therapy. Abdominal cramps, constipation, and diarrhea have been reported. Both anorexia with some weight loss and increased appetite with weight gain have also been reported. The administration of delayed-release divalproex may result in reduction of GI adverse reactions in some patients using oral therapy.

GU – Enuresis and urinary tract infection.

Hematologic – Thrombocytopenia and inhibition of the secondary phase of platelet aggregation may be reflected in altered bleeding time, bruising, epistaxis, frank hemorrhage, hematoma formation, and petechiae. Evidence of bruising, a disorder of hemostasis/coagulation, or hemorrhage is an indication for reduction of the dosage or withdrawal of therapy. Acute intermittent porphyria, agranulocytosis, anemia including macrocytic with or without folate deficiency, aplastic anemia, bone marrow suppression, eosinophilia, hypofibrinogenemia, leukopenia, macrocytosis, relative lymphocytosis, pancytopenia.

Hepatic – Acute pancreatitis, including fatalities, minor elevations of transaminases (eg, ALT, AST) and lactate dehydrogenase are frequent and appear to be dose related. Occasionally, laboratory test results include increases in serum bilirubin and abnormal changes in other liver function tests. These results may reflect potentially serious hepatotoxicity.

Metabolic – Hyperammonemia, hyponatremia, and inappropriate antidiuretic hormone secretion. There have been rare reports of Fanconi syndrome occurring chiefly in children. Decreased carnitine concentrations have been reported, although the clinical relevance is undetermined. Hyperglycinemia has occurred and was associated with a fatal outcome in a patient with preexistent nonketotic hyperglycinemia.

Musculoskeletal – Weakness.

Special senses – Hearing loss, either reversible or irreversible, has been reported; however, a cause-and-effect relationship has not been established. Ear pain has also been reported.

Miscellaneous – Allergic reaction, anaphylaxis, bone pain, bradycardia, cough increased, cutaneous vasculitis, edema of the extremities, fever, hypothermia, lupus erythematosus, otitis media, pneumonia.

Overdosage

➤*Symptoms:* Overdosage with valproate may result in somnolence, heart block, and deep coma. Fatalities have been reported; however, patients have recovered from valproate serum concentrations as high as 2,120 mcg/mL.

➤*Treatment:* In overdose situations, the fraction of drug not bound to protein is high and hemodialysis or tandem hemodialysis plus hemoperfusion may result in significant removal of drug. Apply general supportive measures with particular attention to the maintenance of adequate urinary output.

Naloxone has been reported to reverse the CNS-depressant effects of valproate overdosage. Because naloxone could theoretically also reverse the antiepilepsy effects of valproate, use it with caution in patients with epilepsy.

Patient Information

Warn patients and guardians that abdominal pain, anorexia, nausea, and/or vomiting can be symptoms of pancreatitis and, therefore, require further medical evaluation promptly.

Inform patients of the signs and symptoms associated with hyperammonemic encephalopathy and tell them to inform their health care provider if any of these symptoms occur.

Because valproate injection may produce CNS depression, especially when combined with another CNS depressant (eg, alcohol), advise patients not to engage in hazardous activities, such as driving an automobile or operating dangerous machinery, until it is known that they do not become drowsy from the drug.

Because divalproex has been associated with certain types of birth defects, advise women of childbearing age considering the use of valproate of the risk and of alternative therapeutic options. Tell them to read the patient information section, which appears as the last section of the labeling. This is especially important when the treatment of a spontaneously reversible condition not ordinarily associated with permanent injury or risk of death (eg, migraine) is considered.

Instruct patients that a fever associated with other organ system involvement (eg, lymphadenopathy, rash) may be drug-related and tell them to report such reactions to their health care provider immediately.

Advise diabetic patients that this medication may interfere with urine tests for ketones.

MUSCLE RELAXANTS — ADJUNCTS TO ANESTHESIA

Nondepolarizing Neuromuscular Blockers

ATRACURIUM BESYLATE

Rx	**Atracurium Besylate** (Bedford Labs)	**Injection:** 10 mg/mL[a]	In 5 mL single-dose and 10 mL multi-dose vials.[b]
Rx	**Tracrium** (GlaxoWellcome)		In 5 mL single-use and 10 mL multi-dose vials.[c]

[a] With benzenesulfonic acid.
[b] With 0.9% benzyl alcohol in multi-dose vials.
[c] With 0.9% benzyl alcohol.

ATRACURIUM BESYLATE — INJECTION

Indications

As an adjunct to general anesthesia, to facilitate endotracheal intubation and to provide skeletal muscle relaxation during surgery or mechanical ventilation.

Administration and Dosage

➤*General dosing considerations:* Atracurium should not be administered before unconsciousness has been induced.

Use a peripheral nerve stimulator to monitor twitch suppression and recovery.

ATRACURIUM BESYLATE — INJECTION

➤*Adults:*

Bolus doses for intubation and maintenance of neuromuscular block –

Initial dosage: 0.4 to 0.5 mg/kg (1.7 to 2.2 times the ED_{95}), given as an intravenous (IV) bolus injection. With this dose, good or excellent conditions for nonemergency intubation can be expected in 2 to 2.5 minutes in most patients, with maximum neuromuscular block achieved approximately 3 to 5 minutes after injection. Clinically required neuromuscular block generally lasts 20 to 35 minutes under balanced anesthesia.

Maintenance dosage: 0.08 to 0.10 mg/kg for maintenance of neuromuscular block during prolonged surgical procedures. The first maintenance dose will generally be required 20 to 45 minutes after the initial injection of atracurium, but the need for maintenance doses should be determined by clinical criteria. Because atracurium lacks cumulative effects, maintenance doses may be administered at relatively regular intervals for each patient, ranging approximately from 15 to 25 minutes under balanced anesthesia and slightly longer under isoflurane or enflurane. Higher doses of atracurium (up to 0.2 mg/kg) permit maintenance dosing at longer intervals.

Concomitant therapy with inhalation anesthesia: Atracurium is potentiated by isoflurane or enflurane anesthesia. The same initial dose of atracurium may be used for intubation prior to administration of these inhalation agents; however, if atracurium is first administered under steady state of isoflurane or enflurane, the initial dose of atracurium should be reduced by approximately one-third (ie, to 0.25 to 0.35 mg/kg). With halothane, which has only a marginal (approximately 20%) potentiating effect on atracurium, smaller dosage reductions may be considered.

Recovery from neuromuscular block: Under balanced anesthesia, recovery to 25% of control is achieved approximately 35 to 45 minutes after injection, and recovery is usually 95% complete approximately 60 minutes after injection.

Infusion in the operating room for maintenance of neuromuscular block –

Initial dosage:

Infusion of atracurium should be initiated only after early evidence of spontaneous recovery from the bolus dose. An initial infusion rate of 9 to 10 mcg/kg/min may be required to rapidly counteract the spontaneous recovery of neuromuscular function.

Maintenance dosage: A rate of 5 to 9 mcg/kg/min should be adequate to maintain continuous neuromuscular block in the range of 89% to 99% in most patients under balanced anesthesia. Occasional patients may require infusion rates as low as 2 mcg/kg per minute or as high as 15 mcg/kg per minute.

Dosage adjustment: The rate of administration should be adjusted according to the patient's response as determined by peripheral nerve stimulation. Accurate dosing is best achieved using a precision infusion device.

Cardiopulmonary bypass patients: In patients undergoing cardiopulmonary bypass with induced hypothermia, the rate of infusion of atracurium required to maintain adequate surgical relaxation during hypothermia (25° to 28°C; 77° to 82.4°F) has been shown to be approximately half the rate required during normothermia.

Concomitant therapy with inhalation anesthesia: The neuromuscular-blocking effect of atracurium administered by infusion is potentiated by enflurane or isoflurane and, to a lesser extent, by halothane. Reduction in the infusion rate of atracurium should, therefore, be considered for patients receiving inhalation anesthesia. The infusion rate of atracurium should be reduced by approximately one-third in the presence of steady-state enflurane or isoflurane anesthesia; smaller reductions should be considered in the presence of halothane.

Recovery from neuromuscular block: Spontaneous recovery from neuromuscular block following discontinuation of infusion of atracurium may be expected to proceed at a rate comparable with that following administration of a single bolus dose.

Infusion in the intensive care unit (ICU) – An infusion rate of 11 to 13 mcg/kg/min (range, 4.5 to 29.5) should provide adequate neuromuscular block. There may be wide interpatient variability in dosage requirements and these requirements may increase or decrease with time. Following recovery from neuromuscular block, readministration of a bolus dose may be necessary to quickly reestablish neuromuscular block prior to reinstitution of the infusion.

➤*Children:*

2 years of age or older – See Adults for dosing.

1 month to 2 years of age –

Initial dosage: 0.3 to 0.4 mg/kg under halothane anesthesia.

Maintenance dosage: Maintenance doses may be required with slightly greater frequency in infants and children than in adults.

➤*Patients requiring reduced doses:* An initial dose of atracurium of 0.3 to 0.4 mg/kg, given slowly or in divided doses over 1 minute, is recommended for adults, adolescents, children, or infants with significant cardiovascular disease and for adults, adolescents, children, or infants with any history (eg, severe anaphylactoid reactions or asthma) suggesting a greater risk of histamine release.

Dosage reductions must be considered also in patients with neuromuscular disease, severe electrolyte disorders, or carcinomatosis in which potentiation of neuromuscular block or difficulties with reversal have been demonstrated.

➤*Concomitant use with succinylcholine:*

Adults – An initial dose of atracurium of 0.3 to 0.4 mg/kg is recommended following the use of succinylcholine for intubation under balanced anesthesia. Further reductions may be desirable with the use of potent inhalation anesthetics. The patient should be permitted to recover from the effects of succinylcholine prior to administration of atracurium.

➤*Preparation for administration:* Infusion solutions of atracurium may be prepared by admixing atracurium with an appropriate diluent such as dextrose 5% injection; sodium chloride 0.9% injection; or dextrose 5% and sodium chloride 0.9% injection. Care should be taken during admixture to prevent inadvertent contamination.

➤*Administration:* Administer IV. Do not give by intramuscular (IM) administration. IM administration may result in tissue irritation.

Infusion rate tables – The amount of infusion solution required per minute will depend upon the concentration of atracurium in the infusion solution, the desired dose of atracurium, and the patient's weight.

Infusion Rates of Atracurium Besylate for a Concentration of 0.2 mg/mL

	Drug delivery rate (mcg/kg per minute)								
	5	6	7	8	9	10	11	12	13
Patient weight (kg)	Infusion delivery rate (mL/h)								
30	45	54	63	72	81	90	99	108	117
35	53	63	74	84	95	105	116	126	137
40	60	72	84	96	108	120	132	144	156
45	68	81	95	108	122	135	149	162	176
50	75	90	105	120	135	150	165	180	195
55	83	99	116	132	149	165	182	198	215
60	90	108	126	144	162	180	198	216	234
65	98	117	137	156	176	195	215	234	254
70	105	126	147	168	189	210	231	252	273
75	113	135	158	180	203	225	248	270	293
80	120	144	168	192	216	240	264	288	312
90	135	162	189	216	243	270	297	324	351
100	150	180	210	240	270	300	330	360	390

Infusion Rates of Atracurium Besylate for a Concentration of 0.5 mg/mL

	Drug delivery rate (mcg/kg per minute)								
	5	6	7	8	9	10	11	12	13
Patient weight (kg)	Infusion delivery rate (mL/h)								
30	18	22	25	29	32	36	40	43	47
35	21	25	29	34	38	42	46	50	55
40	24	29	34	38	43	48	53	58	62
45	27	32	38	43	49	54	59	65	70
50	30	36	42	48	54	60	66	72	78
55	33	40	46	53	59	66	73	79	86
60	36	43	50	58	65	72	79	86	94
65	39	47	55	62	70	78	86	94	101
70	42	50	59	67	76	84	92	101	109
75	45	54	63	72	81	90	99	108	117
80	48	58	67	77	86	96	106	115	125
90	54	65	76	86	97	108	119	130	140
100	60	72	84	96	108	120	132	144	156

➤*Admixture compatibility:* Spontaneous degradation of atracurium has been demonstrated to occur more rapidly in Ringer's lactate solution than in sodium chloride 0.9% solution. Therefore, it is recommended that Ringer's lactate injection not be used as a diluent in preparing solutions of atracurium for infusion.

Atracurium, which has an acid pH, should not be mixed with alkaline solutions (eg, barbiturate solutions) in the same syringe or administered simultaneously during intravenous infusion through the same needle. Depending on the resultant pH of such mixtures, atracurium may be inactivated and a free acid may be precipitated.

➤*Storage/Stability:* Atracurium should be refrigerated at 2° to 8°C (36° to 46°F) to preserve potency. Do not freeze. Upon removal from refrigeration to room temperature storage conditions (25°C; 77°F), use atracurium within 14 days even if re-refrigerated.

Infusion solutions should be used within 24 hours of preparation. Unused solutions should be discarded. Solutions containing 0.2 or 0.5 mg/mL atracurium in diluents (See Preparation for administration) may be stored either under refrigeration or at room temperature for 24 hours without significant loss of potency.

Actions

➤*Pharmacology:* Atracurium besylate is a nondepolarizing skeletal muscle relaxant. Nondepolarizing agents antagonize the neurotransmitter action of acetylcholine by binding competitively with cholinergic receptor sites on the motor end-plate. This antagonism is inhibited, and neuromuscular block reversed, by acetylcholinesterase inhibitors such as neostigmine, edrophonium, and pyridostigmine.

The duration of neuromuscular block produced by atracurium besylate is approximately one-third to one-half the duration of block by d-tubocurarine, metocurine, and pancuronium at initially equipotent doses. As with other

ATRACURIUM BESYLATE — INJECTION

nondepolarizing neuromuscular blockers, the time to onset of paralysis decreases and the duration of maximum effect increases with increasing doses of atracurium besylate.

Hemodynamic – Atracurium besylate is a less potent histamine releaser than d-tubocurarine or metocurine. Histamine release is minimal with initial doses of atracurium besylate up to 0.5 mg/kg, and hemodynamic changes are minimal within the recommended dose range. A moderate histamine release and significant falls in blood pressure have been seen following 0.6 mg/kg of atracurium besylate. The histamine and hemodynamic responses were poorly correlated. The effects were generally short-lived and manageable, but the possibility of substantial histamine release in sensitive individuals or in patients in whom substantial histamine release would be especially hazardous (eg, patients with significant cardiovascular disease) must be considered.

➤*Pharmacokinetics:*

Absorption – The pharmacokinetics of atracurium besylate in humans are essentially linear within the 0.3 to 0.6 mg/kg dose range.

Metabolism / Excretion – The duration of neuromuscular block produced by atracurium besylate does not correlate with plasma pseudocholinesterase levels and is not altered by the absence of renal function. This is consistent with the results of in vitro studies that have shown that atracurium besylate is inactivated in plasma via 2 nonoxidative pathways; ester hydrolysis, catalyzed by nonspecific esterases; and Hofmann elimination, a nonenzymatic chemical process that occurs at physiological pH. Some placental transfer occurs in humans.

The elimination half-life is approximately 20 minutes.

Radiolabel studies demonstrated that atracurium besylate undergoes extensive degradation in cats, and that neither kidney nor liver plays a major role in its elimination. Biliary and urinary excretion were the major routes of excretion of radioactivity (totaling greater than 90% of the labeled dose within 7 hours of dosing), of which atracurium besylate represented only a minor fraction. The metabolites in bile and urine were similar, including products of Hofmann elimination and ester hydrolysis.

Contraindications

Known hypersensitivity to atracurium besylate. Use of atracurium besylate from multiple-dose vials containing benzyl alcohol as a preservative is contraindicated in patients with a known hypersensitivity to benzyl alcohol.

Warnings/Precautions

➤*Administration:* Atracurium besylate should be used only by those skilled in airway management and respiratory support. Equipment and personnel must be immediately available for endotracheal intubation and support of ventilation, including administration of positive pressure oxygen. Adequacy of respiration must be assured through assisted or controlled ventilation. Anticholinesterase reversal agents should be immediately available.

Do not give atracurium besylate by intramuscular administration.

➤*Benzyl alcohol:* Atracurium besylate injection 10 mL multiple-dose vials contain benzyl alcohol. In neonates, benzyl alcohol has been associated with an increased incidence of neurological and other complications that are sometimes fatal. Atracurium besylate injection 5 mL single-use vials do not contain benzyl alcohol (see Children).

➤*Long-term use in intensive care unit (ICU):* When there is a need for long-term mechanical ventilation, the benefits-to-risk ratio of neuromuscular block must be considered. The long-term (1 to 10 days) infusion of atracurium besylate during mechanical ventilation in the ICU has been evaluated in several studies. Average infusion rates of 11 to 13 mcg/kg/min (range, 4.5 to 29.5) were required to achieve adequate neuromuscular block. These data suggest that there is wide interpatient variability in dosage requirements. In addition, these studies have shown that dosage requirements may decrease or increase with time. Following discontinuation of infusion of atracurium besylate in these ICU studies, spontaneous recovery of 4 twitches in a train-of-4 occurred in an average of approximately 30 minutes (range, 15 to 75 minutes) and spontaneous recovery to a train-of-4 ratio more than 75% (the ratio of the height of the fourth to the first twitch in a train-of-4) occurred in an average of approximately 60 minutes (range, 32 to 108 minutes).

Little information is available on the plasma levels and clinical consequences of atracurium metabolites that may accumulate during days to weeks of atracurium administration in ICU patients. Laudanosine, a major biologically active metabolite of atracurium without neuromuscular blocking activity, produces transient hypotension and, in higher doses, cerebral excitatory effects (generalized muscle twitching and seizures) when administered to several species of animals. There have been rare spontaneous reports of seizures in ICU patients who have received atracurium or other agents. These patients usually had predisposing causes (such as head trauma, cerebral edema, hypoxic encephalopathy, viral encephalitis, uremia). There are insufficient data to determine whether or not laudanosine contributes to seizures in ICU patients.

Whenever the use of atracurium besylate or any neuromuscular blocking agent is contemplated in the ICU, it is recommended that neuromuscular transmission be monitored continuously during administration with the help of a nerve stimulator. Additional doses of atracurium besylate or any other neuromuscular blocking agent should not be given before there is a definite response to T_1 or to the first twitch. If no response is elicited, infusion administration should be discontinued until a response returns.

Hemofiltration has a minimal effect on plasma levels of atracurium and its metabolites, including laudanosine. The effects of hemodialysis and hemoperfusion on plasma levels of atracurium and its metabolites are unknown.

➤*Risk of bradycardia:* Since atracurium besylate has no clinically significant effects on heart rate in the recommended dosage range, it will not counteract the bradycardia produced by many anesthetic agents or vagal stimulation. As a result, bradycardia during anesthesia may be more common with atracurium besylate than with other muscle relaxants.

➤*Special risk:*

Burn patients – Resistance to nondepolarizing neuromuscular blocking agents may develop in burn patients. Increased doses of nondepolarizing muscle relaxants may be required in burn patients and are dependent on the time elapsed since the burn injury and the size of the burn.

Malignant hyperthermia (MH) – Multiple factors in anesthesia practice are suspected of triggering malignant hyperthermia (MH), a potentially fatal hypermetabolic state of skeletal muscle. Halogenated anesthetic agents and succinylcholine are recognized as the principal pharmacologic triggering agents in MH-susceptible patients; however, since MH can develop in the absence of established triggering agents, the clinician should be prepared to recognize and treat MH in any patient scheduled for general anesthesia. Reports of MH have been rare in cases in which atracurium besylate has been used. In studies of MH-susceptible animals (swine) and in a clinical study of MH-susceptible patients, atracurium besylate did not trigger this syndrome.

Myasthenia gravis, Eaton-Lambert syndrome, or other neuromuscular diseases – Atracurium besylate may have profound effects in patients with myasthenia gravis, Eaton-Lambert syndrome, or other neuromuscular diseases in which potentiation of nondepolarizing agents has been noted. The use of a peripheral nerve stimulator is especially important for assessing neuromuscular block in these patients. Similar precautions should be taken in patients with severe electrolyte disorders or carcinomatosis.

Histamine release – Although atracurium besylate is a less potent histamine releaser than d-tubocurarine or metocurine, the possibility of substantial histamine release in sensitive individuals must be considered. Special caution should be exercised in administering atracurium besylate to patients in whom substantial histamine release would be especially hazardous (eg, patients with clinically significant cardiovascular disease) and in patients with any history (eg, severe anaphylactoid reactions or asthma) suggesting a greater risk of histamine release. In these patients, the recommended initial dose of atracurium besylate is lower (0.3 to 0.4 mg/kg) than for other patients and should be administered slowly or in divided doses over 1 minute.

➤*Pregnancy:* Category C.

Teratogenic – Atracurium besylate has been shown to be potentially teratogenic in rabbits when given in doses up to approximately one-half the human dose. There are no adequate and well-controlled studies in pregnant women. Atracurium besylate should be used during pregnancy only if the potential benefit justifies the potential risk to the fetus.

Atracurium besylate was administered subcutaneously on days 6 through 18 of gestation to nonventilated Dutch rabbits. Treatment groups were given either 0.15 mg/kg once daily or 0.10 mg/kg twice daily. Lethal respiratory distress occurred in 2 animals given 0.15 mg/kg and in 1 animal given 0.10 mg/kg, with transient respiratory distress or other evidence of neuromuscular block occurring in 10 of 19 and in 4 of 20 of the animals given 0.15 mg/kg and 0.10 mg/kg, respectively. There was an increased incidence of certain spontaneously occurring visceral and skeletal anomalies or variations in 1 or both treated groups when compared to nontreated controls. The percentage of male fetuses was lower (41% vs 51%) and the postimplantation losses were increased (15% vs 8%) in the group given 0.15 mg/kg once daily when compared to the controls; the mean numbers of implants (6.5 vs 4.4) and healthy live fetuses (5.4 vs 3.8) were greater in this group when compared to the control group.

Labor and delivery – Atracurium besylate (0.3 mg/kg) has been administered to 26 pregnant women during delivery by cesarean section. No harmful effects were attributable to atracurium besylate in any of the neonates, although small amounts of atracurium besylate were shown to cross the placental barrier. The possibility of respiratory depression in the neonate should always be considered following cesarean section during which a neuromuscular blocking agent has been administered. In patients receiving magnesium sulfate, the reversal of neuromuscular block may be unsatisfactory and the dose of atracurium besylate should be lowered as indicated.

➤*Lactation:* It is not known whether this drug is excreted in human milk. Because many drugs are excreted in human milk, caution should be exercised when atracurium besylate is administered to a nursing woman.

➤*Children:* Safety and effectiveness in pediatric patients below the age of 1 month have not been established.

➤*Elderly:* Since marketing in 1983, uncontrolled clinical experience and limited data from controlled trials have not identified differences in effectiveness, safety, or dosage requirements between healthy elderly and younger patients; however, as with other neuromuscular blocking agents, the use of a peripheral nerve stimulator to monitor neuromuscular function is suggested.

ATRACURIUM BESYLATE — INJECTION

Drug Interactions

Atracurium Drug Interactions

Precipitant drug	Object drug[a]		Description
Diuretics	Atracurium	↑	The neuromuscular blocking effects of atracurium may be increased by thiazide diuretics. Hypokalemia enhances the neuromuscular blockade, possibly by hyperpolarizing the end-plate membrane, increasing resistance to depolarization.
General anesthetics (enflurane, isoflurane, halothane) Antibiotics (eg, aminoglycosides, polypeptide antibiotics) Lithium Verapamil Procainamide Quinidine	Atracurium	↑	These medications may enhance the neuromuscular blocking action of atracurium. Neuromuscular blockade was prolonged 20% by halothane and 35% by enflurane and isoflurane.
Magnesium sulfate	Atracurium	↑	When administered for the management of toxemia of pregnancy, may enhance neuromuscular blockade of pancuronium. However, in one patient, reversal of neuromuscular blockade was not affected by magnesium sulfate.
Other muscle relaxants	Atracurium	↔	If administered during the same procedure, consider the possibility of a synergistic or antagonist effect.
Phenytoin Theophylline	Atracurium	↓	Phenytoin and theophylline may cause resistance to, or reversal of, the neuromuscular blocking action of atracurium.
Succinylcholine	Atracurium	↑	Succinylcholine does not enhance duration, but quickens onset and may increase depth of atracurium-induced neuromuscular blockade.
Acetylcholinesterase inhibitors (eg, neostigmine, edrophonium and pyridostigmine	Atracurium	↓	Antagonism is inhibited and neuromuscular block is reversed by acetylcholinesterase inhibitors.
Corticosteroids	Atracurium	↑	Prolonged weakness may occur.

[a] ↑ = object drug increased; ↓ = object drug decreased; ↔ = undetermined effect.

Adverse Reactions

➤*Observed in controlled clinical studies:* Atracurium besylate was well tolerated and produced few adverse reactions during extensive clinical trials. Most adverse reactions were suggestive of histamine release. In studies including 875 patients, atracurium besylate was discontinued in only 1 patient (who required treatment for bronchial secretions), and 6 other patients required treatment for adverse reactions attributable to atracurium besylate (wheezing in 1, hypotension in 5). Of the 5 patients who required treatment for hypotension, 3 had a history of significant cardiovascular disease. The overall incidence rate for clinically important adverse reactions, therefore, was 7/875 or 0.8%. The table below includes all adverse reactions reported attributable to atracurium besylate during clinical trials with 875 patients.

Atracurium Adverse Reactions

Adverse reaction	Initial dose of atracurium besylate (mg/kg)			
	0 to 0.3 (mg/kg) (n = 485)	0.31 to 0.5[a] (mg/kg) (n = 366)	≥ 0.6 (mg/kg) (n = 24)	Total (mg/kg) (n = 875)
Skin flush	1%	8.7%	29.2%	5%
Erythema	0.6%	0.5%	0%	0.6%
Itching	0.4%	0%	0%	0.2%
Wheezing/bronchial secretions	0.2%	0.3%	0%	0.2%
Hives	0.2%	0%	0%	0.1%

[a] Includes the recommended initial dosage range for most patients.

Most adverse reactions were of little clinical significance unless they were associated with significant hemodynamic changes. The table below summarizes the incidences of substantial vital sign changes noted during clinical trials of atracurium besylate with 530 patients, without cardiovascular disease, in whom these parameters were assessed.

Patients Showing > 30% Vital Sign Changes Following Administration of Atracurium Besylate (%)

Vital sign change	Initial atracurium besylate dose (mg/kg)			
	0 to 0.3 (mg/kg) (n = 365)	0.31 to 0.5[a] (mg/kg) (n = 144)	≥ 0.6 (mg/kg) (n = 21)	Total (mg/kg) (n = 530)
Mean arterial pressure				
Increase	1.9%	2.8%	0%	2.1%
Decrease	1.1%	2.1%	14.3%	1.9%
Heart rate				
Increase	1.6%	2.8%	4.8%	2.1%
Decrease	0.8%	0%	0%	0.6%

[a] Includes the recommended initial dosage range for most patients.

➤*Observed in clinical practice:* Based on initial clinical practice experience in approximately 3 million patients who received atracurium besylate in the US and in the United Kingdom, spontaneously reported adverse reactions were uncommon (approximately 0.01% to 0.02%). The following adverse reactions are among the most frequently reported, but there are insufficient data to support an estimate of their incidence:

Allergic – Allergic reactions (anaphylactic or anaphylactoid responses) which, in rare instances, were severe (eg, cardiac arrest).

Cardiovascular – Hypotension, vasodilatation (flushing), tachycardia, bradycardia.

CNS – There have been rare spontaneous reports of seizures in ICU patients following long-term infusion of atracurium to support mechanical ventilation. There are insufficient data to define the contribution, if any, of atracurium or its metabolite laudanosine.

Local – Rash, urticaria, reaction at injection site.

Musculoskeletal – Inadequate block, prolonged block.

Respiratory – Dyspnea, bronchospasm, laryngospasm.

Overdosage

➤*Symptoms:* There has been limited experience with overdosage of atracurium besylate. The possibility of iatrogenic overdosage can be minimized by carefully monitoring muscle twitch response to peripheral nerve stimulation. Excessive doses of atracurium besylate can be expected to produce enhanced pharmacological effects. Overdosage may increase the risk of histamine release and cardiovascular effects, especially hypotension.

Three pediatric patients (3 weeks, 4 and 5 months of age) unintentionally received doses of 0.8 mg/kg to 1 mg/kg of atracurium besylate. The time to 25% recovery (50 to 55 minutes) following these doses, which were 5 to 6 times the ED_{95} dose, was moderately longer than the corresponding time observed following doses 20 to 2.5 times the atracurium besylate ED_{95} dose in infants (22 to 36 minutes). Cardiovascular changes were minimal. Nonetheless the possibility of cardiovascular changes must be considered in the case of overdose.

An adult patient (17 years of age) unintentionally received an initial dose of 1.3 mg/kg of atracurium besylate. The time from injection to 25% recovery (83 minutes) was approximately twice that observed following maximum recommended doses in adults (35 to 45 minutes). The patient experienced moderate hemodynamic changes (13% increase in mean arterial pressure and 27% increase in heart rate) which persisted for 40 minutes and did not require treatment.

➤*Treatment:* If cardiovascular support is necessary, this should include proper positioning, fluid administration, and the use of vasopressor agents if necessary. The patient's airway should be assured, with manual or mechanical ventilation maintained as necessary. A longer duration of neuromuscular block may result from overdosage and a peripheral nerve stimulator should be used to monitor recovery. Recovery may be facilitated by administration of an anticholinesterase reversing agent such as neostigmine, edrophonium, or pyridostigmine, in conjunction with an anticholinergic agent such as atropine or glycopyrrolate. The appropriate monographs should be consulted for prescribing information.

CISATRACURIUM BESYLATE

Rx	Nimbex (Abbott)	Injection, solution: 2 mg/mL	In 5 mL single-use and 10 mL multiple-use[a] vials.
		10 mg/mL	In 20 mL single-use vials.

[a] Contains benzyl alcohol 0.9%.

CISATRACURIUM BESYLATE — INJECTION

Indications

For inpatients and outpatients as an adjunct to general anesthesia, to facilitate tracheal intubation, and to provide skeletal muscle relaxation during surgery or mechanical ventilation in the ICU.

Administration and Dosage

➤*General dosing considerations:* The use of a peripheral nerve stimulator will permit the most advantageous use of cisatracurium, minimize the possibility of overdosage or underdosage, and assist in the evaluation of recovery.

➤*Adults:*

Adjunct to general anesthesia –

Initial dosage: Doses of 0.15 ($3 \times ED_{95}$) and 0.2 ($4 \times ED_{95}$) mg/kg, as components of a propofol/nitrous oxide/oxygen induction-intubation technique, may produce generally good or excellent conditions for intubation in 2 and 1.5 minutes, respectively. Similar intubation conditions may be expected when these doses of cisatracurium are administered as components of a thiopental/nitrous oxide/oxygen induction-intubation technique.

Maintenance dosage: Maintenance doses of 0.03 mg/kg each sustain neuromuscular block for approximately 20 minutes. Maintenance dosing is generally required 40 to 50 minutes following an initial dose of cisatracurium 0.15 mg/kg and 50 to 60 minutes following an initial dose of cisatracurium 0.2 mg/kg, but the need for maintenance doses should be determined by clinical criteria. For shorter or longer durations of action, smaller or larger maintenance doses may be administered.

Concomitant therapy: Isoflurane or enflurane administered with nitrous oxide/oxygen to achieve 1.25 minimum alveolar concentration (MAC) may prolong the clinically effective duration of action of initial and maintenance doses. The magnitude of these effects may depend on the duration of administration of the volatile agents. Fifteen to 30 minutes of exposure to 1.25 MAC isoflurane or enflurane had minimal effects on the duration of action of initial doses of cisatracurium and, therefore, no adjustment to the initial dose should be necessary when cisatracurium is administered shortly after initiation of volatile agents. In long surgical procedures during enflurane or isoflurane anesthesia, less frequent maintenance dosing or lower maintenance doses of cisatracurium may be necessary.

Continuous infusion in the operating room –

Initial dosage:

Initiate infusion only after early evidence of spontaneous recovery from the initial bolus dose. An initial infusion rate of 3 mcg/kg/min may be required to rapidly counteract the spontaneous recovery of neuromuscular function.

Maintenance dosage: A rate of 1 to 2 mcg/kg/min should be adequate to maintain continuous neuromuscular block in the range of 89% to 99% in most patients under opioid/nitrous oxide/oxygen anesthesia.

Dosage adjustment: Adjust the rate of administration according to the patient's response, as determined by peripheral nerve stimulation. Accurate dosing is best achieved using a precision infusion device.

Concomitant therapy: Consider reduction of the infusion rate by up to 30% to 40% when cisatracurium is administered during stable isoflurane or enflurane anesthesia (administered with nitrous oxide/oxygen at the 1.25 MAC level). Greater reductions in the infusion rate of cisatracurium may be required with longer durations of administration of isoflurane or enflurane.

Coronary artery bypass patients: The rate of infusion of atracurium required to maintain adequate surgical relaxation in patients undergoing coronary artery bypass surgery with induced hypothermia (25° to 28°C; 77° to 82.4°F) is approximately half the rate required during normothermia. Based on the structural similarity between cisatracurium and atracurium, a similar effect on the infusion rate of cisatracurium may be expected.

Recovery from neuromuscular block: Spontaneous recovery from neuromuscular block following discontinuation of infusion of cisatracurium may be expected to proceed at a rate comparable with that following administration of a single bolus dose.

Infusion in the intensive care unit –

An infusion rate of approximately 3 mcg/kg/min (range, 0.5 to 10.2 mcg/kg/min) should provide adequate neuromuscular block. Following recovery from neuromuscular block, readministration of a bolus dose may be necessary to quickly reestablish neuromuscular block prior to reinstitution of the infusion.

➤*Children:*

2 to 12 years of age –

Bolus doses for intubation: 0.1 to 0.15 mg/kg administered over 5 to 10 seconds during halothane or opioid anesthesia. When administered during stable opioid/nitrous oxide/oxygen anesthesia, 0.1 mg/kg produces maximum neuromuscular block in an average of 2.8 minutes (range, 1.8 to 6.7 minutes) and clinically effective block for 28 minutes (range, 21 to 38 minutes). When administered during stable opioid/nitrous oxide/oxygen anesthesia, 0.15 mg/kg produces maximum neuromuscular block in approximately 3 minutes (range, 1.5 to 8 minutes) and clinically effective block (time to 25% recovery) for 36 minutes (range, 29 to 46 minutes).

Continuous infusion in the operating room: See Adults for dosing.

1 to 23 months of age – 0.15 mg/kg administered over 5 to 10 seconds during halothane or opioid anesthesia. When administered during stable opioid/nitrous oxide/oxygen anesthesia, 0.15 mg/kg produces maximum neuromuscular block in approximately 2 minutes (range, 1.3 to 3.4 minutes) and clinically effective block (time to 25% recovery) for approximately 43 minutes (range, 34 to 58 minutes).

➤*Elderly:* Extending the interval between administration of cisatracurium and the intubation attempt for these patients may be required to achieve adequate intubation conditions.

➤*Renal function impairment:* Extending the interval between administration of cisatracurium and the intubation attempt for these patients may be required to achieve adequate intubation conditions.

➤*Preparation for administration:* Do not use solutions that are not clear or that contain visible particulates. Cisatracurium is a colorless to slightly yellow or greenish yellow solution.

➤*Administration:* Cisatracurium should only be administered IV.

Infusion rate tables – The amount of infusion solution required per minute will depend upon the concentration of cisatracurium in the infusion solution, the desired dose of cisatracurium, and the patient's weight. The contribution of the infusion solution to the fluid requirements of the patient also must be considered.

Cistracurium Infusion Rates for a Concentration of 0.1 mg/mL

	Drug delivery rate (mcg/kg/min)				
	1	1.5	2	3	5
Patient weight	Infusion delivery rate (mL/hr)				
10 kg	6	9	12	18	30
45 kg	27	41	54	81	135
70 kg	42	63	84	126	210
100 kg	60	90	120	180	300

Cistracurium Infusion Rates for a Concentration of 0.4 mg/mL

	Drug delivery rate (mcg/kg/min)				
	1	1.5	2	3	5
Patient weight	Infusion delivery rate (mL/hr)				
10 kg	1.5	2.3	3	4.5	7.5
45 kg	6.8	10.1	13.5	20.3	33.8
70 kg	10.5	15.8	21	31.5	52.5
100 kg	15	22.5	30	45	75

➤*Admixture compatibility:*

Compatibility – Cisatracurium is compatible with the following: 5% Dextrose Injection; 0.9% Sodium Chloride Injection; 5% Dextrose and 0.9% Sodium Chloride Injection; sufentanil, alfentanil, fentanyl, midazolam, and droperidol injection, diluted as directed.

Incompatibility – Cisatracurium is acidic (pH = 3.25 to 3.65) and may not be compatible with alkaline solution having a pH greater than 8.5 (eg, barbiturate solutions). Do not dilute in Lactated Ringer's Injection due to chemical instability. Cisatracurium is not compatible with propofol or ketorolac for Y-site administration.

➤*Storage/Stability:* Store at 2° to 8°C (36° to 46°F) in the carton to preserve potency. Protect from light. Do not freeze. Upon removal from refrigeration to room temperature (25°C [77°F]), use within 21 days, even if rerefrigerated.

Cisatracurium injection diluted in 5% Dextrose Injection, 0.9% Sodium Chloride Injection, or 5% Dextrose and 0.9% Sodium Chloride Injection to 0.1 mg/mL may be stored either under refrigeration or at room temperature for 24 hours without significant loss of potency. Dilutions to 0.1 or 0.2 mg/mL in 5% Dextrose and Lactated Ringer's Injection may be stored under refrigeration for 24 hours.

Actions

➤*Pharmacology:*

Pharmacodynamics – Cisatracurium binds competitively to cholinergic receptors on the motor end-plate to antagonize the action of acetylcholine, resulting in block of neuromuscular transmission. This action is antagonized by acetylcholinesterase inhibitors such as neostigmine.

➤*Pharmacokinetics:*

Absorption – Following administration of radiolabeled cisatracurium, 95% of the dose was recovered in the urine; less than 10% of the dose was excreted as unchanged parent drug. Laudanosine, a metabolite of cisatracurium (and atracurium) has been noted to cause transient hypotension and,

CISATRACURIUM BESYLATE — INJECTION

in higher doses, cerebral excitatory effects when administered to several animal species. The relationship between CNS excitation and laudanosine concentrations in humans has not been established. Because cisatracurium is 3 times more potent than atracurium, and lower doses are required, the corresponding laudanosine concentrations following cisatracurium are one-third of those that would be expected following an equipotent dose of atracurium.

Distribution – The volume of distribution of cisatracurium is limited by its large molecular weight and high polarity. The V_{ss} (volume of distribution at steady state) was equal to 145 mL/kg in healthy 19- to 64-year-old surgical patients receiving opioid anesthesia. The V_{ss} was 21% larger in similar patients receiving inhalation anesthesia.

Metabolism – The degradation of cisatracurium is largely independent of liver metabolism. Results from in vitro experiments suggest that cisatracurium undergoes Hofmann elimination (a pH- and temperature-dependent chemical process) to form laudanosine and the monoquaternary acrylate metabolite. The monoquaternary acrylate undergoes hydrolysis by nonspecific plasma esterases to form the monoquaternary alcohol (MQA) metabolite. The MQA metabolite can also undergo Hofmann elimination but at a much slower rate than cisatracurium. Laudanosine is further metabolized to desmethyl metabolites that are conjugated with glucuronic acid and excreted in the urine.

Organ-independent Hofmann elimination is the predominant pathway for the elimination of cisatracurium. The liver and kidney play a minor role in the elimination of cisatracurium but are primary pathways for the elimination of metabolites. Therefore, the t½β values of metabolites (including laudanosine) are longer in patients with kidney or liver dysfunction, and metabolite concentrations may be higher after long-term administration. Most importantly, C_{max} values of laudanosine are significantly lower in healthy surgical patients receiving infusions of cisatracurium than in patients receiving infusions of atracurium (mean ± SD C_{max}: 60 ± 52 and 342 ± 93 ng/mL, respectively).

Excretion – Mean clearance (CL) values for cisatracurium ranged from 4.5 to 5.7 mL/min/kg in studies of healthy surgical patients. Compartmental pharmacokinetic modeling suggests that approximately 80% of the CL is accounted for by Hofmann elimination and the remaining 20% by renal and hepatic elimination. These findings are consistent with the low magnitude of interpatient variability in CL (16%) estimated as part of the population PK/PD analyses and with the recovery of parent and metabolites in urine. Following ^{14}C-cisatracurium administration to 6 healthy male patients, 95% of the dose was recovered in the urine (mostly as conjugated metabolites) and 4% in the feces; less than 10% of the dose was excreted as unchanged parent drug in the urine. In 12 healthy surgical patients receiving nonradiolabeled cisatracurium who had Foley catheters placed for surgical management, approximately 15% of the dose was excreted unchanged in the urine.

In studies of healthy surgical patients, mean t½β values of cisatracurium ranged from 22 to 29 minutes and were consistent with the t½β of cisatracurium in vitro (29 minutes). The mean ± SD t½β values of laudanosine were 3.1 ± 0.4 and 3.3 ± 2.1 hours in healthy surgical patients receiving cisatracurium besylate (n = 10) or atracurium (n = 10), respectively. During IV infusions of cisatracurium besylate, peak plasma concentrations (C_{max}) of laudanosine and the MQA metabolite are approximately 6% and 11% of the parent compound, respectively.

The neuromuscular-blocking activity of cisatracurium besylate is due to parent drug. Cisatracurium plasma concentration-time data following IV bolus administration are best described by a 2-compartment open model (with elimination from both compartments) with an elimination half-life (t½β) of 22 minutes, a plasma clearance (CL) of 4.57 mL/min/kg, and a V_{ss} of 145 mL/kg. Cisatracurium undergoes organ-independent Hofmann elimination (a chemical process dependent on pH and temperature) to form the monoquaternary acrylate metabolite and laudanosine, neither of which has any neuromuscular-blocking activity.

Special populations –

Renal function impairment: Results from a conventional pharmacokinetic study of cisatracurium in 13 healthy adult patients and 15 patients with end-stage renal disease (ESRD) undergoing elective surgery are summarized below. The pharmacokinetic/pharmacodynamic parameters of cisatracurium were similar in healthy adult patients and ESRD patients. The times to 90% block were approximately 1 minute slower in ESRD patients following 0.1 mg/kg cisatracurium. There were no differences in the durations or rates of recovery of cisatracurium between ESRD and healthy adult patients.

The t½β values of metabolites are longer in patients with renal failure and concentrations may be higher after long-term administration.

Population pharmacokinetic analyses revealed that patients with creatinine clearances less than or equal to 70 mL/min had slower rates of equilibration between plasma concentrations and neuromuscular block than patients with normal renal function; this change was associated with slightly slower (approximately 40 seconds) predicted times to 90% T_1 suppression in patients with renal dysfunction following 0.1 mg/kg cisatracurium. There was no clinically significant alteration in the recovery profile of cisatracurium besylate in patients with renal dysfunction. The recovery profile of cisatracurium is unchanged in the presence of renal or hepatic failure, which is consistent with predominantly organ-independent elimination.

Hepatic function impairment: The information summarizes the conventional pharmacokinetic analysis from a study of cisatracurium in 13 patients with end-stage liver disease undergoing liver transplantation and 11 healthy adult patients undergoing elective surgery. The slightly larger volumes of distribution in liver transplant patients were associated with slightly higher plasma clearances of cisatracurium. The parallel changes in these parameters resulted in no difference in t½β values. There were no differences in k_{eo} or EC_{50} between patient groups. The times to maximum block were approximately 1 minute faster in liver transplant patients than in healthy adult patients receiving 0.1 mg/kg cisatracurium. These minor differences in pharmacokinetics were not associated with clinically significant differences in the recovery profile of cisatracurium.

The t½β values of metabolites are longer in patients with hepatic disease, and concentrations may be higher after long-term administration.

Elderly: The results of conventional pharmacokinetic analysis from a study of 12 healthy elderly patients and 12 healthy young adult patients receiving a single IV dose of 0.1 mg/kg cisatracurium are summarized below. Plasma clearances of cisatracurium were not affected by age; however, the volumes of distribution were slightly larger in elderly patients than in young patients, resulting in slightly longer t½β values for cisatracurium. The rate of equilibration between plasma cisatracurium concentrations and neuromuscular block was slower in elderly patients than in young patients (mean ± SD k_{eo}: 0.071 ± 0.036 and 0.105 ± 0.021 minutes^{-1}, respectively); there was no difference in the patient sensitivity to cisatracurium-induced block, as indicated by EC_{50} values (mean ± SD EC_{50}: 91 ± 22 and 89 ± 23 ng/mL, respectively). These changes were consistent with the 1-minute slower times to maximum block in elderly patients receiving 0.1 mg/kg cisatracurium, when compared to young patients receiving the same dose. The minor differences in pharmacokinetic/pharmacodynamic parameters of cisatracurium between elderly patients and young patients were not associated with clinically significant differences in the recovery profile of cisatracurium.

Children: The population pharmacokinetics/pharmacodynamics of cisatracurium were described in 20 healthy children during halothane anesthesia, using the same model developed for healthy adult patients. The CL was higher in healthy children (5.89 mL/min/kg) than in healthy adult patients (4.57 mL/min/kg) during opioid anesthesia. The rate of equilibration between plasma concentrations and neuromuscular block, as indicated by k_{eo}, was faster in healthy children receiving halothane anesthesia (0.133 minutes^{-1}) than in healthy adult patients receiving opioid anesthesia (0.0575 minutes^{-1}). The EC_{50} in healthy children (125 ng/mL) was similar to the value in healthy adult patients (141 ng/mL) during opioid anesthesia. The minor differences in the pharmacokinetic/pharmacodynamic parameters of cisatracurium were associated with a faster time to onset and a shorter duration of cisatracurium-induced neuromuscular block in children.

Other patient factors: Population pharmacokinetic/pharmacodynamic analyses revealed that gender and obesity were associated with statistically significant effects on the pharmacokinetics or pharmacodynamics of cisatracurium; these factors were not associated with clinically significant alterations in the predicted onset or recovery profile of cisatracurium. The use of inhalation agents was associated with a 21% larger V_{ss}, a 78% larger k_{eo}, and a 15% lower EC_{50} for cisatracurium. These changes resulted in a slightly faster (approximately 45 seconds) predicted time to 90% T_1 suppression in patients receiving 0.1 mg/kg cisatracurium during inhalation anesthesia than in patients receiving the same dose of cisatracurium during opioid anesthesia; however, there were no clinically significant differences in the predicted recovery profile of cisatracurium between patient groups.

Contraindications

Hypersensitivities to cisatracurium or other bis-benzylisoquinolinium agents. Use of cisatracurium from vials containing benzyl alcohol as a preservative is contraindicated in patients with a known hypersensitivity to benzyl alcohol.

Warnings/Precautions

➤*Administration:* Administer cisatracurium in carefully adjusted dosage by or under the supervision of experienced clinicians who are familiar with the drug's actions and the possible complications of its use. Do not administer the drug unless personnel and facilities for resuscitation and life support (tracheal intubation, artificial ventilation, oxygen therapy), and an antagonist of cisatracurium besylate are immediately available. It is recommended that a peripheral nerve stimulator be used to measure neuromuscular function during the administration of cisatracurium besylate in order to monitor drug effect, determine the need for additional doses, and confirm recovery from neuromuscular block.

Cisatracurium besylate has no known effect on consciousness, pain threshold, or cerebration. To avoid distress to the patient, do not induce neuromuscular block before unconsciousness.

➤*Benzyl alcohol:* The 10 mL multiple-dose vials of cisatracurium besylate contain benzyl alcohol. In newborn infants, benzyl alcohol has been associated with an increased incidence of neurological and other complications which are sometimes fatal. Single-use vials (5 mL and 20 mL) of cisatracurium besylate do not contain benzyl alcohol.

Because of its intermediate onset of action, cisatracurium is not recommended for rapid sequence endotracheal intubation.

➤*Renal/Hepatic function impairment:* See Actions for more information.

➤*Special risk:* Acid-base or serum electrolyte abnormalities may potentiate or antagonize the action of neuromuscular-blocking agents.

Long-term use in the ICU – Long-term infusion (up to 6 days) of cisatracurium during mechanical ventilation in the ICU has been safely used in 2 studies. Dosage requirements may increase or decrease with time.

Whenever the use of cisatracurium or any other neuromuscular-blocking agent in the ICU is contemplated, monitor neuromuscular function during administration with a nerve stimulator. Do not give additional doses of cisatracurium or any other neuromuscular-blocking agent before there is a definite response to nerve stimulation. If no response is elicited, discontinue infusion administration until a response returns.

CISATRACURIUM BESYLATE — INJECTION

Malignant hyperthermia (MH) – In a study of MH-susceptible pigs, cisatracurium besylate (highest dose 2,000 mcg/kg equivalent to 3 × ED_{95} in pigs and 40 × ED_{95} in humans) did not trigger MH. Cisatracurium has not been studied in MH-susceptible patients. Because MH can develop in the absence of established triggering agents, be prepared to recognize and treat MH in any patient undergoing general anesthesia.

Neuromuscular-blocking agents may have a profound effect in patients with neuromuscular diseases (eg, myasthenia gravis, the myasthenic syndrome). In these and other conditions in which prolonged neuromuscular block is a possibility (eg, carcinomatosis), the use of a peripheral nerve stimulator and a dose of not more than 0.02 mg/kg cisatracurium is recommended to assess the level of neuromuscular block and to monitor dosage requirements.

Burn patients – Patients with burns have been shown to develop resistance to nondepolarizing neuromuscular-blocking agents, including atracurium. The extent of altered response depends upon the size of the burn and the time elapsed since the burn injury. Cisatracurium has not been studied in patients with burns; however, based on its structural similarity to atracurium, the possibility of increased dosing requirements and shortened duration of action must be considered if cisatracurium besylate is administered to burn patients.

Hemiparesis/Paraparesis – Patients with hemiparesis or paraparesis also may demonstrate resistance to nondepolarizing muscle relaxants in the affected limbs. To avoid inaccurate dosing, perform neuromuscular monitoring on a nonparetic limb.

➤*Pregnancy: Category B.*

Teratogenic – There are no adequate and well-controlled studies of cisatracurium in pregnant women. Because animal studies are not always predictive of human response, use cisatracurium during pregnancy only if clearly needed.

➤*Lactation:* It is not known whether cisatracurium besylate is excreted in human milk. Because many drugs are excreted in human milk, exercise caution following administration of cisatracurium besylate to a nursing woman.

➤*Children:* Cisatracurium besylate has not been studied in children below the age of 1 month. Intubation of the trachea in patients 1 to 4 years old was facilitated more reliably when cisatracurium besylate was used in combination with halothane than when opioids and nitrous oxide were used for induction of anesthesia.

➤*Elderly:* Of the total number of subjects in clinical studies of cisatracurium, 57 were 65 years and over, 63 were 70 years and over, and 15 were 80 years and over. The geriatric population included a subset of patients with significant cardiovascular disease. No overall differences in safety or effectiveness were observed between these subjects and younger subjects, and other reported clinical experience has not identified differences in responses between elderly and younger subjects, but greater sensitivity of some older individuals to cisatracurium cannot be ruled out.

See Actions for more information.

➤*Monitoring:* Whenever the use of cisatracurium or any other neuromuscular-blocking agent in the ICU is contemplated, monitor neuromuscular function during administration with a nerve stimulator. Do not give additional doses of cisatracurium or any other neuromuscular-blocking agent before there is a definite response to nerve stimulation. If no response is elicited, discontinue infusion administration until a response returns.

Drug Interactions

➤*Succinylcholine:* Cisatracurium has been used safely following varying degrees of recovery from succinylcholine-induced neuromuscular block. Administration of 0.1 mg/kg (2 × ED_{95}) cisatracurium at 10% or 95% recovery following an intubating dose of succinylcholine (1 mg/kg) produced greater than or equal to 95% neuromuscular block. The time to onset of maximum block following cisatracurium is approximately 2 minutes faster with prior administration of succinylcholine. Prior administration of succinylcholine had no effect on the duration of neuromuscular block following initial or maintenance bolus doses of cisatracurium. Infusion requirements of cisatracurium in patients administered succinylcholine prior to infusions of cisatracurium were comparable to or slightly greater than when succinylcholine was not administered.

➤*General anesthetics:* Isoflurane or enflurane administered with nitrous oxide/oxygen to achieve 1.25 MAC (minimum alveolar concentration) may prolong the clinically effective duration of action of initial and maintenance doses of cisatracurium and decrease the required infusion rate of cisatracurium. The magnitude of these effects may depend on the duration of administration of the volatile agents. Fifteen to 30 minutes of exposure to 1.25 MAC isoflurane or enflurane had minimal effects on the duration of action of initial doses of cisatracurium and, therefore, no adjustment to the initial dose should be necessary when cisatracurium is administered shortly after initiation of volatile agents. In long surgical procedures during enflurane or isoflurane anesthesia, less frequent maintenance dosing, lower maintenance doses, or reduced infusion rates of cisatracurium besylate may be necessary. The average infusion rate requirement may be decreased by as much as 30% to 40%.

➤*Other drugs:* Other drugs which may enhance the neuromuscular-blocking action of nondepolarizing agents such as cisatracurium include certain antibiotics (eg, aminoglycosides, tetracyclines, bacitracin, polymyxins, lincomycin, clindamycin, colistin, sodium colistemethate), magnesium salts, lithium, local anesthetics, procainamide, and quinidine.

➤*Phenytoin and carbamazepine:* Resistance to the neuromuscular-blocking action of nondepolarizing neuromuscular blocking agents has been demonstrated in patients chronically administered phenytoin or carbamazepine. While the effects of chronic phenytoin or carbamazepine therapy on the action of cisatracurium are unknown, slightly shorter durations of neuromuscular block may be anticipated and infusion rate requirements may be higher.

Adverse Reactions

➤*Observed in clinical trials of surgical patients:* Adverse reactions were uncommon among the 945 surgical patients who received cisatracurium in conjunction with other drugs in US and European clinical studies in the course of a wide variety of procedures in patients receiving opioid, propofol, or inhalation anesthesia. The following adverse reactions were judged by investigators during the clinical trials to have a possible causal relationship to administration of cisatracurium:

Incidence less than 1% –
Cardiovascular: Bradycardia (0.4%), hypotension (0.2%), flushing (0.2%).
Dermatologic: Rash (0.1%).
Respiratory: Bronchospasm (0.2%).

➤*Observed in clinical trials of ICU patients:* Adverse reactions were uncommon among the 68 ICU patients who received cisatracurium in conjunction with other drugs in US and European clinical studies. One patient experienced bronchospasm. In 1 of the 2 ICU studies, a randomized and double-blind study of ICU patients using TOF neuromuscular monitoring, there were 2 reports of prolonged recovery (167 and 270 minutes) among 28 patients administered cisatracurium and 13 reports of prolonged recovery (range, 90 minutes to 33 hours) among 30 patients administered vecuronium.

➤*Postmarketing:* In addition to adverse reactions reported from clinical trials, the following reactions have been identified during postapproval use of cisatracurium in conjunction with 1 or more anesthetic agents in clinical practice. Because they are reported voluntarily from a population of unknown size, estimates of frequency cannot be made. These reactions have been chosen for inclusion due to a combination of their seriousness, frequency of reporting, or potential causal connection to cisatracurium.

Hypersensitivity – Histamine release, hypersensitivity reactions including anaphylactic or anaphylactoid responses which, in rare instances, were severe. There are rare reports of wheezing, laryngospasm, bronchospasm, rash, and itching following administration of cisatracurium in children. These reported adverse events were not serious, and their etiology could not be established with certainty.

Musculoskeletal – Prolonged neuromuscular block, inadequate neuromuscular block, muscle weakness, and myopathy.

Overdosage

➤*Treatment:* Overdosage with neuromuscular-blocking agents may result in neuromuscular block beyond the time needed for surgery and anesthesia. The primary treatment is maintenance of a patient airway and controlled ventilation until recovery of normal neuromuscular function is ensured. Once recovery from neuromuscular block begins, further recovery may be facilitated by administration of an anticholinesterase agent (eg, neostigmine, edrophonium) in conjunction with an appropriate anticholinergic agent.

Do not administer antagonists (such as neostigmine and edrophonium) when complete neuromuscular block is evident or suspected. The use of a peripheral nerve stimulator to evaluate recovery and antagonism of neuromuscular block is recommended.

Administration of 0.04 to 0.07 mg/kg neostigmine at approximately 10% recovery from neuromuscular block (range, 0% to 15%) produced 95% recovery of the muscle twitch response and a T_4:T_1 ratio greater than or equal to 70% in an average of 9 to 10 minutes. The times from 25% recovery of the muscle twitch response to a T_4:T_1 ratio greater than or equal to 70% following these doses of neostigmine averaged 7 minutes. The mean 25% to 75% recovery index following reversal was 3 to 4 minutes.

Administration of 1 mg/kg edrophonium at approximately 25% recovery from neuromuscular block (range, 16% to 30%) produced 95% recovery and a T_4:T_1 ratio greater than or equal to 70% in an average of 3 to 5 minutes.

Evaluate patients administered antagonists for evidence of adequate clinical recovery (eg, 5-second head lift and grip strength). Ventilation must be supported until no longer required.

The onset of antagonism may be delayed in the presence of debilitation, cachexia, carcinomatosis, and the concomitant use of certain broad spectrum antibiotics, or anesthetic agents and other drugs that enhance neuromuscular block or separately cause respiratory depression. Under such circumstances the management is the same as that of prolonged neuromuscular block.

ROCURONIUM BROMIDE

Rx	Rocuronium Bromide (Various, eg, Generamedix, Hospira, Sicor Pharmaceuticals)	Injection, solution: 10 mg/mL	In 5 mL and 10 mL multidose vials.
Rx	Zemuron (Organon)		In 5 mL and 10 mL multidose vials.

ROCURONIUM BROMIDE — INJECTION

Indications

➤*Adjunct to general anesthesia:* For inpatients and outpatients as an adjunct to general anesthesia to facilitate both rapid sequence and routine tracheal intubation and to provide skeletal muscle relaxation during surgery or mechanical ventilation.

Administration and Dosage

➤*General dosing considerations:* In patients in whom potentiation of, or resistance to, neuromuscular block is anticipated, consider a dose adjustment (see Special risk patients).

Use a peripheral nerve stimulator to monitor drug effect, need for additional doses, and adequacy of spontaneous recovery or antagonism, and to decrease the complications of overdosage if additional doses are administered.

➤*Adults:*

Continuous infusion –

Initial dosage: 10 to 12 mcg/kg/min only after early evidence of spontaneous recovery from an intubating dose (see Administration for infusion rate tables).

Dosage adjustment: Because of rapid redistribution and the associated rapid spontaneous recovery, initiation of the infusion after substantial return of neuromuscular function (more than 10% of control T_1) may necessitate additional bolus doses to maintain adequate block for surgery. Upon reaching the desired level of neuromuscular block, the infusion of rocuronium must be individualized for each patient. In clinical trials, infusion rates have ranged from 4 to 16 mcg/kg/min.

Rapid sequence intubation – 0.6 to 1.2 mg/kg will provide excellent or good intubating conditions in most appropriately premedicated and adequately anesthetized patients in less than 2 minutes.

Tracheal intubation –

Initial dosage: 0.6 mg/kg. Neuromuscular block sufficient for intubation (80% block or more) is attained in a median time of 1 (0.4 to 6) minute(s), and most patients have intubation completed within 2 minutes. Maximum blockade is achieved in most patients in less than 3 minutes. This dose may be expected to provide 31 (15 to 85) minutes of clinical relaxation under opioid/nitrous oxide/oxygen anesthesia. Under halothane, isoflurane, and enflurane anesthesia, expect some extension of the period of clinical relaxation.

Maintenance dosage: 0.1, 0.15, and 0.2 mg/kg administered at 25% recovery of control T_1 (defined as 3 twitches of train-of-4), provide a median (range) of 12 (2 to 31), 17 (6 to 50), and 24 (7 to 69) minutes of clinical duration under opioid/nitrous oxide/oxygen anesthesia. In all cases, guide dosing based on the clinical duration following initial dose or prior maintenance dose and do not administer until recovery of neuromuscular function is evident. A clinically insignificant cumulation of effect with repetitive maintenance dosing has been observed.

Alternative dosage: 0.45 mg/kg. Neuromuscular block sufficient for intubation (80% block or more) is attained in a median (range) time of 1.3 (0.8 to 6.2) minute(s), and most patients have intubation completed within 2 minutes. Maximum blockade is achieved in most patients in less than 4 minutes. This dose may be expected to provide 22 (12 to 31) minutes of clinical relaxation under opioid/nitrous oxide/oxygen anesthesia. Patients receiving this low dose of 0.45 mg/kg who achieve less than 90% block (about 16% of these patients) may have a more rapid time to 25% recovery, 12 to 15 minutes.

A large bolus dose of 0.9 or 1.2 mg/kg can be administered under opioid/nitrous oxide/oxygen anesthesia without adverse reactions to the cardiovascular system.

➤*Children:*

Tracheal intubation –

17 years of age and younger under sevoflurane (induction) and isoflurane/nitrous oxide (maintenance):

• *Initial dosage* – 0.45 and 0.6 mg/kg generally produce excellent to good intubating conditions within 75 seconds.

• *Maintenance dosage* – Bolus doses of 0.15 mg/kg at reappearance of T_3. Maintenance dosing also can be administered at the reappearance of T_2 at a rate of 7 to 10 mcg/kg/min, with the lowest dose requirement for neonates (birth to younger than 28 days of age) and the highest dose requirement for children (older than 2 years of age to 11 years of age).

3 months to 14 years of age under halothane anesthesia:

• *Initial dosage* – 0.6 mg/kg produces excellent to good intubating conditions within 1 minute.

• *Maintenance dosage* – 0.075 to 0.125 mg/kg, administered on return of T_1 to 25% of control, providing clinical relaxation for 7 to 10 minutes.

• *Alternative dosage* – A continuous infusion initiated at a rate of 12 mcg/kg/min on return of T_1 to 10% of control (1 twitch present in the train-of-4) also may be used.

➤*Hepatic function impairment:* If used for rapid sequence induction in patients with ascites, an increased initial dosage may be necessary to ensure complete block. Duration will be prolonged in these cases. The use of doses higher than 0.6 mg/kg has not been studied.

➤*Obesity:* The initial dose of rocuronium 0.6 mg/kg should be based on the patient's actual body weight.

➤*Prolonged circulation time:* Do not increase the initial dosage in patients with prolonged circulation time to reduce onset time; instead, in these situations, when feasible, allow more time for the drug to achieve onset of effect.

➤*Special risk patients:* Nondepolarizing neuromuscular-blocking agents have been found to exhibit profound neuromuscular-blocking effects in cachectic or debilitated patients, patients with neuromuscular diseases, and patients with carcinomatosis. In these or other patients in whom potentiation of neuromuscular block or difficulty with reversal may be anticipated, consider a decrease from the recommended initial dose. Resistance to nondepolarizing agents is associated with burns, disuse atrophy, denervation, and direct muscle trauma. Resistance sometimes develops in patients with cerebral palsy, or with chronic exposure to nondepolarizing agents. When rocuronium is administered to these patients, shorter durations of neuromuscular block may occur and infusion rates may be higher because of the development of resistance to nondepolarizing muscle relaxants.

➤*Discontinuation of therapy:* Spontaneous recovery and reversal of neuromuscular blockade following discontinuation of rocuronium infusion may be expected to proceed at rates comparable with those following comparable total doses administered by repetitive bolus injections in adults and at rates comparable with that following similar total exposure to single bolus doses in children.

➤*Preparation for administration:* Infusion solutions can be prepared by mixing rocuronium with an appropriate infusion solution such as sodium chloride 0.9% solution, sterile water for injection, glucose 5% in water, Ringer's lactate, and glucose 5% in saline.

➤*Administration:* Rocuronium is for intravenous (IV) use only. The rate of administration should be adjusted according to the patient's twitch response as monitored with the use of a peripheral nerve stimulator.

Infusion rates –

Rocuronium Infusion Rates (0.5 mg/mL)[a]

Patient weight		Drug delivery rate (mcg/kg/min)									
(kg)	(lbs)	4	5	6	7	8	9	10	12	14	16
Infusion delivery rate (mL/h)											
10	22	4.8	6	7.2	8.4	9.6	10.8	12	14.4	16.8	19.2
15	33	7.2	9	10.8	12.6	14.4	16.2	18	21.6	25.2	28.8
20	44	9.6	12	14.4	16.8	19.2	21.6	24	28.8	33.6	38.4
25	55	12	15	18	21	24	27	30	36	42	48
35	77	16.8	21	25.2	29.4	33.6	37.8	42	50.4	58.8	67.2
50	110	24	30	36	42	48	54	60	72	84	96
60	132	28.8	36	43.2	50.4	57.6	64.8	72	86.4	100.8	115.2
70	154	33.6	42	50.4	58.8	67.2	75.6	84	100.8	117.6	134.4
80	176	38.4	48	57.6	67.2	76.8	86.4	96	115.2	134.4	153.6
90	198	43.2	54	64.8	75.6	86.4	97.2	108	129.6	151.2	172.8
100	220	48	60	72	84	96	108	120	144	168	192

[a] Rocuronium 50 mg in 100 mL solution.

Rocuronium Infusion Rates (1 mg/mL)[a]

Patient weight		Drug delivery rate (mcg/kg/min)									
(kg)	(lbs)	4	5	6	7	8	9	10	12	14	16
Infusion delivery rate (mL/h)											
10	22	2.4	3	3.6	4.2	4.8	5.4	6	7.2	8.4	9.6
15	33	3.6	4.5	5.4	6.3	7.2	8.1	9	10.8	12.6	14.4
20	44	4.8	6	7.2	8.4	9.6	10.8	12	14.4	16.8	19.2
25	55	6	7.5	9	10.5	12	13.5	15	18	21	24
35	77	8.4	10.5	12.6	14.7	16.8	18.9	21	25.2	29.4	33.6
50	110	12	15	18	21	24	27	30	36	42	48
60	132	14.4	18	21.6	25.2	28.8	32.4	36	43.2	50.4	57.6
70	154	16.8	21	25.2	29.4	33.6	37.8	42	50.4	58.8	67.2
80	176	19.2	24	28.8	33.6	38.4	43.2	48	57.6	67.2	76.8
90	198	21.6	27	32.4	37.8	43.2	48.6	54	64.8	75.6	86.4
100	220	24	30	36	42	48	54	60	72	84	96

[a] Rocuronium 100 mg in 100 mL solution.

ROCURONIUM BROMIDE — INJECTION

Rocuronium Infusion Rates (5 mg/mL)[a]

Patient weight		Drug delivery rate (mcg/kg/min)									
(kg)	(lbs)	4	5	6	7	8	9	10	12	14	16
Infusion delivery rate (mL/h)											
10	22	0.5	0.6	0.7	0.8	1	1.1	1.2	1.4	1.7	1.9
15	33	0.7	0.9	1.1	1.3	1.4	1.6	1.8	2.2	2.5	2.9
20	44	1	1.2	1.4	1.7	1.9	2.2	2.4	2.9	3.4	3.8
25	55	1.2	1.5	1.8	2.1	2.4	2.7	3	3.6	4.2	4.8
35	77	1.7	2.1	2.5	2.9	3.4	3.8	4.2	5	5.9	6.7
50	110	2.4	3	3.6	4.2	4.8	5.4	6	7.2	8.4	9.6
60	132	2.9	3.6	4.3	5	5.8	6.5	7.2	8.6	10.1	11.5
70	154	3.4	4.2	5	5.9	6.7	7.6	8.4	10.1	11.8	13.4
80	176	3.8	4.8	5.8	6.7	7.7	8.6	9.6	11.5	13.4	15.4
90	198	4.3	5.4	6.5	7.6	8.6	9.7	10.8	13	15.1	17.3
100	220	4.8	6	7.2	8.4	9.6	10.8	12	14.4	16.8	19.2

[a] Rocuronium 500 mg in 100 mL solution.

➤*Admixture compatibility:* Rocuronium is physically incompatible when mixed with the following: amphotericin, amoxicillin, azathioprine, cefazolin, cloxacillin, dexamethasone, diazepam, erythromycin, famotidine, furosemide, hydrocortisone sodium succinate, insulin, intralipid, ketorolac, lorazepam, methohexital, methylprednisolone, thiopental, trimethoprim, and vancomycin.

Do not mix rocuronium with alkaline solutions (eg, barbiturate solutions) in the same syringe, and do not administer simultaneously during IV infusion through the same needle.

If rocuronium is administered via the same infusion line that also is used for other drugs, it is important that this infusion line is adequately flushed between administration of rocuronium and drugs for which incompatibility with rocuronium has been demonstrated or for which compatibility with rocuronium has not been established.

➤*Storage/Stability:* Store at 2° to 8°C (36° to 46°F). Do not freeze. When removed from refrigeration to room temperature storage conditions (25°C; 77°F), use within 60 days. Use opened vials of rocuronium within 30 days. Infusion solutions should be used within 24 hours of mixing. Unused portions of infusion solutions should be discarded.

Rocuronium is compatible in solution at concentrations of up to 5 mg/mL for 24 hours at room temperature in plastic bags, glass bottles, and plastic syringe pumps with the appropriate solution.

Actions

➤*Pharmacology:* Rocuronium is a nondepolarizing, neuromuscular-blocking agent with a rapid to intermediate onset depending on dose and intermediate duration. It acts by competing for cholinergic receptors at the motor end plate. This action is antagonized by acetylcholinesterase inhibitors, such as neostigmine and edrophonium.

➤*Pharmacokinetics:*

Rocuronium Mean (SD[a]) Pharmacokinetic Parameters During Opioid/Nitrous Oxide/Oxygen Anesthesia

Pharmacokinetic parameters	Adults 27 to 58 years of age (n = 22)	Elderly ≥ 65 years of age (n = 20)
Clearance (L/kg/h)	0.25 (0.08)	0.21 (0.06)
V_{ss}[b] (L/kg)	0.25 (0.04)	0.22 (0.03)
Half-life β elimination (h)	1.4 (0.4)	1.5 (0.4)

[a] SD = Standard deviation.
[b] V_{ss} = volume of distribution at steady state.

Distribution – Following IV administration of rocuronium, plasma levels of rocuronium follow a 3-compartment open model. The rapid distribution half-life is 1 to 2 minutes, and the slower distribution half-life is 14 to 18 minutes. Rocuronium is approximately 30% bound to human plasma proteins.

Metabolism/Excretion – Studies of distribution, metabolism, and excretion in cats and dogs indicate that rocuronium is eliminated primarily by the liver. The rocuronium analog 17-desacetyl-rocuronium, a metabolite, has been observed rarely in the plasma or urine of humans administered single doses of 0.5 to 1 mg/kg with or without a subsequent infusion (for up to 12 hours) of rocuronium. In the cat, 17-desacetyl-rocuronium has approximately one-twentieth the neuromuscular-blocking potency of rocuronium.

Special populations –
Children:

Rocuronium Mean (SD) Pharmacokinetic Parameters in Children During Halothane Anesthesia

Pharmacokinetic parameters	Patient age range		
	3 to < 12 months (n = 6)	1 to < 3 years (n = 5)	3 to < 8 years (n = 7)
Clearance (L/kg/h)	0.35 (0.08)	0.32 (0.07)	0.44 (0.16)
V_{ss} (L/kg)	0.3 (0.04)	0.26 (0.06)	0.21 (0.03)
Half-life β elimination (h)	1.3 (0.5)	1.1 (0.7)	0.8 (0.3)

Rocuronium Mean (SD) Pharmacokinetic Parameters in Children During Sevoflurane (Induction) and Isoflurane/Nitrous Oxide (Maintenance) Anesthesia

Pharmacokinetic parameters	Patient age range				
	Birth to < 28 days	28 days to ≤ 3 months	3 months to ≤ 2 years	2 to ≤ 11 years	11 to ≤ 17 years
Clearance (L/kg/h)	0.31 (0.07)	0.3 (0.08)	0.33 (0.1)	0.35 (0.09)	0.29 (0.14)
Volume of distribution (L/kg)	0.42 (0.06)	0.31 (0.03)	0.23 (0.03)	0.18 (0.02)	0.18 (0.01)
Half-life β (h)	1.1 (0.2)	0.9 (0.3)	0.8 (0.2)	0.7 (0.2)	0.8 (0.3)

Renal/Hepatic function impairment: In general, patients undergoing cadaver kidney transplant have a small reduction in clearance, which is offset pharmacokinetically by a corresponding increase in volume, such that the net effect is an unchanged plasma half-life. Patients with demonstrated liver cirrhosis have a marked increase in their volume of distribution, resulting in a plasma half-life approximately twice that of patients with healthy hepatic function.

Rocuronium Mean (SD) Pharmacokinetic Parameters in Adults with Healthy Renal and Hepatic Function, Renal Transplant Patients, and Hepatic Function Impairment Patients During Isoflurane Anesthesia

Pharmacokinetic parameters	Healthy renal and hepatic function (n = 10) (23 to 65 years of age)	Renal transplant patients (n = 10) (21 to 45 years of age)	Hepatic function impairment patients (n = 9) (31 to 67 years of age)
Clearance (L/kg/h)	0.16 (0.05)[a]	0.13 (0.04)	0.13 (0.06)
V_{ss} (L/kg)	0.26 (0.03)	0.34 (0.11)	0.53 (0.14)
Half-life β elimination (h)	2.4 (0.8)[a]	2.4 (1.1)	4.3 (2.6)

[a] Differences in the calculated half-life β and clearance between this study and the study in young adults versus elderly patients (≥ 65 years of age) is related to the different sample populations and aesthetic techniques.

The net result of these findings is that subjects with renal failure have clinical durations that are similar to but somewhat more variable than the duration that is expected in subjects with healthy renal function. Patients with hepatic function impairment, because of the large increase in volume, may demonstrate clinical durations approaching 1.5 times that of subjects with normal hepatic function. In both populations, individualize the dose to the needs of the patient.

Contraindications

Hypersensitivity (eg, anaphylaxis) to rocuroniumor other neuromuscular-blocking agents.

Warnings/Precautions

➤*Administration:* See Administration and Dosage for more information.

Rocuronium has no known effect on consciousness, pain threshold, or cerebration. Therefore, its administration must be accompanied by adequate anesthesia or sedation.

➤*Residual paralysis:* In order to prevent complications resulting from residual paralysis, it is recommended to extubate only after the patient has recovered sufficiently from neuromuscular block. Also consider other factors that could cause residual paralysis after extubation in the postoperative phase (eg, drug interactions, patient condition). If not used as part of standard clinical practice, consider the use of a reversal agent, especially in those cases in which residual paralysis is more likely to occur.

➤*Long-term use:* Rocuronium has not been studied for long-term use in the intensive care unit (ICU). As with other nondepolarizing neuromuscular-blocking drugs, apparent tolerance to rocuronium may develop during chronic administration in the ICU. While the mechanism for development of this resistance is not known, receptor up-regulation may be a contributing factor. It is strongly recommended that neuromuscular transmission be monitored continuously during administration and recovery with the help of a nerve stimulator. Do not give additional doses of rocuronium or any other neuromuscular-blocking agent until there is a definite response (1 twitch of the train-of-4) to nerve stimulation. Prolonged paralysis or skeletal muscle

ROCURONIUM BROMIDE — INJECTION

weakness may be noted during initial attempts to wean patients from the ventilator who have chronically received neuromuscular-blocking drugs in the ICU.

Myopathy – Myopathy after long-term administration of other nondepolarizing neuromuscular-blocking agents in the ICU alone or in combination with corticosteroid therapy has been reported. Therefore, for patients receiving both neuromuscular-blocking agents and corticosteroids, limit the period of use of the neuromuscular-blocking agent as much as possible and use only in the setting where, in the opinion of the prescribing health care provider, the specific advantages of the drug outweigh the risk.

➤*Malignant hyperthermia:* In an animal study in malignant hyperthermia (MH)-susceptible swine, the administration of rocuronium did not appear to trigger MH. Rocuronium has not been studied in MH-susceptible patients. Because rocuronium is always used with other agents, and the occurrence of MH during anesthesia is possible even in the absence of known triggering agents, be familiar with early signs, confirmatory diagnosis, and treatment of MH prior to the start of any anesthetic.

➤*Cardiovascular effects:* The overall analysis of electrocardiogram data in children indicates that the concomitant use of rocuronium with general anesthetic agents can prolong the QTc interval. Conditions associated with increased circulatory delayed time (eg, cardiovascular disease) may be associated with a delay in onset time.

Rocuronium may be associated with increased pulmonary vascular resistance, so caution is appropriate in patients with pulmonary hypertension or valvular heart disease.

➤*Extravasation:* If extravasation occurs, it may be associated with signs or symptoms of local irritation. Immediately terminate the injection or infusion and restart in another vein.

➤*Acid-base/electrolyte abnormalities:* Severe acid-base and/or electrolyte abnormalities may potentiate or cause resistance to the neuromuscular-blocking action of rocuronium. No data are available in such patients and no dosing recommendations can be made. Rocuronium-induced neuromuscular blockade was modified by alkalosis and acidosis in experimental pigs. Both respiratory and metabolic acidosis prolonged the recovery time. The potency of rocuronium was significantly enhanced in metabolic acidosis and alkalosis, but was reduced in respiratory alkalosis. In addition, experience with other drugs has suggested that acute (eg, diarrhea) or chronic (eg, adrenocortical insufficiency) electrolyte imbalance may alter neuromuscular blockade. Because electrolyte imbalance and acid-base imbalance are usually mixed, either enhancement or inhibition may occur.

➤*Myasthenia gravis:* In patients with myasthenia gravis or myasthenic (Eaton-Lambert) syndrome, small doses of nondepolarizing neuromuscular-blocking agents may have profound effects. In such patients, a peripheral nerve stimulator and use of a small test dose may be of value in monitoring the response to administration of muscle relaxants.

➤*Hypersensitivity reactions:* There have been reports of severe anaphylactic reactions to rocuronium, including some that have been life-threatening. Because of the potential severity of these reactions, take the necessary precautions, including the immediate availability of emergency treatment.

➤*Hepatic function impairment:* Because rocuronium is primarily excreted by the liver, use with caution in patients with clinically significant hepatic function impairment. Rocuronium 0.6 mg/kg has been studied in a limited number of patients (n = 9) with clinically significant hepatic function impairment under steady-state isoflurane anesthesia. After rocuronium 0.6 mg/kg, the median (range) clinical duration of 60 (35 to 166) minutes was moderately prolonged, compared with 42 minutes in patients with healthy hepatic function. The median recovery time of 53 minutes was also prolonged in patients with cirrhosis compared with 20 minutes in patients with normal hepatic function. Four of 8 patients with cirrhosis who received rocuronium 0.6 mg/kg under opioid/nitrous oxide/oxygen anesthesia did not achieve complete block. These findings are consistent with the increase in V_{ss} observed in patients with significant hepatic function impairment. If used for rapid sequence induction in patients with ascites, an increased initial dosage may be necessary to ensure complete block. Duration will be prolonged in these cases. The use of doses higher than 0.6 mg/kg has not been studied.

➤*Special risk:* Resistance to nondepolarizing agents, consistent with up-regulation of skeletal muscle acetylcholine receptors, is associated with burns, disuse atrophy, denervation, and direct muscle trauma. Receptor up-regulation may also contribute to the resistance to nondepolarizing muscle relaxants which sometimes develops in patients with cerebral palsy, or with chronic exposure to nondepolarizing agents. When rocuronium is administered to these patients, shorter durations of neuromuscular block may occur and infusion rates may be higher because of the development of resistance to nondepolarizing muscle relaxants.

Nondepolarizing neuromuscular-blocking agents have been found to exhibit profound neuromuscular-blocking effects in cachectic or debilitated patients, patients with neuromuscular diseases, and patients with carcinomatosis.

In these or other patients in whom potentiation of neuromuscular block or difficulty with reversal may be anticipated, consider a decrease from the recommended initial dose.

➤*Pregnancy: Category C.* There are no adequate and well-controlled studies in pregnant women. Use rocuronium during pregnancy only if the potential benefit justifies the potential risk to the fetus.

Labor and delivery – The use of rocuronium in cesarean section has been studied in a limited number of patients. Rocuronium is not recommended for rapid sequence induction in cesarean section patients.

➤*Lactation:* The molecular weight (approximately 610) is low enough for excretion into breast milk, but the amount excreted will be limited because the drug is ionized at physiologic pH. The effects of this exposure on a breast-feeding infant are unknown but are probably not clinically significant.

➤*Children:* The use of rocuronium has been studied in children 3 months to 14 years of age under halothane anesthesia. Of the children anesthetized with halothane who did not receive atropine for induction, about 80% experienced a transient increase (30% or greater) in heart rate after intubation. One of the 19 infants anesthetized with halothane and fentanyl who received atropine for induction experienced this magnitude of change.

Rocuronium also was studied in children 17 years of age and younger, including neonates, under sevoflurane (induction) and isoflurane/nitrous oxide (maintenance) anesthesia. Onset time and clinical duration varied with dose, the age of the patient, and anesthetic technique. The overall analysis of ECG data in children indicates that the concomitant use of rocuronium with general anesthetic agents can prolong the QTc interval. The data also suggest that rocuronium may increase heart rate. However, it was not possible to conclusively identify an effect of rocuronium independent of that of anesthesia and other factors. Additionally, when examining plasma levels of rocuronium in correlation to QTc interval prolongation, no relationship was observed.

Rocuronium is not recommended for rapid sequence intubation in children.

➤*Elderly:* Rocuronium was administered to 140 elderly patients (65 years of age or older) in US clinical trials and 128 elderly patients in European clinical trials. The observed pharmacokinetic profile for elderly patients (n = 20) was similar to that of other adult surgical patients. Onset time and duration of action were slightly longer for elderly patients (n = 43) in clinical trials.

➤*Monitoring:* It is strongly recommended that neuromuscular transmission be monitored continuously during administration and recovery with the help of a nerve stimulator.

Drug Interactions

Rocuronium Drug Interactions

Precipitant drug	Object drug[a]		Description
Antibiotics (eg, aminoglycosides, bacitracin, colistin, lincosamides, polymyxin, sodium colistimethate, tetracyclines, vancomycin)	Rocuronium	↑	Coadministration may enhance the neuromuscular-blocking action of rocuronium.
Carbamazepine	Rocuronium	↓	Rocuronium may have shorter than expected duration or be less effective when given with carbamazepine.
Inhalational anesthetics (eg, enflurane, halothane, isoflurane)	Rocuronium	↑	The use of these drugs with rocuronium will enhance neuromuscular blockade. Potentiation is most prominent with enflurane, followed by isoflurane. It may be necessary to decrease the rate of infusion by 30% to 50% at 45 to 60 minutes after the intubating dose.
Lithium	Rocuronium	↑	Lithium has been shown to increase the duration of neuromuscular block and decrease infusion requirements of neuromuscular-blocking agents.
Local anesthetics	Rocuronium	↑	Local anesthetics have been shown to increase the duration of neuromuscular block and decrease infusion requirements of neuromuscular-blocking agents.
Magnesium	Rocuronium	↑	Magnesium salts, administered for toxemia of pregnancy, may potentiate the actions of rocuronium.
Phenytoin	Rocuronium	↓	Rocuronium may have shorter than expected duration or be less effective when given with phenytoin.

ROCURONIUM BROMIDE — INJECTION

Rocuronium Drug Interactions

Precipitant drug	Object drug[a]		Description
Procainamide	Rocuronium	↑	Procainamide has been shown to increase the duration of neuromuscular block and decrease infusion requirements of neuromuscular-blocking agents.
Quinidine	Rocuronium	↑	The use of quinidine during recovery from use of other muscle relaxants suggests that recurrent paralysis may occur. Consider this possibility for rocuronium.
Succinylcholine	Rocuronium	↑	Prior administration enhances the neuromuscular-blocking effect of rocuronium and its duration of action. If succinylcholine is used before rocuronium, delay administration of rocuronium until recovery from succinylcholine has been observed.

[a] ↑ = object drug increased; ↓ = object drug decreased.

Adverse Reactions

For information on anaphylaxis, residual paralysis, myopathy, or pulmonary vesicular resistance, see Warnings/Precautions.

➤*Common adverse reactions:* In clinical trials, the most common adverse reactions (2%) are transient hypotension and hypertension.

➤*Postmarketing:* In a clinical study in patients with clinically significant cardiovascular disease undergoing coronary artery bypass graft, hypertension and tachycardia were reported in some patients, but these occurrences were less frequent in patients receiving beta or calcium channel-blocking drugs. In some patients, rocuronium was associated with transient increases (30% or greater) in pulmonary vascular resistance. In another clinical study of patients undergoing abdominal aortic surgery, transient increases (30% or greater) in pulmonary vascular resistance were observed in about 24% of patients receiving rocuronium 0.6 or 0.9 mg/kg. In clinical practice, there have been reports of severe allergic reactions (anaphylactic and anaphylactoid reactions and shock) with rocuronium, including some that have been life-threatening and fatal.

Rocuronium Adverse Reactions (< 1%)

Cardiovascular	Arrhythmia, abnormal ECG, tachycardia
GI	Nausea, vomiting
Respiratory	Asthma (bronchospasm, wheezing, or rhonchi), hiccup
Dermatologic	Rash, injection-site edema, pruritus

Children – In pediatric studies worldwide (n = 704), tachycardia occurred at an incidence of 5.3% (n = 37), and it was judged by the investigator as related in 10 cases (1.4%).

Overdosage

➤*Symptoms:* Overdosage with neuromuscular-blocking agents may result in neuromuscular block beyond the time needed for surgery and anesthesia.

➤*Treatment:* The primary treatment is maintenance of a patent airway, controlled ventilation, and adequate sedation until recovery of normal neuromuscular function is ensured. Once evidence of recovery from neuromuscular block is observed, further recovery may be facilitated by administration of an anticholinesterase agent.

Do not administer anticholinesterase agents prior to the demonstration of some spontaneous recovery from neuromuscular blockade. The use of a nerve stimulator to document recovery is recommended.

Evaluate patients for adequate clinical evidence of neuromuscular recovery (eg, 5-second head lift, adequate phonation, ventilation, upper airway patency). Ventilation must be supported while patients exhibit any signs of muscle weakness.

Recovery may be delayed in the presence of debilitation, carcinomatosis, and concomitant use of certain drugs that enhance neuromuscular blockade or separately cause respiratory depression. Under such circumstances, the management is the same as that of prolonged neuromuscular blockade.

Patient Information

Obtain information about your patient's medical history, current medications, and any history of hypersensitivity to rocuronium or other neuromuscular-blocking agents. Inform patients that certain medical conditions and medications might influence how rocuronium works.

Inform the patient that severe anaphylactic reactions to neuromuscular-blocking agents, including rocuronium, have been reported. Because allergic cross-reactivity has been reported in this class, request information from the patient about previous anaphylactic reactions to other neuromuscular-blocking agents.

PANCURONIUM BROMIDE

Rx	**Pancuronium Bromide** (Various, eg, Gensia Sicor)	**Injection:** 1 mg/mL	In 10 mL vials.[a]
		2 mg/mL	In 2 and 5 mL vials, amps.[a]

[a] With benzyl alcohol.

PANCURONIUM BROMIDE — INJECTION

WARNING

This drug should be administered by adequately trained individuals familiar with its actions, characteristics, and hazards.

Indications

➤*Anesthesia, adjunct:* As an adjunct to general anesthesia to facilitate tracheal intubation and to provide skeletal muscle relaxation during surgery or mechanical ventilation.

Administration and Dosage

➤*General dosing considerations:* The dosage information that follows is derived from studies based upon units of drug per unit of body weight and is intended to serve as a guide only.

To obtain maximum clinical benefits of pancuronium and to minimize the possibility of overdosage, the monitoring of muscle twitch response to a peripheral nerve stimulator is advised.

➤*Adults:*

Adjunct to general anesthesia –

Initial dosage: 0.04 to 0.1 mg/kg.

Maintenance dosage: Incremental doses starting at 0.01 mg/kg may be used. These increments slightly increase the magnitude of the blockade and significantly increase the duration of blockade, because a significant number of myoneural junctions are still blocked when there is a clinical need for more drug.

Endotracheal intubation: A bolus dose of 0.06 to 0.1 mg/kg is recommended. Conditions satisfactory for intubation are usually present within 2 to 3 minutes.

➤*Children:*

Adjunct to general anesthesia –

Older than 1 month of age: See Adults for dosing.

Younger than 1 month of age: Neonates are especially sensitive to nondepolarizing neuromuscular blocking agents during the first month of life.

- *Test dose* – 0.02 mg/kg should be given first to measure responsiveness.

➤*Elderly:* Conditions associated with slower circulation time (advanced age) may contribute to a delay in onset time; therefore, dosage should not be increased.

➤*Concomitant therapy with succinylcholine or inhalational anesthetics:* Because potent inhalational anesthetics or prior use of succinylcholine may enhance the intensity and duration of pancuronium, the lower end of the recommended initial dosage range may suffice when pancuronium is first used after intubation with succinylcholine and/or after maintenance doses of volatile liquid inhalational anesthetics are started.

➤*Administration:* For IV use only. This drug should be administered by or under the supervision of experienced clinicians familiar with the use of neuromuscular blocking agents.

➤*Admixture compatibility:* Pancuronium is compatible in solution with sodium chloride 0.9%, dextrose 5%, dextrose 5% and sodium chloride, and Ringer's lactate.

➤*Storage/Stability:* Both concentrations of pancuronium will maintain full clinical potency for 6 months if kept at 18° to 22°C (65° to 72°F); or for 36 months when refrigerated at 2° to 8°C (36° to 46°F). When mixed with the approved solutions in glass or plastic containers, pancuronium will remain stable in solution for 48 hours with no alteration in potency or pH, no decomposition, and no adsorption to either the glass or plastic container.

Actions

➤*Pharmacology:* Pancuronium bromide is a nondepolarizing neuromuscular blocking agent possessing all of the characteristic pharmacological actions of this class of drugs (curariform). It acts by competing for cholinergic receptors at the motor end-plate. The antagonism to acetylcholine is inhibited and neuromuscular block is reversed by anticholinesterase agents such as pyridostigmine, neostigmine, and edrophonium. Pancuronium bromide is ≈ ⅓ less potent than vecuronium and ≈ 5 times as potent as d-tubocurarine: the duration of neuromuscular blockage produced by pancuronium bromide is longer than that of vecuronium at initially equipotent doses.

The most characteristic circulatory effects of pancuronium, studied under halothane anesthesia, are a moderate rise in heart rate, mean arterial pres-

PANCURONIUM BROMIDE — INJECTION

sure, and cardiac output; systemic vascular resistance is not changed significantly and central venous pressure may fall slightly. The heart rate rise is inversely related to the rate immediately before administration of pancuronium, is blocked by prior administration of atropine, and appears unrelated to the concentration of halothane or dose of pancuronium.

➤*Pharmacokinetics:* The elimination half-life of pancuronium has been reported to range between 89 to 161 minutes. The volume of distribution ranges from 241 to 280 mL/kg and plasma clearance is ≈ 1.1 to 1.9 mL/minute/kg. Approximately 40% of the total dose of pancuronium has been recovered in urine as unchanged pancuronium and its metabolites while ≈ 11% has been recovered in bile. As much as 25% of an injected dose may be recovered as 3-hydroxy metabolite, which is half as potent a blocking agent as pancuronium. Less than 5% of the injected dose is recovered as 17-hydroxy metabolite and 3, 17-dihydroxy metabolite, which have been judged to be ≈ 50 times less potent than pancuronium. Pancuronium exhibits strong binding to gamma globulin and moderate binding to albumin. Approximately 13% is unbound to plasma protein. In patients with cirrhosis the volume of distribution is increased by ≈ 50%, the plasma clearance is decreased by ≈ 22% and the elimination half-life is doubled. Similar results were noted in patients with biliary obstruction, except that plasma clearance was less than half the normal rate. The initial total dose to achieve adequate relaxation may thus be high in patients with hepatic and/or biliary tract dysfunction, while the duration of action is greater than usual.

The elimination half-life is doubled and the plasma clearance is reduced by ≈ 60% in patients with renal failure. The volume of distribution is variable, and in some cases elevated. The rate of recovery of neuromuscular blockade, as determined by peripheral nerve stimulation, is variable and sometimes very much slower than normal.

Renal function impairment – A major portion of pancuronium, as well as an active metabolite, are recovered in urine. The elimination half-life is doubled and the plasma clearance is reduced in patients with renal failure; at the same time, the rate of recovery of neuromuscular blockade is variable and sometimes very much slower than normal. This information should be taken into consideration if pancuronium is selected, for other reasons, to be used in a patient with renal failure.

Contraindications

Pancuronium bromide injection is contraindicated in patients known to be hypersensitive to the drug.

Warnings/Precautions

➤*Administration:* See Administration and Dosage for more information.

➤*Long-term use in ICU:* In the intensive care unit, in rare cases, long-term use of neuromuscular blocking drugs to facilitate mechanical ventilation may be associated with prolonged paralysis or skeletal muscle weakness, that may be first noted during attempts to wean such patients from the ventilator. Typically, such patients receive other drugs such as broad spectrum antibiotics, narcotics and steroids and may have electrolyte imbalance and diseases that lead to electrolyte imbalance, hypoxic episodes of varying duration, acid-base imbalance, and extreme debilitation, any of which may enhance the actions of a neuromuscular blocking agent. Additionally, patients immobilized for extended periods frequently develop symptoms consistent with disuse muscle atrophy. Therefore, when there is a need for long-term mechanical ventilation, the benefits-to-risk ratio of neuromuscular blockade must be considered.

Under the above conditions, appropriate monitoring, such as use of a peripheral nerve stimulator, to assess the degree of neuromuscular blockade, may preclude inadvertent excess dosing.

➤*Severe obesity or neuromuscular disease:* Patients with severe obesity or neuromuscular disease may pose airway and ventilatory problems requiring special care before, during, and after the use of neuromuscular blocking agents such as pancuronium bromide.

➤*CNS:* Pancuronium bromide has no known effect on consciousness, the pain threshold, or cerebration. Administration should be accompanied by adequate anesthesia or sedation.

➤*Hepatic function impairment:* The doubled elimination half-life and reduced plasma clearance determined in patients with hepatic and/or biliary tract disease, as well as limited data showing that recovery time is prolonged an average of 65% in patients with biliary tract obstruction, suggests that prolongation of neuromuscular blockage may occur. At the same time, these conditions are characterized by an ≈ 50% increase in volume of distribution of pancuronium, suggesting that the total initial dose to achieve adequate relaxation may in some cases be high. The possibility of slower onset, higher total dosage, and prolongation of neuromuscular blockage must be taken into consideration when pancuronium is used in these patients (see Pharmacokinetics).

➤*Special risk:* Although pancuronium bromide injection has been used successfully in many patients with preexisting pulmonary, hepatic, or renal disease, caution should be exercised in these situations.

In patients who are known to have myasthenia gravis or the myasthenic (Eaton-Lambert) syndrome, small doses of pancuronium bromide may have profound effects. In such patients, a peripheral nerve stimulator and use of a small test dose may be of value in monitoring the response to administration of muscle relaxants.

Conditions associated with slower circulation time (cardiovascular disease, old age, edematous states resulting in increased volume of distribution) may contribute to a delay in onset time; therefore dosage should not be increased.

Electrolyte imbalance and diseases that lead to electrolyte imbalance, such as adrenal cortical insufficiency, have been shown to alter neuromuscular blockade. Depending on the nature of the imbalance, either enhancement or inhibition may be expected.

➤*Pregnancy: Category C.* Animal reproduction studies have not been performed. It is not known whether pancuronium can cause fetal harm when administered to a pregnant woman or can affect reproduction capacity. Theoretically, the combination of relatively high molecular weight (about 733 for the dibromide) and the presence of 2 quaternary ammonium groups that are ionized at physiologic pH should limit the placental transfer of pancuronium. Pancuronium should be given to a pregnant woman only if the administering clinician decides that the benefits outweigh the risks.

Pancuronium may be used in operative obstetrics (Cesarean section), but reversal of pancuronium may be unsatisfactory in patients receiving magnesium sulfate for toxemia of pregnancy, because magnesium salts enhance neuromuscular blockade. Dosage should usually be reduced, as indicated, in such cases. It is also recommended that the interval between use of pancuronium and delivery be reasonably short to avoid clinically significant placental transfer.

➤*Lactation:* No reports describing the use of pancuronium in a lactating woman have been located. Moreover, because pancuronium is a bisquaternary ammonium compound, it is ionized at physiologic pH. Only the nonionized form would be available for excretion into milk, and this would probably be only trace amounts. In addition, compounds of this type are poorly absorbed from the gastrointestinal tract.

➤*Children:* See Administration and Dosage for more information.

The prolonged use of pancuronium bromide for the management of neonates undergoing mechanical ventilation has been associated in rare cases with severe skeletal muscle weakness that may first be noted during attempts to wean such patients from the ventilator; such patients usually receive other drugs such as antibiotics that may enhance neuromuscular blockade. Microscopic changes consistent with disuse atrophy have been noted at autopsy. Although a cause-and-effect relationship has not been established, the benefits-to-risk ratio must be considered when there is a need for neuromuscular blockade to facilitate long-term mechanical ventilation of neonates.

Rare cases of unexplained, clinically significant methemoglobinemia have been reported in premature neonates undergoing emergency anesthesia and surgery that included combined use of pancuronium, fentanyl, and atropine. A direct cause-and-effect relationship between the combined use of these drugs and the reported cases of methemoglobinemia has not been established.

➤*Monitoring:* Use of a peripheral nerve stimulator will usually be of value for monitoring of neuromuscular blocking effect, avoiding overdosage and assisting in evaluation of recovery.

Drug Interactions

➤*Succinylcholine:* Prior administration of succinylcholine may enhance the neuromuscular blocking effect of pancuronium bromide and increase its duration of action. If succinylcholine is used before pancuronium bromide, the administration of pancuronium bromide should be delayed until the patient starts recovering from succinylcholine-induced neuromuscular blockade.

If a small dose of pancuronium bromide is given ≥ 3 minutes prior to the administration of succinylcholine, in order to reduce the incidence and intensity of succinylcholine-induced fasciculations, this dose may induce a degree of neuromuscular block sufficient to cause respiratory depression in some patients.

➤*Other nondepolarizing neuromuscular blocking agents:* Other nondepolarizing neuromuscular blocking agents (vecuronium, atracurium, d-tubocurarine, metocurine, and gallamine) behave in a clinically similar fashion to pancuronium bromide. The combination of pancuronium bromide-metocurine and pancuronium bromide-d-tubocurarine are significantly more potent than the additive effects of each of the individual drugs given alone; however, the duration of blockade of these combinations is not prolonged. There are insufficient data to support concomitant use of pancuronium and the other 3 muscle relaxants mentioned above in the same patient.

➤*Inhalational anesthetics:* Use of volatile inhalational anesthetics such as enflurane, isoflurane, and halothane with pancuronium bromide will enhance neuromuscular blockade. Potentiation is most prominent with use of enflurane and isoflurane.

With the above agents, the intubating dose of pancuronium bromide may be the same as with balanced anesthesia unless the inhalational anesthetic has been administered for a sufficient time at a sufficient dose to have reached clinical equilibrium. The relatively long duration of action of pancuronium should be taken into consideration when the drug is selected for intubation in these circumstances.

Clinical experience and animal experiments suggest that pancuronium should be given with caution to patients receiving chronic tricyclic antidepressant therapy who are anesthetized with halothane because severe ventricular arrhythmias may result from this combination. The severity of the arrhythmias appear in part related to the dose of pancuronium.

➤*Antibiotics:* Parenteral or intraperitoneal administration of high doses of certain antibiotics may intensify, or produce neuromuscular block on their own. The following antibiotics have been associated with various degrees of paralysis: Aminoglycosides (such as neomycin, streptomycin, kanamycin, gentamicin, and dihydrostreptomycin); tetracyclines; bacitracin, polymyxin B, colistin, and sodium colistimethate. If these or other newly introduced

PANCURONIUM BROMIDE — INJECTION

antibiotics are used preoperatively or in conjunction with pancuronium bromide, unexpected prolongation of neuromuscular block should be considered a possibility.

➤*Magnesium salts:* Magnesium salts, administered for the management of toxemia of pregnancy, may enhance the neuromuscular blockade.

➤*Other:* Experience concerning injection of quinidine during recovery from use of other muscle relaxants suggests that recurrent paralysis may occur. This possibility must also be considered for pancuronium bromide.

Adverse Reactions

➤*Cardiovascular:* See discussion of circulatory effects in Pharmacology.

➤*Dermatologic:* An occasional transient rash is noted accompanying the use of pancuronium bromide.

➤*GI:* Salivation is sometimes noted during very light anesthesia, especially if no anticholinergic premedication is used.

➤*Musculoskeletal:* The most frequent adverse reaction to nondepolarizing blocking agents as a class consists of an extension of the drug's pharmacological action beyond the time period needed. This may vary from skeletal muscle weakness to profound and prolonged skeletal muscle paralysis resulting in respiratory insufficiency or apnea (see Warnings, Children).

Inadequate reversal of the neuromuscular blockade is possible with pancuronium bromide as with all curariform drugs. These adverse experiences are managed by manual or mechanical ventilation until recovery is judged adequate.

Prolonged paralysis and skeletal muscle weakness have been reported after long-term use to support mechanical ventilation in the intensive care unit.

➤*Miscellaneous:* Although histamine release is not a characteristic action of pancuronium bromide, rare hypersensitivity reactions such as bronchospasm, flushing, redness, hypotension, tachycardia, and other reactions possibly mediated by histamine release have been reported.

Overdosage

➤*Symptoms:* Residual neuromuscular blockade beyond the time period needed may occur with pancuronium bromide as with other neuromuscular blockers. This may be manifested by skeletal muscle weakness, decreased respiratory reserve, low tidal volume, or apnea.

➤*Treatment:* A peripheral nerve stimulator may be used to assess the degree of residual neuromuscular blockade and help to differentiate residual neuromuscular blockade from other causes of decreased respiratory reserve.

Pyridostigmine bromide, neostigmine, or edrophonium, in conjunction with atropine or glycopyrrolate, will usually antagonize the skeletal muscle relaxant action of pancuronium bromide. Satisfactory reversal can be judged by adequacy of skeletal muscle tone and by adequacy of respiration. A peripheral nerve stimulator may also be used to monitor restoration of twitch response.

Failure of prompt reversal (within 30 minutes) may occur in the presence of extreme debilitation, carcinomatosis, and with concomitant use of certain broad spectrum antibiotics, or anesthetic agents and other drugs that enhance neuromuscular blockade or cause respiratory depression of their own. Under such circumstances, the management is the same as that of prolonged neuromuscular blockade. Ventilation must be supported by artificial means until the patient has resumed control of his respiration. Prior to the use of reversal agents, reference should be made to the specific monograph of the reversal agent.

VECURONIUM BROMIDE

Rx	**Vecuronium Bromide** (Various, eg, Abbott, Baxter, Bedford)	**Powder for Injection:** 10 mg[a]	In 10 mL vials.
Rx	**Norcuron** (Organon)		In 10 mL vials with and without diluent.[b]
Rx	**Vecuronium Bromide** (Various, eg, Abbott, Bedford)	**Powder for Injection:** 20 mg[a]	In 20 mL vials.
Rx	**Norcuron** (Organon)		In 20 mL vials without diluent.

[a] May contain mannitol.

[b] Contains 0.9% benzyl alcohol.

VECURONIUM BROMIDE — INJECTION

WARNING

This drug should be administered by adequately trained individuals familiar with its actions, characteristics, and hazards.

Indications

➤*Anesthesia, adjunct:* As an adjunct to general anesthesia, to facilitate endotracheal intubation, and to provide skeletal muscle relaxation during surgery or mechanical ventilation.

Administration and Dosage

➤*General dosing considerations:* Administer by or under the supervision of an experienced clinician familiar with the use of neuromuscular-blocking agents. (See Administration.)

To obtain maximum clinical benefits of vecuronium and to minimize the possibility of overdosage, the monitoring of muscle twitch response to peripheral nerve stimulation is advised.

If reconstituted with bacteriostatic water for injection, the resultant solution contains benzyl alcohol, which is not for use in newborns.

Long-term intravenous (IV) infusion to support mechanical ventilation in the intensive care unit has not been studied sufficiently to support dosing recommendations (see Warnings/Precautions).

➤*Adults:*

Injection –

Initial dosage: 0.08 to 0.1 mg/kg (1.4 to 1.75 times the ED_{90}), given as an IV bolus injection. Certain situations may require a different initial dosage. (See Administration.)

Maintenance dosage: 0.01 to 0.015 mg/kg of vecuronium 25 to 40 minutes after the initial injection of vecuronium is recommended during prolonged surgical procedures. However, clinical criteria should be used to determine the need for maintenance doses.

Because vecuronium lacks clinically important cumulative effects, subsequent maintenance doses, if required, may be administered at relatively regular intervals for each patient, ranging from approximately 12 to 15 minutes under balanced anesthesia to slightly longer under inhalation agents (if less frequent administration is desired, higher maintenance doses may be administered).

Continuous infusion – Initiate infusions only after there is early evidence of spontaneous recovery from the bolus dose.

Initial dosage: 1 mcg/kg/min IV can be initiated approximately 20 to 40 minutes after intubating dose.

Loading dose: 80 to 100 mcg/kg intubating dose.

Maintenance dosage: Average infusion rates may range from 0.8 to 1.2 mcg/kg/min. The rate of administration should be adjusted according to the patient's twitch response as determined by peripheral nerve stimulation.

Discontinuation of therapy: Spontaneous recovery and reversal of neuromuscular blockade following discontinuation of vecuronium infusion may be expected to proceed at rates comparable with those following a single bolus dose (see Pharmacology).

➤*Children:*

10 years of age and older – See Adults for dosing for children 10 years of age and older.

1 to 10 years of age – May require a slightly higher initial dose and also may require supplementation slightly more often than adults. (See Off-label dosing.)

7 weeks to younger than 1 year of age – Children are moderately more sensitive to vecuronium on a mg/kg basis than adults and may take about 1.5 times as long to recover. (See Off-label dosing.)

Off-label dosing –

Children and infants older than 7 weeks of age: Administer an initial dosage of 0.08 to 0.1 mg/kg/dose IV. Follow with a maintenance dosage of 0.05 to 0.1 mg/kg/dose IV every hour as needed.

For children older than 1 year of age, the dosage for a continuous infusion is 0.05 to 0.07 mg/kg/hour IV.

Neonates: Administer an initial dosage of 0.1 mg/kg/dose IV. Follow with a maintenance dosage of 0.03 to 0.15 mg/kg/dose IV every 1 to 2 hours as needed.

➤*Concomitant therapy:*

Injection – In the presence of potent inhalation anesthetics, the neuromuscular-blocking effect of vecuronium is enhanced. If vecuronium is first administered more than 5 minutes after the start of inhalation agent or when steady state has been achieved, the initial vecuronium dose may be reduced by approximately 15% (ie, 0.06 to 0.085 mg/kg).

Prior administration of succinylcholine may enhance the neuromuscular-blocking effect and duration of action of vecuronium. If intubation is performed using succinylcholine, a reduction of initial dose of vecuronium bromide to 0.04 to 0.06 mg/kg with inhalation anesthesia and 0.05 to 0.06 mg/kg with balanced anesthesia may be required.

If there is reason for the selection of larger doses in individual patients, initial doses ranging from 0.15 mg/kg to 0.28 mg/kg have been administered during surgery under halothane anesthesia without ill effects to the cardiovascular system being noted, as long as ventilation is properly maintained.

Continuous infusion – Inhalation anesthetics, particularly enflurane and isoflurane, may enhance the neuromuscular-blocking action of nondepolarizing muscle relaxants. In the presence of steady-state concentrations of enflurane or isoflurane, it may be necessary to reduce the rate of infusion 25% to 60%, 45 to 60 minutes after the intubating dose. Under halothane anesthesia, it may not be necessary to reduce the rate of infusion.

➤*Preparation for administration:* Vecuronium for injection 10 mg is dissolved by adding 10 mL of sterile water for injection to a vial. Vecuronium

VECURONIUM BROMIDE — INJECTION

for injection 20 mg is dissolved by adding 20 mL of sterile water for injection to a vial, resulting in a solution of 1 mg/mL.

The drug should be completely dissolved before the solution is withdrawn. The solution should then be added to a compatible infusion solution.

➤*Administration:* Vecuronium for injection is for IV use only.

Injection – Administer by or under the supervision of an experienced clinician familiar with the use of neuromuscular-blocking agents. Dosage must be individualized in each case. The dosage information is derived from studies based upon units of drug per unit of body weight and is intended to serve as a guide only, especially regarding enhancement of neuromuscular blockade of vecuronium by volatile anesthetics and by prior use of succinylcholine (see Drug Interactions).

To obtain maximum clinical benefits of vecuronium and to minimize the possibility of overdosage, the monitoring of muscle twitch response to peripheral nerve stimulation is advised.

The recommended initial dose of vecuronium bromide is given as an IV bolus injection. This dose can be expected to produce good or excellent nonemergency intubation conditions in 2.5 to 3 minutes after injection. Under balanced anesthesia, clinically required neuromuscular blockade lasts approximately 25 to 30 minutes, with recovery to 25% of control achieved approximately 25 to 40 minutes after injection and recovery to 95% of control achieved approximately 45 to 65 minutes after injection.

Continuous infusion – The infusion of vecuronium should be individualized for each patient. The rate of administration should be adjusted according to the patient's twitch response as determined by peripheral nerve stimulation. An initial rate of 1 mcg/kg/min is recommended, with the rate of the infusion adjusted thereafter to maintain a 90% suppression of twitch response. Average infusion rates may range from 0.8 to 1.2 mcg/kg/min.

Infusion rates of vecuronium bromide can be individualized for each patient using the following table:

Vecuronium Bromide Delivery Rates

Drug delivery rate (mcg/kg/min)	Infusion delivery rate (mL/kg/min)	
	0.1 mg/mL[a]	0.2 mg/mL[b]
0.7	0.007	0.0035
0.8	0.008	0.004
0.9	0.009	0.0045
1	0.01	0.005
1.1	0.011	0.0055
1.2	0.012	0.006
1.3	0.013	0.0065

[a] 10 mg of vecuronium bromide in 100 mL solution.
[b] 20 mg of vecuronium bromide in 100 mL solution.

The following table is a guideline for mL/min delivery for a solution of 0.1 mg/mL (10 mg in 100 mL) with an infusion pump:

Vecuronium Bromide Infusion Rate (mL/min)

Amount of drug (mcg/kg/min)	Patient weight (kg)						
	40	50	60	70	80	90	100
0.7	0.28	0.35	0.42	0.49	0.56	0.63	0.7
0.8	0.32	0.4	0.48	0.56	0.64	0.72	0.8
0.9	0.36	0.45	0.54	0.63	0.72	0.81	0.9
1	0.4	0.5	0.6	0.7	0.8	0.9	1
1.1	0.44	0.55	0.66	0.77	0.88	0.99	1.1
1.2	0.48	0.6	0.72	0.84	0.96	1.08	1.2
1.3	0.52	0.65	0.75	0.91	1.04	1.17	1.3

Note – If a concentration of 0.2 mg/mL is used (20 mg in 100 mL), the rate should be decreased by one-half.

➤*Admixture compatibility:* Vecuronium is compatible in solution with sodium chloride injection 0.9%, dextrose injection 5%, sterile water for injection, dextrose 5% and sodium chloride injection, and Ringer's lactate injection.

➤*Storage/Stability:* Store at controlled room temperature 15° to 30°C (59° to 86°F). Protect from light.

If reconstituted with bacteriostatic water for injection – Contains benzyl alcohol which is not for use in newborns. Use within 5 days. May be stored at room temperature or refrigerated.

If reconstituted with sterile water for injection or other compatible IV solutions – Refrigerate vial. Single use only. Use within 24 hours. Discard unused portion.

Actions

➤*Pharmacology:* Vecuronium bromide is a nondepolarizing neuromuscular blocking agent possessing all of the characteristic pharmacological actions of this class of drugs (curariform). It acts by competing for cholinergic receptors at the motor-end plate. The antagonism to acetylcholine is inhibited, and neuromuscular block is reversed by acetylcholinesterase inhibitors such as neostigmine, edrophonium, and pyridostigmine. Vecuronium is about ⅓ more potent than pancuronium; the duration of neuromuscular blockade produced by vecuronium is shorter than that of pancuronium at initially equipotent doses. The time to onset of paralysis decreases and the duration of maximum effect increases with increasing vecuronium doses. The use of a peripheral nerve stimulator is recommended in assessing the degree of muscular relaxation with all neuromuscular blocking drugs. The ED_{90} (dose required to produce 90% suppression of the muscle twitch response with balanced anesthesia) has averaged 0.057 mg/kg (0.049 to 0.062 mg/kg in various studies). An initial vecuronium bromide dose of 0.08 to 0.1 mg/kg generally produces first depression of twitch in approximately 1 minute, good or excellent intubation conditions within 2.5 to 3 minutes, and maximum neuromuscular blockade within 3 to 5 minutes of injection in most patients.

➤*Pharmacokinetics:* At clinical doses of 0.04 to 0.1 mg/kg, 60% to 80% of vecuronium is usually bound to plasma protein. The distribution half-life following a single intravenous dose (range 0.025 to 0.28 mg/kg) is approximately 4 minutes. Elimination half-life over this sample dosage range is approximately 65 to 75 minutes in healthy surgical patients and in renal failure patients undergoing transplant surgery.

In late pregnancy, elimination half-life may be shortened to approximately 35 to 40 minutes. The volume of distribution at steady state is approximately 300 to 400 mL/kg; systemic rate of clearance is approximately 3 to 4.5 mL/minute/kg. In man, urine recovery of vecuronium varies from 3% to 35% within 24 hours. Data derived from patients requiring insertion of a T-tube in the common bile duct suggests that 25% to 50% of a total intravenous dose of vecuronium may be excreted in bile within 42 hours. Only unchanged vecuronium has been detected in human plasma following use during surgery. In addition, its 3-desacetylmetabolite has been rarely detected in human plasma following prolonged clinical use in the ICU (see Warnings/Precautions). One metabolite, 3-desacetyl vecuronium, has been recovered in the urine of some patients in quantities that account for up to 10% of injected dose; 3-desacetyl vecuronium has also been recovered by T-tube in some patients accounting for up to 25% of the injected dose.

This metabolite has been judged by animal screening (dogs and cats) to have 50% or more of the potency of vecuronium; equipotent doses are of approximately the same duration as vecuronium in dogs and cats. Biliary excretion accounts for about half the dose of vecuronium within 7 hours in the anesthetized rat. Circulatory bypass of the liver (cat preparation) prolongs recovery from vecuronium. Limited data derived from patients with cirrhosis or cholestasis suggests that some measurements of recovery may be doubled in such patients. In patients with renal failure, measurements of recovery do not differ significantly from similar measurements in healthy patients.

Contraindications

Known hypersensitivity to vecuronium.

Warnings/Precautions

➤*Administration:* Vecuronium should be administered in carefully adjusted dosage by or under the supervision of experienced clinicians who are familiar with its actions and the possible complications that might occur following its use. The drug should not be administered unless facilities for intubation, artificial respiration, oxygen therapy, and reversal agents are immediately available. The clinician must be prepared to assist or control respiration. To reduce the possibility of prolonged neuromuscular blockade and other possible complications that might occur following long-term use in the ICU, vecuronium or any other neuromuscular blocking agent should be administered in carefully adjusted doses by or under the supervision of experienced clinicians who are familiar with its actions and who are familiar with appropriate peripheral nerve stimulator muscle monitoring techniques (see Warnings/Precautions). In patients who are known to have myasthenia gravis or the myasthenic (Eaton-Lambert) syndrome, small doses of vecuronium may have profound effects. In such patients, a peripheral nerve stimulator and use of a small test dose may be of value in monitoring the response to administration of muscle relaxants.

➤*Altered circulation time:* Conditions associated with slower circulation time in cardiovascular disease, old age, edematous states resulting in increased volume of distribution may contribute to a delay in onset time; therefore, dosage should not be increased.

➤*Long-term use in ICU:* In the intensive care unit, long-term use of neuromuscular blocking drugs to facilitate mechanical ventilation may be associated with prolonged paralysis and/or skeletal muscle weakness that may be first noted during attempts to wean such patients from the ventilator. Typically, such patients receive other drugs such as broad spectrum antibiotics, narcotics, and/or steroids and may have electrolyte imbalance and diseases which lead to electrolyte imbalance, hypoxic episodes of varying duration, acid-base imbalance, and extreme debilitation, any of which may enhance the actions of a neuromuscular blocking agent. Additionally, patients immobilized for extended periods frequently develop symptoms consistent with disuse muscle atrophy. The recovery picture may vary from regaining movement and strength in all muscles, to initial recovery of movement of the facial and small muscles of the extremities, and then to the remaining muscles. In rare cases recovery may be over an extended period of time and may even, on occasion, involve rehabilitation. Therefore, when there is a need for long-term mechanical ventilation, the benefits-to-risk ratio of neuromuscular blockade must be considered.

Continuous infusion or intermittent bolus dosing to support mechanical ventilation, has not been studied sufficiently to support dosage recommendations. In the intensive care unit, appropriate monitoring, with the use of a peripheral nerve stimulator to assess the degree of neuromuscular blockade is recommended to help preclude possible prolongation of the blockade. Whenever the use of vecuronium or any other neuromuscular blocking agent is contemplated in the ICU, it is recommended that neuromuscular transmission be monitored continuously during administration and recovery with

VECURONIUM BROMIDE — INJECTION

the help of a nerve stimulator. Additional doses of vecuronium or any other neuromuscular blocking agent should not be given before there is a definite response to t_1 or to the first twitch. If no response is elicited, infusion administration should be discontinued until a response returns.

➤*Severe obesity or neuromuscular disease:* Patients with severe obesity or neuromuscular disease may pose airway and/or ventilatory problems requiring special care before, during, and after the use of neuromuscular blocking agents such as vecuronium.

➤*Malignant hyperthermia:* Many drugs used in anesthetic practice are suspected of being capable of triggering a potentially fatal hypermetabolism of skeletal muscle known as malignant hyperthermia. There are insufficient data derived from screening in susceptible animals (swine) to establish whether or not vecuronium is capable of triggering malignant hyperthermia.

➤*Renal function impairment:* Vecuronium is well tolerated without clinically significant prolongation of neuromuscular blocking effect in patients with renal failure who have been optimally prepared for surgery by dialysis. Under emergency conditions in anephric patients some prolongation of neuromuscular blockade may occur; therefore, if anephric patients cannot be prepared for non-elective surgery, a lower initial dose of vecuronium should be considered.

➤*Hepatic function impairment:* Experience in patients with cirrhosis or cholestasis has revealed prolonged recovery time in keeping with the role the liver plays in vecuronium metabolism and excretion. Data currently available do not permit dosage recommendations in patients with impaired liver function.

➤*Pregnancy: Category C.* Animal reproduction studies have not been conducted with vecuronium. It is also not known whether vecuronium can cause fetal harm when administered to a pregnant woman or can affect reproduction capacity. The molecular weight (about 638) suggests that vecuronium will cross the placenta, but the ionization and low lipid solubility should limit the exposure of the embryo and fetus. Small amounts of vecuronium do cross the human placenta at term. Vecuronium bromide should be given to a pregnant woman only if clearly needed.

➤*Lactation:* The molecular weight (about 638) is low enough, but the low lipid solubility and ionization at physiologic pH would inhibit its excretion into milk. These factors suggest that vecuronium represents no risk to a breast-feeding infant.

➤*Children:* Infants under 1 year of age but older than 7 weeks, also tested under halothane anesthesia, are moderately more sensitive to vecuronium on a mg/kg basis than adults and take about 1-½ times as long to recover. Information presently available does not permit recommendations for usage in neonates.

Drug Interactions

➤*Succinylcholine:* Prior administration of succinylcholine may enhance the neuromuscular blocking effect of vecuronium and its duration of action. If succinylcholine is used before vecuronium, the administration of vecuronium should be delayed until the succinylcholine effect shows signs of wearing off. With succinylcholine as the intubating agent, initial doses of 0.04 to 0.06 mg/kg of vecuronium bromide may be administered to produce complete neuromuscular block with clinical duration of action of 25 to 30 minutes.

➤*Other nondepolarizing neuromuscular blocking agents:* Other nondepolarizing neuromuscular blocking agents (pancuronium, d-tubocurarine, metocurine, and gallamine) act in the same fashion as does vecuronium; therefore, these drugs and vecuronium may manifest an additive effect when used together. There are insufficient data to support concomitant use of vecuronium and other competitive muscle relaxants in the same patient.

➤*Inhalational anesthetics:* Use of volatile inhalational anesthetics such as enflurane, isoflurane, and halothane with vecuronium will enhance neuromuscular blockade. Potentiation is most prominent with use of enflurane and isoflurane. With the above agents, the initial dose of vecuronium may be the same as with balanced anesthesia unless the inhalational anesthetic has been administered for a sufficient time at a sufficient dose to have reached clinical equilibrium (see Pharmacology).

➤*Antibiotics:* Parenteral/intraperitoneal administration of high doses of certain antibiotics may intensify or produce neuromuscular block on their own. The following antibiotics have been associated with various degrees of paralysis: Aminoglycosides (such as neomycin, streptomycin, kanamycin, gentamicin, and dihydrostreptomycin); tetracyclines; bacitracin; polymyxin B; colistin; and sodium colistimethate. If these or other newly introduced antibiotics are used in conjunction with vecuronium, unexpected prolongation of neuromuscular block should be considered a possibility.

➤*Other:* Experience concerning injection of quinidine during recovery from use of other muscle relaxants suggests that recurrent paralysis may occur. This possibility must also be considered for vecuronium. Vecuronium induced neuromuscular blockade has been counteracted by alkalosis and enhanced by acidosis in experimental animals (cats). Electrolyte imbalance and diseases which lead to electrolyte imbalance, such as adrenal cortical insufficiency, have been shown to alter neuromuscular blockade. Depending on the nature of the imbalance, either enhancement or inhibition may be expected. Magnesium salts, administered for the management of toxemia of pregnancy, may enhance the neuromuscular blockade.

Adverse Reactions

Prolonged to profound extensions of paralysis and/or muscle weaknessas well as muscle atrophy have been reported after long-term use to support mechanical ventilation in the intensive care unit (see Warnings/ Precautions). The administration of vecuronium has been associated with rare instances of hypersensitivity reactions(bronchospasm, hypotension and/or tachycardia, sometimes associated with acute urticaria or erythema).

Overdosage

➤*Symptoms:* The possibility of iatrogenic overdosage can be minimized by carefully monitoring muscle twitch response to peripheral nerve stimulation.

Excessive doses of vecuronium produce enhanced pharmacological effects. Residual neuromuscular blockade beyond the time period needed may occur with vecuronium as with other neuromuscular blockers. This may be manifested by skeletal muscle weakness, decreased respiratory reserve, low tidal volume, or apnea. A peripheral nerve stimulator may be used to assess the degree of residual neuromuscular blockade from other causes of decreased respiratory reserve.

Respiratory depression may be due either wholly or in part to other drugs used during the conduct of general anesthesia such as narcotics, thiobarbiturates, and other central nervous system depressants.

➤*Treatment:* Under such circumstances the primary treatment is maintenance of a patent airway and manual or mechanical ventilation until complete recovery of normal respiration is assured. Pyridostigmine, neostigmine, or edrophonium in conjunction with atropine or glycopyrrolate will usually antagonize the skeletal muscle relaxant action of vecuronium. Satisfactory reversal can be judged by adequacy of skeletal muscle tone and by adequacy of respiration. A peripheral nerve stimulator may also be used to monitor restoration of twitch height. Failure of prompt reversal (within 30 minutes) may occur in the presence of extreme debilitation, carcinomatosis, and with concomitant use of certain broad spectrum antibiotics, or anesthetic agents and other drugs which enhance neuromuscular blockade or cause respiratory depression of their own. Under such circumstances, the management is the same as that of prolonged neuromuscular blockade. Ventilation must be supported by artificial means until the patient has resumed control of his respiration. Prior to the use of reversal agents, reference should be made to the specific package insert of the reversal agent.

SUCCINYLCHOLINE CHLORIDE

Rx	**Anectine** (GlaxoWellcome)	**Injection:** 20 mg/ml	In 10 ml vials.[a]
Rx	**Quelicin** (Hospira)		In 5 ml *Abboject* (single-dose) syringe and 10 ml vials.[b]
Rx	**Quelicin-1000** (Hospira)	**Injection, solution:** 100 mg/mL	In 5 and 10 mL single-use, preservative free vials and 20 mL multidose vials.[b]
Rx	**Anectine Flo-Pack** (GlaxoWellcome)	**Powder for infusion:** 500 mg	In vials.
		Powder for infusion: 1 g	In vials.

[a] With methylparaben.

[b] With methyl- and propylparabens.

SUCCINYLCHOLINE CHLORIDE — INJECTION

WARNING

There have been rare reports of acute rhabdomyolysis with hyperkalemia followed by ventricular dysrhythmias, cardiac arrest, and death after the administration of succinylcholine to apparently healthy children who were subsequently found to have undiagnosed skeletal muscle myopathy, most frequently Duchenne's muscular dystrophy.

This syndrome often presents as peaked T-waves and sudden cardiac arrest within minutes after the administration of the drug in healthy appearing children (usually, but not exclusively, males, and most frequently 8 years of age or younger). There have also been reports in adolescents.

Therefore, when a healthy appearing infant or child develops cardiac arrest soon after administration of succinylcholine not felt to be due to inadequate ventilation, oxygenation, or anesthetic overdose, immediate treatment for hyperkalemia should be instituted. This should include administration of intravenous calcium, bicarbonate, and glucose with insulin, with hyperventilation. Due to the abrupt onset of this syndrome, routine resuscitative measures are likely to be unsuccessful. However, extraordinary and prolonged resuscitative efforts have resulted in successful resuscitation in some reported cases. In addition, in the presence of signs of malignant hyperthermia, appropriate treatment should be instituted concurrently.

Since there may be no signs or symptoms to alert the practitioner to which patients are at risk, it is recommended that the use of succinylcholine in children should be reserved for emergency intubation or instances where immediate securing of the airway is necessary, such as laryngospasm, difficult airway, full stomach, or for intramuscular use when a suitable vein is inaccessible.

Indications

➤*Anesthesia, adjunct:* As an adjunct to general anesthesia, to facilitate tracheal intubation, and to provide skeletal muscle relaxation during surgery or mechanical ventilation.

Administration and Dosage

➤*General dosing considerations:* It is recommended that neuromuscular function be carefully monitored with a peripheral nerve stimulator when using succinylcholine by infusion in order to avoid overdose, detect development of phase II block, follow its rate of recovery, and assess the effects of reversing agents.

Intravenous (IV) bolus administration in infants and children may result in malignant ventricular arrhythmias. (See Administration.)

➤*Adults:*

Intramuscular –

Usual dosage: Up to 3 to 4 mg/kg may be given, but not more than 150 mg total dose should be administered by this route. The onset of effect of succinylcholine given intramuscularly (IM) is usually observed in about 2 to 3 minutes.

Maximum dose: 150 mg total dose.

Intravenous –

Short surgical procedures:

• *Usual dosage* – The average dose required to produce neuromuscular blockade and to facilitate tracheal intubation is 0.6 mg/kg given IV. The optimum dose will vary among individuals and may be from 0.3 to 1.1 mg/kg. Following administration of doses in this range, neuromuscular blockade develops in about 1 minute; maximum blockade may persist for about 2 minutes, after which recovery takes place within 4 to 6 minutes. However, very large doses may result in more prolonged blockade.

• *Test dose* – A 5 to 10 mg test dose may be used to determine the sensitivity of the patient and the individual recovery time.

Long surgical procedures:

• *Continuous infusion* – The dose administered by infusion depends upon the duration of the surgical procedure and the need for muscle relaxation. The average rate for an adult ranges between 2.5 and 4.3 mg/min. Solutions containing succinylcholine 1 to 2 mg/mL have commonly been used for continuous infusion. The more dilute solution (1 mg/mL) is probably preferable from the standpoint of ease of control of the rate of administration of the drug and, hence, of relaxation. This IV solution containing 1 mg/mL may be administered at a rate of 0.5 mg (0.5 mL) to 10 mg (10 mL) per minute to obtain the required amount of relaxation. The amount required per minute will depend upon the individual response as well as the degree of relaxation required. Avoid overburdening the circulation with a large volume of fluid.

• *Intermittent intravenous injection* – An IV injection of 0.3 to 1.1 mg/kg may be given initially, followed, at appropriate intervals, by further injections of 0.04 to 0.07 mg/kg to maintain the degree of relaxation required.

➤*Children:*

Intramuscular –

Usual dosage: Up to 3 to 4 mg/kg may be given, but not more than 150 mg total dose should be administered by this route. The onset of effect of succinylcholine given intramuscularly is usually observed in about 2 to 3 minutes.

Maximum dose: 150 mg total dose.

Intravenous –

Older children and adolescents: 1 mg/kg IV.

Infants and small children: 2 mg/kg IV.

Pretreatment: IV bolus administration in infants or children may result in profound bradycardia or, rarely, asystole. The incidence of bradycardia in children is higher following a second dose. The occurrence of bradyarrhythmias may be reduced by pretreatment with atropine.

➤*Preparation for administration:* Admixtures containing 1 to 2 mg/mL may be prepared by adding succinylcholine 1 g (the contents of one succinylcholine sterile powder *Flo-Pack* unit containing succinylcholine 1 g) to 1,000 or 500 mL sterile solution, such as dextrose injection 5% or sodium chloride 0.9% injection. Admixtures of succinylcholine must be used within 24 hours after preparation. Admixtures of succinylcholine should be prepared for single patient use only. The unused portion of diluted succinylcholine should be discarded.

➤*Administration:* For short surgical procedures, the dose is given IV. For long surgical procedures, the dose is given by continuous infusion or intermittent IV injections. If necessary, the dose may be given intramuscularly to infants, older children, or adults when a suitable vein is inaccessible.

Children – Rarely, IV bolus administration in infants and children may result in malignant ventricular arrhythmias and cardiac arrest secondary to acute rhabdomyolysis with hyperkalemia. In such situations, an underlying myopathy should be suspected.

➤*Admixture compatibility:* Succinylcholine is acidic (pH 3.5) and should not be mixed with alkaline solutions having a pH greater than 8.5 (eg, barbiturate solutions).

➤*Storage/Stability:* Store multiple-dose 10 mL vials in the refrigerator at 2° to 8°C (36° to 46°F). The multidose vials are stable for up to 14 days at room temperature without significant loss of potency. Store powder vials at 15° to 25°C (59° to 77°F); refrigeration is not required. Solutions of succinylcholine must be used within 24 hours after preparation. Discard unused solutions.

Actions

➤*Pharmacology:* Succinylcholine is a depolarizing skeletal muscle relaxant. As does acetylcholine, it combines with the cholinergic receptors of the motor end plate to produce depolarization. This depolarization may be observed as fasciculations. Subsequent neuromuscular transmission is inhibited so long as adequate concentration of succinylcholine remains at the receptor site. Onset of flaccid paralysis is rapid (less than 1 minute after IV administration), and with single administration lasts approximately 4 to 6 minutes.

Succinylcholine is rapidly hydrolyzed by plasma cholinesterase to succinylmonocholine (which possesses clinically insignificant depolarizing muscle relaxant properties) and then more slowly to succinic acid and choline (see Precautions). About 10% of the drug is excreted unchanged in the urine. The paralysis following administration of succinylcholine is progressive, with differing sensitivities of different muscles. This initially involves consecutively the levator muscles of the face, muscles of the glottis, and finally, the intercostals and the diaphragm and all other skeletal muscles.

Depending on the dose and duration of succinylcholine administration, the characteristic depolarizing neuromuscular block (Phase I block) may change to a block with characteristics superficially resembling a nondepolarizing block (Phase II block). This may be associated with prolonged respiratory muscle paralysis or weakness in patients who manifest the transition to Phase II block. When this diagnosis is confirmed by peripheral nerve stimulation, it may sometimes be reversed with anticholinesterase drugs such as neostigmine (see Precautions). Anticholinesterase drugs may not always be effective. If given before succinylcholine is metabolized by cholinesterase, anticholinesterase drugs may prolong rather than shorten paralysis.

Succinylcholine has no direct effect on the myocardium. Succinylcholine stimulates both autonomic ganglia and muscarinic receptors which may cause changes in cardiac rhythm, including cardiac arrest. Changes in rhythm, including cardiac arrest, may also result from vagal stimulation, which may occur during surgical procedures, or from hyperkalemia, particularly in children (see Warnings, Children). These effects are enhanced by halogenated anesthetics.

Succinylcholine causes an increase in intraocular pressure immediately after its injection and during the fasciculation phase, and slight increases which may persist after onset of complete paralysis (see Warnings).

Succinylcholine may cause slight increases in intracranial pressure immediately after its injection and during the fasciculation phase (see Precautions).

As with other neuromuscular blocking agents, the potential for releasing histamine is present following succinylcholine administration. Signs and symptoms of histamine-mediated release such as flushing, hypotension, and bronchoconstriction are, however, uncommon in normal clinical usage.

Contraindications

Personal or familial history of malignant hyperthermia; skeletal muscle myopathies; hypersensitivity to the drug; in patients after the acute phase of injury following major burns, multiple trauma, extensive denervation of skeletal muscle, or upper motor neuron injury, because succinylcholine administered to such individuals may result in severe hyperkalemia which may result in cardiac arrest. The risk of hyperkalemia in these patients increases over time and usually peaks at 7 to 10 days after the injury. The risk is dependent on the extent and location of the injury. The precise time of onset and the duration of the risk period are not known.

Warnings/Precautions

➤*Administration:* Succinylcholine should be used only by those skilled in the management of artificial respiration and only when facilities are instantly available for tracheal intubation and for providing adequate ventilation of the patient, including the administration of oxygen under positive

SUCCINYLCHOLINE CHLORIDE — INJECTION

pressure and the elimination of carbon dioxide. The clinician must be prepared to assist or control respiration.

To avoid distress to the patient, succinylcholine should not be administered before unconsciousness has been induced. In emergency situations, however, it may be necessary to administer succinylcholine before unconsciousness is induced.

➤*Hyperkalemia:* Succinylcholine should be administered with *great caution* to patients suffering from electrolyte abnormalities and those who may have massive digitalis toxicity, because in these circumstances succinylcholine may induce serious cardiac arrhythmias or cardiac arrest due to hyperkalemia.

Great caution should be observed if succinylcholine is administered to patients during the acute phase of injury following major burns, multiple trauma, extensive denervation of skeletal muscle, or upper motor neuron injury. The risk of hyperkalemia in these patients increases over time and usually peaks at 7 to 10 days after the injury. The risk is dependent on the extent and location of the injury. The precise time of onset and the duration of the risk period are undetermined. Patients with chronic abdominal infection, subarachnoid hemorrhage, or conditions causing degeneration of central and peripheral nervous systems should receive succinylcholine with *great caution* because of the potential for developing severe hyperkalemia.

➤*Malignant hyperthermia:* Succinylcholine administration has been associated with acute onset of malignant hyperthermia, a potentially fatal hypermetabolic state of skeletal muscle. The risk of developing malignant hyperthermia following succinylcholine administration increases with the concomitant administration of volatile anesthetics. Malignant hyperthermia frequently presents as intractable spasm of the jaw muscles (masseter spasm) which may progress to generalized rigidity, increased oxygen demand, tachycardia, tachypnea and profound hyperpyrexia. Successful outcome depends on recognition of early signs, such as jaw muscle spasm, acidosis, or generalized rigidity to initial administration of succinylcholine for tracheal intubation, or failure of tachycardia to respond to deepening anesthesia. Skin mottling, rising temperature, and coagulopathies may occur later in the course of the hypermetabolic process. Recognition of the syndrome is a signal for discontinuance of anesthesia, attention to increased oxygen consumption, correction of acidosis, support of circulation, assurance of adequate urinary output, and institution of measures to control rising temperature. Intravenous dantrolene sodium is recommended as an adjunct to supportive measures in the management of this problem. Consult literature references and the dantrolene prescribing information for additional information about the management of malignant hyperthermic crisis. Continuous monitoring of temperature and expired CO_2 is recommended as an aid to early recognition of malignant hyperthermia.

➤*Cardiac effects:* In both adults and children, the incidence of bradycardia, which may progress to asystole, is higher following a second dose of succinylcholine. The incidence and severity of bradycardia is higher in children than in adults. Pretreatment with anticholinergic agents (eg, atropine) may reduce the occurrence of bradyarrhythmias.

➤*Ocular effects:* Succinylcholine causes an increase in intraocular pressure. It should not be used in instances in which an increase in intraocular pressure is undesirable (eg, narrow angle glaucoma, penetrating eye injury) unless the potential benefit of its use outweighs the potential risk.

➤*Phase II block:* When succinylcholine is given over a prolonged period of time, the characteristic depolarization block of the myoneural junction (Phase I block) may change to a block with characteristics superficially resembling a nondepolarizing block (Phase II block). Prolonged respiratory muscle paralysis or weakness may be observed in patients manifesting this transition to Phase II block. The transition from Phase I to Phase II block has been reported in 7 of 7 patients studied under halothane anesthesia after an accumulated dose of 2 to 4 mg/kg succinylcholine (administered in repeated, divided doses). The onset of Phase II block coincided with the onset of tachyphylaxis and prolongation of spontaneous recovery. In another study, using balanced anesthesia (N_2O/O_2 /narcotic-thiopental) and succinylcholine infusion, the transition was less abrupt, with great individual variability in the dose of succinylcholine required to produce Phase II block. Of 32 patients studied, 24 developed Phase II block. Tachyphylaxis was not associated with the transition to Phase II block, and 50% of the patients who developed Phase II block experienced prolonged recovery.

When Phase II block is suspected in cases of prolonged neuromuscular blockade, positive diagnosis should be made by peripheral nerve stimulation prior to administration of any anticholinesterase drug. Reversal of Phase II block is a medical decision which must be made upon the basis of the individual, clinical pharmacology, and the experience and judgment of the physician. The presence of Phase II block is indicated by fade of responses to successive stimuli (preferably "train-of-four"). The use of an anticholinesterase drug to reverse Phase II block should be accompanied by appropriate doses of an anticholinergic drug to prevent disturbances of cardiac rhythm. After adequate reversal of Phase II block with an anticholinesterase agent, the patient should be continually observed for at least 1 hour for signs of return of muscle relaxation. Reversal should not be attempted unless: (1) a peripheral nerve stimulator is used to determine the presence of Phase II block (since anticholinesterase agents will potentiate succinylcholine-induced Phase I block), and (2) spontaneous recovery of muscle twitch has been observed for at least 20 minutes and has reached a plateau with further recovery proceeding slowly; this delay is to ensure complete hydrolysis of succinylcholine by plasma cholinesterase prior to administration of the anticholinesterase agent. Should the type of block be misdiagnosed, depolarization of the type initially induced by succinylcholine (ie, Phase I block) will be prolonged by an anticholinesterase agent.

➤*Reduced plasma cholinesterase activity:* Succinylcholine should be used carefully in patients with reduced plasma cholinesterase (pseudocholinesterase) activity. The likelihood of prolonged neuromuscular block following administration of succinylcholine must be considered in such patients (see Administration and Dosage).

Plasma cholinesterase activity may be diminished in the presence of genetic abnormalities of plasma cholinesterase (eg, patients heterozygous or homozygous for atypical plasma cholinesterase gene), pregnancy, severe liver or kidney disease, malignant tumors, infections, burns, anemia, decompensated heart disease, peptic ulcer, or myxedema. Plasma cholinesterase activity may also be diminished by chronic administration of oral contraceptives, glucocorticoids, or certain monoamine oxidase inhibitors, and by irreversible inhibitors of plasma cholinesterase (eg, organophosphate insecticides, echothiophate, and certain antineoplastic drugs).

Patients homozygous for atypical plasma cholinesterase gene (1 in 2500 patients) are extremely sensitive to the neuromuscular blocking effect of succinylcholine. In these patients, a 5- to 10-mg test dose of succinylcholine may be administered to evaluate sensitivity to succinylcholine, or neuromuscular blockade may be produced by the cautious administration of a 1 mg/mL solution of succinylcholine by slow IV infusion. Apnea or prolonged muscle paralysis should be treated with controlled respiration.

➤*Special risk:* Succinylcholine should be employed with caution in patients with fractures or muscle spasm because the initial muscle fasciculations may cause additional trauma.

Succinylcholine may cause a transient increase in intracranial pressure; however, adequate anesthetic induction prior to administration of succinylcholine will minimize this effect.

Succinylcholine may increase intragastric pressure, which could result in regurgitation and possible aspiration of stomach contents.

Neuromuscular blockade may be prolonged in patients with hypokalemia or hypocalcemia.

➤*Pregnancy:* Category C. Animal reproduction studies have not been conducted with succinylcholine chloride. It is also not known whether succinylcholine can cause fetal harm when administered to a pregnant woman or can affect reproduction capacity. Succinylcholine should be given to a pregnant woman only if clearly needed.

Plasma cholinesterase levels are decreased by approximately 24% during pregnancy and for several days postpartum. Therefore, a higher proportion of patients may be expected to show increased sensitivity (prolonged apnea) to succinylcholine when pregnant than when nonpregnant.

Labor and delivery – Succinylcholine is commonly used to provide muscle relaxation during delivery by cesarean section. While small amounts of succinylcholine are known to cross the placental barrier, under normal conditions the quantity of drug that enters fetal circulation after a single dose of 1 mg/kg to the mother should not endanger the fetus. However, since the amount of drug that crosses the placental barrier is dependent on the concentration gradient between the maternal and fetal circulations, residual neuromuscular blockade (apnea and flaccidity) may occur in the neonate after repeated high doses to, or in the presence of atypical plasma cholinesterase in, the mother.

➤*Lactation:* It is not known whether succinylcholine is excreted in human milk. Because many drugs are excreted in human milk, caution should be exercised following succinylcholine administration to a nursing woman.

➤*Children:* See the Warning box for more information.

There may be no signs or symptoms to alert the practitioner to which patients are at risk. A careful history and physical may identify developmental delays suggestive of a myopathy. A preoperative creatine kinase could identify some but not all patients at risk. Due to the abrupt onset of this syndrome, routine resuscitative measures are likely to be unsuccessful. Careful monitoring of the electrocardiogram may alert the practitioner to peaked T-waves (an early sign). Administration of IV calcium, bicarbonate, and glucose with insulin, with hyperventilation have resulted in successful resuscitation in some of the reported cases. Extraordinary and prolonged resuscitative efforts have been effective in some cases. In addition, in the presence of signs of malignant hyperthermia, appropriate treatment should be initiated concurrently. Since it is difficult to identify which patients are at risk, it is recommended that the use of succinylcholine in children should be reserved for emergency intubation or instances where immediate securing of the airway is necessary, such as laryngospasm, difficult airway, full stomach, or for intramuscular use when a suitable vein is inaccessible.

Drug Interactions

Drugs which may enhance the neuromuscular blocking action of succinylcholine include: Promazine, oxytocin, aprotinin, certain non-penicillin antibiotics, quinidine, β-adrenergic blockers, procainamide, lidocaine, trimethaphan, lithium carbonate, magnesium salts, quinine, chloroquine, diethylether, isoflurane, desflurane, metoclopramide, and terbutaline. The neuromuscular blocking effect of succinylcholine may be enhanced by drugs that reduce plasma cholinesterase activity (eg, chronically administered oral contraceptives, glucocorticoids, or certain monoamine oxidase inhibitors) or by drugs that irreversibly inhibit plasma cholinesterase.

If other neuromuscular blocking agents are to be used during the same procedure, the possibility of a synergistic or antagonistic effect should be considered.

Adverse Reactions

Adverse reactions to succinylcholine consist primarily of an extension of its pharmacological actions. Succinylcholine causes profound muscle relaxation resulting in respiratory depression to the point of apnea; this effect may be

SUCCINYLCHOLINE CHLORIDE — INJECTION

prolonged. Hypersensitivity reactions, including anaphylaxis, may occur in rare instances. The following additional adverse reactions have been reported.

➤*Cardiovascular:* Cardiac arrest, arrhythmias, bradycardia, tachycardia, hypertension, hypotension.

➤*Musculoskeletal:* Muscle fasciculation, jaw rigidity, postoperative muscle pain, rhabdomyolysis with possible myoglobinuric acute renal failure.

➤*Respiratory:* Prolonged respiratory depression or apnea.

➤*Miscellaneous:* Increased intraocular pressure, hyperkalemia, malignant hyperthermia, excessive salivation, and rash.

Overdosage

➤*Symptoms:* Overdosage with succinylcholine may result in neuromuscular block beyond the time needed for surgery and anesthesia. This may be manifested by skeletal muscle weakness, decreased respiratory reserve, low tidal volume, or apnea.

➤*Treatment:* The primary treatment is maintenance of a patent airway and respiratory support until recovery of normal respiration is assured. Depending on the dose and duration of succinylcholine administration, the characteristic depolarizing neuromuscular block (Phase I) may change to a block with characteristics superficially resembling a nondepolarizing block (Phase II) (see Precautions).

SKELETAL MUSCLE RELAXANTS

Centrally Acting

BACLOFEN

Rx	**Baclofen** (Various, eg, Ivax, Watson)	**Tablets; oral:** 10 mg	In 30s, 100s, 250s, 500s, and 1000s.
Rx	**Lioresal** (Novartis)		(Lioresal 1010). White, scored, oval. In 100s and UD 100s.
Rx	**Baclofen** (Various, eg, Ivax, Watson)	**Tablets; oral:** 20 mg	In 30s, 100s, 250s, 500s, and 1000s.
Rx	**Lioresal** (Novartis)		(Lioresal 2020). White, scored, capsule shape. In 100s and UD 100s.
Rx	**Kemstro** (Schwarz)	**Tablets, disintegrating; oral:** 10 mg	Mannitol, aspartame, 3.9 mg phenylalanine. (10 SP 351). Scored. Orange flavor. In 100s.
Rx	**Kemstro** (Schwarz)	20 mg	Mannitol, aspartame, 7.9 mg phenylalanine. (20 SP 352). Scored. Orange flavor. In 100s.
Rx	**Gablofen** (CNS Therapeutics)	**Injection, solution; intrathecal:** 0.05 mg per mL (50 mcg/mL)	Preservative free. In single-use syringes.
Rx	**Lioresal Intrathecal** (Medtronic)		Preservative free. In single-use amps.
Rx	**Gablofen** (CNS Therapeutics)	**Injection, solution; intrathecal:** 10 mg per 20 mL (500 mcg/mL)	Preservative free. In single-use vials.
Rx	**Lioresal Intrathecal** (Medtronic)		Preservative free. In single-use amps (1 amp refill kit).
Rx	**Gablofen** (CNS Therapeutics)	**Injection, solution; intrathecal:** 10 mg per 5 mL (2,000 mcg/mL)	Preservative free. In single-use vials.
Rx	**Lioresal Intrathecal** (Medtronic)		Preservative free. In single-use amps (2 or 4 amp refill kits).

BACLOFEN — ORAL

Indications

➤*Spasticity:* For the alleviation of signs and symptoms of spasticity resulting from multiple sclerosis, particularly for the relief of flexor spasms and concomitant pain, clonus, and muscular rigidity. Patients should have reversible spasticity so that baclofen treatment will aid in restoring residual function. Baclofen may also be of some value in patients with spinal cord injuries and other spinal cord diseases.

Baclofen is not indicated in the treatment of skeletal muscle spasm resulting from rheumatic disorders. The efficacy of baclofen in stroke, cerebral palsy, and Parkinson disease has not been established and, therefore, it is not recommended for these conditions.

➤*Off-label uses:*

Alcohol withdrawal – [4] = Insufficient documentation. The role, if any, of baclofen in the suppression of alcohol withdrawal syndrome has not been fully established. A small comparative trial with diazepam suggests that baclofen may be comparable with diazepam in the management of acute withdrawal.

Gastroesophageal reflux disease (adults) – [3] = Safety concerns. Studies have demonstrated consistent findings of decreased transient lower esophageal sphincter relaxation episodes and increased pH after administration of baclofen to patients with gastroesophageal reflux disease (GERD). Clinical benefits, however, were not always measured or observed. In addition, most studies evaluated single bolus doses, whereas multiple daily doses would likely be needed for routine use. American College of Gastroenterology (ACG) guidelines for the management of GERD state that baclofen may be used in select patients as adjunctive therapy with other acid-suppressing agents.

Gastroesophageal reflux disease (children/adolescents) – [4] = Insufficient documentation. Data from a controlled trial in children suggest that baclofen decreased GERD episodes by inhibiting transient lower esophageal sphincter relaxation. Larger, controlled trials are needed to determine the role of baclofen in the treatment of GERD in children.

Hiccups (singultus) – [2] = Fair documentation. Baclofen may be a useful alternative in patients with intractable hiccups from various causes that have been unresponsive to other therapies.

Huntington disease – [5] = Poor documentation. Two small, controlled trials indicate that baclofen does not appear to be effective in delaying the progression of early Huntington disease. Larger trials are needed to confirm this finding, identify appropriate candidates for therapy, and define an optimal dosage.

Idiopathic muscle cramps – [4] = Insufficient documentation. Baclofen is frequently used in clinical practice, but there are no published clinical trials evaluating its efficacy for the management of idiopathic muscle cramps. Guidelines did not recommend baclofen as pharmacologic treatment for muscle cramps.

Nystagmus – [4] = Insufficient documentation. Inconsistent results have been reported with baclofen use for the treatment of nystagmus. It is unclear why some patients with nystagmus benefit from baclofen therapy and others do not. However, given the lack of a definitive symptomatic treatment for this disease, a therapeutic trial of baclofen may be warranted before more invasive or risky approaches such as botulinum toxin injections or surgery are attempted.

Opiate withdrawal – [4] = Insufficient documentation. Baclofen appears to be at least as effective as clonidine in the management of physical symptoms and superior to clonidine for the alleviation of mental symptoms. However, dropout rates were high for baclofen and clonidine when used for the management of opioid withdrawal syndrome.

Parkinson-associated rigidity – [5] = Poor documentation. Most of the published literature on the use of baclofen for the treatment of rigidity associated with Parkinson disease, parkinsonian symptoms, or secondary parkinsonism suggests that the drug has no benefit and may potentially worsen symptoms. Therapy was also frequently associated with adverse effects. The use of baclofen for rigidity associated with Parkinson disease cannot be recommended based on the reported experiences to date.

Prevention of migraine (adults) – [2] = Fair documentation. In 1 small, open-label trial, baclofen was effective for the prevention of migraine headaches in adults. However, other agents have been proven effective for the prevention of migraine and have been recommended in guidelines.

Spasticity of cerebral palsy (children/adolescents) – [4] = Insufficient documentation. Although the guideline authors did not recommend the use of oral baclofen, they acknowledged that it is commonly prescribed in practice for the treatment of spasticity of cerebral palsy in children.

Tourette syndrome (children/adolescents) – [2] = Fair documentation. Baclofen appears to be safe and may provide benefits to pediatric patients with Tourette syndrome by decreasing tic severity and improving the impairment of tics on the patient's life.

Trigeminal neuralgia – [2] = Fair documentation. Small controlled and uncontrolled trials indicate that baclofen provides pain relief in two-thirds to three-fourths of patients with trigeminal neuralgia. Baclofen has also been used in combination with carbamazepine and phenytoin, resulting in better pain relief than single-drug therapy.

Other possible off-label uses – To reduce spasticity in patients with cerebrovascular stroke; neuropathic pain.

Administration and Dosage

➤*General dosing considerations:* The lowest dose compatible with an optimal response is recommended.

If benefits are not evident after a reasonable trial period, patients should be slowly withdrawn from the drug.

BACLOFEN — ORAL

➤*Adults:*

Spasticity –

12 years of age and older:

- *Maximum dose* – 80 mg daily (20 mg 4 times daily).
- *Initial dosage* – 40 to 80 mg daily.
- *Dosage titration* – Start therapy at a low dosage and increase gradually until optimum effect is achieved. The following dosage titration schedule is suggested:

- 5 mg 3 times daily for 3 days;
- 10 mg 3 times daily for 3 days;
- 15 mg 3 times daily for 3 days;
- 20 mg 3 times daily for 3 days.

Off-label dosing –

Alcohol withdrawal: [4] = Insufficient documentation. Initial dose: 10 mg, followed by 10 mg every 8 hours or 3 times daily for 10 to 30 days. In an at-home study, the drug was provided to a family member to administer at home.

Gastroesophageal reflux disease (adults): [3] = Safety concerns. 10 mg orally 4 times/day.

Hiccups (singultus): [2] = Fair documentation. Typical initial doses ranged from 5 to 10 mg 3 times/day, but higher doses have been required for hiccup resolution in some cases (20 to 30 mg 3 times/day). It is recommended that once an effective dose is achieved, dose tapering or withdrawal be attempted to observe if relapse occurs. Some patients may require maintenance or long-term therapy, particularly some patients on dialysis or terminally ill with cancer.

Guidelines for hiccups related to cancer (palliative care) recommend oral doses of 5 to 20 mg, 2 to 3 times daily.

Idiopathic muscle cramps: [4] = Insufficient documentation. 10 mg orally 3 times daily. In a case report, the cessation of daily baclofen therapy resulted in an increase in cramp intensity.

Nystagmus: [4] = Insufficient documentation. 5 mg orally 3 times daily, titrated up at weekly intervals until clinical improvement was achieved or intolerable adverse effects developed. The average final dosage ranged from 15 to 120 mg/day in divided doses.

Opiate withdrawal: [4] = Insufficient documentation. Dosing schedules ranged from 40 mg daily for 2 weeks to 60 mg daily for up to 12 weeks. Initial regimens have started at 10 mg and increased to a maintenance dosage of 20 mg 3 times daily over a 5-day period or 15 mg increased to a maintenance dosage of 40 mg over 4 days.

Prevention of migraine (adults): [2] = Fair documentation. 15 to 30 mg given 3 times a day.

Trigeminal neuralgia: [2] = Fair documentation. 30 to 80 mg/day in 3 to 4 divided doses. The initial dose is typically 5 to 10 mg 3 times daily, but may be as low as 10 mg daily, and is then titrated (10 mg every other day) over 1 to 2 weeks. Study duration has ranged from 1 week to a long-term follow-up of 5 years.

➤*Children:*

Off-label dosing –

Gastroesophageal reflux disease (children/adolescents): [4] = Insufficient documentation. 0.17 or 0.23 mg/kg administered orally or via nasogastric tube 3 times per day. In one study, the drug was administered 30 minutes before meals for 1 week.

Spasticity: Dosage increments may be made every 3 days until desired effect or maximum dosage is reached.

- *2 years of age and older* –
  - *Usual dosage:* 10 to 15 mg per day given in divided doses every 8 hours.
  - *Maximum dose:* 60 mg/day (8 years of age and older); 40 mg/day (less than 8 years of age).

Spasticity of cerebral palsy (children/adolescents): [4] = Insufficient documentation. 5 to 10 mg/day in 3 divided doses. When discontinuing therapy, doses should be tapered gradually to avoid withdrawal symptoms.

Tourette syndrome (children/adolescents): [2] = Fair documentation. 10 to 15 mg orally daily in 3 divided doses (initial), titrated to 60 to 80 mg daily for up to 4 weeks.

➤*Renal function impairment:* Because baclofen is primarily excreted unchanged through the kidneys, it should be given with caution, and it may be necessary to reduce the dosage.

➤*Storage/Stability:* Do not store above 30°C (86°F). Dispense in tight container.

Actions

➤*Pharmacology:* The precise mechanism of action of baclofen is not fully known. Baclofen is capable of inhibiting both monosynaptic and polysynaptic reflexes at the spinal level, possibly by hyperpolarization of afferent terminals, although actions at supraspinal sites may also occur and contribute to its clinical effect. Although baclofen is an analog of the putative inhibitory neurotransmitter gamma-aminobutyric acid (GABA), there is no conclusive evidence that actions on GABA systems are involved in the production of its clinical effects. In studies with animals, baclofen has been shown to have general CNS-depressant properties as indicated by the production of sedation with tolerance, somnolence, ataxia, and respiratory and cardiovascular depression.

➤*Pharmacokinetics:* Baclofen is rapidly and extensively absorbed and eliminated. Absorption may be dose-dependent, being reduced with increasing doses. Baclofen is excreted primarily by the kidney in unchanged form and there is relatively large intersubject variation in absorption and/or elimination.

Contraindications

Hypersensitivity to baclofen.

Warnings/Precautions

➤*Abrupt drug withdrawal:* Hallucinations and seizures have occurred on abrupt withdrawal of baclofen. Therefore, except for serious adverse reactions, the dose should be reduced slowly when the drug is discontinued.

➤*Stroke:* Baclofen has not significantly benefited patients with stroke. These patients have also shown poor tolerability to the drug.

➤*Epilepsy:* In patients with epilepsy, the clinical state and electroencephalogram should be monitored at regular intervals, since deterioration in seizure control and EEG have been reported occasionally in patients taking baclofen.

➤*Spasticity:* Baclofen should be used with caution where spasticity is utilized to sustain upright posture and balance in locomotion or whenever spasticity is utilized to obtain increased function.

➤*Ovarian cysts:* Ovarian cysts have been found by palpation in approximately 4% of the multiple sclerosis patients that were treated with baclofen for up to 1 year. In most cases these cysts disappeared spontaneously while patients continued to receive the drug. Ovarian cysts are estimated to occur spontaneously in approximately 1% to 5% of the healthy female population.

➤*Renal function impairment:* Because baclofen is primarily excreted unchanged through the kidneys, it should be given with caution, and it may be necessary to reduce the dosage.

➤*Hazardous tasks:* Because of the possibility of sedation, patients should be cautioned regarding the operation of automobiles or other dangerous machinery, and activities made hazardous by decreased alertness. Patients should also be cautioned that the CNS effects of baclofen may be additive to those of alcohol and other CNS depressants.

➤*Pregnancy: Category C.* Baclofen has been shown to increase the incidence of omphaloceles (ventral hernias) in fetuses of rats given approximately 13 times the maximum dose recommended for human use, at a dose that caused significant reductions in food intake and weight gain in dams. This abnormality was not seen in mice or rabbits. There was also an increased incidence of incomplete sternebral ossification in fetuses of rats given approximately 13 times the maximum recommended human dose, and an increased incidence of unossified phalangeal nuclei of forelimbs and hindlimbs in fetuses of rabbits given approximately 7 times the maximum recommended human dose. In mice, no teratogenic effects were observed, although reductions in mean fetal weight with consequent delays in skeletal ossification were present when dams were given 17 or 34 times the human daily dose. There are no studies in pregnant women. Baclofen should be used during pregnancy only if the benefit clearly justifies the potential risk to the fetus.

If a woman requires oral baclofen, it should not be withheld because of pregnancy. The lowest possible dose should be used, and offspring should be monitored for late-onset seizures.

➤*Lactation:* It is not known whether this drug is excreted in human milk. As a general rule, nursing should not be undertaken while a patient is on a drug since many drugs are excreted in human milk.

Small amounts of baclofen are excreted into human milk after oral administration. The American Academy of Pediatrics classifies baclofen as compatible with breastfeeding.

➤*Children:* Safety and efficacy in children younger than 12 years of age have not been established.

Adverse Reactions

The most common is transient drowsiness (10% to 63%). In one controlled study of 175 patients, transient drowsiness was observed in 63% of those receiving baclofen compared to 36% of those in the placebo group. Other common adverse reactions are dizziness (5% to 15%), weakness (5% to 15%), and fatigue (2% to 4%). Others reported include the following:

➤*Cardiovascular:* Hypotension (0% to 9%). Rare instances of dyspnea, palpitation, chest pain, and syncope.

➤*GI:* Nausea (4% to 12%), constipation (2% to 6%); and, rarely, dry mouth, anorexia, taste disorder, abdominal pain, vomiting, diarrhea, and positive test for occult blood in stool.

➤*GU:* Urinary frequency (2% to 6%); and, rarely, enuresis, urinary retention, dysuria, impotence, inability to ejaculate, nocturia, and hematuria.

➤*Lab test abnormalities:* Increased AST, elevated alkaline phosphatase, and elevation of blood sugar.

➤*Psychiatric:* Confusion (1% to 11%), headache (4% to 8%), insomnia (2% to 7%); and, rarely, euphoria, excitement, depression, hallucinations, paresthesia, muscle pain, tinnitus, slurred speech, coordination disorder, tremor, rigidity, dystonia, ataxia, blurred vision, nystagmus, strabismus, miosis, mydriasis, diplopia, dysarthria, and epileptic seizure.

➤*Miscellaneous:* Instances of rash, pruritus, ankle edema, excessive perspiration, weight gain, and nasal congestion. Some of the CNS and genitourinary symptoms may be related to the underlying disease rather than to drug therapy.

BACLOFEN — ORAL

Overdosage

➤*Symptoms:* Symptoms of overdosage include vomiting, muscular hypotonia, drowsiness, accommodation disorders, coma, respiratory depression, and seizures.

➤*Treatment:* In the alert patient, empty the stomach promptly by induced emesis followed by lavage. In the obtunded patient, secure the airway with a cuffed endotracheal tube before beginning lavage (do not induce emesis). Maintain adequate respiratory exchange, do not use respiratory stimulants.

BACLOFEN — INTRATHECAL INJECTION

WARNING

Abrupt discontinuation of intrathecal baclofen, regardless of the cause, has resulted in sequelae that include high fever, altered mental status, exaggerated rebound spasticity, and muscle rigidity, which in rare cases has advanced to rhabdomyolysis, multiple organ-system failure, and death.

Prevention of abrupt discontinuation of intrathecal baclofen requires careful attention to programming and monitoring of the infusion system, refill scheduling and procedures, and pump alarms. Advise patients and caregivers of the importance of keeping scheduled refill visits and educate them on the early symptoms of baclofen withdrawal. Give special attention to patients at apparent risk (eg, spinal cord injuries at T-6 or above, communication difficulties, history of withdrawal symptoms from oral or intrathecal baclofen). Consult the technical manual of the implantable infusion system for additional postimplant clinician and patient information (see Warnings).

Indications

➤*Severe spasticity:* For use in the management of severe spasticity. Patients should first respond to a screening dose of intrathecal baclofen prior to consideration for long-term infusion via an implantable pump. For spasticity of spinal cord origin, chronic infusion of baclofen intrathecal injection via an implantable pump should be reserved for patients unresponsive to oral baclofen therapy, or those who experience intolerable CNS side effects at effective doses. Patients with spasticity due to traumatic brain injury should wait at least 1 year after the injury before consideration of long-term intrathecal baclofen therapy. Baclofen intrathecal injection is intended for use by the intrathecal route in single bolus test doses (via spinal catheter or lumbar puncture) and, for chronic use, only in implantable pumps approved by the FDA specifically for the administration of baclofen intrathecal injection into the intrathecal space.

Baclofen intrathecal injection therapy may be considered an alternative to destructive neurosurgical procedures. Prior to implantation of a device for chronic intrathecal infusion of baclofen intrathecal, patients must show a response to it in a screening trial.

➤*Off-label uses:* To reduce spasticity in patients with cerebral palsy; generalized dystonia associated with cerebral palsy.

Administration and Dosage

➤*General dosing considerations:* Patients must be monitored closely in a fully equipped and staffed environment during the screening phase and dose-titration period immediately following implant. Resuscitative equipment should be immediately available for use in case of life-threatening or intolerable side effects.

If there is not a substantive clinical response to increases in the daily dose, check for proper pump function and catheter patency.

Determination of the optimal baclofen intrathecal dose requires individual titration. The lowest dose with an optimal response should be used.

The clinical goal is to maintain muscle tone as close to normal as possible and to minimize the frequency and severity of spasms to the extent possible, without inducing intolerable side effects, or to titrate the dose to the desired degree of muscle tone for optimal functions.

Most patients require gradual increases in dose over time to maintain optimal response during chronic therapy. A sudden large requirement for dose escalation suggests a catheter complication (ie, catheter kink or dislodgment).

Screening phase – Prior to pump implantation and initiation of chronic infusion of baclofen intrathecal injection, patients must demonstrate a positive clinical response to a baclofen intrathecal injection bolus dose administered intrathecally in a screening trial. A positive response consists of a significant decrease in muscle tone and/or frequency and/or severity of spasms. (See Test Dose).

The screening trial employs baclofen intrathecal injection at a concentration of 50 mcg/mL. A 1 mL ampule (50 mcg/mL) is available for use in the screening trial.

➤*Adults:*

Severe spasticity –

Test dose: Initial bolus containing 50 mcg in a volume of 1 mL administered into the intrathecal space by barbotage over a period of not less than 1 minute.

The patient is observed over the ensuing 4 to 8 hours.

If the initial response is less than desired, a second bolus injection may be administered 24 hours after the first. The second screening bolus dose consists of 75 mcg in 1.5 mL. Again, the patient should be observed for an interval of 4 to 8 hours. If the response is still inadequate, a final bolus screening dose of 100 mcg in 2 mL may be administered 24 hours later.

Patients who do not respond to a 100 mcg intrathecal bolus should not be considered candidates for an implanted pump for chronic infusion.

Initial dosage: The screening dose that gave a positive effect should be doubled and administered over a 24-hour period, unless the efficacy of the bolus dose was maintained for more than 8 hours, in which case the starting daily dose should be the screening dose delivered over a 24-hour period.

No dose increases should be given in the first 24 hours (ie, until the steady state is achieved).

Dosage titration:

• *Spasticity of spinal cord region* – After the first 24 hours, the daily dosage should be increased slowly by 10% to 30% increments and only once every 24 hours, until the desired clinical effect is achieved.

• *Spasticity of cerebral region* – After the first 24 hours, the daily dose should be increased slowly by 5% to 15% only once every 24 hours, until the desired clinical effect is achieved.

Maintenance dosage:

• *Spasticity of spinal cord region* – From 12 mcg/day to 2,003 mcg/day, with most patients adequately maintained on 300 to 800 mcg/day. There is limited experience with daily doses more than 1,000 mcg/day.

Often the maintenance dose needs to be adjusted during the first few months of therapy while patients adjust to changes in life style due to the alleviation of spasticity.

• *Spasticity of cerebral region* – From 22 mcg/day to 1,400 mcg/day, with most patients adequately maintained on 90 to 703 mcg/day.

In clinical trials, only 3 of 150 patients required daily doses more than 1,000 mcg/day.

Often the maintenance dose needs to be adjusted during the first few months of therapy while patients adjust to changes in life style due to the alleviation of spasticity.

Dosage adjustment:

• *Spasticity of spinal cord region* – During periodic refills of the pump, the daily dose may be increased by 10% to 40%, but not more than 40%, to maintain adequate symptom control.

The daily dose may be reduced by 10% to 20% if patients experience side effects.

• *Spasticity of cerebral region* – During periodic refills of the pump, the daily dose may be increased by 5% to 20%, but not more than 20%, to maintain adequate symptom control.

The daily dose may be reduced by 10% to 20% if patients experience side effects.

• *Chronic use* – During long-term treatment, approximately 5% of patients become refractory to increasing doses. There is not sufficient experience to make firm recommendations for tolerance treatment; however, this "tolerance" has been treated on occasion, in hospital, by a "drug holiday" consisting of the gradual reduction of baclofen intrathecal over a 2- to 4-week period and switching to alternative methods of spasticity management. After the "drug holiday," baclofen intrathecal may be restarted at the initial continuous infusion dose.

➤*Children:*

Severe spasticity –

12 years of age and older: See Adults for dosing.

4 to 11 years of age: Children should be of sufficient body mass to accommodate the implantable pump for chronic infusion.

Children younger than 12 years of age seemed to require a lower daily dose in clinical trials.

• *Usual dosage* – Average daily dose of 274 mcg/day, with a range of 24 to 1,199 mcg/day. The lowest dose with an optimal response should be used.

• *Test dose* – See Adults for dosing. However for very small patients, a screening dose of 25 mcg may be tried first.

• *Dosage titration* – After the first 24 hours, the daily dose should be increased slowly by 5% to 15% only once every 24 hours, until the desired clinical effect is achieved.

• *Maintenance dosage* – From 22 mcg/day to 1,400 mcg/day, with most patients adequately maintained on 90 to 703 mcg/day.

• *Dosage adjustment* – During periodic refills of the pump, the daily dose may be increased by 5% to 20%, but not more than 20%, to maintain adequate symptom control.

The daily dose may be reduced by 10% to 20% if patients experience side effects.

➤*Renal function impairment:* Because baclofen is primarily excreted unchanged by the kidneys, it should be given with caution in patients with impaired renal function and it may be necessary to reduce the dosage.

➤*Preparation for administration:*

Delivery specifications – The specific concentration that should be used depends upon the total daily dose required and the delivery rate of the pump. Baclofen intrathecal may require dilution when used with certain implantable pumps. Please consult manufacturer's manual for specific recommendations.

Screening – Use the 1 mL screening ampule only (50 mcg/mL) for bolus injection into the subarachnoid space.

For a 50 mcg bolus dose, use 1 mL of the screening ampule. Use 1.5 mL of 50 mcg/mL baclofen intrathecal for a 75 mcg bolus dose.

For the maximum screening dose of 100 mcg, use 2 mL of 50 mcg/mL baclofen intrathecal (2 screening ampules).

BACLOFEN — INTRATHECAL INJECTION

Dilution – For patients who require concentrations other than 500 mcg/mL or 2,000 mcg/mL, baclofen intrathecal must be diluted. Baclofen intrathecal must be diluted with sterile preservative-free sodium chloride for injection.

➤*Administration:* Refer to the manufacturer's manual for the implantable pump approved for intrathecal infusion for specific instructions and precautions for programming the pump and refilling the reservoir.

Delivery regimen – Baclofen intrathecal is most often administered in a continuous infusion mode immediately following implant.

For those patients implanted with programmable pumps who have achieved relatively satisfactory control on continuous infusion, further benefit may be attained using more complex schedules of baclofen intrathecal delivery. For example, patients who have increased spasms at night may require a 20% increase in their hourly infusion rate. Changes in flow rate should be programmed to start 2 hours before the time of desired clinical effect.

Test dose – Direct intrathecal injection by barbotage over no less than 1 minute.

Maintenance regimen – Continuous intrathecal infusion.

➤*Storage/Stability:* Does not require refrigeration. Do not store above 30°C (86°F). Do not freeze or heat sterilize.

Actions

➤*Pharmacology:* The precise mechanism of action of baclofen as a muscle relaxant and antispasticity agent is not fully understood. Baclofen inhibits both monosynaptic and polysynaptic reflexes at the spinal level, possibly by decreasing excitatory neurotransmitter release from primary afferent terminals, although actions at supraspinal sites may also occur and contribute to its clinical effect. Baclofen is a structural analog of the inhibitory neurotransmitter gamma-aminobutyric acid (GABA), and may exert its effects by stimulation of the $GABA^B$ receptor subtype.

Baclofen intrathecal injection when introduced directly into the intrathecal space permits effective CSF concentrations to be achieved with resultant plasma concentrations 100 times less than those occurring with oral administration.

Pharmacodynamics –

Intrathecal bolus:

• *Adults* – The onset of action is generally 30 minutes to 1 hour after an intrathecal bolus. Peak spasmolytic effect is seen at ≈ 4 hours after dosing and effects may last 4 to 8 hours. Onset, peak response, and duration of action may vary with individual patients depending on the dose and severity of symptoms.

• *Children* – The onset, peak response and duration of action is similar to those seen in adult patients.

Continuous infusion: Baclofen intrathecal injection's antispastic action is first seen at 6 to 8 hours after initiation of continuous infusion. Maximum activity is observed in 24 to 48 hours.

➤*Pharmacokinetics:* The pharmacokinetics of CSF clearance of baclofen intrathecal injection calculated from intrathecal bolus or continuous infusion studies approximates CSF turnover, suggesting elimination is by bulk-flow removal of CSF.

Intrathecal bolus – After a bolus lumbar injection of 50 or 100 mcg baclofen intrathecal injection in 7 patients, the average CSF elimination half-life was 1.51 hours over the first 4 hours and the average CSF clearance was approximately 30 mL/hr.

Continuous infusion – The mean CSF clearance for baclofen intrathecal injection was approximately 30 mL/hr in a study involving 10 patients on continuous intrathecal infusion.

Contraindications

Hypersensitivity to baclofen; not recommended for IV, IM, SC, or epidural administration.

Warnings/Precautions

➤*Administration:* Baclofen intrathecal injection is for use in single bolus intrathecal injections (via a catheter placed in the lumbar intrathecal space or injection by lumbar puncture) and in implantable pumps approved by the FDA specifically for the intrathecal administration of baclofen. Because of the possibility of potentially life-threatening CNS depression, cardiovascular collapse, and/or respiratory failure, physicians must be adequately trained and educated in chronic intrathecal infusion therapy.

The pump system should not be implanted until the patient's response to bolus baclofen intrathecal injection is adequately evaluated. Evaluation (consisting of a screening procedure) requires that baclofen intrathecal injection be administered into the intrathecal space via a catheter or lumbar puncture. Because of the risks associated with the screening procedure and the adjustment of dosage following pump implantation, these phases must be conducted in a medically supervised and adequately equipped environment following the instructions outlined in Administration and Dosage.

Resuscitative equipment should be available. Following surgical implantation of the pump, particularly during the initial phases of pump use, the patient should be monitored closely until it is certain that the patient's response to the infusion is acceptable and reasonably stable.

Extreme caution must be used when filling an FDA-approved implantable pump. Such pumps should only be refilled through the reservoir refill septum. However, some pumps are also equipped with a catheter access port that allows direct access to the intrathecal catheter. Direct injection into this catheter access port may cause a life-threatening overdose.

➤*Withdrawal:* Baclofen withdrawal has been identified during postapproval use of baclofen intrathecal injection. Because this reaction is reported simultaneously from a population of uncertain size, it is not possible to reliably estimate the frequency.

Early symptoms of baclofen withdrawal may include pruritus, hypotension, and paresthesias.

Abrupt withdrawal of intrathecal baclofen, regardless of the cause, has, in rare cases, resulted in a life-threatening syndrome that included high fever, altered mental status, exaggerated rebound spasticity, and muscle rigidity that progressed to rhabdomyolysis, multiple organ-system failure, and death.

All patients receiving intrathecal baclofen therapy are potentially at risk. Some clinical characteristics of the advanced intrathecal baclofen withdrawal syndrome may resemble autonomic dysreflexia, or infection (sepsis), malignant hyperthermia, neuroleptic-malignant syndrome, and other conditions associated with a hypermetabolic state or widespread rhabdomyolysis. A rapid and accurate diagnosis is important in an emergency room or intensive care setting before initiating treatment in order to prevent the potentially life-threatening central nervous and systemic effects of intrathecal baclofen withdrawal. The suggested treatment for intrathecal baclofen withdrawal is the restoration of intrathecal baclofen at or near the same dosage as before therapy was interrupted. However, if restoration of intrathecal delivery is delayed, treatment with GABA-ergic agonist drugs, such as oral or enteral baclofen, or oral, enteral, or IV benzodiazepines may prevent potentially fatal sequelae. Because of the phenomenon of $GABA_B$ receptor down-regulation, oral or enteral baclofen alone should not be relied upon to halt the progression of the intrathecal baclofen withdrawal syndrome.

Careful monitoring of infusion pump function and inspection of the catheter for occlusion or dislodgment can help reduce the risk of abrupt withdrawal of intrathecal baclofen.

➤*Hallucinations:* Hallucinations have occurred after abrupt withdrawal of baclofen intrathecal injection.

➤*Seizures:* Seizures have been reported during overdose and with withdrawal from baclofen intrathecal injection and in patients maintained on therapeutic doses of baclofen intrathecal injection.

➤*Fatalities:*

Spasticity of spinal cord origin – There were 16 deaths reported among the 576 US patients treated with baclofen intrathecal injection in pre- and postmarketing studies evaluated as of December 1992. Because these patients were treated under uncontrolled clinical settings, it is impossible to determine definitively what role, if any, baclofen intrathecal injection played in their deaths.

Spasticity of cerebral origin – There were 3 deaths occurring among the 211 patients treated with baclofen intrathecal in premarketing studies as of March 1996. These deaths were not attributed to the therapy.

➤*Screening:* Patients should be infection-free prior to the screening trial with baclofen intrathecal injection because the presence of a systemic infection may interfere with an assessment of the patient's response to bolus baclofen intrathecal injection.

➤*Pump implantation:* Patients should be infection-free prior to pump implantation because the presence of infection may increase the risk of surgical complications. Moreover, a systemic infection may complicate dosing.

➤*Pump dose adjustment and titration:* In most patients, it will be necessary to increase the dose gradually over time to maintain effectiveness; a sudden requirement for substantial dose escalation typically indicates a catheter complication (ie, catheter kink, dislodgment).

➤*Additional considerations pertaining to dosage adjustment:* It may be important to titrate the dose to maintain some degree of muscle tone and allow occasional spasms to:

1.) Help support circulatory function;
2.) possibly prevent the formation of deep vein thrombosis;
3.) optimize activities of daily living and ease of care.

Except in overdose related emergencies, the dose of baclofen intrathecal injection should ordinarily be reduced slowly if the drug is discontinued for any reason.

An attempt should be made to discontinue concomitant oral antispasticity medication to avoid possible overdose or adverse drug interactions, either prior to screening or following implant and initiation of chronic baclofen intrathecal injection infusion. Reduction and discontinuation of oral antispasmotics should be done slowly and with careful monitoring by the physician. Abrupt reduction or discontinuation of concomitant antispastics should be avoided.

➤*Need for spasticity:* Careful dose titration of baclofen intrathecal injection is needed when spasticity is necessary to sustain upright posture and balance in locomotion or whenever spasticity is used to obtain optimal function and care.

➤*Psychotic disorders:* Patients suffering from psychotic disorders, schizophrenia, or confusional states should be treated cautiously with baclofen intrathecal injection and kept under careful surveillance, because exacerbations of these conditions have been observed with oral administration.

➤*Ovarian cysts:* A dose-related increase in incidence of ovarian cysts was observed in female rats treated chronically with oral baclofen. Ovarian cysts have been found by palpation in approximately 4% of the multiple sclerosis patients who were treated with oral baclofen for up to 1 year. In most cases these cysts disappeared spontaneously while patients continued to receive the drug. Ovarian cysts are estimated to occur spontaneously in approximately 1% to 5% of the healthy female population.

BACLOFEN — INTRATHECAL INJECTION

➤*Autonomic dysreflexia:* Baclofen intrathecal injection should be used with caution in patients with a history of autonomic dysreflexia. The presence of nociceptive stimuli or abrupt withdrawal of baclofen intrathecal may cause an autonomic dysreflexic episode.

➤*Renal function impairment:* Because baclofen is primarily excreted unchanged by the kidneys, it should be given with caution in patients with impaired renal function and it may be necessary to reduce the dosage.

➤*Hazardous tasks:* Drowsiness has been reported in patients on baclofen intrathecal injection. Patients should be cautioned regarding the operation of automobiles or other dangerous machinery, and activities made hazardous by decreased alertness.

➤*Pregnancy: Category C.* Baclofen given orally has been shown to increase the incidence of omphaloceles (ventral hernias) in fetuses of rats given ≈ 13 times on a mg/kg basis, or 3 times on a mg/m^2 basis, the maximum oral dose recommended for human use; this dose also caused reductions in food intake and weight gain in the dams.

This abnormality was not seen in mice or rabbits. There are no adequate and well-controlled studies in pregnant women. Baclofen should be used during pregnancy only if the potential benefit justifies the potential risk to the fetus.

The intrathecal route is probably low risk because of the expected very low systemic exposure.

➤*Lactation:* In mothers treated with oral baclofen in therapeutic doses, the active substance passes into the breast milk. It is not known whether detectable levels of drug are present in breast milk of nursing mothers receiving baclofen intrathecal injection. As a general rule, nursing should be undertaken while a patient is receiving baclofen intrathecal injection only if the potential benefit justifies the potential risks to the infant.

The American Academy of Pediatrics classifies baclofen as compatible with breastfeeding.

➤*Monitoring:* On each occasion that the dosing rate of the pump or the concentration of baclofen intrathecal injection in the reservoir is adjusted, close medical monitoring is required until it is certain that the patient's response to the infusion is acceptable and reasonably stable.

Drug Interactions

➤*Alcohol and other CNS depressants:* Patients should also be cautioned that the CNS depressant effects of baclofen intrathecal injection may be additive to those of alcohol and other CNS depressants.

Adverse Reactions

➤*Spasticity of spinal cord origin:*

Commonly observed – In pre- and postmarketing clinical trials, the most commonly observed adverse events associated with use of baclofen intrathecal injection that were not seen at an equivalent incidence among placebo-treated patients were somnolence, dizziness, nausea, hypotension, headache, convulsions, and hypotonia.

Discontinuation of treatment – Eight of 474 patients with spasticity of spinal cord origin receiving long-term infusion of baclofen intrathecal injection in pre- and postmarketing clinical studies in the US discontinued treatment due to adverse events. These include pump pocket infections (3), meningitis (2), wound dehiscence (1), gynecological fibroids (1), and pump overpressurization (1) with unknown, if any, sequela. Eleven patients who developed coma secondary to overdose had their treatment temporarily suspended, but all were subsequently restarted and were not, therefore, considered to be true discontinuations.

Fatalities – See Warnings.

➤*Spasticity of spinal cord origin:*

Incidence in controlled trials – Experience with baclofen intrathecal injection obtained in parallel, placebo-controlled, randomized studies provides only a limited basis for estimating the incidence of adverse events because the studies were of very brief duration (up to 3 days of infusion) and involved only a total of 63 patients. The following events occurred among the 31 patients receiving baclofen intrathecal injection in two randomized, placebo-controlled trials: Hypotension (2), dizziness (2), headache (2), dyspnea (1). No adverse events were reported among the 32 patients receiving placebo in these studies.

Adverse events associated with the use of baclofen intrathecal injection reflect experience gained with 576 patients followed prospectively in the US. They received baclofen intrathecal injection for periods of 1 day (screening) (n = 576) to over 8 years (maintenance) (n = 10). The usual screening bolus dose administered prior to pump implantation in these studies was typically 50 mcg. The maintenance dose ranged from 12 to 2003 mcg/day. Because of the open, uncontrolled nature of the experience, a causal linkage between events observed and the administration of baclofen intrathecal injection cannot be reliably assessed in many cases and many of the adverse events reported are known to occur in association with the underlying conditions being treated. Nonetheless, many of the more commonly reported reactions (eg, hypotonia, somnolence, dizziness, paresthesia, nausea/vomiting, headache) appear clearly drug-related.

Adverse experiences reported during all US studies (both controlled and uncontrolled) are shown in the following table. Eight of 474 patients who received chronic infusion via implanted pumps had adverse experiences, which led to a discontinuation of long-term treatment in the pre- and postmarketing studies.

Baclofen Intrathecal Adverse Reactions (≥ 1%) in Spasticity of Spinal Cord Origin

Adverse reaction	(n = 576)[d] Screening[a]	(n = 474)[d] Titration[b]	(n = 430)[d] Maintenance[c]
Hypotonia	5.4%	13.5%	25.3%
Somnolence	5.7%	5.9%	20.9%
Dizziness	1.7%	1.9%	7.9%
Paresthesia	2.4%	2.1%	6.7%
Nausea and vomiting	1.6%	2.3%	5.6%
Headache	1.6%	2.5%	5.1%
Constipation	0.2%	1.5%	5.1%
Convulsion	0.5%	1.3%	4.7%
Urinary retention	0.7%	1.7%	1.9%
Dry mouth	0.2%	0.4%	3.3%
Accidental injury	0%	0.2%	3.5%
Asthenia	0.7%	1.3%	1.4%
Confusion	0.5%	0.6%	2.3%
Death	0.2%	0.4%	3%
Pain	0%	0.6%	3%
Speech disorder	0%	0.2%	3.5%
Hypotension	1%	0.2%	1.9%
Amblyopia	0.5%	0.2%	2.3%
Diarrhea	0%	0.8%	2.3%
Hypoventilation	0.2%	0.8%	2.1%
Coma	0%	1.5%	0.9%
Impotence	0.2%	0.4%	1.6%
Peripheral edema	0%	0%	2.3%
Urinary incontinence	0%	0.8%	1.4%
Insomnia	0%	0.4%	1.6%
Anxiety	0.2%	0.4%	0.9%
Depression	0%	0%	1.6%
Dyspnea	0.3%	0%	1.2%
Fever	0.5%	0.2%	0.7%
Pneumonia	0.2%	0.2%	1.2%
Urinary frequency	0%	0.6%	0.9%
Urticaria	0.2%	0.2%	1.2%
Anorexia	0%	0.4%	0.9%
Diplopia	0%	0.4%	0.9%
Dysautonomia	0.2%	0.2%	0.9%
Hallucinations	0.3%	0.4%	0.5%
Hypertension	0.2%	0.6%	0.5%

[a] Following administration of test bolus.
[b] 2-month period following implant.
[c] Beyond 2 months following implant.
[d] n = total number of patients entering each period.

In addition to the more common (1% or more) adverse events reported in the prospectively followed 576 domestic patients in pre- and postmarketing studies, experience from an additional 194 patients exposed to baclofen intrathecal injection from foreign studies has been reported. The following adverse events, not described in the table, and arranged in decreasing order of frequency, and classified by body system, were reported:

Cardiovascular – Postural hypotension; bradycardia; palpitations; syncope; arrhythmia ventricular; deep thrombophlebitis; pallor; tachycardia.

CNS – Abnormal gait; thinking abnormal; tremor; amnesia; twitching; vasodilatation; cerebrovascular accident; nystagmus; personality disorder; psychotic depression; cerebral ischemia; emotional lability; euphoria; hypertonia; ileus; drug dependence; incoordination; paranoid reaction; ptosis.

Dermatologic – Alopecia; sweating.

GI – Flatulence; dysphagia; dyspepsia; gastroenteritis.

GU – Hematuria; kidney failure.

Hematologic/Lymphatic – Anemia.

Metabolic/Nutritional – Weight loss; albuminuria; dehydration; hyperglycemia.

Respiratory – Respiratory disorder; aspiration pneumonia; hyperventilation; pulmonary embolus; rhinitis.

Special senses – Abnormal vision; abnormality of accommodation; photophobia; taste loss; tinnitus.

Miscellaneous – Suicide; lack of drug effect; abdominal pain; hypothermia; neck rigidity; chest pain; chills; face edema; flu syndrome; overdose.

BACLOFEN — INTRATHECAL INJECTION

➤*Spasticity of cerebral origin:*

Commonly observed – In premarketing clinical trials, the most commonly observed adverse events associated with use of baclofen intrathecal injection that were not seen at an equivalent incidence among placebo-treated patients included agitation, constipation, somnolence, leukocytosis, chills, urinary retention, and hypotonia.

Discontinuation of treatment – Nine of 211 patients receiving baclofen intrathecal injection in premarketing clinical studies in the US discontinued long-term infusion due to adverse events associated with intrathecal therapy.

The nine adverse events leading to discontinuation were infection (3), CSF leaks (2), meningitis (2), drainage (1), and unmanageable trunk control (1).

Fatalities – See Warnings/Precautions for more information.

Incidence in controlled trials – Experience with baclofen intrathecal injection obtained in parallel, placebo-controlled, randomized studies provides only a limited basis for estimating the incidence of adverse events because the studies involved a total of 62 patients exposed to a single 50 mcg intrathecal bolus. The following events occurred among the 62 patients receiving baclofen intrathecal injection in 2 randomized, placebo-controlled trials involving cerebral palsy and head injury patients, respectively: Agitation, constipation, somnolence, leukocytosis, nausea, vomiting, nystagmus, chills, urinary retention, and hypotonia.

Events observed during the premarketing evaluation – Adverse events associated with the use of baclofen intrathecal injection reflect experience gained with a total of 211 US patients with spasticity of cerebral origin, of whom 112 were children (younger than 16 years of age at enrollment). They received baclofen intrathecal injection for periods of one day (screening) (n = 211) to 84 months (maintenance) (n = 1). The usual screening bolus dose administered prior to pump implantation in these studies was 50 to 75 mcg. The maintenance dose ranged from 22 to 1,400 mcg/day. Doses used in this patient population for long-term infusion are generally lower than those required for patients with spasticity of spinal cord origin.

Because of the open, uncontrolled nature of the experience, a causal linkage between events observed and the administration of baclofen intrathecal injection cannot be reliably assessed in many cases. Nonetheless, many of the more commonly reported reactions (eg, somnolence, dizziness, headache, nausea, hypotension, hypotonia, coma) appear clearly drug-related.

The most frequent (1% or more) adverse events reported during all clinical trials are shown in the following table. Nine patients discontinued long-term treatment due to adverse events.

Baclofen Intrathecal Adverse Reactions (≥ 1%) in Spasticity of Cerebral Origin

Adverse event	(n = 211)[d] Screening[a]	(n = 153)[d] Titration[b]	(n = 150)[d] Maintenance[c]
Hypotonia	2.4%	14.4%	34.7%
Somnolence	7.6%	10.5%	18.7%
Headache	6.6%	7.8%	10.7%
Nausea and vomiting	6.6%	10.5%	4%
Vomiting	6.2%	8.5%	4%
Urinary retention	0.9%	6.5%	8%
Convulsion	0.9%	3.3%	10%
Dizziness	2.4%	2.6%	8%
Nausea	1.4%	3.3%	7.3%
Hypoventilation	1.4%	1.3%	4%
Hypertonia	0%	0.7%	6%
Paresthesia	1.9%	0.7%	3.3%
Hypotension	1.9%	0.7%	2%
Increased salivation	0%	2.6%	2.7%
Back pain	0.9%	0.7%	2%
Constipation	0.5%	1.3%	2%
Pain	0%	0%	4%
Pruritus	0%	0%	4%
Diarrhea	0.5%	0.7%	2%
Peripheral edema	0%	0%	3.3%
Thinking abnormal	0.5%	1.3%	0.7%
Agitation	0.5%	0%	1.3%
Asthenia	0%	0%	2%
Chills	0.5%	0%	1.3%
Coma	0.5%	0%	1.3%
Dry mouth	0.5%	0%	1.3%
Pneumonia	0%	0%	2%
Speech disorder	0.5%	0.7%	0.7%
Tremor	0.5%	0%	1.3%
Urinary incontinence	0%	0%	2%
Urination impaired	0%	0%	2%

[a] Following administration of test bolus.
[b] 2-month period following implant.
[c] Beyond 2 months following implant.
[d] n = total number of patients entering each period. 211 patients received drug; (1 of 212) received placebo only.

The more common (1% or more) adverse events reported in the prospectively followed 211 patients exposed to baclofen intrathecal injection have been reported. In the total cohort, the following adverse events, not described in the table, and arranged in decreasing order of frequency, and classified by body system, were reported:

Cardiovascular – Bradycardia.

CNS – Akathisia; ataxia; confusion; depression; opisthotonos; amnesia; anxiety; hallucinations; hysteria; insomnia; nystagmus; personality disorder; reflexes decreased; vasodilatation.

Dermatologic – Rash; sweating; alopecia; contact dermatitis; skin ulcer.

GI – Dysphagia; fecal incontinence; GI hemorrhage; tongue disorder.

GU – Abnormal ejaculation; kidney calculus; oliguria; vaginitis.

Hematologic/Lymphatic – Leukocytosis; petechial rash.

Respiratory – Apnea; dyspnea; hyperventilation.

Special senses – Abnormality of accommodation.

Miscellaneous – Death; fever; abdominal pain; carcinoma; malaise; hypothermia.

Overdosage

Signs of overdose may appear suddenly or insidiously. Acute massive overdose may present as coma. Less sudden and/or less severe forms of overdose may present with signs of drowsiness, lightheadedness, dizziness, somnolence, respiratory depression, seizures, rostral progression of hypotonia, and loss of consciousness progressing to coma. Should overdose appear likely, the patient should be taken immediately to a hospital for assessment and emptying of the pump reservoir. In cases reported to date, overdose has generally been related to pump malfunction or dosing error.

It is mandatory that the patient, all patient care givers, and the physicians responsible for the patient receive adequate information regarding the risks of this mode of treatment. All medical personnel and care givers should be instructed in 1) the signs and symptoms of overdose, 2) procedures to be followed in the event of overdose and 3) proper home care of the pump and insertion site.

➤*Symptoms:* Drowsiness, lightheadedness, dizziness, somnolence, respiratory depression, seizures, rostral progression of hypotonia, and loss of consciousness progressing to coma of up to 72 hours of duration. In most cases reported, coma was reversible without sequelae after drug was discontinued.

Symptoms of baclofen intrathecal injection overdose were reported in a sensitive adult patient after receiving a 25 mcg intrathecal bolus.

➤*Treatment:* There is no specific antidote for treating overdoses of baclofen intrathecal injection; however, the following steps should ordinarily be undertaken: Residual baclofen intrathecal injection solution should be removed from the pump as soon as possible; patients with respiratory depression should be intubated if necessary, until the drug is eliminated.

Anecdotal reports suggest that IV physostigmine may reverse central side effects, notably drowsiness and respiratory depression. Caution in administering physostigmine is advised, however, because its use has been associated with the induction of seizures, bradycardia, cardiac conduction disturbances.

Adults – Administer 2 mg of physostigmine intramuscularly or intravenously at a slow controlled rate of no more than 1 mg/min. Dosage may be repeated if life-threatening signs, such as arrhythmia, convulsions, or coma.

Children – Administer 0.02 mg/kg physostigmine intramuscularly or intravenously, do not give more than 0.5 mg/min. The dosage may be repeated at 5 to 10 minute intervals until a therapeutic effect is obtained or a maximum dose of 2 mg is attained.

Physostigmine may not be effective in reversing large overdoses and patients may need to be maintained with respiratory support.

If lumbar puncture is not contraindicated, consideration should be given to withdrawing 30 to 40 mL of CSF to reduce CSF baclofen concentration.

Centrally Acting

CARISOPRODOL

Rx	**Carisoprodol** (Wallace)	**Tablets; oral:** 250 mg	Potassium sorbate. (WP 5901). White, round. In 100s.
Rx	**Soma** (MedPointe)		(SOMA 250). In 100s.
Rx	**Carisoprodol** (Various, eg, Caraco, Major, Mutual, UDL, Watson)	**Tablets; oral:** 350 mg	May contain lactose. In 30s, 100s, 500s, 1,000s, and UD 100s.
Rx	**Soma** (MedPointe)		(SOMA 350). In 100s.

CARISOPRODOL — ORAL

Indications

➤*Musculoskeletal conditions:* For the relief of discomfort associated with acute, painful musculoskeletal conditions in adults.

Administration and Dosage

➤*Adults:*

Musculoskeletal conditions –

Usual dosage: 250 to 350 mg 3 times a day and at bedtime.

Duration of therapy: The recommended maximum duration of carisoprodol use is up to 2 or 3 weeks.

➤*Storage/Stability:* Store at 25°C (77°F); excursions are permitted between 15° and 30°C (59° and 86°F).

Actions

➤*Pharmacology:* Carisoprodol is a centrally acting skeletal muscle relaxant that does not directly relax skeletal muscles.

A metabolite of carisoprodol, meprobamate, has anxiolytic and sedative properties. The degree to which these properties of meprobamate contribute to the safety and efficacy of carisoprodol is unknown. In animal studies, muscle relaxation induced by carisoprodol is associated with altered interneuronal activity in the spinal cord and descending reticular formation of the brain.

➤*Pharmacokinetics:*

Absorption – Absolute bioavailability of carisoprodol has not been determined. The mean time to peak plasma concentration (T_{max}) of carisoprodol was approximately 1.5 to 2 hours.

The pharmacokinetics of carisoprodol and its metabolite meprobamate were studied in a crossover study of 24 healthy subjects (12 men and 12 women) who received single doses of carisoprodol 250 and 350 mg (see the following table). The exposure of carisoprodol and meprobamate was dose proportional between the 250 and 350 mg doses. The maximal drug concentration (C_{max}) of meprobamate was 2.5 ± 0.5 mcg/mL (mean ± standard deviation [SD]) after administration of a single 350 mg dose of carisoprodol, which is approximately 30% of the C_{max} of meprobamate (approximately 8 mcg/mL) after administration of a single 400 mg dose of meprobamate.

Pharmacokinetic Parameters of Carisoprodol and Meprobamate (Mean ± SD) (n = 24)

	Carisoprodol 250 mg	Carisoprodol 350 mg
Carisoprodol		
C_{max} (mcg/mL)	1.2 ± 0.5	1.8 ± 1
AUC_{inf}[a] (mcg•h/mL)	4.5 ± 3.1	7 ± 5
T_{max} (h)	1.5 ± 0.8	1.7 ± 0.8
t½[b] (h)	1.7 ± 0.5	2 ± 0.5
Meprobamate		
C_{max} (mcg/mL)	1.8 ± 0.3	2.5 ± 0.5
AUC_{inf} (mcg•h/mL)	32 ± 6.2	46 ± 9
T_{max} (h)	3.6 ± 1.7	4.5 ± 1.9
t½ (h)	9.7 ± 1.7	9.6 ± 1.5

[a] AUC_{inf} = area under the curve.
[b] t½ = half-life.

Effect of food: Coadministration of a high-fat meal with carisoprodol (350 mg tablet) had no effect on the pharmacokinetics of carisoprodol. Therefore, carisoprodol may be administered with or without food.

Metabolism – The major pathway of carisoprodol metabolism is via the liver by cytochrome enzyme CYP2C19 to form meprobamate. This enzyme exhibits genetic polymorphism (see Patients With Reduced CYP2C19 Activity section).

Excretion – Carisoprodol is eliminated by both renal and nonrenal routes, with a terminal elimination half-life of approximately 2 hours. The half-life of meprobamate is approximately 10 hours.

Special populations –

Gender: Exposure of carisoprodol is higher in women than in men (approximately 30% to 50% on a weight-adjusted basis). Overall exposure of meprobamate is comparable between women and men.

Patients with reduced CYP2C19 activity: Use carisoprodol with caution in patients with reduced CYP2C19 activity. Published studies indicate that patients who are poor CYP2C19 metabolizers have a 4-fold increase in exposure to carisoprodol and concomitant 50% reduced exposure to meprobamate compared with normal CYP2C19 metabolizers. The prevalence of poor metabolizers in white and black patients is approximately 3% to 5% and in Asian patients is approximately 15% to 20%.

Contraindications

History of acute intermittent porphyria; hypersensitivity reaction to a carbamate such as meprobamate.

Warnings/Precautions

➤*Sedation:* Carisoprodol may have sedative properties (in the low back pain trials, 13% to 17% of patients who received carisoprodol experienced sedation compared with 6% of patients who received placebo) and may impair the mental and/or physical abilities required for the performance of potentially hazardous tasks, such as driving a motor vehicle or operating machinery.

Because the sedative effects of carisoprodol and other CNS depressants (eg, alcohol, benzodiazepines, opioids, tricyclic antidepressants) may be additive, exercise appropriate caution with patients who take more than one of these CNS depressants simultaneously.

➤*Seizures:* There have been postmarketing reports of seizures in patients who received carisoprodol. Most of these cases have occurred in the setting of multiple-drug overdoses (including drugs of abuse, illegal drugs, and alcohol).

➤*Hypersensitivity reactions:* On very rare occasions, the first dose of carisoprodol has been followed by idiosyncratic symptoms appearing within minutes or hours. Symptoms reported include extreme weakness, transient quadriplegia, dizziness, ataxia, temporary loss of vision, diplopia, mydriasis, dysarthria, agitation, euphoria, confusion, and disorientation. Symptoms usually subside over the course of the next several hours. Supportive and symptomatic therapy, including hospitalization, may be necessary.

➤*Renal function impairment:* Because carisoprodol is excreted by the kidney, exercise caution if carisoprodol is administered to patients with renal function impairment. Carisoprodol is dialyzable by hemodialysis and peritoneal dialysis.

➤*Hepatic function impairment:* Because carisoprodol is metabolized in the liver, exercise caution if carisoprodol is administered to patients with hepatic function impairment.

➤*Drug abuse and dependence:* In the postmarketing experience with carisoprodol, cases of dependence, withdrawal, and abuse have been reported with prolonged use. Most cases of dependence, withdrawal, and abuse occurred in patients who have had a history of addiction or who used carisoprodol in combination with other drugs with abuse potential. Withdrawal symptoms have been reported following abrupt cessation after prolonged use. To reduce the chance of carisoprodol dependence, withdrawal, or abuse, use carisoprodol with caution in addiction-prone patients and in patients taking other CNS depressants, including alcohol, and do not use carisoprodol for more than 2 to 3 weeks for the relief of acute musculoskeletal discomfort.

One of the metabolites of carisoprodol, meprobamate (a controlled substance), may cause dependence.

In dogs, no withdrawal symptoms occurred after abrupt cessation of carisoprodol from doses as high as 1 g/kg/day. In a study in humans, abrupt cessation of 100 mg/kg/day (approximately 5 times the recommended daily adult dose) was followed in some subjects by mild withdrawal symptoms, such as abdominal cramps, insomnia, chilliness, headache, and nausea. Delirium and convulsions did not occur. In clinical use, psychological dependence and abuse have been rare, and there have been no reports of significant abstinence signs. According to the US Drug Enforcement Administration, excessive use of meprobamate (the active metabolite of carisoprodol) can result in psychological and physical dependence. Use the drug with caution in addiction-prone individuals.

➤*Hazardous tasks:* Warn patients that this drug may impair the mental or physical abilities required for the performance of potentially hazardous tasks, such as driving a motor vehicle or operating machinery.

➤*Pregnancy: Category C.* There are no data on the use of carisoprodol during human pregnancy. Animal studies indicate that carisoprodol crosses the placenta and results in adverse effects on fetal growth and postnatal survival. The primary metabolite of carisoprodol, meprobamate, is an approved anxiolytic. Retrospective, postmarketing studies do not show a consistent association between maternal use of meprobamate and an increased risk for particular congenital malformations. The molecular weight (approximately 260) suggests that it will cross to the embryo and fetus (per Briggs' *Drugs in Pregnancy and Lactation*). Moreover, the active metabolite, meprobamate, does cross the placenta (see Meprobamate monograph). Safe use of this drug in pregnancy has not been established. Therefore, use of this drug in pregnancy or in women of childbearing potential requires that the potential benefits of the drug be weighed against the potential hazards to mother and fetus.

Teratogenic – Animal studies have not adequately evaluated the teratogenic effects of carisoprodol. There was no increase in the incidence of congenital malformations noted in reproductive studies in rats, rabbits, and mice treated with meprobamate. Retrospective, postmarketing studies of

CARISOPRODOL — ORAL

meprobamate during human pregnancy were equivocal for demonstrating an increased risk of congenital malformations following first-trimester exposure. Across studies that indicated an increased risk, the types of malformations were inconsistent.

Nonteratogenic – In animal studies, carisoprodol reduced fetal weights, postnatal weight gain, and postnatal survival at maternal doses equivalent to 1 to 1.5 times the human dose (based on a body surface area comparison). Rats exposed to meprobamate in utero showed behavioral alterations that persisted into adulthood. For children exposed to meprobamate in utero, one study found no adverse effects on mental or motor development or IQ scores. Use carisoprodol during pregnancy only if the potential benefit justifies the risk to the fetus.

➤*Lactation:* Very limited data in humans show that carisoprodol is present in breast milk and may reach concentrations 2 to 4 times the maternal plasma concentrations. In one case report, a breast-fed infant received approximately 4% to 6% of the maternal daily dose through breast milk and experienced no adverse reactions. However, milk production was inadequate and the baby was supplemented with formula. In lactation studies in mice, female pup survival and pup weight at weaning were decreased. This information suggests that maternal use of carisoprodol may lead to reduced or less effective infant feeding (because of sedation) and/or decreased milk production. Exercise caution when carisoprodol is administered to a breast-feeding woman.

➤*Children:* The efficacy, safety, and pharmacokinetics of carisoprodol in children younger than 16 years of age have not been established.

➤*Elderly:* The efficacy, safety, and pharmacokinetics of carisoprodol in patients older than 65 years of age have not been established.

Per the Beers list, most muscle relaxants and antispasmodic drugs are poorly tolerated by elderly patients because these cause anticholinergic adverse effects, sedation, and weakness. Additionally, their effectiveness at doses tolerated by elderly patients is questionable. Carisoprodol is also considered a high risk medication for the elderly according to the Centers of Medicare and Medicaid Services.

➤*Monitoring:* Monitor for relief of pain and/or muscle spasm.

Monitor for signs of drug abuse in addiction-prone persons.

Drug Interactions

Carisoprodol Drug Interactions			
Precipitant drug	Object drug[a]		Description
CNS depressants (eg, alcohol, benzodiazepines, opioids, tricyclic antidepressants)	Carisoprodol	↑	The sedative effects of carisoprodol and other CNS depressants may be additive.
Carisoprodol	CNS depressants (eg, alcohol, benzodiazepines, opioids, tricyclic antidepressants)		
CYP2C19 inducers (eg, rifampin, St. John's wort)	Carisoprodol	↑↓	Coadministration of CYP2C19 inducers, such as rifampin or St. John's wort, with carisoprodol could result in decreased exposure of carisoprodol and increased exposure of meprobamate.
CYP2C19 inhibitors (eg, fluvoxamine, omeprazole)	Carisoprodol	↑↓	Coadministration of CYP2C19 inhibitors, such as fluvoxamine or omeprazole, with carisoprodol could result in increased exposure of carisoprodol and decreased exposure of meprobamate.
Meprobamate	Carisoprodol	↑	Concomitant use of meprobamate and carisoprodol, a metabolite of carisoprodol, is not recommended.
Carisoprodol	Meprobamate		

[a] ↑ = object drug increased; ↑↓ = object drug both increased and decreased.

Adverse Reactions

There were no deaths and there were no serious adverse reactions in these 2 trials. In these 2 studies, 2.7%, 2%, and 5.4% of patients treated with placebo, carisoprodol 250 mg, or carisoprodol 350 mg, respectively, discontinued because of adverse reactions; 0.5%, 0.5%, and 1.8% of patients treated with placebo, carisoprodol 250 mg, and carisoprodol 350 mg, respectively, discontinued because of CNS adverse reactions.

The following table displays adverse reactions reported with frequencies greater than 2% and more frequently than placebo in patients treated with carisoprodol in the 2 trials previously described.

Carisoprodol Adverse Reactions (> 2%)			
Adverse reactions	Placebo (n = 560)	Carisoprodol 250 mg (n = 548)	Carisoprodol 350 mg (n = 279)
CNS			
Dizziness	2%	8%	7%
Drowsiness	6%	13%	17%
Headache	2%	5%	3%

➤*Hypersensitivity:* Occasionally, within the period of the first to fourth dose of carisoprodol, allergic reactions have occurred in patients who have had no previous contact with the drug. Eosinophilia, erythema multiforme, fixed-drug eruption, pruritus, and skin rash have been reported with carisoprodol with cross-reaction to meprobamate. Severe reactions have been manifested by anaphylactoid shock, angioneurotic edema, asthmatic episodes, fever, dizziness, hypotension, smarting eyes, and weakness.

➤*Postmarketing:*

Cardiovascular – Facial flushing, postural hypotension, syncope, tachycardia.

CNS – Agitation, ataxia, depressive reactions, dizziness, drowsiness, headache, insomnia, irritability, seizures, tremor, vertigo.

GI – Epigastric discomfort, nausea, vomiting.

Hematologic – Leukopenia, pancytopenia.

Overdosage

➤*Symptoms:* Overdosage of carisoprodol commonly produces CNS depression. Death, coma, respiratory depression, hypotension, seizures, delirium, hallucinations, dystonic reactions, nystagmus, blurred vision, mydriasis, euphoria, muscular incoordination, rigidity, and/or headache have been reported with carisoprodol overdosage. Many of the carisoprodol overdoses have occurred in the setting of multiple-drug overdoses (including drugs of abuse, illegal drugs, and alcohol). The effects of an overdose of carisoprodol and other CNS depressants (eg, alcohol, benzodiazepines, opioids, tricyclic antidepressants) can be additive even when one of the drugs has been taken in the recommended dosage. Fatal accidental and nonaccidental overdoses of carisoprodol have been reported alone or in combination with CNS depressants.

➤*Treatment:* Institute basic life support measures as dictated by the clinical presentation of the carisoprodol overdose. Induced emesis is not recommended because of the risk of CNS and respiratory depression, which may increase the risk of aspiration pneumonia. Consider gastric lavage soon after ingestion (within 1 hour). Administer circulatory support with volume infusion and vasopressor agents if needed. Treat seizures with intravenous benzodiazepines, and the reoccurrence of seizures may be treated with phenobarbital. In cases of severe CNS depression, airway protective reflexes may be compromised; consider tracheal intubation for airway protection and respiratory support.

The following types of treatment have been used successfully with an overdose of meprobamate, a metabolite of carisoprodol: activated charcoal (oral or via nasogastric tube), forced diuresis, peritoneal dialysis, and hemodialysis (carisoprodol is also dialyzable). Careful monitoring of urinary output is necessary; avoid over-hydration. Observe for possible relapse caused by incomplete gastric emptying and delayed absorption. For more information on the management of an overdose of carisoprodol, contact a poison control center.

Patient Information

Advise patients to contact their health care provider if they experience any adverse reactions to carisoprodol (eg, drowsiness, dizziness, irritability, nausea, vomiting).

Because carisoprodol may cause drowsiness and/or dizziness, advise patients to assess their individual response to carisoprodol before engaging in potentially hazardous activities, such as driving a motor vehicle or operating machinery.

Advise patients to avoid alcoholic beverages while taking carisoprodol and to check with their health care provider before taking other CNS depressants, such as benzodiazepines, opioids, tricyclic antidepressants, sedating antihistamines, or other sedatives.

Advise patients that treatment with carisoprodol should be limited to acute use (up to 2 or 3 weeks) for the relief of acute musculoskeletal discomfort. If symptoms still persist, instruct patients to contact their health care provider for further evaluation.

CHLORZOXAZONE

Rx	**Chlorzoxazone** (Various, eg, Goldline)	**Tablets**: 250 mg	In 100s and 1000s.
Rx	**Paraflex Caplets** (McNeil Pharm.)		(Paraflex). Peach, capsule shape. In 100s.
Rx	**Remular-S** (Inter. Ethical)		In 100s.
Rx	**Chlorzoxazone** (Various, eg, Goldline, IDE, Royce, Schein)	**Tablets**: 500 mg	In 100s, 500s and 1000s.
Rx	**Parafon Forte DSC Caplets** (McNeil Pharm.)		(McNeil Parafon Forte DSC). Lt. green, scored. In 100s, 500s and UD 100s.

CHLORZOXAZONE — ORAL

Indications

➤*Musculoskeletal conditions:* As an adjunct to rest, physical therapy, and other measures for the relief of discomfort associated with acute, painful musculoskeletal conditions. The mode of action of this drug has not been clearly identified, but may be related to its sedative properties. Chlorzoxazone does not directly relax tense skeletal muscles.

Administration and Dosage

➤*Adults:*

Musculoskeletal conditions –

Usual dosage: 250 to 500 mg 3 or 4 times daily.

Dosage adjustment: If adequate response is not obtained, the dose may be increased to 750 mg 3 or 4 times daily. As improvement occurs, dosage can usually be reduced.

➤*Storage/Stability:* Store at 15° to 30°C (59° to 86°F).

Actions

➤*Pharmacology:* Chlorzoxazone is a centrally acting agent for painful musculoskeletal conditions. Data available from animal experiments as well as human study indicate that chlorzoxazone acts primarily at the level of the spinal cord and subcortical areas of the brain where it inhibits multisynaptic reflex arcs involved in producing and maintaining skeletal muscle spasm of varied etiology. The clinical result is a reduction of the skeletal muscle spasm with relief of pain and increased mobility of the involved muscles.

➤*Pharmacokinetics:*

Absorption – Blood levels of chlorzoxazone can be detected in people during the first 30 minutes and peak levels may be reached, in the majority of the subjects, in about 1 to 2 hours after oral administration of chlorzoxazone.

Metabolism/Excretion – Chlorzoxazone is rapidly metabolized and is excreted in the urine, primarily in a conjugated form as the glucuronide. Less than 1% of a dose of chlorzoxazone is excreted unchanged in the urine in 24 hours.

Contraindications

Intolerance to the drug.

Warnings/Precautions

➤*Hepatotoxicity:* Serious (including fatal) hepatocellular toxicity has been reported rarely. The mechanism is unknown but appears to be idiosyncratic and unpredictable. Factors predisposing patients to this rare event are not known. Patients should be instructed to report early signs or symptoms of hepatotoxicity (eg, fever, rash, anorexia, nausea, vomiting, fatigue, right upper quadrant pain, dark urine, jaundice). Chlorzoxazone should be discontinued immediately and a physician consulted if any of these signs or symptoms develop. Chlorzoxazone use should also be discontinued if a patient develops abnormal liver enzymes (eg, AST, ALT, alkaline phosphatase, bilirubin.)

➤*Hypersensitivity reactions:* Used with caution in patients with known allergies or with a history of allergic reactions to drugs. If a sensitivity reaction occurs such as urticaria, redness, or itching of the skin, the drug should be stopped.

➤*Pregnancy: Category C.* The safe use of chlorzoxazone has not been established with respect to the possible adverse effects upon fetal development. Therefore, it should be used in women of childbearing potential only when, in the judgment of the physician, the potential benefits outweigh the possible risks.

➤*Lactation:* Per Briggs' *Drugs in Pregnancy and Lactation*, excretion into breast milk is suspected. The effects of this potential exposure on a breast-feeding infant are unknown.

➤*Elderly:* Per the Beers list, most muscle relaxants and antispasmodic drugs are poorly tolerated by elderly patients because these cause anticholinergic adverse effects, sedation, and weakness. Additionally, their effectiveness at doses tolerated by elderly patients is questionable. Chlorzoxazone is also considered a high-risk medication for elderly patients according to the Centers of Medicare and Medicaid Services.

Drug Interactions

➤*CNS agents:* The concomitant use of alcohol or other CNS depressants may have an additive effect.

Adverse Reactions

After extensive clinical use of chlorzoxazone containing products in an estimated 32 million patients, it is apparent that the drug is well tolerated and seldom produces undesirable side effects. Occasional patients may develop gastrointestinal disturbances. It is possible in rare instances that chlorzoxazone may have been associated with GI bleeding. Drowsiness, dizziness, lightheadedness, malaise, or overstimulation may be noted by an occasional patient. Rarely, allergic-type skin rashes, petechiae, or ecchymoses may develop during treatment. Angioneurotic edema or anaphylactic reactions are extremely rare. There is no evidence that the drug will cause renal damage. Rarely, a patient may note discoloration of the urine resulting from a phenolic metabolite of chlorzoxazone. This finding is of no known clinical significance.

Overdosage

➤*Symptoms:* Initially, GI disturbances such as nausea, vomiting, or diarrhea together with drowsiness, dizziness, lightheadedness or headache may occur. Early in the course there may be malaise or sluggishness followed by marked loss of muscle tone, making voluntary movement impossible. The deep tendon reflexes may be decreased or absent. The sensorium remains intact, and there is no peripheral loss of sensation. Respiratory depression may occur with rapid, irregular respiration and intercostal and substernal retraction. The blood pressure is lowered, but shock has not been observed.

➤*Treatment:* Gastric lavage or induction of emesis should be carried out, followed by administration of activated charcoal. Thereafter, treatment is entirely supportive. If respirations are depressed, oxygen and artificial respiration should be employed and a patent airway assured by use of an oropharyngeal airway or endotracheal tube. Hypotension may be counteracted by use of dextran, plasma, concentrated albumin or a vasopressor agent such as norepinephrine. Cholinergic drugs or analeptic drugs are of no value and should not be used.

CYCLOBENZAPRINE HYDROCHLORIDE

Rx	**Cyclobenzaprine Hydrochloride** (Various, eg, Mylan, Sandoz, Watson)	**Tablets; oral**: 5 mg	May contain lactose. In 30s, 100s, 500s, 1,000s, and UD 30s.
Rx	**Flexeril** (McNeil)		Lactose. (FLEX). Yellow-orange, 5-sided, D-shape. Film-coated. In 100s.
Rx	**Cyclobenzaprine Hydrochloride** (Watson)	**Tablets; oral**: 7.5 mg	In 30s, 100s, and 1000s.
Rx	**Fexmid** (Victory)		(Watson 3330). Film-coated. In 100s.
Rx	**Cyclobenzaprine Hydrochloride** (Various, eg, Breckenridge, Jubilant, Mutual, Mylan, Watson, Sandoz)	**Tablets; oral**: 10 mg	May contain lactose. In 30s, 100s, 500s, and 1,000s.
Rx	**Flexeril** (McNeil)		Lactose. (FLEXERIL). Yellow, 5-sided, D-shape. Film-coated. In 100s.
Rx	**Amrix** (ECR)	**Capsules, extended-release; oral**: 15 mg	(ECR 15). Sugar spheres. Orange. In 60s.
		30 mg	(ECR 30). Sugar spheres. Blue/orange. In 60s.

CYCLOBENZAPRINE HYDROCHLORIDE — ORAL

Indications

➤*Muscle spasm:* As an adjunct to rest and physical therapy for relief of muscle spasm associated with acute, painful musculoskeletal conditions.

➤*Off-label uses:* Management of fibromyalgia.

Administration and Dosage

➤*Maximum dose:*

Adults and children 15 years of age and older – 30 mg/day according to the prescribing information.

➤*General dosing considerations:* It is recommended that doses be taken at approximately the same time each day.

➤*Adults:*

Muscle spasm –

Maximum dose: 30 mg/day.

Tablets: 5 mg 3 times a day. The dose may be increased to 7.5 or 10 mg 3 times a day.

Capsules: 15 mg once daily. Some patients may require up to 30 mg/day.

➤*Children:* See Adults for tablet dosing information for children 15 years of age and older.

Safety and efficacy of cyclobenzaprine capsules have not been studied in children.

➤*Elderly:* Capsules should not be used in the elderly.

Muscle spasm –

Tablets: Initiate with a 5 mg dose and titrate slowly upward.

➤*Hepatic function impairment:* Do not use cyclobenzaprine capsules in patients with hepatic impairment.

Muscle spasm –

Tablets:

• *Initial dosage* – Initiate with a 5 mg dose in patients with mild hepatic impairment and titrate slowly upward.

Because of the lack of data in patients with more severe hepatic function impairment, the use of cyclobenzaprine in patients with moderate to severe hepatic function impairment is not recommended.

➤*Duration of therapy:* Use for periods longer than 2 or 3 weeks is not recommended.

➤*Storage / Stability:* Store at 25°C (77°F); excursions between 15° and 30°C (59° and 86°F) are permitted. Dispense capsules in a tight, light-resistant container.

Actions

➤*Pharmacology:* Cyclobenzaprine relieves skeletal muscle spasm of local origin without interfering with muscle function. It is ineffective in muscle spasm due to CNS disease.

➤*Pharmacokinetics:*

Absorption / Distribution –

Tablets: Estimates of mean oral bioavailability of cyclobenzaprine range from 33% to 55%. Cyclobenzaprine exhibits linear pharmacokinetics over the dose range of 2.5 to 10 mg, and is subject to enterohepatic circulation. It is highly bound to plasma proteins. Drug accumulates when dosed 3 times a day, reaching steady state within 3 to 4 days at plasma concentrations about 4-fold higher than after a single dose. At steady state in healthy patients receiving 10 mg 3 times daily (n = 18), peak plasma concentration was 25.9 ng/mL (range, 12.8 to 46.1 ng/mL), and area under the curve (AUC) over an 8-hour dosing interval was 177 ng•h/mL (range, 80 to 319 ng•h/mL).

Capsules: In a single-dose study comprised of healthy adult males (n = 15), the dose-adjusted ratios of the arithmetic means of $AUC_{0\text{-}168}$ and $AUC_{0\text{-}\infty}$ indicated that exposure of cyclobenzaprine 30 mg was about 16% and 10% higher, respectively, than that of cyclobenzaprine 15 mg. The dose-adjusted ratios of the arithmetic means of maximal drug concentration (C_{max}) indicated that the peak plasma concentration of cyclobenzaprine 30 mg was about 20% higher than that of cyclobenzaprine 15 mg. The half-lives and time to peak plasma cyclobenzaprine concentration were similar for both cyclobenzaprine 15 and 30 mg. These data are summarized in the following table.

Cyclobenzaprine Capsules Pharmacokinetic Parameters in Healthy Adult Subjects[a]

Parameter mean ± SD	Cyclobenzaprine 15 mg (n = 15)	Cyclobenzaprine 30 mg (n = 14)
$AUC_{0\text{-}168}$ (ng•h/mL)	318.3 ± 114.7	736.6 ± 259.4
$AUC_{0\text{-}\infty}$ (ng•h/mL)	354.1 ± 119.8	779.9 ± 277.6
C_{max} (ng/mL)	8.3 ± 2.2	19.9 ± 5.9
T_{max} (h)	8.1 ± 2.9	7.1 ± 1.6
t½ (h)	33.4 ± 10.3	32 ± 10.1

[a] SD = standard deviation; T_{max} = time to maximum concentration; t½ = elimination half-life.

In a multiple-dose study utilizing cyclobenzaprine 30 mg administered once daily for 7 days in a group of healthy adult volunteers (n = 35) a 2.5-fold accumulation of plasma cyclobenzaprine levels was noted at steady state.

• *Food effect* – A food effect study conducted in healthy adult subjects (n = 15) utilizing a single dose of cyclobenzaprine 30 mg demonstrated a statistically significant increase in bioavailability when cyclobenzaprine 30 mg was given with food relative to the fasted state. There was a 35% increase in cyclobenzaprine C_{max} and a 20% increase in exposure ($AUC_{0\text{-}168}$ and $AUC_{0\text{-}\infty}$) in the presence of food. No effect, however, was noted in lag time (T_{lag}), T_{max}, or the shape of the mean plasma cyclobenzaprine concentration versus time profile. Cyclobenzaprine in plasma was first detectable in both the fed and fasted states at 1.5 hours.

Metabolism / Excretion – Cyclobenzaprine is extensively metabolized, and is excreted primarily as glucuronides via the kidney. CYP-450 3A4, 1A2, and, to a lesser extent 2D6, mediate N-demethylation, one of the oxidative pathways for cyclobenzaprine. Cyclobenzaprine has an elimination half-life of 18 hours (tablets) and 32 hours (capsules) (range, 8 to 37 hours; n = 18); plasma clearance is 0.7 L/min following single-dose administration.

Special populations –

Hepatic function impairment: In a pharmacokinetic study of 16 patients with hepatic function impairment (15 mild, 1 moderate per Child-Pugh score), both AUC and C_{max} were approximately double the values seen in the healthy control group. Use cyclobenzaprine tablets with caution in patients with mild hepatic function impairment, starting with the 5 mg dose and titrating slowly upward. Because of the lack of data in patients with more severe hepatic function impairment, the use of cyclobenzaprine tablets in patients with moderate to severe impairment is not recommended. Use of cyclobenzaprine capsules is not recommended in subjects with mild, moderate, or severe hepatic function impairment.

Elderly:

• *Tablets* – In a pharmacokinetic study in elderly individuals (65 years of age and older), mean (n = 10) steady-state cyclobenzaprine AUC values were approximately 1.7 fold (171 ng•h/mL; range, 96.1 to 255.3) higher than those seen in a group of 18 younger adults (101.4 ng•h/mL; range, 36.1 to 182.9) from another study. Elderly male patients had the highest observed mean increase, approximately 2.4-fold (198.3 ng•h/mL; range, 155.6 to 255.3 vs 83.2 ng•h/mL; range, 41.1 to 142.5 for younger males) while levels in elderly females were increased to a much lesser extent, approximately 1.2-fold (143.8 ng•h/mL; range, 96.1 to 196.3 vs 115.9 ng•h/mL; range, 36.1 to 182.9 for younger females). In light of these findings, initiate therapy with cyclobenzaprine tablets in the elderly with a 5 mg dose and titrated slowly upward.

• *Capsules* – Although there were no notable differences in C_{max} or T_{max}, cyclobenzaprine plasma AUC is increased by 40% and the plasma half-life of cyclobenzaprine is prolonged in elderly subjects older than 65 years of age (50 hours) after dosing with cyclobenzaprine compared with younger subjects (32 hours).

Contraindications

Hypersensitivity to any component of this product; acute recovery phase of myocardial infarction; arrhythmias; heart block or conduction disturbances; congestive heart failure; hyperthyroidism. Concomitant use of monoamine oxidase inhibitors (MAOIs) or within 14 days after their discontinuation. Hyperpyretic crisis seizures, and deaths have occurred in patients receiving cyclobenzaprine (or structurally similar TCAs) concomitantly with MAOIs.

Warnings/Precautions

➤*Similarity to TCAs:* Cyclobenzaprine is closely related to the TCAs (eg, amitriptyline, imipramine). In short-term studies for indications other than muscle spasm associated with acute musculoskeletal conditions, and usually at doses somewhat greater than those recommended for skeletal muscle spasm, some of the more serious CNS reactions noted with the TCAs have occurred. TCAs have been reported to produce arrhythmias, sinus tachycardia, prolongation of the conduction time leading to myocardial infarction, and stroke.

➤*Hepatic function impairment:* The plasma concentration of cyclobenzaprine is increased in patients with hepatic function impairment.

These patients are generally more susceptible to drugs with potentially sedating effects, including cyclobenzaprine. Use cyclobenzaprine tablets with caution in patients with mild hepatic function impairment starting with a 5 mg dose and titrating slowly upward. Because of the lack of data in patients with more severe hepatic function impairment, the use of cyclobenzaprine tablets in patients with moderate to severe impairment is not recommended. Use of cyclobenzaprine capsules is not recommended in subjects with mild, moderate, or severe hepatic function impairment.

➤*Special risk:* Because of its atropine-like action, use cyclobenzaprine with caution in patients with a history of urinary retention, angle-closure glaucoma, or increased intraocular pressure, and in patients taking anticholinergic medication.

➤*Drug abuse and dependence:* Pharmacologic similarities among the tricyclic drugs require that certain withdrawal symptoms be considered when cyclobenzaprine is administered, even though they have not been reported to occur with this drug. Abrupt cessation of treatment after prolonged administration may rarely produce nausea, headache, and malaise. These are not indicative of addiction.

➤*Hazardous tasks:* Cyclobenzaprine may impair mental and/or physical abilities required for performance of hazardous tasks, such as operating machinery or driving a motor vehicle.

➤*Pregnancy: Category B.* There are no adequate and well-controlled studies in pregnant women. Because animal reproduction studies are not always predictive of human response, use this drug during pregnancy only if clearly needed.

➤*Lactation:* It is not known whether this drug is excreted in human milk. Because cyclobenzaprine is closely related to the TCAs, some of which are

CYCLOBENZAPRINE HYDROCHLORIDE — ORAL

known to be excreted in human milk, exercise caution when cyclobenzaprine is administered to a breast-feeding woman.

➤*Children:* Safety and efficacy of cyclobenzaprine tablets in children younger than 15 years of age have not been established. Safety and efficacy of cyclobenzaprine capsules have not been studied in children.

➤*Elderly:* Per the Beers list, most muscle relaxants and antispasmodic drugs are poorly tolerated by elderly patients because these cause anticholinergic adverse effects, sedation, and weakness. Additionally, their effectiveness at doses tolerated by elderly patients is questionable. Cyclobenzaprine is also considered a high-risk medication for the elderly according to the Centers of Medicare and Medicaid Services.

Tablets – The plasma concentration of cyclobenzaprine is increased in the elderly. The elderly may also be more at risk for CNS adverse reactions such as hallucinations and confusion, cardiac events resulting in falls or other sequelae, drug-drug and drug-disease interactions. For these reasons, in the elderly, use cyclobenzaprine only if clearly needed. In such patients, initiate cyclobenzaprine with a 5 mg dose and titrate slowly upward.

Capsules – The plasma concentration and half-life of cyclobenzaprine are substantially increased in elderly patients when compared with the general patient population. Accordingly, do not use cyclobenzaprine capsules in elderly patients.

Drug Interactions

Cyclobenzaprine Drug Interactions

Precipitant drug	Object drug[a]		Description
MAOIs (eg, isocarboxazid, rasagiline, selegiline)	Cyclobenzaprine	⬆	Concomitant use of cyclobenzaprine with MAOIs or within 14 days after their discontinuation is contraindicated. Hyperpyretic crisis seizures and deaths have occurred.
Cyclobenzaprine	CNS depressants (eg, alcohol, barbiturates)	⬆	Cyclobenzaprine may enhance the effects of CNS depressants.
Cyclobenzaprine	Guanethidine	⬇	Cyclobenzaprine may block the antihypertensive effect of guanethidine and similarly acting compounds.
Cyclobenzaprine	Tramadol	⬆	Coadministration may enhance the seizure risk in patients taking tramadol.

[a] ⬆ = object drug increased; ⬇ = object drug decreased.

➤*Drug/Food interactions:* A single dose of cyclobenzaprine 30 mg demonstrated a statistically significant increase in bioavailability when cyclobenzaprine 30 mg was given with food relative to the fasted state. There was a 35% increase in peak plasma cyclobenzaprine concentration (C_{max}) and a 20% increase in exposure (AUC_{0-168} and $AUC_{0-\infty}$) in the presence of food.

Adverse Reactions

➤*Common adverse reactions:*

Tablets –

Cyclobenzaprine Tablets Adverse Reactions (≥ 3%)

Adverse reaction	Cyclobenzaprine 5 mg (n = 464)	Cyclobenzaprine 10 mg (n = 249)	Placebo (n = 469)
CNS			
Drowsiness	29%	38%	10%
Fatigue	6%	6%	3%
Headache	5%	5%	8%
GI			
Dry mouth	21%	32%	7%

Adverse reactions that were reported in 1% to 3% of patients were abdominal pain, acid regurgitation, constipation, diarrhea, dizziness, nausea, irritability, mental acuity decreased, nervousness, pharyngitis, and upper respiratory tract infection.

Capsules –

Cyclobenzaprine Capsules Adverse Reactions in Clinical Trials (≥ 3%)

Adverse reaction	Cyclobenzaprine 15 mg (n = 127)	Cyclobenzaprine 30 mg (n = 126)	Placebo (n = 128)
GI			
Constipation	1%	3%	0%
Dry mouth	6%	14%	2%
Dyspepsia	0%	4%	1%
Nausea	3%	3%	1%
CNS			
Dizziness	3%	6%	2%
Fatigue	3%	3%	2%
Somnolence	1%	2%	0%

Cyclobenzaprine Capsules Adverse Reactions in a Pharmacokinetic Study (≥ 3%)

Adverse reaction	Cyclobenzaprine 30 mg (N = 36)
Cardiovascular	
Palpitations	6%
CNS	
Disturbance in attention	6%
Dizziness	19%
Headache	17%
Insomnia	0%
Somnolence	100%
Tremor	6%
GI	
Dry mouth	58%
Dry throat	8%
Dysgeusia	6%
Nausea	8%
Miscellaneous	
Acne	6%
Vision blurred	3%

➤*Less frequent adverse reactions:* Adverse reactions that were reported in 1% to 3% of the patients were asthenia, blurred vision, confusion, constipation, dyspepsia, fatigue/tiredness, headache, nausea, nervousness, and unpleasant taste.

Cardiovascular – Arrhythmia, hypotension, palpitation, syncope, tachycardia, vasodilatation (less than 1%).

CNS – Abnormal sensations, abnormal thinking and dreaming, agitation, anxiety, ataxia, convulsions, depressed mood, disorientation, dysarthria, excitement, hallucinations, hypertonia, insomnia, muscle twitching, paresthesia, psychosis, seizures, tremors, vertigo (less than 1%).

GI – Anorexia, diarrhea, edema of the tongue, flatulence, gastritis, GI pain, thirst, vomiting (less than 1%).

GU – Urinary frequency and/or retention (less than 1%).

Hepatic – Abnormal liver function and rare reports of cholestasis, hepatitis, and jaundice (less than 1%).

Hypersensitivity – Anaphylaxis, angioedema, facial edema, pruritus, rash, urticaria (less than 1%).

Special senses – Ageusia, diplopia, tinnitus (less than 1%).

Miscellaneous – Local weakness, malaise, sweating (less than 1%).

Overdosage

➤*Symptoms:* Although rare, deaths may occur from overdosage with cyclobenzaprine. Multiple drug ingestion (including alcohol) is common in deliberate cyclobenzaprine overdose. Signs and symptoms of toxicity may develop rapidly after cyclobenzaprine overdose; therefore, hospital monitoring is required as soon as possible. The acute oral median lethal dose (LD_{50}) of cyclobenzaprine is approximately 338 and 425 mg/kg in mice and rats, respectively.

The most common reactions associated with cyclobenzaprine overdose are drowsiness and tachycardia. Less frequent manifestations include agitation, ataxia, coma, confusion, dizziness, hallucinations, hypertension, nausea, slurred speech, tremor, and vomiting. Rare but potentially critical manifestations of overdose are cardiac arrest, chest pain, cardiac dysrhythmias, severe hypotension, seizures, and neuroleptic malignant syndrome. Changes in the electrocardiogram (ECG), particularly in QRS axis or width, are clinically significant indicators of cyclobenzaprine toxicity.

➤*Treatment:* In order to protect against the rare but potentially critical manifestations previously described, obtain an ECG and immediately initiate cardiac monitoring. Protect the patient's airway, establish an intravenous (IV) line and initiate gastric decontamination. Observation with cardiac monitoring and observation for signs of CNS or respiratory depression, hypotension, cardiac dysrhythmias and/or conduction blocks, and seizures is necessary. If signs of toxicity occur at any time during this period, extended monitoring is required. Monitoring of plasma drug levels should not guide management of the patient. Dialysis is probably of no value because of low plasma concentrations of the drug.

GI decontamination – All patients suspected of an overdose with cyclobenzaprine should receive GI decontamination. This should include large volume gastric lavage followed by activated charcoal. If consciousness is impaired, securing the airway prior to lavage and emesis is contraindicated.

Cardiovascular – A maximal limb-lead QRS duration of at least 0.1 seconds may be the best indication of the severity of the overdose. Institute serum alkalinization to a pH of 7.45 to 7.55, using IV sodium bicarbonate and hyperventilation (as needed), for patients with dysrhythmias and/or QRS widening. A pH more than 7.6 or a pCO_2 less than 20 mm Hg is undesirable. Dysrhythmias unresponsive to sodium bicarbonate therapy/

CYCLOBENZAPRINE HYDROCHLORIDE — ORAL

hyperventilation may respond to lidocaine, bretylium, or phenytoin. Type 1A and 1C antiarrhythmics are generally contraindicated (eg, quinidine, disopyramide, procainamide).

CNS – In patients with CNS depression, early intubation is advised because of the potential for abrupt deterioration. Control seizures with benzodiazepines or, if these are ineffective, other anticonvulsants (eg, phenobarbital, phenytoin). Physostigmine is not recommended except to treat life-threatening symptoms that have been unresponsive to other therapies, and then only in close consultation with a poison control center.

Patient Information

Avoid alcohol and other CNS depressants.

Cyclobenzaprine, especially when used with alcohol or other CNS depressants, may impair mental and/or physical abilities required for performance of hazardous tasks such as operating machinery or driving a motor vehicle.

In the elderly, the frequency and severity of adverse reactions associated with the use of cyclobenzaprine, with or without concomitant medications, is increased. In elderly patients, initiate cyclobenzaprine tablets with a 5 mg dose and titrate slowly upward. Do not use cyclobenzaprine capsules in the elderly.

DIAZEPAM

For complete prescribing information, refer to the Diazepam monograph in the Antianxiety Agents section.

METAXALONE

Rx	**Metaxalone** (Various, eg, Corepharma, Eon Labs)	**Tablets; oral:** 800 mg	In 100s, 500s, and 1,000s.
Rx	**Skelaxin** (King)		(8667 S). Pink, oval, scored. In 100s and 500s.

METAXALONE — ORAL

Indications

➤*Musculoskeletal conditions:* As an adjunct to rest, physical therapy, and other measures for the relief of discomforts associated with acute, painful musculoskeletal conditions.

Administration and Dosage

➤*Adults:*

Musculoskeletal conditions – 800 mg 3 to 4 times a day.

➤*Children:*

Musculoskeletal conditions –

Older than 12 years of age: See Adults for dosing.

➤*Renal function impairment:* Contraindicated in patients with significant renal impairment.

➤*Hepatic function impairment:* Contraindicated in patients with significant hepatic impairment.

➤*Storage/Stability:* Store between 15° and 30°C (59° and 86°F).

Actions

➤*Pharmacology:* The mechanism of action of metaxalone in humans has not been established but may be due to general CNS depression. Metaxalone has no direct action on the contractile mechanism of striated muscle, the motor end plate, or the nerve fiber.

➤*Pharmacokinetics:*

Absorption/Distribution – The pharmacokinetics of metaxalone have been evaluated in healthy adult volunteers after single-dose administration of metaxalone under fasted and fed conditions at doses ranging from 400 to 800 mg.

Peak plasma concentrations of metaxalone occur approximately 3 hours after a 400 mg oral dose under fasted conditions. Doubling the dose of metaxalone from 400 to 800 mg results in a roughly proportional increase in metaxalone exposure, as indicated by peak plasma concentrations (C_{max}) and area under the curve (AUC). Dose proportionality at doses higher than 800 mg has not been studied. The absolute bioavailability of metaxalone is not known.

The single-dose pharmacokinetic parameters of metaxalone in 2 groups of healthy volunteers are shown in the following table.

Mean (% CV) Metaxalone Pharmacokinetic Parameters[a]

Dose (mg)	C_{max} (ng/mL)	T_{max} (h)	AUC_∞ (ng•h/mL)	Half-life (h)	CL/F (L/h)
400[b]	983 (53)	3.3 (35)	7,479 (51)	9 (53)	68 (50)
800[c]	1,816 (43)	3 (39)	15,044 (46)	8 (58)	66 (51)

[a] CV = coefficient of variation; T_{max} = time to maximum concentration; CL/F = apparent oral clearance.
[b] Subjects received 1 × 400 mg tablet under fasted conditions (n = 42).
[c] Subjects received 2 × 400 mg tablets under fasted conditions (n = 59).

Although plasma protein binding and absolute bioavailability of metaxalone are not known, the apparent volume of distribution (approximately 800 L) and lipophilicity (log P = 2.42) of metaxalone suggest that the drug is extensively distributed in the tissues.

Food effects: A randomized, 2-way crossover study was conducted in 42 healthy volunteers (31 men, 11 women) administered one metaxalone 400 mg tablet under fasted conditions and following a standard high-fat breakfast. Subjects ranged in age from 18 to 48 years (mean age, 23.5 ± 5.7 years). Compared with fasted conditions, the presence of a high-fat meal at the time of drug administration increased C_{max} by 177.5% and increased AUC (AUC_{0-t}, AUC_∞) by 123.5% and 115.4%, respectively. T_{max} was also delayed (4.3 vs 3.3 h) and terminal half-life was decreased (2.4 vs 9 h) under fed conditions compared with the fasted state.

In a second food effect study of similar design, two metaxalone 400 mg tablets (800 mg) were administered to healthy volunteers (N = 59; 37 men, 22 women), ranging in age from 18 to 50 years (mean age, 25.6 ± 8.7 years). Compared with fasted conditions, the presence of a high-fat meal at the time of drug administration increased C_{max} by 193.6% and increased AUC (AUC_{0-t}, AUC_∞) by 146.4% and 142.2%, respectively. T_{max} was also delayed (4.9 vs 3 h), and terminal half-life was decreased (4.2 vs 8 h) under fed conditions compared with fasted conditions. The half-life of metaxalone under fed conditions may be more indicative of the disposition half-life of metaxalone, as higher plasma concentrations were achieved. Similar food effect results were observed in the previously described study when one metaxalone 800 mg tablet was administered in place of two metaxalone 400 mg tablets. The increase in metaxalone exposure coinciding with a reduction in half-life may be attributed to more complete absorption of metaxalone in the presence of a high-fat meal.

Metabolism/Excretion – Metaxalone is metabolized by the liver and excreted in the urine as unidentified metabolites. Metaxalone concentrations decline log-linearly, with a terminal half-life of 9 ± 4.8 hours.

Special populations –

Renal function impairment: The impact of renal function impairment on the pharmacokinetics of metaxalone has not been determined. In the absence of such information, use metaxalone with caution in patients with renal function impairment.

Hepatic function impairment: The impact of hepatic function impairment on the pharmacokinetics of metaxalone has not been determined. In the absence of such information, use metaxalone with caution in patients with hepatic function impairment.

Gender: The effect of gender on the pharmacokinetics of metaxalone was assessed in an open-label study in which 48 healthy adult volunteers (24 men, 24 women) were administered two metaxalone 400 mg tablets (800 mg) under fasted conditions. The bioavailability of metaxalone was significantly higher in women compared with men, as evidenced by C_{max} (2,115 vs 1,335 ng/mL) and AUC_∞ (17,884 vs 10,328 ng•h/mL). The mean half-life was 11.1 hours in women and 7.6 hours in men. The apparent volume of distribution of metaxalone was approximately 22% higher in men than in women but not significantly different when adjusted for body weight. Similar findings were also seen when the previously described combined dataset was used in the analysis.

Age: The effects of age on the pharmacokinetics of metaxalone were determined following single administration of two metaxalone 400 mg tablets (800 mg) under fasted and fed conditions. The results were analyzed separately, as well as in combination with the results from 3 other studies. Using the combined data, the results indicate that the pharmacokinetics of metaxalone are significantly more affected by age under fasted conditions than under fed conditions, with bioavailability under fasted conditions increasing with age.

The bioavailability of metaxalone under fasted and fed conditions in the 3 groups of healthy volunteers of varying age is shown in the following table.

Metaxalone Mean (CV) Pharmacokinetics Parameters by Age Group[a]

	Younger volunteers		Older volunteers			
Age (years)	25.6 ± 8.7		39.3 ± 19.8		71.5 ± 5	
n	59		21		23	
Food	Fasted	Fed	Fasted	Fed	Fasted	Fed
C_{max} (ng/mL)	1,816 (43)	3,510 (41)	2,719 (46)	2,915 (55)	3,168 (43)	3,680 (59)
T_{max} (h)	3 (39)	4.9 (48)	3 (40)	8.7 (91)	2.6 (30)	6.5 (67)
AUC_{0-t} (ng•h/mL)	14,531 (47)	20,683 (41)	19,836 (40)	20,482 (37)	23,797 (45)	24,340 (48)
AUC_∞ (ng•h/mL)	15,045 (46)	20,833 (41)	20,490 (39)	20,815 (37)	24,194 (44)	24,704 (47)

[a] Following single administration of two metaxalone 400 mg tablets (800 mg) under fasted and fed conditions.

METAXALONE — ORAL

Contraindications

Hypersensitivity to the drug; tendency to drug-induced, hemolytic, or other anemias; significant renal or hepatic function impairment.

Warnings/Precautions

➤*CNS effects:* Taking metaxalone with food may enhance general CNS depression; elderly patients may be especially susceptible to this CNS effect.

➤*Hepatic function impairment:* Administer metaxalone with great care to patients with preexisting liver damage. Perform serial liver function studies in these patients.

➤*Hazardous tasks:* Metaxalone may impair the mental or physical abilities required for performance of hazardous tasks, such as operating machinery or driving a motor vehicle, especially when used with alcohol or other CNS depressants.

➤*Pregnancy: Category B* (per Briggs' *Drugs in Pregnancy and Lactation*). Postmarketing experience has not revealed evidence of fetal injury, but such experience cannot exclude the possibility of infrequent or subtle damage to the human fetus. Safe use of metaxalone has not been established with regard to possible adverse reactions on fetal development. Therefore, do not use metaxalone tablets in women who are or may become pregnant and particularly during early pregnancy unless in the judgment of the health care provider the potential benefits outweigh the possible hazards.

➤*Lactation:* It is not known whether this drug is secreted in human milk. The molecular weight (about 221) suggests that the drug will be excreted into breast milk. As a general rule, advise patients not to breast-feed while taking a drug because many drugs are excreted in human milk.

➤*Children:* The safety and efficacy in children 12 years of age and younger have not been established.

➤*Elderly:* Per the Beers list, most muscle relaxants and antispasmodics are poorly tolerated by elderly patients because these cause anticholinergic adverse effects, sedation, and weakness. Additionally, their effectiveness at doses tolerated by elderly patients is questionable. Metaxalone is also considered a high-risk medication for the elderly according to the Centers for Medicare and Medicaid Services.

Drug Interactions

➤*CNS depressants:* Metaxalone may enhance the effects of alcohol, barbiturates, and other CNS depressants.

➤*Drug/Lab test interactions:* False-positive Benedict tests, due to an unknown reducing substance, have been noted. A glucose-specific test will differentiate findings.

Adverse Reactions

➤*CNS:* Dizziness, drowsiness, headache, nervousness or "irritability."

➤*Dermatologic:* Rash, with or without pruritus.

➤*GI:* GI upset, nausea, vomiting.

➤*Hematologic:* Hemolytic anemia, leukopenia.

➤*Hepatic:* Jaundice.

➤*Hypersensitivity:* Hypersensitivity reaction. Though rare, anaphylactoid reactions have been reported with metaxalone.

Overdosage

➤*Symptoms:* Deaths by deliberate or accidental overdose have occurred with metaxalone, particularly in combination with antidepressants, and have been reported with this class of drug in combination with alcohol.

➤*Treatment:* Perform gastric lavage and institute supportive therapy. Consultation with a regional poison control center is recommended.

Patient Information

Inform patients that metaxalone may impair the mental or physical abilities required for performance of hazardous tasks, such as operating machinery or driving a motor vehicle, especially when used with alcohol or other CNS depressants.

Inform patients to avoid alcohol and other CNS depressants.

METHOCARBAMOL

Rx	**Methocarbamol** (Various, eg, Geneva, Lederle, Major, Schein, UDL, Zenith-Goldline)	**Tablets:** 500 mg	In 100s, 500s and UD 100s.
Rx	**Robaxin** (Schwarz Pharma)		Saccharin. (Robaxin AHR). Light orange. In 100s, 500s, *Disco-Pak* 100s.
Rx	**Methocarbamol** (Various, eg, Geneva, Lederle, Major, Schein, UDL, Zenith-Goldline)	**Tablets:** 750 mg	In 60s, 100s, 500s and UD 100s.
Rx	**Robaxin-750** (Schwarz Pharma)		Saccharin. (AHR Robaxin-750). Orange. Capsule-shaped. In 100s, 500s and *Disco–Pak* 100s.
Rx	**Robaxin** (Wyeth-Ayerst)	**Injection:** 100 mg/mL	In 10 ml vials.[a]

[a] In solution of polyethylene glycol 300. After mixing with IV infusion fluids, do not refrigerate.

METHOCARBAMOL — ORAL

Indications

➤*Musculoskeletal conditions:* As an adjunct to rest, physical therapy, and other measures for the relief of discomfort associated with acute, painful musculoskeletal conditions.

➤*Tetanus:* There is clinical evidence that suggests that methocarbamol may have a beneficial effect in the control of the neuromuscular manifestations of tetanus. However, it does not replace the usual procedure of debridement, tetanus antitoxin, penicillin, tracheotomy, attention to fluid balance, and supportive care. Add methocarbamol to the regimen as soon as possible.

Administration and Dosage

➤*Adults:*

Musculoskeletal conditions –

Initial dosage: 1,500 mg 4 times a day for the first 48 to 72 hours of treatment. For severe conditions, 8,000 mg/day may be administered. Thereafter, the dosage can usually be reduced to approximately 4,000 mg/day.

Maintenance dosage: 1,000 mg 4 times a day or 750 mg every 4 hours, or 1,500 mg 3 times a day.

Tetanus – After the insertion of a nasogastric tube, crushed methocarbamol tablets suspended in water or saline may then be given through the tube. Total daily oral doses of up to 2,400 mg may be required, as judged by patient response.

➤*Storage/Stability:* Store at 20° to 25°C (68° to 77°F). Protect from light and moisture.

Actions

➤*Pharmacology:* The mechanism of action of methocarbamol in humans has not been established, but may be due to CNS depression. It has no direct action on the contractile mechanism of striated muscle, motor end plate, or nerve fiber.

➤*Pharmacokinetics:*

Absorption – Methocarbamol has an onset of action of 30 minutes. Peak plasma levels occur approximately 2 hours after administration of 2 g.

Metabolism/Excretion – The half-life is from 1 to 2 hours; inactive metabolites are excreted in the urine and small amounts in the feces.

Special populations –

Renal function impairment: The clearance of methocarbamol in 8 renally impaired patients on maintenance hemodialysis was reduced about 40% compared with 17 healthy subjects, although the mean (± SD) elimination half-life in these 2 groups was similar: 1.2 (± 0.6) vs 1.1 (± 0.3) hours, respectively.

Hepatic function impairment: In 8 patients with cirrhosis secondary to alcohol abuse, the mean total clearance of methocarbamol was reduced approximately 70% compared with that obtained in 8 age-and weight-matched healthy subjects. The mean (± SD) elimination half-life in the cirrhotic patients and the healthy subjects was 3.38 (± 1.62) and 1.11 (± 0.27) hours, respectively. The percent of methocarbamol bound to plasma proteins was decreased to approximately 40% to 45% compared with 46% to 50% in the healthy subjects.

Elderly: The mean (± SD) elimination half-life of methocarbamol in elderly healthy volunteers (mean (± SD) age, 69 (± 4) years) was slightly prolonged compared with a younger [mean (± SD) age, 53.3 (± 8.8) years), healthy population (1.5 (± 0.4) vs 1.1 (± 0.27) hours, respectively]. The fraction of bound methocarbamol was slightly decreased in the elderly vs younger volunteers (41% to 43% vs 46% to 50%, respectively).

Contraindications

Hypersensitivity to any of the ingredients.

Warnings/Precautions

➤*Hazardous tasks:* Methocarbamol may impair mental or physical abilities required for performance of hazardous tasks, such as operating machinery or driving a motor vehicle. Caution patients about operating machinery, including automobiles, until they are reasonably certain that methocarbamol therapy does not adversely affect their ability to engage in such activities.

➤*Pregnancy: Category C.* Safe use of methocarbamol has not been established with regard to possible adverse effects upon fetal development. There have been reports of fetal and congenital abnormalities following in utero exposure of methocarbamol. Therefore, do not use methocarbamol tablets in women who are, or may become, pregnant, particularly during early pregnancy, unless, the potential benefits outweigh the possible hazards.

➤*Lactation:* Methocarbamol or its metabolites are excreted in the milk of dogs. It is not known whether methocarbamol or its metabolites are excreted

METHOCARBAMOL — ORAL

in human milk. Because many drugs are excreted in human milk, exercise caution when methocarbamol is administered to a nursing woman. As a general rule, breast-feeding should not be undertaken while a patient is on a drug because many drugs are excreted in human milk.

➤*Children:* Safety and efficacy of methocarbamol in children younger than 16 years of age have not been established.

➤*Elderly:* Per the Beers list, most muscle relaxants and antispasmodics are poorly tolerated by elderly patients because these cause anticholinergic adverse effects, sedation, and weakness. Additionally, their effectiveness at doses tolerated by elderly patients is questionable. Metaxalone is also considered a high-risk medication for the elderly according to the Centers for Medicare and Medicaid Services.

Drug Interactions

➤*Pyridostigmine:* Methocarbamol may inhibit the effect of pyridostigmine bromide. Therefore, use with caution in patients with myasthenia gravis receiving anticholinesterase agents.

➤*CNS agents:* Since methocarbamol may possess a general CNS depressant effect, caution patients receiving methocarbamol about combined effects with alcohol and other CNS depressants.

➤*Drug/Lab test interactions:* Methocarbamol may cause a color interference in certain screening tests for 5-hydroxyindoleacetic acid (5-HIAA) using nitrosonaphthol reagent and in screening tests for urinary vanillylmandelic acid (VMA) using the Gitlow method.

Adverse Reactions

➤*Cardiovascular:* Bradycardia, flushing, hypotension, syncope, thrombophlebitis.

➤*CNS:* Amnesia, confusion, diplopia, dizziness or light-headedness, drowsiness, insomnia, mild muscular incoordination, nystagmus, sedation, seizures (including grand mal), vertigo.

➤*Dermatologic:* Pruritus, rash, urticaria.

➤*GI:* Dyspepsia, jaundice (including cholestatic jaundice), nausea, vomiting.

➤*Hematologic/Lymphatic:* Leukopenia.

➤*Immunologic:* Hypersensitivity reactions.

➤*Special senses:* Blurred vision, conjunctivitis, nasal congestion, metallic taste.

➤*Miscellaneous:* Anaphylactic reaction, angioneurotic edema, fever, headache.

Overdosage

➤*Symptoms:* Limited information is available in the acute toxicity of methocarbamol. Overdose of methocarbamol is frequently in conjunction with alcohol or other CNS depressants and includes the following symptoms: nausea, drowsiness, blurred vision, hypotension, seizures, and coma. One adult survived the deliberate ingestion of 22 to 30 g of methocarbamol without serious toxicity. Another adult survived a dose of 30 to 50 g. The principle symptom in both cases was extreme drowsiness. Treatment was symptomatic and recovery was uneventful.

➤*Treatment:* Management of overdose includes symptomatic and supportive treatment. Supportive measures include maintenance of an adequate airway, monitoring urinary output and vital signs, and administration of IV fluids if necessary. The usefulness of hemodialysis in managing overdose is unknown.

In postmarketing experience, deaths have been reported with an overdose of methocarbamol alone or in the presence of other CNS depressants, alcohol, or psychotropic drugs.

Patient Information

This drug may cause drowsiness, dizziness, or light-headedness. Observe caution while driving or performing other tasks requiring alertness, coordination, or physical dexterity. Avoid alcohol and other CNS depressants.

METHOCARBAMOL — INJECTION

Indications

➤*Musculoskeletal conditions:* As an adjunct to rest, physical therapy, and other measures for the relief of discomfort associated with acute, painful, musculoskeletal conditions.

The mode of action of this drug has not been clearly identified, but may be related to its sedative properties. Methocarbamol does not directly relax tense skeletal muscles.

➤*Tetanus:* There is clinical evidence that suggests that methocarbamol may have a beneficial effect in the control of the neuromuscular manifestations of tetanus. However, it does not replace the usual procedure of debridement, tetanus antitoxin, penicillin, tracheotomy, attention to fluid balance, and supportive care. Add methocarbamol to the regimen as soon as possible.

Administration and Dosage

➤*Adults:*

Moderate musculoskeletal conditions –

Usual dosage: 1,000 mg (10 mL) may be adequate. Ordinarily this injection need not be repeated, as the administration of the oral form will usually sustain the relief initiated by the injection.

Maximum dose: 3,000 mg (30 mL) a day for no more than 3 consecutive days. A like course may be repeated after a lapse of 48 hours if the condition persists.

Severe musculoskeletal conditions –

Usual dosage: 2,000 to 3,000 mg (20 to 30 mL) may be required, if oral administration is not feasible.

Maximum dose: 3,000 mg (30 mL) a day for no more than 3 consecutive days. A like course may be repeated after a lapse of 48 hours if the condition persists.

Tetanus – Inject 1 or 2 vials (1,000 or 2,000 mg) directly into the tubing of the previously inserted indwelling needle. An additional 1,000 (10 mL) or 2,000 mg (20 mL) may be added to the infusion bottle so that a total of up to 3,000 mg (30 mL) is given as the initial dose. This procedure should be repeated every 6 hours until conditions allow for the insertion of a nasogastric tube to continue on oral therapy. (See Oral Methocarbamol monograph.)

➤*Children:*

Tetanus –

Maximum dose: 1.8 g/m^2 for 3 consecutive days.

Initial dosage: A minimum initial dose of 15 mg/kg or 500 mg/m^2. This dosage may be repeated every 6 hours as required.

Maintenance dosage: The maintenance dosage may be given by injection into tubing or by intravenous (IV) infusion with an appropriate quantity of fluid.

➤*Renal function impairment:* Contraindicated in known or suspected renal pathology. This caution is necessary because of the presence of polyethylene glycol 300 in the vehicle. (See Contraindications.)

➤*Hepatic function impairment:* The mean total clearance and plasma protein binding was reduced (70% and 40% to 45%, respectively). The mean elimination half-life was increased. (See Actions.)

➤*Administration:* For IV and intramuscular (IM) use only. Not recommended for subcutaneous administration.

IV use – May be administered undiluted directly into the vein at a maximum rate of 3 mL/min (one 10 mL vial in approximately 3 minutes). It also may be added to an IV drip of sodium chloride injection (sterile isotonic sodium chloride solution for parenteral use) or 5% dextrose injection (sterile 5% dextrose solution); 1 vial given as a single dose should not be diluted to more than 250 mL for IV infusion. Care should be exercised to avoid vascular extravasation of this hypertonic solution, which may result in thrombophlebitis. It is preferable that the patient be in a recumbent position during and for at least 10 to 15 minutes following the injection.

IM use – Not more than 5 mL (one-half vial) should be injected into each gluteal region. The injections may be repeated at 8-hour intervals, if necessary. When satisfactory relief of symptoms is achieved, it usually can be maintained with tablets.

➤*Storage/Stability:* Store between 20° and 25°C (68° and 77°F). After mixing with IV infusion fluids, do not refrigerate.

Actions

➤*Pharmacology:* The mechanism of action in humans has not been established, but may be due to general CNS depression. It has no direct action on the contractile mechanism of striated muscle, the motor end plate, or the nerve fiber.

➤*Pharmacokinetics:*

Special populations

Renal function impairment: The clearance of methocarbamol in renally impaired patients on maintenance hemodialysis was reduced about 40% compared to a healthy population, although the mean elimination half-life in these 2 groups was similar (1.2 vs 1.1 hours, respectively).

Hepatic function impairment: In patients with cirrhosis secondary to alcohol abuse, the mean total clearance of methocarbamol was reduced approximately 70% compared to a healthy population (11.9 L/hr), and the mean elimination half-life was extended to approximately 3.4 hours. The fraction of methocarbamol bound to plasma proteins was decreased to approximately 40% to 45% compared to 46% to 50% in an age- and weight-matched healthy population.

Contraindications

Hypersensitive to methocarbamol or to any of the injection components; known or suspected renal pathology. This caution is necessary because of the presence of polyethylene glycol 300 in the vehicle.

A much larger amount of polyethylene glycol 300 than is present in recommended doses of methocarbamol injectable is known to have increased preexisting acidosis and urea retention in patients with renal impairment. Although the amount present in this preparation is well within the limits of safety, caution dictates this contraindication.

Warnings/Precautions

➤*Administration:* As with other agents administered either intravenously or intramuscularly, careful supervision of dose and rate of injection should be observed. Rate of injection should not exceed 3 mL/min, (one 10 mL vial in approximately 3 minutes). Since methocarbamol injectable is hypertonic, vascular extravasation must be avoided. A recumbent position will reduce the likelihood of side reactions.

METHOCARBAMOL — INJECTION

Blood aspirated into the syringe does not mix with the hypertonic solution. This phenomenon occurs with many other IV preparations. The blood may be safely injected with the methocarbamol, or the injection may be stopped when the plunger reaches the blood, whichever the physician prefers.

The total dosage should not exceed 30 mL (3 vials) a day for more than 3 consecutive days except in the treatment of tetanus.

➤*Special risk:* Caution should be observed in using the injectable form in patients with suspected or known seizure disorders.

➤*Hazardous tasks:* Methocarbamol may impair mental or physical abilities required for performance of hazardous tasks, such as operating machinery or driving a motor vehicle. Patients should be cautioned about operating machinery, including automobiles, until they are reasonably certain that methocarbamol therapy does not adversely affect their ability to engage in such activities.

➤*Pregnancy:* Category C.

Teratogenic – Animal reproduction studies have not been conducted with methocarbamol. It is also not known whether methocarbamol can cause fetal harm when administered to a pregnant woman or can affect reproduction capacity. Methocarbamol should be given to a pregnant woman only if clearly needed.

Safe use of methocarbamol has not been established with regard to possible adverse effects upon fetal development. There have been very rare reports of fetal and congenital abnormalities following in utero exposure to methocarbamol. Therefore, methocarbamol should not be used in women who are or may become pregnant and particularly during early pregnancy unless in the judgment of the physician the potential benefits outweigh the possible hazards.

➤*Lactation:* Methocarbamol or its metabolites are excreted in the milk of dogs; however, it is not known whether methocarbamol or its metabolites are excreted in human milk. Because many drugs are excreted in human milk, caution should be exercised when methocarbamol injectable is administered to a nursing woman.

➤*Children:* Safety and effectiveness of methocarbamol in children have not been established except in tetanus. A minimum initial dose of 15 mg/kg is recommended. This dosage may be repeated every 6 hours as indicated. The maintenance dosage may be given by injection into tubing or by IV infusion with an appropriate quantity of fluid.

➤*Elderly:* Per the Beers list, most muscle relaxants and antispasmodics are poorly tolerated by elderly patients because these cause anticholinergic adverse effects, sedation, and weakness. Additionally, their effectiveness at doses tolerated by elderly patients is questionable. Metaxalone is also considered a high risk medication for the elderly according to the Centers for Medicare and Medicaid Services.

Drug Interactions

➤*CNS agents:* Since methocarbamol may possess a general CNS depressant effect, patients receiving methocarbamol injectable should be cautioned about combined effects with alcohol and other CNS depressants.

➤*Pyridostigmine:* Methocarbamol may inhibit the effect of pyridostigmine bromide. Therefore, use with caution in patients with myasthenia gravis receiving anticholinesterase agents.

➤*Drug/Lab test interactions:* Methocarbamol may cause a color interference in certain screening tests for 5-hydroxy-indoleacetic acid (5-HIAA) using nitrosonaphthol reagent and in screening tests for urinary vanillylmandelic acid (VMA) using the Gitlow method.

Adverse Reactions

The following adverse reactions have been reported coincident with the administration of methocarbamol. Some events may have been due to an overly rapid rate of IV injection.

➤*Cardiovascular:* Bradycardia, flushing, hypotension, syncope, thrombophlebitis .In most cases of syncope there was spontaneous recovery. In others, epinephrine, injectable steroids, or injectable antihistamines were employed to hasten recovery.

➤*CNS:* Amnesia, confusion, diplopia, dizziness or lightheadedness, drowsiness, insomnia, mild muscular incoordination, nystagmus, seizures (including grand mal), vertigo. The onset of convulsive seizures during IV administration of methocarbamol has been reported in patients with seizure disorders. The psychic trauma of the procedure may have been a contributing factor. Although several observers have reported success in terminating epileptiform seizures with methocarbamol injectable, its administration to patients with epilepsy is not recommended.

➤*Dermatologic:* Pruritus, rash, urticaria.

➤*GI:* Dyspepsia, jaundice (including cholestatic jaundice), nausea and vomiting.

➤*Hematologic/Lymphatic:* Leukopenia.

➤*Local:* Pain and sloughing at the site of injection.

➤*Ophthalmic:* Blurred vision, conjunctivitis with nasal congestion.

➤*Special senses:* Metallic taste.

➤*Miscellaneous:* Anaphylactic reaction, fever, headache.

Overdosage

➤*Symptoms:* Limited information is available on the acute toxicity of methocarbamol. Overdose is frequently in conjunction with alcohol or other CNS depressants and includes the following symptoms: Nausea, drowsiness, blurred vision, hypotension, seizures, and coma. One adult survived the deliberate ingestion of 22 to 30 g of methocarbamol without serious toxicity. Another adult survived a dose of 30 to 50 g. The principal symptom in both cases was extreme drowsiness. Treatment was symptomatic and recovery was uneventful.

➤*Treatment:* Management of overdose includes symptomatic and supportive treatment. Supportive measures include maintenance of an adequate airway, monitoring urinary output and vital signs, and administration of IV fluids if necessary. The usefulness of hemodialysis in managing overdose is unknown.

Patient Information

Patients should be cautioned that methocarbamol may cause drowsiness or dizziness, which may impair their ability to operate motor vehicles or machinery.

Because methocarbamol may possess a general CNS-depressant effect, patients should be cautioned about combined effects with alcohol and other CNS depressants.

ORPHENADRINE CITRATE

Rx	**Orphenadrine Citrate** (Various)	**Tablets; oral:** 100 mg	In 30s, 100s, 500s, and 1000s.
Rx	**Orphenadrine Citrate** (Apothecon)	**Tablets, sustained-release; oral:** 100 mg	Lactose. (INV 336). White. In 100s and 500s.
Rx	**Orphenadrine Citrate** (Various)	**Injection, solution:** 30 mg/mL	In 2 mL amps and 10 mL vials.
Rx	**Banflex** (Forest Pharm.)		In 10 mL vials.
Rx	**Flexon** (Various, eg, Keene)		In 10 mL vials.
Rx	**Norflex** (Graceway Pharmaceuticals)		In 2 mL amps.[a]

[a] With sodium bisulfite.

ORPHENADRINE CITRATE — ORAL

Indications

➤*Musculoskeletal conditions:* As an adjunct to rest, physical therapy, and other measures for the relief of discomfort associated with acute painful musculoskeletal conditions.

➤*Off-label uses:* At bedtime in the treatment of quinine-resistant leg cramps.

Administration and Dosage

➤*Adults:*

Musculoskeletal conditions – Two tablets per day; 1 in the morning and 1 in the evening.

➤*Storage/Stability:* Store at 15° to 30°C (59° to 86°F).

Actions

➤*Pharmacology:* The mode of therapeutic action has not been clearly identified, but may be related to its analgesic properties. Orphenadrine also possesses anticholinergic actions.

➤*Pharmacokinetics:*

Absorption – Peak plasma levels occur 2 hours after administration of 100 mg orphenadrine; duration of action is 4 to 6 hours.

Metabolism/Excretion – The half-life is ≈ 14 hours for the parent drug, and 2 to 25 hours for metabolites. Excretion is via urine and feces. Most of orphenadrine is degraded to eight known metabolites.

Contraindications

Glaucoma, pyloric or duodenal obstruction, stenosing peptic ulcers, prostatic hypertrophy or obstruction of the bladder neck, cardiospasm (megaesophagus) and myasthenia gravis; hypersensitivity to the drug.

Warnings/Precautions

➤*Long-term therapy:* Safety of continuous long-term therapy has not been established. Therefore, if orphenadrine is prescribed for prolonged use, periodic monitoring of blood, urine, and liver function values is recommended.

➤*Cardiac disease:* Use with caution in patients with tachycardia, cardiac decompensation, coronary insufficiency, cardiac arrhythmias.

ORPHENADRINE CITRATE — ORAL

➤*Hazardous tasks:* Some patients may experience transient episodes of lightheadedness, dizziness, or syncope. Orphenadrine may impair the ability of the patient to engage in potentially hazardous activities such as operating machinery or driving a motor vehicle; ambulatory patients should therefore be cautioned accordingly.

➤*Pregnancy:* Category C. Animal reproduction studies have not been conducted with orphenadrine. It is also not known whether orphenadrine can cause fetal harm when administered to a pregnant woman or can affect reproduction capacity. Orphenadrine should be given to a pregnant woman only if clearly needed.

➤*Lactation:* There are no data on the use of orphenadrine in breastfeeding women.

➤*Children:* Safety and efficacy in children have not been established.

➤*Elderly:* Per the Beers list, orphenadrine causes more sedation and anticholinergic adverse effects than safer alternatives. Orphenadrine is also considered a high-risk medication for elderly patients according to the Centers of Medicare and Medicaid Services.

Drug Interactions

Orphenadrine Drug Interactions

Precipitant drug	Object drug[a]		Description
Amantadine	Orphenadrine	↑	Anticholinergic effects may be increased.
Orphenadrine	Haloperidol	↔	Worsening of schizophrenic symptoms, decreased haloperidol levels and development of tardive dyskinesia may occur.
Orphenadrine	Phenothiazines	↓	Therapeutic effects of phenothiazines may be decreased.
Orphenadrine	Propoxyphene	↔	Confusion, anxiety, and tremors have been reported in few patients receiving propoxyphene and orphenadrine concomitantly. As these symptoms may be simply due to an additive effect, reduction of dosage or discontinuation of 1 or both agents is recommended in such cases.

[a] ↑ = object drug increased; ↓ = object drug decreased; ↔ = undetermined clinical effect.

Adverse Reactions

Adverse reactions of orphenadrine are mainly due to the mild anticholinergic action of orphenadrine, and are usually associated with higher dosage. Dryness of the mouth is usually the first adverse effect to appear. When the daily dose is increased, possible adverse effects include: Tachycardia, palpitation, urinary hesitancy or retention, blurred vision, dilatation of pupils, increased ocular tension, weakness, nausea, vomiting, headache, dizziness, constipation, drowsiness, hypersensitivity reactions, pruritus, hallucinations, agitation, tremor, gastric irritation, and rarely urticaria and other dermatoses. Infrequently, an elderly patient may experience some degree of mental confusion. These adverse reactions can usually be eliminated by reduction in dosage. Very rare cases of aplastic anemia associated with the use of orphenadrine tablets have been reported. No causal relationship has been established.

ORPHENADRINE CITRATE — INJECTION

Indications

➤*Musculoskeletal conditions:* As an adjunct to rest, physical therapy, and other measures for the relief of discomfort associated with acute painful musculoskeletal conditions.

The mode of action of the drug has not been clearly identified, but may be related to its analgesic properties. Orphenadrine citrate does not directly relax tense skeletal muscles.

Administration and Dosage

➤*Adults:*

Musculoskeletal conditions – One 2 mL ampul (60 mg) IV or IM; may be repeated every 12 hours. Relief may be maintained with 1 orphenadrine extended-release tablet twice daily.

➤*Administration:* Administer IV or IM.

➤*Storage / Stability:* Store at 15° to 30°C (59° to 86°F).

Actions

➤*Pharmacology:* The mode of therapeutic action has not been clearly identified, but may be related to its analgesic properties. Orphenadrine also possesses anticholinergic actions.

Contraindications

Glaucoma, pyloric or duodenal obstruction, stenosing peptic ulcers, prostatic hypertrophy or obstruction of the bladder neck, cardiospasm (megaesophagus) and myasthenia gravis; hypersensitivity to the drug.

Warnings/Precautions

➤*Long-term therapy:* Safety of continuous long-term therapy has not been established. Therefore, if orphenadrine is prescribed for prolonged use, periodic monitoring of blood, urine and liver function values is recommended.

➤*Cardiac disease:* Use with caution in patients with tachycardia, cardiac decompensation, coronary insufficiency, or cardiac arrhythmias.

➤*Sulfite sensitivity:* Orphenadrine injection contains sodium bisulfite, a sulfite that may cause allergic-type reactions including anaphylactic symptoms and life-threatening or less severe asthmatic episodes in certain susceptible people. The overall prevalence of sulfite sensitivity in the general population is unknown and probably low. Sulfite sensitivity is seen more frequently in asthmatic than nonasthmatic people.

➤*Hazardous tasks:* Some patients may experience transient episodes of lightheadedness, dizziness or syncope. Orphenadrine may impair the ability of the patient to engage in potentially hazardous activities such as operating machinery or driving a motor vehicle; ambulatory patients should therefore be cautioned accordingly.

➤*Pregnancy:* Category C. Animal reproduction studies have not been conducted with orphenadrine. It is also not known whether orphenadrine can cause fetal harm when administered to a pregnant woman or can affect reproduction capacity. Orphenadrine should be given to a pregnant woman only if clearly needed.

➤*Lactation:* There are no data on the use of orphenadrine in breastfeeding women.

➤*Children:* Safety and efficacy in children have not been established.

➤*Elderly:* Per the Beers list, orphenadrine causes more sedation and anticholinergic adverse effects than safer alternatives. Orphenadrine is also considered a high-risk medication for elderly patients according to the Centers of Medicare and Medicaid Services.

Drug Interactions

Orphenadrine Drug Interactions

Precipitant drug	Object drug[a]		Description
Amantadine	Orphenadrine	↑	Anticholinergic effects may be increased.
Orphenadrine	Haloperidol	↔	Worsening of schizophrenic symptoms, decreased haloperidol levels and development of tardive dyskinesia may occur.
Orphenadrine	Phenothiazines	↓	Therapeutic effects of phenothiazines may be decreased.
Orphenadrine	Propoxyphene	↔	Confusion, anxiety and tremors have been reported in few patients receiving propoxyphene and orphenadrine concomitantly. As these symptoms may be simply due to an additive effect, reduction of dosage or discontinuation of one or both agents is recommended in such cases.

[a] ↑ = object drug increased; ↓ = object drug decreased; ↔ = undetermined clinical effect.

Adverse Reactions

Adverse reactions of orphenadrine are mainly due to the mild anticholinergic action of orphenadrine, and are usually associated with higher dosage. Dryness of the mouth is usually the first adverse effect to appear. When the daily dose is increased, possible adverse effects include: Tachycardia, palpitation, urinary hesitancy or retention, blurred vision, dilatation of pupils, increased ocular tension, weakness, nausea, vomiting, headache, dizziness, constipation, drowsiness, hypersensitivity reactions, pruritus, hallucinations, agitation, tremor, gastric irritation, and rarely urticaria and other dermatoses. Infrequently, an elderly patient may experience some degree of mental confusion. These adverse reactions can usually be eliminated by reduction in dosage. Very rare cases of aplastic anemia associated with the use of orphenadrine tablets have been reported. No causal relationship has been established.

➤*Hypersensitivity:* Rare instances of anaphylactic reaction have been reported associated with the intramuscular injection of orphenadrine citrate injection.

TIZANIDINE

Rx	**Tizanidine Hydrochloride** (Various, eg, Actav Eliz, Akyma, Eon Labs, Mylan, Par)	**Tablets; oral:** 2 mg	Equiv. to tizanidine hydrochloride 2.29 mg. In 150s, 500s, and 1,000s.
Rx	**Zanaflex** (Acorda Therapeutics)		Equiv. to tizanidine hydrochloride 2.29 mg. Lactose. (A592). Scored. In 150s.
Rx	**Tizanidine Hydrochloride** (Various, eg, Actav Eliz, Akyma, Eon Labs, Mylan, Par)	**Tablets; oral:** 4 mg	Equiv. to tizanidine hydrochloride 4.58 mg. In 150s, 500s, and 1,000s.
Rx	**Zanaflex** (Acorda Therapeutics)		Equiv. to tizanidine hydrochloride 4.58 mg. Lactose. (A594). Scored. In 150s.
Rx	**Zanaflex** (Acorda Therapeutics)	**Capsules; oral:** 2 mg	Equiv. to tizanidine hydrochloride 2.29 mg. Sugar spheres. (2 mg). Blue opaque. In 150s.
		4 mg	Equiv. to tizanidine hydrochloride 4.58 mg. Sugar spheres. (4 mg). White and blue, opaque. In 150s.
		6 mg	Equiv. to tizanidine hydrochloride 6.87 mg. Sugar spheres. (6 mg). Light blue, opaque. In 150s.

TIZANIDINE HYDROCHLORIDE — ORAL

Indications

➤*Muscle spasticity:* For the management of spasticity. Because of the short duration of effect, reserve treatment with tizanidine for daily activities and times when relief of spasticity is most important.

➤*Off-label uses:*

Spasticity of cerebral palsy (children/adolescents) – [2] = Fair documentation. Tizanidine is an effective therapy for spasticity in adults with multiple sclerosis and spinal cord injury. Tizanidine may be considered for the treatment of spasticity of cerebral palsy in children according to American Academy of Neurology guidelines. Use caution if tizanidine is used in children with hepatic impairment because the pharmacokinetic profile of tizanidine can be considerably altered.

Administration and Dosage

➤*General dosing considerations:* Tizanidine tablets and capsules are bioequivalent to each other under fasted conditions but not under fed conditions. (See Administration.)

➤*Adults:*

Muscle spasticity –

Usual dosage: A single oral dose of 8 mg reduces muscle tone in patients with spasticity for a period of several hours. The dose can be repeated at 6- to 8-hour intervals, as needed, to a maximum of 3 doses in 24 hours.

Maximum dose: 36 mg/day.

Initial dosage: Although single doses of less than 8 mg have not been demonstrated to be effective in controlled clinical studies, the dose-related nature of tizanidine common adverse reactions makes it prudent to begin therapy with single oral doses of 4 mg.

Dosage titration: Increase the dose gradually (2 to 4 mg steps) to achieve optimal effect (satisfactory reduction of muscle tone at a tolerated dose).

➤*Children:*

Off-label dosing –

Spasticity of cerebral palsy (children/adolescents): [2] = Fair documentation. 0.05 mg/kg/day orally. This dose has been studied for up to 6 months, but longer-term therapy would be required to maintain symptom control.

➤*Renal function impairment:* Use with caution in patients with renal impairment (CrCl less than 25 mL/min) because clearance is reduced by more than 50%. In these patients, reduce the individual doses during titration. If higher doses are required, increase individual doses rather than dosing frequency. Closely monitor these patients for an onset or increase in severity of the common adverse reactions (eg, asthenia, dizziness, dry mouth, somnolence), which are indicators of potential overdose.

➤*Hepatic function impairment:* Because tizanidine is extensively metabolized in the liver, hepatic impairment would be expected to have significant effects on the pharmacokinetics of tizanidine. Ordinarily avoid tizanidine or use it with extreme caution in patients with hepatic impairment.

➤*Administration:* Food has complex effects on tizanidine pharmacokinetics, which differ between formulations. These pharmacokinetic differences may result in clinically significant differences when switching administration of the tablet or capsule between the fed or fasted state, switching between the tablet and capsule in the fed state, or switching between the intact capsule and sprinkling the contents of the capsule on applesauce. These changes may result in increased adverse reactions or delayed/more rapid onset of activity, depending upon the nature of the switch. For this reason, be thoroughly familiar with the changes in kinetics associated with fed and fasted states.

➤*Storage/Stability:* Store at 25°C (77°F); excursions are permitted to 15° to 30°C (59° to 86°F).

Actions

➤*Pharmacology:* Tizanidine is an agonist at alpha-2 adrenergic receptor sites and presumably reduces spasticity by increasing presynaptic inhibition of motor neurons. In animal models, tizanidine has no direct effect on skeletal muscle fibers or the neuromuscular junction and no major effect on monosynaptic spinal reflexes. The effects of tizanidine are greatest on polysynaptic pathways. The overall effect of these actions is thought to reduce facilitation of spinal motor neurons.

The imidazoline chemical structure of tizanidine is related to that of the antihypertensive drug clonidine and other alpha-2 adrenergic agonists. Pharmacological studies in animals show similarities between the 2 compounds, but tizanidine was found to have 1/10 to 1/50 of the potency of clonidine in lowering blood pressure.

➤*Pharmacokinetics:*

Absorption/Distribution – Following oral administration, tizanidine is essentially completely absorbed. The absolute oral bioavailability of tizanidine is approximately 40% (coefficient of variation [CV] = 24%) because of extensive first-pass hepatic metabolism. Tizanidine is extensively distributed throughout the body, with a mean steady-state volume of distribution of 2.4 L/kg (CV = 21%) following intravenous administration in healthy adult volunteers. Tizanidine is approximately 30% bound to plasma proteins.

Bioequivalency: Tizanidine tablets and capsules are bioequivalent to each other under fasted conditions but not under fed conditions.

Food effects: A single dose of two 4 mg tablets or two 4 mg capsules was administered under fed and fasting conditions in an open-label, 4-period, randomized crossover study in 96 human volunteers, of whom 81 were eligible for the statistical analysis.

Following oral administration of the tablet or capsule (in the fasted state), tizanidine peak plasma concentrations occur 1 hour after dosing, with a half-life of approximately 2 hours.

When two 4 mg tablets are administered with food, the mean maximal plasma concentration (C_{max}) is increased approximately 30%, and the median time to peak plasma concentration is increased from 25 minutes to 1 hour and 25 minutes.

In contrast, when two 4 mg capsules are administered with food, the mean C_{max} is decreased 20%, and the median time to peak plasma concentration is increased from 2 hours to 3 hours. Consequently, the C_{max} for the capsule when administered with food is approximately two-thirds the C_{max} for the tablet when administered with food.

Food also increases the extent of absorption for tablets and capsules. The increase with the tablet (approximately 30%) is significantly greater than with the capsule (approximately 10%). Consequently, when each is administered with food, the amount absorbed from the capsule is about 80% of the amount absorbed from the tablet. Administration of the capsule contents sprinkled on applesauce is not bioequivalent to administration of an intact capsule under fasting conditions. Administration of the capsule contents on applesauce results in a 15% to 20% increase in C_{max} and area under the curve (AUC) of tizanidine compared with administration of an intact capsule while fasting and a 15-minute decrease in the median lag time and time to C_{max}.

Metabolism/Excretion – Tizanidine has linear pharmacokinetics over a dose of 1 to 20 mg. Tizanidine has a half-life of approximately 2.5 hours (CV = 33%). Approximately 95% of an administered dose is metabolized. The primary CYP-450 isoenzyme involved in tizanidine metabolism is CYP1A2. Tizanidine metabolites are not known to be active; their half-lives range from 20 to 40 hours.

Following single- and multiple-oral dosing of ^{14}C-tizanidine, an average of 60% and 20% of total radioactivity was recovered in urine and feces, respectively.

Special populations –

Renal function impairment: Tizanidine clearance is reduced more than 50% in elderly patients with renal function impairment (creatinine clearance [CrCl] less than 25 mL/min) compared with healthy elderly subjects, which would be expected to lead to a longer duration of clinical effect. Use tizanidine with caution in patients with renal function impairment.

Hepatic function impairment: Because tizanidine is extensively metabolized in the liver, hepatic function impairment would be expected to have significant effects on the pharmacokinetics of tizanidine. Ordinarily, avoid tizanidine use or use it with extreme caution in this patient population.

Elderly: Cross-study comparison of pharmacokinetic data following single-dose administration of tizanidine 6 mg showed that younger subjects cleared the drug 4 times faster than elderly subjects.

Contraindications

Known hypersensitivity to tizanidine or to its ingredients; concomitant use of tizanidine with fluvoxamine or ciprofloxacin.

TIZANIDINE HYDROCHLORIDE — ORAL

Warnings/Precautions

➤*Long-term use:* Clinical experience with long-term use of tizanidine at single doses of 8 to 16 mg or total daily doses of 24 to 36 mg is limited. In safety studies, approximately 75 patients have been exposed to individual doses of 12 mg or more for at least 1 year, and approximately 80 patients have been exposed to total daily doses of 30 to 36 mg/day for at least 1 year or more. There is no long-term experience with single daytime doses of 16 mg. Because long-term clinical study experience at high doses is limited, only adverse reactions with a relatively high incidence are likely to have been identified.

➤*Hypotension:* Tizanidine is an alpha-2 adrenergic agonist (like clonidine) and can produce hypotension. In a single-dose study in which blood pressure was monitored closely after dosing, two-thirds of patients treated with tizanidine 8 mg had a 20% reduction in either the diastolic or systolic blood pressure. The reduction was seen within 1 hour after dosing, peaked 2 to 3 hours after dosing, and was associated at times with bradycardia, orthostatic hypotension, light-headedness/dizziness and, rarely, syncope. The hypotensive effect is dose related and has been measured following single doses of 2 mg or more.

The chance of significant hypotension may possibly be minimized by titrating the dose and focusing attention on signs and symptoms of hypotension prior to dose advancement. In addition, patients moving from a supine to a fixed, upright position may be at increased risk for hypotension and orthostatic effects.

➤*Hepatotoxicity:* Tizanidine occasionally causes liver injury, most often hepatocellular in type. In controlled clinical studies, approximately 5% of patients treated with tizanidine had elevations of liver function tests (ALT, AST) to greater than 3 times the upper limit of normal (or 2 times if baseline levels were elevated), compared with 0.4% in control patients. Most cases resolved rapidly upon drug withdrawal, with no reported residual problems. In occasional symptomatic cases, nausea, vomiting, anorexia, and jaundice have been reported. Based upon postmarketing experience, death associated with liver failure has been a rare occurrence reported in patients treated with tizanidine.

Monitoring of aminotransferase levels is recommended during the first 6 months of treatment (eg, baseline, 1, 3, and 6 months) and periodically thereafter, based on clinical status. Because of the potential toxic hepatic effect of tizanidine, ordinarily avoid the drug or use it with extreme caution in patients with hepatic function impairment.

➤*Sedation:* In the multiple-dose, controlled clinical studies, 48% of patients receiving any dose of tizanidine reported sedation as an adverse reaction. The sedation was rated as severe in 10% of these cases, compared with less than 1% in the placebo-treated patients. Sedation may interfere with everyday activity.

The effect appears to be dose related. In a single-dose study, 92% of the patients receiving 16 mg reported drowsiness during the 6-hour study. This compares with 76% of the patients on 8 mg and 35% of the patients on placebo. Patients began noting this effect 30 minutes following dosing. The effect peaked 1.5 hours following dosing. Of the patients who received a single dose of 16 mg, 51% continued to report drowsiness 6 hours following dosing, compared with 13% of the patients receiving placebo or tizanidine 8 mg.

In the multiple-dose studies, the prevalence of patients with sedation peaked following the first week of titration and then remained stable for the duration of the maintenance phase of the study.

➤*Hallucinosis/Psychotic-like symptoms:* Tizanidine use has been associated with hallucinations. Formed, visual hallucinations or delusions have been reported in 5 of 170 (3%) patients in 2 North American controlled clinical studies. These 5 cases occurred within the first 6 weeks. Most of the patients were aware that the events were unreal. One patient developed psychoses in association with the hallucinations. One patient among these 5 continued to have problems for at least 2 weeks following discontinuation of tizanidine.

➤*Cardiovascular effects:* Prolongation of the QT interval and bradycardia were noted in chronic toxicity studies in dogs at doses equal to the maximum human dose on a mg/m^2 basis. Electrocardiogram evaluation was not performed in the controlled clinical studies. Reduction in pulse rate has been noted in association with decreases in blood pressure in the single-dose controlled study.

➤*Ophthalmic effects:* Dose-related retinal degeneration and corneal opacities have been found in animal studies at doses equivalent to approximately the maximum recommended dose on a mg/m^2 basis. There have been no reports of corneal opacities or retinal degeneration in the clinical studies.

➤*Discontinuing therapy:* If therapy needs to be discontinued, especially in patients who have been receiving high doses for long periods, decrease the dose slowly to minimize the risk of withdrawal and rebound hypertension, tachycardia, and hypertonia.

➤*Renal function impairment:* Use tizanidine with caution in patients with renal function impairment (CrCl less than 25 mL/min) because clearance is reduced by greater than 50%. In these patients, reduce the individual doses during titration. If higher doses are required, increase individual doses rather than dosing frequency. Closely monitor these patients for an onset or increase in severity of the common adverse reactions (eg, asthenia, dizziness, dry mouth, somnolence), which are indicators of potential overdose.

➤*Hepatic function impairment:* The influence of hepatic function impairment on the pharmacokinetics of tizanidine has not been evaluated. Because tizanidine is extensively metabolized in the liver, hepatic function impairment would be expected to have significant effects on the pharmacokinetics of tizanidine. Ordinarily avoid tizanidine or use it with extreme caution in patients with hepatic function impairment.

➤*Drug abuse and dependence:* Abuse potential was not evaluated in human studies. Rats were able to distinguish tizanidine from saline in a standard discrimination paradigm after training, but failed to generalize the effects of morphine, cocaine, diazepam, or phenobarbital to tizanidine. Monkeys were shown to self-administer tizanidine in a dose-dependent manner, and abrupt cessation of tizanidine produced transient signs of withdrawal at doses greater than 35 times the maximum recommended human dose (MRHD) on a mg/m^2 basis. These transient withdrawal signs (increased locomotion, body twitching, and aversive behavior toward the observer) were not reversed by naloxone administration.

Tizanidine is closely related to clonidine, which is often abused in combination with narcotics and is known to cause symptoms of rebound upon abrupt withdrawal. Three cases of rebound symptoms on sudden withdrawal of tizanidine have been reported. The case reports suggest that these patients were also misusing narcotics. Withdrawal symptoms included hypertension, tachycardia, hypertonia, tremor, and anxiety. As with clonidine, withdrawal is expected to be more likely in cases in which high doses are used, especially for prolonged periods.

➤*Pregnancy: Category C.* Reproduction studies performed in rats at a dose of 3 mg/kg (equal to the MRHD on a mg/m^2 basis) and in rabbits at 30 mg/kg (16 times the MRHD on a mg/m^2 basis), did not show evidence of teratogenicity.

Tizanidine at doses that are equal to and up to 8 times the MRHD on a mg/m^2 basis increased gestation duration in rats. Prenatal and postnatal pup loss was increased, and developmental retardation occurred. Postimplantation loss was increased in rabbits at doses of 1 mg/kg or greater, greater than or equal to 0.5 times the MRHD on a mg/m^2 basis. Tizanidine has not been studied in pregnant women. Give tizanidine to pregnant women only if clearly needed.

➤*Lactation:* It is not known whether tizanidine is excreted in human milk; although, as a lipid-soluble drug, it might be expected to pass into breast milk.

➤*Children:* There are no adequate and well-controlled studies to document the safety and efficacy of tizanidine in children.

➤*Elderly:* Use tizanidine with caution in elderly patients because clearance is decreased 4-fold.

➤*Monitoring:* Monitoring of aminotransferase levels is recommended during the first 6 months of treatment (eg, baseline, 1, 3, and 6 months) and periodically thereafter, based on clinical status. Because of the potential toxic hepatic effect of tizanidine, use the drug with extreme caution in patients with hepatic function impairment.

Use tizanidine with caution in patients with renal function impairment. Closely monitor these patients for an onset or increase in severity of the common adverse reactions (eg, asthenia, dry mouth, somnolence), which are indicators of potential overdose.

Drug Interactions

➤*QT prolongation:* An additive effect of tizanidine with other drugs that prolong the QT interval cannot be excluded. The following drugs may prolong the QT interval and increase the risk of life-threatening cardiac arrhythmias, including torsades de pointes: Antiarrhythmic agents (eg, amiodarone, bretylium, disopyramide, dofetilide, procainamide, quinidine, and sotalol), arsenic trioxide, chlorpromazine, cisapride, dolasetron, droperidol, mefloquine, mesoridazine, moxifloxacin, pentamidine, pimozide, tacrolimus, thioridazine, and ziprasidone. For a more complete list of drugs that may prolong the QT interval, see the appendix, Drug-Induced Prolongation of the QT Interval and Torsades de Pointes.

Tizanidine Drug Interactions

Precipitant drug	Object drug[a]		Description
Acyclovir	Tizanidine	↑	Avoid concomitant use of tizanidine with acyclovir, a potent CYP1A2 inhibitor. Increased tizanidine plasma concentrations and adverse reactions may occur.
Alcohol	Tizanidine	↑	Alcohol increased the AUC of tizanidine approximately 20% while also increasing its C_{max} approximately 15%. This was associated with an increase in adverse effects of tizanidine. The CNS-depressant effects of tizanidine and alcohol are additive.
Antiarrhythmics (eg, amiodarone, mexiletine, propafenone, verapamil)	Tizanidine	↑	Avoid concomitant use of tizanidine with antiarrhythmics, potent CYP1A2 inhibitors. Increased tizanidine plasma concentrations and adverse reactions may occur.

TIZANIDINE HYDROCHLORIDE — ORAL

Tizanidine Drug Interactions

Precipitant drug	Object drug[a]		Description
Cimetidine	Tizanidine	↑	Avoid concomitant use of tizanidine with cimetidine, a potent CYP1A2 inhibitor. Increased tizanidine plasma concentrations and adverse reactions may occur.
Contraceptives, oral	Tizanidine	↑	Use with caution in women taking oral contraceptives because clearance of tizanidine is reduced approximately 50% in such patients. In these patients, during titration, reduce the individual doses.
Famotidine	Tizanidine	↑	Concomitant use of tizanidine with famotidine, a potent CYP1A2 inhibitor, should be avoided. Increased tizanidine plasma concentrations and adverse reactions may occur.
Fluoroquinolones (eg, ciprofloxacin, norfloxacin)	Tizanidine	↑	Certain fluoroquinolones may inhibit the metabolism (CYP1A2) of tizanidine, causing increased plasma concentrations and increased risk of adverse reactions. Clinically significant hypotension has been reported with coadministration. Concomitant use of tizanidine with ciprofloxacin is contraindicated.
Fluvoxamine	Tizanidine	↑	Concomitant use of tizanidine with fluvoxamine, a potent CYP1A2 inhibitor, is contraindicated. Significant alterations of tizanidine pharmacokinetics, including AUC, half-life, C_{max}, increased oral bioavailability, and decreased plasma clearance have been observed with concomitant use. Clinically significant hypotension has been reported.
Rofecoxib	Tizanidine	↑	Rofecoxib (not available in the United States) may potentiate the adverse effects of tizanidine.
Ticlopidine	Tizanidine	↑	Avoid concomitant use of tizanidine with ticlopidine, a potent CYP1A2 inhibitor. Increased tizanidine plasma concentrations and adverse reactions may occur.
Zileuton	Tizanidine	↑	Avoid concomitant use of tizanidine with zileuton, a potent CYP1A2 inhibitor. Increased tizanidine plasma concentrations and adverse reactions may occur.
Tizanidine	Acetaminophen	↓	Tizanidine delayed the time to C_{max} of acetaminophen by 16 minutes. Acetaminophen did not affect the pharmacokinetics of tizanidine.
Tizanidine	Antihypertensives	↑	Caution is advised when tizanidine is used in patients receiving concurrent antihypertensive therapy. Do not use with other alpha-2 adrenergic agonists.

[a] ↑ = object drug increased; ↓ = object drug decreased.

➤*Drug/Food interactions:* See Actions for more information.

Adverse Reactions

➤*Common adverse reactions leading to discontinuation:* Forty-five of 264 (17%) patients receiving tizanidine and 13 of 261 (5%) patients receiving placebo in 3 multiple-dose, placebo-controlled clinical studies discontinued treatment because of adverse reactions. When patients withdrew from the study, they frequently had more than 1 reason for discontinuing. The adverse reactions most frequently leading to withdrawal of tizanidine-treated patients in the controlled clinical studies were asthenia (weakness, fatigue and/or tiredness) (3%), dry mouth (3%), somnolence (3%), increased spasm or tone (2%), and dizziness (2%).

➤*Most frequent adverse clinical reactions:* In multiple-dose, placebo-controlled, clinical studies involving 264 patients with spasticity, the most frequent adverse reactions were asthenia (weakness, fatigue and/or tiredness), dizziness, dry mouth, and somnolence/sedation. Three-fourths of the patients rated the reactions as mild to moderate, and one-fourth of the patients rated the reactions as being severe. These reactions appeared to be dose related.

➤*Adverse reactions reported in controlled studies:*

Tizanidine Adverse Reactions (> 2%)

Adverse reaction	Placebo (n = 261)	Tizanidine (n = 264)
CNS		
Asthenia[a]	16%	41%
Dizziness	4%	16%
Dyskinesia	0%	3%
Nervousness	< 1%	3%
Somnolence	10%	48%
Speech disorder	0%	3%
GI		
Constipation	1%	4%
Dry mouth	10%	49%
Vomiting	0%	3%
GU		
Urinary frequency	2%	3%
Urinary tract infection	7%	10%
Hepatic		
ALT increased	< 1%	3%
Liver function tests abnormal	< 1%	3%
Respiratory		
Pharyngitis	1%	3%
Rhinitis	2%	3%
Miscellaneous		
Amblyopia (blurred vision)	< 1%	3%
Flu syndrome	2%	3%
Infection	5%	6%

[a] Weakness, fatigue, and/or tiredness.

Common Tizanidine Adverse Reactions in a Single-Dose Study

Adverse reaction	Placebo (n = 48)	Tizanidine tablet 8 mg (n = 45)	Tizanidine tablet 16 mg (n = 49)
Cardiovascular			
Bradycardia	0%	2%	10%
Hypotension	0%	16%	33%
CNS			
Asthenia[a]	40%	67%	78%
Dizziness	4%	22%	45%
Somnolence	31%	78%	92%
GI			
Dry mouth	35%	76%	88%

[a] Weakness, fatigue, and/or tiredness.

➤*Other adverse reactions:*

Cardiovascular – Arrhythmia, postural hypotension, syncope, vasodilatation (0.1% to 1%); angina pectoris, coronary artery disorder, heart failure, myocardial infarction, phlebitis, pulmonary embolus, ventricular extrasystoles, ventricular tachycardia (rare).

CNS – Anxiety, depression, paresthesia (1% or more); abnormal dreams, abnormal thinking, agitation, convulsion, depersonalization, dysautonomia, emotional lability, euphoria, migraine, neuralgia, paralysis, stupor, tremor, vertigo (0.1% to 1%); dementia, hemiplegia, neuropathy (rare).

Dermatologic – Rash, skin ulcer, sweating (1% or more); acne, alopecia, dry skin, pruritus, urticaria (0.1% to 1%); exfoliative dermatitis, herpes simplex, herpes zoster, skin carcinoma (rare).

GI – Abdomen pain, diarrhea, dyspepsia (1% or more); cholelithiasis, dysphagia, fecal impaction, flatulence, GI hemorrhage, hepatitis, melena (0.1% to 1%); gastroenteritis, hematemesis, hepatoma, intestinal obstruction, liver damage (rare).

GU – Cystitis, enlarged uterine fibroids, kidney calculus, menorrhagia, pyelonephritis, urinary retention, urinary urgency, vaginal moniliasis, vaginitis (0.1% to 1%); albuminuria, glycosuria, hematuria, metrorrhagia (rare).

Hematologic/Lymphatic – Anemia, ecchymosis, leukocytosis, leukopenia (0.1% to 1%); petechia, purpura, thrombocythemia, thrombocytopenia (rare).

Centrally Acting

TIZANIDINE HYDROCHLORIDE — ORAL

Metabolic/Nutritional – Edema, hypercholesteremia, hyperlipemia, hypothyroidism, weight loss (0.1% to 1%); adrenal cortex insufficiency, hyperglycemia, hypokalemia, hyponatremia, hypoproteinemia, respiratory acidosis (rare).

Musculoskeletal – Back pain, myasthenia (1% or more); arthralgia, arthritis, bursitis, pathological fracture (0.1% to 1%).

Respiratory – Bronchitis, pneumonia, sinusitis (0.1% to 1%); asthma (rare).

Special senses – Conjunctivitis, deafness, ear pain, eye pain, glaucoma, optic neuritis, otitis media, retinal hemorrhage, tinnitus, visual field defect (0.1% to 1%); iritis, keratitis, optic atrophy (rare).

Miscellaneous – Fever (1% or more); abscess, allergic reaction, cellulitis, death, malaise, moniliasis, neck pain, overdose, sepsis (0.1% to 1%); carcinoma, congenital anomaly, suicide attempt (rare).

Overdosage

➤*Symptoms:* A review of the safety surveillance database revealed cases of intentional and accidental tizanidine overdose. Some of the cases resulted in fatality, and many of the intentional overdoses were with multiple drugs including CNS depressants. The clinical manifestations of tizanidine overdose were consistent with its known pharmacology. In the majority of cases, a decrease in sensorium was observed including lethargy, somnolence, confusion, and coma. Depressed cardiac function has also been observed, most often including bradycardia and hypotension. Respiratory depression is another common feature of tizanidine overdose.

➤*Treatment:* If overdose occurs, undertake basic steps to ensure the adequacy of an airway and monitor cardiovascular and respiratory systems. In general, symptoms resolve within 1 to 3 days following discontinuation of tizanidine and administration of appropriate therapy. Because of the similar mechanism of action, symptoms and management of tizanidine overdose are similar to those following clonidine overdose. For the most recent information concerning the management of overdose, contact a poison control center.

Patient Information

Advise patients of the limited clinical experience with tizanidine in regard to the duration of use and the higher doses required to reduce muscle tone.

Because of the possibility of tizanidine lowering blood pressure, warn patients about the risk of clinically significant orthostatic hypotension.

Because of the possibility of sedation, warn patients about performing activities requiring alertness, such as driving a vehicle or operating machinery.

Instruct patients that the sedation may be additive when tizanidine is taken in conjunction with medicines (eg, baclofen, benzodiazepines) or substances (eg, alcohol) that act as CNS depressants.

Advise patients of the change in the absorption profile of tizanidine if taken with food and of the potential changes in efficacy and adverse reaction profiles that may result.

Advise patients not to stop taking tizanidine suddenly because rebound hypertension and tachycardia may occur.

Use tizanidine with caution when spasticity is utilized to sustain posture and balance in locomotion, or whenever spasticity is utilized to obtain increased function.

Because of the increased risk of serious adverse reactions including severe lowering of blood pressure and sedation when tizanidine and either fluvoxamine or ciprofloxacin are used together, do not use tizanidine with either fluvoxamine or ciprofloxacin. Because of the potential for interaction with other CYP1A2 inhibitors, instruct patients to inform their health care provider and pharmacist when any medication is added or removed from their regimen.

Direct Acting

DANTROLENE SODIUM

Rx	**Dantrolene Sodium** (Various, eg, Actavis Totowa, Global)	**Capsules; oral:** 25 mg	May contain lactose. In 100s, 500s, and UD 100s.
Rx	**Dantrium** (JHP Pharm)		Lactose. Orange/Tan. In 100s and 500s.
Rx	**Dantrolene Sodium** (Various, eg, Actavis Totowa, Global)	**Capsules; oral:** 50 mg	May contain lactose. In 100s, 500s, and UD 100s.
Rx	**Dantrium** (JHP Pharm)		Lactose. Orange/Tan. In 100s.
Rx	**Dantrolene Sodium** (Various, eg, Actavis Totowa, Global)	**Capsules; oral:** 100 mg	May contain lactose. In 100s, 500s, and UD 100s.
Rx	**Dantrium** (JHP Pharm)		Lactose. Orange/Tan. In 100s.
Rx	**Dantrium Intravenous** (JHP Pharm)	**Injection, powder for solution:** 20 mg/vial	Approx 0.32 mg/ml dantrolene sodium after reconstitution. With 3 g mannitol per vial. In 70 ml vials.
Rx	**Revonto** (US Worldmeds)	**Injection, lyophilized powder for solution:** 20 mg/vial	Mannitol 3 g/vial. In 65 mL vials.

DANTROLENE SODIUM — ORAL

WARNING

Dantrolene has a potential for hepatotoxicity; do not use in conditions other than those recommended. Symptomatic hepatitis (fatal and nonfatal) has been reported at various dose levels of the drug. The incidence reported in patients taking up to 400 mg/day is much lower than in those taking doses of 800 mg or more per day. Even sporadic short courses of these higher dose levels within a treatment regimen markedly increased the risk of serious hepatic injury. Liver dysfunction as evidenced by blood chemical abnormalities alone (liver enzyme elevations) has been observed in patients exposed to dantrolene for varying periods of time. Overt hepatitis has occurred at varying intervals after initiation of therapy, but has been most frequently observed between the third and 12th month of therapy. The risk of hepatic injury appears to be greater in females, in patients over 35 years of age, and in patients taking other medication(s) in addition to dantrolene. Use dantrolene only in conjunction with appropriate monitoring of hepatic function including frequent determination of AST or ALT. If no observable benefit is derived from the administration of dantrolene after a total of 45 days, discontinue therapy. Prescribe the lowest possible effective dose for the individual patient.

Indications

➤*Chronic spasticity:* Controlling the manifestations of clinical spasticity resulting from upper motor neuron disorders (eg, spinal cord injury, stroke, cerebral palsy, or multiple sclerosis). It is of particular benefit to the patient whose functional rehabilitation has been retarded by the sequelae of spasticity. Such patients must have presumably reversible spasticity where relief of spasticity will aid in restoring residual function. Dantrolene is not indicated in the treatment of skeletal muscle spasm resulting from rheumatic disorders.

➤*Malignant hyperthermia:* Preoperatively, to prevent or attenuate the development of signs of malignant hyperthermia in known, or strongly suspected, malignant hyperthermia-susceptible patients who require anesthesia and/or surgery. Currently accepted clinical practices in the management of such patients must still be adhered to (careful monitoring for early signs of malignant hyperthermia, minimizing exposure to triggering mechanisms, and prompt use of IV dantrolene and indicated supportive measures should signs of malignant hyperthermia appear); see also the package insert for dantrolene IV.

Administer oral dantrolene following a malignant hyperthermic crisis to prevent recurrence of the signs of malignant hyperthermia.

➤*Off-label uses:*

Neuroleptic malignant syndrome – [4] = Insufficient documentation. The optimal dose, route, and frequency of dantrolene for the treatment of neuroleptic malignant syndrome (NMS) have not been reported. A meta-analysis of more than 200 case reports found that dantrolene use appeared to be associated with a higher rate of mortality than supportive therapy alone. A possible role for dantrolene in the treatment of NMS resulting from use of only one neuroleptic medication was identified. Responses have varied in case reports and the benefits of treatment are unclear.

Other possible off-label uses – Exercise-induced muscle pain, heat stroke.

Administration and Dosage

➤*Adults:*

Chronic spasticity –

Maximum dose: 100 mg 4 times daily.

Initial dosage: 25 mg once daily for 7 days.

Dosage titration: Increase to 25 mg 3 times daily for 7 days; then increase to 50 mg 3 times daily for 7 days with a final dosage of 100 mg 3 times daily. Therapy with a dose 4 times daily may be necessary for some individuals. Some patients will not respond until higher daily dosage is achieved. Maintain each dosage level for 7 days to determine the patient's response. If no further benefit is observed at the next higher dose, decrease the dosage to the previous lower dose.

Discontinuation of therapy: In view of the potential for liver damage in long-term dantrolene use, stop therapy if benefits are not evident within 45 days.

DANTROLENE SODIUM — ORAL

Malignant hyperthermia –

Preoperatively:

• *Usual dosage* – 4 to 8 mg/kg/day in 3 or 4 divided doses for 1 or 2 days prior to surgery, with the last dose being given approximately 3 to 4 hours before scheduled surgery with a minimum of water.

• *Dosage adjustment* – Adjustment can usually be made within the recommended dosage range to avoid incapacitation or excessive GI irritation (including nausea and/or vomiting).

Post-crisis follow-up: 4 to 8 mg/kg/day in 4 divided doses, for a 1- to 3-day period to prevent recurrence.

Off-label dosing –

Neuroleptic malignant syndrome: [4] = Insufficient documentation. Use of oral dantrolene 25 mg/day, gradually increased to 150 mg/day, has been reported, as has conversion to oral therapy with 75 mg/day after initial IV dosing.

➤*Children:*

5 years of age and older –

Chronic spasticity:

• *Maximum dose* – 100 mg 4 times daily.

• *Initial dosage* – 0.5 mg/kg once daily for 7 days.

• *Dosage titration* – Increase to 0.5 mg/kg 3 times daily for 7 days; then increase to 1 mg/kg 3 times daily for 7 days with a final dosage of 2 mg/kg 3 times daily. Therapy with a dose 4 times daily may be necessary for some individuals. Some patients will not respond until higher daily dosage is achieved. Maintain each dosage level for 7 days to determine the patient's response. If no further benefit is observed at the next higher dose, decrease the dosage to the previous lower dose.

Malignant hyperthermia: See Adults for dosing.

➤*Storage/Stability:* Avoid excessive heat (over 40°C [104°F]).

Actions

➤*Pharmacology:* In isolated nerve-muscle preparation, dantrolene has been shown to produce relaxation by affecting the contractile response of the skeletal muscle at a site beyond the myoneural junction, directly on the muscle itself. In skeletal muscle, dantrolene dissociates the excitation-contraction coupling, probably by interfering with the release of Ca^{++} from the sarcoplasmic reticulum. This effect appears to be more pronounced in fast muscle fibers as compared to slow ones, but generally affects both. A CNS effect occurs, with drowsiness, dizziness, and generalized weakness occasionally present. Although dantrolene does not appear to directly affect the CNS, the extent of its indirect effect is unknown.

Clinical experience in the management of fulminant human malignant hyperthermia, as well as experiments conducted in malignant hyperthermia-susceptible swine, have revealed that the administration of IV dantrolene, combined with indicated supportive measures, is effective in reversing the hypermetabolic process of malignant hyperthermia. Known differences between human and swine malignant hyperthermia are minor. The prophylactic administration of oral or IV dantrolene to malignant hyperthermia-susceptible swine will attenuate or prevent the development of signs of malignant hyperthermia in a manner dependent upon the dosage of dantrolene administered and the intensity of the malignant hyperthermia triggering stimulus. Limited clinical experience with the administration of oral dantrolene to patients judged malignant hyperthermia susceptible, when combined with clinical experience in the use of IV dantrolene for the treatment of malignant hyperthermia and data derived from the above cited animal model experiments, suggests that oral dantrolene will also attenuate or prevent the development of signs of human malignant hyperthermia, provided that currently accepted practices in the management of such patients are adhered to; IV dantrolene should also be available for use should the signs of malignant hyperthermia appear.

➤*Pharmacokinetics:* The absorption of dantrolene after oral administration in humans is incomplete and slow but consistent, and dose-related blood levels are obtained. The duration and intensity of skeletal muscle relaxation is related to the dosage and blood levels. The mean biologic half-life of dantrolene in adults is 8.7 hours after a 100 mg dose. Specific metabolic pathways in the degradation and elimination of dantrolene in human subjects have been established. Metabolic patterns are similar in adults and children. In addition to the parent compound, dantrolene, which is found in measurable amounts in blood and urine, the major metabolites noted in body fluids are the 5-hydroxy analog and the acetamido analog. Since dantrolene is probably metabolized by hepatic microsomal enzymes, enhancement of its metabolism by other drugs is possible. However, neither phenobarbital nor diazepam appears to affect dantrolene metabolism.

Contraindications

Active hepatic disease, such as hepatitis and cirrhosis; where spasticity is utilized to sustain upright posture and balance in locomotion or whenever spasticity is utilized to obtain or maintain increased function.

Warnings/Precautions

➤*Long-term use:* Long-term safety has not been established. Chronic studies in rats, dogs, and monkeys at dosages higher than 30 mg/kg/day showed growth or weight depression and signs of hepatopathy and possible occlusion nephropathy, all of which were reversible upon cessation of treatment.

➤*Hepatoxicity:* It is important to recognize that fatal and nonfatal liver disorders of an idiosyncratic or hypersensitivity type may occur with dantrolene therapy.

At the start of dantrolene therapy, it is desirable to do liver function studies (AST, ALT, alkaline phosphatase, total bilirubin) for a baseline or to establish whether there is preexisting liver disease. If baseline liver abnormalities exist and are confirmed, there is a clear possibility that the potential for dantrolene hepatoxicity could be enhanced, although such a possibility has not yet been established.

Perform liver function studies (eg, AST or ALT) at appropriate intervals during dantrolene therapy. If such studies reveal abnormal values, therapy should generally be discontinued. Consider reinitiation or continuation of therapy only where benefits of the drug have been of major importance to the patient. Some patients have revealed a return to normal laboratory values in the face of continued therapy while others have not.

If symptoms compatible with hepatitis, accompanied by abnormalities in liver function tests or jaundice appear, discontinue dantrolene. If caused by dantrolene and detected early, the abnormalities in liver function characteristically have reverted to normal when the drug was discontinued.

Dantrolene therapy has been reinstituted in a few patients who have developed clinical and/or laboratory evidence of hepatocellular injury. If such reinstitution of therapy is done, attempt it only in patients who clearly need dantrolene and only after previous symptoms and laboratory abnormalities have cleared. Hospitalize the patient and restart the drug in very small and gradually increasing doses. Perform laboratory monitoring frequently, and withdraw the drug immediately if there is any indication of recurrent liver involvement. Some patients have reacted with unmistakable signs of liver abnormality upon administration of a challenge dose, while others have not.

Use dantrolene with particular caution in females and in patients over 35 years of age in view of apparent greater likelihood of drug-induced, potentially fatal, hepatocellular disease in these groups.

➤*Special risk:* Use dantrolene with caution in patients with impaired pulmonary function, particularly those with obstructive pulmonary disease, and in patients with severely impaired cardiac function due to myocardial disease. Use with caution in patients with a history of liver disease or dysfunction.

➤*Hazardous tasks:* Caution patients against driving a motor vehicle or participating in hazardous occupations while taking dantrolene. Exercise caution in the concomitant administration of tranquilizing agents.

➤*Photosensitivity:* Dantrolene might possibly evoke a photosensitivity reaction; caution patients about exposure to sunlight while taking it.

➤*Pregnancy: Category C.* Dantrolene has been shown to be embryocidal in the rabbit and has been shown to decrease pup survival in the rat when given at doses 7 times the human oral dose. There are no adequate and well-controlled studies in pregnant women. Use dantrolene capsules during pregnancy only if the potential benefit justifies the potential risk to the fetus.

Labor and delivery – In 1 non-randomized open-label study, 21 term pregnant patients received prophylactic oral dantrolene 100 mg per day for 2 to 10 days prior to delivery. Dantrolene readily crossed the placenta with maternal and fetal whole blood levels approximately equal at delivery; neonatal levels then fell approximately 50% per day for 2 days before declining sharply. No neonatal respiratory and neuromuscular side effects were detected at low dose. More data, at higher doses, are needed before more definitive conclusions can be made.

➤*Lactation:* Do not use dantrolene in nursing mothers.

➤*Children:* The long-term safety of dantrolene in children under the age of 5 years of age has not been established. Because of the possibility that adverse effects of the drug could become apparent only after many years, a benefit-risk consideration of the long-term use of dantrolene is particularly important in children.

Drug Interactions

Dantrolene Drug Interactions

Precipitant drug	Object drug[a]		Description
Dantrolene	CNS agents	↑	Drowsiness may occur with dantrolene therapy, and the concomitant administration of CNS depressants such as sedatives and tranquilizing agents may result in further drowsiness.
Dantrolene	Vecuronium	↑	Administration of dantrolene may potentiate vecuronium-induced neuromuscular block.
Dantrolene	Verapamil	↑	Hyperkalemia and myocardial depression occurred in one patient during concurrent use.
Clofibrate	Dantrolene	↓	Plasma protein binding of dantrolene may be reduced.
Estrogens	Dantrolene	↑	Although a definite drug interaction is not established, hepatotoxicity occurred more often in women older than 35 years of age receiving these agents concurrently.
Warfarin	Dantrolene	↓	Plasma protein binding of dantrolene may be reduced.

[a] ↑ = object drug increased; ↓ = object drug decreased.

DANTROLENE SODIUM — ORAL

Adverse Reactions

The most frequently occurring side effects of dantrolene have been diarrhea, dizziness, drowsiness, fatigue, general malaise, and weakness. These are generally transient, occurring early in treatment, and can often be obviated by beginning with a low dose and increasing dosage gradually until an optimal regimen is established. Diarrhea may be severe and may necessitate temporary withdrawal of dantrolene therapy. If diarrhea recurs upon readministration of dantrolene, therapy should probably be withdrawn permanently.

Other less frequent side effects, listed according to system are:

➤*Cardiovascular:* Erratic blood pressure; heart failure; phlebitis; tachycardia.

➤*CNS:* Alteration of taste; diplopia; drooling; headache; insomnia; lightheadedness; seizure; speech disturbance; visual disturbance.

➤*Dermatologic:* Abnormal hair growth; acne-like rash; eczematoid eruption; pruritus; sweating; urticaria.

➤*GI:* Abdominal cramps; anorexia; constipation, rarely progressing to signs of intestinal obstruction; gastric irritation; GI bleeding; nausea and/or vomiting; swallowing difficulty.

➤*GU:* Crystalluria; difficult erection; difficult urination and/or urinary retention; hematuria; increased urinary frequency; urinary incontinence and/or nocturia.

➤*Hematologic:* Aplastic anemia; leukopenia; lymphocytic lymphoma; thrombocytopenia.

➤*Hepatic:* Hepatitis.

➤*Hypersensitivity:* Anaphylaxis; pleural effusion with pericarditis.

➤*Musculoskeletal:* Backache; myalgia.

➤*Psychiatric:* Increased nervousness; mental confusion; mental depression.

➤*Respiratory:* Feeling of suffocation; respiratory depression.

➤*Special senses:* Excessive tearing.

➤*Miscellaneous:* Chills and fever. The published literature has included some reports of dantrolene use in patients with neuroleptic malignant syndrome (NMS). Dantrolene capsules are not indicated for the treatment of NMS and patients may expire despite treatment with dantrolene capsules.

Overdosage

➤*Symptoms:* Symptoms that may occur in case of overdose include, but are not limited to, muscular weakness and alterations in the state of consciousness (eg, lethargy, coma), vomiting, diarrhea, and crystalluria.

➤*Treatment:* For acute overdosage, employ general supportive measures along with immediate gastric lavage.

Administer IV fluids in fairly large quantities to avert the possibility of crystalluria. Maintain an adequate airway and keep artificial resuscitation equipment at hand. Institute electrocardiographic monitoring, and observe the patient carefully. To date, no experience has been reported with dialysis and its value in dantrolene overdosage is not known.

Patient Information

Caution patients against driving a motor vehicle or participating in hazardous occupations while taking dantrolene. Exercise caution in the concomitant administration of tranquilizing agents.

DANTROLENE SODIUM — INJECTION

WARNING

Dantrolene has a potential for hepatotoxicity. Do not use in conditions other than those recommended. The incidence of symptomatic hepatitis (fatal and nonfatal) reported in patients taking up to 400 mg/day is much lower than in those taking ≥ 800 mg/day. Even sporadic short courses of these higher dose levels within a treatment regimen markedly increased the risk of serious hepatic injury. Liver dysfunction, as evidenced by liver enzyme elevations, has been observed in patients exposed to the drug for varying periods of time. Overt hepatitis has been most frequently observed between the third and twelfth months of therapy. Risk of hepatic injury appears to be greater in females, in patients older than 35 years of age and in patients taking other medications in addition to dantrolene.

Monitor hepatic function, including frequent determinations of AST or ALT. If no observable benefit is derived from therapy after 45 days, discontinue use.

Use the lowest possible effective dose for each patient.

Indications

➤*Malignant hyperthermia:* Along with appropriate supportive measures, for the management of the fulminant hypermetabolism of skeletal muscle characteristic of malignant hyperthermia crises in patients of all ages. Dantrolene IV should be administered by continuous rapid IV push as soon as the malignant hyperthermia reaction is recognized (ie, tachycardia, tachypnea, central venous desaturation, hypercarbia, metabolic acidosis, skeletal muscle rigidity, increased utilization of anesthesia circuit carbon dioxide absorber, cyanosis and mottling of the skin, and, in many cases, fever).

Dantrolene IV is also indicated preoperatively, and sometimes postoperatively, to prevent or attenuate the development of clinical and laboratory signs of malignant hyperthermia in individuals judged to be malignant hyperthermia-susceptible.

➤*Off-label uses:*

Heatstroke – [5] = Poor documentation. Although dantrolene has been used in the treatment of heatstroke in case reports, controlled studies have failed to detect a consistent significant benefit from therapy. European guidelines state that dantrolene is not effective for the treatment of heatstroke.

Neuroleptic malignant syndrome – [4] = Insufficient documentation. The optimal dose, route, and frequency of dantrolene for the treatment of neuroleptic malignant syndrome (NMS) have not been reported. A meta-analysis of more than 200 case reports found that dantrolene use appeared to be associated with a higher rate of mortality than supportive therapy alone. A possible role for dantrolene in the treatment of NMS resulting from use of only one neuroleptic medication was identified. Responses have varied in case reports and the benefits of treatment are unclear.

Other possible off-label uses – Exercise-induced muscle pain.

Administration and Dosage

➤*Adults:*

Malignant hyperthermia –

Usual dosage: Begin at a minimum dose of 1 mg/kg and continue until symptoms subside or the maximum cumulative dose of 10 mg/kg has been reached. If the physiologic and metabolic abnormalities reappear, the regimen may be repeated. It is important to note that administration of dantrolene should be continuous until symptoms subside.

Maximum dose: 10 mg/kg cumulative dose.

Concomitant therapy: As soon as the malignant hyperthermia reaction is recognized, all anesthetic agents should be discontinued; the administration of 100% oxygen is recommended.

Preoperatively: May be administered preoperatively to patients judged malignant hyperthermia-susceptible as part of the overall patient management to prevent or attenuate the development of clinical and laboratory signs of malignant hyperthermia.

• *Prophylactic dosage* – 2.5 mg/kg starting approximately 1 ¼ hours before anticipated anesthesia and infused over approximately 1 hour. Additional doses must be individualized.

Post-crisis follow-up: May be used postoperatively to prevent or attenuate the recurrence of signs of malignant hyperthermia when oral dantrolene administration is not practical. The dose must be individualized, starting with 1 mg/kg or more as the clinical situation dictates.

Off-label dosing –

Neuroleptic malignant syndrome: [4] = Insufficient documentation. 1 to 2 mg/kg IV 1 to 4 times daily, continued until symptom resolution, often in combination with other therapies such as bromocriptine. IV doses varied widely in case reports. Use of oral dantrolene 25 mg/day, gradually increased to 150 mg/day, has also been reported, as has conversion to oral therapy with 75 mg/day after initial IV dosing.

➤*Children:*

Malignant hyperthermia – See Adults for dosing.

➤*Preparation for administration:* Each vial should be reconstituted by adding 60 mL of sterile water for injection (without a bacteriostatic agent), and the vial shaken until the solution is clear. Reconstituted dantrolene should not be transferred to large glass bottles for prophylactic infusion due to precipitate formation observed with the use of some glass bottles as reservoirs. For prophylactic infusion, the required number of individual vials should be reconstituted. The contents of individual vials are then transferred to a larger volume sterile IV plastic bag. While stable for 6 hours, it is recommended that the infusion be prepared immediately prior to the anticipated dosage administration time.

➤*Administration:* Administer by continuous rapid IV push.

➤*Extravasation:* Care must be taken to prevent extravasation of dantrolene solution into the surrounding tissues due to the high pH of the IV formulation. Extravasation resulting in severe tissue damage may occur during administration of dantrolene. If signs or symptoms of extravasation occur, stop the infusion immediately. If possible, withdraw 3 to 5 mL of blood to remove some of the drug. Remove the infusion needle. Delineate the infiltrated area on the patient's skin with a felt-tip marker. Elevate for 48 hours above heart level using a sling or stockinette dressing with an observation window cut in the dressing. Avoid pressure or friction. Do not rub area. Observe for signs of increased erythema, pain, or skin necrosis. If increased symptoms occur, consult a plastic surgeon. Ensure that no medication is given distally to extravasation site. After 48 hours, encourage the patient to use the extremity normally to promote full range of motion.

➤*Admixture compatibility:* Dextrose 5% injection, sodium chloride 0.9% injection, and other acidic solutions are not compatible and should not be used.

➤*Storage / Stability:* Store unreconstituted vials at 15°C to 30°C (59°F to 86°F) and avoid prolonged exposure to light. Store reconstituted solution at 15° to 30°C (59° to 86°F); must be protected from direct light and used within 6 hours after reconstitution.

DANTROLENE SODIUM — INJECTION

Actions

➤*Pharmacology:* In isolated nerve-muscle preparation, dantrolene has been shown to produce relaxation by affecting the contractile response of the muscle at a site beyond the myoneural junction. In skeletal muscle, dantrolene dissociates the excitation-contraction coupling, probably by interfering with the release of Ca^{++} from the sarcoplasmic reticulum. The administration of IV dantrolene to human volunteers is associated with loss of grip strength and weakness in the legs, as well as subjective CNS complaints (see Patient Information). Information concerning the passage of dantrolene across the blood-brain barrier is not available.

In the anesthetic-induced malignant hyperthermia syndrome, evidence points to an intrinsic abnormality of skeletal muscle tissue. In affected humans, it has been postulated that "triggering agents" (eg, general anesthetics and depolarizing neuromuscular blocking agents) produce a change within the cell which results in an elevated myoplasmic calcium. This elevated myoplasmic calcium activates acute cellular catabolic processes that cascade to the malignant hyperthermia crisis.

It is hypothesized that addition of dantrolene to the "triggered" malignant hyperthermic muscle cell re-establishes a normal level of ionized calcium in the myoplasm. Inhibition of calcium release from the sarcoplasmic reticulum by dantrolene re-establishes the myoplasmic calcium equilibrium, increasing the percentage of bound calcium. In this way, physiologic, metabolic, and biochemical changes associated with the malignant hyperthermia crisis may be reversed or attenuated. Experimental results in malignant hyperthermia-susceptible swine show that prophylactic administration of IV or oral dantrolene prevents or attenuates the development of vital sign and blood gas changes characteristic of malignant hyperthermia in a dose-related manner. The efficacy of IV dantrolene in the treatment of human and porcine malignant hyperthermia crisis, when considered along with prophylactic experiments in malignant hyperthermia-susceptible swine, lends support to prophylactic use of oral or IV dantrolene in malignant hyperthermia-susceptible humans. When prophylactic IV dantrolene is administered as directed, whole blood concentrations remain at a near steady state level for greater than or equal to 3 hours after the infusion is completed. Clinical experience has shown that early vital sign and/or blood gas changes characteristic of malignant hyperthermia may appear during or after anesthesia and surgery despite the prophylactic use of dantrolene and adherence to currently accepted patient management practices. These signs are compatible with attenuated malignant hyperthermia and respond to the administration of additional IV dantrolene (see Administration and Dosage). The administration of the recommended prophylactic dose of IV dantrolene to healthy volunteers was not associated with clinically significant cardiorespiratory changes.

➤*Pharmacokinetics:* Specific metabolic pathways for the degradation and elimination of dantrolene in humans have been established. Dantrolene is found in measurable amounts in blood and urine. Its major metabolites in body fluids are 5-hydroxy dantrolene and an acetylamino metabolite of dantrolene. Another metabolite with an unknown structure appears related to the latter. Dantrolene may also undergo hydrolysis and subsequent oxidation forming nitrophenylfuroic acid.

The mean biologic half-life of dantrolene after IV administration is variable, between 4 to 8 hours under most experimental conditions. Based on assays of whole blood and plasma, slightly greater amounts of dantrolene are associated with red blood cells than with the plasma fraction of blood. Significant amounts of dantrolene are bound to plasma proteins, mostly albumin, and this binding is readily reversible.

Contraindications

None.

Warnings/Precautions

➤*Malignant hyperthermia:* The use of dantrolene IV in the management of malignant hyperthermia crisis is not a substitute for previously known supportive measures. These measures must be individualized, but it will usually be necessary to discontinue the suspect triggering agents, attend to increased oxygen requirements, manage the metabolic acidosis, institute cooling when necessary, monitor urinary output, and monitor for electrolyte imbalance.

Since the effect of disease state and other drugs on dantrolene-related skeletal muscle weakness, including possible respiratory depression, cannot be predicted, patients who receive IV dantrolene preoperatively should have vital signs monitored.

If patients judged malignant hyperthermia-susceptible are administered IV or oral dantrolene preoperatively, anesthetic preparation must still follow a standard malignant hyperthermia-susceptible regimen, including the avoidance of known triggering agents. Monitoring for early clinical and metabolic signs of malignant hyperthermia is indicated because attenuation of malignant hyperthermia, rather than prevention, is possible. These signs usually call for the administration of additional IV dantrolene.

➤*Hepatotoxicity:* See the Warning box for more information.

➤*Mannitol:* When mannitol is used for prevention or treatment of late renal complications of malignant hyperthermia, the 3 g of mannitol needed to dissolve each 20 mg vial of IV dantrolene should be taken into consideration.

➤*Extravasation:* See Administration and Dosage for more information.

➤*Pregnancy: Category C.* Dantrolene has been shown to be embryocidal in the rabbit and has been shown to decrease pup survival in the rat when given at doses 7 times the human oral dose. There are no adequate and well-controlled studies in pregnant women. Dantrolene IV should be used during pregnancy only if the potential benefit justifies the potential risk to the fetus.

Labor and delivery – In one uncontrolled study, 100 mg/day of prophylactic oral dantrolene was administered to term pregnant patients awaiting labor and delivery. Dantrolene readily crossed the placenta, with maternal and fetal whole blood levels approximately equal at delivery; neonatal levels then fell approximately 50% per day for 2 days before declining sharply. No neonatal respiratory and neuromuscular side effects were detected at low dose. More data, at higher doses, are needed before more definitive conclusions can be made.

➤*Lactation:* Dantrolene is excreted into human breast milk. Waiting 2 days after the last dantrolene dose to breast-feed would ensure that the exposure of the breast-feeding infant would be negligible.

➤*Elderly:* Clinical studies of dantrolene sodium intravenous did not include sufficient numbers of subjects aged 65 and over to determine whether they respond differently from younger subjects. Other reported clinical experience has not identified differences in response between the elderly and younger patients. In general, dose selection for an elderly patient should be cautious reflecting the greater frequency of decreased hepatic, renal, or cardiac function, and of concomitant disease or other drug therapy.

Drug Interactions

Dantrolene Drug Interactions

Precipitant drug	Object drug[a]		Description
Dantrolene	Verapamil	↑	Hyperkalemia and myocardial depression occurred in one patient during concurrent use.
Dantrolene	Vecuronium	↑	Administration of dantrolene may potentiate vecuronium-induced neuromuscular block.
Clofibrate	Dantrolene	↓	Plasma protein binding of dantrolene may be reduced.
Estrogens	Dantrolene	↑	Although a definite drug interaction is not established, hepatotoxicity occurred more often in women older than 35 years of age receiving these agents concurrently.
Warfarin	Dantrolene	↓	Plasma protein binding of dantrolene may be reduced.

[a] ↑ = object drug increased; ↓ = object drug decreased.

Adverse Reactions

There have been occasional reports of death following malignant hyperthermia crisis even when treated with IV dantrolene; incidence figures are not available (the pre–dantrolene mortality of malignant hyperthermia crisis was approximately 50%). Most of these deaths can be accounted for by late recognition, delayed treatment, inadequate dosage, lack of supportive therapy, intercurrent disease, and/or the development of delayed complications such as renal failure or disseminated intravascular coagulopathy. In some cases there are insufficient data to completely rule out therapeutic failure of dantrolene.

There are rare reports of fatality in malignant hyperthermia crisis, despite initial satisfactory response to IV dantrolene, which involves patients who could not be weaned from dantrolene after initial treatment.

The administration of IV dantrolene to human volunteers is associated with loss of grip strength and weakness in the legs, as well as drowsiness and dizziness.

The following adverse reactions are in approximate order of severity:

- There are rare reports of pulmonary edema developing during the treatment of malignant hyperthermia crisis in which the diluent volume and mannitol needed to deliver IV dantrolene possibly contributed.
- There have been reports of thrombophlebitis following administration of IV dantrolene; actual incidence figures are not available. There have been rare reports of urticaria and erythema possibly associated with the administration of IV dantrolene.
- There has been one case of anaphylaxis.

None of the serious reactions occasionally reported with long-term oral dantrolene use, such as hepatitis, seizures, and pleural effusion with pericarditis, have been reasonably associated with short-term dantrolene IV therapy.

The following events have been reported in patients receiving oral dantrolene: Aplastic anemia, leukopenia, lymphocytic lymphoma, and heart failure.

The published literature has included some reports of dantrolene use in patients with neuroleptic malignant syndrome (NMS). Dantrolene IV is not indicated for the treatment of NMS and patients may expire despite treatment with dantrolene IV.

Overdosage

➤*Symptoms:* Symptoms that may occur in case of overdose include, but are not limited to, muscular weakness and alterations in the state of consciousness (eg, lethargy, coma), vomiting, diarrhea, and crystalluria.

DANTROLENE SODIUM — INJECTION

➤*Treatment:* For acute overdosage, general supportive measures should be employed.

IV fluids should be administered in fairly large quantities to avert the possibility of crystalluria. An adequate airway should be maintained and artificial resuscitation equipment should be at hand. Electrocardiographic monitoring should be instituted, and the patient carefully observed. The value of dialysis in dantrolene overdose is not known.

Patient Information

Based upon data in human volunteers, it will sometimes be appropriate to tell patients who receive dantrolene IV that decrease in grip strength and weakness of leg muscles, especially walking down stairs, can be expected postoperatively. In addition, symptoms such as "lightheadedness" may be noted. Since some of these symptoms may persist for up to 48 hours, patients must not operate an automobile or engage in other hazardous activity during this time. Caution is also indicated at meals on the day of administration because difficulty swallowing and choking has been reported. Caution should be exercised in the concomitant administration of tranquilizing agents.

SKELETAL MUSCLE RELAXANT COMBINATIONS

Rx	**Methocarbamol w/ASA** (Various, eg, Moore, Par)	**Tablets; oral:** 400 mg methocarbamol and 325 mg aspirin. *Dose: 2 tablets 4 times daily*	In 15s, 30s, 40s, 100s, 500s and 1000s.
Rx	**Carisoprodol Compound** (Various, eg, Moore)	**Tablets; oral:** 200 mg carisoprodol and 325 mg aspirin. *Dose: 1 or 2 tablets 4 times daily*	In 15s, 30s, 40s, 100s, 500s and 1000s.
Rx	**Sodol Compound** (Major)		In 100s and 500s.
c-iii	**Carisoprodol, Aspirin, and Codeine Phosphate** (Various, eg, Amide)	**Tablets; oral:** 200 mg carisoprodol, 325 mg aspirin, and 16 mg codeine phosphate. *Dose: 1 or 2 tablets 4 times daily*	In 100s and 500s.
Rx	**Orphenadrine Compound** (Sandoz)	**Tablets; oral:** 25 mg orphenadrine citrate, 385 mg aspirin and 30 mg caffeine. *Dose: 1 or 2 tablets 3 or 4 times daily*	Lactose. (E 713). White/green, round. In 100s.
Rx	**Orphenadrine Compound-DS** (Sandoz)	**Tablets; oral:** 50 mg orphenadrine citrate, 770 mg aspirin and 60 mg caffeine. *Dose: ½ or 1 tablet 3 or 4 times daily*	Lactose. (E 714). White/green, capsule shape. Scored. In 100s.

SKELETAL MUSCLE RELAXANT COMBINATIONS — ORAL

Indications

➤*Uses:* The carisoprodol and aspirin (with or without codeine) combinations are indicated as adjuncts to rest, physical therapy and other measures for relief of discomfort associated with acute, painful musculoskeletal conditions. The other combinations are classified as *"probably effective"* for this indication. Components of these combinations include:

MUSCLE RELAXANTS – Carisoprodol; orphenadrine; (see individual monographs).

ANALGESICS – Aspirin; codeine; (see individual monographs).

CAFFEINE – Caffeine (see individual monograph), used as a CNS stimulant, also has minor analgesic activity.

Warnings/Precautions

➤*Sulfite sensitivity:* Some of these products contain sulfites, which may cause allergic-type reactions (eg, hives, itching, wheezing, anaphylaxis) in certain susceptible people. Although the overall prevalence of sulfite sensitivity in the general population is probably low, it is seen more frequently in asthmatics or in atopic nonasthmatic people. Specific products containing sulfites are identified in the product listings.

➤*Pregnancy: Category B* (caffeine); *Category C* (carisoprodol, orphenadrine, aspirin, codeine); *Category D* (aspirin, if used full-dose at term) (codeine, if used for prolonged periods or in high doses at term) (per Briggs' *Drugs in Pregnancy and Lactation*).

Aspirin consumption during pregnancy may produce adverse reactions in the mother: anemia, antepartum or postpartum hemorrhage, prolonged gestation, and prolonged labor. Premature closure of the ductus arteriosus may occur in the latter part of pregnancy as a result of maternal consumption of full-dose aspirin. Avoid the use of aspirin during pregnancy, especially of chronic or intermittent high doses.

The molecular weight (about 260) of carisprodol suggests that it will cross to the embryo and fetus. Moreover, the active metabolite, meprobamate, does cross the placenta. Although the data do not support a significant risk with carisoprodol, the best course would be to avoid this agent, if possible, during the 1st trimester.

Caffeine crosses the placenta, and fetal blood and tissue levels similar to maternal concentrations are achieved. Use of high doses may be associated with spontaneous abortions, difficulty in becoming pregnant, and infertility.

➤*Lactation:* Caffeine, codeine, carisoprodol, and aspirin are excreted into breast milk.

The American Academy of Pediatrics recommends that aspirin be used cautiously by the mother during lactation because of potential adverse reactions in the breast-feeding infant Women taking carisoprodol who elect to breastfeed should closely monitor their infants for sedation. Avoid long-term consumption of codeine-containing products during breast-feeding. Short-term therapy, such as 1 or 2 days, and close monitoring of the infant should be standard. If the mother or infant demonstrates symptoms of narcotic toxicity, such as sedation, lethargy, or poor milk intake, stop breast-feeding. Although the American Academy of Pediatrics has classified codeine as compatible with breast-feeding, the previous report suggests that, for some women, codeine cannot be considered safe during breast-feeding, especially if the therapy is more than 1 or 2 days.

➤*Parkinson's Disease:* Parkinsonism is a neurological disease with a variety of origins characterized by tremor, rigidity, akinesia, and disorders of posture and equilibrium. The onset is slow and progressive with symptoms advancing over months to years.

Although the biochemical basis of parkinsonism is complex, the primary defect appears to be an imbalance of neurotransmitters (ie, a relative excess of acetylcholine and a deficiency/absence of dopamine in the basal ganglia). Other central neurotransmitters may have some modifying influence on these primary substances. This defect may be part of a more generalized, structural, and enzymatic defect.

Currently, therapy for Parkinson's disease is palliative, as there is no cure for this disease. The goal of therapy is to provide maximum relief from the symptoms and to attempt to maintain the independence and mobility of the patient.

Drug therapy of Parkinson's disease is aimed at correcting or modifying these neurotransmitter defects by inhibiting the effects of acetylcholine or enhancing the effects of dopamine.

➤*Anticholinergic agents:* Centrally-acting anticholinergics tend to diminish the characteristic tremor. Patients with minimal involvement who are functioning relatively well may not require medication. However, as the disease progresses, the anticholinergics may be considered.

➤*Dopaminergic agents:* Dopamine deficiency appears to be the central feature of the pathogenesis of parkinsonism. **Levodopa**, the immediate precursor of dopamine, directly increases dopamine content in the brain; it is currently the most effective treatment for parkinsonism. Other drugs are available that also affect the dopamine content of the brain: **Bromocriptine** and **pergolide** directly stimulate dopamine receptors. Pergolide is 10 to 1000 times more potent than bromocriptine on a milligram per milligram basis; **amantadine** may increase dopamine at the receptor either by releasing intact striatal dopamine stores or by blocking neuronal dopamine reuptake; **selegiline** increases dopaminergic activity through inhibition of monoamine oxidase type B; however, other mechanisms may exist such as interference of dopamine reuptake at the synapse.

Levodopa is used for symptomatic patients with moderate disabilities; therapy is usually initiated with a combination of levodopa and carbidopa (a dopa decarboxylase inhibitor that prevents peripheral metabolism of levodopa). Unfortunately, the response to levodopa gradually diminishes after 2 to 5 years in most patients, at which time the dopaminergic agonists, bromocriptine or pergolide, selegiline, or amantadine may be added to the drug regimen. Amantadine may also be used in patients with minimal involvement when the patients cannot tolerate an anticholinergic drug.

The table below summarizes the drug therapy available for parkinsonism:

Drug Therapy for Parkinsonism						
	Indications					
Drugs	Postencephalitic	Arteriosclerotic	Idiopathic	Drug/chemical induced	Adjunct to Levodopa/Carbidopa	Usual daily dose range (mg)
Anticholinergics						
Benztropine	✓	✓	✓	✓		0.5-6.5
Biperiden	✓	✓	✓	✓		2-8
Diphenhydramine	✓	✓	✓	✓		10-400
Ethopropazine	✓	✓	✓	✓		50-600
Trihexyphenidyl	✓	✓	✓	✓	✓	1-15
Dopaminergic Agents						
Amantadine	✓		✓	✓		200-400
Bromocriptine			✓			12.5-100
Carbidopa/Levodopa	✓		✓	✓[a]		10/100-200/2000
Levodopa	✓	✓	✓	✓[a]		500-8000
Pergolide					✓	1-5
Selegiline					✓	10

[a] Not effective in drug-induced extrapyramidal symptoms.

Anticholinergics

Indications

Refer to individual drug monographs for specific indications of individual agents.

➤*Parkinsonism:* Adjunctive therapy in all forms of parkinsonism (postencephalitic, arteriosclerotic, and idiopathic).

➤*Extrapyramidal disorders:* For the control of drug-induced extrapyramidal disorders.

Administration and Dosage

Dosage depends upon the age of the patient, etiology of the disease, and individual responsiveness. The dosage required for treatment of drug-induced extrapyramidal symptoms will depend on the severity of the side effects. Maintain flexible dosage to permit individualized dosing. In general, younger and postencephalitic patients require and tolerate somewhat higher doses than older patients and those with arteriosclerotic or idiopathic-type parkinsonism.

Give before or after meals, as determined by patient's reaction. Postencephalitic patients (more prone to excessive salivation) may prefer to take it after meals and may, in addition, require small amounts of atropine. If the mouth dries excessively, take before meals, unless it causes nausea. If taken after meals, thirst can be allayed by mint candies, chewing gum, or water.

Actions

➤*Pharmacology:* The anticholinergic agents, although generally less effective than levodopa, are useful in the treatment of all forms of parkinsonism: Postencephalitic, arteriosclerotic, idiopathic, and drug-induced extrapyramidal symptoms. They reduce the incidence and severity of akinesia, rigidity, and tremor by ≈ 20%; secondary symptoms such as drooling are also reduced. In addition to suppressing central cholinergic activity, these agents may also inhibit the reuptake and storage of dopamine at central dopamine receptors, thereby prolonging the action of dopamine.

The naturally occurring belladonna alkaloids (atropine, scopolamine, hyoscyamine) are active anticholinergic agents; however, they have largely been replaced by synthetic agents (eg, benztropine, trihexyphenidyl) with a more selective CNS activity. Peripheral anticholinergic side effects (eg, urinary retention, tachycardia, constipation) frequently limit the size of dosages utilized.

Antihistamines (eg, diphenhydramine) with central anticholinergic effects are also used; they may have a lower incidence of peripheral side effects than the belladonna alkaloids or synthetic derivatives. These agents are generally better tolerated by elderly patients. Some antihistamines provide mild antiparkinson effects, and are useful for initiating therapy in patients with minimal symptoms. Because of their sedative effects, the antihistamines may be useful in certain patients with insomnia.

In spite of limited efficacy, anticholinergics are useful in mild cases of Parkinson's disease where risks and demands of levodopa therapy are not warranted.

➤*Pharmacokinetics:* Little pharmacokinetic data are available for these agents. The following table lists some of the available parameters.

Various Antiparkinson Anticholinergic Pharmacokinetic Parameters				
Anticholinergic	Time to peak concentration (hrs)	Peak concentration (mcg/L)	Half-life (hrs)	Oral bioavailability (%)
Benztropine[a]				
Biperiden	1-1.5	4-5	18.4-24.3	29
Diphenhydramine	2-4	65-90	4-15	50-72
Trihexyphenidyl	1-1.3	87.2	5.6-10.2	≈ 100

[a] No data available.

Contraindications

Hypersensitivity to any component; glaucoma, particularly angle-closure glaucoma (simple type glaucomas do not appear to be adversely affected); pyloric or duodenal obstruction; stenosing peptic ulcers; prostatic hypertrophy or bladder neck obstructions; achalasia (megaesophagus); myasthenia gravis; megacolon.

➤*Benztropine:* Children < 3 years of age; use with caution in older children.

Warnings/Precautions

➤*Ophthalmic:* Incipient narrow-angle glaucoma may be precipitated by these drugs. Perform gonioscopy and closely monitor intraocular pressures at regular intervals.

➤*Concomitant conditions:* Use caution in patients with tachycardia, cardiac arrhythmias, hypertension, hypotension, prostatic hypertrophy (particularly in the elderly), or any tendency toward urinary retention, liver or kidney disorders, and obstructive disease of the GI or GU tract.

➤*CNS:* When used to treat extrapyramidal reactions resulting from phenothiazines in psychiatric patients, antiparkinson agents may exacerbate mental symptoms and precipitate a toxic psychosis. The possibility of antiparkinson agents masking the development of persistent extrapyramidal symptoms with prolonged phenothiazine therapy has not been investigated. Whether to administer prophylactic anticholinergics to prevent drug-induced extrapyramidal effects is controversial.

In addition, 19% to 30% of patients given anticholinergics develop depression, confusion, delusions, or hallucinations. Also, **benztropine** given in large doses or to susceptible patients may cause weakness and inability to move particular muscle groups. Dosage may have to be adjusted.

Tardive dyskinesia – Tardive dyskinesia may appear in some patients on long-term therapy with phenothiazines and related agents, or may occur after therapy has been discontinued. Antiparkinson agents do not alleviate the symptoms of tardive dyskinesia and, in some instances, may aggravate such symptoms.

➤*Heat illness:* Give with caution during hot weather, especially when given concomitantly with other atropine-like drugs to the elderly, the chronically ill, alcoholics, those who have CNS disease, and those who work in a hot environment. Anhidrosis may occur more readily when some disturbance of sweating already exists. Decrease dosage so that the ability to maintain body heat equilibrium by perspiration is not impaired. Severe anhidrosis and fatal hyperthermia have occurred.

➤*Dry mouth:* If dry mouth is so severe that there is difficulty in swallowing or speaking, or if loss of appetite and weight occurs, reduce dosage or discontinue the drug temporarily.

➤*Abuse potential:* Some patients may use these agents for mood elevations or psychedelic experiences. Cannabinoids, barbiturates, opiates, and alcohol may have additive effects with anticholinergics. It is important to be aware of this potential abuse situation.

➤*Hazardous tasks:* May impair mental or physical abilities; patients should observe caution while driving or performing other tasks requiring alertness.

➤*Pregnancy:* *Category C.* Safety for use during pregnancy has not been established. Use only when clearly needed and when the potential benefits outweigh the potential hazards to the fetus.

➤*Lactation:* Safety for use in the nursing mother has not been established. An inhibitory effect on lactation may occur. Although infants are particularly sensitive to anticholinergic agents, no adverse effects have been reported in nursing infants whose mothers were taking atropine.

➤*Children:* Safety and efficacy for use in children have not been established.

➤*Elderly:* Geriatric patients, particularly > 60 years of age, frequently develop increased sensitivity to anticholinergic drugs and require strict dosage regulation. Occasionally, mental confusion and disorientation may occur; agitation, hallucinations, and psychotic-like symptoms may develop.

Drug Interactions

Anticholinergic Drug Interactions

Precipitant drug	Object drug[a]		Description
Amantadine	Anticholinergics	⬆	Amantadine and anticholinergic coadministration may result in an increased incidence of anticholinergic side effects. These effects disappear when the anticholinergic dose is reduced.
Anticholinergics	Digoxin	⬆	Digoxin serum levels may be increased by anticholinergics when digoxin is administered as a slow dissolution oral tablet.
Anticholinergics	Haloperidol	⬇	Haloperidol and anticholinergic coadministration may result in worsening of schizophrenic symptoms, decreased haloperidol serum concentrations, and development of tardive dyskinesia.
Anticholinergics	Levodopa	⬇	Anticholinergics may decrease gastric motility resulting in increased gastric deactivation of levodopa and decreased intestinal absorption, possibly leading to a reduction in levodopa's efficacy. Other reports refute these findings.
Anticholinergics	Phenothiazines	⬇	The pharmacologic/therapeutic actions of phenothiazines may be reduced by concurrent anticholinergics. An increase in the incidence of anticholinergic side effects has occurred.
Phenothiazines	Anticholinergics	⬆	

[a] ⬆ = object drug increased; ⬇ = object drug decreased.

Adverse Reactions

➤*Cardiovascular:* Tachycardia; palpitations; hypotension; postural hypotension; mild bradycardia.

➤*CNS:* Disorientation; confusion; memory loss; hallucinations; psychoses; agitation; nervousness; delusions; delirium; paranoia; euphoria; excitement; lightheadedness; dizziness; headache; listlessness; depression; drowsiness; weakness; giddiness; paresthesia; heaviness of the limbs.

➤*GI:* Dry mouth; acute suppurative parotitis; nausea; vomiting; epigastric distress; constipation; dilation of the colon; paralytic ileus; development of duodenal ulcer.

➤*Hypersensitivity:* Skin rash; urticaria; other dermatoses.

➤*Musculoskeletal:* Muscular weakness; muscular cramping.

➤*Ophthalmic:* Blurred vision; mydriasis; diplopia; increased intraocular tension; angle-closure glaucoma; dilation of pupils.

➤*Renal:* Urinary retention; urinary hesitancy; dysuria.

➤*Miscellaneous:* Elevated temperature; flushing; numbness of fingers; decreased sweating, hyperthermia, heat stroke; difficulty in achieving or maintaining an erection.

Overdosage

➤*Symptoms:* Characterized by the adverse reactions and may also include the following: Circulatory collapse; cardiac arrest; respiratory depression or arrest; CNS depression preceded or followed by stimulation; intensification of mental symptoms or toxic psychosis in mentally ill patients treated with neuroleptic drugs (eg, phenothiazines); shock; coma; stupor; seizures; convulsions; ataxia; anxiety; incoherence; hyperactivity; combativeness; anhidrosis; hyperpyrexia; fever; hot, dry, flushed skin; dry mucous membranes; dysphagia; foul-smelling breath; decreased bowel sounds; dilated and sluggish pupils.

➤*Treatment:* Immediately following acute ingestion, remove remaining drug from stomach by inducing emesis or by gastric lavage (contraindicated in precomatose, convulsive or psychotic states). Activated charcoal is an effective adsorbent.

Treatment of overdosage is symptomatic. To relieve the peripheral effects, 5 mg of pilocarpine may be given orally at repeated intervals.

Artificial respiration and oxygen therapy may be needed for respiratory depression. A short-acting barbiturate or diazepam may be used for CNS excitement or convulsions; use with caution to avoid subsequent depression; institute supportive care for depression. Urinary retention may require catheterization. Hyperpyrexia is best treated with alcohol sponges, ice bags, or other cold applications. To counteract mydriasis and cycloplegia, a local miotic may be used. Darken room for photophobia. Treat circulatory collapse with fluids and vasopressors. The relapse intervals lengthen as the anticholinergic agent is metabolized; observe patient for 8 to 12 hours after last relapse.

Physostigmine salicylate reverses most cardiovascular and CNS effects of overdosage. In *adults*, 1 to 2 mg IM or IV given slowly (no more than 1 mg/min) is effective. In *children*, start with 0.02 mg/kg IM or by slow IV injection (no more than 0.5 mg/min). If necessary, repeat at 5- to 10-minute intervals until a therapeutic effect or a maximum dose of 2 mg is attained. Avoid rapid injection to reduce the possibility of physostigmine-induced convulsions. Give physostigmine cautiously. It can precipitate seizures, cholinergic crisis, bradyarrhythmias, and asystole. Use in a setting where advanced life support is available.

Patient Information

If GI upset occurs, may be taken with food.

May cause drowsiness, dizziness, or blurred vision; observe caution while driving or performing other tasks requiring alertness until response to drug is known.

Avoid alcohol and other CNS depressants.

May cause dry mouth; sucking hard candy, adequate fluid intake, or good oral hygiene may relieve this symptom. Difficult urination or constipation may occur; constipation may be relieved by use of stool softeners. Notify physician if effects persist.

Notify physician if rapid or pounding heartbeat, confusion, eye pain or rash occurs.

Use caution in hot weather. This medication may increase susceptibility to heat stroke.

BELLADONNA ALKALOIDS

Refer to the general discussion in the Antiparkinson Agents introduction. Prescribing information begins in the Antiparkinson Agent Anticholinergics group monograph. For complete prescribing information on the belladonna alkaloids (atropine, scopolamine HBr, hyoscyamine sulfate, and levorotatory alkaloids of belladonna) see the Gastrointestinal Anticholinergics/Antispasmodics monograph.

BENZTROPINE MESYLATE

Rx	**Benztropine Mesylate** (Various, eg, Harber, Moore, Par, Parmed)	**Tablets; oral:** 0.5 mg	In 100s and UD 100s.
Rx	**Cogentin** (MSD)		(MSD 21). White, scored. In 100s.
Rx	**Benztropine Mesylate** (Various, eg, Goldline, Moore, Purepac, Vangard)	**Tablets; oral:** 1 mg	In 100s, 1000s and UD 100s.
Rx	**Benztropine Mesylate** (Various, eg, Goldline, Moore, Purepac, Vangard)	**Tablets; oral:** 2 mg	In 100s, 1000s and UD 100s.
Rx	**Benztropine Mesylate** (West-Ward)	**Injection, solution:** 1 mg/mL	In 2 mL amps.
Rx	**Cogentin** (MSD)		In 2 ml amps.

BENZTROPINE MESYLATE — ORAL

Refer to the general discussion in the Antiparkinson Agents introduction. Complete and comparative prescribing information begins in the Antiparkinson Agent Anticholinergics group monograph.

Indications

➤*Extrapyramidal disorders:* Useful also in the control of extrapyramidal disorders (except tardive dyskinesia; antiparkinsonism agents do not alleviate the symptoms of tardive dyskinesia and, in some instances, may aggravate them. Benztropine is not recommended for use in patients with tardive dyskinesia.) due to neuroleptic drugs (eg, phenothiazines).

➤*Parkinsonism:* For use as an adjunct in the therapy of all forms of parkinsonism.

Administration and Dosage

➤*Adults:*

Drug-induced extrapyramidal disorders –

Usual dosage: 1 to 4 mg once or twice per day orally. Some patients require more than recommended; others do not need as much.

Acute dystonic reactions: 1 to 2 mg of the injection usually relieves the condition quickly. After that, the tablets, 1 to 2 mg twice per day, usually prevent recurrence.

BENZTROPINE MESYLATE — ORAL

Transient extrapyramidal disorders: 1 to 2 mg 2 or 3 times a day usually provides relief within 1 or 2 days. After 1 or 2 weeks, withdraw the drug to determine the continued need for it. If such disorders recur, benztropine can be reinstituted.

Parkinsonism –
Maximum dose: 6 mg/day.
Initial dosage:
• *Idiopathic parkinsonism* – 0.5 to 1 mg daily at bedtime. In some patients, this will be adequate; in others 4 to 6 mg per day may be required.
• *Postencephalitic parkinsonism* – 2 mg a day in 1 or more doses. In highly sensitive patients, therapy may be initiated with 0.5 mg at bedtime and increased as necessary.

Dosage titration: Initiate therapy with a low dose; increase gradually at 5- or 6-day intervals to the smallest amount necessary for optimal relief. Make increases in increments of 0.5 mg, to a maximum of 6 mg, or until optimal results are obtained without excessive adverse reactions.

Maintenance dosage: 1 to 2 mg daily, with a range of 0.5 to 6 mg. Some patients experience greatest relief by taking the entire dose at bedtime; others react more favorably to divided doses 2 to 4 times a day. Frequently, 1 dose per day is sufficient and divided doses may be unnecessary or undesirable.

Concomitant therapy with other antiparkinsonian agents: When benztropine is started, do not abruptly terminate therapy with other antiparkinsonian agents. If the other agents are to be reduced or discontinued, it must be done gradually. Many patients obtain greatest relief with combination therapy.

Concomitant therapy with levodopa: Benztropine may be used concomitantly with carbidopa-levodopa, or with levodopa, in which case periodic dosage adjustment may be required in order to maintain optimum response.

➤*Children:*
3 years of age and older – Because of its atropine-like side effects, use with caution in older children.

➤*Elderly:* Older patients cannot tolerate large doses. Geriatric patients, particularly older than 60 years of age, frequently develop increased sensitivity to anticholinergic drugs and require strict dosage regulation.

➤*Poor candidates for therapy / large doses:* Thin patients cannot tolerate large doses. Most patients with postencephalitic parkinsonism need fairly large doses and tolerate them well. Patients with a poor mental outlook are usually poor candidates for therapy.

➤*Administration:* Give before or after meals, as determined by patient's reaction. Postencephalitic patients (more prone to excessive salivation) may prefer to take it after meals and may, in addition, require small amounts of atropine. If the mouth dries excessively, take before meals unless it causes nausea. If taken after meals, thirst can be allayed by mint candies, chewing gum, or water.

➤*Storage / Stability:* Store at 15° to 30° C (59° to 86° F).

BENZTROPINE MESYLATE — INJECTION

Refer to the general discussion in the Antiparkinson Agents introduction. Complete and comparative prescribing information begins in the Antiparkinson Agent Anticholinergics group monograph.

Indications

➤*Parkinsonism:* This medication is indicated for use as an adjunct in the therapy of all forms of parkinsonism.

➤*Extrapyramidal disorders:* Benztropine mesylate injection is also useful in the control of extrapyramidal disorders (except tardive dyskinesia) due to neuroleptic drugs (eg, phenothiazines). Tardive dyskinesia may appear in some patients on long-term therapy with phenothiazines and related agents, or may occur after therapy with these drugs has been discontinued. Antiparkinsonism agents do not alleviate the symptoms of tardive dyskinesia, and in some instances may aggravate them. Benztropine mesylate is not recommended for use in patients with tardive dyskinesia.

Administration and Dosage

➤*Adults:*
Drug-induced extrapyramidal disorders –
Usual dosage: 1 to 4 mg once or twice a day.
Acute dystonic reactions: 1 to 2 mg.
Transient extrapyramidal disorders: 1 to 2 mg 2 or 3 times a day usually provides relief within 1 or 2 days. After 1 or 2 weeks, the drug should be withdrawn to determine the continued need for it. If such disorders recur, benztropine can be reinstituted.

Parkinsonism –
Maximum dose: 6 mg/day.
Initial dosage:
• *Idiopathic parkinsonism* – 0.5 to 1 mg at bedtime. In some patients, this will be adequate; in others, 4 to 6 mg a day may be required.
• *Postencephalitic parkinsonism* – 2 mg a day in 1 or more doses. In highly sensitive patients, therapy may be initiated with 0.5 mg at bedtime, and increased as necessary.

Dosage titration: Therapy should be initiated with a low dose which is increased gradually at 5- or 6-day intervals to the smallest amount necessary for optimal relief. Increases should be made in increments of 0.5 mg, to a maximum of 6 mg, or until optimal results are obtained without excessive adverse reactions.

Maintenance dosage: 1 to 2 mg daily, with a range of 0.5 to 6 mg. Some patients experience greatest relief when given the entire dose at bedtime; others react more favorably to divided doses, 2 to 4 times a day. Frequently, 1 dose a day is sufficient, and divided doses may be unnecessary or undesirable.

Concomitant therapy with other antiparkinsonian agents: When benztropine is started, do not terminate therapy with other antiparkinsonian agents abruptly. If the other agents are to be reduced or discontinued, it must be done gradually. Many patients obtain greatest relief with combination therapy.

Concomitant therapy with levodopa: Benztropine may be used concomitantly with carbidopa-levodopa, or with levodopa, in which case periodic dosage adjustment may be required in order to maintain optimum response.

➤*Children:*
3 years of age and older – Because of its atropine-like side effects, use with caution in children over 3 years of age.

➤*Elderly:* Older patients cannot tolerate large doses. Geriatric patients, particularly older than 60 years of age, frequently develop increased sensitivity to anticholinergic drugs and require strict dosage regulation.

➤*Emergency situations:* In emergency situations, when the condition of the patient is alarming, 1 to 2 mg will provide quick relief. If the parkinsonian effect begins to return, the dose can be repeated.

➤*Poor candidates for therapy / large doses:* Thin patients cannot tolerate large doses. Most patients with postencephalitic parkinsonism need fairly large doses and tolerate them well. Patients with a poor mental outlook are usually poor candidates for therapy.

➤*Administration:* Since there is no significant difference in onset of effect after IV or IM injection, usually there is no need to use the IV route. The drug is quickly effective after either route, with improvement sometimes noticeable a few minutes after injection.

➤*Storage / Stability:* Store in a dry place.

DIPHENHYDRAMINE

For complete prescribing information and product availability, see the Diphenhydramine monograph in the Antihistamines section and the Antihistamines group monograph. Also refer to the general discussion in the Antiparkinson Agents introduction and the Antiparkinson Agent Anticholinergics group monograph.

TRIHEXYPHENIDYL HYDROCHLORIDE

Rx	**Trihexyphenidyl Hydrochloride** (Various, eg, Balan, Bolar, Danbury, Moore, Raway, Schein)	**Tablets:** 2 mg	In 30s, 100s, 250s, 1000s and UD 100s.
Rx	**Trihexy-2** (Geneva)		White. In 100s and 1000s.
Rx	**Trihexyphenidyl Hydrochloride** (Various, eg, Balan, Bolar, Danbury, Lannett, Moore, Schein)	**Tablets:** 5 mg	In 100s, 250s, 1000s and UD 100s.
Rx	**Trihexy-5** (Geneva)		White. In 100s and 1000s.
Rx	**Trihexyphenidyl Hydrochloride** (Versapharm)	**Elixir:** 2 mg per 5 mL	5% alcohol, parabens, sorbitol. Lime-peppermint flavor. In 473 mL.

TRIHEXYPHENIDYL HYDROCHLORIDE — ORAL

Refer to the general discussion in the Antiparkinson Agents introduction. Complete prescribing information begins in the Antiparkinson Agents Anticholinergics group monograph.

Indications

➤*Parkinsonism:* Trihexyphenidyl HCl is indicated as an adjunct in the treatment of all forms of parkinsonism (postencephalitic, arteriosclerotic, and idiopathic). It is often useful as adjuvant therapy when treating these forms of parkinsonism with levodopa.

➤*Extrapyramidal disorders:* It is indicated for the control of extrapyramidal disorders caused by central nervous system drugs such as the dibenzoxazepines, phenothiazines, thioxanthenes, and butyrophenones.

Administration and Dosage

➤*General dosing considerations:* The size and frequency of the dose of trihexyphenidyl needed to control extrapyramidal reactions to commonly employed tranquilizers, notably the phenothiazines, thioxanthenes, and butyrophenones, must be determined empirically.

Trihexyphenidyl may be substituted, in whole or in part, for other parasympathetic inhibitors. The usual technique is partial substitution initially, with progressive reduction in the other medication as the dose of trihexyphenidyl is increased.

➤*Adults:*

Drug-induced parkinsonism –

Usual dosage: The total daily dosage usually ranges between 5 and 15 mg, although, in some cases, these reactions have been satisfactorily controlled on as little as 1 mg daily.

Initial dosage: The initial dose should be low and then increased gradually. It may be advisable to commence therapy with a single 1 mg dose.

Dosage titration: If the extrapyramidal manifestations are not controlled in a few hours, the subsequent doses may be progressively increased until satisfactory control is achieved. Satisfactory control may sometimes be more rapidly achieved by temporarily reducing the dosage of the tranquilizer on instituting trihexyphenidyl therapy and then adjusting dosage of both drugs until the desired ataractic effect is retained without onset of extrapyramidal reactions.

Maintenance dosage: It is sometimes possible to maintain the patient on a reduced trihexyphenidyl dosage after the reactions have remained under control for several days. Instances have been reported in which these reactions have remained in remission for long periods after trihexyphenidyl therapy was discontinued.

Idiopathic parkinsonism –

Initial dosage: The initial dose should be low and then increased gradually. As initial therapy, trihexyphenidyl 1 mg may be administered the first day.

Dosage titration: The dose may then be increased by 2 mg increments at intervals of 3 to 5 days, until a total of 6 to 10 mg is given daily.

Maintenance dosage: The total daily dose will depend upon what is found to be the optimal level. Many patients derive maximum benefit from this daily total of 6 to 10 mg, but some patients, chiefly those in the postencephalitic group, may require a total daily dose of 12 to 15 mg.

➤*Elderly:* The initial dose should be low and then increased gradually, especially in patients older than 60 years of age. Elderly patients, particularly older than 60 years of age, frequently develop increased sensitivity to the actions of drugs of this type, and, hence, require strict dosage regulation. Incipient glaucoma may be precipitated.

➤*Concomitant therapy with levodopa:* When trihexyphenidyl is used concomitantly with levodopa, the usual dose of each may need to be reduced. Careful adjustment is necessary, depending on adverse reactions and degree of symptom control. Trihexyphenidyl dosage of 3 to 6 mg daily, in divided doses, is usually adequate.

➤*Administration:* The total daily intake of trihexyphenidyl is tolerated best if divided into 3 doses and taken at mealtimes. High doses (more than 10 mg daily) may be divided into 4 parts, with 3 doses administered at mealtimes and the fourth at bedtime.

Whether trihexyphenidyl may best be given before or after meals should be determined by the way the patient reacts. Postencephalitic patients, who are usually more prone to excessive salivation, may prefer to take it after meals and may, in addition, require small amounts of atropine which, under such circumstances, is sometimes an effective adjuvant. If trihexyphenidyl tends to dry the mouth excessively, it may be better to take it before meals, unless it causes nausea. If taken after meals, the thirst sometimes induced can be allayed by mint candies, chewing gum, or water.

➤*Storage / Stability:* Store at 15° to 30°C (59° to 86°F). Do not freeze.

ANTIPARKINSON AGENTS

AMANTADINE HYDROCHLORIDE

For complete prescribing information, refer to the Amantadine HCl monograph in the Antiviral Agents section.

BROMOCRIPTINE MESYLATE

Rx	**Cycloset** (Santarus)	**Tablets; oral:** 0.8 mg	As bromocriptine mesylate. Lactose. (C 9). White, round. In 200s and 600s.
Rx	**Bromocriptine Mesylate** (Various, eg, Mylan, Paddock, Sandoz)	**Tablets; oral:** 2.5 mg	As bromocriptine mesylate. May contain lactose and edetate disodium. In 30s and 100s.
Rx	**Parlodel SnapTabs** (Novartis)		As bromocriptine mesylate. Lactose. (Parlodel 2½). Off-white, scored. In 30s and 100s.
Rx	**Bromocriptine Mesylate** (Various, eg, Mylan, Sandoz, Zydus)	**Capsules; oral:** 5 mg	As bromocriptine mesylate. May contain lactose. In 30s and 100s.
Rx	**Parlodel** (Novartis)		As bromocriptine mesylate. Lactose. (Parlodel 5 mg). Caramel/White. In 30s and 100s.

BROMOCRIPTINE MESYLATE — ORAL

Also refer to the general discussion in the Antiparkinson Agents introduction.

Indications

➤*Acromegaly (except Cycloset)*: For the treatment of acromegaly.

➤*Hyperprolactinemia (except Cycloset)*: For the treatment of dysfunctions associated with hyperprolactinemia including amenorrhea with or without galactorrhea, infertility, or hypogonadism; in patients with prolactin-secreting adenomas, which may be the basic underlying endocrinopathy contributing to the above clinical presentations. Reduction in tumor size has been demonstrated in both men and women with macroadenomas. In cases in which adenectomy is elected, a course of bromocriptine may be used to reduce the tumor mass prior to surgery.

➤*Parkinson disease (except Cycloset)*: In the treatment of the signs and symptoms of idiopathic or postencephalitic Parkinson disease; as adjunctive treatment to levodopa (alone or with a peripheral decarboxylase inhibitor).

Bromocriptine may provide additional therapeutic benefits in those patients who are currently maintained on optimal dosages of levodopa, those who are beginning to deteriorate (develop tolerance) to levodopa therapy, and those who are experiencing "end-of-dose failure" on levodopa. Bromocriptine may permit a reduction of the maintenance dose of levodopa and, thus, may ameliorate the occurrence and/or severity of adverse reactions associated with long-term levodopa, such as abnormal involuntary movements (eg, dyskinesias) and the marked swings in motor function ("on-off" phenomenon).

➤*Type 2 diabetes mellitus (Cycloset only)*: As an adjunct to diet and exercise to improve glycemic control in adults with type 2 diabetes mellitus.

➤*Off-label uses:*

Hepatic encephalopathy – [4] = Insufficient documentation. Despite the recommendation by American College of Gastroenterology guidelines to use bromocriptine in the treatment of hepatic encephalopathy, the effectiveness for this context is not supported by the clinical trial referenced in the guidelines. There are other reports of effectiveness, but overall results are mixed.

Restless legs syndrome – [5] = Poor documentation. The use of bromocriptine for the treatment of restless legs syndrome (RLS) has been limited to fewer than 10 patients in one controlled trial. Although this study suggested some benefit in the management of RLS, the end points were not clearly defined. This drug is not recommended for the treatment of RLS until there is further favorable evidence.

Traumatic brain injury – [1] = Good documentation. The Neurobehavioral Guidelines Working Group assigned different levels to their recommendations for drug therapy of neurobehavioral sequelae of traumatic brain injury. They ranged from "options" to "guidelines" to the highest level of "standards," based on the quality of evidence available and the extent of efficacy observed. Bromocriptine was considered a guideline level recommendation. The authors also noted that bromocriptine was the only drug with evidence of efficacy in improving executive dysfunction.

Administration and Dosage

➤*Adults:*

Acromegaly (except Cycloset) –

Usual dosage: 20 to 30 mg/day.

Maximum dose: 100 mg/day.

Initial dosage: One-half to one 2.5 mg tablet at bedtime (with food) for 3 days.

BROMOCRIPTINE MESYLATE — ORAL

Dosage titration: An additional one-half to 1 tablet should be added to the treatment regimen as tolerated every 3 to 7 days until the patient obtains optimal therapeutic benefit. Patients should be reevaluated monthly, and the dosage should be adjusted based on reductions of growth hormone or clinical response.

Pituitary irradiation: Patients treated with pituitary irradiation should be withdrawn from bromocriptine on a yearly basis to assess both the clinical effects of radiation on the disease process as well as the effects of bromocriptine. Usually a 4- to 8-week withdrawal period is adequate for this purpose. Recurrence of the signs/symptoms or increases in growth hormone indicate the disease process is still active and further courses of bromocriptine should be considered.

Hyperprolactinemia (except Cycloset) –

Initial dosage: One-half to one 2.5 mg tablet daily.

Dosage titration: An additional 2.5 mg tablet may be added to the treatment regimen as tolerated every 2 to 7 days until an optimal therapeutic response is achieved. The therapeutic dosage ranged from 2.5 to 15 mg daily in adults studied clinically.

Parkinson disease (except Cycloset) –

Initial dosage: One-half of a 2.5 mg tablet twice daily with meals. The dosage of levodopa during this introductory period should be maintained, if possible.

Dosage titration: Dosage may be increased every 14 to 28 days by 2.5 mg/day with meals, if necessary. Assessments are advised at 2-week intervals during dosage titration to ensure that the lowest dosage producing an optimal therapeutic response is not exceeded.

Concomitant therapy with levodopa: Should it be advisable to reduce the dosage of levodopa because of adverse reactions, the daily dosage of bromocriptine, if increased, should be accomplished gradually in small (2.5 mg) increments.

Type 2 diabetes mellitus (Cycloset only) –

Usual dosage: 1.6 to 4.8 mg once daily within 2 hours after waking in the morning.

Maximum dose: 4.8 mg (6 tablets) daily.

Initial dosage: 0.8 mg orally once daily initially administered within 2 hours after waking in the morning.

Dosage titration: Increase by one tablet per week until a maximum daily dose of 6 tablets (4.8 mg) or until the maximal tolerated number of tablets between 2 and 6 per day is reached.

Off-label dosing –

Hepatic encephalopathy: [4] = Insufficient documentation. 30 mg twice daily.

Traumatic brain injury: [1] = Good documentation. 2.5 mg/day, continued long-term if response is adequate.

➤*Children:*

Hyperprolactinemia (except Cycloset) –

16 years of age and older: See Adults for dosing.

11 to 15 years of age:

• *Initial dosage* – Based on limited data, the initial dosage is one-half to one 2.5 mg tablet daily.

• *Dosage titration* – Dosing may need to be increased as tolerated until a therapeutic response is achieved. The therapeutic dosage ranged from 2.5 to 10 mg daily in children with prolactin-secreting pituitary adenomas.

➤*Administration:* It is recommended that bromocriptine be taken with food to potentially reduce GI side effects such as nausea.

➤*Storage/Stability:* Store at or below 25°C (77°F) in a tight, light-resistant container.

Actions

➤*Pharmacology:* Bromocriptine is a dopamine receptor agonist, which activates postsynaptic dopamine receptors. The dopaminergic neurons in the tuberoinfundibular process modulate the secretion of prolactin from the anterior pituitary by secreting a prolactin inhibitory factor (thought to be dopamine); in the corpus striatum the dopaminergic neurons are involved in the control of motor function. Clinically, bromocriptine significantly reduces plasma levels of prolactin in patients with physiologically elevated prolactin as well as in patients with hyperprolactinemia. The inhibition of physiological lactation as well as galactorrhea in pathological hyperprolactinemic states is obtained at dose levels that do not affect secretion of other tropic hormones from the anterior pituitary. Experiments have demonstrated that bromocriptine induces long-lasting stereotyped behavior in rodents and turning behavior in rats having unilateral lesions in the substantia nigra. These actions, characteristic of those produced by dopamine, are inhibited by dopamine antagonists and suggest a direct action of bromocriptine on striatal dopamine receptors.

Bromocriptine is a nonhormonal, nonestrogenic agent that inhibits the secretion of prolactin in humans, with little or no effect on other pituitary hormones, except in patients with acromegaly, in which it lowers elevated blood levels of growth hormone in the majority of patients.

In about 75% of cases of amenorrhea and galactorrhea, bromocriptine mesylate therapy suppresses the galactorrhea completely, or almost completely, and reinitiates normal ovulatory menstrual cycles.

Menses are usually reinitiated prior to complete suppression of galactorrhea; the time for this on average is 6 to 8 weeks. However, some patients respond within a few days, and others may take up to 8 months.

Galactorrhea may take longer to control depending on the degree of stimulation of the mammary tissue prior to therapy. At least a 75% reduction in secretion is usually observed after 8 to 12 weeks. Some patients may fail to respond even after 12 months of therapy.

In many acromegalic patients, bromocriptine mesylate produces a prompt and sustained reduction in circulating levels of serum growth hormone.

Bromocriptine mesylate produces its therapeutic effect in the treatment of Parkinson disease, a clinical condition characterized by a progressive deficiency in dopamine synthesis in the substantia nigra, by directly stimulating the dopamine receptors in the corpus striatum. In contrast, levodopa exerts its therapeutic effect only after conversion to dopamine by the neurons of the substantia nigra, which are known to be numerically diminished in this patient population.

Cycloset – The mechanism by which bromocriptine improves glycemic control is unknown. Morning administration of bromocriptine improves glycemic control in patients with type 2 diabetes without increasing plasma insulin concentrations.

Once daily morning administration of bromocriptine to humans increases circulating levels of bromocriptine, a dopamine receptor agonist, for 4 to 5 hours after administration.

Pharmacodynamics –

Postprandial glucose and insulin response to a meal: Patients with type 2 diabetes and inadequate glycemic control on diet alone were randomized to bromocriptine or placebo in a 24-week monotherapy clinical trial. At baseline and study end, plasma samples for insulin and glucose were obtained 1 hour before and 2 hours after standardized meals for breakfast, lunch, and dinner. In this trial, once daily (8 AM) bromocriptine improved post-prandial glucose without increasing plasma insulin concentrations.

➤*Pharmacokinetics:*

Absorption/Distribution – Twenty-eight percent of an oral dose was absorbed from the GI tract. The blood levels following a 2.5 mg dose were in the range of 2 to 3 ng equivalents/mL. Plasma levels were in the range of 4 to 6 ng equivalents/mL, indicating that the red blood cells did not contain appreciable amounts of drug or metabolites. In vitro experiments showed that the drug was 90% to 96% bound to plasma proteins, primarily albumin.

When tablets or standard capsules are administered to healthy volunteers, the absorption half-life is 0.2 to 0.5 hours, and the peak plasma levels of bromocriptine are reached within 1 to 3 hours. An oral dose of 5 mg of bromocriptine results in a maximum plasma concentration (C_{max}) of 0.465 ng/mL. The prolactin-lowering effect begins within 1 to 2 hours of ingestion, reaches its maximum (ie, a reduction of prolactin in the plasma by more than 80%) within 5 to 10 hours and remains close to maximum for 8 to 12 hours.

When *Cycloset* is administered orally, approximately 65% to 95% of the dose is absorbed. Because of extensive hepatic extraction and first-pass metabolism, approximately 7% of the dose reaches the systemic circulation. Under fasting conditions, the time to C_{max} (T_{max}) is 53 minutes.

The volume of distribution is approximately 61 L.

Effect of food: Following a standard high-fat meal, the time to maximum plasma T_{max} increased to approximately 90 to 120 minutes. Also, the relative bioavailability of bromocriptine mesylate is increased under fed as compared with fasting conditions by an average of approximately 55% to 65% (increase in area under the curve $[AUC]_{\infty}$).

Metabolism/Excretion – Bromocriptine undergoes extensive first-pass biotransformation in the liver, reflected by complex metabolite profiles and by almost complete absence of parent drug in urine and feces. It shows a high affinity for CYP3A and hydroxylations at the proline ring of the cyclopeptide moiety constitute a main metabolic pathway. Therefore, inhibitors and/or potent substrates for CYP3A4 might be expected to inhibit the clearance of bromocriptine and lead to increased levels. Bromocriptine is also a potent inhibitor of CYP3A4 with a calculated concentration that inhibits 50% (IC_{50}) value of 1.69 mcM. However, given the low therapeutic concentrations of free bromocriptine in patients, a significant alteration of the metabolism of a second drug whose clearance is medicated by CYP3A4 should not be expected.

The elimination of the parent drug from plasma is biphasic, with a terminal half-life of about 15 hours (range, 8 to 20 hours). Parent drug and metabolites are almost completely excreted via the liver and only 6% eliminated via the kidney.

Cycloset: Bromocriptine is extensively metabolized in the GI tract and liver. Metabolism by CYP3A4 is the major metabolic pathway. Most of the absorbed dose (approximately 93%) undergoes first-pass metabolism. The remaining 7% reaches the systemic circulation.

The major route of excretion of bromocriptine is in the bile with the remaining approximately 2% to 6% of an oral dose excreted via the urine. The elimination half-life is approximately 6 hours. Prior consumption of a standard high-fat meal has little to no effect on the elimination half-life of bromocriptine.

Special populations –

Renal function impairment: Safety and efficacy of bromocriptine have not been established in patients with renal impairment. Use caution in patients with renal impairment.

Hepatic function impairment: Safety and efficacy of bromocriptine have not been established in patients with hepatic impairment. In patients with hepatic impairment, the speed of elimination may be retarded and plasma levels may increase requiring dose adjustments. Because bromocriptine is predominantly metabolized by the liver, use caution in patients with hepatic impairment.

Elderly: No pharmacokinetic studies have been conducted in elderly patients.

Children: Studies characterizing the pharmacokinetics of bromocriptine in children have not been performed.

Gender: The plasma exposure of bromocriptine is increased 18% to 30% in women compared with men.

Race: Studies characterizing the pharmacokinetics of bromocriptine among different ethnic groups have not been performed.

BROMOCRIPTINE MESYLATE — ORAL

Contraindications

Hypersensitivity to bromocriptine or any component of the product; hypersensitivity to ergot alkaloids or ergot-related drugs; women who are breastfeeding, may inhibit lactation and potential for increased risk of stroke.

➤*Parlodel*: Uncontrolled hypertension; pregnancy (risk to benefit evaluation must be performed in women who become pregnant during treatment for acromegaly, prolactinoma, or Parkinson disease; hypertension during treatment should generally result in efforts to withdraw); postpartum period in women with a history of coronary artery disease or severe cardiovascular conditions unless withdrawal is medically contraindicated.

➤*Cycloset*: Syncopal migraine because of increased risk of hypotensive episodes.

Warnings/Precautions

➤*Pituitary tumors:* Because hyperprolactinemia with amenorrhea/galactorrhea and infertility has been found in patients with pituitary tumors, a complete evaluation of the pituitary is indicated before treatment with bromocriptine.

➤*Cardiovascular effects:* Symptomatic hypotension can occur in patients treated with bromocriptine for any indication. In postpartum studies with bromocriptine, decreases in supine systolic and diastolic pressures of greater than 20 mm Hg and 10 mm Hg, respectively, have been observed in almost 30% of patients receiving bromocriptine. On occasion, the drop in supine systolic pressure was as much as 50 to 59 mm Hg. While hypotension during the start of therapy with bromocriptine occurs in some patients, in postmarketing experience in postpartum patients 89 cases of hypertension have been reported, sometimes at the initiation of therapy, but often developing in the second week of therapy; seizures have been reported in 72 cases (including 4 cases of status epilepticus), both with and without the prior development of hypertension; 30 cases of stroke have been reported mostly in postpartum patients whose prenatal and obstetric courses had been uncomplicated. Many of these patients experiencing seizures and/or strokes reported developing a constant and often progressively severe headache hours to days prior to the acute event. Some cases of strokes and seizures were also preceded by visual disturbances (blurred vision and transient cortical blindness). Nine cases of acute myocardial infarction have been reported.

Although a causal relationship between bromocriptine administration and hypertension, seizures, strokes, and myocardial infarction in postpartum women has not been established, use of the drug for prevention of physiological lactation or in patients with uncontrolled hypertension is not recommended. Withdraw bromocriptine when pregnancy is diagnosed in patients being treated for hyperprolactinemia. In the event that bromocriptine is reinstituted to control a rapidly expanding macroadenoma and a patient experiences a hypertensive disorder of pregnancy, weigh the benefit of continuing bromocriptine against the possible risk of its use during a hypertensive disorder of pregnancy. When bromocriptine is being used to treat acromegaly or Parkinson disease in patients who subsequently become pregnant, decide whether the therapy continues to be medically necessary or can be withdrawn. If it is continued, withdraw the drug in those who may experience hypertensive disorders of pregnancy (including eclampsia, preeclampsia, or pregnancy-induced hypertension) unless withdrawal of bromocriptine is considered to be medically contraindicated. Because of the possibility of an interaction between bromocriptine and other ergot alkaloids, the concomitant use of these medications is not recommended. Pay particular attention to patients who have recently been treated or are on concomitant therapy with drugs that can alter the blood pressure. Their concomitant use in the puerperium is not recommended.

Hypotension, including orthostatic hypotension, can occur particularly upon initiation of bromocriptine therapy and with dose escalation. In a 52-week, randomized clinical trial of 3,070 patients, hypotension was reported in 2.2% of patients randomized to bromocriptine compared with 0.8% of patients randomized to placebo. Among bromocriptine-treated patients reporting symptomatic hypotension, 98% were on at least one blood pressure medication compared with 73% on such medication in the total study population. In this trial, 6 bromocriptine-treated patients (0.3%) reported an adverse reaction of orthostatic hypotension compared with 2 (0.2%) placebo-treated patients. All 6 patients were taking antihypertensive medications. Hypotension can result in syncope. In this trial, syncope because of any cause was reported in 1.6% of bromocriptine-treated patients and 0.7% of placebo-treated patients. As a precaution, assessment of orthostatic vital signs is recommended prior to initiation of bromocriptine and periodically thereafter. During early treatment with bromocriptine, advise patients to make slow postural changes and to avoid situations that could lead to serious injury if syncope was to occur. Use caution in patients taking antihypertensive medications.

Periodic monitoring of the blood pressure, particularly during the first weeks of therapy is prudent. If hypertension, severe, progressive, or unremitting headache (with or without visual disturbance), or evidence of CNS toxicity develops, discontinue drug therapy and promptly evaluate the patient.

Pulmonary effects – Among patients on bromocriptine, particularly on long-term and high-dose treatment, pleural and pericardial effusions, as well as pleural and pulmonary fibrosis and constrictive pericarditis, have occasionally been reported. Examine patients with unexplained pleuropulmonary disorders thoroughly and consider discontinuing bromocriptine therapy. In those instances in which bromocriptine was terminated, the changes slowly reverted toward normal.

Macrovascular outcomes – There have been no clinical studies establishing conclusive evidence of macrovascular risk reduction with bromocriptine or any other antidiabetic drug. In a 52-week, randomized clinical trial, bromocriptine use was not associated with an increased risk for adverse cardiovascular reactions.

➤*CNS effects:*

Psychotic disorders – In patients with severe psychotic disorders, treatment with a dopamine receptor agonist such as bromocriptine may exacerbate the disorder or may diminish the effectiveness of drugs used to treat the disorder. Therefore, the use of bromocriptine in patients with severe psychotic disorders is not recommended.

Somnolence – Bromocriptine has been associated with somnolence, and episodes of sudden sleep onset, particularly in patients with Parkinson disease. Sudden onset of sleep during daily activities, in some cases without awareness or warning signs, has been reported very rarely. None of these reactions were reported as serious and the majority of patients reported resolution of somnolence over time. Make patients aware of this potential side effect, particularly when initiating therapy with bromocriptine. Advise patients experiencing somnolence to refrain from driving or operating heavy machinery. Furthermore, consider a reduction of dosage or termination of therapy.

Mental disturbances – High doses of bromocriptine mesylate may be associated with confusion and mental disturbances. Because parkinsonian patients may manifest mild degrees of dementia, use caution when treating such patients.

Hallucinations – Bromocriptine administered alone or concomitantly with levodopa may cause hallucinations (visual or auditory). Hallucinations usually resolve with dosage reduction; occasionally, discontinuation of bromocriptine is required. Rarely, after high doses, hallucinations have persisted for several weeks following discontinuation of bromocriptine.

➤*Ophthalmic effects:* Visual field impairment is a known complication of macroprolactinoma. Effective treatment with bromocriptine leads to a reduction in hyperprolactinaemia and often to a resolution of the visual impairment. In some patients, however, a secondary deterioration of visual fields may subsequently develop despite normalized prolactin levels and tumor shrinkage, which may result from traction on the optic chiasm which is pulled down into the now partially empty sella. In these cases, the visual field defect may improve on reduction of bromocriptine dosage while there is some elevation of prolactin and some tumor re-expansion. Monitoring of visual fields in patients with macroprolactinoma is therefore recommended for an early recognition of secondary field loss caused by chiasmal herniation and adaptation of drug dosage.

The relative efficacy of bromocriptine versus surgery in preserving visual fields is not known. Patients with rapidly progressive visual field loss should be evaluated by a neurosurgeon to help decide on the most appropriate therapy.

➤*Cold-sensitive digital vasospasm:* Cold-sensitive digital vasospasm has been observed in some acromegalic patients treated with bromocriptine. The response, should it occur, can be reversed by reducing the dose of bromocriptine and may be prevented by keeping the fingers warm.

➤*Tumor expansion:* Possible tumor expansion while receiving bromocriptine therapy has been reported in a few acromegaly patients. Because the natural history of growth hormone secreting tumors is unknown, carefully monitor all patients and if evidence of tumor expansion develops, consider discontinuation of treatment and alternative procedures.

➤*GI effects:* Cases of severe GI bleeding from peptic ulcers have been reported, some fatal. Although there is no evidence that bromocriptine increases the incidence of peptic ulcers in acromegalic patients, investigate symptoms suggestive of peptic ulcer thoroughly and treat appropriately. Observe patients with a history of peptic ulcer or GI bleeding carefully during treatment with bromocriptine.

➤*Parkinson disease:* Safety during long-term use for more than 2 years at the doses required for parkinsonism has not been established.

➤*Syncopal migraine:* Bromocriptine is contraindicated in patients with syncopal migraine. In these patients, bromocriptine increases the likelihood of a hypotensive episode. Loss of consciousness during a migraine may reflect dopamine receptor hypersensitivity. Because bromocriptine is a dopamine receptor agonist, it may therefore potentiate the risk for syncope.

➤*Fibrotic-related complicated:* Retroperitoneal fibrosis has been reported in a few patients receiving long-term therapy (2 to 10 years) with bromocriptine in dosages ranging from 30 to 140 mg daily. To ensure recognition of retroperitoneal fibrosis at an early reversible stage, it is recommended to watch its manifestations (eg, back pain, edema of the lower limbs, impaired kidney function) in this category of patients. Withdraw bromocriptine if fibrotic changes in the retroperitoneum are diagnosed or suspected.

➤*Galactose intolerance/Malabsorption:* Advise patients with rare hereditary problems of galactose intolerance, the severe lactase deficiency or glucose-galactose malabsorption to not take this medicine.

➤*Cerebrospinal fluid rhinorrhea:* In some patients with prolactin-secreting adenomas treated with bromocriptine, cerebrospinal fluid rhinorrhea has been observed. The data available suggest that this may result from shrinkage of invasive tumors.

➤*Special risk:* Safety and efficacy of bromocriptine have not been established in patients with renal or hepatic disease. Exercise care when administering bromocriptine therapy concomitantly with other medications known to lower blood pressure.

BROMOCRIPTINE MESYLATE — ORAL

Use the drug with caution in patients with a history of psychosis or cardiovascular disease. If acromegalic patients or patients with prolactinoma or Parkinson disease are being treated with bromocriptine during pregnancy, cautiously observe them, particularly during the postpartum period if they have a history of cardiovascular disease.

As with levodopa, exercise caution when administering bromocriptine to patients with a history of myocardial infarction who have a residual atrial, nodal, or ventricular arrhythmia.

➤*Hazardous tasks:* Because hypotensive reactions may occasionally occur and result in reduced alertness especially during the first days of treatment, exercise particular care when driving a vehicle or operating machinery.

➤*Pregnancy: Category B.* Studies in pregnant women have not shown that bromocriptine increases the risk of abnormalities when administered during pregnancy.

Because the studies in humans cannot rule out the possibility of harm, use bromocriptine during pregnancy only if clearly needed.

A review of 4 different multi-center surveillance programs analyzed 2,351 pregnancies of 2,185 women treated with bromocriptine. In 583 children born of these women and followed for a minimum of 3 to 12 months, there was no suggestion of any adverse effect of intrauterine exposure to bromocriptine on postnatal development. Most (at least 75%) women had taken bromocriptine for 2 to 8 weeks and at 5 to 10 mg per day. Among 86 women having 93 pregnancies and treated with bromocriptine throughout pregnancy or from week 30 of pregnancy onwards (mostly for treatment of prolactinoma), there was only 1 spontaneous abortion. Similar results have been obtained in a Japanese hospital survey of 442 children born to 434 patients treated with bromocriptine during pregnancy and followed for at least 1 year.

If pregnancy occurs during bromocriptine administration, careful observation of these patients is mandatory. Prolactin-secreting adenomas may expand and compression of the optic or other cranial nerves may occur, emergency pituitary surgery becoming necessary. In most cases, the compression resolves following delivery. Reinitiation of bromocriptine treatment has been reported to produce improvement in the visual fields of patients in whom nerve compression has occurred during pregnancy. The safety of bromocriptine treatment during pregnancy to the mother and fetus has not been established.

Because pregnancy is often the therapeutic objective in many hyperprolactinemic patients presenting with amenorrhea/galactorrhea and hypogonadism (infertility), a careful assessment of the pituitary is essential to detect the presence of a prolactin-secreting adenoma. Patients not seeking pregnancy, or those harboring large adenomas, should be advised to use contraceptive measures, other than oral contraceptives, during treatment with bromocriptine.

Because pregnancy may occur prior to reinitiation of menses, a pregnancy test is recommended at least every 4 weeks during the amenorrheic period, and, once menses are reinitiated, every time a patient misses a menstrual period. Discontinue treatment with bromocriptine as soon as pregnancy has been established. Closely monitor patients closely throughout pregnancy for signs and symptoms that may signal the enlargement of a previously undetected or existing prolactin-secreting tumor. Discontinuation of bromocriptine treatment in patients with known macroadenomas has been associated with rapid regrowth of tumor and increase in serum prolactin in most cases.

Information concerning 1,276 pregnancies in women taking bromocriptine has been collected. In the majority of cases, bromocriptine was discontinued within 8 weeks into pregnancy (mean, 28.7 days); however, 8 patients received the drug continuously throughout pregnancy. The mean daily dose for all patients was 5.8 mg (range, 1 to 40 mg).

Of these 1,276 pregnancies, there were 1,088 full-term deliveries (4 stillborn), 145 spontaneous abortions (11.4%), and 28 induced abortions (2.2%). Moreover, 12 extrauterine gravidities and 3 hydatidiform moles (twice in the same patient) caused early termination of pregnancy. These data compare favorably with the abortion rate (11% to 25%) cited for pregnancies induced by clomiphene, menopausal gonadotropin, and chorionic gonadotropin.

Although spontaneous abortions often go unreported, especially prior to 20 weeks of gestation, their frequency has been estimated to be 10% to 15%.

Pregnancy prevention – In order to reduce the likelihood of prolonged exposure to bromocriptine if an unsuspected pregnancy occurs, a mechanical contraceptive should be used in conjunction with bromocriptine until normal ovulatory menstrual cycles have been restored. Contraception may then be discontinued in patients desiring pregnancy. Thereafter, if menstruation does not occur within 3 days of the expected date, bromocriptine should be discontinued and a pregnancy test should be performed.

➤*Lactation:* Bromocriptine is contraindicated in women who are breastfeeding their children because bromocriptine inhibits lactation. The indication for use of bromocriptine for inhibition of postpartum lactation was withdrawn based on postmarketing reports of stroke in this setting; therefore, do not use bromocriptine during lactation in postpartum women.

➤*Children:* The safety and effectiveness of bromocriptine for the treatment of prolactin-secreting pituitary adenomas have been established in patients age 16 years of age and older. No data are available for bromocriptine use in children younger than 8 years of age. A single 8-year-old patient treated with bromocriptine for prolactin-secreting pituitary macroadenoma has been reported without therapeutic response.

The use of bromocriptine for the treatment of prolactin-secreting adenomas in children in the age group 11 to younger than 16 years is supported by evidence from well-controlled trials in adults, with additional data in a limited number (n = 14) of children and adolescents 11 to 15 years of age with prolactin-secreting pituitary macro- and microadenomas who have been treated with bromocriptine. Of the 14 reported patients, 9 had successful outcomes, 3 partial responses, and 2 failed to respond to bromocriptine treatment. Chronic hypopituitarism complicated macroadenoma treatment in 5 of the responders, both in patients receiving bromocriptine alone and in those who received bromocriptine in combination with surgical treatment or pituitary irradiation.

Safety and effectiveness of bromocriptine in children have not been established for any other indication listed.

➤*Elderly:* Even though no variation in efficacy or adverse reaction profile in elderly patients taking bromocriptine has been observed, greater sensitivity of some elderly individuals cannot be categorically ruled out. In general, be cautious in dose selection for an elderly patient, starting at the lower end of the dose range, reflecting the greater frequency of decreased hepatic, renal or cardiac function, and of concomitant disease or other drug therapy in this population.

➤*Monitoring:* Monitoring of visual fields in patients with macroprolactinoma is recommended for an early recognition of secondary field loss caused by chiasmal herniation and adaptation of drug dosage.

As with any chronic therapy, periodic evaluation of hepatic, hematopoietic, cardiovascular, and renal function is recommended.

Closely monitor patients closely throughout pregnancy for signs and symptoms that may signal the enlargement of a previously undetected or existing prolactin-secreting tumor.

Periodic monitoring of the blood pressure, particularly during the first weeks of therapy is prudent.

Drug Interactions

Bromocriptine Drug Interactions

Precipitant drug	Object drug[a]		Description
Alcohol	Bromocriptine	⬆	Alcohol may potentiate the side effects of bromocriptine.
Haloperidol	Bromocriptine	⬇	Coadministration may result in decreased efficacy of bromocriptine.
Macrolide antibiotics (eg, erythromycin)	Bromocriptine	⬆	Bromocriptine levels may be increased, possibly increasing pharmacologic and toxic effects.
Metoclopramide	Bromocriptine	⬇	Coadministration may result in decreased efficacy of bromocriptine.
Phenothiazines (eg, thioridazine)	Bromocriptine	⬇	Efficacy of bromocriptine, when used for prolactin-secreting tumors, may be inhibited.
Pimozide	Bromocriptine	⬇	Coadministration may result in decreased efficacy of bromocriptine.
Protease inhibitors (eg, efavirenz)	Bromocriptine	⬆	Pharmacologic and toxic effects of bromocriptine may be increased. Coadministration is contraindicated.
Sympathomimetics (eg, isometheptene, phenylpropanolamine)	Bromocriptine	⬆	In postmarketing reports, bromocriptine adverse reactions were exacerbated during concurrent use of these agents in hypertension and cardiac dysfunction. Safety of concurrent use for > 10 days is limited.
Triptans (eg, sumatriptan)	Bromocriptine	⬆	Vasoconstrictive effects of triptans and bromocriptine may be additive. Concomitant use is contraindicated, and the drugs should not be used within 24 hours of one another.
Bromocriptine	Triptans (eg, sumatriptan)		
Bromocriptine	Chloramphenicol	⬆	Bromocriptine may increase the unbound fraction of other concomitantly used highly protein-bound drugs such as chloramphenicol. Monitor for an increased risk of adverse reactions.

BROMOCRIPTINE MESYLATE — ORAL

Bromocriptine Drug Interactions			
Precipitant drug	Object drug[a]		Description
Bromocriptine	Dopamine receptor antagonists (neuroleptics [eg, clozapine, olanzapine, ziprasidone])	↓	Other dopamine receptor antagonists, including neuroleptic agents that have dopamine D_2 receptor antagonist properties, may reduce the effectiveness of bromocriptine and bromocriptine may reduce the effects of these agents. Coadministration is not recommended.
Dopamine receptor antagonists (neuroleptics [eg, clozapine, olanzapine, ziprasidone])	Bromocriptine		
Bromocriptine	Ergot drugs (eg, ergotamine)	↑↓	Coadministration may cause an increase in the occurrence of ergot-related adverse reactions such as nausea, vomiting, and fatigue and may also reduce the effectiveness of these ergot therapies when used to treat migraines.
Bromocriptine	Octreotide	↑	Treatment of acromegalic patients with bromocriptine and octreotide led to increased plasma levels of bromocriptine.
Bromocriptine	Probenecid	↑	Bromocriptine may increase the unbound fraction of other concomitantly used highly protein-bound drugs such as probenecid. Monitor for an increased risk of adverse reactions.
Bromocriptine	Methyldopa	↑	Coadministration may cause an increase in hypotensive effects. Consider the dose of methyldopa if hypotension occurs.
Bromocriptine	Salicylates (eg, aspirin, diflunisal)	↑	Bromocriptine may increase the unbound fraction of other concomitantly used highly protein-bound drugs such as salicylates. Monitor for an increased risk of adverse reactions.
Bromocriptine	Sulfonamides	↑	Bromocriptine may increase the unbound fraction of other concomitantly used highly protein-bound drugs such as sulfonamides. Monitor for an increased risk of adverse reactions.

[a] ↑ = object drug increased; ↓ = object drug decreased. ↑↓ = object drug both increased and decreased.

The risk of using bromocriptine mesylate in combination with other drugs has not been systematically evaluated, but alcohol may potentiate the adverse reactions of bromocriptine mesylate. Bromocriptine mesylate may interact with dopamine antagonists, butyrophenones, and certain other agents. Compounds in these categories result in a decreased efficacy of bromocriptine mesylate: Phenothiazines, haloperidol, metoclopramide, pimozide. Concomitant use of bromocriptine mesylate with other ergot alkaloids is not recommended.

Adverse Reactions

➤*Acromegaly:*

Most frequent – The most frequent adverse reactions encountered in acromegalic patients treated with bromocriptine were nausea (18%), constipation (14%), postural/orthostatic hypotension (6%), anorexia (4%), dry mouth/nasal stuffiness (4%), indigestion/dyspepsia (4%), digital vasospasm (3%), drowsiness/tiredness (3%), and vomiting (2%).

Less frequent – Less frequent adverse reactions were GI bleeding, dizziness, exacerbation of Raynaud syndrome, headache and syncope (less than 2%). Rarely hair loss, alcohol potentiation, faintness, lightheadedness, arrhythmia, ventricular tachycardia, decreased sleep requirement, visual hallucinations, lassitude, shortness of breath, bradycardia, vertigo, paresthesia, sluggishness, vasovagal attack, delusional psychosis, paranoia, insomnia, heavy headedness, reduced tolerance to cold, tingling of ears, facial pallor, and muscle cramps (less than 1%) have been reported.

➤*Hyperprolactinemia:* The incidence of adverse effects is quite high (69%) but these are generally mild to moderate in degree. Therapy was discontinued in approximately 5% of patients because of adverse reactions. These in decreasing order of frequency are nausea (49%), headache (19%), dizziness (17%), fatigue (7%), lightheadedness, vomiting (5%), abdominal cramps (4%), nasal congestion, constipation, diarrhea, and drowsiness (3%).

Hypotension: A slight hypotensive effect may accompany bromocriptine mesylate treatment. The occurrence of adverse reactions may be lessened by temporarily reducing dosage to one-half tablet 2 or 3 times daily.

Cerebrospinal fluid rhinorrhea: A few cases of cerebrospinal fluid rhinorrhea have been reported in patients receiving bromocriptine mesylate for treatment of large prolactinomas. This has occurred rarely, usually only in patients who have received previous transsphenoidal surgery, pituitary radiation, or both, and who were receiving bromocriptine mesylate for tumor recurrence. It may also occur in previously untreated patients whose tumor extends into the sphenoid sinus.

➤*Parkinson disease:*

Most common – In clinical trials in which bromocriptine was administered with concomitant reduction in the dose of levodopa/carbidopa, the most common newly appearing adverse reactions were nausea, abnormal involuntary movements, hallucinations, confusion, "on-off" phenomenon, dizziness, drowsiness, faintness/fainting, vomiting, asthenia, abdominal discomfort, visual disturbance, ataxia, insomnia, depression, hypotension, shortness of breath, constipation, and vertigo.

Less common adverse reactions which may be encountered include anorexia, anxiety, blepharospasm, dry mouth, dysphagia, edema of the feet and ankles, erythromelalgia, epileptiform seizure, fatigue, headache, lethargy, mottling of skin, nasal stuffiness, nervousness, nightmares, paresthesia, skin rash, urinary frequency, urinary incontinence, urinary retention, and rarely, signs and symptoms of ergotism such as tingling of fingers, cold feet, numbness, muscle cramps of feet and legs, or exacerbation of Raynaud syndrome.

➤*Postpartum patients:* In postpartum studies with bromocriptine, 23% of postpartum patients treated had at least 1 adverse reaction, but they were generally mild to moderate in degree. Therapy was discontinued in approximately 3% of patients. The most frequently occurring adverse reactions were headache (10%), dizziness (8%), nausea (7%), vomiting (3%), fatigue (1%), syncope (0.7%), diarrhea (0.4%), and cramps (0.4%). Decreases in blood pressure (greater than or equal to 20 mm Hg systolic and greater than or equal to 10 mm Hg diastolic) occurred in 28% of patients at least once during the first 3 postpartum days; these were usually of a transient nature. Reports of fainting in the puerperium may possibly be related to this effect. In postmarketing experience in the United States, serious adverse reactions reported include 72 cases of seizures (including 4 cases of status epilepticus), 30 cases of stroke, and 9 cases of myocardial infarction among postpartum patients. Seizure cases were not necessarily accompanied by the development of hypertension. An unremitting and often progressively severe headache, sometimes accompanied by visual disturbance, often preceded by hours to days many cases of seizure and/or stroke. Most patients had shown no evidence of any of the hypertensive disorders of pregnancy including eclampsia, preeclampsia or pregnancy induced hypertension. One stroke case was associated with sagittal sinus thrombosis, and another was associated with cerebral and cerebellar vasculitis. One case of myocardial infarction was associated with unexplained disseminated intravascular coagulation and a second occurred in conjunction with use of another ergot alkaloid. The relationship of these adverse reactions to bromocriptine mesylate administration has not been established.

➤*Type 2 diabetes (Cycloset only):* Because clinical trials are conducted under widely varying conditions, the adverse reaction rates reported in 1 clinical trial may not be easily compared with those rates reported in another clinical trial, and may not reflect the rates actually observed in clinical practice.

In the pooled bromocriptine phase 3 clinical trials (bromocriptine mesylate, n = 2,298; placebo, n = 1,266), adverse reactions leading to discontinuation occurred in 539 (24%) bromocriptine-treated patients and 118 (9%) placebo-treated patients. This between-group difference was driven mostly by GI adverse reactions, particularly nausea.

The bromocriptine safety trial was a 52-week, placebo-controlled study that included patients treated only with diet therapy or with other antidiabetic medications. A total of 3,070 patients were randomized to bromocriptine (titrated to 1.6 to 4.8 mg daily, as tolerated) or placebo. The study population had a mean baseline age of 60 years of age (range, 27 to 80) and 33% were 65 years of age or older. Approximately 43% of the patients were women, 68% were Caucasian, 17% were black, 13% were Hispanic, and 1% were Asian. The mean baseline body mass index (BMI) was 32 kg/m^2. The mean duration of diabetes at baseline was 8 years and the mean baseline HbA_{1c} was 7% with a mean baseline fasting plasma glucose of 142 mg/dL. At baseline, 12% of patients were treated with diet only, 40% were treated with 1 oral antidiabetic agent, 33% were treated with two oral antidiabetic agents, and 16% were treated with insulin alone or insulin in combination with an oral antidiabetic agent. At baseline, 76% of patients reported a history of hypercholesterolemia, 75% reported a history of hypertension, 11% reported a history of revascularization surgery, 10% reported a history of myocardial infarction, 10% reported a history of angina, and 5% reported a history of stroke. Forty-seven percent of the bromocriptine-treated patients and 32% of the placebo-treated patients prematurely discontinued treatment. Adverse reactions leading to discontinuation of study drug occurred among 24% of the bromocriptine-treated patients and 15% of the placebo-treated patients. This between-group difference was driven mostly by GI adverse reactions, particularly nausea.

The following table summarizes the adverse reactions reported in at least 5% of patients treated with bromocriptine in the phase 3 clinical trials regardless of investigator assessment of causality. The most commonly reported adverse reactions (nausea, fatigue, vomiting, headache, dizziness) lasted a median of 14 days and were more likely to occur during the initial titration of bromocriptine. None of the reports of nausea or vomiting were described as serious. There were no differences in the pattern of common adverse reactions across race groups or age groups (younger than 65 years of age vs older than 65 years of age). In the 52-week bromocriptine safety trial, 11.5% of bromocriptine-treated women compared with 3.6% of placebo-treated women reported vomiting. In this same trial, 5.4% of bromocriptine-treated men compared with 2.8% of placebo-treated men reported vomiting.

Bromocriptine Adverse Reactions (≥ 5%)[a]		
Adverse reactions	Bromocriptine 1.6 mg to 4.8 mg	Placebo
Monotherapy		
N = 159	n = 80	n = 79
CNS		
Asthenia	12.5%	6.3%
Dizziness	12.5%	7.6%
Headache	12.5%	8.9%
GI		
Anorexia	5%	1.3%
Constipation	11.3%	3.8%
Diarrhea	8.8%	5.1%
Dyspepsia	7.5%	2.5%
Nausea	32.5%	7.6%
Vomiting	6.3%	1.3%
Respiratory		
Rhinitis	13.8%	3.8%
Sinusitis	10%	2.5%
Miscellaneous		
Amblyopia	7.5%	1.3%
Infection	6.3%	5.1%
Adjunct to sulfonylurea (2 pooled 24-week studies)		
N = 494	n = 244	n = 250
CNS		
Asthenia	18.9%	8%
Dizziness	11.9%	5.6%
Headache	16.8%	16%
Somnolence	6.6%	2%
GI		
Constipation	9.8%	4.4%
Nausea	25.4%	4.8%
Vomiting	5.3%	3.2%
Respiratory		
Rhinitis	10.7%	4.8%
Sinusitis	7.4%	6.4%
Miscellaneous		
Amblyopia	5.3%	2.4%
Cold	8.2%	8%
Flu syndrome	9.4%	7.6%
52-week safety trial[b]		
N = 3,070	n = 2,054	n = 1,016
CNS		
Dizziness	14.8%	9.2%
Fatigue	13.9%	6.7%
Headache	11.4%	8.3%
GI		
Constipation	5.8%	5.1%
Diarrhea	8.1%	8%
Nausea	32.2%	7.6%
Vomiting	8.1%	3.1%

[a] All randomized subjects receiving ≥ 1 dose of study drug.
[b] The Safety Trial enrolled patients treated with diet or no more than 2 antidiabetic medications (metformin, insulin secretagogues such as a sulfonylurea, thiazolidinediones, alpha glucosidase inhibitors, and/or insulin).

Hypoglycemia – In the monotherapy trial, hypoglycemia was reported in 2 bromocriptine-treated patients (3.7%) and 1 placebo-treated patient (1.3%). In the add-on to sulfonylurea trials, the incidence of hypoglycemia was 8.6% among the bromocriptine-treated patients and 5.2% among the placebo-treated patients. In the bromocriptine safety trial, hypoglycemia was defined as any of the following: 1) symptoms suggestive of hypoglycemia that promptly resolved with appropriate intervention, 2) symptoms with a measured glucose less than 60 mg/dL, or 3) measured glucose below 49 mg/dL regardless of symptoms. In the 52-week safety trial, the incidence of hypoglycemia was 6.9% among the bromocriptine-treated patients and 5.3% among the placebo-treated patients. In the safety trial, severe hypoglycemia was defined as an inability to self-treat neurological symptoms consistent with hypoglycemia that occurred in the setting of a measured blood glucose less than 50 mg/dL (or evidence of prompt resolution of these symptoms with administration of oral carbohydrates, subcutaneous glucagon, or intravenous glucose if blood glucose was not measured). In this trial, severe hypoglycemia was reported among 0.5% of bromocriptine-treated patients and 1% of placebo-treated patients.

Syncope – In combined phase 2 and 3 clinical trials, syncope was reported in 1.4% of the 2,500 bromocriptine-treated patients and 0.6% of the 1,454 placebo-treated patients. Among the 3,070 patients studied in the 52-week safety trial, 33 bromocriptine mesylate-treated patients (1.6%) and 7 placebo-treated patients (0.7%) reported an adverse reaction of syncope. The cause of syncope is not known in all cases. In this trial, electrocardiograms were not available at the time of these events, but an assessment of routine electrocardiograms obtained during the course of the trial did not identify arrhythmias or QTc interval prolongation among the bromocriptine-treated patients reporting syncope.

➤*Cardiovascular:* The primary end point of the 52-week safety trial was the occurrence of all serious adverse reactions. A secondary end point was the occurrence of the composite of myocardial infarction, stroke, coronary revascularization, hospitalization for angina, and hospitalization for congestive heart failure.

All serious adverse reactions and cardiovascular end points were adjudicated by an independent event adjudication committee. Serious adverse reactions occurred in 176 of 2,054 (8.5%) bromocriptine-treated patients and 98 of 1,016 (9.6%) placebo-treated patients. The hazard ratio comparing bromocriptine with placebo for the time to first occurrence of a serious adverse reaction was 1.02 (upper bound of one-sided 96% confidence interval [CI], 1.27). None of the serious adverse reactions grouped by System-Organ-Class occurred more than 0.3 percentage points higher with bromocriptine than with placebo. The composite cardiovascular end point occurred in 31 (1.5%) bromocriptine-treated patients and 30 (3%) placebo-treated patients. The hazard ratio comparing bromocriptine with placebo for the time-to-first occurrence of the prespecified composite cardiovascular end point was 0.58 (2-sided 95% CI, 0.35 to 0.96). Therefore, the incidence of this composite end point was not increased with bromocriptine relative to placebo.

➤*CNS:* In the 52-week safety trial, somnolence and hypoesthesia were the only adverse reactions within the nervous system organ class that were reported at a rate of less than 5% and at least 1% and that occurred at a numerically greater frequency among bromocriptine-treated patients (bromocriptine 4.3% vs placebo 1.3% for somnolence; bromocriptine 1.4% vs placebo 1.1% for hypoesthesia).

➤*Lab test abnormalities:* Abnormalities in laboratory tests may include elevations in blood urea nitrogen, AST, ALT, gamma-glutamyl transpeptidase, creatine phosphokinase, alkaline phosphatase and uric acid, which are usually transient and not of clinical significance.

➤*Postmarketing:* Pleural and pericardial effusions, pleural, and pulmonary fibrosis and retroperitoneal fibrosis and constrictive pericarditis have been reported rarely in patients treated with bromocriptine.

Blurred vision, dyskinesia, and psychomotor agitation/excitation also have occurred in postmarketing experiences.

The active agent in bromocriptine has been used in other formulations and often multiple times per day to treat hyperprolactinemia, acromegaly, and Parkinson disease. The following adverse reactions have been identified during post-approval use of bromocriptine mesylate for these indications, generally at dosages higher than those approved for the treatment of type 2 diabetes. Because these reactions are reported voluntarily from a population of uncertain size, it is generally not possible to reliably estimate their frequency or establish a causal relationship to drug exposure.

➤*Hallucinations:* Hallucinations and mental confusion including delusions have been reported with bromocriptine. To date, there have been no reported cases of hallucinations or delusions among bromocriptine-treated patients (n = 2,500) in combined phase 2 and 3 clinical trials of bromocriptine.

➤*Fibrotic-related complications:* Fibrotic complications, including cases of retroperitoneal fibrosis, pulmonary fibrosis, pleural effusion, pleural thickening, pericarditis and pericardial effusions have been reported. These complications do not always resolve when bromocriptine is discontinued. Among several studies investigating a possible relation between bromocriptine exposure and cardiac valvulopathy, some events of cardiac valvulopathy have been reported, but no definitive association between bromocriptine use and clinically significant (moderate to severe) cardiac valvulopathy could be concluded.

To date, there have been no reported cases of retroperitoneal fibrosis, pulmonary infiltrates, pleural effusion, pleural thickening, pericarditis or pericardial effusions among the bromocriptine-treated patients (n = 2,500) in combined phase 2 and 3 controlled clinical trials of bromocriptine. There was 1 unconfirmed case (0.04% reaction rate) of an adverse reaction of pulmonary fibrosis classified as non-serious in a bromocriptine-treated patient.

No cases of cardiac valvulopathy have been reported in any of the clinical studies to date with bromocriptine.

➤*Psychotic and psychiatric disorders:* Psychotic disorders have been reported with bromocriptine. Additionally, pathological gambling has been reported with bromocriptine used to treat patients with Parkinson disease.

BROMOCRIPTINE MESYLATE — ORAL

To date, there have been no reported cases of psychoses or pathological gambling among the bromocriptine-treated patients (n = 2,500) in combined phase 2 and 3 controlled clinical trials of bromocriptine.

➤*Stroke:* The indication for use of bromocriptine for inhibition of postpartum lactation was withdrawn based on postmarketing reports of stroke. Causality of bromocriptine use and the occurrence of stroke in this patient population have not been proven. Based on the bromocriptine clinical trials, there is no evidence of increased risk for stroke when bromocriptine is used to treat type 2 diabetes.

➤*Neuroleptic-like malignant syndrome:* A neuroleptic-like malignant syndrome (manifested by high fever and increase in creatine phosphokinase) has been reported upon cessation of bromocriptine treatment in patients with advanced Parkinson disease or patients with secondary Parkinsonism. To date, there have been no reported cases of neuroleptic-like malignant syndrome in combined phase 2 and 3 controlled clinical trials of bromocriptine, including the Safety Trial (N = 2,500). In the *Cycloset* Safety Trial, there were no reports of neuroleptic-like malignant syndrome during the 30 days of follow-up after cessation of bromocriptine (N = 2,054).

Overdosage

➤*Symptoms:* The most commonly reported signs and symptoms associated with acute bromocriptine overdose are nausea, vomiting, constipation, diaphoresis, dizziness, pallor, severe hypotension, malaise, confusion, lethargy, drowsiness, delusions, hallucinations, and repetitive yawning. The lethal dose has not been established and the drug has a very wide margin of safety. However, 1 death occurred in a patient who committed suicide with an unknown quantity of bromocriptine and chloroquine.

➤*Treatment:* Treatment of overdose consists of removal of the drug by gastric lavage, activated charcoal, or saline catharsis. Careful supervision and recording of fluid intake and output is essential. Treat hypotension by placing the patient in the Trendelenburg position and administering intravenous fluids. If satisfactory relief of hypotension cannot be achieved by using the above measures to their fullest extent, consider vasopressors.

Patient Information

Inform patients that dizziness, drowsiness, faintness, fainting, and syncope have been reported early in the course of bromocriptine therapy.

Advise patients that bromocriptine has been associated with somnolence, and episodes of sudden sleep onset, particularly in patients with Parkinson disease. Sudden onset of sleep during daily activities, in some cases without awareness or warning signs, has been reported very rarely. Caution all patients receiving bromocriptine with regard to engaging in activities requiring rapid and precise responses, such as driving a car or operating machinery. Patients being treated with bromocriptine and presenting with somnolence and/or sudden sleep episodes must be advised not to drive or engage in activities where impaired alertness may put themselves or others at risk of serious injury or death (eg, operating machinery) until such recurrent episodes and somnolence have resolved.

Inform patients receiving bromocriptine for hyperprolactinemic states associated with macroadenoma or those who have had previous transsphenoidal surgery to report any persistent watery nasal discharge to their health care provider. Patients receiving bromocriptine for treatment of a macroadenoma should be told that discontinuation of drug may be associated with rapid regrowth of the tumor and recurrence of their original symptoms.

Inform patients of the potential risks and benefits of bromocriptine and of alternative therapies. Inform patients about the importance of adherence to dietary instructions, regular physical activity, periodic blood glucose monitoring and HbA_{1c} testing, recognition and management of hypoglycemia and hyperglycemia, and assessment for diabetes complications. During periods of stress such as fever, trauma, infection, or surgery, medication requirements may change and advise patients to seek medical advice promptly.

Advise patients that they may develop postural (orthostatic) hypotension with or without symptoms such as dizziness, nausea, and diaphoresis. Hypotension and syncope may occur more frequently during initial therapy or with an increase in dose at any time. During early treatment with bromocriptine, advise patients to make slow postural changes and to avoid situations that could predispose to serious injury if syncope was to occur.

Advise women who are breast-feeding their children to not take bromocriptine.

Instruct patients to read the Patient Package Insert before starting bromocriptine therapy and to reread it each time the prescription is renewed. Instruct patients to inform their health care provider if they develop any unusual symptoms or if any known symptom persists or worsens.

CARBIDOPA

Rx	**Lodosyn**[a] (Bristol-Myers Squibb Company)	**Tablets:** 25 mg carbidopa	(MSD 129). Orange, scored. In 100s.

[a] Most patients may be maintained on carbidopa/levodopa combination products. *Lodosyn* is available to physicians for use in patients requiring individual titration of carbidopa and levodopa.

CARBIDOPA — ORAL

Carbidopa is used only with levodopa. See levodopa monograph. Also refer to the general discussion in the Antiparkinson Agents introduction.

Indications

➤*Parkinsonism:* For use with carbidopa-levodopa or with levodopa in the treatment of the symptoms of idiopathic Parkinson's disease (paralysis agitans), postencephalitic parkinsonism, and symptomatic parkinsonism which may follow injury to the nervous system by carbon monoxide intoxication and/or manganese intoxication.

For use with carbidopa-levodopa in patients for whom the dosage of carbidopa-levodopa provides less than adequate daily dosage (usually 70 mg daily) of carbidopa.

For use with levodopa in the occasional patient whose dosage requirement of carbidopa and levodopa necessitates separate titration of each entity.

Carbidopa is used with carbidopa-levodopa or with levodopa to permit the administration of lower doses of levodopa with reduced nausea and vomiting, more rapid dosage titration, and with a somewhat smoother response. However, patients with markedly irregular ("on-off") responses to levodopa have not been shown to benefit from the addition of carbidopa.

➤*Off-label uses:* Carbidopa is used to reduce the peripheral metabolism of the L-5-hydroxtryptophan (L-5HTP) when used to treat post-anoxic intention myoclonus.

Administration and Dosage

➤*General dosing considerations:* Since carbidopa prevents the reversal of levodopa effects caused by pyridoxine, supplemental pyridoxine (vitamin B_6), can be given to patients when they are receiving carbidopa and levodopa concomitantly or as carbidopa-levodopa.

Most patients respond to a 1:10 proportion of carbidopa and levodopa, provided the daily dosage of carbidopa is 70 mg or more a day.

➤*Adults:*

Parkinsonism –

Usual dosage:

• *Adding carbidopa to carbidopa-levodopa –*

When patients are taking carbidopa-levodopa 10-100 (which contains 10 mg of carbidopa and 100 mg of levodopa), 25 mg of carbidopa may be given with the first dose of carbidopa-levodopa each day. Additional doses of 12.5 mg or 25 mg may be given during the day with each dose of carbidopa-levodopa. When patients are taking carbidopa-levodopa 25-250 (which contains 25 mg of carbidopa and 250 mg of levodopa) or carbidopa-levodopa 25-100 (which contains 25 mg of carbidopa and 100 mg of levodopa), 25 mg of carbidopa may be given with any dose of carbidopa-levodopa as required for optimum therapeutic response.

• *Individual titration of carbidopa and levodopa –*

Initiate at 25 mg 3 or 4 times a day. The 2 drugs should be given at the same time, starting with no more than one-fifth (20%) to one-fourth (25%) of the previous or recommended daily dosage of levodopa when given without carbidopa. In patients already receiving levodopa therapy, at least 12 hours should elapse between the last dose of levodopa and initiation of therapy with carbidopa and levodopa. A convenient way to initiate therapy in these patients is in the morning following a night when the patient has not taken levodopa for at least 12 hours.

Maximum dose: 200 mg/day given as carbidopa and carbidopa-levodopa.

Dosage adjustment: Dosage of carbidopa may be adjusted by adding or omitting one-half or one tablet a day.

Concomitant therapy: Current evidence indicates other standard antiparkinsonian drugs may be continued while carbidopa and levodopa are being administered. However, the dosage of such other standard antiparkinsonian drugs may require adjustment.

Discontinuation of therapy:

Patients should be observed carefully if abrupt reduction or discontinuation of carbidopa-levodopa or carbidopa-levodopa sustained-release is required, especially if the patient is receiving neuroleptics (see Warnings).

Interruption of therapy: If general anesthesia is required, therapy may be continued as long as the patient is permitted to take fluids and medication by mouth. When therapy is interrupted temporarily, the patient should be observed for symptoms resembling NMS, and the usual daily dosage may be resumed as soon as the patient is able to take medication orally.

➤*Administration:* Administer with food to reduce GI upset.

➤*Storage / Stability:* Store in light-resistant container at room temperature.

Actions

➤*Pharmacology:* Current evidence indicates that symptoms of Parkinson's disease are related to depletion of dopamine in the corpus striatum. Administration of dopamine is ineffective in the treatment of Parkinson's disease apparently because it does not cross the blood-brain barrier. However, levodopa, the metabolic precursor of dopamine, does cross the blood-brain barrier, and presumably is converted to dopamine in the brain. This is thought to be the mechanism whereby levodopa relieves symptoms of Parkinson's disease.

Pharmacodynamics – When levodopa is administered orally it is rapidly decarboxylated to dopamine in extracerebral tissues so that only a small portion of a given dose is transported unchanged to the central nervous system. For this reason, large doses of levodopa are required for adequate therapeutic effect and these may often be accompanied by nausea and other adverse reactions, some of which are attributable to dopamine formed in extracerebral tissues.

CARBIDOPA — ORAL

The incidence of levodopa-induced nausea and vomiting is less when carbidopa is used with levodopa than when levodopa is used without carbidopa. In many patients this reduction in nausea and vomiting will permit more rapid dosage titration.

Carbidopa inhibits decarboxylation of peripheral levodopa. Carbidopa has not been demonstrated to have any overt pharmacodynamic actions in the recommended doses. It does not appear to cross the blood-brain barrier readily and does not affect the metabolism of levodopa within the central nervous system at doses of carbidopa that are recommended for maximum effective inhibition of peripheral decarboxylation of levodopa.

Since its decarboxylase-inhibiting activity is limited primarily to extracerebral tissues, administration of carbidopa with levodopa makes more levodopa available for transport to the brain. However, since levodopa and carbidopa compete with certain amino acids for transport across the gut wall, the absorption of levodopa and carbidopa may be impaired in some patients on a high protein diet.

➤*Pharmacokinetics:* Carbidopa reduces the amount of levodopa required to produce a given response by about 75% and, when administered with levodopa, increases both plasma levels and the plasma half-life of levodopa, and decreases plasma and urinary dopamine and homovanillic acid.

In clinical pharmacologic studies, simultaneous administration of separate tablets of carbidopa and levodopa produced greater urinary excretion of levodopa in proportion to the excretion of dopamine when compared to the two drugs administered at separate times.

Supplemental pyridoxine (vitamin B_6) can be given to patients when they are receiving carbidopa and levodopa concomitantly or as carbidopa-levodopa sustained-release or carbidopa-levodopa. Previous reports in the medical literature cautioned that high doses of vitamin B_6 should not be taken by patients on levodopa therapy alone because exogenously administered pyridoxine would enhance the metabolism of levodopa to dopamine. The introduction of carbidopa to levodopa therapy, which inhibits the peripheral decarboxylation of levodopa to dopamine, counteracts the metabolic-enhancing effect of pyridoxine.

Contraindications

Hypersensitivity to any component of this drug.

Nonselective monoamine oxidase (MAO) inhibitors are contraindicated for use with levodopa or carbidopa-levodopa combination products with or without carbidopa. These inhibitors must be discontinued at least 2 weeks prior to initiating therapy with levodopa. Carbidopa-levodopa or levodopa may be administered concomitantly with the manufacturer's recommended dose of an MAO inhibitor with selectivity for MAO type B (eg, selegiline HCl).

Levodopa or carbidopa-levodopa products, with or without carbidopa, are contraindicated in patients with narrow-angle glaucoma.

Because levodopa or carbidopa-levodopa products, with or without carbidopa, may activate a malignant melanoma, they should not be used in patients with suspicious, undiagnosed skin lesions or a history of melanoma.

Warnings/Precautions

➤*Use with levodopa:* When carbidopa is to be given to patients being treated with levodopa, give the two drugs at the same time, starting with no more than 20% to 25% of the previous daily dosage of levodopa. At least 8 hours should elapse between the last dose of levodopa and initiation of therapy with carbidopa and levodopa.

Carbidopa has no antiparkinsonian effect when given alone. It is indicated for use with carbidopa-levodopa or levodopa. Carbidopa does not decrease adverse reactions due to central effects of levodopa.

Although the administration of carbidopa permits control of parkinsonism and Parkinson's disease with much lower doses of levodopa, there is no conclusive evidence at present that this is beneficial other than in reducing nausea and vomiting, permitting more rapid titration, and providing a somewhat smoother response to levodopa.

Certain patients who responded poorly to levodopa alone have improved when carbidopa and levodopa were given concurrently. This was most likely due to decreased peripheral decarboxylation of levodopa rather than to a primary effect of carbidopa on the peripheral nervous system. Carbidopa has not been shown to enhance the intrinsic efficacy of levodopa.

In considering whether to give carbidopa with carbidopa-levodopa or with levodopa to patients who have nausea or vomiting, the physician should be aware that, while many patients may be expected to improve, some may not. Since one cannot predict which patients are likely to improve, this can only be determined by a trial of therapy. It should be further noted that in controlled trials comparing carbidopa and levodopa with levodopa alone, about half the patients with nausea or vomiting on levodopa alone improved spontaneously despite being retained on the same dose of levodopa during the controlled portion of the trial.

➤*CNS effects:* As with levodopa, concomitant administration of carbidopa and levodopa may cause involuntary movements and mental disturbances. These reactions are thought to be due to increased brain dopamine following administration of levodopa. All patients should be observed carefully for the development of depression with concomitant suicidal tendencies. Patients with past or current psychoses should be treated with caution. Because carbidopa permits more levodopa to reach the brain and, thus, more dopamine to be formed, dyskinesias may occur at lower levodopa dosages and sooner with concomitant use of carbidopa and levodopa or carbidopa-levodopa combination products than with levodopa alone. The occurrence of dyskinesias may require levodopa dosage reduction.

➤*Neuroleptic malignant syndrome (NMS):* Sporadic cases of a symptom complex resembling NMS have been reported in association with dose reductions or withdrawal of certain antiparkinsonian agents such as levodopa, carbidopa-levodopa or carbidopa-levodopa sustained-release. Therefore, patients should be observed carefully when the dosage of levodopa is reduced abruptly or discontinued, especially if the patient is receiving neuroleptics.

NMS is an uncommon but life-threatening syndrome characterized by fever or hyperthermia. Neurological findings, including muscle rigidity, involuntary movements, altered consciousness, mental status changes; other disturbances, such as autonomic dysfunction, tachycardia, tachypnea, sweating, hyper- or hypotension; laboratory findings, such as creatine phosphokinase elevation, leukocytosis, myoglobinuria, and increased serum myoglobin, have been reported.

The early diagnosis of this condition is important for the appropriate management of these patients. Considering NMS as a possible diagnosis and ruling out other acute illnesses (eg, pneumonia, systemic infection) is essential. This may be especially complex if the clinical presentation includes both serious medical illness and untreated or inadequately treated extrapyramidal signs and symptoms (EPS). Other important considerations in the differential diagnosis include central anticholinergic toxicity, heat stroke, drug fever, and primary central nervous system (CNS) pathology.

The management of NMS should include:

1.) Intensive symptomatic treatment and medical monitoring.
2.) Treatment of any concomitant serious medical problems for which specific treatments are available. Dopamine agonists, such as bromocriptine, and muscle relaxants, such as dantrolene, are often used in the treatment of NMS; however, their effectiveness has not been demonstrated in controlled studies.

➤*Special risk:* Patients with chronic wide-angle glaucoma may be treated cautiously with carbidopa and levodopa or carbidopa-levodopa, or any combination of these drugs, just as with levodopa alone, provided the intraocular pressure is well controlled and the patient is monitored carefully for changes in intraocular pressure during therapy.

Levodopa, with or without carbidopa, should be administered cautiously to patients with severe cardiovascular or pulmonary disease, bronchial asthma, renal, hepatic, or endocrine disease.

Care should be exercised in administering levodopa, with or without carbidopa, to patients with a history of myocardial infarction who have residual atrial, nodal, or ventricular arrhythmias. In such patients, cardiac function should be monitored with particular care during the period of initial dosage adjustment, in a facility with provisions for intensive cardiac care.

As with levodopa alone there is a possibility of upper gastrointestinal hemorrhage in patients with a history of peptic ulcer.

➤*Pregnancy: Category C.* There are no adequate and well-controlled studies with carbidopa in pregnant women. It has been reported from individual cases that levodopa crosses the human placental barrier, enters the fetus, and is metabolized. Carbidopa concentrations in fetal tissue appeared to be minimal. Carbidopa should be used during pregnancy only if the potential benefit justifies the potential risk to the fetus.

Carbidopa, at doses as high as 120 mg/kg/day, was without teratogenic effects in the mouse or rabbit. In the rabbit, but not in the mouse, carbidopa-levodopa produced visceral anomalies, similar to those seen with levodopa alone, at approximately 7 times the maximum recommended human dose. The teratogenic effect of levodopa in rabbits was unchanged by the concomitant administration of carbidopa.

➤*Lactation:* It is not known whether carbidopa or levodopa is excreted in human milk. Because many drugs are excreted in human milk, and because of their potential for serious adverse reactions in nursing infants, a decision should be made whether to discontinue nursing or to discontinue the drug, taking into account the importance of the drug to the nursing woman.

➤*Children:* Safety and effectiveness in pediatric patients have not been established, and use of the drug in patients below the age of 18 is not recommended.

➤*Lab test abnormalities:* Abnormalities in laboratory tests may include elevations of liver function tests such as alkaline phosphatase, AST, ALT, lactic dehydrogenase, and bilirubin. Abnormalities in blood urea nitrogen and positive Coombs test have also been reported. Commonly, levels of blood urea nitrogen, creatinine, and uric acid are lower during concomitant administration of carbidopa and levodopa than with levodopa alone.

➤*Monitoring:* As with levodopa alone, periodic evaluations of hepatic, hematopoietic, cardiovascular, and renal function are recommended during extended concomitant therapy with carbidopa and levodopa, or with carbidopa and carbidopa-levodopa, or any combination of these drugs.

Drug Interactions

➤*Antihypertensive agents:* Symptomatic postural hypotension has occurred when carbidopa, given with levodopa or carbidopa-levodopa combination products, was added to the treatment of a patient receiving antihypertensive drugs. Therefore, when therapy with carbidopa, given with or without levodopa or carbidopa-levodopa combination products, is started, dosage adjustment of the antihypertensive drug may be required.

➤*Monoamine oxidase inhibitors:* For patients receiving monoamine oxidase inhibitors. Concomitant therapy with selegiline and carbidopa-levodopa may be associated with severe orthostatic hypotension not attributable to carbidopa-levodopa alone.

CARBIDOPA — ORAL

➤*Tricyclic antidepressants:* There have been rare reports of adverse reactions, including hypertension and dyskinesia, resulting from the concomitant use of tricyclic antidepressants and carbidopa-levodopa preparations.

➤*Dopamine D_2 receptor antagonists and isoniazid:* Dopamine D_2 receptor antagonists (eg, phenothiazines, butyrophenones, risperidone) and isoniazid may reduce the therapeutic effects of levodopa. In addition, the beneficial effects of levodopa in Parkinson's disease have been reported to be reversed by phenytoin and papaverine. Patients taking these drugs with carbidopa and levodopa or carbidopa-levodopa combination products should be carefully observed for loss of therapeutic response.

➤*Iron salts:* Iron salts may reduce the bioavailability of carbidopa and levodopa. The clinical relevance is unclear.

➤*Metoclopramide:* Although metoclopramide may increase the bioavailability of levodopa by increasing gastric emptying, metoclopramide may also adversely affect disease control by its dopamine receptor antagonistic properties.

➤*Drug/Lab test interactions:* Levodopa and carbidopa-levodopa combination products may cause a false-positive reaction for urinary ketone bodies when a test tape is used for determination of ketonuria. This reaction will not be altered by boiling the urine specimen. False-negative tests may result with the use of glucose-oxidase methods of testing for glucosuria.

Adverse Reactions

Carbidopa has not been demonstrated to have any overt pharmacodynamic actions in the recommended doses. The only adverse reactions that have been observed have been with concomitant use of carbidopa with other drugs such as levodopa, and with carbidopa-levodopa combination products.

When carbidopa is administered concomitantly with levodopa or carbidopa-levodopa combination products, the most common adverse reactions have included dyskinesias such as choreiform, dystonic, and other involuntary movements, and nausea. Other adverse reactions reported with carbidopa when administered concomitantly with levodopa alone or carbidopa-levodopa combination products were psychotic episodes including delusions, hallucinations, and paranoid ideation, depression with or without development of suicidal tendencies, and dementia. Convulsions also have occurred; however, a causal relationship with concomitant use of carbidopa and levodopa has not been established.

The following other adverse reactions have been reported with levodopa and carbidopa-levodopa combination products. These same adverse reactions may also occur when carbidopa is administered with these products.

➤*Cardiovascular:* Cardiac irregularities, hypertension, myocardial infarction, hypotension including orthostatic hypotension, palpitation, phlebitis, syncope.

➤*CNS:* Agitation, anxiety, ataxia, blepharospasm (which may be taken as an early sign of excess dosage; consideration of dosage reduction may be made at this time), bradykinetic episodes ("on-off" phenomenon), confusion, decreased mental acuity, disorientation, euphoria, dizziness, dream abnormalities including nightmares, extrapyramidal disorder, falling, gait abnormalities, headache, increased tremor, insomnia, memory impairment, muscle twitching, nervousness, numbness, paresthesia, peripheral neuropathy, somnolence, trismus, activation of latent Horner's syndrome.

➤*Dermatologic:* Flushing, increased sweating, malignant melanoma (see Contraindications), rash, alopecia, dark sweat.

➤*GI:* Anorexia, bruxism, burning sensation of the tongue, constipation, dark saliva, development of duodenal ulcer, diarrhea, dry mouth, dyspepsia, dysphagia, flatulence, gastrointestinal bleeding, gastrointestinal pain, heartburn, hiccups, sialorrhea, taste alterations, vomiting.

➤*GU:* Dark urine, priapism, urinary frequency, urinary incontinence, urinary retention, urinary tract infection.

➤*Hematologic:* Hemolytic and non-hemolytic anemia, leukopenia, thrombocytopenia, agranulocytosis.

➤*Hypersensitivity:* Angioedema, urticaria, pruritus and Henoch-Schonlein purpura, bullous lesions (including pemphigus-like reactions).

➤*Lab test abnormalities:* Abnormalities in alkaline phosphatase, AST, ALT, lactic dehydrogenase, bilirubin, blood urea nitrogen (BUN), Coombs test; elevated serum glucose; decreased hemoglobin and hematocrit; decreased white blood cell count and serum potassium; increased serum creatinine and uric acid; white blood cells, bacteria and blood in the urine; protein and glucose in the urine.

➤*Metabolic:* Edema, weight gain, weight loss.

➤*Musculoskeletal:* Back pain, leg pain, muscle cramps, shoulder pain.

➤*Respiratory:* Upper respiratory tract infection, dyspnea, pharyngeal pain, cough.

➤*Special senses:* Oculogyric crises, diplopia, blurred vision, dilated pupils.

➤*Miscellaneous:* Bizarre breathing patterns, faintness, hoarseness, hot flashes, malaise, neuroleptic malignant syndrome, sense of stimulation, abdominal pain and distress, asthenia, chest pain, fatigue.

Overdosage

No reports of overdose with carbidopa have been received. Management of overdosage with carbidopa is the same as that with levodopa or carbidopa-levodopa preparations.

In the event of overdosage, general supportive measures should be employed, along with immediate gastric lavage. Intravenous fluids should be administered judiciously, and an adequate airway maintained. Electrocardiographic monitoring should be instituted and the patient carefully observed for the development of arrhythmias; if required, appropriate antiarrhythmic therapy should be given. The possibility that the patient may have taken other drugs as well as carbidopa should be taken into consideration. To date, no experience has been reported with dialysis; hence, its value in overdosage is not known. Pyridoxine is not effective in reversing the actions of carbidopa.

Based on studies in which high doses of levodopa or carbidopa were administered, a significant proportion of rats and mice given single oral doses of levodopa of approximately 1500 to 2000 mg/kg are expected to die. A significant proportion of infant rats of both sexes are expected to die at a dose of 800 mg/kg. A significant proportion of rats are expected to die after treatment with similar doses of carbidopa. The addition of carbidopa in a 1:10 ratio with levodopa increases the dose at which a significant proportion of mice are expected to die to 3360 mg/kg.

LEVODOPA/CARBIDOPA

Rx	**Carbidopa and Levodopa** (Various, eg, Endo, Lemmon, Purepac, Teva, UDL)	**Tablets**: 10 mg carbidopa, 100 mg levodopa	In 100s, 500s, and 1,000s.
Rx	**Sinemet-10/100** (Bristol-Myers Squibb)		(647 SINEMET). Dark blue, scored, oval. In 100s and UD 100s.
Rx	**Carbidopa and Levodopa** (Various, eg, Endo, Ivax, Lemmon, Purepac, Teva, UDL)	**Tablets**: 25 mg carbidopa, 100 mg levodopa	In 100s, 500s, and 1,000s.
Rx	**Sinemet-25/100** (Bristol-Myers Squibb)		(650 SINEMET). Yellow, scored, oval. In 100s and UD 100s.
Rx	**Carbidopa and Levodopa** (Various, eg, Endo, Lemmon, Purepac, Teva, UDL)	**Tablets**: 25 mg carbidopa, 250 mg levodopa	In 100s, 500s, and 1,000s.
Rx	**Sinemet-25/250** (Bristol-Myers Squibb)		(654 SINEMET). Light blue, scored, oval. In 100s and UD 100s.
Rx	**Carbidopa and Levodopa** (Mylan)	**Tablets, orally disintegrating**: 10 mg carbidopa, 100 mg levodopa	Aspartame, mannitol, phenylalanine 3.37 mg, sorbitol. (M C51). Green, round. Scored. Peppermint flavor. In 100s and 500s.
Rx	**Parcopa** (Azur Pharma)		Aspartame, mannitol, phenylalanine 3.4 mg. (10/100 SP 341). Blue, scored. Mint flavor. In 100s.
Rx	**Carbidopa and Levodopa** (Mylan)	**Tablets, orally disintegrating**: 25 mg carbidopa, 100 mg levodopa	Aspartame, mannitol, phenylalanine 3.37 mg, sorbitol. (M C52). Blue, round. Scored. Peppermint flavor. In 100s and 500s.
Rx	**Parcopa** (Azur Pharma)		Aspartame, mannitol, phenylalanine 3.4 mg. (25/100 SP 342). Yellow, scored. Mint flavor. In 100s.
Rx	**Carbidopa and Levodopa** (Mylan)	**Tablets, orally disintegrating**: 25 mg carbidopa, 250 mg levodopa	Aspartame, mannitol, phenylalanine 8.42 mg, sorbitol. (M C53). Green, round. Scored. Peppermint flavor. In 100s and 500s.
Rx	**Parcopa** (Azur Pharma)		Aspartame, mannitol, phenylalanine 8.4 mg. (25/250 SP 343). Blue, scored. Mint flavor. In 100s.
Rx	**Carbidopa and Levodopa** (Various, eg, Apotex USA, Mylan, UDL)	**Tablets, extended-release**: 25 mg carbidopa, 100 mg levodopa	In 100s and 500s.
Rx	**Sinemet CR** (Bristol-Myers Squibb)		(601 SINEMET CR). Pink, oval. In 100s, 500s, and UD 100s.

LEVODOPA/CARBIDOPA

Rx	**Carbidopa and Levodopa** (Various, eg, Apotex USA, Mylan, UDL)	**Tablets, extended-release:** 50 mg carbidopa, 200 mg levodopa	In 100s and 500s.
Rx	**Sinemet CR** (Bristol-Myers Squibb)		(521 SINEMET CR). Peach, scored, oval. In 100s, 500s, and UD 100s.

LEVODOPA/CARBIDOPA — ORAL

These agents are used in combination because carbidopa inhibits decarboxylation of levodopa and makes more levodopa available for transport to the brain. For complete information on each of the components, refer to the individual monographs. Also refer to the general discussion in the Antiparkinson Agents introduction.

Indications

➤*Parkinsonism:* Treatment of symptoms of idiopathic Parkinson disease (paralysis agitans), postencephalitic parkinsonism, and symptomatic parkinsonism that may follow injury to the nervous system by carbon monoxide and/or manganese intoxication.

Levodopa and carbidopa are indicated in these conditions to permit the administration of lower doses of levodopa with reduced nausea and vomiting, more rapid dosage titration, a somewhat smoother response, and with supplemental pyridoxine (vitamin B_6).

Administration and Dosage

➤*General dosing considerations:* Determine the optimum daily dose by careful titration in each patient.

Immediate-release tablets of the 2 ratios (eg, 1:4, 25/100 or 1:10, 10/100 and 25/250) may be given separately or combined as needed to provide the optimum dosage.

Immediate-release tablets (25/100 or 10/100) can be added to the dosage regimen of extended-release tablets in selected patients with advanced disease who need additional levodopa.

➤*Adults:*

Parkinsonism –

Patients not receiving levodopa:

• *Maximum dose* – 200 mg/day of the carbidopa component.

• *Initial dosage –*

Immediate-release: Carbidopa 25 mg/levodopa 100 mg 3 times daily, or carbidopa 10 mg/levodopa 100 mg 3 or 4 times daily.

Extended-release: In patients with mild to moderate disease, the initial recommended dose is carbidopa 50 mg/levodopa 200 mg twice daily at intervals of 6 hours or more.

• *Dosage adjustment –*

Immediate-release: Dosage may be increased by 1 tablet every day or every other day, as necessary, until a dosage of 8 tablets a day is reached.

Provide at least 70 to 100 mg carbidopa per day.

When more carbidopa is required, substitute one 25/100 tablet for each 10/100 tablet. When more levodopa is required, substitute the 25/250 tablet for the 25/100 or 10/100 tablet. If necessary, the dosage of 25/250 may be increased by one-half or 1 tablet every day or every other day to a maximum of 8 tablets a day. Experience with total daily dosages of carbidopa greater than 200 mg is limited.

Extended-release: Doses and dosing intervals may be increased or decreased based on response. Most patients have been adequately treated with a dose that provides 400 to 1,600 mg of levodopa per day (divided doses) at intervals of 4 to 8 hours while awake. Higher doses (2,400 mg or more of levodopa per day) and shorter intervals (less than 4 hours) have been used but are not usually recommended. If an interval of less than 4 hours is used and/or if the divided doses are not equal, give the smaller doses at the end of the day. Allow at least a 3-day interval between dosage adjustments.

• *Concomitant therapy* – Other antiparkinson drugs can be given concurrently; dosage adjustment may be necessary.

• *Conversion from immediate-release tablets to extended release tablets* – Substitute dosage with extended-release tablets at an amount that provides approximately 10% more levodopa per day, although this may need to be increased to a dosage that provides up to 30% more levodopa per day. Use intervals of 4 to 8 hours while awake.

Guidelines for Initial Conversion From Immediate-Release to Extended-Release Levodopa

Immediate-release total daily levodopa dose (mg)	Extended-release suggested levodopa dosage regimen
300 to 400	200 mg twice daily
500 to 600	300 mg twice daily or 200 mg 3 times daily
700 to 800	Total of 800 mg in 3 or more divided doses (eg, 300 mg am, 300 mg early pm, and 200 mg later pm)
900 to 1,000	Total of 1,000 mg in 3 or more divided doses (eg, 400 mg am, 400 mg early pm, and 200 mg later pm)

Patients currently treated with levodopa: Discontinue levodopa at least 12 hours before therapy with levodopa/carbidopa. Substitute the combination drug at a dosage that will provide approximately 25% of the previous levodopa dosage.

• *Immediate-release* – Suggested starting dose of 25 mg carbidopa /250 mg levodopa 3 or 4 times daily for patients taking more than 1,500 mg levodopa.

Suggested starting dose of 25 mg carbidopa /100 mg levodopa for patients taking less than 1,500 mg levodopa.

• *Extended-release* – In patients with mild to moderate disease, the initial dose is usually one 50/200 extended-release tablet twice daily.

➤*Administration:*

Immediate-release tablets – Administer 3 or 4 times a day.

Extended-release tablets – Extended-release tablets may be administered as whole or half tablets that should not be crushed or chewed.

Orally disintegrating tablets – Just prior to administration, gently remove the tablet from the bottle with dry hands. Immediately place the tablet on top of the tongue where it will dissolve in seconds, then swallow with saliva. Administration with liquid is not necessary.

➤*Storage/Stability:* Protect from moisture and light. Avoid storing extended-release tablets above 30°C (86°F). Store disintegrating tablets between 20° to 25°C (68° to 86°F); excursions permitted between 15° to 30°C (59° to 86°F).

Actions

➤*Pharmacokinetics:* The extended-release formulation is designed to release the ingredients over a 4- to 6-hour period. There is less variation in plasma levodopa levels than with the conventional formulation. However, the extended-release form is less systemically bioavailable (70% to 75%) and may require increased daily doses to achieve the same level of symptomatic relief. The half-life of levodopa may be prolonged following the extended-release form because of continuous absorption. In elderly subjects, the mean time to peak levodopa concentration was 2 hours for extended-release versus 0.5 hours for conventional. The maximum levodopa concentration of levodopa following the extended-release form was approximately 35% of the conventional form.

Warnings/Precautions

➤*CNS effects:* Certain adverse CNS effects (eg, dyskinesias) will occur at lower dosages and sooner during therapy with levodopa and carbidopa than with levodopa alone.

➤*Pregnancy: Category C.* There are no adequate or well-controlled studies in pregnant women. It has been reported from individual cases that levodopa crosses the human placental barrier, enters the fetus, and is metabolized. Carbidopa concentrations in fetal tissue appeared to be minimal. Use of carbidopa and levodopa extended release tablets in women of childbearing potential requires that the anticipated benefits of the drug be weighed against possible hazards to mother and child.

➤*Lactation:* Levodopa is excreted into breast milk. It is unknown if carbidopa is excreted into breast milk. Use with caution.

Drug Interactions

➤*Drug/Food interactions:* Administration of a single dose of the extended-release form with food increased the extent of levodopa availability by 50% and increased peak levodopa concentrations by 25%.

Adverse Reactions

In clinical trials, the adverse reaction profile of the extended-release form did not differ substantially from that of the conventional form.

ENTACAPONE

Rx	**Comtan** (Novartis)	**Tablets; oral:** 200 mg	Hydrogenated vegetable oil, mannitol, sucrose. (COMTAN). Film-coated. Oval, brownish-orange. In 100s.

ENTACAPONE — ORAL

Indications

➤*Parkinson disease:* As an adjunct to levodopa/carbidopa to treat patients with idiopathic Parkinson disease who experience the signs and symptoms of end-of-dose "wearing-off."

Administration and Dosage

➤*General dosing considerations:* Entacapone should always be administered in association with levodopa/carbidopa. It has no antiparkinsonian effect of its own.

Entacapone may need to be tapered. (See Tapering.)

➤*Adults:*

Parkinson disease –

Usual dosage: 200 mg concomitantly with each levodopa/carbidopa dose.

Maximum dose: 8 times daily (1,600 mg/day).

Concomitant therapy: In clinical trials, the majority of patients required a decrease in daily levodopa dose if their daily dose of levodopa had been at least 800 mg, or if patients had moderate or severe dyskinesias before beginning treatment.

To optimize an individual patient's response, reducing the daily levodopa dose or extending the interval between doses may be necessary. In clinical trials, the average reduction in daily levodopa dose was approximately 25% in those patients requiring a levodopa dose reduction. More than 58% of patients with levodopa doses above 800 mg daily required such a reduction.

Tapering: Rapid withdrawal or abrupt reduction in the entacapone dose could lead to emergence of signs and symptoms of Parkinson disease and may lead to hyperpyrexia and confusion, a symptom complex resembling neuroleptic malignant syndrome (NMS). This syndrome should be considered in the differential diagnosis for any patient who develops a high fever or severe rigidity. If a decision is made to discontinue treatment with entacapone, patients should be monitored closely, and other dopaminergic treatments should be adjusted as needed. Although tapering entacapone has not been systematically evaluated, it seems prudent to withdraw patients slowly if the decision is made to discontinue treatment.

➤*Administration:* May be taken with or without food.

➤*Storage/Stability:* Store at 25°C (77°F); excursions are permitted to 15° to 30°C (59° to 86°F).

Actions

➤*Pharmacology:* Entacapone is a selective and reversible inhibitor of catechol-O-methyltransferase (COMT), used in the treatment of Parkinson disease as an adjunct to levodopa/carbidopa therapy.

The mechanism of action of entacapone is believed to be through its ability to inhibit COMT and alter the plasma pharmacokinetics of levodopa. When entacapone is given in conjunction with levodopa and an aromatic amino acid decarboxylase inhibitor, such as carbidopa, plasma levels of levodopa are greater and more sustained than after administration of levodopa and an aromatic amino acid decarboxylase inhibitor alone. It is believed that at a given frequency of levodopa administration, these more sustained plasma levels of levodopa result in more constant dopaminergic stimulation in the brain, leading to greater effects on the signs and symptoms of Parkinson disease. The higher levodopa levels also lead to increased levodopa adverse effects, sometimes requiring a decrease in the dose of levodopa.

In animals, while entacapone enters the CNS to a minimal extent, it has been shown to inhibit central COMT activity. In humans, entacapone inhibits the COMT enzyme in peripheral tissues. The effects of entacapone on central COMT activity in humans have not been studied.

➤*Pharmacokinetics:*

Absorption – Entacapone is rapidly absorbed, with a time to maximal drug concentration (T_{max}) of approximately 1 hour. The absolute bioavailability following oral administration is 35%. After a single dose of entacapone 200 mg, the maximal drug concentration (C_{max}) is approximately 1.2 mcg/mL.

Effect on levodopa and its metabolites: When entacapone 200 mg is administered together with levodopa/carbidopa, it increases the area under the curve (AUC) of levodopa by approximately 35% and the elimination half-life of levodopa is prolonged from 1.3 to 2.4 hours. In general, the average peak levodopa plasma concentration and the time of its occurrence (T_{max} of 1 hour) are unaffected. The onset of effect occurs after the first administration and is maintained during long-term treatment. Studies in Parkinson disease patients suggest that the maximal effect occurs with entacapone 200 mg. Plasma levels of 3-OMD are markedly and dose-dependently decreased by entacapone when given with levodopa/carbidopa.

Distribution – The volume of distribution of entacapone at steady state after intravenous (IV) injection is small (20 L). Entacapone does not distribute widely into tissues because of its high plasma protein binding. Based on in vitro studies, the plasma protein binding of entacapone is 98% over the concentration range of 0.4 to 50 mcg/mL. Entacapone binds mainly to serum albumin.

Metabolism/Excretion – Entacapone is almost completely metabolized prior to excretion, with only a very small amount (0.2% of dose) found unchanged in urine. The main metabolic pathway is isomerization to the cis-isomer, followed by direct glucuronidation of the parent and cis-isomer; the glucuronide conjugate is inactive. After oral administration of a ^{14}C-labeled dose of entacapone, 10% of labeled parent and metabolite is excreted in urine and 90% in feces.

Entacapone pharmacokinetics are linear over the dose range of 5 to 800 mg and are independent of levodopa/carbidopa coadministration. The elimination of entacapone is biphasic, with an elimination half-life of 0.4 to 0.7 hours based on the beta-phase and 2.4 hours based on the gamma-phase. The gamma-phase accounts for approximately 10% of the total AUC. The total body clearance after IV administration is 850 mL/min.

Special populations –

Hepatic function impairment: A single 200 mg dose of entacapone, without levodopa/dopa decarboxylase inhibitor coadministration, showed approximately 2-fold higher AUC and C_{max} values in patients with a history of alcoholism and hepatic impairment (n = 10) compared with healthy participants (n = 10). All patients had biopsy-proven liver cirrhosis caused by alcohol. According to Child-Pugh grading, 7 patients with liver disease had mild hepatic impairment and 3 patients had moderate hepatic impairment. As only approximately 10% of the entacapone dose is excreted in urine as parent compound and conjugated glucuronide, biliary excretion appears to be the major route of excretion of this drug. Consequently, administer entacapone with care to patients with biliary obstruction.

Contraindications

Hypersensitivity to the drug or its ingredients.

Warnings/Precautions

➤*Hypotension/Syncope:* Dopaminergic therapy in patients with Parkinson disease has been associated with orthostatic hypotension. Entacapone enhances levodopa bioavailability and, therefore, might be expected to increase the occurrence of orthostatic hypotension. However, in entacapone clinical trials, no differences from placebo were seen for measured orthostasis or symptoms of orthostasis. Orthostatic hypotension was documented at least once in 2.7% and 3% of patients treated with entacapone 200 mg and placebo, respectively. A total of 4.3% and 4% of patients treated with entacapone 200 mg and placebo, respectively, reported orthostatic symptoms at some time during their treatment and also had at least 1 episode of orthostatic hypotension documented (however, the episode of orthostatic symptoms itself was not accompanied by vital sign measurements). Neither baseline treatment with dopamine agonists or selegiline, nor the presence of orthostasis at baseline, increased the risk of orthostatic hypotension in patients treated with entacapone compared with patients receiving placebo.

In the large controlled trials, approximately 1.2% and 0.8% of entacapone 200 mg and placebo patients, respectively, reported at least 1 episode of syncope. Reports of syncope were generally more frequent in patients in both treatment groups who had an episode of documented hypotension (although the episodes of syncope, obtained by patient history, were themselves not documented with vital sign measurement).

➤*Diarrhea:* In clinical trials, diarrhea developed in 60 of 603 (10%) and 16 of 400 (4%) patients treated with entacapone 200 mg and placebo, respectively. In patients treated with entacapone, diarrhea was generally mild to moderate in severity (8.6%) but was regarded as severe in 1.3%. Diarrhea resulted in withdrawal in 10 of 603 (1.7%) patients, 7 (1.2%) with mild and moderate diarrhea and 3 (0.5%) with severe diarrhea. Diarrhea generally resolved after discontinuation of entacapone. Two patients with diarrhea were hospitalized. Typically, diarrhea presents within 4 to 12 weeks after entacapone is started, but it may appear as early as the first week and as late as many months after the initiation of treatment.

➤*Hallucinations:* Dopaminergic therapy in patients with Parkinson disease has been associated with hallucinations. In clinical trials, hallucinations developed in approximately 4% of patients treated with entacapone 200 mg or placebo. Hallucinations led to drug discontinuation and premature withdrawal from clinical trials in 0.8% and 0% of patients treated with entacapone 200 mg and placebo, respectively. Hallucinations led to hospitalization in 1% and 0.3% of patients in the entacapone 200 mg and placebo groups, respectively.

➤*Dyskinesia:* Entacapone may potentiate the dopaminergic adverse effects of levodopa and may cause and/or exacerbate preexisting dyskinesia. Although decreasing the dose of levodopa may ameliorate this adverse effect, many patients in controlled trials continued to experience frequent dyskinesias, despite a reduction in their dose of levodopa. The rates of withdrawal for dyskinesia were 1.5% and 0.8% for entacapone 200 mg and placebo, respectively.

➤*Rhabdomyolysis:* Cases of severe rhabdomyolysis have been reported with entacapone use. The complicated nature of these cases makes it impossible to determine what role, if any, entacapone played in their pathogenesis. Severe prolonged motor activity, including dyskinesia, may account for rhabdomyolysis. One case, however, included fever and alteration of consciousness. It is therefore possible that rhabdomyolysis may be a result of the syndrome described in Hyperpyrexia and Confusion in the following section.

➤*Hyperpyrexia and confusion:* Cases of a symptom complex resembling NMS characterized by elevated temperature, muscular rigidity, altered consciousness, and elevated creatine phosphokinase have been reported in association with rapid dose reduction or withdrawal of other dopaminergic drugs. Several cases with similar signs and symptoms have been reported in association with entacapone therapy, although no information about dose

ENTACAPONE — ORAL

manipulation is available. The complicated nature of these cases makes it difficult to determine what role, if any, entacapone may have played in their pathogenesis. No cases have been reported following the abrupt withdrawal or dose reduction of entacapone treatment during clinical studies.

➤*Discontinuation of treatment:* See Administration and Dosage for more information.

➤*Fibrotic complications:* Cases of retroperitoneal fibrosis, pulmonary infiltrates, pleural effusion, and pleural thickening have been reported in some patients treated with ergot-derived dopaminergic agents. These complications may resolve when the drug is discontinued, but complete resolution does not always occur. Although these adverse reactions are believed to be related to the ergoline structure of these compounds, whether other, nonergot-derived drugs (eg, entacapone) that increase dopaminergic activity can cause them is unknown. It should be noted that the expected incidence of fibrotic complications is so low that even if entacapone caused these complications at rates similar to those attributable to other dopaminergic therapies, it is unlikely that it would have been detected in a cohort of the size exposed to entacapone. Four cases of pulmonary fibrosis were reported during clinical development of entacapone; 3 of these patients were also treated with pergolide and one with bromocriptine. The duration of treatment with entacapone ranged from 7 to 17 months.

➤*Melanoma:* Epidemiological studies have shown that patients with Parkinson disease have a higher risk (2-fold to approximately 6-fold higher) of developing melanoma than the general population. Whether the increased risk observed was because of Parkinson disease or other factors, such as drugs used to treat Parkinson disease, is unclear.

For the reasons previously stated, patients and providers are advised to monitor for melanomas frequently and on a regular basis when using entacapone for any indication. Ideally, periodic skin examination should be performed by appropriately qualified individuals (eg, dermatologists).

➤*Renal toxicity:* In a 1-year toxicity study, entacapone (plasma exposure 20 times that in humans receiving the maximum recommended daily dose [MRDD] of 1,600 mg) caused an increased incidence in male rats of nephrotoxicity that was characterized by regenerative tubules, thickening of basement membranes, infiltration of mononuclear cells, and tubular protein casts. These effects were not associated with changes in clinical chemistry parameters, and there is no established method for monitoring for the possible occurrence of these lesions in humans. Although this toxicity could represent a species-specific effect, there is not yet evidence that this is so.

➤*Drugs metabolized by COMT:* When a single dose of entacapone 400 mg was given together with IV isoprenaline (isoproterenol) and epinephrine without coadministered levodopa/dopa decarboxylase inhibitor, the overall mean maximal changes in heart rate during infusion were approximately 50% and 80% higher than with placebo for isoprenaline and epinephrine, respectively.

Ventricular tachycardia was noted in one 32-year-old healthy man in an interaction study after epinephrine infusion and oral entacapone administration. Treatment with propranolol was required. A causal relationship to entacapone administration appears probable but cannot be attributed with certainty.

➤*Hepatic function impairment:* Treat patients with hepatic impairment with caution. The AUC and C_{max} of entacapone approximately doubled in patients with documented liver disease compared with controls.

➤*Pregnancy: Category C.* In embryofetal development studies, entacapone was administered to pregnant animals throughout organogenesis at dosages of up to 1,000 mg/kg/day in rats and 300 mg/kg/day in rabbits. Increased incidences of fetal variations were evident in litters from rats treated with the highest dose, in the absence of overt signs of maternal toxicity. The maternal plasma drug exposure (AUC) associated with this dose was approximately 34 times the estimated plasma exposure in humans receiving the MRDD of 1,600 mg. Increased frequencies of abortions and late/total resorptions and decreased fetal weights were observed in the litters of rabbits treated with maternotoxic dosages of 100 mg/kg/day (plasma AUCs 0.4 times those in humans receiving the MRDD) or greater. There was no evidence of teratogenicity in these studies.

However, when entacapone was administered to female rats prior to mating and during early gestation, an increased incidence of fetal eye anomalies (macrophthalmia, microphthalmia, anophthalmia) was observed in the litters of dams treated with dosages of 160 mg/kg/day (plasma AUCs 7 times those in humans receiving the MRDD) or greater, in the absence of maternotoxicity. Administration of up to 700 mg/kg/day (plasma AUCs 28 times those in humans receiving the MRDD) to female rats during the latter part of gestation and throughout lactation produced no evidence of developmental impairment in offspring.

There is no experience from clinical studies regarding the use of entacapone in pregnant women. Therefore, use entacapone during pregnancy only if the potential benefit justifies the potential risk to the fetus.

➤*Lactation:* It is not known whether entacapone is excreted in human milk; however, the molecular weight (approximately 305) is low enough that embryo and fetal exposure probably occur, but the short elimination half-life will limit the degree of exposure. Because many drugs are excreted in human milk, exercise caution when entacapone is administered to a breast-feeding woman. In animal studies, entacapone was excreted into maternal rat milk.

➤*Children:* There is no identified potential use of entacapone in children.

➤*Monitoring:* If a decision is made to discontinue treatment with entacapone, closely monitor patients and adjust other dopaminergic treatments as needed.

Monitor for melanomas frequently and on a regular basis when using entacapone for any indication.

Drug Interactions

Entacapone Drug Interactions

Precipitant drug	Object drug[a]		Description
Ampicillin Cholestyramine Chloramphenicol Erythromycin Probenecid Rifampin	Entacapone	↑	As most entacapone excretion is via the bile, exercise caution when drugs known to interfere with biliary excretion, glucuronidation, and intestinal beta-glucuronidase are given concurrently with entacapone.
MAOIs[b] (eg, phenelzine)	Entacapone	↑	Monoamine oxidase and COMT are the 2 major enzyme systems involved in catecholamine metabolism. Therefore, it is theoretically possible that the combination of entacapone and a nonselective MAOI (eg, phenelzine, tranylcypromine) would result in inhibition of the majority of the pathways responsible for normal catecholamine metabolism. For this reason, patients should ordinarily not be treated concomitantly with entacapone and a nonselective MAOI. Entacapone may be taken concomitantly with a selective MAO-B inhibitor (eg, selegiline).
Entacapone	Drugs metabolized by COMT (ie, apomorphine, dobutamine, dopamine, epinephrine, isoproterenol, methyldopa, norepinephrine)	↑	Administer drugs known to be metabolized by COMT with caution in patients receiving entacapone regardless of the route of administration (including inhalation), as their interaction may result in increased heart rates, possibly arrhythmias, and excessive changes in blood pressure (see Warnings/Precautions). Closely monitor the clinical response of the patient.

[a] ↑ = object drug increased.
[b] MAOIs = monoamine oxidase inhibitors.

➤*Drug/Lab test interactions:* Entacapone is a chelator of iron. The impact of entacapone on the body's iron stores is unknown; however, a tendency towards decreasing serum iron concentrations was noted in clinical trials. In a controlled clinical study, serum ferritin levels (as marker of iron deficiency and subclinical anemia) were not changed with entacapone compared with placebo after 1 year of treatment, and there was no difference in rates of anemia or decreased hemoglobin levels.

Adverse Reactions

➤*Discontinuation of treatment:* Approximately 14% of the 603 patients given entacapone in the double-blind, placebo-controlled trials discontinued treatment because of adverse reactions compared with 9% of the 400 patients who received placebo. The most frequent causes of discontinuation in decreasing order are psychiatric reasons (2% vs 1%), diarrhea (2% vs 0%), dyskinesia/hyperkinesia (2% vs 1%), nausea (2% vs 1%), abdominal pain (1% vs 0%), and aggravation of Parkinson disease symptoms (1% vs 1%).

➤*Most common adverse reactions:* The most commonly observed adverse reactions (greater than 5%) in the double-blind, placebo-controlled trials (N = 1,003) associated with the use of entacapone and not seen at an equivalent frequency among placebo-treated patients were abdominal pain, diarrhea, dyskinesia/hyperkinesia, nausea, and urine discoloration.

➤*Adverse reactions (at least 1%):*

Entacapone Adverse Reactions (≥ 1%)

Adverse reaction	Entacapone (n = 603)	Placebo (n = 400)
CNS		
Agitation	1%	0%
Anxiety	2%	1%
Asthenia	2%	1%
Dizziness	8%	6%
Dyskinesia	25%	15%
Fatigue	6%	4%
Hyperkinesia	10%	5%

ENTACAPONE — ORAL

Entacapone Adverse Reactions (≥ 1%)		
Adverse reaction	Entacapone (n = 603)	Placebo (n = 400)
Hypokinesia	9%	8%
Somnolence	2%	0%
GI		
Abdominal pain	8%	4%
Constipation	6%	4%
Diarrhea	10%	4%
Dry mouth	3%	0%
Dyspepsia	2%	1%
Flatulence	2%	0%
Gastritis	1%	0%
GI disorders NOS[a]	1%	0%
Nausea	14%	8%
Vomiting	4%	1%
Miscellaneous		
Back pain	4%	2%
Dyspnea	3%	1%
Infection bacterial	1%	0%
Purpura	2%	1%
Sweating increased	2%	1%
Taste perversion	1%	0%
Urine discoloration	10%	0%

[a] NOS = not otherwise specified.

Overdosage

➤*Symptoms:* There have been no reported cases of either accidental or intentional overdose with entacapone tablets. However, COMT inhibition by entacapone treatment is dose dependent. A massive overdose of entacapone may theoretically produce a 100% inhibition of the COMT enzyme in humans, thereby preventing the metabolism of endogenous and exogenous catechols.

The highest single dose of entacapone administered to humans was 800 mg, resulting in a plasma concentration of 14.1 mcg/mL. The highest daily dose given to humans was 2,400 mg, administered in one study as 400 mg 6 times daily with levodopa/carbidopa for 14 days in 15 patients with Parkinson disease, and in another study as 800 mg 3 times daily for 7 days in 8 healthy volunteers. At this daily dose, the peak plasma concentrations of entacapone averaged 2 mcg/mL (at 45 minutes, compared with 1 and 1.2 mcg/mL with entacapone 200 mg at 45 minutes). Abdominal pain and loose stools were the most commonly observed adverse reactions during this study. Daily doses as high as 2,000 mg of entacapone have been administered as 200 mg 10 times daily with levodopa/carbidopa or levodopa/benserazide for at least 1 year in 10 patients, for at least 2 years in 8 patients, and for at least 3 years in 7 patients. However, overall clinical experience with daily doses above 1,600 mg is limited.

The range of lethal plasma concentrations of entacapone based on animal data was 80 to 130 mcg/mL in mice. Respiratory difficulties, ataxia, hypoactivity, and convulsions were observed in mice after high oral (gavage) doses.

➤*Treatment:* Management of entacapone overdose is symptomatic; there is no known antidote to entacapone. Hospitalization is advised, and general supportive care is indicated. There is no experience with hemodialysis or hemoperfusion, but these procedures are unlikely to be of benefit because entacapone is highly bound to plasma proteins. An immediate gastric lavage and repeated doses of charcoal over time may hasten the elimination of entacapone by decreasing its absorption/reabsorption from the GI tract. Carefully monitor the adequacy of the respiratory and circulatory systems and employ appropriate supportive measures. Bear in mind the possibility of drug interactions, especially with catechol-structured drugs.

Patient Information

Instruct patients to take entacapone only as prescribed.

Inform patients that hallucinations can occur.

Advise patients that they may develop postural (orthostatic) hypotension with or without symptoms such as dizziness, nausea, sweating, and syncope. Hypotension may occur more frequently during initial therapy. Accordingly, caution patients against rising rapidly after sitting or lying down, especially if they have been doing so for prolonged periods, and especially at the initiation of treatment with entacapone.

Advise patients that they should neither drive a car nor operate other complex machinery until they have gained sufficient experience on entacapone to gauge whether or not it affects their mental or motor performance adversely. Because of the possible additive sedative effects, use caution when patients are taking other CNS depressants in combination with entacapone.

Inform patients that nausea may occur, especially at the initiation of treatment with entacapone.

Advise patients of the possibility of an increase in dyskinesia.

Advise patients that treatment with entacapone may cause a change in the color of urine (a brownish orange discoloration) that is not clinically relevant. In controlled trials, 10% of patients treated with entacapone reported urine discoloration compared with 0% of placebo patients.

Although entacapone has not been shown to be teratogenic in animals, it is always given in conjunction with levodopa/carbidopa, which is known to cause visceral and skeletal malformations in rabbits. Accordingly, advise patients to notify their health care provider if they become pregnant or intend to become pregnant during therapy.

Entacapone is excreted into maternal milk in rats. Because of the possibility that entacapone may be excreted into human maternal milk, advise patients to notify their health care provider if they intend to breast-feed or are breast-feeding an infant.

Advise patients that there have been reports of patients experiencing intense urges to gamble, increased sexual urges, and other intense urges and the inability to control these urges while taking one or more of the medications that increase central dopaminergic tone and are generally used for the treatment of Parkinson disease, including entacapone. Although it is not proven that the medications caused these events, these urges were reported to have stopped in some cases when the dose was reduced or the medication was stopped. Advise patients to inform their health care provider if they experience new or increased gambling urges, increased sexual urges, or other intense urges while taking entacapone. Consider dose reduction or stopping the medication if the patient develops such urges while taking entacapone.

CARBIDOPA/LEVODOPA/ENTACAPONE

Rx	**Stalevo 50** (Novartis)	**Tablets; oral:** carbidopa 12.5 mg/levodopa 50 mg/entacapone 200 mg	Mannitol, sucrose. (LCE 50). Brownish- or greyish-red. Film-coated. In 100s and 250s.
Rx	**Stalevo 75** (Novartis)	Carbidopa 18.75 mg/levodopa 75 mg/entacapone 200 mg	Mannitol, sucrose. (LCE 75). Lt. brownish-red, oval. Film-coated. In 100s.
Rx	**Stalevo 100** (Novartis)	Carbidopa 25 mg/levodopa 100 mg/entacapone 200 mg	Mannitol, sucrose. (LCE 100). Brownish- or greyish-red, oval. Film-coated. In 100s and 250s.
Rx	**Stalevo 125** (Novartis)	Carbidopa 31.25 mg/levodopa 125 mg/entacapone 200 mg	Mannitol, sucrose. (LCE 125). Lt. brownish-red, oval. Film-coated. In 100s.
Rx	**Stalevo 150** (Novartis)	Carbidopa 37.5 mg/levodopa 150 mg/entacapone 200 mg	Mannitol, sucrose. (LCE 150). Brownish- or greyish-red, elliptical. Film-coated. In 100s and 250s.
Rx	**Stalevo 200** (Novartis)	Carbidopa 50 mg/levodopa 200 mg/entacapone 200 mg	Mannitol, sucrose. (LCE 200). Dk. brownish-red, oval. Film-coated. In 100s.

CARBIDOPA/LEVODOPA/ENTACAPONE — ORAL

For complete prescribing information on each of the components, refer to the individual monographs. Also refer to the general discussion in the Antiparkinson Agents introduction.

Indications

➤*Parkinson disease:* To treat patients with idiopathic Parkinson disease: to substitute (with equivalent strength of each of the 3 components) for immediate-release carbidopa/levodopa and entacapone previously administered as individual products; or to replace immediate-release carbidopa/levodopa therapy (without entacapone) when patients experience the signs and symptoms of end-of-dose "wearing-off" (only for patients taking a total daily dose of levodopa of 600 mg or less and not experiencing dyskinesias).

Administration and Dosage

➤*General dosing considerations:* Carbidopa/levodopa/entacapone should be used as a substitute for patients already stabilized on equivalent doses of carbidopa/levodopa and entacapone. However, some patients who have been stabilized on a given dose of carbidopa/levodopa may be treated with carbidopa/levodopa/entacapone if a decision has been made to add entacapone.

➤*Adults:*

Parkinson disease –

Usual dosage:

• *Current treatment with entacapone –* Patients who are currently treated with entacapone 200 mg tablet with each dose of standard-release

CARBIDOPA/LEVODOPA/ENTACAPONE — ORAL

carbidopa/levodopa can be directly switched to the corresponding strength of the combination tablet containing the same amounts of levodopa and carbidopa.

• *Not currently treated with entacapone* –

More than 600 mg/day of levodopa: Patients with a history of moderate or severe dyskinesias or taking more than 600 mg/day of levodopa are likely to require a reduction in the daily levodopa dose when entacapone is added to their treatment. Because dose adjustment of the individual components is impossible with fixed-dose products, it is recommended that patients first be titrated individually with a carbidopa/levodopa product (1:4 ratio) and an entacapone product, and then transferred to a corresponding dose of the combination tablet once the patient's status has stabilized.

600 mg/day or less of levodopa: In patients who take a total daily levodopa dose of up to 600 mg and who do not have dyskinesias, an attempt can be made to transfer to the corresponding daily dose of the combination tablet. However, even in these patients, a reduction of carbidopa/levodopa or entacapone may be necessary, and this may not be possible with carbidopa/levodopa/entacapone. Because entacapone prolongs and enhances the effects of levodopa, therapy should be individualized and adjusted if necessary according to the desired therapeutic response.

Maximum dose: 8 tablets per day for all strengths except for the carbidopa 50 mg, levodopa 200 mg, and entacapone 200 mg tablet, which is 6 tablets/day.

Dosage titration: When less levodopa is required, the total daily dosage of carbidopa/levodopa should be reduced by decreasing the strength of carbidopa/levodopa/entacapone at each administration or by decreasing the frequency of administration by extending the time between doses.

When more levodopa is required, the next higher strength of carbidopa/levodopa/entacapone should be taken and/or the frequency of doses should be increased, up to a maximum of 8 times daily (6 times daily of carbidopa 50 mg, levodopa 200 mg, and entacapone 200 mg combination).

Concomitant therapy: Standard drugs for Parkinson disease may be used concomitantly while carbidopa/levodopa/entacapone is being administered, although dosage adjustments may be required.

Discontinuation of therapy:

Patients should be observed carefully if abrupt reduction or discontinuation of carbidopa/levodopa/entacapone is required, especially if the patient is receiving neuroleptics.

Interruption of therapy: If general anesthesia is required, carbidopa/levodopa/entacapone may be continued as long as the patient is permitted to take fluids and medication by mouth. If therapy is interrupted temporarily, observe the patient for symptoms resembling NMS, and the usual daily dosage may be administered as soon as the patient is able to take oral medication.

➤*Administration:* Individual tablets should not be fractionated, and only 1 tablet should be administered at each dosing interval.

➤*Storage/Stability:* Store at 25°C (77°F); excursions are permitted between 15° and 30°C (59° and 86°F).

RASAGILINE

Rx	**Azilect** (Teva)	**Tablets:** 0.5 mg (as base)	Mannitol. (GIL 0.5). White. In 30s.
		1 mg (as base)	Mannitol. (GIL 1). White. In 30s.

RASAGILINE — ORAL

Indications

➤*Parkinson disease:* For the treatment of the signs and symptoms of idiopathic Parkinson disease as initial monotherapy and as adjunct therapy to levodopa.

Administration and Dosage

➤*General dosing considerations:* Hypertensive crisis may result if rasagiline is administered with foods and/or beverages with high tyramine content (see Administration).

➤*Adults:*

Parkinson disease –

Monotherapy: 1 mg once daily.

Adjunctive therapy:

• *Initial dosage* – 0.5 mg once daily.

• *Dosage adjustment* – If a sufficient clinical response is not achieved, the dosage may be increased to 1 mg administered once daily.

• *Concomitant therapy with levodopa* – When rasagiline is used in combination with levodopa, a reduction of the levodopa dosage may be considered based upon individual response.

➤*Hepatic function impairment:* Patients with mild hepatic impairment should use rasagiline 0.5 mg/day. Rasagiline should not be used in patients with moderate or severe hepatic impairment.

➤*Concomitant therapy with CYP1A2 inhibitors:* Patients taking concomitant ciprofloxacin or other CYP1A2 inhibitors should use rasagiline 0.5 mg/day.

➤*Administration:* Rasagiline can be administered with or without food. Tyramine-rich foods (eg, aged cheeses, pickled herring, yeast extract), beverages (eg, some red wines, certain beers), or dietary supplements and amines (from nonprescription cough/cold medications) should be avoided to prevent a possible hypertensive crisis/"cheese reaction" during rasagiline treatment (See Warnings/Precautions).

➤*Storage/Stability:* Store at 25°C (77°F); excursions are permitted to 15° to 30°C (59° to 86°F).

Actions

➤*Pharmacology:* Rasagiline is an irreversible monoamine oxidase (MAO) inhibitor indicated for the treatment of idiopathic Parkinson disease. Rasagiline inhibits MAO type B (MAO-B), but adequate studies to establish whether rasagiline is selective for MAO-B in humans have not yet been conducted.

MAO, a flavin-containing enzyme, is classified into 2 major molecular species, A and B, and is localized in mitochondrial membranes throughout the body in nerve terminals, brain, liver, and intestinal mucosa. MAO regulates the metabolic degradation of catecholamines and serotonin in the CNS and peripheral tissues. MAO-B is the major form in the human brain. In ex vivo animal studies in brain, liver, and intestinal tissues, rasagiline was shown to be a potent, irreversible MAO-B selective inhibitor. Rasagiline at the recommended therapeutic dose also was shown to be a potent and irreversible inhibitor of MAO-B in platelets. The selectivity of rasagiline for inhibiting only MAO-B (and not MAO type A [MAO-A]) in humans and the sensitivity to tyramine during rasagiline treatment at any dose have not been sufficiently characterized to avoid restriction of dietary tyramine and amines contained in medications. The precise mechanisms of action of rasagiline are unknown. One mechanism is believed to be related to its MAO-B inhibitory activity, which causes an increase in extracellular levels of dopamine in the striatum. The elevated dopamine level and subsequent increased dopaminergic activity are likely to mediate rasagiline's beneficial effects seen in models of dopaminergic motor dysfunction.

Pharmacodynamics –

Platelet MAO activity in clinical studies: Studies in healthy subjects and patients with Parkinson disease have shown that rasagiline irreversibly inhibits platelet MAO-B. The inhibition lasts at least 1 week after the last dose. Almost 25% to 35% MAO-B inhibition was achieved after a single dose of rasagiline 1 mg/day and more than 55% of MAO-B inhibition was achieved after a single dose of rasagiline 2 mg/day. Over 90% inhibition was achieved 3 days after rasagiline daily dosing at 2 mg/day and this inhibition level was maintained 3 days postdose. Multiple doses of rasagiline 0.5, 1, and 2 mg/day resulted in complete MAO-B inhibition.

➤*Pharmacokinetics:*

Absorption – Rasagiline's pharmacokinetics are linear with doses over the range of 1 to 10 mg. Rasagiline is rapidly absorbed, reaching peak plasma concentration (C_{max}) in approximately 1 hour. The absolute bioavailability of rasagiline is about 36%.

Food effects: Food does not affect the time to reach maximum concentration (T_{max}) of rasagiline, although C_{max} and exposure (AUC) are decreased by approximately 60% and 20%, respectively, when the drug is taken with a high-fat meal. Because AUC is not significantly affected, rasagiline can be administered with or without food.

Distribution – The mean volume of distribution at steady state is 87 L, indicating that the tissue binding of rasagiline is in excess of plasma protein binding. Plasma protein-binding ranges from 88% to 94%, with mean extent of binding 61% to 63% to human albumin over the concentration range of 1 to 100 ng/mL.

Metabolism/Excretion – Rasagiline undergoes almost complete biotransformation in the liver prior to excretion. The metabolism of rasagiline proceeds through 2 main pathways: N-dealkylation and/or hydroxylation to yield 1-aminoindan (AI), 3-hydroxy-N-propargyl-1 aminoindan (3-OH-PAI) and 3-hydroxy-1-aminoindan (3-OH-AI). In vitro experiments indicate that both routes of rasagiline metabolism are dependent on the cytochrome P-450 (CYP) system, with CYP1A2 being the major isoenzyme involved in rasagiline metabolism. Glucuronide conjugation of rasagiline and its metabolites, with subsequent urinary excretion, is the major elimination pathway.

After oral administration of ^{14}C-labeled rasagiline, elimination occurred primarily via urine and secondarily via feces (62% of total dose in urine and 7% of total dose in feces over 7 days), with a total calculated recovery of 84% of the dose over a period of 38 days. Less than 1% of rasagiline was excreted as unchanged drug in urine.

Its mean steady-state half-life is 3 hours, but there is no correlation of pharmacokinetics with its pharmacological effect because of its irreversible inhibition of MAO-B.

Special populations –

Hepatic function impairment: Following repeat dose administration of rasagiline 1 mg/day for 7 days in subjects with mild hepatic function impairment (Child-Pugh score 5 to 6), AUC and C_{max} were increased by 2- and 1.4-fold, respectively, compared with healthy subjects. In subjects with moderate hepatic function impairment (Child-Pugh score 7 to 9), AUC and C_{max} were increased by 7- and 2-fold, respectively, compared with healthy subjects.

Contraindications

Hypersensitivity to the drug; pheochromocytoma; coadministration with meperidine, methadone, propoxyphene, tramadol, dextromethorphan, St. John's wort, mirtazapine, cyclobenzaprine, sympathomimetic amines

RASAGILINE — ORAL

(including amphetamines, nasal and oral decongestants, cold products, and weight-reducing preparations), other MAO inhibitors, cocaine, and local or general anesthetic agents.

Warnings/Precautions

➤*Hypertensive crisis:* Rasagiline treatment at any dose may be associated with a hypertensive crisis/cheese reaction if the patient ingests tyramine-rich foods, beverages, or dietary supplements or amines (from nonprescription medications). Hypertensive crisis, which in some cases may be fatal, consists of marked systemic blood pressure elevation and requires immediate treatment/hospitalization.

MAO in the GI tract and liver (primarily type A) is thought to provide vital protection from exogenous amines (eg, tyramine) that have the capacity, if absorbed intact, to cause a hypertensive crisis, the so-called cheese reaction. If significant amounts of certain exogenous amines gain access to the systemic circulation (eg, tyramine from fermented cheese, red wine, herring, or amines contained in nonprescription cough/cold medications), they can cause release of norepinephrine, which may significantly increase systemic blood pressure. MAO inhibitors that selectively inhibit MAO-B are generally devoid of the potential to cause a hypertensive crisis/cheese reaction at defined relatively low doses at which tyramine sensitivity has been characterized. The selectivity of rasagiline for inhibiting MAO-B (and not MAO-A) in humans has not been sufficiently characterized to permit rasagiline treatment without restriction of dietary tyramine or amines contained in medications. Even for selective MAO-B inhibitors, the selectivity for inhibiting MAO-B typically diminishes and is ultimately lost as the dose is increased beyond particular dose levels.

Instruct patients receiving rasagiline about the tyramine content of foods and beverages (see the following table) and amine-containing medications that should be avoided. Sympathomimetic amines found in nonprescription medicines to be avoided include ephedrine, phenylephrine, phenylpropanolamine, and pseudoephedrine.

It also is necessary to maintain this dietary tyramine restriction and avoidance of exogenous amines contained in medications for 2 weeks following discontinuation of rasagiline because of the irreversible inhibition of the MAO enzyme and the need for new MAO enzyme synthesis.

Instruct patients about the signs and symptoms of marked blood pressure elevation that could represent a hypertensive emergency requiring immediate treatment/hospitalization. These include the following symptoms: blurred vision/visual disturbances, chest pain, difficulty thinking, severe headache, signs or symptoms of a stroke, stupor/coma, seizures, or unexplained nausea or vomiting. Tell patients to immediately contact their health care provider to report any severe headache or other atypical or unusual symptoms not previously experienced that could be caused by a hypertensive crisis.

Acceptable and Unacceptable Tyramine-Containing Foods and Beverages to Consume When Taking Rasagiline

Class of food or beverage[a]	Tyramine-rich foods and beverages to avoid[a]	Acceptable foods, containing little or no tyramine[a]
Meat, poultry, and fish	Air-dried, aged, and fermented meats, sausages, and salamis (including cacciatore, hard salami, and mortadella); pickled herring; any spoiled or improperly stored meat, poultry, and fish (eg, foods that have undergone changes in coloration, odor, or become moldy); spoiled or improperly stored animal livers	Fresh meat, poultry, and fish, including fresh processed meats (eg, lunch meats, hot dogs, breakfast sausage, and cooked, sliced ham)
Vegetables	Broad bean pods (fava bean pods)	All other vegetables
Dairy	Aged cheeses	Processed cheeses, mozzarella, ricotta cheese, cottage cheese, yogurt
Beverages	All varieties of tap beer, beers that have not been pasteurized so as to allow for ongoing fermentation, red wines	Bottled and canned beers and white wines contain little or no tyramine
Miscellaneous	Concentrated yeast extract (eg, Marmite), sauerkraut, most soybean products (including soy sauce and tofu), OTC supplements containing tyramine	Brewer's yeast, baker's yeast, soy milk, commercial chain-restaurant pizzas prepared with cheeses low in tyramine

[a] Adapted from Shulman KI, Walker SE. *Psychiatric Annals*. 2001;31:378-384.

➤*Melanoma:* Comparison of the rates of melanoma in the rasagiline development program with rates in age- and sex-matched populations from 2 epidemiologic databases (Surveillance, Epidemiology, and End Results Registry of the National Cancer Institute and the American Academy of Dermatology Skin Cancer Screening Program) showed a risk of melanoma that was greater in patients treated with rasagiline than in the general population. Some epidemiological studies, however, have shown that patients with Parkinson disease have a higher risk (perhaps 2- to 4-fold higher) of developing melanoma than the general population, although it was unclear whether the observed increased risk was caused by Parkinson disease or drugs used to treat Parkinson disease. The increased incidence of melanoma in the rasagiline development program was comparable with the increased risk observed in the Parkinson disease populations examined in these epidemiological studies. For these reasons, patients and doctors are advised to monitor for melanomas frequently and on a regular basis. Ideally, periodic skin examinations should be performed by appropriately qualified individuals (eg, dermatologists).

➤*Dyskinesia caused by levodopa treatment:* When used as an adjunct to levodopa, rasagiline may potentiate dopaminergic side effects and exacerbate preexisting dyskinesia (treatment-emergent dyskinesia occurred in about 18% of patients treated with rasagiline 0.5 or 1 mg as an adjunct to levodopa, and 10% of patients who received placebo as an adjunct to levodopa). Decreasing the dose of levodopa may ameliorate this side effect.

➤*Postural hypotension:* When used as monotherapy, postural hypotension was reported in approximately 3% of patients treated with rasagiline 1 mg and 5% of patients treated with placebo. In the monotherapy trial, postural hypotension did not lead to drug discontinuation and premature withdrawal in the rasagiline- or placebo-treated patients.

When used as an adjunct to levodopa, postural hypotension was reported in approximately 6% of patients treated with rasagiline 0.5 mg, 9% of patients treated with rasagiline 1 mg, and 3% of patients treated with placebo. Postural hypotension led to drug discontinuation and premature withdrawal from clinical trials in 1 (0.7%) patient treated with rasagiline 1 mg/day, no patients treated with rasagiline 0.5 mg/day, and no placebo-treated patients.

Clinical trial data suggest that postural hypotension occurs most frequently in the first 2 months of rasagiline treatment and tends to decrease over time.

➤*Hallucinations:* In the monotherapy study, hallucinations were reported as an adverse reaction in 1.3% of patients treated with rasagiline 1 mg and in 0.7% of patients treated with placebo. In the monotherapy trial, hallucinations led to drug discontinuation and premature withdrawal from clinical trials in 1.3% of the rasagiline 1 mg–treated patients and none of the placebo-treated patients.

When used as an adjunct to levodopa, hallucinations were reported as an adverse reaction in approximately 5% of patients treated with 0.5 mg/day, 4% of patients treated with rasagiline 1 mg/day, and 3% of patients treated with placebo. Hallucinations led to drug discontinuation and premature withdrawal from clinical trials in about 1% of patients treated with 0.5 or 1 mg/day and none of the placebo-treated patients. Caution patients of the possibility of developing hallucinations and instruct patients to report them to their health care provider promptly if they develop.

➤*Hepatic function impairment:* Rasagiline plasma concentration may increase in patients with mild (up to 2-fold; Child-Pugh score 5 to 6), moderate (up to 7-fold; Child-Pugh score 7 to 9), and severe (Child-Pugh score 10 to 15) hepatic function impairment. Give patients with mild hepatic function impairment the dose of 0.5 mg/day. Do not use rasagiline in patients with moderate or severe hepatic function impairment.

➤*Pregnancy:* *Category C.* In a study in which pregnant rats were dosed with rasagiline 0.1, 0.3, and 1 mg/kg/day orally, from the beginning of organogenesis to day 20 postpartum, offspring survival was decreased and offspring body weight was reduced at doses of 0.3 and 1 mg/kg/day (10 and 16 times the expected plasma rasagiline exposure [AUC] at the MRHD).

No plasma data were available at the no-effect dose (0.1 mg/kg); however, that dose is 1 times the MRHD on a mg/m^2 basis. Rasagiline's effect on physical and behavioral development was not adequately assessed in this study.

Rasagiline may be given as an adjunct therapy to levodopa/carbidopa treatment. In a study in which pregnant rats were dosed with rasagiline 0.1, 0.3, and 1 mg/kg/day, and levodopa/carbidopa 80/20 mg/kg/day (alone and in combination) throughout the period of organogenesis, there was an increased incidence of wavy ribs in fetuses from rats treated with rasagiline in combination with levodopa/carbidopa at 1/80/20 mg/kg/day (approximately 8 times the plasma AUC expected in humans at the MRHD and

RASAGILINE — ORAL

1/1 times the MRHD of levodopa/carbidopa [800/200 mg/day] on a mg/m² basis). In a study in which pregnant rabbits were dosed throughout the period of organogenesis with rasagiline 3 mg/kg alone or in combination with levodopa/carbidopa (rasagiline 0.1, 0.6, and 1.2 mg/kg; levodopa/carbidopa 80/20 mg/kg/day), an increase in embryo fetal death was noted at rasagiline doses of 0.6 and 1.2 mg/kg/day when administered in combination with levodopa/carbidopa (approximately 7 and 13 times, respectively, the plasma rasagiline AUC at the MRHD). There was an increase in cardiovascular abnormalities with levodopa/carbidopa alone (1/1 times the MRHD on a mg/m² basis) and to a greater extent when rasagiline (at all doses; 1 to 13 times the plasma rasagiline AUC at the MRHD) was administered in combination with levodopa/carbidopa.

There are no adequate and well-controlled studies of rasagiline in pregnant women. Therefore, use rasagiline during pregnancy only if the potential benefit justifies the potential risk to the fetus.

➤*Lactation:* In rats, rasagiline was shown to inhibit prolactin secretion and it may inhibit milk secretion in females. It is not known whether rasagiline is excreted in human milk. Because many drugs are excreted in human milk, exercise caution when rasagiline is administered to a breast-feeding woman.

➤*Children:* The safety and efficacy of rasagiline in children have not been studied.

➤*Monitoring:* Patients and doctors are advised to monitor for melanomas frequently and on a regular basis. Qualified individuals (eg, dermatologist) should perform periodic skin examinations.

Drug Interactions

Rasagiline Drug Interactions

Precipitant drug	Object drug[a]		Description
Ciprofloxacin	Rasagiline	↑	Rasagiline AUC increased 83% with coadministration.
CYP1A2 inhibitors (eg, atazanavir, mexiletine, tacrine)	Rasagiline	↑	With coadministration, rasagiline plasma concentrations may increase up to 2-fold in patients, resulting in increased adverse reactions.
Rasagiline	Anesthetics	↑	Patients taking rasagiline should not undergo elective surgery requiring general anesthesia. Do not give cocaine or local anesthesia containing sympathomimetic vasoconstrictors. Discontinue rasagiline at least 14 days prior to elective surgery.
Rasagiline	Antidepressants (eg, tricyclic antidepressants, SSRIs, SNRIs, mirtazapine)	↑	Severe CNS toxicity associated with hyperpyrexia and death has been reported with coadministration of nonselective MAO inhibitors or selective MAO-B inhibitors and antidepressants. This has not been reported with rasagiline; however, in general, avoid this combination. At least 14 days should elapse between discontinuation of rasagiline and initiation of treatment with an antidepressant. At least 5 weeks should elapse between discontinuation of fluoxetine and initiation of rasagiline.
Rasagiline	Cyclobenzaprine	↑	Because cyclobenzaprine is structurally related to tricyclic antidepressants, coadministration with rasagiline is contraindicated.
Rasagiline	Dextromethorphan	↑	The combination of MAO inhibitors and dextromethorphan has been reported to cause brief episodes of psychosis and bizarre behavior. Rasagiline is contraindicated with dextromethorphan.
Rasagiline	Levodopa	↑	Rasagiline may potentiate dopaminergic adverse reactions and exacerbate dyskinesia. May need to reduce the dose of levodopa.
Rasagiline	MAO inhibitors	↑	Rasagiline coadministered with other MAO inhibitors may lead to a hypertensive crisis because of the increased risk of nonselective MAO inhibition. At least 14 days should elapse between discontinuation of rasagiline and initiation of treatment with MAO inhibitors.
Rasagiline	Meperidine, other analgesics (eg, methadone, propoxyphene, tramadol)	↑	Rasagiline is contraindicated with meperidine. Serious reactions (eg, coma, severe hypertension or hypotension, severe respiratory depression, convulsions, death) have been precipitated with coadministration of meperidine with MAO inhibitors. This warning is extended to other analgesics. At least 14 days should elapse between discontinuation of rasagiline and initiation of treatment with meperidine.
Rasagiline	St. John's wort	↑	Coadministration is contraindicated.
Rasagiline	Sympathomimetics	↑	Rasagiline is contraindicated with sympathomimetic amines, including amphetamines, cold products, and anorexiants. Severe hypertensive reactions have followed the coadministration of sympathomimetics and nonselective MAO inhibitors.

[a] ↑ = Object drug increased.

➤*Drug/Food interactions:* Hypertensive crisis may result if rasagiline is administered with foods and/or beverages with high tyramine content.

Adverse Reactions

During the clinical development of rasagiline, 1,361 patients with Parkinson disease received rasagiline as initial monotherapy or as adjunct therapy to levodopa. As these 2 populations differ, not only in the adjunct use of levodopa during rasagiline treatment but also in the severity and duration of their disease, they may have differential risks for various adverse reactions. Therefore, most of the adverse reactions data in this section are presented separately for each population.

➤*Initial monotherapy treatment:*

Discontinuation of treatment – In the double-blind, placebo-controlled trials conducted in patients receiving rasagiline as monotherapy, approximately 5% of the 149 patients treated with rasagiline discontinued treatment because of adverse reactions, compared with 2% of the 151 patients who received placebo. The only adverse reaction that led to the discontinuation of more than 1 patient was hallucinations.

Adverse reaction incidence in controlled clinical studies – The most commonly observed adverse reactions that occurred in at least 5% of patients receiving rasagiline 1 mg as monotherapy (n = 149) participating in the double-blind, placebo-controlled trial and that were at least 1.5 times the incidence in the placebo group (n = 151) were arthralgia, depression, dyspepsia, fall, and flu syndrome.

The following table lists treatment-emergent adverse reactions that occurred in at least 2% of patients receiving rasagiline as monotherapy participating in the double-blind, placebo-controlled trial and that were numerically more frequent than in the placebo group.

Rasagiline Adverse Reactions in Monotherapy Patients (≥ 2%)[a]

Adverse reaction	Rasagiline 1 mg (n = 149)	Placebo (n = 151)
CNS		
Depression	5%	2%
Fall	5%	3%
Headache	14%	12%
Malaise	2%	0%
Paresthesia	2%	1%
Vertigo	2%	1%
Dermatologic		
Ecchymosis	2%	0%
GI		
Dyspepsia	7%	4%
Gastroenteritis	3%	1%

RASAGILINE — ORAL

Rasagiline Adverse Reactions in Monotherapy Patients (≥ 2%)[a]		
Adverse reaction	Rasagiline 1 mg (n = 149)	Placebo (n = 151)
Musculoskeletal		
Arthralgia	7%	4%
Arthritis	2%	1%
Respiratory		
Rhinitis	3%	1%
Miscellaneous		
Conjunctivitis	3%	1%
Fever	3%	1%
Flu syndrome	5%	1%
Neck pain	2%	0%

[a] Incidence at least 2% in the rasagiline 1 mg group and numerically more frequent than in the placebo group.

Adverse reactions (at least 1%) – Other reactions of potential clinical importance reported by 1% or more of patients receiving rasagiline as monotherapy, and at least as frequent as in the placebo group, in descending order of frequency include the following: dizziness, diarrhea, chest pain, albuminuria, allergic reaction, alopecia, angina pectoris, anorexia, asthma, hallucinations, impotence, leukopenia, libido decreased, abnormal liver function tests, skin carcinoma, syncope, vesiculobullous rash, vomiting.

➤*Adjunct to levodopa therapy:*

Discontinuation of treatment – In a double-blind, placebo-controlled trial (study 1) conducted in patients treated with rasagiline as adjunct to levodopa therapy, approximately 9% of the 164 patients treated with rasagiline 0.5 mg/day and 7% of the 149 patients treated with rasagiline 1 mg/day discontinued treatment because of adverse reactions, compared with 6% of the 159 patients who received placebo. Adverse reaction reporting was considered more reliable for study 1 than for the second controlled trial (study 2); therefore, only the adverse reaction data from study 1 are presented in this section.

The adverse reactions that led to discontinuation of more than 1 rasagiline-treated patient were diarrhea, weight loss, hallucination, and rash.

Adverse reactions in controlled clinical studies – The most commonly observed adverse reactions that occurred in at least 5% of patients receiving rasagiline 1 mg (n = 149) as adjunct to levodopa therapy participating in the double-blind, placebo-controlled trial (study 1) and that were at least 1.5 times the incidence in the placebo group (n = 159) in descending order of difference in incidence were dyskinesia, accidental injury, weight loss, postural hypotension, vomiting, anorexia, arthralgia, abdominal pain, nausea, constipation, dry mouth, rash, ecchymosis, somnolence and paresthesia.

The following table lists treatment-emergent adverse reactions that occurred in at least 2% of patients treated with, rasagiline 1 mg/day as adjunct to levodopa therapy participating in the double-blind, placebo-controlled trial (study 1) and that were numerically more frequent than in the placebo group. The table also shows the rates for the 0.5 mg group in study 1.

Rasagiline Adverse Reactions as Adjunct to Levodopa Therapy (≥ 2%)[a]			
Adverse reaction	Rasagiline 1 mg + Levodopa (n = 149)	Rasagiline 0.5 mg + Levodopa (n = 164)	Placebo + Levodopa (n = 159)
Cardiovascular			
Postural hypotension	9%	6%	3%
CNS			
Abnormal dreams	4%	1%	1%
Ataxia	3%	6%	1%
Dyskinesia	18%	18%	10%
Dystonia	3%	2%	1%
Fall	11%	12%	8%
Hallucinations	4%	5%	3%
Headache	11%	8%	10%
Paresthesia	5%	2%	3%
Somnolence	6%	4%	4%
Dermatologic			
Ecchymosis	5%	2%	3%
Rash	6%	3%	3%
Sweating	3%	2%	1%
GI			
Abdominal pain	5%	2%	1%
Anorexia	5%	2%	1%
Constipation	9%	4%	5%
Diarrhea	5%	7%	4%
Dry mouth	6%	2%	3%
Dyspepsia	5%	4%	4%
Nausea	12%	10%	8%
Vomiting	7%	4%	1%
Musculoskeletal			
Arthralgia	8%	6%	4%
Myasthenia	2%	2%	1%
Tenosynovitis	3%	1%	0%
Miscellaneous			
Accidental injury	12%	8%	5%
Dyspnea	3%	5%	2%
Gingivitis	2%	1%	1%
Hemorrhage	2%	1%	1%
Hernia	2%	1%	1%
Infection	3%	2%	2%
Neck pain	3%	1%	1%
Weight loss	9%	2%	3%

[a] Incidence at least 2% in the rasagiline 1 mg group and numerically more frequent than in the placebo group.

Several of the more common adverse reactions seemed dose-related, including weight loss, postural hypotension, and dry mouth.

Adverse reactions (at least 1%): Other reactions of potential clinical importance reported in study 1 by 1% or more of patients treated with rasagiline 1 mg/day as adjunct to levodopa therapy, and at least as frequent as in the placebo group, in descending order of frequency include the following: skin carcinoma, anemia, albuminuria, amnesia, arthritis, bursitis, cerebrovascular accident, confusion, dysphagia, epistaxis, leg cramps, pruritus, skin ulcer.

There were no significant differences in the safety profile based on age or gender.

➤*Cardiovascular:* Bundle branch block (at least 1%); deep thrombophlebitis, heart failure, myocardial infarct, phlebitis, ventricular tachycardia (0.1% to 1%); arterial thrombosis, atrial arrhythmia, AV block complete, AV block second degree, bigeminy, cerebral hemorrhage, cerebral ischemia, ventricular fibrillation (less than 0.1%).

➤*CNS:* Abnormal gait, anxiety, hyperkinesia, hypertonia, neuropathy, tremor (at least 1%); agitation, aphasia, circumoral paresthesia, convulsion, delusions, dementia, dysarthria, dysautonomia, dysesthesia, emotional lability, facial paralysis, foot drop, hemiplegia, hypesthesia, incoordination, manic reaction, migraine, myoclonus, neuritis, neurosis, paranoid reaction, personality disorder, psychosis, wrist drop (0.1% to 1%); apathy, delirium, hostility, manic depressive reaction, myelitis, neuralgia, psychotic depression, stupor (less than 0.1%).

➤*Dermatologic:* Eczema, urticaria (0.1% to 1%); exfoliative dermatitis, leukoderma (less than 0.1%).

➤*GI:* GI hemorrhage (at least 1%); colitis, esophageal ulcer, esophagitis, fecal incontinence, intestinal obstruction, mouth ulceration, stomach ulcer, stomatitis, tongue edema (0.1% to 1%); hematemesis, hemorrhagic gastritis, intestinal perforation, intestinal stenosis, jaundice, large intestine perforation, megacolon, melena (less than 0.1%).

➤*GU:* Hematuria, urinary incontinence (at least 1%); abnormal sexual function, acute kidney failure, dysmenorrhea, dysuria, kidney calculus, nocturia, polyuria, scrotal edema, urinary retention, urination impaired, vaginal hemorrhage, vaginal moniliasis, vaginitis (0.1% to 1%); abnormal ejaculation, amenorrhea, anuria, epididymitis, gynecomastia, hydroureter, leukorrhea, priapism (less than 0.1%).

➤*Hematologic/Lymphatic:* Macrocytic anemia (0.1% to 1%); purpura, thrombocythemia (less than 0.1%).

➤*Musculoskeletal:* Bone necrosis, muscle atrophy (0.1% to 1%); arthrosis (less than 0.1%).

➤*Respiratory:* Increased cough (at least 1%); apnea, emphysema, laryngismus, pleural effusion, pneumothorax (0.1% to 1%); interstitial pneumonia, larynx edema, lung fibrosis (less than 0.1%).

RASAGILINE — ORAL

➤*Special senses:* Blepharitis, deafness, diplopia, eye hemorrhage, eye pain, glaucoma, keratitis, ptosis, retinal degeneration, taste perversion, visual field defect (0.1% to 1%); blindness, parosmia, photophobia, retinal detachment, retinal hemorrhage, strabismus, taste loss, vestibular disorder (less than 0.1%).

➤*Miscellaneous:* Asthenia (at least 1%); chills, face edema, flank pain, hypocalcemia, photosensitivity reaction (0.1% to 1%).

Overdosage

No cases of rasagiline overdose were reported in clinical trials. Rasagiline was well tolerated in a single-dose study in healthy volunteers receiving 20 mg/day and in a 10-day study in healthy volunteers receiving 10 mg/day. Adverse reactions were mild or moderate. In a dose escalation study in patients on chronic levodopa therapy treated with rasagiline 10 mg, there were 3 reports of cardiovascular side effects (including hypertension and postural hypotension), which resolved following treatment discontinuation.

➤*Symptoms:* Symptoms of overdosage, although not observed with rasagiline during clinical development, may resemble those observed with nonselective MAO inhibitors. Although no cases of overdose have been observed with rasagiline, the following description of presenting symptoms and clinical course is based upon overdose descriptions of nonselective MAO inhibitors.

Characteristically, signs and symptoms of nonselective MAO inhibitor overdose may not appear immediately. Delays of up to 12 hours between ingestion of drug and the appearance of signs may occur. Importantly, the peak intensity of the syndrome may not be reached for upwards of a day following the overdose. Death has been reported following overdosage. Therefore, immediate hospitalization, with continuous patient observation and monitoring for a period of at least 2 days following the ingestion of such drugs in overdose, is strongly recommended.

The clinical picture of MAO inhibitor overdose varies considerably; its severity may be a function of the amount of drug consumed. The CNS and cardiovascular system are prominently involved.

Signs and symptoms of overdosage may include, alone or in combination, any of the following: drowsiness, dizziness, faintness, irritability, hyperactivity, agitation, severe headache, hallucinations, trismus, opisthotonos, convulsions, and coma; rapid and irregular pulse, hypertension, hypotension and vascular collapse; precordial pain, respiratory depression and failure, hyperpyrexia, diaphoresis, and cool, clammy skin.

➤*Treatment:* There is no specific antidote for rasagiline overdose. The following suggestions are offered based upon the assumption that rasagiline overdose may be modeled after nonselective MAO inhibitor poisoning. Treatment of overdose with nonselective MAO inhibitors is symptomatic and supportive. Support respiration by appropriate measures, including management of the airway, use of supplemental oxygen, and mechanical ventilatory assistance, as required. Monitor body temperature closely. Intensive management of hyperpyrexia may be required. Maintenance of fluid and electrolyte balance is essential. Call a poison control center for the most current treatment guidelines.

Patient Information

Inform patients and caregivers about which foods and beverages to avoid because of high tyramine content. Inform patients and caregivers that a hypertensive crisis could occur after ingestion of certain foods (eg, aged cheeses, pickled herring, yeast extract) or beverages (eg, some red wines, certain beers) containing significant amounts of tyramine, or amines contained in some medications, including some nonprescription cough/cold medications. Foods high in tyramine content include those that have undergone protein change by aging, fermentation, pickling, or smoking to improve flavor such as aged cheeses, air-dried meats, sauerkraut, soy sauce, tap/draft beers, and red wines. The tyramine content of any protein-rich food may be increased if stored for long periods or improperly refrigerated.

Inform patients and caregivers of the signs and symptoms associated with hypertensive crisis, including severe headache, blurred vision, difficulty thinking, seizures, chest pain, unexplained nausea or vomiting, or signs or symptoms of a stroke. Patients and caregivers should seek immediate medical attention for patients who develop any severe headache or other atypical or unusual symptoms not previously experienced.

Patients should inform health care provider if they are taking, or planning to take, any prescription or nonprescription drugs, especially antidepressants and nonprescription cold medications, because there is a potential for interaction with rasagiline. Patients should not use meperidine with rasagiline.

Advise patients taking rasagiline as adjunct to levodopa that there is the possibility of increased dyskinesia and postural hypotension.

Advise patients to monitor for melanomas frequently and on a regular basis. Ideally, periodic skin examinations should be performed by appropriately qualified individuals (eg, dermatologists).

Instruct patients to take rasagiline as prescribed. If a dose is missed, the patient should not double the dose of rasagiline to catch up. The next dose should be taken at the usual time on the following day.

SELEGILINE

Rx	**Selegiline Hydrochloride** (Various, eg, Apotex)	**Tablets; oral:** 5 mg	May contain lactose. In 60s and 500s.
Rx	**Zelapar** (Valeant Pharmaceuticals)	**Tablets, lyophilized disintegrating; oral:** 1.25 mg	As selegiline hydrochloride. Aspartame, mannitol, phenylalanine 1.25 mg. (V). Pale yellow. Grapefruit flavor. In blister card 60s.
Rx	**Selegiline Hydrochloride** (Various, eg, Apotex)	**Capsules; oral:** 5 mg	May contain lactose. In 60s, 500s, and 1,000s.
Rx	**Eldepryl** (Somerset)		As selegiline hydrochloride. Lactose. (Eldepryl 5 mg). Aqua blue. In 60s.
Rx	**Emsam** (Dey)	**Patch; transdermal:** 6 mg per 24 h	(20 mg per 20 cm^2). In box of 30s.
		9 mg per 24 h	(30 mg per 30 cm^2). In box of 30s.
		12 mg per 24 h	(40 mg per 40 cm^2). In box of 30s.

SELEGILINE HYDROCHLORIDE (L-deprenyl) — ORAL

For more information, refer to the general discussion in the Antiparkinson Agents introduction.

Indications

➤*Parkinson disease:* As an adjunct in the management of patients with Parkinson disease being treated with levodopa/carbidopa who exhibit deterioration in the quality of their response to this therapy.

Administration and Dosage

➤*Adults:*

Parkinson disease –

Capsules/Tablets:

• *Usual dosage* – 5 mg taken at breakfast and lunch (10 mg/day) with concomitant levodopa/carbidopa therapy.

• *Maximum dose* – 10 mg/day.

• *Concomitant therapy with levodopa/carbidopa* – After 2 to 3 days, an attempt may be made to reduce the dose of levodopa/carbidopa. A reduction of 10% to 30% was achieved with the typical participant who was assigned to selegiline treatment in the domestic placebo-controlled trials. Further reductions of levodopa/carbidopa may be possible during continued selegiline therapy.

Orally disintegrating tablets:

• *Maximum dose* – 2.5 mg/day.

• *Initial dosage* – 1.25 mg given once a day for at least 6 weeks with concomitant levodopa/carbidopa.

• *Dosage titration* – After 6 weeks, the dose may be escalated to 2.5 mg given once a day if the desired benefit has not been achieved and the patient is tolerating selegiline.

➤*Children:* The effects of capsules/tablets in children have not been evaluated; the effects of orally disintegrating tablets in children younger than 16 years of age have not been evaluated.

➤*Administration:* Take orally disintegrating tablets in the morning before breakfast, without liquid. Do not attempt to push tablets through the foil backing; peel back the backing of 1 or 2 blisters (as prescribed) with dry hands and gently remove the tablet(s). Immediately place tablet on top of the tongue, where it will disintegrate in seconds. Avoid ingesting food or liquids for 5 minutes before and after administration.

➤*Storage/Stability:* Store capsules and tablets at 20° to 25°C (68° to 77°F). Store orally disintegrating tablets at 25°C (77°F); excursions are permitted between 15° and 30°C (59° and 86°F). Use within 3 months of opening pouch and immediately upon opening individual blister. Store blister tablets in pouch. Potency cannot be guaranteed after 3 months of opening the pouch.

Actions

➤*Pharmacology:* The mechanisms accounting for selegiline's beneficial adjunctive action in the treatment of Parkinson disease are not fully understood. Inhibition of monoamine oxidase type B (MAO-B) activity is generally considered to be of primary importance; in addition, there is evidence that selegiline may act through other mechanisms to increase dopaminergic activity.

Selegiline is best known as an irreversible inhibitor of MAO, an intracellular enzyme associated with the outer membrane of mitochondria. Selegiline inhibits MAO by acting as a "suicide" substrate for the enzyme; that is, it is converted by MAO to an active moiety that combines irreversibly with the active site and/or the enzyme's essential flavin adenine dinucleotide cofactor. Because selegiline has greater affinity for type B than for type A active sites, it can serve as a selective inhibitor of MAO-B if it is administered at the

SELEGILINE HYDROCHLORIDE (L-deprenyl) — ORAL

recommended dose. However, even for "selective" MAO-B inhibitors, the selectivity for inhibiting MAO-B typically diminishes and is ultimately lost as the dose is increased beyond particular dose levels.

Although rare, a few reports of hypertensive reactions have occurred in patients receiving selegiline at the recommended dose (a dose believed to be selective for MAO-B) with tyramine-containing foods. The pathophysiology of the cheese reaction is complicated and, in addition to its ability to inhibit MAO-B selectively, selegiline's relative freedom from this reaction has been attributed to an ability to prevent tyramine and other indirect-acting sympathomimetics from displacing norepinephrine from adrenergic neurons. However, until the pathophysiology of the cheese reaction is more completely understood, it seems prudent to assume that selegiline can ordinarily only be used safely without dietary restrictions in dosages at which it presumably selectively inhibits MAO-B (eg, 10 mg/day [capsules/tablets] or 2.5 mg/day [orally disintegrating tablets]). Safe use of selegiline orally disintegrating tablets at dosages above 2.5 mg/day without dietary tyramine restrictions has not been established.

➤*Pharmacokinetics:*

Absorption – The absolute bioavailability of selegiline following oral dosing is not known. Single oral dose studies do not predict multiple-dose kinetics. At steady state, the peak plasma level of selegiline is 4-fold that obtained following a single dose. Metabolite concentrations increase to a lesser extent, averaging 2-fold that seen after a single dose.

Selegiline orally disintegrating tablets disintegrate within seconds after placement on the tongue and are rapidly absorbed. Detectable levels of selegiline from orally disintegrating tablets have been measured at 5 minutes after administration, the earliest time point examined.

Selegiline is more rapidly absorbed from the 1.25 or 2.5 mg dose of orally disintegrating tablets (time to maximum concentration [T_{max}] range, 10 to 15 minutes) than from the swallowed selegiline 5 mg tablets (T_{max} range, 40 to 90 minutes). Mean (standard deviation [SD]) maximum plasma concentrations of 3.34 (1.68) and 4.47 (2.56) ng/mL are reached after single doses of 1.25 and 2.5 mg orally disintegrating tablets, compared with 1.12 ng/mL (1.48) for the swallowed selegiline 5 mg tablets (given as 5 mg twice daily). On a dose-normalized basis, the relative bioavailability of selegiline from orally disintegrating tablets is greater than from the swallowed formulation.

The pregastric absorption from selegiline orally disintegrating tablets and the avoidance of first-pass metabolism results in higher concentrations of selegiline and lower concentrations of the metabolites compared with the swallowed selegiline 5 mg tablet.

Upon repeat dosing, accumulation in the plasma concentration of selegiline is observed both with selegiline orally disintegrating tablets and the swallowed 5 mg tablet. Steady state is achieved after 8 days.

Effect of food: The bioavailability of selegiline is increased 3- to 4-fold when it is taken with food.

When selegiline orally disintegrating tablets are taken with food, the maximum drug concentration (C_{max}) and area under the curve (AUC) of selegiline are about 60% of those seen when taken in the fasted state. Because selegiline is placed on the tongue and absorbed through the oral mucosa, avoid the intake of food and liquid 5 minutes before and after selegiline administration.

Distribution – Up to 85% of plasma selegiline is reversibly bound to proteins.

Metabolism – Selegiline undergoes extensive metabolism, presumably attributable to presystemic clearance in gut and liver. The major plasma metabolites are N-desmethylselegiline, L-amphetamine, and L-methamphetamine. Only N-desmethylselegiline has MAO-B inhibiting activity. The peak plasma levels of these metabolites following a single oral dose of 10 mg are from 4 to almost 20 times greater than that of the C_{max} of selegiline (1 ng/mL). The maximum concentrations of amphetamine and methamphetamine, however, are far below those ordinarily expected to produce clinically important effects.

Selegiline is metabolized in vivo to 1-methamphetamine and desemthylselegiline, and subsequently to 1-amphetamine; which, in turn, are further metabolized to their hydroxymetabolites.

In vitro metabolism studies indicate that CYP2B6 and CYP3A4 are involved in the metabolism of selegiline. CYP2A6 may play a minor role in the metabolism.

Excretion – The extent of systemic exposure to selegiline at a given dose varies considerably among individuals. Estimates of systemic clearance of selegiline are not available. Following a single oral dose, the mean elimination half-life of selegiline is 2 hours (1.3 hours at the 1.25 mg orally disintegrating dose). Under steady-state conditions, the elimination half-life increases to 10 hours.

Following metabolism in the liver, selegiline is excreted primarily in the urine as metabolites (mainly as L-methamphetamine) and as a small amount in the feces.

Special populations –

Elderly: Although a general conclusion about the effects of age on the pharmacokinetics of selegiline is not warranted because of the size of the sample evaluated (12 subjects older than 60 years of age, 12 subjects between 18 and 30 years of age), systemic exposure was about twice as great in older subjects compared with a younger population given a single oral dose of 10 mg.

Contraindications

Hypersensitivity to any formulation of selegiline or any of the active ingredients in the formulation; use with dextromethorphan, other MAO inhibitors (MAOIs), meperidine, methadone, propoxyphene, and tramadol.

Warnings/Precautions

➤*Maximum dose:* See Administration and Dosage for more information.

The selectivity of selegiline for MAO-B may not be absolute even at the recommended daily dosage of 10 mg/day (capsules/tablets) or 2.5 mg/day (orally disintegrating tablets). Even for "selective" MAO-B inhibitors, the selectivity for inhibiting MAO-B typically diminishes and is ultimately lost as the dose is increased beyond particular dose levels. Rare cases of hypertensive reactions associated with ingestion of tyramine-containing foods have been reported in patients taking the recommended daily dose of selegiline, a dose that is generally believed to be selective for MAO-B. The selectivity is further diminished with increasing daily doses. Obviously, any selectivity is further diminished with increasing daily doses. An increase in tyramine sensitivity for blood pressure responses appears to occur beginning at a 5 mg daily dose. The precise dosage at which selegiline becomes a nonselective inhibitor of all MAO is unknown, but may be in the range of 30 to 40 mg/day.

➤*CNS toxicity:* Severe CNS toxicity associated with hyperpyrexia and death has been reported with the combination of tricyclic antidepressants and nonselective MAOIs (phenelzine, tranylcypromine). A similar reaction has been reported for a patient on amitriptyline and selegiline. Another patient receiving protriptyline and selegiline developed tremors, agitation, and restlessness, followed by unresponsiveness and death 2 weeks after selegiline was added. Related adverse reactions, including hypertension, syncope, asystole, diaphoresis, seizures, changes in behavioral and mental status, muscular rigidity, and death, also have been reported in some patients receiving selegiline and various tricyclic antidepressants.

Serious, sometimes fatal reactions with signs and symptoms that may include hyperthermia, rigidity, myoclonus, autonomic instability with rapid fluctuations of the vital signs, and mental status changes that include extreme agitation progressing to delirium and coma have been reported in patients receiving a combination of selective serotonin reuptake inhibitors (SSRIs), including fluoxetine, fluvoxamine, sertraline, paroxetine, and nonselective MAOIs or the selective MAO-B inhibitor selegiline. Similar reactions have been reported with serotonin norepinephrine reuptake inhibitors (SNRIs), including venlafaxine.

Because the mechanisms of these reactions are not fully understood, it seems prudent, in general, to avoid this combination of selegiline and tricyclic antidepressants, as well as selegiline and SSRIs. At least 14 days should elapse between discontinuation of selegiline and initiation of treatment with a tricyclic antidepressant or SSRIs. Because of the long half-lives of fluoxetine and its active metabolite, at least 5 weeks (perhaps longer, especially if fluoxetine has been prescribed chronically or at higher doses) should elapse between discontinuation of fluoxetine and initiation of treatment with selegiline.

➤*Levodopa adverse reactions:* Some patients given selegiline may experience an exacerbation of levodopa-associated adverse reactions, presumably caused by the increased amounts of dopamine with super-sensitive, postsynaptic receptors. These effects may often be mitigated by reducing the dose of levodopa/carbidopa by approximately 10% to 30%. For example, in the study demonstrating the efficacy of orally disintegrating tablets, there was an average 24% reduction in levodopa/carbidopa dosage in the 17% of patients who experienced a dose reduction during selegiline orally disintegrating tablet treatment.

➤*Atypical responses:* The decision to prescribe selegiline should take into consideration that the MAO system of enzymes is complex and incompletely understood, and there is only a limited amount of carefully documented clinical experience with selegiline. Consequently, the full spectrum of possible responses to selegiline may not have been observed in premarketing evaluation of the drug. Therefore, it is advisable to observe patients closely for atypical responses.

➤*Orthostatic hypotension:* Although the incidence of orthostatic/postural hypotension reported as an adverse reaction was not higher in all patients treated in 2 clinical controlled trials, the incidence of adverse orthostatic hypotension was higher in elderly patients (65 years of age and older) than in nonelderly patients. In elderly patients, this adverse reaction of orthostatic hypotension occurred in about 3% of orally disintegrating tablet–treated patients compared with none (0%) of the placebo-treated elderly patients. Of potential relevance, the risk of dizziness was also greater in the elderly patients. In nonelderly patients, the incidence of adverse orthostatic hypotension was not more frequent with orally disintegrating tablets than with placebo treatment.

It appears that there may be increased risk for orthostatic hypotension in the period after increasing the daily dose of orally disintegrating tablets from 1.25 to 2.5 mg.

➤*Renal effects:* Small increments in serum urea nitrogen (BUN) and creatinine have been observed in patients treated with selegiline 10 mg orally disintegrating tablets daily (4 times the recommended dose). Similar changes were not observed in patients treated with 1.25 or 2.5 mg daily.

➤*Melanoma:* Epidemiological studies have shown that patients with Parkinson disease have a higher risk (2- to approximately 6-fold higher) of developing melanoma than the general population, although it is unclear whether the observed increased risk was caused by Parkinson disease itself or drugs used to treat Parkinson disease. Selegiline is one of the drugs used to treat Parkinson disease. Although selegiline orally disintegrating tablets have not been associated with an increased risk of melanoma specifically,

SELEGILINE HYDROCHLORIDE (L-deprenyl) — ORAL

their potential role as a risk factor has not been systematically studied. Make patients using selegiline orally disintegrating tablets aware of these results and instruct them to undergo periodic dermatologic screening.

Monitor for melanomas frequently and on a regular basis when using selegiline for any indication. Ideally, ensure that periodic skin examinations are performed by appropriately qualified individuals (eg, dermatologist).

➤*Phenylketonurics:* Each orally disintegrating tablet contains phenylalanine 1.25 mg (a component of aspartame). Patients taking the 2.5 mg dose of orally disintegrating tablets will receive phenylalanine 2.5 mg.

➤*Buccal mucosa irritation:* In the controlled clinical trials, periodic examinations of the tongue and oral mucosa were performed. There was an increased frequency of mild oropharyngeal abnormality (eg, swallowing pain, mouth pain, discrete areas of focal reddening, multiple foci of reddening, edema, and/or ulceration) at the end of the study in patients who did not have any abnormality at baseline and who received treatment with orally disintegrating tablets (10%) compared with patients who received placebo (3%). Separate analyses of each oropharyngeal abnormality were also assessed. Selegiline orally disintegrating tablet patients (3%) showed an increased frequency of the development of mild discrete areas of focal reddening compared with placebo patients (0%). Selegiline orally disintegrating tablet patients (2%) also showed an increased frequency of the development of mild ulceration compared with placebo patients (1%).

➤*Dyskinesia:* Selegiline orally disintegrating tablets may potentiate the dopaminergic adverse reactions of levodopa and may cause or exacerbate preexisting dyskinesia. Decreasing the dose of levodopa may ameliorate this adverse reaction.

➤*Withdrawal-emergent hyperpyrexia and confusion:* Although not reported with selegiline orally disintegrating tablets in the clinical development program, a symptom complex resembling neuroleptic malignant syndrome (characterized by elevated temperature, muscular rigidity, altered consciousness, and autonomic instability) with no other obvious etiology has been reported in association with rapid dose reduction or withdrawal of or changes in antiparkinsonian therapy.

➤*Hallucinations:* When used as an adjunct to levodopa, hallucinations were reported as an adverse reaction in approximately 4% of patients treated with selegiline orally disintegrating tablets and 2% of patients treated with placebo. Hallucinations led to drug discontinuation and premature withdrawal from clinical trials in about 1% of patients treated with orally disintegrating tablets and none of the placebo-treated patients.

Caution patients of the possibility of developing hallucinations and instruct them to report them to their health care provider promptly if they develop.

➤*Renal function impairment:* The effect of selegiline orally disintegrating tablets has not been studied in renally impaired patients. Therefore, use selegiline orally disintegrating tablets with caution in patients with a history of, suspected, or known renal function impairment. If such patients experience adverse reactions that seem more frequent or severe than might ordinarily be expected, consider discontinuing the orally disintegrating tablet.

➤*Hepatic function impairment:* The effect of selegiline orally disintegrating tablets have not been studied in patients with hepatic impairment. Therefore, use selegiline orally disintegrating tablets with caution in patients with a history of, suspected, or known hepatic impairment, particularly if the patient has an increased prothrombin time or increased serum bilirubin or decreased serum albumin. If such patients experience adverse reactions that seem more frequent or severe than might ordinarily be expected, consider discontinuing the use of orally disintegrating tablets.

➤*Pregnancy: Category C.* In the rabbit study, increases in total resorptions and percentage of postimplantation loss, and a decrease in the number of live fetuses per dam occurred at the highest dose tested. In a perinatal and postnatal development study in Sprague-Dawley rats (oral doses of 4, 16, and 64 mg/kg, or 4, 15, and 62 times the human therapeutic dose on a mg/m^2 basis), an increase in the number of stillbirths and decreases in the number of pups per dam, pup survival, and pup body weight (at birth and throughout the lactation period) were observed at the 2 highest doses. At the highest dose tested, no pups born alive survived to day 4 postpartum. Postnatal development at the highest dose tested in dams could not be evaluated because of the lack of surviving pups. The reproductive performance of the untreated offspring was not assessed.

There are no adequate and well-controlled studies in pregnant women. It is not known if selegiline crosses the human placenta. The low molecular weight (about 188 for the free base) suggests to expect passage to the embryo and fetus. Use selegiline during pregnancy only if the potential benefit justifies the potential risk to the fetus.

➤*Lactation:* It is not known whether selegiline is excreted in human milk. The low molecular weight (about 188 for the free base) suggests excretion into breast milk. Because many drugs are excreted in human milk and because of the potential for serious adverse reactions in breast-feeding infants from selegiline, decide whether to discontinue breast-feeding or the drug, taking into account the importance of the drug to the mother.

➤*Children:* The effects of selegiline capsules/tablets in children have not been evaluated; the effects of selegiline orally disintegrating tablets in children younger than 16 years of age have not been evaluated.

➤*Elderly:* See Adverse Reactions for more information.

➤*Monitoring:* Periodic routine evaluation of all patients is appropriate. Observe patients closely for atypical responses.

Monitor for melanomas frequently and on a regular basis when using selegiline for any indication. Ideally, periodic skin examinations should be performed by appropriately qualified individuals (eg, dermatologist).

Drug Interactions

➤*Cytochrome P450 system:* Although adequate studies have not been done investigating the effect of CYP3A4-inducers on selegiline, use drugs that induce CYP3A4 (eg, phenytoin, carbamazepine, nafcillin, phenobarbital, rifampin) with caution.

Selegiline Drug Interactions

Precipitant drug	Object drug[a]		Description
Apraclonidine	Selegiline	↑	Coadministration is contraindicated; hypertension may be potentiated. Do not coadminister within 14 days of each other.
Buspirone	Selegiline	↑	Risk of selegiline-induced hypertension may be increased when coadministered with buspirone. Concurrent use is not recommended.
CNS stimulants (eg, atomoxetine, amphetamine, dexmethylphenidate, methylphenidate, sibutramine)	Selegiline	↑	Coadministration is contraindicated. Allow ≥ 2 weeks after discontinuing a CNS stimulant before giving selegiline.
Selegiline	CNS stimulants (eg, atomoxetine, amphetamine, dexmethylphenidate, methylphenidate, sibutramine)		
Contraceptives, hormonal	Selegiline	↑	Plasma selegiline concentrations may be elevated, causing a loss of selective inhibition of MAO-B and increasing the risk of selegiline adverse reactions.
Linezolid	Selegiline	↑	Coadministration is contraindicated. Do not coadminister within 14 days of each other.
Tetrabenazine	Selegiline	↑	Coadministration is contraindicated.
Selegiline	Tetrabenazine		
Selegiline	Alcohol	↑	Severe hypertension may occur when alcoholic beverages, especially those high in tyramine content, are consumed. Concurrent use is not recommended.
Selegiline	Analgesics (eg, meperidine, methadone, propoxyphene, tramadol)	↑	Because of reports of fatal interactions, coadministration is contraindicated. At least 14 days should elapse between selegiline and initiation with meperidine.
Selegiline	Anesthetics	↑	Patients taking selegiline should not undergo elective surgery requiring general anesthesia. Do not give cocaine or local anesthesia containing sympathomimetic vasoconstrictors. Discontinue selegiline ≥ 10 days before elective surgery.
Selegiline	Bupropion	↑	A serotonin syndrome may occur. Coadministration is contraindicated. Allow ≥ 14 days to elapse between discontinuing selegiline and starting bupropion.
Selegiline	Cyclobenzaprine	↑	A serotonin syndrome may occur. Coadministration is contraindicated. A minimum of 14 days should elapse between the discontinuance of MAOIs and the initiation of cyclobenzaprine.
Selegiline	Dextromethorphan	↑	Coadministration is contraindicated. Brief episodes of psychosis and bizarre behavior have occurred with coadministration.

SELEGILINE HYDROCHLORIDE (L-deprenyl) — ORAL

Selegiline Drug Interactions

Precipitant drug	Object drug[a]		Description
Selegiline	Ginseng	↑	Manic-like symptoms, headaches, and tremulousness have been reported. Avoid concurrent use.
Selegiline	Insulin	↑	The hypoglycemic reaction of insulin may be increased.
Selegiline	MAOIs (eg, isocarboxazid, other selegiline products, phenelzine, tranylcypromine)	↑	Do not coadminister because of the increased risk of nonselective MAO inhibition that may lead to hypertensive crisis. Concurrent use is contraindicated. At least 14 days should elapse between discontinuation of selegiline and initiation of another MAOI.
MAOIs (eg, isocarboxazid, other selegiline products, phenelzine, tranylcypromine)	Selegiline		
Selegiline	Maprotiline	↑	Concomitant use is contraindicated. Allow ≥ 14 days after discontinuing selegiline before initiating maprotiline.
Selegiline	Meglitinide antidiabetic agents (eg, nateglinide, repaglinide)	↑	Hypoglycemic effects may be increased.
Selegiline	Serotonin reuptake inhibitors (eg, citalopram, duloxetine, fluoxetine, fluvoxamine, nefazodone, paroxetine, sertraline, venlafaxine)	↑	Concurrent use is contraindicated. During coadministration, serious, sometimes fatal reactions have been reported. At least 5 weeks should elapse between discontinuation of fluoxetine and initiation of an MAOI; ≥ 14 days should elapse between discontinuation of an MAOI and initiation of treatment with a serotonin reuptake inhibitor.
Serotonin reuptake inhibitors (eg, citalopram, duloxetine, fluoxetine, fluvoxamine, nefazodone, paroxetine, sertraline, venlafaxine)	Selegiline		
Selegiline	Sulfonylureas	↑	The hypoglycemic action of sulfonylureas may be increased by selegiline.
Selegiline	Sympathomimetic agents (eg, ephedrine, phenylephrine, pseudoephedrine)	↑	One case of hypertensive crisis has been reported in a patient taking the recommended dose of selegiline and ephedrine.
Selegiline	Tricyclic antidepressants (eg, amitriptyline, protriptyline)	↑	Severe CNS toxicity associated with hyperpyrexia and death has been reported with the combination of tricyclic antidepressants and nonselective MAOIs. Do not coadminister tricyclic antidepressants with or within 2 weeks of selegiline treatment.

[a] ↑ = object drug increased.

➤*Drug/Food interactions:* Warn all patients against eating food with a high tyramine content. Hypertensive crisis may result.

See Actions for more information.

See Actions for more information.

Adverse Reactions

➤*Capsules and tablets:*

Discontinuation – The importance and severity of various reactions reported often cannot be ascertained. However, one index of relative importance is whether or not a reaction caused treatment discontinuation. In prospective premarketing studies, the following reactions led, in decreasing order of frequency, to discontinuation of treatment with selegiline: nausea, hallucinations, confusion, depression, loss of balance, insomnia, orthostatic hypotension, increased akinetic involuntary movements, agitation, arrhythmia, bradykinesia, chorea, delusions, hypertension, new or increased angina pectoris, and syncope. Reactions reported only once as a cause of discontinuation are ankle edema, anxiety, burning lips/mouth, constipation, drowsiness/lethargy, dystonia, excess perspiration, increased freezing, GI bleeding, hair loss, increased tremor, nervousness, and weight loss.

Clinical trials – Experience with selegiline obtained in parallel, placebo-controlled, randomized studies provides only a limited basis for estimates of adverse reaction rates. The following reactions occurred with greater frequency among the 49 patients assigned to selegiline as compared with the 50 patients assigned to placebo in the only parallel, placebo-controlled trial performed in patients with Parkinson disease are shown. None of these adverse reactions led to a discontinuation of treatment.

Selegiline Oral Adverse Reactions

Adverse reactions	Selegiline (n = 49)	Placebo (n = 50)
CNS		
Anxiety, tension	1%	1%
Confusion	3%	0%
Dizziness/light-headedness/fainting	7%	1%
Dyskinesias	2%	5%
Hallucinations	3%	1%
Headache	2%	1%
Insomnia	1%	1%
Lethargy	1%	0%
Vivid dreams	2%	0%
GI		
Abdominal pain	4%	2%
Diarrhea	1%	0%
Dry mouth	3%	1%
Nausea	10%	3%
Miscellaneous		
Ache, generalized	1%	0%
Leg pain	1%	0%
Low back pain	1%	0%
Palpitations	1%	0%
Urinary retention	1%	0%
Weight loss	1%	0%

➤*Other adverse reactions:*

Cardiovascular – Arrhythmia, hypertension, hypotension, new or increased angina pectoris, orthostatic hypotension, palpitations, peripheral edema, sinus bradycardia, syncope, tachycardia.

CNS – Anxiety, apathy, behavior/mood change, blepharospasm, chills, chorea, confusion, delusions, depression, disorientation, dizziness, dreams/nightmares, drowsiness, dyskinesia, dystonic symptoms, facial grimace, falling down, festination, freezing, hallucinations, headache, heavy leg, hollow feeling, impaired memory (reported only at dosages greater than 10 mg/day), increased apraxia, increased bradykinesia, increased energy (reported only at dosages greater than 10 mg/day), increased tremor, involuntary movements, lethargy/malaise, light-headedness, loss of balance, migraine, muscle twitch (reported only at dosages greater than 10 mg/day), myoclonic jerks (reported only at dosages greater than 10 mg/day), numbness of toes/fingers, overstimulation, personality change, restlessness, tiredness, sleep disturbance, speech affected, tardive dyskinesia, transient high (reported only at dosages greater than 10 mg/day), transient irritability, vertigo, weakness.

Dermatologic – Diaphoresis, facial hair, hair loss, hematoma, increased sweating, rash, photosensitivity.

GI – Anorexia, bruxism (reported only at dosages greater than 10 mg/day), constipation, diarrhea, dry mouth, dysphagia, GI bleeding (exacerbation of preexisting ulcer disease), heartburn, nausea/vomiting, poor appetite, rectal bleeding, taste disturbance, weight loss.

GU – Decreased penile sensation (reported only at dosages greater than 10 mg/day), nocturia, prostate hypertrophy, sexual dysfunction, slow urination, transient anorgasmia (reported only at dosages greater than 10 mg/day), urinary frequency, urinary hesitancy, urinary retention.

Musculoskeletal – Back pain, muscle cramps, stiff neck.

Respiratory – Asthma, shortness of breath.

Special senses – Blurred vision, diplopia, supraorbital pain, tinnitus.

Miscellaneous – Chills, generalized ache, leg pain, throat burning.

➤*Orally disintegrating tablets:*

Common adverse reactions – The most commonly observed adverse reactions, which were greater than placebo, reported in the double-blind, placebo-controlled trials during orally disintegrating tablet treatment were dizziness, nausea, pain, headache, insomnia, rhinitis, dyskinesia, back pain, stomatitis, and dyspepsia.

Discontinuation – Of the 194 patients treated with orally disintegrating tablets in the double-blind, placebo-controlled trials, 5.2% discontinued because of adverse reactions compared with 1% of the 98 patients who received placebo. Reactions causing discontinuation of treatment included dizziness, chest pain, accidental injury, and myasthenia.

SELEGILINE HYDROCHLORIDE (L-deprenyl) — ORAL

Clinical trials – The reactions cited reflect experience gained under closely monitored conditions of clinical trials in a highly selected patient population. In actual clinical practice or in other clinical trials, the frequency estimates may not apply.

Selegiline Orally Disintegrating Tablet Adverse Reactions (≥ 2%)[a]

Adverse reactions	Selegiline orally disintegrating tablet[b] 1.25/2.5 mg (n = 194)	Placebo[b] (n = 98)
CNS		
Ataxia	3%	1%
Depression	2%	1%
Dizziness	11%	8%
Dyskinesia	6%	3%
Hallucinations	4%	2%
Headache	7%	6%
Insomnia	7%	4%
Somnolence	3%	2%
Tremor	3%	1%
Dermatologic		
Rash	4%	1%
Skin disorders[c]	6%	2%
GI		
Constipation	4%	0%
Diarrhea	2%	1%
Dry mouth	4%	2%
Dyspepsia	5%	3%
Dysphagia	2%	1%
Flatulence	2%	1%
Nausea	11%	9%
Stomatitis	5%	4%
Tooth disorder	2%	1%
Vomiting	3%	0%
Musculoskeletal		
Leg cramps	3%	1%
Myalgia	3%	0%
Respiratory		
Dyspnea	3%	0%
Pharyngitis	4%	2%
Rhinitis	7%	6%
Miscellaneous		
Back pain	5%	3%
Chest pain	2%	0%
Ecchymosis	2%	0%
Hypertension	3%	2%
Hypokalemia	2%	0%
Pain	8%	7%

[a] Patients may have reported multiple adverse reactions during the study or at discontinuation; thus, patients may be included in > 1 category.
[b] Patients received concomitant levodopa.
[c] Skin disorders represent any new skin abnormality that would not be characterized as rash or neoplastic lesion.

Elderly – Treatment-emergent adverse reactions were reported at a higher frequency by patients 65 years of age and older compared with patients younger than 65 years of age. Analysis of adverse reaction incidence in each group was conducted to calculate and compare relative risk (orally disintegrating tablets percentage/placebo percentage) for each treatment. The relative risk was at least 2-fold higher for orally disintegrating tablet treatment in the elderly patients compared with the nonelderly patients for hypertension, orthostatic/postural hypotension, dizziness, somnolence, echocardiogram abnormality, nausea, dyspepsia, abnormal dreams, anxiety, cheilitis, diarrhea, hyperkalemia, pharyngitis, flu syndrome, and infection.

➤*Other adverse reactions:*

Cardiovascular – Angina pectoris, atrial fibrillation, atrial flutter, bigeminy, cardiomegaly, cardiomyopathy, cerebral ischemia, congestive heart failure, first-degree atrioventricular block, heart arrest, hypotension, myocardial infarct, myocardial ischemia, pallor, sinus bradycardia, supraventricular tachycardia, syncope, vascular disorder, vasodilation.

CNS – Abnormal gait, agitation, akinesia, aphasia, CNS neoplasia, dementia, dystonia, emotional lability, encephalopathy, hyperkinesias, hypertonia, hypokinesia, hypotonia, incoordination, increased salivation, migraine, myoclonus, nervousness, neuralgia, neuropathy, paranoid reaction, paresthesia, peripheral neuritis, personality disorder, psychosis, reflexes decreased, sleep disorder, subdural hematoma, thinking abnormal, vertigo.

Dermatologic – Contact dermatitis, dry skin, eczema, fungal dermatitis, herpes simplex, herpes zoster, pruritus, seborrhea, skin benign neoplasm, skin carcinoma, skin discoloration, skin hypertrophy, skin melanoma, skin ulcer, sweating.

GI – Anorexia, cholecystitis, cholelithiasis, colitis, esophageal ulcer, esophagitis, gamma-glutamyl transpeptidase increased, gastritis, gastroenteritis, gingivitis, hepatitis, intestinal obstruction, liver function tests abnormal, peptic ulcer, tongue edema.

GU – Breast carcinoma, cystitis, epididymitis, kidney calculus, ovarian disorder, prostatic carcinoma, prostatic specific antigen increase, urinary frequency, urinary incontinence, urinary urgency, urination impaired.

Hematologic/Lymphatic – Abnormal platelets, anemia, chronic leukocytosis, cyanosis, eosinophilia, lymphoma-like reaction, myelocytic leukemia, sedimentation rate increased.

Metabolic/Nutritional – Albuminuria, ALT increased, avitaminosis, dehydration, diabetes mellitus, edema, gout, hypercholesteremia, hyperglycemia, hyperkalemia, hyperlipidemia, hyperphosphatemia, hypoglycemia, hyponatremia, hypoproteinemia, .

Musculoskeletal – Arthralgia, arthritis, arthrosis, bone pain, bursitis, leg cramps, tendon rupture, tenosynovitis.

Respiratory – Asthma, bronchitis, carcinoma of the lung, epistaxis, hiccup, lung edema, pleural effusion, pneumonia, pneumothorax, sinusitis, voice alteration.

Special senses – Abnormal vision, amblyopia, blindness, cataract specified, conjunctivitis, deafness, diplopia, dry eyes, eye hemorrhage, glaucoma, otitis externa, retinal artery occlusion, retinal detachment, taste loss, taste perversion, tinnitus.

Miscellaneous – Allergic reaction, cellulitis, cyanosis, cyst, face edema, fever, flank pain, fungal infection, hernia, infection superimposed, infection viral, neck pain, neoplasm.

Postmarketing – Because these reactions are reported voluntarily from a population of uncertain size, it is not always possible to reliably estimate their frequency or establish a causal relationship to drug exposure.

CNS: Seizure in dialyzed chronic renal failure patient on concomitant medications (capsules/tablets).

Miscellaneous: Pathological gambling, increased libido including hypersexuality, and impulse control symptoms (orally disintegrating tablets).

Overdosage

➤*Symptoms:* No specific information is available about clinically significant overdoses with selegiline. However, experience gained during selegiline's development reveal that some individuals exposed to doses of d,l-selegiline 600 mg suffered severe hypotension and psychomotor agitation.

Because the selective inhibition of MAO-B by selegiline is achieved only at doses in the range recommended for the treatment of Parkinson disease (eg, 10 mg/day [capsules or tablets] or 2.5 mg/day [orally disintegrating tablets]), overdoses are likely to cause significant inhibition of both MAO-A and MAO-B. Consequently, the signs and symptoms of overdose may resemble those observed with marketed nonselective MAOIs (eg, isocarboxazide, phenelzine, tranylcypromine). For this reason, in cases of overdose with selegiline, observe dietary tyramine restriction for several weeks to avoid the risk of a hypertensive/cheese reaction.

Nonselective MAO inhibition –

Characteristically, signs and symptoms of nonselective MAOI overdose may not appear immediately. Delays of up to 12 hours between ingestion of drug and the appearance of signs may occur. Importantly, the peak intensity of the syndrome may not be reached for upwards of a day following the overdose. Death has been reported following overdosage. Therefore, immediate hospitalization, with continuous patient observation and monitoring for a period of at least 2 days following the ingestion of such drugs in overdose, is strongly recommended.

Signs and symptoms of overdosage may include, alone or in combination, any of the following: drowsiness, dizziness, faintness, irritability, hyperactivity, agitation, severe headache, hallucinations, trismus, opisthotonus, convulsions, and coma; rapid and irregular pulse, hypertension, hypotension and vascular collapse; precordial pain, respiratory depression and failure, hyperpyrexia, diaphoresis, and cool, clammy skin.

➤*Treatment:* Treatment of overdose with nonselective MAOIs is symptomatic and supportive. Induction of gastric lavage with instillation of charcoal slurry may be helpful in early poisoning, provided the airway has been protected against aspiration. Treat signs and symptom of CNS stimulation, including convulsions, with diazepam, given slowly by IV. Avoid phenothiazine derivatives and CNS stimulants. Treat hypotension and vascular collapse with IV fluids and, if necessary, blood pressure titration with an IV infusion of a dilute pressor agent. It should be noted that adrenergic agents may produce a markedly increased pressor response.

Support respiration by appropriate measures, including management of the airway, use of supplemental oxygen, and mechanical ventilatory, as required.

Monitor body temperature closely. Intensive management of hyperpyrexia may be required. Maintenance of fluid and electrolyte balance is essential.

Patient Information

Advise patients of the possible need to reduce levodopa dosage after the initiation of selegiline.

SELEGILINE HYDROCHLORIDE (L-deprenyl) — ORAL

Advise patients (or their families if the patient is incompetent) not to exceed the daily recommended dose of 10 mg/day (capsules or tablets) or 2.5 mg/day (orally disintegrating tablets). Explain the risk of using higher daily doses of selegiline and provide a brief description of the "cheese reaction." Rare hypertensive reactions with selegiline at recommended doses associated with dietary influences have been reported.

Consequently, it may be useful to inform patients (or their families) about the signs and symptoms associated with MAOI-induced hypertensive reactions. In particular, urge patients to immediately report any severe headache or other atypical or unusual symptoms not previously experienced.

There have been reports of patients experiencing intense urges to gamble, increased sexual urges, and other intense urges and the inability to control these urges while taking one or more of the medications that increase central dopaminergic tone, which are generally used for the treatment of Parkinson disease, including selegiline. Although it is not proven that the medications caused these reactions, these urges were reported to have stopped in some cases when the dose was reduced or the medication was stopped. Ask patients about the development of new or increased gambling urges, sexual urges, or other urges while being treated with selegiline. Inform patients to notify their health care provider if they experience new or increased gambling urges, increased sexual urges, or other intense urges while taking selegiline. Consider dose reduction or stopping the medication if a patient develops such urges while taking selegiline.

Inform patients that hallucinations can occur with the orally disintegrating tablets.

Instruct patients taking the orally disintegrating tablets not to remove the blister from the outer pouch until just prior to dosing. Then peel open the blister park with dry hands and place the orally disintegrating tablet on the tongue, where it will disintegrate. Also, advise patients to avoid drinking liquid or eating food 5 minutes before and after taking orally disintegrating tablets.

Inform phenylketonuric patients that the orally disintegrating tablets contain phenylalanine (a component of aspartame). Each 1.25 mg orally disintegrating tablet contains phenylalanine 1.25 mg.

SELEGILINE — TRANSDERMAL

WARNING

Suicidality and antidepressant drugs – Antidepressants increased the risk compared with placebo of suicidal thinking and behavior (suicidality) in children, adolescents, and young adults in short-term studies of major depressive disorder (MDD) and other psychiatric disorders. Anyone considering the use of selegiline or any other antidepressant in a child, adolescent, or young adult must balance this risk with the clinical need. Short-term studies did not show an increase in the risk of suicidality with antidepressants compared with placebo in adults 24 years of age and older; there was a reduction in risk with antidepressants compared with placebo in adults 65 years of age and older. Depression and certain other psychiatric disorders are themselves associated with increases in the risk of suicide. Patients of all ages who are started on antidepressant therapy should be monitored appropriately and observed closely for clinical worsening, suicidality, or unusual changes in behavior. Families and caregivers should be advised for the need for close observation and communication with the prescriber. Selegiline is not approved for use in children. Furthermore, selegiline at any dose should not be used in children younger than 12 years of age, even when administered with dietary modifications.

Indications

➤*Major depressive disorder:* For the treatment of MDD.

Administration and Dosage

➤*General dosing considerations:* Inform patients that they should avoid tyramine-rich foods and beverages beginning on the first day of 9 mg per 24 hours or 12 mg per 24 hours treatment, and continue to avoid these foods and beverages for 2 weeks after a dose reduction to 6 mg per 24 hours or following the discontinuation of 9 mg per 24 hours or 12 mg per 24 hours treatment.

➤*Adults:*

Major depressive disorder –

Maximum dose: 12 mg per 24 hours.

Initial dosage: 6 mg per 24 hours.

Dosage titration: If dose increases are indicated, they should occur in dose increments of 3 mg per 24 hours (up to a maximum dosage of 12 mg per 24 hours) at intervals of no less than 2 weeks.

Maintenance dosage: 6 mg per 24 hours to 12 mg per 24 hours.

Duration of therapy: It is generally agreed that episodes of depression require several months or longer of sustained pharmacologic therapy. The benefit of maintaining depressed patients on therapy at a dosage of 6 mg per 24 hours after achieving a responder status for an average duration of about 25 days was demonstrated in a controlled trial. Periodically reevaluate the long-term usefulness of the drug for the individual patient.

➤*Children:* Selegiline at any dose should not be used in children younger than 12 years of age, even when administered with dietary modifications. Selegiline is not approved for use in children.

➤*Elderly:*

Usual dosage – 6 mg per 24 hours daily.

Dosage adjustment – Dose increases should be made with caution, and patients should be closely observed for postural changes in blood pressure throughout treatment.

➤*Administration:*

Application – Apply the patch to an area of dry, intact skin on the upper torso (below the neck and above the waist), upper thigh, or the outer surface of the upper arm that is not hairy, oily, irritated, broken, scarred, or calloused. Do not place the patch where your clothing is tight, which could cause the patch to rub off.

Only one patch should be worn at a time. A new application site should be selected with each new patch to avoid reapplication to the same site on consecutive days. Patches should be applied at approximately the same time each day.

➤*Storage/Stability:* Store at 20° to 25°C (68° to 77°F). Do not store outside of the sealed pouch.

Actions

➤*Pharmacology:* Selegiline, an antidepressant, is an irreversible inhibitor of monoamine oxidase (MAO), an intracellular enzyme associated with the outer membrane of mitochondria. MAO exists as 2 isoenzymes, referred to as MAO-A and MAO-B. Selegiline has a greater affinity for MAO-B, compared with MAO-A. However, at antidepressant doses, selegiline inhibits both isoenzymes. The mechanism of action of selegiline as an antidepressant is not fully understood but is presumed to be linked to potentiation of monoamine neurotransmitter activity in the CNS resulting from its inhibition of MAO activity.

In an in vivo animal model used to test for antidepressant activity (forced swim test), selegiline administered by transdermal patch exhibited antidepressant properties only at doses that inhibited both MAO-A and MAO-B activity in brain. In the CNS, MAO-A and MAO-B play important roles in the catabolism of neurotransmitter amines such as norepinephrine, dopamine, and serotonin, as well as neuromodulators such as phenylethylamine. Other molecular sites of action have also been explored, and, in this regard, a direct pharmacological interaction may also occur between selegiline and brain neuronal alpha$_{2B}$ receptors. In in vitro receptor binding assays, selegiline has demonstrated affinity for the human recombinant adrenergic alpha$_{2B}$ receptor (K_i = 284 mcM). No affinity [K_i greater than 10 mcM] was noted at dopamine receptors, adrenergic beta-3, glutamate, muscarinic M_1 to M_5, nicotinic, or rolipram receptor/sites.

➤*Pharmacokinetics:*

Absorption – Following dermal application of selegiline to humans, 25% to 30% of the selegiline content on average is delivered systemically over 24 hours (range, approximately 10% to 40%). Consequently, the degree of drug absorption may be one-third higher than the average amounts of 6 to 12 mg per 24 hours. Transdermal dosing results in substantially higher exposure to selegiline and lower exposure to metabolites, compared with oral dosing, where extensive first-pass metabolism occurs. In a 10-day study with selegiline administered to healthy volunteers, steady-state selegiline plasma concentrations were achieved within 5 days of daily dosing. Absorption of selegiline is similar when selegiline is applied to the upper torso or upper thigh.

Distribution – Following dermal application of radiolabeled selegiline to laboratory animals, selegiline is rapidly distributed to all body tissues. Selegiline rapidly penetrates the blood-brain barrier. In humans, selegiline is approximately 90% bound to plasma protein over a 2 to 500 ng/mL concentration range. Selegiline does not accumulate in the skin.

Metabolism – Transdermally absorbed selegiline is not metabolized in human skin and does not undergo extensive first-pass metabolism. Selegiline is extensively metabolized by several cytochrome P450 (CYP-450)–dependent enzyme systems. Selegiline is metabolized initially via N-dealkylation or N-depropargylation to form N-desmethylselegiline or R(−)-methamphetamine, respectively. Both of these metabolites can be further metabolized to R(−)-amphetamine. These metabolites are all levorotatory (l-)enantiomers and no racemic biotransformation to the dextrorotatory form (ie, S(+)-amphetamine or S(+)-methamphetamine) occurs. R(−)-methamphetamine and R(−)-amphetamine are mainly excreted unchanged in urine.

In vitro studies utilizing human liver microsomes demonstrated that several CYP-450–dependent enzymes are involved in the metabolism of selegiline and its metabolites. CYP2B6, CYP2C9, and CYP3A4/5 appeared to be the major contributing enzymes in the formation of R(−)-methamphetamine from selegiline, with CYP2A6 having a minor role. CYP2A6, CYP2B6, and CYP3A4/5 appeared to contribute to the formation of R(−)-amphetamine from N-desmethylselegiline.

The potential for selegiline or N-desmethylselegiline to inhibit individual CYP-450–dependent enzyme pathways was also examined in vitro with human liver microsomes. Each substrate was examined over a concentration range of 2.5 to 250 mcM. Consistent with competitive inhibition, both selegiline and N-desmethylselegiline caused a concentration-dependent inhibition of CYP2D6 at 10 to 250 mcM and CYP3A4/5 at 25 to 250 mcM. CYP2C19 and CYP2B6 were also inhibited at concentrations of 100 mcM or more. All inhibitory effects of selegiline and N-desmethylselegiline occurred at concentrations that are several orders of magnitude higher than concentrations seen clinically (highest predose concentration observed at a dosage of 12 mg per 24 hours at steady state was 0.046 mcM).

SELEGILINE — TRANSDERMAL

Excretion – Approximately 10% and 2% of a radiolabeled dose applied dermally as a dimethyl sulfoxide solution was recovered in urine and feces respectively, with at least 63% of the dose remaining unabsorbed. The remaining 25% of the dose was unaccounted for. Urinary excretion of unchanged selegiline accounted for 0.1% of the applied dose, with the remainder of the dose recovered in urine being metabolites. The systemic clearance of selegiline after intravenous (IV) administration was 1.4 L/min, and the mean half-lives of selegiline and its 3 metabolites, R(−)-N-desmethylselegiline, R(−)-amphetamine, and R(−)-methamphetamine, ranged from 18 to 25 hours.

Contraindications

Pheochromocytoma; tyramine-rich foods (see Warnings/Precautions); known hypersensitivity to selegiline or to any componenet of the patch; concomitant use with selective serotonin reuptake inhibitors (SSRIs) (eg, fluoxetine, sertraline, paroxetine); dual serotonin and norepinephrine reuptake inhibitors (SNRIs) (eg, duloxetine, venlafaxine); tricyclic antidepressants (TCAs) (eg, amitriptyline, imipramine); bupropion; meperidine and analgesic agents such as tramadol, methadone, and propoxyphene; dextromethorphan; St. John's wort; mirtazapine; cyclobenzaprine; carbamazepine; oxcarbazepine; and sympathomimetic amines, including amphetamines as well as cold products and weight-reducing preparations that contain vasoconstrictors (eg, pseudoephedrine, phenylephrine, phenylpropanolamine, ephedrine); oral selegiline or other MAO inhibitors (MAOIs) (eg, isocarboxazid, phenelzine, tranylcypromine). Patients should not undergo elective surgery requiring general anesthesia; they should not be given cocaine or local anesthesia containing sympathomimetic vasoconstrictors. Discontinue selegiline at least 10 days prior to elective surgery. If surgery is necessary sooner, benzodiazepines, mivacurium, rapacuronium, fentanyl, morphine, and codeine may be used cautiously.

Warnings/Precautions

➤*Clinical worsening and suicide risk:* Patients with MDD, both adults and children, may experience worsening of their depression and/or the emergence of suicidality or unusual changes in behavior, whether or not they are taking antidepressant medications, and this risk may persist until significant remission occurs. Suicide is a known risk of depression and certain other psychiatric disorders, and these disorders themselves are the strongest predictors of suicide. There has been a long-standing concern that antidepressants may have a role in inducing worsening of depression and the emergence of suicidality in certain patients during the early phases of treatment. Pooled analyses of short-term placebo-controlled trials of antidepressant drugs (SSRIs and others) showed that these drugs increase the risk of suicidal thinking and behavior (suicidality) in children, adolescents, and young adults (ages 18 to 24 years) with MDD and other psychiatric disorders. Short-term studies did not show an increase in the risk of suicidality with antidepressants compared with placebo in adults 24 years of age and older; there was a reduction with antidepressants compared with placebo in adults aged 65 years and older.

The pooled analyses of placebo-controlled trials in children and adolescents with MDD, obsessive compulsive disorder (OCD), or other psychiatric disorders included a total of 24 short-term trials of 9 antidepressants in more than 4,400 patients. The pooled analyses of placebo-controlled trials in adults with MDD or other psychiatric disorders included a total of 295 short-term trials (median duration of 2 months) of 11 antidepressant drugs in more than 77,000 patients. There was considerable variation in risk of suicidality among drugs, but a tendency toward an increase in the younger patients for almost all drugs studied. There were differences in absolute risk of suicidality across the different indications, with the highest incidence in MDD. However, the risk differences (drug vs placebo) were relatively stable within age strata and across indications.

No suicides occurred in any of the pediatric trials. There were suicides in the adult trials, but the number was not sufficient to reach any conclusion about drug effect on suicide.

It is unknown whether the suicidality risk extends to longer-term use (ie, beyond several months). However, there is substantial evidence from placebo-controlled maintenance trials in adults with depression that the use of antidepressants can delay the recurrence of depression.

All patients being treated with antidepressants for any indication should be monitored appropriately and observed closely for clinical worsening, suicidality, and unusual changes in behavior, especially during the initial few months of a course of drug therapy, or at times of dose changes, either increases or decreases.

Because of the limited data, selegiline at any dose should not be used in children younger than 12 years of age, even when administered with dietary modifications. Selegiline is not approved for use in children.

Anxiety, agitation, panic attacks, insomnia, irritability, hostility, aggressiveness, impulsivity, akathisia (psychomotor restlessness), hypomania, and mania have been reported in adults and children being treated with antidepressants for MDD as well as for other indications, both psychiatric and nonpsychiatric. Although a causal link between the emergence of such symptoms and either the worsening of depression and/or the emergence of suicidal impulses has not been established, there is concern that such symptoms may represent precursors to emerging suicidality.

Consider changing the therapeutic regimen, including possibly discontinuing the medication, in patients whose depression is persistently worse, or who are experiencing emergent suicidality or symptoms that might be precursors to worsening depression or suicidality, especially if these symptoms are severe, abrupt in onset, or were not part of the patient's presenting symptoms.

Alert families and caregivers of patients being treated with antidepressants for MDD or other indications, both psychiatric and nonpsychiatric, about the need to monitor patients for the emergence of agitation, irritability, unusual changes in behavior, and the other symptoms previously described, as well as the emergence of suicidality, and to report such symptoms immediately to the patient's health care provider. Such monitoring should include daily observation by families and caregivers. Prescribe the smallest quantity consistent with good patient management in order to reduce the risk of overdose.

➤*Screening patients for bipolar disorder:* A major depressive episode may be the initial presentation of bipolar disorder. It is generally believed (though not established in controlled trials) that treating such an episode with an antidepressant alone may increase the likelihood of precipitation of a mixed/manic episode in patients at risk for bipolar disorder. Whether any of the symptoms previously described represent such a conversion is unknown. However, prior to initiating treatment with an antidepressant, adequately screen patients with depressive symptoms to determine if they are at risk for bipolar disorder; such screening should include a detailed psychiatric history, including a family history of suicide, bipolar disorder, and depression. Note that selegiline is not approved for use in treating bipolar depression.

➤*Hypertensive crisis:* Selegiline is an irreversible MAOI. MAO is important in the catabolism of dietary amines (eg, tyramine). In this regard, significant inhibition of intestinal MAO-A activity can impose a cardiovascular safety risk following the ingestion of tyramine-rich foods. As a class, MAOIs have been associated with hypertensive crises caused by the ingestion of foods with a high concentration of tyramine. Hypertensive crises, which in some cases may be fatal, are characterized by some or all of the following symptoms: occipital headache (which may radiate frontally), palpitation, neck stiffness or soreness, nausea, vomiting, sweating (sometimes with fever and sometimes with cold, clammy skin), dilated pupils, and photophobia. Either tachycardia or bradycardia may be present and can be associated with constricting chest pain. Intracranial bleeding has been reported in association with the increase in blood pressure. Instruct patients as to the signs and symptoms of severe hypertension and advise them to seek immediate medical attention if these signs or symptoms are present.

In 6 of the 7 clinical studies conducted with selegiline at doses of 6 to 12 mg per 24 hours, patients were not limited to a modified diet typically associated with this class of compounds. Although no hypertensive crises were reported as part of the safety assessment, the likelihood of developing this reaction cannot be fully determined because the amount of tyramine typically consumed during the course of treatment is not known and blood pressure was not continuously monitored.

To further define the likelihood of hypertensive crises with use of selegiline, several phase 1 tyramine challenge studies were conducted both with and without food. In its entirety, the data for selegiline 6 mg per 24 hours support the recommendation that a modified diet is not required at this dose. Because of the more limited data available for selegiline 9 mg per 24 hours and the results from the phase 1 tyramine challenge study in fed volunteers administered selegiline 12 mg per 24 hours, patients receiving these doses should follow dietary modifications required for patients taking selegiline 9 mg per 24 hours and 12 mg per 24 hours.

If a hypertensive crisis occurs, discontinue selegiline immediately and institute therapy to lower blood pressure immediately. Phentolamine 5 mg or labetalol 20 mg administered slowly IV is the recommended therapy to control hypertension. Alternately, nitroprusside delivered by continuous IV infusion may be used. Manage fever by means of external cooling. Closely monitor patients until symptoms have stabilized.

➤*Required dietary modifications:* Patients should avoid the following foods and beverages beginning on the first day of selegiline 9 mg per 24 hours or 12 mg per 24 hours treatment and should continue to avoid them for 2 weeks after a dosage reduction to selegiline 6 mg per 24 hours or following the discontinuation of selegiline 9 mg per 24 hours or 12 mg per 24 hours.

Acceptable and Unacceptable Tyramine-Containing Foods/Beverages When Taking Selegiline

Class of food and beverage	Tyramine-rich foods and beverages to avoid	Acceptable foods, containing no or little tyramine
Meat, poultry, and fish	Air-dried, aged, and fermented meats, sausages, and salamis (including cacciatore, hard salami, and mortadella); pickled herring; any spoiled or improperly stored meat, poultry, or fish (eg, foods that have undergone changes in coloration or odor, or become moldy); spoiled or improperly stored animal livers	Fresh meat, poultry, and fish, including fresh, processed meats (eg, lunch meats; hot dogs; breakfast sausage; cooked, sliced ham)
Vegetables	Broad bean pods (fava bean pods)	All other vegetables
Dairy	Aged cheeses	Processed cheeses, mozzarella, ricotta cheese, cottage cheese, yogurt

SELEGILINE — TRANSDERMAL

Acceptable and Unacceptable Tyramine-Containing Foods/Beverages When Taking Selegiline		
Class of food and beverage	Tyramine-rich foods and beverages to avoid	Acceptable foods, containing no or little tyramine
Beverages	All varieties of tap beer and beers that have not been pasteurized so as to allow for ongoing fermentation	Concomitant use of alcohol with selegiline transdermal is not recommended. (Bottled and canned beers and wines contain little or no tyramine.)
Miscellaneous	Concentrated yeast extract (eg, *Marmite*), sauerkraut, most soybean products (including soy sauce and tofu), nonprescription supplements containing tyramine	Brewer's yeast, baker's yeast, soy milk, commercial chain restaurant pizzas prepared with cheeses low in tyramine

➤*Serotonin syndrome:* Serious, sometimes fatal, CNS toxicity referred to as the "serotonin syndrome" has been reported with the combination of nonselective MAOIs with certain other drugs, including TCAs or SSRI antidepressants, amphetamines, meperidine, or pentazocine. Serotonin syndrome is characterized by signs and symptoms that may include hyperthermia, rigidity, myoclonus, autonomic instability with rapid fluctuations of the vital signs, and mental status changes that include extreme agitation progressing to delirium and coma. Similar less severe syndromes have been reported in a few patients receiving a combination of oral selegiline with one of these agents.

See Drug Interactions for more information.

Concomitant use of selegiline with buspirone is not advised because several cases of elevated blood pressure have been reported in patients taking MAOIs who were then given buspirone.

After stopping treatment with SSRIs; SNRIs; TCAs; MAOIs; meperidine and analgesics such as tramadol, methadone, and propoxyphene; dextromethorphan; St. John's wort; mirtazapine; bupropion; or buspirone, a time period equal to 4 to 5 half-lives (approximately 1 week) of the drug or any active metabolite should elapse before starting therapy with selegiline. Because of the long half-life of fluoxetine and its active metabolite, at least 5 weeks should elapse between discontinuation of fluoxetine and initiation of treatment with selegiline. At least 2 weeks should elapse after stopping selegiline before starting therapy with buspirone or a drug that is contraindicated with selegiline.

➤*External heat:* The effect of direct heat applied to the selegiline patch on the bioavailability of selegiline has not been studied. However, in theory, heat may result in an increase in the amount of selegiline absorbed from the selegiline patch and produce elevated serum levels of selegiline. Advise patients to avoid exposing the selegiline application site to external sources of direct heat, such as heating pads or electric blankets, heat lamps, saunas, hot tubs, heated water beds, and prolonged direct sunlight.

➤*Hypotension:* As with other MAOIs, postural hypotension, sometimes with orthostatic symptoms, can occur with selegiline therapy. In short-term, placebo-controlled depression studies, the incidence of orthostatic hypotension (ie, a decrease of 10 mm Hg or more in mean blood pressure when changing position from supine or sitting to standing) was 9.8% in selegiline-treated patients and 6.7% in placebo-treated patients. Closely observe elderly patients treated with selegiline for postural changes in blood pressure throughout treatment. Make dose increases cautiously in patients with preexisting orthostasis. Postural hypotension may be relieved by having the patient recline until the symptoms have abated. Caution patients to change positions gradually. Patients displaying orthostatic symptoms should have appropriate dosage adjustments as warranted.

➤*Activation of mania/hypomania:* During phase 3 trials, a manic reaction occurred in 0.4% patients treated with selegiline. Activation of mania/hypomania can occur in a small proportion of patients with a major affective disorder treated with other marketed antidepressants. As with all antidepressants, use selegiline cautiously in patients with a history of mania.

➤*Elective surgery:* As with other MAOIs, patients taking selegiline should not undergo elective surgery requiring general anesthesia. They also should not be given cocaine or local anesthesia containing sympathomimetic vasoconstrictors. Discontinue selegiline at least 10 days prior to elective surgery.

➤*Special risk:* Clinical experience with selegiline in patients with certain concomitant systemic illnesses is limited. Caution is advised when using selegiline in patients with disorders or conditions that can produce altered metabolism or hemodynamic responses.

Selegiline has not been systematically evaluated in patients with a history of recent myocardial infarction or unstable heart disease.

➤*Hazardous tasks:* Selegiline has not been shown to impair psychomotor performance; however, any psychoactive drug may potentially impair judgment, thinking, or motor skills. Caution patients about operating hazardous machinery, including automobiles, until they are reasonably certain that selegiline therapy does not impair their ability to engage in such activities.

➤*Pregnancy: Category C.* In an embryofetal development study in rats, dams were treated with transdermal selegiline during the period of organogenesis at dosages of 10, 30, and 75 mg/kg/day (8, 24, and 60 times the MRHD of selegiline [12 mg per 24 hours] on a mg/m² basis). At the highest dose, there was a decrease in fetal weight and slight increases in malformations, delayed ossification (also seen at the middose), and embryofetal postimplantation lethality. Concentrations of selegiline and its metabolites in fetal plasma were generally similar to those in maternal plasma. In an oral embryofetal development study in rats, a decrease in fetal weight occurred at the highest dose tested (36 mg/kg; no-effect dose, 12 mg/kg); no increase in malformations was seen.

In an embryofetal development study in rabbits, dams were treated with transdermal selegiline during the period of organogenesis at dosages of 2.5, 10, and 40 mg/kg/day (4, 16, and 64 times the MRHD on a mg/m² basis). A slight increase in visceral malformations was seen at the high dose. In an oral embryofetal development study in rabbits, increases in total resorptions and postimplantation loss and a decrease in the number of live fetuses per dam occurred at the highest dose tested (50 mg/kg; no-effect dose, 25 mg/kg).

In a prenatal and postnatal development study in rats, dams were treated with transdermal selegiline at dosages of 10, 30, and 75 mg/kg/day (8, 24, and 60 times the MRHD on a mg/m² basis) on days 6 to 21 of gestation and days 1 to 21 of the lactation period. An increase in postimplantation loss was seen at the mid and high doses, and an increase in stillborn pups was seen at the high dose. Decreases in pup weight (throughout lactation and postweaning periods) and survival (throughout lactation period), retarded pup physical development, and pup epididymal and testicular hypoplasia, were seen at the mid and high doses. Retarded neurobehavioral and sexual development were seen at all doses. Adverse reactions on pup reproductive performance, as evidenced by decreases in implantations and litter size, were seen at the high dose. These findings suggest persistent effects on the offspring of treated dams. A no-effect dose was not established for developmental toxicity. In this study, concentrations of selegiline and its metabolites in milk were approximately 15 and 5 times, respectively, the concentrations in plasma, indicating that the pups were directly dosed during the lactation period.

There are no adequate and well-controlled studies in pregnant women. It is not known if selegiline crosses the human placenta. The low molecular weight (about 188 for the free base) suggests that passage to the embryo and fetus should be expected. Do not use selegiline at any dose in children younger than 12 years of age even when administered with dietary modifications. Selegiline is not approved for use in children. Use selegiline during pregnancy only if the potential benefit justifies the potential risk to the fetus.

➤*Lactation:* In a prenatal and postnatal study of transdermal selegiline in rats, selegiline and metabolites were excreted into the milk of lactating rats. The levels of selegiline and metabolites in milk were approximately 15 and 5 times, respectively, steady-state levels of selegiline and metabolites in maternal plasma. It is not known whether this drug is excreted in human milk. The low molecular weight (about 188 for the free base) suggests that excretion into breast milk should be expected. Because many drugs are excreted in human milk, exercise caution when selegiline is administered to a breast-feeding mother.

➤*Children:* Safety and efficacy in children have not been established. Anyone considering the use of selegiline in a child or adolescent must balance the potential risks with the clinical need.

Because of limited data, do not use selegiline at any dose in children younger than 12 years of age, even when administered with dietary modifications. Selegiline is not approved for use in children.

➤*Elderly:* In short-term, placebo-controlled depression trials, patients 50 years of age and older appeared to be at higher risk for rash (4.4% selegiline vs 0% placebo) than younger patients (3.4% selegiline vs 2.4% placebo).

➤*Monitoring:* Monitor and closely observe all patients appropriately being treated with antidepressants for any indication for clinical worsening, suicidality, and unusual changes in behavior, especially during the initial few months of a course of drug therapy, or at times of dose changes, either increases or decreases.

Closely monitor elderly patients treated with selegiline for postural changes in blood pressure throughout treatment.

Evaluate patients for a history of drug abuse, and closely observe such patients for signs of selegiline misuse or abuse (eg, development of tolerance, increase in dose, drug-seeking behavior).

Drug Interactions

Selegiline Drug Interactions			
Precipitant drug	Object drug[a]		Description
Anticonvulsants (eg, carbamazepine, oxcarbazepine)	Selegiline	↑	A hypertensive crisis may occur. Concurrent use with carbamazepine or oxcarbazepine is contraindicated.
Apraclonidine	Selegiline	↑	Risk of selegiline-induced hypertension may be increased. Coadministration is contraindicated. Do not coadminister within 14 days of each other.
Buspirone	Selegiline	↑	Risk of selegiline-induced hypertension may be increased when coadministered with buspirone. Concurrent use is not recommended.

SELEGILINE — TRANSDERMAL

Selegiline Drug Interactions

Precipitant drug	Object drug[a]		Description
Contraceptives, hormonal	Selegiline	↑	Plasma selegiline concentrations may be elevated, increasing the risk of adverse reactions.
Linezolid	Selegiline	↑	Coadministration is contraindicated. Do not use within 14 days of each other.
Selegiline	Alcohol	↑	Severe hypertension may occur when alcoholic beverages, especially those high in tyramine content are consumed. Concurrent use is not recommended.
Selegiline	Analgesic agents (eg, meperidine, methadone, propoxyphene, tramadol)	↑	A "serotonin syndrome" may occur. Concurrent use is contraindicated. At least 14 days should elapse between discontinuation of selegiline and initiation of meperidine.
Selegiline	Anesthetics	↑	Patients taking selegiline should not undergo elective surgery requiring general anesthesia. Do not give cocaine or local anesthesia containing sympathomimetic vasoconstrictors. Discontinue selegiline at least 10 days before elective surgery.
Selegiline	Bupropion	↑	A "serotonin syndrome" may occur. Concurrent use is contraindicated. Allow at least 14 days to elapse between discontinuing selegiline and starting bupropion.
Selegiline	Buspirone	↑	Several cases of elevated blood pressure have been reported. Concurrent use is not recommended.
Selegiline	CNS stimulants (eg, amphetamine, atomoxetine, dexmethylphenidate, methylphenidate, sibutramine)	↑	Coadministration is contraindicated. Allow at least 2 weeks after discontinuing a CNS stimulant before giving selegiline.
CNS stimulants (eg, amphetamine, atomoxetine, dexmethylphenidate, methylphenidate, sibutramine)	Selegiline		
Selegiline	Cyclobenzaprine	↑	A "serotonin syndrome" may occur. Concurrent use is contraindicated. Discontinue selegiline 14 days before starting cyclobenzaprine.
Selegiline	Dextromethorphan	↑	A "serotonin syndrome" may occur. Concurrent use is contraindicated.
Selegiline	Ginseng	↑	Manic-like symptoms, headaches, and tremulousness have been reported. Avoid concurrent use.
Selegiline	Insulin	↑	The hypoglycemic reaction of insulin may be increased.
Selegiline	MAOIs (eg, oral selegiline, isocarboxazid, phenelzine, tranylcypromine)	↑	A "serotonin syndrome" may occur. Concurrent use is contraindicated. At least 14 days should elapse between discontinuation of selegiline and initiation of another MAOI.
MAOIs (eg, isocarboxazid, phenelzine, tranylcypromine)	Selegiline		
Selegiline	Maprotiline	↑	Selegiline may enhance the sympathomimetic effects of maprotiline. Concomitant use is contraindicated. Allow a minimum of 14 days after discontinuing selegiline before starting maprotiline.
Selegiline	Meglitinide antidiabetic agents (eg, nateglinide, repaglinide)	↑	Hypoglycemic effects may be increased.
Selegiline	Mirtazapine	↑	A "serotonin syndrome" may occur. Concurrent use is contraindicated.
Selegiline	Serotonin reuptake inhibitors (eg, citalopram, duloxetine, fluoxetine, fluvoxamine, nefazodone, paroxetine, sertraline, venlafaxine)	↑	A "serotonin syndrome" may occur. Concurrent use is contraindicated. At least 5 weeks should elapse between discontinuation of fluoxetine and initiation of selegiline; at least 14 days should elapse between discontinuation of selegiline and initiation of treatment with a serotonergic drug.
Serotonin reuptake inhibitors (eg, citalopram, duloxetine, fluoxetine, fluvoxamine, nefazodone, paroxetine, sertraline, venlafaxine)	Selegiline		
Selegiline	St. John's wort	↑	A "serotonin syndrome" may occur. Concurrent use is contraindicated.
Selegiline	Sulfonylureas	↑	The hypoglycemic action of sulfonylureas may be increased by selegiline.
Selegiline	Sympathomimetic agents (eg, ephedrine, phenylephrine, phenylpropanolamine, pseudoephedrine)	↑	A "serotonin syndrome" may occur. Concurrent use is contraindicated.
Selegiline	TCAs (eg, amitriptyline, imipramine)	↑	A "serotonin syndrome" may occur. Concurrent use or use within 2 weeks of selegiline treatment is contraindicated.
Selegiline	Tetrabenazine	↑	Coadministration is contraindicated.
Tetrabenazine	Selegiline		
Selegiline	Triptans (eg, sumatriptan, rizatriptan)	↑	Prolonged vasospastic reactions may occur. Coadminister sumatriptan with an MAOI with caution; concurrent use with rizatriptan within 2 weeks of discontinuation of an MAOI is contraindicated.

[a] ↑ = object drug increased.

➤*Drug/Food interactions:* Warn all patients about eating food with a high tyramine content. Hypertensive crisis may result. (See Warnings/Precautions for more information.)

Adverse Reactions

➤*Discontinuation:* Among 817 depressed patients who received selegiline at doses of either 3 mg per 24 hours (151 patients), 6 mg per 24 hours (550 patients), or 6 mg per 24 hours, 9 mg per 24 hours, and 12 mg per 24 hours (116 patients) in placebo-controlled trials of up to 8 weeks in duration, 7.1% discontinued treatment because of an adverse reaction as compared with 3.6% of 668 patients receiving placebo. The only adverse reaction associated with discontinuation, in at least 1% of selegiline-treated patients at a rate at least twice that of placebo, was application-site reaction (2% selegiline vs 0% placebo).

➤*Adverse reactions (2% or more):* Only one adverse reaction was associated with a reporting of at least 5% in the selegiline group and a rate at least twice that in the placebo group in the pool of short-term, placebo-controlled studies: application site reactions. In one such study, which utilized higher mean doses of selegiline than that in the entire study pool, the following reactions met these criteria: application site reactions, diarrhea, insomnia, and pharyngitis.

SELEGILINE — TRANSDERMAL

Selegiline Transdermal Adverse Reactions (≥ 2%)[a]		
Adverse reactions	Selegiline (n = 817)	Placebo (n = 668)
CNS		
Headache	18%	17%
Insomnia	12%	7%
Dermatologic		
Application-site reaction	24%	12%
Rash	4%	2%
GI		
Diarrhea	9%	7%
Dry mouth	8%	6%
Dyspepsia	4%	3%
Respiratory		
Pharyngitis	3%	2%
Sinusitis	3%	1%

[a] Reactions reported by ≥ 2% of patients treated with selegiline are included, except the following reactions, which had an incidence on placebo treatment greater than or equal to selegiline: abdominal pain, accidental injury, anxiety, asthenia, back pain, dizziness, flu syndrome, infection, nausea, nervousness, pain, palpitations, rhinitis, and somnolence.

➤*Application-site reactions:* In the pool of short-term, placebo-controlled MDD studies, application-site reactions were reported in 24% of selegiline-treated patients and 12% of placebo-treated patients. Most application-site reactions were mild or moderate in severity. None were considered serious. Application-site reactions led to dropout in 2% of selegiline-treated patients and no placebo-treated patients.

In one such study that utilized higher mean doses of selegiline, application-site reactions were reported in 40% of selegiline-treated patients and 20% of placebo-treated patients. Most of the application-site reactions in this study were described as erythema, and most resolved spontaneously, requiring no treatment. When treatment was administered, it most commonly consisted of dermatological preparations of corticosteroids.

➤*Sexual dysfunction:* Although changes in sexual desire, sexual performance, and sexual satisfaction often occur as manifestations of a psychiatric disorder, they may also be a consequence of pharmacologic treatment.

Selegiline Sexual Adverse Reactions		
Adverse reactions	Selegiline	Placebo
Abnormal ejaculation[a]	1%	0%
Anorgasmia[a]	0.2%	0%
Decreased libido, men[a]	0.7%	0%
Decreased libido, women[b]	0%	0.2%
Impotence[a]	0.7%	0.4%

[a] Selegiline, n = 304; placebo, n = 256.
[b] Selegiline, n = 513; placebo, n = 412.

➤*Vital sign changes:* Selegiline and placebo groups were compared with respect to (1) mean change from baseline in vital signs (pulse, systolic blood pressure, and diastolic blood pressure), and (2) the incidence of patients meeting criteria for potentially clinically significant changes from baseline in these variables. In the pool of short-term, placebo-controlled MDD studies, 3% of selegiline-treated patients and 1.5% of placebo-treated patients experienced a low systolic blood pressure, defined as a reading of 90 mm Hg or less with a change from baseline of at least 20 mm Hg. In one study, which utilized higher mean doses of selegiline, 6.2% of selegiline-treated patients and no placebo-treated patients experienced a low standing systolic blood pressure by these criteria.

In the pool of short-term MDD trials, 9.8% of selegiline-treated patients and 6.7% of placebo-treated patients experienced a notable orthostatic change in blood pressure, defined as a decrease of at least 10 mm Hg in mean blood pressure with postural change.

➤*Weight changes:*

Weight Gain/Loss with Selegiline Treatment		
Weight change	Selegiline (n = 757)	Placebo (n = 614)
Gained ≥ 5%	2.1%	2.4%
Lost ≥ 5%	5%	2.8%

In these trials, the mean change in body weight among selegiline-treated patients was −1.2 lbs compared with + 0.3 lbs in placebo-treated patients.

➤*Other adverse reactions:*

Cardiovascular – Hypertension (at least 1%); atrial fibrillation, peripheral vascular disorder, syncope, tachycardia, vasodilatation (0.1% to 1%); myocardial infarction (less than 0.1%).

CNS – Agitation, amnesia, paresthesia, thinking abnormal (at least 1%); circumoral paresthesia, confusion, depersonalization, emotional lability, euphoria, hostility, hyperesthesia, hyperkinesias, hypertonia, increased libido, manic reaction, migraine, myoclonus, neurosis, paranoid reaction, suicide attempt, tremor, twitching, vertigo (0.1% to 1%); ataxia, malaise (less than 0.1%).

Dermatologic – Acne, pruritus, sweating (at least 1%); alopecia, contact dermatitis, dry skin, fungal dermatitis, herpes simplex, herpes zoster, maculopapular rash, skin benign neoplasm, skin hypertrophy, urticaria, vesiculobullous rash (0.1% to 1%); eczema (less than 0.1%).

GI – Anorexia, constipation, flatulence, gastroenteritis, vomiting (at least 1%); colitis, dysphagia, eructation, gastritis, glossitis, increased appetite, increased salivation, melena, periodontal abscess, thirst, tongue disorder, tongue edema, tooth caries (0.1% to 1%); GI neoplasia, rectal hemorrhage (less than 0.1%).

GU – Dysmenorrhea, metrorrhagia, urinary frequency, urinary tract infection (at least 1%); amenorrhea, breast neoplasm (female), breast pain, cystitis (female), dysuria (female), hematuria (female), kidney calculus (female), menorrhagia, pelvic pain, polyuria (female), unintended pregnancy, urinary tract infection (male), urinary urgency (male and female), urination impaired (male), vaginal hemorrhage, vaginal moniliasis, vaginitis (0.1% to 1%).

Hematologic/Lymphatic – Ecchymosis (at least 1%); anemia, lymphadenopathy (0.1% to 1%); leukocytosis, leukopenia, petechia (less than 0.1%).

Hepatic – Abnormal liver function tests, increased ALT, increased AST (0.1% to 1%).

Metabolic/Nutritional – Peripheral edema (at least 1%); alcohol intolerance, dehydration, edema, generalized edema, hypercholesteremia, hyperglycemia, hyponatremia, increased lactic dehydrogenase (0.1% to 1%); bilirubinemia, hypoglycemic reaction, increased alkaline phosphatase (less than 0.1%).

Musculoskeletal – Myalgia, neck pain, pathological fracture (at least 1%); arthralgia, arthritis, arthrosis, flank pain, generalized spasm, leg cramps, myasthenia, neck rigidity, tenosynovitis (0.1% to 1%); osteoporosis (less than 0.1%).

Respiratory – Bronchitis, cough increased (at least 1%); asthma, dyspnea, laryngismus, pneumonia (0.1% to 1%); epistaxis, laryngitis, yawn (less than 0.1%).

Special senses – Taste perversion, tinnitus (at least 1%); conjunctivitis, dry eyes, ear pain, eye pain, otitis media, parosmia (0.1% to 1%); mydriasis, otitis external, visual field defect (less than 0.1%).

Miscellaneous – Chest pain (at least 1%); bacterial infection, chills, cyst, face edema, fever, fungal infection, hernia, intentional injury, neoplasm, overdose, photosensitivity reaction, viral infection (0.1% to 1%); body odor, halitosis, heatstroke, moniliasis, parasitic infection (less than 0.1%).

Overdosage

➤*Overdosage with nonselective MAO inhibition:* Typical signs and symptoms associated with overdosage of nonselective MAOI antidepressants may not appear immediately. Delays of up to 12 hours between ingestion of the drug and the appearance of signs may occur, and peak effects may not be observed for 24 to 48 hours. Because death has been reported following overdosage with MAOI agents, hospitalization with close monitoring during this period is essential.

Overdosage with MAOI agents is typically associated with CNS and cardiovascular toxicity. Signs and symptoms of overdosage may include, alone or in combination, any of the following: drowsiness, dizziness, faintness, irritability, hyperactivity, agitation, severe headache, hallucinations, trismus, opisthotonos, convulsions, coma, rapid and irregular pulse, hypertension, hypotension and vascular collapse, precordial pain, respiratory depression and failure, hyperpyrexia, diaphoresis, and cool, clammy skin. Type and intensity of symptoms may be related to extent of the overdosage.

➤*Symptoms:* Selegiline is considered to be an irreversible MAOI at therapeutic doses and, in overdosage, is likely to cause excessive MAO-A inhibition and may result in the signs and symptoms resembling overdosage with other nonselective, oral MAOI antidepressants (eg, tranylcypromine, phenelzine, isocarboxazide).

➤*Treatment:* Treatment should include supportive measures, with pharmacological intervention as appropriate. Symptoms may persist after drug washout because of the irreversible inhibitory effects of these agents on systemic MAO activity. With overdosage, in order to avoid the occurrence of hypertensive crisis ("cheese reaction"), dietary tyramine should be restricted for several weeks beyond recovery to permit regeneration of the peripheral MAO-A isoenzyme.

There are no specific antidotes for selegiline. If symptoms of overdosage occur, immediately remove selegiline and institute appropriate supportive therapy. For contemporary consultation on the management of poisoning or overdosage, contact the American Association of Poison Control Centers at 1-800-222-1222.

Patient Information

Encourage patients, their families, and their caregivers to be alert to the emergence of anxiety, agitation, panic attacks, insomnia, irritability, hostility, aggressiveness, impulsivity, akathisia (psychomotor restlessness), hypomania, mania, other unusual changes in behavior, worsening of depression, and suicidal ideation, especially early during antidepressant treatment or when the dose is adjusted up or down. Advise families and caregivers of patients to observe for the emergence of such symptoms on a day-to-day basis, since changes may be abrupt. Such symptoms should be reported to the patient's health care provider, especially if they are severe, abrupt in onset, or were not part of the patient's presenting symptoms. Symptoms

SELEGILINE — TRANSDERMAL

such as these may be associated with an increased risk for suicidal thinking and behavior, and indicate a need for very close monitoring and possibly change in the medication.

Advise patients not to use carbamazepine; oxcarbazepine; meperidine; and analgesic agents such as tramadol, methadone, and propoxyphene; or sympathomimetic agents while on selegiline therapy.

Advise patients not to use SSRIs (eg, fluoxetine, sertraline, paroxetine, St. John's wort), SNRIs (eg, venlafaxine, duloxetine), TCAs (eg, amitriptyline, imipramine), mirtazapine, oral selegiline or other MAOIs (eg, isocarboxazid, phenelzine, tranylcypromine), bupropion, or buspirone while on selegiline.

Selegiline has not been shown to impair psychomotor performance; however, any psychoactive drug may potentially impair judgment, thinking, or motor skills. Caution patients about operating hazardous machinery, including automobiles, until they are reasonably certain that selegiline does not impair their ability to engage in such activities.

Tell patients that although selegiline has not been shown to increase the impairment of mental and motor skills caused by alcohol, the concomitant use of selegiline and alcohol in depressed patients is not recommended.

Advise patients to notify their health care provider if they are taking, or planning to take, any prescription or nonprescription drugs, including herbals, because of the potential for drug interactions. Also advise patients to avoid tyramine-containing nutritional supplements and any cough medicine containing dextromethorphan.

Advise patients to use selegiline exactly as prescribed. Explain the need for dietary modifications at higher doses and provide a brief description of hypertensive crisis. Rare hypertensive reactions with oral selegiline at doses recommended for Parkinson disease and associated with dietary influences have been reported. The clinical relevance to selegiline is unknown.

Advise patients to avoid certain tyramine-rich foods and beverages while on selegiline 9 mg per 24 hours or 12 mg per 24 hours, and for 2 weeks following discontinuation of selegiline at these doses.

Instruct patients to immediately report the occurrence of the following acute symptoms: severe headache, neck stiffness, heart racing or palpitations, or other sudden or unusual symptoms.

Advise patients to avoid exposing the selegiline application site to external sources of direct heat, such as heating pads or electric blankets, heat lamps, saunas, hot tubs, heated water beds, and prolonged direct sunlight because heat may result in an increase in the amount of selegiline absorbed from the patch and produce elevated serum levels of selegiline.

Advise patients to change position gradually if light-headed, faint, or dizzy while on selegiline.

Advise patients to notify their health care provider if they become pregnant or intend to become pregnant during selegiline.

Advise patients to notify their health care provider if they are breast-feeding an infant.

While patients may notice improvement with selegiline in 1 to several weeks, advise them of the importance of continuing drug treatment as directed.

Advise patients not to cut the patch into smaller portions.

TOLCAPONE

Rx	**Tasmar** (Roche)	**Tablets**: 100 mg	Lactose. (Tasmar 100 Roche). Beige, hexagonal, biconvex. Film coated. In 90s.
		200 mg	Lactose. (Tasmar 200 Roche). Reddish brown, hexagonal, biconvex. Film coated. In 90s.

TOLCAPONE — ORAL

Refer to the general discussion in the Antiparkinson Agents introduction.

WARNING

Because of the risk of potentially fatal, acute fulminant liver failure, tolcapone should ordinarily be used in patients with Parkinson's disease on l-dopa/carbidopa who are experiencing symptom fluctuations and are not responding satisfactorily to or are not appropriate candidates for other adjunctive therapies.

Because of the risk of liver injury and because tolcapone, when it is effective, provides an observable symptomatic benefit, the patient who fails to show substantial clinical benefit within 3 weeks of initiation of treatment, should be withdrawn from tolcapone.

Tolcapone therapy should not be initiated if the patient exhibits clinical evidence of liver disease or 2 ALT or AST values greater than the upper limit of normal. Patients with severe dyskinesia or dystonia should be treated with caution.

Patients who develop evidence of hepatocellular injury while on tolcapone and are withdrawn from the drug for any reason may be at increased risk for liver injury if tolcapone is reintroduced. Accordingly, such patients should not ordinarily be considered for retreatment.

Cases of severe hepatocellular injury, including fulminant liver failure resulting in death, have been reported in postmarketing use. As of October 1998, 3 cases of fatal fulminant hepatic failure have been reported from approximately 60,000 patients providing about 40,000 patient years of worldwide use. This incidence may be 10- to 100– fold higher than the background incidence in the general population. Underreporting of cases may lead to significant underestimation of the increased risk associated with the use of tolcapone.

A prescriber who elects to use tolcapone in the face of the increased risk of liver injury is strongly advised to monitor patients for evidence of emergent liver injury. Patients should be advised of the need for self-monitoring for both the classical signs of liver disease (eg, clay-colored stools, jaundice) and the nonspecific ones (eg, fatigue, loss of appetite, lethargy).

Although a program of frequent laboratory monitoring for evidence of hepatocellular injury is deemed essential, it is not clear that baseline and periodic monitoring of liver enzymes will prevent the occurrence of fulminant liver failure. However, it is generally believed that early detection of drug-induced hepatic injury along with immediate withdrawal of the suspect drug enhances the likelihood for recovery. It is also widely held, without a robust body of evidence, that patients with preexisting hepatic disease are more vulnerable of hepatotoxins. Accordingly, the following live-monitoring program is recommended.

Before starting treatment with tolcapone, the physician should conduct appropriate tests to exclude the presence of liver disease. In patients determined to be appropriate candidates for treatment with tolcapone, serum glutamic-pyruvic transaminase (ALT) and serum glutamic-oxaloacetic transaminase (AST) levels should be determined at baseline and then every 2 weeks for the first year of therapy, every 4 weeks for the next 6 months, and then every 8 weeks thereafter. If the dose is increased to 200 mg 3 times daily, liver enzyme monitoring should take place before increasing the dose and then be reinitiated at the frequency above.

WARNING (cont.)

Tolcapone should be discontinued if ALT or AST exceeds the upper limit of normal (ULN) or if clinical signs and symptoms suggest the onset of hepatic failure (eg, persistent nausea, fatigue, lethargy, anorexia, jaundice, dark urine, pruritus, right upper quadrant tenderness).

Indications

➤*Parkinsonism:* Tolcapone is indicated as an adjunct to levodopa and carbidopa for the treatment of the signs and symptoms of idiopathic Parkinson's disease. Because of the risk of potentially fatal, acute, fulminant liver failure, tolcapone should ordinarily be used in patients with Parkinson's disease on l-dopa/carbidopa who are experiencing symptom fluctuations and are not responding satisfactorily to or are not appropriate candidates for other adjunctive therapies. Because of the risk of liver injury and because tolcapone, when it is effective, provides an observable symptomatic benefit, the patient who fails to show substantial clinical benefit within 3 weeks of initiation of treatment, should be withdrawn from tolcapone.

Administration and Dosage

➤*Adults:*

Parkinsonism –

Usual dosage: 100 mg 3 times daily, always as an adjunct to levodopa/carbidopa.

In clinical trials, elevations in ALT occurred more frequently at the dose of 200 mg 3 times daily. While it is unknown whether the risk of acute fulminant liver failure is increased at the 200 mg dose, it would be prudent to use 200 mg only if the anticipated incremental clinical benefit is justified. If a patient fails to show the expected incremental benefit on the 200 mg dose after a total of 3 weeks of treatment (regardless of dose), tolcapone should be discontinued.

Concomitant therapy: To optimize an individual patient's response, reductions in daily levodopa dose may be necessary. In clinical trials, the majority of patients required a decrease in their daily levodopa dose if their daily dose of levodopa was over 600 mg or if patients had moderate or severe dyskinesias before beginning treatment. The average reduction in daily levodopa dose was about 30% in those patients requiring a levodopa dose reduction. (greater than 70% of patients with levodopa doses over 600 mg daily required such a reduction).

Discontinuation of therapy: Withdrawal or abrupt reduction in the tolcapone dose may lead to emergence of signs and symptoms of Parkinson disease or hyperpyrexia and confusion, a syndrome complex resembling the neuroleptic malignant syndrome. If a decision is made to discontinue treatment, then it is recommended to closely monitor the patient and adjust other dopaminergic treatments as needed. This syndrome should be considered in the differential diagnosis for any patient who develops a high fever or severe rigidity.

➤*Renal function impairment:* Patients with severe renal impairment should be treated with caution. The safety of tolcapone has not been examined in subjects who had creatinine clearance less than 25 mL/min.

➤*Hepatic function impairment:* Tolcapone should not be initiated if any patient with liver disease or 2 ALT or AST values greater than the ULN.

➤*Administration:* Tolcapone may be taken with or without food. In clinical trials, the first dose of the day of tolcapone was always taken together

TOLCAPONE — ORAL

with the first dose of the day of levodopa/carbidopa, and the subsequent doses of tolcapone were given approximately 6 and 12 hours later.

➤*Storage / Stability:* Store at 20° to 25°C (68° to 77°F).

Actions

➤*Pharmacology:* Tolcapone is a selective and reversible inhibitor of COMT.

The precise mechanism of action of tolcapone is unknown, but it is believed to be related to its ability to inhibit COMT and alter the plasma pharmacokinetics of levodopa. When tolcapone is given in conjunction with levodopa and an aromatic amino acid decarboxylase inhibitor, such as carbidopa, plasma levels of levodopa are more sustained than after administration of levodopa and an aromatic amino acid decarboxylase inhibitor alone. It is believed that these sustained plasma levels of levodopa result in more constant dopaminergic stimulation in the brain, leading to greater effects on the signs and symptoms of Parkinson's disease in patients as well as increased levodopa adverse reactions, sometimes requiring a decrease in the dose of levodopa. Tolcapone enters the CNS to a minimal extent, but has been shown to inhibit central COMT activity in animals.

➤*Pharmacokinetics:* Tolcapone pharmacokinetics are independent of sex, age, body weight, and race (Asian, black and white). Polymorphic metabolism is unlikely based on the metabolic pathways involved.

Absorption – Tolcapone is rapidly absorbed, with a t_{max} of approximately 2 hours. The absolute bioavailability following oral administration is about 65%. Food given within 1 hour before and 2 hours after dosing of tolcapone decreases the relative bioavailability by 10% to 20%.

Distribution – The steady-state volume of distribution of tolcapone is small (9 L). Tolcapone does not distribute widely into tissues due to its high plasma protein binding. The plasma protein binding of tolcapone is approximately 99.9% over the concentration range of 0.32 to 210 mcg/mL. In vitro experiments have shown that tolcapone binds mainly to serum albumin.

Metabolism / Excretion – Tolcapone is almost completely metabolized prior to excretion, with only a very small amount (0.5% of dose) found unchanged in urine. The main metabolic pathway of tolcapone is glucuronidation; the glucuronide conjugate is inactive. In addition, the compound is methylated by COMT to 3-O-methyl-tolcapone. Tolcapone is metabolized to a primary alcohol (hydroxylation of the methyl group), which is subsequently oxidized to the carboxylic acid. In vitro experiments suggest that the oxidation may be catalyzed by cytochrome P450 3A4 and P450 2A6. The reduction to an amine and subsequent N-acetylation occur to a minor extent. After oral administration of a ^{14}C-labeled dose of tolcapone, 60% of labeled material is excreted in urine and 40% in feces.

Tolcapone is a low-extraction-ratio drug (extraction ratio = 0.15) with a moderate systemic clearance of about 7 L/hr.

Tolcapone pharmacokinetics are linear over the dose range of 50 to 400 mg, independent of levodopa/carbidopa coadministration. The elimination half-life of tolcapone is 2 to 3 hours and there is no significant accumulation. With 3-times-daily dosing of 100 or 200 mg, C_{max} is approximately 3 mcg/mL and 6 mcg/mL, respectively.

Special populations –

Hepatic function impairment: A study in patients with hepatic impairment has shown that moderate, noncirrhotic liver disease had no impact on the pharmacokinetics of tolcapone. In patients with moderate cirrhotic liver disease (Child-Pugh class B), however, clearance and volume of distribution of unbound tolcapone was reduced by almost 50%. This reduction may increase the average concentration of unbound drug by 2-fold (see Administration and Dosage). Tolcapone therapy should not be initiated if the patient exhibits clinical evidence of active liver disease or 2 ALT or AST values greater than the ULN.

Contraindications

Liver disease; patients who were withdrawn from tolcapone because of evidence of tolcapone-induced hepatocellular injury; or hypersensitivity to the drug or its ingredients; history of nontraumatic rhabdomyolysis or hyperpyrexia and confusion possibly related to medication.

Warnings/Precautions

➤*Hepatic failure:* In controlled phase 3 trials, increases to greater than 3 times the ULN in ALT or AST occurred in approximately 1% of patients at 100 mg 3 times daily and 3% of patients at 200 mg 3 times daily. Females were more likely than males to have an increase in liver enzymes (approximately 5% vs 2%). Approximately one-third of patients with elevated enzymes had diarrhea. Increases to greater than 8 times the ULN in liver enzymes occurred in 0.3% at 100 mg 3 times daily and 0.7% at 200 mg 3 times daily. Elevated enzymes led to discontinuation in 0.3% and 1.7% of patients treated with 100 mg 3 times daily and 200 mg 3 times daily, respectively. Elevations usually occurred within 6 weeks to 6 months of starting treatment. In about half the cases with elevated liver enzymes, enzyme levels returned to baseline values within 1 to 3 months while patients continued tolcapone treatment. When treatment was discontinued, enzymes generally declined within 2 to 3 weeks but in some cases took as long as 1 to 2 months to return to normal.

➤*Renal toxicity:* When rats were dosed daily for 1 or 2 years (exposures 6 times the human exposure or greater) there was a high incidence of proximal tubule cell damage consisting of degeneration, single cell necrosis, hyperplasia, karyocytomegaly and atypical nuclei. These effects were not associated with changes in clinical chemistry parameters, and there is no established method for monitoring for the possible occurrence of these lesions in humans. Although it has been speculated that these toxicities may occur as the result of a species-specific mechanism, experiments which would confirm that theory have not been conducted.

➤*Hypotension / syncope:* Dopaminergic therapy in Parkinson's disease patients has been associated with orthostatic hypotension. Tolcapone enhances levodopa bioavailability and, therefore, may increase the occurrence of orthostatic hypotension. In tolcapone clinical trials, orthostatic hypotension was documented at least once in 8%, 14% and 13% of the patients treated with placebo, 100, and 200 mg tolcapone 3 times daily, respectively. A total of 2%, 5% and 4% of the patients treated with placebo, 100 and 200 mg tolcapone 3 times daily, respectively, reported orthostatic symptoms at some time during their treatment and also had at least 1 episode of orthostatic hypotension documented (however, the episode of orthostatic symptoms itself was invariably not accompanied by vital sign measurements). Patients with orthostasis at baseline were more likely than patients without symptoms to have orthostatic hypotension during the study, irrespective of treatment group. In addition, the effect was greater in tolcapone-treated patients than in placebo-treated patients. Baseline treatment with dopamine agonists or selegiline did not appear to increase the likelihood of experiencing orthostatic hypotension when treated with tolcapone. Approximately 0.7% of the patients treated with tolcapone (5% of patients who were documented to have had at least one episode of orthostatic hypotension) eventually withdrew from treatment due to adverse events presumably related to hypotension.

In controlled phase 3 trials, approximately 5%, 4%, and 3% of tolcapone 200 mg 3 times daily, 100 mg 3 times daily and placebo patients, respectively, reported at least 1 episode of syncope. Reports of syncope were generally more frequent in patients in all 3 treatment groups who had an episode of documented hypotension (although the episodes of syncope, obtained by history, were themselves not documented with vital sign measurement) compared to patients who did not have any episodes of documented hypotension.

➤*Diarrhea:* In clinical trials, diarrhea developed in approximately 8%, 16%, and 18% of patients treated with placebo, 100 and 200 mg tolcapone 3 times daily, respectively. While diarrhea was generally regarded as mild to moderate in severity, approximately 3% to 4% of patients on tolcapone had diarrhea which was regarded as severe. Diarrhea was the adverse event which most commonly led to discontinuation, with approximately 1%, 5%, and 6% of patients treated with placebo, 100, and 200 mg tolcapone 3 times daily, respectively, withdrawing from the trials prematurely. Discontinuing tolcapone for diarrhea was related to the severity of the symptom. Diarrhea resulted in withdrawal in approximately 8%, 40%, and 70% of patients with mild, moderate and severe diarrhea, respectively. Although diarrhea generally resolved after discontinuation of tolcapone, it led to hospitalization in 0.3%, 0.7%, and 1.7% of patients in the placebo, 100, and 200 mg tolcapone 3-times-daily groups.

Typically, diarrhea presents 6 to 12 weeks after tolcapone is started, but it may appear as early as 2 weeks and as late as many months after the initiation of treatment. Clinical trial data suggested that diarrhea associated with tolcapone use may sometimes be associated with anorexia (decreased appetite).

It is recommended that all cases of persistent diarrhea should be followed up with an appropriate workup (including occult blood samples).

➤*Hallucinations:* In clinical trials, hallucinations developed in approximately 5%, 8%, and 10% of patients treated with placebo, 100 and 200 mg tolcapone 3 times daily, respectively. Hallucinations led to drug discontinuation and premature withdrawal from clinical trials in 0.3%, 1.4%, and 1% of patients treated with placebo, 100 and 200 mg tolcapone 3 times daily, respectively. Hallucinations led to hospitalization in 0%, 1.7%, and 0% of patients in the placebo, 100 mg and 200 mg tolcapone 3 times daily groups, respectively.

In general, hallucinations present shortly after the initiation of therapy with tolcapone (typically within the first 2 weeks). Clinical trial data suggest that hallucinations associated with tolcapone use may be responsive to levodopa dose reduction. Patients whose hallucinations resolved had a mean levodopa dose reduction of 175 to 200 mg (20% to 25%) after the onset of the hallucinations. Hallucinations were commonly accompanied by confusion and to a lesser extent sleep disorder (insomnia) and excessive dreaming.

➤*Dyskinesia:* Tolcapone may potentiate the dopaminergic side effects of levodopa and may cause or exacerbate preexisting dyskinesia. Although decreasing the dose of levodopa may ameliorate this side effect, many patients in controlled trials continued to experience frequent dyskinesias despite a reduction in their dose of levodopa. The rates of withdrawal for dyskinesia were 0%, 0.3%, and 1% for placebo, 100, and 200 mg tolcapone 3 times daily, respectively.

➤*Rhabdomyolysis:* Cases of severe rhabdomyolysis, with 1 case of multiorgan system failure rapidly progressing to death, have been reported. The complicated nature of these cases makes it impossible to determine what role, if any, tolcapone played in their pathogenesis. Severe prolonged motor activity including dyskinesia may account for rhabdomyolysis. Some cases, however, included fever, alteration of consciousness and muscular rigidity. It is possible, therefore, that the rhabdomyolysis may be a result of the syndrome described in Hyperpyrexia and confusion (see Events reported with dopaminergic therapy).

➤*Hematuria:* The rates of hematuria in placebo-controlled trials were approximately 2%, 4%, and 5% in placebo, 100, and 200 mg tolcapone 3 times daily, respectively. The etiology of the increase with tolcapone has not always been explained (for example, by urinary tract infection or warfarin therapy). In placebo-controlled trials in the United States (n = 593) rates of microscopically confirmed hematuria were ≈ 3%, 2%, and 2% in placebo, 100 mg and 200 mg tolcapone 3 times daily, respectively.

TOLCAPONE — ORAL

➤*Events reported with dopaminergic therapy:* The events listed below are known to be associated with the use of drugs that increase dopaminergic activity, although they are most often associated with the use of direct dopamine agonists. While cases of hyperpyrexia and confusion have been reported in association with tolcapone withdrawal (see information below), the expected incidence of fibrotic complications is so low that even if tolcapone caused these complications at rates similar to those attributable to other dopaminergic therapies, it is unlikely that even a single example would have been detected in a cohort of the size exposed to tolcapone.

Hyperpyrexia and confusion – In clinical trials, 4 cases of a symptom complex resembling the neuroleptic malignant syndrome (characterized by elevated temperature, muscular rigidity, and altered consciousness), similar to that reported in association with the rapid dose reduction or withdrawal of other dopaminergic drugs, have been reported in association with the abrupt withdrawal or lowering of the dose of tolcapone. In 3 of these cases, creatine phosphokinase (CPK) was elevated as well. One patient died, and the other 3 patients recovered over periods of approximately 2, 4, and 6 weeks. Rare cases of this symptom complex have been reported during marketed use. These cases are of a complicated nature including the concomitant administration of several medications affecting brain monoaminergic (ie, MAO-I, tricyclic and selective serotonin reuptake inhibitors) and anticholinergic systems. It is difficult, therefore, to determine what role, if any, tolcapone played in the pathogenesis. It may, therefore, be prudent to be particularly cautious if several concomitant medications of these types are used.

Fibrotic complications – Cases of retroperitoneal fibrosis, pulmonary infiltrates, pleural effusion, and pleural thickening have been reported in some patients treated with ergot derived dopaminergic agents. While these complications may resolve when the drug is discontinued, complete resolution does not always occur. Although these adverse events are believed to be related to the ergoline structure of these compounds, whether other, nonergot-derived drugs (eg, tolcapone) that increase dopaminergic activity can cause them is unknown.

Three cases of pleural effusion, one with pulmonary fibrosis, occurred during clinical trials. These patients were also on concomitant dopamine agonists (pergolide or bromocriptine) and had a history of cardiac disease or pulmonary pathology (nonmalignant lung lesion).

➤*Hepatic function impairment:* Because of the risk of liver injury, tolcapone therapy should not be initiated in any patient with liver disease. For similar reasons, treatment should not be initiated in patients who have 2 ALT or AST values greater than the upper limit of normal or any other evidence of hepatocellular dysfunction.

➤*Special risk:* Tolcapone therapy should not be initiated if the patient exhibits clinical evidence of active liver disease or 2 ALT or AST values greater than the ULN. Patients with severe dyskinesia or dystonia should be treated with caution. Patients with severe renal impairment should be treated with caution.

➤*Hazardous tasks:* Patients should be advised that they should neither drive a car nor operate other complex machinery until they have gained sufficient experience on tolcapone to gauge whether or not it affects their mental or motor performance adversely. Because of the possible additive sedative effects, caution should be used when patients are taking other CNS depressants in combination with tolcapone.

➤*Pregnancy: Category C.* Tolcapone, when administered alone during organogenesis, was not teratogenic at doses of up to 300 mg/kg/day in rats or up to 400 mg/kg/day in rabbits (5.7 times and 15 times the recommended daily clinical dose of 600 mg, on a mg/m^2 basis, respectively). In rabbits, however, an increased rate of abortion occurred at a dose of 100 mg/kg/day (3.7 times the daily clinical dose on a mg/m^2 basis) or greater. Evidence of maternal toxicity (decreased weight gain, death) was observed at 300 mg/kg in rats and 400 mg/kg in rabbits. When tolcapone was administered to female rats during the last part of gestation and throughout lactation, decreased litter size and impaired growth and learning performance in female pups were observed at a dose of 250/150 mg/kg/day (dose reduced from 250 to 150 mg/kg/day during late gestation due to high rate of maternal mortality; equivalent to 4.8/2.9 times the clinical dose on a mg/m^2 basis).

Tolcapone is always given concomitantly with levodopa/carbidopa, which is known to cause visceral and skeletal malformations in rabbits. The combination of tolcapone (100 mg/kg/day) with levodopa/carbidopa (80/20 mg/kg/day) produced an increased incidence of fetal malformations (primarily external and skeletal digit defects) compared to levodopa/carbidopa alone when pregnant rabbits were treated throughout organogenesis. Plasma exposures to tolcapone (based on AUC) were 0.5 times the expected human exposure, and plasma exposures to levodopa were 6 times higher than those in humans under therapeutic conditions. In a combination embryofetal development study in rats, fetal body weights were reduced by the combination of tolcapone (10, 30, and 50 mg/kg/day) and levodopa/carbidopa (120/30 mg/kg/day) and by levodopa/carbidopa alone. Tolcapone exposures were 0.5 times expected human exposure or greater: levodopa exposures were 21 times the expected human exposure or greater. The high dose of 50 mg/kg/day of tolcapone given alone was not associated with reduced fetal body weight (plasma exposures of 1.4 times the expected human exposure).

There is no experience from clinical studies regarding the use of tolcapone in pregnant women. Therefore, tolcapone should be used during pregnancy only if the potential benefit justifies the potential risk to the fetus.

➤*Lactation:* In animal studies, tolcapone was excreted into maternal rat milk. It is not known whether tolcapone is excreted in human milk. Because many drugs are excreted in human milk, caution should be exercised when tolcapone is administered to a nursing woman.

➤*Children:* There is no identified potential use of tolcapone in pediatric patients.

➤*Monitoring:* Although a program of frequent laboratory monitoring for evidence of hepatocellular injury is deemed essential, it is not clear that baseline and periodic monitoring of liver enzymes will prevent the occurrence of fulminant liver failure. However, it is generally believed that early detection of drug-induced hepatic injury along with immediate withdrawal of the suspect drug enhances the likelihood for recovery. It is also widely held, without a robust body of evidence, that patients with preexisting hepatic disease are more vulnerable to hepatotoxins. Accordingly, the following liver-monitoring program is recommended.

Before starting treatment with tolcapone, the physician should conduct appropriate tests to exclude the presence of liver disease. In patients determined to be appropriate candidates for treatment with tolcapone, serum glutamic-pyruvic transaminase (ALT) and serum glutamic-oxaloacetic transaminase (AST) levels should be determined at baseline and then every 2 weeks for the first year of therapy, every 4 weeks for the next 6 months and then every 8 weeks thereafter.

If the dose is increased to 200 mg 3 times daily, liver enzyme monitoring should take place before increasing the dose and then be reinitiated at the frequency above.

Tolcapone should be discontinued if ALT or AST exceeds the upper limit of normal or if clinical signs and symptoms suggest the onset of hepatic failure (eg, persistent nausea, fatigue, lethargy, anorexia, jaundice, dark urine, pruritus, right upper quadrant tenderness).

Drug Interactions

➤*Monamine oxidase (MAO) inhibitors:* MAO and COMT are the 2 major enzyme systems involved in the metabolism of catecholamines. It is theoretically possible, therefore, that the combination of tolcapone and a nonselective MAO inhibitor (eg, phenelzine, tranylcypromine) would result in inhibition of the majority of the pathways responsible for normal catecholamine metabolism. For this reason, patients should ordinarily not be treated concomitantly with tolcapone and a nonselective MAO inhibitor.

Tolcapone can be taken concomitantly with a selective MAO-B inhibitor (eg, selegiline).

➤*Drugs metabolized by COMT:* Tolcapone may influence the pharmacokinetics of drugs metabolized by COMT. However, no effects were seen on the pharmacokinetics of the COMT substrate carbidopa. The effect of tolcapone on the pharmacokinetics of other drugs of this class such as a-methyldopa, dobutamine, apomorphine, and isoproterenol has not been evaluated. A dose reduction of such compounds should be considered when they are coadministered with tolcapone.

➤*Effect of tolcapone on the metabolism of other drugs:* Due to its affinity to cytochrome P450 2C9 in vitro, tolcapone may interfere with drugs, whose clearance is dependent on this metabolic pathway, such as tolbutamide and warfarin. However, in an in vivo interaction study, tolcapone did not change the pharmacokinetics of tolbutamide. Therefore, clinically relevant interactions involving cytochrome P450 2C9 appear unlikely. Similarly, tolcapone did not affect the pharmacokinetics of desipramine, a drug metabolized by cytochrome P450 2D6, indicating that interactions with drugs metabolized by that enzyme are unlikely. Since clinical information is limited regarding the combination of warfarin and tolcapone, coagulation parameters should be monitored when these 2 drugs are coadministered.

➤*Drugs that increase catecholamines:* When tolcapone is administered together with levodopa/carbidopa, it increases the relative bioavailability (AUC) of levodopa by approximately 2-fold. This is due to a decrease in levodopa clearance resulting in a prolongation of the terminal elimination half-life of levodopa (from approximately 2 to 3.5 hours). In general, the average peak levodopa plasma concentration (C_{max}) and the time of its occurrence (t_{max}) are unaffected. The onset of effect occurs after the first administration and is maintained during long-term treatment. Studies in healthy volunteers and Parkinson's disease patients have confirmed that the maximal effect occurs with 100 to 200 mg tolcapone. Plasma levels of 3-OMD are markedly and dose-dependently decreased by tolcapone when given with levodopa/carbidopa.

Population pharmacokinetic analyses in patients with Parkinson's disease have shown the same effects of tolcapone on levodopa plasma concentrations that occur in healthy volunteers.

When tolcapone was given together with levodopa/carbidopa and desipramine, there was no significant change in blood pressure, pulse rate and plasma concentrations of desipramine. Overall, the frequency of adverse events increased slightly. These adverse reactions were predictable based on the known adverse reactions to each of the 3 drugs individually. Therefore, caution should be exercised when desipramine is administered to Parkinson's disease patients being treated with tolcapone and levodopa/carbidopa.

Adverse Reactions

Cases of severe hepatocellular injury, including fulminant liver failure resulting in death, have been reported in postmarketing use. As of October, 1998, 3 cases of fatal fulminant hepatic failure have been reported from approximately 60,000 patients providing about 40,000 patient years of worldwide use. This incidence may be 10- to 100-fold higher than the background incidence in the general population.

The most commonly observed adverse reactions (> 5%) in the double-blind, placebo-controlled trials (n = 892) associated with the use of tolcapone not seen at an equivalent frequency among the placebo-treated patients were dyskinesia, nausea, sleep disorder, dystonia, excessive dreaming, anorexia, muscle cramps, orthostatic complaints, somnolence, diarrhea, confusion, dizziness, headache, hallucination, vomiting, constipation, fatigue, upper

TOLCAPONE — ORAL

respiratory tract infection, falling, increased sweating, urinary tract infection, xerostomia, abdominal pain, urine discoloration.

Approximately 16% of the 592 patients who participated in the double-blind, placebo-controlled trials discontinued treatment due to adverse events compared to 10% of the 298 patients who received placebo. Diarrhea was by far the most frequent cause of discontinuation (approximately 6% in tolcapone patients vs 1% on placebo).

➤*Adverse reaction incidence in controlled clinical studies:*

Tolcapone Adverse Reactions after Start of Trial Drug Administration (≥ 1% and at least 1 Tolcapone Dose Group > Placebo)			
	Placebo	Tolcapone 3 times daily	
Adverse reactions	(n = 298)	100 mg (n = 296)	200 mg (n = 298)
Dyskinesia	20%	42%	51%
Nausea	18%	30%	35%
Sleep disorder	18%	24%	25%
Dystonia	17%	19%	22%
Dreaming excessive	17%	21%	16%
Anorexia	13%	19%	23%
Muscle cramps	17%	17%	18%
Orthostatic complaints	14%	17%	17%
Somnolence	13%	18%	14%
Diarrhea	8%	16%	18%
Confusion	9%	11%	10%
Dizziness	10%	13%	6%
Headache	7%	10%	11%
Hallucination	5%	8%	10%
Vomiting	4%	8%	10%
Constipation	5%	6%	8%
Fatigue	6%	7%	3%
Upper respiratory tract infection	3%	5%	7%
Falling	4%	4%	6%
Sweating increased	2%	4%	7%
Urinary tract infection	1%	5%	5%
Xerostomia	2%	5%	6%
Abdominal pain	3%	5%	6%
Syncope	3%	4%	5%
Urine discoloration	1%	2%	7%
Dyspepsia	2%	4%	3%
Influenza	2%	3%	4%
Dyspnea	2%	3%	3%
Balance loss	2%	3%	2%
Flatulence	2%	2%	4%
Hyperkinesia	1%	3%	2%
Chest pain	1%	3%	1%
Hypotension	1%	2%	2%
Paresthesia	2%	3%	1%
Stiffness	1%	2%	2%
Arthritis	1%	2%	1%
Chest discomfort	1%	1%	2%
Hypokinesia	1%	1%	3%
Micturition disorder	1%	2%	1%
Neck pain	1%	2%	2%
Burning	0%	2%	1%
Sinus congestion	0%	2%	1%
Agitation	0%	1%	1%
Dermal bleeding	0%	1%	1%
Irritability	0%	1%	1%
Mental deficiency	0%	1%	1%
Hyperactivity	0%	1%	1%
Malaise	0%	1%	0%
Panic reaction	0%	1%	0%
Tumor, skin	0%	1%	0%
Cataract	0%	1%	0%

Tolcapone Adverse Reactions after Start of Trial Drug Administration (≥ 1% and at least 1 Tolcapone Dose Group > Placebo)			
	Placebo	Tolcapone 3 times daily	
Adverse reactions	(n = 298)	100 mg (n = 296)	200 mg (n = 298)
Euphoria	0%	1%	0%
Fever	0%	0%	1%
Alopecia	0%	1%	0%
Eye inflamed	0%	1%	0%
Hypertonia	0%	0%	1%
Tumor, uterus	0%	1%	0%

Other events reported by greater than or equal to 1% of patients treated with tolcapone but that were equally or more frequent in the placebo group were arthralgia, limb pain, anxiety, micturition frequency, fractures, vision blurred, pneumonia, paresis, lethargy, asthenia, peripheral edema, abnormal gait, taste alteration, weight decrease and sinusitis.

Effects of gender and age on adverse reactions – Experience in clinical trials have suggested that patients older than 75 years of age may be more likely to develop hallucinations than patients younger than 75 years of age, while patients older than 75 may be less likely to develop dystonia. Females may be more likely to develop somnolence than males.

➤*Other adverse reactions observed during all trials in patients with Parkinson's disease:* All reported events that occurred at least twice (or once for serious or potentially serious events), except those already listed above, trivial events and terms too vague to be meaningful are included, without regard to determination of a causal relationship to tolcapone.

Events are further classified within body system categories and enumerated in order of decreasing frequency using the following definitions: Frequent adverse reactions are defined as those occurring in at least 1/100 patients; infrequent adverse reactions are defined as those occurring in between 1/100 and 1/1000 patients; and rare adverse reactions are defined as those occurring in fewer than 1/1000 patients.

Cardiovascular – Palpitation (frequent); hypertension, vasodilation, angina pectoris, heart failure, atrial fibrillation, tachycardia, migraine, aortic stenosis, arrhythmia, arteriospasm, bradycardia, cerebral hemorrhage, coronary artery disorder, heart arrest, myocardial infarct, myocardial ischemia, pulmonary embolus (infrequent); arteriosclerosis, cardiovascular disorder, pericardial effusion, thrombosis (rare).

CNS – Depression, hypesthesia, tremor, speech disorder, vertigo, emotional lability (frequent); neuralgia, amnesia, extrapyramidal syndrome, hostility, increased libido, manic reaction, nervousness, paranoid reaction, cerebral ischemia, cerebrovascular accident, delusions, decreased libido, neuropathy, apathy, choreoathetosis, myoclonus, psychosis, abnormal thinking, twitching (infrequent); antisocial reaction, delirium, encephalopathy, hemiplegia, meningitis (rare).

Dermatologic – Rash (frequent); herpes zoster, pruritus, seborrhea, skin discoloration, eczema, erythema multiforme, skin disorder, furunculosis, herpes simplex, urticaria (infrequent).

Endocrine – Diabetes mellitus (infrequent).

GI – Tooth disorder (frequent); dysphagia, gastrointestinal hemorrhage, gastroenteritis, mouth ulceration, increased salivation, abnormal stools, esophagitis, cholelithiasis, colitis, tongue disorder, rectal disorder (infrequent); cholecystitis, duodenal ulcer, gastrointestinal carcinoma, stomach atony (rare).

GU – Urinary incontinence, impotence (frequent); prostatic disorder, dysuria, nocturia, polyuria, urinary retention, urinary tract disorder, hematuria, kidney calculus, prostatic carcinoma, breast neoplasm, oliguria, uterine atony, uterine disorder, vaginitis (infrequent); bladder calculus, ovarian carcinoma, uterine hemorrhage (rare).

Hematologic/Lymphatic – Anemia (infrequent); leukemia, thrombocytopenia (rare).

Metabolic/Nutritional – Edema, hypercholesteremia, thirst, dehydration (infrequent).

Musculoskeletal – Myalgia (frequent); tenosynovitis, arthrosis, joint disorder (infrequent).

Respiratory – Bronchitis, pharyngitis (frequent); increased cough, rhinitis, asthma, epistaxis, hyperventilation, laryngitis, hiccup (infrequent); apnea, hypoxia, lung edema (rare).

Special senses – Tinnitus (frequent); diplopia, ear pain, eye hemorrhage, eye pain, lacrimation disorder, otitis media, parosmia (infrequent); glaucoma (rare).

Miscellaneous – Flank pain, accidental injury, abdominal pain, infection (frequent); hernia, pain, allergic reaction, cellulitis, infection fungal, viral infection, carcinoma, chills, infection bacterial, neoplasm, abscess, face edema, surgical procedure (infrequent); death (rare).

Overdosage

➤*Symptoms:* The highest dose of tolcapone administered to humans was 800 mg 3 times daily, with and without levodopa/carbidopa coadministration. This was in a 1-week study in elderly, healthy volunteers. The peak plasma concentrations of tolcapone at this dose were on average 30 mcg/mL (compared to 3 mcg/mL and 6 mcg/mL with 100 and 200 mg tolcapone, respectively). Nausea, vomiting and dizziness were observed, particularly in combination with levodopa/carbidopa.

➤*Treatment:* Hospitalization is advised. General supportive care is indicated. Based on the physicochemical properties of the compound, hemodialysis is unlikely to be of benefit.

Patient Information

Tolcapone should not be used by patients until there has been a complete discussion of the risks and the patient has provided written informed consent.

Patients should be informed of the clinical signs and symptoms that suggest the onset of hepatic injury (eg, persistent nausea, fatigue, lethargy, anorexia, jaundice, dark urine, pruritus, right upper quadrant tenderness). If symptoms of hepatic failure occur, patients should be advised to contact their physicians immediately.

Patients should be informed that hallucinations can occur.

Patients should be informed of the need to have regular blood tests to monitor liver enzymes.

Patients should be advised that they may develop postural (orthostatic) hypotension with or without symptoms such as dizziness, nausea, syncope, and sometimes sweating. Hypotension may occur more frequently during initial therapy. Accordingly, patients should be cautioned against rising rapidly after sitting or lying down, especially if they have been doing so for prolonged periods, and especially at the initiation of treatment with tolcapone.

Patients should be advised that they should neither drive a car nor operate other complex machinery until they have gained sufficient experience on tolcapone to gauge whether or not it affects their mental or motor performance adversely. Because of the possible additive sedative effects, caution should be used when patients are taking other CNS depressants in combination with tolcapone.

Patients should be informed that nausea may occur, especially at the initiation of treatment with tolcapone.

Patients should be advised of the possibility of an increase in dyskinesia or dystonia.

Although tolcapone has not been shown to be teratogenic in animals, it is always given in conjunction with levodopa/carbidopa, which is known to cause visceral and skeletal malformations in the rabbit. Accordingly, patients should be advised to notify their physicians if they become pregnant or intend to become pregnant during therapy.

Tolcapone is excreted into maternal milk in rats. Because of the possibility that tolcapone may be excreted into human maternal milk, patients should be advised to notify their physicians if they intend to breastfeed or are breastfeeding an infant.

Dopaminergics

DOPAMINE RECEPTOR AGONISTS, NONERGOT

For additional information, refer to the Antiparkinson Agents introduction.

Indications

➤*Parkinson disease:* For the treatment of the signs and symptoms of idiopathic Parkinson disease.

➤*Restless legs syndrome (pramipexole and ropinirole immediate release only):* For the treatment of moderate to severe primary restless legs syndrome (RLS).

Actions

➤*Pharmacology:* **Pramipexole** and **ropinirole**, nonergot dopamine agonists for Parkinson disease, have high relative in vitro specificity and full intrinsic activity at the D_2 subfamily of dopamine receptors, binding with higher affinity to D_3 than to D_2 or D_4 receptor subtypes. The relevance of D_3 receptor binding in Parkinson disease is unknown. Ropinirole also has moderate in vitro affinity for opioid receptors, and its metabolites have negligible in vitro affinity for dopamine D_1, 5-HT_1, 5-HT_2, benzodiazepine, gamma-aminobutyric acid, muscarinic, $alpha_1$-, $alpha_2$- and beta-adrenoreceptors.

Apomorphine has high in vitro binding affinity for the dopamine D_4 receptor, moderate affinity for the dopamine D_2, D_3, and D_5, and adrenergic $alpha_{1D}$, $alpha_{2B}$, $alpha_{2C}$ receptors, and low affinity for the dopamine D_1, serotonin 5-HT_{1A}, 5-HT_{2A}, 5-HT_{2B}, and 5-HT_{2C} receptors. Apomorphine exhibits no affinity for the adrenergic $beta_1$ and $beta_2$ or histamine H_1 receptors.

The precise mechanism of action as a treatment for Parkinson disease is unknown, although it is believed to be related to stimulation of dopamine receptors in the striatum.

➤*Pharmacokinetics:*

Select Pharmacokinetic Parameters of Nonergot Dopamine Receptor Agonists

	Absolute bioavailability	Protein binding	Half-life	Clearance	Cytochrome P450 metabolism
Pramipexole	> 90%	15%	8 h (12 h)[a]	400 mL/min	None; ≈ 90% excreted unchanged
Ropinirole	55%	30% to 40%	6 h	783 mL/min	Extensive (CYP1A2); 1 to 2% excreted unchanged
Apomorphine	[b]		40 min	223 L/h	Sulfation, N-demethylation, glucuronidation and oxidation

[a] In elderly patients > 65 years of age.
[b] After subcutaneous administration, bioavailability appears equal to that of intravenous (IV) administration.

Absorption – Nonergot dopamine agonists are rapidly absorbed, reaching peak concentrations in approximately 1 to 2 hours.

Apomorphine is a lipophilic compound that is rapidly absorbed (time to peak concentration [T_{max}] ranges from 10 to 60 minutes) following subcutaneous administration into the abdominal wall.

Food effect: Food does not affect the extent of absorption but increases the time to achieve maximum plasma levels by 1 hour for **pramipexole** (2 hours for pramipexole extended release) and 2.5 hours for ropinirole.

Distribution – **Pramipexole** also distributes into red blood cells with an erythrocyte-to-plasma ratio of approximately 2. Steady-state concentrations of nonergot dopamine agonists are achieved within 2 days after dosing.

Nonergot dopamine agonists are extensively distributed throughout the body, with a volume of distribution of approximately 500 L. Mean (range) apparent volume of distribution of **apomorphine** was 218 L (123 to 404 L). Maximum concentrations of **apomorphine** in cerebrospinal fluid are less than 10% of maximum plasma concentrations and occur 10 to 20 minutes later.

Excretion – Urinary excretion is the major route of elimination, with more than 88% of the dose recovered in the urine.

Special populations –

Renal function impairment: The clearance of **pramipexole** was decreased approximately 75% in patients with severe renal impairment (creatinine clearance [CrCl] approximately 20 mL/min) and was 60% lower in patients with moderate renal impairment (CrCl approximately 40 mL/min). Use a lower initial and maintenance dose of pramipexole in these patients.

No dosage adjustment for **ropinirole** is necessary for patients with moderate renal impairment (CrCl 30 to 50 mL/min). The effects of severe renal impairment have not been studied.

In renally impaired patients (moderately impaired, as determined by estimated CrCl) to healthy matched volunteers, the area under the curve (AUC_{0-8}) and maximal drug concentration (C_{max}) values were increased by approximately 16% and 50%, respectively, following a single subcutaneous administration of **apomorphine** into the abdominal wall. Studies in subjects with severe renal impairment have not been conducted.

Hepatic function impairment: Plasma levels of **ropinirole** may increase and clearance may decrease; titrate ropinirole with caution in patients with impaired hepatic function.

In patients with hepatic impairment (moderately impaired, as determined by the Child-Pugh classification method) compared to healthy matched volunteers, the AUC_{0-8} and C_{max} values were increased by approximately 10% and 25%, respectively, following a single subcutaneous administration of **apomorphine** into the abdominal wall. Studies in subjects with severe hepatic impairment have not been conducted.

Smoking: Cigarette smoking is expected to increase the clearance of ropinirole because CYP1A2 is known to be induced by smoking.

Contraindications

Hypersensitivity to the product or any of its components; concomitant use of **apomorphine** with drugs of the 5-HT_3 antagonist class (including, for example, ondansetron, granisetron, dolasetron, palonosetron, and alosetron).

Warnings/Precautions

➤*Cardiovascular effects:*

Coronary events – Four percent of patients treated with **apomorphine** experienced angina, myocardial infarction (MI), cardiac arrest, and/or sudden death; some cases of angina and MI occurred in close proximity to apomorphine dosing (within 2 hours), whereas other cases of cardiac arrest and sudden death were observed at times unrelated to dosing.

Symptomatic hypotension – Dopamine agonists appear to impair the systemic regulation of blood pressure, with resulting orthostatic hypotension, especially during dose escalation. Patients with Parkinson disease appear to have impaired capacity to respond to an orthostatic challenge. Therefore, these patients require careful monitoring for signs and symptoms of orthostatic hypotension while being treated with dopaminergic agonists, especially during dose escalation.

In clinical trials of **apomorphine** in patients with advanced Parkinson disease, 11% had orthostatic hypotension, hypotension, and/or syncope. These events were considered serious in 4 patients (less than 1%) and resulted in withdrawal of apomorphine in 2% of patients. These events occurred both with initial dosing and during long-term treatment.

Syncope – Syncope, sometimes associated with bradycardia, was observed in association with **ropinirole** therapy. In patients with early Parkinson disease treated with ropinirole (without levodopa), 11.5% had syncope compared with 1.4% receiving placebo. Most of these cases occurred more than

DOPAMINE RECEPTOR AGONISTS, NONERGOT

4 weeks after initiation of therapy of ropinirole and were usually associated with a recent increase in dose.

Of 208 patients being treated with both **levodopa** and ropinirole in advanced Parkinson disease trials, syncope was reported in 2.9% versus 1.7% with placebo.

In **apomorphine** clinical studies, approximately 2% of patients experienced syncope.

➤*Hallucinations:* Hallucinations were observed in a greater number of patients receiving dopaminergics than placebo. In early Parkinson disease, hallucinations were observed in approximately 5% to 9% of treated patients versus approximately 1.5% to 2.5% for the placebo group. In patients with advanced Parkinson disease receiving concomitant levodopa, hallucinations were observed in approximately 10% to 16.5% of patients receiving dopaminergics versus approximately 4% receiving placebo. During clinical development of **apomorphine**, hallucinations were reported by 14% of patients. In one randomized, double-blind, placebo-controlled study, hallucinations or confusion occurred in 10% of patients treated with apomorphine and 0% of patients treated with placebo.

Elderly – Age appears to increase the risk of hallucinations attributable to dopaminergics. Elderly patients (older than 65 years of age) with early and advanced Parkinson disease have experienced hallucinations approximately 7 and approximately 5 times more often, respectively, than their younger counterparts when treated with dopaminergics.

➤*Dyskinesia:* Dopamine receptor agonists may potentiate the dopaminergic adverse effects of levodopa and may cause or exacerbate preexisting dyskinesia. Decreasing the dose of levodopa may ameliorate this adverse effect.

Apomorphine may cause dyskinesia or exacerbate preexisting dyskinesia. During clinical development, dyskinesia or worsening of dyskinesia was reported in 24% of patients.

➤*Retinal pathology:* Pathologic changes (degeneration and loss of photoreceptor cells) were observed in the retinas of albino rats receiving dopamine receptor agonists in a 2-year study. The potential significance of this effect in humans has not been established but cannot be disregarded because disruption of a mechanism that is universally present in vertebrates (eg, disk shedding) may be involved.

➤*Withdrawal-emergent hyperpyrexia and confusion:* Although not reported with these specific agents, a symptom complex resembling the neuroleptic malignant syndrome (characterized by elevated temperature, muscular rigidity, altered consciousness, and autonomic instability) with no other obvious cause, has occurred in association with rapid dose reduction, withdrawal of or changes in antiparkinsonian dopaminergic therapy.

➤*Nausea and vomiting:* At the recommended doses of **apomorphine**, severe nausea and vomiting can be expected. Because of this, in domestic clinical studies, 98% of all patients were treated with the antiemetic trimethobenzamide for 3 days prior to beginning apomorphine and were then encouraged to continue trimethobenzamide for at least 6 weeks. In the domestic development of apomorphine, there was no experience with antiemetics other than trimethobenzamide. Some antiemetics with antidopaminergic actions have the potential to worsen the clinical state of patients with Parkinson disease and should be avoided. Concomitant use of apomorphine with the 5–HT_3 antagonist class is contraindicated.

➤*QT prolongation and potential for proarrhythmic effects:* Two patients receiving apomorphine (1 at 2 and 6 mg, 1 at 6 mg) exhibited large QTc increments (greater than 60 msec from predose) and had QTc intervals greater than 500 msec acutely after dosing. Therefore, doses of 6 mg or less are associated with minimal increases in QTc. Doses greater than 6 mg do not provide additional clinical benefit and are not recommended. Although torsades de pointes has not been observed in association with the use of **apomorphine** at recommended doses in premarketing studies, experience is too limited to rule out an increased risk. Palpitations and syncope may signal the occurrence of an episode of torsades de pointes.

➤*Fibrotic complication:* Cases of retroperitoneal fibrosis, pulmonary infiltrates, pleural effusion, and pleural thickening have occurred in some patients treated with ergot-derived dopaminergic agents. While these complications may resolve when the drug is discontinued, complete resolution does not always occur.

Although these adverse events are believed to be related to the ergoline structure of these compounds, whether non–ergot-derived dopamine agonists can cause these reactions is unknown.

➤*CNS effects:* Use concomitant CNS depressants with caution because of the possible additive sedative effects.

There have been reports in the literature of patients treated with **pramipexole** or subcutaneous **apomorphine** injections who suddenly fell asleep without prior warning of sleepiness while engaged in activities of daily living. It is clear that somnolence is commonly associated with pramipexole and apomorphine injection, and many clinical experts believe that falling asleep while engaged in activities of daily living always occurs in a setting of preexisting somnolence even if patients do not give such a history.

After starting or increasing the dose of apomorphine, patients may experience new or worsening mental status and behavioral changes, which may be severe, including psychotic-like behavior. This abnormal thinking and behavior can consist of one or more of a variety of manifestations, including agitation, aggressive behavior, confusion, delirium, delusions, disorientation, hallucinations, and paranoid ideation. Patients with a major psychotic disorder should ordinarily not be treated with apomorphine because of the risk of exacerbating psychosis.

➤*Melanoma:* Some epidemiologic studies have shown that patients with Parkinson disease have a higher risk (perhaps 2- to 4-fold higher) of developing melanoma than the general population. Whether the observed increased risk was because of Parkinson disease or other factors, such as drugs used to treat Parkinson disease, was unclear. Ensure that patients using dopamine agonists for any indication are aware of these results and that they undergo periodic dermatologic screening.

➤*Rebound and augmentation in restless legs syndrome:* Reports in the literature indicate treatment of RLS with dopaminergic medications can result in a shifting of symptoms to the early morning hours, which is referred to as rebound. Rebound was not reported in the clinical trials of pramipexole, but the trials were generally not of sufficient duration to capture this phenomenon. Augmentation has also been described during therapy for RLS. Augmentation refers to the earlier onset of symptoms in the evening (or even the afternoon), increase in symptoms, and spread of symptoms to involve other extremities.

➤*Impulse control/compulsive behavior:* Cases of pathological gambling, hypersexuality, compulsive eating (including binge eating), and compulsive shopping have been reported in patients treated with dopamine agonist therapy. As described in the literature, such behaviors are generally reversible upon dose reduction or treatment discontinuation.

➤*Priapism:* **Apomorphine** may cause prolonged painful erections in some patients.

➤*Rhabdomyolysis:* A single case of rhabdomyolysis occurred in a 49-year-old male with advanced Parkinson disease treated with **pramipexole**. The patient was hospitalized with elevated creatine phosphokinase (CPK) (10,631 units/L). The symptoms resolved with discontinuation of the medication.

➤*Falls:* Patients with Parkinson disease are at risk of falling due to the underlying postural instability and concomitant autonomic instability seen in some patients with Parkinson disease, and from syncope caused by the blood pressure–lowering effects of the drugs used to treat Parkinson disease. Subcutaneous **apomorphine** might increase the risk of falling by simultaneously lowering blood pressure and altering mobility.

➤*Binding to melanin:* **Ropinirole** binds to melanin-containing tissues (eg, eyes, skin) in pigmented rats. After a single dose, long-term retention of the drug was demonstrated in the eye with a half-life of 20 days. It is not known if ropinirole accumulates in these tissues over time.

➤*Sulfite sensitivity:* **Apomorphine** injection may contain sodium metabisulfite, a sulfite that may cause allergic-type reactions, including anaphylactic symptoms and life-threatening or less severe asthmatic episodes in certain susceptible people.

➤*Renal function impairment:* Reduce initial and maintenance doses of **pramipexole** for patients with moderate to severe renal impairment.

Reduce the starting dose to 1 mg when administrating **apomorphine** to patients with mild or moderate renal impairment because the C_{max} and AUC are increased in these patients.

➤*Hepatic function impairment:* Use caution when administering **apomorphine** to patients with mild and moderate hepatic impairment because of increased Cmax and AUC. Studies in patients with severe hepatic impairment have not been conducted.

➤*Drug abuse and dependence:* There are reports of **apomorphine** abuse by patients with Parkinson disease in other countries. These cases are characterized by increasingly frequent dosing leading to hallucinations, dyskinesia, and abnormal behavior. Psychosexual stimulation with increased libido is believed to underlie these cases.

➤*Pregnancy: Category C.* There are no adequate and well-controlled studies in pregnant women. In animals, **ropinirole** has been shown to have adverse effects on embryofetal development, including teratogenic effects, decreased fetal body weight, increased fetal death, and digital malformation. Use during pregnancy only if the potential benefit outweighs the potential risk to the fetus.

➤*Lactation:* Treatment with these agents has resulted in an inhibition of prolactin secretion in humans. It is not known whether these drugs are excreted in breast milk. Decide whether to discontinue breast-feeding or the drug, taking into account the importance of the drug to the mother.

➤*Children:* Safety and efficacy have not been established.

➤*Elderly:* The incidence of hallucinations appears to increase with age (see Hallucinations in Warnings/Precautions).

➤*Monitoring:* Monitor for signs and symptoms of orthostatic hypotension. Continually reassess patients for drowsiness or sleepiness. Monitor for melanoma frequently and on a regular basis.

Drug Interactions

➤*QT prolongation:* An additive effect of **apomorphine** with other drugs that prolong the QT interval cannot be excluded. The following drugs may prolong the QT interval and increase the risk of life-threatening cardiac arrhythmias, including torsades de pointes: antiarrhythmic agents (eg, amiodarone, bretylium, disopyramide, dofetilide, procainamide, quinidine, sotalol), arsenic trioxide, chlorpromazine, cisapride, dolasetron, droperidol, mefloquine, mesoridazine, pentamidine, pimozide, tacrolimus, thioridazine, and ziprasidone. For a more complete list of drugs that may prolong the QT interval, see the appendix Drug-Induced Prolongation of the QT Interval and Torsades de Pointes.

DOPAMINE RECEPTOR AGONISTS, NONERGOT

Nonergot Dopamine Receptor Agonist Drug Interactions

Precipitant drug	Object drug[a]		Description
Alcohol	Nonergot dopamine agonists	↑	Because the chances of falling asleep may be increased, alcohol ingestion should be avoided.
Nonergot dopamine agonists	Alcohol		
Nonergot dopamine agonists	Levodopa	↑	Coadministration increased levodopa C_{max} (20% to 40%); pramipexole C_{max} decreased from 2.5 to 0.5 hours.
Amantadine	Pramipexole	↑	Population pharmacokinetic analyses suggest that amantadine may slightly decrease the oral clearance of pramipexole.
Cimetidine	Pramipexole	↑	Cimetidine caused a 50% increase in pramipexole AUC and a 40% increase in its half-life.
Estrogen	Ropinirole	↑	Estrogens (mainly ethinyl estradiol, 0.6 to 3 mg over a 4-month to 23-year period) reduced the oral clearance of ropinirole by 36% in 16 patients. Dosage adjustment may not be needed because ropinirole is titrated to effect. However, dose adjustment may be required if estrogen therapy is stopped or started during treatment with ropinirole.
Ciprofloxacin	Ropinirole	↑	Coadministration with ciprofloxacin, an inhibitor of CYP1A2, increased ropinirole AUC by 84%, on average, and C_{max} by 60%.
5-HT_3 antagonists (eg, alosetron, dolasetron, granisetron, ondansetron, palonosetron)	Apomorphine	↑	Coadministration of apomorphine with drugs of the 5-HT_3 antagonist class is contraindicated. Profound hypotension and loss of consciousness has been reported.
Dopamine antagonists (eg, butyrophenones, metoclopramide, phenothiazines, thioxanthenes)	Nonergot dopamine agonists	↓	Because these agents are dopamine agonists, it is possible that dopamine antagonists, such as the neuroleptics, may diminish their effectiveness.
Drugs eliminated via renal secretion (eg, cimetidine, diltiazem, quinidine, quinine, ranitidine, triamterene, verapamil)	Pramipexole	↑	Coadministration of drugs that are secreted by the cationic transport system may decrease the oral clearance of pramipexole by approximately 20%.
Inhibitors of CYP1A2 (eg, cimetidine, ciprofloxacin, diltiazem, enoxacin, erythromycin, fluvoxamine, mexiletine, norfloxacin, tacrine)	Ropinirole	↑	Potential exists for substrates or inhibitors of CYP1A2 to alter ropinirole's clearance. If therapy with a potent CYP1A2 inhibitor is stopped or started during ropinirole treatment, dose adjustment may be required.

[a] ↑ = object drug increased; ↓ = object drug decreased.

➤*Drug/Food interactions:* **Pramipexole** and **ropinirole** T_{max} are increased by approximately 1 and 2.5 hours, respectively, when taken with food, although the extent of absorption is not affected.

Adverse Reactions

➤*Early Parkinson disease (without levodopa):* The most commonly observed adverse reactions (greater than 5%) shared by the nonergot dopamine receptor agonists were asthenia, constipation, dizziness, dyspepsia, hallucinations, nausea, and somnolence.

Approximately 24% of **ropinirole**-treated patients discontinued treatment because of adverse reactions versus 13% for placebo. The most common adverse reactions for discontinuing therapy were nausea (6.4%); dizziness (3.8%); and aggravated Parkinson disease, hallucinations, headache, somnolence, and vomiting (1.3%). In **pramipexole** studies, approximately 12% of treated patients versus 11% in the placebo group discontinued therapy because of adverse reactions. The following were the most common reasons for discontinuation: hallucinations (3.1%); dizziness, nausea (2.1%); somnolence, extrapyramidal syndrome (1.6%); headache, confusion (1.3%).

Nonergot Dopamine Receptor Agonist Adverse Reactions in Early Parkinson Disease (Without Levodopa)[a]

Adverse reaction	Pramipexole (n = 388)	Pramipexole extended release (n = 223)	Ropinirole (n = 157)
Cardiovascular			
Atrial fibrillation	—	—	2%
Extrasystoles	—	—	2%
Flushing	—	—	3%
Hypertension	—	—	5%
Hypotension	—	—	2%
Orthostatic symptoms	—	3%	6%
Palpitations	—	—	3%
Syncope	—	—	12%
Tachycardia	—	—	2%
CNS			
Akathisia	2%	—	—
Amnesia	4%	—	3%
Asthenia	14%	3%	6%
Balance disorder	—	2%	—
Confusion	4%	—	5%
Decreased libido	1%	—	—
Depression	—	2%	—
Dizziness	25%	12%	40%
Dystonia	2%	—	—
Fall	—	4%	—
Fatigue	—	6%	11%
Hallucinations[b]	9%	5%	5%
Hyperkinesia	—	—	2%
Hypesthesia	3	—	4%
Impaired concentration	—	—	2%
Insomnia	17%	4%	—
Malaise	2%	—	3%
Myoclonus	1%	—	—
Sleep attacks or sudden onset of sleep	—	3%	—
Sleep disorder	—	2%	—
Somnolence	22%	36%	40%
Yawning	—	—	3%
Thinking abnormalities	2%	—	—
Tremor	—	3%	—
Vertigo	—	4%	2%
GI			
Abdominal discomfort	—	2%	—
Abdominal pain	—	—	6%
Anorexia	4%	—	4%

DOPAMINE RECEPTOR AGONISTS, NONERGOT

Nonergot Dopamine Receptor Agonist Adverse Reactions in Early Parkinson Disease (Without Levodopa)[a]

Adverse reaction	Pramipexole (n = 388)	Pramipexole extended release (n = 223)	Ropinirole (n = 157)
Constipation	14%	14%	—
Dry mouth	—	5%	5%
Dyspepsia	—	3%	10%
Dysphagia	2%	—	—
Flatulence	—	—	3%
Nausea	28%	22%	60%
Upper abdominal pain	—	3%	—
Vomiting	—	4%	12%
Metabolic/Nutritional			
Decreased weight	2%	—	0%
Edema	5%	—	7%
Increased appetite	—	3%	—
Peripheral edema	5%	5%	4%
Respiratory			
Cough	—	3%	—
Bronchitis	—	—	3%
Dyspnea	—	—	3%
Pharyngitis	—	—	6%
Rhinitis	—	—	4%
Sinusitis	—	—	4%
Special senses			
Abnormal vision	3%	—	6%
Eye abnormality	—	—	3%
Xerophthalmia	—	—	2%
Miscellaneous			
Chest pain	—	—	4%
Fever	1%	—	—
Impotence	2%	—	3%
Increased alkaline phosphatase	—	—	3%
Increased sweating	—	—	6%
Muscle spasms	—	5%	—
Pain	—	—	8%
Peripheral ischemia	—	—	3%
Urinary tract infection	—	—	5%
Viral infection	—	—	11%

[a] Data pooled from separate studies; not necessarily comparable.
[b] See Warnings/Precautions.

➤*Advanced Parkinson disease (with levodopa):* The most commonly observed adverse reactions (greater than 5%) shared by the nonergot dopamine receptor agonists were confusion, constipation, dizziness, dry mouth, dyskinesia, extrapyramidal syndrome/aggravated Parkinsonism, hallucinations, injury, insomnia, somnolence, and urinary frequency/infection.

Approximately 24% of patients treated with **ropinirole** and levodopa discontinued therapy because of adverse reactions versus 18% of patients given placebo and levodopa. The most common adverse reactions causing discontinuation of treatment were dizziness (2.9%); confusion, dyskinesia, and vomiting (2.4%); anxiety, hallucinations, and nausea (1.9%); and increased sweating (1.4%). In patients treated with **pramipexole** and levodopa, approximately 12% discontinued therapy as a result of adverse reactions versus 16% in the placebo group. Therapy was discontinued most often because of the following: hallucinations (2.7%); orthostatic hypotension (2.3%); dyskinesia (1.9%); extrapyramidal syndrome (1.5%); dizziness, confusion (1.2%).

Nonergot Dopamine Receptor Agonist Adverse Reactions in Advanced Parkinson Disease (With Levodopa)[a]

Adverse reaction	Pramipexole (n = 260)	Pramipexole extended release (n = 164)	Ropinirole (n = 208)
Cardiovascular			
Postural hypotension	53%	—	2%
Syncope	—	—	3%
CNS			
Akathisia	3%	—	—
Amnesia	6%	—	5%
Asthenia	10%	—	—
Confusion	10%	—	9%
Delusions	1%	—	—
Dizziness	26%	—	26%
Dizziness (postural)		2%	—
Dream abnormalities	11%	—	3%
Dyskinesia	47%	17%	34%
Dystonia	8%	—	—
Extrapyramidal syndrome	28%	—	—
Falls	—	—	10%
Gait abnormalities/hypokinesia	7%	—	5%
Hallucinations	17%	9%	10%
Headache	—	7%	17%
Hypertonia	7%	—	—
Insomnia	27%	4%	—
Malaise	3%	—	—
Nervousness	—	—	5%
Paranoid reaction	2%	—	—
Paresis	—	—	3%
Paresthesia	—	—	5%
Sleep disorders	1%	—	—
Somnolence	9%	—	20%
Thinking abnormalities	3%	—	—
Tremor/Twitching	2%	—	6%
Dermatologic			
Increased sweating	—	—	7%
Skin disorders	2%	—	—
GI			
Abdominal pain	—	—	9%
Constipation	10%	7%	6%
Diarrhea	—	2%	5%
Dry mouth	7%	—	5%
Dysphagia	—	—	2%
Flatulence	—	—	2%
Increased saliva	—	—	2%
Nausea	—	11%	30%
Salivary hypersecretion	—	2%	—
Vomiting	—	—	7%
GU			
Pyuria	—	—	2%
Urinary frequency	6%	—	—
Urinary incontinence	2%	—	2%
Urinary tract infection	4%	—	6%
Metabolic/Nutritional			
General edema	4%	—	—
Increased CPK	1%	—	—
Peripheral edema	2%	—	—
Weight decrease	—	—	2%
Musculoskeletal			
Arthritis	3%	—	3%
Back pain	—	2%	—
Bursitis	2%	—	—
Myasthenia	1%	—	—
Twitching	2%	—	6%

DOPAMINE RECEPTOR AGONISTS, NONERGOT

Nonergot Dopamine Receptor Agonist Adverse Reactions in Advanced Parkinson Disease (With Levodopa)[a]			
Adverse reaction	Pramipexole (n = 260)	Pramipexole extended release (n = 164)	Ropinirole (n = 208)
Respiratory			
Dyspnea	4%		3%
Pneumonia	2%	—	9%
Rhinitis	3%	—	—
Special senses			
Accommodation abnormalities	4%	—	—
Diplopia	1%	—	—
Vision abnormalities	3%	—	—
Miscellaneous			
Accidental injury	17%	—	—
Anemia	—	—	2%
Anorexia	—	5%	—
Chest pain	3%	—	—
Increased drug level	—	—	—
Pain	—	—	—

[a] Data pooled from separate studies; not necessarily comparable.

➤*Apomorphine:* The most common adverse reactions seen in controlled trials were chest pain, dizziness, dyskinesias, edema, flushing, hallucinations, increased sweating, nausea and/or vomiting, pallor, rhinorrhea, somnolence, and yawning.

Apomorphine Adverse Reactions		
Adverse reaction	Apomorphine (n = 20)	Placebo (n = 9)
Any adverse reaction	85%	89%
Chest pain/pressure/angina	15%	11%
Dizziness or postural hypotension	20%	0%
Drowsiness or somnolence	35%	0%
Dyskinesias	35%	11%
Edema/Swelling of extremities	10%	0%
Hallucination or confusion	10%	0%
Nausea and/or vomiting	30%	11%
Rhinorrhea	20%	0%
Yawning	40%	0%

The most common adverse reactions (occurring in at least 5% of the patients and at least plausibly related to treatment) in descending order were injection site complaint, fall, arthralgia, insomnia, headache, depression, urinary tract infection, anxiety, congestive heart failure, limb pain, back pain, Parkinson disease aggravated, pneumonia, confusion, sweating increased, dyspnea, fatigue, ecchymosis, constipation, diarrhea, weakness, and dehydration.

➤*Restless legs syndrome:* The most commonly observed adverse reactions with pramipexole in the treatment of RLS were nausea and somnolence. The adverse reaction most commonly causing discontinuation of therapy was nausea (1%).

Pramipexole Immediate-Release Adverse Reactions in Restless Legs Syndrome[a] (≥ 2%)		
Adverse reaction	Pramipexole 0.125 to 0.75 mg/day (n = 575)	Placebo (n = 223)
CNS		
Headache	16%	15%
Somnolence	6%	3%
GI		
Constipation	4%	1%
Diarrhea	3%	1%
Dry mouth	3%	1%
Nausea	16%	5%
Miscellaneous		
Fatigue	9%	7%
Influenza	3%	1%

[a] Patients may have reported multiple adverse reactions during the study or at discontinuation; thus, patients may be included in more than 1 category.

Overdosage

➤*Symptoms:* There is no clinical experience with massive overdosage. One patient with a 10-year history of schizophrenia took **pramipexole** 11 mg/day for 2 days (2 to 3 times the recommended daily dose). No adverse events were reported related to the increased dose. Blood pressure remained stable, although pulse rate increased to between 100 and 120 beats/min. Of 10 patients ingesting more than 24 mg/day, 1 experienced mild orofacial dyskinesia; another experienced intermittent nausea. Other symptoms reported with accidental overdoses were agitation, increased dyskinesia, grogginess, sedation, orthostatic hypotension, chest pain, confusion, vomiting, and nausea. The largest overdose reported was 435 mg taken over a 7-day period (62.1 mg/day).

An accidental overdose of apomorphine 25 mg injected subcutaneously in a 62 year old man resulted in nausea within 3 minutes and loss of consciousness for 20 minutes. Afterwards, he was alert with a heart rate of 40 beats/minute and supine blood pressure of 90/50. He recovered completely within 1 hour.

➤*Treatment:* There is no known antidote for overdosage of a dopamine agonist. If signs of CNS stimulation are present, a phenothiazine or other butyrophenone neuroleptic agent may be indicated; the efficacy of such drugs in reversing the effects of overdosage has not been assessed. Management of overdose may require general supportive measures along with gastric lavage, IV fluids, and ECG monitoring. A negligible amount of **pramipexole** is removed by dialysis. Refer to General Management of Acute Overdosage.

Patient Information

Inform patients that hallucinations can occur and that elderly patients are at a higher risk than younger patients with Parkinson disease.

Patients may develop postural hypotension with or without symptoms such as dizziness, nausea, fainting or blackouts, and sometimes sweating. Hypotension may occur more frequently during initial therapy. Accordingly, caution patients against rising rapidly after sitting or lying down, especially if they have been doing so for prolonged periods and at the initiation of treatment with pramipexole.

Advise patients that they may experience somnolence and that they should neither drive a car nor operate other complex machinery until they have gained sufficient experience with the drug to gauge whether or not it affects their mental or motor performance adversely. Inform patients of the possible additive sedative effects when taken in combination with other CNS depressants.

Patients should be alerted to the potential sedating effects of **apomorphine** injection and **pramipexole**, including somnolence and the possibility of falling asleep while engaged in daily activities. Because somnolence is a frequent adverse reaction with potentially serious consequences, patients should neither drive a car nor engage in other potentially dangerous activities until they have gained sufficient experience with apomorphine injection or pramipexole to gauge whether or not it affects their mental and/or motor performance adversely.

Inform patients and caregivers that impulse control disorders/compulsive behaviors may occur while taking medicines to treat Parkinson disease or RLS. These include pathological gambling, hypersexuality, compulsive eating (including binge eating), and compulsive shopping. If such behaviors are observed, consider dose reduction or treatment discontinuation.

Because **ropinirole** has been shown to have adverse effects on embryofetal development and because the teratogenic potential of pramipexole has not been completely established and human experience is limited, advise patients to notify their health care provider if they become pregnant or intend to become pregnant during therapy.

Advise patients to notify their health care provider if they intend to breastfeed or are breast-feeding an infant.

If patients develop nausea, advise them that taking this medication with food may reduce the occurrence of nausea.

PRAMIPEXOLE DIHYDROCHLORIDE

Rx	**Pramipexole** (Various, eg, Teva Pharmaceuticals USA, Torrent Pharmaceuticals)	**Tablets; oral:** 0.125 mg	May contain mannitol. In 30s, 63s, 90s, 500s, 5,000s, 6,000s, and UD 100s.
Rx	**Mirapex** (Boehringer Ingelheim)		Mannitol. (BI 83). White, round. In 90s.
Rx	**Pramipexole** (Various, eg, Teva Pharmaceuticals USA, Torrent Pharmaceuticals)	**Tablets; oral:** 0.25 mg	May contain mannitol. In 30s, 90s, 500s, 5,500s, and UD 100s.
Rx	**Mirapex** (Boehringer Ingelheim)		Mannitol. (BI BI 84 84). White, oval, scored. In 90s and UD 100s.

PRAMIPEXOLE DIHYDROCHLORIDE

Rx	**Pramipexole** (Various, eg, Teva Pharmaceuticals USA, Torrent Pharmaceuticals)	**Tablets; oral:** 0.5 mg	May contain mannitol. In 30s, 90s, 500s, 4,000s, and UD 100s.
Rx	**Mirapex** (Boehringer Ingelheim)		Mannitol. (BI BI 85 85). White, oval, scored. In 90s and UD 100s.
Rx	**Pramipexole** (Various, eg, Torrent Pharmaceuticals)	**Tablets; oral:** 0.75 mg	May contain mannitol. In 30s, 90s, 500s, 2,500s, and UD 100s.
Rx	**Mirapex** (Boehringer Ingelheim)		Mannitol. (BI 101). White, oval. In 90s.
Rx	**Pramipexole** (Various, eg, Teva Pharmaceuticals USA, Torrent Pharmaceuticals)	**Tablets; oral:** 1 mg	May contain mannitol. In 30s, 90s, 500s, 2,500s, and UD 100s.
Rx	**Mirapex** (Boehringer Ingelheim)		Mannitol. (BI BI 90 90). White, round, scored. In 90s and UD 100s.
Rx	**Pramipexole** (Various, eg, Teva Pharmaceuticals USA, Torrent Pharmaceuticals)	**Tablets; oral:** 1.5 mg	May contain mannitol. In 30s, 90s, 500s, 1,500s, and UD 100s.
Rx	**Mirapex** (Boehringer Ingelheim)		Mannitol. (BI BI 91 91). White, round, scored. In 90s and UD 100s.
Rx	**Mirapex XR** (Boehringer Ingelheim)	**Tablets, extended-release; oral:** 0.375 mg	(ER 0.375). White to off-white, round. In 30s.
		0.75 mg	(ER 0.75). White to off-white, round. In 30s.
		1.5 mg	(ER 1.5). White to off-white, oval. In 30s.
		3 mg	(ER 3.0). White to off-white, oval. In 30s.
		4.5 mg	(ER 4.5). White to off-white, oval. In 30s.

PRAMIPEXOLE DIHYDROCHLORIDE — ORAL

For complete and comparative prescribing information, refer to the Dopamine Receptor Agonists, Non-Ergot class monograph.

Indications

➤*Parkinson disease:* For the treatment of the signs and symptoms of idiopathic Parkinson disease.

➤*Restless legs syndrome (immediate release only):* For the treatment of moderate to severe primary restless legs syndrome (RLS).

➤*Off-label uses:*

Fibromyalgia – [4] = Insufficient documentation. Preliminary data from a very limited number of patients (approximately 60) indicate that pramipexole may be effective for the treatment of fibromyalgia. (See Administration and Dosage.)

Administration and Dosage

➤*General dosing considerations:* Exercise caution when prescribing pramipexole to patients with renal impairment. Dosage adjustments are required (see Renal function impairment).

If significant interruption in therapy with pramipexole has occurred, retitration of therapy may be warranted.

➤*Adults:*

Parkinson disease –

Immediate-release tablets:

• *Initial dosage* – 0.125 mg 3 times daily for 1 week.

• *Dosage titration* – Gradually titrate in all patients. Do not increase more frequently than every 5 to 7 days. Increase the dosage to achieve a maximum therapeutic effect, balanced against the principal adverse reactions of dyskinesia, hallucinations, somnolence, and dry mouth.

Pramipexole Immediate-Release Dosage Titration Schedule

Week	Dosage	Total daily dose[a]
1	0.125 mg 3 times daily	0.375 mg
2	0.25 mg 3 times daily	0.75 mg
3	0.5 mg 3 times daily	1.5 mg
4	0.75 mg 3 times daily	2.25 mg
5	1 mg 3 times daily	3 mg
6	1.25 mg 3 times daily	3.75 mg
7	1.5 mg 3 times daily	4.5 mg

[a] Taken once daily, 2 to 3 hours before bedtime.

• *Maintenance dosage* – 1.5 to 4.5 mg daily in equally divided doses 3 times per day with or without concomitant levodopa (approximately 800 mg daily).

• *Concomitant therapy* – When used in combination with levodopa, consider a reduction of levodopa dosage. In a controlled study in advanced Parkinson disease, the dosage of levodopa was reduced by an average of 27% from baseline.

• *Discontinuation of therapy* – It is recommended that pramipexole be discontinued over a period of 1 week; however, in some studies, abrupt discontinuation was uneventful.

Extended-release tablets:

• *Maximum dose* – 4.5 mg/day.

• *Initial dosage* – 0.375 mg once per day.

• *Dosage titration* – Based on efficacy and tolerability, dosages may be increased gradually, not more frequently than every 5 to 7 days, first to 0.75 mg/day and then by 0.75 mg increments up to a maximum recommended dosage of 4.5 mg/day.

• *Discontinuation of therapy* – Taper the dose gradually over a period of 1 week.

Restless legs syndrome (immediate-release tablets only) –

Usual dosage: 0.125 mg taken once daily, 2 to 3 hours before bedtime.

Dosage titration: The dose may be increased every 4 to 7 days. Although the dose of pramipexole was increased to 0.75 mg in some patients during long-term, open-label treatment, there is no evidence that the 0.75 mg dose provides additional benefit beyond the 0.5 mg dose.

Pramipexole Immediate-Release Dosage Titration Schedule

Titration step	Duration	Daily dose[a]
1	4 to 7 days	0.125 mg
2 (if needed)	4 to 7 days	0.25 mg
3 (if needed)	4 to 7 days	0.5 mg

[a] Taken once daily, 2 to 3 hours before bedtime.

Discontinuation of therapy: In clinical trials of patients being treated for RLS with dosages of up to 0.75 mg once daily, pramipexole was discontinued without a taper.

Off-label dosing –

Fibromyalgia: [4] = Insufficient documentation. Dose titration in 0.25 mg increments from 0.25 mg nightly to 4.5 mg nightly over a 14-week period.

➤*Renal function impairment:*

Parkinson disease –

Immediate-release tablets:

Pramipexole Immediate-Release Dosage in Parkinson Patients With Renal Impairment

Renal status	Starting dosage	Maximum dosage
Healthy to mild impairment (CrCl[a] > 60 mL/min)	0.125 mg 3 times a day	1.5 mg 3 times a day
Moderate impairment (CrCl = 35 to 59 mL/min)	0.125 mg twice a day	1.5 mg twice a day
Severe impairment (CrCl = 15 to 34 mL/min)	0.125 mg once daily	1.5 mg once daily
Very severe impairment (CrCl < 15 mL/min and hemodialysis patients)	The use of pramipexole has not been adequately studied in this group of patients.	

[a] CrCl = creatinine clearance.

Extended-release tablets:

• *CrCl 30 to 50 mL/min* – In patients with moderate renal impairment (CrCl between 30 and 50 mL/min), pramipexole extended release (ER) should initially be taken every other day. Caution should be exercised and careful assessment of therapeutic response and tolerability should be made before increasing to daily dosing after 1 week and before any additional titration in 0.375 mg increments up to 2.25 mg/day. Dose adjustment should occur no more frequently than at weekly intervals.

• *CrCl less than 30 mL/min* – Pramipexole ER tablets have not been studied in patients with severe renal impairment (CrCl less than 30 mL/min) or patients on hemodialysis and are not recommended in these patients.

Restless legs syndrome –

Immediate-release tablets: The duration between titration steps should be increased to 14 days in patients with RLS with severe and moderate renal impairment (CrCl 20 to 60 mL/min).

PRAMIPEXOLE DIHYDROCHLORIDE — ORAL

➤*Switching from immediate release to extended release:* Patients may be switched overnight from pramipexole immediate release to pramipexole ER at the same daily dose. When switching between ER and immediate release, patients should be monitored to determine if dosage adjustment is necessary.

➤*Administration:* Take with or without food. ER tablets should not be chewed, crushed, or divided.

➤*Storage/Stability:* Store at 25°C (77°F); excursions are permitted to 15° to 30°C (59° to 86°F). Protect from light. Protect ER tablets from exposure to high humidity.

ROPINIROLE

Rx	**Ropinirole** (Various, eg, Corepharma, Roxane, Teva)	**Tablets; oral:** 0.25 mg	As ropinirole hydrochloride. May contain lactose, PEG. In 100s and 1,000s.
Rx	**Requip** (GlaxoSmithKline)		As ropinirole hydrochloride. Lactose, PEG. (SB 4890). White, pentagonal. Film-coated *Tiltab*. In 100s.
Rx	**Ropinirole** (Various, eg, Corepharma, Roxane, Teva)	**Tablets; oral:** 0.5 mg	As ropinirole hydrochloride. May contain lactose, PEG. In 100s and 1,000s.
Rx	**Requip** (GlaxoSmithKline)		As ropinirole hydrochloride. Lactose, PEG. (SB 4891). Yellow, pentagonal. Film-coated *Tiltab*. In 100s.
Rx	**Ropinirole** (Various, eg, Corepharma, Roxane, Teva)	**Tablets; oral:** 1 mg	As ropinirole hydrochloride. May contain lactose, PEG. In 100s and 1,000s.
Rx	**Requip** (GlaxoSmithKline)		As ropinirole hydrochloride. Lactose, PEG. (SB 4892). Green, pentagonal. Film-coated *Tiltab*. In 100s.
Rx	**Ropinirole** (Various, eg, Corepharma, Roxane, Teva)	**Tablets; oral:** 2 mg	As ropinirole hydrochloride. May contain lactose, PEG. In 100s and 1,000s.
Rx	**Requip** (GlaxoSmithKline)		As ropinirole hydrochloride. Lactose, PEG. (SB 4893). Pale yellowish pink, pentagonal. Film-coated *Tiltab*. In 100s.
Rx	**Ropinirole** (Various, eg, Corepharma, Roxane, Teva)	**Tablets; oral:** 3 mg	As ropinirole hydrochloride. May contain lactose, PEG. In 100s and 1,000s.
Rx	**Requip** (GlaxoSmithKline)		As ropinirole hydrochloride. Lactose, PEG. (SB 4895). Pale to moderate reddish-purple, pentagonal. Film-coated *Tiltab*. In 100s.
Rx	**Ropinirole** (Various, eg, Corepharma, Roxane, Teva)	**Tablets; oral:** 4 mg	As ropinirole hydrochloride. May contain lactose, PEG. In 100s and 1,000s.
Rx	**Requip** (GlaxoSmithKline)		As ropinirole hydrochloride. Lactose, PEG. (SB 4896). Pale brown, pentagonal. Film-coated *Tiltab*. In 100s.
Rx	**Ropinirole** (Various, eg, Corepharma, Roxane, Teva)	**Tablets; oral:** 5 mg	As ropinirole hydrochloride. May contain lactose, PEG. In 100s and 1,000s.
Rx	**Requip** (GlaxoSmithKline)		As ropinirole hydrochloride. Lactose, PEG. (SB 4894). Blue, pentagonal. Film-coated *Tiltab*. In 100s.
Rx	**Requip XL** (GlaxoSmithKline)	**Tablets, extended-release; oral:** 2 mg	Equivalent to ropinirole hydrochloride 2.28 mg. Lactose, maltodextrin, mannitol, PEG. (GS 3V2). Pink, capsule-shaped. Film-coated. In 30s and 90s.
		4 mg	Equivalent to ropinirole hydrochloride 4.56 mg. Lactose, maltodextrin, mannitol, PEG. (GS WXG). Light brown, capsule-shaped. Film-coated. In 30s and 90s.
		6 mg	Equivalent to ropinirole hydrochloride 6.84 mg. Lactose, maltodextrin, mannitol, PEG 400. (GS 11F). White, capsule shape. Film-coated. In 30s and 90s.
		8 mg	Equivalent to ropinirole hydrochloride 9.12 mg. Lactose, maltodextrin, mannitol, PEG. (GS 5CC). Red, capsule-shaped. Film-coated. In 30s and 90s.
		12 mg	Equivalent to ropinirole hydrochloride 13.68 mg. Lactose, maltodextrin, mannitol. (GS YX7). Green, capsule shape. Film-coated. In 30s.

ROPINIROLE HYDROCHLORIDE — ORAL

Indications

➤*Parkinson disease:* For the treatment of the signs and symptoms of idiopathic Parkinson disease.

➤*Restless legs syndrome (RLS) (immediate-release only):* For the treatment of moderate to severe primary RLS.

Key diagnostic criteria for RLS are as follows: an urge to move the legs, usually accompanied or caused by uncomfortable and unpleasant leg sensations; symptoms begin or worsen during periods of rest or inactivity such as lying or sitting; symptoms are partially or totally relieved by movement, such as walking or stretching, at least as long as the activity continues; and symptoms are worse or occur only in the evening or night. Difficulty falling asleep may frequently be associated with moderate to severe RLS.

Administration and Dosage

➤*General dosing considerations:* If a significant interruption in therapy with ropinirole has occurred, retitration of therapy may be warranted.

Ropinirole may need to be tapered prior to discontinuation. (See Tapering for Parkinson disease or restless leg syndrome.)

➤*Adults:*

Parkinson disease –

Immediate-release:

• *Initial dosage* – 0.25 mg 3 times daily. In all clinical studies, dosage was initiated at a subtherapeutic level and gradually titrated to therapeutic response. The dosage should be increased to achieve a maximum therapeutic effect, balanced against the principal adverse reactions of nausea, dizziness, somnolence, and dyskinesia.

• *Dosage titration* – Based on individual patient response, dosage should be titrated in weekly increments. After week 4, if necessary, daily dose may be increased by 1.5 mg/day on a weekly basis up to a dose of 9 mg/day, and then by up to 3 mg/day weekly to a total dose of 24 mg/day.

Ropinirole Immediate-Release Ascending Dose Schedule for Parkinson Disease

Week	Dosage	Total daily dose
1	0.25 mg 3 times daily	0.75 mg
2	0.5 mg 3 times daily	1.5 mg
3	0.75 mg 3 times daily	2.25 mg
4	1 mg 3 times daily	3 mg

Extended-release:

• *Maximum dose* – 24 mg/day.

• *Initial dosage* – 2 mg once daily for 1 to 2 weeks.

• *Dosage titration* – Follow initial dosage with increases of 2 mg/day at 1-week or longer intervals, depending on therapeutic response and tolerability, up to a maximum recommended dose of 24 mg/day. Patients should be assessed for therapeutic response and tolerability at a minimal interval of 1 week or longer after each dose increment.

Caution should be exercised during dose titration because a too rapid rate of titration may lead to dose selection that may not provide additional benefit, but that may increase the risk of adverse reactions. Because of the flexible dosing design used in clinical studies, specific dose response information could not be determined.

• *Tapering* – Discontinue gradually over a 7-day period.

Restless leg syndrome –

Immediate-release:

• *Initial dosage* – 0.25 mg once daily, 1 to 3 hours before bedtime. Patients were titrated based on clinical response and tolerability.

• *Dosage titration* – After 2 days, the dosage can be increased to 0.5 mg once daily and to 1 mg once daily at the end of the first week of dosing, then as shown in the following table as needed to achieve efficacy.

ROPINIROLE HYDROCHLORIDE — ORAL

Ropinirole Dose Titration Schedule for Restless Leg Syndrome	
Day/Week	Dose to be taken once daily, 1 to 3 hours before bedtime
Days 1 and 2	0.25 mg
Days 3 to 7	0.5 mg
Week 2	1 mg
Week 3	1.5 mg
Week 4	2 mg
Week 5	2.5 mg
Week 6	3 mg
Week 7	4 mg

• *Tapering* – Discontinue gradually over a 7-day period. The frequency of administration should be reduced from 3 times daily to twice daily for 4 days. For the remaining 3 days, the frequency should be reduced to once daily prior to complete withdrawal of ropinirole.

In clinical trials of patients being treated for RLS with dosages of up to 4 mg once daily, ropinirole was discontinued without a taper.

➤*Concomitant therapy with levodopa:* When ropinirole is administered as adjunct therapy to levodopa, the concurrent dose of levodopa may be decreased gradually as tolerated. Levodopa dosage reduction was allowed during the advanced Parkinson disease (with levodopa) study if dyskinesias or other dopaminergic effects occurred. Overall, reduction of levodopa dosage was sustained in 87% of patients treated with ropinirole immediate-release and in 57% of patients on placebo. On average, the levodopa dose was reduced by 31% in patients treated with ropinirole immediate-release.

In the placebo-controlled advanced Parkinson disease study, the levodopa dose was reduced once patients reached a dose of ropinirole ER 8 mg/day. Overall, levodopa dose reduction was sustained in 93% of patients treated with ropinirole ER and in 72% of patients on placebo. On average, the levodopa dose was reduced by 34% in patients treated with ropinirole ER.

➤*Switching from immediate-release to extended-release:* Patients may be switched directly from immediate-release to ER. The initial dose of ropinirole ER should most closely match the total daily dose of the immediate-release formulation. Following conversion to ER, the dose may be adjusted depending on therapeutic response and tolerability.

Conversion From Ropinirole Immediate-Release to ER	
Immediate-release total daily dose	ER total daily dose
0.75 to 2.25 mg	2 mg
3 to 4.5 mg	4 mg
6 mg	6 mg
7.5 to 9 mg	8 mg
12 mg	12 mg
15 to 18 mg	16 mg
21 mg	20 mg
24 mg	24 mg

➤*Administration:* May be taken with or without food. Patients may be advised that taking ropinirole with food may reduce the occurrence of nausea; however, this has not been established in controlled clinical trials. ER tablets must be swallowed whole and must not be chewed, crushed, or divided.

➤*Storage/Stability:* Store immediate-release tablets at 20° to 25°C (68° to 77°F). Store ER tablets at 25°C (77°F); excursions are permitted between 15° and 30°C (59° and 86°F). Protect from light and moisture. Close container tightly after each use.

APOMORPHINE HYDROCHLORIDE

Rx	Apokyn (Ipsen)	Injection, solution: 10 mg/mL	Benzyl alcohol, sodium metabisulfite. In 3 mL glass cartridges.

APOMORPHINE HYDROCHLORIDE — INJECTION

For complete and comparative prescribing information, refer to the Dopamine Receptor Agonists, Non-Ergot class monograph.

Indications

➤*Parkinson disease:* For the acute, intermittent treatment of hypomobility "off" episodes ("end-of-dose wearing off" and unpredictable "on/off" episodes) associated with advanced Parkinson disease. Apomorphine has been studied as an adjunct to other medications.

Administration and Dosage

➤*General dosing considerations:* The prescribed dose of apomorphine should always be expressed in milliliters to avoid confusion.

➤*Adults:*

Parkinson disease –

Usual dosage: 0.3 to 0.6 mL (3 to 6 mg). The average frequency of dosing was 3 times per day, and there is limited experience with single doses more than 0.6 mL (6 mg), with dosing more than 5 times per day, and with total daily doses greater than 2 mL (20 mg). (See Test Dose.)

If a single dose of apomorphine is ineffective for a particular "off" period, a second dose should not be given for that "off" episode.

Maximum dose: 0.6 mL (6 mg).

Test dose: Patients in an "off" state should be given a 0.2 mL (2 mg) test dose in a setting in which blood pressure can be closely monitored by medical personnel. Both supine and standing blood pressure should be checked predose and at 20, 40, and 60 minutes postdose. Patients who develop clinically significant orthostatic hypotension in response to this test dose should not be considered candidates for treatment with apomorphine. If the patient tolerates the 0.2 mL (2 mg) dose and responds, the starting dose should be 0.2 mL (2 mg), used on an as-needed basis to treat existing "off" episodes. If needed, the dose can be increased in 0.1 mL (1 mg) increments every few days on an outpatient basis.

Beyond this, the general principle guiding dosing is to determine a dose (0.3 or 0.4 mL) that the patient will tolerate as a test dose under monitored conditions and then begin an outpatient dosing trial (periodically assessing both efficacy and tolerability) using a dose 0.1 mL (1 mg) lower than the tolerated test dose.

For patients who tolerate the test dose of 0.2 mL (2 mg) but achieve no response, a dose of 0.4 mL (4 mg) may be administered at the next observed "off" period, but no sooner than 2 hours after the initial test dose of 0.2 mL (2 mg). Both supine and standing blood pressure should be checked predose and at 20, 40, and 60 minutes postdose. If the patient tolerates a test dose of 0.4 mL (4 mg), the starting dose should be 0.3 mL (3 mg), used on an as-needed basis to treat existing "off" episodes. If needed, the dose can be increased in 0.1 mL (1 mg) increments every few days on an outpatient basis. If a patient does not tolerate a test dose of 0.4 mL (4 mg), a test dose of 0.3 mL (3 mg) may be administered during a separate "off" period, no sooner than 2 hours after the test dose of 0.4 mL (4 mg). Both supine and standing blood pressure should be checked predose and at 20, 40, and 60 minutes postdose. If the patient tolerates the 0.3 mL (3 mg) test dose, the starting dose should be 0.2 mL (2 mg), used on an as-needed basis to treat existing "off" episodes. If needed, and the 0.2 mL (2 mg) dose is tolerated, the dose can be increased to 0.3 mL (3 mg) after a few days. In such a patient, the dose ordinarily should not be increased to 0.4 mL (4 mg) on an outpatient basis.

Dosage titration: Titrate the dose on the basis of effectiveness and tolerance, starting at 0.2 mL (2 mg) and increasing up to a maximum recommended dose of 0.6 mL (6 mg). (See Test Dose.)

Concomitant therapy:

• *Concomitant antiemetic therapy* – Apomorphine should not be initiated without use of a concomitant antiemetic. Most antiemetic experience is with trimethobenzamide, and this should generally be used. Trimethobenzamide (300 mg 3 times daily orally) should be started 3 days prior to the initial dose of apomorphine and continued at least during the first 2 months of therapy.

Concomitant therapy with 5-HT_3 antagonists: Based on reports of profound hypotension and loss of consciousness when apomorphine was administered with ondansetron, the concomitant use of apomorphine with drugs of the 5-HT_3 antagonist class (eg, alosetron, dolasetron, granisetron, ondansetron, palonosetron) is contraindicated.

➤*Renal function impairment:*

Mild and moderate renal impairment – The testing dose and, subsequently, the starting dose should be reduced to 0.1 mL (1 mg).

➤*Interruption of therapy:* Patients who have a significant interruption in therapy (more than 1 week) should be restarted on a 0.2 mL (2 mg) dose and gradually titrated to effect.

➤*Administration:* For subcutaneous administration only. Do not administer intravenously (IV).

➤*Storage/Stability:* Store at 25°C (77°F); excursions are permitted to 15° to 30°C (59° to 86°F).

Indications

➤*Myasthenia gravis:* Treatment of myasthenia gravis.

➤*Urinary retention:* The prevention and treatment of postoperative distention and urinary retention after mechanical obstruction has been excluded.

➤*Reversal of nondepolarizing muscle relaxants:* Reversal of nondepolarizing muscle relaxants (**pyridostigmine** and **neostigmine**).

➤*Off-label uses:* Diagnosis of myasthenia gravis (0.022 mg/kg/dose IM × 1).

Actions

➤*Pharmacology:* These drugs facilitate transmission of impulses across the myoneural junction by inhibiting the destruction of acetylcholine by cholinesterase. They differ in duration of action and in adverse effects.

Anticholinesterase Muscle Stimulants Equivalent Doses, Onset, and Duration of Action

Drug	Route	Equivalent Dosage (mg)	Onset (min)	Duration (hours)	Indications
Ambenonium	PO	5-10	20-30	3-8	Myasthenia gravis
Edrophonium	IM	10	2-10	0.17-0.67	Diagnosis myasthenia gravis
	IV	10	< 1	0.08-0.33	Diagnosis myasthenia gravis;[a] Nondepolarizing muscle relaxant antagonist
Neostigmine	PO	15	45-75	2-4	Myasthenia gravis
	IM	1.5	20-30	2-4	Myasthenia gravis
	IV	0.5	4-8	2-4	Diagnosis myasthenia gravis; Nondepolarizing muscle relaxant antagonist
Pyridostigmine	PO	60	20-30	3-6	Myasthenia gravis
	IM	2	< 15	2-4	Myasthenia gravis
	IV	2	2-5	2-4	Myasthenia gravis; Nondepolarizing muscle relaxant antagonist

[a] Also used to evaluate treatment requirements in myasthenia gravis.

Contraindications

Hypersensitivity to anticholinesterases; mechanical intestinal and urinary obstructions; peritonitis (**neostigmine**); history of reaction to bromides (**neostigmine** and **pyridostigmine**).

Warnings/Precautions

➤*Use with caution:* Use with caution in patients with bronchial asthma, epilepsy, bradycardia, recent coronary occlusion, vagotonia, hyperthyroidism, cardiac arrhythmias or peptic ulcer. Treat transient bradycardia with atropine sulfate. Isolated instances of cardiac and respiratory arrest, believed to be vagotonic effects, have occurred. When large doses are given, prior or simultaneous injection of atropine sulfate may be advisable. Use separate syringes.

➤*Cholinergic/Myasthenic crisis:* Overdosage may result in cholinergic crisis, characterized by increasing muscle weakness that, through involvement of the respiratory muscles, may lead to death. Myasthenic crisis because of an increase in disease severity is also accompanied by extreme muscle weakness and may be difficult to distinguish from cholinergic crisis. Differentiation is extremely important; use **edrophonium** and clinical judgment.

Treatment of the two conditions differs radically: Myasthenic crisis requires more intensive anticholinesterase therapy; cholinergic crisis calls for withdrawal of all drugs of this type and immediate use of atropine. Have a syringe containing 1 mg of atropine sulfate immediately available to be given IV to counteract severe cholinergic reactions. Use atropine to abolish or blunt GI side effects or other muscarinic reactions; however, such use may lead to inadvertent induction of cholinergic crisis by masking signs of overdosage.

➤*Used as antagonists to nondepolarizing muscle relaxants:* Obtain adequate recovery of voluntary respiration and neuromuscular transmission prior to discontinuing respiratory assistance. Observe continuously. If there is doubt concerning adequacy of recovery from the nondepolarizing muscle relaxant, continue artificial ventilation.

➤*Supervision:* Great care and supervision are required with **ambenonium chloride**. Because ambenonium has a more prolonged action than other antimyasthenic drugs, simultaneous use with other cholinergics is contraindicated except under strict supervision. Therefore, when a patient is to be given the drug, suspend use of all other cholinergics until the patient has been stabilized.

➤*Anticholinesterase insensitivity:* Anticholinesterase insensitivity may develop for brief or prolonged periods. Carefully monitor the patient; respiratory assistance may be needed. Reduce or withhold dosages until the patient again becomes sensitive.

➤*Hypersensitivity reactions:* Because of possible hypersensitivity in an occasional patient, have atropine and epinephrine readily available when using parenteral therapy.

➤*Pregnancy:* (*Category C* – neostigmine.) Safety for use during pregnancy has not been established. Transient muscular weakness occurred in ≈ 20% of infants born to mothers treated with these drugs during pregnancy. Use only when clearly needed and when the potential benefits outweigh the potential hazards to the fetus.

Anticholinesterase drugs may cause uterine irritability and induce premature labor when given IV to pregnant women near term.

➤*Lactation:* **Pyridostigmine** is excreted in breast milk. Because they are ionized at physiologic pH, **ambenonium chloride** and **neostigmine** would not be expected to be excreted in breast milk.

➤*Children:* Safety and efficacy for use of **neostigmine** in children are not established.

Drug Interactions

Anticholinesterase Muscle Stimulants Drug Interactions

Precipitant drug	Object drug[a]		Description
Anticholinesterase muscle stimulants	Anticholinesterase drugs	↑	Exercise caution in patients with myasthenic symptoms who are receiving other anticholinesterase muscle stimulants. Because symptoms of anticholinesterase overdose (cholinergic crisis) may mimic underdosage (myasthenic weakness), the condition may be worsened.
Anticholinesterase muscle stimulants	Succinylcholine	↑	Neuromuscular blocking effects may be increased. Prolonged respiratory depression with extended periods of apnea may occur. Provide respiratory support as needed.
Aminoglycoside antibiotics (eg, neomycin, streptomycin, kanamycin)	Anticholinesterase muscle stimulants	↑	Aminoglycoside antibiotics have a mild but definite nondepolarizing blocking action which may accentuate neuromuscular block.
Local and general anesthetics Antiarrhythmics	Anticholinesterase muscle stimulants	↓	Use cautiously, if at all, in patients with myasthenia gravis. The neostigmine dose may have to be increased accordingly.
Atropine Belladonna derivatives	Anticholinesterase muscle stimulants	↑	Routine administration of these agents may suppress the parasympathomimetic (muscarinic) symptoms of excessive GI stimulation leaving only the more serious symptoms of fasciculation and paralysis of voluntary muscles as signs of overdosage.
Corticosteroids	Anticholinesterase muscle stimulants	↓	May decrease the anticholinesterase effects of these agents. Conversely, anticholinesterase effects may increase after stopping corticosteroids. Provide respiratory support as needed.
Depolarizing muscle relaxants (eg, succinylcholine, decamethonium)	Anticholinesterase muscle stimulants	↑	Neostigmine may prolong the Phase I block of these drugs. Use these drugs in myasthenic patients only when definitely indicated. Carefully adjust the anticholinesterase dosage.
Magnesium	Anticholinesterase muscle stimulants	↓	Magnesium has a direct depressant effect on skeletal muscle, and it may antagonize the beneficial effects of anticholinesterase therapy.
Mecamylamine	Anticholinesterase muscle stimulants	↑	Do not administer to patients receiving this ganglionic blocking agent.
Methocarbamol	Anticholinesterase muscle stimulants	↓	A single case report indicates this drug may have impaired the effect of **pyridostigmine** in a patient with myasthenia gravis.

[a] ↑ = object drug increased; ↓ = object drug decreased.

Adverse Reactions

➤*Cardiovascular:* Arrhythmias (especially bradycardia); fall in cardiac output leading to hypotension; tachycardia; AV block; nodal rhythm; nonspecific EKG changes; cardiac arrest; syncope.

➤*CNS:* Convulsions; dysarthria; dysphonia; dizziness; loss of consciousness; drowsiness; headache.

➤*Dermatologic:* Skin rash (**pyridostigmine** and **neostigmine**; subsides upon discontinuance); thrombophlebitis (IV).

➤*GI:* Increased salivary, gastric and intestinal secretions; nausea; vomiting; dysphagia; increased peristalsis; diarrhea; abdominal cramps; flatulence.

➤*Hypersensitivity:* Allergic reactions and anaphylaxis.

➤*Musculoskeletal:* Weakness; fasciculations; muscle cramps and spasms; arthralgia.

➤*Respiratory:* Increased tracheobronchial secretions; laryngospasm; bronchiolar constriction; respiratory muscle paralysis; central respiratory paralysis; dyspnea; respiratory depression; respiratory arrest; bronchospasm.

➤*Miscellaneous:* Urinary frequency and incontinence; urinary urgency; diaphoresis; rash; urticaria; flushing; alopecia (**pyridostigmine**).

Overdosage

➤*Symptoms:* When the drug produces overstimulation, the clinical picture is one of increasing parasympathomimetic action that is more or less characteristic when not masked by the use of atropine. Signs and symptoms of overdosage, including cholinergic crises, vary considerably. They are usually manifested by increasing GI stimulation with epigastric distress, abdominal cramps, diarrhea and vomiting, excessive salivation, pallor, cold sweating, urinary urgency, blurring of vision and eventually fasciculation and paralysis of voluntary muscles, including those of the tongue (thick tongue and difficulty in swallowing), shoulder, neck and arms. Miosis, increase in blood pressure with or without bradycardia and subjective sensations of internal trembling, and often severe anxiety and panic may complete the picture. A cholinergic crisis is usually differentiated from the weakness and paralysis of myasthenia gravis insufficiently treated by cholinergic drugs by the fact that myasthenic weakness is not accompanied by any of the above signs and symptoms, except the last two subjective ones (anxiety and panic).

➤*Treatment:* Because the warning of overdosage is minimal, the existence of a narrow margin between the first appearance of side effects and serious toxic effects must be borne in mind constantly. If signs of overdosage occur (excessive GI stimulation, excessive salivation, miosis and more serious fasciculations of voluntary muscles), discontinue temporarily all cholinergic medication and administer from 0.5 to 1 mg (1/120 to 1/60 grain) of atropine IV. A total atropine dose of 5 to 10 mg or more may be required. Give other supportive treatment as indicated (artificial respiration, tracheotomy, oxygen, etc).

Patient Information

Notify physician if nausea, vomiting, diarrhea, sweating, increased salivary secretions, irregular heartbeat, muscle weakness, severe abdominal pain or difficulty in breathing occurs.

AMBENONIUM CHLORIDE

Rx	**Mytelase** (Sanofi Winthrop)	**Tablets:** 10 mg	Scored. In 100s.

AMBENONIUM CHLORIDE — ORAL

For complete and comparative prescribing information, refer to the Anticholinesterase Muscle Stimulants group monograph.

Indications

➤*Myasthenia gravis:* The treatment of myasthenia gravis.

Administration and Dosage

➤*General dosing considerations:* Edrophonium may be used to evaluate the adequacy of the maintenance dose of anticholinesterase medication. (See Evaluation of treatment.)

➤*Adults:*

Myasthenia gravis –

Usual dosage: 5 to 25 mg 3 or 4 times daily. In some patients a 5 mg dose is effective, whereas other patients require as much as 50 to 75 mg per dose.

Dosage titration: Start with a 5 mg dose, carefully observing the effect of the drug on the patient. The dosage may then be increased gradually to determine the effective and safe dose. The longer duration of action of ambenonium makes it desirable to adjust dosage at intervals of 1 to 2 days to avoid drug accumulation and overdosage.

Dosage adjustment: In addition to individual variations in dosage requirements, the amount of cholinergic medication necessary to control symptoms may fluctuate in each patient, depending on his or her activity and the current status of the disease, including spontaneous remission. A few patients have required greater doses for adequate control of myasthenic symptoms, but increasing the dosage above 200 mg daily requires exacting supervision of a health care provider well aware of the signs and treatment of overdosage with cholinergic medication.

➤*Evaluation of treatment:* Edrophonium may be used to evaluate the adequacy of the maintenance dose of anticholinesterase medication. Edrophonium 2 mg is administered intravenously 1 hour after the last anticholinesterase dose. A transient increase in strength occurring about 30 seconds later and lasting 3 to 5 minutes indicates insufficient maintenance dose. If the dose is adequate or excessive, no change or a transient decrease in strength will occur, sometimes accompanied by muscarinic symptoms. (See Edrophonium monograph.)

➤*Administration:* Administration of ambenonium is necessary only every 3 or 4 hours, depending on the clinical response. Usually medication is not required throughout the night, so that the patient can sleep uninterruptedly.

➤*Storage / Stability:* Store at room temperature up to 25° C (77° F).

EDROPHONIUM CHLORIDE

Rx	**Enlon** (Bioniche Pharma)	**Injection, solution:** 10 mg/ml	In 15 mL multidose vials.[a]
Rx	**Reversol** (Organon)		In 10 ml vials (25s).[a]

[a] With 0.45% phenol and 0.2% sodium sulfite.

EDROPHONIUM CHLORIDE — INJECTION

Complete and comparative prescribing information for these products begins in the group monograph.Anticholinesterase Muscle Stimulants

Indications

➤*Myasthenia gravis:* Edrophonium chloride is recommended for the differential diagnosis of myasthenia gravis and as an adjunct in the evaluation of treatment requirements in this disease. It may also be used for evaluating emergency treatment in myasthenic crises. Because of its brief duration of action, it is not recommended for maintenance therapy in myasthenia gravis.

➤*Curare antagonist:* Edrophonium chloride is also useful whenever a curare antagonist is needed to reverse the neuromuscular block produced by curare, tubocurarine, gallamine triethiodide or dimethyl-tubocurarine. It is not effective against decamethonium bromide and succinylcholine chloride. It may be used adjunctively in the treatment of respiratory depression caused by curare overdosage.

Administration and Dosage

➤*General dosing considerations:* Whenever anticholinesterase drugs are used for testing, a syringe containing 1 mg of atropine should be immediately available to be given in aliquots intravenously (IV) to counteract severe cholinergic reactions that may occur in the hypersensitive patient, whether or not the patient is myasthenic.

➤*Adults:*

Curare antagonist –

Usual dosage: 10 mg (1 mL) IV given slowly over 30 to 45 seconds so that the onset of cholinergic reaction can be detected. This dosage may be repeated whenever necessary. Because of its brief effect, edrophonium should not be given prior to the administration of curare, tubocurarine, gallamine triethiodide, or dimethyl-tubocurarine; it should be used at the time when its effect is needed. When given to counteract curare overdosage, the effect of each dose on the respiration should be carefully observed before it is repeated, and assisted ventilation should always be employed.

Maximum dose: 40 mg (4 mL).

Diagnosis of myasthenia gravis –

IV: A tuberculin syringe containing 10 mg (1 mL) of edrophonium is prepared with an IV needle, and 2 mg (0.2 mL) is injected IV within 15 to 30 seconds. The needle is left in situ. The remaining 8 mg (0.8 mL) is injected only if no reaction occurs after 45 seconds. If a cholinergic reaction (muscarinic side effects, skeletal muscle fasciculations, and increased muscle weakness) occurs after injection of 2 mg (0.2 mL), the test is discontinued and atropine 0.4 to 0.5 mg is administered IV. After one-half hour, the test may be repeated.

Intramuscular: 10 mg (1 mL) intramuscularly (IM). Subjects who demonstrate hyper-reactivity to this injection (cholinergic reaction), should be retested after one-half hour with 2 mg (0.2 mL) to rule out false-negative reactions.

Evaluation of treatment in myasthenia gravis – 1 to 2 mg (0.1 mL to 0.2 mL) administered IV 1 hour after oral intake of the drug being used in treatment.

Response will be myasthenic in the undertreated patient, adequate in the controlled patient, and cholinergic in the overtreated patient.

EDROPHONIUM CHLORIDE — INJECTION

Responses to Edrophonium Chloride in Myasthenic and Nonmyasthenic Individuals			
	Myasthenic[a]	Adequate[b]	Cholinergic[c]
Muscle strength (ptosis, diplopia, dysphonia, dysphagia, dysarthria, respiration, limb strength)	Increased	No change	Decreased
Fasciculations (orbicularis oculi, facial muscles, limb muscles)	Absent	Present or absent	Present or absent
Side reactions (lacrimation diaphoresis, salivation, abdominal cramps, nausea, vomiting, diarrhea)	Absent	Minimal	Severe

[a] Myasthenic response occurs in untreated myasthenic patients and may serve to establish diagnosis; in patients under treatment, indicates that therapy is inadequate.
[b] Adequate response is observed in treated patients when therapy is stabilized; a typical response in healthy individuals. In addition to this response in non-myasthenic patients, the phenomenon of forced lid closure is often observed in psychoneurotic patients.
[c] Cholinergic response seen in myasthenic patients who have been overtreated with anticholinesterase drugs.

Evaluating emergency treatment in myasthenic crises – 1 mg (0.1 mL) IV. After an interval of 1 minute, if this dose does not further impair the patient, the remaining 1 mg (0.1 mL) can be injected. If no clear improvement of respiration occurs after 2 mg (0.2 mL) dose, it is usually wise to discontinue all anticholinesterase drug therapy and secure controlled ventilation by tracheostomy with assisted respiration. When the test is performed, there should not be more than 2 mg (0.2 mL) edrophonium in the syringe.

➤*Children:*
Diagnosis of myasthenia gravis –
IV:
• *Maximum dose* –
Weight above 34 kg: 10 mg (1 mL) total dose.
Weight up to 34 kg: 5 mg (0.5 mL) total dose.
• *Usual dosage* –
Weight above 34 kg: 2 mg (0.2 mL); if there is no response after 45 seconds, increments of 1 mg (0.1 mL) every 30 to 45 seconds may be given, up to 10 mg (1 mL).
Weight up to 34 kg: 1 mg (0.1 mL); if there is no response after 45 seconds, increments of 1 mg (0.1 mL) every 30 to 45 seconds may be given, up to 5 mg (0.5 mL).
• *Infants* – 0.5 mg (0.05 mL).
Intramuscular:
• *Usual dosage* –
Weight up to 34 kg: 2 mg (0.2 mL).
Weight more than 34 kg: 5 mg (0.5 mL).
• *Maximum dose* – 10 mg total.
• *Alternative dosage* – 0.04 mg/kg initially as a test dose, then 1 mg increments if no reaction occurs within 1 minute. Total dose is 0.2 mg/kg.

➤*Administration:* IV; IM injection may be used if IV not possible (in adults with inaccessible veins). Because of technical difficulty with IV injection in children, the IM route may be used.

➤*Storage/Stability:* Store at 15° to 30°C (59° to 86°F).

NEOSTIGMINE

Rx	**Prostigmin** (Valeant Pharmaceuticals)	**Tablets; oral:** 15 mg	As neostigmine bromide. Lactose, sugar, talc. (PROSTIGMIN 15 ICN). White, scored. In 100s.
Rx	**Neostigmine Methylsulfate** (Various)	**Injection:** 1:1,000	In 10 mL vials.
Rx	**Prostigmin** (ICN)		As neostigmine methylsulfate. In 10 mL vials.[a]
Rx	**Neostigmine Methylsulfate** (Various)	**Injection:** 1:2,000	In 1 mL amps and 10 mL vials.
Rx	**Prostigmin** (ICN)		As neostigmine methylsulfate. In 1 mL amps[b] and 10 mL vials.[a]
Rx	**Neostigmine Methylsulfate** (Various)	**Injection:** 1:4,000	In 1 mL amps.
Rx	**Prostigmin** (ICN)		As neostigmine methylsulfate. In 1 mL amps.[b]

[a] With phenol 0.45%.
[b] With methyl- and propylparabens 0.2%.

NEOSTIGMINE BROMIDE — ORAL

Indications

➤*Myasthenia gravis:* For the symptomatic treatment of myasthenia gravis.

Administration and Dosage

➤*General dosing considerations:* The onset of action of neostigmine given orally is slower than when given parenterally, but the duration of action is longer and the intensity of action more uniform.

The patient should be encouraged to keep a daily record of his or her condition to assist the health care provider in determining an optimal therapeutic regimen.

As a rule, 15 mg of oral neostigmine bromide is equivalent to 0.5 mg of parenteral neostigmine methylsulfate.

Large doses should be avoided in situations in which there might be an increased absorption rate from the intestinal tract.

➤*Adults:*
Myasthenia gravis –
Usual dosage: The average dose is 10 tablets (150 mg) administered over a 24-hour period. The interval between doses is of paramount importance. Frequently, therapy is required day and night.

Dosage adjustment – The dosage schedule should be adjusted for each patient and changed as the need arises.

Dosage range – Dosage requirements for optimal results vary from 15 to 375 mg per day. In some instances, it may be necessary to exceed these dosages, but the possibility of cholinergic crisis must be recognized.

➤*Children:*
Off-label dosing –
Myasthenia gravis:
• *Usual dose* – 2 mg/kg/h divided every 3 to 4 hours.
• *Maximum dose* – 375 mg per 24 h.

➤*Administration:* Take without regard to food. Larger portions of the total daily dose may be given at times when the patient is more prone to fatigue (eg, afternoon, mealtimes).

➤*Storage/Stability:* Store at 25°C (77°F); excursions permitted to 15°C to 30°C (59°F to 86°F).

NEOSTIGMINE METHYLSULFATE — INJECTION

For complete and comparative prescribing information, refer to the Anticholinesterase Muscle Stimulants group monograph.

Indications

➤*Myasthenia gravis:* For the symptomatic control of myasthenia gravis when oral therapy is impractical.

➤*Postoperative distention/Urinary retention:* The prevention and treatment of postoperative distention and urinary retention after mechanical obstruction has been excluded.

➤*Reversal of nondepolarizing muscle relaxants:* For the reversal of effects of nondepolarizing neuromuscular blocking agents (eg, tubocurarine, metocurine, gallamine, or pancuronium) after surgery.

Administration and Dosage

➤*Adults:*
Myasthenia gravis –
Single dose: 0.5 mg (1 mL of the 1:2,000 solution) subcutaneously or intramuscularly.
Subsequent dosage: Base on the individual patient's response.

Prevention of postoperative distention –
Usual dosage: 0.25 mg (1 mL of the 1:4,000 solution) subcutaneously or intramuscularly as soon as possible after operation; repeat every 4 to 6 hours.
Duration of therapy: 2 or 3 days.

NEOSTIGMINE METHYLSULFATE — INJECTION

Prevention of postoperative urinary retention –
Usual dosage: 0.25 mg (1 mL of the 1:4,000 solution) subcutaneously or intramuscularly as soon as possible after operation; repeat every 4 to 6 hours.
Duration of therapy: 2 or 3 days.

Reversal of effects of nondepolarizing neuromuscular blocking agents –
Usual dosage: 0.5 to 2 mg by slow intravenous (IV) injection. Repeat as required.
Maximum dose: Only in exceptional cases should the total dose of neostigmine exceed 5 mg.
Concomitant therapy: Atropine 0.6 to 1.2 mg IV in a separate syringe.

Treatment of postoperative distention – 0.5 mg (1 mL of the 1:2,000 solution) subcutaneously or intramuscularly.

Treatment of urinary retention – 0.5 mg (1 mL of the 1:2,000 solution) subcutaneously or intramuscularly. If urination does not occur within 1 hour, the patient should be catheterized. After the patient has voided or the bladder has been emptied, continue the 0.5 mg injections every 3 hours for at least 5 injections.

➤*Children:*
Off-label dosing –
Myasthenia gravis diagnosis:
- *Single dose –* 0.025 to 0.04 mg/kg intramuscularly once.
- *Concomitant therapy –* Atropine 0.011 mg/kg IV immediately before or intramuscularly 30 minutes before neostigmine.

Myasthenia gravis treatment: 0.01 to 0.04 mg/kg intramuscularly, IV, or subcutaneously every 2 to 4 hours as needed or 0.1 mg intramuscularly 30 minutes before feeding. Doses should be titrated.

Reversal of nondepolarizing neuromuscular blocking agents:
- *Usual dose –* 0.025 to 0.1 mg/kg IV.
- *Concomitant therapy –* Atropine 0.02 mg/kg or glycopyrrolate.

➤*Administration:*
Myasthenia gravis, postoperative distention, or urinary retention – Administer subcutaneously or intramuscularly.

Reversal of effects of nondepolarizing neuromuscular blocking agents – Administer by slow IV injection with atropine. Some authorities have recommended that the atropine be injected several minutes before the neostigmine rather than concomitantly. It is recommended that the patient be well ventilated and a patent airway maintained until complete recovery of normal respiration is assured. The optimum time for administration of the drug is during hyperventilation when the carbon dioxide level of the blood is low.
Concomitant medications: Never administer in the presence of high concentrations of halothane or cyclopropane.
Cardiac patients: Filtrate the exact dose of neostigmine required using a peripheral nerve stimulator device. In bradycardia, the pulse rate should be increased to about 80 beats/minute with atropine before administering neostigmine.
Severely ill patients: Filtrate the exact dose of neostigmine required using a peripheral nerve stimulator device.

➤*Storage/Stability:* Store at 15° to 30°C (59° to 86°F). Keep injection in carton until ready to use and protect from light.

PYRIDOSTIGMINE BROMIDE

Rx	**Pyridostigmine Bromide** (Various, eg, Geneva, Watson)	**Tablets:** 60 mg	Scored. In 100s and 500s.
Rx	**Mestinon** (ICN)		Lactose. (MESTINON 60 ICN). Scored. In 100s and 500s.
Rx	**Mestinon** (ICN)	**Tablets, extended-release:** 180 mg	(ICN-M180). Scored. In 30s.
Rx	**Mestinon** (ICN)	**Syrup:** 60 mg/5mL	Sucrose, sorbitol, 5% alcohol. Raspberry flavor. In 480 mL.

[a] With 0.2% parabens and 0.02% sodium citrate.

PYRIDOSTIGMINE BROMIDE — ORAL

For complete and comparative prescribing information, refer to the Anticholinesterase Muscle Stimulants group monograph.

Indications

➤*Myasthenia gravis:* Pyridostigmine bromide is useful in the treatment of myasthenia gravis.

➤*Off-label uses:*
Postpoliomyelitis syndrome – [5] = Poor documentation. Evidence from controlled and noncontrolled studies evaluating pyridostigmine for treatment of postpoliomyelitis syndrome have demonstrated conflicting results. International guidelines state that this agent is not effective in the management of fatigue and muscular weakness in postpoliomyelitis syndrome.
Other possible off-label uses –
Treatment of myasthenia gravis in children: 7 mg/kg/24 hours orally divided into 5 or 6 doses.

Administration and Dosage

➤*Adults:*
Myasthenia gravis –
Conventional tablets/syrup: 600 mg/day spaced to provide maximum relief.
Extended-release tablets:
- *Usual dosage –* 180 to 540 mg once or twice daily. Use dosage intervals of 6 hours or more.
- *Concomitant therapy –* For optimum control, rapidly-acting conventional tablets or syrup also may be needed in conjunction with extended-release therapy.

➤*Children:*
Off-label dosing –
Myasthenia gravis:
- *30 days and older –* 7 mg/kg/day in 5 to 6 divided doses.
- *29 days or younger –* 5 mg/dose every 4 to 6 hours.

➤*Administration:* Do not crush or chew extended-release tablets.

➤*Storage/Stability:* Store at 15° to 30°C (59° to 86°F).

EDROPHONIUM CHLORIDE/ATROPINE SULFATE

Rx	**Enlon-Plus** (Bioniche Pharma USA LLC)	**Injection, solution:** edrophonium chloride 10 mg/ atropine sulfate 0.14 mg per mL	Sodium sulfite 2 mg/mL. In 5 mL single-dose amps and 15 mL multiple-dose vials.[a]

[a] Also contains phenol 4.5 mg/mL.

EDROPHONIUM CHLORIDE/ATROPINE SULFATE — INJECTION

For complete and comparative prescribing information, refer to the Anticholinesterase Muscle Stimulants class monograph and the Atropine monograph.

Indications

➤*Adjunct treatment of respiratory depression caused by curare overdosage:* May be used adjunctively for the treatment of respiratory depression caused by curare overdosage.

➤*Reversal of nondepolarizing neuromuscular blocking agents:* As a reversal agent or antagonist of nondepolarizing neuromuscular blocking agents. It is not effective against depolarizing neuromuscular blocking agents.

Administration and Dosage

➤*General dosing considerations:* Response should be monitored carefully and assisted or controlled ventilation secured. Satisfactory reversal permits adequate voluntary respiration and neuromuscular transmission (as tested with a peripheral nerve stimulator). Recurarization has not been reported after satisfactory reversal has been attained.

➤*Adults:*
Curare overdosage –
Usual dosage: 0.05 to 0.1 mL/kg given intravenously (IV) slowly over 45 seconds to 1 minute at a point of at least 5% recovery of twitch response to neuromuscular stimulation (95% block). The dose delivered is edrophonium 0.5 to 1 mg/kg and atropine 0.007 to 0.014 mg/kg.
Maximum dose: A total dose of edrophonium 1 mg/kg should rarely be exceeded.

Reversal of nondepolarizing neuromuscular blocking agents –
Usual dosage: 0.05 to 0.1 mL/kg given IV slowly over 45 seconds to 1 minute at a point of at least 5% recovery of twitch response to neuromuscular stimulation (95% block). The dose delivered is edrophonium 0.5 to 1 mg/kg and atropine 0.007 to 0.014 mg/kg.
Maximum dose: A total dose of edrophonium 1 mg/kg should rarely be exceeded.

➤*Administration:* Administer IV slowly over 45 seconds to 1 minute.

➤*Storage/Stability:* Store between 15° and 26°C (59° and 78°F).

GUANIDINE HYDROCHLORIDE

Rx	**Guanidine HCl** (Schering-Plough)	**Tablets:** 125 mg	Mannitol. (KEY 74). In 100s.

GUANIDINE HYDROCHLORIDE — ORAL

Indications

➤*Myasthenic syndrome of Eaton-Lambert:* Guanidine is indicated for the reduction of the symptoms of muscle weakness and easy fatigability associated with the myasthenic syndrome of Eaton-Lambert. It is not indicated for treating myasthenia gravis. The Eaton-Lambert syndrome is ordinarily differentiated from myasthenia gravis by the usual association of the syndrome with small cell carcinoma of the lung, but myography may be necessary to make the diagnosis.

Administration and Dosage

➤*Adults:*

Myasthenic syndrome of Eaton-Lambert –

Initial dosage: 10 and 15 mg/kg of body weight per day in 3 or 4 divided doses.

Dosage titration: Gradually increase to a total daily dosage of 35 mg/kg of body weight per day or up to the development of side effects. As individual tolerance is highly variable, the dosage must be carefully titrated. Once a tolerable dose has been established, it should be continued.

Discontinuation of therapy: Occasionally removal of the primary neoplastic lesion may result in improvement of symptoms, permitting the discontinuance of guanidine.

➤*Storage/Stability:* Store between 15° and 30°C (59° and 86°F).

Actions

➤*Pharmacology:* Guanidine apparently acts by enhancing the release of acetylcholine following a nerve impulse. It also appears to slow the rates of depolarization and repolarization of muscle cell membranes.

Contraindications

Guanidine is contraindicated in individuals with a history of intolerance or allergy to this drug.

Warnings/Precautions

➤*Bone-marrow suppression:* Fatal bone-marrow suppression, apparently dose related, can occur with guanidine.

➤*Lactation:* Because guanidine is excreted in milk, patients on this drug should discontinue breast feeding.

➤*Children:* Since there is inadequate experience in children who have received this drug, safety and efficacy in children have not been established.

➤*Monitoring:* Baseline blood studies should be followed by frequent red and white blood cell and differential counts. The drug should be discontinued upon appearance of bone-marrow suppression. Concurrent therapy with other drugs that may cause bone-marrow suppression should be avoided.

Renal function may be affected in some patients receiving guanidine. Patients should therefore have regular urine examinations and serum creatinine determinations while taking this drug.

Physicians should be given adequate precautions pertaining to the gastrointestinal side effects and the possibility of induced behavior disorders.

Treatment should not be continued longer than necessary.

Adverse Reactions

Anemia, leukopenia, and thrombocytopenia resulting from bone-marrow depression attributable to guanidine have been reported. Other adverse reactions that have been observed are:

➤*Cardiovascular:* Palpitation, tachycardia, atrial fibrillation, hypotension.

➤*CNS:* Paresthesia of lips, face, hands, feet; cold sensations in hands and feet; nervousness, lightheadedness, jitteriness, increased irritability; tremor, trembling sensation; ataxia.

➤*Dermatologic:* Rash, flushing or pink complexion; folliculitis; petechiae, purpura, ecchymoses; sweating; skin eruptions; dryness and scaling of the skin.

➤*GI:* Dry mouth; gastric irritation; anorexia; nausea; diarrhea; abdominal cramping. Gastrointestinal side effects may preclude the use of guanidine as a desired form of therapy.

➤*Hepatic:* Abnormal liver function tests.

➤*Psychiatric:* Emotional lability; psychotic state; confusion; mood changes and hallucinations.

➤*Renal:* Elevation of blood creatinine; uremia; chronic, interstitial nephritis, acute interstitial nephritis, and renal tubular necrosis.

➤*Miscellaneous:* Sore throat, fever.

Overdosage

Mild gastrointestinal disorders, such as anorexia, increased peristalsis, or diarrhea are early warnings that tolerance is being exceeded. These symptoms may be relieved by atropine, but nevertheless note should be taken of these symptoms and dosage reductions considered. Slight numbness or tingling of the lips and fingertips shortly after taking a dose of guanidine has been reported. This per se is not an indication to discontinue treatment and/or reduce dosage.

Severe guanidine intoxication is characterized by nervous hyperirritability, fibrillary tremors and convulsive contractions of muscle, salivation, vomiting, diarrhea, hypoglycemia, and circulatory disturbances. Administration of intravenous calcium gluconate may control the neuromuscular and convulsive symptoms and provide some relief of other toxic manifestations.

Atropine is more effective than calcium in relieving the G.I. symptoms, circulatory disturbances, and changes in blood sugar.

DISULFIRAM

Rx	**Antabuse** (Duramed)	**Tablets:** 250 mg	Lactose. (OP 706). In 100s.
		500 mg	Lactose. (OP 707). Scored. In 50s, 100s, and 500s.

DISULFIRAM — ORAL

WARNING

Disulfiram should never be administered to a patient when he is in a state of alcohol intoxication, or without his full knowledge. The physician should instruct relatives accordingly.

Indications

➤*Alcoholism:* Disulfiram is an aid in the management of selected chronic alcohol patients who want to remain in a state of enforced sobriety so that supportive and psychotherapeutic treatment may be applied to best advantage.

Administration and Dosage

➤*General dosing considerations:* Disulfiram should never be administered until the patient has abstained from alcohol for at least 12 hours.

➤*Adults:*

Alcoholism –

Maximum dose: 500 mg daily.

Initial dosage: In the first phase of treatment, a maximum of 500 mg daily is given in a single dose for 1 to 2 weeks. To minimize or eliminate the sedative effect, dosage may be adjusted downward.

Maintenance dosage: 250 mg daily (range, 125 to 500 mg).

Duration of therapy: The daily, uninterrupted administration must be continued until the patient is fully recovered socially and a basis for permanent self-control is established. Depending on the individual patient, maintenance therapy may be required for months or years.

➤*Elderly:* Never administer an alcohol-drug test reaction to a patient older than 50 years of age (see Trial With Alcohol).

➤*Management of disulfiram-alcohol reaction:* In severe reactions, whether caused by an excessive test dose or by the patient's unsupervised ingestion of alcohol, supportive measures to restore blood pressure and treat shock should be instituted. Other recommendations include oxygen, carbogen (95% oxygen and 5% carbon dioxide), vitamin C intravenously (IV) in massive doses (1 g), and ephedrine. Antihistamines have also been used IV. Potassium levels should be monitored, particularly in patients on digitalis, because hypokalemia has been reported.

➤*Trial with alcohol:* Where a test reaction is deemed necessary, the suggested procedure is as follows:

After the first 1 to 2 weeks' therapy with 500 mg daily, a drink of 15 mL (½ oz) of 100 proof whiskey or equivalent is taken slowly. This test dose of alcoholic beverage may be repeated once only, so that the total dose does not exceed 30 mL (1 oz) of whiskey. Once a reaction develops, no more alcohol should be consumed. Such tests should be carried out only when the patient is hospitalized or comparable supervision and facilities, including oxygen, are available.

➤*Administration:* Although usually taken in the morning, may be taken on retiring by patients who experience a sedative effect.

➤*Storage/Stability:* Store at 15° to 30°C (59° to 86°F).

DISULFIRAM — ORAL

Actions

➤*Pharmacology:* Disulfiram produces a sensitivity to alcohol which results in a highly unpleasant reaction when the patient under treatment ingests even small amounts of alcohol.

Disulfiram blocks the oxidation of alcohol at the acetaldehyde stage. During alcohol metabolism following disulfiram intake, the concentration of acetaldehyde occurring in the blood may be 5 to 10 times higher than that found during metabolism of the same amount of alcohol alone.

Accumulation of acetaldehyde in the blood produces a complex of highly unpleasant symptoms referred to hereinafter as the disulfiram-alcohol reaction. This reaction, which is proportional to the dosage of both disulfiram and alcohol, will persist as long as alcohol is being metabolized. Disulfiram does not appear to influence the rate of alcohol elimination from the body.

➤*Pharmacokinetics:* Disulfiram is absorbed slowly from the gastrointestinal tract and is eliminated slowly from the body. One (or even 2) weeks after a patient has taken his last dose of disulfiram, ingestion of alcohol may produce unpleasant symptoms.

Prolonged administration of disulfiram does not produce tolerance; the longer a patient remains on therapy, the more exquisitely sensitive he becomes to alcohol.

Contraindications

Patients who are receiving or have recently received metronidazole, paraldehyde, alcohol, or alcohol-containing preparations (eg, cough syrups, tonics and the like); the presence of severe myocardial disease or coronary occlusion, psychoses, and hypersensitivity to disulfiram or to other thiuram derivatives used in pesticides and rubber vulcanization.

Warnings/Precautions

➤*Use with caution:* See the Warning box for more information.

The patient must be fully informed of the disulfiram-alcohol reaction. He must be strongly cautioned against surreptitious drinking while taking the drug, and he must be fully aware of the possible consequences. He should be warned to avoid alcohol in disguised forms (ie, in sauces, vinegars, cough mixtures, and even in aftershave lotions and back rubs). He should also be warned that reactions may occur with alcohol up to 14 days after ingesting disulfiram.

It is suggested that every patient under treatment carry an identification card stating that he is receiving disulfiram and describing the symptoms most likely to occur as a result of the disulfiram-alcohol reaction. In addition, this card should indicate the physician or institution to be contacted in an emergency.

➤*Disulfiram-alcohol reaction:* Disulfiram plus alcohol, even small amounts, produce flushing, throbbing in head and neck, throbbing headache, respiratory difficulty, nausea, copious vomiting, sweating, thirst, chest pain, palpitation, dyspnea, hyperventilation, tachycardia, hypotension, syncope, marked uneasiness, weakness, vertigo, blurred vision, and confusion. In severe reactions there may be respiratory depression, cardiovascular collapse, arrhythmias, myocardial infarction, acute congestive heart failure, unconsciousness, convulsions, and death.

The intensity of the reaction varies with each individual, but is generally proportional to the amounts of disulfiram and alcohol ingested. Mild reactions may occur in the sensitive individual when the blood alcohol concentration is increased to as little as 5 to 10 mg per 100 mL. Symptoms are fully developed at 50 mg per 100 mL, and unconsciousness usually results when the blood alcohol level reaches 125 to 150 mg.

The duration of the reaction varies from 30 to 60 minutes, to several hours in the more severe cases, or as long as there is alcohol in the blood.

➤*Special risk:* Because of the possibility of an accidental disulfiram-alcohol reaction, disulfiram should be used with extreme caution in patients with any of the following conditions: Diabetes mellitus, hypothyroidism, epilepsy, cerebral damage, chronic and acute nephritis, hepatic cirrhosis or insufficiency.

➤*Hepatic toxicity:* Hepatic toxicity including hepatic failure resulting in transplantation or death have been reported. Severe and sometimes fatal hepatitis associated with disulfiram therapy may develop even after many months of therapy. Hepatic toxicity has occurred in patients with or without prior history of abnormal liver function. Patients should be advised to immediately notify their physician of any early symptoms of hepatitis, such as fatigue, weakness, malaise, anorexia, nausea, vomiting, jaundice, or dark urine.

➤*Ethylene dibromide:* Patients taking disulfiram tablets should not be exposed to ethylene dibromide or its vapors. This precaution is based on preliminary results of animal research currently in progress that suggest a toxic interaction between inhaled ethylene dibromide and ingested disulfiram resulting in a higher incidence of tumors and mortality in rats. A correlation between this finding and humans, however, has not been demonstrated.

➤*Hypersensitivity reactions:* Patients with a history of rubber contact dermatitis should be evaluated for hypersensitivity to thiuram derivatives before receiving disulfiram. Hypersensitivity to thiuram derivatives is a containdication for use of disulfiram.

➤*Pregnancy:* Category C. The safe use of this drug in pregnancy has not been established. Therefore, disulfiram should be used during pregnancy only when, in the judgement of the physician, the probable benefits outweigh the possible risks.

➤*Lactation:* It is not known whether this drug is excreted in human milk. Since many drugs are so excreted, disulfiram should not be given to nursing mothers.

➤*Children:* Safety and effectiveness in children have not been established.

➤*Elderly:* A determination has not been made whether controlled clinical studies of disulfiram included sufficient numbers of subjects aged 65 and over to define a difference in response from younger subjects. Other reported clinical experience has not identified differences in responses between the elderly and younger patients. In general, dose selection for an elderly patient should be cautious, usually starting at the low end of the dosing range, reflecting the greater frequency of decreased hepatic, renal or cardiac function, and of concomitant disease or other drug therapy.

➤*Monitoring:* Baseline and follow-up liver function tests (10 to 14 days) are suggested to detect any hepatic dysfunction that may result with disulfiram therapy. In addition, a complete blood count and serum chemistries, including liver function tests, should be monitored.

Drug Interactions

➤*Nitrite:* In rats, simultaneous ingestion of disulfiram and nitrite in the diet for 78 weeks has been reported to cause tumors, and it has been suggested that disulfiram may react with nitrites in the rat stomach to form a nitrosamine, which is tumorigenic. Disulfiram alone in the rat's diet did not lead to such tumors. The relevance of this finding to humans is not known at this time.

Disulfiram Drug Interactions

Precipitant drug	Object drug[a]		Description
Isoniazid	Disulfiram	↑	Observe patients receiving isoniazid and disulfiram for the appearance of unsteady gait or marked changes in behavior; discontinue disulfiram or reduce the dose if such signs appear.
Metronidazole	Disulfiram	↑	Patients may exhibit acute toxic psychosis or confusional state when taking metronidazole in combination with disulfiram, requiring discontinuation of 1 or both of the agents.
Disulfiram	Alcohol	↑	Disulfiram causes a severe alcohol-intolerance reaction (eg, flushing and increased respiration, pulse rate, and cardiac output). Death has been reported. Avoid alcohol in all forms. See Warnings.
Disulfiram	Benzodiazepines	↑	Disulfiram decreases the plasma clearance of benzodiazepines metabolized by oxidation, possibly resulting in increased CNS depressant actions. When benzodiazepine therapy is indicated, use oxazepam, temazepam, or lorazepam since they are metabolized by glucuronidation.
Disulfiram	Caffeine	↑	Cardiovascular and CNS stimulation effects of caffeine may be increased by disulfiram.
Disulfiram	Chlorzoxazone	↑	Disulfiram inhibits the hepatic metabolism of chlorzoxazone. Decrease the dose of chlorzoxazone if increased CNS depression occur.
Disulfiram	Cocaine	↑	Cardiovascular side effects of cocaine may be increased when used concurrently with disulfiram.
Disulfiram	Hydantoins (eg, phenytoin)	↑	Serum hydantoin levels may be increased by disulfiram, resulting in an increase in the pharmacologic and toxic effects. Monitor hydantoin levels and adjust the dosage as needed.
Disulfiram	Theophyllines	↑	Disulfiram may inhibit the metabolism of the theophylline, thus increasing its effects. Monitor the theophylline level and adjust dose accordingly.
Disulfiram	Tricyclic antidepressants	↑	Tricyclic antidepressants and disulfiram coadministration may result in acute organic brain syndrome. The bioavailability of the antidepressant may also be increased.

DISULFIRAM — ORAL

Disulfiram Drug Interactions			
Precipitant drug	Object drug[a]		Description
Disulfiram	Warfarin	↑	Disulfiram may increase the anticoagulant effect of warfarin. Monitor prothrombin time and adjust the warfarin dosage as necessary.

[a] ↑ = object drug increased.

Adverse Reactions

Optic neuritis, peripheral neuritis, polyneuritis, and peripheral neuropathy may occur following administration of disulfiram.

Multiple cases of hepatitis, including both cholestatic and fulminant hepatitis, as well as hepatic failure resulting in transplantation or death, have been reported with administration of disulfiram.

Occasional skin eruptions are, as a rule, readily controlled by concomitant administration of an antihistaminic drug.

In a small number of patients, a transient mild drowsiness, fatigability, impotence, headache, acneform eruptions, allergic dermatitis, or a metallic or garlic-like aftertaste may be experienced during the first 2 weeks of therapy. These complaints usually disappear spontaneously with the continuation of therapy, or with reduced dosage.

Psychotic reactions have been noted, attributable in most cases to high dosage, combined toxicity (with metronidazole or isoniazid), or to the unmasking of underlying psychoses in patients stressed by the withdrawal of alcohol.

➤*Disulfiram-Alcohol interaction:* See Warnings/Precautions for more information.

Overdosage

No specific information is available on the treatment of overdosage with disulfiram. It is recommended that the physician contact the local poison control center.

ACAMPROSATE CALCIUM

Rx	**Campral** (Forest)	**Tablets, delayed release:** 333 mg	(333). White. Enteric-coated. In 180s, 1,080s, and Dose Pak 180s.

ACAMPROSATE CALCIUM — ORAL

Indications

➤*Alcoholism:* For the maintenance of abstinence from alcohol in patients with alcohol dependence who are abstinent at treatment initiation. Treatment with acamprosate should be part of a comprehensive management program that includes psychosocial support.

The efficacy of acamprosate in promoting abstinence has not been demonstrated in subjects who have not undergone detoxification and not achieved alcohol abstinence prior to beginning acamprosate treatment. The efficacy of acamprosate in promoting abstinence from alcohol in polysubstance abusers has not been adequately assessed.

Administration and Dosage

➤*General dosing considerations:* Dosage adjustment is required for patients with renal impairment (See Renal function impairment).

➤*Adults:*

Alcoholism – Two 333 mg tablets (each dose should total 666 mg) given 3 times daily. A lower dose may be effective in some patients.

➤*Elderly:* Because elderly patients are more likely to have decreased renal function, use care in dose selection.

➤*Renal function impairment:* For patients with moderate renal impairment (creatinine clearance [CrCl] 30 to 50 mL/min), a starting dose of one 333 mg tablet taken 3 times daily is recommended. Do not give acamprosate to patients with severe renal impairment (CrCl 30 mL/min or less).

➤*Administration:* Although dosing may be done without regard to meals, dosing with meals was employed during clinical trials and is suggested as an aid to compliance in those patients who regularly eat 3 meals daily.

➤*Storage/Stability:* Store at 25°C (77°F); excursions permitted to 15° to 30°C (59° to 86°F).

Actions

➤*Pharmacology:* The mechanism of action of acamprosate in the maintenance of alcohol abstinence is not completely understood. Chronic alcohol exposure is hypothesized to alter the normal balance between neuronal excitation and inhibition. In vitro and in vivo studies in animals have provided evidence to suggest acamprosate may interact with glutamate and gamma-aminobutyric acid (GABA) neurotransmitter systems centrally, and have led to the hypothesis that acamprosate restores this balance.

Pharmacodynamic studies have shown that acamprosate reduces alcohol intake in alcohol-dependent animals in a dose-dependent manner and that this effect appears to be specific to alcohol and the mechanisms of alcohol dependence.

Acamprosate has negligible observable central nervous system (CNS) activity in animals outside of its effects on alcohol dependence, exhibiting no anticonvulsant, antidepressant, or anxiolytic activity.

Acamprosate is not known to cause alcohol aversion and does not cause a disulfiram-like reaction as a result of ethanol ingestion.

➤*Pharmacokinetics:*

Absorption – The absolute bioavailability of acamprosate after oral administration is approximately 11%. Steady-state plasma concentrations of acamprosate are reached within 5 days of dosing. Steady-state peak plasma concentrations after acamprosate doses of two 333 mg tablets 3 times daily average 350 ng/mL and occur at 3 to 8 hours postdose. Coadministration of acamprosate with food decreases bioavailability as measured by C_{max} and AUC by approximately 42% and 23%, respectively. The food effect on absorption is not clinically significant and no adjustment of dose is necessary.

Distribution – The volume of distribution for acamprosate following intravenous administration is estimated to be 72 to 109 L (approximately 1 L/kg). Plasma protein binding of acamprosate is negligible.

Metabolism – Acamprosate does not undergo metabolism.

Excretion – After oral dosing of two 333 mg acamprosate tablets, the terminal half-life ranges from approximately 20 to 33 hours. Following oral administration of acamprosate, the major route of excretion is via the kidneys as acamprosate.

Special populations –

Renal function impairment: Peak plasma concentrations after administration of a single dose of two 333 mg acamprosate tablets to patients with moderate or severe renal impairment were approximately 2- and 4-fold higher, respectively, compared with healthy subjects. Similarly, elimination half-life was approximately 1.8- and 2.6-fold longer, respectively, compared with healthy subjects. There is a linear relationship between CrCl values and total apparent plasma clearance, renal clearance, and plasma half-life of acamprosate.

See Administration and Dosage for more information.

Elderly: The pharmacokinetics of acamprosate have not been evaluated in an elderly population. However, because renal function diminishes in elderly patients and acamprosate is excreted unchanged in urine, acamprosate plasma concentrations are likely to be higher in the elderly population compared with younger adults.

Contraindications

Hypersensitivity to acamprosate or any of its components; severe renal impairment (CrCl 30 mL/min or less).

Warnings/Precautions

➤*Withdrawal symptoms:* Use of acamprosate does not eliminate or diminish withdrawal symptoms.

➤*Suicide:* In controlled clinical trials of acamprosate, adverse events of a suicidal nature (eg, suicidal ideation, suicide attempts, completed suicides) were infrequent overall, but were more common in acamprosate-treated patients than in patients treated with placebo (1.4% vs 0.5% in studies of 6 months or less; 2.4% vs 0.8% in year-long studies). Completed suicides occurred in 3 of 2,272 (0.13%) patients in the pooled acamprosate group from all controlled studies and 2 of 1,962 patients (0.1%) in the placebo group. Adverse events coded as "depression" were reported at similar rates in acamprosate-treated and placebo-treated patients. Although many of these events occurred in the context of alcohol relapse, no consistent pattern of relationship between the clinical course of recovery from alcoholism and the emergence of suicidality was identified. The interrelationship of alcohol dependence, depression, and suicidality is well-recognized and complex. Monitor alcohol-dependent patients, including those patients being treated with acamprosate, for the development of symptoms of depression or suicidal thinking. Alert families and caregivers of patients being treated with acamprosate of the need to monitor patients for the emergence of symptoms of depression or suicidality, and to report such symptoms to the patient's health care provider.

➤*Renal function impairment:* See Administration and Dosage for more information.

➤*Pregnancy: Category C.* Acamprosate has been shown to be teratogenic in rats when given in doses approximately equal to the human dose (on a mg/m^2 basis) and in rabbits when given in doses approximately 3 times the human dose (on a mg/m^2 basis). Acamprosate produced a dose-related increase in the number of fetuses with malformations in rats at oral doses of 300 mg/kg/day or greater (approximately equal to the daily oral MRHD on a mg/m^2 basis). The malformations included hydronephrosis, malformed iris, retinal dysplasia, and retroesophageal subclavian artery. No findings were observed at an oral dose of 50 mg/kg/day (approximately one fifth the daily oral MRHD on a mg/m^2 basis). An increased incidence of hydronephrosis also was noted in Burgundy Tawny rabbits at oral doses of 400 mg/kg/day or greater (approximately 3 times the daily oral MRHD on a mg/m^2 basis). No developmental effects were observed in New Zealand white rabbits at oral doses up to 1,000 mg/kg/day (approximately 8 times the daily oral MRHD on a mg/m^2 basis). The findings in animals should be considered in relation to known adverse developmental effects of ethyl alcohol, which include the characteristics of fetal alcohol syndrome (eg, craniofacial dysmorphism, intrauterine and postnatal growth retardation, retarded psychomotor and intellectual development) and milder forms of neurological and behavioral

ACAMPROSATE CALCIUM — ORAL

disorders in humans. There are no adequate and well-controlled studies in pregnant women. Use acamprosate during pregnancy only if the potential benefit justifies the potential risk to the fetus.

A study conducted in pregnant mice that were administered acamprosate by the oral route starting on day 15 of gestation through the end of lactation on postnatal day 28 demonstrated an increased incidence of stillborn fetuses at doses of 960 mg/kg/day or greater (approximately 2 times the daily oral MRHD on a mg/m^2 basis). No effects were observed at a dose of 320 mg/kg/day (approximately one half the daily MRHD on a mg/m^2 basis).

➤*Lactation:* In animal studies, acamprosate was excreted in the milk of lactating rats dosed orally with acamprosate. The concentration of acamprosate in milk compared with blood was 1.3:1. It is not known whether acamprosate is excreted in human milk. Because many drugs are excreted in human milk, exercise caution when acamprosate is administered to a woman who is breastfeeding.

➤*Children:* The safety and efficacy of acamprosate have not been established in children.

➤*Elderly:* This drug is known to be substantially excreted by the kidney, and the risk of toxic reactions to this drug may be greater in patients with impaired renal function. Because elderly patients are more likely to have decreased renal function, use care in dose selection; it may be useful to monitor renal function.

Drug Interactions

➤*Naltrexone:* Coadministration of naltrexone with acamprosate produced a 25% increase in AUC and a 33% increase in the C_{max} of acamprosate. No adjustment of dosage is recommended in such patients.

Adverse Reactions

➤*Adverse events leading to discontinuation:* In placebo-controlled trials of 6 months or less, 8% of acamprosate-treated patients discontinued treatment because of an adverse event, compared with 6% of patients treated with placebo. In studies longer than 6 months, the discontinuation rate caused by adverse events was 7% in both the placebo-treated and the acamprosate-treated patients. Only diarrhea was associated with the discontinuation of more than 1% of patients (2% of acamprosate-treated vs 0.7% of placebo-treated patients). Other events, including nausea, depression, and anxiety, while accounting for discontinuation in less than 1% of patients, were nevertheless more commonly cited in association with discontinuation in acamprosate-treated patients than in placebo-treated patients.

➤*Common adverse events reported in controlled trials:*

Acamprosate Adverse Events (≥ 3%)				
Adverse reaction	Acamprosate 1,332 mg/day n = 397	Acamprosate 1,998 mg/day[a] n = 1,539	Acamprosate pooled[b] n = 2,019	Placebo n = 1,706
Number (%) of patients with an AE	248 (62%)	910 (59%)	1,231 (61%)	955 (56%)
CNS	150 (38%)	417 (27%)	598 (30%)	500 (29%)
Anxiety[c]	32 (8%)	80 (5%)	118 (6%)	98 (6%)
Depression	33 (8%)	63 (4%)	102 (5%)	87 (5%)
Dizziness	15 (4%)	49 (3%)	67 (3%)	44 (3%)
Dry mouth	13 (3%)	23 (1%)	36 (2%)	28 (2%)
Insomnia	34 (9%)	94 (6%)	137 (7%)	121 (7%)
Paresthesia	11 (3%)	29 (2%)	40 (2%)	34 (2%)
Dermatologic	26 (7%)	150 (10%)	187 (9%)	169 (10%)
Pruritus	12 (3%)	68 (4%)	82 (4%)	58 (3%)
Sweating	11 (3%)	27 (2%)	40 (2%)	39 (2%)
GI	85 (21%)	440 (29%)	574 (28%)	344 (20%)
Anorexia	20 (5%)	35 (2%)	57 (3%)	44 (3%)
Diarrhea	39 (10%)	257 (17%)	329 (16%)	166 (10%)
Flatulence	4 (1%)	55 (4%)	63 (3%)	28 (2%)
Nausea	11 (3%)	69 (4%)	87 (4%)	58 (3%)
Miscellaneous	121 (30%)	513 (33%)	685 (34%)	517 (30%)
Accidental injury[d]	17 (4%)	44 (3%)	70 (3%)	52 (3%)
Asthenia	29 (7%)	79 (5%)	114 (6%)	93 (5%)
Pain	6 (2%)	56 (4%)	65 (3%)	55 (3%)

[a] Includes 258 patients treated with acamprosate 2,000 mg/day, using a different dosage strength and regimen.
[b] Includes all patients in the first 2 columns as well as 83 patients treated with acamprosate 3,000 mg/day, using a different dosage strength and regimen.
[c] Includes events coded as "nervousness" by sponsor.
[d] Includes events coded as "fracture" by sponsor.

➤*Other adverse events:* Events are further categorized by body system and listed in order of decreasing frequency according to the following definitions: frequent adverse events are those occurring in at least 1/100 patients (only those not already listed in the summary of adverse events in controlled trials appear in this listing); infrequent adverse events are those occurring in 1/100 to 1/1000 patients; rare events are those occurring in fewer than 1/1000 patients.

Cardiovascular – Frequent: hypertension, palpitation, syncope, vasodilatation; Infrequent: angina pectoris, hemorrhage, hypotension, myocardial infarct, phlebitis, postural hypotension, tachycardia, varicose vein; Rare: cardiomyopathy, deep thrombophlebitis, heart failure, mesenteric arterial occlusion, shock.

CNS – Frequent: abnormal thinking, amnesia, headache, libido decrease, somnolence, tremor; Infrequent: abnormal dreams, agitation, apathy, confusion, convulsion, hallucinations, hostility, hypesthesia, libido increase, migraine, neuralgia, neurosis, suicidal ideation, vertigo, withdrawal syndrome; Rare: alcohol craving, depersonalization, encephalopathy, hyperkinesia, increased salivation, manic reaction, paranoid reaction, psychosis, torticollis, twitching.

Dermatologic – Frequent: rash; Infrequent: acne, alopecia, dry skin, eczema, exfoliative dermatitis, maculopapular rash, urticaria, vesiculobullous rash; Rare: psoriasis.

Endocrine – Rare: goiter, hypothyroidism.

GI – Frequent: abdominal pain, constipation, dyspepsia, increased appetite, vomiting; Infrequent: abnormal liver function tests, dysphagia, eructation, esophagitis, gastritis, gastroenteritis, gastrointestinal hemorrhage, hematemesis, hepatitis, liver cirrhosis, nausea and vomiting, pancreatitis, rectal hemorrhage; Rare: carcinoma of liver, cholecystitis, colitis, duodenal ulcer, enlarged abdomen, melena, mouth ulceration, stomach ulcer.

GU – Frequent: impotence; Infrequent: abnormal sexual function, metrorrhagia, urinary frequency, urinary incontinence, urinary tract infection, vaginitis; Rare: abnormal ejaculation, hematuria, kidney calculus, menorrhagia, nocturia, polyuria, urinary urgency.

Hematologic/Lymphatic – Infrequent: anemia, ecchymosis, eosinophilia, lymphocytosis, thrombocytopenia; Rare: leukopenia, lymphadenopathy, monocytosis.

Lab test abnormalities – Infrequent: ALT increase, AST increase; Rare: alkaline phosphatase increase, creatinine increase, lactic dehydrogenase increase.

Metabolic/Nutritional – Frequent: peripheral edema, weight gain; Infrequent: avitaminosis, bilirubinemia, diabetes mellitus, gout, hyperglycemia, hyperuricemia, thirst, weight loss; Rare: hyponatremia.

Musculoskeletal – Frequent: arthralgia, myalgia; Infrequent: leg cramps; Rare: myopathy, rheumatoid arthritis.

Respiratory – Frequent: bronchitis, cough increase, dyspnea, pharyngitis, rhinitis; Infrequent: asthma, epistaxis, pneumonia; Rare: laryngismus, pulmonary embolus.

Special senses – Frequent: abnormal vision, taste perversion; Infrequent: amblyopia, deafness, tinnitus; Rare: diplopia, ophthalmitis, photophobia.

Miscellaneous – Frequent: back pain, chest pain, chills, flu syndrome, infection, suicide attempt; Infrequent: abscess, allergic reaction, fever, hernia, intentional injury, intentional overdose, malaise, neck pain; Rare: ascites, facial edema, photosensitivity reaction, sudden death.

➤*Postmarketing:* Although no causal relationship to acamprosate has been found, the serious adverse event of acute kidney failure has been reported to be temporally associated with acamprosate treatment in at least 3 patients and is not described elsewhere in the labeling.

Overdosage

➤*Symptoms:* In all reported cases of acute overdosage with acamprosate (total reported doses of up to 56 g acamprosate), the only symptom that could be reasonably associated with acamprosate was diarrhea. Hypercalcemia has not been reported in cases of acute overdose. Consider a risk of hypercalcemia in chronic overdosage only.

➤*Treatment:* Treatment of overdose should be symptomatic and supportive.

Patient Information

Any psychoactive drug may impair judgment, thinking, or motor skills. Caution patients about operating hazardous machinery, including automobiles, until they are reasonably certain that acamprosate therapy does not affect their ability to engage in such activities.

Advise patients to notify their physician if they become pregnant or intend to become pregnant during therapy.

Advise patients to notify their physician if they are breastfeeding.

Advise patients to continue acamprosate therapy as directed, even in the event of relapse. Remind them to discuss any renewed drinking with their physician.

Advise patients that acamprosate has been shown to help maintain abstinence only when used as a part of a treatment program that includes counseling and support.

Indications

➤*Smoking cessation:* As an aid to smoking cessation for the relief of nicotine withdrawal symptoms. Use as part of a comprehensive behavioral smoking-cessation program.

Administration and Dosage

Withdrawal from nicotine in addicted individuals is characterized by craving, nervousness, restlessness, irritability, mood lability, anxiety, drowsiness, sleep disturbances, impaired concentration, increased appetite, minor somatic complaints (headache, myalgia, constipation, fatigue), and weight gain. Nicotine toxicity is characterized by nausea, abdominal pain, vomiting, diarrhea, diaphoresis, flushing, dizziness, disturbed hearing/vision, confusion, weakness, palpitations, altered respiration, and hypotension.

The following table includes dosing, duration of therapy, and availability information for nicotine replacement therapy products.

Nicotine Replacement Pharmacotherapy

Type of therapy	Dosage	Duration	Availability
Gum	< 25 cigarettes/day: 2 mg gum up to 24 pieces/day	up to 12 weeks	*otc*
	> 25 cigarettes/day: 4 mg gum up to 24 pieces/day		
Inhaler	6 to 16 cartridges/day	up to 6 months	*Rx* only
Transdermal patch	21 mg/24 hr 14 mg/24 hr 7 mg/24 hr	4 to 6 weeks then 2 weeks then 2 weeks	*otc*
	15 mg/16 hr	6 weeks	
Nasal spray	8 to 40 doses/day	3 to 6 months	*Rx* only

Actions

➤*Pharmacology:* Nicotine, the chief alkaloid in tobacco products, binds stereoselectively to acetylcholine receptors at the autonomic ganglia, in the adrenal medulla, at neuromuscular junctions, and in the brain. Two types of CNS effects are believed to be the basis of nicotine's positively reinforcing properties. A stimulating effect, exerted mainly in the cortex via the locus ceruleus, produces increased alertness and cognitive performance. A "reward" effect via the "pleasure system" in the brain is exerted in the limbic system. At low doses the stimulant effects predominate, while at high doses the reward effects predominate. Intermittent IV administration of nicotine activates neurohormonal pathways, releasing acetylcholine, norepinephrine, dopamine, serotonin, vasopressin, beta-endorphin, growth hormone, and adrenocorticotropic hormone (ACTH).

The cardiovascular effects of nicotine include peripheral vasoconstriction, tachycardia, and elevated blood pressure. Acute and chronic tolerance to nicotine develops from smoking tobacco or ingesting nicotine preparations. Acute tolerance (a reduction in response for a given dose) develops rapidly (< 1 hour), but at distinct rates for different physiologic effects (eg, skin temperature, heart rate, subjective effects). Withdrawal symptoms, such as cigarette craving, can be reduced in some individuals by plasma nicotine levels lower than those for smoking.

Nicotine polacrilex contains nicotine bound to an ion exchange resin in a chewing gum base. The **nicotine transdermal system** is a multilayered unit containing nicotine as the active agent that provides systemic delivery of nicotine for up to 24 hours (*Nicotrol*, up to 16 hours) following its application to intact skin.

➤*Pharmacokinetics:*

Absorption/Distribution –

Nicotine: Nicotine as tobacco smoke is absorbed rapidly through the lungs. Nicotine is a weak base; absorption through mucous membranes depends on pH. Nicotine gum is buffered at an alkaline pH to increase absorption through the buccal mucosa. The volume of distribution of IV nicotine is ≈ 2 to 3 L/kg. Plasma protein binding is < 5%.

Gum: The nicotine is bound to an ion exchange resin and is released only during chewing; nicotine will not be released in significant amounts if the gum is swallowed. The blood level of nicotine will depend upon the vigor and duration of chewing. The trough level of nicotine obtained by smoking 1 cigarette/hour is ≈ 2 times that of chewing one 2 mg piece of gum.

Transdermal: Following application, ≈ 68% of the nicotine released from the system enters the systemic circulation. The remainder of the nicotine released from the system is lost via evaporation from the edge. All systems are labeled by the actual amount of nicotine absorbed by the patient.

After application, plasma concentrations rise rapidly, plateau within 2 to 12 hours, and then slowly decline until the system is removed, after which they decline more rapidly. Following the second daily application, steady-state plasma nicotine concentrations are achieved and are on average 25% to 30% higher compared with single-dose applications. Plasma nicotine concentrations are proportional to dose and are similar for all sites of application on the upper body and upper outer arm.

Half-hourly smoking of cigarettes produces average plasma nicotine concentrations of ≈ 44 ng/mL. Average plasma nicotine concentrations from transdermal nicotine are ≈ 5 to 17 ng/mL.

Inhaler: Most of the nicotine released from the inhaler is deposited in the mouth with only a fraction of the dose released (< 5%) reaching the lower respiratory tract. Eight deep inhalations over 20 minutes releases on average 4 mg of nicotine content from each cartridge, of which 2 mg is systemically absorbed. Peak plasma concentrations are typically reached within 15 minutes after inhalation ends. Absorption of nicotine through the buccal mucosa is relatively slow. Nicotine arterial plasma concentration peaks and declines seen with cigarette smoking are not achieved with the inhaler. After use of a single inhaler, the arterial nicotine concentration rises slowly to an average of 6 ng/mL in contrast to those of a cigarette, which increase rapidly and reach a mean C_{max} of ≈ 49 ng/mL within 5 minutes.

Intermittent use of the nicotine inhaler typically produces nicotine plasma levels of 6 to 8 ng/mL, corresponding to ≈ 33% of those achieved with cigarette smoking.

Nasal spray: Following administration of 2 sprays of nicotine nasal spray (1 mg), ≈ 53% enters the systemic circulation. Plasma concentrations of nicotine rise rapidly, reaching maximum venous concentrations of 12 ng/mL in 15 minutes. The apparent absorption half-life of nicotine is ≈ 3 minutes. There is a wide variation among subjects in the plasma nicotine concentrations for the spray. Peak nicotine concentrations similar to whose seen after smoking 1 cigarette (17 ng/mL) were seen in 20% of subjects after a 1 mg dose of spray.

Metabolism/Excretion –

Nicotine: Nicotine is rapidly and extensively metabolized by the liver. More than 20 metabolites have been identified, all of which are believed to be less active than the parent compound. The primary plasma metabolite, cotinine, has a half-life of 15 to 20 hours, and concentrations that exceed nicotine by 10-fold. About 10% of the nicotine absorbed is excreted unchanged in the urine. This may be increased up to 30% with high urinary flow rates and urine pH < 5. The half-life of nicotine averages 1 to 2 hours. Nicotine accumulates in the body over 6 to 9 hours of regular smoking. Thus, smoking results in a nicotine exposure that lasts 24 hours a day. Persistence of nicotine in the brain results in changes in nicotinic receptors in the brain. Changes in receptor numbers or function are presumably the substrate for nicotine withdrawal syndrome.

Transdermal: Following removal of transdermal nicotine, plasma nicotine concentrations decline exponentially with an apparent mean half-life of 3 to 4 hours due to continued absorption from the skin depot. Most nonsmoking patients will have nondetectable nicotine concentrations in 10 to 12 hours.

Nicotine Pharmacokinetics

Parameter	Smoking	Gum	Transdermal	Nasal spray	Inhaler
Time to peak levels (hours)	ND[a]	0.25 to 0.5	2 to 12	0.25	0.25
Peak plasma level (ng/mL)	44	5 to 10	5 to 17	12	6
Half-life (hours)	15 to 20[b]	3 to 4	3 to 4	1 to 2	ND

[a] No data.
[b] Refers to cotinine, the primary plasma metabolite of nicotine.

Contraindications

Hypersensitivity to nicotine or any components of the products, including menthol.

Warnings/Precautions

➤*Nicotine risks:* Nicotine from any source can be toxic and addictive. Smoking causes lung disease, cancer, and heart disease, and may adversely affect pregnant women or the fetus. For any smoker, with or without concomitant disease or pregnancy, the risk of nicotine replacement in a smoking cessation program should be weighed against the hazard of continued smoking, and the likelihood of achieving cessation of smoking without nicotine replacement.

➤*General:* Urge the patient to stop smoking completely when initiating nicotine replacement therapy. Inform patients that if they continue to smoke while using the product, they may experience adverse effects due to peak nicotine levels higher than those experienced from smoking alone. If there is a clinically significant increase in cardiovascular or other effects attributable to nicotine, the treatment should be discontinued. Physicians should anticipate that concomitant medications may need dosage adjustment (see Drug Interactions). Sustained use (> 6 months) of inhaler or nasal spray by patients who stop smoking has not been studied and is not recommended (see Drug Abuse and Dependence).

➤*Bronchospastic disease:* The **inhaler** has not been specifically studied in asthma or chronic pulmonary disease. Nicotine is an airway irritant and might cause bronchospasm. The inhaler should be used with caution in patients with bronchospastic disease. Other forms of nicotine replacement might be preferable in patients with severe bronchospastic airway disease.

Asthma, bronchospasm, and reactive airway disease exacerbation of bronchospasm in patients with pre-existing asthma has been reported. Use of the **nasal spray** in patients with severe reactive airway disease is not recommended.

➤*Nasal disorders:* Use of the **nasal spray** is not recommended in patients with known chronic nasal disorders (eg, allergy, rhinitis, nasal polyps, sinusitis) because such use has not been adequately studied. The effect of the nasal spray on the nasal mucosa topical application of either nicotine or tobacco products is irritating to the nasal mucosa and physicians should consider both the risks and benefits to the patient before initiating or continuing nasal spray therapy. The effect of the nasal spray on the nasal mucosa was studied in 39 cigarette smokers who used the nasal spray for 1 month. When compared with baseline, random biopsies taken after 4 weeks of treatment revealed 1 patient with persistence of pre-existing dysplasia and 1 patient with a newly found dysplasia. In both, dysplasia was not seen after a recovery period of 8 weeks. Forty-two patients who used the nasal spray for > 6 months underwent follow-up ear, nose, and throat examinations 1 to 3 months after discontinuing the use of the spray. Many reported local irritant effects of the spray during spray use, but none showed persistent mucosal injury that the examining physician could attribute to use of the product. The clinical significance of these findings is not known, but extended use of the product > 6 months is not recommended.

➤*Cardiovascular:* Weigh the benefits against the risks of nicotine in patients with certain cardiovascular and peripheral vascular diseases. Specifically, screen and evaluate patients with coronary heart disease (history of MI or angina pectoris), serious cardiac arrhythmias, or vasospastic diseases (Buerger's disease, Prinzmetal variant angina, Raynaud's phenomena) before nicotine is prescribed. There have been occasional reports of tachycardia and palpitations associated with nicotine replacement therapy; therefore, if cardiovascular symptoms occur, discontinue the drug. Generally, do not use during the immediate post-MI period, nor in patients with serious arrhythmias or with severe or worsening angina pectoris.

Accelerated hypertension – Nicotine therapy constitutes a risk factor for development of malignant hypertension in patients with accelerated hypertension. **Inhaler** therapy should be used with caution in these patients and only when the benefits of including nicotine replacement in a smoking cessation program outweigh the risks.

➤*Endocrine:* Because of the action of nicotine on the adrenal medulla (release of catecholamines), use with caution in patients with hyperthyroidism, pheochromocytoma, or insulin-dependent diabetes.

➤*Oral/GI:* Because nicotine delays healing in peptic ulcer disease, use in patients with active or inactive peptic ulcer only when benefits of including nicotine in a smoking cessation program outweigh risks.

➤*Dental:* When used over an extended time, nicotine **gum** may cause severe occlusal stress due to its heavier viscosity than ordinary chewing gum. Nicotine gum may cause loosening of inlays or fillings, can stick to dentures, and cause damage to oral mucosa and natural teeth. Hard, sugarless candy between doses of gum is recommended to help provide oral stimulation required by some patients. Temporol mandibular joint dysfunction and pain have also been reported with excessive chewing.

➤*Renal/Hepatic function impairment:* Because nicotine is extensively metabolized and its total system clearance is dependent on liver blood flow, anticipate some influence of hepatic impairment on drug kinetics (reduced clearance). Only severe renal impairment should affect clearance of nicotine or its metabolites from circulation.

➤*Drug abuse and dependence:*

Inhaler – The nicotine inhaler is likely to have a low abuse potential based on slower absorption, smaller fluctuations, and lower blood levels of nicotine when compared with cigarettes. However, nicotine withdrawal symptoms were noted in clinical trials during tapering and discontinuation of the nicotine inhaler. Dependence can occur from transference of tobacco-related nicotine dependence to the inhaler. The use of the inhaler for > 6 months is not recommended. Encourage patients to withdraw gradually from therapy after 3 months of usage to minimize the risk of dependence. If necessary, dose reduction can be gradually achieved over a 6- to 12-week period.

Nasal spray – Nicotine nasal spray has a dependence potential intermediate between other nicotine-based therapies and cigarettes. The nasal spray is distinct from other nicotine-based smoking cessation therapies in its greater speed of onset, greater capacity of self-titration of dose, and frequent, rapid fluctuations of plasma nicotine concentration. Dependence on nicotine nasal spray occurred during clinical trials. Feelings of dependency were reported by 32% of active spray users and 13% of placebo spray users. Such dependence may represent transference of tobacco-related nicotine dependence to the nasal spray. Some patients (15% to 20%) used the active spray for longer than recommended (6 to 12 months) and 5% used a higher dose than recommended. Some patients experienced anxiety after discontinuing the spray and some reported craving the spray rather than cigarettes.

➤*Pregnancy: Category D* (**inhaler, spray, transdermal patch**); *Category C* (**gum**). Tobacco smoke contains nicotine, hydrogen cyanide, and carbon monoxide. The harmful effects of cigarette smoking on maternal and fetal health are clearly established. These include low birth weight (21% to 39% of all infants), an increased risk of spontaneous abortion, increased perinatal mortality, and decreased placental perfusion. Smoking causes a decrease in the oxygen-carrying capacity of hemoglobin when carbon monoxide passes through the placenta. Nicotine causes vasoconstriction and decreased placenta blood flow. Smoking interferes with the body's ability to process essential vitamins and minerals, resulting in decreased intestinal synthesis of vitamin B_{12}, calcium loss from bones, and decreased usage of vitamin C. In general, smokers have a nutrient-poor diet. Smoking during pregnancy increases the risk of ectopic pregnancy, spontaneous abortion, preterm birth, premature rupture of membranes, placenta previa, abruptio placenta, and chorioamnionitis.

No association has been found between maternal smoking and congenital anomalies; however, nicotine and cotinine are found in higher concentrations in infants whose mothers smoke.

Second-hand smoking is an increasing concern for its potential effects on infants and siblings. There is an association between maternal smoking and sudden infant death syndrome, but it is unclear whether it is from in utero exposure or postnatal passive exposure, or both.

Nicotine was shown to produce skeletal abnormalities in the offspring of mice when toxic doses were given to the dams.

A nicotine bolus (up to 2 mg/kg) to pregnant rhesus monkeys caused acidosis, hypercarbia, and hypotension (fetal and maternal concentrations were ≈ 20 times those achieved after smoking 1 cigarette in 5 minutes). Fetal breathing movements were reduced in the fetal lamb after IV injection of 0.25 mg/kg nicotine to the ewe (equivalent to smoking 1 cigarette every 20 seconds for 5 minutes). Uterine blood flow was reduced ≈ 30% after infusion of 0.1 mcg/kg/min nicotine to pregnant rhesus monkeys (equivalent to smoking ≈ 6 cigarettes every minute for 20 minutes).

The inhaler and nasal spray do not deliver hydrogen cyanide and carbon monoxide. However, because they do deliver nicotine, it is presumed that the inhaler and the nasal spray can cause fetal harm when administered to a pregnant woman. The effect of nicotine delivered by the inhaler and nasal spray has not been examined in pregnancy and the specific effects of nicotine inhaler and nasal spray therapy on fetal development are unknown. Spontaneous abortion during nicotine replacement therapy has been reported; as with smoking, nicotine as a contributing factor cannot be excluded. Pregnant smokers should be encouraged to attempt cessation using education and behavioral interventions before using pharmacological approaches. If the inhaler or nasal spray are used during pregnancy, or if the patient becomes pregnant while using it, the patient should be apprised of the potential hazard to the fetus. Inhaler and spray therapy should be used during pregnancy only if the likelihood of smoking cessation justifies the potential risk of using it by the pregnant patient who might continue to smoke.

➤*Lactation:* Nicotine and cotinine pass freely into breast milk up to 2 hours after maternal smoking; the milk to plasma ratio averages 2.9. Nicotine is absorbed orally. An infant has the ability to clear nicotine by hepatic first-pass clearance; however, the efficiency of removal is probably lowest at birth. Nicotine concentrations in milk can be expected to be lower with **inhaler** and **nasal spray** nicotine therapy when used as directed than with cigarette smoking, as maternal plasma nicotine concentrations are generally reduced with nicotine replacement. Decide whether to discontinue nursing or to discontinue the drug, weighing the risk of exposure of the infant to nicotine from replacement therapy against the risks associated with the infant's exposure to nicotine from continued smoking by the mother and from nicotine therapy alone or in combination with continued smoking.

➤*Children:* Safety and efficacy in children/adolescents < 18 years of age who smoke have not been evaluated.

Cigarette smoke contains many compounds including carbon monoxide, dioxin, cyanide, and cadmium. Studies have shown residual effects beyond the neonatal period, including growth deficits, and deficiencies in intellectual, emotional, and behavioral development. These manifest as poor auditory responsiveness, fine motor tremors, hypertonicity, and decreases in verbal comprehension.

The amounts of nicotine that are tolerated by adult smokers can produce symptoms of poisoning and could prove fatal if inhaled, ingested, or bucally absorbed by children or pets. An inhaler or nasal spray cartridge container contains ≈ 60% (6 mg) of its initial drug content when discarded. Therefore, caution patients to keep the used and unused systems out of the reach of children and pets.

➤*Elderly:* Nicotine **inhaler** and **nasal spray** therapy appeared to be as effective in elderly patients ≥ 60 years of age as in younger smokers.

Drug Interactions

Smoking cessation, with or without nicotine substitutes, may alter response to concomitant medication in ex-smokers.

Cigarette smoking is an inducer of CYP1A2 enzymes, the primary mechanism for drug interactions. For drugs whose metabolism is stimulated by enzyme inducers, the dose may need to be increased upon initiation of inducer (smoking) therapy and decreased when the inducer (smoking) is discontinued.

Smoking Drug Interactions

Precipitant drug	Object drug[a]		Description
Smoking	Alcohol	⬇	May decrease the rate of absorption and peak serum concentration.
Smoking	Benzodiazepines (diazepam, chlordiazepoxide)	⬇	Smoking may decrease sedation and drowsiness probably by CNS stimulation.
Smoking	Beta adrenergic blockers	⬇	Sympathetic activation by nicotine may decrease end-organ responsiveness. Beta blockers may be less effective for blood pressure and heart rate control in smokers.
Smoking	Caffeine Clozapine Fluvoxamine Olanzapine Tacrine Theophylline	⬇	Smoking is an inducer of CYP1A2 enzymes. It can increase clearance and decrease AUC, mean plasma concentration, half-life, and volume of distribution.
Smoking	Clorazepate Lidocaine (oral)	⬇	Smoking can decrease AUC.
Smoking	Estradiol	⬇	Smoking can increase 2-hydroxylation with possible antiestrogenic effects.
Smoking	Flecanide Imipramine	⬇	Can increase clearance and decrease serum concentrations.

Smoking Drug Interactions			
Precipitant drug	Object drug[a]		Description
Smoking	Heparin	⬇	Smoking can increase clearance and decrease half-life. The smoker may require higher doses of heparin.
Smoking	Insulin	⬇	Smoking can cause decreased SC absorption resulting in higher insulin requirements for smokers.
Smoking	Mexiletine	⬇	Smoking may increase oral clearance and decrease half-life.
Smoking	Opioids (dextropropoxyphene, pentazocine)	⬇	Smoking can decrease the analgesic effect; therefore, smokers may require higher doses for analgesia.
Smoking	Propranolol	⬇	Smoking can increase oral clearance.
Smoking Nicotine	Catecholamines Cortisol	⬆	Smoking and nicotine can increase circulating cortisol and catecholamines. Therapy with adrenergic agonists or adrenergic blockers may need to be adjusted upon changes in nicotine therapy or smoking status.

[a] ⬆ = object drug increased; ⬇ = object drug decreased.

➤*Nasal spray:* The extent of absorption and peak plasma concentration is slightly reduced in patients with the common cold/rhinitis. In addition, the time to peak concentration is prolonged. The use of a nasal vasoconstrictor such as xylometazoline in patients with rhinitis will further prolong the time to peak.

Adverse Reactions

Assessment of adverse events in patients who participated in controlled clinical trials is complicated by the occurrence of signs and symptoms of nicotine withdrawal in some patients and nicotine excess in others. The incidence of adverse events is compounded by the many minor complaints that smokers commonly have, continued smoking by many patients, and the local irritation from the active drug and placebo.

➤*Inhaler:*

Nicotine Inhaler Adverse Reactions (%)		
Adverse reaction	Drug	Placebo
Local irritation (mouth, throat)	40	18
Coughing	32	12
Rhinitis	23	16
Dyspepsia	18	9
Headache	26	15

Local – Taste complaints, pain in jaw and neck, tooth disorders, sinusitis (≥ 3%).

Miscellaneous – Influenza-like symptoms, pain, back pain, allergy, paresthesias, flatulence, fever (≥ 3%).

Withdrawal: Dizziness, anxiety, sleep disorder, depression, withdrawal syndrome, drug dependence, fatigue, myalgia (≥ 3%).

Nicotine-related: Nausea, diarrhea, hiccough (≥ 3%).

Smoking-related: Chest discomfort, bronchitis, hypertension (≥ 3%).

➤*Nasal spray:*

Common smoker complaints: Chest tightness, dyspepsia, paresthesias in limbs, constipation, and stomatitis.

Withdrawal symptoms: Anxiety, irritability, restlessness, cravings, dizziness, impaired concentration, weight increase, emotional lability, somnolence, fatigue, increased sweating, insomnia (≥ 5%); confusion, depression, apathy, tremor, increased appetite, incoordination, increased dreaming (< 5%).

Local irritation: Moderate-to-severe in 94% of patients during the first 2 days of treatment, declining to 81% after 3 weeks of treatment (rated moderate-to-mild); runny nose; throat irritation; watering eyes; sneezing; cough; nasal congestion; subjective comments related to the taste or usage of the dosage form; sinus irritation; transient epistaxis; eye irritation; transient changes in sense of smell; pharyngitis; paresthesias of the nose, mouth, or head; numbness of the nose or mouth; burning of the nose or eyes; earache; facial flushing; transient changes in sense of taste; hoarseness; nasal ulcer or blister.

Dependence: Feelings of dependence and calming were reported by more patients on active spray than placebo.

Others (not attributable to intercurrent illness):

Nicotine Nasal Spray Adverse Reactions (> 1%)		
Adverse reaction	Drug	Placebo
Headache	18	15
Back pain	6	4
Dyspnea	5	6
Nausea	5	5
Arthralgia	5	1
Menstrual disorder	4	4
Palpitation	4	4
Flatulence	4	3
Tooth disorder	4	1
Gum disorder	4	1
Myalgia	3	4
Abdominal pain	3	3
Confusion	3	3
Acne	3	1
Dysmenorrhea	3	0
Pruritus	2	3

CNS – Aphasia, amnesia, migraine, numbness (< 1%).

GI – Dry mouth, hiccough, diarrhea (< 1%).

Respiratory – Bronchitis, bronchospasm, increased sputum (< 1%).

Miscellaneous – Peripheral edema, pain, allergy, purpura, rash, abnormal vision (< 1%).

➤*Gum:*

Miscellaneous – Injury to mouth, teeth, or dental work; belching; increased salivation; mild jaw muscle ache; sore mouth or throat.

➤*Transdermal:*

Miscellaneous – Erythema, pruritus, and/or burning at the application site.

Overdosage

➤*Symptoms:* Signs and symptoms of acute nicotine poisoning include the following: Pallor, cold sweat, nausea, salivation, vomiting, abdominal pain, diarrhea, headache, dizziness, disturbed hearing and vision, tremor, mental confusion, weakness. Prostration, hypotension, and respiratory failure may ensue with large overdoses. Lethal doses produce convulsions quickly; death follows as a result of peripheral or central respiratory paralysis or, less frequently, cardiac failure. The oral minimum acute lethal dose for nicotine in adult humans is reported to be 40 to 60 mg.

➤*Treatment:* Large oral nicotine ingestions cause vomiting, and the consequences of an overdose will vary. Institute gastric lavage and/or activated charcoal (with protected airway) when appropriate. Avoid syrup of ipecac.

Other supportive measures include diazepam or barbiturates for seizures, atropine for excessive bronchial secretions or diarrhea, respiratory support for respiratory failure, and vigorous fluid support for hypotension and cardiovascular collapse.

Nasal spray – A full bottle of nicotine nasal spray contains 100 mg of nicotine and would be expected to be irritating if sprayed in the eyes, mouth, or ears. Treat eye exposure with copious water irrigation for 20 minutes.

Inhaler – One cartridge of nicotine inhaler contains 10 mg of nicotine, of which, ≈ 4 mg is delivered nicotine. It is unlikely that an excessive nicotine overdose will occur via inhalation, but should such an overdose occur, the patient should contact a physician immediately. Refer patients ingesting nicotine inhaler cartridges to a health care facility for management. Administer repeated doses of activated charcoal as long as the cartridge remains in the GI tract because the cartridge will continue to release nicotine for many hours. The cartridge can be identified with a radiogram.

Transdermal – Remove the patch, flush the skin with water, and dry. Do not use soap, which may increase nicotine absorption. If the patch has been ingested, administer activated charcoal. In an unconscious patient, secure an airway before administering activated charcoal via a nasogastric tube. As long as the patch remains in the GI tract, administer repeated doses of charcoal because the patch will continue to release nicotine. A saline cathartic or sorbitol may be added to the first dose of activated charcoal to enhance passage of the patch.

NICOTINE TRANSDERMAL SYSTEM

	Product/Distributor	Dose absorbed in 24 hours (mg/day)	How supplied
otc	**Nicotine Transdermal System Step 1** (Various, eg, Novartis, Watson)	21	In 7 and 30 systems per box.
otc	**Nicotine Transdermal System Step 2** (Various, eg, Novartis, Watson)	14	In 7 and 30 systems per box.
otc	**Nicotine Transdermal System Step 3** (Various, eg, Novartis, Watson)	7	In 7 and 30 systems per box.
otc	**Nicoderm CQ Step 1** (GlaxoSmithKline Consumer)	21	In 7 and 14 systems per box; original and clear patches.
otc	**Nicoderm CQ Step 2** (GlaxoSmithKline Consumer)	14	In 14 systems per box; original and clear patches.
otc	**Nicoderm CQ Step 3** (GlaxoSmithKline Consumer)	7	In 14 systems per box; original and clear patches.
otc	**Nicotrol Step 1** (Pharmacia)	15[a]	In 7s and 14s.
otc	**Nicotrol Step 2** (Pharmacia)	10[a]	In 7s and 14s.
otc	**Nicotrol Step 3** (Pharmacia)	5[a]	In 7s and 14s.

[a] Dose absorbed in 16 hours.

NICOTINE — TRANSDERMAL

For complete and comparative prescribing information, refer to the Nicotine group monograph.

Indications

➤*Smoking cessation:* Nicotine transdermal system is indicated for the reduction of withdrawal symptoms, including nicotine craving, associated with quitting smoking.

➤*Off-label uses:*

Tourette syndrome – [2] = Fair documentation. Data from these initial studies suggest that nicotine in combination with haloperidol but not alone may be effective in reducing tic frequency and severity. (See Administration and Dosage.)

Ulcerative colitis – [4] = Insufficient documentation. The use of transdermal nicotine in the management of ulcerative colitis has demonstrated some benefit. However, additional controlled trials are needed to identify optimal dosage escalation regimens and candidates for treatment. Despite initial evidence, current guidelines state that the place of nicotine therapy in the management of ulcerative colitis is not established. (See Administration and Dosage.)

Administration and Dosage

➤*General dosing considerations:* Patients should stop smoking completely prior to beginning use of the patch.

➤*Adults:*

Smoking cessation –

Persons who smoke greater than 10 cigarettes/day:

Nicotine Transdermal Administration Schedule for 21, 14, and 7 mg Patches		
Step 1	Step 2	Step 3
Use one 21 mg patch/day	Use one 14 mg patch/day	Use one 7 mg patch/day
Weeks 1 to 6	Weeks 7 to 8	Weeks 9 to 10

Nicotine Transdermal Administration Schedule for 15, 10, and 5 mg Patches		
Step 1	Step 2	Step 3
Use one 15 mg patch/day for 6 weeks	Use one 10 mg patch/day for 2 weeks	Use one 5 mg patch/day for 2 weeks
Weeks 1 to 6	Weeks 7 to 8	Weeks 9 to 10

Persons who smoke 10 or fewer cigarettes per day: Do not use step 1. These patients should start with step 2 for 6 weeks, then step 3 for 2 weeks and should then stop. Steps 2 and 3 allow the patient to gradually reduce his or her level of nicotine. Completing the full program will increase the chances of quitting successfully.

Off-label dosing –

Tourette syndrome: [2] = Fair documentation. One 7 or 10 mg patch per day for 2 days.

Ulcerative colitis: [4] = Insufficient documentation. A low-dose patch (such as 11 mg) should be started rather than a high-dose patch (22 mg) to allow for the development of tolerance to adverse effects. Titration of the dose may occur over several days to weeks. In patients with active ulcerative colitis, treatment duration was 4 to 6 weeks in published controlled trials.

➤*Duration of therapy:* Stop using the patch at the end of 10 weeks. When starting the program with step 2, stop using the patch at the end of 8 weeks. If the need to use the patch is still present, consult a health care provider.

➤*Administration:* Patients should apply 1 new patch every 24 hours on skin that is dry, clean, and hairless and should follow these instructions:

1.) Remove backing from patch and immediately press onto skin (upper arm or hip). Hold for 10 seconds.
2.) Wash hands after applying or removing patch. Throw away the patch in the enclosed disposal tray. See user's guide for safety and handling.
3.) Wear the patch for 16 or 24 hours. Patients who crave cigarettes upon awakening should wear the patch for 24 hours.
4.) If vivid dreams or other sleep disturbances occur, remove the patch at bedtime and apply a new one in the morning. The used patch should be removed and a new one applied to a different skin site at the same time each day.
5.) Do not wear more than 1 patch at a time.
6.) Do not cut patch in half or into smaller pieces.
7.) Do not leave patch on for more than 24 hours because it may irritate the skin and lose strength after 24 hours.

➤*Storage/Stability:* Stored at 20° to 25°C (68° to 77°F).

Used patches have enough nicotine to poison children. If swallowed, get medical help or contact a poison control center right away. Dispose of the used patches by folding sticky ends together and inserting in disposal tray supplied with the original packaging.

The amounts of nicotine that are tolerated by adult smokers can produce symptoms of poisoning and could prove fatal if inhaled, ingested, or bucally absorbed by children or pets. Therefore, caution patients to keep the used and unused systems out of the reach of children and pets.

NICOTINE POLACRILEX (Nicotine resin complex)

otc	**Nicorette** (GlaxoSmithKline Consumer)	**Lozenge; oral:** 2 mg	Aspartame,[a] corn syrup, lactose, maltodextrin, mannitol, soy protein. Cherry and mint flavors. In 72s and 168s.
		4 mg	Aspartame,[a] corn syrup, lactose, maltodextrin, mannitol, soy protein. Cherry and mint flavors. In 72s and 168s.
otc	**Nicotine Gum** (Various)	**Gum; oral:** 2 mg	In 48s and 108s.
otc	**Nicorette** (GlaxoSmithKline Consumer)		In orange, mint, and original flavors. In 48s, 108s, and 168s.
otc	**Thrive** (Novartis)		Acesulfame K, glycerin, maltitol, saccharin, sorbitol, sodium 11 mg. Mint flavor. In 110s.
otc	**Nicotine Gum** (Various)	**Gum; oral:** 4 mg	In 48s and 108s.
otc	**Nicorette** (GlaxoSmithKline Consumer)		In orange, mint, and original flavors. In 48s, 108s, and 168s.
otc	**Thrive** (Novartis)		Acesulfame K, glycerin, maltitol, saccharin, sorbitol, sodium 11 mg. Mint flavor. In 110s.

[a] Contains 3.4 mg phenylalanine.

NICOTINE POLACRILEX — ORAL

For complete and comparative prescribing information, refer to the Nicotine group monograph.

Indications

➤*Smoking cessation:* Nicotine polacrilex is indicated for the reduction of withdrawal symptoms, including nicotine craving, associated with quitting smoking.

➤*Off-label uses:*

Tourette syndrome – [2] = Fair documentation. Data from these initial studies suggest that nicotine in combination with haloperidol but not alone may be effective in reducing tic frequency and severity. (See Administration and Dosage.)

Administration and Dosage

➤*General dosing considerations:* Advise the patient to stop smoking completely when beginning to use the gum or lozenges.

To improve the chances of quitting, use at least 9 pieces per day for the first 6 weeks.

➤*Adults:*

Smoking cessation –

Gum:

• *Usual dosage* –

Weeks 1 to 6: 1 piece of gum every 1 to 2 hours.
Weeks 7 to 9: 1 piece of gum every 2 to 4 hours.
Weeks 10 to 12: 1 piece of gum every 4 to 8 hours.

Patients who smoke less than 25 cigarettes a day: Use 2 mg nicotine gum.

Patients who smoke 25 cigarettes a day or more: Start with the 4 mg nicotine gum.

• *Dosage adjustment* – If there are strong and frequent cravings, use a second piece within the hour.

Lozenge:

• *Usual dosage* – If the patient smokes his/her first cigarette more than 30 minutes after waking up, use 2 mg nicotine lozenges. If the patient smokes his/her first cigarette within 30 minutes of waking up, use 4 mg nicotine lozenges.

Weeks 1 to 6: 1 lozenge every 1 to 2 hours.
Weeks 7 to 9: 1 lozenge every 2 to 4 hours.
Weeks 10 to 12: 1 lozenge every 4 to 8 hours.

• *Maximum dose* – Do not use more than 5 lozenges in 6 hours. Do not use more than 20 lozenges/day.

Off-label dosing –

Tourette syndrome: [2] = Fair documentation. 2 mg chewing gum chewed for 30 minutes twice daily or 3 times daily.

➤*Duration of therapy:* Stop using at the end of 12 weeks. If the need to use nicotine is still present, consult a health care provider.

➤*Administration:*

Gum – Instruct the patient to chew gum slowly until it tingles, then park it between the cheek and gum. When the tingle is gone, instruct the patient to begin chewing again until the tingle returns. Repeat the process until most of the tingle is gone (about 30 minutes). Advise the patient not to eat or drink for 15 minutes before chewing the nicotine gum or while chewing a piece. Do not continuously use 1 piece after another because this may cause hiccoughs, heartburn, nausea, or other adverse reactions.

Lozenge –

Instruct the patient to place the lozenge in the mouth and allow it to slowly dissolve (about 20 to 30 minutes). Minimize swallowing. Advise the patient not to chew or swallow the lozenge. The patient may feel a warm or tingling sensation. Advise the patient to occasionally move the lozenge from one side of the mouth to the other until completely dissolved.

Advise the patient not to eat or drink 15 minutes before using or while the lozenge is in the mouth. Do not use more than 1 lozenge at a time or continuously use 1 lozenge after another because this may cause hiccoughs, heartburn, nausea, or other adverse reactions.

➤*Storage/Stability:* Store at 20° to 25°C (68° to 77°F). Protect from light. Place used chewing pieces in a wrapper and dispose of it in such a way to prevent its access by children or pets. If you need to remove the lozenge, wrap it in paper and throw away in the trash. Pieces of nicotine gum may have enough nicotine to make children or pets sick. In case of overdose, contact a medical professional or a poison control center.

NICOTINE INHALATION SYSTEM

Rx	**Nicotrol Inhaler** (Pharmacia)	**Inhaler:** 4 mg delivered (10 mg/cartridge)	Kit contains mouthpiece, storage trays each containing 6 cartridges, plastic storage case, and patient information leaflet. In 42s and 168s.

NICOTINE — INHALATION SYSTEM

For complete prescribing information, refer to the Nicotine class monograph.

Indications

➤*Smoking cessation:* As an aid in smoking cessation for the relief of nicotine withdrawal symptoms. Inhaler therapy is recommended for use as part of a comprehensive behavioral smoking cessation program.

Administration and Dosage

➤*General dosing considerations:* Patients should be instructed to stop smoking completely as they begin using the inhaler.

Regular use of the inhaler during the first week of treatment may help patients adapt to the irritant effects of the product.

If a patient is unable to stop smoking by the fourth week of therapy, discontinue treatment.

➤*Adults:*

Smoking cessation –

Usual dosage: Most successful patients in the clinical trials used between 6 and 16 cartridges per day. Encourage patients to use at least 6 cartridges/day at least for the first 3 to 6 weeks of treatment. In clinical trials, the average daily dose was more than 6 (range, 3 to 18) cartridges for patients who successfully quit smoking. Additional doses may be needed to control the urge to smoke.

Maximum dose: 16 cartridges daily for up to 12 weeks.

Initial dosage: The initial dosage of the nicotine inhaler is individualized. Patients may self-titrate to the level of nicotine they require.

Dosage adjustment: Some patients may exhibit signs or symptoms of nicotine withdrawal or excess that will require an adjustment of the dosage.

Duration of therapy: The recommended duration of treatment is 3 months, after which patients may be weaned from the inhaler by gradual reduction of the daily dose over the following 6 to 12 weeks.

Discontinuation of therapy: Most patients will need to gradually discontinue the use of the inhaler after the initial treatment period. Gradual reduction of dose may begin after 12 weeks of initial treatment and may last for up to 12 weeks. Recommended strategies for discontinuing use include suggesting to patients that they use the product less frequently, keep a tally of daily usage, and try to meet a steadily reducing target, or set a planned quit date for stopping use of the product.

Some patients may not require gradual reduction of dosage and may abruptly stop treatment successfully.

➤*Administration:* Best effect was achieved by frequent continuous puffing (20 minutes).

➤*Storage/Stability:* Store at room temperature not to exceed 25°C (77°F). Protect cartridges from light.

After using the inhaler, carefully separate the mouthpiece, remove the used cartridge, and throw it away, out of the reach of children and pets. Store the mouthpiece in the plastic storage case for further use. The mouthpiece is reusable and should be cleaned regularly with soap and water.

The amounts of nicotine that are tolerated by adult smokers can produce symptoms of poisoning and could prove fatal if inhaled, ingested, or buccally absorbed by children or pets. An inhaler container has about 60% (6 mg) of its initial drug content when discarded. Therefore, caution patients to keep the used and unused systems out of the reach of children and pets.

NICOTINE NASAL SPRAY

Rx	**Nicotrol NS** (Pfizer)	**Spray pump:** 0.5 mg nicotine/actuation (10 mg/mL)	Parabens, EDTA. Each unit has a glass container mounted with a metered spray pump (delivers approximately 200 applications). In 10 mL bottles.

NICOTINE — NASAL SPRAY

For complete prescribing information, refer to the Nicotine group monograph.

Indications

➤*Smoking cessation:* As an aid to smoking cessation for the relief of nicotine withdrawal symptoms. Use the nicotine nasal spray as a part of a comprehensive behavioral smoking cessation program.

Administration and Dosage

➤*General dosing considerations:* Instruct patients to stop smoking completely when they begin using the product.

If a patient is unable to stop smoking by the fourth week of therapy, treatment should probably be discontinued.

Regular use of the spray during the first week of treatment may help patients adapt to the irritant effects of the spray.

NICOTINE — NASAL SPRAY

➤*Adults:*

Smoking cessation –

Usual dosage: For best results, encourage patients to use at least the recommended minimum of 8 doses per day because less is unlikely to be effective. In clinical trials, the patients who successfully quit smoking used the product heavily when nicotine withdrawal was at its peak, sometimes up to the recommended maximum of 40 doses per day (in heavier smokers).

Nicotine Nasal Spray Dosing Recommendations			
Maximum recommended duration of treatment	Recommended doses/h	Maximum doses/h	Maximum doses/day
3 months	1 to 2[a]	5	40

[a] One dose = 2 sprays (1 in each nostril). One dose delivers nicotine 1 mg to the nasal mucosa.

Maximum dose: 40 mg (80 sprays, somewhat less than half of the bottle) per day.

Initial dosage: Patients should be started with 1 or 2 doses per hour, which may be increased up to a maximum recommended dose of 40 mg (80 sprays, somewhat less than half of the bottle) per day.

Dosage adjustment: Dosage can then be adjusted in those subjects with signs or symptoms of nicotine withdrawal or excess. The symptoms of nicotine withdrawal overlap those of nicotine excess. Because patients using the nasal spray therapy may also smoke intermittently, it is sometimes difficult to determine if patients are experiencing nicotine withdrawal or nicotine excess.

Duration of therapy: Treatment with the nasal spray therapy for longer periods has not been shown to improve outcome.

Discontinuation of therapy: Patients who are successfully abstinent on nasal spray therapy should be treated at the selected dosage for up to 8 weeks; use of the spray should be discontinued over the next 4 to 6 weeks. Some patients may not require gradual reduction of dosage and may abruptly stop treatment successfully.

No tapering strategy has been shown to be optimal in clinical studies. Many patients simply stopped using the spray at their last clinic visit. Recommended strategies for discontinuation of use include suggesting the following to patients: Use only half a dose (1 spray) at a time, use the spray less frequently, keep a tally of daily usage, try to meet a steadily reducing usage target, skip a dose by not medicating every hour, or set a planned quit date for stopping use of the spray.

➤*Subsequent attempts:* Patients who fail to quit on any attempt may benefit from interventions to improve their chances for success on subsequent attempts. Patients who were unsuccessful should be counseled and should then probably be given a therapy holiday before the next attempt. A new quit attempt should be encouraged when conditions are more favorable.

➤*Administration:* Patients should be instructed not to sniff, swallow, or inhale through the nose as the spray is being administered. They should also be advised to administer the spray with the head tilted back slightly.

➤*Storage/Stability:* Store at room temperature not to exceed 30°C (86°F).

Take care in handling nicotine nasal spray during periods of opening and closing the container. If it is dropped, it may break. If this occurs, the spill should be cleaned up immediately with an absorbent cloth/paper towel. Care should be taken to avoid contact of the solution with the skin. Broken glass should be picked up carefully, using a broom. The area of the spill should be washed several times. Absorbent material may be disposed of as any other household waste. Should even a small amount of nicotine nasal spray come in contact with the ears, skin, eyes, lips, or mouth, the affected area(s) should be immediately rinsed with water only.

Used bottles of nicotine nasal spray should be disposed of with their child-resistant caps in place. Used bottles should be disposed of in such a way as to prevent access by children or pets.

The amounts of nicotine that are tolerated by adult smokers can produce symptoms of poisoning and could prove fatal if nicotine nasal spray is used or ingested by children or pets. A full bottle of nicotine nasal spray contains nicotine 100 mg, some of which will still be in the bottle when it is discarded. Therefore, caution patients to keep both used and unused containers of nicotine nasal spray out of the reach of children and away from pets.

SMOKING DETERRENTS

BUPROPION HYDROCHLORIDE

Refer to the Antidepressants section for complete prescribing information.

VARENICLINE

Rx	**Chantix** (Pfizer)	**Tablets; oral:** 0.5 mg	Equiv. to varenicline tartrate 0.85 mg. (Pfizer CHX 0.5). White to off-white, capsule shape. Film-coated. In first month of therapy UD 11[a] and 56s.
		1 mg	Equiv. to varenicline tartrate 1.71 mg. (Pfizer CHX 1.0). Lt. blue, capsule shape. Film-coated. In first month of therapy UD pack 42s[a] and continuing months of therapy UD 56s[b] and 56s.

[a] First month of therapy: UD pack includes 1 card (0.5 mg × 11 tablets) and 3 cards (1 mg × 14 tablets).

[b] Continuing months of therapy: UD packs include 4 cards (1 mg × 14 tablets).

VARENICLINE TARTRATE — ORAL

WARNING

Serious neuropsychiatric events, including but not limited to, depression, suicidal ideation, suicide attempt, and completed suicide, have been reported in patients taking varenicline. Some reported cases may have been complicated by the symptoms of nicotine withdrawal in patients who stopped smoking. Depressed mood may be a symptom of nicotine withdrawal. Depression, rarely including suicidal ideation, has been reported in smokers undergoing a smoking cessation attempt without medication. However, some of these symptoms have occurred in patients taking varenicline who continued to smoke.

Observe all patients being treated with varenicline for neuropsychiatric symptoms, including changes in behavior, hostility, agitation, depressed mood, and suicide-related events, including ideation, behavior, and attempted suicide. These symptoms, as well as worsening of preexisting psychiatric illness and completed suicide, have been reported in some patients attempting to quit smoking while taking varenicline in the postmarketing experience. When symptoms were reported, most were during varenicline treatment, but some were following discontinuation of varenicline therapy.

These events have occurred in patients with and without preexisting psychiatric disease. Patients with serious psychiatric illness, such as schizophrenia, bipolar disorder, and major depressive disorder, did not participate in the premarketing studies of varenicline, and safety and efficacy of varenicline in these patients have not been established.

Advise patients and caregivers that the patient needs to stop taking varenicline and contact a health care provider immediately if agitation, hostility, depressed mood, or changes in behavior or thinking that are not typical for the patient are observed, or if the patient develops suicidal ideation or suicidal behavior. In many postmarketing cases, resolution of symptoms after discontinuation of varenicline was reported, although in some cases the symptoms persisted; therefore, provide ongoing monitoring and supportive care until symptoms resolve.

WARNING (cont.)

Weigh the risks of varenicline against the benefits of its use. Varenicline has been demonstrated to increase the likelihood of abstinence from smoking for as long as 1 year compared with treatment with placebo. The health benefits of quitting smoking are immediate and substantial.

Indications

➤*Smoking cessation:* As an aid to smoking cessation treatment.

Administration and Dosage

➤*General dosing considerations:* Smoking cessation therapies are more likely to succeed for patients who are motivated to stop smoking and who are provided additional advice and support. Patients should be provided with appropriate educational materials and counseling to support the attempt to quit.

➤*Adults:*

Smoking cessation treatment – The patient should set a date to stop smoking. Varenicline dosing should start 1 week before this date.

Usual dosage: 1 mg twice daily, following a 1-week titration.

Dosage titration:

Varenicline Dosage Titration	
Days	Dosage
1 through 3	0.5 mg once daily
4 through 7	0.5 mg twice daily
Day 8 through end of treatment	1 mg twice daily

Dosage adjustment: Patients who cannot tolerate the adverse reactions of varenicline may have the dose lowered temporarily or permanently.

Duration of therapy: Patients should be treated with varenicline for 12 weeks. For patients who have successfully stopped smoking at the end of 12 weeks, an additional course of 12 weeks of treatment with varenicline is recommended to further increase the likelihood of long-term abstinence.

Relapse of therapy: Patients who do not succeed in stopping smoking during 12 weeks of initial therapy, or who relapse after treatment, should be

VARENICLINE TARTRATE — ORAL

encouraged to make another attempt once factors contributing to the failed attempt have been identified and addressed.

➤*Renal function impairment:* For patients with severe renal impairment, the recommended starting dosage is 0.5 mg once daily. Patients may then titrate as needed to a maximum dosage of 0.5 mg twice daily.

Hemodialysis – For patients with end-stage renal disease (ESRD) undergoing hemodialysis, a maximum dosage of 0.5 mg once daily may be administered if tolerated well.

➤*Administration:* Varenicline should be taken after eating and with a full glass of water.

➤*Storage/Stability:* Store at 25°C (77°F); excursions are permitted to 15° to 30°C (59° to 86°F).

Actions

➤*Pharmacology:* Varenicline binds with high affinity and selectivity at alpha-4-beta-2 neuronal nicotinic acetylcholine receptors. The efficacy of varenicline in smoking cessation is believed to be the result of varenicline's activity at a subtype of the nicotinic receptor, where its binding produces agonist activity while simultaneously preventing nicotine binding to alpha-4-beta-2 receptors.

Electrophysiology – Electrophysiology studies in vitro and neurochemical studies in vivo have shown that varenicline binds to alpha-4-beta-2 neuronal nicotinic acetylcholine receptors and stimulates receptor-mediated activity, but at a significantly lower level than nicotine. Varenicline blocks the ability of nicotine to activate alpha-4-beta-2 receptors and, thus, to stimulate the central nervous mesolimbic dopamine system, which is believed to be the neuronal mechanism underlying reinforcement and reward experienced when smoking. Varenicline is highly selective and binds more potently to alpha-4-beta-2 receptors than to other common nicotinic receptors (more than 500-fold alpha-3-beta-4, more than 3,500-fold alpha-7, more than 20,000-fold alpha-1-beta-gamma-delta), or to nonnicotinic receptors and transporters (more than 2,000-fold). Varenicline also binds with moderate affinity (Ki = 350 nM) to the 5-HT_3 receptor.

➤*Pharmacokinetics:*

Absorption/Distribution – Maximum plasma concentrations (C_{max}) of varenicline typically occur within 3 to 4 hours after oral administration. Following administration of multiple oral doses of varenicline, steady-state conditions were reached within 4 days. Over the recommended dosing range, varenicline exhibits linear pharmacokinetics after single or repeated doses. In a mass balance study, absorption of varenicline was virtually complete after oral administration, and systemic availability was high.

Oral bioavailability of varenicline is unaffected by time-of-day dosing. Plasma protein binding of varenicline is low (20% or less) and independent of age and renal function.

Metabolism/Excretion – The elimination half-life of varenicline is approximately 24 hours. Varenicline undergoes minimal metabolism, with 92% excreted unchanged in the urine. Renal elimination of varenicline is primarily through glomerular filtration along with active tubular secretion, possibly via the organic cation transporter, OCT2.

Special populations –

Renal function impairment: In patients with moderate renal impairment (estimated creatinine clearance [CrCl] at least 30 mL/min and up to 50 mL/min), varenicline exposure increased 1.5-fold, compared with patients with healthy renal function (estimated CrCl more than 80 mL/min). In subjects with severe renal impairment (estimated CrCl less than 30 mL/min), varenicline exposure was increased 2.1-fold.

• *Hemodialysis* – In patients with ESRD undergoing a 3-hour session of hemodialysis for 3 days per week, varenicline exposure was increased 2.7-fold following 0.5 mg once-daily administration for 12 days. The plasma C_{max} and area under the curve (AUC) of varenicline noted in this setting were similar to healthy subjects receiving about 1 mg twice daily. Caution is warranted with the use of varenicline in subjects with renal impairment. Additionally, in subjects with ESRD, varenicline was efficiently removed by hemodialysis.

Contraindications

None well documented.

Warnings/Precautions

➤*Neuropsychiatric symptoms and suicidality:* Serious neuropsychiatric symptoms have been reported in patients being treated with varenicline. These postmarketing reports have included changes in mood (including depression and mania), psychosis, hallucinations, paranoia, delusions, homicidal ideation, hostility, agitation, anxiety, and panic, as well as suicidal ideation, suicide attempt, and completed suicide. See the Warning box for more information.

These events have occurred in patients with and without preexisting psychiatric disease; some patients have experienced worsening of their psychiatric illnesses. Observe all patients being treated with varenicline for neuropsychiatric symptoms or worsening of preexisting psychiatric illness.

Advise patients and caregivers that the patient should stop taking varenicline and contact a health care provider immediately if agitation, depressed mood, or changes in behavior or thinking that are not typical for the patient are observed, or if the patient develops suicidal ideation or suicidal behavior.

The risks of varenicline should be weighed against the benefits of its use.

For more information on neuropsychiatric symptoms and suicidality, refer to the black box warning.

➤*Skin reactions:* There have been postmarketing reports of rare but serious skin reactions, including Stevens-Johnson syndrome and erythema multiforme, in patients using varenicline. As these skin reactions can be life-threatening, instruct patients to stop taking varenicline and contact their health care provider immediately at the first appearance of a skin rash with mucosal lesions or any other signs of hypersensitivity.

➤*GI effects:* Nausea was the most common adverse reaction associated with varenicline treatment. Nausea was generally described as mild or moderate and often transient; however, for some subjects, it was persistent over several months. The incidence of nausea was dose-dependent. Initial dose titration was beneficial in reducing the occurrence of nausea. Nausea was reported by approximately 30% of patients treated with varenicline 1 mg twice daily after an initial week of dose titration. In patients taking varenicline 0.5 mg twice daily, the incidence of nausea was 16% following initial titration. Approximately 3% of subjects treated with varenicline 1 mg twice daily in studies involving 12 weeks of treatment discontinued treatment prematurely because of nausea. For patients with intolerable nausea, consider dose reduction.

➤*Hypersensitivity reactions:* There have been postmarketing reports of hypersensitivity reactions, including angioedema, in patients treated with varenicline. Clinical signs included swelling of the face, mouth (tongue, lips, and gums), extremities, and neck (throat and larynx). There were infrequent reports of life-threatening angioedema requiring emergent medical attention because of respiratory compromise. Instruct patients to discontinue varenicline and immediately seek medical care if they experience these symptoms.

➤*Drug abuse and dependence:* Fewer than 1 of 1,000 patients reported euphoria in clinical trials with varenicline. At higher doses (more than 2 mg), varenicline produced more frequent reports of GI disturbances, such as nausea and vomiting. There is no evidence of dose escalation to maintain therapeutic effects in clinical studies, which suggests that tolerance does not develop. Abrupt discontinuation of varenicline was associated with an increase in irritability and sleep disturbances in up to 3% of patients. This suggests that, in some patients, varenicline may produce mild physical dependence, which is not associated with addiction.

➤*Hazardous tasks:* There have been postmarketing reports of traffic accidents, near-miss incidents in traffic, or other accidental injuries in patients taking varenicline. In some cases, patients reported somnolence, dizziness, loss of consciousness or difficulty concentrating that resulted in impairment, or concern about potential impairment, in driving or operating machinery. Advise patients to use caution driving or operating machinery or engaging in other potentially hazardous activities until they know how varenicline may affect them.

➤*Pregnancy: Category C.* There are no adequate and well-controlled studies in pregnant women. Use varenicline during pregnancy only if the potential benefit justifies the potential risk to the fetus.

Nonteratogenic – Varenicline has been shown to have adverse effects on the fetus in animal reproduction studies. Administration of varenicline to pregnant rabbits resulted in reduced fetal weights at an oral dosage of 30 mg/kg/day (50 times the human AUC at 1 mg twice daily); this reduction was not evident following treatment with 10 mg/kg/day (23 times the maximum recommended daily human exposure based on AUC). In addition, in the offspring of pregnant rats treated with varenicline, there were decreases in fertility and increases in auditory startle response at an oral dosage of 15 mg/kg/day (36 times the maximum recommended human daily exposure based on AUC at 1 mg twice daily).

➤*Lactation:* Although it is not known whether this drug is excreted in human milk, animal studies have demonstrated that varenicline can be transferred to breast-feeding pups. Because many drugs are excreted in human milk and because of the potential for serious adverse reactions in breast-feeding infants from varenicline, decide whether to discontinue breast-feeding or the drug, taking into account the importance of the drug to the mother. Varenicline's molecular weight (approximately 361), low metabolism, high oral bioavailability, plasma protein binding (20% or less), and long elimination half-life (approximately 24 hours) suggest that the drug will be excreted into breast milk.

➤*Children:* Safety and efficacy of varenicline in children have not been established; therefore, varenicline is not recommended for use in patients younger than 18 years of age.

➤*Elderly:* Varenicline is known to be substantially excreted by the kidney, and the risk of toxic reactions to this drug may be higher in patients with impaired renal function. Because elderly patients are more likely to have decreased renal function, take care in dose selection; it may be useful to monitor renal function.

➤*Monitoring:* Observe patients for neuropsychiatric symptoms, including agitation, changes in behavior, depressed mood, suicidal behavior, and suicidal ideation. Monitoring may also be needed in patients with renal impairment.

Drug Interactions

➤*Effect of smoking cessation:* Physiological changes resulting from smoking cessation, with or without treatment with varenicline, may alter the pharmacokinetics or pharmacodynamics of some drugs, for which dosage adjustment may be necessary (eg, insulin, theophylline, warfarin).

Varenicline Drug Interactions[a]

Precipitant drug	Object drug[a]		Description
Cimetidine	Varenicline	↑	Coadministration increased the systemic exposure of varenicline by 29% because of a reduction in varenicline renal clearance.

VARENICLINE TARTRATE — ORAL

Varenicline Drug Interactions[a]			
Precipitant drug	Object drug[a]		Description
Nicotine transdermal	Varenicline	↑	The incidence of adverse reactions (eg, fatigue, headache, nausea, vomiting) may be increased with coadministration.
Varenicline	Nicotine transdermal		

[a] ↑ = object drug increased.

Adverse Reactions

The following table shows the adverse reactions for varenicline and placebo in the 12-week, fixed-dose studies with titration in the first week (studies 2 [titrated arm only], 4, and 5).

➤*Discontinuation of therapy:* In phase 2 and 3 placebo-controlled studies, the rate of treatment discontinuation because of adverse reactions in patients dosed with 1 mg twice daily was 12% for varenicline compared with 10% for placebo, in studies of 3 months' treatment. In this group, the discontinuation rates for the most common adverse reactions in varenicline-treated patients were nausea (3% vs 0.5% for placebo), headache (0.6% vs 0.9% for placebo), insomnia (1.2% vs 1.1% for placebo), and abnormal dreams (0.3% vs 0.2% for placebo).

➤*Most common:* The most common adverse reactions associated with varenicline (more than 5% and twice the rate seen in placebo-treated patients) were nausea, sleep disturbance, constipation, flatulence, and vomiting.

Smoking cessation, with or without treatment, is associated with nicotine withdrawal symptoms.

The most common adverse reaction associated with varenicline treatment is nausea. For patients treated with the maximum recommended dosage of 1 mg twice daily following initial dosage titration, the incidence of nausea was 30% compared with 10% in patients taking a comparable placebo regimen. In patients taking varenicline 0.5 mg twice daily following initial titration, the incidence was 16%, compared with 11% for placebo. Nausea was generally described as mild or moderate and often transient; however, for some subjects, it was persistent throughout the treatment period.

Varenicline Adverse Reactions			
Adverse reactions	Varenicline 0.5 mg twice daily (n = 129)	Varenicline 1 mg twice daily (n = 821)	Placebo (n = 805)
CNS			
Abnormal dreams	9%	13%	5%
Fatigue/Malaise/Asthenia	4%	7%	6%
Headache	19%	15%	13%
Insomnia[a]	19%	18%	13%
Lethargy	2%	1%	0%
Nightmare	2%	1%	0%
Sleep disorder	2%	5%	3%
Somnolence	3%	3%	2%
Dermatological			
Pruritus	0%	1%	1%
Rash	1%	1%	2%
GI			
Abdominal pain[b]	5%	7%	5%
Constipation	5%	8%	3%
Dry mouth	4%	6%	4%
Dysgeusia	8%	5%	4%
Dyspepsia	5%	5%	3%
Flatulence	9%	6%	3%
Gastroesophageal reflux disease	1%	1%	0%
Nausea	16%	30%	10%
Vomiting	1%	5%	2%
Metabolic/Nutritional			
Decreased appetite/anorexia	1%	2%	1%
Increased appetite	4%	3%	2%
Respiratory			
Dyspnea	2%	1%	1%
Rhinorrhea	0%	1%	0%
Upper respiratory tract disorder	7%	5%	4%

[a] Includes initial insomnia, middle insomnia, and early-morning awakening.
[b] Includes abdominal adverse reactions (pain, pain upper, pain lower, discomfort, tenderness, distension) and stomach discomfort.

The overall pattern and the frequency of adverse reactions during the longer-term trials were very similar to that described in the previous table, though several of the most common reactions were reported by a higher proportion of patients. Nausea, for instance, was reported in 40% of patients treated with varenicline 1 mg twice daily in a 1-year study compared with 8% of placebo-treated patients.

➤*Other adverse reactions:*

Cardiovascular – Hypertension (frequent); angina pectoris, arrhythmia, bradycardia, electrocardiogram abnormal, hypotension, myocardial infarction, palpitations, peripheral ischemia, syncope, tachycardia, thrombosis, ventricular extrasystoles (infrequent); acute coronary syndrome, atrial fibrillation, cardiac flutter, cerebrovascular accident, coronary artery disease, cor pulmonale, transient ischemic attack (rare).

CNS – Anxiety, depression, disturbance in attention, dizziness, emotional disorder, irritability, restlessness, sensory disturbance (frequent); aggression, agitation, amnesia, disorientation, dissociation, libido decreased, migraine, mood swings, parosmia, psychomotor hyperactivity, restless legs syndrome, thinking abnormal, tremor (infrequent); balance disorder, bradyphrenia, convulsion, dysarthria, euphoric mood, facial palsy, hallucination, mental impairment, multiple sclerosis, psychomotor skills impaired, psychotic disorder, suicidal ideation (rare).

Dermatologic – Hyperhidrosis (frequent); acne, dermatitis, dry skin, eczema, erythema, psoriasis, urticaria (infrequent).

GI – Diarrhea, gingivitis (frequent); dysphagia, enterocolitis, eructation, esophagitis, gallbladder disorder, gastritis, GI hemorrhage, mouth ulceration (infrequent); gastric ulcer, intestinal obstruction, pancreatitis acute (rare).

GU – Menstrual disorder, polyuria (frequent); erectile dysfunction, nephrolithiasis, nocturia, urethral syndrome, urine abnormality (infrequent); renal failure acute, sexual dysfunction, urinary retention (rare).

Hematologic/Lymphatic – Anemia, lymphadenopathy (infrequent); leukocytosis, splenomegaly, thrombocytopenia (rare).

Hypersensitivity – Hypersensitivity (infrequent); drug hypersensitivity, photosensitivity reaction (rare).

Lab test abnormalities – Liver function test abnormal (frequent); muscle enzyme increased, urine analysis abnormal (infrequent).

Metabolic/Nutritional – Weight increased (frequent); diabetes mellitus, hyperlipidemia, hypokalemia (infrequent); hyperkalemia, hypoglycemia (rare).

Musculoskeletal – Arthralgia, back pain, muscle cramp, musculoskeletal pain, myalgia (frequent); arthritis, osteoporosis (infrequent); myositis (rare).

Ophthalmic – Conjunctivitis, dry eye, eye irritation, eye pain, vision blurred, visual disturbance (infrequent); acquired night blindness, blindness transient, cataract subcapsular, nystagmus, ocular vascular disorder, photophobia, visual field defect, vitreous floaters (rare).

Respiratory – Epistaxis, respiratory disorder (frequent); asthma (infrequent); pleurisy, pulmonary embolism (rare).

Special senses – Tinnitus, vertigo (infrequent); deafness, Meniere disease (rare).

Miscellaneous – Chest pain, edema, hot flush, influenza-like illness, thirst (frequent); chest discomfort, chills, pyrexia, thyroid gland disorders (infrequent).

➤*Postmarketing:*

CNS – There have been reports of aggression, anxiety, delusions, depression, hallucinations, homicidal ideation, hostility, mania, panic, paranoia, and psychosis, as well as suicidal ideation, suicide attempt, and completed suicide in patients attempting to quit smoking while taking varenicline. Smoking cessation with or without treatment is associated with nicotine withdrawal symptoms and the exacerbation of underlying psychiatric illness. Not all patients had known preexisting psychiatric illness and not all had discontinued smoking.

Hypersensitivity – There have been reports of hypersensitivity reactions, including angioedema.

Dermatologic – There have also been reports of serious skin reactions, including Stevens Johnson syndrome and erythema multiforme, in patients taking varenicline.

Overdosage

➤*Treatment:* In case of overdose, institute standard supportive measures as required.

Varenicline has been shown to be dialyzed in patients with ESRD; however, there is no experience in dialysis following overdose.

Patient Information

Instruct patients to set a date to quit smoking and to initiate varenicline treatment 1 week before the quit date.

Advise patients to take varenicline after eating and with a full glass of water.

Instruct patients on how to titrate varenicline, beginning at a dosage of 0.5 mg/day for the first 3 days. For the next 4 days, one 0.5 mg tablet should be taken in the morning and 1 in the evening.

Advise patients that, after the first 7 days, the dose should be increased to one 1 mg tablet in the morning and 1 in the evening.

Encourage patients to continue to attempt to quit if they have early lapses after the quit date.

Inform patients that nausea and insomnia are side effects of varenicline and are usually transient; however, advise patients to notify their health care provider if they are persistently troubled by these symptoms so that a dose reduction can be considered.

Provide patients with educational materials and necessary counseling to support an attempt at quitting smoking.

VARENICLINE TARTRATE — ORAL

Inform patients that some medications may require dose adjustment after quitting smoking.

Inform patients that they may experience vivid, unusual, or strange dreams during treatment with varenicline.

Inform patients that quitting smoking, with or without varenicline, may be associated with nicotine withdrawal symptoms (agitation, depression) or exacerbation of preexisting psychiatric illness. Some patients have experienced changes in mood (including depression and mania), psychosis, hallucinations, paranoia, delusions, homicidal ideation, aggression, anxiety, and panic, as well as suicidal ideation and suicide, when attempting to quit smoking while taking varenicline. If patients develop agitation, hostility, depressed mood, or changes in behavior or thinking that are not typical for them, or if patients develop suicidal ideation or behavior, urge these patients to discontinue varenicline and report these symptoms to their health care provider immediately.

Advise patients to reveal any history of psychiatric illness prior to initiating treatment.

Advise patients to use caution while driving or operating machinery until they know how quitting smoking with varenicline may affect them.

Advise patients intending to become pregnant or breast-feed an infant of the risks of smoking and the risks and benefits of smoking cessation with varenicline.

Inform patients that there have been reports of angioedema, with swelling of the face, mouth (lip, gum, tongue), and neck (larynx and pharynx), that can lead to life-threatening respiratory compromise. Instruct patients to discontinue varenicline and immediately seek medical care if they experience these symptoms.

Inform patients that serious skin reactions, such as Stevens Johnson syndrome and erythema multiforme, were reported by some patients taking varenicline. Advise patients to stop taking varenicline at the first sign of rash with mucosal lesions or skin reaction and contact a health care provider immediately.

TETRABENAZINE

TETRABENAZINE

Rx	**Xenazine** (Ovation)	**Tablets; oral:** 12.5 mg	Lactose. (CL 12.5). White, cylindrical. In 112s.
		25 mg	Lactose. (CL 25). Yellowish-buff, cylindrical, scored. In 112s.

TETRABENAZINE — ORAL

WARNING

Depression and suicidality – Tetrabenazine can increase the risk of depression and suicidal thoughts and behavior (suicidality) in patients with Huntington disease. Anyone considering the use of tetrabenazine must balance the risks of depression and suicidality with the clinical need for control of choreiform movements. Closely observe patients for the emergence or worsening of depression, suicidality, or unusual changes in behavior. Inform patients, caregivers, and families of the risk of depression and suicidality, and instruct them to report behaviors of concern promptly to the treating health care provider.

Exercise particular caution in treating patients with a history of depression or prior suicide attempts or ideation, which are increased in frequency in Huntington disease. Tetrabenazine is contraindicated in patients who are actively suicidal, and in patients with untreated or inadequately treated depression.

Indications

➤*Chorea associated with Huntington disease:* For the treatment of chorea associated with Huntington disease.

Administration and Dosage

➤*General dosing considerations:* Proper dosing involves careful titration of therapy to determine an individualized dose for each patient. When first prescribed, therapy should be titrated slowly over several weeks to allow the identification of a dose for chronic use that reduces chorea and is well tolerated.

Patients who appear to require doses more than 50 mg/day should be genotyped for CYP2D6.

➤*Adults:*

Chorea associated with Huntington disease –

Maximum dose: 25 mg per dose; 100 mg/day. For CYP2D6 poor metabolizers, 25 mg per dose; 50 mg/day. For CYP2D6 extensive and intermediate metabolizers, 37.5 mg per dose; 100 mg/day.

Initial dosage: 12.5 mg/day given once in the morning.

Dosage titration: After 1 week, the dose should be increased to 25 mg/day given as 12.5 mg twice daily. Titrate up slowly at weekly intervals by 12.5 mg, to allow the identification of a dose that reduces chorea and is well tolerated. If a dose of 37.5 to 50 mg/day is needed, it should be given in a 3-times-daily regimen. If adverse actions such as akathisia, restlessness, parkinsonism, depression, insomnia, anxiety, or intolerable sedation occur, titration should be stopped and the dose should be reduced. If the adverse reaction does not resolve, consider withdrawing treatment or initiating other specific treatment (eg, antidepressants).

• *CYP2D6 extensive, intermediate, and poor metabolizers* – At doses above 50 mg/day, tetrabenazine should be titrated up slowly at weekly intervals by 12.5 mg to allow the identification of a dose that reduces chorea and is well tolerated. Doses above 50 mg/day should be given in a 3-times-daily regimen.

Discontinuation of therapy: Treatment can be discontinued without tapering. Re-emergence of chorea may occur within 12 to 18 hours after the last dose.

Treatment interruption: Following treatment interruption of more than 5 days or a treatment interruption occurring because of a change in the patient's medical condition or concomitant medications, tetrabenazine therapy should be retitrated when resumed. For short-term treatment interruption of less than 5 days, treatment can be resumed at the previous maintenance dose without titration.

➤*Hepatic function impairment:* The use of tetrabenazine in patients with liver disease is contraindicated.

➤*Concomitant therapy with CYP2D6 inhibitors:* Use caution when prescribing a strong CYP2D6 inhibitor (eg, fluoxetine, paroxetine, quinidine) to a patient already receiving a stable dose of tetrabenazine. In patients receiving coadministered strong CYP2D6 inhibitors, the daily dose of tetrabenazine should be halved. To initiate treatment with tetrabenazine in patients on a stable dose of a strong CYP2D6 inhibitor, the dosing recommendations for the CYP2D6 poor metabolizers should be followed. The effect of moderate or weak CYP2D6 inhibitors (eg, amiodarone, duloxetine, sertraline, terbinafine) has not been evaluated.

➤*Administration:* Administer without regard to meals. Doses 37.5 to 50 mg/day should be given in a 3-times-daily regimen.

➤*Storage/Stability:* Store at 25°C (77°F). Excursions are permitted between 15° and 30°C (59° and 86°F).

Actions

➤*Pharmacology:* The precise mechanism by which tetrabenazine exerts its antichorea effects is unknown, but is believed to be related to its effect as a reversible depleter of monoamines, such as dopamine, serotonin, norepinephrine, and histamine, from nerve terminals. Tetrabenazine reversibly inhibits the human vesicular monoamine transporter type 2 (VMAT2) (K_i is approximately 100 nM), resulting in decreased uptake of monoamines into synaptic vesicles and depletion of monoamine stores. Human VMAT2 is also inhibited by dihydrotetrabenazine (HTBZ), a mixture of alpha-HTBZ and beta-HTBZ. Alpha- and beta-HTBZ, major circulating metabolites in humans, exhibit high in vitro binding affinity to bovine VMAT2. Tetrabenazine exhibits weak in vitro binding affinity at the dopamine D2 receptor (K_i = 2,100 nM).

➤*Pharmacokinetics:*

Absorption – Following oral administration of tetrabenazine, the extent of absorption is at least 75%. After single oral doses ranging from 12.5 to 50 mg, plasma concentrations of tetrabenazine are generally below the limit of detection because of the rapid and extensive hepatic metabolism of tetrabenazine to alpha- and beta-HTBZ. Alpha- and beta-HTBZ are metabolized principally by CYP2D6. Peak plasma concentrations (C_{max}) of alpha- and beta-HTBZ are reached within 1 to 1.5 hours postdosing. Alpha- and beta-HTBZ are subsequently metabolized to another major circulating metabolite, O-dealkylated-HTBZ, for which C_{max} is reached approximately 2 hours postdosing.

Distribution – Results of positron emission tonography-scan studies in humans show that radioactivity is rapidly distributed to the brain following intravenous injection of ^{11}C-labeled tetrabenazine or alpha-HTBZ, with the highest binding in the striatum and lowest binding in the cortex.

The in vitro protein binding of tetrabenazine, alpha-HTBZ, and beta-HTBZ was examined in human plasma for concentrations ranging from 50 to 200 ng/mL. Tetrabenazine binding ranged from 82% to 85%, alpha-HTBZ binding ranged from 60% to 68%, and beta-HTBZ binding ranged from 59% to 63%.

Metabolism – Alpha- and beta-HTBZ are formed by carbonyl reductase that occurs mainly in the liver. Alpha-HTBZ is O-dealkylated by CYP-450 enzymes, principally CYP2D6, with some contribution of CYP1A2. Beta-HTBZ is O-dealkylated principally by CYP2D6.

After oral administration in humans, at least 19 metabolites of tetrabenazine have been identified. O-dealkylated HTBZ, alpha-HTBZ, and beta-HTBZ are the major circulating metabolites, and they are subsequently metabolized to sulfate or glucuronide conjugates. CYP1A2, CYP2A6, CYP2C9, CYP2C19, and CYP2E1 do not play a major role in metabolism of alpha- or beta-HTBZ, based on in vitro studies.

Excretion – After oral administration, tetrabenazine is extensively hepatically metabolized, and the metabolites are primarily renally eliminated. Alpha- and beta-HTBZ, major circulating metabolites, have half-lives of 4 to 8 hours and 2 to 4 hours, respectively. In a mass balance study in 6 healthy volunteers, approximately 75% of the dose was excreted in the urine, and fecal recovery accounted for approximately 7% to 16% of the dose. Unchanged tetrabenazine has not been found in human urine. Urinary excretion of alpha- or beta-HTBZ accounted for less than 10% of the administered dose. Circulating metabolites, including the sulfate and glucuronide

TETRABENAZINE — ORAL

conjugates of HTBZ metabolites, as well as products of oxidative metabolism, account for the majority of metabolites in the urine.

Special populations –

Hepatic function impairment: The disposition of tetrabenazine was compared in 12 patients with mild to moderate chronic hepatic function impairment (Child-Pugh scores of 5 to 9) and 12 age- and gender-matched subjects with healthy hepatic function who received a single dose of tetrabenazine 25 mg. In patients with hepatic function impairment, tetrabenazine plasma concentrations were similar to or higher than concentrations of alpha-HTBZ, reflecting the markedly decreased metabolism of tetrabenazine to alpha-HTBZ. The mean tetrabenazine C_{max} in subjects with hepatic function impairment was approximately 7- to 190-fold higher than the detectable peak concentrations in healthy subjects. The elimination half-life of tetrabenazine in subjects with hepatic function impairment was approximately 17.5 hours. The time to peak concentrations (T_{max}) of alpha- and beta-HTBZ was slightly delayed in subjects with hepatic function impairment compared with age-matched controls (1.75 h vs 1 h), and the elimination half-lives of the alpha- and beta-HTBZ were prolonged to approximately 10 and 8 hours, respectively. The exposure to alpha- and beta-HTBZ was approximately 30% to 39% higher in patients with hepatic function impairment than in age-matched controls. The safety and efficacy of this increased exposure to tetrabenazine and other circulating metabolites are unknown, so that it is not possible to adjust the dosage of tetrabenazine in patients with hepatic function impairment to ensure safe use. Therefore, tetrabenazine is contraindicated in patients with hepatic function impairment.

CYP2D6 poor metabolizers: Although the pharmacokinetics of tetrabenazine and its metabolites in subjects who do not express the drug metabolizing enzyme CYP2D6 (poor metabolizers) have not been systematically evaluated, it is likely that the exposure to alpha- and beta-HTBZ would be increased compared with subjects who express the enzyme (extensive metabolizers), with an increase similar to that observed in patients taking strong CYP2D6 inhibitors (3- and 9-fold, respectively). Genotype patients for CYP2D6 prior to treatment with daily doses of tetrabenazine that are more than 50 mg. Do not give patients who are poor metabolizers daily doses of more than 50 mg.

Contraindications

Hepatic function impairment; patients who are actively suicidal or who have untreated or inadequately treated depression; patients taking monoamine oxidase inhibitors (MAOIs) or reserpine.

Warnings/Precautions

➤*Mental and mood changes:* Huntington disease is a progressive disorder characterized by changes in mood, cognition, chorea, rigidity, and functional capacity over time. Although tetrabenazine has been shown to decrease the chorea of Huntington disease in a 12-week controlled trial, it was also shown to cause slight worsening in mood, cognition, rigidity, and functional capacity. Whether these effects persist, resolve, or worsen with continued treatment is unknown. Therefore, proper use of the drug requires attention to all facets of the underlying disease process over time. Periodically reevaluate the need for tetrabenazine by assessing the beneficial effect on choreiform movements and the possible adverse reactions, including depression, cognitive decline, parkinsonism, dysphagia, sedation/somnolence, akathisia, restlessness, and disability. It may be difficult to distinguish between drug-induced adverse reactions and progression of the underlying disease; decreasing the dose or stopping the drug may help the health care provider distinguish between the two possibilities. In some patients, underlying chorea itself may improve over time, decreasing the need for tetrabenazine.

➤*Dosage:* Proper dosing of tetrabenazine involves careful titration of therapy to determine an individualized dose for each patient. When first prescribed, slowly titrate tetrabenazine therapy over several weeks to allow the identification of a dose that both reduces chorea and is well tolerated. Some adverse reactions, such as depression, fatigue, insomnia, sedation/somnolence, parkinsonism, and akathisia, may be dose-dependent and may resolve or lessen with dosage adjustment or specific treatment. If the adverse reaction does not resolve or decrease, consider discontinuing tetrabenazine.

Do not administer doses of more than 50 mg without CYP2D6 genotyping.

➤*Depression and suicidality:* Patients with Huntington disease are at increased risk for depression and suicidal ideation and behavior (suicidality). Tetrabenazine increases these risks. Closely observe all patients treated with tetrabenazine for new or worsening depression or suicidality.

Be alert to the heightened risk of suicide in patients with Huntington disease, regardless of depression indices. Reported rates of completed suicide among individuals with Huntington disease range from 3% to 13%; more than 25% of patients attempt suicide at some point in the illness.

Inform patients, caregivers, and families of the risks of depression, worsening depression, and suicidality associated with tetrabenazine, and instruct them to report behaviors of concern promptly to the treating health care provider. Immediately evaluate patients with Huntington disease who express suicidal ideation.

If depression or suicidality occurs, reduce the dose of tetrabenazine. Initiating treatment with, or increasing the dose of, a concomitant antidepressant may also be useful. In patients with new-onset depression who require antidepressants that are strong CYP2D6 inhibitors, such as paroxetine and fluoxetine, halve the total dose of tetrabenazine. If depression or suicidality does not resolve, consider discontinuing treatment with tetrabenazine.

Exercise caution in treating patients with tetrabenazine who have a history of depression or prior suicide attempts or ideation; these patients may be at increased risk for suicidal behavior. Also exercise caution in using tetrabenazine in patients with diseases, conditions, or treatments that could cause depression or increased suicidality. Do not treat patients who are actively suicidal or who have untreated or inadequately treated depression with tetrabenazine. See the Adverse Reactions section for more information.

➤*Neuroleptic malignant syndrome:* A potentially fatal symptom complex sometimes referred to as neuroleptic malignant syndrome (NMS) has been reported in association with tetrabenazine and other drugs that reduce dopaminergic transmission. Clinical manifestations of NMS are hyperpyrexia, muscle rigidity, altered mental status, and evidence of autonomic instability (irregular pulse or blood pressure, tachycardia, diaphoresis, cardiac dysrhythmia). Additional signs may include elevated creatinine phosphokinase, myoglobinuria, rhabdomyolysis, or acute renal failure. The diagnostic evaluation of patients with this syndrome is complicated. In arriving at the diagnosis, exclude cases where the clinical presentation includes both serious medical illness (eg, pneumonia, systemic infection) and untreated or inadequately treated extrapyramidal signs and symptoms. Other important considerations in the differential diagnosis include central anticholinergic toxicity, heat stroke, drug fever, and primary central nervous system (CNS) pathology.

The management of NMS includes immediate discontinuation of tetrabenazine and other drugs not essential to concurrent therapy, intensive symptomatic treatment and medical monitoring, and treatment of any concomitant serious medical problems for which specific treatments are available. There is no general agreement about specific pharmacological treatment regimens for NMS.

If the patient requires treatment with tetrabenazine after recovery from NMS, carefully consider the potential reintroduction of therapy. Carefully monitor the patient because recurrences of NMS have been reported.

➤*Parkinsonism:* Tetrabenazine can cause parkinsonism. Because rigidity can develop as part of the underlying disease process in Huntington disease, it may be difficult to distinguish between this drug-induced adverse reaction and progression of the underlying disease process. Drug-induced parkinsonism has the potential to cause more functional disability than untreated chorea for some patients with Huntington disease. If a patient develops parkinsonism during treatment with tetrabenazine, consider dose reduction; in some patients, discontinuation of therapy may be necessary. See the Adverse Reactions section for more information.

➤*Dysphagia:* Dysphagia is a component of Huntington disease. However, drugs that reduce dopaminergic transmission have been associated with esophageal dysmotility and dysphagia. The latter symptom may be associated with aspiration pneumonia. Some of the cases of dysphagia were associated with aspiration pneumonia. Whether these events were related to treatment is unknown. Use tetrabenazine and other drugs that reduce dopaminergic with caution in patients with Huntington disease at risk for aspiration pneumonia. See the Adverse Reactions section for more information.

➤*QTc prolongation:* Tetrabenazine causes a small increase (about 8 msec) in the corrected QT (QTc) interval. QT prolongation can lead to development of torsade de pointes–type ventricular tachycardia, with the risk increasing as the degree of prolongation increases. Avoid the use of tetrabenazine in combination with other drugs that are known to prolong QTc. Also avoid tetrabenazine in patients with congenital long QT syndrome and in patients with a history of cardiac arrhythmias. Certain circumstances may increase the risk of the occurrence of torsade de pointes and/or sudden death in association with the use of drugs that prolong the QTc interval, including bradycardia, hypokalemia or hypomagnesemia, concomitant use of other drugs that prolong the QTc interval, and the presence of congenital prolongation of the QT interval. See the Drug Interactions section for more information.

➤*Hypotension:* Tetrabenazine induced postural dizziness in healthy volunteers receiving single doses of 25 or 50 mg. One subject had syncope and one subject with postural dizziness had documented orthostasis. Dizziness occurred in 4% of tetrabenazine-treated patients (vs none on placebo) in the 12-week controlled trial; blood pressure was not measured during these events.

➤*Hyperprolactinemia:* Tetrabenazine elevates serum prolactin concentrations in humans. Following administration of 25 mg to healthy volunteers, peak plasma prolactin levels increased 4- to 5-fold. Tissue culture experiments indicate that approximately one-third of human breast cancers are prolactin-dependent in vitro, a factor of potential importance if tetrabenazine is being considered for a patient with previously detected breast cancer. Although amenorrhea, galactorrhea, gynecomastia, and impotence can be caused by elevated serum prolactin concentrations, the clinical significance of elevated serum prolactin concentrations for most patients is unknown. Chronic increase in serum prolactin levels (although not evaluated in the tetrabenazine development program) has been associated with low levels of estrogen and increased risk of osteoporosis. If there is a clinical suspicion of symptomatic hyperprolactinemia, perform appropriate laboratory testing and consider discontinuation of tetrabenazine.

➤*Tardive dyskinesia:* A potentially irreversible syndrome of involuntary, dyskinetic movements may develop in patients treated with neuroleptic drugs. In an animal model of orofacial dyskinesias, acute administration of reserpine, a monoamine depleter, has been shown to produce vacuous chewing in rats. Although the pathophysiology of tardive dyskinesia remains incompletely understood, the most commonly accepted hypothesis of the mechanism is that prolonged postsynaptic dopamine receptor blockade leads to supersensitivity to dopamine. Neither reserpine nor tetrabenazine, which are dopamine depleters, have been reported to cause clear tardive dyskinesia in humans, but because presynaptic dopamine depletion could theoretically lead to supersensitivity to dopamine, and tetrabenazine can cause the extrapyramidal symptoms also known to be associated with neuroleptics (eg, parkinsonism, akathisia), be aware of the possible risk of tardive dyskinesia. If signs and symptoms of tardive dyskinesia appear in a patient treated with tetrabenazine, consider drug discontinuation.

TETRABENAZINE — ORAL

➤*Ophthalmic effects:* Since tetrabenazine or its metabolites bind to melanin-containing tissues, it could accumulate in these tissues over time. This raises the possibility that tetrabenazine may cause toxicity in these tissues after extended use. Neither ophthalmologic nor microscopic examination of the eye was conducted in the chronic toxicity study in dogs. Ophthalmologic monitoring in humans was inadequate to exclude the possibility of injury occurring after long-term exposure.

The clinical relevance of tetrabenazine's binding to melanin-containing tissues is unknown. Although there are no specific recommendations for periodic ophthalmologic monitoring, be aware of the possibility of long-term ophthalmologic effects.

➤*Special risk:* Clinical experience with tetrabenazine in patients with systemic illnesses is limited. Tetrabenazine has not been evaluated or used to any appreciable extent in patients with a recent history of myocardial infarction or unstable heart disease. Patients with these diagnoses were excluded from premarketing clinical trials.

➤*Drug abuse and dependence:*

Physical and psychological dependence – As with any CNS-active drug, carefully evaluate patients for a history of drug abuse and follow such patients closely, observing them for signs of tetrabenazine misuse or abuse (such as development of tolerance, incrementation of dose, drug-seeking behavior).

➤*Hazardous tasks:* Caution patients about performing activities requiring mental alertness, such as operating a motor vehicle or hazardous machinery, until they are on a maintenance dose of tetrabenazine and know how the drug affects them.

➤*Pregnancy: Category C.* When tetrabenazine was administered to female rats (doses of 5, 15, and 30 mg/kg/day) from the beginning of organogenesis through the lactation period, an increase in stillbirths and offspring postnatal mortality was observed at 15 and 30 mg/kg/day, and delayed pup maturation was observed at all doses. The no-effect dose for stillbirths and postnatal mortality was 0.5 times the MRHD on a mg/m^2 basis.

There are no adequate and well-controlled studies in pregnant women. Use tetrabenazine during pregnancy only if the potential benefit justifies the potential risk to the fetus.

➤*Lactation:* It is not known whether tetrabenazine or its metabolites are excreted in human milk. Since many drugs are excreted into human milk and because of the potential for serious adverse reactions in breast-feeding infants from tetrabenazine, decide whether to discontinue breast-feeding or tetrabenazine, taking into account the importance of the drug to the mother.

➤*Children:* The safety and efficacy of tetrabenazine in children have not been established.

➤*Monitoring:* Before administering a daily dose of more than 50 mg, test patients for the CYP2D6 gene to determine whether they are poor metabolizers or extensive or intermediate metabolizers. When a dose of tetrabenazine is given to poor metabolizers, exposure will be substantially higher (about 3-fold for alpha-HTBZ and 9-fold for beta-HTBZ) than it would be in extensive metabolizers. Therefore, adjust the dosage according to a patient's CYP2D6-metabolizer status by limiting the dose to 50 mg in patients who are CYP2D6 poor metabolizers.

Closely observe patients for the emergence or worsening of depression, suicidality, or unusual changes in behavior.

Periodically reevaluate the need for tetrabenazine by assessing the beneficial effect on choreiform movements and possible adverse reactions, including depression, cognitive decline, parkinsonism, dysphagia, sedation/somnolence, akathisia, restlessness, and disability.

Monitor patients receiving tetrabenazine for the presence of akathisia. Also monitor patients receiving tetrabenazine for signs and symptoms of restlessness and agitation, because these may be indicators of developing akathisia.

Consider monitoring of vital signs on standing in patients who are vulnerable to hypotension.

Monitor patients for signs of NMS and tardive dyskinesia.

Drug Interactions

Tetrabenazine Drug Interactions

Precipitant drug	Object drug[a]		Description
CNS agents (eg, alcohol)	Tetrabenazine	↑	Concomitant use of alcohol or other sedating drugs may have additive effects and worsen sedation and somnolence.
CYP2D6 inhibitors (eg, fluoxetine, paroxetine, quinidine)	Tetrabenazine	↑	Strong CYP2D6 inhibitors markedly increase tetrabenazine exposure. Coadminister with caution. Halve the total dose of tetrabenazine with coadministration.
Dopamine agonists (eg, haloperidol, chlorpromazine, risperidone, olanzapine)	Tetrabenazine	↑	Adverse reactions associated with tetrabenazine, such as QTc prolongation, NMS, and extrapyramidal signs and symptoms, may be exaggerated by concurrent use.
MAOIs (eg, phenelzine)	Tetrabenazine	↑	Coadministration is contraindicated.
Tetrabenazine	MAOIs (eg, phenelzine)		
Reserpine	Tetrabenazine	↑	Coadministration is contraindicated. Allow at least 20 days to elapse after stopping reserpine before starting tetrabenazine.

[a] ↑ = object drug increased.

Adverse Reactions

For more information on NMS, refer to the Warnings/Precautions section.

In a randomized, 12-week, placebo-controlled clinical trial of Huntington disease subjects, adverse reactions were more common in the tetrabenazine group than in the placebo group. Forty-nine of 54 (91%) patients who received tetrabenazine experienced 1 or more adverse reaction at any time during the study. The adverse reactions most commonly reported (more than 10%, and at least 5% greater than placebo) were sedation/somnolence (31% vs 3% for placebo), fatigue (22% vs 13% for placebo), insomnia (22% vs 0% for placebo), depression (19% vs 0% for placebo), akathisia (19% vs 0% for placebo), and nausea (13% vs 7% for placebo). The percentages of the most commonly reported adverse reactions that occurred at any time during the study in 4% or more of tetrabenazine-treated patients, and with a greater frequency than in placebo-treated patients, are presented in the following table.

Tetrabenazine Adverse Reactions

Adverse reaction	Tetrabenazine (n = 54)	Placebo (n = 30)
CNS		
Akathisia[a,b]	19%	0%
Anxiety/Anxiety aggravated	15%	3%
Any extrapyramidal reaction[a]	33%	0%
Appetite decreased	4%	0%
Balance difficulty	9%	0%
Depression	19%	0%
Dizziness	4%	0%
Dysarthria	4%	0%
Extrapyramidal reaction[a,c]	15%	0%
Fatigue	22%	13%
Gait unsteady	4%	0%
Headache	4%	3%
Insomnia	22%	0%
Irritability	9%	3%
Obsessive reaction	4%	0%
Parkinson/Bradykinesia	9%	0%
Sedation/Somnolence	31%	3%
GI		
Nausea	13%	7%
Vomiting	6%	3%
GU		
Dysuria	4%	0%
Respiratory		
Bronchitis	4%	0%
Shortness of breath	4%	0%
Upper respiratory tract infection	11%	7%
Miscellaneous		
Ecchymosis	6%	0%
Fall	15%	13%
Laceration (head)	6%	0%

[a] Patients may have had reactions in more than 1 category.
[b] Patients with the following adverse reaction preferred terms were counted in this category: akathisia, hyperkinesia, restlessness.
[c] Patients with the following adverse reaction preferred terms were counted in this category: bradykinesia, parkinsonism, extrapyramidal disorder, hypertonia.

Dose titration was discontinued or dosage of study drug was reduced because of 1 or more adverse reactions in 28 of 54 (52%) patients randomized to tetrabenazine. These adverse reactions consisted of sedation (15), akathisia (7), parkinsonism (4), depression (3), anxiety (2), fatigue (1), and diarrhea (1). Some patients had more than 1 adverse reaction, and are therefore counted more than once.

➤*Depression/Suicidality:* In a 12-week, double-blind, placebo-controlled study in patients with chorea associated with Huntington disease, 10 of 54 (19%) patients treated with tetrabenazine were reported to have an adverse reaction of depression or worsening depression compared with none of the

TETRABENAZINE — ORAL

30 placebo-treated patients. In 2 open-label studies (in one study, 29 patients received tetrabenazine for up to 48 weeks; in the second study, 75 patients received tetrabenazine for up to 80 weeks), the rate of depression/worsening depression was 35%.

In all of the Huntington disease chorea studies of tetrabenazine (n = 187), 1 patient committed suicide, 1 attempted suicide, and 6 had suicidal ideation.

➤*Akathisia, restlessness, and agitation:* In a 12-week, double-blind, placebo-controlled study in patients with chorea associated with Huntington disease, akathisia was observed in 10 (19%) of tetrabenazine-treated patients and none of placebo-treated patients. In an 80-week, open-label study, akathisia was observed in 20% of tetrabenazine-treated patients. Akathisia was not observed in a 48-week, open-label study. Monitor patients receiving tetrabenazine for the presence of akathisia. Also monitor patients receiving tetrabenazine for signs and symptoms of restlessness and agitation, because these may be indicators of developing akathisia. If a patient develops akathisia, reduce the tetrabenazine dose; however, some patients may require discontinuation of therapy.

➤*Parkinsonism:* In a 12-week, double-blind, placebo-controlled study in patients with chorea associated with Huntington disease, symptoms suggestive of parkinsonism (ie, bradykinesia, hypertonia, rigidity) were observed in 15% of tetrabenazine-treated patients compared with 0% of placebo-treated patients. In 48- and 80-week open-label studies, symptoms suggestive of parkinsonism were observed in 10% and 3% of tetrabenazine-treated patients, respectively.

➤*Dysphagia:* In a 12-week, double-blind, placebo-controlled study in patients with chorea associated with Huntington disease, dysphagia was observed in 4% of tetrabenazine-treated patients and 3% of placebo-treated patients. In 48- and 80-week open-label studies, dysphagia was observed in 10% and 8% of tetrabenazine-treated patients, respectively.

➤*Sedation and somnolence:* Sedation is the most common dose-limiting adverse reaction of tetrabenazine. In a 12-week, double-blind, placebo-controlled trial in patients with chorea associated with Huntington disease, sedation/somnolence was observed in 17 of 54 (31%) tetrabenazine-treated patients and in 1 (3%) placebo-treated patient. Sedation was the reason upward titration of tetrabenazine was stopped and/or the dose of tetrabenazine was decreased in 15 of 54 (28%) patients. In all but one case, decreasing the dose of tetrabenazine resulted in decreased sedation. In 48- and 80-week open-label studies, sedation/somnolence was observed in 17% and 57% of tetrabenazine-treated patients, respectively. In some patients, intolerable sedation occurred at doses that were lower than the efficacious doses.

➤*Laboratory tests:* No clinically significant changes in laboratory parameters were reported in clinical trials with tetrabenazine. In controlled clinical trials, tetrabenazine caused a small mean increase in ALT and AST laboratory values as compared with placebo.

Overdosage

➤*Symptoms:* Three episodes of overdose occurred in the open-label trials performed in support of registration. Eight cases of overdose with tetrabenazine have been reported in the literature. The dose of tetrabenazine in these patients ranged from 100 mg to 1 g. Adverse reactions associated with tetrabenazine overdose included acute dystonia, oculogyric crisis, nausea and vomiting, sweating, sedation, hypotension, confusion, diarrhea, hallucinations, rubor, and tremor.

➤*Treatment:* Treatment consists of those general measures employed in the management of overdosage with any CNS-active drug. General supportive and symptomatic measures are recommended. Monitor cardiac rhythm and vital signs. In managing overdosage, always consider the possibility of multiple drug involvement. Consider contacting a poison control center on the treatment of any overdose. Telephone numbers for certified poison control centers are listed on the American Association of Poison Control Centers Web site, at http://www.aapcc.org.

Patient Information

Inform patients and their families that tetrabenazine may increase the risk of the patient considering or attempting suicide. Encourage patients and their families to be alert to the emergence of suicidal ideation and to report it immediately to the patient's health care provider.

Inform patients and their families that tetrabenazine may cause depression or may worsen preexisting depression. Encourage them to be alert to the emergence of sadness, worsening of depression, withdrawal, insomnia, irritability, hostility (aggressiveness), akathisia (psychomotor restlessness), anxiety, agitation, or panic attacks, and to report such symptoms promptly to the patient's health care provider.

Inform patients and their families that the dose of tetrabenazine will be titrated up slowly to the dose that is best for each patient. Warn them that sedation, akathisia, parkinsonism, depression, and difficulty swallowing may occur. Instruct them to promptly report such symptoms to the health care provider, and inform them that a dose reduction or tetrabenazine discontinuation may be required.

Inform patients that tetrabenazine may induce sedation and somnolence, and may impair the ability to perform tasks that require complex motor and mental skills. Advise patients that, until they learn how they respond to tetrabenazine, they should be careful doing activities that require them to be alert, such as driving a car or operating machinery.

Advise patients and their families that alcohol may potentiate the sedation induced by tetrabenazine.

Advise patients and their families to notify the health care provider if the patient becomes pregnant or intends to become pregnant during tetrabenazine therapy, or is breast-feeding or intending to breast-feed an infant during therapy.

Advise patients and their families to notify the health care provider of all medications the patient is taking and to consult with the health care provider before starting any new medications.

POTASSIUM CHANNEL BLOCKER

DALFAMPRIDINE (4-aminopyridine)

Rx	**Ampyra** (Acorda)	**Tablets, extended-release; oral:** 10 mg	A10 White to off-white, oval-shaped. Film-coated. In 60s.

DALFAMPRIDINE — ORAL

Indications

➤*Multiple sclerosis:* To improve walking in patients with multiple sclerosis (MS).

Administration and Dosage

➤*Adults:*

Multiple sclerosis –

Usual dosage: 10 mg twice daily.
Maximum dose: 20 mg/day.

➤*Renal function impairment:* The risk of seizures in patients with mild renal impairment (creatinine clearance [CrCl] 51 to 80 mL/min) is unknown, but dalfampridine plasma exposure in these patients may approach that seen at a dosage of 15 mg twice daily, a dose that may be associated with an increased risk of seizures. An estimated CrCl should be known before initiating treatment with dalfampridine.

Dalfampridine is contraindicated in patients with moderate or severe renal impairment.

➤*Administration:* May be taken with or without food; doses should be taken approximately 12 hours apart.

Tablets should only be taken whole; do not divide, crush, chew, or dissolve.

➤*Storage/Stability:* Store at 77°F (25°C); excursions are permitted between 59°F and 86°F (15°C and 30°C).

Actions

➤*Pharmacology:* The mechanism by which dalfampridine exerts its therapeutic effect has not been fully elucidated. Dalfampridine is a broad-spectrum potassium channel blocker. In animal studies, dalfampridine has been shown to increase conduction of action potentials in demyelinated axons through inhibition of potassium channels.

➤*Pharmacokinetics:*

Absorption/Distribution – Orally administered dalfampridine is rapidly and completely absorbed from the GI tract. Absolute bioavailability of dalfampridine has not been assessed, but relative bioavailability is 96% when compared with an aqueous oral solution. The extended-release tablet delays absorption of dalfampridine relative to the solution formulation, giving a slower rise to a lower peak concentration (C_{max}), with no effect on the extent of absorption (area under the curve [AUC]). Single dalfampridine tablet 10 mg doses administered to healthy patients in a fasted state gave peak concentrations ranging from 17.3 to 21.6 ng/mL occurring 3 to 4 hours post-administration (T_{max}). In comparison, C_{max} with the same 10 mg dose of dalfampridine in an oral solution was 42.7 ng/mL and occurred approximately 1.3 hours after dosing. Exposure increased proportionally with dose.

Dalfampridine is largely unbound to plasma proteins (97% to 99%). The apparent volume of distribution is 2.6 L/kg.

Effect of food: When dalfampridine is taken with food, there is a slight increase in C_{max} (12% to 17%) and a slight decrease in AUC (4% to 7%). These changes in exposure are not clinically significant; therefore, the drug may be taken with or without food.

Metabolism/Excretion – Dalfampridine and its metabolites' elimination is nearly complete after 24 hours, with 95.9% of the dose recovered in urine and 0.5% recovered in feces. Most of the excreted radioactivity in urine was parent drug (90.3%). Two metabolites were identified: 3-hydroxy-4-aminopyridine (4.3%) and 3- hydroxy-4-aminopyridine sulfate (2.6%). These metabolites have been shown to have no pharmacologic activity on potassium channels.

The elimination half-life of dalfampridine following administration of the extended-release tablet formulation of dalfampridine is 5.2 to 6.5 hours. The plasma half-life of the sulfate conjugate is approximately 7.6 hours and the half-life of 3-hydroxy-4-aminopyridine could not be calculated because concentrations for most subjects were close to or below the limit of quantitation.

In vitro studies with human liver microsomes indicate that CYP2E1 was the major enzyme responsible for the 3-hydroxylation of dalfampridine. The

DALFAMPRIDINE — ORAL

identity of the CYP enzymes suspected of playing a minor role in the 3-hydroxylation of dalfampridine could not be established unequivocally.

Special populations –

Renal function impairment: The pharmacokinetics of dalfampridine were studied in 9 men and 11 women with varying degrees of renal function. Elimination of the drug was significantly correlated with CrCl. Total body clearance of dalfampridine was reduced by about 45% in patients with mild renal impairment (CrCl 51 to 80 mL/min), by about 50% in patients with moderate renal impairment (CrCl = 30 to 50 mL/min), and by about 75% in patients with severe renal impairment (CrCl less than 30 mL/min). The terminal half-life of dalfampridine was about 3.3 times longer in patients with severe renal impairment, but was not prolonged in patients with mild or moderate renal impairment.

Gender: A population pharmacokinetic analysis suggested that women would be expected to have higher C_{max} than men. The magnitude of these differences is small and does not necessitate any dose modification.

Contraindications

History of seizure; moderate or severe renal impairment.

Warnings/Precautions

➤*Seizures:* Dalfampridine is contraindicated in patients with a history of seizures. Increased incidence of seizures has been observed at dalfampridine 20 mg twice daily in controlled clinical studies of 9 to 14 weeks' duration with in patients with MS. There was one seizure seen in the placebo group (0.4%) and at a dose of 10 mg twice daily (0.25%), no seizure seen at 15 mg twice daily, and 2 seizures (3.5%) seen at 20 mg twice daily. In open-label extension trials in patients with MS, the incidence of seizures during treatment with dalfampridine 15 mg twice daily was over 4 times higher than the incidence during treatment with 10 mg twice daily.

Dalfampridine has not been evaluated in patients with a history of seizures or with evidence of epileptiform activity on an EEG because these patients were excluded from clinical trials. The risk of seizures in patients with epileptiform activity on EEG is unknown, and could be substantially higher than that observed in dalfampridine clinical studies. Dalfampridine should be discontinued and not restarted in patients who experience a seizure while on treatment.

➤*Urinary tract infections:* Urinary tract infections (UTIs) were reported more frequently as adverse reactions in controlled studies in patients receiving dalfampridine 10 mg twice daily (12%) compared with placebo (8%).

➤*Renal function impairment:* Dalfampridine is eliminated through the kidneys primarily as unchanged drug.

Because patients with renal impairment would require a dosage lower than 10 mg twice daily and no strength smaller than 10 mg is available, dalfampridine is contraindicated in patients with moderate to severe renal impairment (CrCl 50 mL/min or less). The risk of seizures in patients with mild renal impairment (CrCl 51 to 80 mL/min) is unknown, but dalfampridine plasma levels in these patients may approach those seen at a dosage of 15 mg twice daily, a dosage that may be associated with an increased risk of seizures. If unknown, CrCl should be estimated prior to initiating treatment with dalfampridine.

➤*Pregnancy: Category C.* There are no adequate and well-controlled studies of dalfampridine in pregnant women. Administration of dalfampridine to animals during pregnancy and lactation resulted in decreased offspring viability and growth at dosages similar to the MRHD of 20 mg/day. Use dalfampridine during pregnancy only if the potential benefit justifies the potential risk to the fetus.

➤*Lactation:* It is not known whether dalfampridine is excreted in human milk. Because many drugs are excreted in human milk and because of the potential for serious adverse reactions in nursing infants from dalfampridine, decide whether to discontinue breast-feeding or to discontinue the drug, taking into account the importance of the drug to the mother.

➤*Children:* Safety and effectiveness of dalfampridine in patients younger than 18 years of age have not been established.

➤*Elderly:* A population pharmacokinetics analysis showed that dalfampridine clearance modestly decreased with increasing age, but not sufficiently to necessitate a modification of dose with age. Other reported clinical experience has identified no differences in responses between elderly and younger patients.

Dalfampridine is known to be substantially excreted by the kidney, and the risk of adverse reactions, including seizures, is greater with increasing exposure of dalfampridine. Because elderly patients are more likely to have decreased renal function, it is particularly important to know the estimated CrCl in these patients.

Drug Interactions

➤*Coadministration with other forms of 4-aminopyridine:* Do not administer dalfampridine with other forms of 4-aminopyridine (4-AP, fampridine) because the active ingredient is the same.

➤*Drug/Food interactions:* May administer with or without food; AUC is decreased 4% to 7% and C_{max} is increased 12% to 17% with food.

Adverse Reactions

➤*Discontinuation of therapy:* In 3 placebo-controlled clinical trials of up to 14 weeks' duration, 4% of patients treated with dalfampridine 10 mg twice daily experienced 1 or more treatment-emergent adverse reactions leading to discontinuation, compared with 2% of placebo-treated patients. The treatment-emergent adverse reactions leading to discontinuation of at least 2 patients treated with dalfampridine, and that led to discontinuation more frequently compared with placebo were headache (dalfampridine, 0.5%; placebo 0%), balance disorder (dalfampridine, 0.5%; placebo, 0%), dizziness (dalfampridine, 0.5%; placebo, 0%), and confusional state (dalfampridine, 0.3%; placebo, 0%).

Adverse reactions (at least 2%) – The following table lists adverse reactions that occurred in at least 2% of patients treated with dalfampridine 10 mg twice daily, and more frequently than in placebo-treated patients, in controlled clinical trials.

Dalfampridine Adverse Reactions (≥ 2%)		
Adverse reactions	Dalfampridine 10 mg twice daily (n = 400)	Placebo (n = 238)
CNS		
Asthenia	7%	4%
Balance disorder	5%	1%
Dizziness	7%	4%
Headache	7%	4%
Insomnia	9%	4%
MS relapse	4%	3%
Paresthesia	4%	3%
Eye, Ears, Nose, and Throat		
Nasopharyngitis	4%	2%
Pharyngolaryngeal pain	2%	1%
GI		
Constipation	3%	2%
Dyspepsia	2%	1%
Nausea	7%	3%
Miscellaneous		
Back pain	5%	2%
UTI	12%	8%

➤*Other adverse reactions:* As in controlled clinical trials, a dose-dependent increase in the incidence of seizures has been observed in open-label clinical trials with dalfampridine in patients with MS as follows: dalfampridine 10 mg twice daily 0.41 per 100 person-years (95% confidence interval [CI], 0.13 to 0.96); dalfampridine 15 mg twice daily 1.7 per 100 person-years (95% CI 0.21 to 6.28).

Overdosage

➤*Symptoms:* Three cases of overdose were reported in controlled clinical trials with dalfampridine, involving 2 patients with MS. The first patient took 6 times the currently recommended dose (60 mg) and was taken to the emergency room with altered mental state. The second patient took 40 mg doses on 2 separate occasions. In the first instance, she experienced a complex partial seizure and, in the second instance, a period of confusion. Both patients recovered by the following day without sequelae.

Several cases of overdose are found in the scientific literature in which various formulations of dalfampridine were used, resulting in numerous adverse reactions, including seizure, confusion, tremulousness, diaphoresis, and amnesia. In some instances, patients developed status epilepticus, requiring intensive supportive care and were responsive to standard therapy for seizures. In 1 published case report, a patient with MS who ingested 300 mg of 4- aminopyridine (dalfampridine) developed a condition that resembled limbic encephalitis. This patient developed weakness, reduced awareness, memory loss, hypophonic speech, and temporal lobe hyperintensities on MRI. The patient's speech and language and ambulation improved over time, and an MRI at 4 months after the overdose no longer showed signal abnormalities. At 1 year, the patient continued to have difficulty with short-term memory and learning new tasks.

Patient Information

Inform patients that dalfampridine causes seizures in a dose-dependent fashion, and that they must discontinue use of dalfampridine if they experience a seizure.

Instruct patients to take dalfampridine exactly as prescribed. Instruct patients not to take a double dose after they miss a dose. Instruct patients not take more than 2 tablets in a 24-hour period, and to make sure that there is an approximate 12-hour interval between doses.

RILUZOLE

Rx	**Rilutek** (Sanofi-Aventis)	**Tablets; oral:** 50 mg	(RPR 202). White, capsule shape. Film-coated. In 60s.

RILUZOLE — ORAL

Indications

➤*Amyotrophic lateral sclerosis:* For the treatment of patients with amyotrophic lateral sclerosis (ALS). Riluzole extends survival and/or time to tracheostomy.

Administration and Dosage

➤*Adults:*

Amyotrophic lateral sclerosis – 50 mg every 12 hours. No increased benefit can be expected from higher daily doses, but adverse reactions are increased.

➤*Administration:* Administer at least an hour before or 2 hours after a meal to avoid a food-related decrease in bioavailability.

➤*Storage/Stability:* Store between 20° and 25°C (68° and 77°F); protect from bright light.

Actions

➤*Pharmacology:* The mode of action of riluzole is unknown. Its pharmacological properties include the following, some of which may be related to its effect: an inhibitory effect on glutamate release, inactivation of voltage-dependent sodium channels, and ability to interfere with intracellular events that follow transmitter binding at excitatory amino acid receptors. Riluzole has also been shown, in a single study, to delay median time to death in a transgenic mouse model of ALS. These mice express human superoxide dismutase bearing one of the mutations found in one of the familial forms of human ALS.

It is also neuroprotective in various in vivo experimental models of neuronal injury involving excitotoxic mechanisms. In in vitro tests, riluzole protected cultured rat motor neurons from the excitotoxic effects of glutamic acid and prevented the death of cortical neurons induced by anoxia.

Because of its blockade of glutamatergic neurotransmission, riluzole also exhibits myorelaxant and sedative properties in animal models at doses of 30 mg/kg (about 20 times the recommended human daily dose) and anticonvulsant properties at a dose of 2.5 mg/kg (about 2 times the recommended human daily dose).

➤*Pharmacokinetics:*

Absorption/Distribution – Riluzole is well absorbed (approximately 90%), with average absolute oral bioavailability of about 60% (coefficient of variation [CV], 30%). Pharmacokinetics are linear over a dosage range of 25 to 100 mg given every 12 hours. With multiple-dose administration, riluzole accumulates in plasma by about 2-fold, and steady state is reached in less than 5 days. Riluzole is 96% bound to plasma proteins, mainly to albumin and lipoproteins over the clinical concentration range. The 50 mg tablet was equivalent, with respect to area under the curve (AUC), to the tablet used in the dose-ranging clinical trials, while the maximal concentration (C_{max}) was approximately 30% higher. Both tablets have been used in clinical trials. However, if doses greater than those recommended are given, it is likely that higher plasma levels will be achieved, the safety of which has not been established.

Effect of food: A high-fat meal decreases absorption, reducing AUC by about 20% and peak blood levels by about 45%.

Metabolism/Excretion – Riluzole is extensively metabolized to 6 major metabolites and a number of minor metabolites, not all of which have been identified. Some metabolites appear pharmacologically active in in vitro assays. The metabolism of riluzole is mostly hepatic and consists of cytochrome P450 (CYP-450)–dependent hydroxylation and glucuronidation.

There is marked interindividual variability in the clearance of riluzole, probably attributable to variability of CYP1A2 activity, the principal isozyme involved in N-hydroxylation.

In vitro studies using liver microsomes show that hydroxylation of the primary amine group producing N-hydroxyriluzole is the main metabolic pathway in humans, monkeys, dogs, and rabbits. In humans, CYP1A2 is the principal isozyme involved in N-hydroxylation. In vitro studies predict that CYP2D6, CYP2C19, CYP3A4, and CYP2E1 are unlikely to contribute significantly to riluzole metabolism in humans. Direct glucuroconjugation of riluzole (involving the glucurotransferase isoform UGT-HP4) is very slow in human liver microsomes, whereas N-hydroxyriluzole is readily conjugated at the hydroxylamine group, resulting in the formation of O– (greater than 90%) and N-glucuronides.

The mean elimination half-life of riluzole is 12 hours (CV, 35%) after repeated doses. Following a single dose of ^{14}C-riluzole 150 mg to 6 healthy males, 90% and 5% of the radioactivity was recovered in the urine and feces, respectively, over a period of 7 days. Glucuronides accounted for more than 85% of the metabolites in urine. Only 2% of a riluzole dose was recovered in the urine as unchanged drug.

Special populations –

Hepatic function impairment: The AUC of riluzole after a single 50 mg oral dose increases by about 1.7-fold in patients with mild chronic liver insufficiency (n = 6; Child-Pugh class A) and by about 3-fold in patients with moderate chronic liver insufficiency (n = 6; Child-Pugh class B) compared with healthy volunteers (n = 12). The pharmacokinetics of riluzole have not been studied in patients with severe hepatic impairment.

Gender: In a placebo-controlled clinical trial with population pharmacokinetics, riluzole mean clearance was found to be 30% lower in women (corresponding to an approximate increase in AUC of 45%) compared with men. However, no favorable or adverse effects of riluzole in relation to gender were seen in controlled trials.

Contraindications

History of severe hypersensitivity reactions to riluzole or any of the tablet components.

Warnings/Precautions

➤*Hepatic effects:* Riluzole, even in patients without a history of liver disease, causes serum aminotransferase elevations. Discontinue treatment if ALT levels are 5 or more times the upper limit of normal (ULN) or if clinical jaundice develops.

Experience in almost 800 ALS patients indicates that about 50% of riluzole-treated patients will experience at least one ALT level above the ULN, about 8% will have elevations more than 3 times the ULN, and about 2% of patients will have elevations more than 5 times the ULN. A single non-ALS patient with epilepsy treated with concomitant carbamazepine and phenobarbital experienced marked, rapid elevations of liver enzymes with jaundice (ALT 26 times the ULN, AST 17 times the ULN, and bilirubin 11 times the ULN) 4 months after starting riluzole; these returned to normal 7 weeks after treatment discontinuation.

Maximum increases in serum ALT usually occurred within 3 months after the start of riluzole therapy and were usually transient when less than 5 times the ULN. In trials, if ALT levels were less than 5 times the ULN, treatment continued, and ALT levels usually returned to less than 2 times the ULN within 2 to 6 months. Treatment in studies was discontinued, however, if ALT levels exceeded 5 times the ULN, so there is no experience with continued treatment of ALS patients once ALT values exceed 5 times the ULN. There were rare instances of jaundice. There is limited experience with rechallenge of patients who have had riluzole discontinued for ALT more than 5 times the ULN, but there is the possibility of increased ALT values reoccurring; therefore, rechallenge is not recommended.

In postmarketing experiences, cases of clinical hepatitis associated with riluzole have been reported, including fatal outcomes.

➤*Hematologic effects:* Among approximately 4,000 patients given riluzole for ALS, there were 3 cases of marked neutropenia (absolute neutrophil count less than 500/mm^3), all seen within the first 2 months of riluzole treatment. In 1 case, neutrophil counts rose on continued treatment. In a second case, counts rose after therapy was stopped. A third case was more complex, with marked anemia as well as neutropenia, and the cause of both is uncertain. Warn patients to report any febrile illness to their health care provider. The report of a febrile illness should prompt treating providers to check white blood cell counts.

In the 2 controlled trials in patients with ALS, the frequency with which values for hemoglobin, hematocrit, and erythrocyte counts fell below the lower limit of normal was greater in riluzole-treated patients than in placebo-treated patients; however, these changes were mild and transient. The proportions of patients observed with abnormally low values for these parameters showed a dose-response relationship. Only 1 patient was discontinued from treatment because of severe anemia. The significance of this finding is unknown.

➤*Interstitial lung disease:* Cases of interstitial lung disease have been reported in patients treated with riluzole, some of them severe; upon further investigation, many of these cases were hypersensitivity pneumonitis. If respiratory symptoms (eg, dry cough and/or dyspnea) develop, perform a chest radiography and, in case of findings suggestive of interstitial lung disease or hypersensitivity pneumonitis (eg, bilateral diffuse lung opacities), discontinue riluzole immediately. In the majority of the reported cases, symptoms resolved after drug discontinuation and symptomatic treatment.

➤*Renal/Hepatic function impairment:* Prescribe riluzole with care in patients with current evidence or history of abnormal liver function indicated by significant abnormalities in serum transaminase (ALT, AST), bilirubin, or GGT levels. Ensure that baseline elevations of several liver function tests (especially elevated bilirubin) preclude the use of riluzole.

➤*Special risk:* Use riluzole with caution in patients with concomitant liver insufficiency. In particular, in cases of riluzole-induced hepatic injury manifested by elevated liver enzymes, the effect of the hepatic injury on riluzole metabolism is unknown.

Women may possess a lower metabolic capacity to eliminate riluzole than men.

➤*Hazardous tasks:* Warn patients about the potential for dizziness, vertigo, and somnolence, and advise them not to drive or operate machinery until they have gained sufficient experience on riluzole to gauge whether or not it affects their mental and/or motor performance adversely.

➤*Pregnancy: Category C.* There are no adequate and well-controlled studies in pregnant women. Use riluzole during pregnancy only if the potential benefit justifies the potential risk to the fetus.

Oral administration of riluzole to pregnant animals during the period of organogenesis caused embryotoxicity in rats and rabbits at doses of 27 and 60 mg/kg, respectively, or 2.6 and 11.5 times, respectively, the recommended maximum human daily dose on a mg/m^2 basis. Evidence of maternal toxicity was also observed at these doses.

When administered to rats prior to and during mating (males and females) and throughout gestation and lactation (females), riluzole produced adverse effects on pregnancy (eg, decreased implantations, increased intrauterine

RILUZOLE — ORAL

death) and offspring viability and growth at an oral dose of 15 mg/kg or 1.5 times the maximum daily dose on a mg/m^2 basis.

➤*Lactation:* It is not known whether riluzole is excreted in human breast milk. Because many drugs are excreted in human milk, and because the potential for serious adverse reactions in breast-feeding infants from riluzole is unknown, advise women not to breast-feed during treatment with riluzole. In rat studies, ^{14}C-riluzole was detected in maternal milk.

➤*Children:* The safety and effectiveness of riluzole in children have not been established.

➤*Elderly:* Use riluzole with caution in elderly patients whose hepatic function may be compromised because of age.

Age-related compromised renal and hepatic function may cause a decrease in clearance of riluzole. In controlled clinical trials, about 30% of patients were older than 65 years of age. There were no differences in adverse reactions between younger and older patients.

➤*Monitoring:* Measure serum aminotransferases, including ALT levels, before and during riluzole therapy. Evaluate serum ALT levels every month during the first 3 months of treatment, every 3 months during the remainder of the first year, and periodically thereafter. Evaluate serum ALT levels more frequently in patients who develop elevations.

Drug Interactions

➤*Cytochrome P450 system:* Because riluzole is metabolized mainly by the CYP1A2 enzyme system, substances known to inhibit this enzyme may decrease metabolism or increase bioavailability of riluzole, as indicated by increased whole blood or plasma concentrations. Drugs known to induce these enzyme systems may result in an increased metabolism of riluzole or decreased bioavailability, as indicated by decreased whole blood or plasma concentrations. Monitoring of blood concentrations and appropriate dosage adjustments are essential when such drugs are used concomitantly.

Potential interactions may occur when riluzole is given concurrently with other agents that are also metabolized primarily by CYP1A2 (eg, theophylline, caffeine, tacrine). Currently, it is not known whether riluzole has any potential for enzyme induction in humans.

Riluzole Drug Interactions

Precipitant drug	Object drug[a]		Description
Alcohol	Riluzole	↔	Because it is unknown whether alcohol increases the risk of serious hepatotoxicity with riluzole administration, discourage patients from drinking excessive amounts of alcohol.
Carbamazepine, phenobarbital	Riluzole	↑	Epileptic patients receiving concomitant carbamazepine and phenobarbital experienced marked, rapid elevations of liver enzymes with jaundice and bilirubin 4 months after starting riluzole. Values returned to normal 7 weeks after discontinuation of treatment. Use with caution and carefully monitor liver function.
CYP1A2 inducers (eg, omeprazole, rifampin)	Riluzole	↓	May potentially increase the rate of riluzole elimination. Monitor the response of the patient. If an interaction is suspected, increase the riluzole dose as needed.
CYP1A2 inhibitors (eg, amitriptyline, caffeine, quinolones, theophylline)	Riluzole	↑	May potentially decrease the rate of riluzole elimination. Monitor the response of the patient. If an interaction is suspected, decrease the riluzole dose as needed.
Hepatotoxic drugs (eg, allopurinol, methyldopa, sulfasalazine)	Riluzole	↔	The clinical trials in ALS excluded patients with concomitant medications that were potentially hepatotoxic. Accordingly, there is no information about the safety of administering riluzole in conjunction with such medications. If such a combination is administered, exercise caution.

[a] ↑ = object drug increased; ↓ = object drug decreased; ↔ = undetermined clinical effect.

➤*Drug/Smoking interactions:* Smoking cigarettes increases the elimination of riluzole 20% compared with nonsmokers. However, it is not necessary to adjust the riluzole dose in smokers.

➤*Drugs highly bound to plasma proteins:* Riluzole is highly bound (96%) to plasma proteins, binding mainly to serum albumin and to lipoproteins. The effect of riluzole (up to 5 mcg/mL) on warfarin (5 mcg/mL) binding did not show any displacement of warfarin. Conversely, warfarin binding was unaffected by the addition of warfarin, digoxin, imipramine, and quinine at high therapeutic concentrations.

➤*Drug/Food interactions:* A high-fat meal reduces riluzole absorption, decreasing the AUC and C_{max} 20% and 45%, respectively. Riluzole should be taken 1 hour before or 2 hours after a meal to avoid food-related decreases in bioavailability. Charcoal-broiled foods may increase the rate of riluzole elimination.

Adverse Reactions

➤*Most common adverse reactions:* The most commonly observed adverse reactions associated with the use of riluzole and seen more frequently in riluzole-treated patients than in placebo-treated patients were abdominal pain, anorexia, asthenia, circumoral paresthesia, decreased lung function, diarrhea, dizziness, nausea, pneumonia, somnolence, vertigo, and vomiting. Anorexia, asthenia, circumoral paresthesia, diarrhea, dizziness, nausea, somnolence, and vertigo were dose related.

➤*Discontinuation:* Approximately 14% (n = 141) of the 982 individuals with ALS who received riluzole in premarketing clinical trials discontinued treatment because of an adverse reaction. Of those patients who discontinued because of adverse reactions, the most commonly reported were abdominal pain, ALT elevations, constipation, and nausea. In a dose-response study in ALS patients, the rates of discontinuation of riluzole for abdominal pain, ALT elevation, asthenia, and nausea were dose related.

➤*Adverse reactions (at least 2%):* Treatment-emergent signs and symptoms that occurred in at least 2% of patients with ALS treated with riluzole (n = 794) participating in placebo-controlled trials and were numerically greater in the patients treated with riluzole 100 mg/day than with placebo or for which a dose response relationship is suggested are presented in the following table.

Riluzole Adverse Reactions (≥ 2%)

Adverse reactions	Riluzole 50 mg/day (n = 237)	Riluzole 100 mg/day (n = 313)	Riluzole 200 mg/day (n = 244)	Placebo (n = 320)
Cardiovascular				
Hypertension	6.8%	5.1%	3.3%	4.1%
Palpitation	0.4%	0.6%	1.2%	0.9%
Postural hypotension	0.8%	0%	1.6%	0.6%
Tachycardia	1.3%	2.6%	2%	1.3%
CNS				
Aggravation reaction	0.4%	1.3%	2%	0.9%
Asthenia	14.8%	19.2%	20.1%	12.2%
Circumoral paresthesia	1.3%	1.6%	3.3%	0%
Depression	4.2%	4.5%	6.1%	5%
Dizziness	5.1%	3.8%	12.7%	2.5%
Hypertonia	5.9%	6.1%	5.3%	5.9%
Insomnia	2.1%	3.5%	2.9%	3.4%
Malaise	0.4%	0.6%	1.2%	0%
Somnolence	0.8%	1.9%	4.1%	1.3%
Vertigo	2.5%	1.9%	4.5%	0.9%
Dermatologic				
Alopecia	0%	1%	1.2%	0.6%
Eczema	0.8%	1.6%	1.6%	0.6%
Exfoliative dermatitis	0%	0.6%	1.2%	0%
Pruritus	3.8%	3.8%	2.5%	3.1%
GI				
Abdominal pain	6.8%	5.1%	7.8%	3.8%
Anorexia	3.8%	3.2%	8.6%	3.8%
Diarrhea	5.5%	2.9%	9%	3.1%
Dry mouth	3%	3.5%	2%	3.4%
Dyspepsia	2.5%	3.8%	6.1%	5%
Flatulence	2.5%	2.6%	2%	1.9%
Nausea	12.2%	16.3%	20.5%	10.6%
Oral moniliasis	0.4%	0.6%	1.2%	0.3%
Stomatitis	0.8%	1%	1.2%	0%
Tooth disorder	0%	1%	1.2%	0.3%
Vomiting	4.2%	4.2%	4.5%	1.6%
GU				
Dysuria	0%	1%	1.2%	0.3%
Urinary tract infection	2.5%	2.6%	4.5%	2.2%
Metabolic/Nutritional				
Peripheral edema	4.2%	2.9%	3.3%	2.2%
Weight loss	4.6%	4.8%	3.7%	4.7%
Respiratory				
Decreased lung function	13.1%	10.2%	16%	9.4%
Increased cough	2.1%	2.6%	3.7%	1.6%

RILUZOLE — ORAL

Riluzole Adverse Reactions (≥ 2%)				
Adverse reactions	Riluzole 50 mg/day (n = 237)	Riluzole 100 mg/day (n = 313)	Riluzole 200 mg/day (n = 244)	Placebo (n = 320)
Rhinitis	8.9%	6.4%	7.8%	6.3%
Sinusitis	0.4%	1%	1.6%	0.9%
Miscellaneous				
Arthralgia	5.1%	3.5%	1.6%	3.4%
Back pain	1.7%	3.2%	4.1%	2.5%
Headache	8%	7.3%	7%	6.6%
Phlebitis	0.4%	1%	0.8%	0.3%

Other reactions that occurred in more than 2% of patients treated with riluzole 100 mg/day but equally or more frequently in the placebo group included accidental injury, apnea, bronchitis, constipation, death, dysphagia, dyspnea, flu syndrome, heart arrest, increased sputum, pneumonia, and respiratory disorder.

➤*Gender:* In ALS studies, dizziness occurred more commonly in women (11%) than in men (4%).

➤*Other adverse reactions:* In the following information, a reaction in which the frequency is less than or equal to placebo is marked with an asterisk.

Cardiovascular – Angina pectoris*, atrial fibrillation*, bundle branch block, cerebral hemorrhage, congestive heart failure, heart failure, hypotension, lower extremity embolus, myocardial infarction*, myocardial ischemia*, pericarditis, peripheral vascular disease, shock*, syncope*, ventricular extrasystoles (0.1% to 1%); bradycardia, cerebral ischemia, hemorrhage, mesenteric artery occlusion, subarachnoid hemorrhage, supraventricular tachycardia*, thrombosis, ventricular fibrillation, ventricular tachycardia (less than 0.1%).

CNS – Agitation*, hostility*, tremor (at least 1%); abnormal gait, abnormal thinking*, amnesia, apathy, ataxia, attempted suicide, chills*, coma, confusion*, convulsion, decreased libido, delirium, delusions, depersonalization, dysarthria, emotional lability, extrapyramidal syndrome, facial paralysis, hallucinations, hemiplegia, hypesthesia, hypokinesia, incoordination, increased libido, intentional injury, leg cramps, manic reaction, migraine, myoclonus, paranoid reaction*, personality disorder*, stupor, subdural hematoma (0.1% to 1%); abnormal dreams, acute brain syndrome, cerebral embolism, CNS depression, dementia, euphoria*, hypotonia, peripheral neuritis, psychosis*, psychotic depression, schizophrenic reaction, trismus, wristdrop (less than 0.1%).

Dermatologic – Fungal dermatitis*, psoriasis, seborrhea*, skin disorder, skin ulceration, urticaria (0.1% to 1%); angioedema, contact dermatitis, erythema multiforme, furunculosis*, skin granuloma, skin moniliasis, skin nodule (less than 0.1%).

Endocrine – Diabetes mellitus, thyroid neoplasia (0.1% to 1%); diabetes insipidus, parathyroid disorder (less than 0.1%).

GI – Enlarged abdomen, esophageal stenosis, fecal impaction, fecal incontinence, gastritis*, GI hemorrhage, GI ulceration, glossitis, gum hemorrhage*, hepatitis, increased appetite, intestinal obstruction*, jaundice, pancreatitis, tenesmus (0.1% to 1%); biliary pain, cheilitis*, cholecystitis, enlarged salivary gland, hematemesis, ileus*, melena*, proctitis, pseudomembranous enterocolitis, tooth caries, tongue discoloration (less than 0.1%).

GU – Hematuria, impotence, kidney calculus, kidney pain, metrorrhagia, priapism, prostate carcinoma, urinary incontinence, urinary retention, urinary urgency, urine abnormality (0.1% to 1%); amenorrhea, breast abscess, breast pain, enlarged uterine fibroids, nephritis*, nocturia, pyelonephritis, uterine hemorrhage, vaginal moniliasis (less than 0.1%).

Hematologic / Lymphatic – Anemia*, ecchymosis, leukocytosis, leukopenia (0.1% to 1%); aplastic anemia, cyanosis, hypochromic anemia, iron deficiency anemia, lymphadenopathy, neutropenia, petechiae*, purpura (less than 0.1%).

Lab test abnormalities – Abnormal liver function/tests, increased alkaline phosphatase, increased gamma globulins, increased GGT, positive direct Coombs test (0.1% to 1%); increased lactic dehydrogenase (less than 0.1%).

Metabolic / Nutritional – Edema, gout*, hypokalemia, hyponatremia, thirst*, weight gain* (0.1% to 1%); generalized edema, hypercalcemia, hypercholesteremia (less than 0.1%).

Musculoskeletal – Arthrosis, bone neoplasm, myasthenia* (0.1% to 1%); bone necrosis, osteoporosis, rheumatoid arthritis, tetany (less than 0.1%).

Respiratory – Asthma, epistaxis, hemoptysis, hiccup, hypersensitivity pneumonitis, hyperventilation*, hypoventilation*, hypoxia, interstitial lung disease, laryngitis, lung carcinoma, lung edema*, pleural disorder*, pleural effusion, pneumothorax*, respiratory acidosis, respiratory moniliasis, stridor, yawn (0.1% to 1%).

Special senses – Amblyopia, ophthalmitis (0.1% to 1%); blepharitis, cataract, deafness, diplopia*, ear pain, glaucoma, hyperacusis, photophobia, taste loss, vestibular disorder (less than 0.1%).

Miscellaneous – Abscess*, anaphylactic reaction, anaphylaxis, cellulitis, face edema*, flu syndrome, hernia, injection site reaction, neoplasm, peritonitis, photosensitivity reaction*, sepsis* (0.1% to 1%); acrodynia, hypothermia, moniliasis* (less than 0.1%).

Overdosage

➤*Symptoms:* Experience with riluzole overdose in humans is limited. Neurological and psychiatric symptoms, and acute toxic encephalopathy with stupor, coma, and methemoglobinemia have been observed in isolated cases. The estimated oral median lethal dose is 94 and 39 mg/kg for male mice and rats, respectively.

➤*Treatment:* No specific antidote or information on treatment of overdosage with riluzole is available. In the event of overdose, discontinue riluzole therapy immediately. Ensure that treatment is supportive and directed toward alleviating symptoms. Severe methemoglobinemia may be rapidly reversible after treatment with methylene blue.

Patient Information

Advise patients to report any febrile illness to their health care provider.

Advise patients to report any cough or difficulties in breathing to their health care provider.

Advise patients and caregivers to take riluzole on a regular basis and at the same time of the day (eg, in the morning and evening) each day. If a dose is missed, instruct patients to take the next tablet as originally planned.

Warn patients about the potential for dizziness, vertigo, or somnolence and advise them not to drive or operate machinery until they have gained sufficient experience on riluzole to gauge whether it affects their mental and/or motor performance adversely.

Whether alcohol increases the risk of serious hepatotoxicity with riluzole is unknown; therefore, discourage patients being treated with riluzole from drinking excessive amounts of alcohol.

PHYSICAL ADJUNCTS

Hyaluronic Acid Derivatives

HYALURONIC ACID DERIVATIVES

Rx	**Euflexxa** (Ferring Pharmaceuticals, Inc)	**Injection**: sodium hyaluronate 10 mg/mL	In 2 mL prefilled syringes.[a]
Rx	**Hyalgan** (Sanofi-Synthelabo, Inc)		In 2 mL vials and prefilled syringes.[b]
Rx	**Supartz** (Smith & Nephew)		In 2.5 mL prefilled syringes.[c]
Rx	**Orthovisc** (Anika Therapeutics[d])	**Injection**: hyaluronan 15 mg[e]	Sodium chloride 9 mg per mL. In 2 mL prefilled syringes.
Rx	**Synvisc** (Genzyme Corp)	**Injection**: hylan polymers 8 mg/mL[f]	In 2 mL prefilled syringes.
Rx	**Synvisc-One** (Genzyme Corp)	**Injection**: hylan polymers 8 mg/mL[f]	Sodium chloride 8.5 mg/mL. In 6 mL prefilled syringes.

[a] Molecular weight is 2,400,000 to 3,600,000 Da.
[b] Molecular weight is 500,000 to 730,000 Da.
[c] Molecular weight is 620,000 to 1,170,000 Da.
[d] Anika Therapeutics; 160 New Boston St, Woburn, MA 01801; 1-781-932-6616; http://www.anikatherapeutics.com.
[e] Molecular weight is 1,000,000 to 2,900,000 Da.
[f] Molecular weight is 6,000,000 Da on average.

HYALURONIC ACID DERIVATIVES — INJECTION

Indications

➤*Osteoarthritis symptoms:* For the treatment of pain in osteoarthritis of the knee in patients who have failed to respond adequately to conservative nonpharmacologic therapy and simple analgesics (eg, acetaminophen).

➤*Off-label uses:* Treatment of osteoarthritis of the hand, hip, and temporomandibular joint; treatment of nonradicular pain in the lumbar spine.

Administration and Dosage

➤*Adults:*

Osteoarthritis symptoms –

Euflexxa: Inject 20 mg (2 mL) using a 17- to 21-gauge needle, into the affected knee at weekly intervals for 3 weeks for a total of 3 injections.

Hyalgan: Inject 20 mg (2 mL) once weekly using a 20-gauge needle for a total of 5 injections. Studies with a follow-up period of 60 days have shown that patients may experience benefit with 3 injections given at weekly intervals.

HYALURONIC ACID DERIVATIVES — INJECTION

Orthovisc: Inject 30 mg (2 mL) using an 18- to 21-gauge needle into the knee joint in a series of intra-articular injections 1 week apart for 3 or 4 injections. If symptoms return, repeat courses may be administered. Pain relief may not occur until after the third injection.

Supartz: Inject 25 mg (2.5 mL) once weekly for a total of 5 injections using a 22- to 23-gauge needle. Studies with a follow-up period of 90 days have shown that some patients may experience benefit with 3 injections given at weekly intervals.

Synvisc: Inject 16 mg (2 mL) once weekly for a total of 3 injections using an 18- to 22-gauge needle.

Synvisc-One: Inject 48 mg (6 mL) into one knee only using a 18- to 20-gauge needle.

➤*Joint effusion:* If present, remove joint effusion or synovial fluid before administering therapy. Do not use the same syringe for removing fluid and injecting hyaluronic acid derivatives; however, use the same needle for injecting *Synvisc* and *Synvisc-One*.

➤*Administration:* Administer by intra-articular injection into the affected knee once weekly for the recommended number of injections per treatment cycle. If treatment is bilateral, use a separate vial/syringe for each knee. Do not prepare injection site with skin disinfectants containing quaternary ammonium salts; precipitation of drug can occur. Do not give other intra-articular injectables concomitantly.

Hyalgan and *Supartz* – Injection of a local anesthetic (eg, lidocaine) subcutaneously prior to administration may be recommended.

Synvisc-One – Do not use if the package has been opened or damaged. Using an 18- to 20-gauge needle, remove synovial fluid or effusion before injecting *Synvisc-One*. Do not use the same syringe for removing synovial fluid and for injecting *Synvisc-One*; however, the same 18- to 20-gauge needle should be used. Twist the tip cap before pulling it off; this will minimize product leakage. To ensure a tight seal and prevent leakage during administration, secure the needle tightly while firmly holding the luer hub. Do not over tighten or apply excessive leverage when attaching the needle or removing the needle guard; this may break the syringe tip. Inject the full 6 mL in one knee only.

➤*Storage/Stability:* These products are intended for single use only; use immediately once opened and discard any unused portion. Do not freeze; protect from light. Store *Euflexxa* at 2° to 25°C (36° to 77°F). If refrigerated, remove from refrigeration at least 20 to 30 minutes before use.Store *Hyalgan, Orthovisc*, and *Supartz* in original package below 25°C (77°F). Shelf life for *Supartz* is 42 months. Store *Synvisc* and *Synvisc-One* in the original package below 30°C (86°F).

Actions

➤*Pharmacology:* Hyaluronic acid is a naturally occurring polysaccharide of the glycosaminoglycan family containing repeating disaccharide units of sodium-glucuronate-N-acetylglucosamine. Hyaluronic acid is derived from chicken combs or bacterial cells (*Euflexxa*).

Contraindications

Hypersensitivity to hyaluronan or any components of the product; known allergies to avian or avian-derived products, including eggs, feathers, or poultry (except *Euflexxa*); infections or skin diseases in the area of the injection site or joint; concomitant skin disinfectants containing quarternary ammonium salts.

Warnings/Precautions

➤*Avian allergies:* These products are extracted from chicken/rooster combs (except *Euflexxa*). Use caution in patients allergic to avian proteins, feathers, and egg products.

➤*Immune response:* Patients having repeated exposure to *Euflexxa* have the potential for an immune response; however, this has not been assessed in humans.

➤*Inflamed knee joint:* The safety and efficacy of *Synvisc* in severely inflamed knee joints have not been established.

➤*Inflammatory arthritis:* Transient increases in inflammation in the injected knee following injections with sodium hyaluronate have been reported in some patients with inflammatory arthritis (eg, rheumatoid or gouty arthritis).

➤*Intraarticular administration:* Administer by intraarticular injection only. Avoid intravascular, extra-articular, synovial tissue and capsule administration; rare systemic adverse reactions have been reported. Safety and efficacy of intraarticular administration in locations other than the knee and for conditions other than OA have not been established.

➤*Joint effusion:* Remove joint effusion before using hyaluronic acid derivatives.

➤*Latex sensitivity:* Parts of *Euflexxa* syringe contain natural rubber latex, which may cause allergic reactions. Use caution in patients with a possible history of latex sensitivity.

➤*Lymphatic or venous stasis:* Use *Synvisc* with caution when evidence of lymphatic or venous stasis exists in treatment leg.

➤*Quarternary ammonium salts:* Avoid concomitant use of disinfectants for skin preparation containing quarternary ammonium salts, such as benzalkonium chloride; precipitation of drug may occur.

➤*Treatment cycle:* The efficacy of a single treatment cycle of less than the recommended number of injections has not been established; 3 injections of *Euflexxa*, 3 injections of *Hyalgan*, 3 injections of *Orthovisc*, 3 injections of *Supartz*, 3 injections of *Synvisc*. Safety and efficacy of repeat cycles have not been established.

➤*Hypersensitivity reactions:* Anaphylactoid reactions have occurred with *Supartz*. The incidents resolved with favorable outcomes upon discontinuation of therapy. Five allergic reactions were reported in the *Supartz* group. All 5 reactions were classified as mild to moderate. These were: hay fever, reaction on face and neck, cutaneous reaction on forearms and knees, and an undefined mild allergic reaction. No anaphylactic reactions were observed.

➤*Pregnancy: Category C* (*Hylira*). Safety and efficacy have not been established in pregnant women. Give to a pregnant woman only if potential benefits outweigh the potential risks.

➤*Lactation:* It is not known if hyaluronic acid derivatives are excreted in breast milk. Excretion has been seen in rat milk. Safety and efficacy have not been established in lactating women. Exercise caution when administering to a breast-feeding woman.

➤*Children:* Safety and efficacy have not been established.

Drug Interactions

➤*Concomitant intraarticular injections:* Do not coadminister with other intraarticular injectables. Safety and efficacy have not been established.

➤*Local anesthetic:* Injection of subcutaneous lidocaine or similar local anesthetic may be recommended prior to injection of *Hyalgan* and *Supartz*. Do not inject anesthetics intraarticularly into the knee with *Synvisc* because this may dilute *Synvisc* and affect its safety and efficacy.

Adverse Reactions

➤*Euflexxa:*

Multicenter clinical investigation – A total of 119 patients reported 196 adverse reactions; this number represents 54 patients (33.8%) in the *Euflexxa* group and 65 patients (44.4%) in the active control group. There were no deaths reported during the study. Incidences of each reaction were similar for both groups, except for knee joint effusion, which was reported by 9 patients in the active control group and 1 patient in the *Euflexxa* treatment group. Fifty-two adverse reactions were considered device related. The following table lists the adverse reactions reported during this investigation.

***Euflexxa* Adverse Reactions Reported by > 1% of Patients**

Adverse reaction	*Euflexxa* (n = 160)	Active controlled (n = 161)
Cardiovascular		
Blood pressure increased	6 (3.75%)	1 (0.62%)
Phlebitis	0 (0%)	2 (1.24%)
CNS		
Fatigue	2 (1.25%)	0 (0%)
Headache	1 (0.63%)	3 (1.86%)
Paresthesia	2 (1.25%)	1 (0.62%)
Dermatologic		
Erythema	0 (0%)	2 (1.24%)
Pruritus	0 (0%)	3 (1.86%)
GI		
Nausea	3 (1.88%)	0 (0%)
Musculoskeletal		
Arthralgia	14 (8.75%)	17 (10.6%)
Arthrosis	2 (1.25%)	0 (0%)
Back pain	8 (5%)	11 (6.83%)
Joint disorder	2 (1.25%)	2 (1.24%)
Joint effusion	1 (0.63%)	14 (8.07%)
Joint swelling	3 (1.88%)	3 (1.86%)
Pain in limb	2 (1.25%)	0 (0%)
Tendonitis	3 (1.88%)	2 (1.24%)
Respiratory		
Bronchitis	1 (0.63%)	2 (1.24%)
Rhinitis	5 (3.13%)	7 (4.35%)
Miscellaneous		
Infection	2 (1.25%)	0 (0%)

A total of 160 patients received 478 injections of *Euflexxa*. There were 27 reported adverse reactions considered related to *Euflexxa* injections: arthralgia (11, 6.9%); back pain (1, 0.63%); blood pressure increase (3, 1.88%); joint effusion (1, 0.63%); joint swelling (3, 1.88%); nausea (1, 0.63%); paresthesia (2, 1.25%); feeling of sickness of injection (3, 1.88%); skin irritation (1, 0.63%); and tenderness in study knee (1, 0.63%). The following adverse reactions were reported for the *Euflexxa* group that the relationship to treatment was considered to be unknown: fatigue (3, 1.88%); nausea (1, 0.63%).

HYALURONIC ACID DERIVATIVES — INJECTION

Euflexxa Adverse Reactions Considered Treatment Related		
Adverse reaction	*Euflexxa* (n = 160)	Commercially available hyaluronan product (n = 161)
Cardiovascular		
Blood pressure increase	3	0
CNS		
Paresthesia	2	0
Dermatologic		
Erythema	0	1
Inflammation localized	0	1
Pruritus	0	1
Skin irritation	1	0
GI		
Nausea	1	0
Musculoskeletal		
Arthralgia	11	9
Back pain	1	0
Edema lower limb	0	1
Joint effusion	1	9
Joint swelling	3	2
Tenderness	1	0
Miscellaneous		
Baker cyst	0	1
Sickness	3	0

Single-center study –

Euflexxa Adverse Reactions in Single-Center Study			
Adverse reaction	*Euflexxa*	Placebo	Total
CNS			
Asthenia	1 (3%)	2 (7%)	3
Headache	0 (0%)	1 (3%)	1
Vertigo	0 (0%)	1 (3%)	1
Dermatologic			
Pruritus	0 (0%)	1 (3%)	1
Rash	1 (3%)	1 (3%)	2
GI			
Bitter taste	0 (0%)	1 (3%)	1
Gingivitis	0 (0%)	1 (3%)	1
Peptic ulcer	1 (3%)	0 (0%)	1
Musculoskeletal			
Back pain	2 (6%)	1 (3%)	3
Hip pain	0 (0%)	1 (3%)	1
Hypokinesia of knee	0 (0%)	1 (3%)	1
Knee pain	18 (53%)	11 (35%)	29
Knee swelling	1 (3%)	0 (0%)	1
Knee trauma	0 (0%)	1 (3%)	1
Skeletal pain	1 (3%)	0 (0%)	1
Total knee replacement	1 (3%)	0 (0%)	1
Respiratory			
Rhinitis	1 (3%)	0 (0%)	1
Upper respiratory tract infection	4 (12%)	2 (7%)	6
Special senses			
Sudden sensorial verbal hearing loss	0 (0%)	1 (3%)	1
Swollen eyelids	1 (3%)	0 (0%)	1
Miscellaneous			
Appendicitis	0 (0%)	1 (3%)	1
Chest pain	0 (0%)	1 (3%)	1
Elective nonsurgical procedures	0 (0%)	1 (3%)	1
Herpes simplex	1 (3%)	0 (0%)	1
Herpes zoster	1 (3%)	0 (0%)	1
Surgery	0 (0%)	2 (7%)	2

Of the 65 total reactions reported, 20 were regarded as treatment related. Knee pain, hypokinesia of the knee, knee swelling, and rash were considered to be treatment-related adverse reactions. The following table shows the relation of the treatment-related adverse reactions to the treatment group.

Euflexxa Treatment-Related Adverse Reactions		
Adverse reaction	*Euflexxa* (n = 34)	Placebo (n = 31)
Musculoskeletal		
Hip pain	0	1
Hypokinesia of knee	1	0
Knee pain	10	5
Knee swelling	1	0
Miscellaneous		
Rash	0	1
Taste bitter	0	1

➤*Hyalgan:*

Hyalgan Adverse Reactions in > 5%		
Adverse reaction	*Hyalgan* (n = 164)	Placebo (n = 168)
CNS		
Headache	30 (18%)	29 (17%)
GI		
GI complaints[a]	48 (29%)	59 (36%)
Local		
Injection-site pain[b]	38 (23%)[c]	22 (13%)
Local joint pain and swelling[d]	21 (13%)	22 (13%)
Local skin[e]	23 (14%)	17 (10%)
Pruritus (local)	12 (7%)	7 (4%)

[a] Severe in 4 *Hyalgan*-treated subjects and 4 placebo-treated subjects.
[b] Severe in 5 *Hyalgan*-treated subjects and 2 placebo-treated subjects.
[c] Statistically significant ($P = 0.02$).
[d] Severe in 2 *Hyalgan*-treated subjects (1.2%) and 1 placebo-treated subject.
[e] Includes ecchymosis and rash.

Common adverse reactions reported for the *Hyalgan*-treated subjects were GI complaints, injection-site pain, knee swelling/effusion, local skin reactions (ecchymosis, rash), pruritus, and headache. Swelling and effusion, local skin reactions (ecchymosis and rash), and headache occurred at equal frequency in the *Hyalgan*- and placebo-treated groups.

Two (2/164, 1.2%) *Hyalgan*-treated subjects and 3 of 168 (1.8%) placebo-treated subjects were reported to have positive bacterial cultures of effusion aspirated from the treated knee. The 2 *Hyalgan*-treated subjects and 2 of the placebo-treated subjects did not exhibit evidence of infection clinically or subsequently and were not treated with antibiotics. One of the placebo-treated subjects was hospitalized and received presumptive treatment for septic arthritis.

Hyalgan has been in clinical use in Europe since 1987. Analysis of the adverse reactions that have been reported with the use of *Hyalgan* in Europe reveals that most of the reactions are related to local symptoms such as pain, swelling/effusion, and warmth or redness at the injections site. In the 2 reactions reported as anaphylactoid reactions, *Hyalgan* treatment was discontinued and both had favorable outcomes. Three cases of allergic reactions were reported in which the patients were discontinued from *Hyalgan* treatment and the incidents resolved. Seven cases of fever were reported in which 3 of the cases were reported to be associated with local reactions; pyogenic arthritis was reported to be ruled out in these 3 cases. All the fever patients were discontinued from *Hyalgan* treatment and all incidents resolved. One incident of shock, which was described as hypotensive crisis, was reported. The incident resolved and *Hyalgan* treatment was continued.

➤*Orthovisc:*

Orthovisc Local Individual Adverse Reactions in ITT Populations			
Adverse reaction	*Orthovisc* (n = 562)	Saline (n = 296)	Arthrocentesis (n = 123)
Local			
Injection-site edema	5 (0.9%)	1 (0.3%)	0 (0%)
Injection-site erythema	2 (0.4%)	0 (0%)	0 (0%)
Injection-site pain	14 (2.5%)	6 (2%)	1 (0.8%)
Injection-site reaction NOS[a]	1 (0.2%)	2 (0.7%)	1 (0.8%)
Musculoskeletal			
Aggravated OA	2 (0.4%)	0 (0%)	1 (0.8%)
Arthralgia	71 (12.6%)	51 (17.2%)	1 (0.8%)
Arthritis NOS	4 (0.7%)	5 (1.7%)	0 (0%)
Arthropathy NOS	5 (0.9%)	3 (1%)	0 (0%)
Bursitis	6 (1.1%)	6 (2%)	2 (1.6%)
Joint disorder NOS	2 (0.4%)	0 (0%)	0 (0%)
Joint effusion	2 (0.4%)	1 (0.3%)	1 (0.8%)
Joint stiffness	3 (0.5%)	2 (0.7%)	0 (0%)
Joint swelling	4 (0.7%)	2 (0.7%)	1 (0.8%)

HYALURONIC ACID DERIVATIVES — INJECTION

Orthovisc Local Individual Adverse Reactions in ITT Populations			
Adverse reaction	*Orthovisc* (n = 562)	Saline (n = 296)	Arthrocentesis (n = 123)
Knee arthroplasty	3 (0.5%)	2 (0.7%)	0 (0%)
Localized OA	5 (0.9%)	1 (0.3%)	1 (0.8%)
Miscellaneous			
Any adverse reaction	349 (62.1%)	204 (68.9%)	65 (52.8%)
Baker cyst	2 (0.4%)	2 (0.7%)	0 (0%)
Pain NOS	14 (2.5%)	11 (3.7%)	1 (0.8%)

[a] NOS = Not otherwise specified.

Open-label study –

Orthovisc Local Individual Adverse Reactions			
Adverse reaction	Single treatment (n = 562)	Single treatment (n = 247)	Repeat treatment (n = 127)
Local			
Injection-site edema	5 (0.9%)	1 (0.4%)	0 (0%)
Injection-site erythema	2 (0.4%)	2 (0.8%)	0 (0%)
Injection-site pain	14 (2.5%)	3 (1.2%)	3 (2.4%)
Injection-site reaction NOS	1 (0.2%)	0 (0%)	4 (3.1%)
Musculoskeletal			
Aggravated OA	2 (0.4%)	2 (0.8%)	0 (0%)
Arthralgia	71 (12.6%)	20 (8.1%)	8 (6.3%)
Arthritis NOS	4 (0.7%)	1 (0.4%)	0 (0%)
Arthropathy NOS	5 (0.9%)	0 (0%)	0 (0%)
Bursitis	6 (1.1%)	2 (0.8%)	0 (0%)
Joint disorder NOS	2 (0.4%)	0 (0%)	0 (0%)
Joint effusion	2 (0.4%)	2 (0.8%)	1 (0.8%)
Joint stiffness	3 (0.5%)	0 (0%)	0 (0%)
Joint swelling	4 (0.7%)	2 (0.8%)	2 (1.6%)
Knee arthroplasty	3 (0.5%)	0 (0%)	0 (0%)
Localized OA	5 (0.9%)	3 (1.2%)	1 (0.8%)
Miscellaneous			
Any adverse reaction	349 (62.1%)	136 (55.1%)	39 (30.7%)
Baker cyst	2 (0.4%)	0 (0%)	0 (0%)
Pain NOS	14 (2.5%)	3 (1.2%)	0 (0%)

➤*Supartz*: Five allergic reactions were reported in the *Supartz* group. All 5 reactions were classified as mild to moderate. These were: hay fever (2), reaction on face and neck, cutaneous reaction forearms and knees, and an undefined mild allergy reaction. No anaphylactic reactions were observed in any study patients. Other adverse reactions occurring in 4% or less, but not less than 1%, of the *Supartz*-treated patients included abdominal pain, bronchitis, diarrhea, discomfort in legs, dizziness, dyspepsia, fall, inflicted injury, influenza-like symptoms, leg pain, nausea, rhinitis, sinusitis, upper respiratory tract infection, and urinary tract infection.

Supartz Adverse Reactions (> 4%)		
Adverse reaction	*Supartz* (n = 619)	Control (n = 537)
Local		
Injection-site reaction[a]	35 (5.7%)	18 (3.4%)
Injection-site pain	26 (4.2%)	22 (4.1%)
Musculoskeletal		
Arthralgia	110 (17.8%)	95 (17.7%)
Arthropathy/Arthrosis/Arthritis	68 (11%)	57 (10.6%)
Back pain	40 (6.5%)	26 (4.8%)
Miscellaneous		
Headache	27 (4.4%)	23 (4.3%)
Pain (non-specific)	37 (6%)	26 (4.8%)

[a] Includes application/injection-site reaction, injection-site inflammation, and purpura injection site.

Adverse Reactions Occurring in *Supartz*-treated Patients Receiving 3 Injections		
	French study	
Adverse reaction	Control injections (n = 80)	*Supartz*-3 injections (n = 87)
Local		
Injection-site pain	4 (5%)	3 (3.4%)
Injection-site reaction[a]	0 (0%)	1 (1.1%)
Musculoskeletal		
Arthralgia	12 (15%)	11 (12.6%)
Arthropathy/Arthrosis/Arthritis	3 (3.8%)	1 (1.1%)
Back pain	10 (12.5%)	10 (11.5%)
Miscellaneous		
Headache	4 (5%)	3 (3.4%)
Pain	16 (20%)	16 (18.4%)

[a] Includes application/injection-site reaction, injection-site inflammation, and purpura injection site.

➤*Postmarketing: Supartz* has been in use in Japan since 1987. A prospective postmarketing surveillance study conducted from 1987 to 1993 evaluated safety in 7,404 knees treated from a total of 675 medical institutions. A subset of 7,155 knees was treated with 3 or more consecutive injections. There were 58 cases of adverse reactions in 37 knees (0.5%, 37/7,404). The most frequently observed were 29 cases of pain at the injection site, 16 cases of swelling, and 3 cases of redness. Other adverse reactions were 3 cases of rash, 3 cases of increased serum glutamic-pyruvic transaminase (GPT), 2 cases of increased serum glutamic-oxaloacetic transaminase (GOT), 1 case of itching, and 1 case of increased alkaline phosphatase (Al-P). The incidence of adverse reactions was not related to the number of injections. There was no increase in adverse reactions in patients requiring 3 or more injections.

➤*Synvisc*: A total of 511 patients (559 knees) received 1,771 injections in 7 clinical trials of *Synvisc*. There were 39 reports in 37 patients (2.2% of injections, 7.2% of patients) of knee pain and/or swelling after these injections.

Other adverse reactions – Systemic adverse reactions each occurred in 10 (2%) of the *Synvisc*-treated patients. There was 1 case each of rash (thorax and back) and itching of the skin following *Synvisc* injection in these studies. These symptoms did not recur when these patients received additional *Synvisc* injections. The remaining generalized adverse reactions reported were calf cramps, hemorrhoid problems, ankle edema, muscle pain, tonsillitis with nausea, tachyarrhythmia, phlebitis with varicosities, and low back sprain.

Postmarketing – Other adverse reactions reported include the following: rash, *hives*, itching, *fever*, nausea, *headache*, *dizziness*, *chills*, muscle cramps, *paresthesia*, peripheral edema, *malaise*, *respiratory difficulties*, *flushing*, and *facial swelling*. There have been rare reports of *thrombocytopenia* coincident with *Synvisc* injection. These medical reactions occurred under circumstances where causal relationship to *Synvisc*is uncertain. (Adverse reactions reported only in worldwide postmarketing experience, not seen in clinical trials, are considered more rare and are italicized.)

Patient Information

Provide patients with a copy of the patient information leaflet prior to use.

Inform patients that transient pain and/or swelling of the treated joint may occur after injection.

Advise patients to avoid strenuous or prolonged (more than 1 hour) weight-bearing activities (eg, jogging, tennis) within 48 hours following treatment.

Advise patients that the safety and efficacy of repeated treatment cycles have not been studied with *Euflexxa*, *Orthovisc*, or *Supartz*.

Advise patients receiving *Synvisc* that transient effusion may occur. In some cases the effusion may be considerable and cause pronounced pain; advise patients to consult with their health care provider if swelling is extensive.

HYALURONIC ACID DERIVATIVES, DERMAL INJECTION

Rx	**Perlane** (Medicis)	**Gel for injection:** 20 mg/mL	In single-use, prefilled syringes.
Rx	**Perlane-L** (Medicis Aesthetics)		Lidocaine 0.3%. In single-use, prefilled syringes.
Rx	**Restylane** (Medicis Aesthetics)		In single-use, prefilled syringes.
Rx	**Restylane-L** (Medicis Aesthetics)		Lidocaine 0.3%. In single-use, prefilled syringes.

HYALURONIC ACID DERIVATIVES, DERMAL INJECTION

Rx	**Juvederm Ultra** (Allergan)	**Gel; intradermal**: 24 mg/mL	In single-use, prefilled syringes with 30-gauge needles.
Rx	**Juvederm Ultra Plus** (Allergan)		In single-use, prefilled syringes with 27-gauge needles.
Rx	**Juvederm Ultra XC** (Allergan)		Lidocaine 0.3%. In single-use, prefilled syringes with 30-gauge needles.

HYALURONIC ACID DERMAL — INJECTION

Indications

➤*Facial wrinkles and folds:* For mid-to-deep dermal implantation for the correction of moderate to severe facial wrinkles and folds, such as nasolabial folds.

Administration and Dosage

➤*Adults:*

Facial wrinkles and folds –

Maximum dose: Limit to 1.5 mL per treatment site (limit to 6 mL per treatment for *Perlane*, *Perlane-L*, *Restylane*, and *Restylane-L*).

➤*Preparation for administration:* For safe use, it is important that the needle is properly assembled. Unscrew the tip cap of the syringe carefully. To help avoid needle breakage, do not attempt to straighten a bent needle. Discard it and complete the procedure with a replacement needle. Do not reshield used needles. Recapping by hand is a hazardous practice and should be avoided.

➤*Administration:*

1.) Assess the patient's need for pain management.
2.) Clean the area to be treated with alcohol or another suitable antiseptic solution.
3.) Before injecting, press the rod carefully until a small droplet is visible at the tip of the needle.
4.) Administer using a thin-gauge needle (30 G × ½inch [27 G × ½ inch for *Perlane-L*). The needle is inserted at an approximate angle of 30° parallel to the length of the wrinkle or fold. The bevel of the needle should face upwards and the substance should be injected into the middle of the dermis. Tip: For mid-dermis placement, the contour of the needle should be visible but not the color of it. If injected too deep or intramuscularly, the duration of the effect will be shorter. If injected too superficially this may result in visible lumps and/or grayish discoloration.
5.) Inject applying even pressure on the plunger rod while slowly pulling the needle backward. The wrinkle should be lifted and eliminated by the end of the injection. It is important that the injection is stopped just before the needle is pulled out of the skin to prevent material from leaking out or ending up too superficially in the skin.
6.) Only correct to 100% of the desired volume effect. Do not overcorrect. With cutaneous contour deformities, the best results are obtained if the defect can be manually stretched to the point where it is eliminated. The degree and duration of the correction depend on the character of the defect treated, the tissue stress at the implant site, the depth of the implant in the tissue, and the injection technique. Markedly indurated defects may be difficult to correct.
7.) The injection technique with regard to the depth of injection and the administered quantity may vary. The linear threading technique, serial puncture injections, a combination of the 2, or cross-hatching have been used with success.
8.) When the injection is completed, the treated site should be gently massaged so that it conforms to the contour of the surrounding tissues. If an overcorrection has occurred, massage the area firmly between your fingers or against an underlying superficial bone to obtain optimal results.
9.) If so called "blanching" is observed (ie, the overlying skin turns a whitish color), the injection should be stopped immediately and the area massaged until it returns to a normal color.
10.) If the wrinkle needs further treatment, the same procedure should be repeated with several punctures of the skin until a satisfactory result is obtained. Additional treatment may be necessary to achieve the desired correction. With patients who have localized swelling, the degree of correction is sometimes difficult to judge at the time of treatment. In these cases, it is better to invite the patient to a touch-up session after 1 to 2 weeks.
11.) Typical usage for each treatment session is less than 2 mL per treatment site.
12.) If the treated area is swollen directly after the injection, an ice pack can be applied on the site for a short period.
13.) Patients may have mild to moderate injection site reactions, which typically resolve in few days.

➤*Storage/Stability:* Store up to 25°C (77°F). Do not freeze. Protect from sunlight. Refrigeration is not needed. Do not resterilize as this may damage or alter the product. Do not use if the package is damaged. Immediately return the damaged product to the manufacturer. Discard unshielded needles in approved sharps collectors.

Actions

➤*Pharmacology:* Hyaluronic acid is a naturally occurring polysaccharide of the glycosamin-oglycan family containing repeating disaccharide units of sodium-glucuronate-N-acetyl glucosamine. Exact mechanism(s) of action of hyaluronic acid derivatives is/are not known.

Contraindications

Hyaluronic acid injection is contraindicated for patients with severe allergies manifested by a history of anaphylaxis or history of presence of multiple severe allergies. Hyaluronic acid injection contains trace amounts of gram-positive bacterial proteins and is contraindicated for patients with a history of allergies to such material. Hyaluronic acid injection is contraindicated for use in breast augmentation, and for implantation into bone, tendon, ligament, or muscle. Hyaluronic acid injection must not be implanted into blood vessels. Implantation of hyaluronic acid injection into dermal vessels may cause vascular occlusion, infarction, or embolic phenomena.

➤*Perlane-L* and *Restylane-L*: Patients with bleeding disorders; implantation in anatomical spaces other than the dermis; hypersensitivity to local anesthetics of the amide type, such as lidocaine.

Warnings/Precautions

➤*Skin eruptions:* Use of hyaluronic acid injection at specific sites in which an active inflammatory process (skin eruptions such as cysts, pimples, rashes, or hives) or infection is present should be deferred until the inflammatory process has been controlled.

➤*Injection site reactions:* Injection site reaction to hyaluronic acid injection has been observed as consisting mainly of short-term inflammatory symptoms starting early after treatment and with less than 7 days duration.

➤*Superficial necrosis:* Localized superficial necrosis may occur after injection in the glabellar area. It is thought to result from the injury, obstruction, or compromise of blood vessels.

➤*Treatment of other anatomic regions:* The safety or effectiveness of hyaluronic acid injection for the treatment of anatomic regions other than naso-labial folds has not been established in controlled clinical studies.

➤*Long-term use:* Long-term safety and effectiveness of hyaluronic acid injection beyond 1 year have not been investigated in clinical trials.

➤*Infection:* As with all transcutaneous procedures, hyaluronic acid injection implantation carries a risk of infection. Standard precautions associated with injectable materials should be followed.

➤*Keloid formation and hypertrophic scarring:* The safety of hyaluronic acid injection in patients with increased susceptibility to keloid formation and hypertrophic scarring has not been studied. Hyaluronic acid injection should not be used in patients with known susceptibility to keloid formation or hypertrophic scarring.

➤*Photosensitivity/Cold weather:* The patient should be informed that he or she should minimize exposure of the treated area to excessive sun and UV lamp exposure and extreme cold weather until any initial swelling and redness has resolved.

➤*Other skin treatment:* If laser treatment, chemical peeling or any other procedure based on active dermal response is considered after treatment with hyaluronic acid injection there is a possible risk of eliciting an inflammatory reaction at the implant site. This also applies if hyaluronic acid injection is administered before the skin has healed completely after such a procedure.

➤*Hypersensitivity reactions:* Hypersensitivity as an inflammatory reaction to hyaluronic acid injection has been observed with swelling, redness, tenderness, induration, and, rarely, acneform papules at the injection site.

➤*Special risk:* Hyaluronic acid injection should be used with caution in patients on immunosuppressive therapy.

Patients who are using substances that reduce coagulation, such as aspirin and nonsteroidal anti-inflammatory drugs (NSAIDs) may, as with any injection, experience increased bruising or bleeding at injection sites.

➤*Pregnancy: Category C* (topical). The safety of hyaluronic acid injection for use during pregnancy has not been established.

➤*Lactation:* The safety of hyaluronic acid injection for use in breast-feeding females has not been established.

➤*Children:* The safety of hyaluronic acid injection for use in patients under 18 years has not been established.

Adverse Reactions

In a study of 138 patients at 6 centers, adverse events reported in hyaluronic acid injection patient diaries during 14 days after treatment are reported in the following table. Patients in the study received hyaluronic acid injections in 1 side of the face, and a bovine collagen dermal filler (*Zyplast*) in the other side of the face:

HYALURONIC ACID DERMAL — INJECTION

Hyaluronic Acid Injection vs *Zyplast*: Maximum Intensity of Symptoms after Initial Treatment, Patient Diary (%)

Adverse reaction	Total reporting symptoms		Hyaluronic acid injection side				*Zyplast* side			
	Hyaluronic acid injection side	*Zyplast* side	None	Mild	Moderate	Severe	None	Mild	Moderate	Severe
Bruising	52.2%	48.6%	45.6%	23.2%	25.4%	3.6%	49.3%	31.2%	16.7%	0.7%
Redness	84.8%	84.8%	12.3%	40.6%	39.1%	5.1%	12.3%	52.2%	26.8%	5.8%
Swelling	87%	73.9%	10.1%	39.1%	44.2%	3.6%	23.2%	47.1%	25.4%	1.4%
Pain	57.2%	42%	39.9%	29%	24.6%	3.6%	55.1%	33.3%	7.2%	1.4%
Tenderness	77.5%	64.5%	19.6%	43.5%	31.2%	2.9%	32.6%	50.7%	12.3%	1.4%
Itching	30.4%	23.9%	65.9%	22.5%	8%	0	73.2%	19.6%	4.4%	0
Other	24.6%	23.9%	67.4%	10.1%	10.9%	3.6%	68.1%	14.5%	7.2%	2.2%

Events are reported as local events; because of the design (split-face) of the study, causality of the systemic adverse events cannot be assigned.

Hyaluronic Acid Injection vs *Zyplast*: Duration of Adverse Events After Initial Treatment, Patient Diary

Adverse reaction	Total reporting symptoms		Number of days							
			Hyaluronic acid injection side				*Zyplast* side			
	Hyaluronic acid injection side	*Zyplast* side	1	2 to 7	8 to 13	14+	1	2 to 7	8 to 13	14+
Bruising	52.2%	48.6%	5.1%	40.6%	4.4%	2.2%	5.1%	38.4%	3.6%	1.4%
Redness	84.8%	84.8%	13.8%	49.3%	13%	8.7%	13.8%	51.4%	10.9%	8.7%
Swelling	87%	73.9%	11.6%	60.9%	11.6%	2.9%	10.1%	50.7%	11.6%	1.4%
Pain	57.2%	42%	21%	34.8%	1.4%	0	22.5%	18.1%	0.7%	0.7%
Tenderness	77.5%	64.5%	15.2%	56.5%	4.4%	1.4%	19.6%	39.1%	4.4%	1.4%
Itching	30.4%	23.9%	8%	18.1%	4.4%	0	5.8%	15.9%	2.2%	0
Other	24.6%	23.9%	5.1%	16.7%	2.2%	0.7%	7.2%	10.9%	4.4%	1.4%

Other Hyaluronic Acid Injection Adverse Events Reported in the Randomized Study from Physician Case Report Forms

Adverse reaction	(n = 138)
Inflicted injury	8
Sinusitis	7
Upper respiratory tract infection	6
Acne	5
Back pain	3
Depression	3
Depression aggravated	3
Tooth disorder	4
Bronchitis	2
Pneumonia	2
Dermatitis contact	2
Allergic reaction[a]	2
Arthralgia	2
Osteoporosis	2
Headache	2
Migraine	2
Herpes simplex	2
Hypercholesterolemia	2
Urinary incontinence	2

[a] One case of seasonal allergy, and 1 reaction to make-up in the peri-orbital area.

➤*Postmarketing adverse reactions:* In postmarketing surveillance in other countries, presumptive bacterial infections, inflammatory adverse events, allergic adverse events, and necrosis have been reported. Reported treatments have included systemic steroids, systemic antibiotics, and IV administrations of medications. Additionally, inflammatory reaction to hyaluronic acid injection has been observed with swelling, redness, tenderness, induration, and, rarely, acneform papules at the injection site with onset at 1 to several weeks after the initial treatment in previously unexposed individuals, and in less than 7 days following treatment in patients known to have been previously exposed. Average duration of this effect is 2 weeks. The manufacturer is conducting a post-approval study to determine the likelihood of hypersensitivity reactions for patients receiving hyaluronic acid injections.

Adverse reactions should be reported to the manufacturer at 1-866-222-1480.

SODIUM HYALURONATE TOPICAL

Rx	**Bionect** (JSJ Pharmaceuticals)	**Cream; topical:** 0.2%	As sodium salt. Parabens, PEG. In 25 g.
Rx	**Sodium Hyaluronate** (River's Edge)	**Gel; topical:** 0.2%	Parabens. In 340 g.
Rx	**Bionect** (JSJ Pharmaceuticals)		As sodium salt. Parabens. In 30 g.
Rx	**HyGel** (Aletheia)		Parabens. In 340 mL.
Rx	**Hylira** (Hawthorn)		Parabens. In 113 and 340 g.
Rx	**Bionect** (JSJ Pharmaceuticals)	**Spray; topical:** 0.2%	As sodium salt. Parabens. In 20 mL.
Rx	**Sodium Hyaluronate** (River's Edge Pharm)	**Lotion; topical:** 0.1%	Parabens, trolamine. In 340 and 1,000 g.

SODIUM HYALURONATE — TOPICAL

Indications

➤*Cream, gel, and spray:*

Dermal ulcers/wounds/skin irritations/burns – For the dressing and management of partial to full thickness dermal ulcers (eg, pressure sores, venous stasis ulcers, arterial ulcers, diabetic ulcers); wounds, including cuts, abrasions, donor sites, and postoperative incisions; irritations of the skin; and first- and second-degree burns. The dressing is intended to cover a wound or burn on a patient's skin, and protect against abrasion, friction, and desiccation.

➤*Lotion:*

Xerosis – For treatment of symptoms associated with xerosis (dry, scaly skin).

Administration and Dosage

➤*Adults:*

Burns/dermal ulcers/skin irritation/wounds –

Cream, gel, and spray: Apply a thin layer, without extensive rubbing onto the wound surface, 2 or 3 times per day.

Xerosis –

Lotion: Use a liberal amount 2 to 3 times daily or as directed by a physician.

➤*Administration:*

Cream, gel, and spray – The wounds or ulcers should be cleaned and disinfected prior to treatment. In the event of long-standing ulcers, it may be advisable to clean and/or to debride the wound by surgical or enzymatic means prior to treatment. Cover the lesion area with a sterile gauze pad and, if necessary, with an elastic or compressive bandage.

Lotion – Apply to affected area(s) and rub in thoroughly.

➤*Storage/Stability:* Store at room temperature. Cream and gel may be stored for up to 24 months and spray may be stored for up to 36 months under these conditions.

Actions

➤*Pharmacology:* Hyaluronic acid is a naturally occurring polysaccharide of the glycosamin-oglycan family containing repeating disaccharide units of sodium-glucuronate-N-acetyl glucosamine. The exact mechanism of action of hyaluronic acid derivatives is not known.

Contraindications

Known hypersensitivity to this product.

Warnings/Precautions

➤*Prolonged use:* The prolonged use of the product may give rise to sensitization phenomena. Should this happen, discontinue the treatment and follow a suitable therapy.

➤*Cross-infection:* Each tube of hyaluronic acid should be used by one patient only in order to reduce the risk of cross-infection.

➤*Pregnancy: Category C.* Give to a pregnant patient only if clearly needed.

➤*Lactation:* It is not known if topical sodium hyaluronate is excreted in breast milk. Because many drugs are excreted in breast milk, exercise caution when administering the drug to a nursing woman.

Drug Interactions

Do not use concomitantly with disinfectants containing quaternary ammonium salts because hyaluronic acid can precipitate in their presence.

The concomitant topical treatment of wounds with antibiotics or other local agents has never given rise to interactions or incompatibilities with hyaluronic acid.

Adverse Reactions

All suspected adverse reactions occurring during the treatment with hyaluronic acid should be reported to a health care provider.

SODIUM HYALURONATE — TOPICAL

Patient Information

Advise patients to contact their health care provider immediately if the condition worsens .

HYALURONIDASE

Rx	**Vitrase** (ISTA Pharmaceuticals)	**Powder for injection, lyophilized:** 6,200 units (ovine source)	Lactose 5 mg. Preservative free. In single-use 5 mL vials with 1 mL syringe and 5 mcg filter needle.
Rx	**Amphadase** (Amphastar)	**Solution for injection:** 150 units/mL (bovine source)	Contains no more than 0.1 mg thimerosal. In 2 mL vials.
Rx	**Hylenex** (Baxter Anesthesia)	**Solution for injection:** 150 units/mL (recombinant human)	In 1 mL single-dose vials.[b]
Rx	**Vitrase** (ISTA Pharmaceuticals)	**Solution for injection:** 200 units/mL (ovine source)	Lactose 0.93 mg. Preservative free. In single-use 2 mL vials.

[a] With 8.5 mg sodium chloride, 1 mg EDTA, 0.4 mg calcium chloride, monobasic sodium phosphate buffer, sodium hydroxide.

[b] With 8.5 mg sodium chloride, 1.8 mg sodium phosphate dibasic dihydrate, 4.2 mg sodium hydroxide, 1 mg human serum albumin, 1 mg EDTA, 0.4 mg calcium chloride dihydrate.

HYALURONIDASE — INJECTION

Indications

➤*Absorption and dispersion of injected drugs:* As an adjuvant to increase the absorption and dispersion of other injected drugs.

➤*Hypodermoclysis:* For hypodermoclysis.

➤*Subcutaneous urography:* As an adjunct in subcutaneous urography for improving resorption of radiopaque agents.

➤*Off-label uses:* Treatment of vitreous hemorrhage and diabetic retinopathy.

Administration and Dosage

➤*Adults:*

Absorption and dispersion of injected drugs –

Usual dosage: Add 50 to 300 units, most typically 150 units, to the injection solution.

Concomitant therapy:

When epinephrine is injected along with hyaluronidase, observe precautions for the use of epinephrine in cardiovascular disease, thyroid disease, diabetes, digital nerve block, ischemia of the fingers and toes, etc.

Hypodermoclysis –

Usual dosage: 150 units (Vitrase lyophilized powder and Amphadase solution) or 200 units (Vitrase solution) will facilitate absorption of 1,000 mL or more of solution.

Dosage adjustment: Carefully adjust the dose, the rate of injection, and the type of solution (eg, saline, glucose, Ringer's) to the individual patient.

Urography – When IV administration cannot be successfully accomplished, with the patient prone, inject 75 units subcutaneously over each scapula, followed by injection of the contrast medium at the same sites.

➤*Children:*

Hypodermoclysis –

3 years of age and older: May be added to small volumes of solution (up to 200 mL), such as or solutions of drugs for subcutaneous injection.

Younger than 3 years of age: Limit the volume of a single clysis to 200 mL; in premature infants or during the neonatal period, do not exceed a daily dosage of 25 mL/kg of body weight; the rate of administration should not be greater than 2 mL/min. For older patients, the rate and volume of administration should not exceed those employed for IV infusion.

Urography – When IV administration cannot be successfully accomplished, particularly in infants and small children, with the patient prone, inject 75 units subcutaneously over each scapula, followed by injection of the contrast medium at the same sites.

➤*Preparation for administration:*

Lyophilized powder – Reconstitute in the vial to a concentration of 1,000 units/mL of sodium chloride injection by adding 6.2 mL of solution to the vial. Prior to administration, further dilute the reconstituted solution to the desired concentration, commonly 150 units/mL. Use the resulting solution immediately after preparation.

A 1 mL syringe and a 5 micron filter needle are supplied in the hyaluronidase kit. Following reconstitution, apply the 5 micron filter needle to the 1 mL syringe. Draw the desired amount of hyaluronidase into the syringe, and dilute according to the following table. Remove the filter needle and apply a needle appropriate for the intended injection.

Hyaluronidase Dilution

Desired Concentration	Amount of Hyaluronidase Reconstituted Solution (1,000 units/mL)	Additional Sodium Chloride Injection
50 units/mL	0.05 mL	0.95 mL
75 units/mL	0.075 mL	0.925 mL
150 units/mL	0.15 mL	0.85 mL
300 units/mL	0.3 mL	0.7 mL

Hyaluronidase 200 units/mL solution – Draw the desired amount of hyaluronidase into the syringe to obtain the target hyaluronidase activity.

Amount of Hyaluronidase Solution (200 units/mL) Withdrawn Per Target Hyaluronidase Activity

Target hyaluronidase activity (units)	Volume withdrawn from vial (mL)
50 units	0.25 mL
75 units	0.38 mL
150 units	0.75 mL
200 units	1 mL

➤*Administration:* Insert needle with aseptic precautions. With tip lying free and movable between skin and muscle, begin clysis; fluid should start in readily without pain or lump. Then inject hyaluronidase into rubber tubing close to needle. An alternate method is to inject hyaluronidase under the skin prior to clysis.

When solutions devoid of inorganic electrolytes are given by hypodermoclysis, hypovolemia may occur. This may be prevented by using solutions containing adequate amounts of inorganic electrolytes or controlling the volume and speed of administration.

Administer hyaluronidase only as discussed because its effects relative to absorption and dispersion of other drugs are not produced when it is administered intravenously (IV).

➤*Admixture compatibility:* Furosemide, benzodiazepines, and phenytoin have been found to be incompatible.

➤*Storage/Stability:* Store unopened vial of lyophilized powder in refrigerator at 2° to 8°C (35° to 46°F). After reconstitution, store at 20° to 25°C (68° to 77°F), and use within 6 hours. Protect from light. Store unopened vial of solution in refrigerator at 2° to 8°C (35° to 46°F). Protect from light. Do not freeze.

Actions

➤*Pharmacology:* Hyaluronidase is a spreading or diffusing substance that modifies the permeability of connective tissue through the hydrolysis of hyaluronic acid, a polysaccharide found in the intercellular ground substance of connective tissue, and of certain specialized tissues, such as the umbilical cord and vitreous humor. Hyaluronic acid also is present in the capsules of type A and C hemolytic streptococci. Hyaluronidase hydrolyzes hyaluronic acid by splitting the glucosaminidic bond between C_1 of the glucosamine moiety and C_4 of glucuronic acid. This temporarily decreases the viscosity of the cellular cement and promotes diffusion of injected fluids or of localized transudates or exudates, thus facilitating their absorption.

Hyaluronidase cleaves glycosidic bonds of hyaluronic acid and, to a variable degree, some other acid mucopolysaccharides of the connective tissue. The activity is measured in vitro by monitoring the decrease in the amount of an insoluble serum albumen-hyaluronic acid complex as the enzyme cleaves the hyaluronic acid component.

When no spreading factor is present, material injected subcutaneously spreads very slowly, but hyaluronidase causes rapid spreading, provided local interstitial pressure is adequate to furnish the necessary mechanical impulse. Such an impulse normally is initiated by injected solutions. The rate of diffusion is proportionate to the amount of enzyme, and the extent is proportionate to the volume of solution.

Knowledge of the mechanisms involved in the disappearance of injected hyaluronidase is limited. It is known, however, that the blood of a number of mammalian species brings about the inactivation of hyaluronidase. Studies have demonstrated that hyaluronidase is antigenic; repeated injections of relatively large amounts of this enzyme may result in the formation of neutralizing antibodies.

The reconstitution of the dermal barrier removed by intradermal injection of hyaluronidase (20, 2, 0.2, 0.02, and 0.002 units/mL) to adult humans indicated that, at 24 hours, the restoration of the barrier is incomplete and inversely related to the dosage of enzyme; at 48 hours, the barrier is completely restored in all treated areas.

HYALURONIDASE — INJECTION

Results from an experimental study in humans on the influence of hyaluronidase in bone repair support the conclusion that this enzyme alone, in the usual clinical dosage, does not deter bone healing.

Contraindications

Hypersensitivity to hyaluronidase or any other ingredient in the formulation is a contraindication to the use of this product.

Warnings/Precautions

➤*Uses:* Do not use hyaluronidase to enhance the absorption and dispersion of dopamine and/or alpha-agonist drugs.

Do not use hyaluronidase to reduce the swelling of bites or stings.

➤*Infection/skin inflammation:* Do not inject hyaluronidase into or around an infected or acutely inflamed area because of the danger of spreading a localized infection.

➤*Administration:* Do not use hyaluronidase for IV injections because the enzyme is rapidly inactivated.

Do not apply hyaluronidase directly to the cornea.

➤*Skin testing:* A preliminary skin test for hypersensitivity to hyaluronidase can be performed. This skin test is made by an intradermal injection of approximately 0.02 mL solution (3 or 4 units of a 150 or 200 unit/mL solution, respectively). A positive reaction consists of a wheal with pseudopods appearing within 5 minutes and persisting for 20 to 30 minutes and accompanied by localized itching. Transient vasodilation at the site of the test (ie, erythema) is not a positive reaction.

➤*Hypersensitivity reactions:* Discontinue hyaluronidase if sensitization occurs.

➤*Pregnancy: Category C.* No adequate and well-controlled animal studies have been conducted with hyaluronidase to determine reproductive effects. No adequate and well-controlled studies have been conducted with hyaluronidase in pregnant women. Use hyaluronidase during pregnancy only if clearly needed.

Fertility impairment – It has been reported that testicular degeneration may occur with the production of organ-specific antibodies against this enzyme following repeated injections. Human studies on the effect of intravaginal hyaluronidase in sterility caused by oligospermia indicated that hyaluronidase may have aided conception. Thus, it appears that hyaluronidase may not adversely affect fertility in females.

Labor and delivery – Administration of hyaluronidase during labor was reported to cause no complications: no increase in blood loss or differences in cervical trauma were observed. It is not known whether hyaluronidase has an effect on the fetus if used during labor; the effect of hyaluronidase on the later growth, development, and functional maturation of the infant is unknown.

➤*Lactation:* It is not known whether hyaluronidase is excreted in human milk. Because many drugs are excreted in human milk, exercise caution when hyaluronidase is administered to a breast-feeding woman.

➤*Children:* Hyaluronidase may be added to small volumes of solution (up to 200 mL), such as a small clysis for infants or solutions of drugs for subcutaneous injection. Keep in mind the potential for chemical or physical incompatibilities.

For infants and children younger than 3 years of age, limit the volume of a single clysis to 200 mL; in premature infants or during the neonatal period, do not exceed a daily dosage of 25 mL/kg of body weight; the rate of administration should not be greater than 2 mL/min. For older patients, the rate and volume of administration should not exceed those employed for IV infusion.

During hypodermoclysis, take special care in children to avoid overhydration by controlling the rate and total volume of the clysis.

➤*Elderly:* No overall differences in safety or effectiveness have been observed between elderly and younger adult patients.

Drug Interactions

Patients receiving large doses of salicylates, cortisone, adrenocorticotropic hormone (ACTH), estrogens, or antihistamines may require larger amounts of hyaluronidase for equivalent dispersing effect because these drugs apparently render tissues partly resistant to the action of hyaluronidase.

➤*Local anesthetic:* When hyaluronidase is added to a local anesthetic agent, it hastens the onset of analgesia and tends to reduce the swelling caused by local infiltration. However, the wider spread of the local anesthetic solution increases its absorption; this shortens its duration of action and tends to increase the incidence of systemic reaction.

Adverse Reactions

The most frequently reported adverse reactions have been local injection-site reactions. Hyaluronidase has been reported to enhance the adverse reactions associated with coadministered drug products. Edema has been reported most frequently in association with hypodermoclysis. Allergic reactions (eg, urticaria, angioedema) have been reported in less than 0.1% of patients receiving hyaluronidase. Anaphylactic-like reactions following retrobulbar block or IV injections have occurred rarely.

Overdosage

➤*Symptoms:* Symptoms of toxicity consist of local edema or urticaria, erythema, chills, nausea, vomiting, dizziness, tachycardia, and hypotension.

➤*Treatment:* Discontinue the enzyme and initiate supportive measures immediately.

CALCIUM HYDROXYLAPATITE

Rx	**Radiesse** (BioForm Medical[a])	**Implant; subcutaneous:** calcium hydroxylapatite[b]	In 1.3 and 0.3 mL single-use prefilled syringes.

[a] BioForm Medical, 1875 S. Grant St., Suite 110, San Mateo, CA 94402; 650-286-4000, 866-862-1211; http://www.bioform.com.

[b] Particle size range is 25 to 45 microns.

CALCIUM HYDROXYLAPATITE — IMPLANT

Indications

➤*Facial fat loss (lipoatrophy):* For the restoration and/or correction of the signs of facial fat loss (lipoatrophy) in persons with HIV.

➤*Facial wrinkles and folds:* For subdermal implantation for the correction of moderate to severe facial wrinkles and folds, such as nasolabial folds.

Administration and Dosage

➤*Adults:*

Facial wrinkles and folds and facial fat loss (lipoatrophy) –

Usual dosage: The amount injected will vary depending on the site and extent of the restoration or augmentation desired.

➤*Preparation for administration:* The following are required for the percutaneous injection procedure: calcium hydroxylapatite syringe(s) and 25- to 27-gauge needle with Luer-lock fittings.

Prepare patient for percutaneous injection using standard methods. The treatment injection site should be marked and prepared with a suitable antiseptic. Local or topical anesthesia at the injection site should be used at the discretion of the health care provider.

Prepare the syringes and the injection needle(s) before the percutaneous injection. A new injection needle may be used for each syringe, or the same injection needle may be connected to each new syringe.

Remove the foil pouch from the carton. Open the foil pouch by tearing at the notches (marked 1 and 2), and remove the syringe from the foil pouch. There is a small amount of moisture normally present inside the foil pouch for sterilization purposes; this is not an indication of a defective product.

Remove the Luer syringe cap from the distal end of the syringe prior to attaching the needle. The syringe can then be twisted onto the Luer-lock fitting of the needle. The needle must be tightened securely to the syringe and primed with calcium hydroxylapatite. If excess is on the surface of the Luer-lock fittings, it will need to be wiped clean with sterile gauze. Slowly push the syringe plunger until calcium hydroxylapatite extrudes from the end of the needle. If leakage is noted at the Luer fitting, it may be necessary to tighten the needle or remove the needle and clean the surfaces of the Luer fitting or, in extreme cases, replace both the syringe and the needle.

➤*Administration:* Locate the initial site for the implant. Scar tissue and cartilage may be difficult or impossible to treat. If possible, avoid passing through these tissue types when advancing the injection needle.

Inject subdermally. Use a 1:1 correction factor. No overcorrection is needed.

Insert the needle with bevel down at approximately a 30° angle to the skin. The needle should slide under the dermis to the point you wish to begin the injection. This should be easily palpable with the nondominant hand.

If significant resistance is encountered when pushing the plunger, the injection needle may be moved slightly to allow easier placement of the material, or it may be necessary to change the injection needle. One needle jam occurred in the nasolabial fold clinical study. Needle jams are more likely with use of needles smaller than 27 gauges.

Advance the needle into the subdermis to the starting location. Carefully push the plunger of the syringe to start the injection and slowly inject the calcium hydroxylapatite material in linear threads while withdrawing the needle. Continue placing additional lines of material until the desired level of correction is achieved.

Apply slow, continuous, even pressure to the syringe plunger to inject the implant as you withdraw the needle. The implant material should be completely surrounded by soft tissue without leaving globular deposits. The injected area may be massaged as needed to achieve even distribution of the implant.

➤*Storage/Stability:* Store between 15° and 32°C (59° and 90°F). When stored at these temperatures, the expiration date is 2 years from the manufacture date. Do not use if the expiration date has been exceeded.

Actions

➤*Pharmacology:* Calcium hydroxylapatite stimulates the body to produce new collagen, correcting facial wrinkles.

Contraindications

Severe allergies manifested by a history of anaphylaxis, history or presence of multiple severe allergies, known hypersensitivity to any of the components, known susceptibility to keloid formation or hypertrophic scarring.

CALCIUM HYDROXYLAPATITE — IMPLANT

Warnings/Precautions

➤*Inflammation/Infection:* Use of calcium hydroxylapatite in any person with active skin inflammation or infection in or near the treatment area should be deferred until the inflammatory or infectious process has been controlled.

➤*Local reactions:* Injection procedure reactions to calcium hydroxylapatite have been observed and consisted mainly of short-term (ie, less than 7 days) bruising, redness, and swelling. Refer to the Adverse Reactions section for details.

➤*Administration:* Take special care to avoid injection into the blood vessels. An introduction into the vasculature may occlude the vessels and could cause infarction or embolism.

Calcium hydroxylapatite is packaged for single-patient use. Do not resterilize. Do not use if package is opened or damaged. Do not use if the syringe end cap or syringe plunger is not in place.

Calcium hydroxylapatite should only be used by health care providers with expertise in the correction of volume deficiencies in patients with HIV after fully familiarizing themselves with the product, the product educational materials, and the entire package insert.

Do not overcorrect (overfill) a contour deficiency because the depression should gradually improve within several weeks as the treatment effect of calcium hydroxylapatite occurs.

As with all transcutaneous procedures, calcium hydroxylapatite injection carries a risk of infection. Follow standard precautions associated with injectable materials.

Observe universal precautions when there is a potential for contact with patient body fluids. Conduct the injection session with aseptic technique.

After use, treatment syringes and needles may be potential biohazards. Handle accordingly and dispose of in accordance with accepted medical practice and applicable local, state, and federal requirements.

➤*Use in lips:* The safety and effectiveness of calcium hydroxylapatite for use in lips have not been established. There have been published reports of nodules associated with the use of calcium hydroxylapatite injected into lips.

➤*CT scans/radiography:* The particles of calcium hydroxylapatite are radiopaque and clearly visible on CT scans and may be visible in standard, plain radiography. In a radiographic study of 58 patients, there was no indication that calcium hydroxylapatite potentially masked abnormal tissues or being interpreted as tumors in CT scans. Inform patients of the radiopaque nature of calcium hydroxylapatite so they can inform their primary health care provider as well as radiologists.

➤*Long-term use:* Long-term safety and effectiveness of calcium hydroxylapatite beyond 1 year have not been investigated in clinical trials.

➤*Keloid formation/hypertrophic scarring:* The safety of calcium hydroxylapatite in patients with increased susceptibility to keloid formation and hypertrophic scarring has not been studied.

➤*Periorbital area:* Safety and effectiveness of calcium hydroxylapatite in the periorbital area have not been established.

➤*Photosensitivity:* Inform the patient that he or she should minimize exposure of the treated area to extensive sun or heat exposure for approximately 24 hours after treatment or until any initial swelling and redness have resolved.

➤*Pregnancy:* Safety of calcium hydroxylapatite for use during pregnancy has not been established.

➤*Lactation:* Safety of calcium hydroxylapatite for use in breast-feeding women has not been established.

➤*Children:* Safety of calcium hydroxylapatite in patients younger than 18 years of age has not been established.

Drug Interactions

➤*Anticoagulants:* Patients who are using medications that can prolong bleeding (eg, aspirin, warfarin) may, as with any injection, experience increased bruising or bleeding at the injection site.

Adverse Reactions

➤*Nasolabial folds:* The following tables contain adverse reactions for 117 patients in a randomized, controlled study at 4 US investigational sites. Patients in the study received calcium hydroxylapatite in 1 side of the face and a collagen dermal implant as the control in the other side of the face. Adverse reactions reported in patient diaries during the 14 days after treatment are listed in the first 2 tables. Health care provider–reported adverse reactions are those reported by investigators and patients any time outside the 2-week diaries. Those adverse reactions are presented in the last 2 tables.

Calcium Hydroxylapatite for Nasolabial Folds: Patient-Reported Adverse Reactions Occurring During the 14 Days Posttreatment (N = 117)

Adverse reaction	Calcium hydroxylapatite	Control
Dermatologic		
Ecchymosis	63.2%	42.7%
Erythema	66.7%	71.8%
Pruritus	18%	20.5%
Miscellaneous		
Edema	69.2%	53%
Nodule	0.9%	0.9%
Pain	28.2%	22.2%
Other[a]	29.9%	22.2%

[a] Other adverse reactions for both calcium hydroxylapatite and control include contour irregularity, irritation, numbness, soreness, and tenderness. None of the reports of contour irregularities was determined to be nodules or granulomas.

Calcium Hydroxylapatite for Nasolabial Folds: Health Care Provider–Reported Adverse Reactions Occurring During the 14 Days Posttreatment (N = 117)

Adverse reaction	Calcium hydroxylapatite	Control	Calcium hydroxylapatite				Control			
	Total reporting symptoms		1 to 3 days	4 to 7 days	8 to 14 days	≥14 days	1 to 3 days	4 to 7 days	8 to 14 days	≥14 days
Dermatologic										
Ecchymosis	60.3%	39.7%	10.6%	24.5%	21.9%	3.3%	9.9%	19.2%	7.9%	2.6%
Erythema	45.1%	54.9%	16.7%	11.2%	8.2%	9%	19.3%	15%	6.9%	13.7%
Pruritus	47.1%	52.9%	29.4%	9.8%	5.9%	2%	21.6%	19.6%	5.9%	5.9%
Miscellaneous										
Edema	54.5%	45.5%	17.8%	22.5%	8.9%	5.2%	17.8%	20.4%	5.2%	2.1%
Nodule	50%	50%	0%	0%	0%	50%	0%	0%	0%	50%
Pain	54.8%	45.2%	30.1%	17.8%	5.5%	1.4%	27.4%	13.7%	2.7%	1.4%
Other	56.5%	43.5%	16.3%	18.5%	8.7%	13%	8.7%	10.9%	12%	12%

Calcium Hydroxylapatite for Nasolabial Folds: Health Care Provider–Reported Adverse Reactions Occurring After 14 Days Posttreatment (≥ 1 Adverse Reaction) (N = 117)

Adverse reaction	Calcium hydroxylapatite	Control
Dermatologic		
Ecchymosis	0%	1.7%
Erythema	5.1%	7.7%
Pruritus	0.9%	1.7%

Calcium Hydroxylapatite for Nasolabial Folds: Health Care Provider–Reported Adverse Reactions Occurring After 14 Days Posttreatment (≥ 1 Adverse Reaction) (N = 117)

Adverse reaction	Calcium hydroxylapatite	Control
Miscellaneous		
Edema	4.3%	3.4%
Nodule	0%	1.7%
Pain	1.7%	0.9%
Other[a]	2.6%	2.6%

[a] Other adverse reactions for both calcium hydroxylapatite and control include contour irregularity, irritation, numbness, soreness, and tenderness. None of the reports of contour irregularities was determined to be nodules or granulomas.

CALCIUM HYDROXYLAPATITE — IMPLANT

Calcium Hydroxylapatite for Nasolabial Folds: Health Care Provider–Reported Adverse Reactions Occurring After 14 Days Posttreatment										
	Calcium hydroxylapatite	Control	Calcium hydroxylapatite				Control			
Adverse reaction	Total reporting symptoms		1 to 3 days	4 to 7 days	8 to 14 days	≥14 days	1 to 3 days	4 to 7 days	8 to 14 days	≥14 days
Dermatologic										
Ecchymosis	0%	100%	0%	0%	0%	0%	0%	50%	50%	0%
Erythema	42.9%	57.1%	19%	9.5%	9.5%	4.8%	9.5%	14.3%	19%	14.3%
Pruritus	33.3%	66.7%	0%	0%	33.3%	0%	33.3%	0%	33.3%	0%
Miscellaneous										
Edema	41.7%	58.3%	41.7%	0%	0%	0%	41.7%	0%	0%	16.7%
Needle jamming	100%	0%	100%	0%	0%	0%	0%	0%	0%	0%
Nodule	0%	100%	0%	0%	0%	0%	0%	0%	33.3%	66.7%
Pain	75%	25%	25%	25%	0%	25%	25%	0%	0%	0%
Other	50%	50%	12.5%	0%	25%	12.5%	12.5%	12.5%	0%	25%

➤*HIV-associated facial lipoatrophy:* Adverse reactions reported after calcium hydroxylapatite treatments from a prospective, open-label study of 100 patients at 3 US sites are provided in the following tables. Adverse reactions reported in patient diaries during the 14 days after treatment are listed in the first 2 tables. Health care provider–reported adverse reactions are those reported by investigators and patients any time outside the 2-week diaries. Those adverse reactions are presented in the last 2 tables.

Calcium Hydroxylapatite for HIV-Associated Facial Lipoatrophy: Patient-Reported Adverse Reactions During the 14 Days Posttreatment (N = 100)			
Adverse reaction	Mild	Moderate	Severe
Dermatologic			
Ecchymosis	53.1%	39.1%	7.8%
Erythema	58.2	41.8%	0%
Pruritus	85.7%	14.3%	0%
Miscellaneous			
Edema	46.5%	49.5%	4%
Pain	64.9%	35.1%	0%
Other[a]	62.8%	34.9%	2.3%

[a] Other adverse reactions were those reported that did not fit into the categories detailed in the previous tables. The most common other adverse reaction was contour irregularities. Additional other adverse reactions included burning sensation, dryness, peeling, numbness, rash, and whiteheads.

Calcium Hydroxylapatite for HIV-Associated Facial Lipoatrophy: Duration of the Adverse Reactions Occurring During the 14 Days Posttreatment				
Adverse reaction	1 to 3 days	4 to 7 days	8 to 14 days	>14 days
Dermatologic				
Ecchymosis	20.4%	35.9%	35.2%	8.5%
Erythema	54.3%	32.9%	10.5%	2.4%
Pruritus	51.9%	16.7%	11.1%	20.4%
Miscellaneous				
Edema	47.7%	35.6%	12.1%	4.7%
Pain	49.1%	29.1%	16.4%	5.5%
Other	35.7%	17%	16.1%	31.3%

Calcium Hydroxylapatite for HIV-Associated Facial Lipoatrophy: Severity of Local Adverse Reactions per Health Care Provider (N = 100)			
Adverse reaction	Mild	Moderate	Severe
Dermatologic			
Ecchymosis	66.7%	33.3%	0%
Erythema	100%	0%	0%
Miscellaneous			
Edema	100%	0%	0%
Pain	50%	0%	50%
Other[a]	76.9%	23.1%	0%

[a] Other adverse reactions were those reported that did not fit into the categories detailed in the tables above. The most common other adverse reaction was contour irregularities. Additional other adverse reactions included burning sensation, dryness, peeling, numbness, rash, and whiteheads.

Calcium Hydroxylapatite for HIV-Associated Facial Lipoatrophy: Duration of the Health Care Provider–Reported Adverse Reactions				
Adverse reaction	1 to 3 days	4 to 7 days	8 to 14 days	>14 days
Dermatologic				
Ecchymosis	60%	0%	40%	0%
Erythema	25%	50%	0%	25%
Miscellaneous				
Edema	76.9%	7.7%	7.7%	7.7%
Pain	50%	0%	50%	0%
Other	43.5%	0%	1.6%	54.8%

Patient Information

Inform patients to minimize exposure of the treated area to extensive sun or heat exposure for approximately 24 hours after treatment or until any initial swelling and redness have resolved.

POLY-L-LACTIC ACID

Rx	**Sculptra** (Dermik Laboratories)	**Powder for injection** (freeze dried)	Single-use vials.

POLY-L-LACTIC ACID — INJECTION

Indications

➤*Facial fat loss (lipoatrophy):* For restoration and/or correction of the signs of facial fat loss (lipoatrophy) in people with human immunodeficiency virus.

Administration and Dosage

➤*Adults:*

Facial fat loss (lipoatrophy) – A typical treatment course for severe facial fat loss involves 3 to 6 injection sessions, with the sessions separated by 2 or more weeks. Full effects of the treatment course are evident within weeks to months. Reevaluate the patient no sooner than 2 weeks after each injection session to determine if additional correction is needed. Advise patients that supplemental injection sessions may be required to maintain an optimal treatment effect.

➤*Preparation for administration:* The following supplies are used with poly-L-lactic acid but are to be provided by the end-user: sterile water for injection (SWFI), single-use 5 mL sterile syringe, single-use 1 to 3 mL (depending on physician practitioner preference) sterile syringes (at least 2), 18-gauge sterile needles (at least 2), 26-gauge sterile needles (several should be available), and antiseptic.

Reconstitution

1.) Remove the flip-off cap from the vial and clean the penetrable stopper of the vial with an antiseptic. If the vial, seal, or flip-off cap are damaged, do not use, and call the manufacturer.
2.) Attach an 18-gauge sterile needle to a sterile, single-use 5 mL syringe.
3.) Draw 3 to 5 mL SWFI into the 5 mL syringe.
4.) Introduce the 18-gauge sterile needle into the stopper of the vial and slowly add all SWFI into the vial.
5.) Let the vial stand for at least 2 hours to ensure complete hydration; do not shake during this period.
6.) After waiting at least 2 hours, agitate the vial until a uniform translucent suspension is obtained. A single vial swirling agitator may be used. Agitate product immediately prior to use.
7.) Clean the penetrable stopper of the vial with an antiseptic, and use a new, 18-gauge sterile needle to withdraw an appropriate amount of the suspension (typically 1 mL) into a single-use 1 to 3 mL sterile syringe. Do not store the reconstituted product in the syringe.
8.) Replace the 18-gauge needle with a 26-gauge sterile needle before injecting the product into the deep dermis or subcutaneous layer. Do not inject poly-L-lactic acid using needles of an internal diameter smaller than 26-gauge. 9. To withdraw remaining contents of the vial, repeat steps 6 through 8.

POLY-L-LACTIC ACID — INJECTION

➤*Administration:*

Needle for injections – Inject using a 26-gauge sterile needle. Do not inject with needles smaller than 26-gauge and do not bend the needle. Agitate the product in the syringe as needed to maintain a uniform suspension throughout the procedure. Before injecting, expel some drops of the product from the prepared syringe with 26-gauge needle attached to eliminate air and to check for needle blockage. If the 26-gauge needle becomes occluded or dull during an injection session, replacement may be necessary. Draw a small amount of air into the syringe between needle changes to assist in removing clogged particles.

Dermal plane – Inject into the deep dermis or subcutaneous layer to avoid superficial injections. In order to control the injection depth of poly-L-lactic acid, stretch and pull the skin opposite to the direction of the injection to create a firm injection surface. Introduce the 26-gauge sterile needle, bevel up, into the skin at an angle of approximately 30 to 40 degrees, until the desired skin depth is reached. A change in tissue resistance is evident when the needle traverses the dermal-subcutaneous junction. If the needle is inserted at too shallow an angle (ie, into the mid or superficial [papillary] dermis), the bevel of the needle may be visible through the skin. If the product is injected too superficially, it will be evident as immediate or slightly delayed blanching in the injected area. If this occurs, remove the needle and gently massage the treatment area.

Injecting: threading or tunneling –

Technique: When the appropriate dermal plane is reached, lower the needle angle to advance the needle in that dermal plane. Prior to depositing poly-L-lactic acid in the skin, perform a reflux maneuver to ensure that a blood vessel has not been entered. Using the threading or tunneling technique, deposit a thin trail of poly-L-lactic acid in the tissue plane as the needle is withdrawn. To avoid deposition in the superficial skin, stop deposition before the needle bevel is visible in the skin.

Volume per injection: Limit the volume of poly-L-lactic acid to approximately 0.1 to 0.2 mL per each individual injection. Note that in areas such as the cheek, approximately 20 injections may be required to cover the targeted area.

Volume per treatment area: The volume of product injected per treatment area will vary depending on the surface area to be treated. Treatment of an entire cheek typically requires injection of 1 vial of poly-L-lactic acid per cheek per injection session. Multiple injections (typically administered in a grid or cross-hatched pattern) may be required to cover the targeted area. The total number of injections and, thus, total volume of poly-L-lactic acid injected will vary based on the surface area to be corrected, not on the depth or severity of the deficiency to be corrected.

Depot injection –

Technique: The depot technique is most appropriate for injections into areas of thin skin at the level of the upper zygoma or temples. When using this technique, poly-L-lactic acid is injected as a small bolus. For the upper zygoma, it is injected under the orbicularis oculi muscle. For the temples, it is injected in the temporal fascia.

Volume per injection: Reduce the volume to approximately 0.05 mL/injection. Following each injection, massage the area.

Massage during the injection session – Periodically massage the treatment areas during the injection session to evenly distribute the product.

Degree of correction – The depressed area should never be overcorrected (overfilled) in an injection session. Limited correction of the treatment area allows for the gradual improvement of the depressed area over several weeks as the treatment effect occurs. Typically, patients will experience some degree of edema associated with the injection procedure itself, which will give the appearance of a full correction by the end of the injection session (within approximately 30 minutes). Inform the patient that the injection-related edema typically resolves in several hours to a few days, resulting in the reappearance of the original contour deficiency.

Posttreatment care – Immediately following an injection session, redness, swelling, or bruising may be noted in the treatment area. After the injection session, apply an ice pack (avoiding any direct contact of the ice with the skin) to the treatment area in order to reduce swelling. It is important to thoroughly massage the treatment area to evenly distribute the product. Instruct the patient to periodically massage the treatment area for several days after the injection session to promote a natural-looking correction.

Posttreatment assessment – During the first injection session with poly-L-lactic acid, only a limited correction should be made. Do not overcorrect (overfill). Evaluate the patient no sooner than 2 weeks after the injection session to determine if additional correction is needed. The original skin depression may initially reappear, but the depression should gradually improve within several weeks as the treatment effect of poly-L-lactic acid occurs. Advise the patient of the potential need for additional injection sessions at the first consultation.

➤*Storage / Stability:* Store up to 30°C (86°F). Do not freeze. Refrigeration is not required. Each vial of poly-L-lactic acid is packaged for single-use only. Do not resterilize. Store at room temperature up to 30°C (86°F) during and after hydration. The reconstituted product is usable within 72 hours of reconstitution. Discard any material remaining after use or after 72 hours following reconstitution.

Contraindications

Hypersensitivity to any of the components of the product.

Warnings/Precautions

➤*Skin inflammation / infection:* Defer use of poly-L-lactic acid in any person with active skin inflammation or infection in or near the treatment area until the inflammatory or infectious process has been controlled.

➤*Administration:* Poly-L-lactic acid should only be used by health care providers with expertise in the correction of volume deficiencies in patients with human immunodeficiency virus after fully familiarizing themselves with the product, the product educational materials, and the entire package insert.

Use poly-L-lactic acid in the deep dermis or subcutaneous layer. Avoid superficial injections. Take special care when using poly-L-lactic acid in areas of thin skin.

Safety and effectiveness of treatment in the periorbital area have not been established.

Do not overcorrect (overfill) a contour deficiency because the depression should gradually improve within several weeks as the treatment effect of poly-L-lactic acid occurs.

Take special care to avoid injection into the blood vessels. An introduction into the vasculature may occlude the vessels and could cause infarction or embolism.

As with all injections, patients treated with anticoagulants may run the risk of a hematoma or localized bleeding at the injection site.

➤*Local effects:* Injection procedure reactions to poly-L-lactic acid have been observed, consisting mainly of hematoma, bruising, edema, discomfort, inflammation, and erythema. The most common device-related adverse effect was the delayed occurrence of subcutaneous papules, which were confined to the injection site and were typically palpable, asymptomatic, and nonvisible.

➤*Keloid formation or hypertrophic scarring:* The safety of using poly-L-lactic acid in patients with increased susceptibility to keloid formation and hypertrophic scarring has not been studied. Dermik will conduct a post-approval study to determine the likelihood of keloid formation and hypertrophic scars in patients with human immunodeficiency virus receiving poly-L-lactic acid injections.

➤*Long-term use:* Long-term safety and effectiveness of poly-L-lactic acid beyond 2 years have not been investigated. Dermik is conducting a postapproval study to evaluate the safety and effectiveness of poly-L-lactic acid beyond 2 years.

➤*Risk of infection:* As with all transcutaneous procedures, poly-L-lactic acid injection carries a risk of infection. Follow standard precautions associated with injectable materials.

➤*Photosensitivity:* Inform the patient that he or she should minimize exposure of the treatment area to excessive sun and UV lamp exposure until any initial swelling and redness has resolved.

➤*Pregnancy:* *Category undetermined.*

The safety of poly-L-lactic acid for use during pregnancy has not been established.

➤*Lactation:* The safety of poly-L-lactic acid for use in breast-feeding females has not been established.

➤*Children:* The safety of poly-L-lactic acid for use in patients younger than 18 years of age has not been established.

Drug Interactions

No studies of interactions of poly-L-lactic acid with drugs or other substances or implants have been made.

Adverse Reactions

Adverse event data from 4 clinical studies that included 277 patients are summarized in the following tables.

Poly-L-Lactic Acid Adverse Events Observed in Clinical Studies with 2-Year Follow-Up

	VEGA study (N = 50)	C&W study[c] (N = 29)	Average duration (days)
Injection procedure-related adverse events			
Bruising	3 (6%)	11(38%)	6
Discomfort	0	3 (10%)	3
Edema	2 (4%)	2 (7%)	3
Erythema	0	3 (10%)	3
Hematoma	14 (28%)	0	17
Inflammation	0	3 (10%)	3
Device-related adverse events			Average onset[b] (months)
Injection-site subcutaneous papule[a]	26 (52%)	9 (31%)	7

[a] Subcutaneous papules refer to lesions of 5 mm or less, typically palpable, asymptomatic, and nonvisible.
[b] Onset data available from VEGA study only. Duration not noted for subcutaneous papules because most were ongoing at study completion.
[c] Safety data were collected post hoc for 27 of the patients at approximately 2 years from study start.

POLY-L-LACTIC ACID — INJECTION

Poly-L-Lactic Acid Adverse Events Observed in Clinical Studies with 1-Year Follow-Up		
	APEX 002 study (N = 99)	Blue Pacific study (N = 99)
Injection procedure-related adverse events		
Bruising	1 (1%)	30 (30%)
Discomfort	19 (19%)	15 (15%)
Edema	3 (3%)	17 (17%)
Erythema	0	3 (3%)
Device-related adverse events		
Injection-site subcutaneous papule	6 (6%)	13 (13%)

The duration of the adverse events in the table above was not collected. The most common device-related adverse effect was the delayed occurrence of subcutaneous papules, which were confined to the injection site and were typically palpable, asymptomatic, and nonvisible. The study protocols did not include evaluation of treatment for subcutaneous papules; therefore, no information is available on how the papules were treated. In the VEGA study, the average onset of subcutaneous papules was 7 months after initial injection (range, 0.3 to 25 months). Subcutaneous papules resolved spontaneously in 6 of 26 patients (24%) during the study. No information of onset and duration of papules is available from the Chelsea & Westminster study.

Treatment-related adverse events, not included in the previous 2 tables, observed in clinical studies with a frequency of less than 5% were fever, injection-site bleeding, injection-site induration, injection-site infection, injection-site lesion, and injection-site tenderness.

➤*Postmarketing:*

CNS – Fatigue, lack of effectiveness, malaise.

Dermatologic – Application-site discharge, ectropion, hypertrophy of skin, injection-site abscess, injection-site atrophy, injection-site fat atrophy, injection-site granuloma, injection-site reaction, skin rash, skin roughness, telangiectasias, visible nodules with or without inflammation or dyspigmentation.

Miscellaneous – Aching joints, allergic reaction, angioedema, brittle nails, colitis not otherwise specified, hair breakage, hypersensitivity reaction, photosensitivity reaction, Quincke edema.

Patient Information

To report any adverse reactions, call the manufacturer.

Within the first 24 hours, patients should apply an ice pack (avoiding any direct contact of the ice with the skin) to the treatment area to reduce swelling. Poly-L-lactic acid may cause redness, swelling, or bruising when first injected into the skin, typically resolving in hours to 1 week. Hematoma also may occur, typically resolving in hours to approximately 2 weeks. Instruct patients to report worsening or prolonged symptoms or signs to the health care provider. The original skin depression may initially reappear, but the depression should gradually improve within several weeks as the treatment effect of poly-L-lactic acid occurs. The health care provider will assess the need for additional poly-L-lactic acid injection sessions after 2 or more weeks.

Instruct patients to massage the treatment area daily, for several days following any injection session.

Treatment with poly-L-lactic acid can result in small papules in the treatment area. These subcutaneous papules are typically not visible and asymptomatic and may be noticed only upon pressing on the treatment area. However, visible nodules, sometimes with redness or color change to the skin, have been reported. Advise patients to report any side effects to their health care provider.

Make-up may be applied a few hours posttreatment if no complications are present (eg, open wounds, bleeding, redness, swelling).

Instruct patients to minimize exposure of the treatment area to excessive sun and UV lamp exposure until any initial swelling and redness has resolved.

BOTULINUM TOXINS

Botulinum Toxin Type A

BOTULINUM TOXIN TYPE A

Rx	Botox (Allergan)	**Injection, lyophilized powder for solution:** 100 units of onabotulinumtoxinA[a]	Preservative free. Albumin (human) 0.5 mg, sodium chloride 0.9 mg. In single-use vials.
		200 units of onabotulinumtoxinA[a]	Preservative free. Albumin (human) 1 mg, sodium chloride 1.8 mg. In single-use vials.
Rx	Botox Cosmetic (Allergan)	**Injection, lyophilized powder for solution:** 50 units of onabotulinumtoxinA[a]	Preservative free. Albumin (human) 0.25 mg, sodium chloride 0.45 mg. In single-use vials.
		100 units of onabotulinumtoxinA[a]	Preservative free. Albumin (human) 0.5 mg, sodium chloride 0.9 mg. In single-use vials.
Rx	Dysport (Tercica)	**Injection, lyophilized powder for solution:** 300 units of abobotulinumtoxinA[a]	Preservative free. Albumin (human) 125 mcg, lactose 2.5 mg. In single-use vials.
		500 units of abobotulinumtoxinA[a]	Preservative free. Albumin (human) 125 mcg, lactose 2.5 mg. In single-use vials.
Rx	Xeomin (Merz Pharma)	**Injection, lyophilized powder for solution:** 50 units of incobotulinumtoxinA[a]	Preservative free. Albumin (human) 1 mg, sucrose 4.7 mg. In single-use vials.
		100 units of incobotulinumtoxinA[a]	Preservative free. Albumin (human) 1 mg, sucrose 4.7 mg. In single-use vials.

[a] 1 unit corresponds to the calculated median lethal dose (LD_{50}) in mice when injected intraperitoneally.

BOTULINUM TOXIN TYPE A — INJECTION

WARNING

Botulinum toxin effect – Postmarketing reports indicate that the effects of all botulinum toxin products may spread from the area of injection to produce symptoms consistent with botulinum toxin effects. These may include asthenia, generalized muscle weakness, diplopia, blurred vision, ptosis, dysphagia, dysphonia, dysarthria, urinary incontinence, and breathing difficulties. These symptoms have been reported hours to weeks after injection. Swallowing and breathing difficulties can be life-threatening, and there have been reports of death. The risk of symptoms is probably greatest in children treated for spasticity, but symptoms can also occur in adults treated for spasticity and other conditions, particularly in those patients who have underlying conditions that would predispose them to these symptoms. In unapproved uses, including spasticity in children and adults, and in approved indications, cases of spread of effect have been reported at doses comparable with those used to treat cervical dystonia and at lower doses.

Indications

➤*Axillary hyperhidrosis (Botox only):* For the treatment of severe primary axillary hyperhidrosis that is inadequately managed with topical agents.

➤*Blepharospasm (Xeomin only):* For the treatment of adults with blepharospasm who were previously treated with *Botox*.

➤*Cervical dystonia (Botox, Dysport, and Xeomin only):* For the treatment of cervical dystonia in adults to decrease the severity of abnormal head position and neck pain in botulinum toxin–naive and previously treated patients.

➤*Chronic migraine (Botox only):* For the prophylaxis of headaches in adult patients with chronic migraine (at least 15 days per month with headache lasting 4 hours a day or longer).

➤*Glabellar lines (Botox Cosmetic and Dysport only):* For the temporary improvement in the appearance of moderate to severe glabellar lines associated with corrugator and/or procerus muscle activity in adults 65 years of age and younger.

➤*Strabismus and blepharospasm associated with dystonia (Botox only):* For the treatment of strabismus and blepharospasm associated with dystonia, including benign essential blepharospasm or VII nerve disorders in patients 12 years of age and older.

➤*Upper limb spasticity (Botox only):* For the treatment of upper limb spasticity in adults, to decrease the severity of increased muscle tone in elbow flexors (biceps), wrist flexors (flexor carpi radialis and flexor carpi ulnaris), and finger flexors (flexor digitorum profundus and flexor digitorum sublimis).

➤*Off-label uses:*

Achalasia – [1] = Good documentation. Botulinum toxin is safe and effective for the majority of patients with achalasia and has been recommended for this use by the American College of Gastroenterology for patients who

BOTULINUM TOXIN TYPE A — INJECTION

are at high surgical risk or refuse pneumatic dilatation and surgical myotomy. The primary disadvantage with botulinum toxin for this use is that repeat injections after 6 to 12 months are commonly needed, and the long-term efficacy and safety are not well studied beyond 2 years.

Acquired nystagmus – [4] = Insufficient documentation. Botulinum toxin type A has been found to be objectively and subjectively effective in treating acquired nystagmus and its consequent oscillopsia and impaired vision in a few small case series and case reports. Botulinum toxin type A may be useful in certain patients who have contraindications to other therapies, but it cannot be recommended for routine symptomatic treatment of acquired nystagmus until data from controlled studies enrolling larger numbers of patients can confirm its efficacy and long-term safety.

Cosmetic use (facial lines and wrinkles) – [2] = Fair documentation. Local botulinum toxin injections are approved for the temporary improvement of glabellar lines and appear to be an effective treatment for cosmetic reversal of other types of facial wrinkles. The drug should not be used during pregnancy and/or breast-feeding. Avoid concurrent use with other drugs that affect neurotransmission.

Gustatory sweating (Frey syndrome) – [1] = Good documentation. Local botulinum toxin injections have been very effective in significantly reducing and abolishing gustatory sweating in adult postparotidectomy patients. Onset of action is quick, producing beneficial effects within 1 to 3 days, and sustained effects have been achieved after single injections for up to several months (approximately 27). Reinjection in patients with recurrence has also resulted in similar duration of response.

Hand dystonia – [2] = Fair documentation. Botulinum toxin is safe and effective for the majority of patients with primary dystonia of the hand and has been recommended for consideration for this use by the European Federation of Neurological Societies/Movement Disorder Society-European Section Task Force. Other drug therapies are generally not effective and produce intolerable adverse effects. Larger controlled trials are needed to document optimal dosing, administration techniques, frequency of repeat treatments, and effects of long-term use. Treatment is rarely continued beyond 2 years.

Headache (tension-type) – [4] = Insufficient documentation. The use of botulinum toxin for the treatment of tension-type headache has demonstrated benefit in several noncontrolled settings; however, full publication of data from controlled settings has been conflicting. Data from abstract presentations suggest that this drug may have some benefit.

Hyperhidrosis (palmar) – [2] = Fair documentation. Local botulinum toxin injections appear to be effective for hyperhidrosis of the palms.

Sialorrhea (drooling) in adults – [4] = Insufficient documentation. The use of botulinum toxin for decreasing or controlling severe sialorrhea has been studied in a variety of patients, mostly in noncontrolled settings. Although initial data suggest some benefit, particularly in patients who are unresponsive to anticholinergic therapy, additional information is needed for the expected duration of response, potential candidates, and optimal dosing regimens. Standardization of injection procedures is also needed.

Sialorrhea (drooling) in children – [4] = Insufficient documentation. The use of botulinum toxin type A for decreasing or controlling severe sialorrhea has been studied in approximately 100 children, mostly in noncontrolled settings. Additional information is needed to determine the expected duration of response, potential candidates, and optimal dosing regimens. Standardization of injection procedures also is needed.

Spasticity of cerebral palsy (children/adolescents) – [3] = Safety concerns. Data in children are conflicting. The duration of response is typically 3 to 4 months, and some experts recommend dosing no more frequently than every 3 months. Because the different formulations of botulinum toxin type A are not bioequivalent, caution should be exercised in determining the appropriate dose. The potential for severe generalized weakness should also be considered.

Tourette syndrome – [2] = Fair documentation. Initial data suggest that botulinum toxin A may be beneficial in the treatment of patients with Tourette syndrome.

Other possible off-label uses – Treatment of hemifacial spasms, spasmodic torticollis (ie, clonic twisting of the head), oromandibular dystonia, spasmodic dysphonia (laryngeal dystonia), and for other dystonias (eg, focal task-specific dystonias). Botulinum toxin is being assessed in the treatment of head and neck tremor unresponsive to pharmacologic therapy.

Other reported uses of botulinum toxin type A include the following: oscillopsia, tremor, tics, detrusor sphincter dyssynergia, anismus/vaginismus, cosmesis, myofascial pain, temporomandibular joint dysfunction, and cervicogenic headache.

Administration and Dosage

➤*General dosing considerations:* The potency units of botulinum toxin type A products are specific to the preparation and assay method utilized. They are not interchangeable with other preparations of botulinum toxin products; therefore, units of biological activity of *Dysport*, *Botox*, *Botox Cosmetic*, and *Xeomin* cannot be compared with or converted into units of any other botulinum toxin products assessed with any other specific assay method.

Injection-specific dosage and administration recommendations should be followed.

The safe and effective use of botulinum toxin type A depends on proper storage of the product, selection of the correct dose, and proper reconstitution and administration techniques. Health care providers administering botulinum toxin type A must understand the relevant neuromuscular and/or orbital anatomy of the area involved, as well as any alterations to the anatomy caused by prior surgical procedures. An understanding of standard electromyographic techniques is also required for treatment of strabismus and of upper limb spasticity, and may be useful for the treatment of cervical dystonia.

Use caution when botulinum toxin type A treatment is used in the presence of inflammation at the proposed injection site(s) or when excessive weakness or atrophy is present in the target muscle(s).

➤*Adults:*

Botox –

Blepharospasm:

• *Maximum dose* – Cumulative dose in a 30-day period should not exceed 200 units.

• *Initial dosage* – 1.25 to 2.5 units (0.05 to 0.1 mL volume at each site) injected into the medial and lateral pretarsal orbicularis oculi of the upper lid and into the lateral pretarsal orbicularis oculi of the lower lid.

• *Duration of activity* – The initial effect of the injections is seen within 3 days and reaches a peak at 1 to 2 weeks posttreatment. Each treatment lasts approximately 3 months, following which the procedure can be repeated.

• *Subsequent doses* – Dose may be increased up to 2-fold if the response from the initial treatment is considered insufficient (usually defined as an effect that does not last longer than 2 months). There appears to be little benefit obtainable from injecting more than 5 units per site. Some tolerance may be found when botulinum toxin type A is used in treating blepharospasm if treatments are given any more frequently than every 3 months; it is rare to have the effect be permanent.

Cervical dystonia:

• *Maximum dose* – No more than 50 units per site should be administered.

• *Botulinum toxin–experienced patients* – The mean dose administered to patients in the phase 3 study was 236 units (25th to 75th percentile range, 198 to 300 units). Dose was divided among the affected muscles. Tailor dosing in initial and sequential treatment sessions to the individual patient based on the patient's head and neck position, localization of pain, muscle hypertrophy, patient response, and adverse event history.

• *Botulinum toxin–naive patients* – The initial dose should be at a lower dose, with subsequent dosing adjusted based on individual response. Limiting the total dose injected into the sternocleidomastoid muscles to 100 units or less may decrease the occurrence of dysphagia.

• *Duration of activity* – Clinical improvement generally begins within the first 2 weeks after injection, with maximum clinical benefit at approximately 6 weeks postinjection.

Chronic migraine:

• *Usual dosage* – 155 units administered intramuscularly (IM) as 0.1 mL (5 units) injections per each site. Injections should be divided across 7 specific head/neck muscle areas.

Botox Recommended Dose by Muscle for Chronic Migraine

Head/Neck area	Recommended dose (number of sites[a])
Frontalis[b]	20 units divided in 4 sites
Corrugator[b]	10 units divided in 2 sites
Procerus	5 units in 1 site
Occipitalis[b]	30 units divided in 6 sites
Temporalis[b]	40 units divided in 8 sites
Trapezius[b]	30 units divided in 6 sites
Cerivical paraspinal muscle group[b]	20 units divided in 4 sites
Total dose	155 units divided in 31 sites

[a] Each IM injection site = 0.1 mL = 5 units *Botox*.
[b] Dose distributed bilaterally.

• *Subsequent doses* – The recommended re-treatment schedule is every 12 weeks.

Primary axillary hyperhidrosis:

• *Usual dosage* – 50 units per axilla. Define the hyperhidrotic area to be injected using standard staining techniques (eg, Minor iodine-starch test; see Administration). 50 units of botulinum toxin type A (2 mL) is injected intradermally in 0.1 to 0.2 mL aliquots to each axilla, evenly distributed in multiple sites (10 to 15) approximately 1 to 2 cm apart.

• *Subsequent doses* – Administer repeat injections when the clinical effect of a previous injection diminishes.

Strabismus:

• *Maximum dose* – 25 units for any 1 muscle as a single injection.

• *Initial dosage* – Use the lower listed doses for treatment of small deviations. Use the larger doses only for large deviations.

Vertical muscles, and for horizontal strabismus of less than 20 prism diopters: 1.25 to 2.5 units in any 1 muscle.

Horizontal strabismus of 20 to 50 prism diopters: 2.5 to 5 units in any 1 muscle.

Persistent VI nerve palsy of 1 month or longer duration: 1.25 to 2.5 units in the medial rectus muscle.

• *Duration of activity* – The initial doses create paralysis of injected muscles beginning 1 to 2 days after injection that increases in intensity during the first week. The paralysis lasts for 2 to 6 weeks and gradually resolves over a similar time period. Overcorrections lasting more than 6 months have been rare. About one-half of patients will require subsequent doses because of inadequate paralytic response of the muscle to the initial dose, mechanical factors such as large deviations or restrictions, or lack of binocular motor fusion to stabilize the alignment.

BOTULINUM TOXIN TYPE A — INJECTION

• *Subsequent doses for residual or recurrent strabismus* – Patients should be reexamined 7 to 14 days after each injection to assess the effect of that dose. Patients experiencing adequate paralysis of the target muscle that require subsequent injections should receive a dose comparable with the initial dose. Subsequent doses for patients experiencing incomplete paralysis of the target muscle may be increased up to 2-fold compared with the previously administered dose. Do not administer subsequent injections until the effects of the previous dose have dissipated as evidenced by substantial function in the injected and adjacent muscles.

Upper limb spasticity:

• *Usual dosage* – In clinical trials, doses ranging from 75 to 360 units were divided among selected muscles at a given treatment session.

***Botox* Recommended Dose Ranges Per Muscle**	
	Total dosage (number of sites)
Biceps brachii	100 to 200 units divided in 4 sites
Flexor carpi radialis	12.5 to 50 units in 1 site
Flexor carpi ulnaris	12.5 to 50 units in 1 site
Flexor digitorum profundus	30 to 50 units in 1 site
Flexor digitorum sublimis	30 to 50 units in 1 site

• *Maximum dose* – No more than 50 units per site generally should be administered.

• *Initial dosage* – The lowest recommended starting dose should be used. Dosing in initial and sequential treatment sessions should be tailored to the individual based on the size, number, and location of muscles involved; severity of spasticity; presence of local muscle weakness; and patient's response to previous treatment or adverse event history.

• *Subsequent doses* – Repeat botulinum toxin type A treatment may be administered when the effect of a previous injection has diminished, but generally no sooner than 12 weeks after the previous injection. The degree and pattern of muscle spasticity at the time of reinjection may necessitate alterations in the dose of botulinum toxin type A and muscles to be injected.

Botox Cosmetic –

Glabellar lines:

• *Usual dosage* – An effective dose for facial lines is determined by gross observation of the patient's ability to activate the superficial muscles injected. Inject 0.1 mL into each of 5 sites, 2 in each corrugator muscle and 1 in the procerus muscle for a total dose of 20 units.

• *Duration of activity* – Typically, the initial doses induce a chemical denervation of the injected muscles 1 to 2 days after injection, increasing in intensity during the first week. Duration of activity is approximately 3 to 4 months; more frequent dosing is not recommended.

Dysport –

Cervical dystonia:

• *Usual dosage* – 250 to 1,000 units IM every 12 weeks or longer. Doses higher than 1,000 units have not been systematically evaluated.

• *Initial dosage* – 500 units IM as a divided dose among affected muscles in patients with or without a history of treatment with botulinum toxin.

• *Dosage adjustment* – Make dosage adjustments in 250 unit steps according to the patient's response, with re-treatment every 12 weeks or longer as necessary, based on return of clinical symptoms.

• *Duration of activity* – Clinical studies suggest peak effect occurs between 2 and 4 weeks after injection.

Glabellar lines:

• *Usual dosage* – 50 units IM in 5 equal aliquots of 10 units each.

• *Duration of activity* – The clinical effect may last up to 4 months.

• *Subsequent doses* – Repeat-dose clinical studies demonstrated continued efficacy with up to 4 repeated administrations. Administer no more frequently than every 3 months.

Xeomin –

Blepharospasm:

• *Maximum dose* – 35 units per eye.

• *Initial dosage* – The recommended initial total dose should be the same dose as the patient's previous treatment of *Botox*, although responses may differ in individual patients. If the previous dose of *Botox* is not known, the initial dose should be between 1.25 to 2.5 units per injection site. The number and location of injection sites should be based on severity of blepharospasm, previous dose, and response to *Botox* injections.

The total initial dose in both eyes should not exceed 70 units (35 units per eye).

• *Duration of effect* – The median first onset of effect occurs within 7 days after injection. Typical duration of effect of each treatment is up to 3 months; however, the effect may last significantly longer, or shorter, in individual patients.

• *Subsequent doses* – Subsequent dosing should be tailored to the individual patient, based on response, up to a maximum dose of 35 units per eye. The frequency of repeat treatments should be determined by clinical response, but should generally be no more frequent than every 12 weeks.

Cervical dystonia:

• *Initial dosage* – 120 units IM as the initial total dose. The dose and number of injection sites in each treated muscle should be individualized based on the number and location of the muscle(s) to be treated, the degree of spasticity/dystonia, muscle mass, body weight, and response to any previous botulinum toxin injections. In previously treated patients, their past dose, response to treatment, duration of effect, and adverse reaction history should be taken into consideration when determining the dose.

• *Subsequent doses* – The frequency of repeat treatments should be determined by clinical response, but generally should be no more frequent than every 12 weeks.

• *Duration of effect* – The median first onset of effect occurs within 7 days after injection. Typical duration of effect of each treatment is up to 3 months; however, the effect may last significantly longer, or shorter, in individual patients.

Off-label dosing –

Achalasia: [1] = Good documentation. 20 to 25 units of botulinum toxin injected via endoscopic procedure into each of the 4 quadrants of the lower esophageal sphincter, for a total of 80 to 100 units. Repeated treatment may be needed within the next 6 to 12 months. It is not certain how often or how many total injections will retain efficacy and safety beyond 2 years.

Acquired nystagmus: [4] = Insufficient documentation.

• *Retrobulbar injections* – 10 to 40 units injected retrobulbarly in 1 or both eyes. Some patients received repeat injections every 2 to 4 months as the effects wore off. Repeat injections ranged from 0 to 28 over 5 years.

• *Recti muscle injections* – 2.5 to 3 units injected directly into 1 to 4 of the recti muscles of the eye. One patient received 31 such treatments over the course of 66 months.

Cosmetic use (facial lines and wrinkles): [2] = Fair documentation. It is difficult to assess the optimal dose because dosages varied greatly among reports. Typically, 4 to 5 injection sites at a dose of 2.5 to 5 units per site (total dose, 5 to 25 units) have been used for eliminating muscle tone and voluntary contraction of corrugator muscles. For patients with dominant platysma bands, 3 to 5 injections (0.1 to 0.2 mL) from the jawline to the lower neck have been used to relax the band.

An electromyographic (EMG)–guided injection technique has been recommended to ensure the correct placement of the toxin.

Gustatory sweating (Frey syndrome): [1] = Good documentation. Typical intracutaneous injections have included 2.5 units per site, with mean total dosing ranging from 21.1 to 86.1 units.

Hand dystonia: [2] = Fair documentation. Most patients required injections ranging from 2.5 to 60 units, depending on muscle size, in 2 to 3 muscles.

Headache (tension-type): [4] = Insufficient documentation. Dose has ranged from 5 to 20 units per site to 30 to 50 units divided over 3 to 5 sites.

Hyperhidrosis (palmar): [2] = Fair documentation. Dosages varied greatly (36 to more than 200 mouse units per palm).

Sialorrhea (drooling) in adults: [4] = Insufficient documentation. A detailed report recommends a direct injection of botulinum toxin A (7.5 units of *Botox* or 30 mouse units of the UK product, *Dysport*) via a 29-gauge needle and 1 mL syringe. Gland sites have included parotid, sublingual, and submandibular. Several reports have suggested that the use of ultrasound guidance may reduce the risk of nerve injury. Refer to specific studies prior to dosing.

• *Parkinson disease* – 7.5 to 15 units of *Botox* injected into each parotid gland.

• *Amyotrophic lateral sclerosis* – 5 to 20 units of *Botox* injected into each parotid gland. Mean total doses were 46 units (range, 30 to 72 units).

• *Various causes* – Direct injections into glands with mean doses of 27.7 units per parotid gland (range, 15 to 40 units) and 11.9 units per submandibular gland (range, 10 to 15 units). Mean total *Botox* dose was 76.6 units (range, 50 to 100 units).

Tourette syndrome: [2] = Fair documentation. The dose widely varied, depending on the muscle that was injected, and was reported as similar to doses used for dystonia (range, 1.25 to 300 units). Botulinum toxin was injected directly into the muscle with abnormal movement, often under EMG guidance. The interval between injections varied.

➤*Children:*

Botox –

Blepharospasm: See Adults for dosing for children 12 years of age and older.

Cervical dystonia: See Adults for dosing for children 16 years of age and older

Strabismus: See Adults for dosing for children 12 years of age and older.

Off-label dosing –

Sialorrhea (drooling) in children: [4] = Insufficient documentation. A detailed report recommends direct injection of botulinum toxin A (7.5 units of *Botox* or 30 mouse units of the UK product, *Dysport*) via a 29-gauge needle and 1 mL syringe. Gland sites have included parotid, sublingual, and submandibular. Several reports have suggested that the use of ultrasound guidance may reduce the risk of nerve injury. Refer to specific studies prior to dosing.

• *Various etiologies* – 5 units for parotid gland injections. For submandibular and parotid injections, total dose was 50 to 65 units, typically administered as 22.5 units in each parotid gland, divided into 3 doses of 7.5 units per gland. Each submandibular gland received 10 units.

Spasticity of cerebral palsy (children/adolescents): [3] = Safety concerns.

• *OnabotulinumtoxinA (Botox)* –

Total dose per session: 1 to 30 units/kg.

Total dose per muscle: 0.5 to 6 units/kg.

• *AbobotulinumtoxinA (Dysport)* –

Total dose per session: 8 to 30 units/kg. Botulinum toxin type A has been evaluated for the treatment of spasticity of cerebral palsy in children over a maximum of 16 weeks; however, longer-term treatment may be required for ongoing relief of symptoms.

BOTULINUM TOXIN TYPE A — INJECTION

➤*Elderly:*

Botox Cosmetic – Only indicated in adult patients 65 years of age and younger.

➤*Botulinum toxin assay:* The method utilized for performing the potency assay is specific to the manufacturer's botulinum toxin type A. Because of specific details of this assay, such as the vehicle, dilution scheme, and laboratory protocols for the various potency assays, units of biological activity of botulinum toxin type A cannot be compared with nor converted into units of any other botulinum toxin or any toxin assessed with any other specific assay method. Therefore, differences in species sensitivities to different botulinum neurotoxin serotypes precludes extrapolation of animal dose-activity relationships to human dose relationships.

➤*Preparation for administration:* An injection is prepared by drawing into an appropriately sized sterile syringe an amount of the properly reconstituted toxin (see Dilution Technique) slightly greater than the intended dose. Air bubbles in the syringe barrel are expelled and the syringe is attached to an appropriate injection needle. Confirm patency of the needle. Use a new, sterile needle and syringe to enter the vial on each occasion for removal of botulinum toxin type A.

Botox –

Dilution technique: Prior to injection, reconstitute each vacuum-dried vial of botulinum toxin type A with sterile sodium chloride without a preservative. Draw up the proper amount of diluent in the appropriate size syringe, and slowly inject the diluent into the vial. Discard the vial if a vacuum does not pull the diluent into the vial. Gently mix with the sodium chloride by rotating the vial. Record the date and time of reconstitution on the space on the label.

These dilutions are calculated for an injection volume of 0.1 mL. A decrease or increase in the botulinum toxin type A dose is also possible by administering a smaller or larger injection volume from 0.05 mL (50% decrease in dose) to 0.15 mL (50% increase in dose).

Reconstitute 100 unit vials with 1 mL of diluent to get 10 units per 0.1 mL; add 2 mL of diluent to get 5 units per 0.1 mL; add 4 mL of diluent to get 2.5 units per 0.1 mL; add 8 mL of diluent to get 1.25 units per 0.1 mL.

Reconstitute 200 unit vials with 1 mL of diluent to get 20 units per 0.1 mL; add 2 mL of diluent to get 10 units per 0.1 mL; add 4 mL of diluent to get 5 units per 0.1 mL; add 8 mL of diluent to get 2.5 units per 0.1 mL; add 10 mL of diluent to get 2 units per 0.1 mL.

• *Blepharospasm/Strabismus* – The recommended dilution to achieve 1.25 units is 100 units per 8 mL; for 2.5 units, the recommended dilution is 100 units per 4 mL.

• *Cervical dystonia* – Reconstitute with nonpreserved sterile sodium chloride 0.9% (100 units per 1 mL, 100 units per 2 mL, 200 units per 2 mL, or 200 units per 4 mL).

• *Chronic migraine* – The recommended dilution is 200 units per 4 mL or 100 units per 2 mL, with a final concentration of 5 units per 0.1 mL.

• *Primary axillary hyperhidrosis* – Reconstitute with preservative-free sterile sodium chloride 0.9% (100 units per 4 mL).

• *Upper limb spasticity* – Reconstitute with nonpreserved sterile sodium chloride 0.9% (100 units per 2 mL or 200 units per 4 mL).

Botox Cosmetic –

Dilution technique: Reconstitute only with sterile, nonpreserved sodium chloride prior to IM injection. Using a 21-gauge needle and an appropriately sized syringe, draw up a total of 2.5 mL per 100 unit vial or 1.25 mL per 50 unit vial of sterile sodium chloride 0.9% without a preservative. Insert the needle at a 45-degree angle and slowly inject into the vial. Discard the vial if a vacuum does not pull the diluent into the vial. Gently rotate the vial and record the date and time of reconstitution on the space on the label. The resulting formulation will be 4 units per 0.1 mL and a total treatment dose of 20 units in 0.5 mL.

Draw at least 0.5 mL of the properly reconstituted toxin into the sterile syringe, preferably a tuberculin syringe, and expel any air bubbles in the syringe barrel. Remove the needle used to reconstitute the product and attach a 30- to 33-gauge needle. Confirm the patency of the needle.

Dysport –

Dilution technique: Reconstitution instructions are specific for the 300 unit vial and the 500 unit vial. These volumes yield concentrations specific for the use for each indication.

• *Cervical dystonia* – Each 500 unit vial is to be reconstituted with 1 mL of sodium chloride 0.9% injection without preservative to yield a solution of 500 units/mL. Each 300 unit vial is to be reconstituted with 0.6 mL of sodium chloride 0.9% injection without preservative to yield a solution equivalent to 250 units/mL. Swirl gently to dissolve.

• *Glabellar lines* – Each 300 unit vial is to be reconstituted with 2.5 mL of sterile, preservative-free sodium chloride 0.9% prior to injection. The resulting concentration will be 10 units per 0.08 mL to be delivered in 5 equally divided aliquots of 0.08 mL each. The 300 unit vial may also be reconstituted with 1.5 mL of sterile, preservative-free sodium chloride 0.9% for a solution of 10 units per 0.05 mL to be delivered in 5 equally divided aliquots of 0.05 mL each.

Using a 21-gauge needle, draw up 2.5 or 1.5 mL of sterile, preservative-free sodium chloride 0.9%. Insert needle into the vial at a 45-degree angle and allow sodium chloride diluent to be pulled into the vial by partial vacuum. Discard the vial if the partial vacuum has been lost. Gently rotate the vial (do not shake) until the white substance is fully dissolved.

Draw a single patient dose into a sterile syringe. Expel any air bubbles in the syringe barrel. Remove the needle used to reconstitute the product and attach a 30-gauge needle.

Xeomin –

Dilution technique: Reconstitute each vial with sterile, preservative-free sodium chloride 0.9% injection. Draw up an appropriate amount of sodium chloride 0.9% solution into a syringe. Clean the exposed portion of the rubber stopper of the vial with alcohol (70%) prior to insertion of the needle. Gently inject the sodium chloride solution into the vial. If the vacuum does not pull the solvent into the vial, then the vial must be discarded. Gently mix by rotating the vial.

Diluent Volumes for Reconstitution of *Xeomin*		
Volume of preservative-free sodium chloride 0.9%	50 unit vial: resulting dose in units per 0.1 mL	100 unit vial: resulting dose in units per 0.1 mL
0.25 mL	20 units	—
0.5 mL	10 units	20 units
1 mL	5 units	10 units
2 mL	2.5 units	5 units
4 mL	1.25 units	2.5 units
8 mL	—	1.25 units

➤*Administration:*

Botox –

Blepharospasm: For IM injection only. Inject reconstituted toxin using a sterile, 27- to 30-gauge needle without EMG guidance. Avoiding injection near the levator palpebrae superioris may reduce the complication of ptosis. Avoiding medial lower lid injections and, thereby, reducing diffusion into the inferior oblique may reduce the complication of diplopia. Ecchymosis occurs easily in the soft eyelid tissues. This can be prevented by applying pressure at the injection site immediately after the injection.

Cervical dystonia: For IM injection only. A 25- to 30-gauge needle may be used for superficial muscles, and a longer 22-gauge needle may be used for deeper musculature. Localization of the involved muscles with EMG guidance may be useful.

Chronic migraine: Use a sterile 30-gauge, 0.5 inch needle as 0.1 mL (5 units) injections per each site. Injections should be divided across 7 specific head/neck muscle areas. A 1-inch needle may be needed in the neck region for patients with thick neck muscles. With the exception of the procerus muscle, which should be injected at 1 site (midline), all muscles should be injected bilaterally with half the number of injection sites administered to the left, and half to the right side of the head and neck.

Primary axillary hyperhidrosis: Use a 30-gauge needle. Each dose is injected to a depth of approximately 2 mm and at a 45-degree angle to the skin surface, with the bevel side up to minimize leakage and to ensure the injections remain intradermal. If injection sites are marked in ink, do not inject directly through the ink mark to avoid a permanent tattoo effect. Each injection site has a ring of effect of up to approximately 2 cm in diameter. To minimize the area of no effect, the injection sites should be evenly spaced.

• *Minor iodine-starch test procedure* – Patients should shave underarms and abstain from use of over-the-counter deodorants or antiperspirants for 24 hours prior to the test. Patients should be resting comfortably without exercise or hot drinks for approximately 30 minutes prior to the test. Dry the underarm area and then immediately paint it with iodine solution. Allow the area to dry, then lightly sprinkle the area with starch powder. Gently blow off any excess starch powder. The hyperhidrotic area will develop a deep blue-black color over approximately 10 minutes.

Strabismus: For IM injection only. Intended for injection into extraocular muscles utilizing the electrical activity recorded from the tip of the injection needle as a guide to placement within the target muscle. Injection without surgical exposure or EMG guidance should not be attempted. Health care providers should be familiar with EMG technique. To prepare the eye for injection, it is recommended that several drops of a local anesthetic and an ocular decongestant be given several minutes prior to injection. The volume injected for treatment of strabismus should be between 0.05 to 0.15 mL per muscle.

Upper limb spasticity: For IM injection only. An appropriately sized needle (eg, 25- to 30-gauge) may be used for superficial muscles, and a longer 22-gauge needle may be used for deeper musculature. Localization of the involved muscles with EMG guidance or nerve stimulation techniques is recommended.

Botox Cosmetic – For IM injection only; use a 30- to 33-gauge needle. To reduce the complication of ptosis, take the following steps: avoid injection near the levator palpebrae superioris, particularly in patients with larger brow depressor complexes; place lateral corrugator injections at least 1 cm above the bony supraorbital ridge; ensure the injected volume/dose is accurate and, where feasible, kept to a minimum; do not inject toxin closer than 1 cm above the central eyebrow.

Dysport –

Cervical dystonia: For IM injection. A sterile 23- or 25-gauge needle should be used for administration. Limiting the dose injected into the sternocleidomastoid muscle may reduce the occurrence of dysphagia. Simultaneous EMG-guided application may be helpful in locating active muscle not identified by physical examination alone. Discard any remaining solution after injection.

Glabellar lines:

To inject, advance the needle through the skin into the underlying muscle while applying finger pressure on the superior medial orbital rim. Using a 30-gauge needle, inject 10 units into 5 sites, 2 in each corrugator muscle and 1 in the procerus muscle.

To reduce the complication of ptosis, the following steps should be taken: avoid injection near the levator palpebrae superioris, particularly in

BOTULINUM TOXIN TYPE A — INJECTION

patients with larger brow depressor complexes; medial corrugator injections should be placed at least 1 cm above the bony supraorbital ridge; ensure the injected volume/dose is accurate and, where feasible, kept to a minimum; and do not inject closer than 1 cm above the central eyebrow.

Xeomin – For IM injection only. After reconstitution, use for only 1 injection session and for only 1 patient. A suitable sterile needle (eg, 26-gauge [0.45 mm diameter], 37 mm length for superficial muscles; or 22-gauge [0.7 mm diameter], 75 mm length for injections into deeper muscles) should be used for administration.

Usually injected into the sternocleidomastoid, levator scapulae, splenius capitis, scalenus, and/or the trapezius muscle(s) for the treatment of cervical dystonia. This list is not exhaustive because any of the muscles responsible for controlling head position may require treatment.

Inject carefully when administered at sites close to sensitive structures, such as the carotid artery, lung apices, and esophagus. Before administering, be familiar with the patient's anatomy and any anatomic alterations (eg, due to prior surgical procedures).

Localization of the involved muscles with EMG guidance or nerve stimulation techniques may be useful.

If proposed injection sites are marked with a pen, the product must not be injected through the pen marks; otherwise a permanent tattooing effect may occur.

The number of injection sites is dependent on the size of the muscle to be treated and the volume injected.

➤*Admixture compatibility:* Reconstitute with sterile, nonpreserved sodium chloride only.

➤*Storage/Stability:* Store unopened vials at room temperature at 20° to 25°C (68° to 77°F) or refrigerated at 2° to 8°C (36° to 46°F) (*Xeomin*), in a refrigerator (2° to 8°C [36° to 46°F]) for up to 24 months (*Dysport*, *Botox* 200 unit vial, and *Botox Cosmetic* 50 unit vial) or for up to 36 months (*Botox* 100 unit vial or *Botox Cosmetic* 100 unit vial), or in a freezer at −20° to −10°C (−4° to −14°F) for up to 36 months (*Xeomin*). Because the product and diluent do not contain a preservative, once opened and reconstituted, administer within 4 hours; administer *Xeomin* or the 100 unit vial of *Botox* within 24 hours after reconstitution. During this time period, store reconstituted toxin in a refrigerator (2° to 8°C [36° to 46°F]). Discard any remaining solution. Do not freeze. Protect from light.

Actions

➤*Pharmacology:* Botulinum toxin type A blocks neuromuscular transmission by binding to acceptor sites on motor nerve or sympathetic terminals, entering the nerve terminals, and inhibiting the release of acetylcholine. Toxin activity occurs in the following sequence: toxin heavy chain–mediated binding to specific surface receptors on nerve endings, internalization of the toxin by receptor-mediated endocytosis, pH-induced translocation of the toxin light chain to the cell cytosol and cleavage of synaptosomal-associated protein 25 leading to intracellular blockage of neurotransmitter exocytosis into the neuromuscular junction. This accounts for the therapeutic utility of the toxin in diseases characterized by excessive efferent activity in motor nerves. When injected IM at therapeutic doses, botulinum toxin type A produces partial chemical denervation of the muscle, resulting in a localized reduction in muscle activity. In addition, the muscle may atrophy, axonal sprouting may occur, and extrajunctional acetylcholine receptors may develop. There is evidence that reinnervation of the muscle may occur, thus slowly reversing muscle denervation produced by botulinum toxin type A. When injected intradermally, botulinum toxin type A produces temporary chemical denervation of the sweat gland, resulting in local reduction in sweating.

➤*Pharmacokinetics:* Using currently available analytical technology, it is not possible to detect botulinum toxin type A in the peripheral blood following IM injection at the recommended doses.

Contraindications

Infection at the proposed injection site(s); hypersensitivity to any botulinum toxin preparation or to any of the components in the formulation, including cow's milk protein (*Dysport* only).

Warnings/Precautions

➤*Administration: Botox* and *Botox Cosmetic* contain the same active ingredient in the same formulation. Therefore, adverse reactions observed with the use of *Botox* also have the potential to be associated with the use of *Botox Cosmetic*.

Do not exceed the recommended dosage and frequency of administration for botulinum toxin type A. Risks resulting from administration at higher dosages are not known.

Injection intervals of *Botox Cosmetic* should be no more frequent than every 3 months and should be performed using the lowest effective dose.

➤*Lack of interchangeability:* The potency units of botulinum toxin type A are specific to the preparation and assay method used. They are not interchangeable with other preparations of botulinum toxin products; therefore, units of biological activity of botulinum toxin type A cannot be compared with or converted into units of any other botulinum toxin products assessed with any other specific assay method.

➤*Spread of toxin effect:* See the Warning box for more information.

No definitive serious adverse events of distant spread of toxin effect associated with dermatologic use of *Botox* or *Botox Cosmetic* at the labeled dose of 20 units (for glabellar lines) or 100 units (for severe primary axillary hyperhidrosis) have been reported.

No definitive serious adverse events of distant spread of toxin effect associated with *Botox* for blepharospasm at the recommended dose (30 units and less) or for strabismus at the labeled doses have been reported.

➤*Preexisting neuromuscular disorders:* Closely monitor individuals with peripheral motor neuropathic diseases, amyotrophic lateral sclerosis, or neuromuscular junction disorders (eg, myasthenia gravis, Lambert-Eaton syndrome) when they are given botulinum toxin. Patients with neuromuscular disorders may be at increased risk of clinically significant effects, including severe dysphagia and respiratory compromise, from typical doses of botulinum toxin type A.

➤*Dysphagia and breathing difficulties:* Treatment with botulinum toxin type A and other botulinum toxin products can result in swallowing or breathing difficulties. Patients with preexisting swallowing or breathing difficulties may be more susceptible to these complications. In most cases, this is a consequence of weakening of muscles in the area of injection that are involved in breathing or swallowing. When distant effects occur, additional respiratory muscles may be involved.

Deaths as a complication of severe dysphagia have been reported after treatment with botulinum toxin. Dysphagia may persist for several weeks to months and may require use of a feeding tube to maintain adequate nutrition and hydration. Aspiration may result from severe dysphagia and is a particular risk when treating patients in whom swallowing or respiratory function is already compromised.

Treatment of cervical dystonia with botulinum toxins may weaken neck muscles that serve as accessory muscles of ventilation. This may result in a critical loss of breathing capacity in patients with respiratory disorders who may have become dependent on these accessory muscles. There have been postmarketing reports of serious breathing difficulties, including respiratory failure, in patients with cervical dystonia.

Patients with smaller neck muscle mass and patients who require bilateral injections into the sternocleidomastoid muscle have been reported to be at greater risk for dysphagia. Limiting the dose injected into the sternocleidomastoid muscle may reduce the occurrence of dysphagia. Injections into the levator scapulae may be associated with an increased risk of upper respiratory tract infection and dysphagia.

Patients treated with botulinum toxin may require immediate medical attention if they develop problems with swallowing, speech, or respiratory disorders. These reactions can occur within hours to weeks after injection with botulinum toxin.

➤*Facial anatomy in the treatment of glabellar lines:* Exercise caution when administering botulinum toxin type A to patients with surgical alterations to the facial anatomy, excessive weakness or atrophy in the target muscle(s), marked facial asymmetry, inflammation at the injection site(s), ptosis, excessive dermatochalasis, deep dermal scarring, thick sebaceous skin, or the inability to substantially lessen glabellar lines by physically spreading them apart.

Do not exceed the recommended dosage and frequency of administration of *Dysport*. In clinical trials, subjects who received a higher dose of *Dysport* had an increased incidence of eyelid ptosis.

➤*Cardiovascular events:* There have been reports following administration of botulinum toxin type A of adverse events involving the cardiovascular system, including arrhythmia and myocardial infarction, some with fatal outcomes. Some of these patients had risk factors, including preexisting cardiovascular disease.

➤*Albumin:* This product contains albumin, a derivative of human blood. Based on effective donor screening and product manufacturing processes, it carries an extremely remote risk for transmission of viral diseases. A theoretical risk for transmission of Creutzfeldt-Jakob disease (CJD) also is considered extremely remote. No cases of transmission of viral diseases or CJD have ever been identified for albumin.

➤*Intradermal immune reaction:* The possibility of an immune reaction when injected intradermally is unknown. The safety of *Dysport* for the treatment of hyperhidrosis has not been established.

➤*Safe and effective use:* The safe and effective use of botulinum toxin type A depends on proper storage of the product, selection of the correct dose, and proper reconstitution and administration techniques. When administering botulinum toxin type A, understand the relevant neuromuscular and/or orbital anatomy of the area involved, as well as any alterations to the anatomy caused by prior surgical procedures, and avoid injection into vulnerable anatomic areas. An understanding of standard EMG techniques is also required for treatment of strabismus and may be useful for the treatment of cervical dystonia.

➤*Injection site:* Use caution when botulinum toxin type A treatment is used in the presence of inflammation at the proposed injection site(s) or when excessive weakness or atrophy is present in the target muscle(s).

➤*Corneal exposure and ulceration:* Reduced blinking from botulinum toxin type A injection of the orbicularis muscle can lead to corneal exposure, persistent epithelial defect, and corneal ulceration, especially in patients with VII nerve disorders. One case of corneal perforation in an aphakic eye requiring corneal grafting has occurred because of this effect. Employ careful testing of corneal sensation in eyes previously operated on, avoid injection into the lower lid area to avoid ectropion, and employ vigorous treatment of any epithelial defect. This may require protective drops, ointment, therapeutic soft contact lenses, or closure of the eye by patching or other means. Because of its anticholinergic effects, use botulinum toxin type

BOTULINUM TOXIN TYPE A — INJECTION

A with caution in patients at risk of developing narrow angle glaucoma. To prevent ectropion, do not inject botulinum toxin products into the medial lower eyelid area.

Ecchymosis easily occurs in the soft tissues of the eyelid. Immediate gentle pressure at the injection site can limit that risk.

Inducing paralysis in 1 or more extraocular muscles may produce spatial disorientation, double vision, or past pointing. Covering the affected eye may alleviate these symptoms.

➤*Race:* Exploratory analyses in trials for glabellar lines in black subjects with Fitzpatrick skin types IV, V, or VI and in Hispanic subjects suggested that response rates at day 30 were comparable with and no worse than the overall population

➤*Respiratory effects:* Closely monitor patients with compromised respiratory status treated with *Botox* for upper limb spasticity. In a double-blind, placebo-controlled, parallel-group study in patients with stable reduced pulmonary function (defined as forced expiratory volume at 1 second [FEV_1] 40% to 80% of predicted value and FEV_1/forced vital capacity [FVC] of 0.75 or less), the event rate in change of FVC of 15% or more or 20% or more was generally greater in patients treated with *Botox* than in patients treated with placebo.

***Botox* Event Rate Per Treatment Cycle Among Patients With Reduced Lung Function**[a]

	Botox 360 units		*Botox* 240 units		Placebo	
Decrease in FVC	≥ 15%	≥ 20%	≥ 15%	≥ 20%	≥ 15%	≥ 20%
Week 1	4%	0%	3%	0%	7%	3%
Week 6	7%	4%	4%	2%	2%	2%
Week 12	10%	5%	2%	1%	4%	1%

[a] Differences from placebo were not statistically significant.

In patients with reduced lung function, upper respiratory tract infections were also reported more frequently as adverse reactions in patients treated with *Botox*.

Bronchitis and upper respiratory tract infections – Bronchitis was reported more frequently as an adverse reaction in patients treated for upper limb spasticity with *Botox* (3% at 251 to 360 unit total dose) compared with placebo (1%). In patients with reduced lung function treated for upper limb spasticity, upper respiratory tract infections were also reported more frequently as adverse reactions in patients treated with *Botox* (11% at 360 unit total dose; 8% at 240 unit total dose) compared with placebo (6%).

➤*Retrobulbar hemorrhage:* During the administration of botulinum toxin type A for the treatment of strabismus, retrobulbar hemorrhages sufficient to compromise retinal circulation have occurred. It is recommended that appropriate instruments to decompress the orbit be accessible.

➤*Vasovagal response:* Needle-related pain and/or anxiety may result in vasovagal responses (eg, syncope, hypotension), which may require appropriate medical therapy.

➤*Immunogenicity:* As with all therapeutic proteins, there is a potential for immunogenicity. Formation of neutralizing antibodies to botulinum toxin type A may reduce the effectiveness of botulinum toxin type A treatment by inactivating the biological activity of the toxin. The rate of formation of neutralizing antibodies in patients receiving botulinum toxin type A has not been well studied.

The critical factors for neutralizing antibody formation have not been well characterized. The results from some studies suggest that botulinum toxin type A injections at more frequent intervals or at higher doses may lead to greater incidence of antibody formation. The potential for antibody formation may be minimized by injecting with the lowest effective dose given at the longest feasible intervals between injections.

Botox – In a long-term, open-label study evaluating 326 cervical dystonia patients treated for an average of 9 treatment sessions with the current formulation of botulinum toxin type A, 4 (1.2%) patients had positive antibody tests. All 4 of these patients responded to botulinum toxin type A therapy at the time of the positive antibody test. However, 3 of these patients developed clinical resistance after subsequent treatment, while the fourth patient continued to respond to botulinum toxin type A therapy for the remainder of the study.

One (0.2%) patient among the 445 hyperhidrosis patients and 2 (0.5%) patients among the 380 adult upper limb spasticity patients with analyzed specimens showed the presence of neutralizing antibodies.

The data reflect the patients whose test results were considered positive or negative for neutralizing activity to botulinum toxin type A in a mouse protection assay. The results of these tests are highly dependent on the sensitivity and specificity of the assay. Additionally, the observed incidence of neutralizing activity in an assay may be influenced by several factors, including sample handling, concomitant medications, and underlying disease. For these reasons, comparison of the incidence of neutralizing activity to botulinum toxin type A with the incidence reported to other products may be misleading.

Dysport – Approximately 3% of subjects developed antibodies (binding or neutralizing) over time with botulinum toxin type A treatment. The significance of these antibodies is unknown because in the presence of binding and neutralizing antibodies, some patients may continue to experience clinical benefit.

Testing for antibodies to botulinum toxin type A was performed for 1,554 subjects who had up to 9 cycles of treatment. Two (0.13%) subjects tested positive for binding antibodies at baseline. Three additional subjects tested positive for binding antibodies after receiving botulinum toxin type A treatment. None of the subjects tested positive for neutralizing antibodies.

Xeomin – Neutralizing antibody titers were assessed in all clinical studies of botulinum toxin type A using the hemidiaphragm assay. In the botulinum toxin type A development program, 12 (1.1%) of the 1,080 subjects who were antibody negative at baseline developed neutralizing antibodies to botulinum toxin during the course of their respective study. Each of these 12 subjects had been treated with another botulinum toxin prior to exposure to botulinum toxin type A. Because the majority of patients had previously been exposed to other botulinum toxin neurotoxins, and because most trials were of short duration with controlled intervals between treatments, the potential for antibody formation has not been fully characterized. The significance of these antibodies is unknown because in the presence of neutralizing antibodies, some patients may continue to experience clinical benefit. A single subject with a 20-year history of cervical dystonia who was reported as botulinum toxin–naive and treated with botulinum toxin type A 240 units demonstrated transiently positive neutralizing antibodies that reverted to negative at study termination. This subject was determined to be a primary nonresponder.

The incidence of antibody formation is highly dependent on the sensitivity and specificity of the assay. In addition, the observed incidence of antibody positivity in an assay may be influenced by several factors, including assay methodology, sample handling, timing of sample collection, concomitant medications, and underlying disease. For these reasons, comparison of the incidence of antibodies across products in this class may be misleading.

➤*Hypersensitivity reactions:* Serious and/or immediate hypersensitivity reactions have been rarely reported. These reactions include anaphylaxis, serum sickness, urticaria, soft tissue edema, and dyspnea. One fatal case of anaphylaxis, in which lidocaine was used as the diluent, has been reported and, consequently, the causal agent cannot be reliably determined. If such a reaction occurs, discontinue further injection and institute appropriate medical therapy immediately.

➤*Pregnancy: Category C.* There are no adequate and well-controlled studies of botulinum toxin type A in pregnant women. Administer botulinum toxin type A during pregnancy only if the potential benefit justifies the potential risk to the fetus. If this drug is used during pregnancy, or if the patient becomes pregnant while taking this drug, apprise the patient of the potential risks, including abortion or fetal malformations, which have been observed in rabbits.

Botox – When botulinum toxin type A (4, 8, or 16 units/kg) was administered IM to pregnant mice or rats 2 times during the period of organogenesis (on gestation days 5 and 13), reductions in fetal body weight and decreased fetal skeletal ossification were observed at the 2 highest doses. The no-effect dose for developmental toxicity in these studies (4 units/kg) is approximately 1.5 times the average high human dose for upper limb spasticity of 360 units on a body weight basis (units/kg).

When botulinum toxin type A was administered IM to pregnant rats (0.125, 0.25, 0.5, 1, 4, or 8 units/kg) or rabbits (0.063, 0.125, 0.25, or 0.5 units/kg) daily during the period of organogenesis (total of 12 doses in rats, 13 doses in rabbits), reduced fetal body weights and decreased fetal skeletal ossification were observed at the 2 highest doses in rats and at the highest dose in rabbits. These doses were also associated with significant maternal toxicity, including abortions, early deliveries, and maternal death. The developmental no-effect doses in these studies of 1 unit/kg in rats and 0.25 units/kg in rabbits are less than the average high human dose based on units/kg.

When pregnant rats received single IM injections (1, 4, or 16 units/kg) at 3 different periods of development (prior to implantation, implantation, or organogenesis), no adverse effects on fetal development were observed. The developmental no-effect level for a single maternal dose in rats (16 units/kg) is approximately 3 times the average high human dose based on units/kg.

Botox Cosmetic – In a range-finding study in rabbits, daily injections of 0.125 units/kg/day (days 6 to 18 of gestation) and 2 units/kg (days 6 and 13 of gestation) produced severe maternal toxicity, abortions, and/or fetal malformations. Higher doses resulted in death of the dams. The rabbit appears to be a very sensitive species to botulinum toxin type A.

When pregnant mice and rats were injected IM during the period of organogenesis, the development no observed effect level of botulinum toxin type A was 4 units/kg. Higher doses (8 or 16 units/kg) were associated with reductions in fetal body weights and/or delayed ossification, which may be reversible.

Administration of *Botox Cosmetic* is not recommended during pregnancy.

BOTULINUM TOXIN TYPE A — INJECTION

Dysport – Botulinum toxin type A produced embryofetal toxicity when given to pregnant rats at doses similar to or greater than the maximum recommended human dose (MRHD) of 1,000 units on a body weight (units/kg) basis.

In an embryofetal development study in which pregnant rats received IM injections daily (2.2, 6.6, or 22 units/kg on gestation days 6 through 17) or intermittently (44 units/kg on gestation days 6 and 12 only) during organogenesis, increased early embryonic death was observed with both dosing schedules. The no-effect dose for embryofetal developmental toxicity was 2.2 units/kg (one-tenth the MRHD on a body weight basis). Maternal toxicity was seen at 22 and 44 units/kg. In a pre- and postnatal development study in which female rats received 6 weekly IM injections (4.4, 11.1, 22.2, or 44 units/kg) beginning on day 6 of gestation and continuing through parturition to weaning, an increase in stillbirths was observed at the highest dose, which was maternally toxic. The no-effect dose for pre- and postnatal developmental toxicity was 22.2 units/kg (approximately equal to the MRHD on a body weight basis).

Xeomin – Botulinum toxin type A was embryotoxic in rats and increased abortions in rabbits when given at doses higher than the MRHD for cervical dystonia (120 units) on a body weight basis.

When botulinum toxin type A was administered IM to pregnant rats during organogenesis (3, 10, or 30 units/kg on gestational days 6, 12, and 19; or 7 units/kg on gestational days 6 to 19; or 2, 6, or 18 units/kg on gestational days 6, 9, 12, 16, and 19), decreases in fetal body weight and skeletal ossification were observed at doses that were also maternally toxic. The no-effect level for embryotoxicity in rats was 6 units/kg (3 times the MRHD for cervical dystonia on a body weight basis). IM administration to pregnant rabbits during organogenesis (1.25, 2.5, or 5 units/kg on gestational days 6, 18, and 28) resulted in an increased rate of abortion at the highest dose, which was also maternally toxic. In rabbits, the no-effect level for increased abortion was 2.5 units/kg (similar to the MRHD for cervical dystonia on a body weight basis).

➤*Lactation:* It is not known whether this drug is excreted in human milk. Because many drugs are excreted in human milk, exercise caution when botulinum toxin type A is administered to a breast-feeding woman.

➤*Children:*

Botox – Safety and effectiveness in children younger than 12 years of age have not been established for blepharospasm or strabismus, or younger than 16 years of age for cervical dystonia or 18 years of age for axillary hyperhidrosis, spasticity, or chronic migraine.

Botox Cosmetic – Use of botulinum toxin type A (cosmetic) is not recommended in children.

Dysport –

Cervical dystonia: Safety and effectiveness in children have not been established.

Glabellar lines: Botulinum toxin type A is not recommended for use in children younger than 18 years of age.

Xeomin – Safety and effectiveness in patients younger than 18 years of age have not been established.

➤*Elderly:* There were too few patients older than 75 years of age to enable any comparisons. In general, dose selection for an elderly patient should be cautious, usually starting at the low end of the dosing range, reflecting the greater frequency of decreased hepatic, renal, or cardiac function, and of concomitant disease or other drug therapy.

Dysport –

Glabellar lines: Of the total number of subjects in the placebo-controlled clinical studies of *Dysport*, 1% were 65 years of age and older. Efficacy was not observed in subjects 65 years of age and older. For the entire safety database of elderly patients, although there was no increase in the incidence of eyelid ptosis, elderly patients did have an increase in the number of ocular adverse events compared with younger patients (11% vs 5%).

Xeomin –

Cervical dystonia: In the phase 3 study in cervical dystonia, 29 patients were older than 65 years of age, including 19 patients who received botulinum toxin type A and 10 patients who received placebo. Of these, 53% of patients treated with botulinum toxin type A and 40% of patients treated with placebo experienced an adverse event. For patients older than 65 years of age treated with botulinum toxin type A, the most common adverse events were dysphagia (21%) and asthenia (11%). One botulinum toxin type A–treated patient (5%) experienced severe dizziness.

Blepharospasm: In the phase 3 study in blepharospasm, 41 patients were older than 65 years of age, including 29 of 75 (39%) patients who received botulinum toxin type A and 12 of 34 (35%) patients who received placebo. Of these patients, 76% treated with botulinum toxin type A, compared with 58% of patients treated with placebo, experienced an adverse event. One patient treated with botulinum toxin type A experienced severe dysphagia.

➤*Monitoring:* Closely monitor patients with peripheral motor neuropathic diseases, amyotrophic lateral sclerosis, or neuromuscular junction disorders (eg, myasthenia gravis, Lambert-Eaton syndrome) when they are given botulinum toxin.

Closely monitor patients with compromised respiratory status treated with *Botox* for upper limb spasticity.

Drug Interactions

Botulinum Toxin Type A Drug Interactions

Precipitant drug	Object drug[a]		Description
Aminoglycosides (eg, gentamicin)	Botulinum toxin type A	⬆	Neuromuscular action may be enhanced, resulting in protracted respiratory depression. Use with caution.
Muscle relaxants (eg, metaxalone)	Botulinum toxin type A	⬆	Excessive weakness may be exaggerated. Use with caution.
Nondepolarizing muscle relaxants (eg, tubocurarine), other agents interfering with neuromuscular transmission (eg, anticholinesterases, magnesium sulfate, quinidine)	Botulinum toxin type A	⬆	Neuromuscular action may be enhanced, resulting in protracted respiratory depression. Use with caution.
Other botulinum neurotoxin (botulinum toxin type B)	Botulinum toxin type A		Administration of a different botulinum neurotoxin at the same time or within several months of each other may exacerbate excessive neuromuscular weakness. Use with caution.

[a] ⬆ = object drug increased.

Adverse Reactions

➤*Botox*: In general, adverse reactions occur within the first week following injection of botulinum toxin type A, and while generally transient, may have a duration of several months. Localized bleeding/bruising, erythema, infection, inflammation, pain, swelling, and/or tenderness may be associated with the injection. Needle-related anxiety and/or pain may result in vasovagal responses (eg, hypotension, syncope), which may require appropriate medical therapy. Local weakness of the injected muscle(s) represents the expected pharmacological action of botulinum toxin. However, weakness of adjacent muscles may also occur because of spread of toxin.

Cervical dystonia – In cervical dystonia patients evaluated for safety in double-blind and open-label studies following injection of botulinum toxin type A, the most frequently reported adverse reactions were dysphagia (19%), upper respiratory tract infection (12%), headache (11%), and neck pain (11%).

Other reactions reported in 2% to 10% of patients in any one study in decreasing order of incidence include increased cough, flu syndrome, back pain, rhinitis, dizziness, hypertonia, soreness at injection site, asthenia, oral dryness, speech disorder, fever, nausea, and drowsiness. Stiffness, numbness, diplopia, ptosis, and dyspnea have been reported.

Dysphagia and symptomatic general weakness may be attributable to an extension of the pharmacology of botulinum toxin type A resulting from the spread of the toxin outside the injected muscles.

The most common severe adverse reaction associated with the use of botulinum toxin type A injection in patients with cervical dystonia is dysphagia, with approximately 20% of these cases also reporting dyspnea. Most dysphagia is reported as mild or moderate in severity. However, it may be associated with more severe signs and symptoms.

Additionally, reports in the literature include a case of a female patient who developed brachial plexopathy 2 days after injection of botulinum toxin type A 120 units for the treatment of cervical dystonia, and reports of dysphonia in patients who have been treated for cervical dystonia.

Primary axillary hyperhidrosis – The most frequently reported adverse events (3% to 10% of patients) following injection of botulinum toxin type A in double-blind studies included anxiety, fever, flu syndrome, headache, infection, injection-site pain and hemorrhage, neck or back pain, nonaxillary sweating, pharyngitis, and pruritus.

Blepharospasm – In a study of patients with blepharospasm who received an average dose per eye of 33 units (injected at 3 to 5 sites) of the currently manufactured botulinum toxin type A, the most frequently reported treatment-related adverse reactions were ptosis (21%), eye dryness (6%), and superficial punctate keratitis (6%).

Other reactions reported in prior clinical studies in decreasing order of incidence include irritation, tearing, lagophthalmos, photophobia, ectropion, keratitis, diplopia, entropion, diffuse skin rash, and local swelling of the eyelid skin lasting for several days following eyelid injection.

In 2 cases of VII nerve disorder, reduced blinking from botulinum toxin type A injection of the orbicularis muscle led to serious corneal exposure, persistent epithelial defect, corneal ulceration, and a case of corneal perforation.

Focal facial paralysis, exacerbation of myasthenia gravis, and syncope have also been reported after treatment of blepharospasm.

Strabismus – Extraocular muscles adjacent to the injection site can be affected, causing vertical deviation, especially with higher doses of botulinum toxin type A. The incidence rate of these adverse reactions in 2,058 adults who received 3,650 injections for horizontal strabismus was 17%.

BOTULINUM TOXIN TYPE A — INJECTION

The incidence of ptosis has been reported to be dependent on the location of the injected muscles, 1% after inferior rectus injections, 16% after horizontal rectus injections, and 38% after superior rectus injections.

In a series of 5,587 injections, retrobulbar hemorrhage occurred in 0.3% of cases.

Upper limb spasticity –

Botulinum Toxin Type A Adverse Reactions in Adults With Upper Limb Spasticity (≥ 2%)				
Adverse reactions	Botulinum toxin type A 251 to 360 units (n = 115)	Botulinum toxin type A 150 to 250 units (n = 188)	Botulinum toxin type A < 150 units (n = 54)	Placebo (n = 182)
Musculoskeletal				
Muscular weakness	0%	4%	2%	1%
Pain in extremity	6%	5%	9%	4%
Miscellaneous				
Bronchitis	3%	2%	0%	1%
Fatigue	3%	2%	2%	0%
Nausea	3%	2%	2%	1%

➤*Botox Cosmetic*: A report of acute angle closure glaucoma 1 day after receiving an injection of botulinum toxin for blepharospasm was received, with recovery 4 months later after laser iridotomy and trabeculectomy. Focal facial paralysis, exacerbation of myasthenia gravis, and syncope have also been reported after treatment of blepharospasm.

In general, adverse reactions occur within the first week following injection and, while generally transient, may have a duration of several months or longer. Localized bleeding/bruising, erythema, infection, inflammation, pain, swelling, and/or tenderness may be associated with the injection. Local weakness of the injected muscle(s) represents the expected pharmacological action of botulinum toxin. However, weakness of adjacent muscles may also occur because of the spread of toxin.

Glabellar lines – In clinical trials of botulinum toxin type A, the most frequently reported adverse reactions following injection of botulinum toxin type A were blepharoptosis and nausea. The incidence did not differ from placebo for headache, flu syndrome, and respiratory infection.

Less frequently occurring (less than 3%) adverse reactions included erythema at the injection site and paresthesia, for which the incidence was not different from placebo; muscle weakness; and pain in the face. While local weakness of the injected muscle(s) is representative of the expected pharmacological action of botulinum toxin, weakness of adjacent muscles may occur as a result of the spread of toxin. These reactions are thought to be associated with the injection and occurred within the first week. The reactions were generally transient but may last several months or longer.

In the open-label, repeat injection study, blepharoptosis was reported for 2% of subjects in the first treatment cycle and 1% of subjects in the second treatment cycle. Adverse reactions of any type were reported for 49% of subjects overall. The most frequently reported of these adverse reactions in the open-label study included blepharoptosis, flu syndrome, headache, nausea, pain, and respiratory infection.

Botulinum Toxin Type A Adverse Reactions (> 1%)		
Adverse reactions	Botulinum toxin type A (n = 405)	Placebo (n = 130)
Overall	44%	42%
GI		
Dyspepsia	1%	0%
Nausea	3%	2%
Tooth disorder	1%	0%
Miscellaneous		
Blepharoptosis	3%	0%
Hypertension	1%	0%
Muscle weakness	2%	0%
Pain in face	2%	1%
Skin tightness	1%	0%

➤*Dysport*:

Cervical dystonia –

During the clinical studies, 2 (less than 1%) patients experienced adverse reactions leading to withdrawal. One patient experienced disturbance in attention, eyelid disorder, feeling abnormal, and headache, and 1 patient experienced dysphagia.

Botulinum Toxin Type A Adverse Reactions (> 5%) From a Single Treatment Cycle		
	Double-blind phase	
Adverse reactions	Botulinum toxin type A 500 units (n = 173)	Placebo (n = 182)
Any treatment-emergent reaction	61%	51%
CNS	16%	13%
Fatigue	12%	10%
Headache	11%	9%
GI	28%	15%
Dysphagia	15%	4%
Dry mouth	13%	7%
Local	—	—
Injection-site discomfort	13%	8%
Injection-site pain	5%	4%
Musculoskeletal	30%	18%
Muscular weakness	16%	4%
Musculoskeletal pain	7%	3%
Respiratory	12%	8%
Dysphonia	6%	2%
Miscellaneous	30%	23%
Eye disorders[a]	7%	2%
Infections and infestations	13%	9%

[a] The following preferred terms were reported: accommodation disorder, diplopia, dry eye, eyelid disorder, eye pain, eye pruritus, vision blurred, and visual acuity reduced.

Botulinum Toxin Type A Common Adverse Reactions by Dose in a Fixed-Dose Study				
	Botulinum toxin type A dose			
Adverse reactions	250 units	500 units	1,000 units	Placebo
Any adverse reaction	37%	65%	83%	30%
GI				
Dry mouth	21%	18%	39%	10%
Dysphagia	21%	29%	39%	5%
Miscellaneous				
Dysphonia	0%	18%	28%	0%
Eye disorders	0%	6%	17%	0%
Facial paresis	5%	0%	11%	0%
Injection-site discomfort	5%	18%	22%	10%
Muscular weakness	11%	12%	56%	0%

Local: Injection-site discomfort and injection-site pain were common adverse reactions following botulinum toxin type A administration. These reactions were mainly of mild or moderate intensity.

Less common adverse reactions: The following selected adverse reactions were reported less frequently (less than 5%).

• *Breathing difficulties* – Breathing difficulties were reported by approximately 3% of patients following botulinum toxin type A administration and in 1% of placebo patients in clinical trials during the double-blind phase. These consisted mainly of dyspnea and were generally mild in intensity. The median time to onset from last dose of botulinum toxin type A was approximately 1 week, and the median duration was approximately 3 weeks.

Other selected adverse reactions with incidences of less than 5% in the botulinum toxin type A 500 units group in the double-blind phase of clinical trials included dizziness in 3.5% of subjects treated with botulinum toxin type A and 1% of subjects treated with placebo, and muscle atrophy in 1% of subjects treated with botulinum toxin type A and in none of the subjects treated with placebo.

Lab test abnormalities: Subjects treated with botulinum toxin type A exhibited a small increase from baseline (0.23 mol/L) in mean blood glucose relative to placebo-treated subjects. This was not clinically significant among subjects in the development program but could be a factor in patients whose diabetes is difficult to control.

Electrocardiogram findings: Electrocardiogram measurements were only recorded in a limited number of subjects in an open-label study without a placebo or active control. This study showed a statistically significant reduction in heart rate compared with baseline, averaging approximately 3 beats per minute, observed 30 minutes after injection.

BOTULINUM TOXIN TYPE A — INJECTION

Glabellar lines –

Botulinum Toxin Type A Adverse Reactions (> 1%) in Patients With Glabellar Lines		
Adverse reactions	Botulinum toxin type A (n = 398)[a]	Placebo (n = 496)[a]
Any treatment-emergent adverse reaction	48%	33%
Local		
Injection-site pain	3%	2%
Injection-site reaction	3%	< 1%
Respiratory		
Nasopharyngitis	10%	4%
Sinusitis	2%	1%
Upper respiratory tract infection	3%	2%
Special senses		
Eyelid edema	2%	0%
Eyelid ptosis	2%	< 1%
Miscellaneous		
Blood urine present	2%	< 1%
Headache	9%	5%
Nausea	2%	1%

[a] Subjects who received treatment with placebo and botulinum toxin type A are counted in both treatment columns.

In the overall safety database, where some subjects received up to 12 treatments with botulinum toxin type A, adverse reactions were reported for 57% of subjects. The most frequently reported of these adverse reactions were headache, injection-site bruising, injection-site pain, injection site reaction (numbness, discomfort, erythema, tenderness, tingling, itching, stinging, warmth, irritation, tightness, swelling), nasopharyngitis, sinusitis, and upper respiratory tract infection.

Adverse reactions that emerged after repeated injections in 2% to 3% of the population included bronchitis, contact dermatitis, cough, influenza, injection-site discomfort, injection-site swelling, and pharyngolaryngeal pain.

The incidence of eyelid ptosis did not increase in the long-term safety studies with multiple retreatments at intervals of 3 months or longer. The majority of eyelid ptosis reactions were mild to moderate in severity and resolved over several weeks.

➤*Xeomin:*

Cervical dystonia – Common adverse events (5% or more in any botulinum toxin type A treatment group) observed in patients who received botulinum toxin type A (120 or 240 units) included dysphagia, injection-site pain, muscle weakness, musculoskeletal pain, and neck pain.

Botulinum Toxin Type A Adverse Reactions in Patients With Cervical Dystonia (≥ 5%)			
	Double-blind phase		
Adverse reactions	Botulinum toxin type A 120 units (n = 77)	Botulinum toxin type A 240 units (n = 82)	Placebo (n = 74)
Any adverse reaction	57%	55%	42%
GI	18%	24%	4%
Dysphagia	13%	18%	3%
Musculoskeletal	23%	32%	11%
Muscular weakness	7%	11%	1%
Musculoskeletal pain	7%	4%	1%
Neck pain	7%	15%	4%
Miscellaneous	16%	11%	11%
Infections and infestations	14%	13%	11%
Injection-site pain	9%	4%	7%
Nervous system disorders	16%	17%	7%
Respiratory, thoracic, and mediastinal disorders	13%	10%	3%

Blepharospasm – The adverse events occurring in 5% or more of patients treated with botulinum toxin type A and greater than placebo in the phase 3 study were eyelid ptosis, dry eye, dry mouth, diarrhea, headache, visual impairment, dyspnea, nasopharyngitis, and respiratory tract infection. No serious adverse events occurred in patients who received botulinum toxin type A; 1 patient treated with placebo experienced a serious adverse event (dyspnea).

Botulinum Toxin Type A Adverse Reactions in Patients With Blepharospasm (≥ 5%)		
	Double-blind phase	
Adverse reactions	Botulinum toxin type A (n = 74)	Placebo (n = 34)
Any adverse reaction	70%	62%
CNS	14%	9%
Headache	7%	3%
GI	30%	15%
Diarrhea	8%	—
Dry mouth	16%	3%
Ophthalmologic	38%	21%
Dry eye	16%	12%
Eyelid ptosis	19%	9%
Visual impairment[a]	12%	6%
Respiratory	11%	3%
Dyspnea	5%	3%
Nasopharyngitis	5%	3%
Respiratory tract infection	5%	3%
Miscellaneous	11%	9%
Infections and infestations	20%	15%

[a] Including vision blurred.

➤*Postmarketing:*

Botox – There have been spontaneous reports of death, sometimes associated with dysphagia, pneumonia, and/or other significant debility or anaphylaxis, after treatment with botulinum toxin.

There have also been rare reports of adverse reactions involving the cardiovascular system, including arrhythmia and myocardial infarction, some with fatal outcomes. Some of these patients had risk factors, including cardiovascular disease. The exact relationship of these reactions to the botulinum toxin injection has not been established.

New-onset or recurrent seizures have also been reported, typically in patients who are predisposed to experiencing these events. The exact relationship of these reactions to the botulinum toxin injection has not been established.

The following reactions have been reported since the drug has been marketed: abdominal pain, anorexia, brachial plexopathy, diarrhea, facial palsy, facial paresis, hyperhidrosis, hypoacusis, hypoaesthesia, localized numbness, malaise, myalgia, paresthesia, pyrexia, radiculopathy, skin rash (including erythema multiforme and psoriasiform eruption), tinnitus, vertigo, visual disturbances, and vomiting.

Botox Cosmetic – Transient ptosis, the most frequently reported complication, has been reported in the literature in approximately 5% of patients. There has been a single report of diplopia, which resolved completely in 3 weeks.

CNS: Malaise, vertigo with nystagmus.

Dermatologic: Erythema multiforme, pruritus, psoriasiform eruption, sweating.

GI: Abdominal pain, diarrhea, loss of appetite, vomiting.

Musculoskeletal: Myalgia, myasthenia gravis.

Special senses: Blurred vision, decreased hearing, ear noise, glaucoma, retinal vein occlusion.

Miscellaneous: Brachial plexopathy, fever, focal facial paralysis, localized numbness, syncope.

Dysport – There is extensive postmarketing experience outside the United States for the treatment of glabellar lines. Adverse reactions are reported voluntarily from a population of uncertain size; thus, it is not always possible to estimate their frequency reliably or to establish a causal relationship to drug exposure. The following adverse reactions have been identified during postmarketing use: amyotrophy, burning sensation,diplopia, dizziness, dysphagia, erythema, excessive granulation tissue, eyelid ptosis, facial paresis, headache, hypersensitivity, hypoesthesia, influenza-like illness, injection-site reaction, malaise, nausea, photophobia, sinusitis, vertigo, and vision blurred.

Xeomin – The following adverse reactions have been reported during post-approval use with botulinum toxin type A: eye swelling, eyelid edema, dysphagia, nausea, injection-site pain, injection-site reaction, allergic dermatitis, localized allergic reactions such as swelling, edema, erythema, pruritus or rash, and dysarthria, herpes zoster, hypersensitivity, muscle spasm, muscular weakness, and myalgia.

Overdosage

➤*Symptoms:* Excessive doses of botulinum toxin type A may be expected to produce neuromuscular weakness with a variety of symptoms. In the event of overdose, medically monitor the patient for symptoms of excessive muscle weakness or muscle paralysis.

Symptoms of overdose are likely not to be present immediately following injection. If accidental injection or oral ingestion occur, medically supervise the patient for several weeks for signs and symptoms of excessive muscle weakness or paralysis.

BOTULINUM TOXIN TYPE A — INJECTION

There is no significant information regarding overdose from clinical studies in cervical dystonia and blepharospasm. Doses exceeding 1,000 units of *Dysport* were rarely studied in clinical settings for any indication.

➤*Treatment:* Respiratory support may be required where excessive doses cause paralysis of respiratory muscles. Symptomatic treatment may be necessary.

In the event of overdose, antitoxin raised against botulinum toxin is available from the Centers for Disease Control and Prevention (CDC) in Atlanta, GA. However, the antitoxin will not reverse any botulinum toxin–induced effects already apparent by the time of antitoxin administration. In the event of suspected or actual cases of botulinum toxin poisoning, contact the local or state Health Department to process a request for antitoxin through the CDC. If you do not receive a response within 30 minutes, contact the CDC directly at 1-770-488-7100. More information can be obtained at http://www.cdc.gov/mmwr/preview/mmwrhtml/mm5232a8.htm.

Patient Information

Advise patients to inform their health care provider or pharmacist if they develop any unusual symptoms (including difficulty with swallowing, speaking, or breathing), or if any known symptom persists or worsens.

Counsel patients that if loss of strength, muscle weakness, blurred vision, or drooping eyelids occur, to avoid driving a car or engaging in other potentially hazardous activities.

Advise previously immobile or sedentary patients to gradually resume activities following the injection of botulinum toxin type A.

Inform patients that injections of botulinum toxin type A may cause dyspnea or mild to severe dysphagia, with the risk of aspiration.

Inform patients that injections of botulinum toxin type A may cause reduced blinking or effectiveness of blinking, and advise them to seek immediate medical attention if eye pain or irritation occur following treatment.

RIMABOTULINUMTOXIN B

Rx	**Myobloc** (Solstice Neurosciences)	**Injection, solution**[a]: 5,000 units/mL	Preservative free. In 0.5, 1, and 2 mL single-use vials.[b]

[a] One unit corresponds to the calculated median lethal intraperitoneal dose (LD_{50}) in mice.

[b] With human serum albumin 0.05%, 0.01 M sodium succinate, 0.1 M sodium chloride.

RIMABOTULINUMTOXIN B — INJECTION

WARNING

Distant spread of toxin effect – Postmarketing reports indicate that the effects of rimabotulinumtoxin B and all botulinum toxin products may spread from the area of injection to produce symptoms consistent with botulinum toxin effects. These may include asthenia, generalized muscle weakness, diplopia, blurred vision, ptosis, dysphagia, dysphonia, dysarthria, urinary incontinence, and breathing difficulties. These symptoms have been reported hours to weeks after injection. Swallowing and breathing difficulties can be life-threatening, and there have been reports of death. The risk of symptoms is probably greatest in children treated for spasticity, but symptoms can also occur in adults treated for spasticity and other conditions, particularly in those patients who have underlying conditions that would predispose them to these symptoms. In unapproved uses, including spasticity in children and adults, and in approved indications, cases of spread of effect have occurred at doses comparable with those used to treat cervical dystonia and at lower doses.

Indications

➤*Cervical dystonia:* For the treatment of adults with cervical dystonia to reduce the severity of abnormal head position and neck pain associated with cervical dystonia.

➤*Off-label uses:*

Sialorrhea (drooling) – [4] = Insufficient documentation. The use of rimabotulinumtoxin B for decreasing or controlling severe sialorrhea has been studied in a very small number of patients (approximately 25). Additional information is needed to determine expected duration of response, potential candidates, and optimal dosing regimens. Standardization of injection procedures also is needed to adequately evaluate results. (See Administration and Dosage.)

Administration and Dosage

➤*Adults:*

Cervical dystonia –

Initial dosage:

- *Botulinum toxin–experienced patients* – 2,500 to 5,000 units divided among affected muscles.
- *Botulinum toxin–naive patients* – Patients without a history of tolerating botulinum toxins should receive a lower initial dose.

Maintenance dosage: Optimize subsequent dosing according to the patient's individual response.

Duration of effect: Observed in studies to be between 12 and 16 weeks at doses of 5,000 or 10,000 units.

Off-label dosing –

Sialorrhea (drooling): [4] = Insufficient documentation. One study administered 1,000 units into each parotid gland and 250 units into each submandibular gland (total dose, 2,500 units). Another study administered 1,000 units into each parotid gland (total dose, 2,500 units).

➤*Preparation for administration:* Ready to use; no reconstitution required. Do not shake. Rimabotulinumtoxin B may be diluted with normal saline.

➤*Administration:* For intramuscular (IM) use. The effect of administering different botulinum neurotoxin serotypes at the same time or within less than 4 months of each other is unknown. However, neuromuscular paralysis may be potentiated by coadministration or overlapping administration of different botulinum toxin serotypes.

➤*Storage/Stability:* Store at 2° to 8°C (36° to 46°F). Do not freeze. Protect from light. After dilution with normal saline, the product must be used within 4 hours because the formulation does not contain a preservative. Discard unused portion.

Actions

➤*Pharmacology:* Rimabotulinumtoxin B, a purified neurotoxin, acts at the neuromuscular junction to produce flaccid paralysis.

Rimabotulinumtoxin B specifically has been demonstrated to cleave synaptic vesicle-associated membrane protein (VAMP, also known as synaptobrevin), which is a component of the protein complex responsible for docking and fusion of the synaptic vesicle to the presynaptic membrane, a necessary step for neurotransmitter release.

➤*Pharmacokinetics:* Using currently available analytical technology, it is not possible to detect rimabotulinumtoxin B in the peripheral blood following IM injection at the recommended doses.

Contraindications

Known hypersensitivity to any botulinum toxin preparation or to any of the components in the formulation; infection at the proposed injection site.

Warnings/Precautions

➤*Interchangeability:* The potency units of rimabotulinumtoxin B are specific to the preparation and assay method utilized. They are not interchangeable with other preparations of botulinum toxin products and, therefore, units of biological activity of rimabotulinumtoxin B cannot be compared with or converted into units of any other botulinum toxin products assessed with any other specific assay method.

➤*Spread of toxin effect:* See the Warning box for more information.

➤*Dysphagia and breathing difficulties:* Treatment with rimabotulinumtoxin B and other botulinum toxin products can result in swallowing or breathing difficulties. Patients with preexisting swallowing or breathing difficulties may be more susceptible to these complications. In most cases, this is a consequence of weakening of muscles in the area of injection that are involved in breathing or swallowing. When distant effects occur, additional respiratory muscles may be involved.

Deaths as a complication of severe dysphagia have been reported after treatment with botulinum toxin. Dysphagia may persist for several months and require use of a feeding tube to maintain adequate nutrition and hydration. Aspiration may result from severe dysphagia and is a particular risk when treating patients in whom swallowing or respiratory function is already compromised.

Treatment of cervical dystonia with botulinum toxins may weaken neck muscles that serve as accessory muscles of ventilation. This may result in a critical loss of breathing capacity in patients with respiratory disorders who may have become dependent upon these accessory muscles. There have been postmarketing reports of serious breathing difficulties, including respiratory failure, in cervical dystonia patients. Patients treated with botulinum toxin may require immediate medical attention if they develop problems with swallowing, speech, or respiratory disorders. These reactions can occur within hours to weeks after injection with botulinum toxin.

➤*Neuromuscular disorders:* Patients with peripheral motor neuropathic diseases, amyotrophic lateral sclerosis, or neuromuscular junctional disorders (eg, myasthenia gravis, Lambert-Eaton syndrome) should be monitored particularly closely when given botulinum toxin. Patients with neuromuscular disorders may be at increased risk of clinically significant effects, including severe dysphagia and respiratory compromise from typical doses of rimabotulinumtoxin B.

➤*Albumin:* This product contains albumin, a derivative of human blood. Based on effective donor screening and product manufacturing processes, it carries an extremely remote risk for transmission of viral diseases. A theoretical risk for transmission of Creutzfeldt-Jakob disease (CJD) also is considered extremely remote. No cases of transmission of viral diseases or CJD have ever been identified with albumin.

➤*Botulinum toxin–naive patients:* See Administration and Dosage for more information.

➤*Immunogenicity:* A 2-stage assay was used to test for immunogenicity and neutralizing activity induced by treatment with rimabotulinumtoxin B. In order to account for varying lengths of follow-up, life-table analysis methods were used to estimate the rates of development of immune responses and neutralizing activity. During the repeated treatment studies, 446 subjects were followed with periodic enzyme-linked immunosorbent assay (ELI-

RIMABOTULINUMTOXIN B — INJECTION

SA)–based evaluations for development of antibody responses against rimabotulinumtoxin B. Only patients who showed a positive ELISA were subsequently tested for the presence of neutralizing activity against rimabotulinumtoxin B in the mouse neutralization assay (MNA). Twelve percent of patients had positive ELISA assays at baseline. Patients began to develop new ELISA responses after a single treatment session with rimabotulinumtoxin B. By 6 months after initiating treatment, estimates for ELISA positive rate were 20%, which continued to rise to 36% at 1 year and 50% positive ELISA status at 18 months. Serum neutralizing activity was primarily not seen in patients until after 6 months. Estimated rates of development were 10% at 1 year and 18% at 18 months in the overall group of patients, based on analysis of samples from ELISA-positive patients. The effect of conversion to ELISA or MNA positive status on efficacy was not evaluated in these studies, and the clinical significance of development of antibodies has not been determined.

The data reflect the percentage of patients whose test results were considered positive for antibodies to rimabotulinumtoxin B in an in vitro and in vivo assay. The results of these antibody tests are highly dependent on the sensitivity and specificity of the assays. Additionally, the observed incidence of antibody positivity in an assay may be influenced by several factors, including sample handling, concomitant medications, and underlying disease. For these reasons, comparison of the incidence of antibodies to rimabotulinumtoxin B with the incidence to other products may be misleading.

➤*Pregnancy: Category C.* Animal reproduction studies have not been conducted with rimabotulinumtoxin B. It is also not known whether it can cause fetal harm when administered to a pregnant woman or can affect reproduction capacity. Give rimabotulinumtoxin B to a pregnant woman only if clearly needed.

➤*Lactation:* It is not known if this drug is excreted in human milk. A woman with maternal botulism safely breast-fed her infant; no botulinum toxin was detected in the mother's milk or in the infant. Because doses used medically are lower than those causing botulism, the amount ingested by an infant is expected to be insignificant and not expected to cause adverse effects. Exercise caution when rimabotulinumtoxin B is administered to a breast-feeding woman.

➤*Children:* Safety and efficacy have not been established.

➤*Monitoring:* Patients with peripheral motor neuropathic diseases, amyotrophic lateral sclerosis, or neuromuscular junctional disorders (eg, myasthenia gravis, Lambert-Eaton syndrome) should be monitored particularly closely when given botulinum toxin.

Drug Interactions

Rimabotulinumtoxin B Drug Interactions

Precipitant drug	Object drug[a]		Description
Aminoglycosides (eg, gentamicin)	Rimabotulinumtoxin B	↑	Neuromuscular action may be enhanced, resulting in protracted respiratory depression.
Nondepolarizing muscle relaxants (eg, tubocurarine), other agents interfering with neuromuscular transmission (eg, curare-like compounds)	Rimabotulinumtoxin B	↑	Neuromuscular action may be enhanced, resulting in protracted respiratory depression.
Other botulinum neurotoxin (botulinum toxin type A)	Rimabotulinumtoxin B	↑	Neuromuscular action may be enhanced, resulting in protracted respiratory depression.

[a] ↑ = object drug increased.

Adverse Reactions

➤*Cervical dystonia:*

Rimabotulinumtoxin B Adverse Reactions(≥ 5%)

Adverse reactions	Rimabotulinumtoxin B 2,500 units (n = 31)	Rimabotulinumtoxin B 5,000 units (n = 67)	Rimabotulinumtoxin B 10,000 units (n = 106)	Placebo (n = 104)
CNS				
Asthenia	3%	0%	6%	4%
Dizziness	3%	3%	6%	2%
Headache	10%	16%	11%	8%
Neck pain related to cervical dystonia	0%	16%	17%	16%
Pain related to cervical dystonia/ Torticollis	10%	4%	7%	4%
Torticollis	0%	4%	8%	7%
GI				
Dry mouth	3%	12%	34%	3%
Dyspepsia	3%	0%	10%	5%
Dysphagia	16%	10%	25%	3%
Nausea	10%	3%	8%	5%
Musculoskeletal				
Arthralgia	0%	1%	7%	5%
Back pain	3%	4%	7%	3%
Myasthenia	3%	4%	6%	3%
Respiratory				
Cough increased	3%	6%	7%	3%
Rhinitis	3%	1%	5%	6%
Miscellaneous				
Accidental injury	0%	4%	5%	4%
Flu syndrome	6%	9%	8%	4%
Infection	13%	19%	15%	15%
Injection-site pain	16%	12%	15%	9%
Pain	6%	6%	13%	10%

➤*Dry mouth and dysphagia:* Dry mouth and dysphagia were the adverse reactions most frequently resulting in discontinuation of treatment. There was an increased incidence of dysphagia with increased dose in the sternocleidomastoid muscle. The incidence of dry mouth showed some dose-related increase with doses injected into the splenius capitis, trapezius, and sternocleidomastoid muscles.

In the overall clinical trial experience with rimabotulinumtoxin B (570 patients, including the uncontrolled studies), most cases of dry mouth or dysphagia were reported as mild or moderate in severity. Severe dysphagia was reported by 3% of patients. Severe dry mouth was reported by 6% of patients. Dysphagia and dry mouth were the most frequent adverse reactions reported as a reason for discontinuation from repeated treatment studies. These adverse reactions led to discontinuation from further treatments with rimabotulinumtoxin B in some patients, even when not reported as severe.

➤*Other adverse reactions (2% or more):*

CNS – Anxiety, confusion, headache related to injection, hyperesthesia, migraine, pain related to cervical dystonia/torticollis, somnolence, tremor, vertigo.

Dermatologic – Ecchymosis, pruritus.

GI – GI disorder, glossitis, stomatitis, tooth disorder, vomiting.

GU – Cystitis, urinary tract infection, vaginal moniliasis.

Metabolic / Nutritional – Edema, hypercholesterolemia, peripheral edema.

Musculoskeletal – Arthritis, joint disorder.

Respiratory – Dyspnea, lung disorder, pneumonia.

Special senses – Abnormal vision, amblyopia, otitis media, taste perversion, tinnitus.

Miscellaneous – Abscess, allergic reaction, chest pain, chills, cyst, fever, hernia, malaise, neoplasm, vasodilation, viral infection.

Overdosage

➤*Symptoms:* Excessive doses of rimabotulinumtoxin B may be expected to produce neuromuscular weakness with a variety of symptoms. Symptoms of overdose are not likely to present immediately following injection(s). Should a patient ingest the product or be accidently overdosed, monitor the patient for up to several weeks for signs and symptoms of systemic weakness or paralysis.

➤*Treatment:* Respiratory support may be required where excessive doses cause paralysis of respiratory muscles. Medically monitor the patient for symptoms of excessive muscle weakness or muscle paralysis. Symptomatic treatment may be necessary. In the event of an overdose, antitoxin raised against botulinum toxin is available from the Centers for Disease Control and Prevention (CDC) in Atlanta, GA. However, the antitoxin will not reverse any botulinum toxin-induced effects already apparent by the time of antitoxin administration. In the event of suspected or actual cases of botulinum toxin poisoning, contact your local or state health department to process a request for antitoxin through the CDC. If you do not receive a response within 30 minutes, please contact the CDC directly at 770-488-7100. More information can be obtained at http://www.cdc.gov/ncidod/srp/drugs/drugservice.html.

Patient Information

Provide patients with a copy of the Medication Guide and review the contents with the patient.

Advise patients to inform their health care provider or pharmacist if they develop any unusual symptoms (including difficulty with swallowing, speaking, or breathing), or if any existing symptoms worsen.

Counsel patients to avoid driving a car or engaging in other potentially hazardous activities if loss of strength, muscle weakness, or impaired vision occur.

BISMUTH/METRONIDAZOLE/TETRACYCLINE HYDROCHLORIDE

Rx	**Helidac** (Prometheus Laboratories)	**Tablets, chewable; oral:** bismuth subsalicylate 262.4 mg	Equivalent to bismuth salicylate 102 mg. Mannitol, saccharin. (PG 11). Pink. In 14 blister cards of 8s.
		Tablets; oral: metronidazole 250 mg	Lactose. (Z 2971). In 14 blister cards of 4s.
		Capsules; oral: tetracycline 500 mg	(PG 12). Pale orange and white. In 14 blister cards of 4s.
Rx	**Pylera** (Axcan)	**Capsules; oral:** bismuth subcitrate potassium 140 mg/metronidazole 125 mg/ tetracycline 125 mg	(BMT). In 120s.

BISMUTH/METRONIDAZOLE/TETRACYCLINE HYDROCHLORIDE — ORAL

For more information, refer to the *H. pylori* Treatment Guidelines and individual monographs.

WARNING

Metronidazole has been shown to be carcinogenic in mice and rats. Avoid unnecessary use of the drug. Reserve its use for the conditions listed in the Indications section.

Indications

➤*Helicobacter pylori eradication:*

Helidac – In combination with an H_2 antagonist for the eradication of *Helicobacter pylori* for the treatment of patients with *Helicobacter pylori* infection and duodenal ulcer disease (active or a history of duodenal ulcer). Prescribe appropriate doses of H_2 antagonists for the treatment of active duodenal ulcers in all patients.

Pylera – In combination with omeprazole for the treatment of patients with *H. pylori* infection and duodenal ulcer disease (active or history of within the past 5 years) to eradicate *H. pylori*

Administration and Dosage

➤*Adults:*

Helicobacter pylori eradication –

Helidac:

• *Usual dosage* – Bismuth subsalicylate 525 mg, metronidazole 250 mg, and tetracycline 500 mg four times daily at meals and at bedtime.

• *Duration of therapy* – 14 days.

• *Concomitant therapy* – An H_2 antagonist approved for the treatment of acute duodenal ulcer.

• *Missed dose* – Missed doses can be made up by continuing the normal dosing schedule until the medication is gone. Instruct patients to not take double doses. If more than 4 doses are missed, advise patients to contact their health care provider.

Pylera:

• *Usual dosage* – Each dose of *Pylera* includes 3 capsules. Each dose of all 3 capsules should be taken 4 times a day, after meals and at bedtime.

***Pylera* and Omeprazole Daily Dosing Schedule**

Time of dose	Number of capsules of *Pylera*	Number of capsules of omeprazole 20 mg
After morning meal	3	1
After lunch	3	0
After evening meal	3	1
At bedtime	3	0

• *Duration of therapy* – 10 days.

• *Concomitant therapy* – One omeprazole 20 mg capsule taken twice a day with *Pylera* capsules after the morning or evening meal for 10 days.

➤*Children:* Use is contraindicated in children.

➤*Renal function impairment:* Use is contraindicated in patients with renal function impairment. See Warnings/Precautions for more information.

➤*Hepatic function impairment:* Use is contraindicated in patients with hepatic function impairment. See Warnings/Precautions for more information.

➤*Administration:* Ingestion of adequate amounts of fluid, particularly with the bedtime dose, is recommended to reduce the risk of esophageal irritation and ulceration by tetracycline.

Absorption of tetracycline is impaired by dairy products; give medication at least 1 hour after meals.

Helidac – The metronidazole tablet and tetracycline capsule should be swallowed whole with a full glass of water (8 oz). The bismuth subsalicylate tablets should be chewed and swallowed.

Pylera – Patients should be instructed to swallow capsules whole with a full glass of water (8 oz).

➤*Storage/Stability:* Store at 20° to 25°C (68° to 77°F).

Actions

➤*Pharmacology:* Bismuth, metronidazole, and tetracycline administered individually as combination therapy have been shown to be active against most strains of *H. Pylori* in vitro and in clinical infections.

➤*Pharmacokinetics:* Pharmacokinetics for bismuth subsalicylate, metronidazole, and tetracycline when coadministered have not been studied. There is no information about the gastric mucosal concentrations of bismuth, metronidazole, and tetracycline after administration of these agents concomitantly or in combination with an acid suppressive agent. The systemic pharmacokinetic information presented in this section is based on studies in which each product was administered alone.

Absorption/Distribution –

Bismuth subsalicylate: Upon oral administration, bismuth subsalicylate is almost completely hydrolyzed in the GI tract to bismuth and salicylic acid. Thus, the pharmacokinetics of bismuth subsalicylate following oral administration can be described by the individual pharmacokinetics of bismuth and salicylic acid.

• *Bismuth* – Less than 1% of bismuth from oral doses of bismuth subsalicylate is absorbed from the GI tract into the systemic circulation. Absorbed bismuth is distributed throughout the body. Bismuth is highly bound to plasma proteins (more than 90%). The mean trough blood bismuth concentration after 2 weeks' oral administration of bismuth subsalicylate 787 mg (3 chewable tablets) 4 times daily under fasted condition was 5.1 ± 3.1 ng/mL. In another study, the mean trough blood bismuth concentration after 2 weeks' oral administration of bismuth subsalicylate 525 mg (as *Pepto-Bismol* liquid suspension) 4 times daily was 5 ng/mL, with the highest value being 32 ng/mL.

• *Salicylic acid* – More than 80% of the salicylic acid is absorbed from oral doses of bismuth subsalicylate chewable tablets. Salicylic acid is about 90% plasma protein bound. The volume of distribution is about 170 mL/kg of body weight. After a single oral dose of bismuth subsalicylate 525 mg (2 chewable tablets), the mean peak plasma salicylic acid concentration was 13.1 ± 3.4 mcg/mL under fasted condition. The mean steady-state serum total salicylate concentration after 2 weeks' oral administration of bismuth subsalicylate 525 mg (as *Pepto-Bismol* liquid suspension) 4 times daily was 24 mcg/mL, with the highest value being 70 mcg/mL.

Metronidazole: Following oral administration, metronidazole is well absorbed, with peak plasma concentrations occurring between 1 and 2 hours after administration. Plasma concentrations of metronidazole are proportional to the administered dose, with oral administration of 250 mg producing a peak plasma concentration of 6 mcg/mL.

Tetracycline: Tetracyclines are readily absorbed and are bound to plasma proteins in varying degrees. They are concentrated by the liver in the bile and excreted in the urine and feces at high concentrations in a biologically active form.

Metabolism/Excretion –

Bismuth: Bismuth has multiple disposition half-lives with an intermediate half-life of 5 to 11 days and a terminal half-life of 21 to 72 days. Elimination of bismuth is primarily through urinary and biliary routes with a renal clearance of 50 ± 18 mL/min.

Salicylic acid: Salicylic acid is extensively metabolized, and about 10% is excreted unchanged in the urine. The metabolic clearance of salicylic acid is saturable; accordingly, nonlinear pharmacokinetics are observed as bismuth subsalicylate doses of more than 525 mg. The terminal half-life of salicylic acid upon a single oral dose of bismuth subsalicylate 525 mg is between 2 and 5 hours.

Metronidazole: Metronidazole is the major component appearing in the plasma, with lesser quantities of the 2-hydroxymethyl metabolite also being present. Less than 20% of the circulating metronidazole is bound to plasma proteins. Metronidazole also appears in cerebrospinal fluid, saliva, and human milk in concentrations similar to those found in plasma. The average elimination half-life of metronidazole in healthy volunteers is 8 hours. The major route of elimination of metronidazole and its metabolites is via the urine (60% to 80% of the dose), with fecal excretion accounting for 6% to 15% of the dose. The metabolites that appear in the urine result primarily from side-chain oxidation [1-(β-hydroxyethyl)-2-hydroxymethyl-5-nitroimidazole and 2-methyl-5-nitroimidazole-1-yl-acetic acid] and glucuronide conjugation, with unchanged metronidazole accounting for approximately 20% of the total. Renal clearance of metronidazole is approximately 10 mL/min per 1.73 m^2.

Special populations –

Hepatic function impairment: In patients with decreased hepatic function, plasma clearance of metronidazole is decreased.

Gender: Salicylic acid metabolic clearance is lower in women than in men.

Contraindications

Pregnant or breast-feeding women; children; renal or hepatic function impairment; known hypersensitivity to bismuth subsalicylate, metronidazole, or other nitroimidazole derivatives, or any of the tetracyclines. This product does not contain aspirin but should not be administered to patients who have a known allergy to aspirin or salicylates.

Warnings/Precautions

➤*Reye syndrome:* Children and teenagers who have or who are recovering from chicken pox or flu should not use medications containing bismuth subsalicylate to treat nausea or vomiting. If nausea or vomiting is present, patients are advised to consult a doctor because this could be an early sign of Reye syndrome, a rare but serious illness.

➤*CNS effects:* Convulsive seizures and peripheral neuropathy, the latter characterized mainly by numbness or paresthesia of an extremity, have been reported in patients treated with metronidazole. The prevalence and sever-

BISMUTH/METRONIDAZOLE/TETRACYCLINE HYDROCHLORIDE — ORAL

ity of the neuropathy are directly related to the cumulative dose and duration of therapy; it is most prevalent in patients taking high doses for prolonged treatment periods. The appearance of abnormal neurologic signs demands the prompt discontinuation of metronidazole therapy. Administer with caution to patients with CNS diseases.

There have been rare reports of neurotoxicity associated with excessive doses of bismuth subsalicylate. Effects have been reversible with discontinuation of therapy.

➤*Tooth development:* The use of drugs of the tetracycline class during tooth development (last half of pregnancy, infancy, and childhood up to 8 years of age) may cause permanent discoloration of the teeth (yellow, gray, brown). This adverse reaction is more common during long-term use of the drugs but has been observed following repeated short-term courses. Enamel hypoplasia has also been reported. Tetracycline is a component of therapy; therefore, do not use therapy in these patient populations.

➤*Prophylactic use:* Prescribing therapy in the absence of a proven or strongly suspected bacterial infection or a prophylactic indication is unlikely to provide benefit to the patient and increases the risk of the development of drug-resistant bacteria.

➤*Tongue and/or stool darkening:* Bismuth subsalicylate may cause a temporary and harmless darkening of the tongue and/or black stool. Do not confuse stool darkening with melena.

➤*Blood dyscrasia:* Metronidazole is a nitroimidazole; use it with caution in patients with evidence of or history of blood dyscrasia. A mild leukopenia has been observed; however, no persistent hematologic abnormalities attributable to metronidazole have been observed.

➤*Pseudotumor cerebri:* Pseudotumor cerebri (benign intracranial hypertension) in adults has been associated with the use of tetracyclines. The usual clinical manifestations are headache and blurred vision. While this condition and related symptoms usually resolve soon after discontinuation of the tetracycline, the possibility for permanent sequelae exists.

➤*Renal function impairment:* The antianabolic action of the tetracyclines may cause an increase in serum urea nitrogen (BUN). While this is not a problem in those with healthy renal function, in patients with significant renal function impairment, higher serum levels of tetracycline may lead to azotemia, hyperphosphatemia, and acidosis. See the Contraindications section for more information.

➤*Hepatic function impairment:* Patients with severe hepatic disease metabolize metronidazole slowly, with resultant accumulation of metronidazole and its metabolites in plasma. See the Contraindications section for more information.

➤*Superinfection:* As with other antibiotics, use of tetracycline may result in overgrowth of nonsusceptible organisms, including fungi. If superinfection occurs, discontinue tetracycline and institute appropriate therapy.

Known or previously unrecognized candidiasis may present more prominent symptoms during therapy with metronidazole and requires treatment with a candidacidal agent.

➤*Photosensitivity:* Photosensitivity, manifested by an exaggerated sunburn reaction, has been observed in some patients taking tetracyclines. Advise patients apt to be exposed to direct sunlight or ultraviolet light that this reaction can occur with tetracycline drugs. Discontinue treatment at the first evidence of skin erythema.

➤*Pregnancy: Category D.* Category D is based on the pregnancy category for tetracycline.

Teratogenic – Metronidazole crosses the placental barrier, and its effects on the human fetal organogenesis are not known. No fetotoxicity was observed when metronidazole was administered orally to pregnant mice at 20 mg/kg/day, approximately 1.5 times the most frequently recommended human dose (750 mg/day) based on mg/kg/body weight; however, in a single small study in which the drug was administered intraperitoneally, some intrauterine deaths were observed. The relationship of these findings to the drug is unknown.

There are no adequate and well-controlled studies in pregnant women. Do not use tetracycline as a component of therapy during pregnancy. Results of animal studies indicate that tetracyclines cross the placenta, are found in fetal tissues, and can have toxic effects on the developing fetus (often related to retardation of skeletal development). Evidence of embryotoxicity has also been noted in animals treated early in pregnancy. If this drug is used during pregnancy or if the patient becomes pregnant while taking this drug, apprise the patient of the potential hazard to the fetus.

Nonteratogenic – Pregnant women with renal disease may be more prone to develop tetracycline-associated liver failure.

➤*Lactation:* Metronidazole and tetracycline are both secreted into human milk. Because of the potential for tumorigenicity shown for metronidazole in mouse and rat studies, and because of the potential for serious adverse reactions in breast-feeding infants from tetracyclines, decide whether to discontinue breast-feeding or therapy, taking into account the importance of the therapy to the mother. Metronidazole is secreted in human milk in concentrations similar to those found in plasma.

➤*Children:* Safety and effectiveness in children infected with *H. pylori* have not been established.

Tetracycline use in children may cause permanent discoloration of the teeth. Enamel hypoplasia has also been reported. See the Contraindications section for more information.

➤*Elderly:* In general, consider the greater frequency of decreased hepatic, renal, or cardiac function, and of concomitant disease or other drug therapy in elderly patients when prescribing therapy. This therapy is contraindicated in patients with renal or hepatic function impairment.

Drug Interactions

Bismuth Subsalicylate/Metronidazole/Tetracycline Drug Interactions

Precipitant drug	Object drug[a]		Description
Bismuth subsalicylate	Anticoagulants (eg, warfarin)	↑	Salicylates may cause an increased risk of bleeding when administered with anticoagulant therapy.
Bismuth subsalicylate	Antidiabetic agents (eg, glyburide, tolbutamine)	↑	Possible enhanced hypoglycemic effect.
Aspirin	Bismuth subsalicylate	↑	Bismuth subsalicylate contains salicylate. If taken with aspirin and ringing in the ears occurs, discontinue use.
Bismuth subsalicylate	Aspirin		
Barbiturates (eg, phenobarbital) Phenytoin	Metronidazole	↓	Coadministration may accelerate the elimination of metronidazole, resulting in reduced plasma levels.
Cimetidine	Metronidazole	↑	Decreased metronidazole clearance and increased serum levels may occur; however, data conflict.
Metronidazole	Anticoagulants (eg, warfarin)	↑	The anticoagulant effect of warfarin may be enhanced.
Metronidazole	Disulfiram	↑	Concurrent use may result in an acute psychosis or confusional state. Do not give metronidazole to patients who have taken disulfiram within the last 2 weeks.
Metronidazole	Ethanol	↑	A disulfiram-like reaction, including symptoms of flushing, palpitations, tachycardia, nausea, and vomiting, may occur with concurrent use. Although the risk for most patients may be slight, caution is advised. Advise patients to not consume alcohol during therapy and for ≥ 1 to 3 days afterward.
Metronidazole	Lithium	↑	In patients stabilized on relatively high lithium doses, short-term metronidazole has been associated with increased lithium levels and toxicity in some cases.
Aluminum, calcium, iron, magnesium, zinc salts	Tetracycline	↓	Coadministration of aluminum, calcium, iron, magnesium, or zinc salts, and tetracycline decreases the absorption and serum levels of tetracycline. Absorption of iron salts may also be decreased.
Tetracycline	Iron salts		
Urinary alkalinizers (eg, potassium citrate, sodium bicarbonate, tromethamine)	Tetracycline	↓	Coadministration may result in increased excretion of tetracycline, decreased serum levels, and a decreased therapeutic response. Separate use of these agents by 3 to 4 hours.
Tetracycline	Anticoagulants (eg, warfarin)	↑	Tetracycline has been shown to depress plasma prothrombin activity. Downward adjustment of anticoagulant therapy may be required.
Tetracycline	Contraceptives, oral	↓	Concurrent use of tetracycline may render oral contraceptives less effective.
Tetracycline	Penicillin	↓	Because bacteriostatic drugs such as tetracycline may interfere with the bactericidal effects of penicillin, avoid giving these agents together.

[a] ↑ = object drug increased; ↓ = object drug decreased.

➤*Drug/Lab test interactions:* Bismuth absorbs x-rays and may interfere with x-ray diagnostic procedures of the GI tract.

Metronidazole may interfere with certain types of determinations of serum chemistry values, such as AST, ALT, lactate dehydrogenase, triglycerides, and hexokinase glucose. Values of zero may be observed. All of the assays in which interference has been reported involve enzymatic coupling of the assay to oxidation-reduction of nicotinamide (NAD + ⟷ NADG). Interfer-

BISMUTH/METRONIDAZOLE/TETRACYCLINE HYDROCHLORIDE — ORAL

ence is due to the similarity in absorbance peaks of NADH (340 nm) and metronidazole (322 nm) at pH7.

➤*Drug/Food interactions:* Absorption of tetracycline is impaired by dairy products; give medication at least 1 hour after meals.

Adverse Reactions

➤*Helidac:*

Helidac Adverse Reactions (≥1%)[a]	
Adverse reaction	Bismuth subsalicylate, metronidazole, and tetracycline[b] (N = 266)
CNS	
Asthenia	1.5%
Dizziness	1.5%
Headache	1.5%
Insomnia	1.1%
Paresthesia	1.1%
GI	
Abdominal pain	6.8%
Anal discomfort	1.1%
Anorexia	1.5%
Constipation	1.9%
Diarrhea	6.8%
Discolored tongue	1.5%
Duodenal ulcer	1.1%
Dyspepsia	1.5%
Flatulence	1.1%
GI hemorrhage	1.1%
Melena	3%
Nausea	12%
Stool abnormality	1.1%
Taste perversion	1.1%
Vomiting	1.5%
Miscellaneous	
Pain	1.1%
Sinusitis	1.1%
Upper respiratory tract infection	2.3%

[a] Includes reactions reported at ≥ 1% in patients taking bismuth subsalicylate/metronidazole/tetracycline in Graham, Cutler, and P&GP studies.
[b] In the Graham and Cutler studies (N = 197), most patients were on concomitant acid suppression therapy.

CNS – Nervousness, somnolence, syncope (less than 1%).

Cardiovascular – Cerebral ischemia, chest pain, hypertension, myocardial infarction (less than 1%).

Dermatologic – Acne, ecchymosis, photosensitivity reaction, pruritus, rash (less than 1%).

GI – Dry mouth, dysphagia, eructation, GI monilia, glossitis, intestinal obstruction, rectal hemorrhage, stomatitis, tooth disorder (less than 1%).

GU – Urinary tract infection (less than 1%).

Musculoskeletal – Arthritis, rheumatoid arthritis, tendonitis (less than 1%).

Metabolic/Nutritional – AST increase, ALT increase (less than 1%).

Miscellaneous – Conjunctivitis, flu syndrome, infection, malaise, neoplasm, rhinitis (less than 1%).

➤*Pylera:*

Pylera Adverse Reactions (> 1%)		
Adverse reaction	Pylera plus omeprazole (n = 147)	Omeprazole, amoxicillin, and clarithromycin (n = 152)
Cardiovascular		
Palpitation	1.4%	0%
CNS		
Anxiety	1.4%	0%
Asthenia	4.1%	2.6%
Dizziness	3.4%	2.6%
Headache	8.2%	7.2%
Dermatologic		
Maculopapular rash	1.4%	0%
Pruritus	0%	2.6%
Rash	0.7%	2%
GI		
Abdominal pain	8.8%	9.9%
Diarrhea	8.8%	15.1%
Dry mouth	1.4%	0.7%
Dyspepsia	8.8%	11.2%
Flatulence	0.7%	3.9%
Gastritis	1.4%	0%
Gastroenteritis	1.4%	0%
Glossitis	0%	1.3%
Nausea	8.2%	10.5%
Stool abnormality	15.6%	4.6%
Taste perversion	4.8%	11.8%
Vomit	1.4%	0.7%
GU		
Urinary abnormality	2%	0%
Vaginitis	4.1%	2.6%
Musculoskeletal		
Back pain	2%	1.3%
Respiratory		
Cough	0.7%	2%
Pharyngitis	2%	2.6%
Rhinitis	1.4%	2.6%
Sinusitis	0.7%	1.3%
Miscellaneous		
ALT increased	2%	0%
AST increased	1.4%	0%
Chest pain	1.4%	0%
Flu syndrome	5.4%	3.3%
Infection	2%	3.3%
Lab test abnormality	2.7%	2.6%
Pain	2%	4.6%

Overdosage

➤*Symptoms:* If all 3 components of this therapy are involved in an overdose, acute treatment should focus on the salicylate intoxication. There is neither a pharmacologic basis nor data suggesting an increased toxicity of the combination compared with individual components.

The main concern of an acute bismuth subsalicylate overdose focuses on the salicylate burden and not on bismuth, because less than 1% of the bismuth is normally absorbed. Each 262.4 mg tablet of bismuth subsalicylate contains an amount of salicylate comparable to approximately 130 mg of aspirin. Acute ingestion of less than 150 mg/kg of aspirin (ie, less than 1 tablet of bismuth subsalicylate per kilogram of body weight) is not expected to lead to toxicity. Mild to moderate toxicity may result from the ingestion of 150 to 300 mg/kg, while severe toxicity may occur from ingestions of more than 300 mg/kg. Salicylate intoxication is well described in the literature and presents a complex clinical picture. Multiple respiratory and metabolic effects result in fluid, electrolyte, glucose, and acid-base disturbances. Initial symptoms of salicylate toxicity include hyperpnea, nausea, vomiting, tinnitus, hyperpyrexia, lethargy, tachycardia, and confusion. In severe cases, these symptoms may progress to severe hyperpnea, convulsions, pulmonary or cerebral edema, respiratory failure, cardiovascular collapse, coma, and death.

Single oral doses of metronidazole, up to 19.5 g in adults, have been reported without resultant serious toxicity in suicide attempts and accidental overdoses. Symptoms reported include nausea, vomiting, and ataxia.

Neurotoxic effects, including seizures and peripheral neuropathy, have been reported after 5 to 7 days of doses of 6 to 10.4 g every other day.

The acute toxicity of tetracycline in overdose is not well established in the literature. Therapeutic and overdose quantities of tetracycline can cause GI symptoms such as nausea, vomiting, and diarrhea.

➤*Treatment:* In case of an overdose, patients should contact a health care provider, poison control center, or emergency room.

There is no specific antidote for salicylate poisoning. If there are no contraindications, induce vomiting as soon as possible with syrup of ipecac, or institute gastric lavage, provided that no more than 1 hour has elapsed since ingestion. Activated charcoal and a cathartic may be administered as primary decontamination therapy in cases where more than 1 hour has elapsed since ingestion or to further decontaminate the GI tract in those who have already received ipecac or gastric lavage. Plasma salicylate levels may be useful; a common nomogram can be used to help predict the severity of intoxication. Provide supportive and symptomatic treatment, with emphasis

BISMUTH/METRONIDAZOLE/TETRACYCLINE HYDROCHLORIDE — ORAL

on correcting fluid, electrolyte, blood glucose, and acid-base disturbances. (Note: An acidotic blood pH increases the unionized salicylate form, allowing more to reach the CNS.) Elimination may be enhanced by urinary alkalinization, hemodialysis, or hemoperfusion. Because hemodialysis aids in correcting acid-base disturbances, this method may be preferred over hemoperfusion.

There is no specific antidote for metronidazole or tetracycline overdose. Management of the patient should consist of symptomatic and supportive therapy. Metronidazole and tetracycline are dialyzable.

Patient Information

Missed doses can be made up by continuing the normal dosing schedule until the medication is gone. Patients should not take double doses. If more than 4 doses are missed, instruct patient to contact the health care provider.

Concurrent use of tetracyclines may render oral contraceptives less effective. Advise patients to use a different or additional form of contraception. Breakthrough bleeding has been reported. Advise women who become pregnant while taking these medications to notify their health care provider immediately.

Advise patients to avoid alcoholic beverages while taking metronidazole and for at least 1 day afterward.

Caution patients taking tetracycline to avoid exposure to sun or sun lamps.

Bismuth may cause temporary and harmless darkening of the tongue and/or black stool. Do not confuse stool darkening with melena (blood in the stool).

Counsel patients that antibacterial drugs are only used to treat bacterial infections. They do not treat viral infections (eg, the common cold). When therapy is prescribed to treat a bacterial infection, tell patients that, although it is common to feel better early in the course of therapy, the medication should be taken exactly as directed. Skipping doses or not completing the full course of therapy may decrease the effectiveness of the immediate treatment and increase the likelihood that bacteria will develop resistance and will not be treatable by these or other antibacterial drugs in the future.

Administration of adequate amounts of fluid, particularly with the bedtime dose of tetracycline, is recommended to reduce the risk of esophageal irritation and ulceration.

➤*Helidac*: Each dose of *Helidac* includes 4 pills: 2 pink round chewable tablets (bismuth subsalicylate), 1 white round tablet (metronidazole), and 1 orange and white capsule (tetracycline). Each dose (all 4 pills) should be taken 4 times a day, at mealtimes and bedtime. Instruct patients to chew and sallow the pink, round tablets (bismuth subsalicylate) and to swallow the white, round tablet (metronidazole) and the pale orange and white capsule (tetracycline) whole with a full glass of water (8 oz). Concomitantly prescribed H_2 antagonist therapy should be taken as directed.

The *Helidac* treatment regimen includes salicylates. If taken with aspirin and ringing in the ears occurs, consult the prescriber concerning discontinuation of the aspirin therapy until the *Helidac* therapy is completed.

➤*Pylera*: Each dose of *Pylera* includes 3 capsules. Each dose of 3 capsules should be taking 4 times a day, after meals and at bedtime for 10 days. Instruct patients to swallow capsules whole with a full glass of water (8 oz). One omeprazole 20 mg capsule should be taken twice a day with *Pylera* after the morning and evening meal for 10 days.

LANSOPRAZOLE/AMOXICILLIN/CLARITHROMYCIN

Rx	**Prevpac**[a] (Takeda Pharmaceuticals)	**Capsules; oral**: 500 mg amoxicillin	(AMOX 500 GG849). Yellow. In 4s.
		30 mg lansoprazole	(TAP PREVACID 30). Sugar spheres, sucrose. Black/pink. In 2s.
		Tablets; oral: 500 mg clarithromycin	(Abbott KL). Yellow, oval. Film-coated. In 2s.

[a] Consists of a daily administration pack.

LANSOPRAZOLE/AMOXICILLIN/CLARITHROMYCIN — ORAL

For more information, refer to the *Helicobacter pylori* Treatment Guidelines and individual monographs.

Indications

➤*Eradication of Helicobacter pylori:* Eradication of *H. pylori* to reduce risk of duodenal ulcer recurrence.

Administration and Dosage

➤*Adults:*

Eradication of Helicobacter pylori – Lansoprazole 30 mg, amoxicillin 1 g, and clarithromycin 500 mg administered together twice daily (morning and evening) for 10 or 14 days.

➤*Renal function impairment:* Do not use in patients with creatinine clearance (CrCl) less than 30 mL/min. In the presence of severe renal function impairment with or without coexisting hepatic function impairment, decreased clarithromycin dosage or prolonged dosing intervals may be appropriate.

➤*Hepatic function impairment:* Consider dose reduction of lansoprazole in patients with severe hepatic disease.

➤*Administration:* Each dose should be taken twice per day before eating. Swallow each capsule and tablet whole.

➤*Storage/Stability:* Store between 20° and 25°C (68° and 77°F). Protect from light and moisture.

Actions

➤*Pharmacology:* Lansoprazole suppresses gastric acid secretion by blocking the acid (proton) pump within gastric parietal cells, amoxicillin inhibits bacterial cell wall mucopeptide synthesis, and clarithromycin inhibits microbial protein synthesis.

➤*Pharmacokinetics:*

Absorption –

Lansoprazole: Lansoprazole capsules contain an enteric-coated granule formulation of lansoprazole. Absorption of lansoprazole begins only after the granules leave the stomach. Peak plasma concentrations (C_{max}) of lansoprazole and the area under the plasma concentration curve (AUC) of lansoprazole are approximately proportional in doses from 15 to 60 mg after single-dose oral administration. Lansoprazole does not accumulate and its pharmacokinetics are unaltered by multiple dosing.

The absorption of lansoprazole is rapid, with mean C_{max} occurring approximately 1.7 hours after oral dosing, and relatively complete with absolute bioavailability over 80%.

Amoxicillin: Amoxicillin is rapidly absorbed after oral administration. Orally administered doses of amoxicillin 500 mg result in average peak blood levels 1 to 2 hours after administration in the range of 5.5 to 7.5 mcg/mL. Detectable serum levels are observed up to 8 hours after an orally administered dose of amoxicillin.

Clarithromycin: Clarithromycin is rapidly absorbed from the GI tract after oral administration. The absolute bioavailability of clarithromycin 250 mg tablets was approximately 50%. In nonfasting healthy human subjects (men and women), peak plasma concentrations of clarithromycin were attained within 2 to 3 hours after oral dosing. Steady-state peak plasma clarithromycin concentrations were attained within 3 days and were approximately 3 to 4 mcg/mL with a 500 mg dose administered every 8 to 12 hours. The nonlinearity of clarithromycin pharmacokinetics is slight at the recommended dose of 500 mg administered every 8 to 12 hours. With a 500 mg dosing every 8 to 12 hours, the peak steady-state concentration of 14-OH clarithromycin is up to 1 mcg/mL. The steady-state concentration of 14-OH clarithromycin metabolite is generally attained within 3 to 4 days.

Food effects:

• *Lansoprazole* – The C_{max} and AUC of lansoprazole are diminished by about 50% if the drug is given 30 minutes after food, as opposed to the fasting condition. There is no significant food effect if the drug is given before meals.

• *Amoxicillin* – Amoxicillin is stable in the presence of gastric acid and may be given without regard to meals.

• *Clarithromycin* – For a single clarithromycin 500 mg dose, food slightly delays the onset of clarithromycin absorption, increasing the peak time from approximately 2 to 2.5 hours. Food also increases the clarithromycin peak plasma concentration by about 24% but does not affect the extent of clarithromycin bioavailability. Food does not affect the onset of formation of the antimicrobially active metabolite, 14-OH clarithromycin, or its peak plasma concentration, but it does slightly increase the extent of metabolite formation, indicated by an 11% decrease in AUC. Therefore, clarithromycin may be given without regard to food.

Distribution –

Lansoprazole: Lansoprazole is 97% bound to plasma proteins. Plasma protein binding is consistent over the concentration range of 0.05 to 5 mcg/mL.

Amoxicillin: Amoxicillin diffuses readily into most body tissues and fluids, with the exception of brain and spinal fluid, except when meninges are inflamed. In blood serum, amoxicillin is approximately 20% protein bound.

Metabolism –

Lansoprazole: Lansoprazole is extensively metabolized in the liver. Two metabolites have been identified in measurable quantities in plasma (the hydroxylated sulfinyl and sulfone derivatives of lansoprazole). These metabolites have very little or no antisecretory activity. Lansoprazole is thought to be transformed into 2 active species that inhibit acid secretion by (H^+,K^+)-ATPase within the parietal cell canaliculus but are not present in the systemic circulation.

Excretion –

Lansoprazole: In healthy subjects, the mean (± standard deviation) plasma half-life of lansoprazole was 1.5 (± 1) hours.

The plasma elimination half-life of lansoprazole does not reflect its duration of suppression of gastric acid secretion. Thus, the plasma elimination half-life of lansoprazole is less than 2 hours, while the acid inhibitory effect lasts more than 24 hours.

Following single-dose oral administration of lansoprazole, virtually no unchanged lansoprazole was excreted in the urine. In 1 study, after a single oral dose of ^{14}C-lansoprazole, approximately one third of the administered radiation was excreted in the urine and two thirds was recovered in the feces. This implies a significant biliary excretion of the metabolites of lansoprazole.

Amoxicillin: The half-life of amoxicillin is 61.3 minutes. Most of the amoxicillin is excreted unchanged in the urine; its excretion can be delayed by coadministration of probenecid. Approximately 60% of an orally administered dose of amoxicillin is excreted in the urine within 6 to 8 hours.

Clarithromycin: The elimination half-life of clarithromycin was 5 to 7 hours with 500 mg administered every 8 to 12 hours. The elimination half-life of 14-OH clarithromycin is about 7 to 9 hours. After a 500 mg tablet

LANSOPRAZOLE/AMOXICILLIN/CLARITHROMYCIN — ORAL

every 12 hours, the urinary excretion of clarithromycin is approximately 30%. The renal clearance of clarithromycin approximates the normal glomerular filtration rate. The major metabolite found in urine is 14-OH clarithromycin, which accounts for an additional 10% to 15% of the dose with a 500 mg tablet administered every 12 hours.

Special populations –

Renal function impairment: In patients with severe renal function impairment, plasma protein binding decreased by 1% to 1.5% after administration of lansoprazole 60 mg. Patients with renal function impairment had a shortened elimination half-life and decreased total AUC (free and bound). AUC for free lansoprazole in plasma, however, was not related to the degree of renal function impairment, and C_{max} and time of maximal concentration were not different from subjects with healthy kidneys.

The pharmacokinetics of clarithromycin were also altered in subjects with renal function impairment.

Hepatic function impairment: In patients with various degrees of chronic hepatic disease, the mean plasma half-life of lansoprazole was prolonged from 1.5 hours to 3.2 to 7.2 hours. An increase in mean AUC of up to 500% was observed at steady state in patients with hepatic function impairment compared with healthy subjects. Consider dose reduction in patients with severe hepatic disease.

The steady-state concentrations of clarithromycin in subjects with hepatic function impairment did not differ from those in healthy subjects; however, the 14-OH clarithromycin concentrations were lower in the subjects with hepatic function impairment. The decreased formation of 14-OH clarithromycin was at least partially offset by an increase in renal clearance of clarithromycin in the subjects with hepatic function impairment when compared with healthy subjects.

Elderly: The clearance of lansoprazole is decreased in elderly patients, with elimination half-life increased approximately 50% to 100%. Because the mean half-life in elderly patients remains between 1.9 and 2.9 hours, repeated once-daily dosing does not result in accumulation of lansoprazole. Peak plasma levels were not increased in elderly patients.

Race: The pooled pharmacokinetic parameters of lansoprazole from 12 US phase 1 studies (N = 513) were compared with the mean pharmacokinetic parameters from 2 Asian studies (N = 20). The mean AUCs of lansoprazole in Asian subjects are approximately twice that seen in pooled US data; however, the interindividual variability is high. The C_{max} values are comparable.

➤*Microbiology:* Lansoprazole, clarithromycin, and/or amoxicillin have been shown to be active against most strains of *H. pylori* in vitro and in clinical infections, as described in the Indications section.

Pretreatment resistance – Clarithromycin pretreatment resistance (2 mcg/mL or greater) was 9.5% (91/960) by E-test and 11.3% (12/106) by agar dilution in the dual- and triple-therapy clinical trials (M93-125, M93-130, M93-131, M95-392, and M95-399).

Amoxicillin pretreatment susceptible isolates (0.25 mcg/mL or less) occurred in 97.8% (936/957) and 98% (98/100) of the patients in the dual- and triple-therapy clinical trials by E-test and agar dilution, respectively. Twenty-one of 957 (2.2%) patients by E-test and 2 of 100 (2%) patients by agar dilution had amoxicillin pretreatment minimum inhibitory concentrations (MICs) of greater than 0.25 mcg/mL. One patient on the 14-day triple therapy regimen had an unconfirmed pretreatment amoxicillin MIC of greater than 256 mcg/mL by E-test, and the patient was eradicated of *H. pylori*.

Clarithromycin Susceptibility Test Results and Clinical/Bacteriological Outcomes[a,b]

Clarithromycin pretreatment results		*H. pylori* negative (eradicated)	Clarithromycin posttreatment results: *H. pylori* positive (not eradicated) – Posttreatment susceptibility results: S	I	R	No MIC
14-day triple therapy (lansoprazole 30 mg twice a day/ amoxicillin 1 g twice a day/clarithromycin 500 mg twice a day) (M95-399, M93-131, M95-392)						
Susceptible[c]	112	105				7
Intermediate[c]	3	3				
Resistant[c]	17	6			7	4
10-day triple therapy (lansoprazole 30 mg twice a day/ amoxicillin 1 g twice a day/clarithromycin 500 mg twice a day) (M95-399)						
Susceptible[c]	42	40	1		1	
Intermediate[c]						
Resistant[c]	4	1			3	

[a] Includes only patients with pretreatment clarithromycin susceptibility test results.
[b] S = susceptible; I = intermediate; R = resistant.
[c] S = MIC ≤ 0.25 mcg/mL; I = MIC 0.5 to 1 mcg/mL; R=MIC ≥ 2 mcg/mL.

Patients not eradicated of *H. pylori* following lansoprazole/amoxicillin/clarithromycin triple therapy will likely have clarithromycin-resistant *H. pylori*. Therefore, for those patients who fail therapy, perform clarithromycin susceptibility testing when possible. Do not treat patients with clarithromycin-resistant *H. pylori* with lansoprazole/amoxicillin/clarithromycin triple therapy or with regimens that include clarithromycin as the sole antimicrobial agent.

Contraindications

Known hypersensitivity to any component of the formulation of lansoprazole, any macrolide antibiotic, or any penicillin. Coadministration of this combination therapy (lansoprazole, amoxicillin, and clarithromycin) with astemizole, cisapride, dihydroergotamine, ergotamine, pimozide, or terfenadine is contraindicated. There have been postmarketing reports of drug interactions when clarithromycin and/or erythromycin are coadministered with astemizole, cisapride, pimozide, or terfenadine resulting in cardiac arrhythmias (eg, QT prolongation, torsades de pointes, ventricular fibrillation, ventricular tachycardia) most likely because of inhibition of metabolism of these drugs by erythromycin and clarithromycin. Fatalities have been reported.

Warnings/Precautions

➤*Pseudomembranous colitis:* Pseudomembranous colitis has been reported with nearly all antibacterial agents, including clarithromycin and amoxicillin, and may range in severity from mild to life-threatening. Therefore, it is important to consider this diagnosis in patients who present with diarrhea subsequent to the administration of antibacterial agents. Treatment with antibacterial agents alters the normal flora of the colon and may permit overgrowth of clostridia. Studies indicate that a toxin produced by *Clostridium difficile* is a primary cause of antibiotic-associated colitis.

➤*Gastric malignancy:* Symptomatic response to therapy with lansoprazole does not preclude the presence of gastric malignancy.

➤*Hypersensitivity reactions:* Serious and occasionally fatal hypersensitivity (anaphylactic) reactions have been reported in patients on penicillin therapy. Although anaphylaxis is more frequent following parenteral therapy, it has occurred in patients on oral penicillins. These reactions are more likely to occur in individuals with a history of penicillin hypersensitivity and/or a history of sensitivity to multiple allergens.

There have been reports of individuals with a history of penicillin hypersensitivity who have experienced severe reactions when treated with cephalosporins. Before initiating therapy with amoxicillin, make careful inquiry concerning previous hypersensitivity reactions to penicillins, cephalosporins, or other allergens. If an allergic reaction occurs, discontinue amoxicillin and institute appropriate therapy. Serious anaphylactic reactions require immediate emergency treatment with epinephrine. Also administer oxygen, intravenous (IV) steroids, and airway management, including intubation, as indicated.

➤*Renal/Hepatic function impairment:* Do not use in patients with CrCl less than 30 mL/min. Clarithromycin is principally excreted via the liver and kidney. Clarithromycin may be administered without dosage adjustment to patients with hepatic function impairment and with healthy renal function. However, in the presence of severe renal function impairment with or without coexisting hepatic function impairment, decreased dosage or prolonged dosing intervals may be appropriate. Consider dose reduction of lansoprazole in patients with severe hepatic disease.

➤*Superinfection:* During therapy, keep in mind the possibility of superinfections with mycotic or bacterial pathogens. If superinfections occur, discontinue this combination therapy and institute appropriate therapy.

➤*Pregnancy: Category C.* Category C is based on the pregnancy category for clarithromycin. There were no adequate and well-controlled studies of this combination therapy in pregnant women. Use this combination therapy during pregnancy only if the potential benefit justifies the potential risk to the fetus.

Clarithromycin – Four teratogenicity studies in rats (3 with oral doses and 1 with IV doses of up to 160 mg/kg/day administered during the period of major organogenesis) and 2 in rabbits at oral doses of up to 125 mg/kg/day (approximately 2 times the MRHD based on mg/m^2) or IV doses of 30 mg/kg/day administered during gestation days 6 to 18 failed to demonstrate any teratogenicity from clarithromycin. Two additional oral studies in a different rat strain at similar doses and similar conditions demonstrated a low incidence of cardiovascular anomalies at doses of 150 mg/kg/day administered during gestation days 6 to 15. Plasma levels after 150 mg/kg/day were 2 times the human serum levels. Four studies in mice revealed a variable incidence of cleft palate following oral doses of 1,000 mg/kg/day (2 and 4 times the MRHD based on mg/m^2, respectively) during gestation days 6 to 15. Cleft palate was also seen at 500 mg/kg/day. The 1,000 mg/kg/day exposure resulted in plasma levels of 17 times the human serum levels. In monkeys, an oral dose of 70 mg/kg/day (an approximate equidose of the MRHD based on mg/m^2) produced fetal growth retardation at plasma levels that were 2 times the human serum levels.

Do not use clarithromycin in pregnant women except in clinical circumstances in which no alternative therapy is appropriate. If pregnancy occurs while taking clarithromycin, apprise the patient of the potential hazard to the fetus. Clarithromycin has demonstrated adverse reactions of pregnancy outcome and/or embryofetal development in monkeys, rats, mice, and rabbits at doses that produced plasma levels 2 to 17 times the serum levels achieved in humans treated at the MRHD.

Labor and delivery – Oral ampicillin-class antibiotics are poorly absorbed during labor. Studies in guinea pigs showed that IV administration of ampicillin slightly decreased the uterine tone and frequency of contractions but moderately increased the height and duration of contractions. However, it is not known whether use of these drugs in humans during labor or delivery has immediate or delayed adverse reactions on the fetus, prolongs the duration of labor, or increases the likelihood that forceps delivery or other obstetrical intervention or resuscitation of the newborn will be necessary.

➤*Lactation:* Lansoprazole or its metabolites are excreted in the milk of rats. It is not known whether lansoprazole is excreted in human milk. Penicillins have been shown to be excreted in human milk. Amoxicillin use by

LANSOPRAZOLE/AMOXICILLIN/CLARITHROMYCIN — ORAL

breast-feeding mothers may lead to sensitization of infants. Exercise caution when amoxicillin is administered to a breast-feeding woman. It is not known whether clarithromycin is excreted in human milk. It is known that clarithromycin is excreted in the milk of lactating animals and that other drugs of this class are excreted in human milk.

Because of the potential for serious adverse reactions in breast-feeding infants from this combination therapy and the potential for tumorigenicity shown for lansoprazole in rat carcinogenicity studies, decide whether to discontinue breast-feeding or this combination therapy, taking into account the importance of the therapy to the mother.

➤*Children:* The safety and efficacy of this combination therapy in children infected with *H. pylori* have not been established.

➤*Elderly:* Elderly patients may suffer from asymptomatic renal and hepatic function impairment. Take care when administering this combination therapy to this patient population.

Drug Interactions

➤*Ampicillin, digoxin, iron, ketaconazole:* Lansoprazole causes a profound and long-lasting inhibition of gastric acid secretion; therefore, it is theoretically possible that lansoprazole may interfere with the absorption of drugs in which gastric pH is an important determinant of bioavailability (eg, ampicillin esters, digoxin, iron salts, ketoconazole).

➤*CYP-450 system:* Erythromycin and clarithromycin are substrates and inhibitors of the 3A isoform subfamily of the CYP-450 enzyme system (CYP3A). Coadministration of erythromycin or clarithromycin and a drug primarily metabolized by CYP3A may be associated with elevations in drug concentrations that could increase or prolong the therapeutic and adverse reactions of the concomitant drug. Dosage adjustments may be considered, and, when possible, monitor serum concentrations of drugs primarily metabolized by CYP3A closely in patients concurrently receiving clarithromycin or erythromycin.

Lansoprazole, Amoxicillin, and Clarithromycin Drug Interactions

Precipitant drug	Object drug[a]		Description
Amiloride	Amoxicillin	↓	The therapeutic activity of amoxicillin may be reduced.
Probenecid	Amoxicillin	↑	Probenecid decreases the renal tubular secretion of amoxicillin, which may result in increased and prolonged blood levels of amoxicillin.
Tetracyclines (eg, doxycycline, oxytetracycline)	Amoxicillin	↓	The pharmacologic and therapeutic actions of amoxicillin could be reduced. Avoid this combination if possible.
Amoxicillin	Contraceptives, oral	↓	The efficacy of oral contraceptives may be reduced. Although infrequently reported, contraceptive failure is possible; the use of an additional form of contraception during amoxicillin therapy is advisable.
Amoxicillin	Methotrexate	↑	Serum methotrexate concentrations may be elevated, increasing the risk of toxicity.
Rifamycins (eg, rifabutin, rifampin)	Clarithromycin	↓	The antimicrobial effects of clarithromycin may be decreased, while the frequency of GI adverse effects may be increased.
Antiarrhythmics (eg, disopyramide, quinidine)	Clarithromycin	↑	Torsades de pointes has occurred with coadministration. Monitor electrocardiograms for QTc prolongation during coadministration.
Clarithromycin	Antiarrhythmics (eg, disopyramide, quinidine)	↑	
Clarithromycin	Anticoagulants (eg, warfarin)	↑	Anticoagulant effects may be potentiated. Monitor prothrombin time with coadministration.
Clarithromycin	Benzodiazepines (eg, alprazolam, midazolam, triazolam)	↑	The plasma levels of certain benzodiazepines may be elevated, increasing and prolonging the CNS depressant effects.
Clarithromycin	Buspirone	↑	Plasma buspirone concentrations may be elevated, increasing the pharmacologic and adverse effects.
Clarithromycin	Cabergoline	↑	Cabergoline plasma concentrations may be elevated, increasing the risk of toxicity.
Clarithromycin	Carbamazepine	↑	Increased concentrations of carbamazepine may occur.
Clarithromycin	Cilostazol	↑	Cilostazol plasma concentrations may be elevated, increasing the therapeutic and adverse effects.
Clarithromycin	Astemizole, cisapride, pimozide, terfenadine	↑	Coadministration is contraindicated.
Clarithromycin	Colchicine	↑	There have been postmarketing reports of colchicine toxicity with concomitant use, especially in elderly patients, some of which occurred in patients with renal function impairment. Deaths have been reported in some of these patients.
Clarithromycin	Conivaptan	↑	Conivaptan plasma concentrations may be elevated. Coadministration is contraindicated.
Clarithromycin	Cyclosporine	↑	Elevated cyclosporine levels with increased risk of toxicity may occur.
Clarithromycin	Digoxin	↑	Serum digoxin concentrations may be elevated, resulting in possible digoxin toxicity.
Clarithromycin	Eplerenone	↑	Elevated eplerenone plasma concentrations may increase the risk of hyperkalemia and associated, sometimes fatal, arrhythmias. Coadministration is contraindicated.
Clarithromycin	Ergot alkaloids (eg, dihydroergotamine, ergotamine)	↑	Acute ergot toxicity has occurred with coadministration. Concomitant use is contraindicated.
Clarithromycin	HMG-CoA reductase inhibitors (eg, lovastatin, simvastatin)	↑	The risk of severe myopathy may be increased.
Clarithromycin	Methylprednisolone	↑	The pharmacologic and toxic effects of methylprednisolone may be increased.
Clarithromycin	Ranolazine	↑	Increased risk of life-threatening cardiac arrhythmias. Coadministration is contraindicated.
Clarithromycin	Repaglinide	↑	Clarithromycin may elevate repaglinide plasma levels. Adjust the repaglinide dose as needed.
Clarithromycin	Sildenafil	↑	Sildenafil plasma concentrations may be elevated with coadministration, increasing the risk of adverse reactions.
Clarithromycin	Tacrolimus	↑	Plasma tacrolimus levels may be elevated, increasing the risk of toxicity. Monitor renal function with coadministration.
Clarithromycin	Theophylline	↑	Concurrent use may be associated with increased serum theophylline levels.
Clarithromycin	Verapamil	↑	Increased risk of cardiotoxicity. Monitor cardiac function with coadministration.
Sucralfate	Lansoprazole	↓	Coadministration delayed the absorption and the bioavailability of lansoprazole. Therefore, administer lansoprazole at least 30 minutes prior to sucralfate.
Lansoprazole	Azole antifungals (eg, itraconazole, ketoconazole)	↓	The bioavailability of certain azole antifungals may be decreased because of a possible reduction in tablet dissolution in the presence of a high gastric pH. Avoid coadministration if possible.
Lansoprazole	Protease inhibitors (eg, atazanavir, indinavir)	↓	Do not coadminister because of a significant reduction in protease inhibitor exposure.
Lansoprazole	Salicylates (eg, aspirin)	↑	Enteric-coated salicylates may dissolve more rapidly, increasing gastric adverse reactions.

LANSOPRAZOLE/AMOXICILLIN/CLARITHROMYCIN — ORAL

Lansoprazole, Amoxicillin, and Clarithromycin Drug Interactions			
Precipitant drug	Object drug[a]		Description
Lansoprazole	Warfarin	↑	There have been reports of increased INR[b] and prothrombin time with coadministration.

[a] ↑ = object drug increased; ↓ = object drug decreased.
[b] INR = international normalization ratio.

➤*Drug/Lab test interactions:* High urine concentrations of ampicillin may result in false-positive reactions when testing for the presence of glucose in urine using *Clinitest*, Benedict's solution, or Fehling's solution. Because this effect may also occur with amoxicillin, it is recommended that glucose tests based on enzymatic glucose oxidase reactions (such as *Clinistix*) be used. Following administration of ampicillin to pregnant women, a transient decrease in plasma concentration of total conjugated estriol, estriol-glucuronide, conjugated estrone, and estradiol has been noted. This effect may also occur with amoxicillin.

➤*Drug/Food interactions:* Both C_{max} and AUC of lansoprazole are diminished about 50% if the drug is given 30 minutes after food, as opposed to the fasting condition.

Adverse Reactions

➤*Combination therapy:* The most common adverse reactions (3% or more) reported in clinical trials when all 3 components of this therapy were given concomitantly for 14 days are listed in the following table.

Lansoprazole/Amoxicillin/Clarithromycin Combination Therapy Adverse Reactions (≥ 3%)	
Adverse reaction	Triple therapy (n = 138)
Diarrhea	7%
Headache	6%
Taste perversion	5%

➤*Additional adverse reactions:* The additional adverse reactions reported as possibly or probably related to treatment in clinical trials when all 3 components of this therapy were given concomitantly are listed in the following information.

There were no statistically significant differences in the frequency of reported adverse reactions between the 10- and 14-day triple therapy regimens.

CNS – Confusion, dizziness (less than 3%).

Dermatologic – Skin reactions (less than 3%).

GI – Abdominal pain, dark stools, dry mouth/thirst, glossitis, nausea, oral moniliasis, rectal itching, stomatitis, tongue discoloration, tongue disorder, vomiting (less than 3%).

GU – Vaginal moniliasis, vaginitis (less than 3%).

Musculoskeletal – Myalgia (less than 3%).

Respiratory – Respiratory disorders (less than 3%).

➤*Incidence in clinical trials:* The following adverse reactions were reported by the treating health care provider to have a possible or probable relationship to the drug in 1% or more of lansoprazole-treated patients and occurred at a greater rate in lansoprazole-treated patients than placebo-treated patients.

Lansoprazole Adverse Reactions (≥ 1%)		
Adverse reaction	Lansoprazole (n = 2,768)	Placebo (n = 1,023)
Abdominal pain	2.1%	1.2%
Constipation	1%	0.4%
Diarrhea	3.8%	2.3%
Nausea	1.3%	1.2%

Headache was also seen at a greater than 1% incidence but was more common in the placebo group. The incidence of diarrhea was similar between patients who received placebo and patients who received lansoprazole 15 and 30 mg, but higher in the patients who received lansoprazole 60 mg (2.9%, 1.4%, 4.2%, and 7.4%, respectively).

The most commonly reported possibly or probably treatment-related adverse reaction during maintenance therapy was diarrhea.

➤*Additional lansoprazole adverse reactions:* Additional adverse reactions occurring in less than 1% of patients or subjects in domestic trials are shown in the following information.

Cardiovascular – Angina, arrhythmia, bradycardia, cerebral infarction/cerebrovascular accident, hypertension/hypotension, migraine, myocardial infarction, palpitations, shock (circulatory failure), syncope, tachycardia, vasodilation (less than 1%).

CNS – Abnormal dreams, agitation, amnesia, anxiety, apathy, confusion, convulsion, depersonalization, depression, diplopia, dizziness, emotional lability, hallucinations, hemiplegia, hostility aggravated, hyperkinesia, hypertonia, hypesthesia, insomnia, libido decreased/increased, malaise, nervousness, neurosis, paresthesia, sleep disorder, somnolence, thinking abnormality, tremor, vertigo (less than 1%).

Dermatologic – Acne, alopecia, contact dermatitis, dry skin, fixed eruption, hair disorder, maculopapular rash, nail disorder, pruritus, rash, skin carcinoma, skin disorder, sweating, urticaria (less than 1%).

Endocrine – Diabetes mellitus, goiter, hypothyroidism (less than 1%).

GI – Abdomen enlarged, abnormal stools, anorexia, bezoar, cardiospasm, cholelithiasis, colitis, dry mouth, dyspepsia, dysphagia, enteritis, eructation, esophageal stenosis, esophageal ulcer, esophagitis, fecal discoloration, flatulence, gastric nodules/fundic gland polyps, gastritis, gastroenteritis, GI anomaly, GI disorder, GI hemorrhage, glossitis, gum hemorrhage, hematemesis, increased appetite, increased salivation, melena, mouth ulceration, nausea and vomiting, nausea and vomiting and diarrhea, oral moniliasis, rectal disorder, rectal hemorrhage, stomatitis, tenesmus, thirst, tongue disorder, ulcerative colitis, ulcerative stomatitis (less than 1%).

GU – Abnormal menses, breast enlargement, breast pain, breast tenderness, dysmenorrhea, dysuria, gynecomastia, impotence, kidney calculus, kidney pain, leukorrhea, menorrhagia, menstrual disorder, pelvic pain, penis disorder, polyuria, testis disorder, urethral pain, urinary frequency, urinary tract infection, urinary urgency, urination impaired, vaginitis (less than 1%).

Hematologic/Lymphatic – Anemia, hemolysis, lymphadenopathy (less than 1%).

Metabolic/Nutritional – Gout, dehydration, hyperglycemia/hypoglycemia, peripheral edema, weight gain/loss (less than 1%).

Musculoskeletal – Arthralgia, arthritis, back pain, bone disorder, joint disorder, leg cramps, musculoskeletal pain, myalgia, myasthenia, neck pain, neck rigidity, synovitis (less than 1%).

Respiratory – Asthma, bronchitis, cough increased, dyspnea, epistaxis, hemoptysis, hiccup, laryngeal neoplasia, pharyngitis, pleural disorder, pneumonia, respiratory disorder, rhinitis, sinusitis, stridor, upper respiratory tract inflammation/infection (less than 1%).

Special senses – Abnormal vision, blurred vision, conjunctivitis, deafness, dry eyes, ear disorder, eye pain, otitis media, parosmia, photophobia, retinal degeneration, taste loss, taste perversion, tinnitus, visual field defect (less than 1%).

Miscellaneous – Allergic reaction, asthenia, candidiasis, carcinoma, chest pain (not otherwise specified), chills, edema, fever, flu syndrome, halitosis, infection (not otherwise specified), pain (less than 1%).

➤*Laboratory values:* The following changes in laboratory parameters for lansoprazole were reported as adverse reactions. In the placebo-controlled studies, when AST and ALT were evaluated, 0.4% (4/978) of placebo patients and 0.4% (11/2,677) of lansoprazole patients had enzyme elevations greater than 3 times the upper limit of normal range at the final treatment visit. None of these lansoprazole patients reported jaundice at any time during the study.

Lab test abnormalities – Abnormal albumin-globulin ratio, abnormal liver function tests, abnormal red blood cell count, bilirubinemia, eosinophilia, hyperlipemia, increased alkaline phosphatase, increased creatinine, increased/decreased/abnormal white blood cell count (WBC), increased/decreased/abnormal platelets, increased/decreased cholesterol, increased/decreased electrolytes, increased gastrin levels, increased gamma-glutamyl transpeptidase, increased globulins, increased glucocorticoids, increased lactate dehydrogenase (LDH), increased ALT, increased AST. Urine abnormalities such as albuminuria, glycosuria, and hematuria were also reported. Additional isolated laboratory abnormalities were reported.

➤*Amoxicillin:* The following adverse reactions have been reported in association with the use of penicillins.

CNS – Agitation, anxiety, behavioral changes, confusion, dizziness, insomnia, and/or reversible hyperactivity have been reported rarely.

GI – Nausea, diarrhea, hemorrhagic/pseudomembranous colitis, vomiting.

Onset of pseudomembranous colitis symptoms may occur during or after antibiotic treatment.

Hematologic/Lymphatic – Agranulocytosis, anemia (including hemolytic anemia), eosinophilia, leukopenia, thrombocytopenia, and thrombocytopenic purpura have been reported during therapy with penicillins. These reactions are usually reversible upon discontinuation of therapy and are believed to be hypersensitivity phenomena.

Hepatic – A moderate rise in AST and/or ALT has been noted, but the significance of this finding is unknown. Hepatic function impairment, including acute cytolytichepatitis, cholestatic jaundice, and hepatic cholestasis, has been reported.

Hypersensitivity – Acute generalized exanthematous pustulosis, erythema multiforme, erythematous maculopapular rashes, exfoliative dermatitis, hypersensitivity vasculitis, serum sickness–like reactions, Stevens-Johnson syndrome, toxic epidermal necrolysis, urticaria.

Renal – Crystalluria has also been reported.

Miscellaneous – Tooth discoloration (brown, yellow, or gray staining) has been rarely reported. Most reports occurred in children. Discoloration was reduced or eliminated with brushing or dental cleaning in most cases.

➤*Clarithromycin:* The following adverse reactions from the labeling for clarithromycin are provided for information. The majority of adverse reactions observed in clinical trials were of a mild and transient nature. Fewer than 3% of adult patients without mycobacterial infections discontinued therapy because of drug-related adverse reactions.

The most frequently reported reactions in adults were diarrhea (3%), nausea (3%), abnormal taste (3%), dyspepsia (2%), abdominal pain/discomfort (2%), and headache (2%). Most of these reactions were described as mild or moderate in severity. Of the reported adverse reactions, only 1% was described as severe.

LANSOPRAZOLE/AMOXICILLIN/CLARITHROMYCIN — ORAL

➤*Laboratory values:*

Lab test abnormalities – Elevated ALT less than 1%, AST less than 1%, Gamma-glutamyltransferase (GGT) less than 1%, alkaline phosphatase less than 1%, LDH less than 1%, total bilirubin less than 1%. Decreased WBC less than 1%, elevated prothrombin time 1%.

Elevated serum urea nitrogen 4%, elevated serum creatinine less than 1%. Alkaline phosphatase, GGT, and prothrombin time data are from adult studies only.

➤*Postmarketing:*

Clarithromycin – Allergic reactions ranging from urticaria and mild skin eruptions to rare cases of anaphylaxis, Stevens-Johnson syndrome, and toxic epidermal necrolysis have occurred. Other spontaneously reported adverse reactions include anorexia, dizziness, glossitis, leukopenia, neutropenia, oral moniliasis, pancreatitis, stomatitis, thrombocytopenia, tongue discoloration, and vomiting. There have been reports of tooth discoloration in patients treated with clarithromycin. Tooth discoloration is usually reversible with professional dental cleaning. There have been isolated reports of hearing loss, which is usually reversible, occurring chiefly in elderly women. Reports of alterations of the sense of smell, usually in conjunction with taste perversion or taste loss have also been reported.

Transient CNS reactions, including anxiety, behavioral changes, confusional states, convulsions, depersonalization, disorientation, hallucinations, insomnia, manic behavior, nightmares, psychosis, tinnitus, tremor, and vertigo, have been reported during postmarketing surveillance. Reactions usually resolve with discontinuation of the drug.

Hepatic function impairment, including increased liver enzymes and hepatocellular and/or cholestatic hepatitis, with or without jaundice, has been infrequently reported with clarithromycin. This hepatic function impairment may be severe and is usually reversible. In very rare instances, hepatic failure with a fatal outcome has been reported and generally has been associated with serious underlying diseases and/or concomitant medications.

There have been rare reports of hypoglycemia, some of which have occurred in patients taking oral hypoglycemic agents or insulin. As with other macrolides, clarithromycin has been associated with QT prolongation and ventricular arrhythmias, including ventricular tachycardia and torsades de pointes.

There have been reports of interstitial nephritis coincident with clarithromycin use.

There have been postmarketing reports of colchicine toxicity with concomitant use of clarithromycin and colchicine, especially in elderly patients, some of which occurred in patients with renal function impairment. Deaths have been reported in some of these patients.

Lansoprazole – Additional adverse reactions have been reported since lansoprazole has been marketed. The majority of these cases are foreign-sourced, and a relationship to lansoprazole has not been established. Because these reactions were reported voluntarily from a population of unknown size, estimates of frequency cannot be made. The following reactions are listed by Coding Symbols for a Thesaurus of Adverse Reaction Terms body system.

Dermatologic – Severe dermatologic reactions, including erythema multiforme, Stevens-Johnson syndrome, toxic epidermal necrolysis, (some fatal).

GI – Hepatotoxicity, pancreatitis, vomiting.

GU – Interstitial nephritis, urinary retention.

Hematologic / Lymphatic – Agranulocytosis, aplastic anemia, hemolytic anemia, leukopenia, neutropenia, pancytopenia, thrombocytopenia, and thrombotic thrombocytopenic purpura.

Musculoskeletal – Myositis.

Special senses – Speech disorder.

Miscellaneous – Anaphylactic/anaphylactoid reactions.

Overdosage

In case of an overdose, instruct patients to contact a health care provider, poison control center, or emergency room. There is neither a pharmacologic basis nor data suggesting an increased toxicity of the combination compared with individual components.

➤*Symptoms:*

Lansoprazole – Oral doses of lansoprazole of up to 5,000 mg/kg in rats (approximately 1,300 times the 30 mg human dose based on BSA) and mice (about 675.7 times the 30 mg human dose based on BSA) did not produce deaths or any clinical signs. In 1 reported case of overdose, the patient consumed lansoprazole 600 mg with no adverse reaction.

Amoxicillin – A prospective study of 51 children at a poison control center suggested that overdosages of less than 250 mg/kg of amoxicillin are not associated with significant clinical symptoms and do not require gastric emptying.

Interstitial nephritis resulting in oliguric renal failure has been reported in a small number of patients after overdosage with amoxicillin. Crystalluria, in some cases leading to renal failure, has also been reported after amoxicillin overdosage in adults and children.

Clarithromycin – Overdosage of clarithromycin can cause GI symptoms, such as abdominal pain, diarrhea, nausea, and vomiting.

➤*Treatment:*

Lansoprazole – Lansoprazole is not removed from circulation by hemodialysis.

Amoxicillin – In case of overdosage, discontinue amoxicillin, treat symptomatically, and institute supportive measures as required. If the overdosage is very recent and there is no contraindication, an attempt at emesis or other means of removal of drug from the stomach may be performed.

In case of amoxicillin overdosage, maintain adequate fluid intake and diuresis to reduce the risk of amoxicillin crystalluria. Renal function impairment appears to be reversible with cessation of amoxicillin administration. High blood levels may occur more readily in patients with renal function impairment because of decreased renal clearance of amoxicillin. Amoxicillin can be removed from circulation by hemodialysis.

Clarithromycin – Treat adverse reactions accompanying overdosage of clarithromycin by the prompt elimination of unabsorbed drug and supportive measures. As with other macrolides, clarithromycin serum levels are not expected to be appreciably affected by hemodialysis or peritoneal dialysis.

Patient Information

Each dose of this combination therapy contains 4 pills: 1 pink and black capsule (lansoprazole); 2 opaque, yellow capsules (amoxicillin); and 1 yellow tablet (clarithromycin). Each dose should be taken twice per day before eating. Patients should be instructed to swallow each pill whole.

Clarithromycin may interact with some drugs; therefore, advise patients to report to their health care provider the use of any other medications.

Counsel patients that antibacterial drugs, including this combination therapy, should only be used to treat bacterial infections. They do not treat viral infections (eg, the common cold). When this combination therapy is prescribed to treat a bacterial infection, tell patients that although it is common to feel better early in the course of therapy, the medication should be taken exactly as directed. Skipping doses or not completing the full course of therapy may (1) decrease the efficacy of the immediate treatment, and (2) increase the likelihood that bacteria will develop resistance and will not be treatable by this combination therapy or other antibacterial drugs in the future.

HISTAMINE H_2 ANTAGONISTS

Indications

➤*Benign gastric ulcer:* For the short-term treatment of active, benign gastric ulcer. **Ranitidine** is also indicated for the maintenance therapy after the healing of acute ulcer.

➤*Duodenal ulcer:* For the short-term treatment of active duodenal ulcer and maintenance therapy after the healing of active ulcer.

➤*Gastroesophageal reflux disease (GERD):*

Cimetidine (oral only) – For the treatment of erosive esophagitis diagnosed by endoscopy.

Famotidine – For the short-term treatment of GERD and esophagitis due to GERD, including erosive or ulcerative disease diagnosed by endoscopy.

Nizatidine – For the treatment of endoscopically diagnosed esophagitis, including erosive and ulcerative esophagitis, and associated heartburn due to GERD.

Ranitidine – For the treatment of GERD and endoscopically diagnosed erosive esophagitis; for the maintenance of healing of erosive esophagitis.

➤*GI bleeding (intravenous [IV] cimetidine only):* For the prevention of upper GI bleeding in critically ill patients.

➤*Pathological hypersecretory conditions* (**cimetidine, famotidine, ranitidine**): For the treatment of pathological hypersecretory conditions (eg, Zollinger-Ellison syndrome, systemic mastocytosis, multiple endocrine adenomas).

➤*Heartburn (OTC products only):* For the relief of heartburn associated with acid indigestion and sour stomach; for the prevention of heartburn associated with acid indigestion and sour stomach brought on by certain foods and beverages.

➤*Off-label uses:*

Hirsutism –

Cimetidine (oral): [5] = Poor documentation.

Interstitial cystitis (painful bladder disease) –

Cimetidine: [5] = Poor documentation.

Prevention of aspiration pneumonia –

Cimetidine: [5] = Poor documentation.

Famotidine: [4] = Insufficient documentation.

Ranitidine: [2] = Fair documentation.

Prevention of paclitaxel hypersensitivity reactions –

Famotidine (injection): [2] = Fair documentation.

Urticaria –

Cimetidine: [4] = Insufficient documentation.

Famotidine: [4] = Insufficient documentation.

Ranitidine: [5] = Poor documentation.

Warts (cutaneous, nongenital) –

Cimetidine (oral): [5] = Poor documentation.

Weight loss –
Cimetidine: [5] = Poor documentation.

Weight loss (antipsychotic-induced weight gain) –
Nizatidine: [4] = Insufficient documentation.

Other possible off-label uses – As part of a multidrug regimen to eradicate *Helicobacter pylori* in the treatment of peptic ulcer; in the perioperative setting to suppress gastric acid secretion, and prevent stress ulcers.

Cimetidine: Prevention of paclitaxel hypersensitivity (IV cimetidine); to reduce the incidence of GI hemorrhage associated with stress-related ulcers (IV cimetidine).

Famotidine: Prevention of recurrent bleeding after successful endoscopic treatment of bleeding peptic ulcer (IV famotidine); to reduce the incidence of GI hemorrhage associated with stress-related ulcers (IV famotidine).

Nizatidine: Prevention of nonsteroidal anti-inflammatory drug–induced gastroduodenal ulcer.

Ranitidine: Prevention of paclitaxel hypersensitivity (IV ranitidine); as prophylaxis to reduce the incidence of nonsteroidal anti-inflammatory drug (NSAID)-induced duodenal ulcer; to reduce the incidence of GI hemorrhage associated with stress-related ulcers (IV ranitidine).

Histamine H_2 Antagonists: Summary of Indications[a]

✓ – Labeled x – Unlabeled	Cimetidine	Famotidine	Nizatidine	Ranitidine
Benign gastric ulcer Treatment	✓	✓	✓	✓
Maintenance				✓
Duodenal ulcer Treatment	✓	✓	✓	✓
Maintenance	✓	✓	✓	✓
Erosive esophagitis, maintenance				✓
GERD (including erosive esophagitis)	✓	✓	✓	✓
Pathological hypersecretory conditions	✓	✓		✓
Peptic ulcer[c]	x[g]	x[g]	x[g]	x[g]
Prevent aspiration pneumonitis		x[f]	x[g]	x[e]
Prevent NSAID-induced duodenal ulcer			x[g]	x[g]
Prevent paclitaxel hypersensitivity	x (IV)[g]	x (IV)[e]		x (IV)[g]
Prevent stress ulcers	x[g]	x[g]	x[g]	x[g]
Prevent upper GI bleeding	✓ (IV)			
Reduce incidence of GI hemorrhage associated with stress-related ulcers	x (IV)[g]	x (IV)[g]		x (IV)[g]
Reduce recurrent peptic ulcer bleeding (after endoscopy)		x (IV)[g]		
Relieve and prevent heartburn/acid indigestion/sour stomach	✓[b]	✓[b]	✓[b]	✓[b]
Suppress gastric acid secretion perioperatively	x[g]	x[g]	x[g]	x[g]
Treat certain types of urticaria[d]		x[f]		
Weight loss (antipsychotic-induced weight gain)			x[f]	

[a] For more detailed information, see the preceding paragraphs and individual drug monographs.
[b] OTC use only.
[c] As part of a multidrug regimen to eradicate *H. pylori.*
[d] In combination with histamine H_1 antagonists.
[e] Fair documentation.
[f] Insufficient documentation.
[g] Not rated.

Actions

➤*Pharmacology:* Histamine H_2 antagonists (also known as H_2 blockers) competitively and reversibly inhibit the action of histamine at the histamine H_2 receptors, including receptors on the gastric parietal cells. These agents are not anticholinergic.

Cimetidine –

Antisecretory activity:

• *Nocturnal* – Cimetidine 800 mg at bedtime reduces mean hourly hydrogen ion (H^+) activity by more than 85% over 8 hours in duodenal ulcer patients, with no effect on daytime acid secretion. The 1600 mg bedtime dose produces 100% inhibition of mean hourly H^+ activity over an 8-hour period in duodenal ulcer patients, but also reduces H^+ activity by 35% for an additional 5 hours the next morning. Both the 400 mg twice daily and 300 mg 4 times daily dosages decrease nocturnal acid secretion in a dose-related manner, 47% to 83% over 6 to 8 hours and 54% over 9 hours, respectively.

• *Food stimulated* – By the first hour after a standard meal, 300 mg inhibited gastric acid secretion in duodenal ulcer patients by at least 50% and during the next 2 hours by at least 75%. A 300 mg breakfast dose continued for at least 4 hours, with partial suppression of the rise in gastric acid secretion following lunch in duodenal ulcer patients.

Total pepsin output is also reduced as a result of the decrease in volume of gastric juice. Cimetidine 300 mg inhibited the rise in intrinsic factor concentration produced by betazole, but some intrinsic factor was secreted at all times.

• *24-Hour mean activity* – Dosages of 800 mg at bedtime, 400 mg twice daily, and 300 mg 4 times daily all provide a similar, moderate (less than 60%) level of 24-hour acid suppression. However, the 800 mg at bedtime regimen exerts its entire effect on nocturnal acid, and does not affect daytime gastric physiology.

Famotidine – The acid concentration and volume of gastric secretion are suppressed, while changes in pepsin secretion are proportional to volume output. Exocrine pancreatic function is not affected. After oral use, the onset of antisecretory effect occurred within 1 hour; the maximum effect was dose-dependent, occurring within 1 to 3 hours. Duration of secretion inhibition by doses of 20 and 40 mg was 10 and 12 hours, respectively.

After IV administration, the maximum effect was achieved within 30 minutes. Single IV doses of 10 and 20 mg inhibited nocturnal secretion for 10 and 12 hours, respectively.

There is no cumulative effect with repeated doses. The nocturnal intragastric pH was raised by evening doses of 20 and 40 mg to mean values of 5 and 6.4, respectively. When famotidine was given after breakfast, the basal daytime interdigestive pH at 3 and 8 hours after 20 or 40 mg was raised to about 5.

Nizatidine – Nizatidine significantly inhibited nocturnal gastric acid secretion for up to 12 hours. Total pepsin output was reduced in proportion to the reduced volume of gastric secretions. Oral administration of 75 to 300 mg of nizatidine increased betazole-stimulated secretion of intrinsic factor.

Ranitidine – Basal, nocturnal, and betazole-stimulated secretion are most sensitive to inhibition by ranitidine, responding almost completely to doses of 100 mg or less. Ranitidine does not affect pepsin secretion or pentagastrin-stimulated intrinsic factor secretion. Other pharmacological actions include an increase in gastric nitrate-reducing organisms; small, transient, dose-related increases in serum prolactin after IV bolus injections of 100 mg or more, and possible impairment of vasopressin release. No effect on prolactin levels has been noted with recommended oral or IV doses.

➤*Pharmacokinetics:*

Pharmacokinetic Properties of Histamine H_2 Antagonists

H_2 receptor antagonist	Bioavailability (%)	T_{max} (h)[a]	Peak plasma concentration[b] (mcg/mL)	Half-life (h)	Protein binding (%)	Volume of distribution (L/kg)	Elimination (%) Urine, unchanged Oral	IV
Cimetidine	≈ 60 (oral)	0.75 to 1.5 (oral)	2 to 3 (400 mg oral dose)	≈ 2[c]	13 to 25	≈ 1	48	75
Famotidine	40 to 45 (oral)	1 to 3	–	2.5 to 3.5[d]	15 to 20	≈ 1.3	25 to 30	65 to 70
Nizatidine	> 70	0.5 to 3	0.7 to 1.8/ 1.4 to 3.6 (150/300 mg dose)	1 to 2[d]	≈ 35	0.8 to 1.5	60	NA[e]
Ranitidine	50 (oral) (90 to 100 IM)[f]	2 to 3 (oral) (0.25 IM)	0.44 to 0.55 (oral) (0.58 IM)	2.5 to 3 (oral)[d] 2 to 2.5 (IV)[d]	15	1.3	30	≈70

[a] T_{max} = time to maximum concentration.
[b] Dose-dependent.
[c] Increased in renal and hepatic impairment and in the elderly.
[d] Increased in renal impairment.
[e] NA = not applicable.
[f] IM = intramuscular. Additional pharmacokinetic data for these agents are discussed individually.

Cimetidine – Absorption may be decreased by antacids. Both oral and parenteral administration provide comparable periods of effective serum levels. Blood concentrations remain above those required to provide 80% inhibition of basal gastric acid secretion for 4 to 5 hours following a 300 mg dose. Cimetidine is widely distributed. Following oral administration, the drug is extensively metabolized, the sulfoxide being the major metabolite. Hemodialysis reduces the level of circulating cimetidine.

Famotidine – Plasma levels after multiple doses of famotidine are similar to those after single doses. Famotidine is eliminated by renal (65% to 70%) and metabolic (30% to 35%) routes. The only metabolite identified is the S-oxide.

Nizatidine – Plasma concentrations 12 hours after administration are less than 10 mcg/L. Plasma clearance is 40 to 60 L/h. Because of the short half-life and rapid clearance, drug accumulation would not be expected in individuals with normal renal function who take either 300 mg at bedtime or 150 mg twice daily. Nizatidine exhibits dose proportionality over the recommended dose range.

Antacids consisting of aluminum and magnesium hydroxides with simethicone decrease nizatidine absorption by about 10%. With food, area under the curve (AUC) and maximum concentration increase by about 10%.

In humans, less than 7% of an oral dose is metabolized as N2-monodesmethylnizatidine, an H_2-receptor antagonist. Other likely metabolites are the N2-oxide (less than 5% of the dose) and the S-oxide (less than 6% of the dose). More than 90% of an oral dose of nizatidine is excreted in the urine within 12 hours. Renal clearance is approximately 500 mL/min, which indicates excretion by active tubular secretion. Less than 6% is eliminated in the feces.

Ranitidine – Absorption of oral ranitidine is not significantly impaired by the administration of food or antacids. Hepatic metabolism results in 3 metabolites. Maintenance of serum concentrations necessary to inhibit 50% of stimulated gastric acid secretion (36 to 94 ng/mL) is 12 hours orally (6 to 8 hours IV). However, blood levels bear no consistent relationship to dose or degree of acid inhibition.

Contraindications

Hypersensitivity to individual agents or to other histamine H_2 antagonists (cross-sensitivity has been observed).

Warnings/Precautions

➤*Carcinogenesis:* A statistically significant increase in benign Leydig cell tumor incidence was seen in rats that received 378 and 950 mg/kg/day **cimetidine**. The tumors were common in control groups as well as treated groups, and the difference became apparent only in aged rats.

➤*Benzyl alcohol:* Benzyl alcohol contained in some of these products as a preservative, has been associated with a fatal "gasping syndrome" in premature infants.

➤*Phenylketonuria:* Inform patients with phenylketonuria that some of these products contain phenylalanine.

➤*Gastric malignancy:* Symptomatic response to these agents does not preclude gastric malignancy. Rare reports of transient healing of gastric ulcers has occurred with **cimetidine** despite subsequently documented malignancy. Follow gastric ulcer patients closely.

➤*CNS effects:* Reversible CNS effects (eg, mental confusion, agitation, psychosis, depression, anxiety, hallucinations, disorientation) have occurred. For **cimetidine**, these confusional states usually developed within 2 to 3 days after initiation of therapy and cleared within 3 to 4 days following discontinuation. Advancing age (50 years of age and older) and preexisting liver and/or renal disease appear to be contributing factors.

➤*Hepatic effects:* Occasionally, reports of hepatocellular, cholestatic, or mixed hepatitis, with or without jaundice, have occurred with **ranitidine**. In such circumstances, immediately discontinue ranitidine. These events are usually reversible, but in rare circumstances death has occurred. Rare cases of hepatic failure have also been reported. In normal volunteers, ALT values were increased to at least twice the pretreatment levels in 6 of 12 subjects receiving 100 mg 4 times daily IV for 7 days, and in 4 of 24 subjects receiving 50 mg 4 times a day IV for 5 days. In patients receiving IV ranitidine at dosages of 100 mg 4 times daily or higher for periods of 5 days or longer, monitor ALT daily (from day 5) for the remainder of IV therapy. For more information regarding other histamine H_2 antagonists causing hepatic effects, see Adverse Reactions.

Laboratory test monitoring – Laboratory test monitoring for liver abnormalities is appropriate.

➤*Porphyria:* Rare reports suggest that **ranitidine** may precipitate acute porphyric attacks in patients with acute porphyria. Avoid using ranitidine in patients with a history of acute porphyria.

➤*Rapid IV administration:* Rapid IV administration of **cimetidine** has been followed by rare instances of cardiac arrhythmias and hypotension. Bradycardia in association with rapid administration of IV **ranitidine** may occur rarely, usually in patients predisposed to cardiac rhythm disturbances.

➤*Antiandrogenic effect:* **Cimetidine** has a weak antiandrogenic effect. Gynecomastia in patients treated for 1 month or more may occur. In patients with pathological hypersecretory states, this occurred in approximately 4% of cases; in all others, the incidence was approximately 0.3% to 1%. No evidence of endocrine dysfunction was found; the condition remained unchanged or returned to normal with continuing treatment. (Also see Adverse Reactions.)

➤*Immunocompromised patients:* Decreased gastric acidity, including that produced by acid-suppressing agents such as histamine H_2 antagonists, may increase the possibility of strongyloidiasis.

➤*Hypersensitivity reactions:* Rare cases of anaphylaxis have occurred, as well as rare episodes of hypersensitivity (eg, bronchospasm, laryngeal edema, rash, eosinophilia). Refer to Management of Acute Hypersensitivity Reactions.

➤*Renal function impairment:* Because these agents are excreted primarily via the kidneys, decreased clearance may occur; reduced dosage may be necessary (see Administration and Dosage). Since CNS adverse effects have been reported in patients with moderate and severe renal insufficiency, longer intervals between doses or lower doses may need to be used in patients with moderate (creatinine clearance [Ccr] less than 50 mL/min) or severe (Ccr less than 10 mL/min) renal insufficiency to adjust for the longer elimination half-life of famotidine.

➤*Hepatic function impairment:* Observe caution. Decreased clearance may occur; these agents are partly metabolized in the liver. In normal renal function with uncomplicated hepatic dysfunction, **nizatidine** disposition is similar to that in healthy individuals.

➤*Pregnancy: Category B.* Cimetidine crosses the placenta. There are no adequate and well controlled studies with these agents in pregnant women. Use only when clearly needed and when the potential benefits outweigh the potential hazards to the fetus.

➤*Lactation:*

Cimetidine – Cimetidine is excreted in breast milk. However, the American Academy of Pediatrics considers cimetidine to be compatible with breast-feeding.

Famotidine – Famotidine is excreted in the breast milk of rats. Transient growth depression was seen in young rats suckling from mothers treated with maternotoxic doses of at least 600 times the usual human dose. Famotidine is detectable in human milk. Because of the potential for serious adverse reactions in breast-feeding infants, decide whether to discontinue breast-feeding or the drug, taking into account the importance of the drug to the mother.

Nizatidine – Studies have shown that 0.1% of an oral dose of nizatidine is excreted in breast milk in proportion to plasma concentrations. Because of the growth depression in pups reared by lactating rats treated with nizatidine, decide whether to discontinue breast-feeding or the drug, taking into account the importance of the drug to the mother.

Ranitidine – Ranitidine is excreted in breast milk. Exercise caution when administering to a breast-feeding mother.

➤*Children:*

Cimetidine – Safety and efficacy are limited. **Cimetidine** is not recommended for children younger than 16 years of age, unless anticipated benefits outweigh potential risks. In very limited experience, cimetidine 20 to 40 mg/kg/day has been used. OTC use is not recommended in children younger than 12 years of age.

Famotidine – Efficacy has been established. See individual monograph for suggested dosages.

Nizatidine – Efficacy in patients younger than 12 years of age has not been established.

Ranitidine – Safety and efficacy of ranitidine have been established in infants and children from 1 month to 16 years of age for treatment of duodenal and gastric ulcers, GERD, and erosive esophagitis; and for the maintenance of healed duodenal and gastric ulcer. Safety and efficacy in pediatric patients for the treatment of pathological hypersecretory conditions or the maintenance of healing of erosive esophagitis have not been established. Safety and efficacy in neonates (younger than 1 month of age) have not been established.

➤*Elderly:* Safety and efficacy appear similar to those of younger patients; however, the elderly may have reduced renal function. Exercise caution in dose selection.

Per the Beers list, cimetidine may cause CNS adverse reactions including confusion.

Drug Interactions

➤*Cytochrome P-450:* **Cimetidine** reduces the hepatic metabolism of drugs metabolized via the cytochrome P-450 pathway, delaying elimination and increasing serum levels. Drugs metabolized by hepatic microsomal enzymes, particularly those of low therapeutic ratio or in patients with renal or hepatic impairment, may require dosage adjustment. **Ranitidine** (which weakly binds to cytochrome P-450 in vitro), **famotidine**, and **nizatidine** do not inhibit the cytochrome P-450–linked oxygenase enzyme system in the liver. Drug interactions with these agents mediated by inhibition of hepatic metabolism are not expected. However, some interactions may occur with these agents (see table).

Histamine H_2 Antagonist Drug Interactions			
Precipitant drug	Object drug[a]		Description
H_2 antagonists Cimetidine	Amiodarone	↑	Coadministration may increase amiodarone and its active metabolite. Monitor closely.
H_2 antagonists Cimetidine Ranitidine	Benzodiazepines	↑	Coadministration of cimetidine or ranitidine with benzodiazepines that undergo oxidative metabolism may increase the serum levels of these benzodiazepines (eg, alprazolam, chlordiazepoxide, clorazepate, diazepam, flurazepam, midazolam, triazolam). Ranitidine has been shown to increase triazolam plasma concentrations.
H_2 antagonists Cimetidine	Beta-blockers (ie, metoprolol, propranolol, timolol)	↑	Cimetidine may reduce the hepatic metabolism of beta-blockers metabolized by CYP-450 (ie, metoprolol, propranolol, timolol). Monitor closely and adjust the beta-blocker dose accordingly.
H_2 antagonists Cimetidine Ranitidine	Calcium channel blockers (ie, diltiazem, nifedipine)	↑	Cimetidine may reduce the hepatic metabolism of nifedipine. Monitor closely and adjust the nifedipine dose accordingly. Cimetidine and ranitidine increased diltiazem concentrations.
H_2 antagonists Cimetidine	Carbamazepine	↑	Cimetidine may inhibit carbamazepine hepatic metabolism. Monitor carbamazepine levels and adjust dose as needed.
H_2 antagonists Cimetidine	Carmustine	↑	Cimetidine may enhance the myelosuppressive effects of carmustine. Avoid coadministration if possible.
H_2 antagonists	Cephalosporins (ie, cefpodoxime, cefuroxime, cephalexin)	↓	H_2 antagonists may possibly decrease the bioavailability of certain cephalosporins.
H_2 antagonists Cimetidine	Chloroquine	↑	Cimetidine may inhibit the hepatic metabolism of chloroquine.
H_2 antagonists Cimetidine	Dofetilide	↑	Cimetidine may increase dofetilide concentrations, increasing the risk of ventricular arrhythmias including torsades de pointes. Coadministration is contraindicated.
H_2 antagonists	Ethanol	↑	Coadministration may increase ethanol concentrations. Data are conflicting.
H_2 antagonists Cimetidine	Hydantoins (eg, phenytoin)	↑	Cimetidine may reduce the hepatic metabolism of hydantoins, thereby increasing blood levels. Monitor closely and adjust the hydantoin dose accordingly.
H_2 antagonists	Iron Salts	↓	Oral absorption of iron may be impaired. Consider administering iron preparations at least 1 hour before H_2 antagonists.
H_2 antagonists	Ketoconazole	↓	Alteration of gastric pH may affect the absorption of ketoconazole.
H_2 antagonists Cimetidine	Lidocaine	↑	Cimetidine may reduce the hepatic metabolism of lidocaine, causing increased adverse effects.
H_2 antagonists Cimetidine	Metformin	↑	Coadministration may increase metformin concentrations. Monitor closely.
H_2 antagonists Cimetidine	Metronidazole	↑	Cimetidine may reduce the hepatic metabolism of metronidazole, thereby increasing blood levels. Data are conflicting.
H_2 antagonists Cimetidine	Moricizine	↑	Cimetidine may inhibit the hepatic metabolism of moricizine. Monitor closely, especially electrocardiogram.
H_2 antagonists Cimetidine	Pentoxifylline	↑	Cimetidine may inhibit the hepatic metabolism of pentoxifylline.
H_2 antagonists Cimetidine	Praziquantel	↑	Plasma concentrations of praziquantel may be elevated. Observe closely.
H_2 antagonists Cimetidine Ranitidine	Procainamide	↑	Increased procainamide concentrations may occur. Avoid coadministration with cimetidine if possible. Monitor closely.
H_2 antagonists Cimetidine	Quinidine	↑	Increased quinidine concentrations may occur. Avoid coadministration if possible. Monitor closely.
H_2 antagonists Nizatidine	Salicylates	↑	Increased serum salicylate levels occurred when nizatidine was coadministered to patients receiving very high daily doses of aspirin (3,900 mg).
H_2 antagonists Cimetidine	Sildenafil	↑	Sildenafil plasma concentrations may be elevated.
H_2 antagonists Cimetidine	Selective serotonin reuptake inhibitors (SSRIs)	↑	Serum levels of certain SSRIs may be increased.
H_2 antagonists Cimetidine	St. John's wort	↑	Cimetidine may increase the levels of hypericin.
H_2 antagonists Cimetidine Ranitidine	Sulfonylureas	↑	Reduced clearance of sulfonylureas may occur. Monitor blood glucose and adjust dose as needed.
H_2 antagonists Cimetidine	Theophyllines	↑	Cimetidine may reduce the hepatic metabolism of theophyllines. Monitor theophylline levels closely and adjust dose as needed.
H_2 antagonists Cimetidine	Tricyclic antidepressants	↑	Cimetidine may reduce the hepatic metabolism of certain tricyclic antidepressants. Monitor closely and adjust the dose as needed.
H_2 antagonists Cimetidine Ranitidine	Warfarin	↑	The effects of warfarin may be increased. Monitor anticoagulation parameters closely and adjust warfarin dose as needed.

[a] ↑ = Object drug increased. ↓ = Object drug decreased.

➤*Drug/Lab test interactions:* False-positive tests for urobilinogen with *Multistix* may occur during **nizatidine** therapy. False-positive tests for urine protein with *Multistix* may occur during **ranitidine** therapy; testing with sulfosalicylic acid is recommended.

➤*Drug/Food interactions:* Food may increase bioavailability of **famotidine** and **nizatidine**; this is of no clinical consequence.

Adverse Reactions

Histamine H_2 Antagonist Adverse Reactions[a]

Adverse reaction	Cimetidine	Famotidine	Nizatidine	Ranitidine
CNS				
Agitation/ Anxiety	[b]	[b]	1.8%	rare
Confusional states[c]	[b]	[b]	rare	rare
Depression	[b]	[b]		rare
Dizziness	1%	1.3%	4.6%	rare
Hallucinations	[b]	[b]		rare
Headache	2.1% to 3.5%[d]	4.7%	16.6%	[b,d]
Insomnia		[b]	2.7%	rare
Somnolence/ Fatigue	1%	[b]	1.9%	rare
Dermatologic				
Alopecia	rare[c]	[b]		rare
Erythema multiforme	rare			rare
Exfoliative dermatitis/ erythroderma	rare		[b]	
Pruritus/ Urticaria		[b]	1.7%/0.5%	
Rash	[b]	[b]	1.9%	[b]
GI				
Abdominal discomfort		[b]		[b]
Cholestatic/ Hepatocellular effects	rare[c]	[b]	rare	[b]
Constipation		1.2%		[b]
Diarrhea	1%	1.7%	7.2%	[b]
Nausea		[b]	[b]	[b]
Pancreatitis	rare[c]			rare
Vomiting		[b]		[b]
Hematologic				
Agranulocytosis	rare	rare		rare
Granulocytopenia				rare[c]
Immune hemolytic/ aplastic anemia	rare			rare
Leukopenia		rare		rare[c]
Pancytopenia	rare	rare		rare
Thrombocytopenia	rare	rare	[b]	[b,c]
Miscellaneous				
Arthralgia	rare[c]	[b]		rare
Decreased libido		[b]	[b]	[b]
Gynecomastia	0.3% to 4%	rare	rare	[b]
Hypersensitivity reactions	rare[c]	[b]	rare	rare
Impotence	[b,c]	rare	[b]	[b]
Transient pain at injection site		[b]	NA	[b]

[a] Data are pooled from separate studies and are not necessarily comparable.
[b] Occurs, no incidence reported, or not well established.
[c] Reversible.
[d] May be severe.

In addition to the adverse reactions listed in the table, the following have been reported:

Cimetidine –

Cardiovascular: Rare cases of bradycardia, tachycardia and atrioventricular (AV) heart block have been reported with histamine H_2 antagonists. Rare instances of cardiac arrhythmias and hypotension have been reported following the rapid administration of cimetidine injection by IV bolus.

CNS: Reversible confusional states (see Warnings/Precautions).

Dermatologic: Very rarely, cases of severe generalized skin reactions including Stevens-Johnson syndrome, epidermal necrolysis, erythema multiforme, exfoliative dermatitis and generalized exfoliative erythroderma have been reported with histamine H_2 antagonists.

GU: Gynecomastia (see Warnings/Precautions). Reversible impotence has been reported in patients with pathological hypersecretory disorders (eg, Zollinger-Ellison syndrome) receiving cimetidine, particularly in high doses, for at least 12 months (range, 12 to 79 months; mean, 38 months). However, in large-scale surveillance studies at regular dosage, the incidence has not exceeded that commonly reported in the general population.

Small, possibly dose-related increases in plasma creatinine, presumably due to competition for renal tubular secretion, are not uncommon and do not signify deteriorating renal function. Rare cases of interstitial nephritis and urinary retention, which cleared on withdrawal of the drug, have been reported.

Hematologic: Decreased white blood cell counts (approximately 1 per 100,000 patients), including agranulocytosis (approximately 3 per million patients), have been reported, including a few reports of recurrence on rechallenge. Most of these reports were in patients who had serious concomitant illnesses and received drugs and/or treatment known to produce neutropenia.

Hepatic: Dose-related increases in serum transaminase have been reported. In most cases they did not progress with continued therapy and returned to normal at the end of therapy. There have been rare reports of cholestatic or mixed cholestatic-hepatocellular effects. These were usually reversible. Because of the predominance of cholestatic features, severe parenchymal injury is considered highly unlikely. However, as in the occasional liver injury with other histamine H_2 antagonists, in exceedingly rare circumstances fatal outcomes have been reported. There has been reported a single case of biopsy-proven periportal hepatic fibrosis in a patient receiving cimetidine.

Musculoskeletal: There have been rare reports of reversible myalgia; exacerbation of joint symptoms in patients with preexisting arthritis has also been reported. Such symptoms have usually been alleviated by a reduction in the dosage of cimetidine. Rare cases of polymyositis have been reported, but no causal relationship has been established.

Miscellaneous: Rare cases of fever and allergic reactions including anaphylaxis and hypersensitivity vasculitis, which cleared on withdrawal of the drug, have been reported. There have been extremely rare reports of strongyloidiasis hyperinfection in immunocompromised patients.

Famotidine –

Cardiovascular: Arrhythmia, AV block, palpitation.

CNS: Generalized tonic-clonic seizure; paresthesia; psychic disturbances, which were reversible in cases for which follow-up was obtained (see Warnings/Precautions).

Dermatologic: Acne, dry skin, flushing; toxic epidermal necrolysis (very rare).

GI: Anorexia, cholestatic jaundice, dry mouth, liver enzyme abnormalities.

Hypersensitivity: Anaphylaxis, angioedema, conjunctival injection, orbital or facial edema, rash, urticaria.

Musculoskeletal: Musculoskeletal pain including muscle cramps.

Respiratory: Bronchospasm.

Special Senses: Taste disorder, tinnitus.

Miscellaneous: Asthenia, fatigue, fever.

• ***Children*** – In a clinical study in 35 pediatric patients younger than 1 year of age with GERD symptoms (eg, vomiting [spitting up], irritability [fussing]), agitation was observed in 5 patients on famotidine that resolved when the medication was discontinued.

Nizatidine –

Cardiovascular: In clinical pharmacology studies, short episodes of asymptomatic ventricular tachycardia occurred in 2 individuals administered nizatidine and in 3 untreated subjects.

CNS: Rare cases of reversible mental confusion have been reported (see Warnings/Precautions).

Dermatologic: Sweating; vasculitis has been reported rarely.

GU: Clinical pharmacology studies and controlled clinical trials showed no evidence of antiandrogenic activity due to nizatidine.

Hematologic: Anemia; fatal thrombocytopenia was reported in a patient who was treated with nizatidine and another histamine H_2 antagonist. On previous occasions, this patient had experienced thrombocytopenia while taking other drugs. Rare cases of thrombocytopenic purpura have been reported.

Hepatic: Hepatocellular injury, evidenced by elevated liver enzyme tests (AST, ALT, or alkaline phosphatase), occurred in some patients and was possibly or probably related to nizatidine. In some cases, there was marked elevation of AST, ALT enzymes (greater than 500 units/L) and, in a single instance, ALT was greater than 2,000 units/L. The overall rate of occurrences ofelevated liver enzymes and elevations to 3 times the upper limit of normal, however, did not significantly differ from the rate of liver enzyme abnormalities in placebo-treated patients. All abnormalities were reversible after discontinuation of nizatidine. Since market introduction, hepatitis and jaundice have been reported. Rare cases of cholestatic or mixed hepatocellular and cholestatic injury with jaundice have been reported with reversal of the abnormalities after discontinuation of nizatidine.

Miscellaneous: As with other histamine H_2 antagonists, rare cases of anaphylaxis following administration of nizatidine have been reported. Rare episodes of hypersensitivity reactions (eg, bronchospasm, laryngeal edema, rash, eosinophilia) have been reported. Serum sickness–like reactions have occurred rarely in conjunction with nizatidine use. Hyperuricemia unassociated with gout or nephrolithiasis was reported. Eosinophilia and fever have been reported.

• ***Children*** – In controlled clinical trials in pediatric patients (2 to 18 years of age), nizatidine was found to be generally safe and well tolerated. The principal adverse reactions (greater than 5%) were pyrexia, nasopharyngitis, diarrhea, vomiting, irritability, nasal congestion, and cough. Most adverse reactions were mild or moderate in severity. Mild elevations in serum transaminase (1 to 2 times the upper limit of normal) were noted in some patients. One subject experienced a seizure by electroencephalogram diagnosis after taking nizatidine oral solution 2.5 mg/kg twice daily for 23 days.

Ranitidine –

Cardiovascular: As with other histamine H_2 antagonists, rare reports of arrhythmias such as tachycardia, bradycardia, AV block, and premature ventricular beats. Bradycardia in association with rapid administration of ranitidine injection has been reported rarely, usually in patients with factors predisposing to cardiac rhythm disturbances.

CNS: Rarely, malaise and vertigo. Rare cases of reversible mental confusion (see Warnings/Precautions), agitation, depression, and hallucinations have been reported, predominantly in severely ill elderly patients. Rare cases of reversible blurred vision suggestive of a change in accommodation have been reported. Rare reports of reversible involuntary motor disturbances have been received.

Dermatologic: Rare cases of vasculitis.

Endocrine: Controlled studies in animals and humans have shown no stimulation of any pituitary hormone by ranitidine and no antiandrogenic activity, and cimetidine-induced gynecomastia and impotence in hypersecretory patients have resolved when ranitidine has been substituted.

Hepatic: There have been occasional reports of hepatocellular, cholestatic, or mixed hepatitis, with or without jaundice. In such circumstances, immediately discontinue ranitidine. These events are usually reversible, but in rare circumstances death has occurred. Rare cases of hepatic failure have also been reported. In normal volunteers, ALT values were increased to at least twice the pretreatment levels in 6 of 12 subjects receiving 100 mg 4 times daily IV for 7 days, and in 4 of 24 subjects receiving 50 mg 4 times daily IV for 5 days (see Warnings/Precautions).

Musculoskeletal: Rare reports of myalgias.

Miscellaneous: Rare cases of hypersensitivity reactions(eg, bronchospasm, fever, rash, eosinophilia), anaphylaxis, angioneurotic edema, and small increases in serum creatinine. Transient pain at the site of IM injection has been reported. Transient local burning or itching has been reported with IV administration of ranitidine.

Overdosage

➤*Symptoms:* Toxic doses in animals are associated with rapid respiration or respiratory failure, tachycardia, muscular tremors, vomiting, restlessness, pallor of mucous membranes or redness of mouth and ears, hypotension, and collapse.

Reported ingestions of up to 20 g of **cimetidine** have been associated with transient adverse reactions similar to those encountered in normal clinical experience. Two deaths have occurred in adults who reportedly ingested more than 40 g on a single occasion.

Famotidine dosages of up to 640 mg/day have been given to patients with pathological hypersecretory conditions with no serious adverse effects.

Reported acute ingestions of up to 18 g of **ranitidine** have been associated with transient adverse reactions similar to those encountered in normal clinical experience. In addition, abnormalities of gait and hypotension have been reported.

➤*Treatment:* Symptomatic and supportive. Remove unabsorbed material from the GI tract, monitor the patient, and employ supportive therapy. Refer to General Management of Acute Overdosage.

The ability of hemodialysis to remove **nizatidine** from the body has not been conclusively demonstrated; however, due to its large volume of distribution, nizatidine is not expected to be efficiently removed from the body by this method.

Patient Information

Advise patients to inform their health care provider or pharmacist of any concomitant drug therapy, especially when taking **cimetidine**.

These agents may be taken without regard to meals.

➤*OTC:* Patients should not take maximum daily dose for longer than 2 weeks continuously except under the advice and supervision of a health care provider.

CIMETIDINE

otc	**Cimetidine** (Various, eg, Ivax, Mylan, Teva)	**Tablets**: 200 mg	In 30s and 50s.
otc	**Acid Reducer 200** (Major)		In 30s.
otc	**Tagamet HB 200** (GlaxoSmith-Kline Consumer)		In 6s, 30s, and 50s.
Rx	**Cimetidine** (Various, eg, Endo, Major, Mylan, Novopharm, Schein)	**Tablets**: 200 mg	In 100s, 500s, and 1,000s.
Rx	**Cimetidine** (Various, eg, Ivax, Major, Mylan)	**Tablets**: 300 mg	In 100s, 500s, and 1,000s.
Rx	**Cimetidine** (Various, eg, Endo, Ivax, Major, Mylan)	**Tablets**: 400 mg	In 60s, 100s, 500s, and 1,000s.
Rx	**Tagamet** (GlaxoSmithKline)		(Tagamet 400 SB). Light green. Capsule shape. In 60s.
Rx	**Cimetidine** (Various, eg, Mylan)	**Tablets**: 800 mg	In 30s, 100s, and 250s.
Rx	**Tagamet** (GlaxoSmithKline)		(Tagamet 800 SB). Light green. Oval. In 30s.
Rx	**Cimetidine** (Various, eg, Roxane, Teva)	**Oral solution**: 300 mg (as hydrochloride) per 5 mL	May contain alcohol, parabens, saccharin, sorbitol. In 240 and 480 mL and UD 5 mL.
Rx	**Cimetidine** (Various, eg, Hospira, Stada)	**Injection**: 150 mg (as hydrochloride) per mL	In 2 mL single-dose vials and 8 mL multidose vials.[a]
Rx	**Cimetidine in 0.9% Sodium Chloride** (Hospira)	**Injection (premixed)**: 6 mg (as hydrochloride) per mL	In 50 mL single-dose flexible container.

[a] May contain 9 mg/mL benzyl alcohol as a preservative.

CIMETIDINE — ORAL

For complete and comparative prescribing information, refer to the Histamine H_2 Antagonists group monograph.

Indications

➤*Benign gastric ulcer:* For short-term treatment of active, benign gastric ulcer.

➤*Duodenal ulcer:* For short-term treatment of active duodenal ulcer and maintenance therapy after the healing of active ulcer.

➤*Gastroesophageal reflux disease (GERD), erosive:* For the treatment of erosive esophagitis diagnosed by endoscopy.

➤*Pathological hypersecretory conditions:* For the treatment of pathological hypersecretory conditions (eg, Zollinger-Ellison syndrome, systemic mastocytosis, multiple endocrine adenomas).

➤*Heartburn (OTC only):* For the relief of heartburn associated with acid indigestion and sour stomach; for the prevention of heartburn associated with acid indigestion and sour stomach brought on by certain foods and beverages.

➤*Off-label uses:*

Hirsutism – [5] = Poor documentation. Other more potent antiandrogens, such as spironolactone, have produced better results in reducing hair growth in hirsutes. Cimetidine does not appear effective for this use.

Interstitial cystitis (painful bladder disease) – [4] = Insufficient documentation. The published literature examining the use of cimetidine in the treatment of painful bladder disease or interstitial cystitis is limited to 1 controlled trial and 2 open trials. Most data reveal a moderate to complete benefit in some patients. It is not clear which patients are optimal candidates. In addition, the dose has not been standardized. At the current time, cimetidine is not recommended as first-line treatment for these patients, but may be considered in refractory patients. (See Administration and Dosage.)

Prevention of aspiration pneumonia – [5] = Poor documentation. No evidence was found to support the use of cimetidine for preventing aspiration pneumonia caused by normal flora. In fact, acid suppressive therapy has been linked to increased susceptibility of respiratory infection by raising gastric pH, which serves as a barrier to pathogenic colonization of the GI tract. In American Society of Anesthesiologists guidelines, routine use of cimetidine, other H_2-antagonists, or proton pump inhibitors is not recommended.

Urticaria – [4] = Insufficient documentation. Data from a limited number of patients suggest that cimetidine, administered orally or as an injection, may have a role in the management of acute urticaria. Further study is required in larger controlled settings before this drug can be recommended. (See Administration and Dosage.)

Warts (cutaneous, nongenital) – [4] = Insufficient documentation. Cimetidine use for the treatment of warts has produced varied results in controlled and noncontrolled trials. It is not clear why results varied, but it may be due to differences in doses, mixed populations (children and adults), and varied wart types and location. Further studies are needed with cimetidine in the treatment as monotherapy or adjunctive therapy in specific warts types/locations and in segregated age groups to determine if this agent has a beneficial role in the management of warts therapy. (See Administration and Dosage.)

Weight loss – [5] = Poor documentation. The majority of study in this area has been investigated by 1 group, and results have not been verified by another study group. Thus, it is unclear if cimetidine significantly promotes weight loss.

Other possible off-label uses – As part of a multidrug regimen to eradicate *Helicobacter pylori* in the treatment of peptic ulcer; in the perioperative setting to suppress gastric acid secretion and prevent stress ulcers.

Administration and Dosage

➤*Adults:*

Benign gastric ulcer –

Short-term therapy: 800 mg at bedtime or 300 mg 4 times per day with meals and at bedtime. The preferred regimen is 800 mg at bedtime, based on convenience and lowered potential for drug interaction.

Duration of therapy: There is no information concerning the usefulness of treatment periods longer than 8 weeks.

CIMETIDINE — ORAL

Duodenal ulcer –

Short-term therapy: 800 mg at bedtime, or 300 mg 4 times per day with meals and at bedtime, or 400 mg twice per day.

Maintenance dosage: 400 mg at bedtime.

Duration of therapy: While healing often occurs during the first few weeks, continue treatment for 4 to 6 weeks unless healing is demonstrated by endoscopy.

It has been shown that patients who have an endoscopically demonstrated ulcer larger than 1 cm and who are also heavy smokers (1 pack of cigarettes or more a day) are more difficult to heal. There is some evidence that suggests more rapid healing can be achieved in this subpopulation with a dose of 1,600 mg at bedtime.

Concomitant therapy: Give antacids as needed for pain relief. However, simultaneous administration with antacids is not recommended, since antacids have been reported to interfere with the absorption of cimetidine.

Gastroesophageal reflux disease, erosive –

Usual dosage: 1,600 mg daily in divided doses (800 mg twice daily or 400 mg 4 times per day) for 12 weeks.

Duration of therapy: Use beyond 12 weeks has not been established.

Heartburn (over the counter only) –

Maximum dose: 400 mg/day. Patients should not take the maximum dose for longer than 2 weeks continuously unless otherwise directed by a health care provider.

To relieve symptoms: 200 mg with water as symptoms occur or as directed, up to twice daily (up to 400 mg in 24 hours).

To prevent symptoms: 200 mg with a glass of water right before or any time up to 30 minutes before eating food or drinking beverages that cause heartburn.

Pathological hypersecretory conditions –

Usual dosage: 300 mg 4 times per day with meals and at bedtime. If necessary, give higher doses more often. Individualize dosage.

Maximum dose: 2,400 mg/day.

Duration of therapy: Continue as long as clinically indicated.

Off-label dosing –

Interstitial cystitis (painful bladder disease): [4] = Insufficient documentation. 600 to 800 mg/day in divided doses as 200 mg 3 times/day, up to 400 mg twice daily.

Urticaria: [4] = Insufficient documentation. 800 to 1,200 mg daily for 7 days.

Warts (cutaneous, nongential): [4] = Insufficient documentation. 400 or 800 mg 3 times daily for 12 weeks or 30 to 40 mg/kg/day divided in 3 daily doses for 3 months.

➤*Children:* See Adults for dosing in children older than 16 years of age for prescription dosing. See Adults for dosing for children older than 12 years of age for OTC dosing.

Off-label dosing –

General dosing:

Cimetidine Off-Label Pediatric Dosing	
Neonates	5 to 20 mg/kg given in divided doses every 6 to 12 hours
Infants	10 to 20 mg/kg given in divided doses every 6 to 12 hours
Children	20 to 40 mg/kg given in divided doses every 6 hours

Warts (cutaneous, nongential): [4] = Insufficient documentation. 20 to 40 mg/kg/day given in 2 divided doses, 3 divided doses, or 4 divided doses for 2 months.

➤*Renal function impairment:* In severe renal impairment, accumulation may occur. Use the lowest dose; 300 mg every 12 hours orally or IV has been recommended. According to the patient's condition, dosage frequency may be increased to every 8 hours or even further with caution. When liver impairment is also present, further dosage reductions may be necessary.

Hemodialysis – Give the dose at the end of hemodialysis.

➤*Storage/Stability:* Store between 15° and 30°C (59° and 86°F); dispense in a tight, light-resistant container.

CIMETIDINE — INJECTION

For complete and comparative prescribing information, refer to the Histamine H_2 Antagonists group monograph.

Indications

➤*Benign gastric ulcer:* For short-term treatment of active, benign gastric ulcer.

➤*Duodenal ulcer:* For short-term treatment of active duodenal ulcer and maintenance therapy after the healing of active ulcer.

➤*GI bleeding (intravenous [IV] only):* For the prevention of upper GI bleeding in critically ill patients.

➤*Pathological hypersecretory conditions:* For the treatment of pathological hypersecretory conditions (ie, Zollinger-Ellison syndrome, systemic mastocytosis, multiple endocrine adenomas).

➤*Off-label uses:*

Prevention of aspiration pneumonia – [5] = Poor documentation. No evidence was found to support the use of cimetidine for preventing aspiration pneumonia caused by normal flora. In fact, acid suppressive therapy has been linked to increased susceptibility of respiratory infection by raising gastric pH, which serves as a barrier to pathogenic colonization of the GI tract. In American Society of Anesthesiologists guidelines, routine use of cimetidine, other H_2-antagonists, or proton pump inhibitors is not recommended.

Urticaria – [4] = Insufficient documentation. Data from a limited number of patients suggest that cimetidine, administered orally or as an injection, may have a role in the management of acute urticaria. Further study is required in larger controlled settings before this drug can be recommended. (See Administration and Dosage.)

Other possible off-label uses – As part of a multidrug regimen to eradicate *Helicobacter pylori* in the treatment of peptic ulcer; in the perioperative setting to suppress gastric acid secretion and prevent stress ulcers; treatment of cutaneous warts (data are conflicting); prevention of paclitaxel hypersensitivity (IV only); to reduce the incidence of GI hemorrhage associated with stress-related ulcers(IV only).

Administration and Dosage

➤*General dosing considerations:* Antacids should be given as needed for relief of pain.

➤*Adults:*

Benign gastric ulcer –

Usual dosage: 300 mg IV or IM every 6 to 8 hours.

Dosage adjustment: If it is necessary to increase dosage, do so by more frequent administration of a 300 mg dose, not to exceed 2,400 mg/day.

Duodenal ulcer –

Usual dosage: 300 mg IV or IM every 6 to 8 hours.

Dosage adjustment: If it is necessary to increase dosage, do so by more frequent administration of a 300 mg dose, not to exceed 2,400 mg/day.

GI bleeding –

Usual dosage: Continuous IV infusion of 50 mg/hour.

Duration of therapy: Treatment beyond 7 days has not been studied.

Pathological hypersecretory conditions –

Usual dosage: 300 mg IV or IM every 6 to 8 hours.

Dosage adjustment: If it is necessary to increase dosage, do so by more frequent administration of a 300 mg dose, not to exceed 2,400 mg/day.

Off-label dosing –

Urticaria: [4] = Insufficient documentation. Single intramuscular (IM) or IV dose (300 mg) in the emergency room.

➤*Children:* See Adults for dosing in children 16 years of age and older.

Off-label dosing –

General dosing:

Cimetidine Off-Label Pediatric Dosing	
Neonates	5 to 20 mg/kg IV or IM given in divided doses every 6 to 12 hours
Infants	10 to 20 mg/kg IV or IM given in divided doses every 6 to 12 hours
Children	20 to 40 mg/kg IV or IM given in divided doses every 6 hours

➤*Renal function impairment:* In severe renal impairment, accumulation may occur. Use the lowest dose; 300 mg every 12 hours orally or IV has been recommended. According to the patient's condition, dosage frequency may be increased to every 8 hours or even further with caution. When liver impairment also is present, further dosage reductions may be necessary.,

Gastrointestinal bleeding – Patients with creatinine clearance less than 30 mL/min should receive half the recommended dose. Treatment beyond 7 days has not been studied.

Hemodialysis – Give the dose at the end of hemodialysis.

➤*Preparation for administration:*

Cimetidine injection (150 mg/mL) –

Intravenous injection: Dilute 300 mg injection in 0.9% sodium chloride injection or other compatible IV solution to a total volume of 20 mL.

Intermittent intravenous infusion: Dilute 300 mg injection in at least 50 mL of 5% dextrose injection or another compatible IV solution.

Continuous intravenous infusion: Dilute 900 mg injection in a compatible IV solution. Injection may be diluted in 100 to 1,000 mL.

➤*Administration:*

Intramuscular – Administer cimetidine 150 mg/mL undiluted.

Intravenous injection – Inject over a period of at least 5 minutes.

Intermittent intravenous infusion – Infuse over a period of 15 to 20 minutes.

Continuous intravenous infusion – 37.5 mg/h (900 mg/day). For patients requiring more rapid elevation of gastric pH, continuous infusion may be preceded by a 150 mg loading dose administered by IV infusion. Administer by constant infusion over a 24-hour period. If volume is less than 250 mL, a volumetric pump is recommended.

➤*Admixture compatibility:*

Compatibility – 0.9% sodium chloride injection, 5% or 10% dextrose injection, Ringer's lactate solution, 5% sodium bicarbonate injection.

Incompatibility – Do not add other drugs to premixed cimetidine in 0.9% sodium chloride injection.

CIMETIDINE — INJECTION

➤*Storage/Stability:*

Cimetidine injection – Store vials at controlled room temperature, 15° to 30°C (59° to 86°F). Do not refrigerate. When added to or diluted, cimetidine injection should not be used after more than 48 hours of storage at room temperature.

Cimetidine in 0.9% sodium chloride – Avoid excessive heat. Store at room temperature (25°C [77°F]).

RANITIDINE

otc	**Ranitidine** (Various, eg, Ivax)	**Tablets; oral:** 75 mg	As ranitidine hydrochloride. In 10s, 20s, 30s, and 60s.
otc sf	**Zantac 75** (Boehringer Ingelheim)		Sugar free, sodium free. As ranitidine hydrochloride. (Z 75). In 4s, 10s, 20s, 30s, 60s, and 80s.
Rx	**Ranitidine** (Various, eg, Apotex Inc., Ivax, Ranbaxy, Teva, UDL, Watson)	**Tablets; oral:** 150 mg	As ranitidine hydrochloride. In 60s, 100s, 500s, 1,000s, 5,000s, and UD 100s.
Rx	**Zantac** (GlaxoSmithKline)		As ranitidine hydrochloride. (Zantac 150 Glaxo). Peach, 5-sided. Film-coated. In 60s, 180s, 500s, 1,000s, and UD 100s.
otc sf	**Zantac 150 Maximum Strength** (Boehringer Ingelheim)		Sugar free, sodium free. As ranitidine hydrochloride. (Z). 90s.
Rx	**Ranitidine** (Various, eg, Apotex USA, Ivax, Ranbaxy, Teva, Watson)	**Tablets; oral:** 300 mg	As ranitidine hydrochloride. In 30s, 100s, 250s.
Rx	**Zantac** (GlaxoSmithKline)		As ranitidine hydrochloride. (Zantac 300 Glaxo). Yellow, capsule shape. Film-coated. In 30s, 250s, and UD 100s.
Rx	**Zantac EFFERdose** (GlaxoSmithKline)	**Tablets, effervescent; oral:** 25 mg	As ranitidine hydrochloride. (GS 25C). White/pale yellow. In 60s.[a]
Rx	**Ranitidine** (Various, eg, Par)	**Capsules; oral:** 150 mg	As ranitidine hydrochloride. In 60s and 500s.
		300 mg	As ranitidine hydrochloride. In 30s and 100s.
Rx	**Ranitidine Hydrochloride** (Various, eg, Actavis Mid Atlantic, Apotex, Par)	**Solution; oral:** 15 mg per mL	May contain alcohol, parabens, saccharin, sorbitol. Peppermint flavor. In 473 mL.
Rx	**Zantac** (GlaxoSmithKline)		As ranitidine hydrochloride. 7.5% alcohol, saccharin, sorbitol, parabens. Peppermint flavor. In 480 mL.
Rx	**Zantac** (GlaxoSmithKline)	**Injection (premixed):** 1 mg per mL	As ranitidine hydrochloride. Preservative free. In premixed 50 mL single-dose plastic containers.[c]
Rx	**Ranitidine** (Bedford)	**Injection:** 25 mg per mL	As ranitidine hydrochloride. In 2 mL single-dose vials and 6 mL multidose vials.[d]
Rx	**Zantac** (GlaxoSmithKline)		As ranitidine hydrochloride. In 2 mL single-dose vials and 6 mL multidose vials.[d]

[a] With aspartame, 2.81 mg phenylalanine, and 30.52 mg sodium/tablet.
[b] With aspartame, 16.84 mg phenylalanine, and 183.12 mg sodium/tablet.
[c] Premixed in 0.45% sodium chloride.
[d] With 5 mg/mL phenol.

RANITIDINE HYDROCHLORIDE — ORAL

For complete and comparative prescribing information, refer to the Histamine H_2 Antagonists group monograph.

Indications

➤*Benign gastric ulcer:* For the short-term treatment of active, benign gastric ulcer and maintenance therapy after the healing of acute ulcer.

➤*Duodenal ulcer:* For the short-term treatment of active duodenal ulcer and maintenance therapy after the healing of acute ulcers.

➤*Erosive esophagitis:* For the treatment of endoscopically diagnosed erosive esophagitis; for the maintenance of healing of erosive esophagitis.

➤*Gastroesophageal reflux disease (GERD):* For the treatment of GERD.

➤*Pathological hypersecretory conditions:* For the treatment of pathological hypersecretory conditions (eg, Zollinger-Ellison syndrome, systemic mastocytosis).

➤*Heartburn (OTC only):* For the relief of heartburn associated with acid indigestion and sour stomach; for the prevention of heartburn associated with acid indigestion and sour stomach brought on by certain foods and beverages.

➤*Off-label uses:*

Aspiration pneumonia – [2] = Fair documentation. Current data suggest that ranitidine decreases gastric fluid volume and acidity compared with placebo when used preoperatively. However, these studies evaluated patients receiving general anesthesia, which does not include all populations at risk for aspiration. Although it is possible to show that these agents increase gastric pH and reduce gastric volumes, no evidence to prove a reduction in morbidity and mortality exists to support their routine use because the incidence of aspiration is so infrequent. Recent anesthesiology practice guidelines do not recommend the routine use of H_2 antagonists to decrease the risk of pulmonary aspiration in patients who have no apparent increased risk for pulmonary aspiration. Further studies are needed to evaluate the effects on the incidence of pulmonary aspiration, as well as effects on morbidity or mortality, in patients who have aspirated gastric contents. (See Administration and Dosage.)

Urticaria – [5] = Poor documentation. Data from a limited number of patients demonstrated varied results when ranitidine was added to antihistamine therapy in the management of chronic refractory urticaria. Further study is required in larger controlled settings with newer antihistamines before this drug can be recommended based on evidence.

Other possible off-label uses – As part of a multidrug regimen to eradicate *Helicobacter pylori* in the treatment of peptic ulcer; in the perioperative setting to suppress gastric acid secretion and prevent stress ulcers,and as prophylaxis to reduce the incidence of nonsteroidal anti-inflammatory drug –induced duodenal ulcer.

Administration and Dosage

➤*General dosing considerations:* Decrease dose to 150 mg every 24 hours in patients with creatinine clearance (CrCl) less than 50 mL/min (see Renal function impairment).

Zantac EFFERdose tablets should not be chewed, swallowed whole, or dissolved on the tongue.

Give concomitant antacids as needed for pain relief to patients with active duodenal ulcer; active, benign gastric ulcer; hypersecretory states; GERD; and erosive esophagitis.

➤*Adults:*

Benign gastric ulcer –

Initial dosage: 150 mg twice daily for treatment.
Maintenance dosage: 150 mg at bedtime.

Duodenal ulcer –

Initial dosage: 150 mg orally twice daily for treatment.
Maintenance dosage: 150 mg at bedtime.
Alternative dosage: 300 mg once daily after the evening meal or at bedtime can be used for patients in whom dosing convenience is important; 100 mg twice daily is as effective as the 150 mg dose in inhibiting gastric acid secretion.

Erosive esophagitis –

Initial dosage: 150 mg 4 times daily for treatment.
Maintenance dosage: 150 mg twice daily.

Gastroesophageal reflux disease – 150 mg twice daily.

Pathological hypersecretory conditions –

Usual dosage: 150 mg orally twice a day.
Dosage adjustment: More frequent doses may be necessary. Individualize dosage and continue as long as indicated. Dosages up to 6 g/day have been used for severe disease.

Heartburn (OTC only) –

Initial dosage: For relief of symptoms, swallow 1 tablet with a glass of water.
Maintenance dosage: Can be used up to twice daily (up to 2 tablets in 24 hours).
Prophylactic dosage: To prevent symptoms, swallow 1 tablet with a glass of water 30 to 60 minutes before eating food or drinking beverages that cause heartburn.

Off-label dosing –

Aspiration pneumonia: [2] = Fair documentation. Oral ranitidine 150 mg the evening before and again 2 to 3 hours before surgery, or a single 50 mg intravenous (IV) dose 1 hour prior to surgery.

RANITIDINE HYDROCHLORIDE — ORAL

➤*Children:* The safety and efficacy of ranitidine have been established in children from 1 month to 16 years of age. Do not give OTC ranitidine to children younger than 12 years of age unless directed by a health care provider.

1 month of age and older –

Active duodenal and gastric ulcers:

- *Maximum dose* – Maximum dose for treatment is 300 mg/day; maximum dose for maintenance is 150 mg/day.
- *Initial dosage* – 2 to 4 mg/kg twice daily for treatment.
- *Maintenance dosage* – 2 to 4 mg/kg once daily.

Gastroesophageal reflux disease and erosive esophagitis: Although limited data exist for these conditions in pediatric patients, published literature supports a dosage of 5 to 10 mg/kg/day, usually given as 2 divided doses.

Off-label dosing –

Neonates (0 to 29 days): 2 to 4 mg/kg/day in divided doses every 8 to 12 hours.

➤*Renal function impairment:* Decrease dose to 150 mg orally every 24 hours in patients with CrCl less than 50 mL/min. The frequency of dosing may be increased to every 12 hours or further with caution.

Hemodialysis – Hemodialysis reduces the level of circulating ranitidine. Adjust dosage timing so that a scheduled dose coincides with the end of hemodialysis.

➤*Preparation for administration:*

Zantac EFFERdose 25 mg tablets – Dissolve 1 tablet in no less than 5 mL (1 teaspoonful) of water in an appropriate measuring cup. Wait until the tablet is completely dissolved before administering the solution to the infant/child. The solution may be administered by medicine dropper for infants.

Zantac EFFERdose 150 mg tablets – Dissolve each dose in approximately 6 to 8 oz of water before drinking.

➤*Administration:*

Zantac EFFERdose tablets – Tablet should not be chewed, swallowed whole, or dissolved on the tongue.

➤*Storage/Stability:*

Tablets – Store between 15° and 30°C (59° and 86°F) in a dry place. Protect from light. Replace cap securely after each opening.

Effervescent tablets and granules – Store between 2° and 30°C (36° and 86°F).

Syrup – Store between 4° and 25°C (39° and 77°F). Dispense in a tight, light-resistant container.

RANITIDINE — INJECTION

For complete and comparative prescribing information, refer to the Histamine H_2 Antagonists group monograph.

Indications

➤*Alternative to oral ranitidine:* As an alternative to the oral dosage form for short-term use in patients who are unable to take oral medication.

➤*Duodenal ulcers:* Indicated in some hospitalized patients with intractable duodenal ulcers.

➤*Pathological hypersecretory conditions:* Indicated in some hospitalized patients with pathological hypersecretory conditions (eg, Zollinger-Ellison).

➤*Off-label uses:* As part of a multidrug regimen to eradicate *Helicobacter pylori* in the treatment of peptic ulcer; in the perioperative setting to suppress gastric acid secretion, prevent stress ulcers, and prevent aspiration pneumonitis; in combination with histamine H_1 antagonists in the treatment of certain types of urticaria; prevention of paclitaxel hypersensitivity (IV ranitidine); as prophylaxis to reduce the incidence of nonsteroidal anti-inflammatory drug (NSAID)-induced duodenal ulcer; reduce the incidence of GI hemorrhage associated with stress-related ulcers(IV ranitidine).

Administration and Dosage

➤*General dosing considerations:* Give concomitant antacids as needed for pain relief to patients with active duodenal ulcer; active, benign gastric ulcer; hypersecretory states; gastroesophageal reflux disease; and erosive esophagitis.

➤*Adults:*

Alternative to oral ranitidine –

Usual dosage: 50 mg (2 mL) administered IM or as an intermittent IV bolus or infusion every 6 to 8 hours.

Maximum dose: 400 mg/day administered IM or by intermittent IV bolus or infusion.

Alternative dosage: Administer as a continuous infusion delivered at a rate of 6.25 mg/hour.

Duodenal ulcers – See Alternative to Oral Ranitidine for dosing.

Pathological hypersecretory conditions – See Alternative to Oral Ranitidine for dosing.

Zollinger-Ellison:

- *Initial dosage* – Administer as a continuous IV infusion at a rate of 1 mg/kg/hour.
- *Dosage adjustment* – After 4 hours if either the measured gastric acid output is greater than 10 mEq/hour or the patient becomes symptomatic, adjust the dose upwards in 0.5 mg/kg/hour increments and remeasure the acid output. Doses up to 2.5 mg/kg/hour and infusion rates as high as 220 mg/hour have been used.

➤*Children:*

1 month of age and older –

Usual dosage: 2 to 4 mg/kg/day, divided every 6 to 8 hours.

Maximum dose: 50 mg given every 6 to 8 hours.

Neonates younger than 1 month of age – Limited data in neonatal patients receiving extracorporeal membrane oxygenation (ECMO) have shown that a dose of 2 mg/kg is usually sufficient to increase gastric pH to greater than 4 for at least 15 hours. Therefore, consider doses of 2 mg/kg given every 12 to 24 hours or as a continuous infusion.

Off-label dosing –

Prophylaxis against dexamethasone-associated ulceration in premature infants with bronchopulmonary dysplasia:

- *Neonates (0 to 29 days)* – 0.031 to 1.25 mg/kg/hour during dexamethasone therapy to maintain gastric pH above 4.

Prophylaxis against stress ulceration:

- *Neonates (0 to 29 days)* –

Term neonates: 2 mg/kg every 12 hours or 1.5 mg/kg every 8 hours. 2 mg/kg over 10 minutes, then a continuous infusion of 0.083 mg/kg/hour.

Preterm neonates: 0.5 mg/kg every 12 hours.

➤*Renal function impairment:* Decrease dose to 50 mg parenterally every 18 to 24 hours in patients with CrCl less than 50 mL/min. The frequency of dosing may be increased to every 12 hours or further with caution.

Hemodialysis – Hemodialysis reduces the level of circulating ranitidine. Adjust dosage timing so that a scheduled dose coincides with the end of hemodialysis.

➤*Preparation for administration:*

Intermittent bolus – Dilute 50 mg in 0.9% sodium chloride or other compatible IV solution to a concentration no greater than 2.5 mg/mL (20 mL).

Intermittent IV infusion – Dilute 50 mg in 5% dextrose injection or other compatible IV solution to a concentration no greater than 0.5 mg/mL (100 mL).

Continuous IV infusion – Add ranitidine injection to 5% dextrose injection or other compatible IV solution.

For Zollinger-Ellison patients, dilute ranitidine injection in 5% dextrose injection or other compatible IV solution to a concentration of 2.5 mg/mL or less.

Premixed injection – Do not introduce additives into the premixed injection solution.

Do not use flexible plastic container in series connections.

➤*Administration:*

Adults –

Intermittent bolus: Inject at a rate no greater than 4 mL/min (5 minutes).

Intermittent IV infusion: Infuse at a rate no greater than 5 to 7 mL/min (15 to 20 minutes), or use 50 mL of 1 mg/mL premixed solution and infuse over 15 to 20 minutes.

Premixed injection: Requires no dilution and should be infused over 15 to 20 minutes. Administer by slow IV drip infusion only. If used with a primary IV fluid system, discontinue primary solution during premixed infusion.

Continuous IV infusion: Deliver at a rate of 6.25 mg/hour (eg, 150 mg [6 mL] ranitidine injection in 250 mL of 5% dextrose injection at 10.7 mL/hour).

➤*Admixture compatibility:* Ranitidine injection is stable for 48 hours at room temperature when added to or diluted with most commonly used IV solutions (eg, sodium chloride 0.9% injection, dextrose 5% or 10% injection, Ringer's lactate injection, sodium bicarbonate 5% injection).

➤*Storage/Stability:* Undiluted ranitidine injection tends to exhibit a yellow color that may intensify over time without adversely affecting potency. Ranitidine injection is stable for 48 hours at room temperature when added to or diluted with most commonly used IV solutions (eg, 0.9% sodium chloride injection, 5% or 10% dextrose injection, Ringer's lactate injection, 5% sodium bicarbonate injection).

Store the premixed injection between 2° and 25°C (36° and 77°F) and the injection between 4° and 25°C (39° and 77°F). Protect from light. Ranitidine injection premixed in flexible plastic containers is sterile through the expiration date on the label when stored under recommended conditions.

Ranitidine injection premixed, 50 mg/50 mL, in 0.45% sodium chloride, is available as a sterile, premixed solution for IV administration in single-dose, flexible plastic containers. It contains no preservatives.

Minimize exposure of pharmaceutical products to heat. Avoid excessive heat; however, brief exposure up to 40°C (104°F) does not adversely affect the product. Protect from freezing.

NIZATIDINE

otc	**Axid AR** (Wyeth Consumer)	**Tablets:** 75 mg	(AXID AR). In 12s and 30s.
Rx	**Nizatidine** (Various, eg, Eon, Ivax, Mylan, Par)	**Capsules:** 150 mg	In 60s, 100s, 500s, 1000s, and UD 100s.
Rx	**Axid Pulvules** (GlaxoSmithKline)		(AXID Reliant/150). Yellow. In 60s.
Rx	**Nizatidine** (Various, eg, Eon, Ivax, Mylan, Par)	**Capsules:** 300 mg	In 30s, 100s, and 500s.
Rx	**Axid** (Braintree)	**Oral solution:** 15 mg/mL	Parabens, saccharin, sucrose. Clear yellow. Bubble gum flavor. In 480 mL.

NIZATIDINE — ORAL

For complete and comparative prescribing information, refer to the Histamine H_2 Antagonists group monograph.

Indications

➤*Benign gastric ulcer:* For the treatment of active benign ulcer for up to 8 weeks. Before initiating therapy, exclude the possibility of malignant gastric ulceration.

➤*Duodenal ulcer:* For the treatment of active ulcer for up to 8 weeks and maintenance therapy after healing of active ulcer. The consequences of continuous therapy with nizatidine for longer than 1 year are not known.

➤*Gastroesophageal reflux disease (GERD):* For the treatment of endoscopically diagnosed esophagitis, including erosive and ulcerative esophagitis, and associated heartburn due to GERD for up to 12 weeks in adults and up to 8 weeks in children (12 years of age and older).

➤*Heartburn (OTC product only):* For the relief of heartburn, acid indigestion, and sour stomach and the prevention of these symptoms brought on by certain foods and beverages.

➤*Off-label uses:*

Antipsychotic-induced weight gain – [4] = Insufficient documentation. Preliminary data with nizatidine in a single case report suggest a possible relationship with H_2 antagonism and weight loss. (See Administration and Dosage.)

Other possible off-label uses – Prevention of nonsteroidal anti-inflammatory drug–induced gastroduodenal ulcer; in combination with amoxicillin and clarithromycin for *Helicobacter pylori* infection.

Administration and Dosage

➤*Adults:*

Benign gastric ulcer – 300 mg given either as 150 mg twice daily or 300 mg once daily at bedtime.

Duodenal ulcer –

Initial dosage: 300 mg once daily at bedtime for treatment of an active ulcer. An alternative dosage regimen is 150 mg twice daily. Most heal in 4 weeks.

Maintenance dosage: 150 mg once daily at bedtime for maintenance of healed ulcer.

GERD – 150 mg twice daily.

Heartburn, acid indigestion, and sour stomach (OTC products only) –

Maximum dose: 150 mg/day.

Prevention of symptoms: 75 mg with a full glass of water right before eating or up to 60 minutes before consuming food and beverages that cause heartburn. May be used up to twice daily (150 mg/day).

Relief of symptoms: 75 mg with a full glass of water. May be used up to twice daily (150 mg/day).

Off-label dosing –

Antipsychotic-induced weight gain: [4] = Insufficient documentation. 150 mg twice daily.

➤*Children:*

Erosive esophagitis – See Adults for dosing for children 12 years of age and older.

GERD – See Adults for dosing for children 12 years of age and older.

Heartburn, acid indigestion, and sour stomach (OTC products only) – See Adults for dosing for children 12 years of age and older.

➤*Elderly:* Dosage should be adjusted according to renal function.

➤*Renal function impairment:*

Adults –

Nizatidine Dosage in Renal Function Impairment

	Dosage	
Creatinine clearance (CrCl)	Active duodenal ulcer, GERD, benign gastric ulcer	Maintenance therapy
20 to 50 mL/min	150 mg/day	150 mg every other day
< 20 mL/min	150 mg every other day	150 mg every 3 days

Children – Children with CrCl of less than 50 mL/min should have their dose of nizatidine reduced accordingly.

➤*Storage/Stability:* Store at 25°C (77°F); excursions are permitted to 15° to 30°C (59° to 86°F). Dispense in a tight, light-resistant container.,

FAMOTIDINE

otc	**Famotidine** (Ivax)	**Tablets; oral:** 10 mg	In 18s, 30s, 50s, and 70s.
otc	**Pepcid AC** (J & J Merck)		(Pepcid AC). In 2s, 6s, 18s, 30s, 60s, and 90s.
Rx	**Famotidine** (Various, eg, Ivax, Teva, UDL)	**Tablets; oral:** 20 mg	May contain lactose. In 30s, 100s, 500s, 1,000s, UD 100s, and *Robot-Ready* 25s.
Rx	**Pepcid** (Merck)		(MSD 963 PEPCID). Beige, U-shape. Film-coated. In 1,000s, 10,000s, unit-of-use 30s, 90s, and 100s, UD 100s, and *Uniblister* 31s.
otc	**Pepcid AC Maximum Strength** (J & J Merck)		In 25s.
Rx	**Famotidine** (Various, eg, Ivax, Par, Teva)	**Tablets; oral:** 40 mg	May contain lactose. In 30s, 100s, 500s, 1,000s, and UD 100s.
Rx	**Pepcid** (Merck)		(MSD 964 PEPCID). Lt. brownish orange, U-shape. Film-coated. In 1,000s, 10,000s, unit-of-use 30s, 90s, and 100s, UD 100s, and *Uniblister* 31s.
otc	**Pepcid AC** (J & J Merck)	**Gelcaps; oral:** 10 mg	(PEPCID AC). In 30s, 50s, 60s, and 90s.
otc	**Pepcid AC** (J & J Merck)	**Tablets, chewable; oral:** 10 mg	Aspartame, lactose, mannitol, 1.4 mg phenylalanine. (PEPCID AC). In 6s, 18s, 30s, 50s, 60s, and 68s.
otc	**Pepcid AC Maximum Strength EZ Chews** (J & J Merck)	**Tablets, chewable; oral:** 20 mg	Dextrose, lactose, sucralose. Cool mint and berries and cream flavors. In 25s and 50s.
Rx	**Pepcid RPD** (Merck)	**Tablets, orally disintegrating; oral:** 20 mg	Aspartame, mannitol, 1.05 mg phenylalanine. Mint flavor. Pale rose, hexagonal. In UD 30s and 100s.
		40 mg	Aspartame, mannitol, 2.1 mg phenylalanine. Mint flavor. Pale rose, hexagonal. In UD 30s and 100s.
Rx	**Famotidine** (Various, eg, Lupin Pharmaceuticals, ZyGenerics)	**Powder for suspension; oral:** 40 mg per 5 mL	May contain parabens, sodium benzoate, sucrose, sugar. In 50 mL.
Rx	**Pepcid** (Merck)		Parabens, sucrose. Cherry-banana-mint flavor. In bottles of 400 mg.
Rx	**Famotidine** (Various, eg, Baxter, Bedford, Hospira)	**Injection:** 10 mg/mL	May contain mannitol or benzyl alcohol. In 1 and 2 mL single-dose vials and 4, 20, and 50 mL multidose vials.
Rx	**Famotidine** (Baxter)	**Injection (premixed):** 20 mg per 50 mL	In 50 mL single-dose *Galaxy* containers.

[a] Preservative free.

[b] With 0.9% benzyl alcohol.

FAMOTIDINE — ORAL

For complete and comparative prescribing information, refer to the Histamine H_2 Antagonists group monograph.

Indications

➤*Benign gastric ulcer:* For the short-term treatment (up to 8 weeks) of active benign gastric ulcer.

➤*Duodenal ulcer:* For the short-term treatment (up to 8 weeks) of active duodenal ulcer and maintenance therapy after healing of active ulcer.

➤*Gastroesophageal reflux disease (GERD):* For the short-term treatment (up to 6 weeks) of GERD and esophagitis due to GERD, including erosive or ulcerative disease diagnosed by endoscopy.

➤*Pathological hypersecretory conditions:* For the treatment of pathological hypersecretory conditions (eg, Zollinger-Ellison syndrome).

➤*Heartburn (OTC only):* For the relief of heartburn associated with acid indigestion and sour stomach; for the prevention of heartburn associated with acid indigestion and sour stomach brought on by certain foods and beverages.

➤*Off-label uses:*

Aspiration pneumonia – [4] = Insufficient documentation. Several trials have shown that famotidine is effective in reducing gastric volume and increasing gastric pH. However, evidence that proves that altering gastric volume and pH is clinically significant in reducing morbidity and mortality associated with aspiration pneumonitis is lacking. Additional trials are needed to further evaluate this causal relationship. Moreover, the routine use of H_2 antagonists, such as famotidine, is not recommended by the American Society of Anesthesiologists. (See Administration and Dosage.)

Urticaria – [4] = Insufficient documentation. Data from a limited number of patients suggest that famotidine, administered orally or as an injection, may have a role in the management of acute urticaria. Further study is required in larger controlled settings before this drug can be recommended. (See Administration and Dosage.)

Other possible off-label uses – As part of a multidrug regimen to eradicate *Helicobacter pylori* in the treatment of peptic ulcer; in the perioperative setting to suppress gastric acid secretion and prevent stress ulcers.

Administration and Dosage

➤*General dosing considerations:* Famotidine oral suspension may be substituted for famotidine tablets in any of these indications.

➤*Adults:*

Benign gastric ulcer – As acute therapy, 40 mg once a day at bedtime.

Duodenal ulcer –

Usual dosage: As acute therapy, 40 mg/day at bedtime. Most heal in 4 weeks; there is rarely reason to use full dosage for more than 6 to 8 weeks. 20 mg twice daily is also effective.

Maintenance dosage: 20 mg once a day at bedtime.

Gastroesophageal reflux disease –

Usual dosage: 20 mg twice daily for up to 6 weeks.

• *For esophagitis, including erosions and ulcerations, and accompanying symptoms due to gastroesophageal reflux disease* – Usual dosage is 20 or 40 mg twice daily for up to 12 weeks.

Heartburn, acid indigestion, and sour stomach (OTC only) –

Maximum dose: Up to twice daily (up to 2 tablets in 24 hours). Patients should not take the maximum dose for more than 2 weeks continuously unless otherwise directed by their health care provider.

Acute therapy: 10 or 20 mg with water up to twice daily (up to 2 tablets in 24 hours).

Prevention: 10 or 20 mg 15 to 60 minutes before eating food or drinking a beverage that is expected to cause symptoms. May take up to twice daily (up to 2 tablets in 24 hours).

Pathological hypersecretory conditions – Individualize dosage.

Initial dosage: 20 mg every 6 hours; some patients may require a higher starting dose.

Duration of therapy: Continue as long as clinically indicated.

Severe Zollinger-Ellison syndrome: Up to 160 mg every 6 hours.

Off-label dosing –

Aspiration pneumonia: [4] = Insufficient documentation. Usual dosage is 40 mg the night before and/or the morning of elective surgery.

Urticaria: [4] = Insufficient documentation. Usual dosage is 20 mg twice daily for 7 days.

➤*Children:* While published uncontrolled studies suggest efficacy of famotidine in the treatment of GERD and peptic ulcer, data in pediatric patients are insufficient to establish percent response with dose and duration of therapy. Therefore, individualize treatment duration (initially based on adult duration recommendations) and dose based on clinical response and/or pH determination (gastric or esophageal) and endoscopy. Published uncontrolled clinical studies in pediatric patients 1 to 16 years of age have employed dosages up to 1 mg/kg/day for peptic ulcer and 2 mg/kg/day for GERD with or without esophagitis including erosions and ulcerations.

Gastroesophageal reflux disease with or without esophagitis including erosions and ulcerations –

1 to 16 years of age:

• *Initial dosage* – 1 mg/kg/day orally divided twice daily up to 40 mg twice daily.

• *Alternative dosage* – 2 mg/kg/day.

3 months to younger than 1 year of age: The usual dosage is 0.5 mg/kg/dose of oral suspension twice daily for up to 8 weeks.

Infants should also be receiving conservative measures (eg, thickened feedings).

Younger than 3 months of age: The usual dosage is 0.5 mg/kg/dose of oral suspension for up to 8 weeks once daily. Infants should also be receiving conservative measures (eg, thickened feedings).

Heartburn, acid indigestion, and sour stomach (OTC only) –

12 years of age and older: See Adults for dosing for children 12 years of age and older.

Peptic ulcer –

1 to 16 years of age:

• *Initial dosage* – 0.5 mg/kg/day orally at bedtime or divided twice daily, up to 40 mg/day.

• *Alternative dosage* – Up to 1 mg/kg/day.

➤*Elderly:* Dosage reduction may be required in elderly patients with underlying renal impairment. (See Renal Function Impairment.)

➤*Renal function impairment:* In adult patients with moderate (creatinine clearance [CrCl] less than 50 mL/min) or severe (CrCl less than 10 mL/min) renal insufficiency, the elimination half-life of famotidine is increased. For patients with severe renal insufficiency, elimination half-life may exceed 20 hours, reaching approximately 24 hours in anuric patients. Since CNS adverse reactions have been reported in patients with moderate and severe renal insufficiency, to avoid excess accumulation of the drug in patients with moderate or severe renal insufficiency, the dose of famotidine may be reduced by half or the dosing interval may be prolonged to 36 to 48 hours as indicated by the patient's clinical response.

Based on the comparison of pharmacokinetic parameters for famotidine in adults and pediatric patients, dosage adjustment in pediatric patients with moderate or severe renal insufficiency should be considered.

➤*Concomitant therapy:* Antacids may be given concomitantly if needed.

➤*Preparation for administration:*

Directions for preparing famotidine oral suspension – Prepare suspension at time of dispensing. Slowly add 46 mL of purified water. Shake vigorously for 5 to 10 seconds immediately after adding the water and immediately before use. Unused constituted oral suspension should be discarded after 30 days.

➤*Administration:* Patients should not swallow the chewable tablets whole; they should be chewed completely.

➤*Storage/Stability:*

Tablets/Oral suspension dry powder and suspension – Store at 25°C (77°F); excursions are permitted between 15° and 30°C (59° and 86°F). Protect suspension from freezing. Discard unused suspension after 30 days.

OTC products – Store at 20° to 30°C (68° to 86°F). Protect from moisture.

FAMOTIDINE — INJECTION

For complete and comparative prescribing information, refer to the Histamine H_2 Antagonists group monograph.

Indications

➤*Benign gastric ulcer:* For the short-term treatment (up to 8 weeks) of active benign gastric ulcer.

➤*Duodenal ulcer:* For the short-term treatment (up to 8 weeks) of active duodenal ulcer and maintenance therapy after healing of active ulcer.

➤*Gastroesophageal reflux disease (GERD):* For the short-term treatment (up to 6 weeks) of GERD and esophagitis due to GERD, including erosive or ulcerative disease diagnosed by endoscopy.

➤*Pathological hypersecretory conditions:* For the treatment of pathological hypersecretory conditions (eg, Zollinger-Ellison syndrome).

➤*Intravenous (IV):* For use in some hospitalized patients with pathological hypersecretory conditions or intractable ulcers, or as an alternative to the oral dosage forms for short-term use in patients who are unable to take oral medication.

➤*Off-label uses:* As part of a multidrug regimen to eradicate *Helicobacter pylori* in the treatment of peptic ulcer; in the perioperative setting to suppress gastric acid secretion, prevent stress ulcers, and prevent aspiration pneumonitis; prevention of recurrent bleeding after successful endoscopic treatment of bleeding peptic ulcer (IV famotidine); to reduce the incidence of GI hemorrhage associated with stress-related ulcers (IV famotidine).

Prevention of paclitaxel hypersensitivity reactions – [2] = Fair documentation. Initial data indicate that famotidine is effective in a premedication regimen to reduce or prevent paclitaxel-related hypersensitivity reactions. A very small kinetic trial also indicated that there was no difference between cimetidine and famotidine for this use. (See Administration and Dosage.)

Urticaria – [4] = Insufficient documentation. Data from a limited number of patients suggest that famotidine, administered orally or as an injection, may have a role in the management of acute urticaria. Further study is required in larger controlled settings before this drug can be recommended. (See Administration and Dosage.)

Administration and Dosage

➤*General dosing considerations:* Antacids may be given concomitantly if needed.

FAMOTIDINE — INJECTION

➤*Adults:*

Usual dosage – 20 mg IV every 12 hours. Doses and regimen for GERD are not established.

Off-label dosing –

Prevention of paclitaxel hypersensitivity reactions: [2] = Fair documentation. 20 mg administered IV 30 minutes prior to infusion. Other drugs also coadministered (at 30 minutes prior to chemotherapy) have included IV dexamethasone (20 mg) and diphenhydramine (50 mg). In some patients, oral dexamethasone was administered on the night prior to chemotherapy.

Urticaria: [4] = Insufficient documentation. Single 50 mg intramuscular (IM) dose.

➤*Children:*

Benign gastric ulcer –

1 to 16 years of age: The initial dosage is 0.25 mg/kg IV (injected over a period of at least 2 minutes or as a 15-minute infusion) every 12 hours, up to 40 mg/day.

Duodenal ulcer –

1 to 16 years of age: The initial dosage is 0.25 mg/kg IV (injected over a period of at least 2 minutes or as a 15-minute infusion) every 12 hours, up to 40 mg/day.

Gastroesophageal reflux disease – Doses and regimen for GERD are not established. The use of IV famotidine in children younger than 1 year of age with GERD has not been adequately studied.

Pathological hypersecretory conditions –

1 to 16 years of age: The initial dosage is 0.25 mg/kg IV (injected over a period of at least 2 minutes or as a 15-minute infusion) every 12 hours, up to 40 mg/day.

➤*Elderly:* Dosage reduction may be required in elderly patients with underlying renal impairment. (See Renal Function Impairment.)

➤*Renal function impairment:* To avoid excess accumulation of the drug in patients with moderate (creatinine clearance [CrCl] less than 50 mL/min) or severe renal insufficiency (CrCl less than 10 mL/min) the dose may be reduced to half the dose or the dosing interval may be prolonged to 36 to 48 hours, as indicated by patient response.

➤*Preparation for administration:*

IV solutions – Dilute 2 mL famotidine IV (solution containing 10 mg/mL) with sodium chloride 0.9% injection or other compatible IV solution to a total volume of 5 or 10 mL.

IV infusion solutions – Famotidine IV may also be administered as an infusion of 2 mL of famotidine diluted with 100 mL of dextrose 5% or other compatible solution and infused over 15 to 30 minutes. A premixed solution is also available containing famotidine premixed with sodium chloride 0.9%.

➤*Administration:*

IV solutions – Administer over not less than 2 minutes.

IV infusion solutions – Infuse over 15 to 30 minutes.

➤*Storage/Stability:* Store injection vials (non-premixed) at 2° to 8°C (36° to 46°F). Store premixed injection at room temperature (25°C; 77°F). Avoid exposure of the premixed product to excessive heat; brief exposure to temperatures up to 35°C (95°F) does not adversely affect the product. If solution freezes, bring to room temperature; allow sufficient time to solubilize all the components.

Solution is stable for 7 days at room temperature when added to or diluted with most commonly used IV solutions (eg, water for injection, sodium chloride 0.9% injection, dextrose 5% or 10% injection, Ringer's lactate injection, sodium bicarbonate 5% injection). When added to or diluted with sodium bicarbonate 5% injection, a precipitate may form at higher concentrations of famotidine injection (more than 0.2mg/mL). Although diluted famotidine injection has been shown to be stable for 7 days at room temperature, there are no data on the maintenance of sterility after dilution. Therefore, it is recommended that if not used immediately after preparation, diluted solutions of famotidine injection should be refrigerated and used within 48 hours.

HISTAMINE H_2 ANTAGONIST COMBINATIONS

otc	**Dual Action Complete** (Major Pharmaceuticals)	**Tablets, chewable; oral:** 10 mg famotidine, 800 mg calcium carbonate, 165 mg magnesium hydroxide	Aspartame, dextrates, lactose, phenylalanine 2.2 mg. In 25s.
otc	**Pepcid Complete** (J & J Merck)		Lactose, sugar. (P). Mint flavor. In 5s, 15s, 25s, and 50s.
otc	**Tums Dual Action** (GlaxoSmithKline)		Aspartame, glyceryl, lactose, phenylalanine 2.2 mg, polysorbate 80. Berry flavor. In 25s.

HISTAMINE H_2 ANTAGONIST COMBINATIONS — ORAL

For complete prescribing information, refer to the Histamine H_2 Antagonists class monograph.

Indications

➤*Heartburn:* For the relief of heartburn associated with acid indigestion and sour stomach.

Administration and Dosage

➤*Maximum dose:*

12 years of age and older – 2 tablets/day.

➤*Adults:*

Heartburn –

Usual dosage: 1 tablet to relieve symptoms. Chew before swallowing.

➤*Children:*

Heartburn – See Adults for dosing in children 12 years of age and older.

➤*Administration:* Tablets should be chewed completely; do not swallow tablets whole.

➤*Storage/Stability:* Store between 25° and 30°C (77° and 86°F). Protect from moisture.

PROTON PUMP INHIBITORS

Indications

Proton Pump Inhibitors: Summary of Indications[a]

Indication ✔ = Labeled X = Unlabeled	Dexlansoprazole	Esomeprazole	Lansoprazole	Omeprazole	Pantoprazole	Rabeprazole
Duodenal ulcer			✔[b]	✔	X	✔
Duodenal ulcer associated with *Helicobacter pylori* (in combination with antibiotics)		✔[b]	✔[b]	✔	X	✔
Gastric ulcer		✔[b]	✔[b]	✔	X	X
Erosive esophagitis	✔	✔[b]	✔	✔	✔	✔
GERD[c] in adults	✔	✔[b]	✔[b]	✔	✔	✔
GERD in children		✔[b]	X	✔		
H. pylori gastritis in children[d]			X	X[e]		
Hypersecretory conditions (eg, Zollinger-Ellison syndrome)		✔[b]	✔[b]	✔	✔	✔
GERD-related laryngitis				X[f]		
Laryngitis			X[g]		X[g]	
To improve pancreatic enzyme absorption in cystic fibrosis patients with intestinal malabsorption			X[e]	X[e]		

[a] For more detailed information, see the following information and the individual drug monographs.
[b] Oral only.
[c] GERD = gastroesophageal reflux disease.
[d] In combination with amoxicillin and clarithromycin.
[e] Not rated.
[f] Fair documentation.
[g] Insufficient documentation.

➤*Duodenal ulcer (lansoprazole, omeprazole, rabeprazole):* For short-term treatment of active duodenal ulcer. Lansoprazole also is indicated to maintain the healing of duodenal ulcers.

➤*Duodenal ulcer associated with H. pylori infection:* For the treatment of patients with *H. pylori* infection and duodenal ulcer to eradicate *H. pylori*.

Dual therapy – In combination with clarithromycin (**omeprazole**) or amoxicillin (**lansoprazole**).

Triple therapy (esomeprazole, lansoprazole, omeprazole, rabeprazole) – In combination with clarithromycin and amoxicillin.

➤*Erosive esophagitis (dexlansoprazole, esomeprazole, lansoprazole, omeprazole, pantoprazole, rabeprazole):* For short-term treatment and maintenance of healing of erosive esophagitis.

➤*Gastric ulcer (esomeprazole, lansoprazole, omeprazole):* Lansoprazole and omeprazole are indicated for short-term treatment of active benign gastric ulcer. Esomeprazole and lansoprazole are indicated for reducing the risk of and healing nonsteroidal anti-inflammatory agent (NSAID)–associated gastric ulcers in patients who continue NSAID use.

➤*GERD (dexlansoprazole, esomeprazole, lansoprazole, omeprazole, pantoprazole, rabeprazole):* For the treatment of heartburn and other symptoms associated with GERD.

➤*Hypersecretory conditions (esomeprazole, lansoprazole, omeprazole, pantoprazole, rabeprazole):* For the long-term treatment of pathological hypersecretory conditions (eg, Zollinger-Ellison syndrome, multiple endocrine adenomas, systemic mastocytosis).

➤*Off-label uses:* Refer to individual monographs for further information.

Laryngitis –

Lansoprazole: [4] = Insufficient documentation.
Omeprazole: [2] = Fair documentation.
Pantoprazole: [4] = Insufficient documentation.

Other possible off-label uses –

Prevention of GI bleeding in patients receiving antiplatelets: The American College of Cardiology, the American College of Gastroenterology, and the American Heart Association recommend the use of proton pump inhibitors (PPIs) to reduce the risk of GI bleeding in patients who are at high risk for GI bleeding and are receiving anti-platelet therapy. Patients at high risk for GI bleeding are defined as those with a history of GI bleeding; advanced age; concurrent use of anticoagulants, steroids, or NSAIDs, including aspirin; and *H. pylori* infection. However, patients who are not at high risk for bleeding achieve little benefit from concurrent use of a PPI with clopidogrel. If a PPI is needed in a patient at lower risk for GI bleeding, a drug that is not a strong or moderate cytochrome P450 2C19 (CYP2C19) inhibitor, such as pantoprazole, should be considered, because omeprazole may interfere with the metabolic (CYP2C19) conversion of clopidogrel to its active metabolite. There are conflicting data on the clinical impact of concurrent use of clopidogrel and PPIs. However, the prescribing information recommends against concurrent use of omeprazole and clopidogrel.

Actions

➤*Pharmacology:* **Omeprazole**, **esomeprazole**, **lansoprazole**, **dexlansoprazole**, **rabeprazole**, and **pantoprazole** belong to a class of antisecretory compounds, the substituted benzimidazoles, that do not exhibit anticholinergic or histamine H_2 antagonistic properties, but that suppress gastric acid secretion by specific inhibition of the H^+/K^+ ATPase enzyme system at the secretory surface of the gastric parietal cell. Because this enzyme system is the "acid (proton) pump" within the gastric mucosa, these agents have been characterized as gastric acid pump inhibitors; they block the final step of acid production. This effect is dose-related and inhibits basal and stimulated acid secretion regardless of the stimulus.

Serum gastrin levels increase parallel with inhibition of acid secretion. No further increase in serum gastrin occurs with continued treatment. Gastrin values usually returned to pretreatment levels within 24 hours (intravenous [IV] pantoprazole), 1 to 2 weeks (omeprazole), 4 weeks (esomeprazole, lansoprazole), 1 month (dexlansoprazole), or 3 months (oral pantoprazole) after discontinuation of therapy.

➤*Pharmacokinetics:*

Absorption/Distribution – Most of these oral agents contain enteric-coated granules. Absorption of these agents is rapid and begins only after the granules leave the stomach.

Peak plasma concentrations of AUC and **omeprazole** are approximately proportional with doses of up to 40 mg, but because of saturable first-pass effect, a more than linear response occurs with doses more than 40 mg.

The **esomeprazole** maximal concentration (C_{max}) increases proportionally when the dose is increased, and there is a 3-fold increase in the area under the curve (AUC) from 20 to 40 mg. The AUC after administration of a single 40 mg dose of esomeprazole is decreased by 43% to 53% after food intake compared with fasting conditions.

C_{max} and AUC of **lansoprazole** are diminished by approximately 50% to 70% if the drug is given 30 minutes after food as opposed to the fasting condition. Increases in C_{max} ranged from 12% to 55%, increases in AUC ranged from 9% to 37%, and time to C_{max} (T_{max}) varied (ranging from a decrease of 0.7 hours to an increase of 3 hours) when **dexlansoprazole** was administered with food compared with fasting. The AUC after administration of a single 40 mg dose of esomeprazole is decreased by 43% to 53% after food intake compared with fasting conditions. Esomeprazole should be taken at least 1 hour before meals. When **pantoprazole** is given with food, its T_{max} is highly variable and may increase significantly. Absorption may be delayed up to 2 hours or longer; however, the C_{max} and AUC of pantoprazole are not altered. When **rabeprazole** is administered with a high-fat meal, its T_{max} is variable and may delay its absorption up to 4 hours or longer; however, the C_{max} and AUC are not significantly altered.

Metabolism/Excretion – These agents are extensively metabolized by the liver. Several metabolites have been identified. These metabolites have very little or no antisecretory activity. The plasma elimination half-life of PPIs does not reflect duration of suppression of gastric acid secretion. Thus, the plasma elimination half-life is less than 2 hours while the acid inhibitory effect lasts more than 24 hours, apparently because of prolonged binding to the parietal H^+/K^+ ATPase enzyme. When the drug is discontinued, secretory activity returns over 1 to 5 days.

Little unchanged drug is excreted in urine. Approximately 33% of **lansoprazole**, 50.7% of **dexlansoprazole**, and the majority of **omeprazole** (approximately 77%), **esomeprazole** (approximately 80%), **rabeprazole** (approximately 90%), and **pantoprazole** (approximately 71%) is eliminated in urine. The remainder of the dose is excreted in feces. This implies a significant biliary excretion of the metabolites of omeprazole and lansoprazole.

Proton Pump Inhibitors Pharmacokinetics

Parameter	Dexlansoprazole	Esomeprazole	Lansoprazole	Omeprazole[a]	Pantoprazole	Rabeprazole
Bioavailability (%)		≈ 64 (single dose) ≈ 90 (multiple dose)	> 80	30 to 40	≈ 77 (oral)	≈ 52
T_{max} (h)	1 to 2 (1st peak) 4 to 5 (2nd peak)	≈ 1.5	1.7	0.5 to 3.5	≈ 2.5 (oral)	2 to 5
Protein binding (%)	96.1 to 98.8	97	97	≈ 95	≈ 98	96.3
Half-life (h)	1 to 2	≈ 1 to 1.5	≈ 1.5 (oral) ≈ 1.3 (IV)	0.5 to 1	≈ 1	1 to 2
Total body clearance (mL/min)	≈ 190		≈ 185 (IV)	500 to 600	≈ 127 to 233 (IV)	
Onset (h)			1 to 3	≤ 1		≤ 1
Duration (h)			> 24	72	> 24	

[a] Capsules.

Special populations –

Renal function impairment: In patients with chronic renal impairment (creatinine clearance [CrCl], 10 to 62 mL/min per 1.73 m²), the disposition of **omeprazole** was similar to that in healthy volunteers but with a slight increase in bioavailability. Because urinary excretion is a primary route of elimination of omeprazole metabolites, their elimination slowed in proportion to the decreased CrCl. However, no dosage adjustment is necessary.

In patients with severe renal insufficiency, plasma protein binding decreased by 1% to 1.5% after administration of **lansoprazole** 60 mg. Patients with renal insufficiency had a shortened elimination half-life and decreased total AUC (free and bound). However, AUC for free lansoprazole in plasma was not related to the degree of renal impairment, and C_{max} and T_{max} were not different from subjects with healthy kidneys.

Hepatic function impairment: In patients with moderate hepatic impairment, AUC of **dexlansoprazole** was approximately 2 times greater compared with subjects with healthy hepatic function.

In patients with severe hepatic insufficiency, the **esomeprazole** AUC was 2 to 3 times higher.

In patients with chronic hepatic disease, the bioavailability of **omeprazole** increased to approximately 100%, reflecting decreased first-pass effect; plasma half-life increased to nearly 3 hours. Plasma clearance averaged 70 mL/min, compared with 500 to 600 mL/min in healthy subjects.

In patients with various degrees of chronic hepatic disease, the mean plasma half-life of **lansoprazole** was prolonged from 1.5 hours to 3.2 to 7.2 hours. An increase in mean AUC of up to 500% was observed at steady state in hepatically impaired patients compared with healthy subjects. Consider dose reduction in patients with severe hepatic disease.

In patients with chronic, mild to moderate hepatic disease, the AUC of **rabeprazole** doubled, the elimination half-life increased 2- to 3-fold, and the total body clearance decreased to less than half compared with healthy patients after a 20 mg oral dose.

In patients with mild to severe hepatic impairment, maximum **pantoprazole** concentrations increased 1.5-fold, serum half-life increased 7 to 9 hours, and AUC increased 5- to 7-fold compared with healthy subjects; however, these values were no greater than those observed in slow CYP2C19 metabolizers.

Elderly: In elderly patients, the elimination rate of **omeprazole** was somewhat decreased and bioavailability was increased. Omeprazole was 76% bioavailable with a 40 mg oral dose in elderly volunteers versus 58% in younger volunteers. Nearly 70% of the dose was recovered in urine as metabolites; no unchanged drug was detected. The plasma clearance of omeprazole was 250 mL/min and its plasma half-life averaged 1 hour. However, no dosage adjustment is necessary.

The elimination half-life and AUC of **dexlansoprazole** are increased in elderly patients. However, no dosage adjustment is needed.

The **esomeprazole** AUC and C_{max} values were slightly higher (25% and 18%, respectively) in elderly patients compared with younger subjects.

The clearance of **lansoprazole** is decreased in elderly patients, with elimination half-life increased by approximately 50% to 100%. Because the mean half-life in elderly patients remains between 1.9 to 2.9 hours, repeated once-daily dosing does not result in accumulation of lansoprazole.

In healthy elderly subjects receiving **rabeprazole** 20 mg once daily for 7 days, AUC values doubled and C_{max} increased by 60% compared with a younger control group.

In elderly subjects receiving **pantoprazole**, the AUC increased by 43% and the C_{max} increased by 26% compared with younger subjects.

Gender: The AUC of **dexlansoprazole** was 42.8% higher in women than in men. No dosage adjustment is necessary based on gender.

The AUC and C_{max} values of **esomeprazole** were 13% higher in women than in men at steady state. Dosage adjustment based on gender is not necessary.

Race: An increase in AUC of **omeprazole** of approximately 4-fold was noted in Asian subjects compared with white subjects. Consider dose adjustment for Asian subjects, particularly where maintenance of healing of erosive esophagitis is indicated.

The mean AUCs of **lansoprazole** in Asian subjects were approximately twice those seen in pooled US data; however, the interindividual variability was high. The C_{max} values were comparable.

In healthy Japanese men, the **rabeprazole** AUC was approximately 50% to 60% greater than values derived from pooled data from healthy men in the United States.

CYP2C19 polymorphism: Mean C_{max} and AUC of **dexlansoprazole** were up to 4 and 12 times higher, respectively, in poor metabolizers and 2 times higher in intermediate metabolizers.

Contraindications

Hypersensitivity to any component of the formulation; substituted benzimidazoles (**rabeprazole**, **esomeprazole**, **omeprazole**).

Warnings/Precautions

➤*Bone fracture:* Several published observational studies suggest that PPI therapy may be associated with an increased risk for osteoporosis-related fractures of the hip, wrist, or spine. The risk of fracture was increased in patients who received high-dose (defined as multiple daily doses) and long-term PPI therapy (1 year or longer). Use the lowest dose and shortest duration of PPI therapy appropriate to the condition being treated. Manage patients at risk for osteoporosis-related fractures according to the established treatment guidelines.

➤*Gastritis:* Atrophic gastritis has been noted occasionally in gastric corpus biopsies from patients treated long term with **esomeprazole** and **omeprazole**.

Patients with healed GERD were treated for up to 40 months with **rabeprazole** and monitored with serial gastric biopsies. Patients with *H. pylori* infection at baseline had mild or moderate inflammation of the gastric body or mild inflammation in the gastric antrum. At baseline, 8% of patients had atrophy of glands in the gastric body and 15% had atrophy in the gastric antrum. At end point, 15% of patients had atrophy of glands in the gastric body and 11% had atrophy in the gastric antrum. Approximately 4% of patients had intestinal metaplasia at some point during follow-up, but no consistent changes were seen.

➤*Hepatic effects:* Mild, transient transaminase elevations have been observed in IV **pantoprazole** clinical studies. The clinical significance is unknown.

➤*Gastric malignancy:* Symptomatic response to therapy with PPIs does not preclude the presence of gastric malignancy.

➤*Vitamin B_{12} deficiency:* Generally, daily treatment with any acid-suppressing medications over a long period of time (ie, longer than 3 years) may lead to malabsorption of cyanocobalamin (vitamin B_{12}) caused by hypochlorhydria or achlorhydria. Rare reports of cyanocobalamin deficiency occurring with acid-suppressing therapy have been reported in the literature. Consider this possibility if clinical symptoms consistent with cyanocobalamin deficiency are observed.

➤*Hypersensitivity reactions:* Anaphylaxis has been reported with the use of IV **pantoprazole**. Hypersensitivity and anaphylaxis has been reported with **dexlansoprazole** and **esomeprazole** use. This may require emergency medical treatment.

➤*Hepatic function impairment:* In patients with various degrees of chronic hepatic disease, the mean plasma half-life of **lansoprazole** was prolonged from 1.5 hours to 3.2 to 7.2 hours, and an increase in the mean AUC of up to 500% was observed at steady state.

In patients with moderate hepatic impairment, AUC of **dexlansoprazole** was approximately 2 times greater compared with subjects with healthy hepatic function. No studies have been conducted in patients with severe hepatic impairment.

In patients with chronic hepatic disease, the bioavailability and plasma half-life of **omeprazole** increased and the plasma clearance decreased.

In patients with chronic mild to moderate compensated cirrhosis of the liver, **rabeprazole** AUC was approximately doubled, elimination half-life was 2- to 3-fold higher, and the total body clearance was decreased to less than half.

In patients with severe hepatic insufficiency, the **esomeprazole** AUC was 2 to 3 times higher.

➤*Pregnancy: Category B* (**dexlansoprazole**, **esomeprazole**, **lansoprazole**, **rabeprazole**, **pantoprazole**); *Category C* (**omeprazole**). In rabbits, doses 5.5 to 56 times the human dose of omeprazole produced dose-related increases in embryolethality, fetal resorptions, and pregnancy disruptions. In rats, dose-related embryo/fetal toxicity and postnatal developmental toxicity were observed in offspring of parents treated with approximately 5.6 to 56 times the human dose.

Sporadic reports have been received of congenital abnormalities occurring in infants born to women who received omeprazole during pregnancy.

An expert review of published data on experiences with omeprazole use during pregnancy by the Teratogen Information System (TERIS) concluded that therapeutic doses during pregnancy are unlikely to pose a substantial teratogenic risk (the quantity and quality of data were assessed as fair).

However, there are no adequate and well-controlled studies in pregnant women. Use during pregnancy only if the potential benefit justifies the risk to the fetus.

➤*Lactation:* The excretion of **esomeprazole** in milk has not been studied; however, **omeprazole** concentrations have been measured in the breast milk of women. The peak concentration of omeprazole in breast milk was less than 7% of the peak serum concentration. It is unknown if **dexlansoprazole** is excreted in human milk. **Lansoprazole** and **pantoprazole** and their metabolites are excreted in the milk of rats. Decreased body weight gain of rat pups was observed when **rabeprazole** was administered to rats in late gestation and during lactation at doses of approximately 195 times the human dose for body surface area. Because of the potential for serious adverse reactions in breast-feeding infants, and because of the potential for tumorigenicity shown in rat carcinogenicity studies, decide whether to discontinue breast-feeding or the drug, taking into account the importance of the drug to the mother.

➤*Children:* The safety and efficacy of **dexlansoprazole**, **esomeprazole** injection, **pantoprazole**, and **rabeprazole** in children have not been established. The safety and efficacy of oral esomeprazole in children 1 to 17 years of age for short-term treatment of GERD have been established; safety and efficacy have not been established in children younger than 1 year of age. The safety and efficacy of oral esomeprazole for other indications have not been established. The safety and efficacy of **lansoprazole** have been established in patients 1 to 17 years of age for short-term treatment of symptomatic GERD and erosive esophagitis. The safety and efficacy of lansoprazole in patients younger than 1 year of age have not been established. The safety and efficacy of **omeprazole** have been established in patients 1 to 16 years of age for the treatment of acid-related GI diseases, including the treatment of symptomatic GERD and the treatment and maintenance of healing of erosive esophagitis. The safety and efficacy of omeprazole have not been established for children younger than 1 year of age.

➤*Elderly:* The elimination rate of **omeprazole** was somewhat decreased in elderly patients and the bioavailability increased (see Pharmacokinetics).

The clearance of **lansoprazole** is decreased in elderly patients, with an approximately 50% to 100% increase of elimination half-life (see Pharmacokinetics).

The elimination half-life and AUC of **dexlansoprazole** are increased in elderly patients. However, no dosage adjustment is needed.

AUC values and C_{max} of **esomeprazole**, **rabeprazole**, and oral **pantoprazole** were increased in elderly subjects compared with healthy controls (see Pharmacokinetics), but no dosage adjustment is recommended.

Drug Interactions

➤*Antiplatelets (eg, clopidogrel):* The American College of Cardiology, the American College of Gastroenterology, and the American Heart Association recommend the use of PPIs to reduce the risk of GI bleeding in patients who are at high risk for GI bleeding and are receiving antiplatelet therapy. Patients at high risk for GI bleeding are defined as those with a history of GI bleeding; advanced age; concurrent use of anticoagulants, steroids, or NSAIDs, including aspirin; and *H. pylori* infection. However, patients who are not at high risk for bleeding achieve little benefit from concurrent use of a PPI with clopidogrel. If a PPI is needed in a patient at lower risk for GI bleeding, consider a drug that is not a strong or moderate CYP2C19 inhibitor, such as pantoprazole, because omeprazole may interfere with the metabolic (CYP2C19) conversion of clopidogrel to its active metabolite. There are conflicting data on the clinical impact of concurrent use of clopidogrel and PPIs. However, the prescribing information recommends against concurrent use of omeprazole and clopidogrel.

➤*Gastric pH-dependent drugs:* PPIs cause a profound and long-lasting inhibition of gastric acid secretion; therefore, **dexlansoprazole**, **esomeprazole**, **lansoprazole**, **omeprazole**, **pantoprazole**, and **rabeprazole** may interfere with the absorption of drugs where gastric pH is an important determinant of bioavailability (eg, ketoconazole, ampicillin, iron salts, digoxin, cyanocobalamin).

➤*CYP450 system:* There have been reports of interactions between **omeprazole** and certain drugs metabolized via the CYP450 system (eg, cyclosporine, disulfiram, benzodiazepines). **Dexlanzoprazole**, **esomeprazole**, **lansoprazole**, **pantoprazole**, and **rabeprazole** are extensively metabolized by CYP2C19 and CYP3A4. In clinical trials, antacids were used concomitantly with these agents.

Proton Pump Inhibitor Drug Interactions

Precipitant drug	Object drug[a]		Description
Clarithromycin	PPIs Dexlansoprazole Esomeprazole Omeprazole Rabeprazole	↑	Serum concentrations of clarithromycin and the PPI may be increased. Based on available data, no special action is needed.
PPIs Esomeprazole Omeprazole	Clarithromycin		
Fluvoxamine	PPIs	↑	Plasma levels of PPIs may be elevated. Monitor for an increase in adverse reactions.
Sucralfate	PPIs Lansoprazole	↓	Coadministration delayed the absorption and the bioavailability of the PPI. Give the PPI at least 30 minutes prior to sucralfate.
Voriconazole	PPIs	↑	PPI plasma concentrations may be elevated, increasing the pharmacologic effects and risk of adverse reactions. Close clinical monitoring is warranted. An initial reduction in the dexlansoprazole dose may be needed when voriconazole is added.
PPIs	Azole antifungals (eg, itraconazole, ketoconazole)	↓	The bioavailability of certain azole antifungals may be decreased because of a possible reduction in tablet dissolution in the presence of a high gastric pH. Avoid coadministration if possible.
PPIs Esomeprazole Omeprazole	Benzodiazepines	↑	The oxidative metabolism of certain benzodiazepines (eg, diazepam, triazolam) may be decreased, thus reducing the clearance, prolonging the half-life, and increasing the serum levels of the benzodiazepine. Reduce the benzodiazepine dosage or increase the dosing interval.
PPIs Omeprazole	Carbamazepine	↑	Carbamazepine plasma concentrations may be elevated, increasing the risk of toxicity. Additional carbamazepine concentration and clinical monitoring is warranted. Adjust the carbamazepine dose as needed when starting or stopping omeprazole.
PPIs Esomeprazole Omeprazole	Cilostazol	↑	Concurrent use may increase cilostazol plasma concentrations, increasing the therapeutic and adverse effects. Consider dosage adjustment of cilostazol.
PPIs	Clopidogrel	↓	Controlled studies are needed to determine the magnitude of this interaction with each PPI and clopidogrel. The antiplatelet activity of clopidogrel may be decreased by PPIs. Certain PPIs (eg, omeprazole) may interfere with the metabolic (CYP2C19) conversion of clopidogrel to its active metabolite. If a PPI is clearly indicated in a patient receiving clopidogrel, use with caution. According to the prescribing information, avoid coadministration of omeprazole with clopidogrel. For more information, see the "Antiplatelets" paragraph that preceeds the drug interaction table. An antacid or H_2-receptor antagonist (eg, ranitidine) may be a safer alternative.
PPIs Omeprazole	Clozapine	↑	Clozapine plasma concentrations and pharmacologic effects may be increased. Clozapine toxicity may occur. Close clinical and laboratory monitoring is warranted. Adjust the clozapine dose as needed.
PPIs	Digoxin	↑	Coadministration may increase serum digoxin levels. The magnitude of this change would not be expected to be clinically important in most patients.
PPIs Omeprazole	Disulfiram	↑	The neuropsychiatric toxicity of disulfiram may be increased. The clinical importance of this interaction is not known. If an interaction is suspected, it may be necessary to discontinue both drugs.
PPIs	Erlotinib	↓	Esomeprazole may interfere with the absorption of erlotinib. Plasma concentration and pharmacologic effects of erlotinib may be decreased. Avoid coadministration.
PPIs Omeprazole	Hydantoins (eg, phenytoin)	↑	Serum hydantoin levels may be increased because of omeprazole inhibiting the oxidative hepatic metabolism of hydantoins. Consider monitoring serum hydantoin levels and adjust dosage as needed.
PPIs	Methotrexate	↑	PPIs may decrease the renal elimination of methotrexate, increasing methotrexate concentrations and the risk of toxicity. Closely monitor methotrexate concentrations and monitor for signs of methotrexate toxicity. Longer duration of leucovorin rescue, systemic hydration, and urinary alkalinization may be required for high-dose methotrexate. Consider discontinuing or suspending the PPI.
PPIs	Mycophenolate	↓	Mycophenolate plasma concentrations and pharmacologic effects may be decreased. Larger mycophenolate doses may be needed during coadministration of dexlansoprazole. Monitor the clinical response and adjust the mycophenolate dose as needed.
PPIs Dexlansoprazole Esomeprazole	Protease inhibitors (eg, atazanavir, indinavir, nelfinavir)	↓	Dexlansoprazole may decrease the systemic concentrations of atazanavir, which is dependent on the presence of gastric acid for absorption. May result in loss of therapeutic effect of atazanavir and the development of HIV resistance. Do not administer PPIs in patients receiving atazanavir or nelfinavir.
PPIs Dexlanzoprazole Lansoprazole Omeprazole	Tacrolimus	↑	Tacrolimus whole blood levels may be elevated, increasing the pharmacologic effects and risk of adverse reactions, especially in intermediate and poor CYP2C19 metabolizers. Closely monitor tacrolimus plasma trough concentrations when the PPI is started or stopped. Clinical monitoring for signs and symptoms of toxicity is also warranted. Rabeprazole may be a potential alternative.
PPIs Omeprazole	Theophylline	↑	The rate of theophylline absorption from slow-release forms of theophylline may be increased. In addition, interactions have been reported with other drugs metabolized by the CYP-450 system. Clinical and laboratory monitoring is warranted. Adjust the theophylline dose as needed.

Proton Pump Inhibitor Drug Interactions

Precipitant drug	Object drug[a]		Description
PPIs	Tolterodine extended release	↑	An increase in the release of tolterodine from the extended-release dosage form may occur as a result of the increase in gastric pH associated with PPI administration. Plasma concentrations of tolterodine and its active metabolite may be elevated, increasing the pharmacologic effects and risk of adverse reactions. Monitor the clinical response and for adverse reactions. Adjust the tolterodine dose as needed.
PPIs	Tyrosine kinase receptor inhibitor (eg, dasatinib, nilotinib)	↓	Esomeprazole may interfere with the absorption of dasatinib and nilotinib. Plasma concentration and pharmacologic effects of dasatinib and nilotinib may be decreased. Avoid coadministration.
PPIs	Salicylates, enteric-coated	↑	Enteric-coated salicylates may dissolve more rapidly, increasing gastric adverse effects.
PPIs Omeprazole	Sulfonylureas	↑	Concurrent use may increase the serum sulfonylurea concentration, increasing the hypoglycemic effects. Based on available data, no special action is needed.
PPIs	Warfarin	↑	Postmarketing reports of changes in prothrombin measures have been received in patients on concomitant warfarin and a PPI. Monitor INR[b] and prothrombin time, and adjust the warfarin dose as needed.

[a] ↑ = object drug increased; ↓ = object drug decreased.
[b] INR = international normalized ratio.

➤*Drug/Food interactions:* When **omeprazole** 20 mg capsules were administered with applesauce, the C_{max} was reduced 25% without a significant change in AUC; however, the clinical significance is unknown. When omeprazole oral suspension is administered 1 hour after a meal, C_{max} and AUC are reduced by 63% and 24%, respectively. It is recommended that omeprazole capsules are administered before meals and the oral suspension administered on an empty stomach 1 hour before a meal. The AUC after administration of a single 40 mg dose of **esomeprazole** is decreased by 43% to 53% after food intake compared with fasting conditions. Esomeprazole should be taken at least 1 hour before eating. Both C_{max} and AUC of **lansoprazole** are diminished by approximately 50% to 70% if the drug is given 30 minutes after food as opposed to the fasting condition; therefore, lansoprazole should be taken before eating. Increases in C_{max} ranged from 12% to 55%, increases in AUC ranged from 9% to 37%, and T_{max} varied (ranging from a decrease of 0.7 hours to an increase of 3 hours) when **dexlansoprazole** was administered with food compared with fasting. Dexlansoprazole may be taken without regard to food. When **pantoprazole** is given with food, its T_{max} is highly variable and may increase significantly. Absorption may be delayed up to 2 hours or longer; however, the C_{max} and AUC of pantoprazole are not altered and pantoprazole may be taken without regard to timing of meals. When **rabeprazole** is administered with a high-fat meal, its T_{max} is variable and may delay its absorption up to 4 hours or longer; however, the C_{max} and AUC are not significantly altered and rabeprazole may be taken without regard to timing of meals.

Adverse Reactions

Safety data reflect exposure to **omeprazole** capsules in 3,096 patients with duodenal ulcer, resistant ulcer, and Zollinger-Ellison syndrome. The most common adverse reactions reported (incidence of at least 2%) included headache (6.9%), abdominal pain (5.2%), nausea (4%), diarrhea (3.7%), vomiting (3.2%), and flatulence (2.7%). Additional adverse reactions that occurred in at least 1% of patients included acid regurgitation, upper respiratory tract infection (1.9%); constipation, dizziness, rash (1.5%); asthenia (1.3%); back pain (1.1%); and cough (1.1%). Fever was reported frequently in children 1 to 2 years of age (33%).

The following adverse reactions occurred in at least 2% of patients treated with **dexlansoprazole**.

Dexlansoprazole Adverse Reactions (≥ 2%)

Adverse reactions	Dexlansoprazole 30 mg (n = 455)	Dexlansoprazole 60 mg (n = 2,218)	Dexlansoprazole (n = 2,621)	Placebo (n = 896)
GI				
Abdominal pain	3.5%	4%	4%	3.5%
Diarrhea	5.1%	4.7%	4.8%	2.9%
Flatulence	2.6%	1.4%	1.6%	0.6%
Nausea	3.3%	2.8%	2.9%	2.6%
Vomiting	2.2%	1.4%	1.6%	0.8%
Respiratory				
Upper respiratory tract infection	2.9%	1.7%	1.9%	0.8%

In general, **lansoprazole** treatment has been well tolerated in short- and long-term trials. The following adverse events were reported in 1% or more of patients: diarrhea (3.8%); abdominal pain (2.1%); nausea (1.3%); constipation (1%). Headache occurred at a greater than 1% incidence but was more common with placebo. The incidence of diarrhea is similar between placebo and lansoprazole 15 and 30 mg patients (2.9%, 1.4%, and 4.2%, respectively), but higher with lansoprazole 60 mg (7.4%). The most commonly reported adverse event during maintenance therapy was diarrhea.

In clinical trials with **rabeprazole**, the only adverse event occurring in greater than 1% of patients and appearing with greater frequency than placebo was headache (2.4% vs placebo 1.6%).

The following adverse events occurred in 1% or more of patients treated with **pantoprazole**: abdominal pain, ALT increased, anxiety, arthralgia, asthenia, back pain, bronchitis, chest pain, constipation, cough increased, diarrhea, dizziness, dyspepsia, dyspnea, eructation, flatulence, flu syndrome, gastroenteritis, GI disorder, headache, hyperglycemia, hyperlipemia, hypertonia, infection, insomnia, liver function tests abnormal, migraine, nausea, neck pain, pain, pharyngitis, rash, rectal disorder, rhinitis, sinusitis, upper respiratory tract infection, urinary frequency, urinary tract infection, and vomiting. The following adverse events occurred in greater than 1% of patients treated with IV pantoprazole: Abdominal pain, constipation, diarrhea, dyspepsia, headache, injection-site reaction (including thrombophlebitis and abscess), insomnia, nausea, rhinitis.

The following adverse reactions occurred in more than 1% of patients treated with **esomeprazole** IV: reactions associated with test procedures (23.1%); headache (10.9%); flatulence (10.3%); dyspepsia, nausea (6.4%); abdominal pain (5.8%); diarrhea, dry mouth (3.9%); constipation, dizziness (2.5%); application-site reaction (including mild focal erythema and pruritus at IV insertion site), sinusitis (1.7%); pruritus, respiratory tract infection (1.1%).

The following adverse reactions occurred in less than 1% of patients:

➤*Cardiovascular:*

Dexlansoprazole – Angina, arrhythmia, bradycardia, chest pain, deep vein thrombosis, edema, hot flush, hypertension, myocardial infarction (MI), palpitation, tachycardia (less than 2%).

Esomeprazole – Hypertension, tachycardia.

Lansoprazole – Angina, arrhythmia, bradycardia, cerebrovascular accident/cerebral infarction, hypertension/hypotension, MI, palpitations, shock (circulatory failure), syncope, tachycardia, vasodilation.

Pantoprazole – Abnormal electrocardiogram, angina pectoris, arrhythmia, atrial fibrillation/flutter, cardiovascular disorder, congestive heart failure, hemorrhage, hypertension, hypotension, MI, myocardial ischemia, palpitation, syncope, tachycardia, thrombophlebitis, thrombosis, vasodilatation.

Rabeprazole – Angina pectoris, bradycardia, bundle branch block, electrocardiogram abnormal, hypertension, MI, palpitation, sinus bradycardia, syncope, tachycardia; pulmonary embolus, QTc prolongation, supraventricular tachycardia, thrombophlebitis, vasodilation, and ventricular tachycardia (less than or equal to 0.1%).

➤*CNS:*

Dexlansoprazole – Abnormal dreams, altered taste, anxiety, asthenia, convulsion, depression, dizziness, feeling abnormal, headache, insomnia, libido changes, memory impairment, migraine, paresthesia, psychomotor hyperactivity, tremor, trigeminal neuralgia (less than 2%).

Esomeprazole – Apathy, appetite increased, asthenia, confusion, depression aggravated, dizziness, fatigue, hypertonia, hypesthesia, insomnia, migraine, migraine aggravated, nervousness, paresthesia, sleep disorder, somnolence, tremor, vertigo.

Lansoprazole – Abnormal dreams, agitation, amnesia, anxiety, apathy, asthenia, confusion, convulsion, depersonalization, depression, diplopia, dizziness, emotional lability, hallucinations, hemiplegia, hostility aggravated, hyperkinesia, hypertonia, hypesthesia, insomnia, libido decreased/increased, migraine, nervousness, neurosis, paresthesia, sleep disorder, somnolence, thinking abnormality, tremor, vertigo.

Pantoprazole – Abnormal dreams, confusion, convulsion, depression, dysarthria, emotional lability, hallucinations, hyperkinesia, hypesthesia, libido decreased, nervousness, neuralgia, neuritis, neuropathy, paresthesia, reflexes decreased, sleep disorder, somnolence, thinking abnormal, tremor, vertigo.

Rabeprazole – Abnormal dreams, anxiety, asthenia, convulsion, depression, dizziness, hypertonia, insomnia, libido decreased, migraine, nervousness, neuralgia, neuropathy, paresthesia, somnolence, tremor, vertigo; agitation, amnesia, confusion, extrapyramidal syndrome, hyperkinesia (less than or equal to 0.1%).

➤*Dermatologic:*

Dexlansoprazole – Acne, dermatitis, erythema, rash, skin lesion, sunburn, urticaria (less than 2%).

Esomeprazole – Acne, angioedema, dermatitis, pruritus, pruritus ani, rash, rash erythematous, rash maculopapular, skin inflammation, sweating increased, urticaria.

Lansoprazole – Acne, alopecia, contact dermatitis, dry skin, fixed eruption, hair disorder, maculopapular rash, nail disorder, pruritus, rash, skin carcinoma, skin disorder, sweating, urticaria.

Pantoprazole – Acne, alopecia, contact dermatitis, dry skin, eczema, fungal dermatitis, hemorrhage, herpes simplex, herpes zoster, lichenoid dermatitis, maculopapular rash, pruritus, skin disorder, skin ulcer, sweating, urticaria.

Rabeprazole – Alopecia, pruritus, rash, sweating, urticaria; dry skin, herpes zoster, psoriasis, skin discoloration (less than or equal to 0.1%).

➤*GI:*

Dexlansoprazole – Abdominal discomfort, abdominal tenderness, abnormal bowel sounds, abnormal feces, anal discomfort, Barrett esophagus, bezoar, breath odor, colonic polyp, constipation, dry mouth, duodenitis, dyspepsia, dysphagia, enteritis, eructation, esophagitis, gastric polyp, gastritis, gastroenteritis, GERD, GI disorders, GI hypermotility disorders, GI ulcers and perforation, hematemesis, hematochezia, hemorrhoids, impaired gastric emptying, irritable bowel syndrome, microscopic colitis, mucus stools, nausea and vomiting, oral herpes, oral mucosal blistering, oral paresthesia, painful defecation, proctitis, rectal hemorrhage (less than 2%).

Esomeprazole – Abdomen enlarged, anorexia, bowel irregularity, constipation aggravated, dyspepsia, dysphagia, epigastric pain, eructation, esophageal disorder, frequent stools, gastroenteritis, GI dysplasia, GI hemorrhage, GI symptoms not otherwise specified, melena, mouth disorder, pharynx disorder, rectal disorder, tongue disorder, tongue edema, ulcerative stomatitis, vomiting.

Lansoprazole – Abdomen enlarged, abnormal stools, anorexia, bezoar, cardiospasm, cholelithiasis, colitis, diarrhea, dry mouth, dyspepsia, dysphagia, enteritis, eructation, esophageal stenosis, esophageal ulcer, esophagitis, fecal discoloration, flatulence, gastric nodules/fundic gland polyps, gastritis, gastroenteritis, GI anomaly, GI disorder, GI hemorrhage, glossitis, gum hemorrhage, hematemesis, increased appetite, increased salivation, melena, mouth ulceration, nausea, oral moniliasis, rectal disorder, rectal hemorrhage, stomatitis, tenesmus, tongue disorder, ulcerative colitis, ulcerative stomatitis, vomiting.

Pantoprazole – Anorexia, aphthous stomatitis, cardiospasm, colitis, dry mouth, duodenitis, dysphagia, enteritis, esophageal hemorrhage, esophagitis, GI carcinoma, GI hemorrhage, GI moniliasis, gingivitis, glossitis, halitosis, hematemesis, increased appetite, melena, mouth ulceration, oral moniliasis, periodontal abscess, periodontitis, rectal hemorrhage, stomach ulcer, stomatitis, stools abnormal, tongue discoloration, ulcerative colitis.

Rabeprazole – Abdomen enlarged, abdominal pain, abnormal stools, anorexia, cholecystitis, cholelithiasis, colitis, constipation, diarrhea, dry mouth, dyspepsia, dysphagia, eructation, esophagitis, flatulence, gastroenteritis, gingivitis, glossitis, increased appetite, melena, mouth ulceration, nausea, pancreatitis, proctitis, rectal hemorrhage, stomatitis, vomiting; bloody diarrhea, cholangitis, duodenitis, GI hemorrhage, salivary gland enlargement (less than or equal to 0.1%).

➤*GU:*

Dexlansoprazole – Dysmenorrhea, dyspareunia, dysuria, menorrhagia, menstrual disorder, micturition urgency, vulvovaginal infection (less than 2%).

Esomeprazole – Abnormal urine, albuminuria, cystitis, dysmenorrhea, dysuria, fungal infection, genital moniliasis, glycosuria, hematuria, impotence, menstrual disorder, micturition frequency, moniliasis, polyuria, vaginitis.

Lansoprazole – Abnormal menses, albuminuria, breast enlargement, breast pain, breast tenderness, dysmenorrhea, dysuria, glycosuria, gynecomastia, hematuria, impotence, kidney calculus, kidney pain, leukorrhea, menorrhagia, menstrual disorder, penis disorder, polyuria, testis disorder, urethral pain, urinary frequency, urinary tract infection, urinary urgency, urination impaired, vaginitis.

Pantoprazole – Albuminuria, balanitis, breast pain, cystitis, dysmenorrhea, dysuria, epididymitis, glycosuria, hematuria, impotence, kidney calculus, kidney pain, nocturia, prostatic disorder, pyelonephritis, scrotal edema, urethral pain, urethritis, urinary tract disorder, urination impaired, vaginitis.

Rabeprazole – Cystitis, dysmenorrhea, dysuria, kidney calculus, metrorrhagia, polyuria, urinary frequency; breast enlargement, hematuria, impotence, leukorrhea, menorrhagia, orchitis, urinary incontinence, urine abnormality (less than or equal to 0.1%).

➤*Hematologic / Lymphatic:*

Dexlansoprazole – Anemia, lymphadenopathy (less than 2%).

Esomeprazole – Anemia, anemia hypochromic, cervical lymphadenopathy, epistaxis, leukocytosis, leukopenia, thrombocytopenia.

Lansoprazole – Anemia, hemolysis, lymphadenopathy.

Pantoprazole – Anemia, ecchymosis, eosinophilia, hypochromic anemia, iron deficiency anemia, leukocytosis, leukopenia, thrombocytopenia.

Rabeprazole – Anemia, ecchymosis, hypochromic anemia, lymphadenopathy.

➤*Hepatic:*

Dexlansoprazole – Biliary colic, cholelithiasis, hepatomegaly (less than 2%).

Esomeprazole – Bilirubinemia, hepatic function abnormal.

Pantoprazole – Biliary pain, cholecystitis, cholelithiasis, cholestatic jaundice, hepatitis, hyperbilirubinemia.

Rabeprazole – Hepatic encephalopathy, hepatitis, hepatoma, liver fatty deposit.

➤*Lab test abnormalities:*

Dexlansoprazole – Alkaline phosphatase increased, ALT increased, AST increased, bilirubin decreased/increased, blood creatinine increased, blood gastrin increased, blood glucose increased, blood potassium increased, liver function test abnormal, platelet count decreased, total protein increased (less than 2%).

Esomeprazole – Increased alkaline phosphatase, ALT, AST, creatinine, hemoglobin, platelets, potassium, serum gastrin, sodium, thyroid stimulating hormone, thyroxine, total bilirubin, uric acid, and white blood cell count (WBC).

Decreased hemoglobin, platelets, potassium, sodium, thyroxine, and WBC.

Lansoprazole – Abnormal bilirubinemia, eosinophilia, hyperlipemia, liver function tests, red blood cell count (RBC); increased AST, ALT, alkaline phosphatase, creatinine, gastrin levels, gamma-glutamyl transpeptidase (GGTP), globulins, glucocorticoids, lactic acid dehydrogenase; increased/decreased/abnormal WBC, platelets; increased/decreased cholesterol electrolytes.

Urine abnormalities such as albuminuria, glycosuria, and hematuria also were reported.

Pantoprazole – Abnormal laboratory test; increased alkaline phosphatase, ALT, AST, creatinine, glycosuria, hypercholesterolemia, hyperuricemia, GGTP.

Rabeprazole – Abnormal erythrocytes, liver function tests, platelets, urine, WBC; increased ALT, creatine phosphokinase, prostatic specific antigen; albuminuria, hypercholesteremia, hyperglycemia, hyperlipemia, hypokalemia, hyponatremia, leukocytosis, leukorrhea.

➤*Metabolic / Nutritional:*

Dexlansoprazole – Appetite changes, hypercalcemia, hypokalemia, weight increased (less than 2%).

Esomeprazole – Facial edema, generalized edema, goiter, hyperuricemia, hyponatremia, leg edema, peripheral edema, thirst, vitamin B_{12} deficiency, weight gain/loss.

Lansoprazole – Dehydration, diabetes mellitus, edema, goiter, gout, hyperglycemia/hypoglycemia, hypothyroidism, peripheral edema, thirst, weight gain/loss.

Pantoprazole – Dehydration, diabetes mellitus, facial edema, generalized edema, goiter, gout, peripheral edema, thirst, weight gain/loss.

Rabeprazole – Dehydration, edema, facial edema, gout, hyperthyroidism, hypothyroidism, peripheral edema, thirst, weight gain/loss.

➤*Musculoskeletal:*

Dexlansoprazole – Arthralgia, arthritis, joint sprains, muscle cramps, musculoskeletal pain, myalgia (less than 2%).

Esomeprazole – Arthralgia, arthritis aggravated, arthropathy, cramps, fibromyalgia syndrome, hernia, polymyalgia rheumatica.

Lansoprazole – Arthralgia, arthritis, bone disorder, joint disorder, leg cramps, musculoskeletal pain, myalgia, myasthenia, synovitis.

Pantoprazole – Arthritis, arthrosis, bone disorder/pain, bursitis, joint disorder, leg cramps, myalgia, tenosynovitis.

Rabeprazole – Arthritis, arthrosis, bone pain, bursitis, leg cramps, myalgia; twitching (less than or equal to 0.1%).

➤*Respiratory:*

Dexlansoprazole – Aspiration, asthma, bronchitis, cough, dyspnea, hiccups, hyperventilation, nasopharyngitis, pharyngitis, respiratory tract congestion, sinusitis, sore throat (less than 2%).

Esomeprazole – Asthma aggravated, coughing, dyspnea, hiccup, larynx edema, pharyngitis, rhinitis, sinusitis.

Lansoprazole – Asthma, bronchitis, cough increased, dyspnea, epistaxis, hemoptysis, hiccup, laryngeal neoplasia, pharyngitis, pleural disorder, pneumonia, respiratory disorder, rhinitis, sinusitis, stridor, upper respiratory tract inflammation/infection.

Pantoprazole – Asthma, epistaxis, hiccup, laryngitis, lung disorder, pneumonia, voice alteration.

Rabeprazole – Asthma, dyspnea, epistaxis, hiccup, hyperventilation, laryngitis; apnea, hypoventilation (less than or equal to 0.1%).

➤*Special senses:*

Dexlansoprazole – Ear pain, eye irritation, eye swelling, tinnitus, vertigo (less than 2%).

Esomeprazole – Conjunctivitis, earache, otitis media, parosmia, taste loss, taste perversion, tinnitus, visual field defect, vision abnormal.

Lansoprazole – Abnormal vision, blurred vision, conjunctivitis, deafness, dry eyes, ear disorder, eye pain, otitis media, parosmia, photophobia, retinal degeneration, taste loss, taste perversion, tinnitus, visual field defect.

Pantoprazole – Abnormal vision, amblyopia, cataract specified, deafness, diplopia, ear pain, extraocular palsy, glaucoma, otitis externa, retinal vascular disorder, taste perversion, tinnitus.

Rabeprazole – Abnormal vision, amblyopia, cataract, dry eyes, glaucoma, otitis media, tinnitus; blurred vision, corneal opacity, diplopia, deafness, eye pain, retinal degeneration, strabismus (less than or equal to 0.1%).

➤*Miscellaneous:*

Dexlansoprazole – *Candida* infections, chills, falls, fractures, goiter, hypersensitivity, inflammation, influenza, nodule, overdose, pain, procedural pain, pyrexia, viral infection (less than 2%).

Esomeprazole – Allergic reaction, back pain, chest pain, chest pain substernal, fever, flu-like disorder, flushing, hot flushes, malaise, pain, rigors.

Lansoprazole – Allergic reaction, back pain, candidiasis, carcinoma, chest pain (not otherwise specified), chills, fever, flu syndrome, halitosis, infection (not otherwise specified), malaise, neck pain, neck rigidity, pain, pelvic pain.

Pantoprazole – Abscess, allergic reaction, chest pain substernal, chills, cyst, fever, heat stroke, hernia, malaise, moniliasis, neck rigidity, neoplasm, nonspecified drug reaction, photosensitivity reaction.

Rabeprazole – Allergic reaction, asthenia, chest pain substernal, chills, fever, malaise, neck rigidity, photosensitivity reaction; face edema, hangover effect (less than or equal to 0.1%).

➤*Postmarketing:*

Dexlansoprazole – Anaphylactic shock requiring emergency intervention, blurred vision, facial edema, generalized rash, leukocytoclastic vasculitis, oral edema, pharyngeal edema, Stevens-Johnson syndrome, throat tightness, toxic epidermal necrolysis (TEN) (some fatal).

Esomeprazole – Aggression, agitation, agranulocytosis, alopecia, anaphylactic reaction, bone fracture, blurred vision, bronchospasm, erythema multiforme, GI candidiasis, gynecomastia, hallucination, hepatic encephalopathy, hepatic failure, hepatitis (with or without jaundice), hyperhidrosis, hypomagnesemia, interstitial nephritis, muscular weakness, myalgia, pancreatitis, pancytopenia, photosensitivity, shock, Stevens-Johnson syndrome, stomatitis, taste disturbance, TEN.

Lansoprazole – Agranulocytosis, anaphylactoid-like reaction, aplastic anemia, hemolytic anemia, hepatotoxicity, leukopenia, neutropenia, pancreatitis, pancytopenia, severe dermatologic reactions including erythema multiforme, Stevens-Johnson syndrome, thrombocytopenia, thrombotic thrombocytopenic purpura, TEN (some fatal); speech disorder, urinary retention, vomiting.

Omeprazole – Abdominal swelling; aggression; agitation; agranulocytosis (some fatal); allergic reactions, including anaphylaxis, anaphylactic shock, bronchospasm, interstitial nephritis, and urticaria; alopecia; anemia; angioedema; anorexia; anxiety; apathy; anterior ischemic optic neuropathy; blurred vision; bone fracture; bradycardia; chest pain or angina; confusion; depression; double vision; dream abnormalities; dry eye syndrome; dry mouth; dry skin; elevated blood pressure; elevated serum creatinine and GGTP; epistaxis; esophageal candidiasis; fatigue; fecal discoloration; fever; gastric fundic gland polyps; glycosuria; gynecomastia; hallucinations; hematuria; hemolytic anemia; hyperhidrosis; hypomagnesemia; hyponatremia; hypoglycemia; insomnia; interstitial nephritis; increased alkaline phosphatase, ALT, AST, and bilirubin; irritable colon; joint pain; leg pain; leukocytosis; malaise; microscopic pyuria; mucosal atrophy of the tongue; muscle cramps; muscle weakness; myalgia; nervousness; neutropenia; pancreatitis (some fatal); ocular irritation; optic atrophy; optic neuritis; overt liver disease has occurred rarely, including hepatocellular, cholestatic, or mixed hepatitis, liver necrosis (some fatal), hepatic failure (some fatal), jaundice, and hepatic encephalopathy; pain; palpitation; pancytopenia; paresthesia; peripheral edema; pharyngeal pain; photosensitivity; proteinuria; pruritus; purpura and/or petechiae; rash and, rarely, cases of severe generalized skin reactions including TEN (some fatal), Stevens-Johnson syndrome, and erythema multiforme; skin inflammation; somnolence; stomatitis; tachycardia; taste perversion; testicular pain; thrombocytopenia; tinnitus; tremors; urinary tract infection; urinary frequency; urticaria; vertigo; weight gain.

Pantoprazole – Anaphylaxis (including anaphylactic shock); angioedema (Quincke edema); anterior ischemic optic neuropathy; elevated creatine phosphokinase; severe dermatologic reactions, including erythema multiforme, Stevens-Johnson syndrome, and TEN (some fatal); hepatocellular damage leading to jaundice and hepatic failure; interstitial nephritis; pancreatitis; pancytopenia; and rhabdomyolysis. Confusion, hypokinesia, speech disorder, increased salivation, vertigo, nausea, tinnitus, and blurred vision.

Rabeprazole – Agranulocytosis, anaphylaxis, angioedema, bullous and other drug eruptions of the skin, coma, delirium, disorientation, erythema multiforme, hemolytic anemia, hyperammonemia, interstitial nephritis, interstitial pneumonia, jaundice, leukopenia, pancytopenia, rhabdomyolysis, severe dermatologic reactions including TEN (some fatal), Stevens-Johnson syndrome, sudden death, thrombocytopenia, thyroid-stimulating hormone elevations; increases in prothrombin time/INR in patients treated with concomitant warfarin have been reported.

Overdosage

➤*Symptoms:* Overdosage with **omeprazole** has been reported. Doses ranged up to 2,400 mg (120 times the usual recommended dose). Symptoms were transient and included blurred vision, confusion, diaphoresis, drowsiness, dry mouth, flushing, headache, nausea, tachycardia, and vomiting. No serious clinical outcome has been reported. No specific antidote for omeprazole overdosage is known.

In 1 overdose case, a patient consumed 600 mg of **lansoprazole** with no adverse reaction.

Multiple doses of **dexlansoprazole** 120 mg and a single dose of 300 mg did not result in death or other severe adverse reactions.

There has been no experience with large overdoses of **rabeprazole**. The maximum reported overdose was 80 mg. There were no signs or symptoms associated with any overdose. Patients with Zollinger-Ellison syndrome have been treated with up to 120 mg/day.

Two reports of overdose with 400 and 600 mg of **pantoprazole** have been reported with no adverse effects observed. There has been 1 report of suicide involving an overdose of pantoprazole 560 mg; however, the death was more reasonably attributed to other drugs ingested.

➤*Treatment:* **Omeprazole**, **esomeprazole**, **dexlansoprazole**, **lansoprazole**, **pantoprazole**, and **rabeprazole** are extensively protein bound and are not readily dialyzable. Treatment should be symptomatic and supportive. Refer to General Management of Acute Overdosage.

Patient Information

Advise patients to take **omeprazole**, **esomeprazole**, and **lansoprazole** before meals. Advise patients to take **dexlansoprazole**, **rabeprazole**, and **pantoprazole** without regard to meals.

Advise patients not to open, crush, or chew omeprazole or esomeprazole capsules; do not chew or crush dexlansoprazole or omeprazole tablets or lansoprazole products; do not chew, crush, or split rabeprazole or pantoprazole tablets.

Antacids may be used while taking PPIs.

Advise patients that **dexlansoprazole** and **esomeprazole** capsules can be opened and intact granules sprinkled on 1 tablespoon of applesauce, and then swallowed immediately.

ESOMEPRAZOLE

Rx	**Nexium** (AstraZeneca)	**Capsules, delayed-release; oral**[a]: 20 mg	Equiv. to esomeprazole magnesium 22.3 mg. Sugar spheres. (NEXIUM 20 mg). Opaque amethyst. In 90s, 1,000s, unit-of-use 30s, and UD 100s.
		40 mg	Equiv. to esomeprazole magnesium 44.5 mg. Sugar spheres. (NEXIUM 40 mg). Opaque amethyst. In 90s, 1,000s, UD 30s, and UD 100s.
Rx	**Nexium** (AstraZeneca)	**Powder for suspension, delayed-release; oral**[a]: 10 mg	As esomeprazole magnesium. Dextrose. In UD 30s.
		20 mg	As esomeprazole magnesium. Dextrose. In UD 30s.
		40 mg	As esomeprazole magnesium. Dextrose. In UD 30s.
Rx	**Nexium I.V.** (AstraZeneca)	**Injection, freeze-dried powder for solution:** 20 mg	Equiv. to esomeprazole sodium 21.3 mg. Edetate disodium. In single-use vials.
		40 mg	Equiv. to esomeprazole 42.5 mg. Edetate disodium. In single-use vials.

[a] Contains enteric-coated granules.

ESOMEPRAZOLE MAGNESIUM — ORAL

For complete and comparative prescribing information, refer to the Proton Pump Inhibitors class monograph.

Indications

➤*Gastroesophageal reflux disease:*

Healing of erosive esophagitis – For the short-term (4 to 8 weeks) treatment in the healing and symptomatic resolution of diagnostically confirmed erosive esophagitis. For patients who have not healed after 4 to 8 weeks of treatment, consider an additional 4- to 8-week course of esomeprazole.

Maintenance of healing of erosive esophagitis – To maintain symptom resolution and healing of erosive esophagitis. Controlled studies do not extend beyond 6 months.

Symptomatic gastroesophageal reflux disease – For short-term (4 to 8 weeks) treatment of heartburn and other symptoms associated with gastroesophageal reflux disease (GERD) in adults and children 1 year of age and older.

➤*Helicobacter pylori eradication:*

Triple therapy (esomeprazole plus amoxicillin and clarithromycin) – In combination with amoxicillin and clarithromycin for the treatment of patients with *H. pylori* infection and duodenal ulcer disease (active or within the past 5 years) to eradicate *H. pylori*. Eradication of *H. pylori* has been shown to reduce the risk of duodenal ulcer recurrence.

➤*Pathological hypersecretory conditions, including Zollinger-Ellison syndrome:* For the long-term treatment of pathological hypersecretory conditions, including Zollinger-Ellison syndrome.

➤*Risk reduction of nonsteroidal anti-inflammatory drug–associ-*

ESOMEPRAZOLE MAGNESIUM — ORAL

ated gastric ulcer: For the reduction in the occurrence of gastric ulcers associated with continuous nonsteroidal anti-inflammatory drug (NSAID) therapy in patients at risk of developing gastric ulcers. Patients are considered to be at risk because of their age (60 years of age and older) and/or documented history of gastric ulcers. Controlled studies do not extend beyond 6 months.

➤*Off-label uses:* Non-GERD dyspepsia; Barrett esophagus; stress ulcer prophylaxis.

Administration and Dosage

➤*Adults:*

Gastroesophageal reflux disease –

Healing of erosive esophagitis:

- *Initial dosage* – 20 or 40 mg daily for 4 to 8 weeks.
- *Maintenance dosage* – 20 mg daily.
- *Duration of therapy* – The majority of patients heal within 4 to 8 weeks.

For patients who do not heal after 4 to 8 weeks, consider an additional 4 to 8 weeks of treatment.

Symptomatic gastroesophageal reflux disease:

- *Usual dosage* – 20 mg daily.
- *Duration of therapy* – 4 weeks. If symptoms do not resolve completely after 4 weeks, consider an additional 4 weeks of treatment.

H. pylori eradication –

Triple therapy:

- *Esomeprazole* – 40 mg once daily for 10 days.
- *Amoxicillin* – 1,000 mg twice daily for 10 days.
- *Clarithromycin* – 500 mg twice daily for 10 days.

Pathological hypersecretory conditions, including Zollinger-Ellison syndrome –

Initial dosage: 40 mg twice daily.

Maintenance dosage: Dosages vary with the individual patient. Dosage regimens should be adjusted to individual patient needs. Dosages of up to 240 mg daily have been administered.

Risk reduction of NSAID-associated gastric ulcer –

Usual dosage: 20 or 40 mg daily.

Duration of therapy: Up to 6 months.

➤*Children:*

Esomeprazole Oral Dosage Schedule for Children

Indication	Recommended dosage	Frequency
Children 12 to 17 years of age		
Short-term treatment of GERD	20 or 40 mg	Once daily for up to 8 weeks
Children 1 to 11 years of age[a]		
Healing of erosive esophagitis weight ≥ 20 kg	10 or 20 mg	Once daily for 8 weeks
Healing of erosive esophagitis weight < 20 kg	10 mg	Once daily for 8 weeks
Short-term treatment of symptomatic GERD	10 mg	Once daily for up to 8 weeks

[a] Dosages > 1 mg/kg/day have not been studied.

➤*Hepatic function impairment:*

Severe liver impairment (Child-Pugh class C) – Do not exceed a dose of esomeprazole 20 mg.

➤*Administration:* Esomeprazole should be taken at least 1 hour before eating.

Delayed-release capsules – Capsules can be swallowed whole or can be opened and mixed with applesauce.

Difficulty swallowing: Add 1 tablespoon of applesauce to an empty bowl and open the capsule. Carefully empty the granules inside the capsule onto the applesauce. Granules should be mixed with the applesauce and then swallowed immediately. The applesauce should not be hot and should be soft enough to be swallowed without chewing. Do not chew or crush the granules. Do not store the granules/applesauce mixture for future use.

Nasogastric tube administration: The delayed-release capsules can be opened and the intact granules emptied into a 60 mL catheter-tipped syringe and mixed with 50 mL of water. It is important to only use a catheter-tipped syringe when administering esomeprazole through a nasogastric tube. Replace the plunger and shake the syringe vigorously for 15 seconds. Hold the syringe with the tip up and check for granules remaining in the tip. Attach the syringe to a nasogastric tube and deliver the contents of the syringe through the nasogastric tube into the stomach. After administering the granules, flush the nasogastric tube with additional water. Do not administer the granules if they have dissolved or disintegrated. The suspension must be used immediately after preparation.

Delayed-release oral suspension – Empty the contents of a 10, 20, or 40 mg packet into a container with 15 mL of water. Stir, then leave 2 to 3 minutes to thicken. Stir and drink within 30 minutes. If any material remains after drinking, add more water, stir, and drink immediately.

Nasogastric/Gastric tube administration – Add 15 mL of water to a catheter-tipped syringe and then add the contents of a 10, 20, or 40 mg packet. It is important to only use a catheter-tipped syringe when administering esomeprazole through a nasogastric or gastric tube. Immediately shake the syringe and leave 2 to 3 minutes to thicken. Shake the syringe and inject through the nasogastric or gastric tube (French size 6 or larger) into the stomach within 30 minutes. Refill the syringe with 15 mL of water. Shake and flush any remaining contents from the nasogastric or gastric tube into the stomach.

➤*Storage/Stability:* Store at 25°C (77°F); excursions are permitted between 15° and 30°C (59° and 86°F). Keep the container tightly closed. Dispense in a tight container if the product package is subdivided.

ESOMEPRAZOLE SODIUM — INJECTION

For complete and comparative prescribing information, refer to the Proton Pump Inhibitors class monograph.

Indications

➤*Gastroesophageal reflux disease:* For short-term treatment of gastroesophageal reflux disease (GERD) with erosive esophagitis in adults and children 1 month to 17 years, inclusively as an alternative to oral therapy when therapy with oral esomeprazole is not possible or appropriate.

➤*Off-label uses:* Stress ulcer prophylaxis.

Administration and Dosage

➤*Adults:*

Gastroesophageal reflux disease –

Usual dosage: 20 or 40 mg given once daily by intravenous (IV) injection or IV infusion.

➤*Children:*

Gastroesophageal reflux disease with erosive esophagitis –

1 year to 17 years of age: See also off-label dosing.

- *Weight 55 kg or more* – 20 mg once daily by IV infusion.
- *Weight less than 55 kg* – 10 mg once daily by IV infusion.

1 month to younger than 1 year:

- *Usual dose* – 0.5 mg/kg once daily by IV infusion.

Off-label dosing –

12 to 17 years of age: 20 to 40 mg daily for up to 8 weeks.

➤*Hepatic function impairment:* In patients with severe liver impairment (Child-Pugh class C), a dose of 20 mg should not be exceeded.

➤*Preparation for administration:*

Adults –

IV injection: The freeze-dried powder should be reconstituted with 5 mL of sodium chloride 0.9% injection. Withdraw 5 mL of the reconstituted solution and administer as an IV injection.

IV infusion: A solution for IV infusion is prepared by first reconstituting the contents of 1 vial with 5 mL of sodium chloride 0.9% injection, Ringer's lactate injection, or dextrose 5% injection, and then further diluting the resulting solution to a final volume of 50 mL.

Children –

IV infusion:

- *1 month to less than 1 year* – First reconstitute the contents of 1 vial with 5 mL of sodium chloride 0.9% injection and further dilute the resulting solution to a final volume of 50 mL. The resultant concentration after diluting to a final volume of 50 mL is as follows: 40 mg vial: 0.8 mg/mL; 20 mg vial: 0.4 mg/mL.

Withdraw appropriate amount of volume for desired dose (0.5 mg/kg) and administer as an IV infusion over 10 to 30 minutes.

- *1 to 17 years of age* –

40 mg vial: First reconstitute the contents of 1 vial with 5 mL of sodium chloride 0.9% injection and further dilute the resulting solution to a final volume of 50 mL. The resultant concentration after diluting to a final volume of 50 mL is 0.8 mg/mL. For a 20 mg dose, withdraw 25 mL of the final solution and administer as an IV infusion over 10 to 30 minutes. For a 10 mg dose, withdraw 12.5 mL of the final solution and administer as an IV infusion over 10 to 30 minutes.

20 mg vial: First reconstitute the contents of 1 vial with 5 mL of sodium chloride 0.9% injection and further diluting the resulting solution to a final volume of 50 mL. The resultant concentration after diluting to a final volume of 50 mL is 0.4 mg/mL. For a 20 mg dose, administer the final solution (50 mL) as an IV infusion over 10 to 30 minutes. For a 10 mg dose, withdraw 25 mL of the final solution and administer as an IV infusion over 10 to 30 minutes.

Following reconstitution and administration, discard any unused portion.

➤*Administration:* Administer IV injections over no less than 3 minutes.

Administer IV infusions over a period of 10 to 30 minutes.

➤*Admixture compatibility:* Esomeprazole should not be administered with any other medications through the same IV site and/or tubing. The IV line should always be flushed with sodium chloride 0.9% injection, Ringer's lactate injection, or dextrose 5% injection prior to and after administration of esomeprazole.

➤*Storage/Stability:* Store vials at 25°C (77°F); excursions are permitted between 15° and 30°C (59° and 86°F). Protect from light. Store in carton until time of use.

ESOMEPRAZOLE SODIUM — INJECTION

IV injection – Store the reconstituted solution at room temperature, up to 30°C (86°F), and administer within 12 hours after reconstitution. No refrigeration is required.

IV infusion – Store the admixture at room temperature, up to 30°C (86°F), and administer within the designated time period. No refrigeration is required.

Recommended Esomeprazole IV Infusion Storage Time	
Diluent	Administer within:
Sodium chloride 0.9% injection	12 hours
Ringer's lactate injection	12 hours
Dextrose 5% injection	6 hours

LANSOPRAZOLE

otc	**Prevacid 24 Hour** (Novartis)	**Capsules, delayed-release; oral:**[a] 15 mg	PEG, sugar spheres, sucrose. 14s, 28s, and 42s.
Rx	**Lansoprazole** (Various, eg, Mylan, Sandoz)		May contain PEG, sugar spheres, sucrose. In 30s, 100s, and 1,000s.
Rx	**Lansoprazole** (Various, eg, Mylan, Sandoz)	**Capsules, delayed-release; oral:**[a] 30 mg	May contain PEG, sugar spheres, sucrose. In 90s, 100s, 500s, and 1,000s.
Rx	**Prevacid** (Takeda Pharmaceuticals)	**Tablets, disintegrating, delayed-release; oral:**[a] 15 mg	Mannitol, lactose, aspartame, phenylalanine 2.5 mg. White to yellowish-white with orange to dark brown speckles. Strawberry flavor. In UD 30s.
		30 mg	Mannitol, lactose, aspartame, phenylalanine 5.1 mg. White to yellowish-white with orange to dark brown speckles. Strawberry flavor. In UD 30s.
		Capsules, delayed-release; oral:[a] 15 mg	Sugar spheres, sucrose. (PREVACID 15). Pink/Green. In 1,000s, unit-of-use 30s, and UD 100s.
		30 mg	Sugar spheres, sucrose. (PREVACID 30). Pink/Black. In 100s, 1,000s, and UD 100s.
		Granules for suspension, delayed-release; oral:[a] 15 mg	Sugar, mannitol, docusate sodium. Strawberry flavor. In UD 30s.
		30 mg	Sugar, mannitol, docusate sodium. Strawberry flavor. In UD 30s.

[a] Contains enteric-coated granules.

LANSOPRAZOLE — ORAL

For complete and comparative prescribing information, refer to the Proton Pump Inhibitors class monograph. Refer to the Penicillins and Macrolides class monographs for complete prescribing information for amoxicillin and clarithromycin.

Indications

➤*Short-term treatment of active duodenal ulcer:* Short-term treatment (up to 4 weeks) for healing and symptom relief of active duodenal ulcer.

➤*Helicobacter pylori eradication to reduce the risk of duodenal ulcer recurrence:*

Triple therapy –

Lansoprazole/Amoxicillin/Clarithromycin: For the treatment of patients with *H. pylori* infection and duodenal ulcer disease (active or 1-year history of a duodenal ulcer) to eradicate *H. pylori*. Eradication of *H. pylori* has been shown to reduce the risk of duodenal ulcer recurrence.

Dual therapy –

Lansoprazole/Amoxicillin: For the treatment of patients with *H. pylori* infection and duodenal ulcer disease (active or 1-year history of a duodenal ulcer) who are either allergic or intolerant to clarithromycin or in whom resistance to clarithromycin is known or suspected. Eradication of *H. pylori* has been shown to reduce the risk of duodenal ulcer recurrence.

➤*Maintenance of healed duodenal ulcers:* To maintain healing of duodenal ulcers. Controlled studies do not extend beyond 12 months.

➤*Short-term treatment of active benign gastric ulcer:* For short-term treatment (up to 8 weeks) for healing and symptom relief of active benign gastric ulcer.

➤*Healing of nonsteroidal anti-inflammatory drug–associated gastric ulcer:* For the treatment of nonsteroidal anti-inflammatory drug (NSAID)–associated gastric ulcer in patients who continue NSAID use. Controlled studies did not extend beyond 8 weeks.

➤*Risk reduction of NSAID-associated gastric ulcer:* For reducing the risk of NSAID-associated gastric ulcers in patients with a history of a documented gastric ulcer who require the use of an NSAID. Controlled studies did not extend beyond 12 weeks.

➤*Gastroesophageal reflux disease:*

Short-term treatment of symptomatic gastroesophageal reflux disease – For the treatment of heartburn and other symptoms associated with symptomatic gastroesophageal reflux disease (GERD).

Erosive esophagitis – For short-term treatment (up to 8 weeks) for healing and symptomatic relief of all grades of erosive esophagitis; to maintain healing of erosive esophagitis.

➤*Maintenance of healing of erosive esophagitis:* To maintain healing of erosive esophagitis. Controlled studies did not extend beyond 12 months.

➤*Pathological hypersecretory conditions, including Zollinger-Ellison syndrome:* For the long-term treatment of pathological hypersecretory conditions, including Zollinger-Ellison syndrome.

➤*Heartburn (Prevacid 24 Hour only):* For the treatment of frequent heartburn (2 or more days per week).

➤*Off-label uses:*

Alternate-day dosing in the long-term management of reflux esophagitis – [4] = Insufficient documentation. Data from 1 study suggest that alternate-day therapy is as effective as daily dosing in maintaining remission rates during long-term treatment after patients have been healed via a shorter course (8 weeks) of therapy.

Laryngitis – [4] = Insufficient documentation. Initial data on lansoprazole in the treatment of chronic laryngitis appear promising. However, larger controlled trials are needed before clear benefit may be established. In addition, comparative studies with omeprazole may help establish which agent may be preferred.

Other possible off-label uses –

Prevention of GI bleeding in patients receiving antiplatelets: The American College of Cardiology, the American College of Gastroenterology, and the American Heart Association recommend the use of proton pump inhibitors (PPIs) to reduce the risk of GI bleeding in patients who are at high risk for GI bleeding and are receiving antiplatelet therapy. Patients at high risk for GI bleeding are defined as those with a history of GI bleeding; advanced age; concurrent use of anticoagulants, steroids, or NSAIDs, including aspirin; and *H. pylori* infection. However, patients who are not at high risk for bleeding achieve little benefit from concurrent use of a PPI with clopidogrel. If a PPI is needed in a patient at lower risk for GI bleeding, a drug that is not a strong or moderate CYP2C19 inhibitor, such as pantoprazole, should be considered, because omeprazole may interfere with the metabolic (CYP2C19) conversion of clopidogrel to its active metabolite.

Administration and Dosage

➤*Adults:*

Duodenal ulcer –

Initial dosage: 15 mg once daily for 4 weeks.

Maintenance dosage: 15 mg once daily for maintenance of healing.

Duodenal ulcer associated with H. pylori –

Dual therapy (lansoprazole/amoxicillin): Lansoprazole 30 mg plus amoxicillin 1 g both taken 3 times/day (every 8 hours) for 14 days for patients intolerant or resistant to clarithromycin.

Triple therapy (lansoprazole/clarithromycin/amoxicillin): Lansoprazole 30 mg plus clarithromycin 500 mg and amoxicillin 1 g all taken twice daily (every 12 hours) for 10 or 14 days.

Erosive esophagitis –

Initial dosage: 30 mg once daily for up to 8 weeks. For adults who do not heal within 8 weeks (5% to 10%), it may be helpful to give an additional 8 weeks of treatment. If there is a recurrence of erosive esophagitis, consider an additional 8-week course.

Maintenance dosage: 15 mg once daily.

Gastric ulcer – 30 mg once daily for up to 8 weeks.

Gastric ulcer associated with NSAIDs –

Healing: 30 mg once daily for up to 8 weeks.

Risk reduction: 15 mg once daily for up to 12 weeks.

Gastroesophageal reflux disease – 15 mg once daily for up to 8 weeks.

Heartburn –

Usual dosage: 1 capsule with a glass of water before eating in the morning, taken every day for 14 days. A 14-day course may be repeated every 4 months.

Maximum dose: Patients should not take more than 1 capsule per day. Patients should not use for more than 14 days unless directed by their health care provider.

Hypersecretory conditions, including Zollinger-Ellison syndrome –

Initial dosage: 60 mg once daily.

Maintenance dosage: Individualize dosage. Dosages of up to 90 mg twice daily have been administered. Administer daily doses greater than 120 mg in divided doses.

Duration of therapy: Some patients with Zollinger-Ellison syndrome have been treated with lansoprazole for longer than 4 years.

LANSOPRAZOLE — ORAL

Off-label dosing –

Alternate-day dosing in the long-term management of reflux esophagitis: [4] = Insufficient documentation. 15 to 30 mg every other day after healing was achieved by an 8-week course of 30 mg daily.

Laryngitis: [4] = Insufficient documentation. 30 mg twice daily for 3 months.

➤*Children:*

Erosive esophagitis –

12 years of age and older: See Adults for dosing.

1 to 11 years of age:

- *Weighing more than 30 kg –*
  - *Initial dosage:* 30 mg once daily.
  - *Dosage adjustment:* Dosage was increased (up to 30 mg twice daily) in some children after 2 or more weeks of treatment if they remained symptomatic.
  - *Duration of therapy:* Up to 12 weeks.
- *Weighing 30 kg or less –*
  - *Initial dosage:* 15 mg once daily.
  - *Dosage adjustment:* Dosage was increased (up to 30 mg twice daily) in some children after 2 or more weeks of treatment if they remained symptomatic.
  - *Duration of therapy:* Up to 12 weeks.

Gastroesophageal reflux disease –

12 years of age and older: 15 mg once daily for up to 8 weeks.

1 to 11 years of age:

- *Weighing more than 30 kg –*
  - *Initial dosage:* 30 mg once daily.
  - *Dosage adjustment:* Dosage was increased (up to 30 mg twice daily) in some children after 2 or more weeks of treatment if they remained symptomatic.
  - *Duration of therapy:* Up to 12 weeks.
- *Weighing 30 kg or less –*
  - *Initial dosage:* 15 mg once daily.
  - *Dosage adjustment:* Dosage was increased (up to 30 mg twice daily) in some children after 2 or more weeks of treatment if they remained symptomatic.
  - *Duration of therapy:* Up to 12 weeks.

Off-label dosing –

Reflux esophagitis:

- *Neonates* – 0.73 to 1.66 mg/kg once daily.

➤*Hepatic function impairment:* Consider dosage adjustment in patients with severe liver disease.

➤*Administration:* Administer before meals. Do not crush or chew lansoprazole oral products.

Capsules – For patients who have difficulty swallowing capsules, lansoprazole can be opened and the intact granules contained within can be sprinkled on 1 tablespoon of applesauce, *Ensure* pudding, cottage cheese, yogurt, or strained pears and swallowed immediately. Alternatively, the capsules may be emptied into a small volume of apple, orange, or tomato juice (60 mL; approximately 2 oz), mixed briefly, and swallowed immediately. To ensure complete delivery of the dose, the glass should be rinsed with 2 or more volumes of juice and the contents should be swallowed immediately. Use in other foods and liquids has not been studied clinically and, therefore, is not recommended.

Oral suspension – The packet contents should be emptied into 2 tablespoons of water. Other liquids or foods should not be used. After stirring well, the patient should drink the suspension immediately. If any material remains after drinking, the patient can add more water, stir, and drink immediately again. The suspension should not be given through enteral administration tubes.

Orally disintegrating tablets – The orally disintegrating tablet should be placed on the tongue and allowed to disintegrate with or without water until the particles can be swallowed. The tablet typically disintegrates in less than 1 minute. *SoluTabs* are not designed to be swallowed intact or chewed.

For administration via oral syringe, a 15 mg tablet should be placed in an oral syringe and approximately 4 mL of water should be drawn in, or a 30 mg tablet can be placed in an oral syringe and approximately 10 mL of water should be drawn in. The syringe should be shaken gently to allow for quick dispersal. After the tablet has dispersed, the contents should be administered within 15 minutes. The syringe should be refilled with approximately 2 mL (5 mL for the 30 mg tablet) of water, shaken gently, and any remaining contents should be administered.

Nasogastric tube –

Capsules: Lansoprazole capsules can be opened and the intact granules mixed in 40 mL apple juice. Other liquids should not be used. This mixture should be injected through the nasogastric (NG) tube into the stomach. After administering the granules, the NG tube should be flushed with additional apple juice to clear the tube.

Orally disintegrating tablets: A 15 mg tablet should be placed in a syringe and 4 mL of water should be drawn in, or a 30 mg tablet should be placed in the syringe and 10 mL of water should be drawn in. The syringe should be shaken gently to allow for quick dispersal. After the tablet has dispersed, this mixture should be injected through the NG tube into the stomach within 15 minutes. The syringe should be refilled with approximately 5 mL of water, shaken gently, and flushed through the NG tube.

➤*Storage/Stability:* Store at 25°C (77°F); excursions are permitted between 15° and 30°C (59° and 86°F). Store in a tight container protected from moisture.

OMEPRAZOLE

otc	**Prilosec OTC** (Procter & Gamble)	**Tablets, delayed-release; oral:** 20 mg	Equiv. to omeprazole magnesium 20.6 mg. Polyethylene glycol, sucrose. In 14s, 28s, and 42s.
otc	**Omeprazole** (Various, eg, Major, Wal-Mart)		May contain lactose. In 14s.
Rx	**Omeprazole** (Various, eg, Kremers-Urban, Mylan)	**Capsules, delayed-release; oral**[a]: 10 mg	May contain sugar spheres. In 30s and 100s.
Rx	**Prilosec** (AstraZeneca)		Lactose, mannitol. (606 PRILOSEC 10). Apricot/Amethyst opaque. In unit-of-use 30s.
Rx	**Omeprazole** (Various, eg, Kremers-Urban, Mylan)	**Capsules, delayed-release; oral**[a]: 20 mg	May contain sugar spheres. In 30s, 90s, 100s, 500s, and 1,000s.
Rx	**Prilosec** (AstraZeneca)		Lactose, mannitol. (742 PRILOSEC 20). Amethyst opaque. In 1,000s and unit-of-use 30s.
Rx	**Omeprazole** (Various, eg, Kremers-Urban, Mylan)	**Capsules, delayed-release; oral**[a]: 40 mg	May contain sugar spheres. In 30s, 100s, 500s, 1,000s, and UD 30s.
Rx	**Prilosec** (AstraZeneca)		Lactose, mannitol. (743 PRILOSEC 40). Apricot/Amethyst opaque. In 100s and unit-of-use 30s.
Rx	**Prilosec** (AstraZeneca)	**Granules for suspension, delayed-release; oral**[a]: 2.5 mg	Equiv. to omeprazole magnesium 2.8 mg. Sugar spheres, dextrose. In UD 30s.
		10 mg	Equiv. to omeprazole magnesium 11.2 mg. Sugar spheres, dextrose. In UD 30s.

[a] Contains enteric-coated granules.

OMEPRAZOLE — ORAL

For complete and comparative prescribing information, refer to the Proton Pump Inhibitors class monograph.

Indications

➤*Duodenal ulcer (Rx only):* For short-term treatment of active duodenal ulcer in adults. Most patients heal within 4 weeks. Some patients may require an additional 4 weeks of therapy.

➤*Duodenal ulcer associated with Helicobacter pylori (Rx only):* In combination with clarithromycin to eradicate *H. pylori*. In patients with a 1-year history of duodenal ulcers or active duodenal ulcers, use in combination with clarithromycin and amoxicillin to eradicate *H. pylori* in adults. Eradication of *H. pylori* has been shown to reduce the risk of duodenal ulcer recurrence.

➤*Erosive esophagitis (Rx only):* For short-term treatment (4 to 8 weeks) of erosive esophagitis diagnosed by endoscopy in children and adults; to maintain healing of erosive esophagitis in children and adults.

➤*Gastric ulcer (Rx only):* For short-term treatment (4 to 8 weeks) of active benign gastric ulcer in adults.

➤*Gastroesophageal reflux disease (Rx only):* For the treatment of heartburn and other symptoms associated with gastroesophageal reflux disease (GERD) in children and adults.

➤*Heartburn (OTC):* To treat frequent heartburn (occurring 2 or more days a week); not intended for immediate relief. This drug may take 1 to 4 days to reach full effect.

➤*Hypersecretory conditions (Rx only):* For long-term treatment of pathological hypersecretory conditions (eg, Zollinger-Ellison syndrome, multiple endocrine adenomas, systemic mastocytosis) in adults.

OMEPRAZOLE — ORAL

➤*Off-label uses:*

Extended-interval dosing (alternate-day dosing) – [2] = Fair documentation. Data from studies suggest that alternate-day therapy is effective in maintaining ulcer or GERD remission rates during long-term treatment after patients have healed via a shorter course (4 to 8 weeks) of daily therapy. (See Administration and Dosage.)

Laryngitis – [2] = Fair documentation. Based on the available evidence from several noncontrolled trials, it appears that omeprazole may be beneficial in the treatment of GERD-related laryngitis symptoms in patients who have not responded to antireflux measures alone. (See Administration and Dosage.)

Other possible off-label uses – In combination with antibiotics (eg, amoxicillin, clarithromycin) for the eradication of *H. pylori* in children with *H. pylori*–induced gastritis; to improve pancreatic enzyme absorption in patients with cystic fibrosis and intestinal malabsorption.

Administration and Dosage

➤*General dosing considerations:* Administer daily doses more than 80 mg in divided doses.

May open capsules for patients who have difficulty swallowing. (See Administration.)

➤*Adults:*

Duodenal ulcer –

Usual dosage: 20 mg/day.

Duration of therapy: Most patients heal within 4 weeks, although some may require an additional 4 weeks of therapy.

Duodenal ulcer associated with H. pylori –

Triple therapy (omeprazole / clarithromycin / amoxicillin):

• *Usual dosage* – Omeprazole 20 mg plus clarithromycin 500 mg plus amoxicillin 1,000 mg, each given twice daily.

• *Duration of therapy* – 10 days. If an ulcer is present at the initiation of therapy, continue omeprazole 20 mg once daily for an additional 18 days.

Dual therapy (omeprazole / clarithromycin):

• *Usual dosage* – Omeprazole 40 mg once daily plus clarithromycin 500 mg 3 times daily.

• *Duration of therapy* – 14 days. If an ulcer is present at the initiation of therapy, continue omeprazole 20 mg for an additional 14 days.

Resistance: Among patients who fail to respond to therapy, omeprazole with clarithromycin is more likely to be associated with the development of clarithromycin resistance, as compared with triple therapy. In patients who fail to respond to therapy, perform susceptibility testing. If resistance to clarithromycin is demonstrated or if susceptibility testing is not possible, institute alternative antimicrobial therapy.

Gastric ulcer –

Usual dosage: 40 mg once daily.

Duration of therapy: 4 to 8 weeks.

Gastroesophageal reflux disease –

Gastroesophageal reflux disease without esophageal lesions: 20 mg once daily for up to 4 weeks.

Gastroesophageal reflux disease with erosive esophagitis:

• *Initial dosage* – 20 mg once daily for 4 to 8 weeks.

• *Maintenance dosage* – 20 mg once daily.

• *Duration of therapy* –

Healing of erosive esophagitis: The efficacy of omeprazole used for more than 8 weeks in patients with GERD has not been established. If a patient does not respond to 8 weeks of treatment, an additional 4 weeks of treatment may be given. If there is recurrence of erosive esophagitis or GERD, an additional 4- to 8-week course of omeprazole may be considered.

Maintenance: Controlled studies do not extend beyond 12 months.

Heartburn (nonprescription) –

Maximum dose: 20 mg once daily.

Duration of therapy: 14 days. It may take 1 to 4 days for full effect, although some patients get complete relief within 24 hours. The 14-day course may be repeated every 4 months.

Pathological hypersecretory conditions –

Initial dosage: 60 mg daily.

Maintenance dosage: Individualize dosage and continue for as long as clinically indicated. Dosages of up to 120 mg 3 times per day have been administered. Some patients with Zollinger-Ellison syndrome have been treated continuously for more than 5 years.

Off-label dosing –

Extended-interval dosing (alternate-day dosing): [2] = Fair documentation. 20 to 40 mg every other day.

Laryngitis: [2] = Fair documentation. 20 to 40 mg at bedtime for 6 to 24 weeks or 20 mg twice daily for 4 to 12 weeks.

➤*Children:*

1 to 16 years of age –

Gastroesophageal reflux disease:

• *20 kg or more* – 20 mg once daily.

• *10 to less than 20 kg* – 10 mg once daily.

• *5 to less than 10 kg* – 5 mg once daily.

Erosive esophagitis: On a per kg basis, the doses of omeprazole required to heal erosive esophagitis are greater than those for adults.

See Gastroesophageal reflux disease for dosing.

Off-label dosing –

Neonates:

• *Duodenal ulcer (refractory)* – 0.5 to 1.5 mg/kg once daily for up to 8 weeks.

• *Reflux esophagitis (documented)* – 0.5 to 1.5 mg/kg once daily for up to 8 weeks.

➤*Hepatic function impairment:* Consider dose adjustment for patients with hepatic impairment, particularly when maintenance of healing of erosive esophagitis is indicated.

➤*Race:* Consider dose adjustment in Asian patients, particularly when maintenance of healing of erosive esophagitis is indicated.

➤*Administration:*

Prescription – Omeprazole should be taken on an empty stomach at least 1 hour before a meal. Instruct patients not to crush or chew the capsule but to swallow it whole. Instruct patients not to chew or crush the tablets.

Daily doses of more than 80 mg should be administered in divided doses.

For patients who have difficulty swallowing capsules, instruct them to add 1 tablespoon of applesauce to an empty bowl, open the omeprazole capsule, and empty the pellets onto the applesauce. Advise patients to mix the pellets with the applesauce and swallow immediately with cool water to ensure complete swallowing of the pellets. Advise patients not to heat or chew the applesauce and not to chew or crush the pellets. The pellet/applesauce mixture should not be stored for future use.

Nonprescription – Administer with a glass of water once daily in the morning before eating. Do not chew or crush tablets.

Oral suspension – Empty the contents of a 2.5 mg packet into a container containing 5 mL of water, or empty the contents of a 10 mg packet into a container containing 15 mL of water. Stir. Leave 2 to 3 minutes to thicken. Stir and drink within 30 minutes. If any material remains after drinking, add more water, stir, and drink immediately.

Patients with a nasogastric or gastric tube: Add 5 mL of water to a catheter tipped syringe and then add the contents of a 2.5 mg packet (or 15 mL of water for the 10 mg packet). It is important to only use a catheter tipped syringe when administering omeprazole through a nasogastric tube or gastric tube. Immediately shake the syringe and leave 2 to 3 minutes to thicken. Shake the syringe and inject through the nasogastric or gastric tube, French size 6 or larger, into the stomach within 30 minutes. Refill the syringe with an equal amount of water. Shake and flush any remaining contents from the nasogastric tube into the stomach.

➤*Storage / Stability:*

Capsules – Store capsules between 15° and 30°C (59° and 86°F) in a tightly closed container. Protect from light and moisture.

Tablets – Store tablets between 20° and 25°C (68° and 77°F). Keep product out of high heat and humidity; protect from moisture.

Oral suspension – Store at 25°C (77°F); excursions are permitted between 15° and 30°C (59° and 86°F).

PANTOPRAZOLE

Rx	**Pantoprazole Sodium** (Teva)	**Tablets, delayed-release; oral:** 20 mg	As pantoprazole sodium 22.6 mg. May contain lactose. In 90s.
Rx	**Protonix** (Wyeth-Ayerst)		As pantoprazole sodium 22.6 mg. Mannitol. (P20). Yellow, oval. In 90s.
Rx	**Pantoprazole Sodium** (Teva)	**Tablets, delayed-release; oral:** 40 mg	As pantoprazole sodium 45.1 mg. May contain lactose. In 90s.
Rx	**Protonix** (Wyeth-Ayerst)		As pantoprazole sodium 45.1 mg. Mannitol. (PROTONIX). Yellow, oval. In 90s and UD 100s.
Rx	**Protonix** (Wyeth-Ayerst)	**Granules for suspension, delayed-release; oral:** 40 mg	As pantoprazole sodium 45.1 mg. Pale yellow to dark brown enteric-coated granules. In UD 30s.
Rx	**Protonix I.V.** (Wyeth-Ayerst)	**Injection, lyophilized powder for solution:** 40 mg	As pantoprazole sodium. Edetate disodium. In vials.

PANTOPRAZOLE SODIUM — ORAL

For comparative prescribing information, refer to the Proton Pump Inhibitors group monograph.

Indications

➤*Maintenance of healing of erosive esophagitis:* For maintenance of healing of erosive esophagitis and reduction in relapse rates of daytime and nighttime heartburn symptoms in patients with gastroesophageal reflux disease (GERD). Controlled studies did not extend beyond 12 months.

➤*Pathological hypersecretory conditions, including Zollinger-Ellison syndrome:* For the long-term treatment of pathological hypersecretory conditions, including Zollinger-Ellison syndrome.

PANTOPRAZOLE SODIUM — ORAL

➤*Short-term treatment of erosive esophagitis associated with gastroesophageal reflux disease:* For the short-term treatment (up to 8 weeks) in the healing and symptomatic relief of erosive esophagitis.

➤*Off-label uses:*

Laryngitis – [4] = Insufficient documentation. Initial data on pantoprazole in the treatment of chronic laryngitis appear promising. (See Administration and Dosage.)

Other possible off-label uses –

Prevention of GI bleeding in patients receiving antiplatelets: The American College of Cardiology, the American College of Gastroenterology, and the American Heart Association recommend the use of proton pump inhibitors (PPIs) to reduce the risk of GI bleeding in patients who are at high risk for GI bleeding and are receiving antiplatelet therapy. Patients at high risk for GI bleeding are defined as those with a history of GI bleeding; advanced age; concurrent use of anticoagulants, steroids, or nonsteroidal anti-inflammatory drugs (NSAIDs), including aspirin; and patients with *Helicobacter pylori* infection. However, patients who are not at high risk for bleeding achieve little benefit from concurrent use of a PPI with clopidogrel. If a PPI is needed in a patient at lower risk for GI bleeding, a drug that is not a strong or moderate CYP2C19 inhibitor, such as pantoprazole, should be considered because omeprazole may interfere with the metabolic (CYP2D19) conversion of clopidogrel to its active metabolite.

Administration and Dosage

➤*General dosing considerations:* Administer without regard to meals, but administer with food if GI upset occurs.

May be used concomitantly with antacids.

Instruct the patient to swallow the tablet whole and not to split, chew, or crush the tablet.

Administer the delayed-release oral suspension only in apple juice or applesauce, not in water or other liquids or foods.

➤*Adults:*

Maintenance of healing of erosive esophagitis – 40 mg orally daily.

Pathological hypersecretory conditions, including Zollinger-Ellison syndrome – The dosage of pantoprazole in patients with pathological hypersecretory conditions varies with the individual patient. The recommended starting dosage is 40 mg twice daily. Adjust dosage regimens to individual patient needs and continue for as long as clinically indicated. Dosages of up to 240 mg daily have been administered. Some patients have been treated continuously with pantoprazole for more than 2 years.

Short-term treatment of erosive esophagitis associated with gastroesophageal reflux disease – 40 mg once daily for up to 8 weeks in adults. For patients who have not healed after 8 weeks of treatment, an additional 8-week course of pantoprazole may be considered.

Off-label dosing –

Laryngitis: [4] = Insufficient documentation. Pantoprazole 40 mg was dosed once daily for 6 weeks as monotherapy or twice daily (30 minutes prior to meals) for 4 weeks in combination with cisapride.

➤*Administration:*

Tablets – Patients should swallow whole, with or without food in the stomach. If patients are unable to swallow a 40 mg tablet, two 20 mg tablets may be taken. Coadministration of antacids does not affect the absorption of pantoprazole. Caution patients that pantoprazole tablets should not be split, chewed, or crushed.

Oral suspension – Delayed-release oral suspension should be administered in applesauce or apple juice approximately 30 minutes prior to a meal. Patients should be cautioned that the granules should not be split, chewed, or crushed. The oral suspension should only be administered in apple juice or applesauce, not in water or other liquids or foods.

Oral administration in applesauce: Open the packet. Sprinkle intact granules on 1 teaspoonful of applesauce. Patients should swallow within 10 minutes of preparation.

Oral administration in apple juice: Open the packet. Empty intact granules into a small cup containing 5 mL of apple juice (approximately 1 teaspoonful). Stir for 5 seconds and swallow immediately. To ensure complete delivery of the dose, rinse the container once or twice with apple juice to remove any remaining granules and swallow immediately.

Nasogastric tube administration – For patients who have a nasogastric (NG) tube in place, the delayed-release oral suspension can be administered as follows: separate the plunger from the barrel of a 2 oz (60 mL) catheter tip syringe. Connect the catheter tip of the syringe to a 16 French (or larger) NG tube. Hold the syringe attached to the tubing as high as possible during application steps to prevent any bending of the tubing in order to provide smooth flow of contents under gravity. Empty the contents of the packet into the barrel of the syringe. Add 10 mL of apple juice and gently tap and/or shake the barrel of the syringe to help empty the syringe. Add an additional 10 mL of apple juice and gently tap and/or shake the barrel of the syringe to help rinse the syringe and NG tube. Repeat with at least 2 additional 10 mL aliquots of apple juice. No granules should remain in the syringe. Make sure the NG tube is not clogged to ensure that the patient receives the full dose.

➤*Storage/Stability:* Store between 20° and 25°C (68° to 77°F); excursions are permitted between 15° and 30°C (59° and 86°F).

PANTOPRAZOLE SODIUM — INJECTION

For complete and comparative prescribing information, refer to the Proton Pump Inhibitors group monograph.

Indications

➤*Gastroesophageal reflux disease associated with a history of erosive esophagitis:* For short-term treatment (7 to 10 days) of patients with gastroesophageal reflux disease (GERD) and a history of erosive esophagitis.

➤*Pathological hypersecretion associated with Zollinger-Ellison syndrome:* For the treatment of pathological hypersecretory conditions associated with Zollinger-Ellison syndrome or other neoplastic conditions.

➤*Off-label uses:*

Prevention of GI bleeding in patients receiving antiplatelets – The American College of Cardiology, the American College of Gastroenterology and the American Heart Association recommend the use of proton pump inhibitors (PPIs) to reduce the risk of GI bleeding in patients who are at high risk for GI bleeding and are receiving antiplatelet therapy. Patients at high risk for GI bleeding are defined as those with a history of GI bleeding; advanced age; concurrent use of anticoagulants, steroids, or nonsteroidal anti-inflammatory drugs (NSAIDs), including aspirin; and in those with *Helicobacter pylori* infection. However, patients who are not at high risk for bleeding achieve little benefit from concurrent use of a PPI with clopidogrel. If a PPI is needed in a patient at lower risk for GI bleeding, a drug that is not a strong or moderate CYP2C19 inhibitor, such as pantoprazole, should be considered, since omeprazole may interfere with the metabolic (CYP2C19) conversion of clopidogrel to its active metabolite.

Administration and Dosage

➤*General dosing considerations:* Data on safe and effective dosing for conditions other than those described, such as life-threatening upper GI bleeds, are not available. Pantoprazole 40 mg intravenously (IV) once daily does not raise gastric pH to levels sufficient to contribute to the treatment of such life-threatening conditions.

➤*Adults:*

Gastroesophageal reflux disease associated with a history of erosive esophagitis –

Usual dosage: 40 mg given once daily by IV infusion for 7 to 10 days.

Duration of therapy: Safety and efficacy of pantoprazole IV as a treatment of patients with GERD and a history of erosive esophagitis for more than 10 days have not been demonstrated.

Pathological hypersecretion associated with Zollinger-Ellison syndrome –

Usual dosage: 80 mg IV every 12 hours. The dosage varies with individual patients. The frequency of dosing can be adjusted to individual patient needs based on acid output measurements. In those patients who need a higher dosage, 80 mg every 8 hours is expected to maintain acid output below 10 mEq/h. Daily doses higher than 240 mg or administered for more than 6 days have not been studied.

Conversion: Transition from oral to IV and from IV to oral formulations of gastric acid inhibitors should be performed in such a manner to ensure continuity of effect of suppression of acid secretion. Patients with Zollinger-Ellison syndrome may be vulnerable to serious clinical complications of increased acid production, even after a short period of loss of effective inhibition.

➤*Children:*

Off-label dosing –

Gastroesophageal reflux disease associated with erosive esophagitis:

• *2 to 16 years of age –*

Usual dosage: 0.32 to 1.88 mg/kg/dose IV given up to twice daily, based upon limited pharmacokinetic data.

Maximum dose: 80 mg per dose IV.

➤*Duration of therapy:* Treatment with pantoprazole IV should be discontinued as soon as the patient is able to be treated with pantoprazole tablets.

➤*Preparation for administration:*

Gastroesophageal reflux disease associated with a history of erosive esophagitis –

15-minute infusion: Pantoprazole IV should be reconstituted with 10 mL of sodium chloride 0.9% injection and further diluted (admixed) with 100 mL of dextrose 5% injection, sodium chloride 0.9% injection, or Ringer's lactate injection, to a final concentration of approximately 0.4 mg/mL. The reconstituted solution may be stored for up to 6 hours at room temperature prior to further dilution. The admixed solution may be stored at room temperature and must be used within 24 hours from the time of initial reconstitution. Neither the reconstituted solution nor the admixed solution needs to be protected from light.

2-minute infusion: Pantoprazole IV should be reconstituted with 10 mL of sodium chloride 0.9% injection to a final concentration of approximately 4 mg/mL. The reconstituted solution may be stored for up to 24 hours at room temperature prior to IV infusion and does not need to be protected from light.

Pathological hypersecretion associated with Zollinger-Ellison syndrome –

15-minute infusion: Each vial of pantoprazole IV should be reconstituted with 10 mL of sodium chloride 0.9% injection. The contents of the 2 vials should be combined and further diluted (admixed) with 80 mL of dextrose 5% injection, sodium chloride 0.9% injection, or Ringer's lactate injection, to a total volume of 100 mL, with a final concentration of approximately 0.8 mg/mL. The reconstituted solution may be stored for up to 6 hours at room temperature prior to further dilution. The admixed solution may be stored at room temperature and must be used within 24 hours from the time of initial reconstitution. Neither the reconstituted solution nor the admixed solution needs to be protected from light.

PANTOPRAZOLE SODIUM — INJECTION

2-minute infusion: Pantoprazole IV should be reconstituted with 10 mL of sodium chloride 0.9% injection per vial to a final concentration of approximately 4 mg/mL. The reconstituted solution may be stored for up to 24 hours at room temperature prior to IV infusion and does not need to be protected from light. The total volume from both vials should be administered IV over a period of at least 2 minutes.

➤*Administration:* Parenteral routes of administration other than IV are not recommended.

Pantoprazole injection may be administered IV through a dedicated line or a Y-site. The IV line should be flushed before and after administration of pantoprazole IV with either dextrose 5% injection, sodium chloride 0.9% injection, or Ringer's lactate injection.

15-minute infusion – Pantoprazole IV admixtures should be administered IV over a period of approximately 15 minutes at a rate of approximately 7 mL/min.

2-minute infusion – Pantoprazole IV should be administered IV over a period of at least 2 minutes.

➤*Admixture compatibility:*

Compatibility – When administered through a Y-site, pantoprazole IV is compatible with the following solutions: dextrose 5% injection, sodium chloride 0.9% injection, or Ringer's lactate injection.

Incompatibility – Midazolam has been shown to be incompatible with Y-site administration of pantoprazole IV. Pantoprazole IV may not be compatible with products containing zinc. When pantoprazole IV is administered through a Y-site, immediately stop use if precipitation or discoloration occurs.

➤*Storage/Stability:* Store pantoprazole IV vials between 20° and 25°C (68° and 77°F); excursions are permitted between 15° and 30°C (59° and 86°F). Protect from light. The reconstituted product should not be frozen.

The reconstituted solution for the 15-minute infusion may be stored for up to 6 hours at room temperature prior to further dilution. The admixed solution may be stored at room temperature and must be used within 24 hours from the time of initial reconstitution. Neither the reconstituted solution nor the admixed solution need to be protected from light.

The reconstituted solution for the 2-minute infusion may be stored for up to 24 hours at room temperature prior to IV infusion and does not need to be protected from light.

RABEPRAZOLE SODIUM

Rx	**AcipHex** (Eisai)	**Tablets, delayed-release; oral:** 20 mg	Mannitol. (ACIPHEX 20). Lt. yellow. Enteric-coated. In 30s, 90s, and UD 100s.

RABEPRAZOLE SODIUM — ORAL

For complete and comparative prescribing information, refer to the Proton Pump Inhibitors group monograph.

Indications

➤*Healing of duodenal ulcers:* For short-term (4 weeks or less) treatment in the healing and symptomatic relief of duodenal ulcers. Most patients heal within 4 weeks.

➤*Healing of erosive or ulcerative gastroesophageal reflux disease:* For short-term (4 to 8 weeks) treatment in the healing and symptomatic relief of erosive or ulcerative gastroesophageal reflux disease (GERD). For those patients who have not healed after 8 weeks of treatment, an additional 8-week course may be considered.

➤*Helicobacter pylori eradication:* In combination with amoxicillin and clarithromycin as a 3-drug regimen for the treatment of patients with *H. pylori* infection and duodenal ulcer disease (active or history of within the past 5 years) to eradicate *H. pylori*. Eradication of *H. pylori* has been shown to reduce the risk of duodenal ulcer recurrence.

➤*Maintenance of healing of erosive or ulcerative gastroesophageal reflux disease:* For maintaining healing and reduction in relapse rates of heartburn symptoms in patients with erosive or ulcerative GERD. Controlled studies do not extend beyond 12 months.

➤*Treatment of pathological hypersecretory conditions, including Zollinger-Ellison syndrome:* For the long-term treatment of pathological hypersecretory conditions, including Zollinger-Ellison syndrome.

➤*Treatment of symptomatic gastroesophageal reflux disease:* For the treatment of daytimeand nighttime heartburn and other symptoms associated with GERD in adults and adolescents 12 years of age and older.

➤*Off-label uses:*

Prevention of GI bleeding in patients receiving antiplatelets – The American College of Cardiology, the American College of Gastroenterology, and the American Heart Association recommend the use of proton pump inhibitors (PPIs) to reduce the risk of GI bleeding in patients who are at high risk for GI bleeding and are receiving antiplatelet therapy. Patients at high risk for GI bleeding are defined as those with a history of GI bleeding; with advanced age; concurrently using anticoagulants, steroids, or nonsteroidal anti-inflammatory drugs (NSAIDs), including aspirin; and with *Helicobactor pylori* infection. However, patients who are not a high risk for bleeding achieve little benefit from concurrent use of a PPI with clopidogrel.

If a PPI is needed in a patient at lower risk for GI bleeding, consider a drug that is not a strong or moderate CYP3C19 inhibitor, such as pantoprazole, because omeprazole may interfere with the metabolic (CYP2C19) conversion of clopidogrel to its active metabolite.

Administration and Dosage

➤*Adults:*

Usual dosage – 20 mg/day.

Duodenal ulcer – 20 mg once daily after the morning meal for up to 4 weeks. Most patients with duodenal ulcer heal within 4 weeks. A few patients may require additional therapy to achieve healing.

Gastroesophageal reflux disease (erosive or ulcerative) –

Initial dosage: 20 mg once daily for 4 to 8 weeks. For patients who have not healed after 8 weeks of treatment, an additional 8-week course may be considered.

Maintenance dosage: 20 mg once daily for maintenance of healing.

Gastroesophageal reflux disease (symptomatic) – 20 mg once daily for 4 weeks. If symptoms do not resolve completely after 4 weeks, an additional course of treatment may be considered.

H. pylori eradication – Rabeprazole 20 mg plus amoxicillin 1,000 mg and clarithromycin 500 mg, each given twice daily (with the morning and evening meals) for 7 days.

Pathological hypersecretory conditions –

Initial dosage: 60 mg once daily.

Maintenance dosage: Adjust to individual patient needs. Some patients may require divided doses. Dosages of up to 100 mg daily and 60 mg twice daily have been administered.

Duration of therapy: Continue for as long as clinically indicated. Some patients with Zollinger-Ellison syndrome have been treated continuously with rabeprazole for up to 1 year.

➤*Children:*

Gastroesophageal reflux disease (symptomatic) –

12 years of age and older: 20 mg once daily for up to 8 weeks.

➤*Administration:* Do not chew, crush, or split tablets; swallow whole. May be taken with or without food.

➤*Storage/Stability:* Store at 25°C (77°F); excursions are permitted between 15° and 30°C (59° and 86°F). Protect from moisture.

DEXLANSOPRAZOLE

Rx	**Dexilant** (Takeda Pharmaceuticals America)	**Capsules, delayed-release; oral:** 30 mg	PEG, sucrose, sugar spheres. (TAP 30). Blue, blue/gray opaque. In 30s, 90s, 1,000s, and UD 100s.
		60 mg	PEG, sucrose, sugar spheres. (TAP 60). Blue, opaque. In 30s, 90s, 1,000s, and UD 100s.

DEXLANSOPRAZOLE — ORAL

For complete and comparative prescribing information, refer to the Proton Pump Inhibitors class monograph.

Indications

➤*Gastroesophageal disease:*

Healing of erosive esophagitis – Healing of all grades of erosive esophagitis for up to 8 weeks.

Maintenance of healed erosive esophagitis – Maintain healing of erosive esophagitis for up to 6 months.

Symptomatic nonerosive gastroesophageal reflux disease – Treatment of heartburn associated with nonerosive gastroesophageal reflux disease (GERD) for 4 weeks.

Administration and Dosage

➤*Adults:*

Gastroesophageal disease –

Healing of erosive esophagitis:

- *Initial dosage* – 60 mg once daily.
- *Maintenance dosage* – 30 mg once daily.
- *Duration of therapy* – For up to 8 weeks for the healing of erosive esophagitis; controlled studies did not extend beyond 6 months for the maintenance of healed erosive esophagitis.

Symptomatic nonerosive gastroesophageal reflux disease:

- *Usual dosage* – 30 mg once daily.
- *Duration of therapy* – 4 weeks.

DEXLANSOPRAZOLE — ORAL

➤*Hepatic function impairment:* Consider a maximum daily dose of 30 mg for patients with moderate hepatic impairment (Child-Pugh class B).

➤*Administration:* May be taken without regard to food. Some patients may benefit from administering the dose prior to a meal if postmeal symptoms do not resolve under postfed conditions.

Dexlansoprazole should be swallowed whole. Alternatively, dexlansoprazole capsules can be opened and the intact granules sprinkled on 1 tablespoon of applesauce, and swallowed immediately. Granules should not be chewed.

➤*Storage/Stability:* Store at 25°C (77°F); excursions are permitted between 15° and 30°C (59° and 86°F).

PROTON PUMP INHIBITOR COMBINATION

otc	**Zegerid OTC** (Schering-Plough)	**Capsules, immediate-release; oral:** 20 mg omeprazole/1,100 mg sodium bicarbonate	Sodium 303 mg. White and blue. In 14s and 42s.
Rx	**Zegerid** (Santarus)		(Santarus 20). Light blue and white. In 30s.
Rx	**Zegerid** (Santarus)	**Capsules, immediate-release; oral:** 40 mg omeprazole/1,100 mg sodium bicarbonate	(Santarus 40). Dark blue and white. In 30s.
		Powder for suspension; oral: 20 mg omeprazole/1,680 sodium bicarbonate	Sucrose, sucralose, xylitol, xanthan gum. In 30 unit-dose packets.
		40 mg omeprazole/1,680 sodium bicarbonate	Sucrose, sucralose, xylitol, xanthan gum. In 30 unit-dose packets.

OMEPRAZOLE/SODIUM BICARBONATE — ORAL

For complete and comparative prescribing information, refer to the Proton Pump Inhibitors group monograph.

Indications

➤*Benign gastric ulcer:* For short-term treatment (4 to 8 weeks) of active benign gastric ulcer

➤*Duodenal ulcer:* For short-term treatment of active duodenal ulcer. Most patients heal within 4 weeks. Some patients may require an additional 4 weeks of therapy.

➤*Gastroesophageal reflux disease (GERD):*

Symptomatic GERD – For the treatment of heartburn and other symptoms associated with GERD.

Erosive esophagitis – For the short-term treatment (4 to 8 weeks) of erosive esophagitis that has been diagnosed by endoscopy.

The efficacy of omeprazole/sodium bicarbonate used for longer than 8 weeks in these patients has not been established. In the rare instance of a patient not responding to 8 weeks of treatment, it may be helpful to give up to an additional 4 weeks of treatment. If there is recurrence of erosive esophagitis or GERD symptoms (eg, heartburn), additional 4 to 8 week courses of omeprazole may be considered.

➤*Maintenance of healing of erosive esophagitis:* To maintain healing of erosive esophagitis. Controlled studies do not extend beyond 12 months.

➤*Reduction of risk of upper GI bleeding in critically ill patients:* Omeprazole/sodium bicarbonate 40 mg/1,680 mg powder for oral suspension is indicated for the reduction of risk of upper GI bleeding in critically ill patients.

Administration and Dosage

➤*General dosing considerations:* Because the 20 and 40 mg oral suspension packets contain the same amount of sodium bicarbonate (1,680 mg), 2 packets of 20 mg are not equivalent to one 40 mg packet of omeprazole/sodium bicarbonate; therefore, two 20 mg packets should not be substituted for one 40 mg packet.

Because the 20 and 40 mg capsules contain the same amount of sodium bicarbonate (1,100 mg), 2 capsules of 20 mg are not equivalent to one 40 mg capsule of omeprazole/sodium bicarbonate; therefore, two 20 mg capsules should not be substituted for one 40 mg capsule.

➤*Adults:* The following dosages are provided as mg of omeprazole.

Active duodenal ulcer – 20 mg once daily for 4 weeks. Most patients heal within 4 weeks. Some patients may require an additional 4 weeks of therapy.

Benign gastric ulcer – 40 mg once daily for 4 to 8 weeks.

Erosive esophagitis –

Initial dosage: 20 mg once daily for 4 to 8 weeks.

Maintenance dosage: 20 mg once daily.

GERD (with no esophageal erosions) – 20 mg once daily for up to 4 weeks.

Reduction of risk of upper GI bleeding in critically ill patients (40 mg oral suspension only) – 40 mg initially followed by 40 mg 6 to 8 hours later and 40 mg daily thereafter for 14 days.

➤*Preparation for administration:*

Suspension – Empty packet contents into a small cup containing 1 to 2 tablespoons of water. Do not use other liquids or foods. Stir well. If omeprazole/sodium bicarbonate is to be administered through a NG/OG tube, the suspension should be constituted with approximately 20 mL of water. Do not use other liquids or foods. Stir well.

➤*Administration:* Omeprazole/sodium bicarbonate should be taken on an empty stomach at least 1 hour before a meal.

Capsules – Capsules should be swallowed intact with water. Do not use other liquids. Do not open capsule and sprinkle contents onto food.

Suspension –

Oral: Drink immediately after mixed. Refill cup with water and drink.

NG/OG tube feeding: Administer immediately after mixed. An appropriately-sized syringe should be used to instill the suspension in the tube. The suspension should be washed through the tube with 20 mL of water.

For patients receiving continuous nasogastric/orogastric (NG/OG) tube feeding, enteral feeding should be suspended approximately 3 hours before and 1 hour after administration of omeprazole/sodium bicarbonate.

➤*Storage/Stability:* Store at 25°C (77°F); excursions are permitted to 15° to 30°C (59° to 86°F).

SUCRALFATE

SUCRALFATE

Rx	**Sucralfate** (Various, eg, Eon Labs, Major, Martec, Teva)	**Tablets:** 1 g	In 100s and 500s.
Rx	**Carafate** (Axcan Scandipharm)		(Carafate 1712). Light pink, oblong, scored. In 100s, 120s, and 500s.
Rx	**Sucralfate** (Precision Dose)	**Suspension:** 1 g/10 mL	Methylparaben, sorbitol. In 10 mL unit dose cups.
Rx	**Carafate** (Axcan Scandipharm)		Sorbitol, methylparaben. In 415 mL.

SUCRALFATE — ORAL

Indications

➤*Active duodenal ulcer:* Short-term treatment (up to 8 weeks) of active duodenal ulcer.

➤*Maintenance therapy for duodenal ulcer:* For duodenal ulcer patients at reduced dosage after healing of acute ulcers.

➤*Off-label uses:*

Prevention of mucositis (oral) – [5] = Poor documentation. Current guidelines recommend against the use of oral sucralfate for the prevention of mucositis in patients receiving radiation therapy. Sucralfate does not prevent acute diarrhea in patients receiving pelvic radiation and is associated with increased GI adverse effects, including acute bleeding.

Prevention of mucositis (rectal) – [5] = Poor documentation. Current guidelines recommend against the use of sucralfate for the prevention of GI mucositis in patients receiving radiation therapy. Rectal sucralfate does not prevent acute or late diarrhea, and the risk of bleeding is unknown at this time.

Other possible off-label uses – Sucralfate has been used in the following conditions: Accelerating healing of gastric ulcers; long-term treatment of gastric ulcers; treatment of reflux and peptic esophagitis; treatment of NSAID- and aspirin-induced GI symptoms and mucosal damage; prevention of stress ulcers and GI bleeding in critically ill patients. Because increased gastric pH may be implicated in causing nosocomial infections in critically ill patients, sucralfate may offer an advantage over antacids and histamine H_2 antagonists in stress ulcer prophylaxis.

SUCRALFATE — ORAL

Sucralfate in suspension has also been used in treatment of oral and esophageal ulcers due to radiation, chemotherapy and sclerotherapy.

Administration and Dosage

➤*Adults:*

Active duodenal ulcer –

Usual dosage: 1 g (10 mL of the oral suspension) 4 times a day on an empty stomach.

Maintenance dosage: 1 g twice a day.

Duration of therapy: While healing with sucralfate may occur during the first week or two, treatment should be continued for 4 to 8 weeks unless healing has been demonstrated by x-ray or endoscopic examination.

Concomitant therapy: Antacids may be prescribed as needed for relief of pain, but should not be taken within one-half hour before or after sucralfate.

Maintenance therapy for duodenal ulcer – 1 g twice a day.

Off-label dosing –

➤*Elderly:* No dosage adjustment is required.

➤*Renal function impairment:* Sucralfate should be used with caution in patients with chronic renal failure. See Warnings/Precautions.

➤*Hepatic function impairment:* No dosage adjustment is required.

➤*Administration:* Take on an empty stomach. Shake the oral suspension well before using.

➤*Storage/Stability:*

Oral suspension – Store at 20° to 25°C (68° to 77°F).

Tablets – Store at 20° to 25°C (68° to 77°F). Dispense in a tight, light-resistant container.

Actions

➤*Pharmacokinetics:* Sucralfate is only minimally absorbed from the gastrointestinal tract. The small amounts of the sulfated disaccharide that are absorbed are excreted primarily in the urine.

Although the mechanism of sucralfate's ability to accelerate healing of duodenal ulcers remains to be fully defined, it is known that it exerts its effect through a local, rather than systemic, action. The following observations also appear pertinent:

1.) Studies in human subjects and with animal models of ulcer disease have shown that sucralfate forms an ulcer-adherent complex with proteinaceous exudate at the ulcer site.
2.) In vitro, a sucralfate-albumin film provides a barrier to diffusion of hydrogen ions.
3.) In human subjects, sucralfate given in doses recommended for ulcer therapy inhibits pepsin activity in gastric juice by 32%.
4.) In vitro, sucralfate absorbs bile salts.

These observations suggest that sucralfate's antiulcer activity is the result of formation of an ulcer-adherent complex that covers the ulcer site and protects it against further attack by acid, pepsin, and bile salts. There are approximately 14 to 16 mEq of acid-neutralizing capacity per 1 g dose of sucralfate.

Contraindications

There are no known contraindications to the use of sucralfate.

Warnings/Precautions

➤*Ulcer recurrence:* Duodenal ulcer is a chronic, recurrent disease. While short-term treatment with sucralfate can result in complete healing of the ulcer, a successful course of treatment with sucralfate should not be expected to alter the posthealing frequency or severity of duodenal ulceration.

➤*Renal function impairment:* When sucralfate is administered orally, small amounts of aluminum are absorbed from the gastrointestinal tract. Concomitant use of sucralfate with other products that contain aluminum, such as aluminum-containing antacids, may increase the total body burden of aluminum. Patients with normal renal function receiving the recommended doses of sucralfate and aluminum-containing products adequately excrete aluminum in the urine. Patients with chronic renal failure or those receiving dialysis have impaired excretion of absorbed aluminum. In addition, aluminum does not cross dialysis membranes because it is bound to albumin and transferrin plasma proteins. Aluminum accumulation and toxicity (aluminum osteodystrophy, osteomalacia, encephalopathy) have been described in patients with renal impairment. Sucralfate should be used with caution in patients with chronic renal failure.

➤*Pregnancy: Category B.*

There are no adequate and well-controlled studies in pregnant women. Because animal reproduction studies are not always predictive of human response, this drug should be used during pregnancy only if clearly needed.

➤*Lactation:* It is not known whether this drug is excreted in human milk. Because many drugs are excreted in human milk, caution should be exercised when sucralfate is administered to a nursing woman.

➤*Children:* Safety and effectiveness in pediatric patients have not been established.

Drug Interactions

Sucralfate Drug Interactions

Precipitant drug	Object drug[a]		Description
Sucralfate	Antacids, aluminum-containing	⬆	The total body burden of aluminum may be increased with sucralfate coadministration. See Warnings.
Sucralfate	Anticoagulants	⬇	A decrease in the hypoprothrombinemic effect of warfarin may occur.
Sucralfate	Diclofenac	⬇	The pharmacologic effects of diclofenac may be decreased.
Sucralfate	Digoxin	⬇	Serum digoxin levels may be reduced, decreasing the therapeutic effects.
Sucralfate	Histamine H_2 antagonists Cimetidine Ranitidine	⬇	Bioavailability of the histamine H_2 antagonists may be decreased. Administering the histamine H_2 antagonist ≥ 2 hours before sucralfate may eliminate the interaction.
Sucralfate	Hydantoins	⬇	Phenytoin absorption may be decreased.
Sucralfate	Ketoconazole	⬇	Ketoconazole bioavailability may be decreased.
Sucralfate	Levothyroxine	⬇	The effects of levothyroxine may be decreased.
Sucralfate	Penicillamine	⬇	Penicillamine's effectiveness may be lessened or negated.
Sucralfate	Quinidine	⬇	Serum quinidine levels may be reduced, decreasing the therapeutic effects.
Sucralfate	Quinolones	⬇	Bioavailability of the quinolones may be decreased. Administering the quinolone ≥ 2 hours before sucralfate may eliminate the interaction.
Sucralfate	Tetracycline	⬇	Tetracycline bioavailability may be decreased.
Sucralfate	Theophylline	⬇	Theophylline bioavailability may be decreased.

[a] ⬆ = object drug increased; ⬇ = object drug decreased.

Adverse Reactions

Constipation was the most frequent complaint (2%). Other adverse effects reported in less than 0.5% of the patients are listed below by body system:

➤*CNS:* Dizziness, insomnia, sleepiness, vertigo.

➤*Dermatologic:* Pruritus, rash.

➤*GI:* Diarrhea, nausea, vomiting, gastric discomfort, indigestion, flatulence, dry mouth.

➤*Miscellaneous:* Back pain, headache.

➤*Postmarketing experience with sucralfate:* Postmarketing reports of hypersensitivity reactions, including urticaria (hives), angioedema, respiratory difficulty, rhinitis, laryngospasm, and facial swelling have been reported in patients receiving sucralfate tablets. Similar events were reported with sucralfate suspension. However, a causal relationship has not been established.

Bezoars have been reported in patients treated with sucralfate. The majority of patients had underlying medical conditions that may predispose to bezoar formation (such as delayed gastric emptying) or were receiving concomitant enteral tube feedings.

Inadvertent injection of insoluble sucralfate and its insoluble excipients has led to fatal complications, including pulmonary and cerebral emboli. Sucralfate is not intended for intravenous administration.

Overdosage

➤*Symptoms:* Acute oral toxicity studies in animals, however, using doses up to 12 g/kg body weight, could not find a lethal dose. Sucralfate is only minimally absorbed from the gastrointestinal tract. Risks associated with acute overdosage should, therefore, be minimal. In rare reports describing sucralfate overdose, most patients remained asymptomatic. Those few reports where adverse events were described included symptoms of dyspepsia, abdominal pain, nausea, and vomiting.

➤*Treatment:* Due to limited experience in humans with overdosage of sucralfate, no specific treatment recommendations can be given.

MISOPROSTOL

Rx	**Misoprostol** (Various, eg, Greenstone)	**Tablets:** 100 mcg	(G 5007). White. In unit-of-use 60s and 120s.
Rx	**Cytotec** (Pfizer)		(SEARLE 1451). White. In UD 100s and unit-of-use 60s and 120s.
Rx	**Misoprostol** (Various, eg, Greenstone)	**Tablets:** 200 mcg	(G 5008). White, hexagonal. In unit-of-use 60s and 100s.
Rx	**Cytotec** (Pfizer)		(SEARLE 1461). White, hexagonal. In UD 100s and unit-of-use 60s and 100s.

MISOPROSTOL — ORAL

WARNING

Misoprostol administration to women who are pregnant can cause abortion, premature birth, or birth defects. Uterine rupture has been reported when misoprostol was administered in pregnant women to induce labor or to induce abortion beyond the eighth week of pregnancy (see Warnings, Pregnancy, Labor and delivery). Misoprostol should not be taken by pregnant women to reduce the risk of ulcers induced by nonsteroidal anti-inflammatory drugs (NSAIDs) (see Contraindications, Warnings, and Precautions).

Patients must be advised of the abortifacient property and warned not to give the drug to others.

Misoprostol should not be used for reducing the risk of NSAID-induced ulcer in women of childbearing potential unless the patient is at high risk of complications from gastric ulcers associated with use of the NSAID, or is a high risk of developing gastric ulceration. In such patients, misoprostol may be prescribed if the patient:

- Has had a negative serum pregnancy test within 2 weeks prior to beginning therapy.
- Is capable of complying with effective contraceptive measures.
- Has received both oral and written warnings of the hazards of misoprostol, the risk of possible contraception failure, and the danger to other women of childbearing potential should the drug be taken by mistake.
- Will begin misoprostol only on the second or third day of the next normal menstrual period.

Indications

➤*Prevention of NSAID-induced gastric ulcers:* Misoprostol is indicated for the prevention of NSAID-induced gastric ulcers in patients at high risk of complications from gastric ulcer (eg, the elderly and patients with concomitant debilitating disease) as well as patients at high risk of developing gastric ulceration, such as patients with a history of ulcer. Misoprostol has not been shown to prevent duodenal ulcers in patients taking NSAIDs. Misoprostol should be taken for the duration of NSAID therapy. Misoprostol has been shown to prevent gastric ulcers in controlled studies of 3 months' duration. It had no effect, compared to placebo, on GI pain or discomfort associated with NSAID use.

➤*Off-label uses:*

Constipation (chronic) – [4] = Insufficient documentation. Initial results from 2 small trials suggest that misoprostol has beneficial effects in patients with severe chronic constipation. However, some patients may be unable to tolerate the GI cramping. (See Administration and Dosage.)

Postpartum hemorrhage – [5] = Poor documentation. Rectal misoprostol could have potential advantages in the management of postpartum bleeding. However, current data are insufficient to support the use of rectal misoprostol for postpartum hemorrhage.

Prevention of radiation proctitis – [5] = Poor documentation. Data from a limited number of controlled trials evaluating the use of rectal misoprostol for the prevention of radiation proctitis are conflicting.

Other possible off-label uses –

Cervical ripening and labor induction: Vaginal misoprostol has been proven safe and effective for cervical ripening and labor induction. However, vaginal misoprostol is associated with a higher frequency of excessive uterine contractility and intervention (see Warnings/Precautions).

Pregnancy termination: Misoprostol has been used in combination with mifepristone for pregnancy termination. Patients taking mifepristone must take 400 mcg misoprostol orally 2 days after taking mifepristone unless a complete abortion has already been confirmed before that time.

Administration and Dosage

➤*Adults:*

Prevention of NSAID-induced gastric ulcers –

Usual dosage: 200 mcg 4 times daily with food. If this dose cannot be tolerated, a dose of 100 mcg can be used.

Duration of therapy: Misoprostol should be taken for the duration of NSAID therapy.

Off-label dosing –

Constipation (chronic): [4] = Insufficient documentation.

- *Short-term* – 400 mcg 3 times/day for 1 week.
- *Long-term* – 200 mcg 3 times/day for 2 weeks, then titrated to effect and tolerance to a minimum daily dose of 400 mcg and maximum daily dose of 2,400 mcg.

➤*Renal function impairment:* Adjustment of the dosing schedule in renally impaired patients is not routinely needed, but dosage can be reduced if the 200 mcg dose is not tolerated.

➤*Administration:* Take with meals, and the last dose of the day should be at bedtime.

➤*Storage/Stability:* Store at or below 25°C (77°F), in a dry area.

Actions

➤*Pharmacology:* Misoprostol has both antisecretory (inhibiting gastric acid secretion) and (in animals) mucosal protective properties. NSAIDs inhibit prostaglandin synthesis, and a deficiency of prostaglandins within the gastric mucosa may lead to diminishing bicarbonate and mucus secretion and may contribute to the mucosal damage caused by these agents. Misoprostol can increase bicarbonate and mucus production, but in man this has been shown at doses 200 mcg and above that are also antisecretory. It is therefore not possible to tell whether the ability of misoprostol to prevent gastric ulcer is the result of its antisecretory effect, its mucosal protective effect, or both.

In vitro studies on canine parietal cells using tritiated misoprostol acid as the ligand have led to the identification and characterization of specific prostaglandin receptors. Receptor binding is saturable, reversible, and stereospecific. The sites have a high affinity for misoprostol, for its acid metabolite, and for other E type prostaglandins, but not for F or I prostaglandins and other unrelated compounds, such as histamine or cimetidine. Receptor-site affinity for misoprostol correlates well with an indirect index of antisecretory activity. It is likely that these specific receptors allow misoprostol taken with food to be effective topically, despite the lower serum concentrations attained.

Misoprostol produces a moderate decrease in pepsin concentration during basal conditions, but not during histamine stimulation. It has no significant effect on fasting or postprandial gastrin nor on intrinsic factor output.

Effects on gastric acid secretion – Misoprostol, over the range of 50 to 200 mcg, inhibits basal and nocturnal gastric acid secretion, and acid secretion in response to a variety of stimuli, including meals, histamine, pentagastrin, and coffee. Activity is apparent 30 minutes after oral administration and persists for at least 3 hours. In general, the effects of 50 mcg were modest and shorter-lived, and only the 200 mcg dose had substantial effects on nocturnal secretion or on histamine and meal-stimulated secretion.

Uterine effects – Misoprostol has been shown to produce uterine contractions that may endanger pregnancy (see Warning Box). In studies in women undergoing elective termination of pregnancy during the first trimester, misoprostol caused partial or complete expulsion of the uterine contents in 11% of the subjects and increased uterine bleeding in 41%.

Other pharmacologic effects – Misoprostol does not produce clinically significant effects on serum levels of prolactin, gonadotropins, thyroid-stimulating hormone, growth hormone, thyroxine, cortisol, gastrointestinal hormones (somatostatin, gastrin, vasoactive intestinal polypeptide, and motilin), creatinine, or uric acid. Gastric emptying, immunologic competence, platelet aggregation, pulmonary function, or the cardiovascular system are not modified by recommended doses of misoprostol.

➤*Pharmacokinetics:*

Absorption – Misoprostol is extensively absorbed, and undergoes rapid de-esterification to its free acid, which is responsible for its clinical activity and, unlike the parent compound, is detectable in plasma. The alpha side chain undergoes beta oxidation and the beta side chain undergoes omega oxidation followed by reduction of the ketone to give prostaglandin F analogs.

In healthy volunteers, misoprostol is rapidly absorbed after oral administration with a t_{max} of misoprostol acid of 12 ± 3 minutes and a terminal half-life of 20 to 40 minutes.

Distribution – There is high variability of plasma levels of misoprostol acid between and within studies but mean values after single doses show a linear relationship with dose over the range of 200 to 400 mcg. No accumulation of misoprostol acid was noted in multiple dose studies; plasma steady state was achieved within 2 days.

The serum protein binding of misoprostol acid is less than 90% and is concentration-independent in the therapeutic range.

Metabolism – Maximum plasma concentrations of misoprostol acid are diminished when the dose is taken with food, and total availability of misoprostol acid is reduced by use of concomitant antacid. Clinical trials were conducted with concomitant antacid, however, so this effect does not appear to be clinically important.

Misoprostol Pharmacokinetics

Mean ± SD	C_{max} (pg/mL)	$AUC_{(0-4)}$ (pg•hr/mL)	t_{max} (min)
Fasting	811 ± 317	417 ± 135	14 ± 8
With antacid	689 ± 315	349 ± 108[a]	20 ± 14
With high-fat breakfast	303 ± 176[a]	373 ± 111	64 ± 79[a]

[a] Comparisons with fasting results statistically significant, $P < 0.05$.

Excretion – After oral administration of radiolabeled misoprostol, about 80% of detected radioactivity appears in urine. Pharmacokinetic studies in patients with varying degrees of renal impairment showed an approximate doubling of $t_{1/2}$, C_{max}, and AUC compared to healthy patients, but no clear

MISOPROSTOL — ORAL

correlation between the degree of impairment and AUC. In subjects over 64 years of age, the AUC for misoprostol acid is increased. No routine dosage adjustment is recommended in older patients or patients with renal impairment, but dosage may need to be reduced if the usual dose is not tolerated.

Misoprostol does not affect the hepatic mixed function oxidase (cytochrome P450) enzyme systems in animals.

Contraindications

See Warning Box. Misoprostol should not be taken by pregnant women to reduce the risk of ulcers induced by NSAIDs.

Misoprostol should not be taken by anyone with a history of allergy to prostaglandins.

Warnings/Precautions

➤*Women of child-bearing potential and pregnant women:* See Warning Box.

➤*Pregnancy: Category X.*

Fertility impairment – There is a possibility of a general adverse effect on fertility in males and females.

Teratogenic – See Warning Box. Congenital anomalies sometimes associated with fetal death have been reported subsequent to the unsuccessful use of misoprostol as an abortifacient but the drug's teratogenic mechanism has not been demonstrated. Several reports in the literature associate the use of misoprostol during the first trimester of pregnancy with skull defects, cranial nerve palsies, facial malformations, and limb defects.

Misoprostol in not fetotoxic or teratogenic in rats and rabbits at doses 625 and 63 times the human dose, respectively.

Nonteratogenic – See Warning Box. Misoprostol may endanger pregnancy (may cause abortion) and thereby cause harm to the fetus when administered to a pregnant woman. Misoprostol may produce uterine contractions, uterine bleeding, and expulsion of the products of conception. Abortions caused by misoprostol may be incomplete. If a woman is or becomes pregnant while taking this drug to reduce the risk of NSAID-induced ulcers, the drug should be discontinued and the patient apprised of the potential hazard to the fetus.

Labor and delivery – Misoprostol can induce or augment uterine contractions. Vaginal administration of misoprostol, outside of its approved indication, has been used as a cervical ripening agent, for the induction of labor and for treatment of serious postpartum hemorrhage in the presence of uterine atony. A major adverse effect of the obstetrical use of misoprostol is hyperstimulation of the uterus that may progress to uterine tetany with marked impairment of uteroplacental blood flow, uterine rupture (requiring surgical repair, hysterectomy, or salpingo-oophorectomy), or amniotic fluid embolism. Pelvic pain, retained placenta, severe genital bleeding, shock, fetal bradycardia, and fetal and maternal death have been reported.

There may be an increased risk of uterine tachysystole, uterine rupture, meconium passage, meconium staining of amniotic fluid, and Cesarean delivery due to uterine hyperstimulation with the use of higher doses of misoprostol; including the manufactured 100 mcg tablet. The risk of uterine rupture increases with advancing gestational ages and with prior uterine surgery, including Cesarean delivery. Grand multiparity also appears to be a risk factor for uterine rupture.

The effect of misoprostol on the later growth, development, and functional maturation of the child when misoprostol is used for cervical ripening or induction of labor have not been established. Information on misoprostol's effect on the need for forceps delivery or other intervention is unknown.

➤*Lactation:* It is unlikely that misoprostol is excreted in human milk since it is rapidly metabolized throughout the body. However, it is not known if the active metabolite (misoprostol acid) is excreted in human milk. Therefore, misoprostol should not be administered to nursing mothers because the potential excretion of misoprostol acid could cause significant diarrhea in nursing infants.

➤*Children:* Safety and effectiveness of misoprostol in pediatric patients have not been established.

➤*Elderly:* There were no significant differences in the safety profile of misoprostol in approximately 500 ulcer patients who were 65 years of age or older compared with younger patients.

Drug Interactions

Misoprostol has not been shown to interfere with the beneficial effects of aspirin on signs and symptoms of rheumatoid arthritis. Misoprostol does not exert clinically significant effects on the absorption, blood levels, and antiplatelet effects of therapeutic doses of aspirin. Misoprostol has no clinically significant effect on the kinetics of diclofenac or ibuprofen.

Adverse Reactions

The following have been reported as adverse reactions in subjects receiving misoprostol:

➤*GI:* In subjects receiving misoprostol 400 or 800 mcg daily in clinical trials, the most frequent gastrointestinal adverse reactions were diarrhea and abdominal pain. The incidence of diarrhea at 800 mcg in controlled trials in patients on NSAIDs ranged from 14% to 40% and in all studies (over 5,000 patients) averaged 13%. Abdominal pain occurred in 13% to 20% of patients in NSAID trials and about 7% in all studies, but there was no consistent difference from placebo.

Diarrhea was dose-related and usually developed early in the course of therapy (after 13 days), usually was self-limiting (often resolving after 8 days), but sometimes required discontinuation of misoprostol (2% of the patients). Rare instances of profound diarrhea leading to severe dehydration have been reported. Patients with an underlying condition such as inflammatory bowel disease, or those in whom dehydration, were it to occur, would be dangerous, should be monitored carefully if misoprostol is prescribed. The incidence of diarrhea can be minimized by administering after meals and at bedtime, and by avoiding coadministration of misoprostol with magnesium-containing antacids.

➤*GU:* Women who received misoprostol during clinical trials reported the following gynecological disorders: Spotting (0.7%), cramps (0.6%), hypermenorrhea (0.5%), menstrual disorder (0.3%) and dysmenorrhea (0.1%). Postmenopausal vaginal bleeding may be related to misoprostol administration. If it occurs, diagnostic workup should be undertaken to rule out gynecological pathology. There have been reports in which intravaginal administration of misoprostol in pregnant women resulted in rupture of the uterus and death of the infant (see Warning Box).

➤*Additional adverse reactions (incidence greater than 1%):*

Miscellaneous – In clinical trials, the following adverse reactions were reported by more than 1% of the subjects receiving misoprostol and may be causally related to the drug: Nausea (3.2%), flatulence (2.9%), headache (2.4%), dyspepsia (2%), vomiting (1.3%), and constipation (1.1%). However, there were no significant differences between the incidences of these events for misoprostol and placebo.

➤*Adverse reactions (infrequent):* The following adverse reactions were infrequently reported. Causal relationships between misoprostol and these reactions have not been established but cannot be excluded:

Cardiovascular – Chest pain, edema, diaphoresis, hypotension, hypertension, arrhythmia, phlebitis, increased cardiac enzymes, and syncope.

CNS – Anxiety, change in appetite, depression, drowsiness, dizziness, thirst, impotence, loss of libido, sweating increase, neuropathy, neurosis, and confusion.

Dermatologic – Dermatitis, alopecia, and pallor.

GI – GI bleeding, GI inflammation/infection, rectal disorder, abnormal hepatobiliary function, gingivitis, reflux, dysphagia, and amylase increase.

GU – Polyuria, dysuria, hematuria, and urinary tract infection.

Hypersensitivity – Anaphylaxis.

Metabolic – Glycosuria, gout, increased nitrogen, and increased alkaline phosphatase.

Respiratory – Upper respiratory tract infection, bronchitis, bronchospasm, dyspnea, pneumonia, and epistaxis.

Special senses – Abnormal taste, abnormal vision, conjunctivitis, deafness, tinnitus, and earache.

Miscellaneous – Aches/pains, asthenia, fatigue, fever, rigors, weight changes, and breast pain.

Musculoskeletal – Arthralgia, myalgia, muscle cramps, stiffness, and back pain.

Hematologic – Anemia, abnormal differential, thrombocytopenia, purpura, and ESR increased.

Overdosage

➤*Symptoms:* The toxic dose of misoprostol in humans has not been determined. Cumulative total daily doses of 1600 mcg have been tolerated, with only symptoms of GI discomfort being reported. In animals, the acute toxic effects are diarrhea, gastrointestinal lesions, focal cardiac necrosis, hepatic necrosis, renal tubular necrosis, testicular atrophy, respiratory difficulties, and depression of the CNS. Clinical signs that may indicate an overdose are sedation, tremor, convulsions, dyspnea, abdominal pain, diarrhea, fever, palpitations, hypotension, or bradycardia. Symptoms should be treated with supportive therapy.

➤*Treatment:* It is not known if misoprostol acid is dialyzable. However, because misoprostol is metabolized like a fatty acid, it is unlikely that dialysis would be appropriate treatment for overdosage.

Patient Information

See Warning Box.

Women of childbearing potential using misoprostol to decrease the risk of NSAID-induced ulcers should be told that they must not be pregnant when misoprostol therapy is initiated, and they must use an effective contraception method while taking misoprostol.

Misoprostol is intended for administration along with NSAIDs, including aspirin, to decrease the chance of developing an NSAID-induced gastric ulcer.

Misoprostol should be taken only according to the directions given by a physician.

If the patient has questions about or problems with misoprostol, the physician should be contacted promptly.

The patient should not give misoprostol to anyone else. Misoprostol has been prescribed for the patient's specific condition, may not be the correct treatment for another person, and may be dangerous to the other person if she is or were to become pregnant.

The misoprostol package the patient receives from the pharmacist will include information containing patient information. The patient should read this information before taking misoprostol and each time the prescription is renewed because the information may have been revised.

Keep out of reach of children.

➤*Special note for women:* Misoprostol may cause abortion (sometimes incomplete), premature labor, or birth defects if given to pregnant women.

MISOPROSTOL — ORAL

Misoprostol is available only as a unit-of-use package that includes patient information.

Misoprostol is being prescribed by your doctor to decrease the chance of getting stomach ulcers related to the arthritis/pain medication that you take.

Do not take misoprostol to reduce the risk of NSAID-induced ulcers if you are pregnant (see Warning Box). Misoprostol can cause abortion (sometimes incomplete that could lead to dangerous bleeding and require hospitalization and surgery), premature birth, or birth defects. It is also important to avoid pregnancy while taking this medication and for at least 1 month or through 1 menstrual cycle after you stop taking it. Misoprostol has been reported to cause the uterus to rupture (tear) when given after the eighth week of pregnancy. Rupturing (tearing) of the uterus can result in severe bleeding, hysterectomy, or maternal or fetal death.

If you become pregnant during misoprostol therapy, stop taking misoprostol and contact your physician immediately. Remember than even if you are on a means of birth control it is still possible to become pregnant. Should this occur, stop taking misoprostol and contact your physician immediately.

Misoprostol may cause diarrhea, abdominal cramping, or nausea in some people. In most cases these problems develop during the first few weeks of therapy and stop after about a week. You can minimize possible diarrhea by making sure you take misoprostol with food.

Because these side effects are usually mild to moderate and usually go away in a matter of days, most patients can continue to take misoprostol. If you have prolonged difficulty (more than 8 days), or if you have severe diarrhea, cramping or nausea, call your doctor.

Take misoprostol only according to the directions given by your physician.

Do not give misoprostol to anyone else. It has been prescribed for your specific condition, may not be the correct treatment for another person, and would be dangerous if the other person were pregnant.

The information does not cover all possible side effects of misoprostol. The patient information does not address the side effects of your arthritis/pain medication. See your doctor if you have questions.

ANTACIDS

Indications

➤*Hyperacidity:* Symptomatic relief of upset stomachassociated with hyperacidity (heartburn, gastroesophageal reflux, acid indigestion, and sour stomach); hyperacidity associated with peptic ulcer and gastric hyperacidity.

➤*Aluminum carbonate:* Treatment, control, or management of hyperphosphatemia or for use with a low phosphate diet to prevent formation of phosphate urinary stones.

➤*Calcium carbonate:* Treating calcium deficiency states (ie, postmenopausal/senile osteoporosis). See Calcium monograph in Minerals and Electrolytes, Oral section.

➤*Magnesium oxide:* Treatment of magnesium deficiencies or magnesium depletion from malnutrition, restricted diet, alcoholism, or magnesium-depleting drugs.

➤*Off-label uses:* Antacids with aluminum and magnesium hydroxides or aluminum hydroxide alone effectively prevent significant stress ulcer bleeding. Antacids are also effective in treatment and maintenance of duodenal ulcer and may be effective in treating gastric ulcer. Antacids are also recommended, initially, for gastroesophageal reflux disease.

Aluminum hydroxide has been used to reduce phosphate absorption in hyperphosphatemia in patients with chronic renal failure.

Calcium carbonate may also be used to bind phosphate.

Administration and Dosage

Administration and dosage depends on the condition being treated and the agent being used. See individual products for specific information.

Liquid doseforms are usually preferred because of their rapid action and greater activity; however, tablets may be more acceptable and convenient, particularly when patients are away from home or where the liquid would be inconvenient to carry. Other doseforms are available but do not appear to offer any significant advantage.

Actions

➤*Pharmacology:* Antacids neutralize gastric acidity, resulting in an increase in the pH of the stomach and duodenal bulb. Additionally, by increasing the gastric pH above 4, they inhibit the proteolytic activity of pepsin. Antacids do not "coat" the mucosal lining, but may have a local astringent effect. Antacids also increase the lower esophageal sphincter tone. Aluminum ions inhibit smooth muscle contraction, thus inhibiting gastric emptying. Use aluminum-containing products with caution in patients with gastric outlet obstruction.

A systemic antacid (eg, sodium bicarbonate) is readily absorbed and capable of producing systemic electrolyte disturbances and alkalosis. A nonsystemic antacid forms compounds that are not absorbed to a significant extent and thus does not exert an appreciable systemic effect unless use is chronic, high-dose, or the patient has confounding pathology. However, nonsystemic antacids may alter urinary pH in some patients.

Acid neutralizing capacity (ANC) – ANC is a consideration in selecting an antacid. It varies for commercial antacid preparations and is expressed as mEq/mL. Milliequivalents of ANC is defined by the mEq of HCl required to keep an antacid suspension at pH 3.5 for 10 minutes in vitro. An antacid must neutralize ≥ 5 mEq/dose. Also, any ingredient must contribute ≥ 25% of the total ANC of a given product to be considered an antacid. Antacids with high ANC are usually more effective in vivo. Sodium bicarbonate and calcium carbonate have the greatest neutralizing capacity but are not suitable for chronic therapy because of systemic effects. Suspensions have greater neutralizing capacity than powders or tablets. For maximum effectiveness, chew tablets thoroughly. If ingested in the fasting state, antacids reduce acidity for approximately 20 to 40 minutes because of rapid gastric emptying. If ingested 1 hour after meals, they reduce gastric acidity for at least 3 hours.

Alginic acid – Alginic acid, an ingredient found with sodium bicarbonate in some antacid products, is not an antacid; however, in the presence of saliva, it reacts with sodium bicarbonate to form sodium alginate. Its protective effect is due to its foaming, viscous, and floating properties.

Phosphate binding – Aluminum-containing antacids bind with phosphate ions in the intestine to form insoluble aluminum phosphate, which is excreted in the feces. This is of value in treating hyperphosphatemia of chronic renal failure. Calcium carbonate can also suppress phosphate concentrations. The aluminum salt with useful phosphate binding capacity is aluminum hydroxide.

Warnings/Precautions

➤*Sodium content:* Sodium content of antacids may be significant. Patients with hypertension, CHF, marked renal failure, or those on restricted or low-sodium diets should use a low-sodium preparation. The sodium content of most commercial antacid preparations is found in the product listings.

➤*"Acid rebound":* Antacids may cause dose-related rebound hyperacidity because they may increase gastric secretion or serum gastrin levels. Early data implicated calcium carbonate as the only agent that caused "acid rebound;" however, it is now clear that most antacids may result in this effect. In addition, the effect may not be clinically significant because the "acid rebound" may be compensated for by buffers in the antacid.

➤*Milk-alkali syndrome:* Milk-alkali syndrome, an acute illness with symptoms of headache, nausea, irritability, and weakness, or a chronic illness with alkalosis, hypercalcemia, and possibly, renal impairment, has occurred following the concurrent use of high-dose calcium carbonate and sodium bicarbonate.

➤*Hypophosphatemia:* Prolonged use of aluminum-containing antacids may result in hypophosphatemia in normophosphatemic patients if phosphate intake is not adequate. In its more severe forms, hypophosphatemia can lead to anorexia, malaise, muscle weakness, and osteomalacia.

➤*GI hemorrhage:* Use aluminum hydroxide with care in patients who have recently suffered massive upper GI hemorrhage.

➤*Lipid effects:* In 1 study, administration of an aluminum hydroxide-containing antacid reduced LDL cholesterol by 18.5% after 4 months in hypercholesterolemic patients. Although HDL was also reduced (to a lesser extent), the HDL/LDL ratio increased by 13%. Similar results were noted in a smaller pilot study. In another study, calcium carbonate reduced LDL by 4.4% and increased HDL by 4.1%. Further studies are needed to determine the role of antacids in hypercholesterolemia.

➤*Buffered aspirin solutions:* Caution against use of these antacid/analgesic combinations in chronic pain syndromes. Alkalinization of urine accelerates aspirin excretion, and systemic alkalosis and increased sodium load may occur.

➤*Renal function impairment:* Use magnesium-containing products with caution, particularly when more than 50 mEq magnesium is given daily. Hypermagnesemia and toxicity may occur because of decreased clearance of the magnesium ion. Approximately 5% to 20% of orally administered magnesium salts can be systemically absorbed.

Prolonged use of aluminum-containing antacids in patients with renal failure may result in or worsen dialysis osteomalacia. Elevated tissue aluminum levels contribute to the development of the dialysis encephalopathy and osteomalacia syndromes. Small amounts of aluminum are absorbed from the GI tract and renal excretion of aluminum is impaired in renal failure. Aluminum is not well removed by dialysis because it is bound to albumin and transferrin, which do not cross dialysis membranes. As a result, aluminum is deposited in bone, and dialysis osteomalacia may develop when large amounts of aluminum are ingested orally by patients with impaired renal function.

➤*Pregnancy: Category A* (magnesium). A pregnant woman should consult a physician before using an antacid.

➤*Lactation:* Breast-feeding women should consult a physician before using an antacid.

Drug Interactions

Antacid Drug Interactions

Drug	Antacid[a]				
	Aluminum salts	Calcium salts	Magnesium salts	Sodium bicarbonate	Magnesium-aluminum combinations
Allopurinol	↓				
Amphetamines				↑	
Benzodiazepines	↑		↓	↓	↓
Captopril					↓
Chloroquine	↓		↓		

Antacid Drug Interactions

Drug	Antacid[a] Aluminum salts	Calcium salts	Magnesium salts	Sodium bicarbonate	Magnesium-aluminum combinations
Corticosteroids	↓		↓		↓
Dicumarol			↑		
Diflunisal	↓				
Digoxin	↓		↓		
Ethambutol	↓				
Flecainide				↑	
Fluoroquinolones		↓			↓
Histamine H_2 antagonists	↓		↓		
Hydantoins	↓	↓	↓		
Iron salts	↓	↓	↓	↓	↓
Isoniazid	↓				
Ketoconazole				↓	↓
Levodopa					↑
Lithium				↓	
Methenamine				↓	
Methotrexate				↓	
Nitrofurantoin			↓		
Penicillamine	↓		↓		↓
Phenothiazines	↓		↓		↓
Quinidine		↑	↑	↑	↑
Salicylates		↓		↓	↓
Sodium polystyrene sulfonate					‡[b]
Sulfonylureas			↑	↓	↑
Sympathomimetics				↑	
Tetracyclines	↓	↓	↓	↓	↓
Thyroid hormones	↓				
Ticlopidine	↓		↓		↓
Valproic acid					↑

[a] Pharmacologic effect increased (↑) or decreased (↓) by antacids.
[b] Concomitant use may cause metabolic alkalosis in patients with renal impairment.

Antacids may interfere with drugs by:

1.) Increasing the gastric pH altering disintegration, dissolution, solubility, ionization and gastric emptying time. Absorption of weakly acidic drugs is decreased, possibly resulting in decreased drug effect (eg, digoxin, phenytoin, chlorpromazine, isoniazid). Weakly basic drug absorption is increased possibly resulting in toxicity or adverse reactions (eg, pseudoephedrine, levodopa).
2.) Adsorbing or binding drugs to their surface resulting in decreased bioavailability (eg, tetracycline). Magnesium trisilicate and magnesium hydroxide have the greatest ability to adsorb drugs; calcium carbonate and aluminum hydroxide have an intermediate ability to adsorb drugs.
3.) Increasing urinary pH affecting the rate of drug elimination. The effect is inhibition of the excretion of basic drugs (eg, quinidine, amphetamines) and enhanced excretion of acidic drugs (eg, salicylates). Sodium bicarbonate has the most pronounced effect on urinary pH.

Staggering the administration times of the interacting drug and the antacid by ≥ 2 hours will often help avoid undesirable drug interactions. Refer to individual product monographs for information.

Adverse Reactions

Magnesium-containing antacids – Laxative effect as saline cathartic may cause diarrhea; hypermagnesemia in renal failure patients (see Warnings).

Aluminum-containing antacids – Constipation (may lead to intestinal obstruction); aluminum-intoxication, osteomalacia and hypophosphatemia (see Precautions); accumulation of aluminum in serum, bone and the CNS (aluminum accumulation may be neurotoxic); encephalopathy.

Antacids – Dose-dependent rebound hyperacidity and milk-alkali syndrome (see Warnings).

Patient Information

➤*Chewable tablets:* Thoroughly chew before swallowing. Follow with a glass of water.

➤*Effervescent tablets:* Allow to completely dissolve in water. Allow most of the bubbling to stop before drinking.

➤*Drug interaction precaution:* Antacids may interact with certain prescription drugs. If you are presently taking a prescription drug, do not take an antacid without checking with your physician or pharmacist.

Magnesium-containing products may act as a saline cathartic in larger doses and produce a laxative effect and may cause diarrhea; aluminum and calcium-containing products may cause constipation. Magnesium/aluminum antacid mixtures are used to avoid bowel function changes.

Notify physician if relief is not obtained or if there are any symptoms that suggest bleeding, such as black tarry stools or "coffee ground" vomitus.

Taking too much of these products can cause the stomach to secrete excess stomach acid. Consult your physician or pharmacist about the appropriate dose. Do not use the maximum dosage of antacids for more than 2 weeks, except under the supervision of a physician.

MAGNESIA (Magnesium Hydroxide)

otc	**Phillips' Chewable** (Bayer Consumer)	**Tablets, chewable; oral:** 311 mg	Sucrose. Mint flavor. In 100s and 200s.
otc	**Pedia-Lax** (Fleet)	**Tablets, chewable; oral:** 400 mg	Magnesium 170 mg, maltodextrin, mannitol, sorbitol, sucralose. Watermelon flavor. In 30s.
otc	**Milk of Magnesia** (Various, eg, Geneva, Goldline, UDL)	**Liquid; oral:** 400 mg per 5 mL	In 360 mL, pt and gal, UD 15 and 30 mL.
otc	**Phillips' Milk of Magnesia** (Sterling Health)		Original, mint and cherry flavors. In 120, 360 and 780 mL.
otc sf	**Dulcolax** (Boehringer Ingelheim)		Original and mint flavors. In 355 mL.
otc	**Phillips' Milk of Magnesia** (Sterling Health)	**Liquid, concentrate; oral:** 800 mg per 5 mL	Sorbitol, sugar. Strawberry flavor. In 240 mL.
otc	**Milk of Magnesia** (Roxane)	**Liquid, concentrate; oral:** 1,200 mg per 5 mL	Benzyl alcohol, sorbitol, sugar. Lemon flavor. In 400 mL.

MAGNESIUM HYDROXIDE — ORAL

For complete prescribing information, refer to the Laxatives group monograph.

Indications

➤*Laxative:* For relief of occasional constipation. This product generally produces bowel movement in 30 minutes to 6 hours.

➤*Antacid:* For the temporary relief of heartburn, upset stomach, sour stomach, or acid indigestion.

Administration and Dosage

➤*General dosing considerations:* Magnesium hydroxide should not be used by patients on a magnesium-restricted diet unless directed by a health care provider.

➤*Adults:*

Antacid –

Chewable tablets (Phillips'): Chew 2 to 4 tablets up to 4 times per day.

Laxative –

Chewable tablets (Phillips'): Chew 8 tablets as a single daily dose taken at bedtime or in divided doses.

Milk of magnesia liquid (400 mg per 5 mL): 30 to 60 mL taken as a single daily dose at bedtime or in divided doses.

Milk of magnesia concentrated liquid:

• *800 mg per 5 mL* – 15 to 30 mL taken as a single daily dose at bedtime or in divided doses.

• *1,200 mg per 5 mL* – 10 to 20 mL taken as a single daily dose at bedtime or in divided doses.

Off-label dosing –

Opioid-induced constipation: 30 mL orally every 6 hours as needed. Consider milk of magnesia if senna in combination with docusate is ineffective.

➤*Children:*

Antacid – See Adults for dosing for children 12 years of age and older.

MAGNESIUM HYDROXIDE — ORAL

Laxative – See Adults for dosing for children 12 years of age and older.

Chewable tablets (Phillips'):

- *6 to 11 years of age* – Chew 4 tablets as a single daily dose taken at bedtime or in divided doses.
- *3 to 5 years of age* – Chew 2 tablets as a single daily dose taken at bedtime or in divided doses.

Milk of magnesia liquid (400 mg per 5 mL):

- *6 to 11 years of age* – 15 to 30 mL taken as a single daily dose at bedtime or in divided doses.
- *2 to 5 years of age* – 5 to 15 mL taken as a single daily dose or in 2 to 4 divided doses.
- *Younger than 2 years of age* – 0.5 mL/kg/day as a single daily dose or in 2 to 4 divided doses.

Chewable tablets (Pedia-Lax):

- *6 to 11 years of age* – Chew 3 to 6 tablets as a single dose or in divided doses, maximum 6 tablets/day.
- *2 to 5 years of age* – Chew 1 to 3 tablets as a single dose or in divided doses, maximum 3 tablets/day.
- *Younger than 2 years of age* – Consult a doctor.

Milk of magnesia concentrated liquid:

- *800 mg per 5 mL* –
  - *6 to 11 years of age:* 7.5 to 15 mL taken as a single daily dose at bedtime or in divided doses.
  - *2 to 5 years of age:* 2.5 to 7.5 mL taken as a single daily dose at bedtime or in divided doses.
- *1,200 mg per 5 mL* –
- *6 to 11 years of age* – 5 to 10 mL taken as a single daily dose at bedtime or in divided doses.

➤*Renal function impairment:* Magnesium hydroxide should not be used by patients with kidney disease.

➤*Duration of therapy:*

Antacid – Do not use the maximum dosage for more than 2 weeks.

Laxative – Do not use longer than 1 week.

➤*Administration:* Shake liquids well before using. Take with a full glass (240 mL; 8 ounces) of water.

➤*Storage/Stability:* Keep tightly closed. Store at 20° to 25°C (68° to 77°F). Protect from freezing.

ALUMINUM HYDROXIDE

				Sodium[a] (mg)	ANC[a] (mEq)
otc	**Amphojel** (Wyeth-Ayerst)	**Tablets:** 600 mg	(Wyeth). Saccharin. In 100s.		
otc	**Aluminum Hydroxide Gel** (Various, eg, Goldline, Pharm Assoc,, UDL)	**Suspension:** 320 mg per 5 mL	In 360 and 480 mL, UD 15 and 30 mL.		
otc	**Concentrated Aluminum Hydroxide Gel** (Roxane)	**Suspension:** 450 mg per 5 mL	Peppermint flavor. In 500 mL and UD 30 mL.	1-2	
		675 mg per 5 mL	Creamsicle flavor. In 180 and 500 mL, UD 20 and 30 mL.		
otc	**Concentrated Aluminum Hydroxide Gel** (Various, eg, Pharm Assoc, Roxane)	**Liquid:** 600 mg per 5 mL	In 30, 180 and 480 mL.		
otc	**AlternaGEL** (J & J-Merck)		Parabens, sorbitol. In 150 and 360 mL.		

[a] Acid neutralizing capacity and sodium content per capsule, tablet, or 5 mL.

ALUMINUM HYDROXIDE — ORAL

For complete and comparative prescribing information, refer to the Antacids group monograph.

Indications

➤*Peptic ulcer and gastric hyperacidity:* For uncomplicated peptic ulcer and gastric hyperacidity.

Administration and Dosage

➤*Maximum dose:*

Capsules/Tablets – 9 capsules or tablets per day.

Suspension – 30 mL as needed between meals and at bedtime.

➤*Adults:*

Gastric hyperacidity –

Capsules/Tablets:

- *Usual dosage* – 500 to 1,500 mg 3 to 6 times daily, between meals and at bedtime.

Liquid:

- *Usual dosage* – 5 to 10 mL between meals, at bedtime or as directed by a physician.

Peptic ulcer (uncomplicated) –

Capsules/Tablets:

- *Usual dosage* – 500 to 1,500 mg 3 to 6 times daily, between meals and at bedtime.

Liquid:

- *Usual dosage* – 5 to 10 mL between meals, at bedtime or as directed by a physician.

➤*Duration of therapy:* Do not take for more than 2 weeks, except under the advice and supervision of a physician.

➤*Preparation for administration:* Shake the suspension well.

➤*Storage/Stability:* Store at 20° to 25°C (68° to 77°F).

CALCIUM CARBONATE

For complete prescribing information, refer to the Calcium monograph in the Nutritionals chapter.

MAGNESIUM OXIDE

For prescribing information, refer to the Magnesium Oxide monograph in the Nutritionals chapter.

MAGALDRATE (Aluminum Magnesium Hydroxide Sulfate)

otc	**Magaldrate** (Various, eg, Moore)	**Liquid:** 540 mg per 5 mL	In 355 mL.
otc	**Iosopan** (Goldline)		In 355 mL.

MAGALDRATE — ORAL

For complete and comparative prescribing information, refer to the Antacids group monograph.

Indications

➤*Heartburn/indigestion/upset stomach:* For the relief of heartburn, sour stomach, acid indigestion, and upset stomach associated with these symptoms.

➤*Hyperphosphatemia/hypocalcemia/hypomagnesemia:* It is also indicated for treating hyperphosphatemia, hypocalcemia, and hypomagnesemia.

Administration and Dosage

➤*Adults:*

Antacid –

Usual dosage: 5 to 10 mL between meals and at bedtime.

Hyperphosphatemia, hypocalcemia, hypomagnesemia –

Usual dosage: 5 to 10 mL between meals and at bedtime.

➤*Children:*

Antacid – See Adults for dosing for children 12 years of age and older.

Hyperphosphatemia, hypocalcemia, hypomagnesemia – See Adults for dosing for children 12 years of age and older.

➤*Duration of therapy:* Do not use the maximum dosage for more than 2 weeks.

➤*Administration:* Shake well before use.

➤*Storage/Stability:* Store at room temperature or refrigerate. Protect from freezing. Keep tightly closed.

SODIUM BICARBONATE

For complete prescribing information for oral Sodium Bicarbonate, refer to the Systemic Alkalinizers section of the Nutritionals chapter. For complete prescribing information for injectable Sodium Bicarbonate, refer to the IV nutritionals section.

SODIUM CITRATE

otc	**Citra pH** (ValMed)	**Solution:** 450 mg per 5 mL	As sodium citrate dihydrate. With sodium 105.67 mg per 5 mL, sucrose. Clear In 30 mL.

SODIUM CITRATE DIHYDRATE — ORAL

For complete and comparative prescribing information, refer to the Antacids group monograph.

Indications

➤*Heartburn/indigestion/upset stomach:* Sodium citrate dihydrate is indicated for the quick relief of acid indigestion, sour stomach or heartburn.

Administration and Dosage

➤*Maximum dose:*

Adults – 120 mL/day according to the prescribing information.

➤*General dosing considerations:* This product may have a laxative effect. Sodium citrate should not be used by patients on a sodium-restricted diet unless directed by a health care provider.

➤*Adults:*

Antacid –

Usual dosage: 30 mL/day.

Maximum dose: 120 mL/day.

Duration of therapy: Do not use the maximum dosage of this product for more than 2 weeks.

➤*Administration:* Taste is enhanced if chilled before use.

ANTACID CAPSULES AND TABLETS

Content given in mg per tablet or gelcap. 23 mg sodium = 1 mEq.

	Product & distributor	Aluminum Hydroxide	Magnesium Hydroxide	Calcium Carbonate	Other Content	Sodium (mg)	How supplied
otc	**Rolaids Tablets** (Pfizer Consumer)		110	550	Dextrose, sucrose		Chewable. Peppermint, spearmint, and cherry flavors. In 12s, 36s, 150s, 250s, and 300s.
otc	**Mylanta Antacid Gelcaps** (J&J/Merck)		125	550	Benzyl alcohol, parabens		In 24s, 50s, and 100s.
otc	**Rolaids Extra Strength Tablets** (Pfizer Consumer)		135	675	Dextrose, sucrose		Chewable. Cool strawberry, freshmint, fruit, and tropical punch flavors. In 10s, 30s, and 100s.
otc	**Rolaids Multi-Symptom Tablets** (Pfizer Consumer)		135	675	60 mg simethicone, dextrose, sucrose		Chewable. Cool mint and berry flavors. In 10s, 30s, and 60s.
otc	**Mylanta Ultra Tabs** (J&J/Merck)		300	700	Sugar, sorbitol		Chewable. Cool mint and cherry creme flavors. In 35s and 70s and 3 roll packs.
otc	**Mintox Tablets** (Major)	200	200		Saccharin		Chewable. Mint flavor. In 100s.
otc	**Mintox Tablets** (Major)	300	150		Aspartame, phenylalanine, sorbitol		Chewable. In 24s.
otc *sf*	**Titralac Extra Strength Tablets** (3M Pharm.)			750	Saccharin	0.6	Chewable. Spearmint flavor. In 100s.
otc	**Maalox Advanced Maximum Strength Tablets** (Novartis)			1,000	60 mg simethicone, acesulfame K, dextrose, maltodextrin, mannitol		Chewable. In assorted fruit flavor. In 35s.
otc	**Maalox Max Maximum Strength Tablets** (Novartis)			1,000	60 mg simethicone, 400 mg calcium, dextrose		Chewable. In wild berry, lemon, and assorted fruit flavors. In 35s, 65s, and 90s.
otc	**Mylagen Gelcaps** (Goldline)			311	232 mg magnesium carbonate		In 24s.
otc	**Gas-Ban** (Roberts Med)			300	40 mg simethicone		In UD 8s and 1000s.
otc	**Maalox Plus Antigas Junior** (Novartis Consumer Health			400	24 mg simethicone		Acesulfame K, dextrose, maltodextrin, mannitol. Wild berry flavor. In 24s.
otc	**Gas-X with Maalox Extra Strength Tablets** (Novartis)			500	125 mg simethicone, dextrose		Chewable. Wild berry and orange flavors. In 8s and 24s.
otc *sf*	**Titralac Tablets** (3M Pharm.)			420	Saccharin	0.3	Chewable. Spearmint flavor. In 40s, 100s and 1000s.
otc	**Titralac Plus Tablets** (3M Pharm.)				21 mg simethicone, saccharin	1.1	Chewable. (TITRALAC PLUS). Spearmint flavor. In 100s.
otc	**Rolaids Plus Gas Relief Softchews** (Pfizer)			1177	510 mg calcium, 5 mg magnesium, 80 mg simethicone, corn syrup, maltodextrin, sorbitol, sucrose	2	Chewable. Tropical fruit flavor. In 6s, 12s, and 36s.
otc	**Gaviscon Tablets** (GlaxoSmithKline)	80			Alginic acid, 5 mg magnesium, 14.2 mg magnesium trisilicate, sodium bicarbonate, sucrose	21	Chewable. In 100s.
otc	**Double Strength Gaviscon-2 Tablets** (SK-Beecham)	160			Alginic acid, sodium bicarbonate, 40 mg magnesium trisilicate, sucrose	36.8	Chewable. In 48s.
otc	**Gaviscon Extra Strength Antacid** (GlaxoSmithKline Consumer Healthcare)				105 mg magnesium carbonate, acesulfame K, alginic acid, corn syrup, mannitol, sodium bicarbonate, sucrose, calcium stearate	29.9	Chewable. Cherry flavor. In 30s and 100s.
otc	**Extra Strength Genaton Tablets** (Goldline)				105 mg magnesium carbonate, alginic acid, sodium bicarbonate, sucrose, calcium stearate	29.9	Chewable. In 100s.

ANTACID CAPSULES AND TABLETS

	Product & distributor	Aluminum Hydroxide	Magnesium Hydroxide	Calcium Carbonate	Other Content	Sodium (mg)	How supplied
otc	**Almacone** Tablets (Rugby)	200	200		20 mg simethicone		Chewable. Yellow/white. Peppermint flavor. In 100s and 1000s.
otc	**Trial AG Tablets** (Zee Medical)				25 mg simethicone, sucrose, mannitol		Lemon flavor. In 20s.
otc	**Gelusil Tablets** (Parke-Davis)				25 mg simethicone, sorbitol, sugar	< 5	Chewable. (P-D GELUSIL 034). Peppermint flavor. In 100s.
otc	**Mintox Plus Tablets** (Major)				25 mg simethicone, saccharin, sucrose		Chewable. In 100s.
otc	**Calcium Rich Rolaids Tablets** (Warner-Lambert)		80	412		0.4	Chewable. Original, cherry, spearmint and assorted fruit flavors. In 12s, 36s, 75s and 150s.
otc	**Advanced Formula Di-Gel** Tablets (Schering-Plough)		128	280	20 mg simethicone, sucrose		Chewable. Mint and lemon-orange flavors. In 30s, 60s. and 90s.
otc	**Riopan Plus** Tablets (Whitehall)				480 mg magaldrate, 20 mg simethicone, sorbitol, sucrose		Chewable. Cool mint flavor. In 50s and 100s.
otc	**Riopan Plus Double Strength Tablets** (Whitehall)				1080 mg magaldrate, 20 mg simethicone, saccharin, sorbitol, sucrose		Chewable. Cool mint flavor. In 60s

Refer to the general discussion of these products in the Antacids group monograph.

ANTACID LIQUIDS

Content given in mg per 5 mL. 23 mg sodium = 1 mEq.

	Product & Distributor	Aluminum Hydroxide	Magnesium Hydroxide	Calcium Carbonate	Other Content	Sodium (mg)	How Supplied
otc	**Maalox Advanced Regular Strength Liquid** (Novartis Consumer Health)	200	200		20 mg simethicone, 5 mg potassium, parabens, saccharin, sorbitol		Mint flavor. In 355 mL.
otc	**Maalox Regular Strength Liquid** (Novartis)				20 mg simethicone, parabens, saccharin, sorbitol		In mint and cherry flavors. In 148, 355, and 769 mL.
otc	**Mi-Acid Fast Acting Regular Strength Suspension** (Major Pharmaceuticals)				20 mg simethicone, 85 mg magnesium, benzyl alcohol, parabens, saccharin, sorbitol.	1	In 355 mL.
otc	**Mintox Suspension** (Major Pharmaceuticals)				20 mg simethicone, 85 mg magnesium, benzyl alcohol, parabens, saccharin, sorbitol.	1	Mint creme flavor. In 355 mL.
otc	**Mylanta Regular Strength Liquid** (J&J Merck)				20 mg simethicone, parabens, saccharin, sorbitol		In original, cherry, and mint flavors. In 150 mL (original), 360 mL (all flavors), and 720 mL (original and cherry).
otc	**Alamag Suspension** (Goldline)	225	200		Sorbitol, sucrose, parabens	< 1.25	Mint flavor. In 355 mL.
otc	**Alamag Plus Suspension** (Goldline)				25 mg simethicone, parabens, saccharin, sorbitol		Lemon flavor. In 355 mL.
otc	**RuLox Suspension** (Rugby)				Parabens, saccharin, sorbitol		Mint flavor. In 360 and 769 mL and gal.
otc	**Aludrox Suspension** (Wyeth-Ayerst)	307	103		Simethicone, saccharin, sorbitol, parabens		In 355 mL.
otc	**Maalox Maximum Strength Multi-Symptom Liquid** (Novartis Consumer Health)	400	400		40 mg simethicone, parabens, saccharin, sorbitol		Wild berry flavor. In 769 mL.
otc	**Mi-Acid Maximum Strength Liquid** (Major)				40 mg simethicone, parabens, saccharin, sorbitol	1	Lemon/Mint flavor. In 360 mL.
otc	**Mylanta Extra Strength Liquid** (J&J/Merck)				40 mg simethicone, parabens, saccharin, sorbitol	2	Cherry and mint flavors. In 360 and 480 mL.

ANTACID LIQUIDS

	Product & Distributor	Aluminum Hydroxide	Magnesium Hydroxide	Calcium Carbonate	Other Content	Sodium (mg)	How Supplied
otc	**Maalox Advanced Maximum Strength Liquid** (Novartis Consumer Health)	400	400		40 mg simethicone, 5 mg potassium, parabens, saccharin, sorbitol		Cherry flavor. In 355 mL.
otc	**Extra Strength Mintox Plus Liquid** (Major)	500	450		40 mg simethicone, parabens, saccharin, sorbitol		Lemon Swiss creme flavor. In 355 mL.
otc	**Gaviscon Extra Strength Relief Formula Liquid** (SK-Beecham)	254			237.5 mg magnesium carbonate, parabens, EDTA, saccharin, sorbitol, simethicone, sodium alginate		Cool mint flavor. In 355 mL.
otc	**Alenic Alka Liquid** (Rugby)	31.7			137.3 mg magnesium carbonate, sodium alginate, EDTA, saccharin, sorbitol, parabens	13	Spearmint flavor. In 355 mL.
otc	**Gaviscon Liquid** (SK-Beecham)				119.3 mg magnesium carbonate, sodium alginate, EDTA, saccharin, sorbitol, parabens	13	Cool mint flavor. In 177 and 355 mL.
otc	**Acid Gone Antacid Suspension** (Major Pharmaceuticals)	31.7			119.33 mg magnesium carbonate, benzyl alcohol, edetate disodium, glycerin, saccharin, sodium alginate, sorbitol	13	In 355 mL.
otc	**Marblen Liquid** (Fleming)			520	400 mg magnesium carbonate		Peach/Apricot flavor. In 473 mL.
otc sf	**Titralac Plus Liquid** (3M Personal Health Care)			500	20 mg simethicone, parabens, saccharin, sorbitol	0.15	Mint flavor. In 360 mL.
otc	**Almacone Liquid** (Rugby)	200	200		20 mg simethicone		In 360 mL and gal.
otc	**Di-Gel Liquid** (Schering-Plough)				20 mg simethicone, saccharin, sorbitol, parabens		Mint and lemon-orange flavors. In 180 and 360 mL.
otc	**Mi-Acid Liquid** (Major)				20 mg simethicone, parabens, sorbitol		In 355 and 780 mL.
otc	**Mylagen Liquid** (Goldline)				20 mg simethicone, parabens, sorbitol, sucrose	< 1.25	In 355 mL.
otc	**Mygel Suspension** (Geneva)				20 mg simethicone		In 360 mL.
otc	**Mylanta** (J&J-Merck)				20 mg simethicone, sorbitol, parabens, saccharin (lemon, mint, cherry only)		Original, lemon, mint, and cherry flavors. In 150 (original), 355 (original, cherry, lemon, mint), and 720 (original, cherry) mL.
otc	**Alumina, Magnesia, and Simethicone Suspension** (Roxane)	213	200		20 mg simethicone, parabens, sorbitol		In UD 15 and 30 mL.
otc	**Almacone Double Strength Liquid** (Rugby)	400	400		40 mg simethicone, saccharin, sorbitol		In 360 mL and gal.
otc	**Gas Ban DS Liquid** (Roberts)				40 mg simethicone		In 150 mL.
otc	**Mi-Acid II Liquid** (Major)				40 mg simethicone, parabens, sorbitol		In 355 mL.
otc	**Mintox Maximum Strength Suspension** (Major Pharmaceuticals)				40 mg simethicone, 165 mg magnesium, benzyl alcohol, glycerin, parabens, saccharin, sorbitol	1	Lemon creme flavor. In 355 mL.
otc	**Mygel II Suspension** (Geneva)				40 mg simethicone		In 360 mL.
otc	**Mylagen II Liquid** (Goldline)				40 mg simethicone, parabens, sorbitol, sucrose	< 1.25	In 355 mL.
otc	**Isopan Plus Liquid** (Goldline)	500	450		540 mg magaldrate, 40 mg simethicone		In 355 mL.
otc	**Magaldrate Plus Suspension** (Various, eg, Moore)				540 mg magaldrate, 40 mg simethicone		In 360 mL.
otc	**Mylanta Supreme** (Johnson & Johnson/Merck)		135	400	Saccharin, sorbitol		Mint, lemon, and cherry flavors. In 355 mL.

Refer to the general discussion of these products in the Antacids group monograph.

ANTACIDS

Antacid Combinations

ANTACID POWDERS AND EFFERVESCENT TABLETS

Content given per dose or tablet.

	Product and Distributor	Sodium Bicarbonate (mg)	Other Content	Sodium (mg)	How Supplied
otc	**Bromo Seltzer Effervescent Granules** (Warner-Lambert)	2781	325 mg acetaminophen, 2224 mg citric acid (when dissolved, forms 2848 mg sodium citrate), sugar	761	In 127.5 g.
otc	**E-Z-Gas II Effervescent Granules** (EZ EM)	2210	1,530 mg citric acid, 40 mg simethicone, 2210 mg sodium bicarbonate		Saccharin. Orange flavor. In 4 g packets. In 50s.
otc	**Sparkles Effervescent Granules** (Lafayette)	2000	1500 mg citric acid, simethicone		In UD 50s.
otc	**Alka-Seltzer Gold Effervescent Tablets** (Bayer Consumer)	1050[a]	1,000 mg citric acid, 344 mg potassium bicarbonate	309	Mannitol. In 36s.
otc	**Alka-Seltzer Effervescent Tablets** (Bayer Consumer)	1700	325 mg aspirin, 1000 mg citric acid	504	Aspartame, phenylalanine 9 mg per tablet. Lemon-lime flavor. In 24s.
otc	**Zee-Seltzer Effervescent Tablets** (Zee Medical)	1916	325 mg aspirin, 1000 mg citric acid	524	In 12s.
otc	**Original Alka-Seltzer Effervescent Tablets** (Bayer Consumer)	1916[a]	325 mg aspirin, 1000 mg citric acid	567	In 24s.
otc	**Alka-Seltzer Heartburn Relief** (Bayer)	1940[a]	1000 mg citric acid	575	Acesulfame K, aspartame, phenylalanine 5.6 mg per tablet, mannitol. Lemon lime flavor. In 24s, 36s.
otc	**Extra Strength Alka-Seltzer Effervescent Tablets** (Bayer Consumer)	1985[a]	500 mg aspirin, 1000 mg citric acid	588	In 12s and 24s.

[a] Heat-treated.

Refer to the general discussion of these products in the Antacids group monograph.

Indications

The general uses for these agents are listed below. Refer to the individual product listings for specific indications.

➤*Peptic ulcer:* Adjunctive therapy for peptic ulcer. These agents suppress gastric acid secretion. There is no conclusive evidence they aid in the healing of a peptic ulcer, decrease the rate of recurrence or prevent complications. Anticholinergics are used much less frequently in modern ulcer management.

➤*Other GI conditions:* Functional GI disorders (diarrhea, pylorospasm, hypermotility, neurogenic colon), irritable bowel syndrome (spastic colon, mucous colitis), acute enterocolitis, ulcerative colitis, diverticulitis, mild dysenteries, pancreatitis, splenic flexure syndrome and infant colic.

➤*Biliary tract:* For spastic disorders of the biliary tract. Given in conjunction with a narcotic analgesic.

➤*Urogenital tract:* Uninhibited hypertonic neurogenic bladder.

➤*Bradycardia:* Atropine is used in the suppression of vagally mediated bradycardias.

➤*Preoperative medication:* Atropine, scopolamine, hyoscyamine and glycopyrrolate are used as preanesthetic medication to control bronchial, nasal, pharyngeal, and salivary secretions; and to block cardiac vagal inhibitory reflexes during induction of anesthesia and intubation. Scopolamine is used for preanesthetic sedation and for obstetric amnesia.

➤*Antidotes for poisoning by cholinergic drugs:* Atropine is used for poisoning by organophosphorus insecticides, chemical warfare nerve gases and as an antidote for mushroom poisoning due to muscarine in certain species such as *Amanita muscaria* (see Pralidoxime Chloride monograph).

➤*Miscellaneous uses:* Calming delirium; motion sickness (scopolamine), see Antiemetic/Antivertigo Agents group monograph; parkinsonism, see Antiparkinson Agents group monograph.

➤*Off-label uses:*

Bronchial asthma – Atropine and related agents are effective in some patients with cholinergic-mediated bronchospasm. Use in chronic lung disease is not generally recommended; these agents reduce bronchial secretions resulting in decreased fluidity and thickening of residual secretion.

Glycopyrrolate may be effective in the treatment of bronchial asthma; doses of 1 mg (nebulization) and 1.3 mg (solution) have been used.

Actions

➤*Pharmacology:* Anticholinergics are also known as antimuscarinic drugs. In addition to the Anticholinergics/Antispasmodics discussed below, related drugs include: Anticholinergic Antiparkinson Agents, Cycloplegic Mydriatics and Urinary Anticholinergics. See specific monographs.

GI anticholinergics are used primarily to decrease motility (smooth muscle tone) in GI, biliary and urinary tracts and for antisecretory effects. Antispasmodics, related compounds, decrease GI motility by acting on smooth muscle.

Gastrointestinal Anticholinergic/Antispasmodic Dosage

Drug	Adult Dosage	
	Oral	Parenteral
Anticholinergics Atropine	0.4-0.6 mg	0.4-0.6 mg
Scopolamine		0.32-0.65 mg
L-hyoscyamine	0.125-0.25 mg tid-qid (0.375 to 0.7 mg q 12 h – sustained release)	0.25-0.5 mg q 4 h
L-alkaloids of belladonna	0.25-0.5 mg tid	
Belladonna alkaloids	0.18-0.3 mg tid-qid	
Quaternary Anticholinergics Methscopolamine bromide	2.5 mg ac; 2.5-5 mg hs	
Clidinium bromide	2.5-5 mg tid-qid	
Glycopyrrolate	1-2 mg bid-tid	0.1-0.2 mg tid-qid
Mepenzolate bromide	25-50 mg qid	
Methantheline bromide	50-100 mg q 4-6 h	
Propantheline bromide	7.5-15 mg tid; 30 mg hs	
Tridihexethyl chloride	25-50 mg tid-qid	
Antispasmodics Dicyclomine HCl	20-40 mg qid	20 mg qid

These agents inhibit the muscarinic actions of acetylcholine at postganglionic parasympathetic neuroeffector sites including smooth muscle, secretory glands and CNS sites. Large doses may block nicotinic receptors at the autonomic ganglia and at the neuromuscular junction.

Specific anticholinergic responses are dose-related. Small doses inhibit salivary and bronchial secretions and sweating; moderate doses dilate the pupil, inhibit accommodation and increase heart rate (vagolytic effect); larger doses decrease motility of GI and urinary tracts; very large doses inhibit gastric acid secretion.

➤*Pharmacokinetics:*

Absorption / Distribution –

Belladonna alkaloids: Belladonna alkaloids are rapidly absorbed after oral use. They readily cross blood-brain barrier, and affect the CNS. The major difference between these agents is that atropine at usual therapeutic doses is a stimulant, whereas scopolamine is a CNS depressant. Undesirable peripheral and central effects occur at doses sufficient to control GI motility and gastric acid secretion.

Atropine has a half-life of about 2.5 hours; 94% of a dose is eliminated through the urine in 24 hours.

Quaternary anticholinergics: Synthetic or semisynthetic derivatives structurally related to the belladonna alkaloids, they are poorly and unreliably absorbed orally. Because they do not cross the blood-brain barrier, CNS effects are negligible. They are also less likely to affect the pupil or ciliary muscle of the eye. Duration of action is more prolonged than alkaloids. In addition, they may cause some degree of ganglionic blockade; neuromuscular blockade may occur at toxic doses.

Antispasmodics: The tertiary ammonium compounds have little or no antimuscarinic activity, and therefore, no significant effect on gastric acid secretion. They exhibit a nonspecific direct relaxant effect on smooth muscle.

Contraindications

➤*Hypersensitivity:* Hypersensitivity to anticholinergic drugs; patients hypersensitive to belladonna or to barbiturates may be hypersensitive to **scopolamine**.

➤*Ocular:* Narrow-angle glaucoma; adhesions (synechiae) between the iris and lens.

➤*Cardiovascular:* Tachycardia; unstable cardiovascular status in acute hemorrhage; myocardial ischemia.

➤*GI:* Obstructive disease (eg, achalasia, pyloroduodenal stenosis or pyloric obstruction, cardiospasm); paralytic ileus; intestinal atony of the elderly or debilitated; severe ulcerative colitis; toxic megacolon complicating ulcerative colitis; hepatic disease.

➤*GU:* Obstructive uropathy (eg, bladder neck obstruction due to prostatic hypertrophy); renal disease.

➤*Musculoskeletal:* Myasthenia gravis.

➤*Asthma:* **Atropine** is contraindicated in asthma patients.

➤*Dicyclomine:* Infants younger than 6 months of age (see Warnings).

Warnings/Precautions

➤*Heat prostration:* Heat prostration can occur with anticholinergic drug use (fever and heat stroke due to decreased sweating) in the presence of a high environmental temperature.

➤*Diarrhea:* Diarrhea may be an early symptom of incomplete intestinal obstruction, especially in patients with ileostomy or colostomy. Treatment of diarrhea with these drugs is inappropriate and possibly harmful.

➤*Parkinsonism:* Vomiting, malaise, sweating and salivation may occur in patients with parkinsonism upon sudden withdrawal of large doses of **scopolamine**.

➤*Anticholinergic psychosis:* Anticholinergic psychosis has been reported in sensitive individuals given anticholinergic drugs. CNS signs and symptoms include confusion, disorientation, short-term memory loss, hallucinations, dysarthria, ataxia, coma, euphoria, decreased anxiety, fatigue, insomnia, agitation and mannerisms, and inappropriate affect. These CNS signs and symptoms usually resolve 12 to 24 hours after drug discontinuation.

➤*Gastric ulcer:* Gastric ulcer may produce a delay in gastric emptying time and may complicate therapy (antral stasis).

➤*Use with caution in the following:*

Cardiovascular – Coronary heart disease; CHF; cardiac arrhythmias; tachycardia; hypertension.

GI – Hepatic disease; early evidence of ileus, as in peritonitis; ulcerative colitis (large doses may suppress intestinal motility and precipitate or aggravate toxic megacolon); hiatal hernia associated with reflux esophagitis (anticholinergics may aggravate it).

GU – Renal disease; prostatic hypertrophy. Patients with prostatism can have dysuria and may require catheterization.

Ocular – Glaucoma; light irides. If there is mydriasis and photophobia, wear dark glasses. Use caution in the elderly because of increased incidence of glaucoma.

Pulmonary – Debilitated patients with chronic lung disease; reduction in bronchial secretions can lead to inspissation and formation of bronchial plugs. Use cautiously in patients with asthma or allergies.

Miscellaneous – Autonomic neuropathy; hyperthyroidism.

In pain or severe anxiety, scopolamine is usually given with analgesics or sedatives to avoid behavioral disturbances. Risk of hyperpyrexia is increased in patients with fever. In elderly patients, confusional states are more common.

➤*Tartrazine sensitivity:* Some of these products contain tartrazine (FD&C Yellow No. 5), which may cause allergic-type reactions (including bronchial asthma) in susceptible individuals. Although the incidence of sensitivity is low, it is frequently seen in patients who also have aspirin hypersensitivity. Specific products containing tartrazine are identified in the product listings.

➤*Sulfite sensitivity:* Some of these products contain sulfites that may cause allergic-type reactions (including anaphylactic symptoms and life-threatening or less severe asthmatic episodes) in certain susceptible persons. The overall prevalence of sulfite sensitivity in the general population is unknown and probably low. It is seen more frequently in asthmatic or atopic nonasthmatic persons.

➤*Special risk:* Use cautiously in infants, small children, and people with Down's syndrome, brain damage, or spastic paralysis.

➤*Hazardous tasks:* Patients should use caution while driving or performing other tasks requiring alertness, coordination, or physical dexterity.

➤*Pregnancy:* *Category B* – **glycopyrrolate**; **mepenzolate** per manufacturer's prescribing information). *Category C* – **Hyoscyamine**; **atropine**; **belladonna**; **scopolamine**; **isopropamide**; **propantheline**; **methantheline**; **mepenzolate** per Briggs' *Drugs in Pregnancy and Lactation*. Hyoscyamine crosses the placenta; atropine and scopolamine cross the placenta rapidly after IV use. Effects on the fetus depend on maturity of its parasympathetic nervous system. In neonates, scopolamine may depress respiration and contribute to neonatal hemorrhage due to reduction in vitamin K-dependent clotting factors.

Safety for use during pregnancy has not been established. Use only when clearly needed and when the potential benefits outweigh the potential hazards to the fetus.

Glycopyrrolate has been recommended as the anticholinergic of choice during anesthesia for electroconvulsive therapy in pregnant patients

Labor and delivery – **Scopolamine** does not affect uterine contractions during labor or increase duration of labor. It crosses the placenta but has not been reported to affect the fetus adversely.

➤*Lactation:* **Hyoscyamine** is excreted in breast milk; other anticholinergics (especially **atropine**) may be excreted in milk, causing infant toxicity, and may reduce milk production. Documentation is lacking or conflicting. Generally, do not use in nursing women. The American Academy of Pediatrics classifies atropine and **scopolamine** as compatible with breast-feeding.

➤*Children:* Safety and efficacy are not established. **Hyoscyamine** has been used in infant colic. Safety and efficacy of **glycopyrrolate** in children younger than 12 years of age are not established for peptic ulcer.

There are reports of infants in the first 3 months of life, administered **dicyclomine** syrup, who experienced respiratory distress, seizures, syncope, asphyxia, pulse rate fluctuations, muscular hypotonia, and coma. These symptoms occurred within minutes of ingestion and lasted 20 to 30 minutes; this suggests that they were a consequence of local irritation or aspiration rather than a pharmacologic effect. A few deaths have been reported in infants ≤ 3 months of age. Two of these were associated with excessively high dicyclomine blood levels. Dicyclomine is contraindicated in infants younger than 6 months of age.

➤*Elderly:* Elderly patients may react with excitement, agitation, drowsiness and other untoward manifestations to even small doses of anticholinergic drugs.

Per the Beers list, **dicyclomine**, **hyoscyamine**, **propantheline**, and **belladonna** are highly anticholinergic and have uncertain effectiveness. These drugs should be avoided (especially for long term use). Dicyclomine, hyoscyamine, propantheline, and belladonna are also considered a high risk medication for the elderly according to the Centers of Medicare and Medicaid Services.

Drug Interactions

➤*Amantadine:* Coadministration of anticholinergics may result in an increase in anticholinergic side effects. Consider decreasing the anticholinergic dose.

➤*Atenolol:* The pharmacologic effects may be increased by concurrent anticholinergic administration. **Metoprolol** and **propranolol** were not affected in 2 studies.

➤*Digoxin:* Pharmacologic effects may be increased by anticholinergic coadministration. This may be product specific, (ie, slow-dissolving digoxin tablets interact whereas digoxin capsules and elixir are not affected). However, because USP standards require a minimum dissolution rate, tablets available in the US are not likely to be affected.

➤*Phenothiazines:* The antipsychotic effectiveness may be decreased by anticholinergic coadministration. Anticholinergic side effects may also be increased by concurrent therapy. Adjust the phenothiazine dose as necessary.

➤*Tricyclic antidepressants:* Anticholinergic coadministration may increase anticholinergic side effects (eg, dry mouth, constipation, urinary retention) because of an additive effect. A tricyclic antidepressant with less anticholinergic activity may be beneficial.

Adverse Reactions

➤*Cardiovascular:* Palpitations; bradycardia (following low doses of **atropine**); tachycardia (after higher doses).

➤*CNS:* Headache; flushing; nervousness; drowsiness; weakness; dizziness; confusion; insomnia; fever (especially in children); mental confusion or excitement especially in elderly patients with even small doses. Large doses may produce CNS stimulation (restlessness, tremor). In the presence of pain, **scopolamine** may produce excitement, restlessness, hallucinations, or delirium. Parenteral **dicyclomine** may cause temporary lightheadedness.

➤*Dermatologic:* Severe allergic reactions including anaphylaxis, urticaria, and other dermal manifestations. Local irritation may occur with parenteral **dicyclomine.**

➤*GI:* Xerostomia; altered taste perception; nausea; vomiting; dysphagia; heartburn; constipation; bloated feeling; paralytic ileus.

➤*GU:* Urinary hesitancy and retention; impotence.

➤*Ophthalmic:* Blurred vision; mydriasis; photophobia; cycloplegia; increased intraocular pressure; dilated pupils.

➤*Miscellaneous:* Suppression of lactation; nasal congestion; decreased sweating.

Overdosage

➤*Symptoms:*

GI – Dry mouth; thirst; vomiting; nausea; abdominal distention; difficulty swallowing.

CNS – Theoretically, a curare-like action may occur (ie, neuromuscular blockade leading to muscular weakness and paralysis); CNS stimulation; delirium; drowsiness; restlessness; anxiety; stupor; fever; disorientation; dizziness; headache; seizures; hallucinations; ataxia; convulsions; coma; psychotic behavior; other signs of an acute organic psychosis.

Cardiovascular – Circulatory failure; rapid pulse and respiration; vasodilation; tachycardia with weak pulse; hypertension; hypotension; respiratory depression; palpitations.

GU – Urinary urgency with difficulty in micturition.

Ocular – Blurred vision; photophobia; dilated pupils.

Miscellaneous – Leukocytosis; flushed hot dry skin; rash; respiratory failure.

Children – Children, especially those with Down's syndrome, spastic paralysis, or brain damage, are more sensitive than adults to toxic effects.

➤*Treatment:* Induce emesis or perform gastric lavage, then administer activated charcoal slurry, and supportive and symptomatic therapy, as indicated. See also General Management of Acute Overdosage.

Physostigmine by slow IV injection of 0.2 to 4 mg has been used to reverse anticholinergic effects. Because physostigmine is rapidly metabolized, the patient may relapse into coma after 1 to 2 hours; repeat doses as necessary to a total of 6 mg (2 mg in children). However, profound bradycardia, asystole, and seizures may occur (see Antidotes monograph). The role of physostigmine is not clear; avoid it if other therapeutic agents successfully reverse cardiac dysrhythmias.

Neostigmine methylsulfate 0.25 to 2.5 mg IV, repeated as needed, may be given.

Diazepam, short-acting barbiturates, IV sodium thiopental (2% solution), or chloral hydrate (100 to 200 mL of a 2% solution) by rectal infusion may control excitement. **Hyoscyamine** is dialyzable, but hemodialysis is ineffective for atropine poisoning. Treat hyperpyrexia with physical cooling measures.

If the curare-like effect progresses to paralysis of respiratory muscles, institute artificial respiration and maintain until effective respiratory action returns.

Patient Information

Usually taken 30 to 60 minutes before a meal.

May cause drowsiness, dizziness, or blurred vision; patients should observe caution while driving or performing other tasks requiring alertness.

Notify physician if rash, flushing, or eye pain occurs.

May cause dry mouth, difficulty in urination, constipation or increased sensitivity to light; notify physician if these effects persist or become severe.

HYOSCYAMINE SULFATE

Rx	**Hyoscyamine Sulfate** (Franklin Pharmaceutical)	**Tablets; oral:** 0.125 mg	Lactose, mannitol. (AP 112). Blue, round. In 100s.
Rx	**HyoMax** (Aristos)		Lactose, mannitol. (AP). Green, round. In 100s.
Rx	**Levsin** (Alaven)		(SCHWARZ 531). White, scored. In 100s and 500s.
Rx	**Cystospaz** (PolyMedica)	**Tablets; oral:** 0.15 mg	(W 2225). Blue. In 100s.
Rx	**HyoMax-FT** (Aristos Pharmaceutical[a])	**Tablets, chewable; oral:** 0.125 mg	Lactose, mannitol. (FT). Green. Mint flavor. In 100s.
Rx	**Hyoscyamine Sulfate** (Kremers Urban)	**Tablets, sublingual; oral:** 0.125 mg	(KU 102). White, scored, beveled. Peppermint flavor. In 100s.
Rx	**Levsin/SL** (Alaven)		(Schwarz 532). Blue-green, scored. Octagonal. Peppermint flavor. In 100s and 500s.
Rx	**Symax-SL** (Capellon)		(SL 125). Green. In 100s.
Rx	**Hyoscyamine Sulfate** (River's Edge)	**Tablets, extended-release; oral:** 0.25 mg (0.125 mg immediate-release)	(RE 251). Yellow and white, capsule shape. In 90s.
Rx	**Hyoscyamine Sulfate** (Various, eg, Econolab, Ethex, Global, Goldline)	**Tablets, extended-release; oral:** 0.375 mg	In 100s and 1000s.
Rx	**Levbid** (Alaven)		(AP 115). In 50s and 100s.
Rx	**Symax-SR** (Capellon)	**Tablets, extended- release; oral:** 0.375 mg	(SR 375). Green, scored, capsule shape. In 100s.
Rx	**Symax Duotab** (Capellon)	**Tablets, extended-release; oral:** 0.375 mg (0.125 mg immediate-release, 0.25 mg extended-release)	(SYMAX DUOTAB). Purple/White, capsule-shape, bilayered. In 90s.
Rx	**Hyoscyamine Sulfate** (Vision Pharmaceuticals)	**Tablets, disintegrating; oral:** 0.125 mg	Aspartame, mannitol, 2.2 mg phenylananine per tablet. (VP 3). White. Mint flavor. In 90s and 100s.
Rx	**ED-SPAZ** (Edwards)		Mannitol. (634). White, round, scored. In 100s.
Rx	**Neosol** (Breckenridge)		Mint flavor. White. In 100s.
Rx	**NuLev** (Schwarz Pharma)		Aspartame, mannitol. 1.7 mg phenylalanine. (SP 111). White. Mint flavor. In 100s.
Rx	**Symax FasTab** (Capellon)		Lactose. mannitol. (FT). Green. Peppermint flavor. In 100s.
Rx	**Mar-Spas** (Marnel)	**Tablets, disintegrating; oral:** 0.25 mg	Aspartame, 3.5 mg phenylalanine. (4 4). Spearmint flavor. White, scored, capsule-shape. In 100s.
Rx	**Hyoscyamine Sulfate** (Ethex)	**Capsules, extended release; oral:** 0.375 mg	In 100s.
Rx	**Hyoscyamine Sulfate** (Various, eg, Breckenridge)	**Capsules, timed release; oral:** 0.375 mg	In 100s.
Rx	**Levsinex Timecaps** (Alaven)		(SCHWARZ 537). Brown/clear. In 100s and 500s.
Rx	**Hyoscyamine Sulfate** (Goldline)	**Solution; oral:** 0.125 mg/mL	5% alcohol. In 15 mL w/dropper.
Rx	**IB-Stat** (InKine)	**Spray; oral:** 0.125 mg/mL (0.125 mg/ spray)	5.3% alcohol, liquid sugar, methylparaben, sorbitol. In 30 mL.
Rx	**Levsin** (Alaven)	**Injection:** 0.5 mg/mL	In 1 mL amps and 10 mL[b] vials.

[a] Aristos Pharmaceutical, Cary NC 27518, 1–866–280–5755

[b] With 1.5% benzyl alcohol and 0.1% sodium metabisulfite.

HYOSCYAMINE SULFATE — ORAL

For complete and comparative prescribing information, refer to the Gastrointestinal Anticholinergics/Antispasmodics group monograph.

Indications

➤*GI:* To aid in the control of gastric secretion, visceral spasm, hypermotility in spastic colitis, spastic bladder, pylorospasm, and associated abdominal cramps. To relieve symptoms in functional intestinal disorders (eg, mild dysenteries and diverticulitis), infant colic, and biliary colic. As adjunctive therapy in peptic ulcer; irritable bowel syndrome (irritable colon, spastic colon, mucous colitis, acute enterocolitis, functional GI disorders); neurogenic bowel disturbances including splenic flexure syndrome and neurogenic colon; to reduce pain and hypersecretion in pancreatitis.

➤*Respiratory tract:* As a "drying agent" in the relief of symptoms of acute rhinitis.

➤*CNS:* In parkinsonism to reduce rigidity and tremors and to control associated sialorrhea and hyperhidrosis. May be used for poisoning by anticholinesterase agents.

➤*GU:* Cystitis; renal colic.

➤*Cardiovascular:* Certain cases of partial heart block associated with vagal activity.

Administration and Dosage

➤*Maximum dose:*

Adults – 1.5 mg (1.8 mg for the 0.15 mg tablet) according to the prescribing information.

Children –

12 years of age and over: 1.5 mg (1.8 mg for the 0.15 mg tablet) according to the prescribing information.

2 years of age to younger than 12 years: 0.75 mg according to the prescribing information.

Younger than 2 years of age: 0.0825 mg to 0.16 mg based upon weight according to the prescribing information for the oral solution. There are no well-established maximum doses for the other dose forms according to the prescribing information.

➤*Adults:*

Acute rhinitis, anticholinesterase poisoning, GI disorders, GU disorders (cystitis, renal colic), parkinsonism –

Regular tablets and sublingual tablets:
- *Usual dose* – 1 to 2 tablets every 4 hours or as needed.
- *Maximum dose* – 12 tablets in 24 hours.

Orally disintegrating tablets:
- *Mar-Spas* (only) – ½ to 1 tablet 3 to 4 times a day, 30 minutes to 1 hour before meals and at bedtime.
- *All other disintegrating tablets* –
  Usual dosage: 1 to 2 tablets every 4 hours or as needed.
  Maximum dose: 12 tablets in 24 hours.

Extended-release tablets:
- *Usual dose* – 1 to 2 tablets every 12 hours.
- *Maximum dose* – Do not exceed 4 tablets in 24 hours.

Extended-release and timed-release capsules:
- *Usual dose* – 1 to 2 capsules every 12 hours. Dosage may be adjusted to 1 capsule every 8 hours if needed.
- *Maximum dose* – Do not exceed 4 capsules in 24 hours.

Oral solution:
- *Usual dose* – 1 to 2 mL every 4 hours or as needed.
- *Maximum dose* – Do not exceed 12 mL in 24 hours.

Elixir:
- *Usual dose* – 1 to 2 teaspoonfuls every 4 hours or as needed.
- *Maximum dose* – Do not exceed 12 teaspoonfuls in 24 hours.

Oral spray:
- *Usual dose* – 1 to 2 mL (1 to 2 sprays) every 4 hours or as needed.
- *Maximum dose* – Do not exceed 12 mL (12 sprays) in 24 hours.

HYOSCYAMINE SULFATE — ORAL

➤*Children:*

Acute rhinitis, anticholinesterase poisoning, GI disorders, GU disorders (cystitis, renal colic), parkinsonism –

Regular tablets and sublingual tablets:

- *12 years of age and older* – See Adults for dosing.
- *2 years of age to younger than 12 years of age* –

  Usual dosage: ½ to 1 tablet every 4 hours or as needed.

  Maximum dose: Do not exceed 6 tablets in 24 hours.

Mar-Spas orally disintegrating tablets:

- *12 years of age and older* – See Adults for dosing.

All other disintegrating tablets:

- *12 years of age and older* – See Adults for dosing
- *2 years of age to younger than 12 years of age* –

  Usual dosage: ½ to 1 tablet every 4 hours or as needed.

  Maximum dose: Do not exceed 6 tablets in 24 hours.

Extended-release tablets:

- *12 years of age and older* – See Adults for dosing.

Extended-release and timed-release capsules:

- *12 years of age and older* – See Adults for dosing.

Oral solution:

- *12 years of age and older* – See Adults for dosing.
- *2 years of age to younger than 12 years of age* –

  Usual dosage: 0.25 to 1 mL every 4 hours or as needed.

  Maximum dose: Do not exceed 6 mL in 24 hours.

- *Younger than 2 years of age* – The following dosage guide is based upon body weight. The doses may be repeated every 4 hours or as needed.

Hyoscyamine Oral Solution Pediatric Dosing

Body weight	Usual dose	Do not exceed in 24 hours
3.4 kg (7.5 lb)	4 drops	24 drops
5 kg (11 lb)	5 drops	30 drops
7 kg (15 lb)	6 drops	36 drops
10 kg (22 lb)	8 drops	48 drops

Elixir:

- *12 years of age and older* – See Adults for dosing.
- *2 years of age to younger than 12 years of age* – Please see the following dosage guide based on body weight. The doses may be repeated every 4 hours or as needed. Do not exceed 6 teaspoonfuls in 24 hours.

Hyoscyamine Elixir Pediatric Dosing

Body weight	Usual dose
10 kg (22 lb)	1/4 tsp (1.25 mL)
20 kg (44 lb)	1/2 tsp (2.5 mL)
40 kg (88 lb)	3/4 tsp (3.75 mL)
50 kg (110 lb)	1 tsp (5 mL)

Oral spray:

- *12 years of age and older* – See Adults for dosing.

➤*Administration:*

Extended-release and timed-release capsules – Do not crush or chew capsules.

Extended-release tablets – Tablets are scored and may be broken to allow for dose titration if needed. Do not crush or chew tablets.

Orally disintegrating tablets – Place orally disintegrating tablets on tongue, allowing the tablet to rapidly disintegrate and be swallowed; may be taken with or without water.

Sublingual tablets – Sublingual tablets are formulated for sublingual administration; however, the tablets may be chewed or taken orally.

➤*Storage/Stability:* Store at controlled room temperature 15° to 30°C (59° to 86°F).

Orally disintegrating tablets – Store at 25°C (77°F); excursions permitted to 15° to 30°C (59° to 86°F). Protect from moisture. Dispense in tight, light-resistant container.

Oral spray – Dispense in original container with metered sprayer.

HYOSCYAMINE SULFATE — INJECTION

For complete and comparative prescribing information, refer to the Gastrointestinal Anticholinergics/Antispasmodics group monograph.

Indications

➤*GI:* To aid in the control of gastric secretion, visceral spasm, hypermotility in spastic colitis, spastic bladder, pylorospasm, and associated abdominal cramps. To relieve symptoms in functional intestinal disorders (eg, mild dysenteries and diverticulitis), infant colic, and biliary colic. As adjunctive therapy in peptic ulcer; irritable bowel syndrome (irritable colon, spastic colon, mucous colitis, acute enterocolitis, functional GI disorders); neurogenic bowel disturbances including splenic flexure syndrome and neurogenic colon; to reduce pain and hypersecretion in pancreatitis.

➤*Respiratory tract:* As a "drying agent" in the relief of symptoms of acute rhinitis.

➤*CNS:* In parkinsonism to reduce rigidity and tremors and to control associated sialorrhea and hyperhidrosis. May be used for poisoning by anticholinesterase agents.

➤*GU:* Cystitis; renal colic.

➤*Cardiovascular:* Certain cases of partial heart block associated with vagal activity.

➤*Parenteral:* Reduces duodenal motility to facilitate the diagnostic radiologic procedure, hypotonic duodenography. May also improve radiologic visibility of the kidneys.

➤*Preoperative medication:* Parenteral hyoscyamine is indicated as a preoperative antimuscarinic to reduce salivary, tracheobronchial, and pharyngeal secretions; to reduce volume and acidity of gastric secretions; to block cardiac vagal inhibitory reflexes during induction of anesthesia and intubation. Hyoscyamine protects against peripheral muscarinic effects such as bradycardia and excessive secretions produced by halogenated hydrocarbons and cholinergic agents such as physostigmine, neostigmine, and pyridostigmine given to reverse actions of curariform agents.

Administration and Dosage

➤*Adults:*

Anesthesia –

Preanesthetic medication: 5 mcg (0.005 mg) per kg of body weight given subcutaneously, IV, or IM 30 to 60 minutes prior to the anticipated time of induction of anesthesia or at the time the preanesthetic narcotic or sedatives are administered.

Reduce drug-induced bradycardia during surgery: Administer IV in increments of 0.125 mg (0.25 mL undiluted) and repeat as needed.

Reversal of neuromuscular blockade: 0.2 mg (0.4 mL undiluted) administered subcutaneously, IV, or IM for every 1 mg neostigmine or the equivalent dose of physostigmine or pyridostigmine.

Diagnostic procedures – 0.25 to 0.5 mg (0.5 to 1 mL undiluted) administered IV 5 to 10 minutes prior to the diagnostic procedure.

Gastrointestinal disorders – 0.25 to 0.5 mg (0.5 to 1 mL undiluted) administered subcutaneously, IV, or IM. Some patients may need only a single dose, others may require administration 2, 3, or 4 times a day at 4-hour intervals.

➤*Children:* As a preanesthetic medication, see Adults for dosing for children older than 2 years of age.

➤*Administration:* The dose may be administered subcutaneously, IM, or IV without dilution.

➤*Storage/Stability:* Store at controlled room temperature, 15° to 30°C (59° to 86°F).

ATROPINE SULFATE

Rx	**Sal-Tropine** (Hope)	**Tablets:** 0.4 mg	In 100s.
Rx	**Atropine Sulfate** (Hospira)	**Injection:** 0.05 mg/mL	In 5 mL Abboject syringes.
Rx	**Atropine Sulfate** (Hospira)	**Injection:** 0.1 mg/mL	In 5 and 10 mL Abboject syringes.
Rx	**Atropine Sulfate** (Various, eg, GlaxoWellcome, Loch, Moore, Schein, Vortech)	**Injection:** 0.3 mg/mL	In 1 and 30 mL vials.
		0.4 mg/mL	In 1 mL amps and 1, 20, and 30 mL vials.
		0.5 mg/mL	In 1 and 30 mL vials and 5 mL syringes.
		0.8 mg/mL	In 0.5 and 1 mL amps and 0.5 mL syringes.
		1 mg/mL	In 1 mL amps and vials and 10 mL syringes.
Rx	**AtroPen** (Meridian Medical Technologies)	**Injection:** 0.5 mg	Glycerin, phenol. In pre-filled auto-injectors.
		1 mg	Glycerin, phenol. In pre-filled auto-injectors.
		2 mg	Glycerin, phenol. In pre-filled auto-injectors.

ATROPINE SULFATE — ORAL

For complete and comparative prescribing information, refer to the Gastrointestinal Anticholinergics/Antispasmodics group monograph.

Indications

➤*Salivation / bronchial secretion reduction:* Atropine sulfate is used to reduce salivation and bronchial secretions.

➤*GI tract spasms:* The antispasmodic action of atropine sulfate is useful in pylorospasm and other spastic conditions of the gastrointestinal tract.

➤*Ureteral and biliary colic:* For ureteral and biliary colic, concomitant use of atropine and morphine may be indicated.

Administration and Dosage

➤*Adults:*

Antispasmodic – 0.4 mg. Repeat every 4 to 6 hours as needed. This dose may be exceeded in certain cases.

Reduce salivation and bronchial secretions – 0.4 mg. Repeat every 4 to 6 hours as needed. This dose may be exceeded in certain cases.

➤*Children:*

Reduce salivation and bronchial secretions –

Usual dosage: These doses may be exceeded in certain cases.

- *3.12 to 7.26 kg (7 to 16 lb)* – 0.1 mg.
- *7.71 to 10.89 kg (17 to 24 lb)* – 0.15 mg.
- *10.89 to 18.14 kg (24 to 40 lb)* – 0.2 mg.
- *18.14 to 29.48 kg (40 to 65 lb)* – 0.3 mg.
- *29.48 to 40.82 kg (65 to 90 lb)* – 0.4 mg.
- *Over 40.82 kg (90 lb)* – 0.4 mg.

Antispasmodic –

Usual dosage: These doses may be exceeded in certain cases.

- *3.12 to 7.26 kg (7 to 16 lb)* – 0.1 mg.
- *7.71 to 10.89 kg (17 to 24 lb)* – 0.15 mg.
- *10.89 to 18.14 kg (24 to 40 lb)* – 0.2 mg.
- *18.14 to 29.48 kg (40 to 65 lb)* – 0.3 mg.
- *29.48 to 40.82 kg (65 to 90 lb)* – 0.4 mg.
- *Over 40.82 kg (90 lb)* – 0.4 mg.

➤*Storage / Stability:* Store at 15° to 30°C (59° to 86°F).

ATROPINE SULFATE — INJECTION

For complete and comparative prescribing information, refer to the Gastrointestinal Anticholinergics/Antispasmodics group monograph.

Indications

➤*Respiratory tract:* Antisialagogue for preanesthetic medication to prevent or reduce secretions of the respiratory tract.

To control rhinorrhea of acute rhinitis or hay fever.

➤*CNS conditions:* Treatment of parkinsonism. Rigidity and tremor are relieved by the apparently selective depressant action.

In cases of closed head injuries that cause acetylcholine to be released or to be present in cerebrospinal fluid, which in turn causes abnormal EEG patterns, stupor, and neurological signs.

To control the crying and laughing episodes in patients with brain lesions.

➤*Cardiovascular conditions:* Restore cardiac rate and arterial pressure during anesthesia when vagal stimulation produced by intra-abdominal surgical traction causes a sudden decrease in pulse rate and cardiac action.

Lessen the degree of atrioventricular heart block when increased vagal tone is a major factor in the conduction defect as in some cases due to digitalis.

Overcome severe bradycardia and syncope due to a hyperactive carotid sinus reflex.

➤*Antidote:* Antidote (with external cardiac massage) for cardiovascular collapse from the injudicious use of a choline ester (cholinergic) drug, pilocarpine, physostigmine, or isoflurophate.

➤*GI conditions:* Relieve pylorospasm, hypertonicity of small intestine, and hypermotility of colon; relaxation of the upper GI tract and colon during hypertonic radiography; relax the spasm of biliary and ureteral colic and bronchial spasm; for the management of peptic ulcer.

➤*GU conditions:* Diminish the tone of the detrusor muscle of the urinary bladder in the treatment of urinary tract disorders; relieve hypertonicity of the uterine muscle.

➤*Poisoning:* Treatment of anticholinesterase poisoning from organophosphorus insecticides; as an antidote for mushroom poisoning due to muscarine, in certain species such as *Amanita muscaria*.

For the treatment of poisoning by susceptible organophosphorus nerve agents having cholinesterase activity as well as organophosphorus or carbamate insecticides. Also intended as initial treatment of the muscarinic symptoms of insecticide or nerve agent poisonings (generally breathing difficulties due to increased secretions). Pralidoxime chloride may serve as an important adjunct to atropine therapy.

Administration and Dosage

➤*Adults:*

Antimuscarinic – The usual dosage is 0.4 to 0.6 mg IM, IV, or subcutaneous. See Indications for complete list of uses.

Bradyarrhythmias –

Usual dosage: 0.4 to 1 mg IV every 1 to 2 hours as needed; larger doses, up to a maximum of 2 mg, may be required.

Maximum dose: 2 mg/dose.

Hypotonic radiography – 1 mg IM.

Poisoning –

Anticholinesterase poisoning: At least 2 to 3 mg parenterally; repeat until signs of atropine intoxication appear.

Muscarinic mushroom poisoning: Give in doses sufficient to control parasympathomimetic signs before coma and cardiovascular collapse supervene.

AtroPen: *AtroPen* 2 mg is typically used for adults and patients weighing more than 90 lbs.

The *AtroPen* auto-injector should be administered as soon as symptoms of organophosphorus or carbamate poisoning appear (eg, usually tearing, excessive oral secretions, wheezing, muscle fasciculations).

More than 1 *AtroPen* may be required until atropinization is achieved (flushing, mydriasis, tachycardia, dryness of the mouth and nose). No more than 3 *AtroPen* injections should be used unless the patient is under the supervision of a trained medical provider. Different dose strengths of the *AtroPen* are available depending on the recipient's age and weight.

• *Mild symptoms* – One *AtroPen* is recommended if 2 or more of the following mild symptoms of nerve agent (nerve gas) or insecticide exposure appear in situations where exposure is known or suspected: blurred vision, miosis, excessive unexplained teary eyes, excessive unexplained runny nose, increased salivation such as sudden unexplained excessive drooling, chest tightness or difficulty breathing, tremors throughout the body or muscular twitching, nausea and/or vomiting, unexplained wheezing or coughing, acute onset of stomach cramps, tachycardia, or bradycardia.

• *Severe symptoms* – Two additional *AtroPen* injections given in rapid succession are recommended 10 minutes after receiving the first *AtroPen* injection if the victim develops any of the following severe symptoms. If possible, a person other than the victim should administer the second and third *AtroPen* injections. If a victim is encountered who is unconscious or has any of the severe symptoms, immediately administer 3 *AtroPen* injections into the victim's midlateral thigh in rapid succession using the appropriate weight-based *AtroPen* dose. Symptoms include: strange or confused behavior, severe difficulty breathing or severe secretions from the lungs/airway, severe muscular twitching and general weakness, involuntary urination and defecation (feces), convulsions, or unconsciousness.

• *Concomitant therapy* – Administer an anticonvulsant (eg, diazepam) if seizure is suspected in the unconscious individual since the classic tonic-clonic jerking may not be apparent due to the effects of the poison.

Pralidoxime (if used) is most effective if administered immediately or soon after the poisoning. Generally, little is accomplished if pralidoxime is given more than 36 hours after termination of exposure unless the poison is known to age slowly or re-exposure is possible, such as in delayed continuing GI absorption of ingested poisons. Fatal relapses, thought to be due to delayed absorption, have been reported after initial improvement. Continued administration for several days may be useful in such patients.

Emergency care of the severely poisoned individual should include removal of oral and bronchial secretions, maintenance of a patent airway, supplemental oxygen and, if necessary, artificial ventilation. In general, atropine should not be used until cyanosis has been overcome because atropine may produce ventricular fibrillation and possible seizures in the presence of hypoxia.

Close supervision of all moderately to severely poisoned patients is indicated for at least 48 to 72 hours.

Surgery – 0.5 mg (range, 0.4 to 0.6 mg) subcutaneously, IM, or IV. As an antisialagogue, it is usually injected IM prior to induction of anesthesia. During surgery, the drug is given IV when reduction in pulse rate and cessation of cardiac action are due to increased vagal activity. However, if the anesthetic is cyclopropane, use doses less than 0.4 mg and give slowly to avoid production of ventricular arrhythmia. Usual doses reduce severe bradycardia and syncope associated with hyperactive carotid sinus reflex.

➤*Children:*

Antimuscarinic – See Indications for complete list of uses.

Atropine Injection Dosage Recommendations in Children

Weight		Dose
7 to 16 lb	3.2 to 7.3 kg	0.1 mg
16 to 24 lb	7.3 to 10.9 kg	0.15 mg
24 to 40 lb	10.9 to 18.1 kg	0.2 mg
40 to 65 lb	18.1 to 29.5 kg	0.3 mg
65 to 90 lb	29.5 to 40.8 kg	0.4 mg
> 90 lb	40.8 kg	0.4 to 0.6 mg

Bradyarrhythmias – 0.01 to 0.03 mg/kg IV.

Poisoning –

Anticholinesterase poisoning: Give doses parenterally; repeat until signs of atropine intoxication appear.

Muscarinic mushroom poisoning: Give in doses sufficient to control parasympathomimetic signs before coma and cardiovascular collapse supervene.

AtroPen: The *AtroPen* auto-injector should be administered as soon as symptoms of organophosphorus or carbamate poisoning appear (eg, usually tearing, excessive oral secretions, wheezing, muscle fasciculations).

More than 1 *AtroPen* may be required until atropinization is achieved (flushing, mydriasis, tachycardia, dryness of the mouth and nose). No more

ATROPINE SULFATE — INJECTION

than 3 *AtroPen* injections should be used, unless the patient is under the supervision of a trained medical provider. Different dose strengths of the *AtroPen* are available depending on the recipient's age and weight.

AtroPen Dosing	
Patient group	Dose strength
Adults and children weighing more than 90 lbs (generally over 10 years of age)	2 mg IM
Children weighing 40 to 90 lbs (generally 4 to 10 years of age)	1 mg IM
Children weighing 15 to 40 lbs (generally 6 months to 4 years of age)[a]	0.5 mg IM

[a] Children weighing less than 15 lbs (generally younger than 6 months of age) should ordinarily not be treated with the *AtroPen* auto-injector. Atropine doses for these children should be individualized at doses of 0.05 mg/kg.

See Adults for additional dosing information.

Surgery – During surgery, the drug is given IV when reduction in pulse rate and cessation of cardiac action are due to increased vagal activity. However, if the anesthetic is cyclopropane, use lower doses and give slowly to avoid production of ventricular arrhythmia. Usual doses reduce severe bradycardia and syncope associated with hyperactive carotid sinus reflex.

Children:

- *Usual dosage* – 0.01 mg/kg up to a maximum of 0.4 mg subcutaneous, IM, or IV, repeated every 4 to 6 hours as needed.
- *Maximum dose* – 0.4 mg/dose.

Infants:

- *Less than 5 kg* – 0.04 mg/kg subcutaneous, IM, or IV repeated every 4 to 6 hours as needed.
- *More than 5 kg* – 0.03 mg/kg subcutaneous, IM, or IV repeated every 4 to 6 hours as needed.

➤*Administration:* For IV use, but may be given IM or subcutaneously.

AtroPen administration –

1.) Snap the grooved end of the plastic sleeve down and over the yellow safety cap. Remove the *AtroPen* from the plastic sleeve. Do not place fingers on the green tip.
2.) Firmly grasp the *AtroPen* with the green tip pointed down.
3.) Pull off the yellow safety cap with your other hand.
4.) Aim and firmly jab the green tip straight down (a 90° angle) against the outer thigh. The *AtroPen* device will then activate and deliver the medicine. It is okay to inject through clothing, but make sure pockets at the injection site are empty. Very thin people and small children also should be injected in the thigh, but before giving the *AtroPen*, bunch up the thigh to provide a thicker area for injection.
5.) Hold the auto-injector firmly in place for at least 10 seconds to allow the injection to finish.
6.) Remove the *AtroPen* and massage the injection site for several seconds. If the needle is not visible, check to be sure the yellow safety cap has been removed, and repeat steps 3 and 5, but press harder.

➤*Storage/Stability:* Store at 15° to 30°C (59° to 86°F).

AtroPen – Store at 25°C (77°F); excursions permitted between 15° and 30°C (59° and 86°F). Keep from freezing; protect from light.

SCOPOLAMINE HYDROBROMIDE (Hyoscine HBr)

Rx	**Scopace** (Hope Pharm)	**Tablets, soluble:** 0.4 mg	(Hope 301). White. In 100s.
Rx	**Scopolamine HBr** (Various, eg, Loch)	**Injection:** 0.3 mg/mL	In 1 mL vials.
Rx	**Scopolamine HBr** (Various, eg, GlaxoWellcome)	**Injection:** 0.4 mg/mL	In 0.5 mL amps and 1 mL vials.
Rx	**Scopolamine HBr** (GlaxoWellcome)	**Injection:** 0.86 mg/mL	In 0.5 mL amps.[1]
Rx	**Scopolamine HBr** (Various, eg, Loch)	**Injection:** 1 mg/mL	In 1 mL vials.

[1] With alcohol and mannitol.

SCOPOLAMINE HYDROBROMIDE — ORAL

For complete and comparative prescribing information, refer to the Gastrointestinal Anticholinergics/Antispasmodics group monograph. See also the Antiemetic/Antivertigo Agents monograph.

Indications

➤*Postencephalitic parkinsonism:* Scopolamine HBr tablets are used as an anticholinergic, CNS depressant; in the symptomatic treatment of postencephalitic parkinsonism and paralysis agitans; in spastic states.

➤*Ophthalmic:* May be used locally as a substitute for atropine in ophthalmology.

➤*GI tract disorders:* Scopolamine hydrobromide inhibits excessive motility and hypertonus of the GI tract in such conditions as the irritable colon syndrome, mild dysentery, diverticulitis, pylorospasm, and cardiospasm.

➤*Motion sickness:* May be used to prevent motion sickness.

➤*Off-label uses:* Treatment of postoperative and chemotherapy-induced nausea and vomiting.

Administration and Dosage

➤*Adults:*

Usual dosage – 0.4 to 0.8 mg.

➤*Renal function impairment:* Should not be administered to patients with impaired renal function.

➤*Hepatic function impairment:* Should not be administered to patients with impaired hepatic function.

➤*Storage/Stability:* Store at 15° to 30°C (59° to 86°F).

SCOPOLAMINE HYDROBROMIDE — INJECTION

For complete and comparative prescribing information, refer to the Gastrointestinal Anticholinergics/Antispasmodics group monograph. See also the Antiemetic/Antivertigo Agents monograph.

Indications

➤*Sedation/tranquilization:* For use as a sedative and tranquilizing depressant to the central nervous system.

In addition to the usual uses for antimuscarinic drugs, scopolamine is employed for its central depressant actions as a sedative. Frequently, it is given as a preanesthetic medicament for both its sedative-tranquilizing and antisecretory actions.

➤*Antiemetic:* For use as an antiemetic.

➤*Maniacal states:* For use in maniacal states.

➤*Delirium tremens:* For use in delirium tremens.

➤*Obstetrics:* For use in obstetrics.

➤*Mydriatic/cycloplegic:* For use as a mydriatic and cycloplegic. It has a somewhat shorter duration (3 to 7 days) and intraocular pressure is affected less markedly than with atropine.

Administration and Dosage

➤*General dosing considerations:* Close supervision is recommended for infants, blondes, people with Down syndrome, and children with spastic paralysis or brain damage because an increased responsiveness to belladonna alkaloids has been reported in these patients and dosage adjustments are often required.

Belladonna alkaloids provide a therapeutic effect in approximately 1 or 2 hours with a duration of approximately 4 hours.

➤*Adults:*

Antiemetic – 0.6 to 1 mg subcutaneously.

Obstetric amnesia – 0.32 to 0.65 mg.

Preoperative sedation – 0.32 to 0.65 mg.

Sedation/Tranquilization – 0.6 mg 3 or 4 times a day.

➤*Children:*

Antiemetic – 0.006 mg/kg subcutaneously.

Preoperative sedation –

3 to 6 years of age: 0.2 to 0.3 mg.
6 months to 3 years of age: 0.1 to 0.15 mg.

Sedation/Tranquilization –

3 to 6 years of age: 0.2 to 0.3 mg.
6 months to 3 years of age: 0.1 to 0.15 mg.

➤*Elderly:* Elderly and debilitated patients may respond to the usual doses with excitement, agitation, drowsiness, or confusion; lower doses may be required in such patients.

➤*Administration:* For IM, IV or subcutaneous use.

Administration of belladonna alkaloids and barbiturates 30 to 60 minutes before meals is recommended to maximize absorption and, when issued for reducing stomach acid formation, to allow its effect to coincide better with antacid administration following the meal.

Use only if solution is clear and seal is intact.

➤*Storage/Stability:* Store at 15° to 30°C (59° to 86°F). Protect from light.

METHSCOPOLAMINE BROMIDE

Rx	**Methscopolamine Bromide** (Boca Pharmacal)	**Tablets; oral:** 2.5 mg	(BOCA/603). In 100s.
Rx	**Pamine** (Kenwood/Bradley)		In 100s and 500s.
Rx	**Methscopolamine Bromide** (Boca Pharmacal)	**Tablets; oral:** 5 mg	(BOCA/604). Oval. In 60s and 5 blisters of 12 tablets.
Rx	**Pamine Forte** (Kenwood Therapeutics)		(PAMINE 5). Oval. In 60s.
Rx	**Pamine FQ Kit** (Kenwood Therapeutics)		With 30 **Flora-Q** capsules.[a] (PAMINE 5). Oval. In 60s.

[a] *Flora-Q* capsules contain 8 million CFUs of *Lactobacillus acidophilus, L. paracasei, Bifidobacterium, Streptococcus thermophilus.*

METHSCOPOLAMINE BROMIDE — ORAL

For complete and comparative prescribing information, refer to the Gastrointestinal Anticholinergics/Antispasmodics group monograph.

Indications

➤*Peptic ulcer:* Adjunctive therapy for the treatment of peptic ulcer.

Methscopolamine bromide has not been shown to be effective in contributing to the healing of peptic ulcer, decreasing the rate of recurrence or preventing complications.

➤*Off-label uses:* Atropine and related agents are effective in some patients with cholinergic-mediated bronchospasm. Use in chronic lung disease is not generally recommended; these agents reduce bronchial secretions resulting in decreased fluidity and thickening of residual secretions.

Administration and Dosage

➤*General dosing considerations:* Patients whose dosage has been reduced to eliminate or modify adverse effects often continue to show adequate response both subjectively in relief of symptoms and objectively as measured by antisecretory effects.

The ultimate aim of therapy is to arrive at a dosage that provides maximal clinical effectiveness with a minimum of unpleasant adverse effects. Many patients report no adverse effects on a dosage that gives complete relief of symptoms. On the other hand, some patients have reported severe adverse effects without appreciable symptomatic relief. Such patients must be considered unsuited for this therapy. Usually they have been or will prove to be similarly intolerant to other anticholinergic drugs. If methscopolamine is to be used in a patient who gives a history of such intolerance, it should be started at a low dosage.

➤*Adults:*

Peptic ulcer –

Usual dosage: 2.5 mg taken 30 minutes before meals and 2.5 to 5 mg taken at bedtime. A starting dose of 12.5 mg/day will be clinically effective in most patients without the production of appreciable side effects.

Alternative dosage: If the patient is having severe symptoms which demand prompt relief, the drug may be started on a dosage of 20 mg/day, administered in doses of 5 mg taken 30 minutes before meals and at bedtime. If very unpleasant adverse effects develop promptly, the daily dosage should be reduced. If neither symptomatic relief nor adverse effects appear, the daily dosage may be increased. Some patients have tolerated 30 mg/day with no unpleasant reactions.

➤*Storage/Stability:* Store at 15° to 30°C (59° to 86°F).

GLYCOPYRROLATE

Rx	**Glycopyrrolate** (Rising)	**Tablets; oral:** 1 mg	Lactose. (cor 155). White. In 100s and 1,000s.
Rx	**Robinul** (Horizon)		Lactose. (HPC 200). White, scored. In 100s and 500s.
Rx	**Glycopyrrolate** (Rising)	**Tablets; oral:** 2 mg	Lactose. (cor 156). White. In 100s and 1,000s.
Rx	**Robinul Forte** (Horizon)		Lactose. (Horizon 205). White, scored. In 100s.
Rx	**Cuvposa** (Shionogi Pharma)	**Solution; oral:** 1 mg/5 mL	Cherry flavored. Parabens, sorbitol, propylene glycol, saccharin. In 16 oz bottles.
Rx	**Glycopyrrolate** (Various, eg, American Regent, Schein, Texas Drug, VHA)	**Injection:** 0.2 mg/mL	In 1, 2, 5, and 20 mL vials.
Rx	**Robinul** (Robins)		In 1, 2, 5, and 20 mL vials.[a]

[a] With benzyl alcohol 0.9%.

GLYCOPYRROLATE — ORAL

For complete and comparative prescribing information, refer to the Gastrointestinal Anticholinergics/Antispasmodics class monograph.

Indications

➤*Drooling (oral solution only):* To reduce chronic, severe drooling in children 3 to 16 years of age with neurologic conditions associated with problem drooling (eg, cerebral palsy).

➤*Peptic ulcer (tablets only):* For use as adjunctive therapy in the treatment of peptic ulcer.

➤*Off-label uses:*

Drooling – [2] = Fair documentation. Glycopyrrolate has been studied primarily in retrospective reviews of children and young adults with severe drooling due to cerebral palsy and other developmental disabilities. (See Administration and Dosage.)

Administration and Dosage

➤*General dosing considerations:* The dosage of glycopyrrolate should be adjusted to the needs of the individual patient to ensure symptomatic control with a minimum of adverse reactions.

➤*Adults:*

Peptic ulcer –

1 mg tablets:

• *Initial dosage* – 1 mg three times daily (in the morning, early afternoon, and at bedtime). Some patients may require 2 mg at bedtime to ensure overnight control of symptoms.

• *Maintenance dosage* – 1 mg twice a day.

2 mg tablets:

• *Usual dosage* – 2 mg two or three times daily at equally spaced intervals.

Off-label dosing –

Drooling: [2] = Fair documentation. 1 to 4 mg/day, or 0.2 to 0.4 mg three times per day.

➤*Children:*

Drooling –

3 to 16 years of age:

• *Maximum dose* – 0.1 mg/kg three times daily not to exceed 1.5 to 3 mg per dose based upon weight.

• *Initial dosage* – 0.02 mg/kg orally 3 times daily.

• *Dosage titration* – Titrate in increments of 0.02 mg/kg every 5 to 7 days based on therapeutic response and adverse reactions.

Glycopyrrolate Oral Solution Recommended Dose Titration Schedule (Each Dose to be Given 3 Times Daily)

Weight	Dose level 1 (−0.02 mg/kg)		Dose level 2 (−0.04 mg/kg)		Dose level 3 (−0.06 mg/kg)		Dose level 4 (−0.08 mg/kg)		Dose level 5 (−0.1 mg/kg)	
13 to 17 kg	0.3 mg	1.5 mL	0.6 mg	3 mL	0.9 mg	4.5 mL	1.2 mg	6 mL	1.5 mg	7.5 mL
18 to 22 kg	0.4 mg	2 mL	0.8 mg	4 mL	1.2 mg	6 mL	1.6 mg	8 mL	2 mg	10 mL
23 to 27 kg	0.5 mg	2.5 mL	1 mg	5 mL	1.5 mg	7.5 mL	2 mg	10 mL	2.5 mg	12.5 mL
28 to 32 kg	0.6 mg	3 mL	1.2 mg	6 mL	1.8 mg	9 mL	2.4 mg	12 mL	3 mg	15 mL
33 to 37 kg	0.7 mg	3.5 mL	1.4 mg	7 mL	2.1 mg	10.5 mL	2.8 mg	14 mL	3 mg	15 mL
38 to 42 kg	0.8 mg	4 mL	1.6 mg	8 mL	2.4 mg	12 mL	3 mg	15 mL	3 mg	15 mL
43 to 47 kg	0.9 mg	4.5 mL	1.8 mg	9 mL	2.7 mg	13.5 mL	3 mg	15 mL	3 mg	15 mL
≥ 48 kg	1 mg	5 mL	2 mg	10 mL	3 mg	15 mL	3 mg	15 mL	3 mg	15 mL

GLYCOPYRROLATE — ORAL

Peptic ulcer – See Adults for dosing for children 12 years of age and older.

➤*Administration:* Glycopyrrolate oral solution must be measured and administered with an accurate measuring device.

Glycopyrrolate should be dosed at least 1 hour before or 2 hours after meals. The presence of high-fat food reduces the oral bioavailability of glycopyrrolate if taken shortly after a meal.

➤*Storage/Stability:* Store tablets between 15°and 30°C (59° and 86°F). Dispense in tight container.

Store oral solution between 20° and 25°C (68° and 77°F); excursions are permitted between 15° and 30°C (59° and 86°F).

GLYCOPYRROLATE — INJECTION

For complete and comparative prescribing information, refer to the Gastrointestinal Anticholinergics/Antispasmodics group monograph.

Indications

➤*Anesthesia:* Use as a preoperative antimuscarinic to reduce salivary, tracheobronchial, and pharyngeal secretions; to reduce the volume and free acidity of gastric secretions; and to block cardiac vagal inhibitory reflexes during induction of anesthesia and intubation. When indicated, glycopyrrolate injection may be used intraoperatively to counteract drug-induced or vagal traction reflexes with the associated arrhythmias. Glycopyrrolate protects against the peripheral muscarinic effects (eg, bradycardia, excessive secretions) of cholinergic agents such as neostigmine and pyridostigmine given to reverse the neuromuscular blockade due to nondepolarizing muscle relaxants.

➤*Peptic ulcer:* For use in adults as adjunctive therapy for the treatment of peptic ulcer when rapid anticholinergic effect is desired or when oral medication is not tolerated.

➤*Off-label uses:*

Cholelithiasis pain – [5] = Poor documentation. There are limited data available regarding the use of glycopyrrolate in the management of cholelithiasis pain. Only 1 small controlled study has been published to date, which demonstrated no benefit or relief in pain when glycopyrrolate was compared with placebo. It is recommended that this drug not be used to treat this condition until evidence of its benefit is apparent.

Sialorrhea (drooling) – [2] = Fair documentation. This drug has been studied primarily in retrospective reviews of children and young adults with severe drooling due to cerebral palsy or other developmental disabilities. (See Administration and Dosage.)

Administration and Dosage

➤*General dosing considerations:* Because of the long duration of action of glycopyrrolate injection, if used as preanesthetic medication, additional glycopyrrolate for anticholinergic effect intraoperatively is rarely needed.

➤*Adults:*

Anesthesia –

Preanesthetic medication: 0.004 mg/kg IM, given 30 to 60 minutes prior to the anticipated time of induction of anesthesia or at the time the preanesthetic narcotic or sedative is administered.

Intraoperative medication: 0.1 mg IV as a single dose and repeated, as needed, at intervals of 2 to 3 minutes.

Reversal of neuromuscular blockade: 0.2 mg IV for each 1 mg of neostigmine or 5 mg of pyridostigmine. In order to minimize the appearance of cardiac side effects, the drugs may be administered simultaneously by IV injection and may be mixed in the same syringe.

Peptic ulcer –

Usual dosage: 0.1 mg IV or IM at 4-hour intervals, 3 or 4 times daily. Where more profound effect is required, 0.2 mg may be given. Some patients may need only a single dose and frequency of administration should be dictated by patient response up to a maximum of 4 times daily.

Off-label dosing –

➤*Children:*

Anesthesia –

Preanesthetic medication:

- *2 years of age and older* – 0.004 mg/kg IM, given 30 to 60 minutes prior to the anticipated time of induction of anesthesia or at the time the preanesthetic narcotic or sedative is administered.
- *1 month to 2 years of age* – Up to 0.009 mg/kg may be required.

Intraoperative medication:

- *Older than 1 month of age* –
  Usual dosage: 0.004 mg/kg IV, not to exceed 0.1 mg, in a single dose which may be repeated, as needed, at intervals of 2 to 3 minutes.

Reversal of neuromuscular blockade: See Adults for dosing for children 1 month of age and older.

Off-label dosing –

Sialorrhea (drooling): [2] = Fair documentation. 0.1 mg subcutaneously in the morning and 0.2 mg in the evening.

➤*Administration:* Glycopyrrolate may be administered IM or IV without dilution.

➤*Admixture compatibility:* Glycopyrrolate stability is generally dependent upon pH. The pH of the USP product ranges between 2 and 3. Stability decreases rapidly above pH 6.

Compatibility – Glycopyrrolate injection is stable for 48 hours in IV infusion solutions of 5% Dextrose, 10% Dextrose, 0.45% Sodium Chloride, 0.9% Sodium Chloride or Ringer's Injection.

Glycopyrrolate injection is generally physically compatible with drugs having an acid pH (less than 6); however, this would also be dependent on concentration of the drugs and temperature as well as pH.

Incompatibility – Glycopyrrolate injection would be expected to be incompatible with drugs having a more alkaline pH (more than 6) such as the barbiturates, diazepam, or buffered Lactated Ringer's injection. The latter may be used for administration via the tubing of a running IV infusion.

➤*Storage/Stability:* Store at 15° to 30°C (59° to 86°F).

MEPENZOLATE BROMIDE

Rx	**Cantil** (Hoechst Marion Roussel)	**Tablets:** 25 mg	Tartrazine. (Merrell 37). Yellow. In 100s.

MEPENZOLATE BROMIDE — ORAL

For complete and comparative prescribing information, refer to the Gastrointestinal Anticholinergics/Antispasmodics group monograph.

Indications

➤*Peptic ulcer:* Adjunctive therapy in the treatment of peptic ulcer. It has not been shown to be effective in contributing to the healing of peptic ulcer, decreasing the rate of recurrence, or preventing complications.

Administration and Dosage

➤*Adults:*

Peptic ulcer – 25 or 50 mg 4 times a day, preferably with meals and at bedtime. Begin with the lower dosage when possible and adjust subsequently according to the patient's response.

➤*Storage/Stability:* Keep tightly closed. Store below 30°C (86°F). Protect from excessive heat. Dispense in tight containers with child-resistant closure.

PROPANTHELINE BROMIDE

Rx	**Propantheline Bromide** (Various, eg, Goldline, Harber, Moore, Par, Richlyn, Roxane)	**Tablets:** 15 mg	In 100s, 500s, 1000s, and UD 100s.

PROPANTHELINE BROMIDE — ORAL

For complete and comparative prescribing information, refer to the Gastrointestinal anticholinergics/Antispasmodics group monograph.

Indications

➤*Peptic ulcer:* Adjunctive therapy in the treatment of peptic ulcer.

Administration and Dosage

➤*Adults:*

Peptic ulcer –

Usual dosage: 15 mg taken 30 minutes before each meal and 30 mg at bedtime (a total of 75 mg daily).

Dosage adjustment: Subsequent dosage adjustment should be made according to the patient's individual response and tolerance.

➤*Storage/Stability:* Store at 20° to 25°C (68° to 77°F). Dispense in tight, light-resistant container.

DICYCLOMINE HYDROCHLORIDE

Rx	**Dicyclomine HCl** (Various, eg, Bolar, Goldline, Lederle, Major)	**Capsules:** 10 mg	In 30s, 100s, 120s, 1000s, and UD 100s.
Rx	**Bentyl** (Axcan Scandipharm)		(Bentyl 10). In 100s, 500s, and UD 100s.
Rx	**Dicyclomine HCl** (Various, eg, Bolar, Goldline, Lederle, Major)	**Tablets:** 20 mg	In 15s, 20s, 30s, 100s, 120s, 250s, 1000s, and UD 100s.
Rx	**Bentyl** (Axcan Scandipharm)		(Bentyl 20) In 100s, 500s, 1000s, and UD 100s.
Rx	**Dicyclomine HCl** (Various, eg, Moore, Ritchie)	**Capsules** : 20 mg	In 100s, and 1000s.
Rx	**Dicyclomine HCl** (Various, eg, Gen-King, Goldline, Harber, Moore, Qualitest)	**Syrup:** 10 mg/5 mL	In 118 mL, pt, and gal.
Rx	**Bentyl** (Axcan Scandipharm)		Saccharin in pt.
Rx	**Dicyclomine HCl** (Various, eg, Goldline, Major, Moore, Ritchie, Steris)	**Injection:** 10 mg/mL	In 2 and 10 mL vials.
Rx	**Bentyl** (Axcan Scandipharm)		In 2 mL amps and 10 mL vials.

DICYCLOMINE HYDROCHLORIDE — ORAL

For complete and comparative prescribing information, refer to the Gastrointestinal Anticholinergics/Antispasmodics group monograph.

Indications

➤*Irritable bowel syndrome:* For the treatment of functional bowel/irritable bowel syndrome (irritable colon, spastic colon, mucous colitis).

Administration and Dosage

➤*Adults:*

Functional Bowel/Irritable Bowel Syndrome –

Initial dosage: 80 mg/day (in 4 equally divided doses).

Dosage titration: Depending upon the patient's response during the first week of therapy, the dose should be increased to 160 mg/day unless side effects limit dosage escalation.

Maintenance dosage: 160 mg/day (in 4 equally divided doses).

Discontinuation of therapy: If efficacy is not achieved within 2 weeks or side effects require dosages below 80 mg/day, the drug should be discontinued.

➤*Elderly:* Use should be avoided in elderly patients.

➤*Storage/Stability:* Store between 15° and 30°C (59° and 86°F). Protect from light, freezing, and moisture.

Dispense in a tight, light-resistant container with a child-resistant closure.

DICYCLOMINE HYDROCHLORIDE — INJECTION

For complete and comparative prescribing information, refer to the Gastrointestinal Anticholinergics/Antispasmodics group monograph.

Indications

➤*Irritable bowel syndrome:* For the treatment of functional bowel/irritable bowel syndrome.

Administration and Dosage

➤*General dosing considerations:* The IM dosage form is to be used temporarily when the patient cannot take oral medication.

IM injection is about twice as bioavailable as oral dosage forms.

➤*Adults:*

Functional Bowel/Irritable Bowel Syndrome –

Usual dosage: 80 mg IM daily (in 4 equally divided doses).

Duration of therapy: The IM form should not be used for periods of longer than 1 or 2 days. Oral dicyclomine should be started as soon as possible.

➤*Elderly:* Use should be avoided in elderly patients.

➤*Administration:* Give by IM injection. Not for IV use.

➤*Storage/Stability:* Store preferably below 30°C (86°F). Protect from freezing.

GASTROINTESTINAL ANTICHOLINERGIC COMBINATIONS

Content given per tablet, capsule, 5 mL liquid, or 1 mL drops.

	Product and Distributor	Anticholinergic	Sedative, Antianxiety Agent or Other	Other	Daily Dose	How Supplied
Rx sf	**Antrocol Elixir** (ECR)	0.195 mg atropine sulfate	16 mg phenobarbital	20% alcohol	15 to 40 mL. *Children* - 0.5 mL per 15 lbs every 4 to 6 hours	In 473 mL.
Rx	**Belladonna Alkaloids w/ PhenobarbitalTablets** (Various, eg, Goldline, Major, Westward)	0.0194 mg atropine sulfate, 0.0065 mg scopolamine HBr, 0.1037 mg hyoscyamine HBr or sulfate	16.2 mg phenobarbital		3 to 8 tablets	In 50s, 100s, 1,000s and UD 100s.
Rx	**Antispasmodic Elixir**[a] (Various, eg, Goldline, Qualitest, RID, UDL)			23% alcohol, sugar, sorbitol		In 120 mL, 473 mL, and gal.
Rx	**Donnatal Tablets** (PBM Pharm)				3 to 8 tablets	Lactose. (D Donnatal). White, D shape. In 100s and 1,000s.
Rx	**Donnatal Elixir** (PBM Pharm)			Ethyl alcohol, saccharin, sucrose, sorbitol	5 to 10 mL tid or qid. *Children: 4.5 kg* - 0.5 mL every 4 h or 0.75 mL every 6 h; *9.1 kg* - 1 mL every 4 h or 1.5 mL every 6 h; *13.6 kg* - 1.5 mL every 4 h or 2 mL every 6 h; *22.7 kg* - 2.5 mL every 4 h or 3.75 mL every 6 h; *34 kg* - 3.75 mL every 4 h or 5 mL every 6 h; *45 kg* - 5 mL every 4 h or 7.5 mL every 6 h.	Grape flavor. In 118 and 473 mL.
c-iv	**Quadrapax Elixir** (Acella Pharmaceuticals)			Alcohol 23%, glycerin, saccharin, sorbitol, sucrose		Grape flavor. In 473 mL.
Rx	**Spasmolin Tablets** (Various, eg, Global)				3 to 8 tablets	In 100s and 1,000s.
Rx	**Donnatal Extentabs Extended-Release Tablets** (PBM Pharm)	0.0582 mg atropine sulfate, 0.0195 mg scopolamine HBr, 0.3111 mg hyoscyamine sulfate	48.6 mg phenobarbital		2 to 3 tablets	Lactose, polydextrose. (P421). Green. Film coated. In 100s and 500s.
Rx	**Digex NF** (Pronova Corp)	0.0625 mg hyoscyamine sulfate	15 mg phenyltoloxamine citrate		4 to 8 capsules	Lactose. (GEX001). In 100s.
Rx	**Digex Capsules** (Pronova Corp)	0.0625 mg hyoscyamine sulfate	15 mg phenyltoloxamine citrate	Amylase 30 mg, cellulase 2 mg, lipase 1,200 units, protease 6 mg	1 or 2 capsules	(DIGEX). In 100s.
Rx	**Butibel Tablets** (Wallace)	15 mg belladonna extract	15 mg butabarbital sodium		4 to 8 tablets	(Butibel 37/046). Red. In 100s.
Rx	**Butibel Elixir** (Wallace)			7% alcohol, sucrose, saccharin	20 to 40 mL. *Children ≥ 6* - 10 mL; *Children < 6* - 5 to 10 mL	Orange flavor. In 473 mL.
Rx	**Chlordiazepoxide w/ Clidinium Bromide Capsules** (Various, eg, Eon, Goldline, Moore, Schein)	2.5 mg clidinium bromide	5 mg chlordiazepoxide hydrochloride		1 to 2 capsules 3 to 4 times a day	In 100s, 500s, 1,000s, and UD 100s.
Rx	**RE Chlordiazepoxide/Clidinium Capsules** (River's Edge)					Lactose. (RE 369). Yellow. In 100s.
Rx	**Librax Capsules** (Valeant)					Lactose, parabens. Green. In 100s.

[a] May contain alcohol.

Refer to the general discussion of these products in the GI Anticholinergics/Antispasmodics group monograph.

MESALAMINE (5-aminosalicylic acid, 5-ASA)

Rx	**Lialda** (Shire US)	**Tablets, delayed-release; oral**: 1.2 g	(S476). Red-brown, ellipsoidal. Film-coated. In 120s.
Rx	**Asacol** (Procter & Gamble Pharmaceuticals)	**Tablets, delayed-release; oral**: 400 mg	Lactose. (Asacol NE). Red-brown, capsule shape. In 180s.
Rx	**Asacol HD** (Warner Chilcott)	**Tablets, delayed-release; oral**: 800 mg	Lactose, PEG. (PG 800). Red-brown, capsule shape. In 180s.
Rx	**Pentasa** (Shire US)	**Capsules, controlled-release; oral**: 250 mg	Sugar. (2010 PENTASA 250 mg). Green/blue. In 240s and UD 80s.
		500 mg	Sugar. (PENTASA 500 mg). Blue. In 120s and UD 80s.
Rx	**Apriso** (Salix)	**Capsules,[a] extended-release; oral**: 375 mg	Aspartame, phenylalanine. (G/M). Lt. blue. Enteric-coated granules. In 4s and 120s.
Rx	**Canasa** (Axcan Scandipharm)	**Suppositories; rectal**: 1,000 mg	Hard fat base. Lt. tan. In 30s.
Rx	**Mesalamine** (Various, eg, Clay Park, Prasco, Teva)	**Enema; rectal**: 4 g per 60 mL	May contain EDTA, potassium metabisulfite. In 7s in disposable bottles.
Rx	**Rowasa** (Alaven)		EDTA, potassium metabisulfite, white petrolatum. In 7s and 28s with lubricated applicator tip in disposable bottles.
Rx	**sfRowasa** (Alaven)	**Suspension; rectal**: 4 g per 60 mL	Sulfite free. Edetate disodium. In 7s, 14s, and 28s.

[a] Capsule is a delayed- and extended-release dosage form.

MESALAMINE — ORAL

Indications

➤*Ulcerative colitis:*

Apriso – For the maintenance of remission of ulcerative colitis in patients 18 years of age and older.

Asacol – For the treatment of mildly to moderately active ulcerative colitis and for the maintenance of remission of ulcerative colitis.

Asacol HD – For the treatment of moderately active ulcerative colitis.

Lialda – For the induction of remission in patients with active, mild to moderate ulcerative colitis.

Pentasa – For the induction of remission and for the treatment of patients with mildly to moderately active ulcerative colitis.

Administration and Dosage

➤*General dosing considerations:* Monitor renal function in all patients prior to initiation and periodically while on mesalamine therapy. Closely monitor blood cell counts during drug therapy.

One *Asacol HD* 800 mg tablet has not been shown to be bioequivalent to 2 *Asacol* 400 mg tablets.

➤*Adults:*

Induction of remission in patients with active, mild to moderate ulcerative colitis –

Lialda:

• *Usual dosage* – Two to four 1.2 g tablets taken once daily with food for a total daily dose of 2.4 or 4.8 g.

• *Duration of therapy* – Treatment duration in controlled clinical trials was up to 8 weeks.

Pentasa:

• *Usual dosage* – 1 g (four 250 mg capsules or two 500 mg capsules) 4 times daily for a total dose of 4 g.

• *Duration of therapy* – Treatment duration in controlled trials was up to 8 weeks.

Maintenance of remission of ulcerative colitis –

Apriso:

• *Usual dosage* – 1.5 g (4 capsules) orally once daily in the morning. May be taken without regard to meals.

• *Duration of therapy* – Treatment duration in controlled trial was 6 months.

• *Concomitant therapy* – Mesalamine should not be coadministered with antacids.

Asacol:

• *Usual dosage* – 1.6 g daily in divided doses.

• *Duration of therapy* – Treatment duration in the prospective, well-controlled trial was 6 months.

Treatment of mildly to moderately active ulcerative colitis –

Asacol: Two 400 mg tablets to be taken 3 times daily for a total daily dose of 2.4 g for a duration of 6 weeks.

Pentasa:

• *Usual dosage* – 1 g (four 250 mg capsules or two 500 mg capsules) 4 times daily for a total dose of 4 g.

• *Duration of therapy* – Treatment duration in controlled trials was up to 8 weeks.

Treatment of moderately active ulcerative colitis –

Asacol HD:

• *Usual dosage* – Two 800 mg tablets 3 times daily with or without food, for a total daily dose of 4.8 g.

• *Duration of therapy* – 6 weeks. Safety and effectiveness beyond 6 weeks have not been established.

➤*Elderly:* Dose selection for an elderly patient should be cautious, usually starting at the low end of the dosing range. See Adults for dosing.

➤*Administration:* Swallow tablets whole, taking care not to break the outer coating. Do not cut or chew tablets. Take *Lialda* with food.

➤*Storage/Stability:*

Apriso – Store at 20° to 25°C (68° to 77°F); excursions are permitted between 15° and 30°C (59° and 86°F)

Asacol and *Asacol HD* – Store at controlled room temperature, 20° to 25°C (68° to 77°F).

Lialda and *Pentasa* – Store at 15° to 25°C (59° to 77°F); excursions are permitted between 15° and 30°C (59° and 86°F).

Actions

➤*Pharmacology:* Mesalamine is thought to be the major therapeutically active part of the sulfasalazine molecule in the treatment of ulcerative colitis. Sulfasalazine is converted to equimolar amounts of sulfapyridine and mesalamine by bacterial action in the colon. The usual oral dose of sulfasalazine for active ulcerative colitis in adults is 3 to 4 g daily in divided doses, which provides 1.2 to 1.6 g of mesalamine to the colon. The mechanism of action of mesalamine (and sulfasalazine) is unknown, but it appears to be topical rather than systemic. Mucosal production of arachidonic acid metabolites, both through the cyclooxygenase pathways (ie, prostanoids), and through the lipoxygenase pathways (ie, leukotrienes) and hydroxyeicosatetraenoic acids, is increased in patients with chronic inflammatory bowel disease, and it is possible that mesalamine diminishes inflammation by blocking cyclooxygenase and inhibiting prostaglandin production in the colon. Recent data also suggest that mesalamine can inhibit the activation of NFKB, a nuclear transcription factor that regulates the transcription of many genes for proinflammatory proteins.

➤*Pharmacokinetics:*

Absorption/Distribution –

Asacol: *Asacol* tablets are coated with an acrylic-based resin that delays release of mesalamine until it reaches the terminal ileum and beyond. This has been demonstrated in human studies conducted with radiological and serum markers. Approximately 28% of the mesalamine in *Asacol* tablets is absorbed after oral ingestion, leaving the remainder available for topical action and excretion in the feces. Absorption of mesalamine is similar in fasted and fed subjects. Mesalamine from orally administered *Asacol* tablets appears to be more extensively absorbed than the mesalamine released from sulfasalazine. Maximum plasma levels of mesalamine and N-acetyl-5-aminosalicylic acid following multiple *Asacol* tablet doses are about 1.5 to 2 times higher than those following an equivalent dose of mesalamine in the form of sulfasalazine. Combined mesalamine and N-acetyl-5-aminosalicylic acid areas under the plasma concentration time curve (AUCs) and urine drug dose recoveries following multiple doses of *Asacol* tablets are about 1.3 to 1.5 times higher than those following an equivalent dose of mesalamine in the form of sulfasalazine. The T_{max} for mesalamine and its metabolite, N-acetyl-5-aminosalicylic acid, is usually delayed, reflecting the delayed release, and ranges from 4 to 12 hours.

Pentasa: *Pentasa* capsules are an ethylcellulose-coated, controlled-release formulation of mesalamine designed to release therapeutic quantities of mesalamine throughout the GI tract. Based on urinary excretion data, 20% to 30% of the mesalamine in *Pentasa* capsules is absorbed. In contrast, when mesalamine is administered orally as an unformulated 1 g aqueous suspension, mesalamine is approximately 80% absorbed. Plasma mesalamine concentration peaked at approximately 1 mcg/mL 3 hours following a *Pentasa* 1 g dose and declined in a biphasic manner. N-acetylmesalamine peaked at approximately 3 hours at 1.8 mcg/mL, and its concentration followed a biphasic decline.

Lialda: The total absorption of mesalamine from *Lialda* 2.4 or 4.8 g given once daily for 14 days to healthy volunteers was found to be approximately 21% to 22% of the administered dose.

Gamma-scintigraphy studies have shown that a single dose of *Lialda* 1.2 g (1 tablet) passed intact through the upper GI tract of fasted healthy volunteers. Scintigraphic images showed a trail of radio-labeled tracer in the colon, suggesting that mesalamine had distributed throughout this region of the GI tract. Mesalamine is approximately 43% bound to plasma proteins at the concentration of 2.5 mcg/mL.

In a single-dose study, *Lialda* 1.2, 2.4, and 4.8 g were administered in the fasted state to healthy subjects. Plasma concentrations of mesalamine were detectable after 2 hours and reached a maximum by 9 to 12 hours on average for the doses studied. The pharmacokinetic parameters are highly variable among subjects. Mesalamine systemic exposure in terms of AUC was slightly more than dose proportional between 1.2 and 4.8 g. Maximum plasma concentrations (C_{max}) of mesalamine increased approximately dose proportionately between 1.2 and 2.4 g and subproportionately between 2.4 and 4.8 g, with the dose normalized value at 4.8 g representing, on average, 74% of that at 2.4 g on geometric means.

MESALAMINE — ORAL

Mean (SD) Pharmacokinetic Parameters For *Lialda* (Single-Dose) Under Fasting Conditions[a]			
Parameter[b] of mesalamine	*Lialda* 1.2 g (n = 47)	*Lialda* 2.4 g (n = 48)	*Lialda* 4.8 g (n = 48)
AUC_{0-1} (ng•h/mL)	9,039[c] (5,054)	20,538 (12,980)	41,434 (26,640)
$AUC_{0-\infty}$ (ng•h/mL)	9,578[d] (5,214)	21,084 (13,185)	44,775[e] (30,302)
C_{max} (ng/mL)	857 (638)	1,595 (1,484)	2,154 (1,140)
T_{max}[f] (h)	9[g] (4 to 32.1)	12 (4 to 34.1)	12 (4 to 34)
T_{lag}[f] (h)	2[g] (0 to 8)	2 (1 to 4)	2 (1 to 4)
$t_{1/2}$ (h) (terminal phase)	8.56 (6.38)	7.05[h] (5.54)	7.25[e] (8.32)

[a] SD = standard deviation; T_{lag} = lag time; $t_{1/2}$ = half-life.
[b] Arithmetic mean of parameter values are presented except for T_{max} and T_{lag}.
[c] n = 43.
[d] n = 27.
[e] n = 36.
[f] Median (min, max).
[g] n = 46.
[h] n = 33.

• *Food effects* – Administration of a single dose of *Lialda* 4.8 g with a high-fat meal resulted in further delay in absorption, and plasma concentrations of mesalamine were detectable 4 hours following dosing. However, a high-fat meal increased systemic exposure of mesalamine (mean C_{max} increased 91%; mean AUC increased 16%) compared with results in the fasted state. *Lialda* was administered with food in the phase 3 trials.

In a single- and multiple-dose pharmacokinetic study of *Lialda* 2.4 or 4.8 g was administered once daily with standard meals to 28 healthy volunteers per dose group. Plasma concentrations of mesalamine were detectable after 4 hours and were maximal by 8 hours after the single dose. Steady state was achieved generally by 2 days after dosing. Mean AUC at steady state was only modestly greater (1.1- to 1.4-fold) than predictable from single-dose pharmacokinetics.

Metabolism / Excretion – The major metabolite of mesalamine (5-aminosalicylic acid) is N-acetyl-5-aminosalicylic acid. Its formation is brought about by N-acetyltransferase activity in the liver and intestinal mucosa. Elimination of mesalamine is mainly via the renal route following metabolism to N-acetyl-5-aminosalicylic acid (acetylation).

Pharmacological activities of N-acetylmesalamine are unknown, and other metabolites have not been identified.

Asacol: The absorbed mesalamine is rapidly acetylated in the gut mucosal wall and by the liver. It is excreted mainly by the kidney as N-acetyl-5-aminosalicylic acid. The half-lives of elimination for mesalamine and N-acetyl-5-aminosalicylic acid are usually about 12 hours, but are variable, ranging from 2 to 15 hours. There is a large intersubject variability in the plasma concentrations of mesalamine and N-acetyl-5-aminosalicylic acid and in their elimination half-lives following administration of *Asacol* tablets.

Pentasa: The literature describes a mean terminal half-life of 42 minutes for mesalamine following intravenous (IV) administration. Because of the continuous release and absorption of mesalamine from *Pentasa* capsules throughout the GI tract, the true elimination half-life cannot be determined after oral administration.

Oral mesalamine pharmacokinetics were nonlinear when *Pentasa* capsules were dosed from 250 mg to 1 g 4 times daily, with steady-state mesalamine plasma concentrations increasing about 9 times, from 0.14 to 1.21 mcg/mL, suggesting saturable first-pass metabolism. N-acetylmesalamine pharmacokinetics were linear.

About 130 mg of free mesalamine was recovered in the feces following a single 1 g *Pentasa* dose, which was comparable with the 140 mg of mesalamine recovered from the molar equivalent sulfasalazine tablet dose of 2.5 g. Elimination of free mesalamine and salicylates in feces increased proportionately with *Pentasa* dose. N-acetylmesalamine was the primary compound excreted in the urine (19% to 30%) following *Pentasa* dosing.

Lialda: There is limited excretion of the parent drug in urine. Of the approximately 21% to 22% of the dose absorbed, less than 8% of the dose was excreted unchanged in the urine, compared with more than 13% for N-acetyl-5-aminosalicylic acid. The apparent terminal half-lives for mesalamine and its major metabolite after administration of *Lialda* 2.4 and 4.8 g were, on average, 7 to 9 hours and 8 to 12 hours, respectively.

Contraindications

Hypersensitivity to mesalamine, salicylates, or any of the component of the formulation.

Warnings/Precautions

➤*Cardiac hypersensitivity:* Mesalamine-induced cardiac hypersensitivity reactions (myocarditis and pericarditis) have been reported with mesalamine medications. Take caution in prescribing mesalamine to patients with conditions predisposing to the development of myocarditis or pericarditis.

➤*Pyloric stenosis:* Patients with pyloric stenosis may have prolonged gastric retention of mesalamine delayed-release tablets, which could delay the release of mesalamine in the colon.

➤*Intolerance / Colitis exacerbation:* Mesalamine has been associated with an acute intolerance syndrome that may be difficult to distinguish from a flare of inflammatory bowel disease. Although the exact frequency of occurrence cannot be ascertained, it has occurred in 3% of patients in controlled clinical trials of mesalamine or sulfasalazine. Symptoms include cramping, acute abdominal pain, and bloody diarrhea, and sometimes fever, headache, malaise, pruritus, conjunctivitis, and rash. If acute intolerance syndrome is suspected, prompt withdrawal is required. Symptoms usually abate when mesalamine is discontinued. If a rechallenge is performed later in order to validate the hypersensitivity, carry it out under close medical supervision at reduced dose and only if clearly needed.

➤*Hypersensitivity reactions:* Some patients who have experienced a hypersensitivity reaction to sulfasalazine may have a similar reaction to mesalamine or to other compounds that are converted to mesalamine. The majority of patients who are intolerant or hypersensitive to sulfasalazine can take mesalamine medications without risk of similar reactions. However, exercise caution when treating patients allergic to sulfasalazine.

➤*Renal function impairment:* Renal function impairment, including minimal change nephropathy, nephrotic syndrome, acute and chronic interstitial nephritis, and, rarely, renal failure, has been reported in patients taking mesalamine medications and prodrugs of mesalamine. Therefore, exercise caution and use only if the benefits outweigh the risks when using mesalamine (or other compounds that are converted to mesalamine or its metabolites) in patients with known renal function impairment or history of renal disease. It is recommended that all patients have an evaluation of renal function prior to initiation of mesalamine and periodically while on treatment.

Therefore, exercise caution and only use mesalamine (or other compounds that are converted to mesalamine or its metabolites) in patients with known renal function impairment or history of renal disease if the benefits outweigh the risks. It is recommended that all patients have an evaluation of renal function prior to initiation of mesalamine periodically while on treatment.

Carefully monitor patients with preexisting renal disease, increased blood urea nitrogen (BUN) or serum creatinine, or proteinuria, especially during the initial phase of treatment. Expect mesalamine-induced nephrotoxicity in patients developing renal function impairment during treatment.

➤*Pregnancy: Category B*. Mesalamine is known to cross the placental barrier. There are no adequate and well-controlled studies in pregnant women. Because animal reproduction studies are not always predictive of human response, use this drug only if clearly needed.

➤*Lactation:* Low concentrations of mesalamine and higher concentrations of its N-acetyl metabolite have been detected in human breast milk. While the clinical significance of this had not been determined, exercise caution when administering mesalamine to a breast-feeding woman and use only if the benefits outweigh the risks. Hypersensitivity reactions like diarrhea in the infant cannot be excluded.

Minute quantities of mesalamine were distributed to breast milk and amniotic fluid of pregnant women following sulfasalazine therapy. When treated with sulfasalazine at a dose equivalent to 1.25 g/day of mesalamine, 0.02 to 0.08 mcg/mL and trace amounts of mesalamine were measured in amniotic fluid and breast milk, respectively. N-acetylmesalamine, in quantities of 0.07 to 0.77 mcg/mL and 1.13 to 3.44 mcg/mL, was identified in the same fluids, respectively.

➤*Children:* Safety and efficacy of mesalamine in children 18 years of age and younger have not been established.

➤*Elderly:* In general, dose selection for an elderly patient should be cautious, usually starting at the low end of the dosing range, reflecting the greater frequency of decreased hepatic, renal, or cardiac function, and of concomitant disease or other drug therapy in elderly patients. Reports from uncontrolled clinical studies and postmarketing reporting systems suggest a higher incidence of blood dyscrasias (ie, agranulocytosis, neutropenia, pancytopenia) in subjects receiving mesalamine who are 65 years of age and older. Use caution to closely monitor blood cell counts during drug therapy.

This drug is known to be substantially excreted by the kidney, and the risk of toxic reactions to this drug may be greater in patients with renal function impairment. Because elderly patients are more likely to have decreased renal function, take care when prescribing this drug therapy. As previously stated, it is recommended that all patients have an evaluation of renal function prior to initiation of mesalamine and periodically while on therapy.

➤*Monitoring:* Monitor renal function in all patients prior to initiation and periodically while on mesalamine therapy. Closely monitor blood cell counts during drug therapy.

Drug Interactions

Mesalamine Drug Interactions			
Precipitant drug	Object drug[a]		Description
Nephrotoxic drugs (eg, NSAIDs[b])	Mesalamine	↑	Concurrent use may increase the risk of renal reactions.
Mesalamine	Nephrotoxic drugs (eg, NSAIDs)		
Mesalamine	Azathioprine Mercaptopurine	↑	Concurrent use of mesalamine can increase the potential for blood disorders. Monitor blood cell counts and adjust therapy as needed.

MESALAMINE — ORAL

Mesalamine Drug Interactions			
Precipitant drug	Object drug[a]		Description
Mesalamine	Warfarin	⬇	The anticoagulant effect of warfarin may be decreased. Monitor anticoagulant parameters when starting, stopping, or changing the dose of mesalamine.

[a] ⬆ = object drug increased; ⬇ = object drug decreased.
[b] NSAIDs = nonsteroidal antiinflammatory drugs.

➤*Drug/Food interactions:* Administration of a single dose of *Lialda* 4.8 g with a high-fat meal resulted in further delay in absorption, and plasma concentrations of mesalamine were detectable 4 hours following dosing. However, the high-fat meal increased systemic exposure of mesalamine (mean C_{max} increased 91%; mean AUC increased 16%) compared with results in the fasted state. *Lialda* was administered with food in the phase 3 trials.

Adverse Reactions

➤*Asacol:* In 2 short-term (6-week), placebo-controlled clinical studies involving 245 patients, 155 of whom were randomized to *Asacol* tablets, 5 (3.2%) of the *Asacol* patients discontinued therapy because of adverse reaction, compared with 2 (2.2%) of the placebo patients. Adverse reactions leading to withdrawal from *Asacol* tablets included the following (each in 1 patient): diarrhea and colitis flare; dizziness, nausea, joint pain, and headache; rash, lethargy and constipation; dry mouth, malaise, lower back discomfort, mild disorientation, mild indigestion and cramping; headache, nausea, malaise, aching, vomiting, muscle cramps, a stuffy head, plugged ears, and fever.

Adverse reactions occurring in *Asacol*-treated patients at a frequency of 2% or more in the 2 short-term, double-blind, placebo-controlled clinical trials previously mentioned are listed in the following table. Overall, the incidence of adverse reactions seen with *Asacol* tablets was similar to placebo.

Asacol Adverse Reactions (≥ 2%)		
Adverse reaction	Placebo (n = 87)	*Asacol* (n = 152)
CNS		
Asthenia	15%	7%
Dizziness	8%	8%
Headache	36%	35%
Insomnia	0%	2%
Malaise	1%	2%
Dermatologic		
Acne	1%	2%
Pruritus	0%	3%
Rash	3%	6%
Sweating	1%	3%
GI		
Abdominal pain	14%	18%
Colitis exacerbation	0%	3%
Constipation	1%	5%
Diarrhea	9%	7%
Dyspepsia	1%	6%
Eructation	15%	16%
Flatulence	7%	3%
Nausea	15%	13%
Vomiting	2%	5%
Musculoskeletal		
Arthralgia	3%	5%
Arthritis	0%	2%
Back pain	5%	7%
Hypertonia	3%	5%
Myalgia	1%	3%
Respiratory		
Increased cough	1%	2%
Pharyngitis	9%	11%
Rhinitis	5%	5%
Miscellaneous		
Chest pain	2%	3%
Chills	2%	3%
Conjunctivitis	0%	2%
Dysmenorrhea	3%	3%
Fever	8%	6%
Flu syndrome	2%	3%
Pain	8%	14%
Peripheral edema	2%	3%

Of these adverse reactions, only rash showed a consistently higher frequency with increasing *Asacol* dose in these studies.

Other clinical trials – In a 6-month, placebo-controlled, maintenance trial involving 264 patients, 177 of whom were randomized to *Asacol* tablets, 6 (3.4%) of the *Asacol* patients discontinued therapy because of adverse reactions, compared with 4 (4.6%) of the placebo patients. Adverse reactions leading to withdrawal from *Asacol* included the following (each in 1 patient): anxiety; headache; pruritus; decreased libido; rheumatoid arthritis; and stomatitis and asthenia.

In the 6-month, placebo-controlled, maintenance trial, the incidence of adverse reactions seen with *Asacol* was similar to that seen with placebo. In addition to reactions listed in the previous table, the following adverse reactions occurred in *Asacol*-treated patients at a frequency of at least 2% in this study: abdominal enlargement, anxiety, bronchitis, ear disorder, ear pain, gastroenteritis, GI hemorrhage, infection, joint disorder, migraine, nervousness, paresthesia, rectal disorder, rectal hemorrhage, sinusitis, stool abnormalities, tenesmus, urinary frequency, vasodilation, and vision abnormalities.

In 3,342 patients in uncontrolled clinical trials, the following adverse reactions occurred at a frequency of at least 5% and appeared to increase in frequency with increasing dose: asthenia, fever, flu syndrome, pain, abdominal pain, back pain, flatulence, GI bleeding, arthralgia, and rhinitis.

➤*Pentasa:* In 2 domestic placebo-controlled trials involving more than 600 patients with ulcerative colitis, adverse reactions were fewer in *Pentasa*-treated patients than in the placebo-treated group (*Pentasa* capsules 14% vs placebo 18%) and were not dose related. Of these, only nausea and vomiting were more frequent in the *Pentasa* capsules group. Withdrawal from therapy because of adverse reactions was more common on placebo than *Pentasa* (7% vs 4%).

Reactions occurring in at least 1% of patients are shown in the following table. Generally, *Pentasa* therapy was well tolerated. The most common reactions (ie, 1% or more) were diarrhea (3.4%), headache (2%), nausea (1.8%) abdominal pain (1.7%), dyspepsia (1.6%), vomiting (1.5%), and rash (1%).

Pentasa Adverse Reactions (> 1%)		
Adverse reaction	*Pentasa* (n = 451)	Placebo (n = 173)
CNS		
Headache	2.2%	3.5%
Dermatologic		
Acne	0.2%	1.2%
Rash	1.3%	1.2%
GI		
Abdominal pain	1.1%	4%
Anorexia	1.1%	1.2%
Diarrhea	3.5%	7.5%
Melena (bloody diarrhea)	0.9%	3.5%
Nausea	3.1%	—
Nausea/vomiting	1.1%	—
Rectal urgency	0.2%	2.3%
Worsening of ulcerative colitis	0.4%	1.2%
Miscellaneous		
Fever	0.9%	1.2%

Lab test abnormalities – Clinical laboratory measurements showed no significant abnormal trends for any test, including measurement of hematologic, liver, and kidney function.

➤*Other adverse reactions (less than 1%) (Pentasa):* The following adverse reactions, presented by body system, were reported infrequently (ie, less than 1%) during domestic ulcerative colitis and Crohn disease trials. In many cases, the relationship to *Pentasa* has not been established.

Cardiovascular – Palpitations, pericarditis, vasodilation.

CNS – Asthenia, depression, dizziness, insomnia, malaise, paresthesia, somnolence.

Dermatologic – Acne, alopecia, dry skin, eczema, erythema nodosum, nail disorder, photosensitivity, pruritus, sweating, urticaria.

GI – Abdominal distention, ALT increase, anorexia, AST increase, constipation, duodenal ulcer, dysphagia, eructation, esophageal ulcer, fecal incontinence, gamma-glutamyl transpeptidase increase, GI bleeding, increased alkaline phosphatase, lactate dehydrogenase (LDH) increase, mouth ulcer, oral moniliases, pancreatitis, rectal bleeding, stool abnormalities (color or texture change), thirst.

GU – Albuminuria, amenorrhea, breast pain, hematuria, hypomenorrhea, menorrhagia, metrorrhagia, urinary frequency.

MESALAMINE — ORAL

Musculoskeletal – Arthralgia, leg cramps, myalgia.

Respiratory – Pulmonary infiltrates.

One week after completion of an 8-week ulcerative colitis study, a man 72 years of age, with no history of pulmonary problems, developed dyspnea. The patient was subsequently diagnosed with interstitial pulmonary fibrosis without eosinophilia by one health care provider and bronchiolitis obliterans with organizing pneumonitis by a second health care provider. A causal relationship between this event and mesalamine therapy has not been established.

Miscellaneous – Amylase increase, conjunctivitis, ecchymosis, edema, fever, Kawasaki-like syndrome, lichen planus, lipase increase, thrombocythemia, thrombocytopenia.

Published case reports and/or spontaneous postmarketing surveillance have described infrequent instances of pericarditis, fatal myocarditis, chest pain and T-wave abnormalities, hypersensitivity pneumonitis, pancreatitis, nephrotic syndrome, interstitial nephritis, hepatitis, aplastic anemia, pancytopenia, leukopenia, agranulocytosis, or anemia while receiving mesalamine therapy. Anemia can be a part of the clinical presentation of inflammatory bowel disease. Allergic reactions, which could involve eosinophilia, can be seen in connection with *Pentasa* therapy.

➤*Lialda:* A lower percentage of *Lialda* patients discontinued therapy because of adverse reactions compared with placebo (2.2% vs 7.3%). The most frequent adverse reaction leading to discontinuation from *Lialda* therapy was exacerbation of ulcerative colitis (0.8%).

The majority of adverse reactions in the double-blind, placebo-controlled trials were mild or moderate in severity. The percentage of patients with severe adverse reactions was higher in the placebo group (6.1% in placebo, 1.1% in 2.4 g/day, 2.2% in 4.8 g/day).

The most common severe adverse reactions were GI disorders, which were mainly symptoms associated with ulcerative colitis. Pancreatitis occurred in less than 1% of patients during clinical trials and resulted in discontinuation of therapy with *Lialda* in patients experiencing this event. The most common treatment-related adverse reactions with *Lialda* 2.4 and 4.8 g/day were headache (5.6% and 3.4%, respectively) and flatulence (4% and 2.8%, respectively).

Overall, the percentage of patients who experienced any adverse reaction was similar across treatment groups. Treatment-emergent adverse reactions occurring in *Lialda* or placebo groups at a frequency of at least 1% in 2 phase 3, 8-week, double-blind, placebo-controlled trials are listed in the following table.

***Lialda* Adverse Reactions (≥ 1%)**			
Adverse reaction	*Lialda* 2.4 g/day (n = 177)	*Lialda* 4.8 g/day (n = 179)	Placebo (n = 179)
CNS			
Headache	5.6%	3.4%	0.6%
Dermatologic			
Alopecia	0%	1.1%	0%
Pruritus	0.6%	1.1%	0%
GI			
Flatulence	4%	2.8%	2.8%
Hepatic			
Increased ALT	0.6%	1.1%	0%

➤*Other adverse reactions (Lialda):*

Cardiovascular – Hypertension, hypotension, tachycardia.

CNS – Asthenia, fatigue, somnolence, tremor.

Dermatologic – Acne, prurigo, rash, urticaria.

GI – Abdominal distention, diarrhea, pancreatitis, rectal polyp, vomiting.

Hematologic – Decreased platelet count.

Hepatic – Elevated total bilirubin.

Musculoskeletal – Arthralgia, back pain.

Respiratory – Pharyngolaryngeal pain.

Special senses – Ear pain.

Miscellaneous – Face edema, pyrexia.

➤*Postmarketing:* The following events have been reported in clinical studies, literature reports, and postmarketing use of products that contain (or have been metabolized to) mesalamine. Because many of these reactions were reported voluntarily from a population of unknown size, estimates of frequency cannot be made. These reactions have been chosen for inclusion because of their seriousness, frequency of reporting, or potential causal connection to mesalamine:

➤*Asacol*:

Cardiovascular – Myocarditis (rare), pericarditis (rare).

CNS – Confusion, depression, emotional lability, Guillain-Barré syndrome (rare), hyperesthesia, peripheral neuropathy (rare), somnolence, transverse myelitis (rare), tremor, vertigo.

Dermatologic – Alopecia, dry skin, erythema nodosum, psoriasis (rare), pyoderma gangrenosum (rare), urticaria.

GI – Anorexia, bloody diarrhea, cholecystitis, dry mouth, gastritis, increased appetite, pancreatitis, perforated peptic ulcer (rare), oral ulcers.

GU – Dysuria, epididymitis, hematuria, interstitial nephritis, menorrhagia, minimal change nephropathy, renal failure (acute and chronic) (rare), urinary urgency.

Hematologic – Agranulocytosis (rare), anemia, aplastic anemia (rare), eosinophilia, granulocytopenia, leukopenia, lymphadenopathy, thrombocytopenia.

Lab test abnormalities – Elevated alkaline phosphatase, elevated ALT or AST, elevated bilirubin, elevated serum creatinine and BUN, elevated gamma-glutamyltransferase, elevated LDH.

Musculoskeletal – Gout.

Respiratory – Asthma exacerbation, eosinophilic pneumonia, interstitial pneumonitis, pleuritis, pneumonitis.

Special senses – Blurred vision, eye pain, taste perversion, tinnitus.

Miscellaneous – Drug fever (rare), edema, facial edema, lupus-like syndrome, neck pain.

➤*Pentasa*:

Hepatic – Reports of hepatotoxicity, including elevated liver enzymes (AST, ALT, GGT, LDH, alkaline phosphatase, bilirubin), hepatitis, jaundice, cholestatic jaundice, cirrhosis, and possible hepatocellular damage including liver necrosis and liver failure. Asymptomatic elevations of liver enzymes usually resolved during continued use or with discontinuation of the drug. Some of these cases were fatal. One case of Kawasaki-like syndrome, which included hepatic function changes, was also reported.

Miscellaneous – Systemic lupus erythematosis, angioedema.

Overdosage

➤*Symptoms:* Two cases of pediatric overdosage have been reported. A 3-year-old boy who ingested 2 g of mesalamine delayed-release tablets was treated with ipecac and activated charcoal; no adverse reactions occurred. Another 3-year-old boy, approximately 16 kg, ingested an unknown amount of a maximum of 24 g of mesalamine delayed-release tablets crushed in solution (ie, uncoated mesalamine); he was treated with orange juice and activated charcoal, and experienced no adverse reactions.

Mesalamine is an aminosalicylate, and symptoms of salicylate toxicity may include confusion, diarrhea, drowsiness, headache, hyperventilation, sweating, tinnitus, vertigo, and vomiting. Severe intoxication may lead to disruption of electrolyte balance and blood pH, hyperthermia, and dehydration.

➤*Treatment:* Because mesalamine is an aminosalicylate, conventional therapy for salicylate toxicity may be beneficial in the event of acute overdosage. This includes prevention of further GI tract absorption by emesis and, if necessary, by gastric lavage. Correct fluid and electrolyte imbalance by the administration of appropriate IV therapy. Maintain adequate renal function.

Patient Information

Instruct patients to swallow tablets whole, taking care not to break the outer coating. The outer coating is designed to remain intact to protect the active ingredient and ensure mesalamine availability for action in the colon. In 2% to 3% of patients in clinical studies, intact or partially intact tablets have been reported in the stool. If this occurs repeatedly, patients should contact their health care provider.

Inform patients with ulcerative colitis that ulcerative colitis rarely remits completely and that the risk of relapse can be substantially reduced by continued administration of mesalamine therapy at a maintenance dosage.

MESALAMINE — RECTAL

Indications

➤*Enema:* For the treatment of active mild to moderate distal ulcerative colitis, proctosigmoiditis, or proctitis.

➤*Suppository:* For the treatment of active ulcerative proctitis.

Administration and Dosage

➤*General dosing considerations:* Carefully monitor renal function (ie, urinalysis, BUN, serum creatinine) in patients with preexisting renal disease and on mesalamine, especially those on concurrent oral mesalamine products.

➤*Adults:*

Enema – One rectal instillation (4 g per 60 mL) once a day, preferably at bedtime, and retained for approximately 8 hours.

While the effect may be seen within 3 to 21 days, the usual course of therapy would be from 3 to 6 weeks, depending on symptoms and sigmoidoscopic findings. Studies available to date have not assessed if the enema will modify relapse rates after the 6-week, short-term treatment.

Suppository – For the treatment of active ulcerative proctitis, one 1,000 mg suppository daily at bedtime. Retain the suppository in the rectum for 1 to 3 hours or more if possible to achieve maximum benefit.

While the effect may be seen within 3 to 21 days, the usual course of therapy is 3 to 6 weeks, depending on symptoms and sigmoidoscopic findings. Studies have suggested the suppositories will delay relapse after the 6-week, short-term treatment.

➤*Administration:*

Suppository – Detach 1 suppository from the strip of suppositories. Hold the suppository upright and carefully remove the plastic wrapper. Avoid excessive handling of the suppository, which is designed to melt at body tem-

MESALAMINE — RECTAL

perature. Insert the suppository completely into rectum with gentle pressure, pointed end first. A small amount of lubricating gel may be used on the tip of the suppository to assist insertion.

Enema – Patients should be instructed to shake the bottle well to make sure the suspension is homogeneous. The patient should remove the protective sheath from the applicator tip. Holding the bottle at the neck will not cause any of the medication to be discharged. The position most often used is obtained by lying on the left side (to facilitate migration into the sigmoid colon), with the lower leg extended and the upper right leg flexed forward for balance. An alternative is the knee-chest position. The applicator tip should be gently inserted in the rectum pointing toward the umbilicus. A steady squeezing of the bottle will discharge most of the preparation. The preparation should be used at bedtime with the objective of retaining it all night.

Note – Mesalamine enema or suppositories will cause staining of direct contact surfaces, including but not limited to fabrics, flooring, painted surfaces, marble, granite, vinyl, and enamel. Take care in choosing a suitable location for administration of this product.

➤*Storage/Stability:*

Suppository – Store below 25°C (77°F). Do not freeze. Keep away from direct heat, light, or humidity.

Enema – Store at controlled room temperature, 20° to 25°C (68° to 77°F). Once the foil-wrapped unit of 7 bottles is opened, all enemas should be used promptly as directed by the health care provider. Contents of enemas removed from the foil pouch may darken with time. Slight darkening will not affect potency; however, enemas with dark brown contents should be discarded.

Actions

➤*Pharmacology:* Sulfasalazine is split by bacterial action in the colon into sulfapyridine and mesalamine. It is thought that the mesalamine component only is therapeutically active in ulcerative colitis. The usual oral dose of sulfasalazine for active ulcerative colitis in adults is 2 to 4 g/day in divided doses. Sulfasalazine 4 g provides free mesalamine 1.6 g to the colon.

The mechanism of action of mesalamine (and sulfasalazine) is unknown, but appears to be topical rather than systemic. Although the pathology of inflammatory bowel disease is uncertain, both prostaglandins and leukotrienes have been implicated as mediators of mucosal injury and inflammation. Recently, however, the role of mesalamine as a free radical scavenger or inhibitor of tumor necrosis factor (TNF) has also been postulated. Mucosal production of arachidonic acid metabolites, both through the cyclooxygenase pathways (ie, prostanoids) and through the lipoxygenase pathways (ie, leukotrienes, hydroxyeicosatetraenoic acids), is increased in patients with chronic inflammatory bowel disease, and it is possible that mesalamine diminishes inflammation by blocking cyclooxygenase and inhibiting prostaglandin production in the colon.

➤*Pharmacokinetics:*

Absorption/Distribution –

Enema: Mesalamine is poorly absorbed from the colon. The extent of absorption is dependent upon the retention time of the drug product, and there is considerable individual variation. At steady state, approximately 10% to 30% of the daily 4 g dose can be recovered in cumulative 24-hour urine collections. Other than the kidney, the organ distribution and other bioavailability characteristics of absorbed mesalamine in humans are not known.

Suppository: In patients with ulcerative colitis treated with mesalamine 500 mg rectal suppositories administered once every 8 hours for 6 days, the mean mesalamine peak plasma concentration (C_{max}) was 353 ng/mL (coefficient of variation [CV], 55%) following the initial dose and 361 ng/mL (CV, 67%) at steady state. The mean minimum steady-state plasma concentration (C_{min}) was 89 ng/mL (CV, 89%). Absorbed mesalamine does not accumulate in the plasma.

Mesalamine administered as rectal suppositories distributes in rectal tissue to some extent. In patients with ulcerative proctitis treated with mesalamine 1,000 mg rectal suppositories, rectal tissue concentrations for mesalamine and N-acetyl-5-aminosalicylic acid have not been rigorously quantified.

Metabolism/Excretion – Mesalamine is extensively metabolized, mainly to N-acetyl-5-aminosalicylic acid. It is known that the compound undergoes acetylation, but whether this process takes place at colonic or systemic sites has not been elucidated. Mesalamine is eliminated from plasma mainly by urinary excretion, predominantly as N-acetyl-5-aminosalicylic acid.

Enema: Mesalamine is excreted principally in the feces during subsequent bowel movements. The poor colonic absorption of rectally administered mesalamine is substantiated by the low serum concentration of mesalamine and N-acetyl-5-aminosalicylic acid seen in ulcerative colitis patients after dosage with mesalamine. Under clinical conditions, patients demonstrated plasma levels 10 to 12 hours post-mesalamine administration of 2 mcg/mL, about two-thirds of which was the N-acetyl metabolite. While the elimination half-life of mesalamine is short (0.5 to 1.5 hours), the acetylated metabolite exhibits a half-life of 5 to 10 hours. In addition, steady-state plasma levels demonstrated a lack of accumulation of either free or metabolized drug during repeated daily administrations.

Suppository: In patients with ulcerative proctitis treated with 1 mesalamine 500 mg rectal suppository every 8 hours for 6 days, 12% or less of the dose was eliminated in urine as unchanged mesalamine and 8% to 77% as N-acetyl-5-aminosalicylic acid following the initial dose. At steady state, 11% or less of the dose was eliminated as unchanged mesalamine and 3% to 35% as N-acetyl-5-aminosalicylic acid. The mean elimination half-life was 5 hours (CV, 73%) for 5-aminosalicylic acid and 6 hours (CV, 63%) for mesalamine following the initial dose. At steady state, the mean elimination half-life was 7 hours for both mesalamine and N-acetyl-5-aminosalicylic acid (CV, 102% for mesalamine and 82% for N-acetyl-5-aminosalicylic acid).

Contraindications

Hypersensitivity to mesalamine, salicylates (including aspirin), or to any component of this medication (ie, suppository vehicle of vegetable fatty acid esters).

Warnings/Precautions

➤*Pancolitis:* While using mesalamine, some patients have developed pancolitis. However, extension of upper disease boundary and/or flare-ups occurred less often in the mesalamine-treated group than in the placebo-treated group.

➤*Pericarditis:* Rare instances of pericarditis have been reported with mesalamine-containing products, including sulfasalazine. Cases of pericarditis have also been reported as manifestations of inflammatory bowel disease. In the cases reported, there have been positive rechallenges with mesalamine or mesalamine-containing products. In one of these cases, however, a second rechallenge with sulfasalazine was negative throughout a 2-month follow-up. Investigate chest pain or dyspnea in patients treated with mesalamine with this information in mind. Discontinuation of mesalamine may be warranted in some cases, but rechallenge with mesalamine can be performed under careful clinical observation should the continued therapeutic need for mesalamine be present.

➤*Intolerance/Colitis exacerbation:* Worsening of colitis or symptoms of inflammatory bowel disease, including melena and hematochezia, may occur after commencing mesalamine.

Mesalamine has been implicated in the production of an acute intolerance syndrome characterized by cramping, acute abdominal pain, and bloody diarrhea, sometimes fever, headache, and a rash; in such cases, prompt withdrawal is required. Reevaluate the patient's history of sulfasalazine intolerance, if any. If a rechallenge is performed later in order to validate the hypersensitivity, carry it out under close supervision and only if clearly needed, giving consideration to reduced dosage. In the literature, one patient previously sensitive to sulfasalazine was rechallenged with 400 mg of oral mesalamine; within 8 hours, she experienced headache, fever, intensive abdominal colic, and profuse diarrhea and was readmitted as an emergency. She responded poorly to steroid therapy, and, 2 weeks later, a pancolectomy was required.

➤*Hypersensitivity reactions:* In a clinical trial, most patients who were hypersensitive to sulfasalazine were able to take mesalamine without evidence of any allergic reaction. Nevertheless, exercise caution when mesalamine is initially used in patients known to be allergic to sulfasalazine. Instruct these patients to discontinue therapy if signs of rash or fever become apparent.

There have been 2 reports in the literature of additional serious adverse reactions: 1 patient who developed leukopenia and thrombocytopenia after 7 months of treatment with one 500 mg suppository nightly, and 1 patient with rash and fever, which was a similar reaction to sulfasalazine.

➤*Sulfite sensitivity:* Mesalamine enema contains potassium metabisulfite, a sulfite that may cause allergic-type reactions, including anaphylactic symptoms and life-threatening or less severe asthmatic episodes, in certain susceptible people. The overall prevalence of sulfite sensitivity in the general population is unknown but probably low. Sulfite sensitivity is seen more frequently in asthmatic or in atopic nonasthmatic persons. Epinephrine is the preferred treatment for serious allergic or emergency situations even though epinephrine injection contains sodium or potassium metabisulfite with the previously mentioned potential liabilities. The alternatives to using epinephrine in a life-threatening situation may not be satisfactory. The presence of a sulfite(s) in epinephrine injection should not deter the administration of the drug for treatment of serious allergic or other emergency situations.

➤*Renal function impairment:* Although renal abnormalities were not noted in the clinical trials with mesalamine, the possibility of increased absorption of mesalamine and concomitant renal tubular damage, as noted in the preclinical studies, must be kept in mind. Carefully monitor patients on mesalamine enema or suppositories, especially those on concurrent oral products that liberate mesalamine and those with preexisting renal disease, with urinalysis, blood urea nitrogen (BUN), and creatinine studies.

➤*Pregnancy: Category B.*

There are no adequate and well-controlled studies in pregnant women for either sulfasalazine or mesalamine. Because animal reproduction studies are not always predictive of human response, use mesalamine during pregnancy only if clearly needed.

➤*Lactation:* It is not known whether mesalamine or its metabolite(s) are excreted in human milk. Because many drugs are excreted in human milk, exercise caution if administering mesalamine to a breast-feeding woman.

➤*Children:* Safety and efficacy in children have not been established.

➤*Elderly:* In general, dose selection for an elderly patient should be cautious, reflecting the greater frequency of decreased hepatic, renal, or cardiac function, and of concomitant disease or other drug therapy.

Mesalamine is known to be substantially excreted by the kidney, and the risk of toxic reactions to this drug may be greater in patients with renal function impairment. Because elderly patients are more likely to have decreased renal function, it may be useful to monitor renal function.

➤*Monitoring:* Carefully monitor renal function (ie, urinalysis, BUN, serum creatinine) in patients with preexisting renal disease and on mesalamine, especially those on concurrent oral mesalamine products.

Drug Interactions

Not known.

MESALAMINE — RECTAL

Adverse Reactions

➤*Enema:* Mesalamine is usually well tolerated. Most adverse reactions have been mild and transient.

Mesalamine Enema Adverse Reactions (> 0.1%)

Adverse reaction	Mesalamine (n = 815)	Mesalamine (n = 128)
CNS		
Asthenia	0.1%	3.1%
Dizziness	1.8%	2.3%
Headache	6.5%	12.5%
Insomnia	0.1%	2.3%
Tiredness/weakness/malaise/fatigue	3.4%	6.3%
Dermatologic		
Itching	1.2%	0.8%
Rash/spots	2.8%	3.1%
GI		
Abdominal pain/cramps/discomfort	8.1%	7.8%
Bloating	1.5%	1.6%
Constipation	0.98%	3.1%
Diarrhea	2.1%	3.9%
Gas/flatulence	6.1%	3.9%
Hemorrhoids	1.4%	0%
Nausea	5.8%	9.48%
Rectal pain	1.2%	0%
Rectal pain/soreness/burning	0.6%	2.3%
Musculoskeletal		
Back pain	1.45%	0.8%
Leg/joint pain	2.1%	0.8%
Miscellaneous		
Cold/sore throat	2.3%	7%
Fever	3.2%	0%
Flu	5.3%	0.8%
Hair loss	0.9%	0%
Pain on insertion of enema tip	1.4%	0.8%
Peripheral edema	0.6%	8.6%
UTI/urinary burning	0.6%	3.1%

➤*Suppository:* The most frequent adverse reactions observed in the double-blind, placebo-controlled trials are summarized in the following table.

Mesalamine Suppository Adverse Reactions (> 1%)

Adverse reaction	Mesalamine (n = 177)	Placebo (n = 84)
CNS		
Dizziness	3%	2.4%
Dermatologic		
Acne	1.2%	0%
Rash	1.2%	0%
Miscellaneous		
Colitis	1.2%	0%
Fever	1.2%	0%
Rectal pain	1.8%	0%

In the multicenter, open-label, randomized, parallel-group study comparing the 1,000 mg suppository (at bedtime) with the 500 mg suppository (twice daily), there were no differences between the 2 treatment groups in the adverse reaction profile. The most frequent adverse reactions were headache (14.4%), flatulence (5.2%), abdominal pain (5.2%), diarrhea (3.1%), and nausea (3.1%). Three patients had to discontinue medication because of a treatment-emergent adverse reaction; one of these adverse reactions (headache) was deemed possibly related to study medication.

➤*Postmarketing:*

GI – Elevated liver enzymes, pancreatitis.

GU – Infertility in men, nephrotoxicity, oligospermia

Hematologic – Agranulocytosis, aplastic anemia, eosinophilia, neutropenia, pancytopenia, thrombocytopenia (rare). Anemia, leukocytosis, and thrombocytosis can be part of the clinical presentation of inflammatory bowel disease.

Respiratory – Fibrosing alveolitis.

Miscellaneous – Mild hair loss characterized by "more hair in the comb" but no withdrawal from clinical trials has been observed in 7 of 815 mesalamine patients but none of the placebo-treated patients. In the literature, there are at least 6 additional patients with mild hair loss who received either mesalamine or sulfasalazine. Retreatment is not always associated with repeated hair loss.

Overdosage

➤*Symptoms:* There have been no documented reports of serious toxicity in humans resulting from massive overdosing with mesalamine. Under ordinary circumstances, mesalamine absorption from the colon is limited.

Patient Information

Advise patients that the enema and suppository will cause staining of direct contact surfaces, including but not limited to fabrics, flooring, painted surfaces, marble, granite, vinyl, and enamel. Take care in choosing a suitable location for administration of this product.

Advise patients to report to their health care provider any sharp abdominal pain or cramps, bloody diarrhea, fever, headache, or rash.

➤*Suppository:* Remove the foil wrapper. Avoid excessive handling of the suppository, which is designed to melt at body temperature. Insert completely into rectum with gentle pressure, pointed end first.

➤*Enema:* Shake the bottle well to make sure the suspension is homogeneous. The patient should remove the protective sheath from the applicator tip. Holding the bottle at the neck will not cause any of the medicine to be discharged. The position most often used is obtained by lying on the left side (to facilitate migration into the sigmoid colon), with the lower leg extended and the upper right leg flexed forward for balance. An alternative is the knee-chest position. The applicator tip should be gently inserted in the rectum pointing toward the umbilicus. A steady squeezing of the bottle will discharge most of the preparation. The preparation should be taken at bedtime with the objective of retaining it all night.

Inform patients that the enema may contain sulfites and may cause an allergic reaction in some patients.

OLSALAZINE SODIUM

Rx	**Dipentum** (UCB Pharma)	**Capsules; oral:** 250 mg	(Dipentum 250 mg). Beige. In 100s and 500s.

OLSALAZINE SODIUM — ORAL

Indications

➤*Ulcerative colitis:* Maintenance of remission of ulcerative colitis in patients who are intolerant of sulfasalazine.

Administration and Dosage

➤*Adults:*

Ulcerative colitis – 1 g/day in 2 divided doses.

➤*Administration:* Take with food.

➤*Storage/Stability:* Store at 25°C (77°F). Excursions are permitted to 15° to 30°C (59° to 86°F).

Actions

➤*Pharmacology:* The conversion of olsalazine to mesalamine (5-ASA) in the colon is similar to that of sulfasalazine, which is converted into sulfapyridine and mesalamine. It is thought that the mesalamine component is therapeutically active in ulcerative colitis. The usual dose of sulfasalazine for maintenance of remission in patients with ulcerative colitis is 2 g daily, which would provide approximately 0.8 g of mesalamine to the colon. More than 0.9 g of mesalamine would usually be made available in the colon from 1 g of olsalazine.

The mechanism of action of mesalamine (and sulfasalazine) is unknown, but appears to be topical rather than systemic. Mucosal production of arachidonic acid (AA) metabolites, both through the cyclooxygenase pathways (ie, prostanoids) and through the lipoxygenase pathways (ie, leukotrienes [LTs] and hydroxyelcosatetraenoic acids [HETEs]) is increased in patients with chronic inflammatory bowel disease, and it is possible that mesalamine diminishes inflammation by blocking cyclooxygenase and inhibiting prostaglandin (PG) production in the colon.

➤*Pharmacokinetics:*

Absorption – After oral administration, olsalazine has limited systemic bioavailability. Based on oral dosing studies, approximately 2.4% of a single 1 g oral dose is absorbed.

OLSALAZINE SODIUM — ORAL

Distribution – The pharmacokinetics of olsalazine are similar in both healthy volunteers and in patients with ulcerative colitis. Maximum serum concentrations of olsalazine appear after approximately 1 hour, and are low (eg, 1.6 to 6.2 mcmol/L) even after a 1 g single dose. Olsalazine has a very short serum half-life, approximately 0.9 hours. Olsalazine is greater than 99% bound to plasma proteins. It does not interfere with protein binding of warfarin.

Total recovery of oral ^{14}C-labeled olsalazine in animals and humans ranges from 90% to 97%.

Metabolism – Approximately 0.1% of an oral dose of olsalazine is metabolized in the liver to olsalazine-O-sulfate (olsalazine-S). Olsalazine-S, in contrast to olsalazine, has a half-life of 7 days. Olsalazine-S accumulates to steady state within 2 to 3 weeks.

Patients on daily doses of 1 g olsalazine for 2 to 4 years show a stable plasma concentration of olsalazine-S (3.3 to 12.4 mcmol/L). Olsalazine-S is greater than 99% bound to plasma proteins. Its long half-life is mainly due to slow dissociation from the protein binding site. Less than 1% of both olsalazine and olsalazine-S appears undissociated in plasma.

5-aminosalicylic acid (5-ASA): Serum concentrations of 5-ASA are detected after 4 to 8 hours. The peak levels of 5-ASA after an oral dose of 1 g olsalazine are low (ie, 0 to 4.3 mcmol/L). Of the total 5-ASA found in the urine, more than 90% is in the form of N-acetyl-5-ASA (Ac-5-ASA). Only small amounts of 5-ASA are detected.

N-acetyl-5-ASA (Ac-5-ASA), the major metabolite of 5-ASA found in plasma and urine, is acetylated (deactivated) in at least 2 sites, the colonic epithelium and the liver. Ac-5-ASA is found in the serum, with peak values of 1.7 to 8.7 mcmol/L after a single 1 g dose.

Excretion – Less than 1% of olsalazine is recovered in the urine. The remaining 98% to 99% of an oral dose will reach the colon where each molecule is rapidly converted into 2 molecules of 5-aminosalicylic acid (5-ASA) by colonic bacteria and the low prevailing redox potential found in this environment. The liberated 5-ASA is absorbed slowly resulting in very high local concentrations in the colon.

Approximately 20% of the total 5-ASA is recovered in the urine, where it is found almost exclusively as Ac-5-ASA. The remaining 5-ASA is partially acetylated and is excreted in the feces. From fecal dialysis, the concentration of 5-ASA in the colon following olsalazine has been calculated to be 18 to 49 mmol/L. No accumulation of 5-ASA or Ac-5-ASA in plasma has been detected. 5-ASA and Ac-5-ASA are 74% and 81%, respectively, bound to plasma proteins.

Contraindications

Hypersensitivity to salicylates.

Warnings/Precautions

➤*Diarrhea:* Overall, approximately 17% of subjects receiving olsalazine in clinical studies reported diarrhea sometime during therapy. This diarrhea resulted in withdrawal of treatment in 6% of patients. This diarrhea appears to be dose related, although it may be difficult to distinguish from the underlying symptoms of the disease.

➤*Exacerbation of colitis symptoms:* Exacerbation of the symptoms of colitis thought to have been caused by mesalamine or sulfasalazine has been noted.

➤*Renal function impairment:* Although renal abnormalities were not reported in clinical trials with olsalazine, there have been rare reports from postmarketing experience. Therefore, the possibility of renal tubular damage due to absorbed mesalamine or its n-acetylated metabolite must be kept in mind, particularly for patients with preexisting renal disease. In these patients, monitoring with urinalysis, BUN, and creatinine determinations is advised.

➤*Pregnancy:* Category C.

Olsalazine has been shown to produce fetal developmental toxicity as indicated by reduced fetal weights, retarded ossifications, and immaturity of the fetal visceral organs when given during organogenesis to pregnant rats in doses 5 to 20 times the human dose (100 to 400 mg/kg). There are no adequate and well-controlled studies in pregnant women. Olsalazine should be used during pregnancy only if the potential benefit justifies the potential risk to the fetus.

➤*Lactation:* Oral administration of olsalazine to lactating rats in doses 5 to 20 times the human dose produced growth retardation in their pups. It is not known whether this drug is excreted in human milk. Because many drugs are excreted in human milk, caution should be exercised when olsalazine is administered to a breast-feeding woman.

➤*Children:* Safety and efficacy in children have not been established.

➤*Elderly:* In general, elderly patients should be treated with caution due to the greater frequency of decreased hepatic, renal, or cardiac function, coexistence of other diseases, as well as concomitant drug therapy.

➤*Monitoring:* Monitoring with urinalysis, BUN, and creatinine determinations is advised in patients with preexisting renal disease.

Drug Interactions

➤*Warfarin:* Increased prothrombin time in patients taking concomitant warfarin has been reported.

Adverse Reactions

Olsalazine Adverse Reactions Resulting in Withdrawal from Controlled Studies

Adverse reaction	Olsalazine (n = 441)	Placebo (n = 208)
Diarrhea/loose stools	26 (5.9%)	10 (4.8%)
Nausea	3	2
Abdominal pain	5 (1.1%)	0
Rash/itching	5 (1.1%)	0
Headache	3	0
Heartburn	2	0
Rectal bleeding	1	0
Insomnia	1	0
Dizziness	1	0
Anorexia	1	0
Light-headedness	1	0
Depression	1	0
Miscellaneous	4 (0.9%)	3 (1.4%)
Total number of patients withdrawn	46 (10.4%)	14 (6.7%)

Olsalazine Adverse Reactions in Ulcerative Colitis Patients in Double-Blind Controlled Studies

Adverse reaction	Olsalazine (n = 441)	Placebo (n = 208)
GI		
Abdominal pain/cramps	10.1%	7.2%
Anorexia	1.3%	1.9%
Bloating	1.5%	1.4%
Diarrhea	11.1%	6.7%
Dyspepsia	4%	4.3%
Increased blood in stools	-	3.4%
Nausea	5%	3.9%
Stomatitis	1%	-
Vomiting	1%	-
CNS		
Fatigue/drowsiness/lethargy	1.8%	2.9%
Headache	5%	4.8%
Insomnia	-	2.4%
Vertigo/dizziness	1%	-
Psychiatric		
Depression	1.5%	-
Dermatologic		
Itching	1.3%	-
Rash	2.3%	1.4%
Musculoskeletal		
Arthralgia/joint pain	4%	2.9%
Miscellaneous		
Upper respiratory tract infection	1.5%	-

➤*Other clinical trials:* Over 2500 patients have been treated with olsalazine in various controlled and uncontrolled clinical studies. In these as well as in the postmarketing experience, olsalazine was administered mainly to patients intolerant to sulfasalazine. There have been rare reports of the following adverse reactions in patients receiving olsalazine. These were often difficult to distinguish from possible symptoms of the underlying disease or from the effects of prior or concomitant therapy. A causal relationship to the drug has not been demonstrated for some of these reactions.

Cardiovascular – Pericarditis; second-degree heart block; interstitial pulmonary disease; hypertension; orthostatic hypotension; peripheral edema; chest pains; tachycardia; palpitations; bronchospasm; shortness of breath.

A patient who developed thyroid disease 9 days after starting olsalazine was given propranolol and radioactive iodine and subsequently developed shortness of breath and nausea. The patient died 5 days later with signs and symptoms of acute diffuse myocarditis.

CNS – Chills; depression; fatigue; headache; insomnia; irritability; mood swings; paresthesia; tremors; fever; rigors; vertigo; dizziness; drowsiness; lethargy.

Dermatologic – Erythema nodosum; photosensitivity; erythema; hot flashes; rash/itching; alopecia.

GI – Pancreatitis; diarrhea with dehydration; increased blood in stool; rectal bleeding; flare in symptoms; rectal discomfort; epigastric discomfort; flatulence.

In a double-blind, placebo-controlled study, increased frequency and severity of diarrhea were reported in patients randomized to olsalazine 500 mg twice daily with concomitant pelvic radiation.

GU – Frequency; dysuria; hematuria; proteinuria; nephrotic syndrome; interstitial nephritis; impotence; menorrhagia.

OLSALAZINE SODIUM — ORAL

Hematologic – Leukopenia; neutropenia; lymphopenia; eosinophilia; thrombocytopenia; anemia; hemolytic anemia; reticulocytosis.

Hepatic – Rare cases of granulomatous hepatitis and nonspecific, reactive hepatitis have been reported in patients receiving olsalazine. Additionally, a patient developed mild cholestatic hepatitis during treatment with sulfasalazine and experienced the same symptoms 2 weeks later after the treatment was changed to olsalazine. Withdrawal of olsalazine led to complete recovery in these cases.

Lab test abnormalities – ALT or AST elevated beyond the normal range.

Musculoskeletal – Muscle cramps.

Respiratory – Upper respiratory tract infection.

Special senses – Tinnitus; dry mouth; dry eyes; watery eyes; blurred vision.

➤*Postmarketing reports:* The following events have been identified during postapproval use of products that contain (or are metabolized to) mesalamine in clinical practice. Because they are reported voluntarily from a population of unknown size, estimates of frequency cannot be made. These events have been chosen for inclusion due to a combination of seriousness, frequency of reporting, or potential causal connection to mesalamine.

Reports of hepatotoxicity, including elevated liver function tests (AST, ALT, GGT, LDH, alkaline phosphatase, bilirubin), jaundice, cholestatic jaundice, cirrhosis, and possible hepatocellular damage including liver necrosis and liver failure. Some of these cases were fatal. One case of Kawasaki-like syndrome that included hepatic function changes was also reported.

Overdosage

Symptoms of acute toxicity were decreased motor activity and diarrhea in all species tested and in addition, vomiting in dogs.

➤*Animal toxicology:* Preclinical subacute and chronic toxicity studies in rats have shown the kidney to be the major target organ of olsalazine toxicity. At an oral daily dose of greater than or equal to 400 mg/kg, olsalazine treatment produced nephritis and tubular necrosis in a 4-week study; interstitial nephritis and tubular calcinosis in a 6-month study, and renal fibrosis, mineralization, and transitional cell hyperplasia in a 1-year study.

Patient Information

Patients should be instructed to take olsalazine with food. The drug should be taken in evenly divided doses. Patients should be informed that approximately 17% of subjects receiving olsalazine during clinical studies reported diarrhea sometime during therapy. If diarrhea occurs, patients should contact their physician.

BALSALAZIDE DISODIUM

BALSALAZIDE DISODIUM

Rx	**Balsalazide Disodium** (Various, eg, Apotex USA, Mylan, Roxane)	**Capsule; oral:** 750 mg	Equiv. to mesalamine 267 mg. In 30s, 280s, 350s, 500s, and blister packs of 100s.
Rx	**Colazal** (Salix)		Equiv. to mesalamine 267 mg. ≈ 86 mg sodium. (CZ). Beige. In 280s and 500s.

BALSALAZIDE DISODIUM — ORAL

Indications

➤*Ulcerative colitis:* For the treatment of active mild to moderate ulcerative colitis in patients 5 years of age and older.

Safety and efficacy of balsalazide beyond 8 weeks in children 5 to 17 years of age and 12 weeks in adults have not been established.

Administration and Dosage

➤*Adults:*

Ulcerative colitis – 2,250 mg (3 capsules) 3 times daily (6.75 g/day) for up to 8 weeks. Some patients in the adult clinical trials required treatment for up to 12 weeks.

➤*Children:*

Ulcerative colitis –

5 to 17 years of age: 2,250 mg (3 capsules) 3 times daily (6.75 g/day) for up to 8 weeks, or 750 mg (1 capsule) 3 times daily (2.25 g/day) for up to 8 weeks.

➤*Administration:* For patients who have difficulty swallowing, administer by carefully opening the capsule and sprinkling the contents on applesauce. The entire drug/applesauce mixture should be swallowed immediately; the contents may be chewed, if necessary, because they are not coated beads/granules. Do not store the drug/applesauce mixture for future use.

If the capsules are opened for sprinkling, color variation of the powder inside the capsules ranges from orange to yellow and is expected because of color variation of the active pharmaceutical ingredient.

Teeth and/or tongue staining may occur in some patients who sprinkle balsalazide on applesauce.

➤*Storage/Stability:* Store between 20° to 25° C (68° to 77°F); excursions are permitted between 15° and 30°C (59° and 86°F).

Actions

➤*Pharmacology:* Balsalazide is delivered intact to the colon, where it is cleaved by bacterial azoreduction to release equimolar quantities of mesalamine, which is the therapeutically active portion of the molecule, and the 4-aminobenzoyl-β-alanine carrier moiety. The carrier moiety released when balsalazide is cleaved is only minimally absorbed and is largely inert.

The mechanism of action of 5-aminosalicylic acid is unknown but appears to be local to the colonic mucosa rather than systemic. Mucosal production of arachidonic acid metabolites through the cyclooxygenase pathways (ie, prostanoids) and through the lipoxygenase pathways (ie, leukotrienes and hydroxyeicosatetraenoic acids) is increased in patients with chronic inflammatory bowel disease. It is possible that 5-aminosalicylic acid diminishes inflammation by blocking production of arachidonic acid metabolites in the colon.

➤*Pharmacokinetics:*

Absorption – Balsalazide is insoluble in acid and is designed to be delivered to the colon as the intact prodrug. Upon reaching the colon, bacterial azoreductases cleave the compound to release equimolar quantities of 5-aminosalicylic acid (the therapeutically active portion of the molecule) and 4-aminobenzoyl-β-alanine. 5-aminosalicylic acid is further metabolized to yield N-acetyl-5-aminosalicylic acid, a second key metabolite.

In a study of adults with ulcerative colitis, patients received balsalazide 1.5 g twice daily for longer than 1 year. Systemic drug exposure, based on mean area under the curve (AUC) values, was up to 60 times greater (8 to 480 ng•h/mL) when compared with healthy subjects who received the same dose.

Effect of food: The plasma pharmacokinetics of balsalazide and its key metabolites from a crossover study in healthy volunteers are summarized in the following table. In this study, a single oral dose of balsalazide 2.25 g was administered to healthy volunteers as intact capsules (3 × 750 mg) under fasting conditions, as intact capsules (3 × 750 mg) after a high-fat meal, and unencapsulated (3 × 750 mg) as sprinkles on applesauce.

Plasma Pharmacokinetics for Balsalazide and Key Metabolites Following a Fast, a High-Fat Meal, and Contents Sprinkled on Applesauce (Mean ± Standard Deviation)

	Fasting (n = 17)	High-fat meal (n = 17)	Sprinkled (n = 17)
C_{max}[a] (mcg/mL)			
Balsalazide	0.51 ± 0.32	0.45 ± 0.39	0.21 ± 0.12
5-aminosalicylic acid	0.22 ± 0.12	0.11 ± 0.136	0.29 ± 0.17
N-acetyl-5-aminosalicylic acid	0.88 ± 0.39	0.64 ± 0.534	1.04 ± 0.57
AUC_{last} (mcg•h/mL)			
Balsalazide	1.35 ± 0.73	1.52 ± 1.01	0.87 ± 0.48
5-aminosalicylic acid	2.59 ± 1.46	2.1 ± 2.58	2.99 ± 1.7
N-acetyl-5-aminosalicylic acid	17.8 ± 8.14	17.7 ± 13.7	20 ± 11.4
T_{max}[a] (h)			
Balsalazide	0.8 ± 0.85	1.2 ± 1.11	1.6 ± 0.44
5-aminosalicylic acid	8.2 ± 1.98	22 ± 8.23	8.7 ± 1.99
N-acetyl-5-aminosalicylic acid	9.9 ± 2.49	20.2 ± 8.94	10.8 ± 5.39

[a] C_{max} = maximal drug concentration; T_{max} = time of maximal concentration.

A relatively low systemic exposure was observed under all 3 administered conditions (fasting, fed with high-fat meal, sprinkled on applesauce), which reflects the variable, but minimal absorption of balsalazide and its metabolites. The data indicate that C_{max} and AUC_{last} were lower, while T_{max} was markedly prolonged under fed (high-fat meal), compared with fasted, conditions. Moreover, the data suggest that dosing balsalazide as a sprinkle or as a capsule provides highly variable, but relatively similar, mean pharmacokinetic parameter values. No inference can be made as to how the systemic exposure differences of balsalazide and its metabolites in this study might predict the clinical efficacy under different dosing conditions (ie, fasted, fed with high-fat meal, or sprinkled on applesauce) because clinical efficacy after balsalazide administration is presumed to be primarily caused by the local effects of 5-aminosalicylic acid on the colonic mucosa.

Distribution – The binding of balsalazide to human plasma proteins was at least 99%.

Metabolism – The products of the azoreduction of this compound, 5-aminosalicylic acid and 4-aminobenzoyl-β-alanine, and their N-acetylated metabolites have been identified in plasma, urine, and feces.

Excretion – Following single-dose administration of balsalazide 2.25 g (three 750 mg capsules) under fasting conditions in healthy subjects, mean urinary recovery of balsalazide, 5-aminosalicylic acid, and N-acetyl-5-aminosalicylic acid was 0.2%, 0.22%, and 10.2%, respectively.

In a multiple-dose study in healthy subjects receiving a dosage of 2 balsalazide 750 mg capsules twice daily (3 g/day) for 10 days, mean urinary recovery of balsalazide, 5-aminosalicylic acid, and N-acetyl-5-aminosalicylic acid was 0.1%, 0%, and 11.3%, respectively. During this study, subjects received their morning dose 0.5 hours after being fed a standard meal, and subjects received their evening dose 2 hours after being fed a standard meal.

BALSALAZIDE DISODIUM — ORAL

In a study with 10 healthy volunteers, 65% of a single dose of balsalazide 2.25 g was recovered as 5-aminosalicylic acid, 4-aminobenzoyl-β-alanine, and the N-acetylated metabolites in feces, while less than 1% of the dose was recovered as parent compound.

In a study that examined the disposition of balsalazide in patients who were taking balsalazide 3 to 6 g daily for more than 1 year and were in remission from ulcerative colitis, less than 1% of an oral dose was recovered as intact balsalazide in the urine. Less than 4% of the dose was recovered as 5-aminosalicylic acid, while virtually no 4-aminobenzoyl-β-alanine was detected in urine. The mean urinary recovery of N-acetyl-5-aminosalicylic acid and N-acetyl-4-aminobenzoyl-β-alanine comprised less than 16% to less than 12% of the balsalazide dose, respectively. No fecal recovery studies were performed in this population.

All pharmacokinetic studies with balsalazide are characterized by large variability in the plasma concentration versus time profiles for balsalazide and its metabolites, thus half-life estimates of these analytes are indeterminate.

Special populations –

Children: In studies of children with active mild to moderate ulcerative colitis receiving 3 balsalazide 750 mg capsules 3 times daily (6.75 g/day) for 8 weeks, steady state was reached within 2 weeks, as observed in adult patients. Likewise, the pharmacokinetics of balsalazide, 5-aminosalicylic acid, and N-acetyl-5-aminosalicylic acid were characterized by very large interpatient variability, which is also similar to that seen in adult patients.

The prodrug moiety, balsalazide, appeared to exhibit dose-independent (ie, dose-linear) kinetics in children, and the systemic exposure parameters (C_{max} and $AUC_{0\ to\ 8}$) increased in an almost dose-proportional fashion after the 6.75 g/day versus the 2.25 g/day doses. However, the absolute magnitude of these exposure parameters was greater, relative to adults. The C_{max} and $AUC_{0\ to\ 8}$ observed in children were 26% and 102% greater than those observed in adult patients at the 6.75 g/day dosage level. In contrast, the systemic exposure parameters for the active metabolites, 5-aminosalicylic acid and N-acetyl-5-aminosalicylic acid, in children increased in a less than dose-proportional manner after the 6.75 g/day dose versus the 2.25 g/day dose. Additionally, the magnitude of these exposure parameters was decreased for both metabolites relative to adults. For the metabolite of key safety concern from a systemic exposure perspective, 5-aminosalicylic acid, the C_{max} and $AUC_{0\ to\ 8}$ observed in children were 67% and 64% lower than those observed in adult patients at the 6.75 g/day dosage level. Likewise, for N-acetyl-5-aminosalicylic acid, the C_{max} and $AUC_{0\ to\ 8}$ observed in children were 68% and 55% lower than those observed in adult patients at the 6.75 g/day dosage level.

Contraindications

Hypersensitivity to salicylates, any of the components of balsalazide, or balsalazide metabolites.

Warnings/Precautions

➤*Ulcerative colitis exacerbation:* In the adult clinical trials, 3 out of 259 patients reported exacerbation of the symptoms of ulcerative colitis. In clinical trials, 4 out of 68 children reported exacerbation of the symptoms of ulcerative colitis.

Observe patients closely for worsening of these symptoms while on treatment.

➤*Pyloric stenosis:* Patients with pyloric stenosis may have prolonged gastric retention of balsalazide.

➤*Renal toxicity:* Renal toxicity has been observed in animals and patients given other mesalamine products. Exercise caution when administering balsalazide to patients with known renal function impairment or a history of renal disease.

➤*Pregnancy: Category B.*

There are no adequate and well-controlled studies in pregnant women. Because animal reproduction studies are not always predictive of human response, use this drug during pregnancy only if clearly needed.

➤*Lactation:* It is not known whether balsalazide is excreted in human milk. Because many drugs are excreted in human milk, exercise caution when administering balsalazide to a breast-feeding woman.

➤*Children:* Safety and efficacy of balsalazide in children younger than 5 years of age have not been established. A clinical trial of 68 patients 5 to 17 years of age has been conducted comparing 2 doses of balsalazide (6.75 and 2.25 g/day). Based on limited data available, dosing can be initiated at either 6.75 or 2.25 g/day.

➤*Monitoring:* Monitor colitis symptoms, including rectal bleeding, stool frequency and character, abdominal pain, and overall functional status.

Drug Interactions

None known.

Adverse Reactions

➤*Adults:* In 4 controlled clinical trials, patients receiving balsalazide 6.75 g/day most frequently reported the following reactions: headache (8%); abdominal pain (6%); diarrhea, nausea (5%); arthralgia, respiratory tract infection, vomiting (4%). Withdrawal from therapy because of adverse reactions was comparable among patients taking balsalazide and placebo.

Adverse reactions reported by 1% or more of patients who participated in the 4 well-controlled phase 3 trials are presented by the treatment group in the following table.

Balsalazide Adverse Reactions (≥ 1%)[a]		
Adverse reaction	Balsalazide 6.75 g/day (n = 259)	Placebo (n = 35)
CNS		
Fatigue	2%	0%
Insomnia	2%	0%
GI		
Abdominal pain	6%	3%
Anorexia	2%	0%
Constipation	1%	0%
Cramps	1%	0%
Diarrhea	5%	3%
Dry mouth	1%	0%
Dyspepsia	2%	0%
Flatulence	2%	0%
Musculoskeletal		
Arthralgia	4%	0%
Myalgia	1%	0%
Respiratory		
Coughing	2%	0%
Pharyngitis	2%	0%
Rhinitis	2%	0%
Miscellaneous		
Fever	2%	0%
Flu-like disorder	1%	0%
Urinary tract infection	1%	0%

[a] Adverse reactions occurring in at least 1% of balsalazide patients that were less frequent than placebo for the same event were not included in the table.

The number of placebo patients is too small for valid comparisons. Some adverse reactions (eg, abdominal pain, fatigue, nausea) were reported more frequently in women than in men. Abdominal pain, anemia, and rectal bleeding can be part of the clinical presentation of ulcerative colitis.

➤*Children:* In a clinical trial in 68 children 5 to 17 years of age with active mild to moderate ulcerative colitis who received balsalazide 6.75 or 2.25 g/day for 8 weeks, the most frequently reported adverse reactions were as follows: headache (15%); upper abdominal pain (13%); abdominal pain (12%); vomiting (10%); diarrhea (9%); nasopharyngitis, pyrexia, ulcerative colitis (6%).

One patient who received balsalazide 6.75 g/day and 3 patients who received balsalazide 2.25 g/day discontinued treatment because of adverse reactions. In addition, 2 patients in each dose group discontinued the study because of lack of efficacy.

Adverse reactions reported by 3% or more of children within either treatment group in the phase 3 trial are presented in the following table.

Balsalazide Adverse Reactions in Children (≥ 3%)			
Adverse reaction	Balsalazide 6.75 g/day (n = 33)	Balsalazide 2.25 g/day (n = 35)	Total (N = 68)
CNS			
Fatigue	6%	3%	4%
Headache	15%	14%	15%
GI			
Abdominal pain	12%	11%	12%
Abdominal pain, upper	9%	17%	13%
Diarrhea	6%	11%	9%
Hematochezia	0%	9%	4%
Nausea	0%	9%	4%
Stomatitis	0%	6%	3%
Ulcerative colitis	6%	6%	6%
Vomiting	3%	17%	10%
Respiratory			
Cough	0%	6%	3%
Nasopharyngitis	9%	3%	6%
Pharyngolaryngeal pain	6%	0%	3%
Miscellaneous			
Dysmenorrhea	6%	0%	3%
Influenza	3%	6%	4%
Pyrexia	0%	11%	6%

➤*Postmarketing:* The following adverse reactions have been identified during postapproval use in clinical practice of products that contain (or are

BALSALAZIDE DISODIUM — ORAL

metabolized to) mesalamine. Because they are reported voluntarily from a population of unknown size, it is not always possible to reliably estimate their frequency or establish a causal relationship to drug exposure. These adverse reactions have been chosen for inclusion because of a combination of seriousness, frequency of reporting, or potential causal connection to mesalamine.

Postmarketing adverse reactions of hepatotoxicity have been reported, including elevated liver function tests (AST, ALT, gamma-glutamyl transferase, lactate dehydrogenase, alkaline phosphatase, bilirubin), jaundice, cholestatic jaundice, cirrhosis, and hepatocellular damage, including liver necrosis and liver failure. Some of these cases were fatal; however, no fatalities associated with these adverse reactions were reported in balsalazide clinical trials. One case of Kawasaki-like syndrome, which included hepatic function changes, was also reported; however, this adverse reaction was not reported in balsalazide clinical trials.

Several cases of alopecia in patients taking balsalazide have been reported.

Overdosage

➤*Symptoms:* No case of overdose has occurred with balsalazide. A boy 3 years of age was reported to have ingested 2 g of another mesalamine product. He was treated with ipecac and activated charcoal with no adverse reactions.

➤*Treatment:* If an overdose occurs with balsalazide use, initiate supportive treatment, with particular attention to correction of electrolyte abnormalities.

Patient Information

Instruct patients not to take balsalazide if they have a hypersensitivity to salicylates (eg, aspirin). Instruct patients to contact their health care provider under the following circumstances: if they experience a worsening of ulcerative colitis symptoms, if they are diagnosed with pyloric stenosis (balsalazide capsules may be slow to pass through their digestive tract), or if they are diagnosed with renal function impairment. Damage to the kidney has been observed in people given medications similar to balsalazide.

Inform patients that in adult clinical trials, the most common adverse reactions were headache, abdominal pain, arthralgia, diarrhea, nausea, vomiting, and respiratory tract infection. In children, the most common adverse reactions were abdominal pain, diarrhea, headache, nasopharyngitis, pyrexia, ulcerative colitis, and vomiting.

Inform patients that this listing of adverse reactions is not complete and not all adverse reactions can be anticipated. If appropriate, discuss a more comprehensive list of adverse reactions with patients.

Advise the patient to swallow the balsalazide capsule whole. Advise the patient that balsalazide capsules may also be opened and the contents sprinkled on applesauce. The entire drug/applesauce mixture should be swallowed immediately; the contents may be chewed, if necessary. Advise the patient not to save the drug/applesauce mixture for future use.

Inform the patient that the usual course of therapy is 8 to 12 weeks.

SULFASALAZINE

SULFASALAZINE

Rx	**Sulfasalazine** (Various, eg, Mutual Pharm, Watson)	**Tablets:** 500 mg	In 50s, 100s, 500s, and 1,000s.
Rx	**Azulfidine** (Pfizer)		(101 KPh). Gold, scored. In 100s, 300s, and UD 100s.
Rx	**Sulfasalazine** (Greenstone)	**Tablets, delayed-release:** 500 mg	(104). Gold, elliptical. Enteric coated. In 100s and 300s.
Rx	**Azulfidine EN-tabs** (Pfizer)		(102 KPh). Gold, elliptical. Enteric coated. In 100s and 300s.

SULFASALAZINE — ORAL

Indications

➤*Tablets and delayed-release tablets:* Treatment of mild-to-moderate ulcerative colitis, and as adjunctive therapy in severe ulcerative colitis, and for the prolongation of the remission period between acute attacks of ulcerative colitis.

➤*Delayed-release tablets:* Treatment of patients with rheumatoid arthritis who have responded inadequately to salicylates or other nonsteroidal anti-inflammatory drugs (NSAIDs) (eg, an insufficient therapeutic response to, or intolerance of, an adequate trial of full doses of 1 or more nonsteroidal anti-inflammatory drugs).

Sulfasalazine delayed-release tablets are also indicated in the treatment of pediatric patients with polyarticular-course juvenile rheumatoid arthritis who have responded inadequately to salicylates or other NSAIDs.

Sulfasalazine enteric-coated, delayed-release tablets are particularly indicated in patients with ulcerative colitis who cannot take uncoated sulfasalazine tablets because of GI intolerance, and in whom there is evidence that this intolerance is not primarily the result of high blood levels of sulfapyridine and its metabolites (eg, patients experiencing nausea and vomiting with the first few doses of the drug, or patients in whom a reduction in dosage does not alleviate the adverse GI effects).

In patients with rheumatoid arthritis or juvenile rheumatoid arthritis, continue rest and physiotherapy as indicated. Unlike anti-inflammatory drugs, sulfasalazine delayed-release tablets do not produce an immediate response. Concurrent treatment with analgesics or NSAIDs is recommended at least until the effect of sulfasalazine delayed-release tablets is apparent.

➤*Off-label uses:*

Multiple sclerosis – [5] = Poor documentation. Sulfasalazine has been studied for the treatment of multiple sclerosis (MS) in a randomized, controlled trial. Based on the results of this study, it was determined that sulfasalazine provides no therapeutic benefit in patients with MS. Its use for this indication is not recommended.

Psoriasis – [2] = Fair documentation. According to the American Academy of Dermatology guidelines, methotrexate, cyclosporine, and acitretin are considered first-line systemic agents for psoriasis, but sulfasalazine may be an appropriate alternative for certain patients. Sulfasalazine is contraindicated in patients with porphyria, urinary or intestinal obstruction, and hypersensitivity to sulfasalazine, its metabolites, sulfonamides, or salicylates.

Other possible off-label uses – Ankylosing spondylitis; Crohn disease; granulomatous colitis; regional enteritis.

Administration and Dosage

➤*General dosing considerations:* If symptoms of gastric intolerance (eg, anorexia, nausea, vomiting) occur after the first few doses of sulfasalazine, they are probably due to increased serum levels of total sulfapyridine, and may be alleviated by halving the daily dose of sulfasalazine and subsequently increasing it gradually over several days. If gastric intolerance continues, stop the drug for 5 to 7 days, then reintroduce at a lower daily dose.

Sulfasalazine enteric-coated delayed-release tablets are particularly indicated in patients who cannot take uncoated sulfasalazine tablets because of GI intolerance (eg, anorexia, nausea).

Some patients may be sensitive to treatment with sulfasalazine. Various desensitization-like regimens have been reported to be effective. See Desensitization.

The response of acute ulcerative colitis to sulfasalazine can be evaluated by clinical criteria, including the presence of fever, weight changes, and degree and frequency of diarrhea and bleeding, as well as by sigmoidoscopy and the evaluation of biopsy samples. It is often necessary to continue medication even when clinical symptoms, including diarrhea, have been controlled.

➤*Adults:*

Rheumatoid arthritis –

Delayed-release tablets:

• *Initial dosage* – 0.5 to 1 g daily.

• *Maintenance dosage* – 2 g/day in 2 evenly divided doses. A suggested dosing schedule is given below.

Sulfasalazine Dosing Schedule for Adult Rheumatoid Arthritis		
	Number of sulfasalazine delayed-release tablets	
Week of treatment	Morning	Evening
1	-	1
2	1	1
3	1	2
4	2	2

• *Dosage adjustment* – Consideration can be given to increasing the dose to 3 g/day if the clinical response after 12 weeks is inadequate. Careful monitoring is recommended for doses over 2 g/day.

Ulcerative colitis –

Initial dosage: 3 to 4 g/day in evenly divided doses with dosage intervals not exceeding 8 hours. It may be advisable to initiate therapy with a lower dosage (eg, 1 to 2 g/day) to reduce possible GI intolerance.

Maintenance dosage: 2 g/day. If doses exceeding 4 g/day are required to achieve the desired therapeutic effect, keep in mind the increased risk of toxicity.

Dosage adjustment: When endoscopic examination confirms satisfactory improvement, reduce dosage of sulfasalazine to a maintenance level. If diarrhea recurs, increase dosage to previously effective levels.

Off-label dosing –

Psoriasis: [2] = Fair documentation. The recommended starting dosage is 500 mg orally twice daily. Dosages may be increased up to a total of 3 to 4 g/day as tolerated. Because there are no known cumulative toxicities, the duration of use is for as long as needed.

SULFASALAZINE — ORAL

➤*Children:*

Juvenile rheumatoid arthritis (polyarticular course) –

Delayed-release tablets:

- *6 years of age and older* –

  Initial dosage: To reduce possible GI intolerance, begin with a quarter to a third of the planned maintenance dose.

  Dosage titration: Increase weekly until reaching the maintenance dose at 1 month.

  Maintenance dosage: 30 to 50 mg/kg daily in 2 evenly divided doses.

Ulcerative colitis –

6 years of age and older:

- *Initial dosage* – 40 to 60 mg/kg per day, divided into 3 to 6 doses.
- *Maintenance dosage* – 30 mg/kg per day, divided into 4 doses.
- *Dosage adjustment* – When endoscopic examination confirms satisfactory improvement, reduce dosage of sulfasalazine to a maintenance level. If diarrhea recurs, increase dosage to previously effective levels.

➤*Desensitization:* Some patients may be sensitive to treatment with sulfasalazine. Various desensitization-like regimens have been reported to be effective in 34 of 53 patients, 7 of 8 patients, and 19 of 20 patients. These regimens suggest starting with a total daily dose of 50 to 250 mg sulfasalazine initially, and doubling it every 4 to 7 days thereafter until the desired therapeutic level is achieved. If the symptoms of sensitivity recur, discontinue sulfasalazine. Do not attempt desensitization in patients who have a history of agranulocytosis or who have experienced an anaphylactoid reaction while on a previous course of sulfasalazine therapy.

➤*Administration:* Take sulfasalazine in evenly divided doses, preferably after meals. Swallow the delayed-release tablets whole.

➤*Storage/Stability:* Store at 25°C (77°F); excursions are permitted to 15° to 30°C (59° to 86°F).

Actions

➤*Pharmacokinetics:*

Absorption – In vivo studies have indicated that the absolute bioavailability of orally administered SSZ is less than 15% for parent drug. In the intestine, SSZ is metabolized by intestinal bacteria to SP and 5-ASA. Of the 2 species, SP is relatively well absorbed from the intestine and highly metabolized, while 5-ASA is much less well absorbed.

Following oral administration of 1 g of SSZ to 9 healthy males, less than 15% of a dose of SSZ is absorbed as parent drug. Detectable serum concentrations of SSZ have been found in healthy subjects within 90 minutes after the ingestion. Maximum concentrations of SSZ occur between 3 and 12 hours postingestion, with the mean peak concentration (6 mcg/mL) occurring at 6 hours.

In comparison, peak plasma levels of both SP and 5-ASA occur approximately 10 hours after dosing. This longer time to peak is indicative of GI transit to the lower intestine, where bacteria-mediated metabolism occurs. SP apparently is well absorbed from the colon, with an estimated bioavailability of 60%. In this same study, 5-ASA is much less well absorbed from the GI tract, with an estimated bioavailability of 10% to 30%.

Distribution – Following IV injection, the calculated volume of distribution (Vd_{ss}) for SSZ was 7.5 ± 1.6 L. SSZ is highly bound to albumin (greater than 99.3%), while SP is only about 70% bound to albumin. Acetylsulfapyridine (AcSP), the principal metabolite of SP, is approximately 90% bound to plasma proteins.

Metabolism – As mentioned above, SSZ is metabolized by intestinal bacteria to SP and 5-ASA. Approximately 15% of a dose of SSZ is absorbed as parent and is metabolized to some extent in the liver to the same 2 species. The observed plasma half-life for IV sulfasalazine is 7.6 ± 3.4 hours. The primary route of metabolism of SP is via acetylation to form AcSP. The rate of metabolism of SP to AcSP is dependent upon acetylator phenotype. In fast acetylators, the mean plasma half-life of SP is 10.4 hours, while in slow acetylators, it is 14.8 hours. SP can also be metabolized to 5-hydroxysulfapyridine (SPOH) and N-acetyl-5-hydroxy-sulfapyridine. 5-ASA is primarily metabolized in both the liver and intestine to N-acetyl-5-aminosalicylic acid via a nonacetylation, phenotype-dependent route. Due to low plasma levels produced by 5-ASA after oral administration, reliable estimates of plasma half-life are not possible.

Excretion – Absorbed SP and 5-ASA and their metabolites are primarily eliminated in the urine either as free metabolites or as glucuronide conjugates. The majority of 5-ASA stays within the colonic lumen and is excreted as 5-ASA and acetyl-5-ASA with the feces. The calculated clearance of SSZ following IV administration was 1 L/h. Renal clearance was estimated to account for 37% of total clearance.

Special populations –

Elderly: Elderly patients with rheumatoid arthritis showed a prolonged plasma half-life for SSZ, SP, and their metabolites. The clinical impact of this is unknown.

Children: Small studies have been reported in the literature in children down to the age of 4 years with ulcerative colitis and inflammatory bowel disease. In these populations, relative to adults, the pharmacokinetics of SSZ and SP correlated poorly with either age or dose.

Acetylator status: The metabolism of SP to AcSP is mediated by polymorphic enzymes such that 2 distinct populations of slow and fast metabolizers exist. Approximately 60% of the white population can be classified as belonging to the slow acetylator phenotype. These subjects will display a prolonged plasma half-life for SP (14.8 vs 10.4 hours) and an accumulation of higher plasma levels of SP than fast acetylators. The clinical implication of this is unclear; however, in a small pharmacokinetic trial where acetylator status was determined, subjects who were slow acetylators of SP showed a higher incidence of adverse reactions.

Contraindications

Hypersensitivity to sulfasalazine, its metabolites, sulfonamides, or salicylates; intestinal or urinary obstruction; porphyria.

Warnings/Precautions

➤*Deaths:* Deaths associated with the administration of sulfasalazine have been reported from hypersensitivity reactions, agranulocytosis, aplastic anemia, other blood dyscrasias, renal and liver damage, irreversible, neuromuscular and CNS changes, and fibrosing alveolitis.

➤*Blood dyscrasis:* Only administer sulfasalazine to patients with blood dyscrasia after critical appraisal.

The presence of clinical signs such as sore throat, fever, pallor, purpura, or jaundice may be indications for serious blood disorders.

➤*Undisintegrated tablets:* Isolated instances have been reported when sulfasalazine delayed-release tablets have passed undisintegrated. If this is observed, discontinue the administration of sulfasalazine delayed-release tablets immediately.

➤*Hypersensitivity reactions:* Give sulfasalazine with caution to patients with severe allergy or bronchial asthma. Adequate fluid intake must be maintained in order to prevent crystalluria and stone formation. Observe patients with glucose-6-phosphate dehydrogenase deficiency closely for signs of hemolytic anemia. This reaction is frequently dose related. If toxic or hypersensitivity reactions occur, discontinue the drug immediately.

➤*Renal/Hepatic function impairment:* Use sulfasalazine only after a critical appraisal in patients with hepatic or renal damage.

➤*Pregnancy:* *Category B.*

Teratogenic – Reproduction studies have been performed in rats and rabbits at doses up to 6 times the human dose and have revealed no evidence of impaired female fertility or harm to the fetus due to sulfasalazine. There are, however, no adequate and well-controlled studies in pregnant women. Because animal reproduction studies are not always predictive of human response, use this drug during pregnancy only if clearly needed.

Nonteratogenic – Sulfasalazine and sulfapyridine pass the placental barrier. Although sulfapyridine has been shown to have poor bilirubin-displacing capacity, keep in mind the potential for kernicterus in newborns.

A case of agranulocytosis has been reported in an infant whose mother was taking both sulfasalazine and prednisone throughout pregnancy.

➤*Lactation:* Exercise caution when sulfasalazine is administered to a breast-feeding mother. Sulfonamides are excreted in the milk. In the newborn, they compete with bilirubin for binding sites on the plasma proteins and may cause kernicterus. Insignificant amounts of uncleaved sulfasalazine have been found in milk, whereas the sulfapyridine levels in milk are about 30% to 60% of those in the maternal serum. Sulfapyridine has been shown to have a poor bilirubin-displacing capacity.

➤*Children:* The safety and efficacy of sulfasalazine in pediatric patients below the age of 2 years with ulcerative colitis have not been established.

Delayed-release tablets – The safety and efficacy of sulfasalazine for the treatment of the signs and symptoms of polyarticular-course juvenile rheumatoid arthritis in pediatric patients aged 6 to 16 years is supported by evidence from adequate and well-controlled studies in adult rheumatoid arthritis patients. The extrapolation from adults with rheumatoid arthritis to children with polyarticular-course juvenile rheumatoid arthritis is based on similarities in disease and response to therapy between these 2 patient populations. Published studies support the extrapolation of safety and efficacy for sulfasalazine to polyarticular-course juvenile rheumatoid arthritis.

It has been reported that the frequency of adverse reactions in patients with systemic-course of juvenile arthritis is high. Use in children with systemic-course juvenile rheumatoid arthritis has frequently resulted in a serum sickness-like reaction. This reaction is often severe and presents as fever, nausea, vomiting, headache, rash, and abnormal liver function tests. Treatment of systemic-course juvenile rheumatoid arthritis with sulfasalazine is not recommended.

➤*Monitoring:* Perform complete blood counts, including differential white cell count and liver function tests, before starting sulfasalazine and every second week during the first 3 months of therapy. During the second 3 months, do the same tests once monthly and thereafter once every 3 months, and as clinically indicated. Do urinalysis and an assessment of renal function periodically during treatment with sulfasalazine.

The determination of serum sulfapyridine levels may be useful since concentrations greater than 50 mcg/mL appear to be associated with an increased incidence of adverse reactions.

Drug Interactions

Sulfasalazine Drug Interactions

Precipitant drug	Object drug[a]		Description
Sulfasalazine	Cyclosporine	↓↑	Cyclosporine serum levels may be decreased. The risk of nephrotoxicity may be increased.
Sulfasalazine	Digoxin	↓	Reduced absorption of digoxin has been reported when coadministered with sulfasalazine.

SULFASALAZINE — ORAL

Sulfasalazine Drug Interactions

Precipitant drug	Object drug[a]		Description
Sulfasalazine	Folic acid	⬇	Reduced GI absorption of folic acid has been reported when coadministered with sulfasalazine. Periodically monitor patients taking sulfasalazine. If folate deficiency is noted, potential treatment measures include increasing dietary folate, giving sulfasalazine between meals, and administering additional folic acid or folinic acid.
Sulfasalazine	Methotrexate	⬆	Sulfonamides (eg, sulfasalazine) may displace methotrexate from protein binding and decrease renal clearance, therefore increasing the risk of methotrexate-induced bone marrow suppression. Monitor for hematologic toxicity. In addition, the overall toxicity profile of this combination revealed an increased incidence of GI adverse reactions, especially nausea.
Sulfasalazine	Sulfonylureas (eg, glipizide)	⬆	Sulfonamides (eg, sulfasalazine) may impair hepatic metabolism of sulfonylureas or alter plasma protein binding. Monitor blood glucose and decrease the sulfonylurea dose as necessary.
Sulfasalazine	Thiopurines (eg, azathioprine, mercaptopurine)	⬆	The risk of leukopenia may be increased due to inhibition of the thiopurine-metabolizing enzyme by sulfasalazine. Closely monitor leukocyte counts.
Sulfasalazine	Warfarin	⬆	Anticoagulant effect of warfarin may be increased. Monitor closely.

[a] ⬆ = Object drug increased. ⬇ = Object drug decreased.

Adverse Reactions

➤*Most common adverse reactions:*

Miscellaneous – The most common adverse reactions associated with sulfasalazine in ulcerative colitis are anorexia, headache, nausea, vomiting, gastric distress, and apparently reversible oligospermia. These occur in about one-third of the patients. Less frequent adverse reactions are skin rash, pruritus, urticaria, fever, Heinz body anemia, hemolytic anemia, and cyanosis which may occur at a frequency of 1 in every 30 patients or less. Experience suggests that with a daily dosage of 4 g or more, or total serum sulfapyridine levels above 50 mcg/mL, the incidence of adverse reactions tends to increase.

Delayed-release tablets: Similar adverse reactions are associated with sulfasalazine use in adult rheumatoid arthritis, although there was a greater incidence of some reactions. In rheumatoid arthritis studies, the following common adverse reactions were noted: nausea (19%), dyspepsia (13%), rash (13%), headache (9%), abdominal pain (8%), vomiting (8%), fever (5%), dizziness (4%), stomatitis (4%), pruritus (4%), abnormal liver function tests (4%), leukopenia (3%), and thrombocytopenia (1%). One report showed a 10% rate of immunoglobulin suppression, which was slowly reversible and rarely accompanied by clinical findings.

In general, the adverse reactions in juvenile rheumatoid arthritis patients are similar to those seen in patients with adult rheumatoid arthritis except for a high frequency of serum sickness-like syndrome in systemic-course juvenile rheumatoid arthritis (see Warnings, Children). One clinical trial showed an approximate 10% rate of immunoglobulin suppression.

➤*Less common or rare adverse reactions:* Although the following listing includes a few adverse reactions that have not been reported with this specific drug, the pharmacological similarities among the sulfonamides require that each of these reactions be considered when sulfasalazine is administered.

CNS – Transverse myelitis, convulsions, meningitis, transient lesions of the posterior spinal column, cauda equina syndrome, Guillain-Barre syndrome, peripheral neuropathy, mental depression, vertigo, hearing loss, insomnia, ataxia, hallucinations, tinnitus and drowsiness.

GI – Hepatitis, pancreatitis, bloody diarrhea, impaired folic acid absorption, impaired digoxin absorption, stomatitis, diarrhea, abdominal pains, and neutropenic enterocolitis.

Hematologic –

Blood dyscrasias: Aplastic anemia, agranulocytosis, leukopenia, megaloblastic (macrocytic) anemia, purpura, thrombocytopenia, hypoprothrombinemia, methemoglobinemia, congenital neutropenia, and myleodysplastic syndrome.

Hypersensitivity – Erythema multiforme (Stevens-Johnson syndrome); exfoliative dermatitis; epidermal necrolysis (Lyell's syndrome) with corneal damage; anaphylaxis; serum sickness syndrome; pneumonitis with or without eosinophilia; vasculitis; fibrosing alveolitis; pleuritis; pericarditis with or without tamponade; allergic myocarditis; polyarteritis nodosa; lupus erythematosus-like syndrome; hepatitis and hepatic necrosis with or without immune complexes; fulminant hepatitis, sometimes leading to liver transplantation; parapsoriasis varioliformis acuta (Mucha-Haberman syndrome); rhabdomyolysis; photosensitization; arthralgia; periorbital edema; conjunctival and scleral injection; and alopecia.

Renal – Toxic nephrosis with oliguria and anuria, nephritis, nephrotic syndrome, hematuria, crystalluria, proteinuria, and hemolytic-uremic syndrome.

Miscellaneous – Urine discoloration and skin discoloration.

The sulfonamides bear certain chemical similarities to some goitrogens, diuretics (acetazolamide and the thiazides), and oral hypoglycemic agents. Goiter production, diuresis, and hypoglycemia have occurred rarely in patients receiving sulfonamides. Cross-sensitivity may exist with these agents. Rats appear to be especially susceptible to the goitrogenic effects of sulfonamides, and long-term administration has produced thyroid malignancies in this species.

➤*Postmarketing reports:*

GI – Reports of hepatotoxicity, including elevated liver function tests (AST, ALT, gamma-glutamyl transferase [GGT], lactic dehydrogenase [LDH], alkaline phosphatase, bilirubin), jaundice, cholestatic jaundice, cirrhosis, and possible hepatocellular damage including liver necrosis and liver failure. Some of these cases were fatal. One case of Kawasaki-like syndrome, which included hepatic function changes, was also reported.

Overdosage

➤*Symptoms:* There is evidence that the incidence and severity of toxicity following overdosage are directly related to the total serum sulfapyridine concentration. Symptoms of overdosage may include nausea, vomiting, gastric distress, and abdominal pains. In more advanced cases, CNS symptoms (eg, drowsiness, convulsions) may be observed. Serum sulfapyridine concentrations may be used to monitor the progress of recovery from overdosage.

There are no documented reports of deaths due to ingestion of large single doses of sulfasalazine. It has not been possible to determine the LD_{50} in laboratory animals such as mice, since the highest oral daily dose of sulfasalazine which can be given (12 g/kg) is not lethal; a single oral dose of 12 g/kg was not lethal to mice. Doses of regular sulfasalazine tablets of 16 g/day have been given to patients without mortality.

➤*Treatment:* Gastric lavage or emesis plus catharsis as indicated. Alkalinize urine. If kidney function is normal, force fluids. If anuria is present, restrict fluids and salt, and treat appropriately. Catherization of the ureters may be indicated for complete renal blockage by crystals. The low molecular weight of sulfasalazine and its metabolites may facilitate their removal by dialysis.

Patient Information

Inform patients of the possibility of adverse reactions and of the need for careful medical supervision. The occurrence of sore throat, fever, pallor, purpura, or jaundice may indicate a serious blood disorder. Should any of these occur, the patient should seek medical advice.

Instruct patients to take sulfasalazine in evenly divided doses preferably after meals. Swallow the enteric-coated tablets whole. Additionally, advise patients that sulfasalazine may produce an orange-yellow discoloration of the urine or skin.

➤*Ulcerative colitis:* Patients with ulcerative colitis should be made aware that ulcerative colitis rarely remits completely, and that the risk of relapse can be substantially reduced by continued administration of sulfasalazine tablets at a maintenance dosage.

➤*Delayed-release tablets:*

Rheumatoid arthritis – Rheumatoid arthritis rarely remits. Therefore, continued administration of sulfasalazine is indicated. Patients requiring sulfasalazine should follow up with their physicians to determine the need for continued administration.

LUBIPROSTONE

Rx	Amitiza (Sucampo Pharm/Takeda Pharm)[a]	Capsules; oral: 8 mcg	Sorbitol. (SPI). Pink, oval. In 60s.
		24 mcg	Sorbitol. (SPI). Orange, oval. In 60s.

[a] Sucampo Pharmaceuticals Inc., 4733 Bethesda Ave., Ste. 450, Bethesda, MD 20814; 301-961-3400; http://www.sucampo.com.

LUBIPROSTONE — ORAL

Indications

➤*Chronic idiopathic constipation:* For the treatment of chronic idiopathic constipation in adults.

➤*Irritable bowel syndrome (IBS) with constipation:* For the treatment of IBS with constipation in women 18 years of age and older.

Administration and Dosage

➤*Adults:*

Chronic idiopathic constipation – 24 mcg twice daily with food and water.

IBS with constipation – 8 mcg twice daily with food and water.

➤*Administration:* Take with food and water to reduce potential symptoms of nausea. Swallow the capsule whole; do not break it apart or chew it.

➤*Storage/Stability:* Store at 25°C (77°F); excursions are permitted to 15° to 30°C (59° to 86°F).

Actions

➤*Pharmacology:* Lubiprostone is a locally acting chloride channel activator that enhances a chloride-rich intestinal fluid secretion without altering sodium and potassium concentrations in the serum. Lubiprostone acts by specifically activating ClC-2, which is a normal constituent of the apical membrane of the human intestine, in a protein kinase A–independent fashion. By increasing intestinal fluid secretion, lubiprostone increases motility in the intestine, thereby increasing the passage of stool and alleviating symptoms associated with chronic idiopathic constipation. Patch clamp cell studies in human cell lines have indicated that the majority of the beneficial biological activity of lubiprostone and its metabolites is observed only on the apical (luminal) portion of the GI epithelium. Additionally, activation of ClC-2 by lubiprostone has been shown to stimulate recovery of mucosal barrier function via the restoration of tight junction protein complexes in ex vivo studies of ischemic porcine intestine.

Pharmacodynamics – Although the pharmacologic effects of lubiprostone in humans have not been fully evaluated, animal studies have shown that oral administration of lubiprostone increases chloride ion transport into the intestinal lumen, enhances fluid secretion into the bowels, and improves fecal transit.

➤*Pharmacokinetics:*

Absorption – Lubiprostone has low systemic availability following oral administration, and concentrations of lubiprostone in plasma are below the level of quantitation (10 pg/mL). Therefore, standard pharmacokinetic parameters, such as the area under the curve (AUC), maximum effective plasma concentration (C_{max}), and half-life, cannot be reliably calculated. However, the pharmacokinetic parameters of the only measurable active metabolite (M3) have been characterized.

Peak plasma levels of M3 after a single, oral dose of lubiprostone 24 mcg occur at approximately 1.1 hours. The C_{max} is 41.5 pg/mL, and the mean $AUC_{0\text{-}t}$ is 57.1 pg•h/mL. The $AUC_{0\text{-}t}$ of M3 increases dose-proportionally after single doses of lubiprostone 24 and 144 mcg.

Food effect: A study was conducted with a single dose of ^{3}H-labeled lubiprostone 72 mcg to evaluate the potential of a food effect on lubiprostone absorption, metabolism, and excretion. Pharmacokinetic parameters of total radioactivity demonstrated that C_{max} decreased by 55%, while $AUC_{0\text{-}\infty}$ was unchanged when lubiprostone was administered with a high-fat meal. The clinical relevance of the effect of food on the pharmacokinetics of lubiprostone is not clear. However, lubiprostone was administered with food in a majority of clinical trials.

Distribution – In vitro protein-binding studies indicate that lubiprostone is approximately 94% bound to human plasma proteins. Studies in rats with radiolabeled lubiprostone indicate minimal distribution beyond the GI tissues. Concentrations of radiolabeled compound at 48 hours postadministration were minimal in all tissues.

Metabolism – The results of human and animal studies indicate that lubiprostone is rapidly and extensively metabolized by 15-position reduction, α-chain β-oxidation, and ω-chain ω-oxidation. These biotransformations are not mediated by the hepatic cytochrome P-450 system; rather, they appear to be mediated by the ubiquitously expressed carbonyl reductase. M3, a metabolite of lubiprostone in humans and animals, is formed by the reduction of the carbonyl group at the 15-hydroxy moiety that consists of α-hydroxy and β-hydroxy epimers. M3 makes up less than 10% of the dose of radiolabeled lubiprostone. Animal studies have shown that metabolism of lubiprostone rapidly occurs within the stomach and jejunum, most likely in the absence of any systemic absorption. This is presumed to be the case in humans as well.

Excretion – Lubiprostone could not be detected in plasma; however, M3 has a half-life ranging from 0.9 to 1.4 hours. After a single, oral dose of ^{3}H-labeled lubiprostone 72 mcg, 60% of total administered radioactivity was recovered in the urine within 24 hours and 30% of total administered radioactivity was recovered in the feces by 168 hours. Lubiprostone and M3 are only detected in trace amounts of human feces.

Contraindications

Known hypersensitivity to the drug or any of its excipients; a history of mechanical GI obstruction.

Warnings/Precautions

➤*GI effects:* Lubiprostone may cause nausea. If this occurs, coadministration of food with lubiprostone may reduce symptoms of nausea. Do not administer lubiprostone to patients who have severe diarrhea. Make patients aware of the possible occurrence of diarrhea during treatment.

➤*Dyspnea:* There were reports of dyspnea in clinical trials conducted to study lubiprostone in the treatment of chronic idiopathic constipation and IBS with constipation. This was reported in 2.5% of the treated chronic idiopathic constipation population and in 0.4% of the treated IBS with constipation population. Although not classified as a serious adverse reaction, some patients discontinued treatment because of this reaction. There have been postmarketing reports of dyspnea when using lubiprostone 24 mcg. Most have not been characterized as serious adverse reactions, but some patients have discontinued therapy because of dyspnea. These reactions have usually been described as a sensation of chest tightness and difficulty taking in a breath, and generally have an acute onset within 30 to 60 minutes after taking the first dose. They generally resolve within a few hours after taking the dose, but recurrence has been frequently reported with subsequent doses.

➤*GI obstruction:* Evaluate patients with symptoms suggestive of mechanical GI obstruction prior to initiating lubiprostone treatment.

➤*Pregnancy:* Category C.

Teratogenic – Teratology studies with lubiprostone have been conducted in rats at oral doses up to 2,000 mcg/kg/day (approximately 332 times the recommended human dose, based on BSA), and in rabbits at oral doses of up to 100 mcg/kg/day (approximately 33 times the recommended human dosage, based on BSA). Lubiprostone was not teratogenic in rats and rabbits.

In guinea pigs, lubiprostone caused fetal loss at repeated doses of 10 and 25 mcg/kg/day (approximately 2 and 6 times the human dosage, respectively, based on BSA) administered on days 40 to 53 of gestation.

There are no adequate and well-controlled studies in pregnant women. However, during clinical testing of lubiprostone, 6 women became pregnant. Per protocol, lubiprostone was discontinued upon pregnancy detection. Four of the 6 women delivered healthy babies. The fifth woman was monitored for 1 month following discontinuation of study drug, at which time the pregnancy was progressing as expected; the patient was subsequently lost to follow-up. The sixth pregnancy was electively terminated.

Only use lubiprostone during pregnancy if the potential benefit justifies the potential risk to the fetus. If a woman is or becomes pregnant while taking the drug, apprise the patient of the potential hazard to the fetus. Women who could become pregnant should have a negative pregnancy test prior to beginning therapy with lubiprostone and should be capable of complying with effective contraceptive measures.

➤*Lactation:* It is not known whether lubiprostone is excreted in human milk. Because many drugs are excreted in human milk and because of the potential for serious adverse reactions in breast-feeding infants from lubiprostone, decide whether to discontinue breast-feeding or the drug, taking into account the importance of the drug to the mother.

➤*Children:* Safety and effectiveness in children have not been studied.

➤*Elderly:*

Chronic idiopathic constipation – The efficacy of lubiprostone in elderly patients (65 years of age and older) was consistent with the efficacy in the overall study population. Of the total number of constipated patients treated in the dose-finding, efficacy, and long-term studies of lubiprostone, 15.5% were 65 years of age and older and 4.2% were 75 years of age and older. Elderly patients taking lubiprostone at any dosage experienced a lower incidence rate of associated nausea compared with the overall study population taking lubiprostone (18% vs 29%, respectively).

IBS with constipation – The safety profile of lubiprostone in the elderly patient (65 years of age and older) subpopulation (8% were 65 years of age and older and 1.8% were 75 years of age and older) was consistent with the safety profile in the overall study population. Clinical studies of lubiprostone did not include sufficient numbers of patients 65 years of age and older to determine whether they respond differently from younger patients.

Adverse Reactions

➤*Chronic idiopathic constipation:*

Lubiprostone Adverse Reactions in Patients With Chronic Idiopathic Constipation (≥ 1%)

Adverse reactions[a]	Placebo (n = 316)	Lubiprostone 24 mcg once daily (n = 29)	Lubiprostone 24 mcg twice daily (n = 1,113)
CNS			
Dizziness	< 1%	3%	3%
Fatigue	< 1%	—	2%
Headache	5%	3%	11%

LUBIPROSTONE — ORAL

Lubiprostone Adverse Reactions in Patients With Chronic Idiopathic Constipation (≥ 1%)			
Adverse reactions[a]	Placebo (n = 316)	Lubiprostone 24 mcg once daily (n = 29)	Lubiprostone 24 mcg twice daily (n = 1,113)
GI			
Abdominal discomfort[b]	< 1%	3%	2%
Abdominal distension	2%	—	6%
Abdominal pain	3%	3%	8%
Diarrhea	< 1%	7%	12%
Dry mouth	< 1%	—	1%
Dyspepsia	< 1%	—	2%
Flatulence	2%	3%	6%
Loose stools	—	—	3%
Nausea	3%	17%	29%
Stomach discomfort	< 1%	—	1%
Vomiting	—	—	3%
Respiratory			
Dyspnea	—	3%	2%
Miscellaneous			
Chest discomfort/pain	—	3%	2%
Edema	< 1%	—	3%

[a] Includes only those reactions associated with treatment (possibly, probably, or definitely related, as assessed by the investigator).
[b] This term combines "abdominal discomfort," "abdominal rigidity," "abdominal tenderness," and "GI discomfort."

Nausea – Approximately 29% of patients who received lubiprostone 24 mcg twice daily experienced an adverse reaction of nausea; 4% of patients had severe nausea and 9% of patients discontinued treatment because of nausea. The rate of nausea associated with lubiprostone at any dosage was substantially lower among men (7%) and elderly patients (18%). Further analysis of the safety data revealed that long-term exposure to lubiprostone does not appear to place patients at an elevated risk for experiencing nausea. The incidence of nausea increased in an dose-dependent manner with the lowest overall incidence for nausea reported at the 24 mcg once-daily dose (17%). In open-label, long-term studies, patients were allowed to adjust the dose of lubiprostone to 24 mcg once daily from 24 mcg twice daily if experiencing nausea. Nausea decreased when lubiprostone was administered with food. No patients in the clinical studies were hospitalized because of nausea.

Diarrhea – Approximately 12% of patients who received lubiprostone 24 mcg twice daily experienced an adverse reaction of diarrhea; 2% of patients had severe diarrhea, and 2% of patients discontinued treatment because of diarrhea.

Electrolytes – No serious adverse reactions of electrolyte imbalance were reported in clinical studies, and no clinically significant changes were seen in serum electrolyte levels in patients receiving lubiprostone.

➤*Other adverse reactions (less than 1%):*
Cardiovascular – Syncope.
CNS – Anxiety, tremor.
Dermatologic – Cold sweat, hyperhidrosis.
GI – Constipation, defecation urgency, dysgeusia, eructation, fecal incontinence, frequent bowel movements, intestinal functional disorder.
Metabolic/Nutritional – Decreased appetite.
Musculoskeletal – Joint swelling, muscle cramp, myalgia.
Respiratory – Cough, influenza, pharyngolaryngeal pain.
Miscellaneous – Pain.

➤*IBS with constipation:*

Lubiprostone Adverse Reactions in Patients With IBS With Constipation Studies (≥ 1%)		
Adverse reactions[a]	Placebo (n = 435)	Lubiprostone 8 mcg twice daily (n = 1,011)
GI		
Abdominal distension	2%	3%
Abdominal pain	5%	5%
Diarrhea	4%	7%
Nausea	4%	8%

[a] Includes only those reactions associated with treatment (possibly or probably related, as assessed by the investigator).

➤*Other adverse reactions (less than 1%):*
Cardiovascular – Palpitations.
CNS – Anxiety, depression, fatigue, fibromyalgia, lethargy.
Dermatologic – Erythema.
GI – Constipation, dry mouth, dyspepsia, eructation, fecal incontinence, gastritis, gastroesophageal reflux disease, hard feces, loose stools, rectal hemorrhage, vomiting.
GU – Pollakiuria, urinary tract infection.
Lab test abnormalities – Increased ALT, increased AST.
Metabolic/Nutritional – Anorexia, edema, increased weight.
Respiratory – Dyspnea.

➤*Postmarketing:* Voluntary reports of adverse reactions occurring with the use of lubiprostone include the following: allergic-type reactions (including rash, swelling, and throat tightness), asthenia, increased heart rate, malaise, muscle cramps or spasms, rash, and syncope.

Overdosage

➤*Symptoms:* There have been 2 confirmed reports of overdosage with lubiprostone. The first report involved a child 3 years of age who accidentally ingested 7 to 8 capsules of lubiprostone 24 mcg and fully recovered. The second report was a study subject who self-administered a total of lubiprostone 96 mcg daily for 8 days. The subject experienced no adverse reactions during this time. Additionally, in a definitive phase 1 cardiac repolarization study, 51 patients administered a single, oral dose of lubiprostone 144 mcg, which is 6 times the normal single administration dose. Thirty-eight of the 51 patients experienced an adverse reaction.

The adverse reactions reported in at least 1% of these patients included the following: nausea (45%); diarrhea (35%); vomiting (27%); dizziness (14%); headache (12%); abdominal pain (8%); flushing or hot flash (8%); retching (8%); dyspnea, pallor, stomach discomfort (4%); anorexia, asthenia, chest discomfort, dry mouth, hyperhidrosis, syncope (2%).

Patient Information

Advise patients to take lubiprostone twice daily, once in the morning and once in the evening as prescribed, with food and water to reduce potential symptoms of nausea. Advise patients to swallow the capsule whole, and not to break it apart or chew it. Periodically assess the need for continued therapy.

Advise patients to inform their health care provider if they experience severe diarrhea, dyspnea, or nausea. Patients taking lubiprostone may experience dyspnea within an hour of the first dose. This symptom generally resolves within 3 hours but may recur with repeat dosing.

Instruct patients with chronic idiopathic constipation to take a single lubiprostone 24 mcg capsule twice daily with food and water.

Instruct patients with IBS with constipation to take a single lubiprostone 8 mcg capsule twice daily with food and water.

ALVIMOPAN

Rx	**Entereg** (GlaxoSmithKline)	**Capsules; oral:** 12 mg	PEG. (ADL2698). Blue. In UD 30s.

ALVIMOPAN — ORAL

WARNING

For short-term hospital use only – Alvimopan is available only for short-term (15 doses) use in hospitalized patients. Only hospitals that have registered in and met all of the requirements for the *Entereg* Access Support and Education (E.A.S.E.) program may use alvimopan.

Indications

➤*Postoperative ileus:* To accelerate the time to upper and lower GI recovery following partial large or small bowel resection surgery with primary anastomosis.

Administration and Dosage

➤*General dosing considerations:* For hospital use only.
➤*Adults:*
Postoperative ileus –
Usual dosage: 12 mg 30 minutes to 5 hours prior to surgery, followed by 12 mg twice daily beginning the day after surgery.
Maximum dose: 15 doses (180 mg total).
Duration of therapy: Maximum of 7 days or until discharge.

➤*Renal function impairment:* Alvimopan is not recommended for use in patients with end-stage renal disease.

ALVIMOPAN — ORAL

➤*Hepatic function impairment:* Alvimopan is not recommended for use in patients with severe hepatic function impairment (Child-Pugh class C).

➤*Storage/Stability:* Store at 25°C (77°F); excursions are permitted to 15° to 30°C (59° to 86°F).

Actions

➤*Pharmacology:* Alvimopan is a selective antagonist of the cloned human mu-opioid receptor with a Ki of 0.4 nM (0.2 ng/mL) and no measurable opioid-agonist effects in standard pharmacologic assays. The dissociation of [^{3}H]-alvimopan from the human mu-opioid receptor is slower than that of other opioid ligands, consistent with its higher affinity for the receptor. At concentrations of 1 to 10 mcM, alvimopan demonstrated no activity at any of more than 70 non-opioid receptors, enzymes, and ion channels.

Postoperative ileus is the impairment of GI motility after intra-abdominal surgery or other nonabdominal surgeries. Postoperative ileus affects all segments of the GI tract and may last from 5 to 6 days or longer. This may delay GI recovery and hospital discharge until its resolution. It is characterized by abdominal distention and bloating, nausea, vomiting, pain, accumulation of gas and fluids in the bowel, and delayed passage of flatus and defecation. Postoperative ileus is the result of a multifactorial process that includes inhibitory sympathetic input, release of hormones, neurotransmitters, and other mediators (eg, endogenous opioids). A component of postoperative ileus also results from an inflammatory reaction and the effects of opioid analgesics. Morphine and other mu-opioid receptor agonists are universally used for the treatment of acute postsurgical pain; however, they are known to have an inhibitory effect on GI motility and may prolong the duration of postoperative ileus.

Following oral administration, alvimopan antagonizes the peripheral effects of opioids on GI motility and secretion by competitively binding to GI tract mu-opioid receptors. The antagonism produced by alvimopan at opioid receptors is evident in isolated guinea pig ileum preparations where alvimopan competitively antagonizes the effects of morphine on contractility. Alvimopan achieves this selective GI opioid antagonism without reversing the central analgesic effects of mu-opioid agonists.

Pharmacodynamics – In exploratory studies in healthy volunteers, alvimopan 3 mg 3 times daily appeared to reduce the delay in GI transit produced by morphine 30 mg twice daily as measured by radiopaque markers.

In a study designed to evaluate potential effects on cardiac conduction, alvimopan did not cause clinically significant QTc prolongation at dosages of up to 24 mg twice daily for 7 days. The potential for QTc effects at higher doses has not been studied.

➤*Pharmacokinetics:*

Absorption – Following oral administration of alvimopan capsules in healthy volunteers, plasma alvimopan concentration peaked at approximately 2 hours postdose. No significant accumulation in alvimopan concentration was observed following twice daily dosing. The mean peak plasma concentration was 10.98 (± 6.43) ng/mL and mean area under the curve (AUC_{0-12h}) was 40.2 (± 22.5) ng•h/mL after alvimopan 12 mg twice daily for 5 days. The absolute bioavailability was estimated to be 6% (range, 1% to 19%). Plasma concentrations of alvimopan increased approximately proportionally with increasing doses between 6 and 18 mg, but less than proportionally from 18 to 24 mg.

There was a delay in the appearance of the metabolite, which had a median time to maximum plasma concentration (T_{max}) of 36 hours following administration of a single dose of alvimopan. Intersubject and intrasubject metabolite concentrations were highly variable. The metabolite accumulated after multiple doses of alvimopan. The mean maximum plasma concentration (C_{max}) for the metabolite after alvimopan 12 mg twice daily for 5 days was 35.73 ± 35.29 ng/mL.

Concentrations of alvimopan and its metabolite are higher (approximately 1.9-fold and 1.4-fold, respectively) in postoperative ileus patients than in healthy volunteers.

Food effects: A high-fat meal decreased the extent and rate of alvimopan absorption. The C_{max} and AUC were decreased by approximately 38% and 21%, respectively, and the T_{max} was prolonged by approximately 1 hour. The clinical significance of this decreased bioavailability is unknown. In postoperative ileus clinical trials, the preoperative dose of alvimopan was administered in a fasting state. Subsequent doses were given without regard to meals.

Distribution – The steady-state volume of distribution of alvimopan was estimated to be 30 ± 10 L. Plasma protein binding of alvimopan and its metabolite was independent of concentration over ranges observed clinically, and averaged 80% and 94%, respectively. Both alvimopan and the metabolite were bound to albumin and not to alpha-1 acid glycoprotein.

Metabolism/Excretion – Following oral administration of alvimopan, an amide hydrolysis compound is present in the systemic circulation, which is considered a product exclusively of intestinal flora metabolism. This compound is referred to as the metabolite. It is also a mu-opioid receptor antagonist with a Ki of 0.8 nM (0.3 ng/mL).

The average plasma clearance for alvimopan was 402 (± 89) mL/min. Renal excretion accounted for approximately 35% of total clearance. There was no evidence that hepatic metabolism was a significant route for alvimopan elimination. Biliary secretion was considered the primary pathway for alvimopan elimination. Unabsorbed drug and unchanged alvimopan resulting from biliary excretion were then hydrolyzed to its metabolite by gut microflora. The metabolite was eliminated in the feces and urine as unchanged metabolite, the glucuronide conjugate of the metabolite, and other minor metabolites. The mean terminal phase half-life of alvimopan after multiple oral doses ranged from 10 to 17 hours. The terminal half-life of the metabolite ranged from 10 to 18 hours.

Special populations –

Renal function impairment: There was no relationship between renal function (eg, creatinine clearance [CrCl]) and plasma alvimopan pharmacokinetics (C_{max}, AUC, or half-life) in patients with mild (CrCl, 51 to 80 mL/min), moderate (CrCl, 31 to 50 mL/min), or severe (CrCl less than 30 mL/min) renal function impairment (n = 6 each). Renal clearance of alvimopan was related to renal function; however, because renal clearance was only a small fraction (35%) of the total clearance, renal function impairment had a small effect on the apparent overall clearance of alvimopan. The half-lives of alvimopan were comparable in the mild, moderate, and control renal function impairment groups but longer in the severe renal function impairment group. Exposure to the metabolite tended to be 2- to 5-fold higher in patients with moderate or severe renal function impairment compared with patients with mild renal function impairment or control subjects. Thus, there may be accumulation of alvimopan and metabolite in patients with severe renal function impairment receiving multiple doses of alvimopan. Patients with end-stage renal disease were not studied.

Hepatic function impairment: Exposure to alvimopan following a single 12-mg dose tended to be higher (1.5- to 2-fold, on average) in patients with mild or moderate hepatic function impairment (as defined by Child-Pugh Class A and B; n = 8 each) compared with healthy controls (n = 4). There were no consistent effects on the C_{max} or half-life of alvimopan in patients with hepatic function impairment. However, 2 of 16 patients with mild to moderate hepatic function impairment had longer than expected alvimopan half-lives, indicating that some accumulation may occur upon multiple dosing. The C_{max} of the metabolite tended to be more variable in patients with mild or moderate hepatic function impairment than in matched healthy subjects. A study of 3 patients with severe hepatic function impairment (Child-Pugh Class C), indicated similar alvimopan exposure in 2 patients and an approximately 10-fold increase in C_{max} and exposure in 1 patient with severe hepatic function impairment when compared with healthy control volunteers.

Race: Race had no effect on the pharmacokinetics of alvimopan. Plasma metabolite concentrations were lower in black and Hispanic patients (by 43% and 82%, respectively) than in white patients following alvimopan administration. These changes are not considered to be clinically significant in surgical patients; therefore, dosage adjustment based on race is not required.

Crohn disease: There was no relationship between disease activity in patients with Crohn disease (measured as Crohn Disease Activity Index or bowel movement frequency) and alvimopan pharmacokinetics (AUC or C_{max}). Patients with active or quiescent Crohn disease had increased variability in alvimopan pharmacokinetics, and exposure tended to be 2-fold higher in patients with quiescent disease than in those with active disease or healthy subjects. Concentrations of the metabolite were lower in patients with Crohn disease.

Contraindications

Patients who have taken therapeutic doses of opioids for more than 7 consecutive days immediately prior to taking alvimopan.

Warnings/Precautions

➤*Myocardial infarction (MI):* There were more reports of MI in patients treated with alvimopan 0.5 mg twice daily compared with placebo-treated patients in a 12-month study of patients treated with opioids for chronic pain. In this study, the majority of MIs occurred between 1 and 4 months after initiation of treatment. This imbalance has not been observed in other studies of alvimopan, including studies in patients undergoing bowel resection surgery who received alvimopan 12 mg twice daily for up to 7 days. A causal relationship with alvimopan has not been established.

➤*Distribution program:* Alvimopan is available only to hospitals that enroll in the E.A.S.E. program. To enroll in this program, the hospital must acknowledge that the hospital staff who prescribe, dispense, or administer alvimopan have been provided the educational materials on the need to limit use of alvimopan to short-term inpatient use; that patients will not receive more than 15 doses of alvimopan; and that alvimopan will not be dispensed to patients after they have been discharged from the hospital. For more information, contact the E.A.S.E. program at 1-866-423-6567.

➤*Opioid tolerance and GI adverse reactions:* Patients recently exposed to opioids are expected to be more sensitive to the effects of mu-opioid receptor antagonists. Because alvimopan acts peripherally, clinical signs and symptoms of increased sensitivity would likely be limited to the GI tract (eg, abdominal pain, diarrhea, nausea and vomiting). Patients receiving more than 3 doses of an opioid within the week prior to surgery were not studied in the postoperative ileus clinical trials; therefore, administer alvimopan 12 mg capsules to these patients with caution.

➤*Bowel obstruction:* Use of alvimopan in patients undergoing surgery for correction of complete bowel obstruction is not recommended.

➤*Renal function impairment:* Patients with mild to severe renal function impairment do not require dosage adjustment, but monitor these patients for adverse reactions. Closely monitor patients with severe renal function impairment for possible adverse reactions (eg, cramping, diarrhea, GI pain) that could indicate high drug or metabolite levels, and discontinue alvimopan if adverse reactions occur.

No studies have been conducted in patients with end-stage renal disease. Alvimopan is not recommended for use in these patients.

➤*Hepatic function impairment:* Although there is a potential for higher plasma levels of drug in patients with mild to moderate hepatic function impairment, dosage adjustment in these patients is not required. Closely monitor patients with mild to moderate hepatic function impairment for possible adverse reactions (eg, cramping, diarrhea, GI pain) that could indicate high drug or metabolite levels, and discontinue alvimopan if adverse reactions occur. Alvimopan is not recommended for use in patients with severe hepatic function impairment.

ALVIMOPAN — ORAL

In patients with severe hepatic function impairment, there is a potential for 10-fold higher plasma levels of drug. There are no studies of alvimopan in patients with severe hepatic function impairment undergoing bowel resection. Because of the limited data available, alvimopan is not recommended for use in patients with severe hepatic function impairment.

➤*Pregnancy: Category B.* Reproduction studies have been performed in pregnant rats at about 68 to 136 times the recommended human oral dose based on BSA and IV doses of about 3.4 to 6.8 times the recommended human oral dose based on BSA, and in pregnant rabbits at IV doses at about 5 to 10 times the recommended human oral dose based on BSA, and have revealed no evidence of impaired fertility or harm to the fetus from alvimopan.

There are, however, no adequate and well-controlled studies in pregnant women. Because animal reproduction studies are not always predictive of human response, use this drug during pregnancy only if clearly needed.

➤*Lactation:* Alvimopan and its metabolite are detected in the milk of lactating rats. It is not known whether alvimopan is excreted in human milk. Because many drugs are excreted in human milk, exercise caution when administering alvimopan to breast-feeding women.

➤*Children:* Safety and effectiveness in children have not been established.

➤*Elderly:* Of the total number of patients in 5 clinical efficacy studies treated with alvimopan or placebo, 45% were 65 years of age and older, while 18% were 75 years of age and older. No overall differences in safety or effectiveness were observed between these patients and younger patients, and other reported clinical experience has not identified differences in responses between elderly and younger patients, but greater sensitivity of some elderly individuals cannot be ruled out. No dosage adjustment based on age is required in elderly patients.

Drug Interactions

None known.

Adverse Reactions

The following table presents treatment-emergent adverse reactions reported in at least 3% of patients treated with alvimopan and for which the rate for alvimopan was at least 1% higher than placebo. Treatment-emergent adverse reactions are those reactions occurring after the first dose of study medication treatment and within 7 days of the last dose of study medication, or those reactions present at baseline that increased in severity after the start of study medication treatment.

Alvimopan Adverse Reactions (≥ 3%)

Adverse reaction	Bowel resection patients		All surgical patients	
	Placebo (n = 986)	Alvimopan (n = 999)	Placebo (n = 1,365)	Alvimopan (n = 1,650)
Hematologic				
Anemia	4.2%	5.2%	5.4%	5.4%
GI				
Constipation	3.9%	4%	7.6%	9.7%
Dyspepsia	4.6%	7%	4.8%	5.9%
Flatulence	4.5%	3.1%	7.7%	8.7%
GU				
Urinary retention	2.1%	3.2%	2.3%	3.5%
Metabolic and nutritional				
Hypokalemia	8.5%	9.5%	7.5%	6.9%
Musculoskeletal				
Back pain	1.7%	3.3%	2.6%	3.4%

Overdosage

➤*Treatment:* There is no specific antidote for overdosage with alvimopan. Manage patients with appropriate supportive therapy. Single doses of up to 120 mg and multiple doses of up to 48 mg for 7 days have been administered to healthy subjects in clinical studies and were well-tolerated.

Patient Information

Inform patients that they must disclose long-term or intermittent opioid pain therapy, including any use of opioids in the week prior to receiving alvimopan. Ensure that they understand that recent use of opioids may make them more susceptible to adverse reactions to alvimopan, primarily those limited to the GI tract (eg, abdominal pain, diarrhea, nausea and vomiting).

Inform patients that alvimopan is for hospital use only for no more than 7 days after bowel resection surgery.

Inform patients that the most common adverse reactions with alvimopan in patients undergoing bowel resection are constipation, dyspepsia, and flatulence.

LAXATIVES

Indications

➤*Constipation:* Treatment of constipation.

➤*Rectal/Bowel examinations:* Certain stimulant, lubricant, and saline laxatives are used to evacuate the colon for rectal and bowel examinations.

➤*Prophylaxis:* Laxatives, generally **fecal softeners** or **mineral oil**, are useful prophylactically in patients who should not strain during defecation(ie, following anorectal surgery, MI).

➤*Psyllium:* Useful in patients with irritable bowel syndrome and diverticular disease.

➤*Polycarbophil:* For constipation or diarrhea associated with conditions such as irritable bowel syndrome and diverticulosis; acute nonspecific diarrhea.

➤*Mineral oil (enema):* Relief of fecal impaction.

➤*Docusate sodium:* Prevention of dry, hard stools.

➤*Off-label uses:*

Hepatic encephalopathy (adults) –

Lactulose: [1] = Good documentation.

Other possible off-label uses – **Psyllium** appears to be useful in the reduction of cholesterol levels as an adjunct to a dietary program.

Actions

➤*Pharmacology:* Laxatives function by promoting active electrolyte secretion, decreasing water and electrolyte absorption, increasing intraluminal osmolarity, or increasing hydrostatic pressure in the gut.

Pharmacologic Actions of Laxatives

	Laxatives	Onset of action (h)	Site of action	Mechanism of action	Comments
Saline	Dibasic sodium phosphate[a,b] Magnesium citrate Magnesium hydroxide Magnesium sulfate Monobasic sodium phosphate[a,b] Sodium biphosphate[a]	0.5 to 3	Small and large intestine	Attract/Retain water in intestinal lumen, increasing intraluminal pressure; cholecystokinin release.	May alter fluid and electrolyte balance. Sulfate salts are considered the most potent.
Stimulant/Irritant	Cascara	6 to 8	Colon	Direct action on intestinal mucosa or nerve plexus; alters water and electrolyte secretion.	May prefer castor oil when more complete evacuation is required.
	Bisacodyl tablets Casanthranol Senna	6 to 10			
	Bisacodyl suppository	0.25 to 1			
Bulk-producing	Methylcellulose Polycarbophil Psyllium	12 to 72	Small and large intestine	Holds water in stool to increase bulk-stimulating peristalsis; forms emollient gel.	Safe; minimal side effects. Take with plenty of water (240 mL/dose).
Emollient	Mineral oil	6 to 8	Colon	Retards colonic absorption of fecal water; softens stool.	May decrease absorption of fat-soluble vitamins.

Pharmacologic Actions of Laxatives

	Laxatives	Onset of action (h)	Site of action	Mechanism of action	Comments
Fecal softeners/ Surfactants	Docusate[c]	12 to 72	Small and large intestine	Facilitates admixture of fat and water to soften stool.	Beneficial in anorectal conditions in which passage of a firm stool is painful.
Hyperosmotic	Glycerin suppository	0.25 to 1	Colon	Local irritation; hyperosmotic action.	Sodium stearate in preparation causes local irritation.
	Lactulose	24 to 48	Colon	Osmotic effect retains fluid in the colon, lowering the pH and increasing colonic peristalsis.	Also indicated in portal-systemic encephalopathy.
Miscellaneous	Castor oil	2 to 6	Small intestine	Direct action on intestinal mucosa or nerve plexus; alters water and electrolyte secretion.	Castor oil is converted to ricinoleic acid (active component) in the gut.

[a] Onset of action for rectal preparations is 2 to 15 minutes.
[b] Colon is site of action for rectal preparations.
[c] Site of action for potassium salt is in the colon.

Calcium polycarbophil is a hydrophilic agent. As a bulk laxative, it retains free water within the intestinal lumen and indirectly opposes dehydrating forces of the bowel, promoting well-formed stools. In diarrhea, when the intestinal mucosa is incapable of absorbing water at normal rates, it absorbs free fecal water, forming a gel and producing formed stools. Thus, in diarrhea and constipation, it works by restoring a more normal moisture level and providing bulk.

Lactulose, a synthetic disaccharide analog of lactose containing galactose and fructose, decreases blood ammonia concentrations and reduces the degree of portal-systemic encephalopathy.

The human GI tissue does not have an enzyme capable of hydrolysis of this disaccharide; as a result, oral doses pass to the colon virtually unchanged. After reaching the colon, lactulose is metabolized by bacteria resulting in the formation of lactic acid, formic acid, acetic acid, and carbon dioxide. These products produce an increased osmotic pressure and slightly acidify the colonic contents, resulting in an increase in stool water content and stool softening. Because the colonic contents are more acidic than the blood, ammonia can migrate from the blood into the colon. The acid colonic contents convert NH_3 to the ammonium ion $[NH_4]^+$, trapping it and preventing its absorption. The laxative action of the lactulose metabolites then expels the trapped ammonium ion from the colon.

➤*Pharmacokinetics:* **Lactulose** is poorly absorbed. When given orally, only small amounts reach the blood. Urinary excretion is ≤ 3% and is essentially complete within 24 hours. Lactulose does not exert its effect until it reaches the colon. Transit time through the colon may be slow; therefore, 24 to 48 hours may be required to produce a normal bowel movement.

Contraindications

Hypersensitivity to any ingredient; nausea, vomiting, or other symptoms of appendicitis; fecal impaction; intestinal obstruction; undiagnosed abdominal pain; patients who require a low galactose diet (**lactulose**).

Do not give **docusate sodium** if **mineral oil** is being given.

Warnings/Precautions

➤*Constipation:* Prior to using laxatives, consider living habits affecting bowel function, including disease state and drug history. Treatment and prevention of constipation include the following: Adequate fluid intake (4 to 6 glasses [8 oz] of water daily), proper dietary habits including increasing fiber intake, responding to the urge to defecate, and daily exercise. Restrict self-medication to short-term therapy of constipation; chronic use of laxatives (particularly stimulants) may lead to dependence.

Agents That May Cause Constipation

Prostaglandin synthesis inhibitors	Non-potassium sparing diuretics
Anticholinergics	Ganglionic blockers
Antihistamines	Iron preparations
Phenothiazines	Barium sulfate
Tricyclic antidepressants	Clonidine
Benztropine	Polystyrene sodium sulfonate
Trihexyphenidyl	Antacids containing either calcium carbonate or aluminum hydroxide
Opiates	

➤*Fluid and electrolyte balance:* Excessive laxative use may lead to significant fluid and electrolyte imbalance. Monitor patients periodically.

Preparations containing sodium should be used cautiously by individuals on a sodium-restricted diet, and in the presence of edema, CHF, renal failure, or borderline hypertension.

Megacolon, bowel obstruction, imperforate anus, or CHF – Do not use **sodium phosphate** and **sodium biphosphate** in these patients; hypernatremic dehydration may occur.

Abuse/Dependency – Chronic use of laxatives may result in fluid and electrolyte imbalances, steatorrhea, osteomalacia, diarrhea, cathartic colon, and liver disease. Also known as laxative abuse syndrome (LAS), it is difficult to diagnose. It is often seen in women with depression, personality disorders, or anorexia nervosa. Many agents can be detected in urine or stool samples; however, it is important to follow up negative test results if LAS is suspected, because patients may be intermittent abusers or change laxative products frequently.

Cathartic colon – Cathartic colon, a poorly functioning colon, results from the chronic abuse of stimulant cathartics.

➤*Melanosis coli:* Melanosis coli is a darkened pigmentation of the colonic mucosa resulting from chronic use of anthraquinone derivatives (**casanthrol**, **cascara sagrada**, **senna**).

➤*Lipid pneumonitis:* Lipid pneumonitis may result from oral ingestion and aspiration of **mineral oil**, especially when patient reclines. The young, elderly, and debilitated are at greatest risk.

➤*Electrocautery procedures:* A theoretical hazard may exist for patients being treated with **lactulose** who may undergo electrocautery procedures during proctoscopy or colonoscopy. Accumulation of H_2 gas in significant concentration in the presence of an electrical spark may result in an explosion. Although this complication has not been reported with lactulose, patients should have a thorough bowel cleansing with a nonfermentable solution. Insufflation of CO_2 as an additional safeguard may be pursued, but is considered a redundant measure.

➤*Diabetic patients:* **Lactulose** syrup contains galactose (less than 1.6 g/15 mL) and lactose (less than 1.2 g/15 mL). Use with caution in these individuals.

➤*Concomitant laxative use:* Do not use other laxatives, especially during the initial phase of therapy for portal-systemic encephalopathy; the resulting loose stools may falsely suggest adequate lactulose dosage.

➤*Rectal bleeding or failure to respond:* Rectal bleeding or failure to respond to therapy may indicate a serious condition, which may require further medical attention.

➤*Urine discoloration:* Discoloration of acidic urine to yellow-brown or black may occur with **cascara sagrada** or **senna**. Pink-red, red-violet, or red-brown discoloration of alkaline urine may occur with cascara sagrada or senna.

➤*Impaction or obstruction:* Impaction or obstruction may be caused by bulk-forming agents if temporarily arrested in their passage through the alimentary canal (eg, patients with esophageal strictures). Administer bulk-forming agents with plenty of fluid (240 mL/dose).

➤*Melanosis coli:* Anthraquinone derivatives (**casanthrol**, **cascara sagrada**, and **senna**) may cause melanosis coli, a harmless discoloring of colonic mucosa, persisting ≤ 6 months following discontinuation.

➤*Tartrazine sensitivity:* Some of these products contain tartrazine, which may cause allergic-type reactions (including bronchial asthma) in susceptible individuals. Although the incidence of tartrazine sensitivity in the general population is low, it is frequently seen in patients who also have aspirin hypersensitivity. Specific products containing tartrazine are identified in the product listings.

➤*Renal function impairment:* Up to 20% of the magnesium in magnesium salts may be absorbed. Use caution with products containing phosphate, sodium, magnesium, or potassium salts in the presence of renal dysfunction. Use **sodium phosphate** and **sodium biphosphate** with caution in these patients; hyperphosphatemia, hypernatremia, acidosis, and hypocalcemia may occur.

➤*Pregnancy: Category B.* (**Lactulose**, **magnesium sulfate**). *Category C.* (**Bisacodyl** [per Briggs' *Drugs in Pregnancy and Lactation*], **casanthranol**, **cascara sagrada**, **castor oil** [per Briggs' *Drugs in Pregnancy and Lactation*], **danthron**, **docusate sodium**, **docusate calcium**, **docusate potassium**, **glycerin** [per Briggs' *Drugs in Pregnancy and Lactation*], **mineral oil**, **senna**). Do not use **castor oil** during pregnancy; its irritant effect may induce premature labor. Mineral oil may decrease absorption of fat-soluble vitamins. Improper use of saline cathartics can lead to dangerous electrolyte imbalance. If needed, limit use to bulk-forming or surfactant laxatives.

➤*Lactation:* Anthraquinone derivatives (eg, **casanthranol**, **cascara sagrada**, **danthron**) are excreted in breast milk resulting in a potential increased incidence of diarrhea in the nursing infant. Magnesium emulsions administered orally did not affect the stools of nursing infants, although magnesium content in breast milk was slightly elevated compared with untreated patients. Sennosides A and B (eg, **senna**) are not excreted in breast milk. It is not known whether **bisacodyl**, **docusate calcium**, **docusate potassium**, **docusate sodium**, **lactulose**, and **mineral oil** are excreted in breast milk. The active ingredient in castor oil, ricinoleic acid, is absorbed systemically and could be excreted into milk.

➤*Children:* Administer with caution. Dosage is product specific. Do not administer enemas to children younger than 2 years of age. Infants receiving **lactulose** may develop hyponatremia and dehydration.

➤*Elderly:* Per the Beers list, long-term use of **bisacodyl**, **cascara sagrada**, or **castor oil**, except in the presence of opiate analgesic use, may exacerbate bowel dysfunction.

Per the Beers list, **mineral oil** has the potential for aspiration and adverse effects. Safer alternatives are available.

➤*Monitoring:* In the overall management of portal-systemic encephalopathy, there is serious underlying liver disease with complications such as electrolyte disturbance (eg, hypokalemia, hypernatremia), which may require other specific therapy. Elderly, debilitated patients who receive **lactulose** for more than 6 months should have serum electrolytes (potassium, chloride) and carbon dioxide measured periodically.

Drug Interactions

Laxative Drug Interactions

Precipitant drug	Object drug[a]		Description
Surfactants (eg, docusate)	Mineral oil	↑	When concomitantly administered, surfactants (eg, docusate) may increase mineral oil absorption.
Milk Antacids H_2 antagonists Protein pump inhibitors	Bisacodyl	↑	Avoid administration 1 to 2 hours before bisacodyl tablets; concomitant administration may cause the enteric coating to dissolve, resulting in gastric lining irritation or dyspepsia.
Mineral oil	Lipid-soluble vitamins	↓	Absorption of lipid-soluble vitamins may decrease during prolonged mineral oil administration.
Neomycin and other anti-infectives	Lactulose	↔	Reports conflict about concomitant use of lactulose syrup. The elimination of certain colonic bacteria may interfere with desired degradation of lactulose and prevent acidification of colonic contents. Monitor patient if concomitant oral anti-infectives are given.
Antacids	Lactulose	↓	Nonabsorbable antacids given concurrently with lactulose may inhibit the desired lactulose-induced drop in colonic pH.

[a] ↑ = Object drug increased. ↓ = Object drug decreased. ↔ = Undetermined clinical effect.

Adverse Reactions

Diarrhea; nausea; vomiting; perianal irritation; fainting; bloating; flatulence; cramps.

Obstruction of the esophagus, stomach, small intestine, and colon has occurred when bulk-forming laxatives are administered without adequate fluids or in patients with intestinal stenosis.

Large doses of **mineral oil** may cause anal seepage, resulting in itching (pruritus ani), rectal inflammation, and perianal discomfort.

Lactulose – Gaseous distention with flatulence, belching, abdominal discomfort such as cramping (≈ 20%); nausea; vomiting. Excessive dosage can lead to diarrhea.

Overdosage

There have been no reports of accidental **lactulose** overdose. It is expected that diarrhea and abdominal cramps would be the major symptoms; discontinue the drug.

Patient Information

Direct attention to proper dietary fiber intake, adequate fluids, and regular exercise.

Do not use in the presence of abdominal pain, nausea, or vomiting.

Laxative use is only a temporary measure; do not use more than 1 week. When regularity returns, discontinue use. Prolonged, frequent, or excessive use may result in dependence or electrolyte imbalance.

Notify physician if unrelieved constipation, rectal bleeding, or symptoms of electrolyte imbalance (eg, muscle cramps or pain, weakness, dizziness) occur.

Pink-red, red-violet, red-brown, yellow-brown, or black discoloration of urine may occur with **cascara sagrada** or **senna**.

Refrigerate **magnesium citrate** solutions to improve taste.

➤*Mineral oil:* Preferably administered on an empty stomach.

➤*Bisacodyl tablets:* Swallow whole; do not take within 1 to 2 hours of antacids, prescription or *otc* H_2 antagonists, proton pump inhibitors, or milk.

➤*Lactulose:* May be mixed with fruit juice, water, or milk to increase palatability.

May cause belching, flatulence, or abdominal cramps; notify physician if these effects become bothersome or if diarrhea occurs.

Do not take other laxatives while on lactulose therapy.

In the event that unusual diarrheal condition occurs, contact your physician.

SALINE LAXATIVES

otc	**Phillips'** (Bayer Consumer)	**Tablets:** 500 mg magnesium (as oxide)	Polyvinyl alcohol. In 24s.
otc	**Pedia-Lax** (Fleet)	**Tablets, chewable; oral:** 400 mg magnesium as hydroxide	Watermelon flavor. In 30s.
otc	**Epsom Salt** (Various, eg, Humco)	**Granules:** Magnesium sulfate. *Dose:* Adults ≥ 12 years - 5 to 10 mL in ½ glass of water. Children 6 to 12 years - 2.5 to 5 mL in ½ glass of water.	In 120 g and 1 and 4 lbs.
otc	**Milk of Magnesia – Concentrated** (Roxane)	**Suspension:** Equiv. to 30 mL milk of magnesia *Dose:* 10 to 20 mL.	In 100 and 400 mL and UD 10 mL.
otc	**Phillips' Milk of Magnesia, Concentrated** (Bayer Consumer)	**Suspension:** Magnesium hydroxide 800 mg/5 mL *Dose:* Adults and children ≥ 12 years – 15 to 30 mL. Children 6 to 11 years - 7.5 to 15 mL Children 2 to 5 years - 2.5 to 7.5 mL	Sorbitol, sugar. Strawberry creme flavor. In 240 mL.
otc	**Milk of Magnesia** (Various, eg, Geneva, Goldline, Humco, Roxane, URL)	**Suspension:** Magnesium hydroxide 400 mg/5 mL *Dose:* Adults and children ≥ 12 years - 30 to 60 mL/day, taken with liquid. Children 6 to 11 years - 15 to 30 mL/day Children 2 to 5 years - 5 to 15 mL/day	In 180, 360, 480 mL and UD 30 mL, gallon
otc	**Phillips' Milk of Magnesia** (Bayer Consumer)		Saccharin (mint); sorbitol, sugar (cherry). Mint, cherry, and regular flavors. In 120, 360, and 780 mL.
otc sf	**Magnesium Citrate Solution** (Humco)	**Solution:** 1.75 g magnesium citrate/30 mL *Dose:* Adults and children ≥ 12 years - ½ to 1 bottle Children 6 to 12 years - ⅓ to ½ bottle	Saccharin. Cherry and lemon flavors. In 296 mL.

For complete and comparative prescribing information, refer to the Laxatives group monograph.

Irritant or Stimulant Laxatives

CASCARA SAGRADA

otc	**Aromatic Cascara Fluidextract** (Various, eg, Goldline)	**Liquid:** *Dose:* Adults and children ≥ 12 years - 2 to 6 mL single daily dose	19% alcohol. In 473 mL.

Irritant or Stimulant Laxatives

SENNOSIDES

otc	**Dr. Edwards' Olive** (Oakhurst)	**Tablets; oral:** 8.6 mg sennosides (from senna concentrate) *Dose:* Adults - 2 tablets a day, not to exceed 4 tablets twice daily Children 6 to 12 y -1 tablet a day, not to exceed 2 tablets twice daily	In 75s.
otc	**Senexon** (Rugby)	**Tablets; oral:** 8.6 mg sennosides *Dose:* Adults and children ≥ 12 y - 2 tablets once or twice daily Children 6 to younger than 12 y - 1 tablet once or twice/day	Lactose. In 100s and 1,000s.
otc	**Senna-Gen** (Zenith-Goldline)	**Tablets; oral:** 8.6 mg sennosides *Dose:* Adults and children ≥ 12 y - 2 to 4 tablets once or twice daily Children 6 to younger than 12 y - 1 to 2 tablets once or twice daily Children 2 to younger than 6 y - ½ to 1 tablet once or twice daily	Lactose. In 100s and 1,000s.
otc	**ex•lax** (Novartis Consumer)	**Tablets; oral:** 15 mg sennosides *Dose:* Adults and children ≥ 12 y - 2 tablets once or twice daily with water Children 6 to younger than 12 y - 1 tablet once or twice daily with water	Sucrose. (ex-lax 1). In 8s, 30s, and 60s.
otc	**ex•lax chocolated** (Novartis Consumer)	**Tablets; oral:** 15 mg sennosides *Dose:* Adults and children ≥ 12 y - 2 tablets once or twice daily with water Children 6 to younger than 12 y - 1 tablet once or twice daily with water	Sugar, oil, dry milk. Chocolated. In 6s, 18s, and 48s.
otc	**Lax-Pills** (G & W Labs)	**Tablets; oral:** 15 mg sennosides *Dose:* Adults and children ≥ 12 y - 2 tablets once or twice daily with water Children 6 to younger than 12 y - 1 tablet once or twice daily with water	In blister pack 30s and 60s.
otc	**Senna Smooth** (Novartis Consumer Health)	**Tablets; oral:** 15 mg sennosides *Dose:* Adults and children ≥ 12 y - 1 tablet once or twice daily	Sucrose. In 24s.
otc	**SenokotXTRA** (Purdue Frederick)	**Tablets; oral:** 17 mg sennosides *Dose:* Adults and children ≥ 12 y - Start with 1 tablet/day, not to exceed 2 tablets twice/day Children 6 to younger than 12 y - Start with ½ tablet/day, not to exceed 1 tablet twice/day	Lactose. In 12s and 36s.
otc	**Lax-Pills** (G & W Labs)	**Tablets; oral:** 25 mg sennosides *Dose:* Adults and children ≥ 12 years - 2 tablets once or twice daily with water Children 6 to younger than 12 years - 1 tablet once or twice daily with water	In blister pack 24s and 48s.
otc	**Maximum Relief ex•lax** (Novartis Consumer)	**Tablets; oral:** 25 mg sennosides *Dose:* Adults and children ≥ 12 y - 2 tablets once or twice daily with water Children 6 to younger than 12 y - 1 tablet once or twice daily with water	Sucrose. (ex-lax 1). In 24s and 48s.
otc	**Black Draught** (Lee Pharmaceuticals)	**Tablets; oral:** 6 mg sennosides *Dose:* Adults and children ≥ 12 y - 2 tablets once or twice/day Children 6 to younger than 12 y - 1 tablet once or twice/day	Sucrose. In 30s.
		Tablets, chewable; oral: 10 mg sennosides *Dose:* Adults and children ≥ 12 y - 2 tablets once or twice daily Children 6 to younger than 12 y - 1 tablet once or twice/day	Sugar. In 30s.
		Granules; oral: 20 mg sennosides/5 mL *Dose:* Adults and children ≥ 12 y - As a tea: ¼ to ½ cup	Tartrazine, sucrose. In 22.5 g.
otc	**Senokot** (Purdue Frederick)	**Tablets; oral:** 8.6 mg sennosides *Dose:* Adults and children ≥ 12 y - Start with 2 tablets/day, not to exceed 4 tablets twice/day Children 6 to younger than 12 y - Start with 1 tablet/day, not to exceed 2 tablets twice/day Children 2 to younger than 6 y - ½ tablet/day, not to exceed 1 tablet twice/day	Lactose. In 10s, 20s, 50s, 100s, 1,000s, and UD 100s.
		Granules; oral: 15 mg/5 mL sennosides *Dose:* Adults and children ≥ 12 y - Start with 5 mL/day, not to exceed 10 mL twice/day Children 6 to younger than 12 y - 2.5 mL/day, not to exceed 5 mL twice/day Children 2 to younger than 6 y - 1.25 mL/day, not to exceed 2.5 mL twice/day	Sucrose. In 56, 170, and 340 g.
otc	**Senna** (SDA Labs)	**Syrup; oral:** 8.8 mg/5 mL sennosides *Dose:* Adults and children ≥ 12 y - 10 to 15 mL/day, not to exceed 15 mL twice/day Children 6 to younger than 12 y - 5 to 7.5 mL/day, not to exceed 7.5 mL twice/day Children 2 to younger than 6 y - 2.5 to 3.75 mL/day, not to exceed 3.75 mL twice/day	Parabens, sucrose. In 236 mL.
	Senokot (Purdue Frederick)		Alcohol free. Parabens, sucrose. In 59 and 237 mL.
otc	**Senna** (Pharmaceutical Associates)	**Syrup; oral:** 176 mg/5 mL senna leaf extract *Dose:* Adults and children ≥ 12 y - 10 to 15 mL once/day not to exceed 15 mL twice/day Children 6 to younger than 12 y - 5 to 7.5 mL once/day not to exceed 7.5 mL twice/day Children 2 to younger than 6 y - 2.5 to 3.75 mL once/day not to exceed 3.75 mL twice/day	Glycerin, parabens, sucrose. In 237 mL.
otc	**Evac-u-gen** (Lee Pharmaceuticals)	**Tablets, chewable; oral:** 10 mg sennosides *Dose:* Adults - 2 tablets once or twice daily Children ≥ 6 y - 1 tablet once or twice/day	Sugar. In 35s.
otc	**Senexon** (Rugby)	**Liquid; oral:** 8.8 mg sennosides/5 mL *Dose:* Adults and children ≥ 12 y - 10 to 15 mL once a day, not to exceed 15 mL twice a day Children 6 to younger than 12 y - 5 to 7.5 mL once a day, not to exceed 7.5 mL twice a day Children 2 to younger than 6 y - 2.5 to 3.75 mL once a day, not to exceed 3.75 mL twice a day	Parabens, sucrose. In 237 mL.
otc	**Fletcher's Castoria** (Mentholatum)	**Liquid; oral:** 33.3 mg/mL senna concentrate *Dose:* Children 6 to 15 y -10 to 15 mL ≤ 2 times/day Children 2 to 5 y - 5 to 10 mL ≤ 2 times/day	Alcohol free. Sucrose, parabens. In 74 and 150 mL.
otc	**Agoral** (Numark Labs)	**Liquid; oral:** 8.3 mg/5 mL sennosides *Dose:* Adults and children ≥ 12 y - 15 to 25 mL 2 times/day	Parabens, potassium sorbate, propylene glycol, sucrose. Marshmallow flavor. In 237 mL.
otc	**Little Tummys Laxative Drops** (Vetco Inc.)	**Drops; oral:** 8.8 mg/mL sennosides *Dose:* Children 6 to younger than 12 y - 1 to 1.5 mL once a day, not to exceed 1.5 mL twice a day Children 2 to younger than 6 y - 0.5 to 0.75 mL once a day, not to exceed 0.75 mL twice a day	Alcohol free. Parabens, sorbitol. In 30 mL with dropper.

SENNOSIDES — ORAL

For complete and comparative prescribing information, refer to the Laxatives group monograph.

Irritant or Stimulant Laxatives

BISACODYL

otc	**Bisacodyl** (Various, eg, Global Source, Major, UDL, URL)	**Tablets, delayed release; oral:** 5 mg	In 25s, 50s, 100s, 1,000s, and UD 100s.
otc	**Alophen** (Numark)		Sugar. In 100s.
otc	**Bisa-Lax** (Bergen Brunswig)		In 25s and 50s.
otc	**Dulcolax** (Boehringer Ingelheim)		Lactose, sucrose, parabens. (BI 12). In 10s, 25s, 50s, and 100s.
otc	**Ex-Lax Ultra** (Novartis Consumer Health)		Lactose, methylparaben, PEG. In 24s.
otc	**Fleet Laxative** (Fleet)		Sucrose. In 25s and 100s.
otc	**Modane** (Savage Labs)		Lactose. In 100s.
otc	**Bisac-Evac** (G & W Labs)		In 25s.
otc	**Caroid** (Mentholatum Co.)		Sugar. In 100s.
otc	**Correctol** (Schering-Plough)		Talc, lactose, sugar. (Correctol). In 30s, 60s, and 90s.
otc	**Feen-a-mint** (Schering-Plough)		Talc, lactose, sugar. (Feen-a-mint). In 30s.
otc	**Bisacodyl** (Various, eg, Global Source, URL)	**Suppositories; rectal:** 10 mg	In 12s, 16s, and 100s.
otc	**Bisacodyl Uniserts** (Upsher-Smith)		In 12s.
otc	**Bisa-Lax** (Bergen Brunswig)		Hydrogenated vegetable oil. In 50s.
otc	**Bisac-Evac** (G & W Labs)		In 8s, 12s, 50s, 100s, 500s, and 1,000s.
otc	**Dulcolax** (Boehringer Ingelheim)		In 4s, 8s, 16s, and 50s.
otc	**Fleet Laxative** (Fleet)		In 4s, 12s, 50s, and 100s.
otc	**Dulcolax Bowel Prep Kit** (Boehringer Ingelheim)	**Tablets delayed release; oral:** 5 mg	Docusate sodium, lactose, parabens, sucrose. In 4s.
		Suppository; rectal: 10 mg	Hydrogenated vegetable oil. In 1s.

BISACODYL — ORAL

For complete and comparative prescribing information, refer to the Laxatives group monograph.

Indications

➤*Constipation:* This medication is used to relieve occasional constipation (irregularity).

➤*Enteric-coated tablets:* Expect results in 8 to 12 hours if taken at bedtime or within 6 hours if taken before breakfast.

➤*Regular tablets:* Bisacodyl generally causes a bowel movement in 6 to 12 hours.

Administration and Dosage

➤*Adults:*

Constipation – 5 to 15 mg in a single dose once daily.

➤*Children:*

Constipation –

12 years of age and older: 5 to 15 mg in a single dose once daily.

6 to younger than 12 years of age: 5 mg once daily.

➤*Duration of therapy:* Laxative products should not be used for longer than 1 week unless told to do so by a health care provider.

➤*Administration:* Do not chew or crush tablets. Take with water. Do not administer tablets within 1 hour after taking an antacid or milk.

➤*Storage/Stability:* Store at 15° to 30°C (59° to 86°F). Avoid excessive humidity.

BISACODYL — RECTAL

For complete and comparative prescribing information, refer to the Laxatives group monograph.

Indications

➤*Suppositories:* This medication is indicated for relief of occasional constipation and irregularity. This medication stimulates bowel movement in 15 minutes to 1 hour.

➤*Enema:* This preparation is indicated for relief of occasional constipation or bowel cleansing before rectal examinations in adults and children 12 years of age and older.

Administration and Dosage

➤*Adults:*

Bowel cleansing –

Enema: 1 bottle as a single daily dose.

Constipation –

Enema: 1 bottle as a single daily dose.

Suppositories: Use 1 suppository.

Off-label dosing –

Opioid-induced constipation: Consider bisacodyl suppositories if senna in combination with docusate is ineffective.

1 suppository every 6 hours as needed.

➤*Children:* See Adults for dosing for children older than 12 years of age.

Constipation –

Suppositories:

• *6 to younger than 12 years of age* – One-half suppository. Some products are not approved for use in children younger than 12 years of age. See product labeling.

Off-label dosing –

Opioid-induced constipation: Consider bisacodyl suppositories if senna in combination with docusate is ineffective.

• *Younger than 2 years of age* – 5 mg/day (single dose) given as a rectal suppository as needed.

• *2 to 11 years of age* – 5 to 10 mg/day (single dose) given as a rectal suppository as needed.

➤*Administration:*

Enema –

Left side position: Lie on left side with knee bent and arms resting comfortably.

Knee-chest position: Kneel, then lower head and chest forward until left side of face is resting on surface with left arm folded comfortably.

How to use enema:

1.) Remove protective shield from enema tip before inserting.
2.) With steady pressure, gently insert enema tip into rectum with a slight side-to-side movement, with tip pointing toward navel. Insertion may be easier if the person receiving enema bears down, as if having a bowel movement. This helps relax the muscles around the anus.
3.) Do not force the enema tip into the rectum, as this may cause injury.
4.) Squeeze bottle until nearly all the liquid is gone. It is not necessary to empty the bottle completely, as it contains more liquid than needed.
5.) Remove enema tip from rectum and maintain position until urge to evacuate is strong, 5 to 20 minutes, if possible.

Suppositories – Remove foil wrap. Lie on side and gently insert suppository pointed end first towards the navel and well up into rectum. Make sure suppository touches the bowel wall. Retain suppository for at least 15 to 20 minutes.

➤*Storage/Stability:*

Enemas – Store at temperatures not above 30°C (86°F).

Suppositories – Bisacodyl suppositories should be stored below 25°C (77°F). Therefore, they may be stored in the refrigerator if the room temperature exceeds 25°C (77°F) in order to help keep suppositories from softening. Allow the product to return to room temperature before using.

Bulk-Producing Laxatives

PSYLLIUM

otc	**Metamucil** (Procter & Gamble Co.)	**Capsules:** 0.52 g psyllium husk *Dose:* Adults 12 years of age and older - 2 to 6 capsules for increasing daily fiber intake; 6 capsules for cholesterol-lowering use. Take with 8 oz liquid (swallow 1 capsule at a time) up to tid.	In 100s and 160s.
otc *sf*	**Fiberall Tropical Fruit Flavor** (Heritage Consumer)	**Powder:** 3.5 g psyllium hydrophilic mucilloid per dose *Dose:* 1 rounded teaspoon (5 to 5.9 g) in 6 oz cool water or juice once daily followed immediately by ½ glass of water. After 1 week, may take ≤ 3 servings/day.	Aspartame. In 454 g and UD 10 g packets.
otc	**Fiberall Orange Flavor** (Heritage Consumer)		Aspartame. In 480 g.
otc	**Genfiber** (Goldline Consumer)	**Powder:** 3.4 g psyllium hydrophilic mucilloid fiber and 14 calories per dose. *Dose:* Adults - 1 rounded teaspoon in 8 oz liquid 1 to 3 times/day. Children 6 to 12 years of age - ½ rounded teaspoon in 8 oz liquid 1 to 3 times/day.	Dextrose. In 595 g.
otc	**Genfiber, Orange Flavor** (Goldline Consumer)	**Powder:** 3.4 g psyllium hydrophilic mucilloid per dose. *Dose:* Adults - 1 rounded tablespoon in 8 oz liquid 1 to 3 times/day. Children 6 to 12 years of age - ½ rounded tablespoon in 8 oz liquid 1 to 3 times/day.	Sucrose. Orange flavor. In 397 g.
otc	**Natural Psyllium Fiber** (Plus Pharma)	**Powder:** 3.4 g psyllium hydrophilic mucilloid fiber, 3 mg sodium, and 25 calories per dose. *Dose*: Adults - 1 rounded teaspoon in 8 oz liquid 2 to 3 times/day.	Dextrose. In 368 g.
otc	**Natural Psyllium Fiber, Orange** (Plus Pharma)	**Powder:** 3.4 g psyllium hydrophilic mucilloid fiber, 3 mg sodium, and 25 calories per dose. *Dose*: Adults - 1 rounded teaspoon in 8 oz liquid 2 to 3 times/day.	Sucrose. Orange flavor. In 368 g.
otc *sf*	**Hydrocil Instant** (Numark)	**Powder:** 3.5 g psyllium hydrophilic mucilloid/dose *Dose:* 1 level scoopful (3.7 g) in liquid	In 250 g.
otc *sf*	**Konsyl Orange Sugar Free** (Konsyl Pharm.)	**Powder:** 3.5 g psyllium hydrophilic mucilloid/tsp *Dose:* Adults and children 12 years and over - 1 level teaspoon mixed in 8 oz liquid 1 to 3 times/day; Children 6 to under 12 - ½ adult dose in 8 oz liquid up to 3 times/day	Sugar free. Aspartame, calcium 6 mg, maltodextrin, phenylalanine 21 mg, potassium 32 mg, sodium 3 mg per tsp. Orange flavor. In 450 g.
otc *sf*	**Konsyl** (Konsyl Pharm.)	**Powder:** 6 g psyllium. *Dose:* 1 packet or rounded teaspoon (6 g) in liquid	In 300 and 450 g and UD 6 g packets.
otc *sf*	**Konsyl Easy Mix Formula** (Konsyl Pharm.)	**Powder:** 6 g psyllium, 4.4 mg Na, 48 mg Ca, 4 mg P, 0.06 mg Zn, 42 mg K, 0.35 g carbohydrates, 4 calories/5 mL *Dose:* 1 teaspoon (5 mL) or 6.3 g packet	In 200 g and packets.
otc	**Geri-Mucil** (Geri-Care)	**Powder:** 3.4 g psyllium husk, 10 mg sodium, and 14 calories per dose *Dose:* Adults and children 12 years of age or older - 1 teaspoon in 8 oz liquid, 1 to 3 times a day.	Dextrose. In 368 g.
otc	**Metamucil Orange Flavor, Smooth Texture** (Procter & Gamble Co.)	**Powder:** ≈ 3.4 g psyllium husk, 5 mg sodium, 12 g carbohydrates, and 45 calories per dose *Dose:* Adults and children 12 years of age or older - 1 rounded tablespoon in liquid, 1 to 3 times a day. Children 6 to 12 years of age - ½ adult dose	Sucrose. In 420, 630, and 1368 g, and 100 UD single-dose packs (100s).
otc *sf*	**Metamucil, Sugar Free, Smooth Texture** (Procter & Gamble Co.)	**Powder:** ≈ 3.4 g psyllium husk, 5 g carbohydrates, 4 mg sodium, and 20 calories per dose *Dose:* Adults and children 12 years of age and older - 1 rounded teaspoon in liquid, 1 to 3 times a day. Children 6 to 12 years of age - ½ adult dose	In 425 g and packets of 30s or 100s.
otc *sf*	**Metamucil, Sugar Free, Orange Flavor, Smooth Texture** (Procter & Gamble Co.)	**Powder:** ≈ 3.4 g psyllium husk, 5 g carbohydrates, 5 mg sodium, 20 calories per dose. *Dose:* Adults and children 12 years of age and older - 1 rounded teaspoon in liquid 1 to 3 times a day. Children 6 to 12 years of age - ½ adult dose	Aspartame, 25 mg phenylalanine per dose. In 210, 420, 630, and 660 g.
otc	**Metamucil Orange Flavor, Original Texture** (Procter & Gamble Co.)	**Powder:** ≈ 3.4 g psyllium husk, 10 g carbohydrates, 5 mg sodium, 40 calories/dose *Dose:* Adults and children 12 years of age and older - 1 rounded tablespoon in 8 oz liquid ≤ 3 times/day Children 6 to 12 years of age - ½ adult dose	Sucrose. In 210, 420, 538, and 630 g.
otc	**Metamucil Original Texture** (Procter & Gamble Co.)	**Powder:** ≈ 3.4 g psyllium husk, 6 g carbohydrates, 3 mg sodium, 25 calories/dose *Dose:* Adults and children 12 years of age and older - 1 rounded teaspoon in 8 oz liquid ≤ 3 times/day Children 6 to 12 years of age - ½ adult dose	Sucrose. In 822 g and packets of 30.
otc	**Reguloid, Orange** (Rugby)	**Powder:** ≈ 3.4 g psyllium mucilloid/tablespoon *Dose:* Adults and children 12 years of age and older - 1 rounded tablespoon, 1 to 3 times daily in 8 oz liquid. Children 6 to 12 years of age - ½ adult dose	Sucrose. Orange flavor. In 369 and 540 g.
otc *sf*	**Reguloid, Sugar Free Orange** (Rugby)	**Powder:** ≈ 3.4 g psyllium hydrophilic mucilloid per rounded teaspoon *Dose:* Adults and children 12 years of age and older - 1 rounded teaspoon in 8 oz liquid, 1 to 3 times/day. Children 6 to 12 years of age - ½ adult dose in 8 oz liquid 1 to 3 times/day	Aspartame, 30 mg phenylalanine per dose. In 284 and 426 g.
otc *sf*	**Reguloid, Sugar Free Regular** (Rugby)	**Powder:** ≈ 3.4 g psyllium hydrophilic mucilloid per dose *Dose:* Adults and children 12 years of age and older - 1 rounded teaspoon in 8 oz liquid, 1 to 3 times/day. Children 6 to 12 years of age - ½ adult dose in 8 oz liquid 1 to 3 times a day.	Aspartame, 6 mg phenylalanine per dose. In 284 and 426 g.
otc	**Natural Fiber Laxative** (Apothecary)	**Powder:** ≈ 3.4 g psyllium hydrophilic mucilloid/7 g dose. 14 calories/dose. *Dose:* Adults and children 12 years of age and older - 7 g 1 to 3 times/day Children 6 to 12 years of age - ½ adult dose	Sodium free. In 390 g.
otc	**Syllact** (Wallace)	**Powder:** 3.3 g psyllium seed husks and ≈ 14 calories per rounded teaspoon *Dose:* Adults and children 12 years of age and older - 1 rounded teaspoon in 8 oz liquid, 1 to 3 times daily. Children 6 to younger than 12 years of age – ½ to 1 rounded teaspoon in 8 oz liquid 1 to 3 times/day	Dextrose, saccharin, parabens. Fruit flavor. In 284 g.
otc	**Konsyl-D** (Konsyl Pharm.)	**Powder:** 3.4 g psyllium, 14 calories per rounded teaspoon *Dose:* Adults and children 12 years of age and older - 1 teaspoon 1 to 3 times/day Children 6 to younger than 12 years of age - ½ teaspoon 1 to 3 times/day	Dextrose. In 325 and 500 g and UD 6.5 g.
otc	**Reguloid** (Rugby)	**Powder:** ≈ 3.4 g of 95% pure psyllium husk fiber/5 ml *Dose:* Adults and children ≥ 12 years - 1 rounded tsp in 8 oz liquid, 1 to 3 times a day. Children 6 to 12 years - ½ rounded tsp in 8 oz liquid, 1 to 3 times a day.	Dextrose. 14 calories per rounded teaspoon. In 369 and 540 g.

Bulk-Producing Laxatives

PSYLLIUM

otc	**Perdiem Fiber Therapy** (Novartis Consumer Health)	**Granules**: 4.03 g psyllium, 1.8 mg sodium, 36.1 mg potassium and 4 calories/rounded teaspoon (6 g) *Dose:* Adults - 1 to 2 rounded teaspoons with 8 oz liquid, once or twice daily. Do not chew. Children 7 to 11 years of age - 1 rounded teaspoon with 8 oz liquid once or twice daily	Sucrose. Dye free. Mint flavor. In 100 and 250 g.
otc	**Serutan** (Menley & James)	**Granules**: 2.5 g psyllium and less than 0.03 g sodium per heaping teaspoon *Dose:* Adults - 1 to 3 heaping teaspoon on cereal or other food, 1 to 3 times daily. Children 6 to 12 years of age - ½ to 1½ heaping teaspoon with 8 oz liquid.	Saccharin, sugar. In 170 and 540 g.
otc	**Metamucil** (Procter & Gamble Co.)	**Wafers**: ≈ 3.4 g psyllium husk/dose, 17 g carbohydrates, 20 mg sodium, 5 g fat, 120 calories/dose *Dose:* Adults and children 12 years of age and older - 2 wafers w/8 oz liquid ≤ 3 times/day Children 6 to 12 years of age - 1 wafer w/8 oz liquid ≤ 3 times/day	Sugar, fructose, molasses, sucrose. Cinnamon spice and apple crisp flavors. In 24s.

PSYLLIUM — ORAL

For complete and comparative prescribing information, refer to the Laxatives group monograph.

CALCIUM POLYCARBOPHIL

otc	**Equalactin** (Numark)	**Tablets, chewable**: 625 mg calcium polycarbophil (equivalent to 500 mg polycarbophil)	Citrus flavor. In 24s and 48s.
otc	**Konsyl Fiber** (Konsyl)	**Tablets**: 500 mg polycarbophil	In 90s.
otc	**Fiber-Lax** (Rugby)	**Tablets**: 625 mg calcium polycarbophil (equivalent to 500 mg polycarbophil)	In 60s, 90s, and 500s.
otc	**Bulk Forming Fiber Laxative** (Goldline Consumer)		Film-coated. In 60s.
otc	**FiberCon** (Lederle)		Calcium carbonate. (LL F66). In 36s, 60s, 90s, and 150s.

CALCIUM POLYCARBOPHIL — ORAL

For complete and comparative prescribing information, refer to the Laxatives group monograph.

Indications

➤*Constipation:* Polycarbophil promotes normal function of the bowel by increasing bulk volume and water content of the stool. This product generally produces a bowel movement in 12 to 72 hours.

Administration and Dosage

➤*Adults:*

Bowel regularity – 2 tablets 1 to 4 times per day.

➤*Children:*

Bowel regularity –

12 years of age and older: 2 tablets 1 to 4 times per day.

6 to 12 years of age: 1 tablet 1 to 4 times per day. Some products are not approved for use in children younger than 12 years of age. See package insert.

➤*Duration of therapy:* Continued use for 1 to 3 days normally is required to provide full benefit. Laxative products should not be used for longer than 1 week unless directed by a health care provider.

➤*Administration:* A full glass (240 mL [8 fl oz]) of liquid should be taken with each dose. Taking this product without adequate fluid may cause it to swell and block your throat or esophagus and may cause choking. Do not take this product if you have difficulty swallowing. Do not take more than the maximum daily dose.

➤*Storage/Stability:* Store at 15° to 30°C (59° to 86°F). Protect contents from moisture.

MISCELLANEOUS BULK-PRODUCING LAXATIVES

otc	**Citrucel** (GlaxoSmithKline)	**Powder**: 2 g methylcellulose per heaping tablespoon	Sucrose. Orange flavor. In 480 and 846 g.
otc sf	**Citrucel Sugar Free** (GlaxoSmithKline)	**Powder**: 2 g methylcellulose, 52 mg phenylalanine per leveled scoop	Aspartame. Orange flavor. In 245 and 480 g.
otc	**Citrucel** (GlaxoSmithKline)	**Tablets**: 500 mg methylcellulose	Maltodextrin. (CIT). Capsule shape. In 164s.
otc	**Unifiber** (Niche)	**Powder**: Powdered cellulose	In 150, 270, and 480 g.
otc	**Maltsupex** (Wallace)	**Powder**: 8 g malt soup extract per level scoop	In 227 and 454 g.
otc sf	**Benefiber Ultra Caplets** (Novartis)	**Tablets; oral**: Fiber 1 g	Gluten free, sugar free. Wheat dextrin. Capsule shape. In 72s and 114s.
otc sf	**Benefiber Plus Heart Health Caplets** (Novartis)		Gluten free, sugar free. Folic acid 44.7 mcg, vitamin B_6 0.23 mg, B_{12} 0.67 mcg, wheat dextrin. Capsule shape. In 60s.
otc sf	**Benefiber** (Novartis)	**Tablets, chewable; oral**: Fiber 1 g	Gluten free, sugar free. Acesulfame K, aspartame, dextrates, phenylalanine, sorbitol, sucralose, wheat dextrin. In assorted fruit and orange creme flavors. In 100s.
otc sf	**Benefiber Plus Calcium** (Novartis)		Gluten free, sugar free. Acesulfame K, aspartame, calcium 100 mg, dextrates, maltodextrin, phenylalanine, sorbitol, sucralose, wheat dextrin. In berry flavor. In 90s.
otc sf	**Benefiber** (Novartis)	**Powder; oral**: Fiber 1.5 g per teaspoon	Gluten free, sugar free. Wheat dextrin. In 70, 133, 217, 315, 437.5, and 665 g.
otc sf	**Benefiber for Children** (Novartis)		Gluten free, sugar free. Wheat dextrin. In 153 g.
otc sf	**Benefiber Plus Heart Health** (Novartis)		Gluten free, sugar free. Folic acid 67 mg, vitamin B_6 0.35 mg, B_{12} 1 mcg, wheat dextrin. In 181.4 g.
otc sf	**Benefiber Plus Calcium** (Novartis)	**Powder; oral**: Fiber 3 g per tablespoon	Gluten free, sugar free. Calcium 300 mg, wheat dextrin. In 423.8 g.

Bulk-Producing Laxatives

MISCELLANEOUS BULK-PRODUCING LAXATIVES

otc sf	**Benefiber Sticks** (Novartis)	**Powder; oral**: Fiber 3 g per packet	Sugar free. Acesulfame K, aspartame, maltodextrin, phenylalanine (all except unflavored); tartrazine (citrus punch flavor); wheat dextrin. In unflavored, cherry pomegranate, citrus punch, kiwi strawberry, and raspberry tea flavors. In 8s, 16s, and 28s.
otc sf	**Benefiber Drink Mix** (Novartis)		Sugar free. Acesulfame K, aspartame, maltodextrin, phenylalanine, potassium citrate, wheat dextrin. In cherry pomegranate, citrus punch, kiwi strawberry, and raspberry tea flavors. In 8s and 16s.

METHYLCELLULOSE — ORAL

For complete and comparative prescribing information, refer to the Laxatives group monograph.

MISCELLANEOUS BULK-PRODUCING LAXATIVES — ORAL

For complete and comparative prescribing information, refer to the Laxatives group monograph.

Administration and Dosage

➤*Adults:*

Bowel regularity –

Benefiber:

- *Chewable tablets* – 3 tablets up to 3 times per day.
- *Tablets* – 3 tablets up to 3 times per day with liquid. Do not exceed 9 per day.
- *Powder, Powder for Children, Plus Heart Health* – 2 teaspoons up to 3 times daily. Do not exceed 6 teaspoons per day. Stir into 120 to 240 mL of beverage or soft food.
- *Powder Plus Calcium* – 1 level tablespoon per day. Do not exceed 1 tablespoon per day. Stir into 240 mL of beverage or soft food.

Citrucel: 1 heaping tablespoon (19 g) or 1 packet (10.7 g) in 8 oz of cold water, 1 to 3 times daily.

Maltsupex: Up to 32 g twice daily for 3 or 4 days, then 16 to 32 g at bedtime.

Unifiber: 1 tablespoon in 3 or 4 oz. of fruit juice, milk, or water, or mix with soft foods such as applesauce, mashed potatoes, or pudding. Can be taken up to 3 times daily if needed or as recommended by a doctor.

➤*Children:*

Bowel regularity – See Adults for dosing for children 12 years of age and older.

Benefiber:

- *Chewable tablets* –
  6 to 11 years of age: 1½ tablets up to 3 times per day. Do not exceed 4½ tablets per day.
- *Powder, Powder for Children, Plus Heart Health* –
  6 to 11 years of age: 1 teaspoon up to 3 times daily. Do not exceed 3 teaspoons per day. Stir into 120 to 240 mL of beverage or soft food.
- *Powder Plus Calcium* –
  6 years of age and older: 1 level tablespoon per day. Do not exceed 1 tablespoon per day. Stir into 240 mL of beverage or soft food.

Citrucel:

- *6 to 11 years of age* – ½ the adult dose in 8 oz of cold water once daily.

Maltsupex:

- *6 to 12 years of age* – Up to 16 g twice daily for 3 or 4 days.
- *2 to 6 years of age* – 8 g twice daily for 3 or 4 days.

Unifiber: 1 tablespoon in 3 or 4 oz of fruit juice, milk, or water, or mix with soft foods such as applesauce, mashed potatoes, or pudding. Can be taken up to 3 times daily if needed or as recommended by a doctor.

➤*Preparation for administration:*

Benefiber Powder, Powder for Children, Plus Heart Health – Stir into 120 to 240 mL of beverage or soft food. Stir well until dissolved. Not recommended for carbonated beverages.

Benefiber Powder Plus Calcium – Stir into 240 mL of beverage or soft food. Stir well until dissolved. Not recommended for carbonated beverages.

Benefiber Stick Packs –

Flavored packs: Take a sip from 500 mL bottle of water if filled to the top. Empty contents of 1 packet into bottle. Shake well until dissolved. Not recommended for carbonated beverages.

Unflavored packs: Stir 1 packet into 120 to 240 mL beverage or soft food. Stir until well dissolved. Not recommended for carbonated beverages.

Benefiber Drink Mix – Empty contents of one stick pack into 500 mL bottle of water. Shake well until dissolved.

Citrucel – Mix powder in at least 8 oz of cold water or other fluid; stir briskly and drink promptly.

Unifiber – Stir into any beverage (water, fruit juice, milk, etc.) or soft food (cereals, applesauce, mashed potatoes, pudding, etc.). Not recommended for carbonated beverages.

➤*Administration:* Take with a full glass of water; encourage additional fluid intake.

Emollients

MINERAL OIL

otc	**Mineral Oil** (Various, eg, Fleet, Paddock)	**Liquid**: Mineral oil	In 180 and 473 mL.
otc	**Kondremul Plain** (Heritage Consumer Prod.)	**Emulsion**: Mineral oil	Irish moss, acacia, glycerin. In 480 mL.

MINERAL OIL — ORAL

For complete and comparative prescribing information, refer to the Laxatives group monograph.

Indications

➤*Constipation:* Mineral oil acts only as a non-irritating intestinal lubricant for relief of occasional constipation. This product generally produces a bowel movement in 6 to 8 hours.

➤*Prophylaxis:* Mineral oil may be useful prophylactically in patients who should not strain during defecation (ie, following anorectal surgery, MI).

Administration and Dosage

➤*Adults:*

Constipation – 15 to 45 mL as a single daily dose or in divided doses.

➤*Children:*

Constipation –

Older than 12 years of age: 15 to 45 mL as a single daily dose or in divided doses.

6 to 12 years of age: 5 to 15 mL as a single daily dose or in divided doses.

Younger than 6 years of age: Do not administer to children under 6 years of age.

➤*Duration of therapy:* Do not use more than 1 week.

➤*Administration:* Do not take with meals. Administer on an empty stomach.

➤*Storage/Stability:* Keep tightly closed. Protect from sunlight.

Fecal Softeners/Surfactants

DOCUSATE SODIUM (Dioctyl Sodium Sulfosuccinate; DSS)

otc	**ex-lax Stool Softener** (Novartis Consumer Health)	**Tablets; oral**: 100 mg *Dose:* Adults and children ≥ 12 years - 100 to 300 mg/day Children 2 to younger than 12 years - 100 mg/day	Methylparabens. Caplet shape. In 40s.
otc	**Dioctyn** (Dixon-Shane)	**Tablets; oral**: 100 mg *Dose:* Adults and children ≥ 12 years - 100 to 200 mg at bedtime Children 6 to 12 years - 100 mg at bedtime	Sorbitol. In 1,000s.
otc	**Colace** (Purdue)	**Capsules; oral**: 50 mg *Dose:* Adults and children ≥ 12 years - 50 to 300 mg/day Children 6 to 12 years - 50 to 150 mg/day	(RPC 052). In 30s, 60s, and UD 100s.

Fecal Softeners/Surfactants

DOCUSATE SODIUM (Dioctyl Sodium Sulfosuccinate; DSS)

otc	**Colace** (Purdue)	**Capsules; oral:** 100 mg *Dose:* Adults and children ≥ 12 years - 100 to 300 mg/day Children 6 to 12 years - 100 mg/day Children 2 to 6 years - Products vary. Consult product labeling for specific guidelines.	In 30s, 60s, 250s, 1,000s, and UD 100s.
otc	**D-S-S** (Magno-Humphries)		In 100s.
otc	**Non-Habit Forming Stool Softener** (Rugby)		Sorbitol, parabens. In 100s and 1,000s.
otc	**Stool Softener** (Rugby)		Lactose, tartrazine. In 1,000s.
otc	**Docusate Sodium** (Various, eg, Geneva, UDL, URL)	**Capsules; oral:** 250 mg *Dose:* Adults and children ≥ 12 years - 250 mg/day	In 100s and 1,000s, and UD 100s.
otc	**Stool Softener** (Rugby)		Lactose. In 1,000s.
otc	**Docusate Sodium** (UDL)	**Capsules, softgel; oral:** 50 mg *Dose:* Adults and children ≥ 12 years - 50 to 300 mg/day Children 2 to younger than 12 years - 50 mg/day	In 100s and UD 100s.
otc	**Docusate Sodium** (Various, eg, Goldline Consumer, UDL, URL)	**Capsules, softgel; oral:** 100 mg *Dose:* Adults and children ≥ 12 years - 100 to 300 mg/day Children 6 to younger than 12 years - 100 mg/day Children 2 to 6 years - Products vary. Consult product labeling for specific guidelines.	In 100s, 1,000s, and UD 100s and 300s.
otc	**D.O.S.** (Goldline Consumer)		Parabens. In 100s and 1,000s.
otc	**Dulcolax Stool Softener** (Boehringer Ingelheim)		Sorbitol, glycerin. In 25s.
otc	**Phillips' Liqui-Gels** (Bayer Consumer)		Parabens, sorbitol. (Phillips). In 10s, 30s, and 50s.
otc	**Sof-lax** (Fleet)		5 mg sodium/capsule. In 60s.
otc	**Docusate Sodium** (Various, eg, Schein)	**Capsules, softgel; oral:** 250 mg *Dose:* Adults and children ≥ 12 years - 250 mg/day	In 100s.
otc	**Stool Softener** (Rugby)		Sorbitol, parabens. In 100s and 1,000s.
otc	**D.O.S.** (Goldline Consumer)		Oblong. Red-orange. In 100s and 500s.
otc	**Docusate Sodium** (Roxane)	**Syrup; oral:** 50 mg per 15 mL *Dose:* Adults and children ≥ 12 years - 50 to 100 mg Children 6 to 12 years - 50 mg Children 3 to 5 years - 33 mg	Saccharin, sucrose, parabens. In UD 15 and 30 mL (100s).
otc	**Docu** (Hi-Tech Pharmacal Co.)	**Syrup; oral:** 20 mg per 5 mL *Dose:* Adults and children ≥ 12 years - 60 to 180 mg/day Children 6 to 12 years - 40 mg 1 to 3 times/day Children 3 to 6 years - 20 to 60 mg/day	5% alcohol. In 480 mL.
otc	**Diocto** (Various, eg, Alpharma)	**Syrup; oral:** 60 mg per 15 mL	In 480 mL. *Dose:* Adults and children ≥ 12 years - 60 to 360 mg/day Children 2 to 12 years - Dosage varies. Consult product labeling for specific guidelines. Generally, 40 to 150 mg/day.
otc	**Colace** (Purdue)		≤ 1% alcohol. Menthol, parabens, sucrose. In 237 and 473 mL. *Dose:* Adults and children ≥ 12 years - 60 to 300 mg/day Children 6 to 12 years - 40 to 120 mg/day Children 3 to 6 years - 20 to 60 mg/day Children younger than 3 years of age - 10 to 40 mg/day
otc	**Silace** (Silarx)		≤ 1% alcohol. In 473 mL. *Dose:* Adults and children ≥ 12 years - 60 to 180 mg/day Children 6 to 12 years - 40 mg 1 to 3 times/day
otc	**Docusate Sodium** (Roxane)	**Syrup; oral:** 100 mg/30 mL *Dose:* Adults and children ≥ 12 years - 50 to 100 mg Children 6 to 12 years - 50 mg Children 3 to 5 years - 33 mg	Saccharin, sucrose, parabens. In UD 15 and 30 mL (100s).
otc	**Silace** (Silarx)	**Liquid; oral:** 10 mg/mL *Dose:* Adults and children ≥ 12 years - 50 to 200 mg/day (5 to 20 mL) Children 6 to younger than 12 years - 40 to 120 mg/day (4 to 12 mL) Children 3 to younger than 6 years - 20 to 60 mg/day (2 to 6 mL)	Parabens. In 473 mL.
otc	**Diocto** (Various, eg, Goldline Consumer)	**Liquid; oral:** 150 mg per 15 mL	In 480 mL. *Dose:* Adults and children ≥ 12 years - 50 to 350 mg/day Children 2 to younger than 12 years - Dosage varies. Consult product labeling for specific guidelines. Generally, 20 to 150 mg/day.
otc	**Colace** (Purdue)		Parabens. In 30 and 480 mL. *Dose:* Children 3 to 6 years - 20 mg 1 to 3 times/day
otc	**Docu** (Hi-Tech Pharmacal Co.)		In 480 mL. *Dose:* Adults and children older than 12 years - 50 to 200 mg/day Children 6 to 12 years - 40 to 120 mg/day Children 3 to 6 years - 20 to 60 mg/day
otc	**DocuSol** (Alliance Labs)	**Enema; rectal:** 283 mg	*Dose:* Adults and children older than 12 years - 1 to 3 units/day Children 6 to 12 years - 1 unit/day

DOCUSATE SODIUM — ORAL

For complete and comparative prescribing information, refer to the Laxatives group monograph.

Indications

➤*Docusate sodium tablets and capsules:* Relief of occasional constipation (irregularity), especially for sensitive systems. This stimulant-free formula generally works within 12 to 72 hours after the first dose.

➤*Docusate sodium syrup and liquid:* Useful in constipation due to hard stools in painful anorectal conditions, in cardiac and other conditions in which maximum ease of passage is desirable to avoid difficult or painful defecation, and when peristaitic stimulants are contraindicated.

Administration and Dosage

➤*General dosing considerations:* Dosage varies according to product; see product labeling.

➤*Adults:*

Constipation – 50 to 300 mg/day taken as a single daily dose or in divided doses. The higher doses are recommended for initial therapy. Dosage should be adjusted to individual response.

Retention or flushing enemas – Add 5 to 10 mL of a docusate rectal solution to the enema fluid and administer rectally.

➤*Children:*

Constipation –

2 to younger than 12 years of age: 20 to 150 mg/day taken as a single daily dose or in divided doses.

➤*Administration:*

Tablets – Take tablets with a glass of water at any time.

Liquid – Shake well before using. Give in glass of milk or fruit juice, or in infant formula.

Syrup – Shake well before using. Take each dose with a full glass of water or liquid (may be taken with fruit juice). Drink increased fluids. To mask taste, the syrup may be given in a half a glass of milk or fruit juice, or in infant formula.

➤*Storage/Stability:*

Tablets and capsules – Store in a dry place between 15° and 30°C (59° and 86°F). Protect from moisture.

Syrup and liquid – Store between 15° and 30°C (59° and 86°F). Protect from excessive temperatures. Dispense in tight, light-resistant container.

DOCUSATE SODIUM — RECTAL

Indications

➤*Constipation:* For the relief of occasional constipation (irregularity). This product usually produces a bowel movement in 2 to 15 minutes.

Administration and Dosage

➤*Maximum dose:* There is no well-established maximum dose according to the product label.

➤*Adults:*

Adults – 1 to 3 units/day.

➤*Children:*

12 years of age and older – See Adults for dosing.

6 to 12 years of age – 1 unit/day.

Younger than 6 years of age – Consult health care provider.

➤*Duration of therapy:* Do not use laxative products for longer than 1 week unless directed otherwise by a health care provider.

➤*Administration:* Twist off and remove tip.

Lubricate tip prior to insertion. Place a few drops of water or a few drops of the product on the shaft prior to insertion. Also apply one of these lubricants to the anus before inserting the enema.

In the knee-chest position, kneel, then lower head and chest forward until the side of the face is resting on the surface with arm folded comfortably.

With steady pressure, gently insert the enema into the rectum. Insert the enema up to the shoulder of the tube. Make sure tube is in a gravity flow position prior to squeezing. Forcing the tip can cause injury to the rectal wall.

Squeeze the tube to empty the contents.

Slowly remove the disposable tube after the contents have been emptied.

Discard the unit.

➤*Storage/Stability:* Store at room temperature, between 15° and 30°C (59° and 86°F). Keep out of the reach of children.

Warnings/Precautions

➤*GI problems:* Do not use product when abdominal pain, nausea, or vomiting are present.

➤*Rectal issues:* Rectal bleeding and sudden changes in bowel habits that persist have been reported. Advise patients to notify health care provider if these occur. Failure to have a bowel movement after use of this product may be an indication of a serious condition.

➤*Pregnancy: Category C* (per Briggs' *Drugs in Pregnancy and Lactation*). No reports linking the use of docusate with congenital defects have been located. As with any drug, if you are pregnant, seek the advice of a health care provider before using this product.

➤*Lactation:* As with any drug, if you are breast-feeding a baby, seek the advice of a health care provider before using this product. Docusate is minimally absorbed from the GI tract and, therefore, is unlikely to be found in breast milk.

Patient Information

Advise patients to stop using this product and consult a health care provider if they experience rectal bleeding; notice a sudden change in bowel habits that persists over a period of 2 weeks; or fail to have a bowel movement after use because this may indicate a serious condition.

Instruct patients not to use this product if they have abdominal pain, nausea, or vomiting.

Instruct patients not to use this product for longer than 1 week.

DOCUSATE CALCIUM (Dioctyl Calcium Sulfosuccinate)

otc	**Docusate Calcium** (Various)	**Capsules**: 240 mg	In 100s, 500s, and UD 100s and 300s.
otc	**Stool Softener** (Apothecary)		In 50s.
otc	**Stool Softener DC** (Rugby)		Sorbitol, parabens. In 100s, 500s, and 1000s.
otc	**Life-Line** (National Vitamin)	**Capsules, soft gel**: 240 mg	Sorbitol. In 100s.
otc	**Sulfolax** (Major)		Sorbitol, parabens. In 100s.
otc	**Surfak Stool Softener** (Chattem)		Corn oil, glycerin, propylene glycol, sorbitol. (Kao SS). In 10s.
otc	**DC Softgels** (Goldline)		In 100s and 500s.

DOCUSATE CALCIUM — ORAL

For complete and comparative prescribing information, refer to the Laxatives group monograph.

Indications

➤*Constipation:* Docusate calcium, a stool softener, is indicated for the relief of occasional constipation. It is used for the prevention of dry, hard stools.

➤*Prophylaxis:* Fecal softeners are useful prophylactically in patients who should not strain during defecation (ie, following anorectal surgery, MI).

Administration and Dosage

➤*Adults:*

Constipation – 240 mg/day for several days or until bowel movements are normal.

➤*Children:* See Adults for dosing for children 12 years of age and older.

➤*Storage/Stability:* Store at room temperature in a dry place.

Hyperosmotic Agents

GLYCERIN

otc	**Glycerin** (Various, eg, Apothecary)	**Suppositories**: Glycerin	**Adults:** In 10s, 12s, 25s, 50s, and 100s. **Pediatric:** In 10s, 12s, and 25s.
otc	**Sani-Supp** (G & W Labs)		**Adults:** In 10s, 25s, and 50s. **Pediatric:** In 10s and 25s.
otc	**Colace** (Purdue)		**Adults:** In 12s, 24s, 48s, and 100s.
otc	**Colace Infant/Child** (Purdue)		**Pediatric:** In 12s and 24s.
otc	**Fleet Babylax** (Fleet)	**Liquid:** 4 mL per applicator	In 6 applicators.

GLYCERIN — RECTAL

For complete and comparative prescribing information, refer to the Laxatives group monograph.

Indications

➤*Constipation:* For relief of occasional constipation. This product generally produces a bowel movement within 15 minutes to 1 hour.

Administration and Dosage

➤*Adults:*

Constipation –

Usual dosage: Insert 1 suppository into rectum and retain for about 15 minutes.

➤*Children:*

Constipation –

Pediatric rectal liquid:

- *2 years to younger than 6 years of age* – 1 unit daily.

Suppositories:

- *2 years of age and older –*

Usual dosage: Insert 1 suppository into rectum and retain for about 15 minutes.

➤*Duration of therapy:* Laxative products should not be used longer than 1 week unless directed by a health care provider.

➤*Administration:* For rectal use only. May cause rectal discomfort or a burning sensation.

Pediatric rectal liquid – Hold unit upright, grasping bulb of unit with fingers. Grasp orange protective shield with the other hand and pull gently to remove. With steady pressure, gently insert tip into rectum with a slight side-to-side movement, with tip pointing toward the navel. Discontinue use if resistance is encountered. Forcing the tip can result in injury. Squeeze the bulb until nearly all the liquid is expelled. While continuing to squeeze the bulb, remove the tip from the rectum and discard unit. It is not necessary to empty the unit completely. The unit contains more than the amount of liquid needed for effective use. A small amount of liquid will remain in the unit after squeezing.

Suppositories – Remove foil wrapper. Insert 1 suppository into rectum and retain for about 15 minutes. It need not melt to produce laxative action.

Left side position – Place child on left side with knees bent and arms resting comfortably.

Knee-chest position – Have child kneel, then lower head and chest forward until left side of face is resting on the surface with left arm folded comfortably.

➤*Storage/Stability:* Avoid excessive heat.

LACTULOSE

Rx	**Lactulose** (Various, eg, Zenith Goldline)	**Solution; oral:** 10 g per 15 mL (< 1.6 g galactose, < 1.2 g lactose, and ≤ 1.2 g of other sugars)	In 237, 473, 960, and 1893 mL.
Rx	**Cephulac** (Hoechst-Marion Roussel)		In 473 mL, 1.9 L, and UD 30 mL.
Rx	**Constulose** (Alpharma)		In 237 and 946 mL.
Rx	**Enulose** (Alpharma)		In 473 mL and 1.89 L.
Rx	**Generlac** (Morton Grove Pharmaceuticals)	**Solution; oral or rectal:** 10 g per 15 mL	In 473 and 1,892 mL.
Rx	**Kristalose** (Bertek)	**Solution, crystals; oral:** Lactulose (< 0.3 g galactose and lactose/10 g)	In 10 g (30s) and 20 g (30s).

LACTULOSE — ORAL

For complete and comparative prescribing information, refer to the Laxatives group monograph.

Indications

➤*Constipation:* For the treatment of constipation. In patients with a history of chronic constipation, lactulose therapy increases the number of bowel movements per day and the number of days on which bowel movements occur.

➤*Portal-systemic encephalopathy (solution only):* For the prevention and treatment of portal-systemic encephalopathy, including the stages of hepatic precoma and coma.

➤*Off-label uses:*

Hepatic encephalopathy (adults) – [1] = Good documentation. Evidence-based guidelines and randomized, controlled trials confirm the effectiveness of lactulose in the treatment of subclinical hepatic encephalopathy. If diarrhea develops, the drug should be stopped and reinstituted at a lower dose.

Administration and Dosage

➤*Adults:*

Constipation – Twenty-four to 48 hours may be required to produce a normal bowel movement.

Solution: 15 to 30 mL, containing 10 to 20 g of lactulose daily. May be increased to 60 mL daily if necessary.

Crystals: 10 to 20 g of lactulose daily. May be increased to 40 g daily if necessary.

Prevention and treatment of portal-systemic encephalopathy –

Usual dosage: 30 to 45 mL containing 20 to 30 g of lactulose 3 or 4 times daily.

Dosage adjustment: May be adjusted every day or two (as needed) to produce 2 or 3 soft stools daily. Hourly doses of 30 to 45 mL may be used to induce the rapid laxation indicated in the initial phase of the therapy of portal-systemic encephalopathy. When the laxative effect has been achieved, the dose of lactulose may then be reduced to the recommended daily dose. Improvement in the patient's condition may occur within 24 hours, but may not begin before 48 hours or even later.

Continuous long-term therapy: To lessen the severity and prevent the recurrence of portal-systemic encephalopathy, the dose of lactulose is the same as the recommended daily dose.

Off-label dosing –

Hepatic encephalopathy (adults): [1] = Good documentation. 30 to 60 mL/day orally in 2 to 3 divided doses to maintain bowel movements between 2 and 3 times daily for up to 3 months.

➤*Children:*

Prevention and treatment of portal-systemic encephalopathy – Very little information on the use of lactulose in young children and adolescents has been recorded. As with adults, the subjective goal in proper treatment is to produce 2 or 3 soft stools daily.

Usual dosage:

- *Infants* – The initial daily oral dose is 2.5 to 10 mL in divided doses.
- *Older children and adolescents* – The total daily dose is 40 to 90 mL in divided doses.

Dosage adjustment: If the initial dose causes diarrhea, reduce the dose immediately.

Discontinuation of therapy: If diarrhea persists, discontinue lactulose.

Off-label dosing –

Constipation: 7.5 mL/day. One reference suggests administering the dose preferably after breakfast.

➤*Preparation for administration:*

Crystals for reconstitution – Dissolve contents of packet in half a glass (120 mL) of water. When lactulose crystals are dissolved in water, the resulting solution may be colorless to a slightly pale yellow.

➤*Administration:* Some patients have found that lactulose solution may be more acceptable when mixed with fruit juice, water, or milk.

➤*Storage/Stability:* Store at controlled room temperature, 15° to 30°C (59° to 86°F), preferably below 30°C (86°F). Do not freeze.

Solution – Dispense in a tightly closed, light-resistant container with a child-resistant closure.

Under recommended storage conditions, a normal darkening of color may occur. Such darkening is characteristic of sugar solutions and does not affect therapeutic action. Prolonged exposure to temperatures greater than 30°C (86°F) or to direct light may cause extreme darkening and turbidity, which may be pharmaceutically objectionable. If this condition develops, do not use.

Prolonged exposure to freezing temperatures may cause change to a semisolid, too viscous to pour. Viscosity will return to normal upon warming to room temperature.

Hyperosmotic Agents

LACTULOSE — RECTAL

For complete and comparative prescribing information, refer to the Laxatives group monograph.

Indications

➤*Portal-systemic encephalopathy:* For the prevention and treatment of portal-systemic encephalopathy, including the stages of hepatic precoma and coma.

Administration and Dosage

➤*General dosing considerations:* When the adult patient is in the impending coma or coma stage of portal-systemic encephalopathy and the danger of aspiration exists, or when the necessary endoscopic or intubation procedures physically interfere with the administration of the recommended oral doses, lactulose solution may be given as a retention enema via a rectal balloon catheter. Do not use cleansing enemas containing soap suds or other alkaline agents.

➤*Adults:*

Portal-systemic encephalopathy –

Usual dosage: Mix lactulose solution 300 mL with water or physiologic saline 700 mL and retain for 30 to 60 minutes. This lactulose enema may be repeated every 4 to 6 hours. If this lactulose enema is inadvertently evacuated too promptly, it may be repeated immediately.

The goal of treatment should be a reversal of the coma stage in order that the patient may be able to take oral medication. Reversal of coma may take place within 2 hours of the first enema in some patients.

Conversion: Start lactulose given orally in the recommended doses before lactulose by enema is stopped entirely.

➤*Storage/Stability:* Store at controlled room temperature, 2° to 30°C (36° to 86°F). Do not freeze.

Under recommended storage conditions, a normal darkening of color may occur. Such darkening is characteristic of sugar solutions and does not affect therapeutic action. Prolonged exposure to temperatures above 30°C (86°F) or to direct light may cause extreme darkening and turbidity that may be pharmaceutically objectionable. If this condition develops, do not use.

Prolonged exposure to freezing temperatures may cause change to a semisolid, too viscous to pour. Viscosity will return to normal upon warming to room temperature.

Enemas

MISCELLANEOUS ENEMAS

otc	**Docusol Mini-Enema** (Alliance Labs)	**Enema; rectal:** 283 mg docusate sodium, polyethylene glycol, and glycerin *Dose:* Adults and children ≥ 12 years – 1 to 3 units/day Children 6 to < 12 years – 1 unit/day.	In 5s.
otc	**Fleet** (Fleet)	**Enema; rectal:** 7 g dibasic sodium phosphate and 19 g monobasic sodium phosphate per 118 mL delivered dose (4.4 g sodium per dose) *Dose:* Adults – 118 mL. Children 2 to younger than 12 years – 59 mL.	In squeeze bottles. **Pediatric:** In 66 mL. **Adult:** In 133 mL.
otc	**Fleet Bisacodyl** (Fleet)	**Enema; rectal:** 10 mg bisacodyl per 30 mL delivered dose *Dose:* Adults and children ≥ 12 years – 30 mL.	In 37 mL squeeze bottles.
otc	**Fleet Mineral Oil** (Fleet)	**Enema; rectal:** Mineral oil *Dose:* Adults and children ≥ 12 years – 118 mL. Children 2 to younger than 12 years – 59 mL.	In 133 mL plastic squeeze bottles.
otc	**Therevac-SB** (Jones Medical)	**Enema; rectal:** 283 mg docusate sodium in a base of soft soap, polyethylene glycol, and 275 mg glycerin per 4 mL ampule *Dose:* 4 mL.	In UD 30s.
otc	**Therevac-Plus** (Jones Medical)	**Enema; rectal:** 283 mg docusate sodium, 275 mg glycerin, and 20 mg benzocaine in a base of soft soap, polyethylene glycol per 4 mL ampule *Dose:* 4 mL.	In 50s and UD 30s.

For complete prescribing information, refer to the Laxatives group monograph. For Bisacodyl prescribing information, see the Bisacodyl Rectal monograph in the Irritant or Stimulant Laxatives section.

MINERAL OIL — RECTAL

For complete and comparative prescribing information, refer to the Laxatives group monograph.

CO_2-RELEASING SUPPOSITORIES

otc	**Ceo-Two** (Beutlich)	**Suppositories:** Sodium bicarbonate and potassium bitartrate in a water-soluble polyethylene glycol base. Before inserting, moisten suppository with warm water.	In 10s.

For complete prescribing information, refer to the Laxatives group monograph.

Bowel Evacuants

POLYETHYLENE GLYCOL-ELECTROLYTE SOLUTION (PEG-ES)

Rx	**CoLyte** (Alaven Pharmaceuticals)	**Powder for solution; oral:** 1 gal: 227.1 g PEG 3350, 21.5 g sodium sulfate, 6.36 g sodium bicarb, 5.53 g NaCl, 2.82 g KCl	Regular and pineapple flavors. In bottles.
		4 L: 240 g PEG 3350, 22.72 g sodium sulfate, 6.72 g sodium bicarb, 5.84 g NaCl, 2.98 g KCl	Citrus berry, lemon lime, cherry, and pineapple flavors. In bottles.
Rx	**Polyethylene Glycol 3350 and Electrolytes** (Mylan)	**Powder for solution; oral:** 236 g PEG 3350, 22.74 g sodium sulfate, 6.74 g sodium bicarbonate, 5.86 g NaCl, 2.97 g KCl	In disposable jugs.
Rx	**GoLYTELY** (Braintree Labs)		In disposable jugs.
Rx	**GoLYTELY** (Braintree Labs)	**Powder for solution; oral:** 227.1 g PEG 3350, 21.5 g sodium sulfate, 6.36 g sodium bicarb, 5.53 g NaCl, 2.82 g KCl	In packets.
Rx	**MoviPrep** (Salix)	**Powder for solution; oral:** 100 g PEG 3350, 7.5 g sodium sulfate, 2.691 g NaCl, 1.015 KCl	Aspartame, 4.7 ascorbic acid, 5.9 g sodium ascorbate. 2.33 mg phenylalanine. Lemon flavor. In cartons w/ disposable container and 4 pouches.
Rx	**PEG-3350, Sodium Chloride, Sodium Bicarbonate, Potassium Chloride** (Mylan)	**Powder for solution; oral:** 420 g PEG 3350, 5.72 g sodium bicarbonate, 11.2 g NaCl, 1.48 g KCl	In 4 L disposable jugs with cherry, lemon-lime, orange, and pineapple flavor packs.
Rx	**NuLytely** (Braintree Labs)		Cherry, lemon-lime, and orange flavors. In 4 L disposable jugs.
Rx	**TriLyte** (Alaven Pharmaceuticals)		In 4 L bottles with flavor packs.
Rx	**GaviLyte-C** (Gavis Pharmaceuticals)	**Powder for solution; oral:** 240 g PEG 3350, 6.72 g sodium bicarbonate, 5.84 g sodium chloride, 22.72 g sodium sulfate, 2.98 g potassium chloride	In 4 L with lemon flavor pack.

POLYETHYLENE GLYCOL-ELECTROLYTE SOLUTION (PEG-ES)

Rx	**GaviLyte-G** (Gavis Pharmaceuticals)	**Powder for solution; oral**: 236 g PEG 3350, 6.74 g sodium bicarbonate, 5.86 g sodium chloride, 22.74 g sodium sulfate, 2.97 g potassium chloride	In 4 L with lemon flavor pack.
Rx	**GaviLyte-N** (Gavis)	**Powder for solution; oral**: 420 g PEG 3350, 5.72 g sodium bicarbonate, 11.2 g sodium chloride, 1.48 g potassium chloride	In 4 L with lemon flavor pack.
Rx	**OCL** (Abbott)	**Solution; oral**: 146 mg NaCl, 168 mg sodium bicarb, 1.29 g sodium sulfate decahydrate, 75 mg KCl, 6 g PEG 3350, 30 mg polysorbate 80/100 mL	In 1500 mL (3 pack).

POLYETHYLENE GLYCOL-ELECTROLYTE SOLUTION (PEG-ES) — ORAL

For complete prescribing information, refer to the Laxatives group monograph.

Indications

➤*Bowel evacuation:* For bowel cleansing prior to GI examination.

➤*Off-label uses:* PEG electrolyte solutions are useful in the management of acute iron overdose in children. In a 33-month-old, 2,953 mL/kg was administered over 5 days.

Administration and Dosage

➤*General dosing considerations:* The first bowel movement should occur in approximately 1 hour.

One method is to schedule patients for a midmorning exam, allowing 3 hours for drinking and 1 hour to complete bowel evacuation. Another method is to give the solution the evening before the exam, particularly if the patient is to have a barium enema.

➤*Adults:*

Bowel cleansing prior to GI examination – Dosage is 4 L of oral solution prior to GI exam. Patients should drink 240 mL every 10 minutes until 4 L are consumed or until the rectal effluent is clear. May be given via a nasogastric tube to patients unwilling or unable to drink the preparation. (See also Administration.)

➤*Preparation for administration:* Tap water may be used to reconstitute the solution. Shake container vigorously several times to ensure that the powder is completely dissolved. Do not add flavorings or additional ingredients to solution before use. Chilling before administration improves palatability.

➤*Administration:* The patient should fast 3 to 4 hours prior to ingestion of the solution; do not give solid foods less than 2 hours before solution is administered. No foods, except clear liquids, are permitted after solution administration.

Rapid drinking of each portion is preferred to drinking small amounts continuously. Nasogastric tube rate of administration is 20 to 30 mL/min (1.2 to 1.8 L/hour).

➤*Storage / Stability:* Refrigerate reconstituted solution; use within 24 hours.

Actions

➤*Pharmacology:* Oral solution induces diarrhea, which rapidly cleanses the bowel, usually within 4 hours. Polyethylene glycol 3350 (PEG 3350) and the electrolyte concentration result in virtually no net absorption or excretion of ions or water. Large volumes may be given without significant changes in water or electrolyte balance.

Contraindications

GI obstruction; gastric retention; bowel perforation; toxic colitis, megacolon, or ileus.

Warnings/Precautions

➤*Regurgitation / Aspiration:* Observe unconscious or semiconscious patients with impaired gag reflex and those who are otherwise prone to regurgitation or aspiration during use, especially if given via a nasogastric tube. If GI obstruction or perforation is suspected, rule out these contraindications before administration.

➤*GI problems:* If a patient experiences severe bloating, distention, or abdominal pain, slow or temporarily discontinue administration until symptoms abate.

➤*Severe ulcerative colitis:* Use with caution.

➤*Pregnancy:* *Category C*. Safety has not been established. Polyethylene glycol is completely non-absorbed from the adult GI tract. Use only when clearly needed and when the benefits outweigh the potential hazards to the fetus.

➤*Children:* Safety and efficacy for use in children have not been established.

Several studies in infants and children from 3 to 14 years of age showed PEG-electrolyte solutions are safe and effective in bowel evacuation.

Drug Interactions

Oral medication given within 1 hour of start of therapy may be flushed from the GI tract and not absorbed.

Adverse Reactions

Nausea, abdominal fullness, and bloating are the most common adverse reactions (occurring in up to 50% of patients). Abdominal cramps, vomiting, and anal irritation occur less frequently. These adverse reactions are transient. Isolated cases of urticaria, rhinorrhea, and dermatitis have been reported, which may represent allergic reactions.

POLYETHYLENE GLYCOL (PEG) SOLUTION

otc	**Dulcolax Balance** (Boehringer Ingelheim Consumer)	**Powder for solution; oral**: 17 g PEG 3350	In 238 g.
otc	**GaviLAX** (Gavis)		In 238 and 510 g.
Rx	**GlycoLax** (Kremers Urban)		In 14 single-dose packets.
otc	**MiraLax** (Schering-Plough)	**Powder for solution; oral**: 17 g PEG 3350	In 12 single-dose packets.
		119 g PEG 3350	In 119 g.
		238 g	In 239 g.
Rx	**Polyethylene Glycol** (Braintree)	**Powder for solution; oral**: 255 g PEG 3350	In 16 oz.
Rx	**GlycoLax** (Kremers Urban)		In 16 oz w/dosing cup.
otc	**MiraLax** (Schering-Plough)	**Powder for solution; oral**: 510 g PEG 3350	In 510 g.
Rx	**Polyethylene Glycol** (Braintree)	**Powder for solution; oral**: 527 g PEG 3350	In 32 oz.

POLYETHYLENE GLYCOL 3350 — ORAL

For complete and comparative prescribing information, refer to the Laxatives group monograph.

Indications

➤*Constipation:* For the treatment of occasional constipation. This product should be used for 2 weeks or less or as directed by a physician.

Administration and Dosage

➤*General dosing considerations:* To produce a bowel movement, 2 to 4 days (48 to 96 hours) may be required.

➤*Adults:*

Constipation – Usual dosage is 17 g (approximately 1 heaping Tbsp) of powder per day (or as directed by a health care provider) in 8 oz of water.

➤*Storage / Stability:* Store at 25°C (77°F); excursions are permitted from 15° to 30°C (59° to 86°F).

MISCELLANEOUS BOWEL EVACUANTS

otc	**Tridrate Bowel Cleansing System** (Lafayette)	**Liquid; oral**: magnesium citrate 19 g. With 3 bisacodyl 5 mg **tablets** and 1 bisacodyl 10 mg **suppository**.
otc	**Fleet Prep Kit 3** (Fleet)	**Liquid; oral**: 45 mL of **Fleet Phospho-soda** (monobasic sodium phosphate 21.6 g and dibasic sodium phosphate 8.1 g) with 4 bisacodyl 5 mg **enteric-coated tablets** and One 30 mL bisacodyl 10 mg **enema.**
Rx	**Visicol** (Salix)	**Tablets; oral**: sodium phosphate monobasic monohydrate 1.102 g, sodium phosphate dibasic anhydrous 0.398 g (total of sodium phosphate 1.5 g). Gluten free. White to off-white. I. In 40s and 100s.
Rx	**OsmoPrep** (Salix)	**Tablets; oral**: sodium phosphate monobasic monohydrate 1.102 g, sodium phosphate dibasic 0.398 g (total of sodium phosphate 1.5 g). Gluten free. PEG 8000. White to off-white. SLX 102. In 100s.
Rx	**HalfLytely** (Braintree)	**Solution, powder for reconstitution; oral**: 2 L bottle (210 g of PEG 3350, 5.6 g of sodium chloride, 2.86 g of sodium bicarbonate, 0.74 g of potassium chloride, lemon-lime flavor). With 4 bisacodyl 5 mg **delayed-release enteric-coated tablets** (lactose, sugar, sucrose).
Rx	**Suprep Bowel Prep Kit** (Braintree Labs)	**Solution; oral**: Sodium sulfate 17.5 g, potassium sulfate 3.13 g, magnesium sulfate 1.6 g per 180 mL. Sodium benzoate, sucralose. In kits with 2s and mixing container.

For complete prescribing information, refer to the Laxatives class monograph.

SODIUM PHOSPHATE — ORAL

WARNING

There have been rare but serious reports of acute phosphate nephropathy in patients who received oral sodium phosphate products for colon cleansing prior to colonoscopy. Some cases have resulted in permanent impairment of renal function and some patients required long-term dialysis. While some cases have occurred in patients without identifiable risk factors, patients at increased risk of acute phosphate nephropathy may include those with increased age, hypovolemia, increased bowel transit time (such as bowel obstruction), active colitis, or baseline kidney disease, and those using medicines that affect renal perfusion or function (such as diuretics, angiotensin-converting enzyme [ACE] inhibitors, angiotensin receptor blockers, and possibly nonsteroidal anti-inflammatory drugs [NSAIDs]).

It is important to use the dose and dosing regimen as recommended (pm/am split dose).

Indications

➤*Colon cleansing:* For cleansing of the colon as a preparation for colonoscopy in adults 18 years of age and older.

Administration and Dosage

➤*General dosing considerations:* Patients should be advised of the importance of taking the recommended fluid regimen. It is recommended that patients be advised to adequately hydrate before, during, and after use.

Patients should not use this medication within 7 days of previous administration. No additional enema or laxative is required, and patients should be advised not to take additional agents, particularly those containing sodium phosphate.

➤*Adults:*

Colon cleansing –

OsmoPrep: 32 tablets (48 g of sodium phosphate) with a total of 2 quarts of clear liquids in the following manner: the evening before the procedure, take 4 tablets with 8 ounces of clear liquids every 15 minutes for a total of 20 tablets. On the day of the procedure, starting 3 to 5 hours before the procedure, take 4 tablets with 8 ounces of clear liquids every 15 minutes for a total of 12 tablets.

Suprep Bowel Prep Kit: 2 bottles of solution (sodium sulfate 17.5 g, potassium sulfate 3.13 g, magnesium sulfate 1.6 g per 180 mL) with a total of 3 quarts of clear liquids in the following manner: the evening before the procedure, pour the contents of 1 bottle of *Suprep Bowel Prep Kit* into the mixing container provided. Fill the container with water to the 480 mL fill line, and drink the entire amount. Drink 2 additional containers filled to the 480 mL line with water over the next hour. On the day of the procedure, pour the contents of the second bottle of *Suprep Bowel Prep Kit* into the mixing container provided. Fill the container with water to the 480 mL fill line, and drink the entire amount. Drink 2 additional containers filled to the 480 mL line with water over the next hour. Complete all *Suprep Bowel Prep Kit* and required water at least 1 hour prior to the procedure. On the day before the procedure, consume either a light breakfast or only clear liquids, and avoid red and purple liquids, milk, and alcoholic beverages. Have only clear liquids until after the procedure, and avoid red and purple liquids, milk, and alcoholic beverages.

Visicol: 40 tablets (60 g of sodium phosphate) with a total of 3.6 quarts of clear liquids in the following manner: the evening before the procedure, take 3 tablets (the last dose will be 2 tablets) with 8 ounces of clear liquids every 15 minutes for a total of 20 tablets. On the day of the procedure, starting 3 to 5 hours before the procedure, take 3 tablets (the last dose will be 2 tablets) with 8 ounces of clear liquids every 15 minutes for a total of 20 tablets.

➤*Renal function impairment:* Exercise caution in patients with renal impairment. Considerable caution should be advised before use in patients with severe renal insufficiency (creatinine clearance [CrCl] less than 30 mL/min).

➤*Administration:* Take orally with clear liquids.

➤*Storage/Stability:* Store at 25°C (77°F); excursions are permitted between 15° and 30° C (59° and 86°F). Discard any unused portion.

Actions

➤*Pharmacology:* Sodium phosphate induces diarrhea, which effectively cleanses the entire colon. Each administration has a purgative effect for approximately 1 to 3 hours. The primary mode of action is thought to be through the osmotic effect of sodium, causing large amounts of water to be drawn into the colon, promoting evacuation.

➤*Pharmacokinetics:*

Absorption – Serum phosphorus level rose from a mean (± standard deviation) baseline of 4 (± 0.7) mg/dL to 7.7 (± 1.6 mg/dL), at a median of 3 hours after the administration of the first 30 g dose of sodium phosphate tablets. Serum phosphorus level rose to a mean of 8.4 (± 1.9) mg/dL, at a median of 4 hours after the administration of the second 30 g dose of sodium phosphate tablets. Serum phosphorus level remained above baseline for a median of 24 hours after the administration of the initial dose of sodium phosphate tablets (range, 16 to 48 hours).

Special populations –

Renal function impairment: See Warnings/Precautions for more information.

Elderly: In a single pharmacokinetic study of sodium phosphate, which included 6 elderly volunteers, plasma half-life increased 2-fold in subjects older than 70 years of age compared with subjects younger than 50 years of age (3 subjects and 5 subjects, respectively).

Contraindications

Biopsy-proven acute phosphate nephropathy; known allergy or hypersensitivity to sodium phosphate salts or any of its ingredients.

Warnings/Precautions

➤*Hydration:* Administration of sodium phosphate products prior to colonoscopy for colon cleansing has resulted in fatalities because of significant fluid shifts, severe electrolyte abnormalities, and cardiac arrhythmias. These fatalities have been observed in patients with renal insufficiency, in patients with bowel perforation, and in patients who misused or overdosed sodium phosphate products. It is recommended that patients receiving sodium phosphate be advised to adequately hydrate before, during, and after the use of the medicine.

➤*Cardiovascular effects:* Use with considerable caution in patients with congestive heart failure or unstable angina.

QT prolongation – Prolongation of the QT interval has been observed in some patients who were dosed with sodium phosphate. QT prolongation with sodium phosphate has been associated with electrolyte imbalances such as hypokalemia and hypocalcemia. Use with caution in patients who are taking medications known to prolong the QT interval because serious complications may occur.

Cardiac arrhythmias – There have been rare, but serious, reports of arrhythmias associated with the use of sodium phosphate products. Use sodium phosphate tablets with caution in patients with higher risk of arrhythmias (patients with a history of cardiomyopathy, patients with prolonged QT, patients with a history of uncontrolled arrhythmias, and patients with a recent history of a myocardial infarction). Consider predose and post-colonoscopy electrocardiograms (ECGs) in patients with high risk of serious cardiac arrhythmias.

Cardiac surgery – Because *Visicol* was not studied in patients who recently had cardiac surgery (including coronary artery bypass graft surgery), use with caution in these patients.

➤*Bulimia:* Laxatives and purgatives have the potential for abuse by bulimia nervosa patients who frequently binge eat and vomit.

➤*GI effects:* Use with considerable caution in patients with ascites, gastric retention, ileus, acute bowel obstruction, pseudo-obstruction of the bowel, severe chronic constipation, bowel perforation, acute colitis, toxic megacolon, gastric bypass or stapling surgery, or hypomotility syndrome.

Aphthous ulcers – Administration of sodium phosphate tablets may induce colonic mucosal aphthous ulcerations, because this endoscopic finding was observed with other sodium phosphate cathartic preparations.

Consider this colonoscopic finding in patients with known or suspected inflammatory bowel disease.

Bowel Evacuants

SODIUM PHOSPHATE — ORAL

Inflammatory bowel disease – Because published data suggest that sodium phosphate absorption may be enhanced in patients experiencing an acute exacerbation of chronic inflammatory bowel disease, use sodium phosphate with caution in such patients.

➤*Renal toxicity:* There have been rare, but serious, reports of renal failure, acute phosphate nephropathy, and nephrocalcinosis in patients who received oral sodium phosphate products (including oral sodium phosphate solutions and tablets) for colon cleansing prior to colonoscopy. These cases often resulted in permanent impairment of renal function and several patients required long-term dialysis. The time to onset is typically within days; however, in some cases, the diagnosis of these reactions has been delayed up to several months after the ingestion of these products. Patients at increased risk of acute phosphate nephropathy may include patients with the following: hypovolemia, baseline kidney disease, increased age, and patients using medicines that affect renal perfusion or function (such as diuretics, ACE inhibitors, angiotensin receptor blockers, and possibly NSAIDs).

➤*Electrolyte disturbances:* Use sodium phosphate tablets with caution in patients a history of acute phosphate nephropathy, known or suspected electrolyte disturbances (such as dehydration), or patients taking concomitant medications that may affect electrolyte levels (such as diuretics). Correct electrolyte abnormalities such as hypernatremia, hyperphosphatemia, hypokalemia, or hypocalcemia before treatment with sodium phosphate.

➤*Seizures:* There have been rare reports of generalized tonic-clonic seizures and/or loss of consciousness associated with use of sodium phosphate products in patients with no prior history of seizures. The seizure cases were associated with electrolyte abnormalities (eg, hyponatremia, hypokalemia, hypocalcemia, hypomagnesemia) and low serum osmolality. The neurologic abnormalities resolved with correction of fluid and electrolyte abnormalities. Use sodium phosphate with caution in patients with a history of seizures and in patients at higher risk of seizure (patients using concomitant medications that lower the seizure threshold [eg, tricyclic antidepressants], patients withdrawing from alcohol or benzodiazepines, or patients with known or suspected hyponatremia).

➤*Dysphagia:* Patients with a history of swallowing difficulties or anatomic narrowing of the esophagus, such as stricture, may have difficulty swallowing *Visicol* tablets. Undigested or partially digested tablets from other medications may be seen in the stool or during colonoscopy.

➤*Renal function impairment:* Use with considerable caution in patients with severe renal insufficiency (CrCl less than 30 mL/min).

➤*Pregnancy: Category C.* Animal reproduction studies have not been conducted with sodium phosphate. It is not known whether sodium phosphate can cause fetal harm when administered to a pregnant woman, or can affect reproduction capacity. Give sodium phosphate to a pregnant woman only if clearly needed.

➤*Children:* The safety and efficacy of sodium phosphate have not been demonstrated in patients younger than 18 years of age.

➤*Elderly:* Sodium phosphate is known to be substantially excreted by the kidney, and the risk of adverse reactions with sodium phosphate may be greater in patients with impaired renal function. Because elderly patients are more likely to have impaired renal function, consider performing baseline and postcolonoscopy labs (phosphate, calcium, potassium, sodium, creatinine, and serum urea nitrogen [BUN]) in these patients.

➤*Monitoring:* Consider performing baseline and postcolonoscopy labs (phosphate, calcium, potassium, sodium, creatinine, and BUN) in patients who may be at increased risk for serious adverse events, including those with history of renal insufficiency, history of or at greater risk for acute phosphate nephropathy, known or suspected electrolyte disorders (such as dehydration), seizures, arrhythmias, cardiomyopathy, prolonged QT, recent history of a MI, and those with known or suspected hyperphosphatemia, hypocalcemia, hypokalemia, and hypernatremia. Also, if patient develops vomiting and/or signs of dehydration, measure postcolonoscopy labs (phosphate, calcium, potassium, sodium, creatinine, and BUN). Consider predose and postcolonoscopy ECGs in patients with prolonged QT and/or in patients with high risk of serious cardiac arrhythmias.

Drug Interactions

Medications administered in close proximity to sodium phosphate may not be absorbed from the GI tract because of the rapid intestinal peristalsis and watery diarrhea induced by the purgative agent.

➤*QT prolongation:* An additive effect of sodium phosphate with other drugs that prolong the QT interval cannot be excluded. The following drugs may prolong the QT interval and increase the risk of life-threatening cardiac arrhythmias, including torsades de pointes: antiarrhythmic agents (eg, amiodarone, bretylium, disopyramide, dofetilide, procainamide, quinidine, sotalol), arsenic trioxide, chlorpromazine, cisapride, dolasetron, droperidol, mefloquine, mesoridazine, moxifloxacin, pentamidine, pimozide, tacrolimus, thioridazine, and ziprasidone. For a more complete list of drugs that may prolong the QT interval, see the appendix Drug-Induced Prolongation of the QT Interval and Torsades de Pointes.

Adverse Reactions

➤*OsmoPrep:*

***OsmoPrep* Adverse Reactions (≥ 3%)**

GI adverse reactions	*OsmoPrep* 32 tablets (48 g) (n = 272)	*OsmoPrep* 40 tablets (60 g) (n = 265)	*Visicol* 40 tablets (60 g) (n = 268)
Abdominal pain	23%	24%	25%
Bloating	31%	39%	41%
Nausea	26%	37%	30%
Vomiting	4%	10%	9%

➤*Visicol:*

***Visicol* Adverse Reactions (≥ 2%) (Studies A and B)[a]**

GI adverse reactions	*Visicol* (n = 427)	*NuLYTELY*[b] (n = 432)
Abdominal pain	30%	36%
Bloating	47%	61%
Nausea	35%	54%
Vomiting	7%	18%

[a] Drug-related adverse reactions were adverse reaction possibly or probably drug related.
[b] PEG-3350, sodium chloride, sodium bicarbonate, and potassium chloride for oral solution.

Electrolyte changes – See Warnings/Precautions for more information.

➤*Postmarketing:*

Renal – Renal impairment, increased BUN, increased creatinine, acute renal failure, acute phosphate nephropathy, nephrocalcinosis, renal tubular necrosis.

Miscellaneous – Arrhythmias; hypersensitivity reactions, including anaphylaxis, rash, pruritus, urticaria, throat tightness, bronchospasm, dyspnea, pharyngeal edema, dysphagia, paresthesia and swelling of the lips and tongue, and facial swelling; seizures.

Overdosage

➤*Symptoms:* There have been no reported cases of overdosage with sodium phosphate. Purposeful or accidental ingestion of more than the recommended dosage of sodium phosphate might be expected to lead to severe electrolyte disturbances, including hyperphosphatemia, hypocalcemia, hypernatremia, or hypokalemia, as well as dehydration and hypovolemia, with attendant signs and symptoms of these disturbances. Certain severe electrolyte disturbances resulting from overdose may lead to cardiac arrhythmias, seizure, renal failure, and death.

➤*Treatment:* Monitor the patient who has taken an overdosage, and treat symptomatically for complications until stable.

Patient Information

Instruct patients to drink 8 ounces of clear liquids with each 4-tablet dose of *OsmoPrep* or each 3-tablet (or each 2-tablet) dose of *Visicol*. Patients should take a total of 2 quarts of clear liquids with *OsmoPrep* or 3.6 quarts of clear liquids with *Visicol*. Inadequate fluid intake, as with any effective purgative, may lead to excessive fluid loss, hypovolemia, and dehydration. Dehydration from purgation may be exacerbated by inadequate oral fluid intake, vomiting, and/or use of diuretics.

Instruct patients not to administer additional laxative or purgative agents, particularly additional sodium phosphate–based purgative or enema products.

Advise patients with swallowing difficulties or anatomic narrowing of the esophagus that they may have difficult swallowing *Visicol* tablets.

Advise patients that undigested or partially digested tablets from other medications may be seen in the stool.

Miscellaneous Laxatives

CASTOR OIL

otc	**Castor Oil** (Various, eg, Humco, Paddock)	**Liquid:** *Dose:* Adults and children ≥ 12 years - 15 to 60 mL/day. Children 2 to younger than 12 years - 5 to 15 mL/day.	In 60, 120, and 480 mL.
otc	**Emulsoil** (Paddock)	**Emulsion:** 95% castor oil with emulsifying agents. *Dose:* Adults and children ≥ 12 years - 15 to 60 mL/day mixed with ½ to 1 glass liquid. Children 2 to younger than 12 years - 5 to 15 mL mixed with ½ to 1 glass liquid.	Butylparaben. In 63 mL.

CASTOR OIL — ORAL

For complete and comparative prescribing information, refer to the Laxatives group monograph.

Laxative Combinations

LAXATIVE COMBINATIONS, CAPSULES/TABLETS

		Docusate (mg)	Senna Concentrate (mg)	Casanthranol (mg)	Cascara sagrada (mg)	Psyllium (mg)	Other Content and How Supplied
otc	**Dok Plus Tablets** (Major)	50[a]	8.6[b]				PEG-400. In 100s.
otc	**Senna Plus Tablets** (Contract Pharmacal)	50[a]	8.6[b]				Tartrazine. In 100s.
otc	**Senna-S** (Akyma)	50[a]	8.6[b]				In 1,000s.
otc	**Senokot-S Tablets** (Purdue Frederick)	50[a]	8.6[b]				Lactose. In 10s, 30s, 60s, 1,000s, and UD 100s.
otc	**Peri-Colace Tablets** (Purdue)	50[a]	8.6[b]				In 10s, 30s, and 60s.
otc	**Docusate w/Casanthranol Caps** (Various, eg, Paddock, Schein, URL)	100[a]		30			In 100s, 1,000s, and UD 100s, 300s, and 600s.
otc	**DSS 100 Plus Capsules** (Magno-Humphries)						In 60s.
otc	**Senna Prompt Capsules** (Konsyl)		9			500	In 90s.

[a] As sodium.
[b] As sennosides.

LAXATIVE COMBINATIONS — CAPSULES, TABLETS

For complete prescribing information, refer to the Laxatives class monograph.

Administration and Dosage

➤*General dosing considerations:* Products vary. Consult product labeling for specific guidelines.

➤*Adults:*

Constipation –

Docusate/Senna: Usual dosage is 2 to 4 tablets/day.

Senna/Psyllium: 5 capsules 1 or 2 times per day.

Off-label dosing –

Opioid-induced constipation: 2 tablets (sennoside 8.6 mg/docusate 50 mg) every morning.

➤*Children:*

Constipation – See Adults for dosing for children 12 years of age and older.

6 to younger than 12 years of age:

• *Docusate/Senna* – Usual dosage is 1 to 2 tablets/day.

2 to younger than 6 years of age:

• *Docusate/Senna* – Usual dosage is to 1 tablet/day.

Off-label dosing –

Opioid-induced constipation:

• *Older than 12 years of age* – 1 tablet (sennoside 8.6 mg/docusate 50 mg) twice daily.

• *6 to 12 years of age* – ½ tablet (sennoside 8.6 mg/docusate 50 mg) twice daily.

• *2 to 5 years of age* – ¼ tablet (sennoside 8.6 mg/docusate 50 mg) twice daily.

➤*Storage/Stability:* Store at 25°C (77 °F); excursions are permitted between 15° and 30°C (59° to 86° F). Keep tightly closed.

LAXATIVE COMBINATIONS, LIQUIDS

otc	**Haley's M-O** (Bayer)	**Liquid:** ≈ 900 mg magnesium hydroxide and 3.75 mL mineral oil per 15 mL	Saccharin (vanilla creme only). Regular or vanilla creme. In 360 (both) and 780 mL (vanilla creme only).
otc	**Black Draught** (Monticello)	**Syrup:** 90 mg per 15 mL casanthranol with senna extract, rhubarb, methyl salicylate, and menthol	5% alcohol. Tartrazine, parabens, sucrose, saccharin. In 60 and 150 mL.
otc	**Sorbitol Solution** (Various, eg, Geritrex, Humco, Spectrum, Upsher-Smith)	**Solution:** 70% w/w D-sorbitol	In 454 mL.

LAXATIVE COMBINATIONS — LIQUIDS

For complete prescribing information, refer to the Laxatives group monograph.

Administration and Dosage

➤*General dosing considerations:* Products vary. Consult product labeling for specific guidelines.

➤*Adults:*

Constipation –

Casanthranol: Usual dosage is 5 to 15 mL/day.

Magnesium hydroxide/mineral oil: Usual dosage is 45 to 60 mL taken as a single dose or in divided doses.

➤*Children:*

Constipation – See Adults for dosing for children 12 years of age and older.

6 to 11 years of age:

• *Magnesium hydroxide/mineral oil* – Usual dosage is 20 to 30 mL taken as a single dose or in divided doses.

➤*Administration:* Shake well. Take doses with 8 oz of liquid.

ANTIDIARRHEALS

DIFENOXIN HYDROCHLORIDE WITH ATROPINE SULFATE

c-iv	**Motofen**[a] (Valeant)	**Tablets; oral:** 1 mg difenoxin (as hydrochloride) and 0.025 mg atropine sulfate	Dye free. (C 8674). White, scored. Five-sided. In 50s and 100s.

[a] Currently unavailable, but the manufacturer is planning on reintroducing this product in late 2009.

DIFENOXIN HYDROCHLORIDE WITH ATROPINE SULFATE — ORAL

Indications

➤*Diarrhea:* Adjunctive therapy in management of acute nonspecific diarrhea and acute exacerbations of chronic functional diarrhea.

Administration and Dosage

➤*Maximum dose:*

Adults and children 12 years of age and older – 8 tablets/day.

➤*General dosing considerations:* Difenoxin with atropine is not innocuous; strictly adhere to dosage recommendations.

➤*Adults:*

Diarrhea –

Usual dosage: 2 tablets, then 1 tablet after each loose stool or 1 tablet every 3 to 4 hours as needed.

Duration of therapy: For diarrhea in which clinical improvement is not observed in 48 hours, continued administration is not recommended. For acute diarrhea and acute exacerbations of functional diarrhea, treatment beyond 48 hours is usually not necessary.

➤*Children:*

Diarrhea – See Adults for dosing for children 12 years of age and older.

DIFENOXIN HYDROCHLORIDE WITH ATROPINE SULFATE — ORAL

➤*Renal function impairment:* Use with extreme caution in patients with advanced hepato-renal disease.

➤*Hepatic function impairment:* Use with extreme caution in patients with advanced hepato-renal disease and in all patients with abnormal liver function tests because hepatic coma may be precipitated.

➤*Storage/Stability:* Store at 20° to 25°C (68° to 77°F).

Actions

➤*Pharmacology:* Difenoxin is an antidiarrheal agent chemically related to meperidine. Atropine sulfate is present to discourage deliberate overdosage.

Animal studies have shown that difenoxin manifests its antidiarrheal effect by slowing intestinal motility. The mechanism of action is by a local effect on the gastrointestinal wall.

Difenoxin is the principal active metabolite of diphenoxylate and is effective at one-fifth the dosage of diphenoxylate.

➤*Pharmacokinetics:* Difenoxin is rapidly and extensively absorbed orally. Mean peak plasma levels of 160 ng/mL occur within 40 to 60 minutes in most patients following a 2 mg dose. Plasma levels decline to less than 10% of their peak values within 24 hours and to less than 1% of their peak values within 72 hours. This decline parallels the appearance of difenoxin and its metabolites in the urine. Difenoxin is metabolized to an inactive hydroxylated metabolite. Both the drug and its metabolites are excreted, mainly as conjugates, in urine and feces.

Contraindications

Diarrhea associated with organisms that penetrate the intestinal mucosa (eg, toxigenic *E. coli*, *Salmonella* sp, *Shigella*;) and pseudomembranous colitis associated with broad-spectrum antibiotics. Antiperistaltic agents may prolong or worsen diarrhea.

Children younger than 2 years of age because of the decreased margin of safety of drugs in this class in younger age groups.

Hypersensitivity to difenoxin, atropine or any of the inactive ingredients; jaundice.

Warnings/Precautions

➤*Fluid and electrolyte balance:* The use of this drug does not preclude the administration of appropriate fluid and electrolyte therapy. Dehydration, particularly in children, may further influence the variability of response and may predispose to delayed difenoxin intoxication. Drug-induced inhibition of peristalsis may result in fluid retention in the colon, and this may further aggravate dehydration and electrolyte imbalance. If severe dehydration or electrolyte imbalance is manifested, withhold the drug until appropriate corrective therapy has been initiated.

➤*Ulcerative colitis:* Agents which inhibit intestinal motility or delay intestinal transit time have induced toxic megacolon. Consequently, carefully observe patients with acute ulcerative colitis. Discontinue promptly if abdominal distention occurs or if other untoward symptoms develop.

➤*Liver and kidney disease:* Use with extreme caution in patients with advanced hepato-renal disease and in all patients with abnormal liver function tests since hepatic coma may be precipitated.

➤*Atropine:* A subtherapeutic dose of atropine has been added to difenoxin to discourage deliberate overdosage. A recommended dose is not likely to cause prominent anticholinergic side effects, but avoid in patients in whom anticholinergic drugs are contraindicated. Observe the warnings and precautions for use of anticholinergic agents. In children, signs of atropinism may occur even with recommended doses, particularly in patients with Down's syndrome.

➤*Drug abuse and dependence:* Addiction to (dependence on) difenoxin is theoretically possible at high dosage. Therefore, do not exceed recommended dosage. Because of the structural and pharmacological similarities of difenoxin to drugs with definite addiction potential, administer with caution to patients receiving addicting drugs, to addiction-prone individuals, or to those whose histories suggest they may increase the dosage on their own initiative.

➤*Pregnancy: Category C.* Reproduction studies in rats and rabbits with doses up to 75 times the human therapeutic dose demonstrated no evidence of teratogenesis. Pregnant rats receiving oral doses 20 times the maximum human dose had an increase in delivery time as well as a significant increase in the percent of stillbirths. Neonatal survival in rats was also reduced with most deaths occurring within 4 days of delivery. There are no well controlled studies in pregnant women. Use during pregnancy only if the potential benefit justifies the potential risk to the fetus.

➤*Lactation:* Because of the potential for serious adverse reactions in nursing infants, decide whether to discontinue nursing or to discontinue the drug, taking into account the importance of the drug to the mother.

➤*Children:* Contraindicated in children under 2 years of age. Safety and efficacy in children below the age of 12 have not been established. See Overdosage section for information on hazards from accidental poisoning in children.

➤*Elderly:* Atropine is considered a high risk medication for the elderly according to the Centers of Medicare and Medicaid Services.

Drug Interactions

Difenoxin Drug Interactions

Precipitant drug	Object drug[a]		Description
Difenoxin	Barbiturates, tranquilizers, narcotics, and alcohol	↑	Barbiturates, tranquilizers, narcotics, and alcohol may be potentiated by coadministration of difenoxin. Closely monitor patients.
Difenoxin	MAOIs	↑	Because the chemical structure of difenoxin is similar to meperidine, concurrent use with MAOIs may, in theory, precipitate a hypertensive crisis.

[a] ↑ = Object drug increased.

Adverse Reactions

Anticholinergic – In view of the small amount of atropine present (0.025 mg/tablet), effects such as dryness of the skin and mucous membranes, flushing, hyperthermia, tachycardia and urinary retention are very unlikely to occur, except perhaps in children.

Many adverse effects reported during clinical investigation are difficult to distinguish from symptoms of diarrheal syndrome. However, the following events have occurred:

➤*CNS:* Dizziness, lightheadedness (5%); drowsiness (4%); headache (2.5%); tiredness, nervousness, insomnia, confusion (less than 1%).

➤*GI:* Nausea (7%), vomiting, dry mouth (3%); epigastric distress, constipation (≤ 1%).

➤*Ophthalmic:* Burning eyes, blurred vision (infrequent).

Overdosage

➤*Symptoms:* Initial signs may include dryness of the skin and mucous membranes, flushing, hyperthermia and tachycardia followed by lethargy or coma, hypotonic reflexes, nystagmus, pinpoint pupils and respiratory depression. Overdosage may result in severe respiratory depression and coma, possibly leading to permanent brain damage or death.

➤*Treatment:* Gastric lavage, establishment of a patent airway and, possibly, mechanically assisted respiration are advised. Refer to General Management of Acute Overdosage.

Naloxone may be used in the treatment of respiratory depression. When administered IV, the onset is generally apparent within 2 minutes. Naloxone may also be administered SC or IM providing a slightly less rapid onset but a more prolonged effect.

Because the duration of action of difenoxin is longer than that of naloxone, improvement of respiration following administration may be followed by recurrent respiratory depression. Continuous observation is necessary until the effect of difenoxin on respiration (which may persist for many hours) has passed. Supplemental IM naloxone doses may be used to produce a longer lasting effect. Treat all possible overdosages as serious; observe for at least 48 hours, preferably under continuous hospital care.

Although signs of overdosage and respiratory depression may not be evident soon after ingestion of difenoxin, respiratory depression may occur 12 to 30 hours later.

Patient Information

Adhere strictly to recommended dosage schedules. Keep out of reach of children since accidental overdosage may result in severe, even fatal, respiratory depression.

May cause dizziness or drowsiness; use caution while driving or performing other tasks requiring alertness, coordination or physical dexterity.

DIPHENOXYLATE HYDROCHLORIDE/ATROPINE SULFATE

c-v	**Diphenoxylate hydrochloride w/Atropine Sulfate** (Various, eg, Mylan, Purepac, Schein)	**Tablets:** 2.5 mg diphenoxylate hydrochloride and 0.025 mg atropine sulfate	In 100s, 500s, 1000s, 2500s and UD 100s.
c-v	**Logen** (Goldline)		White. In 100s, 500s & 1000s.
c-v	**Lomotil** (Searle)		Sorbitol, sucrose. (Searle 61). White. In 100s, 500s, 1000s, 2500s, UD 100s.
c-v	**Lonox** (Sandoz)		(GG 4). White. In 30s, 100s, 500s, 1,000s & UD 100s.
c-v	**Diphenoxylate hydrochloride w/ Atropine Sulfate** (Various, eg, Goldline, Roxane)	**Liquid:** 2.5 mg diphenoxylate hydrochloride and 0.025 mg atropine sulfate per 5 mL	In 60 mL, UD 4 and 10 mL.
c-v	**Lomanate** (Qualitest)		In 60 mL.
c-v	**Lomotil** (Searle)		15% alcohol. Sorbitol. Cherry flavor. In 60 mL w/dropper.

DIPHENOXYLATE HYDROCHLORIDE/ATROPINE SULFATE — ORAL

Indications

➤*Diarrhea:* Adjunctive therapy in the management of diarrhea.

Administration and Dosage

➤*Adults:*

Diarrhea –

Initial dosage: 5 mg (based on diphenoxylate) 4 times per day.

Maintenance dosage: Reduce dosage as soon as initial control of symptoms is achieved. Maintenance dosage may be as low as one-fourth of the initial daily dosage.

Duration of therapy: Clinical improvement of acute diarrhea is usually observed within 48 hours. If clinical improvement of chronic diarrhea is not seen within 10 days after a maximum daily dose of 20 mg, symptoms are unlikely to be controlled by further use.

➤*Children:*

Diarrhea – See Adults for dosing for children 12 years of age and older.

2 to 12 years of age: In children 2 to 12 years of age, use liquid form only.

• *Initial dosage* – 0.3 to 0.4 mg/kg/day (based on diphenoxylate) in 4 divided doses.

Diphenoxylate With Atropine Pediatric Initial Dosage			
	Approximate weight		
Age (years)	kg	lb	Dosage[a] (mL) (4 times daily)
9 to 12	23 to 55	51 to 121	3.5 to 5
6 to 8	17 to 32	38 to 71	2.5 to 5
5	16 to 23	35 to 51	2.5 to 4.5
4	14 to 20	31 to 44	2 to 4
3	12 to 16	26 to 35	2 to 3
2	11 to 14	24 to 31	1.5 to 3

[a] Based on diphenoxylate 2.5 mg and atropine 0.025 mg per 5 mL.

• *Maintenance dosage* – Reduce dosage as soon as initial control of symptoms is achieved. Maintenance dosage may be as low as one-fourth of the initial daily dosage. Do not exceed recommended dosage.

• *Dosage adjustment* – The dosage may be adjusted downwards according to the overall nutritional status and degree of dehydration encountered in the sick child.

• *Duration of therapy* – Clinical improvement of acute diarrhea is usually observed within 48 hours. If no response occurs within 48 hours, diphenoxylate/atropine is unlikely to be effective.

Younger than 2 years of age: Not recommended.

➤*Renal function impairment:* Use with extreme caution in patients with advanced hepato-renal disease.

➤*Hepatic function impairment:* Use with extreme caution in patients with advanced hepato-renal disease or abnormal liver function; hepatic coma may be precipitated.

➤*Storage/Stability:* Store at 20° to 25°C (68° to 77°F).

Actions

➤*Pharmacology:* Diphenoxylate, a constipating meperidine congener, lacks analgesic activity. High doses (40 to 60 mg) cause opioid activity, (eg, euphoria, suppression of morphine abstinence syndrome, physical dependence after chronic use).

➤*Pharmacokinetics:* Bioavailability of tablet vs liquid is ≈ 90%. Diphenoxylate is rapidly, extensively metabolized to diphenoxylic acid (difenoxine), the active major metabolite. Elimination half-life is ≈ 12 to 14 hrs. An average of 14% of drug and metabolites are excreted over 4 days in urine, 49% in feces. Urinary excretion of unmetabolized drug is less than 1%; difenoxine plus its glucuronide conjugate constitutes ≈ 6%.

Contraindications

Children younger than 2 years of age, due to greater variability of response; hypersensitivity to diphenoxylate or atropine; obstructive jaundice; diarrhea associated with pseudomembranous enterocolitis or enterotoxin-producing bacteria (see Warnings).

Warnings/Precautions

➤*Diarrhea:* Diphenoxylate may prolong or aggravate diarrhea associated with organisms that penetrate intestinal mucosa (ie, toxigenic *Escherichia coli, Salmonella, Shigella*) or in pseudomembranous enterocolitis associated with broad-spectrum antibiotics. Do not use diphenoxylate in these conditions. In some patients with acute ulcerative colitis, diphenoxylate may induce toxic megacolon. Discontinue therapy if abdominal distention or other untoward symptoms develop.

➤*Fluid/electrolyte balance:* Dehydration, particularly in younger children, may influence variability of response and may predispose to delayed diphenoxylate intoxication. Inhibition of peristalsis may result in fluid retention in the intestine, which may further aggravate dehydration and electrolyte imbalance. If severe dehydration or electrolyte imbalance occurs, withhold the drug until initiating corrective therapy.

➤*Hepatic function impairment:* Use with extreme caution in patients with advanced hepato-renal disease or abnormal liver function; hepatic coma may be precipitated.

➤*Drug abuse and dependence:* In recommended doses, diphenoxylate has not produced addiction and is devoid of morphine-like subjective effects. At high doses, it exhibits codeine-like subjective effects; therefore, addiction to diphenoxylate is possible. A subtherapeutic dose of atropine may discourage deliberate abuse.

➤*Hazardous tasks:* Patients should use caution while driving or performing other tasks requiring alertness, coordination or physical dexterity.

➤*Pregnancy: Category C.* There are no adequate and well controlled studies in pregnant women. Use in women of childbearing potential only when clearly needed and when the potential benefits outweigh the potential hazards to the fetus.

➤*Lactation:* Exercise caution when administering to a nursing mother. Diphenoxylic acid may be excreted in breast milk and atropine is excreted in breast milk.

➤*Children:* Use with caution; signs of atropinism may occur with recommended doses, particularly in Down's syndrome patients. Use with caution in young children due to variable response. Not recommended in children younger than 2 years of age.

➤*Elderly:* Atropine is considered a high risk medication for the elderly according to the Centers of Medicare and Medicaid Services.

Long-term use of diphenoxylate to treat diarrhea should be avoided in the elderly because of the risk for drowsiness, cognitive impairment and dependence. Consideration should be given to using nondrug therapy and modification of diet or loperamide.

Drug Interactions

Diphenoxylate Drug Interactions			
Precipitant drug	Object drug[a]		Description
Diphenoxylate	MAOIs	↑	Since the chemical structure of diphenoxylate is similar to meperidine, concurrent use may precipitate hypertensive crises.
Diphenoxylate	Barbiturates, tranquilizers, and alcohol	↑	Diphenoxylate may potentiate the depressant action. Closely observe the patient when these medications are used concomitantly.

[a] ↑ = Object drug increased.

Adverse Reactions

Atropine effects – Dry skin and mucous membranes, flushing, hyperthermia, tachycardia, urinary retention, especially in children.

➤*CNS:* Dizziness; drowsiness; sedation; headache; malaise; lethargy; restlessness; euphoria; depression; numbness of extremities; confusion.

➤*GI:* Anorexia; nausea; vomiting; abdominal discomfort; paralytic ileus; toxic megacolon; pancreatitis.

➤*Hypersensitivity:* Pruritus; gum swelling; angioneurotic edema; urticaria; anaphylaxis.

Overdosage

➤*Symptoms:* Initial signs include dry skin and mucous membranes, mydriasis, restlessness, flushing, hyperthermia and tachycardia followed by lethargy or coma, hypotonic reflexes, nystagmus and pinpoint pupils. Severe, even fatal, respiratory depression may result. Signs of overdosage and respiratory depression may not be evident soon after ingestion; respiratory depression may occur 12 to 30 hours later.

DIPHENOXYLATE HYDROCHLORIDE/ATROPINE SULFATE — ORAL

➤*Treatment:* includes usual supportive measures. Refer to General Management of Acute Overdosage. Gastric lavage, induction of emesis, establishment of a patent airway, and, possibly, mechanically assisted respiration are advised. Use naloxone for respiratory depression (see individual monograph). Diphenoxylate's duration of action is longer than that of naloxone; improved respiration after administration may be followed by recurrent respiratory depression. Consequently, continuous observation for at least 48 hours is necessary until diphenoxylate's effect on respiration has passed. Activated charcoal may significantly decrease bioavailability of diphenoxylate. In non-comatose patients, 100 g activated charcoal slurry can be given immediately after induction of vomiting or gastric lavage.

Patient Information

Do not exceed prescribed dosage. Avoid alcohol and other CNS depressants.

May cause drowsiness or dizziness; use caution while driving or performing other tasks requiring alertness, coordination or physical dexterity.

May cause dry mouth.

Notify physician if diarrhea persists or if fever, palpitations or abnormal distention occur.

LOPERAMIDE HYDROCHLORIDE

otc	**Loperamide** (Geri-Care)	**Tablets; oral:** 2 mg	Capsule shape. In 24s.
otc	**Diar-aid Caplets** (Thompson)		In 12s.
otc	**Imodium A-D Caplets** (McNeil-CPC)		Lactose. (Imodium Janssen). In 6s and 12s.
otc	**K-Pek II** (Rugby)		Lactose. (122). Capsule shape. In 12s.i
Rx	**Loperamide** (Various, eg, Mylan, Novopharm)	**Capsules; oral:** 2 mg	In 100s, 500s, and 1,000s.
otc	**Neo-Diaral** (Roberts)		In UD 8s and 250s.
otc	**Loperamide** (Various, eg, Barre-National, Roxane)	**Liquid; oral:** 1 mg per 5 mL	In 60 and 118 mL.
otc	**Imodium A-D** (McNeil-CPC)		5.25% alcohol. Cherry/licorice flavor. In 60, 90 and 120 mL.
otc	**Imodium A-D** (McNeil Consumer)	**Liquid; oral:** 1 mg per 7.5 mL	Mint flavor. In 120 mL.

LOPERAMIDE HYDROCHLORIDE — ORAL

Indications

➤*Rx:* Loperamide is indicated for the control and symptomatic relief of acute nonspecific diarrhea and of chronic diarrhea associated with inflammatory bowel disease. Loperamide is also indicated for reducing the volume of discharge from ileostomies.

➤*OTC:* Control of symptoms of diarrhea, including traveler's diarrhea.

➤*Off-label uses:*

Traveler's diarrhea – [1] = Good documentation. Current guidelines suggest that mild cases of traveler's diarrhea should be managed with adequate hydration and bismuth subsalicylate or loperamide. (See Administration and Dosage.)

Administration and Dosage

➤*Adults:*

Diarrhea –

Usual dosage: 4 mg after the first loose stool then 2 mg after each subsequent loose stool. Clinical improvement is usually observed within 48 hours. See also the dosing table in the Children section.

Maintenance dosage: For chronic diarrhea, the dosage of loperamide should be reduced to meet individual requirements after the diarrhea is controlled. When the optimal daily dosage has been established, this amount may then be administered as a single dose or in divided doses. The average maintenance dosage in clinical trials was 4 to 8 mg daily. A dosage of 16 mg was rarely exceeded. If clinical improvement is not observed after treatment with 16 mg per day for at least 10 days, symptoms are unlikely to be controlled by further administration. Loperamide administration may be continued if diarrhea cannot be adequately controlled with diet or specific treatment.

Off-label dosing –

Traveler's diarrhea: [1] = Good documentation. Loperamide 4 mg followed by 2 mg after each loose stool (maximum, 16 mg/day) for symptomatic management, particularly in situations in which restrooms are inaccessible.

➤*Children:*

Diarrhea –

OTC products: For dosing of OTC products, see the following table. If possible, use weight to dose, otherwise use age.

OTC Loperamide Dosing by Doseform

Age	Dose after first loose stool	Dose after each subsequent loose stool	Daily dosage limit
Liquid 1 mg/5 mL			
Adults and children ≥ 12 years of age	20 mL (4 tsp)	10 mL (2 tsp)	40 mL (8 tsp)[a]
Children 9 to 11 years of age (60 to 95 lbs)	10 mL (2 tsp)	5 mL (1 tsp)	30 mL (6 tsp)[a]
Children 6 to 8 years of age (48 to 59 lbs)	10 mL (2 tsp)	5 mL (1 tsp)	20 mL (4 tsp)[a]
Children < 6 years of age (up to 47 lbs)	Consult health care provider. Not intended for use in children younger than 6 years of age		

OTC Loperamide Dosing by Doseform

Age	Dose after first loose stool	Dose after each subsequent loose stool	Daily dosage limit
Liquid (1 mg/7.5 mL)			
Adults and children ≥ 12 years of age	30 mL (6 tsp)	15 mL (3 tsp)	60 mL (12 tsp) in 24 hours
Children 9 to 11 years of age (60 to 95 lbs)	15 mL (3 tsp)	7.5 mL (1.5 tsp)	45 mL (9 tsp) in 24 hours
Children 6 to 8 years of age (48 to 59 lbs)	15 mL (3 tsp)	7.5 mL (1.5 tsp)	30 mL (6 tsp) in 24 hours
Children < 6 years of age (up to 47 lbs)	Consult health care provider. Not intended for use in children younger than 6 years of age		
Tablets			
Adults and children ≥ 12 years of age	2	1	4
Children 9 to 11 years of age (60 to 95 lbs)	1	½	3
Children 6 to 8 years of age (45 to 59 lbs)	1	½	2
Children < 6 years of age (up to 47 lbs)	Consult health care provider. Not intended for use in children younger than 6 years of age		

[a] Limit use to no more than 2 days.

Rx products: See Adults for dosing for children 12 years of age and older. In children 2 to 5 years of age (20 kg or less), a nonprescription liquid formulation should be used; for children ages 6 to 12, either loperamide capsules or liquid may be used.

- *8 to 12 years of age (greater than 30 kg)* –
  Initial dosage: 2 mg 3 times a day (6 mg daily dose) for the first day.
  Maintenance dosage: Following the first treatment day, it is recommended that subsequent loperamide doses (1 mg/10 kg body weight) be administered only after a loose stool. Total daily dosage should not exceed recommended dosages for the first day.
- *6 to 8 years (20 to 30 kg)* –
  Initial dosage: 2 mg twice a day (4 mg daily dose) for the first day.
  Maintenance dosage: Following the first treatment day, it is recommended that subsequent loperamide doses (1 mg/10 kg body weight) be administered only after a loose stool. Total daily dosage should not exceed recommended dosages for the first day.
- *2 to 5 years (13 to 20 kg)* –
  Initial dosage: 1 mg 3 times a day (3 mg daily dose) for the first day.
  Maintenance dosage: Following the first treatment day, it is recommended that subsequent loperamide doses (1 mg/10 kg body weight) be administered only after a loose stool. Total daily dosage should not exceed recommended dosages for the first day.
- *Younger than 2 years of age* – Use is not recommended.

➤*Preparation for administration:* Shake the oral liquids well before using.

➤*Administration:* Drink plenty of clear fluids to help prevent dehydration, which may accompany diarrhea. The chewable tablets should be taken on an empty stomach (1 hour before or 2 hours after a meal).

➤*Storage/Stability:* Store at 15° to 25°C (59° to 77°F).

LOPERAMIDE HYDROCHLORIDE — ORAL

Actions

➤*Pharmacology:* In vitro and animal studies show that loperamide acts by slowing intestinal motility and by affecting water and electrolyte movement through the bowel. Loperamide inhibits peristaltic activity by a direct effect on the circular and longitudinal muscles of the intestinal wall.

In man, loperamide prolongs the transit time of the intestinal contents. It reduces the daily fecal volume, increases the viscosity and bulk density, and diminishes the loss of fluid and electrolytes. Tolerance to the antidiarrheal effect has not been observed.

➤*Pharmacokinetics:* Clinical studies have indicated that the apparent elimination half-life of loperamide in man is 10.8 hours with a range of 9.1 to 14.4 hours. Plasma levels of unchanged drug remain below 2 ng/mL after the intake of a 2 mg capsule of loperamide. Plasma levels are highest approximately 5 hours after administration of the capsule and 2.5 hours after the liquid. The peak plasma levels of loperamide were similar for both formulations. Of the total excreted in urine and feces, most of the administered drug was excreted in feces.

In those patients in whom biochemical and hematological parameters were monitored during clinical trials, no trends toward abnormality during loperamide therapy were noted. Similarly, urinalyses, EKG and clinical ophthalmological examinations did not show trends toward abnormality.

Contraindications

Loperamide is contraindicated in patients with known hypersensitivity to the drug and in those in whom constipation must be avoided.

Warnings/Precautions

➤*Acute dysentery:* Loperamide should not be used in the case of acute dysentery, which is characterized by blood in stools and high fever.

➤*Fluid and electrolyte depletion:* Fluid and electrolyte depletion may occur in patients who have diarrhea. In such cases, administration of appropriate fluid and electrolytes is very important. The use of loperamide does not preclude the administration of appropriate fluid and electrolyte therapy.

➤*Toxic megacolon:* In some patients with acute ulcerative colitis, and in pseudomembranous colitis associated with broad-spectrum antibiotics, agents which inhibit intestinal motility or delay intestinal transit time have been reported to induce toxic megacolon.

➤*Discontinue use:* Loperamide therapy should be discontinued promptly if abdominal distention, constipation, or ileus occurs.

In acute diarrhea, if clinical improvement is not observed in 48 hours, the administration of loperamide should be discontinued.

➤*Hepatic function impairment:* Patients with hepatic dysfunction should be monitored closely for signs of CNS toxicity because of the apparent large first-pass biotransformation.

➤*Drug abuse and dependence:*

Abuse – A specific clinical study designed to assess the abuse potential of loperamide at high doses resulted in a finding of extremely low abuse potential.

Dependence – Studies in morphine-dependent monkeys demonstrated that loperamide hydrochloride at doses above those recommended for humans prevented signs of morphine withdrawal. However, in humans, the naloxone challenge pupil test, which when positive indicates opiate-like effects, performed after a single high dose, or after more than 2 years of therapeutic use of loperamide, was negative. Orally administered loperamide (loperamide formulated with magnesium stearate) is both highly insoluble and penetrates the CNS poorly.

➤*Pregnancy: Category B.* Reproduction studies in rats and rabbits have revealed no evidence of impaired fertility or harm to the fetus at doses up to 30 times the human dose. Higher doses impaired the survival of mothers and nursing young. The studies offered no evidence of teratogenic activity. There are, however, no adequate and well controlled studies in pregnant women. Because animal reproduction studies are not always predictive of human response, this drug should be used during pregnancy only if clearly needed.

➤*Lactation:* It is not known whether this drug is excreted in human milk. Because many drugs are excreted in human milk, caution should be exercised when loperamide is administered to a nursing woman.

➤*Children:* Loperamide should be used with special caution in young children because of the greater variability of response in this age group. Dehydration, particularly in younger children, may further influence the variability of response to loperamide.

➤*Monitoring:* Patients with hepatic dysfunction should be monitored closely for signs of CNS toxicity because of the apparent large first-pass biotransformation.

Drug Interactions

There was no evidence in clinical trials of drug interactions with concurrent medications.

Adverse Reactions

The adverse effects reported during clinical investigations of loperamide are difficult to distinguish from symptoms associated with the diarrheal syndrome. Adverse experiences recorded during clinical studies with loperamide were generally of a minor and self-limiting nature. They were more commonly observed during the treatment of chronic diarrhea.

The following patient complaints have been reported and are listed in decreasing order of frequency with the exception of hypersensitivity reactions, which is listed first since it may be the most serious:

- Hypersensitivity reactions (including skin rash) have been reported with loperamide use.
- Abdominal pain, distention or discomfort.
- Nausea and vomiting.
- Constipation.
- Tiredness.
- Drowsiness or dizziness.
- Dry mouth.

In postmarketing experiences, there have been rare reports of paralytic ileus associated with abdominal distention. Most of these reports occurred in the setting of acute dysentery, overdose, and with very young children of less than 2 years of age.

Overdosage

➤*Symptoms:* In cases of overdosage, paralytic ileus and CNS depression may occur. Children may be more sensitive to CNS effects than adults.

➤*Treatment:* Clinical trials have demonstrated that a slurry of activated charcoal administered promptly after ingestion of loperamide hydrochloride can reduce the amount of drug which is absorbed into the systemic circulation by as much as 9-fold. If vomiting occurs spontaneously upon ingestion, a slurry of 100 g of activated charcoal should be administered orally as soon as fluids can be retained.

If vomiting has not occurred, gastric lavage should be performed followed by administration of 100 g of activated charcoal slurry through the gastric tube. In the event of overdosage, patients should be monitored for signs of CNS depression for at least 24 hours. Children may be more sensitive to central nervous system effects than adults. If CNS depression is observed, naloxone may be administered. If responsive to naloxone, vital signs must be monitored carefully for recurrence of symptoms of drug overdose for at least 24 hours after the last dose of naloxone.

In view of the prolonged action of loperamide and the short duration (1 to 3 hours) of naloxone, the patient must be monitored closely and treated repeatedly with naloxone as indicated. Since relatively little drug is excreted in the urine, forced diuresis is not expected to be effective for loperamide overdosage.

In clinical trials an adult who took three 20 mg doses within a 24 hour period was nauseated after the second dose and vomited after the third dose. In studies designed to examine the potential for side effects, intentional ingestion of up to 60 mg of loperamide hydrochloride in a single dose to healthy subjects resulted in no significant adverse effects.

Patient Information

Patients should be advised to check with their physician if their diarrhea does not improve after a couple of days or if they note blood in their stools or develop a fever.

Do not use if you have ever had a rash or other allergic reaction to loperamide hydrochloride. Do not use if you have bloody or black stool. Ask a doctor before use if you have high fever (greater than 38.3°C; 101°F), mucus present in your stool, a history of liver disease, or are taking antibiotics. Stop use and ask a doctor if diarrhea lasts for more than 2 days. If pregnant or breastfeeding, ask a health professional before use. In case of overdose, get medical help or contact a poison control center right away. Do not use for more than 2 days unless directed by a physician.

➤*OTC tablets:* Do not use if you have ever had a rash or other allergic reaction to loperamide hydrochloride. Do not use if you have bloody or black stool.

Ask a doctor of pharmacist before use if you are taking antibiotics. Stop use and ask a doctor if diarrhea lasts for more than 2 days. If pregnant or breastfeeding, ask a health professional before use.

Keep out of reach of children. In case of overdose, get medical help or contact a poison control center right away.

BISMUTH SUBSALICYLATE (BSS)

otc	**Kaopectate** (Pfizer Consumer Health)	**Tablets; oral:** 262 mg	Capsule shape. In 12s and 20s.
otc sf	**Bismuth** (Contract Pharmacal Corporation)	**Tablets, chewable; oral:** 262 mg	Sugar free. Cherry flavoring, mannitol, saccharin, sorbitol, wintergreen oil flavoring. In 30s.
otc	**Bismatrol** (Major)		Sodium 0.1 mg, saccharin, mannitol. In 30s.
otc	**Peptic Relief** (Rugby)		Dextrose, sorbitol. In 30s.
otc sf	**Pepto-Bismol** (Procter & Gamble)		< 2 mg sodium/tablet. Saccharin, mannitol. (Pepto-Bismol). Pink. Original and cherry flavors. In 30s and 42s (cherry). In 24s and 42s (original).
otc	**Kaopectate Children's** (Pharmacia)	**Liquid; oral:** 87 mg per 5 mL	Sucrose. Cherry flavor. In 236 mL.
otc	**Pink Bismuth** (Various, eg, Goldline)	**Liquid; oral:** 130 mg per 15 mL	In 240 mL.
otc	**Pink Bismuth** (Various, eg, Goldline)	**Liquid; oral:** 262 mg per 15 mL	In 240 mL.
otc	**Kao-Tin** (Major)		Saccharin, sorbitol. In 236 and 473 mL.
otc	**Kaopectate** (Pharmacia)		Sucrose. In 236 and 355 mL (regular flavor) and 236 and 355 mL (peppermint flavor).
otc	**Peptic Relief** (Rugby)		Saccharin, sorbitol. In 237 mL.
otc sf	**Pepto-Bismol** (Procter & Gamble)		5 mg sodium/15 mL. Saccharin. In 120, 240, 360, and 480 mL.
otc sf	**Pepto-Bismol Maximum Strength** (Procter & Gamble)	**Liquid; oral:** 524 mg per 15 mL	< 5 mg sodium/15 mL. Saccharin. In 120, 240, and 360 mL.
otc	**Bismatrol Maximum Strength** (Major)	**Liquid; oral:** 525 mg per 15 mL	Saccharin, sodium 6 mg. In 237 mL.
otc	**Kaopectate Extra Strength** (Pharmacia)		Sucrose. Peppermint flavor. In 236 mL.
otc	**Maalox Total Stomach Relief Liquid** (Novartis)	**Suspension; oral:** 525 mg per 15 mL	Parabens, sorbitol, sucralose, and alcohol (peppermint only). In strawberry and peppermint flavors. In 355 mL.

BISMUTH SUBSALICYLATE — ORAL

Indications

➤*Diarrhea:* To control diarrhea, reduce number of bowel movements, and help firm stool.

➤*Gas/indigestion/heartburn/nausea:* To control gas, upset stomach, indigestion, heartburn, and nausea.

➤*Off-label uses:*

Traveler's diarrhea – [1] = Good documentation. Current guidelines suggest that mild cases of traveler's diarrhea should be managed with adequate hydration and bismuth subsalicylate or loperamide. (See Administration and Dosage.)

Administration and Dosage

➤*Maximum dose:* 8 doses/day (regular strength); 4 doses/day (maximum strength).

➤*General dosing considerations:* Drink plenty of clear fluids to help prevent dehydration, which may accompany diarrhea.

This medication may cause a temporary and harmless darkening of the tongue or stool.

➤*Adults:*

Gastrointestinal conditions – See Indications for the specific uses.

Usual dosage: 2 tablets or 30 mL. Repeat dosage every 30 minutes to 1 hour, as needed, up to 8 doses/day (regular strength) or 4 doses/day (maximum strength).

Off-label dosing –

Traveler's diarrhea: [1] = Good documentation. 1 ounce every 30 minutes for 8 doses.

➤*Children:*

Gastrointestinal conditions – See Indications for the specific uses.

See Adults for dosing for children 12 years of age and older.

Some products are not approved for use in children younger than 12 years of age. See product labeling.

9 to 11 years of age:

- *Usual dosage* – 15 mL or one chewable tablet. Repeat dosage every 30 minutes to 1 hour, as needed, up to 8 doses in 24 hours.

6 to 8 years of age:

- *Usual dosage* – 10 mL or ⅔ chewable tablet. Repeat dosage every 30 minutes to 1 hour, as needed, up to 8 doses in 24 hours.

3 to 5 years of age:

- *Usual dosage* – 5 mL or ⅓ chewable tablet. Repeat dosage every 30 minutes to 1 hour, as needed, up to 8 doses in 24 hours.

➤*Duration of therapy:* Use until diarrhea stops but not more than 2 days.

➤*Administration:* Shake the liquids well immediately before each use. Chew or dissolve the chewable tablets in mouth. Swallow the conventional tablets with water; do not chew.

➤*Storage/Stability:* Store at 20° to 25°C (68° to 77°F). Avoid excessive heat, 40°C (104°F).

Actions

➤*Pharmacology:* BSS appears to have antisecretory and antimicrobial effects in vitro and may have some anti-inflammatory effects. The salicylate moiety provides the antisecretory effect, while the bismuth moiety may exert direct antimicrobial effects against bacterial and viral enteropathogens.

➤*Pharmacokinetics:*

Absorption/Distribution – BSS undergoes chemical dissociation in the GI tract. Two BSS tablets yield 204 mg salicylate. Following ingestion, salicylate is absorbed, with greater than 90% recovered in the urine; plasma levels are similar to levels achieved after a comparable dose of aspirin. Absorption of bismuth is negligible.

Warnings/Precautions

➤*Reye syndrome:* Children and teenagers who have or are recovering from chicken pox, flu symptoms, or flu should not use this product. If nausea, vomiting, or fever occur, consult a doctor because these symptoms could be an early sign of Reye's syndrome, a rare but serious illness.

➤*Ringing in the ears:* This product contains salicylates. If taken with other salicylate-containing preparations (such as aspirin) and ringing in the ears occurs, discontinue use.

➤*Impaction:* Impaction may occur in infants and debilitated patients.

➤*Radiologic examinations:* May interfere with radiologic examinations of GI tract. Bismuth is radiopaque.

➤*Pregnancy: Category C* (per Briggs' *Drugs in Pregnancy and Lactation*). The use of bismuth subsalicylate during gestation should be restricted to the first half of pregnancy, and then only in amounts that do not exceed the recommended dose.

➤*Lactation:* The excretion of significant amounts of bismuth obtained from bismuth subsalicylate into breast milk is not expected because of the poor absorption of bismuth into the systemic circulation. Salicylates, however, are excreted in milk and are eliminated more slowly from milk than from plasma with milk:plasma ratios rising from 0.03 to 0.08 at 3 hours to 0.34 at 12 hours. Because of the potential for adverse effects in the breast-feeding infant, the American Academy of Pediatrics recommends that salicylates should be used cautiously during breast-feeding.

Drug Interactions

Bismuth Subsalicylate (BSS) Drug Interactions

Precipitant drug	Object drug[a]		Description
BSS	Aspirin	↑	BSS contains salicylate. If taken with aspirin and ringing of the ears occurs, discontinue use.
BSS	Tetracyclines	↓	BSS may decrease GI absorption and bioavailability of tetracyclines, reducing their efficacy.

[a] ↑ = object drug increased; ↓ = object drug decreased.

BISMUTH SUBSALICYLATE — ORAL

Ask a doctor or pharmacist before use if you are taking a prescription drug for anticoagulation (thinning the blood), diabetes, gout, or arthritis.

Patient Information

Shake liquid well before using. Chew tablets or allow to dissolve in mouth.

Stool may temporarily appear gray-black.

If diarrhea is accompanied by high fever or continues for more than 2 days, consult physician.

Do not use if you are allergic to salicylates (including aspirin) unless directed by a doctor.

Ask a doctor or pharmacist before use if you are taking a prescription drug for anticoagulation (thinning the blood), diabetes, gout, or arthritis.

Do not use for more than 2 days or in the presence of fever, or in children under 3 years of age unless directed by a doctor.

If pregnant or breastfeeding, ask a health professional before use.

ANTIDIARRHEAL COMBINATION PRODUCTS

otc	**Kaolin w/Pectin** (Various, eg, Roxane, Wyeth-Ayerst)	**Suspension**: 90 g kaolin, 2 g pectin/30 mL. *Dose:* After each bowel movement. *Adults* - 60 to 120 mL/dose. *Children - 6 to 12 years:* 30 to 60 mL/dose. *3 to 6 years:* 15 to 30 mL/dose.	In 180 mL, pt and UD 30 mL.
otc	**Kapectolin** (Various, eg, Goldline, Major)		In 360 mL.
otc	**K-Pec** (Rugby)	**Suspension**: 750 mg attapulgite/15 mL. *Dose:* After each bowel movement up to 6 doses/day. ≥ *12* – 30 mL. *Children - 6 to younger than 12 years of age:* 15 mL/dose. *3 to younger than 6 years of age:* 7.5 mL/dose.	EDTA, methylparaben. sucrose. In 237 and 473 mL.
otc	**Kaodene Non-Narcotic** (Pfeiffer)	**Liquid**: 3.9 g kaolin, 194.4 mg pectin/30 mL, bismuth subsalicylate. *Dose:* 1 to 3 doses/day or after each loose stool. *Adults* – 45 mL/dose. *Children - 6 to 12 years:* 22.5 mL/dose. *3 to 6 years:* 15 mL/dose.	Alcohol free. Sucrose. In 120 mL.
otc	**Diasorb** (Columbia)	**Tablets**: 750 mg activated attapulgite. *Dose:* After each bowel movement up to 3 doses/day. *Adults* - 4/dose. *Children – 6 to 12 years:* 2/dose. *3 to 6 years:* 1/dose.	Sorbitol. In 24s.
		Liquid: 750 mg activated attapulgite/ 5 mL. *Dose:* After each bowel movement up to 3 doses/day. *Adults* – 20 mL/dose. *Children – 6 to 12 years:* 10 mL/dose. *3 to 6 years:* 5 mL/dose.	Sugar free. Sorbitol, saccharin. Cola flavor. In 120 mL.
otc	**Kaopectate Maximum Strength** (Upjohn)	**Caplets**: 750 mg attapulgite. *Dose:* After each bowel movement up to 6 doses/day. *Adults* - 2/dose. *Children - 6 to 12 years:* 1/dose.	Sucrose. In 12s and 20s.
otc	**Imodium Multi-Symptom Relief** (McNeil Consumer)	**Tablets; oral**: 2 mg loperamide HCl, 125 mg simethicone. *Dose:* After each loose bowel movement. ≥ *12 years* - 2 tablets 1 time, then 1 tablet/dose up to 4/day. *Children - 9 to 11 years:* 1 tablet 1 time, then ½ tablet/dose up to 3/day. *Children - 6 to 8 years:* 1 tablet 1 time, then ½ tablet/dose up to 2/day.	Acesulfame K, 165 mg calcium, 4 mg sodium. Capsule shape. In 12s, 18s, 30s, and 42s.
otc	**Imodium Multi-Symptom Relief** (McNeil Consumer)	**Tablets, chewable; oral**: 2 mg loperamide HCl, 125 mg simethicone. *Dose:* After each loose bowel movement. ≥ *12 years* - 2 tablets 1 time, then 1 tablet/dose up to 4/day. *Children - 9 to 11 years:* 1 tablet 1 time, then ½ tablet/dose up to 3/day. *Children - 6 to 8 years:* 1 tablet 1 time, then ½ tablet/dose up to 2/day.	50 mg calcium, saccharin, sorbitol, sugar. Mint flavor. In 18s and 42s.

Indications

➤*Diarrhea:* For the symptomatic treatment of diarrhea by reducing intestinal motility or adsorbing fluid.

Warnings/Precautions

➤*Diarrhea from other causes:* Do not use antiperistaltic agents for diarrhea associated with pseudomembranous enterocolitis or in diarrhea caused by toxigenic bacteria.

➤*Salicylate absorption:* Salicylate absorption may occur from bismuth subsalicylate; therefore, observe caution in patients with bleeding disorders or salicylate sensitivity and in children.

➤*Ingredients:* The use of the ingredients in combination in the following products as nonspecific antidiarrheal agents has, to a large extent, been empiric. Adequate controlled clinical studies demonstrating the efficacy of these antidiarrheal combinations are lacking. The FDA has determined that the following ingredients are *not* generally recognized as safe and effective and are misbranded when present in *otc* antidiarrheal preparations: Aluminum hydroxide, atropine sulfate, calcium carbonate, carboxymethylcellulose, glycine, homatropine methylbromide, hyoscyamine sulfate, *Lactobacillus acidophilus* and *bulgaricus*, opium (powdered and tincture), paregoric, phenyl salicylate, scopolamine hydrobromide and zinc phenolsulfonate.

In 1986, in the tentative final monograph for these agents, the FDA considered attapulgite a Category I agent (safe and effective) and placed kaolin and pectin in Category III (insufficient data to permit classification). Recently, however, an FDA advisory committee recommended that the FDA reverse the classifications, making attapulgite Category III and kaolin and pectin Category I. Further studies are pending.

Activated **attapulgite**, **kaolin** and **pectin** are used for their adsorbent and protectant actions.

Bismuth salts have antacid and adsorbent properties.

➤*Pregnancy: Category C* ([**kaolin**, **pectin**, **bismuth**] per Briggs' *Drugs in Pregnancy and Lactation*). Seek the advise of a health care provider before using in pregnant women. The use of bismuth subsalicylate during gestation should be restricted to the first half of pregnancy, and then only in amounts that do not exceed the recommended doses.

➤*Lactation:* **Bismuth**, **kaolin**, and **pectin** are not absorbed into the systemic circulation. Seek the advise of a health care provider before using in breast-feeding women. Bismuth subsalicylate should be avoided during lactation because of systemic salicylate absorption.

SIMETHICONE

otc	**Phazyme** (Reed & Carnrick)	**Tablets; oral:** 60 mg	Enteric coated inner core. In 50s, 100s and 1000s.
otc	**Bicarsim** (Kramer-Novis)	**Tablets; oral:** 80 mg	Sugar. In 60s.
otc	**Phazyme 95** (GlaxoSmithKline Consumer)	**Tablets; oral:** 95 mg	Enteric coated inner core. In 50s, 100s, 500s and Consumer Pak 10s.
otc	**Bicarsim Forte** (Kramer-Novis)	**Tablets; oral:** 125 mg	Sugar. In 60s.
otc	**Gas Relief** (Rugby)	**Tablets, chewable; oral:** 80 mg	In 100s.
otc	**Gas-X** (Novartis Consumer Health)		(Gas-X). White, scored. In 12s, 30s.
otc	**Genasyme** (Goldline)		In 100s.
otc	**Mylanta Gas** (J&J/Merck)		Mint flavor. In 100s.
otc	**Gas-X Extra Strength** (Novartis Consumer Health)	**Tablets, chewable; oral:** 125 mg	(Gas-X). Yellow, scored. In 18s.
otc	**Gas Relief** (Rugby)		Dextrose, sugar, sorbitol. In 60s and 100s.
otc	**Mylanta Gas Maximum Strength** (J&J/Merck)		Mint and cherry flavors. In 12s, 24s, and 60s.
otc	**Phazyme 125** (GlaxoSmithKline Consumer)	**Capsules; oral:** 125 mg	(Phazyme 125). Red. In 50s.
otc	**Phazyme** (GlaxoSmithKline Consumer)	**Capsules; oral:** 180 mg	In 12s.
otc	**Gas-X Extra Strength** (Novartis Consumer Health)	**Capsules, softgel; oral:** 125 mg	Sorbitol. In 10s and 30s.
otc	**Mylanta Gas Maximum Strength** (J&J/Merck)		Peppermint oil. In 24s.
otc	**Gas-X Infant Drops** (Novartis Consumer Health)	**Drops; oral:** 20 mg per 0.3 mL	In 30 mL w/calibrated dropper.
otc	**Simethicone** (Various)	**Drops; oral:** 40 mg per 0.6 mL	In 30 mL w/calibrated oral syringe.
otc	**Flatulex** (Dayton)		In 30 mL w/calibrated dropper.
otc	**Genasyme Drops** (Goldline)		Hydroxypropyl methylcellulose, saccharin calcium, sodium benzoate, sodium citrate. In 30 mL.
otc	**Mylicon** (J&J/Merck)		In 30 mL dropper bottle.
otc	**Gas-X Thin Strips** (Novartis Consumer Health)	**Strip, orally disintegrating; oral:** 62.5 mg	Maltodextrin, menthol, sorbitol, sucralose. In 18s.

SIMETHICONE — ORAL

Indications

➤*Gas retention:* For relief of painful symptoms (ie, pressure, bloating, discomfort) of excess gas in the stomach and intestines. Used as an adjunct in the treatment of many conditions in which gas retention may be a problem, such as postoperative gaseous distention, air swallowing, functional dyspepsia, peptic ulcer, spastic or irritable colon, or diverticulosis.

➤*Off-label uses:* Simethicone has been used for treating the symptoms of infant colic. It is generally administered with meals.

Administration and Dosage

➤*Maximum dose:*

Adults and children older than 2 years of age – 500 mg/day.

Younger than 2 years of age – 240 mg/day.

➤*Adults:*

Gas retention –

Usual dosage: 40 to 360 mg as needed after meals and at bedtime.

➤*Children:*

Gas retention – See Adults for dosing for children 12 years of age and older.

2 to 12 years of age or greater than 24 pounds:

• *Usual dosage* – 40 mg as needed after meals and at bedtime.

Younger than 2 years of age or less than 24 pounds:

• *Usual dosage* – 20 mg as needed after meals and at bedtime.

➤*Administration:*

Chewable tablets – Chew thoroughly and swallow.

Drops – Shake well before using. Fill enclosed dropper to recommended dosage level and dispense liquid slowly into the infant's mouth, toward the inner cheek. The dosage can also be mixed with 1 oz of cool water, infant formula, or other suitable liquids.

Strips – Allow to dissolve on tongue.

➤*Storage/Stability:* Store at 15° to 30°C (59° to 86°F). Protect from excessive moisture and heat.

ALPHA-D-GALACTOSIDASE

otc	**Beano** (AK Pharma)	**Liquid:** Alpha-D-galactosidase-derived from *Aspergillus niger* (≥ 175 galactose units per 5 drop dosage)	Glycerol. In 75 serving size at 5 drops per dose.
		Tablets: Alpha-galactosidase enzyme derived from *Aspergillus niger*	Cornstarch, sucrose, hydrogenated cottonseed oil, sorbitol. In 12s, 30s and 100s.

ALPHA-D-GALACTOSIDASE — ORAL

Indications

➤*Intestinal gas/bloating:* Treatment of gassiness or bloating as a result of eating a variety of grains, cereals, nuts, seeds, or vegetables containing the sugars raffinose, stachyose, or verbascose. This includes all or most legumes and all or most cruciferous vegetables (eg, oats, wheats, beans, peas, lentils, peanuts, soy-content foods, pistachios, broccoli, brussels sprouts, cabbage, carrots, corn, onions, squash, cauliflower).

Administration and Dosage

➤*General dosing considerations:* The patient should use a higher or lower amount depending on the quantity of food eaten, levels of alpha-linked sugars in the food, and the gas-producing propensity and tolerance of the person.

➤*Adults:*

Intestinal gas/bloating –

Capsules (Gax-X Prevention): 1 capsule taken right before a problem food.

Liquid (Beano): 5 drops of liquid per ½ cup serving of gassy food. A typical meal consists of 2 or 3 servings of food, so the patient should take 15 drops with each meal. Adjust the number of drops according to the number of servings.

Tablets (Beano): 1 tablet per ½ cup of gassy food. A typical meal consists of 2 or 3 servings of food, so the patient should take 2 or 3 tablets at the start of each meal. Adjust the number of tablets according to the number of servings.

➤*Children:*

Intestinal gas/bloating –

12 years of age and older: Gax-X Prevention is not intended for children.

• *Liquid (Beano)* – 5 drops of liquid per ½ cup serving of gassy food. A typical meal consists of 2 or 3 servings of food, so the patient should take 15 drops with each meal. The patient should adjust the number of drops according to the number of servings.

ALPHA-D-GALACTOSIDASE — ORAL

• *Tablets (Beano)* – 1 tablet per ½ cup of gassy food. A typical meal consists of 2 or 3 servings of food, so the patient should take 3 tablets with each meal. The patient should adjust the number of tablets according to the number of servings.

➤*Administration:* Take right before the first bite of problem food.

➤*Storage/Stability:* Store below 25° C (77° F). Avoid heat to protect product freshness.

Actions

➤*Pharmacology:* Alpha-D-galactosidase enzyme hydrolyzes raffinose, verbascose and stachyose into the digestible sugars sucrose, fructose, glucose, and galactose.

Warnings/Precautions

➤*Galactosemics:* Galactosemics should not use this supplement without physician advice since one of the breakdown sugars is galactose.

➤*Pregnancy: Category: Undetermined.* Alpha-d-galactosidase has not been tested on pregnant women. There is, however, no information to indicate that alpha-d-galactosidase is unsafe for use during pregnancy.

➤*Lactation:* There is no information to indicate that alpha-d-galactosidase is unsafe for use while breast-feeding.

LIPASE INHIBITORS

ORLISTAT

otc	**Alli** (GlaxoSmithKline)	**Capsules**: 60 mg	Opaque blue. In 60s, 90s, 120s, and 150s.
Rx	**Xenical** (Roche)	**Capsules**: 120 mg	(Roche XENICAL 120). Dark blue. In 90s.

ORLISTAT — ORAL

Indications

➤*Obesity management (Rx):* For obesity management, including weight loss and weight maintenance, when used in conjunction with a reduced-calorie diet. Orlistat is also indicated to reduce the risk for weight regain after prior weight loss. Orlistat is indicated for obese patients with an initial body mass index (BMI) of 30 kg/m^2 or more or 27 kg/m^2 or more in the presence of other risk factors (eg, hypertension, diabetes, dyslipidemia).

BMI is calculated by dividing weight in kilograms by height in meters squared. For example, a person who weighs 180 lbs and is 5'5" would have a BMI of 30.

➤*Obesity management (OTC):* For weight loss in overweight adults, 18 years of age and older, when used along with a reduced-calorie and low-fat diet.

➤*Off-label uses:*

Chylous ascites – [4] = Insufficient documentation. To date, there is limited published information available regarding the use of orlistat in the treatment of chylous ascites. Theoretically, it appears this agent may have some benefit; however, further data are needed before its place in therapy can be established. (See Administration and Dosage.)

Administration and Dosage

➤*General dosing considerations:* Orlistat should be taken with a reduced-calorie, low-fat diet and exercise program until patient's weight-loss goal is reached. Most weight loss occurs in the first 6 months.

If discontinuing orlistat, a diet and exercise program should be continued. If weight gain occurs after discontinuation of orlistat, orlistat therapy may be restarted along with a diet and exercise program.

The patient should be on a nutritionally balanced, reduced-calorie diet that contains approximately 30% of calories from fat. The daily intake of fat, carbohydrate, and protein should be distributed over 3 main meals. If a meal is occasionally missed or contains no fat, the dose of orlistat can be omitted.

Because orlistat has been shown to reduce the absorption of some fat-soluble vitamins and beta-carotene, counsel patients to take a multivitamin containing fat-soluble vitamins to ensure adequate nutrition. The supplement should be taken at least 2 hours before or after the administration of orlistat, such as at bedtime.

Based on fecal fat measurements, the effect of orlistat is seen as soon as 24 to 48 hours after dosing. Upon discontinuation of therapy, fecal fat content usually returns to pretreatment levels within 48 to 72 hours.

➤*Adults:*

Obesity management –

OTC:

• *Usual dosage* – 60 mg with each meal containing fat.

Rx: 120 mg 3 times daily with each main meal containing fat (during or up to 1 hour after the meal).

Off-label dosing –

Chylous ascites: [4] = Insufficient documentation. 120 mg 3 times daily.

➤*Children:*

Obesity management – The OTC product is not approved for use in children younger than 18 years of age. The Rx product is approved for use in children 12 years of age and older. See Adults for dosing.

➤*Storage/Stability:*

OTC – Store at 20° to 25°C (68° to 77°F).Protect drug from excessive light, humidity, and temperatures higher than 30°C (86°F).

Rx – Store at 25°C (77°F); excursions are permitted to 15° to 30°C (59° to 86°F). Keep the bottle tightly closed.

Actions

➤*Pharmacology:* Orlistat is a reversible inhibitor of lipases. It exerts its therapeutic activity in the lumen of the stomach and small intestine by forming a covalent bond with the active serine residue site of gastric and pancreatic lipases. The inactivated enzymes are thus unavailable to hydrolyze dietary fat in the form of triglycerides into absorbable free fatty acids and monoglycerides. As undigested triglycerides are not absorbed, the resulting caloric deficit may have a positive effect on weight control. Systemic absorption of the drug is therefore not needed for activity. At the recommended therapeutic dose of 120 mg 3 times daily, orlistat inhibits dietary fat absorption by approximately 30%.

➤*Pharmacokinetics:*

Absorption – Systemic exposure to orlistat is minimal. Following oral dosing with 360 mg ^{14}C-orlistat, plasma radioactivity peaked at approximately 8 hours; plasma concentrations of intact orlistat were near the limits of detection (less than 5 ng/mL). In therapeutic studies involving monitoring of plasma samples, detection of intact orlistat in plasma was sporadic and concentrations were low (less than 10 ng/mL or 0.02 mcM), without evidence of accumulation, and consistent with minimal absorption.

The average absolute bioavailability of intact orlistat was assessed in studies with male rats at oral doses of 150 and 1,000 mg/kg/day and in male dogs at oral doses of 100 and 1,000 mg/kg/day and found to be 0.12%, 0.59% in rats and 0.7%, 1.9% in dogs, respectively.

Distribution – In vitro orlistat was greater than 99% bound to plasma proteins (lipoproteins and albumin were major binding proteins). Orlistat minimally partitioned into erythrocytes.

Metabolism – Based on animal data, it is likely that the metabolism of orlistat occurs mainly within the gastrointestinal wall. Based on an oral ^{14}C-orlistat mass balance study in obese patients, 2 metabolites, M1 (4-member lactone ring hydrolyzed) and M3 (M1 with N-formyl leucine moiety cleaved), accounted for approximately 42% of total radioactivity in plasma. M1 and M3 have an open beta-lactone ring and extremely weak lipase inhibitory activity (1,000- and 2,500-fold less than orlistat, respectively). In view of this low inhibitory activity and the low plasma levels at the therapeutic dose (average of 26 ng/mL and 108 ng/mL for M1 and M3, respectively, 2 to 4 hours after a dose), these metabolites are considered pharmacologically inconsequential. The primary metabolite M1 had a short half-life (approximately 3 hours) whereas the secondary metabolite M3 disappeared at a slower rate (half-life approximately 13.5 hours). In obese patients, steady-state plasma levels of M1, but not M3, increased in proportion to orlistat doses.

Excretion – Following a single oral dose of 360 mg ^{14}C-orlistat in both healthy weight and obese subjects, fecal excretion of the unabsorbed drug was found to be the major route of elimination. Orlistat and its M1 and M3 metabolites were also subject to biliary excretion. Approximately 97% of the administered radioactivity was excreted in feces; 83% of that was found to be unchanged orlistat. The cumulative renal excretion of total radioactivity was less than 2% of the given dose of 360 mg ^{14}C-orlistat. The time to reach complete excretion (fecal plus urinary) was 3 to 5 days. The disposition of orlistat appeared to be similar between healthy weight and obese subjects. Based on limited data, the half-life of the absorbed orlistat is in the range of 1 to 2 hours.

Contraindications

Chronic malabsorption syndrome or cholestasis; hypersensitivity to orlistat or to any component of this product.

Warnings/Precautions

➤*Causes of obesity:* Exclude organic causes of obesity (eg, hypothyroidism) before prescribing orlistat.

➤*Dietary guidelines:* Advise patients to adhere to dietary guidelines. Gastrointestinal events may increase when orlistat is taken with a diet high in fat (greater than 30% total daily calories from fat). The daily intake of fat should be distributed over 3 main meals. If orlistat is taken with any one meal very high in fat, the possibility of gastrointestinal effects increases.

➤*Multivitamin supplement:* Strongly encourage patients to take a multivitamin supplement that contains fat-soluble vitamins to ensure adequate nutrition because orlistat has been shown to reduce the absorption of some fat-soluble vitamins and beta-carotene. In addition, the levels of vitamin D and beta-carotene may be low in obese patients compared with nonobese subjects. Give the supplement once a day at least 2 hours before or after the administration of orlistat, such as at bedtime.

ORLISTAT — ORAL

Incidence of Low Vitamin Values on ≥ 2 Consecutive Visits in Nonsupplemented Orlistat-Treated Adult Patients with Normal Baseline Values (First and Second Year)		
	Placebo[a]	Orlistat[a]
Vitamin A	1%	2.2%
Vitamin D	6.6%	12%
Vitamin E	1%	5.8%
Beta-carotene	1.7%	6.1%

[a] Treatment designates placebo plus diet or orlistat plus diet.

Incidence of Low Vitamin Values on ≥ 2 Consecutive Visits in Orlistat-Treated Pediatric Patients with Normal Baseline Values[a]		
	Placebo[b]	Orlistat[b]
Vitamin A	0%	0%
Vitamin D	0.7%	1.4%
Vitamin E	0%	0%
Beta-carotene	0.8%	1.5%

[a] All patients were treated with vitamin supplementation throughout the course of the study.
[b] Treatment designates placebo plus diet or orlistat plus diet.

➤*Special risk:* Some patients may develop increased levels of urinary oxalate following treatment with orlistat. Exercise caution when prescribing orlistat to patients with a history of hyperoxaluria or calcium oxalate nephrolithiasis.

Diabetic patients – Weight-loss induction by orlistat may be accompanied by improved metabolic control in diabetics, which might require a reduction in dose of oral hypoglycemic medication (eg, sulfonylureas, metformin) or insulin.

➤*Drug abuse and dependence:* As with any weight-loss agent, the potential exists for misuse of orlistat in inappropriate patient populations (eg, patients with anorexia nervosa or bulimia).

➤*Pregnancy: Category B.*

Teratogenic – The incidence of dilated cerebral ventricles was increased in the mid- and high-dose groups of the rat teratology study. These doses were 6 and 23 times the daily human dose calculated on a body surface area (mg/m^2) basis for the mid- and high-dose levels, respectively. This finding was not reproduced in 2 additional rat teratology studies at similar doses.

There are no adequate and well-controlled studies of orlistat in pregnant women. Because animal reproductive studies are not always predictive of human response, orlistat is not recommended for use during pregnancy.

➤*Lactation:* It is not known if orlistat is secreted in human milk. Therefore, orlistat should not be taken by nursing women.

➤*Children:* The safety and efficacy of orlistat have been evaluated in obese adolescent patients aged 12 to 16 years. Orlistat has not been studied in pediatric patients younger than 12 years of age.

Drug Interactions

Orlistat Drug Interactions			
Precipitant drug	Object drug[a]		Description
Orlistat	Cyclosporine	⟷	Because changes in cyclosporine absorption have been reported with variations in dietary intake, caution is advised in the concomitant use of orlistat plus diet in patients receiving cyclosporine therapy.
Orlistat	Fat-soluble vitamins	⬇	A pharmacokinetic interaction study showed a 30% reduction in beta-carotene supplement absorption when concomitantly administered with orlistat. Orlistat inhibited absorption of a vitamin E acetate supplement by ≈ 60%. The effect on the absorption of supplemental vitamin D, vitamin A, and nutritionally derived vitamin K is not known at this time.
Orlistat	Warfarin	⟷	In 12 healthy-weight subjects, administration of orlistat 120 mg 3 times a day for 16 days did not result in any change in either warfarin pharmacokinetics or pharmacodynamics. Although undercarboxylated osteocalcin, a marker of vitamin K nutritional status, was unaltered with orlistat administration, vitamin K levels tended to decline in subjects taking orlistat. Therefore, as vitamin K absorption may be decreased with orlistat, monitor patients on chronic stable doses of warfarin who are prescribed orlistat closely for changes in coagulation parameters.

[a] ⬇ = object drug decreased; ⟷ = undetermined clinical effect.

Adverse Reactions

➤*Commonly observed adverse reactions (based on first-year and second-year data orlistat 120 mg 3 times daily vs placebo):* Gastrointestinal symptoms were the most commonly observed treatment-emergent adverse events associated with the use of orlistat in double-blind, placebo-controlled clinical trials and are primarily a manifestation of the mechanism of action. (Commonly observed is defined as an incidence of greater than or equal to 5% and an incidence in the orlistat 120 mg group that is at least twice that of placebo.)

Commonly Observed Orlistat Adverse Reactions				
	Year 1		Year 2	
Adverse reaction	Orlistat (n = 1,913)[a]	Placebo (n = 1,466)[a]	Orlistat (n = 613)[a]	Placebo (n = 524)[a]
Fatty/oily stool	20%	2.9%	5.5%	0.6%
Fecal incontinence	7.7%	0.9%	1.8%	0.2%
Fecal urgency	22.1%	6.7%	2.8%	1.7%
Flatus with discharge	23.9%	1.4%	2.1%	0.2%
Increased defecation	10.8%	4.1%	2.6%	0.8%
Oily evacuation	11.9%	0.8%	2.3%	0.2%
Oily spotting	26.6%	1.3%	4.4%	0.2%

[a] Treatment designates orlistat 3 times daily plus diet or placebo plus diet.

These and other commonly observed adverse reactions were generally mild and transient, and they decreased during the second year of treatment. In general, the first occurrence of these events was within 3 months of starting therapy. Overall, approximately 50% of all episodes of GI adverse events associated with orlistat treatment lasted for less than 1 week, and a majority lasted for no more than 4 weeks. However, GI adverse events may occur in some individuals over a period of 6 months or longer.

➤*Discontinuation of treatment:* In controlled clinical trials, 8.8% of patients treated with orlistat discontinued treatment due to adverse events, compared with 5% of placebo-treated patients. For orlistat, the most common adverse events resulting in discontinuation of treatment were gastrointestinal.

➤*Incidence in controlled clinical trials:*

Orlistat Treatment-Emergent Adverse Reactions from 7 Placebo-Controlled Clinical Trials (≥ 2%)				
	Year 1		Year 2	
Adverse reaction	Orlistat (n = 1,913)[a]	Placebo (n = 1,466)[a]	Orlistat (n = 613)[a]	Placebo (n = 524)[a]
Cardiovascular				
Pedal edema	-	-	2.8%	1.9%
CNS				
Dizziness	5.2%	5%	-	-
Headache	30.6%	27.6%	-	-
Dermatological				
Dry skin	2.1%	1.4%	-	-
Rash	4.3%	4%	-	-
GI				
Abdominal pain/ discomfort	25.5%	21.4%	-	-
Gingival disorder	4.1%	2.9%	2%	1.5%
Infectious diarrhea	5.3%	4.4%	-	-
Nausea	8.1%	7.3%	3.6%	2.7%
Rectal pain/ discomfort	5.2%	4%	3.3%	1.9%
Tooth disorder	4.3%	3.1%	2.9%	2.3%
Vomiting	3.8%	3.5%	-	-
GU				
Menstrual irregularity, female	9.8%	7.5%	-	-
Urinary tract infection	7.5%	7.3%	5.9%	4.8%
Vaginitis, female	3.8%	3.6%	2.6%	1.9%
Hearing and vestibular disorders				
Otitis	4.3%	3.4%	2.9%	2.5%
Musculoskeletal				
Arthritis	5.4%	4.8%	-	-
Back pain	13.9%	12.1%	-	-
Joint disorder	2.3%	2.2%	-	-
Myalgia	4.2%	3.3%	-	-
Pain, lower extremities	-	-	10.8%	10.3%
Tendonitis	-	-	2%	1.9%

ORLISTAT — ORAL

Orlistat Treatment-Emergent Adverse Reactions from 7 Placebo-Controlled Clinical Trials (≥ 2%)

	Year 1		Year 2	
Adverse reaction	Orlistat (n = 1,913)[a]	Placebo (n = 1,466)[a]	Orlistat (n = 613)[a]	Placebo (n = 524)[a]
Psychiatric				
Depression	-	-	3.4%	2.5%
Psychiatric anxiety	4.7%	2.9%	2.8%	2.1%
Respiratory				
Ear, nose, and throat symptoms	2%	1.6%	-	-
Influenza	39.7%	36.2%	-	-
Lower respiratory tract infection	7.8%	6.6%	-	-
Upper respiratory tract infection	38.1%	32.8%	26.1%	25.8%
Miscellaneous				
Fatigue	7.2%	6.4%	3.1%	1.7%
Sleep disorder	3.9%	3.3%	-	-

[a] Treatment designates orlistat 120 mg 3 times daily plus diet or placebo plus diet. None reported at a frequency greater than or equal to 2% and greater than placebo.

➤*Other clinical studies or postmarketing surveillance:* Rare cases of hypersensitivity have been reported with the use of orlistat. Signs and symptoms have included pruritus, rash, urticaria, angioedema, and anaphylaxis.

Preliminary data from a orlistat and cyclosporine drug interaction study indicate a reduction in cyclosporine plasma levels when orlistat was coadministered with cyclosporine.

➤*Pediatric patients:* In clinical trials with orlistat in adolescent patients ages 12 to 16 years, the profile of adverse reactions was generally similar to that observed in adults.

Overdosage

Single doses of 800 mg orlistat and multiple doses of up to 400 mg 3 times daily for 15 days have been studied in healthy-weight and obese subjects without significant adverse findings.

Should a significant overdose of orlistat occur, it is recommended that the patient be observed for 24 hours. Based on human and animal studies, systemic effects attributable to the lipase-inhibiting properties of orlistat should be rapidly reversible.

Patient Information

Read the patient information before starting treatment with orlistat and each time your prescription is renewed.

GI STIMULANTS

METOCLOPRAMIDE

Rx	**Metoclopramide Hydrochloride** (Various, eg, Teva, Watson)	**Tablets; oral:** 5 mg	As monohydrochloride. In 60s, 100s, 500s, and 1,000s.
Rx	**Reglan** (Alaven)		As monohydrochloride. Lactose. (REGLAN 5 SP). Green, elliptical. In 100s.
Rx	**Metoclopramide Hydrochloride** (Various, eg, Teva, Watson)	**Tablets; oral:** 10 mg	As monohydrochloride. In 60s, 100s, 500s, 1,000s, and UD 100s.
Rx	**Reglan** (Alaven)		As monohydrochloride. Mannitol. (REGLAN SP 10). White, scored. Capsule shape. In 100s.
Rx	**Metozolv ODT** (Salix)	**Tablets, disintegrating; oral:** 5 mg	Equiv. to metoclopramide hydrochloride 5.91 mg. Acesulfame K, gelatin, mannitol. (5). White, round. Mint flavor. In UD 100s.
Rx	**Metozolv ODT** (Salix)	**Tablets, disintegrating; oral:** 10 mg	Equiv. to metoclopramide hydrochloride 11.82 mg. Acesulfame K, gelatin, mannitol. (10). White, round. Mint flavor. In UD 100s.
Rx	**Metoclopramide Hydrochloride** (Various, eg, Ani Pharma, Morton Grove)	**Solution; oral:** 1 mg/mL	As monohydrochloride. May contain alcohol. In 473 mL and UD 10 mL.
Rx	**Metoclopramide Hydrochloride** (Various, eg, Baxter, Hospira, Sicor)	**Injection, solution:** 5 mg/mL	As monohydrochloride. In 2, 10, 20, and 30 mL vials, 2 mL amps, and 2 mL prefilled syringes.
Rx	**Reglan** (Baxter)		As monohydrochloride. Preservative free. In single-dose 2, 10, and 30 mL vials.

METOCLOPRAMIDE HYDROCHLORIDE — ORAL

See also the Antiemetic/Antivertigo monograph.

WARNING

Treatment with metoclopramide can cause tardive dyskinesia, a serious movement disorder that is often irreversible. The risk of developing tardive dyskinesia increases with duration of treatment and total cumulative dose.

Discontinue metoclopramide therapy in patients who develop signs or symptoms of tardive dyskinesia. There is no known treatment for tardive dyskinesia. In some patients, symptoms lessen or resolve after metoclopramide treatment is stopped.

Avoid treatment with metoclopramide for longer than 12 weeks in all but rare cases in which therapeutic benefit is thought to outweigh the risk of developing tardive dyskinesia. (See also Warnings/Precautions.)

Indications

➤*Diabetic gastroparesis (diabetic gastric stasis):* For the relief of symptoms associated with acute and recurrent diabetic gastric stasis in adults.

➤*Gastroesophageal reflux:* Short-term (4 to 12 weeks) therapy for adults with documented symptomatic gastroesophageal reflux disease (GERD) who fail to respond to conventional therapy.

➤*Off-label uses:*

Adjunctive treatment for migraine – [3] = Safety concerns. US-based guidelines support the use of intravenous (IV) metoclopramide for the adjunctive treatment of migraines, specifically in patients who experience nausea associated with an attack. Rational combinations include metoclopramide and a nonopioid analgesic with or without the addition of a triptan or ergotamine. European-based guidelines also support the use of oral metoclopramide. Rectal use of metoclopramide has inconsistent or conflicting data.

Gastric bezoars – [4] = Insufficient documentation. Limited data are available regarding the use of metoclopramide for treatment of gastric bezoars. Noncontrolled studies and case reports have demonstrated efficacy. However, without more robust controlled studies, a definitive role of metoclopramide for this use cannot be determined.

Gastric ulcers – [5] = Poor documentation. Newer agents, such as histamine H_2-receptor antagonists and proton pump inhibitors, have been shown to be safe and efficacious for the treatment of gastric ulceration. Additionally, with the discovery of *Helicobacter pylori* as an infectious etiological agent for gastric ulcers, the approach to therapy has been significantly impacted to include the addition of antibiotics. Recent evidence supporting newer approaches and limited older data with mixed results provide little justification for the use of metoclopramide for the treatment of gastric ulcers.

Gastroparesis (adults) – [1] = Good documentation. Based on the American Gastroenterological Association Institute (AGAI) guidelines, metoclopramide 10 to 20 mg given 30 minutes before meals and at bedtime for up to 8 weeks along with dietary changes and an antiemetic for nausea and vomiting are effective in the short-term management of delayed gastric emptying.

Hiccups – [1] = Good documentation. In the limited published experience, metoclopramide has been effective for prevention and treatment of hiccups. Of note, the drug is not universally efficacious in this setting. When used as a preventive measure, some patients still experience hiccups. As a treatment, cases of delayed onset of efficacy and only partial efficacy have been reported. Nevertheless, the generally benign adverse reaction profile, including in elderly patients and patients with serious underlying medical conditions, suggests a risk-benefit ratio favoring a therapeutic trial of metoclopramide in the absence of contraindications of therapy.

Improving lactation – [3] = Safety concerns. Metoclopramide is a widely accepted treatment for improving lactation in postpartum mothers. The use of metoclopramide has been shown to be effective in improving lactation in mothers delivering full-term infants. Evidence supporting the use of metoclopramide in mothers delivering preterm infants has not been

METOCLOPRAMIDE HYDROCHLORIDE — ORAL

established. The risks associated with metoclopramide are minimal; therefore, it may be a potential option for improving lactation.

Nausea and vomiting of pregnancy – [2] = Fair documentation. Metoclopramide was included among the therapies recommended by the American College of Obstetrics and Gynecology for the management of nausea and vomiting during pregnancy in its practice bulletin. Metoclopramide use in this setting was also endorsed by the AGAI.

Tardive dyskinesia – [5] = Poor documentation. There is no current information regarding the use of metoclopramide in the management of tardive dyskinesia. In addition, metoclopramide has a black box warning regarding tardive dyskinesia. Based on a lack of efficacy data and safety considerations, the use of this drug for the management of tardive dyskinesia is not recommended.

Tourette syndrome – [4] = Insufficient documentation. Data from initial studies suggest that metoclopramide may be effective in reducing tic frequency and severity. Metoclopramide may be advantageous in that it does not induce the weight gain associated with some antipsychotics also used to treat this disorder (eg, haloperidol). Currently, the majority of data are in children, with larger controlled trials needed to confirm these results and to establish optimal dosing regimens.

Other possible off-label uses – Studies have indicated some potential value of metoclopramide in the following conditions: nausea and vomiting of a variety of causes, including radiation-induced emesis and chemotherapy-induced nausea/vomiting (See Administration and Dosage); anorexia nervosa (due to GI stimulation); improvement in patient response to ergotamine and analgesics, perhaps by enhancing absorption of the other medications; diabetic cystoparesis (atonic bladder).

Administration and Dosage

➤*General dosing considerations:* Discontinue metoclopramide therapy in patients who develop signs or symptoms of tardive dyskinesia. There is no known treatment for tardive dyskinesia. In some patients, symptoms lessen or resolve after metoclopramide treatment is stopped.

Avoid treatment with metoclopramide for longer than 12 weeks in all but rare cases in which therapeutic benefit is thought to outweigh the risk of developing tardive dyskinesia. (See also Black Box Warning.)

➤*Adults:*

Diabetic gastroparesis (diabetic gastric stasis) –

Usual dosage: 10 mg administered 30 minutes before each meal and at bedtime (up to 4 times daily).

The initial route of administration should be determined by the severity of the presenting symptoms. If only the earliest manifestations of diabetic gastric stasis are present, oral administration of metoclopramide may be initiated. However, if severe symptoms are present, therapy should begin with metoclopramide injection. Administration of metoclopramide injection for up to 10 days may be required before symptoms subside, at which time oral administration may be instituted. Because diabetic gastric stasis is frequently recurrent, therapy should be reinstituted at the earliest manifestation.

Duration of therapy: 2 to 8 weeks, depending on response and the likelihood of continued well-being upon drug discontinuation. Should not exceed 12 weeks.

Gastroesophageal reflux –

Usual dosage: 10 to 15 mg up to 4 times daily administered 30 minutes before each meal and at bedtime.

Single dose: If symptoms occur only intermittently or at specific times of the day, use of metoclopramide in single doses of up to 20 mg prior to the provoking situation may be preferred rather than continuous treatment.

Duration of therapy: Prolonged treatment (longer than 12 weeks) with metoclopramide should be avoided in all but rare cases in which therapeutic benefit is thought to outweigh the risks to the patient of developing tardive dyskinesia.

Off-label dosing –

Adjunctive treatment for migraine: [3] = Safety concerns. 10 to 20 mg orally or 5 to 10 mg IV or intramuscularly (IM), generally given as a 1-time dose as adjunctive therapy with an analgesic.

Chemotherapy-induced nausea and vomiting:

- *Nausea and vomiting due to highly emetogenic chemotherapy* – 2 mg/kg administered 1 hour before chemotherapy, followed by 3 more doses at 2-hour intervals. If vomiting persists, 2 additional doses may be given every 3 hours (total daily dose of 12 mg/kg).
- *Prevention of delayed nausea and vomiting due to chemotherapy* – 20 to 40 mg (or 0.5 mg/kg) given 2 to 4 times daily for 3 to 4 days beginning 16 to 24 hours after chemotherapy given in combination with dexamethasone. May be given IV in patients unable to take oral medications.

Gastric bezoars: [4] = Insufficient documentation. 5 to 10 mg administered 4 times daily until resolution of gastric bezoar. Long-term treatment was used in one study in which 1 patient received treatment for 16 months.

Gastroparesis (adults): [1] = Good documentation. 10 to 20 mg administered 4 times daily (30 minutes before meals and at bedtime for 2 to 8 weeks), as adjunctive therapy.

Hiccups: [1] = Good documentation.

- *Prevention* – 10 mg every 6 to 8 hours starting the day of or 1 day before the anticipated hiccup-precipitating event.
- *Treatment* – 10 mg every 6 to 8 hours. Therapy may begin with parenteral dosing (5 to 10 mg IV or IM every 8 hours) and transition to oral dosing when hiccups are controlled. Treatment usually continues until metoclopramide can be withdrawn without provoking a recurrence.

Improving lactation: [3] = Safety concerns. As monotherapy, metoclopramide 10 to 15 mg 3 times per day for 2 weeks.

Nausea and vomiting of pregnancy: [2] = Fair documentation. 5 to 10 mg every 8 hours.

Tourette syndrome: [4] = Insufficient documentation.

- *Maximum dose* – 240 mg daily.
- *Initial dosage* – Initial dosing in clinical studies ranged from 10 to 20 mg daily or 40 mg 3 times daily.
- *Duration of therapy* – 8 weeks to several months (up to 22 months).

➤*Children:*

Off-label dosing –

Chemotherapy-induced nausea and vomiting: Metoclopramide is not usually considered as a first-line antiemetic agent in children because of the high incidence of extrapyramidal effects. Some clinicians routinely administer diphenhydramine concomitantly to reduce this incidence.

- *Nausea and vomiting due to highly emetogenic chemotherapy* – 1 to 2 mg/kg. One reference suggests administering metoclopramide 1 hour before chemotherapy, followed by 3 more doses at 2- to 4-hour intervals. Maximum total dose is 5 doses/day.
- *Prevention of delayed nausea and vomiting due to chemotherapy* – 0.5 mg/kg administered 4 times daily for 4 days beginning 16 to 24 hours after chemotherapy given in combination with dexamethasone. May be given IV in patients unable to take oral medications.

Gastroesophageal reflux or GI dysmotility:

- *30 days and older* –

  Usual dosage: 0.1 to 0.2 mg/kg up to 4 times daily.

  Maximum dose: 0.8 mg/kg/day.

Tourette syndrome: [4] = Insufficient documentation.

- *Usual dose* – Mean dosages were 36.2 mg daily.
- *Maximum dose* – 60 mg daily.
- *Initial dosage* – 5 mg daily, with increases every 3 days as tolerated.
- *Duration of therapy* – 8 weeks to several months (up to 22 months).

➤*Elderly:* Occasionally, patients who are more sensitive to the therapeutic or adverse effects of metoclopramide will require 5 mg/dose.

➤*Renal function impairment:* According to the manufacturer, in patients whose creatinine clearance (CrCl) is less than 40 mL/min, therapy should be initiated at approximately one-half the recommended dosage. Depending upon clinical efficacy and safety considerations, the dosage may be increased or decreased as appropriate.

According to another reference, the adult dosage should be decreased to 75% of the usual dose in patients with a glomerular filtration rate (GFR) of 10 to 50 mL/min. In patients with a GFR of less than 10 mL/min, the dosage should be decreased to 50% of the usual dose.

Dialysis – For adult patients receiving continuous renal replacement therapy, decrease the metoclopramide dose to 75% of the usual dose.

➤*Special risk patients:* Occasionally, patients who are more sensitive to the therapeutic or adverse effects of metoclopramide will require only 5 mg/dose when treating GERD.

➤*Administration:* Give 30 minutes before meals and at bedtime when being used for gastroparesis and GERD.

Orally disintegrating tablets – Take on an empty stomach at least 30 minutes before eating because food can decrease the peak concentrations (C_{max}) of drug in the bloodstream and/or the time it takes to achieve the maximum drug level (T_{max}) in the bloodstream. Do not repeat dose if inadvertently taken with food.

Because the tablet absorbs moisture rapidly, only remove each dose from the packaging just prior to taking. Handle the tablet with dry hands and place on the tongue. If the tablet should break or crumble while handling, discard and remove a new tablet.

Metoclopramide orally disintegrating tablets disintegrate on the tongue in approximately 1 minute (range, 10 seconds to 14 minutes). Metoclopramide orally disintegrating tablets are designed to be taken without liquid.

➤*Storage/Stability:* Store between 20° and 25°C (68° and 77°F).

Actions

➤*Pharmacology:* Metoclopramide stimulates motility of the upper GI tract without stimulating gastric, biliary, or pancreatic secretions. Its mode of action is unclear. It seems to sensitize tissues to the action of acetylcholine. The effect of metoclopramide on motility is not dependent on intact vagal innervation, but it can be abolished by anticholinergic drugs.

Metoclopramide increases the tone and amplitude of gastric (especially antral) contractions, relaxes the pyloric sphincter and the duodenal bulb, and increases peristalsis of the duodenum and jejunum, resulting in accelerated gastric emptying and intestinal transit. It increases the resting tone of the lower esophageal sphincter. It has little, if any, effect on the motility of the colon or gallbladder.

In patients with gastroesophageal reflux and lower esophageal sphincter pressure (LESP), single oral doses of metoclopramide produce dose-related increases in LESP. Effects begin at approximately 5 mg and increase through 20 mg (the largest dose tested). The increase in LESP from a 5 mg dose lasts about 45 minutes and that of 20 mg lasts between 2 and 3 hours. Increased rate of stomach emptying has been observed with single oral doses of metoclopramide 10 mg.

The antiemetic properties of metoclopramide appear to be a result of its antagonism of central and peripheral dopamine receptors. Dopamine produces nausea and vomiting by stimulation of the medullary chemoreceptor trigger zone, and metoclopramide blocks stimulation of the chemoreceptor trigger zone by agents like levodopa or apomorphine, which are known to increase dopamine levels or to possess dopamine-like effects. Metoclopramide also abolishes the slowing of gastric emptying caused by apomorphine.

METOCLOPRAMIDE HYDROCHLORIDE — ORAL

Like the phenothiazines and related drugs, which are also dopamine antagonists, metoclopramide produces sedation and may produce extrapyramidal reactions, although these are comparatively rare. Metoclopramide inhibits the central and peripheral effects of apomorphine, induces release of prolactin, and causes a transient increase in circulating aldosterone levels, which may be associated with transient fluid retention.

Pharmacodynamics – The onset of pharmacological action of metoclopramide is 30 to 60 minutes following an oral dose; pharmacological effects persist for 1 to 2 hours.

In children, the pharmacodynamics of metoclopramide following oral administration are highly variable and a concentration-effect relationship has not been established.

➤*Pharmacokinetics:*

Absorption / Distribution – Metoclopramide is rapidly and well absorbed. Relative to an IV dose of 20 mg, the absolute oral bioavailability of metoclopramide is 80% ± 15.5% as demonstrated in a crossover study of 18 subjects. C_{max} occurs at approximately 1 to 2 hours after a single oral dose. Similar T_{max} is observed after individual doses at steady state.

In a single-dose study of 12 subjects, the area under the curve (AUC) increases linearly with doses from 20 to 100 mg. C_{max} increases linearly with dose, T_{max} remains the same, whole body clearance is unchanged, and the elimination rate remains the same.

The drug is not extensively bound to plasma proteins (approximately 30%). The whole body volume of distribution (Vd) is high (approximately 3.5 L/kg), which suggests extensive distribution of drug to the tissues.

For the orally disintegrating tablets, the in vivo disintegrating time (time reported between placing the tablet on the tongue and it completely disintegrating into fine particles) was approximately 1 minute (range, 10 seconds to 14 minutes). In 2 clinical trials (N = 96), the a mean ± standard deviation was 76.8 ± 110.6 seconds and the median was 53.5 seconds.

In a randomized, 2-arm, 2-way crossover study in 44 healthy adult (men and women) fasted subjects, metoclopramide orally disintegrating tablets were bioequivalent to metoclopramide tablets.

Food effects: In a food-effect study with 28 subjects, metoclopramide orally disintegrating tablets taken immediately after a high-fat meal had a 17% lower peak blood level than when taken after an overnight fast. The time to peak blood levels increased from approximately 1.75 hours under fasted conditions to 3 hours when taken immediately after a high-fat meal. The extent of metoclopramide absorbed (AUC) was comparable whether the orally disintegrating tablets were administered with or without food. The clinical effect of the decrease in C_{max} if metoclopramide orally disintegrating tablets are inadvertently taken with food is unknown.

Metabolism / Excretion – The average elimination half-life in individuals with healthy renal function is 5 to 6 hours.

Approximately 85% of the radioactivity of an orally-administered dose appears in the urine within 72 hours. Of the 85% eliminated in the urine, approximately half is present as free or conjugated metoclopramide.

Special populations –

Renal function impairment: Renal impairment affects the clearance of metoclopramide. In a study of patients with varying degrees of renal impairment, a reduction in CrCl was correlated with a reduction in plasma clearance, renal clearance, and nonrenal clearance and an increase in elimination half-life; however, the kinetics of metoclopramide in the presence of renal impairment remained linear. The reduction in clearance as a result of renal impairment suggests having a downward adjustment maintenance dosage to avoid drug accumulation.

Children: In an open-label study, 6 children (age range, 3.5 weeks to 5.4 months) with GERD received metoclopramide 0.15 mg/kg oral solution every 6 hours for 10 doses. The mean C_{max} of metoclopramide after the 10th dose was 2-fold (56.8 mcg/L) higher compared with that observed after the first dose (29 mcg/L), indicating drug accumulation with repeated dosing. After the 10th dose, the mean T_{max} (2.2 hours), half-life (4.1 hours), clearance (0.67 L/h/kg), and Vd (4.4 L/kg) of metoclopramide were similar to those observed after the first dose. In the youngest patient (3.5 weeks of age), metoclopramide half-life after the first and the 10th dose (23.1 and 10.3 hours, respectively) was significantly longer compared with other infants because of reduced clearance. This may be attributed to immature hepatic and renal systems at birth.

Contraindications

Metoclopramide should not be used whenever stimulation of GI motility might be dangerous (eg, in the presence of GI hemorrhage, mechanical obstruction, or perforation).

Patients with pheochromocytoma because the drug may cause a hypertensive crisis, probably caused by release of catecholamines from the tumor.

Known sensitivity or intolerance to the drug; patients with epilepsy or those receiving other drugs that are likely to cause extrapyramidal reactions because the frequency and severity of seizures or extrapyramidal reactions may be increased.

Warnings/Precautions

➤*Depression:* Mental depression has occurred in patients with and without a history of depression. Symptoms have ranged from mild to severe and have included suicidal ideation and suicide. Give metoclopramide to patients with a history of depression only if the expected benefits outweigh the potential risks.

➤*Extrapyramidal symptoms:* Extrapyramidal symptoms, manifested primarily as acute dystonic reactions, occur in approximately 1 in 500 patients treated with the usual adult dosages of metoclopramide 30 to 40 mg/day. These usually are seen during the first 24 to 48 hours of treatment with metoclopramide, occur more frequently in children and adults younger than 30 years of age, and are even more frequent at the higher doses. These symptoms may include involuntary movements of limbs and facial grimacing, torticollis, oculogyric crisis, rhythmic protrusion of tongue, bulbar type of speech, trismus, or dystonic reactions resembling tetanus. Rarely, dystonic reactions may present as stridor and dyspnea, possibly due to laryngospasm. If these symptoms occur, inject diphenhydramine 50 mg IM and they usually will subside. Benztropine 1 to 2 mg IM may also be used to reverse these reactions.

➤*Parkinson-like symptoms:* Parkinson-like symptoms have occurred, more commonly within the first 6 months after beginning treatment with metoclopramide, but occasionally after longer periods. These symptoms generally subside within 2 to 3 months following discontinuance of metoclopramide. Give metoclopramide cautiously to patients with preexisting Parkinson disease, if at all, because such patients may experience exacerbation of Parkinsonian symptoms when taking metoclopramide.

➤*Tardive dyskinesia:* Treatment with metoclopramide can cause tardive dyskinesia, a potentially irreversible and disfiguring disorder characterized by involuntary movements of the face, tongue, or extremities. Although the risk of tardive dyskinesia with metoclopramide has not been extensively studied, one published study reported a tardive dyskinesia prevalence of 20% among patients treated for at least 12 weeks. Avoid treatment with metoclopramide for longer than 12 weeks in all but rare cases in which therapeutic benefit is thought to outweigh the risk of developing tardive dyskinesia.

Although the risk of developing tardive dyskinesia in the general population may be increased among the elderly, women, and diabetic individuals, it is not possible to predict which patients will develop metoclopramide-induced tardive dyskinesia. Both the risk of developing tardive dyskinesia and the likelihood that it will become irreversible increase with duration of treatment and total cumulative dose.

Discontinue metoclopramide in patients who develop signs or symptoms of tardive dyskinesia. There is no known effective treatment for established cases of tardive dyskinesia, although in some patients, tardive dyskinesia may remit partially or completely within several weeks to months after metoclopramide is withdrawn.

Metoclopramide itself may suppress or partially suppress the signs of tardive dyskinesia, thereby masking the underlying disease process. The effect of this symptomatic suppression on the long-term course of tardive dyskinesia is unknown; therefore, do not use metoclopramide for the symptomatic control of tardive dyskinesia.

➤*Neuroleptic malignant syndrome:* There have been rare reports of an uncommon but potentially fatal symptom complex sometimes referred to as neuroleptic malignant syndrome (NMS) associated with metoclopramide. Clinical manifestations of NMS include hyperthermia, muscle rigidity, altered consciousness, and evidence of autonomic instability (irregular pulse or blood pressure, tachycardia, diaphoresis, and cardiac arrhythmias).

The diagnostic evaluation of patients with this syndrome is complicated. In arriving at a diagnosis, it is important to identify cases in which the clinical presentation includes serious medical illness (eg, pneumonia, systemic infection) and untreated or inadequately treated extrapyramidal signs and symptoms. Other important considerations in the differential diagnosis include central anticholinergic toxicity, heat stroke, malignant hyperthermia, drug fever, and primary CNS pathology.

Include in the management of NMS immediate discontinuation of metoclopramide and other drugs not essential to concurrent therapy; intensive symptomatic treatment and medical monitoring; and treatment of any concomitant serious medical problems for which specific treatments are available. Bromocriptine and dantrolene have been used in treatment of NMS, but their effectiveness has not been established.

➤*Hypertension:* In one study in hypertensive patients, IV-administered metoclopramide was shown to release catecholamines; therefore, exercise caution when metoclopramide is used in patients with hypertension. There are also clinical reports of hypertensive crises in some patients with undiagnosed pheochromocytoma. Any rapid rise in blood pressure associated with metoclopramide use should result in immediate cessation of metoclopramide in those patients. Such hypertensive crises may be controlled by phentolamine.

➤*Withdrawal:* Adverse reactions, especially those involving the nervous system, may occur after stopping the use of metoclopramide. A small number of patients may experience withdrawal symptoms after stopping metoclopramide, which could include dizziness, nervousness, and/or headaches.

➤*Renal function impairment:* Metoclopramide is known to be substantially excreted by the kidney, and the risk of toxic reactions to this drug may be greater in patients with impaired renal function. Dosage adjustment may be required. (See Administration and Dosage.)

➤*Special risk:* Because metoclopramide produces a transient increase in plasma aldosterone, certain patients, especially those with cirrhosis or congestive heart failure, may be at risk of developing fluid retention and volume overload. If these adverse reactions occur at any time during metoclopramide therapy, discontinue the drug.

Patients with reduced nicotinamide adenine dinucleotide (NADH)–cytochrome b_5 reductase deficiency are at an increased risk of developing methemoglobinemia and/or sulfhemoglobinemia when metoclopramide is administered. In patients with glucose-6-phosphate dehydrogenase (G6PD) deficiency who experience metoclopramide-induced methemoglobinemia, methylene blue treatment is not recommended.

➤*Hazardous tasks:* Metoclopramide may impair the mental and/or physical abilities required for the performance of hazardous tasks such as operating machinery or driving a motor vehicle.

METOCLOPRAMIDE HYDROCHLORIDE — ORAL

➤*Pregnancy: Category B.* Metoclopramide has been used for decades for the treatment of nausea and vomiting in pregnant women. It has also been used during pregnancy to decrease gastric emptying time. (See Administration and Dosage.) Metoclopramide has been used during all stages of pregnancy, and there has been no evidence of embryo, fetal, or newborn harm found in human and animal studies. According to a retrospective cohort study, the use of metoclopramide during the first trimester did not result in significantly increased risks of any adverse effects on the fetus. Use this drug during pregnancy only if clearly needed.

➤*Lactation:* Metoclopramide has been used as a lactation stimulant. (See Administration and Dosage.) Metoclopramide is excreted in human milk. Exercise caution when metoclopramide is administered to a breast-feeding mother.

Metoclopramide apparently represents a small risk to the breast-feeding infant with maternal dosages of 45 mg/day or less. Mild adverse reactions have only been reported in 2 breast-feeding infants. One review stated that the drug should not be used during breast-feeding because of the potential risks to the neonate, but there are no published studies to substantiate this caution. The American Academy of Pediatrics classifies metoclopramide as a drug for which the effect on a breast-feeding infant is unknown but may be of concern because it is a dopaminergic-blocking agent.

Because of the potential for serious adverse reactions from metoclopramide in breast-feeding infants and because of the potential for tumorigenicity (including tumor-promoting potential in rats), decide whether to discontinue breast-feeding or the drug, taking into account the importance of the drug to the mother.

➤*Children:* According to the manufacturer, safety and effectiveness in children have not been established.

Exercise care in administering metoclopramide to neonates because prolonged clearance may produce excessive serum concentrations. In addition, neonates have reduced levels of NADH-cytochrome b_5 reductase that, in combination with the aforementioned pharmacokinetic factors, make neonates more susceptible to methemoglobinemia.

The safety profile of metoclopramide in adults cannot be extrapolated to children. Dystonias and other extrapyramidal reactions associated with metoclopramide are more common in children than in adults.

➤*Elderly:* Clinical studies of metoclopramide did not include sufficient numbers of subjects 65 years of age and older to determine whether elderly subjects respond differently from younger subjects.

The risk of developing drug-induced Parkinsonism due to metoclopramide is dose related. Elderly patients should receive the lowest dose that is effective. If drug-induced Parkinsonism symptoms develop in an elderly patient, discontinue metoclopramide. Elderly patients may be at greater risk of tardive dyskinesia.

Sedation is a potential adverse reaction associated with metoclopramide use in elderly patients.

Metoclopramide is known to be substantially excreted by the kidney, and the risk of toxic reactions to this drug may be greater in patients with impaired renal function. Use caution in dose selection for an elderly patient, starting at the low end of the dosing range because of the greater frequency of decreased renal function, concomitant disease, or other drug therapy in elderly patients.

Drug Interactions

➤*Extrapyramidal symptoms:* Metoclopramide is contraindicated in patients receiving other drugs likely to cause extrapyramidal reactions because the frequency and severity of extrapyramidal reactions may be increased.

Metoclopramide Oral Drug Interactions

Precipitant drug	Object drug[a]		Description
Anticholinergics Narcotic analgesics	Metoclopramide	↓	The effects of metoclopramide on GI motility are antagonized by these agents. Observe patients for a decrease or loss of metoclopramide effects. Adjust the metoclopramide dose as needed.
CNS depressants (eg, sedatives)	Metoclopramide	↑	Additive sedative effects can occur when metoclopramide is given with hypnotics, narcotics, sedatives, or tranquilizers. If excessive sedation occurs, the dose of one or both drugs may need to be reduced.
Metoclopramide	CNS depressants (eg, sedatives)		
Disulfiram	Metoclopramide	↑	Because metoclopramide syrup contains a small amount of alcohol, there is a possibility of an acute and severe alcohol intolerance reaction. Avoid coadministration of metoclopramide syrup in patients receiving disulfiram.

Metoclopramide Oral Drug Interactions

Precipitant drug	Object drug[a]		Description
Metoclopramide	Alcohol	↑	Metoclopramide increases the rate of absorption of alcohol by decreasing the time it takes alcohol to reach the small intestine, where it is rapidly absorbed. In addition, sedative effects of metoclopramide and alcohol are additive. Warn patients of possible excessive sedation. If excessive sedation occurs, the dose of one or both drugs may need to be reduced.
Metoclopramide	Cabergoline	↓	Metoclopramide may decrease the hypoprolactinemic effects of cabergoline. Avoid coadministration.
Metoclopramide	Cimetidine	↓	Bioavailability of cimetidine may be reduced because of decreased absorption as a result of faster gastric transit time. Consider administering cimetidine at least 2 hours before metoclopramide.
Metoclopramide	Cyclosporine	↑	A faster gastric emptying time may allow for an increase in cyclosporine absorption, possibly increasing its immunosuppressive and toxic effects. Measure cyclosporine concentrations when starting or stopping metoclopramide. Adjust the cyclosporine dose as needed.
Metoclopramide	Digoxin	↓	Digoxin absorption, plasma levels, and therapeutic effects may be decreased. The capsule, elixir, and tablets with a high dissolution rate are least affected and are less likely to interact.
Metoclopramide	Insulin	↑	Gastroparesis (gastric stasis) may be responsible for poor diabetic control in some patients. Exogenously administered insulin may begin to act before food has left the stomach and lead to hypoglycemia. Because the action of metoclopramide will influence the delivery of food to the intestines and, thus, the rate of absorption, insulin dosage or timing of dosage may require adjustment.
Metoclopramide	Levodopa	↑	These agents have opposite effects on dopamine receptors. The bioavailability of levodopa may be increased, and levodopa may decrease the effects of metoclopramide on gastric emptying and lower esophageal pressure. Metoclopramide is relatively contraindicated in patients with Parkinson disease.
Levodopa	Metoclopramide	↓	
Metoclopramide	MAOIs[b]	↑	Because metoclopramide releases catecholamines in patients with essential hypertension, use cautiously, if at all, in patients receiving MAOIs.
Metoclopramide	Pergolide	↓	Metoclopramide may decrease the pharmacologic effects of pergolide. Avoid coadministration.
Metoclopramide	Serotonin reuptake inhibitors (eg, sertraline, venlafaxine)	↑	Metoclopramide plasma concentrations may be elevated because of enzyme inhibition, increasing the pharmacologic effects and adverse reactions. In addition, the risk of serotonin syndrome may be increased. Observe the patient for an increase in adverse reactions. If serotonin syndrome occurs, immediate medical attention is required.
Serotonin reuptake inhibitors (eg, sertraline, venlafaxine)	Metoclopramide		

METOCLOPRAMIDE HYDROCHLORIDE — ORAL

Metoclopramide Oral Drug Interactions			
Precipitant drug	Object drug[a]		Description
Metoclopramide	Succinylcholine	↑	By inhibiting plasma cholinesterase, metoclopramide may increase the neuromuscular-blocking effects of succinylcholine. Use with caution, closely monitoring neuromuscular function. Provide mechanical respiratory support if needed.

[a] ↑ = object drug increased; ↓ = object drug decreased.
[b] MAOIs = monoamine oxidase inhibitors.

Adverse Reactions

For more information on acute dystonic reactions, NMS, tardive dyskinesia, Parkinsonian-like symptoms, depression, and hypertension, see Warnings/Precautions.

➤*Adverse reactions (2% or more):*

Metoclopramide Oral Adverse Reactions (≥ 2%)		
Adverse reactions	Metoclopramide orally disintegrating tablets (n = 96[a])	Metoclopramide tablets (n = 72[b])
CNS		
Dizziness	1%	4.2%
Fatigue	2.1%	2.8%
Headache	5.2%	4.2%
Somnolence	2.1%	2.8%
GI		
Nausea	4.2%	5.6%
Vomiting	2.1%	1.4%

[a] n = 68 patients under fasted conditions and 28 patients under fed conditions.
[b] n = 44 patients under fasted conditions and 28 patients under fed conditions.

➤*Other adverse reactions:*

Cardiovascular – Acute congestive heart failure, bradycardia, fluid retention, hypertension, hypotension, possible atrioventricular block, supraventricular tachycardia.

CNS – Drowsiness, fatigue, lassitude, and restlessness occur in approximately 10% of patients receiving the most commonly prescribed dosage of 10 mg 4 times daily. Confusion, dizziness, headache, insomnia, or mental depression with suicidal ideation occur less frequently. The incidence of drowsiness is greater at higher doses. There are isolated reports of convulsive seizures without clear-cut relationship to metoclopramide. Rarely, hallucinations have been reported.

Extrapyramidal symptoms: Acute dystonic reactions, the most common type of extrapyramidal symptoms associated with metoclopramide, occur in approximately 0.2% of patients (1 in 500) treated with 30 to 40 mg/day. Symptoms include bulbar type of speech, facial grimacing, involuntary movements of limbs, oculogyric crisis, opisthotonus (tetanus-like reactions), rhythmic protrusion of tongue, torticollis, trismus, and, rarely, stridor and dyspnea, possibly due to laryngospasm; ordinarily, these symptoms are readily reversed by diphenhydramine.

Parkinsonian-like symptoms may include bradykinesia, cogwheel rigidity, mask-like facies, and tremor.

Tardive dyskinesia most frequently is characterized by involuntary movements of the tongue, face, mouth, or jaw, and sometimes by involuntary movements of the trunk and/or extremities; movements may be choreoathetotic in appearance.

Motor restlessness (akathisia) may consist of feelings of agitation, anxiety, insomnia, and jitteriness, as well as the inability to sit still, pacing, and foot-tapping. These symptoms may disappear spontaneously or respond to a reduction in dosage.

Neuroleptic malignant syndrome: Rare occurrences of NMS have been reported. This potentially fatal syndrome is comprised of the symptom complex of altered consciousness, autonomic dysfunction, hyperthermia, and muscular rigidity.

Endocrine – Amenorrhea, galactorrhea, gynecomastia, and impotence secondary to hyperprolactinemia. Fluid retention secondary to transient elevation of aldosterone.

GI – Bowel disturbances, primarily diarrhea; nausea.

Hematologic – A few cases of agranulocytosis, leukopenia, or neutropenia, generally without clear-cut relationship to metoclopramide. Methemoglobinemia, especially with overdosage in neonates. Sulfhemoglobinemia in adults.

Hepatic – Rarely, cases of hepatotoxicity, characterized by such findings as jaundice and altered liver function tests when metoclopramide was administered with other drugs with known hepatotoxic potential.

Hypersensitivity – A few cases of bronchospasm, rash, or urticaria, especially in patients with a history of asthma. Rarely, angioneurotic edema, including glossal or laryngeal edema.

Renal – Urinary frequency, urinary incontinence.

Miscellaneous – Porphyria, visual disturbances.

Overdosage

➤*Symptoms:* Symptoms of overdosage may include drowsiness, disorientation, and extrapyramidal reactions.

Unintentional overdose due to misadministration has been reported in infants and children with the use of metoclopramide oral solution. While there was no consistent pattern to the reports associated with these overdoses, events included seizures, extrapyramidal reactions, and lethargy.

Methemoglobinemia has occurred in premature and full-term neonates who were given overdoses of metoclopramide (1 to 4 mg/kg/day orally, IM, or IV for 1 to 3 or more days).

➤*Treatment:* Anticholinergic or anti-Parkinson drugs or antihistamines with anticholinergic properties may be helpful in controlling the extrapyramidal reactions. Symptoms are self-limiting and usually disappear within 24 hours.

Hemodialysis removes relatively little metoclopramide, probably because of the small amount of the drug in blood relative to tissues. Similarly, continuous ambulatory peritoneal dialysis does not remove significant amounts of drug. Dialysis is not likely to be an effective method of drug removal in overdose situations.

Methemoglobinemia can be reversed by the IV administration of methylene blue. However, methylene blue may cause hemolytic anemia in patients with G6PD deficiency, which may be fatal.

Patient Information

Instruct patients to take metoclopramide at least 30 minutes before eating and at bedtime when used for gastroparesis or gastroesophageal reflux.

Instruct patients to take metoclopramide orally disintegrating tablets 30 minutes before food. Do not repeat dose if inadvertently taken with food.

Inform patients or their caregivers of serious potential issues associated with metoclopramide use, such as tardive dyskinesia, extrapyramidal symptoms, and NMS. Advise patients to inform their health care provider if symptoms associated with these disorders occur during or after treatment with metoclopramide.

Inform patients that metoclopramide may cause drowsiness, dizziness, or otherwise impair the mental and/or physical abilities required for the performance of hazardous tasks, such as operating machinery or driving a motor vehicle. Sedation may be more pronounced in elderly patients. Caution the ambulatory patient.

Inform patients that the most common adverse reactions in patients treated with metoclopramide are headache, nausea, vomiting, tiredness, sleepiness, dizziness, or restlessness.

METOCLOPRAMIDE HYDROCHLORIDE — INJECTION

See also the Antiemetic/Antivertigo monograph.

WARNING

Treatment with metoclopramide can cause tardive dyskinesia, a serious movement disorder that is often irreversible. The risk of developing tardive dyskinesia increases with duration of treatment and total cumulative dose.

Discontinue metoclopramide therapy in patients who develop signs or symptoms of tardive dyskinesia. There is no known treatment for tardive dyskinesia. In some patients, symptoms lessen or resolve after metoclopramide treatment is stopped.

Avoid treatment with metoclopramide for longer than 12 weeks in all but rare cases in which therapeutic benefit is thought to outweigh the risk of developing tardive dyskinesia. (See also Warnings/Precautions.)

Indications

➤*Diabetic gastroparesis (diabetic gastric stasis):* For the relief of symptoms associated with acute and recurrent diabetic gastric stasis.

➤*Prevention of nausea and vomiting associated with emetogenic cancer chemotherapy:* For the prophylaxis of vomiting associated with emetogenic cancer chemotherapy.

➤*Prevention of postoperative nausea and vomiting:* For the prophylaxis of postoperative nausea and vomiting in those circumstances where nasogastric suction is undesirable.

➤*Radiological examination:* To stimulate gastric emptying and intestinal transit of barium in cases where delayed emptying interferes with radiological examination of the stomach and/or small intestine.

➤*Small bowel intubation:* To facilitate small bowel intubation in adults and children in whom the tube does not pass the pylorus with conventional maneuvers.

➤*Off-label uses:*

Adjunctive treatment for vascular headache – [2] = Fair documentation. Data from controlled trials support the use of metoclopramide injection as an effective adjunctive treatment for vascular headache. Published studies have demonstrated efficacy and safety. Administering metoclopramide by slow intravenous (IV) infusion over 15 minutes has been shown to reduce the occurrence of akathisia.

METOCLOPRAMIDE HYDROCHLORIDE — INJECTION

Gastric bezoars – [4] = Insufficient documentation. Limited data are available regarding the use of metoclopramide for treatment of gastric bezoars. Noncontrolled studies and case reports have demonstrated efficacy. However, without more robust controlled studies, a definitive role of metoclopramide for this use cannot be determined.

Gastroparesis (adults) – [1] = Good documentation. Based on the American Gastroenterological Association Institute (AGAI) guidelines, metoclopramide along with dietary changes and an antiemetic for nausea and vomiting are effective in the short-term management of delayed gastric emptying.

Gastroparesis (preterm infants) – [4] = Insufficient documentation. Data from case reports in a limited number of patients show inconsistent results of metoclopramide use for improving gastroparesis in preterm infants. The most recent published case report was from 1989. Controlled trials are needed to establish benefit, optimal dosing, and appropriate candidates for metoclopramide use in preterm infants with gastroparesis.

Hiccups – [1] = Good documentation. In the limited published experience, metoclopramide has been effective for prevention and treatment of hiccups. Of note, the drug is not universally efficacious in this setting. When used as a preventive measure, some patients still experience hiccups. As a treatment, cases of delayed onset of efficacy and cases of only partial efficacy have been reported. Nevertheless, the generally benign adverse reaction profile, including in elderly patients and patients with serious underlying medical conditions, suggests a risk-benefit ratio favoring a therapeutic trial of metoclopramide in the absence of contraindications of therapy.

Nausea and vomiting of pregnancy – [2] = Fair documentation. Metoclopramide was included among the therapies recommended by the American College of Obstetrics and Gynecology for the management of nausea and vomiting during pregnancy in its practice bulletin. Metoclopramide use in this setting was also endorsed by the AGAI.

Tardive dyskinesia – [5] = Poor documentation. There is no current information regarding the use of metoclopramide in the management of tardive dyskinesia. In addition, metoclopramide has a black box warning regarding tardive dyskinesia. Based on a lack of efficacy data and safety considerations, the use of this drug for the management of tardive dyskinesia is not recommended.

Treatment of migraine (adults) – [2] = Fair documentation. The efficacy of IV metoclopramide for the treatment of an acute migraine attack has been shown in several controlled trials. American Academy of Neurology clinical practice guidelines for the pharmacologic treatment of migraine headache in adults consider IV metoclopramide to be effective as adjunctive therapy to control nausea (grade C evidence) and note that it may be considered as monotherapy for migraine pain relief (grade B evidence). Additional studies are needed to determine the optimal dose.

Variceal bleeding – [5] = Poor documentation. Use of metoclopramide for variceal bleeding has been studied in only one small, controlled trial that did not provide rebleeding outcome data. Until there is bleeding outcome data in an adequately sized sample, metoclopramide cannot be recommended for routine treatment of esophageal vophyariceal bleeding.

Other possible off-label uses – Used to improve lactation. Dosages of 30 to 45 mg/day have increased milk secretion, possibly by elevating serum prolactin levels.

Studies have indicated some potential value of metoclopramide in nausea and vomiting of a variety of causes (uncontrolled studies report 80% to 90% efficacy), including radiation-induced emesis; gastric ulcer; anorexia nervosa (due to GI stimulation); improving patient response to ergotamine, analgesics, and sedatives in migraine, perhaps by enhancing absorption of the other medications; and diabetic cystoparesis (atonic bladder).

Administration and Dosage

➤*General dosing considerations:* For adults, if acute dystonic reactions occur, inject diphenhydramine 50 mg intramuscular (IM) and symptoms usually subside.

Discontinue metoclopramide therapy in patients who develop signs or symptoms of tardive dyskinesia. There is no known treatment for tardive dyskinesia. In some patients, symptoms may lessen or resolve after metoclopramide treatment is stopped.

Avoid treatment with metoclopramide for longer than 12 weeks in all but rare cases in which therapeutic benefit is thought to outweigh the risk of developing tardive dyskinesia. (See also Black Box Warning.)

➤*Adults:*

Diabetic gastroparesis (diabetic gastric stasis) –

Usual dosage: 10 mg administered slowly IV over a 1- to 2-minute period.

Duration of therapy: Up to 10 days may be required before symptoms subside, at which time oral administration of metoclopramide may be instituted.

Prevention of nausea and vomiting associated with emetogenic cancer chemotherapy – The initial 2 doses should be 2 mg/kg if highly emetogenic drugs, such as cisplatin or dacarbazine, are used alone or in combination. For less emetogenic regimens, 1 mg/kg dose may be adequate. Administer by IV infusion over a period of not less than 15 minutes. Administer 30 minutes before beginning cancer chemotherapy and repeat every 2 hours for 2 doses, then every 3 hours for 3 doses.

Prevention of postoperative nausea and vomiting – 10 mg IM near the end of surgery; doses of 20 mg may also be used.

Radiological examinations – 10 mg (undiluted) as a single dose administered IV over 1 to 2 minutes in patients for whom delayed gastric emptying interferes with radiological examination of the stomach and/or small intestine.

Small bowel intubation – 10 mg (undiluted) as a single dose administered IV over 1 to 2 minutes if the tube has not passed the pylorus with conventional maneuvers in 10 minutes.

Off-label dosing –

Adjunctive treatment for vascular headache: [2] = Fair documentation. 10 mg given as a 1-time dose by slow IV infusion over 15 minutes or as an IV bolus over 2 minutes in combination with another agent. The incidence of akathisia may be significantly reduced when given by slow IV infusion.

Gastric bezoars: [4] = Insufficient documentation. 5 to 10 mg IV 4 times daily until resolution of gastric bezoar. Long-term treatment was used in one study in which one patient received treatment for 16 months.

Gastroparesis (adults): [1] = Good documentation. 10 to 20 mg IV 4 times daily (30 minutes before meals and at bedtime for 2 to 8 weeks), as adjunctive therapy.

Hiccups: [1] = Good documentation.

- *Prevention* – 0.17 mg/kg IV for one dose starting the day of or 1 day before the anticipated hiccup-precipitating event.
- *Treatment* – 5 to 10 mg IV or IM every 8 hours. Therapy may begin with parenteral dosing and transition to oral dosing (10 mg orally every 6 to 8 hours) when hiccups are controlled. Treatment usually continues until metoclopramide can be withdrawn without provoking a recurrence.

Nausea and vomiting of pregnancy: [2] = Fair documentation. 5 to 10 mg IM or IV.

Opioid-induced nausea and vomiting: 10 mg IV every 6 hours as needed.

Treatment of migraine (adults): [2] = Fair documentation. 10 mg IV infused over 15 minutes. A more recent study evaluated the efficacy of metoclopramide 20 mg IV infused over 15 minutes to determine if increased dose improved outcomes.

➤*Children:*

Small bowel intubation – If the tube has not passed the pylorus with conventional maneuvers in 10 minutes, administer the following dose according to age.

14 years of age and older: 10 mg (undiluted) as a single dose administered slowly IV over a 1- to 2-minute period.

6 to 14 years of age: 2.5 to 5 mg (undiluted) as a single dose administered slowly IV over a 1- to 2-minute period.

Younger than 6 years of age: 0.1 mg/kg (undiluted) as a single dose administered slowly IV over a 1- to 2-minute period.

Off-label dosing –

Chemotherapy-induced emesis: 1 to 2 mg/kg/dose IV over 60 minutes every 2 to 4 hours, up to a maximum of 5 doses/day. Premedicate with diphenhydramine to reduce extrapyramidal symptoms.

Gastroesophageal reflux or GI dysmotility:

- *Children 30 days and older* –
  - *Usual dosage:* 0.1 to 0.2 mg/kg IV or IM up to 4 times daily.
  - *Maximum dose:* 0.8 mg/kg/day.

Gastroparesis (preterm infants): [4] = Insufficient documentation. 0.1 to 0.2 mg/kg/day IV in 3 divided doses for up to 14 days used as monotherapy.

Postoperative nausea and vomiting:

- *Older than 14 years of age* – 10 mg IV after induction of anesthesia or upon arrival in recovery room. Repeat every 6 to 8 hours as needed.
- *14 years of age and younger* – 0.1 to 0.2 mg/kg (up to 10 mg) IV after induction of anesthesia or upon arrival in recovery room. Repeat every 6 to 8 hours as needed.

Opioid-induced nausea and vomiting: 0.15 to 0.25 mg/kg IV every 6 hours as needed. The maximum dose is 10 mg. For severe nausea and vomiting, metoclopramide may be alternated with ondansetron.

➤*Renal function impairment:* According to the manufacturer, in patients whose creatinine clearance (CrCl) is less than 40 mL/min, therapy should be initiated at approximately one-half the recommended dosage. Depending on clinical efficacy and safety considerations, the dosage may be increased or decreased as appropriate.

According to another reference, the adult dosage should be decreased to 75% of the usual dose in patients with a glomerular filtration rate (GFR) of 10 to 50 mL/min. In patients with a GFR of less than 10 mL/min, the dosage should be decreased to 50% of the usual dose.

Dialysis – For adult patients receiving continuous renal replacement therapy, decrease metoclopramide dose to 75% of the usual dose.

➤*Preparation for administration:* For doses in excess of 10 mg, metoclopramide should be diluted in 50 mL of a parenteral solution. The preferred parenteral solution is sodium chloride injection (normal saline).

➤*Administration:* May be administered IM, by IV injection (10 mg or less), or by IV infusion.

IV infusions of metoclopramide, diluted in a parenteral solution, should be made slowly over a period of not less than 15 minutes.

IV injections of undiluted metoclopramide should be made slowly, allowing 1 to 2 minutes for 10 mg because a transient but intense feeling of anxiety and restlessness followed by drowsiness may occur with rapid administration.

➤*Admixture compatibility:*

Physically and chemically compatible up to 48 hours – Cimetidine, mannitol, potassium acetate, potassium phosphate.

Physically compatible up to 48 hours – Ascorbic acid, benztropine, cytarabine, dexamethasone sodium phosphate, diphenhydramine, doxorubicin, heparin, hydrocortisone sodium phosphate, lidocaine, multivitamin infusion (must be refrigerated), vitamin B complex with ascorbic acid.

Physically compatible up to 24 hours (do not use if precipitation occurs) – Clindamycin phosphate, cyclophosphamide, insulin.

METOCLOPRAMIDE HYDROCHLORIDE — INJECTION

Conditionally compatible (use within 1 hour after mixing or may be infused directly into the same running IV line) – Ampicillin, cisplatin, erythromycin lactobionate, methotrexate, penicillin G potassium, tetracycline.

Incompatible (do not mix) – Cephalothin, chloramphenicol, sodium bicarbonate.

➤*Storage/Stability:* Store at 20° to 25°C (68° to 77°F). Store vials in carton until used. Do not store open single-dose vials for later use, as they contain no preservative. This product is light sensitive. It should be inspected before use and discarded if either color or particulate is observed. Dilutions may be stored unprotected from light under normal light conditions up to 24 hours after preparation.

Sodium chloride injection (normal saline), when combined with metoclopramide injection, can be stored frozen for up to 4 weeks. Metoclopramide injection is degraded when admixed and frozen with dextrose 5% in water. Metoclopramide injection diluted in sodium chloride injection, dextrose 5% in water, dextrose 5% in sodium chloride 0.45%, Ringer's injection, or Ringer's lactate injection may be stored up to 48 hours (without freezing) after preparation if protected from light. All dilutions may be stored unprotected from light under normal light conditions up to 24 hours after preparation.

Actions

➤*Pharmacology:* Metoclopramide stimulates motility of the upper GI tract without stimulating gastric, biliary, or pancreatic secretions. Its mode of action is unclear. It seems to sensitize tissues to the action of acetylcholine. The effect of metoclopramide on motility is not dependent on intact vagal innervation, but it can be abolished by anticholinergic drugs.

Metoclopramide increases the tone and amplitude of gastric (especially antral) contractions, relaxes the pyloric sphincter and the duodenal bulb, and increases peristalsis of the duodenum and jejunum, resulting in accelerated gastric emptying and intestinal transit. It increases the resting tone of the lower esophageal sphincter. It has little, if any, effect on the motility of the colon or gallbladder.

In patients with gastroesophageal reflux and low lower esophageal sphincter pressure, single oral doses of metoclopramide produce dose-related increases in lower esophageal sphincter pressure. Effects begin at approximately 5 mg and increase through 20 mg (the largest dose tested). The increase in lower esophageal sphincter pressure from a 5 mg dose lasts approximately 45 minutes, and that of 20 mg lasts between 2 and 3 hours. Increased rate of stomach emptying has been observed with single oral doses of 10 mg.

The antiemetic properties of metoclopramide appear to be a result of its antagonism of central and peripheral dopamine receptors. Dopamine produces nausea and vomiting by stimulation of the medullary chemoreceptor trigger zone, and metoclopramide blocks stimulation of the chemoreceptor trigger zone by agents like levodopa or apomorphine, which are known to increase dopamine levels or to possess dopamine-like effects. Metoclopramide also abolishes the slowing of gastric emptying caused by apomorphine.

Like the phenothiazines and related drugs, which are also dopamine antagonists, metoclopramide produces sedation and may produce extrapyramidal reactions, although these are comparatively rare. Metoclopramide inhibits the central and peripheral effects of apomorphine, induces release of prolactin, and causes a transient increase in circulating aldosterone levels, which may be associated with transient fluid retention.

Pharmacodynamics – The onset of pharmacological action of metoclopramide is 1 to 3 minutes following an IV dose and 10 to 15 minutes following IM administration. Similar time to peak drug concentration (T_{max}) is observed after individual doses at steady state. Pharmacological effects persist for 1 to 2 hours.

➤*Pharmacokinetics:*

Absorption/Distribution – In a single-dose study of 12 subjects, the area under the curve increases linearly with doses from 20 to 100 mg. Peak drug concentrations (C_{max}) increase linearly with dose, T_{max} remains the same, whole body clearance is unchanged, and the elimination rate remains the same.

The drug is not extensively bound to plasma proteins (approximately 30%). The whole body volume of distribution (Vd) is high (approximately 3.5 L/kg), which suggests extensive distribution of drug to the tissues.

Metabolism/Excretion – The average elimination half-life in individuals with healthy renal function is 5 to 6 hours.

Approximately 85% of the radioactivity of an orally administered dose appears in the urine within 72 hours. Of the 85% eliminated in the urine, approximately half is present as free or conjugated metoclopramide.

Special populations –

Renal function impairment: Renal impairment affects the clearance of metoclopramide. In a study with patients with varying degrees of renal impairment, a reduction in CrCl was correlated with a reduction in plasma clearance, renal clearance, nonrenal clearance, and increase in elimination half-life. However, the kinetics of metoclopramide in the presence of renal impairment remained linear. The reduction in clearance as a result of renal impairment suggests that the maintenance dosage should be adjusted downward to avoid drug accumulation.

Children: In children, the pharmacodynamics of metoclopramide following oral and IV administration are highly variable and a concentration-effect relationship has not been established.

Single IV doses of metoclopramide 0.22 to 0.46 mg/kg (mean, 0.35 mg/kg) were administered over 5 minutes to 9 pediatric cancer patients receiving chemotherapy (mean age, 11.7 years; range, 7 to 14 years) for prophylaxis of cytotoxic-induced vomiting. The metoclopramide plasma concentrations extrapolated to time zero ranged from 65 to 395 mcg/L (mean, 152 mcg/L). The mean elimination half-life, clearance, and Vd of metoclopramide were 4.4 hours (range, 1.7 to 8.3 hours), 0.56 L/h/kg (range, 0.12 to 1.2 L/h/kg), and 3 L/kg (range, 1 to 4.8 L/kg), respectively.

In another study, 9 pediatric cancer patients (age range, 1 to 9 years) received 4 to 5 IV infusions (over 30 minutes) of metoclopramide at a dose of 2 mg/kg to control emesis. After the last dose, the C_{max} of metoclopramide ranged from 1,060 to 5,680 mcg/L. The mean elimination half-life, clearance, and Vd of metoclopramide were 4.5 hours (range, 2 to 12.5 hours), 0.37 L/h/kg (range, 0.1 to 1.24 L/h/kg), and 1.93 L/kg (range, 0.95 to 5.5 L/kg), respectively.

Contraindications

Known sensitivity or intolerance to the drug; whenever stimulation of GI motility might be dangerous (eg, in the presence of GI hemorrhage, mechanical obstruction, perforation); patients with pheochromocytoma because the drug may cause a hypertensive crisis, probably due to release of catecholamines from the tumor (such hypertensive crises may be controlled by phentolamine); in epileptic patients or patients receiving other drugs that are likely to cause extrapyramidal reactions, because the frequency and severity of seizures or extrapyramidal reactions may be increased.

Warnings/Precautions

➤*Administration:* Make IV injections of undiluted metoclopramide slowly, allowing 1 to 2 minutes for 10 mg because a transient but intense feeling of anxiety and restlessness followed by drowsiness may occur with rapid administration.

IV administration of metoclopramide diluted in a parenteral solution should be made slowly over a period of not less than 15 minutes.

➤*Neuroleptic malignant syndrome:* There have been rare reports of an uncommon but potentially fatal symptom complex sometimes referred to as neuroleptic malignant syndrome (NMS) associated with metoclopramide. Clinical manifestations of NMS include hyperthermia, muscle rigidity, altered consciousness, and evidence of autonomic instability (irregular pulse or blood pressure, tachycardia, diaphoresis, and cardiac arrhythmias).

The diagnostic evaluation of patients with this syndrome is complicated. In arriving at a diagnosis, it is important to identify cases in which the clinical presentation includes both serious medical illness (eg, pneumonia, systemic infection) and untreated or inadequately treated extrapyramidal signs and symptoms. Other important considerations in the differential diagnosis include central anticholinergic toxicity, heat stroke, malignant hyperthermia, drug fever, and primary CNS pathology.

The management of NMS includes the following: immediate discontinuation of metoclopramide and other drugs not essential to concurrent therapy; intensive symptomatic treatment and medical monitoring; and treatment of any concomitant serious medical problems for which specific treatments are available. Bromocriptine and dantrolene have been used in treatment of NMS, but their effectiveness is not established.

➤*Extrapyramidal symptoms:* Acute dystonic reactions occur in approximately 1 in 500 patients treated with the usual adult dosages of metoclopramide 30 to 40 mg/day. These usually are seen during the first 24 to 48 hours of treatment with metoclopramide, occur more frequently in children and adults younger than 30 years of age, and are even more frequent at the higher doses used in prophylaxis of vomiting due to cancer chemotherapy. These symptoms may include involuntary movements of limbs and facial grimacing, torticollis, oculogyric crisis, rhythmic protrusion of tongue, bulbar type of speech, trismus, or dystonic reactions resembling tetanus. Rarely, dystonic reactions may present as stridor and dyspnea, possibly due to laryngospasm. If these symptoms occur, inject diphenhydramine 50 mg IM, and they will usually subside. Benztropine 1 to 2 mg IM may also be used to reverse these reactions.

➤*Tardive dyskinesia:* Treatment with metoclopramide can cause tardive dyskinesia, a potentially irreversible and disfiguring disorder characterized by involuntary movements of the face, tongue, or extremities. Although the risk of tardive dyskinesia with metoclopramide has not been extensively studied, one published study reported a tardive dyskinesia prevalence of 20% among patients treated for at least 12 weeks. Avoid treatment with metoclopramide for longer than 12 weeks in all but rare cases in which the therapeutic benefit is thought to outweigh the risk of developing tardive dyskinesia.

Although the risk of developing tardive dyskinesia in the general population may be increased among elderly patients, women, and individuals with diabetes, it is not possible to predict which patients will develop metoclopramide-induced tardive dyskinesia. Both the risk of developing tardive dyskinesia and the likelihood that it will become irreversible increase the duration of treatment and total cumulative dose.

Discontinue metoclopramide in patients who develop signs or symptoms of tardive dyskinesia. There is no known effective treatment for established cases of tardive dyskinesia, although in some patients, tardive dyskinesia may remit partially or completely within several weeks to months after metoclopramide is withdrawn.

Metoclopramide itself may suppress or partially suppress the signs of tardive dyskinesia, thereby masking the underlying disease process. The effect of this symptomatic suppression on the long-term course of tardive dyskinesia is unknown. Therefore, do not use metoclopramide for the symptomatic control of tardive dyskinesia.

➤*Parkinsonian-like symptoms:* Parkinsonian-like symptoms, including bradykinesia, tremor, cogwheel rigidity, or mask-like facies, have occurred, more commonly within the first 6 months after beginning treatment with metoclopramide, but occasionally after longer periods. These symptoms generally subside within 2 to 3 months following discontinuance of metoclopramide. Give patients with preexisting Parkinson disease metoclopramide

METOCLOPRAMIDE HYDROCHLORIDE — INJECTION

cautiously, if at all, because such patients may experience exacerbation of Parkinsonian symptoms when taking metoclopramide.

➤*Depression:* Mental depression has occurred in patients with and without history of depression. Symptoms have ranged from mild to severe and have included suicidal ideation and suicide. Give metoclopramide to patients with a history of depression only if the expected benefits outweigh the potential risks.

➤*Anastomosis or closure of the gut:* Giving a promotility drug, such as metoclopramide, could theoretically put increased pressure on suture lines following a gut anastomosis or closure. Consider and weigh the possibility when deciding whether to use metoclopramide or nasogastric suction in the prevention of postoperative nausea and vomiting.

➤*Hypertension:* In one study in patients with hypertension, IV-administered metoclopramide was shown to release catecholamines; therefore, exercise caution when metoclopramide is used in patients with hypertension.

➤*Renal function impairment:* Metoclopramide is known to be substantially excreted by the kidney, and the risk of toxic reactions to this drug may be greater in patients with impaired renal function. Dosage adjustment may be required. (See Administration and Dosage.)

➤*Special risk:* Because metoclopramide produces a transient increase in plasma aldosterone, certain patients, especially those with cirrhosis or congestive heart failure, may be at risk of developing fluid retention and volume overload. If these adverse reactions occur at any time during metoclopramide therapy, discontinue the drug.

Patients with reduced nicotinamide adenine dinucleotide (NADH)—cytochrome b_5 reductase deficiency are at an increased risk of developing methemoglobinemia and/or sulfhemoglobinemia when metoclopramide is administered. In patients with glucose-6-phosphate dehydrogenase (G6PD) deficiency who experience metoclopramide-induced methemoglobinemia, methylene blue treatment is not recommended.

➤*Hazardous tasks:* Metoclopramide may impair the mental and/or physical abilities required for the performance of hazardous tasks such as operating machinery or driving a motor vehicle.

➤*Pregnancy: Category B.* Metoclopramide has been used for decades for the treatment of nausea and vomiting in pregnant women. It has also been used during pregnancy to decrease gastric emptying time. (See Administration and Dosage.) Metoclopramide has been used during all stages of pregnancy, and there has been no evidence of embryo, fetal, or newborn harm found in human and animal studies. According to a retrospective cohort study, the use of metoclopramide during the first trimester did not result in significantly increased risks of any adverse effects on the fetus. Use this drug during pregnancy only if clearly needed.

➤*Lactation:* Metoclopramide has been used as a lactation stimulant. (See Metoclopramide oral monograph.) Metoclopramide is excreted in human milk. Exercise caution when metoclopramide is administered to a breast-feeding mother.

Metoclopramide apparently represents a small risk to the breast-feeding infant with maternal dosages of 45 mg/day or less. Mild adverse reactions only have been reported in 2 breast-feeding infants. One review stated that the drug should not be used during breast-feeding because of the potential risks to the neonate, but there are no published studies to substantiate this caution. The American Academy of Pediatrics classifies metoclopramide as a drug for which the effect on a breast-feeding infant is unknown but may be of concern because it is a dopaminergic-blocking agent.

➤*Children:* According to the manufacturer, safety and efficacy in children have not been established except as stated to facilitate small bowel intubation.

Exercise care in administering metoclopramide to neonates because prolonged clearance may produce excessive serum concentrations.

In addition, neonates have reduced levels of NADH-cytochrome b_5 reductase that, in combination with the aforementioned pharmacokinetic factors, make neonates more susceptible to methemoglobinemia.

The safety profile of metoclopramide in adults cannot be extrapolated to children. Dystonias and other extrapyramidal reactions associated with metoclopramide are more common in children than in adults.

➤*Elderly:* The risk of developing Parkinsonian-like adverse reactions increases with ascending dose. Elderly patients should receive the lowest dose of metoclopramide that is effective. If Parkinsonian-like symptoms develop in an elderly patient receiving metoclopramide, generally discontinue metoclopramide before initiating any specific anti-Parkinsonian agent.

Elderly patients may be at greater risk of tardive dyskinesia.

Sedation has been reported in metoclopramide users. Sedation may cause confusion and manifest as oversedation in elderly.

Dose selection for an elderly patient should be cautious, usually starting at the low end of the dosing range, reflecting the greater frequency of decreased renal function, concomitant disease, or other drug therapy in the elderly.

Drug Interactions

Metoclopramide Injection Drug Interactions

Precipitant drug	Object drug[a]		Description
Anticholinergics Narcotic analgesics	Metoclopramide	↓	The effects of metoclopramide on GI motility are antagonized by these agents. Observe patients for a decrease or loss of metoclopramide effects. Adjust the metoclopramide dose as needed.
CNS depressants (eg, sedatives)	Metoclopramide	↑	Additive sedative effects can occur when metoclopramide is given with hypnotics, narcotics, sedatives, or tranquilizers. If excessive sedation occurs, the dose of one or both drugs may need to be reduced.
Metoclopramide	CNS depressants (eg, sedatives)		
Metoclopramide	Alcohol	↑	Metoclopramide increases the rate of absorption of alcohol by decreasing the time it takes alcohol to reach the small intestine where it is rapidly absorbed. In addition, sedative effects of metoclopramide and alcohol are additive. If excessive sedation occurs, the dose of one or both drugs may need to be reduced.
Metoclopramide	Cabergoline	↓	Metoclopramide may decrease the hypoprolactinemic effects of cabergoline. Avoid coadministration.
Metoclopramide	Cimetidine	↓	Bioavailability of cimetidine may be reduced due to decreased absorption as a result of faster gastric transit time. Consider administering cimetidine at least 2 hours before metoclopramide.
Metoclopramide	Cyclosporine	↑	A faster gastric emptying time may allow for an increase in cyclosporine absorption, possibly increasing its immunosuppressive and toxic effects. Measure cyclosporine concentrations when starting or stopping metoclopramide. Adjust the cyclosporine dose as needed.
Metoclopramide	Digoxin	↓	Digoxin absorption, plasma levels, and therapeutic effects may be decreased. The capsule, elixir, and tablets with a high dissolution rate are least affected and are less likely to interact.
Metoclopramide	Insulin	↑	Gastroparesis (gastric stasis) may be responsible for poor diabetic control in some patients. Exogenously administered insulin may begin to act before food has left the stomach and lead to hypoglycemia. Because the action of metoclopramide will influence the delivery of food to the intestines and thus the rate of absorption, insulin dosage or timing of dosage may require adjustment.
Metoclopramide	Levodopa	↑	These agents have opposite effects on dopamine receptors. The bioavailability of levodopa may be increased, and levodopa may decrease the effects of metoclopramide on gastric emptying and lower esophageal pressure. Metoclopramide is relatively contraindicated in Parkinson disease patients.
Levodopa	Metoclopramide	↓	

METOCLOPRAMIDE HYDROCHLORIDE — INJECTION

Metoclopramide Injection Drug Interactions

Precipitant drug	Object drug[a]		Description
Metoclopramide	MAOIs[b]	↑	Because metoclopramide releases catecholamines in patients with essential hypertension, use cautiously, if at all, in patients receiving MAOIs.
Metoclopramide	Pergolide	↓	Metoclopramide may decrease the pharmacologic effects of pergolide. Avoid coadministration.
Metoclopramide	Serotonin reuptake inhibitors (eg, sertraline, venlafaxine)	↑	Metoclopramide plasma concentrations may be elevated due to enzyme inhibition, increasing the pharmacologic effects and adverse reactions. In addition, the risk of serotonin syndrome may be increased. Observe the patient for an increase in adverse reactions. If serotonin syndrome occurs, immediate medical attention is required.
Serotonin reuptake inhibitors (eg, sertraline, venlafaxine)	Metoclopramide		
Metoclopramide	Succinylcholine	↑	By inhibiting plasma cholinesterase, metoclopramide may increase the neuromuscular-blocking effects of succinylcholine. Use with caution, closely monitoring neuromuscular function. Provide mechanical respiratory support if needed.

[a] ↑ = object drug increased; ↓ = object drug decreased.
[b] MAOIs = monoamine oxidase inhibitors.

Adverse Reactions

For more information on acute dystonic reactions, NMS, tardive dyskinesia, Parkinsonian-like symptoms, depression, and hypertension, see Warnings/Precautions.

➤*Cardiovascular:* Acute congestive heart failure, bradycardia, fluid retention, hypertension, hypotension, possible atrioventricular block, supraventricular tachycardia.

➤*CNS:* Drowsiness, fatigue, lassitude, and restlessness may occur in patients receiving the recommended prescribed dose of metoclopramide injection. Confusion, dizziness, headache, insomnia, or mental depression with suicidal ideation also may occur. In cancer chemotherapy patients being treated with 1 to 2 mg/kg per dose, incidence of drowsiness is approximately 70%. There are isolated reports of convulsive seizures without clear-cut relationship to metoclopramide. Rarely, hallucinations have been reported.

Extrapyramidal symptoms – Acute dystonic reactions, the most common type of extrapyramidal symptoms associated with metoclopramide, occur in approximately 0.2% of patients (1/500) treated with metoclopramide 30 to 40 mg/day. In cancer chemotherapy patients receiving 1 to 2 mg/kg per dose, the incidence is 2% in patients older than 30 to 35 years of age and 25% or higher in children and adults younger than 30 years of age who have not had prophylactic administration of diphenhydramine. Symptoms include involuntary movements of limbs, facial grimacing, torticollis, oculogyric crisis, rhythmic protrusion of tongue, bulbar type of speech, trismus, opisthotonus (tetanus-like reactions) and, rarely, stridor and dyspnea, possibly due to laryngospasm; ordinarily these symptoms are readily reversed by diphenhydramine.

Parkinsonian-like symptoms may include bradykinesia, tremor, cogwheel rigidity, mask-like facies.

Tardive dyskinesia most frequently is characterized by involuntary movements of the tongue, face, mouth, or jaw, and sometimes by involuntary movements of the trunk and/or extremities; movements may be choreoathetotic in appearance.

Motor restlessness (akathisia) may consist of feelings of anxiety, agitation, jitteriness, and insomnia, as well as inability to sit still, pacing, and foot tapping. These symptoms may disappear spontaneously or respond to a reduction in dosage.

Neuroleptic malignant syndrome – Rare occurrences of NMS have been reported. This potentially fatal syndrome is comprised of the symptom complex of hyperthermia, muscular rigidity, altered consciousness, and autonomic instability.

➤*Endocrine:* Amenorrhea, galactorrhea, gynecomastia, impotence secondary to hyperprolactinemia. Fluid retention secondary to transient elevation of aldosterone.

➤*GI:* Bowel disturbances, primarily diarrhea; nausea.

➤*Hematologic:* A few cases of neutropenia, leukopenia, or agranulocytosis, generally without clear-cut relationship to metoclopramide. Methemoglobinemia in adults and especially with overdosage in neonates. Sulfhemoglobinemia in adults.

➤*Hepatic:* Rarely, cases of hepatotoxicity, characterized by such findings as jaundice and altered liver function tests, when metoclopramide was administered with other drugs with known hepatotoxic potential.

➤*Hypersensitivity:* A few cases of bronchospasm, rash, or urticaria, especially in patients with a history of asthma. Rarely, angioneurotic edema, including glossal or laryngeal edema.

➤*Renal:* Urinary frequency, urinary incontinence.

➤*Miscellaneous:* Porphyria, visual disturbances.

Transient flushing of the face and upper body, without alterations in vital signs, following high IV doses.

Overdosage

➤*Symptoms:* Symptoms of overdosage may include drowsiness, disorientation, and extrapyramidal reactions.

Unintentional overdose due to misadministration has been reported in infants and children with the use of metoclopramide syrup. While there was no consistent pattern to the reports associated with these overdoses, events included seizures, extrapyramidal reactions, and lethargy.

Methemoglobinemia has occurred in premature and full-term neonates who were given overdoses of metoclopramide (1 to 4 mg/kg/day orally, IM, or IV for 1 to 3 or more days).

➤*Treatment:* Anticholinergic or anti-Parkinson drugs or antihistamines with anticholinergic properties may be helpful in controlling the extrapyramidal reactions. Symptoms are self-limiting and usually disappear within 24 hours.

Dialysis is not likely to be an effective method of drug removal in overdose situations.

Methemoglobinemia can be reversed by the IV administration of methylene blue. However, methylene blue may cause hemolytic anemia in patients with G6PD deficiency, which may be fatal.

Patient Information

Metoclopramide may impair the mental and/or physical abilities required for the performance of hazardous tasks such as operating machinery or driving a motor vehicle. Caution the ambulatory patient accordingly.

DEXPANTHENOL (Dextro-Pantothenyl Alcohol)

Rx	**Dexpanthenol** (Various)	**Injection**: 250 mg per mL	In 10 mL and 2 mL vials.
Rx	**Ilopan** (Adria)		In UD *Stat-Pak* 2 mL disp. syringes.[1]

[1] Syringes contain no more than 0.5% chlorobutanol.

DEXPANTHENOL — INJECTION

Indications

➤*Prevention of postoperative paralytic ileus:* Prophylactic use immediately after major abdominal surgery to minimize the possibility of paralytic ileus.

➤*Intestinal atony:* Intestinal atony causing abdominal distention.

➤*Decreased intestinal motility:* For the treatment of postoperative or postpartum retention of flatus, or postoperative delay in resumption of intestinal motility.

➤*Paralytic ileus:* For the treatment of paralytic ileus.

Administration and Dosage

➤*Adults:*

Prevention of postoperative adynamic ileus – 250 or 500 mg IM. May repeat in 2 hours and then every 6 hours until all danger of adynamic ileus has passed.

Treatment of adynamic ileus – 500 mg IM. May repeat in 2 hours and then every 6 hours as needed.

➤*Preparation for administration:* For IV administration, dexpanthenol 2 mL (500 mg) injection may be mixed with bulk IV solutions such as glucose or Ringer's lactate and slowly infused by IV.

➤*Administration:* Give by IM or slowly infused IV injection. Administration of dexpanthenol injection directly into the vein is not advised.

➤*Storage/Stability:* Store at 15° to 30°C (59° to 86°F). Protect from freezing or excessive heat.

Actions

➤*Pharmacology:* Pantothenic acid is a precursor of coenzyme A, which serves as a cofactor for a variety of enzyme-catalyzed reactions involving transfer of acetyl groups. The final step in the synthesis of acetylcholine consists of the choline acetylase transfer of acetyl group from acetylcoenzyme A to choline. Acetylcholine is the neurohumoral transmitter in the parasym-

DEXPANTHENOL — INJECTION

pathetic system and as such maintains the normal functions of the intestine. Decrease in acetylcholine content would result in decreased peristalsis and in extreme cases adynamic ileus. The pharmacological mode of action of the drug is unknown.

➤*Pharmacokinetics:* Pharmacokinetics data in humans is unavailable.

Contraindications

There are no known contraindications to the use of dexpanthenol injection.

Warnings/Precautions

➤*Administration:* Administration of dexpanthenol injection directly into the vein is not advised (See Dosage and Administration).

➤*Mechanical obstruction:* If ileus is a secondary consequence of mechanical obstruction, primary attention should be directed to the obstruction. The management of adynamic ileus includes the correction of any fluid and electrolyte imbalance (especially hypokalemia), anemia and hypoproteinemia, treatment of infection, avoidance where possible of drugs which are known to decrease gastrointestinal motility and decompression of the GI tract when considerably distended by nasogastric suction or use of a long intestinal tube.

➤*Hypersensitivity reactions:* If any signs of a hypersensitivity reaction appear, dexpanthenol injection should be discontinued.

There have been rare instances of allergic reactions of unknown cause during the concomitant use of dexpanthenol injection with drugs such as antibiotics, narcotics and barbiturates.

➤*Pregnancy: Category C.*

Dexpanthenol injection should be given to a pregnant woman only if clearly needed.

➤*Lactation:* It is not known whether this drug is excreted in human milk. Because many drugs are excreted in human milk, caution should be exercised when dexpanthenol injection is administered to a nursing woman.

➤*Children:* Safety and effectiveness in children have not been established.

Drug Interactions

The effects of succinylcholine appeared to have been prolonged in a woman administered dexpanthenol. (See Warnings).

Dexpanthenol Drug Interactions			
Precipitant drug	Object drug[a]		Description
Dexpanthenol	Antibiotics, barbiturates, or narcotics	↑	Allergic reactions have occurred rarely during concomitant use of dexpanthenol.
Dexpanthenol	Succinylcholine	↑	Temporary respiratory difficulty occurred following dexpanthenol administration 5 minutes after succinylcholine was discontinued. Succinylcholine's effects appeared to have been prolonged. Do not administer within 1 hour of succinylcholine.

[a] ↑ = object drug increased.

Adverse Reactions

➤*Allergic:* There have been a few reports of allergic reactions and single reports of several other adverse events in association with the administration of dexpanthenol. A causal relationship is uncertain. One patient experienced itching, tingling, difficulty in breathing. Another patient had red patches of skin. Two patients had generalized dermatitis and one patient urticaria.

➤*Cardiovascular:* One patient experienced a noticeable but slight drop in blood pressure after administration of dexpanthenol while in the recovery room.

➤*GI:* One patient experienced intestinal colic ½ hr after the drug was administered.

➤*Respiratory:* One patient experienced temporary respiratory difficulty following administration of dexpanthenol injection 5 minutes after succinylcholine was discontinued.

➤*Miscellaneous:* Two patients vomited following administration and two patients had diarrhea 10 days post-surgery and after dexpanthenol injection.

One elderly patient became agitated after administration of the drug.

DIGESTIVE ENZYMES

DIGESTIVE ENZYMES

Content given per capsule, tablet, or 0.7 g powder.

	Product and Distributor[a]	Lipase (USP units)	Protease (USP units)	Amylase (USP units)	How Supplied
			PANCREATIN		
otc sf	**Hi-Vegi-Lip Tablets** (Freeda)	4,800	60,000	60,000	Gluten free, lactose free, sugar free. Mannitol. In 100s and 250s.
			PANCRELIPASE		
Rx	**Pancreaze Delayed-Release Capsules** (McNeil)	4,200	10,000	17,500	(McNEIL MT 4). Yellow opaque/clear. Enteric-coated microtablets. In 100s.
Rx	**Pancrelipase Delayed-Release Capsules** (X-Gen Pharmaceuticals)	5,000	17,000	27,000	(PAN 5). White/blue, opaque. Enteric-coated beads. In 100s.
Rx	**Zenpep Delayed-Release Capsules**[b] (Eurand Pharmaceuticals)				(EURAND5). White. Enteric-coated beads. In 12s and 100s.
Rx	**Creon Delayed-Release Capsules**[b] (Abbott)	6,000	19,000	30,000	(CREON 1206). Orange/Blue. Enteric-coated spheres. In 100s and 250s.
Rx	**Tri-Pase 8** (Acella)	8,000	30,000	30,000	Lactose. (309). Tan, round. In 100s.
Rx	**Zenpep Delayed-Release Capsules**[b] (Eurand Pharmaceuticals)	10,000	34,000	55,000	(EURAND10). Yellow/White. Enteric-coated beads. In 12s and 100s.
Rx	**Pancreaze Delayed-Release Capsules** (McNeil)	10,500	25,000	43,750	(McNEIL MT 10). Pink opaque clear. Enteric-coated microtablets. In 100s.
Rx	**Creon Delayed-Release Capsules**[b] (Abbott)	12,000	38,000	60,000	(CREON 1212). Brown/Transparent. Enteric-coated spheres. In 100s and 250s.
Rx	**Zenpep Delayed-Release Capsules**[b] (Eurand Pharmaceuticals)	15,000	51,000	82,000	(EURAND 15). Red/White. Enteric-coated beads. In 12s and 100s.
Rx	**Tri-Pase 16** (Acella)	16,000	60,000	60,000	Lactose. (310). Tan, oval. In 100s.
Rx	**Zenpep Delayed-Release Capsules**[b] (Eurand Pharmaceuticals)	20,000	68,000	109,000	(EURAND 20). Green/White. Enteric-coated beads. In 12s, 100s, and 500s.
Rx	**Creon Delayed-Release Capsules**[b] (Abbott)	24,000	76,000	120,000	(CREON 1224). Orange/Transparent. Enteric-coated spheres. In 100s and 250s.

[a] Product tables do not imply bioequivalence (see page xi). Also refer to Bioequivalency (in Administration and Dosage).

[b] Porcine-derived enzymes.

DIGESTIVE ENZYMES — ORAL

Indications

➤*Rx:*

Pancreatic insufficiency – Enzyme replacement therapy in patients with deficient exocrine pancreatic secretions, such as in cystic fibrosis, chronic pancreatitis, postpancreatectomy, ductal obstructions caused by cancer of the pancreas or common bile duct, and pancreatic insufficiency, and for steatorrhea of malabsorption syndrome and postgastrectomy (Billroth II and total) or post-GI surgery (eg, Billroth II gastroenterostomy).

Presumptive test for pancreatic function, especially in pancreatic insufficiency caused by chronic pancreatitis.

➤*otc:*

Digestive aid – For use as a digestive enzyme aid.

Administration and Dosage

➤*Bioequivalency:* These products are not bioequivalent and cannot be interchanged without health care provider supervision. Variability not only occurs at the product level, but may also be clinically significant from one batch of product to the next.

Pancrelipase capsules and tablets are required to contain between 90% and 150% of the labeled lipase activity. Pancrelipase delayed-release capsules are required to contain between 90% and 165% of the labeled lipase activity, and not less than 90% of amylase and protease labeled activities. No USP standards have currently been identified for pancreatin capsules.

➤*Administration:* Capsules or tablets should be taken with meals or snacks with sufficient liquid. Adjust dosage based on severity of the exocrine pancreatic enzyme deficiency. The number of tablets, capsules, or dosage given with meals or snacks should be estimated by assessing which dose minimizes steatorrhea and maintains good nutritional status. Dose

DIGESTIVE ENZYMES — ORAL

increases, if required, should be made slowly, with careful monitoring of response and symptomatology.

To protect enteric coating, do not crush or chew the microspheres or microtablets; they should be swallowed whole. Where swallowing of capsules is difficult, they may be opened and shaken onto a small quantity of soft non-hot food (eg, applesauce, gelatin) that does not require chewing. Swallow immediately without chewing or crushing as the proteolytic action may cause irritation of the mucosa. Follow with a glass of juice or water to ensure complete swallowing of the microspheres/microtablets. Take care to ensure that no drug is retained in the mouth. Microsphere contact with foods having a pH greater than 5.5 can dissolve the enteric coating.

Creon (infants up to 12 months of age) – The drug should be administered immediately prior to each feeding using a dosage of lipase 2,000 to 4,000 units per 120 mL of formula or per breast-feeding. Contents of the capsule may be administered directly to the mouth or with a small amount of applesauce. Administration should be followed by breast milk or formula. Contents of the capsule should not be mixed directly into formula or breast milk as this may diminish efficacy. Care should be taken to ensure than *Creon* is not crushed or chewed or retained in the mouth to avoid irritation of the oral mucosa.

➤*Hi-Vegi-Lip*:

Adults – 1 tablet daily preferably with each meal.

➤*Pancrelipase:*

Adults – Lipase 4,000 to 20,000 units with each meal and with snacks.

Children 7 to 12 years of age – Lipase 4,000 to 12,000 units with each meal and with snacks.

Children 1 to 6 years of age – Lipase 4,000 to 8,000 units with each meal and 4,000 units with snacks.

Children 6 months to younger than 1 year of age – Lipase 2,000 units/meal.

➤*Creon*: Initiate therapy at the lowest recommended dose and gradually increase. Individualize the dosage based on clinical symptoms, the degree of steatorrhea present, and the fat content of the diet.

Dosage recommendations for pancreatic enzyme replacement therapy were published following the Cystic Fibrosis Foundation Consensus Conferences. Administer in a manner consistent with the recommendations of the Conferences provided in the following paragraphs. Patients may be dosed on a fat ingestion–based or actual body weight–based dosing scheme.

Adults and children 4 years of age and older – Dosing should begin with lipase 500 units/kg body weight per meal for those older than 4 years of age to a maximum of lipase 2,500 units/kg body weight per meal (or up to lipase 10,000 units/kg body weight per day), or less than lipase 4,000 units/g fat ingested per day.

Usually half the prescribed dose for an individualized full meal should be given with each snack. The total daily dose should reflect approximately 3 meals plus 2 or 3 snacks per day.

Enzyme doses expressed as lipase units/kg body weight per meal should be decreased in older patients because they weigh more but tend to ingest less fat per kilogram body weight.

Children older than 12 months and younger than 4 years of age – Begin with lipase 1,000 units/kg body weight per meal for children younger than 4 years of age to a maximum of lipase 2,500 units/kg body weight per meal (or up to lipase 10,000 units/kg body weight per day), or less than lipase 4,000 units/g fat ingested per day.

Infants (up to 12 months of age) – Infants may be given lipase 2,000 to 4,000 units per 120 mL of formula or per breast-feeding. Do not mix *Creon* capsule contents directly into formula or breast milk prior to administration.

Limitations on dosing – Dosing should not exceed the recommended maximum dosage set forth by the Cystic Fibrosis Foundation Consensus Conferences Guidelines. If symptoms and signs of steatorrhea persist, the dosage may be increased by a health care provider. Patients should be instructed not to increase the dosage on their own. There is great interindividual variation in response to enzymes; thus, a range of doses is recommended. Changes in dosage may require an adjustment period of several days. If doses are to exceed lipase 2,500 units/kg of body weight per meal, further investigation is warranted. Use caution in doses greater than lipase 2,500 units/kg of body weight per meal (or greater than lipase 10,000 units/kg of body weight per day) and only if they are documented to be effective by 3-day fecal fat measures that indicate a significantly improved coefficient of fat absorption. Doses greater than lipase 6,000 units/kg of body weight per meal have been associated with colonic stricture, indicative of fibrosing colonopathy, in children younger than 12 years of age. Patients currently receiving doses higher than lipase 6,000 units/kg of body weight per meal should be examined, and the dosage either immediately decreased or titrated downward to a lower range.

➤*Pancreaze, Zenpep*: Initiate therapy at the lowest recommended dose and gradually increase. Individualize the dosage based on clinical symptoms, the degree of steatorrhea present, and the fat content of the diet.

Dosage recommendations for pancreatic enzyme replacement therapy were published following the Cystic Fibrosis Foundation Consensus Conferences. Administer in a manner consistent with the recommendations of the Conferences provided in the following paragraphs. Patients may be dosed on a fat ingestion–based or actual body weight–based dosing scheme.

Adults and children 4 years of age and older – Begin enzyme dosing with lipase 500 units/kg of body weight per meal for those older than 4 years of age to a maximum of lipase 2,500 units/kg of body weight per meal (or less than or equal to lipase 10,000 units/kg of body weight per day), or less than lipase 4,000 units/g fat ingested per day.

Usually, give half of the prescribed dose for an individualized full meal with each snack. The total daily dose should reflect approximately 3 meals plus 2 or 3 snacks per day.

Enzyme doses expressed as lipase units/kg of body weight per meal should be decreased in older patients because they weigh more, but tend to ingest less fat per kilogram of body weight.

Children older than 12 months and younger than 4 years of age – Begin enzyme dosing with lipase 1,000 units/kg of body weight per meal for children younger than 4 years of age to a maximum of lipase 2,500 units/kg of body weight per meal (or less than or equal to lipase 10,000 units/kg of body weight per day), or less than lipase 4,000 units/g fat ingested per day.

Infants (up to 12 months of age) – Infants may be given lipase 2,000 to 4,000 units per 120 mL of formula or per breast-feeding. Give immediately prior to feedings. Do not mix capsule contents directly into formula or breast milk prior to administration. Administration should be followed by breast milk or formula. Contents of the capsule may also be administered directly in the mouth.

Limitations on dosing – Dosing should not exceed the recommended maximum dosage set forth by the Cystic Fibrosis Foundation Consensus Conferences Guidelines.

If symptoms and signs of steatorrhea persist, the dosage may be increased by a health care provider. Patients should be instructed not to increase the dosage on their own. There is great interindividual variation in response to enzymes; thus, a range of doses is recommended. Changes in dosage may require an adjustment period of several days. If doses are to exceed lipase 2,500 units/kg of body weight per meal, further investigation is warranted.

Use caution in doses greater than lipase 2,500 units/kg of body weight per meal (or greater than lipase 10,000 units/kg of body weight per day) and only if they are documented to be effective by 3-day fecal fat measures that indicate a significantly improved coefficient of fat absorption. Doses greater than lipase 6,000 units/kg of body weight per meal have been associated with colonic strictures, indicative of fibrosing colonopathy, in children with cystic fibrosis younger than 12 years of age. Patients currently receiving doses higher than lipase 6,000 units/kg of body weight per meal should be examined, and the dosage either immediately decreased or titrated downward to a lower range.

➤*Administration:*

Pancreaze –

Children and adults: Administer during meals or snacks, with sufficient fluid. Capsules and capsule contents should not be crushed or chewed. Capsules should be swallowed whole.

For patients who are unable to swallow intact capsules, the capsules may be carefully opened and the contents sprinkled on small amounts of acidic soft food with a pH of 4.5 or less (eg, applesauce). The mixture should be swallowed immediately without crushing or chewing and followed with water or juice to ensure complete ingestion. Care should be taken to ensure that no drug is retained in the mouth.

Infants (up to 12 months): Contents of the capsule may be sprinkled on small amounts of acidic soft food with a pH of 4.5 or less (eg, applesauce) and given to the infant within 15 minutes. Contents of the capsule should not be mixed directly into formula or breast milk as this may diminish efficacy. Care should be taken to ensure that it is not crushed or chewed or retained in the mouth, to avoid irritation of the oral mucosa.

➤*Storage/Stability:*

Creon – Store at 25°C (77°F) and protect from moisture. Temperature excursions are permitted between 25° and 40°C (77° to 104°F) for up to 30 days. Discard if exposed to higher temperature and moisture conditions higher than 70%. After opening, keep bottle tightly closed between uses to protect from moisture.

Hi-Vegi-Lip – Store at room temperature. Do not expose to excessive heat or moisture.

Pancreaze, pancrelipase – Store at room temperature not exceeding 25°C (77°F) in a dry place. Protect from high humidity. Store in tight containers. Do not refrigerate.

Zenpep – Store at 20° to 25°C (68° to 77°F); brief excursions are permitted to 15° to 40°C (59° to 104°F). Protect from moisture. After opening, keep bottle tightly closed between uses to protect from moisture. Avoid excessive heat.

Actions

➤*Pharmacology:* Digestive enzymes (pancreatic enzymes) hydrolyze fats to glycerol and fatty acids, change proteins into peptides and amino acids, and starch into dextrins and maltose. These agents exert their primary actions in the duodenum and upper jejunum. Once the digestive enzymes accomplish their catalytic function to hydrolyze food, the digestive enzymes may be inactivated by anti-enzymes, excreted by intestinal mucosa, or by protease digestion. The digested enzyme fragments may be absorbed from the intestine and subsequently excreted in the urine. The inactivated enzymes are excreted in the feces. Fat malabsorption (steatorrhea) and protein maldigestion occur when the pancreas loses more than 90% of its ability to produce digestive enzymes. The resultant diarrhea and malabsorption can be reasonably managed if 30,000 lipase units are delivered to the duodenum during a 4-hour period with and after a meal, representing approximately 10% of the normal pancreatic output.

The USP defines standards for 2 pancreatic enzyme preparations, pancreatin and pancrelipase. Pancreatin (a substance containing principally amylase, lipase, and protease) contains not less than 2 USP units of lipase activity, and not less than 25 USP units of amylase as well as protease activity. Pancrelipase (a substance containing principally lipase, and also con-

DIGESTIVE ENZYMES — ORAL

taining amylase and protease) contains not less than 24 USP units of lipase activity, and not less than 100 USP units of amylase as well as protease activity.

Contraindications

Hypersensitivity to pork protein or enzymes; acute pancreatitis; acute exacerbations of chronic pancreatic diseases.

Warnings/Precautions

➤*Colonic strictures:* Cases of fibrotic strictures in the colon have been reported primarily in cystic fibrosis patients with the use of enzyme supplements, generally at dosages above the recommended range. Some cases required surgery, including resection of the bowel. If symptoms suggestive of GI obstruction occur, consider the possibility of bowel strictures.

➤*Treatment failure:* Treatment failures have been reported in cystic fibrosis patients when brand name products were replaced by a generic substitution. Use care and monitor closely when switching patients from one product to another.

➤*Replacement therapy:* Pancreatic exocrine replacement therapy should not delay or supplant treatment of the primary disorder.

➤*Excessive doses:* Excessive doses may cause nausea, abdominal cramps, or diarrhea. Extremely high doses have been associated with hyperuricosuria and hyperuricemia.

➤*Pork sensitivity:* Use pork products with caution in patients sensitive to pork. Discontinue use if symptoms of sensitivity appear and initiate symptomatic and supportive treatment if necessary. Individuals previously sensitized to trypsin, pancreatin, or pancrelipase may have allergic reactions.

➤*Irritation of skin/mucous membranes:* Do not spill powder on hands because it may irritate skin. The dust of finely powdered concentrates irritates the nasal mucosa and the respiratory tract. Inhalation of airborne powder can precipitate an asthma attack. Asthma also can occur in patients sensitized to pancreatic enzyme concentrates.

➤*Pregnancy: Category C (Creon, Pancrelipase).* It is not known whether the drug can cause fetal harm when administered to a pregnant woman or can affect reproduction capacity. Give to a pregnant woman only if clearly needed. The enteric coating component, diethyl phthalate, has been teratogenic in rats with high intraperitoneal dosing.

➤*Lactation:* It is not known whether pancreatin is excreted in breast milk. Exercise caution when administering to a nursing mother.

➤*Children:* Colonic strictures, particularly in children with cystic fibrosis, have been associated with doses generally above the recommended dosing range (see Warnings). Patients currently receiving doses above 2,500 lipase units/kg/meal or 4,000 lipase units/g fat/day should be re-evaluated and the dosage either immediately decreased or titrated downward to the lowest effective clinical dose as assessed by 3-day fecal fat excretion.

Drug Interactions

Digestive Enzymes Drug Interactions

Precipitant drug	Object drug[a]		Description
Antacids	Digestive enzymes	⬇	Calcium carbonate or magnesium hydroxide may negate the beneficial effect of the enzymes.
Digestive enzymes	Folic acid	⬇	Impaired folic acid absorption by oral pancreatic enzymes may lead to folic acid deficiency.
Digestive enzymes	Iron	⬇	The serum iron response to oral iron may be decreased by concomitant pancreatic extracts.

[a] ⬇ = object drug decreased.

Adverse Reactions

The most frequently reported adverse reactions are GI in nature. Less frequently, allergic-type reactions also have been observed. Other adverse reactions reported include the following: Colonic strictures; diarrhea; abdominal pain; intestinal obstruction; vomiting; intestinal stenosis; constipation; dermatitis; flatulence; nausea; melena; weight decrease; pain; bloating; cramping. Perianal irritation and, rarely, inflammation with large doses may occur with pancreatin. Extremely high doses have been associated with hyperuricemia and hyperuricosuria.

Overdosage

Overdosage may cause diarrhea or transient intestinal upset. No acute toxic reactions have been reported.

Patient Information

Take before or with meals. Take with plenty of fluids.

Do not inhale powder dosage form or powder from capsules because it may irritate skin or mucous membranes.

To protect enteric coating, do not crush or chew the microspheres/tablets in the enteric-coated capsule formulations.

Do not switch products without consulting your physician.

GALLSTONE SOLUBILIZING AGENTS

URSODIOL (Ursodeoxycholic acid)

Rx	**Ursodiol** (Watson)	**Capsules; oral:** 300 mg	(Watson 3159). White. In 100s.
Rx	**Actigall** (Watson)		(ACTIGALL 300 mg). White and pink. In 100s.
Rx	**Ursodiol** (Teva)	**Tablets; oral:** 250 mg	PEG. (93 5360). White to off-white, oval. Film-coated. In 100s.
Rx	**URSO 250** (Axcan Scandipharm)		(URS785). Elliptical, white. Film-coated. In 100s and 500s.
Rx	**Ursodiol** (Teva)	**Tablets; oral:** 500 mg	PEG. (9 3 53 61). White to off-white, scored. oval. Film-coated. In 100s.
Rx	**URSO Forte** (Axcan Scandipharm)		(URS790). Elliptical, white. Film-coated. In 100s and 500s.

URSODIOL — ORAL

Indications

➤*Gallstones (capsules only):* For patients with radiolucent, noncalcified gallbladder stones less than 20 mm in greatest diameter in whom elective cholecystectomy would be undertaken except for the presence of increased surgical risk caused by systemic disease, advanced age, idiosyncratic reaction to general anesthesia, or for those patients who refuse surgery. Safety for use of ursodiol beyond 24 months is not established.

For the prevention of gallstone formationin obese patients experiencing rapid weight loss.

➤*Primary biliary cirrhosis (tablets only):* For the treatment of patients with primary biliary cirrhosis (PBC).

➤*Off-label uses:*

Other possible off-label uses – Treatment of biliary atresia in infants; enhance fatty acid metabolism in children with cystic fibrosis. (See Administration and Dosage.)

Administration and Dosage

➤*General dosing considerations:*

Gallstone dissolution – Obtain ultrasound images of the gallbladder at 6-month intervals for the first year of ursodiol therapy to monitor gallstone response. If gallstones appear to have dissolved, continue ursodiol therapy and confirm dissolution on a repeat ultrasound examination within 1 to 3 months. Most patients who eventually achieve complete stone dissolution will show partial or complete dissolution at the first on-treatment reevaluation. If partial stone dissolution is not seen by 12 months of ursodiol therapy, the likelihood of success is greatly reduced.

➤*Adults:*

Gallstone dissolution –

Capsules: 8 to 10 mg/kg/day given in 2 or 3 divided doses.

Gallstone prevention –

Capsules: 600 mg/day (300 mg twice daily) in patients undergoing rapid weight loss.

Primary biliary cirrhosis (PBC) –

Tablets: 13 to 15 mg/kg/day administered in 2 to 4 divided doses with food. Adjust dosing regimen according to each patient's need.

➤*Children:*

Off-label dosing –

Biliary atresia:

• *Infants* – A dosage of 10 to 15 mg/kg once daily has been used but is based on limited data.

• *Enhance fatty acid metabolism in children with cystic fibrosis* – 15 to 30 mg/kg, given once daily or in 3 divided doses per day.

➤*Storage/Stability:*

Capsules – Store at 25°C (77°F); excursions permitted between 15° and 30°C (59° and 86°F). Dispense in a tight container.

Tablets – Store between 20°C and 25°C (68° and 77°F). Dispense in a tight container.

Actions

➤*Pharmacology:* Ursodiol is normally present as a minor fraction of the total bile acids in humans (5%).

Ursodiol suppresses hepatic synthesis and secretion of cholesterol and also inhibits intestinal absorption of cholesterol. It appears to have little inhibitory effect on synthesis and secretion into bile of endogenous bile acids and does not appear to affect secretion of phospholipids into bile.

Although insoluble in aqueous media, cholesterol can be solubilized in at least 2 different ways in the presence of dihydroxy bile acids. In addition to solubilizing cholesterol in micelles, ursodiol acts by an apparently unique mechanism to cause dispersion of cholesterol as liquid crystals in aqueous

URSODIOL — ORAL

media. Thus, even though administration of high doses (eg, 15 to 18 mg/kg/day) does not result in a concentration of ursodiol higher than 60% of the total bile acid pool, ursodiol-rich bile effectively solubilizes cholesterol. The overall effect of ursodiol is to increase the concentration level at which saturation of cholesterol occurs.

The various actions of ursodiol combine to change the bile of patients with gallstones from cholesterol-precipitating to cholesterol-solubilizing, thus resulting in bile conducive to cholesterol stone dissolution.

➤*Pharmacokinetics:*

Absorption/Distribution –

Capsules: About 90% of a therapeutic dose of ursodiol is absorbed in the small bowel after oral administration. After absorption, ursodiol enters the portal vein and undergoes efficient extraction from portal blood by the liver (there is a large "first-pass" effect) where it is conjugated with either glycine or taurine and is then secreted into the hepatic bile ducts. Ursodiol in bile is concentrated in the gallbladder and expelled into the duodenum in gallbladder bile via the cystic and common ducts by gallbladder contractions provoked by physiologic responses to eating. Only small quantities of ursodiol appear in the systemic circulation and very small amounts are excreted into urine. The sites of the drug's therapeutic actions are in the liver, bile, and gut lumen. With repeated dosing, bile ursodeoxycholic acid concentrations reach steady state in about 3 weeks.

After ursodiol dosing is stopped, the concentration of the bile acid in bile falls exponentially, declining to about 5% to 10% of its steady-state level in about 1 week.

Tablets: Following oral administration, the majority of ursodiol is absorbed by passive diffusion and its absorption is incomplete. Once absorbed, ursodiol undergoes hepatic extraction to the extent of about 50% in the absence of liver disease. As the severity of liver disease increases, the extent of extraction decreases. In the liver, ursodiol is conjugated with glycine or taurine, then secreted into bile. These conjugates of ursodiol are absorbed in the small intestine by passive and active mechanisms. The conjugates also can be deconjugated in the ileum by intestinal enzymes, leading to the formation of free ursodiol that can be reabsorbed and reconjugated in the liver.

In healthy subjects, at least 70% of ursodiol (unconjugated) is bound to plasma protein. No information is available on the binding of conjugated ursodiol to plasma protein in healthy subjects or PBC patients. Its volume of distribution has not been determined, but is expected to be small because the drug is mostly distributed in the bile and small intestine.

Metabolism/Excretion –

Capsules: Beyond conjugation, ursodiol is not altered or catabolized appreciably by the liver or intestinal mucosa. A small proportion of orally administered drug undergoes bacterial degradation with each cycle of enterohepatic circulation. Ursodiol can be both oxidized and reduced at the 7-carbon, yielding either 7-keto-lithocholic acid or lithocholic acid, respectively. Further, there is some bacterially catalyzed deconjugation of glyco- and tauro-ursodeoxycholic acid in the small bowel. Free ursodiol, 7-keto-lithocholic acid, and lithocholic acid are relatively insoluble in aqueous media and larger proportions of these compounds are lost from the distal gut into the feces. Reabsorbed free ursodiol is reconjugated by the liver. Eighty percent (80%) of lithocholic acid formed in the small bowel is excreted in the feces, but the 20% that is absorbed is sulfated at the 3-hydroxyl group in the liver to relatively insoluble lithocholyl conjugates that are excreted into bile and lost in feces. Absorbed 7-keto-lithocholic acid is stereospecifically reduced in the liver to chenodiol.

Lithocholic acid, when administered chronically to animals, causes cholestatic liver injury and can cause death from liver failure in certain species unable to form sulfate conjugates. Lithocholic acid is formed by 7-dehydroxylation of the dihydroxy bile acids (ursodiol and chenodiol) in the gut lumen. The 7-dehydroxylation reaction appears to be alpha-specific (chenodiol is more efficiently 7-dehydroxylated than ursodiol) and, for equimolar doses of ursodiol and chenodiol, levels of lithocholic acid appearing in bile are lower with the former. Humans and chimpanzees can sulfate lithocholic acid. Although liver injury has not been associated with ursodiol therapy, a reduced capacity to sulfate may exist in some individuals. Nonetheless, such a deficiency has not yet been clearly demonstrated and must be extremely rare, given the several thousand patient-years of clinical experience with ursodiol.

Tablets: Nonabsorbed ursodiol passes into the colon where it is mostly 7-dehydroxylated to lithocholic acid. Some ursodiol is epimerized to chenodiol (CDCA) via a 7-oxa intermediate. Chenodiol also undergoes 7-dehydroxylation to lithocholic acid. These metabolites are poorly soluble and excreted in the feces. A small portion of lithocholic acid is reabsorbed, conjugated in the liver with glycine or taurine, and sulfated at the 3 position. The resulting sulfated lithocholic acid conjugates are excreted in bile and then lost in feces.

Ursodiol is excreted primarily in the feces. With treatment, urinary excretion increases, but remains lower than 1% except in severe cholestatic liver disease.

During chronic administration of ursodiol, it becomes a major biliary and plasma bile acid. At a chronic dose of 13 to 15 mg/kg/day, ursodiol constitutes 30% to 50% of biliary and plasma bile acids.

Contraindications

Hypersensitivity or intolerance to ursodiol or any of the components of the formulations.

Ursodiol will not dissolve calcified cholesterol stones, radiopaque stones, or radiolucent bile pigment stones. Hence, patients with such stones are not candidates for ursodiol therapy.

Patients with compelling reasons for cholecystectomy including unremitting acute cholecystitis, cholangitis, biliary obstruction, gallstone pancreatitis, or biliary-GI fistula are not candidates for ursodiol therapy.

Allergy to bile acids.

Warnings/Precautions

➤*Pregnancy: Category B.* There have been no adequate and well-controlled studies of the use of ursodiol in pregnant women, but inadvertent exposure of 4 women to therapeutic doses of the drug in the first trimester of pregnancy during the ursodiol trials led to no evidence of effects on the fetus or newborn baby. Although it seems unlikely, the possibility that ursodiol can cause fetal harm cannot be ruled out; hence, the drug is not recommended for use during pregnancy.

➤*Lactation:* It is not known whether ursodiol is excreted in human milk. Because many drugs are excreted in human milk, exercise caution when ursodiol is administered to a breastfeeding mother.

➤*Children:* The safety and effectiveness of ursodiol in pediatric patients have not been established.

➤*Elderly:*

Capsules – Small differences in efficacy and greater sensitivity of some elderly individuals taking ursodiol cannot be ruled out. Therefore, it is recommended that dosing proceed with caution in this population.

➤*Monitoring:* Abnormalities in liver enzymes have not been associated with ursodiol therapy and, in fact, ursodiol has been shown to decrease liver enzyme levels in liver disease. However, patients given ursodiol should have AST and ALT measured at the initiation of therapy and thereafter as indicated by the particular clinical circumstances.

Patients with variceal bleeding, hepatic encephalopathy, ascites, or in need of an urgent liver transplant should receive appropriate specific treatment.

Hepatic effects – Ursodiol therapy has not been associated with liver damage. Lithocholic acid, a naturally occurring bile acid, is known to be a liver-toxic metabolite. This bile acid is formed in the gut from ursodiol less efficiently and in smaller amounts than that seen from chenodiol. Lithocholic acid is detoxified in the liver by sulfation and, although man appears to be an efficient sulfater, it is possible that some patients may have a congenital or acquired deficiency in sulfation, thereby predisposing them to lithocholate-induced liver damage.

Drug Interactions

Ursodiol Drug Interactions

Precipitant drug	Object drug[a]		Description
Antacids	Ursodiol	⬇	Aluminum-based antacids adsorb bile acids in vitro and interfere with the action of ursodiol by reducing its absorption.
Bile acid sequestrants	Ursodiol	⬇	Cholestyramine and colestipol may interfere with the action of ursodiol by reducing its absorption.
Clofibrate Estrogens Oral Contraceptives	Ursodiol	⬇	These agents (and perhaps other lipid-lowering drugs) increase hepatic cholesterol secretion, and encourage cholesterol gallstone formation and hence may counteract the effectiveness of ursodiol.

[a] ⬇ = Object drug decreased.

Adverse Reactions

➤*Capsules:*

Adverse Reactions with the Use of Ursodiol in Gallstone Dissolution (≥ 5%)

	Ursodiol 8 to 10 mg/kg/day (n = 155)	Placebo (n = 159)	
Adverse reactions	n	n	%
CNS			
Fatigue	7	8	5%
Headache	28	34	21.4%
Insomnia	3	8	5%
GI			
Abdominal pain	67	70	44%
Cholecystitis	8	7	4.4%
Constipation	15	14	8.8%
Diarrhea	42	34	21.4%
Dyspepsia	26	18	11.3%
Flatulence	12	12	7.5%
GI disorder	6	8	5%
Nausea	22	27	17%
Vomiting	15	11	6.9%
GU			
Urinary tract infection	10	7	4.4%
Musculoskeletal			
Arthralgia	12	24	15.1%
Arthritis	9	4	2.5%
Back pain	11	18	11.3%
Myalgia	9	9	5.7%
Respiratory			
Bronchitis	10	6	3.8%
Coughing	11	7	4.4%
Pharyngitis	13	5	3.1%

URSODIOL — ORAL

Adverse Reactions with the Use of Ursodiol in Gallstone Dissolution (≥ 5%)				
	Ursodiol 8 to 10 mg/kg/day (n = 155)		Placebo (n = 159)	
Adverse reactions	n		n	%
Rhinitis	8		11	6.9%
Sinusitis	17		18	11.3%
Upper respiratory tract infection	24		21	13.2%
Miscellaneous				
Allergy	8		7	4.4%
Chest pain	5		10	6.3%
Infection, viral	30		41	25.8%

Adverse Reactions with the Use of Ursodiol for Gallstone Prevention				
	Ursodiol 600 mg (n = 322)		Placebo (n = 325)	
Adverse reactions	n	%	n	%
CNS				
Dizziness	53	16.5%	42	12.9%
Fatigue	25	7.8%	33	10.2%
Headache	80	24.8%	78	24%
Dermatologic				
Alopecia	17	5.3%	8	2.5%
GI				
Abdominal pain	20	6.2%	39	12%
Constipation	85	26.4%	72	22.2%
Diarrhea	81	25.2%	68	20.9%
Flatulence	15	4.7%	24	7.4%
Nausea	56	17.4%	43	13.2%
Vomiting	44	13.7%	44	13.5%
GU				
Dysmenorrhea	18	5.6%	19	5.8%
Musculoskeletal				
Back pain	38	11.8%	21	6.5%
Musculoskeletal pain	19	5.9%	15	4.6%
Respiratory				
Pharyngitis	10	3.1%	19	5.8%
Sinusitis	17	5.3%	18	5.5%
Upper respiratory tract infection	40	12.4%	35	10.8%
Miscellaneous				
Infection viral	29	9%	29	8.9%
Influenza-like symptoms	21	6.5%	19	5.8%

➤*Tablets:* The following table summarizes the adverse reactions observed in the 2 placebo-controlled clinical trials.

Adverse Reactions With the Use of Ursodiol Tablets				
	Visit at 12 months		Visit at 24 months	
Adverse reactions[a]	UDCA n (%)[b]	Placebo n (%)	UDCA n (%)[b]	Placebo n (%)
Diarrhea			1 (1.32%)	
Elevated creatinine	-	-	1 (1.32%)	-
Elevated blood glucose	1 (1.18%)	-	1 (1.32%)	-
Leukopenia			2 (2.63%)	-
Peptic ulcer			1 (1.32%)	-
Skin rash			2 (2.63%)	-

[a] Those adverse reactions occurring at the same or higher incidence in the placebo group as in the UDCA group have been deleted from this table (this includes diarrhea and thrombocytopenia at 12 months, nausea/vomiting, fever, and other toxicity).
[b] UDCA = Ursodeoxycholic acid = ursodiol.

In a randomized, crossover study in 60 PBC patients, 4 patients (6.7%) experienced 1 serious adverse reaction each (diabetes mellitus, cyst, and breast neoplasm [experienced by 2 patients]). No deaths occurred in the study. Forty-three patients (71.7%) experienced at least 1 treatment-emergent adverse reaction (TEAE) during the study. The most common (greater than 5%) TEAEs were asthenia (11.7%), dyspepsia (10%), peripheral edema (8.3%), hypertension (8.3%), nausea (8.3%), GI disorders, chest pain, and pruritus (5%). Seven patients (11.6%) reported 9 events that were judged as possibly or probably related to study medication. These 9 TEAEs included abdominal pain and asthenia (1 patient), nausea (3 patients), dyspepsia (2 patients) and anorexia and esophagitis (1 patient each). One patient on the twice-daily regimen (total dose 1,000 mg) withdrew due to nausea. All of these 9 TEAEs except esophagitis were observed with the twice-daily regimen at a total daily dose of 1,000 mg or greater.

Overdosage

➤*Symptoms:* Neither accidental nor intentional overdosage with ursodiol has been reported. Doses of ursodiol in the range of 16 to 20 mg/kg/day have been tolerated by 7 patients for 6 to 37 months without symptoms. The LD_{50} for ursodiol in rats is over 5,000 mg/kg given over 7 to 10 days and over 7,500 mg/kg for mice.

Single oral doses of ursodiol at 10, 5, and 10 g/kg in mice, rats, and dogs, respectively, were not lethal. A single oral dose of ursodiol at 1.5 g/kg was lethal in hamsters. Symptoms of acute toxicity were salivation and vomiting in dogs, and ataxia, dyspnea, ptosis, agonal convulsions, and coma in hamsters.

➤*Treatment:* The most likely manifestation of severe overdose with ursodiol would likely be diarrhea, which should be treated symptomatically.

CHENODIOL

Rx	**Chenodal** (Manchester Pharmaceuticals)	**Tablets; oral:** 250 mg	(MP 250). White. Film-coated. In 100s.

CHENODIOL — ORAL

WARNING

Chenodiol is not an appropriate treatment for many patients with gallstones because of the potential hepatotoxicity of chenodiol, poor response rate in some subgroups of chenodiol-treated patients, and an increased rate of a need for cholecystectomy in other chenodiol-treated subgroups. Reserve chenodiol for carefully selected patients, and treatment must be accompanied by systematic monitoring for liver function alterations. Aspects of patient selection, response rates, and risks versus benefits are given in the monograph.

Indications

➤*Radiolucent gallstones:* For patients with radiolucent stones in well-opacifying gallbladders, in whom selective surgery would be undertaken except for the presence of increased surgical risk because of systemic disease or age.

Administration and Dosage

➤*Adults:*

Radiolucent gallstones –

Usual dosage: 13 to 16 mg/kg/day in 2 divided doses, morning and night.

Initial dosage: 250 mg twice daily the first 2 weeks.

Dosage titration: Increase by 250 mg/day each week thereafter until the recommended or maximum tolerated dose is reached.

Dosage adjustment: If diarrhea occurs during dosage buildup or later in treatment, it usually can be controlled by temporary dosage adjustment until symptoms abate, after which the previous dosage usually is tolerated. Dosage less than 10 mg/kg usually is ineffective and may be associated with increased risk of cholecystectomy, so is not recommended.

Duration of therapy: Oral cholecystograms or ultrasonograms are recommended at 6 to 9 month intervals to monitor response. Complete dissolutions should be confirmed by a repeat test after 1 to 3 months continued chenodiol administration. After confirmed dissolution, treatment generally should be stopped.

Most patients who eventually achieve complete dissolution will show partial (or complete) dissolution at the first on-treatment test. If partial dissolution is not seen by 9 to 12 months, the likelihood of success of treating longer is greatly reduced; chenodiol should be discontinued if there is no response by 18 months. Safety of use beyond 24 months is not established.

Recurrence: Stone recurrence can be expected within 5 years in 50% of cases. After confirmed dissolution, treatment generally should be stopped. Serial cholecystograms or ultrasonograms are recommended to monitor for recurrence, keeping in mind that radiolucency and gallbladder function should be established before starting another course of chenodiol. A prophylactic dosage is not established; reduced doses cannot be recommended; stones have recurred on 500 mg/day. Low cholesterol or carbohydrate diets, and dietary bran, have been reported to reduce biliary cholesterol; maintenance of reduced weight is recommended to forestall stone recurrence.

➤*Storage/Stability:* Store at 20° to 25°C (68° to 77°F).

Actions

➤*Pharmacology:* At therapeutic doses, chenodiol suppresses hepatic synthesis of both cholesterol and cholic acid, gradually replacing the latter and its metabolite, deoxycholic acid in an expanded bile acid pool. These actions contribute to biliary cholesterol desaturation and gradual dissolution of radiolucent cholesterol gallstones in the presence of a gallbladder visualized by oral cholecystography. Chenodiol has no effect on radiopaque (calcified) gallstones or on radiolucent bile pigment stones.

➤*Pharmacokinetics:*

Absorption/Distribution – Chenodiol is well absorbed from the small intestine. Owing to 60% to 80% first-pass hepatic clearance, the body pool of chenodiol resides mainly in the enterohepatic circulation; serum and urinary bile acid levels are not significantly affected during chenodiol therapy.

Metabolism/Excretion – Chenodiol is taken up by the liver where it is converted to its taurine and glycine conjugates and secreted in bile. At steady state, an amount of chenodiol near the daily dose escapes to the colon and is converted by bacterial action to lithocholic acid. About 80% of the lithocholate is excreted in the feces; the remainder is absorbed and converted in the liver to its poorly absorbed sulfolithocholyl conjugates. During chenodiol therapy there is only a minor increase in biliary lithocholate, while fecal bile acids are increased 3- to 4-fold.

CHENODIOL — ORAL

Contraindications

Known hepatocyte dysfunction or bile ductal abnormalities such as intrahepatic cholestasis, primary biliary cirrhosis, or sclerosing cholangitis; a gallbladder confirmed as nonvisualizing after 2 consecutive single doses of dye; radiopaque stones; gallstone complications or compelling reasons for gallbladder surgery, including unremitting acute cholecystitis, cholangitis, biliary obstruction, gallstone pancreatitis, or biliary GI fistula; women who are or may become pregnant.

Warnings/Precautions

➤*Hepatic effects:* Safe use of chenodiol depends upon selection of patients without preexisting liver disease and upon faithful monitoring of serum aminotransferase levels to detect drug-induced liver toxicity. Aminotransferase elevations over 3 times the upper limit of normal (ULN) have required discontinuation of chenodiol in 2% to 3% of patients. Although clinical and biopsy studies have not shown fulminant lesions, the possibility remains that an occasional patient may develop serious hepatic disease. Three patients with biochemical and histologic pictures of chronic active hepatitis while on chenodiol, 375 or 750 mg/day, have been reported. The biochemical abnormalities returned spontaneously to normal in 2 of the patients within 13 and 17 months; and after 17 months treatment with prednisone in the third. Follow-up biopsies were not done; and the causal relationship of the drug could not be determined. Another biopsied patient was terminated from therapy because of elevated aminotransferase levels and a liver biopsy was interpreted as showing active drug hepatitis.

One patient with sclerosing cholangitis, biliary cirrhosis, and history of jaundice died during chenodiol treatment for hepatic duct stones. Before treatment, serum aminotransferase and alkaline phosphate levels were over twice the ULN; within 1 month they rose to over 10 times. Chenodiol was discontinued at 7 weeks, when the patient was hospitalized with advanced hepatic failure and *Escherichia coli* peritonitis; death ensued at the eighth week. A contribution of chenodiol to the fatal outcome could not be ruled out.

➤*Colon cancer:* Epidemiologic studies suggest that bile acids might contribute to human colon cancer, but direct evidence is lacking. Bile acids, including chenodiol and lithocholic acid, have no carcinogenic potential in animal models, but have been shown to increase the number of tumors when administered with certain known carcinogens. The possibility that chenodiol therapy might contribute to colon cancer in otherwise susceptible individuals cannot be ruled out.

➤*Hepatic function impairment:* Safe use of chenodiol depends on selection of patients without preexisting liver disease.

➤*Pregnancy: Category X.* Chenodiol is contraindicated in women who are or may become pregnant. Chenodiol may cause fetal harm when administered to a pregnant woman. No human data are available at this time. If this drug is used during pregnancy, or if the patient becomes pregnant while taking this drug, the patient should be apprised of the potential hazard to the fetus.

Serious hepatic, renal, and adrenal lesions occurred in fetuses of female Rhesus monkeys given 60 to 90 mg/kg/day (4 to 6 times the MRHD) from day 21 to day 45 of pregnancy. Hepatic lesions also occurred in neonatal baboons whose mothers had received 18 to 38 mg/kg (1 to 2 times the MRHD), all during pregnancy. Fetal malformations were not observed. Neither fetal liver damage nor fetal abnormalities occurred in reproduction studies in rats and hamsters.

➤*Lactation:* It is not known whether chenodiol is excreted in human milk. Because many drugs are excreted in human milk, caution should be exercised when chenodiol is administered to a breast-feeding mother.

➤*Children:* The safety and effectiveness of chenodiol in children have not been established.

➤*Monitoring:*

Liver function – The optimal frequency of monitoring liver function tests is not known. It is suggested that serum aminotransferase levels should be monitored monthly for the first 3 months and every 3 months thereafter during chenodiol administration. Under National Cooperative Gallstone Study (NCGS) guidelines, if a minor, usually transient elevations (1½ to 3 times the ULN) persisted longer than 3 to 6 months. Chenodiol was discontinued and resumed only after the aminotransferase level returned to normal; however, allowing the elevations to persist over such an interval is not known to be safe. Elevations over 3 times the ULN require immediate discontinuation of chenodiol and usually reoccur on challenge.

Cholesterol – Serum cholesterol should be monitored at 6 month intervals. It may be advisable to discontinue chenodiol if cholesterol rises above the acceptable age-adjusted limit for a given patient

Drug Interactions

Chenodiol Drug Interactions

Precipitant drug	Object drug[a]		Description
Aluminum-based antacids (eg, aluminum-hydroxide)	Chenodiol	⬇	Chenodiol absorption may be reduced, decreasing the pharmacologic effect. Coadminister with caution. Consider separating the administration times by as much as possible. If an interaction is still suspected, consider discontinuing one of the drugs.
Bile acid sequestrants (eg, cholestyramine, colestipol)	Chenodiol	⬇	Chenodiol absorption may be reduced, decreasing the pharmacologic effect. Coadminister with caution. Consider separating the administration times by as much as possible. If an interaction is still suspected, consider discontinuing one of the drugs.
Clofibrate	Chenodiol	⬇	Because clofibrate increases biliary cholesterol secretion and the incidence of cholesterol gallstones, chenodiol effectiveness may be counteracted. Coadminister with caution. If an interaction is suspected, consider discontinuing one of the drugs.
Contraceptives, hormonal	Chenodiol	⬇	Because estrogens increase biliary cholesterol secretion and the incidence of cholesterol gallstones, chenodiol effectiveness may be counteracted. Coadminister with caution. If an interaction is suspected, consider discontinuing one of the drugs.
Chenodiol	Warfarin	⬆	Because chenodiol is hepatotoxic, warfarin pharmacodynamics may be affected, resulting in prothrombin time prolongation and hemorrhage. Carefully monitor anticoagulant parameters. Adjust the warfarin dose as needed or discontinue chenodiol therapy.

[a] ⬆ = object drug increased; ⬇ = object drug decreased.

Adverse Reactions

➤*GI:* Dose-related diarrhea has been encountered in 30% to 40% of chenodiol-treated patients and may occur at any time during treatment, but is most commonly encountered when treatment is initiated. Usually, the diarrhea is mild, translucent, and well-tolerated and does not interfere with therapy. Dose reduction has been required in 10% to 15% of patients, and in a controlled trial about half of these required a permanent reduction in dose. Antidiarrhea agents have proven useful in some patients.

Discontinuation of chenodiol because of failure to control diarrhea is to be expected in approximately 3% of patients treated. Steady epigastric pain with nausea typical of lithiasis (biliary colic) usually is easily distinguishable from the crampy abdominal pain of drug-induced diarrhea.

Other less frequent GI adverse effects reported include urgency, cramps, heartburn, constipation, nausea and vomiting, anorexia, epigastric distress, dyspepsia, flatulence, and nonspecific abdominal pain.

➤*Hematologic:* Decreases in white blood cell count, never below 3,000, have been noted in a few patients treated with chenodiol; the drug was continued in all patients without incident.

➤*Hepatic:* Dose-related serum aminotransferase (mainly alanine aminotransferase [ALT]) elevations, usually not accompanied by rises in alkaline phosphatase or bilirubin, occurred in 30% or more of patients treated with the recommended dose of chenodiol. In most cases, these elevations were minor (1½ to 3 times the upper limit of laboratory normal) and transient, returning to within the normal range within 6 months despite continued administration of the drug. In 2% to 3% of patients, ALT levels rose to over 3 times the upper limit of laboratory normal, recurred on rechallenge with the drug, and required discontinuation of chenodiol treatment. Enzyme levels have returned to normal following withdrawal of chenodiol.

Morphologic studies of liver biopsies taken before and after 9 and 24 months of treatment with chenodiol have shown that 63% of the patients prior to chenodiol treatment had evidence of intrahepatic cholestasis. Almost all pretreatment patients had electron microscopic abnormalities. By the ninth month of treatment, reexamination of two-thirds of the patients showed an 89% incidence of the signs of intrahepatic cholestasis. Two of 89 patients at the ninth month had lithocholate-like lesions in the canalicular membrane, although there were not clinical enzyme abnormalities in the face of continued treatment and no change in type 2 light microscopic parameters.

➤*Lab test abnormalities:* Serum total cholesterol and low-density lipoprotein cholesterol may rise 10% or more during administration of chenodiol; no change has been seen in the high-density lipoprotein fraction; small decreases in serum triglyceride levels for females have been reported.

➤*Miscellaneous:* NCGS patients with a history of biliary pain prior to treatment had higher cholecystectomy rates during the study if assigned to low-dosage chenodiol (375 mg/day) than if assigned to either placebo or high dosage chenodiol (750 mg/day). The association with low-dosage chenodiol though not clearly a causal one, suggests that patients unable to take higher doses of chenodiol may be at greater risk of cholecystectomy.

Overdosage

Accidental or intentional overdoses of chenodiol have not been reported. One patient tolerated 4 g/day (58 mg/kg/day) for 6 months without incident.

CHENODIOL — ORAL

Patient Information

Counsel patients on the importance of periodic visits for liver function tests and oral cholecystograms (or ultrasonograms) for monitoring stone dissolution; inform patients of the symptoms of gallstone complications and warn them to report immediately such symptoms to the health care provider.

Instruct patients on ways to facilitate faithful compliance with the dosage regimen throughout the usual long term of therapy, and on temporary dose reduction if episodes of diarrhea occur.

MOUTH AND THROAT PRODUCTS

NYSTATIN

For prescribing information, see the Nystatin monograph in the Antifungal Agents section of the Anti-Infective Agents chapter.

CLOTRIMAZOLE

Rx	**Clotrimazole** (Various, eg, Roxane)	**Troches:** 10 mg	In 70s, 140s, 500s, and UD 70s.
Rx	**Mycelex** (Bayer)		(MYCELEX 10). White. In 70s and 140s.

CLOTRIMAZOLE — ORAL

For information on topical and vaginal clotrimazole, refer to individual monographs.

Indications

➤*Treatment of oropharyngeal candidiasis:* For the local treatment of oropharyngeal candidiasis. The diagnosis should be confirmed by a KOH smear or culture prior to treatment.

➤*Prophylaxis of oropharyngeal candidiasis:* Prophylactically to reduce the incidence of oropharyngeal candidiasis in patients immunocompromised by conditions that include chemotherapy, radiotherapy, or steroid therapy utilized in the treatment of leukemia, solid tumors, or renal transplantation. There are no data from adequate and well-controlled trials to establish the safety and efficacy of this product for prophylactic use in patients immunocompromised by etiologies other than those listed in the previous sentence.

Administration and Dosage

➤*Adults:*

Oropharyngeal candidiasis –

Prophylactic dosage: 1 troche 3 times daily for the duration of chemotherapy or until steroids are reduced to maintenance levels.

Treatment dosage: 1 troche 5 times a day for 14 consecutive days.

➤*Children:*

Oropharyngeal candidiasis –

3 years of age and older:

- *Treatment dosage* – 1 troche 5 times a day for 14 consecutive days.

➤*Administration:* Clotrimazole troches are administered only as a lozenge that must be slowly dissolved in the mouth.

➤*Storage/Stability:* Store below 30°C (86°F). Avoid freezing.

Actions

➤*Pharmacology:* Clotrimazole is a broad-spectrum antifungal agent that inhibits the growth of pathogenic yeasts by altering the permeability of cell membranes. The action of clotrimazole is fungistatic at concentrations of drug up to 20 mcg/mL and may be fungicidal in vitro against *Candida albicans* and other species of the genus *Candida* at higher concentrations. No single-step or multiple-step resistance to clotrimazole has developed during successive passages of *Candida albicans* in the laboratory; however, individual organism tolerance has been observed during successive passages in the laboratory. Such in vitro tolerance has resolved once the organism has been removed from the antifungal environment.

After oral administration of a 10 mg clotrimazole troche to healthy volunteers, concentrations sufficient to inhibit most species of *Candida* persist in saliva for up to three hours following the ≈ 30 minutes needed for a troche to dissolve. The long term persistence of drug in saliva appears to be related to the slow release of clotrimazole from the oral mucosa to which the drug is apparently bound. Repetitive dosing at three hour intervals maintains salivary levels above the minimum inhibitory concentrations of most strains of *Candida*; however, the relationship between in vitro susceptibility of pathogenic fungi to clotrimazole and prophylaxis or cure of infections in humans has not been established.

In another study, the mean serum concentrations were 4.98 ± 3.7 and 3.23 ± 1.4 nanograms/mL of clotrimazole at 30 and 60 minutes, respectively, after administration as a troche.

Contraindications

Hypersensitivity to clotrimazole or any of its components.

Warnings/Precautions

➤*Systemic mycoses:* Clotrimazole troches are not indicated for the treatment of systemic mycoses including systemic candidiasis.

➤*Administration:* Since patients must be instructed to allow each troche to dissolve slowly in the mouth in order to achieve maximum effect of the medication, they must be of such an age and physical or mental condition to comprehend such instructions.

➤*Pregnancy: Category C* (per manufacturer's prescribing information. *Category B* (per *Briggs' Drugs in Pregnancy and Lactation*). Clotrimazole has been shown to be embryotoxic in rats and mice when given in doses 100 times the adult human dose (in mg/kg), possibly secondary to maternal toxicity. The drug was not teratogenic in mice, rabbits, and rats when given in doses up to 200, 180, and 100 times the human dose.

Clotrimazole given orally to mice from nine weeks before mating through weaning at a dose 120 times the human dose was associated with impairment of mating, decreased number of viable young, and decreased survival to weaning. No effects were observed at 60 times the human dose. When the drug was given to rats during a similar time period at 50 times the human dose, there was a slight decrease in the number of pups per litter and decreased pup viability.

There are no adequate and well controlled studies in pregnant women. Clotrimazole troches should be used during pregnancy only if the potential benefit justifies the potential risk to the fetus.

➤*Lactation:* The absorption of clotrimazole from the skin and vagina is minimal. It is doubtful that measurable amounts of clotrimazole appear in milk.

➤*Children:* Safety and effectiveness of clotrimazole in children below the age of 3 years have not been established; therefore, its use in such patients is not recommended.

The safety and efficacy of the prophylactic use of clotrimazole troches in children have not been established.

➤*Monitoring:* Abnormal liver function tests have been reported in patients treated with clotrimazole troches; elevated SGOT levels were reported in about 15% of patients in the clinical trials. In most cases the elevations were minimal and it was often impossible to distinguish effects of clotrimazole from those of other therapy and the underlying disease (malignancy in most cases). Periodic assessment of hepatic function is advisable particularly in patients with preexisting hepatic impairment.

Adverse Reactions

Abnormal liver function tests have been reported in patients treated with clotrimazole troches; elevated SGOT levels were reported in about 15% of patients in the clinical trials.

Nausea, vomiting, unpleasant mouth sensations and pruritus have also been reported with the use of the troche.

CHLORHEXIDINE GLUCONATE

Rx	**PerioChip** (Adrian Pharmaceuticals)	**Chip; oral:** 2.5 mg	Glycerin, hydrolyzed gelatin. Orange-brown, rectangular (rounded at 1 end). In blister pack 10s.
Rx	**Chlorhexidine Gluconate** (Various, eg, Xttrium)	**Rinse; oral:** 0.12%	In 473 mL.[a]
Rx	**Peridex** (Procter & Gamble)		In 480 mL.[a]
Rx	**PerioGard** (Colgate Oral)		In 473 mL with 15 mL dose cup.[a]

[a] With alcohol 11.6%, saccharin.

CHLORHEXIDINE GLUCONATE — ORAL

Indications

➤*Chip:* As an adjunct to scaling and root planing procedures for reduction of pocket depth in patients with adult periodontitis. Chlorhexidine gluconate chip may be used as a part of a periodontal maintenance program, which includes good oral hygiene and scaling and root planing.

➤*Rinse:* For use between dental visits as part of a professional program for the treatment of gingivitis as characterized by redness and swelling of the gingivae, including gingival bleeding upon probing. Chlorhexidine gluconate oral rinse has not been tested among patients with acute necrotizing ulcerative gingivitis (ANUG). For patients having coexisting gingivitis and periodontitis, see Precautions.

CHLORHEXIDINE GLUCONATE — ORAL

➤*Off-label uses:*

Mucositis – [5] = Poor documentation. Current guidelines recommend that chlorhexidine not be used for the treatment of oral mucositis in patients with established oral mucositis.

Prevention of mucositis (chemotherapy-induced) – [4] = Insufficient documentation. Guidelines recommend that chlorhexidine not be used for the prevention of oral mucositis in patients receiving radiation therapy but do not address its use in patients receiving chemotherapy. Several small studies and a large, randomized study suggest chlorhexidine is no more effective than placebo in patients receiving chemotherapy. Results of a more recent controlled trial suggest a role for chlorhexidine in the prevention of oral mucositis in patients receiving high-dose chemotherapy with 5-fluorouracil.

Prevention of mucositis (radiation-induced) – [5] = Poor documentation. Guidelines recommend that chlorhexidine not be used for the prevention of oral mucositis in patients with solid head and neck tumors receiving radiation therapy.

Administration and Dosage

➤*Adults:*

Gingivitis –

Rinse:

• *Usual dosage* – ½ fl. oz. (marked on dosage cup) of undiluted chlorhexidine gluconate oral rinse twice daily for 30 seconds. (See Administration.)

• *Duration of therapy* – Therapy should be initiated directly following a dental prophylaxis. Patients should be reevaluated and given a thorough prophylaxis at intervals no longer than 6 months.

Periodontitis –

Chip: One chip is inserted into a periodontal pocket with probing pocket depth (PD) ≥ 5 mm. Up to 8 chips may be inserted in a single visit. Treatment is recommended to be administered once every 3 months in pockets with PD remaining ≥ 5 mm.

Off-label dosing –

Prevention of mucositis (chemotherapy-induced): [4] = Insufficient documentation. Oral doses of chlorhexidine mouthwash ranged from 10 to 20 mL of a 0.1% solution rinsed for 30 seconds to 1 minute and expectorated 2 to 4 times daily to 0.3% solution rinsed for 30 seconds and expectorated 3 times daily.

➤*Administration:*

Chip – The periodontal pocket should be isolated and the surrounding area dried prior to chip insertion. The chip should be grasped using forceps (such that the rounded end points away from the forceps) and inserted into the periodontal pocket to its maximum depth. If necessary, the chip can be further maneuvered into position using the tips of the forceps or a flat instrument. The chip does not need to be removed since it biodegrades completely.

In the unlikely event of chip dislodgment (in the 2 pivotal clinical trials, only 8 chips were reported lost), several actions are recommended, depending on the day of chip loss. If dislodgment occurs ≥ 7 days after placement, the dentist should consider the subject to have received a full course of treatment. If dislodgment occurs within 48 hours after placement, a new chip should be inserted. If dislodgment occurs more than 48 hours after placement, the dentist should not replace the chip, but reevaluate the patient at 3 months and insert a new chip if the pocket depth has not been reduced to less than 5 mm.

Rinse – Use morning and evening after toothbrushing. Patients should be instructed not to rinse with water or other mouthwashes, brush teeth, or eat immediately after using the rinse. The rinse is not intended for ingestion and should be expectorated after rinsing.

➤*Storage/Stability:*

Chip – Store in a refrigerator between 2° and 8°C (36° and 46°F).

Rinse – Store above freezing (0°C; 32°F).

Actions

➤*Pharmacology:*

Rinse – Chlorhexidine gluconate oral rinse provides antimicrobial activity during oral rinsing. The clinical significance of 0.12% chlorhexidine gluconate oral rinse's antimicrobial activities is not clear. Microbiological sampling of plaque has shown a general reduction of counts of certain assayed bacteria, both aerobic and anaerobic, ranging from 54% to 97% through 6 months of use.

Use of a chlorhexidine gluconate oral rinse in a 6-month clinical study did not result in any significant changes in bacterial resistance, overgrowth of potentially opportunistic organisms or other adverse changes in the oral microbial ecosystem. Three months after chlorhexidine gluconate use was discontinued, the number of bacteria in plaque had returned to baseline levels and the resistance of plaque bacteria to chlorhexidine gluconate was equal to that at baseline.

➤*Pharmacokinetics:*

Chip – Chlorhexidine gluconate chip releases chlorhexidine in vitro in a biphasic manner, initially releasing ≈ 40% of the chlorhexidine within the first 24 hours and then releasing the remaining chlorhexidine in an almost linear fashion for 7 to 10 days. This enzymatic release rate assay is an experimental collagenase assay that differs from the Regulatory Specification's Agar Release Rate Assay. This release profile may be explained as an initial burst effect, dependent on diffusion of chlorhexidine from the chip, followed by a further release of chlorhexidine as a result of enzymatic degradation.

In an in vivo study of 18 evaluable adult patients, there were no detectable plasma or urine levels of chlorhexidine following the insertion of 4 chlorhexidine gluconate chips under clinical conditions. The concentration of chlorhexidine released from the chlorhexidine gluconate chip was determined in the gingival crevicular fluid (GCF) of these same subjects. In these subjects, a highly variable biphasic release profile for chlorhexidine was demonstrated, with GCF levels 4 hours after chip insertion (mean: 1444 ± 783 mcg/mL), followed by a second peak at 72 hours (mean: 1902 ± 1073 mcg/mL). In a second study involving the insertion of 1 chlorhexidine gluconate chip under clinical conditions, the mean GCF level of chlorhexidine peaked at 1088 ± 678 mcg/mL at 4 hours. The mean GCF levels then declined in a highly erratic fashion to levels of 482 ± 447 mcg/mL at 72 hours without producing a true second peak. The results of these studies confirm a high degree of intersubject variability in chlorhexidine release from the chlorhexidine gluconate chip matrix in vivo that was not seen in vitro. Due to the nature and clinical use of the chlorhexidine gluconate chip dosage form, dose proportionality was not and would not be expected to be demonstrated between the 2 studies.

Rinse – Pharmacokinetic studies with a 0.12% chlorhexidine gluconate oral rinse indicate ≈ 30% of the active ingredient is retained in the oral cavity following rinsing. This retained drug is slowly released into the oral fluids. Studies conducted on human subjects and animals demonstrate chlorhexidine gluconate is poorly absorbed from the GI tract. The mean plasma level of chlorhexidine gluconate reached a peak of 0.206 mcg/g in humans 30 minutes after they ingested a 300 mg dose of the drug. Detectable levels of chlorhexidine gluconate were not present in the plasma of these subjects 12 hours after the compound was administered. Excretion of chlorhexidine gluconate occurred primarily through the feces (≈ 90%). Less than 1% of the chlorhexidine gluconate ingested by these subjects was excreted in the urine.

➤*Microbiology:* Chlorhexidine gluconate is active against a broad spectrum of microbes. The chlorhexidine molecule, due to its positive charge, reacts with the microbial cell surface, destroys the integrity of the cell membrane, penetrates into the cell, precipitates the cytoplasm, and the cell dies. Studies with chlorhexidine gluconate chip showed reductions in the numbers of the putative periodontopathic organisms *Porphyromonas (Bacteriodes) gingivalis*, *Prevotella (Bacteriodes) intermedia*, *Bacteriodes forsythus*, and *Campylobacter rectus* (*Wolinella recta*) after placement of the chip. No overgrowth of opportunistic organisms or other adverse changes in the oral microbial ecosystem were noted. The relationship of the microbial findings to clinical outcome has not been established.

Contraindications

Hypersensitivity to chlorhexidine gluconate or other formula ingredients.

Warnings/Precautions

➤*Calculus deposits:* The effect of chlorhexidine gluconate oral rinse on periodontitis has not been determined. An increase in supragingival calculus was noted in clinical testing with users of chlorhexidine gluconate oral rinse compared with control users. It is not known if chlorhexidine gluconate use results in an increase in subgingival calculus. Calculus deposits should be removed by a dental prophylaxis at intervals not greater than 6 months. Hypersensitivity and generalized allergic reactions have occurred (see Contraindications).

➤*Abscessed periodontal pocket:* The use of chlorhexidine gluconate chip in an acutely abscessed periodontal pocket has not been studied and therefore is not recommended. Management of patients with periodontal disease should include consideration of potentially contributing medical disorders, such as cancer, diabetes, and immunocompromised status.

➤*Gingivitis and periodontitis:* For patients having coexisting gingivitis and periodontitis, the presence or absence of gingival inflammation following treatment with chlorhexidine gluconate oral rinse should not be used as a major indicator of underlying periodontitis.

➤*Staining:* Chlorhexidine gluconate oral rinse can cause staining of oral surfaces, such as tooth surfaces, restorations, and the dorsum of the tongue. Not all patients will experience a visually significant increase in tooth staining. In clinical testing, 56% of the chlorhexidine gluconate oral rinse users exhibited a measurable increase in facial anterior stain, compared to 35% of control users after 6 months; 15% of the chlorhexidine gluconate users developed what was judged to be heavy stain, compared to 1% of control users after 6 months. Stain will be more pronounced in patients who have heavier accumulations of unremoved plaque.

Stain resulting from the use of chlorhexidine gluconate oral rinse does not adversely affect health of the gingivae or other oral tissues. Stain can be removed from most tooth surfaces by conventional professional prophylactic techniques. Additional time may be required to complete the prophylaxis.

Discretion should be used when prescribing to patients with anterior facial restorations with rough surfaces or margins. If natural stain cannot be removed from these surfaces by a dental prophylaxis, patients should be excluded from chlorhexidine gluconate oral rinse treatment if permanent discoloration is unacceptable. Stain in these areas may be difficult to remove by dental prophylaxis and on rare occasions may necessitate replacement of these restorations.

➤*Taste perception alteration:* Some patients may experience an alteration in taste perception while undergoing treatment with a chlorhexidine gluconate oral rinse. Rare instances of permanent taste alteration following chlorhexidine gluconate oral rinse use have been reported via postmarketing surveillance.

➤*Pregnancy:*

Chip – *Category C.* While chlorhexidine is known to be very poorly absorbed from the GI tract, it may be absorbed following placement within a periodontal pocket. Therefore, it is unclear whether these data are relevant

CHLORHEXIDINE GLUCONATE — ORAL

to clinical use of chlorhexidine gluconate chip. In clinical studies, placement of 4 chlorhexidine gluconate chips within periodontal pockets resulted in plasma concentrations of chlorhexidine that were at or below the limit of detection. However, it is not known whether chlorhexidine gluconate chip can cause fetal harm when administered to a pregnant woman or can affect reproductive capacity. Chlorhexidine gluconate chip should be used in a pregnant woman only if clearly needed.

Rinse – Category B. Adequate and well-controlled studies in pregnant women have not been done. Because animal reproduction studies are not always predictive of human response, this drug should be used during pregnancy only if clearly needed.

➤*Lactation:* It is not known whether this drug is excreted in human milk. Because many drugs are excreted in human milk, caution should be exercised when chlorhexidine gluconate is administered to a nursing woman.

➤*Children:* Clinical safety and efficacy of chlorhexidine gluconate oral rinse have not been established in children younger than 18 years of age.

Adverse Reactions

➤*Chip:* The most frequently observed adverse events in the 2 pivotal clinical trials were toothache, upper respiratory tract infection, and headache. Toothache was the only adverse reaction that was significantly higher (P = 0.042) in the chlorhexidine gluconate chip group when compared to placebo. Most oral pain or sensitivity occurred within the first week of the initial chip placement following SRP procedures, was mild to moderate in nature, and spontaneously resolved within days. These reactions were observed less frequently with subsequent chip placement at 3 and 6 months.

Chlorhexidine Gluconate Chip Adverse Reactions From 2 Five-Center US Clinical Trials (≥ 1%)

	Chlorhexidine gluconate chip (n = 225)		Placebo chip (n = 222)	
Adverse reaction	n	%	n	%
All patients with adverse events	193	85.8%	189	85.1%
Toothache[a]	114	50.7%	92	41.4%
Upper respiratory tract infection	64	28.4%	58	26.1%
Headache	61	27.1%	61	27.5%
Sinusitis	31	13.8%	29	13.1%
Influenza-like symptoms	17	7.6%	21	9.5%
Back pain	15	6.7%	25	11.3%
Tooth disorder[b]	14	6.2%	15	6.8%
Bronchitis	14	6.2%	7	3.2%
Abscess	13	5.8%	13	5.9%
Pain	11	4.9%	11	5%
Allergy	9	4%	13	5.9%
Myalgia	9	4%	9	4.1%
Gum hyperplasia	8	3.6%	5	2.3%
Pharyngitis	8	3.6%	5	2.3%
Arthralgia	7	3.1%	13	5.9%
Dysmenorrhea	7	3.1%	13	5.9%
Dyspepsia	7	3.1%	6	2.7%
Rhinitis	6	2.7%	11	5%
Coughing	6	2.7%	7	3.2%
Arthrosis	6	2.7%	4	1.8%
Hypertension	5	2.2%	6	2.7%
Stomatitis ulcerative	5	2.2%	1	0.5%
Tendinitis	5	2.2%	1	0.5%

[a] Includes dental, gingival or mouth pain, tenderness, aching, throbbing, soreness, discomfort or sensitivity.
[b] Includes broken, cracked or fractured teeth, mobile teeth, and lost bridges, crowns, or fillings.

➤*Rinse:* The most common side effects associated with chlorhexidine gluconate oral rinses are an increase in staining of teeth and other oral surfaces, an increase in calculus formation, and an alteration in taste perception (see Precautions). Oral irritation and local allergy-type symptoms have been spontaneously reported as side effects associated with use of chlorhexidine gluconate rinse. The following oral mucosal side effects were reported during placebo-controlled adult clinical trials: Aphthous ulcer, grossly obvious gingivitis, trauma, ulceration, erythema, desquamation, coated tongue, keratinization, geographic tongue, mucocele, and short frenum. Each occurred at a frequency of less than 1%.

Among postmarketing reports, the most frequently reported oral mucosal symptoms associated with chlorhexidine gluconate oral rinse are stomatitis, gingivitis, glossitis, ulcer, dry mouth, hypesthesia, glossal edema, and paresthesia.

Minor irritation and superficial desquamation of the oral mucosa have been noted in patients using chlorhexidine gluconate oral rinses.

There have been cases of parotid gland swelling and inflammation of the salivary glands (sialadenitis) reported in patients using chlorhexidine gluconate oral rinse.

Overdosage

Ingestion of 1 or 2 ounces of chlorhexidine gluconate oral rinse by a small child (≈ 10 kg body weight) might result in gastric distress, including nausea, or signs of alcohol intoxication. Medical attention should be sought if more than 4 ounces of chlorhexidine gluconate oral rinse is ingested by a small child or if signs of alcohol intoxication develop.

Patient Information

Patients should avoid dental floss at the site of chlorhexidine gluconate chip insertion for 10 days after placement, because flossing might dislodge the chip. All other oral hygiene may be continued as usual. No restrictions regarding dietary habits are needed. Dislodging of the chlorhexidine gluconate chip is uncommon; however, patients should be instructed to notify the dentist promptly if the chlorhexidine gluconate chip dislodges. Patients should also be advised that, although some mild to moderate sensitivity is normal during the first week after placement of chlorhexidine gluconate chip, they should notify the dentist promptly if pain, swelling, or other problems occur.

CARBAMIDE PEROXIDE (Urea Peroxide)

otc	**Cankaid Liquid** (Dickinson)	**Solution:** 10% in anhydrous glycerol	EDTA. In 22.5 mL.
otc	**Gly-Oxide Liquid** (GlaxoSmithKline)	**Solution:** 10%	In 15 and 60 mL.
otc	**Orajel Perioseptic** (Del)	**Liquid:** 15%	Saccharin, sorbitol, EDTA, methylparaben, ethyl alcohol. In 240 mL.

CARBAMIDE PEROXIDE — ORAL

Indications

➤*Liquid:*

Oral hygiene – For everyday use, to improve oral hygiene as an aid to regular brushing or when regular brushing is inadequate or impossible (eg, total care geriatrics). Carbamide peroxide kills germs to reduce mouth odors and odors on dental appliances. Carbamide peroxide penetrates between teeth and other areas of the mouth to flush out food particles ordinary brushing can miss. Carbamide peroxide also helps remove stains on dental appliances to improve appearance.

Specific dental problems – For temporary (problem) use, carbamide peroxide cleanses canker sores and minor wounds or gum inflammation resulting from minor dental procedures, dentures, orthodontic appliances, accidental injury or other irritations of the mouth and gums. Carbamide peroxide can also be used to guard against the risk of infections in the mouth and gums.

Administration and Dosage

➤*Adults:*

Oral hygiene – For everyday use, apply carbamide peroxide to the toothbrush (it will sink into the brush), cover with toothpaste, brush normally, and spit out.

Specific dental problems – For temporary (problem) use, apply several drops directly from bottle onto affected area; spit out after 2 to 3 minutes. Use up to 4 times daily after meals and at bedtime or as directed, or place 10 drops on tongue, mix with saliva, swish for several minutes, and then spit out.

➤*Children:* See Adults for dosing for children 2 years of age and older.

➤*Administration:* Do not dilute.

➤*Storage/Stability:* Protect from excessive heat and direct sunlight.

CARBAMIDE PEROXIDE — ORAL

Actions

➤*Pharmacology:* Carbamide peroxide releases oxygen to help gently remove unhealthy tissue, then cleanse and soothe canker sores and minor wounds and inflammations. It also inhibits odor-forming bacteria.

Warnings/Precautions

➤*Monitoring:* Severe or persistent oral inflammation, denture irritation, or gingivitis may be serious. If these conditions or unexpected side effects occur, consult a dentist or health care provider immediately. Avoid contact with eyes.

➤*Pregnancy:* Category C (per Hale's *Medications and Mothers' Milk*). Carbamide peroxide's transfer to the plasma is minimal, if at all.

➤*Lactation:* According to Hale's *Medications and Mothers' Milk*, it would be impossible for carbamide peroxide to reach breast milk unless under extreme overdose.

➤*Children:* Do not use for children younger than 2 years of age unless directed by a dentist or health care provider. Supervise children younger than 12 years of age in the use of this product.

Keep out of reach of children. In case of accidental overdose, seek professional assistance or contact poison control immediately.

Patient Information

Severe or persistent oral inflammation, denture irritation, or gingivitis may be serious. If these or unexpected side effects occur, consult health care provider or dentist promptly.

Discontinue use if condition persists or worsens.

PILOCARPINE HYDROCHLORIDE

Rx	**Pilocarpine Hydrochloride** (Various, eg, Actavis Elizabeth, Purepac, Sandoz)	**Tablets; oral:** 5 mg	In 100s.
Rx	**Salagen** (Eisai)		(MGI 705). White. Film-coated. In 100s.
Rx	**Pilocarpine Hydrochloride** (Actavis Elizabeth)	**Tablets; oral:** 7.5 mg	(SAL 7.5). Blue. Film-coated. In 100s.
Rx	**Salagen** (Eisai)		(SAL 7.5). Blue. Film-coated. In 100s.

PILOCARPINE HYDROCHLORIDE — ORAL

Indications

➤*Dry mouth:* Treatment of symptoms of dry mouth from salivary gland hypofunction caused by radiotherapy for cancer of the head and neck; treatment of symptoms of dry mouth in patients with Sjögren's syndrome.

➤*Off-label uses:*

Keratoconjunctivitis sicca (dry eye syndrome) – [2] = Fair documentation. Controlled clinical trials of oral pilocarpine suggest that it can effectively reduce keratoconjunctivitis sicca in patients with Sjögren syndrome, although not all patients respond to treatment. Most studies show that a total daily dose of 20 mg is effective, but some patients may require 30 mg per day. Sweating occurs with a high incidence, appears to be dose-related, and may lead to discontinuation in some patients. (See Administration and Dosage.)

Other possible off-label uses – Relief of dry mouth in patients with graft-versus-host disease.

Administration and Dosage

➤*Adults:*

Dry mouth –

Head and neck cancer patients:

- *Initial dosage* – 5 mg 3 times/day.
- *Maintenance dosage* – 15 to 30 mg/day (not to exceed 2 tablets/dose).

Use the lowest dose that is tolerated and effective.

- *Dosage adjustment* – Adjust dosage according to therapeutic response and tolerability. The incidence of the most common adverse events increases with dose.
- *Duration of therapy* – Although early improvement may be realized, at least 12 weeks of uninterrupted therapy may be necessary to assess whether a beneficial response will be achieved.

Sjogren syndrome: 5 mg 4 times/day. Efficacy was established by 6 weeks of use.

Off-label dosing –

Keratoconjunctivitis sicca (dry eye syndrome): [2] = Fair documentation. 5 mg orally 4 times per day. Some patients may require 30 mg/day. Total daily doses of 10 to 30 mg in divided doses 2 to 4 times per day have been studied for short-term use of up to 12 weeks' duration. Pilocarpine also has been evaluated as a 5 mg buccal insert used 3 times per day.

➤*Hepatic function impairment:*

Severe hepatic function impairment (Child-Pugh score of 10 to 15) – Use is not recommended.

Moderate hepatic function impairment (Child-Pugh score of 7 to 9) – The starting dose should be 5 mg twice daily, followed by adjustment based on therapeutic response and tolerability.

Mild hepatic function impairment (Child-Pugh score of 5 to 6) – Dosage reduction not required.

➤*Storage/Stability:* Store at 15° to 30°C (59° to 86°F).

Actions

➤*Pharmacology:* Pilocarpine is a cholinergic parasympathomimetic agent exerting a broad spectrum of pharmacologic effects with predominant muscarinic action. Pilocarpine in appropriate dosage can increase secretion by the exocrine glands. The sweat, salivary, lacrimal, gastric, pancreatic, intestinal glands, and the mucous cells of the respiratory tract may be stimulated. Dose-related smooth muscle stimulation of the intestinal tract may cause increased tone, increased motility, spasm, and tenesmus. Bronchial smooth muscle tone may increase. The tone and motility of urinary tract, gallbladder, and biliary duct smooth muscle may be enhanced. Pilocarpine may have paradoxical effects on the cardiovascular system. The expected effect of a muscarinic agonist is vasodepression, but administration of pilocarpine may produce hypertension after a brief episode of hypotension. Bradycardia and tachycardia have been reported with use of pilocarpine.

➤*Pharmacokinetics:*

Absorption – In a multiple-dose pharmacokinetic study in male volunteers following 2 days of 5 or 10 mg oral pilocarpine given at 8 am, noon, and 6 pm, the t_{max} was 1.25 and 0.85 hours and C_{max} was 15 and 41 ng/mL, respectively. The AUC was 33 and 108 ng•h/mL, respectively, following the last 6-hour dose.

In a study in 12 healthy male volunteers, there was a dose-related increase in unstimulated salivary flow following single 5 and 10 mg oral doses. The stimulatory effect was time-related with an onset at 20 minutes and peak at 1 hour with a duration of 3 to 5 hours.

Effect of food: When taken with a high-fat meal, there was a decrease in the rate of absorption of pilocarpine. Mean T_{max} was 1.47 and 0.87 hours and mean C_{max} was 51.8 and 59.2 ng/mL for fed and fasted states, respectively.

Excretion – In a multiple-dose pharmacokinetic study in male volunteers following 2 days of 5 or 10 mg oral pilocarpine given at 8 am, noon, and 6 pm, the mean elimination half-life was 0.76 and 1.35 hours for the 5 and 10 mg doses, respectively.

Inactivation of pilocarpine is thought to occur at neuronal synapses and probably in plasma. Pilocarpine and its minimally active or inactive degradation products, including pilocarpic acid, are excreted in the urine.

Special populations –

Hepatic function impairment: In patients with mild to moderate hepatic function impairment (n = 12), administration of a single 5 mg dose resulted in a 30% decrease in total plasma clearance and a doubling of exposure (as measured by AUC). Peak plasma levels also were increased by about 30% and half-life was increased to 2.1 hours.

Elderly: In 5 healthy elderly female volunteers, the mean C_{max} and AUC were approximately twice that of elderly males and young healthy male volunteers.

Contraindications

Uncontrolled asthma; hypersensitivity to pilocarpine; when miosis is undesirable (eg, in acute iritis and in narrow-angle [angle closure] glaucoma).

Warnings/Precautions

➤*Cardiovascular disease:* Patients with significant cardiovascular disease may be unable to compensate for transient changes in hemodynamics or rhythm induced by pilocarpine. Pulmonary edema has been reported as a complication of pilocarpine toxicity from high ocular doses given for acute angle-closure glaucoma. Administer pilocarpine with caution and under close medical supervision in patients with significant cardiovascular disease.

The dose-related cardiovascular effects of pilocarpine include hypotension, hypertension, bradycardia, and tachycardia.

➤*Ocular effects:* Ocular formulations of pilocarpine have caused visual blurring, which may result in decreased visual acuity, especially at night and in patients with central lens changes, and impairment of depth perception. Advise caution while driving at night or performing hazardous activities in reduced lighting.

➤*Pulmonary disease:* Pilocarpine increases airway resistance, bronchial smooth muscle tone, and bronchial secretions. Administer with caution and under close medical supervision in patients with controlled asthma, chronic bronchitis, or chronic obstructive pulmonary disease requiring pharmacologic therapy.

➤*Toxicity:* Pilocarpine toxicity is characterized by an exaggeration of its parasympathomimetic effects. These may include the following: Headache; visual disturbance; lacrimation; sweating; respiratory distress; GI spasm; nausea; vomiting; diarrhea; AV block; tachycardia; bradycardia; hypotension; hypertension; shock; mental confusion; cardiac arrhythmia; tremors.

➤*Biliary tract:* Administer with caution to patients with known or suspected cholelithiasis or biliary tract disease. Contractions of the gallbladder

PILOCARPINE HYDROCHLORIDE — ORAL

or biliary smooth muscle could precipitate complications including cholecystitis, cholangitis, and biliary obstruction.

➤*Renal colic:* Pilocarpine may increase ureteral smooth muscle tone and could theoretically precipitate renal colic (or ureteral reflux), particularly in patients with nephrolithiasis.

➤*Psychiatric disorder:* Cholinergic agonists may have dose-related CNS effects. Consider this when treating patients with underlying cognitive or psychiatric disturbances.

➤*Hepatic function impairment:* Based on decreased plasma clearance observed in patients with moderate hepatic impairment, the starting dose in these patients should be 5 mg twice daily, followed by adjustment based on therapeutic response and tolerability. Patients with mild hepatic insufficiency (Child-Pugh score of 5 to 6) do not require dosage reductions. To date, pharmacokinetic studies in subjects with severe hepatic impairment (Child-Pugh score of 10 to 15) have not been carried out. The use of pilocarpine in these patients is not recommended.

➤*Pregnancy: Category C.* Pilocarpine was associated with a reduction in mean fetal body weight and an increase in the incidence of skeletal variations when given to pregnant rats at a dosage of 90 mg/kg/day (approximately 26 times the maximum recommended dose for a 50 kg human). These effects may have been secondary to maternal toxicity. In another study, oral administration of pilocarpine to female rats during gestation and lactation at a dosage of 36 mg/kg/day (approximately 10 times the maximum recommended dose for a 50 kg human when compared on the basis of body surface area (mg/m^2) estimates) resulted in an increased incidence of stillbirths; decreased neonatal survival and reduced mean body weight of pups were observed at dosages of 18 mg/kg/day (approximately 5 times the maximum recommended dose for a 50 kg human when compared on the basis of body surface area (mg/m^2) estimates) and above. There are no adequate and well-controlled studies in pregnant women. Use during pregnancy only if the potential benefit justifies the potential risk to the fetus.

Fertility impairment – The data obtained in animal studies suggest that pilocarpine may impair the fertility of male and female humans. Administer pilocarpine tablets to individuals who are attempting to conceive a child only if the potential benefit justifies potential fertility impairment.

➤*Lactation:* It is not known whether this drug is excreted in breast milk. Because of the potential for serious adverse reactions in nursing infants, decide whether to discontinue nursing or to discontinue the drug, taking into account the importance of the drug to the mother.

➤*Children:* Safety and efficacy in children have not been established.

➤*Elderly:* In placebo-controlled trials in Sjogren's syndrome patients, the mean age of patients was approximately 55 years of age (range, 21 to 85 years of age). The adverse events reported by those over 65 years of age and those 65 years of age and younger were comparable except for notable trends for urinary frequency, diarrhea, and dizziness.

Drug Interactions

Pilocarpine Oral Drug Interactions			
Precipitant drug	Object drug[a]		Description
Pilocarpine	Anticholinergics	⬇	Pilocarpine may antagonize the anticholinergic effects of drugs used concomitantly. Consider these effects when anticholinergic properties may be contributing to the therapeutic effect of concomitant medication (eg, atropine, inhaled ipratropium).
Pilocarpine	Beta blockers	⬆	Use coadministration with caution because of possible conduction disturbances.

[a] ⬆ = Object drug increased. ⬇ = Object drug decreased.

➤*Drug/Food interactions:* The rate of absorption of pilocarpine is decreased when taken with a high-fat meal. Maximum concentration is decreased and time to reach maximum concentration is increased.

Adverse Reactions

➤*Head and neck cancer patients:*

Pilocarpine Adverse Reactions (%)				
		Pilocarpine		
Adverse reaction	Placebo (n = 152)	5 mg tid (n = 141)	10 mg tid (n = 121)	5 or 10 mg tid (n = 212)
Sweating	9	29	68	-
Nausea	4	6	15	-
Rhinitis	7	5	14	-
Diarrhea	5	4	7	-
Chills	< 1	3	15	-
Flushing	3	8	13	-
Urinary frequency	7	9	12	-
Dizziness	4	5	12	-
Asthenia	3	6	12	-
Headache	8	-	-	11
Dyspepsia	5	-	-	7
Lacrimation	8	-	-	6
Edema	4	-	-	5
Abdominal pain	4	-	-	4
Amblyopia	2	-	-	4
Vomiting	1	-	-	4
Pharyngitis	8	-	-	3
Hypertension	1	-	-	3

The following events were reported at dosages of 7.5 to 30 mg/day (1% to 2%) – Abnormal vision, conjunctivitis, dysphagia, epistaxis, myalgias, pruritus, rash, sinusitis, tachycardia, taste perversion, tremor, voice alteration.

The following events also were reported (less than 1%). Causal relation is unknown. –

Cardiovascular: Bradycardia; ECG abnormality; palpitations; syncope.
CNS: Anxiety; confusion; depression; abnormal dreams; hyperkinesia; hypesthesia; nervousness; paresthesias; speech disorder; twitching.
GI: Anorexia; increased appetite; esophagitis; GI disorder; tongue disorder.
GU: Dysuria; metrorrhagia; urinary impairment.
Hematologic: Leukopenia; lymphadenopathy.
Respiratory: Increased sputum; stridor; yawning.
Special senses: Deafness; eye pain; glaucoma.
Miscellaneous: Body odor; hypothermia; mucous membrane abnormality; seborrhea. In long-term treatment of 2 patients with underlying cardiovascular disease, 1 experienced an MI and the other an episode of syncope.

➤*Sjogren's syndrome patients:* The adverse events reported by those over 65 years of age and those 65 years of age and younger were comparable except for notable trends for urinary frequency, diarrhea, and dizziness. The incidences of urinary frequency and diarrhea in the elderly were about double those in the nonelderly. The incidence of dizziness was about 3 times as high in the elderly as in the nonelderly. These adverse experiences were not considered to be serious. In the 2 placebo-controlled studies, the most common adverse events related to drug use were sweating, urinary frequency, chills, and vasodilation (flushing). The most commonly reported reason for patient discontinuation of treatment was sweating. Expected pharmacologic effects of pilocarpine include the following adverse experiences.

Pilocarpine Adverse Experiences (%)		
Adverse event	5 mg qid (20 mg/day) (n = 255)	Placebo qid (n = 253)
Sweating	40	7
Urinary frequency	10	4
Nausea	9	9
Flushing	9	2
Rhinitis	7	8
Diarrhea	6	7
Chills	4	2
Increased salivation	4	0
Asthenia	2	2
Headache	13	19
Flu syndrome	9	9
Dyspepsia	7	7
Dizziness	6	7
Pain	4	2
Sinusitis	4	5
Abdominal pain	3	4
Vomiting	3	1
Pharyngitis	2	5
Rash	2	3
Infection	2	6

The following events were reported in Sjogren's syndrome patients at incidences of 1% to 2% at dosing of 20 mg/day: Accidental injury; allergic reaction; back pain; blurred vision; constipation; increased cough; edema; epistaxis; face edema; fever; flatulence; glossitis; lab test abnormalities, including chemistry, hematology, and urinalysis; myalgia; palpitation; pruritus; somnolence; stomatitis; tachycardia; tinnitus; urinary incontinence, urinary tract infection; vaginitis.

The following events were reported rarely in Sjogren's syndrome patients (fewer than 1%) at dosing of 10 to 30 mg/day. Causal relation is unknown.

Cardiovascular: Angina pectoris, arrhythmia, ECG abnormality, hypotension, hypertension, intracranial hemorrhage, migraine, MI.
CNS: Abnormal dreams, abnormal thinking, aphasia, confusion, depression, emotional lability, hyperkinesia, hypesthesia, insomnia, leg cramps, nervousness, paresthesias, tremor.
Dermatologic: Alopecia, contact dermatitis, dry skin, eczema, erythema nodosum, exfoliative dermatitis, herpes simplex, skin ulcer, vesiculobullous rash.
GI: Abnormal liver function tests, anorexia, bilirubinemia, cholelithiasis, colitis, dry mouth, eructation, gastritis, gastroenteritis, GI disorder, gingivi-

PILOCARPINE HYDROCHLORIDE — ORAL

tis, hepatitis, increased sputum, melena, nausea and vomiting, pancreatitis, parotid gland enlargement, salivary gland enlargement, taste loss, tongue disorder, tooth disorder.

GU: Breast pain, dysuria, mastitis, menorrhagia, metrorrhagia, ovarian disorder, pyuria, salpingitis, urethral pain, urinary urgency, vaginal hemorrhage, vaginal moniliasis.

Hematologic: Abnormal WBC, abnormal platelets, hematuria, lymphadenopathy, thrombocythemia, thrombocytopenia, thrombosis.

Metabolic/Nutritional: Hypoglycemia, peripheral edema.

Musculoskeletal: Arthralgia, arthritis, bone disorder, myasthenia, pathological fracture, spontaneous bone fracture, tendon disorder, tenosynovitis.

Respiratory: Bronchitis, dyspnea, hiccough, laryngismus, laryngitis, pneumonia, viral infection, voice alteration.

Special senses: Abnormal vision, cataract, conjunctivitis, dry eyes, ear disorder, ear pain, eye disorder, eye hemorrhage, glaucoma, lacrimation disorder, retinal disorder, taste perversion.

Miscellaneous: Chest pain, cyst, death, moniliasis, neck pain, neck rigidity, photosensitivity reaction.

The following adverse experiences have been reported rarely with ocular pilocarpine: AV block, agitation, ciliary congestion, confusion, delusion, depression, dermatitis, eyelid twitching, iris cysts, macular hole, malignant glaucoma, middle ear disturbance, shock, and visual hallucination.

Overdosage

Pilocarpine fatal overdosage resulting from poisoning has been reported at doses presumed to be greater than 100 mg in 2 hospitalized patients; 100 mg is considered potentially fatal. Treat overdosage with atropine titration (0.5 to 1 mg SC or IV) and use supportive measures to maintain respiration and circulation. Epinephrine (0.3 to 1 mg SC or IM) also may be of value in the presence of severe cardiovascular depression or bronchoconstriction. Refer to General Management of Acute Overdosage. It is not known if pilocarpine is dialyzable.

Patient Information

Inform patients that pilocarpine may cause visual disturbances, especially at night, that could impair their ability to drive safely.

If a patient sweats excessively while taking pilocarpine and cannot drink enough liquid, have the patient consult a physician. Dehydration may develop.

MAGIC MOUTHWASH

Rx	**First Mouthwash BLM** (CutisPharma)	**Suspension; oral:** diphenhydramine hydrochloride 0.2 g, lidocaine hydrochloride 1.6 g, aluminum hydroxide 3.15 g, magnesium hydroxide 3.15 g, simethicone 0.315 g	Benzyl alcohol, parabens, saccharin, sorbitol. In compounding kits.
Rx	**First BXN Mouthwash** (CutisPharma)	**Suspension; oral:** diphenhydramine hydrochloride 0.2 g, lidocaine hydrochloride 1.6 g, nystatin 1.6 g	Alcohol, benzyl alcohol, FD&C yellow #5, propylparaben, saccharin, sorbitol. In compounding kits.
Rx	**First Duke's Mouthwash** (Cutis Pharma)	**Suspension; oral:** 0.525 g diphenhydramine hydrochloride, 0.06 g hydrocortisone, 0.6 g nystatin	Benzyl alcohol, propylene glycol, propylparabens, saccharin, sorbitol. In 237 mL compounding kits.
Rx	**First Mary's Mouthwash** (Cutis Pharma)	**Suspension; oral:** 0.45 g diphenhydramine hydrochloride, 0.06 g hydrocortisone, 1.2 g nystatin, 1.5 g tetracycline hydrochloride	Benzyl alcohol, propylene glycol, propylparabens, saccharin, sorbitol. In 237 mL compounding kits.

MAGIC MOUTHWASH — ORAL

Indications

This product is not Food and Drug Administration approved.

➤*Off-label uses:* Palliation of generalized oral mucositis.

Administration and Dosage

➤*General dosing considerations:* There are numerous formulations for "magic mouthwash." Verify the desired formulation and dosage with the prescribing health care provider.

The most common ingredients used to compound "magic mouthwash" are diphenhydramine, lidocaine 2% viscous, magnesium hydroxide/aluminum hydroxide, nystatin, and corticosteroids (eg, hydrocortisone, prednisone). According to one study, the inclusion of nystatin is not rational, and the efficacy of corticosteroids has not been adequately studied.

➤*Adults:* Dosage depends on the prescribed formulation.

Usual dosage – For diphenhydramine/lidocaine 2%/antacid (1:1:1), the dosage is 15 mL swished in the mouth for 30 seconds, then spit out. May be used every 2 to 3 hours. According to one study, "magic mouthwash" has been prescribed to be given every 4 hours, every 6 hours, every 8 hours, every 1 to 2 hours, every 12 hours, and as needed.

➤*Children:* No well-established guidelines are available.

Palliation of generalized oral mucositis –

Maximum dose: The maximum recommended topical dose of lidocaine 2% viscous is 3 mg/kg/dose at intervals of at least 2 hours.

➤*Preparation for administration:* Prior to dispensing, tap the top and bottom of the bottles to loosen the powder. Shake the bottle of the mouthwash liquid suspension for a few minutes. Empty the contents of one bottle into the mouthwash liquid suspension. Residual quantities remaining in the bottles after emptying need not be rinsed out. Close the bottle and shake for 20 to 30 seconds. Repeat with the remaining bottles.

Extemporaneous compounding – To compound a suspension containing diphenhydramine (12.5 mg per 5 mL), an antacid, and lidocaine 2% viscous solution, mix in equal proportions (1:1:1). Shake well.

Diphenhydramine syrup may be preferred over diphenhydramine elixir because the syrup contains less alcohol, which may irritate the oral mucosa.

Antacids that are commonly used include the following:

- Magnesium hydroxide 200 mg per 5 mL, aluminum hydroxide 225 mg per 5 mL
- Magnesium hydroxide 200 mg per 5 mL, aluminum hydroxide 200 mg per 5 mL, simethicone 20 mg per 5 mL.

➤*Administration:* For oral use only. Shake suspension well before each use. Generally, instruct the patient to swish the suspension in the mouth for 30 seconds then spit out.

➤*Storage/Stability:*

First Mouthwash BLM – Prior to compounding, store at 15° to 30°C (59° to 86°F). Store final compounded formulation at 15° to 30°C (59° to 86°F). The compounded product is stable for at least 6 months at room temperature. Protect from light and freezing.

First BXN Mouthwash – Prior to compounding, store at room temperature, not to exceed 25°C (77°F). Store final compounded formulation at 2° to 8°C (36° to 46°F). The compounded product is stable for at least 15 days when stored in the refrigerator. Keep container tightly closed. Protect from light and freezing.

Extemporaneous compounding – Store at room temperature. Protect from light. No stability information is available for this preparation. When a manufactured final dosage-form product is used as a source of active ingredient, it may be appropriate to assign an expiration date of up to 25% of the manufacturer's remaining date, or 6 months, whichever method gives the shortest expiry.

Actions

➤*Pharmacology:* Diphenhydramine and lidocaine provide local analgesia. The antacid (magnesium hydroxide/aluminum hydroxide) component is thought to coat the oral mucosa. Tetracycline is an anti-infective that inhibits protein synthesis and hydrocortisone is a corticosteroid that depresses formation, release, and activity of endogenous mediators of inflammation. Some formulations also contain nystatin, but nystatin has not shown efficacy and fungal infections are not common in patients with chemotherapy-induced oral mucositis.

Contraindications

Hypersensitivity to any component of the product; hypersensitivity to local anesthetics of the amide type (lidocaine only). Oral diphenhydramine is contraindicated in newborns or premature infants and breast-feeding women.

Warnings/Precautions

➤*Local anesthesia:* Lidocaine is a local anesthetic that can impair the gag reflex. This increases the risk of aspiration when eating. Advise patients to be careful when eating; the numbness this drug produces may cause them to bite their tongues or the inside of their mouths. It may also cause decreased heat sensation. Caution patients to avoid eating for at least 1 hour after the administration of viscous lidocaine.

➤*Traumatized mucosa:* Advise patients to use lidocaine with extreme caution if the mucosa in the area of application has been traumatized because under such conditions there is the potential for rapid systemic absorption.

➤*Excessive doses:* Excessive dosage, or short intervals between doses, can result in high plasma levels and serious adverse effects. Instruct patients to strictly adhere to the recommended administration and dosage guidelines.

➤*Hypersensitivity reactions:* Use lidocaine with caution in patients with known drug sensitivities. Patients allergic to para-aminobenzoic acid derivatives (eg, procaine, tetracaine, benzocaine) have not shown cross-sensitivity to lidocaine.

➤*Pregnancy: Category B* (diphenhydramine, lidocaine); *Category C* (nystatin).

Diphenhydramine – Both the animal data and the published human experience suggest that diphenhydramine is safe for use during human pregnancy. The exception is a case-control study showing an association with cleft palate. In addition, premature infants exposed within 2 weeks of

MAGIC MOUTHWASH — ORAL

birth may be at risk for toxicity. At least one review has concluded that diphenhydramine is the drug of choice if parenteral antihistamines are indicated in pregnancy.

Lidocaine – Lidocaine is considered to be compatible with pregnancy. Lidocaine may produce CNS depression in the newborn with high serum levels. The Collaborative Perinatal Project monitored 50,282 mother-child pairs, 293 of whom had exposure to lidocaine during the first trimester. No evidence of an association with large classes of malformations was found. Greater than expected risks were found for anomalies of the respiratory tract (3 cases), tumors (2 cases), and inguinal hernias (8 cases), but the statistical significance is unknown and independent confirmation is required. For use any time during pregnancy, 947 exposures were recorded. From these data, no evidence of an association with large categories of major or minor malformations or to individual defects was found.

Nystatin – Nystatin is poorly absorbed after oral administration and from intact skin and mucous membranes.

➤*Lactation:*

Diphenhydramine – Diphenhydramine is excreted into human breast milk, but levels have not been reported. Although the levels are not thought to be sufficiently high to affect the infant after therapeutic doses, most manufacturers consider the drug contraindicated in breast-feeding mothers. The reason given for this is the increased sensitivity of newborn or premature infants to antihistamines.

Lidocaine – Small amounts of lidocaine are excreted into breast milk. The American Academy of Pediatrics classifies lidocaine as compatible with breast-feeding.

Nystatin – Because nystatin is poorly absorbed, if at all, serum and milk levels would not occur.

➤*Children:* No well-established pediatric dosage guidelines are available.

Drug Interactions

No known interactions.

Adverse Reactions

➤*CNS:* Drowsiness or any CNS adverse effects (11%).

➤*GI:* Constipation, diarrhea, nausea (11%); dry mouth.

➤*Special senses:* Taste disturbances (49%); burning/tingling in the oral cavity (29%).

➤*Miscellaneous:* Hypersensitivity reactions.

Overdosage

➤*Symptoms:* Excessive use or overdose of lidocaine may result in systemic toxicity. Children younger than 2 years of age are at increased risk of overdose with therapeutic use. Symptoms include initial drowsiness followed by CNS excitation or depression, seizures, tinnitus, blurred vision, bradycardia, and hypotension. Seizures have occurred with doses as low as 5 to 30 mL of lidocaine 2% to 4% viscous.

Patient Information

Advise patients to shake the suspension well before each use.

Advise patients that lidocaine is a local anesthetic that can impair the gag reflex. This increases the risk of aspiration when eating. Advise patients to be careful when eating; the numbness this drug produces may cause them to bite their tongue or the inside of their mouth.

Advise patients that lidocaine may also cause decreased heat sensation. Caution patients to avoid eating for at least 1 hour after the administration of viscous lidocaine.

CEVIMELINE HYDROCHLORIDE

Rx	**Evoxac** (Daiichi Pharm.)	**Capsules:** 30 mg	Lactose. White. In 100s and 500s.

CEVIMELINE HYDROCHLORIDE — ORAL

Indications

➤*Dry mouth:* For the treatment of symptoms of dry mouth in patients with Sjögren's syndrome.

Administration and Dosage

➤*Adults:*

Dry mouth associated with Sjögren's syndrome – 30 mg 3 times a day.

➤*Storage/Stability:* Store at 25°C (77°F); excursion is permitted to 15° to 30°C (59°to 86° F).

Actions

➤*Pharmacology:*

Pharmacodynamics – Cevimeline hydrochloride is a cholinergic agonist which binds to muscarinic receptors. Muscarinic agonists in sufficient dosage can increase secretion of exocrine glands, such as salivary and sweat glands and increase tone of the smooth muscle in the GI and urinary tracts.

➤*Pharmacokinetics:*

Absorption – After administration of a single 30 mg capsule, cevimeline hydrochloride was rapidly absorbed with a mean time to peak concentration of 1.5 to 2 hours. No accumulation of active drug or its metabolites was observed following multiple-dose administration. When administered with food, there is a decrease in the rate of absorption, with a fasting T_{max} of 1.53 hours and a T_{max} of 2.86 hours after a meal; the peak concentration is reduced by 17.3%. Single oral doses across the clinical dose range are dose proportional.

Distribution – Cevimeline hydrochloride has a volume of distribution of ≈ 6 L/kg and is less than 20% bound to human plasma proteins. This suggests that cevimeline hydrochloride is extensively bound to tissues; however, the specific binding sites are unknown.

Metabolism – Isozymes CYP2D6 and CYP3A3/4 are responsible for the metabolism of cevimeline hydrochloride. After 24 hours, 86.7% of the dose was recovered (16% unchanged, 44.5% as cis and trans-sulfoxide, 22.3% of the dose as glucuronic acid conjugate and 4% of the dose as N-oxide of cevimeline hydrochloride). Approximately 8% of the trans-sulfoxide metabolite is then converted into the corresponding glucuronic acid conjugate and eliminated. Cevimeline hydrochloride did not inhibit cytochrome P450 isozymes 1A2, 2A6, 2C9, 2C19, 2D6, 2E1, and 3A4.

Excretion – The mean half-life of cevimeline is 5 ± 1 hours. After 24 hours, 84% of a 30 mg dose of cevimeline hydrochloride was excreted in urine. After 7 days, 97% of the dose was recovered in the urine and 0.5% was recovered in the feces.

Contraindications

Uncontrolled asthma, hypersensitivity to cevimeline hydrochloride, and when miosis is undesirable (eg, in acute iritis and in narrow-angle [angle-closure] glaucoma).

Warnings/Precautions

➤*Cardiovascular disease:* Cevimeline hydrochloride can potentially alter cardiac conduction or heart rate. Patients with significant cardiovascular disease may potentially be unable to compensate for transient changes in hemodynamics or rhythm induced by cevimeline hydrochloride. Cevimeline hydrochloride should be used with caution and under close medical supervision in patients with a history of cardiovascular disease evidenced by angina pectoris or myocardial infarction (MI).

➤*Pulmonary disease:* Cevimeline hydrochloride can potentially increase airway resistance, bronchial smooth muscle tone, and bronchial secretions. Cevimeline hydrochloride should be administered with caution and with close medical supervision to patients with controlled asthma, chronic bronchitis, or chronic obstructive pulmonary disease.

➤*Ocular:* Ophthalmic formulations of muscarinic agonists have been reported to cause visual blurring which may result in decreased visual acuity, especially at night and in patients with central lens changes, and to cause impairment of depth perception. Caution should be advised while driving at night or performing hazardous activities in reduced lighting.

➤*Toxicity:* Cevimeline hydrochloride toxicity is characterized by an exaggeration of its parasympathomimetic effects. These may include headache, visual disturbance, lacrimation, sweating, respiratory distress, GI spasm, nausea, vomiting, diarrhea, atrioventricular block, tachycardia, bradycardia, hypotension, hypertension, shock, mental confusion, cardiac arrhythmia, and tremors.

➤*Special risk:* Cevimeline hydrochloride should be administered with caution to patients with a history of nephrolithiasis or cholelithiasis. Contractions of the gallbladder or biliary smooth muscle could precipitate complications such as cholecystitis, cholangitis and biliary obstruction. An increase in the ureteral smooth muscle tone could theoretically precipitate renal colic or ureteral reflux in patients with nephrolithiasis.

➤*Hazardous tasks:* Ophthalmic formulations of muscarinic agonists have been reported to cause visual blurring which may result in decreased visual acuity, especially at night and in patients with central lens changes, and to cause impairment of depth perception. Caution should be advised while driving at night or performing hazardous activities in reduced lighting.

➤*Pregnancy:* Category C.

Cevimeline hydrochloride was associated with a reduction in the mean number of implantations when given to pregnant Sprague-Dawley rats from 14 days prior to mating through day 7 of gestation at a dosage of 45 mg/kg/day (≈ 5 times the maximum recommended dose for a 60 kg human when compared on the basis of body surface area estimates). This effect may have been secondary to maternal toxicity. There are no adequate and well-controlled studies in pregnant women. Cevimeline hydrochloride should be used during pregnancy only if the potential benefit justifies the potential risk to the fetus.

➤*Lactation:* It is not known whether this drug is secreted in human milk. Because many drugs are excreted in human milk, and because of the potential for serious adverse reactions in nursing infants from cevimeline hydrochloride, a decision should be made whether to discontinue nursing or discontinue the drug, taking into account the importance of the drug to the mother.

➤*Children:* Safety and effectiveness in pediatric patients have not been established.

➤*Elderly:* Although clinical studies of cevimeline hydrochloride included subjects over the age of 65, the numbers were not sufficient to determine whether they respond differently from younger subjects. Special care should

CEVIMELINE HYDROCHLORIDE — ORAL

be exercised when cevimeline hydrochloride treatment is initiated in an elderly patient, considering the greater frequency of decreased hepatic, renal, or cardiac function, and of concomitant disease or other drug therapy in the elderly.

Drug Interactions

Drugs which inhibit CYP2D6 and CYP3A3/4 also inhibit the metabolism of cevimeline hydrochloride. Cevimeline hydrochloride should be used with caution in individuals known or suspected to be deficient in CYP2D6 activity, based on previous experience, as they may be at a higher risk of adverse events. In an in vitro study cytochrome P450 isozymes 1A2, 2A6, 2C9, 2C19, 2D6, 2E1, and 3A4 were not inhibited by exposure to cevimeline hydrochloride.

Cevimeline Drug Interactions

Precipitant drug	Object drug[a]		Description
Cevimeline	Beta blockers	↑	Administer cevimeline with caution to patients taking beta adrenergic antagonists because of the possibility of conduction disturbances.
Cevimeline	Parasympathomimetics	↑	Drugs with parasympathomimetic effects administered concurrently with cevimeline may be expected to have additive effects.
Cevimeline	Antimuscarinics	↓	Cevimeline might interfere with desirable antimuscarinic effects of drugs used concomitantly.

[a] ↑ = Object drug increased. ↓ = Object drug decreased.

➤*Drug/Food interactions:* See Actions for more information.

Adverse Reactions

The following adverse events associated with muscarinic agonism were observed in the clinical trials of cevimeline hydrochloride in Sjögren's syndrome patients:

Cevimeline Adverse Reactions Associated with Muscarinic Agonism

Adverse reaction	Cevimeline 30 mg (3 times daily) n = 533[a]	Placebo (3 times daily) n = 164
Excessive sweating	18.7%	2.4%
Nausea	13.8%	7.9%
Rhinitis	11.2%	5.4%
Diarrhea	10.3%	10.3%
Excessive salivation	2.2%	0.6%
Urinary frequency	0.9%	1.8%
Asthenia	0.5%	0%
Flushing	0.3%	0.6%
Polyuria	0.1%	0.6%

[a] N is the total number of patients exposed to the dose at any time during the study.

In addition, the following adverse events (≥ 3% incidence) were reported in the Sjögren's clinical trials:

Cevimeline Adverse Reactions (≥ 3%)

Adverse reaction	Cevimeline 30 mg (3 times daily) n = 533[a]	Placebo (3 times daily) n = 164
Headache	14.4%	20.1%
Sinusitis	12.3%	10.9%
Upper respiratory tract infection	11.4%	9.1%
Dyspepsia	7.8%	8.5%
Abdominal pain	7.6%	6.7%
Urinary tract infection	6.1%	3%
Coughing	6.1%	3%
Pharyngitis	5.2%	5.4%
Vomiting	4.6%	2.4%
Injury	4.5%	2.4%
Back pain	4.5%	4.2%
Rash	4.3%	6%
Conjunctivitis	4.3%	3.6%
Dizziness	4.1%	7.3%
Bronchitis	4.1%	1.2%
Arthralgia	3.7%	1.8%
Surgical intervention	3.3%	3%
Fatigue	3.3%	1.2%
Pain	3.3%	3%
Skeletal pain	2.8%	1.8%
Insomnia	2.4%	1.2%
Hot flushes	2.4%	0%
Rigors	1.3%	1.2%
Anxiety	1.3%	1.2%

[a] N is the total number of patients exposed to the dose at any time during the study.

The following events were reported in Sjögren's patients at incidences of less than 3% and ≥ 1%: Constipation, tremor, abnormal vision, hypertonia, peripheral edema, chest pain, myalgia, fever, anorexia, eye pain, ear ache, dry mouth, vertigo, salivary gland pain, pruritus, influenza-like symptoms, eye infection, post-operative pain, vaginitis, skin disorder, depression, hiccup, hyporeflexia, infection, fungal infection, sialoadenitis, otitis media, erythematous rash, pneumonia, edema, salivary gland enlargement, allergy, gastroesophageal reflux, eye abnormality, migraine, tooth disorder, epistaxis, flatulence, tooth ache, ulcerative stomatitis, anemia, hypoesthesia, cystitis, leg cramps, abscess, eructation, moniliasis, palpitation, increased amylase, xerophthalmia, allergic reaction.

The following events were reported rarely in treated Sjögren's patients (less than 1%) (causal relation is unknown):

➤*Cardiovascular:* Abnormal ECG, heart disorder, heart murmur, aggravated hypertension, hypotension, arrhythmia, extrasystoles, t wave inversion, tachycardia, supraventricular tachycardia, angina pectoris, myocardial infarction, pericarditis, pulmonary embolism, peripheral ischemia, superficial phlebitis, purpura, deep thrombophlebitis, vascular disorder, vasculitis, hypertension.

➤*CNS:* Carpal tunnel syndrome, coma, abnormal coordination, dysesthesia, dyskinesia, dysphonia, aggravated multiple sclerosis, involuntary muscle contractions, neuralgia, neuropathy, paresthesia, speech disorder, agitation, confusion, depersonalization, aggravated depression, abnormal dreaming, emotional lability, manic reaction, paroniria, somnolence, abnormal thinking, hyperkinesia, hallucination.

➤*Dermatologic:* Acne, alopecia, burn, dermatitis, contact dermatitis, lichenoid dermatitis, eczema, furunculosis, hyperkeratosis, lichen planus, nail discoloration, nail disorder, onychia, onychomycosis, paronychia, photosensitivity reaction, rosacea, scleroderma, seborrhea, skin discoloration, dry skin, skin exfoliation, skin hypertrophy, skin ulceration, urticaria, verruca, bullous eruption, cold clammy skin, basal cell carcinoma, squamous carcinoma.

➤*Endocrine:* Increased glucocorticoids, goiter, hypothyroidism.

➤*GI:* Appendicitis, increased appetite, ulcerative colitis, diverticulitis, duodenitis, dysphagia, enterocolitis, gastric ulcer, gastritis, gastroenteritis, gastrointestinal hemorrhage, gingivitis, glossitis, rectum hemorrhage, hemorrhoids, ileus, irritable bowel syndrome, melena, mucositis, esophageal stricture, esophagitis, oral hemorrhage, peptic ulcer, periodontal destruction, rectal disorder, stomatitis, tenesmus, tongue discoloration, tongue disorder, geographic tongue, tongue ulceration, dental caries.

➤*GU:* Epididymitis, prostatic disorder, abnormal sexual function, amenorrhea, female breast neoplasm, malignant female breast neoplasm, female breast pain, positive cervical smear test, dysmenorrhea, endometrial disorder, intermenstrual bleeding, leukorrhea, menorrhagia, menstrual disorder, ovarian cyst, ovarian disorder, genital pruritus, uterine hemorrhage, vaginal hemorrhage, atrophic vaginitis, albuminuria, bladder discomfort, increased blood urea nitrogen, dysuria, hematuria, micturition disorder, nephrosis, nocturia, increased nonprotein nitrogen, pyelonephritis, renal calculus, abnormal renal function, renal pain, strangury, urethral disorder, abnormal urine, urinary incontinence, decreased urine flow, pyuria.

➤*Hematologic:* Thrombocytopenic purpura, thrombocythemia, thrombocytopenia, hypochromic anemia, eosinophilia, granulocytopenia, leucopenia, leukocytosis, cervical lymphadenopathy, lymphadenopathy.

➤*Hepatic:* Cholelithiasis, increased gamma-glutamyl transferase, increased hepatic enzymes, abnormal hepatic function, viral hepatitis, increased serum AST, increased serum ALT.

➤*Immunologic:* Cellulitis, herpes simplex, herpes zoster, bacterial infection, viral infection, genital moniliasis, sepsis.

➤*Metabolic/Nutritional:* Dehydration, diabetes mellitus, hypercalcemia, hypercholesterolemia, hyperglycemia, hyperlipemia, hypertriglyceridemia, hyperuricemia, hypoglycemia, hypokalemia, hyponatremia, thirst.

➤*Musculoskeletal:* Arthritis, aggravated arthritis, arthropathy, femoral head avascular necrosis, bone disorder, bursitis, costochondritis, plantar fasciitis, muscle weakness, osteomyelitis, osteoporosis, synovitis, tendinitis, tenosynovitis, aggravated rheumatoid arthritis, lupus erythematosus rash, lupus erythematosus syndrome.

➤*Respiratory:* Asthma, bronchospasm, chronic obstructive airway disease, dyspnea, hemoptysis, laryngitis, nasal ulcer, pleural effusion, pleurisy, pulmonary congestion, pulmonary fibrosis, respiratory disorder.

➤*Special senses:* Deafness, decreased hearing, motion sickness, parosmia, taste perversion, blepharitis, cataract, corneal opacity, corneal ulceration, diplopia, glaucoma, anterior chamber eye hemorrhage, keratitis, keratoconjunctivitis, mydriasis, myopia, photopsia, retinal deposits, retinal disorder, scleritis, vitreous detachment, tinnitus.

CEVIMELINE HYDROCHLORIDE — ORAL

➤*Miscellaneous:* Aggravated allergy, precordial chest pain, abnormal crying, hematoma, leg pain, edema, periorbital edema, activated pain trauma, pallor, changed sensation temperature, weight decrease, weight increase, choking, mouth edema, syncope, malaise, face edema, substernal chest pain, fall, food poisoning, heat stroke, joint dislocation, post-operative hemorrhage.

In 1 subject with lupus erythematosus receiving concomitant multiple drug therapy, a highly elevated ALT level was noted after the fourth week of cevimeline hydrochloride therapy. In 2 other subjects receiving cevimeline hydrochloride in the clinical trials, very high AST levels were noted. The significance of these findings is unknown.

Additional adverse events – Additional adverse events (relationship unknown) which occurred in other clinical studies (patient population different from Sjögren's patients) are as follows:

Cholinergic syndrome, blood pressure fluctuation, cardiomegaly, postural hypotension, aphasia, convulsions, abnormal gait, hyperesthesia, paralysis, abnormal sexual function, enlarged abdomen, change in bowel habits, gum hyperplasia, intestinal obstruction, bundle branch block, increased creatine phosphokinase, electrolyte abnormality, glycosuria, gout, hyperkalemia, hyperproteinemia, increased lactic dehydrogenase (LDH), increased alkaline phosphatase, failure to thrive, abnormal platelets, aggressive reaction, amnesia, apathy, delirium, delusion, dementia, illusion, impotence, neurosis, paranoid reaction, personality disorder, hyperhemoglobinemia, apnea, atelectasis, yawning, oliguria, urinary retention, distended vein, lymphocytosis.

Overdosage

➤*Treatment:* Management of the signs and symptoms of acute overdosage should be handled in a manner consistent with that indicated for other muscarinic agonists; general supportive measures should be instituted. If medically indicated, atropine, an anticholinergic agent, may be of value as an antidote for emergency use in patients who have had an overdose of cevimeline hydrochloride. If medically indicated, epinephrine may also be of value in the presence of severe cardiovascular depression or bronchoconstriction. It is not known if cevimeline hydrochloride is dialyzable.

Patient Information

Patients should be informed that cevimeline hydrochloride may cause visual disturbances, especially at night, that could impair their ability to drive safely.

If a patient sweats excessively while taking cevimeline hydrochloride, dehydration may develop. The patient should drink extra water and consult a health care provider.

SALIVA SUBSTITUTES

otc	**Saliva Substitute** (Roxane)	**Solution; oral:** Sorbitol, sodium carboxymethylcellulose, methylparaben	In 120 mL bottle.
otc	**Moi-Stir** (Kingswood)	**Solution; oral:** Dibasic sodium phosphate, magnesium, calcium chloride, sodium chloride, and potassium chlorides, sorbitol, sodium carboxymethylcellulose, parabens	In 120 mL spray.
otc	**Moi-Stir Swabsticks** (Kingswood)	**Swabsticks; oral:** Dibasic sodium phosphate, magnesium, calcium chloride, sodium chloride, and potassium chlorides, sorbitol, sodium carboxymethylcellulose, parabens	In packets (3s).
otc	**Entertainer's Secret** (KLI Corp)	**Solution; oral:** Sodium carboxymethylcellulose, potassium chloride, dibasic sodium phosphate, parabens, aloe vera gel, glycerin	In 60 mL spray.
otc	**Salivart** (Gebauer)	**Solution; oral:** Sodium carboxymethylcellulose, sorbitol, sodium chloride, potassium chloride, calcium chloride, magnesium chloride, dibasic potassium phosphate, nitrogen (as propellant)	Preservative-free. In 75 mL aerosol spray cans.
otc	**MouthKote** (Parnell)	**Solution; oral:** Xylitol, sorbitol, yerba santa, citric acid, ascorbic acid, sodium benzoate, saccharin	Lemon-lime flavor. In 60 and 240 mL spray.
Rx	**Caphosol** (EUSA Pharma)	**Solution; oral:** Dibasic sodium phosphate 3.2 g, monobasic sodium phosphate 0.9 g, calcium chloride 5.2 g, sodium chloride 56.9 g	Vanilla flavor. In 30 and 120 dose boxes (1 dose = two 15 mL amps mixed together).
Rx	**Aquoral** (Bi-Coastal Pharmaceutical)	**Spray, solution; oral:** Aspartame, oxidized glycerol triesters, phenylalanine, silicon dioxide	In 40 mL spray pump (400 sprays per pump).
Rx	**Numoisyn** (Align)	**Solution; oral:** Sorbitol, linseed (flaxseed) extract, *Chondrus crispus*, parabens, sodium benzoate, potassium sorbate, dipotassium phosphate	In 30 and 300 mL.
		Lozenges; oral: 0.3 g sorbitol, polyethylene glycol, malic acid, sodium citrate, calcium phosphate dibasic, hydrogenated cottonseed oil, citric acid, magnesium stearate, silicon dioxide	In 100s.
otc sf	**Salese** (Nuvora)	**Lozenges; oral:** Eucalyptus oil, glyceryl, lemon oil, sucralose, thymol, wintergreen oil, xylitol, zinc	Alcohol free, sugar free. In 12s.
otc	**SalivaSure** (Scandinavian Formulas)	**Lozenges; oral:** Apple acid, citric acid, dibasic calcium phosphate, xylitol	Citrus flavor. In 90s.
otc	**NeutraSal** (Invado Pharmaceuticals)	**Powder; oral:** 50 mg calcium chloride, 10 mg dibasic sodium phosphate, 10 mg monobasic sodium phosphate, 2 mg silicon dioxide, 450 mg sodium chloride, 16 mg sodium bicarbonate	In individual packets of 30s and 120s.

SALIVA SUBSTITUTES — ORAL

Indications

➤*Dry mouth and throat:* These products are used as saliva substitutes to relieve dry mouth and throat in xerostomia, which may be caused by the following: Surgery or radiation near the salivary glands; chemotherapy; Sjogren syndrome; Bell palsy; HIV/AIDS; lupus; diabetes; aging; emotional factors; dry throat; scratchy, hoarse voice; medications (eg, antidepressants, antihistamines, antihypertensives); infection or dysfunction of the salivary glands.

Administration and Dosage

➤*Maximum dose:*
Lozenges – 16/day.

➤*Adults:*
Dry mouth and throat –
Lozenges:
• *Usual dosage* – Dissolve slowly in the mouth when needed. To obtain optimal effect, move the lozenge around in the mouth. Repeat as necessary.

Spray: Hold close to mouth and spray for one-half second or less to relieve dryness. May be used as often as needed to moisten and lubricate; may swallow or expectorate.

Swabsticks: Swab and cleanse all intraoral surfaces for 2 to 3 minutes using all 3 disposable swabsticks. Repeat procedure every 3 to 4 hours while awake or more frequently if needed.

➤*Storage/Stability:* Store at 15° to 30°C (59° to 86°F). Protect from direct sunlight and heat greater than 38°C (100°F).

DOXYCYCLINE

For complete prescribing information, refer to the Doxycycline monograph in the Tetracycline section of the Systemic Anti-Infectives chapter.

MINOCYCLINE HYDROCHLORIDE

For prescribing information, refer to the Minocycline monograph in the Tetracyclines in the Anti-infective chapter.

AMLEXANOX

Rx	**Aphthasol** (Discus Dental)	**Paste; oral:** 5%	Benzyl alcohol, mineral oil, petrolatum. In 5 g.

AMLEXANOX — ORAL

Indications

➤*Aphthous ulcers:* For the treatment of aphthous ulcers in people with normal immune systems.

Administration and Dosage

➤*General dosing considerations:* The paste should be applied as soon as possible after noticing the symptoms of an aphthous ulcer.

AMLEXANOX — ORAL

➤*Adults:*

Aphthous ulcers –

Usual dosage: Apply approximately ¼ inch (0.5 cm) of paste onto a finger tip and apply to the ulcer. Repeat for each ulcer. Use 4 times daily, preferably following oral hygiene after breakfast, lunch, dinner, and at bedtime. (See Administration for more information.)

Duration of therapy: Use of the medication should be continued until the ulcer heals. If significant healing or pain reduction has not occurred in 10 days, consult the dentist or physician.

➤*Administration:*

1.) Dry the ulcer(s) by gently patting it with a soft, clean cloth.
2.) Wash hands before applying amlexanox oral paste.
3.) Moisten the tip of the index finger.
4.) Squeeze a dab of paste approximately ¼ inch (0.5 cm) onto a finger tip.
5.) Gently dab the oral paste onto the ulcer. Repeat the process onto each ulcer.
6.) Wash hands immediately after applying amlexanox oral paste.

➤*Storage / Stability:* Store at 15° to 30°C (59° to 86°F).

Actions

➤*Pharmacology:* The mechanism of action by which amlexanox accelerates healing of aphthous ulcers is unknown. In vitro studies have demonstrated amlexanox to be a potent inhibitor of the formation or release of inflammatory mediators (histamine and leukotrienes) from mast cells, neutrophils and mononuclear cells. Given orally to animals, amlexanox has demonstrated antiallergenic and anti-inflammatory activities and has been shown to suppress both immediate and delayed type hypersensitivity reactions. The relevance of these activities of amlexanox to its effects on aphthous ulcers has not been established.

➤*Pharmacokinetics:* After a single oral application of 100 mg of paste (5 mg amlexanox), maximal serum levels of approximately 120 ng/mL are observed at 2.4 hours. Most of the systemic absorption of amlexanox is via the gastrointestinal tract, and the amount absorbed directly through the active ulcer is not a significant portion of the applied dose. The half-life for elimination was 3.5 ± 1.1 hours in healthy individuals. Approximately 17% of the dose is eliminated into the urine as unchanged amlexanox, a hydroxylated metabolite, and their conjugates. With multiple applications 4 times daily, steady-state levels were reached within 1 week, and no accumulation was observed with up to 4 weeks of use.

Contraindications

Hypersensitivity to amlexanox or other ingredients in the formulation.

Warnings/Precautions

➤*Local irritation:* Wash hands immediately after applying amlexanox oral paste directly to ulcers with the finger tips. In the event that a rash or contact mucositis occurs, discontinue use.

➤*Pregnancy: Category B.* There are no adequate and well-controlled studies in pregnant women. Because animal reproduction studies are not always predictive of human response, this drug should be used during pregnancy only if clearly needed.

➤*Lactation:* Amlexanox was found in the milk of lactating rats; therefore, caution should be exercised when administering amlexanox oral paste to a nursing woman.

➤*Children:* Safety and effectiveness of amlexanox oral paste in pediatric patients have not been established.

➤*Elderly:* Clinical studies of amlexanox oral paste did not include sufficient numbers of subjects aged 65 and over to determine whether they respond differently from younger subjects. Other reported clinical experience has not identified differences in responses between the elderly and younger patients. In general, dose selection for an elderly patient should be cautious, usually starting at the low end of the dosing range, reflecting the greater frequency of decreased hepatic, renal, or cardiac function, and of concomitant disease or other drug therapy.

Adverse Reactions

Adverse reactions considered related or possibly related to amlexanox oral paste were not reported by more than 5% of patients. Adverse reactions reported by 1% to 2% of patients were transient pain, stinging or burning at the site of application. Infrequent (less than 1%) adverse reactions in the clinical studies were contact mucositis, nausea, and diarrhea.

Overdosage

There are no reports of human ingestion overdosage. Ingestion of a full tube of 5 g of paste would result in systemic exposure well below the maximum nontoxic dose of amlexanox in animals. Gastrointestinal upset such as diarrhea and vomiting could result from an overdose.

SULFURIC ACID/SULFONATED PHENOLICS

Rx	**Debacterol** (Epien Medical[a])	**Liquid**: 30% sulfuric acid and 50% sulfonated phenolics	In 1.5 mL.

[a] Epien Medical, Inc., 4225 White Bear Parkway, Suite 600, St. Paul, MN 55110-3389; (888) 884-4675, (651) 653-3380, fax (651) 653-8569

SULFURIC ACID/SULFONATED PHENOLICS — ORAL

Indications

➤*Ulcerating lesions:* Topical treatment of ulcerating lesions of the oral cavity, such as recurrent aphthous stomatitis (canker sores). Provides relief from pain and discomfort of oral mucosal ulcers.

Not intended for the treatment of vesicular lesions, such as cold sores or fever blisters.

Administration and Dosage

➤*Adults:*

Ulcerating lesions – One application per ulcer treatment is usually sufficient. However, if the ulcer pain returns shortly after rinsing with water, it is an indication that some part of the ulcer was not covered with the sulfuric acid/sulfonated phenolics liquid. A second application should then be applied to the ulcer immediately during the same treatment session until the patient remains pain-free after the ulcer rinsing. It is not recommended that more than 1 treatment session be performed on any individual mucosal ulcer. Do not reapply the product to the same lesion after the patient is free of pain. See Administration for more information.

➤*Children:* See Adults for dosing for children 12 years of age and older.

➤*Administration:* Immediately before applying, thoroughly dry the ulcerated area of oral mucosa that is to be treated using a sterile cotton-tipped applicator or some similar method. After drying the lesion, hold swab with the colored ring end up. Bend the colored ring tip gently to the side until it snaps to release the liquid inside. Liquid flows down into the white tip applicator. Then apply the coated applicator directly to the dried ulcer bed. A very brief stinging sensation is experienced immediately upon application of the liquid to the ulcer. Hold the cotton-tipped applicator in contact with the ulcer for at least 5 seconds while using a rolling motion to thoroughly coat the entire ulcer bed, the ulcer rim, and the surrounding halo of normal mucosa. Do not hold the applicator on the ulcer for more than 10 seconds. The sulfuric acid/sulfonated phenolics liquid will not harm the normal oral mucosa when used as directed. Then thoroughly rinse out the mouth with water and spit out the rinse water. The stinging sensation and ulcer pain will subside almost immediately after the water rinse.

If excess irritation occurs during use, a rinse with sodium bicarbonate (baking soda) solution will neutralize the reaction (use 2.5 mL in 120 mL of water).

➤*Storage / Stability:* Store at 15° to 30°C (59° to 86°F).

Actions

➤*Pharmacology:* The liquid contains sulfonated phenolics, which are antiseptic agents with topical analgesic properties, and sulfuric acid, which is a tissue denaturant and sterilizing agent, in an aqueous solution.

Contraindications

Known allergy to sulfonated phenolics.

Warnings/Precautions

➤*Allergy:* Do not use if allergic to sulfonated phenolics.

➤*Prolonged use:* Because of its nature, prolonged use on normal tissue should be avoided. The sulfuric acid/sulfonated phenolics liquid will eventually necrotize and slough all tissue to which it is applied in sufficient volume; apply carefully.

➤*External use only:* Avoid eye contact.

➤*Pregnancy: Category C.* Safety and efficacy in pregnant women has not been established.

➤*Lactation:* There is no information regarding the use of this drug in breast-feeding women.

➤*Children:* Safety and efficacy in children younger than 12 years of age have not been established. Keep out of the reach of children.

Adverse Reactions

May cause local irritation upon administration. If excess irritation occurs during use, a rinse with sodium bicarbonate (baking soda) solution will neutralize the reaction (use 2.5 mL in 120 mL of water).

Indications

➤*Sore throat and irritation:* Minor sore throat and minor irritation of the throat or mouth.

Administration and Dosage

Do not use for more than 2 days or in children younger than 2 years of age, unless directed by physician. For dosage guidelines, refer to the specific package labeling.

Actions

➤*Pharmacology:*

Benzocaine and dyclonine – Benzocaine and dyclonine are local anesthetics.

Cetylpyridinium chloride, eucalyptus oil, thymol and hexylresorcinol – Cetylpyridinium chloride, eucalyptus oil, thymol, and hexylresorcinol have antiseptic activity.

Menthol, camphor, capsicum, dyclonine and phenol – Menthol, camphor, capsicum, dyclonine, and phenol are used for their antipruritic, local anesthetic and counterirritant activities.

Hydrocortisone and triamcinolone (corticosteroids) – Hydrocortisone and triamcinolone (corticosteroids) are used for their anti-inflammatory activities.

Warnings/Precautions

➤*Severe/Persistent sore throat:* Severe and persistent sore throat or sore throat accompanied by high fever, headache, nausea and vomiting may be serious. Consult physician promptly.

➤*Tartrazine sensitivity:* Some of these products contain tartrazine (FD&C Yellow No. 5), which may cause allergic-type reactions (including bronchial asthma) in susceptible individuals. Although the incidence of sensitivity is low, it is frequently seen in patients who also have aspirin hypersensitivity. Specific products containing tartrazine are identified in the product listings.

LOZENGES AND TROCHES

otc sf	**Sucrets Defense Kid's Formula** (Insight)	**Lozenges; oral:** 3.9 mg vitamin C, 0.93 mg zinc, 20 mg glutathione	Acesulfame K, tartrazine. Tropical fruit and grape flavors. In 18s.
otc	**Vicks Children's Chloraseptic** (Richardson-Vicks)	**Lozenges; oral:** 5 mg benzocaine	Corn syrup, sucrose. Grape flavor. In 18s.
otc	**Spec-T** (Apothecon)	**Lozenges; oral:** 10 mg benzocaine	Sucrose. In 10s.
otc	**Cēpacol Sore Throat** (Combe)	**Lozenges; oral:** 10 mg benzocaine, 2 mg menthol	Glucose, sucrose. Menthol flavor. In 18s.
otc	**Cēpacol Sore Throat** (Combe)	**Lozenges; oral:** 10 mg benzocaine, 2.1 mg menthol	Glucose, sucrose. Citrus flavor. In 18s.
otc	**Cēpacol Sore Throat** (Combe)	**Lozenges; oral:** 10 mg benzocaine, 2.6 mg menthol	Glucose, sucrose. Honey-lemon flavor. In 18s.
otc	**Cēpacol Sore Throat** (Combe)	**Lozenges; oral:** 10 mg benzocaine, 3.6 mg menthol	Glucose, sucrose. Cherry flavor. In 18s.
otc sf	**Cēpacol Sore Throat** (Combe)	**Lozenges; oral:** 10 mg benzocaine, 4.5 mg menthol	Sorbitol. Cherry flavor. In 16s.
otc sf	**Mycinettes** (Pfeiffer)	**Lozenges; oral:** 15 mg benzocaine	Sorbitol, saccharin, menthol. Cherry flavor. In 12s.
otc	**Chloraseptic Sore Throat Maximum Numbing** (Prestige)	**Lozenges; oral:** 6 mg benzocaine, 10 mg menthol	Acesulfame K, glucose, sucrose. Honey lemon, cherry, and menthol flavors. In 18s.
otc	**Cēpacol Sore Throat** (Combe)	**Lozenges; oral:** 15 mg benzocaine, 3.6 mg menthol	Sucrose. Cherry flavor. In 18s.
otc sf	**Cēpacol Sore Throat Maximum Strength** (Combe)	**Lozenges; oral:** 15 mg benzocaine, 4 mg menthol	Sugar free. Acesulfame K, maltitol. Cherry flavor. In 16s.
otc sf	**Cēpacol Sore Throat + Coating Relief Maximum Numbing** (Combe)	**Lozenges; oral:** 15 mg benzocaine, 5 mg pectin	Sugar free. Acesulfame K. Lemon lime flavor. In 18s.
otc sf	**Cylex** (Pharmakon)	**Lozenges; oral:** 15 mg benzocaine, 5 mg cetylpyridinium chloride	Sorbitol. Cherry flavor. In 12s.
otc	**Cēpacol Throat** (J.B. Williams)	**Lozenges; oral:** 0.07% cetylpyridinium chloride, 0.3% benzyl alcohol	Tartrazine. In 27s and 40s.
otc	**Sucrets Children's Formula** (Insight Pharmaceuticals)	**Lozenges; oral:** 1.2 mg dyclonine hydrochloride	Corn syrup, menthol, sucrose. Cherry flavor. In 18s.
otc	**Sucrets Original Formula Sore Throat Wild Cherry** (Insight Pharmaceuticals)	**Lozenges; oral:** 2 mg dyclonine hydrochloride	Corn syrup, menthol, sucrose. Cherry flavor. In 24s.
otc	**Sucrets Maximum Strength Sore Throat** (Insight Pharmaceuticals)	**Lozenges; oral:** 3 mg dyclonine hydrochloride	Corn syrup, menthol, sucrose. Black cherry flavor. In 18s.
otc	**Sucrets Complete** (Insight Pharmaceuticals)	**Lozenges; oral:** 3 mg dyclonine hydrochloride, 3 mg menthol	Acesulfame K, corn syrup, sucrose. Cool citrus and vapor cherry flavors. In 18s.
otc	**Sucrets Original Formula Sore Throat Mint** (Insight Pharmaceuticals)	**Lozenges; oral:** 2.4 mg hexylresorcinol	Corn syrup, menthol, sucrose. Original mint flavor. In 18s.
otc	**Cēpacol Menthol Regular Strength** (Combe)	**Lozenges; oral:** 3 mg menthol	Glucose, peppermint oil, propylene glycol, sucrose. In blister pack 648s.
otc	**Cēpacol Sore Throat** (Combe)		Mint flavor. In 18s.
otc sf	**N'ice 'n Clear** (SK-Beecham)	**Lozenges; oral:** 5 mg menthol	Sorbitol. Cool peppermint, cherry eucalyptus, and menthol eucalyptus flavors. In 16s.
otc	**Robitussin Honey Cough** (Whitehall-Robins)		Herbal with natural honey center. Corn syrup, sorbitol, sucrose. In 20s.
			Honey lemon tea flavor: Corn syrup, sucrose. In 25s.
otc	**Sucrets Herbal** (Insight Pharmaceuticals)	**Lozenges; oral:** 5 mg menthol, 6 mg pectin	Acesulfame K, corn syrup, sucrose. Honey lemon ginseng and berry pomegranate flavors. In 18s.
otc	**Cēpacol Sore Throat Post Nasal Drip** (Combe)	**Lozenges; oral:** 5.4 mg menthol	Glucose, sucrose. Cherry flavor. In 18s.
otc	**Kof-Eze** (Roberts Med)	**Lozenges; oral:** 6 mg menthol	In 4s and 500s.
otc	**Menthol Cough Drops** (Major)	**Lozenges; oral:** 6.5 mg menthol	Eucalyptus oil, glucose syrup, sucrose. In 30s.
otc	**Extra Strength Vicks Cough Drops** (Richardson-Vicks)	**Lozenges; oral:** 8.4 mg menthol	Corn syrup, sucrose. Menthol flavor. In 9s and 30s.
otc	**Extra Strength Vicks Cough Drops** (Richardson-Vicks)	**Lozenges; oral:** 10 mg menthol	Corn syrup, sucrose. Cherry and honey lemon flavors. In 9s and 30s.
otc	**Maximum Strength Halls-Plus** (Warner-Lambert)	**Lozenges; oral:** 10 mg menthol	Corn syrup, sucrose. In regular, cherry, mentholyptus, and honey-lemon flavors. In 10s and 25s.
otc	**Robitussin Cough Drops** (Robins)	**Lozenges; oral:** 7.4 mg menthol, eucalyptus oil	Sucrose, corn syrup. (R). In cherry and menthol eucalyptus flavors. In 9s and 25s.
		10 mg menthol, eucalyptus oil	Sucrose, corn syrup. (R). Honey-lemon flavor. In 9s and 25s.

LOZENGES AND TROCHES

otc	**Vicks Menthol Cough Drops** (Richardson-Vicks)	**Lozenges; oral**: Menthol, thymol, eucalyptus oil, camphor, tolu balsam	Benzyl alcohol. Menthol flavor. In 14s and 40s.
otc sf	**Cepastat Cherry** (Heritage Consumer Prod.)	**Lozenges; oral**: 14.5 mg phenol, menthol	Saccharin, sorbitol. Cherry flavor. In 18s.
otc sf	**Cepastat Extra Strength** (Heritage Consumer Prod.)	**Lozenges; oral**: 29 mg phenol, menthol, eucalyptus oil	Sorbitol. In 18s.
otc	**Get Better Bear Sore Throat Pops** (Whitehall)	**Lozenge on a stick; oral**: 19 mg pectin	Corn syrup, sucrose, parabens. Cherry and grape flavors. In 10s.
otc sf	**Hall's Sugar Free Mentho-Lyptus** (Warner-Lambert)	**Tablets; oral**: 5 mg menthol, 2.8 mg eucalyptus oil	Citrus blend and black cherry flavors. In 25s.
		6 mg menthol, 2.8 mg eucalyptus oil	Mountain menthol flavor. In 25s.
otc	**Cēpacol Maximum Numbing Sore Throat** (Combe)	**Lozenges; oral**: 15 mg benzocaine, 3.6 mg menthol	Glucose, sucrose, potassium acesulfame, sodium bicarbonate. Cherry flavor. In 18s.
		Lozenges; oral: 15 mg benzocaine, 2.1 mg menthol	Maltitol, sucralose. Citrus flavor. In 18s.
		Lozenges; oral: 15 mg benzocaine, 2.6 mg menthol	Maltitol, sucralose. Honey lemon flavor. In 18s.
otc	**Cēpacol Sore Throat Post Nasal Drip** (Combe)	**Lozenges; oral**: 4.5 mg menthol	Glucose, sucrose. Cherry flavor. In 18s.
otc sf	**Cēpacol Sugar Free Maximum Numbing Sore Throat** (Combe)	**Lozenges; oral**: 15 mg benzocaine, 4 mg menthol	Sugar free. Maltitol, potassium acesulfame, sodium bicarbonate. Cherry flavor. In 16s.
otc	**Cēpacol Fizzlers** (Combe)	**Tablets, disintegrating; oral**: 6 mg benzocaine	Corn syrup, mannitol, sucralose, sodium bicarbonate. Grape flavor. In 12s.

MOUTHWASHES AND SPRAYS

otc	**TiSol** (Parnell)	**Solution**: 1% benzyl alcohol, 0.04% menthol, 0.9% isotonic NaCl	EDTA, sorbitol. In 237 mL.
Rx	**OraMagicRx** (MPM Medical)	**Powder for oral rinse**: *AloemannonPlus* (high molecular weight complex carbohydrates, mannons, and low molecular weight constituents extracted from aloe vera L), citric acid, lemon/lime flavor, maltodextrin, potassium benzoate, potassium sorbate, xanthan, xylitol	Alcohol free. In 25 and 37.5 g.
otc	**FreshBurst Listerine** (GlaxoWellcome)	**Rinse**: 0.064% thymol, 0.092% eucalyptol, 0.06% methyl salicylate, 0.042% menthol, 21.6% alcohol	Sorbitol, saccharin. In 250 mL.
otc	**Scope** (Procter & Gamble)	**Rinse**: Cetylpyridinium chloride, 67.9% SD alcohol 38-F	Tartrazine, saccharin. Original mint and wintergreen flavors. In 90, 180, 360, 720, 1,080, and 1,440 mL.
otc sf	**Sucrets** (SK-Beecham)	**Throat spray**: 0.1% dyclonine hydrochloride, 10% alcohol	Sorbitol. Mint and cherry flavors. In 90 and 180 mL.
otc sf	**Cepacol Dual Relief Sore Throat + Coating** (Combe)	**Spray**: 5% benzocaine, 33% glycerin	Sugar free. Acesulfame K, alcohol, castor oil. Cherry flavor. In 22.2 mL.
otc	**Cepacol Sore Throat** (Combe)	**Spray**: 0.1% dyclonine hydrochloride, 33% glycerin	Menthol. Cherry, honey-lemon, citrus, menthol, and sugar-free cherry flavors. In 118 mL.
otc	**N'ice** (SK-Beecham)	**Throat spray**: 0.12% menthol, 25% glycerin, 23% alcohol	Glucose, saccharin, sorbitol. Peppermint flavor. In 180 mL.
otc sf	**Chloraseptic Kids Sore Throat** (Prestige)	**Throat spray**: 0.5% phenol	Saccharin. Alcohol free. Grape flavor. In 177 mL.
otc sf	**Triaminic Sore Throat** (Novartis Consumer Health)		Alcohol free. Saccharin, sorbitol. Grape flavor. In 118 mL.
otc sf	**Chloraseptic Sore Throat** (Prestige)	**Throat spray**: 1.4% phenol	Saccharin. Alcohol free. Cherry, soothing citrus, menthol, and cool mint flavors. In 177 mL.
otc sf	**Sore Throat Spray** (Major)		Alcohol free. Saccharin. Cherry and menthol flavors. In 177 mL.
otc sf	**Phenaseptic** (Rugby)		Saccharin. Cherry flavor. In 177 mL.
otc sf	**Green Throat Spray** (Clay-Park Labs)		Alcohol free. Glycerin, saccharin. In 473 mL.
otc sf	**Red Throat Spray** (Clay-Park Labs)		Alcohol free. Glycerin, saccharin. In 177 mL.
otc	**Cheracol Sore Throat** (Roberts)	**Throat spray**: 1.4% phenol, 12.5% alcohol	Sorbitol, saccharin. Cherry flavor. In 180 mL.
otc sf	**Mycinette** (Pfeiffer)	**Throat spray**: 1.4% phenol, 0.3% alum (aluminum ammonium sulfate)	Alcohol free. Regular, cherry, mint, and cool blue menthol flavors. In 180 mL.
otc	**Throto-Ceptic** (S.S.S. Company)	**Spray/Gargle**: 1.4% phenol, 0.5% alum (aluminum ammonium sulfate)	Mint, cherry, cool blue menthol, or regular flavors. In 171 mL.
otc sf	**Vicks Chloraseptic** (Procter & Gamble)	**Mouthrinse/Gargle**: 1.4% phenol	Alcohol free. Saccharin. Menthol flavor. In 355 mL.
otc	**Bioténe with Calcium** (Laclede)	**Mouthwash**: Propylene glycol, xylitol, hydrogenated starch hydrosylate, poloxamer 407, hydroxyethylcellulose, sodium benzoate, peppermint, benzoic acid, zinc gluconate, aloe vera, calcium lactate, lactoferrin, lysozyme, lactoperoxidase, potassium thiocyanate, glucose oxidase	Alcohol free. In 474 mL.
otc sf	**Choice DM Gentle Care** (Bristol-Myers Squibb)	**Mouthwash**: Sorbitol, poloxamer 407, sodium, saccharin, flavor, cetylpyridinium chloride, citric acid, blue 1, yellow 5	Alcohol free. Fresh mint flavor. In 500 mL.
otc	**Listerine, Natural Citrus** (Pfizer Consumer)	**Mouthwash**: 0.064% thymol, 0.092% eucalyptol, 0.06% methyl salicylate, 0.042% menthol, 21.6% alcohol	Sorbitol, sucralose. In 250 and 500 mL and 1 and 1.5 L.
otc	**Listerine, Tartar Control** (Pfizer Consumer)	**Mouthwash**: 0.064% thymol, 0.092% eucalyptol, 0.06% methyl salicylate, 0.042% menthol, 21.6% alcohol	Sorbitol, sucrose. Wintermint flavor. In 250 and 500 mL and 1 and 1.5 L.

MOUTHWASHES AND SPRAYS

otc	**Listermint** (J & J Consumer)	**Mouthwash**: Glycerin, poloxamer 335, PEG 600, sodium lauryl sulfate, sodium benzoate, benzoic acid, zinc chloride	Alcohol free. Saccharin. In 960 mL.
otc	**Cepacol** (Combe)	**Mouthwash**: 0.05% cetylpyridinium chloride, 14% alcohol	Tartrazine, saccharin. In 360, 540, 720, and 960 mL.
otc	**Plax** (Pfizer Consumer Health)	**Mouthwash**: Sorbitol solution, 8.7% alcohol, tetrasodium pyrophosphate, benzoic acid, flavor, poloxamer 407, sodium benzoate, sodium lauryl sulfate, sodium saccharin, xanthan gum	Original, mint sensation, and softmint flavors. In 118, 237, 473, and 710 mL.
otc	**Listerine** (GlaxoWellcome)	**Mouthwash**: 0.06% thymol, 0.09% eucalyptol, 0.06% methyl salicylate, 0.04% menthol, 26.9% alcohol (regular flavor), 21.6% alcohol (cool mint flavor)	Sorbitol, saccharin (Cool Mint). Regular, cool mint flavors. In 90, 180, 360, 540, 720, 960, and 1,440 mL.
otc	**Phylorinol** (Schaffer)	**Mouthwash**: 0.6% phenol, methyl salicylate	Alcohol free. Sorbitol. In 240 mL.
otc	**Oral Wound Rinse** (Carrington Laboratories)	**Mouthwash**: Acemannan hydrogel	Fructose. In 7.4 g
otc	**Tonsiline** (Oakhurst)	**Mouthwash**: 4% alcohol, glycerin, sucrose, iron chloride, flavor, magnesium carbonate, tolu balsam, sodium saccharide	In 118 mL.
Rx	**MuGard** (Access Pharmaceuticals)	**Rinse; oral**: Benzyl alcohol, carbomer homopolymer A, citric acid, glycerin, potassium hydroxide, saccharin	In 237 mL.

MISCELLANEOUS MOUTH AND THROAT PREPARATIONS

otc sf	**Dentiva** (Nuvora)	**Lozenges; oral**: Eucalyptus oil, glycerol, menthol, peppermint oil, sucralose, wintergreen, xylitol, zinc	Alcohol free, sugar free. In 12s.
otc sf	**Salese** (Nuvora)	**Lozenges; oral**: Eucalyptus oil, glycerin, sucralose, peppermint oil, wintergreen oil, xylitol, zinc	Alcohol free, sugar free. Peppermint and wintergreen flavors. In 12s.
otc	**Zilactin-L** (Blairex Labs)	**Liquid; oral**: 10% benzyl alcohol	SD alcohol 37. In 539 mL.
otc	**Red Cross Toothache** (Mentholatum)	**Liquid; oral**: 85% eugenol, sesame oil	In 3.7 mL with cotton pellets and tweezers.
otc sf	**Ulcerease** (Med-Derm)	**Liquid; oral**: 0.6% liquefied phenol, glycerin, sodium bicarbonate, sodium borate	Alcohol free. In 180 mL.
otc	**Phylorinol** (Schaffer)	**Liquid; oral**: 0.6% phenol, boric acid, strong iodine solution, sodium copper chlorophyll	Sorbitol. In 240 mL.
otc	**Curasore** (S.S.S. Company)	**Liquid; oral**: 1% pramoxine hydrochloride	Ethyl alcohol, ethyl ether. In 15 mL.
otc	**Orasept** (Pharmakon Labs)	**Liquid; oral**: 12.16% tannic acid, 1.53% methylbenzethonium Cl, 53.31% denatured ethyl alcohol, camphor, menthol, benzyl alcohol, spearmint oil and oil of Cassia	In 15 mL.
otc	**Blistex** (Blistex)	**Ointment; oral**: 0.5% camphor, 0.5% phenol, 1% allantoin, lanolin	Mineral oil base. In 4.2 and 10.5 g.
otc	**Lip Medex** (Blistex)	**Ointment; oral**: Petrolatum, 1% camphor, 0.54% phenol, cocoa butter, lanolin	In 210 g.
otc	**Abreva** (SmithKline Beecham Consumer)	**Cream; oral**: 10% docosanol, benzyl alcohol, light mineral oil	In 2 g.
otc	**Pfeiffer's Cold Sore** (Pfeiffer)	**Lotion; oral**: 7% gum benzoin, camphor, menthol, eucalyptol, 85% alcohol	In 15 mL.
otc	**Banadyne-3** (Norstar)	**Solution; oral**: 4% lidocaine, menthol 1%, 45% alcohol	In 7.5 mL.
otc	**Peroxyl Dental Rinse** (Colgate)	**Solution; oral**: 1.5% hydrogen peroxide, 6% alcohol	Mint flavor. In 240 mL and pint.
otc	**Amosan** (Oral-B)	**Powder; oral**: Sodium peroxyborate monohydrate (derived from sodium perborate)	Saccharin. Peppermint, menthol, and vanilla flavors. In 1.7 g UD packets (20s and 40s).
otc	**Baby Orajel Tooth & Gum Cleanser** (Del Pharm)	**Gel; oral**: 2% poloxamer 407, 0.12% simethicone	Parabens, saccharin, sorbitol. In 14.2 g.
Rx	**Gelclair** (EKR Therapeutics)	**Gel; oral**: Maltodextrin, propylene glycol, polyvinylpyrrolidone, sodium hyaluronate, potassium sorbate, sodium benzoate, hydroxyethylcellulose, PEG-40 hydrogenated castor oil, benzalkonium chloride	EDTA, saccharin. In 15 mL single-use packets.
otc	**Probax** (Fischer)	**Gel; oral**: 2% propolis, petrolatum, mineral oil, lanolin	In 3.5 g.
otc	**Tanac** (Del Pharm)	**Gel; oral**: 1% dyclonine hydrochloride, 0.5% allantoin, petrolatum, lanolin	In 9.45 g.
otc	**Zilactin** (Blairex Labs)	**Gel; oral**: 10% benzyl alcohol	Salicylic acid, hydroxypropylcellulose. In 7 g.
otc	**Rembrandt Canker Pain Relief Kit** (Den-Mat Corp.)	**Gel; oral**: 5% benzocaine **Rinse; oral**: Methylparaben, saccharin **Paste; oral**: 0.15% fluoride ion from sodium monofluorophosphate w/v ½.	In 28 g. In 37 mL. In 34 g.
Rx	**Orabase HCA** (Colgate)	**Paste; oral**: 0.5% hydrocortisone acetate, 5% polyethylene, mineral oil	In 5 g.
Rx	**Kenalog in Orabase** (Apothecon)	**Paste; oral**: 0.1% triamcinolone acetonide	In 5 g.
Rx	**Oralone Dental** (Taro)	**Paste; oral**: 0.1% triamcinolone acetonide	In 5 g.
otc	**Orabase-Plain** (Colgate)	**Paste; oral**: Plasticized hydrocarbon gel	In 5 and 15 g.
otc	**Tanac Dual Core** (Del Pharm)	**Stick; oral**: 7.5% benzocaine, 6% tannic acid, 0.75% octyl dimethyl PABA, 0.2% allantoin, 0.12% benzalkonium chloride	Cetyl alcohol, butylparaben. In 2.84 g stick.
otc	**Blistex** (Blistex)	**Lip balm; oral**: 0.5% camphor, 0.5% phenol, 1% allantoin, 2% dimethicone, 6.6% padimate O, 2.5% oxybenzone, petrolatum	SPF 10. Parabens. In 4.5 g.

MISCELLANEOUS MOUTH AND THROAT PREPARATIONS

otc	**Herpecin-L** (Chattem)	**Lip balm; oral:** 1% dimethicone, 5% meradimate, 7.5% octinoxate, 5% octisalate, 6% oxybenzone	SPF 30. *Helianthus annuus* (hybrid sunflower) oil, petrolatum mineral oil, talc, titanium dioxide. In 1 tube per package.
otc	**Blistex** (Blistex)	**Lip balm; oral:** 1% camphor, 1% menthol, 0.5% phenol, petrolatum, cocoa butter, lanolin, mixed waxes, oil of cloves	In 0.25 and 0.38 oz.
otc	**Chap Stick Medicated Lip Balm** (Robins)	**Lip balm; oral:** 1% camphor, 0.6% menthol, 0.5% phenol, petrolatum, mineral oil, cocoa butter, lanolin	Parabens. In jars (7 g), squeezable tubes (10 g), and sticks (4.2 g).
otc	**Chloraseptic Kids Sore Throat** (Medtech)	**Strips; oral:** 2 mg benzocaine, 2 mg menthol	Glycerin, sucralose. In 20s.

PREPARATIONS FOR SENSITIVE TEETH

otc	**Denquel Sensitive Teeth** (Procter & Gamble)	**Paste; dental:** 5% potassium nitrate	Mint flavor. In 48, 90 and 135 g.
Rx	**Fluoridex Daily Defense Sensitivity Relief** (Discus Dental)	**Paste; dental:** 5% Potassium nitrate, 1.1% sodium fluoride	Saccharin, sorbitol. Mint flavor. In 112 g.
otc	**Sensodyne Cool Gel** (Block)		Saccharin, sorbitol, parabens. In 28.3 g.
otc	**Sensodyne-F** (Block)	**Paste; dental:** Potassium nitrate, sodium monofluorophosphate	Saccharin, sorbitol. In 72 and 138 g.
otc	**Sensodyne-SC** (Block)	**Paste; dental:** 10% strontium Cl hexahydrate	Saccharin, sorbitol, parabens. In 26 g.
otc	**Sensitivity Protection Crest** (Procter & Gamble)	**Paste; dental:** Sodium fluoride, potassium nitrate	Mint flavor. In 175 g.
otc	**Sensodyne Fresh Mint** (Block)	**Paste; dental:** Potassium nitrate, sodium monofluorophosphate	Sorbitol, saccharin. In 26 g.
Rx	**Triamcinolone Acetonide Dental 0.1%** (Various, eg, Qualitest, Taro)	**Paste; dental:** 0.1% triamcinolone acetonide	In 5 g.

DENTAL PREPARATIONS FOR SENSITIVE TEETH — ORAL

Administration and Dosage

➤*General dosing considerations:* These toothpastes are specially formulated to replace regular toothpaste for people with sensitive teeth.

➤*Adults:*

Cavity prevention and sensitive teeth – Use daily as in regular dental care. Expectorate after use.

SYSTEMIC DEODORIZERS

CHLOROPHYLL DERIVATIVES (Chlorophyllin)

otc sf	**Chlorophyll** (Freeda)	**Tablets:** 20 mg chlorophyll	In 100s, 250s and 500s.
otc	**PALS** (Palisades)	**Tablets:** 100 mg chlorophyllin copper complex	In 100s.
otc	**Derifil** (Integra LifeSciences)	**Tablets:** 100 mg chlorophyllin copper complex sodium	6 mg sodium, dextrose. (D). Dark green, scored. Film coated. In 30s, 100s, and 1,000s.

CHLOROPHYLL DERIVATIVES (Chlorophyllin)

Refer to the Dermatologicals chapter for additional information.

Indications

To control fecal odors in colostomy, ileostomy or incontinence; also for certain breath and body odors.

Administration and Dosage

➤*Adults:*

Fecal odors, certain breath and body odors – 1 to 2 tablets/day; may be increased to 3 tablets/day. In ostomies, take tablets orally or place in the appliance.

➤*Children:*

Fecal odors, certain breath and body odors – See Adults for dosing for children 12 years of age and older.

Warnings/Precautions

➤*Diarrhea:* If cramping or diarrhea occur, reduce the dosage.

➤*Pregnancy: Category: Undetermined.* Consult a health care provider before using in pregnant women.

➤*Lactation:* Consult a health care provider before using in a breast-feeding woman.

Adverse Reactions

No toxic effects have been reported. A temporary mild laxative effect may occur; the stool is commonly stained dark green.

BISMUTH SUBGALLATE

otc	**Devrom** (Parthenon)	**Tablets:** 200 mg	Lactose, sugar. Chewable. In 100s.

BISMUTH SUBGALLATE — ORAL

Indications

To control fecal odors in colostomy, ileostomy or incontinence.

Administration and Dosage

➤*Adults:*

Control of fecal odors – 1 or 2 tablets 3 times daily with meals. Chew or swallow whole.

➤*Administration:* Tablets may be chewed or swallowed whole.

Warnings/Precautions

➤*Pregnancy: Category: Undetermined.* The data available for bismuth in pregnancy are poor, and the actual fetal risks cannot be determined.

➤*Lactation:* Bismuth is poorly absorbed into the systemic circulation.

Adverse Reactions

A temporary darkening of the tongue or stool may occur.

The anorectal preparations are used primarily for the symptomatic relief of the discomfort associated with hemorrhoids and perianal itching or irritation. In addition to the products specifically listed in this section, many of the Topical Local Anesthetics and Topical Corticosteroids may also be used locally in anorectal therapy (see specific monographs in the Dermatologics chapter).

Active Ingredients

The various components of these products are briefly discussed below. For complete information on specific indications, contraindications, precautions and adverse effects of ingredients, refer to the appropriate monographs as indicated.

➤*Hydrocortisone:* Hydrocortisone (see additional monographs in the Endocrine/Metabolic and Dermatologics chapters) reduces inflammation, itching and swelling.

➤*Local anesthetics:* Local anesthetics (benzocaine, pramoxine) temporarily relieve pain, itching and irritation. The most frequent adverse effects of topical local anesthetic use are allergic reactions (eg, burning, itching). Their safety and efficacy when used intrarectally require further evaluation (see additional monographs in the Dermatologics chapter).

➤*Vasoconstrictors:* Vasoconstrictors (ephedrine, phenylephrine) reduce swelling and congestion of anorectal tissues. They relieve local itching by a slight anesthetic effect. These agents are not effective in stopping bleeding from venous tissues.

➤*Astringents:* Astringents (witch hazel, zinc oxide) coagulate the protein in skin cells, protecting the underlying tissue and decreasing the cell volume. They lessen mucus and other secretions, and relieve anorectal irritation and inflammation.

➤*Antiseptics:* Antiseptics (benzalkonium chloride, phenylmercuric nitrate) are not of therapeutic value when applied to the anorectal area. There is no convincing evidence that they prevent infection in the anorectal area. Many are present as preservatives.

➤*Emollients/protectants:* Emollients (glycerin, lanolin, mineral oil, petrolatum, zinc oxide, cocoa butter, shark liver oil, bismuth salts) form a physical barrier on the skin and lubricate tissues, preventing irritation of the anorectal area and water loss from the stratum corneum. Many of these substances are used as bases and carriers of pharmacologically active compounds.

➤*Counterirritants:* Counterirritants (camphor) evoke a feeling of comfort, cooling, tingling or warmth and distract the perception of pain and itching.

➤*Keratolytics:* Keratolytics (resorcinol) cause desquamation and sloughing of epidermal surface cells and may help to expose underlying tissue to therapeutic agents.

➤*Wound-healing agents:* Wound-healing agents (balsam peru, skin respiratory factor or srf, yeast cell derivative) are claimed to promote wound healing or tissue repair. Effectiveness of these compounds has not been conclusively demonstrated.

➤*Anticholinergic agents:* Anticholinergic agents inhibit the action of acetylcholine. Because these agents produce their action systemically, they are not effective in ameliorating local symptoms of anorectal disease.

Patient Information

Maintain normal bowel function by proper diet, adequate fluid intake and regular exercise.

Products for external use only are not to be used intrarectally. Apply external products sparingly after, rather than before, a bowel movement. If possible, wash, rinse and dry the area before use.

Avoid excessive laxative use.

Stool softeners or bulk laxatives may be useful adjunctive therapy.

In general, patients with conditions such as diabetes, hypertension, hyperthyroidism or cardiovascular disease should not use products containing vasoconstrictors.

Products containing resorcinol should not be used on open wounds.

If anorectal symptoms do not improve in 7 days, or if bleeding, protrusion, seepage or pain occurs, consult a physician.

STEROID-CONTAINING PRODUCTS

Rx	**Lidocaine/Hydrocortisone Rectal** (River's Edge)	**Cream; rectal:** 0.5% hydrocortisone acetate, 3% lidocaine hydrochloride	Alcohols, aluminum sulfate, glycerin, lt. mineral oil, parabens, petrolatum. In 7 g single-use units with applicator.
Rx	**Lidocaine HCl 3%/Hydrocortisone Acetate 0.5%** (Kylemore Pharmaceuticals)		Alcohols, mineral oil, parabens, propylene glycol, white petrolatum. In 14 and 20 single-use 7 g tubes and applicators.
Rx	**Proctocort** (Salix)	**Cream; rectal:** 1% hydrocortisone	Stearyl and cetyl alcohols. In 28.35 g.
Rx	**Lidocaine HCl 3%/Hydrocortisone Acetate 1%** (Kylemore Pharmaceuticals)	**Cream; rectal:** 1% hydrocortisone acetate, 3% lidocaine hydrochloride	Alcohols, glycerin, mineral oil, parabens, propylene glycol, trolamine, urea, white petrolatum. In 20 single-use 7 g tubes, applicators, and cleansing wipes.
Rx	**Xyralid RC** (Auriga Pharmaceuticals)		Cetyl alcohol, glycerin, mineral oil, parabens, stearyl alcohol, urea, white petrolatum. In 7 g with applicators and cleansing wipes.
Rx	**Analpram-HC** (Ferndale)	**Cream; rectal:** 1% hydrocortisone acetate, 1% pramoxine hydrochloride	Cetyl alcohol, 0.1% potassium sorbate, 0.1% sorbic acid. In 30 g.
Rx	**EndaRoid** (Larken Labs)		In 28 g.
Rx	**Lidocaine HCl 2%/Hydrocortisone Acetate 2%** (Kylemore Pharmaceuticals)	**Cream; rectal:** 2% hydrocortisone acetate, 2% lidocaine hydrochloride	Alcohols, glycerin, mineral oil, parabens, propylene glycol, trolamine, urea, white petrolatum. In 24 single-use 7 g tubes, applicators, and cleansing wipes.
Rx	**Analpram-HC** (Ferndale)	**Cream; rectal:** 2.5% hydrocortisone acetate, 1% pramoxine hydrochloride	0.1% potassium sorbate, 0.1 % sorbic acid, cetyl alcohol. In 30 g.
Rx	**Anusol-HC** (Salix)	**Cream; rectal:** 2.5% hydrocortisone	Petrolatum, EDTA, benzyl and stearyl alcohols. In 30 g.
Rx	**ProctoCream-HC** (Alaven Pharmaceutical)	**Cream; rectal:** 2.5% hydrocortisone	Benzyl alcohol, glycerin, stearyl alcohol. In 30 g.
Rx	**HC Pramoxine** (Veracity[a])	**Cream; rectal:** 2.5% hydrocortisone acetate and 1% pramoxine hydrochloride	Cetyl alcohol. In 28 g.
Rx	**Proctozone-HC** (Actavis)	**Cream; rectal:** 2.5% hydrocortisone	Alcohols, glyceryl, parabens, propylene glycol, white wax. In 20, 30, and 453.6 g.
otc	**Balneol for Her** (Alaven Consumer Healthcare)	**Lotion; rectal:** 0.25% hydrocortisone	Lanolin oil, mineral oil, parabens, PEG-4, PEG-40, PEG-100. In 89 mL and 2 g convenience packs.
Rx	**Analpram-HC** (Ferndale)	**Lotion; rectal:** 2.5% hydrocortisone acetate, 1% pramoxine hydrochloride	Hydrophilic. Alcohol, glycerin. In 60 mL.
Rx	**Lidocaine HCl/ Hydrocortisone Acetate with Aloe** (River's Edge)	**Gel; rectal:** 0.55% hydrocortisone acetate, 2.8% lidocaine	Aloe, parabens, PEG-4. In 100 g with 15 single-use applicators.

STEROID-CONTAINING PRODUCTS

Rx	**Lidocaine/Hydrocortisone** (River's Edge)	**Gel; rectal:** 2.5% hydrocortisone acetate, 3% lidocaine hydrochloride	Cetyl alcohol, mineral oil, parabens, petrolatum, stearyl alcohol, urea. In 20 single use 7 g tubes with applicators and cleansing wipes.
Rx	**AnaMantle HC 2.5%** (Kenwood Therapeutics)		Parabens, stearyl alcohol, urea. In 20 single-use 7 g tubes with built-in applicator and single-use cleansing wipes.
Rx	**Lidocaine HCl 3%/Hydrocortisone Acetate 2.5%** (Kylemore Pharmaceuticals)		Alcohols, glycerin, glyceryl, mineral oil, parabens, propylene glycol, urea, white petrolatum. In 20 single-use 7 g tubes, applicators, and cleansing wipes.
Rx	**LidoCort** (Aristos)		Mineral oil, parabens, petrolatum. In 20 single-use 7 g tubes with applicators and cleansing wipes.
Rx	**Cortifoam** (Schwarz Pharma)	**Aerosol, Foam; rectal:** 10% hydrocortisone acetate	Parabens. 90 mg/applicatorful. In 14 applications.
Rx	**Proctofoam-HC** (Alaven Pharmaceuticals)	**Aerosol, Foam; rectal:** 1% hydrocortisone acetate, 1% pramoxine hydrochloride	Parabens, cetyl alcohol, stearyl alcohol. In 10 g (≥ 14 applications) w/applicator.
Rx	**Proctocort** (Salix)	**Suppositories; rectal:** 30 mg hydrocortisone acetate	In hydrogenated vegetable oil base. In 12s and 24s.
Rx	**Hydrocortisone Acetate** (Various, eg, Able, Clay-Park, Cypress, Major, Paddock)	**Suppositories; rectal:** 25 mg hydrocortisone acetate	In 12s and 24s.
Rx	**Anucort-HC** (G & W)		Vegetable oil. In 12, 24s and 100s.
Rx	**Anusol-HC** (Salix)		In a hydrogenated vegetable oil base. In 12s and 24s.
Rx	**Cort-Dome High Potency** (Bayer)		In 12s.
Rx	**Hemril-HC Uniserts** (Upsher-Smith)		Vegetable oil. In 12s.
Rx	**Hemorrhoidal HC** (Various, eg, Schein, Geneva, Goldline)		In 12s, 24s, 50s, 100s & UD 12s.
Rx	**LidaMantle HC Relief** (Doak)	**Pads; topical:** 2% hydrocortisone acetate, 2% lidocaine HCl	Mineral oil, parabens, urea. In 60s.
Rx	**Hydrocortisone Rectal Suspension** (Various, eg, Bay Pharma, Teva)	**Enema; rectal:** 100 mg/60 mL	May contain parabens. In 60 mL single-use bottles.
Rx	**Cortenema** (Ani)		Parabens. In 60 mL single-use bottles.
Rx	**Colocort** (Paddock)		Parabens. In 60 mL single-use bottles.

[a] Veracity Pharmaceuticals, 6601 Lyons Road, Suite E-7, Coconut Creek, FL 33073; (954) 426-4199, fax (954) 426-1905

Refer to the general discussion of these products in the Anorectal Preparations Introduction.

LOCAL ANESTHETIC-CONTAINING PRODUCTS

otc	**Tronolane** (Lee)	**Cream; topical:** 1% pramoxine hydrochloride	5% zinc oxide, cetyl alcohol, parabens. In 30 and 60 g.
otc	**Americaine** (Insight Pharmaceuticals)	**Ointment; topical:** 20% benzocaine	PEG-300, PEG-3350. In 28 g.
otc	**Tucks** (Pfizer Consumer Health)	**Ointment; topical:** 1% pramoxine hydrochloride	12.5% zinc oxide, 46.6% mineral oil and cocoa butter. In 30 g with applicator.
otc	**ProctoFoam NS** (Schwarz Pharma)	**Aerosol Foam; topical:** 1% pramoxine hydrochloride	In 15 g with applicator.
otc	**Fleet Pain Relief** (Fleet)	**Pads; topical:** 1% pramoxine hydrochloride, 12% glycerin	In 100s.

Refer to the general discussion of these products in the Anorectal Preparations Introduction. Also see Benzocaine and Pramoxine Hydrochloride monographs in the Local Anesthetics, Topical, section of the Dermatological Agents chapter.

PERIANAL HYGIENE PRODUCTS

otc	**Balneol** (Alaven)	**Lotion; topical:** Glyceryl, lanolin oil, mineral oil, methylparaben, PEG-4, PEG-40, PEG-100, propylene glycol	In 88 mL.
otc	**Balneol For Her** (Alaven)	**Lotion; topical:** Glyceryl, lanolin oil, mineral oil, methylparaben, PEG-4, PEG-40, PEG-100, propylene glycol	In 89 mL.
otc	**Balneol For Her Convenience Packets** (Alaven)	**Lotion; topical:** Glyceryl, hydrocortisone 0.25%, lanolin oil, methylparaben, mineral oil, PEG-4, PEG-40, PEG-100, propylene glycol	In 20s.
otc	**Sensi-Care Perineal Skin Cleanser Solution** (ConvaTec)	**Solution; topical:** Sodium C_{12-14} olefin sulfonate, disodium cocoamphodiacetate.	Aloe vera. In 120 and 240 mL.
otc	**Bodi Kleen** (Geritrex)	**Spray; topical:** Triethanolamine lauryl sulfate, 2-phenoxy-ethanol, hexylene glycol, aloe vera gel	In 8 oz.
otc	**Aloe Vesta** (ConvaTec)	**Foam; topical:** Aloe, disodium cocoamphodiacetate, sodium C_{14-16} olefin sulfonate	In 236 mL.
otc	**Tucks Take-Alongs** (Parke-Davis)	**Pads; topical:** 50% witch hazel and 10% glycerin with 0.003% benzalkonium Cl	In 12s.
otc	**Fleet Medicated Wipes** (Fleet)	**Pads; topical:** 50% hamamelis water, 7% alcohol, 10% glycerin, benzalkonium chloride and methylparaben	In 100s.
otc	**Preparation H Cleansing** (Whitehall)	**Tissues; topical:** Propylene glycol, phenoxyethanol	Alcohol free. Parabens, citric acid. In 15s and 40s.
otc	**Aloe Vesta** (ConvaTec)	**Cloth; topical:** Aloe barbadensis leaf juice, dimethicone, parabens, urea	In 24s.

PERIANAL HYGIENE PRODUCTS

Refer to the general discussion of these products in the Anorectal Preparations Introduction.

MISCELLANEOUS ANORECTAL COMBINATION PRODUCTS

otc	**Preparation H Cooling Gel** (Whitehall-Robins)	**Gel; rectal:** 50% witch hazel, 0.25% phenylephrine hydrochloride. 7.5% alcohol, EDTA, parabens.	In 51 g.
otc	**Preparation H** (Whitehall-Robins)	**Cream ; rectal:** 18% petrolatum, 12% glycerin, 3% shark liver oil, 0.25% phenylephrine hydrochloride, cetyl alcohol, stearyl alcohol, EDTA, lanolin, parabens	In 27 and 54 g.
		Ointment; rectal: 71.9% petrolatum, 14% mineral oil, 3% shark liver oil, 0.25% phenylephrine hydrochloride, corn oil, glycerin, lanolin, lanolin alcohol, parabens, tocopherol	In 30 and 60 g.
otc	**Formulation R** (G & W)	**Cream; rectal:** 18% petrolatum, 12% glycerin, 0.25% phenylephrine hydrochloride, shark liver oil	Cetyl alcohol, edetate disodium, parabens, stearyl alcohol. In 54 g.
		Ointment; rectal: 71.9% petrolatum, 14% mineral oil, 0.25% phenylephrine hydrochloride, shark liver oil	Corn oil, lanolin alcohol, parabens. In 30 and 60 g.
otc	**Hem-Prep** (G & W)	**Ointment; rectal:** 0.025% phenylephrine hydrochloride, 11% zinc oxide, white petrolatum	In 42.5 g
otc	**Hemorrhoidal Ointment** (Cardinal Health)	**Ointment; rectal:** 0.25% phenylephrine hydrochloride, 3% shark liver oil, 71.9% petrolatum, 14% mineral oil	Benzoic acid, glycerin, lanolin, lanolin alcohol, parabens, thyme oil. In 57 g.
otc	**Preparation H** (Wyeth)	**Suppositories; rectal:** 3% shark liver oil, 79% cocoa butter, corn oil, EDTA, parabens and tocopherol	In 12s, 24s, 36s, and 48s.
otc	**Preparation H** (Wyeth)	**Cream; rectal:** 14.4% glycerin, 0.25% phenylephrine hydrochloride, 1% pramoxine hydrochloride, 15% white petrolatum.	Aloe, cetyl alcohol, EDTA, mineral oil, parabens, stearyl alcohol. In 15 and 26 g.
otc	**Wyanoids Relief Factor** (Wyeth)	**Suppositories; rectal:** 79% cocoa butter, 3% shark liver oil, corn oil, EDTA, parabens and tocopherol	In 12s.
otc	**Tucks** (Pfizer Consumer Health)	**Suppositories; rectal:** 51% topical starch	Benzyl alcohol, hydrogenated vegetable oil, vitamin E. In 12s and 24s.
otc	**Hemril Uniserts** (Upsher-Smith)	**Suppositories; rectal:** 2.25% bismuth subgallate, 1.75% bismuth resorcin compound, 1.2% benzyl benzoate, 11% zinc oxide, 1.8% balsam peru in hydrolyzed vegetable oil base	In 12s and 50s.
otc	**Rectagene** (Pfeiffer)	**Suppositories; rectal:** Live yeast cell derivative supplying 2,000 units Skin Respiratory Factor per ounce and shark liver oil in a cocoa butter base	In 12s.
otc	**Rectagene II** (Pfeiffer)	**Suppositories; rectal:** 2.25% bismuth subgallate, 1.75% bismuth resorcin compound, 1.2% benzyl benzoate, 1.8% peruvian balsam, 11% zinc oxide, bismuth subiodide, calcium phosphate in a hydrogenated vegetable oil base	In 12s.
otc	**Pazo Hemorrhoid** (Bristol-Myers Products)	**Suppositories; rectal:** 3.8 mg ephedrine sulfate, 96.5 mg zinc oxide, vegetable oil	In 12s and 24s.
otc	**Hem-Prep** (G & W)	**Suppositories; rectal:** 0.25% phenylephrine hydrochloride, 11% zinc oxide	In 12s.
otc	**Anu-Med** (Major)	**Suppositories; rectal:** 0.25% phenylephrine hydrochloride, 88.7% hard fat	Corn starch, parabens. In 12s.
otc	**Tronolane** (Monticello)	**Suppositories; rectal:** 0.25% phenylephrine hydrochloride, 88.7% hard fat	Parabens. In 12s.
otc	**Hemorid For Women** (Thompson Medical)	**Cream; rectal:** 30% white petrolatum, 20% mineral oil, 1% pramoxine hydrochloride, 0.25% phenylephrine hydrochloride, aloe vera gel, parabens, cetyl and stearyl alcohols	In 28.3 g.

Refer to the general discussion of these products in the Anorectal Preparations Introduction.

Indications

➤*Oral:* In the treatment of mildly to moderately severe infections caused by penicillin-sensitive microorganisms.

➤*Penicillinase-resistant penicillins:* The percentage of staphylococcal isolates resistant to **penicillin G** outside the hospital is increasing, approximating the high percentage found in the hospital. Therefore, use a penicillinase-resistant penicillin as initial therapy for any suspected staphylococcal infection until culture and sensitivity results are known.

When treatment is initiated before definitive culture and sensitivity results are known, consider that these agents are only effective in the treatment of infections caused by pneumococci, group A beta-hemolytic streptococci, and penicillin G-resistant and penicillin G-sensitive staphylococci.

➤*Parenteral:* In patients with severe infection or when there is nausea, vomiting, gastric dilatation, cardiospasm, or intestinal hypermotility. Parenteral aqueous **penicillin G** (eg, potassium, sodium) is the dosage form of choice in severe infections caused by penicillin-sensitive microorganisms when rapid and high penicillin serum levels are required.

For specific labeled indications, refer to individual drug monographs.

Administration and Dosage

Therapy may be initiated prior to obtaining results of bacteriologic studies when there is reason to believe the causative organisms may be susceptible. Once results are known, adjust therapy.

Dosage for any individual patient must take into consideration the severity of infection, the susceptibility of the organisms causing the infection and the status of the patient's host defense mechanism. Duration of therapy depends on the severity of the infection.

Continue treatment of all infections for a minimum of 48 to 72 hours beyond the time that the patient becomes asymptomatic or evidence of bacterial eradication has been obtained, unless single-dose therapy is employed. A minimum of 10 days treatment is recommended for any infection caused by group A beta-hemolytic streptococci to prevent the occurrence of acute rheumatic fever or acute glomerulonephritis.

Patients with a history of rheumatic fever or chorea and receiving continuous prophylaxis may harbor increased numbers of penicillin-resistant organisms.

Actions

➤*Pharmacology:* Penicillins are bactericidal antibiotics that include natural and semisynthetic derivatives. These agents contain the 6-β-aminopenicillanic acid nucleus and have a similar mechanism of action. All penicillins share cross-allergenicity. Significant differences among agents include: resistance to gastric acid inactivation; resistance to inactivation by penicillinase; spectrum of antimicrobial activity. In addition to the prototype **penicillin G**, this class includes an acid-stable penicillin G derivative (**penicillin V**), penicillinase-resistant penicillins, the aminopenicillins, and the extended spectrum derivatives. Several of these penicillins also are available in combination with agents that inactivate β-lactamase enzymes (eg, clavulanic acid, sulbactam), thereby extending the antibiotic spectrum to include many bacteria normally resistant to it and to other β-lactam antibiotics (see Pharmacokinetics). The available combinations include ampicillin/sulbactam, amoxicillin/clavulanate potassium, ticarcillin/clavulanate potassium, and piperacillin/tazobactam sodium.

Penicillins

	Routes of administration	Penicillinase-resistant	Acid stable	% Protein bound	May be taken with meals
Natural					
Penicillin G	IM-IV	no	no	60%	†[a]
Penicillin V	Oral	no	no	80%	yes
Penicillinase-resistant					
Dicloxacillin	Oral	yes	yes	98%	no
Nafcillin	IM-IV-Oral	yes	yes	87% to 90%	no
Oxacillin	IM-IV-Oral	yes	yes	94%	no
Aminopenicillins					
Amoxicillin	Oral	no	yes	20%	yes
Amoxicillin/potassium clavulanate	Oral	yes	yes	18%/25%	yes
Ampicillin	IM-IV-Oral	no	yes	20%	no
Ampicillin/sulbactam	IM-IV	yes	†[a]	28%/38%	†[a]
Extended-spectrum					
Carbenicillin	Oral	no	yes	50%	no
Piperacillin	IM-IV	no	†[a]	16%	†[a]
Piperacillin/tazobactam sodium	IV	yes	†[a]	30%/30%	†[a]
Ticarcillin/potassium clavulanate	IV	yes	†[a]	45%/9%	†[a]

[a] Available only for intramuscular (IM) or intravenous (IV) use.

Mechanism – Penicillins inhibit the biosynthesis of cell wall mucopeptide. They are bactericidal against sensitive organisms when adequate concentrations are reached, and they are most effective during the stage of active multiplication. Inadequate concentrations may produce only bacteriostatic effects.

➤*Pharmacokinetics:*

Absorption – Because gastric acidity, stomach emptying time and other factors affecting absorption may vary considerably, serum levels may be reduced to nontherapeutic levels in certain individuals. **Penicillin V** shows less individual variation than **penicillin G** and has become the only natural penicillin available for oral administration. **Nafcillin**'s oral absorption is inferior to **oxacillin** and **dicloxacillin**. **Ampicillin** and **carbenicillin** indanyl have good GI absorption, but amoxicillin is more completely absorbed.

Absorption of most penicillins is affected by food; these medications are best taken on an empty stomach, 1 hour before or 2 hours after meals. Penicillin V may be given with meals; however blood levels may be slightly higher when given on an empty stomach. Amoxicillin tablets and amoxicillin/clavulanate potassium may be given without regard to meals.

Peak serum levels occur approximately 1 hour after oral use. After a 500 mg oral dose, peak serum concentrations for oxacillin and dicloxacillin range from 5 to 7, 7.5 to 14.4, and 10 to 17 mcg/mL, respectively. One hour after a 1 g oral nafcillin dose, average serum concentration was 1.19 mcg/mL (range, 0 to 3.12). IM injections of 1 g nafcillin, 560 mg oxacillin, and 1 g **methicillin** produced peak serum levels in 0.5 to 1 hour of 7.61, 15, and 17 mcg/mL, respectively.

Parenteral penicillin G (sodium and potassium) gives rapid and high but transient blood levels; derivatives provide prolonged penicillin blood levels with IM use. **Procaine penicillin G**, an equimolecular suspension of procaine and penicillin G, must be given IM; it dissolves slowly at the injection site and plateaus in about 4 hours; levels decline gradually over 15 to 20 hours. **Benzathine penicillin G** also must be given IM only; is absorbed very slowly from the injection site and is hydrolyzed to penicillin G; hence, serum levels are much lower but more prolonged, sustaining serum levels for up to 4 weeks.

Clavulanic acid is well absorbed orally.

Distribution – Penicillins are bound to plasma proteins, primarily albumin, in varying degrees (see table in Pharmacology section). They diffuse readily into most body tissues and fluids, including kidneys, liver, lungs, heart, skin, synovial fluid, intestines, bile, peritoneal fluid, bronchial and wound secretions, bone, prostate, pericardial and ascitic fluids, spleen and other tissues. Penetration into cerebrospinal fluid (CSF), the brain, and the eye occurs only with inflammation. CSF levels usually do not exceed 5% of penicillin G's peak serum concentration. Penicillins cross the placenta and appear in amniotic fluid and cord serum.

Clavulanic acid is widely distributed to many body tissues.

Excretion – Penicillins are excreted largely unchanged in the urine by glomerular filtration and active tubular secretion. Nonrenal elimination includes hepatic inactivation and excretion in bile; this is only a minor route for all penicillins except **nafcillin** and oxacillin. Excretion by renal tubular secretion can be delayed by coadministration of probenecid. Excretion is delayed in neonates and infants. Elimination half-life of most penicillins is short (1.4 h or less). Impaired renal function prolongs the serum half-life of penicillins eliminated primarily by renal excretion. The half-life is not greatly affected for nafcillin, oxacillin, and **dicloxacillin** because of increased biotransformation and biliary excretion. Because **piperacillin** is excreted by biliary and renal routes, it can be used safely in appropriate dosage in patients with severe renal impairment and in the treatment of hepatobiliary infections.

Half-life is approximately 1 hour; 35% to 45% is excreted unchanged in the urine during the first 6 hours after administration. Probenecid does not alter renal excretion of clavulanic acid.

➤*Microbiology:*

β-lactamase inhibitors – (Clavulanic acid, sulbactam, and tazobactam). These have weak antimicrobial activity but irreversibly inactivate bacterial β-lactamase enzymes. Used with β-lactam antibiotics, they protect antibiotics from inactivation by β-lactamase-producing organisms.

Clavulanic acid – Used in combination with **amoxicillin** and **ticarcillin**, it inhibits plasmid-mediated β-lactamases (eg, *Haemophilus influenzae*, *Neisseria gonorrheae*, *Escherichia coli*, *Salmonella*, *Shigella*, staphylococci) and chromosomal-mediated β-lactamases (eg, *Klebsiella*, *Bacteroides fragilis*, *Legionella*). It does not inhibit β-lactamases produced by *Enterobacter*, *Serratia*, *Morganella*, *Citrobacter*, *Pseudomonas*, or *Acinetobacter* species.

Sulbactam – Another β-lactamase inhibitor, this extends the bacterial spectrum of ampicillin to include such β-lactamase-producing organisms as *S. aureus*, *H. influenzae*, *B. fragilis*, and most strains of *E. coli*.

Tazobactam – This is a penicillanic acid sulfone β-lactamase inhibitor and has poor activity against chromosomal β-lactamases of Enterobacteriaceae but has good activity against many of the plasmid β-lactamases. Tazobactam extends the spectrum but does not increase the activity of **piperacillin** against *Pseudomonas aeruginosa*. The currently recommended piperacillin dose in **piperacillin/tazobactam** is less than the recommended dose of piperacillin when used alone for serious infections and may prove ineffective in the treatment of some *P. aeruginosa* infections. The manufacturer recommends concomitant aminoglycoside therapy when treating *P. aeruginosa* nosocomial pneumonia. The following table indicates the organisms that are generally susceptible to the penicillins in vitro:

Organisms Generally Susceptible to Penicillins

	Organisms	Natural penicillins		Penicillinase-resistant			Aminopenicillins				Extended spectrum			
	✓ = Generally susceptible	Penicillin G	Penicillin V	Dicloxacillin	Nafcillin	Oxacillin	Amoxicillin	Ampicillin	Amoxicillin/potassium clavulanate	Ampicillin/ subactam	Carbenicillin	Piperacillin	Ticarcillin/potassium clavulanate	Piperacillin/tazobactam sodium
Gram-positive	Staphylococci	✓[a]	✓[a]	✓	✓	✓	✓[a]	✓[a]	✓	✓	✓[a]	✓[a]	✓	
	Staphylococcus aureus	✓[a]	✓[a]	✓	✓	✓			✓	✓	✓[a]	✓[a]	✓	✓
	Staphylococcus epidermidis													✓[b]
	Streptococci	✓	✓					✓		✓				
	Streptococcus pneumoniae	✓	✓	✓	✓	✓	✓	✓	✓	✓	✓	✓	✓	✓[c]
	Beta-hemolytic streptococci	✓	✓		✓		✓	✓	✓	✓	✓	✓	✓	
	Enterococcus (Streptococcus) faecalis	✓[d]					✓	✓	✓	✓	✓	✓	✓	✓
	Streptococcus viridans	✓	✓		✓		✓	✓	✓	✓		✓	✓	
	Corynebacterium diphtheriae	✓	✓											
	Bacillus anthracis	✓	✓					✓		✓				
	Streptococcus agalactiae												✓	
	Streptococcus pyogenes												✓	
	Erysipelothrix rhusiopathiae	✓												
	Listeria monocytogenes	✓	✓				✓	✓		✓				
Gram-negative	*Escherichia coli*	✓					✓	✓	✓	✓	✓	✓	✓	✓
	Haemophilus influenzae						✓	✓	✓	✓	✓	✓[c]	✓	✓
	Haemophilus parainfluenzae													
	Eikenella corrodens								✓					
	Bacteroides melaninogenicus													✓
	Pseudomonas sp.												✓	
	Klebsiella sp.								✓	✓		✓	✓	✓
	Neisseria gonorrhoeae	✓[a]	✓				✓	✓	✓	✓	✓	✓	✓	✓
	Neisseria meningitidis	✓						✓	✓	✓		✓	✓	✓[c]
	Proteus mirabilis	✓					✓	✓	✓	✓	✓	✓	✓	✓
	Salmonella sp.	✓						✓		✓	✓	✓	✓	
	Shigella sp.	✓						✓		✓		✓		
	Morganella morganii									✓	✓	✓	✓	✓
	Proteus vulgaris									✓	✓	✓	✓	✓
	Providencia rettgeri									✓	✓	✓	✓	
	Providencia stuartii									✓				
	Enterobacter sp.	✓							✓	✓	✓	✓	✓	
	Citrobacter sp.										✓	✓	✓	
	Pseudomonas aeruginosa										✓	✓	✓	✓
	Serratia sp.										✓	✓	✓	✓
	Acinetobacter sp.									✓		✓	✓	
	Streptobacillus moniliformis	✓	✓											
	Moraxella (Branhamella) catarrhalis								✓	✓		✓	✓	✓
Anaerobic	*Clostridium* sp.	✓	✓				✓	✓	✓	✓	✓	✓	✓	✓
	Peptococcus sp.	✓	✓				✓	✓	✓	✓	✓	✓	✓	
	Peptostreptococcus sp.	✓	✓				✓		✓	✓	✓	✓	✓	
	Bacteroides sp.	✓[e]							✓	✓	✓	✓	✓	✓
	Fusobacterium sp.	✓							✓	✓	✓	✓	✓	✓
	Eubacterium sp.	✓										✓	✓	
	Treponema pallidum	✓	✓											
	Actinomyces bovis	✓	✓									✓		
	Veillonella sp.											✓	✓	

[a] Nonpenicillinase-producing.
[b] Nonmethicillin/oxacillin-resistant strains.
[c] Nonbeta-lactamase-producing.
[d] Bacteriostatic effect.
[e] Many strains of *B. fragilis* are resistant.

Contraindications

History of hypersensitivity to penicillins, cephalosporins, imipenem, or β-lactamase inhibitors (**piperacillin/tazobactam**).

Do not treat severe pneumonia, empyema, bacteremia, pericarditis, meningitis and purulent or septic arthritis with an oral penicillin during the acute stage.

History of amoxicillin/**clavulanate potassium**-associated cholestatic jaundice/hepatic dysfunction (amoxicillin/clavulanate potassium only).

Warnings/Precautions

➤*Bleeding abnormalities:* **Piperacillin** may induce hemorrhagic manifestations associated with abnormalities of coagulation tests (eg, bleeding time, prothrombin time, platelet aggregation). Upon withdrawal of the drug, bleeding should cease and coagulation abnormalities revert to normal. Observe patients with renal impairment, in whom excretion of these drugs is delayed, for prolonged bleeding manifestations.

➤*Cystic fibrosis:* These patients have a higher incidence of side effects (eg, fever, rash) when treated with extended spectrum penicillins (eg, **piperacillin**, **carbenicillin**). This may be caused by the higher IgE, IgG and eosinophil levels in this population.

➤*Streptococcal infections:* Therapy must be sufficient to eliminate the organism (a minimum of 10 days); otherwise, sequelae (eg, endocarditis, rheumatic fever) may occur. Take cultures after treatment to confirm that streptococci have been eradicated.

➤*Sexually transmitted diseases:* When treating gonococcal infections in which primary and secondary syphilis are suspected, perform proper diagnostic procedures, including darkfield examinations and monthly serological tests for at least 4 months. All cases of penicillin-treated syphilis should receive clinical and serological examinations every 6 months for 2 to 3 years. Test all syphilis patients for HIV infection.

➤*Resistance:* The number of strains of staphylococci resistant to penicillinase-resistant penicillins has been increasing; widespread use of penicillinase-resistant penicillins may result in an increasing number of resistant staphylococcal strains. Interpret resistance to any penicillinase-resistant penicillin as evidence of clinical resistance to all. Cross-resistance with cephalosporin derivatives also occurs frequently.

➤*Pseudomembranous colitis:* This has occurred with the use of broad spectrum antibiotics because of overgrowth of *Clostridia* sp; therefore, it is important to consider its diagnosis in patients who develop diarrhea in association with antibiotic use. Mild cases may respond to drug discontinuation alone. Manage moderate to severe cases with fluid, electrolyte, and protein supplementation. If it is not relieved by drug withdrawal, or when it is severe, oral vancomycin is the treatment of choice.

➤*Procaine sensitivity:* If sensitivity to the procaine in **penicillin G procaine** is suspected, inject 0.1 mL of a 1% to 2% procaine solution intradermally. Development of erythema, wheal, flare, or eruption indicates procaine sensitivity; treat by the usual methods. Do not use procaine penicillin preparations.

➤*Parenteral administration:* Inadvertent intravascular administration, including direct intra-arterial injection or injection immediately adjacent to arteries, has resulted in severe neurovascular damage, including transverse myelitis with permanent paralysis, gangrene requiring amputation of digits and more proximal portions of extremities, and necrosis and sloughing at and surrounding the injection site. Such severe effects have occurred following injections into the buttock, thigh, and deltoid areas. Other serious complications include immediate pallor, mottling, or cyanosis of the extremity, both distal and proximal to the injection site, followed by bleb formation; severe edema requiring anterior or posterior compartment fasciotomy in the lower extremity. These severe effects have most often occurred in infants and small children. Promptly consult a specialist if any evidence of a compromise of the blood supply occurs at, proximal to, or distal to the site of injection.

Quadriceps femoris fibrosis and atrophy have occurred following repeated IM injections of penicillin preparations into the anterolateral thigh.

Take particular care with IV administration because of the possibility of thrombophlebitis. Higher than recommended IV doses of most of the penicillins may cause neuromuscular excitability or convulsions.

Avoid subcutaneous and fat layer injections; pain and induration may occur. If these occur, apply an ice pack.

➤*Electrolyte imbalance:* Administer **aqueous penicillin G** IV in high doses (more than 10 million units) slowly because of electrolyte imbalance from either the potassium or sodium content. When sodium restriction is necessary (eg, cardiac patients), make periodic electrolyte determinations and monitor cardiac status.

Patients given continuous IV therapy with **potassium penicillin G** in high dosage (more than 10 million units daily) may suffer severe or even fatal potassium poisoning, particularly if renal insufficiency is present. Hyperreflexia, convulsions, coma, cardiac arrhythmias, and cardiac arrest may be indicative of this syndrome. High dosage of **sodium salts of penicillins** may result in or aggravate congestive heart failure because of high sodium intake. Individuals with liver disease or those receiving cytotoxic therapy or diuretics rarely demonstrated a decrease in serum potassium concentrations with high doses of **piperacillin**.

Sodium penicillin G contains 2 mEq sodium per million units, **potassium penicillin G** contains 1.7 mEq potassium and 0.3 mEq sodium per million units. The sodium content of other IV penicillin derivatives is listed below:

Sodium Content of IV Penicillins

Penicillin	Maximum recommended daily dose (g)	Sodium content (mEq/g)[a]	Sodium (mEq/day)[a,b]
Ampicillin sodium	14	2.9 to 3.1	40.6 to 43.4
Nafcillin sodium	6	2.9	17.4
Oxacillin sodium	6	2.5 to 3.1	15 to 18.6
Piperacillin sodium	24	1.85	44.4
Piperacillin/ tazobactam sodium	12	2.35	28.2

[a] 1 mEq sodium equals 23 mg.
[b] Based on maximum daily dose.

Hypokalemia – This has occurred in a few patients receiving **piperacillin**. It may also occur in patients with low potassium reserves and in patients receiving cytotoxic therapy or diuretics. Monitor serum potassium and supplement when necessary.

➤*Hypersensitivity reactions:* Serious and occasionally fatal immediate hypersensitivity reactions have occurred. The incidence of anaphylactic shock is between 0.015% and 0.04%. Anaphylactic shock resulting in death has occurred in approximately 0.002% of the patients treated. Although anaphylaxis is more frequent following parenteral therapy, it may occur with oral use. Accelerated reactions (including urticaria and laryngeal edema) and delayed reactions (serum sickness-like reactions) may also occur. These reactions are likely to be immediate and severe in penicillin-sensitive individuals with a history of atopic conditions (see Adverse Reactions).

Hypersensitivity myocarditis – This is not dose-dependent and may occur at any time during treatment. The initial reaction involves rash, fever, and eosinophilia. The second stage reflects cardiac involvement: Sinus tachycardia, ST-T changes, slight increase in cardiac enzymes (creatine phosphokinase), and cardiomegaly.

An urticarial rash, not representing a true penicillin allergy, occasionally occurs with **ampicillin** (9%). This reaction is more frequent in patients on allopurinol (14% to 22.4%), patients with lymphatic leukemia (90%), and in those with infectious mononucleosis (43% to 100%). Typically, the rash appears 7 to 10 days after the start of oral ampicillin therapy and remains for a few days to a week after drug discontinuance. In most cases, the rash is maculopapular, pruritic, and generalized.

Before therapy, inquire about previous hypersensitivity reactions to penicillins, cephalosporins, and other allergens.

Desensitization: Patients with a positive skin test to one of the penicillin determinants can be desensitized, which is a relatively safe procedure. This is recommended in instances when penicillin must be given (eg, neurosyphilis, congenital syphilis, syphilis in pregnancy) where no proven alternatives exist. This can be done orally, IV, or subcutaneously; however, oral is thought to be safest and easiest. Various protocols are described, but each protocol utilizes the same principles, which involve gradually increasing doses of penicillin, increasing each dose every 15 to 20 minutes. For example, one oral protocol using **penicillin V** uses 14 total doses, each dose given 15 minutes apart. The units per dose are doubled at each interval (eg, 100, 200, 400, 800) for a total cumulative dose of 1.3 million units over 4 hours. After desensitization, maintain patients on penicillin for the duration of therapy.

Cross-allergenicity with cephalosporins: Individuals with a history of penicillin hypersensitivity have experienced severe reactions when treated with a cephalosporin. The incidence of cross-allergenicity between penicillins and cephalosporins is estimated to range from 5% to 16%; however, it is possible the incidence is much lower, possibly 3% to 7%.

Urticaria, other skin rashes and serum sickness-like reactions may be controlled by antihistamines and, if necessary, corticosteroids. Discontinue use unless the condition being treated is life-threatening and amenable only to penicillin therapy. Serious anaphylactoid reactions require emergency measures. (See Management of Acute Hypersensitivity Reactions).

➤*Tartrazine sensitivity:* Some of these products contain tartrazine, which may cause allergic-type reactions (including bronchial asthma) in susceptible individuals. Although the incidence of tartrazine sensitivity in the general population is low, it is frequently seen in patients who also have aspirin hypersensitivity. Specific products containing tartrazine are identified in the product listings.

➤*Sulfite sensitivity:* Some of these products contain sodium formaldehyde sulfoxylate, a sulfite that may cause allergic-type reactions including anaphylactic symptoms and life-threatening or less severe asthmatic episodes in certain susceptible people. The overall prevalence of sulfite sensitivity in the general population is unknown and probably low. Sulfite sensitivity is seen more frequently in asthmatic than in nonasthmatic people.

➤*Renal function impairment:* Because **carbenicillin** is primarily excreted by the kidney, patients with severe renal impairment (creatinine clearance [Ccr] less than 10 mL/min) will not achieve the therapeutic urine levels of carbenicillin.

In patients with Ccr 10 to 20 mL/min, it may be necessary to adjust dosage to prevent accumulation of the drug.

Reduce the dosage of **penicillin G** in patients with severe renal impairment, with additional modifications when hepatic disease accompanies the renal impairment.

➤*Superinfection:* Use of antibiotics (especially prolonged or repeated therapy) may result in bacterial or fungal overgrowth of nonsusceptible organisms. Such overgrowth may lead to a secondary infection. Take appropriate measures if this occurs.

Indwelling IV catheters encourage superinfections.

➤*Pregnancy: Category B*. There are no adequate or well-controlled studies in pregnant women. Penicillins cross the placenta. Use during pregnancy only if clearly needed.

Labor and delivery – Oral aminopenicillins are poorly absorbed during labor. It is not known whether use has immediate or delayed adverse effects on the fetus or alters normal labor.

➤*Lactation:* Penicillins are excreted in breast milk in low concentrations; use may cause diarrhea, candidiasis, or allergic response in the nursing infant. **Ampicillin** use by breast-feeding mothers may lead to sensitization of infants; therefore, decide whether to discontinue breast-feeding or ampicillin, taking into account the importance of the drug to the mother.

➤*Children:* Safety and efficacy of **carbenicillin**, **piperacillin**, and the β-lactamase inhibitor/penicillin combinations have not been established in infants and children younger than 12 years of age. Penicillins are excreted largely unchanged by the kidney. Because of incompletely developed renal function in infants, the rate of elimination will be slow. Penicillinase-resistant penicillins (especially **methicillin**) may not be completely excreted, with abnormally high blood levels resulting. Oral aminopenicillins are not absorbed as well in neonates as in adults. Use caution in administering to newborns and evaluate organ system function frequently. Frequent blood levels are advisable, with dosage adjustments when necessary. Monitor all newborns closely for clinical and laboratory evidence of toxic or adverse effects.

➤*Monitoring:* Perform bacteriologic studies to determine causative organisms and their susceptibility so that appropriate therapy is administered.

Obtain blood cultures, white blood cell (WBC) and differential cell counts prior to initiation of therapy and at least weekly during therapy with penicillinase-resistant penicillins. Measure AST and ALT during therapy to monitor for liver function abnormalities.

Perform periodic urinalysis, blood-urea nitrogen (BUN), and creatinine determinations during therapy with penicillinase-resistant penicillins, and consider dosage alterations if these values become elevated. If renal impairment is known or suspected, reduce the total dosage and monitor blood levels to avoid possible neurotoxic reactions.

Monitoring is particularly important in newborns, infants and when high dosages are used.

Drug Interactions

Penicillin Drug Interactions

Precipitant drug	Object drug[a]		Description
Penicillins, parenteral	Aminoglycosides, parenteral	↔	Although these agents are often used together to achieve a synergistic action, certain penicillins may inactivate certain aminoglycosides in vitro. Do not mix in the same IV solution. Also, oral neomycin may reduce the serum concentrations of oral penicillin.
Penicillins, parenteral	Anticoagulants	↑	Large IV doses of penicillins can increase bleeding risks of anticoagulants by prolonging bleeding time. Conversely, nafcillin and dicloxacillin have been associated with warfarin resistance.
Penicillins, oral	Beta blockers	↔	Ampicillin may reduce the bioavailability of atenolol. Case reports indicated that beta blockers may potentiate anaphylactic reactions of penicillin.
Penicillins	Contraceptives, oral	↓	The efficacy of oral contraceptives may be reduced and increased breakthrough bleeding may occur. Although infrequently reported, contraceptive failure is possible; the use of an additional form of contraception during penicillin therapy is advisable.
Penicillins, parenteral	Heparin	↑	An increased risk of bleeding may occur, possibly because of additive effects.
Penicillin	Methotrexate	↑	Serum concentrations and pharmacologic effects of methotrexate may be increased by penicillins (oral). Toxicity may occur.
Allopurinol	Ampicillin	↑	The rate of ampicillin-induced skin rash appears much higher when coadministered with allopurinol than with either drug by itself (see Warnings).
Chloramphenicol	Penicillins	↔	Synergistic effects may develop, but antagonism has been reported in animal studies.
Erythromycin	Penicillins	↔	In vitro tests and clinical studies have demonstrated both antagonism and synergism with coadministration.
Tetracyclines	Penicillins	↓	The bacteriostatic action of tetracycline derivatives may impair the bactericidal effects of penicillins.
Nafcillin	Cyclosporine	↓	Administered concomitantly subtherapeutic cyclosporine levels have been reported. When used concomitantly in organ transplant patients, the cyclosporine levels should be monitored.
Piperacillin	Vecuronium	↑	Piperacillin when used concomitantly with vecuronium has been implicated in the prolongation of the neuromuscular blockade of vecuronium. It is expected that the neuromuscular blockade produced by any of the nondepolarizing muscle relaxants could be prolonged in the presence of piperacillin.
Aspirin, phenylbutazone, sulfonamides, indomethacin, thiazide diuretics, furosemide, ethacrynic acid	Penicillin G	↑	These drugs may compete with penicillin G for renal tubular secretion and thus prolong the serum half-life of penicillin.
Probenecid	Penicillins (renally excreted)	↑	Probenecid administered concomitantly with piperacillin/tazobactam prolongs the half-life of piperacillin by 21% and tazobactam by 71%. Carbenicillin indanyl sodium blood levels may be increased and prolonged by concurrent administration of probenecid.

[a] ↑ = object drug increased; ↓ = object drug decreased; ↔ = undetermined clinical effect.

➤*Drug/Lab test interactions:* False-positive **urine glucose** reactions may occur with penicillin therapy if Clinitest, Benedict's Solution or Fehling's Solution are used. It is recommended that enzymatic glucose oxidase tests (such as *Clinistix* or *Tes-Tape*) be used. Positive *Coombs' tests* have occurred. Positive direct antiglobulin tests (DAT) have been reported after large IV doses of **piperacillin**; **clavulanic acid** has also been reported to cause a positive DAT. High urine concentrations of some penicillins may produce false-positive protein reactions (pseudoproteinuria) with the following methods: Sulfosalicylic acid and boiling test, acetic acid test, biuret reaction, and nitric acid test. The bromphenol blue (*Multi-Stix*) reagent strip test has been reported to be reliable.

➤*Drug/Food interactions:* Absorption of most penicillins is affected by food; these medications are best taken on an empty stomach, 1 hour before or 2 hours after meals. **Penicillin V** may be given with meals; however, blood levels may be slightly higher when taken on an empty stomach. **Amoxicillin** and amoxicillin/clavulanate potassium tablets may be given without regard to meals.

Adverse Reactions

➤*Cardiovascular:* Cardiac arrest, cerebrovascular accident, hypotension, palpitations, pulmonary embolism, pulmonary hypertension, syncope, tachycardia, vasovagal reaction, vasodilation.

➤*CNS:* Penicillins have caused neurotoxicity (manifested as convulsions and seizures, hallucinations, lethargy, neuromuscular hyperirritability) when given in large IV doses, especially in patients with renal failure. Mental disturbances including agitation, anxiety, combativeness, confusion, depression, hallucinations, seizures, weakness, and expressed fear of impending death have been reported in individuals following single-dose therapy for gonorrhea with **penicillin G procaine**, which may have been a reaction to procaine. Reactions have been transient, lasting from 15 to 30 minutes. Dizziness, fatigue, insomnia, reversible hyperactivity, and prolonged muscle relaxation have occurred.

➤*GI:* Abdominal pain or cramp, abnormal taste sensation, black "hairy" tongue, diarrhea or bloody diarrhea, dry mouth, enterocolitis, epigastric distress, flatulence, furry tongue, gastritis, glossitis, nausea, sore mouth or tongue, rectal bleeding, stomatitis, vomiting; pseudomembranous colitis, intestinal necrosis (see Precautions). Incidence of symptoms, particularly diarrhea, is less with **amoxicillin** than with **ampicillin**.

➤*GU:* Hematuria, impotence, neurogenic bladder, priapism, proteinuria, renal failure, vaginitis.

➤*Hematologic/Lymphatic:*

Bleeding abnormalities – Hemorrhagic manifestations associated with abnormalities of coagulation tests such as clotting and prothrombin time have occurred and are more likely to occur in patients with renal failure (see Warnings). Agranulocytosis; anemia; bone marrow depression; decrease in WBC and lymphocyte counts; eosinophilia; granulocytopenia; hemolytic anemia; increase in lymphocytes, monocytes, basophils, and platelets; leukopenia; lymphadenopathy; neutropenia; prolongation of bleeding and prothrombin time; reduction in hemoglobin or hematocrit; thrombocytopenia; thrombocytopenic purpura. These reactions are usually reversible on discontinuation of therapy and are believed to be hypersensitivity phenomena. A slight thrombocytosis occurred in less than 1% of patients treated with amoxicillin/clavulanate potassium. Atypical lymphocytosis has been observed in one pediatric patient receiving ampicillin/sulbactam sodium.

➤*Hypersensitivity:* Adverse reactions (estimated incidence, 0.7% to 10%) are more likely to occur in individuals with previously demonstrated hypersensitivity. In penicillin-sensitive individuals with a history of allergy, asthma, or hay fever, the reactions may be immediate and severe (see Warnings).

Allergic symptoms include allergic vasculitis, angioneurotic edema, asthenia, bronchospasm, death, erythema multiforme (rarely, Stevens-Johnson syndrome), headache, hypotension, laryngeal edema, laryngospasm, maculopapular to exfoliative dermatitis, pain, prostration, pruritus, reactions resembling serum sickness (arthralgia, arthritis, chills, edema, fever, malaise), skin rashes, urticaria, vascular collapse, vesicular eruptions.

➤*Local:* Atrophy; deep vein thrombosis; ecchymosis; hematomas; pain (accompanied by induration) at the site of injection; skin ulcer; neurovascular reactions including warmth, vasospasm, pallor, mottling, gangrene, numbness of the extremities, cyanosis of the extremities and neurovascular damage. Vein irritation and phlebitis can occur, particularly when undiluted solution is injected directly into the vein. Tissue necrosis due to extravasated **nafcillin** has been successfully modified with hyaluronidase.

➤*Renal:* Interstitial nephritis (eg, hematuria, hyaline casts, oliguria, proteinuria, pyuria) and nephropathy are infrequent and usually associated with high doses of parenteral penicillins; however, this has occurred with all of the penicillins. Such reactions are hypersensitivity responses and are usually associated with fever, skin rash, and eosinophilia. Elevations of creatinine or BUN may occur.

➤*Lab test abnormalities:* Elevations of AST, ALT, bilirubin, and LDH have been noted in patients receiving semisynthetic penicillins (particularly **oxacillin**); such reactions are more common in infants. Elevations of serum alkaline phosphatase and hypernatremia, and reduction in serum potassium, albumin, total proteins, and uric acid may occur. Decreased hemoglobin, hematocrit, red blood cell counts, WBC, neutrophils, lymphocytes, platelets, and increased lymphocytes, monocytes, basophils, eosinophils and platelets; increased BUN and creatinine; presence of RBCs and hyaline casts in urine (ampicillin sodium/sulbactam sodium). Evidence indicates glutamic oxaloacetic transaminase (GOT) is released at the site of IM injection of **ampicillin**. Increased amounts of this enzyme in the blood do not necessarily indicate liver involvement.

Hemorrhagic manifestations associated with abnormalities of coagulation tests such as clotting and prothrombin time have occurred and are more likely to occur in patients with renal failure (see Warnings).

➤*Miscellaneous:* Anorexia; apnea; blindness; blurred vision; diaphoresis; dyspnea; exacerbation of arthritis; hypoxia; joint disorder; myoglobinuria; periostitis; rhabdomyolysis; hyperthermia, itchy eyes, transient hepatitis, and cholestatic jaundice (rare); sciatic neuritis caused by IM injection of penicillin. The Jarisch-Herxheimer reaction has been reported in the treatment of syphilis.

Overdosage

➤*Symptoms:* Penicillin overdosage can result in neuromuscular hyperexcitability or convulsive seizures. Dose-related toxicity may arise with the use of massive doses of IV penicillins (40 to 100 million units/day), particularly in patients with severe renal impairment. Manifestations may include agitation, confusion, asterixis, hallucinations, stupor, coma, multifocal myoclonus, seizures and encephalopathy. Hyperkalemia is also possible.

➤*Treatment:* In case of overdosage, discontinue penicillin, treat symptomatically and institute supportive measures as required. Refer to General Management of Acute Overdosage. If necessary, hemodialysis may be used to reduce blood levels of **penicillin**, although the degree of effectiveness of this procedure is questionable. Hemodialysis does not accelerate the rate of clearance of **nafcillin** from the blood. The metabolic by-products of **carbenicillin indanyl sodium**, **indanyl sulfate** and **glucuronide**, as well as free **carbenicillin**, are dialyzable. In renal function impairment, aminopenicillins can be removed by hemodialysis, but not peritoneal dialysis. The molecular weight, degree of protein binding and pharmacokinetic profile of **sulbactam** and **clavulanic acid** suggest these compounds may also be removed by hemodialysis.

Patient Information

Complete full course of therapy.

Take on an empty stomach 1 hour before or 2 hours after meals. Absorption of **penicillin V** and **amoxicillin** tablets and amoxicillin/clavulanate potassium is not significantly affected by food.

Take at even intervals, preferably around the clock.

Notify physician if skin rash, itching, hives, severe diarrhea, shortness of breath, wheezing, black "hairy"tongue, sore throat, nausea, vomiting, fever, swollen joints, or any unusual bleeding or bruising occurs.

Discard any liquid forms of **penicillin** after 7 days if stored at room temperature or after 14 days if refrigerated.

Natural Penicillins

PENICILLIN G

Rx	**Penicillin G Potassium** (Baxter)	**Injection, solution**: 1,000,000 units	In premixed, frozen 50 mL *Galaxy* containers.
		2,000,000 units	In premixed, frozen 50 mL *Galaxy* containers.
		3,000,000 units	In premixed, frozen 50 mL *Galaxy* containers.
Rx	**Penicillin G Sodium** (Sandoz)	**Injection, powder for solution**: 5,000,000 units	1.68 mEq sodium/million units. In vials.
Rx	**Pfizerpen** (Pfizer)		≈ 6.8 mg sodium (0.3 mEq), 65.6 mg potassium (1.68 mEq)/million units. In vials.
Rx	**Pfizerpen** (Pfizer)	**Injection, powder for solution**: 20,000,000 units per vial	≈ 6.8 mg sodium (0.3 mEq), 65.6 mg potassium (1.68 mEq)/million units. In vials.
Rx	**Penicillin G Procaine** (Monarch)	**Injection; suspension**: 600,000 units/vial	In 1 mL *Tubex*.[a]
		1,200,000 units/vial	In 2 mL *Tubex*.[a]
Rx	**Bicillin L-A** (Monarch)	**Injection; suspension**: 600,000 units/dose	As penicillin G benzathine. In 1 mL *Tubex*[b]
		1,200,000 units/dose	As penicillin G benzathine. In 2 mL *Tubex*[b]
		2,400,000 units/dose	As penicillin G benzathine. In 4 mL prefilled syringe.[b]
Rx	**Permapen** (Roerig)	**Injection; suspension**: 1,200,000 units/dose	As penicillin G benzathine. In 2 mL *Isoject*[c]

[a] With parabens and povidone.
[b] With povidone and parabens.
[c] With polyvinylpyrrolidone and parabens.

PENICILLIN G (AQUEOUS) — INJECTION

For complete and comparative prescribing information, refer to the Penicillins class monograph.

Administration and Dosage

➤*Infants:* Preferably administered IV as 15- to 30-minute infusions.

Older than 7 days old – 75,000 units/kg/day in divided doses every 8 hours (meningitis – 200,000 to 300,000 units/kg/day every 6 hours).

Younger than 7 days old – 50,000 units/kg/day in divided doses every 12 hours; group B streptococcus – 100,000 units/kg/day; meningitis – 100,000 to 150,000 units/kg/day).

Streptococci in groups A, C, G, H, L and M are very sensitive to penicillin G. Some group D organisms are sensitive to the high serum levels obtained with aqueous penicillin G.

Penicillin G injection should be administered by IV infusion.

Parenteral Penicillin G Use and Dosages in Adults

Indications	Adult dosage
Labeled uses:	
Meningococcal meningitis/septicemia:	24 million units/day; 1 to 2 million units IM every 2 hours; or 20 to 30 million units/day continuous IV drip for 14 days or until afebrile for 7 days; or 200,000 to 300,000 units/kg/day every 2 to 4 hours in divided doses for a total of 24 doses
Actinomycosis:	
For cervicofacial cases	1 to 6 million units/day
For thoracic and abdominal disease	10 to 20 million units/day IV every 4 to 6 hours for 6 weeks. May be followed by oral penicillin V, 500 mg 4 times daily for 2 to 3 months

PENICILLIN G (AQUEOUS) — INJECTION

Parenteral Penicillin G Use and Dosages in Adults

Indications	Adult dosage
Clostridial infections:	
Botulism (adjunctive therapy to antitoxin), gas gangrene and tetanus (adjunctive therapy to human tetanus immune globulin)	20 million units/day every 4 to 6 hours as adjunct to antitoxin
Fusospirochetal infections: Severe infections of oropharynx, lower respiratory tract and genital area	5 to 10 million units/day every 4 to 6 hours
Rat-bite fever (Spirillum minus, Streptobacillus moniliformis), Haverhill fever:	12 to 20 million units/day every 4 to 6 hours for 3 to 4 weeks
Listeria infections (Listeria monocytogenes):	
Meningitis (adults)	15 to 20 million units/day every 4 to 6 hours for 2 weeks
Endocarditis (adults)	15 to 20 million units/day every 4 to 6 hours for 4 weeks
Pasteurella infections (Pasteurella multocida): Bacteremia and meningitis	4 to 6 million units/day every 4 to 6 hours for 2 weeks
Erysipeloid (Erysipelothrix rhusiopathiae): Endocarditis	12 to 20 million units/day every 4 to 6 hours for 4 to 6 weeks
Diphtheria: Adjunct to antitoxin to prevent carrier state	2 to 3 million units/day in divided doses every 4 to 6 hours for 10 to 12 days
Anthrax: (B. anthracis is often resistant)	Minimum 5 million units/day; 12 to 20 million units/day have been used
Serious streptococcal infections (S. pneumoniae):	
Empyema, pneumonia, pericarditis, endocarditis, meningitis	5 to 24 million units/day in divided doses every 4 to 6 hours
Syphilis:[a]	
Neurosyphilis[a]	18 to 24 million units/day IV (3 to 4 million units every 4 hours) for 10 to 14 days. Many recommend benzathine penicillin G 2.4 million units IM weekly for 3 weeks following the completion of this regimen
Disseminated gonococcal infections: (eg, meningitis, endocarditis, arthritis)	10 million units/day every 4 to 6 hours, with the exception of meningococcal meningitis/septicemia, ie, every 2 hours

[a] CDC 1998 Sexually Transmitted Diseases Treatment Guidelines. *Morbidity and Mortality Weekly Report* 1997 Jan 23;47 (No. RR-1):1-118.

Parenteral Penicillin G Use and Dosages in Children

Indications	Pediatric dosage
Serious streptococcal infections, such as pneumonia and endocarditis (*S. pneumoniae*) and meningococcus:	150,000 units/kg/day divided in equal doses every 4 to 6 hours; duration depends on infecting organism and type of infection
Meningitis caused by susceptible strains of pneumococcus and meningococcus:	250,000 units/kg/day divided in equal doses every 4 hours for 7 to 14 days depending on the infecting organism (maximum dose of 12 to 20 million units/day)
Disseminated gonococcal infections (penicillin-susceptible strains):	*Weight < 45 kg:*
Arthritis	100,000 units/kg/day in 4 equally divided doses for 7 to 10 days
Meningitis	250,000 units/kg/day in equal doses every 4 hours for 10 to 14 days
Endocarditis	250,000 units/kg/day in equal doses every 4 hours for 4 weeks
	Weight ≥ 45 kg:
Arthritis, meningitis, endocarditis	10 million units/day in 4 equally divided doses with the duration of therapy depending on the type of infection
Syphilis (congenital and neurosyphilis) after the newborn period:	200,000 to 300,000 units/kg/day (administered as 50,000 units/kg every 4 to 6 hours) for 10 to 14 days
Congenital syphilis:[a] Symptomatic or asymptomatic infants	*Infants:* 50,000 units/kg/dose IV every 12 hours the first 7 days, thereafter every 8 hours for total of 10 days. *Children:* 50,000 units/kg every 4 to 6 hours for 10 days.
Diphtheria (adjunctive therapy to antitoxin and for prevention of carrier state):	150,000 to 250,000 units/kg/day in equal doses every 6 hours for 7 to 10 days
Rat-bite fever; Haverhill fever (with endocarditis caused by S. moniliformis):	150,000 to 250,000 units/kg/day in equal doses every 4 hours for 4 weeks

[a] CDC 1998 Sexually Transmitted Diseases Treatment Guidelines. *Morbidity and Mortality Weekly Report* 1997 Jan 23;47 (No. RR-1):1-118.

➤*Renal function impairment:* Penicillin G is relatively nontoxic and dosage adjustments are generally required only in cases of severe renal impairment. The recommended dosage regimen is as follows:

Creatinine clearance less than 10 mL/min; administer a full loading dose followed by one-half of the loading dose every 8 to 10 hours.

Uremic patients with a creatinine clearance more than 10 mL/min; administer a full loading dose followed by one-half of the loading dose every 4 to 5 hours.

➤*Rheumatic fever:* Because alpha-hemolytic streptococci resistant to penicillin may be found when patients are receiving continuous oral penicillin for secondary prevention of rheumatic fever, prophylactic agents other than penicillin may be prescribed in addition to their continuous rheumatic fever prophylactic regimen.

➤*Potassium and sodium content:* Penicillin G potassium contains 1.7 mEq potassium and 0.3 mEq sodium per million units; penicillin G sodium contains 2 mEq sodium per million units.

Give recommended daily dosage IM or by continuous IV infusion.

➤*IM:* Keep total volume of injection small. The IM route is the preferred route of administration. Solutions containing ≤ 100,000 units/mL may be used with a minimum of discomfort. Use greater concentrations as required.

➤*Continuous IV infusion:* When larger doses are required, administer aqueous solutions by means of continuous IV infusion. Determine volume and rate of fluid administration required by the patient in a 24-hour period. Add appropriate daily dosage to this fluid.

➤*Intrapleural or other local infusion:* If fluid is aspirated, give infusion in a volume equal to one fourth or one half the amount of fluid aspirated; otherwise, prepare as for the IM injection.

➤*Intrathecal use:* Must be highly individualized. Use only with full consideration of the possible irritating effects of penicillin when used by this route. The preferred route of therapy in bacterial meningitis is IV, supplemented by IM injection. It has been suggested that intrathecal use has no place in therapy.

➤*Admixture compatibility/incompatibility:* Depending on the route of administration, use sterile water for injection, isotonic sodium chloride injection, or dextrose injection. Penicillins are rapidly inactivated in the presence of carbohydrate solutions at alkaline pH.

➤*Off-label dosing:*

Lyme neuroborreliosis – [1] = Good documentation.

Adults: 18 to 24 million units per day in divided doses every 4 hours administered IV for 14 days. In studies, outcomes were similar with regimens lasting between 10 and 28 days. Dosage should be reduced in patients with renal dysfunction.

PENICILLIN G (AQUEOUS) — INJECTION

Children: 200,000 to 400,000 units/kg/day divided every 4 hours (maximum, 18 to 24 million units/day) administered IV for 14 days. In studies, outcomes were similar with regimens lasting between 10 and 28 days. Dosage should be reduced in patients with renal dysfunction.

➤*Storage / Stability:* The dry powder is stable and does not require refrigeration. Sterile solutions may be kept in the refrigerator for 1 week without loss of potency. Solutions prepared for IV infusion are stable at room temperature for at least 24 hours.

Premixed, frozen solution – Thaw frozen container at room temperature (25°C; 77°F) or in a refrigerator (5°C; 41°F). Do not force thaw by immersion in water baths or by microwave irradiation.

The thawed solution is stable for 24 hours at room temperature or for 14 days under refrigeration. Do not refreeze thawed antibiotics.

PENICILLIN G PROCAINE — INJECTION

For complete and comparative prescribing information, refer to the Penicillins group monograph.

Indications

➤*General information:* In the treatment of moderately severe infections in both adults and pediatric patients due to penicillin-G-susceptible microorganisms that are susceptible to the low and persistent serum levels common to this particular dosage form in the indications listed below. Therapy should be guided by bacteriological studies (including susceptibility tests) and by clinical response.

When high, sustained serum levels are required, aqueous penicillin G, either IM or IV, should be used. The following infections will usually respond to adequate dosages of IM penicillin G procaine: Moderately severe to severe infections of the upper respiratory tract, skin and soft-tissue infections, scarlet fever, and erysipelas due to susceptible streptococci (group A, without bacteremia).

Severe pneumonia, empyema, bacteremia, pericarditis, meningitis, peritonitis, and arthritis of pneumococcal etiology are better treated with aqueous penicillin G during the acute stage.

➤*Streptococcal infections:* Streptococci in groups A, C, G, H, L, and M are very sensitive to penicillin G. Other groups, including group D (enterococcus), are resistant. Aqueous penicillin is recommended for streptococcal infections with bacteremia.

➤*Respiratory tract infection:* Moderately severe infections of the respiratory tract due to susceptible pneumococci.

➤*Skin and soft tissue infection:* Moderately severe infections of the skin and soft tissues due to susceptible staphylococci (penicillin G-susceptible).

Reports indicate an increasing number of strains of staphylococci resistant to penicillin G, emphasizing the need for culture and sensitivity studies in treating suspected staphylococcal infections. Indicated surgical procedures should be performed.

➤*Fusospirochetosis:* Fusospirochetosis (Vincent's gingivitis and pharyngitis). Moderately severe infections of the oropharynx due to susceptible fusiform bacilli and spirochetes.

Necessary dental care should be accomplished in infections involving the gum tissue.

➤*Syphilis:* Syphilis (all stages) due to susceptible *Treponema pallidum*.

➤*Beta-lactamase producing bacteria:* This drug should not be used in the treatment of beta-lactamase producing organisms that include most strains of *Neisseria gonorrhea*.

➤*Yaws, bejel, and pinta:* Yaws, bejel, and pinta due to susceptible organisms.

➤*Diphtheria:* Penicillin G procaine is an adjunct to antitoxin for prevention of the carrier stage of diphtheria due to susceptible *C. diphtheriae*.

➤*Anthrax:* To reduce the incidence or progression of the disease following exposure to aerosolized *Bacillus anthracis*.

➤*Rat-bite fever:* Rat-bite fever due to susceptible *Streptobacillus moniliformis* and *Spirillum minus* organisms.

➤*Erysipeloid:* Erysipeloid due to susceptible *Erysipelothrix rhusiopathiae*.

➤*Endocarditis:* Subacute bacterial endocarditis, only in extremely sensitive infections, due to susceptible group A streptococci.

Administration and Dosage

➤*General dosing considerations:* For IM injection only. Do not inject into or near an artery or nerve. Injection into or near a nerve may result in permanent neurologic damage (see Administration).

➤*Adults:*

Anthrax, cutaneous – 600,000 to 1 million units/day IM.

Anthrax, inhalational (postexposure) –

Usual dosage: 1.2 million units IM every 12 hours.

Duration of therapy: The available safety data for penicillin G procaine at this dose would best support a duration of therapy of 2 weeks or less. Treatment for inhalational anthrax (postexposure) must be continued for a total of 60 days. Health care providers must consider the risks and benefits of continuing administration of penicillin G procaine for more than 2 weeks or switching to an effective alternative treatment.

Bacterial endocarditis (group A streptococci), only in extremely sensitive infections – 600,000 to 1 million units/day IM.

Penicillin G procaine is not recommended for prophylaxis against bacterial endocarditis. For prophylaxis against bacterial endocarditis in patients with congenital heart disease or rheumatic or other acquired valvular heart disease when undergoing dental procedures or surgical procedures of the upper respiratory tract, use penicillin V. For patients unable to take oral medications, aqueous penicillin G procaine is recommended.

Diphtheria –

Adjunctive therapy with antitoxin: 300,000 to 600,000 units/day IM.

Diphtheria carrier state: 300,000 units/day IM for 10 days.

Erysipeloid – 600,000 to 1 million units/day IM.

Fusospirochetosis (Vincent's infection) – 600,000 to 1 million units/day IM.

Pneumonia (pneumococcal), moderately severe (uncomplicated) – 600,000 to 1 million units/day IM.

Rat-bite fever (Streptobacillus moniliformis and Spirillum minus) – 600,000 to 1 million units/day IM.

Scarlet fever – 600,000 to 1 million units/day IM for a 10-day minimum.

Skin and soft tissue infections – 600,000 to 1 million units/day IM for a 10-day minimum.

Staphylococcal infections, moderately severe to severe – 600,000 to 1 million units/day IM.

Streptococcal infections (group A) – 600,000 to 1 million units/day IM for a 10-day minimum.

Syphilis –

Primary, secondary, and latent with a negative spinal fluid: 600,000 units/day IM for 8 days; total, 4.8 million units.

Late (tertiary, neurosyphilis, and latent syphilis with positive spinal-fluid examination or no spinal-fluid examination): 600,000 units/day IM for 10 to 15 days; total, 6 to 9 million units.

Congenital syphilis under 70 lb body weight: 50,000 units/kg/day IM for 10 days.

Yaws, bejel, and pinta: Treatment as for syphilis in corresponding stage of disease.

Tonsillitis, moderately severe to severe – 600,000 to 1 million units/day IM for 10-day minimum.

Upper respiratory tract infections – 600,000 to 1 million units/day IM for 10-day minimum.

➤*Children:*

Anthrax, inhalational (postexposure) – 25,000 units/kg of body weight (maximum, 1,200,000 units) every 12 hours.

The available safety data for penicillin G procaine at this dose would best support a duration of therapy of 2 weeks or less. Treatment for inhalational anthrax (postexposure) must be continued for a total of 60 days. Health care providers must consider the risks and benefits of continuing administration of penicillin G procaine for more than 2 weeks or switching to an effective alternative treatment.

Pneumonia – For children weighing under 60 lbs, 300,000 units/day IM.

Staphylococcal infections – For children weighing under 60 lbs, 300,000 units/day IM.

Streptococcal (group A) infections – For children weighing under 60 lbs, 300,000 units/day IM.

Syphilis (primary, secondary, and latent with a negative spinal fluid) – For children over 12 years of age, 600,000 units/day IM for 8 days; total, 4.8 million units.

➤*Administration:* For IM injection only. Do not inject into or near an artery or nerve. Injection into or near a nerve may result in permanent neurologic damage.

Inadvertent intravascular administration, including inadvertent direct intra-arterial injection or injection immediately adjacent to arteries, of penicillin G procaine and other penicillin preparations has resulted in severe neurovascular damage, including transverse myelitis with permanent paralysis, gangrene requiring amputation of digits and more proximal portions of extremities, and necrosis and sloughing at and surrounding the injection site. Such severe effects have been reported following injections into the buttock, thigh, and deltoid areas. Other serious complications of suspected intravascular administration that have been reported include immediate pallor, mottling, or cyanosis of the extremity, both distal and proximal to the injection site, followed by bleb formation; and severe edema requiring anterior or posterior compartment fasciotomy in the lower extremity. The previously-described severe effects and complications have most often occurred in infants and small children. Prompt consultation with an appropriate specialist is indicated if any evidence of compromise of the blood supply occurs at, proximal to, or distal to the site of injection.

Quadriceps femoris fibrosis and atrophy have been reported following repeated IM injections of penicillin preparations into the anterolateral thigh.

PENICILLIN G PROCAINE — INJECTION

Administer by deep IM injection in the upper, outer quadrant of the buttock. In neonates, infants, and small children, the midlateral aspect of the thigh may be preferable. When doses are repeated, vary the injection site.

➤*Storage/Stability:* Store in a refrigerator, 2° to 8°C (36° to 46°F). Keep from freezing.

PENICILLIN G BENZATHINE — INTRAMUSCULAR

For complete and comparative prescribing information, refer to the Penicillins group monograph.

Indications

➤*General information:* Treatment of infections due to penicillin G-sensitive microorganisms that are susceptible to the low and very prolonged serum levels common to this particular dosage form. Therapy should be guided by bacteriological studies (including sensitivity tests) and by clinical response.

The following infections will usually respond to adequate dosage of IM penicillin G benzathine:

➤*Respiratory infections:* Mild-to-moderate infections of the upper respiratory tract due to susceptible streptococci.

➤*Venereal infections:* Syphilis, yaws, bejel, and pinta.

➤*Prophylaxis of rheumatic fever and chorea:* Prophylaxis with penicillin G benzathine has proven effective in preventing recurrence of these conditions. It has also been used as follow-up prophylactic therapy for rheumatic heart disease and acute glomerulonephritis.

Administration and Dosage

➤*General dosing considerations:* For IM injection only. Do not inject into or near an artery or nerve, or intravenously. See Administration.

➤*Adults:*

Prophylaxis for rheumatic fever and glomerulonephritis – Following an acute attack, penicillin G benzathine (parenteral) may be given in doses of 1.2 million units once a month or 600,000 units every 2 weeks.

Streptococcal (group A) upper respiratory tract infections (eg, pharyngitis) – 1.2 million units IM (single dose).

Syphilis –

Primary, secondary, and latent: 2.4 million units IM (single dose).

Late (tertiary and neurosyphilis): 2.4 million units IM at 7-day intervals for 3 doses. See also Off-label uses for alternative dosing.

Yaws, bejel, and pinta: 1.2 million units IM (single dose).

Off-label dosing –

Other possible off-label uses:

• *Neurosyphilis* – Aqueous penicillin G 18 to 24 million units/day IV (3 to 4 million units every 4 hours) for 10 to 14 days. Many recommend benzathine penicillin G 2.4 million units IM once/week for up to 3 weeks following completion of this regimen.

Alternatively, procaine penicillin G 2.4 million units/day IM plus probenecid 500 mg orally 4 times daily, both for 10 to 14 days. Many recommend benzathine penicillin G 2.4 million units IM once/week for up to 3 weeks following completion of this regimen.

➤*Children:*

Streptococcal (group A) upper respiratory tract infections (eg, pharyngitis) –

Older children: 900,000 units IM (single dose).

Infants and children weighing less than 27 kg: 300,000 to 600,000 units IM (single dose).

Syphilis, congenital –

2 to 12 years of age: Adjust dosage based on adult dosage schedule.

Younger than 2 years of age: 50,000 units/kg, up to adult dosage.

Off-label dosing –

Other possible off-label uses:

• *Gummas and cardiovascular syphilis (latent)* – 50,000 units/kg IM, up to adult dosage.

➤*Administration:* Penicillin G benzathine is intended for IM injection only. Do not inject into or near an artery or nerve, or IV or admix with other IV solutions (see Warnings/Precautions).

Administer by deep IM injection in the upper, outer quadrant of the buttock. In neonates, infants, and small children, the midlateral aspect of the thigh may be preferable. When doses are repeated, vary the injection site.

Because of the high concentration of suspended material in this product, the needle may be blocked if the injection is not made at a slow, steady rate.

➤*Admixture compatibility:* Do not admix with other IV solutions.

➤*Storage/Stability:* Store in a refrigerator 2° to 8°C (36° to 46°F). Keep from freezing.

PENICILLIN G BENZATHINE/PENICILLIN G PROCAINE

Rx	**Bicillin C-R** (Monarch)	**Injection:** 600,000 units/dose (300,000 units each penicillin G benzathine and penicillin G procaine)	In 1 mL *Tubex*[a]
		1,200,000 units/dose (600,000 units each penicillin G benzathine and penicillin G procaine)	In 2 mL *Tubex*[a]
Rx	**Bicillin C-R 900/300** (Monarch)	**Injection:** 1,200,000 units/dose (900,000 units penicillin G benzathine and 300,000 units penicillin G procaine)	In 2 mL *Tubex*[a]

[a] With parabens, lecithin, and povidone.

PENICILLIN G BENZATHINE/PENICILLIN G PROCAINE — INJECTION

For complete and comparative prescribing information, refer to the Penicillins group monograph.

WARNING

Not for intravenous (IV) use. Do not inject IV or admix with other IV solutions. There have been reports of inadvertent IV administration of penicillin G benzathine, which has been associated with cardiorespiratory arrest and death. Prior to administration of this drug, carefully read the labeling.

Indications

➤*General information:* Treatment of moderately severe infections due to penicillin G–susceptible microorganisms that are susceptible to serum levels common to this particular dosage form. Therapy should be guided by bacteriological studies (including susceptibility testing) and by clinical response.

Treatment of the following in adults and children (*Bicillin C-R 900/300* is only indicated in children):

➤*Streptococcal infections:* Moderately severe to severe infections of the upper respiratory tract, scarlet fever, erysipelas, and skin and soft tissue infections due to susceptible streptococci.

Streptococci in groups A, C, G, H, L, and M are very sensitive to penicillin G. Other groups, including group D (enterococci), are resistant. Penicillin G sodium or potassium is recommended for streptococcal infections with bacteremia.

➤*Pneumococcal infections:* Moderately severe pneumonia and otitis media due to susceptible pneumococci.

Severe pneumonia, empyema, bacteremia, pericarditis, meningitis, peritonitis, and arthritis of pneumococcal etiology are better treated with penicillin G sodium or potassium during the acute stage.

➤*High serum levels:* When high, sustained serum levels are required, use penicillin G sodium or potassium, either intramuscular (IM) or IV.

➤*Venereal diseases:* Do not use this drug in the treatment of venereal diseases, including syphilis, gonorrhea, yaws, bejel, and pinta.

Administration and Dosage

➤*General dosing considerations:* For IM injection only. Do not inject into or near an artery or nerve or IV. See Administration.

➤*Adults:*

Pneumococcal infections (except pneumococcal meningitis) – 1.2 million units IM every 2 or 3 days until the temperature is normal for 48 hours. Other forms of penicillin may be necessary for severe cases.

Streptococcal infections group A –

Bicillin C-R:

• *Usual dosage* – 2.4 million units IM. Treatment is usually given at a single session using multiple IM sites when indicated.

• *Alternative dosage* – One-half the total dose on day 1 and one-half on day 3. This will also ensure the penicillinemia that is required over a 10-day period; however, this alternate schedule should be used only when the health care provider can be assured of the patient's cooperation.

➤*Children:*

Pneumococcal infections (except pneumococcal meningitis) –

Bicillin C-R: 600,000 units IM every 2 or 3 days until the temperature is normal for 48 hours. Other forms of penicillin may be necessary for severe cases.

Bicillin C-R 900/300: 1.2 million units IM every 2 or 3 days until the temperature is normal for 48 hours. Other forms of penicillin may be necessary for severe cases.

Streptococcal infections group A –

Bicillin C-R: Treatment is usually given at a single session using multiple IM sites when indicated.

• *Usual dosage* –

Over 60 lbs (27 kg): 2.4 million units IM.

30 to 60 lbs (14 to 27 kg): 900,000 to 1.2 million units IM.

Under 30 lbs (14 kg): 600,000 units IM.

• *Alternative dosage* – One-half the total dose on day 1 and one-half on day 3. This will also ensure the penicillinemia required over a 10-day period; however, this alternate schedule should be used only when the health care provider can be assured of the patient's cooperation.

Natural Penicillins

PENICILLIN G BENZATHINE/PENICILLIN G PROCAINE — INJECTION

Bicillin C-R 900/300: 1.2 million units IM. A single injection is usually sufficient for the treatment of group A streptococcal infections in children.

➤*Administration:* For IM injection only. Do not inject into or near an artery or nerve or IV. Administer by deep IM injection in the upper, outer quadrant of the buttock. In neonates, infants, and small children, the mid-lateral aspect of the thigh may be preferable. When doses are repeated, vary the injection site.

Because of the high concentration of suspended material in this product, the needle may be blocked if the injection is not made at a slow, steady rate.

➤*Admixture compatibility:* Do not admix with other IV solutions.

➤*Storage/Stability:* Store in a refrigerator at 2° to 8°C (36° to 46°F). Keep from freezing.

PENICILLIN V (Phenoxymethyl Penicillin)

Rx	**Penicillin VK** (Various, eg, Teva)	**Tablets:** 250 mg	In 100s, and 1000s.
Rx	**Penicillin VK** (Various, eg, Teva)	**Tablets:** 500 mg	In 100s and 500s.
Rx	**Penicillin VK** (Various, eg, Teva)	**Powder for Oral Solution:** 125 mg/5 mL when reconstituted	In 100 and 200 mL.
Rx	**Penicillin VK** (Various, eg, Teva)	**Powder for Oral Solution:** 250 mg/5 mL when reconstituted	In 100 and 200 mL.

PENICILLIN V POTASSIUM — ORAL

For complete and comparative prescribing information, refer to the Penicillins group monograph.

Indications

➤*General information:* Treatment of mild to moderately severe infections due to penicillin G-sensitive microorganisms. Therapy should be guided by bacteriologic studies (including sensitivity tests) and by clinical response.

Severe pneumonia, empyema, bacteremia, pericarditis, meningitis, and arthritis should not be treated with penicillin V during the acute stage.

Indicated surgical procedures should be performed.

➤*Streptococcal infections (without bacteremia):* The following infections will usually respond to adequate dosage of penicillin V. Mild-to-moderate infections of the upper respiratory tract, scarlet fever, and mild erysipelas due to susceptible streptococci.

Streptococci in groups A, C, G, H, L, and M are very sensitive to penicillin. Other groups, including group D (*enterococcus*), are resistant.

➤*Pneumococcal infections:* Mild to moderately severe infections of the respiratory tract, including otitis media, due to susceptible pneumococci.

➤*Staphylococcal infections-penicillin G-sensitive:* Mild infections of the skin and soft tissues due to susceptible staphylococci.

➤*Fusospirochetosis (Vincent's gingivitis and pharyngitis):* Reports indicate an increasing number of strains of staphylococci resistant to penicillin G, emphasizing the need for culture and sensitivity studies in treating suspected staphylococcal infections.

➤*For the prevention of recurrence following rheumatic fever and/or chorea:* Prophylaxis with oral penicillin on a continuing basis has proven effective in preventing recurrence of these conditions.

Penicillin V Uses and Dosages

Organisms/Infections	Dosage
Labeled uses:	
Streptococcal infections: Mild to moderately severe infections of the upper respiratory tract, including scarlet fever and mild erysipelas	125 to 250 mg orally every 6 to 8 hours for 10 days
Pharyngitis in children	25 to 50 mg/kg/day divided every 6 hours for 10 days
Pneumococcal infections: Mild to moderately severe respiratory tract infections including otitis media	250 to 500 mg orally every 6 hours until afebrile at least 2 days
Staphylococcal infections: Mild infections of skin and soft tissue	250 to 500 mg orally every 6 to 8 hours
Fusospirochetosis (Vincent's infection) of the oropharynx: Mild to moderately severe infections	250 to 500 mg orally every 6 to 8 hours
For prevention of recurrence following rheumatic fever or chorea	125 to 250 mg orally 2 times/day on a continuing basis
Unlabeled uses:	
Prophylactic treatment of children with sickle cell anemia or splenectomy: To reduce the incidence of *S. pneumoniae* septicemia	*3 months to 5 years of age:* 125 mg orally 2 times/day *> 5 years of age:* 250 mg BID
Actinomycosis	Penicillin G 10 to 20 mg/day IV for 4 to 6 week, then Penicillin V 2 to 4 g/day for 6 to 12 months
Early Lyme disease (Borrelia burgdorferi): Erythema migrans	500 mg orally 4 times a day for 10 to 20 days
Anthrax: Postexposure prophylaxis - Confirmed or suspected exposure to *Bacillus anthracis*	*Adults:* 7.5 mg/kg orally 4 times/day *Children < 9 years of age:* 50 mg/kg/day orally divided 4 times/day Continue prophylaxis until exposure to *B. anthracis* has been excluded. If exposure is confirmed and vaccine is available, continue prophylaxis for 4 weeks and until 3 doses of vaccine have been administered or for 30 to 60 days if vaccine if not available.

Administration and Dosage

➤*Adults:*

Fusospirochetosis (Vincent's infection) of the oropharynx – 250 to 500 mg (400,000 to 800,000 units) by mouth every 6 to 8 hours.

Pneumococcal infections – 250 to 500 mg (400,000 to 800,000 units) by mouth every 6 hours until the patient has been afebrile for at least 2 days.

Prevention of rheumatic fever/chorea – 125 to 250 mg (200,000 to 400,000 units) by mouth twice daily on a continuing basis.

Staphylococcal infections – 250 to 500 mg (400,000 to 800,000 units) by mouth every 6 to 8 hours.

Streptococcal infections – 125 to 250 mg (200,000 to 400,000 units) by mouth every 6 to 8 hours for 10 days.

➤*Children:*

12 years of age and older –

Fusospirochetosis (Vincent's infection) of the oropharynx: 250 to 500 mg (400,000 to 800,000 units) by mouth every 6 to 8 hours.

Pneumococcal infections: 250 to 500 mg (400,000 to 800,000 units) by mouth every 6 hours until the patient has been afebrile for at least 2 days.

Prevention of rheumatic fever/chorea: 125 to 250 mg (200,000 to 400,000 units) by mouth twice daily on a continuing basis.

Staphylococcal infections: 250 to 500 mg (400,000 to 800,000 units) by mouth every 6 to 8 hours.

Streptococcal infections: 125 to 250 mg (200,000 to 400,000 units) by mouth every 6 to 8 hours for 10 days.

Off-label dosing –

Group A streptococcal infection:

- *Younger than 12 years of age* –
  - *Less than 27 kg (60 lb):* 250 mg 2 or 3 times daily for 10 days.
  - *27 kg (60 lb) or more:* 500 mg 2 or 3 times daily for 10 days.

Mild to moderate infections:

- *Younger than 12 years of age (excluding newborns)* – 25 to 50 mg/kg/24 hours divided every 6 to 8 hours (max, 3 g/24 hours).

Prevention of pneumococcal disease in sickle cell disease or children with asplenia:

- *5 years of age and older* – 250 mg twice daily.
- *Younger than 5 years of age* – 125 mg twice daily.

Secondary prevention of rheumatic fever: 250 mg twice daily.

➤*Administration:* May be given with meals; however, blood levels are slightly higher when the drug is given on an empty stomach.

➤*Storage/Stability:*

Solution – After reconstitution, solution must be stored in a refrigerator. Discard any unused portion after 14 days.

Tablets – Dispense in a tight container. Keep tightly closed.considerably delayed.

NAFCILLIN SODIUM

Rx	**Nafcillin Sodium** (Sandoz)	**Powder for injection:** 1 g	In *Add-Vantage* vials.
		2 g	In *Add-Vantage* vials.
Rx	**Nafcillin Injection** (Baxter)	**Injection:** 1 g	In premixed, frozen 50 mL single-dose *Galaxy* containers.
		2 g	In premixed, frozen 100 mL single-dose *Galaxy* containers.
Rx	**Nafcillin Injection** (Baxter)	**Injection, solution:** 1 g	Dextrose 1.8 g. In premixed, frozen 50 mL single-dose *Galaxy* containers.
		2 g	Dextrose 3.6 g. In premixed, frozen 100 mL in single-dose *Galaxy* containers.

NAFCILLIN SODIUM — INJECTION

For complete and comparative prescribing information, refer to the Penicillins group monograph.

Indications

➤*Staphylococcal infections:* Treatment of infections caused by penicillinase-producing staphylococci which have demonstrated susceptibility to the drug. Culture and susceptibility tests should be performed initially to determine the causative organism and its susceptibility to the drug.

To initiate therapy in suspected cases of resistant staphylococcal infections prior to the availability of susceptibility test results. Nafcillin should not be used in infections caused by organisms susceptible to penicillin G. If the susceptibility tests indicate that the infection is due to an organism other than a resistant *Staphylococcus*, therapy should not be continued with nafcillin sodium.

➤*Off-label uses:*

Catheter-related bloodstream infections (children) – [2] = Fair documentation. Nafcillin is recommended by the Infectious Diseases Society of America (IDSA) clinical practice guidelines as a first-line agent for the treatment of catheter-related infections due to methicillin-susceptible *Staphylococcus aureus* in pediatric patients.

Administration and Dosage

➤*Adults:*

Staphylococcal infections –

Usual dosage: 500 mg intravenously (IV) every 4 hours. For severe infections, 1 g every 4 hours is recommended.

Duration of therapy:

In severe staphylococcal infections, continue therapy for at least 14 days. Continue therapy for at least 48 hours after the patient has become afebrile and asymptomatic, and cultures are negative. The treatment of endocarditis and osteomyelitis may require a longer duration of therapy.

➤*Children:*

Off-label dosing –

Catheter-related bloodstream infections (children): [2] = Fair documentation.

- *Maximum dose* – 12 g/day.
- *Neonates* – 50 to 100 mg/kg/day administered IV every 6 to 12 hours in divided doses for a minimum of 14 days.
- *Infants and children* – 100 to 200 mg/kg/day administered IV every 4 to 6 hours for a minimum of 14 days.

➤*Renal function impairment:* For patients with renal failure, measure nafcillin serum levels and adjust dosage accordingly.

According to the prescribing information, renal failure does not appreciably affect the serum half-life of nafcillin; therefore, no modification of the usual nafcillin dosage is necessary in patients with renal failure with or without hemodialysis. Hemodialysis does not accelerate the rate of nafcillin clearance from the blood.

Adults receiving continuous renal replacement therapy (CRRT) – A dosage of 2 g IV every 4 to 6 hours is recommended for patients receiving continuous venovenous hemofiltration (CVVH), continuous venovenous hemodialysis (CVVHD), or continuous venovenous hemodialfiltration (CVVHDF). This recommendation assumes ultrafiltration and dialysis flow rates of 1 to 2 L/h.

Adults receiving intermittent hemodialysis (IHD) – 2 g IV every 4 to 6 hours. This recommendation assumes the patient is receiving standard IHD 3 times per week and completes the full dialysis sessions.

➤*Hepatic function impairment:* For patients with hepatic insufficiency, measure nafcillin serum levels and adjust dosage accordingly.

➤*Preparation for administration:*

Nafcillin in Galaxy containers – Thaw frozen container at room temperature, 25°C (77°F), or under refrigeration, 5°C (41°F). Do not forcefully thaw by immersion in water baths or microwave irradiation. Components of the solution may precipitate in the frozen state and will dissolve upon reaching room temperature with little or no agitation. Agitate after solution has reached room temperature. After visual inspection, discard the container if the solution remains cloudy, an insoluble precipitate is noted, or any seals or outlet ports are not intact.

Nafcillin powder for injection – Vials in the *ADD-Vantage Drug Delivery System* are to be used with *ADD-Vantage* diluent containers of sodium chloride 0.9% injection 50 and 100 mL. See the manufacturer's instructions for reconstitution and administration instructions.

➤*Administration:* With IV administration, particularly in elderly patients, take care because of the possibility of thrombophlebitis.

Nafcillin in Galaxy containers – Administer slowly over at least 30 to 60 minutes to minimize the risk of vein irritation and extravasation.

Do not use plastic containers in series connections. Such use could result in air embolism because of residual air being drawn from the primary container before administration of the fluid from the secondary container is complete.

Nafcillin powder for injection – For IV use only. The drug concentration and the rate and volume of the infusion should be adjusted so that the total dose of nafcillin is administered before the drug loses its stability in the solution in use. This route of administration should be used for relatively short-term therapy (24 to 48 hours) because of the occasional occurrence of thrombophlebitis, particularly in elderly patients.

➤*Extravasation:* Extravasation may occur during administration of nafcillin. If signs or symptoms of extravasation occur, stop the infusion immediately. If possible, withdraw 3 to 5 mL of blood to remove some of the drug. Remove the infusion needle. Delineate the infiltrated area on the patient's skin with a felt-tip marker. Hyaluronidase is an effective antidote for hyperosmolar drug infiltrations; administer promptly within the first few minutes to 1 hour after extravasation. Higher doses (150 units) have primarily been used in adults while lower doses (15 units) have been used in children. Administer hyaluronidase according to the following steps. Dilute hyaluronidase to desired concentration, depending on the dose and product used. (Note: Some products do not require dilution.) For example, if the total dose is 15 units, make 15 units/mL dilution. If the total dose is 150 units, make 150 units/mL dilution. Cleanse area with povidone-iodine. Inject hyaluronidase locally, subcutaneously or intradermally, using a 25-gauge needle or smaller. The dose is given as five 0.2 mL injections at the leading edge of the extravasation site. Change needle after each injection. Elevate for 48 hours above heart level using a sling or stockinette dressing with an observation window cut in the dressing. Avoid pressure or friction. Do not rub area. Observe for signs of increased erythema, pain, or skin necrosis. If increased symptoms occur, consult a plastic surgeon. Ensure that no medication is given distally to extravasation site. After 48 hours, encourage the patient to use the extremity normally to promote full range of motion.

➤*Admixture compatibility:* Do not add supplementary medication to the nafcillin injection.

➤*Storage/Stability:*

Galaxy containers – Store at or below −20°C (−4°F). The thawed 1 and 2 g solutions are stable for 21 days under refrigeration, 5°C (41°F), or 72 hours at room temperature, 25°C (77°F). Do not refreeze.

Vials – Store between 20° and 25°C (68° and 77°F). At concentrations ranging from 10 to 40 mg/mL in sodium chloride 0.9% injection or dextrose 5% injection, nafcillin will have utility times of 24 hours at room temperature, 25°C (77°F).

OXACILLIN SODIUM

Rx	**Oxacillin Sodium** (Various, eg, Geneva)	**Powder for Injection:** 500 mg	In vials.
		Powder for Injection: 1 g	In vials, *ADD-Vantage* vials, and piggyback vials.
		Powder for Injection: 2 g	In vials, *ADD-Vantage* vials, and piggyback vials.
		Powder for Injection: 10 g	In bulk vials.

Penicillinase-Resistant Penicillins

OXACILLIN SODIUM — INJECTION

For complete and comparative prescribing information, refer to the Penicillins group monograph.

Indications

➤*Staphylococcal infections:* In the treatment of infections caused by penicillinase-producing staphylococci which have demonstrated susceptibility to the drug. Cultures and susceptibility tests should be performed initially to determine the causative organism and their susceptibility to the drug.

To initiate therapy in suspected cases of resistant staphylococcal infections prior to the availability of laboratory test results. Oxacillin should not be used in infections caused by organisms susceptible to penicillin G. If the susceptibility tests indicate that the infection is due to an organism other than a resistant staphylococcus, therapy should not be continued with oxacillin.

➤*Off-label uses:*

Catheter-related bloodstream infections – [2] = Fair documentation. Guidelines suggest that oxacillin may be used as first-line therapy for the treatment of catheter-related bloodstream infections caused by methicillin-susceptible *Staphylococcus aureus* or methicillin-susceptible, coagulase-negative *Staphylococcus* species.

Administration and Dosage

➤*Adults:*

Staphylococcal infections –

Mild to moderate infections: 250 to 500 mg IV every 4 to 6 hours.

Severe infections: 1 g IV every 4 to 6 hours.

Off-label dosing –

Catheter-related bloodstream infections: [2] = Fair documentation. 2 g administered IV every 4 hours.

➤*Children:* Because of incompletely developed renal function in pediatric patients, oxacillin may not be completely excreted, with abnormally high blood levels resulting. Frequent blood levels are advisable in this group with dosage adjustments when necessary.

Staphylococcal infections –

Patients weighing less than 40 kg (88 lbs):

• *Mild to moderate infections* – 50 mg/kg/day IV in equally divided doses every 6 hours.

• *Severe infections* – 100 mg/kg/day IV in equally divided doses every 4 to 6 hours.

Off-label dosing –

Catheter-related bloodstream infections: [2] = Fair documentation.

• *Infants and children* – 150 to 200 mg/kg/day administered IV in divided doses every 4 to 6 hours.

• *Neonates* – 50 to 200 mg/kg/day administered IV in divided doses every 6 to 12 hours.

➤*Concomitant therapy:* Coadministration of oxacillin and probenecid increases and prolongs serum penicillin levels. Probenecid decreases the apparent volume of distribution and slows the rate of excretion by competitively inhibiting renal tubular secretion of penicillin. Penicillin-probenecid therapy is generally limited to those infections where very high serum levels of penicillin are necessary.

➤*Duration of therapy:* In severe staphylococcal infections, therapy with oxacillin should be continued for at least 14 days. Therapy should be continued for at least 48 hours after the patient has become afebrile, asymptomatic, and cultures are negative. Treatment of endocarditis and osteomyelitis may require a longer term of therapy.

➤*Preparation for administration:*

Directions for use of Galaxy plastic container – Thaw at room temperature (25°C; 77°F) or under refrigeration (5°C; 41°F). [Do not force thaw by immersion in water baths or by microwave irradiation]. Components of the solution may precipitate in the frozen state and will dissolve upon reaching room temperature with little or no agitation. Potency is not affected. Mix after solution has reached room temperature. Check for minute leaks by squeezing bag firmly. If leaks are found, discard solution as sterility may be impaired. Do not use if the solution is cloudy or precipitated or if seals are not intact. The thawed solution is stable for 21 days under refrigeration or 48 hours at room temperature. Do not refreeze.

➤*Administration:* Oxacillin injection is to be administered as a continuous or intermittent IV infusion. With IV administration, particularly in elderly patients, care should be taken because of the possibility of thrombophlebitis.

Do not use plastic containers in series connections. Such use could result in air embolism due to residual air being drawn from the primary container before administration of the fluid from the secondary container is complete.

➤*Admixture compatibility:* Do not add supplementary medication to oxacillin injection.

➤*Storage/Stability:* Store in a freezer capable of maintaining a temperature at or below −20°C (−4°F). The thawed solution from *Galaxy* plastic containers is stable for 21 days under refrigeration or 48 hours at room temperature.

DICLOXACILLIN SODIUM

Rx	**Dicloxacillin Sodium** (Various, eg, Teva)	**Capsules**: 250 mg	In 40s, 100s, 500s, and UD 100s.
		500 mg	In 30s, 40s, 50s, 100s, 500s, and UD 100s.

DICLOXACILLIN SODIUM — ORAL

For complete and comparative prescribing information, refer to the Penicillins group monograph.

Indications

➤*Staphylococcal infections:* Treatment of infections caused by penicillinase-producing staphylococci. May be used to initiate therapy when a staphylococcal infection is suspected (see Indications in the group monograph concerning use of penicillinase-resistant penicillins).

Administration and Dosage

➤*General dosing considerations:* Do not use oral preparations of the penicillinase-resistant penicillins as initial therapy in serious, life-threatening infections.

➤*Adults:*

Staphylococcal infections –

Mild to moderate infections: 125 mg every 6 hours.

Severe infections: 250 mg every 6 hours.

➤*Children:* Frequent blood level monitoring is advisable in newborns with dosage adjustments made accordingly.

Staphylococcal infections –

Patients weighing less than 40 kg (88 lbs):

• *Mild to moderate infections* – 12.5 mg/kg/day in equally divided doses every 6 hours.

• *Severe infections* – 25 mg/kg/day in equally divided doses every 6 hours.

➤*Concomitant therapy:* Penicillin-probenecid therapy generally is limited to those infections where very high serum levels of penicillin are necessary.

➤*Duration of therapy:* In severe staphylococcal infections, continue therapy with penicillinase-resistant penicillins for at least 14 days. Continue therapy for at least 48 hours after the patient has become afebrile and asymptomatic and cultures are negative. The treatment of endocarditis and osteomyelitis may require a longer term of therapy.

Treat infections caused by group A beta-hemolytic streptococci for at least 10 days to help prevent the occurrence of acute rheumatic fever or acute glomerulonephritis.

➤*Administration:* Dicloxacillin is best absorbed when taken on an empty stomach, preferably 1 to 2 hours before meals.

Aminopenicillins

AMPICILLIN

Rx	**Ampicillin** (Various, eg, Teva)	**Capsules; oral:** 250 mg (as trihydrate)	In 100s and 500s.
Rx	**Principen** (Geneva)		Lactose. (BRISTOL 7992). Lt. gray/scarlet. In 100s, 500s, and UD 100s.
Rx	**Ampicillin** (Various, eg, Teva)	**Capsules; oral:** 500 mg (as trihydrate)	In 100s and 500s.
Rx	**Principen** (Geneva)		Lactose. (BRISTOL 7993). Lt. gray/scarlet. In 100s, 500s, and UD 100s.
Rx	**Principen** (Geneva)	**Powder for suspension; oral:** 125 mg/5 mL (as trihydrate) when reconstituted	Sucrose. Fruit flavor. In 100, 150, and 200 mL.
Rx	**Principen** (Geneva)	**Powder for suspension; oral:** 250 mg/5 mL (as trihydrate) when reconstituted	Sucrose. Fruit flavor. In 100 and 200 mL.
Rx	**Ampicillin Sodium** (Sandoz)	**Injection, powder for solution**[a]: 125 mg	In vials.

AMPICILLIN

Rx	**Ampicillin Sodium** (Various, eg, APP, Geneva)	**Injection, powder for solution**[a]: 250 mg	In vials.
Rx	**Ampicillin Sodium** (Various, eg, APP, Geneva)	**Injection, powder for solution**[a]: 500 mg	In vials.
Rx	**Ampicillin Sodium** (Various, eg, APP)	**Injection, powder for solution**[a]: 1 g	In vials.
Rx	**Ampicillin Sodium** (Various, eg, APP)	**Injection, powder for solution**[a]: 2 g	In vials.
Rx	**Ampicillin Sodium** (Sandoz)	**Injection, powder for solution**[a]: 10 g	In vials.

[a] Contains approximately 2.9 mEq of sodium/g.

AMPICILLIN — ORAL

For complete and comparative prescribing information, refer to the Penicillins group monograph.

Indications

➤*Genitourinary tract infections, including gonorrhea:* *E. coli*, *P. mirabilis*, enterococci, *Shigella*, *S. typhosa* and other *Salmonella*, and nonpenicillinase-producing *N. gonorrhoeae*.

➤*Respiratory tract infections:* Nonpenicillinase-producing *H. influenzae* and staphylococci, and streptococci including *streptococcus pneumoniae*.

➤*GI tract infections:* *Shigella*, *S. typhosa* and other *Salmonella*, *E. coli*, *P. mirabilis*, and enterococci.

➤*Meningitis:* Due to *N. meningitides*.

Administration and Dosage

➤*General dosing considerations:* Larger doses may be required for severe or chronic infections. Smaller doses than those indicated in the following sections should not be used.

➤*Adults:*

Genitourinary tract infections (excluding gonorrhea) – 500 mg 4 times/day in equally spaced doses; severe or chronic infections may require larger doses.

GI tract infections – 500 mg 4 times/day in equally spaced doses; severe or chronic infections may require larger doses.

Gonorrhea – A single dose of 3.5 g of ampicillin administered simultaneously with 1 g of probenecid.

Health care providers are cautioned to use no less than the previously recommended dosage for the treatment of gonorrhea. Follow-up cultures should be obtained from the original site(s) of infection 7 to 14 days after therapy. In women, it is also desirable to obtain culture test-of-cure from both the endocervical and anal canals. Prolonged intensive therapy is needed for complications such as prostatitis and epididymitis.

Respiratory tract infections – 250 mg 4 times/day in equally spaced doses.

➤*Children:* Doses for children should not exceed doses recommended for adults. Administration to neonates and young infants should be limited to the lowest dosage compatible with an effective therapeutic regimen.

See Adults for dosing for children weighing more than 20 kg.

Genitourinary tract infections –

Children weighing 20 kg or less: 100 mg/kg/day total in equally divided and spaced doses given 4 times a day.

GI tract infections –

Children weighing 20 kg or less: 100 mg/kg/day total in equally divided and spaced doses given 4 times a day.

Respiratory tract infections –

Children weighing 20 kg or less: 50 mg/kg/day total in equally divided and spaced doses given 3 to 4 times a day.

➤*Duration of therapy:* Except for the single-dose regimen for gonorrhea referred to previously, therapy should be continued for a minimum of 48 to 72 hours after the patient becomes asymptomatic or evidence of bacterial eradication has been obtained. In infections caused by hemolytic strains of streptococci, a minimum of 10 days of treatment is recommended to guard against the risk of rheumatic fever of glomerulonephritis. In the treatment of chronic urinary or gastrointestinal infections, frequent bacteriologic and clinical appraisal is necessary during therapy and may be necessary for several months afterwards. Stubborn infections may require treatment for several weeks.

➤*Administration:* Although ampicillin is resistant to degradation by gastric acid, it should be administered at least 30 minutes before or 2 hours after meals for maximal absorption. Ampicillin should be taken with a full glass (8 oz) of water.

➤*Storage/Stability:*

Capsules – Store at room temperature; avoid excessive heat; keep tightly closed.

Powder for oral suspension – Store at room temperature; after constitution, discard unused portion after 7 days if kept at room temperature or after 14 days if refrigerated; keep bottles tightly closed.

AMPICILLIN — INJECTION

For complete and comparative prescribing information, refer to the Penicillins group monograph.

Indications

➤*General information:* It is advisable to reserve the parenteral form of this drug for moderately severe and severe infections and for patients who are unable to take the oral forms. A change to oral ampicillin may be made as soon as appropriate.

Indicated surgical procedures should be performed.

➤*Respiratory tract infections:* Caused by *S. pneumoniae*, *Staphylococcus aureus* (penicillinase and non-penicillinase producing), *H. influenzae*, and group A beta-hemolytic streptococci.

➤*Bacterial meningitis:* Caused by *E. coli*, group B streptococci, and other Gram-negative bacteria (*Listeria monocytogenes*, *N. meningitidis*). The addition of an aminoglycoside with ampicillin may increase its effectiveness against gram-negative bacteria.

➤*Septicemia and endocarditis:* Caused by susceptible Gram-positive organisms including *Streptococcus* sp., penicillin G-susceptible staphylococci, and enterococci. Gram-negative sepsis caused by *E. coli*. *Proteus mirabilis*, and *Salmonella* sp. respond to ampicillin. Endocarditis due to enterococcal strains usually respond to IV therapy. The addition of an aminoglycoside may enhance the effectiveness of ampicillin when treating streptococcal endocarditis.

➤*Urinary tract infections:* Caused by sensitive strains of *E. coli* and *Proteus mirabilis*.

➤*GI infections:* Caused by *Salmonella typhosa* (typhoid fever), other *Salmonella* sp. and *Shigella* sp. (dysentery) usually respond to oral or IV therapy.

Administration and Dosage

➤*General dosing considerations:* In the treatment of chronic urinary tract and intestinal infections, frequent bacteriologic and clinical appraisal is necessary. Smaller doses than those recommended above should not be used. Higher doses should be used for stubborn or severe infections. In stubborn infections, therapy may be required for several weeks. It may be necessary to continue clinical or bacteriologic follow-up for several months after cessation of therapy.

➤*Adults:*

Bacterial meningitis – 150 to 200 mg/kg/day in equally divided doses every 3 to 4 hours. (Treatment may be initiated with IV infusion therapy and continued with IM injections.)

Genitourinary tract infections (including those caused by Neisseria gonorrhoeae in females) –

Patients weighing 40 kg (88 pounds) or more: 500 mg IV or IM every 6 hours.

Patients weighing less than 40 kg (88 pounds): 50 mg/kg/day IV or IM in equally divided doses at 6- to 8-hour intervals.

GI tract infections –

Patients weighing 40 kg (88 pounds) or more: 500 mg IV or IM every 6 hours.

Patients weighing less than 40 kg (88 pounds): 50 mg/kg/day IV or IM in equally divided doses at 6- to 8-hour intervals.

Respiratory tract infections –

Patients weighing 40 kg (88 pounds) or more: 250 to 500 mg IV or IM every 6 hours.

Patients weighing less than 40 kg (88 pounds): 25 to 50 mg/kg/day IV or IM in equally divided doses at 6- to 8-hour intervals.

Septicemia – 150 to 200 mg/kg/day. Start with IV administration for at least 3 days and continue with the IM route every 3 to 4 hours.

Soft tissue infections –

Patients weighing 40 kg (88 pounds) or more: 250 to 500 mg IV or IM every 6 hours.

Patients weighing less than 40 kg (88 pounds): 25 to 50 mg/kg/day IV or IM in equally divided doses at 6- to 8-hour intervals.

Urethritis in males due to N. gonorrhoeae – Two doses of 500 mg each IV or IM at an interval of 8 to 12 hours. Treatment may be repeated if necessary or extended if required.

In the treatment of complications of gonorrheal urethritis, such as prostatitis and epididymitis, prolonged and intensive therapy is recommended. Cases of gonorrhea with a suspected primary lesion of syphilis should have darkfield examinations before receiving treatment. In all other cases where concomitant syphilis is suspected, monthly serological tests should be made for a minimum of 4 months.

➤*Children:* See Adults for dosing.

AMPICILLIN — INJECTION

➤*Renal function impairment:*

CrCl 10 to 50 mL/min – Give dose every 6 to 12 hours.

CrCl less than 10 mL/min – Give dose every 12 to 16 hours.

Hemodialysis – Give dose after dialysis.

Adults receiving continuous renal replacement therapy (CRRT): One reference suggests a dosage of 250 mg to 2 g every 6 to 12 hours.

The following alternative recommendations assume ultrafiltration and dialysis flow rates of 1 to 2 L/h.

- *Loading dose* – 2 g IV.
- *Maintenance dosage* –
  - *Continuous venovenous hemofiltration (CVVH):* 1 to 2 g IV every 8 to 12 hours.
  - *Continuous venovenous hemodialysis (CVVHD):* 1 to 2 g IV every 8 hours.
  - *Continuous venovenous hemodialfiltration (CVVHDF):* 1 to 2 g IV every 6 to 8 hours.

Adults receiving intermittent hemodialysis (IHD): 1 to 2 g IV every 12 to 24 hours. If the dose is given every 24 hours, then administer the dose after the dialysis session. This dosing recommendation assumes the patient is receiving standard IHD 3 times per week and completes the full dialysis sessions.

Continuous ambulatory peritoneal dialysis – 250 mg every 12 hours.

➤*Duration of therapy:* Treatment of all infections should be continued for a minimum of 48 to 72 hours beyond the time that the patient becomes asymptomatic or evidence of bacterial eradication has been obtained. A minimum of 10 days of treatment is recommended for any infection caused by group A beta-hemolytic streptococci to help prevent the occurrence of acute rheumatic fever or acute glomerulonephritis.

➤*Preparation for administration:* Use only freshly prepared solutions. IM and IV injections should be administered within 1 hour after preparation because the potency may decrease significantly after this period.

For IM use – Dissolve contents of a vial with the amount of sterile water for injection or bacteriostatic water for injection listed in the following table.

Preparation of Ampicillin IM Solution

Vial strength	Diluent (mL)	Withdrawable volume (mL)	Concentration (mg/mL)
250 mg	0.9 mL	1 mL	250 mg/mL
500 mg	1.7 mL	2 mL	250 mg/mL
1 g	3.4 mL	4 mL	250 mg/mL
2 g	6.8 mL	8 mL	250 mg/mL

While ampicillin for injection 1 and 2 g vials are primarily for IV use, the contents may be administered IM when the 250 or 500 mg vials are unavailable. In such instances, dissolve in 3.4 or 6.8 mL of sterile water for injection or bacteriostatic water for injection, respectively. The resulting solution will provide a concentration of 250 mg/mL.

For direct IV use – Add 5 mL of sterile water for injection or bacteriostatic water for injection to the 250 and 500 mg vials. Ampicillin for injection, 1 or 2 g, may also be given by direct IV administration. Dissolve in 7.4 or 14.8 mL of sterile water for injection or bacteriostatic water for injection, respectively.

For administration by IV drip – Reconstitute as previously directed (See For direct IV use) prior to diluting with IV solution. Stability studies on ampicillin at several concentrations in various IV solutions indicate the drug will lose less than 10% activity at the temperatures noted for the time periods stated in the tables in the Admixture compatibility section. (See Admixture compatibility.)

Only those solutions listed in the tables in Admixture compatibility (See Admixture compatibility) should be used for the IV infusion of ampicillin. The concentrations should fall within the range specified. The drug concentration and the rate and volume of the infusion should be adjusted so that the total dose of ampicillin is administered before the drug loses its stability in the solution in use.

➤*Administration:* Treatment for bacterial meningitis may be initiated with IV infusion therapy and continued with IM injections. The doses for other infections may be given by either by the IV or IM route. A change to oral ampicillin may be made when appropriate.

Ampicillin 250 and 500 mg should be administered slowly by IV over a 3-to 5-minute period. Ampicillin 1 or 2 g may also be given by direct IV administration and administered slowly over at least 10 to 15 minutes. More rapid administration may result in convulsive seizures.

➤*Admixture compatibility:*

Stability of Ampicillin Infusion Solutions at Room Temperature (25°C; 77°F)

Diluent	Concentrations up to (mg/mL)	Stability periods (h)
Sterile water for injection	30	8
Sodium chloride 0.9% injection	30	8
M/6 sodium lactate injection	30	8
Dextrose 5% in water	10 to 20	2
Dextrose 5% in water	2	4
Dextrose 5% and 0.45 NaCl injection	2	4
Invert sugar 10% in water	2	4
Lactated Ringer's injection	30	8

Stability of Ampicillin Solution Refrigerated (4°C; 39°F)

Diluent	Concentrations up to (mg/mL)	Stability periods (h)
Sterile water for injection	30	48
Sterile water for injection	20	72
Sodium chloride 0.9% injection	30	48
Sodium chloride 0.9% injection	20	72
Lactated Ringer's injection	30	24
M/6 sodium lactate injection	30	8
Dextrose 5% in water	20	4
Dextrose 5% and 0.45 NaCl injection	10	4
Invert sugar 10%	20	3

➤*Storage/Stability:* Store at 15° to 30°C (59° to 86°F). IM and IV injections should be administered within 1 hour after preparation because the potency may decrease significantly after this period.

AMPICILLIN/SULBACTAM

Rx	**Ampicillin/Sulbactam** (Various, APP, Hospira, Sandoz)	**Injection, powder for solution**: 1.5 g (ampicillin 1 g/sulbactam 0.5 g)	As ampicillin sodium/sulbactam sodium. In vials.
Rx	**Unasyn** (Roerig)		As ampicillin sodium/sulbactam sodium. In vials, bottles, and *ADD-Vantage* vials.
Rx	**Ampicillin/Sulbactam** (Various, APP, Hospira, Sandoz)	**Injection, powder for solution**: 3 g (ampicillin 2 g/sulbactam 1 g)	As ampicillin sodium/sulbactam sodium. In vials.
Rx	**Unasyn** (Roerig)		As ampicillin sodium/sulbactam sodium. In vials, bottles, and *ADD-Vantage* vials.
Rx	**Ampicillin/Sulbactam** (Various, APP, Hospira, Sandoz)	**Injection, powder for solution**: 15 g (ampicillin 10 g/sulbactam 5 g)	As ampicillin sodium/sulbactam sodium. In bulk package.
Rx	**Unasyn** (Roerig)		

AMPICILLIN SODIUM/SULBACTAM SODIUM — INJECTION

For complete and comparative prescribing information, refer to the Penicillins class monograph.

Indications

➤*Gynecological infections:* For gynecological infections caused by beta-lactamase–producing strains of *Escherichia coli* and *Bacteroides* species (including *Bacteroides fragilis*). The efficacy for these organisms in this organ system was studied in fewer than 10 infections.

➤*Intra-abdominal infections:* For intra-abdominal infections caused by beta-lactamase–producing strains of *E. coli*, *Bacteroides* species (including *B. fragilis*), *Klebsiella* species (including *Klebsiella pneumoniae*, and *Enterobacter* species (the efficacy for these organisms in this organ system was studied in fewer than 10 infections).

➤*Skin and skin structure infections:* For skin and skin structure infections caused by beta-lactamase–producing strains of *E. coli*, *Klebsiella* species (including *K. pneumoniae*), *Proteus mirabilis*, *B. fragilis*, *Enterobacter* species, *Acinetobacter calcoaceticus* (the efficacy for these organisms in this organ system was studied in fewer than 10 infections), and *Staphylococcus aureus*.

➤*Off-label uses:*

Community-acquired pneumonia – [1] = Good documentation. Infectious Diseases Society of America/American Thoracic Society (IDSA/ATS) guidelines confirm ampicillin/sulbactam plus azithromycin or a fluoroquinolone as an option for empiric treatment of community-acquired pneumonia in intensive care unit inpatients and as an alternative treatment to carbapenems for susceptible *Acinetobacter* species.

Hospital-acquired pneumonia – [1] = Good documentation. According to the IDSA/ATS consensus guidelines on the management of hospital-acquired pneumonia in adults, ampicillin/sulbactam is recommended as initial empiric treatment of hospital-acquired pneumonia in patients with early-onset hospital-acquired pneumonia, ventilator-associated pneumonia, or health care–associated pneumonia, and no known risk factors of multidrug-resistant pathogens.

Infective endocarditis – Recommendations for the use of ampicillin/sulbactam to treat infective endocarditis depend on the bacterial cause of the infection. Ampicillin/sulbactam is recommended to treat infective endocarditis caused by enterococcal infections with a strain that is penicillin resistant, susceptible to aminoglycosides and vancomycin, and produces beta-lactamase; *Haemophilus parainfluenzae*, *Haemophilus aphrophilus*, *Haemophilus paraphrophilus*, *Haemophilus influenzae*, *Actinobacillus actinomycetemcomitans*, *Cardiobacterium hominis*, *Eikenella corrodens*, *Kingella kingae*, and *Kingella denitrificans* (HACEK) organisms; and suspected *Bartonella* infection with a negative culture.

Infective endocarditis (adults): [1] = Good documentation.

Infective endocarditis (children/adolescents): [1] = Good documentation.

Pelvic inflammatory disease – [1] = Good documentation. The Centers for Disease Control and Prevention (CDC) guidelines recommend the use of ampicillin/sulbactam in conjunction with doxycycline as an alternative regimen in treating pelvic inflammatory disease (PID) when treatment with cefotetan, cefoxitin, or clindamycin plus gentamicin is not appropriate.

Administration and Dosage

➤*General dosing considerations:* Dosage adjustment is required for patients with renal impairment. (See Renal Function Impairment.)

➤*Adults:*

Usual dosage – 1.5 to 3 g intravenously (IV) or intramuscularly (IM) every 6 hours.

Off-label dosing –

Community-acquired pneumonia: [1] = Good documentation. Empirically, 3 g IV twice daily in combination with azithromycin or a fluoroquinolone. Patients should be treated for a minimum of 5 days and should be afebrile for 48 to 72 hours and have no more than 1 community-acquired pneumonia–associated sign of clinical instability before discontinuation of therapy.

Hospital-acquired pneumonia: [1] = Good documentation. 1.5 to 3 g IV every 6 hours. The recommended duration of treatment is 7 to 8 days for uncomplicated hospital-acquired pneumonia infections with good clinical response.

Infective endocarditis: [1] = Good documentation. 12 g/day administered IV in 4 equally divided doses; duration depends on causative agent.

• *Enterococcal infection with a strain that is penicillin resistant, susceptible to aminoglycosides and vancomycin, and produces beta-lactamase* – 12 g/day, administered IV in 4 equally divided doses for 6 weeks in combination with gentamicin. If the bacteria are also gentamicin resistant, treatment duration should be longer than 6 weeks.

• *HACEK infections* – 12 g/day, administered IV in 4 equally divided doses for 4 weeks.

• *Patients with native valves and suspected Bartonella infection with a negative culture* – 12 g/day, administered IV in 4 equally divided doses for 4 to 6 weeks in combination with gentamicin. Patients with culture-negative endocarditis should be treated with consultation with an infectious diseases specialist.

Pelvic inflammatory disease: [1] = Good documentation. 3 g IV every 6 hours, given in conjunction with doxycycline. Ampicillin/sulbactam IV therapy should continue until 24 hours after clinical improvement is noted; at this time, oral doxycycline should be continued for a total of 14 days of treatment.

➤*Children:*

Skin and skin structure infections –

1 year of age and older:

• *Patients weighing 40 kg or more* –

Usual dosage: 1.5 g to 3 g IV or IM every 6 hours.

Maximum dose: Sulbactam 4 g daily.

Duration of therapy: Do not routinely exceed 14 days of IV therapy.

Patients weighing less than 40 kg:

• *Usual dosage* – 300 mg/kg/day (ampicillin 200 mg/sulbactam 100 mg) by IV infusion in divided doses every 6 hours.

• *Duration of therapy* – Do not routinely exceed 14 days of IV therapy.

Off-label dosing –

Older than 1 month of age:

• *Mild to moderate infections* –

Usual dosage: Ampicillin 100 to 150 mg/kg/day given IV in divided doses every 6 hours.

Maximum dose: Ampicillin 8 g/sulbactam 4 g per day.

• *Meningitis* –

Usual dosage: Ampicillin 200 to 400 mg/kg/day given IV in divided doses every 4 to 6 hours.

Maximum dose: Ampicillin 8 g/sulbactam 4 g per day.

• *Severe infections* –

Usual dosage: Ampicillin 200 to 400 mg/kg/day given IV in divided doses every 6 hours.

Maximum dose: Ampicillin 8 g/sulbactam 4 g per day.

Infective endocarditis: [1] = Good documentation. 300 mg/kg/day administered IV in 4 or 6 equally divided doses; duration depends on causative agent.

• *Enterococcal infection with a strain that is penicillin resistant, susceptible to aminoglycosides and vancomycin, and produces beta-lactamase* – 300 mg/kg/day administered IV in 4 equally divided doses for 6 weeks in combination with gentamicin. If the bacteria are also gentamicin resistant, treatment duration should be longer than 6 weeks.

• *HACEK infections* – 300 mg/kg/day administered IV in 4 or 6 equally divided doses for 4 weeks.

• *Patients with native valves and suspected Bartonella infection with a negative culture* – 300 mg/kg/day administered IV in 4 or 6 equally divided doses for 4 to 6 weeks in combination with gentamicin. Patients with culture-negative endocarditis should be treated with consultation with an infectious diseases specialist.

Pelvic inflammatory disease: [1] = Good documentation.

• *Adolescents* – 3 g IV every 6 hours, given in conjunction with doxycycline. Ampicillin/sulbactam IV therapy should continue until 24 hours after clinical improvement is noted; at this time, oral doxycycline should be continued for a total of 14 days of treatment.

➤*Renal function impairment:*

Adults –

Ampicillin/Sulbactam Dosage Guide for Adults With Renal Impairment

CrCl (mL/min per 1.73 m²)	Ampicillin/Sulbactam half-life	Recommended dosage
≥ 30	1 h	1.5 to 3 g every 6 to 8 h
15 to 29	5 h	1.5 to 3 g every 12 h
5 to 14	9 h	1.5 to 3 g every 24 h

[a] CrCl = creatinine clearance.

Hemodialysis: Give dose after dialysis.

• *Continuous renal replacement therapy* – The following recommendations assume ultrafiltration and dialysis flow rates of 1 to 2 L/h.

Loading dose: 3 g IV.

Maintenance dosage:

➤*Continuous venovenous hemofiltration:* 1.5 to 3 g IV every 8 to 12 hours.

➤*Continuous venovenous hemodialysis:* 1.5 to 3 g IV every 8 hours.

➤*Continuous venovenous hemodiafiltration:* 1.5 to 3 g IV every 6 to 8 hours.

• *Intermittent hemodialysis* – 1.5 to 3 g IV every 12 to 24 hours. If the dose is given every 24 hours, administer the dose after the dialysis session. This dosing recommendation assumes the patient is receiving standard intermittent hemodialysis 3 times per week and completes the full dialysis sessions.

Continuous ambulatory peritoneal dialysis: Give dose every 24 hours.

➤*Preparation for administration:* Reconstitute powder for IV and IM use with any of the compatible diluents described as follows. Allow solutions to stand after dissolution so that any foaming will dissipate. This permits visual inspection for complete solubilization.

Preparation for IV use –

1.5 and 3 g bottles: Reconstitute to desired concentrations (3 to 45 mg/mL) with any of the following diluents. Discard unused solutions after indicated times.

AMPICILLIN SODIUM/SULBACTAM SODIUM — INJECTION

Ampicillin/Sulbactam Reconstituted for IV Use		
Diluent	Maximum concentration	Stability
Sterile water for injection	45 mg/mL	8 h at 25°C[a]
	45 mg/mL	48 h at 4°C
	30 mg/mL	72 h at 4°C
Sodium chloride 0.9% injection	45 mg/mL	8 h at 25°C[a]
	45 mg/mL	48 h at 4°C
	30 mg/mL	72 h at 4°C
Dextrose 5% injection	30 mg/mL	2 h at 25°C[a]
	30 mg/mL	4 h at 4°C
	3 mg/mL	4 h at 25°C[a,b]
Ringer's lactate injection	45 mg/mL	8 h at 25°C[a]
	45 mg/mL	24 h at 4°C
M/6 sodium lactate injection	45 mg/mL	8 h at 25°C[a]
	45 mg/mL	8 h at 4°C[c]
Dextrose 5% in saline 0.45%	3 mg/mL	4 h at 25°C
	15 mg/mL	4 h at 4°C
Invert sugar 10%	3 mg/mL	4 h at 25°C
	30 mg/mL	3 h at 4°C

[a] 21°C for pharmacy bulk package.
[b] 4 h for pharmacy bulk package.
[c] 8 h for pharmacy bulk package.

Vials: Initially, reconstitute with sterile water for injection to yield 375 mg/mL. Immediately dilute to yield 3 to 45 mg/mL.

ADD-Vantage vials: The *ADD-Vantage* system is intended as single-dose for IV administration after dilution with the *ADD-Vantage Flexible Diluent Container* containing 50 mL (1.5 g vial only), 100 or 250 mL of sodium chloride 0.9% injection. Once diluted, the solution is stable at a maximum concentration of 30 mg/mL for 8 hours at 25°C (77°F). Therefore, the final diluted solution should be completely administered within 8 hours to assure proper potency.

Pharmacy bulk package: The 15 g vial may be reconstituted with 92 mL of sterile water for injection or sodium chloride injection 0.9%. The diluent should be added in 2 separate aliquots in a suitable work area, such as a laminar flow hood. Add 50 mL of solution, shake to dissolve; add an additional 42 mL and shake. The solution should be allowed to stand after dissolution to allow any foaming to dissipate in order to permit visual inspection for complete solubilization. The resultant solution will have a final concentration of approximately ampicillin 100 mg/mL and sulbactam 50 mg/mL. The closure may be penetrated only 1 time after reconstitution, if needed, using a suitable sterile transfer device or dispensing set that allows for measured dispensing of the contents.

After reconstitution, use within 2 hours if stored at room temperature, or within 4 hours if stored under refrigeration.

Reconstituted bulk solution should not be used for direct infusion.

If the reconstituted bulk solution is stored for less than 1 hour at room temperature (20°C [68°F]) prior to further dilution, the use periods indicated in the previous table apply for the diluted solutions.

If the bulk solution is stored for 1 to 2 hours at room temperature (20°C) and then diluted with sterile water for injection or sodium chloride 0.9% injection to the following concentrations, the use periods indicated in the following table apply.

Any unused portions of solution that remain after the indicated time periods should be discarded.

Ampicillin/Sulbactam Diluted Bulk Solution Stability		
IV solution	Maximum concentration	Use period
Sterile water for injection	45 mg/mL	4 h at 21°C
	45 mg/mL	24 h at 4°C
Sodium chloride 0.9% injection	45 mg/mL	4 h at 21°C
	45 mg/mL	24 h at 4°C

Preparation for IM injection –

Vials: Reconstitute 1.5 and 3 g vials with sterile water for injection or lidocaine 0.5% or 2% injection. Consult the following table for recommended volumes needed to obtain 375 mg/mL solutions. Use only freshly prepared solutions; give within 1 hour after preparation.

Ampicillin/Sulbactam Reconstitution for IM Use		
Vial size	Volume of diluent to be added	Withdrawal volume
1.5 g	3.2 mL	4 mL
3 g	6.4 mL	8 mL

➤*Administration:* May be given IV or IM. For IV administration, the dose can be given by slow IV injection over at least 10 to 15 minutes, or can be delivered in greater dilutions with 50 to 100 mL of a compatible diluent as an IV infusion over 15 to 30 minutes. Administration by IV push may cause seizures.

May also be administered by deep IM injection. IM administration is painful; administer deep into a large muscle mass. Safety and efficacy of IM administration in children have not been established.

➤*Admixture compatibility:* When concomitant aminoglycosides are indicated, reconstitute and administer this product and aminoglycosides separately; aminopenicillins inactivate aminoglycosides in vitro.

➤*Storage/Stability:* Store at or below 30°C (86°F) prior to reconstitution. (See Preparation for Administration.)

AMOXICILLIN

Rx	**Amoxicillin** (Various, eg, Ranbaxy, Teva)	**Tablets; oral:** 500 mg	In 20s and 100s.
Rx	**Amoxicillin** (Various, eg, Ranbaxy, Teva)	**Tablets; oral:** 875 mg	In 20s, 100s, and 500s.
Rx	**Amoxil** (GlaxoSmithKline)		(Amoxil 875). Pink, capsule shape, scored. Film-coated. In 20s, 100s, 500s.
Rx	**Amoxicillin** (Various, eg, Ranbaxy, Teva)	**Tablets, chewable; oral:** 125 mg	In 100s.
Rx	**Amoxicillin** (Ranbaxy)	**Tablets, chewable; oral:** 200 mg	In 20s.
Rx	**Amoxicillin** (Various, eg, Ranbaxy, Teva)	**Tablets, chewable; oral:** 250 mg	In 100s, 250s, and 500s.
Rx	**Amoxicillin** (Ranbaxy)	**Tablets, chewable; oral:** 400 mg	In 20s and 100s.
Rx	**DisperMox** (Ranbaxy)	**Tablets for suspension; oral:** 200 mg	Aspartame, phenylalanine 5.6 mg. (RX565). Lt. pink, mottled. Strawberry flavor. In 20s, 60s, 1,000s, and UD 100s.
		400 mg	Aspartame, 5.6 mg phenylalanine. (RX567). Lt. pink, mottled. Strawberry flavor. In 20s, 60s, 500s, and UD 100s.
Rx	**Amoxicillin** (Various, eg, Ranbaxy, Teva)	**Capsules; oral:** 250 mg	In 100s, 500s, and 1,000s.
Rx	**Amoxicillin** (Various, eg, Ranbaxy, Teva)	**Capsules; oral:** 500 mg	In 50s, 100s, and 500s.
Rx	**Amoxil** (GlaxoSmithKline)		(Amoxil 500). Blue/Pink. In 500s.
Rx	**Amoxicillin** (Various, eg, Teva)	**Powder for suspension; oral:** 125 mg per 5 mL when reconstituted	In 80, 100, and 150 mL.
Rx	**Amoxil** (GlaxoSmithKline)		Sucrose. Strawberry flavor. In 80 and 150 mL.
Rx	**Trimox** (Sandoz)		Sucrose. Raspberry-strawberry flavor. In 80, 100, and 150 mL.
Rx	**Amoxicillin** (Ranbaxy)	**Powder for suspension; oral:** 200 mg per 5 mL when reconstituted	Fruit flavor. In 50, 75, and 100 mL.
Rx	**Amoxicillin** (Various, eg, Teva)	**Powder for suspension; oral:** 250 mg per 5 mL when reconstituted	In 80, 100, and 150 mL.
Rx	**Amoxicillin** (Ranbaxy)	**Powder for suspension; oral:** 400 mg per 5 mL when reconstituted	Fruit flavor. In 50, 75, and 100 mL.
Rx	**Moxatag** (Middlebrook)	**Tablets, extended-release; oral:** 775 mg	(MB-111). Blue, oval. Film-coated. In 30s and UD 10s.

AMOXICILLIN — ORAL

Indications

➤*General information:* In the treatment of infections due to susceptible (only beta-lactamase-negative) strains of the designated microorganisms in the following conditions.

Perform indicated surgical procedures.

➤*Ear, nose, and throat infections:* Infections of the ear, nose, and throat due to *Streptococcus* sp. (alpha- and beta-hemolytic strains only), *Streptococcus pneumoniae*, *Staphylococcus* sp., or *Haemophilus influenzae*. (Also see Off-label uses below.)

➤*Gonorrhea:* Gonorrhea, acute uncomplicated (anogenital and urethral infections) due to *Neisseria gonorrhoeae* (males and females).

➤*GU tract infections:* Infections of the GU tract due to *Escherichia coli*, *Proteus mirabilis*, or *Enterobacter faecalis*.

➤*H. pylori infections: H. pylori* eradication to reduce the risk of duodenal ulcer recurrence.

➤*Lower respiratory tract infections:* Infections of the lower respiratory tract due to *Streptococcus* sp. (alpha- and beta-hemolytic strains only), *Streptococcus pneumoniae*, *Staphylococcus* sp. or *H. influenzae*.

➤*Skin and skin structure infections:* Infections of the skin and skin structure due to *Streptococcus* sp. (alpha- and beta-hemolytic strains only), *Staphylococcus* sp., or *E. coli*.

➤*Dual therapy (amoxicillin/lansoprazole):* Amoxicillin, in combination with lansoprazole delayed-release capsules as dual therapy, is indicated for the treatment of patients with *H. pylori*infection and duodenal ulcer disease (active or 1-year history of a duodenal ulcer) who are either allergic or intolerant to clarithromycin or in whom resistance to clarithromycin is known or suspected. Eradication of *H. pylori* has been shown to reduce the risk of duodenal ulcer recurrence.

➤*Triple therapy (amoxicillin/clarithromycin/lansoprazole):* Amoxicillin, in combination with clarithromycin plus lansoprazole as triple therapy, is indicated for the treatment of patients with *H. pylori* infection and duodenal ulcer disease (active or 1-year history of a duodenal ulcer) to eradicate *H. pylori*. Eradication of *H. pylori* has been shown to reduce the risk of duodenal ulcer recurrence.

➤*Extended-release tablets:* Amoxicillin extended-release tablets are indicated for the treatment of tonsillitis and/or pharyngitis secondary to *Streptococcus pyogenes* in adults and children 12 years of age and older.

➤*Off-label uses:*

Acute otitis media (children) – [1] = Good documentation. According to American Academy of Pediatrics guidelines on the management of acute otitis media, high-dose amoxicillin is recommended as first-line treatment for most children when an antibiotic is considered necessary.

Lyme neuroborreliosis – [2] = Fair documentation. For the treatment of nervous system Lyme disease, guidelines from the Quality Standards Subcommittee of the American Academy of Neurology recommend oral amoxicillin as an alternative to doxycycline in cases for which doxycycline was contraindicated.

Other possible off-label uses – Lyme disease; subacute bacterial endocarditis prophylaxis.

Administration and Dosage

➤*General dosing considerations:* Dosing for infections caused by less susceptible organisms should follow the recommendations for severe infections.

➤*Adults:*

Ear, nose and throat infections –
Mild to moderate: 500 mg every 12 hours or 250 mg every 8 hours.
Severe: 875 mg every 12 hours or 500 mg every 8 hours.

Genitourinary tract infection –
Mild to moderate: 500 mg every 12 hours or 250 mg every 8 hours.
Severe: 875 mg every 12 hours or 500 mg every 8 hours.

Gonorrhea, acute uncomplicated (anogenital and urethral infections) – 3 g as a single dose.

H. pylori eradication to reduce the risk of duodenal ulcer recurrence –
Dual therapy: Amoxicillin 1 g and lansoprazole 30 mg, each given 3 times daily (every 8 hours) for 14 days.
Triple therapy: Amoxicillin 1 g, clarithromycin 500 mg, and lansoprazole 30 mg, all given twice daily (every 12 hours) for 14 days.

Lower respiratory tract infection – 875 mg every 12 hours or 500 mg every 8 hours.

Pharyngitis – 775 mg (extended-release tablets) once daily for 10 days.

Skin and skin structure infections –
Mild to moderate: 500 mg every 12 hours or 250 mg every 8 hours.
Severe: 875 mg every 12 hours or 500 mg every 8 hours.

Tonsillitis – 775 mg (extended-release tablets) once daily for 10 days.

Off-label dosing –
Lyme neuroborreliosis: [2] = Fair documentation. 500 mg 3 times per day for 14 days. In studies, outcomes were similar with regimens lasting between 10 and 28 days.

➤*Children:* The children's dose is intended for individuals who weigh less than 40 kg. Children weighing 40 kg or more should be dosed according to the adult recommendations.

Ear, nose and throat infections –
3 months of age and older (less than 40 kg):
• *Mild to moderate* – 25 mg/kg/day in divided doses every 12 hours or 20 mg/kg/day in divided doses every 8 hours (also see Off-label dosing below for alternative dosing.)
• *Severe* – 45 mg/kg/day in divided doses every 12 hours or 40 mg/kg/day in divided doses every 8 hours (also see Off-label dosing below for alternative dosing.)
Neonates and infants 12 weeks (3 months) of age and younger: Up to 30 mg/kg/day divided every 12 hours.

Genitourinary tract infections –
3 months of age and older (less than 40 kg):
• *Mild to moderate* – 25 mg/kg/day in divided doses every 12 hours or 20 mg/kg/day in divided doses every 8 hours.
• *Severe* – 45 mg/kg/day in divided doses every 12 hours or 40 mg/kg/day in divided doses every 8 hours.
Neonates and infants 12 weeks (3 months) of age and younger: Up to 30 mg/kg/day divided every 12 hours.

Gonorrhea, acute uncomplicated (anogenital and urethral infections) in males and females –
Prepubertal children: Amoxicillin 50 mg/kg combined with probenecid 25 mg/kg as a single dose.
Younger than 2 years of age: Probenecid is contraindicated in children younger than 2 years of age. Do not use this regimen in these cases.

Lower respiratory tract infections –
3 months of age and older (less than 40 kg): 45 mg/kg/day in divided doses every 12 hours or 40 mg/kg/day in divided doses every 8 hours.
Neonates and infants 12 weeks (3 months) of age and younger: Up to 30 mg/kg/day divided every 12 hours.

Skin/skin structure infections –
3 months of age and older (less than 40 kg):
• *Mild to moderate* – 25 mg/kg/day in divided doses every 12 hours or 20 mg/kg/day in divided doses every 8 hours.
• *Severe* – 45 mg/kg/day in divided doses every 12 hours or 40 mg/kg/day in divided doses every 8 hours.
Neonates and infants 12 weeks (3 months) of age and younger: Up to 30 mg/kg/day divided every 12 hours.

Off-label dosing –
Acute otitis media (children): [1] = Good documentation. Oral amoxicillin 80 to 90 mg/kg daily for 10 days in children younger than 6 years of age or for those with severe disease. In children 6 years of age and older with mild to moderate disease, a 5- to 7-day course is recommended.
Early Lyme disease:
• *Usual dose* – 50 mg/kg/day divided every 8 hours for 14 to 21 days.
• *Maximum dose* – 1.5 g/day.
Subacute bacterial endocarditis prophylaxis:
• *Usual dose* – One time dose of 50 mg/kg 1 hour before procedure.
• *Maximum dose* – 2 g.
Lyme neuroborreliosis: [2] = Fair documentation. 50 mg/kg/day in 3 divided doses (maximum, 500 mg/dose) for 14 days. In studies, outcomes were similar with regimens lasting between 10 and 28 days.

➤*Renal function impairment:* Severely impaired patients with a glomerular filtration rate (GFR) of less than 30 mL/min should not receive the 875 mg tablet.

Patients with a GFR of 10 to 30 mL/min should receive 500 or 250 mg every 12 hours, depending on the severity of the infection.

Patients with a less than 10 mL/min GFR should receive 500 or 250 mg every 24 hours, depending on severity of the infection.

There are currently no dosing recommendations for pediatric patients with impaired renal function.

Hemodialysis – 500 or 250 mg every 24 hours, depending on severity of the infection. Hemodialysis patients should receive an additional dose both during and at the end of dialysis.

➤*Administration:*

Capsules, chewable tablets, and oral suspension – May be given without regard to meals. The 400 mg suspension, 400 mg chewable tablet, and 875 mg tablet have been studied only when administered at the start of a light meal. However, food-effect studies have not been performed with the 200 mg and 500 mg formulations.

Extended-release tablets – Do not chew or crush tablets. Take within 1 hour of finishing a meal.

➤*Storage/Stability:* Store 250 and 500 mg capsules and 125 and 250 mg unreconstituted powder at or below 20°C (68°F).

Store 200 and 400 mg unreconstituted powder, 200 and 400 mg chewable tablets, and 500 and 875 mg tablets at or below 25°C (77°F). Dispense in a tight container. Any unused portion of the reconstituted suspension must be discarded after 14 days. Refrigeration is preferable but not required.

Store extended-release tablets at 25°C (77°F); excursions are permitted between 15° and 30°C (59° and 86° F).

AMOXICILLIN/CLAVULANATE POTASSIUM

Rx	**Amoxicillin/Clavulanate Potassium** (Various)	**Tablets; oral**: 250 mg amoxicillin and 125 mg clavulanic acid[a]	In 30s.
Rx	**Augmentin** (GlaxoSmithKline)		PEG. 0.63 mEq potassium. (Augmentin 250/125). Oval. Film-coated. In 30s and UD 100s.
Rx	**Amoxicillin/Clavulanate Potassium** (Various, eg, Ranbaxy, Teva)	**Tablets; oral**: 500 mg amoxicillin and 125 mg clavulanic acid[a]	In 20s, 100s, and UD 100s.
Rx	**Augmentin** (GlaxoSmithKline)		PEG. 0.63 mEq potassium. (Augmentin 500/125). Oval. Film-coated. In 20s and UD 100s.
Rx	**Amoxicillin/Clavulanate Potassium** (Various, eg, Ranbaxy, Teva)	**Tablets; oral**: 875 mg amoxicillin and 125 mg clavulanic acid[a]	In 20s, 100s, and UD 100s.
Rx	**Augmentin** (GlaxoSmithKline)		PEG. 0.63 mEq potassium. (Augmentin 875). Capsule shape, scored. In 20s and UD 100s.
Rx	**Amoxicillin/Clavulanate Potassium** (Sandoz)	**Tablets, extended-release; oral**: 1,000 mg amoxicillin and 62.5 mg clavulanic acid	PEG. 0.31 mEq potassium, 1.25 mEq sodium. White to cream, oval, scored. Film-coated. In 28s (7-day XR pack) and 40s (10-day XR pack).
Rx	**Augmentin XR** (GlaxoSmithKline)		PEG. 0.32 mEq potassium, 1.27 mEq sodium. (AUGMENTIN XR). Oval. Bilayered, scored. Film-coated. In 28s (7-day XR pack) and 40s (10-day XR pack).
Rx	**Amoxicillin/Clavulanate Potassium** (Various, eg, Teva)	**Tablets, chewable; oral**: 200 mg amoxicillin and 28.5 mg clavulanic acid[a]	In 20s and UD 20s.
Rx	**Augmentin** (GlaxoSmithKline)		0.14 mEq potassium, saccharin, mannitol, aspartame.[b] Pink, mottled. Cherry-banana flavor. In 20s.
Rx	**Amoxicillin/Clavulanate Potassium** (Various, eg, Teva)	**Tablets, chewable; oral**: 400 mg amoxicillin and 57 mg clavulanic acid[a]	In 20s and UD 20s.
Rx	**Augmentin** (GlaxoSmithKline)		0.29 mEq potassium, saccharin, mannitol, aspartame.[c] Pink, mottled. Cherry-banana flavor. In 20s.
Rx	**Augmentin** (GlaxoSmithKline)	**Powder for suspension; oral**: 125 mg amoxicillin and 31.25 mg clavulanic acid[a] per 5 mL (after reconstitution)	0.16 mEq per 5 mL potassium, saccharin, mannitol. Banana flavor. In 75, 100, and 150 mL.
Rx	**Amoxicillin/Clavulanate Potassium** (Various, eg, Teva)	**Powder for suspension; oral**: 200 mg amoxicillin and 28.5 mg clavulanic acid[a] per 5 mL (after reconstitution)	In 100 mL.
Rx	**Amoclan** (West-ward)		0.143 mEq per 5 mL potassium, aspartame.[d] Golden syrup and orange flavor. In 50, 75, and 100 mL.
Rx	**Augmentin** (GlaxoSmithKline)	**Powder for suspension; oral**: 250 mg amoxicillin and 62.5 mg clavulanic acid[a] per 5 mL (after reconstitution)	0.32 mEq per 5 mL potassium, saccharin, mannitol. Orange flavor. In 75, 100, and 150 mL.
Rx	**Amoxicillin/Clavulanate Potassium** (Various, eg, Teva)	**Powder for suspension; oral**: 400 mg amoxicillin and 57 mg clavulanic acid[a] per 5 mL (after reconstitution)	In 100 mL.
Rx	**Amoclan** (West-ward)		0.286 mEq per 5 mL potassium, aspartame.[d] Golden syrup and orange flavor. In 50, 75, and 100 mL.
Rx	**Augmentin** (GlaxoSmithKline)		0.29 mEq per 5 mL potassium, saccharin, mannitol, aspartame.[d] Orange flavor. In 50, 75, and 100 mL.
Rx	**Amoxicillin/Clavulanate Potassium** (Various, eg, Ivax, Ranbaxy, Teva)	**Powder for suspension; oral**: 600 mg amoxicillin and 42.9 mg clavulanic acid[a] per 5 mL (after reconstitution)	May contain aspartame or saccharin. In 50, 75, 100, 125, 150, and 200 mL.
Rx	**Augmentin ES-600** (GlaxoSmithKline)		0.23 mEq per 5 mL potassium, aspartame.[d] Strawberry cream flavor. In 75, 125, and 200 mL.

[a] As the potassium salt.
[b] Contains 2.1 mg phenylalanine.
[c] Contains 4.2 mg phenylalanine.
[d] Contains 7 mg of phenylalanine per 5 mL.

AMOXICILLIN/CLAVULANATE POTASSIUM — ORAL

For complete and comparative prescribing information, refer to the Penicillins group monograph.

Indications

Amoxicillin/Clavulanate Potassium Indications					
X = Labeled use	Amoxicillin/ Clavulanate potassium tablets	Amoxicillin/ Clavulanate potassium extended-release tablets (*Augmentin* extended-release 1,000 mg)	Amoxicillin/ Clavulanate potassium chewable tablets	Amoxicillin/ Clavulanate potassium oral suspension (125/31.25, 200/28.5, 250/62.5, 400/57 mg per 5 mL)	Amoxicillin/ Clavulanate potassium oral suspension (*Augmentin ES-600* 600/42.9 mg per 5 mL)
Acute otitis media[a,b]					X
Acute bacterial sinusitis[c,d]		X			
Community-acquired pneumonia[c,d]		X			
Lower respiratory tract infection[e]	X		X	X	

AMOXICILLIN/CLAVULANATE POTASSIUM — ORAL

Amoxicillin/Clavulanate Potassium Indications					
X = Labeled use	Amoxicillin/ Clavulanate potassium tablets	Amoxicillin/ Clavulanate potassium extended-release tablets (*Augmentin*) extended-release 1,000 mg)	Amoxicillin/ Clavulanate potassium chewable tablets	Amoxicillin/ Clavulanate potassium oral suspension (125/31.25, 200/28.5, 250/62.5, 400/57 mg per 5 mL)	Amoxicillin/ Clavulanate potassium oral suspension (*Augmentin ES-600* 600/42.9 mg per 5 mL)
Otitis media[e]	X		X	X	
Sinusitis[e]	X		X	X	
Skin and skin structure infections[f]	X		X	X	
Urinary tract infections[g]	X		X	X	

[a] Recurrent or persistent acute otitis media caused by *Streptococcus pneumoniae* (penicillin minimum inhibitory concentration [MIC] 2 mcg/mL or less), *Haemophilus influenzae* (including beta-lactamase–producing strains), and *Moraxella catarrhalis* (including beta-lactamase–producing strains) in patients with a history of antibiotic exposure for acute otitis media in the preceding 3 months and who are either 2 years of age or younger or attend day care).
[b] *Augmentin ES-600* is not indicated for the treatment of acute otitis media caused by *S. pneumoniae* with penicillin MIC of 4 mcg/mL or greater.
[c] For the treatment of patients with community-acquired pneumonia or acute bacterial sinusitis caused by confirmed or suspected beta-lactamase–producing pathogens (ie, *H. influenzae, M. catarrhalis, Haemophilus parainfluenzae, Klebsiella pneumoniae,* methicillin-susceptible *Staphylococcus aureus*) and *S. pneumoniae* with reduced susceptibility to penicillin (penicillin MIC = 2 mcg/mL).
[d] *Augmentin XR* is not indicated for the treatment of infections caused by *S. pneumoniae* with penicillin MIC of 4 mcg/mL or greater. Data are limited with regard to infections caused by *S. pneumoniae* with penicillin MIC of 4 mcg/mL or greater.
[e] Caused by beta-lactamase–producing strains of *H. influenzae* and *M. catarrhalis.*
[f] Caused by beta-lactamase–producing strains of *S. aureus, Escherichia coli,* and *Klebsiella* spp.
[g] Caused by beta-lactamase–producing strains of *E. coli, Klebsiella* spp., and *Enterobacter* spp.

While amoxicillin/clavulanate potassium is indicated only for the conditions previously listed, infections caused by ampicillin-susceptible organisms are also amenable to this drug because of its amoxicillin content. Therefore, mixed infections caused by ampicillin-susceptible organisms and beta-lactamase–producing organisms susceptible to amoxicillin/clavulanate potassium should not require an additional antibiotic. Therapy may be instituted prior to obtaining the results from bacteriologic and susceptibility studies when there is reason to believe the infection may involve both *S. pneumoniae* (penicillin MIC 2 mcg/mL or less) and any of the beta-lactamase–producing organisms previously listed. Once the results are known, adjust therapy.

➤*Off-label uses:*

Acute otitis media (children) – [1] = Good documentation. According to American Academy of Pediatrics guidelines on the management of acute otitis media, high-dose amoxicillin/clavulanate is recommended for severe illness (severe otalgia and/or temperature of 39°C or higher). (See Administration and Dosage.)

Administration and Dosage

➤*General dosing considerations:* The 200 and 400 mg formulations (suspension and chewable tablets) contain aspartame and should not be used by patients with phenylketonuria.

Interchangeability –

Tablets: Because the 250 and 500 mg tablets contain the same amount of clavulanic acid (125 mg as potassium salt), two 250 mg tablets are not equivalent to one 500 mg tablet. The 875 mg tablet also contains clavulanate potassium 125 mg. In addition, the 250 mg tablet and 250 mg chewable tablet do not contain the same amount of clavulanate potassium; do not substitute them for each other because they are not interchangeable.

Amoxicillin/clavulanate potassium tablets (250 or 500 mg) cannot be used to provide the same dosages as extended-release tablets. This is because extended-release tablets contain clavulanic acid 62.5 mg, while the 250 and 500 mg tablets each contain clavulanic acid 125 mg. In addition, the extended-release tablet provides an extended time course of plasma amoxicillin concentrations compared with immediate-release tablets. Therefore, two 500 mg tablets are not equivalent to 1 extended-release tablet.

Suspensions: Amoxicillin/clavulanate potassium ES-600 suspension, 600 mg per 5 mL, does not contain the same amount of clavulanic acid (as the potassium salt) as any of the other suspensions. Amoxicillin/clavulanate potassium ES-600 suspension contains clavulanic acid 42.9 mg per 5 mL, whereas the 200 mg per 5 mL suspension contains clavulanic acid 28.5 mg per 5 mL and the 400 mg per 5 mL suspension contains clavulanic acid 57 mg per 5 mL. Therefore, do not substitute the 200 mg per 5 mL and 400 mg per 5 mL suspensions for amoxicillin/clavulanate potassium ES-600 suspension because they are not interchangeable.

➤*Adults:*

Tablets, chewable tablets, standard oral suspensions –

Infections: For a list of infections, see Indications.

• *Usual dosage* – 500 mg every 12 hours or 250 mg every 8 hours. For more severe infections, 875 mg every 12 hours or 500 mg every 8 hours.

Extended-release tablets –

Acute bacterial sinusitis: 2,000 mg (2 tablets) every 12 hours for 10 days.

Community-acquired pneumonia: 2,000 mg (2 tablets) every 12 hours for 7 to 10 days.

➤*Children:* Children weighing 40 kg or more should be dosed according to the adult recommendations. (See Adults for dosing recommendations.)

The every-12-hour regimen is associated with significantly less diarrhea.

3 months of age or older (weighing less than 40 kg) – See also Off-label dosing for dosing recommendations from the American Academy of Pediatrics guidelines on the management of acute otitis media.

Chewable tablets and standard oral suspensions: The children's dose is based on amoxicillin content. Refer to the following table. Because of the different amoxicillin to clavulanic acid ratios in the 250 mg tablets (250/125) versus the 250 mg chewable tablets (250/62.5), do not use the 250 mg tablet until the child weighs 40 kg or more.

Amoxicillin/Clavulanate Potassium Dosing in Children ≥ 3 Months of Age (Weighing		
	Dosing regimen	
Infections	200 or 400 mg chewable tablets or 200 or 400 mg per 5 mL (divided every 12 h)	125 mg per 5 mL or 250 mg per 5 mL (divided every 8 h)
Lower respiratory tract infections, otitis media,[a] severe infections, sinusitis	45 mg/kg/day	40 mg/kg/day[b]
Less severe infections	25 mg/kg/day	20 mg/kg/day

[a] Recommended duration is 10 days.
[b] See also Off-label dosing for dosing recommendations from the American Academy of Pediatrics guidelines on the management of acute otitis media.

Oral suspension ES-600/42.9 mg per 5 mL: Based on the amoxicillin component (600 mg per 5 mL), the recommended dosage is 90 mg/kg/day divided every 12 hours, administered for 10 days (see the following table).

Experience with amoxicillin/clavulanate potassium ES-600 suspension in children weighing 40 kg or more is not available.

Amoxicillin/Clavulanate Potassium ES-600 Suspension Dosage in Children ≥ 3 Months of Age (Weighing < 40 kg)	
Body weight (kg)	Volume of amoxicillin/clavulanate potassium ES-600 suspension providing 90 mg/kg/day
8	3 mL twice daily
12	4.5 mL twice daily
16	6 mL twice daily
20	7.5 mL twice daily
24	9 mL twice daily
28	10.5 mL twice daily
32	12 mL twice daily
36	13.5 mL twice daily

Younger than 3 months of age –

Chewable tablets and standard oral suspensions: 30 mg/kg/day divided every 12 hours, based on the amoxicillin component. Use of the 125 mg per 5 mL oral suspension is recommended.

Off-label dosing –

Acute otitis media (children): [1] = Good documentation. Amoxicillin/clavulanate (amoxicillin 90 mg/kg daily with clavulanate 6.4 mg/kg daily) in divided doses for 10 days is recommended for severe illness (moderate to severe otalgia and/or temperature of 39°C or higher).

Aminopenicillins

AMOXICILLIN/CLAVULANATE POTASSIUM — ORAL

➤*Renal function impairment:* A dose reduction is generally not required unless renal impairment is severe. Severely impaired patients with a glomerular filtration rate (GFR) of less than 30 mL/min should not receive the 875 mg tablet. Give patients with a GFR of 10 to 30 mL/min 500 or 250 mg every 12 hours, depending on the severity of infection. Give patients with a GFR of less than 10 mL/min 500 or 250 mg every 24 hours, depending on severity of infection.

Amoxicillin/clavulanate potassium extended-release is contraindicated in patients with severe renal impairment (creatinine clearance [CrCl] of less than 30 mL/min).

Hemodialysis – Give patients who require hemodialysis 500 or 250 mg every 24 hours and an additional dose both during and at the end of dialysis. Amoxicillin/clavulanate potassium extended-release is contraindicated in patients who require hemodialysis.

➤*Hepatic function impairment:* Dose with caution and monitor hepatic function.

➤*Administration:* Amoxicillin/clavulanate potassium (tablets, chewable tablets, and standard and ES-600 suspensions) may be taken without regard to meals; however, absorption of clavulanate potassium is enhanced when amoxicillin/clavulanate potassium is administered at the start of a meal. To minimize the potential for GI intolerance, amoxicillin/clavulanate potassium should be taken at the start of a meal.

Amoxicillin/clavulanate potassium extended-release should be taken at the start of a meal to enhance the absorption of amoxicillin and minimize the potential for GI intolerance. Absorption of the amoxicillin component is decreased when amoxicillin/clavulanate potassium extended-release is taken on an empty stomach.

The scored amoxicillin/clavulanate potassium extended-release tablets are available for greater convenience for adults who have difficulty swallowing. The scored amoxicillin/clavulanate potassium extended-release tablet may be broken in half at the score line. The scored tablet is not intended to reduce the dosage of medication taken.

Adults who have difficulty swallowing may be given the 125 mg per 5 mL or 250 mg per 5 mL suspension in place of the 500 mg tablet, or given the 200 mg per 5 mL or 400 mg per 5 mL suspension in place of the 875 mg tablet.

Experience with amoxicillin/clavulanate potassium ES-600 suspension in adults is not available, and adults who have difficulty swallowing should not be given amoxicillin/clavulanate potassium ES-600 suspension in place of the 500 or 875 mg tablet.

➤*Storage/Stability:* Store tablets and dry powder at or below 25°C (77°F); dispense in the original container. Refrigerate reconstituted suspension and discard after 10 days. Shake well before using.

Extended-Spectrum Penicillins

TICARCILLIN/CLAVULANATE

Rx	**Timentin** (GlaxoSmithKline)	**Injection, powder for reconstitution:** 3 g ticarcillin and 0.1 g clavulanic acid[a]	In 3.1 g vials, *ADD-Vantage* vials, and pharmacy bulk packages.[b]
		Injection, solution: 3 g ticarcillin and 0.1 g clavulanic acid per 100 mL[c]	In 100 mL single-dose, premixed, frozen *Galaxy* plastic containers.

[a] Contains 4.51 mEq/g sodium and 0.15 mEq/g potassium.
[b] Pharmacy bulk package contains 30 g ticarcillin (as disodium) and 1 g clavulanic acid.
[c] Contains 18.7 mEq sodium and 0.5 mEq potassium per 100 mL.

TICARCILLIN/CLAVULANATE — INJECTION

For complete and comparative prescribing information, refer to the Penicillins group monograph.

Indications

➤*General information:* For the treatment of infections caused by susceptible β-lactamase–producing strains of these designated organisms in the following conditions:

➤*Septicemia:* Includes bacteremia caused by *Klebsiella* species, *Escherichia coli*, *Staphylococcus aureus*, or *Pseudomonas aeruginosa* (or other *Pseudomonas* species) (efficacy for these organisms in this organ system was studied in fewer than 10 infections).

➤*Lower respiratory tract infections:* Caused by *S. aureus*; *Haemophilus influenzae*, or *Klebsiella* species (efficacy for these organisms in this organ system was studied in fewer than 10 infections).

➤*Bone and joint infections:* Caused by *S. aureus*.

➤*Skin and skin structure infections:* Caused by *S. aureus*; *Klebsiella* species, or *E. coli* (efficacy for these organisms in this organ system was studied in fewer than 10 infections).

➤*Urinary tract infections:* Complicated and uncomplicated infections caused by *E. coli*, *Klebsiella* species; *P. aeruginosa* (and other *Pseudomonas* species), *Citrobacter* species, *Enterobacter cloacae*, *Serratia marcescens*, or *S. aureus* (efficacy for these organisms in this organ system was studied in fewer than 10 infections).

➤*Gynecologic infections:* Endometritis caused by *Prevotella melaninogenicus*, *Enterobacter* species (including *E. cloacae*) *K. pneumoniae* (efficacy for these organisms in this organ system was studied in fewer than 10 infections); *E. coli*, *S. aureus*, or *Staphylococcus epidermidis*.

➤*Intra-abdominal infections:* Peritonitis caused by *E. coli*, *K. pneumoniae*; or *Bacteroides fragilis* group (efficacy for this organism in this organ system was studied in fewer than 10 infections).

➤*Mixed infections:* While ticarcillin/clavulanate is indicated only for the conditions previously listed, infections caused by ticarcillin-susceptible organisms also are amenable to treatment with ticarcillin/clavulanate because of its ticarcillin content. Therefore, mixed infections caused by ticarcillin-susceptible organisms and β-lactamase–producing organisms susceptible to ticarcillin/clavulanate should not require the addition of another antibiotic.

➤*Culture and susceptibility tests:* Appropriate culture and susceptibility tests should be performed before treatment in order to isolate and identify organisms causing infection and to determine their susceptibility to ticarcillin/clavulanate. Because of its broad spectrum of bactericidal activity against gram-positive and gram-negative bacteria, ticarcillin/clavulanate is particularly useful for the treatment of mixed infections and for presumptive therapy prior to the identification of the causative organisms. Ticarcillin/clavulanate has been shown to be effective as single drug therapy in the treatment of some serious infections in which normally combination antibiotic therapy might be employed. Therapy with ticarcillin/clavulanate may be initiated before results of such tests are known when there is reason to believe the infection may involve any of the β-lactamase–producing organisms previously listed.

➤*Drug-resistant bacteria:* To reduce the development of drug-resistant bacteria and maintain the efficacy of ticarcillin/clavulanate and other antibacterial drugs, use ticarcillin/clavulanate only to treat or prevent infections that are proven or strongly suspected to be caused by susceptible bacteria. When culture and susceptibility information are available, they should be considered in selecting or modifying antibacterial therapy. In the absence of such data, local epidemiology and susceptibility patterns may contribute to the empiric selection of therapy.

Administration and Dosage

➤*General dosing considerations:* Frequent bacteriologic and clinical appraisal is necessary during therapy of chronic urinary tract infections and may be required for several months after therapy has been completed; persistent infections may require treatment for several weeks; do not use doses smaller than those indicated.

➤*Adults:*

Infections – For a list of infections, refer to Indications.

Ticarcillin/Clavulanate Dosage in Adults			
	Systemic and urinary tract infections	Gynecological infections	
		Moderate	Severe
Adults ≥ 60 kg	3.1 g every 4 to 6 h	200 mg/kg/day in divided doses every 6 h	300 mg/kg/day in divided doses every 4 h
Adults < 60 kg	200 to 300 mg/kg/day in divided doses every 4 to 6 h		

➤*Children:*

Infections – For a list of infections, refer to Indications.

3 months of age and older:

Ticarcillin/Clavulanate Dosage in Children (≥ 3 Months of Age)		
	Mild to moderate infections	Severe infections
Children ≥ 60 kg	3.1 g every 6 h	3.1 g every 4 h
Children < 60 kg (dosed at 50 mg/kg/dose)	200 mg/kg/day IV in divided doses every 6 h	300 mg/kg/day IV in divided doses every 4 h

➤*Renal function impairment:* The following dosage recommendations are according to the prescribing information.

Ticarcillin/Clavulanate Administration in Renal Function Impairment[a,b]	
Ccr (mL/min)	Dosage
60	3.1 g every 4 h
30 to 60	2 g every 4 h
10 to 30	2 g every 8 h
< 10	2 g every 12 h
< 10 with hepatic function impairment	2 g every 24 h

TICARCILLIN/CLAVULANATE — INJECTION

Ticarcillin/Clavulanate Administration in Renal Function Impairment[a,b]	
Ccr (mL/min)	Dosage
Patients on peritoneal dialysis	3.1 g every 12 h
Patients on hemodialysis	2 g every 12 h supplemented with 3.1 g after each dialysis

[a] Ccr = creatinine clearance.
[b] Initial loading dose is 3.1 g. Follow with doses based on Ccr and type of dialysis.

Adults receiving continuous renal replacement therapy (CRRT) –

The following recommendations assume ultrafiltration and dialysis flow rates of 1 to 2 L/h.

Loading dose: 3.1 g IV.

Maintenance dosage:

• *Continuous venovenous hemofiltration (CVVH)* – 2 g IV every 6 to 8 hours.

• *Continuous venovenous hemodialysis (CVVHD)* – 3.1 g IV every 6 to 8 hours.

• *Continuous venovenous hemodialfiltration (CVVHDF)* – 3.1 g IV every 6 hours.

Adults receiving intermittent hemodialysis (IHD) – 2 g IV every 12 hours and also administer a supplemental dose of 3.1 g after dialysis. For infections difficult to eradicate, an alternative dosage of 2 g IV every 8 hours (without a supplemental dose after dialysis) has been recommended. These recommendations assume the patient is receiving standard IHD 3 times per week and completes the full dialysis sessions.

➤*Duration of therapy:* The duration of therapy depends upon the severity of infection. Generally, continue treatment for at least 2 days after signs and symptoms of infection have disappeared. The usual duration is 10 to 14 days; however, difficult and complicated infections may require more prolonged therapy. Persistent urinary tract infections may require treatment for several weeks.

➤*Administration:* Administer over 30 minutes by direct infusion or through a Y-type IV infusion set. If this method of administration is used, temporarily discontinue administering any other solutions during the infusion of ticarcillin/clavulanate.

Do not use plastic containers in series connections. Such use could result in an embolism because of residual air being drawn from the primary container before administration of the fluid from the secondary container is complete.

➤*Admixture compatibility:* Incompatible with sodium bicarbonate.

When administering in combination with another antimicrobial (eg, an aminoglycoside), administer each drug separately. As with other penicillins, the mixing of ticarcillin/clavulanate with an aminoglycoside in solutions for parenteral administration can result in substantial inactivation of the aminoglycoside.

➤*Storage/Stability:*

IV solution – The concentrated stock solution (200 mg/mL) is stable for up to 6 hours at room temperature (21° to 24°C; 70° to 75°F) or up to 72 hours refrigerated (4°C; 40°F). If the solution is further diluted to a concentration between 10 and 100 mg/mL with any of the recommended diluents, the following stability periods apply.

Stability and Storage for Ticarcillin/Clavulanate IV Solutions				
		Stability		
Concentration	Compatible diluents	Controlled room temp (21° to 24°C; 70° to 75°F)	Refrigerated (4°C; 40°F)	Frozen (−18°C; 0°F)
IV solution: 10 mg/mL to	Sodium chloride injection	24 h	7 days	30 days
100 mg/mL	Dextrose 5% injection	24 h	3 days	7 days
	Ringer's lactate injection	24 h	7 days	30 days
ADD-Vantage solution: 30 mg/mL to	Sodium chloride injection	24 h		
60 mg/mL	Dextrose 5% in water	12 h		

Unused solutions must be discarded after the time period stated above. Use all thawed solutions within 8 hours or discard. Do not refreeze thawed solutions. Avoid excess heat. Protect vials, *ADD-vantage* vials, and pharmacy bulk package from freezing.

Premixed, frozen solutions – Avoid unnecessary handling of bags. Store at less than −20°C (−4°F). Thaw at room temperature 22°C (72°F) or refrigerate at 4°C (39°F). Do not force thaw by immersion in water baths or by microwave irradiation. Check for minute leaks by squeezing bag firmly. If leaks are detected, discard solution. Thawed solution is stable for 7 days if refrigerated or for 24 hours at room temperature. Do not refreeze.

Pharmacy bulk package – Aliquots of the reconstituted stock solution at 300 mg/mL are stable for up to 6 hours between 21° and 24°C (70° and 75°F) or up to 72 hours refrigerated at 4°C (40°F). Refrigerate the reconstituted stock solution at 4°C (40°F).

If the aliquots of the reconstituted stock solution (300 mg/mL) are held up to 6 hours between 21° and 24°C (70° and 75°F) or up to 72 hours refrigerated at 4°C (40°F) and further diluted to a concentration between 10 and 100 mg/mL with any of the diluents listed below, then the following stability periods apply.

Stability and Storage of Ticarcillin/Clavulanate Pharmacy Bulk Packages		
IV solution (ticarcillin concentrations of 10 to 100 mg/mL)	Room temperature (21° to 24°C; 70° to 75°F)	Refrigerated (4°C; 40°F)
Dextrose 5% injection	24 h	3 days
Sodium chloride injection 0.9%	24 h	4 days
Ringer's lactate injection	24 h	4 days
Sterile water for injection	24 h	4 days

If an aliquot of concentrated stock solution (300 mg/mL) is stored for up to 6 hours between 21° and 24°C (70° and 75°F) and then further diluted to a concentration between 10 and 100 mg/mL, solutions of sodium chloride injection, Ringer's lactate injection, and sterile water for injection may be stored frozen at −18°C (0°F) for up to 30 days. Solutions prepared with dextrose 5% injection may be stored frozen at −18°C (0°F) for up to 7 days. All thawed solutions should be used within 8 hours or discarded. Once thawed, solutions should not be refrozen.

PIPERACILLIN SODIUM

Rx	**Piperacillin Sodium** (American Pharmaceutical Partners)	**Powder for injection:** 2 g (as base)	In vials.[a]
		3 g (as base)	In vials.[a]
		4 g (as base)	In vials.[a]
		40 g	In pharmacy bulk vials.[a]

[a] Contains 1.85 mEq (42.5 mg) sodium/g.

PIPERACILLIN SODIUM — INJECTION

For complete and comparative prescribing information, refer to the Penicillins group monograph.

Indications

➤*General information:* For the treatment of serious infections caused by susceptible strains of the designated organisms in the conditions listed below.

➤*Combination therapy:* May be administered as single-drug therapy in some situations where normally 2 antibiotics might be employed.

Successfully used with aminoglycosides, especially in patients with impaired host defenses. Both drugs should be used in full therapeutic doses.

➤*Intra-abdominal infections (including hepatobiliary and surgical infections):* Those caused by *Escherichia coli*, *Pseudomonas aeruginosa*, enterococci, *Clostridium* sp, anaerobic cocci, and *Bacteroides* sp, including *B. fragilis*.

➤*Urinary tract infections (UTIs):* Those caused by *E. coli*, *Klebsiella* sp, *P. aeruginosa*, *Proteus* sp, including *P. mirabilis*, and enterococci.

➤*Gynecologic infections (including endometritis, pelvic inflammatory disease, pelvic cellulitis):* Those caused by *Bacteroides* sp including *B. fragilis*, anaerobic cocci, *Neisseria gonorrhoeae*, and enterococci (*S. faecalis*).

➤*Septicemia (including bacteremia):* Caused by *E. coli*, *Klebsiella* sp, *Enterobacter* sp, *Serratia* sp, *P. mirabilis*, *S. pneumoniae*, enterococci, *P. aeruginosa*, *Bacteroides* sp, and anaerobic cocci.

➤*Lower respiratory tract infections:* Those caused by *E. coli*, *Klebsiella* sp, *Enterobacter* sp, *P. aeruginosa*, *Serratia* sp, *Haemophilus influenzae*, *Bacteroides* sp, and anaerobic cocci.

Although improvement has been noted in patients with cystic fibrosis, lasting bacterial eradication may not necessarily be achieved.

➤*Skin and skin structure infections:* Those caused by *E. coli*, *Klebsiella* sp, *Serratia* sp, *Acinetobacter* sp, *Enterobacter* sp, *P. aeruginosa*, indole-positive *Proteus* sp, *P. mirabilis*, *Bacteroides* sp, including *B. fragilis*, anaerobic cocci, and enterococci.

➤*Bone and joint infections:* Those caused by *P. aeruginosa*, enterococci, *Bacteroides* sp, and anaerobic cocci.

PIPERACILLIN SODIUM — INJECTION

➤*Gonococcal infections:* Treatment of uncomplicated gonococcal urethritis.

➤*Streptococcal infections:* Clinically effective for the treatment of infections at various sites caused by *Streptococcus* species including group A β-hemolytic *Streptococcus* and *S. pneumoniae*; however, infections caused by these organisms are ordinarily treated with more narrow spectrum penicillins. Because of its broad spectrum of bactericidal activity against gram-positive and gram-negative aerobic and anaerobic bacteria, piperacillin is particularly useful for the treatment of mixed infections and presumptive therapy prior to the identification of the causative organisms.

➤*Prophylaxis:* For prophylactic use in surgery, including intra-abdominal (GI and biliary) procedures, vaginal hysterectomy, abdominal hysterectomy, and cesarean section. Effective prophylactic use depends on the time of administration, and piperacillin should be given 30 minutes to 1 hour before the operation so that effective levels can be achieved in the site prior to the procedure.

Stop the prophylactic use of piperacillin within 24 hours, since continuing administration of any antibiotic increases the possibility of adverse reactions, but in the majority of surgical procedures, does not reduce the incidence of subsequent infections. If there are signs of infection, obtain specimens for culture for identification of the causative organism so that appropriate therapy can be instituted.

➤*Off-label uses:*

Infective endocarditis (adults) – [1] = Good documentation. The American Heart Association (AHA) recommends piperacillin in combination with tobramycin to treat endocarditis caused by *P. aeruginosa*.

Administration and Dosage

➤*Adults:*

Maximum dose – 24 g/day, although higher doses have been used.

Usual dosage – 3 to 4 g every 4 to 6 hours as a 20- to 30-minute infusion.

Infections –

Piperacillin Dosage Recommendations

Type of infection	Usual total daily dose
Complicated UTIs	8 to 16 g/day IV (125 to 200 mg/kg/day) in divided doses every 6 to 8 hours
Serious infections such as septicemia, nosocomial pneumonia, intra-abdominal infections, aerobic and anaerobic gynecologic infections, and skin and soft tissue infections	12 to 18 g/day IV (200 to 300 mg/kg/day) in divided doses every 4 to 6 hours
Uncomplicated UTIs and most community-acquired pneumonia	6 to 8 g/day IM or IV (100 to 125 mg/kg/day) in divided doses every 6 to 12 hours
Uncomplicated gonorrhea infections	2 g IM[a] as a 1-time dose

[a] 1 g of probenecid given orally one-half hour prior to injection.

Prophylaxis –

Piperacillin Prophylactic Dosing

Indication	First Dose	Second Dose	Third Dose
Intra-abdominal surgery	2 g IV just prior to surgery	2 g during surgery	2 g every 6 h post-op for no more than 24 h
Vaginal hysterectomy	2 g IV just prior to surgery	2 g 6 h after the first dose	2 g 12 h after the first dose
Cesarean section	2 g IV after the cord is clamped	2 g 4 h after the first dose	2 g 8 h after the first dose
Abdominal hysterectomy	2 g IV just prior to surgery	2 g on return to the recovery room	2 g after 6 h

Off-label dosing –

Infective endocarditis (adults): [1] = Good documentation. 12 to 18 g IV in divided doses every 4 to 6 hours in combination with high-dose tobramycin for at least 6 weeks for patients with *P. aeruginosa*.

➤*Children:*

12 years of age and older – See Adults for dosing.

Off-label dosing –

Piperacillin Off-Label Dosing in Children

Indication	Usual dosage
Cystic fibrosis	300 to 600 mg/kg/day IM or IV divided every 4 to 6 hours.
Infections	
Children and infants	200 to 300 mg/kg/day IM or IV divided every 4 to 6 hours.
Neonates 8 to 29 days of age (more than 36 weeks of gestation)	300 mg/kg/day IV divided every 6 hours.
Neonates 8 to 29 days of age (36 weeks of gestation or less)	225 mg/kg/day IV divided every 8 hours.
Neonates 7 days of age or younger (more than 36 weeks of gestation)	225 mg/kg/day IV divided every 8 hours.
Neonates 7 days of age or younger (36 weeks of gestation or less)	150 mg/kg/day IV divided every 12 hours.
Perforated appendectomy	200 mg/kg/day IM or IV divided every 8 hours.

Maximum dose: 18 to 24 g/day in patients with cystic fibrosis and children and infants with infections.

➤*Renal function impairment:*

CrCl greater than 50 mL/min – No adjustment. 3 to 4 g every 4 to 6 hours.

CrCL 10 to 50 mL/min – 3 to 4 g every 6 to 8 hours.

CrCL less than 10 mL/min – 3 to 4 g every 8 hours.

HD/AD/CAPD – 3 to 4 g every 8 hours.

➤*Concomitant therapy:* When piperacillin is given concurrently with aminoglycosides, use both drugs in full therapeutic doses.

➤*Duration of therapy:* The average duration of treatment is from 7 to 10 days, except in the treatment of gynecologic infections, in which it is from 3 to 10 days; the duration should be guided by the patient's clinical and bacteriological progress. For most acute infections, continue treatment for at least 48 to 72 hours after the patient becomes asymptomatic. Maintain antibiotic therapy for *S. pyogenes* infections for at least 10 days to reduce the risk of rheumatic fever.

➤*Preparation for administration:*

Reconstitution directions for bulk vial – Reconstitute the 40 g vial with 172 mL of suitable diluent (except lidocaine hydrochloride 0.5% to 1% without epinephrine) to achieve a concentration of 1 g per 5 mL.

1.) For hanger use, grasp top portion of the bottle label. Peel the laminated film (sling) away from the printed portion of the pressure sensitive label. Invert bottle and pull sling over the base of the bottle. Hang bottle using sling portion of the label.
2.) During use, container must be stored and all manipulations performed in an appropriate laminar flow hood.
3.) Remove cover from closure and cleanse with antiseptic.
4.) The container closure may be penetrated only one time, utilizing a suitable sterile transfer device or dispensing set that allows measured distribution of its contents. Use of a single syringe with needle is not recommended as it may cause leakage. Use of this product is restricted to a suitable work area, such as a laminar flow hood.

Withdraw container contents without delay. If this is not possible, a maximum of 4 hours from initial closure entry is permitted to complete fluid transfer operations. Begin this time limit with the introduction of solvent or diluent into the PBP.

Reconstituting directions conventional vials – Reconstitute each gram of piperacillin for injection with at least 5 mL of suitable diluent (except lidocaine hydrochloride 0.5% to 1% without epinephrine). Shake well until dissolved. Reconstituted solution may be further diluted to the desired volume (eg, 50 or 100 mL) in suitable IV solutions and admixture.

➤*Administration:* Administered IM (except pharmacy bulk package) or IV as a 20- to 30-minute infusion. For serious infections, use the IV route.

Limit IM injections to 2 g/injection site. This route of administration has been used primarily in the treatment of patients with uncomplicated gonorrhea and UTIs.

Intermittent IV infusion – Infuse diluted solution over a period of approximately 30 minutes. During infusion, it is desirable to discontinue the primary IV solution.

IV injection (bolus) – Inject reconstituted solution from conventional vials slowly over a 3- to 5-minute period to help avoid vein irritation.

➤*Admixture compatibility:* Do not mix piperacillin with an aminoglycoside in a syringe or infusion bottle since this can result in inactivation of the aminoglycoside.

Diluents for reconstitution – Sterile water for injection, bacteriostatic water for injection, sodium chloride injection, bacteriostatic sodium chloride injection, dextrose 5% in water, dextrose 5% and sodium chloride 0.9%, lidocaine hydrochloride 0.5% to 1% (without epinephrine).

For IM use only. Lidocaine is contraindicated in patients with a known history of hypersensitivity to local anesthetics of the amide type.

IV admixtures – Normal saline [+ KCl 40 mEq], dextrose 5% in water [+ KCl 40 mEq], dextrose 5%/normal saline [+ KCl 40 mEq], Ringer's injection [+ KCl 40 mEq], lactated Ringer's injection [+ KCl 40 mEq].

When piperacillin for injection is further diluted with lactated Ringer's injection, the diluted solution must be administered within 2 hours.

IV solutions – Dextrose 5% in water, sodium chloride 0.9%, dextrose 5% and sodium chloride 0.9%, lactated Ringer's injection, dextran 6% in sodium chloride 0.9%.

When piperacillin for injection is further diluted with lactated Ringer's injection, the diluted solution must be administered within 2 hours.

➤*Storage/Stability:* Store at 20° to 25°C (68° to 77°F).

PIPERACILLIN SODIUM — INJECTION

Conventional vials – Piperacillin is stable in both glass and plastic containers when reconstituted with recommended diluents and when diluted with suitable IV solutions and IV admixtures.

Use pharmacy vials immediately after reconstitution. Discard any unused portion after 24 hours if stored at 20° to 25°C (68° to 77°F), or after 48 hours if stored at 2° to 8°C (36° to 46°F). Do not freeze vials after reconstitution.

Pharmacy bulk package – After entry, use entire contents of vial promptly. Dispense the entire contents of the vial within 4 hours of initial entry. Never freeze the pharmacy bulk vial after reconstitution.

PIPERACILLIN/TAZOBACTAM

Rx	**Piperacillin/Tazobactam** (Various, eg, Hospira, Sandoz)	**Injection, powder for solution, concentrate**: 2.25 g (piperacillin 2 g and tazobactam 0.25 g)	Preservative free. As piperacillin sodium/tazobactam sodium. Sodium 108 mg. In single-dose vials.
		3.375 g (piperacillin 3 g and tazobactam 0.375 g)	Preservative free. As piperacillin sodium/tazobactam sodium. Sodium 162 mg. In single-dose vials.
		4.5 g (piperacillin 4 g and tazobactam 0.5 g)	Preservative free. As piperacillin sodium/tazobactam sodium. Sodium 216 mg. In single-dose vials.
Rx	**Zosyn** (Wyeth)	**Injection, powder for solution, concentrate**: 2.25 g (piperacillin 2 g and tazobactam 0.25 g)	As piperacillin sodium/tazobactam sodium. Preservative free. In single-dose vials and *ADD-Vantage* vials.[a]
		3.375 g (piperacillin 3 g and tazobactam 0.375 g)	As piperacillin sodium/tazobactam sodium. Preservative free. In single-dose vials and *ADD-Vantage* vials.[a]
		4.5 g (piperacillin 4 g and tazobactam 0.5 g)	As piperacillin sodium/tazobactam sodium. Preservative free. In single-dose vials and *ADD-Vantage* vials.[a]
		40.5 g (piperacillin 36 g and tazobactam 4.5 g)	As piperacillin sodium/tazobactam sodium.[a] Preservative free. In bulk vials.
		Injection, solution: 2.25 g per 50 mL (piperacillin 2 g and tazobactam 0.25 g)	As piperacillin sodium/tazobactam sodium. In 50 mL single-dose, premixed, frozen *Galaxy* containers.[a,b]
		3.375 g per 50 mL (piperacillin 3 g and tazobactam 0.375 g)	As piperacillin sodium/tazobactam sodium. In 50 mL single-dose, premixed, frozen *Galaxy* containers.[a,b]
		4.5 g per 100 mL (piperacillin 4 g and tazobactam 0.5 g)	As piperacillin sodium/tazobactam sodium. In 100 mL single-dose, premixed, frozen *Galaxy* containers.[a,b]

[a] Contains approximately 2.79 mEq (64 mg) of sodium per gram of piperacillin. Also contains edetate disodium dihydrate (EDTA).

[b] Also contains dextrose.

PIPERACILLIN SODIUM/TAZOBACTAM SODIUM — INJECTION

For complete and comparative prescribing information, refer to the Penicillins group monograph.

Indications

➤*General information:* For the treatment of patients with moderate to severe infections caused by piperacillin-resistant, piperacillin/tazobactam–susceptible, beta-lactamase–producing strains of the designated microorganisms in the following conditions.

➤*Appendicitis (complicated by rupture or abscess):* Caused by piperacillin-resistant, beta-lactamase–producing strains of *Escherichia coli* or these members of the *Bacteroides fragilis* group: *B. fragilis, Bacteroides ovatus, Bacteroides thetaiotaomicron,* or *Bacteroides vulgatus*. The individual organisms of this group were studied in fewer than 10 cases.

➤*Community-acquired pneumonia (moderate severity only):* Caused by piperacillin-resistant, beta-lactamase–producing strains of *Haemophilus influenzae*.

➤*Nosocomial pneumonia (moderate to severe):* Caused by piperacillin-resistant, beta-lactamase–producing strains of *Staphylococcus aureus* and by piperacillin/tazobactam-susceptible *Acinetobacter baumanii, H. influenzae, Klebsiella pneumoniae,* and *Pseudomonas aeruginosa* (nosocomial pneumonia caused by *P. aeruginosa* should be treated in combination with an aminoglycoside).

➤*Pelvic inflammatory disease:* Caused by piperacillin-resistant, beta-lactamase–producing strains of *E. coli*.

➤*Peritonitis:* Caused by piperacillin-resistant, beta-lactamase–producing strains of *E. coli* or these members of the *B. fragilis* group: *B. fragilis, B. ovatus, B. thetaiotaomicron,* or *B. vulgatus*. The individual members of this group were studied in fewer than 10 cases.

➤*Postpartum endometritis:* Caused by piperacillin-resistant, beta-lactamase–producing strains of *E. coli*.

➤*Uncomplicated and complicated skin and skin structure infections:* Including cellulitis, cutaneous abscesses, and ischemic/diabetic foot infections caused by piperacillin-resistant, beta-lactamase–producing strains of *S. aureus*.

➤*Off-label uses:*

Catheter-related bloodstream infections (adults) – [2] = Fair documentation. Current guidelines for the treatment of catheter-related bloodstream infections recommend piperacillin/tazobactam alone or in combination with other agents for the treatment of *P. aeruginosa* in adults. Piperacillin/tazobactam can also be used as empiric coverage for infections caused by gram-negative bacilli in neutropenic or severely ill patients. Limited evidence also shows a place in therapy for infections caused by *Enterobacter* species or extended-spectrum beta-lactamase–producing *E. coli*, although additional controlled studies are needed to confirm these initial results. In patients with renal dysfunction, the dosage of piperacillin/tazobactam should be adjusted accordingly. Currently, there are no recommendations regarding the use of piperacillin/tazobactam in pediatric patients with catheter-related bloodstream infections.

Administration and Dosage

➤*Adults:*

Infections – For a list of infections, refer to Indications.

Usual dosage: 3.375 g intravenously (IV) every 6 hours, totaling 13.5 g (piperacillin 12 g per 1.5 g of tazobactam) daily for 7 to 10 days. Administer by IV infusion over 30 minutes.

Duration of therapy: 7 to 10 days. In all conditions, the duration of therapy should be guided by the severity of the infection and the patient's clinical and bacteriologic progress.

Nosocomial pneumonia –

Initial dosage: 4.5 g IV every 6 hours plus an aminoglycoside, totaling 18 g (piperacillin 16 g per tazobactam 2 g) for 7 to 14 days. Administer by IV infusion over 30 minutes.

Duration of therapy: 7 to 14 days. The duration of therapy should be guided by the severity of the infection and the patient's clinical and bacteriologic progress.

Continue the aminoglycoside in patients from whom *P. aeruginosa* is isolated. If it is not isolated, the aminoglycoside may be discontinued at the discretion of the treating health care provider.

Off-label dosing –

Catheter-related bloodstream infections (adults): [2] = Fair documentation. 4.5 g IV every 6 hours for 7 to 14 days. Renal dosing is required with piperacillin/tazobactam, and the package insert should be referred to for specific dosing recommendations in renal insufficiency.

➤*Children:*

Appendicitis –

Children weighing more than 40 kg:

• *Usual dosage* – 3.375 g IV every 6 hours, totaling 13.5 g (piperacillin 12 g per 1.5 g of tazobactam) daily for 7 to 10 days. Administer by IV infusion over 30 minutes.

• *Duration of therapy* – 7 to 10 days. In all conditions, the duration of therapy should be guided by the severity of the infection and the patient's clinical and bacteriologic progress.

9 months of age and older (weighing up to 40 kg):

• *Usual dosage* – Piperacillin 100 mg/tazobactam 12.5 mg per kilogram of body weight, every 8 hours in patients with healthy renal function.

• *Duration of therapy* – 7 to 10 days. In all conditions, the duration of therapy should be guided by the severity of the infection and the patient's clinical and bacteriologic progress.

2 to 9 months of age:

• *Usual dosage* – Piperacillin 80 mg/tazobactam 10 mg per kilogram of body weight, every 8 hours.

• *Duration of therapy* – 7 to 10 days. In all conditions, the duration of therapy should be guided by the severity of the infection and the patient's clinical and bacteriologic progress.

Peritonitis – See dosing listed under Appendicitis.

➤*Elderly:* Initial dosage should be at the low end of the dosing range. Adjust dosage in the presence of renal function impairment.

➤*Renal function impairment:* In patients with renal function impairment (creatinine clearance [CrCl] 40 mL/min or less), the IV dose of

PIPERACILLIN SODIUM/TAZOBACTAM SODIUM — INJECTION

piperacillin/tazobactam should be adjusted to the degree of actual renal function impairment. In patients with nosocomial pneumonia receiving concomitant aminoglycoside therapy, the aminoglycoside dosage should be adjusted according to the manufacturer's recommendations.

Piperacillin/Tazobactam Dosage Recommendations for Adults With Renal Function Impairment[a]		
CrCl (mL/min)	All indications (except nosocomial pneumonia)	Nosocomial pneumonia
> 40	3.375 g every 6 h	4.5 g every 6 h
20 to 40[b]	2.25 g every 6 h	3.375 g every 6 h
< 20[b]	2.25 g every 8 h	2.25 g every 6 h
Hemodialysis[c]	2.25 g every 12 h[c]	2.25 g every 8 h[c]
CAPD[d]	2.25 g every 12 h	2.25 g every 8 h

[a] Dosage provided is "total" combined piperacillin/tazobactam.
[b] CrCl for patients not receiving hemodialysis.
[c] Administer 0.75 g following each hemodialysis session on hemodialysis days.
[d] CAPD = continuous ambulatory peritoneal dialysis.

Adults receiving dialysis – The maximum dosage is 2.25 g every 12 hours for all indications other than nosocomial pneumonia and 2.25 g every 8 hours for nosocomial pneumonia. In addition, because hemodialysis removes 30% to 40% of a dose, the manufacturer recommends administering 1 additional 0.75 g dose following each dialysis period on hemodialysis days. Another reference suggests administering 2.25 g every 8 hours plus 1.125 g after the hemodialysis session for mild/moderate infections. Higher doses should be used for pseudomonal or severe/life-threatening infections. No additional dosage of piperacillin/tazobactam is necessary for patients with CAPD.

Adults receiving continuous renal replacement therapy (CRRT) – One reference suggests a dosage of 4.5 g every 8 hours.

The following alternative recommendations assume ultrafiltration and dialysis flow rates of 1 to 2 L/hr.

Continuous venovenous hemofiltration (CVVH) – 2.25 to 3.375 g every 6 to 8 hours.

Continuous venovenous hemodialysis (CVVHD) or continuous venovenous hemodialfiltration (CVVHDF) – 2.25 to 3.375 g every 6 hours.

➤*Preparation for administration:*

Powder for solution –

Conventional vials: Reconstitute conventional vials with 5 mL of compatible diluent per gram of piperacillin. Piperacillin/tazobactam 2.25, 3.375, and 4.5 g should be reconstituted with 10, 15, and 20 mL, respectively. Swirl until dissolved. Use immediately after reconstitution. Reconstituted piperacillin/tazobactam should be further diluted (recommended volume per dose of 50 to 150 mL) in a compatible IV solution. (See Admixture Compatibility.)

ADD-Vantage vials: Admixtures include dextrose 5% in water (50 or 100 mL) or sodium chloride 0.9% (50 or 100 mL).

Solution for injection (Galaxy containers) – Thaw frozen containers at room temperature, 20° to 25°C (68° to 77°F) or under refrigeration, 2° to 8°C (36° to 46°F). Do not force thaw by immersion in water baths or by microwave irradiation.

Check for minute leaks by squeezing container firmly. If leaks are detected, discard solution because sterility may be impaired.

The container should be visually inspected. Components of the solution may precipitate in the frozen state and will dissolve upon reaching room temperature with little or no agitation. Potency is not affected. Agitate after solution has reached room temperature. If after visual inspection the solution remains cloudy, an insoluble precipitate is noted, or if any seals or outlet ports are not intact, the container should be discarded.

Do not use plastic containers in series connections. Such use could result in air embolism because of residual air being drawn from the primary container before administration of the fluid from the secondary container is complete.

➤*Administration:* Administer by IV infusion over a period of at least 30 minutes. During infusion, it is desirable to discontinue the primary infusion solution.

Piperacillin/tazobactam in vials/bulk containers can be used in ambulatory IV infusion pumps.

In order to prevent unintentional overdose, piperacillin/tazobactam in *Galaxy* containers should not be used in children who require less than the full adult dose of piperacillin/tazobactam. The other available formulations of piperacillin/tazobactam can be used in this population.

Concurrent aminoglycoside administration – Because of the in vitro inactivation of the aminoglycoside by beta-lactam antibiotics, piperacillin/tazobactam and the aminoglycoside are recommended for separate administration. Piperacillin/tazobactam and the aminoglycoside should be reconstituted, diluted, and administered separately when concomitant therapy with aminoglycosides is indicated.

➤*Admixture compatibility:*

Compatibility –

Conventional vials:

• *Reconstitution diluents* – Compatible reconstitution diluents include sodium chloride 0.9% injection, sterile water for injection (maximum recommended volume per dose is 50 mL), dextrose 5%, bacteriostatic saline/parabens, bacteriostatic water/parabens, bacteriostatic saline/benzyl alcohol, and bacteriostatic water/benzyl alcohol.

• *IV solutions* – Compatible IV solutions include sodium chloride 0.9% injection, sterile water for injection (maximum recommended volume per dose is 50 mL), dextrose 5%, dextran 6% in saline, and Ringer's lactate solution (only with piperacillin/tazobactam containing EDTA).

Y-site compatibility with aminoglycosides: In circumstances in which coadministration via Y-site is necessary, reformulated piperacillin/tazobactam containing EDTA is compatible for simultaneous coadministration via Y-site infusion only with the following aminoglycosides and under the following conditions (the following compatibility information does not apply to the piperacillin/tazobactam formulation not containing EDTA).

Piperacillin/Tazobactam + Aminoglycoside Compatibility				
Aminoglycoside	Piperacillin/ tazobactam dose (g)	Piperacillin/ tazobactam diluent volume[a] (mL)	Aminoglycoside concentration range[b] (mg/mL)	Acceptable diluents
Amikacin	2.25, 3.375, 4.5	50, 100, 150	1.75 to 7.5	Sodium chloride 0.9% or dextrose 5%
Gentamicin	2.25, 3.375,[a] 4.5	100, 150	0.7 to 3.32	Sodium chloride 0.9%

[a] For vials and bulk containers.
[b] The concentration ranges in this table are based on administration of the aminoglycoside in divided doses (10 to 15 mg/kg/day in 2 daily doses for amikacin and 3 to 5 mg/kg/day in 3 daily doses for gentamicin). Administration of amikacin or gentamicin in a single daily dose or in doses exceeding those previously stated via Y-site with piperacillin/tazobactam containing EDTA has not been evaluated. See the individual monographs for each aminoglycoside for complete dosage and administration instructions.

Compatibility of piperacillin/tazobactam with other aminoglycosides has not been established. Only the concentration and diluents for amikacin or gentamicin with the dosages of piperacillin/tazobactam previously listed have been established as compatible for coadministration via Y-site infusion. Simultaneous coadministration via Y-site infusion in any manner other than previously listed may result in inactivation of the aminoglycoside by piperacillin/tazobactam.

Incompatibility – Piperacillin/tazobactam should not be mixed with other drugs in a syringe or infusion bottle because compatibility has not been established. Piperacillin/tazobactam is not chemically stable in solutions that contain only sodium bicarbonate and solutions that significantly alter pH. Piperacillin/tazobactam should not be added to blood products or albumin hydrolysates.

Piperacillin/tazobactam 3.375 g per 50 mL *Galaxy* containers are not compatible with gentamicin for coadministration via a Y-site because of the higher concentrations of piperacillin and tazobactam.

Piperacillin/tazobactam is not compatible with tobramycin for simultaneous coadministration via Y-site infusion.

➤*Storage/Stability:*

Vials and ADD-Vantage vials – Reconstituted piperacillin/tazobactam is stable in glass and plastic containers (plastic syringes, IV, bags, and tubing) when used with compatible diluents.

Store at 20° to 25°C (68° to 77°F) prior to reconstitution. Use single-dose vials immediately after reconstitution. Discard any unused portion after 24 hours if stored at room temperature or after 48 hours if stored at refrigerated temperature, 2° to 8°C (36° to 46°F). Do not freeze vials after reconstitution.

Stability in the IV bags has been demonstrated for up to 24 hours at room temperature and up to 1 week at refrigerated temperature. Piperacillin/tazobactam contains no preservatives. Appropriate consideration of aseptic technique should be used.

Stability of piperacillin/tazobactam is not affected when administered using an ambulatory IV infusion pump. Stability in an ambulatory IV infusion pump has been demonstrated for a period of 12 hours at room temperature. Each dose was reconstituted and diluted to a volume of 37.5 or 25 mL. One-day supplies of dosing solution were aseptically transferred into the medication reservoir (IV bags or cartridge). The reservoir was fitted to a preprogrammed ambulatory IV infusion pump per the manufacturer's instructions.

Stability with the admixed *ADD-Vantage* system has been demonstrated through 24 hours at room temperature. Do not refrigerate or freeze the admixed *ADD-Vantage* after reconstitution.

Galaxy containers – Store in a freezer capable of maintaining a temperature of −20°C (−4°F).

The thawed solution is stable for 14 days under refrigeration, 2° to 8°C (36° to 46°F) or 24 hours at room temperature, 20° to 25°C (68° to 77°F). Do not refreeze thawed antibiotics.

Unused portions of piperacillin/tazobactam should be discarded.

Indications

➤*Infections:* For specific approved indications, refer to individual drug monographs.

➤*Off-label uses:* Refer to individual monographs for further information.

Catheter-related bloodstream infections –

Cefazolin: [2] = Fair documentation.
Cefepime: [2] = Fair documentation.
Ceftazidime: [2] = Fair documentation.

Chancroid –

Ceftriaxone: [1] = Good documentation.

Epididymitis –

Ceftriaxone: [1] = Good documentation.

Gonococcal meningitis and endocarditis –

Ceftriaxone: [1] = Good documentation.

Infective endocarditis (adults) –

Ceftriaxone: [1] = Good documentation.

Infective endocarditis (children / adolescents) –

Ceftriaxone: [1] = Good documentation.

Lyme neuroborreliosis –

Cefotaxime: [1] = Good documentation.
Ceftriaxone: [1] = Good documentation.
Cefuroxime: [2] = Fair documentation.

Proctitis, proctocolitis, enteritis – [1] = Good documentation.

Administration and Dosage

➤*Duration of therapy:* Continue administration for a minimum of 48 to 72 hours after fever abates or after evidence of bacterial eradication has been obtained. A minimum of 10 days treatment is recommended for group A β-hemolytic streptococci infections to guard against the risk of rheumatic fever or glomerulonephritis.

➤*Perioperative prophylaxis:* Discontinue prophylactic use within 24 hours after the surgical procedure. In surgery where infection may be particularly devastating (eg, open heart surgery, prosthetic arthroplasty), may continue prophylactic use for 3 to 5 days following surgery completion. If there are signs of infection, obtain cultures and perform sensitivity tests so appropriate therapy may be instituted.

Actions

➤*Pharmacology:* Cephalosporins are structurally and pharmacologically related to penicillins. **Cefoxitin** and **cefotetan** (cephamycins) are included because of their similarity.

Most cephalosporins and related compounds are divided into first, second and third generation agents (see table). Within each group, differentiation is primarily by pharmacokinetics; groups are divided by antibacterial spectrum. In general, progression from first to third generation reveals broadening gram-negative spectrum, loss of efficacy against gram-positive organisms, greater efficacy against resistant organisms and increased cost. However, this classification scheme is becoming less clearly defined as newer agents enter the market. The decision to use a specific agent in the clinical setting should be primarily based on bacterial spectrum, route of administration, side effect profile and indications.

Mechanism – Cephalosporins inhibit mucopeptide synthesis in the bacterial cell wall, making it defective and osmotically unstable. The drugs are usually bactericidal, depending on organism susceptibility, dose, tissue concentrations and the rate at which organisms are multiplying. They are more effective against rapidly growing organisms forming cell walls.

➤*Pharmacokinetics:*

Pharmacokinetic Parameters of Cephalosporins

	Drug	Routes	Half-Life: Normal renal function (minutes)	Half-Life: ESRD[a] (hours)	Hemodialysis (hours)	Protein bound (%)	Recovered unchanged in urine (%)	Peak serum level 1 g IV dose (mcg/mL)	Sodium (mEq/g)
First	Cefadroxil	Oral	78-96	20-25	3-4	20	> 90	—	—
	Cefazolin	IM-IV	90-120	3-7	9-14	80-86	60-80	185	2-2.1
	Cephalexin	Oral	50-80	19-22	4-6	10	> 90	—	—
	Cephradine	Oral/IM-IV	48-80	8-15		8-17	> 90	86	6[b]
Second	Cefaclor	Oral	35-54	2-3	1.6-2.1	25	60-85	—	—
	Cefotetan	IM-IV	180-276	13-35	5	88-90	51-81	158	3.5
	Cefoxitin	IV	40-60	20	4	73	85	110	2.3
	Cefprozil	Oral	78	5.2-5.9	decreased	36	60	—	—
	Cefuroxime	Oral/IM-IV	80	16-22[c]	3.5	50	66-100	100[d]	2.4[c]
Third	Cefdinir	Oral	100	16	3.2	60-70	12-18	—	—
	Cefixime	Oral	180-240	11.5	—	65	50	—	—
	Cefoperazone	IM-IV	120	1.3-2.9	2	82-93	20-30	73-153	1.5
	Cefotaxime	IM-IV	60	3-11	2.5	30-40	60	42-102	2.2
	Cefpodoxime[e]	Oral	120-180	9.8	—	21-29	29-33	—	—
	Ceftazidime	IM-IV	114-120	14-30	—	< 10	80-90	69-90	2.3
	Ceftibuten	Oral	144	13.4-22.3	2-4	65	56	—	—
	Ceftizoxime	IM-IV	102	25-30	6	30	80	60-87	2.6
	Ceftriaxone	IM-IV	348-522	15.7	14.7	85-95	33-67	151	3.6
Fourth	Cefepime	IM-IV	102-138	17-21	11-16	20	85	79	—
Fifth	Ceftaroline	IV	96-160	—	—	20	64	19-21[f]	—

[a] ESRD = end-stage renal disease (creatinine clearance [CrCl] ^{2}).
[b] Also available in sodium-free form.
[c] Injection only.
[d] Following 1.5 g IV dose.
[e] Extended-spectrum agent.
[f] Following 600 mg IV dose.

CEPHALOSPORINS AND RELATED ANTIBIOTICS

✓ = generally susceptible
‡ = demonstrated in vitro activity

Organisms Generally Susceptible to Cephalosporins																					
Organisms		First Generation				Second Generation					Third Generation									Fourth Generation	Fifth Generation
		Cefadroxil	Cefazolin	Cephalexin	Cephradine	Cefaclor	Cefoxitin	Cefuroxime	Cefotetan	Cefprozil	Cefdinir	Cefixime	Cefoperazone	Cefotaxime	Cefpodoxime[b]	Ceftazidime	Ceftibuten	Ceftizoxime	Ceftriaxone	Cefepime[a]	Ceftaroline
Gram-positive	Staphylococci[c]	✓	✓	✓[d]	✓	✓[d]	✓	✓	✓	✓	✓[e]		✓	✓[e]	✓[d]	✓		✓	✓	✓[f]	
	Staphylococcus aureus										✓✓[e]										✓
	Staphylococcus epidermidis							‡			‡[f]										
	Staphylococcus saprophyticus							‡													
	Streptococci, beta-hemolytic	✓	✓	✓	✓	✓	✓	✓	✓	✓		✓	✓	✓	✓	✓		✓	✓	‡	
	Streptococcus agalactiae							‡			‡										✓
	Streptococcus dysgalactial																				‡
	Streptococcus bovis																				
	Streptococcus pneumoniae	✓	✓	✓	✓	✓	✓	✓	✓	✓	✓[g]	✓	✓	✓	✓	✓	✓[g]	✓	✓	✓	
	Streptococcus pyogenes					✓		✓	✓	✓	✓	✓	✓	✓	✓	✓	✓	✓	✓	✓[h]	✓
	Streptococcus viridans										‡										
Gram-negative	*Acinetobacter* sp.												✓[d]	✓		‡		✓	‡	‡	
	Citrobacter sp.							✓[d]	‡	‡	‡	‡	✓	✓	‡	✓		‡	‡	‡	‡
	Enterobacter sp.		✓[d]					✓[d]	✓				✓	✓		✓		✓	✓	✓	‡
	Escherichia coli	✓	✓	✓	✓	✓	✓	✓	✓	‡	‡	✓	✓	✓	✓	✓		✓	✓	✓	✓
	Haemophilus influenzae		✓	✓	✓	✓[e]	✓[e]	✓[e]	✓[e]	✓[e]	✓[e]	✓[e]	✓[e]	✓[e]	✓[e]	✓[e]	✓[e]	✓[e]	✓[e]	‡[e]	✓
	Haemophilus parainfluenzae					‡		‡			✓[e]	‡[e]		✓	‡	‡			✓		‡
	Hafnia alvei																			‡	
	Klebsiella sp.	✓	✓	✓	✓	✓	✓		✓	‡	‡	‡	✓	✓	✓	✓		✓	✓	✓	
	Klebsiella pneumoniae					‡															✓
	Klebsiella oxytoca																				✓
	Moraxella (Branhamella) catarrhalis	‡		‡		✓[e]		‡	‡	✓[e]	✓[e]	✓[e]			✓	✓	✓[e]	‡		‡[e]	‡
	Morganella (Proteus) morganii						✓	✓[d]	✓				✓	✓		‡		✓	✓	‡	‡
	Neisseria catarrhalis			✓																	
	Neisseria gonorrhoeae					‡	✓	✓	‡	‡		‡	✓[e]	✓	✓[d]	‡		✓	✓		
	Neisseria meningitidis							✓					‡	✓		✓		‡	✓		
	Pasteurella multocida																				
	Proteus inconstans							‡													
	Proteus mirabilis	✓	✓	✓	✓	✓	✓	✓	✓	‡	‡	✓	✓	✓	✓	✓		✓	✓	✓	‡
	Proteus vulgaris						✓		✓			‡	✓	✓	‡	✓		✓	✓	‡	
	Providencia sp.						✓	✓	✓			‡		‡		‡		‡	‡	‡	
	Providencia rettgeri						✓	✓	✓			‡	✓	✓	‡	‡		✓	‡	‡	
	Pseudomonas aeruginosa												✓	✓[d]		✓		✓[d]	✓[d]	✓	
	Salmonella sp.							✓	‡	‡		‡	‡	‡		‡		‡	‡		
	Salmonella typhi													‡				‡	‡		
	Serratia sp.								‡			‡	✓	✓		✓		✓	✓	‡	
	Shigella sp.							✓	‡	‡		‡	‡	‡		‡		‡	‡		
	Yersinia enterocolitica								✓												

CEPHALOSPORINS AND RELATED ANTIBIOTICS

	Organisms Generally Susceptible to Cephalosporins																				
Organisms		First Generation				Second Generation					Third Generation									Fourth Generation	Fifth Generation
✓ = generally susceptible ‡ = demonstrated in vitro activity		Cefadroxil	Cefazolin	Cephalexin	Cephradine	Cefaclor	Cefoxitin	Cefuroxime	Cefotetan	Cefprozil	Cefdinir	Cefixime	Cefoperazone	Cefotaxime	Cefpodoxime[b]	Ceftazidime	Ceftibuten	Ceftizoxime	Ceftriaxone	Cefepime[a]	Ceftaroline
Anaerobes	*Bacteroides* sp.					✓	✓	✓	✓[d]	‡			✓	✓		✓[d]		‡	✓		
	Bacteroides fragilis						✓		✓				✓	✓				✓	‡		
	Clostridium sp.						✓	✓	✓	‡			✓	✓		‡		‡	‡		
	Clostridium difficile								‡	‡			‡								
	Eubacterium sp.												‡						‡		
	Fusobacterium sp.							✓	✓	‡			‡	✓				‡	‡		
	Peptococcus sp.					‡	✓	✓	✓				✓	✓		‡		✓	‡		
	Peptococcus niger					‡															
	Peptostreptococcus sp.					‡	✓	✓	✓	‡			✓	✓	‡	‡		✓	‡		
	Porphyromonas asaccharolytica								‡												
	Prevotella bivia								✓												
	Prevotella digiens								✓												
	Prevotella melaninogenica								‡												
	Prevotella oralis								‡												
	Propionibacterium acnes					‡															
	Propionibacterium sp.								‡												
	Veillonella sp.								‡												
Other	*Borrelia burgdorferi*							✓													

[a] Including some beta-lactamase-producing strains.
[b] Extended-spectrum agent.
[c] Methicillin-susceptible strains only.
[d] Some strains are resistant.
[e] Penicillin-susceptible strains only.
[f] Lancefield's group *A streptococci*.
[g] Some other references consider this fourth generation.
[h] Coagulase-positive, coagulase-negative, and penicillinase-producing.

Absorption – **Cephalexin**, **cephradine**, **cefaclor**, **cefixime**, **cefprozil**, **cefadroxil**, and **ceftibuten** are well absorbed from the GI tract; absorption of these agents (except **cefadroxil** and **cefprozil**) may be delayed by food, but the amount absorbed is not affected. After oral administration, **cefuroxime axetil** is absorbed from the GI tract and rapidly hydrolyzed in the intestinal mucosa and blood to cefuroxime. **Cefpodoxime proxetil** is a pro-drug that is absorbed from the GI tract and de-esterified to its active metabolite, cefpodoxime. The absorption of oral cefuroxime and cefpodoxime is increased when given with food. **Cefdinir** may be taken without regard to meals.

Distribution – Cephalosporins are widely distributed to most tissues and fluids. First and second generation agents do not readily enter cerebrospinal fluid (CSF), except **cefuroxime**, even when meninges are inflamed. Third generation compounds (little data for **cefixime**) and cefuroxime readily diffuse into the CSF of patients with inflamed meninges. However, CSF levels of **cefoperazone** are relatively low. No data are available for **cefdinir** human CSF penetration. Therapeutic levels are reached in bone after usual doses of most agents. **Cefazolin** penetrates acutely inflamed bone at higher concentrations than in normal bone.

High concentrations of **ceftriaxone** and **cefoperazone** are attained in bile. Therapeutic levels of **ceftizoxime**, **cefuroxime**, **cefotetan**, **ceftazidime**, and **cefoxitin** are attained in bile. Bile levels of **cefazolin** can reach or exceed serum levels by up to five times in patients without obstructive biliary disease.

Metabolism/Excretion – **Cefuroxime axetil** is metabolized to free cefuroxime plus acetaldehyde and acetic acid. Desacetylcefotaxime, a major metabolite of **cefotaxime**, contributes to the bactericidal activity and increases the spectrum to include anaerobes, specifically *Bacteroides* sp; the synergy with the parent drug appears to extend the dosing interval to 8 to 12 hours because of the prolonged metabolite half-life. **Cefpodoxime proxetil** is a pro-drug that is de-esterified to its active metabolite, cefpodoxime. **Ceftaroline fosamil** is converted to bioactive ceftaroline by a phosphatase enzyme. **Cefdinir** is not appreciably metabolized and is primarily excreted renally. Most cephalosporins and metabolites are primarily excreted renally. **Cefoperazone** is excreted mainly in the bile; peak serum levels and serum half-lives are unchanged, even in patients with severe renal insufficiency. In hepatic dysfunction, serum half-life and urinary excretion are increased.

➤*Microbiology:* Refer to the previous tables for organisms generally susceptible to cephalosporins.

Beta-lactamase resistance – First generation cephalosporins are generally inactivated by beta-lactamase-producing organisms. Newer agents are distinguished by an increasing resistance to beta-lactamase inactivation. **Cefdinir** and **cefixime** have a high degree of stability to some beta-lactamases. **Cefoxitin**, **cefuroxime**, **ceftriaxone**, **cefotaxime**,**ceftizoxime**, and **cefotetan** have a high degree of stability in the presence of both penicillinases and cephalosporinases produced by gram-negative and gram-positive bacteria. **Cefoperazone**, **cefpodoxime** and **ceftazidime** are highly stable in the presence of beta-lactamases produced by most gram-negative pathogens and are active against some organisms that are resistant to other beta-lactam antibiotics because of beta-lactamase production. **Cefepime** has a broad spectrum of activity against gram-positive and gram-negative bacteria but has a low affinity for chromosomally encoded beta-lactamases. **Ceftaroline** is not active against gram-negative bacteria producing extended-spectrum beta-lactamases from the TEM, SHV**Cefaclor** is stable in the presence of some β-lactamases. **Cefprozil** has in vitro activity against a broad range of gram-positive and gram-negative bacteria.

Contraindications

Hypersensitivity to cephalosporins or related antibiotics (see Warnings/Precautions); hyperbilirubinemic neonates, especially premature neonates (**ceftriaxone**); concomitant use with calcium-containing IV solutions (including total parenteral nutrition [TPN] agents) in neonates because of the risk of precipitation of ceftriaxone-calcium salt (**ceftriaxone**).

Warnings/Precautions

➤*Cross-allergenicity with penicillin:* Administer cautiously to **penicillin**-sensitive patients. There is evidence of partial cross-allergenicity; cephalosporins cannot be assumed to be an absolutely safe alternative to **penicillin** in the penicillin-allergic patient. The estimated incidence of cross-sensitivity is 5% to 16%; however, it is possibly as low as 3% to 7%.

➤*Serum sickness-like reactions:* Erythema multiforme or skin rashes accompanied by polyarthritis, arthralgia and, frequently, fever have been reported; these reactions usually occurred following a second course of therapy. Signs and symptoms occur after a few days of therapy and resolve a few days after drug discontinuation with no serious sequelae. Antihistamines and corticosteroids may be of benefit in managing symptoms.

➤*Seizures:* Several cephalosporins have been implicated in triggering seizures, particularly in patients with renal impairment when the dosage was not reduced. If seizures associated with drug therapy occur, discontinue the drug. Anticonvulsant therapy can be given if clinically indicated.

➤*Calcium-containing products:* Do not use diluents containing calcium, such as Ringer's solution or Hartmann's solution, to reconstitute **ceftriaxone** vials or to further dilute a reconstituted vial for IV administration because a precipitate can form. Precipitation of **ceftriaxone**-calcium can also occur when **ceftriaxone** is mixed with calcium-containing solutions in the same IV administration line. **Ceftriaxone** must not be administered simultaneously with calcium-containing IV solutions, including continuous calcium-containing infusions, such as parenteral nutrition through a Y-site. However, in patients other than neonates, **ceftriaxone** and calcium-containing solutions may be administered sequentially if the infusion lines are thoroughly flushed between infusions with a compatible fluid. In vitro studies using adult and neonatal plasma from umbilical cord blood demonstrated that neonates have an increased risk of precipitation of **ceftriaxone**-calcium.

No data are available on the potential interaction between **ceftriaxone** and oral calcium-containing products or the interaction between IM **ceftriaxone** and calcium-containing products (IV or oral).

➤*Coagulation abnormalities:* **Cefoperazone**, **cefotetan** and **ceftriaxone** may be associated with a fall in prothrombin activity. Those at risk include patients with renal impairment, cancer, impaired vitamin K synthesis or low vitamin K stores (eg, chronic hepatic disease or malnutrition), as well as patients receiving a protracted course of antimicrobial therapy. Monitor prothrombin time for patients at risk and administer exogenous vitamin K as indicated. Vitamin K administration may be necessary if the prothrombin time is prolonged before therapy.

➤*Clostridium difficile–associated diarrhea:* *C. difficile*–associated diarrhea has been reported for nearly all systemic antibacterial agents, including cephalosporins, and may range in severity from mild diarrhea to fatal colitis.

Treatment with antibacterial agents alters the normal flora of the colon and may permit overgrowth of *C. difficile*.

C. difficile produces toxins A and B, which contribute to the development of *C. difficile*–associated diarrhea. Hypertoxin-producing strains of *C. difficile* cause increased morbidity and mortality because these infections can be refractory to antimicrobial therapy and may require colectomy. *C. difficile*–associated diarrhea must be considered in all patients who present with diarrhea following antibiotic use. Careful medical history is necessary because *C. difficile*–associated diarrhea has been reported to occur more than 2 months after the administration of antibacterial agents.

If *C. difficile*–associated diarrhea is suspected or confirmed, discontinue antibacterials not directed against *C. difficile*, if possible. Institute appropriate fluid and electrolyte management, protein supplementation, antibiotic treatment of *C. difficile*, and surgical evaluation as clinically indicated.

➤*Immune hemolytic anemia:* This has been observed in patients receiving cephalosporin class antibiotics. Rare cases of severe hemolytic anemia, including fatalities, have been reported in association with cephalosporins. If a patient develops anemia any time within 2 to 3 weeks subsequent to the start of therapy, the diagnosis of cephalosporin-associated anemia should be considered and the drug stopped until the etiology is determined with certainty. Blood transfusions may be administered as needed. Patients who receive prolonged courses of cephalosporins for treatment of infections should have periodic monitoring for signs and symptoms of hemolytic anemia, including a measurement of hematological parameters where appropriate.

➤*Parenteral use:* Inject IM preparations deep into musculature; properly dilute IV preparations and administer over an appropriate time interval. See individual product monographs. Prolonged or high dosage IV use may be associated with thrombophlebitis; use small IV needles, larger veins and alternate infusion sites.

➤*Gonorrhea:* In the treatment of gonorrhea, all patients should have a serologic test for syphilis. Patients with incubating syphilis (seronegative without clinical signs of syphilis) are likely to be cured by the regimens used for gonorrhea.

➤*Gallbladder disease:* There have been reports of sonographic abnormalities in the gallbladder of patients treated with **ceftriaxone**; some of these patients also had symptoms of gallbladder disease. These abnormalities appear on sonography as an echo without acoustical shadowing, suggesting sludge, or as an echo with acoustical shadowing that may be misinterpreted as gallstones. The chemical nature of the sonographically detected material is predominantly **ceftriaxone**-calcium salt. The condition appears to be transient and reversible upon discontinuation of **ceftriaxone** and institution of conservative management. Therefore, discontinue **ceftriaxone** in patients who develop signs and symptoms suggestive of gallbladder disease or the sonographic findings described previously.

➤*Pancreatitis:* Cases of pancreatitis, possibly secondary to biliary obstruction, have been reported rarely in patients treated with **ceftriaxone**. Most patients presented with risk factors of biliary stasis and biliary sludge (preceding major therapy, severe illness, TPN). A cofactor role of **ceftriaxone**-related biliary precipitation cannot be ruled out.

➤*Benzyl alcohol:* Some cephalosporin products contain benzyl alcohol. In neonates, benzyl alcohol has been associated with neurological and other complications which are sometimes fatal. Benzyl alcohol-containing cephalosporin products should not be used in neonates.

➤*Renal function impairment:* Cephalosporins may be nephrotoxic; use with caution in the presence of markedly impaired renal function (CrCl rate of < 50 mL/min/1.73 m^2). In the elderly and in patients with known or suspected renal impairment, monitor carefully prior to and during therapy.

Some cephalosporins require a reduced total daily dosage in patients with transient or persistent reduction of urinary output caused by renal insufficiency; high and prolonged serum concentrations can occur in such patients from usual doses. See individual product monographs for information on dosage adjustments in impaired renal function.

➤*Hepatic function impairment:* **Cefoperazone** is extensively excreted in bile. Serum half-life increases 2-fold to 4-fold in patients with hepatic disease or biliary obstruction. If higher dosages are used (> 4 g), monitor serum concentrations.

➤*Special risk:* Prescribe **ceftriaxone** with caution in individuals with a history of GI disease, especially colitis. Prescribe products with dextrose with caution in patients with overt or known subclinical diabetes mellitus or carbohydrate intolerance for any reason.

➤*Superinfection:* Use of antibiotics (especially prolonged or repeated therapy) may result in overgrowth of nonsusceptible organisms. Such overgrowth may lead to a secondary infection. Take appropriate measures if this occurs.

➤*Pregnancy: Category B.* Safety for use during pregnancy is not established. Use only when potential benefits outweigh potential hazards to the fetus. Cephalosporins appear safe for pregnant patients, but relatively few controlled studies exist.

These agents cross the placenta; peak umbilical cord concentrations for the various agents range from 3 to 29 mcg/mL following doses of 0.5 to 2 g. These data yielded a maternal:fetal serum ratio range of 0.16 to 1. Drug levels in cord blood after administration of **cefazolin** are approximately ¼ to ⅓ maternal drug levels. **Cefotetan** reaches therapeutic levels in cord blood.

In addition, the pharmacokinetic parameters of these drugs appear to change in the pregnant woman; tendencies are toward shorter half-lives, lower serum levels, larger volumes of distribution and increased clearance.

➤*Lactation:* Most of these agents are excreted in breast milk in small quantities. Levels range from 0.16 to 4 mcg/mL, or a breast milk:maternal serum ratio of 0.01 to 0.5 following 0.5 to 2 g doses. **Cefdinir** was not detected in breast milk following single 600 mg doses. It is not known whether **ceftaroline** is excreted in breast milk. However, consider these problems for the nursing infant: modification/alteration of bowel flora; pharmacological effects; interference with interpretation of culture results if a fever/infection workup is needed. **Ceftibuten** has not been studied.

➤*Children:* When using cephalosporins in infants, consider the relative benefit to risk. In neonates, accumulation of cephalosporin antibiotics, with resulting prolongation of drug half-life, has occurred.

Do not treat hyperbilirubinemic neonates, especially premature neonates, with **ceftriaxone**. In vitro studies have shown that ceftriaxone can displace bilirubin from its binding to serum albumin, and bilirubin encephalopathy can possibly develop in these patients.

In children 3 months of age or older, higher doses of **cefoxitin** have been associated with an increased incidence of eosinophilia and elevated AST.

In children 6 months of age or older, **ceftizoxime** has been associated with transient elevated levels of eosinophils, AST, ALT and creatine phosphokinase (CPK).

Safety and efficacy in children younger than 1 month of age (**cefazolin** and **cefaclor** capsule and suspension), younger than 3 months (**cefuroxime** and **cefoxitin**), younger than 5 months (**cefpodoxime**), younger than 6 months (**cefdinir, cefixime, ceftozoxime** and **cefprozil**), younger than 9 months (**oral cephradine**) and younger than 1 year (**cefepime** and **parenteral cephradine**) have not been established.

Safety and efficacy of **cefaclor** extended release tablets in children younger than 16 years of age have not been established.

Safety and efficacy of **ceftaroline, cefoperazone, cephalexin** and **cefotetan** in children have not been established.

➤*Elderly:* In elderly patients, dosage adjustments based on decreased renal function may be necessary.

Drug Interactions

Cephalosporin Drug Interactions

Precipitant drug	Object drug[a]		Description
Cephalosporins Cefazolin Cefoperazone Cefotetan	Ethanol	↑	Alcoholic beverages consumed concurrently with or ≤ 72 hours after cefoperazone, cefazolin, or cefotetan may produce acute alcohol intolerance (disulfiram-like reaction). These antibiotics possess a methyltetrazolethiol side chain that may inhibit aldehyde dehydrogenase. The reaction begins within 30 minutes after alcohol ingestion and may subside 30 minutes to several hours afterwards; the reaction may occur ≤ 3 days after the last dose of the antibiotic.
Aminoglycosides (eg, gentamicin, tobramycin)	Cephalosporins	↑	Aminoglycoside nephrotoxicity may be potentiated by concurrent use of some cephalosporins, specifically cephalothin.[b] Bactericidal activity against certain pathogens may be enhanced. Monitor aminoglycoside concentrations and renal function closely. If renal dysfunction develops, reduce the dosage or discontinue one or both drugs and use alternative agents.
Cephalosporins	Aminoglycosides (eg, gentamicin, tobramycin)		

Cephalosporin Drug Interactions

Precipitant drug	Object drug[a]		Description
Calcium-containing solutions	Cephalosporins Ceftriaxone	↑	Neonatal deaths have been reported due to pulmonary and renal precipitation with calcium-ceftriaxone. Ceftriaxone is contraindicated in neonates needing, or expected to need, calcium-containing IV solutions, including TPN. Avoid simultaneous administration of calcium-containing solutions and ceftriaxone in the same IV line. However, in patients other than neonates, ceftriaxone and calcium may be administered sequentially if the infusion lines are thoroughly flushed between products with a compatible solution. Additionally, a potential risk exists for calcium-ceftriaxone precipitation leading to gallbladder sludging, as well as precipitation in the lungs and kidney.
Cephalosporins Ceftriaxone	Calcium-containing solutions		
Cephalosporins Cefazolin Cefoperazone Cefotetan	Anticoagulants (eg, warfarin)	↑	The anticoagulant effect of warfarin may be increased by cephalosporins with a methyltetrazolethiol side chain. Warfarin doses may need to be reduced during administration with cephalosporins. Monitor coagulation parameters and adjust the warfarin dose as needed. The concurrent use of heparin may also theoretically increase the risk of bleeding.
Cephalosporins Ceftriaxone	Cyclosporine	↑	Elevated cyclosporine levels with an increased risk of toxicity may occur. However, clinical significance is unknown. Monitor serum cyclosporine and creatinine concentrations. Adjust the cyclosporine dose as needed.
Probenecid	Cephalosporins	↑	Probenecid may increase and prolong cephalosporin plasma levels by competitively inhibiting renal tubular secretion. This is most significant for cephalosporins eliminated primarily by tubular secretion.
Antacids	Cephalosporins Cefaclor Cefdinir Cefpodoxime	↓	Plasma concentrations of cefaclor extended-release tablets, cefdinir and cefpodoxime may be reduced by coadministration of antacids. If antacids are required during administration of these antibiotics, the cephalosporin should be taken 2 hours before or after the antacid. Cefprozil and ceftibuten do not appear to be affected by coadministration of antacids.
H_2 antagonists	Cephalosporins Cefpodoxime Cefuroxime	↓	Plasma concentrations of cefpodoxime and cefuroxime may be reduced by coadministration of H_2 antagonists, decreasing the antibiotic effect. Cefaclor extended-release tablets do not appear to be affected by coadministration of H_2 antagonists.
Iron supplements	Cephalosporins Cefdinir	↓	Iron supplements and foods fortified with iron reduce the absorption of cefdinir by 80% and 30%, respectively. If iron supplements are needed during cefdinir therapy, cefdinir should be taken 2 hours before or after the supplement. Iron-fortified infant formula (2.2 mg elemental iron/6 oz) has no effect on cefdinir absorption.
Loop diuretics	Cephalosporins	↑	Use cephalosporins with caution in patients receiving potent diuretics (eg, loop diuretics). The risk of nephrotoxicity may be increased. Monitor renal function.

[a] ↑ = object drug increased; ↓ = object drug decreased.
[b] No longer marketed in the United States.

➤*Drug/Lab test interactions:* A false-positive reaction for **urine glucose** may occur with Benedict's solution, Fehling's solution or with *Clinitest* tablets, but not with enzyme-based tests such as *Clinistix* and *Tes-Tape*.

Cephradine may cause false-positive reactions in urinary protein tests that use sulfosalicylic acid.

Cefuroxime may cause a false-negative reaction in the ferricyanide test for **blood glucose**.

Cefdinir may cause a false-positive reaction for ketones in urine when measured using nitroprusside but not nitroferricynide.

A false-positive direct Coombs test has occurred in some patients receiving cephalosporins, particularly those with azotemia, in hematologic studies, in transfusion cross-matching procedures when **antiglobulin tests** are performed on the minor side or in Coombs testing of newborns of mothers receiving cephalosporins before parturition. This reaction is nonimmunological.

Cephalosporins may falsely elevate **urinary 17-ketosteroid** values.

High concentrations of **cephalothin** or **cefoxitin** (> 100 mcg/mL) may interfere with measurement of creatinine levels by the Jaffe reaction and produce false results. Serum samples from patients on cefoxitin should not be analyzed for creatinine if obtained within 2 hours of drug use. **Cefotetan** may affect these measurements.

➤*Drug/Food interactions:* Food increases absorption of **cefpodoxime** and oral **cefuroxime**.

Adverse Reactions

For more information on serum sickness-like reactions, seizures, coagulation abnormalities, CDAD, immune hemolytic anemia, hypersensitivity, and nephrotoxicity, refer to Warnings/Precautions.

➤*Cardiovascular:* Bradycardia (**ceftaroline**), chest pain, hypotension, palpitations, syncope, vasodilation.

➤*CNS:* Anxiety, confusion, convulsions (**ceftaroline**), dizziness, fatigue, headache, hyperactivity, hypertonia, insomnia, lethargy, nervousness, paresthesia, somnolence, vertigo. Generalized tonic-clonic seizures, mild hemiparesis, and extreme confusion after large doses in renal failure (**cefazolin**).

➤*Dermatologic:* Cutaneous moniliasis, diaphoresis, erythema, flushing, maculopapular rash, pruritus, urticaria; allergic dermatitis (postmarketing).

➤*GI:* Nausea; vomiting; diarrhea; constipation; anorexia; thirst; glossitis; oral candidiasis and moniliasis; abdominal pain; flatulence; heartburn; gastritis; stomach cramps; eructation; melena; bleeding peptic ulcer; ileus; gallbladder sludge; dyspepsia; colitis, including *C. difficile* colitis, can appear during or after treatment (see Warnings/Precautions); adverse GI effects after parenteral use of some cephalosporins; glossitis, stomatitis (postmarketing).

➤*GU:* Acute renal failure (rare), dysuria, genital candidiasis and moniliasis, genito-anal pruritus, hematuria, pyuria, reversible interstitial nephritis, transitory elevations in serum urea nitrogen with and without elevated serum creatinine, toxic nephropathy, vaginal discharge, vaginitis; casts in urine, hematuria, nephrolithiasis, renal precipitations (**ceftriaxone**), oliguria (postmarketing).

➤*Hematologic:* Eosinophilia; transient neutropenia; lymphocytosis; leukocytosis; leukopenia; thrombocythemia; thrombocytopenia; agranulocytosis; granulocytopenia; hemolytic anemia; bone marrow depression; pancytopenia; decreased platelet function; bleeding in association with hypoprothrombinemia; anemia; aplastic anemia; hemorrhage; transient thrombocytosis; neutropenia caused by an immunologic reaction and characterized by rapid destruction of peripheral neutrophils may require drug discontinuation; transient fluctuations in leukocyte counts, predominantly lymphocytosis; slight decreases in neutrophil count; decreased hemoglobin or hematocrit; disturbances in vitamin K-dependent clotting function (increased prothrombin time); increased platelet and increased bleeding. Lymphopenia, monocytosis, basophilia.

➤*Hepatic:* Elevated AST, ALT, total bilirubin, alkaline phosphatase, lactate dehydrogenase; hepatomegaly; hepatitis; jaundice; cholestasis; cholestatic jaundice; hepatic failure; hepatic dysfunction (including cholestasis); biliary lithiasis.

➤*Hypersensitivity:* Anaphylaxis; angioedema; Stevens-Johnson syndrome; erythema multiforme; toxic epidermal necrolysis.

➤*Local:* Pain; induration; temperature elevation and tenderness from IM injection; sterile abscesses from accidental subcutaneous injection; local swelling; inflammation; burning, cellulitis, paresthesia, phlebitis and thrombophlebitis following IV or IM administration.

➤*Musculoskeletal:* Arthralgia, exacerbation of myasthenia gravis (**cefoxitin**), myalgia, rhabdomyolysis.

➤*Respiratory:* Asthma, bronchitis, bronchospasm, dyspnea, interstitial pneumonitis, laryngeal edema, pneumonia, respiratory failure; allergic pneumonitis, epistaxis (**ceftriaxone**, rare).

➤*Miscellaneous:* Facial edema; swollen tongue; fever; chills; malaise; asthenia; dysgeusia; glucosuria; drug fever; serum sickness–like reaction; superinfection; encephalopathy in renally impaired patients receiving unadjusted dosage regiment (**cefepime**); hyperglycemia, hyperkalemia, hypokalemia (**ceftaroline**); Jarisch-Herxheimer reaction (**cefuroxime**); muscle cramps, stiffness, spasms of neck, pain/tightness in chest, pain/bleeding in urethra, kidney pain, tachycardia, lockjaw-type reaction (**cefuroxime**, single dose for gonorrhea); elevated CPK (IM **ceftizoxime** or **cefaclor** extended release tablets); mild to moderate hearing loss reported in some pediatric patients (**cefuroxime**).

Cases of fatal reactions with ceftriaxone-calcium precipitates in the lungs and kidneys in neonates have been described. In some cases, the infusion lines and the times of administration of ceftriaxone and calcium-containing solutions were different.

Overdosage

➤*Parenteral cephalosporins:* Inappropriately large doses may cause seizures, particularly in renal impairment. Reduce dosage when renal function is impaired. If seizures occur, promptly discontinue drug; administer anticonvulsants if clinically indicated; consider hemodialysis in cases of overwhelming overdosage.

Patient Information

Counsel patients that antibacterial drugs are only used to treat bacterial infections. They do not treat viral infections (eg, the common cold). Although it is common to feel better early in the course of therapy, tell patients to take the medication exactly as directed. Skipping doses or not completing the full course of therapy may decrease the effectiveness of the immediate treatment and increase the likelihood that bacteria will develop resistance and will not be treatable by ceftriaxone or other antibacterial drugs in the future.

Diarrhea is a common problem caused by antibiotics that usually ends when the antibiotic is discontinued. Sometimes after starting treatment with antibiotics, patients can develop watery and bloody stools (with or without stomach cramps and fever) as late as 2 months or longer after taking the last dose of the antibiotic. If this occurs, advise patients to contact their health care provider as soon as possible.

➤*For oral preparations:* Complete full course of therapy.

May cause GI upset; may take with food or milk. Take **cefpodoxime** and **cefuroxime** with food to increase absorption.

A false-positive reaction for urine glucose may occur with the nonspecific urine tests. Use an enzyme-based test.

➤*Cephradine:*

Diabetics – Notify physician before changing diet or dosage of medication.

➤*Phenylketonurics:* **Cefprozil** oral suspension contains phenylalanine 28 mg/5 mL.

➤*Antacids:* Those containing magnesium or aluminum interfere with the absorption of **cefdinir**. If this type of antacid is required during **cefdinir** therapy, take **cefdinir** 2 hours before or after the antacid.

CEFPODOXIME PROXETIL

Rx	**Cefpodoxime Proxetil** (Aurobindo)	**Tablets; oral:** 100 mg	Lactose. (C 61). Lt. yellowish-orange, elliptical. Film-coated. In 20s.
Rx	**Vantin** (Pharmacia & Upjohn)		Lactose. (U3617). Orange. Film coated. In 20s, 100s and UD 100s.
Rx	**Cefpodoxime Proxetil** (Aurobindo)	**Tablets; oral:** 200 mg	Lactose. (C 62). Coral red, elliptical. Film-coated. In 20s.
Rx	**Vantin** (Pharmacia & Upjohn)		Lactose. (U3618). Coral red. Film coated. In 20s, 100s and UD 100s.
Rx	**Cefpodoxime Proxetil** (Aurobindo)	**Granules for suspension; oral:** 50 mg/5 mL	Lactose, sucrose. In 50, 75, and 100 mL bottles.
		100 mg/5 mL	Lactose, sucrose. In 50, 75, and 100 mL bottles.

CEFPODOXIME PROXETIL — ORAL

For complete and comparative prescribing information, refer to the Cephalosporins group monograph.

Indications

➤*Acute otitis:* Caused by *Streptococcus pneumoniae*, (excluding penicillin-resistant strains). *Streptococcus pyogenes*, *Haemophilus influenzae* (including beta-lactamase-producing strains), or *Moraxella* (*Branhamella*) *catarrhalis* (including beta-lactamase producing strains).

➤*Pharyngitis or tonsillitis:* Caused by *Streptococcus pyogenes*. Only penicillin by the IM route of administration has been shown to be effective in the prophylaxis of rheumatic fever. Cefpodoxime proxetil is generally effective in the eradication of streptococci from the oropharynx. However, data

CEFPODOXIME PROXETIL — ORAL

establishing the efficacy of cefpodoxime proxetil for the prophylaxis of subsequent rheumatic fever are not available.

➤*Community-acquired pneumonia:* Caused by *S. pneumoniae* or *H. influenzae* (including beta-lactamase-producing strains).

➤*Acute bacterial exacerbation of chronic bronchitis:* Caused by *S. pneumoniae, H. influenzae* (non-beta-lactamase-producing strains only), or *M. catarrhalis*. Data are insufficient at this time to establish efficacy in patients with acute bacterial exacerbations of chronic bronchitis caused by beta-lactamase-producing strains of *H. influenzae*.

➤*Acute, uncomplicated urethral and cervical gonorrhea:* Caused by *Neisseria gonorrhoeae* (including penicillinase-producing strains).

➤*Acute, uncomplicated anorectal infections in women:* Due to *Neisseria gonorrhoeae* (including penicillinase-producing strains).

The efficacy of cefpodoxime in treating male patients with rectal infections caused by *N. gonorrhoeae* has not been established. Data do not support the use of cefpodoxime proxetil in the treatment of pharyngeal infections due to *N. gonorrhoeae* in men or women.

➤*Uncomplicated skin and skin structure infections:* Caused by *Staphylococcus aureus* (including penicillinase-producing strains) or *Streptococcus pyogenes*. Abscesses should be surgically drained as clinically indicated.

In clinical trials, successful treatment of uncomplicated skin and skin structure infections was dose related. The effective therapeutic dose for skin infections was higher than those used in other recommended indications (see Administration and Dosage).

➤*Acute maxillary sinusitis:* Caused by *Haemophilus influenzae* (including beta-lactamase producing strains), *Streptococcus pneumoniae*, and *Moraxella catarrhalis*.

➤*Uncomplicated urinary tract infections (cystitis):* Caused by *Escherichia coli, Klebsiella pneumoniae, Proteus mirabilis*, or *Staphylococcus saprophyticus*.

In considering the use of cefpodoxime proxetil in the treatment of cystitis, cefpodoxime proxetil's lower bacterial eradication rates should be weighed against the increased eradication rates and different safety profiles of some other classes of approved agents.

Administration and Dosage

➤*Adults:*

Infections – Cefpodoxime oral suspension is not indicated for acute bacterial exacerbations of chronic bronchitis.

Cefpodoxime Dosing in Patients 12 Years of Age and Older

Type of infection	Total daily dose	Dose frequency	Duration
Acute bacterial exacerbations of chronic bronchitis	400 mg	200 mg every 12 hours	10 days
Acute community-acquired pneumonia	400 mg	200 mg every 12 hours	14 days

Cefpodoxime Dosing in Patients 12 Years of Age and Older

Type of infection	Total daily dose	Dose frequency	Duration
Acute maxillary sinusitis	400 mg	200 mg every 12 hours	10 days
Pharyngitis and/ or tonsillitis	200 mg	100 mg every 12 hours	5 to 10 days
Skin and skin structure	800 mg	400 mg every 12 hours	7 to 14 days
Uncomplicated gonorrhea (men and women) and rectal gonococcal infections (women)	200 mg	single dose	
Uncomplicated urinary tract infection	200 mg	100 mg every 12 hours	7 days

➤*Children:*

Infections – Cefpodoxime oral suspension is not indicated for acute bacterial exacerbations of chronic bronchitis.

See Adults for dosing for children 12 years of age and older.

2 months to 12 years of age: The following dosing is for cefpodoxime oral suspension.

Cefpodoxime Dosing in Patients 2 Months to 12 Years of Age

Infection	Total daily dose	Dose frequency	Duration
Acute maxillary sinusitis	10 mg/kg/day (max 400 mg/day)	5 mg/kg every 12 hours (max 200 mg/dose)	10 days
Acute otitis media	10 mg/kg/day (max 400 mg/day)	5 mg/kg every 12 hours (max 200 mg/dose)	5 days
Pharyngitis and/ or tonsillitis	10 mg/kg/day (max 200 mg/day)	5 mg/kg/dose every 12 hours (max 100 mg/dose)	5 to 10 days

➤*Renal function impairment:* For patients with severe renal impairment (< 30 mL/min creatinine clearance), the dosing intervals should be increased to every 24 hours. In patients maintained on hemodialysis, the dose frequency should be 3 times/week after hemodialysis.

➤*Administration:* Cefpodoxime tablets should be administered orally with food to enhance absorption. Cefpodoxime oral suspension may be given without regard to food.

➤*Storage/Stability:* Store tablets at 20° to 25°C (68° to 77°F). Protect unit dose packs from excessive moisture.

Store unsuspended granules at 20° to 25°C (68° to 77°F). After mixing, suspension should be stored in a refrigerator, 2° to 8°C (36° to 46°F). The mixture may be used for 14 days. Discard unused portion after 14 days.

CEFACLOR

Rx	**Raniclor** (Ranbaxy)	**Tablets, chewable**: 125 mg	2.8 mg phenylalanine, aspartame, mannitol, tartrazine. (RX 555). Yellow, scored. Fruity flavor. In 20s, 30s, 250s, and UD 100s.
		187 mg	4.2 mg phenylalanine, aspartame, mannitol, tartrazine. (RX 556). Yellow, scored. Fruity flavor. In 20s, 250s, and UD 100s.
		250 mg	5.6 mg phenylalanine, aspartame, mannitol, tartrazine. (RX 557). Yellow, scored. Fruity flavor. In 20s, 30s, 250s, and UD 100s.
		375 mg	8.4 mg phenylalanine, aspartame, mannitol, tartrazine. (RX 558). Yellow, scored. Fruity flavor. In 20s, 250s, and UD 100s.
Rx	**Cefaclor** (Zenith Goldline)	**Tablets, extended release**: 375 mg	(X 4194 500). Blue, oval. In 100s.
		500 mg	
Rx	**Cefaclor** (Various, eg, Apothecon, Mylan, URL)	**Capsules**: 250 mg	In 30s, 100s, 500s, and 1000s.
Rx	**Ceclor Pulvules** (Eli Lilly)		(3061). White and purple. In 15s, 100s and UD 100s.
Rx	**Cefaclor** (Various, eg, Apothecon, Mylan, URL)	**Capsules**: 500 mg	In 15s, 100s and 500s.
Rx	**Cefaclor** (Various, eg, Apothecon, Mylan, URL, Zenith Goldline)	**Powder for oral suspension**: 125 mg/5 mL	In 75 and 150 mL.
	Ceclor (Eli Lilly)		Sucrose. Strawberry flavor. In 75 and 150 mL.
Rx	**Cefaclor** (Various, eg, Apothecon, Mylan, URL, Zenith Goldline)	**Powder for oral suspension**: 187 mg/5 mL	In 50 and 100 mL.
	Ceclor (Eli Lilly)		Sucrose. Strawberry flavor. In 50 and 100 mL.
Rx	**Cefaclor** (Various, eg, Apothecon, Mylan, URL, Zenith Goldline)	**Powder for oral suspension**: 250 mg/5 mL	In 75 and 150 mL.
	Ceclor (Eli Lilly)		Sucrose. Strawberry flavor. In 75 and 150 mL.
Rx	**Cefaclor** (Various, eg, Apothecon, Mylan, URL, Zenith Goldline)	**Powder for oral suspension**: 375 mg/5 mL	In 50 and 100 mL.
	Ceclor (Eli Lilly)		Sucrose. Strawberry flavor. In 50 and 100 mL.

CEFACLOR — ORAL

For complete and comparative prescribing information, refer to the Cephalosporins group monograph.

Indications

➤*Extended-release tablets:*

Pharyngitis and tonsillitis – Pharyngitis and tonsillitis due to *Streptococcus pyogenes*.

Uncomplicated skin and skin structure infections – Uncomplicated skin and skin structure infections due to *Staphylococcus aureus* (methicillin-susceptible).

Acute bacterial exacerbations of chronic bronchitis – Acute bacterial exacerbations of chronic bronchitis due to *Haemophilus influenzae* (non-β-lactamase-producing strains only), *Moraxella catarrhalis* (including β-lactamase-producing strains) or *Streptococcus pneumoniae*.

Secondary bacterial infections of acute bronchitis – Secondary bacterial infections of acute bronchitis due to *Haemophilus influenzae* (non-β-lactamase-producing strains only), *Moraxella catarrhalis* (including β-lactamase-producing strains), or *Streptococcus pneumoniae*.

➤*Capsules, chewable tablets, and oral suspension:*

Otitis media – Caused by *Streptococcus pneumoniae*, *Haemophilus influenzae*, staphylococci, and *Streptococcus pyogenes*.

Pharyngitis and tonsillitis – Due to *Streptococcus pyogenes*.

Lower respiratory tract infections – Including pneumonia, caused by *Streptococcus pneumoniae*, *Haemophilus influenzae*, and *Streptococcus pyogenes*.

Urinary tract infections – Including pyelonephritis and cystitis, caused by *Escherichia coli*, *Proteus mirabilis*, *Klebsiella* spp, and coagulase-negative staphylococci.

Administration and Dosage

➤*General dosing considerations:*

Equivalence – 500 mg twice daily of cefaclor extended-release tablets is clinically equivalent to 250 mg 3 times daily of cefaclor immediate-release as a capsule. 500 mg twice daily of cefaclor extended-release tablets is not equivalent to 500 mg 3 times daily of other cefaclor formulations.

➤*Adults:*

Infections – For a list of infections, refer to Indications.

Capsules, chewable tablets, and oral suspension: The usual dosage is 250 mg every 8 hours. For more severe infections (such as pneumonia) or those caused by less susceptible organisms, doses may be doubled.

Extended-release tablets:

Cefaclor Extended-Release Tablets Dosing in Patients 16 Years of Age and Older			
Infection	Total daily dose	Dose and frequency	Duration
Acute bacterial exacerbations of chronic bronchitis due to *H. influenzae* (non-β-lactamase-producing strains only), *Moraxella catarrhalis* (including β-lactamase producing strains) or *Streptococcus pneumoniae*	1,000 mg	500 mg every 12 hours	7 days
Secondary bacterial infection of acute bronchitis due to *H. influenzae* (non-β-lactamase-producing strains only), *Moraxella catarrhalis* (including β-lactamase producing strains) or *S. pneumoniae* (see Indications)	1,000 mg	500 mg every 12 hours	7 days
Pharyngitis or tonsillitis due to *S. pyogenes*	750 mg	375 mg every 12 hours	10 days
Uncomplicated skin and skin structure infections due to *S. aureus* (methicillin-susceptible strains) (see Indications)	750 mg	375 mg every 12 hours	7 to 10 days

➤*Children:*

Infections – For a list of infections, refer to Indications.

Capsules, chewable tablets, and oral suspension:

• *1 month of age and older* –

Usual dosage: 20 mg/kg/day in divided doses every 8 hours. In more serious infections, otitis media, and infections caused by less susceptible organisms, 40 mg/kg/day are recommended.

For the treatment of otitis media and pharyngitis, the total daily dosage may be divided and administered every 12 hours.

Cefaclor Suspension Every 8 Hour Dosing		
Weight	125 mg/5 mL	250 mg/5 mL
20 mg/kg/day		
9 kg	2.5 mL 3 times daily	
18 kg	5 mL 3 times daily	2.5 mL 3 times daily
40 mg/kg/day		
9 kg	5 mL 3 times daily	2.5 mL 3 times daily
18 kg		5 mL 3 times daily

Cefaclor Suspension Twice-Daily Dosing		
Weight	187 mg/5 mL	375 mg/5 mL
20 mg/kg/day (pharyngitis)		
9 kg	2.5 mL twice daily	
18 kg	5 mL twice daily	2.5 mL twice daily
40 mg/kg/day (otitis media)		
9 kg	5 mL twice daily	2.5 mL twice daily
18 kg		5 mL twice daily

Maximum dose: 1 g/day.

Extended-release tablets: See Adults for dosing for children 16 years of age and older.

➤*Duration of therapy:* Continue administration for a minimum of 48 to 72 hours after fever abates or after evidence of bacterial eradication has been obtained. In the treatment of beta-hemolytic streptococcal infections, a therapeutic dosage of cefaclor should be administered for at least 10 days to guard against the risk of rheumatic fever or glomerulonephritis.

➤*Administration:* May cause GI upset; may take with food or milk.

Capsules – Food does not affect the extent of absorption.

Extended-release tablets – Cefaclor extended-release tablets should be administered with meals (ie, at least within 1 hour of eating). The extended-release tablets should not be cut, crushed, or chewed.

➤*Storage/Stability:* Store at 15° to 30°C (59° to 86°F). Refrigerate suspension after reconstitution; discard after 14 days.

CEPHALEXIN

Rx	**Cephalexin** (Teva)	**Tablets; oral:** 250 mg	In 100s.
Rx	**Cephalexin** (Teva)	**Tablets; oral:** 500 mg	In 100s.
Rx	**Cephalexin** (Various, eg, Teva, UDL, West-Ward)	**Capsules; oral:** 250 mg	In 100s and 500s.
Rx	**Keflex** (Victory Pharma)		(Keflex 250 mg). White/dark green. In 20s and 100s.
Rx	**Cephalexin** (Various, eg, Teva, UDL, West-Ward)	**Capsules; oral:** 500 mg	In 100s and 500s.
Rx	**Keflex** (Victory Pharma)		(Keflex 500 mg). Light green and dark green. In 20s and 100s.
Rx	**Keflex** (Victory Pharma)	**Capsules; oral:** 750 mg	(Keflex 750 mg). Dark green. In 50s.
Rx	**Cephalexin** (Various, eg, Par, Ranbaxy, Teva)	**Powder for suspension; oral:** 125 mg per 5 mL (after reconstitution)	In 100 and 200 mL.
Rx	**Cephalexin** (Various, eg, Par, Ranbaxy, Teva)	**Powder for suspension; oral:** 250 mg per 5 mL (after reconstitution)	In 100 and 200 mL.

CEPHALEXIN — ORAL

For complete and comparative prescribing information, refer to the Cephalosporins group monograph.

Indications

➤*Bone infections:* Caused by *Staphylococcus aureus* and/or *Proteus mirabilis*.

➤*Genitourinary tract infections:* Including acute prostatitis caused by *Escherichia coli, P. mirabilis*, and *Klebsiella pneumoniae*.

➤*Otitis media:* Caused by *Streptococcus pneumoniae, Haemophilus influenzae, S. aureus, Streptococcus pyogenes*, and *Moraxella catarrhalis*.

➤*Respiratory tract infections:* Caused by *S. pneumoniae* and *S. pyogenes*.

➤*Skin and skin structure infections:* Caused by *S. aureus* and/or *S. pyogenes*.

➤*Off-label uses:* Bacterial endocarditis prophylaxis for dental and upper airway procedures.

Administration and Dosage

➤*Maximum dose:* 4 g/day.

➤*General dosing considerations:* For more severe infections, or for those caused by less susceptible organisms, larger doses may be needed. If daily doses of cephalexin more than 4 g are required, consider parental cephalosporins in appropriate doses.

➤*Adults:*

Usual dosage – Usual dosage is 250 mg every 6 hours; 500 mg every 12 hours may be administered for streptococcal pharyngitis, skin and skin structure infections, and uncomplicated cystitis. Doses range from 1 to 4 g daily in divided oral doses. The 333 and 750 mg strengths should be administered so that the daily dose is within 1 to 4 g/day.

➤*Children:*

Beta-hemolytic streptococcal infections –
Usual dosage: 25 to 50 mg/kg/day in divided doses.
Maximum dose: 4 g/day.
Duration of therapy: At least 10 days.

Bone infections –
Usual dosage: 25 to 50 mg/kg/day in divided doses.
Maximum dose: 4 g/day.

Genitourinary tract infections –
Usual dosage: 25 to 50 mg/kg/day in divided doses.
Maximum dose: 4 g/day.

Otitis media –
Usual dosage: 75 to 100 mg/kg/day in 4 divided doses.
Maximum dose: 4 g/day.

Respiratory tract infections –
Usual dosage: 25 to 50 mg/kg/day in divided doses.
Maximum dose: 4 g/day.

Skin and skin structure infections –
Usual dosage: 25 to 50 mg/kg/day in divided doses. Total daily dose may be divided and administered every 12 hours. In severe infections, the dose may be doubled.
Maximum dose: 4 g/day.

Streptococcal pharyngitis –
Usual dosage: 25 to 50 mg/kg/day in divided doses. For children older than 1 year of age, the total daily dose may be divided and administered every 12 hours. In severe infections, the dose may be doubled.
Maximum dose: 4 g/day.

Uncomplicated cystitis –
15 years of age and older:
- *Usual dosage* – 250 mg every 6 hours; 500 mg every 12 hours may be administered. Doses range from 1 to 4 g daily in divided oral doses. The 333 and 750 mg strengths should be administered so that the daily dose is within 1 to 4 g/day.
- *Duration of therapy* – 7 to 14 days.

Younger than 15 years of age:
- *Usual dosage* – 25 to 50 mg/kg/day in divided doses.
- *Maximum dose* – 4 g/day.

Off-label dosing –
Bacterial endocarditis prophylaxis:
- *Usual dose* – One time dose of 50 mg/kg 1 hour before the procedure.
- *Maximum dose* – 2 g.

➤*Renal function impairment:* In patients with marked renal impairment, safe dosage may be lower than that usually recommended.

➤*Administration:* May be given without regard to meals.

➤*Storage/Stability:* Store the tablets and capsules at controlled room temperature, 20° to 25°C (68° to 77°F). Store the powder for oral suspension at controlled room temperature, 15° to 30°C (59° to 86°F). Shake the reconstituted suspension well and refrigerate; discard after 14 days.

CEFADROXIL

Rx	**Cefadroxil** (Various, eg, Major)	**Capsules:** 500 mg[1]	In 100s.
Rx	**Cefadroxil** (Various, eg, Major)	**Tablets:** 1 g[1]	In 24s, 50s, 100s and 500s.
Rx	**Cefadroxil** (Various, eg, Major)	**Powder for oral suspension:** 125 mg/5 mL	Orange-pineapple flavor. In 50 and 100 mL.
		250 mg/5 mL	Sucrose. Orange-pineapple flavor. In 50 and 100 mL.
		500 mg/5 mL	Sucrose. Orange-pineapple flavor. In 75 and 100 mL.

[1] As monohydrate.

CEFADROXIL — ORAL

For complete and comparative prescribing information, refer to the Cephalosporins group monograph.

Indications

➤*Urinary tract infections:* Caused by *E. coli, P. mirabilis*, and *Klebsiella* species.

➤*Skin and skin structure infections:* Caused by staphylococci or streptococci.

➤*Pharyngitis or tonsillitis:* Caused by *Streptococcus pyogenes* (group A beta-hemolytic streptococci).

Administration and Dosage

➤*Adults:*

Pharyngitis – 1 g/day in single or divided doses (twice daily) for 10 days.

Skin and skin structure infections – 1 g/day in single or divided (twice daily) doses.

Tonsillitis – 1 g/day in single or divided (twice daily) doses for 10 days.

Urinary tract infections – For uncomplicated lower urinary tract infections (ie, cystitis) the usual dosage is 1 or 2 g/day in single or divided (twice daily) doses.

For all other urinary tract infections the usual dosage is 2 g/day in divided doses (twice daily).

➤*Children:*

Pharyngitis – 30 mg/kg/day in a single dose or in equally divided doses every 12 hours. In the treatment of beta-hemolytic streptococcal infections, dosage should be administered for at least 10 days.

Skin and skin structure infections –
Impetigo: 30 mg/kg/day in a single dose or in equally divided doses every 12 hours.
Other infections: 30 mg/kg/day in equally divided doses every 12 hours.

Tonsillitis – 30 mg/kg/day in a single dose or in equally divided doses every 12 hours. In the treatment of beta-hemolytic streptococcal infections, dosage should be administered for at least 10 days.

Urinary tract infections – 30 mg/kg/day in divided doses every 12 hours.

Oral suspension –

Cefadroxil Oral Suspension Daily Dosage

Child's weight				
lbs	kg	125 mg/5 mL	250 mg/5 mL	500 mg/5 mL
10	4.5	5 mL	-	-
20	9.1	10 mL	5 mL	
30	13.6	15 mL	7.5 mL	
40	18.2	20 mL	10 mL	5 mL
50	22.7	25 mL	12.5 mL	6.25 mL
60	27.3	30 mL	15 mL	7.5 mL
70 and above	31.8+	-	-	10 mL

➤*Renal function impairment:* In patients with renal impairment, the dosage of cefadroxil should be adjusted according to creatinine clearance rates to prevent drug accumulation. In adults, the initial dose is 1 g of cefadroxil, and the maintenance dose (based on the creatinine clearance rate [mL/min/1.73 m^2]) is 500 mg at the time intervals listed below.

Cefadroxil Dosage in Adults with Renal Impairment

Creatinine clearances	Dosage interval
0 to 10 mL/min	36 hours
10 to 25 mL/min	24 hours
25 to 50 mL/min	12 hours

CEFADROXIL — ORAL

➤*Preparation for administration:* Directions for mixing are included on the label. Shake well before using.

➤*Administration:* Cefadroxil is acid-stable and may be administered orally without regard to meals. Administration with food may be helpful in diminishing potential GI complaints occasionally associated with oral cephalosporin therapy.

➤*Storage/Stability:* Store at 15° to 30°C (59° to 86°F). After reconstitution of oral suspension, store in the refrigerator. Keep container tightly closed. Discard unused portion of oral suspension after 14 days.

CEFPROZIL

Rx	**Cefprozil** (Various, eg, Lupin, Sandoz, Teva)	**Tablets**: 250 mg (as anhydrous)	In 100s.
Rx	**Cefprozil** (Various, eg, Lupin, Sandoz, Teva)	**Tablets**: 500 mg (as anhydrous)	In 50s and 100s.
Rx	**Cefprozil** (Various, eg, Lupin, Sandoz, Teva)	**Powder for oral suspension**: 125 mg per 5 mL (as anhydrous)	May contain aspartame, sucrose, phenylalanine. In 50, 75, and 100 mL.
Rx	**Cefprozil** (Various, eg, Lupin, Sandoz, Teva)	**Powder for oral suspension**: 250 mg per 5 mL (as anhydrous)	May contain aspartame, sucrose, phenylalanine. In 50, 75, and 100 mL.

CEFPROZIL — ORAL

For complete and comparative prescribing information, refer to the Cephalosporins group monograph.

Indications

➤*Pharyngitis/tonsillitis:* Caused by *Streptococcus pyogenes*.

➤*Otitis media:* Caused by *Streptococcus pneumoniae, Haemophilus influenzae* (including β-lactamase-producing strains) and *Moraxella (Branhamella) catarrhalis* (including β-lactamase-producing strains.

In the treatment of otitis media due to β-lactamase-producing organisms, cefprozil had bacteriologic eradication rates somewhat lower than those observed with a product containing a specific β-lactamase inhibitor. In considering the use of cefprozil, lower overall eradication rates should be balanced against the susceptibility patterns of the common microbes in a given geographic area and the increased potential for toxicity with products containing β-lactamase inhibitors.

➤*Acute sinusitis:* Caused by *Streptococcus pneumoniae, Haemophilus influenzae* (including β-lactamase-producing strains), and *Moraxella (Branhamella) catarrhalis* (including β-lactamase-producing strains).

➤*Secondary bacterial infection of acute bronchitis and acute bacterial exacerbation of chronic bronchitis:* Caused by *Streptococcus pneumoniae, Haemophilus influenzae* (including β-lactamase-producing strains), and *Moraxella (Branhamella) catarrhalis* (including β-lactamase-producing strains).

➤*Uncomplicated skin and skin structure infections:* Caused by *Staphylococcus aureus* (including penicillinase-producing strains) and *Streptococcus pyogenes*. Abscesses usually require surgical drainage.

Administration and Dosage

➤*Adults:*

Infections –

Cefprozil Dosing For Patients 13 Years of Age and Older

Infection	Dosage	Duration (days)
Acute sinusitis (for moderate to severe infections, the higher dose should be used)	250 or 500 mg every 12 hours	10
Pharyngitis/tonsillitis	500 mg every 24 hours	10[a]
Secondary bacterial infection of acute bronchitis and acute bacterial exacerbation of chronic bronchitis	500 mg every 12 hours	10
Uncomplicated skin and skin structure infections	250 or 500 mg every 12 hours or	10
	500 mg every 24 hours	

[a] In the treatment of infections due to *Streptococcus pyogenes*, cefprozil should be administered for at least 10 days.

➤*Children:*

Infections – See Adults for dosing for children 13 years of age and older.

2 to 12 years of age:

Cefprozil Dosing for Children 2 to 12 Years of Age

Infection	Dosage	Duration (days)
Pharyngitis/tonsillitis	7.5 mg/kg every 12 hours[a]	10[b]
Uncomplicated skin and skin structure infections	20 mg/kg every 24 hours[a]	10

[a] Not to exceed recommended adult doses.
[b] In the treatment of infections due to *Streptococcus pyogenes*, cefprozil should be administered for at least 10 days.

6 months to 12 years of age:

Cefprozil Dosing for Children 6 months to 12 Years of Age

Infection	Dosage	Duration (days)
Acute sinusitis[a] (for moderate to severe infections, the higher dose should be used)	7.5 mg/kg or 15 mg/kg every 12 hours[b]	10
Otitis media[a] (see Indications)	15 mg/kg every 12 hours[b]	10

[a] Acute sinusitis and otitis media are the only infections indicated in children younger than 2 years of age.
[b] Not to exceed recommended adult doses.

➤*Renal function impairment:* The following dosage schedule should be used.

Cefprozil Dosing in Renal Impairment

Creatinine clearance (mL/min)	Dosage	Dosing interval
30 to 120	standard	standard
0 to 29[a]	50% of standard	standard

[a] Cefprozil is in part removed by hemodialysis; therefore, cefprozil should be administered after the completion of hemodialysis.

➤*Administration:* May cause GI upset; may take with food or milk.

➤*Storage/Stability:*

Tablets – Store at 15° to 30°C (59° to 86°F).

Oral suspension – Store at 15° to 25° C (59° to 77°F) prior to constitution. After mixing, store in a refrigerator and discard unused portion after 14 days.

CEFTIBUTEN

Rx	**Cedax** (Pernix Therapeutics)	**Capsules; oral**: 400 mg	Parabens. (Cedax 400). White. In 20s.
		Powder for suspension; oral: 90 mg per 5 mL	Cherry flavoring, polysorbate 80, sodium benzoate, sucrose. . In 60, 90, and 120 mL.
		180 mg per 5 mL	Cherry flavoring, polysorbate 80, sodium benzoate, sucrose. In 30 and 60 mL.

CEFTIBUTEN — ORAL

For complete and comparative prescribing information, refer to the Cephalosporins group monograph.

Indications

➤*Acute bacterial exacerbations of chronic bronchitis:* Acute bacterial exacerbations of chronic bronchitis due to *Haemophilus influenzae* (including β-lactamase-producing strains), *Moraxella catarrhalis* (including β-lactamase-producing strains), or *Streptococcus pneumoniae* (penicillin-susceptible strains only).

In acute bacterial exacerbations of chronic bronchitis clinical trials where *Moraxella catarrhalis* was isolated from infected sputum at baseline, ceftibuten clinical efficacy was 22% less than control.

➤*Acute bacterial otitis media:* Acute bacterial otitis media due to *Haemophilus influenzae* (including β-lactamase-producing strains), *Moraxella catarrhalis* (including β-lactamase-producing strains), or *Streptococcus pyogenes*.

Although ceftibuten used empirically was equivalent to comparators in the treatment of clinically or microbiologically documented acute otitis media,

CEFTIBUTEN — ORAL

the efficacy against streptococcus pneumoniae was 23% less than control. Therefore, ceftibuten should be given empirically only when adequate antimicrobial coverage against *Streptococcus pneumoniae* has been previously administered.

➤*Pharyngitis and tonsillitis:* Pharyngitis and tonsillitis due to *Streptococcus pyogenes*.

Administration and Dosage

➤*Maximum dose:* 400 mg/day.

➤*Adults:*

Infections – For a list of infections, refer to Indications.
Usual dosage: 400 mg once daily for 10 days.
Maximum dose: 400 mg/day according to the prescribing information.

➤*Children:*

Infections – For a list of infections, refer to Indications.

See Adults for dosing for children 12 years of age and older.

6 months to 12 years of age: Ceftibuten is not indicated for the treatment of acute bacterial exacerbations of chronic bronchitis in children.

• *Usual dosage* – 9 mg/kg once daily for 10 days. Children weighing more than 45 kg should receive 400 mg/day.

Ceftibuten Oral Suspension Pediatric Dosage Chart

Weight	90 mg per 5 mL	180 mg per 5 mL
10 kg	5 mL once daily	2.5 mL once daily
20 kg	10 mL once daily	5 mL once daily
40 kg	20 mL once daily	10 mL once daily

• *Maximum dose* – 400 mg/day.

➤*Renal function impairment:*

Ceftibuten Dosing in Renal Impairment

Creatinine clearance (mL/min)	Recommended dosing schedule
> 50	9 mg/kg or 400 mg every 24 hours (normal dosing schedule)
30 to 49	4.5 mg/kg or 200 mg every 24 hours
5 to 29	2.25 mg/kg or 100 mg every 24 hours

Hemodialysis – In patients undergoing hemodialysis 2 or 3 times weekly, a single 400 mg dose of ceftibuten capsules, or a single dose of 9 mg/kg (maximum, ceftibuten 400 mg) oral suspension may be administered at the end of each hemodialysis session.

➤*Administration:* Ceftibuten oral suspension must be administered at least 2 hours before or 1 hour after a meal.

➤*Storage/Stability:*

Capsules – Store between 2° and 25°C (36° and 77°F). Replace cap securely after each opening.

Oral suspension – Prior to reconstitution, the powder must be stored between 2° and 25°C (36° and 77°F). Once it is reconstituted, the oral suspension is stable for 14 days when stored in the refrigerator between 2° and 8°C (36° and 46°F).

CEFDINIR

Rx	**Cefdinir** (Various, eg, Dava, Lupin, Sandoz, Teva)	**Capsules; oral:** 300 mg	In 60s, 100s, and UD 10s and 50s.
Rx	**Omnicef** (Abbott)		(OMNICEF). Lavender and turquoise. In 60s.
Rx	**Cefdinir** (Various, eg, Dava, Lupin, Sandoz, Teva)	**Powder for suspension; oral:** 125 mg per 5 mL (after reconstitution)	May contain sucrose. Strawberry or cherry flavor. In 60 and 100 mL.
Rx	**Omnicef** (Abbott)		Sucrose. Strawberry-flavored. In 60 and 100 mL.
Rx	**Cefdinir** (Various, eg, Dava, Lupin, Sandoz, Teva)	**Powder for suspension; oral:** 250 mg per 5 mL (after reconstitution)	May contain sucrose. Strawberry or cherry flavor. In 60 and 100 mL.
Rx	**Omnicef** (Abbott)		Sucrose. Strawberry-flavored. In 60 and 100 mL.

CEFDINIR — ORAL

For complete and comparative prescribing information, refer to the Cephalosporins group monograph.

Indications

➤*Adults and adolescents:*

Community-acquired pneumonia – Caused by *Haemophilus influenzae* (including β-lactamase-producing strains), *H. parainfluenzae* (including β-lactamase-producing strains), *Streptococcus pneumoniae* (penicillin-susceptible strains only) and *Moraxella catarrhalis* (including β-lactamase-producing strains).

Acute exacerbations of chronic bronchitis – Caused by *H. influenzae* (including β-lactamase producing strains), *H. parainfluenzae* (including β-lactamase-producing strains), *S. pneumoniae* (penicillin-susceptible strains only) and *M. catarrhalis* (including β-lactamase-producing strains).

Acute maxillary sinusitis – Caused by *H. influenzae* (including β-lactamase-producing strains), *S. pneumoniae* (penicillin-susceptible strains only) and *M. catarrhalis* (including β-lactamase-producing strains).

Pharyngitis/Tonsillitis – Caused by *S. pyogenes*.

Uncomplicated skin and skin structure infections – Caused by *Staphylococcus aureus* (including β-lactamase-producing strains) and *S. pyogenes*.

➤*Children:*

Acute bacterial otitis media – Caused by *H. influenzae* (including β-lactamase-producing strains), *S. pneumoniae* (penicillin-susceptible strains only) and *M. catarrhalis* (including β-lactamase-producing strains).

Pharyngitis/Tonsillitis – Caused by *S. pyogenes*.

Uncomplicated skin and skin structure infections – Caused by *S. aureus* (including β-lactamase-producing strains) and *S. pyogenes*.

Administration and Dosage

➤*General dosing considerations:* Once-daily dosing for 10 days is as effective as twice-daily dosing. Once-daily dosing has not been studied in pneumonia or skin infections; therefore, administer cefdinir twice daily in these infections.

➤*Adults:*

Infections –

Cefdinir Dosage in Adults

Type of infection	Dosage	Duration
Acute exacerbations of chronic bronchitis	300 mg q 12 h or 600 mg q 24 h	5 to 10 days 10 days
Acute maxillary sinusitis	300 mg q 12 h or 600 mg q 24 h	10 days 10 days
Community-acquired pneumonia	300 mg q 12 h	10 days
Pharyngitis/Tonsillitis	300 mg q 12 h or 600 mg q 24 h	5 to 10 days 10 days
Uncomplicated skin and skin structure infections	300 mg q 12 h	10 days

➤*Children:*

13 years of age and older – See Adults for dosing.

6 months to 12 years of age –
Usual dosage: 14 mg/kg/day, up to a maximum dose of 600 mg/day.

Cefdinir Dosage in Pediatric Patients (6 Months Through 12 Years of Age)

Type of infection	Dosage	Duration
Acute bacterial otitis media	7 mg/kg q 12 h or 14 mg/kg q 24 h	5 to 10 days 10 days
Acute maxillary sinusitis	7 mg/kg q 12 h or 14 mg/kg q 24 h	10 days 10 days
Pharyngitis/Tonsillitis	7 mg/kg q 12 h or 14 mg/kg q 24 h	5 to 10 days 10 days
Uncomplicated skin and skin structure infections	7 mg/kg q 12 h	10 days

CEFDINIR — ORAL

Maximum dose: 600 mg/day.
Oral suspension:

Cefdinir Oral Suspension Pediatric Dosage

Weight			
kg	lb	125 mg per 5 mL	250 mg per 5 mL
9	20	2.5 mL (½ tsp) q 12 h or 5 mL (1 tsp) q 24 h	Use 125 mg per 5 mL product
18	40	5 mL (1 tsp) q 12 h or 10 mL (2 tsp) q 24 h	2.5 mL q 12 h or 5 mL q 24 h
27	60	7.5 mL (1½ tsp) q 12 h or 15 mL (3 tsp) q 24 h	3.75 mL q 12 h or 7.5 mL q 24 h
36	80	10 mL (2 tsp) q 12 h or 20 mL (4 tsp) q 24 h	5 mL q 12 h or 10 mL q 24 h
≥ 43[a]	95	12 mL (2½ tsp) q 12 h or 24 mL (5 tsp) q 24 h	6 mL q 12 h or 12 mL q 24 h

[a] Pediatric patients who weigh ≥ 43 kg should receive the maximum daily dose of 600 mg.

➤*Renal function impairment:*

Adults – For adult patients with creatinine clearance (Ccr) less than 30 mL/min, the dose of cefdinir should be 300 mg given once daily.

Children – For pediatric patients with a Ccr of less than 30 mL/min/1.73 m², the dose of cefdinir should be 7 mg/kg (300 mg or less) given once daily.

Hemodialysis – Hemodialysis removes cefdinir from the body. In patients maintained on chronic hemodialysis, the recommended initial dosage regimen is a 300 mg or 7 mg/kg dose every other day. At the conclusion of each hemodialysis session, 300 mg (or 7 mg/kg) should be given. Subsequent doses (300 mg or 7 mg/kg) are then administered every other day.

➤*Administration:* Cefdinir may be taken without regard to meals.

➤*Storage/Stability:*

Capsules and powder for oral suspension – Store at 25°C (77°F); excursions permitted to 15° to 30°C (59° to 86°F).

Reconstituted oral suspension – After mixing, the suspension can be stored at room temperature (25°C [77°F]). The suspension may be used for 10 days, after which any unused portion must be discarded.

CEFAZOLIN SODIUM

Rx	**Cefazolin Sodium** (Apothecon)	**Powder for Injection**: 500 mg[a]	In vials and piggyback vials.
		1 g[a]	In vials and piggyback vials.
		5 g[a]	In vials and piggyback vials.
		10 g[a]	In pharmacy bulk packages.
		20 g[a]	In pharmacy bulk packages.

[a] Contains 2.1 mEq sodium/g.

CEFAZOLIN — INJECTION

Indications

➤*General information:* Cefazolin is indicated in the treatment of the following serious infections due to susceptible organisms:

➤*Respiratory tract infections:* Due to *Streptococcus pneumoniae, Klebsiella* species, *Haemophilus influenzae, Staphylococcus aureus* (penicillin-sensitive and penicillin-resistant) and group A beta-hemolytic streptococci.

Injectable benzathine penicillin is considered to be the drug of choice in treatment and prevention of streptococcal infections, including the prophylaxis of rheumatic fever.

Cefazolin is effective in the eradication of streptococci from the nasopharynx; however, data establishing the efficacy of cefazolin in the subsequent prevention of rheumatic fever are not available at present.

➤*Urinary tract infections:* Due to *Escherichia coli, Proteus mirabilis, Klebsiella* species and some strains of enterobacter and enterococci.

➤*Skin and skin structure infections:* Due to *S. aureus* (penicillin-sensitive and penicillin-resistant), group A beta-hemolytic streptococci and other strains of streptococci.

➤*Biliary tract infections:* Due to *Escherichia coli*, various strains of streptococci, *Proteus mirabilis, Klebsiella* species and *S. aureus.*

➤*Bone and joint infections:* Due to *S. aureus.*

➤*Genital infections (ie, prostatitis, epididymitis):* Due to *Escherichia coli, Proteus mirabilis, Klebsiella* species and some strains of enterococci.

➤*Septicemia:* Due to *Streptococcus pneumoniae, S. aureus* (penicillin-sensitive and penicillin-resistant), *Proteus mirabilis, Escherichia coli* and *Klebsiella* species.

➤*Endocarditis:* Due to *S. aureus* (penicillin-sensitive and penicillin-resistant) and group A beta-hemolytic streptococci.

➤*Perioperative prophylaxis:* The prophylactic administration of cefazolin preoperatively, intraoperatively and postoperatively may reduce the incidence of certain postoperative infections in patients undergoing surgical procedures which are classified as contaminated or potentially contaminated (eg, vaginal hysterectomy, and cholecystectomy in high-risk patients such as those greater than 70 years of age, with acute cholecystitis, obstructive jaundice or common duct bile stones).

The perioperative use of cefazolin may also be effective in surgical patients in whom infection at the operative site would present a serious risk (eg, during open-heart surgery and prosthetic arthroplasty).

The prophylactic administration of cefazolin should usually be discontinued within a 24-hour period after the surgical procedure. In surgery where the occurrence of infection may be particularly devastating (eg, open-heart surgery and prosthetic arthroplasty), the prophylactic administration of cefazolin may be continued for 3 to 5 days following the completion of surgery.

➤*Off-label uses:*

Catheter-related bloodstream infections (adults) – [2] = Fair documentation. According to Infectious Diseases Society of America (IDSA) guidelines, the preferred agents to treat methicillin-susceptible *S. aureus* are nafcillin or oxacillin, but cefazolin may be chosen as an alternative agent. Also, a first-generation cephalosporin, which includes cefazolin, may be appropriate therapy in patients with methicillin-susceptible, coagulase-negative *Staphylococcus* species from a catheter-related bloodstream infection.

Administration and Dosage

➤*General dosing considerations:* Reduced doses are required in patients with renal function impairment. (See Renal Function Impairment).

➤*Adults:*

Infection –

Cefazolin Usual Adult Dosage

Type of infection	Dose IM or IV	Frequency
Acute, uncomplicated urinary tract infections	1 g	every 12 hours
Mild infections caused by susceptible gram and cocci	250 to 500 mg	every 8 hours
Moderate to severe infections	500 mg to 1 g	every 6 to 8 hours
Pneumococcal pneumonia	500 mg	every 12 hours
Severe, life-threatening infections (eg, endocarditis, septicemia)[a]	1 to 1.5 g	every 6 hours

[a] In rare instances, doses of up to 12 g of cefazolin injection per day have been used.

Perioperative prophylaxis –

Preoperative: 1 g intravenously (IV) or intramuscularly (IM) administered one-half hour to 1 hour prior to the start of surgery.

Intraoperative: For procedures 2 hours or more, 500 mg to 1 g IV or IM during surgery (administration modified depending on the duration of the operative procedure).

Postoperative: 500 mg to 1 g IV or IM every 6 to 8 hours for 24 hours postoperatively.

In surgery where the occurrence of infection may be particularly devastating (eg, open-heart surgery, prosthetic arthroplasty), the prophylactic administration of cefazolin injection may be continued for 3 to 5 days following the completion of surgery.

It is important that the preoperative dose be given just prior (one-half to 1 hour) to the start of surgery, so that adequate antibiotic levels are present in the serum and tissues at the time of initial surgical incision; cefazolin injection should be administered, if necessary, at appropriate intervals during surgery to provide sufficient levels of the antibiotic at the anticipated moments of greatest exposure to infective organisms.

Off-label dosing –

Catheter-related bloodstream infections (adults): [2] = Fair documentation. 2 g IV every 8 hours.

➤*Children:*

30 days and older –

Infections: 25 to 50 mg/kg daily IV or IM divided in 3 or 4 doses. May increase to 100 mg/kg daily IV or IM divided in 3 or 4 doses for severe infections.

CEFAZOLIN — INJECTION

Cefazolin Pediatric Dosage Guidelines					
Weight		25 mg/kg/day divided into 3 doses		25 mg/kg/day divided into 4 doses	
lbs	kg	Approximate single dose (mg) every 8 hours	Volume (mL) needed with dilution of 125 mg/mL	Approximate single dose (mg) every 6 hours	Volume (mL) needed with dilution of 125 mg/mL
10	4.5	40 mg	0.35 mL	30 mg	0.25 mL
20	9	75 mg	0.6 mL	55 mg	0.45 mL
30	13.6	115 mg	0.9 mL	85 mg	0.7 mL
40	18.1	150 mg	1.2 mL	115 mg	0.9 mL
50	22.7	190 mg	1.5 mL	140 mg	1.1 mL
Weight		50 mg/kg/day divided into 3 doses		50 mg/kg/day divided into 4 doses	
lbs	kg	Approximate single dose (mg) every 8 hours	Volume (mL) needed with dilution of 225 mg/mL	Approximate single dose (mg) every 6 hours	Volume (mL) needed with dilution of 225 mg/mL
10	4.5	75 mg	0.35 mL	55 mg	0.25 mL
20	9	150 mg	0.7 mL	110 mg	0.5 mL
30	13.6	225 mg	1 mL	170 mg	0.75 mL
40	18.1	300 mg	1.35 mL	225 mg	1 mL
50	22.7	375 mg	1.7 mL	285 mg	1.25 mL

Off-label dosing –

Neonates 0 to 29 days old:

Cefazolin Off-Label Dosing in Neonates	
Infection	
Age	Dosage
Postnatal age older than 7 days and body weight greater than 2,000 g	20 mg/kg IV or IM every 8 hours
Postnatal age older than 7 days and body weight 2,000 g or less	20 mg/kg IV or IM every 12 hours
Postnatal age 7 days or younger	20 mg/kg IV or IM every 12 hours
Perioperative prophylaxis	
20 to 30 mg/kg IV or IM 30 to 60 minutes prior to surgery. May need to redose for procedures longer than 2 hours.	

➤*Renal function impairment:*

Adults –

Cefazolin Dosage in Renal Impairment				
		Dose		
Serum creatinine (mg/dL)	CrCl (mL/min)	Mild to moderate infection (mg)	Moderate to severe infection (mg)	Dosage interval (h)
≤ 1.5	≥ 55	250 to 500	500 to 1,000	6 to 8
1.6 to 3	35 to 54	250 to 500	500 to 1,000	≥ 8
3.1 to 4.5	11 to 34	125 to 250	250 to 500	12
≥ 4.6	≤ 10	125 to 250	250 to 500	18 to 24

Continuous renal replacement therapy: One reference suggests a dosage of 250 mg to 2 g IV every 12 hours.

The following alternative recommendations assume ultrafiltration and dialysis flow rates of 1 to 2 L/h.

- *Loading dose* – 2 g IV.
- *Maintenance dosage* –

Continuous venovenous hemofiltration: 1 to 2 g IV every 12 hours.

Continuous venovenous hemodialysis or continuous venovenous hemodialfiltration: 1 g IV every 8 hours or 2 g IV every 12 hours.

Intermittent hemodialysis: One reference suggests a dosage of 15 to 20 mg/kg administered after dialysis.

Another reference suggests a dosage of 500 mg to 1 g IV every 24 hours administered after dialysis on dialysis days. Alternatively, administer 1 to 2 g IV every 48 to 72 hours after dialysis. These dosing recommendations assume the patient is receiving standard intermittent hemodialysis (IHD) 3 times per week and completes the full dialysis sessions.

Peritoneal dialysis: In patients undergoing peritoneal dialysis (2 L/h), cefazolin produced mean serum levels of approximately 10 and 30 mcg/mL after 24 hours' instillation of a dialyzing solution containing 50 mg/L and 150 mg/L, respectively. Mean peak levels were 29 mcg/mL (range, 13 to 44 mcg/mL) with 50 mg/L (3 patients) and 72 mcg/mL (range, 26 to 142 mcg/mL) with 150 mg/L (6 patients). Intraperitoneal administration of cefazolin is usually well tolerated.

One reference suggests a dosage of 500 mg every 12 hours.

Children –

CrCl 70 to 40 mL/min: 60% of normal daily dose divided every 12 hours.
CrCl 40 to 20 mL/min: 25% of normal daily dose divided every 12 hours.
CrCl 20 to 5 mL/min: 10% of normal daily dose every 24 hours.

➤*Preparation for administration:* Reconstituted solutions may range in color from pale yellow to yellow without a change in potency.

For IM injection, IV direct (bolus) injection or IV infusion, reconstitute with sterile water for injection according to the table. Shake well until dissolved.

Cefazolin Single Dose Vial Reconstitution			
Vial size	Amount of diluent	Approximate concentration	Approximate available volume
500 mg	2 mL	225 mg/mL	2.2 mL
1 g	2.5 mL	330 mg/mL	3 mL

For infusion bottles, dilute reconstituted cefazolin with 50 to 100 mL of sodium chloride injection, dextrose 5% or 10% injection, dextrose 5% in Ringer's lactate injection, dextrose 5% and sodium chloride 0.9% injection, dextrose 5% and sodium chloride 0.45% injection, dextrose 5% and sodium chloride 0.2% injection, Ringer's lactate injection, invert sugar 5% or 10% in sterile water for injection, Ringer's injection, sodium bicarbonate 5% injection. When adding diluent to vial, allow air to escape by using a small vent needle or by pumping the syringe. Shake well. Administer with primary IV fluids, as a single dose.

For direct (bolus) injection, further dilute vials with approximately 5 mL sterile water for injection.

➤*Administration:*

Intramuscular administration – Inject cefazolin into a large muscle mass. Pain on injection is infrequent with cefazolin.

Intravenous administration –

Direct (bolus) injection: Inject the solution slowly over 3 to 5 minutes, directly or through tubing for patients receiving compatible parenteral fluids.

➤*Storage/Stability:* Prior to reconstitution, store at 25°C (77°F); excursions are permitted to 15° to 30°C (59° to 86°F). Protect from light.

As with other cephalosporins, cefazolin tends to darken depending on storage conditions; within the stated recommendations, however, product potency is not adversely affected.

When reconstituted or diluted according to the instructions, cefazolin is stable for 24 hours at room temperature or for 10 days if stored under refrigeration (5°C or 41°F).

CEFOXITIN SODIUM

Rx	**Cefoxitin** (American Pharmaceutical Partners)	**Injection, powder for solution:** 1 g	In vials and infusion bottles.
Rx	**Cefoxitin and Dextrose** (B. Braun McGaw)	**Injection, powder for solution:** 1 g	Preservative free. Dextrose 50 mL. In single-use *Duplex* drug delivery system.
Rx	**Cefoxitin** (American Pharmaceutical Partners)	**Injection, powder for solution:** 2 g	In vials and infusion bottles.
Rx	**Cefoxitin and Dextrose** (B. Braun McGaw)	**Injection, powder for solution:** 2 g	Preservative free. Dextrose 50 mL. In single-use *Duplex* drug delivery system.
Rx	**Cefoxitin** (American Pharmaceutical Partners)	**Injection, powder for solution:** 10 g	In pharmacy bulk packages.

CEFOXITIN SODIUM — INJECTION

For complete and comparative prescribing information, refer to the Cephalosporins group monograph.

Indications

➤*Lower respiratory tract infections:* Including pneumonia and lung abscess, caused by *S. pneumoniae*, other streptococci (excluding enterococci; eg, *E. faecalis* [formerly *Streptococcus faecalis*]), *S. aureus* (including penicillinase-producing strains), *E. coli*, *Klebsiella* species, *Haemophilus influenzae*, and *Bacteroides* species.

➤*Urinary tract infections:* Caused by *E. coli*, *Klebsiella* species, *P. mirabilis*, *Morganella morganii*, *Proteus vulgaris* and *Providencia* species (including *Providencia rettgeri*).

➤*Intra-abdominal infections:* Including peritonitis and intra-abdominal abscess, caused by *E. coli*, *Klebsiella* species, *Bacteroides* species (including *Bacteroides fragilis*), and *Clostridium* species.

➤*Gynecological infections:* Including endometritis, pelvic cellulitis, and pelvic inflammatory disease caused by *E. coli*, *Neisseria gonorrhoeae* (includ-

CEFOXITIN SODIUM — INJECTION

ing penicillinase-producing strains), *Bacteroides* species including *B. fragilis*, *Clostridium* species, *P. niger*, *Peptostreptococcus* species, and *Streptococcus agalactiae*.

➤*Chlamydia trachomatis:* See Administration and Dosage for more information.

➤*Septicemia:* Caused by *S. pneumoniae*, *S. aureus* (including penicillinase-producing strains), *E. coli*, *Klebsiella* species, and *Bacteroides* species including *B. fragilis*.

➤*Bone and joint infections:* Caused by *S. aureus* (including penicillinase-producing strains).

➤*Skin and skin structure infections:* Caused by *S. aureus* (including penicillinase-producing strains), *Staphylococcus epidermidis*, *Streptococcus pyogenes* and other streptococci (excluding enterococci [eg, *E. faecalis*] [formerly *S. faecalis*]), *E. coli*, *P. mirabilis*, *Klebsiella* species, *Bacteroides* species including *B. fragilis*, *Clostridium* species, *P. niger*, and *Peptostreptococcus* species.

➤*Perioperative prophylaxis:* For the prophylaxis of infection in patients undergoing uncontaminated GI surgery, vaginal hysterectomy, abdominal hysterectomy, or cesarean section.

Administration and Dosage

➤*General dosing considerations:* If *C. trachomatis* is a suspected pathogen, appropriate antichlamydial coverage should be added, because cefoxitin has no activity against this organism.

➤*Adults:*

Infections – For a list of infections, refer to Indications.

Usual dosage: 1 to 2 g IV every 6 to 8 hours. Dosage should be determined by susceptibility of the causative organisms, severity of infection, and the condition of the patient (see the following table).

Cefoxitin Dosage Guidelines for Adults

Type of infection	Daily dosage	Frequency and route
Uncomplicated forms[a] of infection such as pneumonia, urinary tract infection, cutaneous infection	3 to 4 g	1 g IV every 6 to 8 hours
Moderately severe or severe infections	6 to 8 g	1 g IV every 4 hours or 2 g IV every 6 to 8 hours
Infections commonly requiring antibiotics in higher dosage (eg, gas gangrene)	12 g	2 g IV every 4 hours or 3 g IV every 6 hours

[a] Including patients in whom bacteremia is absent or unlikely.

Prophylactic dosage: Effective surgical prophylactic use depends on the time of administration. Cefoxitin usually should be given 30 minutes to 1 hour before the operation, which is sufficient time to achieve effective levels in the wound during the procedure. Prophylactic administration should usually be stopped within 24 hours because continuing administration of any antibiotic increases the possibility of adverse reactions, but, in the majority of surgical procedures, does not reduce the incidence of subsequent infection.

• *GI surgery (uncontaminated), vaginal or abdominal hysterectomy* – 2 g IV just prior to surgery (approximately 30 minutes to 1 hour before the initial incision) followed by 2 g every 6 hours after the first dose for no more than 24 hours.

• *Cesarean section* – Either a single 2 g dose IV as soon as the umbilical cord is clamped or a 3-dose regimen consisting of 2 g given IV as soon as the umbilical cord is clamped followed by 2 g 4 and 8 hours after the initial dose is recommended.

➤*Children:* In children 3 months of age and older, higher doses of cefoxitin have been associated with an increased incidence of eosinophilia and elevated AST.

Infections – For a list of infections, refer to Indications.

3 months of age and older:

• *Usual dosage* – 80 to 160 mg/kg/day IV divided into 4 to 6 equal doses. The higher dosages should be used for more severe or serious infections.

• *Maximum dose* – 12 g/day.

• *Prophylactic dosage* – Effective surgical prophylactic use depends on the time of administration. Cefoxitin usually should be given 30 minutes to 1 hour before the operation, which is sufficient time to achieve effective levels in the wound during the procedure. Prophylactic administration should usually be stopped within 24 hours because continuing administration of any antibiotic increases the possibility of adverse reactions, but, in the majority of surgical procedures, does not reduce the incidence of subsequent infection.

For prophylactic use in uncontaminated GI surgery, vaginal hysterectomy, or abdominal hysterectomy, the dosage is 30 to 40 mg/kg given at the times previously designated.

➤*Renal function impairment:*

Adults –

Loading dose: 1 to 2 g IV for adults with renal insufficiency.

Maintenance dosage: After a loading dose, the recommendations for maintenance dosage (see the following table) may be used as a guide.

Maintenance Cefoxitin Dosage in Adults with Renal Impairment

Renal function	CrCl (mL/min)	Dose (g)	Frequency
Mild impairment	30 to 50	1 to 2	every 8 to 12 hours
Moderate impairment	10 to 29	1 to 2	every 12 to 24 hours
Severe impairment	5 to 9	0.5 to 1	every 12 to 24 hours
Essentially no function	< 5	0.5 to 1	every 24 to 48 hours

Children: In children with renal insufficiency, the dosage and frequency of dosage should be modified consistent with the recommendations for adults.

Hemodialysis: In patients undergoing hemodialysis, the loading dose of 1 to 2 g should be given after each hemodialysis, and the maintenance dose should be given as indicated in the previous table.

Continuous ambulatory peritoneal dialysis: Give 1 g every 24 hours.

➤*Duration of therapy:* Antibiotic therapy for group A beta-hemolytic streptococcal infections should be maintained for at least 10 days to guard against the risk of rheumatic fever or glomerulonephritis.

➤*Preparation for administration:*

Powder for injection –

Preparation of Cefoxitin Solution for IV Administration

Strength	Amount of diluent to be added (mL)[a]	Approximate withdrawable volume (mL)	Approximate average concentration (mg/mL)
1 g vial	10	10.5	95
2 g vial	10 or 20	11.1 or 21	180 or 95
1 g infusion bottle	50 or 100	50 or 100	20 or 10
2 g infusion bottle	50 or 100	50 or 100	40 or 20
10 g bulk	43 or 93	49 or 98.5	200 or 100

[a] Shake to dissolve and let stand until clear.

Vials: 1 g should be constituted with at least 10 mL, and 2 g with 10 or 20 mL, of sterile water for injection, bacteriostatic water for injection, sodium chloride 0.9% injection, or dextrose 5% injection.

Bulk packages: The 10 g bulk packages should be constituted with 43 or 93 mL of sterile water for injection, bacteriostatic water for injection, sodium chloride 0.9% injection, or dextrose 5% injection. Caution: The 10 g bulk stock solution is not for direct infusion.

Dilution: These primary solutions may be further diluted in 50 to 1,000 mL of the following diluents: sodium chloride 0.9% injection, dextrose 5% or 10% injection, dextrose 5% and sodium chloride 0.9% injection, dextrose 5% injection with saline 0.2% or 0.45% solution, Ringer's lactate injection, dextrose 5% in Ringer's lactate injection, sodium bicarbonate 5% injection, M/6 sodium lactate solution, or mannitol 5% and 10%.

• *Infusion bottles* – 1 or 2 g of cefoxitin for infusion may be constituted with 50 or 100 mL of sodium chloride 0.9% injection, or dextrose 5% or 10% injection.

• *ADD-Vantage* vials – Cefoxitin in *ADD-Vantage* vials should be constituted with *ADD-Vantage* diluent containers containing 50 mL or 100 mL of either sodium chloride 0.9% injection or dextrose 5% injection. Cefoxitin in *ADD-Vantage* vials is for IV use only.

Duplex drug delivery system – To avoid inadvertent activation, *Duplex* container should remain in the folded position until activation is intended. Apply patient-specific label on foil side of container. use care to avoid activation. Do not cover any portion of foil strip with patient label. Unlatch side tab and unfold *Duplex* container. Visually inspect diluent chamber for particulate matter. Use only if container and seals are intact. To inspect the drug powder for foreign matter or discoloration, peel foil strip from drug chamber. Protect from light after removal of foils trip. If foil is removed, product must be used within 7 days, but not beyond the labeled expiration date. the product should be refolded and the side tab latched until ready to activate. Do not use directly after storage refrigeration, allow the product to equilibrate to room temperature before patient use. Unfold the *Duplex* container and point the set port in a downward direction. Starting at the hanger tab end, fold the *Duplex* container just below the diluent meniscus trapping all air above the fold. To activate, squeeze the folded diluent chamber until the seal between the diluent and powder opens, releasing diluent into the drug powder. Agitate the liquid-powder mixture until the drug powder is completely dissolved. Following reconstitution (activation), product must be used within 12 hour if stored at room temperature or within 7 days if stored under refrigeration. Visually inspect the reconstituted solution for particulate matter.

Premixed IV solution – Thaw frozen container at room temperature, 25°C (77°F), or under refrigeration, 2° to 8°C (36° to 46°F). Do not force thaw by immersion in water baths or by microwave irradiation. After thawing, check for minute leaks by squeezing container firmly. If leaks are detected, discard solution because sterility may be impaired.

The container should be visually inspected for particulate matter and discoloration prior to administration. Components of the solution may precipi-

CEFOXITIN SODIUM — INJECTION

tate in the frozen state and will dissolve upon reaching room temperature with little or no agitation. Agitate after solution has reached room temperature.

Do not use if the solution is cloudy or if a precipitate has formed. If any seals or outlet ports are not intact, the container should be discarded. Solutions of cefoxitin tend to darken depending on storage conditions; however, product potency is not adversely affected.

Additives should not be introduced into this solution.

➤*Administration:* Cefoxitin is to be administered IV. The IV route is preferable for patients with bacteremia, bacterial septicemia, or other severe or life-threatening infections, or for patients who may be poor risks because of lowered resistance resulting from such debilitating conditions as malnutrition, trauma, surgery, diabetes, heart failure, or malignancy, particularly if shock is present or impending.

Intermittent IV administration – A solution containing 1 or 2 g in 10 mL of sterile water for injection can be injected over a period of 3 to 5 minutes. Using an infusion system, it may also be given over a longer period of time through the tubing system by which the patient may be receiving other IV solutions. However, during infusion of the solution containing cefoxitin, it is advisable to temporarily discontinue administration of any other solutions at the same site.

Continuous IV infusion – For higher doses, solution of cefoxitin may be added to an IV bottle containing dextrose 5% injection, sodium chloride 0.9% injection, or dextrose 5% and sodium chloride 0.9% injection. *Butterfly* or scalp vein-type needles are preferred for this type of infusion.

Duplex drug delivery system – Point the set port in a downward direction. Starting at the hanger tab end, fold the *Duplex* container just below the solution meniscus trapping all air above the fold. Squeeze the folded *Duplex* container until the seal between reconstituted drug solution and set port opens, releasing liquid to set port. Prior to attaching the IV set, check for minute leaks by squeezing the container firmly. If leaks are found, discard container and solution as sterility may be impaired. Using aseptic technique, remove the set port cover from the set port and attach sterile administration set. Refer to Directions for Use accompanying the administration set. As with other cephalosporins, reconstituted cefoxitin for injection and dextrose injection tends to darken depending on storage conditions, within the stated recommendations. However, product potency is not adversely affected. Use only if prepared solution is clear and free from particulate matter. Do not use in series connection. Do not introduce additives into the *Duplex* container. Do not freeze.

Premixed IV solution – Cefoxitin premixed IV solution in *Galaxy* containers (PL 2040 plastic) is to be administered either as a continuous or intermittent infusion using sterile equipment. Scalp vein-type needles are preferred for this type of infusion. It is recommended that the IV administration apparatus be replaced at least once every 48 hours.

Cefoxitin premixed IV solution may be administered through the tubing system by which the patient may be receiving other IV solutions. However, during infusion of the solution containing cefoxitin premixed IV solution, it is advisable to temporarily discontinue administration of any other solutions at the same site.

➤*Admixture compatibility:* Solutions of cefoxitin, like those of most beta-lactam antibiotics, should not be added to aminoglycoside solutions (eg, gentamicin sulfate, tobramycin sulfate, amikacin sulfate) because of potential interaction. However, cefoxitin and aminoglycosides may be administered separately to the same patient.

See also Storage/Stability for more compatibility information.

➤*Storage/Stability:* Cefoxitin in the dry state should be stored between 2° and 25°C (36° and 77°F). Avoid exposure to temperatures higher than 50°C (122°F). The dry material, as well as solutions, tend to darken depending on storage conditions; however, product potency is not adversely affected.

Vials and bulk packages – Cefoxitin powder for injection, as supplied in vials or the bulk package and constituted to 1 g per 10 mL with sterile water for injection, bacteriostatic water for injection, sodium chloride 0.9% injection, or dextrose 5% injection, maintains satisfactory potency for 6 hours at room temperature or for 1 week under refrigeration (less than 5°C; 43°F).

Infusion bottles – Cefoxitin, as supplied in infusion bottles and constituted with 50 to 100 mL of sodium chloride 0.9% injection, or dextrose 5% or 10% injection, maintains satisfactory potency for 24 hours at room temperature or for 1 week under refrigeration (less than 5°C; 43°F).

ADD-Vantage vials – Cefoxitin is supplied in single-dose *ADD-Vantage* vials and should be prepared as directed in the manufacturers instructions for use of cefoxitin in *ADD-Vantage* vials using *ADD-Vantage* diluent containers containing 50 mL or 100 mL of either sodium chloride 0.9% injection or dextrose 5% injection. When prepared with either of these diluents, cefoxitin maintains satisfactory potency for 24 hours at room temperature. After the time periods mentioned previously, any unused solutions should be discarded.

Duplex drug delivery system – Store the inactivated unit at 20° to 25°C (68° to 77°F).

Cefoxitin premixed IV solution – Store at or below −20°C (−4°F). Cefoxitin, supplied as frozen, premixed, iso-osmotic solution in *Galaxy* containers (PL 2040 plastic), maintains satisfactory potency after thawing for 24 hours at a room temperature of 25°C (77°F) or 21 days under refrigeration, 2° to 8°C (36° to 46°F). After these periods, any unused solutions should be discarded. Do not refreeze.

CEFUROXIME

Rx	**Cefuroxime Axetil** (Ranbaxy)	**Tablets; oral:** (as axetil) 125 mg	(RX 750). Blue, capsule shape. In 60s and 100s.
Rx	**Ceftin** (GlaxoWellcome)		(Glaxo 395). White. Capsule shape. Film coated. In 20s and UD 100s.
Rx	**Cefuroxime Axetil** (Ranbaxy)	**Tablets; oral:** (as axetil) 250 mg	(RX 751). Blue, capsule shape. In 20s, 60s, and 100s.
Rx	**Ceftin** (GlaxoWellcome)		(Glaxo 387). Light blue. Capsule shape. Film coated. In 10s, 20s, 60s and UD 100s.
Rx	**Cefuroxime Axetil** (Ranbaxy)	**Tablets; oral:** (as axetil) 500 mg	(RX 752). Blue, capsule shape. In 20s, 60s, and 100s.
Rx	**Ceftin** (GlaxoWellcome)		(Glaxo 394). Dark blue. Capsule shape. Film coated. In 20s, 60s and UD 50s.
Rx	**Cefuroxime Axetil** (Ranbaxy Pharmaceuticals)	**Suspension; oral:** 125 mg/5 mL (as axetil) when reconstituted	Aspartame, mannitol, phenylalanine 45 mg per 5 mL, sucrose. Fruit flavor. In 50 and 100 mL.
Rx	**Cefuroxime Axetil** (Ranbaxy Pharmaceuticals)	**Suspension; oral:** 250 mg/5 mL (as axetil) when reconstituted	Aspartame, mannitol, phenylalanine 45 mg per 5 mL, sucrose. Fruit flavor. In 50 and 100 mL.
Rx	**Ceftin** (GlaxoWellcome)		Sucrose. Tutti-frutti flavor. In 50 and 100 mL bottles.
Rx	**Cefuroxime Sodium** (Various, eg, Cura Pharm)	**Powder for Injection**[a]: 750 mg (as sodium).	In 10 mL vials and 100 mL piggyback vials.
Rx	**Zinacef** (GlaxoWellcome)		In vials, infusion pack and *ADD-Vantage* vials.
Rx	**Cefuroxime Sodium** (Various, eg, Cura Pharm)	**Powder for Injection**[a]: 1.5 g (as sodium)	In 20 mL vials and 100 mL piggyback vials.
Rx	**Zinacef** (GlaxoWellcome)		In vials, infusion packs and *ADD-Vantage* vials.
Rx	**Cefuroxime Sodium** (Various, eg, Cura Pharm)	**Powder for Injection**[a]: 7.5 g (as sodium)	In pharmacy bulk package.
Rx	**Zinacef** (GlaxoWellcome)		In pharmacy bulk package.
Rx	**Zinacef** (GlaxoWellcome)	**Injection**[a]: 750 mg (as sodium)	Premixed, frozen. In 50 mL.
		1.5 g (as sodium)	Premixed, frozen. In 50 mL.

[a] Contains 2.4 mEq sodium/g.

CEFUROXIME AXETIL — ORAL

For complete and comparative prescribing information, refer to the Cephalosporins group monograph.

Indications

➤*Tablets:*

Pharyngitis/tonsillitis – Caused by *Streptococcus pyogenes*. The usual drug of choice in the treatment and prevention of streptococcal infections, including the prophylaxis of rheumatic fever, is penicillin given by the IM route. Cefuroxime axetil tablets are generally effective in the eradication of streptococci from the nasopharynx; however, substantial data establishing the efficacy of cefuroxime in the subsequent prevention of rheumatic fever are not available. Please also note that in all clinical trials, all isolates had to be sensitive to both penicillin and cefuroxime. There are no data from adequate and well-controlled trials to demonstrate the effectiveness of cefuroxime in the treatment of penicillin-resistant strains of *Streptococcus pyogenes*.

Acute bacterial otitis media – Caused by *Streptococcus pneumoniae*, *Haemophilus influenzae* (including beta-lactamase-producing strains), *Moraxella catarrhalis* (including beta-lactamase-producing strains), or *Streptococcus pyogenes*.

Acute bacterial maxillary sinusitis – Caused by *Streptococcus pneumoniae* or *Haemophilus influenzae* (non-beta-lactamase-producing strains only). In view of the insufficient numbers of isolates of beta-lactamase-producing strains of *Haemophilus influenzae* and *Moraxella catarrhalis* that were obtained from clinical trials with cefuroxime axetil tablets for patients

CEFUROXIME AXETIL — ORAL

with acute bacterial maxillary sinusitis, it was not possible to adequately evaluate the effectiveness of cefuroxime axetil tablets for sinus infections known, suspected, or considered potentially to be caused by beta-lactamase-producing *Haemophilus influenzae* or *Moraxella catarrhalis*.

Acute bacterial exacerbations of chronic bronchitis and secondary bacterial infections of acute bronchitis – Caused by *Streptococcus pneumoniae*, *Haemophilus influenzae* (beta-lactamase negative strains), or *Haemophilus parainfluenzae* (beta-lactamase negative strains).

Uncomplicated skin and skin-structure infections – Caused by *Staphylococcus aureus* (including beta-lactamase-producing strains) or *Streptococcus pyogenes*.

Uncomplicated urinary tract infections – Caused by *Escherichia coli* or *Klebsiella pneumoniae*.

Uncomplicated gonorrhea, urethral and endocervical – Caused by penicillinase-producing and non-penicillinase-producing strains of *Neisseria gonorrhoeae* and uncomplicated gonorrhea, rectal, in females, caused by non-penicillinase-producing strains of *Neisseria gonorrhoeae*.

Early Lyme disease (erythema migrans) – Caused by *Borrelia burgdorferi*.

➤*Powder for oral suspension:* For the treatment of pediatric patients 3 months to 12 years of age with mild-to-moderate infections caused by susceptible strains of the designated microorganisms in the conditions listed below. The safety and efficacy of cefuroxime axetil for oral suspension in the treatment of infections other than those specifically listed below have not been established either by adequate and well-controlled trials or by pharmacokinetic data with which to determine an effective and safe dosing regimen.

Pharyngitis/tonsillitis – Caused by *Streptococcus pyogenes*. The usual drug of choice in the treatment and prevention of streptococcal infections, including the prophylaxis of rheumatic fever, is penicillin given by the IM route. Cefuroxime axetil for oral suspension is generally effective in the eradication of streptococci from the nasopharynx; however, substantial data establishing the efficacy of cefuroxime in the subsequent prevention of rheumatic fever are not available. Please also note that in all clinical trials, all isolates had to be sensitive to both penicillin and cefuroxime. There are no data from adequate and well-controlled trials to demonstrate the effectiveness of cefuroxime in the treatment of penicillin-resistant strains of *Streptococcus pyogenes*.

Acute bacterial otitis media – Caused by *Streptococcus pneumoniae*, *Haemophilus influenzae* (including beta-lactamase-producing strains), *Moraxella catarrhalis* (including beta-lactamase-producing strains), or *Streptococcus pyogenes*.

Impetigo – Caused by *Staphylococcus aureus* (including beta-lactamase-producing strains) or *Streptococcus pyogenes*.

➤*Off-label uses:*

Lyme neuroborreliosis – [2] = Fair documentation. For the treatment of nervous system Lyme disease, guidelines from the Quality Standards Subcommittee of the American Academy of Neurology recommend oral cefuroxime as an alternative to doxycycline in cases for which doxycycline is contraindicated.

Other possible off-label uses – Acrodermatitis chronica atrophicans and lyme arthritis (see Administration and Dosage).

Administration and Dosage

➤*General dosing considerations:* Cefuroxime tablets and suspension are not bioequivalent and are not substitutable on a mg/mg basis.

➤*Adults:*

Tablets –

Dosage for Cefuroxime Axetil Tablets in Adults

Indication	Dosage	Duration (days)
Acute bacterial maxillary sinusitis	250 mg twice daily	10
Acute bacterial exacerbations of chronic bronchitis	250 or 500 mg twice daily	10[a]
Early Lyme disease	500 mg twice daily	20
Pharyngitis/tonsillitis	250 mg twice daily	10
Secondary bacterial infections of acute bronchitis	250 or 500 mg twice daily	5 to 10
Uncomplicated skin and skin-structure infections	250 or 500 mg twice daily	10
Uncomplicated urinary tract infections	250 mg twice daily	7 to 10
Uncomplicated gonorrhea	1000 mg once	single dose

[a] The safety and effectiveness of cefuroxime administered for less than 10 days in patients with acute exacerbations of chronic bronchitis have not been established.

Off-label dosing –

Acrodermatitis chronica atrophicans: 500 mg twice daily for 21 days.

Lyme arthritis: 500 mg twice daily for 28 days for patients without clinical evidence of neurologic disease.

Lyme neuroborreliosis: [2] = Fair documentation. 500 mg orally twice daily for 14 days. In studies, outcomes of regimens lasting between 10 and 28 days were similar.

➤*Children:*

Tablets –

Dosage for Cefuroxime Axetil Tablets in Children

Indication	Dosage	Duration (days)
Adolescents and adults (13 years and older)		
Acute bacterial maxillary sinusitis	250 mg twice daily	10
Acute bacterial exacerbation of chronic bronchitis	250 or 500 mg twice daily	10[a]
Early Lyme disease	500 mg twice daily[b]	20
Pharyngitis/tonsillitis	250 mg twice daily[b]	10
Secondary bacterial infections of acute bronchitis	250 or 500 mg twice daily	5 to 10
Uncomplicated skin and skin-structure infections	250 or 500 mg twice daily	10
Uncomplicated urinary tract infections	250 mg twice daily	7 to 10
Uncomplicated gonorrhea	1000 mg once	single dose
Children who can swallow tablets whole		
Acute otitis media	250 mg twice daily	10
Acute bacterial maxillary sinusitis	250 mg twice daily	10

[a] The safety and effectiveness of cefuroxime administered for less than 10 days in patients with acute exacerbations of chronic bronchitis have not been established.
[b] See Off-Label Dosing for dosage in children 3 months to 12 years of age.

Oral suspension –

Dosage for Cefuroxime Axetil Suspension in Children 3 Months to 12 Years of Age[a]

Indication	Dosage	Daily maximum dose	Duration (days)
Acute bacterial maxillary sinusitis	30 mg/kg/day divided twice daily	1000 mg	10
Acute otitis media	30 mg/kg/day divided twice daily	1000 mg	10
Impetigo	30 mg/kg/day divided twice daily[b]	1000 mg	10
Pharyngitis/tonsillitis	20 mg/kg/day divided twice daily[b]	500 mg	10

[a] See also Off-Label Dosing for dosing in Lyme disease.
[b] See also Off-Label Dosing for dosage of tablet formulation.

Off-label dosing –

Acrodermatitis chronica atrophicans:

- *Usual dose* – 30 mg/kg/day divided twice daily for 21 days.
- *Maximum dose* – 500 mg/dose (1,000 mg/day).

Impetigo:

- *3 months to 12 years of age* – 250 mg (tablets) twice daily.

Lyme arthritis:

- *Usual dose* – 30 mg/kg/day divided twice daily for 28 days in patients without clinical evidence of neurologic disease.
- *Maximum dose* – 500 mg/dose (1,000 mg/day).

Lyme disease (early):

- *Usual dose* – 30 mg/kg/day (oral suspension) divided twice daily for 14 to 21 days.
- *Maximum dose* – 500 mg/dose (1,000 mg/day).

Lyme neuroborreliosis: [2] = Fair documentation. 30 mg/kg/day in 2 divided doses (up to 500 mg/dose) for 14 days. In studies, outcomes of regimens lasting between 10 and 28 days were similar.

Pharyngitis/tonsillitis:

- *3 months to 12 years of age* – 125 mg (tablets) twice daily.

➤*Renal function impairment:* The safety and efficacy of cefuroxime in patients with renal failure have not been established. Since cefuroxime is renally eliminated, its half-life will be prolonged in patients with renal failure.

➤*Preparation for administration:*

Reconstitution of oral suspension – Prepare a suspension at the time of dispensing.

1.) Shake the bottle to loosen the powder.
2.) Remove the cap.
3.) Add the total amount of water for reconstitution and replace the cap.

CEFUROXIME AXETIL — ORAL

4.) Invert the bottle and vigorously rock the bottle from side to side so that water rises through the powder.
5.) Once the sound of the powder against the bottle disappears, turn the bottle upright and vigorously shake it in a diagonal direction.

Amount of Water Required for Reconstituting Cefuroxime Axetil Suspension		
Cefuroxime suspension	Labeled volume after reconstitution	Amount of water required for reconstitution
125 mg/5 mL	100 mL	37 mL
250 mg/5 mL	50 mL	19 mL
	100 mL	35 mL

➤*Administration:*

Tablets – Administer without regard to meals.

Oral suspension – Take with food. Shake well each time before using. Replace cap securely after each opening.

➤*Storage/Stability:*

Tablets – Store the tablets between 15° and 30°C (59° and 86°F). Replace cap securely after each opening. Protect unit-dose packs from excessive moisture.

Oral suspension – Before reconstitution, store dry powder between 2° and 30°C (36° and 86°F). After reconstitution, store suspension between 2° and 25°C (36° and 77°F), in a refrigerator or at room temperature. Discard after 10 days.

CEFUROXIME SODIUM — INJECTION

For complete and comparative prescribing information, refer to the Cephalosporins group monograph.

Indications

➤*Lower respiratory tract infections:* Including pneumonia, caused by *Streptococcus pneumoniae, Haemophilus influenzae* (including ampicillin-resistant strains), *Klebsiella* sp., *Staphylococcus aureus* (penicillinase- and non-penicillinase-producing strains), *Streptococcus pyogenes,* and *Escherichia coli.*

➤*Urinary tract infections:* Caused by *E. coli* and *Klebsiella* sp.

➤*Skin and skin structure infections:* Caused by *S. aureus* (penicillinase- and non-penicillinase-producing strains), *S. pyogenes, E. coli, Klebsiella* sp., and *Enterobacter* sp.

➤*Septicemia:* Caused by *S. aureus* (penicillinase- and non-penicillinase-producing strains), *S. pneumoniae, E. coli, H. influenzae* (including ampicillin-resistant strains), and *Klebsiella* sp.

➤*Meningitis:* Caused by *S. pneumoniae, H. influenzae* (including ampicillin-resistant strains), *Neisseria meningitidis,* and *S. aureus* (penicillinase- and non-penicillinase-producing strains).

➤*Gonorrhea:* Uncomplicated and disseminated gonococcal infections due to *Neisseria gonorrhoeae* (penicillinase- and non-penicillinase-producing strains) in both men and women.

➤*Bone and joint infections:* Caused by *S. aureus* (penicillinase- and non-penicillinase-producing strains).

➤*Mixed infections:* Clinical microbiological studies in skin and skin-structure infections frequently reveal the growth of susceptible strains of both aerobic and anaerobic organisms. Cefuroxime sodium has been used successfully in these mixed infections in which several organisms have been isolated.

In certain cases of confirmed or suspected gram-positive or gram-negative sepsis or in patients with other serious infections in which the causative organism has not been identified, cefuroxime sodium injection may be used concomitantly with an aminoglycoside. The recommended doses of both antibiotics may be given, depending on the severity of the infection and the patient's condition.

➤*Preoperative prophylaxis:* The preoperative prophylactic administration of cefuroxime sodium may prevent the growth of susceptible disease-causing bacteria and thereby may reduce the incidence of certain postoperative infections in patients undergoing surgical procedures (eg, vaginal hysterectomy) that are classified as clean-contaminated or potentially contaminated procedures. Effective prophylactic use of antibiotics in surgery depends on the time of administration. Cefuroxime sodium should usually be given one-half to 1 hour before the operation to allow sufficient time to achieve effective antibiotic concentrations in the wound tissues during the procedure. Repeat the dose intraoperatively if the surgical procedure is lengthy.

Prophylactic administration is usually not required after the surgical procedure ends and should be stopped within 24 hours. In the majority of surgical procedures, continuing prophylactic administration of any antibiotic does not reduce the incidence of subsequent infections but will increase the possibility of adverse reactions and the development of bacterial resistance.

The perioperative use of cefuroxime sodium has also been effective during open heart surgery for surgical patients in whom infections at the operative site would present a serious risk. For these patients it is recommended that therapy with cefuroxime sodium be continued for at least 48 hours after the surgical procedure ends. If an infection is present, obtain specimens for culture for the identification of the causative organism, and institute appropriate antimicrobial therapy.

Administration and Dosage

➤*Adults:*

Usual dosage – 750 mg to 1.5 g every 8 hours, usually for 5 to 10 days.

Bacterial meningitis – Do not exceed 3 g every 8 hours.

Bone and joint infections – 1.5 g every 8 hours. In clinical trials, surgical intervention was performed when indicated as an adjunct to therapy with cefuroxime. A course of oral antibiotics was administered when appropriate following the completion of parenteral administration of cefuroxime.

Disseminated gonococcal infections – 750 mg every 8 hours.

Life-threatening infections or infections due to less susceptible organisms – 1.5 g every 6 hours may be required.

Preventive use – 1.5 g IV just before surgery (approximately 30 minutes to 1 hour before the initial incision) is recommended. Thereafter, give 750 mg IV or IM every 8 hours when the procedure is prolonged.

Preventive use during open heart surgery – 1.5 g IV at the induction of anesthesia and every 12 hours thereafter for a total of 6 g is recommended.

Severe or complicated infections – 1.5 g every 8 hours.

Skin and skin structure infections – 750 mg every 8 hours.

Uncomplicated gonococcal infection – 1.5 g given IM as a single dose at 2 different sites together with 1 g of oral probenecid.

Uncomplicated pneumonia – 750 mg every 8 hours.

Uncomplicated urinary tract infections – 750 mg every 8 hours.

➤*Children:*

Three months of age and older –

Infections: For a list of infections, refer to Indications.

50 to 100 mg/kg/day in equally divided doses every 6 to 8 hours has been successful for most infections susceptible to cefuroxime.

Bacterial meningitis: 200 to 240 mg/kg/day IV in divided doses every 6 to 8 hours. However, cefuroxime is not recommended by the American Academy of Pediatrics for the treatment of meningitis.

Bone and joint infections: 150 mg/kg/day (not to exceed the maximum adult dosage) in equally divided doses every 8 hours.

Severe or serious infections: 100 mg/kg/day (not to exceed the maximum adult dosage).

Off-label dosing –

Younger than 3 months of age:

- *6 days and younger and less than 2,000 g* – 100 mg/kg/day divided every 12 hours.
- *6 days and younger and more than 2,000 g* – 150 mg/kg/day divided every 8 hours.
- *7 days and older* – 150 mg/kg/day divided every 8 hours.

➤*Renal function impairment:*

Adults – Creatinine clearance (CrCl) greater than 20 mL/min, administer a dose of 750 mg to 1.5 g every 8 hours; CrCl 10 to 20 mL/min, administer 750 mg every 12 hours; CrCl less than 10 mL/min, administer 750 mg every 24 hours. Since cefuroxime is dialyzable, give patients on hemodialysis a further dose at the end of the dialysis.

Children – The frequency of dosing should be modified consistent with the recommendations for adults.

➤*Duration of therapy:* Administration of cefuroxime should be continued for a minimum of 48 to 72 hours after the patient becomes asymptomatic or after evidence of bacterial eradication has been obtained; a minimum of 10 days of treatment is recommended in infections caused by *S. pyogenes* in order to guard against the risk of rheumatic fever or glomerulonephritis; frequent bacteriologic and clinical appraisal is necessary during therapy of chronic urinary tract infection and may be required for several months after therapy has been completed; persistent infections may require treatment for several weeks; and doses smaller than those indicated above should not be used. In staphylococcal and other infections involving a collection of pus, carry out surgical drainage where indicated.

➤*Preparation for administration:*

Preparation of Cefuroxime Sodium Injection Solution and Suspension			
Strength	Amount of diluent to be added (mL)	Volume to be withdrawn	Approximate cefuroxime sodium concentration (mg/mL)
750 mg vial	3 (IM)	Total[a]	220
750 mg vial	8 (IV)	Total	90
1.5 g vial	16 (IV)	Total	90
750 mg infusion pack	100 (IV)	-	7.5
1.5 g infusion pack	100 (IV)	-	15
7.5 g pharmacy bulk package	77 (IV)	Amount needed[b]	95

[a] Note: Cefuroxime is a suspension at IM concentrations.
[b] 8 mL of solution contains 750 mg of cefuroxime; 16 mL of solution contains 1.5 g of cefuroxime.

Constitute each 750 mg vial with sterile water for injection. Constitute each 750 mg and 1.5 g infusion pack with 100 mL of sterile water for injection, 5% dextrose injection, 0.9% sodium chloride injection, 1/6 M sodium lactate

CEFUROXIME SODIUM — INJECTION

injection, Ringers injection, Ringers lactate injection, 5% dextrose and 0.9% sodium chloride injection, 5% dextrose injection, 5% dextrose and 0.45% sodium chloride injection, 5% dextrose and 0.225% sodium chloride injection, 10% dextrose injection, and 10% invert sugar in water for injection. Shake gently to disperse.

GALAXY plastic containers – Use sterile equipment. Do not use plastic containers in series connections. Such use could result in air embolism due to residual air being drawn from the primary container before administration of the fluid from the secondary container is complete.

Preparation for administration
1.) Suspend container from eyelet support.
2.) Remove protector from outlet port at bottom of container.
3.) Attach administration set. Refer to complete directions accompanying set.

ADD-Vantage vials – *ADD-Vantage* vials are to be constituted only with 50 or 100 mL of 5% dextrose injection, 0.9% sodium chloride injection, or 0.45% sodium chloride injection in the manufacturer's *ADD-Vantage* flexible diluent containers.

To open diluent container: Peel the corner of the *ADD-Vantage* diluent overwrap and remove flexible diluent container. Some opacity of the plastic flexible container due to moisture absorption during the sterilization process may be observed. This is normal and does not affect the solution quality or safety. The opacity will diminish gradually.

To assemble vial and flexible diluent container (use aseptic technique): Remove the protective covers from the top of the vial and the vial port on the diluent container as follows
1.) To remove the breakaway vial cap, swing the pull ring over the top of the vial and pull down far enough to start the opening, then pull straight up to remove the cap. Once the breakaway cap has been removed, do not access vial with syringe.
2.) Recheck the vial to ensure that it is tight by trying to turn it further in the direction of assembly.
3.) Label appropriately.

To prepare admixture
1.) Squeeze the bottom of the diluent container gently to inflate the portion of the container surrounding the end of the drug vial.
2.) With the other hand, push the drug vial down into the container, telescoping the walls of the container. Grasp the inner cap of the vial through the walls of the container.
3.) Pull the inner cap from the drug vial. Verify that the rubber stopper has been pulled out, allowing the drug and diluent to mix.
4.) Mix container contents thoroughly and use within the specified time.

➤*Administration:* Cefuroxime may be given IV or by deep IM injection into a large muscle mass (eg, gluteus, lateral part of the thigh). Before injecting IM, aspiration is necessary to avoid inadvertent injection into a blood vessel.

IV administration – The IV route may be preferable for patients with bacterial septicemia or other severe or life-threatening infections or for patients who may be poor risks because of lowered resistance, particularly if shock is present or impending.

Direct intermittent IV administration – Slowly inject the solution into a vein over a period of 3 to 5 minutes or give it through the tubing system by which the patient is also receiving other IV solutions.

Intermittent IV infusion – For intermittent IV infusion with a Y-type administration set, dosing can be accomplished through the tubing system by which the patient may be receiving other IV solutions. However, during infusion of the solution containing cefuroxime sodium injection, it is advisable to temporarily discontinue administration of any other solutions at the same site.

Continuous IV infusion – A solution of cefuroxime may be added to an IV infusion pack containing 1 of the following fluids: 0.9% sodium chloride injection, 5% dextrose injection, 10% dextrose injection, 5% dextrose and 0.9% sodium chloride injection, 5% dextrose and 0.45% sodium chloride injection, or 1/6 M sodium lactate injection.

ADD-Vantage vials
1.) Confirm the activation and admixture of vial contents.
2.) Check for leaks by squeezing container firmly. If leaks are found, discard unit as sterility may be impaired.
3.) Close flow-control clamp of administration set.
4.) Remove cover from outlet port at bottom of container.
5.) Insert piercing pin of administration set into port with a twisting motion until the pin is firmly seated. Note: See full directions on administration set carton.
6.) Lift the free end of the hanger loop on the bottom of the vial, breaking the 2 tie strings. Bend the loop outward to lock it in the upright position, then suspend container from hanger.
7.) Squeeze and release drip chamber to establish proper fluid level in chamber.
8.) Open flow-control clamp and clear air from set. Close clamp.
9.) Attach set to venipuncture device. If device is not indwelling, prime and make venipuncture.
10.) Regulate rate of administration with flow-control clamp

Warning: Do not use flexible container in series connections.

➤*Admixture compatibility:* Solutions of cefuroxime should not be added to solutions of aminoglycoside antibiotics because of potential interaction. However, if concurrent therapy with cefuroxime and an aminoglycoside is indicated, each of these antibiotics can be administered separately to the same patient.

➤*Storage/Stability:* Cefuroxime in the dry state should be stored between 15° and 30°C (59° and 86°F) and protected from light.

IM – When constituted as directed, cefuroxime maintains satisfactory potency for 24 hours at room temperature and for 48 hours under refrigeration (5° C; 41° F). Any unused suspensions should be discarded.

IV – When the 750 mg, 1.5 g, and 7.5 g pharmacy bulk vials are constituted as directed with sterile water for injection, the solutions maintain satisfactory potency for 24 hours at room temperature and for 48 hours (750 mg and 1.5 g vials) or for 7 days (7.5 mg pharmacy bulk vial) under refrigeration (5°C; 44°F). These solutions may be further diluted to concentrations of between 1 and 30 mg/mL in the approved solutions and will lose not more than 10% activity for 24 hours at room temperature or for at least 7 days under refrigeration. Discard unused solutions after the time periods previously mentioned.

Cefuroxime has also been found compatible for 24 hours at room temperature when admixed in IV infusion with heparin (10 and 50 units/mL) in 0.9% sodium chloride injection and potassium chloride (10 and 40 mEq/L) in 0.9% sodium chloride injection. Sodium bicarbonate injection is not recommended for the dilution of cefuroxime.

The 750 mg and 1.5 g cefuroxime sodium *ADD-Vantage* vials, when diluted in 50 or 100 mL of 5% dextrose injection, 0.9% sodium chloride injection, or 0.45% sodium chloride injection, may be stored for up to 24 hours at room temperature or for 7 days under refrigeration. Joined vials that have not been activated may be used within a 14-day period; this period corresponds to that for use of the manufacturer's *ADD-Vantage* containers following removal of the outer packaging (overwrap). Freezing solutions of cefuroxime in the *ADD-Vantage* system is not recommended.

Cefuroxime supplied as a frozen, sterile, iso-osmotic, nonpyrogenic solution in plastic containers is to be administered after thawing either as a continuous or intermittent IV infusion. The thawed solution of the premixed product is stable for 28 days if stored under refrigeration (5°C; 41°F) or for 24 hours if stored at room temperature (25°C; 77°F). Do not refreeze. Thaw container at room temperature (25°C; 77°F) or under refrigeration (5°C; 41°F). Do not force thaw by immersion in water baths or by microwave irradiation. Components of the solution may precipitate in the frozen state and will dissolve upon reaching room temperature with little or no agitation. Potency is not affected. Mix after solution has reached room temperature. Check for minute leaks by squeezing bag firmly. Discard bag if leaks are found as sterility may be impaired. Do not add supplementary medication. Do not use unless solution is clear and seal is intact.

Frozen stability – Constitute the 750 mg, 1.5 g, or 7.5 g vial as directed for IV administration in the Preparation of Solution and Suspension table. Immediately withdraw the total contents of the 750 mg or 1.5 g vial or 8 or 16 mL from the 7.5 g bulk vial and add to a Baxter *Viaflex Mini-Bag* containing 50 or 100 mL of 0.9% sodium chloride injection or 5% dextrose injection and freeze. Frozen solutions are stable for 6 months when stored at −20°C (4°F). Frozen solutions should be thawed at room temperature and not refrozen. Do not force thaw by immersion in water baths or by microwave irradiation. Thawed solutions may be stored for up to 24 hours at room temperature or for 7 days in a refrigerator.

Directions for dispensing (pharmacy bulk package [not for direct infusion]) – The pharmacy bulk package is for use in a pharmacy admixture service only under a laminar flow hood. Entry into the vial must be made with a sterile transfer set or other sterile dispensing device, and the contents dispensed in aliquots using aseptic technique. The use of syringe and needle is not recommended as it may cause leakage. After initial withdrawal use entire contents of vial promptly. Any unused portion must be discarded within 24 hours.

CEFTRIAXONE

Rx	**Ceftriaxone Sodium** (Various, eg, Cephazone, Lupin, Sicor)	**Injection, powder for solution:** 250 mg	As ceftriaxone sodium.[a] In vials.
Rx	**Ceftriaxone Sodium** (Various, eg, Cephazone, Lupin, Sicor)	**Injection, powder for solution:** 500 mg	As ceftriaxone sodium.[a] In vials.
Rx	**Rocephin** (Roche)		As ceftriaxone sodium.[a] In vials.
Rx	**Ceftriaxone Sodium** (Various, eg, Baxter, B. Braun/McGaw, Cephazone, Lupin, Sicor, West-Ward)	**Injection, powder for solution:** 1 g	As ceftriaxone sodium.[a] In vials and single-use 50 mL *Duplex* container.[b]
Rx	**Ceftriaxone Sodium** (Various, eg, Baxter, B. Braun/McGaw, Cephazone, Lupin, Sicor, West-Ward)	**Injection, powder for solution:** 2 g	As ceftriaxone sodium.[a] In vials and single-use 50 mL *Duplex* container.[b]
Rx	**Rocephin** (Roche)		As ceftriaxone sodium.[a] In vials.

CEFTRIAXONE

Rx	Ceftriaxone Sodium (Various, eg, Sandoz)	Injection, powder for solution: 10 g	As ceftriaxone sodium.[a] In bulk containers.

[a] Contains approximately 3.6 mEq of sodium per gram of ceftriaxone activity.

[b] *Duplex drug delivery system* is a flexible dual chamber. The drug chamber is filled with ceftriaxone, and the diluent chamber contains approximately 50 mL of dextrose injection.

CEFTRIAXONE SODIUM — INJECTION

For complete and comparative prescribing information, refer to the Cephalosporins group monograph.

Indications

➤*Acute bacterial otitis media:* Caused by *Streptococcus pneumoniae*, *Haemophilus influenzae* (including beta-lactamase–producing strains), or *Moraxella catarrhalis* (including beta-lactamase–producing strains).

In one study, lower clinical cure rates were observed with a single dose of ceftriaxone compared with 10 days of oral therapy. In a second study, comparable cure rates were observed between single-dose ceftriaxone and the comparator. Balance the potentially lower clinical cure rate of ceftriaxone against the potential advantages of parenteral therapy.

➤*Bacterial septicemia:* Caused by *Staphylococcus aureus*, *S. pneumoniae*, *Escherichia coli*, *H. influenzae*, or *Klebsiella pneumoniae*.

➤*Bone and joint infections:* Caused by *S. aureus*, *S. pneumoniae*, *E. coli*, *Proteus mirabilis*, *K. pneumoniae*, or *Enterobacter* species.

➤*Intra-abdominal infections:* Caused by *E. coli*, *K. pneumoniae*, *Bacteriosides fragilis*, *Clostridium* species (most strains of *Clostridium difficile* are resistant), or *Peptostreptococcus* species.

➤*Lower respiratory tract infections:* Caused by *S. pneumoniae*, *S. aureus*, *H. influenzae*, *Haemophilus parainfluenzae*, *K. pneumoniae*, *E. coli*, *Enterobacter aerogenes*, *P. mirabilis*, or *Serratia marcescens*.

➤*Meningitis:* Caused by *H. influenzae*, *Neisseria meningitidis*, or *S. pneumoniae*. Ceftriaxone has also been used successfully in a limited number of cases of meningitis and shunt infection caused by *Staphylococcus epidermidis* and *E. coli* (efficacy for these 2 organisms in this organ system was studied in less than 10 infections).

➤*Pelvic inflammatory disease:* Caused by *Neisseria gonorrhoeae*. Ceftriaxone, like other cephalosporins, has no activity against *Chlamydia trachomatis*. Therefore, when cephalosporins are used in the treatment of patients with pelvic inflammatory disease and *C. trachomatis* is one of the suspected pathogens, appropriate antichlamydial coverage should be added.

➤*Skin and skin structure infections:* Caused by *S. aureus*, *S. epidermidis*, *Streptococcus pyogenes*, viridans group streptococci, *E. coli*, *Enterobacter cloacae*, *Klebsiella oxytoca*, *K. pneumoniae*, *P. mirabilis*, *Morganella morganii* (efficacy for this organism in this organ system was studied in less than 10 infections), *Pseudomonas aeruginosa*, *S. marcescens*, *Acinetobacter calcoaceticus*, or *B. fragilis* (efficacy for this organism in this organ system was studied in less than 10 infections), or *Peptostreptococcus* species.

➤*Surgical prophylaxis:* The preoperative administration of a single dose of ceftriaxone 1 g may reduce the incidence of postoperative infections in patients undergoing surgical procedures classified as contaminated or potentially contaminated (eg, vaginal or abdominal hysterectomy or cholecystectomy for chronic calculous cholecystitis in high-risk patients, such as those older than 70 years of age, with acute cholecystitis not requiring therapeutic antimicrobials, obstructive jaundice, or common duct bile stones) and in surgical patients for whom infection at the operative site would present serious risk (eg, during coronary artery bypass surgery). Although ceftriaxone has been shown to have been as effective as cefazolin in the prevention of infection following coronary artery bypass surgery, no placebo-controlled trials have been conducted to evaluate any cephalosporin antibiotic in the prevention of infection following coronary artery bypass surgery.

When administered prior to surgical procedures for which it is indicated, a single dose of ceftriaxone 1 g provides protection from most infections caused by susceptible organisms throughout the course of the procedure.

➤*Uncomplicated gonorrhea (cervical/urethral and rectal):* Caused by *N. gonorrhoeae*, including both penicillinase- and nonpenicillinase-producing strains, and pharyngeal gonorrhea caused by nonpenicillinase-producing strains of *N. gonorrhoeae*.

➤*Urinary tract infections (complicated and uncomplicated):* Caused by *E. coli*, *P. mirabilis*, *Proteus vulgaris*, *M. morganii*, or *K. pneumoniae*.

➤*Off-label uses:*

Chancroid – [1] = Good documentation. Based on Centers for Disease Control and Prevention (CDC) guidelines, ceftriaxone is a recommended therapy for treatment of chancroid.

Epididymitis – [1] = Good documentation. Centers for Disease Control and Prevention (CDC) guidelines recommend ceftriaxone in combination with doxycycline as a regimen for acute epididymitis caused by suspected or confirmed gonococcal or chlamydial infections.

Gonococcal meningitis and endocarditis – [1] = Good documentation. Based on CDC guidelines, ceftriaxone is a recommended therapy for gonococcal meningitis or endocarditis.

Lyme neuroborreliosis – [1] = Good documentation. Parenteral regimens for Lyme disease of the nervous system have a greater potential for morbidity. For severe neurologic disease, class 1 and 2 studies suggested that parenteral treatment (ie, cefotaxime, ceftriaxone, penicillin) was probably safe and effective, but class 2 and 3 studies also indicated that oral therapy (and doxycycline specifically) was comparably safe and effective for patients without parenchymal involvement.

Proctitis, proctocolitis, enteritis – [1] = Good documentation. CDC guidelines recommend ceftriaxone in combination with doxycycline as a regimen for known or presumptive therapy of proctitis, proctocolitis, or enteritis.

Administration and Dosage

➤*General dosing considerations:* If *C. trachomatis* is a suspected pathogen, appropriate antichlamydial coverage should be added because ceftriaxone has no activity against this organism.

➤*Adults:*

Maximum dose – 4 g/day.

Usual dosage – 1 to 2 g given intramuscularly (IM) or intravenously (IV) once a day or in equally divided doses twice daily, depending on the type and severity of infection. Continue for at least 2 days after the signs and symptoms of infection have disappeared. The usual duration of therapy is 4 to 14 days; in complicated infections, longer therapy may be required. When treating infections caused by *S. pyogenes*, therapy should be continued for at least 10 days.

Surgical prophylaxis – A single dose of 1 g administered IV 30 minutes to 2 hours before surgery.

Uncomplicated gonococcal infections – A single IM dose of 250 mg.

Off-label dosing –

Chancroid: [1] = Good documentation. 250 mg IM in a single dose.

Epididymitis: [1] = Good documentation. A single IM dose of 250 mg. Ceftriaxone should be given in conjunction with twice-daily oral doxycycline.

Gonococcal meningitis and endocarditis: [1] = Good documentation.

• *Gonococcal meningitis* – 1 g IV every 12 hours. Continue therapy for 10 to 14 days.

• *Gonococcal endocarditis* – 1 g IV every 12 hours. Continue therapy for a minimum of 4 weeks.

Lyme neuroborreliosis: [1] = Good documentation. 2 g/day IV for 14 days. In studies, outcomes of regimens lasting between 10 and 28 days were similar.

Pelvic inflammatory disease (mild to moderately severe): 250 mg given IM as a single dose with doxycycline 100 mg orally twice daily for 14 days, with or without metronidazole 500 mg orally twice daily for 14 days.

Proctitis, proctocolitis, enteritis: [1] = Good documentation. Single IM dose of 125 mg. Ceftriaxone should be given in conjunction with twice-daily oral doxycycline.

Uncomplicated gonococcal infections: 125 mg given IM as a single dose.

➤*Children:* Hyperbilirubinemic neonates, especially premature neonates, should not be treated with ceftriaxone.

Acute bacterial otitis media –

Usual dosage: A single IM dose of 50 mg/kg (not to exceed 1 g) is recommended.

Maximum dose: 1 g.

Meningitis –

Usual dosage: It is recommended that the initial therapeutic dose be 100 mg/kg (not to exceed 4 g) given IM or IV. Thereafter, a total daily dose of 100 mg/kg/day (not to exceed 4 g daily) is recommended. The daily dose may be administered once a day (or in equally divided doses every 12 hours).

Maximum dose: 4 g/day.

Duration of therapy: 7 to 14 days.

Serious infections other than meningitis –

Usual dosage: 50 to 75 mg/kg given IM or IV in divided doses every 12 hours.

Maximum dose: 2 g/day.

Duration of therapy: Continue for at least 2 days after the signs and symptoms of infection have disappeared. The usual duration of therapy is 4 to 14 days; in complicated infections, longer therapy may be required. When treating infections caused by *S. pyogenes*, therapy should be continued for at least 10 days.

Skin and skin structure infections –

Usual dosage: 50 to 75 mg/kg given once a day (or in equally divided doses twice daily).

Maximum dose: 2 g/day.

Duration of therapy: Ceftriaxone therapy should be continued for at least 2 days after the signs and symptoms of infection have disappeared. The usual duration of therapy is 4 to 14 days; in complicated infections, longer therapy may be required. When treating infections caused by *S. pyogenes*, therapy should be continued for at least 10 days.

Off-label dosing –

Acute bacterial otitis media, persistent/treatment failure: 50 mg/kg IM or IV (not to exceed 1 g) daily for 3 days.

Lyme neuroborreliosis: [1] = Good documentation. 50 to 75 mg/kg/day (as a single daily dose, up to 2 g) for 14 days. In studies, outcomes of regimens lasting between 10 and 28 days were similar.

➤*Renal function impairment:* No dosage adjustment is necessary for patients with renal function impairment; however, blood levels should be

CEFTRIAXONE SODIUM — INJECTION

monitored in patients with severe renal function impairment (eg, dialysis patients) and in patients with both renal and hepatic function impairment.

Maximum dose – The dose should not exceed 2 g/day without closely monitoring serum concentrations.

Adults receiving continuous renal replacement therapy – The following recommendations assume ultrafiltration and dialysis flow rates of 1 to 2 L/hr.

Loading dose: 2 g IV.

Maintenance dosage: 1 to 2 g IV every 12 to 24 hours for patients receiving continuous venovenous hemofiltration, continuous venovenous hemodialysis, or continuous venovenous hemodialfiltration.

Adults receiving intermittent hemodialysis – 1 to 2 g IV every 24 hours administered after the dialysis session. This recommendation assumes the patient is receiving standard intermittent hemodialysis 3 times per week and completes the full dialysis sessions.

➤*Hepatic function impairment:* No dosage adjustment is necessary for patients with hepatic function impairment; however, blood levels should be monitored in patients with both renal and hepatic function impairment.

Maximum dose – The dose should not exceed 2 g/day without closely monitoring serum concentrations.

➤*Duration of therapy:* Generally, ceftriaxone therapy should be continued for at least 2 days after the signs and symptoms of infection have disappeared. The usual duration of therapy is 4 to 14 days; in complicated infections, longer therapy may be required. When treating infections caused by *S. pyogenes*, therapy should be continued for at least 10 days.

➤*Preparation for administration:*

IM – Reconstitute ceftriaxone powder with the appropriate diluent. Inject the diluent into the vial and shake the vial thoroughly to form the solution. Withdraw the entire contents of the vial into the syringe to equal the total labeled dose.

After reconstitution, each 1 mL of solution contains an approximately 250 or 350 mg equivalent of ceftriaxone according to the amount of diluent indicated in the following table. If required, more dilute solutions could be utilized. A 350 mg/mL concentration is not recommended for the 250 mg vial because it may not be possible to withdraw the entire contents.

IM Ceftriaxone Reconstitution

Vial dosage size	Amount of diluent to add: 250 mg/mL	350 mg/mL
250 mg	0.9 mL	–
500 mg	1.8 mL	1 mL
1 g	3.6 mL	2.1 mL
2 g	7.2 mL	4.2 mL

IV – Concentrations between 10 and 40 mg/mL are recommended; however, lower concentrations may be used if desired. Reconstitute vials with an appropriate IV diluent.

IV Ceftriaxone Reconstitution

Vial dosage size	Amount of diluent to add
250 mg	2.4 mL
500 mg	4.8 mL
1 g	9.6 mL
2 g	19.2 mL

After reconstitution, each 1 mL of solution contains an approximately 100 mg equivalent of ceftriaxone. Withdraw entire contents and dilute to the desired concentration with the appropriate IV diluent.

Pharmacy bulk package – The 10 g vial should be reconstituted with 95 mL of an appropriate IV diluent in a suitable work area, such as a laminar flow hood. The resulting solution will contain approximately 100 mg/mL of ceftriaxone. The container closure may be penetrated only 1 time after reconstitution, using a suitable sterile transfer device or dispensing set that allows measured dispensing of the contents. A sterile substance that must be reconstituted prior to use may require a separate closure entry. Use of this product is restricted to a suitable work area, such as a laminar flow hood.

Withdraw the container contents without delay. If this is not possible, a maximum time of 4 hours from initial closure entry is permitted to complete fluid transfer operations. If reconstitution is necessary, begin this time limit with the introduction of solvent or diluent into the pharmacy bulk package.

Unused portions of solution held longer than the recommended time periods should be discarded.

Transfer individual dose to appropriate IV solutions as soon as possible following reconstitution of the bulk package. The stability of the solution that has been transferred into a container varies according to diluent, concentration, and temperature. Concentrations between 10 and 40 mg/mL are recommended; however, lower concentrations may be used if desired.

Duplex drug delivery system – To avoid inadvertent activation, the *Duplex* container should remain in the folded position until activation is intended. Apply the patient-specific label on the foil side of the container. Use care to avoid activation. Do not cover any portion of the foil strip with the patient label. Unlatch the side tab and unfold the *Duplex* container. Visually inspect the diluent chamber for particulate matter. Use only if the container and seals are intact. To inspect the drug powder for foreign matter or discoloration, peel the foil strip from the drug chamber. Protect from light after removal of the foil strip. If the foil strip is removed, the product must be used within 7 days but not beyond the labeled expiration date. The product should be refolded and the side tab latched until ready to activate.

Do not use directly after storage by refrigeration; allow the product to equilibrate to room temperature before patient use.

Unfold the *Duplex* container and point the set port in a downward direction. Starting at the hanger tab end, fold the *Duplex* container just below the diluent meniscus, trapping all air above the fold. To activate, squeeze the folded diluent chamber until the seal between the diluent and powder opens, releasing the diluent into the drug powder chamber. Agitate the liquid-powder mixture until the drug powder is completely dissolved.

➤*Administration:* Reconstituted bulk solutions should not be used for direct infusion. Ceftriaxone may be administered IV or IM.

IM – As with all IM preparations, ceftriaxone should be injected well within the body of a relatively large muscle; aspiration helps to avoid unintentional injection into a blood vessel.

IV – Ceftriaxone should be administered IV by infusion over a period of 30 minutes.

➤*Admixture compatibility:*

Compatibility – Ceftriaxone has been shown to be compatible with metronidazole injection. The concentration should not exceed metronidazole 5 to 7.5 mg/mL with ceftriaxone 10 mg/mL as an admixture. The admixture is stable for 24 hours at room temperature only in sodium chloride 0.9% injection or dextrose 5% in water. No compatibility studies have been conducted with the metronidazole injection formulation or use of other diluents. Metronidazole at concentrations of more than 8 mg/mL will precipitate. Do not refrigerate the admixture because precipitation will occur.

After the indicated stability time periods, unused portions of solutions should be discarded.

Incompatibility – Vancomycin and fluconazole are physically incompatible with ceftriaxone in admixtures. When either of these drugs is to be coadministered with ceftriaxone by intermittent IV infusion, it is recommended that they be given sequentially, with thorough flushing of the IV lines (with one of the compatible fluids) between the administrations.

To avoid possible incompatibility, ceftriaxone solutions should not be physically mixed with or piggybacked into solutions containing other antimicrobial drugs or into diluent solutions other than those previously listed.

Do not use diluents containing calcium, such as Ringer's lactate solution or Hartmann solution, to reconstitute ceftriaxone. vials or to further dilute a reconstituted vial for IV administration because a precipitate can form. Precipitation of ceftriaxone-calcium can occur when ceftriaxone is mixed with calcium-containing solutions in the same IV administration line. Ceftriaxone must not be administered simultaneously with calcium-containing IV solutions, including continuous calcium-containing infusions such as parenteral nutrition via a Y-site in any age group. However, in patients other than neonates (less than or equal to 28 days of age), ceftriaxone and calcium-containing solutions may be administered sequentially of one another if the infusion lines are thoroughly flushed between infusions with a compatible fluid.

Do not introduce additives into the *Duplex* container. Do not use plastic containers in series connections. Such use would result in air embolism caused by residual air being drawn from the primary container before administration of the fluid from the secondary container is complete.

➤*Storage/Stability:* Store ceftriaxone sterile powder at room temperature (20° to 25°C [68° to 77°F]) or below. Protect from light. After reconstitution, protection from normal light is not necessary. The color of solutions ranges from light yellow to amber, depending on the length of storage and the concentration and diluent used.

After the indicated stability time periods, unused portions of solutions should be discarded.

IM solutions – Ceftriaxone IM solutions remain stable (loss of potency less than 10%) for the following time periods:

Storage/Stability of Ceftriaxone IM

Diluent	Concentration (mg/mL)	Storage: Room temperature (25°C [77°F])	Refrigerated (4°C [39°F])
Sterile water for injection	100	2 d	10 d
	250, 350	24 h	3 d
Sodium chloride 0.9% solution	100	2 d	10 d
	250, 350	24 h	3 d
Dextrose 5% solution	100	2 d	10 d
	250, 350	24 h	3 d
Bacteriostatic water + benzyl alcohol 0.9%	100	24 h	10 d
	250, 350	24 h	3 d
Lidocaine 1% solution (without epinephrine)	100	24 h	10 d
	250, 350	24 h	3 d

IV solutions – Ceftriaxone IV solutions at concentrations of 10, 20, and 40 mg/mL remain stable (loss of potency less than 10%) for the following time periods stored in glass or polyvinyl chloride (PVC) containers:

CEFTRIAXONE SODIUM — INJECTION

Storage/Stability of Ceftriaxone IV		
	Storage	
Diluent	Room temperature (25°C [77°F])	Refrigerated (4°C [39°F])
Sterile water	2 d	10 d
Sodium chloride 0.9% solution	2 d	10 d
Dextrose 5% solution	2 d	10 d
Dextrose 10% solution	2 d	10 d
Dextrose 5% + sodium chloride 0.9% solution[a]	2 d	Incompatible
Dextrose 5% + sodium chloride 0.45% solution	2 d	Incompatible

[a] Data available for 10 to 40 mg/mL concentrations in this diluent in PVC containers only.

The following ceftriaxone IV solutions are stable at room temperature (25°C [77°F]) for 24 hours at concentrations between 10 and 40 mg/mL: sodium lactate (PVC container), invert sugar 10% (glass container), sodium bicarbonate 5% (glass container), *FreAmine III* (glass container), *Normosol-M* in dextrose 5% (glass and PVC containers), *Ionosol-B* in dextrose 5% (glass container), mannitol 5% (glass container), and mannitol 10% (glass container).

Ceftriaxone reconstituted with dextrose 5% or sodium chloride 0.9% solution at concentrations between 10 and 40 mg/mL and then stored in frozen state (−20°C [−4°F]) in PVC or polyolefin containers remains stable for 26 weeks.

All frozen solutions of ceftriaxone should be thawed at room temperature before use. After thawing, discard unused portions. Do not refreeze.

Duplex drug delivery system – As with other cephalosporins, reconstituted ceftriaxone for injection and dextrose injection tends to darken, depending on storage conditions within the stated recommendations. However, the product potency is not adversely affected. Use only if the prepared solution is clear and free from particulate matter. Following reconstitution (activation), the product must be used within 24 hours if stored at room temperature or within 7 days if stored under refrigeration.

CEFIXIME

Rx	**Suprax** (Lupin Pharma)	**Powder for suspension; oral**: 100 mg per 5 mL	Sucrose. Strawberry flavored. In 50, 75, and 100 mL.
		200 mg per 5 mL	Sucrose. Strawberry flavored. In 25, 37.5, 50, 75, and 100 mL.

CEFIXIME — ORAL

For complete and comparative prescribing information, refer to the Cephalosporins group monograph.

Indications

➤*Acute bronchitis and acute exacerbations of chronic bronchitis:* Caused by *Streptococcus pneumoniae* and *Haemophilus influenzae* (beta-lactamase positive and negative strains).

➤*Otitis media:* Caused by *H. influenzae* (beta-lactamase positive and negative strains), *Moraxella (Branhamella) catarrhalis*, (most of which are beta-lactamase positive) and *Streptococcus pyogenes*. Efficacy for this organism in this organ system was studied in fewer than 10 infections.

➤*Pharyngitis and tonsillitis:* Caused by *S. pyogenes*.

➤*Uncomplicated gonorrhea (cervical/urethral):* Caused by *Neisseria gonorrhoeae* (penicillinase- and non-penicillinase-producing strains).

➤*Uncomplicated urinary tract infections:* Caused by *Escherichia coli* and *Proteus mirabilis*.

Administration and Dosage

➤*Adults:*

Usual dosage – 400 mg/day. For the treatment of uncomplicated gonorrhea (cervical/urethral), the dose is 400 mg as a single dose.

➤*Children:* See Adults for dosing for children older than 12 years of age (weighing 50 kg or more).

6 months to 12 years of age (weighing 50 kg or less) –

Usual dosage: 8 mg/kg/day as a single daily dose, or may be given in 2 divided doses as 4 mg/kg every 12 hours.

Cefixime Children Dosage Chart					
		100 mg per 5 mL suspension		200 mg per 5 mL suspension	
Patient weight (kg)	Dose/day (mg)	Dose/day (mL)	Dose/day (teaspoonful of suspension)	Dose/day (mL)	Dose/day (teaspoonful of suspension)
6.25	50	2.5	0.5	1.25	0.25
12.5	100	5	1	2.5	0.5
18.75	150	7.5	1.5	3.75	0.75
25	200	10	2	5	1
31.25	250	12.5	2.5	6.25	1.25
37.5	300	15	3	7.5	1.5

Off-label dosing –

Acute urinary tract infection:

• *6 months to 12 years of age* –

Usual dosage: 16 mg/kg/day in divided doses every 12 hours on day 1, followed by 8 mg/kg once daily for 13 days.

Maximum dose: 400 mg/day.

Sexual victimization prophylaxis:

• *Older than 12 years of age* – One time dose of cefixime 400 mg, azithromycin 1 g orally, and metronidazole 2 g orally. Doxycycline 100 mg orally twice daily for 7 days may be used in place of azithromycin.

• *6 months to 12 years of age* –

Usual dosage: One time dose of cefixime 8 mg/kg and azithromycin 20 mg/kg orally.

Maximum dose: Cefixime 400 mg and azithromycin 1 g.

➤*Renal function impairment:*

Cefixime Dosage in Renal Function Impairment	
CrCl[a] (mL/min)	Dosage
> 60	Standard
21 to 60 or renal hemodialysis	75% of standard
< 20 or continuous ambulatory peritoneal dialysis	50% of standard

[a] CrCl = creatinine clearance.

Neither hemodialysis nor peritoneal dialysis removes significant amounts of drug from the body.

➤*Duration of therapy:* In the treatment of infections due to *S. pyogenes*, a therapeutic dosage of cefixime should be administered for at least 10 days.

➤*Administration:* Cefixime, given orally, is about 40% to 50% absorbed whether administered with or without food. Shake well before using.

➤*Storage/Stability:* Store drug powder at 20° to 25°C (68° to 77°F). After reconstitution, the suspension may be kept for 14 days at room temperature or under refrigeration without significant loss of potency. Discard unused portion after 14 days. Keep tightly closed.

CEFOTAXIME SODIUM

Rx	**Cefotaxime** (Various, eg, Cura)	**Powder for Injection**[a]: 500 mg	In vials, packages of 10.
Rx	**Claforan** (Hoechst Marion Roussel)		In vials, packages of 10.
Rx	**Cefotaxime** (Various, eg, Cura)	**Powder for Injection**[a]: 1 g	In vials, packages of 25.
Rx	**Claforan** (Hoechst Marion Roussel)		In vials, packages of 10s, 25s, 50s. Infusion bottles in 10s. *ADD-Vantage* system vials in 25s and 50s.
Rx	**Cefotaxime** (Various, eg, Cura)	**Powder for Injection**[a]: 2 g	In vials, packages of 25.
Rx	**Claforan** (Hoechst Marion Roussel)		In vials, packages of 10s, 25s, 50s. Infusion bottles in 10s. *ADD-Vantage* system vials in 25s and 50s.
Rx	**Cefotaxime** (Various, eg, Cura)	**Powder for Injection**[a]: 10 g	In bottles.
Rx	**Claforan** (Hoechst Marion Roussel)		In bottles.

CEFOTAXIME SODIUM

Rx	**Cefotaxime** (Cura)	**Injection**[a]: 1 g	In infusion bottles, packages of 25.
Rx	**Claforan** (Hoechst Marion Roussel)		Premixed, frozen. In 50 mL, package of 12s.
Rx	**Cefotaxime** (Cura)	**Injection**[a]: 2 g	In infusion bottles, packages of 25.
Rx	**Claforan** (Hoechst Marion Roussel)		Premixed, frozen. In 50 mL, package of 12s.

[a] Contains 2.2 mEq sodium/g.

CEFOTAXIME SODIUM — INJECTION

Complete and comparative prescribing information for these products begins in the Cephalosporins group monograph.

Indications

➤*General information:* Although many strains of enterococci (eg, *Streptococcus faecalis*) and *Pseudomonas* species are resistant to cefotaxime in vitro, cefotaxime has been used successfully in treating patients with infections caused by susceptible organisms.

➤*Lower respiratory tract infections:* Including pneumonia, caused by *Streptococcus pneumoniae* (formerly *Diplococcus pneumoniae*), *Streptococcus pyogenes* (efficacy for this organism, in this organ system, has been studied in less than 10 infections [group A streptococci]) and other streptococci (excluding enterococci, [eg, *Enterococcus faecalis*]), *Staphylococcus aureus* (penicillinase and nonpenicillinase producing), *Escherichia coli*, *Klebsiella* species, *Haemophilus influenzae* (including ampicillin-resistant strains), *Haemophilus parainfluenzae*, *Proteus mirabilis*, *Serratia marcescens* (efficacy for this organism, in this organ system, has been studied in less than 10 infections), *Enterobacter species*, and *indole-positive Proteus* and *Pseudomonas species* (including *Pseudomonas aeruginosa*).

➤*Genitourinary infections:* Caused by *Enterococcus* species, *Staphylococcus epidermidis*, *S. aureus* (penicillinase and nonpenicillinase producing; efficacy for this organism, in this organ system, has been studied in less than 10 infections), *Citrobacter* species, *Enterobacter* species, *E. coli*, *Klebsiella* species, *P. mirabilis*, *Proteus vulgaris* (efficacy for this organism, in this organ system, has been studied in less than 10 infections), *Providencia stuartii*, *Morganella morganii* (efficacy for this organism, in this organ system, has been studied in less than 10 infections), *Providencia rettgeri* (efficacy for this organism, in this organ system, has been studied in less than 10 infections), *Serratia marcescens*, and *Pseudomonas* species (including *P. aeruginosa*). Also, uncomplicated gonorrhea (cervical/urethral and rectal) caused by *Neisseria gonorrhoeae*, including penicillinase-producing strains.

➤*Gynecologic infections:* Including pelvic inflammatory disease, endometritis, and pelvic cellulitis, caused by *S. epidermidis*, *Streptococcus* species, *Enterococcus* species, *Enterobacter* species (efficacy for this organism, in this organ system, has been studied in less than 10 infections), *Klebsiella* species (efficacy for this organism, in this organ system, has been studied in less than 10 infections), *E. coli*, *P. mirabilis*, *Bacteroides* species (including *Bacteroides fragilis*; efficacy for this organism, in this organ system, has been studied in less than 10 infections), *Clostridium* species, and anaerobic cocci (including *Peptostreptococcus* and *Peptococcus* species) and *Fusobacterium* species (including *Fusobacterium nucleatum*; efficacy for this organism, in this organ system, has been studied in less than 10 infections).

Cefotaxime, like other cephalosporins, has no activity against *Chlamydia trachomatis*. Therefore, when cephalosporins are used in the treatment of patients with pelvic inflammatory disease and *C. trachomatis* is 1 of the suspected pathogens, add appropriate antichlamydial coverage.

➤*Bacteremia/Septicemia:* Caused by *E. coli*, *Klebsiella* species, and *S. marcescens*, *S. aureus* and *Streptococcus* species (including *S. pneumoniae*).

➤*Skin and skin structure infections:* Caused by *S. aureus* (penicillinase and nonpenicillinase producing), *S. epidermidis*, *S. pyogenes* (group A streptococci) and other streptococci, *Enterococcus* species, *Acinetobacter* species (efficacy for this organism, in this organ system, has been studied in less than 10 infections), *E. coli*, *Citrobacter* species (including *Citrobacter freundii*; efficacy for this organism, in this organ system, has been studied in less than 10 infections), *Enterobacter* species, *Klebsiella* species, *P. mirabilis*, *P. vulgaris* (efficacy for this organism, in this organ system, has been studied in less than 10 infections), *M. morganii*, *P. rettgeri* (efficacy for this organism, in this organ system, has been studied in less than 10 infections), *Pseudomonas* species, *S. marcescens*, *Bacteroides* species, and anaerobic cocci (including *Peptostreptococcus*; efficacy for this organism, in this organ system, has been studied in less than 10 infections) species and *Peptococcus* species.

➤*Intra-abdominal infections:* Including peritonitis caused by *Streptococcus* species (efficacy for this organism, in this organ system, has been studied in less than 10 infections), *E. coli*, *Klebsiella* species, *Bacteroides* species, and anaerobic cocci (including *Peptostreptococcus*; efficacy for this organism, in this organ system, has been studied in less than 10 infections) species and *Peptococcus* (efficacy for this organism, in this organ system, has been studied in less than 10 infections) species, *P. mirabilis* (efficacy for this organism, in this organ system, has been studied in less than 10 infections), and *Clostridium* species (efficacy for this organism, in this organ system, has been studied in less than 10 infections).

➤*Bone or joint infections:* Caused by *S. aureus* (penicillinase and nonpenicillinase producing strains), *Streptococcus* species (including *S. pyogenes*; efficacy for this organism, in this organ system, has been studied in less than 10 infections), *Pseudomonas* species (including *P. aeruginosa*; efficacy for this organism, in this organ system, has been studied in less than 10 infections), and *P. mirabilis* (efficacy for this organism, in this organ system, has been studied in less than 10 infections).

➤*CNS infections:* Caused by *Neisseria meningitidis*, *H. influenzae*, *S. pneumoniae*, *K. pneumoniae* (efficacy for this organism, in this organ system, has been studied in less than 10 infections), and *E. coli* (efficacy for this organism, in this organ system, has been studied in less than 10 infections).

➤*Concomitant aminoglycoside therapy:* In certain cases of confirmed or suspected gram-positive or gram-negative sepsis, or in patients with other serious infections in which the causative organism has not been identified, cefotaxime may be used concomitantly with an aminoglycoside. The dosage recommended in the labeling of both antibiotics may be given and depends on the severity of the infection and the patient's condition. Carefully monitor renal function, especially if higher dosages of the aminoglycosides are to be administered or if therapy is prolonged, because of the potential nephrotoxicity and ototoxicity of aminoglycoside antibiotics. It is possible that nephrotoxicity may be potentiated if cefotaxime is used concomitantly with an aminoglycoside.

➤*Perioperative prophylaxis:* The administration of cefotaxime preoperatively reduces the incidence of certain infections in patients undergoing surgical procedures (eg, abdominal or vaginal hysterectomy, GI and GU tract surgery) that may be classified as contaminated or potentially contaminated.

For patients undergoing GI surgery, preoperative bowel preparation by mechanical cleansing, as well as with a nonabsorbable antibiotic (eg, neomycin), is recommended.

➤*Cesarean section:* In patients undergoing cesarean section, intraoperative (after clamping the umbilical cord) and postoperative use of cefotaxime may also reduce the incidence of certain postoperative infections. The first dose of 1 g is administered intravenously (IV) as soon as the umbilical cord is clamped. The second and third doses should be given as 1 g IV or intramuscularly (IM) at 6 and 12 hours after the first dose.

➤*Off-label uses:*

Lyme neuroborreliosis – [1] = Good documentation. Parenteral regimens for Lyme disease of the nervous system have a greater potential for morbidity. For severe neurologic disease, class 1 and 2 studies suggested that parenteral treatment (ie, cefotaxime, ceftriaxone, penicillin) was probably safe and effective, but class 2 and 3 studies also indicated that oral therapy (and doxycycline specifically) was comparably safe and effective for patients without parenchymal involvement.

Administration and Dosage

➤*General dosing considerations:* If *C. trachomatis* is a suspected pathogen, appropriate antichlamydial coverage should be added because cefotaxime has no activity against this organism.

➤*Adults:*

Infections – For a list of infections, refer to Indications.

Maximum dose: 12 g/day.

Gonococcal urethritis/cervicitis: 0.5 g IM (single dose).

Gonorrhea, rectal (men): 1 g IM (single dose).

Gonorrhea, rectal (women): 0.5 g IM (single dose).

Moderate to severe infections: 1 to 2 g IM or IV every 8 hours.

More severe infections: For infections commonly needing antibiotics in higher dosage (eg, septicemia), 2 g IV every 6 to 8 hours.

Life-threatening infections: 2 g IV every 4 hours up to 12 g/day.

Perioperative prophylaxis: To prevent postoperative infection in contaminated or potentially contaminated surgery, the recommended dose is a single 1 g IM or IV administered 30 to 90 minutes prior to start of surgery.

For Cesarean section patients, the first dose of 1 g is administered IV as soon as the umbilical cord is clamped. The second and third doses should be given as 1 g IV or IM at 6 and 12 hours after the first dose.

Uncomplicated infections: 1 g IM or IV every 12 hours.

Off-label dosing –

CDC recommended treatment schedules for gonorrhea (MMWR. 2002;51[RR06]:1-80.):

- *Disseminated gonococcal infection* – 1 g IV every 8 hours.

Lyme neuroborreliosis: [1] = Good documentation. 2 g IV every 8 hours for 14 days. In studies, outcomes were similar with regimens lasting between 10 and 28 days.

➤*Children:*

Infections – For a list of infections, refer to Indications.

Usual dosage:

Cefotaxime Dosing for Children			
Age	Weight (kg)	Dosage schedule	Route
0 to 1 week	—	50 mg/kg every 12 hours	IV
1 to 4 weeks	—	50 mg/kg every 8 hours	IV

CEFOTAXIME SODIUM — INJECTION

Cefotaxime Dosing for Children			
Age	Weight (kg)	Dosage schedule	Route
1 month to 12 years	< 50[a]	50 to 180 mg/kg/day in 4 to 6 divided doses[b]	IV or IM

[a] For children ≥ 50 kg, use adult dosage. Do not exceed adult recommended doses. (See Adults).
[b] Use higher doses for more severe or serious infections, including meningitis.

Maximum dose: 12 g/day for children weighing 50 kg or more.

Off-label dosing –

CDC recommended treatment schedules for gonorrhea (MMWR. 2002;51[RR06]:1-80.):

- *Disseminated gonococcal infection and gonococcal scalp abscesses in newborns* – 25 mg/kg IV or IM every 12 hours for 7 days, with a duration of 10 to 14 days if meningitis is documented.

Lyme neuroborreliosis: [1] = Good documentation. 150 to 200 mg/kg/day in 3 to 4 divided doses (maximum, 6 g/day) for 14 days. In studies, outcomes were similar with regimens lasting between 10 and 28 days.

➤*Renal function impairment:* Because high and prolonged serum antibiotic concentrations can occur from usual doses in patients with transient or persistent reduction of urinary output because of renal insufficiency, the total daily dose should be reduced when cefotaxime is administered to such patients. Continued dosage should be determined by degree of renal impairment, severity of infection, and susceptibility of the causative organism.

Although there is no clinical evidence supporting the necessity of changing the dosage of cefotaxime in patients with even profound renal dysfunction, it is suggested that, until further data are obtained, the dose of cefotaxime be halved in patients with estimated creatinine clearances (CrCl) of less than 20 mL/min/1.73 m^2.

Alternatively, the following dosage adjustments have been recommended

CrCl 10 to 50 mL/min – Give doses every 12 to 24 hours.

CrCl less than 10 mL/min – Give doses every 24 hours.

Adults receiving continuous renal replacement therapy (CRRT) – One reference suggests a dosage of 1 g every 12 hours.

The following alternative recommendations assume ultrafiltration and dialysis flow rates of 1 to 2 L/h.

Continuous venovenous hemofiltration (CVVH): 1 to 2 g IV every 8 to 12 hours.

Continuous venovenous hemodialysis (CVVHD): 1 to 2 g IV every 8 hours.

Continuous venovenous hemodialfiltration (CVVHDF): 1 to 2 g IV every 6 to 8 hours.

Adults receiving intermittent hemodialysis (IHD) – One dosing recommendation is to administer a 0.5 to 2 g supplement after dialysis.

Alternatively, administer 1 to 2 g IV every 24 hours after dialysis on dialysis days. This dosing recommendation assumes the patient is receiving standard IHD 3 times per week and completes the full dialysis sessions.

Continuous ambulatory peritoneal dialysis – 0.5 to 1 g every 24 hours.

➤*Duration of therapy:* As with antibiotic therapy in general, administration of cefotaxime should be continued for a minimum of 48 to 72 hours after the patient defervescence or after evidence of bacterial eradication has been obtained. A minimum of 10 days of treatment is recommended for infections caused by group A beta-hemolytic streptococci to guard against the risk of rheumatic fever or glomerulonephritis. Frequent bacteriologic and clinical appraisal is necessary during therapy of chronic urinary tract infection and may be required for several months after therapy has been completed. Persistent infections may require treatment of several weeks. Doses smaller than those previously indicated should not be used.

➤*Preparation for administration:*

Powder for injection – Cefotaxime sterile powder for IM or IV administration should be reconstituted as follows:

Cefotaxime Reconstitution			
Strength	Diluent (mL)	Withdrawable volume (mL)	Approximate concentration (mg/mL)
500 mg vial[a] (IM)	2	2.2	230
1 g vial[a] (IM)	3	3.4	300
2 g vial[a] (IM)	5	6	330
500 mg vial[a] (IV)	10	10.2	50
1 g vial[a] (IV)	10	10.4	95
2 g vial[a] (IV)	10	11	180
1 g infusion	50 to 100	50 to 100	10 to 20
2 g infusion	50 to 100	50 to 100	20 to 40

[a] In conventional vials.

Shake to dissolve; inspect for particulate matter and discoloration prior to use. Solutions of cefotaxime range from very pale yellow to light amber, depending on concentration, diluent used, and length and condition of storage.

A solution of cefotaxime 1 g in 14 mL of sterile water for injection is isotonic.

Preparation for IM administration: Reconstitute vials with sterile water for injection or bacteriostatic water for injection as previously described.

Preparation for IV administration: Reconstitute vials with at least 10 mL of sterile water for injection. Reconstitute infusion bottles with 50 or 100 mL of 0.9% sodium chloride injection or 5% dextrose injection. Reconstituted solutions may be further diluted up to 1,000 mL. For other diluents, see Admixture Compatibility.

Preparation of cefotaxime in ADD-Vantage system: Cefotaxime sterile powder for injection 1 or 2 g may be reconstituted in 50 or 100 mL of 5% dextrose or 0.9% sodium chloride in the *ADD-Vantage* diluent container. Refer to the manufacturer's instructions for *ADD-Vantage* system.

Premixed solution for injection (in Galaxy container) – Cefotaxime injection in *Galaxy* containers (PL 2040 plastic) is for continuous or intermittent infusion using sterile equipment.

Thaw frozen container at room temperature or under refrigeration (at or below 5°C [41°F]). Do not force thaw by immersion in water baths or by microwave irradiation. Check for minute leaks by squeezing container firmly. If leaks are detected, discard solution because sterility may be impaired. Do not add supplementary medication.

Visually inspect the container. Components of the solution may precipitate in the frozen state and will dissolve upon reaching room temperature with little or no agitation. Potency is not affected. Agitate after solution has reached room temperature. If the solution remains cloudy after visual inspection, an insoluble precipitate is noted, or any seals or outlet ports are not intact, discard the container.

Caution: Do not use plastic containers in series connections. Such use could result in air embolism caused by residual air being drawn from the primary container before administration of the fluid from the secondary container is complete.

➤*Administration:* Dosage and route of administration should be determined by susceptibility of the causative organisms, severity of the infection, and the condition of the patient. Premixed cefotaxime injection is intended for IV administration after thawing. Cefotaxime sterile powder for injection may be administered IM or IV after reconstitution.

IM administration – Cefotaxime should be injected well within the body of a relatively large muscle, such as the upper outer quadrant of the buttock (ie, gluteus maximus); aspiration is necessary to avoid inadvertent injection into a blood vessel. Individual IM doses of 2 g may be given if the dose is divided and administered in different IM sites.

IV administration – The IV route is preferable for patients with bacteremia, bacterial septicemia, peritonitis, meningitis, or other severe or life-threatening infections, or for patients who may be poor risks because of lowered resistance resulting from such debilitating conditions as malnutrition, trauma, surgery, diabetes, heart failure, or malignancy, particularly if shock is present or impending.

Intermittent IV: For intermittent IV administration, a solution containing 1 or 2 g in 10 mL of sterile water for injection can be injected over a period of 3 to 5 minutes. Cefotaxime should not be administered over a period of less than 3 minutes. With an infusion system, it may also be given over a longer period of time through the tubing system by which the patient may be receiving other IV solutions. However, during infusion of the solution containing cefotaxime, it is advisable to temporarily discontinue the administration of other solutions at the same site.

Continuous IV: For the administration of higher doses by continuous IV infusion, a solution of cefotaxime may be added to IV bottles containing the solutions discussed in this section.

➤*Admixture compatibility:*

Compatibility – Reconstituted solutions may be further diluted up to 1,000 mL with the following solutions and maintain satisfactory potency for 24 hours at or below 22°C (71.6°F), and at least 5 days under refrigeration (at or below 5°C; 41°F): 0.9% sodium chloride injection; 5% or 10% dextrose injection; 5% dextrose and 0.9% sodium chloride injection, 5% dextrose and 0.45% sodium chloride injection; 5% dextrose and 0.2% sodium chloride injection; Ringer's lactate solution; sodium lactate injection (M/6); 10% invert sugar injection, 8.5% *Travasol* amino acid injection without electrolytes.

Solutions of cefotaxime sterile powder for injection reconstituted in 0.9% sodium chloride injection or 5% dextrose injection in *Viaflex* plastic containers maintain satisfactory potency for 24 hours at or below 22°C (71.6°F), 5 days under refrigeration (at or below 5°C; 41°F) and 13 weeks frozen. Solutions of cefotaxime sterile powder for injection sterile reconstituted in 0.9% sodium chloride injection or 5% dextrose injection in the *ADD-Vantage* flexible containers maintain satisfactory potency for 24 hours at or below 22°C (71.6°F). Do not freeze.

Incompatibility – Solution of cefotaxime must not be admixed with aminoglycoside solutions. If cefotaxime and aminoglycosides are to be administered to the same patient, they must be administered separately and not as mixed injection.

Cefotaxime solutions exhibit maximum stability in the pH 5 to 7 range. Do not prepare solutions of cefotaxime with diluents having a pH greater than 7.5, such as sodium bicarbonate injection.

➤*Storage/Stability:* Store cefotaxime in the dry state below 30°C (86°F). The dry material as well as solutions tend to darken depending on storage conditions; and protect from elevated temperatures and excessive light.

Store premixed cefotaxime injection at or below −20°C (−4°F). The thawed solution is stable for 10 days under refrigeration at or below 5°C (41°F) or 24 hours at or below 22°C (72°F). Do not refreeze thawed antibiotics.

Solutions of cefotaxime sterile powder for injection reconstituted as previously described remain chemically stable (potency remains greater than 90%) as follows when stored in original containers and disposable plastic syringes:

CEFOTAXIME SODIUM — INJECTION

Cefotaxime Storage/Stability				
Strength	Reconstituted concentration mg/mL	Stability ≤ 22°C; 71.6°F	Stability under refrigeration (≤ 5°C; 41°F) Original containers	Plastic syringes
500 mg vial (IM)	230	12 hours	7 days	5 days
1 g vial (IM)	300	12 hours	7 days	5 days
2 g vial (IM)	330	12 hours	7 days	5 days
500 mg vial (IV)	50	24 hours	7 days	5 days
1 g vial (IV)	95	24 hours	7 days	5 days

Cefotaxime Storage/Stability				
Strength	Reconstituted concentration mg/mL	Stability ≤ 22°C; 71.6°F	Stability under refrigeration (≤ 5°C; 41°F) Original containers	Plastic syringes
2 g vial (IV)	180	12 hours	7 days	5 days
1 g infusion bottle	10 to 20	24 hours	10 days	
2 g infusion bottle	20 to 40	24 hours	10 days	

Reconstituted solutions stored in original containers and plastic syringes remain stable for 13 weeks frozen.

CEFTIZOXIME SODIUM

Rx	Cefizox (Fujisawa)	**Powder for Injection:**[a,b] 500 mg	In 10 mL single-dose fliptop vials.
		1 g	In 20 mL single-dose fliptop vials and 100 mL piggyback vials.
		2 g	In 20 mL single-dose fliptop vials and 100 mL piggyback vials.
		10 g	In pharmacy bulk package.
		Injection:[b] 1 g	Frozen, premixed. In 50 mL single-dose plastic containers.
		2 g	Frozen, premixed. In 50 mL single-dose plastic containers.

[a] Contains 2.6 mEq sodium/g.

[b] As sodium.

CEFTIZOXIME SODIUM — INJECTION

For complete and comparative prescribing information, refer to the Cephalosporins group monograph.

Indications

➤*Lower respiratory tract infections:* Caused by *Klebsiella* spp.; *Proteus mirabilis*; *Escherichia coli*; *Haemophilus influenzae* including ampicillin-resistant strains; *Staphylococcus aureus* (penicillinase- and nonpenicillinase-producing); *Serratia* spp.; *Enterobacter* spp.; *Bacteroides* spp.; and *Streptococcus* spp. including *S. pneumoniae*, but excluding enterococci.

➤*Urinary tract infections:* Caused by *Staphylococcus aureus* (penicillinase- and nonpenicillinase-producing); *Escherichia coli*; *Pseudomonas* spp. including *P. aeruginosa*; *Proteus mirabilis*; *P. vulgaris*; *Providencia rettgeri* (formerly *Proteus rettgeri*) and *Morganella morganii* (formerly *Proteus morganii*); *Klebsiella* spp.; *Serratia* spp. including *S. marcescens*; and *Enterobacter* spp.

➤*Gonorrhea:* Including uncomplicated cervical and urethral gonorrhea caused by *Neisseria gonorrhoeae*.

➤*Pelvic inflammatory disease:* Caused by *Neisseria gonorrhoeae*, *Escherichia coli* or *Streptococcus agalactiae*.

Ceftizoxime, like other cephalosporins, has no activity against *Chlamydia trachomatis*. Therefore, when cephalosporins are used in the treatment of patients with pelvic inflammatory disease and *C. trachomatis* is one of the suspected pathogens, appropriate anti-chlamydial coverage should be added.

➤*Intra-abdominal infections:* Caused by *Escherichia coli*; *Staphylococcus epidermidis*; *Streptococcus* spp. (excluding enterococci); *Enterobacter* spp.; *Klebsiella* spp.; *Bacteroides* spp. including *B. fragilis*; and anaerobic cocci, including *Peptococcus* spp. and *Peptostreptococcus* spp.

➤*Septicemia:* Caused by *Streptococcus* spp. including *S. pneumoniae* (but excluding enterococci); *Staphylococcus aureus* (penicillinase- and nonpenicillinase-producing); *Escherichia coli*; *Bacteroides* spp. including *B. fragilis*; *Klebsiella* spp.; and *Serratia* spp.

➤*Skin and skin structure infections:* Caused by *Staphylococcus aureus* (penicillinase- and nonpenicillinase-producing); *Staphylococcus epidermidis*; *Escherichia coli*; *Klebsiella* spp.; *Streptococcus* spp. including *Streptococcus pyogenes* (but excluding enterococci); *Proteus mirabilis*; *Serratia* spp.; *Enterobacter* spp.; *Bacteroides* spp. including *B. fragilis*; and anaerobic cocci, including *Peptococcus* spp. and *Peptostreptococcus* spp.

➤*Bone and joint infections:* Caused by *Staphylococcus aureus* (penicillinase- and nonpenicillinase-producing); *Streptococcus* spp. (excluding enterococci); *Proteus mirabilis*; *Bacteroides* spp.; and anaerobic cocci, including *Peptococcus* spp. and *Peptostreptococcus* spp.

➤*Meningitis:* Caused by *Haemophilus influenzae*. Ceftizoxime has also been used successfully in the treatment of a limited number of pediatric and adult cases of meningitis caused by *Streptococcus pneumoniae*.

➤*Mixed infections:* Infections caused by aerobic gram-negative and by mixtures of organisms resistant to other cephalosporins, aminoglycosides, or penicillins have responded to treatment with ceftizoxime.

Administration and Dosage

➤*General dosing considerations:* If *C. trachomatis* is a suspected pathogen in pelvic inflammatory disease, appropriate anti-chlamydial coverage should be added because ceftizoxime has no action against this organism.

Because of the serious nature of urinary tract infections caused by *P. aeruginosa* and because many strains of *Pseudomonas* species are only moderately susceptible to ceftizoxime, higher dosage is recommended. Other therapy should be instituted if the response is not prompt.

➤*Adults:*

Infections – For a list of infections, refer to Indications.

Usual dosage: 1 or 2 g IM or IV every 8 to 12 hours. Proper dosage and route of administration should be determined by the condition of the patient, severity of the infection, and susceptibility of the causative organisms.

Ceftizoxime Dosage for Adults		
Type of infection	Daily dose (g)	Frequency and route
Gonorrhea (uncomplicated)	1	1 g IM (single) dose
Pelvic inflammatory disease	6	2 g every 8 h IV
Urinary tract infection (uncomplicated)	1	500 mg every 12 h IM or IV
Other sites	2-3	1 g every 8 to 12 h IM or IV
Severe or refractory	3-6	1 g every 8 h IM or IV 2 g every 8 to 12 h IM[a] or IV
Life-threatening[b]	9-12	3 to 4 g every 8 h IV

[a] Divide 2 g IM doses and give in different large muscle masses.

[b] Dosages ≤ 2 g every 4 hours have been given.

Severe or life-threatening infections: Dosages of up to 2 g IV every 4 hours have been given for life-threatening infections.

The IV route may be preferable for patients with bacterial septicemia, localized parenchymal abscesses (such as intra-abdominal abscess), peritonitis, or other severe or life-threatening infections. The IV dosage for such infections is 2 to 12 g/day. In conditions such as bacterial septicemia, 6 to 12 g/day may be given initially by the IV route for several days, and the dosage may then be gradually reduced according to clinical response and laboratory findings.

➤*Children:*

Infections – For a list of infections, refer to Indications.

6 months of age and older:

• *Usual dosage* – 50 mg/kg/dose every 6 to 8 hours. Dosage may be increased to a total daily dose of 200 mg/kg.

• *Maximum dose* – 200 mg/kg/day (up to the maximum adult dose for serious infection).

➤*Renal function impairment:* Modification of ceftizoxime dosage is necessary in patients with impaired renal function.

Loading dose – 500 mg to 1 g IM or IV.

Maintenance dosage – Further dosing should be determined by therapeutic monitoring, severity of the infection, and susceptibility of the causative organisms.

Mild impairment (CrCl 50 to 79 mL/min): 500 mg every 8 hours for less severe infections; 750 mg to 1.5 g every 8 hours for life-threatening infections.

Moderate to severe impairment (CrCl 5 to 49 mL/min): 250 to 500 mg every 12 hours for less severe infections; 500 mg to 1 g every 12 hours for life-threatening infections.

Dialysis (CrCl less than 4 mL/min): 500 mg every 48 hours or 250 mg every 24 hours for less severe infections; 500 mg to 1 g every 48 hours, or 500 mg every 24 hours for life-threatening infections. In patients undergoing hemodialysis, no additional supplemental dosing is required following hemodialysis; however, dosing should be timed so that the patient receives the dose at the end of the dialysis.

➤*Preparation for administration:* Reconstituted solutions may range from yellow to amber without changes in potency.

CEFTIZOXIME SODIUM — INJECTION

Reconstitution –

Pharmacy bulk vials: Pharmacy bulk vials are not for direct infusion. Reconstitute before using sterile water for injection. Shake well. Add to parenteral fluids listed under Preparation for IV Infusion.

When 30 mL of diluent is added to a 10 g bulk vial, the approximate available volume is 37 mL, yielding an approximate concentration of 1 g in 3.5 mL. The stability of this solution at room temperature is 16 hours. When 45 mL of diluent is added to a 10 g bulk vial, the approximate available volume is 51 mL, yielding an approximate concentration of 1 g in 5 mL. The stability of this solution at room temperature is 24 hours.

These reconstituted solutions of ceftizoxime are stable for 96 hours if refrigerated (5°C; 41°F).

Pharmacy bulk packages:

The withdrawal of reconstituted transfer fluid from a pharmacy bulk vial should be accomplished without delay. However, if this is not possible, a maximum time of 4 hours from the initial introduction of the solvent, or diluent, into the pharmacy bulk vial is permitted to complete fluid transfer operations.

Although the ceftizoxime in the transfer fluid is stable for 16 or 24 hours at room temperature, depending on dilution or 96 hours if refrigerated (5°C; 41°F), it is recommended that the transfer fluid/admixture be used promptly.

Preparation for IV infusion – For intermittent or continuous infusion, dilute reconstituted ceftizoxime in 50 to 100 mL of 1 of the following solutions: sodium chloride injection, dextrose 5% or 10% injection, dextrose 5% and sodium chloride 0.9%, 0.45%, or 0.2% injection, Ringer's injection, Ringer's lactate injection, invert sugar 10% in sterile water for injection, sodium bicarbonate 5% in sterile water for injection, dextrose 5% in Ringer's lactate injection (only when reconstituted with 4% sodium bicarbonate injection). In these fluids, ceftizoxime is stable 24 hours at room temperature or 96 hours if refrigerated (5°C; 41°F).

➤*Administration:*

IM injection – Inject well within the body of a relatively large muscle. When administering 2 g IM doses, the dose should be divided and given in different large muscle masses.

IV administration – Direct (bolus) injection, slowly over 3 to 5 minutes, directly or through tubing for patients receiving parenteral fluids (see list in Preparation for administration).

The IV route may be preferable for patients with bacterial septicemia, localized parenchymal abscesses (such as intra-abdominal abscess), peritonitis, or other severe or life-threatening infections.

➤*Storage / Stability:* Unreconstituted ceftizoxime should be protected from excessive light, and stored at controlled room temperature 15° to 30°C (59° to 86°F) in the original package until used. Also see Preparation for Administration.

CEFOTETAN DISODIUM

Rx	**Cefotetan Disodium** (Abraxis)	**Injection, powder for solution:** 1 g	3.5 mEq sodium/mL. In 10 mL vials.
		Injection, powder for solution: 2 g	3.5 mEq/mL. In 20 mL vials.
		Injection, powder for solution: 10 g	3.5 mEq/mL. In 20 mL vials.

CEFOTETAN — INJECTION

For complete and comparative prescribing information, refer to the Cephalosporins class monograph.

Indications

➤*Urinary tract infections:* Caused by *E. coli, Klebsiella* sp. (including *K. pneumoniae*), *Proteus mirabilis* and *Proteus* sp. (which may include the organisms now called *Proteus vulgaris, Providencia rettgeri*, and *Morganella morganii*).

➤*Lower respiratory tract infections:* Caused by *Streptococcus pneumoniae, Staphylococcus aureus* (penicillinase- and non-penicillinase-producing strains), *Haemophilus influenzae* (including ampicillin-resistant strains), *Klebsiella* species (including *K. pneumoniae*), *E. coli, Proteus mirabilis*, and *Serratia marcescens* (efficacy for this organism in this organism system was studied in < 10 infections).

➤*Skin and skin structure infections:* Due to *Staphylococcus aureus* (penicillinase- and non-penicillinase-producing strains), *Staphylococcus epidermidis, Streptococcus pyogenes, Streptococcus* species (excluding enterococci), *Escherichia coli, Klebsiella pneumoniae, Peptococcus niger* (efficacy for this organism in this organism system was studied in < 10 infections), *Peptostreptococcus* species.

➤*Gynecologic infections:* Caused by *Staphylococcus aureus*, (including penicillinase- and non-penicillinase-producing strains), *Staphylococcus epidermidis, Streptococcus* species (excluding enterococci), *Streptococcus agalactiae, E. coli, Proteus mirabilis, Neisseria gonorrhoeae, Bacteroides* species (excluding *B. distasonis, B. ovatus, B. thetaiotaomicron*), *Fusobacterium* species (efficacy for this organism in this organism system was studied in < 10 infections), and gram-positive anaerobic cocci (including *Peptococcus* and *Peptostreptococcus* species).

Cefotetan, like other cephalosporins, has no activity against *Chlamydia trachomatis*. Therefore, when cephalosporins are used in the treatment of pelvic inflammatory disease, and *C. trachomatis* is 1 of the suspected pathogens, appropriate antichlamydial coverage should be added.

➤*Intra-abdominal infections:* Caused by *E. coli, Klebsiella* species (including *K. pneumoniae*), *Streptococcus* species (excluding enterococci), *Bacteroides* species (excluding *B. distasonis, B. ovatus, B. thetaiotaomicron*) and *Clostridium* species (efficacy for this organism in this organ system was studied in < 10 infections).

➤*Bone and joint infections:* Caused by *Staphylococcus aureus* (efficacy for this organism in this organ system was studied in < 10 infections).

➤*Preoperative prophylaxis:* The preoperative administration of cefotetan may reduce the incidence of certain postoperative infections in patients undergoing surgical procedures that are classified as clean contaminated or potentially contaminated (eg, cesarean section, abdominal or vaginal hysterectomy, transurethral surgery, biliary tract surgery, and GI surgery).

Administration and Dosage

➤*General dosing considerations:* If *Chlamydia trachomatis* is a suspected pathogen in gynecologic infections, appropriate antichlamydial coverage should be added because cefotetan has no activity against this organism.

➤*Adults:*

Infections – For a list of infections, refer to Indications.

Usual dosage: 1 or 2 g every 12 hours for 5 to 10 days. Cefotetan disodium for injection may be administered IV or IM.

Cefotetan Dosage Guidelines

Infection	Daily dose	Frequency and route
Skin and skin structure (mild to moderate)[a]	2 g	2 g every 24 hours IV 1 g every 12 hours IV or IM
Skin and skin structure (severe)	4 g	2 g every 12 hours IV
Urinary tract	1 to 4 g	500 mg every 12 hours IV or IM 1 or 2 g every 24 hours IV or IM 1 or 2 g every 12 hours IV or IM
Other sites	2 to 4 g	1 or 2 g every 12 hours IV or IM
Severe	4 g	2 g every 12 hours IV
Life-threatening	6 g[b]	3 g every 12 hours IV

[a] *Klebsiella pneumoniae* skin and skin structure infections should be treated with 1 or 2 g every 12 hours IV or IM.
[b] Maximum daily dosage should not exceed 6 g.

Maximum dose: 6 g/day.

Prophylactic dosage: To prevent postoperative infection in clean contaminated or potentially contaminated surgery, the recommended dosage is 1 or 2 g administered IV once, 30 to 60 minutes prior to surgery. In patients undergoing cesarean section, the dose should be administered as soon as the umbilical cord is clamped.

➤*Renal function impairment:*

Cefotetan Dosage in Patients With Renal Function Impairment

CrCl[a] (mL/min)	Dose	Frequency
> 30	Usual recommended dosage[b]	Every 12 hours
10 to 30	Usual recommended dosage[b]	Every 24 hours
< 10	Usual recommended dosage[b]	Every 48 hours

[a] CrCl = creatinine clearance.
[b] Dose determined by the type and severity of infection, and susceptibility of the causative organism.

Alternatively, the dosing interval may remain constant at 12-hour intervals, but with the dose reduced to 50% the usual recommended dose for patients with a CrCl of 10 to 30 mL/min and 25% the usual recommended dose for patients with a CrCl of less than 10 mL/min.

Hemodialysis – Cefotetan is dialyzable, and it is recommended that for patients undergoing intermittent hemodialysis, 25% of the usual recommended dose should be given every 24 hours on days between dialysis and 50% of the usual recommended dose on the day of dialysis.

Alternatively, give a 1 g supplement after dialysis.

Continuous ambulatory peritoneal dialysis – Give 1 g every 24 hours.

CEFOTETAN — INJECTION

➤*Preparation for administration:*

Powder for solution –

Preparation for IV administration: Reconstitute with sterile water for injection. Shake to dissolve, and let stand until clear.

Volume and Concentration Following Reconstitution of IV Cefotetan			
Vial size	Amount of diluent to add (mL)	Approximate withdrawable volume (mL)	Approximate average concentration (mg/mL)
1 g	10	10.5	95
2 g	10 to 20	11 to 21	182 to 95

Infusion bottles (100 mL) may be reconstituted with 50 to 100 mL of dextrose injection 5% or sodium chloride injection 0.9%.

Preparation for IM administration – Reconstitute with sterile water for injection; bacteriostatic water for injection; sodium chloride injection 0.9%; 0.5% lidocaine hydrochloride; or 1% lidocaine hydrochloride. Shake to dissolve and let stand until clear.

Volume and Concentration Following Reconstitution of IM Cefotetan			
Vial size	Amount of diluent to add (mL)	Approximate withdrawable volume (mL)	Approximate average concentration (mg/mL)
1 g	2	2.5	400
2 g	3	4	500

➤*Administration:* Proper dosage and route of administration should be determined by the condition of the patient, severity of the infection, and susceptibility of the causative organism.

IV administration – The IV route is preferable for patients with bacteremia, bacterial septicemia, or other severe or life-threatening infections, or for patients who may be high risk because of lowered resistance resulting from such debilitating conditions as malnutrition, trauma, surgery, diabetes, heart failure, or malignancy, particularly if shock is present or impending.

Butterfly or scalp vein-type needles are preferred for this type of infusion. However, during infusion of cefotetan, it is advisable to temporarily discontinue the administration of other solutions at the same site.

Intermittent IV administration: For intermittent IV administration, a solution containing 1 or 2 g of cefotetan in sterile water for injection can be injected over a period of 3 to 5 minutes. Using an infusion system, the solution may also be given over a longer period of time through the tubing system by which the patient may be receiving other IV solutions.

IM administration – As with all IM preparations, cefotetan should be injected well within the body of a relatively large muscle, such as the upper outer quadrant of the buttock (ie, gluteus maximus); aspiration is necessary to avoid inadvertent injection into a blood vessel.

➤*Admixture compatibility:* Solutions of cefotetan must not be admixed with solutions containing aminoglycosides. If cefotetan and aminoglycosides are to be administered to the same patient, they must be administered separately and not as a mixed injection. Do not add supplementary medications.

See also Preparation for Administration for more compatibility information.

➤*Storage / Stability:*

Cefotetan disodium for injection (powder) – Cefotetan reconstituted as previously described maintains satisfactory potency for 24 hours at room temperature (25°C; 77°F), for 96 hours under refrigeration (5°C; 41°F), and for at least 1 week in the frozen state (−20°C; −4°F). After reconstitution and subsequent storage in disposable glass or plastic syringes, cefotetan is stable for 24 hours at room temperature and 96 hours under refrigeration.

CEFTAZIDIME

Rx	**Fortaz** (GlaxoWellcome)	**Injection, powder for solution:** 500 mg	In vials.[a]
Rx	**Ceftazidime** (Sandoz)	**Injection, powder for solution:** 1 g	In vials.[a]
Rx	**Ceptaz** (GlaxoWellcome)		In vials and infusion packs.[b]
Rx	**Fortaz** (GlaxoWellcome)		In vials, *ADD-Vantage* vials and infusion packs.[a]
Rx	**Tazicef** (Hospira)		In vials, *ADD-Vantage* vials and piggyback vials.[a]
Rx	**Tazidime** (Eli Lilly)		In 20 mL, 100 mL and *ADD-Vantage* vials.[b]
Rx	**Ceftazidime** (Sandoz)	**Injection, powder for solution:** 2 g	In vials.[a]
Rx	**Ceptaz** (GlaxoWellcome)		In vials and infusion packs.[b]
Rx	**Fortaz** (GlaxoWellcome)		In vials, *ADD-Vantage* vials and infusion packs.[a]
Rx	**Tazicef** (Hospira)		In vials, *ADD-Vantage* vials and piggyback vials.[a]
Rx	**Tazidime** (Eli Lilly)		In 50 mL, 100 mL and *ADD-Vantage* vials.[2]
Rx	**Ceftazidime** (Sandoz)	**Injection, powder for solution:** 6 g	In bulk packages.[a]
Rx	**Fortaz** (GlaxoWellcome)		In bulk package.[a]
Rx	**Tazicef** (Hospira)		In bulk package.[a]
Rx	**Tazidime** (Eli Lilly)		In 100 mL vial.[b]
Rx	**Fortaz** (GlaxoWellcome)	**Injection:** 1 g	Premixed, frozen. In 50 mL.[c]
		2 g	Premixed, frozen. In 50 mL.[d]
Rx	**Tazicef** (Hospira)	**Injection:** 1 g	In *Galaxy* containers.
		2 g	In *Galaxy* containers.

[a] Contains 2.3 mEq sodium/g.
[b] As pentahydrate with L-arginine.
[c] With 2.2 g dextrose hydrous.
[d] With 1.6 g dextrose hydrous.

CEFTAZIDIME — INJECTION

For complete and comparative prescribing information, refer to the Cephalosporins group monograph.

Indications

➤*Lower respiratory tract infections:* Including pneumonia, caused by *Pseudomonas aeruginosa* and other *Pseudomonas* spp.; *Haemophilus influenzae*, including ampicillin-resistant strains; *Klebsiella* spp.; *Enterobacter* spp.; *Proteus mirabilis*; *Escherichia coli*; *Serratia* spp.; *Citrobacter* spp.; *Streptococcus pneumoniae*; and *Staphylococcus aureus* (methicillin-susceptible strains).

➤*Skin and skin-structure infections:* Caused by *Pseudomonas aeruginosa*; *Klebsiella* spp.; *Escherichia coli*; *Proteus* spp.; including *Proteus mirabilis* and indole-positive *Proteus*; *Enterobacter* spp.; *Serratia* spp.; *Staphylococcus aureus* (methicillin-susceptible strains); and *Streptococcus pyogenes* (group A beta-hemolytic streptococci).

➤*Urinary tract infections, complicated and uncomplicated:* Caused by *Pseudomonas aeruginosa*; *Enterobacter* spp.; *Proteus* spp., including *Proteus mirabilis* and indole-positive *Proteus*; *Klebsiella* spp.; and *Escherichia coli*.

➤*Bacterial septicemia:* Caused by *Pseudomonas aeruginosa*, *Klebsiella* spp., *Haemophilus influenzae*, *Escherichia coli*, *Serratia* spp., *Streptococcus pneumoniae*, and *Staphylococcus aureus* (methicillin-susceptible strains).

➤*Bone and joint infections:* Caused by *Pseudomonas aeruginosa*, *Klebsiella* spp., *Enterobacter* spp., and *Staphylococcus aureus* (methicillin-susceptible strains).

➤*Gynecologic infections:* Including endometritis, pelvic cellulitis, and other infections of the female genital tract caused by *Escherichia coli*.

➤*Intra-abdominal infections:* Including peritonitis caused by *Escherichia coli*, *Klebsiella* spp., and *Staphylococcus aureus* (methicillin-susceptible strains) and polymicrobial infections caused by aerobic and anaerobic organisms and *Bacteroides* spp. (many strains of *Bacteroides fragilis* are resistant).

➤*CNS infections:* Including meningitis, caused by *Haemophilus influenzae* and *Neisseria meningitidis*. Ceftazidime has also been used successfully in a limited number of cases of meningitis due to *Pseudomonas aeruginosa* and *Streptococcus pneumoniae*.

➤*Concomitant therapy:* Ceftazidime may also be used concomitantly with other antibiotics, such as aminoglycosides, vancomycin, and clindamycin; in severe and life-threatening infections; and in the immunocompromised patient. When such concomitant treatment is appropriate, prescribing information in the labeling for the other antibiotics should be followed. The dose depends on the severity of the infection and the patient's condition.

➤*Off-label uses:*

Catheter-related bloodstream infections (children / adolescents) – [2] = Fair documentation. A third-generation cephalosporin, such as ceftazidime, is recommended by Infectious Diseases Society of America (IDSA) clinical practice guidelines as a first-line agent for the treatment of catheter-related infections due to susceptible extended-spectrum beta-lactamase–negative *E. coli* and *Klebsiella* species in children. The

CEFTAZIDIME — INJECTION

recommended pediatric dosage in IDSA guidelines is slightly higher than that in the prescribing information for ceftazidime.

Administration and Dosage

➤*Adults:*

Infections – The usual adult dosage is 1 g IV or IM every 8 to 12 hours. The dosage and route should be determined by the susceptibility of the causative organisms, the severity of infection, and the condition and renal function of the patient.

The guidelines for dosage of ceftazidime are listed in the following table.

Ceftazidime Dosing for Patients Older Than 12 Years of Age		
Infection	Dose	Frequency
Usual recommended dosage	1 g IV or IM	every 8 to 12 hours
Bone and joint infections	2 g IV	every 12 hours
Gynecologic and intra-abdominal infections (serious)	2 g IV	every 8 hours
Lung infections caused by *Pseudomonas* spp. in patients with cystic fibrosis with healthy renal function[a]	30 to 50 mg/kg IV (maximum, 6 g per day)	every 8 hours
Meningitis	2 g IV	every 8 hours
Pneumonia (uncomplicated)	500 mg to 1 g IV or IM	every 8 hours
Skin and skin structure infections (mild)	500 mg to 1 g IV or IM	every 8 hours
Urinary tract infections (complicated)	500 mg IV or IM	every 8 to 12 hours
Urinary tract infections (uncomplicated)	250 mg IV or IM	every 12 hours
Very severe life-threatening infections, especially in immunocompromised patients	2 g IV	every 8 hours

[a] Although clinical improvement has been shown, bacteriologic cures cannot be expected in patients with chronic respiratory disease and cystic fibrosis.

➤*Children:*

Infections – See Adults for dosing for children older than 12 years of age.

1 month to 12 years of age:

• *Usual dosage* – 30 to 50 mg/kg IV every 8 hours. The higher dose should be reserved for immunocompromised pediatric patients or pediatric patients with cystic fibrosis or meningitis.

• *Maximum dose* – 6 g/day.

0 to 4 weeks of age: The usual dosage is 30 mg/kg IV every 12 hours.

Off-label dosing –

Catheter-related bloodstream infections (children/adolescents): [2] = Fair documentation.

• *Neonates* – 100 to 150 mg/kg/day administered IV every 8 to 12 hours in divided doses for 7 to 14 days.

• *Infants and children younger than 12 years of age* – 100 to 150 mg/kg/day administered IV every 8 hours in divided doses for 7 to 14 days.

• *Maximum dose* – 6 g/day.

➤*Renal function impairment:* Ceftazidime is excreted by the kidneys, almost exclusively by glomerular filtration. Therefore, in patients with impaired renal function (glomerular filtration rate [GFR] less than 50 mL/min), it is recommended that the dosage of ceftazidime be reduced to compensate for its slower excretion.

Adults –

Loading dose: 1 g in patients with suspected renal insufficiency.

Maintenance dosage: An estimate of GFR should be made to determine the appropriate maintenance dosage. The recommended dosages are presented in the following table.

If the dose recommended in the previous table (see Adults) is lower than that recommended for patients with renal insufficiency as outlined in the following table, the lower dose should be used.

Ceftazidime Dosage in Renal Impairment		
Creatinine clearance (mL/min)	Dose	Frequency of dosing
31 to 50	1 g	every 12 hours
16 to 30	1 g	every 24 hours
6 to 15	500 mg	every 24 hours
< 5	500 mg	every 48 hours

In patients with severe infections who would normally receive ceftazidime 6 g daily were it not for renal insufficiency, the unit dose given in the previous information for maintenance dosing in renal insufficiency may be increased by 50%, or the dosing frequency may be increased appropriately. Further dosing should be determined by therapeutic monitoring, severity of the infection, and susceptibility of the causative organism.

Children – In children, as for adults, the creatinine clearance should be adjusted for body surface area or lean body mass, and the dosing frequency should be reduced in cases of renal insufficiency.

Hemodialysis –

Adults receiving continuous renal replacement therapy (CRRT): One reference suggests a dosage of 1 to 2 g every 12 hours, or a loading dose of 2 g followed by a maintenance dosage of 3 g/day as a continuous infusion.

The following alternative recommendations assume ultrafiltration and dialysis flow rates of 1 to 2 L/h. A higher dosage is recommended when treating viral meningoencephalitis and varicella-zoster virus infections.

• *Loading dose* – 2 g IV.

• *Maintenance dosage* –

Continuous venovenous hemofiltration (CVVH): 1 to 2 g IV every 12 hours.

Continous venovenous hemodialysis (CVVHD) or continuous venovenous hemodialfiltration (CVVHDF): 1 g IV every 8 hours or 2 g IV every 12 hours. For patients infected with gram-negative rods with an MIC of 4 mg/L or higher, a dosage of 2 g IV every 8 hours may be needed.

Adults receiving intermittent hemodialysis (IHD): According to the prescribing information, in patients undergoing hemodialysis, a loading dose of 1 g is recommended followed by 1 g after each hemodialysis period.

An alternative dosage is 500 mg to 1 g IV every 24 hours administered after dialysis on dialysis days, or alternatively 1 to 2 g IV every 48 to 72 hours administered after dialysis. This recommendation assumes the patient is receiving standard IHD 3 times per week and completes the full dialysis sessions.

Peritoneal dialysis – Ceftazidime can also be used in patients undergoing intraperitoneal dialysis and continuous ambulatory peritoneal dialysis. In such patients, a loading dose of 1 g of ceftazidime may be given, followed by 500 mg every 24 hours. In addition to IV use, ceftazidime can be incorporated in the dialysis fluid at a concentration of 250 mg for 2 L of dialysis fluid.

➤*Duration of therapy:* Generally, ceftazidime should be continued for 2 days after the signs and symptoms of infection have disappeared, but in complicated infections, longer therapy may be required.

➤*Preparation for administration:* All vials of ceftazidime as supplied are under reduced pressure. When ceftazidime is dissolved, carbon dioxide is released and a positive pressure develops. For ease of use, follow the recommended techniques of constitution.

IM administration – For IM administration, ceftazidime should be constituted with one of the following diluents: Sterile Water for Injection, Bacteriostatic Water for Injection, or 0.5% or 1% Lidocaine Hydrochloride Injection.

Intermittent IV administration – Reconstitute ceftazidime as directed below with Sterile Water for Injection.

IV infusion – Reconstitute the 1 g infusion pack with 100 mL of Sterile Water for Injection or one of the compatible IV fluids listed under the Storage/Stability section. (See Storage/Stability.) Alternatively, constitute the 500 mg, 1 or 2 g vial and add an appropriate quantity of the resulting solution to an IV container with one of the compatible IV fluids.

Intermittent IV infusion – *ADD-Vantage* vials are to be constituted only with 50 or 100 mL of 5% Dextrose Injection, 0.9% Sodium Chloride Injection, or 0.45% Sodium Chloride Injection in Abbott *ADD-Vantage* flexible diluent containers.

Preparation of Ceftazidime Solutions			
Size	Amount of diluent to be added (mL)	Approximate available volume (mL)	Approximate ceftazidime concentration (mg/mL)
IM			
500 mg vial	1.5	1.8	280
1 g vial	3	3.6	280
IV			
500 mg vial	5	5.3	100
1 g vial	10	10.6	100
2 g vial	10	11.5	170
Infusion pack			
1 g vial	100[a]	100	10
2 g vial	100[a]	100	20
Pharmacy bulk package			
6 g vial	26	30	200

[a] Addition should be in 2 stages.

Galaxy containers – Ceftazidime supplied as a frozen, sterile, iso-osmotic, nonpyrogenic solution in plastic containers is to be administered after thawing either as a continuous or intermittent IV infusion. The thawed solution is stable for 24 hours at room temperature or for 7 days if stored under refrigeration. Do not refreeze.

Thaw container at room temperature (25°C [77°F]) or under refrigeration (5°C [41°F]). Do not force thaw by immersion in water baths or by microwave irradiation. Components of the solution may precipitate in the frozen state and will dissolve upon reaching room temperature with little or no agitation. Potency is not affected. Mix after solution has reached room temperature. Check for minute leaks by squeezing the bag firmly. Discard the bag if

CEFTAZIDIME — INJECTION

leaks are found, as sterility may be impaired. Do not add supplementary medication. Do not use unless solution is clear and seal is intact. Use sterile equipment.

➤*Administration:* Ceftazidime may be given IV or by deep IM injection into a large muscle mass such as the upper outer quadrant of the gluteus maximus or lateral part of the thigh. Intra-arterial administration should be avoided.

The IV route is preferable for patients with bacterial septicemia, bacterial meningitis, peritonitis, or other severe or life-threatening infections, or for patients who may be poor risks because of lowered resistance resulting from such debilitating conditions as malnutrition, trauma, surgery, diabetes, heart failure, or malignancy, particularly if shock is present or pending.

Intermittent IV administration – Slowly inject directly into the vein over a period of 3 to 5 minutes or give through the tubing of an administration set while the patient is also receiving one of the compatible IV fluids.

Intermittent IV infusion – Intermittent IV infusion with a Y-type administration set can be accomplished with compatible solutions. However, during infusion of a solution containing ceftazidime, it is desirable to discontinue the other solution.

➤*Admixture compatibility:* Solutions of ceftazidime, like those of most beta-lactam antibiotics, should not be added to solutions of aminoglycoside antibiotics because of potential interaction. However, if concurrent therapy with ceftazidime and an aminoglycoside is indicated, each of these antibiotics can be administered separately to the same patient.

Ceftazidime is less stable in Sodium Bicarbonate Injection than in other IV fluids. It is not recommended as a diluent.

Vancomycin solution exhibits a physical incompatibility when mixed with a number of drugs, including ceftazidime. The likelihood of precipitation with ceftazidime is dependent on the concentrations of vancomycin and ceftazidime present. It is therefore recommended, when both drugs are to be administered by intermittent IV infusion, that they be given separately, flushing the IV lines (with one of the compatible IV fluids) between the administration of these two agents.

See also Storage/Stability for more compatibility information.

➤*Storage/Stability:* Ceftazidime in the dry state should be stored between 15° and 30°C (59° and 86°F) and protected from light.

As with other cephalosporins, ceftazidime powder as well as solutions tend to darken, depending on storage conditions; within the stated recommendations, however, product potency is not adversely affected.

IM – Ceftazidime, when constituted as directed with Sterile Water for Injection, Bacteriostatic Water for Injection, or 0.5% or 1% Lidocaine Hydrochloride Injection, maintains satisfactory potency for 24 hours at room temperature or for 7 days under refrigeration. Solutions in Sterile Water for Injection that are frozen immediately after constitution in the original container are stable for 3 months when stored at −20°C (−4°F). Once thawed, solutions should not be refrozen. Thawed solutions may be stored for up to 8 hours at room temperature or for 4 days in a refrigerator.

IV – Ceftazidime, when constituted as directed with Sterile Water for Injection, maintains satisfactory potency for 24 hours at room temperature or for 7 days under refrigeration. Solutions in Sterile Water for Injection in the infusion vial or in 0.9% Sodium Chloride Injection in *Viaflex* small-volume containers that are frozen immediately after constitution are stable for 6 months when stored at −20°C (−4°F). Once thawed, solutions should not be refrozen. Thawed solutions may be stored for up to 24 hours at room temperature or for 7 days in a refrigerator. More concentrated solutions in Sterile Water for Injection in the original container that are frozen immediately after constitution are stable for 3 months when stored at −20°C (−4°F). Once thawed, solutions should not be refrozen. Thawed solutions may be stored for up to 8 hours at room temperature or for 4 days in a refrigerator.

Ceftazidime is compatible with the more commonly used IV infusion fluids. Solutions at concentrations between 1 and 40 mg/mL in 0.9% Sodium Chloride Injection, 1/6 M Sodium Lactate Injection, 5% Dextrose Injection, 5% Dextrose and 0.225% Sodium Chloride Injection, 5% Dextrose and 0.45% Sodium Chloride Injection, 5% Dextrose and 0.9% Sodium Chloride Injection, 10% Dextrose Injection, Ringer's Injection, Lactated Ringer's Injection, 10% Invert Sugar in Water for Injection, and *Normosol-M* in 5% Dextrose Injection may be stored for up to 24 hours at room temperature or for 7 days if refrigerated.

The 1 and 2 g ceftazidime *ADD-Vantage* vials, when diluted in 50 or 100 mL of 5% Dextrose Injection, 0.9% Sodium Chloride Injection, or 0.45% Sodium Chloride Injection, may be stored for up to 24 hours at room temperature or for 7 days under refrigeration.

Ceftazidime is less stable in Sodium Bicarbonate Injection than in other IV fluids. It is not recommended as a diluent. Solutions of ceftazidime in 5% Dextrose Injection and 0.9% Sodium Chloride Injection are stable for at least 6 hours at room temperature in plastic tubing, drip chambers, and volume control devices of common IV infusion sets.

Ceftazidime at a concentration of 4 mg/mL has been found compatible for 24 hours at room temperature or for 7 days under refrigeration in 0.9% Sodium Chloride Injection or 5% Dextrose Injection when admixed with cefuroxime sodium 3 mg/mL, heparin 10 or 50 U/mL, or potassium chloride 10 or 40 mEq/L.

ADD-Vantage vials – ADD-Vantage vials that have been joined to Abbott *ADD-Vantage* diluent containers and activated to dissolve the drug are stable for 24 hours at room temperature or for 7 days under refrigeration. Freezing solutions of ceftazidime in the *ADD-Vantage* system is not recommended. Joined vials that have not been activated may be used within a 14-day period; this period corresponds to that for use of Abbott *ADD-Vantage* containers following removal of the outer packaging (overwrap).

CEFEPIME HYDROCHLORIDE

Rx	**Cefepime** (Apotex USA)	**Injection, powder for solution**[a]: 500 mg	In vials (1s and 10s).
Rx	**Cefepime** (Apotex USA)	**Injection, powder for solution**[a]: 1 g	In vials (1s and 10s).
Rx	**Cefepime** (Apotex USA)	**Injection, powder for solution**[a]: 2 g	In vials (1s and 10s).
Rx	**Cefepime** (Baxter)	**Injection, solution:** 1 g	Dextrose 1.03 g. In 50 mL single-dose *Galaxy* containers.
		Injection, solution: 2 g	Dextrose 2.06 g. In 100 mL single-dose *Galaxy* containers.

[a] Contains arginine.

CEFEPIME HYDROCHLORIDE — INJECTION

For complete and comparative prescribing information, refer to the Cephalosporins group monograph.

Indications

➤*Pneumonia (moderate to severe):* Caused by *Streptococcus pneumoniae*, including cases associated with concurrent bacteremia, *Pseudomonas aeruginosa*, *Klebsiella pneumoniae*, or *Enterobacter* species.

➤*Empiric therapy for febrile neutropenic patients:* As monotherapy for empiric treatment of febrile neutropenic patients. In patients at high risk for severe infection (including patients with a history of recent bone marrow transplantation, with hypotension at presentation, with an underlying hematologic malignancy, or with severe or prolonged neutropenia), antimicrobial monotherapy may not be appropriate. Insufficient data exist to support the efficacy of cefepime monotherapy in such patients.

➤*Uncomplicated and complicated urinary tract infections (including pyelonephritis):* Caused by *Escherichia coli* or *Klebsiella pneumoniae*, when the infection is severe, or caused by *Escherichia coli*, *Klebsiella pneumoniae*, or *Proteus mirabilis*, when the infection is mild to moderate, including cases associated with concurrent bacteremia with these microorganisms.

➤*Uncomplicated skin and skin structure infections:* Caused by *Staphylococcus aureus* (methicillin-susceptible strains only) or *Streptococcus pyogenes*.

➤*Complicated intra-abdominal infections (used in combination with metronidazole):* Caused by *Escherichia coli*, viridans group streptococci, *P. aeruginosa*, *Klebsiella pneumoniae*, *Enterobacter* species, or *Bacteroides fragilis*.

➤*Off-label uses:*

Catheter-related bloodstream infections – [2] = Fair documentation. Guidelines suggest that cefepime may be used for treatment of catheter-related bloodstream infections caused by *P. aeruginosa* and as an alternative agent for the treatment of *Enterobacter* species and *Serratia marcescens*.

Cefepime can be used empirically for infections thought to be caused by gram-negative bacilli or used in combination with other antimicrobial agents when *P. aeruginosa* is thought to be the pathogen, especially in neutropenic or severely ill patients.

Administration and Dosage

➤*Adults:*

Infections –

Cefepime Dosing in Patients 16 Years of Age and Older With CrCl > 60 mL/min

Infection	Dose	Frequency	Duration (days)
Empiric therapy for febrile neutropenic patients	2 g IV	q 8 h	7[a]
Intra-abdominal infections (complicated, used in combination with metronidazole) caused by *E. coli*, viridans group streptococci, *P. aeruginosa*, *K. pneumoniae*, *Enterobacter* species, or *B. fragilis*	2 g IV	q 12 h	7 to 10
Pneumonia (moderate to severe) due to *S. pneumoniae*,[b] *P. aeruginosa*, *K. pneumoniae*, or *Enterobacter* species	1 to 2 g IV	q 12 h	10
Skin and skin structure infections (moderate to severe uncomplicated) due to *S. aureus* or *S. pyogenes*	2 g IV	q 12 h	10

CEFEPIME HYDROCHLORIDE — INJECTION

Cefepime Dosing in Patients 16 Years of Age and Older With CrCl > 60 mL/min			
Infection	Dose	Frequency	Duration (days)
Urinary tract infections (mild to moderate uncomplicated or complicated), including pyelonephritis, due to *E. coli, K. pneumoniae*, or *P. mirabilis*[b]	0.5 to 1 g IV/IM[c]	q 12 h	7 to 10
Urinary tract infections (severe uncomplicated or complicated), including pyelonephritis, due to *E. coli* or *K. pneumoniae*[b]	2 g IV	q 12 h	10

[a] Or until resolution of neutropenia. In patients whose fever resolves but who remain neutropenic for more than 7 days, the need for continued antimicrobial therapy should be reevaluated frequently.
[b] Including cases associated with concurrent bacteremia.
[c] IM route of administration is indicated only for mild to moderate, uncomplicated, or complicated UTIs due to *E. coli* when the IM route is considered to be a more appropriate route of drug administration.

Off-label dosing –

Catheter-related bloodstream infections: [2] = Fair documentation. 2 g IV every 8 hours for 7 to 10 days.

➤*Children:* The maximum dose for children should not exceed the recommended adult dose.

Infections – See Adults for dosing for children 16 years of age and older.

2 months of age up to 16 years of age (up to 40 kg):

• *Empiric therapy for febrile neutropenic patients –*

Usual dosage: 50 mg/kg every 8 hours for 7 days or until resolution of neutropenia. In patients whose fever resolves but who remain neutropenic for more than 7 days, the need for continued antimicrobial therapy should be reevaluated frequently.

Maximum dose: 2 g.

• *Pneumonia –*

Usual dosage: 50 mg/kg every 12 hours for 10 days.

Maximum dose: 2 g.

• *Skin and skin structure infections (uncomplicated) –*

Usual dosage: 50 mg/kg every 12 hours for 10 days.

Maximum dose: 2 g.

• *Urinary tract infections (uncomplicated and complicated, including pyelonephritis) –*

Usual dosage: 50 mg/kg every 12 hours for 7 to 10 days.

Maximum dose: 2 g.

Off-label dosing –

Catheter-related bloodstream infections: [2] = Fair documentation.

• *Infants older than 2 weeks of age and children weighing 40 kg or less* – 50 mg/kg IV every 12 hours for 7 to 10 days, not to exceed the adult maximum daily dose.

• *Infants younger than 2 weeks of age* – 30 mg/kg IV every 12 hours for 7 to 10 days.

➤*Renal function impairment:*

Adults – In patients with impaired renal function (CrCl of 60 mL/min or less), the dose of cefepime should be adjusted to compensate for the slower rate of renal elimination. The recommended initial dose should be the same as in patients with healthy renal function, except in patients undergoing hemodialysis. The recommended doses of cefepime in patients with renal insufficiency are presented in the following table.

Cefepime Maintenance Dosing for Adults With Renal Function Impairment				
CrCl (mL/min)	Recommended maintenance schedule			
> 60 normal recommended dosing schedule	500 mg q 12 h	1 g q 12 h	2 g q 12 h	2 g q 8 h
30 to 60	500 mg q 24 h	1 g q 24 h	2 g q 24 h	2 g q 12 h
11 to 29	500 mg q 24 h	500 mg q 24 h	1 g q 24 h	2 g q 24 h
< 11	250 mg q 24 h	250 mg q 24 h	500 mg q 24 h	1 g q 24 h
CAPD[a]	500 mg q 48 h	1 g q 48 h	2 g q 48 h	2 g q 48 h
Hemodialysis[b]	1 g on day 1, then 500 mg q 24 h thereafter			1 g q 24 h

[a] CAPD = continuous ambulatory peritoneal dialysis.
[b] On hemodialysis days, cefepime should be administered following hemodialysis. Whenever possible, cefepime should be administered at the same time each day.

Hemodialysis: In patients undergoing hemodialysis, approximately 68% of the total amount of cefepime present in the body at the start of dialysis will be removed during a 3-hour dialysis period.

• *Continuous renal replacement therapy* – One reference suggests a dosage of 1 to 2 g every 12 hours.

The following alternative recommendations assume ultrafiltration and dialysis flow rates of 1 to 2 L/h.

Loading dose: 2 g IV.

Continuous venovenous hemofiltration: 1 to 2 g IV every 12 hours.

Continuous venovenous hemodialysis or continuous venous hemodialfiltration: 1 g IV every 8 hours or 2 g IV every 12 hours. Consider 2 g IV every 8 hours for gram-negative pathogens with MIC of 4 mg/L or higher.

• *Intermittent hemodialysis* – According to the prescribing information, the dosage of cefepime for hemodialysis patients is 1 g on day 1, follwed by 500 mg every 24 hours for the treatment of all infections except febrile neutropenia, which is 1 g every 24 hours. Administer cefepime at the same time each day and following the completion of hemodialysis on hemodialysis days.

One reference suggests a 25% to 50% dosage reduction of the usual dosage administered every 24 hours.

The following are other alternative dosage regimens: administer 500 mg to 1 g IV every 24 hours administered after dialysis on dialysis days, or administer 1 to 2 g IV every 48 to 72 hours after dialysis. These dosing recommendations assume the patient is receiving standard IHD 3 times per week and completes the full dialysis sessions.

CAPD: In patients undergoing CAPD, cefepime may be administered at normally recommended doses at a dosage interval of every 48 hours.

➤*Preparation for administration:*

Preparation for IV administration – For IV infusion, constitute the 1 or 2 g piggyback (100 mL) bottle with 50 or 100 mL of a compatible IV fluid listed in Admixture compatibility. (See Admixture compatibility). Alternatively, constitute the 500 mg, 1 g, or 2 g vial, and add an appropriate quantity of the resulting solution to an IV container with one of the compatible IV fluids. The resulting solution should be administered over approximately 30 minutes.

ADD-Vantage vials are to be constituted only with 50 or 100 mL of 5% Dextrose Injection or 0.9% Sodium Chloride Injection in Abbott *ADD-Vantage* flexible diluent containers. (See *ADD-Vantage* vial instructions for use.)

Preparation for IM administration – For IM administration, cefepime should be constituted with 1 of the following diluents: Sterile Water for Injection, 0.9% Sodium Chloride, 5% Dextrose Injection, 0.5% or 1% lidocaine HCl, or Sterile Bacteriostatic Water for Injection with parabens or benzyl alcohol.

Preparation of cefepime solutions is presented in the following table:

Preparation of Cefepime			
Single-dose vials for IV/IM administration	Amount of diluent to be added (mL)	Approximate available volume (mL)	Approximate cefepime concentration (mg/mL)
Cefepime vial content			
500 mg (IV)	5	5.6	100
500 mg (IM)	1.3	1.8	280
1 g (IV)	10	11.3	100
1 g (IM)	2.4	3.6	280
2 g (IV)	10	12.5	160
Piggyback (100 mL)			
1 g bottle	50	50	20
1 g bottle	100	100	10
2 g bottle	50	50	40
2 g bottle	100	100	20
ADD-Vantage			
1 g vial	50	50	20
1 g vial	100	100	10
2 g vial	50	50	40
2 g vial	100	100	20

➤*Administration:* Cefepime should be administered IV over approximately 30 minutes. Intermittent IV infusion with a Y-type administration set can be accomplished with compatible solutions. However, during infusion of a solution containing cefepime, it is desirable to discontinue the other solution.

Cefepime may also be administered IM. The IM route of administration is indicated only for mild to moderate, uncomplicated, or complicated UTIs due to *E. coli* when the IM route is considered to be a more appropriate route of drug administration.

➤*Admixture compatibility:*

Compatibility –

Preparation for IV administration: Cefepime is compatible at concentrations between 1 and 40 mg/mL with the following IV infusion fluids: 0.9% Sodium Chloride Injection, 5% and 10% Dextrose Injection, M/6 Sodium Lactate Injection, 5% Dextrose and 0.9% Sodium Chloride Injection, Lactated Ringers and 5% Dextrose Injection, *Normosol-R*, and *Normosol-M* in 5% Dextrose Injection. These solutions may be stored up to 24 hours at controlled room temperature, 20° to 25°C (68° to 77°F), or 7 days in a refrigerator, 2° to 8°C (36° to 46°F). Cefepime in *ADD-Vantage* vials is stable at concentrations of 10 to 40 mg/mL in 5% Dextrose Injection or 0.9% Sodium Chloride Injection for 24 hours at controlled room temperature, 20° to 25°C (68° to 77°F), or 7 days in a refrigerator, 2° to 8°C (36° to 46°F).

CEFEPIME HYDROCHLORIDE — INJECTION

Cefepime Admixture Stability				
			Stability time for	
Cefepime concentration	Admixture and concentration	IV infusion solutions	RT/L[a] (20° to 25°C; 68° to 77°F)	Refrigeration (2° to 8°C; 36° to 46°F)
40 mg/mL	Amikacin 6 mg/mL	NS[b] or D5W[c]	24 hours	7 days
40 mg/mL	Ampicillin 1 mg/mL	D5W[c]	8 hours	8 hours
40 mg/mL	Ampicillin 10 mg/mL	D5W[c]	2 hours	8 hours
40 mg/mL	Ampicillin 1 mg/mL	NS[b]	24 hours	48 hours
40 mg/mL	Ampicillin 10 mg/mL	NS[b]	8 hours	48 hours
4 mg/mL	Ampicillin 40 mg/mL	NS[b]	8 hours	8 hours
4 to 40 mg/mL	Clindamycin phosphate 0.25 to 6 mg/mL	NS[b] or D5W[c]	24 hours	7 days
4 mg/mL	Heparin 10 to 50 units/mL	NS[b] or D5W[c]	24 hours	7 days
4 mg/mL	Potassium chloride 10 to 40 mEq/L	NS[b] or D5W[c]	24 hours	7 days
4 mg/mL	Theophylline 0.8 mg/mL	D5W[c]	24 hours	7 days
1 to 4 mg/mL	na[d]	*Aminosyn* II 4.25% with electrolytes and calcium	8 hours	3 days
0.125 to 0.25 mg/mL	na[d]	*Inpersol* with 4.25% dextrose	24 hours	7 days

[a] RT/L = ambient room temperature and light.
[b] NS = 0.9% sodium chloride injection.
[c] D5W = 5% dextrose injection.
[d] na = not applicable.

Preparation for IM administration: Cefepime constituted as directed is stable for 24 hours at controlled room temperature, 20° to 25°C (68° to 77°F), or for 7 days in a refrigerator, 2° to 8°C (36° to 46°F), with the following diluents: Sterile Water for Injection, 0.9% Sodium Chloride Injection, 5% Dextrose Injection, Sterile Bacteriostatic Water for Injection with parabens or benzyl alcohol, or 0.5% or 1% lidocaine HCl.

Incompatibility – Solutions of cefepime, like those of most beta-lactam antibiotics, should not be added to solutions of ampicillin at a concentration greater than 40 mg/mL, and should not be added to metronidazole, vancomycin, gentamicin, tobramycin, netilmicin sulfate, or aminophylline because of potential interaction. However, if concurrent therapy with cefepime is indicated, each of these antibiotics can be administered separately.

➤*Storage/Stability:* Cefepime in the dry state should be stored between 2° and 25°C (36° and 77°F) and protected from light.

As with other cephalosporins, the color of cefepime powder, as well as its solutions, tend to darken depending on storage conditions; however, when stored as recommended, the product potency is not adversely affected.

CEFDITOREN

Rx	**Cefditoren Pivoxil** (Aristos)	**Tablets; oral:** 200 mg	As cefditoren pivoxil. May contain mannitol, sodium caseinate. In blister pack 20s.
Rx	**Spectracef** (Cornerstone)		As cefditoren pivoxil. Mannitol. (CBP 200). White, elliptical. Film-coated. In 60s.
Rx	**Cefditoren Pivoxil** (Aristos)	**Tablets; oral:** 400 mg	As cefditoren pivoxil. May contain mannitol, sodium caseinate. In blister pack 20s and 28s.
Rx	**Spectracef** (Cornerstone)		As cefditoren pivoxil. Mannitol. (CBP 400). White, elliptical. Film-coated. In blister pack 20s and 28s.

CEFDITOREN PIVOXIL — ORAL

For complete and comparative prescribing information, refer to the Cephalosporins group monograph.

Indications

➤*General information:* For the treatment of mild-to-moderate infections in adults and adolescents (12 years of age or older) that are caused by susceptible strains of the designated microorganisms in the following conditions:

➤*Acute bacterial exacerbation of chronic bronchitis:* Caused by *Haemophilus influenzae* (including β-lactamase-producing strains), *Haemophilus parainfluenzae* (including β-lactamase-producing strains), *Streptococcus pneumoniae* (penicillin-susceptible strains only), or *Moraxella catarrhalis* (including β-lactamase-producing strains).

➤*Community-acquired pneumonia:* Caused by *Haemophilus influenzae* (including β-lactamase-producing strains), *Haemophilus parainfluenzae* (including β-lactamase-producing strains), *Streptococcus pneumoniae* (penicillin-susceptible strains only), or *Moraxella catarrhalis* (including β-lactamase-producing strains).

➤*Pharyngitis/tonsillitis:* Caused by *Streptococcus pyogenes*.

➤*Uncomplicated skin and skin-structure infections:* Caused by *Staphylococcus aureus* (including β-lactamase-producing strains) or *Streptococcus pyogenes*.

Administration and Dosage

➤*Adults:*

Infections –

Cefditoren Dosage in Patients ≥ 12 Years of Age		
Type of infection	Dosage	Duration (days)
Acute bacterial exacerbation of chronic bronchitis	400 mg twice daily	10
Community-acquired pneumonia	400 mg twice daily	14
Pharyngitis/Tonsillitis	200 mg twice daily	10
Uncomplicated skin and skin structure infections		

➤*Children:*

Infections – See Adults for dosing for children 12 years of age and older.

➤*Renal function impairment:*

Moderate renal impairment (Ccr, 30 to 49 mL/min/1.73 m^2) – Not more than 200 mg twice daily should be administered.

Severe renal impairment (Ccr, less than 30 mL/min/1.73 m^2) – 200 mg once daily. The appropriate dose in patients with end-stage renal disease has not been determined.

➤*Administration:* Take cefditoren with meals to enhance absorption.

➤*Storage/Stability:* Store at 25°C (77°F); excursions are permitted to 15° to 30°C (59° to 86°F). Protect from light and moisture. Dispense in a tight, light-resistant container.

CEFTAROLINE FOSAMIL

Rx	**Teflaro** (Forest Pharmaceuticals)	**Injection, powder for solution**: 400 mg	As ceftaroline fosamil monoacetate. In single-use vials.
		600 mg	As ceftaroline fosamil monoacetate. In single-use vials.

CEFTAROLINE FOSAMIL MONOACETATE — INJECTION

Indications

➤*Acute bacterial skin and skin structure infections:* For the treatment of acute bacterial skin and skin structure infections caused by susceptible isolates of the following gram-positive and gram-negative microorganisms: *Staphylococcus aureus* (including methicillin-susceptible and methicillin-resistant isolates), *Streptococcus pyogenes*, *Streptococcus agalactiae*, *Escherichia coli*, *Klebsiella pneumoniae*, and *Klebsiella oxytoca*.

➤*Community-acquired bacterial pneumonia:* For the treatment of community-acquired bacterial pneumonia caused by susceptible isolates of the following gram-positive and gram-negative microorganisms: *Streptococcus pneumoniae* (including cases with concurrent bacteremia), *S. aureus* (methicillin-susceptible isolates only), *Haemophilus influenzae*, *Klebsiella pneumoniae*, *Klebsiella oxytoca*, and *E. coli*.

Administration and Dosage

➤*Adults:*

Acute bacterial skin and skin structure infection – 600 mg intravenous (IV) every 12 hours for 5 to 14 days.

Community-acquired bacterial pneumonia – 600 mg IV every 12 hours for 5 to 7 days.

➤*Elderly:* Dosage adjustment for elderly patients should be based on renal function.

➤*Renal function impairment:*

Ceftaroline Fosamil Injection Dosage in Renal Impairment

Estimated CrCl[a] (mL/min)	Ceftaroline fosamil recommended dosage regimen
> 50 mL/min	No dosage adjustment necessary
> 30 to ≤ 50 mL/min	400 mg IV every 12 hours
≥ 15 to ≤ 30 mL/min	300 mg IV every 12 hours
ESRD including hemodialysis[b]	200 mg IV every 12 hours[c]

[a] Creatinine clearance (CrCl) estimated using the Cockcroft-Gault formula.
[b] End-stage renal disease (ESRD) is defined as CrCl < 15 mL/min.
[c] Ceftaroline fosamil is hemodialyzable; therefore, ceftaroline should be administered after hemodialysis on hemodialysis days.

➤*Preparation for administration:* The contents of the ceftaroline fosamil vial should be reconstituted with 20 mL of sterile water for injection.

Ceftaroline Fosamil Preparation for IV Administration

Dosage strength	Volume of diluent to be added	Approximate ceftaroline fosamil concentration	Amount to be withdrawn
400 mg	20 mL	20 mg/mL	Total volume
600 mg	20 mL	30 mg/mL	Total volume

Reconstitution time is less than 2 minutes. Mix gently to reconstitute, and check to see that the contents have dissolved completely.

The color of ceftaroline fosamil infusion solutions ranges from clear, to light to dark yellow, depending on the concentration and storage conditions. When stored as recommended, the product potency is not affected.

Dilution – The reconstituted solution must be further diluted in at least 250 mL before infusion. Appropriate infusion solutions include sodium chloride 0.9% injection (normal saline); dextrose 5% injection; dextrose 2.5% injection and sodium chloride 0.45% injection; or Ringer's lactate injection.

➤*Administration:* Administer by IV infusion over 1 hour.

➤*Admixture compatibility:* The compatibility of ceftaroline fosamil with other drugs has not been established. Ceftaroline fosamil should not be mixed with or physically added to solutions containing other drugs.

➤*Storage/Stability:* Vials should be stored refrigerated at 2° to 8°C (36° to 46°F). Reconstituted solution in the infusion bag should be used within 6 hours when stored at room temperature or within 24 hours when stored under refrigeration at 2° to 8°C (36° to 46°F).

CARBAPENEM

MEROPENEM

Rx	**Meropenem** (Hospira)	**Injection, powder for solution**: 500 mg	Sodium 45.1 mg. In 20 and 30 mL vials.
Rx	**Merrem I.V.** (AstraZeneca)		Sodium 45.1 mg. In 20 and 30 mL vials.
Rx	**Meropenem** (Hospira)	**Injection, powder for solution**: 1 g	Sodium 90.2 mg. In 20 and 30 mL vials.
Rx	**Merrem I.V.** (AstraZeneca)		Sodium 90.2 mg. In 20 and 30 mL vials.

MEROPENEM — INJECTION

Indications

➤*Bacterial meningitis:* As single agent therapy for the treatment of bacterial meningitis in children 3 months of age and older caused by *Streptococcus pneumoniae* (the efficacy of meropenem as monotherapy in the treatment of meningitis caused by penicillin nonsusceptible isolates of *S. pneumoniae* has not been established), *Haemophilus influenzae* (beta-lactamase- and non–beta-lactamase-producing isolates), and *Neisseria meningitidis*.

Meropenem has been found to be effective in eliminating concurrent bacteremia in association with bacterial meningitis.

➤*Complicated skin and skin structure infections:* As single agent therapy for the treatment of complicated skin and skin structure infections (SSSIs) caused by *Staphylococcus aureus* (beta-lactamase- and non–beta-lactamase-producing, methicillin-susceptible isolates only), *Streptococcus pyogenes*, *Streptococcus agalactiae*, viridans group streptococci, *Enterococcus faecalis* (excluding vancomycin-resistant isolates), *Pseudomonas aeruginosa*, *Escherichia coli*, *Proteus mirabilis*, *Bacteroides fragilis*, and *Peptostreptococcus* species.

➤*Intra-abdominal infections:* As single agent therapy for the treatment of complicated appendicitis and peritonitis caused by viridans group streptococci, *E. coli*, *Klebsiella pneumoniae*, *P. aeruginosa*, *B. fragilis*, *Bacteroides thetaiotaomicron*, and *Peptostreptococcus* species.

➤*Culture and susceptibility testing:* To reduce the development of drug-resistant bacteria and maintain the effectiveness of meropenem and other antibacterial drugs, meropenem should only be used to treat or prevent infections that are proven or strongly suspected to be caused by susceptible bacteria. When culture and susceptibility information are available, they should be considered in selecting or modifying antibacterial therapy. In the absence of such data, local epidemiology and susceptibility patterns may contribute to the empiric selection of therapy.

➤*Off-label uses:*

Catheter-related bloodstream infection – [2] = Fair documentation. Guidelines suggest that meropenem may be used to treat catheter-related bloodstream infections caused by *P. aeruginosa*, gram-negative bacilli that are extended-spectrum beta-lactamase–positive, *Enterobacter* species, *Serratia marcescens*, *Acinetobacter* species, and *Burkholderia cepacia*. Meropenem can also be used as an alternative antimicrobial agent for the treatment of catheter-related bloodstream infections caused by *Chryseobacterium* species and *Ochrobactrum anthropi*.

Community-acquired pneumonia – [1] = Good documentation. According to the Infectious Diseases Society of America (IDSA)/American Thoracic Society (ATS) consensus guidelines on the management of community-acquired pneumonia (CAP) in adults, meropenem in combination with a fluoroquinolone is recommended as empiric treatment of CAP in adult inpatients admitted to the intensive care unit with risk factors for *Pseudomonas* infection.

Hospital-acquired pneumonia – [1] = Good documentation. According to ATS/IDSA consensus guidelines on the management of hospital-acquired pneumonia in adults, meropenem is recommended as empiric treatment of hospital-acquired pneumonia in adult patients with risk factors for multidrug-resistant pathogens or late-onset disease. Additionally, the British Society for Antimicrobial Chemotherapy best practice recommendations based on clinical experience include meropenem as an option for treating patients who have suspected or confirmed hospital-acquired pneumonia caused by *P. aeruginosa*.

Administration and Dosage

➤*Adults:*

Complicated skin and skin structure infections – 500 mg intravenously (IV) every 8 hours.

Intra-abdominal infections – 1 g IV every 8 hours.

MEROPENEM — INJECTION

Off-label dosing –

Catheter-related bloodstream infection: [2] = Fair documentation. 1 g IV infused over 15 to 30 minutes every 8 hours.

Community-acquired pneumonia: [1] = Good documentation. Empirically, 500 mg infused IV every 8 hours for a minimum of 5 days, used in combination with a fluoroquinolone.

Empiric therapy in febrile neutropenic patients: In a study of 101 cancer patients with 120 febrile neutropenic episodes, a dosage of 1 g IV every 8 hours was shown to be as effective and well tolerated as ceftazidime.

Hospital-acquired pneumonia: [1] = Good documentation. 1 g infused every 8 hours. Duration of treatment is 7 to 8 days for uncomplicated hospital-acquired pneumonia infections.

Nosocomial pneumonia: As an initial empirical therapy, meropenem in a dosage of 1 g IV every 8 hours has been shown to be effective for adults with hospital-acquired pneumonia (HAP), ventilator-associated pneumonia (VAP), and health care-associated pneumonia (HCAP). It should be used in patients with late-onset disease or risk factors for multidrug-resistant pathogens.

➤*Children:*

3 months of age and older –

Bacterial meningitis:

- *Weighing more than 50 kg* – 2 g IV every 8 hours.
- *Weighing 50 kg or less* –
  Usual dosage: 40 mg/kg IV every 8 hours.
  Maximum dose: 2 g IV every 8 hours.

Complicated skin and skin structure infections:

- *Weighing more than 50 kg* – 500 mg IV every 8 hours.
- *Weighing 50 kg or less* –
  Usual dosage: 10 mg/kg IV every 8 hours.
  Maximum dose: 500 mg IV every 8 hours.

Intra-abdominal infections:

- *Weighing more than 50 kg* – 1 g IV every 8 hours.
- *Weighing 50 kg or less* –
  Usual dosage: 20 mg/kg IV every 8 hours.
  Maximum dose: 1 g IV every 8 hours.

Off-label dosing –

Catheter-related bloodstream infection: [2] = Fair documentation.

- *Infants 3 months of age and older and children* – 20 mg/kg infused over 15 to 30 minutes every 8 hours.
- *Neonates* – Postnatal age 0 to 7 days, 20 mg/kg infused over 15 to 30 minutes every 12 hours; postnatal older than 7 days of age and 1,200 to 2,000 g, 20 mg/kg infused over 15 to 30 minutes every 12 hours; postnatal older than 7 days of age and more than 2,000 g, 20 mg/kg infused over 15 to 30 minutes every 8 hours.

Neonates: 15 to 20 mg/kg IV every 12 hours. For neonates weighing more than 2 kg, a dosage of 20 mg/kg IV every 8 hours has been suggested. Administer dose over 15 to 30 minutes.

➤*Elderly:* Because elderly patients are more likely to have decreased renal function, take care in dose selection; it may be useful to monitor renal function.

➤*Renal function impairment:*

Adults –

Meropenem Dosing for Adults With Renal Impairment

CrCl[a]	Dose (dependent on type of infection)	Dosing interval
≥ 51 mL/min	Recommended dose (500 mg complicated SSSI and 1 g intra-abdominal)	Every 8 hours
26 to 50 mL/min	Recommended dose (500 mg complicated SSSI and 1 g intra-abdominal	Every 12 hours
10 to 25 mL/min	½ recommended dose	Every 12 hours
< 10 mL/min	½ recommended dose	Every 24 hours

[a] CrCl = creatinine clearance.

➤*Administration:* Meropenem should be administered by IV infusion over approximately 15 to 30 minutes. Doses of 1 g also may be administered as an IV bolus injection (5 to 20 mL) over approximately 3 to 5 minutes.

➤*Admixture compatibility:* Compatibility of meropenem with other drugs has not been established. Meropenem should not be mixed with or physically added to solutions containing other drugs. (See Storage/Stability for more information.)

➤*Storage/Stability:*

Dry powder – Store the dry powder at 20° to 25°C (68° to 77°F).

Reconstituted solution – Freshly prepared solutions of meropenem should be used whenever possible. However, constituted solutions of meropenem maintain satisfactory potency at 15° to 25°C (59° to 77°F), or under refrigeration at 4°C (39°F) as described in the following sections. Solutions of meropenem should not be frozen.

Solutions for IV bolus: Meropenem injection vials constituted with sterile water for injection for bolus administration (meropenem up to 50 mg/mL) may be stored for up to 2 hours at 15° to 25°C (59° to 77°F), or for up to 12 hours at 4°C (39°F).

Solutions for IV infusion:

- *Stability in infusion vials* – Meropenem infusion vials constituted with sodium chloride 0.9% injection (meropenem concentrations ranging from 2.5 to 50 mg/mL) are stable for up to 2 hours at 15° to 25°C (59° to 77°F), or for up to 18 hours at 4°C (39°F). Infusion vials of meropenem constituted with dextrose 5% injection (meropenem concentrations ranging from 2.5 to 50 mg/mL) are stable for up to 1 hour at 15° to 25°C (59° to 77°F), or for up to 8 hours at 4°C (39°F).
- *Stability in plastic IV bags* – Solutions prepared for infusion (meropenem concentrations ranging from 1 to 20 mg/mL) may be stored in plastic IV bags with diluents as shown in the following table.

Meropenem Stored in IV Plastic Bags: Stability With Diluents

Diluent	Number of hours stable at 15° to 25°C (59° to 77°F)	Number of hours stable at 4°C (39°F)
Dextrose 5% injection	1	4
Dextrose 10% injection	1	2
Dextrose 5% and sodium chloride 0.9% injection	1	2
Dextrose 5% and sodium chloride 0.2% injection	1	4
Dextrose 2.5% and sodium chloride 0.45% injection	3	12
Dextrose 5% injection in *Normosol-M*	1	8
Dextrose 5% injection in Ringer's lactate injection	1	4
Mannitol 2.5% injection	2	16
Potassium chloride 0.15% in dextrose 5% injection	1	6
Ringer's injection	4	24
Ringer's lactate injection	4	12
Sodium bicarbonate 5% injection	1	4
Sodium bicarbonate 0.02% in dextrose 5% injection	1	6
Sodium chloride 0.9% injection	4	24
Sodium lactate injection 1/6 N	2	24

- *Stability in Baxter Minibag Plus* – Solutions of meropenem (concentrations ranging from 2.5 to 20 mg/mL) in *Baxter Minibag Plus* bags with sodium chloride 0.9% injection may be stored for up to 4 hours at 15° to 25°C (59° to 77°F), or for up to 24 hours at 4°C (39°F). Solutions of meropenem (concentrations ranging from 2.5 to 20 mg/mL) in *Baxter Minibag Plus* bags with dextrose 5% injection may be stored up to 1 hour at 15° to 25°C (59° to 77°F), or for up to 6 hours at 4°C (39°F).
- *Stability in plastic syringes, tubing, and IV infusion sets* – Solutions of meropenem (concentrations ranging from 1 to 20 mg/mL) in water for injection or sodium chloride 0.9% injection (for up to 4 hours) or in dextrose 5% injection (for up to 2 hours) at 15° to 25°C (59° to 77°F), are stable in plastic tubing and volume-control devices of common IV infusion sets.

Solutions of meropenem (concentrations ranging from 1 to 20 mg/mL) in water for injection or sodium chloride 0.9% injection (for up to 48 hours) or in dextrose 5% injection (for up to 6 hours) are stable at 4°C (39°F) in plastic syringes.

Actions

➤*Pharmacology:* Meropenem is a broad-spectrum carbapenem antibiotic. It is active against gram-positive and gram-negative bacteria. Meropenem exerts its action by penetrating bacterial cells readily and interfering with the synthesis of vital cell wall components, which leads to cell death. The bactericidal activity of meropenem results from the inhibition of cell wall synthesis. Meropenem readily penetrates the cell wall of most gram-positive and gram-negative bacteria to reach penicillin-binding protein (PBP) targets.

➤*Pharmacokinetics:*

Absorption – At the end of a 30-minute IV infusion of a single dose of meropenem in healthy volunteers, mean peak plasma concentrations are approximately 23 mcg/mL (range, 14 to 26 mcg/mL) for the 500 mg dose and 49 mcg/mL (range, 39 to 58 mcg/mL) for the 1 g dose. A 5-minute IV bolus injection of meropenem in healthy volunteers results in mean peak plasma concentrations of approximately 45 mcg/mL (range, 18 to 65 mcg/mL) for the 500 mg dose and 112 mcg/mL (range, 83 to 140 mcg/mL) for the 1 g dose.

Following IV doses of 500 mg, mean plasma concentrations of meropenem usually decline to approximately 1 mcg/mL 6 hours after administration.

Distribution – Plasma protein binding of meropenem is approximately 2%.

Meropenem penetrates well into most body fluids and tissues, including cerebrospinal fluid (CSF), achieving concentrations matching or exceeding those required to inhibit most susceptible bacteria. After a single IV dose of meropenem, the highest mean concentrations of meropenem were found in tissues and fluids at 1 hour (0.5 to 1.5 hours) after the start of infusion.

Metabolism – There is 1 metabolite that is microbiologically inactive.

Excretion – In subjects with healthy renal function, the elimination half-life of meropenem is approximately 1 hour. Approximately 70% of the IV

MEROPENEM — INJECTION

dose is recovered as unchanged meropenem in the urine over 12 hours, after which little further urinary excretion is detectable. Urinary concentrations of meropenem in excess of 10 mcg/mL are maintained for up to 5 hours after a 500 mg dose. No accumulation of meropenem in plasma or urine was observed with regimens using 500 mg administered every 8 hours or 1 g administered every 6 hours in volunteers with healthy renal function.

Special populations –

Renal function impairment: Pharmacokinetic studies with meropenem in patients with renal insufficiency have shown that the plasma clearance of meropenem correlates with CrCl. Dosage adjustments are necessary in subjects with renal impairment.

Elderly: A pharmacokinetic study with meropenem in elderly patients with renal insufficiency has shown a reduction in plasma clearance of meropenem that correlates with age-associated reduction in CrCl.

➤*Microbiology:*

Resistance – There are several mechanisms of resistance to carbapenems: decreased permeability of the outer membrane of gram-negative bacteria (because of diminished production of porins) causing reduced bacterial uptake, reduced affinity of the target PBP, increased expression of efflux pump components, and production of antibiotic-destroying enzymes (carbapenemases, metallo-beta-lactamases). Cross-resistance is sometimes observed with strains resistant to other carbapenems.

Meropenem has been shown to be active against most isolates of the following microorganisms, both in vitro and in clinical infections.

Aerobic and facultative gram-positive microorganisms – *E. faecalis* (excluding vancomycin-resistant isolates); *S. aureus* (beta-lactamase- and non–beta-lactamase-producing, methicillin-susceptible isolates only); *S. agalactiae*; *S. pyogenes*; Viridans group streptococci; *S. pneumoniae* (penicillin-susceptible isolates only). Penicillin-resistant isolates had meropenem minimum inhibitory concentration (MIC_{90}) values of 1 or 2 mcg/mL, which is above the 0.12 mcg/mL susceptible breakpoint for this species.

Aerobic and facultative gram-negative microorganisms – *E. coli*; *H. influenzae* (beta-lactamase- and non–beta-lactamase-producing); *K. pneumoniae*; *N. meningitidis*; *P. aeruginosa*; *P. mirabilis*.

Anaerobic microorganisms – *B. fragilis*; *B. thetaiotaomicron*; *Peptostreptococcus* species.

Contraindications

Known hypersensitivity to any component of this product or to other drugs in the same class, or in patients who have demonstrated anaphylactic reactions to beta-lactams.

Warnings/Precautions

➤*Seizures:* Seizures and other CNS adverse reactions have been reported during treatment with meropenem. These experiences have occurred most commonly in patients with CNS disorders (eg, brain lesions, history of seizures) or with bacterial meningitis and/or compromised renal function.

During clinical investigations, 2,904 immunocompetent adult patients were treated for non-CNS infections, with the overall seizure rate being 0.7% (based on 20 patients with this adverse reaction). All meropenem-treated patients with seizures had preexisting contributing factors. Among these were history of seizures or CNS abnormality and concomitant medications with seizure potential. Dosage adjustment is recommended in patients with advanced age and/or reduced renal function.

Close adherence to the recommended dosage regimens is urged, especially in patients with known factors that predispose to convulsive activity. Continue anticonvulsant therapy in patients with known seizure disorders. If focal tremors, myoclonus, or seizures occur, evaluate patients neurologically, place them on anticonvulsant therapy if it has not already been instituted, and re-examine the dosage of IV meropenem to determine whether to decrease it or to discontinue the antibiotic.

➤*Clostridium difficile–associated diarrhea:* *Clostridium difficile*–associated diarrhea (CDAD) has been reported with use of nearly all antibacterial agents, including meropenem, and may range in severity from mild diarrhea to fatal colitis. Treatment with antibacterial agents alters the normal flora of the colon and may permit overgrowth of *C. difficile*.

C. difficile produces toxins A and B, which contribute to the development of CDAD. Hypertoxin-producing strains of *C. difficile* cause increased morbidity and mortality because these infections can be refractory to antimicrobial therapy and may require colectomy. CDAD must be considered in all patients who present with diarrhea following antibiotic use. Careful medical history is necessary because CDAD has been reported to occur more than 2 months after the administration of antibacterial agents.

If CDAD is suspected or confirmed, ongoing antibiotic use not directed against *C. difficile* may need to be discontinued. Institute appropriate fluid and electrolyte management, protein supplementation, antibiotic treatment of *C. difficile*, and surgical evaluation as clinically indicated.

➤*Reducing drug resistance:* Prescribing meropenem in the absence of a proven or strongly suspected bacterial infection or a prophylactic indication is unlikely to provide benefit to the patient and increases the risk of the development of drug-resistant bacteria.

➤*Hypersensitivity reactions:* Serious and occasionally fatal hypersensitivity (anaphylactic) reactions have been reported in patients receiving therapy with beta-lactams. These reactions are more likely to occur in individuals with a history of sensitivity to multiple allergens.

There have been reports of individuals with a history of penicillin hypersensitivity who have experienced severe hypersensitivity reactions when treated with another beta-lactam. Before initiating therapy with meropenem, make careful inquiry concerning previous hypersensitivity reactions to penicillins, cephalosporins, other beta-lactams, and other allergens. If an allergic reaction to meropenem occurs, discontinue the drug immediately. Serious anaphylactic reactions require immediate emergency treatment with epinephrine, oxygen, IV steroids, and airway management, including intubation. Other therapy may also be administered as indicated.

➤*Renal function impairment:* Dosage should be reduced in patients with a CrCl less than 51 mL/min.

In patients with renal dysfunction, thrombocytopenia has been observed, but no clinical bleeding has been reported.

See Administration and Dosage for more information.

➤*Superinfection:* As with other broad-spectrum antibiotics, prolonged use of meropenem may result in overgrowth of nonsusceptible organisms. Repeated evaluation of the patient is essential. If superinfection does occur during therapy, take appropriate measures.

➤*Pregnancy: Category B.* Use this drug during pregnancy only if clearly needed. There are no adequate and well-controlled studies in pregnant women. Although the placental passage in humans or animals has not been studied, placental transfer to the fetus may occur because of the molecular weight (about 438) of meropenem. Meropenem penetrates well into most body fluids and tissues, including the endometrium, fallopian tubes, and ovaries.

Reproductive studies have been performed with meropenem in rats at dosages of up to 1,000 mg/kg/day, and cynomolgus monkeys at dosages of up to 360 mg/kg/day (on the basis of AUC comparisons, approximately 1.8 and 3.7 times, respectively, to the human exposure at the usual dosage of 1 g every 8 hours). These studies revealed no evidence of impaired fertility or harm to the fetus caused by meropenem, although there were slight changes in fetal body weight at dosages of 250 mg/kg/day (on the basis of AUC comparisons, 0.4 times the human exposure at a dosage of 1 g every 8 hours) and more in rats. Because animal reproduction studies are not always predictive of human response, use this drug during pregnancy only if clearly needed.

➤*Lactation:* It is not known whether this drug is excreted in human milk. However, the molecular weight of meropenem (about 438) is low enough for excretion into breast milk. Because many drugs are excreted in human milk, exercise caution when meropenem is administered to a breast-feeding woman.

➤*Children:* The safety and efficacy of meropenem have been established for children 3 months of age and older.

➤*Elderly:* Meropenem is known to be substantially excreted by the kidney, and the risk of toxic reactions to this drug may be greater in patients with impaired renal function. Because elderly patients are more likely to have decreased renal function, take care in dose selection; it may be useful to monitor renal function.

➤*Monitoring:* While meropenem possesses the characteristic low toxicity of the beta-lactam group of antibiotics, periodic assessment of organ system functions, including renal, hepatic, and hematopoietic, is advisable during prolonged therapy.

Drug Interactions

➤*Probenecid:* Probenecid competes with meropenem for active tubular secretion and thus inhibits the renal excretion of meropenem. This led to statistically significant increases in the elimination half-life (38%) and in the extent of systemic exposure (56%). Therefore, the coadministration of probenecid with meropenem is not recommended.

➤*Valproic acid:* A clinically significant reduction in serum valproic acid concentration has been reported in patients receiving carbapenem antibiotics and may result in loss of seizure control. When taken concomitantly with carbapenems, valproic acid concentrations were noted to be reduced by 45% to 95%, and seizures occurred in greater than 50% of patients. Frequently monitor serum valproic acid concentrations after initiating carbapenem therapy. Consider an alternative antibacterial or anticonvulsant therapy if serum valproic acid concentrations drop below the therapeutic range or a seizure occurs.

Adverse Reactions

➤*Non-CNS infections (adults):*

Cardiovascular – Bradycardia, heart arrest, heart failure, hypertension, hypotension, myocardial infarction, pulmonary embolus, syncope, tachycardia (0.1% to 1%).

CNS – Headache (2.3%); agitation/delirium, anxiety, asthenia, chills, confusion, depression, dizziness, hallucinations, insomnia, nervousness, paresthesia, seizure (see Warnings/Precautions), somnolence (0.1% to 1%).

Dermatologic – Rash (1.9%); pruritus (1.2%); skin ulcer, sweating, urticaria (0.1% to 1%).

GI – Diarrhea (4.8%); nausea/vomiting (3.6%); constipation (1.4%); GI hemorrhage (0.5%); melena (0.3%); hemoperitoneum (0.2%); abdominal enlargement, abdominal pain, anorexia, cholestatic jaundice/jaundice, dyspepsia, flatulence, hepatic failure, ileus, intestinal obstruction, oral moniliasis (0.1% to 1%).

GU – Dysuria, kidney failure, urinary incontinence, vaginal moniliasis (0.1% to 1%).

Hematologic – Anemia, hypervolemia, hypochromic anemia (0.1% to 1%).

Local – Inflammation at the injection site (2.4%); injection-site reaction (0.9%); phlebitis/thrombophlebitis (0.8%); pain at the injection site (0.4%); edema at the injection site (0.2%).

MEROPENEM — INJECTION

Respiratory – Apnea (1.3%); epistaxis (0.2%); asthma, cough increased, dyspnea, hypoxia, lung edema, pleural effusion, respiratory disorder (0.1% to 1%).

Miscellaneous – Sepsis (1.6%); shock (1.2%); back pain, chest pain, fever, pain, pelvic pain, peripheral edema (0.1% to 1%).

➤*Complicated skin and skin structure infections (adults):*

CNS – Headache (7.8%).

GI – Nausea (7.8%); constipation, diarrhea (7%); GI disorder (more than 1%).

Respiratory – Pharyngitis, pneumonia (more than 1%).

Miscellaneous – Anemia (5.5%); pain (5.1%); accidental injury, hypoglycemia, peripheral vascular disorder (more than 1%).

➤*Children:*

Serious bacterial infections (excluding meningitis) – Meropenem was studied in 515 children (3 months to younger than 13 years of age) with serious bacterial infections (excluding meningitis) at dosages of 10 to 20 mg/kg every 8 hours. The types of clinical adverse reactions seen in these patients are similar to the adults, with the most common adverse reactions reported as possibly, probably, or definitely related to meropenem and their rates of occurrence as follows: diarrhea (3.5%), rash (1.6%), and nausea and vomiting (0.8%).

Bacterial meningitis – Meropenem was studied in 321 pediatric patients (3 months to younger than 17 years of age) with meningitis at a dosage of 40 mg/kg every 8 hours. The types of clinical adverse reactions seen in these patients are similar to the adults, with the most common adverse reactions reported as possibly, probably, or definitely related to meropenem and their rates of occurrence as follows: diarrhea (4.7%), rash (mostly diaper area moniliasis) (3.1%), oral moniliasis (1.9%), glossitis (1%).

Seizures: In the meningitis studies, the rates of seizure activity during therapy were comparable between patients with no CNS abnormalities who received meropenem and those who received comparator agents (either cefotaxime or ceftriaxone). In the meropenem-treated group, 12 of 15 patients with seizures had late-onset seizures (defined as occurring on day 3 or later) versus 7 of 20 in the comparator arm.

➤*Lab test abnormalities (adults):*

Hematologic – Eosinophils increased, hematocrit decreased, hemoglobin decreased, hypokalemia, leukocytosis, platelets increased/decreased, shortened prothrombin time, shortened partial thromboplastin time, white blood cell count decreased (more than 0.2%).

Hepatic – Increased alkaline phosphatase, ALT, AST, bilirubin, lactate dehydrogenase (more than 0.2%).

Renal – Increased serum urea nitrogen (BUN), increased creatinine, presence of red blood cells in the urine (more than 0.2%).

For patients with varying degrees of renal impairment, the incidence of heart failure, kidney failure, seizure, and shock reported irrespective of relationship to meropenem increased in patients with moderately severe renal impairment (CrCl more than 10 to 26 mL/min).

➤*Postmarketing:*

Dermatologic – Angioedema, erythema multiforme, Stevens-Johnson syndrome, toxic epidermal necrolysis.

Hematologic – Agranulocytosis, hemolytic anemia, leukopenia, neutropenia.

Miscellaneous – Positive direct or indirect Coombs test.

Overdosage

➤*Symptoms:* Limited postmarketing experience indicates that if adverse reactions occur following overdosage, they are consistent with the adverse reaction profile described in the Adverse Reactions section and are generally mild in severity and resolve on withdrawal or dose reduction.

➤*Treatment:* Consider symptomatic treatments. In individuals with healthy renal function, rapid renal elimination takes place. Meropenem and its metabolite are readily dialyzable and effectively removed by hemodialysis; however, no information is available on the use of hemodialysis to treat overdosage.

Patient Information

Counsel patients only to use antibacterial drugs, including meropenem, to treat bacterial infections. Antibacterial drugs do not treat viral infections (eg, the common cold). When meropenem is prescribed to treat a bacterial infection, tell patients that although it is common to feel better early in the course of therapy, the medication should be taken exactly as directed. Skipping doses or not completing the full course of therapy may decrease the efficacy of the immediate treatment and increase the likelihood that bacteria will develop resistance and will not be treatable by meropenem or other antibacterial drugs in the future.

Diarrhea is a common problem caused by antibiotics that usually ends when the antibiotic is discontinued. Sometimes after starting treatment with antibiotics, patients can develop watery and bloody stools (with or without stomach cramps and fever) even as late as 2 or more months after having taken the last dose of the antibiotic. If this occurs, instruct patients to contact their health care provider as soon as possible.

IMIPENEM/CILASTATIN

Rx	**Primaxin I.V.** (Merck)	**Powder for Injection**: 250 mg imipenem equivalent and 250 mg cilastatin equivalent. Contains 0.8 mEq sodium.	In vials, infusion bottles, and *ADD-Vantage* vials.
		500 mg imipenem equivalent and 500 mg cilastatin equivalent. Contains 1.6 mEq sodium.	In vials, infusion bottles, and *ADD-Vantage* vials.
Rx	**Primaxin I.M.** (Merck)	**Powder for Injection**: 500 mg imipenem equivalent and 500 mg cilastatin equivalent. Contains 1.4 mEq sodium.	In vials.

IMIPENEM/CILASTATIN — INJECTION

Indications

➤*General information:* Infections resistant to other antibiotics (eg, cephalosporins, penicillins, aminoglycosides) have responded to treatment with imipenem.

➤*IV:* Treatment of serious infections caused by susceptible strains of the designated microorganisms in the conditions listed below:

Lower respiratory tract infections – *Staphylococcus aureus* (penicillinase-producing), *Escherichia coli*, *Klebsiella* sp., *Enterobacter* sp., *Haemophilus influenzae*, *Haemophilus parainfluenzae*, *Acinetobacter* sp., *Serratia marcescens*.

Urinary tract infections (complicated and uncomplicated) – *Enterococcus faecalis*, *S. aureus* (penicillinase-producing), *E. coli*, *Klebsiella* sp., *Enterobacter* sp., *Proteus vulgaris*, *Providencia rettgeri*, *M. morganii*, *P. aeruginosa*.

Intra-abdominal infections – *E. faecalis*, *S. aureus* (penicillinase-producing), *Staphylococcus epidermidis*, *E. coli*, *Klebsiella* sp., *Enterobacter* sp., *Proteus* sp., *Morganella morganii*, *P. aeruginosa*, *Citrobacter* sp., *Clostridium* sp., *Bacteroides* sp. including *B. fragilis*, *Fusobacterium* sp., *Peptococcus* sp., *Peptostreptococcus* sp., *Eubacterium* sp., *Propionibacterium* sp., *Bifidobacterium* sp.

Gynecologic infections – *E. faecalis*; *S. aureus* (penicillinase-producing), *S. epidermidis*, *Streptococcus agalactiae* (group B streptococcus), *E. coli*, *Klebsiella* sp., *Proteus* sp., *Enterobacter* sp., *Bifidobacterium* sp., *Bacteroides* sp. including *B. fragilis*, *Gardnerella vaginalis*; *Peptococcus* sp., *Peptostreptococcus* sp., *Propionibacterium* sp.

Bacterial septicemia – *E. faecalis*, *S. aureus* (penicillinase-producing), *E. coli*, *Klebsiella* sp., *P. aeruginosa*, *Serratia* sp., *Enterobacter* sp., *Bacteroides* sp.

Bone and joint infections – *E. faecalis*; *S. aureus* (penicillinase-producing), *S. epidermidis*, *Enterobacter* sp., *P. aeruginosa*.

Skin and skin structure infections – *E. faecalis*, *S. aureus* (penicillinase-producing), *S. epidermidis*, *E. coli*, *Klebsiella* sp., *Enterobacter* sp., *P. vulgaris*, *P. rettgeri*, *M. morganii*, *P. aeruginosa*, *Serratia* sp., *Citrobacter* sp., *Acinetobacter* sp., *Bacteroides* sp., *Fusobacterium* sp., *Peptococcus* sp., *Peptostreptococcus* sp.

Endocarditis – *S. aureus* (penicillinase-producing).

Polymicrobic infections – Including those in which *S. pneumoniae* (pneumonia, septicemia), *S. pyogenes* (skin and skin structure) or nonpenicillinase-producing *S. aureus* is one of the causative organisms. However, these monobacterial infections are usually treated with narrower spectrum antibiotics (eg, penicillin G). Although clinical improvement has been observed in patients with cystic fibrosis, chronic pulmonary disease, and lower respiratory tract infections caused by *P. aeruginosa*, bacterial eradication may not be achieved.

➤*IM:* Treatment of serious infections of mild-to-moderate severity where IM therapy is appropriate. Not intended for severe or life-threatening infections, including bacterial sepsis or endocarditis, or in major physiological impairments (eg, shock).

Lower respiratory tract infections – Including pneumonia and bronchitis as an exacerbation of COPD that are caused by *S. pneumoniae* and *H. influenzae*.

Intra-abdominal infections – Including acute gangrenous or perforated appendicitis and appendicitis with peritonitis that are caused by group D streptococcus including *E. faecalis*; *Streptococcus* (viridans group); *E. coli*; *Klebsiella pneumoniae*; *P. aeruginosa*; *Bacteroides* sp. including *B. fragilis*, *B. distasonis*, *B. intermedius*, and *B. thetaiotaomicron*; *Fusobacterium* sp; *Peptostreptococcus* sp.

Skin and skin structure infections – Including abscesses, cellulitis, infected skin ulcers, and wound infectionscaused by *S. aureus* (including penicillinase-producing strains); *Streptococcus pyogenes*; group D streptococcus including *E. faecalis*; *Acinetobacter* sp. including *A. calcoaceticus*; *Citrobacter* sp; *E. coli*; *Enterobacter cloacae*; *K. pneumoniae*; *P. aeruginosa*; *Bacteroides* sp. including *B. fragilis*.

Gynecologic infections – Including postpartum endomyometritis that are caused by group D streptococcus such as *E. faecalis*; *E. coli*; *K. pneumoniae*; *B. intermedius*; *Peptostreptococcus* sp.

IMIPENEM/CILASTATIN — INJECTION

➤*Off-label uses:*

Catheter-related bloodstream infections (children/adolescents) – [2] = Fair documentation. The use of imipenem/cilastatin in children with catheter-related bloodstream infections is appropriate for empiric coverage based on local antimicrobial susceptibility data and severity of disease. Imipenem/cilastatin can be used to treat catheter-related bloodstream infections caused by gram-negative bacilli that are extended-spectrum beta-lactamase positive, *Enterobacter* species, and *S. marcescens*. Imipenem/cilastatin may also be used to treat catheter-related bloodstream infections caused by *Ochrobactrum anthropi*.

Infective endocarditis – The use of imipenem/cilastatin to treat endocarditis caused by *E. faecalis* infection is recommended based on conflicting evidence of efficacy and expert opinion.

Infective endocarditis (adults): [1] = Good documentation.

Infective endocarditis (children/adolescents): [1] = Good documentation.

Administration and Dosage

➤*Maximum dose:*

Adults –

IV: 50 mg/kg/day or 4 g/day, whichever is lower, according to the prescribing information.

IM: 1,500 mg/day according to the prescribing information.

Children 3 months of age and older – The following maximum doses are according to the prescribing information.

Fully susceptible organisms: 2 g/day IV.

Moderately susceptible organisms: 4 g/day IV.

➤*General dosing considerations:* Dosage recommendations represent the quantity of imipenem to be administered. An equivalent amount of cilastatin is also present in the solution.

Base the initial dosage on the type or severity of infection and administer in equally divided doses. Base subsequent dosing on severity of illness, degree of susceptibility of the pathogen(s), renal function, weight, and creatinine clearance.

➤*Adults:*

IM –

Maximum dose: 1,500 mg/day.

Duration of therapy: Duration of therapy depends on the type and severity of the infection. Generally, continue for greater than or equal to 2 days after signs and symptoms of infection have resolved. Safety and efficacy of treatment more than 14 days have not been established.

Imipenem-Cilastatin IM Dosage Guidelines in Adults

Type/Location of infection	Severity	Dosage regimen
Intra-abdominal	Mild/Moderate	750 mg every 12 h
Lower respiratory tract Skin and skin structure Gynecologic	Mild/Moderate	500 or 750 mg every 12 h depending on the severity of infection

IV –

Maximum dose: Because of high antimicrobial activity, do not exceed 50 mg/kg/day or 4 g/day, whichever is lower. There is no evidence that higher doses provide greater efficacy.

Patients weighing at least 70 kg:

Imipenem-Cilastatin IV Dosing Schedule for Adults with Normal Renal Function

Type or severity of infection	Fully susceptible organisms[a]	Total daily dose	Moderately susceptible organisms, primarily some strains of *P. aeruginosa*	Total daily dose
Mild	250 mg every 6 h	1 g	500 mg every 6 h	2 g
Moderate	500 mg every 8 h or 500 mg every 6 h	1.5 or 2 g	500 mg every 6 h or 1 g every 8 h	2 or 3 g
Severe, life-threatening	500 mg every 6 h	2 g	1 g every 8 h or 1 g every 6 h	3 or 4 g
Uncomplicated UTI	250 mg every 6 h	1 g	250 mg every 6 h	1 g
Complicated UTI	500 mg every 6 h	2 g	500 mg every 6 h	2 g

[a] Including gram-positive and -negative aerobes and anaerobes.

Patients weighing less than 70 kg:

Reduced Imipenem-Cilastatin IV Dosage in Adult Patients with Body Weight < 70 kg

≥ 70 kg	60 kg	50 kg	40 kg	30 kg
If total daily dose for normal renal function is 1 g/day, use:				
250 q 6 h	250 q 8 h	125 q 6 h	125 q 6 h	125 q 8 h
If total daily dose for normal renal function is 1.5 g/day, use:				
500 q 8 h	250 q 6 h	250 q 6 h	250 q 8 h	125 q 6 h
If total daily dose for normal renal function is 2 g/day, use:				
500 q 6 h	500 q 8 h	250 q 6 h	250 q 6 h	250 q 8 h
If total daily dose for normal renal function is 3 g/day, use:				
1,000 q 8 h	750 q 8 h	500 q 6 h	500 q 8 h	250 q 6 h
If total daily dose for normal renal function is 4 g/day, use:				
1,000 q 6 h	1,000 q 8 h	750 q 8 h	500 q 6 h	500 q 8 h

Off-label dosing –

Infective endocarditis (adults): [1] = Good documentation.

• *E. faecalis infections resistant to penicillin, aminoglycosides, and vancomycin* – 2 g IV every 24 hours in 4 divided doses in combination with ampicillin for at least 8 weeks.

➤*Children:* IV use is not recommended in pediatric patients with CNS infections because of the risk of seizures, or in pediatric patients less than 30 kg with impaired renal function because no data are available.

IM –

12 years of age and older: 10 to 15 mg/kg IM every 6 hours for mild to moderate infections.

IV –

3 months of age and older:

• *Usual dosage* – 15 to 25 mg/kg/dose IV every 6 hours for non-CNS infections.

• *Maximum dose* – 2 g/day for fully susceptible organisms; 4 g/day for infections with moderately susceptible organisms (primarily some strains of *P. aeruginosa*).

• *Cystic fibrosis patients* – Higher doses (up to 90 mg/kg/day in older children) have been used in cystic fibrosis patients.

4 weeks to 3 months of age (weighing at least 1,500 g): 25 mg/kg IV every 6 hours for non-CNS infections.

1 to 4 weeks of age (weighing at least 1,500 g): 25 mg/kg IV every 8 hours for non-CNS infections.

Younger than 1 week of age (weighing at least 1,500 g): 5 mg/kg IV every 12 hours for non-CNS infections.

Off-label dosing –

Catheter-related bloodstream infections (children/adolescents): [2] = Fair documentation.

• *Infants older than 3 months of age and children* – 60 to 100 mg/kg/day IV divided every 6 hours.

• *Infants younger than 3 months of age* – 100 mg/kg/day IV divided every 6 hours.

• *Neonates* – 0 to 4 weeks of age and less than 1,200 g, 20 mg/kg IV every 18 to 24 hours; postnatal age 7 days and younger and 1,200 to 1,500 g, 40 mg/kg/day IV divided every 12 hours; postnatal age 7 days and younger and more than 1,500 g, 50 mg/kg/day IV divided every 12 hours; postnatal age older than 7 days and 1,200 to 1,500 g, 40 mg/kg/day IV divided every 12 hours; postnatal age older than 7 days and more than 1,500 g, 75 mg/kg/day IV divided every 8 hours.

Infective endocarditis (children/adolescents): [1] = Good documentation.

• *E. faecalis infections resistant to penicillin, aminoglycosides, and vancomycin* – 60 to 100 mg/kg/day IV in 4 equally divided doses in combination with ampicillin for at least 8 weeks.

➤*Renal function impairment:* For IV administration, patients with creatinine clearance (CrCl) less than 70 mL/min per 1.73 m^2 require dosage adjustment (see table). For IM administration, safety and efficacy of patients with CrCl less than 20 mL/min per 1.73 m^2 have not been studied.

Reduced Imipenem-Cilastatin IV Dosage in Adult Patients with Impaired Renal Function

Body weight	≥ 70 kg	60 kg	50 kg	40 kg	30 kg
CrCl (mL/min/1.73 m^2)	If total daily dose for normal renal function is 1 g/day, use:				
≥ 71	250 q 6 h	250 q 8 h	125 q 6 h	125 q 6 h	125 q 8 h
41 to 70	250 q 8 h	125 q 6 h	125 q 6 h	125 q 8 h	125 q 8 h
21 to 40	250 q 12 h	250 q 12 h	125 q 8 h	125 q 12 h	125 q 12 h
6 to 20	250 q 12 h	125 q 12 h	125 q 12 h	125 q 12 h	125 q 12 h

IMIPENEM/CILASTATIN — INJECTION

Reduced Imipenem-Cilastatin IV Dosage in Adult Patients with Impaired Renal Function					
Body weight	≥ 70 kg	60 kg	50 kg	40 kg	30 kg
If total daily dose for normal renal function is 1.5 g/day, use:					
≥ 71	500 q 8 h	250 q 6 h	250 q 6 h	250 q 8 h	125 q 6 h
41 to 70	250 q 6 h	250 q 8 h	250 q 8 h	125 q 6 h	125 q 8 h
21 to 40	250 q 8 h	250 q 8 h	250 q 12 h	125 q 8 h	125 q 8 h
6 to 20	250 q 12 h	250 q 12 h	250 q 12 h	125 q 12 h	125 q 12 h
If total daily dose for normal renal function is 2 g/day, use:					
≥ 71	500 q 6 h	500 q 8 h	250 q 6 h	250 q 6 h	250 q 8 h
41 to 70	500 q 8 h	250 q 6 h	250 q 6 h	250 q 8 h	125 q 6 h
21 to 40	250 q 6 h	250 q 8 h	250 q 8 h	250 q 12 h	125 q 8 h
6 to 20	250 q 12 h	250 q 12 h	250 q 12 h	250 q 12 h	125 q 12 h
If total daily dose for normal renal function is 3 g/day, use:					
≥ 71	1,000 q 8 h	750 q 8 h	500 q 6 h	500 q 8 h	250 q 6 h
41 to 70	500 q 6 h	500 q 8 h	500 q 8 h	250 q 6 h	250 q 8 h
21 to 40	500 q 8 h	500 q 8 h	250 q 6 h	250 q 8 h	250 q 8 h
6 to 20	500 q 12 h	500 q 12 h	250 q 12 h	250 q 12 h	250 q 12 h
If total daily dose for normal renal function is 4 g/day, use:					
≥ 71	1,000 q 6 h	1,000 q 8 h	750 q 8 h	500 q 6 h	500 q 8 h
41 to 70	750 q 8 h	750 q 8 h	500 q 6 h	500 q 8 h	250 q 6 h
21 to 40	500 q 6 h	500 q 8 h	500 q 8 h	250 q 6 h	250 q 8 h
6 to 20	500 q 12 h	500 q 12 h	500 q 12 h	250 q 12 h	250 q 12 h

Hemodialysis – Imipenem-cilastatin is cleared by hemodialysis. According to the prescribing information, administer after hemodialysis and at 12-hour intervals timed from the end of that dialysis session. For patients on hemodialysis, imipenem-cilastatin is recommended only when the benefits outweigh the potential risk of seizures. Carefully monitor dialysis patients, especially those with CNS diseases.

Adults receiving continuous renal replacement therapy (CRRT): One reference suggests a dosage of 500 mg IV every 6 hours.

The following alternative recommendations assume ultrafiltration and dialysis flow rates of 1 to 2 L/h.

- *Loading dose* – 1 g IV.
- *Maintenance dosage* – According to one study, a maintenance dosage regimen of 500 mg IV every 6 hours should be considered for those Gram-negative rods with an MIC of 4 to 8 mg/L or for infections difficult to eradicate.

Continuous venovenous hemofiltration (CVVH): 500 mg IV every 8 hours.

Continuous venovenous hemodialysis (CVVHD): 500 mg IV every 6 to 8 hours.

Continuous venovenous hemodiafiltration (CVVHDF): 500 mg IV every 6 hours.

Adults receiving intermittent hemodialysis (IHD): 250 to 500 mg IV every 12 hours. This recommendation assumes the patient is receiving standard IHD 3 times per week and completes the full dialysis sessions.

Continuous ambulatory peritoneal dialysis – Dose as for CrCl less than 10 mL/min.

➤*Preparation for administration:*

IM – Prepare with 1% lidocaine solution (without epinephrine). Prepare the 500 mg vial with 2 mL and the 750 mg vial with 3 mL lidocaine.

IV – Reconstitute contents of infusion bottles with 100 mL diluent (see Compatibility).

➤*Administration:*

IM – Administer by deep IM injection into a large muscle mass (such as the gluteal muscles or lateral part of the thigh) with a 21-gauge 2-inch needle. Aspiration is necessary to avoid inadvertent injection into a blood vessel.

IV – Give a 125, 250, or 500 mg dose by IV infusion over 20 to 30 min. Infuse a 750 mg or 1 g dose over 40 to 60 min. If nausea develops, slow the infusion rate.

For children, give doses less than or equal to 500 mg by IV infusion over 15 to 30 minutes. Give doses more than 500 mg by IV infusion over 40 to 60 minutes.

➤*Admixture compatibility:*

Compatibility – 0.9% Sodium Chloride Injection; 5% or 10% Dextrose Injection; 5% Dextrose and 0.9% Sodium Chloride Injection; 5% Dextrose Injection with 0.225% or 0.45% saline solution; 5% Dextrose Injection with 0.15% potassium chloride solution; Mannitol 5% and 10%.

Incompatibility – Do not mix with or physically add to antibiotics. However, it may be administered concomitantly with other antibiotics (eg, aminoglycosides).

➤*Storage / Stability:* Store dry powder at less than 25°C (77°F).

Imipenem-cilastatin in infusion bottles and vials, reconstituted as directed with the following diluents, maintains satisfactory potency for 4 hours at room temperature and for 24 hours when refrigerated (5°C; 41°F): 0.9% Sodium Chloride Injection; 5% or 10% Dextrose Injection; 5% Dextrose and 0.9% Sodium Chloride Injection; 5% Dextrose Injection with 0.225% or 0.45% saline solution; 5% Dextrose Injection with 0.15% potassium chloride solution; Mannitol 5% and 10%. Do not freeze solutions.

Actions

➤*Pharmacology:* This product is a formulation of imipenem, a thienamycin antibiotic, and cilastatin sodium, the inhibitor of dehydropeptidase 1, which inactivates imipenem when it is administered alone. Cilastatin thereby increases urinary recovery of imipenem and decreases possible renal toxicity associated with excessive intracellular antibiotic accumulation. The bactericidal activity of imipenem results from the inhibition of cell wall synthesis with a high affinity for penicillin binding proteins (PBPs) 1A, 1B, 2, 4, 5, and 6 of *Escherichia coli* and 1A, 1B, 2, 4, and 5 of *Pseudomonas aeruginosa*. The lethal effect is related to binding to PBP 2 and PBP 1B.

➤*Pharmacokinetics:*

Absorption / Distribution –

IV: IV infusion over 20 minutes results in peak plasma levels of imipenem antimicrobial activity of 14 to 24 mcg/ml for the 250 mg dose, 21 to 58 mcg/ml for the 500 mg dose, and 41 to 83 mcg/ml for the 1 g dose. Plasma levels declined to less than 1 mcg/mL in 4 to 6 hours. Peak plasma levels of cilastatin following a 20-minute IV infusion range from 15 to 25 mcg/mL for the 250 mg dose, 31 to 49 mcg/mL for the 500 mg dose, and 56 to 88 mcg/mL for the 1 g dose.

The plasma half-life of each component is approximately 1 hour. Protein binding is 20% for imipenem and 40% for cilastatin. Urine imipenem concentrations more than 10 mcg/mL can be maintained for up to 8 hours at the 500 mg dose.

After a 1 g dose, the following average levels (mcg/ml or mcg/g) of imipenem were measured (usually 1 hour post-dose except where indicated) in the following tissues and fluids: peritoneal 23.9 (2 hours); pleural 22; interstitial 16.4; fallopian tubes 13.6; endometrium 11.1; lung 5.6; bile 5.3 (2.25 hours); myometrium 5; skin, fascia 4.4; vitreous humor 3.4 (3.5 hours); aqueous humor 2.99 (2 hours); CSF (inflamed) 2.6 (2 hours); bone 2.6; sputum 2.1; CSF (uninflamed) 1 (4 hours).

IM: Following IM administration of 500 or 750 mg doses, peak plasma levels of imipenem antimicrobial activity occur within 2 hours and average 10 and 12 mcg/ml, respectively. For cilastatin, peak plasma levels average 24 and 33 mcg/ml, respectively, and occur within 1 hour. When compared with IV administration, imipenem is approximately 75% bioavailable following IM administration while cilastatin is approximately 95% bioavailable. The absorption of imipenem from the IM injection site continues for 6 to 8 hours while that for cilastatin is essentially complete within 4 hours. This prolonged absorption of imipenem following IM use results in an effective plasma half-life of approximately 2 to 3 hours and plasma levels which remain above 2 mcg/ml for at least 6 or 8 hours following a 500 or 750 mg dose, respectively. This plasma profile for imipenem permits IM administration every 12 hours with no accumulation of cilastatin and only slight accumulation of imipenem. Imipenem urine levels remain above 10 mcg/ml for the 12-hour dosing interval following IM administration of 500 or 750 mg doses. Total urinary excretion of imipenem and cilastatin averages 50% and 75%, respectively, following either dose.

Metabolism / Excretion – Imipenem, when administered alone, is metabolized in the kidneys by dehydropeptidase 1 resulting in relatively low levels in urine. Cilastatin, an inhibitor of this enzyme, prevents renal metabolism of imipenem. Within 10 hours of administration, approximately 70% of imipenem and cilastatin is recovered in urine.

➤*Microbiology:* Imipenem has in vitro activity against a wide range of gram-positive and gram-negative organisms. It has a high degree of stability in the presence of beta-lactamases, including penicillinases and cephalosporinases produced by gram-negative and gram-positive bacteria. It is a potent

IMIPENEM/CILASTATIN — INJECTION

inhibitor of β-lactamases from certain gram-negative bacteria resistant to many beta-lactam antibiotics (eg, *Pseudomonas aeruginosa*, *Serratia* sp., *Enterobacter* sp.).

In vitro, imipenem is active against most strains of clinical isolates in the following microorganisms: Gram-positive aerobes; streptococcus; gram-negative aerobes; gram-positive anaerobes; gram-negative anaerobes.

In vitro tests show imipenem to act synergistically with aminoglycoside antibiotics against some isolates of *Pseudomonas aeruginosa*.

Contraindications

Hypersensitivity to any component of this product.

➤*IM:* Hypersensitivity to local anesthetics of the amide type and in patients with severe shock or heart block due to the use of lidocaine HCl diluent.

➤*IV:* Patients with meningitis (safety and efficacy have not been established).

Warnings/Precautions

➤*Benzyl alcohol:* As a preservative, it has been associated with toxicity in neonates. While toxicity has not been demonstrated in children more than 3 months old, small pediatric patients in this age range may also be at risk for benzyl alcohol toxicity. Therefore, do not use diluents containing benzyl alcohol when imipenem-cilastatin IV is constituted for administration to pediatric patients in this age range.

➤*Resistance:* As with other beta-lactam antibiotics, some strains of *Pseudomonas aeruginosa* may develop resistance fairly rapidly during treatment with imipenem-cilastatin. During therapy of *P. aeruginosa* infections, perform periodic susceptibility testing when clinically appropriate.

➤*Pseudomembranous colitis:* Consider this diagnosis in patients who present with diarrhea because it has occurred with nearly all antibacterial agents. Treatment with antibacterial agents alters the normal flora of the colon and may permit overgrowth of clostridia. Studies show that a toxin produced by *Clostridium difficile* is a primary cause of "antibiotic-associated colitis." Initiate therapeutic measures after the diagnosis of pseudomembranous colitis has been established. Mild cases respond to the discontinuation of the drug alone. In moderate-to-severe cases, consider management with fluids and electrolytes, protein supplementation, and treatment with an antibacterial drug effective against *C. difficile* colitis.

➤*CNS effects:* Adverse reactions (eg, myoclonic activity, confusional states, seizures) have occurred with the IV formulation, especially when recommended dosages were exceeded. They are most common in patients with CNS disorders (eg, brain lesions, history of seizures) who may also have compromised renal function. However, CNS adverse experiences have been reported in patients who had no recognized or documented underlying CNS disorder or compromised renal function. Closely adhere to recommended dosage and dosage schedules, especially in patients with known factors that predispose to convulsive activity. Continue anticonvulsants in patients with a known seizure disorder. If focal tremors, myoclonus, or seizures occur, neurologically evaluate patient, institute anticonvulsants, re-examine the dose, and determine whether to decrease dosage or discontinue the drug. If these effects occur with the IM formulation, discontinue the drug.

➤*Cross-allergenicity:* Use caution when administering to patients with a history of penicillin allergy due to a possible cross-sensitivity to imipenem-cilastatin.

➤*Hypersensitivity reactions:* Serious and occasionally fatal hypersensitivity (anaphylactic) reactions have occurred with β-lactam therapy and are more apt to occur in people with a sensitivity history to multiple allergens. Patients with a history of penicillin hypersensitivity have experienced severe reactions when treated with another β-lactam. If a reaction occurs, discontinue the drug. Serious reactions require immediate emergency measures (see Management of Acute Hypersensitivity Reactions).

➤*Renal function impairment:* Do not give imipenem-cilastatin IV to patients with creatinine clearance (CrCl) of less than or equal to 5 mL/min per 1.73 m^2 unless hemodialysis is instituted within 48 hours. For patients on hemodialysis, imipenem-cilastatin IV is recommended only when the benefit outweighs the potential risk of seizures.

➤*Superinfection:* Use of antibiotics (especially prolonged or repeated therapy) may result in bacterial or fungal overgrowth of nonsusceptible organisms. Such overgrowth may lead to secondary infection. Take appropriate measures if superinfection occurs.

➤*Pregnancy: Category C.* There are no adequate and well-controlled studies in pregnant women. Use only when potential benefits outweigh potential hazards.

➤*Lactation:* It is not known whether this drug is excreted in breast milk. Exercise caution when administering to a breast-feeding woman.

➤*Children:*

IM – Safety and efficacy in children younger than 12 years old have not been established.

IV – Use in neonates to 16 years of age (with non-CNS infections) is supported by evidence from adequate and well controlled studies. IV use is not recommended in pediatric patients with CNS infections because of the risk of seizures, or in pediatric patients less than 30 kg with impaired renal function because no data are available.

➤*Monitoring:* While imipenem-cilastatin has the characteristic low toxicity of the beta-lactam group of antibiotics, periodically assess organ system functions, including renal, hepatic, and hematopoietic, during prolonged therapy.

Drug Interactions

Imipenem-Cilastatin Drug Interactions

Precipitant drug	Object drug[a]		Description
Cyclosporine	Imipenem-Cilastatin	↑	The CNS side effects of both agents may be increased possibly because of additive or synergistic toxicity.
Imipenem-Cilastatin	Cyclosporine	↑	
Imipenem-Cilastatin	Ganciclovir	↑	Generalized seizures have occurred with coadministration. Do not use concomitantly.
Probenecid	Imipenem	↑	Coadministration results in only minimal increases in imipenem levels and half-life; do not give probenecid concurrently.

[a] ↑ = object drug increased.

Adverse Reactions

➤*IV:*

Lab test abnormalities –

Hepatic: Increased AST, ALT, alkaline phosphatase, bilirubin, and LDH.

Hemic: Increased eosinophils, monocytes, lymphocytes, basophils; decreased neutrophils, agranulocytosis, hemoglobin, hematocrit; increased/decreased WBCs and platelets; positive Coombs' test; abnormal prothrombin time.

Electrolytes: Decreased serum sodium; increased potassium and chloride.

Renal: Increased BUN and creatinine.

Urinalysis: Presence of protein, RBCs, WBCs, casts, bilirubin, or urobilinogen.

Cardiovascular – Hypotension (0.4%); palpitations, tachycardia (less than 0.2%).

CNS – Fever (0.5%); seizures (0.4%); dizziness (0.3%); somnolence (0.2%); encephalopathy, tremor, confusion, myoclonus, paresthesia, vertigo, headache, psychic disturbances including hallucinations (less than 0.2%).

Dermatologic – Rash (0.9%); pruritus (0.3%); urticaria (0.2%); erythema multiforme, Stevens-Johnson syndrome, angioneurotic edema, toxic epidermal necrolysis, flushing, cyanosis, skin texture changes, candidiasis, hyperhidrosis, pruritus vulvae (less than 0.2%).

GI – Nausea (2%); diarrhea (1.8%); vomiting (1.5%); pseudomembranous colitis, hemorrhagic colitis, hepatitis, jaundice, staining of the teeth or tongue, gastroenteritis, abdominal pain, glossitis, tongue papillar hypertrophy, heartburn, pharyngeal pain, increased salivation (less than 0.2%).

Hematologic – Pancytopenia, bone marrow depression, thrombocytopenia, neutropenia, leukopenia, hemolytic anemia (less than 0.2%).

Local – Phlebitis/thrombophlebitis (3.1%); pain (0.7%) and erythema at injection site (0.4%); vein induration (0.2%); infused vein infection (0.1%).

Respiratory – Chest discomfort, dyspnea, hyperventilation, thoracic spine pain (less than 0.2%).

Miscellaneous – Hearing loss, tinnitus, polyarthralgia, taste perversion, asthenia/weakness, drug fever, oliguria/anuria, polyuria, acute renal failure, urine discoloration (less than 0.2%).

Children –

Children greater than or equal to 3 months old: Diarrhea (3.9%); rash, phlebitis (2.2%); gastroenteritis, vomiting, IV site irritation, urine discoloration (1.1%).

Newborn to 3 months old: Convulsions (5.9%); diarrhea (3%); oliguria/anuria (2.2%); oral candidiasis, rash, tachycardia (1.5%).

➤*IM:*

Lab test abnormalities –

Hemic: Decreased hemoglobin and hematocrit; eosinophilia; increased/decreased WBCs and platelets; decreased erythrocytes; increased prothrombin time.

Hepatic: Increased AST, ALT, alkaline phosphatase and bilirubin.

Renal: Increased BUN and creatinine.

Urinalysis: Presence of RBCs, WBCs, casts and bacteria in the urine.

Miscellaneous – Pain at the injection site (1.2%); nausea, diarrhea (0.6%); rash (0.4%); vomiting (0.3%).

Overdosage

➤*Treatment:* In the case of overdosage, discontinue the drug. Treat symptomatically and institute supportive measures as required. Refer to General Management of Acute Overdosage. Imipenem-cilastatin is hemodialyzable; however, usefulness of this procedure in the overdosage setting is questionable.

ERTAPENEM

Rx	**Invanz** (Merck)	**Injection, lyophilized powder for solution:** 1 g	Equiv. to ertapenem sodium 1.046 g. Sodium 6 mEq, sodium bicarbonate 175 mg. In single-dose vials and single-dose *ADD-Vantage* vials.

ERTAPENEM SODIUM — INJECTION

Indications

➤*Moderate to severe infections:*

Acute pelvic infections – For the treatment of acute pelvic infections, including postpartum endomyometritis, septic abortion, and postsurgical gynecologic infections caused by *Streptococcus agalactiae, Escherichia coli, Bacteroides fragilis, Porphyromonas asaccharolytica, Peptostreptococcus* sp., or *Prevotella bivia*.

Community-acquired pneumonia – For the treatment of community-acquired pneumonia (CAP) caused by *Streptococcus pneumoniae* (penicillin-susceptible isolates only), including cases with concurrent bacteremia, *Haemophilus influenzae* (beta-lactamase–negative isolates only), or *Moraxella catarrhalis*.

Complicated intra-abdominal infections – For the treatment of complicated intra-abdominal infections (IAI) caused by *E. coli, Clostridium clostridioforme, Eubacterium lentum, Peptostreptococcus* sp., *B. fragilis, Bacteroides distasonis, Bacteroides ovatus, Bacteroides thetaiotaomicron*, or *Bacteroides uniformis*.

Complicated skin and skin structure infections – For the treatment of complicated skin and skin structure infections (SSSIs), including diabetic foot infections without osteomyelitis caused by *Staphylococcus aureus* (methicillin-susceptible isolates only), *S. agalactiae, Streptococcus pyogenes, E. coli, Klebsiella pneumoniae, Proteus mirabilis, B. fragilis* , *Peptostreptococcus* sp., *P. asaccharolytica*, or *P. bivia*. Ertapenem has not been studied in diabetic foot infections with concomitant osteomyelitis.

Complicated urinary tract infections – For the treatment of complicated urinary tract infections (UTIs), including pyelonephritis caused by *E. coli*, including cases with concurrent bacteremia or *K. pneumoniae*.

➤*Prophylaxis of surgical-site infection:*

Colorectal surgery – For the prophylaxis of surgical site infection in adults following elective colorectal surgery in adults.

➤*Off-label uses:*

Catheter-related bloodstream infections – [1] = Good documentation. Guidelines suggest that empiric use of ertapenem should be based on local antimicrobial susceptibility data and severity of disease. Ertapenem can be used to treat catheter-related bloodstream infections caused by gram-negative bacilli that are extended-spectrum beta-lactamase (ESBL)–positive, *Enterobacter* species, and *Serratia marcescens*. Ertapenem may also be used as an alternative antimicrobial agent for the treatment of catheter-related bloodstream infections caused by *Ochrobactrum anthropi*. There is a lack of information supporting the use of ertapenem in children.

Hospital-acquired pneumonia – [1] = Good documentation. According to American Thoracic Society/Infectious Diseases Society of America practice guidelines, ertapenem has proved useful in the treatment of hospital-acquired pneumonia, ventilator-associated pneumonia, and health care–associated pneumonia as both empiric therapy in patients without known risk factors for multidrug-resistant pathogens and infections caused by extended-spectrum, beta-lactamase–producing gram-negative bacteria. The use of ertapenem is considered more convenient because of its once-daily dosing schedule.

Administration and Dosage

➤*Adults:*

Acute pelvic infections –

Usual dosage: 1 g once daily.

Duration of therapy: 3 to 10 days.

Community-acquired pneumonia –

Usual dosage: 1 g once daily.

Duration of therapy: 10 to 14 days. Duration includes a possible switch to an appropriate oral therapy after at least 3 days of parenteral therapy, once clinical improvement has been demonstrated.

Complicated intra-abdominal infections –

Usual dosage: 1 g once daily.

Duration of therapy: 5 to 14 days.

Complicated skin and skin structure infections –

Usual dosage: 1 g once daily.

Duration of therapy: 7 to 14 days. Adults with diabetic foot infections received up to 28 days of treatment (parenteral or parenteral plus oral switch therapy).

Complicated urinary tract infections –

Usual dosage: 1 g once daily.

Duration of therapy: 10 to 14 days. Duration includes a possible switch to an appropriate oral therapy after at least 3 days of parenteral therapy, once clinical improvement has been demonstrated.

Prophylaxis of surgical-site infection following colorectal surgery – 1 g administered by intravenous (IV) infusion 1 hour prior to surgical incision.

Off-label dosing –

Catheter-related bloodstream infections: [1] = Good documentation. 1 g IV infused over 30 minutes once a day for up to 14 days.

Hospital-acquired pneumonia: [1] = Good documentation. Empiric therapy should begin with ertapenem 1 g IV daily, infused over 30 minutes, for a total duration of 7 to 14 days.

➤*Children:*

13 years of age and older – See Adults for dosing.

3 months to 12 years of age –

Acute pelvic infections:
- *Usual dosage* – 15 mg/kg twice daily.
- *Maximum dose* – 1 g/day.
- *Duration of therapy* – 3 to 10 days.

Community-acquired pneumonia:
- *Usual dosage* – 15 mg/kg twice daily.
- *Maximum dose* – 1 g/day.
- *Duration of therapy* – 10 to 14 days. Duration includes a possible switch to an appropriate oral therapy after at least 3 days of parenteral therapy, once clinical improvement has been demonstrated.

Complicated intra-abdominal infections:
- *Usual dosage* – 15 mg/kg twice daily.
- *Maximum dose* – 1 g/day.
- *Duration of therapy* – 5 to 14 days.

Complicated skin and skin structure infections:
- *Usual dosage* – 15 mg/kg twice daily.
- *Maximum dose* – 1 g/day.
- *Duration of therapy* – 7 to 14 days.

Complicated urinary tract infections:
- *Usual dosage* – 15 mg/kg twice daily.
- *Maximum dose* – 1 g/day.
- *Duration of therapy* – 10 to 14 days. Duration includes a possible switch to an appropriate oral therapy after at least 3 days of parenteral therapy, once clinical improvement has been demonstrated.

➤*Renal function impairment:*

Adults –

Creatinine clearance 30 mL/min/1.73 m² or less and end-stage renal impairment (Creatinine clearance 10 mL/min/1.73 m² or less: 500 mg daily.

Hemodialysis: 500 mg within 6 hours prior to hemodialysis, a supplementary dose of 150 mg is recommended following the hemodialysis session. If ertapenem is given at least 6 hours prior to hemodialysis, no supplementary dose is needed.

➤*Preparation for administration:*

IV – Ertapenem must be reconstituted and then diluted prior to administration.

Reconstitute the contents of a 1 g vial of ertapenem with 10 mL of one of the following: water for injection, sodium chloride 0.9% injection, or bacteriostatic water for injection. Shake well to dissolve. For adults and children 13 years of age and older, immediately transfer the contents of the reconstituted vial to sodium chloride 0.9% injection 50 mL. For children 3 months to 12 years of age, immediately withdraw a volume equal to 15 mg/kg of body weight (not to exceed 1 g/day) and dilute in sodium chloride 0.9% injection to a final concentration of 20 mg/mL or less. Complete the infusion within 6 hours of reconstitution.

ADD-Vantage vials: Ertapenem in *ADD-Vantage* vials should be reconstituted with *ADD-Vantage* diluent containers containing 50 or 100 mL of 0.9% sodium chloride injection.

Intramuscular – Ertapenem must be reconstituted prior to administration. Reconstitute the contents of a 1 g vial of ertapenem with 3.2 mL of lidocaine hydrochloride 1% injection (without epinephrine). Shake the vial thoroughly to form the solution. For adults, immediately withdraw the contents of the vial and administer by deep intramuscular (IM) injection. For children, immediately withdraw a volume equal to 15 mg/kg of body weight (not to exceed 1 g/day) and administer by deep IM injection. The reconstituted IM solution should be used within 1 hour after preparation. The reconstituted solution should not be administered IV.

➤*Administration:* Administer by IV infusion for up to 14 days or IM injection for up to 7 days.

IV – Infuse over a period of 30 minutes.

IM – IM administration may be used as an alternative to IV in the treatment of those infections for which IM therapy is appropriate. Administer by deep IM injection into a large muscle mass (eg, the gluteal muscles, lateral part of the thigh).

➤*Admixture compatibility:* Do not mix or coinfuse ertapenem with other medications. Do not use diluents containing dextrose (alpha-D-glucose).

➤*Storage/Stability:* Do not store the powder above 25°C (77°F). The reconstituted IM solution should be used within 1 hour after preparation. The reconstituted solution, immediately diluted in sodium chloride 0.9% injection, may be stored at room temperature (25°C [77°F]) and used within 6 hours, or stored for 24 hours under refrigeration (5°C [41°F]) and used within 4 hours after removal from refrigeration. Do not freeze.

Actions

➤*Pharmacology:* Ertapenem is structurally related to beta-lactam antibiotics. The bactericidal activity of ertapenem results from the inhibition of

ERTAPENEM SODIUM — INJECTION

cell wall synthesis and is mediated through ertapenem's binding to penicillin-binding proteins (PBPs).

➤*Pharmacokinetics:*

Absorption – Ertapenem, reconstituted with lidocaine 1% injection (in saline without epinephrine), is almost completely absorbed following IM administration at the recommended dose of 1 g. The mean bioavailability is approximately 90%. Following 1 g daily IM administration, mean peak plasma concentrations (C_{max}) are achieved in approximately 2.3 hours (time to maximal concentration [T_{max}]).

Adults:

Ertapenem Plasma Concentrations in Adults After Single-Dose Administration									
	Average plasma concentrations (mcg/mL)								
Dose/Route	0.5 h	1 h	2 h	4 h	6 h	8 h	12 h	18 h	24 h
1 g IV[a]	155	115	83	48	31	20	9	3	1
1 g IM	33	53	67	57	40	27	13	4	2

[a] Infused at a constant rate over 30 minutes.

The area under the curve (AUC) of ertapenem in adults increased less than dose proportional based on total ertapenem concentrations over the 0.5 to 2 g dose range, whereas the AUC increased more than dose proportional based on unbound ertapenem concentrations. Ertapenem exhibits nonlinear pharmacokinetics because of concentration-dependent plasma protein binding at the proposed therapeutic dose.

There is no accumulation of ertapenem following multiple IV or IM 1 g daily doses in healthy adults.

Children:

Ertapenem Plasma Concentrations in Children After Single-Dose IV[a] Administration									
		Average plasma concentrations (mcg/mL)							
Age group	Dose	0.5 h	1 h	2 h	4 h	6 h	8 h	12 h	24 h
3 to 23 months									
	15 mg/kg[b]	103.8	57.3	43.6	23.7	13.5	8.2	2.5	—
	20 mg/kg[b]	126.8	87.6	58.7	28.4	—	12	3.4	0.4
	40 mg/kg[c]	199.1	144.1	95.7	58	—	20.2	7.7	0.6
2 to 12 years									
	15 mg/kg[b]	113.2	63.9	42.1	21.9	12.8	7.6	3	—
	20 mg/kg[b]	147.6	97.6	63.2	34.5	—	12.3	4.9	0.5
	40 mg/kg[c]	241.7	152.7	96.3	55.6	—	18.8	7.2	0.6
13 to 17 years									
	20 mg/kg[b]	170.4	98.3	67.8	40.4	—	16	7	1.1
	1 g[d]	155.9	110.9	74.8	—	24	—	6.2	—
	40 mg/kg[c]	255	188.7	127.9	76.2	—	31	15.3	2.1

[a] Infused at a constant rate over 30 minutes.
[b] Up to a maximum dose of 1 g/day.
[c] Up to a maximum dose of 2 g/day.
[d] Based on 3 patients receiving ertapenem 1 g who volunteered for pharmacokinetic assessment in 1 of the 2 safety and efficacy studies.

Distribution – Ertapenem is highly bound to human plasma proteins, primarily albumin. In healthy young adults, the protein binding of ertapenem decreases as plasma concentrations increase, from approximately 95% bound at an approximate plasma concentration of less than 100 mcg/mL to approximately 85% bound at an approximate plasma concentration of 300 mcg/mL.

The apparent volume of distribution at steady state (V_{ss}) of ertapenem in adults is approximately 0.12 L/kg, approximately 0.2 L/kg in children 3 months to 12 years of age, and approximately 0.16 L/kg in children 13 to 17 years of age.

Ertapenem Concentrations (mcg/mL) in Adult Skin Blister Fluid[a]						
0.5 h	1 h	2 h	4 h	8 h	12 h	24 h
7	12	17	24	24	21	8

[a] Concentrations from day 3 of 1 g once daily IV dosing.

The ratio of AUC_{0-24} in skin blister fluid/AUC_{0-24} in plasma is 0.61.

The concentration of ertapenem in breast milk from 5 lactating women with pelvic infections (5 to 14 days postpartum) was measured at random time points daily for 5 consecutive days following the last 1 g dose of IV therapy (3 to 10 days of therapy). The concentration of ertapenem in breast milk within 24 hours of the last dose of therapy in all 5 women ranged from less than 0.13 (lower limit of quantitation) to 0.38 mcg/mL; peak concentrations were not assessed. By day 5 after discontinuation of therapy, the level of ertapenem was undetectable in the breast milk of 4 women and below the lower limit of quantitation (less than 0.13 mcg/mL) in 1 woman.

Metabolism – In healthy young adults, after infusion of IV radiolabeled ertapenem 1 g, the plasma radioactivity consisted predominantly (94%) of ertapenem. The major metabolite of ertapenem is the inactive ring-opened derivative formed by hydrolysis of the beta-lactam ring.

Excretion – Ertapenem is eliminated primarily by the kidneys. The mean plasma half-life in healthy young adults is approximately 4 hours, and the plasma clearance is approximately 1.8 L/h. The mean plasma half-life in children 13 to 17 years of age is approximately 4 hours and approximately 2.5 hours in children 3 months to 12 years of age.

Following the administration of IV radiolabeled ertapenem 1 g to healthy young adults, approximately 80% is recovered in urine and 10% in feces. Of the 80% recovered in urine, approximately 38% is excreted as unchanged drug and approximately 37% as the ring-opened metabolite.

In healthy young adults given a 1 g IV dose, the mean percentage of the administered dose excreted in urine was 17.4% during 0 to 2 hours postdose, 5.4% during 4 to 6 hours postdose, and 2.4% during 12 to 24 hours postdose.

Special populations –

Renal function impairment: The unbound AUC increased 4.4- and 7.6-fold in subjects with advanced renal insufficiency (CrCl = 5 to 30 mL/min/1.73 m^2) and end-stage renal insufficiency (CrCl less than 10 mL/min/1.73 m^2), respectively, compared with healthy young subjects. The effects of renal insufficiency on AUC of total drug were of smaller magnitude. The recommended dose of ertapenem in adults with a CrCl of 30 mL/min/1.73 m^2 or less is 0.5 g every 24 hours.

Following a single 1 g IV dose given immediately prior to a 4-hour hemodialysis session in 5 patients with end-stage renal insufficiency, approximately 30% of the dose was recovered in the dialysate. A supplementary dose of 150 mg is recommended if ertapenem is administered within 6 hours prior to hemodialysis.

Elderly: The total and unbound AUC increased 37% and 67%, respectively, in elderly adults relative to young adults. These changes were attributed to age-related changes in CrCl.

Children: The plasma clearance (mL/min/kg) of ertapenem in patients 3 months to 12 years of age is approximately 2-fold higher compared with that in adults. At the 15 mg/kg dose, the AUC value (doubled to model a twice-daily dosing regimen [ie, 30 mg/kg/day exposure]) in patients 3 months to 12 years of age was comparable with the AUC value in young healthy adults receiving a 1 g IV dose of ertapenem.

➤*Microbiology:* Ertapenem has in vitro activity against gram-positive and gram-negative aerobic and anaerobic bacteria. The bactericidal activity of ertapenem results from the inhibition of cell wall synthesis and is mediated through ertapenem's binding to PBPs. In *E. coli*, it has strong affinity toward PBPs 1a, 1b, 2, 3, 4, and 5, with preference for PBPs 2 and 3. Ertapenem is stable against hydrolysis by a variety of beta-lactamases, including penicillinases, cephalosporinases, and ESBL. Ertapenem is hydrolyzed by metallo-beta–lactamases.

Aerobic and facultative gram-positive microorganisms – *S. aureus* (methicillin-susceptible isolates only), *S. agalactiae*, *S. pneumoniae* (penicillin-susceptible isolates only), and *S. pyogenes*.

Note: Methicillin-resistant staphylococci and *Enterococcus* species are resistant to ertapenem.

Aerobic and facultative gram-negative microorganisms – *E. coli*, *H. influenzae* (beta-lactamase–negative strains only), *K. pneumoniae*, *M. catarrhalis*, and *P. mirabilis*.

Anaerobic microorganisms – *B. fragilis*, *B. distasonis*, *B. ovatus*, *B. thetaiotaomicron*, *B. uniformis*, *C. clostridioforme*, *E. lentum*, *Peptostreptococcus* species, *P. asaccharolytica*, and *P. bivia*.

The following in vitro data are available, but their clinical significance is unknown.

At least 90% of the following microorganisms exhibit an in vitro minimum inhibitory concentration (MIC) less than or equal to the susceptible breakpoint for ertapenem; however, the safety and efficacy of ertapenem in treating clinical infections caused by these microorganisms have not been established in adequate and well-controlled clinical studies:

Aerobic and facultative gram-positive microorganisms – *Staphylococcus epidermidis* (methicillin-susceptible isolates only) and *S. pneumoniae* (penicillin-intermediate isolates only).

Aerobic and facultative gram-negative microorganisms – *Citrobacter freundii*, *Citrobacter koseri*, *Enterobacter aerogenes*, *Enterobacter cloacae*, *H. influenzae* (beta-lactamase–positive isolates), *Haemophilus parainfluenzae*, *Klebsiella oxytoca* (excluding ESBL-producing isolates), *Morganella morganii*, *Proteus vulgaris*, *Providencia rettgeri*, *Providencia stuartii*, and *S. marcescens*.

Contraindications

Known hypersensitivity to any component of this product or to other drugs in the same class or in patients who have demonstrated anaphylactic reactions to beta-lactams; known hypersensitivity to local anesthetics of the amide type (IM use only).

Warnings/Precautions

➤*Clostridium difficile–associated diarrhea:* *Clostridum difficile*–associated diarrhea (CDAD) has been reported with use of nearly all antibacterial agents, including ertapenem, and may range in severity from mild diarrhea to fatal colitis. Treatment with antibacterial agents alters the normal flora of the colon, leading to overgrowth of *C. difficile*.

C. difficile produces toxins A and B, which contribute to the development of CDAD. Hypertoxin-producing strains of *C. difficile* cause increased morbidity and mortality, as these infections can be refractory to antimicrobial therapy and may require colectomy. CDAD must be considered in all patients who present with diarrhea following antibiotic use. Careful medical history is necessary because CDAD has been reported to occur over 2 months after the administration of antibacterial agents.

If CDAD is suspected or confirmed, ongoing antibiotic use not directed against *C. difficile* may need to be discontinued. Institute appropriate fluid and electrolyte management, protein supplementation, antibiotic treatment of *C. difficile*, and surgical evaluation as clinically indicated.

ERTAPENEM SODIUM — INJECTION

➤*IM administration:* Use caution when administering ertapenem IM to avoid inadvertent injection into a blood vessel.

Lidocaine is the diluent for IM administration of ertapenem.

➤*Drug resistance:* Prescribing ertapenem in the absence of a proven or strongly suspected bacterial infection or a prophylactic indication is unlikely to provide benefit to the patient and increases the risk of the development of drug-resistant bacteria.

➤*Seizures:* Seizures and other CNS adverse reactions have been reported during treatment with ertapenem.

Case reports have shown that coadministration of carbapenems, including ertapenem, to patients receiving valproic acid or divalproex sodium results in a reduction in valproic acid concentrations. The valproic acid concentrations may drop below the therapeutic range as a result of this interaction, therefore increasing the risk of breakthrough seizures. Increasing the dose of valproic acid or divalproex sodium may not be sufficient to overcome this interaction. The concomitant use of ertapenem and valproic acid/divalproex sodium is generally not recommended. Consider antibacterials other than carbapenems to treat infections in patients whose seizures are well controlled on valproic acid or divalproex sodium. If administration of ertapenem is necessary, consider supplemental anticonvulsant therapy

During clinical investigations in adults treated with ertapenem 1 g once a day, seizures, irrespective of drug relationship, occurred in 0.5% of patients during study therapy plus a 14-day follow-up period. These reactions have occurred most commonly in patients with CNS disorders (eg, brain lesions, history of seizures) and/or compromised renal function. Close adherence to the recommended dosage regimen is urged, especially in patients with known factors that predispose to convulsive activity. Continue anticonvulsant therapy in patients with known seizure disorders. If focal tremors, myoclonus, or seizures occur, evaluate patients neurologically, place them on anticonvulsant therapy if not already instituted, and reexamine the dosage of ertapenem to determine whether it should be decreased or the antibiotic discontinued.

➤*Hypersensitivity reactions:* Serious and occasionally fatal hypersensitivity (anaphylactic) reactions have been reported in patients receiving therapy with beta-lactams. These reactions are more likely to occur in individuals with a history of sensitivity to multiple allergens. There have been reports of individuals with a history of penicillin hypersensitivity who have experienced severe hypersensitivity reactions when treated with another beta-lactam. Before initiating therapy with ertapenem, make careful inquiry concerning previous hypersensitivity reactions to penicillins, cephalosporins, other beta-lactams, and other allergens. If an allergic reaction to ertapenem occurs, discontinue the drug immediately. Serious anaphylactic reactions require immediate emergency treatment with epinephrine, oxygen, IV steroids, and airway management, including intubation. Other therapy may also be administered as indicated.

➤*Renal function impairment:* Dosage adjustment of ertapenem is recommended in patients with reduced renal function.

➤*Superinfection:* As with other antibiotics, prolonged use of ertapenem may result in overgrowth of nonsusceptible organisms. Repeated evaluation of the patient's condition is essential. If superinfection occurs during therapy, take appropriate measures.

➤*Pregnancy: Category B.* There are no adequate and well-controlled studies in pregnant women. Because animal reproduction studies are not always predictive of human response, use this drug during pregnancy only if clearly needed. It is not known if ertapenem crosses the human placenta. The molecular weight (about 498) is low enough that passage to the fetus should be expected.

In mice given 700 mg/kg/day, slight decreases in average fetal weights and an associated decrease in the average number of ossified sacrocaudal vertebrae were observed. Ertapenem crosses the placental barrier in rats.

➤*Lactation:* Ertapenem is excreted in human breast milk. Exercise caution when administering ertapenem to a breast-feeding women. Administer ertapenem to breast-feeding mothers only when the expected benefit outweighs the risk.

➤*Children:* Ertapenem is not recommended in infants younger than 3 months of age. No data are available.

Ertapenem is not recommended in the treatment of meningitis in children because of a lack of sufficient cerebrospinal fluid penetration.

➤*Elderly:* This drug is known to be substantially excreted by the kidney, and the risk of toxic reactions to this drug may be greater in patients with impaired renal function. Because elderly patients are more likely to have decreased renal function, take care in dose selection and consider monitoring renal function.

➤*Monitoring:* While ertapenem possesses toxicity similar to the beta-lactam group of antibiotics, periodic assessment of organ system function, including renal, hepatic, and hematopoietic, is advisable during prolonged therapy.

Drug Interactions

Ertapenem Drug Interactions

Precipitant drug	Object drug[a]		Description
Probenecid	Ertapenem	⬆	Probenecid increased ertapenem's AUC by 25% and reduced plasma and renal clearances 20% and 35%, respectively. Ertapenem's half-life increased from 4 to 4.8 hours. Because of the small effect on half-life, coadministration of probenecid to extend the half-life of ertapenem is not recommended.
Ertapenem	Valproic acid	⬇	Valproic acid plasma levels may be decreased, leading to a loss of seizure control. Monitor valproic acid plasma concentrations and observe the patient for seizure activity. Consider adjusting the valproic acid dose as needed or using an alternative antibiotic.

[a] ⬆ = object drug increased; ⬇ = object drug decreased.

Adverse Reactions

➤*Moderate to severe infections in adults:* Clinical studies enrolled 1,954 patients treated with ertapenem; in some of the clinical studies, parenteral therapy was followed by a switch to an appropriate oral antimicrobial. Most adverse reactions reported in these clinical studies were described as mild to moderate in severity. Ertapenem was discontinued because of adverse reactions in 4.7% of patients.

Common adverse reactions – The most common drug-related adverse reactions in patients treated with ertapenem, including those who were switched to therapy with an oral antimicrobial, were diarrhea (5.5%), infused vein complication (3.7%), nausea (3.1%), headache (2.2%), vaginitis in women (2.1%), phlebitis/thrombophlebitis (1.3%), and vomiting (1.1%).

Adverse reactions (1% or more):

Ertapenem Adverse Reactions in Adults (≥ 1%)

Adverse reactions	Ertapenem[a] 1 g daily (n = 802)	Piperacillin/ tazobactam[a] 3.375 g every 6 h (n = 774)	Ertapenem[b] 1 g daily (n = 1,152)	Ceftriaxone[b] 1 or 2 g daily (n = 942)
Cardiovascular				
Hypertension	1.6%	1.4%	0.7%	1%
Hypotension	2%	1.4%	1%	1.2%
Tachycardia	1.6%	1.3%	1.3%	0.7%
CNS				
Altered mental status[c]	5.1%	3.4%	3.3%	2.5%
Anxiety	1.4%	1.3%	0.8%	1.2%
Asthenia/fatigue	1.2%	0.9%	1.2%	1.1%
Dizziness	2.1%	3%	1.5%	2.1%
Headache	5.6%	5.4%	6.8%	6.9%
Insomnia	3.2%	5.2%	3%	4.1%
Dermatologic				
Erythema	1.6%	1.7%	1.2%	1.2%
Pruritus	2%	2.6%	1%	1.9%
Rash	2.5%	3.1%	2.3%	1.5%
GI				
Abdominal pain	3.6%	4.8%	4.3%	3.9%
Acid regurgitation	1.6%	0.9%	1.1%	0.6%
Constipation	4%	5.4%	3.3%	3.1%
Diarrhea	10.3%	12.1%	9.2%	9.8%
Dyspepsia	1.1%	0.6%	1%	1.6%
Nausea	8.5%	8.7%	6.4%	7.4%
Oral candidiasis	0.1%	1.3%	1.4%	1.9%
Vomiting	3.7%	5.3%	4%	4%
Local				
Extravasation	1.9%	1.7%	0.7%	1.1%
Infused vein complication	7.1%	7.9%	5.4%	6.7%
Phlebitis/ thrombophlebitis	1.9%	2.7%	1.6%	2%

ERTAPENEM SODIUM — INJECTION

Ertapenem Adverse Reactions in Adults (≥ 1%)				
Adverse reactions	Ertapenem[a] 1 g daily (n = 802)	Piperacillin/tazobactam[a] 3.375 g every 6 h (n = 774)	Ertapenem[b] 1 g daily (n = 1,152)	Ceftriaxone[b] 1 or 2 g daily (n = 942)
Respiratory				
Cough	1.6%	1.7%	1.3%	0.5%
Dyspnea	2.6%	1.8%	1%	2.4%
Pharyngitis	0.7%	1.4%	1.1%	0.6%
Rales/rhonchi	1.1%	1%	0.5%	1%
Respiratory distress	1%	0.4%	0.2%	0.2%
Miscellaneous				
Chest pain	1.5%	1.4%	1%	2.5%
Death	2.5%	1.6%	1.3%	1.6%
Edema/swelling	3.4%	2.5%	2.9%	3.3%
Fever	5%	6.6%	2.3%	3.4%
Leg pain	1.1%	0.5%	0.4%	0.3%
Vaginitis	1.4%	1%	3.3%	3.7%

[a] Includes phase 2b/3 complicated IAI, complicated SSSI, and acute pelvic infections studies.
[b] Includes phase 2b/3 CAP and complicated UTI, and phase 2a studies.
[c] Includes agitation, changed mental status, confusion, decreased mental acuity, disorientation, somnolence, or stupor.

Mortality: In patients treated for complicated IAI, death occurred in 4.7% of patients receiving ertapenem and 2.6% of patients receiving comparator drug. These deaths occurred in patients with significant comorbidity and/or severe baseline infections. Deaths were considered unrelated to study drugs by investigators.

Seizures: In clinical studies, seizure was reported during study therapy plus a 14-day follow-up period in 0.5% of patients treated with ertapenem, 0.3% of patients treated with piperacillin/tazobactam, and 0% of patients treated with ceftriaxone.

Additional adverse reactions (more than 0.1%) –

Cardiovascular: Arrhythmia, asystole, atrial fibrillation, bradycardia, cardiac arrest, heart failure, heart murmur, hematoma, subdural hemorrhage, syncope, ventricular tachycardia.

CNS: Aggressive behavior, depression, hypesthesia, malaise, nervousness, paresthesia, seizure, spasm, tremor, vertigo.

Dermatologic: Dermatitis, desquamation, flushing, sweating, urticaria.

GI: Abdominal distention, anorexia, CDAD, cholelithiasis, duodenitis, dysphagia, esophagitis, flatulence, gastritis, GI hemorrhage, hemorrhoids, ileus, jaundice, mouth ulcer, pancreatitis, pyloric stenosis, stomatitis.

GU: Bladder dysfunction, hematuria, oliguria/anuria, renal insufficiency, urinary retention, vaginal candidiasis, vaginal pruritus, vulvovaginitis.

Local: Injection-site induration, injection-site pain.

Respiratory: Asthma, bronchoconstriction, epistaxis, hemoptysis, hiccups, hypoxemia, pharyngeal discomfort, pleural effusion, pleuritic pain, voice disturbance.

Miscellaneous: Candidiasis, chills, dehydration, facial edema, flank pain, gout, necrosis, pain, septic shock, septicemia, taste perversion, weight loss.

Prophylaxis of surgical-site infection in adults –

Ertapenem Adverse Reactions in Adults for Prophylaxis of Surgical-Site Infections (≥ 1%)		
Adverse reactions	Ertapenem 1 g (n = 476)	Cefotetan 2 g (n = 476)
Dermatologic		
Wound complication	2.9%	2.3%
Wound dehiscence	1.3%	1.5%
Wound infection	6.5%	12.4%
Wound secretion	1.9%	2.1%
GI		
C. difficile infection or colitis	1.7%	0.6%
Small intestinal obstruction	2.1%	1.9%
GU		
Dysuria	1.1%	1.3%
UTI	3.8%	5.5%
Local		
Cellulitis	1.5%	1.5%
Seroma	1.3%	1.9%
Respiratory		
Atelectasis	3.4%	1.9%
Pneumonia	2.1%	4%
Miscellaneous		
Anastomatic leak	1.5%	1.3%
Anemia	5.7%	6.9%
Postoperative infection	2.3%	4%

Additional adverse reactions (more than 0.5% to less than 1%) –

GI: Abdominal abscess, dry mouth, hematochezia, intestinal stoma complication.

Local: Incision-site complication, incision-site hemorrhage.

Respiratory: Lung crackles, lung infiltration, pulmonary congestion, pulmonary embolism, wheezing.

Miscellaneous: Cerebrovascular accident, crepitations, fungal rash, muscle spasms, pelvic abscess, pollakiuria.

➤*Children:*

Common adverse reactions – The most common drug-related adverse reactions in children treated with ertapenem, including those who were switched to therapy with an oral antimicrobial, were diarrhea (6.5%), infusion-site pain (5.5%), infusion-site erythema (2.6%), and vomiting (2.1%).

Ertapenem Adverse Reactions in Children (≥ 1%)			
Adverse reactions	Ertapenem[a,b] (n = 384)	Ceftriaxone[a] (n = 100)	Ticarcillin/clavulanate[b] (n = 24)
CNS			
Dizziness	1.6%	0%	0%
Headache	4.4%	4%	0%
Dermatologic			
Dermatitis	1%	1%	0%
Diaper dermatitis	4.7%	4%	0%
Pruritus	1.6%	0%	0%
Rash	2.9%	2%	8.3%
GI			
Abdominal abscess	1%	0%	4.2%
Abdominal pain	4.7%	3%	4.2%
Constipation	2.3%	0%	0%
Diarrhea	11.7%	17%	4.2%
Loose stools	2.1%	0%	0%
Nausea	1.6%	0%	0%
Upper abdominal pain	1%	2%	0%
Vomiting	10.2%	11%	8.3%
Local			
Infusion-site erythema	3.9%	3%	8.3%
Infusion-site induration	1%	1%	0%
Infusion-site pain	7%	4%	20.8%
Infusion-site phlebitis	1.8%	3%	0%
Infusion-site swelling	1.8%	1%	4.2%
Infusion-site warmth	1.3%	1%	4.2%
Respiratory			
Cough	4.4%	3%	0%
Nasopharyngitis	1.6%	6%	0%
Upper respiratory tract infection	2.3%	3%	0%
Viral pharyngitis	1%	0%	0%
Wheezing	1%	0%	0%

ERTAPENEM SODIUM — INJECTION

Ertapenem Adverse Reactions in Children (≥ 1%)

Adverse reactions	Ertapenem[a,b] (n = 384)	Ceftriaxone[a] (n = 100)	Ticarcillin/ clavulanate[b] (n = 24)
Miscellaneous			
Herpes simplex	1%	1%	4.2%
Hypothermia	1.6%	1%	0%
Pyrexia	4.9%	6%	8.3%

[a] Includes phase 2b complicated SSSI, CAP, and complicated UTI studies in which patients 3 months to 12 years of age received ertapenem 15 mg/kg IV twice daily up to a maximum of 1 g or ceftriaxone 50 mg/kg/day IV in 2 divided doses up to a maximum of 2 g, and patients 13 to 17 years of age received ertapenem 1 g IV daily or ceftriaxone 50 mg/kg/day IV in a single daily dose.

[b] Includes phase 2b acute pelvic infections and complicated IAI studies in which patients 3 months to 12 years of age received ertapenem 15 mg/kg IV twice daily up to a maximum of 1 g and patients 13 to 17 years of age received ertapenem 1 g IV daily or ticarcillin/clavulanate 50 mg/kg for patients < 60 kg or ticarcillin/clavulanate 3 g 4 or 6 times a day for patients > 60 kg.

Additional adverse reactions (more than 0.5% to less than 1%) –

Cardiovascular: Chest pain, phlebitis.
CNS: Insomnia, somnolence.
Dermatologic: Atopic dermatitis, erythematous rash, skin lesion.
Respiratory: Pleural effusion, rhinitis, rhinorrhea.
Miscellaneous: Arthralgia, candidiasis, decreased appetite, ear infection, genital rash, infusion-site pruritus, oral candidiasis.

➤*Lab test abnormalities:*

Treatment of moderate to severe infections in adults – Drug-related laboratory adverse reactions that were reported during therapy in at least 1% of adults treated with ertapenem, including those who were switched to therapy with an oral antimicrobial, in clinical studies were ALT increased (6%), AST increased (5.2%), serum alkaline phosphatase increased (3.4%), platelet count increased (2.8%), and eosinophils increased (1.1%). Ertapenem was discontinued because of laboratory adverse reactions in 0.3% of patients.

Ertapenem Lab Test Abnormalities in Adults (≥ 1%)[a]

Lab test abnormalities	Ertapenem[b] 1 g daily (n = 766)[c]	Piperacillin/ tazobactam[b] 3.375 g every 6 h (n = 755)[c]	Ertapenem[d] 1 g daily (n = 1,122)[b]	Ceftriaxone[d] 1 or 2 g daily (n = 920)[b]
ALT increased	8.8%	7.3%	8.3%	6.9%
AST increased	8.4%	8.3%	7.1%	6.5%
Eosinophils increased	1.1%	1.1%	2.1%	1.8%
Hematocrit decreased	3%	2.9%	3.4%	2.4%
Hemoglobin decreased	4.9%	4.7%	4.5%	3.5%
Platelet count decreased	1.1%	1.2%	1.1%	1%
Platelet count increased	6.5%	6.3%	4.3%	3.5%
Prothrombin time increased	1.2%	2%	0.3%	0.9%
Segmented neutrophils decreased	1%	0.3%	1.5%	0.8%
Serum albumin decreased	1.7%	1.5%	0.9%	1.6%
Serum alkaline phosphatase increased	6.6%	7.2%	4.3%	2.8%
Serum creatinine increased	1.1%	2.7%	0.9%	1.2%
Serum glucose increased	1.2%	2.3%	1.7%	2%
Serum potassium decreased	1.7%	2.8%	1.8%	2.4%
Serum potassium increased	1.3%	0.5%	0.5%	0.7%
Total serum bilirubin increased	1.7%	1.4%	0.6%	1.1%
Urine red blood cells increased	2.5%	2.9%	1.1%	1%
Urine white blood cells increased	2.5%	3.2%	1.6%	1.1%
White blood cells decreased	0.8%	0.7%	1.5%	1.4%

[a] Number of patients with laboratory adverse reactions/number of patients with the laboratory test.
[b] Includes phase 2b/3 complicated IAI, complicated SSSI, and acute pelvic infections studies.
[c] Number of patients with 1 or more laboratory tests.
[d] Includes phase 2b/3 CAP and complicated UTI, and phase 2a studies.

Additional laboratory adverse reactions (more than 0.1% to less than 1%) – Increases in direct and indirect serum bilirubin, monocytes, partial thromboplastin time, serum sodium, serum urea nitrogen (BUN), and urine epithelial cells and decreases in serum bicarbonate.

Prophylaxis of surgical-site infection in adults – In a clinical study in adults for the prophylaxis of surgical-site infection following elective colorectal surgery, in which 476 patients received a dose of ertapenem 1 g one hour prior to surgery and were then followed for safety 14 days postsurgery, the overall laboratory adverse reaction profile was generally comparable with that observed for ertapenem in previous clinical trials. Additional laboratory adverse reactions that were reported during therapy and the 14 days postsurgery period in more than 1% of patients, regardless of causality, include white blood cell count increased and urine protein present.

Children – Drug-related laboratory adverse reactions that were reported during therapy in at least 2% of children treated with ertapenem, including those who were switched to therapy with an oral antimicrobial, in clinical studies were neutrophil count decreased (3%), ALT increased (2.2%), and AST increased (2.1%).

Ertapenem Lab Test Abnormalities in Children (≥ 1%)[a]

Lab test abnormalities	Ertapenem (n = 379)[b]	Ceftriaxone (n = 97)[b]	Ticarcillin/ clavulanate (n = 24)[b]
Alkaline phosphatase increased	1.1%	0%	0%
ALT increased	3.8%	1.1%	4.3%
AST increased	3.8%	1.1%	4.3%
Eosinophil count increased	1.1%	2.1%	0%
Neutrophil count decreased	5.8%	3.1%	0%
Platelet count increased	1.3%	0%	8.7%

[a] Number of patients with laboratory adverse reactions/number of patients with the laboratory test; at least 300 patients had the test.
[b] Number of patients with 1 or more laboratory tests.

Additional laboratory adverse reactions (more than 0.5% to less than 1%): Protein urine present and white blood cell count decreased.

➤*Postmarketing:*

CNS – Altered mental status (including aggression, delirium), dyskinesia, hallucinations, myoclonus, tremor.

Hypersensitivity – Anaphylaxis, including anaphylactoid reactions.

Overdosage

➤*Symptoms:* IV administration of ertapenem 2 g over 30 minutes or 3 g over 1 to 2 hours in healthy volunteers resulted in an increased incidence of nausea. In clinical studies in adults, inadvertent administration of three 1 g doses of ertapenem in a 24-hour period resulted in diarrhea and transient dizziness in 1 patient. In pediatric clinical studies, a single IV dose of 40 mg/kg up to a maximum of 2 g did not result in toxicity.

➤*Treatment:* In the event of an overdose, discontinue ertapenem and give general supportive treatment until renal elimination takes place.

Ertapenem can be removed by hemodialysis; the plasma clearance of the total fraction of ertapenem was increased 30% in subjects with end-stage renal insufficiency when hemodialysis (4-hour session) was performed immediately following administration. However, no information is available on the use of hemodialysis to treat overdosage.

Patient Information

Counsel patients to inform their health care provider if they are taking valproic acid or divalproex. Valproic acid concentrations in the blood may drop below the therapeutic range upon coadministration with ertapenem. If treatment with ertapenem is necessary and continued, alternative or supplemental anticonvulsant medication to prevent and/or treat seizures may be needed.

Counsel patients that antibacterial drugs including ertapenem should be used only to treat bacterial infections. They do not treat viral infections (eg, common cold). When ertapenem is prescribed to treat a bacterial infection, tell patients that, although it is common to feel better early in the course of therapy, to take the medication exactly as directed. Skipping doses or not completing the full course of therapy may decrease the efficacy of the imme-

ERTAPENEM SODIUM — INJECTION

diate treatment and increase the likelihood that bacteria will develop resistance and will not be treatable by ertapenem or other antibacterial drugs in the future.

Diarrhea is a common problem caused by antibiotics that usually ends when the antibiotic is discontinued. Sometimes after starting treatment with antibiotics, patients can develop watery and bloody stools (with or without stomach cramps and fever) even as late as 2 or more months after having taken the last dose of the antibiotic. If this occurs, instruct patients to contact their health care provider as soon as possible.

DORIPENEM

Rx	Doribax (Janssen)	Injection, powder for solution, concentrate: 500 mg	Preservative free. In single-use vials.

DORIPENEM — INJECTION

Indications

➤*Complicated intra-abdominal infections:* As a single agent for the treatment of complicated intra-abdominal infections caused by *Escherichia coli*, *Klebsiella pneumoniae*, *Pseudomonas aeruginosa*, *Bacteroides caccae*, *Bacteroides fragilis*, *Bacteroides thetaiotaomicron*, *Bacteroides uniformis*, *Bacteroides vulgatus*, *Streptococcus intermedius*, *Streptococcus constellatus*, and *Peptostreptococcus micros*.

➤*Complicated urinary tract infections, including pyelonephritis:* As a single agent for the treatment of complicated urinary tract infections (UTIs), including pyelonephritis, caused by *E. coli* including cases with concurrent bacteremia, *K. pneumoniae*, *Proteus mirabilis*, *P. aeruginosa*, and *Acinetobacter baumannii*.

➤*Off-label uses:*

Catheter-related bloodstream infection (adults) – [2] = Fair documentation. Doripenem is recommended by Infectious Diseases Society of America (IDSA) clinical practice guidelines as a first-line agent for the treatment of catheter-related infections caused by extended-spectrum beta-lactamase–producing *E. coli* and *Klebsiella* species in adults. The guidelines also list doripenem as an appropriate alternative agent given with an aminoglycoside for catheter-related infections caused by *Ochrobactrum anthropi*. Doripenem may also be used in the treatment of catheter-related infections caused by susceptible *Enterobacter* species, *Serratia marcescens*, *Acinetobacter* species, *P. aeruginosa*, and *Burkholderia cepacia*.

Community-acquired pneumonia – [2] = Fair documentation. The use of doripenem for empiric treatment of severe community-acquired pneumonia in adult inpatients with risk factors for *Pseudomonas* is supported by virtue of its antimicrobial spectrum of activity. According to the IDSA/American Thoracic Society consensus guidelines on the management of community-acquired pneumonia in adults, carbapenems (imipenem, meropenem) are recommended as empiric treatment of community-acquired pneumonia in adult inpatients admitted to the intensive care unit with risk factors for *Pseudomonas* infection.

Hospital-acquired pneumonia – [1] = Good documentation. Initial data from 2 controlled trials suggest that doripenem is well tolerated and noninferior to piperacillin/tazobactam and, thus, has a place in the treatment of adults with early-onset hospital-acquired pneumonia, ventilator-associated pneumonia, and health care–associated pneumonia.

Administration and Dosage

➤*Adults:*

Intra-abdominal infection (complicated) –

Usual dosage: 500 mg every 8 hours by intravenous (IV) infusion over 1 hour.

Duration of therapy: 5 to 14 days. Duration includes a possible switch to an appropriate oral therapy after at least 3 days of parenteral therapy, once clinical improvement has been demonstrated.

Urinary tract infections, including pyelonephritis (complicated) –

Usual dosage: 500 mg every 8 hours by IV infusion over 1 hour.

Duration of therapy: 10 days. Duration includes a possible switch to an appropriate oral therapy after at least 3 days of parenteral therapy, once clinical improvement has been demonstrated. Duration can be extended up to 14 days in patients with concurrent bacteremia.

Off-label dosing –

Catheter-related bloodstream infection: [2] = Fair documentation. 500 mg administered IV every 8 hours for 7 to 14 days, infused over 1 hour.

Community-acquired pneumonia: [2] = Fair documentation. The most common dose studied was 500 mg infused every 8 hours for a minimum of 5 days.

Hospital-acquired pneumonia: [1] = Good documentation. 500 mg administered IV over 1 to 4 hours every 8 hours for a total duration of 7 to 14 days.

➤*Renal function impairment:*

Doripenem Dosage in Patients With Renal Function Impairment

Estimated CrCl[a] (mL/min)	Recommended dosage regimen of doripenem
> 50	No dosage adjustment necessary
≥ 30 to ≤ 50	250 mg IV (over 1 h) every 8 h
> 10 to < 30	250 mg IV (over 1 h) every 12 h

[a] CrCl = creatinine clearance.

➤*Preparation for administration:* Reconstitute the vial with 10 mL of sterile water for injection or sodium chloride 0.9% injection and gently shake to form a suspension. The resulting concentration is 50 mg/mL. Caution: the reconstituted suspension is not for direct injection. Withdraw the suspension using a syringe with a 21-gauge needle and add it to an infusion bag containing 100 mL of sodium chloride 0.9% or dextrose 5%; gently shake until clear. The infusion solution concentration is 4.5 mg/mL.

For a 250 mg dose, remove 55 mL of this solution from the bag and discard. Infuse the remaining solution, which contains 250 mg (4.5 mg/mL).

To prepare doripenem infusions in Baxter *Minibag Plus* infusion bags, consult the infusion bag manufacturer's instructions.

➤*Administration:* Doripenem should be administered by IV infusion over 1 hour.

➤*Admixture compatibility:* The compatibility of doripenem with other drugs has not been established. Doripenem should not be mixed with or physically added to solutions containing other drugs.

➤*Storage/Stability:*

Vials – Store vials at 25°C (77°F); excursions are permitted to 15° to 30°C (59° to 86°F).

Reconstituted solutions – Upon reconstitution with sterile water for injection or sodium chloride 0.9% injection, doripenem suspension in the vial may be held for 1 hour prior to transfer and dilution in the infusion bag.

Following dilution of the suspension with sodium chloride 0.9% or dextrose 5%, doripenem infusions stored at controlled room temperature or under refrigeration should be completed according to the times in the following table.

Doripenem Storage and Stability Times of Infusion Solutions Prepared in Sodium Chloride 0.9% or Dextrose 5%

Infusion prepared in	Stability time at room temperature[a]	Stability time at 2° to 8°C (refrigeration)[b]
Sodium chloride 0.9%	12 h	72 h
Dextrose 5%	4 h	24 h

[a] Includes room temperature storage and infusion time.
[b] Includes refrigerator storage and infusion time.

Reconstituted doripenem suspension or doripenem infusion should not be frozen. This storage information applies also to doripenem diluted in Baxter *Minibag Plus*.

Actions

➤*Pharmacology:* Doripenem belongs to the carbapenem class of antimicrobials with in vitro antibacterial activity against aerobic and anaerobic gram-positive and gram-negative bacteria. Doripenem exerts its bactericidal activity by inhibiting bacterial cell wall biosynthesis. Doripenem inactivates multiple essential penicillin-binding proteins, resulting in inhibition of cell wall synthesis with subsequent cell death. In *E. coli* and *P. aeruginosa*, doripenem binds to penicillin-binding protein 2, which is involved in the maintenance of cell shape, as well as to penicillin-binding proteins 3 and 4.

➤*Pharmacokinetics:*

Absorption – The pharmacokinetics of doripenem (maximal drug concentration [C_{max}] and area under the curve [AUC]) are linear over a dose range of 500 mg to 1 g when IV infused over 1 hour. There is no accumulation of doripenem following multiple IV infusions of 500 mg or 1 g administered every 8 hours for 7 to 10 days in subjects with healthy renal function.

Distribution – The average binding of doripenem to plasma proteins is approximately 8.1% and is independent of plasma drug concentrations. The median (range) volume of distribution at steady state in healthy subjects is 16.8 L (8.09 to 55.5 L), similar to extracellular fluid volume (18.2 L).

Doripenem penetrates into several body fluids and tissues, including those at the site of infection for the approved indications. Doripenem concentrations in peritoneal and retroperitoneal fluid match or exceed those required to inhibit most susceptible bacteria; however, the clinical relevance of this finding has not been established.

Metabolism – Metabolism of doripenem to a microbiologically inactive ring-opened metabolite (doripenem-M1) occurs primarily via dehydropeptidase-I. The mean (standard deviation [SD]) plasma doripenem-M1 to doripenem AUC ratio following single 500 mg and 1 g doses in healthy subjects is 18% (7.2%).

Excretion – Doripenem is primarily eliminated unchanged by the kidneys. The mean plasma terminal elimination half-life of doripenem in healthy nonelderly adults is approximately 1 hour and mean (SD) plasma clearance is 15.9 (5.3) L/h. Mean (SD) renal clearance is 10.8 (3.5) L/h. The magnitude of this value, coupled with the significant decrease in the elimination of doripenem with concomitant probenecid administration, suggests that doripenem undergoes both glomerular filtration and active tubular secretion. In healthy adults given a single 500 mg dose of doripenem, a mean of 70% and 15% of the dose was recovered in urine as unchanged drug and the ring-opened metabolite, respectively, within 48 hours. Following the admin-

DORIPENEM — INJECTION

istration of a single 500 mg dose of radiolabeled doripenem to healthy adults, less than 1% of the total radioactivity was recovered in feces after 1 week.

Special populations –

Renal function impairment: Following a single 500 mg dose of doripenem, the mean AUC of doripenem in subjects with mild (CrCl 50 to 79 mL/min), moderate (CrCl 31 to 50 mL/min), and severe renal function impairment (CrCl 30 mL/min or less) was 1.6, 2.8, and 5.1 times that of age-matched healthy subjects with healthy renal function (CrCl 80 mL/min or more), respectively. Dosage adjustment is necessary in patients with moderate and severe renal function impairment.

A single 500 mg dose of doripenem was administered to subjects with end-stage renal disease 1 hour prior to or 1 hour after hemodialysis. The mean doripenem AUC following the posthemodialysis infusion was 7.8 times that of healthy subjects with healthy renal function. The mean total recovery of doripenem and doripenem-M1 in the dialysate following a 4-hour hemodialysis session was 231 and 28 mg, respectively, or a total of 259 mg (52% of the dose). There is insufficient information to make dose adjustment recommendations in patients on hemodialysis.

Elderly: See Warnings/Precautions for more information.

Race: The effect of race on doripenem pharmacokinetics was examined using a population pharmacokinetic analysis of data from phase 1 and 2 studies. Compared with white subjects, mean doripenem clearance was 14% greater in Hispanic/Latino subjects, whereas no difference in clearance was observed for black subjects.

➤*Microbiology:* Doripenem has been shown to be active against most isolates from the following microorganisms, both in vitro and in clinical infections.

Facultative gram-negative microorganisms – A. baumannii, E. coli, K. pneumoniae, P. mirabilis, P. aeruginosa.

Facultative gram-positive microorganisms – S. constellatus, S. intermedius.

Anaerobic microorganisms – B. caccae, B. fragilis, B. thetaiotaomicron, B. uniformis, B. vulgatus, P. micros.

Contraindications

Known serious hypersensitivity to doripenem or other drugs in the same class or in patients who have demonstrated anaphylactic reactions to beta-lactams.

Warnings/Precautions

➤*Clostridium difficile–associated diarrhea:* *C. difficile*–associated diarrhea has been reported with nearly all antibacterial agents and may range in severity from mild diarrhea to fatal colitis.

Treatment with antibacterial agents alters the normal flora of the colon and may permit overgrowth of *C. difficile*.

C. difficile produces toxins A and B, which contribute to the development of *C. difficile*–associated diarrhea. Hypertoxin-producing strains of *C. difficile* cause increased morbidity and mortality, as these infections can be refractory to antimicrobial therapy and may require colectomy. *C. difficile*–associated diarrhea must be considered in all patients who present with diarrhea following antibiotic use. Careful medical history is necessary since *C. difficile*–associated diarrhea has been reported to occur more than 2 months after the administration of antibacterial agents.

If *C. difficile*–associated diarrhea is suspected or confirmed, ongoing antibiotic use not directed against *C. difficile* may need to be discontinued. Institute appropriate fluid and electrolyte management, protein supplementation, antibiotic treatment of *C. difficile*, and surgical evaluation, as clinically indicated.

➤*Drug-resistant bacteria:* Prescribing doripenem in the absence of a proven or strongly suspected bacterial infection is unlikely to provide benefit to the patient and increases the risk of the development of drug-resistant bacteria.

➤*Pneumonitis with inhalational use:* When doripenem has been used investigationally via inhalation, pneumonitis has occurred. Do not administer doripenem by this route.

➤*Hypersensitivity reactions:* Serious and occasionally fatal hypersensitivity (anaphylactic) and serious skin reactions have been reported in patients receiving beta-lactam antibiotics. These reactions are more likely to occur in individuals with a history of sensitivity to multiple allergens. Before therapy with doripenem is instituted, inquire carefully to determine whether the patient has had previous hypersensitivity reaction to other carbapenems, cephalosporins, penicillins, or other allergens. If this product is to be given to a penicillin-allergic or other beta-lactam–allergic patient, exercise caution because cross-hyperreactivity among beta-lactam antibiotics has been clearly documented.

If an allergic reaction to doripenem occurs, discontinue the drug. Serious acute hypersensitivity (anaphylactic) reactions require emergency treatment with epinephrine and other emergency measures, including oxygen, IV fluids, IV antihistamines, corticosteroids, pressor amines, and airway management, as clinically indicated.

➤*Renal function impairment:* See Administration and Dosage for more information.

➤*Pregnancy:* *Category B.* There are no adequate and well-controlled studies in pregnant women. Because animal reproduction studies are not always predictive of human response, use this drug during pregnancy only if clearly needed.

➤*Lactation:* It is not known whether this drug is excreted in human milk. Because many drugs are excreted in human milk, exercise caution when doripenem is administered to a breast-feeding woman.

➤*Children:* Safety and effectiveness in children have not been established.

➤*Elderly:* Clinical cure rates in complicated intra-abdominal and complicated UTIs were slightly lower in patients 65 years of age and older and also in the subgroup of patients 75 years of age and older versus patients younger than 65 years of age. These results were similar between doripenem and comparator treatment groups.

Elderly subjects had greater doripenem exposure relative to nonelderly subjects; however, this increase in exposure was mainly attributed to age-related changes in renal function.

Doripenem is known to be excreted substantially by the kidney, and the risk of adverse reactions to this drug may be greater in patients with renal function impairment or prerenal azotemia. Because elderly patients are more likely to have decreased renal function or prerenal azotemia, take care in dose selection. It may be useful to monitor renal function.

➤*Monitoring:* Monitor renal function in patients with moderate to severe renal function impairment.

Drug Interactions

Doripenem Drug Interactions

Precipitant drug	Object drug[a]		Description
Probenecid	Doripenem	⬆	Probenecid interferes with the active tubular secretion of doripenem, resulting in increased plasma concentrations of doripenem. Coadministration is not recommended.
Doripenem	Valproic acid	⬇	Doripenem may reduce serum valproic acid concentrations to subtherapeutic levels, resulting in loss of seizure control. Monitor serum valproic acid levels frequently after initiating doripenem therapy.

[a] ⬆ = object drug increased; ⬇ = object drug decreased.

Adverse Reactions

➤*Discontinuation:* During clinical trials, adverse drug reactions that led to doripenem discontinuation were nausea (0.2%), vulvomycotic infection (0.1%), and rash (0.1%).

Doripenem Adverse Reactions[a,b] (≥ 1%)

	Complicated UTIs (1 trial)		Complicated intra-abdominal infections (2 trials)	
Adverse reaction	Doripenem 500 mg every 8 h (n = 376)	Levofloxacin 250 mg IV every 24 h (n = 372)	Doripenem 500 mg every 8 h (n = 477)	Meropenem 1g every 8 h (n = 469)
Cardiovascular				
Phlebitis	4%	4%	8%	6%
CNS				
Headache	16%	15%	4%	5%
Dermatologic				
Pruritus	< 1%	1%	3%	2%
Rash[c]	1%	1%	5%	2%
GI				
Diarrhea	6%	10%	11%	11%
Nausea	4%	6%	12%	9%
Hematologic/Lymphatic				
Anemia[b]	2%	1%	10%	5%
Hepatic				
Hepatic enzyme elevation[d]	2%	3%	1%	3%
Renal				
Renal function impairment/ renal failure[b]	< 1%	0%	1%	< 1%

DORIPENEM — INJECTION

Doripenem Adverse Reactions[a,b] (≥ 1%)				
	Complicated UTIs (1 trial)		Complicated intra-abdominal infections (2 trials)	
Adverse reaction	Doripenem 500 mg every 8 h (n = 376)	Levofloxacin 250 mg IV every 24 h (n = 372)	Doripenem 500 mg every 8 h (n = 477)	Meropenem 1g every 8 h (n = 469)
Miscellaneous				
Oral candidiasis	1%	0%	1%	2%
Vulvomycotic infection	2%	1%	1%	< 1%

[a] An adverse drug reaction was defined as an undesirable effect, reasonably associated with the use of doripenem, that may occur as part of its pharmacological action or may be unpredictable in its occurrence.
[b] An adverse reaction refers to any untoward medical reaction associated with the use of the drug in humans, whether or not considered drug related.
[c] Includes reactions reported as allergic and bullous dermatitis, erythema, erythema multiforme, macular/papular eruptions, and urticaria.
[d] Includes reactions reported as ALT increased, AST increased, hepatic enzyme increased, and transaminases increased.

➤*Postmarketing:*

Hypersensitivity – Anaphylaxis.

CNS – Seizure.

Dermatologic – Stevens Johnson syndrome, toxic epidermal necrolysis.

Respiratory – Interstitial pneumonia.

Overdosage

➤*Treatment:* In the event of overdose, discontinue doripenem and give general supportive treatment.

Doripenem can be removed by hemodialysis. In subjects with end-stage renal disease administered doripenem 500 mg, the mean total recovery of doripenem and doripenem-M1 in the dialysate following a 4-hour hemodialysis session was 259 mg (52% of the dose). However, no information is available on the use of hemodialysis to treat overdosage.

Patient Information

Advise patients that allergic reactions, including serious allergic reactions, could occur and that serious reactions require immediate treatment. Tell patients to report any previous hypersensitivity reactions to doripenem, other carbapenems, beta-lactams, or other allergens.

Counsel patients that antibacterial drugs, including doripenem, should only be used to treat bacterial infections. They do not treat viral infections (eg, the common cold). When doripenem is prescribed to treat a bacterial infection, tell patients that although it is common to feel better early in the course of therapy, the medication should be taken exactly as directed. Skipping doses or not completing the full course of therapy may decrease the effectiveness of the immediate treatment and increase the likelihood that bacteria will develop resistance and will not be treatable by doripenem or other antibacterial drugs in the future.

MONOBACTAMS

AZTREONAM

Rx	**Aztreonam** (APP Pharmaceutical)	**Injection, lyophilized cake for solution:** 500 mg[a]	In single-dose vials.
Rx	**Azactam** (Squibb)		In single-dose 15 mL vials.
Rx	**Aztreonam** (APP Pharmaceutical)	**Injection, lyophilized cake for solution:** 1 g[a]	In single-dose vials.
Rx	**Azactam** (Squibb)		In single-dose 15 mL vials and single-dose 100 mL infusion bottles.
Rx	**Aztreonam** (APP Pharmaceutical)	**Injection, lyophilized cake for solution:** 2 g[a]	In single-dose vials.
Rx	**Azactam** (Squibb)		In single-dose 30 mL vials and single-dose 100 mL infusion bottles.
Rx	**Cayston** (Gilead Sciences)	**Powder for solution, lyophilized; inhalation:** 75 mg	Preservative free, arginine free. Lysine 46.7 mg. In 2 mL single-dose vials with 1 mL ampule of sodium chloride 0.17% diluent.

[a] With approximately 780 mg of L-arginine per gram of aztreonam.

AZTREONAM — INJECTION

Indications

➤*Urinary tract infections (complicated and uncomplicated):* Including pyelonephritis and cystitis (initial and recurrent) caused by *Escherichia coli*; *Klebsiella pneumoniae*; *Proteus mirabilis*; *Pseudomonas aeruginosa*; *Enterobacter cloacae*; *Klebsiella oxytoca*, *Citrobacter* species and *Serratia marcescens* (efficacy of these organisms in this organ system was studied in less than 10 infections).

➤*Lower respiratory tract infections:* Including pneumonia and bronchitis caused by *Escherichia coli*, *Klebsiella pneumoniae*, *Pseudomonas aeruginosa*, *Haemophilus influenzae*, *Proteus mirabilis*, *Enterobacter* and *Serratia marcescens* (efficacy of this organism in this organ system was studied in less than 10 infections).

➤*Septicemia:* *Enterobacter* species; caused by *Escherichia coli*; *Klebsiella pneumoniae*; *Pseudomonas aeruginosa*; *Proteus mirabilis*, *Serratia marcescens* (efficacy for these organisms in this organ system was studied in less than 10 infections).

➤*Skin and skin-structure infections:* Including those associated with postoperative wounds, ulcers and burns caused by *Escherichia coli*, *Proteus mirabilis*, *Serratia marcescens*, *Enterobacter species*, *Pseudomonas aeruginosa*, *Klebsiella pneumoniae* and *Citrobacter* species (efficacy for these organisms in this organ system was studied in fewer than 10 infections).

➤*Intra-abdominal infections:* Including peritonitis caused by *Escherichia coli*; *Klebsiella* species including *K. pneumoniae*; *Enterobacter* species including *E. cloacae* (efficacy for E. cloacae in this organ system was studied in less than 10 infections); *Pseudomonas aeruginosa*; *Citrobacter* species including *C. freundii*, and *Serratia* species including *S. marcescens* (efficacy for the specified organisms and their species in this organ system was studied in less than 10 infections).

➤*Gynecologic infections:* Including endometritis and pelvic cellulitis caused by *Escherichia coli*; *Klebsiella pneumoniae*, *Enterobacter*species including *E. cloacae*, *Proteus mirabilis*.

➤*Surgery:* Aztreonam is indicated for adjunctive therapy to surgery in the management of infections caused by susceptible organisms, including abscesses, infections complicating hollow viscus perforations, cutaneous infections and infections of serous surfaces. Aztreonam is effective against most of the commonly encountered gram-negative aerobic pathogens seen in general surgery.

➤*Concurrent therapy:* Concurrent initial therapy with other antimicrobial agents and aztreonam for injection is recommended before the causative organism(s) is known in seriously ill patients who are also at risk of having an infection due to gram-positive aerobic pathogens. If anaerobic organisms are also suspected as etiologic agents, therapy should be initiated using an anti-anaerobic agent concurrently with aztreonam (see Administration and Dosage). Certain antibiotics (eg, cefoxitin, imipenem) may induce high levels of beta-lactamase in vitro in some gram-negative aerobes such as *Enterobacter* and *Pseudomonas* species, resulting in antagonism to many beta-lactam antibiotics including aztreonam. These in vitro findings suggest that such beta-lactamase inducing antibiotics not be used concurrently with aztreonam. Following identification and susceptibility testing of the causative organism(s), appropriate antibiotic therapy should be continued.

➤*Off-label uses:*

Surgical prophylaxis – [2] = Fair documentation. Clinical guidelines recommend the use of aztreonam for surgical prophylaxis in patients with a documented beta-lactam allergy undergoing procedures with a high risk of infection from gram-negative bacteria, such as abdominal or vaginal hysterectomy or colorectal procedures.

Other possible off-label uses – 1 g IM may be beneficial for acute uncomplicated gonorrhea in patients with penicillin-resistant gonococci, as an alternative to spectinomycin.

Administration and Dosage

➤*Adults:*

Infections – For a list of infections, refer to Indications.

Maximum dose: 8 g/day.

Moderately severe systemic infections: 1 or 2 g IV or IM every 8 or 12 hours

Severe systemic or life-threatening infections: 2 g IV or IM every 6 or 8 hours.

Pseudomonal infections: 2 g IV or IM every 6 or 8 hours, at least upon initiation of therapy.

Urinary tract infections: 500 mg or 1 g IV or IM every 8 or 12 hours.

Off-label dosing –

Surgical prophylaxis: [2] = Fair documentation. 1 to 2 g IV administered over 20 to 60 minutes 1 hour prior to incision. Redosing may be necessary every 3 to 5 hours, with discontinuation within 24 hours after operation.

➤*Children:*

Infections – For a list of infections, refer to Indications.

Maximum dose: 120 mg/kg/day.

9 months of age and older:

- *Mild to moderate infections* – 30 mg/kg IV every 8 hours.
- *Moderate to severe infections* – 30 mg/kg IV every 6 or 8 hours.

➤*Renal function impairment:*

CrCl 10 to 30 mL/min/1.73 m^2 – The dosage of aztreonam should be halved after an initial loading dose of 1 or 2 g.

CrCl less than 10 mL/min/1.73 m^2 and patients on hemodialysis – The usual dose of 500 mg, 1 g or 2 g should be given initially. The maintenance dose should be one-fourth of the usual initial dose given at the usual fixed interval of 6, 8, or 12 hours. For serious or life-threatening infec-

AZTREONAM — INJECTION

tions, in addition to the maintenance doses, one-eighth of the initial dose should be given after each hemodialysis session.

Continuous ambulatory peritoneal dialysis – Administer 25% of the usual dose at the usual interval.

➤*Duration of therapy:* The duration of therapy depends on the severity of infection. Generally, aztreonam should be continued for at least 48 hours after the patient becomes asymptomatic or evidence of bacterial eradication has been obtained. Persistent infections may require treatment for several weeks. Doses smaller than those indicated should not be used.

➤*Preparation for administration:* Upon the addition of the diluent to the container, contents should be shaken immediately and vigorously. Constituted solutions are not for multiple-dose use; should the entire volume in the container not be used for a single-dose, the unused solution must be discarded.

Depending upon the concentration of aztreonam and diluent used, constituted aztreonam yields a colorless to light straw-yellow solution, which may develop a slight pink tint on standing (potency is not affected).

IV solutions –

For bolus injection: The contents of an aztreonam 15 mL capacity vial should be constituted with 6 to 10 mL sterile water for injection.

For infusion: Contents of the 100 mL capacity bottle should be constituted to a final concentration not exceeding 2% w/v (at least 50 mL of any appropriate infusion solution listed in the next paragraph per gram aztreonam). These solutions may be frozen immediately after constitution in the original container (see Stability of IV and IM Solutions).

If the contents of a 15 or 30 mL capacity vial are to be transferred to an appropriate infusion solution, each gram of aztreonam should be initially constituted with at least 3 mL sterile water for injection. Further dilution may be obtained with one of the following IV infusion solutions: sodium chloride 0.9% injection; Ringer's injection; Ringer's lactate injection; dextrose 5% or 10% injection; dextrose and sodium chloride 5%:0.9%, 5%:0.45%, or 5%:0.2% injection; sodium lactate injection (M/6 sodium lactate); *Ionosol* B and dextrose 5%; *Isolyte* E; *Isolyte* E with dextrose 5%; *Isolyte* M with dextrose 5%; *Normosol*-R; Normosol-R and dextrose 5%; *Normosol*-M and dextrose 5%; mannitol injection 5% or 10%; lactated Ringer's and dextrose 5% injection; *Plasma-Lyte* M and dextrose 5%; *Travert* 10% injection; *Travert* 10% and Electrolyte No. 1 injection; *Travert* 10% and Electrolyte No. 2 injection; *Travert* 10% and Electrolyte No. 3 injection.

IM solutions – The contents of an aztreonam 15 mL capacity vial should be constituted with at least 3 mL of an appropriate diluent per gram aztreonam. The following diluents may be used: sterile water for injection; sterile bacteriostatic water for injection (with benzyl alcohol or with methyl- and propylparabens); sodium chloride 0.9% injection; bacteriostatic sodium chloride injection (with benzyl alcohol).

➤*Administration:*

Adults – Aztreonam may be administered IV or by IM injection. Dosage and route of administration should be determined by susceptibility of the causative organisms, severity and site of infection, and the condition of the patient.

Children – Aztreonam should be administered IV to pediatric patients with healthy renal function. There are insufficient data regarding IM administration to children.

IV administration – The IV route is recommended for patients requiring single doses greater than 1 g or those with bacterial septicemia, localized parenchymal abscess (eg, intra-abdominal abscess), peritonitis, or other severe systemic or life-threatening infections.

Bolus injection: A bolus injection may be used to initiate therapy. The dose should be slowly injected directly into a vein, or the tubing of a suitable administration set, over a period of 3 to 5 minutes (see the Infusion section for information regarding flushing of tubing).

Infusion: With any intermittent infusion of aztreonam and another drug with which it is not pharmaceutically compatible, the common delivery tube should be flushed before and after delivery of aztreonam with any appropriate infusion solution compatible with both drug solutions; the drugs should not be delivered simultaneously. Any aztreonam infusion should be completed within a 20- to 60-minute period. With use of a Y-type administration set, careful attention should be given to the calculated volume of aztreonam solution required so that the entire dose will be infused. A volume control administration set may be used to deliver an initial dilution of aztreonam (see Preparation for Administration) into a compatible infusion solution during administration; in this case, the final dilution of aztreonam should provide a concentration not exceeding 2% w/v.

IM administration – The dose should be given by deep injection into a large muscle mass (such as the upper outer quadrant of the gluteus maximus or lateral part of the thigh). Aztreonam is well tolerated and should not be admixed with any local anesthetic agent.

➤*Admixture compatibility:*

Compatibility – IV infusion solutions of aztreonam not exceeding 2% w/v prepared with sodium chloride 0.9% injection or dextrose 5% injection, to which clindamycin phosphate, gentamicin sulfate, tobramycin sulfate, or cefazolin sodium have been added at concentrations usually used clinically, are stable for up to 48 hours at room temperature or 7 days under refrigeration. Ampicillin sodium admixtures with aztreonam in sodium chloride 0.9% injection are stable for 24 hours at room temperature and 48 hours under refrigeration; stability in dextrose 5% injection is 2 hours at room temperature and 8 hours under refrigeration.

Aztreonam-cloxacillin sodium and aztreonam-vancomycin hydrochloride admixtures are stable in peritoneal dialysis solution (with dextrose 4.25%) for up to 24 hours at room temperature.

Incompatibility – Aztreonam is incompatible with nafcillin sodium, cephradine, and metronidazole. Other admixtures are not recommended since compatibility data are not available.

➤*Storage / Stability:* Store original packages at room temperature; avoid excessive heat.

Stability of IV and IM solutions – Aztreonam solutions for IV infusion at concentrations not exceeding 2% w/v must be used within 48 hours following constitution if kept at controlled room temperature (15° to 30°C; 59° to 86°F) or within 7 days if refrigerated (2° to 8°C; 36° to 46°F).

Aztreonam solutions at concentrations exceeding 2% w/v, except those prepared with sterile water for injection or sodium chloride injection, should be used promptly after preparation; the 2 excepted solutions must be used within 48 hours if stored at controlled room temperature or within 7 days if refrigerated.

Frozen aztreonam infusion solutions may be stored for up to 3 months at −20°C (−4°F); frozen solutions may be thawed at controlled room temperature or by overnight refrigeration. Solutions that have been thawed and maintained at controlled room temperature or under refrigeration should be used within 24 or 72 hours after removal from the freezer, respectively. Solutions should not be refrozen.

Actions

➤*Pharmacokinetics:*

Absorption / Distribution – Single 30-minute IV infusions of 500 mg, 1 g, and 2 g doses of aztreonam for injection in healthy subjects produced aztreonam peak serum levels of 54, 90, and 204 mcg/mL, respectively, immediately after administration; at 8 hours, serum levels were 1, 3, and 6 mcg/mL, respectively. Single 3-minute IV injections of the same doses resulted in serum levels of 58, 125, and 242 mcg/mL at 5 minutes following completion of injection.

Serum concentrations of aztreonam in healthy subjects following completion of single IM injections of 500 mg and 1 g doses are depicted in the figure below; maximum serum concentrations occur at about 1 hour. After identical single IV or IM doses of aztreonam, the serum concentrations of aztreonam are comparable at 1 hour (1.5 hours from start of IV infusion) with similar slopes of serum concentrations thereafter.

When aztreonam pharmacokinetics were assessed for adult and pediatric patients, they were found to be comparable (down to 9 months old). The serum half-life of aztreonam averaged 1.7 hours (1.5 to 2) in subjects with normal renal function, independent of the dose and route of administration. In healthy subjects, based on a 70 kg person, the serum clearance was 91 mL/min and renal clearance was 56 mL/min; the apparent mean volume of distribution at steady-state averaged 12.6 L, approximately equivalent to extracellular fluid volume.

Average urine concentrations of aztreonam were approximately 1,100, 3,500, and 6,600 mcg/mL within the first 2 hours following single 500 mg, 1 and 2 g IV doses of aztreonam (30 minute infusions), respectively. The range of average concentrations for aztreonam in the 8 to 12 hour urine specimens in these studies was 25 to 120 mcg/mL. After IM injection of single 500 mg and 1 g doses of aztreonam for injection, urinary levels were approximately 500 and 1,200 mcg/mL, respectively, within the first 2 hours, declining to 180 and 470 mcg/mL in the 6 to 8 hour specimens. In healthy subjects, aztreonam is excreted in the urine about equally by active tubular secretion and glomerular filtration. Approximately 60% to 70% of an IV or IM dose was recovered in the urine by 8 hours. Urinary excretion of a single parenteral dose was essentially complete by 12 hours after injection. About 12% of a single IV radiolabeled dose was recovered in the feces. Unchanged aztreonam and the inactive beta-lactam ring hydrolysis product of aztreonam were present in feces and urine.

IV or IM administration of a single 500 mg or 1 g dose of aztreonam every 8 hours for 7 days to healthy subjects produced no apparent accumulation of aztreonam or modification of its disposition characteristics; serum protein binding averaged 56% and was independent of dose. An average of about 6% of a 1 g IM dose was excreted as a microbiologically inactive open beta-lactam ring hydrolysis product (serum half-life approximately 26 hours) of aztreonam in the 0 to 8 hour urine collection on the last day of multiple dosing.

Special populations –

Renal function impairment: In patients with impaired renal function, the serum half-life of aztreonam is prolonged.

Hepatic function impairment: The serum half-life of aztreonam is only slightly prolonged in patients with hepatic function impairment since the liver is a minor pathway of excretion.

Elderly: In a study of healthy elderly male subjects (65 to 75 years of age), the average elimination half-life of aztreonam was slightly longer than in young healthy males.

➤*Microbiology:* Aztreonam exhibits potent and specific activity in vitro against a wide spectrum of gram-negative aerobic pathogens including *Pseudomonas aeruginosa*. The bactericidal action of aztreonam results from the inhibition of bacterial cell wall synthesis due to a high affinity of aztreonam for penicillin binding protein 3 (PBP3). Aztreonam, unlike the majority of beta-lactam antibiotics, does not induce beta-lactamase activity and its molecular structure confers a high degree of resistance to hydrolysis by beta-lactamases (ie, penicillinases, cephalosporinases) produced by most gram-negative and gram-positive pathogens; it is, therefore, usually active against gram-negative aerobic microorganisms that are resistant to antibiotics hydrolyzed by beta-lactamases. It is active against many strains that are multiply-resistant to other antibiotics, such as certain cephalosporins, penicillin, and aminoglycosides. Aztreonam maintains its antimicrobial activity over a pH range of 6 to 8 in vitro, as well as in the presence of human serum and under anaerobic conditions.

AZTREONAM — INJECTION

Aztreonam has been shown to be active against most strains of the following microorganisms, both in vitro and in clinical infections as described in the Indications section.

Aerobic gram-negative microorganisms – *Citrobacter* species, including *C. freundii*, *Enterobacter* species, including *E. cloacae*, *Escherichia coli*, *Haemophilus influenzae* (including ampicillin-resistant and other penicillinase-producing strains), *Klebsiella oxytoca*, *Klebsiella pneumoniae*, *Proteus mirabilis*, *Pseudomonas aeruginosa*, *Serratia* species, including *S. marcescens*.

Aerobic gram-negative microorganisms – Aztreonam and aminoglycosides have been shown to be synergistic in vitro against most strains of *P. aeruginosa*, many strains of *Enterobacteriaceae*, and other gram-negative aerobic bacilli.

Alterations of the anaerobic intestinal flora by broad spectrum antibiotics may decrease colonization resistance, thus permitting overgrowth of potential pathogens (eg, Candida and *Clostrium* species). Aztreonam has little effect on the anaerobic intestinal microflora in in vitro studies. *Clostridium difficile* and its cytotoxin were not found in animal models following administration of aztreonam. (See Adverse Reactions.)

Contraindications

Hypersensitivity to aztreonam or any other component in the formulation.

Warnings/Precautions

➤*Pseudomembranous colitis:* Pseudomembranous colitis has been reported with nearly all antibacterial agents, including aztreonam, and may range in severity from mild to life-threatening. Therefore, it is important to consider this diagnosis in patients who present with diarrhea subsequent to the administration of antibacterial agents.

Treatment with antibacterial agents alters the normal flora of the colon and may permit overgrowth of clostridia. Studies indicate that a toxin produced by *Clostridium difficile* is one primary cause of "antibiotic-associated colitis."

After the diagnosis of pseudomembranous colitis has been established, therapeutic measures should be initiated. Mild cases of pseudomembranous colitis usually respond to drug discontinuation alone. In moderate to severe cases, consideration should be given to management with fluids and electrolytes, protein supplementation, and treatment with an antibacterial drug clinically effective against *C. difficile* colitis.

➤*Toxic epidermal necrolysis:* Rare cases of toxic epidermal necrolysis have been reported in association with aztreonam in patients undergoing bone marrow transplant with multiple risk factors including sepsis, radiation therapy and other concomitantly administered drugs associated with toxic epidermal necrolysis.

➤*Hypersensitivity reactions:* Careful inquiry should be made to determine whether the patient has any history of hypersensitivity reactions to any allergens.

While cross-reactivity of aztreonam with other beta-lactam antibiotics is rare, this drug should be administered with caution to any patient with a history of hypersensitivity to beta-lactams (eg, penicillins, cephalosporins, carbapenems). Treatment with aztreonam can result in hypersensitivity reactions in patients with or without prior exposure to aztreonam. If an allergic reaction to aztreonam occurs, discontinue the drug and institute supportive treatment as appropriate (eg, maintenance of ventilation, pressor amines, antihistamines, corticosteroids). Serious hypersensitivity reactions may require epinephrine and other emergency measures.

➤*Superinfection:* The use of antibiotics may promote the overgrowth of nonsusceptible organisms, including gram-positive organisms (*Staphylococcus aureus* and *Streptococcus faecalis*) and fungi. Should superinfection occur during therapy, appropriate measures should be taken.

➤*Pregnancy: Category B.* Aztreonam crosses the placenta and enters the fetal circulation.

There are no adequate and well-controlled studies in pregnant women. Because animal reproduction studies are not always predictive of human response, aztreonam should be used during pregnancy only if clearly needed.

➤*Lactation:* Aztreonam is excreted in human milk in concentrations that are less than 1% of concentrations determined in simultaneously obtained maternal serum; consideration should be given to temporary discontinuation of nursing and use of formula feedings.

➤*Children:* The safety and efficacy of IV aztreonam for injection have been established in the age groups 9 months to 16 years. Use of aztreonam in these age groups is supported by evidence from adequate and well-controlled studies of aztreonam in adults with additional efficacy, safety, and pharmacokinetic data from noncomparative clinical studies in pediatric patients. Sufficient data are not available for children less than 9 months of age or for the following treatment indications/pathogens: Septicemia and skin and skin-structure infections (where the skin infection is believed or known to be due to *H. influenzae* type B). In children with cystic fibrosis, higher doses of aztreonam may be warranted.

➤*Monitoring:* In patients with impaired hepatic or renal function, appropriate monitoring is recommended during therapy. If an aminoglycoside is used concurrently with aztreonam, especially if high dosages of the former are used or if therapy is prolonged, renal function should be monitored because of the potential nephrotoxicity and ototoxicity of aminoglycoside antibiotics.

Drug Interactions

Aztreonam Drug Interactions			
Precipitant drug	Object drug[a]		Description
Probenecid Furosemide	Aztreonam	↑	Concomitant administration causes clinically insignificant increases in aztreonam serum levels.
Antibiotics (eg, cefoxitin, imipenem)	Aztreonam	↓	Antibiotics may induce high levels of β-lactamase in vitro in some gram-negative aerobes such as *Enterobacter* and *Pseudomonas* sp, resulting in antagonism to many β-lactam antibiotics including aztreonam. Do not use β-lactamase-inducing antibiotics concurrently with aztreonam.
Aztreonam	Aminoglycosides	↑	If an aminoglycoside is used concurrently with aztreonam, especially if high dosages of the former are used or if therapy is prolonged, monitor renal function because of potential nephrotoxicity and ototoxicity of aminoglycoside antibiotics.

[a] ↑ = object drug increased; ↓ = object drug decreased.

Adverse Reactions

➤*Local:* Local reactions such as phlebitis/thrombophlebitis following IV administration, and discomfort/swelling at the injection site following IM administration occurred at rates of approximately 1.9% and 2.4%, respectively.

➤*Systemic:* Systemic reactions (considered to be related to therapy or of uncertain etiology) occurring at an incidence of 1% to 1.3% include diarrhea, nausea and/or vomiting, and rash. Reactions occurring at an incidence of less than 1% are listed within each body system in order of decreasing severity:

➤*Cardiovascular:* Hypotension; transient ECG changes (ventricular bigeminy and PVC); flushing.

➤*CNS:* Seizure; confusion; vertigo; paresthesia; insomnia; dizziness.

➤*Dermatologic:* Toxic epidermal necrolysis (see Warnings); purpura; erythema multiforme; exfoliative dermatitis; urticaria; petechiae; pruritus; diaphoresis.

➤*GI:* Abdominal cramps; rare cases of *C. difficile*-associated diarrhea, including pseudomembranous colitis, or gastrointestinal bleeding have been reported. Onset of pseudomembranous colitis symptoms may occur during or after antibiotic treatment. (See Warnings.)

➤*GU:* Vaginal candidiasis; vaginitis; breast tenderness.

➤*Hematologic:* Pancytopenia; neutropenia; thrombocytopenia; anemia; eosinophilia; leukocytosis; thrombocytosis.

➤*Hepatic:* Hepatitis; jaundice.

➤*Hypersensitivity:* Anaphylaxis; angioedema; bronchospasm.

➤*Musculoskeletal:* Muscular aches.

➤*Respiratory:* Wheezing; dyspnea; chest pain.

➤*Special senses:* Tinnitus; diplopia; mouth ulcer; altered taste; numb tongue; sneezing; nasal congestion; halitosis.

➤*Miscellaneous:* Weakness; headache; fever; malaise.

➤*Children:* Of the 612 children who were treated with aztreonam for injection in clinical trials, less than 1% required discontinuation of therapy due to adverse events. The following systemic adverse events, regardless of drug relationship, occurred in greater than or equal to 1% of treated patients in domestic clinical trials: Rash (4.3%), diarrhea (1.4%), and fever (1%). These adverse events were comparable to those observed in adult clinical trials.

In 343 children receiving IV therapy, the following local reactions were noted: Pain (12%), erythema (2.9%), induration (0.9%), and phlebitis (2.1%). In the US patient population, pain occurred in 1.5% of patients, while each of the remaining three local reactions had an incidence of 0.5%.

➤*Laboratory adverse reactions:* The following laboratory adverse reactions, regardless of drug relationship, occurred in greater than or equal to 1% of treated patients: increased ALT (6.5%), increased eosinophils (6.3%), increased serum creatinine (5.8%), increased platelets (3.6%), increased AST (3.8%), and neutropenia (3.2%).

Adverse laboratory changes without regard to drug relationship that were reported during clinical trials were:

Hematologic – Increases in prothrombin and partial thromboplastin times, positive Coombs' test.

Hepatic – Elevations of AST, ALT, and alkaline phosphatase; signs or symptoms of hepatobiliary dysfunction occurred in less than 1% of recipients (see above).

Renal – Increases in serum creatinine.

➤*Children:* In US pediatric clinical trials, neutropenia (absolute neutrophil count less than 1,000/mm^3) occurred in 11.3% of patients (8 of 71) less

AZTREONAM — INJECTION

than 2 years of age receiving 30 mg/kg every 6 hours. AST and ALT elevations to greater than 3 times the upper limit of normal were noted in 15% to 20% of patients greater than or equal to 2 years of age receiving 50 mg/kg every 6 hours. The increased frequency of these reported laboratory adverse events may be due to either increased severity of illness treated or higher doses of aztreonam administered.

Overdosage

➤*Treatment:* If necessary, aztreonam may be cleared from the serum by hemodialysis or peritoneal dialysis.

AZTREONAM — INHALATION

Indications

➤*Cystic fibrosis:* To improve respiratory symptoms in cystic fibrosis patients with *Pseudomonas aeruginosa*.

Administration and Dosage

➤*General dosing considerations:* Patients should use a bronchodilator before administration of aztreonam. (See Concomitant Therapy.)

➤*Adults:*

Cystic fibrosis –

Usual dosage: 75 mg 3 times a day. Doses should be taken at least 4 hours apart.

Duration of therapy: 28 days (followed by 28 days off aztreonam therapy).

➤*Children:*

Cystic fibrosis –

7 years of age and older: See Adults for dosing.

➤*Concomitant therapy:* Patients should use a bronchodilator before administration. Short-acting bronchodilators can be taken between 15 minutes and 4 hours prior to each dose of aztreonam. Alternatively, long-acting bronchodilators can be taken between 30 minutes and 12 hours prior to administration of aztreonam. For patients taking multiple inhaled therapies, the recommended order of administration is as follows: bronchodilator, mucolytics, and, lastly, aztreonam.

➤*Preparation for administration:* Do not reconstitute aztreonam until ready to administer a dose. Take 1 amber glass vial containing aztreonam and 1 diluent ampule from the carton. To open the glass vial, carefully remove the metal ring by pulling the tab and remove the gray rubber stopper. Twist the tip off the diluent ampule and squeeze the liquid into the glass vial. Replace the rubber stopper, then gently swirl the vial until the contents have completely dissolved. Administer immediately after reconstitution. Do not reconstitute more than 1 dose at a time.

➤*Administration:* For inhalation use only; not for intravenous (IV) or intramuscular (IM) administration. Aztreonam is administered by inhalation using an *Altera Nebulizer System*. Aztreonam should not be administered with any other nebulizer. Aztreonam should not be mixed with any other drugs in the *Altera Nebulizer Handset*.

To administer, pour the reconstituted solution into the handset of the nebulizer system. Turn the unit on. The patient should place the mouthpiece of the handset in the mouth and breathe normally only through the mouth. Administration typically takes between 2 and 3 minutes.

➤*Storage / Stability:* Store at 2° to 8°C (36° to 46°F); may be stored at up to 25°C (77°F) for up to 28 days. Do not separate the aztreonam vials from the diluent ampules. Aztreonam should be protected from light. Do not use aztreonam if it has been stored at room temperature for more than 28 days.

Actions

➤*Pharmacology:* Aztreonam is a monobactam antibacterial drug. Aztreonam exhibits activity in vitro against gram-negative aerobic pathogens, including *P. aeruginosa*. Aztreonam binds to penicillin-binding proteins of susceptible bacteria, which leads to inhibition of bacterial cell-wall synthesis and death of the cell. Aztreonam activity is not decreased in the presence of cystic fibrosis lung secretions.

➤*Pharmacokinetics:*

Absorption – The mean plasma concentration 1 hour following the first dose of aztreonam (at approximately the peak plasma concentration [C_{max}]) was 0.59 mcg/mL. Mean C_{max} in patients receiving aztreonam 3 times a day for 28 days was 0.55, 0.67, and 0.65 mcg/mL on days 0, 14, and 28, respectively, indicating no systemic accumulation of aztreonam. In contrast, the serum concentration of aztreonam following administration of an aztreonam 500 mg injection is approximately 54 mcg/mL. Evaluation of plasma and urine aztreonam concentrations following administration of aztreonam indicates low systemic absorption of aztreonam.

Sputum concentrations: Sputum aztreonam concentrations exhibited considerable variability among patients receiving aztreonam 75 mg in clinical trials. The mean sputum concentration 10 minutes following the first dose of aztreonam in patients with cystic fibrosis (N = 195) was 726 mcg/g. Mean sputum concentrations of aztreonam in patients receiving aztreonam 3 times a day for 28 days were 984, 793, and 715 mcg/g 10 minutes after dose administration on days 0, 14, and 28, respectively, indicating no accumulation of aztreonam in sputum.

Distribution – The protein binding of aztreonam in serum is approximately 56% and is independent of dose.

Metabolism – Following IM administration of aztreonam 500 mg injection every 8 hours for 7 days, approximately 6% of the dose was excreted as a microbiologically inactive open beta-lactam ring hydrolysis product in an 8-hour urine collection on the last day of multiple dosing.

Excretion – The elimination half-life of aztreonam from plasma is approximately 2.1 hours following administration of aztreonam to adult patients with cystic fibrosis. Approximately 10% of the total aztreonam dose is excreted in the urine as unchanged drug, compared with 60% to 65% following IV administration of aztreonam injection. Systemically absorbed aztreonam is eliminated approximately equally by active tubular secretion and glomerular filtration. Following administration of a single IV dose of radiolabeled aztreonam injection, approximately 12% of the dose was recovered in the feces.

Contraindications

Known allergy to aztreonam.

Warnings/Precautions

➤*Bronchospasm:* Bronchospasm is a complication associated with nebulized therapies, including aztreonam. Reduction of 15% or more in FEV_1 immediately following administration of study medication after pretreatment with a bronchodilator was observed in 3% of patients treated with aztreonam.

➤*Pulmonary exacerbation:* In clinical trials, patients with increases in FEV_1 during a 28-day course of aztreonam were sometimes treated for pulmonary exacerbations when FEV_1 declined after the treatment period. Consider a patient's baseline FEV_1 measured prior to aztreonam therapy and the presence of other symptoms when evaluating whether posttreatment changes in FEV_1 are caused by a pulmonary exacerbation.

➤*Development of drug-resistant bacteria:* Prescribing aztreonam in the absence of known *P. aeruginosa* infection in patients with cystic fibrosis is unlikely to provide benefit and increases the risk of development of drug-resistant bacteria.

➤*Hypersensitivity reactions:* Severe allergic reactions have been reported following administration of aztreonam injection to patients with no known history of exposure to aztreonam. In addition, allergic reaction with facial rash, facial swelling, and throat tightness was reported with aztreonam in clinical trials. If an allergic reaction to aztreonam occurs, stop administration of aztreonam and initiate treatment as appropriate.

Caution is advised when administering aztreonam to patients if they have a history of beta-lactam allergy, although patients with a known beta-lactam allergy have received aztreonam in clinical trials and no severe allergic reactions were reported. A history of allergy to beta-lactam antibiotics, such as penicillins, cephalosporins, and/or carbapenems, may be a risk factor because cross-reactivity may occur.

➤*Pregnancy: Category B.* No adequate and well-controlled studies of aztreonam injection or aztreonam inhalation in pregnant women have been conducted. Because animal reproduction studies are not always predictive of human response, use aztreonam during pregnancy only if clearly needed.

➤*Lactation:* Following administration of aztreonam injection, aztreonam is excreted in human milk at concentrations that are less than 1% of those determined in simultaneously obtained maternal serum. C_{max} of aztreonam following administration of inhaled aztreonam is approximately 1% of peak concentrations observed following IV aztreonam. Therefore, use of aztreonam during breast-feeding is unlikely to pose a risk to infants.

➤*Children:* Safety and effectiveness in children younger than 7 years of age have not been established.

➤*Monitoring:* Obtain baseline FEV_1 prior to initiating therapy and as needed during therapy. Monitor patients for signs and symptoms of an allergic reaction (eg, facial rash, facial swelling, throat tightness).

Drug Interactions

None known.

Adverse Reactions

➤*Adverse reactions (greater than 5%):*

Aztreonam Inhalation Adverse Reactions (> 5%)		
Adverse reactions	Aztreonam 75 mg 3 times a day (n = 146)	Placebo (n = 160)
GI		
Abdominal pain	7%	5%
Vomiting	6%	4%
Respiratory		
Cough	54%	51%
Wheezing	16%	10%
Special senses		
Nasal congestion	16%	12%
Pharyngolaryngeal pain	12%	11%
Miscellaneous		
Chest discomfort	8%	6%
Pyrexia	13%	6%

AZTREONAM — INHALATION

➤*Other adverse reactions (less than 5%):*

Dermatologic – Rash (2%).

Respiratory – Bronchospasm (3%).

Overdosage

➤*Symptoms:* No overdoses have been reported with aztreonam in clinical trials to date. In clinical trials, 225 mg doses of aztreonam were associated with higher rates of drug-related respiratory adverse reactions, particularly cough. Because the C_{max} of aztreonam following administration of aztreonam 75 mg is approximately 0.6 mcg/mL, compared with a serum concentration of 54 mcg/mL following administration of aztreonam 500 mg injection, no systemic safety issues associated with aztreonam overdose are anticipated.

Patient Information

Advise patients that aztreonam is for inhalation use only and should only be administered using the *Altera Nebulizer System*. Instruct patients only to reconstitute aztreonam with the provided diluent and not mix other drugs with aztreonam in the *Altera Nebulizer System*.

Advise patients to complete the full 28-day course of aztreonam even if they are feeling better. Inform patients that if they miss a dose to take all 3 daily doses as long as the doses are at least 4 hours apart.

Advise patients to use a bronchodilator prior to administration of aztreonam. Advise patients taking several inhaled medications to use the medications in the following order of administration: bronchodilator, mucolytics, and, lastly, aztreonam.

Advise patients to tell their health care provider if they have new or worsening symptoms. Advise patients who believe they are experiencing an allergic reaction to aztreonam to contact their health care provider immediately.

Counsel patients that antibacterial drugs, including aztreonam, should only be used to treat bacterial infections. They do not treat viral infection (eg, the common cold). When aztreonam is prescribed to treat a bacterial infection, tell patients that, although it is common to feel better early in the course of therapy, the medication should be taken as directed. Skipping doses or not completing the full course of therapy may decrease the effectiveness of the immediate treatment and increase the likelihood that bacteria will develop resistance and will not be treatable by aztreonam or other antibacterial drugs in the future.

CHLORAMPHENICOL

CHLORAMPHENICOL

Rx	**Chloramphenicol Sodium Succinate** (Various)	**Powder for Injection:** 100 mg/mL (as sodium succinate) when reconstituted	1 g in 15 mL vials.

CHLORAMPHENICOL SODIUM SUCCINATE — INJECTION

WARNING

Serious and fatal blood dyscrasias (aplastic anemia, hypoplastic anemia, thrombocytopenia, and granulocytopenia) are known to occur after the administration of chloramphenicol. In addition, there have been reports of aplastic anemia attributed to chloramphenicol which later terminated in leukemia. Blood dyscrasias have occurred after both short-term and prolonged therapy with this drug. Chloramphenicol must not be used when less potentially dangerous agents will be effective, as described in Indications. It must not be used in the treatment of trivial infections or where it is not indicated, as in colds, influenza, infections of the throat; or as a prophylactic agent to prevent bacterial infections.

It is essential that adequate blood studies be made during treatment with the drug. While blood studies may detect early peripheral blood changes, such as leukopenia, reticulocytopenia, or granulocytopenia, before they become irreversible, such studies cannot be relied on to detect bone marrow depression prior to development of aplastic anemia. To facilitate appropriate studies and observation during therapy, it is desirable that patients be hospitalized.

Indications

➤*Serious infections:* In accord with the concepts in the Warning Box, chloramphenicol must be used only in those serious infections for which less potentially dangerous drugs are ineffective or contraindicated. However, chloramphenicol may be chosen to initiate antibiotic therapy on the clinical impression that one of the conditions below is believed to be present; in vitro sensitivity tests should be performed concurrently so that the drug may be discontinued as soon as possible if less potentially dangerous agents are indicated by such tests. The decision to continue use of chloramphenicol rather than another antibiotic when both are suggested by in vitro studies to be effective against a specific pathogen should be based upon severity of the infection, susceptibility of the pathogen to the various antimicrobial drugs, efficacy of the various drugs in the infection, and the important additional concepts contained in the Warning Box above.

Serious infections caused by susceptible strains in accordance with the concepts expressed above:

1.) *Salmonella* species.
2.) *H. influenzae*, specially meningeal infections.
3.) Rickettsia.
4.) Lymphogranuloma-psittacosis group.
5.) Various gram-negative bacteria causing bacteremia, meningitis, or other serious gram-negative infections.
6.) Other susceptible organisms which have been demonstrated to be resistant to all other appropriate antimicrobial agents.

➤*Acute infections caused by Salmonella typhi:* It is not recommended for the routine treatment of the typhoid carrier state.

In treatment of typhoid fever some authorities recommend that chloramphenicol be administered at therapeutic levels for 8 to 10 days after the patient has become afebrile to lessen the possibility of relapse.

➤*Cystic fibrosis:* Cystic fibrosis regimens.

Administration and Dosage

➤*General dosing considerations:* Patients started on intravenous (IV) chloramphenicol sodium succinate should be changed to the oral form of another appropriate antibiotic as soon as practical.

➤*Adults:*

Infections – For a list of infections, refer to Indications.

Usual dosage: 50 mg/kg/day IV in divided doses at 6-hour intervals. In exceptional cases, patients with infections due to moderately resistant organisms may require increased dosage up to 100 mg/kg/day to achieve blood levels inhibiting the pathogen, but these high doses should be decreased as soon as possible.

➤*Children:*

Infections – For a list of infections, refer to Indications.

Infants and children: 50 mg/kg/day IV in divided doses at 6-hour intervals. Severe infections (eg, bacteremia, meningitis), especially when adequate cerebrospinal fluid concentrations are desired, may require dosage up to 100 mg/kg/day; however, it is recommended that dosage be reduced to 50 mg/kg/day as soon as possible.

Infants and children with suspected immature metabolic functions: 25 mg/kg/day will usually produce therapeutic concentrations of the drug in the blood. In this group particularly, the concentration of the drug in the blood should be carefully followed by microtechniques.

Neonates: (See also Adverse Reactions for information regarding "Gray syndrome.")

• *Usual dosage* – 25 mg/kg/day IV in divided doses at 6-hour intervals. Increased dosage in these individuals, demanded by severe infections, should be given only to maintain the blood concentration within a therapeutically effective range.

• *Dosage adjustment* – After the first 2 weeks of life, full-term neonates ordinarily may receive up to a total of 50 mg/kg/day in divided doses at 6-hour intervals. These dosage recommendations are extremely important because blood concentration in all premature and full-term neonates younger than 2 weeks of age differs from that of other infants neonates. This difference is due to variations in the maturity of the metabolic functions of the liver and the kidneys. When these functions are immature (or seriously impaired in adults), high concentrations of the drug are found, which tend to increase with succeeding doses.

➤*Renal function impairment:* Excessive blood levels may result from administration of the recommended dose to patients with impaired kidney function. The dosage should be adjusted accordingly, or preferably, the blood concentration should be determined at appropriate intervals.

➤*Hepatic function impairment:* Excessive blood levels may result from administration of the recommended dose to patients with impaired liver function. The dosage should be adjusted accordingly, or preferably, the blood concentration should be determined at appropriate intervals.

➤*Preparation for administration:* Chloramphenicol is considered a potential teratogen and mutagen. Follow safe handling procedures when preparing, administering, or dispensing chloramphenicol.

A 10% (100 mg/mL) solution is prepared by the addition of 10 mL of an aqueous diluent such as water for injection or dextrose 5% injection.

➤*Administration:* Chloramphenicol sodium succinate is intended for IV use only. As a 10% (100 mg/mL) solution, it should be injected IV over at least a 1-minute interval. It has been demonstrated to be ineffective when given intramuscularly.

➤*Storage/Stability:* Store between 15° and 25°C (59° and 77°F).

Actions

➤*Pharmacokinetics:*

Absorption – Chloramphenicol administered orally is absorbed rapidly from the intestinal tract. In controlled studies in adult volunteers using the recommended dosage of 50 mg/kg/day, a dosage of 1 g every 6 hours for 8 doses was given. Using the microbiological assay method, the average peak serum level was 11.2 mcg/mL 1 hour after the first dose. A cumulative effect gave a peak rise to 18.4 mcg/mL after the fifth dose of 1 g. Mean serum levels ranged from 8 to 14 mcg/mL over the 48-hour period.

Distribution – Chloramphenicol diffuses rapidly, but its distribution is not uniform. Highest concentrations are found in liver and kidney, and lowest concentrations are found in brain and cerebrospinal fluid. Chloramphenicol enters cerebrospinal fluid even in the absence of meningeal inflammation, appearing in concentrations about half of those found in the

CHLORAMPHENICOL SODIUM SUCCINATE — INJECTION

blood. Measurable levels are also detected in pleural and in ascitic fluids, saliva, milk, and in the aqueous and vitreous humors. Transport across the placental barrier occurs with somewhat lower concentration in cord blood of neonates than in maternal blood.

Excretion – Total urinary excretion of chloramphenicol in these studies ranged from a low of 68% to a high of 99% over a 3-day period. From 8% to 12% of the antibiotic excreted is in the form of free chloramphenicol; the remainder consists of microbiologically inactive metabolites, principally the conjugate with glucuronic acid. Since the glucuronide is excreted rapidly, most chloramphenicol detected in the blood is in the microbiologically active free form. Despite the small proportion of unchanged drug excreted in the urine, the concentration of free chloramphenicol is relatively high, amounting to several hundred mcg/mL in patients receiving divided doses of 50 mg/kg/day. Small amounts of active drug are found in bile and feces.

➤*Microbiology:* Chloramphenicol is a broad-spectrum antibiotic originally isolated from *Streptomyces venezuelae*. It inhibits bacterial protein synthesis by interfering with the transfer of activated amino acids from soluble RNA to ribosomes. In vitro, chloramphenicol exerts mainly a bacteriostatic effect on a wide range of gram-negative and gram-positive bacteria. Bacteriological studies should be performed to determine the causative organisms and their susceptibilities to chloramphenicol.

Chloramphenicol has been shown to be active against most strains of the following microorganisms, both in vitro and in clinical infections as described in the Indications.

Aerobic gram-negative microorganisms – *Haemophilus influenzae*; *Salmonella* species, including *Salmonella typhi*.

Other microorganisms – Lymphogranuloma-psittacosis group; Rickettsia.

Contraindications

History of previous hypersensitivity or toxic reaction to it. It must not be used in the treatment of trivial infections or where it is not indicated, as in colds, influenza, infections of the throat; or as a prophylactic agent to prevent bacterial infections.

Warnings/Precautions

➤*Duration of therapy:* Repeated courses of chloramphenicol treatment should be avoided if at all possible. Treatment should not be continued longer than required to produce a cure with little or no risk or relapse of the disease.

➤*Renal/Hepatic function impairment:* Excessive blood levels may result from administration of the recommended dose to patients with impaired liver or kidney function. The dosage should be adjusted accordingly, or preferably, the blood concentration should be determined at appropriate intervals.

➤*Superinfection:* The use of this antibiotic, as with other antibiotics, may result in an overgrowth of nonsusceptible organisms, including fungi. If infections caused by nonsusceptible organisms appear during therapy, appropriate measures should be taken.

➤*Pregnancy: Category C.* Animal reproduction studies have not been conducted with chloramphenicol. There are no adequate and well-controlled studies to establish safety of this drug in pregnancy. It is not known whether chloramphenicol can cause fetal harm when administered to a pregnant woman. Orally administered chloramphenicol has been shown to cross the placental barrier. Because of potential toxic effects on the fetus, chloramphenicol should be given to a pregnant woman only if the potential benefit justifies the potential risk to the fetus.

➤*Lactation:* Chloramphenicol is excreted in human milk following oral administration of the drug. Because of the potential for serious adverse reactions in nursing infants from chloramphenicol, a decision should be made whether to discontinue nursing or to discontinue the drug, taking into account the importance of the drug to the mother.

➤*Children:* Precaution should be used in therapy of premature and full-term neonates and infants to avoid Gray syndrome toxicity. Due to immature metabolic processes in the neonate and infant, excessive blood levels may result from administration of the recommended dose. The dosage should be adjusted accordingly or, preferable, the blood concentration should be determined at appropriate intervals (see Adverse Reactions, Gray syndrome).

See Administration and Dosage for dosing information in the pediatric population.

➤*Monitoring:* Baseline blood studies should be followed by periodic blood studies approximately every 2 days during therapy. The drug should be discontinued upon appearance of reticulocytopenia, leukopenia, thrombocytopenia, anemia or any other blood study findings attributable to chloramphenicol. However, it should be noted that such studies do not exclude the possible later appearance of the irreversible type of bone marrow depression.

Drug Interactions

Chloramphenicol Drug Interactions

Precipitant drug	Object drug[a]		Description
Barbiturates	Chloramphenicol	↓	Decreased chloramphenicol serum levels may occur, and barbiturate clearance may be decreased, resulting in increased levels or toxicity.
Chloramphenicol	Barbiturates	↑	
Rifampin	Chloramphenicol	↓	Concomitant administration may reduce serum chloramphenicol levels, presumably through hepatic enzyme induction.
Chloramphenicol	Anticoagulants	↑	Anticoagulant action may be enhanced.
Chloramphenicol	Cyclophosphamide	↓	Decreased or delayed activation of cyclophosphamide may occur, although it is unclear if a significant decrease in its effect would occur.
Chloramphenicol	Hydantoins	↑	Serum hydantoin levels may be increased, possibly resulting in toxicity. In addition, chloramphenicol levels may be increased or decreased.
Hydantoins	Chloramphenicol	↔	
Chloramphenicol	Iron salts	↑	Serum iron levels may be increased.
Chloramphenicol	Penicillins	↔	Synergistic effects may develop in the treatment of certain microorganisms, but antagonism may also occur.
Chloramphenicol	Sulfonylureas		Clinical manifestations of hypoglycemia may occur with concurrent use.
Chloramphenicol	Vitamin B_{12}	↓	Hematologic effects of vitamin B_{12} may be decreased in patients with pernicious anemia by concurrent chloramphenicol.

[a] ↑ = object drug increased; ↓ = object drug decreased; ↔ = undetermined effect.

Concurrent therapy with other drugs that may cause bone marrow depression should be avoided.

Adverse Reactions

➤*CNS:* Headache, mild depression, mental confusion, and delirium have been described in patients receiving chloramphenicol. Optic and peripheral neuritis have been reported, usually following long-term therapy. If this occurs, the drug should be promptly withdrawn.

➤*GI:* Nausea, vomiting, glossitis and stomatitis, diarrhea and enterocolitis may occur in low incidence.

➤*Hematologic:* The most serious adverse effect of chloramphenicol is bone marrow depression. Serious and fatal blood dyscrasias (aplastic anemia, hypoplastic anemia, thrombocytopenia, and granulocytopenia) are known to occur after the administration of chloramphenicol. An irreversible type of marrow depression leading to aplastic anemia with a high rate of mortality is characterized by the appearance weeks or months after therapy of bone marrow aplastic or hypoplasia. Peripherally, pancytopenia is most often observed, but in a small number of cases only 1 or 2 of the 3 major cell types (erythrocytes, leukocytes, platelets) may be depressed.

A reversible type of bone marrow depression, which is dose related, may occur. This type of marrow depression is characterized by vacuolization of the erythroid cells, reduction of reticulocytes and leukopenia, and responds promptly to the withdrawal of chloramphenicol.

An exact determination of the risk of serious and fatal blood dyscrasias is not possible because of lack of accurate information regarding the size of the population at risk, the total number of drug-associated dyscrasias, and the total number of non-drug associated dyscrasias.

Aplastic anemia – In a report to the California State Assembly by the California Medical Association and the State Department of Public Health in January 1967, the risk of fatal aplastic anemia was estimated at 1:24,200 to 1:40,500 based on 2 dosage levels.

There have been reports of aplastic anemia attributed to chloramphenicol which later terminated in leukemia.

Hemoglobinuria – Paroxysmal nocturnal hemoglobinuria has been reported.

➤*Hypersensitivity:* Fever, macular and vesicular rashes, angioedema, urticaria, and anaphylaxis may occur. Herxheimer's reactions have occurred during therapy for typhoid fever.

➤*Miscellaneous:* Toxic reactions including fatalities have occurred in the premature and neonate; the signs and symptoms associated with these reactions have been referred to as the Gray syndrome. One case of Gray syndrome has been reported in a neonate born to a mother having received chloramphenicol during labor. One case has been reported in a 3-month-old infant. The following summarizes the clinical and laboratory studies that have been made on these patients:

1.) In most cases, therapy with chloramphenicol had been instituted within the first 48 hours of life.
2.) Symptoms first appeared after 3 to 4 days of continued treatment with high doses of chloramphenicol.

CHLORAMPHENICOL SODIUM SUCCINATE — INJECTION

3.) The symptoms appeared in the following order:
 a.) Abdominal distension with or without emesis.
 b.) Progressive pallid cyanosis.
 c.) Vasomotor collapse, frequently accompanied by irregular respiration.
 d.) Death within a few hours of onset of these symptoms.

4.) The progression of symptoms from onset to exitus was accelerated with higher dose schedules.
5.) Preliminary blood serum level studies revealed unusually high concentrations of chloramphenicol (over 90 mcg/mL after repeated doses).
6.) Termination of therapy upon early evidence of the associated symptomatology frequently reversed the process with complete recovery.

FLUOROQUINOLONES

WARNING

Tendonitis and tendon rupture – Fluoroquinolones are associated with an increased risk of tendinitis and tendon rupture in all ages. This risk is further increased in older patients usually older than 60 years of age, in patients taking corticosteroid drugs, and in patients with kidney, heart, or lung transplants.

Myasthenia gravis – Fluoroquinolones may exacerbate muscle weakness in persons with myasthenia gravis. Avoid fluoroquinolones in patients with known history of myasthenia gravis.

Indications

For specific approved indications, refer to individual drug monographs.

➤*Off-label uses:* Refer to individual monographs for further information.

Anthrax prophylaxis(adults) –
 Ciprofloxacin: [1] = Good documentation.

Catheter-related bloodstream infections –
 Ciprofloxacin: [3] = Safety concerns.

Chancroid –
 Ciprofloxacin: [1] = Good documentation.

Epididymitis –
 Levofloxacin: [1] = Good documentation.
 Ofloxacin: [1] = Good documentation.

Granuloma inguinale (donovanosis) –
 Ciprofloxacin: [1] = Good documentation.

Hospital-acquired pneumonia –
 Moxifloxacin: [1] = Good documentation.

Infective endocarditis (adults) –
 Ciprofloxacin: [1] = Good documentation.
 Levofloxacin: [1] = Good documentation.
 Moxifloxacin: [1] = Good documentation.

Infective endocarditis (children/adolescents) –
 Ciprofloxacin: [1] = Good documentation.
 Levofloxacin: [1] = Good documentation.

Pelvic inflammatory disease –
 Levofloxacin: [1] = Good documentation.
 Ofloxacin: [1] = Good documentation.

Plague –
 Ciprofloxacin (adults): [1] = Good documentation.
 Ciprofloxacin (children): [1] = Good documentation.

Surgical prophylaxis –
 Ciprofloxacin: [1] = Good documentation.

Traveler's diarrhea –
 Ciprofloxacin: [1] = Good documentation.
 Levofloxacin: [1] = Good documentation.
 Norfloxacin: [1] = Good documentation.
 Ofloxacin: [1] = Good documentation.

Tuberculosis –
 Levofloxacin: [1] = Good documentation.
 Moxifloxacin: [1] = Good documentation.

Tularemia –
 Ciprofloxacin (adults): [1] = Good documentation.
 Ciprofloxacin (children): [1] = Good documentation.

Other possible off-label uses –

Ciprofloxacin: Ciprofloxacin has been used in children with cystic fibrosis for periods of 10 days to 6 months without documented adverse effects or intolerance.

Multidrug-resistant tuberculosis, alternative regimen for cutaneous and GI anthrax.

• *Disseminated gonorrhea (alternative regimen)* – 400 mg IV every 12 hours for 24 to 48 hours after improvement begins, then 500 mg orally twice daily for 7 days.

Gatifloxacin, and moxifloxacin: Gatifloxacin, and moxifloxacin are effective against multidrug-resistant strains of *S. pneumoniae* and, therefore, may be used in pediatric patients who fail initial treatment for acute otitis media and sinusitis.

Levofloxacin: An alternative regimen for disseminated gonococcal infections if antimicrobial susceptibility exists and can be documented by culture. Administer 250 mg once daily IV for 24 to 48 hours (after improvement begins, administer 500 mg/day orally for 7 days).

Ciprofloxacin and norfloxacin: Ciprofloxacin and norfloxacin have been used for the treatment of gastroenteritis in children.

Mycobacterial infections: In children, atypical mycobacterial infections have been satisfactorily treated with ciprofloxacin as part of combination therapy; in vitro, gatifloxacin has been shown to be active against *M. leprae*.

Fluoroquinolones: Fluoroquinolones are used as empiric therapy for low-risk febrile neutropenic pediatric patients. Regimens including fluoroquinolones for tuberculosis have been shown to be equivalent to standard antituberculosis regimens, and these agents are currently suggested for the management of multidrug-resistant infections or in patients with adverse reactions to other agents. The outcome of regimens including quinolones has been poorer in HIV-seropositive patients. Ciprofloxacin and ofloxacin are the quinolones most often evaluated and recommended in mycobacterial diseases.

Actions

➤*Pharmacology:* The fluoroquinolones are synthetic, broad-spectrum antibacterial agents that inhibit DNA gyrase and topoisomerase IV. DNA gyrase is an essential enzyme that is involved in the replication, transcription, and repair of bacterial DNA. Topoisomerase IV is an enzyme known to play a key role in the partitioning of the chromosomal DNA during bacterial cell division. The basic molecule has been modified at the N-1 position, with different groups added to the C-6, C-7, and C-8 positions. The addition of a fluorine atom at position C-6 enhances DNA gyrase inhibitory activity and provides activity against *staphylococci*; addition of a second fluorine group at position C-8 increases absorption and longer half-life; the addition of a piperazine group at position C-7 provides the best gram-negative activity; ring alkylation improves gram-positive activity and half-life; substitution of a methyl group for the piperazine group increases absorption and a longer half-life; and addition of acyclopropyl group at position N-1 and amino group at position C-5 and a fluorine group at C-8 increases activity against mycoplasma and chlamydia.

➤*Pharmacokinetics:*

Pharmacokinetics of Fluoroquinolones

Fluoroquinolone	Bioavailability (%)	Max urine concentration (mcg/mL) (dose)	Mean peak plasma concentration (mcg/mL) (dose)	Area under curve (AUC) (mcg • hr/mL) (dose)	Protein binding (%)	t½ (hr)	Urine recovery unchanged (%)
Ciprofloxacin Oral	≈ 70-80	> 200 (250 mg)	1.2 (250 mg) 2.4 (500 mg) 4.3 (750 mg) 5.4 (1000 mg)	4.8 (250 mg) 11.6 (500 mg) 20.2 (750 mg) 30.8 (1000 mg)	20-40	≈ 4	≈ 40-50
IV		> 200 (200 mg) > 400 (400 mg)	4.4 (400 mg)	4.8 (200 mg) 11.6 (400 mg)		≈ 5-6	≈ 50-70

Pharmacokinetics of Fluoroquinolones							
Fluoroquinolone	Bio-availability (%)	Max urine concentration (mcg/mL) (dose)	Mean peak plasma concentration (mcg/mL) (dose)	Area under curve (AUC) (mcg • hr/mL) (dose)	Protein binding (%)	t½ (hr)	Urine recovery unchanged (%)
Gatifloxacin[a] Oral	≈ 96		≈ 2 (200 mg single dose) ≈ 3.8 (400 mg single dose) ≈ 4.2 (400 mg multiple dose)	≈ 14.2 (200 mg single dose) ≈ 33 (400 mg single dose) ≈ 34.4 (400 mg multiple dose)	≈ 20	≈ 7.8 (400 mg single dose) ≈7.1 (400 mg multiple dose)	≈ 73.8 (200 mg single dose) ≈72.4 (400 mg single dose) ≈ 80.2 (400 mg multiple dose)
IV			≈ 2.2 (200 mg single dose) ≈ 2.4 (200 mg multiple dose) ≈ 5.5 (400 mg single dose) ≈ 4.6 (400 mg multiple dose)	≈ 15.9 (200 mg single dose) ≈ 16.8 (200 mg multiple dose) ≈ 35.1 (400 mg single dose) ≈ 35.4 (400 mg multiple dose)		≈ 11.1 (200 mg single dose) ≈ 12.3 (200 mg multiple dose) ≈ 7.4 (400 mg single dose) ≈ 13.9 (400 mg multiple dose)	≈ 71.7 (200 mg single dose) ≈ 72.4 (200 mg multiple dose) ≈ 62.3 (400 mg single dose) ≈ 83.5 (400 mg multiple dose)
Levofloxacin	≈ 99		≈ 2.8-11.5 (single dose oral or IV) ≈ 5.7-12.1 (multiple dose oral or IV)	≈ 27.2-110 (single dose oral or IV) ≈ 47.5-108 (multiple dose oral or IV)	≈ 24-38	≈ 6.3-7.5 (single dose oral or IV) ≈ 7-8.8 (multiple dose oral or IV)	≈ 87 (oral)
Lomefloxacin	≈ 95-98	> 300 (400 mg)	0.8 (100 mg) 1.4 (200 mg) 3.2 (400 mg)	5.6 (100 mg) 10.9 (200 mg) 26.1 (400 mg)	≈ 10	≈ 8	≈ 65
Moxifloxacin	≈ 90		3.1 to 4.5 (400 mg)	36.1 to 49.3 (400 mg)	30 to 50	≈ 12	≈ 20
Norfloxacin	30-40	≥ 200 (400 mg)	0.8 (200 mg) 1.5 (400 mg) 2.4 (800 mg)		10-15	3-4	26-32
Ofloxacin Oral	≈ 98	≈ 220 (200 mg)	1.5 (200 mg) 2.4 (300 mg) 2.9 (400 mg) 4.6 (400 mg steady-state)	14.1 (200 mg) 21.2 (300 mg) 31.4 (400 mg) 61 (400 mg steady-state)	≈ 32	≈ 9	65-80
IV		nd[b]	2.7 (200 mg) 4 (400 mg)	43.5 (400 mg)	≈ 32	5-10	≈ 65
Sparfloxacin	92	> 12 (400 mg)[c]	≈ 1.3 (400 mg)	≈ 34 (400 mg)	≈ 45	≈ 20	≈ 10

[a] Single dose: AUC (0-∞); Multiple dose: AUC (0-24).
[b] nd = no data.
[c] Following a 400 mg loading dose of sparfloxacin, the mean urine concentration 4 hours postdose was in excess of 12 mcg/mL.

Norfloxacin –

Absorption/Distribution: Absorption is rapid. Food or dairy products may decrease absorption. Steady-state norfloxacin levels will be attained within 2 days of dosing. Urinary concentrations of ≥ 200 mcg/mL are attained 2 to 3 hours after a single 400 mg dose. Mean urinary concentrations of norfloxacin remain above 30 mcg/mL for at least 12 hours following a 400 mg dose. Norfloxacin is least soluble at urinary pH of 7.5; greater solubility occurs at pHs above and below this value.

Metabolism/Excretion: Norfloxacin is eliminated through metabolism, biliary excretion, and renal excretion. Renal excretion occurs by glomerular filtration and tubular secretion, as evidenced by the high rate of renal clearance (≈ 275 mL/min). Within 24 hours of administration, 5% to 8% of the dose is recovered in the urine as 6 less-active metabolites. Fecal recovery accounts for another 30%. In healthy elderly volunteers (65 to 75 years of age), norfloxacin is eliminated more slowly because of decreased renal function. Drug absorption appears unaffected. Disposition of norfloxacin in patients with creatinine clearance (Ccr) rates > 30 mL/min/1.73 m^2 is similar to that in healthy volunteers. In patients with Ccr rates ≤ 30 mL/min/1.73 m^2, the renal elimination decreases so that the effective serum half-life is 6.5 hours; dosage alteration is necessary. See Administration and Dosage.

Ciprofloxacin –

Absorption/Distribution: Ciprofloxacin is rapidly and well absorbed from the GI tract after oral administration with no substantial loss by first-pass metabolism. When given concomitantly with food, there is a delay in the absorption of the drug, resulting in peak concentrations that are closer to 2 hours after dosing rather than 1 hour. However, the overall absorption is not substantially affected. Maximum serum concentrations are attained 1 to 2 hours after oral dosing. Mean concentrations 12 hours after dosing with 250, 500, or 750 mg are 0.1, 0.2, and 0.4 mcg/mL, respectively. Following 60-minute IV infusions of 200 and 400 mg, mean maximum serum concentrations achieved were 2.1 and 4.6 mcg/mL, respectively; concentrations at 12 hours were 0.1 and 0.2 mcg/mL, respectively. Ciprofloxacin is widely distributed throughout the body. Tissue concentrations often exceed serum concentrations in men and women, particularly in genital tissue. The drug diffuses into the cerebrospinal fluid (CSF); however, CSF concentrations are generally < 10% of peak serum concentrations.

Metabolism/Excretion: Four metabolites have been identified in urine which, together, account for ≈ 15% of an oral dose. The metabolites have antimicrobial activity, but are less active than unchanged ciprofloxacin. After IV administration, 3 metabolites have been identified in urine, which account for ≈ 10% of the IV dose. After a 250 mg oral dose, urine concentrations usually exceed 200 mcg/mL during the first 2 hours and are ≈ 30 mcg/mL at 8 to 12 hours after dosing. Following a 200 or 400 mg IV dose, urine concentrations usually exceed 200 and 400 mcg/mL, respectively, during the first 2 hours and are generally > 15 and > 30 mcg/mL, respectively, at 8 to 12 hours after dosing. Urinary ciprofloxacin excretion is virtually complete within 24 hours after dosing. Renal clearance is ≈ 300 mL/min; active tubular secretion plays a significant role. Although bile concentrations are several-fold higher than serum after oral dosing, only a small amount is recovered from the bile. Approximately 20% to 35% of an oral dose is recovered from feces within 5 days after dosing. In patients with reduced renal function, the half-life is slightly prolonged; dosage adjustments may be required. See Administration and Dosage.

Ofloxacin –

Absorption/Distribution: Maximum serum concentrations are achieved 1 to 2 hours after an oral dose. The amount absorbed increases proportionately with the dose. Elimination is biphasic; half-lives are ≈ 4 to 5 hours and 20 to 25 hours, although accumulation at steady state can be estimated using a half-life of 9 hours. Steady-state concentrations are achieved after

4 doses and are ≈ 40% higher than concentrations after single doses. Ofloxacin is widely distributed to body tissues and fluids.

Metabolism/Excretion: Ofloxacin has a pyridobenzoxazine ring that appears to decrease the extent of parent compound metabolism; < 5% of a dose is recovered in the urine as the desmethyl or N-oxide metabolites. Elimination is mainly by renal excretion; 4% to 8% is excreted in the feces. A longer plasma half-life of ≈ 6.4 to 7.4 hours was observed in elderly subjects, compared with 4 to 5 hours for young subjects. Slower elimination is observed in elderly subjects as compared with younger subjects, which may be attributable to the reduced renal function and renal clearance observed in the elderly subjects. Because ofloxacin is known to be substantially excreted by the kidney, and elderly patients are more likely to have decreased renal function, dosage adjustment is necessary for elderly patients with impaired renal function as recommended for all patients. Clearance is reduced in patients with renal function impairment (Ccr ≤ 50 mL/min); dosage adjustment is necessary. See Administration and Dosage.

Lomefloxacin –

Absorption/Distribution: Absorption is rapid. Following coadministration with food, rate of absorption is delayed (time to reach maximum plasma concentration delayed by 41%, maximum concentration decreased by 18%), and the extent of absorption (AUC) is decreased by 12%. At 24 hours postdose, single doses of 200 or 400 mg result in mean plasma levels of 0.1 and 0.24 mcg/mL, respectively. Steady-state concentrations are achieved within 48 hours of initiating once-daily dosing. The mean urine concentration exceeds 35 mcg/mL for ≥ 24 hours after dosing. Urine pH appears to affect the solubility of lomefloxacin, with solubilities ranging from 7.8 mg/mL at pH 5.2, to 2.4 mg/mL at pH 6.5, and 3.03 mg/mL at pH 8.12.

Metabolism/Excretion: Mean renal clearance is 145 mL/min in subjects with normal renal function, which may indicate tubular secretion. Approximately 9% of a dose is recovered in the urine as the glucuronide metabolite; 4 other metabolites have been identified and account for < 0.5% of the dose. Approximately 10% of a dose is recovered unchanged in the feces. In healthy elderly volunteers, plasma clearance was reduced by ≈ 25% and the AUC was increased by ≈ 33%, which may be caused by decreased renal function in this population. In patients with Ccr between 10 and 40 mL/min/1.73 m^2, the mean AUC after a single dose increased 335% over the AUC in patients with Ccr > 80 mL/min/1.73 m^2, and mean half-life increased to 21 hours. In patients with Ccr < 10 mL/min/1.73 m^2, AUC increased 700% and half-life increased to 45 hours. Adjustment of dosage is necessary. See Administration and Dosage.

Levofloxacin –

Absorption: Levofloxacin is rapidly and completely absorbed after oral administration. Peak plasma concentrations are usually attained 1 to 2 hours after oral dosing. Levofloxacin pharmacokinetics are linear and predictable after single and multiple oral/IV dosing regimens. Steady-state is reached within 48 hours following a 500 or 750 mg once-daily dosage regimen. The mean peak and trough concentrations attained following multiple once-daily oral dosage regimens were ≈ 5.7 and 0.5 mcg/mL after the 500 mg doses, and 8.6 and 1.1 mcg/mL after the 750 mg doses, respectively. The mean peak and trough plasma concentrations attained following multiple once-daily IV regimens were ≈ 6.4 and 0.6 mcg/mL after the 500 mg doses and 12.1 and 1.3 mcg/mL after the 750 mg doses, respectively. Oral administration of 500 mg levofloxacin tablet with food slightly prolongs the time to peak concentration by ≈ 1 hour and slightly decreases the peak concentration by ≈ 14%. Therefore, levofloxacin tablets can be administered without regard to food. The plasma concentration profile of levofloxacin after IV administration is similar and comparable in extent of exposure (AUC) to that observed for levofloxacin tablets when equal doses (mg/mg) are administered. Therefore, the oral and IV routes of administration can be considered interchangeable.

Distribution: The mean volume of distribution of levofloxacin generally ranges from 74 to 112 L after single and multiple 500 or 750 mg doses, indicating widespread distribution into body tissues. It reaches peak levels in skin tissues and in blister fluid at ≈ 3 hours after dosing. Levofloxacin also penetrates well into the lung tissues. Lung tissue concentrations were generally 2- to 5-fold higher than plasma concentrations. Levofloxacin is mainly bound to serum albumin and is independent of the drug concentration.

Metabolism: Levofloxacin undergoes limited metabolism and is primarily excreted as unchanged drug in the urine. Less than 4% of the dose was recovered in the feces in 72 hours. Less than 5% of an administered dose was recovered in the urine as the desmethyl and N-oxide metabolites. These metabolites have little relevant pharmacological activity.

Excretion: Levofloxacin is excreted largely as unchanged drug in the urine. The mean apparent total body clearance and renal clearance range from ≈ 144 to 226 mL/min and 96 to 142 mL/min, respectively. Renal clearance in excess of the glomerular filtration rate suggest the tubular secretion of levofloxacin occurs in addition to glomerular filtration.

Sparfloxacin –

Absorption: Sparfloxacin is well absorbed following oral administration. Steady-state concentration was achieved on the first day by giving a loading dose that was double the daily dose. Maximum plasma concentrations for the initial oral 400 mg loading dose were typically achieved between 3 to 6 hours following administration with a mean value of ≈ 4 hours. Maximum plasma concentrations for a 200 mg dose were also achieved between 3 to 6 hours after administration with a mean of ≈ 4 hours. Oral absorption of sparfloxacin is unaffected by administration with milk or food, including high-fat meals.

Distribution: Upon reaching general circulation, it distributes well into the body. The volume of distribution is 3.9 L/kg. It has low plasma protein binding. It penetrates well into body fluids and tissues. The concentrations in the lower respiratory tract tissues and fluids generally exceed the corresponding plasma concentrations.

Metabolism: Sparfloxacin is metabolized by the liver, primarily by phase II glucuronidation, to form a glucuronide conjugate. It does not utilize or interfere with cytochrome P450.

Excretion: The total body clearance and renal clearance of sparfloxacin were 11.4 and 1.5 L/hr respectively. It is excreted in the feces (50%) and urine (50%). The half-life is independent of the administered dose, suggesting the sparfloxacin elimination kinetics is linear.

Moxifloxacin –

Absorption: Moxifloxacin is well absorbed from the GI tract. Coadministration with a high-fat meal (eg, 500 calories from fat) does not affect the absorption of moxifloxacin. Plasma concentrations increase proportionally. Steady state is achieved after ≥ 3 days with a 400 mg once-daily regimen.

Distribution: The volume of distribution ranges from 1.7 to 2.7 L/kg. Moxifloxacin is widely distributed throughout the body, with tissue concentrations often exceeding plasma concentrations. The rates of elimination of moxifloxacin from tissue generally parallel the elimination from plasma.

Metabolism/Excretion: Moxifloxacin is metabolized via glucuronide and sulfate conjugation. The sulfate conjugate (M1) accounts for ≈ 38% of the dose and is eliminated primarily in the feces. Approximately 14% of an oral or IV dose are converted to a glucuronide conjugate (M2), which is excreted exclusively in the urine. A total of 96% of an oral dose is excreted as either unchanged drug or known metabolites. The mean apparent total body clearance and renal clearance are ≈ 12 L/hr and 2.6 L/hr, respectively.

Gatifloxacin –

Absorption: Gatifloxacin is well absorbed from the GI tract after oral administration and can be given without regard to food. Peak plasma concentrations usually occur 1 to 2 hours after oral dosing. The oral and IV routes of administration can be considered interchangeable since the pharmacokinetics of gatifloxacin after 1 hour IV administration are similar to those observed for orally administered gatifloxacin when equal doses are administered. Gatifloxacin pharmacokinetics are linear and time-independent at doses ranging from 200 to 800 mg administered over a period of up to 14 days. Steady-state concentrations are achieved by the third daily oral or IV dose. The mean steady-state peak and trough plasma concentrations attained are ≈ 4.2 mcg/mL and 0.4 mcg/mL, respectively for oral administration 4.6 mcg/mL and 0.4 mcg/mL, respectively for IV administration.

Distribution: Serum protein binding is ≈ 20% and is concentration-independent. Concentrations of gatifloxacin in saliva were approximately equal to those in plasma. The mean volume of distribution of gatifloxacin at steady-state ranged from 1.5 to 2 L/kg. Gatifloxacin was widely distributed throughout the body into many body tissues and fluids. Rapid distribution of gatifloxacin into tissues results in higher gatifloxacin concentrations in most target tissues than in serum.

Metabolism: Gatifloxacin undergoes limited biotransformation in humans with

Excretion: Gatifloxacin is excreted as unchanged drug primarily by the kidney. Less than 1% of the dose is recovered in the urine as 2 metabolites. The mean elimination half-life ranges from 7 to 14 hours and is independent of dose and route of administration. Renal clearance is independent of dose with mean value ranging from 124 to 161 mL/min. Gatifloxacin undergoes glomerular filtration and tubular secretion. It may also undergo minimal biliary or intestinal elimination, since 5% of the dose was recovered in the feces as unchanged drug.

➤*Microbiology:*

	Organisms Generally Susceptible to Fluoroquinolones In Vitro								
	Organism	Ciprofloxacin	Gatifloxacin	Levofloxacin	Lomefloxacin	Moxifloxacin	Norfloxacin	Ofloxacin	Sparfloxacin
Gram-negative	*Acinetobacter anitritus*								✓[a]
	Acinetobacter iwoffi	✓[a]	✓[a]	✓[a]					✓[a]
	Acinetobacter calcoaceticus							✓[a]	
	Aeromonas hydrophilia	✓[a]			✓[a]				
	Bacteroides distasonis								
	Bacteroides ovatus								
	Bordetella pertussis			✓[a]				✓[a]	
	Campylobacter jejuni	✓[b]							
	Chlamydia trachamotis							✓	
	Citrobacter diversus	✓	✓[a]	✓[a]	✓		✓[a]	✓	✓[a]
	Citrobacter freundii	✓	✓[a]		✓[a]	✓[a]	✓	✓[a]	
	Citrobacter koseri		✓[a]						
	Enterobacter cloacae	✓	✓[a]	✓	✓	✓[a]	✓	✓[a]	✓
	Enterobacter aerogenes	✓[a]	✓[a]	✓[a]	✓[a]		✓	✓	✓[a]
	Enterobacter agglomerans			✓[a]	✓[a]		✓[a]		
	Enterobacter sakazakii			✓[a]					
	Escherichia coli	✓	✓	✓	✓	✓[a]	✓	✓	✓
	Edwardsiella tarda	✓[a]					✓[a]		
	Gardenella vaginalis							✓	
	Haemophilus ducreyi						✓[a]	✓[a]	
	Haemophilus influenzae	✓	✓	✓	✓	✓		✓	✓
	Haemophilus parainfluenzae	✓	✓	✓	✓[a]	✓			
	Hafnia alvei				✓[a]				
	Klebsiella pneumoniae	✓	✓	✓	✓	✓	✓	✓	✓
	Klebsiella oxytoca	✓[a]	✓[a]	✓[a]	✓[a]	✓[a]	✓[a]	✓[a]	✓[a]
	Klebsiella ozaenae				✓[a]				
	Moraxella-catarrhalis	✓[b]	✓	✓	✓			✓[a]	✓
	Morganella morganii	✓	✓[a]	✓[a]	✓[a]		✓[a]	✓[a]	✓[a]
	Mycoplasma hominis							✓[a]	
	Neisseria gonorrhoeae	✓[b]	✓				✓	✓	
	Pasteurella multocida	✓[a]							
	Proteus mirabilis	✓		✓	✓	✓[a]	✓	✓	✓[a]
	Proteus vulgaris	✓	✓[a]	✓[a]	✓		✓	✓[a]	✓[a]
	Providencia alcalifaciens			✓[a]	✓[a]		✓[a]		
	Providencia rettgeri			✓[a]	✓[a]		✓[a]	✓[a]	
	Providencia stuartii	✓		✓[a]			✓[a]	✓[a]	
	Pseudomonas aeruginosa	✓		✓[c]	✓[d]		✓	✓[c]	
	Pseudomonas fluorescens			✓[a]					
	Pseudomonas stutzeri						✓[a]		
	Salmonella sp.	✓[e]						✓	✓
	Salmonella typhi	✓							
	Salmonella enteritidis	✓[a]							
	Serratia marcescens	✓		✓[a]	✓[a]		✓	✓[a]	
	Serratia proteomaculans				✓[a]				
	Shigella sp.	✓[e]		✓				✓	✓
	Shigella boydii	✓[b]							
	Shigella dysenteriae	✓[b]							
	Shigella flexneri	✓[b]							
	Shigella sonnei	✓[b]							
	Ureoplasma urealtycium						✓[a]	✓[a]	
	Vibrio parahemolyticus	✓[a]							
	Vibrio vulnificus	✓[a]							
	Vibrio cholerae	✓[a]							
	Yersinia enterocolitica	✓[a]							

Organisms Generally Susceptible to Fluoroquinolones In Vitro									
	Organism	Ciprofloxacin	Gatifloxacin	Levofloxacin	Lomefloxacin	Moxifloxacin	Norfloxacin	Ofloxacin	Sparfloxacin
Gram-positive	*Staphylococcus aureus* methicillin susceptible		✓	✓	✓[a]	✓	✓[f]	✓	✓[f]
	Staphylococcus aureus methicillin resistant				✓[a]				
	Staphylococcus epidermidis methicillin susceptible	✓[a]	✓	✓[a]	✓[a]	✓[a]	✓[f]	✓[a]	✓
	Staphylococcus epidermidis methicillin resistant		✓		✓[a]				
	Staphylococcus hemolyticus	✓							
	Staphylococcus hominis	✓							
	S. saprophyticus	✓	✓[a]	✓	✓		✓	✓[a]	
	Streptococci pyogenes	✓	✓[a]	✓		✓[a]		✓	✓[a]
	Streptococcus viridans			✓[a]		✓[a]			✓[a]
	Streptococcus anginosus					✓			
	Streptococcus constellatus					✓			
	Streptococcus pneumoniae					✓			
	Streptococcus group c/f, g			✓[a]					
	Streptococcus milleri			✓[a]					
	S. agalactiae			✓[a]		✓[a]	✓		✓[a]
	Enteroccus faecalis	✓[g]		✓[g]		✓	✓		
	Penicillin susceptible		✓	✓				✓	✓
	Penicillin resistant		✓[a]	✓				✓[a]	✓[a]
Atypical bacteria	*Legionella pneumophilia*	✓[a]	✓	✓	✓[a]	✓[a]		✓[a]	✓[a]
	Mycoplasma pneumoniae		✓	✓		✓		✓[a]	✓
	Chlamydia pneumoniae		✓	✓	✓	✓		✓[a]	✓
Anaerobe bacteria	*Bacteroides fragilis*								
	Peptostreptococcus sp.		✓[a]						
	Clostridium perfringes			✓[a]			✓	✓[a]	
	Bacteroides thetaiotaomicron				✓				
	Fusobacterium sp.				✓[a]				
	Prevotella sp.				✓[a]				

[a] Exhibits in vitro MIC of ≤ 1 mcg/mL (ciprofloxacin, sparfloxacin); ≤ 2 mcg/mL (gatifloxacin, levofloxacin, lomefloxacin, moxifloxacin and ofloxacin); ≤ 4 mcg/mL norfloxacin against most (≥ 90%) strains of microorganisms; however, the safety and effectiveness in treating clinical infections due to these microorganisms have not been established in adequate and well-controlled clinical trials.
[b] Oral ciprofloxacin.
[c] As with other drugs in this class, some strains of *P. aeruginosa* may develop resistance fairly rapidly during treatment.
[d] Urinary tract only.
[e] See following text for individual microorganisms.
[f] Does not specify susceptible or resistant.
[g] Many strains are moderately susceptible.

Ciprofloxacin – Most strains of streptococci are only moderately susceptible, as are *Mycobacterium tuberculosis*, *M. fortuitum*, and *Chlamydia trachomatis* (moderate activity). Some strains of *Pseudomonas aeruginosa* may develop resistance fairly rapidly.

Ciprofloxacin does not cross-react with other antimicrobial agents such as beta-lactams or aminoglycosides; however, additive activity may result when it is combined with beta-lactams, aminoglycosides, clindamycin, or metronidazole.

Most strains of *Burkholderia cepacia* and some strains of *Stenotrophomonas maltophilia* are resistant to ciprofloxacin as are most anaerobic bacteria, including *Bacteroides fragilis* and *Clostridium difficile*.

Gatifloxacin – The activity of gatifloxacin against *T. pallidum* has not been evaluated; however, other quinolones are not active against *T. pallidum*.

Levofloxacin – As with other drugs in this class, some strains of *P. aeruginosa* may develop resistance fairly rapidly during treatment with levofloxacin.

Norfloxacin – *Ureoplasma urealyticum* is susceptible in vitro. Resistance to norfloxacin due to spontaneous mutation in vitro is rare (< 1%). Development of resistance is greatest in the following: *P. aeruginosa*; *Klebsiella pneumoniae*; *Acinetobacter* sp.; *Enterococcus* sp. Norfloxacin is not generally active against obligate anaerobes.

Norfloxacin has not been shown to be active against *T. pallidum*.

Ofloxacin – The following organisms are susceptible in vitro:
Anaerobes: Clostridium perfringens; *Gardnerella vaginalis*.
Other: Chlamydia pneumoniae; *C. trachomatis*; *Mycoplasma pneumoniae*; *M. hominis*; *U. urealyticum*.

Many strains of other streptococcal sp, enterococcus sp, and anaerobes are resistant. It is not active against *T. pallidum*. Although cross-resistance has been observed between ofloxacin and other fluoroquinolones, some organisms resistant to other quinolones may be susceptible to ofloxacin.

Lomefloxacin – Most group A, B, D, and G streptococci, *S. pneumoniae*, *Pseudomonas cepacia*, *U. urealyticum*, *M. hominis* and anaerobic bacteria are resistant.

Cross-resistance has occurred between lomefloxacin and other quinolone-class antimicrobial agents, but not between lomefloxacin and other antimicrobials, such as aminoglycosides, penicillins, tetracyclines, cephalosporins, or sulfonamides. Lomefloxacin is active in vitro against some strains of cephalosporin- and aminoglycoside-resistant gram-negative bacteria.

Contraindications

Hypersensitivity to fluoroquinolones or the quinolone group; tendinitis or tendon rupture associated with quinolone use; patients receiving disopyramide and amiodarone as well as other QT_c-prolonging antiarrhythmic drugs reported to cause torsade de pointes, such as class IA antiarrhythmic agents (eg, quinidine, procainamide), class III antiarrhythmic agents (eg, sotalol), and bepridil (**sparfloxacin** only); patients with known QT_c prolongation or in patients being treated concomitantly with medications known to produce an increase in the QT_c interval or torsades de pointes (**sparfloxacin**); patients whose lifestyle or employment will not permit compliance with required safety precautions concerning phototoxicity (**sparfloxacin**).

Warnings/Precautions

➤*Phototoxicity:* Moderate-to-severe phototoxic reactions have occurred in patients exposed to direct or indirect sunlight or to artificial ultraviolet light (eg, sunlamps) during or following treatment with **lomefloxacin**, **sparfloxacin** or **ofloxacin**. These reactions also have occurred in patients exposed to shaded or diffused light, including exposure through glass. Advise patients to discontinue therapy of any fluoroquinolone antibiotic at the first signs or symptoms of a phototoxicity reaction such as a sensation of skin burning, redness, swelling, blisters, rash, itching, or dermatitis.

These reactions have occurred with and without the use of sunscreens or sunblocks and with single doses of lomefloxacin. In a few cases, recovery was prolonged for several weeks. As with some other types of phototoxicity, there is the potential for exacerbation of the reaction on re-exposure to sunlight or artificial ultraviolet light prior to complete recovery from the reaction. In rare cases, reactions have recurred up to several weeks after stopping therapy.

Avoid direct exposure to direct or indirect sunlight (even when using sunscreens or sunblocks) while taking lomefloxacin and other fluoroquinolones for several days following therapy. Discontinue therapy at first signs or symptoms of phototoxicity.

➤*Cardiac toxicity:* **Moxifloxacin** and **gatifloxacin** have been shown to prolong the QT interval of the electrocardiogram in some patients. Avoid in patients with known prolongation of the QT interval, patients with uncorrected hypokalemia, and patients receiving class IA (eg, quinidine, procainamide) or class III (eg, amiodarone, sotalol) antiarrhythmic agents, due to the lack of clinical experience with these drugs in these patient populations.

Use with caution in patients with ongoing proarrhythmic conditions, such as significant bradycardia or acute myocardial ischemia.

Increases in the QT_c interval have been observed in healthy volunteers treated with **sparfloxacin**. After a single loading dose of 400 mg, a mean increase in the QT_c interval of 11 msec (2.9%) is seen; at steady-state the mean increase is 7 msec (1.9%). The magnitude of the QT_c effect does not increase with repeated administration, and the QT_c returns to baseline within 48 hours of the last dose.

Avoid the concomitant prescription of medications known to prolong the QT_c interval (eg, erythromycin, terfenadine, astemizole, cisapride, pentamidine, tricyclic antidepressants, some antipsychotics including phenothiazines). **Sparfloxacin** is not recommended for use in patients with proarrhythmic conditions (eg, hypokalemia, significant bradycardia, CHF, myocardial ischemia, atrial fibrillation).

➤*Convulsions:* Increased intracranial pressure, convulsions, and toxic psychosis have occurred. CNS stimulation may also occur, which may lead to tremor, restlessness, nervousness, nightmares, insomnia, paranoia, agitation, anxiety, lightheadedness, confusion, dizziness, depression, hallucinations, and rarely, suicidal thoughts or acts. Use with caution in patients with known or suspected CNS disorders (eg, severe cerebral arteriosclerosis, epilepsy) or other factors that predispose to seizures or lower the seizure threshold, or in the presence of other risk factors that may predispose to seizures or lower the seizure threshold (eg, certain drug therapy, renal dysfunction). If these reactions occur, stop the drug, and institute appropriate measures.

➤*Tendon effects:* Ruptures of the shoulder, hand, and Achilles tendons that required surgical repair or resulted in prolonged disability have been reported with fluoroquinolone antimicrobials. The risk is further increased in patients older than 60 years of age, those using corticosteroids, and in patients with kidney, heart, or lung transplants. Tendon rupture can occur during or after completion of therapy; cases occurring up to several months after completion of therapy have been reported. Discontinue therapy if the patient experiences pain, inflammation, or rupture of a tendon. Patients should rest and refrain from exercise until the diagnosis of tendinitis or tendon rupture has been confidently excluded. Tendon rupture can occur at any time during or after therapy.

➤*Peripheral neuropathy:* Rare cases of sensory or sensorimotor axonal polyneuropathy affecting small and/or large axons resulting in dysesthesias, hypesthesias, paresthesia, and weakness have been reported in patients receiving quinolones.

➤*Syphilis:* **Ofloxacin**, **ciprofloxacin**, **norfloxacin** and **gatifloxacin** are not effective for syphilis. High doses of antimicrobial agents for short periods of time to treat gonorrhea may mask or delay symptoms of incubating syphilis. All patients should have a serologic test for syphilis at the time of gonorrhea diagnosis. Patients treated with ofloxacin, ciprofloxacin, norfloxacin and gatifloxacin should have a follow-up serologic test after 3 months.

➤*Chronic bronchitis due to S. pneumoniae:* **Lomefloxacin** is not indicated for the empiric treatment of acute bacterial exacerbation of chronic bronchitis when it is probable that *S. pneumoniae* is a causative pathogen because it exhibits in vitro resistance to lomefloxacin. Use only if sputum gram stain demonstrates an adequate quality of specimen and there is a predominance of gram-negative and not gram-positive organisms.

➤*Pseudomonas aeruginosa:* In clinical trials of complicated UTIs due to *P. aeruginosa*, 12 of 16 patients had the microorganism eradicated from the urine after therapy with **lomefloxacin**. No patients had concomitant bacteremia. Serum levels of lomefloxacin do not reliably exceed the MIC of *Pseudomonas* isolates. The safety and efficacy of lomefloxacin in treating patients with *Pseudomonas* bacteremia have not been established.

➤*Clostridium difficile–associated diarrhea: Clostridium difficile*–associated diarrhea (CDAD) has been reported with nearly all antibacterial agents, including fluoroquinolones, and may range from mild diarrhea to fatal colitis. Therefore, it is important to consider this diagnosis in patients who present with diarrhea subsequent to the administration of antibacterial agents. Careful medical history is necessary because CDAD has been reported to occur more than 2 months after the administration of antibacterial agents.

➤*Crystalluria:* Needle-shaped crystals were found in the urine of some volunteers who received either placebo or 800 or 1,600 mg **norfloxacin**. While crystalluria is not expected to occur under usual conditions with 400 mg twice daily, do not exceed the daily recommended dosage. Crystalluria related to **ciprofloxacin** has occurred only rarely in humans because human urine is usually acidic. Advise the patient to drink sufficient fluids to ensure proper hydration and adequate urinary output. Avoid alkalinity of the urine and do not exceed the recommended daily dose.

➤*Resistance:* Prescribing antibacterial agents in the absence of a proven or strongly suspected bacterial infection or a prophylactic indication is unlikely to provide benefit and increases the risk of the development of drug-resistant bacteria.

➤*Hemolytic reactions:* Rarely, hemolytic reactions have been reported in patients with latent or actual defects in glucose-6-phosphate dehydrogenase activity who take quinolone antibacterial agents, including **norfloxacin**.

➤*Myasthenia gravis:* Fluoroquinolones have neuromuscular blocking activity and may exacerbate muscle weakness in persons with myasthenia gravis. Postmarketing serious adverse events, including deaths and requirement for ventilatory support, have been associated with fluoroquinolone use in persons with myasthenia gravis. Avoid fluoroquinolones in patients with known history of myasthenia gravis.

➤*Blood glucose abnormalities:* As with other quinolones, disturbances of blood glucose, including symptomatic hyper- and hypoglycemia, have been reported, usually in diabetic patients receiving concomitant treatment with an oral hypoglycemic agent (eg, glyburide) or with insulin. In these patients, careful monitoring of blood glucose is recommended. If a hypoglycemic reaction occurs, initiate appropriate therapy immediately.

➤*Hypersensitivity reactions:* Serious and occasionally fatal reactions have occurred in patients receiving quinolone therapy, some following the first dose. Some reactions were accompanied by cardiovascular collapse, loss of consciousness, tingling, pharyngeal or facial edema, dyspnea, urticaria, and itching. If an allergic reaction occurs, discontinue the drug. Refer to Management of Acute Hypersensitivity Reactions.

➤*Renal function impairment:* The pharmacokinetic parameters of **moxifloxacin** are not significantly altered by mild, moderate, or severe renal impairment. No dosage adjustment is necessary in patients with renal impairment.

Total **gatifloxacin** clearance was reduced 57% in moderate renal insufficiency and 77% with severe renal insufficiency following administration of a single oral 400 mg dose. Systemic exposure was ≈ 2 times higher in moderate renal insufficiency and 4 times higher in severe renal insufficiency. Reduce the dose of gatifloxacin in patients with a Ccr < 40 mL/min, including patients requiring hemodialysis or continuous ambulatory peritoneal dialysis (CAPD).

In patients with renal impairment, the terminal elimination half-life is lengthened. Single or multiple doses of **sparfloxacin** in patients with varying degrees of renal impairment typically produce plasma concentrations that are twice those observed in patients with normal renal function. Adjust the dosage accordingly.

Clearance of **levofloxacin** is substantially reduced and plasma elimination half-life is prolonged in patients with impaired renal function, requiring dosage adjustments in such patients to avoid accumulation. Neither hemodialysis nor CAPD is effective in removal of levofloxacin from the body, indicating that supplemental doses of levofloxacin are not required following hemodialysis or CAPD.

➤*Hepatic function impairment:* **Moxifloxacin** should be used with caution in mild, moderate, or severe hepatic insufficiency (Child-Pugh class A, B, or C) because the metabolic disturbances associated with hepatic insufficiency may lead to QT prolongation.

➤*Superinfection:* Use of antibiotics (especially prolonged or repeated therapy) may result in bacterial or fungal overgrowth of nonsusceptible organisms. Such overgrowth may lead to a secondary infection. Take appropriate measures if superinfection occurs.

➤*Pregnancy: Category C.* There are no adequate and well-controlled studies in pregnant women. Use during pregnancy only if the potential benefit justifies the potential risk to the fetus.

Norfloxacin – Produces embryonic loss in monkeys when given in doses 10 times the maximum human dose.

Ciprofloxacin, moxifloxacin, sparfloxacin, gatifloxacin, levofloxacin, and norfloxacin – Caused lameness in immature dogs due to permanent cartilage lesions, and caused arthropathy in immature animals.

Ofloxacin – Doses equivalent to 10 to 50 times the recommended maximum dose were fetotoxic (ie, decreased fetal body weight, increased fetal mortality) in rats and rabbits, and minor skeletal variations occurred in rats; it also caused arthropathy in immature animals.

Lomefloxacin – Increased incidence of fetal loss in monkeys at ≈ 3 to 6 times the recommended human dose. In rabbits, maternal toxicity and associated fetotoxicity, decreased placental weight and variations of the coccygeal vertebrae occurred at doses 2 times the recommended human dose.

➤*Lactation:* **Norfloxacin** was not detected in breast milk following the administration of 200 mg to nursing mothers; however, this was a low dose. **Ciprofloxacin** is excreted in breast milk. **Ofloxacin**, as a single 200 mg dose, resulted in breast milk concentrations in nursing females that were similar to those found in plasma. **Levofloxacin** has not been measured in breast milk. Based upon data from ofloxacin, it can be presumed that levofloxacin will be excreted in breast milk. **Sparfloxacin** is excreted in breast milk. **Gatifloxacin** and **moxifloxacin** are excreted in the breast milk of rats; moxifloxacin may also be excreted in human milk. It is not known whether **lomefloxacin** or **gatifloxacin** are excreted in breast milk. Because of the potential for serious adverse reactions in nursing infants, decide whether to discontinue nursing or to discontinue the drug, taking into account the importance of the drug to the mother.

➤*Children:* Safety and efficacy of **gatifloxacin**, **levofloxacin**, **moxifloxacin**, **norfloxacin**, **lomefloxacin**, **sparfloxacin**, and **ofloxacin** in children younger than 18 years of age have not been established. **Ciprofloxacin**, **sparfloxacin**, **gatifloxacin**, **levofloxacin**, **moxifloxacin**, **lomefloxacin**, and **ofloxacin** cause arthropathy and osteochondrosis in immature animals. Administration of **norfloxacin**, **moxifloxacin**, and **ciprofloxacin** caused lameness in immature dogs due to permanent cartilage lesions.

➤*Elderly:* Elderly patients may be more susceptible to drug-associated effects of QT interval and 7 tendon disorders. Use with caution, especially in those on corticosteroids. **Norfloxacin** is eliminated more slowly because of decreased renal function; absorption appears unaffected. The apparent half-life of **ofloxacin** is 6.4 to 7.4 hours, compared with 4 to 5 hours in younger adults; absorption is unaffected. **Lomefloxacin** plasma clearance was reduced by ≈ 25% and the AUC was increased by ≈ 33% in the elderly, which may be due to decreased renal function in this population.

➤*Monitoring:* Periodic assessment of organ system functions, including renal, hepatic, and hematopoietic, is advisable during prolonged therapy.

Drug Interactions

➤*QT prolongation:* An additive effect of moxifloxacin, gatifloxacin, and sparfloxacin with other drugs that prolong the QT interval cannot be excluded. The following drugs may prolong the QT interval and increase the risk of life-threatening cardiac arrhythmias, including torsades de pointes: antiarrhythmic agents (eg, amiodarone, bretylium, disopyramide, dofetilide, procainamide, quinidine, sotalol), arsenic trioxide, bepridil, chloroquine, chlorpromazine, cisapride, dolasetron, droperidol, fluconazole, H_1 antagonists (eg, fexofenadine), halofantrine, haloperidol, histone deacetylase inhibitors (eg, romidepsin), lithium, maprotiline, mefluoquine, mesoridazine, methasone, nilotinib, pentamidine, perflutren, pimozide, tacrolimus, tetrabenazine, thioridazine, tyrosine-kinase receptor inhibitors (eg, dasatinib), and ziprasidone. For a more complete list of drugs that may prolong the QT interval, see the appendix Drug-Induced Prolongation of the QT Interval and Torsades de Pointes.

➤*Vaccines:* Moxifloxacin may decrease the effectiveness of live vaccines. Concurrent use is not recommended.

Fluoroquinolone Drug Interactions

Precipitant drug	Object drug[a]		Description
Antacids (aluminum or magnesium-containing)	Fluoroquinolones	↓	Decreased GI absorption of quinolones resulting in decreased serum levels. Avoid simultaneous use. Give quinolone at least 4 hours before or 8 hours after antacids.
Azlocillin	Ciprofloxacin	↑	The clearance of ciprofloxacin is decreased by azlocillin resulting in a higher and prolonged ciprofloxacin serum concentration.
Calcium	Moxifloxacin	↓	The moxifloxacin C_{max} was slightly reduced, and the time to maximum plasma concentration was prolonged when moxifloxacin was given with calcium. These differences are not considered to be clinically significant.
Cimetidine	Fluoroquinolones	↑	Cimetidine may interfere with the elimination of the fluoroquinolones.
Corticosteroids (eg, prednisone)	Fluoroquinolones	↑	Because of additive or synergestic effects, the risk of tendon rupture may be increased.
Fluoroquinolones	Corticosteroids (eg, prednisone)		
Didanosine (chewable/buffered tablets or pediatric powder for oral solution)	Fluoroquinolones	↓	The magnesium and aluminum cations in the buffers present in didanosine tablets decrease the GI absorption of quinolones via chelation. Avoid simultaneous use. Give quinolone at least 4 hours before or 8 hours after these products.
Iron salts, zinc salts	Fluoroquinolones	↓	GI absorption of certain quinolones may be decreased by formation of an iron-quinolone complex. Avoid coadministration of these drugs. Give quinolone at least 4 hours before or 8 hours after these products.
Nitrofurantoin	Norfloxacin	↓	Antibacterial effect of norfloxacin in the urinary tract may be antagonized.
NSAIDs (eg, indomethacin)	Fluoroquinolones	↑	The concurrent administration of NSAIDs with a quinolone may increase the risk of CNS stimulation and convulsive seizures. Seizures have been reported in patients taking NSAIDs.
Rifamycin (eg, rifampin)	Moxifloxacin	↓	Moxifloxacin plasma concentrations may be reduced, decreasing the efficacy.
Sucralfate	Fluoroquinolones	↓	Decreased GI absorption of quinolones. Avoid simultaneous use; administer at least 4 hours before or 8 hours after sucralfate.
Tramadol	Moxifloxacin	↑	The risk of seizures may be increased.
Tretinoin	Moxifloxacin	↑	Concurrent use may increase the risk of photosensitization. Avoid concurrent use.
Moxifloxacin	Tretinoin		
Sparfloxacin Gatifloxacin Moxifloxacin	Antiarrhythmic agents (amiodarone, bretylium, disopyramide, procainamide, quinidine, sotalol)	↑	The risk of life-threatening cardiac arrhythmias including torsades de pointes may be increased. The mechanism is unknown. Avoid coadministration. Sparfloxacin is contraindicated in patients receiving class IA and III antiarrhythmic agents.
Fluoroquinolones	Anticoagulants (eg, warfarin)	↑	Quinolones decrease the clearance of the R-warfarin, the less active isomer of racemic warfarin. Enoxacin does not affect the clearance of the active S-isomer, and changes in clotting time have not been observed when coadministered. Nevertheless, monitor the prothrombin time when given concomitantly.
Moxifloxacin	Antidiabetic agents (eg, glyburide)	↓	Mean AUC and C_{max} were 12% and 21% lower, respectively, during coadministration. Nonetheless, blood glucose levels were decreased slightly, suggesting no interference by moxifloxacin on the activity of glyburide.
Moxifloxacin Sparfloxacin	Antipsychotics (eg, iloperidone, paliperidone, phenothiazines, ziprasidone)	↑	The risk of life-threatening cardiac arrhythmias including torsades de pointes may be increased. Concurrent use with sparfloxacin is contraindicated. Concurrent use with moxifloxacin and ziprasidone is not recommended. Use with phenothiazines with caution.
Moxifloxacin	Atenolol	↓	The mean C_{max} of a single dose of atenolol decreased by approximately 10% following coadministration of a single dose of moxifloxacin.
Sparfloxacin	Astemizole Terfenadine[b]	↑	The risk of life-threatening cardiac arrythmias, including torsades de pointes may be increased. Sparfloxacin is contraindicated in patients receiving astemizole.
Moxifloxacin Sparfloxacin	Bepridil	↑	The risk of life-threatening cardiac arrhythmias, including torsades de pointes may be increased. Sparfloxacin is contraindicated in drugs that prolong the QTc interval.
Moxifloxacin Sparfloxacin	Macrolide-related antibiotics (eg, erythromycin)	↑	The risk of life-threatening cardiac arrythmias, including torsades de pointes may be increased. Concurrent use with sparfloxacin is contraindicated.
Ciprofloxacin Norfloxacin	Caffeine	↑	The hepatic metabolism of caffeine is decreased by certain quinolones; therefore, the pharmacologic effects of caffeine may be increased.
Gatifloxacin Moxifloxacin Sparfloxacin	Cisapride	↑	The risk of cardiovascular adverse effects may be increased. Concurrent use is contraindicated.
Ciprofloxacin Norfloxacin	Cyclosporine	↑	Increased cyclosporine toxicity. The mechanism is unknown.
Moxifloxacin	Digoxin	↑	The mean digoxin C_{max} increased by approximately 50% during the distribution phase of digoxin. This transient increase is not viewed to be clinically significant.
Ofloxacin	Procainamide	↑	Plasma procainamide concentrations may be increased. Monitor plasma procainamide concentrations and adjust dose accordingly.
Ciprofloxacin Norfloxacin Ofloxacin	Theophyllines	↑	Administration of theophylline with ciprofloxacin has decreased theophylline clearance and increased plasma levels and symptoms of toxicity, including seizures.

Fluoroquinolone Drug Interactions			
Precipitant drug	Object drug[a]		Description
Moxifloxacin Sparfloxacin	TCAs[c] (eg, amitriptyline)	↑	The risk of life-threatening cardiac arrythmias, including torsades de pointes, may be increased. Concurrent use with sparfloxacin is contraindicated.

[a] ↑ = object drug increased; ↓ = object drug decreased.
[b] Withdrawn from market.
[c] TCAs = tricyclic antidepressants.

➤*Drug/Lab test interactions:* **Sparfloxacin** therapy may produce false-negative culture results for *Mycobacterium tuberculosis* by suppression of mycobacterial growth.

➤*Drug/Food interactions:* Food may decrease the absorption of **norfloxacin**. Food delays the absorption of **ciprofloxacin**, resulting in peak concentrations that are closer to 2 hours after dosing rather than 1 hour; however, overall absorption is not substantially affected. Dairy products such as milk and yogurt reduce the absorption of ciprofloxacin; avoid concurrent use. The bioavailability of ciprofloxacin may also be decreased by enteral feedings. Food delays the rate of absorption of **lomefloxacin** (time-to-reach maximum plasma concentration delayed by 41%, maximum concentration decreased by 18%) and decreases the extent of absorption (AUC) by 12%.

Adverse Reactions

Fluoroquinolone Adverse Reactions (%)

	Adverse reaction	Ciprofloxacin[a]	Gatifloxacin	Levofloxacin	Lomefloxacin	Moxifloxacin	Norfloxacin[b]	Ofloxacin[a]	Sparfloxacin
CNS	Headache	1.2	3	0.1-6.4	3.6	< 2	2-2.8	1-9	4.2-8.1
	Dizziness	< 1	3	0.3-2.7	2.1	2	1.7-2.6	1-5	2-3.8
	Fatigue/Lethargy/Malaise	< 1		< 1-1.2	< 1		0.3-1	1-3	< 1
	Somnolence/Drowsiness	< 1	< 0.1	< 1	< 1	< 2	0.3-1	1-3	< 1-1.5
	Depression	< 1	< 0.1	< 1	< 1	< 0.1	0.1-0.2	< 1	< 1
	Insomnia	< 1	≥ 0.1-< 3	0.5-4.6	< 1	< 2	0.3-1	3-7	1.9
	Seizures/Convulsions[c]	< 1	< 0.1	< 1	< 1	< 0.1	✓[d]	< 1	
	Confusion	≤ 1	< 0.1	< 1	< 1	< 0.1	✓[d]	< 1	< 1
	Psychotic reactions	< 1				PM[e]	✓[d]		
	Paresthesia	< 1	≥ 0.1-< 3	< 1	< 1	< 0.1	✓[d]	< 1	< 1
	Hallucinations	< 1	< 0.1	< 1		< 0.1		< 1	< 1
Dermatologic	Photosensitivity[c]	< 1			2.3	< 0.1	✓[d]	✓[d]	
	Rash	1.1	≥ 0.1-< 3	0.3-1.2	< 1	< 2	0.3-1	1-3	1.1
	Pruritus	< 1	< 0.1	0.4-1.3	< 1	< 2	0.3-1	1-3	1.8-3.3
	Toxic epidermal necrolysis	< 1				PM	✓[d]		
	Stevens-Johnson syndrome	< 1				PM	✓[d]		
	Exfoliative dermatitis	< 1					✓[d]		
	Hypersensitivity[c]	< 1			< 1		✓[d]	✓[c]	
GI	Nausea	5.2	8	1.3-7.2	3.5	6	2.6-4.2	3-10	4.3-7.6
	Abdominal pain/discomfort/cramping	≤ 1-1.7	≥ 0.1-< 3	0.4-2.5	1.2	< 2	0.3-1.6	1-3	1.8-2.4
	Diarrhea	2.3	4	1-5.6	1.4	5	0.3-1	1-4	3.2-4.6
	Vomiting	≤ 1-2	≥ 0.1-< 3	0.2-2.3	< 1	< 2	0.3-1	1-4	< 1-1.3
	Dry/painful mouth	< 1	< 1	< 1	< 1	< 2	0.3-1	1-3	< 1-1.4
	Dyspepsia/Heartburn	< 1	≥ 0.1-< 3	0.3-2.4	< 1	< 2	0.3-1	< 1	1.6-2.3
	Constipation	< 1	≥ 0.1-< 3	0.1-3.2	< 1	< 2	0.3-1	1-3	< 1
	Flatulence	< 1	< 0.1	0.4-1.5	< 1	< 2	0.3-1	1-3	< 1-1.1
	Pseudomembranous colitis[c]	< 1	< 0.1	< 1	✓[d]	< 0.1	✓[d]	✓[c]	
Miscellaneous	Visual disturbances	< 1			< 1		0.1-0.2	1-3	
	Hearing loss	< 1					✓[d]	< 1	
	Vaginitis	< 1	6	0.7-1.8	< 1	< 2		1-5	< 1
	Hypertension	< 1	< 0.1	< 1	< 1	< 0.1		< 1	< 1
	Palpitations	< 1	≥ 0.1-< 3	< 1	< 1	< 2		< 1	< 1
	Syncope	< 1		< 1	< 1	< 0.1		< 1	
	Chills	< 1	≥ 0.1-< 3		< 1		0.1-0.2	< 1	
	Edema	< 1	< 0.1	< 1	< 1		0.1-0.2	< 1	
	Fever	< 1	≥ 0.1-< 3	< 1			0.3-1	1-3	< 1

	Fluoroquinolone Adverse Reactions (%)								
	Adverse reaction	Ciprofloxacin[a]	Gatifloxacin	Levofloxacin	Lomefloxacin	Moxifloxacin	Norfloxacin[b]	Ofloxacin[a]	Sparfloxacin
Abnormal laboratory values	↑ ALT/↑ AST	1.9/1.7	< 1		≤ 0.4		1.4/1.4-1.6	≥ 1	2-2.3
	↑ Alkaline phosphatase	0.8	< 1		0.1		1.1	≥ 1	< 1
	↑ LDH	0.4		< 1		< 2	✓[d]		
	↑ or ↓ Bilirubin	0.3	< 1		0.1				< 1
	Eosinophilia	0.6			0.1	< 2	0.6-1.5	≥ 1	
	Leukopenia	0.4		< 1	0.1	< 2	1.4	≥ 1	
	↑ or ↓ Platelets	0.1			< 1		1		< 1
	Pancytopenia	0.1							
	↑ ESR/Lymphocytopenia				< 0.1			≥ 1	
	Neutropenia		< 1				1.4	≥ 1	
	↑ Serum creatinine	1.1			0.1		✓[d]	≥ 1	
	↑ BUN	0.9			0.1		✓[d]	≥ 1	
	Crystalluria/Cylinduria/Candiduria	✓[d]					✓[d]		
	Hematuria	✓[d]						≥ 1	
	Glucosuria/Pyuria						✓[d]	≥ 1	
	Proteinuria/Albuminuria				< 0.1		1	≥ 1	
	↑ γ-glutamyltransferase	< 0.1			< 0.1				
	↑ Serum amylase	< 0.1	< 1			< 2			< 1
	↑ Uric acid	< 0.1							
	↑ or ↓ Blood glucose	< 0.1		2.2	< 0.1			≥ 1	< 1
	↓ Hemoglobin/Hematocrit	< 0.1			< 0.1		0.6		
	↑ or ↓ Potassium	✓[d]			0.1				< 1
	Anemia	< 0.1			< 0.1			≥ 1	
	Bleeding/↑ PT	< 0.1			< 0.1				
	↑ Monocytes	< 0.1			0.2				< 1
	Leukocytosis	< 0.1		< 1	0.1			≥ 1	
	↑ Triglycerides/Cholesterol	✓[d]							

[a] Includes data for oral and IV formulations.
[b] From single- and multiple-dose studies.
[c] See Warnings and Precautions.
[d] ✓ = Adverse reaction observed; incidence not reported.
[e] PM = postmarketing.

Other adverse reactions listed only for the individual agents:

➤*Ciprofloxacin:*

Cardiovascular – Cardiovascular collapse, arrhythmia, tachycardia, cardiac murmur, hypotension (≤ 1%); angina pectoris, atrial flutter, cardiopulmonary arrest, cerebral thrombosis, MI, ventricular ectopy (< 1%); postural hypotension.

CNS – Restlessness (1.1%); paranoia, toxic psychosis, dysphasia, phobia, depersonalization, unresponsiveness, lightheadedness, anxiety, weakness, manic reaction (≤ 1%); nightmares, irritability, tremor, ataxia, anorexia (< 1%).

Dermatologic – Anaphylactic reactions, erythema multiforme, vasculitis, angioedema, edema of the lips, face, neck, conjunctivae, hands or lower extremities, purpura, cutaneous candidiasis, vesicles, increased perspiration; urticaria, flushing, hyperpigmentation, erythema nodosum (< 1%).

GI – Ileus, jaundice, *C. difficile*-associated diarrhea, pancreatitis, hepatic necrosis, oral ulceration, anorexia (≤ 1%); painful oral mucosa (< 1%).

GU – Renal calculi, hemorrhagic cystitis, frequent urination, gynecomastia, candiduria, crystalluria, cylindruria, hematuria, albuminuria (≤ 1%); acidosis, interstitial nephritis, nephritis, renal failure, polyuria, urinary retention, urethral bleeding (< 1%); vaginal candidiasis.

Hypersensitivity – Hyperpigmentation (< 1%)

Musculoskeletal – Arthralgia, jaw, arm, or back pain, joint stiffness, neck and chest pain, achiness, flare-up of gout (≤ 1%).

Respiratory – Respiratory arrest, respiratory distress, pleural effusion (≤ 1%); bronchospasm, dyspnea, epistaxis, hemoptysis, hiccoughs, laryngeal/pulmonary edema, pulmonary embolism (< 1%).

Special senses – Nystagmus, decreased visual acuity, blurred vision, anosmia (≤ 1%); bad taste in mouth, eye pain, tinnitus, diplopia (< 1%).

Miscellaneous – Thrombophlebitis, injection site burning, pain, pruritus, paresthesia, erythema, swelling (≤ 1%); oral candidiasis, intestinal perforation, GI bleeding, (< 1%); exacerbation of myasthenia gravis; dysphasia; agranulocytosis; cholestatic jaundice.

➤*Gatifloxacin:*

CNS – Abnormal dream, tremor, vasodilatation, vertigo (≥ 0.1% to < 3%); abnormal thinking, agitation, alcohol intolerance, anorexia, anxiety, ataxia, depersonalization, euphoria, hostility, migraine, nervousness, panic attack, paranoia, psychosis, stress (< 0.1%).

Cardiovascular – Bradycardia, breast pain, substernal chest pain, tachycardia (< 0.1%).

Dermatologic – Cheilitis, dry skin, ecchymosis, epistaxis, face edema, hyperesthesia, lymphadenopathy, maculopapular rash, vesiculobullous rash (< 0.1%).

Endocrine – Diabetes mellitus, hyperglycemia, hypoglycemia (< 0.1%).

GI – Glossitis, oral moniliasis, stomatitis, mouth ulcer (≥ 0.1% to < 3%); colitis, dysphagia, gastritis, GI hemorrhage, gingivitis, halitosis, hematemesis, mouth edema, rectal hemorrhage, thirst, tongue edema (< 0.1%).

GU – Dysuria, hematuria (≥ 0.1% to

Musculoskeletal – Arthralgia, arthritis, asthenia, bone pain, hypertonia, leg cramp, myalgia, myasthenia, neck pain (< 0.1%).

Respiratory – Dyspnea, pharyngitis (≥ 0.1% to

Special senses – Abnormal vision, taste perversion, tinnitus (≥ 0.1% to < 3%); ear pain, eye pain, parosmia, ptosis, taste loss (< 0.1%).

Miscellaneous – Local injection site reaction (redness at injection site) (5%); allergic reaction, back pain, chest pain, peripheral edema, sweating (≥ 0.1% to < 3%); electrolyte abnormalities (

➤*Levofloxacin:*

Cardiovascular – Cardiac failure, circulatory failure, hypotension, arrhythmia, atrial fibrillation, bradycardia, cardiac arrest, heart block, supraventricular tachycardia, tachycardia, ventricular fibrillation, angina pectoris, coronary thrombosis, MI, postural hypotension (< 1%).

CNS – Abnormal coordination, coma, hyperkinesia, hypertonia, hypoaesthesia, involuntary muscle contractions, paralysis, speech disorder, stupor, tremor, vertigo (< 1%).

Dermatologic – Erythema nodosum, genital pruritus, increased sweating, skin disorder, skin exfoliation, skin ulceration (< 1%); rash erythematous (0.1%); urticaria (< 1% to 0.1%).

GI – Dysphagia, gastroenteritis, GI hemorrhage, pancreatitis, tongue edema (< 1%).

GU – Abnormal renal function, acute renal failure, face edema, hematuria (< 1%).

Hematologic – Abnormal platelets, embolism (blood clot), epistaxis, purpura, thrombocytopenia, anemia (< 1%).

Hepatic – Abnormal hepatic function, cholelithiasis, hepatic coma, jaundice (< 1%).

Lab test abnormalities – Granulocytopenia, lymphadenopathy, WBC abnormal (not otherwise specified) (< 1%).

Metabolic/Nutritional – Aggravated diabetes mellitus, dehydration, hyperglycemia, hyperkalemia, hypoglycemia, hypokalemia, weight decrease (< 1%).

Musculoskeletal – Arthralgia, arthritis, arthrosis, muscle weakness, myalgia, osteomyelitis, rhabdomyolysis, synovitis, tendinitis (< 1%).

Psychiatric – Abnormal dreaming, aggressive reaction, agitation, anorexia, anxiety, delirium, emotional lability, impaired concentration, impotence, manic reaction, mental deficiency, paranoia, sleep disorder, withdrawal syndrome (< 1%); nervousness (0.1% to < 1%).

Respiratory – ARDS, asthma, coughing, dyspnea, hemoptysis, hypoxia, pleural effusion, respiratory insufficiency (< 1%).

Special senses – Taste perversion (0.2% to 1%); ear disorder (not otherwise specified), tinnitus, abnormal vision, conjunctivitis, diplopia (< 1%).

Miscellaneous – Injection site reaction (3.5%); decreased lymphocytes (2.2%); injection site pain (1.7%); pain (1.4%); sinusitis (1.3%); chest pain (1.2%); back pain, injection site inflammation (1.1%); rhinitis (0.2% to 1%); asthenia, rigors, substernal chest pain, carcinoma, parosmia, ejaculation failure, cerebrovascular disorder, phlebitis (

➤*Lomefloxacin:*

Cardiovascular – Hypotension, tachycardia, bradycardia, arrhythmia, extrasystoles, cyanosis, cardiac failure, angina pectoris, MI, pulmonary embolism, cerebrovascular disorder, cardiomyopathy, phlebitis (< 1%).

CNS – Coma, hyperkinesia, tremor, vertigo, nervousness, anorexia, anxiety, agitation, increased appetite, depersonalization, paranoid reaction, paroniria, twitching, hypertonia, confusion, abnormal thinking, concentration impairment (< 1%).

Dermatologic – Urticaria, eczema, skin exfoliation, skin disorder, bullous eruption, acne, skin discoloration, skin ulceration, angioedema (< 1%).

GI – GI inflammation/bleeding, dysphagia, tongue discoloration, stomatitis (< 1%).

GU – Dysuria, hematuria, strangury, micturition disorder, anuria, leukorrhea, intermenstrual bleeding, perineal pain, vaginal moniliasis, orchitis, epididymitis, menstrual disorder (< 1%).

Hematologic – Thrombocythemia, thrombocytopenia, anemia (< 1%).

Respiratory – Dyspnea, respiratory tract infection, epistaxis, respiratory disorder, bronchospasm, cough, increased sputum, stridor, rhinitis, pharyngitis, respiratory depression (

Special senses – Earache, tinnitus, conjunctivitis, eye pain, abnormal lacrimation, taste perversion (< 1%).

Miscellaneous – Flushing, increased sweating, back/chest pain, asthenia, facial edema, influenza-like symptoms, decreased heat tolerance, purpura, lymphadenopathy, increased fibrinolysis, thirst, gout, hypoglycemia, leg cramps, arthralgia, myalgia, hot flashes, abnormal liver function, hyperglycemia, viral infection, moniliasis, fungal infection, allergic reaction, anaphylactoid reaction (< 1%); abnormalities of urine specific gravity or serum electrolytes (≤ 0.1%); increased albumin, macrocytosis (< 0.1%).

➤*Moxifloxacin:*

Cardiovascular – Cardiac arrythmias (not otherwise specified), prolonged QT interval, tachycardia (> 0.1% to < 2%); abnormal ECG, atrial fibrillation, chest pain, hypotension, supraventricular tachycardia, ventricular tachycardia (< 0.1%); ventricular tachyarrhythmias including, in very rare cases, cardiac arrest and torsades de pointes, and usually in patients with concurrent severe underlying proarrhythmic conditions (postmarketing).

CNS – Anxiety, nervousness, tremor, vertigo (> 0.1% to < 2%); abnormal dreams, abnormal thinking, amnesia, aphasia, depersonalization, emotional lability, hypesthesia, incoordination, sleep disorders, speech disorders (< 0.1%); altered coordination, abnormal gait, exacerbation of myasthenia gravis (postmarketing).

Dermatologic – Sweating, urticaria (> 0.1% to

GI – Anorexia, oral moniliasis, stomatitis, glossitis, GGTP increased (> 0.1% to < 2%); dysphagia, gastritis, GI disorder (< 0.1%).

Hematologic/Lymphatic – Prothrombin decrease (PT prolonged/INR increased), thrombocythemia (> 0.1% to

Lab test abnormalities – Abnormal liver function test (> 0.1% to < 2%); increased MCH, neutrophils, WBCs, PT ratio, ionized calcium, chloride, albumin, globulin, bilirubin (≥ 2%); decreases in hemoglobin, RBCs, neutrophils, eosinophils, basophils, PT ratio, glucose, pO_2, bilirubin, amylase (≥ 2%).

Musculoskeletal – Arthralgia, myalgia (> 0.1% to < 2%); arthritis, back pain, leg pain, pelvic pain, tendon disorder (< 0.1%); tendon rupture (postmarketing).

Renal – Abnormal kidney function (< 0.1%); renal dysfunction, renal failure (postmarketing).

Respiratory – Asthma, dyspnea (< 0.1%).

Special senses – Taste perversion (> 0.1% to < 2%); abnormal vision, amblyopia, parosmia, taste loss, tinnitus (< 0.1%).

Miscellaneous – Asthenia, malaise, moniliasis, pain, allergic reaction, dehydration, vaginal moniliasis (> 0.1% to < 2%); abnormal lab tests (not specified), jaundice, face edema, hypertonia, peripheral edema, tongue discoloration (< 0.1%); anaphylactic reaction, anaphylactic shock, angioedema, hepatic failure, hepatitis (postmarketing).

➤*Norfloxacin (single- and multiple-dose studies):*

Cardiovascular – Chest pain, MI, palpitation (0.1% to 0.2%).

CNS – Myoclonus; tingling of the fingers (0.3% to 1%); anxiety, sleep disturbances (0.1% to 0.2%).

Dermatologic – Erythema multiforme; erythema, urticaria (0.1% to 0.2%).

GI – Hepatitis; pancreatitis; stomatitis; anorexia, anal/rectal pain, loose stools (0.3% to 1%); abdominal swelling, bitter taste, anorexia, mouth ulcer, renal colic (0.1% to 0.2%).

Musculoskeletal – Arthralgia; back pain (0.3% to 1%); bursitis (0.1% to 0.2%).

Miscellaneous – Hyperhidrosis (0.3% to 1%); asthenia (0.3% to 1.3%); allergies, dysmenorrhea, pruritus ani (0.1% to 0.2%).

➤*Ofloxacin:*

Cardiovascular – Chest pain (1% to 3%); vasodilation, cardiac arrest, hypotension (< 1%).

CNS – Sleep disorders, nervousness (1% to 3%); anxiety, cognitive change, dream abnormality, euphoria, vertigo, tremor (< 1%).

Dermatologic – Angioedema, urticaria, vasculitis (< 1%).

GU – Vaginal discharge (1% to 3%); external genital pruritus in women (1% to 6%); burning/irritation/pain/rash of female genitalia, dysmenorrhea, menorrhagia, metrorrhagia, urinary frequency/pain/retention, dysuria (< 1%).

Respiratory – Cough, rhinorrhea, respiratory arrest (< 1%).

Special senses – Dysgeusia (1% to 3%); photophobia, tinnitus, decreased hearing acuity (< 1%).

Miscellaneous – Decreased appetite, GI distress, pharyngitis, trunk pain (1% to 3%); hyperglycemia, hypoglycemia (≥ 1%); arthralgia, asthenia, diaphoresis, myalgia, thirst, vasculitis, weight loss, extremity pain, epistaxis, pain (< 1%).

➤*Sparfloxacin:*

Cardiovascular – QT_c interval prolongation (1.3%); chest pain, electrocardiogram abnormal , tachycardia, sinus bradycardia, PR interval shortened, angina pectoris, arrhythmia, atrial fibrillation, atrial flutter, complete AV block, first degree AV block, second degree AV block, cardiovascular disorder, hemorrhage, migraine, peripheral vascular disorder, supraventricular extrasystoles, ventricular extrasystoles, postural hypotension (< 1%).

CNS – Hypesthesia, nervousness, abnormal dreams, tremor, anxiety, hyperesthesia, hyperkinesia, sleep disorder, hypokinesia, vertigo, abnormal gait, agitation, lightheadedness, emotional lability, euphoria, abnormal thinking, amnesia, twitching (< 1%).

Dermatologic – Photosensitivity reaction (3.6% to 7.9%); rash, cellulitis, face edema, maculopapular rash, dry skin, herpes simplex, sweating, urticaria, vesiculobullous rash, exfoliative dermatitis, acne, alopecia, angioedema, contact dermatitis, fungal dermatitis, furunculosis, pustular rash, skin discoloration, herpes zoster, petechial rash (< 1%).

GI – Anorexia, gingivitis, oral moniliasis, stomatitis, tongue disorder, tooth disorder, gastroenteritis, increased appetite, mouth ulceration (< 1%).

GU – Dysuria, breast pain, dysmenorrhea, hematuria, menorrhagia, nocturia, polyuria, urinary tract infection, kidney pain, leukorrhea, metorrhagia, vulvovaginal disorder (< 1%).

Hematologic – Cyanosis, ecchymosis, lymphadenopathy (< 1%).

Lab test abnormalities – Elevated white blood cells (1.1%); increased/decreased white blood cells, increased aPTT, increased blood urea nitrogen, increased calcium, increased creatinine, increased eosinophils, increased serum lipase, increased neutrophils, increased urine glucose, increased urine protein, increased urine red blood cells, increased urine white blood cells, decreased albumin, decreased creatinine clearance, decreased hematocrit, decreased hemoglobin, decreased lymphocytes, decreased phosphorus, decreased red blood cells, decreased sodium (< 1%).

Metabolic/Nutritional – Gout, peripheral edema, thirst (< 1%).

Musculoskeletal – Arthralgia, arthritis, joint disorder, myalgia, neck pain, rheumatoid arthritis (< 1%).

Respiratory – Asthma, epistaxis, pneumonia, rhinitis, pharyngitis, bronchitis, hemoptysis, sinusitis, cough increased, dyspnea, laryngismus, lung disorder, pleural disorder (< 1%).

Special senses – Taste perversion (1.4%); ear pain, amblyopia, photophobia, tinnitus, conjunctivitis, diplopia, abnormality of accommodation, blepharitis, ear disorder, eye pain, lacrimation disorder, otitis media (< 1%).

Miscellaneous – Vaginal moniliasis (2.8%); asthenia (1.7%); vasodilatation (1%); generalized pain, allergic reaction, back pain, accidental injury, anaphylactoid reaction, infection, mucous membrane disorder (< 1%).

Overdosage

➤*Symptoms:* One patient developed oliguric acute renal failure following ingestion of 21 g of **ciprofloxacin** (serum concentration, 12 mcg/mL). The patient responded to prednisone therapy.

Information on overdosage with **ofloxacin** is limited. One incident of accidental overdosage has been reported. In this case, an adult female received 3 g of ofloxacin IV over 45 minutes. A blood sample obtained 15 minutes after the completion of the infusion revealed an ofloxacin level of 39.3 mcg/mL. In 7 hours, the level had fallen to 16.2 mcg/mL and by 24 hours to 2.7 mcg/mL. During the infusion, the patient developed drowsiness, nausea, dizziness, hot and cold flushes, subjective facial swelling and numbness, slurring of speech, and mild to moderate disorientation. All complaints, except the dizziness, subsided within 1 hour after discontinuation of the infusion. The dizziness, most bothersome while standing, resolved in ≈ 9 hours. Laboratory testing reportedly revealed no clinically significant changes in routine parameters in this patient.

Levofloxacin exhibits a low potential for acute toxicity. Mice, rats, dogs, and monkeys exhibited the following clinical signs after receiving a single high dose of levofloxacin: Ataxia, ptosis, decreased locomotor activity, dyspnea, prostration, tremors, and convulsions. Doses in excess of 1500 mg/kg orally and 250 mg/kg IV produced significant mortality in rodents. In the event of an acute overdosage, the stomach should be emptied. Observe the patient and maintain appropriate hydration. Levofloxacin is not efficiently removed by hemodialysis or peritoneal dialysis.

In case of overdosage, monitor the patient in a suitably equipped medical facility and advise to avoid sun exposure for 5 days. ECG monitoring is recommended because of the possible prolongation of the QT_c interval. There is no known antidote for **sparfloxacin** overdosage. It is not known whether sparfloxacin is dialyzable.

➤*Treatment:* Empty the stomach by inducing vomiting or by gastric lavage. Observe patient carefully and give symptomatic and supportive treatment. Maintain adequate hydration. Refer to General Management of Acute Overdosage.

Only a small amount of **ciprofloxacin** (< 10%) is removed from the body after hemodialysis or peritoneal dialysis. In the event of acute **moxifloxacin** overdosage, the stomach should be emptied and ECG monitoring is recommended because of the possible prolongation of the QT interval. Carefully observe the patient and give supportive treatment. Adequate hydration must be maintained. It is not known whether moxifloxacin is dialyzable. **Ofloxacin**, **norfloxacin**, **gatifloxacin**, **levofloxacin**, and **lomefloxacin** are not efficiently removed by dialysis.

Patient Information

Advise patients to drink fluids liberally.

Advise patients to not take antacids containing magnesium, calcium, or aluminum or products containing citric acid buffered with sodium citrate, iron, magnesium, zinc, or didanosine chewable/buffered tablets or buffered solution, or the pediatric powder for oral solution simultaneously or within 6 hours before or 2 hours (8 hours with **moxifloxacin**) after dosing.

Advise patients to take **norfloxacin** 1 hour before or 2 hours after meals. **Ciprofloxacin**, **ofloxacin**, **levofloxacin**, **moxifloxacin**, **gatifloxacin**, and **lomefloxacin** can be taken without regard to meals.

Inform patients that **sparfloxacin** can be taken with food, milk, or caffeine-containing products.

Inform patients that **ciprofloxacin** may increase the effects of theophylline and caffeine. There is a possibility of caffeine accumulation when products containing caffeine are consumed while taking quinolones.

Inform patients that these drugs may cause dizziness or lightheadedness; observe caution while driving or performing other tasks requiring alertness, coordination, or physical dexterity. CNS stimulation may occur (eg, tremor, restlessness, confusion); use with caution in patients predisposed to seizures or with other CNS disorders.

Inform patients that hypersensitivity reactions may occur, even following the first dose; discontinue the drug at the first sign of skin rash or other allergic reaction.

Advise patients to avoid excessive sunlight/artificial ultraviolet light; discontinue drug if phototoxicity occurs. Avoid re-exposure to sunlight and ultraviolet light. Reactions may recur up to several weeks after stopping therapy. See Warnings.

Advise patients to discontinue treatment and inform their health care provider if experiencing pain, inflammation, or rupture of a tendon, and to rest and refrain from exercise until the diagnosis of tendinitis or tendon rupture has been confidently excluded.

Advise patients to discontinue **levofloxacin**, **ofloxacin**, or **gatifloxacin** and consult a health care provider if patient is diabetic and being treated with insulin or an oral hypoglycemic agent and a hypoglycemic reaction occurs.

Advise patients that diarrhea is a common problem caused by antibiotics that usually ends when the antibiotic is discontinued. Sometimes after starting treatment with antibiotics, patients can develop watery and bloody stools (with or without stomach cramps and fever), even as late as 2 or more months after having taken the last dose of the antibiotic. If this occurs, advise patients to contact their health care provider as soon as possible.

Advise patients to notify their health care provider if they are taking warfarin; concurrent administration of warfarin and **levofloxacin** has been associated with increases of the International Normalized Ratio (INR) or prothrombin time and clinical episodes of bleeding.

Inform patients that convulsions have been reported in patients taking quinolones. Notify a health care provider before taking quinolones if there is a history of this condition.

Advise patients to inform their health care provider if development of symptoms suggestive of pancreatitis including abdominal pain or nausea and vomiting occurs.

Inform patients that **gatifloxacin** and **moxifloxacin** may produce changes in the electrocardiogram (QT_c interval prolongation).

Avoid **gatifloxacin** and **moxifloxacin** in patients receiving Class IA (eg, quinidine, procainimide) or Class III (eg, amiodarone, sotalol) antiarrhythmic agents.

Advise patients to use **gatifloxacin** and **moxifloxacin** with caution if they are receiving drugs that may affect the QT_c interval such as cisapride, erythromycin, antipsychotics, and tricyclic antidepressants.

Advise patients to inform their health care provider of any personal or family history of QT_c prolongation or proarrhythmic condition such as recent hypokalemia, significant bradycardia, or recent myocardial ischemia.

Advise patients to inform health care providers of any other medications when taken concurrently with fluoroquinolones, including OTC medications.

Advise patients to contact their health care providers if palpitations or fainting spells occur while taking **gatifloxacin** or **moxifloxacin**.

CIPROFLOXACIN

Rx	**Ciprofloxacin** (Dr. Reddy's)	**Tablets; oral:** 100 mg	As ciprofloxacin hydrochloride. In 6s.
Rx	**Ciprofloxacin** (Various, eg, Dr. Reddy's, Ivax)	**Tablets; oral:** 250 mg	As ciprofloxacin hydrochloride. In 50s, 100s, 500s, and UD 100s.
Rx	**Cipro** (Schering-Plough)		As ciprofloxacin hydrochloride. Polyethylene glycol. (BAYER/CIP 250). White to yellowish. Film-coated. In 50s, 100s, and UD 100s.
Rx	**Ciprofloxacin** (Various, eg, Dr. Reddy's, Ivax)	**Tablets; oral:** 500 mg	As ciprofloxacin hydrochloride. In 50s, 100s, 500s, and UD 100s.
Rx	**Cipro** (Schering-Plough)		As ciprofloxacin hydrochloride. Polyethylene glycol. (BAYER/CIP 500). White to yellowish, capsule shape. Film-coated. In 50s, 100s, and UD 100s.
Rx	**Ciprofloxacin** (Various, eg, Apotex, Dr. Reddy's, Ivax)	**Tablets; oral:** 750 mg	As ciprofloxacin hydrochloride. In 50s, 100s, 500s, and UD 100s.
Rx	**Cipro** (Schering-Plough)		As ciprofloxacin hydrochloride. Polyethylene glycol. (BAYER/CIP 750). White to yellowish, capsule shape. Film-coated. In 50s, 100s, and UD 100s.
Rx	**Ciprofloxacin** (Various, eg, Dr. Reddy's, Mylan)	**Tablets, extended-release; oral:** 500 mg	As a bilayer tablet containing both ciprofloxacin base and ciprofloxacin hydrochloride. In 30s, 50s, 100s, 500s, and UD 100s.
Rx	**Cipro XR** (Schering-Plough)		As a bilayer tablet containing both ciprofloxacin base and ciprofloxacin hydrochloride. Polyethylene glycol. (BAYER C500 QD). White to yellowish, oblong. Film-coated. In 50s.
Rx	**Proquin XR** (Depomed)		As ciprofloxacin hydrochloride. (500 DMI). Blue, oval. Film-coated. In 30s and UD 3s.
Rx	**Ciprofloxacin** (Various, eg, Dr. Reddy's, Mylan)	**Tablets, extended-release; oral:** 1,000 mg	As a bilayer tablet containing both ciprofloxacin base and ciprofloxacin hydrochloride. In 30s, 50s, 100s, 250s, 500s, and UD 100s.
Rx	**Cipro XR** (Schering-Plough)		As a bilayer tablet containing both ciprofloxacin base and ciprofloxacin hydrochloride. Polyethylene glycol. (BAYER C1000 QD). White to yellowish, oblong. Film-coated. In 50s and UD 30s.
Rx	**Cipro** (Schering-Plough)	**Microcapsules for suspension; oral:** 250 mg per 5 mL (5%) (when reconstituted)	Sucrose. Strawberry flavor. In 100 mL with diluent.
Rx	**Cipro** (Schering-Plough)	**Microcapsules for suspension; oral:** 500 mg per 5 mL (10%) (when reconstituted)	Sucrose. Strawberry flavor. In 100 mL with diluent.
Rx	**Ciprofloxacin** (Various, eg, Bedford, Hospira, Sicor)	**Injection, solution, concentrate:** 10 mg/mL (1%)	May contain lactic acid. In 20 and 40 mL vials.
Rx	**Cipro I.V.** (Schering-Plough)		Latex free. Lactic acid. In 20 and 40 mL vials.

CIPROFLOXACIN

Rx	**Ciprofloxacin** (Various, eg, Hospira, Teva)	**Injection, solution**: 2 mg/mL (0.2%)	May contain lactic acid. In 100 and 200 mL premix flexible containers with dextrose 5%.
Rx	**Cipro I.V.** (Schering-Plough)		Latex free. Lactic acid. In 100 and 200 mL premix flexible containers with dextrose 5%.

CIPROFLOXACIN HYDROCHLORIDE — ORAL

For complete and comparative prescribing information, refer to the Fluoroquinolones class monograph.

WARNING

Tendonitis and tendon rupture – Fluoroquinolones, including ciprofloxacin, are associated with an increased risk of tendinitis and tendon rupture in all ages. This risk is further increased in older patients (usually older than 60 years of age), in patients taking corticosteroid drugs, and in patients with kidney, heart, or lung transplants.

Myasthenia gravis – Fluoroquinolones, including ciprofloxacin, may exacerbate muscle weakness in persons with myasthenia gravis. Avoid ciprofloxacin in patients with known history of myasthenia gravis.

Indications

➤*Immediate-release tablets and oral suspension:*

Adults –

Acute sinusitis: Caused by *Haemophilus influenzae*, *Streptococcus pneumoniae* (penicillin-susceptible), or *Moraxella catarrhalis*.

Acute uncomplicated cystitis (in women): Caused by *Escherichia coli* or *Staphylococcus saprophyticus*.

Bone and joint infections: Caused by *Enterobacter cloacae*, *Serratia marcescens*, or *Pseudomonas aeruginosa*.

Chronic bacterial prostatitis: Caused by *E. coli* or *Proteus mirabilis*.

Complicated intra-abdominal infections: Used in combination with metronidazole, caused by *E. coli*, *P. aeruginosa*, *P. mirabilis*, *Klebsiella pneumoniae*, or *Bacteroides fragilis*.

Infectious diarrhea: Caused by *E. coli* (enterotoxigenic strains), *Campylobacter jejuni*, *Shigella boydii* (although treatment of infections caused by this organism in this organ system demonstrated a clinically significant outcome, efficacy was studied in fewer than 10 patients), *Shigella dysenteriae*, *Shigella flexneri*, or *Shigella sonnei* (although treatment of infections caused by this organism in this organ system demonstrated a clinically significant outcome, efficacy was studied in fewer than 10 patients) when antibacterial therapy is indicated.

Lower respiratory tract infections: Caused by *E. coli*, *K. pneumoniae*, *E. cloacae*, *P. mirabilis*, *P. aeruginosa*, *H. influenzae*, *Haemophilus parainfluenzae*, or *S. pneumoniae* (penicillin-susceptible). Also, *M. catarrhalis* for the treatment of acute exacerbations of chronic bronchitis.

Although effective in clinical trials, ciprofloxacin is not a drug of first choice in the treatment of presumed or confirmed pneumonia secondary to *S. pneumoniae*.

Skin and skin structure infections: Caused by *E. coli*, *K. pneumoniae*, *E. cloacae*, *P. mirabilis*, *Proteus vulgaris*, *Providencia stuartii*, *Morganella morganii*, *Citrobacter freundii*, *P. aeruginosa*, *Staphylococcus aureus* (methicillin-susceptible), *Staphylococcus epidermidis* (methicillin-susceptible), or *Streptococcus pyogenes*.

Typhoid fever (enteric fever): Caused by *Salmonella typhi*. The efficacy of ciprofloxacin in the eradication of the chronic typhoid carrier state has not been demonstrated.

Uncomplicated cervical and urethral gonorrhea: Caused by *Neisseria gonorrhoeae*.

Urinary tract infections: Caused by *E. coli*, *K. pneumoniae*, *E. cloacae*, *S. marcescens*, *P. mirabilis*, *Providencia rettgeri*, *M. morganii*, *Citrobacter diversus*, *C. freundii*, *P. aeruginosa*, *S. epidermidis* (methicillin-susceptible), *S. saprophyticus*, or *Enterococcus faecalis*.

Children (1 to 17 years of age) –

Complicated urinary tract infections and pyelonephritis: Caused by *E. coli*.

Adults and children –

Inhalational anthrax (postexposure): To reduce the incidence or progression of disease following exposure to aerosolized *Bacillus anthracis*.

➤*Extended-release tablets:* Ciprofloxacin extended-release (ER) and immediate-release tablets are not interchangeable.

Cipro XR –

Acute uncomplicated pyelonephritis: Caused by *E. coli*.

Complicated urinary tract infections: Caused by *E. coli*, *K. pneumoniae*, *E. faecalis*, *P. mirabilis*, or *P. aeruginosa* (treatment of infections caused by this organism in the organ system was studied in fewer than 10 patients).

Uncomplicated urinary tract infections (acute cystitis): Caused by *E. coli*, *P. mirabilis*, *E. faecalis*, or *S. saprophyticus* (treatment of infections caused by this organism in this organ system was studied in fewer than 10 patients).

Proquin XR – *Proquin XR* is not interchangeable with other ciprofloxacin ER or immediate-release oral formulations.

Uncomplicated urinary tract infections (acute cystitis): Caused by susceptible strains of *E. coli* and *K. pneumoniae*.

➤*Off-label uses:*

Anthrax prophylaxis (adults) – [1] = Good documentation. Ciprofloxacin is recommended by the Centers for Disease Control and Prevention (CDC) as 1 of 2 possible first-line agents for bioterrorism postexposure prophylaxis of anthrax in adults. It should be used as part of a multidrug regimen with 1 or 2 other antimicrobials that show in vitro activity to *Bacillus anthracis* (rifampin, vancomycin, penicillin, ampicillin, chloramphenicol, imipenem, clindamycin, or clarithromycin) plus a corticosteroid and a 3-dose series of anthrax vaccine, adsorbed (AVA). Because of the limited data and no known controlled trials, current recommendations are based on in vitro and primate studies.

Chancroid – [1] = Good documentation. Based on CDC guidelines, ciprofloxacin is a recommended therapy for the treatment of chancroid. However, intermediate resistance to ciprofloxacin has been reported in several isolates. Potential resistance issues should be considered when initiating therapy for the treatment of chancroid.

Granuloma inguinale (donovanosis) – [1] = Good documentation. CDC guidelines recommend ciprofloxacin as an alternative regimen for treatment of granuloma inguinale when doxycycline is not appropriate. The use of ciprofloxacin in pregnant women is contraindicated.

Infective endocarditis (adults) – [1] = Good documentation. According to American Heart Association (AHA) guidelines, ciprofloxacin may be considered for treatment of *Haemophilus parainfluenzae*, *Haemophilus aphrophilus*, *Haemophilus paraphrophilus*, *Haemophilus influenzae*, *Actinobacillus actinomycetemcomitans*, *Cardiobacterium hominis*, *Eikenella corrodens*, *Kingella kingae*, and *Kingella denitrificans* (HACEK) and culture-negative endocarditis, including *Bartonella* infection in patients with a native valve.

Infective endocarditis (children/adolescents) – [1] = Good documentation. Fluoroquinolones are not generally recommended for patients younger than 18 years of age. According to AHA guidelines, fluoroquinolone therapy is recommended only for patients unable to tolerate cephalosporin and ampicillin therapy. Ciprofloxacin may be considered for treatment of HACEK and culture-negative endocarditis, including *Bartonella* infection in patients with a native valve.

Plague – Plague is sufficiently uncommon to preclude large, controlled studies of appropriate therapies. Ciprofloxacin is among several agents that may be appropriate for prophylaxis or treatment of naturally occurring or bioterrorism-related plague. Plague is a notifiable disease in the United States. Any suspected case should be reported immediately to local and state health departments, which will in turn notify the CDC. If an outbreak is thought to be potentially related to a bioterrorism event, the local and state health departments, Federal Bureau of Investigation field office, and CDC should all be contacted. Treatment and prophylaxis choices should be guided by the recommendations of these health authorities.

Plague (adults): [1] = Good documentation.

Plague (children): [1] = Good documentation.

Surgical prophylaxis – [1] = Good documentation. The use of ciprofloxacin as a prophylaxis is suitable as monotherapy for urologic surgical procedures and in combination with metronidazole or clindamycin for abdominal or vaginal hysterectomies, cesarean sections, and colorectal surgical procedures in patients with a beta-lactam allergy.

Traveler's diarrhea – [1] = Good documentation. Antibiotics have been shown to shorten the duration of traveler's diarrhea and also may be used in moderate to severe cases; however, because of increased antibiotic resistance, doxycycline is no longer recommended for the treatment of traveler's diarrhea. Current guidelines suggest that mild cases of traveler's diarrhea should be managed with adequate hydration and bismuth subsalicylate or loperamide.

Tularemia – Although streptomycin has long been considered the drug of choice for tularemia, alternative agents, such as ciprofloxacin, may play a greater role when streptomycin is not commercially available. Tularemia is a notifiable disease; inform local and state health departments when cases are identified. The choice of treatment may be guided by the most current recommendations of these health authorities. In mass exposures, treatment choices may also depend on the drugs provided from the Strategic National Stockpile.

Tularemia (adults): [1] = Good documentation.

Tularemia (children): [1] = Good documentation.

Other possible off-label uses – Ciprofloxacin has been used in children with cystic fibrosis for periods of 10 days to 6 months without documented adverse reactions or intolerance.

Ciprofloxacin has been used for the treatment of gastroenteritis in children.

Atypical mycobacterial infections have been satisfactorily treated with ciprofloxacin as part of combination therapy.

Ciprofloxacin is recommended for mycobacterial diseases.

Multidrug-resistant tuberculosis.

Disseminated gonorrhea (alternative regimen): 400 mg intravenously (IV) every 12 hours for 24 to 48 hours after improvement begins, then 500 mg orally twice daily for 7 days.

Administration and Dosage

➤*General dosing considerations:* Ciprofloxacin ER, ciprofloxacin immediate release, and *Proquin XR* are not interchangeable.

CIPROFLOXACIN HYDROCHLORIDE — ORAL

➤*Adults:*

Immediate-release tablets and oral suspension –

Usual dosage:

Ciprofloxacin Immediate-Release Tablets and Oral Suspension for Adults

Infection	Severity	Dose	Frequency	Usual duration[a]
Acute sinusitis	Mild/Moderate	500 mg	Every 12 h	10 days
Bone and joint	Mild/Moderate	500 mg	Every 12 h	≥ 4 to 6 wk
	Severe/Complicated	750 mg	Every 12 h	≥ 4 to 6 wk
Chronic bacterial prostatitis	Mild/Moderate	500 mg	Every 12 h	28 days
Infectious diarrhea	Mild/Moderate/Severe	500 mg	Every 12 h	5 to 7 days
Inhalational anthrax (postexposure)[b]		500 mg	Every 12 h	60 days
Intra-abdominal[c]	Complicated	500 mg	Every 12 h	7 to 14 days
Lower respiratory tract	Mild/Moderate	500 mg	Every 12 h	7 to 14 days
	Severe/Complicated	750 mg	Every 12 h	7 to 14 days
Skin and skin structure	Mild/Moderate	500 mg	Every 12 h	7 to 14 days
	Severe/Complicated	750 mg	Every 12 h	7 to 14 days
Typhoid fever	Mild/Moderate	500 mg	Every 12 h	10 days
Urethral and cervical gonococcal infections	Uncomplicated	250 mg	Single dose	Single dose
UTI	Acute uncomplicated	250 mg	Every 12 h	3 days
	Mild/Moderate	250 mg	Every 12 h	7 to 14 days
	Severe/Complicated	500 mg	Every 12 h	7 to 14 days

[a] Generally, ciprofloxacin should be continued for at least 2 days after the signs and symptoms of infection have disappeared, except for inhalational anthrax (postexposure).

[b] Drug administration should begin as soon as possible after suspected or confirmed exposure. This indication is based on a surrogate end point, ciprofloxacin serum concentrations achieved in humans, reasonably likely to predict clinical benefit.

[c] Used in conjunction with metronidazole.

Conversion: Patients whose therapy is started with IV ciprofloxacin may be switched to ciprofloxacin tablets or oral suspension at the discretion of the health care provider when clinically indicated.

Ciprofloxacin Equivalent AUC[a] Dosing Regimens

Ciprofloxacin oral dosage	Equivalent ciprofloxacin IV dosage
250 mg tablet every 12 h	200 mg IV every 12 h
500 mg tablet every 12 h	400 mg IV every 12 h
750 mg tablet every 12 h	400 mg IV every 8 h

[a] AUC = area under the curve.

Ciprofloxacin ER tablets –

Usual dosage: Ciprofloxacin ER tablets should be administered orally once daily as described in the following table.

Ciprofloxacin ER Dosing for Adults

Indication	Dose	Frequency	Usual duration
Acute uncomplicated pyelonephritis	1,000 mg	Every 24 h	7 to 14 days
Complicated UTIs	1,000 mg	Every 24 h	7 to 14 days
Uncomplicated UTIs (acute cystitis)	500 mg	Every 24 h	3 days

Conversion: Patients whose therapy is started with ciprofloxacin IV for UTIs may be switched to ciprofloxacin ER tablets at the discretion of the health care provider when clinically indicated.

Proquin XR –

Uncomplicated urinary tract infections (acute cystitis): 500 mg once daily for 3 days with a main meal of the day, preferably the evening meal.

Off-label dosing –

Anthrax prophylaxis: [1] = Good documentation.

- *Zoonotic cutaneous anthrax, excluding involvement of the head or neck* – 500 mg orally twice daily for 7 to 10 days.
- *Inhalational, GI, or oropharyngeal anthrax/cutaneous anthrax with systemic, edematous, or head/neck involvement* – 400 mg IV every 12 hours, switch to oral 500 mg twice daily. Continue treatment for a total of 60 days. Initiate ciprofloxacin as part of a multidrug regimen with 1 or 2 other antimicrobials with in vitro activity to *B. anthracis* (rifampin, vancomycin, penicillin, ampicillin, chloramphenicol, imipenem, clindamycin, or clarithromycin) plus a corticosteroid. Start with IV therapy until susceptibility is known, and switch to oral dosing when clinically appropriate.

Chancroid: [1] = Good documentation. 500 mg orally twice daily for 3 days.

Granuloma inguinale (donovanosis): [1] = Good documentation. 750 mg orally twice daily for at least 3 weeks. Treatment should continue until all lesions have completely healed.

Infective endocarditis (adults): [1] = Good documentation.

- *HACEK infections* – 1,000 mg orally daily in 2 divided doses for 4 weeks in native valve infections and for 6 weeks in prosthetic valve infections or other cardiac prosthetic materials. Fluoroquinolone therapy is recommended only for patients unable to tolerate cephalosporin and ampicillin therapy; levofloxacin, gatifloxacin, or moxifloxacin may be substituted.
- *Culture-negative endocarditis, including Bartonella infection in patients with a native valve* – 1,000 mg orally daily in 2 divided doses for 4 to 6 weeks in combination with vancomycin and gentamicin.

Plague: [1] = Good documentation. 500 mg orally twice daily. Prophylaxis should continue for 7 days after the last known or suspected exposure or until exposure has been excluded. Treatment of suspected or confirmed clinical cases should continue for 10 to 14 days.

Surgical prophylaxis: [1] = Good documentation. 500 mg every 12 hours or a 1-time dose of 1,500 mg.

Traveler's diarrhea: [1] = Good documentation. 500 mg twice daily for 3 days.

Tularemia: [1] = Good documentation.

- *Mass casualty management and postexposure prophylaxis* – 500 mg orally twice daily for 14 days.

➤*Children:* The dosing and initial route of therapy (ie, IV, oral) for complicated UTIs or pyelonephritis should be determined by the severity of the infection. In the clinical trial, children with moderate to severe infection were initiated on 6 to 10 mg/kg IV every 8 hours and allowed to switch to oral therapy (10 to 20 mg/kg every 12 hours) at the discretion of the health care provider.

An increased incidence of adverse reactions compared with controls, including reactions related to the joints and/or surrounding tissues, has been observed in ciprofloxacin-treated children.

Immediate-release tablets and oral suspension –

Ciprofloxacin Immediate-Release Tablets and Oral Suspension for Children

Infection	Route of administration	Dose	Frequency	Total duration
Complicated UTIs or pyelonephritis (patients 1 to 17 years of age)	IV	6 to 10 mg/kg (maximum, 400 mg/dose; not to be exceeded even in patients weighing > 51 kg)	Every 8 h	10 to 21 days[a]
	Oral	10 to 20 mg/kg (maximum, 750 mg/dose; not to be exceeded even in patients weighing > 51 kg)	Every 12 h	
Inhalational anthrax (postexposure)[b]	IV	10 mg/kg (maximum, 400 mg/dose)	Every 12 h	60 days
	Oral	15 mg/kg (maximum, 500 mg/dose)	Every 12 h	

[a] The total duration of therapy for complicated UTIs and pyelonephritis in the clinical trial was determined by the health care provider. The mean duration of treatment was 11 days (range, 10 to 21 days).

[b] Drug administration should begin as soon as possible after suspected or confirmed exposure to *B. anthracis* spores. This indication is based on a surrogate end point, ciprofloxacin serum concentration achieved in humans, reasonably likely to predict clinical benefit.

Off-label dosing –

Children: 10 to 15 mg/kg every 12 hours. Maximum dosage is 1.5 g/day.

Anthrax: For treatment of inhalational/systemic/cutaneous anthrax, start with 10 to 15 mg/kg IV every 12 hours. Maximum IV dosage is 800 mg/day.

CIPROFLOXACIN HYDROCHLORIDE — ORAL

Convert to oral ciprofloxacin (10 to 15 mg/kg every 12 hours) when clinically indicated. Maximum oral dosage is 1 g/day. Duration of ciprofloxacin therapy is 60 days.

Cystic fibrosis: 20 mg/kg every 12 hours. Maximum dosage is 2 g/day.

Infective endocarditis (children / adolescents): [1] = Good documentation.

- *HACEK infections* – 20 to 30 mg/kg/day in 2 divided doses administered orally for 4 weeks in native valve infections and for 6 weeks in prosthetic valve infections or other cardiac prosthetic materials. Fluoroquinolone therapy is recommended only for patients unable to tolerate cephalosporin and ampicillin therapy; levofloxacin, gatifloxacin, or moxifloxacin may be substituted. Fluoroquinolones are not generally recommended for patients younger than 18 years of age.
- *Culture-negative endocarditis, including Bartonella infection in patients with a native valve* – 20 to 30 mg/kg/day in 2 divided doses administered orally for 4 to 6 weeks in combination with vancomycin and gentamicin.

Plague: [1] = Good documentation. 10 to 20 mg/kg orally twice daily. Prophylaxis should continue for 7 days after the last known or suspected exposure or until exposure has been excluded. Treatment of suspected or confirmed clinical cases should continue for 10 to 14 days.

Tularemia: [1] = Good documentation.

- *Mass casualty management and postexposure prophylaxis* – 15 mg/kg orally twice daily, not to exceed 1 g/day, for 14 days.

➤*Renal function impairment:*

Adults –

Immediate-release tablets and oral suspension: Some modification of dosage is recommended, particularly for patients with severe renal function impairment. The following table provides dosage guidelines for use in adults with renal function impairment.

In patients with severe infections and severe renal function impairment, a unit dose of 750 mg may be administered at the intervals previously noted. Patients should be carefully monitored.

Ciprofloxacin Oral Dosing in Adults With Renal Function Impairment

CrCl[a] (mL/min)	Dosage
> 50	See usual dosage
30 to 50	250 to 500 mg every 12 h
5 to 29	250 to 500 mg every 18 h
Patients on hemodialysis or peritoneal dialysis	250 to 500 mg every 24 h (after dialysis)

[a] CrCl = creatinine clearance.

ER tablets and Proquin XR – No dosage adjustment is required for patients with uncomplicated UTIs receiving ciprofloxacin ER 500 mg or *Proquin XR* with mild to moderate renal impairment. The efficacy of *Proquin XR* has not been studied in patients with severe renal impairment.

In patients with complicated UTIs and acute uncomplicated pyelonephritis who have a CrCl of less than 30 mL/min, the dose of ciprofloxacin ER should be reduced from 1,000 to 500 mg daily. For patients on hemodialysis or peritoneal dialysis, administer ciprofloxacin ER after the dialysis procedure is completed.

➤*Concomitant therapy:* Ciprofloxacin should be administered at least 2 hours before or 6 hours after magnesium/aluminum antacids, sucralfate, didanosine chewable/buffered tablets or pediatric powder for oral solution, or other highly buffered drugs, and multivitamin preparations or other products containing calcium, iron, or zinc.

Proquin XR should be administered at least 4 hours before or 2 hours after antacids containing magnesium or aluminum, sucralfate, didanosine chewable/buffered tablets or pediatric powder, metal cations such as iron, and multivitamin preparations containing zinc.

➤*Duration of therapy:* The duration of treatment depends upon the severity of infection. The usual duration is 7 to 14 days; however, for severe and complicated infections, more prolonged therapy may be required.

➤*Administration:* Take ciprofloxacin with or without meals and drink fluids liberally. *Proquin XR* should be administered with a main meal of the day, preferably the evening meal.

Ciprofloxacin should not be taken with dairy product (eg, milk, yogurt) or calcium-fortified juices alone because ciprofloxacin absorption may be significantly reduced; however, ciprofloxacin may be taken with a meal that contains these products. A 2-hour window between substantial calcium intake (more than 800 mg) and dosing with ciprofloxacin ER is recommended.

Ciprofloxacin ER should be swallowed whole. Do not split, crush, or chew the ER tablets or *Proquin XR* tablets.

Instruct the patient to shake ciprofloxacin oral suspension vigorously each time before use for approximately 15 seconds and not to chew the microcapsules. Ciprofloxacin oral suspension should not be administered through feeding tubes because of its physical characteristics.

Ciprofloxacin ER, ciprofloxacin immediate-release, and *Proquin XR* are not interchangeable.

➤*Storage / Stability:*

Immediate-release tablets – Store below 30°C (86°F).

Oral suspension – Store microcapsules and diluent below 25°C (77°F) and protect from freezing. The reconstituted product may be stored below 30°C (86°F) for 14 days. Protect from freezing.

ER tablets and Proquin XR – Store at 25°C (77°F); excursions are permitted to 15° to 30°C (59° to 86°F).

CIPROFLOXACIN — INJECTION

For complete and comparative prescribing information, refer to the Fluoroquinolones class monograph.

WARNING

Tendinitis and tendon rupture – Fluoroquinolones, including ciprofloxacin, are associated with an increased risk of tendinitis and tendon rupture in all ages. This risk is further increased in older patients (usually older than 60 years), in patients taking corticosteroid drugs, and in patients with kidney, heart, or lung transplants.

Myasthenia gravis – Fluoroquinolones, including ciprofloxacin, may exacerbate muscle weakness in persons with myasthenia gravis. Avoid ciprofloxacin in patients with known history of myasthenia gravis.

Indications

For the treatment of infections caused by susceptible strains of the designated microorganisms in the following conditions and patient populations when the intravenous (IV) administration offers a route of administration advantageous to the patient. If anaerobic organisms are suspected of contributing to the infection, administer appropriate therapy.

➤*Adults:*

Acute sinusitis – Caused by *Haemophilus influenzae*, *Streptococcus pneumoniae* (penicillin-susceptible), or *Moraxella catarrhalis*.

Bone and joint infections – Caused by *Enterobacter cloacae*, *Serratia marcescens*, or *Pseudomonas aeruginosa*.

Chronic bacterial prostatitis – Caused by *Escherichia coli* or *Proteus mirabilis*.

Complicated intra-abdominal infections – Used in conjunction with metronidazole, caused by *E. coli*, *P. aeruginosa*, *P. mirabilis*, *Klebsiella pneumoniae*, or *Bacteroides fragilis*.

Empirical therapy for febrile neutropenic patients – In combination with piperacillin.

Lower respiratory tract infections – Caused by *E. coli*, *K. pneumoniae* subspecies *pneumoniae*, *E. cloacae*, *P. mirabilis*, *P. aeruginosa*, *H. influenzae*, *Haemophilus parainfluenzae*, or *S. pneumoniae* (penicillin-susceptible). Also, *M. catarrhalis* for the treatment of acute exacerbations of chronic bronchitis.

Although effective in clinical trials, ciprofloxacin is not a drug of first choice in the treatment of presumed or confirmed pneumonia secondary to *S. pneumoniae*.

Nosocomial pneumonia – Caused by *H. influenzae* or *K. pneumoniae*.

Skin and skin structure infections – Caused by *E. coli*, *K. pneumoniae* subspecies *pneumoniae*, *E. cloacae*, *P. mirabilis*, *Proteus vulgaris*, *Providencia stuartii*, *Morganella morganii*, *Citrobacter freundii*, *P. aeruginosa* (methicillin-susceptible), *Staphylococcus aureus* (methicillin-susceptible), *Staphylococcus epidermidis*, or *Streptococcus pyogenes*.

Urinary tract infections – Caused by *E. coli* (including cases with secondary bacteremia), *K. pneumoniae* subspecies *pneumoniae*, *E. cloacae*, *S. marcescens*, *P. mirabilis*, *Providencia rettgeri*, *M. morganii*, *Citrobacter diversus*, *C. freundii*, *P. aeruginosa* (methicillin-susceptible), *S. epidermidis*, *Staphylococcus saprophyticus*, or *Enterococcus faecalis*.

➤*Children (1 to 17 years of age):*

Complicated urinary tract infections and pyelonephritis – Caused by *E. coli*.

See Warnings/Precautions for more information.

➤*Adults and children:*

Inhalational anthrax (postexposure) – To reduce the incidence or progression of disease following exposure to aerosolized *Bacillus anthracis*.

➤*Off-label uses:*

Anthrax prophylaxis(adults) – [1] = Good documentation. Ciprofloxacin is recommended by the Centers for Disease Control and Prevention (CDC) as 1 of 2 possible first-line agents for bioterrorism postexposure prophylaxis of anthrax in adults. It should be used as part of a multidrug regimen with 1 or 2 other antimicrobials that show in vitro activity to *Bacillus anthracis* (rifampin, vancomycin, penicillin, ampicillin, chloramphenicol, imipenem, clindamycin, or clarithromycin) plus a corticosteroid and a 3-dose series of anthrax vaccine, adsorbed. Because of the limited data and no known controlled trials, current recommendations are based on in vitro and primate studies.

Catheter-related bloodstream infections – [3] = Safety concerns. Guidelines recommend that ciprofloxacin not be used as the first choice to treat catheter-related bloodstream infections in pediatric patients because of increased incidence of adverse events related to joints and/or surrounding tissues. Experience in neonates is limited. The risks and benefits of fluoroquinolones in children should be assessed prior to use. Ciprofloxacin is not recommended as first-line therapy for children younger than 18 years of age.

Conservative treatment using antibiotic lock therapy is shown to be useful in catheter-related bloodstream infection treatment, but there is scarce evidence supporting its impact in clinical practice.

CIPROFLOXACIN — INJECTION

Infective endocarditis (adults) – [1] = Good documentation. According to American Heart Association (AHA) guidelines, ciprofloxacin may be considered for treatment of *Haemophilus parainfluenzae*, *Haemophilus aphrophilus*, *Haemophilus paraphrophilus*, *Haemophilus influenzae*, *Actinobacillus actinomycetemcomitans*, *Cardiobacterium hominis*, *Eikenella corrodens*, *Kingella kingae*, and *Kingella denitrificans* (HACEK) and culture-negative endocarditis, including *Bartonella* infection in patients with a native valve.

Infective endocarditis (children/adolescents) – [1] = Good documentation. Fluoroquinolones are not generally recommended for patients younger than 18 years of age. According to AHA guidelines, fluoroquinolone therapy is recommended only for patients unable to tolerate cephalosporin and ampicillin therapy. Ciprofloxacin may be considered for treatment of HACEK and culture-negative endocarditis, including *Bartonella* infection in patients with a native valve.

Plague – Plague is sufficiently uncommon to preclude large, controlled studies of appropriate therapies. Ciprofloxacin is among several agents that may be appropriate for prophylaxis or treatment of naturally occurring or bioterrorism-related plague. Plague is a notifiable disease in the United States. Any suspected case should be reported immediately to local and state health departments, which will in turn notify the CDC. If an outbreak is thought to be potentially related to a bioterrorism event, the local and state health departments, Federal Bureau of Investigation field office, and CDC should all be contacted. Treatment and prophylaxis choices should be guided by the recommendations of these health authorities.

Plague (adults): [1] = Good documentation.

Plague (children): [1] = Good documentation.

Surgical prophylaxis – [1] = Good documentation. The use of ciprofloxacin as a prophylaxis is suitable as monotherapy for urologic surgical procedures and in combination with metronidazole or clindamycin for abdominal or vaginal hysterectomies, cesarean deliveries, and colorectal surgical procedures in patients with a beta-lactam allergy.

Tularemia – Although streptomycin has long been considered the drug of choice for tularemia, alternative agents, such as ciprofloxacin, may play a greater role when streptomycin is not commercially available. Tularemia is a notifiable disease, and local and state health departments should be informed when cases are identified. The choice of treatment may be guided by the most current recommendations of these health authorities. In mass exposures, treatment choices may also depend on the drugs provided from the Strategic National Stockpile.

Tularemia (adults): [1] = Good documentation.

Tularemia (children): [1] = Good documentation.

Other possible off-label uses – Multidrug-resistant tuberculosis; alternative regimen for cutaneous, oropharyngeal, and GI anthrax.

Ciprofloxacin has been used in children with cystic fibrosis for periods of 10 days to 6 months without documented adverse reactions or intolerance.

Disseminated gonorrhea (alternative regimen): 400 mg IV every 12 hours for 24 to 48 hours after improvement begins, then 500 mg orally twice daily for 7 days.

Administration and Dosage

➤*Adults:*

Infections –

Usual dosage:

Ciprofloxacin Injection Dosing for Adults

Infection[a]	Severity	Dose	Frequency	Usual duration
Acute sinusitis	Mild/Moderate	400 mg	Every 12 h	10 days
Bone and joint	Mild/Moderate	400 mg	Every 12 h	≥ 4 to 6 weeks
	Severe/Complicated	400 mg	Every 8 h	≥ 4 to 6 weeks
Chronic bacterial prostatitis	Mild/Moderate	400 mg	Every 12 h	28 days
Empirical therapy in febrile neutropenic patients	Severe	Ciprofloxacin 400 mg	Every 8 h	7 to 14 days
		Piperacillin 50 mg/kg, not to exceed 24 g/day	Every 4 h	
Inhalational anthrax (postexposure)[b]		400 mg	Every 12 h	60 days
Intra-abdominal[c]	Complicated	400 mg	Every 12 h	7 to 14 days
Lower respiratory tract	Mild/Moderate	400 mg	Every 12 h	7 to 14 days
	Severe/Complicated	400 mg	Every 8 h	7 to 14 days
Nosocomial pneumonia	Mild/Moderate/Severe	400 mg	Every 8 h	10 to 14 days
Skin and skin structure	Mild/Moderate	400 mg	Every 12 h	7 to 14 days
	Severe/Complicated	400 mg	Every 8 h	7 to 14 days

Ciprofloxacin Injection Dosing for Adults

Infection[a]	Severity	Dose	Frequency	Usual duration
UTI[d]	Mild/Moderate	200 mg	Every 12 h	7 to 14 days
	Severe/Complicated	400 mg	Every 12 h	7 to 14 days

[a] Due to the designated pathogens.
[b] Begin drug administration as soon as possible after suspected or confirmed exposure. This indication is based on a surrogate end point, ciprofloxacin serum concentrations achieved in humans, reasonably likely to predict clinical benefit. Total duration of ciprofloxacin administration (IV or oral) for inhalational anthrax (postexposure) is 60 days.
[c] Used in conjunction with metronidazole.
[d] UTI = urinary tract infection.

Conversion:

Ciprofloxacin Equivalent AUC[a] Dosing Regimens

Ciprofloxacin oral dosage	Equivalent ciprofloxacin IV dosage
250 mg tablet every 12 h	200 mg IV every 12 h
500 mg tablet every 12 h	400 mg IV every 12 h
750 mg tablet every 12 h	400 mg IV every 8 h

[a] AUC = area under the curve.

Off-label dosing –

Anthrax prophylaxis: [1] = Good documentation.

• *Inhalational, GI, or oropharyngeal anthrax/cutaneous anthrax with systemic, edematous, or head/neck involvement* – 400 mg IV every 12 hours, switch to oral 500 mg twice daily. Continue treatment for a total of 60 days. Initiate ciprofloxacin as part of a multidrug regimen with 1 or 2 other antimicrobials with in vitro activity to *B. anthracis* (rifampin, vancomycin, penicillin, ampicillin, chloramphenicol, imipenem, clindamycin, or clarithromycin) plus a corticosteroid. Start with IV therapy until susceptibility is known, and switch to oral dosing when clinically appropriate.

Catheter-related bloodstream infections: [3] = Safety concerns. 400 mg IV every 12 hours for 10 to 14 days. Continuation of therapy for 4 to 6 weeks in patients with persistent bacteremia is recommended.

Infective endocarditis (adults): [1] = Good documentation.

• *HACEK infections* – 800 mg IV daily in 2 divided doses for 4 weeks in native valve infections and for 6 weeks in prosthetic valve infections or other cardiac prosthetic materials. Fluoroquinolone therapy is recommended only for patients unable to tolerate cephalosporin and ampicillin therapy; levofloxacin, gatifloxacin, or moxifloxacin may be substituted.

• *Culture-negative endocarditis, including Bartonella infection in patients with a native valve* – 800 mg IV daily in 2 divided doses for 4 to 6 weeks in combination with vancomycin and gentamicin.

Plague: [1] = Good documentation. 400 mg IV twice daily. Prophylaxis should continue for 7 days after the last known or suspected exposure or until exposure has been excluded. Treatment of suspected or confirmed clinical cases should continue for 10 to 14 days.

Surgical prophylaxis: [1] = Good documentation. 400 mg infused over 60 minutes and repeated every 4 to 10 hours.

Tularemia: [1] = Good documentation.

• *Individual medical management* – 400 mg IV twice daily for 10 days.

➤*Children:* Dosing and initial route of therapy (ie, IV or oral) for complicated UTI or pyelonephritis should be determined by the severity of the infection. In the clinical trial, children with moderate to severe infection were initiated on 6 to 10 mg/kg IV every 8 hours and allowed to switch to oral therapy (10 to 20 mg/kg every 12 hours), at the discretion of the health care provider.

Infections –

Ciprofloxacin Dosing for Children

Infection	Route of administration	Dose	Frequency	Total duration
Complicated UTIs or pyelonephritis (patients 1 to 17 years of age)	IV	6 to 10 mg/kg (maximum, 400 mg/dose; not to be exceeded even in patients weighing > 51 kg)	Every 8 h	10 to 21 days[a]
	Oral	10 to 20 mg/kg (maximum, 750 mg/dose; not to be exceeded even in patients weighing > 51 kg)	Every 12 h	

CIPROFLOXACIN — INJECTION

Ciprofloxacin Dosing for Children				
Infection	Route of administration	Dose	Frequency	Total duration
Inhalational anthrax (postexposure)[b]	IV	10 mg/kg (maximum, 400 mg/dose)	Every 12 h	60 days
	Oral	15 mg/kg (maximum, 500 mg/dose)	Every 12 h	

[a] The total duration of therapy for complicated UTIs and pyelonephritis in the clinical trial was determined by the health care provider. The mean duration of treatment was 11 days (range, 10 to 21 days).
[b] Begin drug administration as soon as possible after suspected or confirmed exposure to *B. anthracis* spores. This indication is based on a surrogate end point, ciprofloxacin serum concentrations achieved in humans, reasonably likely to predict clinical benefit.

Off-label dosing –

Children: 10 to 15 mg/kg IV every 12 hours. Maximum dosage is 800 mg/day.

Anthrax: For treatment of inhalational/systemic/cutaneous anthrax, start with 10 to 15 mg/kg IV every 12 hours. Maximum IV dosage is 800 mg/day. Convert to oral ciprofloxacin (10 to 15 mg/kg every 12 hours) when clinically indicated. Maximum oral dosage is 1 g/day. Duration of ciprofloxacin therapy is 60 days.

Catheter-related bloodstream infections: [3] = Safety concerns.
- *Infants and children* – 20 to 30 mg/kg/day IV divided every 12 hours.
- *Neonates* – 7 to 40 mg/kg/day IV divided every 12 hours.

Cystic fibrosis: 20 to 30 mg/kg/day IV given in divided doses every 8 to 12 hours. Maximum dosage is 1.2 g/day.

Infective endocarditis (children/adolescents): [1] = Good documentation.
- *HACEK infections* – 20 to 30 mg/kg/day in 2 divided doses administered IV for 4 weeks in native valve infections and for 6 weeks in prosthetic valve infections or other cardiac prosthetic materials. Fluoroquinolone therapy is recommended only for patients unable to tolerate cephalosporin and ampicillin therapy; levofloxacin, gatifloxacin, or moxifloxacin may be substituted. Fluoroquinolones are not generally recommended for patients younger than 18 years of age.
- *Culture-negative endocarditis, including Bartonella infection in patients with a native valve* – 20 to 30 mg/kg/day in 2 divided doses administered IV for 4 to 6 weeks in combination with vancomycin and gentamicin.

Plague: [1] = Good documentation. 10 to 15 mg/kg IV twice daily. Prophylaxis should continue for 7 days after the last known or suspected exposure or until exposure has been excluded. Treatment of suspected or confirmed clinical cases should continue for 10 to 14 days.

Tularemia: [1] = Good documentation.

- *Individual medical management* – 15 mg/kg IV twice daily (maximum, 1 g/day) for 10 days.

➤*Renal function impairment:*

Adults –

Ciprofloxacin Injection Dosing in Adults With Renal Function Impairment	
CrCl[a] (mL/min)	Dosage
> 30	Usual dosage
5 to 29	200 to 400 mg every 18 to 24 h

[a] CrCl = creatinine clearance.

➤*Preparation for administration:*

Vials (concentrated solution) – This preparation must be diluted before use. Prepare the IV dose by aseptically withdrawing the concentrate from the vial of ciprofloxacin IV. This should be diluted with a suitable IV solution to a final concentration of 1 to 2 mg/mL. (See Admixture Compatibility.)

Premixed solutions – The solutions in flexible containers do not need to be diluted.

➤*Administration:* Ciprofloxacin should be administered by IV infusion over a period of 60 minutes by direct infusion or through a Y-type IV infusion set, which may already be in place. Slow infusion of a dilute solution into a larger vein will minimize patient discomfort and reduce the risk of venous irritation.

If the Y-type or the piggyback method of administration is used, it is advisable to temporarily discontinue the administration of any other solutions during the infusion of ciprofloxacin. If the concomitant use of ciprofloxacin and another drug is necessary, each drug should be given separately in accordance with the recommended dosage and route of administration for each drug.

➤*Admixture compatibility:* Ciprofloxacin injection 1% (10 mg/mL), when diluted with the following IV solutions to concentrations of 0.5 to 2 mg/mL, is stable for up to 14 days at refrigerated or room temperature storage: sodium chloride 0.9% injection, dextrose 5% injection, sterile water for injection, dextrose 10% for injection, dextrose 5% and sodium chloride 0.225% for injection, dextrose 5% and sodium chloride 0.45% for injection, or Ringer's lactate for injection are compatible IV solutions for diluting ciprofloxacin in vials.

➤*Storage/Stability:* Store vials between 5° and 30°C (41° and 86°F) and flexible containers between 5° and 25°C (41° and 77°F). Protect from light, avoid excessive heat, and protect from freezing.

Ciprofloxacin 1% (10 mg/mL), when diluted with compatible IV solution (see Admixture Compatibility) to concentrations of 0.5 to 2 mg/mL, is stable for up to 14 days when refrigerated or stored at room temperature.

LEVOFLOXACIN

Rx	Levaquin (Ortho-McNeil-Janssen)	**Tablets; oral:** 250 mg	Polyethylene glycol. (LEVAQUIN 250). Terra cotta pink, capsule shape. Film-coated. In 50s and UD 100s.
		500 mg	Polyethylene glycol. (LEVAQUIN 500). Peach, capsule shape. Film-coated. In 50s and UD 100s.
		750 mg	Polyethylene glycol. (LEVAQUIN 750). White, capsule shape. Film-coated. In 20s and UD 100s.
		Solution; oral: 25 mg/mL	Benzyl alcohol, glycerin, propylene glycol, sucralose, sucrose. In 480 mL.
		Injection, solution: 5 mg/mL	Preservative free. In 50, 100, and 150 mL premix flexible containers in dextrose 5% solution.
		Injection, solution, concentrate: 25 mg/mL	Preservative free. In 20 and 30 mL single-use vials.

LEVOFLOXACIN — ORAL

For complete and comparative prescribing information, refer to the Fluoroquinolones class monograph.

WARNING

Tendinitis and tendon rupture – Fluoroquinolones, including levofloxacin, are associated with an increased risk of tendinitis and tendon rupture in all ages. This risk is further increased in older patients (usually older than 60 years), in patients taking corticosteroid drugs, and in patients with kidney, heart, or lung transplants (see also Warnings/Precautions).

Myasthenia gravis – Fluoroquinolones, including levofloxacin, may exacerbate muscle weakness in persons with myasthenia gravis. Avoid levofloxacin use in patients with a known history of myasthenia gravis (see also Warnings/Precautions).

Indications

➤*Acute bacterial exacerbation of chronic bronchitis:* Caused by methicillin-susceptible *Staphylococcus aureus, Streptococcus pneumoniae, Haemophilus influenzae, Haemophilus parainfluenzae*, or *Moraxella catarrhalis*.

➤*Acute bacterial sinusitis (5-day or 10- to 14-day treatment regimen):* Caused by *S. pneumoniae, H. influenzae*, or *M. catarrhalis*.

➤*Acute pyelonephritis (5- or 10-day treatment regimen):* Caused by *Escherichia coli*, including cases with concurrent bacteremia.

➤*Chronic bacterial prostatitis:* Caused by *E. coli, Enterococcus faecalis*, or methicillin-susceptible *Staphylococcus epidermidis*.

➤*Community-acquired pneumonia (5-day treatment regimen):* Caused by *S. pneumoniae* (excluding multidrug-resistant strains), *H. influenzae, H. parainfluenzae, Mycoplasma pneumoniae*, or *Chlamydophila pneumoniae*.

➤*Community-acquired pneumonia (7- to 14-day treatment regimen):* Caused by methicillin-susceptible *S. aureus, S. pneumoniae* (including multidrug-resistant *S. pneumoniae* [MDRSP]), *H. influenzae, H. parainfluenzae, Klebsiella pneumoniae, M. catarrhalis, C. pneumoniae, Legionella pneumophila*, or *M. pneumoniae*.

MDRSP isolates are strains resistant to 2 or more of the following antibacterials: penicillin (minimum inhibitory concentration [MIC] of 2 mcg/mL or more), second-generation cephalosporins (eg, cefuroxime), macrolides, tetracyclines, and trimethoprim/sulfamethoxazole.

➤*Inhalational anthrax (postexposure):* To reduce the incidence or progression of disease following exposure to aerosolized *Bacillus anthracis*.

➤*Nosocomial pneumonia:* Caused by methicillin-susceptible *S. aureus, Pseudomonas aeruginosa, Serratia marcescens, E. coli, K. pneumoniae, H. influenzae*, or *S. pneumoniae*. Use adjunctive therapy as clinically indicated.

LEVOFLOXACIN — ORAL

Combination therapy with an antipseudomonal beta-lactam is recommended when *P. aeruginosa* is a documented or presumptive pathogen.

➤*Skin and skin structure infections, complicated:* Caused by methicillin-susceptible *S. aureus*, *E. faecalis*, *Streptococcus pyogenes*, or *Proteus mirabilis*.

➤*Skin and skin structure infections, uncomplicated (mild to moderate):* Including abscesses, cellulitis, furuncles, impetigo, pyoderma, and wound infections caused by methicillin-susceptible *S. aureus* or *S. pyogenes*.

➤*Urinary tract infections, complicated (5-day treatment regimen):* Caused by *E. coli*, *K. pneumoniae*, or *P. mirabilis*.

➤*Urinary tract infections, complicated (mild to moderate) (10-day treatment regimen):* Caused by *E. faecalis*, *Enterobacter cloacae*, *E. coli*, *K. pneumoniae*, *P. mirabilis*, or *P. aeruginosa*.

➤*Urinary tract infections, uncomplicated (mild to moderate):* Caused by *E. coli*, *K. pneumoniae*, or *Staphylococcus saprophyticus*.

➤*Off-label uses:*

Epididymitis – [1] = Good documentation. Centers for Disease Control and Prevention (CDC) guidelines recommend levofloxacin as a regimen for cases of epididymitis likely to be caused by enteric organisms, or those confirmed negative for gonococcal infection.

Infective endocarditis (adults) – [1] = Good documentation. According to American Heart Association (AHA) guidelines, levofloxacin may be considered as an alternative treatment to ciprofloxacin in the management of endocarditis due to *H. parainfluenzae*, *Haemophilus aphrophilus*, *Haemophilus paraphrophilus*, *H. influenzae*, *Actinobacillus actinomycetemcomitans*, *Cardiobacterium hominis*, *Eikenella corrodens*, *Kingella kingae*, and *Kingella denitrificans* (HACEK) organisms.

Infective endocarditis (children/adolescents) – [1] = Good documentation. Fluoroquinolones are not generally recommended for patients younger than 18 years. According to AHA guidelines, levofloxacin may be considered as an alternative treatment to ciprofloxacin in the management of endocarditis due to HACEK organisms.

Pelvic inflammatory disease – [1] = Good documentation. CDC guidelines advise use of levofloxacin as a recommended regimen for cases of pelvic inflammatory disease (PID) in which parenteral cephalosporin therapy is not feasible. Low risk of gonococcal infection and specific testing for gonorrhea are mandatory with the use of levofloxacin for PID because of concerns of fluoroquinolone-resistant infections.

Traveler's diarrhea – [1] = Good documentation. Antibiotics have been shown to shorten the duration of traveler's diarrhea and may also be used in moderate to severe cases; however, because of increased antibiotic resistance, doxycycline is no longer recommended for the treatment of traveler's diarrhea. Current guidelines suggest that mild cases of traveler's diarrhea should be managed with adequate hydration and bismuth subsalicylate or loperamide.

Tuberculosis – [1] = Good documentation. The American Thoracic Society, CDC, and Infectious Diseases Society of America joint guidelines on the treatment of tuberculosis (TB) recommend oral levofloxacin 500 to 1,000 mg daily as a second-line agent. The Food and Drug Administration (FDA) has not approved levofloxacin for the treatment of TB. The guideline states that on the basis of cumulative experience suggesting a good safety profile with long-term use of levofloxacin, it is the preferred oral agent for treating drug-resistant TB caused by organisms known or presumed to be sensitive to fluoroquinolones or when first-line drugs cannot be used because of intolerance. This recommendation is based on expert opinion.

Other possible off-label uses –

Gonococcal infections, disseminated: As an alternative regimen if antimicrobial susceptibility exists and can be documented by culture. Administer 250 mg once daily intravenously (IV) for 24 to 48 hours (after improvement begins, administer 500 mg/day orally for 7 days).

Administration and Dosage

➤*General dosing considerations:* The oral and IV routes of administration can be considered interchangeable. Levofloxacin oral solution and tablet formulations are bioequivalent.

Adequate hydration of patients receiving levofloxacin should be maintained to prevent the formation of highly concentrated urine. Crystalluria and cylindruria have been reported with quinolones.

➤*Adults:*

Infections – The usual dosage is 250, 500, or 750 mg every 24 hours, as indicated by infection and described by the following dosing recommendations.

Levofloxacin Dosage in Patients With Healthy Renal Function ($CrCl \geq 50$ mL/min)[a]

Type of infection[b]	Dosed every 24 h	Duration (days)[c]
Acute bacterial exacerbation of chronic bronchitis	500 mg	7
Acute bacterial sinusitis	750 mg	5
	500 mg	10 to 14
Chronic bacterial prostatitis	500 mg	28
Community-acquired pneumonia[d]	500 mg	7 to 14
Community-acquired pneumonia[e]	750 mg	5
Inhalational anthrax (postexposure)[f,g]	500 mg	60[g]
Nosocomial pneumonia	750 mg	7 to 14
Skin and skin structure infections, complicated	750 mg	7 to 14
Skin and skin structure infections, uncomplicated	500 mg	7 to 10
UTI (complicated) or acute pyelonephritis[h]	750 mg	5
UTI (complicated) or acute pyelonephritis[i]	250 mg	10
UTI, uncomplicated	250 mg	3

[a] CrCl = creatinine clearance; UTI = urinary tract infection.
[b] Because of the designated pathogens (see Indications).
[c] Sequential therapy (IV to oral) may be instituted at the discretion of the health care provider.
[d] Caused by methicillin-susceptible *S. aureus*, *S. pneumoniae* (including MDRSP), *H. influenzae*, *H. parainfluenzae*, *K. pneumoniae*, *M. catarrhalis*, *C. pneumoniae*, *L. pneumophila*, or *M. pneumoniae*.
[e] Caused by *S. pneumoniae* (excluding MDRSP), *H. influenzae*, *H. parainfluenzae*, *M. pneumoniae*, or *C. pneumoniae*.
[f] Drug administration should begin as soon as possible after suspected or confirmed exposure to aerosolized *B. anthracis*. This indication is based on a surrogate end point. Levofloxacin plasma concentrations achieved in humans are reasonably likely to predict clinical benefit.
[g] The safety of levofloxacin in adults for durations of therapy beyond 28 days has not been studied. Prolonged levofloxacin therapy should only be used when the benefit outweighs the risk.
[h] This regimen is indicated for complicated UTIs caused by *E. coli*, *K. pneumoniae*, or *P. mirabilis*, and acute pyelonephritis caused by *E. coli*, including cases with concurrent bacteremia.
[i] This regimen is indicated for complicated UTIs caused by *E. faecalis*, *E. cloacae*, *E. coli*, *K. pneumoniae*, *P. mirabilis*, or *P. aeruginosa*; and for acute pyelonephritis caused by *E. coli*.

Concomitant therapy – Use adjunctive therapy as clinically indicated. Combination therapy with an antipseudomonal beta-lactam is recommended when *P. aeruginosa* is a documented or presumptive pathogen.

Off-label dosing –

Epididymitis: [1] = Good documentation. 500 mg orally once daily for 10 days.

Infective endocarditis (adults): [1] = Good documentation.

• *HACEK infections* – Levofloxacin can be substituted for ciprofloxacin for 4 weeks in native valve infections and for 6 weeks in prosthetic valve infections. Specific dosing for levofloxacin is not provided in AHA guidelines. In patients with healthy renal function, the usual dosage of levofloxacin is 500 or 750 mg daily.

Pelvic inflammatory disease: [1] = Good documentation. 500 mg orally once daily for 14 days. May be given in conjunction with metronidazole 500 mg orally twice daily for 14 days if concerns of anaerobic infection exist.

Traveler's diarrhea: [1] = Good documentation. 500 mg once daily for 3 days.

Tuberculosis: [1] = Good documentation. 500 to 1,000 mg orally daily.

➤*Children:*

Inhalational anthrax (postexposure) –

6 months and older:

• *Usual dosage* –

Weighing at least 50 kg: 500 mg once every 24 hours.

Weighing less than 50 kg: 8 mg/kg (not to exceed 250 mg/dose) once every 12 hours.

• *Maximum dose* – 250 mg/dose for children weighing less than 50 kg.

• *Duration of therapy* – 60 days. The safety of levofloxacin in children for durations of therapy beyond 14 days has not been studied. An increased incidence of musculoskeletal adverse reactions compared with controls has been observed in children. Prolonged levofloxacin therapy should only be used when the benefit outweighs the risk.

• *Conversion* – Sequential therapy (IV to oral) may be instituted at the discretion of the health care provider.

Off-label dosing –

Acute otitis media (recurrent or persistent):

• *6 months to younger than 5 years* – 10 mg/kg every 12 hours for 10 days. Maximum dosage is 500 mg/day.

Community-acquired pneumonia:

• *5 to 12 years of age* – 10 mg/kg every 24 hours. Maximum dosage is 500 mg/day.

• *6 months to younger than 5 years* – 10 mg/kg every 12 hours.

Infective endocarditis (children/adolescents): [1] = Good documentation.

• *HACEK infections* – Levofloxacin can be substituted for ciprofloxacin for 4 weeks in native valve infections and for 6 weeks in prosthetic valve infections. Specific dosing for levofloxacin is not provided in AHA guidelines. Fluoroquinolones are not generally recommended for patients younger than 18 years.

Pelvic inflammatory disease: [1] = Good documentation.

• *Adolescents* – 500 mg orally once daily for 14 days. May be given in conjunction with metronidazole 500 mg orally twice daily for 14 days if concerns of anaerobic infection exist.

➤*Elderly:* Because elderly patients are more likely to have decreased renal function, take care in dose selection; it may be useful to monitor renal function.

LEVOFLOXACIN — ORAL

➤*Renal function impairment:* Administer levofloxacin with caution in the presence or renal insufficiency. Careful clinical observation and appropriate laboratory studies should be performed prior to and during therapy because elimination of levofloxacin may be reduced.

Levofloxacin Dosage in Adults With Renal Function Impairment (CrCl < 50 mL/min)

Dosage in healthy renal function every 24 h	CrCl 20 to 49 mL/min	CrCl 10 to 19 mL/min	Hemodialysis or CAPD[a]
750 mg	750 mg every 48 h	750 mg initial dose, then 500 mg every 48 h	750 mg initial dose, then 500 mg every 48 h
500 mg	500 mg initial dose, then 250 mg every 24 h	500 mg initial dose, then 250 mg every 48 h	500 mg initial dose, then 250 mg every 48 h
250 mg	No dosage adjustment required	250 mg every 48 h; if treating uncomplicated UTI, no dosage adjustment is required.	No information on dosing adjustment is available.

[a] CAPD = chronic ambulatory peritoneal dialysis.

➤*Administration:* Levofloxacin tablets can be administered without regard to food. It is recommended that levofloxacin oral solution be taken 1 hour before or 2 hours after eating. Levofloxacin oral solution and tablet formulations are bioequivalent.

Administer levofloxacin tablets and oral solution at least 2 hours before or after antacids containing magnesium or aluminum, as well as sucralfate, metal cations (eg, iron), multivitamins with zinc, or didanosine chewable/buffered tablets or the pediatric powder for oral solution.

➤*Storage/Stability:*

Tablets – Store at 15° to 30°C (59° to 86°F) in well-closed containers.

Oral solution – Store at 25°C (77°F); excursions are permitted from 15° to 30°C (59° to 86°F).

LEVOFLOXACIN — INJECTION

For complete and comparative prescribing information, refer to the Fluoroquinolones class monograph.

WARNING

Tendinitis and tendon rupture – Fluoroquinolones, including levofloxacin, are associated with an increased risk of tendinitis and tendon rupture in all ages. This risk is further increased in older patients (usually older than 60 years), in patients taking corticosteroid drugs, and in patients with kidney, heart, or lung transplants (see also Warnings/Precautions).

Myasthenia gravis – Fluoroquinolones, including levofloxacin, may exacerbate muscle weakness in persons with myasthenia gravis. Avoid levofloxacin use in patients with a known history of myasthenia gravis (see also Warnings/Precautions).

Indications

➤*General information:* For the treatment of adults 18 years and older with mild, moderate, and severe infections caused by susceptible strains of the designated microorganisms in the following conditions listed.

Levofloxacin injection is indicated when intravenous (IV) administration offers a route of administration advantageous to the patient (eg, patient cannot tolerate an oral dosage regimen).

➤*Acute bacterial exacerbation of chronic bronchitis:* Caused by methicillin-susceptible *Staphylococcus aureus, Streptococcus pneumoniae, Haemophilus influenzae, Haemophilus parainfluenzae,* or *Moraxella catarrhalis.*

➤*Acute bacterial sinusitis (5-day or 10- to 14-day treatment regimen):* Caused by *S. pneumoniae, H. influenzae,* or *M. catarrhalis.*

➤*Acute pyelonephritis (5- or 10-day treatment regimen):* Caused by *Escherichia coli,* including cases with concurrent bacteremia.

➤*Chronic bacterial prostatitis:* Caused by *E. coli, Enterococcus faecalis,* or methicillin-susceptible *Staphylococcus epidermidis.*

➤*Community-acquired pneumonia (5-day treatment regimen):* Caused by *S. pneumoniae* (excluding multidrug-resistant strains), *H. influenzae, H. parainfluenzae, Mycoplasma pneumoniae,* or *Chlamydophila pneumoniae.*

➤*Community-acquired pneumonia (7- to 14-day treatment regimen):* Caused by methicillin-susceptible *S. aureus, S. pneumoniae* (including multidrug-resistant *S. pneumoniae* [MDRSP]), *H. influenzae, H. parainfluenzae, Klebsiella pneumoniae, M. catarrhalis, C. pneumoniae, Legionella pneumophila,* or *M. pneumoniae.*

MDRSP isolates are strains resistant to 2 or more of the following antibacterials: penicillin (minimal inhibitory concentration [MIC] of 2 mcg/mL or more), second-generation cephalosporins (eg, cefuroxime), macrolides, tetracyclines, and trimethoprim/sulfamethoxazole.

➤*Inhalational anthrax (postexposure):* To reduce the incidence or progression of disease following exposure to aerosolized *Bacillus anthracis.*

➤*Nosocomial pneumonia:* Caused by methicillin-susceptible *S. aureus, Pseudomonas aeruginosa, Serratia marcescens, E. coli, K. pneumoniae, H. influenzae,* or *S. pneumoniae.* Use adjunctive therapy as clinically indicated. Combination therapy with an antipseudomonal beta-lactam is recommended where *P. aeruginosa* is a documented or presumptive pathogen.

➤*Skin and skin structure infections, complicated:* Caused by methicillin-susceptible *S. aureus, E. faecalis, Streptococcus pyogenes,* or *Proteus mirabilis.*

➤*Skin and skin structure infections, uncomplicated (mild to moderate):* Including abscesses, cellulitis, furuncles, impetigo, pyoderma, and wound infections caused by methicillin-susceptible *S. aureus* or *S. pyogenes.*

➤*Urinary tract infections, complicated (5-day treatment regimen):* Caused by *E. coli, K. pneumoniae,* or *P. mirabilis.*

➤*Urinary tract infections, complicated (mild to moderate) (10-day treatment regimen):* Caused by *E. faecalis, Enterobacter cloacae, E. coli, K. pneumoniae, P. mirabilis,* or *P. aeruginosa.*

➤*Urinary tract infections, uncomplicated (mild to moderate):* Caused by *E. coli, K. pneumoniae,* or *Staphylococcus saprophyticus.*

➤*Off-label uses:*

Infective endocarditis (adults) – [1] = Good documentation. According to American Heart Association (AHA) guidelines, levofloxacin may be considered as an alternative treatment to ciprofloxacin in the management of endocarditis due to *H. parainfluenzae, Haemophilus aphrophilus, Haemophilus paraphrophilus, H. influenzae, Actinobacillus actinomycetemcomitans, Cardiobacterium hominis, Eikenella corrodens, Kingella kingae,* and *Kingella denitrificans* (HACEK) organisms.

Infective endocarditis (children/adolescents) – [1] = Good documentation. Fluoroquinolones are not generally recommended for patients younger than 18 years. According to AHA guidelines, levofloxacin may be considered as an alternative treatment to ciprofloxacin in the management of endocarditis due to HACEK organisms.

Other possible off-label uses –

Gonococcal infections, disseminated: As an alternative regimen if antimicrobial susceptibility exists and can be documented by culture. Administer 250 mg once daily IV for 24 to 48 hours (after improvement begins, administer 500 mg/day orally for 7 days).

Administration and Dosage

➤*General dosing considerations:* The oral and IV routes of administration can be considered interchangeable.

Adequate hydration of patients receiving levofloxacin should be maintained to prevent the formation of highly concentrated urine. Crystalluria and cylindruria have been reported with quinolones.

➤*Adults:*

Infections – The usual dose is 250 or 500 mg administered by slow IV infusion over 60 minutes every 24 hours or 750 mg administered by slow IV infusion over 90 minutes every 24 hours, as indicated by infection and described by the following dosing recommendations.

Levofloxacin Dosage in Adults With Healthy Renal Function (CrCl ≥ 50 mL/min)[a]

Type of infection[b]	Dosed every 24 h	Duration (days)[c]
Acute bacterial exacerbation of chronic bronchitis	500 mg	7
Acute bacterial sinusitis	750 mg	5
	500 mg	10 to 14
Chronic bacterial prostatitis	500 mg	28
Community-acquired pneumonia[d]	500 mg	7 to 14

LEVOFLOXACIN — INJECTION

Levofloxacin Dosage in Adults With Healthy Renal Function (CrCl ≥ 50 mL/min)[a]		
Type of infection[b]	Dosed every 24 h	Duration (days)[c]
Community-acquired pneumonia[e]	750 mg	5
Inhalational anthrax (postexposure)[f,g]	500 mg	60[g]
Nosocomial pneumonia	750 mg	7 to 14
Skin and skin structure infections, complicated	750 mg	7 to 14
Skin and skin structure infections, uncomplicated	500 mg	7 to 10
UTI (complicated) or acute pyelonephritis[h]	750 mg	5
UTI (complicated) or acute pyelonephritis[i]	250 mg	10
UTI, uncomplicated	250 mg	3

[a] CrCl = creatinine clearance; UTI = urinary tract infection.
[b] Caused by the designated pathogens (see Indications).
[c] Sequential therapy (IV to oral) may be instituted at the discretion of the health care provider.
[d] Caused by methicillin-susceptible *S. aureus, S. pneumoniae* (including MDRSP), *H. influenzae, H. parainfluenzae, K. pneumoniae, M. catarrhalis, C. pneumoniae, L. pneumophila*, or *M. pneumoniae*.
[e] Caused by *S. pneumoniae* (excluding MDRSP), *H. influenzae, H. parainfluenzae, M. pneumoniae*, or *C. pneumoniae*.
[f] Drug administration should begin as soon as possible after suspected or confirmed exposure to aerosolized *B. anthracis* occurs. This indication is based on a surrogate end point. Levofloxacin plasma concentrations achieved in humans are reasonably likely to predict clinical benefit.
[g] The safety of levofloxacin in adults for durations of therapy beyond 28 days has not been studied. Prolonged levofloxacin therapy should be used only when the benefit outweighs the risk.
[h] This regimen is indicated for complicated UTIs caused by *E. coli, K. pneumoniae*, or *P. mirabilis*, and acute pyelonephritis caused by *E. coli*, including cases with concurrent bacteremia.
[i] This regimen is indicated for complicated UTIs caused by *E. faecalis, E. cloacae, E. coli, K. pneumoniae, P. mirabilis*, or *P. aeruginosa*; and for acute pyelonephritis caused by *E. coli*.

Off-label dosing –

Infective endocarditis (adults): [1] = Good documentation.

• *HACEK infections* – Levofloxacin can be substituted for ciprofloxacin for 4 weeks in native valve infections and for 6 weeks in prosthetic valve infections. Specific dosing for levofloxacin is not provided in AHA guidelines. In patients with healthy renal function, the usual dosage of levofloxacin is 500 or 750 mg daily.

• *Concomitant therapy* – Use adjunctive therapy as clinically indicated. Combination therapy with an antipseudomonal beta-lactam is recommended where *P. aeruginosa* is a documented or presumptive pathogen.

➤*Children:*

Inhalational anthrax (postexposure) –

6 months and older:

• *Usual dosage* –

Weighing at least 50 kg: 500 mg by slow IV infusion over 60 minutes once every 24 hours.

Weighing less than 50 kg: 8 mg/kg (not to exceed 250 mg/dose) by slow IV infusion over 60 minutes once every 12 hours.

• *Maximum dose* – 250 mg/dose for children weighing less than 50 kg.

• *Duration of therapy* – 60 days. The safety of levofloxacin in children for durations of therapy beyond 14 days has not been studied. An increased incidence of musculoskeletal adverse reactions compared with controls has been observed in children. Prolonged levofloxacin therapy should be used only when the benefit outweighs the risk.

• *Conversion* – Sequential therapy (IV to oral) may be instituted at the discretion of the health care provider.

Off-label dosing –

Community-acquired pneumonia:

• *5 to 12 years of age* – 10 mg/kg IV every 24 hours. Maximum dosage is 500 mg/day.

• *6 months to younger than 5 years* – 10 mg/kg IV every 12 hours.

Infective endocarditis (children / adolescents): [1] = Good documentation.

• *HACEK infections* – Levofloxacin can be substituted for ciprofloxacin for 4 weeks in native valve infections and for 6 weeks in prosthetic valve infections. Specific dosing for levofloxacin is not provided in AHA guidelines. Fluoroquinolones are not generally recommended for patients younger than 18 years.

➤*Elderly:* Because elderly patients are more likely to have renal function impairment, take care in dose selection; it may be useful to monitor renal function.

➤*Renal function impairment:* Administer levofloxacin with caution in the presence of renal insufficiency. Careful clinical observation and appropriate laboratory studies should be performed prior to and during therapy because elimination of levofloxacin may be reduced.

The following dosage adjustments are according to the prescribing information:

Levofloxacin Dosage in Adults With Renal Function Impairment (CrCl < 50 mL/min)			
Dosage in healthy renal function every 24 h	CrCl 20 to 49 mL/min	CrCl 10 to 19 mL/min	Hemodialysis or CAPD[a]
750 mg	750 mg every 48 h	750 mg initial dose, then 500 mg every 48 h	750 mg initial dose, then 500 mg every 48 h
500 mg	500 mg initial dose, then 250 mg every 24 h	500 mg initial dose, then 250 mg every 48 h	500 mg initial dose, then 250 mg every 48 h
250 mg	No dosage adjustment required.	250 mg every 48 h. If treating uncomplicated UTI, no dosage adjustment is required.	No information on dosing adjustment is available.

[a] CAPD = chronic ambulatory peritoneal dialysis.

Adults receiving continuous renal replacement therapy (CRRT) – One reference suggests a dosage of 500 mg every 48 hours.

The following alternative recommendations assume ultrafiltration and dialysis flow rates of 1 to 2 L/h.

Loading dose: 500 to 750 mg IV.

Maintenance dosage:

• *Continuous venovenous hemofiltration (CVVH)* – 250 mg IV every 24 hours.

• *Continuous venovenous hemodialysis (CVVHD)* – 250 to 500 mg IV every 24 hours.

• *Continuous venovenous hemodialfiltration (CVVHDF)* – 250 to 750 mg IV every 24 hours.

Adults receiving intermittent hemodialysis (IHD) – See the previous table for recommendations according to the prescribing information. An alternative dosage is 250 to 500 mg IV every 48 hours administered after the dialysis session. This recommendation assumes the patient is receiving standard IHD 3 times per week and completes the full dialysis sessions.

➤*Preparation for administration:* Samples containing visible particles should be discarded.

Single-use vials – The single-use vials require dilution prior to administration. The concentration of the resulting diluted solution should be 5 mg/mL prior to administration (see Admixture Compatibility).

Because no preservative or bacteriostatic agent is present in this product, aseptic technique must be used in preparation of the final IV solution. Because the vials are for single-use only, discard any unused portion remaining in the vial. When used to prepare two 250 mg doses from the 20 mL vial containing levofloxacin 500 mg, withdraw the full content of the vial at once using a single-entry procedure, and a second dose should be prepared and stored for subsequent use.

Prepare the desired dosage of levofloxacin according to the following table.

Levofloxacin IV Preparation			
Desired dosage strength	Withdraw volume from appropriate vial	Volume of diluent	Infusion time (min)
250 mg	10 mL (20 mL vial)	40 mL	60
500 mg	20 mL (20 mL vial)	80 mL	60
750 mg	30 mL (30 mL vial)	120 mL	90

For example, to prepare a 500 mg dose using the 20 mL vial (25 mg/mL), withdraw 20 mL and dilute with a compatible IV solution to a total volume of 100 mL.

Premix in single-use flexible containers – Levofloxacin is also supplied in flexible containers within a foil overwrap. These contain a premixed, ready-to-use levofloxacin solution in dextrose 5% for single use. The concentration of each premixed levofloxacin container is 5 mg/mL. No further dilution of these preparations is necessary. Because the premix flexible containers are for single use only, any unused portion should be discarded.

➤*Administration:* Levofloxacin injection should be slowly infused IV over a period of at least 60 or 90 minutes, depending on the dosage. Rapid or bolus IV infusion of levofloxacin has been associated with hypotension and must be avoided. It is not for intramuscular (IM), intrathecal, intraperitoneal, or subcutaneous administration.

➤*Admixture compatibility:*

Compatibility – Any of the following IV solutions may be used to prepare levofloxacin 5 mg/mL solution with the following approximate pH values:

Levofloxacin-Compatible IV Solutions	
IV fluids	Final pH of levofloxacin solution
Sodium chloride 0.9% injection	4.71
Dextrose 5% injection	4.58
Dextrose 5%/Sodium chloride 0.9% injection	4.62

LEVOFLOXACIN — INJECTION

Levofloxacin-Compatible IV Solutions	
IV fluids	Final pH of levofloxacin solution
Dextrose 5% in Ringer's lactate	4.92
Plasma-Lyte 56/Dextrose 5% injection	5.03
Dextrose 5%, sodium chloride 0.45%, and potassium chloride 0.15% injection	4.61
Sodium lactate injection (M/6)	5.54

Incompatibility – Because only limited data are available on the compatibility of levofloxacin IV with other IV substances, additives or other medications should not be added to levofloxacin in single-use vials/flexible containers or infuse simultaneously through the same IV line. If the same IV line is used for sequential infusion of several different drugs, flush the line before and after infusion of levofloxacin with an infusion solution compatible with levofloxacin and with any other drug administered via this common line.

Levofloxacin injection should not be coadministered with any solution containing multivalent cations (eg, magnesium) through the same line.

➤*Storage/Stability:*

Single-use vials – Store at 15° to 30°C (59° to 86°F); protect from light.

Stability of levofloxacin following dilution: Levofloxacin, when diluted in a compatible IV fluid to a concentration of 5 mg/mL, is stable for 72 hours when stored at or below 25°C (77°F) and for 14 days when stored under refrigeration at 5°C (41°F) in plastic IV containers. Solutions that are diluted in a compatible IV solution and frozen in glass bottles or plastic IV containers are stable for 6 months when stored at −20°C (−4°F). Thaw frozen solutions at room temperature (25°C [77°F]) or in a refrigerator (8°C [46°F]). Do not force thaw by microwave irradiation or water bath immersion. Do not refreeze after initial thawing.

Premix flexible containers – Store at or below 25°C (77°F); however, brief exposure of up to 40°C (104°F) does not adversely affect the product. Avoid excessive heat and protect from freezing and light.

MOXIFLOXACIN

Rx	**Avelox** (Schering-Plough)	**Tablets; oral:** 400 mg	As moxifloxacin hydrochloride. Lactose, PEG. (BAYER M400). Red, oblong. Film-coated. In 30s, UD 50s, and *ABC* packs of 5.
Rx	**Avelox I.V.** (Schering-Plough)	**Injection, solution:** 400 mg per 250 mL	As moxifloxacin hydrochloride. With sodium chloride 0.8% (34.2 mEq in 250 mL). Preservative free. In 250 mL single-use latex-free flexible premix bags.[a]

[a] No further dilution of this preparation is necessary.

MOXIFLOXACIN HYDROCHLORIDE — ORAL

For complete and comparative prescribing information, refer to the Fluoroquinolones class monograph.

WARNING

Fluoroquinolones, including moxifloxacin, are associated with an increased risk of tendinitis and tendon rupture in patients of all ages. This risk is further increased in older patients (usually older than 60 years), patients taking corticosteroid drugs, and patients with kidney, heart, or lung transplants.

Fluoroquinolones, including moxifloxacin, may exacerbate muscle weakness in persons with myasthenia gravis. Avoid moxifloxacin in patients with known history of myasthenia gravis.

Indications

Moxifloxacin is for the treatment of adults (18 years and older) with infections caused by susceptible strains of the designated microorganisms in the following conditions:

➤*Acute bacterial exacerbation of chronic bronchitis:* Caused by *Haemophilus influenzae, Haemophilus parainfluenzae, Klebsiella pneumoniae,* methicillin-susceptible *Staphylococcus aureus, Moraxella catarrhalis,* or *Streptococcus pneumoniae.*

➤*Acute bacterial sinusitis:* Caused by *H. influenzae, M. catarrhalis,* or *S. pneumoniae.*

➤*Community-acquired pneumonia:* Caused by *Chlamydia pneumoniae, H. influenzae, K. pneumoniae, M. catarrhalis,* methicillin-susceptible *S. aureus, S. pneumoniae* (including multidrug-resistant strains), or *Mycoplasma pneumoniae.* Multidrug-resistant *S. pneumoniae* (MDRSP) includes isolates previously known as penicillin-resistant *S. pneumoniae* (PRSP), and are strains resistant to 2 or more of the following antibiotics: penicillin (minimum inhibitory concentration [MIC], 2 mcg/mL or more), second-generation cephalosporins (eg, cefuroxime), macrolides, tetracyclines, and trimethoprim/sulfamethoxazole.

➤*Complicated intra-abdominal infections:* Including polymicrobial infections, such as abscess caused by *Bacteroides fragilis, Bacteroides thetaiotaomicron, Clostridium perfringens, Enterococcus faecalis, Escherichia coli, Peptostreptococcus* species, *Proteus mirabilis, Streptococcus anginosus,* or *Streptococcus constellatus.*

➤*Complicated skin and skin structure infections:* Caused by *E. coli, Enterobacter cloacae, K. pneumoniae,* or methicillin-susceptible *S. aureus.*

➤*Uncomplicated skin and skin structure infections:* Caused by methicillin-susceptible *S. aureus* or *Streptococcus pyogenes.*

➤*Off-label uses:*

Hospital-acquired pneumonia – [1] = Good documentation. According to American Thoracic Society (ATS)/Infectious Diseases Society of America (IDSA) practice guidelines for the management of adults with early-onset hospital-acquired pneumonia, ventilator-associated pneumonia, or health care–associated pneumonia and no known risk factors for multidrug-resistant pathogens, moxifloxacin is recommended as initial empiric therapy.

Infective endocarditis (adults) – [1] = Good documentation. Moxifloxacin can be used as a substitute for ciprofloxacin to treat endocarditis due to *H. parainfluenzae, Haemophilus aphrophilus, Haemophilus paraphrophilus, H. influenza, Actinobacillus actinomycetemcomitans, Cardiobacterium hominis, Eikenella corrodens, Kingella kingae,* and *Kingella denitrificans* (HACEK) organisms; however, fluoroquinolones are only recommended if patients are not able to tolerate cephalosporins or ampicillin.

Tuberculosis – [1] = Good documentation. The ATS, Centers for Disease Control and Prevention (CDC), and IDSA joint guidelines on the treatment of tuberculosis (TB) recommend oral or intravenous (IV) moxifloxacin 400 mg daily as a second-line agent. The Food and Drug Administration (FDA) has not approved moxifloxacin for the treatment of TB. The guideline states that, of the fluoroquinolones, levofloxacin, moxifloxacin, and gatafloxacin have the most activity against *Mycobacterium tuberculosis.* Data on long-term safety and tolerability of moxifloxacin, especially at dosages above 400 mg/day, are limited. Moxifloxacin can be used for resistant TB caused by organisms known or presumed to be sensitive to fluoroquinolones or when first-line drugs cannot be used because of intolerance. This recommendation is based on expert opinion.

Administration and Dosage

➤*Adults:*

Usual dosage – 400 mg once every 24 hours. The duration of therapy depends on the type of infection.

Moxifloxacin Dosing Recommendations		
Infection[a]	Dosage	Duration[b]
Acute bacterial exacerbation of chronic bronchitis	400 mg once daily	5 days
Acute bacterial sinusitis	400 mg once daily	10 days
Community-acquired pneumonia	400 mg once daily	7 to 14 days
Complicated intra-abdominal infections[c]	400 mg once daily	5 to 14 days
Complicated skin and skin-structure infections	400 mg once daily	7 to 21 days
Uncomplicated skin and skin-structure infections	400 mg once daily	7 days

[a] Caused by the designated pathogens (see Indications).
[b] Sequential therapy (IV to oral) may be instituted at the discretion of the health care provider.
[c] For complicated intra-abdominal infections, therapy should be initiated with the IV formulation.

Off-label dosing –

Hospital-acquired pneumonia: [1] = Good documentation. 400 mg IV once daily administered over 60 minutes, followed by a switch to 400 mg orally once daily. The switch to oral medication may be made at the health care provider's discretion, and the recommended duration of treatment is 7 to 8 days.

Infective endocarditis (adults): [1] = Good documentation.

• *HACEK infections* – Moxifloxacin can be substituted for ciprofloxacin for 4 weeks in native valve infections and for 6 weeks in prosthetic valve infections. Specific dosing for moxifloxacin is not provided in guidelines. The usual dosage of moxifloxacin is 400 mg daily.

Tuberculosis: [1] = Good documentation. 400 mg orally daily.

➤*Administration:* Moxifloxacin may be taken with or without food; drink fluids liberally. Administer oral doses of moxifloxacin at least 4 hours before or 8 hours after products, including antacids, containing magnesium or aluminum, iron or zinc, sucralfate, metal cations (eg, iron), multivitamins , and didanosine chewable/buffered tablets or pediatric powder for oral solution.

➤*Storage/Stability:* Store at 25°C (77°F); excursions are permitted to 15° to 30°C (59° to 86°F). Avoid high humidity.

MOXIFLOXACIN HYDROCHLORIDE — INJECTION

For complete and comparative prescribing information, refer to the Fluoroquinolones class monograph.

WARNING

Fluoroquinolones, including moxifloxacin, are associated with an increased risk of tendinitis and tendon rupture in all ages. This risk is further increased in older patients usually older than 60 years, patients taking corticosteroid drugs, and patients with kidney, heart, or lung transplants.

Fluoroquinolones, including moxifloxacin, may exacerbate muscle weakness in persons with myasthenia gravis. Avoid moxifloxacin in patients with known history of myasthenia gravis.

Indications

➤*Acute bacterial exacerbation of chronic bronchitis:* Caused by *Haemophilus influenzae*, *Haemophilus parainfluenzae*, *Klebsiella pneumoniae*, methicillin-susceptible *Staphylococcus aureus*, *Moraxella catarrhalis*, or *Streptococcus pneumoniae*.

➤*Acute bacterial sinusitis:* Caused by *H. influenzae*, *M. catarrhalis*, or *S. pneumoniae*.

➤*Community-acquired pneumonia:* Caused by *Chlamydia pneumoniae*, *H. influenzae*, *K. pneumoniae*, *M. catarrhalis*, methicillin-susceptible *S. aureus*, *S. pneumoniae* (including multidrug-resistant strains), or *Mycoplasma pneumoniae*. Multidrug-resistant *S. pneumoniae* (MDRSP) includes isolates previously known as penicillin-resistant *S. pneumoniae* (PRSP), and are strains resistant to 2 or more of the following antibiotics: penicillin (minimum inhibitory concentration [MIC], 2 mcg/mL or more), second-generation cephalosporins (eg, cefuroxime), macrolides, tetracyclines, and trimethoprim/sulfamethoxazole.

➤*Complicated intra-abdominal infections:* Including polymicrobial infections, such as abscess caused by *Bacteroides fragilis*, *Bacteroides thetaiotaomicron*, *Clostridium perfringens*, *Enterococcus faecalis*, *Escherichia coli*, *Peptostreptococcus* species, *Proteus mirabilis*, *Streptococcus anginosus*, or *Streptococcus constellatus*.

➤*Complicated skin and skin structure infections:* Caused by *E. coli*, *Enterobacter cloacae*, *K. pneumoniae*, or methicillin-susceptible *S. aureus*.

➤*Uncomplicated skin and skin-structure infections:* Caused by methicillin-susceptible *S. aureus* or *Streptococcus pyogenes*.

➤*Off-label uses:*

Hospital-acquired pneumonia – [1] = Good documentation. According to American Thoracic Society (ATS)/Infectious Diseases Society of America (IDSA) practice guidelines for the management of adults with early-onset hospital-acquired pneumonia, ventilator-associated pneumonia, or healthcare-associated pneumonia and no known risk factors for multidrug-resistant pathogens, moxifloxacin is recommended as initial empiric therapy.

Infective endocarditis (adults) – [1] = Good documentation. Moxifloxacin can be used as a substitute for ciprofloxacin to treat endocarditis due to *Haemophilus parainfluenzae*, *Haemophilus aphrophilus*, *Haemophilus paraphrophilus*, *Haemophilus influenza*, *Actinobacillus actinomycetemcomitans*, *Cardiobacterium hominis*, *Eikenella corrodens*, *Kingella kingae*, and *Kingella denitrificans* (HACEK) organisms; however, fluoroquinolones are only recommended if patients are not able to tolerate cephalosporins or ampicillin.

Tuberculosis – [1] = Good documentation. The ATS, Centers for Disease Control and Prevention (CDC), and IDSA joint guidelines on the treatment of tuberculosis (TB) recommend oral or intravenous (IV) moxifloxacin 400 mg daily as a second-line agent. The Food and Drug Administration (FDA) has not approved moxifloxacin for the treatment of TB. The guideline states that, of the fluoroquinolones, levofloxacin, moxifloxacin, and gatafloxacin have the most activity against *Mycobacterium tuberculosis*. Data on long-term safety and tolerability of moxifloxacin, especially at dosages above 400 mg/day, are limited. Moxifloxacin can be used for resistant TB caused by organisms known or presumed to be sensitive to fluoroquinolones or when first-line drugs cannot be used because of intolerance. This recommendation is based on expert opinion.

Administration and Dosage

➤*Adults:*

Usual dosage – 400 mg as an IV infusion once every 24 hours. The duration of therapy depends on the type of infection.

Moxifloxacin Dosing Recommendations

Infection[a]	Dosage	Duration[b]
Acute bacterial exacerbation of chronic bronchitis	400 mg once daily	5 days
Acute bacterial sinusitis	400 mg once daily	10 days
Community-acquired pneumonia	400 mg once daily	7 to 14 days
Complicated intra-abdominal infections[c]	400 mg once daily	5 to 14 days
Complicated skin and skin-structure infections	400 mg once daily	7 to 21 days
Uncomplicated skin and skin-structure infections	400 mg once daily	7 days

[a] Caused by the designated pathogens (see Indications).
[b] Sequential therapy (IV to oral) may be instituted at the discretion of the health care provider.
[c] For complicated intra-abdominal infections, therapy should be initiated with the IV formulation.

Off-label dosing –

Hospital-acquired pneumonia: [1] = Good documentation. 400 mg IV once daily administered over 60 minutes, followed by a switch to 400 mg orally once daily. The switch to oral medication may be made at the health care provider's discretion, and the recommended duration of treatment is 7 to 8 days.

Infective endocarditis (adults): [1] = Good documentation.

• *HACEK infections* – Moxifloxacin can be substituted for ciprofloxacin for 4 weeks in native valve infections and for 6 weeks in prosthetic valve infections. Specific dosing for moxifloxacin is not provided in guidelines. The usual dosage of moxifloxacin is 400 mg daily.

Tuberculosis: [1] = Good documentation. 400 mg IV daily.

➤*Preparation for administration:* No further dilution of this preparation is necessary. To prepare moxifloxacin premixed containers for administration, close flow-control clamp of administration set; remove cover from port at bottom of container; insert piercing pin from an appropriate transfer set (ie, one that does not require excessive force [eg, ISO-compatible administration set]) into port with a gentle twisting motion until pin is firmly seated. Refer to the complete directions that have been provided with the administration set.

➤*Administration:* Administer by IV infusion only, over a period of 60 minutes by direct infusion or through a Y-type IV infusion set that may already be in place. It is not intended for intra-arterial, intramuscular (IM), intrathecal, intraperitoneal, or subcutaneous administration. Rapid or bolus IV infusion must be avoided.

➤*Admixture compatibility:*

Compatibility – Moxifloxacin IV is compatible with the following IV solutions at ratios from 1:10 to 10:1: sodium chloride 0.9% injection, 1M sodium chloride injection, dextrose 5% injection, sterile water for injection, dextrose 10% for injection, Ringer's lactate for injection.

Incompatibility – Because only limited data are available on the compatibility of moxifloxacin with other IV substances, do not add additives or other medications to moxifloxacin or infuse them simultaneously through the same IV line. If the same IV line or a Y-type line is used for sequential infusion of other drugs, or if the "piggyback" method is used, flush the line before and after infusion of moxifloxacin with an infusion solution compatible with moxifloxacin as well as with other drug(s) administered via this common line.

➤*Storage/Stability:* Store at 25°C (77°F); excursions permitted to 15° to 30°C (59° to 86°F). Discard any unused portion. Do not refrigerate; product precipitates upon refrigeration.

GEMIFLOXACIN

Rx	**Factive** (Cornerstone)	**Tablets; oral:** 320 mg	As gemifloxacin mesylate. PEG. (GE 320). White to off-white, oval, scored. Film-coated. In UD 5s and 7s.

GEMIFLOXACIN MESYLATE — ORAL

For complete prescribing information, refer to the Fluoroquinolones group monograph.

WARNING

Fluoroquinolones, including gemifloxacin, are associated with an increased risk of tendinitis and tendon rupture in all ages. This risk is further increased in patients older than 60 years; in patients taking corticosteroid drugs; and in patients with kidney, heart, or lung transplants.

Fluoroquinolones, including gemifloxacin, may exacerbate muscle weakness in individuals with myasthenia gravis. Avoid gemifloxacin in patients with known history of myasthenia gravis.

Indications

➤*General information:* For the treatment of infections caused by susceptible strains of the designated microorganisms in the following conditions.

➤*Acute bacterial exacerbation of chronic bronchitis:* Caused by *Streptococcus pneumoniae, Haemophilus influenzae, Haemophilus parainfluenzae*, or *Moraxella catarrhalis*.

➤*Community-acquired pneumonia (mild to moderate):* Caused by *H. influenzae, M. catarrhalis, Mycoplasma pneumoniae, Chlamydia pneumoniae, Klebsiella pneumoniae*, or *S. pneumoniae* (including multidrug-resistant strains of *S. pneumoniae* [MDRSP]). MDRSP includes isolates previously known as penicillin-resistant *S. pneumoniae* (PRSP), and are strains resistant to 2 or more of the following antibiotics: penicillin (minimum inhibitory concentration [MIC] 2 mcg/mL or greater), second-generation cephalosporins (eg, cefuroxime), macrolides, tetracyclines, and trimethoprim/sulfamethoxazole.

Administration and Dosage

➤*Adults:*

Gemifloxacin Dosage Guidelines

Indication	Dose	Duration
Acute bacterial exacerbation of chronic bronchitis	One 320 mg tablet daily	5 days
Community-acquired pneumonia (mild to moderate severity)		
Caused by known or suspected *S. pneumoniae, H. influenzae, M. pneumoniae*, or *C. pneumoniae* infection	One 320 mg tablet daily	5 days
Caused by known or suspected MDRSP[a], *K. pneumoniae*, or *M. catarrhalis* infection	One 320 mg tablet daily	7 days

[a] MDRSP includes isolates previously known as PRSP, and are strains resistant to 2 or more of the following antibiotics: penicillin (MIC ≥ 2 mcg/mL), second-generation cephalosporins (eg, cefuroxime), macrolides, tetracyclines, and trimethoprim/sulfamethoxazole.

➤*Renal function impairment:* Dose adjustment in patients with creatinine clearance (CrCl) greater than 40 mL/min is not required. Modification of the dosage is recommended for patients with CrCl 40 mL/min or less.

Recommended Gemifloxacin Doses in Renal Function Impairment

CrCl	Dose
> 40 mL/min	See usual dosage
≤ 40 mL/min	160 mg every 24 hours

Dialysis – Patients requiring routine hemodialysis or continuous ambulatory peritoneal dialysis (CAPD) should receive 160 mg every 24 hours.

➤*Administration:* Gemifloxacin may be taken with or without food and should be swallowed whole with a liberal amount of liquid.

➤*Storage/Stability:* Store at 25°C (77°F); excursions are permitted to 15° to 30°C (59° to 86°F). Protect from light.

NORFLOXACIN

Rx	**Noroxin** (Merck)	**Tablets; oral:** 400 mg	(705). White to off-white, oval. Film-coated. In 100s and UD 20s.

NORFLOXACIN — ORAL

For complete and comparative prescribing information, refer to the Fluoroquinolones class monograph.

WARNING

Tendinitis and tendon rupture – Fluoroquinolones, including norfloxacin, are associated with an increased risk of tendinitis and tendon rupture in all ages. This risk is further increased in older patients, usually older than 60 years, in patients taking corticosteroid drugs, and in patients with kidney, heart, or lung transplants.

Myasthenia gravis – Fluoroquinolones, including norfloxacin, may exacerbate muscle weakness in persons with myasthenia gravis. Avoid norfloxacin in patients with known history of myasthenia gravis.

Indications

➤*General information:* For the treatment of adults with the following infections caused by susceptible strains of the designated microorganisms:

➤*Prostatitis:* Prostatitis caused by *Escherichia coli*.

➤*Sexually transmitted diseases:* Uncomplicated urethral and cervical gonorrhea caused by *Neisseria gonorrhoeae*.

➤*Urinary tract infections:* Uncomplicated urinary tract infections (UTIs) (including cystitis) caused by *Enterococcus faecalis, E. coli, Klebsiella pneumoniae, Proteus mirabilis, Pseudomonas aeruginosa, Staphylococcus epidermidis, Staphylococcus saprophyticus, Citrobacter freundii, Enterobacter aerogenes, Enterobacter cloacae, Proteus vulgaris, Staphylococcus aureus*, or *Streptococcus agalactiae*.

Complicated UTIs caused by *Enterococcus faecalis, E. coli, K. pneumoniae, P. mirabilis, P. aeruginosa*, or *Serratia marcescens*.

➤*Off-label uses:*

Traveler's diarrhea – [1] = Good documentation. Antibiotics have been shown to shorten the duration of traveler's diarrhea and may also be used in moderate or severe cases; however, because of increased antibiotic resistance, doxycycline is no longer recommended for the treatment of traveler's diarrhea. Current guidelines suggest that mild cases of traveler's diarrhea should be managed with adequate hydration and bismuth subsalicylate or loperamide. (See Administration and Dosage.)

Administration and Dosage

➤*General dosing considerations:* Norfloxacin should be taken with a glass of water. Patients receiving norfloxacin should be well hydrated.

Norfloxacin should not be taken within 2 hours of multivitamins, other products containing iron or zinc, antacids containing magnesium and aluminum, sucralfate, or didanosine chewable/buffered tablets or the powder for oral solution.

➤*Adults:*

Norfloxacin Recommended Adult Dosage

Infection	Description	Unit dose	Frequency	Duration	Daily dose
Prostatitis	Acute or chronic	400 mg	every 12 h	28 days	800 mg
Sexually transmitted diseases	Uncomplicated gonorrhea	800 mg	single dose	1 day	800 mg
Urinary tract	Uncomplicated UTIs (cystitis) caused by *E. coli, K. pneumoniae*, or *P. mirabilis*	400 mg	every 12 h	3 days	800 mg
	Uncomplicated UTIs caused by other indicated organisms	400 mg	every 12 h	7 to 10 days	800 mg
	Complicated UTIs	400 mg	every 12 h	10 to 21 days	800 mg

Concomitant therapy – Multivitamins, other products containing iron or zinc, antacids, sucralfate, or didanosine chewable/buffered tablets or the powder for oral solution should not be taken within 2 hours of administration of norfloxacin.

Off-label dosing –

Traveler's diarrhea: [1] = Good documentation. 400 mg twice daily for 3 days.

➤*Elderly:* Elderly patients being treated for UTIs who have a creatinine clearance (CrCl) of 30 mL/min per 1.73 m^2 or less should receive 400 mg once daily.

➤*Renal function impairment:* In patients with CrCl rate of 30 mL/min per 1.73 m^2 or less, the recommended dosage is one 400 mg tablet once daily for the duration previously specified. At this dosage, the urinary concentration exceeds the minimal inhibitory concentrations (MICs) for most urinary pathogens susceptible to norfloxacin, even when the CrCl is less than 10 mL/min per 1.73 m^2.

➤*Administration:* Administer norfloxacin at least 1 hour before or at least 2 hours after a meal or ingestion of milk or other dairy products. Patients should take norfloxacin with a glass of water. Patients receiving norfloxacin should be well hydrated.

➤*Storage/Stability:* Store at 25°C (77°F); excursions are permitted to between 15° and 30°C (59° and 86°F). Keep container tightly closed.

OFLOXACIN

Rx	**Ofloxacin** (Various, eg, Par, Ranbaxy)	**Tablets; oral:** 200 mg	May contain lactose, PEG 400. Lt. yellow, oval. Film-coated. In 100s.
Rx	**Floxin** (Ortho-McNeil)		Lactose. (Floxin 200). Lt. yellow. Film-coated. In 50s and UD 6s and 100s.
Rx	**Ofloxacin** (Various, eg, Par, Ranbaxy)	**Tablets; oral:** 300 mg	May contain lactose, PEG 400. White to off-white, oval. Film-coated. In 100s.
Rx	**Floxin** (Ortho-McNeil)		Lactose. (Floxin 300). White. Film-coated. In 50s and UD 100s.
Rx	**Ofloxacin** (Various, eg, Par, Ranbaxy)	**Tablets; oral:** 400 mg	(93 7182). Pale gold, oval. Film-coated. In 100s.
Rx	**Floxin** (Ortho-McNeil)		Lactose. (Floxin 400). Pale gold. Film-coated. In 100s and UD 100s.

OFLOXACIN — ORAL

For complete and comparative prescribing information, refer to the Fluoroquinolones group monograph.

WARNING

Tendonitis and tendon rupture – Fluoroquinolones, including ofloxacin, are associated with an increased risk of tendinitis and tendon rupture in all ages. This risk is further increased in older patients (usually older than 60 years), patients taking corticosteroid drugs, and patients with kidney, heart, or lung transplants.

Myasthenia gravis – Fluoroquinolones, including ofloxacin, may exacerbate muscle weakness in persons with myasthenia gravis. Avoid ofloxacin in patients with a known history of myasthenia gravis.

Indications

➤*General information:* To reduce the development of drug-resistant bacteria and maintain the effectiveness of ofloxacin tablets and other antibacterial drugs, use ofloxacin tablets only to treat or prevent infections that are proven or strongly suspected to be caused by susceptible bacteria. When culture and susceptibility information are available, consider them in selecting or modifying antibacterial therapy. In the absence of such data, local epidemiology and susceptibility patterns may contribute to the empiric selection of therapy.

For the treatment of adults with mild to moderate infections (unless otherwise indicated) caused by susceptible strains of the following designated microorganisms in the infections listed.

➤*Acute bacterial exacerbations of chronic bronchitis:* Due to *Haemophilus influenzae* or *Streptococcus pneumoniae*.

➤*Acute pelvic inflammatory disease (including severe infection):* Due to *Chlamydia trachomatis* and/or *Neisseria gonorrhoeae*.

➤*Acute, uncomplicated urethral and cervical gonorrhea:* Due to *N. gonorrhoeae*.

➤*Community-acquired pneumonia:* Due to *H. influenzae* or *S. pneumoniae*.

➤*Complicated urinary tract infections:* Due to *Escherichia coli, Klebsiella pneumoniae, Proteus mirabilis, Citrobacter diversus*, or *Pseudomonas aeruginosa*. Although treatment of infections due to *C. diversus* and *P. aeruginosa* in this organ system demonstrated a clinically significant outcome, efficacy was studied in fewer than 10 patients.

➤*Mixed infections of the urethra and cervix:* Due to *C. trachomatis* and *N. gonorrhoeae*.

➤*Nongonococcal urethritis and cervicitis:* Due to *C. trachomatis*.

➤*Prostatitis:* Due to *E. coli*.

➤*Uncomplicated cystitis:* Due to *C. diversus, Enterobacter aerogenes, E. coli, K. pneumoniae, P. mirabilis*, or *P. aeruginosa*.

➤*Uncomplicated skin and skin structure infections:* Due to *Staphylococcus aureus* (methicillin-susceptible), *S. pyogenes*, or *P. mirabilis*.

➤*Off-label uses:*

Epididymitis – [1] = Good documentation. Centers for Disease Control and Prevention (CDC) guidelines recommend ofloxacin as a regimen for cases of epididymitis likely to be caused by enteric organisms, or those confirmed negative for gonococcal infection.

Pelvic inflammatory disease – [1] = Good documentation. The CDC guidelines advise ofloxacin as a recommended regimen for cases of pelvic inflammatory disease (PID) in which parenteral cephalosporin therapy is not feasible. Low risk of gonococcal infection and specific testing for gonorrhea are mandatory with the use of ofloxacin for PID because of concerns of fluoroquinolone-resistant infections.

Traveler's diarrhea – [1] = Good documentation. Antibiotics have been shown to shorten the duration of traveler's diarrhea and may also be used in moderate or severe cases; however, because of increased antibiotic resistance, doxycycline is no longer recommended for the treatment of traveler's diarrhea. Current guidelines suggest that mild cases of traveler's diarrhea should be managed with adequate hydration and bismuth subsalicylate or loperamide.

Administration and Dosage

➤*Adults:*

Usual dosage – 200 mg to 400 mg orally every 12 hours.

Infections – For a list of infections, see Indications.

Usual dosage:

Ofloxacin Oral Dosage Guidelines[a]

Infection[b]	Unit dose	Frequency	Duration	Daily dose
Acute bacterial exacerbation of chronic bronchitis	400 mg	every 12 h	10 days	800 mg
Acute pelvic inflammatory disease	400 mg	every 12 h	10 to 14 days	800 mg
Acute, uncomplicated urethral and cervical gonorrhea	400 mg	single dose	1 day	400 mg
Community-acquired pneumonia	400 mg	every 12 h	10 days	800 mg
Complicated UTIs	200 mg	every 12 h	10 days	400 mg
Mixed infection of the urethra and cervix due to *C. trachomatis* and *N. gonorrhoeae*	300 mg	every 12 h	7 days	600 mg
Nongonococcal cervicitis/urethritis due to *C. trachomatis*	300 mg	every 12 h	7 days	600 mg
Prostatitis due to *E. coli*	300 mg	every 12 h	6 weeks	600 mg
Uncomplicated cystitis due to *E. coli* or *K. pneumoniae*	200 mg	every 12 h	3 days	400 mg
Uncomplicated cystitis due to other approved pathogens	200 mg	every 12 h	7 days	400 mg
Uncomplicated skin and skin structure infections	400 mg	every 12 h	10 days	800 mg

[a] Dosing recommendations in patients with healthy renal function (creatinine clearance [CrCl] 50 mL/min or less).
[b] Due to the designated pathogens. See Indications.

Concomitant therapy: Antacids containing calcium, magnesium, or aluminum; sucralfate; divalent or trivalent cations such as iron; multivitamins containing zinc; or didanosine chewable/buffered tablets or the powder for oral solution should not be taken within 2 hours before or 2 hours after taking ofloxacin.

Off-label dosing –

Epididymitis: [1] = Good documentation. 300 mg orally twice daily for 10 days.

Pelvic inflammatory disease: [1] = Good documentation. 400 mg orally twice daily for 14 days. May be given in conjunction with metronidazole 500 mg orally twice daily for 14 days when concerns of anaerobic infection exist.

Traveler's diarrhea: [1] = Good documentation. 200 mg twice daily for 3 days.

➤*Children:*

Off-label dosing –

Pelvic inflammatory disease: [1] = Good documentation.

• *Adolescents* – 400 mg orally twice daily for 14 days. May be given in conjunction with metronidazole 500 mg orally twice daily for 14 days when concerns of anaerobic infection exist.

➤*Elderly:* Dosage adjustment is necessary for elderly patients with impaired renal function.

➤*Renal function impairment:* Dosage should be adjusted for patients with a CrCl of 50 mL/min or less. After a normal initial dose, dosage should be adjusted as follows:

CrCl 20 to 50 mL/min – Usual maintenance dose administered every 24 hours.

CrCl less than 20 mL/min – Half the usual recommended dose administered every 24 hours.

OFLOXACIN — ORAL

➤*Hepatic function impairment:* The excretion of ofloxacin may be reduced in patients with severe hepatic function disorders (eg, cirrhosis with or without ascites). A maximum dosage of ofloxacin 400 mg/day should therefore not be exceeded.

➤*Storage/Stability:* Dispense in a tight, light-resistant container. Store at 20° to 25°C (68° to 77°F).

TETRACYCLINES

Refer to the Gastrointestinal Agents chapter for additional information regarding tetracycline use in periodontitis.

Indications

➤*General information:* Refer to individual agents for more specific information.

➤*Gram-negative organisms:* *Haemophilus ducreyi* (chancroid); *Francisella tularensis* (tularemia); *Yersinia pestis* (plague); *Bartonella bacilliformis* (bartonellosis); *Campylobacter fetus*; *Vibrio cholerae* (cholera); *Brucella* sp. (brucellosis, may be in conjunction with streptomycin); *Calymmatobacterium granulomatis* (granuloma inguinale).

➤*Infections caused by the following miscellaneous microorganisms:* *Rickettsiae* (Rocky Mountain spotted fever, typhus fever and the typhus group, Q fever, rickettsialpox, and tick fevers); *Mycoplasma pneumoniae* (PPLO, Eaton agent, respiratory tract infections); *Chlamydia trachomatis* (lymphogranuloma venereum, trachoma [infectious agent not always eliminated], inclusion conjunctivitis, uncomplicated urethral, endocervical, or rectal infections); *Chlamydia psittaci* (psittacosis [ornithosis]); *Borrelia* sp. (relapsing fever); *Ureaplasma urealyticum* (nongonococcal urethritis).

➤*Following susceptibility testing (resistance has been documented):* *Escherichia coli*; *Enterobacter aerogenes*; *Acinetobacter* sp.; *Haemophilus influenzae* (respiratory tract infections); *Klebsiella* sp. (respiratory and urinary infections); *Streptococcus pneumoniae* (upper respiratory tract infections); *S. pyogenes*, *S. pneumoniae*, *Mycoplasma pneumoniae* (Eaton agent), and *Klebsiella* sp. (lower respiratory tract infections); *Staphylococcus aureus*, *S. pyogenes* (skin and skin structure infections); *Bacteroides* and *Shigella* sp.

➤*Alternative therapy for the following infections when penicillin is contraindicated:* Uncomplicated gonorrhea due to *Neisseria gonorrhoeae*; syphilis due to *Treponema pallidum*; yaws due to *T. pertenue*; *Listeria monocytogenes*; anthrax due to *Bacillus anthracis*; Vincent's infection due to *Fusobacterium fusiforme*; actinomycosis due to *Actinomyces* sp.; *Clostridium* sp.

➤*Acute intestinal amebiasis:* Due to *Entamoeba histolytica* as adjunct to amebicides.

➤*Severe acne (tetracycline, doxycycline, minocycline only):* As adjunctive therapy.

➤*Anthrax, including inhalational anthrax (doxycline only):* To reduce the incidence or progression of disease following exposure to aerosolized *Bacillus anthracis*.

➤*Malaria (doxycycline only):* Prophylaxis of malaria due to *Plasmodium falciparum* in short-term travelers (less than 4 months) to areas with chloroquine and/or pyrimethamine-sulfadoxine resistant strains.

➤*Neisseria meningitidis (minocycline only):* Treatment of asymptomatic meningococcal carriers of *N. meningitidis*.

➤*Note:* Do not use tetracyclines for streptococcal disease unless organism has been shown to be susceptible. Tetracyclines are not the drugs of choice in treatment of any type of staphylococcal infection.

➤*Off-label uses:* Refer to individual monographs for further information.

Inappropriate secretion of antidiuretic hormone –
Demeclocycline: [1] = Good documentation.

Infective endocarditis (adults) –
Doxycycline: [1] = Good documentation.
Minocycline: [2] = Fair documentation.

Infective endocarditis (children/adolescents) –
Doxycycline: [1] = Good documentation.

Lyme disease –
Doxycycline: [1] = Good documentation.

Pelvic inflammatory disease – [1] = Good documentation.

Proctitis, proctocolitis, enteritis –
Doxycycline: [1] = Good documentation.

Rheumatoid arthritis –
Doxycycline: [4] = Insufficient documentation.
Minocycline: [2] = Fair documentation.

Traveler's diarrhea –
Doxycycline: [5] = Poor documentation.

Other possible off-label uses –
Tetracycline: In conjunction with metronidazole for the treatment of extraintestinal amebiasis caused by *E. histolytica*; gonococcal arthritis; early Lyme disease; malaria; ocular rosacea; adjunctive therapy for peptic ulcers due to *Helicobacter pylori* (500 mg 4 times/day).

Doxycycline: Treatment of malaria (100 mg twice daily for 7 days in combination with other antimalarial agents), pleural malignant effusions, alternative agent for nocardiosis in patients who cannot take sulfa medications, ocular rosacea, treatment of traveler's diarrhea, prophylaxis of pneumothorax.

• *CDC-recommended treatment schedules for sexually transmitted diseases –*
Granuloma inguinale (donovanosis): 100 mg twice daily for at least 3 weeks.
Early syphilis: 100 mg twice daily for 14 days.
Latent syphilis: 100 mg twice daily for 28 days.
Chlamydial infections:
Adults and children (8 years of age and older) – 100 mg twice daily for 7 days.
Epididymitis most likely caused by gonococcal or chlamydial infection: 100 mg twice daily for 10 days plus a single dose of ceftriaxone 250 mg intramuscularly (IM).
Sexual assault prophylaxis: 100 mg twice daily for 7 days plus ceftriaxone and metronidazole.

Minocycline: Gallbladder infections caused by *E. coli*, alternative agent for nocardiosis in patients who cannot take sulfa medications, chronic malignant pleural effusion.

Administration and Dosage

Avoid rapid IV administration. Thrombophlebitis may result from prolonged IV therapy.

Continue therapy at least 24 to 48 hours after symptoms and fever subside. Treat all infections caused by group A β-hemolytic streptococci for 10 days or more.

Take on an empty stomach, at least 2 hours before or after meals. Absorption and peak plasma levels may be reduced when administered with meals or with dairy products, including milk.

Administer oral tetracyclines with plenty of fluids.

Actions

➤*Pharmacology:* The tetracyclines are bacteriostatic. They exert their antimicrobial effect by reversibly binding to the 30S subunit of the bacterial ribosome, preventing the binding of aminoacyl transfer RNA and inhibiting protein synthesis and thus cell growth. Tetracyclines are active against a wide range of gram-positive and gram-negative organisms and have similar antimicrobial spectra, and cross-resistance is common.

➤*Pharmacokinetics:*

Absorption/Distribution – Tetracyclines are adequately but incompletely absorbed from the GI tract. The percentage absorbed when taken on an empty stomach is lowest for **demeclocycline**, and **tetracycline**, and highest for **doxycycline** and **minocycline**. The extent of absorption is usually decreased by the presence of divalent and trivalent cations and to a variable degree by milk or food (see Drug Interactions). Tetracyclines are bound to plasma proteins in varying degrees.

Penetration of the tetracyclines into most body fluids and tissues is excellent. Tetracyclines are distributed in varying amounts into bile, liver, lung, kidney, prostate, urine, CSF, synovial fluid, mucosa of the maxillary sinus, brain, sputum, and bone. Inflammation of the meninges is not required for passage into the CSF, but concentrations may increase in the presence of inflamed meninges. Tetracyclines cross the placenta and enter the fetal circulation and amniotic fluid.

Metabolism/Excretion – The tetracyclines are concentrated in the bile by the liver. They are excreted in the urine and feces at high concentrations in a biologically active form. Because renal clearance of tetracyclines is by glomerular filtration, excretion is significantly affected by the state of renal function. The renal clearance of **demeclocycline** has been shown to be about half of that of tetracycline. The urinary and fecal recovery of **minocycline** is one half to one third that of other tetracyclines, and minocycline also appears to undergo some metabolism, largely to 9-hydroxyminocycline. **Doxycycline** appears to be excreted extensively by the digestive tract.

Tetracyclines Pharmacokinetics

Tetracyclines	Absorption (%)	C_{max} (mcg/mL)	T_{max} (h)	Protein binding (%)	Serum half-life (h)	Excreted in urine (%)
Demeclocycline	60% to 80%	1.5 to 1.7[a]	3 to 4[a]	35% to 90%	16	nd[b]
Doxycycline	90% to 100%	2.6 (hyclate)[c] 3.61 (monohydrate)[c] 3.6 (IV)[d]	2 (hyclate)[c] 2.6 (monohydrate)[c]	80% to 95%	18 to 22	40%

Tetracyclines Pharmacokinetics						
Tetracyclines	Absorption (%)	C_{max} (mcg/mL)	T_{max} (h)	Protein binding (%)	Serum half-life (h)	Excreted in urine (%)
Minocycline	90% to 100%	2.1 to 5.1[e]	1 to 4	75%	11 to 22 (oral) 15 to 23 (IV)	5% to 10%
Tetracycline	60% to 80%	nd	2 to 4	20% to 65%	6 to 12	20% to 55%

[a] 300 mg single oral dose.
[b] nd = no data
[c] 200 mg single oral dose.
[d] 200 mg administered IV over 2 hours.
[e] Single oral dose of two 100 mg pellet-filled capsules.

➤*Microbiology:*

Organisms Generally Susceptible to Tetracyclines[a]					
	Organism	Demeclocycline	Doxycycline	Minocycline	Tetracycline
Gram-positive	*Actinomyces* sp.	✓	✓		✓
	Alpha-hemolytic streptococci (Viridans group)		✓	✓	✓
	Bacillus anthracis	✓	✓	✓	✓
	Clostridium sp.	✓	✓	✓	✓
	Enterococcus faecalis[b,c]		✓	✓	✓
	E. faecium		✓	✓	✓
	Listeria monocytogenes	✓	✓	✓	✓
	Propionibacterium acnes		✓	✓	✓
	Staphylococcus aureus[d]	✓	✓	✓	✓
	Streptococcus pneumoniae[b]	✓	✓	✓	✓
	S. pyogenes[b,e]	✓	✓	✓	✓
	Treponema pallidum	✓	✓	✓	✓
	T. pertenue	✓	✓	✓	✓
Gram-negative	*Acinetobacter* sp.[b]	✓	✓	✓	✓
	Bacteroides sp.[b]	✓	✓	✓	✓
	Bartonella bacilliformis	✓	✓	✓	✓
	Borrelia recurrentis	✓	✓	✓	✓
	Brucella sp.	✓	✓	✓	✓
	Calymmatobacterium granulomatis	✓	✓	✓	✓
	Campylobacter fetus	✓	✓	✓	✓
	Enterobacter aerogenes[b]	✓	✓	✓	✓
	Escherichia coli[b]	✓	✓	✓	✓
	Francisella tularensis	✓	✓	✓	✓
	Fusobacterium fusiforme	✓	✓	✓	✓
	Haemophilus ducreyi	✓	✓	✓	✓
	H. influenzae[b]	✓	✓	✓	✓
	Klebsiella sp.[b]	✓	✓	✓	✓
	Neisseria gonorrhoeae	✓	✓	✓	✓
	N. meningitides		✓	✓	
	Shigella sp.[b]	✓	✓	✓	✓
	Vibrio cholerae	✓	✓	✓	✓
	Yersinia pestis	✓	✓	✓	✓
Miscellaneous	*Balantidium coli*				✓
	Chlamydia psittaci	✓	✓	✓	✓
	C. trachomatis	✓	✓	✓	✓
	Entamoeba sp.	✓	✓	✓	✓
	Mycobacterium marinum			✓	
	Mycoplasma pneumoniae	✓	✓	✓	✓
	Plasmodium falciparum[f]		✓		
	Rickettsiae sp.	✓	✓	✓	✓
	Ureaplasma urealyticum		✓	✓	✓

[a] Cross-resistance of these organisms to tetracyclines is common.
[b] Because many strains of gram-negative micro-organisms have been shown to be resistant to tetracyclines, culture and susceptibility testing are recommended.
[c] Up to 74% of *Enterococcus faecalis* have been found to be resistant to tetracyclines.
[d] Tetracyclines are not the drugs of choice in the treatment of any type of staphylococcal infections.
[e] Up to 44% of *Streptococcus pyogenes* have been found to be resistant to tetracycline drugs.
[f] Doxycycline has been found to be active against the asexual erythrocytic form of *Plasmodium falciparum* but not against the gametocytes of *P. falciparum*.

Contraindications

Hypersensitivity to any of the tetracyclines or components of product formulations.

Warnings/Precautions

➤*Malaria prophylaxis (doxycycline only):* **Doxycycline** offers substantial, but not complete, suppression of the asexual stages of *Plasmodium* strains. It does not suppress *P. falciparum*'s sexual blood stage gametocytes, and patients completing this prophylactic regimen may still transmit the infection to mosquitos outside endemic areas. Advise patients taking doxycycline for malaria prophylaxis as to when prophylaxis should begin and end; that no present-day antimalarial, including doxycycline, guarantees protection against malaria; and to avoid being bitten by mosquitos (eg, wear protective clothing, use effective insect-repellent and mosquito nets).

➤*Pseudomembranous colitis:* Treatment with antibacterial agents alters the normal flora of the colon and may permit overgrowth of clostridia. Pseudomembranous colitis has been reported with nearly all antibacterial agents and may range in severity from mild to life-threatening. It is important to consider this diagnosis in patients who present with diarrhea following subsequent administration of antibacterial agents. Once the diagnosis is established, initiate therapeutic measures. Mild cases usually respond to discontinuation of the drug. Moderate to severe cases may require management with fluids, electrolytes, protein supplementation, and treatment with an antibacterial agent effective against *Clostridium difficile* colitis.

➤*Parenteral therapy:* Reserve for situations in which oral therapy is not indicated. Institute oral therapy as soon as possible. If given IV over prolonged periods, thrombophlebitis may result. IM use produces lower blood levels than recommended oral dosages. If high blood levels are needed rapidly, administer IV.

➤*Nephrogenic diabetes insipidus:* Administration of **demeclocycline** has resulted in appearance of the diabetes insipidus syndrome (eg, polyuria, polydipsia, weakness) in some patients on long-term therapy. The syndrome has been shown to be nephrogenic, dose-dependent, and reversible on discontinuation of therapy.

➤*CNS effects:* In adults, pseudotumor cerebri (benign intracranial hypertension) has been associated with tetracycline use. Usual clinical manifestations are headache and blurred vision. Bulging fontanels have been associated with tetracycline use in infants. While both conditions and related symptoms usually resolve soon after tetracycline discontinuation, the possibility for permanent sequelae exists.

➤*Outdated products:* Under no circumstances should outdated tetracyclines be administered; the degradation products of tetracyclines are highly nephrotoxic and have, on occasion, produced a Fanconi-like syndrome.

➤*Hypersensitivity reactions:* Sensitivity reactions are more likely to occur in patients with a history of allergy, asthma, hay fever, or urticaria. Use tetracyclines with caution in these patients. Cross-sensitivity among the tetracyclines is extremely common.

➤*Sulfite sensitivity:* Some of these products contain sulfites that may cause allergic-type reactions (eg, anaphylactic symptoms, life-threatening or less severe asthmatic episodes) in certain susceptible people. The overall prevalence of sulfite sensitivity in the general population is unknown and probably low. It is seen more frequently in asthmatic or atopic nonasthmatic people. Specific products containing sulfites are identified in the product listings.

➤*Renal function impairment:* Use tetracyclines with caution in patients with impaired renal function.

If renal impairment exists, even usual doses may lead to excessive systemic accumulation of the tetracyclines (with the exception of **doxycycline**) and possible liver toxicity. Use lower than usual doses; if therapy is prolonged, drug serum level determinations may be advisable. Concurrent use of tetracycline and methoxyflurane has resulted in fatal renal toxicity.

The antianabolic action of tetracyclines may cause an increase in blood urea nitrogen. In significantly impaired renal function, higher serum tetracycline levels may lead to azotemia, hyperphosphatemia, and acidosis. This does not seem to occur with doxycycline.

➤*Hepatic function impairment:* Use tetracyclines with caution in patients with impaired liver function.

In the presence of renal dysfunction, and particularly in pregnancy, IV tetracycline more than 2 g/day has been associated with death secondary to liver failure. When need for intensive treatment outweighs its potential dangers (especially during pregnancy or in known or suspected renal and liver impairment), monitor renal and liver function tests. Serum tetracycline concentrations should not exceed 15 mcg/mL. Do not prescribe other potentially hepatotoxic drugs concomitantly.

Hepatotoxicity has been reported with **minocycline**; therefore, minocycline should be used with caution in patients with hepatic dysfunction and in conjunction with other hepatotoxic drugs.

The hazard of liver toxicity is of particular importance in parenteral administration to pregnant or postpartum patients with pyelonephritis.

➤*Hazardous tasks:* Light-headedness, dizziness, or vertigo may occur with tetracyclines. Advise patients to observe caution while driving or performing other tasks requiring alertness. These symptoms may disappear during therapy and always disappear rapidly when the drug is discontinued.

➤*Superinfection:* Use of antibiotics (especially prolonged or repeated therapy) may result in bacterial or fungal overgrowth of nonsusceptible organisms. Such overgrowth may lead to a secondary infection. Take appropriate measures if superinfection occurs. Superinfection of the bowel by staphylococci may be life-threatening.

➤*Photosensitivity:* Photosensitivity manifested by an exaggerated sunburn reaction has been observed in some individuals taking tetracyclines. Advise patients who are apt to be exposed to direct sunlight or ultraviolet light that this reaction can occur with tetracycline drugs, and discontinue treatment at the first evidence of skin erythema.

Exaggerated sunburn reactions are characterized by severe burns of exposed surfaces, resulting from direct exposure to sunlight during therapy with moderate or large doses. Phototoxic reactions are most frequent with demeclocycline and occur less frequently with the other tetracyclines.

➤*Pregnancy:* *Category D.* Tetracyclines readily cross the placenta, are found in fetal tissues, and can have toxic effects on the developing fetus (retardation of skeletal development). Evidence of embryotoxicity has also been noted in animals treated early in pregnancy.

A case-control study (18,515 mothers of infants with congenital anomalies and 32,804 mothers of infants with no congenital anomalies) shows a weak but marginally statistically significant association with total malformations and use of **doxycycline** any time during pregnancy. Sixty-three (0.19%) of the controls and 56 (0.3%) of the cases were treated with doxycycline. This association was not seen when the analysis was confined to maternal treatment during the period of organogenesis with the exception of a marginal relationship with neural tube defect based on only 2 exposed cases.

➤*Lactation:* Tetracyclines are excreted in breast milk. Milk:plasma ratios vary between 0.25 and 1.5. Because of the potential for serious adverse reactions, decide whether to discontinue nursing or the drug.

➤*Children:* Generally, do not use tetracyclines in children younger than 8 years of age (except for anthrax, including inhalational) unless other drugs are not likely to be effective or are contraindicated.

Teeth – The use of tetracyclines during the period of tooth development (from the last half of pregnancy through 8 years of age) may cause permanent discoloration (yellow, gray, brown) of teeth. This adverse reaction is more common during long-term use of the drugs, but has been observed following repeated short-term courses. Enamel hypoplasia has also been reported.

Bone – Tetracyclines form a stable calcium complex in any bone-forming tissue. Decreased fibula growth rate occurred in premature infants given oral tetracycline 25 mg/kg every 6 hours. This was reversible when the drug was discontinued.

➤*Monitoring:* In sexually transmitted diseases when coexistent syphilis is suspected, perform darkfield examination before starting treatment and repeat the blood serology monthly for at least 4 months.

In long-term therapy, perform periodic laboratory evaluation of organ systems, including hematopoietic, renal, and hepatic studies.

Drug Interactions

Tetracyclines Drug Interactions

Precipitant drug	Object drug[a]		Description
Antacids (containing aluminum, calcium or magnesium salts) Iron salts Zinc salts	Tetracyclines	⬇	Tetracyclines administered with aluminum, calcium, magnesium, iron, or zinc salts form an insoluble chelate, thereby decreasing the absorption and serum levels of the tetracycline. Administer tetracyclines at least 2 hours before or after these agents.
Barbiturates	Doxycycline	⬇	Barbiturates increase the hepatic metabolism of doxycycline, therefore decreasing doxycycline's half-life and serum levels. Adjust doxycycline dose as needed. Consider using an alternative tetracycline.
Bismuth salts	Tetracyclines	⬇	Coadministration of bismuth salts in liquid formulations may decrease the serum levels of tetracyclines. Give the bismuth salt 2 hours after the tetracycline.
Carbamazepine	Doxycycline	⬇	Carbamazepine may decrease the half-life and serum levels of doxycycline because of increased hepatic metabolism. Adjust doxycycline dose as needed. Consider using an alternative tetracycline.
Cholestyramine Colestipol	Tetracyclines	⬇	Coadministration may decrease or delay the absorption of tetracyclines, therefore decreasing the serum concentrations. Adjust the tetracycline dose if needed.
Phenytoin Rifamycins	Doxycycline	⬇	Phenytoin and rifamycins appear to induce the metabolism of doxycycline, causing the half-life to be significantly decreased. Increased doxycycline dosage may be needed.
Urinary alkalinizers (eg, sodium lactate, potassium citrate)	Tetracyclines	⬇	Coadministration may result in increased excretion of the tetracyclines and decreased serum levels. Separate administration by 3 to 4 hours; however, this may not be effective, and an increase in tetracycline dose may be necessary if the pH of the urine remains increased.

Tetracyclines Drug Interactions			
Precipitant drug	Object drug[a]		Description
Tetracyclines	Anticoagulants, oral	↑	The action of oral anticoagulants may be increased because of the elimination of vitamin K-producing gut bacteria by tetracyclines. Monitor coagulation parameters and adjust anticoagulant dose as needed.
Tetracyclines	Contraceptives, oral	↓	Tetracyclines may interfere with the enterohepatic recirculation of certain contraceptive steroids, leading to reduced efficacy. Although infrequently reported, contraceptive failure is possible.
Tetracyclines	Digoxin	↑	Coadministration may result in increased serum levels of digoxin in a small subset of patients (≈ 10%). Monitor digoxin levels and signs of toxicity.
Tetracyclines	Insulin	↑	The ability of insulin to produce hypoglycemia may be potentiated. In diabetic patients, monitor blood glucose concentrations closely and tailor the insulin regimen as needed.
Tetracyclines	Isotretinoin	↑	Isotretinoin use has been associated with a number of cases of pseudotumor cerebri, some of which involved coadministration of tetracyclines. Therefore, avoid concomitant use.
Tetracyclines	Methoxyflurane	↑	Coadministration may enhance the risk for renal toxicity; deaths have been reported. Do not coadminister. If possible seek alternative agents.
Tetracyclines	Penicillins	↓	The bacteriostatic action of tetracyclines may interfere with the bactericidal activity of penicillins. Consider avoiding this combination if at all possible.
Tetracyclines	Theophyllines	↑	The incidence of adverse reactions to theophyllines may be increased. Monitor theophylline levels and adjust dose as needed.

[a] ↑ = object drug increased; ↓ = object drug decreased.

➤*Drug/Lab test interactions:* During **doxycycline** or **minocycline** therapy, false elevations of urinary catecholamine levels may occur because of interference with the fluorescence test.

➤*Drug/Food interactions:* The administration of **demeclocycline** and **tetracycline** with milk and dairy products forms poorly absorbed chelates. A number of studies have reported the serum levels of these tetracyclines, when administered with milk products, to be 50% to 80% lower. Administer the interacting tetracyclines at least 2 hours before or after meals. The inhibitory effect of food and milk on the absorption of **doxycycline** and **minocycline** is considerably less than that observed with the other tetracycline derivatives. These 2 drugs are often administered without regard to meals, but the potential risk of decreased drug efficacy must be weighed against the benefit of treating the infection. The administration of doxycycline with a high-fat meal has been shown to delay the time to peak plasma concentrations by an average 1 hour 20 minutes. Peak plasma concentrations of doxycycline were also decreased by up to 20% with simultaneous ingestion of dairy products or a high-fat, high-protein meal. The peak plasma concentration of minocycline was slightly decreased and delayed by 1 hour when administered with food, compared with dosing under fasting conditions.

Adverse Reactions

The following adverse reactions have been reported with the tetracyclines.

➤*Oral:*

CNS – Bulging fontanel, convulsions, dizziness, headache, hypesthesia, paresthesia, pseudotumor cerebri, sedation, vertigo; myasthenic syndrome (**demeclocycline**; rare).

Dermatologic – Alopecia, balanitis, erythema multiforme, erythema nodosum, fixed drug eruptions, hyperpigmentation of the nails, maculopapular and erythematous rashes, photosensitivity, pruritus, skin and mucus membrane pigmentation, Stevens-Johnson syndrome, toxic epidermal necrolysis, vasculitis; exfoliative dermatitis (rare).

GI – Anorexia, diarrhea, dyspepsia, dysphagia, enamel hypoplasia, enterocolitis, esophageal ulcerations, esophagitis, glossitis, inflammatory lesions (with monilial overgrowth) in the anogenital region, nausea, pancreatitis, pseudomembranous colitis, stomatitis, vomiting; black hairy tongue, bulky loose stools, hoarseness, sore throat (**tetracycline**).

Due to oral **minocycline** and **doxycycline**'s virtually complete absorption, adverse reactions of the lower bowel, particularly diarrhea, have been infrequent.

Hematologic – Anemia, eosinophilia, hemolytic anemia, neutropenia, thrombocytopenia.

Hepatic – Hepatic cholestasis, hepatic toxicity, hyperbilirubinemia, increased liver enzymes; hepatic failure, hepatitis (rare).

Hypersensitivity – Anaphylactoid purpura, anaphylaxis, angioneurotic edema, pericarditis, polyarthralgia, pulmonary infiltrates with eosinophilia, systemic lupus erythematous exacerbation, urticaria.

Musculoskeletal – Arthralgia, arthritis, bone discoloration, joint stiffness and swelling, myalgia.

Renal – Acute renal failure, dose-related increase in BUN, interstitial nephritis; nephrogenic diabetes insipidus (**demeclocycline**).

Respiratory – Asthma exacerbation, bronchospasm, cough, dyspnea.

Miscellaneous – Brown-black microscopic discoloration of thyroid glands (prolonged therapy), decreased hearing, fever, lupus-like syndrome, secretion discoloration, serum sickness-like syndrome, tooth discoloration, tinnitus, vulvovaginitis.

➤*Parenteral:*

CNS – Bulging fontanels, convulsions, dizziness, headache, hypesthesia, paresthesia, pseudotumor cerebri, sedation, vertigo.

Dermatologic – Alopecia, balanitis, erythema multiforme, erythema nodosum, fixed drug eruptions, hyperpigmentation of the nails, injection site erythema and injection site pain, maculopapular and erythematous rashes, photosensitivity, pruritus, skin and mucus membrane pigmentation, Stevens-Johnson syndrome, toxic epidermal necrolysis, vasculitis; exfoliative dermatitis (rare).

GI – Anorexia, diarrhea, dyspepsia, dysphagia, enamel hypoplasia, enterocolitis, glossitis, inflammatory lesions (with monilial overgrowth) in the anogenital region, pancreatitis, pseudomembranous colitis, nausea, stomatitis, vomiting.

Hematologic – Agranulocytosis, eosinophilia, hemolytic anemia, leukopenia, neutropenia, thrombocytopenia, pancytopenia.

Hepatic – Hepatic cholestasis, hepatitis, hyperbilirubinemia, increased liver enzymes, jaundice, liver failure.

Hypersensitivity – Anaphylactoid purpura, anaphylaxis, angioneurotic edema, exacerbation of systemic lupus erythematous, myocarditis, pericarditis, pulmonary infiltrates, urticaria.

Musculoskeletal – Arthralgia, arthritis, bone discoloration, joint stiffness and swelling, myalgia, polyarthralgia.

Renal – Dose-related increase in BUN; acute renal failure, interstitial nephritis (**minocycline**).

Respiratory – Asthma exacerbation, bronchospasm, cough, dyspnea.

Miscellaneous – Brown-black microscopic discoloration of thyroid glands (prolonged therapy); hypersensitivity syndrome (cutaneous reaction, eosinophilia, and one or more of the following: fever, hepatitis, lymphadenopathy, myocarditis, nephritis, pericarditis, pneumonitis), lupus-like syndrome, secretion discoloration, serum sickness-like syndrome, tinnitus, tooth discoloration, vulvovaginitis.

Overdosage

➤*Symptoms:* Dizziness, nausea, and vomiting are the most commonly seen adverse reactions in overdosage situations.

➤*Treatment:* Discontinue medication and institute appropriate symptomatic treatment and supportive measures. Tetracyclines are not significantly removed by hemodialysis or peritoneal dialysis.

Patient Information

Advise patients to take medicine on an empty stomach, at least 2 hours before or after meals, with full glass of water (240 mL).

Instruct patients to avoid simultaneous dairy products (milk, cheese), antacids, laxatives, or iron-containing products. If these items must be taken, instruct them to take at least 2 hours before or 2 hours after tetracyclines.

Concurrent use of tetracyclines with oral contraceptives may render oral contraceptives less effective (see Drug Interactions).

Advise patients to avoid prolonged exposure to sunlight or sunlamps; tetracyclines may cause photosensitivity.

Caution patients who experience CNS symptoms about driving vehicles or using hazardous machinery while receiving therapy.

Advised patients to discard unused supplies of tetracycline antibiotics by the expiration date.

TETRACYCLINE HYDROCHLORIDE

Rx	**Tetracycline** (Various, eg, Ivax)	**Capsules:** 250 mg	In 100s, 1000s, and UD 100s.
Rx	**Sumycin '250'** (Par)		Mineral oil, lactose. (SQUIBB 655). Pink. In 100s and 1000s.
Rx	**Tetracycline HCl** (Various, eg, Ivax)	**Capsules:** 500 mg	In 100s, 1000s, and UD 100s.
Rx	**Sumycin '500'** (Par)		Mineral oil, lactose. (SQUIBB 763). Pink/White. In 100s and 500s.
Rx	**Sumycin Syrup** (Par)	**Oral Suspension:** 125 mg/5 mL	Saccharin, sodium metabisulfite, sorbitol, sucrose. Fruit flavor. In 473 mL.

TETRACYCLINE HYDROCHLORIDE — ORAL

Complete and comparative prescribing information for these products begins in the Tetracyclines group monograph.

Indications

➤*Gram-negative organisms:* *Haemophilus ducreyi* (chancroid); *Francisella tularensis* (tularemia); *Yersinia pestis* (plague); *Bartonella bacilliformis* (bartonellosis); *Campylobacter fetus*; *Vibrio cholerae* (cholera); *Brucella* sp. (in conjunction with streptomycin); *Calymmatobacterium granulomatis* (granuloma inguinale).

➤*Infections caused by the following miscellaneous organisms:* *Rickettsiae* (Rocky Mountain spotted fever, typhus fever and the typhus group, Q fever, rickettsialpox, tick fevers); *Mycoplasma pneumoniae* (respiratory tract infections); *Chlamydia trachomatis* (lymphogranuloma venereum, trachoma [infectious agent not always eliminated], inclusion conjunctivitis, uncomplicated urethral, endocervical, or rectal infections); *Chlamydia psittaci* (psittacosis [ornithosis]); *Borellia* sp. (relapsing fever); *Ureaplasma urealyticum* (nongonococcal urethritis).

➤*Following susceptibility testing (resistance has been documented):* *Escherichia coli*; *Enterobacter aerogenes*; *Acinetobacter* sp.; *Haemophilus influenzae* (upper respiratory tract infections); *Klebsiella* sp. (respiratory and urinary tract infections); *Streptococcus pneumoniae* (upper respiratory infections); *Streptococcus pyogenes*, *S. pneumoniae*, *Mycoplasma pneumoniae* (Eaton agent), and *Klebsiella* sp. (lower respiratory tract infections); *Staphylococcus aureus*, *S. pyogenes* (skin and skin structure infections); *Bacteroides* and *Shigella* sp.

➤*Alternative therapy for the following infections when penicillin is contraindicated:* Uncomplicated gonorrhea due to *Neisseria gonorrhoeae*; syphilis due to *Treponema pallidum*; yaws due to *Treponema pertenue*; *Listeria monocytogenes*; anthrax due to *Bacillus anthracis*; Vincent's infection due to *Fusobacterium fusiforme*; actinomycosis due to *Actinomyces* sp.; *Clostridium* sp.

➤*Acute intestinal amebiasis:* As adjunct to amebicides.

➤*Severe acne:* As adjunctive therapy.

➤*Off-label uses:* In conjunction with metronidazole for the treatment of extraintestinal amebiasis caused by *E. histolytica*; gonococcal arthritis; early Lyme disease; malaria; ocular rosacea; adjunctive therapy for peptic ulcers caused by *Helicobacter pylori* (500 mg 4 times/day).

Administration and Dosage

➤*Adults:*

Infections – For a list of infections, see Indications.

Usual dosage: 1 to 2 g/day in 2 or 4 equal doses.

Mild to moderate infections: 500 mg 2 times/day or 250 mg 4 times/day.

Severe infections: 500 mg 4 times/day.

Acne (severe, long-term therapy): Initially, 1 g/day in divided doses. For maintenance, give 125 to 500 mg/day. (Alternate-day or intermittent therapy may be adequate in some patients.)

Brucellosis: 500 mg 4 times/day for 3 weeks, accompanied by streptomycin 1 g IM twice daily the first week and once daily the second week.

Gonorrhea (uncomplicated): 500 mg every 6 hours for 7 days.

Syphilis:

• *Sumycin* only – A total of 30 to 40 g in equally divided doses over 10 to 15 days. Perform close follow-up and laboratory tests.

• *All except Sumycin* –

Early (less than 1 year): 500 mg 4 times/day for 15 days.

More than 1 year's duration: 500 mg 4 times/day for 30 days.

Urethral, endocervical, or rectal infections caused by C. trachomatis (uncomplicated): 500 mg 4 times/day for at least 7days.

➤*Children:*

Infections – For a list of infections, see Indications.

Older than 8 years of age: 25 to 50 mg/kg/day in 4 equally divided doses.

➤*Renal function impairment:* Decrease recommended dosages and/or extend dosing intervals in patients with renal impairment.

➤*Concomitant therapy:* Absorption is impaired by antacids containing aluminum, calcium, or magnesium, and preparations containing iron, zinc, or sodium bicarbonate.

➤*Duration of therapy:* Treat streptococcal infections for at least 10 days.

➤*Administration:* Take with plenty of fluids. Food and some dairy products interfere with the absorption of tetracycline. Take on an empty stomach at least 2 hours before or after meals.

➤*Storage/Stability:* Store below 30°C (86°F). Keep tightly closed. Protect from light; avoid excessive heat.

Outdated products – Under no circumstances should outdated tetracyclines be administered because the degradation of tetracyclines is highly nephrotoxic and has, on occasion, produced a Fanconi-like syndrome.

DEMECLOCYCLINE HYDROCHLORIDE

Rx	**Demeclocycline HCl** (Impax)	**Tablets:** 150 mg	Lactose. (G 2111). In 100s and 500s.
Rx	**Declomycin** (ESP Pharma)		(LL D11). Red. Film-coated. In 100s.
Rx	**Demeclocycline HCl** (Impax)	**Tablets:** 300 mg	Lactose. (G 2122). In 48s, 100s, and 500s.
Rx	**Declomycin** (ESP Pharma)		(LL D12). Red. Film-coated. In 48s.

DEMECLOCYCLINE HYDROCHLORIDE — ORAL

Complete and comparative prescribing information for these products begins in the Tetracyclines group monograph.

Indications

➤*Gram-negative organisms:* *Haemophilus ducreyi* (chancroid); *Francisella tularensis*; *Yersinia pestis*; *Bartonella bacilliformis*; *Campylobacter fetus*; *Vibrio cholerae*; *Brucella* sp. (in conjunction with streptomycin); *Calymmatobacterium granulomatis* (granuloma inguinale).

➤*Infections caused by the following miscellaneous organisms:* *Rickettsiae* (Rocky Mountain spotted fever, typhus fever and the typhus group, Q fever, rickettsialpox, tick fevers); *Mycoplasma pneumoniae* (PPLO, Eaton agent); *Chlamydia trachomatis* (lymphogranuloma venereum, trachoma [infectious agent not always eliminated], inclusion conjunctivitis); *Chlamydia psittaci* (psittacosis [ornithosis]); *Calymmatobacterium granulomatis* (granuloma inguinale); *Borellia recurrentis* (relapsing fever); *Bacteroides* sp.

➤*Following susceptibility testing (resistance has been documented):* *Escherichia coli*; *Enterobacter aerogenes*; *Acinetobacter* sp.; *Haemophilus influenzae* (respiratory tract infections); *Klebsiella* sp. (respiratory and urinary tract infections); *Streptococcus pneumoniae* (upper respiratory infections); *Streptococcus pyogenes*, *S. pneumoniae*, *Mycoplasma pneumoniae* (Eaton agent) and *Klebsiella* sp. (lower respiratory tract infections); *Staphylococcus aureus* (skin and skin structure infections); *Streptococcus pyogenes*; *Shigella* sp.

➤*Alternative therapy for the following infections when penicillin is contraindicated:* *Neisseria gonorrhoeae*; syphilis due to *Treponema pallidum*; yaws due to *Treponema pertenue*; *Listerial monocytogenes*; anthrax due to *Bacillus anthracis*; Vincent's infection due to *Fusobacterium fusiforme*; *Actinomyces* sp.; *Clostridium* sp.

➤*Acute intestinal amebiasis:* As an adjunct to amebicides.

➤*Off-label uses:*

Inappropriate secretion of antidiuretic hormone – [1] = Good documentation. Demeclocycline is recommended for patients who are refractory to fluid restriction. Although the medication has demonstrated efficacy, the risks associated with use require close monitoring by health care providers.

Administration and Dosage

➤*Adults:*

Infections – For a list of infections, see Indications.

Usual dosage: 150 mg 4 times daily or 300 mg twice daily.

Gonorrhea: For patients sensitive to penicillin, initial dose is 600 mg, followed by 300 mg every 12 hours for 4 days to a total of 3 g.

Off-label dosing –

Inappropriate secretion of antidiuretic hormone: [1] = Good documentation. 600 to 1,200 mg daily given in divided doses.

➤*Children:*

Infections – For a list of infections, see Indications.

Older than 8 years of age: 6.6 to 13.2 mg/kg (3 to 6 mg/lb), depending upon the severity of the disease, divided into 2 or 4 doses.

➤*Renal function impairment:* Administer tetracyclines cautiously with renal impairment; reduce the recommended dosage and/or extend the dosing interval.

DEMECLOCYCLINE HYDROCHLORIDE — ORAL

➤*Hepatic function impairment:* Administer tetracyclines cautiously with hepatic impairment; reduce the recommended dosage and/or extend the dosing interval.

➤*Concomitant therapy:* Absorption is impaired by antacids containing aluminum, calcium, or magnesium and by preparations containing iron. Take demeclocycline at least 1 hour before or 2 hours after these products.

➤*Duration of therapy:* Treat streptococcal infections for at least 10 days.

➤*Administration:* Take with plenty of fluids. Foods and some dairy products interfere with absorption; take demeclocycline at least 1 hour before or 2 hours after meals or dairy products.

➤*Storage/Stability:* Store at 20° to 25°C (68° to 77°F).

DOXYCYCLINE

Rx	**Doxycycline** (Various, eg, Ivax, Lannett Company, Inc)	**Tablets; oral:** 20 mg	As hyclate. May contain lactose. Film-coated. In 60s, 100s, and 1,000s.
Rx	**Alodox Convenience Kit** (OCuSOFT, Inc[a])		As hyclate. Lactose, polydextrose Film-coated. (MP 573). In 60s.
Rx	**Periostat** (CollaGenex)		As hyclate. Lactose. (PS 20). White. In 60s, 100s, and 1,000s.
Rx	**Doxycycline** (Various, eg, Lannett Company, Inc, Par)	**Tablets; oral:** 50 mg	As monohydrate. May contain corn starch, lactose. Yellow. Film-coated. In 100s.
Rx	**Doxycycline** (Par)	**Tablets; oral:** 75 mg	As monohydrate. Lactose. (par 092). Lt. orange. Film-coated. In 100s and 500s.
Rx	**Adoxa** (Doak)		As monohydrate. Lactose. (D 75). Lt. orange. Film-coated. In ADOXA Pak 31s.
Rx	**Doxycycline** (Various, eg, Lannett Company, Inc, Par)	**Tablets; oral:** 100 mg	As monohydrate. May contain corn starch, lactose. Yellow. Film-coated. In 50s and 250s.
Rx	**Doxycycline** (Various, eg, Ivax, Watson)		As hyclate. In 50s, 100s, 200s, 500s, and UD 100s.
Rx	**Adoxa** (Doak)		As monohydrate. Lactose. (D 100). Yellow. Film-coated. In ADOXA Pak 31s and 60s.
Rx	**Vibra-Tabs** (Pfizer)		As hyclate. (VIBRA-TABS PFIZER 099). Salmon. Film-coated. In 50s.
Rx	**Doxycycline** (Mylan)	**Tablets; oral:** 150 mg	As monohydrate. (M D 24). Orange. Film-coated. In 30s, 100s, and 500s.
Rx	**Adoxa** (Doak)		As monohydrate. Lactose. (D/D 150). Peach, scored. Film-coated. In ADOXA Pak 30s.
Rx	**Adoxa TT Kit** (Doak)		As monohydrate. Lactose. (D/D 150). Peach, scored. Film-coated. In ADOXA Pak 30s with 30 **Tersaseptic** facial cleansing pads.
Rx	**Doxycycline** (Mylan)	**Tablets, delayed-release; oral:** 75 mg	As hyclate. Lactose. (M D 31). White, round, scored. In 60s and 500s.
Rx	**Doryx** (Warner Chilcott)		As hyclate. Lactose. (D75). White, oval. In 60s.
Rx	**Doxycycline** (Mylan)	**Tablets, delayed-release; oral:** 100 mg	As hyclate. Lactose. (M D 32). White, round, scored. In 100s and 500s.
Rx	**Doryx** (Warner Chilcott)		As hyclate. Lactose. (D100). White, oval. In 100s and 500s.
Rx	**Doryx** (Warner Chilcott)	**Tablets, delayed-release; oral:** 150 mg	As hyclate. (D150). Lactose. White, oval, scored. In 60s.
Rx	**Oraxyl** (E5 Pharma)	**Capsules; oral:** 20 mg	As hyclate. (e5 131). Ivory. In 100s.
Rx	**Oracea** (Galderma)	**Capsules; oral:** 40 mg (30 mg immediate-release and 10 mg delayed-release)	Sugar spheres. (CGPI 40). Beige opaque. In 30s.
Rx	**Doxycycline** (Various, eg, Ivax, Watson)	**Capsules; oral:** 50 mg	As hyclate. In 50s and 500s.
Rx	**Doxycycline Monohydrate** (Watson)		As monohydrate. (WATSON 410 50 mg). White/ivory opaque. In 100s.
Rx	**Monodox** (Oclassen)		As monohydrate. (MONODOX 50 M 260). White/yellow. In 100s.
Rx	**NutriDox** (Advanced Vision Research)	**Capsules; oral:** 75 mg	As monohydrate. (75 mg RX615). Blue, opaque. In 30s and blister 1s, and in convenience kits with *TheraTears Nutrition* softgels and *iHeat* portable warm compress system.
Rx	**Doxycycline** (Various, eg, Ivax, Watson)	**Capsules; oral:** 100 mg	As hyclate. In 50s, 500s, and UD 100s.
Rx	**Doxycycline Monohydrate** (Watson)		As monohydrate. (WATSON 411 100 mg). Ivory/brown opaque. In 50s and 250s.
Rx	**Monodox** (Oclassen)		As monohydrate. (MONODOX 100 M 259). Yellow/brown. In 50s and 250s.
Rx	**Vibramycin** (Pfizer)		As hyclate. (VIBRA PFIZER 095). Lt. blue. In 50s.
Rx	**Adoxa** (Doak)	**Capsules; oral:** 150 mg	As monohydrate. (ADOXA 150 mg). Peach. In 60s.
Rx	**Adoxa CK Kit** (Doak)		As monohydrate. (ADOXA 150 mg). Peach. In 60s with 30 **Tersaseptic** facial cleansing pads.
Rx	**Doxycycline** (Eon)	**Capsules, coated pellets; oral:** 75 mg	As hyclate. Sugar spheres. (E 814). In 60s and 100s.
Rx	**Doryx** (Warner Chilcott)		As hyclate. (DORYX 75). Orange/Green. In 60s.
Rx	**Doxycycline** (Eon)	**Capsules, coated pellets; oral:** 100 mg	As hyclate. Sugar spheres. (E 815). In 50s and 100s.
Rx	**Doryx** (Warner Chilcott)		As hyclate. (DORYX WC). Dk. yellow/lt. blue. In 50s.
Rx	**Doxycycline** (Teva)	**Powder for suspension; oral:** 25 mg per 5 mL	As monohydrate. Parabens, maltodextrin, sucrose. Raspberry flavor. In 60 mL.
Rx	**Vibramycin** (Pfizer)		As monohydrate. Parabens, sucrose. Raspberry flavor. In 60 mL.
Rx	**Vibramycin** (Pfizer)	**Syrup; oral:** 50 mg per 5 mL	As calcium. Parabens, sodium metabisulfite, sorbitol. Apple-raspberry flavor. In 473 mL.

DOXYCYCLINE

Rx	**Atridox** (CollaGenex)	**Injection:** 42.5 mg (10%)	As hyclate. In 2 syringe mixing system and blunt cannula.
Rx	**Doxycycline** (Various, eg, Bedford)	**Injection, lyophilized, powder for solution:** 100 mg	As hyclate. In vials.
Rx	**Doxy 100** (APP)		As hyclate. 300 mg mannitol. In vials.
Rx	**Doxy 200** (APP)	**Injection, lyophilized, powder for solution:** 200 mg	As hyclate. 600 mg mannitol. In vials.

[a] OCuSOFT, Inc, P.O. Box 429, Richmond, TX 77406–0429; 1–800–233–5469; http://www.ocusoft.com

DOXYCYCLINE CALCIUM — ORAL

Complete and comparative prescribing information for these products begins in the Tetracyclines group monograph.

Indications

➤*Treatment of infections caused by miscellaneous organisms:* Rocky mountain spotted fever, typhus fever and the typhus group; Q fever, rickettsialpox, and tick fevers caused by Rickettsiae; respiratory tract infections caused by *Mycoplasma pneumoniae*; lymphogranuloma venereum caused by *Chlamydia trachomatis*; psittacosis (ornithosis) caused by *Chlamydia psittaci*; trachoma caused by *Chlamydia trachomatis*, although the infectious agent is not always eliminated as judged by immunofluorescence; inclusion conjunctivitis caused by *Chlamydia trachomatis*; uncomplicated urethral, endocervical or rectal infections in adults caused by *Chlamydia trachomatis*; nongonococcal urethritis caused by *Ureaplasma urealyticum*; and relapsing fever due to *Borrelia recurrentis*.

➤*Treatment of infections caused by gram-negative microorganisms:* Chancroid caused by *Haemophilus ducreyi*; plague due to *Yersinia pestis*; tularemia due to *Francisella tulerensis*; cholera caused by *Vibrio cholerae*; campylobacter fetus infections caused by *Campylobacter fetus*; brucellosis due to *Brucella* species (in conjunction with streptomycin); bartonellosis due to *Bartonella bacilliformis*; and granuloma inguinale caused by *Calymmatobacterium granulomatis*.

➤*Following susceptibility testing (resistance has been documented):* *Escherichia coli*; *Enterobacter aerogenes*; *Shigella* species; *Acinetobacter* species; respiratory tract infections caused by *Haemophilus influenzae*; respiratory tract and urinary tract infections caused by *Klebsiella* species; and upper respiratory tract infections caused by *Streptococcus pneumoniae*.

➤*Anthrax including inhalational anthrax:* Due to *Bacillus anthracis*, including inhalational anthrax (postexposure), to reduce the incidence or progression of disease following exposure to aerosolized *Bacillus anthracis*.

➤*Alternative therapy for infections when penicillin is contraindicated:* Uncomplicated gonorrhea caused by *Neisseria gonorrhoeae*; syphilis caused by *Treponema pallidum*; yaws caused by *Treponema pertenue*; listeriosis due to *Listeria monocytogenes*; Vincent's infection caused by *Fusobacterium fusiforme*; actinomycosis caused by *Actinomyces israelii*; and infections caused by *Clostridium* species

➤*Acute intestinal amebiasis:* In acute intestinal amebiasis, doxycycline may be a useful adjunct to amebicides.

➤*Severe acne:* In severe acne, doxycycline may be useful adjunctive therapy.

➤*Malaria prophylaxis:* Doxycycline is indicated for the prophylaxis of malaria due to *Plasmodium falciparum* in short-term travelers (under 4 months) to areas with chloroquine or pyrimethamine-sulfadoxine resistant strains. For adults, the recommended dose is 100 mg daily. For children over 8 years of age, the recommended dose is 2 mg/kg given once daily up to the adult dose. Prophylaxis should begin 1 to 2 days before travel to the malarious area. Prophylaxis should be continued daily during travel in the malarious area and for 4 weeks after the traveler leaves the malarious area.

➤*Off-label uses:*

Infective endocarditis – According to American Heart Association (AHA) guidelines, doxycycline is preferred in combination with gentamicin or rifampin for the treatment of confirmed *Bartonella* endocarditis.

Infective endocarditis (adults): [1] = Good documentation.

Infective endocarditis (children/adolescents): [1] = Good documentation.

Pelvic inflammatory disease – [1] = Good documentation. Centers for Disease Control and Prevention (CDC) guidelines advise use of doxycycline in treating pelvic inflammatory disease as part of a recommended regimen that includes a third-generation cephalosporin or ampicillin/sulbactam.

Proctitis, proctocolitis, enteritis – [1] = Good documentation. CDC guidelines recommend doxycycline in combination with ceftriaxone as a regimen for known or presumptive therapy of proctitis, proctocolitis, or enteritis. Cases of lymphogranuloma venereum (LGV)–associated disease will require a longer duration of therapy.

Rheumatoid arthritis – [4] = Insufficient documentation. Although in vitro and in vivo trials have demonstrated that doxycycline produces beneficial inhibition of collagenase activity, clinical benefit has not been firmly established. Results with oral doxycycline in the treatment of rheumatoid arthritis (RA) have been variable, demonstrating beneficial effects in 2 small studies but no clinical benefit in a more recent placebo-controlled trial. In addition, no trial has shown benefit in disease progression based on radiographic assessment. Optimal use with or without disease-modifying antirheumatic drugs has yet to be determined. Further studies are required to establish doxycycline's role, if any, in the management of RA. It should be noted that doxycycline therapy was not included in the most recent American College of Rheumatology Subcommittee on Rheumatoid Arthritis Guidelines.

Traveler's diarrhea – [5] = Poor documentation. Antibiotics have been shown to shorten the duration of traveler's diarrhea and may also be used in moderate to severe cases; however, because of increased antibiotic resistance, doxycycline is no longer recommended for the treatment of traveler's diarrhea. Current guidelines suggest that mild cases of traveler's diarrhea should be managed with adequate hydration and bismuth salicylate or loperamide.

Other possible off-label uses – Treatment of malaria (100 mg twice daily for 7 days in combination with other antimalarial agents); pleural malignant effusions; alternative agent for nocardiosis in patients who cannot take sulfa medications; ocular rosacea; prophylaxis of pneumothorax.

Lyme disease:

- *Arthritis* – 100 mg twice daily for 30 to 60 days.
- *Carditis (first degree AV block)* – 100 mg twice daily for 14 to 21 days.
- *Early Lyme disease* – 100 mg twice daily for 14 to 21 days.
- *Facial nerve paralysis* – 100 mg twice daily for 14 to 21 days.
- *Tick bite from endemic area* – 200 mg once.

CDC-recommended treatment schedules for sexually transmitted diseases:

- *Chlamydial infections (adults and children 8 years of age and older)* – 100 mg twice daily for 7 days.
- *Early syphilis* – 100 mg twice daily for 14 days.
- *Epididymitis most likely caused by gonococcal or chlamydial infection* – 100 mg twice daily for 10 days plus a single dose of ceftriaxone 250 mg intramuscularly (IM).
- *Granuloma inguinale (donovanosis)* – 100 mg twice daily for at least 3 weeks.
- *Latent syphilis* – 100 mg twice daily for 28 days.
- *Sexual assault prophylaxis* – 100 mg twice daily for 7 days plus ceftriaxone and metronidazole.

Administration and Dosage

➤*Adults:*

Infections – For a list of infections, refer to Indications.

Usual dosage: 200 mg on the first day of treatment (administered 100 mg by mouth every 12 hours) followed by a maintenance dose of 100 mg/day. The maintenance dose may be administered as a single dose or as 50 mg by mouth every 12 hours.

Severe infections: In the management of more severe infections (particularly chronic infections of the urinary tract), 100 mg every 12 hours is recommended.

Acute epididymo-orchitis caused by C. trachomatis or N. gonorrhoeae: 100 mg, by mouth, twice a day for at least 10 days.

Inhalational anthrax (postexposure): 100 mg, by mouth, twice a day for 60 days.

Malaria prophylaxis: 100 mg by mouth daily. Prophylaxis should begin 1 to 2 days before travel to the malarious area. Prophylaxis should be continued daily during travel in the malarious area and for 4 weeks after the traveler leaves the malarious area.

Nongonococcal urethritis caused by C. trachomatis or U. urealyticum: 100 mg by mouth twice a day for 7 days.

Syphilis (early): Patients who are allergic to penicillin should be treated with doxycycline 100 mg by mouth twice a day for 2 weeks.

Syphilis of more than 1 year's duration: Patients who are allergic to penicillin should be treated with doxycycline 100 mg by mouth twice a day for 4 weeks.

Uncomplicated gonococcal infections (except anorectal infections in men): 100 mg, by mouth, twice a day for 7 days. As an alternate single visit dose, administer 300 mg immediately followed in 1 hour by a second 300 mg dose.

Uncomplicated urethral, endocervical, or rectal infection caused by Chlamydia trachomatis: 100 mg by mouth twice a day for 7 days.

Off-label dosing –

Infective endocarditis (adults): [1] = Good documentation.

- *Suspected Bartonella infection with a negative culture* – 200 mg orally every 24 hours in 2 equally divided doses for 6 weeks in combination with gentamicin and ceftriaxone.
- *Documented Bartonella infection with a positive culture* – 200 mg orally every 24 hours in 2 equally divided doses for 6 weeks in combination with gentamicin or rifampin.

Pelvic inflammatory disease: [1] = Good documentation. 100 mg orally twice daily for 14 days in conjunction with a single dose of ceftriaxone, cefoxitin, or another third-generation parenteral cephalosporin. Metronidazole 500 mg orally twice daily may be added to the regimen if concerns of anaerobic infection exist.

Proctitis, proctocolitis, enteritis: [1] = Good documentation. 100 mg orally twice daily for 7 days. Doxycycline should be given in conjunction with a 1-time IM dose of ceftriaxone 125 mg. Persons diagnosed with LGV should receive 21 days of doxycycline therapy.

Rheumatoid arthritis: [4] = Insufficient documentation. 100 mg by mouth twice daily for 3 or 6 months. Doses of 150 mg/day also have been used.

DOXYCYCLINE CALCIUM — ORAL

Other possible off-label uses:

• *CDC recommended treatment schedules for sexually transmitted diseases (MMWR.* 2002 May 10;51 [No. RR-6]:1-84.) –

Epididymitis most likely caused by gonococcal or chlamydial infection: 100 mg by mouth twice daily for 10 days plus a single dose of ceftriaxone 250 mg IM.

Granuloma inguinale (donovanosis): 100 mg by mouth twice daily for at least 3 weeks.

Lymphogranuloma venereum: 100 mg by mouth twice daily for at least 21 days.

Sexual assault prophylaxis: 100 mg by mouth twice daily for 7 days plus ceftriaxone and metronidazole.

➤*Children:* For children 8 years of age and older weighing more than 100 lbs, the usual adult dose should be used. See Adults for dosing.

Infections – For a list of infections, see the Indications section.

8 years of age and older:

• *Usual dosage* – For children weighing less than or equal to 100 pounds, the dosage is 2 mg/lb of body weight divided into 2 doses on the first day of treatment, followed by 1 mg/lb of body weight given as a single daily dose or divided into 2 doses, on subsequent days.

• *Severe infections* – Up to 2 mg/lb of body weight may be used.

• *Malaria prophylaxis* – 2 mg/kg given once daily up to the adult dose. Prophylaxis should begin 1 to 2 days before travel to the malarious area. Prophylaxis should be continued daily during travel in the malarious area and for 4 weeks after the traveler leaves the malarious area.

Inhalational anthrax (postexposure): For children weighing less than 100 lbs (45 kg), the dosage is 1 mg/lb (2.2 mg/kg), by mouth, twice daily for 60 days. Children weighing 100 lb or more should receive the adult dose.

Off-label dosing –

Infective endocarditis (children/adolescents): [1] = Good documentation.

• *Suspected Bartonella infection with a negative culture* – 2 to 4 mg/kg orally every 24 hours in 2 equally divided doses for 6 weeks in combination with gentamicin and ceftriaxone.

• *Documented Bartonella infection with a positive culture* – 2 to 4 mg/kg orally every 24 hours in 2 equally divided doses for 6 weeks in combination with gentamicin or rifampin.

Pelvic inflammatory disease: [1] = Good documentation.

• *Adolescents* – 100 mg orally twice daily for 14 days in conjunction with a single dose of ceftriaxone, cefoxitin, or another third-generation parenteral cephalosporin. Metronidazole 500 mg orally twice daily may be added to the regimen if concerns of anaerobic infection exist.

CDC recommended treatment schedules for sexually transmitted diseases (MMWR. 2002 May 10;51 [No. RR-6]:1-84.):

• *Chlamydial infections* – For children 8 years of age and older, 100 mg by mouth twice daily for 7 days.

• *Anthrax* –

Younger than 8 years of age: 2.2 mg/kg/day divided twice daily. 200 mg/day.

➤*Duration of therapy:* When used in streptococcal infections, therapy should be continued for 10 days.

➤*Administration:* Administration of adequate amounts of non-dairy fluid along with capsule and tablet forms of drugs in the tetracycline class is recommended to wash down the drugs and reduce the risk of esophageal irritation and ulceration.

Absorption and peak plasma levels may be reduced when administered with meals or with dairy products, including milk.

If GI upset occurs, administration with a small amount of a low-fat, low-protein, non-dairy food may reduce upset, but the potential risk of decreased drug efficacy must be weighed against the benefit of treating the infection with this antibiotic.

➤*Storage/Stability:* Store below 30°C (86°F) and dispense in tight, light-resistant containers.

DOXYCYCLINE HYCLATE — ORAL

Complete and comparative prescribing information for these products begins in the Tetracyclines group monograph.

Indications

➤*Treatment of infections caused by miscellaneous organisms:* Rocky mountain spotted fever, typhus fever and the typhus group, Q fever, rickettsialpox, and tick fevers caused by Rickettsiae; *Mycoplasma pneumoniae* (PPLO, Eaton's agent); respiratory tract infections caused by *Mycoplasma pneumoniae*; lymphogranuloma venereum caused by *Chlamydia trachomatis* and granuloma inguinale; psittacosis (ornithosis) caused by *Chlamydia psittaci*; trachoma caused by *Chlamydia trachomatis*, although the infectious agent is not always eliminated as judged by immunofluorescence; inclusion conjunctivitis caused by *Chlamydia trachomatis*; uncomplicated urethral, endocervical or rectal infections in adults caused by *Chlamydia trachomatis*; nongonococcal urethritis caused by *Ureaplasma urealyticum*; and relapsing fever due to *Borrelia recurrentis*.

➤*Treatment of the following infections caused by gram-negative microorganisms:* Chancroid caused by *Haemophilus ducreyi*; plague due to *Yersinia pestis* (formerly *Pasteurella pestis*); tularemia due to *Francisella tularensis* (formerly *Pasteurella tularensis*); cholera caused by *Vibrio cholerae* (formerly *Vibrio comma*); campylobacter fetus infections caused by *Campylobacter fetus* (formerly *Vibrio fetus*); brucellosis due to *Brucella* species (in conjunction with streptomycin); Bartonellosis due to *Bartonella bacilliformis*; *Bacteroides* species; and granuloma inguinale caused by *Calymmatobacterium granulomatis*.

➤*Following susceptibility testing (resistance has been documented):* *Escherichia coli*; *Enterobacter aerogenes* (formerly *Aerobacter aerogenes*); *Shigella* species; *Acinetobacter* species (formerly *Mima* species and *Herellea* species); respiratory tract infections caused by *Haemophilus influenzae*; Respiratory tract and urinary tract infections caused by *Klebsiella* species; upper respiratory tract infections caused by *Streptococcus pneumoniae* (formerly *Diplococcus pneumoniae*); and*Streptococcus* species. Up to 44% of strains of *Streptococcus pyogenes* and 74% of *Streptococcus faecalis* have been found to be resistant to tetracycline drugs. Therefore, tetracyclines should not be used for streptococcal disease unless the organism has been demonstrated to be susceptible. For upper respiratory tract infections due to group A beta-hemolytic streptococci, penicillin is the usual drug of choice, including prophylaxis of rheumatic fever. *Staphylococcus aureus* (respiratory, skin and soft-tissue infections); tetracyclines are not the drug of choice in the treatment of any type of staphylococcal infection.

➤*Anthrax, including inhalational anthrax:* Due to *Bacillus anthracis*, including inhalational anthrax (postexposure), to reduce the incidence or progression of disease following exposure to aerosolized *Bacillus anthracis*.

➤*Alternative therapy when penicillin is contraindicated:* Uncomplicated gonorrhea caused by *Neisseria gonorrhoeae*; syphilis caused by *Treponema pallidum*; yaws caused by *Treponema pertenue*; listeriosis due to *Listeria monocytogenes*; anthrax due to *Bacillus anthracis*; Vincent's infection caused by *Fusobacterium fusiforme*; actinomycosis caused by *Actinomyces israelii*; and infections caused by *Clostridium* species.

➤*Acute intestinal amebiasis:* In acute intestinal amebiasis, doxycycline may be a useful adjunct to amebicides.

➤*Severe acne:* In severe acne, doxycycline may be useful adjunctive therapy.

➤*Trachoma:* Treatment of trachoma, although the infectious agent is not always eliminated, as judged by immunofluorescence.

➤*Inclusion conjunctivitis:* Inclusion conjunctivitis may be treated with oral doxycycline alone, or with a combination of topical agents.

➤*Uncomplicated urethral, endocervical or rectal infections:* Doxycycline is indicated for the treatment of uncomplicated urethral, endocervical or rectal infections in adults caused by *Chlamydia trachomatis*.

➤*Nongonococcal urethritis:* Doxycycline is indicated for the treatment of nongonococcal urethritis caused by *Chlamydia trachomatis* and *Ureaplasma urealyticum* and for the treatment of acute epididymo-orchitis caused by *Chlamydia trachomatis*.

➤*Uncomplicated gonococcal infections:* For the treatment of uncomplicated gonococcal infections in adults (except for anorectal infections in men), the gonococcal arthritis-dermatitis syndrome and acute epididymo-orchitis caused by *N. gonorrhoeae*.

➤*Malaria prophylaxis:* Doxycycline is indicated for the prophylaxis of malaria due to *Plasmodium falciparum* in short-term travelers (under 4 months) to areas with chloroquine or pyrimethamine-sulfadoxine resistant strains.

➤*Periostat* tablets: Doxycycline hyclate is indicated for use as an adjunct to scaling and root planing to promote attachment level gain and to reduce pocket depth in patients with adult periodontitis.

➤*Oraxyl* capsules: As an adjunct to scaling and root planing to promote attachment level gain and to reduce pocket depth in patients with adult periodontitis.

➤*Off-label uses:*

Infective endocarditis – According to American Heart Association (AHA) guidelines, doxycycline is preferred in combination with gentamicin or rifampin for the treatment of confirmed *Bartonella* endocarditis.

Infective endocarditis (adults): [1] = Good documentation.

Infective endocarditis (children/adolescents): [1] = Good documentation.

Pelvic inflammatory disease – [1] = Good documentation. Centers for Disease Control and Prevention (CDC) guidelines advise use of doxycycline in treating pelvic inflammatory disease as part of a recommended regimen that includes a third-generation cephalosporin or ampicillin/sulbactam.

Proctitis, proctocolitis, enteritis – [1] = Good documentation. CDC guidelines recommend doxycycline in combination with ceftriaxone as a regimen for known or presumptive therapy of proctitis, proctocolitis, or enteritis. Cases of lymphogranuloma venereum (LGV)–associated disease will require a longer duration of therapy.

Rheumatoid arthritis – [4] = Insufficient documentation. Although in vitro and in vivo trials have demonstrated that doxycycline produces beneficial inhibition of collagenase activity, clinical benefit has not been firmly established. Results with oral doxycycline in the treatment of rheumatoid arthritis (RA) have been variable, demonstrating beneficial effects in 2 small studies but no clinical benefit in a more recent placebo-controlled trial. In addition, no trial has shown benefit in disease progression based on radiographic assessment. Optimal use with or without disease-modifying antirheumatic drugs has yet to be determined. Further studies are required to establish doxycycline's role, if any, in the management of RA. It should be noted that doxycycline therapy was not included in the most recent American College of Rheumatology Subcommittee on Rheumatoid Arthritis Guidelines.

DOXYCYCLINE HYCLATE — ORAL

Traveler's diarrhea – [5] = Poor documentation. Antibiotics have been shown to shorten the duration of traveler's diarrhea and may also be used in moderate to severe cases; however, because of increased antibiotic resistance, doxycycline is no longer recommended for the treatment of traveler's diarrhea. Current guidelines suggest that mild cases of traveler's diarrhea should be managed with adequate hydration and bismuth subsalicylate or loperamide.

Other possible off-label uses – Treatment of malaria (100 mg twice daily for 7 days in combination with other antimalarial agents); pleural malignant effusions; alternative agent for nocardiosis in patients who cannot take sulfa medications; ocular rosacea; prophylaxis of pneumothorax.

Lyme disease:

• *Arthritis* – 100 mg twice daily for 30 to 60 days.

• *Carditis (first-degree atrioventricular [AV] block)* – 100 mg twice daily for 14 to 21 days.

• *Early Lyme disease* – 100 mg twice daily for 14 to 21 days.

• *Facial nerve paralysis* – 100 mg twice daily for 14 to 21 days.

• *Tick bite from endemic area* – 200 mg once.

CDC-recommended treatment schedules for sexually transmitted diseases:

• *Chlamydial infections (adults and children 8 years of age and older)* – 100 mg twice daily for 7 days.

• *Early syphilis* – 100 mg twice daily for 14 days.

• *Epididymitis most likely caused by gonococcal or chlamydial infection* – 100 mg twice daily for 10 days plus a single dose of ceftriaxone 250 mg intramuscularly (IM).

• *Granuloma inguinale (donovanosis)* – 100 mg twice daily for at least 3 weeks.

• *Latent syphilis* – 100 mg twice daily for 28 days.

• *Sexual assault prophylaxis* – 100 mg twice daily for 7 days plus ceftriaxone and metronidazole.

Administration and Dosage

➤*General dosing considerations:* The dosage of *Periostat* and *Oraxyl* differ from that of doxycycline used to treat infections. Exceeding the recommended dosage may result in an increased incidence of adverse reaction, including the development of resistant microorganisms.

➤*Adults:*

Infections – For a list of infections, see Indications.

Usual dosage: 200 mg on the first day of treatment (administered 100 mg every 12 hours) followed by a maintenance dose of 100 mg/day. The maintenance dose may be administered as a single dose or as 50 mg every 12 hours.

Severe infections: In the management of more severe infections (particularly chronic infections of the urinary tract), 100 mg every 12 hours is recommended.

Acute epididymo-orchitis caused by C. trachomatis or N. gonorrhoeae: 100 mg orally twice a day for at least 10 days.

Inhalational anthrax (postexposure): 100 mg orally twice a day for 60 days.

Nongonococcal urethritis caused by C. trachomatis or U. urealyticum: 100 mg orally twice a day for 7 days.

Periodontitis:

• *Periostat* and *Oraxyl* – 20 mg twice daily as an adjunct following scaling and root planing may be administered for up to 9 months. *Periostat* should be taken twice daily at 12-hour intervals, usually in the morning and evening.

Prophylaxis of malaria: 100 mg daily. Prophylaxis should begin 1 to 2 days before travel to the malarious area. Prophylaxis should be continued daily during travel in the malarious area and for 4 weeks after the traveler leaves the malarious area.

Syphilis (early): Patients who are allergic to penicillin should be treated with doxycycline 100 mg by mouth twice a day for 2 weeks.

• *Coated pellets* – 300 mg/day in divided doses for at least 10 days for the treatment of primary and secondary syphilis.

Syphilis of more than 1 year's duration: Patients who are allergic to penicillin should be treated with doxycycline 100 mg by mouth twice a day for 4 weeks.

Uncomplicated gonococcal infections (except anorectal infections in men): 100 mg orally twice a day for 7 days. As an alternate single-visit dose, administer 300 mg immediately followed in 1 hour by a second 300 mg dose. The dose may be administered with food, including carbonated beverage, as required.

Uncomplicated urethral, endocervical, or rectal infection caused by Chlamydia trachomatis: 100 mg orally twice a day for 7 days.

Off-label dosing –

Infective endocarditis (adults): [1] = Good documentation.

• *Suspected Bartonella infection with a negative culture* – 200 mg orally every 24 hours in 2 equally divided doses for 6 weeks in combination with gentamicin and ceftriaxone.

• *Documented Bartonella infection with a positive culture* – 200 mg orally every 24 hours in 2 equally divided doses for 6 weeks in combination with gentamicin or rifampin.

Pelvic inflammatory disease: [1] = Good documentation. 100 mg orally twice daily for 14 days in conjunction with a single dose of ceftriaxone, cefoxitin, or another third-generation parenteral cephalosporin. Metronidazole 500 mg orally twice daily may be added to the regimen if concerns of anaerobic infection exist.

Proctitis, proctocolitis, enteritis: [1] = Good documentation. 100 mg orally twice daily for 7 days. Doxycycline should be given in conjunction with a 1-time IM dose of ceftriaxone 125 mg. Persons diagnosed with LGV should receive 21 days of doxycycline therapy.

Rheumatoid arthritis: [4] = Insufficient documentation. 100 mg twice daily for 3 or 6 months. Doses of 150 mg/day also have been used.

Other possible off-label uses:

• *CDC recommended treatment schedules for sexually transmitted diseases (MMWR.* 2002 May 10;51 [No. RR-6]:1-84.) –

Epididymitis most likely caused by gonococcal or chlamydial infection: 100 mg twice daily for 10 days plus a single dose of 250 mg ceftriaxone IM.

Granuloma inguinale (donovanosis): 100 mg twice daily for at least 3 weeks.

Lymphogranuloma venereum: 100 mg twice daily for at least 21 days.

Sexual assault prophylaxis: 100 mg twice daily for 7 days plus ceftriaxone and metronidazole.

➤*Children:* For children 8 years of age and older weighing more than 100 lbs, the usual adult dose should be used. See Adults for dosing.

Infections – For a list of infections, see Indications.

8 years of age and older:

• *Usual dosage* – The recommended dosage schedule for children weighing less than or equal to 100 pounds is 2 mg/lb of body weight divided into 2 doses on the first day of treatment, followed by 1 mg/lb of body weight given as a single daily dose or divided into 2 doses, on subsequent days.

• *Severe infections* – Up to 2 mg/lb of body weight may be used.

• *Malaria prophylaxis* – 2 mg/kg given once daily up to the adult dose. Prophylaxis should begin 1 to 2 days before travel to the malarious area. Prophylaxis should be continued daily during travel in the malarious area and for 4 weeks after the traveler leaves the malarious area.

Inhalational anthrax (postexposure): For children weighing less than 100 lbs (45 kg), the dosage is 1 mg/lb (2.2 mg/kg), by mouth, twice a day for 60 days. Children weighing 100 lb or more should receive the adult dose.

Off-label dosing –

Infective endocarditis (children/adolescents): [1] = Good documentation.

• *Suspected Bartonella infection with a negative culture* – 2 to 4 mg/kg orally every 24 hours in 2 equally divided doses for 6 weeks in combination with gentamicin and ceftriaxone.

• *Documented Bartonella infection with a positive culture* – 2 to 4 mg/kg orally every 24 hours in 2 equally divided doses for 6 weeks in combination with gentamicin or rifampin.

Pelvic inflammatory disease: [1] = Good documentation.

• *Adolescents* – 100 mg orally twice daily for 14 days in conjunction with a single dose of ceftriaxone, cefoxitin, or another third-generation parenteral cephalosporin. Metronidazole 500 mg orally twice daily may be added to the regimen if concerns of anaerobic infection exist.

CDC recommended treatment schedules for sexually transmitted diseases (MMWR. 2002 May 10;51 [No. RR-6]:1-84.):

• *Chlamydial infections* – For children 8 years of age and older, 100 mg by mouth twice daily for 7 days.

• *Anthrax* –

Younger than 8 years of age: 2.2 mg/kg/day divided twice daily. 200 mg/day.

➤*Concomitant therapy:* Antacids containing aluminum, calcium or magnesium, sodium bicarbonate and iron-containing preparations should not be given to patients using oral tetracyclines.

➤*Duration of therapy:* The therapeutic antibacterial serum activity will usually persist for 24 hours following recommended dosage. When used in streptococcal infections, therapy should be continued for 10 days.

➤*Administration:* Administration of adequate amounts of non-dairy fluid with capsule and tablet forms of drugs in the tetracycline class is recommended to wash down the drugs and reduce the risk of esophageal irritation and ulceration.

Absorption and peak plasma levels may be reduced when administered with meals or with dairy products, including milk.

If GI upset occurs, administration with a small amount of a low-fat, low-protein, non-dairy food may reduce upset, but the potential risk of decreased drug efficacy must be weighed against the benefit of treating the infection with this antibiotic.

Capsules containing coated pellets – Doxycycline hyclate-coated pellet capsules may also be administered by carefully opening the capsules and sprinkling the capsule contents onto a spoonful of applesauce. However, any loss of pellets in the transfer would prevent using the dose. The applesauce should be swallowed immediately without chewing and followed with a cool 240 mL glass of water to ensure complete swallowing of the capsule contents. The applesauce should not be hot, and it should be just enough to be swallowed without chewing. In the event that a prepared dose of applesauce and doxycycline hyclate-coated pellet capsules cannot be taken immediately, the mixture should be discarded and not stored for later use.

Oraxyl capsules – *Oraxyl* should be administered at least 1 hour prior to morning and evening meals. Administration of adequate amounts of fluid along with the capsules is recommended to wash down the drug and reduce the risk of esophageal irritation and ulceration.

Periostat tablets – It is recommended that if *Periostat* tablets are taken close to meal times, patients should allow at least 1 hour prior to or 2 hours after meals.

➤*Storage/Stability:*

Capsules and tablets – Store below 30°C (86°F).

Coated pellets – Store below 25°C (77°F).

Periostat tablets – Store at 15° to 30°C (59° to 86°F).

Oraxyl capsules – Store at 20° to 25°C (68° to 77°F). Protect from moisture.

DOXYCYCLINE MONOHYDRATE — ORAL

Complete and comparative prescribing information for these products begins in the Tetracyclines group monograph.

Indications

➤*General information:* Doxycycline is not the drug of choice in the treatment of any type of staphylococcal infections.

➤*Treatment of infections caused by miscellaneous organisms:* Rocky mountain spotted fever, typhus fever and the typhus group, Q fever, rickettsialpox, and tick fevers caused by Rickettsiae; respiratory tract infections caused by *Mycoplasma pneumoniae*; lymphogranuloma venereum caused by *Chlamydia trachomatis*; psittacosis (ornithosis) caused by *Chlamydia psittaci*; trachoma caused by *Chlamydia trachomatis*, although the infectious agent is not always eliminated as judged by immunofluorescence; inclusion conjunctivitis caused by *Chlamydia trachomatis*; uncomplicated urethral, endocervical, or rectal infections in adults caused by *Chlamydia trachomatis*; nongonococcal urethritis caused by *Ureaplasma urealyticum*; and relapsing fever due to *Borrelia recurrentis*.

➤*Treatment of the following infections caused by gram-negative microorganisms:* Chancroid caused by *Haemophilus ducreyi*; plague due to *Yersinia pestis* (formerly *Pasteurella pestis*); tularemia due to *Francisella tularensis* (formerly *Pasteurella tularensis*); cholera caused by *Vibrio cholerae* (formerly *Vibrio comma*); campylobacter fetus infections caused by *Campylobacter fetus* (formerly *Vibrio fetus*); brucellosis due to *Brucella* species (in conjunction with streptomycin); bartonellosis due to *Bartonella bacilliformis*; and granuloma inguinale caused by *Calymmatobacterium granulomatis*.

➤*For the treatment of infections caused by the following gram-negative microorganisms, when bacteriologic testing indicates appropriate susceptibility to the drug:* *Escherichia coli*; *Enterobacter aerogenes* (formerly *Aerobacter aerogenes*); *Shigella* species and *Acinetobacter* species (formerly *Mima* species and *Herellea* species); respiratory tract infections caused by *Haemophilus influenzae*; respiratory tract and urinary tract infections caused by *Klebsiella* species.

➤*For the treatment of infections caused by the following gram-positive microorganisms, when bacteriologic testing indicates appropriate susceptibility to the drug:* Upper respiratory tract infections caused by *Streptococcus pneumoniae* (formerly Diplococcus pneumoniae); and skin and skin structure infections caused by *Staphylococcus aureus*.

➤*Anthrax, including inhalational anthrax:* Due to *Bacillus anthracis*, including inhalational anthrax (postexposure): To reduce the incidence or progression of disease following exposure to aerosolized *Bacillus anthracis*.

➤*Alternative therapy when penicillin is contraindicated:* Uncomplicated gonorrhea caused by *Neisseria gonorrhoeae*; syphilis caused by *Treponema pallidum*; yaws caused by *Treponema pertenue*; listeriosis due to *Listeria monocytogenes*; Vincent's infection caused by *Fusobacterium fusiforme*; actinomycosis caused by *Actinomyces israelii*; and infections caused by *Clostridium* species.

➤*Acute intestinal amebiasis:* Doxycycline may be a useful adjunct to amebicides.

➤*Severe acne:* In severe acne, doxycycline may be useful adjunctive therapy.

➤*Oracea:* For the treatment of only inflammatory lesions (papules and pustules) of rosacea in adult patients. No meaningful effect was demonstrated for generalized erythema (redness) of rosacea. Doxycycline has not been evaluated for the treatment of erythematous, telangiectatic, or ocular components of rosacea. Efficacy of doxycycline beyond 16 weeks and safety beyond 9 months have not been established.

This formulation of doxycycline has not been evaluated in the treatment or prevention of infections. Doxycycline should not be used for treating bacterial infections, providing antibacterial prophylaxis, or reducing the numbers or eliminating microorganisms associated with any bacterial disease.

To reduce the development of drug-resistant bacteria as well as to maintain the effectiveness of other antibacterial drugs, use doxycycline only as indicated.

➤*Off-label uses:*

Infective endocarditis – According to American Heart Association (AHA) guidelines, doxycycline is preferred in combination with gentamicin or rifampin for the treatment of confirmed *Bartonella* endocarditis.

Infective endocarditis (adults): [1] = Good documentation.

Infective endocarditis (children/adolescents): [1] = Good documentation.

Pelvic inflammatory disease – [1] = Good documentation. Centers for Disease Control and Prevention (CDC) guidelines advise use of doxycycline in treating pelvic inflammatory disease as part of a recommended regimen that includes a third-generation cephalosporin or ampicillin/sulbactam.

Proctitis, proctocolitis, enteritis – [1] = Good documentation. CDC guidelines recommend doxycycline in combination with ceftriaxone as a regimen for known or presumptive therapy of proctitis, proctocolitis, or enteritis. Cases of lymphogranuloma venereum (LGV)–associated disease will require a longer duration of therapy.

Rheumatoid arthritis – [4] = Insufficient documentation. Although in vitro and in vivo trials have demonstrated that doxycycline produces beneficial inhibition of collagenase activity, clinical benefit has not been firmly established. Results with oral doxycycline in the treatment of rheumatoid arthritis (RA) have been variable, demonstrating beneficial effects in 2 small studies but no clinical benefit in a more recent placebo-controlled trial. In addition, no trial has shown benefit in disease progression based on radiographic assessment. Optimal use with or without disease-modifying antirheumatic drugs has yet to be determined. Further studies are required to establish doxycycline's role, if any, in the management of RA. It should be noted that doxycycline therapy was not included in the most recent American College of Rheumatology Subcommittee on Rheumatoid Arthritis Guidelines.

Traveler's diarrhea – [5] = Poor documentation. Antibiotics have been shown to shorten the duration of traveler's diarrhea and may also be used in moderate to severe cases; however, because of increased antibiotic resistance, doxycycline is no longer recommended for the treatment of traveler's diarrhea. Current guidelines suggest that mild cases of traveler's diarrhea should be managed with adequate hydration and bismuth subsalicylate or loperamide.

Other possible off-label uses – Treatment of malaria (100 mg twice daily for 7 days in combination with other antimalarial agents); pleural malignant effusions; alternative agent for nocardiosis in patients who cannot take sulfa medications; ocular rosacea; prophylaxis of pneumothorax.

Lyme disease:
- *Arthritis* – 100 mg twice daily for 30 to 60 days.
- *Carditis (first-degree atrioventricular block)* – 100 mg twice daily for 14 to 21 days.
- *Early Lyme disease* – 100 mg twice daily for 14 to 21 days.
- *Facial nerve paralysis* – 100 mg twice daily for 14 to 21 days.
- *Tick bite from endemic area* – 200 mg once.

CDC-recommended treatment schedules for sexually transmitted diseases:
- *Chlamydial infections (adults and children 8 years of age and older)* – 100 mg twice daily for 7 days.
- *Early syphilis* – 100 mg twice daily for 14 days.
- *Epididymitis most likely caused by gonococcal or chlamydial infection* – 100 mg twice daily for 10 days plus a single dose of ceftriaxone 250 mg intramuscularly (IM).
- *Granuloma inguinale (donovanosis)* – 100 mg twice daily for at least 3 weeks.
- *Latent syphilis* – 100 mg twice daily for 28 days.
- *Sexual assault prophylaxis* – 100 mg twice daily for 7 days plus ceftriaxone and metronidazole.

Administration and Dosage

➤*General dosing considerations:* The dosage of *Oracea* differs from that of doxycycline used to treat infections. Exceeding the recommended dosage may result in an increased incidence of adverse reactions, including the development of resistant microorganisms.

➤*Adults:*

Infections – For a list of infections, see Indications.

Usual dosage: 200 mg on the first day of treatment (administered 100 mg every 12 hours or 50 mg every 6 hours) followed by a maintenance dose of 100 mg/day. The maintenance dose may be administered as a single dose or as 50 mg every 12 hours.

More severe infections: In the management of more severe infections (particularly chronic infections of the urinary tract), 100 mg every 12 hours is recommended

Acne (severe): 150 mg daily or as directed by a health care provider.

Acute epididymo-orchitis caused by C. trachomatis or N. gonorrhoeae: 100 mg orally twice a day for at least 10 days.

Inhalational anthrax (postexposure): 100 mg orally twice a day for 60 days.

Nongonococcal urethritis caused by C. trachomatis or U. urealyticum: 100 mg orally twice a day for at least 7 days.

Rosacea:
- *Oracea* – 40 mg taken once daily in the morning on an empty stomach, preferably at least 1 hour prior or 2 hours after meals.

Syphilis, primary and secondary: 300 mg a day in divided doses for at least 10 days.

Uncomplicated gonococcal infections (except anorectal infections in men): 100 mg orally twice a day for 7 days. As an alternate single visit dose, administer 300 mg immediately followed in 1 hour by a second 300 mg dose.

Uncomplicated urethral, endocervical, or rectal infection caused by C. trachomatis: 100 mg orally twice a day for at least 7 days.

Off-label dosing –

Infective endocarditis (adults): [1] = Good documentation.
- *Suspected Bartonella infection with a negative culture* – 200 mg orally every 24 hours in 2 equally divided doses for 6 weeks in combination with gentamicin and ceftriaxone.
- *Documented Bartonella infection with a positive culture* – 200 mg orally every 24 hours in 2 equally divided doses for 6 weeks in combination with gentamicin or rifampin.

Pelvic inflammatory disease: [1] = Good documentation. 100 mg orally twice daily for 14 days in conjunction with a single dose of ceftriaxone, cefoxitin, or another third-generation parenteral cephalosporin. Metronidazole 500 mg orally twice daily may be added to the regimen if concerns of anaerobic infection exist.

Proctitis, proctocolitis, enteritis: [1] = Good documentation. 100 mg orally twice daily for 7 days. Doxycycline should be given in conjunction with a 1-time IM dose of ceftriaxone 125 mg. Persons diagnosed with LGV should receive 21 days of doxycycline therapy.

Rheumatoid arthritis: [4] = Insufficient documentation. Dosages used in studies were 100 mg twice daily for 3 or 6 months. Doses of 150 mg/day also have been used.

DOXYCYCLINE MONOHYDRATE — ORAL

Other possible off-label uses:

• *CDC recommended treatment schedules for sexually transmitted diseases (Centers for Disease Control and Prevention [CDC]. Sexually transmitted diseases treatment guidelines 2002. MMWR Recomm Rep.* 2002;51[RR-6]:1-78.) –

Epididymitis most likely caused by gonococcal or chlamydial infection: 100 mg twice daily for 10 days plus a single dose of ceftriaxone 250 mg IM.

Granuloma inguinale (donovanosis): 100 mg twice daily for at least 3 weeks.

Lymphogranuloma venereum: 100 mg twice daily for at least 21days.

Sexual assault prophylaxis: 100 mg twice daily for 7 days plus ceftriaxone and metronidazole.

➤*Children:* For children 8 years of age and older weighing more than 100 lbs, the usual adult dose should be used. See Adults for dosing.

Infections – For a list of infections, see Indications.

8 years of age and older:

• *Usual dosage* – For children weighing 100 lbs or less is 2 mg/lb of body weight divided into 2 doses on the first day of treatment, followed by 1 mg/lb of body weight given as a single daily dose or divided into 2 doses, on subsequent days.

• *Severe infections* – Up to 2 mg/lb of body weight may be used.

Inhalational anthrax (postexposure): For children weighing less than 100 lbs (45 kg), the dosage is 1 mg/lb (2.2 mg/kg) of body weight orally twice a day for 60 days. Children weighing 100 lbs or more should receive the adult dose.

Off-label dosing –

Infective endocarditis (children/adolescents): [1] = Good documentation.

• *Suspected Bartonella infection with a negative culture* – 2 to 4 mg/kg orally every 24 hours in 2 equally divided doses for 6 weeks in combination with gentamicin and ceftriaxone.

• *Documented Bartonella infection with a positive culture* – 2 to 4 mg/kg orally every 24 hours in 2 equally divided doses for 6 weeks in combination with gentamicin or rifampin.

Pelvic inflammatory disease: [1] = Good documentation.

• *Adolescents* – 100 mg orally twice daily for 14 days in conjunction with a single dose of ceftriaxone, cefoxitin, or another third-generation parenteral cephalosporin. Metronidazole 500 mg orally twice daily may be added to the regimen if concerns of anaerobic infection exist.

CDC recommended treatment schedules for sexually transmitted diseases (MMWR. 2002 May 10;51 [No. RR-6]:1-84.):

• *Chlamydial infections* – For children 8 years of age and older, 100 mg by mouth twice daily for 7 days.

• *Anthrax –*

Younger than 8 years of age: 2.2 mg/kg/day divided twice daily. 200 mg/day.

➤*Duration of therapy:* When used in streptococcal infections, therapy should be continued for 10 days.

➤*Administration:* Administration of adequate amounts of fluid along with capsule and tablet forms of drugs in the tetracycline class is recommended to wash down the drugs and reduce the risk of esophageal irritation and ulceration. If gastric irritation occurs, doxycycline may be given with food. Ingestion of a high-fat meal has been shown to delay the time to peak plasma concentrations by an average of 1 hour and 20 minutes. However, in the same study, food enhanced the average peak concentration by 7.5% and the area under the curve by 5.7%.

➤*Storage/Stability:*

Tablets – Store at 20° to 25°C (68° to 77°F). Protect from light.

Capsules – Store at controlled room temperature, 15° to 30°C (59° to 86°F).

DOXYCYCLINE HYCLATE — INJECTION

Complete and comparative prescribing information for these products begins in the Tetracyclines group monograph.

Indications

➤*Infections caused by miscellaneous organisms: Rickettsiae* (Rocky Mountain spotted fever, typhus fever, and the typhus group, Q fever, rickettsialpox and tick fevers); *Mycoplasma pneumoniae* (PPLO, Eaton Agent); agents of psittacosis and ornithosis; agents of lymphogranuloma venereum and granuloma inguinale; and the spirochetal agent of relapsing fever (*Borrelia recurrentis*).

➤*Infections caused by gram-negative microorganisms: Haemophilus ducreyi* (chancroid); *Pasteurella pestis* and *Pasteurella tularensis*; *Bartonella bacilliformis*; *Bacteroides* species; *Vibrio comma* and *Vibrio fetus*; and *Brucella* species (in conjunction with streptomycin).

➤*Infections following susceptibility testing (resistance has been documented): Escherichia coli*; *Enterobacter aerogenes* (formerly *Aerobacter aerogenes*); *Shigella* species; *Mima* species and *Herellea* species; *Haemophilus influenzae* (respiratory infections); *Klebsiella* species (respiratory and urinary infections); *Diplococcus pneumoniae*.

Staphylococcus aureus, respiratory, skin and soft tissue infections. Tetracyclines are not the drugs of choice in the treatment of any type of staphylococcal infections.

Streptococcus species – Up to 44% of strains of *Streptococcus pyogenes* and 74% of *Streptococcus faecalis* have been found to be resistant to tetracycline drugs. Therefore, tetracyclines should not be used for streptococcal disease unless the organism has been demonstrated to be sensitive.

For upper respiratory tract infections due to group A beta-hemolytic streptococci, penicillin is the usual drug of choice, including prophylaxis of rheumatic fever.

➤*Alternative therapy when penicillin is contraindicated: Neisseria gonorrhoeae* and *N. meningitidis*; *Treponema pallidum* and *Treponema pertenue* (syphilis and yaws); *Listeria monocytogenes*; *Clostridium* species; *Bacillus anthracis*; *Fusobacterium fusiforme* (Vincent's infection); and *Actinomyces* species.

➤*Acute intestinal amebiasis:* In acute intestinal amebiasis, doxycycline may be a useful adjunct to amebicides.

➤*Trachoma:* Doxycycline is indicated in the treatment of trachoma, although the infectious agent is not always eliminated, as judged by immunofluorescence.

➤*Atridox* only: For chronic adult periodontitis for a gain in clinical attachment, reduction in probing depth, and reduction in bleeding on probing.

➤*Off-label uses:*

Infective endocarditis – According to American Heart Association (AHA) guidelines, doxycycline is preferred in combination with gentamicin or rifampin for the treatment of confirmed *Bartonella* endocarditis.

Infective endocarditis (adults): [1] = Good documentation.

Infective endocarditis (children/adolescents): [1] = Good documentation.

Pelvic inflammatory disease – [1] = Good documentation. Centers for Disease Control and Prevention (CDC) guidelines advise use of doxycycline in treating pelvic inflammatory disease as part of a recommended regimen that includes a third-generation cephalosporin or ampicillin/sulbactam.

Rheumatoid arthritis (RA) – [4] = Insufficient documentation. Although in vitro and in vivo trials have demonstrated that doxycycline produces beneficial inhibition of collagenase activity, clinical benefit has not been firmly established. Results with oral doxycycline in the treatment of RA have been variable, demonstrating beneficial effects in 2 small studies but no clinical benefit in a more recent placebo-controlled trial. In addition, no trial has shown benefit in disease progression based on radiographic assessment. Optimal use with or without disease-modifying antirheumatic drugs has yet to be determined. Further studies are required to establish doxycycline's role, if any, in the management of RA. It should be noted that doxycycline therapy was not included in the most recent American College of Rheumatology Subcommittee of Rheumatoid Arthritis Guidelines.

Administration and Dosage

➤*General dosing considerations:* Rapid administration is to be avoided. See Administration.

➤*Adults:*

Infections – For a list of infections, see the Indications section.

Usual dosage: 200 mg on the first day of treatment administered in 1 or 2 IV infusions. Subsequent daily dosage is 100 to 200 mg depending upon the severity of infection, with 200 mg administered in 1 or 2 infusions.

Chronic periodontitis:

• *Atridox* only – Doxycycline injection is a variable-dose product dependent on the size, shape, and number of pockets being treated. May repeat application 4 months after initial treatment.

Inhalational anthrax (postexposure): 100 mg IV twice daily for 60 days.

Syphilis: 300 mg IV daily for at least 10 days for the treatment of primary and secondary syphilis.

Off-label dosing –

Infective endocarditis (adults): [1] = Good documentation.

• *Suspected Bartonella infection with a negative culture* – 200 mg IV every 24 hours in 2 equally divided doses for 6 weeks in combination with gentamicin and ceftriaxone.

• *Documented Bartonella infection with a positive culture* – 200 mg IV every 24 hours in 2 equally divided doses for 6 weeks in combination with gentamicin or rifampin.

Pelvic inflammatory disease: [1] = Good documentation. 100 mg IV every 12 hours in conjunction with cefotetan, cefoxitin, or ampicillin/sulbactam. Parenteral therapy may be discontinued 24 hours after clinical improvement, with oral doxycycline continued for a total of 14 days of treatment. Because of pain associated with the administration of IV doxycycline, oral administration is the preferred route when possible.

Rheumatoid arthritis: [4] = Insufficient documentation. IV therapy was administered as 200 mg/day for 2 weeks, followed by 200 mg/week for a total of 11 weeks.

Other possible off-label uses:

• *CDC recommended treatment schedules for sexually transmitted diseases (MMWR.* 2002 May 10;51 [No. RR-6]:1-84. –

Chlamydial infections: 100 mg twice daily for 7 days.

Epididymitis most likely caused by gonococcal or chlamydial infection: 100 mg twice daily for 10 days plus a single dose of ceftriaxone 250 mg IM.

Granuloma inguinale (donovanosis): 100 mg twice daily for at least 3 weeks.

Lymphogranuloma venereum: 100 mg twice daily for at least 21 days.

Nongonococcal urethritis: 100 mg twice daily for 7 days.

Sexual assault prophylaxis: 100 mg twice daily for 7 days plus ceftriaxone and metronidazole.

DOXYCYCLINE HYCLATE — INJECTION

➤*Children:* For children 8 years of age and older weighing more than 100 lbs, the usual adult dose should be used. See Adults for dosing.

Infections –

8 years of age and older:

• *Usual dosage* – For children weighing 100 pounds or less, the dosage is 2 mg/lb of body weight on the first day of treatment administered in 1 or 2 IV infusions. Subsequent daily dosage is 1 to 2 mg/lb of body weight given as 1 or 2 infusions, depending on the severity of the infection.

• *Inhalational anthrax (postexposure)* – For children weighing less than 100 lbs (45 kg), the dosage is 1 mg/lb (2.2 mg/kg) administered IV twice daily for 60 days.

Off-label dosing –

Infective endocarditis (children / adolescents): [1] = Good documentation.

• *Suspected Bartonella infection with a negative culture* – 2 to 4 mg/kg IV every 24 hours in 2 equally divided doses for 6 weeks in combination with gentamicin and ceftriaxone.

• *Documented Bartonella infection with a positive culture* – 2 to 4 mg/kg IV every 24 hours in 2 equally divided doses for 6 weeks in combination with gentamicin or rifampin.

Pelvic inflammatory disease: [1] = Good documentation.

• *Adolescents* – 100 mg IV every 12 hours in conjunction with cefotetan, cefoxitin, or ampicillin/sulbactam. Parenteral therapy may be discontinued 24 hours after clinical improvement, with oral doxycycline continued for a total of 14 days of treatment. Because of pain associated with the administration of IV doxycycline, oral administration is the preferred route when possible.

CDC recommended treatment schedules for sexually transmitted diseases (MMWR. 2002 May 10;51 [No. RR-6]:1-84.):

• *Chlamydial infections* – For children 8 years of age and older, 100 mg by mouth twice daily for 7 days.

• *Anthrax* –

Younger than 8 years of age: 2.2 mg/kg/day divided twice daily. 200 mg/day.

➤*Duration of therapy:* Therapy should be continued for at least 24 to 48 hours after symptoms and fever have subsided. The therapeutic antibacterial serum activity will usually persist for 24 hours following recommended dosage.

➤*Preparation for administration:* To prepare a solution containing 10 mg/mL, the contents of the vial should be reconstituted with 10 mL (for the 100 mg/vial container) of sterile water for injection or any of the following 10 IV infusion solutions. Each 100 mg of doxycycline (ie, withdraw entire solution from the 100 mg vial) is further diluted with 100 to 1,000 mL of the following IV solutions: 0.9% sodium chloride injection; 5% dextrose injection; Ringer's injection; invert sugar, 10% in water; Ringer's lactated injection; dextrose 5% in Ringer's lactated; *Normosol-M* in dextrose 5% in water injection; *Normosol-R* in dextrose 5% in water injection; *Plasma-Lyte* 56 in 5% dextrose; and *Plasma-Lyte* 148 in 5% dextrose.

This will result in desired concentrations of 0.1 to 1 mg/mL. Concentrations lower than 0.1 mg/mL or higher than 1 mg/mL are not recommended.

➤*Administration:* Rapid administration is to be avoided. Parenteral therapy is indicated only when oral therapy is not indicated. Oral therapy should be instituted as soon as possible. If IV therapy is given over prolonged periods of time, thrombophlebitis may result. IV solutions should not be injected IM or subcutaneously. Caution should be taken to avoid the inadvertent introduction of the IV solution into the adjacent soft tissue.

The duration of infusion may vary with the dose (100 to 200 mg/day), but is usually 1 to 4 hours. A recommended minimum infusion time for 100 mg of a 0.5 mg/mL solution is 1 hour.

➤*Storage / Stability:* Store lyophilized product at or below 25°C (77°F) and protect from light.

Atridox – Store at 2° to 8°C (36° to 46°F).

Stability – Doxycycline is stable for 48 hours in solution when diluted with sodium chloride injection or 5% dextrose injection to concentrations between 1 and 0.1 mg/mL and stored at 25°C (77°F). Doxycycline in these solutions is stable under fluorescent light for 48 hours, but must be protected from direct sunlight during storage and infusion. Reconstituted solutions (1 to 0.1 mg/mL) may be stored up to 72 hours prior to start of infusion if refrigerated and protected from sunlight and artificial light. Infusion must then be completed within 12 hours. Solutions must be used within these time periods or discarded.

Doxycycline, when diluted with Ringer's injection or invert sugar, 10% in water, or *Normosol-M* in dextrose 5% in water injection, or *Normosol-R* in dextrose 5% in water injection, or *Plasma-Lyte* 56 in 5% dextrose, or *Plasma-Lyte* 148 in 5% dextrose to a concentration between 1 and 0.1 mg/mL, must be completely infused within 12 hours after reconstitution to ensure adequate stability. During infusion, the solution must be protected from direct sunlight. Reconstituted solutions (1 to 0.1 mg/mL) may be stored up to 72 hours prior to start of infusion if refrigerated and protected from sunlight and artificial light. Infusion must then be completed within 12 hours. Solutions must be used within these time periods or discarded.

When diluted with Ringer's lactate injection or dextrose 5% in Ringer's lactate, infusion of the solution (ca. 1 mg/mL) or lower concentrations (not less than 0.1 mg/mL) must be completed within 6 hours after reconstitution to ensure adequate stability. During infusion, the solution must be protected from direct sunlight. Solutions must be used within this time period or discarded.

Solutions of doxycycline hyclate for injection at a concentration of 10 mg/mL in sterile water for injection, when frozen immediately after reconstitution are stable for 8 weeks when stored at −20°C (−44°F). If the product is warmed, care should be taken to avoid heating it after the thawing is complete. Once thawed, the solution should not be refrozen.

MINOCYCLINE

Rx	**Minocycline** (Par)	**Tablets; oral:** 50 mg	As minocycline hydrochloride. Lactose. (Par 511). White, capsule shape. Film-coated. In 100s and 1,000s.
Rx	**Dynacin** (Medicis)		As minocycline hydrochloride. Lactose. (DYN-50 747). White, capsule shape. Film-coated. In 100s and 1,000s.
Rx	**Myrac** (Glades)		As minocycline hydrochloride. Lactose. (STIEFEL 7338). Yellow, oval. Film-coated. In 100s.
Rx	**Minocycline** (Par)	**Tablets; oral:** 75 mg	As minocycline hydrochloride. Lactose. (Par 512). White, capsule shape. Film-coated. In 100s and 1,000s.
Rx	**Dynacin** (Medicis)		As minocycline hydrochloride. Lactose. (DYN-75 748). Gray, capsule shape. Film-coated. In 100s and 1,000s.
Rx	**Myrac** (Glades)		As minocycline hydrochloride. Lactose. (STIEFEL 7339). Yellow, oval. Film-coated. In 100s.
Rx	**Minocycline Hydrochloride** (Par)	**Tablets; oral:** 100 mg	As minocycline hydrochloride. Lactose. (Par 513). White, capsule shape. Film-coated. In 50s and 1,000s.
Rx	**Dynacin** (Medicis)		As minocycline hydrochloride. Lactose. (DYN-100 749). Dark gray, capsule shape. Film-coated. In 50s and 1,000s.
Rx	**Myrac** (Glades)		As minocycline hydrochloride. Lactose. (STIEFEL 7340). Yellow, oval, bisected. Film-coated. In 50s.
Rx	**Minocycline Hydrochloride** (Teva)	**Tablets, extended-release; oral:** 45 mg	As minocycline hydrochloride. Lactose. (b 178). Gray, capsule shape. Film-coated. In 30s, 100s, and 1,000s.
Rx	**Solodyn** (Medicis)		As minocycline hydrochloride. Lactose. (DYN 045). Gray. Film-coated. In 30s and 100s.
Rx	**Solodyn** (Medicis)	**Tablets, extended-release; oral:** 65 mg	As minocycline hydrochloride. Lactose. (DYN 065). Blue. Film-coated. In 30s.
Rx	**Minocycline Hydrochloride** (Teva)	**Tablets, extended-release; oral:** 90 mg	As minocycline hydrochloride. Lactose. (b 179). Yellow, capsule shape. Film-coated. In 30s, 100s, and 1,000s.
Rx	**Solodyn** (Medicis)		As minocycline hydrochloride. Lactose. (DYN 090). Yellow. Film-coated. In 30s and 100s.
Rx	**Solodyn** (Medicis)	**Tablets, extended-release; oral:** 115 mg	As minocycline hydrochloride. Lactose. (DYN 115). Green. Film-coated. In 30s.
Rx	**Minocycline Hydrochloride** (Teva)	**Tablets, extended-release; oral:** 135 mg	As minocycline hydrochloride. Lactose. (b 190). Orange-brown, capsule shape. Film-coated. In 30s, 100s, and 1,000s.
Rx	**Solodyn** (Medicis)		As minocycline hydrochloride. Lactose. (DYN 135). Pink. Film-coated. In 30s and 100s.

MINOCYCLINE

Rx	**Minocycline Hydrochloride** (Various, eg, Danbury, Global, Ranbaxy, Teva)	**Capsules; oral:** 50 mg	As minocycline hydrochloride. In 100s.
Rx	**Dynacin** (Medicis)		As minocycline hydrochloride. 0497 DYNACIN 50 mg). White. In 100s, 500s, and 1,000s.
Rx	**Minocycline Hydrochloride** (Various, eg, Global, Ranbaxy)	**Capsules; oral:** 75 mg	As minocycline hydrochloride. In 100s.
Rx	**Dynacin** (Medicis)		As minocycline hydrochloride. (0499 DYNACIN 75 mg). Lt. gray. In 100s and 1,000s.
Rx	**Minocycline Hydrochloride** (Various, eg, Danbury, Global, Ranbaxy, Teva)	**Capsules; oral:** 100 mg	As minocycline hydrochloride. In 50s.
Rx	**Dynacin** (Medicis)		As minocycline hydrochloride. (0498 DYNACIN 100 mg). Dk. gray/white. In 50s, 500s, and 1,000s.
Rx	**Minocin** (Lederle)	**Capsules, pellet-filled; oral:** 50 mg	As minocycline hydrochloride. (M45 Lederle 50 mg). Yellow/green. In 100s.
		100 mg	As minocycline hydrochloride. (M46 Lederle 100 mg). Lt. green/green. In 50s.
		Suspension; oral: 50 mg per 5 mL	As minocycline hydrochloride. 5% alcohol, parabens, EDTA, saccharin. Custard flavor. In 60 mL.
Rx	**Arestin** (Cord Logistics)	**Powder, extended-release; dental:** 1 mg	As minocycline hydrochloride. As microspheres. In UD 12s.
Rx	**Minocin** (Triax)	**Injection, lyophilized powder for solution:** 100 mg	As minocycline hydrochloride. In vials.

MINOCYCLINE HYDROCHLORIDE — ORAL

Complete and comparative prescribing information for these products begins in the Tetracyclines group monograph.

Indications

➤*Gram-negative organisms (not extended release): Haemophilus ducreyi* (chancroid); *Francisella tularensis* (tularemia); *Yersinia pestis* (plague); *Bartonella bacilliformis* (bartonellosis); *Campylobacter fetus*; *Vibrio cholerae* (cholera); *Brucella* sp. (in conjunction with streptomycin); *Neisseria gonorrhoeae* (uncomplicated urethritis in men).

➤*Infections caused by the following miscellaneous organisms (not extended release): Rickettsiae* (Rocky Mountain spotted fever, typhus fever and the typhus group, Q fever, rickettsialpox, tick fevers); *Mycoplasma pneumoniae* (respiratory tract infections); *C. trachomatis* (lymphogranuloma venereum, trachoma [infectious agent not always eliminated], inclusion conjunctivitis); *C. psittaci* (psittacosis [ornithosis]); *Borellia recurrentis* (relapsing fever); *Ureaplasma urealyticum* (nongonococcal urethritis).

➤*Following susceptibility testing (resistance has been documented): Escherichia coli*; *Enterobacter aerogenes*; *Acinetobacter* and *Shigella* sp.; *Haemophilus influenzae* (respiratory tract infections); *Klebsiella* sp. (respiratory and urinary tract infections); *Streptococcus pneumoniae* (upper respiratory infections); *Staphylococcus aureus* (skin and skin structure infections).

➤*Alternative therapy for the following infections when penicillin is contraindicated (not extended release): Neisseria gonorrhoeae* infections; syphilis caused by *Treponema pallidum*; yaws caused by *Treponema pertenue*; listeriosis caused by *Listeria monocytogenes*; anthrax caused by *Bacillus anthracis*; Vincent's infection caused by *Fusobacterium fusiforme*; actinomycosis caused by *Actinomyces israelii*; infections caused by *Clostridium* sp.

➤*Acute intestinal amebiasis (not extended release):* As adjunct to amebicides.

➤*Severe acne:* As adjunctive therapy.

➤*Neisseria meningitidis (not extended release):* Treatment of asymptomatic meningococcal carriers of *N. meningitidis*.

➤*Off-label uses:*

Infective endocarditis (adults) – [2] = Fair documentation. The use of minocycline to treat endocarditis is only recommended in patients with oxacillin-resistant staphylococcal infections. This recommendation is based on limited experimental data and clinical experience.

Rheumatoid arthritis – [2] = Fair documentation. Results with minocycline in the treatment of rheumatoid arthritis (RA) have been variable, demonstrating beneficial effects on laboratory parameters but modest clinical effects in patients with chronic active disease. In addition, the largest trial to date has failed to show benefit in disease progression based on radiographic assessment. Optimal use with or without disease-modifying antirheumatic drugs has yet to be determined. However, data from the most recent study suggest that minocycline may best be used as therapy in patients with recent-onset disease.

Other possible off-label uses – Treatment of gallbladder infections caused by *E. coli*; alternative agent for nocardiosis in patients who cannot take sulfa medications; chronic malignant pleural effusion. *Mycobacterium marinum* infections (100 mg every 12 hours for 6 to 8 weeks).

Administration and Dosage

➤*Adults:*

Immediate-release –

Infections: For a list of infections, refer to Indications.

- *Usual dosage* – 200 mg initially, followed by 100 mg every 12 hours. If more frequent doses are preferred, give 100 or 200 mg initially; follow with 50 mg 4 times per day.
- *Gonococcal infections (except urethritis and anorectal infections in men, uncomplicated)* – 200 mg initially, followed by 100 mg every 12 hours for at least 4 days, with posttherapy cultures within 2 to 3 days.
- *Gonococcal urethritis in men (uncomplicated)* – 100 mg every 12 hours for 5 days.
- *Meningococcal carrier state* – 100 mg every 12 hours for 5 days.
- *Syphilis* – 200 mg initially, followed by 100 mg every 12 hours for 10 to 15 days. Close follow-up, including laboratory tests, is recommended.
- *Urethral infections caused by C. trachomatis or Ureaplasma urealyticum (uncomplicated)* – 100 mg every 12 hours for at least 7 days.

Extended-release tablets –

Acne vulgaris: 1 mg/kg daily for 12 weeks.

Minocycline Extended-Release Tablet Dosing			
Patients weight (lbs)	Patients weight (kg)	Tablet strength (mg)	Actual mg/kg dose
99 to 131	45 to 59	45	1 to 0.76
132 to 199	60 to 90	90	1.5 to 1
200 to 300	91 to 136	135	1.48 to 0.99

Off-label dosing –

Infective endocarditis (adults): [2] = Fair documentation. 100 mg orally twice daily for at least 6 weeks.

Rheumatoid arthritis: [2] = Fair documentation. 100 mg twice a day for up to 48 weeks.

➤*Children:*

Immediate-release –

Infections: For a list of infections, refer to Indications.

- *Older than 8 years of age* –
  - *Usual dosage:* Initially, 4 mg/kg; follow with 2 mg/kg every 12 hours.
  - *Maximum dose:* 200 mg/day.

Extended-release tablets – See Adults for dosing for children 12 years of age and older.

Off-label dosing –

Children 12 years of age and older:

- *Chlamydia trachomatis* – 100 mg every 12 hours for 7 days.
- *Ureaplasma urealyticum* – 100 mg every 12 hours for 7 days.
- *Acne (immediate release)* – 50 to 100 mg once or twice daily.

➤*Renal function impairment:* Decrease the recommended dosage and/or increase the dosing intervals in patients with renal impairment. Do not exceed *Minocin* 200 mg in 24 hours in patients with renal impairment.

➤*Administration:* Take minocycline with plenty of fluids. Capsules and extended-release tablets may be taken with or without food. Ingestion of food may help reduce the risk of esophageal irritation and ulceration.

Take minocycline tablets and pellet-filled capsules 1 hour before or 2 hours after a meal.

Capsules should be swallowed whole.

➤*Storage/Stability:* Store at 15° to 30°C (59° to 86°F). Do not freeze. Protect from light, moisture, and excessive heat.

MINOCYCLINE — INJECTION

Indications

➤*Infections caused by susceptible strains of the designated microorganisms:* Rocky Mountain spotted fever; typhus fever and the typhus group; Q fever; rickettsialpox and tick fevers caused by rickettsiae; respiratory tract infections caused by *Mycoplasma pneumoniae*; lymphogranuloma venereum caused by *Chlamydia trachomatis*; psittacosis (ornithosis) caused by *Chlamydia psittaci*; trachoma caused by *C. trachomatis*, although the infectious agent is not always eliminated, as judged by immunofluorescence; inclusion conjunctivitis caused by *C. trachomatis*; nongonococcal urethritis, endocervical, or rectal infections in adults caused by *Ureaplasma urealyticum* or *C. trachomatis*; relapsing fever caused by *Borrelia recurrentis*; chancroid caused by *Haemophilus ducreyi*; plague caused by *Yersinia pestis*; tularemia caused by *Francisella tularensis*; cholera caused by *Vibrio cholerae*; *Campylobacter fetus* infections caused by *C. fetus*; brucellosis caused by *Brucella* species (in conjunction with streptomycin); bartonellosis caused by *Bartonella bacilliformis*; granuloma inguinale caused by *Calymmatobacterium granulomatis*.

➤*Infections caused by the following gram-negative microorganisms when bacteriologic testing indicates appropriate susceptibility to the drug: Escherichia coli*; *Enterobacter aerogenes*; *Shigella* species; *Acinetobacter* species; respiratory tract infections caused by *Haemophilus influenzae*; respiratory tract and urinary tract infections caused by *Klebsiella* species.

➤*Infections caused by the following gram-positive microorganisms when bacteriologic testing indicates appropriate susceptibility to the drug:* Upper respiratory tract infections caused by *Streptococcus pneumoniae*; skin and skin structure infections caused by *Staphylococcus aureus* (note: minocycline is not the drug of choice in the treatment of any type of staphylococcal infection).

➤*As an alternative drug in the treatment of the following infections when penicillin is contraindicated:* Uncomplicated urethritis in men caused by *Neisseria gonorrhoeae* and for the treatment of other gonococcal infections; infections in women caused by *N. gonorrhoeae*; meningitis caused by *Neisseria meningitidis*; syphilis caused by *Treponema pallidum* subspecies *pallidum*; yaws caused by *T. pallidum* subspecies *pertenue*; listeriosis caused by *Listeria monocytogenes*; anthrax caused by *Bacillus anthracis*; Vincent infection caused by *Fusobacterium fusiforme*; actinomycosis caused by *Actinomyces israelii*; infections caused by *Clostridium* species.

In acute intestinal amebiasis, minocycline may be a useful adjunct to amebicides.

In severe acne, minocycline may be useful adjunctive therapy.

To reduce the development of drug-resistant bacteria and maintain the efficacy of minocycline and other antibacterial drugs, minocycline should be used only to treat or prevent infections that are proven or strongly suspected to be caused by susceptible bacteria. When culture and susceptibility information is available, it should be considered in selecting or modifying antibacterial therapy. In the absence of such data, local epidemiology and susceptibility patterns may contribute to the empiric selection of therapy.

➤*Off-label uses:*

Infective endocarditis (adults) – [2] = Fair documentation. The use of minocycline to treat endocarditis is only recommended in patients with oxacillin-resistant staphylococcal infections. This recommendation is based on limited experimental data and clinical experience.

Administration and Dosage

➤*Dosage:* The usual dosage and frequency of administration of minocycline differs from that of the other tetracyclines. Exceeding the recommended dosage may result in an increased incidence of adverse reactions.

➤*Adults:* 200 mg followed by 100 mg every 12 hours, not to exceed 400 mg in 24 hours.

Off-label dosing –

Infective endocarditis (adults): [2] = Fair documentation. 100 mg IV twice daily for at least 6 weeks.

➤*Children:* 4 mg/kg initially followed by 2 mg/kg every 12 hours, not to exceed the usual adult dose.

➤*Renal function impairment:* The pharmacokinetics of minocycline in patients with renal function impairment (creatinine clearance [Ccr] less than 80 mL/min) have not been fully characterized. Current data are insufficient to determine if a dosage adjustment is warranted. The total daily dosage should not exceed 200 mg in 24 hours. However, because of the antianabolic effect of tetracyclines, serum urea nitrogen (BUN) and creatinine should be monitored.

➤*Dilution:* The cryodesiccated powder should be reconstituted with sterile water for injection 5 mL and immediately further diluted to 500 to 1,000 mL with sodium chloride injection, dextrose injection, dextrose and sodium chloride injection, Ringer's injection, or Ringer's lactate injection, but not with other solutions containing calcium because a precipitate may form, especially in neutral and alkaline solutions. When further diluted in 500 to 1,000 mL of compatible solutions (except Ringer's lactate), the pH usually ranges from 2.5 to 4. The pH of intravenous (IV) minocycline 100 mg in Ringer's lactate 500 to 1,000 mL usually ranges from 4.5 to 6.

Final dilutions (500 to 1,000 mL) should be administered immediately, but product and diluents are compatible at room temperature for 24 hours without a significant loss of potency. Any unused portions must be discarded after that period.

➤*Administration:* Avoid rapid administration. Parenteral therapy is indicated only when oral therapy is not adequate or tolerated. Oral therapy should be instituted as soon as possible. If IV therapy is given over prolonged periods of time, thrombophlebitis may result.

➤*Admixture compatibility:*

Incompatibilities – Minocycline IV should not be mixed before or during administration with any solutions containing the following: adrenocorticotropic hormone, aminophylline, amobarbital sodium, amphotericin B, bicarbonate infusion mixtures, calcium gluconate or chloride, carbenicillin, cefazolin sodium, cephalothin sodium, chloramphenicol succinate, colistin sulfate, heparin sodium, hydrocortisone sodium succinate, iodine sodium, methicillin sodium, novobiocin, penicillin, pentobarbital, phenytoin sodium, polymyxin, prochlorperazine, sodium ascorbate, sulfadiazine, sulfisoxazole, thiopental sodium, vitamin K (sodium bisulfate or sodium salt), or whole blood.

➤*Storage/Stability:* Store at controlled room temperature, 20° to 25°C (68° to 77°F).

MINOCYCLINE — DENTAL

Indications

➤*Adult periodontitis:* As an adjunct to scaling and root planing procedures for reduction of pocket depth in patients with adult periodontitis; may be used as part of a periodontal maintenance program that includes good oral hygiene and scaling and root planing.

Administration and Dosage

➤*Adults:*

Adult periodontitis – Minocycline is a variable dose product dependent on the size, shape, and number of pockets being treated. In US clinical trials, up to 121 unit-dose cartridges were used in a single visit, and up to 3 treatments, at 3-month intervals, were administered in pockets with a depth of 5 mm or greater.

➤*Preparation for administration:* Minocycline microspheres are provided as a dry powder and packaged in a unit-dose cartridge, which is inserted into a cartridge handle for administration. The oral health care provider removes the disposable cartridge from its pouch and connects the cartridge to the handle mechanism.

➤*Administration:* Minocycline microspheres administration does not require local anesthesia. Professional subgingival administration is accomplished by inserting the unit-dose cartridge into the base of the periodontal pocket and then pressing the thumb ring in the handle mechanism to expel the powder while gradually withdrawing the tip from the base of the pocket. The handle mechanism should be sterilized between patients. Minocycline microspheres do not have to be removed because they are bioresorbable; an adhesive or dressing is not required.

➤*Storage/Stability:* Store at 20° to 25°C (68° to 77°F)/60% relative humidity. Excursions permitted to 15° to 30°C (59° to 86°F). Avoid exposure to excessive heat.

GLYCYLCLYCLINES

TIGECYCLINE

Rx	**Tygacil** (Wyeth)	**Injection, lyophilized powder for solution:** 50 mg	Preservative free. Lactose. In 10 mL single-dose vials.

TIGECYCLINE — INJECTION

Indications

➤*Community-acquired bacterial pneumonia:* Caused by *Streptococcus pneumoniae* (penicillin-susceptible isolates), including cases with concurrent bacteremia, *Haemophilus influenzae* (beta-lactamase negative isolates), and *Legionella pneumophila*.

➤*Complicated intra-abdominal infections:* Caused by *Citrobacter freundii*, *Enterobacter cloacae*, *Escherichia coli*, *Klebsiella oxytoca*, *Klebsiella pneumoniae*, *Enterococcus faecalis* (vancomycin-susceptible isolates), *Staphylococcus aureus* (methicillin-susceptible and methicillin-resistant isolates), *Streptococcus anginosus* group (includes *S. anginosus*, *Streptococcus intermedius*, and *Streptococcus constellatus*), *Bacteroides fragilis*, *Bacteroides thetaiotaomicron*, *Bacteroides uniformis*, *Bacteroides vulgatus*, *Clostridium perfringens*, and *Peptostreptococcus micros*.

TIGECYCLINE — INJECTION

➤*Complicated skin and skin structure infections:* Caused by *E. coli*, *E. faecalis* (vancomycin-susceptible isolates), *S. aureus* (methicillin-susceptible and methicillin-resistant isolates), *Streptococcus agalactiae*, *S. anginosus* group (includes *S. anginosus*, *S. intermedius*, and *S. constellatus*), *Streptococcus pyogenes*, *E. cloacae*, *K. pneumoniae*, and *B. fragilis*.

➤*Off-label uses:*

Hospital-acquired pneumonia – [2] = Fair documentation. Data from observational studies and case series enrolling fewer than 100 patients suggest that tigecycline may be a beneficial therapy option in patients with hospital-acquired pneumonia, ventilator-associated pneumonia, and healthcare-associated pneumonia associated with multidrug-resistant (MDR) gram-negative bacteria, specifically cases associated with *Acinetobacter* species. Larger randomized, controlled trials are needed to confirm these findings and specify the role of tigecycline in patients with hospital-acquired pneumonia.

Administration and Dosage

➤*Adults:*

Community-acquired bacterial pneumonia –
Initial dosage: 100 mg intravenous (IV).
Maintenance dosage: 50 mg IV every 12 hours.
Duration of therapy: 7 to 14 days.

Complicated intra-abdominal infections –
Initial dosage: 100 mg IV.
Maintenance dosage: 50 mg IV every 12 hours.
Duration of therapy: 5 to 14 days.

Complicated skin and skin structure infections – See Complicated Intra-Abdominal Infections.

Off-label dosing –
Hospital-acquired pneumonia: [2] = Fair documentation. Loading dose of 100 mg IV, followed by 50 mg IV every 12 hours. Recommended duration of treatment ranges from 13 to 20 days.

➤*Children:*

Off-label dosing –
12 years of age and older:
- *Usual dose* – 1 mg/kg IV every 12 hours.
- *Maximum dose* – 50 mg/dose.
- *Initial dosage* – 1.5 mg/kg IV.
- *Alternative dosage* –
  8 years of age and older:
- *Usual dosage* – 1 mg/kg IV every 12 hours.
- *Maximum dose* – 50 mg/dose.

➤*Hepatic function impairment:*

Severe hepatic function impairment –
Initial dosage: 100 mg IV.
Maintenance dosage: 25 mg IV every 12 hours.

➤*Preparation for administration:* Each vial should be reconstituted with 5.3 mL of sodium chloride 0.9% injection, dextrose 5% injection, or Ringer's lactate injection to achieve a concentration of tigecycline 10 mg/mL. Each vial contains a 6% overage; therefore, 5 mL of reconstituted solution is equivalent to 50 mg of the drug. The vial should be gently swirled until the drug dissolves.

Reconstituted solution must be transferred and further diluted for IV infusion. Immediately withdraw 5 mL of the reconstituted solution from the vial and add to a 100 mL IV bag for infusion (for a 100 mg dose, reconstitute 2 vials; for a 50 mg dose, reconstitute 1 vial). The maximum concentration in the IV bag should be 1 mg/mL. The reconstituted solution should be yellow to orange in color. If it is not, the solution should be discarded.

➤*Administration:* Administer IV over 30 to 60 minutes through a dedicated line or through a Y-site. If the same IV line is used for sequential infusion of several drugs, the line should be flushed before and after infusion of tigecycline with sodium chloride 0.9% injection, dextrose 5% injection, or Ringer's lactate injection. The injection should be made with an infusion solution compatible with tigecycline and with any other drug(s) administered via this common line.

➤*Admixture compatibility:*

Compatibility – Compatible IV solutions include sodium chloride 0.9% injection, dextrose 5% injection, and Ringer's lactate injection. When administered through a Y-site, tigecycline is compatible with the following drugs or diluents when used with sodium chloride 0.9% injection or dextrose 5% injection: amikacin, dobutamine, dopamine, gentamicin, haloperidol, lidocaine, metoclopramide, morphine, norepinephrine, piperacillin/tazobactam (EDTA formulation), potassium chloride, propofol, ranitidine, Ringer's lactate, theophylline, and tobramycin.

Incompatibility – The following drugs should not be administered simultaneously through the same Y-site with tigecycline: amphotericin B, amphotericin B lipid complex, diazepam, esomeprazole, and omeprazole.

➤*Storage/Stability:* Prior to reconstitution, store tigecycline at 20° to 25°C (68° to 77°F); excursions are permitted between 15° and 30°C (59° and 86°F). Once reconstituted, tigecycline may be stored at room temperature for up to 24 hours (up to 6 hours in the vial, and the remaining time in the IV bag). Alternatively, tigecycline mixed with sodium chloride 0.9% injection or dextrose 5% may be stored refrigerated at 2° to 8°C (36° to 46°F) for up to 48 hours following immediate transfer of the reconstituted solution into the IV bag.

Actions

➤*Pharmacology:* Tigecycline, a glycylcycline antibacterial, inhibits protein translation in bacteria by binding to the 30S ribosomal subunit and blocking entry of amino-acyl tRNA molecules into the A site of the ribosome. This prevents incorporation of amino acid residues into elongating peptide chains. In general, tigecycline is considered bacteriostatic; however, tigecycline has demonstrated bactericidal activity against isolates of *S. pneumoniae* and *L. pneumophila*.

➤*Pharmacokinetics:*

Absorption/Distribution – Following the administration of tigecycline 100 mg followed by 50 mg every 12 hours to 33 healthy volunteers, the tigecycline area under the curve ($AUC_{0\text{-}12h}$) (134 mcg•h/mL) in alveolar cells was approximately 78-fold higher than the $AUC_{0\text{-}12h}$ in the serum, and the $AUC_{0\text{-}12h}$ (2.28 mcg•h/mL) in epithelial lining fluid was approximately 32% higher than the $AUC_{0\text{-}12h}$ in the serum. The $AUC_{0\text{-}12h}$ (1.61 mcg•h/mL) of tigecycline in skin blister fluid was approximately 26% lower than the $AUC_{0\text{-}12h}$ in the serum of 10 healthy subjects.

The in vitro plasma protein binding of tigecycline ranges from approximately 71% to 89% at concentrations observed in clinical studies (0.1 to 1 mcg/mL). The steady-state volume of distribution of tigecycline averaged 500 to 700 L (7 to 9 L/kg), indicating tigecycline is extensively distributed beyond the plasma volume and into the tissues.

Metabolism/Excretion – Tigecycline is not extensively metabolized. In vitro studies with tigecycline using human liver microsomes, liver slices, and hepatocytes led to the formation of only trace amounts of metabolites. In healthy men receiving ^{14}C-tigecycline, tigecycline was the primary ^{14}C-labeled material recovered in urine and feces, but a glucuronide, an N-acetyl metabolite, and a tigecycline epimer (each at no more than 10% of the administered dose) were also present.

The recovery of total radioactivity in feces and urine following administration of ^{14}C-tigecycline indicates that 59% of the dose is eliminated by biliary/fecal excretion and 33% is excreted in urine. Approximately 22% of the total dose is excreted as unchanged tigecycline in urine. Overall, the primary route of elimination for tigecycline is biliary excretion of unchanged tigecycline and its metabolites. Glucuronidation and renal excretion of unchanged tigecycline are secondary routes.

Special populations –
Hepatic function impairment: Systemic clearance of tigecycline was reduced by 25% and the half-life of tigecycline was prolonged by 23% in patients with moderate hepatic impairment (Child-Pugh class C). Systemic clearance of tigecycline was reduced by 55% and the half-life was prolonged by 43% in patients with severe hepatic impairment (Child-Pugh class C). Dosage adjustment is necessary in patients with severe hepatic impairment (Child-Pugh class C) (see Administration and Dosage).

➤*Microbiology:* Tigecycline has been shown to be active against most strains of the following microorganisms, both in vitro and in clinical infections.

Facultative gram-positive bacteria – *E. faecalis* (vancomycin-susceptible isolates), *S. aureus* (methicillin-susceptible and methicillin-resistant isolates), *S. agalactiae*, *S. anginosus* group (includes *S. anginosus*, *S. intermedius*, and *S. constellatus*), *S. pneumoniae* (penicillin-susceptible isolates), *S. pyogenes*.

Facultative gram-negative bacteria – *C. freundii*, *E. cloacae*, *E. coli*, *H. influenzae* (beta-lactamase negative isolates), *K. oxytoca*, *K. pneumoniae*, *L. pneumophila*.

Anaerobic bacteria – *B. fragilis*, *B. thetaiotaomicron*, *B. uniformis*, *B. vulgatus*, *C. perfringens*, *P. micros*.

Contraindications

Known hypersensitivity to tigecycline.

Warnings/Precautions

➤*All-cause mortality:* An increase in all-cause mortality has been observed across phase 3 and 4 clinical trials in tigecycline-treated patients versus comparator-treated patients. In all 13 phase 3 and 4 trials that included a comparator, death occurred in 4% of patients receiving tigecycline and 3% of patients receiving comparator drugs. In a pooled analysis of these trials, based on a random effects model by trial weight, an adjusted risk difference of all-cause mortality was 0.6% (95% confidence interval [CI], 0.1 to 1.2) between tigecycline- and comparator-treated patients. The cause of this increase has not been established. Consider this increase in all-cause mortality when selecting among treatment options.

➤*Hepatic effects:* Increases in total bilirubin concentration, prothrombin time, and transaminases have been seen in patients treated with tigecycline. Isolated cases of significant hepatic dysfunction and hepatic failure have been reported in patients being treated with tigecycline. Some of these patients were receiving multiple concomitant medications. Monitor patients who develop abnormal liver function tests during tigecycline therapy for evidence of worsening hepatic function and evaluate for risk/benefit of continuing tigecycline therapy. Adverse events may occur after the drug has been discontinued.

➤*Ventilator-associated pneumonia:* A study of patients with hospital-acquired pneumonia failed to demonstrate the efficacy of tigecycline. In this study, patients were randomized to received tigecycline (100 mg initially, then 50 mg every 12 hours) or a comparator. In addition, patients were allowed to receive specified adjunctive therapies. The subgroup of patients with ventilator-associated pneumonia who received tigecycline had lower cure rates (47.9% vs 70.1% for the clinically evaluable population).

In this study, greater mortality was seen in patients with ventilator-associated pneumonia who received tigecycline (19.1% vs 12.3% in

TIGECYCLINE — INJECTION

comparator-treated patients). Particularly high mortality was seen among tigecycline-treated patients with ventilator-associated pneumonia and bacteremia at baseline (50% vs 7.7% in comparator-treated patients).

➤*Pancreatitis:* Acute pancreatitis, including fatal cases, has occurred in association with tigecycline treatment. Consider the diagnosis of acute pancreatitis in patients taking tigecycline who develop clinical symptoms, signs, or laboratory abnormalities suggestive of acute pancreatitis. Cases have been reported in patients without known risk factor for pancreatitis. Patients usually improve after tigecycline discontinuation. Consider the cessation of the treatment with tigecycline in patients suspected of having developed pancreatitis.

➤*Tooth development:* The use of tigecycline during tooth development (last half of pregnancy, infancy, and childhood until 8 years of age) may cause permanent discoloration of the teeth (yellow/gray/brown). Results of studies in rats with tigecycline have shown bone discoloration. Do not use tigecycline during tooth development unless other drugs are not likely to be effective or are contraindicated.

➤*Clostridium difficile–associated diarrhea: C. difficile*–associated diarrhea (CDAD) has been reported with use of nearly all antibacterial agents, including tigecycline, and may range in severity from mild diarrhea to fatal colitis. Treatment with antibacterial agents alters the flora of the colon, leading to overgrowth of*C. difficile*.

C. difficile produces toxins A and B, which contribute to the development of CDAD. Hypertoxin-producing strains of *C. difficile* cause increased morbidity and mortality because these infections can be refractory to antimicrobial therapy and may require colectomy. CDAD must be considered in all patients who have diarrhea following antibiotic use. Careful medical history assessment is necessary because CDAD has been reported to occur more than 2 months after the administration of antibacterial agents.

➤*Intestinal perforation:* Exercise caution when considering tigecycline monotherapy in patients with complicated intra-abdominal infections secondary to clinically apparent intestinal perforation. In complicated intra-abdominal infection studies (n = 1,642), 6 patients treated with tigecycline and 2 patients treated with imipenem/cilastatin had intestinal perforations and developed sepsis/septic shock. The 6 patients treated with tigecycline had higher Acute Physiology and Chronic Health Evaluation II (APACHE II) scores (median, 13) versus the 2 patients treated with imipenem/cilastatin (APACHE II scores of 4 and 6). Because of differences in baseline APACHE II scores between treatment groups and small overall numbers, the relationship of this outcome to treatment cannot be established.

➤*Tetracycline antibiotics:* Tigecycline is structurally similar to tetracycline class antibiotics and may have similar adverse reactions. Such effects may include photosensitivity, pseudotumor cerebri, and antianabolic action (which has led to increased serum urea nitrogen [BUN], azotemia, acidosis, and hypophosphatemia). As with tetracyclines, pancreatitis has been reported with the use of tigecycline.

➤*Resistance:* Prescribing tigecycline in the absence of a proven or strongly suspected bacterial infection is unlikely to provide benefit to the patient and increases the risk of the development of drug-resistant bacteria.

➤*Hypersensitivity reactions:* Anaphylaxis/anaphylactoid reactions have been reported with nearly all antibacterial agents, including tigecycline, and may be life-threatening. Tigecycline is structurally similar to tetracycline class antibiotics; administer with caution in patients with known hypersensitivity to tetracycline class antibiotics.

➤*Hepatic function impairment:* Treat patients with severe hepatic impairment with caution and monitor them for treatment response. See Administration and Dosage for more information.

➤*Superinfection:* As with other antibacterial drugs, use of tigecycline may result in overgrowth of nonsusceptible organisms, including fungi. Carefully monitor patients during therapy. If superinfection occurs, take appropriate measures.

➤*Pregnancy: Category D.* Tigecycline may cause fetal harm when administered to a pregnant woman. If the patient becomes pregnant while taking tigecycline, inform her of the potential hazard to the fetus. Results of animal studies indicate that tigecycline crosses the placenta and is found in fetal tissues. Decreased fetal weights in rats and rabbits (with associated delays in ossification) and fetal loss in rabbits have been observed with tigecycline.

Tigecycline was not teratogenic in the rat or rabbit. In preclinical safety studies, ^{14}C-labeled tigecycline crossed the placenta and was found in fetal tissues, including fetal bony structures. The administration of tigecycline was associated with slight reductions in fetal weights and an increased incidence of minor skeletal anomalies (delays in bone ossification) at exposures of 5 and 1 times the human daily dose based on AUC in rats and rabbits, respectively (28 and 6 mcg•h/mL at 12 and 4 mg/kg/day). An increased incidence of fetal loss was observed at maternotoxic doses in the rabbits with exposure equivalent to human dose.

There are no adequate and well-controlled studies of tigecycline in pregnant women. It is not known if tigecycline crosses the human placenta. The molecular weight (approximately 586), prolonged elimination half-life, and wide distribution in tissues suggest that the antibiotic will cross to the embryo/fetus. Inadvertent or planned use in the first trimester probably does not represent a major risk to the embryo or fetus, but avoid use in later trimesters. Use tigecycline during pregnancy only if the potential benefit justifies the potential risk to the fetus.

➤*Lactation:* Results from animal studies using ^{14}C-labeled tigecycline indicate that tigecycline is excreted readily via the milk of lactating rats. Consistent with the limited oral bioavailability of tigecycline, there is little or no systemic exposure to tigecycline in breast-feeding pups as a result of exposure via maternal milk.

It is not known whether this drug is excreted in human milk. The molecular weight (about 586), prolonged elimination half-life, and wide distribution in tissues suggest that tigecycline will be excreted into breast milk. Even if the oral bioavailability in infants is negligible, the presence of the antibiotic in milk could cause 3 potential problems: modification of bowel flora, direct effects on the infant's gut, and interference with the interpretation of culture results if a fever workup is required. Thus, the best option if a woman is receiving this antibiotic is not to breast-feed. Because many drugs are excreted in human milk, exercise caution when tigecycline is administered to a breast-feeding woman.

➤*Children:* Safety and efficacy in children younger than 18 years of age have not been established. Because of effects on tooth development, use in patients younger than 8 years of age is not recommended.

➤*Elderly:* Of the total number of subjects who received tigecycline in phase 3 clinical studies (N = 2,514), 664 were 65 years of age and older, while 228 were 75 years of age and older. No unexpected overall differences in safety or efficacy were observed between these subjects and younger subjects, but greater sensitivity to adverse reactions of some older individuals cannot be ruled out.

➤*Monitoring:* Monitor prothrombin time or another suitable anticoagulation test if tigecycline is administered with warfarin. Monitor patients for superinfection during therapy. Monitor patients who develop abnormal liver function tests during tigecycline therapy for evidence of worsening hepatic function and evaluate for risk/benefit of continuing tigecycline therapy.

Drug Interactions

Tigecycline Drug Interactions

Precipitant drug	Object drug[a]		Description
Tigecycline	Contraceptives, hormonal	⬇	Concurrent use may render oral contraceptives less effective. Advise patients wishing to avoid even a slight increase in the risk of pregnancy to use an additional nonhormonal method of contraception.
Tigecycline	Cyclosporine	⬆	Cyclosporine concentrations and risk of adverse reactions may be increased. Closely monitor cyclosporine trough whole blood concentrations when tigecycline is started or stopped. Adjust the cyclosporine dose as needed.
Tigecycline	Warfarin	⬆	Coadministration resulted in a decrease in clearance of R-warfarin and S-warfarin by 40% and 23%, an increase in C_{max}[b] by 38% and 43%, and an increase in AUC by 68% and 29%, respectively. Monitor prothrombin time or other suitable anticoagulant tests if tigecycline and warfarin are given concurrently. Adjust the warfarin dose as needed.

[a] ⬆ = object drug increased; ⬇ = object drug decreased.
[b] C_{max} = maximum plasma concentration.

Adverse Reactions

➤*Serious adverse reactions:* In comparative clinical studies, infection-related serious adverse reactions were more frequently reported for subjects treated with tigecycline (7%) versus comparators (6%). Serious adverse reactions of sepsis/septic shock were more frequently reported for subjects treated with tigecycline (2%) versus comparators (1%). Because of baseline differences between treatment groups in this subset of patients, the relationship of this outcome to treatment cannot be established.

➤*Common adverse reactions:* The most common treatment-emergent adverse reactions were nausea and vomiting, which generally occurred during the first 1 to 2 days of therapy. The majority of cases of nausea and vomiting associated with tigecycline and comparators were either mild or moderate in severity. In patients treated with tigecycline, nausea incidence was 26% (17% mild, 8% moderate, 1% severe) and vomiting incidence was 18% (11% mild, 6% moderate, 1% severe).

In patients treated for complicated skin and skin structure infections, nausea incidence was 35% for tigecycline and 9% for vancomycin/aztreonam; vomiting incidence was 20% for tigecycline and 4% for vancomycin/aztreonam. In patients treated for complicated intra-abdominal infections, nausea incidence was 25% for tigecycline and 21% for imipenem/cilastatin; vomiting incidence was 20% for tigecycline and 15% for imipenem/cilastatin. In patients treated for community-acquired bacterial pneumonia, nausea incidence was 24% for tigecycline and 8% for levofloxacin; vomiting incidence was 16% for tigecycline and 6% for levofloxacin.

➤*Discontinuation:* Tigecycline was discontinued because of adverse reactions in 7% of patients compared with 6% for all comparators. Discontinuation from tigecycline was most frequently associated with nausea (1%) and vomiting (1%). For comparators, discontinuations were most frequently associated with nausea (less than 1%).

➤*Mortality:* In all 13 phase 3 and 4 trials that included a comparator, death occurred in 4% of patients receiving tigecycline and 3% of patients receiving comparator drugs. In a pooled analysis of these trials, based on a

TIGECYCLINE — INJECTION

random effects model by trial weight, an adjusted risk difference of all-cause mortality was 0.6% (95% CI, 0.1 to 1.2) between tigecycline- and comparator-treated patients. The cause of the imbalance has not been established. Generally, deaths were the result of worsening infection, complications of infection, or underlying comorbidities.

Tigecycline Adverse Reactions of Death by Infection Type					
	Tigecycline		Comparator		Risk difference[a]
Infection type	n	%	n	%	% (95% CI)
Complicated skin and skin structure infection	834	1.4%	813	0.7%	0.7 (−0.3 to 1.7)
Complicated intra-abdominal infection	1,382	3%	1,393	2.2%	0.8 (−0.4 to 2)
Community-acquired pneumonia	424	2.8%	422	2.6%	0.2 (−2 to 2.4)
Hospital-acquired pneumonia	467	14.1%	467	12.2%	1.9 (−2.4 to 6.3)
Nonventilator-associated pneumonia[b]	336	12.2%	345	12.2%	0 (−4.9 to 4.9)
Ventilator-associated pneumonia[b]	131	19.1%	122	12.3%	6.8 (−2.1 to 15.7)
Resistant pathogens	128	8.6%	43	4.7%	0.7 (−4 to 11.9)
Diabetic foot infections	553	1.3%	508	0.6%	0.7 (−0.5 to 1.8)
Overall adjusted	3,788	4%	3,646	3%	0.6 (0.1 to 1.2)[c]

[a] The difference between the percentage of patients who died in tigecycline and comparator treatment groups. The 95% CI for each infection type was calculated using the normal approximation method without continuity correction.
[b] These are subgroups of the hospital-acquired pneumonia population. The phase 3 studies include 300, 305, and 900 patients with complicated skin and skin structure infection; 301, 306, 315, 316, and 400 patients with complicated intra-abdominal infection; 308 and 313 patients with community-acquired pneumonia; 311 patients with hospital-acquired pneumonia; 307 patients with resistant gram-positive pathogen study in patients with methicillin-resistant *S. aureus* or vancomycin-resistant *Enterococcus*; and 319 patients with diabetic foot infections with and without osteomyelitis.
[c] Overall adjusted (random effects model by trial weight) risk-difference estimate and 95% CI.

➤*Adverse reactions (2% or more):*

Tigecycline Adverse Reactions (≥ 2%)		
Adverse reactions	Tigecycline (n = 2,514)	Comparators[a] (n = 2,307)
CNS		
Asthenia	3%	2%
Dizziness	3%	3%
Headache	6%	7%
GI		
Abdominal pain	6%	4%
Diarrhea	12%	11%
Dyspepsia	2%	2%
Nausea	26%	13%
Vomiting	18%	9%
Hepatic		
Alkaline phosphatase increased	4%	3%
ALT increased[b]	5%	5%
AST increased[b]	4%	5%
Bilirubinemia	2%	1%
Metabolic/Nutritional		
Amylase increased	3%	2%
BUN increased	3%	1%
Hypoproteinemia	5%	3%
Miscellaneous		
Abnormal healing	4%	3%
Abscess	3%	3%
Anemia	4%	5%
Infection	8%	5%
Phlebitis	3%	4%
Rash	3%	4%

[a] Vancomycin/aztreonam, imipenem/cilastatin, levofloxacin, linezolid.
[b] Liver function test abnormalities in tigecycline-treated patients were reported more frequently in the posttherapy period than those in comparator-treated patients, which occurred more often during therapy.

➤*Adverse reactions (less than 2%):*

GI – Abnormal stools, anorexia.

GU – Leukorrhea, vaginal moniliasis, vaginitis.

Hematologic/Lymphatic – Eosinophilia, increased international normalized ratio, prolonged activated partial thromboplastin time, prolonged prothrombin time, thrombocytopenia.

Local – Injection-site edema, injection-site inflammation, injection-site pain, injection-site phlebitis, injection-site reaction.

Metabolic/Nutritional – Hypocalcemia, hypoglycemia, hyponatremia, increased creatinine.

Miscellaneous – Allergic reaction, chills, jaundice, pruritus, septic shock, taste perversion, thrombophlebitis.

➤*Postmarketing:*

Hepatic – Acute pancreatitis, hepatic cholestasis, jaundice.

Hypersensitivity – Anaphylaxis/anaphylactoid reactions.

Overdosage

➤*Symptoms:* IV administration of tigecycline at a single dose of 300 mg over 60 minutes in healthy volunteers resulted in an increased incidence of nausea and vomiting.

➤*Treatment:* No specific information is available on the treatment of overdosage with tigecycline. Tigecycline is not removed in significant quantities by hemodialysis.

Patient Information

Counsel patients that antibacterial drugs, including tigecycline, should only be used to treat bacterial infections. Antibacterial drugs do not treat viral infections (eg, the common cold). When tigecycline is prescribed to treat a bacterial infection, tell patients that although it is common to feel better early in the course of therapy, to take the medication exactly as directed. Skipping doses or not completing the full course of therapy may decrease the efficacy of the immediate treatment and increase the likelihood that bacteria will develop resistance and not be treatable by tigecycline or other antibacterial drugs in the future.

Inform patients that diarrhea is a common problem caused by antibiotics, which usually ends when the antibiotic is discontinued. Sometimes after starting treatment with antibiotics, they can develop watery and bloody stools (with or without stomach cramps and fever) even as late as 2 months or more after having taken the last dose of the antibiotic. If this occurs, instruct patients to contact their health care provider as soon as possible.

Indications

Refer to individual product monographs for specific indications.

To reduce the development of drug-resistant bacteria and maintain the effectiveness, only use macrolides to treat or prevent infections that are proven, or strongly suspected, to be caused by susceptible bacteria. When culture and susceptibility information are available, consider them when selecting or modifying antibacterial therapy. In the absence of such data, local epidemiology and susceptibility patterns may contribute to the empiric selection of therapy.

Macrolides — Summary of Indications[a,b]

Indications ✓ = FDA approved X = off-label use	Azithromycin				Clarithromycin			Erythromycin	
	Tablets (250 and 500 mg) and oral suspension (100 and 200 mg/5 mL)	Tablets (600 mg) and oral suspension (1 g)	ER oral suspension	Injection	Tablets	Oral suspension	ER tablets	Oral	Injection
Adults									
Acne vulgaris								X[c]	
Acne vulgaris (topical)				X[d]					
Acute bacterial exacerbation of chronic bronchitis	✓				✓	✓	✓		
Acute maxillary sinusitis	✓		✓		✓	✓	✓		
Babesiosis	X[e]								
Bacillary angiomatosis (immunocompromised patients)								X[c]	
Campylobacter enteritis								X[c]	
Cellulitis, erysipelas								X[c]	
Chancroid (genital ulcer disease)	✓[f]							X[c]	
Chlamydial infections	X[c]								
Cholera	X[c]								
Community-acquired pneumonia	✓		✓	✓	✓	✓	✓		
Diphtheria								✓	✓
Disseminated mycobacterial infections		✓			✓	✓			
Erythrasma								✓	✓
Granuloma inguinale (donovanosis)	X[e]	X[e]						X[e]	
Helicobacter pylori infection and duodenal ulcer[g]					✓				
Hospital-acquired pneumonia				X[e]					
Impetigo, ecthyma								X[c]	
Inclusion conjunctivitis								X[c]	
Infected wounds of the extremities								X[c]	
Intestinal amebiasis								✓	
Legionnaire disease								✓	✓
Leptospirosis								X[c]	
Listeriosis								✓	
Lyme disease (early)	X[c]				X[c]	X[c]		X[c]	
Lymphogranuloma venereum								X[c]	
Nongonococcal urethritis								✓	
Nongonococcal urethritis/cervicitis	✓	✓							
Pelvic inflammatory disease				✓				✓	✓
Pertussis (whooping cough)								✓	
Pharyngitis/Tonsillitis	✓				✓	✓			
Prevention of disseminated *Mycobacterium avium* complex (MAC) in patients with advanced HIV infection		✓			✓	✓			
Prevention of rheumatic fever								✓	✓
Primary syphilis								✓	
Prophylaxis after a sexual assault	X[c]	X[c]							
Relapsing fever								X[c]	
Respiratory tract infections due to *Mycoplasma pneumoniae*								✓	✓
Rosacea	X[d]								
Skin and skin structure infections	✓				✓	✓		✓	✓
Traveler's diarrhea	X[e]								
Uncomplicated urethral, endocervical, or rectal infections								✓	
Upper/Lower respiratory tract infections								✓	✓
Urethritis/Cervicitis	✓								
Urogenital infections during pregnancy								✓	
Children									
Acute maxillary sinusitis					✓	✓			
Acute otitis media	✓				✓	✓			
Babesiosis	X[e]								
Chlamydial infections	X[c]								

Macrolides — Summary of Indications[a,b]									
	Azithromycin				Clarithromycin			Erythromycin	
Indications ✓ = FDA approved X = off-label use	Tablets (250 and 500 mg) and oral suspension (100 and 200 mg/5 mL)	Tablets (600 mg) and oral suspension (1 g)	ER oral suspension	Injection	Tablets	Oral suspension	ER tablets	Oral	Injection
Community-acquired pneumonia	✓		✓		✓	✓			
Conjunctivitis of the newborn								✓	
Disseminated mycobacterial infections					✓	✓			
Impetigo, ecthyma								X[c]	
Lyme disease (early)	X[c]				X[c]	X[c]		X[c]	
Pharyngitis/ Tonsillitis	✓				✓	✓			
Pneumonia of infancy								✓	
Prevention of acute otitis media	X[h]								
Prevention of disseminated MAC in patients with advanced HIV infection					✓	✓			
Skin and skin structure infections, uncomplicated					✓	✓			

[a] Causative organisms may vary for each indication for specific macrolides. Refer to individual monographs for this information.
[b] FDA = Food and Drug Administration; ER = extended-release.
[c] Not rated.
[d] Insufficient documentation.
[e] Good documentation.
[f] Approved for use in men only.
[g] In combination with amoxicillin and lansoprazole or omeprazole to eradicate *H. pylori* infection in patients with *H. pylori* infection and duodenal ulcer disease (active or 5-year history of duodenal ulcer); also indicated in combination with omeprazole or ranitidine bismuth citrate for active duodenal ulcer associated with *H. pylori* infection.
[h] Fair documentation.

➤*Off-label uses:* Refer to individual monographs for further information.

Acne vulgaris (topical) –
Azithromycin: [4] = Insufficient documentation.

Acute pharyngitis or tonsillitis (group A streptococcal) (children), 3-day regimen –
Azithromycin: [5] = Poor documentation.

Acute skin and soft tissue infections (children), 3-day regimen –
Azithromycin: [1] = Good documentation.

Babesiosis –
Azithromycin: [1] = Good documentation.

Chancroid –
Erythromycin (base): [1] = Good documentation.

Granuloma inguinale (donovanosis) –
Azithromycin: [1] = Good documentation.
Erythromycin: [1] = Good documentation.

H. pylori infection –
Azithromycin: [4] = Insufficient documentation.

Hospital-acquired pneumonia –
Azithromycin: [1] = Good documentation.

Lower respiratory tract infections (children), 3-day regimen –
Azithromycin: [2] = Fair documentation.

Prevention of acute otitis media (children), once-weekly regimen –
Azithromycin: [2] = Fair documentation.

Prevention of coronary events –
Azithromycin: [5] = Poor documentation.

Rosacea –
Azithromycin: [4] = Insufficient documentation.

Rosacea (topical) –
Azithromycin: [5] = Poor documentation.

Traveler's diarrhea –
Azithromycin: [1] = Good documentation.

Other possible off-label uses –
Azithromycin:
• *Cholera* – Treatment of cholera in adults.
• *Chlamydial infections caused by Chlamydia trachomatis* – The Centers for Disease Control and Prevention (CDC) recommends azithromycin 1 g orally in a single dose.

For children who have chlamydial infections and weigh 45 kg or more but are younger than 8 years of age, the CDC recommends azithromycin 1 g orally in a single dose.

For children 8 years of age and older with chlamydial infection, the CDC recommends azithromycin 1 g orally in a single dose.
• *Lyme disease (early)* – IDSA guidelines recommend macrolides as second-line therapy in patients who are intolerant of or should not take first-line therapy (eg, amoxicillin, cefuroxime axetil, doxycycline).
• *Prophylaxis after a sexual assault* – The CDC recommends azithromycin 1 g orally in a single dose plus ceftriaxone and metronidazole.

Clarithromycin:
• *Lyme disease (early)* – IDSA guidelines recommend macrolides as second-line therapy in patients who are intolerant of or should not take first-line therapy (eg, amoxicillin, cefuroxime axetil, doxycycline).

Erythromycin:
• *Acne vulgaris* – Helpful in decreasing the population of lipophilic bacteria and may also have an anti-inflammatory effect.
• *Bacillary angiomatosis (immunocompromised patients)* – Caused by *Bartonella henselae* or *Bartonella quintana*; as an alternative agent, erythromycin 500 mg 4 times/day.
• *Campylobacter enteritis* – Caused by *Campylobacter jejuni*.
• *Cellulitis, erysipelas* – As an alternative agent for the treatment of cellulitis (erysipelas) of the extremities that is not associated with venous catheter and is not diabetes related.
• *Granuloma inguinale (donovanosis)* – Caused by *Calymmatobacterium granulomatis*; as an alternative to doxycycline or trimethoprim-sulfamethoxazole.
• *Impetigo, ecthyma* – As an alternative agent for the treatment of nonbullous lesions.
• *Inclusion conjunctivitis (adults)* – Caused by *C. trachomatis*; as an alternative agent.
• *Infected wounds of the extremities* – As an alternative agent for the treatment of mild to moderate, uncomplicated, infected wounds of the extremities.
• *Leptospirosis* – Caused by *Leptospira* species; for the treatment of moderate to severe leptospirosis.
• *Lyme disease (early)* – IDSA guidelines recommend macrolides as second-line therapy in patients who are intolerant of or should not take first-line therapy (eg, amoxicillin, cefuroxime axetil, doxycycline).
• *Lymphogranuloma venereum* – Genital, inguinal or anorectal.
• *Relapsing fever* – For the treatment of tick- and louse-borne relapsing fever.

Other uses: Prior to elective colorectal surgery, to reduce wound complications, erythromycin base with oral neomycin is a popular preoperative combination. Other uses, as an alternative to penicillins, include anthrax, Vincent gingivitis, erysipeloid, actinomycosis, *Nocardia* infections (with a sulfonamide), *Eikenella corrodens* infections, and *Borrelia* infections.

Actions

➤*Pharmacology:* Macrolide antibiotics, which include **azithromycin**, **clarithromycin**, and **erythromycin**, are bacteriostatic agents that exert their antibacterial action by binding to the 50S ribosomal subunit of susceptible organisms, resulting in inhibition of protein synthesis. Nucleic acid synthesis is not affected. For adult dosage calculation, use a ratio of 400 mg of **erythromycin** activity as the ethylsuccinate to 250 mg of erythromycin activity as the stearate or base.

➤*Pharmacokinetics:*

Macrolides — Summary of Pharmacokinetics[a]

Macrolide	Oral bioavailability	C_{max} (mcg/mL)	T_{max}	Protein binding	Volume of distribution	Effect of food	Half-life	Metabolism	Elimination
Azithromycin		0.5 mcg/mL (single 500 mg dose)	≈ 2 to 2.5 h (≈ 5 h for ER oral suspension)	51% (at 0.02 mcg/mL); 7% (at 2 mcg/mL)	31.1 L/kg (oral); 33.3 L/kg (IV)	*Tablets and oral suspension*: Take with or without food. Food increased C_{max} by 23% (tablets) and by 56% (oral suspension); no effect on AUC. *ER oral suspension*: Take on an empty stomach (≥ 1 h before or 2 h following a meal). Administration with food increased C_{max} by 115% to 119% and the AUC by 12% to 23%.	68[b] h	Some hepatic metabolism to inactive metabolites	Primarily excreted unchanged in bile; ≈ 6% of dose is excreted unchanged in urine
Clarithromycin	≈ 50% (tablets)	1 to 2 mcg/mL (after doses of 250 mg every 12 h); 3 to 4 mcg/mL (after doses of 500 mg every 8 to 12 h)	*Tablets*: 2 to 3 h *Oral suspension*: ≈ 3 h *ER tablets*: 5 to 8 h	40% to 70%		*Tablets and oral suspension*: Take without regard to food. Food slightly delays onset of absorption; does not affect extent of bioavailability. *ER tablets*: Administer with food. Administration under fasting conditions lowers clarithromycin AUC by ≈ 30%.	3 to 7[c] h (5 to 9[c] h for 14-OH clarithromycin)	Metabolized in the liver to active metabolite (14-OH clarithromycin)	Renal clearance approximates the normal GFR. *Tablets*: ≈ 20% to 30% of dose is excreted in urine as clarithromycin and ≈ 10% to 15% as 14-OH clarithromycin. *Oral suspension*: ≈ 40% of dose is excreted in urine as clarithromycin
Erythromycin		*Base*: 0.3 to 1.9 mcg/mL *Ethylsuccinate*: 1.5 mcg/mL *IV*: 10 mcg/mL	*Base*: 4 h *Ethylsuccinate*: 1 to 2 h *IV*: 1 h	70% to 80%		*Erythromycin base film-coated tablets and delayed-release capsules and erythromycin stearate*: Take on an empty stomach. *Erythromycin base delayed-release tablets and erythromycin ethylsuccinate*: Take without regard to food.	1.6 h[d]	Metabolized in the liver to inactive metabolites	< 5% (oral) and 12% to 15% (IV) excreted unchanged in urine; significant quantity excreted in bile

[a] C_{max} = maximum plasma concentration; T_{max} = time to reach maximum concentration; AUC = area under the curve; GFR = glomerular filtration rate; IV = intravenous.
[b] Terminal elimination half-life.
[c] Elimination half-life.
[d] Serum half-life.

Absorption/Distribution – **Azithromycin** is widely distributed throughout the body with tissue concentrations exceeding serum concentrations by 10- to 100-fold.

Clarithromycin is rapidly absorbed from the GI tract after oral administration. First-pass metabolism decreases the bioavailability by 50% to 55%. Clarithromycin and the 14-OH clarithromycin metabolite distribute readily into body tissues and fluids. Because of high intracellular concentrations, tissue concentrations are higher than serum concentrations.

Erythromycin base is inactivated by gastric acid, but is absorbed from the upper small intestine when administered with enteric coating. Orally administered erythromycin base and its salts are readily absorbed in the microbiologically active form. Interindividual variations in the absorption of erythromycin are, however, observed, and some patients do not achieve optimal serum levels. After absorption, erythromycin diffuses readily into most body fluids. In the absences of meningeal inflammation, low concentrations are normally achieved in the spinal fluid, but the passage of the drug across the blood-brain barrier increases in meningitis. Erythromycin is largely bound to plasma proteins.

Metabolism/Excretion – **Azithromycin** is slowly released from tissues to allow for once daily dosing and a shortened duration of treatment.

Clarithromycin is metabolized in the liver to several metabolites with the major metabolite, 14-hydroxyclarithromycin (14-OH clarithromycin), possessing antibacterial activity.

Erythromycin is concentrated in the liver and excreted in the bile. After oral administration, less than 5% of the administered dose can be recovered in the active form in the urine.

Special populations –

Renal function impairment: Following the oral administration of a single 1,000 mg dose of **azithromycin**, mean C_{max} and AUC_{0-120} increased by 5.1% and 4.2%, respectively, in subjects with mild to moderate renal function impairment (GFR 10 to 80 mL/min) compared with subjects with healthy renal function (GFR more than 80 mL/min). The mean C_{max} and AUC_{0-120} increased by 61% and 35%, respectively, in subjects with severe renal function impairment (GFR less than 10 mL/min) compared with subjects with healthy renal function (GFR more than 80 mL/min). No dosage adjustment is recommended.

The pharmacokinetics of **clarithromycin** are altered in patients with renal function impairment. In the presence of severe renal function impairment with or without coexisting hepatic function impairment, decreased dosage or prolonged dosing intervals may be appropriate.

The serum half-life of **erythromycin** in patients with anuria is 5 hours.

Hepatic function impairment: The steady-state concentrations of **clarithromycin** in patients with hepatic function impairment did not differ from those in healthy patients; however, the 14-OH clarithromycin concentrations were lower in patients with hepatic function impairment.

Elderly: In elderly women, higher **azithromycin** concentrations (increased by 30% to 50%) were observed; no significant accumulation occurred.

C_{max} and AUC of **clarithromycin** and 14-OH clarithromycin were increased in healthy elderly patients. These changes in pharmacokinetics parallel known age-related decreases in renal function.

➤*Microbiology:*

Organisms Generally Susceptible to Macrolides In Vitro				
	Organisms	Azithromycin	Clarithromycin	Erythromycin
Gram-positive aerobes	*Staphylococcus aureus*	✓	✓	✓[a]
	Streptococcus pyogenes	✓	✓	✓
	Streptococcus pneumoniae	✓	✓	✓
	Streptococcus agalactiae	✓	✓[b]	
	Streptococci (Groups C, F, G)	✓[b]	✓[b]	
	Viridans group streptococci	✓[b]	✓[b]	✓[b]
	Listeria monocytogenes			✓
	Corynebacterium diphtheriae			✓
	Corynebacterium minutissimum			✓
Gram-negative aerobes	*C. jejuni*	✓[b]		
	Haemophilus influenzae	✓	✓	✓[c]
	Haemophilus parainfluenzae		✓	
	Haemophilus ducreyi	✓		
	Moraxella catarrhalis	✓	✓	✓[b]
	Bordetella pertussis	✓[b]	✓[b]	✓
	Legionella pneumophila	✓	✓[b]	✓
	Neisseria gonorrhoeae	✓		✓
	Pasteurella multocida		✓[b]	
Anaerobes	*Prevotella* (formerly *Bacteroides*) *bivius*	✓[b]		
	Prevotella (formerly *Bacteroides*) *melaninogenicus*		✓[b]	
	Clostridium perfringens	✓[b]	✓[b]	
	Propionibacterium acnes		✓[b]	
	Peptococcus niger		✓[b]	
	Peptostreptococcus sp.	✓[b]		
Other	*Borrelia burgdorferi*	✓[b]		
	C. trachomatis	✓		✓
	M. pneumoniae	✓	✓	✓
	Treponema pallidum	✓[b]		✓
	Ureaplasma urealyticum	✓[b]		✓
	Entamoeba histolytica			✓
	Chlamydia pneumoniae (TWAR strain)	✓	✓	
	Mycoplasma hominis	✓		
	M. avium	✓	✓	
	Mycobacterium intracellulare	✓	✓	
	H. pylori		✓	
	C. tetani			✓

[a] Resistant *S. aureus* may emerge during a course of erythromycin treatment.
[b] Safety and effectiveness in treating clinical infections due to this microorganism have not been established in adequate and well-controlled clinical trials; clinical significance if unknown.
[c] Many strains are resistant to erythromycin alone, but are susceptible to erythromycin and sulfonamides used concomitantly.

Contraindications

Hypersensitivity to any of the macrolide antibiotics.

Azithromycin is also contraindicated in patients with a hypersensitivity to a ketolide antibiotic (eg, telithromycin).

Clarithromycin is contraindicated in patients receiving any of the following drugs: cisapride, pimozide, astemizole, terfenadine, and ergotamine or dihydroergotamine (See Drug Interactions).

Erythromycin is contraindicated in patients receiving any of the following drugs: cisapride, pimozide, astemizole, or terfenadine (See Drug Interactions).

Warnings/Precautions

➤*Clostridium difficile–associated diarrhea: Clostridium difficile*–associated diarrhea (CDAD) has been reported with use of nearly all antibacterial agents and may range in severity from mild diarrhea to fatal colitis. Therefore, it is important to consider this diagnosis in patients who present with diarrhea subsequent to the administration of antibacterial agents.

Treatment with antibacterial agents alters the normal flora of the colon and may permit overgrowth of clostridia. *C. difficile* produces toxins A and B, which contribute to the development of CDAD. Hypertoxin-producing strains of *C. difficile* cause increased morbidity and mortality, because these infections can be refractory to antimicrobial therapy and may require colectomy. CDAD must be considered in all patients who present with diarrhea following antibiotic use. Careful medical history is necessary since CDAD has been reported to occur more than 2 months after the administration of antibacterial agents.

If CDAD is suspected or confirmed, ongoing antibiotic use not directed against *C. difficile* may need to be discontinued. Institute appropriate fluid and electrolyte management, protein supplementation, antibiotic treatment of *C. difficile*, and surgical evaluation as clinically indicated.

➤*Acute porphyria:* Do not use **clarithromycin** in combination with ranitidine bismuth citrate in patients with a history of acute porphyria.

➤*Pneumonia:* In the treatment of pneumonia, **azithromycin** has only been shown to be safe and effective in the treatment of community-acquired pneumonia due to *C. pneumoniae*, *H. influenzae*, *M. pneumonia*, or *S. pneumoniae* in patients appropriate for oral therapy. Do not use azithromycin in patients with pneumonia who are judged to be inappropriate for oral therapy because of moderate to severe illness or risk factors such as nosocomially acquired infections, known or suspected bacteremia, conditions requiring hospitalization, cystic fibrosis, significant underlying health problems that may compromise the patient's ability to respond to his/her illness (including immunodeficiency or functional asplenia), or elderly or debilitated patients.

➤*Cardiac effects:* Prolonged cardiac repolarization and QT interval, imparting a risk of developing cardiac arrhythmia and torsades de pointes, have been seen in treatment with macrolides. A similar effect with **azithromycin** cannot be completely ruled out in patients at increased risk for prolonged cardiac repolarization.

➤*Hepatic effects:* There have been reports of hepatic function impairment, including increased liver enzymes, and hepatocellular and/or cholestatic hepatitis, with or without jaundice, occurring in patients receiving oral **erythromycin**.

➤*Syphilis:* There have been reports suggesting that **erythromycin** does not reach the fetus in adequate concentration to prevent congenital syphilis. Use an appropriate penicillin regimen to treat infants born to women treated with oral erythromycin during pregnancy for early syphilis.

➤*Myasthenia gravis:* There have been reports that **azithromycin** and **erythromycin** may aggravate the weakness of patients with myasthenia gravis. New onset of myasthenic syndrome have been reported in patients receiving azithromycin therapy.

➤*Drug-resistant bacteria:* Prescribing macrolides in the absence of a proven or strongly suspected bacterial infection or a prophylactic indication is unlikely to provide benefit to the patient and increases the risk of the development of drug-resistant bacteria.

➤*Superinfection:* Prolonged or repeated use of macrolides may result in an overgrowth of nonsusceptible bacteria or fungi. If superinfection occurs, discontinue the macrolide and institute appropriate therapy.

➤*Infantile hypertrophic pyloric stenosis:* There have been reports of infantile hypertrophic pyloric stenosis (IHPS) occurring in infants following **erythromycin** therapy. In one cohort of 157 newborns who were given erythromycin for pertussis prophylaxis, 7 (5%) neonates developed symptoms of nonbilious vomiting or irritability with feeding and were subsequently diagnosed as having IHPS requiring surgical pyloromyotomy. A possible dose-response effect was described with an absolute risk of IHPS of 5.1% for infants who took erythromycin for 8 to 14 days and 10% for infants who took erythromycin for 15 to 21 days. Since erythromycin may be used in the treatment of conditions in infants that are associated with significant mortality or morbidity (such as pertussis or neonatal *C. trachomatis* infections), the benefit of erythromycin therapy needs to be weighed against the potential risk of developing IHPS. Inform parents to contact their health care provider if vomiting or irritability with feeding occurs.

➤*Local IV-site reactions:* Local IV-site reactions have been reported with the IV administration of **azithromycin**. The incidence and severity of these reactions were the same when 500 mg was given over 1 hour (2 mg/mL as 250 mL infusion) or 3 hours (1 mg/mL as 500 mL infusion). All volunteers who received infusate concentrations more than 2 mg/mL experienced local IV site reactions; therefore, avoid higher concentrations.

➤*Hypersensitivity reactions:* Serious allergic reactions, including angioedema, anaphylaxis, and dermatologic reactions, including Stevens-Johnson syndrome and toxic epidermal necrolysis, have been reported rarely in patients on **azithromycin** therapy. Although rare, fatalities have occurred. Despite initially successful symptomatic treatment of the allergic symptoms, when symptomatic therapy was discontinued, the allergic symptoms recurred soon thereafter in some patients without further azithromycin exposure. These patients required prolonged periods of observation and symptomatic treatment. The relationship of these episodes to the long tissue half-life of azithromycin and subsequent prolonged exposure to antigen is unknown at present. If an allergic reaction occurs with azithromycin, discontinue and institute appropriate therapy. Be aware that the reappearance of the allergic symptoms may occur when symptomatic therapy is discontinued.

Allergic reactions ranging from urticaria and mild skin eruptions to rare cases of anaphylaxis, Stevens-Johnson syndrome, and toxic epidermal necrolysis have occurred with **clarithromycin**.

Allergic reactions ranging from urticaria to anaphylaxis have occurred with **erythromycin**. Skin reactions ranging from mild eruptions to erythema multiforme, Stevens-Johnson syndrome, and toxic epidermal necrolysis have been reported rarely.

➤*Renal / Hepatic function impairment:* Because **azithromycin** is principally eliminated via the liver, exercise caution when administering to patients with hepatic function impairment. Because of the limited data in subjects with GFR less than 10 mL/min, exercise caution when prescribing azithromycin to these patients.

Clarithromycin is principally excreted via the liver and kidney, and may be administered without dosage adjustment to patients with hepatic function impairment and healthy renal function. However, in the presence of severe renal function impairment (creatinine clearance [CrCl] less than 30 mL/min) with or without coexisting hepatic function impairment, the dosage should be halved or the dosing intervals doubled. Clarithromycin in combination with ranitidine bismuth citrate therapy is not recommended in patients with CrCl less than 25 mL/min.

Erythromycin is principally excreted by the liver. Exercise caution in administering to patients with hepatic function impairment. There have been isolated reports of reversible hearing loss occurring chiefly in patients with renal function impairment and in patients receiving high doses of erythromycin.

➤*Pregnancy: Category B* (**azithromycin**, **erythromycin**); *Category C* (**clarithromycin**). There are no adequate and well-controlled studies of macrolides in pregnant women. Use **azithromycin** and **erythromycin** only when clearly needed. Azithromycin and erythromycin cross the placental barrier in humans, but fetal plasma levels are generally low. Do not use **clarithromycin** in pregnant women except in clinical circumstances when no alternative therapy is appropriate. Use clarithromycin during pregnancy only if the potential benefit justifies the potential risk to the fetus. If pregnancy occurs while taking clarithromycin, apprise the patient of the hazard to the fetus. Clarithromycin has demonstrated adverse effects on pregnancy outcome and/or embryo-fetal development in monkeys, rats, mice, and rabbits at doses that produced plasma levels 2 to 17 times the serum levels achieved in humans treated at the maximum recommended human doses.

There have been reports suggesting that **erythromycin** does not reach the fetus in adequate concentration to prevent congenital syphilis. Use an appropriate penicillin regimen to treat infants born to women treated with oral erythromycin during pregnancy for early syphilis.

➤*Lactation:* **Erythromycin** is excreted in breast milk and may concentrate (observed milk:plasma ratio of 0.5). Although no infant adverse reactions are reported, potential problems for breast-feeding infants include modification of bowel flora, pharmacological effects, and interference with fever work-ups (ie, interference of culture results). Erythromycin is considered by the American Academy of Pediatrics to be compatible with breast-feeding. According to one case report, **azithromycin** accumulates in breast milk, but is considered to be probably compatible with breast-feeding. It is not known whether **clarithromycin** is excreted in breast milk. Clarithromycin is excreted in the milk of lactating animals. Exercise caution when administering to a breast-feeding woman.

➤*Children:* Safety and efficacy of **clarithromycin** in children younger than 6 months of age have not been established. The safety of clarithromycin has not been studied in MAC patients younger than 20 months of age.

Safety and efficacy of **azithromycin** in children younger than 6 months of age have not been established for acute bacterial sinusitis, acute otitis media, or community-acquired pneumonia. Safety and efficacy of azithromycin in children younger than 2 years of age have not been established for pharyngitis/tonsillitis. Safety and efficacy of azithromycin for IV injection in children or adolescents younger than 16 years of age have not been established. Safety and effectiveness of azithromycin extended-release oral suspension in children younger than 6 months of age for the treatment of community-acquired pneumonia or in children of any age for the treatment of acute bacterial sinusitis have not been established. Azithromycin oral suspension 1 g single-dose are not approved for children.

Erythromycin is approved for use in children.

➤*Elderly:* C_{max} and AUC of **clarithromycin** and 14-OH clarithromycin were increased in healthy elderly patients. These changes in pharmacokinetics parallel known age-related decreases in renal function. In clinical trials, elderly patients did not have an increased incidence of adverse reactions compared with younger patients. Consider dosage adjustment in elderly patients with severe renal function impairment.

Elderly patients, particularly those with reduced renal or hepatic function, may be at increased risk for developing **erythromycin**-induced hearing loss. Elderly patients may be more susceptible to the development of torsades de pointes arrhythmias than younger patients. Elderly patients may experience increased effects of oral anticoagulant therapy while undergoing treatment with erythromycin.

Drug Interactions

➤*CYP-450 system:* **Erythromycin** and **clarithromycin** are substrates and inhibitors of the 3A isoform subfamily of the CYP-450 enzyme system (CYP3A). Coadministration of erythromycin or clarithromycin and a drug primarily metabolized by CYP3A may be associated with elevations in drug concentrations that could increase or prolong both the therapeutic effects and adverse reactions of the concomitant drug. Consider dosage adjustments and, when possible, closely monitor serum concentrations of drugs primarily metabolized by CYP3A in patients concurrently receiving clarithromycin or erythromycin.

➤*QT prolongation:* An additive effect of macrolides with other drugs that prolong the QT interval cannot be excluded. The following drugs may prolong the QT interval and increase the risk of life-threatening cardiac arrhythmias, including torsades de pointes: antiarrhythmic agents (eg, amiodarone, bretylium, disopyramide, dofetilide, procainamide, quinidine, sotalol), arsenic trioxide, chlorpromazine, cisapride, dolasetron, droperidol, gatifloxacin, halofantrine, levomethadyl, mefloquine, mesoridazine, moxifloxacin, pentamidine, pimozide, probucol, sparfloxacin, tacrolimus, thioridazine, and ziprasidone.

Macrolides Drug Interactions

Precipitant drug	Object drug[a]		Description
Alcohol	Macrolides Erythromycin	↑↓	The effects of erythromycin ethylsuccinate may be decreased and delayed. Advise patients to avoid ingestion of erythromycin ethylsuccinate with ethanol.
Antacids (eg, aluminum- and magnesium-containing)	Macrolides Azithromycin	↓	Coadministration may decrease the absorption of azithromycin. Do not take aluminum- and magnesium-containing antacids and azithromycin simultaneously.
Antiarrhythmic agents (eg, amiodarone, bretylium, disopyramide, dofetilide, procainamide, quinidine, sotalol)	Macrolides	↑	The risk of life-threatening cardiac arrhythmias, including torsades de pointes, may be increased. An additive or synergistic increase in the QT interval may result with coadministration.
Macrolides	Antiarrhythmic agents (eg, amiodarone, bretylium, disopyramide, dofetilide, procainamide, quinidine, sotalol)		
Cimetidine	Macrolides Clarithromycin	↓	The antimicrobial effects of clarithromycin may be decreased.
Diltiazem	Macrolides Clarithromycin Erythromycin	↑	Coadministration may cause elevated plasma concentrations of macrolides, increasing the risk of cardiotoxicity. Avoid coadministration.
Fluconazole	Macrolides Clarithromycin	↑	Coadministration resulted in increases in the mean steady-state clarithromycin minimum plasma concentration and AUC of 33% and 18%, respectively.
Fluoroquinolones (eg, levofloxacin, moxifloxacin, sparfloxacin)	Macrolides	↑	Coadministration of macrolides with fluoroquinolones known to prolong the QT interval may increase the risk of life-threatening cardiac arrhythmias, including torsades de pointes. Avoid coadministration with levofloxacin and use moxifloxacin with caution. Coadministration with sparfloxacin[b] is contraindicated.
Macrolides	Fluoroquinolones (eg, levofloxacin, moxifloxacin, sparfloxacin)		
Nelfinavir	Macrolides Azithromycin	↑	Coadministration resulted in increased azithromycin serum concentrations. Monitor for adverse reactions of azithromycin (eg, liver abnormalities, hearing impairment).
Proton pump inhibitors (eg, esomeprazole, lansoprazole, omeprazole)	Macrolides Clarithromycin	↑	Coadministration of clarithromycin and omeprazole may increase the serum concentrations of both drugs. Plasma levels of other proton pump inhibitors (ie, esomeprazole, lansoprazole) may be elevated when given with clarithromycin.
Macrolides Clarithromycin	Proton pump inhibitors (eg, esomeprazole, lansoprazole, omperazole)		

Macrolides Drug Interactions

Precipitant drug	Object drug[a]		Description
Rifamycins (eg, rifabutin, rifampin)	Macrolides Clarithromycin Erythromycin	↑↓	Coadministration may decrease antimicrobial effects of macrolides and may also increase the frequency of GI and rifamycin adverse reactions. Azithromycin may be a safer alternative.
Macrolides Clarithromycin Erythromycin	Rifamycins (eg, rifabutin, rifampin)		
Ritonavir	Macrolides Clarithromycin	↑↓	Concurrent use resulted in a 77% increase in clarithromycin AUC and a 100% decrease in the AUC of the clarithromycin active metabolite. For patients with a CrCl of 30 to 60 mL/min, decrease the clarithromycin dose by 50%. For patients with CrCl of less than 30 mL/min, decrease the clarithromycin dose by 75%.
Theophyllines (eg, aminophylline, theophylline)	Macrolides Erythromycin	↓	Coadministration may decrease erythromycin levels. Macrolides may increase the serum levels of the theophylline; toxicity may occur. Monitor theophylline levels.
Macrolides	Theophyllines (eg, aminophylline, theophylline)	↑	
Verapamil	Macrolides Clarithromycin Erythromycin	↑	Coadministration may increase the plasma levels of both the macrolide and verapamil, increasing the risk of cardiotoxicity. Closely monitor cardiac function.
Macrolides Clarithromycin Erythromycin	Verapamil		
Macrolides Clarithromycin Erythromycin	Alfentanil	↑	Pharmacologic effects of alfentanil may be increased.
Macrolides Clarithromycin Erythromycin	Antihistamines (ie, astemizole[b], terfenadine[b])	↑	There have been postmarketing reports of drug interactions when clarithromycin or erythromycin are coadministered with terfenadine, resulting in cardiac arrhythmias (QT prolongation, ventricular tachycardia, ventricular fibrillation, and torsades de pointes) most likely due to inhibition of hepatic metabolism by the macrolide. Fatalities have been reported. Coadministration is contraindicated.
Macrolides	Benzodiazepines (ie, alprazolam, diazepam, midazolam, triazolam)	↑	Coadministration may decrease the metabolism of certain benzodiazepines, resulting in increased CNS depression and prolonged sedation.
Macrolides Clarithromycin Erythromycin	Bromocriptine	↑	Bromocriptine serum levels may be increased, resulting in an increase in the pharmacologic and toxic effects.
Macrolides Clarithromycin Erythromycin	Buspirone	↑	Coadministration may increase buspirone concentrations, increasing the pharmacologic effects and adverse reactions.
Macrolides Clarithromycin Erythromycin	Cabergoline[b]	↑	Coadministration may increase cabergoline concentrations, increasing the risk of toxicity.
Macrolides Clarithromycin Erythromycin	Carbamazepine	↑	Carbamazepine concentration/toxicity may be increased. Avoid this combination if possible; otherwise, monitor carbamazepine levels closely. Azithromycin is unlikely to interact.
Macrolides Clarithromycin Erythromycin	Cilostazol	↑	Coadministration may increase cilostazol concentrations, increasing the therapeutic and adverse reactions.

Macrolides Drug Interactions

Precipitant drug	Object drug[a]		Description
Macrolides Clarithromycin Erythromycin	Cisapride[c]	↑	Coadministration has resulted in cardiac arrhythmias (QT prolongation, ventricular tachycardia, ventricular fibrillation, and torsades de pointes) most likely due to the inhibition of hepatic metabolism of cisapride by the macrolide. Coadministration is contraindicated. Azithromycin may be a safer alternative.
Macrolides Clarithromycin Erythromycin	Clopidogrel	↓	The antiplatelet effect of clopidogrel may be inhibited by certain macrolides. Carefully monitor platelet function and adjust the clopidogrel dose as needed. Azithromycin may be a safer alternative.
Macrolides Erythromycin	Clozapine	↑	Serum clozapine concentrations may be elevated, increasing the pharmacologic and toxic effects.
Macrolides Clarithromycin Erythromycin	Colchicine	↑	Increased colchicine serum concentrations with toxicity may occur. Deaths have been reported. Avoid this combination.
Macrolides Clarithromycin	Conivaptan	↑	Coadministration may cause elevated conivaptan plasma concentrations, increasing the risk of adverse reactions. Coadministration is contraindicated.
Macrolides	Cyclosporine	↑	Elevated cyclosporine levels, increasing the risk of toxicity (nephrotoxicity, neurotoxicity), may occur. Monitor cyclosporine levels and serum creatinine; adjust cyclosporine dose as needed.
Macrolides	Digoxin	↑	Coadministration may increase digoxin serum levels; toxicity may occur. The effects of this interaction may persist for several weeks following erythromycin administration. Monitor digoxin levels and adjust dose as needed.
Macrolides Clarithromycin Erythromycin	Eletriptan	↑	Plasma levels of eletriptan may be elevated, increasing the pharmacologic and toxic effects. Eletriptan should not be taken within 72 hours of potent CYP 3A4 inhibitors (eg, clarithromycin).
Macrolides Clarithromycin	Eplerenone	↑	Coadministration may cause elevated eplerenone plasma concentrations, which may increase the risk of hyperkalemia and associated serious, sometimes fatal, arrhythmias. Coadministration is contraindicated.
Macrolides	Ergot derivatives (ie, dihydroergotamine, ergotamine)	↑	Acute ergotism manifested as peripheral ischemia has been reported with concomitant use of these agents. Coadministration of ergot derivatives with clarithromycin is contraindicated.
Macrolides Erythromycin	Felodipine	↑	The pharmacologic effects and adverse reactions of felodipine may be increased.
Macrolides	Hexobarbital	↑	Coadministration may elevate the serum levels of hexobarbital.
Macrolides	HMG-CoA reductase inhibitors (ie, atorvastatin, lovastatin, simvastatin)	↑	Severe myopathy or rhabdomyolysis may occur because of increased HMG-CoA reductase inhibitor levels.
Macrolides Clarithromycin	Lapatinib	↑	Coadministration may increase the plasma concentrations of lapatinib, increasing the risk of toxicity. If coadministration cannot be avoided, then decrease the lapatinib dose to 500 mg/day.

Macrolides Drug Interactions			
Precipitant drug	Object drug[a]		Description
Macrolides Clarithromycin Erythromycin	Methylprednisolone	↑	The pharmacologic and toxic effects of methylprednisolone may be increased.
Macrolides	Phenytoin	↑	Coadministration may elevate the serum levels of phenytoin.
Macrolides	Pimozide	↑	Increased pimozide plasma concentrations with cardiotoxicity may occur. Coadministration is contraindicated.
Macrolides Clarithromycin Erythromycin	Quetiapine	↑	Quetiapine plasma concentrations may be elevated, increasing the pharmacologic effects and adverse reactions.
Macrolides	Ranolazine	↑	Increased ranolazine plasma concentrations with cardiotoxicity may occur. Coadministration is contraindicated.
Macrolides Clarithromycin Erythromycin	Repaglinide	↑	Coadministration may increase repaglinide plasma levels, increasing the pharmacologic effects and adverse reactions. Monitor blood glucose levels carefully and adjust the repaglinide dose as needed.
Macrolides Clarithromycin Erythromycin	Sildenafil	↑	Sildenafil plasma concentrations may be elevated, increasing the risk of adverse reactions. Consider a lower dose of sildenafil. Azithromycin may be a safer alternative.
Macrolides Clarithromycin Erythromycin	Tacrolimus	↑	Tacrolimus plasma levels may be elevated, increasing the risk of toxicity. Monitor renal function and tacrolimus blood levels and adjust the tacrolimus dose as needed.
Macrolide	Valproic acid	↑	Concurrent use with macrolide antibiotics may elevate the serum levels of valproic acid, producing valproic acid toxicity.
Macrolides Erythromycin	Vinblastine	↑	The risk of vinblastine toxicity (eg, constipation, myalgia, neutropenia) may be increased. Avoid coadministration.
Macrolides	Warfarin	↑	The anticoagulant effect of warfarin may be increased. Hemorrhage has occurred. Monitor anticoagulant parameters and adjust the warfarin dose as needed.
Macrolides Clarithromycin	Zidovudine	↑↓	Coadministration has resulted in both decreased and increased concentrations of zidovudine.

[a] ↑ = object drug increased; ↓ = object drug decreased; ↑↓ = object drug increased and decreased.
[b] No longer marketed in the US.
[c] Available from the manufacturer on a limited-access protocol.

➤*Drug/Lab test interactions:* **Erythromycin** interferes with the fluorometric determination of urinary catecholamines.

➤*Drug/Food interactions:* Grapefruit juice may inhibit the metabolism of **clarithromycin** and **erythromycin**, resulting in elevated plasma levels of the macrolide. Avoid coadministration.

Azithromycin tablets and oral suspension can be taken with or without food. Following administration of azithromycin extended-release oral suspension with food, the C_{max} increased by 115% to 119%, and the AUC increased by 12% to 23%. Advise patient to only take the extended-release oral suspension on an empty stomach (at least 1 hour before or 2 hours following a meal).

Clarithromycin tablets and oral suspension may be given without regard to food. While the extent of formation of 14-OH clarithromycin following administration of clarithromycin extended-release tablets (2 × 500 mg once daily) is not affected by food, administration under fasting conditions is associated with approximately 30% lower clarithromycin AUC relative to administration with food. Therefore, advise the patient to take clarithromycin extended-release tablets with food.

Antimicrobial effectiveness of **erythromycin** stearate and certain formulations of erythromycin base may be reduced when taken with food. Erythromycin ethylsuccinate and the base in a delayed release tablet form may be administered without regard to meals (See Patient Information).

Adverse Reactions

Macrolides Adverse Reactions[a,b]					
Adverse reactions	Azithromycin		Clarithromycin		Erythromycin
	Adults	Children	Adults	Children	
Cardiovascular					
Chest pain	≤ 1%	< 1%			
Palpitations	≤ 1%				
QT prolongation	✓[c]	✓[c]	✓[c]		✓
Torsades de pointes	✓[c]	✓[c]	✓[c]		✓
Ventricular arrhythmias			✓[c]		✓
Ventricular tachycardia	✓[c]	✓[c]	✓[c]		✓
CNS					
Agitation	✓[c]	≤ 1%			
Asthenia	≤ 1%	✓[c]			
Convulsions	✓[c]	✓[c]	✓[c]		Rare
Dizziness	≤ 1%	≤ 1%	✓[c]		
Fatigue	≤ 1%	≤ 1%			
Headache	≤ 1%	≤ 1.1%	2% to 2.7%	2%	
Hyperkinesia		≤ 1%			
Insomnia		≤ 1%	✓[c]		
Malaise	✓[c]	≤ 1%			
Nervousness	✓[c]	≤ 1%			
Somnolence	≤ 1%	✓[c]			
Vertigo	≤ 1%	✓[c]	✓[c]		
Dermatologic					
Eczema		≤ 1%			
Fungal dermatitis		≤ 1%			
Pruritus	≤ 1.9%	≤ 1%			
Rash	≤ 1.9%	≤ 1.6%	3.2%	3%	
Sweating		≤ 1%			
Urticaria	< 1%	≤ 1%	✓[c]		✓
Vesiculobullous rash		≤ 1%			
GI					
Abdominal pain/discomfort	1.9% to 7%	1.2% to 3.4%	2% to 5%	3%	✓
Abnormal taste	≤ 1%	✓[c]	3%, 7%[d]		
Anorexia	1.9%	≤ 1%	✓[c]		✓
Constipation	< 1%	≤ 1%			
Diarrhea/Loose stools	4% to 14%	1.8% to 5.8%	3%, 6%[d]	6%	✓
Dyspepsia	≤ 1%	≤ 1%	2% to 3.8%		
Enteritis		≤ 1%			
Flatulence	≤ 1%	≤ 1%	2.4%		
Gastritis	≤ 1%	≤ 1%			
Melena	≤ 1%				
Mucositis	≤ 1%				
Nausea	3% to 18%	0.4% to 1.9%	3% to 11.2%, 3%[d]		✓
Oral moniliasis	≤ 1%	≤ 1%	✓[c]		
Pancreatitis	✓[c]	✓[c]	✓[c]		Rare
Pseudomembranous colitis/CDAD	✓[c]	✓[c]		✓	✓
Stomatitis	1.9%				
Taste perversion	≤ 1%		8%		
Vomiting	≤ 7%	1.1% to 5.6%	5.9%	6%	✓

Macrolides Adverse Reactions[a,b]

Adverse reactions	Azithromycin		Clarithromycin		
	Adults	Children	Adults	Children	Erythromycin
GU					
Interstitial nephritis	≤ 1%	✓[c]	✓[c]		
Monilia	≤ 1%				
Vaginitis	≤ 2.8%	✓[c]			
Hematologic					
Anemia		≤ 1%			
Leukopenia	≤ 1%	≤ 1%	✓[c]		
Neutropenia	< 1%		✓[c]		
Hepatic					
Cholestatic jaundice	≤ 1%	✓[c]			
Hepatic function impairment	✓[c]	✓[c]	✓[c]		✓
Hepatitis symptoms	✓[c]	✓[c]			✓
Hepatocellular and/or cholestatic hepatitis (with or without jaundice)			✓[c]		✓
Jaundice		≤ 1%			
Hypersensitivity[e]					
Allergic reactions	✓	≤ 1%	✓[c]		✓
Anaphylaxis	✓	✓	Rare[c]		✓
Angioedema	≤ 1%	✓[c]			
Bronchospasm	≤ 1%				
Erythema multiforme	✓[c]	✓[c]			Rare
Photosensitivity	≤ 1%				✓
Skin reactions	✓[c]	✓[c]	✓[c]		✓
Stevens-Johnson syndrome	Rare[c]	Rare[c]	Rare[c]		Rare
Toxic epidermal necrolysis	Rare[c]	Rare[c]	Rare[c]		Rare
Injection-site reactions					
Application-site reaction	1.9%				
Local inflammation	3.1%				
Pain at injection site	6.5%				
Venous irritation					✓
Lab test abnormalities					
Alkaline phosphatase, elevated	< 1%		< 1% to 2%		
ALT, elevated	> 1%		< 1% to 3%	< 1%	
AST, elevated	> 1%		< 1% to 4%	< 1%	
Basophils, elevated	< 1%				
Bicarbonate, decreased	≥ 1%				
Bilirubin, elevated	< 3%		< 1%	< 1%	
BUN, elevated	> 1%		4%	4%	
Eosinophils, increased	≥ 1%				
GGT, elevated	> 1%		< 1%		
Glucose (blood), decreased	> 1%				
Hematocrit, decreased	> 1%				
Hemoglobin, decreased	> 1%		3%		
LDH, elevated	< 3%		< 1%	< 1%	
Liver enzymes, increased			✓[c]		✓
Lymphocytes, decreased	> 1%				
Lymphocytes, elevated	> 1%				
Monocytes, elevated	< 1%				
Neutrophils, decreased	> 1%	✓			
Neutrophils, elevated	> 1%				
Phosphate, elevated	< 1%				
Platelet count, decreased	< 1%		4%		
Platelet count, increased	> 1%				
Potassium, decreased	< 1%				
Potassium, elevated	> 1%				
Prothrombin time, elevated			1%		
Serum CPK, elevated	> 1%				
Serum creatinine, elevated	> 1%		< 1%	< 1%	
Sodium, decreased	< 1%				
WBC, decreased			< 1% to 4%	< 1%	
Respiratory					
Bronchospasm	≤ 1%				
Cough increased		≤ 1%			
Pharyngitis		≤ 1%			
Pleural effusions		≤ 1%			
Rhinitis		≤ 1%			
Miscellaneous					
Conjunctivitis		≤ 1%			
Face edema		≤ 1%			
Fever		≤ 1%			
Fungal infection		≤ 1%			
Hearing loss	✓[c]	✓[c]	✓[c]		✓[e]
Pain		≤ 1%			

[a] ✓ = Event occurred, but incidence is unknown; BUN = serum urea nitrogen; GGT = gamma-glutamyltransferase; LDH = lactate dehydrogenase; CPK = creatine phosphokinase; WBC = white blood cell count.
[b] Data are pooled from separate studies and are not necessarily comparable.
[c] Postmarketing.
[d] Clarithromycin extended-release tablets.
[e] See Warnings for more details.

➤*Postmarketing:*

Azithromycin –

Cardiovascular: Arrhythmias, hypotension, syncope.
CNS: Aggressive reaction, anxiety, hyperactivity, paresthesia, syncope.
GI: Oral candidiasis, tongue discoloration (rare).
GU: Acute renal failure.
Hematologic: Thrombocytopenia.
Hepatic: Cholestatic jaundice, rare cases of hepatic necrosis and hepatic failure (some of which have resulted in death).
Special senses: Hearing disturbances, including deafness and/or tinnitus, and rare reports of taste loss and smell perversion and/or loss.
Miscellaneous: Arthralgia, edema.

Clarithromycin –

CNS: Anxiety, behavioral changes, confusional states, depersonalization, disorientation, hallucinations, manic behavior, nightmares, psychosis, tremor.

GI: Glossitis, stomatitis, tongue discoloration, tooth discoloration (reversible); clarithromycin extended-release tablets found in the stool, many of which have occurred in patients with anatomic (including ileostomy or colostomy) or functional GI disorders with shortened GI transit times.

Hematologic: Thrombocytopenia.

Hepatic: In very rare instances, hepatic failure with fatal outcome has been reported and generally has been associated with serious underlying diseases and/or concomitant medications.

Special senses: Alterations of the sense of smell, taste loss, tinnitus.

Miscellaneous: Hypoglycemia (rare).

Overdosage

➤*Symptoms:* The toxic symptoms following an overdose of a macrolide antibiotic may include abdominal pain, diarrhea, nausea, and vomiting. There have been isolated reports of reversible hearing loss occurring chiefly in patients with renal function impairment and in patients receiving high doses of **erythromycin**.

➤*Treatment:* Treatment includes usual supportive measures. Hemodialysis and peritoneal dialysis are not particularly effective. Refer to General Management of Acute Overdosage.

Patient Information

Counsel patients that antibacterial drugs, including macrolides, should only be used to treat bacterial infections. They do not treat viral infections (eg, the common cold). When a macrolide is prescribed to treat a bacterial infection, inform patients that although it is common to feel better early in the course of therapy, to take the medication exactly as directed. Skipping doses or not completing the full course of therapy may (1) decrease the effectiveness of the immediate treatment and (2) increase the likelihood that bacteria will develop resistance and will not be treatable by macrolides or other antibacterial drugs in the future.

Diarrhea is a common problem caused by antibiotics that usually ends when the antibiotic is discontinued. Sometimes after starting treatment with antibiotics, patients can develop watery and bloody stools (with or without stomach cramps and fever), even as late as two or more months after having taken the last dose of the antibiotic. If this occurs, advise patients to contact their health care provider as soon as possible.

Patients should discontinue the drug immediately and contact a health care provider if any signs of an allergic reaction occur.

➤*Azithromycin:* Azithromycin tablets and oral suspension may be taken with or without food. However, increased tolerability has been observed when tablets are taken with food. The reconstituted oral suspension does not need to be refrigerated. Caution patients not to take aluminum- and magnesium-containing antacids and azithromycin tablets or oral suspension simultaneously.

Instruct patients to take azithromycin extended-release oral suspension on an empty stomach (at least 1 hour before or 2 hours following a meal). Store at room temperature and use within 12 hours of constitution. Shake well before use. The entire contents of the bottle should be consumed. Instruct patients who vomit within the first hour to contact their health care provider about further treatment. Azithromycin extended-release suspension may be taken without regard to antacids containing magnesium hydroxide and/or aluminum hydroxide.

➤*Clarithromycin:* Clarithromycin tablets and oral suspension can be taken with or without food and can be taken with milk; however, instruct patients to take clarithromycin extended-release tablets with food. Do not refrigerate the suspension. Swallow the extended-release tablets whole. Do not chew, break, or crush the tablets.

➤*Erythromycin:*

Erythromycin base – In most patients, erythromycin particles in tablets and delayed-release capsules are well absorbed and may be taken without regard to meals. However, optimal blood levels are obtained when the tablets are taken on an empty stomach (at least a half hour, preferably 2 hours, before meals).

Erythromycin base delayed-release tablets may be given without regard to meals. Instruct patients to take erythromycin base film-coated tablets on an empty stomach (at least a half hour, preferably 2 hours, before meals).

Erythromycin ethylsuccinate – May be administered without regard to meals. Refrigeration is not required for *Ery-Ped*. Refrigerate reconstituted *E.E.S.Granules*.

Erythromycin stearate – Take in the fasting state or immediately before meals.

CLARITHROMYCIN

Rx	**Clarithromycin** (Various, eg, Dava, Roxane, Sandoz, Teva, Wockhard)	**Tablets; oral:** 250 mg	In 60s, 100s, and UD 100s.
Rx	**Biaxin** (Abbott)		(KT). Yellow, oval. Film-coated. In 60s and *ABBO-PAC* UD 100s.
Rx	**Clarithromycin** (Various, eg, Dava, Roxane, Sandoz, Teva, UDL)	**Tablets; oral:** 500 mg	In 60s, 100s, and UD 100s.
Rx	**Biaxin** (Abbott)		(KL). Yellow, oval. Film-coated. In 60s and *ABBO-PAC* UD 100s.
Rx	**Clarithromycin** (Watson)	**Tablets, extended-release; oral:** 500 mg	May contain lactose. In 60s.
Rx	**Biaxin XL** (Abbott)		Lactose. (KJ). Yellow, oval. Film-coated. In 60s and *BIAXIN XL PAC* blister pack 4 × 14s, and *ABBO-PAC* UD 100s.
Rx	**Clarithromycin** (Various, eg, Dava, Ranbaxy, Sandoz)	**Granules for suspension; oral:** 125 mg per 5 mL (after reconstitution)	May contain maltodextrin, sucrose. In 50 and 100 mL.
Rx	**Biaxin** (Abbott)		Sucrose. Fruit punch flavor. In 50 and 100 mL.
Rx	**Clarithromycin** (Various, eg, Dava, Ranbaxy, Sandoz)	**Granules for suspension; oral:** 250 mg per 5 mL (after reconstitution)	May contain maltodextrin, sucrose. In 50 and 100 mL.
Rx	**Biaxin** (Abbott)		Sucrose. Fruit punch flavor. In 50 and 100 mL.

CLARITHROMYCIN — ORAL

For complete and comparative prescribing information, refer to the Macrolides group monograph.

Indications

Clarithromycin Indications

Infection	Adults		Children (≥ 6 months of age)
X = Approved indication	Tablets and oral suspension	ER[a] tablets	Tablets and oral suspension
Pharyngitis/Tonsillitis caused by:	X		X
Streptococcus pyogenes[b]			
Acute maxillary sinusitis caused by:	X	X	X
Haemophilus influenzae			
Moraxella catarrhalis			
Streptococcus pneumoniae			
Acute bacterial exacerbation of chronic bronchitis caused by:	X	X	
H. influenzae			
Haemophilus parainfluenzae			
M. catarrhalis			
S. pneumoniae			
Acute otitis media caused by:			X
H. influenzae			
M. catarrhalis			
S. pneumoniae			
Community-acquired pneumonia caused by:			
H. parainfluenzae		X	
H. influenzae	X	X	
Mycoplasma pneumoniae	X	X	X
S. pneumoniae	X	X	X
Chlamydia pneumoniae Taiwan acute respiratory (TWAR) virus	X	X	X

CLARITHROMYCIN — ORAL

Clarithromycin Indications			
Infection	Adults		Children (≥ 6 months of age)
X = Approved indication	Tablets and oral suspension	ER[a] tablets	Tablets and oral suspension
Disseminated mycobacterial infections caused by: *Mycobacterium avium* *Mycobacterium intracellulare*	X		X[c]
Prevention of disseminated *M. avium* complex (MAC) disease in patients with advanced HIV infection	X		X[c]
Uncomplicated skin and skin structure infection[d] caused by: *Staphylococcus aureus* *S. pyogenes*	X		X
Helicobacter pylori infection and duodenal ulcer disease (active or 5-year history[e])	X		

[a] ER = extended release.
[b] The usual drug of choice in the treatment and prevention of streptococcal infections and the prophylaxis of rheumatic fever is oral/intramuscular penicillin. Clarithromycin is generally effective in the eradication of *S. pyogenes* from the nasopharynx; however, data establishing the efficacy of clarithromycin in the subsequent prophylaxis of rheumatic fever are not available.
[c] The safety of clarithromycin has not been studied in MAC patients
[d] Abscesses usually require surgical drainage.
[e] In combination with amoxicillin and lansoprazole or omeprazole, or in combination with omeprazole or ranitidine bismuth citrate. Regimens that contain clarithromycin as the single antimicrobial agent are more likely to be associated with the development of clarithromycin resistance among patients who fail therapy. Do not use clarithromycin-containing regimens in patients with known or suspected clarithromycin-resistant isolates because the efficacy of treatment is reduced in this setting.

Administration and Dosage

➤*General dosing considerations:*

Mycobacterial infections – Clarithromycin is recommended as the primary agent for the treatment of disseminated MAC. Clarithromycin should be used in combination with other antimycobacterial drugs that have shown in vitro activity against MAC or clinical benefit in MAC treatment. Clarithromycin therapy should continue for life if clinical and mycobacterial improvements are observed.

➤*Adults:*

Infections –

Clarithromycin Dosing for Adults				
	Tablets		Extended-release tablets	
Infection	Dosage (every 12 h)	Duration (days)	Dosage (every 24 h)	Duration (days)
M. catarrhalis	250 mg	7 to 14	1,000 mg	7
H. influenzae	500 mg	7 to 14	1,000 mg	7
Community-acquired pneumonia caused by:				
M. pneumoniae	250 mg	7 to 14	1,000 mg	7
S. pneumoniae	250 mg	7 to 14	1,000 mg	7
H. parainfluenzae	—	—	1,000 mg	7
H. influenzae	250 mg	7	1,000 mg	7
M. catarrhalis	—	—	1,000 mg	7
C. pneumoniae	250 mg	7 to 14	1,000 mg	7
Disseminated mycobacterial infections (prevention and treatment)	500 mg	[a]	—	—
Acute maxillary sinusitis caused by: *H. influenzae* *M. catarrhalis* *S. pneumoniae*	500 mg	14	1,000 mg	14
H. parainfluenzae	500 mg	7	1,000 mg	7
S. pneumoniae	250 mg	7 to 14	1,000 mg	7
Acute exacerbation of chronic bronchitis caused by:				
Pharyngitis/Tonsillitis caused by: *S. pyogenes*	250 mg	10	—	—
Uncomplicated skin and skin structure infection caused by: *S. aureus* *S. pyogenes*	250 mg	7 to 14	—	—

[a] Clarithromycin therapy should continue for life if clinical and mycobacterial improvements are observed.

Duodenal ulcer associated with H. pylori – For *H. pylori* eradication to reduce the risk of duodenal ulcer recurrence.

Triple therapy:

• *Clarithromycin/Lansoprazole/Amoxicillin* – Clarithromycin 500 mg, lansoprazole 30 mg, and amoxicillin 1 g every 12 hours for 10 or 14 days.

• *Clarithromycin/Omeprazole/Amoxicillin* – Clarithromycin 500 mg, omeprazole 20 mg, and amoxicillin 1 g every 12 hours for 10 days. In patients with an ulcer present at the time of therapy initiation, an additional 18 days of omeprazole 20 mg once daily is recommended for ulcer healing and symptom relief.

Dual therapy:

• *Clarithromycin/Omeprazole* – Clarithromycin 500 mg 3 times/day (every 8 hours) and omeprazole 40 mg once daily (every morning) for 14 days. An additional 14 days of omeprazole 20 mg once daily is recommended for ulcer healing and symptom relief.

• *Clarithromycin/Ranitidine bismuth citrate* – Clarithromycin 500 mg 2 times/day (every 12 hours) or 3 times/day (every 8 hours) and ranitidine bismuth citrate 400 mg given 2 times/day (every 12 hours) for 14 days. An additional 14 days of ranitidine bismuth citrate 400 mg 2 times/day is recommended for ulcer healing and symptom relief.

➤*Children:*

Infections – For a list of infections, refer to Indications.

6 months of age and older:

• *Usual dosage* – 7.5 mg/kg every 12 hours for 10 days.

Clarithromycin Dosage Guidelines for Children				
Dosing calculated on 7.5 mg/kg every 12 h				
Weight		Dose	Oral suspension 125 mg per 5 mL	Oral suspension 250 mg per 5 mL
kg	lbs	(every 12 h)	(every 12 h)	(every 12 h)
9	20	62.5 mg	2.5 mL	1.25 mL
17	37	125 mg	5 mL	2.5 mL
25	55	187.5 mg	7.5 mL	3.75 mL
33	73	250 mg	10 mL	5 mL

Mycobacterial infections –

20 months of age and older: 7.5 mg/kg twice daily up to 500 mg twice daily for treatment and prevention.

Off-label dosing –

Bacterial endocarditis prophylaxis in patients allergic to penicillin:

• *Usual dose* – 15 mg/kg/day orally 1 hour before dental and/or respiratory tract procedure.

• *Maximum dose* – 500 mg.

Infections:

• *Usual dose* – 15 mg/kg/day every 12 hours.

• *Maximum dose* – 1 g/day.

Mycobacterial infections:

• *Usual dose* – 15 mg/kg/day every 12 hours for MAC treatment and prevention.

• *Maximum dose* – 1 g per 24 hours.

• *Concomitant therapy* – Clarithromycin is taken with other antimycobacterial drugs for MAC treatment.

➤*Elderly:* Consider dosage adjustment in elderly patients with severe renal impairment.

➤*Renal function impairment:* In the presence of severe renal impairment (CrCl less than 30 mL/min), with or without coexisting hepatic impairment, the dose should be halved or the dosing interval doubled.

Clarithromycin in combination with ranitidine bismuth citrate therapy is not recommended in patients with CrCl less than 25 mL/min.

➤*Administration:* Tablets and oral suspension may be given with or without food and can be taken with milk. Clarithromycin extended-release tablets should be taken with food. The extended-release tablets should be swallowed whole and not chewed, broken, or crushed.

➤*Storage/Stability:*

Tablets and granules for oral suspension – Store at 15° to 30°C (59° to 86°F) in a well-closed container. Protect the 250 mg tablets from light.

Extended-release tablets – Store at 20° to 25°C (68° to 77°F); excursions are permitted to 15° to 30°C (59° to 86°F).

Reconstituted suspension – Shake well before each use. Keep tightly closed. Do not refrigerate. After mixing, store at 15° to 30°C (59° to 86°F) and use within 14 days.

AZITHROMYCIN

Rx	**Azithromycin** (Various, eg, Greenstone, Teva, Wockhardt)	**Tablets; oral:** 250 mg	May contain lactose. In 1s, 3s, 6s, 30s, and UD 18s, 50s, and 100s.
Rx	**Zithromax** (Pfizer)		Lactose, sodium 0.9 mg. (PFIZER 306). Pink, capsule shape. Film-coated. In 30s, UD 50s, and *Z-Pak* 6s.
Rx	**Azithromycin** (Various, eg, Greenstone, Teva, Wockhardt)	**Tablets; oral:** 500 mg	May contain lactose. In 3s, 6s, 30s, and UD 9s, 50s, and 100s.
Rx	**Zithromax** (Pfizer)		Lactose, sodium 1.8 mg. (PFIZER ZTM500). Pink, capsule shape. Film-coated. In 30s, UD 50s, and *TRI-PAK* 3s.
Rx	**Azithromycin** (Various, eg, Greenstone, Teva, Wockhardt)	**Tablets; oral:** 600 mg	May contain lactose. In 30s.
Rx	**Zithromax** (Pfizer)		Lactose, sodium 2.1 mg. (PFIZER 308). White, oval. Film-coated. In 30s.
Rx	**Azithromycin** (Various, eg, Greenstone, Teva)	**Powder for suspension; oral:** 100 mg per 5 mL (after reconstitution)	May contain sugar, sucrose. In 15 mL bottles.
Rx	**Zithromax** (Pfizer)		Sodium 3.7 mg per 5 mL, sucrose. Cherry/Banana/Creme de vanilla flavors. In 15 mL bottles.
Rx	**Azithromycin** (Various, eg, Greenstone, Teva)	**Powder for suspension; oral:** 200 mg per 5 mL (after reconstitution)	May contain sucrose. In 15, 22.5, and 30 mL bottles.
Rx	**Zithromax** (Pfizer)		Sodium 7.4 mg per 5 mL, sucrose. Cherry/Banana/Creme de vanilla flavors. In 15, 22.5, and 30 mL bottles.
Rx	**Azithromycin** (Greenstone)	**Powder for suspension; oral:** 1 g/packet	May contain sucrose. Cherry/Banana flavors. In single-dose packets of 3s and 10s.
Rx	**Zithromax** (Pfizer)		Sodium 37 mg, sucrose. Cherry/Banana flavors. In single-dose packets of 3s and 10s.
Rx	**Zmax** (Pfizer)	**Powder for suspension, extended-release; oral:** 2 g	Contains microspheres. Sucrose, sodium 148 mg. Cherry/Banana flavors. In single-dose bottles.
Rx	**Azithromycin** (Various, eg, APP, Hospira, Sicor)	**Injection, lyophilized powder for solution:** 500 mg	May contain sodium. In vials.
Rx	**Zithromax** (Pfizer)		Sodium 114 mg (4.96 mEq). In vials with 1 *Vial-Mate* adapter.
Rx	**Azithromycin** (Various, eg, Sicor, Teva)	**Injection, lyophilized powder for solution:** 2.5 g	May contain sodium. In pharmacy bulk packages.

AZITHROMYCIN — ORAL

For complete and comparative prescribing information, refer to the Macrolides class monograph.

Indications

Azithromycin Oral Indications

Infection	Adults			Children (≥ 6 months of age, except when noted)	
X = Approved indication	Tablets (250 and 500 mg) and oral suspension (100 mg per 5 mL and 200 mg per 5 mL)	Tablets (600 mg) and oral suspension (1 g)	Extended-release oral suspension	Tablets (250 and 500 mg) and oral suspension (100 mg per 5 mL and 200 mg per 5 mL)	Extended-release oral suspension
Acute bacterial exacerbations of chronic obstructive pulmonary disease caused by: *Haemophilus influenzae*, *Moraxella catarrhalis*, *Streptococcus pneumoniae*	X				
Acute bacterial sinusitis caused by: *H. influenzae*, *M. catarrhalis*, *S. pneumoniae*	X		X	X	
Acute otitis media caused by: *H. influenzae*, *M. catarrhalis*, *S. pneumoniae*				X	
CAP[a] caused by: *H. influenzae*, *M. pneumoniae*, *S. pneumoniae*, *Chlamydophila pneumoniae*	X		X	X	X
Genital ulcer disease (chancroid) in men caused by: *Haemophilus ducreyi*	X				
Pharyngitis/Tonsillitis caused by: *Streptococcus pyogenes*[b]	X			X[c]	
Prevention/Treatment of disseminated MAC[d] disease in patients with advanced HIV infection		X			
Uncomplicated skin and skin structure infections[e] caused by: *Staphylococcus aureus*, *S. pyogenes*, *Streptococcus agalactiae*	X				

AZITHROMYCIN — ORAL

Azithromycin Oral Indications					
Infection	Adults			Children (≥ 6 months of age, except when noted)	
X = Approved indication	Tablets (250 and 500 mg) and oral suspension (100 mg per 5 mL and 200 mg per 5 mL)	Tablets (600 mg) and oral suspension (1 g)	Extended-release oral suspension	Tablets (250 and 500 mg) and oral suspension (100 mg per 5 mL and 200 mg per 5 mL)	Extended-release oral suspension
Urethritis and cervicitis caused by: *Chlamydia trachomatis*	X	X			
Urethritis and cervicitis caused by: *Neisseria gonorrhoeae*	X				

[a] CAP = community-acquired pneumonia. Do not use azithromycin in patients with pneumonia who are judged to be inappropriate for oral therapy because of moderate to severe illness or risk factors, such as any of the following: patients with cystic fibrosis, nosocomially acquired infections, known or suspected bacteremia, or significant underlying health problems that may compromise their ability to respond to their illness (including immunodeficiency or functional asplenia); patients requiring hospitalization; or elderly or debilitated patients.

[b] Azithromycin is an alternative to first-line therapy in individuals who cannot use first-line therapy. Penicillin by the intramuscular (IM) route is the usual drug of choice in the treatment of *S. pyogenes* infection and the prophylaxis of rheumatic fever. Azithromycin is often effective in the eradication of susceptible strains of *S. pyogenes* from the nasopharynx. Because some strains are resistant to azithromycin, perform susceptibility tests when patients are treated with azithromycin. Data establishing efficacy of azithromycin in subsequent prevention of rheumatic fever are not available.

[c] Approved for use in children ≥ 2 years of age.

[d] MAC = *Mycobacterium avium* complex.

[e] Abscesses usually require surgical drainage.

➤*Gonorrhea or syphilis:* Do not rely on azithromycin at the recommended dose to treat gonorrhea or syphilis. Antimicrobial agents used in high doses for short periods of time to treat nongonococcal urethritis may mask or delay the symptoms of incubating gonorrhea or syphilis. Administer a serologic test for syphilis and perform appropriate cultures for gonorrhea at the time of diagnosis to all patients with sexually transmitted urethritis or cervicitis. Initiate appropriate antimicrobial therapy and follow-up tests for these diseases if infection is confirmed.

➤*Off-label uses:*

Acute pharyngitis or tonsillitis (group A streptococcal) (children), 3-day regimen – [5] = Poor documentation. Although azithromycin 3-day regimens appear to produce good initial clinical results in some studies, poor eradication rates and higher relapse rates need to be further evaluated. Consider the higher dose and longer duration regimen as recommended by the manufacturer (12 mg/kg for 5 days) to be the alternative to first-line treatment with penicillin.

Acute skin and soft tissue infections (children), 3-day regimen – [1] = Good documentation. In 2 studies, 3-day regimens of azithromycin produced comparable efficacy compared with conventional regimens of cefaclor or cloxacillin esters for the treatment of acute skin infections in children.

Babesiosis – [1] = Good documentation. Guidelines based on randomized, controlled trials recommend the use of azithromycin and atovaquone for the treatment of active babesiosis.

Granuloma inguinale (donovanosis) – [1] = Good documentation. Centers for Disease Control and Prevention (CDC) guidelines recommend azithromycin as an alternative regimen for treatment of granuloma inguinale when doxycycline is not appropriate. World Health Organization (WHO) guidelines provide additional support for this recommendation.

Helicobacter pylori infection – [4] = Insufficient documentation. Several trials have evaluated the use of azithromycin in combination with other agents for the treatment of *H. pylori* infection and noted conflicting results. Current guidelines do not address its use. Considering the large body of evidence supporting the efficacy of other available agents, azithromycin cannot be recommended for routine inclusion in *Helicobacter* eradication regimens until controlled studies can unequivocally demonstrate its place in therapy.

Lower respiratory tract infections (children), 3-day regimen – [2] = Fair documentation. The majority of published information has been manufacturer sponsored and suggests comparable efficacy with the conventional regimens studied. The issue of possible resistance with a shorter antibiotic regimen has not been fully addressed by these trials. Some studies have noted persistence rates approximating 20%. Although safety data indicate no differences in incidence of adverse events, it should be noted that the 10 mg/kg/day regimen is double the conventional doses on days 2 and 3, and thus, GI events should be expected.

Prevention of acute otitis media (children), once-weekly regimen – [2] = Fair documentation. This regimen may be a useful alternative, but appropriate selection of patients should be considered to avoid the risk of promoting resistance.

Prevention of coronary events – [5] = Poor documentation. The usefulness of azithromycin in the prevention of secondary cardiac events in patients with coronary syndromes is questionable. Large, controlled trials have not proven a consistent relationship between the use of the drug and improved cardiac outcomes. Routine use of azithromycin for this indication cannot be recommended until a consistent therapeutic benefit is established.

Rosacea – [4] = Insufficient documentation. In the limited published data available, oral azithromycin appears to be as effective as oral doxycycline in the management of rosacea. This agent may be considered an alternative in patients who are not responsive to or who cannot tolerate doxycycline.

Traveler's diarrhea – [1] = Good documentation. Antibiotics have been shown to shorten the duration of traveler's diarrhea and may also be used in moderate to severe cases; however, because of increased antibiotic resistance, doxycycline is no longer recommended for the treatment of traveler's diarrhea. Current guidelines suggest that mild cases of traveler's diarrhea should be managed with adequate hydration and bismuth subsalicylate or loperamide.

Other possible off-label uses – Anti-inflammatory agent in cystic fibrosis; *Mycobacterium avium* complex prophylaxis; treatment in children with HIV; treatment of cholera in adults.

Chlamydial infections caused by C. trachomatis: The CDC recommends azithromycin 1 g orally in a single dose.

For children who have chlamydial infection and weigh 45 kg or more but are younger than 8 years of age, the CDC recommends azithromycin 1 g orally in a single dose.

For children 8 years of age and older with chlamydial infection, the CDC recommends azithromycin 1 g orally in a single dose.

Lyme disease (early): Infectious Diseases Society of America (IDSA) guidelines recommend azithromycin as second-line therapy in patients who are intolerant of or should not take first-line therapy (eg, amoxicillin, cefuroxime axetil, doxycycline).

Prophylaxis after a sexual assault: The CDC recommends azithromycin 1 g orally in a single dose plus ceftriaxone and metronidazole.

Administration and Dosage

➤*General dosing considerations:* Single-dose 1 g packets are not for pediatric use.

Azithromycin extended-release oral suspension provides a full course of antibacterial therapy in a single oral dose.

The single 2 g doses of *Zmax* and azithromycin powder for oral suspension are not bioequivalent and are not interchangeable.

➤*Adults:*

Immediate-release tablets and oral suspension –

Acute bacterial exacerbations of chronic obstructive pulmonary disease (mild to moderate severity):

- *Usual dosage* – 500 mg/day.
- *Alternative dosage* – 500 mg as a single dose on the first day followed by 250 mg once daily on days 2 through 5.
- *Duration of therapy* – 3 days.

Acute bacterial sinusitis:

- *Usual dosage* – 500 mg/day.
- *Duration of therapy* – 3 days.

Community-acquired pneumonia (mild severity): 500 mg as a single dose on the first day followed by 250 mg once daily on days 2 through 5.

Genital ulcer disease (chancroid): Single 1 g dose.

Gonococcal urethritis/cervicitis: Single 2 g dose.

Nongonococcal urethritis/cervicitis: Refer to Genital Ulcer Disease for dosing.

Pharyngitis/tonsillitis (as second-line therapy): Refer to Community-Acquired Pneumonia for dosing.

Prevention of disseminated M. avium complex disease: 1,200 mg taken once weekly.

Treatment of disseminated M. avium complex disease: 600 mg/day in combination with ethambutol at the recommended daily dose of 15 mg/kg.

Uncomplicated skin/skin structure infections: Refer to Community-Acquired Pneumonia for dosing.

Zmax –

Acute bacterial sinusitis: A single 2 g dose.

Community-acquired pneumonia (mild severity): Refer to Acute Bacterial Sinusitis for dosing.

Off-label dosing –

Babesiosis: [1] = Good documentation. 500 to 1,000 mg orally on day 1, followed by 250 mg orally daily thereafter for 7 to 10 days; higher dosages

AZITHROMYCIN — ORAL

may be required in immunocompromised patients (600 to 1,000 mg daily). IDSA recommends the combination of azithromycin and atovaquone for 7 to 10 days as initial therapy for the treatment of active babesiosis.

Granuloma inguinale (donovanosis): [1] = Good documentation. 1 g once weekly for at least 3 weeks. Treatment should continue until all lesions have completely healed. WHO guidelines suggest a dosage of 1 g on day 1, followed by 500 mg once daily until complete epithelization.

Helicobacter pylori infection: [4] = Insufficient documentation. 500 mg/day for 3 to 7 days in combination with an acid-reducing medication and other antibiotic(s).

Rosacea: [4] = Insufficient documentation. In 2 small, open trials, 250 mg 3 times weekly (Mondays, Wednesdays, and Fridays) for up to 32 weeks was studied.

A tapering regimen over a 3-month period was also used with oral azithromycin 500 mg 3 times weekly for the first month and 250 mg 3 times weekly during the second month (Mondays, Wednesdays, and Saturdays). During the third month, dosing was 250 mg twice weekly (Tuesdays and Saturdays).

Traveler's diarrhea: [1] = Good documentation. 1,000 mg given as 1 dose.

➤*Children:*

2 years of age and older –

Immediate-release oral suspension:

• *Pharyngitis / Tonsillitis –*

Azithromycin Oral Children Dosage Guidelines for Pharyngitis/Tonsillitis: 5-Day Regimen[a]

Weight		Amount of 200 mg per 5 mL suspension	Total mL per treatment course	Total mg per treatment course
kg	lbs	Days 1 to 5		
8	18	2.5 mL	12.5 mL	500 mg
17	37	5 mL	25 mL	1,000 mg
25	55	7.5 mL	37.5 mL	1,500 mg
33	73	10 mL	50 mL	2,000 mg
40	88	12.5 mL	62.5 mL	2,500 mg

[a] Dosing calculated on 12 mg/kg/day for 5 days.

Usual dosage: 12 mg/kg once daily.

Maximum dose: 500 mg/day.

Duration of therapy: 5 days.

6 months of age and older –

Immediate-release oral suspension:

• *Acute bacterial sinusitis –*

Usual dosage: 10 mg/kg oral suspension once daily.

Duration of therapy: 3 days.

• *Acute otitis media –*

Usual dosage: 30 mg/kg oral suspension given as a single dose.

Alternative dosage: 10 mg/kg once daily for 3 days or 10 mg/kg as a single dose on the first day, followed by 5 mg/kg on days 2 through 5.

• *Community-acquired pneumonia –* 10 mg/kg oral suspension as a single dose on the first day followed by 5 mg/kg on days 2 through 5.

Azithromycin Oral Children Dosage Guidelines for Otitis Media and Community-Acquired Pneumonia: 5-Day Regimen[a,b]

Weight		Amount of 100 mg per 5 mL suspension		Amount of 200 mg per 5 mL suspension		Total mL per treatment course	Total mg per treatment course
kg	lbs	Day 1	Days 2 to 5	Day 1	Days 2 to 5		
5	11	2.5 mL	1.25 mL			7.5 mL	150 mg
10	22	5 mL	2.5 mL			15 mL	300 mg
20	44			5 mL	2.5 mL	15 mL	600 mg
30	66			7.5 mL	3.75 mL	22.5 mL	900 mg
40	88			10 mL	5 mL	30 mL	1,200 mg
≥ 50	≥ 110			12.5 mL	6.25 mL	37.5 mL	1,500 mg

[a] Dosing calculated on 10 mg/kg/day on day 1, followed by 5 mg/kg/day on days 2 to 5.
[b] Efficacy of the 1- or 3-day regimen in children with community-acquired pneumonia has not been established.

Azithromycin Oral Children Dosage Guidelines for Otitis Media and Acute Bacterial Sinusitis: 3-Day Regimen[a,b]

Weight		Amount of 100 mg per 5 mL suspension	Amount of 200 mg per 5 mL suspension	Total mL per treatment course	Total mg per treatment course
kg	lbs	Days 1 to 3	Days 1 to 3		
5	11	2.5 mL		7.5 mL	150 mg
10	22	5 mL		15 mL	300 mg
20	44		5 mL	15 mL	600 mg
30	66		7.5 mL	22.5 mL	900 mg
40	88		10 mL	30 mL	1,200 mg
≥ 50	≥ 110		12.5 mL	37.5 mL	1,500 mg

[a] Dosing calculated on 10 mg/kg/day.
[b] Efficacy of the 1- or 5-day regimen in children with acute bacterial sinusitis has not been established.

Azithromycin Oral Children Dosage Guidelines for Otitis Media: 1-Day Regimen[a]

Weight		Amount of 200 mg per 5 mL suspension	Total mL per treatment course	Total mg per treatment course
kg	lbs	Day 1		
5	11	3.75 mL	3.75 mL	150 mg
10	22	7.5 mL	7.5 mL	300 mg
20	44	15 mL	15 mL	600 mg
30	66	22.5 mL	22.5 mL	900 mg
40	88	30 mL	30 mL	1,200 mg
≥ 50	≥ 110	37.5 mL	37.5 mL	1,500 mg

[a] Dosing calculated on 30 mg/kg as a single dose.

Zmax:

• *Community-acquired pneumonia – Zmax* should be taken as a single dose of 60 mg/kg body weight. Children weighing 75 lb (34 kg) or more should receive the adult dose.

The dose in milliliters is equivalent to the child's weight in pounds (1 mL/lb dose) for a body weight of less than 75 lb (34 kg).

***Zmax* Children Dosage Guidelines: 1-Dose Regimen[a]**

Weight		1 mL/lb dose	
kg	lbs	Dose (mg)	Volume (mL)
5	10	270 mg	10 mL
7	15	405 mg	15 mL
9	20	540 mg	20 mL
11	25	675 mg	25 mL
14	30	810 mg	30 mL
16	35	945 mg	35 mL
18	40	1,080 mg	40 mL
20	45	1,215 mg	45 mL
23	50	1,350 mg	50 mL
25	55	1,485 mg	55 mL
27	60	1,620 mg	60 mL
30	65	1,755 mg	65 mL
32	70	1,890 mg	70 mL
34	≥ 75	2,000 mg	Consume entire contents of bottle

[a] To ensure accurate dosing, a dosing spoon, medicine syringe, or cup is recommended.

Off-label dosing –

Acute pharyngitis or tonsillitis (group A streptococcal) (children), 3-day regimen: [3] = Safety concerns. Use is not recommended. Dose used in clinical trials was 10 mg/kg once daily for 3 days (administered 1 hour before meals or 2 hours after meals) as oral suspension.

Acute skin and soft tissue infections (children), 3-day regimen: [2] = Fair documentation. 10 mg/kg once daily for 3 days (administered 1 hour before meals or 2 hours after meals) as oral suspension.

Anti-inflammatory agent in cystic fibrosis:

• *40 kg or more –* 500 mg 3 times per week (eg, Monday, Wednesday, Friday).

• *25 to 39 kg –* 250 mg 3 times per week (eg, Monday, Wednesday, Friday).

Babesiosis: [2] = Fair documentation. 10 mg/kg orally on day 1 (up to a maximum of 500 mg), followed by 5 mg/kg orally daily thereafter (up to a maximum of 250 mg per dose). IDSA recommends the combination of azithromycin and atovaquone for up to 7 to 10 days as initial therapy for the treatment of active babesiosis.

Lower respiratory tract infections (children), 3-day regimen (off-label): [1] = Good documentation. 10 mg/kg once daily for 3 days (administered 1 hour before meals or 2 hours after meals) as oral suspension.

AZITHROMYCIN — ORAL

Mycobacterium avium complex prophylaxis in HIV patients:
- *First episode –*
  Usual dosage: 20 mg/kg once weekly.
  Maximum dose: 1,200 mg.
  Alternative dosage: 5 mg/kg once daily (max, 250 mg) with or without rifabutin.
- *Recurrence –*
  Usual dosage: 5 mg/kg once daily plus ethambutol with or without rifabutin.
  Maximum dose: 250 mg once daily.

Mycobacterium avium complex treatment in HIV patients:
- *Usual dose* – 10 to 12 mg/kg once daily plus ethambutol with or without rifabutin.
- *Maximum dose* – 500 mg once daily.
- *Duration of therapy* – 1 month or longer.

Prevention of acute otitis media (children), once-weekly regimen: [1] = Good documentation. 10 mg/kg once weekly for 6 months.

➤*Re-dosing azithromycin:*

Children – The safety of re-dosing azithromycin in children who vomit after receiving 30 mg/kg as a single dose has not been established. In clinical studies involving 487 patients with acute otitis media given a single dose of azithromycin 30 mg/kg, 8 patients who vomited within 30 minutes of dosing were re-dosed at the same total dose.

Zmax – In the event that a patient vomits within 5 minutes of administration, consider additional antibiotic treatment because there would be minimal absorption of azithromycin. Because insufficient data exist on absorption of azithromycin, if a patient vomits between 5 and 60 minutes following administration, consider alternative therapy. Neither a second dose of *Zmax* nor alternative treatment is warranted if vomiting occurs at least 60 minutes following administration in patients with normal gastric emptying. In patients with delayed gastric emptying, alternative therapy should be considered.

➤*Preparation for administration:*

Oral suspension –

Reconstitution of Azithromycin Oral Suspension

Amount of water to be added	Total volume after reconstitution (azithromycin content)	Azithromycin concentration after reconstitution
9 mL (300 mg)	15 mL (300 mg)	100 mg per 5 mL

Reconstitution of Azithromycin Oral Suspension

Amount of water to be added	Total volume after reconstitution (azithromycin content)	Azithromycin concentration after reconstitution
9 mL (600 mg)	15 mL (600 mg)	200 mg per 5 mL
12 mL (900 mg)	22.5 mL (900 mg)	200 mg per 5 mL
15 mL (1,200 mg)	30 mL (1,200 mg)	200 mg per 5 mL

1 g packet – Thoroughly mix the entire contents of the packet with approximately 60 mL (2 oz) of water. Do not use the single-dose packet to administer doses other than azithromycin 1,000 mg. The packet is not for pediatric use.

Zmax – Reconstitute with 60 mL water. Shake well before dispensing. Patients should consume suspension within 12 hours.

➤*Administration:* Tablets and immediate-release oral suspension can be taken with or without food; however, increased tolerability has been observed when tablets are taken with food. It is recommended that *Zmax* be taken on an empty stomach (at least 1 hour before or 2 hours following a meal).

1 g packet – The patient should drink the entire contents immediately and then add an additional 60 mL of water, mix, and drink to ensure complete consumption of dosage.

Zmax – For dosing in children weighing less than 75 lb (34 kg), use of a dosing device is recommended. The pharmacist should inform the patient's caregiver that any suspension remaining after dosing must be discarded.

➤*Storage / Stability:*

Tablets – Store tablets between 15° and 30°C (59° and 86°F).

Oral suspension – Store dry powder below 30°C (86°F).

Store single-dose packets between 5° and 30°C (41° and 86°F). Store reconstituted oral suspension between 5° and 30°C (41° and 86°F) and use within 10 days. Shake well before each use. Discard after full dosing is completed.

Store *Zmax* dry powder at or below 30°C (86°F). Store reconstituted *Zmax* suspension at 25°C (77°F); excursions are permitted between 15° and 30°C (59° and 86°F). Do not refrigerate or freeze. Patients should consume suspension within 12 hours.

AZITHROMYCIN — INJECTION

For complete prescribing information, refer to the Macrolides class monograph.

Indications

➤*Community-acquired pneumonia:* In patients requiring initial intravenous (IV) therapy with community-acquired pneumonia caused by *Chlamydia pneumoniae*, *Haemophilus influenzae*, *Streptococcus pneumoniae*, *Mycoplasma pneumoniae*, *Legionella pneumophila*, *Moraxella catarrhalis*, and *Staphylococcus aureus*.

➤*Pelvic inflammatory disease:* In patients requiring initial IV therapy with pelvic inflammatory disease (PID) caused by *Chlamydia trachomatis*, *Neisseria gonorrhoeae*, or *Mycoplasma hominis*. If anaerobic microorganisms are suspected of contributing to the infection, administer an antimicrobial agent with anaerobic activity in combination with azithromycin.

➤*Off-label uses:*

Acne vulgaris (topical) – [4] = Insufficient documentation. In the limited published data available, topical azithromycin caused improvement in only the noninflammatory lesions of acne vulgaris.

Hospital-acquired pneumonia – [1] = Good documentation. Azithromycin is recommended as add-on therapy by the American Thoracic Society/Infectious Diseases Society of America practice guidelines for the treatment of hospital-acquired pneumonia, ventilator-associated pneumonia, and healthcare-associated pneumonia in adults with suspected *Legionella pneumophila* infiltrates. Current literature evaluating azithromycin use in hospital-acquired pneumonia, ventilator-associated pneumonia, or healthcare-associated pneumonia is lacking. Future controlled clinical trials are necessary to further evaluate azithromycin's place in therapy, and dosage and duration in the treatment of hospital-acquired pneumonia, ventilator-associated pneumonia, or healthcare-associated pneumonia.

Rosacea (topical) – [5] = Poor documentation. In the limited published data available, topical azithromycin did not have a significant effect in the management of rosacea and was less effective than topical erythromycin. Use is not recommended.

Administration and Dosage

➤*Adults:*

Community-acquired pneumonia –

Initial dosage: 500 mg IV as a single daily dose for at least 2 days in adults.

Maintenance dosage: Follow IV therapy by the oral route at a single daily dose of 500 mg to complete a 7- to 10-day course of therapy. The timing of the switch to oral therapy should be done at the discretion of the health care provider and in accordance with clinical response.

Pelvic inflammatory disease –

Initial dosage: 500 mg IV as a single daily dose for 1 or 2 days in adults.

Maintenance dosage: Follow IV therapy by the oral route at a single daily dose of 250 mg to complete a 7-day course of therapy. The timing of the switch to oral therapy should be done at the discretion of the health care provider and in accordance with clinical response.

Concomitant therapy: If anaerobic microorganisms are suspected of contributing to the infection, administer an antimicrobial agent with anaerobic activity in combination with azithromycin.

Off-label dosing –

Acne vulgaris (topical): [4] = Insufficient documentation. Topical azithromycin 2% was applied each evening for 12 weeks.
- *Extemporaneous formulation* – Azithromycin 2% (20 mg/mL) in a 60% ethanol/40% water solution as prepared using 500 mg vials of IV azithromycin diluted to a final volume of 25 mL. This mixture was stable at room temperature for up to 6 months as measured by high-performance liquid chromatography.

Hospital-acquired pneumonia: [1] = Good documentation. 500 mg IV once daily added to the current antibiotic regimen. A switch to oral azithromycin may be made at the prescriber's discretion. The recommended duration of treatment is 7 to 14 days.

➤*Children:*

16 years of age and older – See Adults for dosing.

➤*Preparation for administration:* Prepare the initial solution of azithromycin for injection by adding 4.8 mL of sterile water for injection to the 500 mg vial and shaking the vial until all of the drug is dissolved. Because azithromycin for injection is supplied under vacuum, it is recommended that a standard 5 mL (nonautomated) syringe be used to ensure that the exact amount of sterile water, 4.8 mL, is dispensed.

Each milliliter of reconstituted solution contains azithromycin 100 mg.

To provide azithromycin over a concentration range of 1 to 2 mg/mL, transfer 5 mL of the azithromycin 100 mg/mL solution into the appropriate amount of any of the following diluents: sodium chloride 0.9%, sodium chloride 0.45%, dextrose 5% in water, Ringer's lactate solution, dextrose 5% in sodium chloride 0.45% with potassium chloride 20 mEq, dextrose 5% in Ringer's lactate solution, 5% dextrose in sodium chloride 0.3%, dextrose 5% in sodium chloride 0.45%, *Normosol-M* in dextrose 5%, *Normosol-R* in dextrose 5%.

➤*Administration:* Infuse injections over a period of at least 60 minutes. The infusate concentration and rate of infusion for azithromycin IV should be 1 mg/mL over 3 hours or 2 mg/mL over 1 hour.

Do not administer azithromycin injection as a bolus or intramuscular (IM) injection.

➤*Admixture compatibility:* Do not add other IV substances, additives, or medications to azithromycin injection or infuse simultaneously through the same IV line.

➤*Storage / Stability:* Reconstituted solution and the diluted solution (1 to 2 mg/mL) are stable for 24 hours when stored below 30°C (86°F). The diluted solution is stable for 7 days when refrigerated at 5°C (41°F).

ERYTHROMYCIN BASE

Rx	**Ery-Tab** (Abbott)	**Tablets, delayed-release ; oral:** 250 mg	(EC). White, oval. Enteric-coated. In 100s and 500s.
Rx	**Ery-Tab** (Abbott)	**Tablets, delayed-release; oral:** 333 mg	(EH). White, oval. Enteric-coated. In 100s and 500s.
Rx	**PCE Dispertab** (Abbott)		Contains coated erythromycin particles. Lactose. (PCE). White with pink speckles, oval. Enteric-coated. In 60s.
Rx	**Ery-Tab** (Abbott)	**Tablets, delayed-release ; oral:** 500 mg	(ED). White, oval. Enteric-coated. In 100s.
Rx	**PCE Dispertab** (Abbott)		Contains coated erythromycin particles. (EK). White, oval. Enteric-coated. In 100s.
Rx	**Erythromycin Filmtab** (Abbott)	**Tablets, film-coated; oral:** 250 mg	(EB). Pink, oval. In 100s and 500s.
Rx	**Erythromycin Filmtab** (Abbott)	**Tablets, film-coated ; oral:** 500 mg	(EA). Pink, oval. In 100s.
Rx	**Erythromycin** (Abbott)	**Capsules, delayed-release ; oral:** 250 mg	(ER) Clear, opaque, maroon, with pink and yellow particles. Contains enteric-coated pellets. In 100s and 500s.

ERYTHROMYCIN BASE — ORAL

For complete and comparative prescribing information, refer to the Macrolides group monograph.

Indications

➤*General information:* For the treatment of infections caused by susceptible strains of the designated organisms in the following diseases:

➤*Acute pelvic inflammatory disease caused by Neisseria gonorrhoeae:* Erythromycin lactobionate for injection followed by erythromycin base orally as an alternative drug in treatment of acute pelvic inflammatory disease caused by *N. gonorrhoeae* in female patients with a history of sensitivity to penicillin. Patients should have a serologic test for syphilis before receiving erythromycin as treatment of gonorrhea and a follow-up serologic test for syphilis after 3 months.

➤*Diphtheria:* Infections caused by *Corynebacterium diphtheriae*, as an adjunct to antitoxin, to prevent establishment of carriers, and to eradicate the organism in carriers.

➤*Erythrasma:* In the treatment of infections caused by *Corynebacterium minutissimum*.

➤*Infections caused by Chlamydia trachomatis:* Conjunctivitis of the newborn, pneumonia of infancy, and urogenital infections during pregnancy. When tetracyclines are contraindicated or not tolerated, erythromycin is indicated for the treatment of uncomplicated urethral, endocervical, or rectal infections in adults caused by *C. trachomatis*.

➤*Intestinal amebiasis:* Intestinal amebiasis caused by *Entamoeba histolytica*. Extraenteric amebiasis requires treatment with other agents.

➤*Legionnaire disease:* Legionnaire disease caused by *Legionella pneumophila*. Although no controlled clinical efficacy studies have been conducted, in vitro and limited preliminary clinical data suggest that erythromycin may be effective in treating Legionnaire disease.

➤*Listeriosis:* Listeriosis caused by *Listeria monocytogenes*.

➤*Lower respiratory tract infections:* Lower respiratory tract infections of mild to moderate severity caused by *Streptococcus pneumoniae* or *Streptococcus pyogenes*.

➤*Nongonococcal urethritis:* When tetracyclines are contraindicated or not tolerated, erythromycin is indicated for the treatment of nongonococcal urethritis caused by *Ureaplasma urealyticum*.

➤*Pertussis (whooping cough):* Pertussis (whooping cough) caused by *Bordetella pertussis*. Erythromycin is effective in eliminating the *B. pertussis* from the nasopharynx of infected individuals rendering them noninfectious. Some clinical studies suggest that erythromycin may be helpful in the prophylaxis of pertussis in exposed susceptible individuals.

➤*Prophylaxis of rheumatic fever:*

Prevention of initial attacks of rheumatic fever – Penicillin is considered by the American Heart Association to be the drug of choice in the prevention of initial attacks of rheumatic fever (treatment of *S. pyogenes* infections of the upper respiratory tract) (eg, pharyngitis, tonsillitis). Erythromycin is indicated for the treatment of penicillin-allergic patients.

Prevention of recurrent attacks of rheumatic fever – Penicillin or sulfonamides are considered by the American Heart Association to be the drugs of choice in the prevention of recurrent attacks of rheumatic fever. In patients who are allergic to penicillin and sulfonamides, oral erythromycin is recommended by the American Heart Association in the long-term prophylaxis of streptococcal pharyngitis (for the prevention of recurrent attacks of rheumatic fever).

➤*Respiratory tract infections:* Respiratory tract infections caused by *Mycoplasma pneumoniae*.

➤*Skin and skin-structure infections:* Skin and skin-structure infections of mild to moderate severity caused by *S. pyogenes* or *Staphylococcus aureus* (resistant staphylococci may emerge during treatment).

➤*Syphilis caused by Treponema pallidum:* Erythromycin is an alternate choice of treatment for primary syphilis in penicillin-allergic patients. In the treatment of primary syphilis, perform spinal fluid examinations before treatment and as part of follow-up after therapy.

➤*Upper respiratory tract infections:* Upper respiratory tract infections of mild to moderate severity caused by *S. pyogenes*, *S. pneumoniae*, or *Haemophilus influenzae* (when used concomitantly with adequate doses of sulfonamides, since many strains of *H. influenzae* are not susceptible to the erythromycin concentrations ordinarily achieved).

➤*Off-label uses:*

Chancroid – [1] = Good documentation. Based on Centers for Disease Control and Prevention (CDC) guidelines, erythromycin is a recommended therapy for treatment of chancroid. However, intermediate resistance to erythromycin has been reported in several isolates. Potential resistance issues should be considered when initiating therapy for the treatment of chancroid.

Granuloma inguinale (donovanosis) – [1] = Good documentation. CDC guidelines recommend erythromycin as an alternative regimen for the treatment of granuloma inguinale when doxycycline is not appropriate. It is the recommended treatment for pregnant women. World Health Organization guidelines provide additional support for this recommendation.

Other possible off-label uses –

Acne vulgaris: Erythromycin base is helpful in decreasing the population of lipophilic bacteria and may also have an anti-inflammatory effect.

Bacillary angiomatosis (immunocompromised patients): Caused by *Bartonella henselae* or *Bartonella quintana*; as an alternative agent, erythromycin 500 mg 4 times/day.

Campylobacter enteritis: Caused by *Campylobacter jejuni*.

Cellulitis, erysipelas: As an alternative agent for the treatment of cellulitis (erysipelas) of the extremities that is not associated with venous catheter and not diabetes related.

Impetigo, ecthyma: As an alternative agent for the treatment of nonbullous lesions.

Inclusion conjunctivitis (adults): Caused by *C. trachomatis*; as an alternative agent.

Infected wounds, extremity: As an alternative agent for the treatment of mild to moderate, uncomplicated, infected wounds of the extremities.

Leptospirosis: Caused by *Leptospira*; for the treatment of moderate to severe leptospirosis.

Lyme disease (early): Caused by *Borrelia burgorferi*; as an alternative agent.

Lymphogranuloma venereum: Caused by *C. trachomatis*; as an alternative to doxycycline.

Relapsing fever: For the treatment of tick- and louse-borne relapsing fever.

Tetanus: Caused by *Clostridium tetani*; as an alternative agent.

Administration and Dosage

➤*Adults:*

Infections – For a list of infections, refer to Indications.

Usual dosage: 250 mg every 6 hours, 333 mg every 8 hours, or 500 mg every 12 hours. Dosage may be increased up to 4 g/day, according to the severity of the infection. However, twice-a-day dosing is not recommended when doses larger than 1 g daily are administered.

Maximum dose: 4 g/day.

Acute pelvic inflammatory disease caused by N. gonorrhoeae: 500 mg erythromycin lactobionate for injection every 6 hours for 3 days, followed by 500 mg erythromycin base orally every 12 hours, or 333 mg erythromycin base orally every 8 hours for 7 days; or 250 mg orally every 6 hours for 7 days.

Intestinal amebiasis: 500 mg every 12 hours, 333 mg every 8 hours, or 250 mg every 6 hours for 10 to 14 days.

Legionnaire disease: Although optimal dosage has not been established, doses utilized in reported clinical data were 1 to 4 g daily in divided doses.

Nongonococcal urethritis caused by U. urealyticum: 500 mg 4 times a day or two 333 mg tablets every 8 hours for at least 7 days when tetracycline is contraindicated or not tolerated.

Pertussis: Although optimal dosage and duration have not been established, dosages of erythromycin utilized in reported clinical studies were 40 to 50 mg/kg/day, given in divided doses for 5 to 14 days.

Preoperative prophylaxis for elective colorectal surgery (Ery-Tab only): The following is an example of a recommended bowel preparation regimen. A proposed surgery time of 8:00 am has been used.

- *Pre-op day 3* – Minimum residue or clear liquid diet. Bisacodyl, 1 tablet orally at 6:00 pm.
- *Pre-op day 2* – Minimum residue or clear liquid diet. Magnesium sulfate, 30 mL, 50% solution (15 g) orally at 10:00 am, 2:00 pm, and 6:00 pm. Enema at 7:00 pm and 8:00 pm.
- *Pre-op day 1* – Clear liquid diet. Supplemental intravenous (IV) fluids as needed. Magnesium sulfate, 30 mL, 50% solution (15 g) orally at 10:00 am and 2:00 pm. Neomycin sulfate (1 g) and erythromycin base (two 500 mg tablets, three 333 mg tablets, or four 250 mg tablets) orally at 1:00 pm, 2:00 pm, and 11:00 pm. No enema.
- *Day of operation* – Patient evacuates rectum at 6:30 am for scheduled operation at 8:00 am.

ERYTHROMYCIN BASE — ORAL

Primary syphilis: 30 to 40 g given in divided doses over a period of 10 to 15 days.

Streptococcal infections: In the treatment of streptococcal infections of the upper respiratory tract (eg, pharyngitis, tonsillitis), administer the therapeutic dosage of erythromycin for at least 10 days.

The American Heart Association suggests a dosage of 250 mg of erythromycin orally, twice a day in long-term prophylaxis of streptococcal upper respiratory tract infections for the prevention of recurring attacks of rheumatic fever in patients allergic to penicillin and sulfonamides.

Urethral, endocervical, or rectal infections caused by C. trachomatis (uncomplicated): 500 mg 4 times a day or two 333 mg tablets every 8 hours for at least 7 days when tetracycline is contraindicated or not tolerated.

Urogenital infections during pregnancy caused by C. trachomatis: Although the optimal dose and duration of therapy have not been established, the suggested treatment is erythromycin 500 mg 4 times a day or 2 erythromycin 333 mg tablets every 8 hours on an empty stomach for at least 7 days. For women who cannot tolerate this regimen, a decreased dose of 1 erythromycin 500 mg tablet every 12 hours, one 333 mg tablet every 8 hours, or 250 mg 4 times a day should be used for at least 14 days.

Off-label dosing –

Chancroid: [1] = Good documentation. 500 mg (base) 3 times per day for 7 days.

Granuloma inguinale (donovanosis): [1] = Good documentation. 500 mg 4 times daily for at least 3 weeks. Treatment should continue until all lesions have completely healed.

➤*Children:*

Infections – For a list of infections, refer to Indications.

Usual dosage: 30 to 50 mg/kg/day, in equally divided doses. For the treatment of more severe infections, this dosage may be doubled but should not exceed 4 g/day.

Maximum dose: 4 g/day.

Conjunctivitis of the newborn caused by C. trachomatis: Oral erythromycin suspension 50 mg/kg/day in 4 divided doses for at least 2 weeks. (For erythromycin suspension, see the Erythromycin Ethylsuccinate monograph.)

Intestinal amebiasis: 30 to 50 mg/kg/day in divided doses for 10 to 14 days.

Pertussis: Although optimal dosage and duration have not been established, dosages of erythromycin utilized in reported clinical studies were 40 to 50 mg/kg/day, given in divided doses for 5 to 14 days.

Pneumonia of infancy caused by C. trachomatis: Although the optimal duration of therapy has not been established, the recommended therapy is oral erythromycin suspension 50 mg/kg/day in 4 divided doses for at least 3 weeks. (For erythromycin suspension, see the Erythromycin Ethylsuccinate monograph.)

➤*Administration:* Erythromycin base is inactivated by gastric acids; therefore, it is administered as enteric-coated tablets or capsules containing enteric-coated pellets.

In most patients, *PCE Dispertab* tablets and erythromycin delayed-release capsules are well absorbed and may be taken without regard to meals. However, optimal blood levels are obtained when they are taken on an empty stomach (at least 30 minutes and preferably 2 hours before meals).

Ery-Tab may be given without regard to meals.

Erythromycin base filmtab should be taken on an empty stomach (at least 30 minutes and preferably 2 hours before meals).

➤*Storage/Stability:* Store below 30°C (86°F). Keep tightly closed.

Protect the capsules from moisture and excessive heat.

ERYTHROMYCIN

Rx	**Erythrocin Stearate** (Abbott)	**Tablets; oral:** 250 mg	PEG. (ES). Pink. Film-coated. In 100s and 500s.
			(ET). Pink. Film-coated. In 100s.

ERYTHROMYCIN STEARATE — ORAL

For complete and comparative prescribing information, refer to the Macrolides group monograph.

Indications

➤*General information:* To reduce the development of drug-resistant bacteria and maintain the effectiveness of erythromycin and other antibacterial drugs, use erythromycin only to treat or prevent infections that are proven or strongly suspected to be caused by susceptible bacteria. When culture and susceptibility information is available, consider it in selecting or modifying antibacterial therapy. In the absence of such data, local epidemiology and susceptibility patterns may contribute to the empiric selection of therapy.

➤*Acute pelvic inflammatory disease:* Erythromycin for injection, followed by erythromycin orally, as an alternative drug for treatment of acute pelvic inflammatory disease caused by *Neisseria gonorrhoeae* in female patients with a history of sensitivity to penicillin. Patients should have a serologic test for syphilis before receiving erythromycin as treatment of gonorrhea and a follow-up serologic test for syphilis after 3 months.

➤*Diphtheria:* Infections caused by *Corynebacterium diphtheriae*, as an adjunct to antitoxin, to prevent establishment of carriers and to eradicate the organism in carriers.

➤*Erythrasma:* For the treatment of infections caused by *Corynebacterium minutissimum*.

➤*Infections caused by Chlamydia trachomatis:* Conjunctivitis of the newborn, pneumonia of infancy, and urogenital infections during pregnancy. When tetracyclines are contraindicated or not tolerated, erythromycin is indicated for the treatment of uncomplicated urethral, endocervical, or rectal infections in adults caused by *C. trachomatis*.

➤*Intestinal amebiasis:* For the treatment of intestinal amebiasis caused by *Entamoeba histolytica*. Extraenteric amebiasis requires treatment with other agents.

➤*Legionnaire disease:* For the treatment of Legionnaire disease caused by *Legionella pneumophila*. Although no controlled clinical efficacy studies have been conducted, in vitro and limited preliminary clinical data suggest that erythromycin may be effective in treating Legionnaire disease.

➤*Listeriosis:* For the treatment of listeriosis caused by *Listeria monocytogenes*.

➤*Lower respiratory tract infections:* For the treatment of lower respiratory tract infections of mild to moderate severity caused by *Streptococcus pyogenes* or *Streptococcus pneumoniae*.

➤*Nongonococcal urethritis:* For the treatment of nongonococcal urethritis caused by *Ureaplasma urealyticum* when tetracyclines are contraindicated or not tolerated.

➤*Pertussis (whooping cough):* For the treatment of pertussis caused by *Bordetella pertussis*. Erythromycin is effective in eliminating the organism from the nasopharynx of infected individuals, rendering them noninfectious. Some clinical studies suggest that erythromycin may be helpful in the prophylaxis of pertussis in exposed, susceptible individuals.

➤*Primary syphilis:* For the treatment of primary syphilis caused by *Treponema pallidum*. Erythromycin is an alternative choice of treatment for primary syphilis in patients allergic to the penicillins. For the treatment of primary syphilis, examine spinal fluid before treatment and as part of the follow-up after therapy.

➤*Prophylaxis of rheumatic fever:*

Prevention of initial attacks of rheumatic fever – Penicillin is considered by the American Heart Association (AHA) to be the drug of choice in the prevention of initial attacks of rheumatic fever (treatment of *S. pyogenes* infections of the upper respiratory tract [eg, tonsillitis, pharyngitis]). Erythromycin is indicated for the treatment of penicillin-allergic patients.

Prevention of recurrent attacks of rheumatic fever – Penicillin or sulfonamides are considered by the AHA to be the drugs of choice in the prevention of recurrent attacks of rheumatic fever. In patients who are allergic to penicillin and sulfonamides, erythromycin is recommended by the AHA in the long-term prophylaxis of streptococcal pharyngitis (for the prevention of recurrent attacks of rheumatic fever).

➤*Respiratory tract infections:* For the treatment of respiratory tract infections caused by *Mycoplasma pneumoniae*.

➤*Skin and skin structure infections:* For the treatment of skin and skin structure infections of mild tomoderate severity caused by *S. pyogenes* or *Staphylococcus aureus* (resistant staphylococci may emerge during treatment).

➤*Upper respiratory tract infections:* For the treatment of upper respiratory tract infections of mild to moderate degree caused by *S. pyogenes*, *S. pneumoniae*, or *Haemophilus influenzae* (when used concomitantly with adequate doses of sulfonamides, because many strains of *H. influenzae* are not susceptible to the erythromycin concentrations ordinarily achieved).

➤*Off-label uses:*

Granuloma inguinale (donovanosis) – [1] = Good documentation. Centers for Disease Control and Prevention guidelines recommend erythromycin as an alternative regimen for the treatment of granuloma inguinale when doxycycline is not appropriate. It is the recommended treatment for pregnant women. World Health Organization guidelines provide additional support for this recommendation.

Other possible off-label uses –

T. pallidum: For treatment of early syphilis (primary or secondary) for nonpregnant patients for whom compliance with therapy and follow-up can be ensured. For the treatment of primary syphilis, examine spinal fluid before treatment and as part of the follow-up after therapy. The use of erythromycin for the treatment of in utero syphilis is not recommended.

Lymphogranuloma venereum: Genital, inguinal, or anorectal.

Haemophilus ducreyi (chancroid): Treat until ulcers or lymph nodes are healed.

• *Other uses* – Prior to elective colorectal surgery erythromycin base with oral neomycin is a popular preoperative combination to reduce wound complications. Other uses, as alternative to penicillins, include the following: anthrax; Vincent gingivitis; erysipeloid; tetanus; actinomycosis; *Nocardia* infections (with a sulfonamide); *Eikenella corrodens* infections; *Borrelia* infections (including early Lyme disease).

ERYTHROMYCIN STEARATE — ORAL

Administration and Dosage

➤*Adults:*

Infections – For a list of infections, refer to Indications.

Usual dosage: 250 mg every 6 hours or 500 mg every 12 hours. Dosage may be increased up to 4 g/day according to the severity of the infection. However, twice-a-day dosing is not recommended when doses larger than 1 g daily are administered.

Maximum dose: 4 g/day.

Acute pelvic inflammatory disease: Erythromycin 500 mg for injection every 6 hours for 3 days, followed by 500 mg orally every 12 hours, or 333 mg orally every 8 hours, or 250 mg orally every 6 hours for 7 days. (For erythromycin 333 mg tablets, see the Erythromycin Base monograph.)

Intestinal amebiasis: 500 mg every 12 hours, 333 mg every 8 hours, or 250 mg every 6 hours for 10 to 14 days. (For erythromycin 333 mg tablets, see the Erythromycin Base monograph.)

Legionnaire disease: Although optimal dosage has not been established, dosages utilized in reported clinical data were 1 to 4 g daily in divided dosages.

Nongonococcal urethritis caused by U. urealyticum: 500 mg 4 times a day or two 333 mg tablets every 8 hours for at least 7 days when tetracycline is contraindicated or not tolerated. (For erythromycin 333 mg tablets, see the Erythromycin Base monograph.)

Pertussis: Although optimal dosage and duration have not been established, dosages of erythromycin utilized in reported clinical studies were 40 to 50 mg/kg/day given in divided doses for 5 to 14 days.

Primary syphilis: 30 to 40 g given in divided doses over a period of 10 to 15 days.

Streptococcal infections of the upper respiratory tract (eg, pharyngitis, tonsillitis): The therapeutic dosage of erythromycin should be administered for at least 10 days.

The AHA suggests a dosage of erythromycin 250 mg orally twice a day for long-term prophylaxis of streptococcal upper respiratory tract infections for the prevention of recurring attacks of rheumatic fever in patients allergic to penicillin and sulfonamides.

Urethral, endocervical, or rectal infections caused by C. trachomatis (uncomplicated): 500 mg 4 times a day or two 333 mg tablets every 8 hours for at least 7 days when tetracycline is contraindicated or not tolerated. (For erythromycin 333 mg tablets, see the Erythromycin Base monograph.)

Urogenital infections during pregnancy: Although the optimal dose and duration of therapy have not been established, the suggested treatment is erythromycin 500 mg 4 times a day or 2 erythromycin 333 mg tablets every 8 hours on an empty stomach for at least 7 days. For women who cannot tolerate this regimen, a decreased dosage of erythromycin 500 mg every 12 hours, one 333 mg tablet every 8 hours, or 250 mg 4 times a day should be used for at least 14 days. (For erythromycin 333 mg tablets, see the Erythromycin Base monograph).

Off-label dosing –

Granuloma inguinale (donovanosis): [1] = Good documentation. 500 mg 4 times daily for at least 3 weeks. Treatment should continue until all lesions have completely healed.

➤*Children:*

Infections – For a list of infections, refer to Indications.

Usual dosage: 30 to 50 mg/kg/day in equally divided doses. For more severe infections, this dosage may be doubled, but it should not exceed 4 g/day.

Maximum dose: 4 g/day.

Conjunctivitis of the newborn caused by C. trachomatis: Oral erythromycin suspension 50 mg/kg/day in 4 divided doses for at least 2 weeks. (For erythromycin suspension, see the Erythromycin Ethylsuccinate monograph.)

Intestinal amebiasis: 30 to 50 mg/kg/day in divided doses for 10 to 14 days.

Pertussis: Although optimal dosage and duration have not been established, dosages of erythromycin utilized in reported clinical studies were 40 to 50 mg/kg/day given in divided doses for 5 to 14 days.

Pneumonia of infancy caused by C. trachomatis: Although the optimal duration of therapy has not been established, the recommended therapy is oral erythromycin suspension 50 mg/kg/day in 4 divided doses for at least 3 weeks. (For erythromycin suspension, see the Erythromycin Ethylsuccinate monograph.)

➤*Administration:* Optimal serum levels of erythromycin are reached when erythromycin is taken in the fasting state or immediately before meals.

➤*Storage / Stability:* Store below 30°C (86°F).

ERYTHROMYCIN ETHYLSUCCINATE

Rx	**Erythromycin Ethylsuccinate** (Abbott)	**Tablets; oral**: 400 mg of erythromycin activity[a]	Sugar. (74 ZE). Pink, oval. In 100s and 500s.
Rx	**E.E.S. 400 Filmtab** (Abbott)		Sugar. (EE). Pink, oval. Film-coated. In 100s and 500s.
Rx	**Erythromycin Ethylsuccinate** (Abbott)	**Suspension; oral**: 200 mg of erythromycin activity[b] per 5 mL	Parabens, sucrose. Cherry flavor. In 473 mL.
Rx	**Erythromycin Ethylsuccinate** (Abbott)	**Suspension; oral**: 400 mg of erythromycin activity[a] per 5 mL	Parabens, sucrose. Cherry flavor. In 473 mL.
Rx	**E.E.S. 400 Liquid** (Abbott)		Sodium 117.5 mg (5.1 mEq) per dose. Parabens, sucrose. Orange flavor. In 100 and 473 mL bottles.
Rx	**EryPed Drops** (Abbott)	**Powder for suspension; oral**: 100 mg of erythromycin activity [c] per 2.5 mL (after reconstitution)	Sodium 58.8 mg (2.6 mEq) per dose. Sucrose. Fruit flavor. In 50 mL.
Rx	**EryPed 200** (Abbott)	**Powder for suspension; oral**: 200 mg of erythromycin activity[b] per 5 mL (after reconstitution)	Sucrose. Fruit flavor. In 100 and 200 mL.
Rx	**E.E.S. Granules** (Abbott)	**Granules for suspension ; oral**: 200 mg of erythromycin activity[b] per 5 mL (after reconstitution)	Sucrose. Cherry flavor. In 100 and 200 mL.
Rx	**EryPed 400** (Abbott)	**Powder for suspension; oral**: 400 mg of erythromycin activity[a] per 5 mL (after reconstitution)	Sucrose. Banana flavor. In 100, 200, and UD 5 mL (100s).

[a] Equivalent to 250 mg of erythromycin activity as the stearate or base.
[b] Equivalent to 125 mg of erythromycin activity as the stearate or base.
[c] Equivalent to 62.5 mg of erythromycin activity as the stearate or base.

ERYTHROMYCIN ETHYLSUCCINATE — ORAL

For complete and comparative prescribing information, refer to the Macrolides group monograph.

Indications

➤*General information:* In the treatment of infections caused by susceptible strains of the designated organisms in the following diseases:

➤*Acute pelvic inflammatory disease caused by Neisseria gonorrhoeae:* As an alternative drug in treatment of acute pelvic inflammatory disease caused by *N. gonorrhoeae* in female patients with a history of sensitivity to penicillin. Patients should have a serologic test for syphilis before receiving erythromycin as treatment of gonorrhea and a follow-up serologic test for syphilis after 3 months.

➤*Diphtheria:* Infections caused by *Corynebacterium diphtheriae*, as an adjunct to antitoxin, to prevent establishment of carriers and to eradicate the organism in carriers.

➤*Erythrasma:* In the treatment of infections caused by*Corynebacterium minutissimum*.

➤*Infections caused by Chlamydia trachomatis:* Conjunctivitis of the newborn, pneumonia of infancy, and urogenital infections during pregnancy. When tetracyclines are contraindicated or not tolerated, erythromycin is indicated for the treatment of uncomplicated urethral, endocervical, or rectal infections in adults caused by *C. trachomatis*.

➤*Intestinal amebiasis:* Intestinal amebiasis caused by *Entamoeba histolytica*. Extraenteric amebiasis requires treatment with other agents.

➤*Legionnaire disease:* Legionnaire disease caused by *Legionella pneumophila*. Although no controlled clinical efficacy studies have been conducted, in vitro and limited preliminary clinical data suggest that erythromycin may be effective in treating Legionnaire disease.

➤*Listeriosis:* Listeriosis caused by *Listeria monocytogenes*.

➤*Lower respiratory tract infections:* Lower respiratory tract infections of mild to moderate severity caused by *Streptococcus pneumoniae* or *Streptococcus pyogenes*.

➤*Nongonococcal urethritis:* When tetracyclines are contraindicated or not tolerated, erythromycin is indicated for the treatment of nongonococcal urethritis caused by *Ureaplasma urealyticum*.

➤*Pertussis (whooping cough):* Pertussis caused by *Bordetella pertussis*. Erythromycin is effective in eliminating the organism from the nasopharynx of infected individuals, rendering them noninfectious. Some clinical studies suggest that erythromycin may be helpful in the prophylaxis of pertussis in exposed susceptible individuals.

➤*Prevention of recurrent attacks of rheumatic fever:* Penicillin or sulfonamides are considered by the American Heart Association to be the drugs of choice in the prevention of recurrent attacks of rheumatic fever. In patients who are allergic to penicillin and sulfonamides, oral erythromycin is recommended by the American Heart Association in the long-term prophylaxis of streptococcal pharyngitis (for the prevention of recurrent attacks of rheumatic fever).

ERYTHROMYCIN ETHYLSUCCINATE — ORAL

➤*Primary syphilis:* Primary syphilis caused by *Treponema pallidum*. Erythromycin is an alternate choice of treatment for primary syphilis in penicillin-allergic patients. In the treatment of primary syphilis, spinal fluid examinations should be done before treatment and as part of follow-up after therapy.

➤*Prophylaxis of rheumatic fever:*

Prevention of initial attacks of rheumatic fever – Penicillin is considered by the American Heart Association to be the drug of choice in the prevention of initial attacks of rheumatic fever (treatment of *S. pyogenes* infections of the upper respiratory tract [eg, tonsillitis, pharyngitis]). Erythromycin is indicated for the treatment of penicillin-allergic patients.

➤*Respiratory tract infections:* Respiratory tract infections due to *Mycoplasma pneumoniae*.

➤*Skin and skin structure infections:* Skin and skin structure infections of mild to moderate severity caused by *S. pyogenes* or *Staphylococcus aureus* (resistant staphylococci may emerge during treatment).

➤*Upper respiratory tract infections:* Upper respiratory tract infections of mild to moderate degree caused by *S. pyogenes*, *S. pneumoniae*, or *Haemophilus influenzae* (when used concomitantly with adequate doses of sulfonamides, because many strains of *H. influenzae* are not susceptible to the erythromycin concentrations ordinarily achieved).

Administration and Dosage

➤*General dosing considerations:* For adult dosage calculation, use a ratio of 400 mg of erythromycin activity as the ethylsuccinate to 250 mg of erythromycin activity as the stearate or base.

➤*Adults:*

Infections – For a list of infections, refer to Indications.

Usual dosage: 400 mg every 6 hours. Dosage may be increased up to 4 g/day according to the severity of the infection. If twice-a-day dosage is desired, one-half of the total daily dose may be given every 12 hours. Doses also may be given 3 times daily by administering one-third of the total daily dose every 8 hours.

Maximum dose: 4 g/day.

Intestinal amebiasis: 400 mg 4 times daily for 10 to 14 days.

Legionnaire disease: Although optimal doses have not been established, doses utilized in reported clinical data were those recommended previously (1.6 to 4 g daily in divided doses).

Pertussis: Although optimal dosage and duration have not been established, dosages of erythromycin utilized in reported clinical studies were 40 to 50 mg/kg/day, given in divided doses for 5 to 14 days.

Primary syphilis: 48 to 64 g given in divided doses over a period of 10 to 15 days.

Streptococcal infections: A therapeutic dosage of erythromycin ethylsuccinate should be administered for at least 10 days. In continuous prophylaxis against recurrences of streptococcal infections in persons with a history of rheumatic heart disease, the usual dosage is 400 mg twice a day.

Urethritis caused by C. trachomatis or U. urealyticum: 800 mg 3 times a day for 7 days.

➤*Children:*

Infections – For a list of infections, refer to Indications.

Usual dosage: 30 to 50 mg/kg/day in equally divided doses every 6 hours for mild to moderate infections. For more severe infections, this dosage may be doubled. If twice-a-day dosage is desired, one-half of the total daily dose may be given every 12 hours. Doses also may be given 3 times daily by administering one-third of the total daily dose every 8 hours.

Erythromycin Ethylsuccinate Dosing in Children

Body weight	Total daily dose
< 4.5 kg (< 10 lbs)	30 to 50 mg/kg/day 15 to 25 mg/kg every 12 hours
4.5 to 6.8 kg (10 to 15 lbs)	200 mg
7.3 to 11.4 kg (16 to 25 lbs)	400 mg
11.8 to 22.7 kg (26 to 50 lbs)	800 mg
23.2 to 45.5 kg (51 to 100 lbs)	1,200 mg
> 45.5 kg (> 100 lbs)	1,600 mg

Intestinal amebiasis: 30 to 50 mg/kg/day in divided doses for 10 to 14 days.

Pertussis: Although optimal dosage and duration have not been established, dosages of erythromycin utilized in reported clinical studies were 40 to 50 mg/kg/day, given in divided doses for 5 to 14 days.

Off-label dosing –

Infections:

• *Neonates* –

Weight less than 1.2 kg: 20 mg/kg/day in divided doses twice daily.

Weight 1.2 kg or more0 to 7 days old: 20 mg/kg/day in divided doses twice daily.Older than 7 days 30 mg/kg/day in divided doses every 8 hours.

Chlamydial conjunctivitis and pneumonia:

• *Neonates* – 50 mg/kg/day in divided doses every 6 hours for 14 days.

➤*Administration:* May be administered without regard to meals. To avoid unpleasant taste, the tablets should not be chewed.

➤*Storage/Stability:*

Granules for oral suspension – Prior to mixing, store below 30°C (86°F). After mixing, refrigerate and use within 10 days.

Powder for oral suspension – Prior to mixing, store below 30°C (86°F). After reconstitution, store at or below 25°C (77°F) and use within 35 days; refrigeration is not required.

Suspension – Refrigerate to preserve taste. Refrigeration by patient is not required if used within 14 days.

Tablets – Store below 30°C (86°F).

ERYTHROMYCIN

Rx	**Erythrocin Lactobionate** (Hospira)	**Injection, lyophilized powder for solution:** 500 mg	In vials.
		1 g	In vials.

ERYTHROMYCIN LACTOBIONATE — INJECTION

For complete and comparative prescribing information, refer to the Macrolide group monograph.

Indications

➤*Acute pelvic inflammatory disease:* Intravenous (IV) erythromycin followed by oral erythromycin, as an alternative drug in the treatment of acute pelvic inflammatory disease caused by *Neisseria gonorrhoeae* in female patients with a history of sensitivity to penicillin.

Before treatment of gonorrhea, patients who are suspected of also having syphilis should have a microscopic examination for *Treponema pallidum* (by immunofluorescence or darkfield) before receiving erythromycin and monthly serologic tests for a minimum of 4 months thereafter.

➤*Diphtheria:* As an adjunct to antitoxin infections caused by *Corynebacterium diphtheriae* to prevent establishment of carriers and to eradicate the organism in carriers.

➤*Erythrasma:* In the treatment of infections caused by *Corynebacterium minutissimum*.

➤*Legionnaire disease:* Legionnaire disease caused by *Legionella pneumophilia*. Although no controlled clinical efficacy studies have been conducted, in vitro and limited preliminary clinical data suggest that erythromycin may be effective in treating Legionnaire disease.

➤*Lower respiratory tract infections:* Lower respiratory tract infections of mild to moderate severity caused by *Streptococcus pyogenes* (group A beta-hemolytic streptococci) or *Streptococcus pneumoniae* (*Diplococcus pneumoniae*).

➤*Prophylaxis of rheumatic fever:*

Prevention of initial attacks of rheumatic fever – Penicillin is considered by the American Heart Association (AHA) to be the drug of choice in the prevention of initial attacks of rheumatic fever (treatment of group A beta-hemolytic streptococcal infections of the upper respiratory tract [eg, tonsillitis, pharyngitis]). Erythromycin is indicated for the treatment of penicillin-allergic patients.

Prevention of recurrent attacks of rheumatic fever – Penicillin or sulfonamides are considered by the AHA to be the drugs of choice in the prevention of recurrent attacks of rheumatic fever. In patients who are allergic to penicillin and sulfonamides, oral erythromycin is recommended by the AHA in the long-term prophylaxis of streptococcal pharyngitis (for the prevention of recurrent attacks of rheumatic fever).

➤*Respiratory tract infections:* Respiratory tract infections caused by *Mycoplasma pneumoniae*.

➤*Skin and skin structure infections:* Skin and skin structure infections of mild to moderate severity caused by *S. pyogenes* and *Staphylococcus aureus* (resistant staphylococci may emerge during treatment).

➤*Upper respiratory tract infections:* Upper respiratory tract infections of mild to moderate degree caused by *S. pyogenes* (group A beta-hemolytic streptococci), *S. pneumoniae* (*D. pneumoniae*), or *Haemophilus influenzae* (when used concomitantly with adequate doses of sulfonamides, because many strains of *H. influenzae* are not susceptible to the erythromycin concentrations ordinarily achieved).

Administration and Dosage

➤*Adults:*

Infections – For a list of infections, refer to Indications.

ERYTHROMYCIN LACTOBIONATE — INJECTION

Usual dosage: 15 to 20 mg/kg/day given IV. Higher dosages, up to 4 g/day, may be given for severe infections.

Maximum dose: 4 g/day.

Acute pelvic inflammatory disease: 500 mg IV every 6 hours for 3 days, followed by 500 mg orally every 12 hours, 333 mg orally every 8 hours, or 250 mg orally every 6 hours for 7 days.

Legionnaire disease: Although optimal dosage has not been established, doses utilized in reported clinical data were 1 to 4 g daily in divided doses.

Streptococcal infections: In the treatment of streptococcal infections of the upper respiratory tract (eg, tonsillitis, pharyngitis), the therapeutic dosage of erythromycin should be administered for at least 10 days.

The AHA suggests a dosage of erythromycin 250 mg orally twice a day in long-term prophylaxis of streptococcal upper respiratory tract infections for the prevention of recurring attacks of rheumatic fever in patients allergic to penicillin and sulfonamides.

➤*Children:*

Infections – For a list of infections, refer to Indications.

Usual dosage: 15 to 20 mg/kg/day given IV. Higher dosages, up to 4 g/day, may be given for severe infections.

Maximum dose: 4 g/day.

➤*Preparation for administration:*

- Prepare the initial solution of erythromycin IV by adding 10 mL of sterile water for injection to the 500 mg vial or 20 mL of sterile water for injection to the 1 g vial. Use only sterile water for injection because other diluents may cause precipitation during reconstitution. Do not use diluents containing preservatives or inorganic salts. After reconstitution, each mL contains 50 mg of erythromycin activity.
- Add the initial dilution to one of the following diluents before administration to give a concentration of 1 g of erythromycin activity per liter (1 mg/mL) for continuous infusion or 1 to 5 mg/mL for intermittent infusion: sodium chloride 0.9% injection; Ringer's lactate injection; *Normosol-r*.
- The following solutions may also be used providing they are first buffered with sodium bicarbonate 4% by adding 1 mL of sodium bicarbonate 4% per 100 mL of solution: dextrose 5% injection; dextrose 5% and Ringer's lactate injection; dextrose 5% and sodium chloride 0.9% injection. Sodium bicarbonate 4% must be added to these solutions so that their pH is in the optimal range for erythromycin stability. Acidic solutions of erythromycin are unstable and lose their potency rapidly. A pH of at least 5.5 is desirable for the final diluted solution of erythromycin.

➤*Administration:* IV erythromycin must be administered by continuous or intermittent IV infusion only. Because of the irritative properties of erythromycin, IV push is an unacceptable route of administration. Continuous infusion of erythromycin is preferable because of the slower infusion rate and lower concentration of erythromycin; however, intermittent infusion at 6-hour intervals is also effective. IV erythromycin should be replaced by oral erythromycin as soon as possible.

For slow continuous infusion – The final diluted solution of erythromycin is prepared to give a concentration of 1 g/L (1 mg/mL).

For intermittent infusion – Administer one-fourth the total daily dose of erythromycin by IV infusion over 20 to 60 minutes at intervals no greater than every 6 hours. The final diluted solution of erythromycin is prepared to give a concentration of 1 to 5 mg/mL. No less than 100 mL of IV diluent should be used. Infusion should be sufficiently slow to minimize pain along the vein.

➤*Admixture compatibility:* No drug or chemical agent should be added to an erythromycin IV fluid admixture unless its effect on the chemical and physical stability of the solution has first been determined.

➤*Storage/Stability:* The initial solution is stable at refrigerator temperature for 2 weeks, or for 24 hours at room temperature. The final diluted solution of erythromycin should be completely administered within 8 hours because it is not suitable for storage. Store the vials at 20° to 25°C (68° to 77°F).

KETOLIDES

TELITHROMYCIN

Rx	**Ketek** (Sanofi-Aventis)	**Tablets; oral:** 300 mg	(38AV). Lt. orange, oval. In 20s. Film-coated
		400 mg	(H3647 400). Lt. orange, oval. In 60s. **Ketek** *Pak,* 10-tablet cards (2 tablets per blister cavity). Film-coated.

TELITHROMYCIN — ORAL

WARNING

Telithromycin is contraindicated in patients with myasthenia gravis. There have been reports of fatal and life-threatening respiratory failure in patients with myasthenia gravis associated with the use of telithromycin.

Indications

➤*Community-acquired pneumonia (CAP) (of mild to moderate severity):* Due to *Streptococcus pneumoniae* (including multidrug-resistant *S. pneumoniae* [MDRSP] isolates, including isolates known as penicillin-resistant *S. pneumoniae* [PRSP], and are isolates resistant to 2 or more of the following antibiotics: penicillin, second-generation cephalosporins [eg, cefuroxime], macrolides, tetracyclines, and trimethoprim/sulfamethoxazole), *Haemophilus influenzae, Moraxella catarrhalis, Chlamydophila pneumoniae,* or *Mycoplasma pneumoniae.*

➤*Off-label uses:*

Sinusitis (adults) – [1] = Good documentation. The use of telithromycin is recommended by evidence-based guidelines published by the American Academy of Allergy, Asthma and Immunology and the American College of Allergy, Asthma and Immunology. Results from a limited number of controlled trials have shown telithromycin to be equivalent to the initial treatment options amoxicillin/clavulanic acid and cefuroxime. Because of its once-daily dosing and possible shorter treatment duration, telithromycin treatment can provide a benefit in patients with medication compliance issues. Larger, controlled trials are needed to further evaluate the efficacy of telithromycin for treating multidrug-resistant infections.

Administration and Dosage

➤*Adults:*

Community-acquired pneumonia (mild to moderate severity) – 800 mg orally once every 24 hours for 7 to 10 days.

Off-label dosing –

Sinusitis (adults): [1] = Good documentation. 800 mg orally once daily for 5 to 14 days or for 7 days after symptom resolution.

➤*Renal function impairment:* In the presence of severe renal function impairment (creatinine clearance [CrCl] less than 30 mL/min), including patients who need dialysis, the dosage should be reduced to telithromycin 600 mg once daily.

In the presence of severe renal function impairment (CrCl less than 30 mL/min) with coexisting hepatic function impairment, the dosage should be reduced to telithromycin 400 mg once daily.

Hemodialysis – In patients undergoing hemodialysis, telithromycin should be given after the dialysis session on dialysis days.

➤*Administration:* Telithromycin can be administered with or without food.

➤*Storage/Stability:* Store at 25°C (77°F); excursions are permitted to 15° to 30°C (59° to 86°F).

Actions

➤*Pharmacology:* Telithromycin belongs to the ketolide class of antibacterials and is structurally related to the macrolide family of antibiotics. Telithromycin blocks protein synthesis by binding to domains II and V of 23S RNA of the 50S ribosomal subunit. By binding at domain II, telithromycin retains activity against gram-positive cocci (eg, *S. pneumoniae*) in the presence of resistance mediated by methylases (erythromycin resistance methylase genes) that alter the domain V binding site of telithromycin. Telithromycin may also inhibit the assembly of nascent ribosomal units.

➤*Pharmacokinetics:*

Absorption – Following oral administration, telithromycin reached maximal concentration at about 1 hour (range, 0.5 to 4 hours). It has an absolute bioavailability of 57% in both younger and elderly subjects. The rate and extent of absorption are unaffected by food intake; thus, telithromycin tablets can be given without regard to food.

In healthy adult subjects, peak plasma telithromycin concentrations of approximately 2 mcg/mL are attained at a median of 1 hour after an 800 mg oral dose. Steady-state plasma concentrations are reached within 2 to 3 days of once-daily dosing with telithromycin 800 mg. The pharmacokinetics of telithromycin after administration of single and multiple (7 days) once-daily 800 mg doses to healthy adult subjects are shown in the following table.

Telithromycin Pharmacokinetic Parameters

Parameter	Mean (SD[a]) Single dose (n = 18)	Multiple dose (n = 18)
C_{max}[a] (mcg/mL)	1.9 (0.8)	2.27 (0.71)
T_{max}[a] (h) median (min, max)[b]	1 (0.5, 4)	1 (0.5, 3)
$AUC_{(0-24)}$[a] (mcg•h/mL)	8.25 (2.6)	12.5 (5.4)
Terminal $t_{½}$[a] (h)	7.16 (1.3)	9.81 (1.9)
$C_{24\ h}$[a] (mcg/mL)	0.03 (0.013)	0.07 (0.051)

[a] C_{max} = maximum plasma concentration; SD = standard deviation; T_{max} = time to C_{max}; AUC = area under concentration vs time curve; $t_{½}$ = terminal plasma half-life; $C_{24\ h}$ = plasma concentration at 24 hours postdose.
[b] Median (min, max) values.

In a patient population, mean peak and trough plasma concentrations were 2.9 mcg/mL (± 1.55; n = 219) and 0.2 mcg/mL (± 0.22; n = 204), respectively, after 3 to 5 days of telithromycin 800 mg once daily.

TELITHROMYCIN — ORAL

Distribution – Total in vitro protein binding is approximately 60% to 70% and is primarily because of human serum albumin. Protein binding is not modified in elderly subjects or in patients with hepatic function impairment. The volume of distribution of telithromycin after intravenous infusion is 2.9 L/kg.

Telithromycin concentration in white blood cells exceeds the concentration in plasma and it is eliminated more slowly from white blood cells than from plasma. Mean white blood cell concentrations of telithromycin peaked at 72.1 mcg/mL at 6 hours, and remained at 14.1 mcg/mL 24 hours after 5 days of repeated dosing of 600 mg once daily. After 10 days of repeated dosing of 600 mg once daily, white blood cell concentrations remained at 8.9 mcg/mL 48 hours after the last dose.

Metabolism/Excretion – In total, metabolism accounts for approximately 70% of the dose. In plasma, the main circulating compound after administration of an 800 mg radiolabeled dose was parent compound, representing 56.7% of the total radioactivity. The main metabolite represented 12.6% of the AUC of telithromycin. Three other plasma metabolites were quantified, each representing 3% or less of the AUC of telithromycin. It is estimated that approximately 50% of its metabolism is mediated by CYP-450 3A4 and the remaining 50% is CYP-450 independent.

The systemically available telithromycin is eliminated by multiple pathways as follows: 7% of the dose is excreted unchanged in feces by biliary and/or intestinal secretion, 13% of the dose is excreted unchanged in urine by renal excretion, and 37% of the dose is metabolized by the liver.

Special populations –

Renal function impairment: In a multiple-dose study, 36 subjects with varying degrees of renal function impairment received telithromycin 400, 600, or 800 mg once daily for 5 days. There was a 1.4-fold increase in C_{max} in the steady state and a 1.9-fold increase in AUC from 0 to 24 hours in the steady state at 800 mg multiple doses in the severely renally impaired group (CrCl less than 30 mL/min), compared with healthy volunteers. Renal excretion may serve as a compensatory elimination pathway for telithromycin in situations in which metabolic clearance is impaired. Patients with severe renal function impairment are prone to conditions that may impair their metabolic clearance. Therefore, in the presence of severe renal function impairment (CrCl less than 30 mL/min), a reduced dosage of telithromycin is recommended.

Hepatic function impairment: An increase in renal elimination was observed in hepatically impaired patients, indicating that this pathway may compensate for some of the decrease in metabolic clearance. No dosage adjustment is recommended in cases of hepatic function impairment.

Elderly: Pharmacokinetic data show that there is a 1.4-fold increase in exposure (AUC) in 20 patients 65 years of age and older with CAP in a phase 3 study, and a 2-fold increase in exposure (AUC) in 14 subjects 65 years of age and older compared with subjects younger than 65 years of age in a phase 1 study. No dosage adjustment is required based on age alone.

Multiple insufficiency: The effects of coadministration of ketoconazole in 12 subjects (60 years of age and older) with impaired renal function were studied (CrCl, 24 to 80 mL/min). In this study, when severe renal function impairment (CrCl less than 30 mL/min; n = 2) and concomitant impairment of the CYP3A4 metabolism pathway were present, telithromycin exposure (AUC_{0-24}) was increased by approximately 4- to 5-fold, compared with the exposure in healthy subjects with healthy renal function receiving telithromycin alone. In the presence of severe renal function impairment (CrCl less than 30 mL/min) with coexisting hepatic function impairment, a reduced dosage of telithromycin is recommended.

➤*Microbiology:* Telithromycin concentrates in phagocytes, where it exhibits activity against intracellular respiratory pathogens. In vitro, telithromycin has been shown to demonstrate concentration-dependent bactericidal activity against isolates of *S. pneumoniae* (including MDRSP).

Resistance – *Staphylococcus aureus* and *Streptococcus pyogenes* with the constitutive macrolide-lincosamide-streptogramin B ($cMLS_B$) phenotype are resistant to telithromycin.

Mutants of *S. pneumoniae* derived in the laboratory by serial passage in subinhibitory concentrations of telithromycin have demonstrated resistance based on L22 riboprotein mutations (telithromycin minimum inhibitory concentrations [MICs] are elevated but still within the susceptible range), 1 of 2 reported mutations affecting the L4 riboprotein, and production of K-peptide. The clinical significance of these laboratory mutants is not known.

Microorganisms – Telithromycin has been shown to be active against most strains of the following microorganisms, both in vitro and in clinical settings.

Aerobic gram-positive microorganisms: S. pneumoniae (including multidrug-resistant isolates [MDRSP]).

Aerobic gram-negative microorganisms: H. influenzae, M. catarrhalis.

Other microorganisms: C. pneumoniae, M. pneumoniae.

Contraindications

History of hypersensitivity to telithromycin and/or any components of telithromycin tablets, or any macrolide antibiotic; coadministration with cisapride or pimozide; in patients with myasthenia gravis; previous history of hepatitis and/or jaundice associated with the use of telithromycin, or any macrolide antibiotic.

Warnings/Precautions

➤*Hepatotoxicity:* Acute hepatic failure and severe liver injury, in some cases fatal, have been reported in patients treated with telithromycin. These hepatic reactions included fulminant hepatitis and hepatic necrosis leading to liver transplant, and were observed during or immediately after treatment. In some of these cases, liver injury progressed rapidly and occurred after administration of a few doses of telithromycin. Health care providers and patients should monitor for the appearance of signs or symptoms of hepatitis, such as fatigue, malaise, anorexia, nausea, jaundice, bilirubinuria, acholic stools, liver tenderness, or hepatomegaly. Patients with signs or symptoms of hepatitis must be advised to discontinue telithromycin and immediately seek medical evaluation, which should include liver function tests. If clinical hepatitis or transaminase elevations combined with other systemic symptoms occur, permanently discontinue telithromycin.

Telithromycin must not be readministered to patients with a history of hepatitis and/or jaundice associated with the use of telithromycin tablets, or any macrolide antibiotic.

In addition, less severe hepatic dysfunction associated with increased liver enzymes, hepatitis, and, in some cases, jaundice was reported with the use of telithromycin. These events associated with less severe forms of liver toxicity were reversible.

➤*Myasthenia gravis:* Telithromycin is contraindicated in patients with myasthenia gravis. Exacerbations of myasthenia gravis have been reported in patients with myasthenia gravis treated with telithromycin. This has sometimes occurred within a few hours after intake of the first dose of telithromycin. Reports have included fatal and life-threatening acute respiratory failure with a rapid onset and progression.

➤*Cardiac effects:* Telithromycin has the potential to prolong the QTc interval of the electrocardiogram (ECG) in some patients. QTc prolongation may lead to an increased risk for ventricular arrhythmias, including torsades de pointes. Thus, avoid telithromycin use in patients with congenital prolongation of the QTc interval, and in patients with ongoing proarrhythmic conditions, such as uncorrected hypokalemia or hypomagnesemia, those with clinically significant bradycardia, and in patients receiving class IA (eg, quinidine, procainamide) or class III (eg, dofetilide) antiarrhythmic agents.

No cardiovascular morbidity or mortality attributable to QTc prolongation occurred with telithromycin treatment in 4,780 patients in clinical efficacy trials, including 204 patients who had a prolonged QTc at baseline. Cases of torsades de points have been reported in postmarketing with telithromycin.

➤*Visual disturbances:* Telithromycin may cause visual disturbances, particularly in slowing the ability to accommodate and the ability to release accommodation. Visual disturbances included blurred vision, difficulty focusing, and diplopia. Most events were mild to moderate; however, severe cases have been reported.

➤*Loss of consciousness:* There have been postmarketing adverse reaction reports of transient loss of consciousness, including some cases associated with vagal syndrome.

➤*Clostridium difficile– associated diarrhea (CDAD):* CDAD has been reported with nearly all antibacterial agents, including telithromycin, and may range in severity from mild diarrhea to fatal colitis. Treatment with antibacterial agents alters the normal flora of the colon leading to overgrowth of *C. difficile*. *C. difficile* produces toxins A and B, which contribute to the development of CDAD. Hypertoxin-producing strains of *C. difficile* cause increased morbidity and mortality, as these infections can be refractory to antimicrobial therapy and may require colectomy. CDAD must be considered in all patients who present with diarrhea following antibiotic use. Careful medical history is necessary because CDAD has been reported to occur over 2 months after the administration of antibacterial agents.

If CDAD is suspected or confirmed, ongoing antibiotic use not directed against *C. difficile* may need to be discontinued. Institute appropriate fluid and electrolyte management, protein supplementation, antibiotic treatment of *C. difficile*, and surgical evaluation as clinically indicated.

➤*Renal/Hepatic function impairment:* Telithromycin is principally excreted via the liver and kidney. In the presence of severe renal function impairment (CrCl less than 30 mL/min), a reduced dosage of telithromycin is recommended. Telithromycin may be administered without dosage adjustment in the presence of hepatic function impairment.

➤*Hazardous tasks:* Because of potential visual difficulties or loss of consciousness, advise patients to minimize activities, such as driving a motor vehicle, operating heavy machinery, or engaging in other hazardous activities during treatment with telithromycin. If patients experience visual disorders or loss of consciousness while taking telithromycin, advise patients not to drive a motor vehicle, operate heavy machinery, or engage in other hazardous activities.

➤*Superinfection:* Prescribing telithromycin in the absence of a proven or strongly suspected bacterial infection or a prophylactic indication is unlikely to provide benefit to the patient and increases the risk of the development of drug-resistant bacteria.

➤*Pregnancy: Category C.* At doses higher than the 900 and 240 mg/m² in rats and rabbits, respectively, maternal toxicity may have resulted in delayed fetal maturation.

There are no adequate and well-controlled studies in pregnant women. Use telithromycin during pregnancy only if the potential benefit justifies the potential risk to the fetus.

➤*Lactation:* Telithromycin is excreted in breast milk of rats. Telithromycin may also be excreted in human milk. Because many drugs are excreted in human milk, exercise caution when telithromycin is administered to a breast-feeding mother.

➤*Children:* The safety and efficacy of telithromycin in children have not been established.

➤*Elderly:* Efficacy and safety in elderly patients 65 years of age and older were generally similar to those observed in younger patients; however, greater sensitivity of some older individuals cannot be ruled out. No dosage adjustment is required based on age alone.

TELITHROMYCIN — ORAL

➤*Monitoring:* Monitor for the appearance of signs or symptoms of hepatitis, such as fatigue, malaise, anorexia, nausea, jaundice, bilirubinuria, acholic stools, liver tenderness, or hepatomegaly.

Drug Interactions

➤*QT prolongation:* An additive effect of telithromycin with other drugs that prolong the QT interval cannot be excluded. The following drugs may prolong the QT interval and increase the risk of life-threatening cardiac arrhythmias, including torsades de pointes: Antiarrhythmic agents (eg, amiodarone, bretylium, disopyramide, dofetilide, procainamide, quinidine, and sotalol), arsenic trioxide, chlorpromazine, cisapride, dolasetron, droperidol, mefloquine, mesoridazine, moxifloxacin, pentamidine, pimozide, tacrolimus, thioridazine, and ziprasidone. For a more complete list of drugs that may prolong the QT interval, see the appendix, Drug-Induced Prolongation of the QT Interval and Torsades de Pointes.

Telithromycin Drug Interactions

Precipitant drug	Object drug[a]		Description
Azole antifungals (eg, itraconazole, ketoconazole)	Telithromycin	↑	Coadministration with itraconazole resulted in an increase in telithromycin C_{max} and AUC of 22% and 54%, respectively. Coadministration with ketoconazole resulted in an increase in telithromycin C_{max} and AUC of 51% and 95%, respectively.
CYP3A4 inducers (eg, carbamazepine, phenobarbital, phenytoin, rifampin)	Telithromycin	↓	Coadministration with CYP3A4 inducers (eg, carbamazepine, phenobarbital, phenytoin) is likely to result in subtherapeutic levels of telithromycin and loss of effect. Avoid coadministration of telithromycin and rifampin.
Telithromycin	Antiarrhythmic agents (eg, amiodarone, bretylium, disopyramide, dofetilide, procainamide, quinidine, sotalol)	↑	The risk of life-threatening cardiac arrhythmias, including torsades de pointes, may be increased. Avoid coadministration with class IA and class III antiarrhythmic agents.
Telithromycin	Benzodiazepines (eg, midazolam)	↑	Coadministration resulted in an increase in midazolam AUC. Monitor closely and adjust midazolam dose as needed. Use with caution with other benzodiazepines that are metabolized by CYP3A4 and undergo a high first-pass effect (eg, triazolam).
Telithromycin	Carbamazepine, cyclosporine, hexobarbital, phenytoin, sirolimus, tacrolimus	↑	Elevation of serum levels of these drugs may be observed when coadministered with telithromycin. Increases or prolongation of the therapeutic and/or adverse reactions of the concomitant drug may be observed.
Telithromycin	Cisapride	↑	Coadministration resulted in a 95% increase in cisapride peak plasma concentrations, resulting in significant increases in QTc interval. Coadministration is contraindicated.
Telithromycin	Colchicine	↑	Increased serum colchicine concentrations with toxicity may occur.
Telithromycin	CYP3A4 inhibitors (eg, buspirone, cabergoline, ranolazine, repaglinide)	↑	Coadministration with CYP3A4 inhibitors is likely to increase plasma concentrations, increasing the pharmacologic and adverse reactions.
Telithromycin	Digoxin	↑	Coadministration resulted in a 73% and 21% increase in digoxin plasma peak and trough levels, respectively. Monitor digoxin levels and adverse reactions during use with telithromycin therapy.
Telithromycin	Ergot alkaloids	↑	Acute ergot toxicity characterized by severe peripheral vasospasm and dysesthesia has occurred when an ergot alkaloid was given with a macrolide. Without further data, the coadministration of telithromycin and ergot alkaloids is not recommended.
Telithromycin	HMG-CoA reductase inhibitors (eg, atorvastatin, lovastatin, simvastatin)	↑	Coadministration resulted in a 5.3- and 8.9-fold increase in simvastatin C_{max} and AUC, respectively. Avoid concurrent use of telithromycin with atorvastatin, lovastatin, or simvastatin.
Telithromycin	Metoprolol	↑	Coadministration resulted in an approximate 38% increase in metoprolol C_{max} and AUC; however, there was no effect on metoprolol elimination half-life. Coadminister with caution in heart failure patients.
Telithromycin	Oral anticoagulants (eg, warfarin)	↑	The anticoagulant effect of oral anticoagulants may be increased. Hemorrhage has occurred. Monitor prothrombin time/international normalized ratio when coadministering.
Telithromycin	Oral contraceptives	↑	When oral contraceptives containing ethinyl estradiol and levonorgestrel were coadministered with telithromycin, the steady-state AUC of ethinyl estradiol did not change but the steady-state AUC of levonorgestrel was increased 50%.
Telithromycin	Pimozide	↑	Coadministration may lead to increased pimozide plasma levels. Coadministration is contraindicated.
Telithromycin	Sotalol	↓	Coadministration resulted in a decrease in sotalol C_{max} and AUC of 34% and 20%, respectively.
Telithromycin	Theophylline	↑	Coadministration resulted in an approximate 16% and 17% increase in theophylline C_{max} and AUC, respectively. Coadministration may worsen GI effects, such as nausea and vomiting. Take telithromycin and theophylline 1 hour apart to decrease the risk of GI side effects.
Telithromycin	Verapamil	↑	Increased risk of cardiotoxicity. Closely monitor cardiac function.

[a] ↑ = object drug increased; ↓ = object drug decreased.

Adverse Reactions

In phase 3 clinical trials, 4,780 patients (n = 2,702 in controlled trials) received daily oral doses of telithromycin 800 mg once daily for 5 days or 7 to 10 days. Most adverse reactions were mild to moderate in severity. In the combined phase 3 studies, discontinuation because of treatment-emergent adverse reactions occurred in 4.4% of telithromycin-treated patients and 4.3% of combined comparator-treated patients. Most discontinuations in the telithromycin group were because of treatment-emergent adverse reactions in the GI body system, primarily diarrhea (0.9% for telithromycin vs 0.7% for comparators) and nausea (0.7% for telithromycin vs 0.5% for comparators).

Telithromycin Adverse Reactions (≥2%)

Adverse reaction[a]	All treatment-emergent adverse reactions		Possibly related treatment-emergent adverse reactions	
	Telithromycin (n = 2,702)	Comparator[b] (n = 2,139)	Telithromycin (n = 2,702)	Comparator[b] (n = 2,139)
CNS				
Dizziness (excluding vertigo)	3.7%	2.7%	2.8%	1.5%
Headache	5.5%	5.8%	2%	2.5%
GI				
Diarrhea	10.8%	8.6%	10%	8%
Dysgeusia	1.6%	3.6%	1.5%	3.6%

TELITHROMYCIN — ORAL

Telithromycin Adverse Reactions (≥2%)				
	All treatment-emergent adverse reactions		Possibly related treatment-emergent adverse reactions	
Adverse reaction[a]	Telithromycin (n = 2,702)	Comparator[b] (n = 2,139)	Telithromycin (n = 2,702)	Comparator[b] (n = 2,139)
Loose stools	2.3%	1.5%	2.1%	1.4%
Nausea	7.9%	4.6%	7%	4.1%
Vomiting	2.9%	2.2%	2.4%	1.4%

[a] Based on a frequency of all and possibly related treatment-emergent adverse reactions of 2% or more in telithromycin or comparator groups.
[b] Includes comparators from all controlled phase 3 studies.

➤*Adverse reactions (at least 0.2% and less than 2%):*

CNS – Dry mouth, fatigue, increased sweating, insomnia, somnolence, vertigo.

Dermatologic – Rash.

GI – Abdominal distension, abdominal pain, anorexia, constipation, dyspepsia, flatulence, gastritis, gastroenteritis, GI upset, glossitis, oral candidiasis, stomatitis, upper abdominal pain, watery stools.

GU – Vaginal candidiasis, vaginitis, vaginosis fungal.

Hematologic – Increased platelet count.

Hepatic – Hepatitis, with or without jaundice, occurred in 0.07% of patients treated with telithromycin and was reversible.

Lab test abnormalities – Abnormal liver function tests including the following: increased liver enzymes (eg, ALT, AST) and increased transaminases were usually asymptomatic and reversible; ALT elevations above 3 times the upper limit of normal were observed in 1.6% and 1.7% of patients treated with telithromycin and comparators, respectively.

Special senses – Visual adverse reactions most often included blurred vision, diplopia, or difficulty focusing. Most reactions were mild to moderate; however, severe cases have been reported. Some patients discontinued therapy because of these adverse reactions. Visual adverse reactions were reported as having occurred after any dose during treatment, but most visual adverse reactions (65%) occurred following the first or second dose. Visual events lasted several hours and recurred upon subsequent dosing in some patients. For patients who continued treatment, some resolved on therapy while others continued to have symptoms until they completed the full course of treatment.

Women and patients younger than 40 years of age experienced a higher incidence of telithromycin-associated visual adverse reactions.

➤*Adverse reactions (less than 0.2%):* Other possibly related clinically relevant reactions occurring in less than 0.2% of patients treated with telithromycin from the controlled phase 3 studies included anxiety, bradycardia, eczema, elevated blood bilirubin, erythema multiforme, flushing, hypotension, increased blood alkaline phosphatase, increased eosinophil count, paresthesia, pruritus, and urticaria.

➤*Postmarketing:*

Cardiovascular – Atrial arrhythmias, palpitations.

CNS – Loss of consciousness, in some cases associated with vaginal syndrome.

GI – Pancreatitis.

Hepatic – Severe and, in some cases, fatal hepatotoxicity, including fulminant hepatitis, hepatic necrosis, and hepatic failure, have been reported in some patients treated with telithromycin. These hepatic reactions were observed during or immediately after treatment. In some cases, liver injury progressed rapidly and occurred after administration of only a few doses of telithromycin. Severe reactions, in some cases but not all cases, have been associated with serious underlying diseases or concomitant medications.

Data from postmarketing reports and clinical trials show that most cases of hepatic function impairment were mild to moderate.

Hypersensitivity – Face edema, rare reports of severe allergic reactions, including angioedema and anaphylaxis.

Musculoskeletal – Muscle cramps, rare reports of exacerbation of myasthenia gravis.

Overdosage

➤*Treatment:* In the event of acute overdosage, empty the stomach by gastric lavage. Carefully monitor the patient (eg, ECG, electrolytes) and give symptomatic and supportive treatment. Maintain adequate hydration. The efficacy of hemodialysis in an overdose situation with telithromycin is unknown.

Patient Information

Inform patients that telithromycin may cause problems with vision, particularly when looking quickly between objects nearby and objects far away. These reactions include blurred vision, difficulty focusing, and objects looking doubled. Most events were mild to moderate; however, severe cases have been reported. Problems with vision were reported as having occurred after any dose during treatment, but most occurred following the first or second dose. These problems lasted several hours and, in some patients, came back with the next dose.

Advise patients that avoiding quick changes in viewing between objects in the distance and objects nearby may help to decrease the effects of these visual difficulties.

Because of potential visual difficulties or loss of consciousness, advise patients to minimize activities such as driving a motor vehicle, operating heavy machinery, or engaging in otherwise hazardous activities during treatment with telithromycin.

If patients experience visual difficulties, loss of consciousness, or fainting, advise them to avoid driving a motor vehicle, operating heavy machinery, or engaging in otherwise hazardous activities, and to seek advice from their health care provider before taking another dose.

Advise patients:

- of the possibility of liver injury associated with telithromycin, which in rare cases may be severe. Instruct patients that if they develop signs or symptoms of liver injury to discontinue telithromycin and seek medical attention immediately. Symptoms of liver injury may include nausea, fatigue, anorexia, jaundice, dark urine, light-colored stools, pruritus, or tender abdomen. Telithromycin must not be taken by patients with a previous history of hepatitis/jaundice associated with the use of telithromycin or macrolide antibiotics.
- that diarrhea is a common problem caused by antibiotics, which usually ends when the antibiotic is discontinued. Sometimes after starting treatment with antibiotics, patients can develop watery and bloody stools (with or without stomach cramps and fever) even as late as 2 or more months after having taken the last dose of the antibiotic. If this occurs, advise patients to contact their health care provider as soon as possible.
- that antibacterial drugs, including telithromycin, should only be used to treat bacterial infections. They do not treat viral infections (eg, the common cold). When telithromycin is prescribed to treat a bacterial infection, tell patients that although it is common to feel better early in the course of therapy, take the medication exactly as directed. Skipping doses or not completing the full course of therapy may (1) decrease the efficacy of the immediate treatment, and (2) increase the likelihood that bacteria will develop resistance and will not be treatable by telithromycin or other antibacterial drugs in the future.
- that telithromycin has the potential to produce changes in the ECG (QTc interval prolongation), and to report any fainting occurring during drug treatment.
- to avoid taking telithromycin if receiving class 1A (eg, quinidine, procainamide) or class 3 (eg, dofetilide) antiarrhythmic agents.
- to inform their health care provider of any personal or family history of QTc prolongation or proarrhythmic conditions such as uncorrected hypokalemia, or clinically significant bradycardia.
- that telithromycin is contraindicated in patients with myasthenia gravis. Advise patients to inform their health care provider if they have myasthenia gravis.
- to avoid simvastatin, lovastatin, or atorvastatin if receiving telithromycin. If telithromycin is prescribed, stop therapy with simvastatin, lovastatin, or atorvastatin during the course of treatment.
- that telithromycin tablets can be taken with or without food.
- to inform their health care provider of any other medications taken concurrently with telithromycin, including over-the-counter medications and dietary supplements.

QUINUPRISTIN/DALFOPRISTIN

Rx	**Synercid** (Monarch)	**Injection, lyophilized**: 500 mg (150 mg quinupristin; 350 mg dalfopristin)/10 mL	In 10 mL vials.

QUINUPRISTIN/DALFOPRISTIN — INJECTION

WARNING

One of quinupristin/dalfopristin's approved indications is for the treatment of patients with serious or life-threatening infections associated with vancomycin-resistant *Enterococcus faecium* (VREF) bacteremia. Quinupristin/dalfopristin has been approved for marketing in the US for this indication under the FDA's accelerated approval regulations that allow marketing of products for use in life-threatening conditions when other therapies are not available. Approval of drugs for marketing under these regulations is based upon a demonstrated effect on a surrogate endpoint that is likely to predict clinical benefit.

Approval of this indication is based upon quinupristin/dalfopristin's ability to clear VREF from the bloodstream with clearance of bacteremia considered to be a surrogate end point. No results from well-controlled clinical studies confirm the validity of this surrogate marker. However, a study to verify the clinical benefit of therapy with quinupristin/dalfopristin on traditional clinical endpoints (such as cure of the underlying infection) is presently underway.

Indications

➤*Life-threatening infections:* Treatment of patients with serious or life-threatening infections associated with vancomycin-resistant *Enterococcus faecium* (VREF) bacteremia.

➤*Complicated skin and skin structure infections:* Caused by *Staphylococcus aureus* (methicillin-susceptible) or *Streptococcus pyogenes*.

➤*Off-label uses:*

Infective endocarditis – Quinupristin/dalfopristin may be used to treat native or prosthetic valve endocarditis due to *E. faecium* infections that are resistant to penicillin, aminoglycosides, and vancomycin.

Infective endocarditis (adults): [1] = Good documentation.

Infective endocarditis (children/adolescents): [1] = Good documentation.

Administration and Dosage

➤*Adults:*

Complicated skin and skin structure infections – 7.5 mg/kg IV every 12 hours.

Vancomycin-resistant Enterococcus faecium – 7.5 mg/kg IV every 8 hours.

Off-label dosing –

Infective endocarditis (adults): [1] = Good documentation. 22.5 mg/kg IV in 3 divided doses daily for at least 8 weeks.

➤*Children:* See Adults for dosing for children 16 years of age and older.

Younger than 16 years of age – A dosage of 7.5 mg/kg IV every 8 or 12 hours has been used in a limited number of children under emergency-use conditions. However, the safety and efficacy in patients younger than 16 years of age have not been established.

Off-label dosing –

Infective endocarditis (children/adolescents): [1] = Good documentation. 22.5 mg/kg IV in 3 divided doses daily for at least 8 weeks.

➤*Concomitant therapy:* If quinupristin/dalfopristin is to be given concomitantly with another drug, give each drug separately in accordance with the recommended dosage and route of administration for each drug.

➤*Duration of therapy:* The minimum recommended treatment duration for complicated skin and skin structure infections is 7 days. For vancomycin-resistant *E. faecium* infection, base treatment duration on the site and severity of the infection.

➤*Preparation for administration:* Reconstitute the single-dose vial by slowly adding 5 ml of dextrose 5% in water or sterile water for injection. Gently swirl the vial by manual rotation without shaking to ensure dissolution of contents while limiting foam formation. Allow the solution to sit for a few minutes until all the foam has disappeared. The resulting solution should be clear. Vials reconstituted in this manner will give a solution of 100 mg/mL. Caution: further dilution required before infusion.

According to the patient's weight, add the reconstituted solution to 250 mL of dextrose 5% solution (approximately 2 mg/ml). An infusion volume of 100 mL may be used for central line infusions.

➤*Administration:* Administer by IV infusion in dextrose 5% in water solution over a 60-minute period. An infusion pump or device may be used to control the rate of infusion. If necessary, central venous access (eg, peripherally inserted central catheter [PICC]) can be used to administer quinupristin/dalfopristin to decrease the incidence of venous irritation. If moderate to severe venous irritation occurs following peripheral administration of quinupristin/dalfopristin diluted in 250 mL of dextrose 5% in water, consider increasing the infusion volume to 500 or 750 mL, changing the infusion site, or infusing by a PICC or a central venous catheter.

Following completion of a peripheral infusion, flush the vein with dextrose 5% in water solution to minimize venous irritation. Do not flush with saline or heparin because of incompatibility concerns.

With intermittent infusion of quinupristin/dalfopristin and other drugs through a common IV line, flush the line before and after administration with dextrose 5% in water solution.

➤*Admixture compatibility:*

Compatibility – The following table lists compatibility by Y-site injection.

Y-Site Injection Compatibility of Quinupristin/Dalfopristin at 2 mg/mL Concentration

Admixture and concentration	IV infusion solutions for admixture
Aztreonam 20 mg/mL	D5W[a]
Ciprofloxacin 1 mg/mL	D5W
Fluconazole 2 mg/mL	Used as the undiluted solution
Haloperidol 0.2 mg/mL	D5W
Metoclopramide 5 mg/mL	D5W
Potassium chloride 40 mEq/L	D5W

[a] D5W = dextrose 5% injection.

Incompatibility – Do not dilute with saline solutions because quinupristin/dalfopristin is not compatible with these agents. Do not mix quinupristin/dalfopristin with or physically add to other drugs except for the drugs listed previously in Compatibility.

➤*Storage/Stability:*

Before reconstitution – Refrigerate the unopened vials at 2° to 8°C (36° to 46°F).

Reconstituted and infusion solutions – Because quinupristin/dalfopristin contains no antibacterial preservative, reconstitute under strict aseptic conditions (eg, Laminar Air Flow Hood). Dilute the reconstituted solution within 30 minutes. Vials are for single use. The storage time of the diluted solution should be as short as possible to minimize the risk of microbial contamination. Stability of the diluted solution prior to the infusion is established as 5 hours at room temperature or 54 hours if refrigerated 2° to 8°C (36° to 46°F). Do not freeze the solution.

Actions

➤*Pharmacology:* Quinupristin/dalfopristin, a streptogramin antibacterial agent for IV administration, is a sterile, lyophilized formulation of 2 semisynthetic pristinamycin derivatives, quinupristin (derived from pristinamycin I) and dalfopristin (derived from pristinamycin IIA).

The streptogramin components of quinupristin/dalfopristin are present in a ratio of 30 parts quinupristin to 70 parts dalfopristin. These 2 components act synergistically so that quinupristin/dalfopristin's microbiologic in vitro activity is greater than that of the components individually. Quinupristin's and dalfopristin's metabolites also contribute to the antimicrobial activity of quinupristin/dalfopristin. In vitro synergism of the major metabolites with the complementary parent compound has been demonstrated.

Quinupristin/dalfopristin is bacteriostatic against *E. faecium* and bactericidal against strains of methicillin-susceptible and methicillin-resistant staphylococci.

The site of action of quinupristin and dalfopristin is the bacterial ribosome. Dalfopristin inhibits the early phase of protein synthesis while quinupristin inhibits the late phase of protein synthesis.

Resistance – In non-comparative studies, emerging resistance to quinupristin/dalfopristin during treatment of VREF infections occurred. Resistance to quinupristin/dalfopristin is associated with resistance to both components.

➤*Pharmacokinetics:* Pharmacokinetic profiles of quinupristin and dalfopristin in combination with their metabolites were determined using a bioassay following multiple 60-minute infusions in 2 groups of healthy young adult male volunteers. Each group received 7.5 mg/kg of quinupristin/dalfopristin IV every 12 hours or every 8 hours for a total of 9 or 10 doses, respectively. The pharmacokinetic parameters were proportional with every-12-hour and every-8-hour dosing: Those of the every-8-hour regimen are shown in the following table.

Mean Steady-State Pharmacokinetic Parameters of Quinupristin and Dalfopristin in Combination with Their Metabolites (Dose = 7.5 mg/kg every 8 h; n = 10)

	C_{max} (mcg/mL)	AUC (mcg•h/mL)	$t_{1/2}$ (h)
Quinupristin and metabolites	3.2	7.2	3.07
Dalfopristin and metabolite	7.96	10.57	1.04

Obesity (body mass index at least 30) – In obese patients, the C_{max} and AUC of quinupristin increased approximately 30% and those of dalfopristin approximately 40%.

Distribution – The clearances of unchanged quinupristin and dalfopristin are similar (0.72 L/h/kg), and the steady-state volume of distribution is 0.45 and 0.24 L/kg, respectively. The protein binding is moderate.

Penetration of unchanged quinupristin and dalfopristin in noninflammatory blister fluid corresponds to approximately 19% and 11%, respectively, of that

QUINUPRISTIN/DALFOPRISTIN — INJECTION

estimated in plasma. The penetration into blister fluid of quinupristin and dalfopristin in combination with their major metabolites was in total approximately 40% compared with that in plasma.

Metabolism – Quinupristin and dalfopristin are the main active components circulating in the plasma. They are converted to several active major metabolites: 2 conjugated metabolites for quinupristin (1 with glutathione and 1 with cysteine) and 1 non-conjugated metabolite for dalfopristin (formed by drug hydrolysis).

In vitro, the transformation of the parent drugs into their major active metabolites occurs by non-enzymatic reactions and is not dependent on cytochrome-P450 or glutathione-transferase enzyme activities. Quinupristin/dalfopristin is a major inhibitor of the activity of cytochrome P450 3A4 isoenzyme. Quinupristin/dalfopristin can interfere with the metabolism of other drug products that are associated with QTc prolongation. However, electrophysiologic studies confirm that quinupristin/dalfopristin does not itself induce QTc prolongation.

Excretion – The elimination half-life of quinupristin and dalfopristin is approximately 0.85 and 0.7 hours, respectively.

Fecal excretion constitutes the main elimination route for both parent drugs and their metabolites (75% to 77% of dose). Urinary excretion accounts for approximately 15% of the quinupristin dose and 19% of the dalfopristin dose. Preclinical data in rats demonstrated that approximately 80% of the dose is excreted in the bile and suggest that in humans, biliary excretion is probably the principal route for fecal elimination.

Special populations –

Renal function impairment: In patients with creatinine clearance 6 to 28 mL/min, the AUC of quinupristin and dalfopristin in combination with their major metabolites increased approximately 40% and 30%, respectively.

In patients undergoing continuous ambulatory peritoneal dialysis, dialysis clearance for quinupristin, dalfopristin, and their metabolites is negligible. The plasma AUC of unchanged quinupristin and dalfopristin increased approximately 20% and 30%, respectively. Because of the high molecular weight of both components, it is unlikely to be removed by hemodialysis.

Hepatic function impairment: In patients with hepatic dysfunction (Child-Pugh scores A and B), the terminal half-life of quinupristin and dalfopristin was not modified. However, the AUC of quinupristin and dalfopristin in combination with their major metabolites increased ≈ 180% and 50%, respectively (see Administration and Dosage).

➤*Microbiology:* Quinupristin/dalfopristin is active against most strains of the following microorganisms both in vitro and in clinical infections.

Aerobic gram-positive microorganisms – *Enterococcus faecium* (vancomycin-resistant and multi-drug resistant strains only); *Staphylococcus aureus* (methicillin-susceptible strains); *Streptococcus pyogenes*.

Note: Quinupristin/dalfopristin is not active against *Enterococcus faecalis*. Differentiation of enterococcal species is important to avoid misidentification of *E. faecalis* as *E. faecium*.

Contraindications

Hypersensitivity to quinupristin/dalfopristin or prior hypersensitivity to other streptogramins (eg, pristinamycin, virginiamycin).

Warnings/Precautions

➤*Pseudomembranous colitis:* Pseudomembranous colitis has been reported with nearly all antibacterial agents, including quinupristin/dalfopristin, and may range in severity from mild to life-threatening. Therefore, consider this diagnosis in patients who present with diarrhea subsequent to the administration of antibacterial agents. After the diagnosis of pseudomembranous colitis has been established, initiate therapeutic measures. Mild cases usually respond to drug discontinuation alone. In moderate-to-severe cases, consider managing with fluids and electrolytes, protein supplementation, and treatment with an antibacterial drug clinically effective against *C. difficile* colitis.

➤*Venous irritation:* Following completion of a peripheral infusion, flush the vein with 5% Dextrose in Water solution to minimize venous irritation. Do not flush with saline or heparin after quinupristin/dalfopristin administration because of incompatibility concerns. If moderate-to-severe venous irritation occurs following peripheral administration of quinupristin/dalfopristin diluted in 250 mL of Dextrose 5% in Water, consider increasing the infusion volume to 500 or 750 mL, changing the infusion site, or infusing by a peripherally inserted central catheter (PICC) or a central venous catheter. In clinical trials, concomitant administration of hydrocortisone or diphenhydramine did not appear to alleviate venous pain or inflammation.

➤*Rate of infusion:* In animal studies, toxicity was higher when quinupristin/dalfopristin was administered as a bolus compared with slow infusion. However, the safety of an IV bolus has not been studied in humans. Clinical trial experience has been exclusively with an IV duration of 60 minutes and, thus, other infusion rates cannot be recommended.

➤*Arthralgias/Myalgias:* Episodes of arthralgia and myalgia, some severe, have been reported in patients treated with quinupristin/dalfopristin. In some patients, improvement has been noted with a reduction in dose frequency to every 12 hours. In those patients available for follow-up, symptoms resolved following discontinuation of treatment. The etiology of these myalgias and arthralgias is under investigation.

➤*Hyperbilirubinemia:* Elevations of total bilirubin more than 5 times the upper limit of normal were noted in approximately 25% of patients in the noncomparative studies. In some patients, isolated hyperbilirubinemia (primarily conjugated) can occur during treatment, possibly resulting from competition between quinupristin/dalfopristin and bilirubin for excretion. In the comparative trials, elevations in ALT and AST occurred at a similar frequency in both the quinupristin/dalfopristin and comparator groups.

➤*Hepatic function impairment:* Following a single 1-hour infusion of quinupristin/dalfopristin (7.5 mg/kg) to patients with hepatic insufficiency, plasma concentrations were significantly increased. However, the effect of dose reduction or increase in dosing interval on the pharmacokinetics of quinupristin/dalfopristin in these patients has not been studied. Therefore, no recommendations can be made at this time regarding the appropriate dose modification.

➤*Superinfection:* Use of antibiotics (especially prolonged or repeated therapy) may result in bacterial or fungal overgrowth of nonsusceptible organisms. Such overgrowth may lead to a secondary infection. Appropriate measures should be taken if superinfection occurs.

➤*Pregnancy:* Category B. There are no adequate and well-controlled studies in pregnant women. Use during pregnancy only if clearly needed.

➤*Lactation:* In lactating rats, quinupristin/dalfopristin was excreted in milk. It is not known whether quinupristin/dalfopristin is excreted in human breast milk. Exercise caution when administering to a breastfeeding woman.

➤*Children:* Quinupristin/dalfopristin has been used in a limited number of pediatric patients under emergency-use conditions at a dose of 7.5 mg/kg every 8 or 12 hours. However, the safety and efficacy in patients younger than 16 years of age have not been established.

Drug Interactions

➤*Cytochrome P450 3A4 inhibition:* It is reasonable to expect that the concomitant administration of quinupristin/dalfopristin and other drugs primarily metabolized by the cytochrome P450 3A4 enzyme system may result in increased plasma concentrations of these drugs that could increase or prolong their therapeutic effect or increase adverse reactions (see the following table). Therefore, coadministration with drugs that are cytochrome P450 3A4 substrates and possess a narrow therapeutic window requires caution and monitoring of these drugs whenever possible. Avoid concomitant medications metabolized by the cytochrome P450 3A4 enzyme system that may prolong the QTc interval.

Cyclosporine – Twenty-four subjects given quinupristin/dalfopristin 7.5 mg/kg every 8 hours for 2 days and 300 mg of cyclosporine on day 3 showed an increase of 63% in the AUC of cyclosporine, a 30% increase in C_{max}, a 77% increase in the half-life, and a 34% decrease in clearance. Perform therapeutic level monitoring of cyclosporine when cyclosporine must be used concomitantly with quinupristin/dalfopristin.

Nifedipine/Midazolam – Coadministration of quinupristin/dalfopristin and nifedipine (repeated oral doses) and midazolam (IV bolus dose) in healthy volunteers led to elevated plasma concentrations of these drugs. The C_{max} increased by 18% and 14% (median values) and the AUC increased by 44% and 33% for nifedipine and midazolam, respectively.

Selected Drugs That are Predicted to Have Plasma Concentrations Increased by Quinupristin/Dalfopristin[a]
Anti-HIV (NNRTIs and protease inhibitors): Delavirdine, nevirapine, indinavir, ritonavir
Antineoplastic agents: Vinca alkaloids (eg, vinblastine), docetaxel, paclitaxel
Benzodiazepines: Midazolam, diazepam
Calcium channel blockers: Dihydropyridines (eg, nifedipine), verapamil, diltiazem
Cholesterol-lowering agents: HMG-CoA reductase inhibitors
GI motility agents: Cisapride
Immunosuppressive agents: Cyclosporine, tacrolimus
Steroids: Methylprednisolone
Other: Carbamazepine, quinidine, lidocaine, disopyramide

[a] This list of drugs is not all inclusive.

Adverse Reactions

➤*Comparative trials:* Safety data are available from 5 comparative clinical studies (n = 1,099 quinupristin/dalfopristin; n = 1,095 comparator). One of the deaths in the comparative studies was assessed as possibly related to quinupristin/dalfopristin. The most frequent reasons for discontinuation because of drug-related adverse reactions were as follows:

Patients Discontinuing Quinupristin/Dalfopristin Therapy (%): All Comparative Studies		
Type	Quinupristin/Dalfopristin (n = 1099)	Comparator (n = 1095)
Venous	9.2	2
Non-venous	9.6	4.3
Rash	1	0.5
Nausea	0.9	0.6
Vomiting	0.5	0.5
Pain	0.5	0
Pruritus	0.5	0.3

QUINUPRISTIN/DALFOPRISTIN — INJECTION

Quinupristin/Dalfopristin Adverse Reactions (≥ 1%): All Comparative Studies		
Adverse reaction	Quinupristin/Dalfopristin (n = 1099)	Comparator (n = 1095)
Inflammation at infusion site	42	25
Pain at infusion site	40	23.7
Edema at infusion site	17.3	9.5
Infusion site reaction	13.4	10.1
Nausea	4.6	7.2
Diarrhea	2.7	3.2
Vomiting	2.7	3.8
Rash	2.5	1.4
Thrombophlebitis	2.4	0.3
Headache	1.6	0.9
Pruritus	1.5	1.1
Pain	1.5	0.1

Additional adverse reactions that were possibly or probably related to quinupristin/dalfopristin with an incidence less than 1% are listed below.

Cardiovascular – Palpitation; phlebitis.

CNS – Anxiety; confusion; dizziness; hypertonia; insomnia; leg cramps; paresthesia; vasodilation.

Dermatologic – Maculopapular rash; sweating; urticaria.

GI – Constipation; dyspepsia; oral moniliasis; pancreatitis; pseudomembranous enterocolitis; stomatitis.

GU – Hematuria; vaginitis.

Metabolic – Gout; peripheral edema.

Musculoskeletal – Arthralgia; myalgia; myasthenia.

Respiratory – Dyspnea; pleural effusion.

Miscellaneous – Abdominal pain; worsening of underlying illness; allergic reaction; chest pain; fever; infection.

Patients Discontinuing Quinupristin/Dalfopristin Therapy (%): Skin/Skin Structure Studies		
Type	Quinupristin/Dalfopristin (n = 1,099)	Comparator[a] (n = 1,095)
Venous	12	2
Non-venous	11.8	4
Rash	2	0.9
Nausea	1.1	0
Vomiting	0.9	0
Pain	0.9	0
Pruritus	0.9	0.5

[a] Comparator regimens were oxacillin/vancomycin or cefazolin/vancomycin.

Quinupristin/Dalfopristin Adverse Reactions (%): Skin/Skin Structure Studies		
Adverse reaction	Quinupristin/Dalfopristin (n = 1,099)	Comparator (n = 1,095)
Venous	68	32.7
Pain at infusion site	44.7	17.8
Inflammation at infusion site	38.2	14.7
Edema at infusion site	18	7.2
Infusion site reaction	11.6	3.6
Non-venous	24.7	13.1
Nausea	4	2
Vomiting	3.7	1
Rash	3.1	1.3
Pain	3.1	0.2

There were 8 (1.7%) episodes of thrombus or thrombophlebitis in the quinupristin/dalfopristin arms and none in the comparator arms.

Lab test abnormalities – The following table shows the percentage of patients exhibiting laboratory values above or below the clinically relevant "critical" values during treatment phase.

Lab Test Abnormalities: Quinupristin/Dalfopristin vs Comparator (≥ 0.1%): All Comparative Studies			
Parameter	Critically high or low value	Quinupristin/ Dalfopristin critically high or low	Comparator critically high or low
AST	> 10 × ULN	0.9	0.2
ALT	> 10 × ULN	0.4	0.4
Total bilirubin	> 5 × ULN	0.9	0.2
Conjugated bilirubin	> 5 × ULN	3.1	1.3
LDH	> 5 × ULN	2.6	2.1
Alkaline phosphatase	> 5 × ULN	0.3	0.7
Gamma-GT	> 10 × ULN	1.9	1
CPK	> 10 × ULN	1.6	1.4
Creatinine	≥ 440 mcmol/L	0.1	0.1
BUN	≥ 35.5 mmol/L	0.3	1.2
Blood glucose	> 22.2 mmol/L	1.3	1.3
Blood glucose	< 2.2mmol/L	0.1	0.1
Bicarbonates	> 40 mmol/L	0.3	0.5
Bicarbonates	< 10 mmol/L	0.5	0.5
CO_2	> 50 mmol/L	0	0
CO_2	< 15 mmol/L	0.2	0
Sodium	> 160 mmol/L	0	0
Sodium	< 120 mmol/L	0.5	0.3
Potassium	> 6 mmol/L	0.3	0.6
Potassium	< 2 mmol/L	0	0.1
Hemoglobin	< 8 g/dl	2.6	1.6
Hematocrit	> 60%	0.2	0
Platelets	> 1,000,000/ mm^3	0.2	0.2
Platelets	< 50,000/mm^3	0.6	0.7

➤*Noncomparative trials:* Approximately 33% of patients discontinued therapy in these trials because of adverse events. However, the discontinuation rate because of adverse reactions assessed by the investigator as possibly or probably related to quinupristin/dalfopristin therapy was approximately 5%.

There were 3 prospectively designed non-comparative clinical trials in patients (n = 972) treated with quinupristin/dalfopristin. One of these studies (301) had more complete documentation than the other two (398 and 398B). The most common events probably or possibly related to therapy were the following.

Quinupristin/Dalfopristin Adverse Reactions (%): Noncomparative Studies	
Adverse reaction	
Arthralgia	4.3-7.8
Arthralgia and myalgia	3.3-7.4
Nausea	2.8-4.9
Myalgia	0.95-5.1

The percentage of patients who experienced severe related arthralgia and myalgia was 3.3% and 3.1%, respectively. The percentage of patients who discontinued treatment because of related arthralgia and myalgia was 2.3% and 1.8%, respectively.

Lab test abnormalities – The most frequently observed abnormalities in laboratory studies were in total and conjugated bilirubin, with increases more than 5 times the ULN, regardless of relationship to quinupristin/dalfopristin, reported in 25% and 34.6% of patients, respectively. The percentage of patients who discontinued treatment because of increased total and conjugated bilirubin was 2.7% and 2.3%, respectively. Notably, 46.5% and 59% of patients had high baseline total and conjugated bilirubin levels before study entry.

Miscellaneous – Serious adverse reactions in clinical trials, including non-comparative studies, considered possibly or probably related to quinupristin/dalfopristin administration with an incidence of less than 0.1% include the following: Acidosis; anaphylactoid reaction; apnea; arrhythmia; bone pain; cerebral hemorrhage; cerebrovascular accident; coagulation disorder; convulsion; dysautonomia; encephalopathy; grand mal convulsion; hemolysis; hemolytic anemia; heart arrest; hepatitis; hypoglycemia; hyponatremia; hypoplastic anemia; hypoventilation; hypovolemia; hypoxia; jaundice; mesenteric arterial occlusion; neck rigidity; neuropathy; pancytopenia; paraplegia; pericardial effusion; pericarditis; respiratory distress syndrome; shock; skin ulcer; supraventricular tachycardia; syncope; tremor; ventricular extrasystoles; ventricular fibrillation. Cases of hypotension and GI hemorrhage were reported in less than 0.2% of patients.

Overdosage

➤*Symptoms:* There are 4 reports of patients receiving quinupristin/dalfopristin at doses up to 3 times that recommended (7.5 mg/kg). No adverse events were considered possibly or probably related to quinupristin/dalfopristin overdose. Signs of acute overdosage may include dyspnea, emesis, tremors, and ataxia as seen in animals given extremely high doses (50 mg/kg) of quinupristin/dalfopristin.

➤*Treatment:* Carefully observe patients who receive an overdose, and give them supportive treatment. Refer to the General Management of Acute Overdosage. Quinupristin/dalfopristin is not removed by peritoneal dialysis or by hemodialysis.

DAPTOMYCIN

Rx	**Cubicin** (Cubist)	**Injection, lyophilized powder for solution:** 500 mg	Preservative free. Single-use vials.

DAPTOMYCIN — INJECTION

Indications

➤*Complicated skin and skin structure infections:* For the treatment of complicated skin and skin structure infections caused by susceptible isolates of the following gram-positive bacteria: *Staphylococcus aureus* (including methicillin-resistant isolates), *Streptococcus pyogenes*, *Streptococcus agalactiae*, *Streptococcus dysgalactiae* subspecies *equisimilis*, and *Enterococcus faecalis* (vancomycin-susceptible strains only).

➤*S. aureus bloodstream infections:* For the treatment of *S. aureus* bloodstream infections (bacteremia), including those with right-sided infective endocarditis, caused by methicillin-susceptible and methicillin-resistant isolates.

Administration and Dosage

➤*General dosing considerations:* In phase 1 and 2 clinical studies, serum creatine phosphokinase (CPK) elevations appeared to be more frequent when daptomycin was dosed more frequently than once daily. Therefore, daptomycin should not be dosed more than once per day.

➤*Adults:*

Complicated skin and skin structure infections –
Usual dosage: 4 mg/kg intravenous (IV) once every 24 hours.
Duration of therapy: 7 to 14 days.

S. aureus bloodstream infections (bacteremia) –
Usual dosage: 6 mg/kg IV once every 24 hours.
Duration of therapy: Give for a minimum of 2 to 6 weeks.

➤*Renal function impairment:*

Daptomycin Dosage in Adult Patients Based on Renal Function[a]

CrCl	Dosage regimen: Complicated skin and skin structure infections	Dosage regimen: *S. aureus* bloodstream infections
≥ 30 mL/min	4 mg/kg once every 24 hours	6 mg/kg once every 24 hours
< 30 mL/min, including hemodialysis and CAPD	4 mg/kg once every 48 hours[b]	6 mg/kg once every 48 hours[b]

[a] CrCl = creatinine clearance; CAPD = continuous ambulatory peritoneal dialysis.
[b] When possible, administer daptomycin following the completion of hemodialysis on hemodialysis days.

Adults receiving continuous renal replacement therapy – A dosage of 4 to 6 mg/kg IV every 48 hours is recommended for patients receiving continuous venovenous hemofiltration (CVVH), continuous venovenous hemodialysis (CVVHD), or continuous venovenous hemodiafiltration (CVVHDF). This recommendation assumes ultrafiltration and dialysis flow rates of 1 to 2 L/h.

According to 2 studies, there is concern for underdosing when 4 to 6 mg/kg IV every 48 hours is administered to patients receiving continuous renal replacement therapy (CRRT) or slow extended daily dialysis. For critically ill patients receiving CRRT who have severe infections, consider decreasing the dosing interval to every 24 hours (ie, 4 to 6 mg/kg IV every 24 hours) or administering 8 mg/kg IV every 48 hours. Additional monitoring (eg, CPK) may be warranted.

Adults receiving intermittent hemodialysis – One source recommends 4 to 6 mg/kg IV every 48 to 72 hours administered after the dialysis session. This recommendation assumes the patient is receiving standard intermittent hemodialysis 3 times per week and completes the full dialysis session.

➤*Preparation for administration:* The contents of a vial should be reconstituted, using aseptic technique, to 50 mg/mL as follows:

Remove the polypropylene flip-off cap from the daptomycin vial to expose the central portion of the rubber stopper. Slowly transfer 10 mL of sodium chloride 0.9% injection through the center of the rubber stopper into the daptomycin vial, pointing the transfer needle toward the wall of the vial. Ensure that all of the daptomycin powder is wetter by gently rotating the vial. Allow the wetted product to stand undisturbed for 10 minutes. Gently rotate or swirl the vial contents for a few minutes as needed to obtain a completely reconstituted solution. To minimize foaming, avoid vigorous agitation or shaking of the vial during or after reconstitution.

For IV injection over 2 minutes, administer the appropriate volume of the reconstituted daptomycin (concentration of 50 mg/mL).

For IV infusion over 30 minutes, the appropriate volume of the reconstituted daptomycin (concentration of 50 mg/mL) should be further diluted using aseptic technique into a 50 mL IV infusion bag containing sodium chloride 0.9% injection.

➤*Administration:* Administer IV by injection over 2 minutes or by infusion over 30 minutes.

➤*Admixture compatibility:*

Compatibility – Daptomycin is compatible with sodium chloride 0.9% injection and Ringer's lactate injection.

Incompatibility – Daptomycin is not compatible with dextrose-containing diluents. Because only limited data are available about the compatibility of daptomycin with other IV substances, additives or other medications should not be added to daptomycin single-use vials or infusion bags, or infused simultaneously through the same IV line. If the same IV line is used for sequential infusion of different drugs, the line should be flushed with a compatible IV solution before and after infusion with daptomycin.

Daptomycin should not be used in conjunction with *ReadyMED* elastomeric infusion pumps (Cardinal Health, Inc). Stability studies of daptomycin solutions stored in *ReadyMED* elastomeric infusion pumps identified an impurity (2-mercaptobenzothiazole) leaching from this pump system into the daptomycin solution.

➤*Storage/Stability:* Refrigerate original packages at 2° to 8°C (36° to 46°F); avoid excessive heat. Daptomycin vials are for single use only.

Stability studies have shown that the reconstituted solution is stable in the vial for 12 hours at room temperature or up to 48 hours if refrigerated at 2° to 8°C (36° to 46°F). The diluted solution is stable in the infusion bag for 12 hours at room temperature or 48 hours if refrigerated. The combined time (vial and infusion bag) should not exceed 12 hours at room temperature or 48 hours refrigerated.

Actions

➤*Pharmacology:* Daptomycin is an antibacterial drug belonging to the cyclic lipopeptide class.

The mechanism of action of daptomycin is distinct from any other antibiotic. Daptomycin binds to bacterial membranes and causes a rapid depolarization of membrane potential. The loss of membrane potential leads to inhibition of protein, DNA, and RNA synthesis, which results in bacterial cell death.

➤*Pharmacokinetics:*

Absorption –

30-minute infusion:

Daptomycin 30-Minute Infusion Mean (SD) Pharmacokinetic Parameters in Healthy Volunteers at Steady State[a]

Dose[b] mg/kg	AUC_{0-24} (mcg•h/mL)	t½ (h)	V_{ss} (L/kg)	CL_T (mL/h/kg)	C_{max} (mcg/mL)
4 mg/kg (n = 6)	494 (75)	8.1 (1)	0.096 (0.009)	8.3 (1.3)	57.8 (3)
6 mg/kg (n = 6)	632 (78)	7.9 (1)	0.101 (0.007)	9.1 (1.5)	93.9 (6)
8 mg/kg (n = 6)	858 (213)	8.3 (2.2)	0.101 (0.013)	9 (3)	123.3 (16)
10 mg/kg (n = 9)	1,039 (178)	7.9 (0.6)	0.098 (0.017)	8.8 (2.2)	141.1 (24)
12 mg/kg (n = 9)	1,277 (253)	7.7 (1.1)	0.097 (0.018)	9 (2.8)	183.7 (25)

[a] AUC_{0-24} = area under the curve from 0 to 24 hours; t½ = elimination half-life; V_{ss} = volume of distribution at steady state; CL_T = total plasma clearance; C_{max} = maximum plasma concentration.
[b] Doses of daptomycin in excess of 6 mg/kg have not been approved.

Daptomycin pharmacokinetics were generally linear and time-independent at dosages of 4 to 12 mg/kg once daily administered for up to 14 days. Steady-state trough concentrations were achieved by the third daily dose. The mean (SD) steady-state trough concentrations attained following administration of 4, 6, 8, 10, and 12 mg/kg once daily were 5.9 (1.6), 6.7 (1.6), 10.3 (5.5), 12.9 (2.9), and 13.7 (5.2) mcg/mL, respectively.

2-minute injection: Following IV administration of daptomycin over a 2-minute period to healthy volunteers at doses of 4 mg/kg (n = 8) and 6 mg/kg (n = 12), the mean (SD) steady-state systemic exposure (AUC) values were 475 (71) and 701 (82) mcg•h/mL, respectively. Values for a C_{max} at the end of the 2-minute period could not be determined adequately in this study. However, using pharmacokinetic parameters from 14 healthy volunteers who received a single dose of daptomycin 6 mg/kg IV administered over a 30-minute period in a separate study, steady-state C_{max} values were simulated for daptomycin 4 and 6 mg/kg IV administered over a 2-minute period. The simulated mean (SD) steady-state C_{max} values were 77.7 (8.1) and 116.6 (12.2) mcg/mL, respectively.

Distribution – Daptomycin is reversibly bound to human plasma proteins, primarily to serum albumin, in a concentration-independent manner. The overall mean binding ranged from 90% to 93%.

In clinical studies, mean serum protein binding in subjects with a CrCl of 30 mL/min or more was comparable with that observed in healthy subjects with normal renal function. However, there was a trend toward decreasing serum protein binding among subjects with CrCl less than 30 mL/min (88%), including hemodialysis (86%) and CAPD (84%) patients. The protein binding of daptomycin in subjects with moderate hepatic impairment (Child-Pugh class B) was similar to healthy adult subjects. The V_{ss} of daptomycin in healthy adult subjects was approximately 0.1 L/kg and was independent of dose.

Metabolism – In 5 healthy younger adults, after infusion of radiolabeled ^{14}C-daptomycin, the plasma total radioactivity was similar to the concentration determined by microbiological assay. Inactive metabolites of daptomycin were detected in the urine, as determined by the difference in total radioactive concentrations and microbiologically active concentrations. In a separate study, no metabolites were observed in plasma on day 1 following the administration of daptomycin 6 mg/kg to subjects. Minor amounts of 3

DAPTOMYCIN — INJECTION

oxidative metabolites and 1 unidentified compound were detected in urine. The site of metabolism has not been identified.

Excretion – Daptomycin is excreted primarily by the kidney. In a mass balance study of 5 healthy subjects using radiolabeled daptomycin, approximately 78% of the administered dose was recovered from urine based on total radioactivity (approximately 52% of the dose based on microbiologically active concentrations) and 5.7% of the dose was recovered from feces (collected for up to 9 days) based on total radioactivity.

Special populations –

Renal function impairment: Population-derived pharmacokinetic parameters were determined for infected patients (complicated skin and skin structure infections and *S. aureus* bacteremia) and noninfected subjects with varying degrees of renal function. CL_T, elimination half-life, and V_{ss} were similar in patients with complicated skin and skin structure infections compared with those with *S. aureus* bacteremia. Following the IV administration of daptomycin 4 mg/kg once daily, the mean CL_T was 9%, 22%, and 46% lower among subjects and patients with mild (CrCl from 50 to 80 mL/min), moderate (CrCl from 30 to less than 50 mL/min), and severe (CrCl less than 30 mL/min) renal impairment, respectively, than those with healthy renal function (CrCl greater than 80 mL/min). The mean steady-state systemic exposure (AUC), $t_{½}$, and V_{ss} increased with decreasing renal function, although the mean AUC was not markedly different for patients with CrCl from 30 to 80 mL/min compared with those with healthy renal function. The mean AUC values for patients with CrCl less than 30 mL/min and patients on dialysis (CAPD and on hemodialysis dosed postdialysis) were approximately 2 and 3 times higher, respectively, than the values in individuals with healthy renal function. The mean C_{max} ranged from 60 to 70 mcg/mL in subjects with a CrCl of 30 mL/min or more, while the mean C_{max} for those with a CrCl of less than 30 mL/min ranged from 41 to 58 mcg/mL. The mean C_{max} ranged from 80 to 114 mcg/mL in patients with mild to moderate renal impairment and was similar to that of patients with healthy renal function after the administration of daptomycin 6 mg/kg once daily.

Daptomycin 30-Minute Infusion Mean (SD) Pharmacokinetic Parameters in Patients With Renal Impairment[a]

	Parameters obtained following a single dose from patients with complicated skin and skin structure infections and healthy subjects				Parameters obtained at steady state from patients with *S. aureus* bacteremia	
Renal function	$t_{½}$ (h) 4 mg/kg	V_{ss} (L/kg) 4 mg/kg	CL_T (mL/h/kg) 4 mg/kg	$AUC_{0-\infty}$ (mcg•h/mL) 4 mg/kg	AUC_{ss} (mcg•h/mL) 6 mg/kg	$C_{min,ss}$ (mcg/mL) 6 mg/kg
Normal (CrCl > 80 mL/min)	9.39 (4.74) n = 165	0.13 (0.05) n = 165	10.9 (4) n = 165	417 (155) n = 165	545 (296) n = 62	6.9 (3.5) n = 61
Mild renal impairment (CrCl 50 to 80 mL/min)	10.75 (8.36) n = 64	0.12 (0.05) n = 64	9.9 (4) n = 64	466 (177) n = 64	637 (215) n = 29	12.4 (5.6) n = 29
Moderate renal impairment (CrCl 30 to	14.7 (10.5) n = 24	0.15 (0.06) n = 24	8.5 (3.4) n = 24	560 (258) n = 24	868 (349) n = 15	19 (9) n = 14
Severe renal impairment (CrCl < 30 mL/min)	27.83 (14.85) n = 8	0.2 (0.15) n = 8	5.9 (3.9) n = 8	925 (467) n = 8	1050, 892 n = 2	24.4, 21.4 n = 2
Hemodialysis	30.51 (6.51) n = 16	0.16 (0.04) n = 16	3.9 (2.1) n = 16	1,193 (399) n = 16	NA[b]	NA
CAPD	27.56 (4.53) n = 5	0.11 (0.02) n = 5	2.9 (0.4) n = 5	1,409 (238) n = 5	NA	NA

[a] CrCl = creatinine clearance estimated using the Cockroft-Goult equation with actual body weight; $AUC_{0-\infty}$ = area under the curve extrapolated to infinity; AUC_{ss} = area under the curve calculated over the 24-hour dosing interval at steady state; $C_{min,ss}$ = trough concentration at steady state.
[b] NA = not applicable.

See Administration and Dosage for more information.

Elderly: The pharmacokinetics of daptomycin were evaluated in 12 healthy elderly subjects (75 years of age and older) and 11 healthy younger matched controls (18 to 30 years of age). Following administration of a single 4 mg/kg IV dose, the mean total clearance of daptomycin was reduced approximately 35%, and the mean $AUC_{0-\infty}$ increased approximately 58% in elderly subjects compared with younger healthy subjects. There were no differences in C_{max}.

Obesity: The pharmacokinetics of daptomycin were evaluated in 6 moderately obese (body mass index [BMI] 25 to 39.9 kg/m^2) and 6 extremely obese (BMI 40 kg/m^2 or more) subjects and controls matched for age, gender, and renal function. Following administration of a single 4 mg/kg IV dose based on total body weight, the plasma clearance of daptomycin normalized to total body weight was approximately 15% lower in moderately obese subjects and 23% lower in extremely obese subjects compared with nonobese controls. The $AUC_{0-\infty}$ of daptomycin increased approximately 30% in moderately obese and 31% in extremely obese subjects compared with nonobese controls. The differences were most likely due to differences in the renal clearance of daptomycin. No dosage adjustment of daptomycin is warranted in obese subjects.

➤*Microbiology:* Daptomycin belongs to the cyclic lipopeptide class of antibiotics. Daptomycin has clinical utility in the treatment of infections caused by aerobic gram-positive bacteria. The in vitro spectrum of activity of daptomycin encompasses most clinically relevant gram-positive pathogenic bacteria.

Daptomycin exhibits rapid, concentration-dependent bactericidal activity against gram-positive bacteria in vitro. This has been demonstrated by time-kill curves and by minimum bactericidal concentration/MIC ratios using broth dilution methodology. Daptomycin maintained bactericidal activity in vitro against stationary phase *S. aureus* in simulated endocardial vegetations. The clinical significance of this is not known.

In vitro studies have investigated interactions of daptomycin with other antibacterials. Antagonism, as determined by kill curve studies, has not been observed. In vitro synergistic interactions occurred with aminoglycosides, beta-lactam antibacterials, and rifampin against some isolates of staphylococci (including some methicillin-resistant isolates) and enterococci (including some vancomycin-resistant isolates).

Resistance –

Complicated skin and skin structure infection trials: The emergence of daptomycin nonsusceptible isolates occurred in 2 infected patients across the set of phase 2 and pivotal phase 3 clinical trials of complicated skin and skin structure infections. In 1 case, a nonsusceptible *S. aureus* was isolated from a patient in a phase 2 trial who received daptomycin at less than the protocol-specified dose for the initial 5 days of therapy. In the second case, a nonsusceptible *E. faecalis* was isolated from a patient with an infected chronic decubitus ulcer enrolled in a salvage trial.

S. aureus bacteremia/endocarditis and other postapproval trials: In subsequent clinical trials, nonsusceptible isolates were recovered. *S. aureus* was isolated from a patient in a compassionate use trial and from 7 patients in the *S. aureus* bacteremia/endocarditis trial. An *Enterococcus faecium* was isolated from a patient in a vancomycin-resistant enterococcus trial.

Contraindications

Hypersensitivity to daptomycin.

Warnings/Precautions

➤*Myopathy and rhabdomyolysis:* Myopathy, defined as muscle aching or muscle weakness in conjunction with increases in CPK values to greater than 10 times the upper limit of normal (ULN), has been reported with the use of daptomycin. Rhabdomyolysis, with or without acute renal failure, has been reported.

Monitor patients receiving daptomycin for the development of muscle pain or weakness, particularly of the distal extremities. In patients who receive daptomycin, monitor CPK levels weekly and more frequently in patients who received recent prior or concomitant therapy with an HMG-CoA reductase inhibitor or in whom elevations in CPK occur during treatment with daptomycin.

In patients with renal impairment, monitor renal function and CPK more frequently than once weekly.

In phase 1 studies and phase 2 clinical trials, CPK elevations appeared to be more frequent when daptomycin was dosed more than once daily. Therefore, daptomycin should not be dosed more frequently than once a day.

Discontinue daptomycin in patients with unexplained signs and symptoms of myopathy in conjunction with CPK elevations to levels more than 1,000 units/L (approximately 5 × ULN), and in patients without reported symptoms who have marked elevations in CPK, with levels more than 2,000 units/L (at least 10 × ULN). In addition, consider suspending agents associated with rhabdomyolysis, such as HMG-CoA reductase inhibitors, temporarily in patients receiving daptomycin.

➤*Eosinophilic pneumonia:* Eosinophilic pneumonia has been reported in patients receiving daptomycin. In reported cases associated with daptomycin, patients developed fever, dyspnea with hypoxic respiratory insufficiency, and diffuse pulmonary infiltrates. In general, patients developed eosinophilic pneumonia 2 to 4 weeks after starting daptomycin and improved when daptomycin was discontinued and steroid therapy was initiated. Recurrence of eosinophilic pneumonia upon re-exposure has been reported. Patients who develop these signs and symptoms while receiving daptomycin should undergo prompt medical evaluation, and daptomycin should be discontinued immediately. Treatment with systemic steroids is recommended.

➤*Peripheral neuropathy:* Cases of peripheral neuropathy have been reported during the daptomycin postmarketing experience. Therefore, be alert to signs and symptoms of peripheral neuropathy in patients receiving daptomycin.

➤*Clostridium difficile–associated diarrhea: C. difficile*–associated diarrhea has been reported with the use of nearly all systemic antibacterial agents, including daptomycin, and may range in severity from mild diarrhea to fatal colitis. Treatment with antibacterial agents alters the normal flora of the colon, leading to overgrowth of *C. difficile*.

C. difficile produces toxins A and B, which contribute to the development of *C. difficile*–associated diarrhea. Hypertoxin-producing strains of *C. difficile* cause increased morbidity and mortality because these infections can be refractory to antimicrobial therapy and may require colectomy. *C. difficile*–associated diarrhea must be considered in all patients who present with diarrhea following antibacterial use. Careful medical history is necessary because *C. difficile*–associated diarrhea has been reported to occur more than 2 months after the administration of antibacterial agents.

If *C. difficile*–associated diarrhea is suspected or confirmed, ongoing antibacterial use not directed against *C. difficile* may need to be discontinued. Insti-

DAPTOMYCIN — INJECTION

tute appropriate fluid and electrolyte management, protein supplementation, antibacterial treatment of *C. difficile*, and surgical evaluation as clinically indicated.

➤*Persisting or relapsing S. aureus bacteremia/endocarditis:* Patients with persisting or relapsing *S. aureus* bacteremia/endocarditis or poor clinical response should have repeat blood cultures. If a culture is positive for *S. aureus*, perform MIC susceptibility testing of the isolate using a standardized procedure, as well as diagnostic evaluation to rule out sequestered foci of infection. Appropriate surgical intervention (eg, debridement, removal of prosthetic devices, valve replacement surgery) and/or consideration of a change in antibacterial regimen may be required.

Failure of treatment because of persisting or relapsing *S. aureus* bacteremia/endocarditis may be due to reduced daptomycin susceptibility (as evidenced by increasing MIC of the *S. aureus* isolate).

➤*Hypersensitivity reactions:* Anaphylaxis/hypersensitivity reactions have been reported with the use of antibacterial agents, including daptomycin, and may be life-threatening. If an allergic reaction to daptomycin occurs, discontinue the drug and institute appropriate therapy.

➤*Renal function impairment:* Daptomycin is eliminated primarily by the kidneys; therefore, a modification of daptomycin dosage is recommended for patients with CrCl less than 30 mL/min, including patients receiving hemodialysis or continuous ambulatory peritoneal dialysis (CAPD). In patients with renal impairment, monitor renal function and CPK more frequently than once weekly.

There are limited data available from the complicated skin and skin structure infections clinical trials regarding clinical efficacy of daptomycin treatment in patients with CrCl less than 50 mL/min; only 6% of patients treated with daptomycin in the intent-to-treat (ITT) population had a baseline CrCl less than 50 mL/min. The following table shows the number of patients by CrCl and treatment group who were clinical successes in the complicated skin and skin structure infections trials.

Daptomycin Clinical Success Rates by Treatment Group and Renal Function in the Complicated Skin and Skin Structure Infection Clinical Trials (Population: ITT)

CrCl	Success rate (%) Daptomycin 4 mg/kg every 24 hours		Comparator	
50 to 70 mL/min	n = 38	66%	n = 48	63%
30 to < 50 mL/min	n = 15	47%	n = 35	57%

In a subgroup analysis of the ITT population in the *S. aureus* bacteremia/endocarditis trial, clinical success rates, as determined by a treatment-blind adjudication committee, in the daptomycin-treated patients were lower in patients with baseline CrCl less than 50 mL/min. A decrease of the magnitude shown in the following table was not observed in comparator-treated patients.

Daptomycin Adjudication Committee Success Rates at Test of Cure by Baseline CrCl in the *S. aureus* Bacteremia/Endocarditis Trial (Population: ITT)

	Success rate (%)							
	Daptomycin				Comparator			
Baseline CrCl	Bacteremia		Right-sided infective endocarditis		Bacteremia		Right-sided infective endocarditis	
>80 mL/min	n = 50	60%	n = 14	50%	n = 42	45%	n = 11	46%
50 to 80 mL/min	n = 26	46%	n = 4	25%	n = 31	42%	n = 2	50%
30 to 50 mL/min	n = 14	14%	n = 1	0%	n = 17	41%	n = 1	100%

Consider these data when selecting antibacterial therapy for use in patients with baseline moderate to severe renal impairment.

➤*Superinfection:* The use of antibiotics may promote the overgrowth of nonsusceptible organisms. If superinfection occurs during therapy, take appropriate measures.

➤*Pregnancy: Category B.* There are no adequate and well-controlled studies in pregnant women. Because animal reproduction studies are not always predictive of human response, use daptomycin during pregnancy only if the potential benefit outweighs the possible risk.

The high molecular weight of daptomycin might limit exposure of the embryo and fetus. Most antibiotics can be classified as low risk in gestation; therefore, if daptomycin is required, it should not be withheld because of pregnancy.

➤*Lactation:* It is not known if daptomycin is excreted in human milk. The high molecular weight (approximately 1,621) should limit excretion into breast milk. Because many drugs are excreted in human milk, exercise caution when administering daptomycin to a breast-feeding woman.

Limited data indicate daptomycin is excreted in low levels in breast milk.

The risk to the breast-fed infant appears to be low. Modification of the infant's bowel flora resulting in diarrhea and other GI complaints are potential concerns. Therefore, if a lactating woman requires treatment with the antibiotic, her breast-fed infant should be closely observed for changes in bowel function.

➤*Children:* Safety and efficacy of daptomycin in patients younger than 18 years of age have not been established.

➤*Elderly:* In the phase 3 clinical studies of complicated skin and skin structure infection and *S. aureus* bacteremia/endocarditis, lower clinical success rates were seen in patients 65 years of age and older compared with those younger than 65 years of age. In addition, treatment-emergent adverse reactions were more common in patients 65 years of age and older than in patients younger than 65 years of age.

➤*Monitoring:* Monitor patients receiving daptomycin for the development of muscle pain or weakness, particularly of the distal extremities. Monitor CPK levels weekly and more frequently in patients who have received recent, prior, or concomitant therapy with an HMG-CoA reductase inhibitor or in whom elevations in CPK occur during treatment. In patients with renal impairment, monitor renal function and CPK more frequently than once weekly.

Drug Interactions

➤*HMG-CoA reductase inhibitors:* Coadministration of daptomycin and HMG-CoA reductase inhibitors may increase the risk of rhabdomyolysis. Consider a temporary suspension of the HMG-CoA reductase inhibitor. Monitor CPK levels weekly and more frequently in patients receiving recent prior or concomitant therapy with HMG-CoA reductase inhibitors. Discontinue daptomycin in patients with unexplained signs and symptoms of myopathy in conjunction with CPK elevations to levels greater than 1,000 units/L.

Daptomycin Injection Drug Interactions

Precipitant drug	Object drug[a]		Description
HMG-CoA reductase inhibitors (eg, simvastatin)	Daptomycin	↑	Coadministration of daptomycin and HMG-CoA reductase inhibitors may increase the risk of rhabdomyolysis. Consider a temporary suspension of the HMG-CoA reductase inhibitor. Monitor CPK levels weekly and more frequently in patients receiving recent prior or concomitant therapy with HMG-CoA reductase inhibitors. Discontinue daptomycin in patients with unexplained signs and symptoms of myopathy in conjunction with CPK elevations to levels greater than 1,000 units/L.
Daptomycin	HMG-CoA reductase inhibitors (eg, simvastatin)		
Tobramycin	Daptomycin	↑	In a study in which 6 healthy adult men received a single dose of daptomycin 2 mg/kg IV and tobramycin 1 mg/kg IV, and both in combination, the mean C_{max} and $AUC_{0-\infty}$ of daptomycin increased 12.7% and 8.7%, respectively, when coadministered with tobramycin. The mean C_{max} and $AUC_{0-\infty}$ of tobramycin decreased 10.7% and 6.6%, respectively, when administered with daptomycin. None of these differences was statistically significant. The interaction between daptomycin and tobramycin with a clinical dose of daptomycin (4 mg/kg) is unknown. Caution is warranted when daptomycin is coadministered with tobramycin.
Daptomycin	Tobramycin	↓	

[a] ↑ = object drug increased; ↓ = object drug decreased.

➤*Minimally or noninteracting drugs:*

Aztreonam – In a study in which 15 healthy adult subjects received a single dose of daptomycin 6 mg/kg IV, aztreonam 1,000 mg IV, and both in combination, the C_{max} and $AUC_{0-\infty}$ of daptomycin were not significantly altered by aztreonam; the C_{max} and $AUC_{0-\infty}$ of aztreonam were not significantly altered by daptomycin. No dosage adjustment of either antibiotic is warranted when coadministered.

Simvastatin – In 20 healthy subjects on a stable daily dosage of simvastatin 40 mg, administration of daptomycin 4 mg/kg IV once daily for 14 days (n = 10) was not associated with a higher incidence of adverse reactions than subjects receiving placebo once daily (n = 10).

Probenecid – Coadministration of probenecid (500 mg 4 times daily) and a single dose of daptomycin 4 mg/kg IV did not significantly alter the C_{max} and $AUC_{0-\infty}$ of daptomycin. No dosage adjustment of daptomycin is warranted when daptomycin is coadministered with probenecid.

Warfarin – Coadministration of daptomycin 6 mg/kg once daily for 5 days and a single oral dose of warfarin 25 mg had no significant effect on the pharmacokinetics of either drug, and the international normalized ratio (INR) was not significantly altered.

➤*Drug/Lab test interactions:* Clinically relevant daptomycin plasma concentrations have caused a concentration-dependent false prolongation of prothrombin time (PT) and elevation of INR when certain recombinant thromboplastin reagents are utilized for assay. The possibility of an erroneous PT/INR result may be minimized by drawing specimens for PT or INR testing near the time of daptomycin trough plasma concentrations. However,

DAPTOMYCIN — INJECTION

sufficient daptomycin concentrations may be present at trough to cause a laboratory test interaction.

Adverse Reactions

➤*Complicated skin and skin structure infection:*

Discontinuation of therapy – In phase 3 complicated skin and skin structure infection trials, daptomycin was discontinued in 2.8% of patients because of an adverse reaction, while comparator was discontinued in 3% of patients.

➤*Adverse reactions (2% or more):*

Daptomycin Adverse Reactions in Phase 3 Complicated Skin and Skin Structure Infection Trials Studies (≥ 2%)

Adverse reaction	Daptomycin 4 mg/kg (n = 534)	Comparator[a] (n = 558)
CNS		
Dizziness	2.2%	2%
Headache	5.4%	5.4%
Lab test abnormalities		
Abnormal liver function tests	3%	1.6%
Elevated CPK	2.8%	1.8%
Miscellaneous		
Diarrhea	5.2%	4.3%
Dyspnea	2.1%	1.6%
Hypotension	2.4%	1.4%
Rash	4.3%	3.8%
Urinary tract infections	2.4%	0.5%

[a] Comparators included vancomycin (1 g IV every 12 hours) or an anti-staphylococcal semisynthetic penicillin (nafcillin, oxacillin, cloxacillin, flucloxacillin; 4 to 12 g IV every 24 hours in divided doses).

Adverse reactions (less than 1%) –

CNS: Fatigue, mental status change, paresthesia, vertigo, weakness (less than 1%).

GI: Abdominal distension, increased serum lactate dehydrogenase, jaundice, stomatitis (less than 1%).

Hematologic/Lymphatic: Eosinophilia, increased INR, leukocytosis, thrombocytopenia, thrombocytosis (less than 1%).

Metabolic/Nutritional: Electrolyte disturbance, hypomagnesemia, increased serum bicarbonate (less than 1%).

Musculoskeletal: Arthralgia, myalgia, muscle cramps, muscle weakness (less than 1%).

Special senses: Eye irritation, taste disturbance (less than 1%).

Miscellaneous: Eczema, flushing, hypersensitivity, rigors, supraventricular arrhythmia (less than 1%).

➤*S. aureus bacteremia/endocarditis:*

Gram-negative infections – Serious gram-negative infections (including bloodstream infections) were reported in 8.3% of daptomycin-treated and 0 of 115 comparator-treated patients. Comparator patients received dual therapy that included initial gentamicin for 4 days. Infections were reported during treatment and during early and late follow-up. Gram-negative infections included cholangitis, alcoholic pancreatitis, sternal osteomyelitis/mediastinitis, bowel infarction, recurrent Crohn disease, recurrent line sepsis, and recurrent urosepsis caused by a number of different gram-negative bacteria.

Adverse reactions (5% or more) –

Daptomycin Adverse Reactions (≥ 5%) in the *S. aureus* Bacteremia/Endocarditis Trial

Adverse reactions	Daptomycin 6 mg/kg (n = 120)	Comparator[a] (n = 116)
Dermatologic		
Pruritus	6%	5%
Sweating increased	5%	0%
Miscellaneous		
Abdominal pain NOS[b]	6%	3%
Bacteremia	5%	0%
Blood CPK increased	7%	1%
Chest pain	7%	6%
Edema NOS	7%	4%
Hypertension NOS	6%	3%
Insomnia	9%	7%
Pharyngolaryngeal pain	8%	2%
Sepsis NOS	5%	3%

[a] Vancomycin (1 g IV ever 12 hours) or an anti-staphylococcal semisynthetic penicillin (eg, nafcillin, oxacillin, cloxacillin, flucloxacillin; 2 g IV every 4 hours), each with initial low-dose gentamicin.

[b] NOS = not otherwise specified.

Other adverse reactions –

Cardiovascular: Atrial fibrillation, atrial flutter, cardiac arrest.

CNS: Dyskinesia, hallucination NOS, paresthesia.

Dermatologic: Pruritus generalized, rash vesicular.

GI: Appetite decreased NOS, dry mouth, epigastric discomfort, gingival pain, oral candidiasis, oral hypoesthesia.

GU: Proteinuria, renal impairment NOS, urinary tract infection fungal, vaginal candidiasis.

Hematologic/lymphatic: Eosinophilia, lymphadenopathy, thrombocythemia, thrombocytopenia.

Lab test abnormalities: Alanine aminotransferase increased, aspartate aminotransferase increased, blood alkaline phosphatase increased, blood phosphorus increased, INR increased, liver function test abnormal, prothrombin time prolonged.

Special senses: Vision blurred, tinnitus.

Miscellaneous: Candidal infection NOS, fungemia, myalgia.

➤*Other trials:* In phase 3 trials of community-acquired pneumonia, the death rate and rates of serious cardiorespiratory adverse events were higher in daptomycin-treated patients than in comparator-treated patients. These differences were due to lack of therapeutic effectiveness of daptomycin in the treatment of CAP in patients experiencing these adverse events.

➤*Lab test abnormalities:*

Complicated skin and skin structure infection – In phase 3 complicated skin and skin structure infection trials of daptomycin at a dose of 4 mg/kg, elevations in CPK were reported as clinical adverse events in 2.8% of daptomycin-treated patients, compared with 1.8% of comparator-treated patients. Of the 534 patients treated with daptomycin, 0.2% had symptoms of muscle pain or weakness associated with CPK elevations to greater than 4 times the ULN. The symptoms resolved within 3 days and CPK returned to normal within 7 to 10 days after treatment was discontinued.

Daptomycin CPK Elevations in Phase 3 Complicated Skin and Skin Structure Infection Trials Studies (%)

	All patients		Patients with normal CPK at baseline	
	Daptomycin (n = 430)	Comparator[a] (n = 459)	Daptomycin (n = 374)	Comparator[a] (n = 392)
No increase	90.7%	91.1%	91.2%	91.1%
Maximum value > 1 × ULN[b]	9.3%	8.9%	8.8%	8.9%
> 2 × ULN	4.9%	4.8%	3.7%	3.1%
> 4 × ULN	1.4%	1.5%	1.1%	1%
> 5 × ULN	1.4%	0.4%	1.1%	0%
> 10 × ULN	0.5%	0.2%	0.2%	0%

[a] Vancomycin (1 g IV every 12 hours) or an anti-staphylococcal semisynthetic penicillin (eg, nafcillin, oxacillin, cloxacillin, or flucloxacillin; 4 to 12 g/day IV in divided doses).

[b] ULN is defined as 200 units/L.

Elevations in CPK observed in patients treated with daptomycin or comparator were not clinically or statistically significantly different.

S. aureus bacteremia/endocarditis – In the *S. aureus* bacteremia/endocarditis trial, at a dose of 6 mg/kg, 9.2% of daptomycin-treated patients, including 2 patients with baseline CPK levels more than 500 units/L, had CPK elevations to levels more than 500 units/L, compared with 0.9% of comparator-treated patients. Of the 11 daptomycin-treated patients, 4 had prior or concomitant treatment with an HMG-CoA reductase inhibitor. Three of these 11 daptomycin-treated patients discontinued therapy because of CPK elevation, while the 1 comparator-treated patient did not discontinue therapy.

➤*Postmarketing:*

Dermatologic – Serious skin reactions, including Stevens-Johnson syndrome and vesiculobullous rash (with or without mucous membrane involvement).

Hypersensitivity – Anaphylaxis; hypersensitivity reactions including difficulty swallowing, hives, pruritus, pulmonary eosinophilia, shortness of breath, and truncal erythema.

GI – Nausea, vomiting.

Musculoskeletal – Myoglobin increased; rhabdomyolysis (some reports involved patients treated concurrently with daptomycin and HMG-CoA reductase inhibitors).

Respiratory – Cough, eosinophilic pneumonia.

Miscellaneous – *C. difficile*–associated diarrhea, peripheral neuropathy.

DAPTOMYCIN — INJECTION

Overdosage

➤*Treatment:* Supportive care is advised with maintenance of glomerular filtration. Daptomycin is slowly cleared from the body by hemodialysis or by peritoneal dialysis. The use of high-flux dialysis membranes during 4 hours of hemodialysis may increase the percentage of dose removed compared with that removed by low-flux membranes.

Patient Information

Advise patients that allergic reactions, including serious allergic reactions, could occur and that serious reactions require immediate treatment. Advise patients to report any previous allergic reactions to daptomycin.

Advise patients to report muscle pain or weakness, especially in the forearms and lower legs, as well as tingling or numbness.

Advise patients to report any symptoms of cough, breathlessness, or fever.

Diarrhea is a common problem caused by antibacterials that usually ends when the antibacterial is discontinued. Sometimes after starting treatment with antibacterials, patients can develop watery and bloody stools (with or without stomach cramps and fever), even as late as 2 or more months after having received the last dose of the antibacterial. If this occurs, advise patients to contact their health care provider as soon as possible.

Counsel patients that antibacterial drugs, including daptomycin, are for the use of treating bacterial infections. They do not treat viral infections (eg, the common cold). When daptomycin is prescribed to treat a bacterial infection, tell patients that although it is common to feel better early in the course of therapy, administer the medication exactly as directed. Skipping doses or not completing the full course of therapy may decrease the effectiveness of the immediate treatment and increase the likelihood that bacteria will develop resistance and will not be treatable by daptomycin or other antibacterial drugs in the future.

VANCOMYCIN

Rx	**Vancocin** (ViroPharma)	**Capsules; oral:** 125 mg	As vancomycin hydrochloride. PEG. (3125 Vancocin HCl 125 mg). Opaque blue and opaque brown. In *Identi-Dose* 20s.
		250 mg	As vancomycin hydrochloride. PEG. (3126 Vancocin HCl 250 mg). Opaque blue and opaque lavender. In *Identi-Dose* 20s.
Rx	**Vancomycin Hydrochloride** (Various, eg, Akorn, American Pharmaceutical Partners, Hospira)	**Injection, powder for solution:** 500 mg	As vancomycin hydrochloride. Preservative free. In single-dose vials.
Rx	**Vancomycin Hydrochloride** (Hospira)	**Injection, powder for solution:** 750 mg	As vancomycin hydrochloride. Preservative free. In single-dose vials.
Rx	**Vancomycin Hydrochloride** (Various, eg, Akorn, American Pharmaceutical Partners, Hospira)	**Injection, powder for solution:** 1 g	Preservative free. In single-dose vials.
Rx	**Vancomycin Hydrochloride** (Akorn, American Pharmaceutical Partners)	**Injection, powder for solution:** 5 g	In 100 mL pharmacy bulk packages.
Rx	**Vancomycin Hydrochloride** (American Pharmaceutical Partners, Hospira)	**Injection, powder for solution:** 10 g	In 100 mL pharmacy bulk packages.
Rx	**Vancomycin Hydrochloride** (Baxter)	**Injection, solution:** 500 mg	In premixed 100 mL *Galaxy* containers.
Rx		1 g	In premixed 200 mL *Galaxy* containers.

VANCOMYCIN HYDROCHLORIDE — ORAL

Indications

➤*Pseudomembranous colitis:* For the treatment of antibiotic-associated pseudomembranous colitis caused by *Clostridium difficile*.

➤*Staphylococcal enterocolitis:* For treatment of enterocolitis caused by *Staphylococcus aureus* (including methicillin-resistant strains).

➤*Off-label uses:*

Rectal administration – [4] = Insufficient documentation. The lack of controlled trials and varied information from case reports makes it difficult to provide guidelines or recommendations.

Administration and Dosage

➤*Maximum dose:*

Adults – There are no well-established maximum doses for the approved indications according to the prescribing information.

Children – 2 g/day according to the prescribing information.

➤*General dosing considerations:* Certain parenteral products may be administered orally. See the Vancomycin injection monograph for more information.

➤*Adults:*

Usual dosage – 500 mg to 2 g orally in 3 or 4 divided doses for 7 to 10 days.

Off-label dosing –

Rectal administration: [4] = Insufficient documentation. Varied doses ranging from initial doses of 1 to 2 g and maintenance dosing of 100 to 500 mg every 6 hours. In a review of pseudomembranous colitis, one author recommends intravenous (IV) vancomycin (at least 2 g/day) along with vancomycin enemas every 8 hours (500 mg/L of normal saline solution). Administration is recommended as an enema or with a *Bardex* catheter (as with a barium enema) if the patient is unable to retain the enema.

➤*Children:*

Usual dosage – 40 mg/kg/day in 3 or 4 divided doses for 7 to 10 days. The total daily dosage should not exceed 2 g.

➤*Elderly:* Exercise caution in dose selection for an elderly patient, usually starting at the low end of the dosing range, reflecting the greater frequency of decreased hepatic, renal, or cardiac function, and of concomitant disease or other drug therapy.

➤*Administration:* May be taken with or without food.

➤*Storage/Stability:* Store at 15° to 30°C (59° to 86°F).

Actions

➤*Pharmacology:* Vancomycin is a tricyclic glycopeptide antibiotic. The bactericidal action of vancomycin results primarily from inhibition of cell-wall biosynthesis. In addition, vancomycin alters bacterial cell membrane permeability and RNA synthesis.

➤*Pharmacokinetics:*

Absorption – Vancomycin is poorly absorbed after oral administration. During multiple dosing of 250 mg every 8 hours for 7 doses, fecal concentrations of vancomycin in volunteers exceeded 100 mg/kg in the majority of samples. No blood concentrations were detected and urinary recovery did not exceed 0.76%. With dosages of 2 g daily, very high concentrations of drug can be found in the feces (more than 3,100 mg/kg) and very low concentrations (less than 1 mcg/mL) can be found in the serum of patients with healthy renal function who have pseudomembranous colitis. Orally administered vancomycin does not usually enter the systemic circulation even when inflammatory lesions are present. After multiple-dose oral administration of vancomycin, measurable serum concentrations may infrequently occur in patients with active *Clostridium difficile*–induced pseudomembranous colitis.

Special populations –

Renal function impairment: In the presence of renal impairment, the possibility of accumulation exists.

Elderly: Total systemic and renal clearances of vancomycin are reduced in elderly patients.

Anephric patients: In anephric patients with no inflammatory bowel disease, blood concentrations of vancomycin were barely measurable (0.66 mcg/mL) in 2 of 5 subjects who received vancomycin 2 g for oral solution daily for 16 days. No measurable blood concentrations were attained in the other 3 patients.

➤*Microbiology:* The oral form of vancomycin is effective only for the infections noted in the Indications section. The oral form is not effective for any other type of infection.

Aerobic gram-positive microorganisms – *S. aureus* (including methicillin-resistant strains) associated with enterocolitis.

Anaerobic gram-positive microorganisms – *C. difficile* antibiotic–associated pseudomembranous colitis.

Resistance – There is no cross-resistance between vancomycin and other antibiotics.

Contraindications

Hypersensitivity to vancomycin.

Warnings/Precautions

➤*Systemic absorption:* Some patients with inflammatory disorders of the intestinal mucosa may have significant systemic absorption of vancomycin and, therefore, may be at risk for the development of adverse reactions associated with the parenteral administration of vancomycin. The risk is greater if renal impairment is present.

VANCOMYCIN HYDROCHLORIDE — ORAL

➤*Ototoxicity:* Ototoxicity has occurred in patients receiving vancomycin. It may be transient or permanent. It has been reported mostly in patients who have been given excessive IV doses, who have an underlying hearing loss, or who are receiving concomitant therapy with another ototoxic agent, such as an aminoglycoside. Serial tests of auditory function may be helpful to minimize the risk of ototoxicity.

➤*Renal function impairment:* When patients with underlying renal dysfunction are being treated, perform serial monitoring of renal function. The risk of significant systemic absorption of vancomycin is greater in patients with renal impairment.

➤*Superinfection:* Use of vancomycin may result in the overgrowth of nonsusceptible organisms. If superinfection occurs during therapy, take appropriate measures.

➤*Pregnancy: Category B.* The human pregnancy experience with vancomycin is adequate to demonstrate that the embryofetal risk is very low or nonexistent. In a controlled clinical study, the potential ototoxic and nephrotoxic effects of vancomycin on infants were evaluated when the drug was administered IV to pregnant women for serious staphylococcal infections complicating IV drug abuse. Vancomycin was found in cord blood. No sensorineural hearing loss or nephrotoxicity attributable to vancomycin was noted. One infant whose mother received vancomycin in the third trimester experienced conductive hearing loss that was not attributed to the administration of vancomycin. Because the number of patients treated in this study was limited and vancomycin was administered only in the second and third trimesters, manufacturers state that it is not known whether vancomycin causes fetal harm. Because animal reproduction studies are not always predictive of human response, give vancomycin to a pregnant woman only if clearly needed.

➤*Lactation:* Vancomycin is excreted in human milk based on information obtained with the IV administration of vancomycin. However, systemic absorption of vancomycin is very low following oral administration of vancomycin capsules. It is not known whether oral vancomycin is excreted in human milk, as no studies of vancomycin concentration in human milk after oral administration have been done. Exercise caution when vancomycin is administered to a breast-feeding woman. Based on limited human data, vancomycin is probably compatible with breast-feeding. Because of the potential for adverse reactions, decide whether to discontinue breast-feeding or the drug, taking into account the importance of the drug to the mother.

➤*Children:* Safety and effectiveness in children have not been established. However, see Administration and Dosage for dosing.

➤*Elderly:* Total systemic and renal clearance are reduced in elderly patients. Exercise caution in dose selection for an elderly patient, usually starting at the low end of the dosing range, reflecting the greater frequency of decreased hepatic, renal, or cardiac function, and of concomitant disease or other drug therapy.

➤*Monitoring:* Clinically significant serum concentrations have been reported in some patients who have taken multiple oral doses of vancomycin for active *C. difficile*–induced pseudomembranous colitis; therefore, monitoring of serum concentrations may be appropriate in some instances (eg, in patients with renal insufficiency and/or colitis).

Serial tests of auditory function may be helpful to minimize the risk of ototoxicity.

When patients with underlying renal dysfunction or those receiving concomitant therapy with an aminoglycoside are being treated, perform serial monitoring of renal function.

Drug Interactions

➤*Aminoglycosides (eg, gentamicin):* The risk of nephrotoxicity may be increased with coadministration. Monitor renal function and serum drug concentrations with coadministration.

➤*Nondepolarizing muscle relaxants (eg, vecuronium):* The neuromuscular blockade of nondepolarizing muscle relaxants may be enhanced. Avoid this combination if possible. When necessary, monitor neuromuscular function closely, titrate the dose of nondepolarizing muscle relaxants, and be prepared to provide mechanical respiratory support as needed.

Adverse Reactions

For more information on ototoxicity, see Warnings/Precautions.

➤*Hematologic:* Reversible neutropenia, usually starting 1 week or more after onset of IV therapy with vancomycin or after a total dose of more than 25 g, has been reported for several dozen patients. Neutropenia appears to be promptly reversible when vancomycin is discontinued. Thrombocytopenia has rarely been reported.

➤*Hypersensitivity:* A condition has been reported that is similar to the IV-induced syndrome with symptoms consistent with anaphylactoid reactions, including dyspnea, flushing of the upper body ("red man syndrome"), hypotension, pain and muscle spasm of the chest and back, pruritus, urticaria, and wheezing. These reactions usually resolve within 20 minutes but may persist for several hours.

➤*Renal:* Rarely, renal failure, principally manifested by increased serum creatinine or serum urea nitrogen concentrations, especially in patients given large IV doses of vancomycin has been reported. Rare cases of interstitial nephritis have been reported. Most of these have occurred in patients who were given aminoglycosides concomitantly or who had preexisting kidney dysfunction. When vancomycin was discontinued, azotemia resolved in most patients.

➤*Special senses:* A few dozen cases of hearing loss associated with vancomycin IV have been reported. Most of these patients had kidney dysfunction or a preexisting hearing loss or were receiving concomitant treatment with an ototoxic drug. Dizziness, tinnitus, and vertigo have been reported rarely.

➤*Miscellaneous:* Infrequently, patients have been reported to have had anaphylaxis, drug fever, chills, nausea, eosinophilia, rashes (including exfoliative dermatitis), Stevens-Johnson syndrome, toxic epidermal necrolysis, and rare cases of vasculitis in association with the administration of vancomycin.

Overdosage

➤*Treatment:* Supportive care is advised, with maintenance of glomerular filtration. Vancomycin is poorly removed by dialysis. Hemofiltration and hemoperfusion with polysulfone resin have been reported to result in increased vancomycin clearance.

Patient Information

Counsel patients that antibacterial drugs, including vancomycin, should only be used to treat bacterial infections. Antibacterial drugs do not treat viral infections (eg, the common cold).

When vancomycin is prescribed to treat a bacterial infection, tell patients that although it is common to feel better early in the course of therapy, the medication should be taken exactly as directed. Skipping doses or not completing the full course of therapy may decrease the effectiveness of the immediate treatment, and increase the likelihood that bacteria will develop resistance and will not be treatable by vancomycin or other antibacterial drugs in the future.

VANCOMYCIN HYDROCHLORIDE — INJECTION

Indications

➤*Endocarditis:*

Staphylococcal – In the treatment of staphylococcal endocarditis.

Streptococcal – Alone or in combination with an aminoglycoside for endocarditis caused by *Streptococcus viridans* or *Streptococcus bovis*. For endocarditis caused by enterococci (eg, *Enterococcus faecalis*), vancomycin has been reported to be effective only in combination with an aminoglycoside.

Diphtheroid – For the treatment of diphtheroid endocarditis. Vancomycin has been used successfully in combination with either rifampin, an aminoglycoside, or both in early-onset prosthetic valve endocarditis caused by *Staphylococcus epidermidis* or diphtheroids.

➤*Pseudomembranous colitis/Staphylococcal enterocolitis:* Certain parenteral products of vancomycin may be administered orally for treatment of antibiotic-associated pseudomembranous colitis caused by *Clostridium difficile* and for staphylococcal enterocolitis. Parenteral administration of vancomycin alone is of unproven benefit for these indications. Vancomycin is not effective by the oral route for other types of infection.

➤*Staphylococcal infections:* For the treatment of serious or severe infections caused by susceptible strains of methicillin-resistant (beta-lactam–resistant) staphylococci. It is indicated for patients who are allergic to penicillin, for patients who cannot receive or who have failed to respond to other drugs, including the penicillins or cephalosporins, and for infections caused by vancomycin-susceptible organisms that are resistant to other antimicrobial drugs. Vancomycin is indicated for initial therapy when methicillin-resistant staphylococci are suspected, but after susceptibility data are available, adjust therapy accordingly.

Its effectiveness has been documented in other infections due to staphylococci, including septicemia, bone infections, lower respiratory tract infections, and skin and skin structure infections. When staphylococcal infections are localized and purulent, antibiotics are used as adjuncts to appropriate surgical measures.

➤*Off-label uses:*

Aerosolization – [4] = Insufficient documentation. Further clinical trials are needed to evaluate the utility and safety of this route of administration. Prior dosing with terbutaline or albuterol may decrease the risk of vancomycin-induced bronchospasm.

Rectal administration – [4] = Insufficient documentation. The lack of controlled trials and varied information from case reports makes it difficult to provide guidelines or recommendations.

Surgical prophylaxis – [3] = Safety concerns. The use of vancomycin as prophylaxis is suitable as monotherapy for surgical procedures, including joint replacement, cardiothoracic operations, or general, vascular, and neurosurgical operations with implants in patients with a beta-lactam allergy or when exposure to methicillin-resistant *Staphylococcus aureus* and/or *S. epidermidis* is suspected. Reports of emerging resistance have significantly altered attitudes toward the use of vancomycin prophylaxis in surgery. As a consequence, recent guidelines for prevention of surgical-site infections strongly recommend avoiding the routine use of vancomycin as a first-line agent. Further study and research are needed to determine strategies to minimize the emergence of vancomycin-resistant bacteria.

VANCOMYCIN HYDROCHLORIDE — INJECTION

Administration and Dosage

➤*General dosing considerations:* Administer over at least 60 minutes. Infusion-related events are related to concentration and rate of administration of vancomycin. Concentrations of no more than 5 mg/mL and rates of no more than 10 mg/min are recommended in adults. In selected patients in need of fluid restriction, a concentration of up to 10 mg/mL may be used; use of such higher concentrations may increase the risk of infusion-related events. Infusion-related events may occur, however, at any rate or concentration.

Other patient factors, such as age or obesity, may call for modification of the usual daily dose.

➤*Adults:*

Endocarditis – 2 g intravenously (IV) divided as 500 mg every 6 hours or 1 g every 12 hours. Administer at a rate of no faster than 10 mg/min, or over at least 60 minutes, whichever is longer.

Pseudomembranous colitis/Staphylococcal enterocolitis –500 mg to 2 g orally daily given in 3 or 4 divided doses for 7 to 10 days. (See Preparation for Administration and Administration.)

Staphylococcal infections – 2 g IV divided as 500 mg every 6 hours or 1 g every 12 hours. Administer at a rate of no faster than 10 mg/min, or over at least 60 minutes, whichever is longer.

Off-label dosing –

Aerosolization: [4] = Insufficient documentation.

• *Dosage* – 120 mg (1 mL) every 6 hours via face mask.

Alternative dosing: [1] = Good documentation. The use of vancomycin has been included in therapeutic monitoring guidelines published in a consensus review of the American Society of Health-System Pharmacists, the Infectious Diseases Society of America, and the Society of Infectious Diseases Pharmacists. (Also see Therapeutic Drug Monitoring for more information.)

• *Usual dose* – Per consensus guidelines, IV daily doses of 15 to 20 mg/kg (as actual body weight) should be administered every 8 to 12 hours in patients with healthy renal function when the minimum inhibitory concentration (MIC) is 1 mg/L or less.

• *Complicated infections* – In complicated infections, consensus guidelines recommend a loading dose of 25 to 30 mg/kg (based on actual body weight) to rapidly achieve target trough serum concentrations of vancomycin.

• *Hospital-acquired pneumonia* – American Thoracic Society guidelines recommend 15 mg/kg every 12 hours in adults with healthy renal function.

Preoperative antimicrobial prophylaxis: For genitourinary and GI tract (excluding esophageal) procedures, the preoperative dose of vancomycin is 1 g IV given over 1 to 2 hours plus gentamicin 1.5 mg/kg (up to 120 mg) IV or intramuscularly (IM). Complete the infusion/injection within 30 minutes of starting the procedure. This regimen is indicated for high-risk patients allergic to ampicillin or amoxicillin. For moderate-risk patients allergic to ampicillin or amoxicillin, the regimen excludes gentamicin.

Rectal administration: [4] = Insufficient documentation. Varied doses ranging from initial doses of 1 to 2 g and maintenance dosing of 100 to 500 mg every 6 hours. In a review of pseudomembranous colitis, one author recommends vancomycin IV (at least 2 g/day) along with vancomycin enemas every 8 hours (500 mg/L of normal saline solution). Administration is recommended as an enema or with a *Bardex* catheter (as with a barium enema) if the patient is unable to retain the enema.

Surgical prophylaxis: [3] = Safety concerns. 1 g IV over 60 minutes, administered 60 to 120 minutes before incision.

➤*Children:*

Endocarditis –

1 month of age and older: 10 mg/kg/dose IV given every 6 hours. Administer over at least 60 minutes.

Up to 1 month of age: The total daily IV dosage may be lower. An initial dose of 15 mg/kg is suggested, followed by 10 mg/kg every 12 hours for neonates in the first week of life and every 8 hours thereafter up to the age of 1 month. Administer over 60 minutes. In premature infants, vancomycin clearance decreases as postconceptional age decreases. Therefore, longer dosing intervals may be necessary in premature infants.

Pseudomembranous colitis/Staphylococcal enterocolitis –

Usual dosage: 40 mg/kg/day given orally in 3 or 4 divided doses for 7 to 10 days. (See Preparation for Administration and Administration.)

Maximum dose: 2 g/day.

Staphylococcal infections –

1 month of age and older: 10 mg/kg/dose IV given every 6 hours. Administer over at least 60 minutes.

Up to 1 month of age: The total daily IV dosage may be lower. An initial dose of 15 mg/kg is suggested, followed by 10 mg/kg every 12 hours for neonates in the first week of life and every 8 hours thereafter up to the age of 1 month. Administer over 60 minutes. In premature infants, vancomycin clearance decreases as postconceptional age decreases. Therefore, longer dosing intervals may be necessary in premature infants.

Off-label dosing –

Infants and children:

• *Severe infections including CNS infections (meningitis)* –

Usual dosage: 10 to 15 mg/kg IV every 6 hours. For meningitis, the dosage is 15 mg/kg IV every 6 hours.

Maximum dose: 1 g/dose (4 g/day).

• *Mild to moderate infections* –

Usual dosage: 40 mg/kg/day IV in divided doses every 6 to 8 hours.

Maximum dose: 1 g/dose (2 g/day).

Neonates: Optimal dosage should be based on serum concentrations, especially in neonates with low birth weight (less than 1.5 kg). For neonates with very low birth weight (less than 1.2 kg), dosing every 18 to 24 hours may be appropriate for the first 7 days of life.

• *0 to 4 weeks of age and weighing less than 1.2 kg* – 15 mg/kg IV every 24 hours.

• *Younger than 1 week of age* –

Body weight 1.2 to 2 kg: 10 to 15 mg/kg IV every 12 to 18 hours.

Body weight more than 2 kg: 10 to 15 mg/kg IV every 8 to 12 hours.

• *1 week of age and older* –

Body weight 1.2 to 2 kg: 10 to 15 mg/kg IV every 8 to 12 hours.

Body weight more than 2 kg: 10 to 15 mg/kg IV every 6 or 8 hours.

Aerosolization: [4] = Insufficient documentation.

• *Dosage* – 250 mg per 4 mL per 10 minutes every 12 hours, 40 mg 3 times/day for 72 hours, 4 mg/kg/dose 4 times/day for 5 days.

Central venous catheter infection: Add 25 mg/mL of vancomycin to the parenteral nutrition solution and administer as a continuous infusion or as a flush/lock.

Preoperative antimicrobial prophylaxis: For cardiac surgery (prosthetic valve or pacemaker), neurosurgery (craniotomy), and orthopedic surgery (internal fixation of fractures or prosthetic joints), the preoperative dose of vancomycin is 10 mg/kg IV if the likely pathogens include methicillin-resistant *Staphylococcal aureus* or methicillin-resistant *S. epidermidis*.

For genitourinary and GI tract (excluding esophageal) procedures, the preoperative dose of vancomycin is 20 mg/kg IV given over 1 to 2 hours plus gentamicin 1.5 mg/kg IV or IM. Complete the infusion/injection within 30 minutes of starting the procedure. This regimen is indicated for high-risk patients allergic to ampicillin or amoxicillin. For moderate-risk patients allergic to ampicillin or amoxicillin, the regimen excludes gentamicin.

Ventricular shunt infection: Systemic vancomycin is generally given at a dosage of 15 mg/kg IV every 6 hours. Also, administer vancomycin 10 mg/day (50 mg/mL diluted with normal saline to a final concentration of 5 mg/mL) directly into the ventricle (if the shunt is not externalized) or into the externalized shunt, which is then clamped for 1 hour after administration.

➤*Elderly:* Vancomycin dosage schedules should be adjusted in elderly patients. Greater dosage reductions than expected may be necessary because of decreased renal function.

➤*Renal function impairment:* Dosage adjustment must be made in patients with impaired renal function. In premature infants and elderly patients, greater dosage reductions than expected may be necessary because of decreased renal function. Measurement of vancomycin serum concentrations can be helpful in optimizing therapy, especially in seriously ill patients with changing renal function.

Vancomycin is not effectively removed by hemodialysis or peritoneal dialysis; there have been no reports of vancomycin clearance with hemoperfusion.

If creatinine clearance (CrCl) can be measured or estimated accurately, the dosage for most patients with renal impairment can be calculated using the following data. The dosage of vancomycin hydrochloride/day in milligrams is about 15 times the glomerular filtration rate (GFR) in mL/min.

Vancomycin Dosage for Patients With Impaired Renal Function

CrCl	Dose
100 mL/min	1,545 mg per 24 h
90 mL/min	1,390 mg per 24 h
80 mL/min	1,235 mg per 24 h
70 mL/min	1,080 mg per 24 h
60 mL/min	925 mg per 24 h
50 mL/min	770 mg per 24 h
40 mL/min	620 mg per 24 h
30 mL/min	465 mg per 24 h
20 mL/min	310 mg per 24 h
10 mL/min	155 mg per 24 h

In patients with marked renal impairment, it may be more convenient to give maintenance doses of 250 to 1,000 mg once every several days rather than administering the drug on a daily basis.

Initial dosage – The initial dose should be no less than 15 mg/kg, even in patients with mild to moderate renal insufficiency.

Alternative dosage –

Adults:

• *GFR more than 50 mL/min* – 1 g every 12 to 24 h.

• *GFR 10 to 50 mL/min* – 1 g every 24 to 96 h.

• *GFR less than 10 mL/min* – 1 g every 4 to 7 days.

• *Hemodialysis/Peritoneal dialysis* – 1 g every 4 to 7 days.

• *Continuous renal replacement therapy* – 1 g every 12 to 24 h.

Children:

• *GFR 30 to 50 mL/min per 1.73 m^2* – 10 mg/kg every 12 h.

• *GFR 10 to 29 mL/min per 1.73 m^2* – 10 mg/kg every 18 to 24 h.

• *GFR less than 10 mL/min per 1.73 m^2* – 10 mg/kg as needed per serum concentration monitoring.

• *Hemodialysis* – 10 mg/kg as needed per serum concentration monitoring.

• *Peritoneal dialysis* – 10 mg/kg as needed per serum concentration monitoring or loading dose 500 mg/L and maintenance dose 30 mg/L.

• *Continuous renal replacement therapy* – 10 mg/kg every 12 to 24 h as needed per serum concentration monitoring.

VANCOMYCIN HYDROCHLORIDE — INJECTION

Anephric patients – For functionally anephric patients, an initial dose of 15 mg/kg should be given to achieve prompt therapeutic serum concentrations. The dose required to maintain stable concentrations is 1.9 mg/kg every 24 hours.

Anuria – 1,000 mg every 7 to 10 days has been recommended.

➤*Preparation for administration:*

Powder for IV infusion solution – At the time of use, reconstitute by adding 10 mL of sterile water for injection to the 500 mg vial, 15 mL of sterile water for injection to the 750 mg vial, 20 mL of sterile water for injection to the 1 g vial, 100 mL of sterile water for injection to the 5 g pharmacy bulk package, or 95 mL of sterile water for injection to the 10 g pharmacy bulk package of dry, sterile vancomycin powder. Reconstituted solutions of the 5 g pharmacy bulk package contain 500 mg per 10 mL and reconstituted solutions of the 10 g pharmacy bulk package contain 1 g per 10 mL. Further dilution is required.

Reconstituted solutions containing 500 mg of vancomycin must be diluted with at least 100 mL of diluent. Reconstituted solutions containing 750 mg of vancomycin must be diluted with at least 150 mL of diluent. Reconstituted solutions containing 1 g of vancomycin must be diluted with at least 200 mL of diluent. The desired dose, diluted in this manner, should be administered by intermittent IV infusion over a period of at least 60 minutes.

Pharmacy bulk packages: Pharmacy bulk package is for use in the hospital pharmacy admixture service. Use of this product is restricted to a suitable work area, such as a laminar flow hood. Using aseptic technique, the closure should be penetrated 1 time using a suitable sterile transfer device or dispensing set, which allows measured distribution of the contents. Use of a syringe and needle is not recommended as it may cause leakage. Once the sterile dispensing set has been inserted into the container, withdrawal of the contents of the pharmacy bulk package bottle should be completed within 4 hours after entry. This time limit should begin with the introduction of solvent or dilution into the pharmacy bulk package bottle.

Galaxy containers – Thaw frozen containers at room temperature (25°C [77°F]) or under refrigeration (5°C [41°F]). Do not force thaw by immersion in water baths or by microwave irradiation. Check for minute leaks by squeezing the bag firmly. If leaks are detected, discard solution because sterility may be impaired. Do not add supplementary medication. Visually inspect the container for particulate matter and discoloration. Components of the solution may precipitate in the frozen state and should dissolve with little or no agitation after the solution has reached room temperature. Potency is not affected. If, after visual inspection, the solution is discolored or remains cloudy, an insoluble precipitate is noted, or any seals or outlet ports are not intact, the container should be discarded.

Oral administration – Certain parenteral products may be administered orally (check the manufacturers' package inserts). The appropriate dose may be diluted in 1 oz of water and given to the patient to drink. Common flavoring syrups may be added to the solution to improve the taste. The diluted solution may also be administered via a nasogastric tube. Vancomycin in the *Galaxy* container is not to be administered orally.

➤*Administration:* Intermittent infusion is the recommended method of administration. Vancomycin is irritating to tissue and must be given by a secure IV route of administration. Pain, tenderness, and necrosis occur with IM injection of vancomycin or with inadvertent extravasation. Thrombophlebitis may occur, the frequency and severity of which can be minimized by administering the drug slowly and by rotating the sites of venous access. Vancomycin has been administered by intravitreal injection (off-label use).

The safety and efficacy of vancomycin administration by the intraperitoneal and intrathecal (intralumbar or intraventricular) routes have not been assessed. Chemical peritonitis has been reported following intraperitoneal administration of vancomycin during continuous ambulatory peritoneal dialysis. (See also Warnings/Precautions.)

During or soon after rapid infusion of vancomycin, patients may develop anaphylactoid reactions, including hypotension, wheezing, dyspnea, urticaria, or pruritus. Rapid infusion may also cause flushing of the upper body ("red neck" or "red man syndrome") or pain and muscle spasms of the chest and back. These reactions usually resolve within 20 minutes but may persist for several hours. Such events are infrequent if vancomycin is given by a slow infusion over 60 minutes. To help prevent "red man syndrome," consider lengthening the infusion time to 120 minutes and/or administer an antihistamine (eg, diphenhydramine) prior to the vancomycin infusion.

Adults – Administer vancomycin in concentrations of no more than 5 mg/mL and at rates of no more than 10 mg/min or over a period of at least 60 minutes, whichever is longer. In selected patients in need of fluid restriction, a concentration of up to 10 mg/mL may be used; use of such higher concentrations may increase the risk of infusion-related events.

Children – Administer over at least 60 minutes.

➤*Admixture compatibility:*

Compatibility – The following diluents are physically and chemically compatible with vancomycin: dextrose 5% injection, dextrose 5% injection and sodium chloride 0.9% injection, Ringer's lactate injection, dextrose 5% and Ringer's lactate injection, *Normosol-M* and dextrose 5%, sodium chloride 0.9% injection, and*Isolyte E*. (See also Storage/Stability.)

Incompatibility – Mixtures of solutions of vancomycin and beta-lactam antibiotics have been shown to be physically incompatible. The likelihood of precipitation increases with higher concentrations of vancomycin. It is recommended to adequately flush the IV lines between the administration of these antibiotics. It is also recommended to dilute solutions of vancomycin to 5 mg/mL or less.

Vancomycin solution has a low pH and may cause physical instability of other compounds.

Although intravitreal injection is not an approved route of administration for vancomycin, precipitation has been reported after intravitreal injection of vancomycin and ceftazidime for endophthalmitis using different syringes and needles. The precipitates dissolved gradually, with complete clearing of the vitreous cavity over 2 months and with improvement of visual acuity. To screen for specific compatibilities, see *Trissel's IV-Chek*.

➤*Storage / Stability:*

Galaxy containers – Store *Galaxy* containers in a freezer capable of maintaining a temperature at or below −20°C (−4°F). The thawed solution in *Galaxy* plastic containers remains chemically stable for 72 hours at room temperature (25°C [77°F]) or for 30 days when stored under refrigeration (5°C [41°F]). Do not refreeze thawed antibiotics.

Vials – Store at 20° to 25°C (68° to 77°F). After initial reconstitution with sterile water for injection, dextrose 5% injection, or sodium chloride 0.9% injection, solutions are stable for 14 days if refrigerated. After further dilution with dextrose 5% injection or sodium chloride 0.9% injection, the solution may be stored in a refrigerator for 14 days without significant loss of potency. Solutions diluted with dextrose 5% and sodium chloride 0.9% injection, Ringer's lactate injection, Ringer's lactate injection and dextrose 5% injection, *Isolyte E*, or *Normosol-M* and dextrose 5% may be stored in a refrigerator for 96 hours.

Pharmacy bulk packages – Store at 20° to 25°C (68° to 77°F). Discard pharmacy bulk packages no later than 4 hours after initial closure puncture.

Actions

➤*Pharmacology:* The bactericidal action of vancomycin results primarily from inhibition of cell-wall biosynthesis. In addition, vancomycin alters bacterial cell membrane permeability and RNA synthesis. There is no cross-resistance between vancomycin and other antibiotics.

➤*Pharmacokinetics:*

Absorption – Vancomycin is poorly absorbed after oral administration. In subjects with healthy kidney function, multiple IV dosing of vancomycin 1 g (15 mg/kg) infused over 60 minutes produces mean plasma concentrations of approximately 63 mcg/mL immediately after the completion of infusion, mean plasma concentrations of approximately 23 mcg/mL 2 hours after infusion, and mean plasma concentrations of approximately 8 mcg/mL 11 hours after the end of the infusion. Multiple dosing of 500 mg infused over 30 minutes produces mean plasma concentrations of about 49 mcg/mL at the completion of infusion, mean plasma concentrations of about 19 mcg/mL 2 hours after infusion, and mean plasma concentrations of about 10 mcg/mL 6 hours after infusion. The plasma concentrations during multiple dosing are similar to those after a single dose.

Distribution – Vancomycin is approximately 55% serum protein bound as measured by ultrafiltration at vancomycin serum concentrations of 10 to 100 mcg/mL. After IV administration of vancomycin, inhibitory concentrations are present in pleural, pericardial, ascitic, and synovial fluids; in urine; in peritoneal dialysis fluid; and in atrial appendage tissue. Vancomycin does not readily diffuse across healthy meninges into the spinal fluid, but, when the meninges are inflamed, penetration into the spinal fluid occurs.

Metabolism / Excretion – The mean elimination half-life of vancomycin from plasma is 4 to 6 hours in subjects with healthy renal function. In the first 24 hours, about 75% of an administered dose of vancomycin is excreted in urine by glomerular filtration. Mean plasma clearance is about 0.058 L/kg/h, and mean renal clearance is about 0.048 L/kg/h. The distribution coefficient is from 0.3 to 0.43 L/kg. There is no apparent metabolism of the drug.

Special populations –

Renal function impairment: Renal dysfunction slows excretion of vancomycin. In anephric patients, the average half-life of elimination is 7.5 days. About 60% of an intraperitoneal dose of vancomycin administered during peritoneal dialysis is absorbed systemically in 6 hours. Vancomycin is not effectively removed by hemodialysis or peritoneal dialysis; there have been no reports of vancomycin clearance with hemoperfusion. Dosage adjustment required in patients with renal function impairment.

Elderly: Total systemic and renal clearance of vancomycin may be reduced in elderly patients.

Intraperitoneal injection: Serum concentrations of about 10 mcg/mL are achieved by intraperitoneal injection of vancomycin 30 mg/kg. However, the safety and efficacy of the intraperitoneal use of vancomycin have not been established in adequate and well-controlled trials.

➤*Microbiology:*

Synergy – The combination of vancomycin and an aminoglycoside acts synergistically in vitro against many strains of *Staphylococcus aureus*, *S. bovis*, enterococci, and the viridans group streptococci.

Vancomycin has been shown to be active against most strains of the following microorganisms, in vitro and in clinical infections described in the Indications section.

Aerobic gram-positive microorganisms – Diphtheroids, enterococci (eg, *Enterococcus faecalis*), staphylococci, including *S. aureus* and *S. epidermidis* (including heterogeneous methicillin-resistant strains), *S. bovis*, and viridans group streptococci.

Contraindications

Hypersensitivity to vancomycin; solutions containing dextrose may be contraindicated in patients with known allergy to corn or corn products (premixed *Galaxy* containers only).

Warnings/Precautions

➤*Resistance:* Prescribing vancomycin in the absence of a proven or strongly suspected bacterial infection or a prophylactic indication is unlikely to provide benefit to the patient and increases the risk of the development of drug-resistant bacteria.

VANCOMYCIN HYDROCHLORIDE — INJECTION

➤*Administration:* Rapid bolus administration (eg, over several minutes) may be associated with exaggerated hypotension, including shock and, rarely, cardiac arrest. (See also Hypersensitivity.)

Administer vancomycin over a period of not less than 60 minutes to avoid rapid-infusion-related reactions. Stopping the infusion usually results in prompt cessation of these reactions.

➤*Ototoxicity:* Ototoxicity has occurred in patients receiving vancomycin. It may be transient or permanent. It has been reported mostly in patients who have been given excessive doses, who have an underlying hearing loss, or who are receiving concomitant therapy with another ototoxic agent, such as an aminoglycoside. Serial tests of auditory function may be helpful in order to minimize the risk of ototoxicity.

➤*C. difficile-associated diarrhea:* *C. difficile*–associated diarrhea has been reported with nearly all antibacterial agents, including vancomycin, and may range in severity from mild diarrhea to fatal colitis. Therefore, it is important to consider this diagnosis in patients who present with diarrhea subsequent to the administration of antibacterial agents.

C. difficile produces toxins A and B, which contribute to the development of *C. difficile*–associated diarrhea. Hypertoxin-producing strains of *C. difficile* cause increased morbidity and mortality because these infections can be refractory to antimicrobial therapy and may require colectomy. Careful medical history is necessary because *C. difficile*–associated diarrhea has been reported to occur over 2 months after administration of antibacterial agents.

If *C. difficile*–associated diarrhea is suspected or confirmed, ongoing antibiotic use not directed against *C. difficile* may need to be discontinued. Institute appropriate fluid and electrolyte management, protein supplementation, antibiotic treatment of *C. difficile*, and surgical evaluation, as clinically indicated.

In rare instances, there have been reports of pseudomembranous colitis because of *C. difficile* developing in patients who received IV vancomycin.

Clinically significant serum concentrations have been reported in some patients being treated for active *C. difficile*–induced pseudomembranous colitis after multiple oral doses of vancomycin.

➤*Neutropenia:* Reversible neutropenia, usually starting 1 week or more after onset of therapy with vancomycin or after a total dosage of more than 25 g, has been reported in patients receiving vancomycin. Periodically monitor the leukocyte count of patients who will undergo prolonged therapy with vancomycin or those who are receiving concomitant drugs that may cause neutropenia.

➤*Tissue irritation:* Vancomycin is irritating to tissue and must be given by a secure IV route of administration. Pain, tenderness, and necrosis occur with IM injection of vancomycin or with inadvertent extravasation. Thrombophlebitis may occur, the frequency and severity of which can be minimized by administering the drug slowly and by rotating the sites of venous access.

➤*Intraperitoneal and intrathecal routes:* The safety and efficacy of vancomycin administration by the intraperitoneal and intrathecal (intralumbar or intraventricular) routes have not been established by adequate and well-controlled trials.

Although the safety and efficacy of sterile vancomycin by the intraperitoneal route have not been established, reports reveal that the product has been given by this route during continuous ambulatory peritoneal dialysis (CAPD). Administration of sterile vancomycin by the intraperitoneal route during CAPD has resulted in more than 50 reports of chemical peritonitis that developed in some patients within the 12-hour period after administration. To date, all have been self-limited and ranged from cloudy dialysate alone to severe abdominal pain and fever. Most cloudy dialysates were sterile, and some contained increased numbers of white blood cells and polymorphonuclear cells. Fluids usually cleared promptly after discontinuation of the sterile vancomycin.

➤*Hypersensitivity reactions:* During or soon after the rapid infusion of vancomycin, patients may develop anaphylactoid reactions, including dyspnea, hypotension, pruritus, urticaria, or wheezing. Rapid infusion may also cause flushing of the upper body ("red neck") or pain and muscle spasm of the chest and back. These reactions usually resolve within 20 minutes but may persist for several hours. Such reactions are infrequent if vancomycin is given by a slow infusion over 60 minutes. In studies of healthy volunteers, infusion-related reactions did not occur when vancomycin was administered at a rate of 10 mg/min or less.

➤*Renal function impairment:* Use vancomycin with caution in patients with renal insufficiency because the risk of toxicity is appreciably increased by high, prolonged blood concentrations.

See Administration and Dosage for more information.

To minimize the risk of nephrotoxicity when treating patients with underlying renal dysfunction or patients receiving concomitant therapy with an aminoglycoside, perform serial monitoring of renal function and take particular care in following appropriate dosing schedules.

➤*Superinfection:* Prolonged use of vancomycin may result in the overgrowth of nonsusceptible organisms. Careful observation of the patient is essential. If superinfection occurs during therapy, take appropriate measures.

➤*Pregnancy:* *Category C* per manufacturer's prescribing information, *Category B* per Briggs' *Drugs in Pregnancy and Lactation*. The human pregnancy experience with vancomycin is adequate to demonstrate that the embryofetal risk is very low or nonexistent. In a controlled clinical study, the potential ototoxic and nephrotoxic effects of vancomycin on infants were evaluated when the drug was administered to pregnant women for serious staphylococcal infections that were complications of their IV drug abuse. Vancomycin was found in cord blood. No sensorineural hearing loss or nephrotoxicity attributable to vancomycin was noted. One infant whose mother received vancomycin in the third trimester experienced conductive hearing loss that was not attributed to the administration of vancomycin. Because the number of patients treated in this study was limited and vancomycin was administered only in the second and third trimesters, manufacturers state that it is not known whether vancomycin causes fetal harm. Give vancomycin to a pregnant woman only if clearly needed.

➤*Lactation:* Vancomycin is excreted in human milk. Vancomycin is poorly absorbed from the GI tract and, therefore, systemic absorption is not likely. According to the manufacturers, exercise caution when vancomycin is administered to a breast-feeding woman. However, according to limited data, vancomycin is not expected to cause adverse effects on a breast-feeding infant and special precautions are not required. Because of the potential for adverse reactions, decide whether to discontinue breast-feeding or the drug, taking into account the importance of the drug to the mother.

➤*Children:* In children, it may be appropriate to confirm desired vancomycin serum concentrations. Coadministration of vancomycin and anesthetic agents has been associated with erythema and histamine-like flushing in children. The potential for toxic effects in children from chemicals that may leach from the plastic containers into the single-dose, premixed IV preparation has not been determined.

➤*Elderly:* See Administration and Dosage for more information.

➤*Monitoring:* To minimize the risk of nephrotoxicity when treating patients with underlying renal dysfunction or patients receiving concomitant therapy with an aminoglycoside, perform serial monitoring of renal function and take particular care in following appropriate dosing schedules.

Serial tests of auditory function may be helpful in order to minimize the risk of ototoxicity.

Periodically monitor the leukocyte count of patients who will undergo prolonged therapy with vancomycin or those who are receiving concomitant drugs that may cause neutropenia.

Consensus review monitoring guidelines state that trough serum concentrations are the most reliable and recommended method for monitoring efficacy and toxicity and should be obtained immediately prior to the next dose at steady-state conditions (approximately after the fourth dose). Always maintain trough concentrations above 10 mg/L to avoid development of resistance. However, the minimum trough concentration should be higher (at least 15 mg/L) to generate a target AUC/MIC of 400 when the MIC is 1 mg/L. In complicated infections (eg, endocarditis, osteomyelitis, meningitis, hospital-acquired pneumonia related to *S. aureus*), higher serum trough concentrations (15 to 20 mg/L) are recommended to improve penetrations and optimize clinical outcomes.

Close monitoring of serum concentrations may be warranted in children.

ATS guidelines recommend trough levels of 15 to 20 mg/L for hospital-acquired pneumonia.

Drug Interactions

Vancomycin Drug Interactions

Precipitant drug	Object drug[a]		Description
Indomethacin	Vancomycin	⬆	Indomethacin may increase the effects of vancomycin in neonates. Monitor closely.
Nephrotoxic/ Neurotoxic drugs (eg, aminoglycosides, amphotericin B, bacitracin, cisplatin, colistin,[b] polymyxin B, viomycin[b])	Vancomycin	⬆	The risk of toxicity may be increased with coadministration. Monitor renal function and serum drug concentrations with coadministration.
Vancomycin	Nephrotoxic/ Neurotoxic drugs (eg, aminoglycosides, amphotericin B, bacitracin, cisplatin, colistin,[b] polymyxin B, viomycin[b])		
Vancomycin	Anesthetics	⬆	Concomitant use has been associated with erythema and histamine-like flushing in children. Infusion-related reactions may be minimized by the administration of vancomycin as a 60-minute infusion prior to anesthetic induction.
Vancomycin	Methotrexate	⬆	Plasma concentration and pharmacologic effects of methotrexate may be increased by vancomycin. Monitor renal function and adjust methotrexate dosage as needed.

VANCOMYCIN HYDROCHLORIDE — INJECTION

Vancomycin Drug Interactions			
Precipitant drug	Object drug[a]		Description
Vancomycin	Nondepolarizing muscle relaxants (eg, vecuronium)	↑	Neuromuscular blockade of nondepolarizing muscle relaxants may be enhanced. Avoid this combination if possible. When necessary, monitor neuromuscular function closely, titrate the dose of nondepolarizing muscle relaxant, and be prepared to provide mechanical respiratory support as needed.

[a] ↑ = object drug increased.
[b] Drug is no longer marketed in the United States.

Adverse Reactions

For more information on administration-related adverse reactions, ototoxicity, *C. difficile*–associated diarrhea, neutropenia, tissue irritation, or hypersensitivity, see Warnings/Precautions.

➤*GI:* See Warnings/Precautions for more information.

➤*Hematologic:* Reversible neutropenia, usually starting 1 week or more after onset of therapy with vancomycin or after a total dosage of more than 25 g, has been reported for several dozen patients. Neutropenia appears to be promptly reversible when vancomycin is discontinued. Thrombocytopenia has rarely been reported.

Although a causal relationship has not been established, reversible agranulocytosis (granulocytes less than 500/mm^3) has been reported rarely.

➤*Hypersensitivity:* See Warnings/Precautions for more information.

➤*Local:* Inflammation at the injection site has been reported.

➤*Renal:* Rarely, renal failure, principally manifested by increased serum creatinine or serum urea nitrogen concentrations, especially in patients given large doses of vancomycin, has been reported. Rare cases of interstitial nephritis have been reported. Most of these have occurred in patients who were given aminoglycosides concomitantly or who had preexisting kidney dysfunction. When vancomycin was discontinued, azotemia resolved in most patients.

➤*Special senses:* A few dozen cases of hearing loss associated with vancomycin have been reported. Most of these patients had kidney dysfunction or a preexisting hearing loss or were receiving concomitant treatment with an ototoxic drug. Dizziness, tinnitus, and vertigo have been reported rarely.

➤*Miscellaneous:* Infrequently, patients have been reported to have had anaphylaxis, chills, drug fever, eosinophilia, nausea, rashes (including exfoliative dermatitis), Stevens-Johnson syndrome, toxic epidermal necrolysis, and vasculitis in association with administration of vancomycin. See Warnings/Precautions for more information.

➤*Postmarketing:*

Dermatologic – Drug rash with eosinophilia and systemic symptoms.

Overdosage

➤*Treatment:* Supportive care is advised, with maintenance of glomerular filtration. Vancomycin is poorly removed by dialysis. Hemofiltration and hemoperfusion with polysulfone resin have been reported to result in increased vancomycin clearance.

Patient Information

Counsel patients that antibacterial drugs, including vancomycin, should only be used to treat bacterial infections. They do not treat viral infections (eg, the common cold). When vancomycin is prescribed to treat a bacterial infection, tell patients that although it is common to feel better early in the course of therapy, they should take the medication exactly as directed. Skipping doses or not completing the full course of therapy may decrease the effectiveness of the immediate treatment, and increase the likelihood that bacteria will develop resistance and will not be treatable by vancomycin or other antibacterial drugs in the future.

Diarrhea is a common problem caused by antibiotics which usually ends when the antibiotic is discontinued. Sometimes after starting treatment with antibiotics, patients can develop watery and bloody stools (with or without stomach cramps and fever) even as late as 2 or more months after having taken the last dose of the antibiotic. If this occurs, advise patients to contact their health care provider as soon as possible.

LIPOGLYCOPEPTIDES

TELAVANCIN

Rx	**Vibativ** (Astellas)	**Injection, lyophilized powder for solution:** 250 mg[a]	As telavancin hydrochloride. Preservative free. In single-dose vials.
		Injection, lyophilized powder for solution: 750 mg[b]	As telavancin hydrochloride. Preservative free. In single-dose vials.

[a] Contains hydroxypropyl-beta-cyclodextrin 2,500 mg and mannitol 312.5 mg per vial.
[b] Contains hydroxypropyl-beta-cyclodextrin 7,500 mg and mannitol 937.5 mg per vial.

TELAVANCIN HYDROCHLORIDE — INJECTION

WARNING

Fetal risk – Women of childbearing potential should have a serum pregnancy test prior to administration of telavancin.

Avoid use of telavancin during pregnancy unless the potential benefit to the patient outweighs the potential risk to the fetus.

Adverse developmental outcomes observed in 3 animal species at clinically relevant doses raise concerns about potential adverse developmental outcomes in humans.

Indications

➤*Complicated skin and skin structure infections:* For the treatment of adults with complicated skin and skin structure infections caused by susceptible isolates of the following gram-positive microorganisms: *Staphylococcus aureus* (including methicillin-susceptible and methicillin-resistant isolates), *Streptococcus pyogenes*, *Streptococcus agalactiae*, *Streptococcus anginosus* group (includes *S. anginosus*, *S. intermedius*, and *S. constellatus*), or *Enterococcus faecalis* (vancomycin-susceptible isolates only).

Combination therapy may be clinically indicated if the documented or presumed pathogens include gram-negative organisms.

Administration and Dosage

➤*General dosing considerations:* The duration of therapy should be guided by the severity and site of the infection and the patient's clinical and bacteriological progress.

Dosage adjustment required in patients whose creatinine clearance (CrCl) is 50 mL/min or less. (See Renal Function Impairment.)

➤*Adults:*

Complicated skin and skin structure infections – 10 mg/kg administered by intravenous (IV) infusion over 60 minutes once every 24 hours for 7 to 14 days.

➤*Renal function impairment:*

Telavancin Dosage Adjustment in Adults With Renal Impairment	
CrCl[a] (mL/min)	Telavancin dosage regimen
> 50	10 mg/kg every 24 hours
30 to 50	7.5 mg/kg every 24 hours
10 to ≤ 30	10 mg/kg every 48 hours

[a] As calculated using the Cockcroft-Gault formula.

➤*Preparation for administration:*

250 mg vial – Reconstitute the contents of a telavancin 250 mg vial with 15 mL of dextrose 5% injection, sterile water for injection, or sodium chloride 0.9% injection. The resultant solution has a concentration of 15 mg/mL (total volume of approximately 17 mL).

750 mg vial – Reconstitute the contents of a telavancin 750 mg vial with 45 mL of dextrose 5% injection, sterile water for injection, or sodium chloride 0.9% injection. The resultant solution has a concentration of 15 mg/mL (total volume of approximately 50 mL).

For doses of 150 to 800 mg, the appropriate volume of reconstituted solution must be further diluted in 100 to 250 mL prior to infusion. Doses less than 150 mg or greater than 800 mg should be further diluted in a volume resulting in a final concentration of 0.6 to 8 mg/mL. Appropriate infusion solutions include dextrose 5% injection, sodium chloride 0.9% injection, or lactated Ringer's injection.

Reconstitution time is generally less than 2 minutes, but can sometimes take up to 20 minutes. Mix thoroughly to reconstitute and check to see if the contents have dissolved completely. Discard the vial if the vacuum did not pull the diluent into the vial.

➤*Administration:* Administer by IV infusion over a period of 60 minutes.

➤*Admixture compatibility:* Additives or other medications should not be added to telavancin single-use vials or infused simultaneously through the same IV line. If the same IV line is used for sequential infusion of additional medications, the line should be flushed before and after infusion of telavancin with dextrose 5% injection, sodium chloride 0.9% injection, or lactated Ringer's injection.

➤*Storage/Stability:* Store at 2° to 8°C (35° to 46°F). Excursions up to 25°C (77°F) are acceptable. Avoid excessive heat. The reconstituted solution in the vial should be used within 4 hours when stored at room temperature or within 72 hours under refrigeration at 2° to 8°C (36° to 46°F). The diluted (dosing) solution in the infusion bag should be used within 4 hours when stored at room temperature or used within 72 hours when stored under refrigeration at 2° to 8°C (36° to 46°F). The total time in the vial plus the

TELAVANCIN HYDROCHLORIDE — INJECTION

time in the infusion bag should not exceed 4 hours at room temperature and 72 hours under refrigeration at 2° to 8°C (36° to 46°F).

Actions

➤*Pharmacology:* Telavancin is a semisynthetic lipoglycopeptide antibacterial that is a synthetic derivative of vancomycin. Telavancin inhibits bacterial cell wall synthesis by interfering with the polymerization and cross-linking of peptidoglycan. Telavancin binds to the bacterial membrane and disrupts membrane barrier function.

➤*Pharmacokinetics:*

Telavancin Pharmacokinetic Parameters[a]		
	10 mg/kg single dose (n = 42)	10 mg/kg multiple dose (n = 36)
C_{max} (mcg/mL)	93.6 ± 14.2	108 ± 26
$AUC_{0-\infty}$ (mcg•h/mL)	747 ± 129	—[b]
AUC_{0-24h} (mcg•h/mL)	666 ± 107	780 ± 125
Half-life (h)	8 ± 1.5	8.1 ± 1.5
Cl (mL/h/kg)	13.9 ± 2.9	13.1 ± 2
V_{ss} (mL/kg)	145 ± 23	133 ± 24

[a] C_{max} = maximum plasma concentration; Cl = clearance; V_{ss} = apparent volume of distribution at steady state.
[b] Data not available.

Absorption – In healthy young adults, the pharmacokinetics of telavancin administered IV were linear following single doses from 5 to 12.5 mg/kg and multiple doses from 7.5 to 15 mg/kg administered once daily for up to 7 days. Steady-state concentrations were achieved by the third daily dose.

Distribution – Telavancin binds to human plasma proteins, primarily to serum albumin, in a concentration-independent manner. The mean binding is approximately 90% and is not affected by renal or hepatic impairment.

Concentrations of telavancin in skin blister fluid were 40% of those in plasma (AUC_{0-24h} ratio) after 3 daily doses of telavancin 7.5 mg/kg in healthy young adults.

Metabolism –

In a mass balance study in men using radiolabeled telavancin, 3 hydroxylated metabolites were identified with the predominant metabolite (THRX-651540) accounting for less than 10% of the radioactivity in urine and less than 2% of the radioactivity in plasma. The metabolic pathway for telavancin has not been identified.

Excretion – Telavancin is primarily eliminated by the kidney. In a mass balance study, approximately 76% of the administered dose was recovered from urine and less than 1% of the dose was recovered from feces (collected up to 216 hours) based on total radioactivity.

Special populations –

Renal function impairment: The pharmacokinetics of telavancin were evaluated in subjects with normal renal function and subjects with varying degrees of renal impairment following administration of a single dose of telavancin 7.5 mg/kg (n = 28). The mean $AUC_{0-\infty}$ values were approximately 13%, 29%, and 118% higher for subjects with CrCl greater than 50 to 80 mL/min, CrCl 30 to 50 mL/min, and CrCl 30 mL/min or less, respectively, compared with subjects with normal renal function. Dosage adjustment is required in patients with CrCl 50 mL/min or less.

Following administration of a single dose of telavancin 7.5 mg/kg to subjects with end-stage renal disease, approximately 5.9% of the administered dose of telavancin was recovered in the dialysate following 4 hours of hemodialysis. The effects of peritoneal dialysis have not been studied.

Following a single IV dose of telavancin 7.5 mg/kg, the clearance of hydroxypropyl-beta-cyclodextrin was reduced in subjects with renal impairment, resulting in a higher exposure to hydroxypropyl-beta-cyclodextrin. In subjects with mild, moderate, and severe renal impairment, the mean clearance values were 38%, 59%, and 82% lower, respectively, compared with subjects with normal renal function. Multiple infusions of telavancin may result in accumulation of hydroxypropyl-beta-cyclodextrin.

Hepatic function impairment: The pharmacokinetics of telavancin were not altered in subjects with moderate hepatic impairment (n = 8, Child-Pugh class B) compared with healthy subjects with normal hepatic function matched for gender, age, and weight. The pharmacokinetics of telavancin have not been evaluated in patients with severe hepatic impairment (Child-Pugh class C).

➤*Microbiology:* Telavancin exerts concentration-dependent, bactericidal activity against gram-positive organisms in vitro, as demonstrated by time-kill assays and minimum bactericidal concentration/minimum inhibitory concentration (MBC/MIC) ratios using broth dilution methodology. In vitro studies demonstrated a telavancin postantibiotic effect ranging from 1 to 6 hours against *S. aureus* and other gram-positive pathogens.

Antibacterial activity – Telavancin has been shown to be active against most isolates of the following microorganisms in in vitro and clinical infections as described in Indications.

Facultative gram-positive microorganisms: S. aureus (including methicillin-resistant isolates), *S. pyogenes, E. faecalis* (vancomycin-susceptible isolates only), *S. agalactiae*, and *S. anginosus* group (includes *S. anginosus, S. intermedius*, and *S. constellatus*).

Contraindications

None known.

Warnings/Precautions

➤*Women of childbearing potential:* See the Warning box for more information. If not already pregnant, instruct women of childbearing potential to use effective contraception during telavancin treatment.

➤*Nephrotoxicity:* Increases in serum creatinine to 1.5 times baseline occurred more frequently among telavancin-treated patients with normal baseline serum creatinine (15%) compared with vancomycin-treated patients with normal baseline serum creatinine (7%).

In 3.1% of telavancin-treated patients compared with 1.1% vancomycin-treated patients, renal adverse events indicative of renal impairment occurred, as defined by the following terms: increased serum creatinine, renal impairment, renal insufficiency, and/or renal failure. In 17 of the 30 telavancin-treated patients, these adverse events had not completely resolved by the end of the trials, compared with 6 of the 10 vancomycin-treated patients. Serious adverse events indicative of renal impairment occurred in 1.2% telavancin-treated patients compared with 0.3% vancomycin-treated patients. Twelve patients treated with telavancin discontinued treatment because of adverse events indicative of renal impairment compared with 2 patients treated with vancomycin. Adverse events were more likely to occur in patients with baseline comorbidities known to predispose patients to kidney dysfunction (eg, congestive heart failure, diabetes mellitus, hypertension, preexisting renal disease). The renal adverse event rate was also higher in patients who received concomitant medications known to affect kidney function (eg, angiotensin-converting enzyme [ACE] inhibitors, loop diuretics, nonsteroidal anti-inflammatory drugs [NSAIDs]). Adverse events indicative of renal impairment occurred in 8.6% of patients 65 years of age and older compared with 1.9% of patients younger than 65 years of age.

Monitor renal function (ie, serum creatinine, CrCl) in all patients receiving telavancin. Obtain values prior to initiation of treatment, during treatment (at 48- to 72-hour intervals or more frequently, if clinically indicated), and at the end of therapy. If renal function decreases, assess the benefit of continuing telavancin versus discontinuing and initiating therapy with an alternative agent.

In patients with renal dysfunction, accumulation of the solubilizer hydroxypropyl-beta-cyclodextrin can occur.

➤*Infusion-related reactions:* Telavancin is a lipoglycopeptide antibacterial agent; administer over a period of 60 minutes to reduce the risk of infusion-related reactions. Rapid IV infusions of the glycopeptide class of antimicrobial agents can cause "red-man syndrome"–like reactions, including flushing of the upper body, urticaria, pruritus, or rash. Stopping or slowing the infusion may result in cessation of these reactions.

➤*Clostridium difficile–associated diarrhea: Clostridium difficile*–associated diarrhea (CDAD) has been reported with nearly all antibacterial agents and may range in severity from mild diarrhea to fatal colitis. Treatment with antibacterial agents alters the flora of the colon and may permit overgrowth of *C. difficile*.

C. difficile produces toxins A and B, which contribute to the development of CDAD. Hypertoxin-producing strains of *C. difficile* cause increased morbidity and mortality because these infections can be refractory to antimicrobial therapy and may require colectomy. CDAD must be considered in all patients who present with diarrhea following antibiotic use. Careful medical history is necessary because CDAD has been reported to occur over 2 months after the administration of antibacterial agents.

If CDAD is suspected or confirmed, ongoing antibiotic use not directed against *C. difficile* may need to be discontinued. Institute appropriate fluid and electrolyte management, protein supplementation, antibiotic treatment of *C. difficile*, and surgical evaluation as clinically indicated.

➤*Resistance:* Prescribing telavancin in the absence of a proven or strongly suspected bacterial infection is unlikely to provide benefit to the patient and increases the risk of the development of drug-resistant bacteria.

➤*QTc prolongation:* In a study involving healthy volunteers, doses of telavancin 7.5 and 15 mg/kg prolonged the QTc interval. Patients with congenital long QT syndrome, known prolongation of the QTc interval, uncompensated heart failure, or severe left ventricular hypertrophy were not included in clinical trials of telavancin. Avoid use of telavancin in patients with these conditions. Caution is warranted when prescribing telavancin to patients taking drugs known to prolong the QT interval. See Drug Interactions for more information.

➤*Renal function impairment:* The complicated skin and skin structure infections trials included patients with normal renal function and patients with varying degrees of renal impairment. Patients with underlying renal dysfunction or risk factors for renal dysfunction had a higher incidence of renal adverse events. Patients with CrCl 50 mL/min or less also had lower clinical cure rates. Consider these data when selecting antibacterial therapy in patients with baseline moderate/severe renal impairment (CrCl 50 mL/min or less).

See Administration and Dosage for more information.

Hydroxypropyl-beta-cyclodextrin is excreted in urine and may accumulate in patients with renal impairment. Closely monitor serum creatinine and, if renal toxicity is suspected, consider an alternative agent.

Decreased efficacy – In a subgroup analysis of the pooled complicated skin and skin structure infections studies, clinical cure rates in the telavancin-treated patients were lower in patients with baseline CrCl 50 mL/min or less compared with those with CrCl greater than 50 mL/min. A decrease of this magnitude was not observed in vancomycin-treated patients. Consider these data when selecting antibacterial therapy for use in patients with baseline moderate/severe renal impairment.

TELAVANCIN HYDROCHLORIDE — INJECTION

➤*Superinfection:* As with other antibacterial drugs, use of telavancin may result in overgrowth of nonsusceptible organisms, including fungi. Carefully monitor patients during therapy. If superinfection occurs, take appropriate measures.

➤*Pregnancy: Category C.* There are no data on telavancin use in pregnant women. In 3 animal species, telavancin exposure during pregnancy at clinically relevant doses caused reduced fetal weights and increased rates of digit and limb malformations in offspring. These data raise concern about potential adverse developmental outcomes in humans.

In embryo-fetal development studies in rats, rabbits, and minipigs, telavancin demonstrated the potential to cause limb and skeletal malformations when given IV during the period of organogenesis at dosages of up to 150, 45, or 75 mg/kg/day, respectively. These doses resulted in exposure levels approximately 1- to 2-fold the human exposure (AUC) at the maximum clinical recommended dose. Malformations observed at less than 1% (but absent or at lower rates in historical or concurrent controls), included brachymelia (rats and rabbits), syndactyly (rats, minipigs), adactyly (rabbits), and polydactyly (minipigs). Additional findings in rabbits included flexed front paw and absent ulna, and in the minipigs included misshapen digits and deformed front leg. Fetal body weights were decreased in rats.

In a prenatal/perinatal development study, pregnant rats received IV telavancin at up to 150 mg/kg/day (approximately the same AUC as observed at the maximum clinical dose) from the start of organogenesis through lactation. Offspring showed decreases in fetal body weight and an increase in the number of stillborn pups. Brachymelia was also observed. Developmental milestones and fertility of the pups were unaffected.

Given the lack of human data and the risks suggested by animal data, avoid using telavancin in pregnant women unless the benefits to the patient outweigh the potential risks to the fetus.

Pregnancy exposure registry – There is a pregnancy registry that monitors pregnancy outcomes in women exposed to telavancin during pregnancy. Health care providers are encouraged to register pregnant patients, or pregnant women may enroll themselves in the telavancin pregnancy registry by calling 1-888-658-4228.

➤*Lactation:* It is not known whether telavancin is excreted in human milk. The molecular weight (about 1,756 for the free base) and moderately high plasma protein binding (about 90%) may partially inhibit excretion into breast milk, but the high fat solubility and long elimination half-life (8 hours) suggest that some drug will cross into milk. Because telavancin is a weak base, ion trapping in the more acidic milk may occur that results in a milk:plasma ratio > 1. Because many drugs are excreted in human milk, exercise caution when telavancin is administered to a breast-feeding woman.

➤*Children:* The safety and effectiveness have not been studied.

➤*Elderly:* Telavancin is substantially excreted by the kidney, and the risk of adverse reactions may be greater in patients with impaired renal function. Because elderly patients are more likely to have decreased renal function, take care in dose selection in this age group.

➤*Monitoring:* Monitor renal function (ie, serum creatinine, CrCl) in all patients receiving telavancin. Obtain values prior to initiation of treatment, during treatment (at 48- to 72-hour intervals or more frequently, if clinically indicated), and at the end of therapy. Carefully monitor patients for superinfection during therapy.

Drug Interactions

➤*QT prolongation:* An additive effect of telavancin with other drugs that prolong the QT interval cannot be excluded. The following drugs may prolong the QT interval and increase the risk of life-threatening cardiac arrhythmias, including torsades de pointes: antiarrhythmic agents (eg, amiodarone, bretylium, disopyramide, dofetilide, procainamide, and quinidine), arsenic trioxide, chlorpromazine, cisapride, dolasetron, droperidol, mefloquine, mesoridazine, moxifloxacin, pentamidine, pimozide, tacrolimus, thioridazine, and ziprasidone. For a more complete list of drugs that may prolong the QT interval, see Drug Interaction table for additional agents and see the appendix Drug-Induced Prolongation of the QT Interval and Torsades de Pointes.

Telavancin Drug Interactions

Precipitant drug	Object drug[a]		Description
Drugs affecting kidney function (eg, ACE inhibitors, loop diuretics, NSAIDs)	Telavancin	↑	Risk of renal adverse events may be increased. Use with caution. Observe the patient for adverse renal events. Monitor renal function.
Telavancin	Drugs affecting kidney function (eg, ACE inhibitors, loop diuretics, NSAIDs)		
QT-prolonging drugs (eg, amiodarone, pimozide, ziprasidone)	Telavancin	↑	Possible additive effects with other drugs that prolong the QT interval. Use with caution.
Telavancin	QT-prolonging drugs (eg, amiodarone, pimozide, zipras-idone)		

[a] ↑ = object drug increased.

➤*Drug/Lab test interactions:* Telavancin does not interfere with coagulation; however, it interferes with certain tests used to monitor coagulation, including activated clotting time, activated partial thromboplastin time, coagulation-based factor Xa tests, international normalized ratio, and prothrombin time. Collect blood samples for these coagulation tests as close as possible prior to a patient's next dose of telavancin. No evidence of increased risk of bleeding has been observed.

Telavancin interferes with urine qualitative dipstick protein assays and quantitative dye methods (eg, pyrogallol red-molybdate). However, microalbumin assays are not affected and can be used to monitor urinary protein excretion during telavancin treatment.

Adverse Reactions

➤*Discontinuation:* Treatment discontinuations because of adverse reactions occurred in 8% of patients treated with telavancin, the most common reactions being nausea and rash (approximately 1% each). Treatment discontinuations caused by adverse reactions occurred in 6% of vancomycin-treated patients, the most common reactions being pruritus and rash (approximately 1% each).

➤*Serious adverse reactions:* In the complicated skin and skin structure infections clinical trials, less than 1% of patients who received telavancin died and less than 1% of patients treated with vancomycin died. Serious adverse reactions were reported in 7% of patients treated with telavancin and most commonly included cardiac, renal, or respiratory events.

➤*Adverse reactions (≥ 2%):*

Telavancin Adverse Reactions (≥ 2%)

	Telavancin (n = 929)	Vancomycin (n = 938)
CNS		
Dizziness	6%	6%
Rigors	4%	2%
Taste disturbance[a]	33%	7%
Dermatologic		
Generalized pruritus	3%	6%
Pruritus	6%	13%
Rash	4%	5%
GI		
Abdominal pain	2%	2%
Diarrhea	7%	8%
Nausea	27%	15%
Vomiting	14%	7%
Local		
Infusion-site erythema	3%	3%
Infusion-site pain	4%	4%
Miscellaneous		
Decreased appetite	3%	2%
Foamy urine	13%	3%

[a] Described as a metallic or soapy taste.

Overdosage

➤*Treatment:* In the event of overdosage, discontinue telavancin and advise supportive care with maintenance of glomerular filtration and careful monitoring of renal function. Following administration of a single dose of telavancin 7.5 mg/kg to subjects with end-stage renal disease, approximately 5.9% of the administered dose of telavancin was recovered in the dialysate following 4 hours of hemodialysis. However, no information is available on the use of hemodialysis to treat an overdosage.

The clearance of telavancin by continuous venovenous hemofiltration (CVVH) was evaluated in an in vitro study. Telavancin was cleared by CVVH and the clearance of telavancin increased with increasing ultrafiltration rate. However, the clearance of telavancin by CVVH has not been evaluated in a clinical study; thus, the clinical significance of this finding and use of CVVH to treat an overdosage is unknown.

Patient Information

Advise patients to read the Medication Guide before initiation of therapy.

TELAVANCIN HYDROCHLORIDE — INJECTION

Inform women of childbearing potential (those who have not had complete absence of menses for at least 24 months or medically confirmed menopause, medically confirmed primary ovarian failure, a history of hysterectomy, bilateral oophorectomy, or tubal ligation) about the potential risk of fetal harm if telavancin is used during pregnancy.

Instruct women of childbearing potential to have a pregnancy test prior to administration of telavancin.

Educate patients on the use of effective contraceptive methods to prevent pregnancy during telavancin treatment.

Inform patients to notify their health care provider if they become pregnant during telavancin treatment.

Inform patients of the pregnancy registry that monitors pregnancy outcomes in women exposed to telavancin during pregnancy. Pregnant women may enroll themselves in the pregnancy registry by calling 1-888-658-4228.

Inform patients that diarrhea is a common problem caused by antibiotics that usually ends when the antibiotic is discontinued. Sometimes after starting treatment with antibiotics, patients can develop watery and bloody stools (with or without stomach cramps and fever) even as late as 2 or more months after having received the last dose of the antibiotic. If this occurs, patients should contact their health care provider as soon as possible.

Counsel patients that antibacterial drugs, including telavancin, should only be used to treat bacterial infections. They do not treat viral infections (eg, the common cold).

Educate patients that although it is common to feel better early in the course of therapy, the medication should be taken exactly as directed. Skipping doses or not completing the full course of therapy may decrease the effectiveness of immediate treatment, and increase the likelihood that the bacteria will develop resistance and will not be treatable by telavancin or other antibacterial drugs in the future.

Inform patients about the common adverse effects of telavancin, including foamy urine, headache, nausea, taste disturbance, and vomiting.

Inform patients that telavancin has been associated with elevations in serum creatinine and changes in the electrocardiogram (prolongation of the QTc interval).

Inform patients that telavancin may interfere with the results of some coagulation tests.

Instruct patients to inform their health care provider if they develop any unusual symptom, or if any known symptom persists or worsens.

Instruct patients to inform their health care provider of any other medications they are currently taking with telavancin, including nonprescription medications.

OXAZOLIDINONES

LINEZOLID

Rx	**Zyvox** (Pfizer)	**Tablets; oral:** 600 mg[a]	PEG. (ZYVOX 600 mg). White, capsule shape. Film-coated. In 20s, 100s, and UD 30s.
		Powder for suspension; oral: 100 mg per 5 mL[b]	Aspartame, mannitol, phenylalanine 20 mg per 5 mL, sodium benzoate, sucrose. Orange flavor. In 150 mL.
		Injection, solution: 2 mg/mL[c]	Dextrose, sodium citrate. In 100, 200, and 300 mL single-use, ready-to-use bags.

[a] Sodium content is 2.92 mg per tablet (0.1 mEq/tablet).
[b] Sodium content is 8.52 mg per 5 mL (0.4 mEq per 5 mL).
[c] Sodium content is 0.38 mg/mL (5 mEq per 300 mL bag, 3.3 mEq per 200 mL bag, 1.7 mEq per 100 mL bag).

LINEZOLID — ORAL

Indications

➤*Community-acquired pneumonia:* Caused by *Streptococcus pneumoniae* (including multidrug-resistant strains), including cases with concurrent bacteremia, or *Staphylococcus aureus* (methicillin-susceptible strains only).

➤*Complicated skin and skin structure infections:* Complicated skin and skin structure infections, including diabetic foot infections, without concomitant osteomyelitis, caused by *S. aureus* (methicillin-susceptible and -resistant strains), *Streptococcus pyogenes*, or *Streptococcus agalactiae*.

➤*Nosocomial pneumonia:* Caused by *S. aureus* (methicillin-susceptible and -resistant strains), or *S. pneumoniae* (including multidrug-resistant strains).

➤*Uncomplicated skin and skin structure infections:* Caused by *S. aureus* (methicillin-susceptible strains only) or *S. pyogenes*.

➤*Vancomycin-resistant enterococcal infections:* Vancomycin-resistant *Enterococcus faecium* infections, including cases with concurrent bacteremia.

➤*Off-label uses:*

Infective endocarditis – According to American Heart Association (AHA) guidelines, linezolid is one of the preferred treatments for endocarditis caused by multidrug-resistant enterococci.

Infective endocarditis (adults): [1] = Good documentation.

Infective endocarditis (children/adolescents): [1] = Good documentation.

Administration and Dosage

➤*Maximum dose:* There are no well-established maximum doses for the approved indications according to the prescribing information.

➤*Adults:*

Linezolid Oral Adult Dosage Guidelines

Infection[a]	Dosage and route of administration	Recommended duration of treatment (consecutive days)
Complicated skin and skin structure infections	600 mg[b] every 12 h	10 to 14 days
Community-acquired pneumonia, including concurrent bacteremia	600 mg[b] every 12 h	10 to 14 days
Methicillin-resistant staphylococcal infections	600 mg[b] every 12 h	
Nosocomial pneumonia	600 mg[b] every 12 h	10 to 14 days
Uncomplicated skin and skin structure infections	400 mg[b] every 12 h	10 to 14 days
Vancomycin-resistant *E. faecium* infections, including concurrent bacteremia	600 mg[b] every 12 h	14 to 28 days

[a] Caused by the designated pathogens (see Indications).
[b] Oral dosing using either tablets or oral suspension.

Off-label dosing –

Infective endocarditis (adults): [1] = Good documentation.

• *E. faecium infections resistant to penicillin, aminoglycosides, and vancomycin* – 1,200 mg/day orally in 2 equally divided doses for at least 8 weeks.

➤*Children:*

Linezolid Oral Dosage Guidelines for Children

Infection[a]	Dosage and route of administration: Children[b] (birth through 11 years of age)	Adolescents (12 years of age and older)	Recommended duration of treatment (consecutive days)
Complicated skin and skin structure infections	10 mg/kg[c] every 8 h	600 mg[c] every 12 h	10 to 14 days
Community-acquired pneumonia, including concurrent bacteremia			
Nosocomial pneumonia			
Uncomplicated skin and skin structure infections	< 5 years: 10 mg/kg[c] every 8 h; 5 to 11 years: 10 mg/kg[c] every 12 h	600 mg[c] every 12 h	10 to 14 days
Vancomycin-resistant *E. faecium* infections, including concurrent bacteremia	10 mg/kg[c] every 8 h	600 mg[c] every 12 h	14 to 28 days

[a] Caused by the designated pathogens.
[b] For neonatal dosing, see the following Neonates section.
[c] Oral dosing using either tablets or oral suspension.

Neonates – Most preterm neonates younger than 7 days of age (gestational age younger than 34 weeks) have lower systemic linezolid clearance

LINEZOLID — ORAL

values and larger area under the curve (AUC) values than many full-term neonates and older infants. These neonates should be initiated with a dosing regimen of 10 mg/kg every 12 hours. Consideration may be given to the use of a 10 mg/kg every 8 hours regimen in neonates with a suboptimal clinical response. All neonatal patients should receive 10 mg/kg every 8 hours by 7 days of life.

Off-label dosing –

Infective endocarditis (children/adolescents): [1] = Good documentation.

• *E. faecium infections resistant to penicillin, aminoglycosides, and vancomycin* – 30 mg/kg/day orally in 3 equally divided doses for at least 8 weeks.

➤*Renal function impairment:*

Hemodialysis – Both linezolid and the 2 metabolites are eliminated by dialysis. Linezolid should be given after hemodialysis.

➤*Preparation for administration:*

Oral suspension – Gently tap bottle to loosen powder. Add a total of 123 mL of distilled water in 2 portions. After adding the first half, shake vigorously to wet all of the powder. Then add the second half of the water and shake vigorously to obtain a uniform suspension. After constitution, each 5 mL of the suspension contains linezolid 100 mg.

➤*Administration:* Linezolid may be taken with or without food. Large quantities of foods or beverages with high tyramine content should be avoided while taking linezolid.

Oral suspension – Before using, gently mix by inverting the bottle 3 to 5 times. Do not shake.

➤*Storage/Stability:* Store at 25°C (77°F); excursions are permitted to 15° to 30°C (59° to 86°F). Protect from light. Keep bottles tightly closed to protect from moisture.

Store constituted suspension at room temperature. Use within 21 days after constitution.

Actions

➤*Pharmacology:* Linezolid is a synthetic antibacterial agent of a new class of antibiotics, the oxazolidinones, which has clinical utility in the treatment of infections caused by aerobic gram-positive bacteria. The in vitro spectrum of activity of linezolid also includes certain gram-negative bacteria and anaerobic bacteria. Linezolid inhibits bacterial protein synthesis through a mechanism of action different from that of other antibacterial agents; therefore, cross-resistance between linezolid and other classes of antibiotics is unlikely. Linezolid binds to a site on the bacterial 23S ribosomal RNA of the 50S subunit and prevents the formation of a functional 70S initiation complex, which is an essential component of the bacterial translation process. The results of time-kill studies have shown linezolid to be bacteriostatic against enterococci and staphylococci. For streptococci, linezolid was found to be bactericidal for the majority of strains.

➤*Pharmacokinetics:*

Absorption – Linezolid is rapidly and extensively absorbed after oral dosing. C_{max} are reached approximately 1 to 2 hours after dosing, and the absolute bioavailability is approximately 100%. Therefore, linezolid may be given orally or IV without dose adjustment.

Effect of food: Linezolid may be administered without regard to the timing of meals. The T_{max} is delayed from 1.5 hours to 2.2 hours, and C_{max} is decreased by approximately 17% when high-fat food is given with linezolid. However, the total exposure measured as $AUC_{0-\infty}$ values is similar under both conditions.

Distribution – Animal and human pharmacokinetic studies have demonstrated that linezolid readily distributes to well-perfused tissues. The plasma protein binding of linezolid is approximately 31% and is concentration-independent. The volume of distribution of linezolid at steady state averaged 40 to 50 L in healthy adult volunteers.

Metabolism – Linezolid is primarily metabolized by oxidation of the morpholine ring, which results in 2 inactive ring-opened carboxylic acid metabolites, the aminoethoxyacetic acid metabolite (A) and the hydroxyethyl glycine metabolite (B). Formation of metabolite A is presumed to be formed via an enzymatic pathway, whereas metabolite B is mediated by a nonenzymatic chemical oxidation mechanism in vitro. In vitro studies have demonstrated that linezolid is minimally metabolized and may be mediated by human cytochrome P450 (CYP-450). However, the metabolic pathway of linezolid is not fully understood. Linezolid is not an inducer of CYP-450 in rats, and it does not inhibit the activities of clinically significant human CYP isoforms (1A2, 2C9, 2C19, 2D6, 2E1, 3A4).

Excretion – Nonrenal clearance accounts for approximately 65% of the total clearance of linezolid. Under steady-state conditions, approximately 30% of the dose appears in the urine as linezolid, 40% as metabolite B, and 10% as metabolite A. The renal clearance of linezolid is low (average 40 mL/min) and suggests net tubular reabsorption. Virtually no linezolid appears in the feces, while approximately 6% of the dose appears in the feces as metabolite B and 3% as metabolite A.

A small degree of nonlinearity in clearance was observed with increasing doses of linezolid, which appears to be caused by lower renal and nonrenal clearance of linezolid at higher concentrations. However, the difference in clearance was small and not reflected in the apparent elimination half-life.

Special populations –

Renal function impairment: Because similar plasma concentrations of linezolid are achieved regardless of renal function, no dose adjustment is recommended for patients with renal insufficiency. However, given the absence of information on the clinical significance of accumulation of the primary metabolites, weigh use of linezolid in patients with renal insufficiency against the potential risks of accumulation of these metabolites.

• *Dialysis* – Both linezolid and the 2 metabolites are eliminated by dialysis. No information is available on the effect of peritoneal dialysis on the pharmacokinetics of linezolid. Approximately 30% of a dose was eliminated in a 3-hour dialysis session beginning 3 hours after the dose of linezolid was administered; therefore, give linezolid after hemodialysis.

Children: The C_{max} and the volume of distribution (V_{ss}) of linezolid are similar regardless of age in children. However, clearance of linezolid varies as a function of age. With the exclusion of preterm neonates younger than 1 week of age, clearance is most rapid in the youngest age groups, ranging from older than 1 week of age to 11 years of age, resulting in lower single-dose systemic exposure (AUC) and shorter half-life compared with adults. As age of children increases, the clearance of linezolid gradually decreases, and by adolescence, mean clearance values approach those observed for the adult population. There is wider intersubject variability in linezolid clearance and systemic drug exposure (AUC) across all pediatric age groups compared with adults.

Pharmacokinetic information generated in children with ventriculoperitoneal shunts showed variable cerebrospinal fluid (CSF) linezolid concentrations following single and multiple dosing of linezolid; therapeutic concentrations were not consistently achieved or maintained in the CSF. Therefore, the use of linezolid for the empiric treatment of children with CNS infections is not recommended.

➤*Microbiology:*

Resistance – Reports of vancomycin-resistant *E. faecium* becoming resistant to linezolid during its clinical use have been published. In one report, nosocomial spread of vancomycin- and linezolid-resistant *E. faecium* occurred. There has been a report of *S. aureus* (methicillin-resistant) developing resistance to linezolid during its clinical use. The linezolid resistance in these organisms was associated with a point mutation in the 23S rRNA (substitution of thymine for guanine at position 2576) of the organism. When antibiotic-resistant organisms are encountered in the hospital, it is important to emphasize infection control policies. Resistance to linezolid has not been reported in *Streptococcus* spp., including *S. pneumoniae*.

Susceptible organisms –

Aerobic and facultative gram-positive microorganisms: E. faecium (vancomycin-resistant strains only), *S. aureus* (including methicillin-resistant strains), *S. agalactiae*, *S. pneumoniae* (including multidrug-resistant isolates), *S. pyogenes*.

The following in vitro data are available, but their clinical significance is unknown. At least 90% of the following microorganisms exhibit an in vitro minimum inhibitory concentration (MIC) less than or equal to the susceptible break point for linezolid. However, the safety and efficacy of linezolid in treating clinical infections caused by these microorganisms have not been established in adequate and well-controlled clinical trials.

Aerobic and facultative gram-positive microorganisms: E. faecalis (including vancomycin-resistant strains), *E. faecium* (vancomycin-susceptible strains), *Staphylococcus epidermidis* (including methicillin-resistant strains), *Staphylococcus haemolyticus*, Viridans group streptococci.

Aerobic and facultative gram-negative microorganisms – *Pasteurella multocida*.

Contraindications

Known hypersensitivity to linezolid or any other product components; patients taking any medicinal product that inhibits monoamine oxidases A or B (eg, isocarboxazid, phenelzine) or within 2 weeks of taking any such medicinal product; uncontrolled hypertension, pheochromocytoma, thyrotoxicosis, and/or patients taking any of the following types of medications: directly and indirectly acting sympathomimetic agents (eg, pseudoephedrine), vasopressive agents (eg, epinephrine, norepinephrine), or dopaminergic agents (eg, dopamine, dobutamine), unless monitored for potential increase in blood pressure; carcinoid syndrome and/or patients taking any of the following medications: serotonin reuptake inhibitors, tricyclic antidepressants, serotonin 5-HT_1 receptor agonists (triptans), meperidine, or buspirone, unless carefully observed for signs and/or symptoms of serotonin syndrome.

Warnings/Precautions

➤*Myelosuppression:* Myelosuppression (including anemia, leukopenia, pancytopenia, and thrombocytopenia) has been reported in patients receiving linezolid. In cases where the outcome is known, when linezolid was discontinued, the affected hematologic parameters have risen toward pretreatment levels. Monitor complete blood cell counts weekly in patients who receive linezolid, particularly in those who receive linezolid for longer than 2 weeks, those with preexisting myelosuppression, those receiving concomitant drugs that produce bone marrow suppression, or those with a chronic infection who have received previous or concomitant antibiotic therapy. Consider discontinuation of therapy with linezolid in patients who develop or have worsening myelosuppression.

➤*Catheter-related infections:* An imbalance in mortality was seen in patients treated with linezolid relative to vancomycin/dicloxacillin/oxacillin in an open-label study in seriously ill patients with intravascular catheter-related infections (21.5% vs 16%; odds ratio, 1.426; 95% confidence interval [CI], 0.97 to 2.098). While causality has not been established, this observed imbalance occurred primarily in linezolid-treated patients in whom either gram-negative pathogens, mixed gram-negative and gram-positive pathogens, or no pathogen were identified at baseline, but was not seen in patients with gram-positive infections only.

Linezolid is not approved and should not be used for the treatment of patients with catheter-related bloodstream infections or catheter-site infections.

LINEZOLID — ORAL

➤*Gram-negative infections:* Linezolid has no clinical activity against gram-negative pathogens and is not indicated for the treatment of gram-negative infections. It is critical that specific gram-negative therapy be initiated immediately if a concomitant gram-negative pathogen is documented or suspected.

➤*Clostridium difficile–associated diarrhea: C. difficile*–associated diarrhea has been reported with use of nearly all antibacterial agents, including linezolid, and may range in severity from mild diarrhea to fatal colitis. Treatment with antibacterial agents alters the normal flora of the colon, leading to overgrowth of *C. difficile*.

C. difficile produces toxins A and B, which contribute to the development of *C. difficile*–associated diarrhea. Hypertoxin-producing strains of *C. difficile* cause increased morbidity and mortality because these infections can be refractory to antimicrobial therapy and may require colectomy. *C. difficile*–associated diarrhea must be considered in all patients who present with diarrhea following antibiotic use.

Careful medical history is necessary because *C. difficile*–associated diarrhea has been reported to occur over 2 months after the administration of antibacterial agents.

If *C. difficile*–associated diarrhea is suspected or confirmed, ongoing antibiotic use not directed against *C. difficile* may need to be discontinued. Institute appropriate fluid and electrolyte management, protein supplementation, antibiotic treatment of *C. difficile*, and surgical evaluation as clinically indicated.

➤*Lactic acidosis:* Lactic acidosis has been reported with the use of linezolid. In reported cases, patients experienced repeated episodes of nausea and vomiting. Institute an immediate medical evaluation for patients who develop recurrent nausea or vomiting, unexplained acidosis, or a low bicarbonate level while receiving linezolid.

➤*Serotonin syndrome:* Spontaneous reports of serotonin syndrome associated with the coadministration of linezolid and serotonergic agents, including antidepressants such as selective serotonin reuptake inhibitors (SSRIs), have been reported.

Where administration of linezolid and concomitant serotonergic agents is clinically appropriate, closely observe patients for signs and symptoms of serotonin syndrome, such as cognitive dysfunction, hyperpyrexia, hyperreflexia, and incoordination. If signs or symptoms occur, consider discontinuation of either one or both agents. If the concomitant serotonergic agent is withdrawn, discontinuation symptoms can be observed.

➤*Peripheral and optic neuropathy:* Peripheral and optic neuropathy have been reported in patients treated with linezolid, primarily those patients treated for longer than the maximum recommended duration of 28 days. In cases of optic neuropathy that progressed to loss of vision, patients were treated for extended periods beyond the maximum recommended duration. Visual blurring has been reported in some patients treated with linezolid for fewer than 28 days.

If patients experience symptoms of visual impairment, such as changes in visual acuity, changes in color vision, blurred vision, or visual field defect, prompt ophthalmic evaluation is recommended. Monitor visual function in all patients taking linezolid for extended periods (at least 3 months) and in all patients reporting new visual symptoms, regardless of length of therapy with linezolid. If peripheral or optic neuropathy occurs, weigh the continued use of linezolid against the potential risks in these patients.

➤*Convulsions:* Convulsions have been reported in patients when treated with linezolid. In some cases, a history of seizures or risk factors for seizures were reported.

➤*Resistance:* Prescribing linezolid in the absence of a proven or strongly suspected bacterial infection or a prophylactic indication is unlikely to provide benefit to the patient and increases the risk of the development of drug-resistant bacteria.

➤*Duration of therapy:* The safety and efficacy of linezolid formulations given for greater than 28 days have not been evaluated in controlled clinical trials.

➤*Special risk:* Linezolid has not been studied in patients with uncontrolled hypertension, pheochromocytoma, carcinoid syndrome, or untreated hyperthyroidism.

➤*Superinfection:* The use of antibiotics may promote the overgrowth of nonsusceptible organisms. If superinfection occurs during therapy, take appropriate measures.

➤*Pregnancy: Category C.* Linezolid was not teratogenic in mice or rats at exposure levels 6.5-fold (in mice) or equivalent (in rats) to the expected human exposure level, based on AUCs. However, embryo and fetal toxicities were seen. There are no adequate and well-controlled studies in pregnant women. It is not known if linezolid crosses the human placenta. The molecular weight (approximately 337) is low enough to expect transfer to the fetus. Use linezolid during pregnancy only if the potential benefit justifies the potential risk to the fetus.

In mice, embryo and fetal toxicities were seen only at doses that caused maternal toxicity (clinical signs and reduced body weight gain). A dosage of 450 mg/kg/day (6.5-fold the estimated human exposure level based on AUCs) correlated with increased postimplantational embryo death, including total litter loss, decreased fetal body weights, and an increased incidence of costal cartilage fusion.

In rats, mild fetal toxicity was observed at 15 and 50 mg/kg/day (exposure levels 0.22-fold to approximately equivalent to the estimated human exposure, respectively, based on AUCs). The effects consisted of decreased fetal body weights and reduced ossification of sternebrae, a finding often seen in association with decreased fetal body weights. Slight maternal toxicity, in the form of reduced body weight gain, was seen at 50 mg/kg/day.

In rabbits, reduced fetal body weight occurred only in the presence of maternal toxicity (clinical signs, reduced body weight gain, and food consumption) when administered at a dose of 15 mg/kg/day (0.06-fold the estimated human exposure based on AUCs).

When female rats were treated with 50 mg/kg/day (approximately equivalent to the estimated human exposure based on AUCs) of linezolid during pregnancy and lactation, survival of pups was decreased on postnatal days 1 to 4. Male and female pups permitted to mature to reproductive age, when mated, showed an increase in preimplantation loss.

➤*Lactation:* Linezolid and its metabolites are excreted in the milk of lactating rats. Concentrations in milk were similar to those in maternal plasma. It is not known whether linezolid is excreted in human milk. The molecular weight (approximately 337) is low enough to expect excretion into breast milk. Because many drugs are excreted in human milk, exercise caution when linezolid is administered to a breast-feeding woman.

➤*Children:* See Administration and Dosage for more information.

➤*Monitoring:* Monitor complete blood cell counts weekly, particularly in those who receive linezolid for longer than 2 weeks, those with preexisting myelosuppression, those receiving concomitant drugs that produce bone marrow suppression, or those with a chronic infection who have received previous or concomitant antibiotic therapy.

Where administration of linezolid and concomitant serotonergic agents is clinically appropriate, closely observe patients for signs and symptoms of serotonin syndrome, such as cognitive dysfunction, hyperpyrexia, hyperreflexia, and incoordination.

Monitor visual function in all patients taking linezolid for extended periods (at least 3 months) and in all patients reporting new visual symptoms, regardless of length of therapy with linezolid.

Drug Interactions

Linezolid Drug Interactions

Precipitant drug	Object drug[a]		Description
Apraclonidine	Linezolid	↑	Linezolid is a reversible, nonselective MAOI[b]. Apraclonidine is contraindicated in patients receiving MAOIs. The risk of hypertension may be increased. Do not coadminister linezolid and apraclonidine within 14 days of each other.
Ginseng	Linezolid	↑	Use of linezolid with ginseng may produce unexpected toxic effects (eg, manic-like symptoms, headache). Avoid concomitant use of linezolid and ginseng.
MAOIs (eg, phenelzine)	Linezolid	↑	Linezolid is a reversible, nonselective MAOI; do not coadminister with any medicinal product that inhibits MAO-A or MAO-B or within 2 weeks of use of such products.
Linezolid	MAOIs (eg, phenelzine)		
Rifamycins (eg, rifampin)	Linezolid	↓	Administration of linezolid 600 mg twice daily for 5 days with and without rifampin 600 mg once daily for 8 days decreased the linezolid maximum concentration and AUC 21% and 32%, respectively. Monitor the patient for a decreased response to linezolid. Be prepared to adjust therapy as needed.
Sibutramine	Linezolid	↑	The risk of serotonin syndrome may be increased. Serotonergic effects of these agents may be additive. MAOIs are contraindicated in patients receiving sibutramine.
Linezolid	Sibutramine		
Tetrabenazine	Linezolid	↑	The combination of linezolid and tetrabenazine may produce severe unexpected toxicity (eg, confusion, restlessness, behavioral changes). Coadministration of linezolid and tetrabenazine is contraindicated.
Tryptophan	Linezolid	↑	The risk of serotonin syndrome may be increased. Serotonergic effects of these agents may be additive. Carefully monitor patients for adverse reactions, including signs and symptoms of serotonin syndrome.
Linezolid	Tryptophan		

LINEZOLID — ORAL

Linezolid Drug Interactions			
Precipitant drug	Object drug[a]		Description
Linezolid	Atomoxetine	↑	Risk of serious or fatal reactions, including hyperthermia and rapid fluctuations in vital signs, may be increased. Coadministration of linezolid and atomoxetine within 14 days of each other is contraindicated.
Linezolid	Beta-2 agonists (eg, albuterol)	↑	Coadministration of linezolid and beta-2 agonists may result in adverse cardiovascular effects characterized by hypertension. Use caution within 14 days of coadministration of linezolid and beta-2 agonists. Monitor for potential increases in blood pressure with coadministration of these agents.
Linezolid	Bupropion	↑	The risk of hypertensive crisis is increased. Do not coadminister bupropion and linezolid within 14 days of each other.
Linezolid	Buspirone	↑	Unless patients are carefully observed for signs and symptoms of serotonin syndrome, do not coadminister linezolid with buspirone.
Linezolid	COMT[b] inhibitors (eg, entacapone)	↑	Coadministration of linezolid and COMT inhibitors may result in inhibition of the majority of pathways responsible for normal catecholamine metabolism. Excessive sympathetic stimulation may result. Use of linezolid with COMT inhibitors is not recommended.
Linezolid	Cyclobenzaprine	↑	The risk of hypertensive crisis, convulsions, and death is increased. Do not coadminister cyclobenzaprine and linezolid within 14 days of each other.
Linezolid	Dopaminergic agents (eg, dobutamine, dopamine)	↑	Unless patients are monitored for increases in blood pressure, do not coadminister linezolid with dopaminergic agents.
Linezolid	Levodopa	↑	Linezolid may increase the pharmacologic and toxic effects (flushing, headache, hypertension) of levodopa. Hypertensive crisis may occur. Avoid coadministration. If inadvertently given and hypertension occurs, administer phentolamine.
Linezolid	Meperidine	↑	Unless patients are carefully observed for signs and symptoms of serotonin syndrome, do not coadminister linezolid with meperidine.
Linezolid	Methylphenidate	↑	The risk of hypertensive crisis is increased. Do not coadminister methylphenidate and linezolid within 14 days of each other.
Linezolid	Propoxyphene	↑	A severe reaction potentially involving the respiratory, cardiac, and central nervous systems may occur shortly after administering propoxyphene to patients receiving linezolid. Use propoxyphene with caution in patients receiving linezolid.
Linezolid	Selective 5-HT_1 receptor agonists (eg, sumatriptan)	↑	Unless patients are carefully observed for signs and symptoms of serotonin syndrome, do not coadminister linezolid with selective 5-HT_1 receptor agonists.
Linezolid	Serotonin reuptake inhibitors (eg, fluoxetine, paroxetine, sertraline, venlafaxine)	↑	Linezolid has the potential to interact with serotonergic agents. Unless patients are carefully observed for signs and symptoms of serotonin syndrome, do not coadminister linezolid with serotonin reuptake inhibitors.
Linezolid	Sympathomimetic agents (eg, pseudoephedrine)	↑	Unless patients are monitored for increases in blood pressure, do not coadminister linezolid with sympathomimetic agents.
Linezolid	Tricyclic antidepressants (eg, amitriptyline)	↑	Unless patients are carefully observed for signs and symptoms of serotonin syndrome, do not coadminister linezolid with tricyclic antidepressants.
Linezolid	Vasopressive agents (eg, epinephrine, norepinephrine)	↑	Unless patients are monitored for increases in blood pressure, do not coadminister linezolid with vasopressive agents.

[a] ↑ = object drug increased. ↓ = object drug decreased.
[b] MAOI = monoamine oxidase inhibitor; COMT = catechol-O-methyl transferase.

➤*Drug/Food interactions:* See Actions for more information.

Avoid large quantities of foods or beverages with high tyramine content while taking linezolid. Quantities of tyramine consumed should be less than 100 mg per meal.

Adverse Reactions

➤*Adults:*

Most common adverse reactions – The most common adverse reactions in patients treated with linezolid were diarrhea (incidence across studies, 2.8% to 11%), headache (incidence across studies, 0.5% to 11.3%), and nausea (incidence across studies, 3.4% to 9%).

Adverse reactions (2% or more) –

Linezolid Adverse Reactions (≥ 2%)		
Adverse reaction	Linezolid (n = 2,046)	All comparators[a] (n = 2,001)
CNS		
Dizziness	2%	1.9%
Headache	6.5%	5.5%
Insomnia	2.5%	1.7%
GI		
Constipation	2.2%	2.1%
Diarrhea	8.3%	6.3%
Nausea	6.2%	4.6%
Vomiting	3.7%	2%
Miscellaneous		
Fever	1.6%	2.1%
Rash	2%	2.2%

[a] Comparators included cefpodoxime proxetil 200 mg orally every 12 hours; ceftriaxone 1 g IV every 12 hours; clarithromycin 250 mg orally every 12 hours; dicloxacillin 500 mg orally every 6 hours; oxacillin 2 g IV every 6 hours; vancomycin 1 g IV every 12 hours.

Other adverse reactions – Other adverse reactions reported in phase 2 and phase 3 studies included oral moniliasis, vaginal moniliasis, hypertension, dyspepsia, localized abdominal pain, pruritus, and tongue discoloration.

Adverse reactions by dose –

Linezolid Adverse Reactions (> 1%) by Dose				
	Uncomplicated skin and skin structure infections		All other indications	
Adverse reactions	Linezolid 400 mg orally every 12 h (n = 548)	Clarithromycin 250 mg orally every 12 h (n = 537)	Linezolid 600 mg every 12 h (n = 1498)	All other comparators[a] (n = 1,464)
Patients with 1 drug-related adverse reaction	25.4%	19.6%	20.4%	14.3%
Patients discontinuing because of drug-related adverse reactions[b]	3.5%	2.4%	2.1%	1.7%

Linezolid Adverse Reactions (> 1%) by Dose

Adverse reactions	Uncomplicated skin and skin structure infections: Linezolid 400 mg orally every 12 h (n = 548)	Uncomplicated skin and skin structure infections: Clarithromycin 250 mg orally every 12 h (n = 537)	All other indications: Linezolid 600 mg every 12 h (n = 1498)	All other indications: All other comparators[a] (n = 1,464)
CNS				
Dizziness	1.1%	1.5%	0.4%	0.3%
Headache	2.7%	2.2%	1.9%	1%
GI				
Diarrhea	5.3%	4.8%	4%	2.7%
Nausea	3.5%	3.5%	3.3%	1.8%
Oral moniliasis	0.4%	0%	1.1%	0.4%
Taste alteration	1.8%	2%	0.9%	0.2%
Tongue discoloration	1.1%	0%	0.2%	0%
Vomiting	0.9%	0.4%	1.2%	0.4%
Miscellaneous				
Abnormal liver function tests	0.4%	0%	1.3%	0.5%
Fungal infection	1.5%	0.2%	0.1%	< 0.1%
Vaginal moniliasis	1.6%	1.3%	1%	0.4%

[a] Comparators included cefpodoxime proxetil 200 mg orally every 12 hours; ceftriaxone 1 g IV every 12 hours; dicloxacillin 500 mg orally every 6 hours; oxacillin 2 g IV every 6 hours; vancomycin 1 g IV every 12 hours.

[b] The most commonly reported drug-related adverse reactions leading to discontinuation in patients treated with linezolid were diarrhea, headache, nausea, and vomiting.

➤*Children:*

Mortality – In the study of hospitalized children (birth through 11 years of age) with gram-positive infections who were randomized 2 to 1 (linezolid:vancomycin), mortality was 6% in the linezolid arm and 3% in the vancomycin arm. However, given the severe underlying illness in the patient population, no causality could be established.

Adverse reactions (2% or more)

Linezolid Adverse Reactions (≥ 2%) in Children

Adverse reaction	Uncomplicated skin and skin structure infections[a]: Linezolid (n = 248)	Uncomplicated skin and skin structure infections[a]: Cefadroxil (n = 251)	All other indications[b]: Linezolid (n = 215)	All other indications[b]: Vancomycin (n = 101)
CNS				
Convulsion	0%	0%	2.8%	2%
Headache	6.5%	4%	0.9%	0%
Dermatologic				
Rash	1.6%	1.2%	7%	15.2%
Skin disorder	2%	0%	0.9%	1%
GI				
Diarrhea	7.8%	8%	10.8%	12.1%
Generalized abdominal pain	2.4%	2.8%	0.9%	2%
GI bleeding	0%	0%	2.3%	1%
Localized abdominal pain	2.4%	2.8%	0.5%	1%
Loose stools	1.6%	0.8%	2.3%	3%
Nausea	3.7%	3.2%	1.9%	0%
Vomiting	2.9%	6.4%	9.4%	9.1%
Hematologic				
Anemia	0%	0%	5.6%	7.1%
Thrombocythemia	0%	0%	2.8%	2%
Thrombocytopenia	0%	0%	4.7%	2%
Respiratory				
Apnea	0%	0%	2.3%	2%
Cough	2.4%	4%	0.9%	0%
Dyspnea	0%	0%	3.3%	1%
Pharyngitis	2.9%	1.6%	0.5%	1%
Pneumonia	0%	0%	2.8%	2%
Upper respiratory tract infection	3.7%	5.2%	4.2%	1%
Miscellaneous				
Fever	2.9%	3.6%	14.1%	14.1%
Generalized edema	0%	0%	2.3%	1%
Hypokalemia	0%	0%	2.8%	3%
Localized pain	2%	1.6%	0.9%	0%
Reaction at site of injection or of vascular catheter	0%	0%	3.3%	5.1%
Sepsis	0%	0%	8%	7.1%
Trauma	3.3%	4.8%	2.8%	2%

[a] Patients 5 through 11 years of age received linezolid 10 mg/kg orally every 12 hours or cefadroxil 15 mg/kg orally every 12 hours. Patients 12 years of age and older received linezolid 600 mg orally every 12 hours or cefadroxil 500 mg orally every 12 hours.

[b] Patients from birth through 11 years of age received linezolid 10 mg/kg IV/orally every 8 hours or vancomycin 10 to 15 mg/kg IV every 6 to 24 hours, depending on age and renal clearance.

Adverse reactions (more than 1%) –

Linezolid Adverse Reactions in Children (> 1% and > 1 Patient)

Adverse reaction	Uncomplicated skin and skin structure infections[a]: Linezolid (n = 248)	Uncomplicated skin and skin structure infections[a]: Cefadroxil (n = 251)	All other indications[b]: Linezolid (n = 215)	All other indications[b]: Vancomycin (n = 101)
Patients with ≥ 1 drug-related adverse reaction	19.2%	14.1%	18.8%	34.3%
Patients discontinuing because of a drug-related adverse reaction	1.6%	2.4%	0.9%	6.1%
CNS				
Headache	2.4%	0.8%	0%	0%
Vertigo	1.2%	0.4%	0%	0%
Dermatologic				
Pruritus at nonapplication site	0.4%	0%	0%	2%
Rash	0.4%	1.2%	1.4%	7.1%
Hematologic				
Anemia	0%	0%	1.4%	1%
Eosinophilia	0.4%	0.4%	1.4%	0%
Thrombocytopenia	0%	0%	1.9%	0%
GI				
Diarrhea	5.7%	5.2%	3.8%	6.1%
Generalized abdominal pain	1.6%	1.2%	0%	0%
Localized abdominal pain	1.6%	1.2%	0%	0%
Loose stools	1.2%	0.8%	1.9%	0%
Nausea	3.3%	2%	1.4%	0%
Oral moniliasis	0%	0%	0.9%	4%
Vomiting	1.2%	2.4%	1.9%	1%
Miscellaneous				
Anaphylaxis	0%	0%	0%	10.1%[c]
Fever	0%	0%	0.5%	3%

[a] Patients 5 through 11 years of age received linezolid 10 mg/kg orally every 12 hours or cefadroxil 15 mg/kg orally every 12 hours. Patients 12 years of age and older received linezolid 600 mg orally every 12 hours or cefadroxil 500 mg orally every 12 hours.

[b] Patients from birth through 11 years of age received linezolid 10 mg/kg IV/orally every 8 hours or vancomycin 10 to 15 mg/kg IV every 6 to 24 hours, depending on age and renal clearance.

[c] These reports were of "red-man syndrome," which were coded as anaphylaxis.

➤*Thrombocytopenia:* Linezolid has been associated with thrombocytopenia when used in doses of up to and including 600 mg every 12 hours for up to 28 days. In phase 3 comparator-controlled trials, the percentage of adults who developed a substantially low platelet count (defined as less than 75% of lower limit of normal and/or baseline) was 2.4% (range among studies, 0.3% to 10%) with linezolid and 1.5% (range among studies, 0.4% to 7%) with a comparator. In a study of hospitalized children ranging in age from birth through 11 years, the percentage of patients who developed a substantially

LINEZOLID — ORAL

low platelet count (defined as less than 75% of lower limit of normal and/or baseline) was 12.9% with linezolid and 13.4% with vancomycin. In an outpatient study of children 5 through 17 years of age, the percentage of patients who developed a substantially low platelet count was 0% with linezolid and 0.4% with cefadroxil. Thrombocytopenia associated with the use of linezolid appears to be dependent on duration of therapy (generally more than 2 weeks of treatment). The platelet counts for most patients returned to the normal range/baseline during the follow-up period. No related clinical adverse reactions were identified in phase 3 clinical trials in patients developing thrombocytopenia. Bleeding reactions were identified in thrombocytopenic patients in a compassionate use program for linezolid; the role of linezolid in these reactions cannot be determined.

➤*Lab test abnormalities:*

Adults –

Linezolid Hematologic Adverse Reactions in Adults[a]

Hematologic adverse reaction	Uncomplicated skin and skin structure infections		All other indications	
	Linezolid 400 mg every 12 h	Clarithromycin 250 mg every 12 h	Linezolid 600 mg every 12 h	All other comparators[b]
Hemoglobin (g/dL)	0.9%	0%	7.1%	6.6%
Platelet count (× 10^3/mm^3	0.7%	0.8%	3%	1.8%
WBC[c] (× 10^3/mm^3)	0.2%	0.6%	2.2%	1.3%
Neutrophils (× 10^3/mm^3)	0%	0.2%	1.1%	1.2%

[a] Less than 75% (less than 50% for neutrophils) of lower limit of normal for values normal at baseline; less than 75% (less than 50% for neutrophils) of lower limit of normal and of baseline for values abnormal at baseline.
[b] Comparators included cefpodoxime proxetil 200 mg orally every 12 hours; ceftriaxone 1 g IV every 12 hours; dicloxacillin 500 mg orally every 6 hours; oxacillin 2 g IV every 6 hours; vancomycin 1 g IV every 12 hours.
[c] WBC = white blood cell count.

Linezolid Laboratory Abnormality in Adults[a]

Laboratory abnormality	Uncomplicated skin and skin structure infections		All other indications	
	Linezolid 400 mg every 12 h	Clarithromycin 250 mg every 12 h	Linezolid 600 mg every 12 h	All other comparators[b]
AST (U/L)	1.7%	1.3%	5%	6.8%
ALT (U/L)	1.7%	1.7%	9.6%	9.3%
LDH[c] (U/L)	0.2%	0.2%	1.8%	1.5%
Alkaline phosphatase (U/L)	0.2%	0.2%	3.5%	3.1%
Lipase (U/L)	2.8%	2.6%	4.3%	4.2%
Amylase (U/L)	0.2%	0.2%	2.4%	2%
Total bilirubin (mg/dL)	0.2%	0%	0.9%	1.1%
BUN[c] (mg/dL)	0.2%	0%	2.1%	1.5%
Creatinine (mg/dL)	0.2%	0%	0.2%	0.6%

[a] Greater than 2 times the upper limit of normal (ULN) for values normal at baseline; greater than 2 times ULN and greater than 2 times baseline for values abnormal at baseline.
[b] Comparators included cefpodoxime proxetil 200 mg orally every 12 hours; ceftriaxone 1 g IV every 12 hours; dicloxacillin 500 mg orally every 6 hours; oxacillin 2 g IV every 6 hours; vancomycin 1 g IV every 12 hours.
[c] LDH = lactate dehydrogenase; BUN = serum urea nitrogen.

Children –

Linezolid Hematologic Abnormality in Children[a]

Hematologic abnormality	Uncomplicated skin and skin structure infections[b]		All other indications[c]	
	Linezolid	Cefadroxil	Linezolid	Vancomycin
Hemoglobin (g/dL)	0%	0%	15.7%	12.4%
Platelet count (× 10^3/mm^3)	0%	0.4%	12.9%	13.4%
WBC (× 10^3/mm^3)	0.8%	0.8%	12.4%	10.3%
Neutrophils (× 10^3/mm^3)	1.2%	0.8%	5.9%	4.3%

[a] Less than 75% (less than 50% for neutrophils) of lower limit of normal for values normal at baseline; less than 75% (less than 50% for neutrophils) of lower limit of normal and less than 75% (less than 50% for neutrophils, less than 90% for hemoglobin if baseline is less than lower limit of normal) of baseline for values abnormal at baseline.
[b] Patients 5 through 11 years of age received linezolid 10 mg/kg orally every 12 hours or cefadroxil 15 mg/kg orally every 12 hours. Patients 12 years of age and older received linezolid 600 mg orally every 12 hours or cefadroxil 500 mg orally every 12 hours.
[c] Patients from birth through 11 years of age received linezolid 10 mg/kg IV/orally every 8 hours or vancomycin 10 to 15 mg/kg IV every 6 to 24 hours, depending on age and renal clearance.

Linezolid Laboratory Abnormality in Children[a]

Laboratory abnormality	Uncomplicated skin and skin structure infections[b]		All other indications[c]	
	Linezolid	Cefadroxil	Linezolid	Vancomycin
ALT (U/L)	0%	0%	10.1%	12.5%
Lipase (U/L)	0.4%	1.2%	—	—
Amylase (U/L)	—	—	0.6%	1.3%
Total bilirubin (mg/dL)	—	—	6.3%	5.2%
Creatinine (mg/dL)	0.4%	0%	2.4%	1%

[a] Greater than 2 times the ULN for values normal at baseline; greater than 2 times ULN and greater than 2 (greater than 1.5 for total bilirubin) times baseline for values abnormal at baseline.
[b] Patients 5 through 11 years of age received linezolid 10 mg/kg orally every 12 hours or cefadroxil 15 mg/kg orally every 12 hours. Patients 12 years of age and older received linezolid 600 mg orally every 12 hours or cefadroxil 500 mg orally every 12 hours.
[c] Patients from birth through 11 years of age received linezolid 10 mg/kg IV/orally every 8 hours or vancomycin 10 to 15 mg/kg IV every 6 to 24 hours, depending on age and renal clearance.

➤*Postmarketing:*

CNS – Convulsions, peripheral neuropathy, and optic neuropathy sometimes progressing to loss of vision. Serotonin syndrome has been reported in patients receiving concomitant serotonergic agents, including antidepressants, such as selective serotonin reuptake inhibitors (SSRIs), and linezolid.

Hematologic – Myelosuppression (including anemia, leukopenia, pancytopenia, and thrombocytopenia).

Miscellaneous – Anaphylaxis, angioedema, bullous skin disorders, such as those described as Stevens-Johnson syndrome, lactic acidosis, superficial tooth discoloration, and tongue discoloration.

The tooth discoloration was removable with professional dental cleaning (manual descaling) in cases with known outcome.

Overdosage

➤*Treatment:* In the event of overdosage, supportive care is advised, with maintenance of glomerular filtration. Hemodialysis may facilitate more rapid elimination of linezolid. In a phase 1 clinical trial, approximately 30% of a dose of linezolid was removed during a 3-hour hemodialysis session beginning 3 hours after the dose of linezolid was administered. Data are not available for removal of linezolid with peritoneal dialysis or hemoperfusion.

Patient Information

Inform patient that linezolid may be taken with or without food.

Advise patients to inform their health care provider of any history of hypertension.

Inform patients to avoid large quantities of foods or beverages with high tyramine content while taking linezolid. Quantities of tyramine consumed should be less than 100 mg per meal. Foods high in tyramine content include those that may have undergone protein changes by aging, fermentation, pickling, or smoking to improve flavor, such as aged cheeses (tyramine 0 to 15 mg per 30 mL); fermented or air-dried meats (tyramine 0.1 to 8 mg per 30 mL); sauerkraut (tyramine 8 mg per 237 mL); soy sauce (tyramine 5 mg/teaspoon); tap beers (tyramine 4 mg per 355 mL); and red wines (tyramine 0 to 6 mg per 237 mL). The tyramine content of any protein-rich food may be increased if stored for long periods or improperly refrigerated.

Instruct patients to inform health care provider if they are taking medications containing pseudoephedrine or phenylpropanolamine, such as cold remedies and decongestants, or if they are taking serotonin reuptake inhibitors or other antidepressants.

Inform phenylketonuric patients that each linezolid 5 mL oral suspension contains phenylalanine 20 mg (a component of aspartame).

Instruct patients to inform their health care provider if they experience changes in vision.

Instruct patients to inform their health care provider of any history of seizures.

LINEZOLID — ORAL

Advise patients that diarrhea is a common problem caused by antibiotics that usually ends when the antibiotic is discontinued. Sometimes after starting treatment with antibiotics, patients can develop watery and bloody stools (with or without stomach cramps and fever), even as late as 2 or more months after having taken the last dose of the antibiotic. If this occurs, contact the health care provider as soon as possible.

Counsel patients to only use antibacterial drugs, including linezolid, to treat bacterial infections. They do not treat viral infections (eg, the common cold).

When linezolid is prescribed to treat a bacterial infection, advise patients that although it is common to feel better early in the course of therapy, to take the medication exactly as directed. Skipping doses or not completing the full course of therapy may decrease the effectiveness of the immediate treatment and increase the likelihood that bacteria will develop resistance and will not be treatable by linezolid or other antibacterial drugs in the future.

LINEZOLID — INJECTION

Indications

➤*Community-acquired pneumonia:* Caused by *Streptococcus pneumoniae* (including multidrug-resistant strains), including cases with concurrent bacteremia, or *Staphylococcus aureus* (methicillin-susceptible strains only).

➤*Complicated skin and skin structure infections:* Complicated skin and skin structure infections, including diabetic foot infections, without concomitant osteomyelitis, caused by *S. aureus* (methicillin-susceptible and -resistant strains), *Streptococcus pyogenes*, or *Streptococcus agalactiae*.

➤*Nosocomial pneumonia:* Caused by *S. aureus* (methicillin-susceptible and -resistant strains), or *S. pneumoniae* (including multidrug-resistant strains).

➤*Vancomycin-resistant enterococcal infections:* Vancomycin-resistant *Enterococcus faecium* infections, including cases with concurrent bacteremia.

➤*Off-label uses:*

Infective endocarditis – According to American Heart Association (AHA) guidelines, linezolid is one of the preferred treatments for endocarditis caused by multidrug-resistant enterococci.

Infective endocarditis (adults): [1] = Good documentation.

Infective endocarditis (children / adolescents): [1] = Good documentation.

Administration and Dosage

➤*Adults:*

Linezolid Injection Adult Dosage Guidelines[a]

Infection[b]	Dosage and route of administration	Recommended duration of treatment (consecutive days)
Complicated skin and skin structure infections	600 mg IV every 12 h	10 to 14 days
Community-acquired pneumonia, including concurrent bacteremia		
Methicillin-resistant staphylococcal infections	600 mg IV every 12 h	
Nosocomial pneumonia	600 mg IV every 12 h	10 to 14 days
Vancomycin-resistant *E. faecium* infections, including concurrent bacteremia	600 mg IV every 12 h	14 to 28 days

[a] IV = intravenous.
[b] Caused by the designated pathogens (see Indications).

Off-label dosing –

Infective endocarditis (adults): [1] = Good documentation.

- *E. faecium infections resistant to penicillin, aminoglycosides, and vancomycin* – 1,200 mg/day IV in 2 equally divided doses for at least 8 weeks.

➤*Children:*

Linezolid Injection Dosage Guidelines for Children

Infection[a]	Dosage and route of administration: Children[b] (birth through 11 years of age)	Dosage and route of administration: Adolescents (12 years of age and older)	Recommended duration of treatment (consecutive days)
Complicated skin and skin structure infections	10 mg/kg IV every 8 h	600 mg IV every 12 h	10 to 14 days
Community-acquired pneumonia, including concurrent bacteremia			
Nosocomial pneumonia			
Vancomycin-resistant *E. faecium* infections, including concurrent bacteremia	10 mg/kg IV every 8 h	600 mg IV every 12 h	14 to 28 days

[a] Caused by the designated pathogens (see Indications).
[b] For neonatal dosing, see the following Neonates section.

Neonates – Most preterm neonates younger than 7 days of age (gestational age younger than 34 weeks) have lower systemic linezolid clearance values and larger area under the curve (AUC) values than many full-term neonates and older infants. These neonates should be initiated with a dosing regimen of 10 mg/kg every 12 hours. Consideration may be given to the use of a 10 mg/kg every-8-hours regimen in neonates with a suboptimal clinical response. All neonatal patients should receive 10 mg/kg every 8 hours by 7 days of life.

Off-label dosing –

Infective endocarditis (children / adolescents): [1] = Good documentation.

- *E. faecium infections resistant to penicillin, aminoglycosides, and vancomycin* – 30 mg/kg/day IV in 3 equally divided doses for at least 8 weeks.

➤*Renal function impairment:*

Hemodialysis – Both linezolid and the 2 metabolites are eliminated by dialysis. Linezolid should be given after hemodialysis. Patients receiving continuous renal replacement therapy or intermittent hemodialysis should receive the normal dosage regimen (ie, 600 mg IV every 12 hours).

➤*Administration:* Linezolid should be administered by IV infusion over a period of 30 to 120 minutes. Do not use this IV infusion bag in series connections.

➤*Admixture compatibility:* Additives should not be introduced into this solution. If linezolid IV injection is to be given concomitantly with another drug, each drug should be given separately in accordance with the recommended dosage and route of administration for each product. In particular, physical incompatibilities resulted when linezolid IV injection was combined with the following drugs during simulated Y-site administration: amphotericin B, chlorpromazine hydrochloride, diazepam, pentamidine isethionate, erythromycin lactobionate, phenytoin sodium, and trimethoprim/sulfamethoxazole. Additionally, chemical incompatibility resulted when linezolid IV injection was combined with ceftriaxone sodium.

If the same IV line is used for sequential infusion of several drugs, the line should be flushed before and after infusion of linezolid IV injection with an infusion solution compatible with linezolid IV injection and with any other drug or drugs administered via the common line. Linezolid is compatible with dextrose 5% injection, sodium chloride 0.9% injection, and lactated Ringer's injection.

➤*Storage / Stability:* Store at 25°C (77°F); excursions are permitted between 15° and 30°C (59° and 86°F). Protect from light. Keep the infusion bags in the overwrap until ready to use. Protect from freezing.

Actions

➤*Pharmacology:* Linezolid is a synthetic antibacterial agent of a new class of antibiotics, the oxazolidinones, which has clinical utility in the treatment of infections caused by aerobic gram-positive bacteria. The in vitro spectrum of activity of linezolid also includes certain gram-negative bacteria and anaerobic bacteria. Linezolid inhibits bacterial protein synthesis through a mechanism of action different from that of other antibacterial agents; therefore, cross-resistance between linezolid and other classes of antibiotics is unlikely. Linezolid binds to a site on the bacterial 23S ribosomal RNA of the 50S subunit and prevents the formation of a functional 70S initiation complex, which is an essential component of the bacterial translation process. The results of time-kill studies have shown linezolid to be bacteriostatic against enterococci and staphylococci. For streptococci, linezolid was found to be bactericidal for the majority of strains.

➤*Pharmacokinetics:*

Distribution – Animal and human pharmacokinetic studies have demonstrated that linezolid readily distributes to well-perfused tissues. The plasma protein binding of linezolid is approximately 31% and is concentration-independent. The volume of distribution of linezolid at steady state averaged 40 to 50 L in healthy adult volunteers.

Metabolism – Linezolid is primarily metabolized by oxidation of the morpholine ring, which results in 2 inactive, ring-opened carboxylic acid metabolites: the aminoethoxyacetic acid metabolite (A) and the hydroxyethyl glycine metabolite (B). Formation of metabolite A is presumed to be formed via an enzymatic pathway, whereas metabolite B is mediated by a nonenzymatic chemical oxidation mechanism in vitro. In vitro studies have demonstrated that linezolid is minimally metabolized and may be mediated by human cytochrome P450 (CYP-450); however, the metabolic pathway of linezolid is not fully understood. Linezolid is not an inducer of CYP-450 in rats and it does not inhibit the activities of clinically significant human CYP isoforms (1A2, 2C9, 2C19, 2D6, 2E1, 3A4).

Excretion – Nonrenal clearance accounts for approximately 65% of the total clearance of linezolid. Under steady-state conditions, approximately 30% of the dose appears in the urine as linezolid, 40% as metabolite B, and 10% as metabolite A. The renal clearance of linezolid is low (average, 40 mL/min) and suggests net tubular reabsorption. Virtually no linezolid appears in the feces, while approximately 6% of the dose appears in the feces as metabolite B and 3% as metabolite A.

LINEZOLID — INJECTION

A small degree of nonlinearity in clearance was observed with increasing doses of linezolid, which appears to be caused by lower renal and nonrenal clearance of linezolid at higher concentrations. However, the difference in clearance was small and was not reflected in the apparent elimination half-life.

Special populations –

Renal function impairment: Because similar plasma concentrations of linezolid are achieved regardless of renal function, no dose adjustment is recommended for patients with renal insufficiency. However, given the absence of information on the clinical significance of accumulation of the primary metabolites, weigh the use of linezolid in patients with renal insufficiency against the potential risks of accumulation of these metabolites.

• *Dialysis* – Both linezolid and the 2 metabolites are eliminated by dialysis. No information is available on the effect of peritoneal dialysis on the pharmacokinetics of linezolid. Approximately 30% of a dose was eliminated in a 3-hour dialysis session beginning 3 hours after the dose of linezolid was administered; therefore, give linezolid after hemodialysis.

Hepatic function impairment: The pharmacokinetics of linezolid are not altered in patients (n = 7) with mild to moderate hepatic insufficiency (Child-Pugh class A or B). On the basis of the available information, no dose adjustment is recommended for patients with mild to moderate hepatic function impairment. The pharmacokinetics of linezolid in patients with severe hepatic insufficiency have not been evaluated.

Children: The C_{max} and the volume of distribution (V_{ss}) of linezolid are similar regardless of age in children. However, clearance of linezolid varies as a function of age. With the exclusion of preterm neonates younger than 1 week of age, clearance is most rapid in the youngest age groups ranging from older than 1 week to 11 years of age, resulting in lower single-dose systemic exposure (AUC) and shorter half-life compared with adults. As the age of children increases, the clearance of linezolid gradually decreases, and by adolescence, mean clearance values approach those observed for the adult population. There is wider intersubject variability in linezolid clearance and systemic drug exposure (AUC) across all pediatric age groups compared with adults.

Pharmacokinetic information generated in children with ventriculoperitoneal shunts showed variable cerebrospinal fluid (CSF) linezolid concentrations following single and multiple dosing of linezolid; therapeutic concentrations were not consistently achieved or maintained in the CSF. Therefore, the use of linezolid for the empiric treatment of children with CNS infections is not recommended.

➤*Microbiology:*

Resistance – Reports of vancomycin-resistant *E. faecium* becoming resistant to linezolid during its clinical use have been published. In 1 report, nosocomial spread of vancomycin- and linezolid-resistant *E. faecium* occurred. There has been a report of *S. aureus* (methicillin-resistant) developing resistance to linezolid during its clinical use. The linezolid resistance in these organisms was associated with a point mutation in the 23S rRNA (substitution of thymine for guanine at position 2576) of the organism. When antibiotic-resistant organisms are encountered in the hospital, it is important to emphasize infection control policies. Resistance to linezolid has not been reported in *Streptococcus* spp., including *S. pneumoniae*.

Aerobic and facultative gram-positive microorganisms – *E. faecium* (vancomycin-resistant strains only); *S. aureus* (including methicillin-resistant strains); *S. agalactiae*; *S. pneumoniae* (including multidrug-resistant isolates); *S. pyogenes*.

The following in vitro data are available, but their clinical significance is unknown. At least 90% of the following microorganisms exhibit an in vitro minimum inhibitory concentration (MIC) less than or equal to the susceptible break point for linezolid. However, the safety and effectiveness of linezolid in treating clinical infections caused by these microorganisms have not been established in adequate and well-controlled clinical trials.

Aerobic and facultative gram-positive microorganisms:

- *E. faecalis* (including vancomycin-resistant strains).
- *E. faecium* (vancomycin-susceptible strains).
- *Staphylococcus epidermidis* (including methicillin-resistant strains).
- *Staphylococcus haemolyticus.*
- Viridans group streptococci.

Aerobic and facultative gram-negative microorganisms –

- *Pasteurella multocida.*

Contraindications

Known hypersensitivity to linezolid or any of the other product components; patients taking any medicinal product that inhibits monoamine oxidases (MAO) A or B (eg, phenelzine, isocarboxazid) or within 2 weeks of taking any such medicinal product; uncontrolled hypertension, pheochromocytoma, thyrotoxicosis, and/or patients taking any of the following types of medications: directly and indirectly acting sympathomimetic agents (eg, pseudoephedrine), vasopressive agents (eg, epinephrine, norepinephrine), or dopaminergic agents (eg, dopamine, dobutamine); unless monitored for potential increase in blood pressure; carcinoid syndrome and/or patients taking any of the following medications: serotonin reuptake inhibitors, tricyclic antidepressants, serotonin 5-HT_1 receptor agonists (triptans), meperidine, or buspirone, unless carefully observed for signs/symptoms of serotonin syndrome.

Warnings/Precautions

➤*Myelosuppression:* Myelosuppression (including anemia, leukopenia, pancytopenia, and thrombocytopenia) has been reported in patients receiving linezolid. In cases where the outcome is known, when linezolid was discontinued, the affected hematologic parameters have risen toward pretreatment levels. Monitor complete blood cell counts weekly in patients who receive linezolid, particularly in those who receive linezolid for longer than 2 weeks, those with preexisting myelosuppression, those receiving concomitant drugs that produce bone marrow suppression, or those with a chronic infection who have received previous or concomitant antibiotic therapy. Consider discontinuation of therapy with linezolid in patients who develop or have worsening myelosuppression.

➤*Catheter-related infections:* An imbalance in mortality was seen in patients treated with linezolid relative to vancomycin/dicloxacillin/oxacillin in an open-label study in seriously ill patients with intravascular catheter-related infections (21.5% vs 16%; odds ratio 1.426; 95% confidence interval [CI], 0.97 to 2.098). While causality has not been established, this observed imbalance occurred primarily in linezolid-treated patients in whom gram-negative pathogens, mixed gram-negative and gram-positive pathogens, or no pathogen were identified at baseline but was not seen in patients with gram-positive infections only.

Linezolid is not approved and should not be used for the treatment of patients with catheter-related bloodstream infections or catheter-site infections.

➤*Gram-negative infections:* Linezolid has no clinical activity against gram-negative pathogens and is not indicated for the treatment of gram-negative infections. It is critical that specific gram-negative therapy be initiated immediately if a concomitant gram-negative pathogen is documented or suspected.

➤*Clostridium difficile–associated diarrhea: C. difficile*–associated diarrhea has been reported with use of nearly all antibacterial agents, including linezolid, and may range in severity from mild diarrhea to fatal colitis. Treatment with antibacterial agents alters the normal flora of the colon, leading to overgrowth of *C. difficile*.

C. difficile produces toxins A and B, which contribute to the development of *C. difficile*–associated diarrhea. Hypertoxin-producing strains of *C. difficile* cause increased morbidity and mortality, as these infections can be refractory to antimicrobial therapy and may require colectomy. *C. difficile*–associated diarrhea must be considered in all patients who present with diarrhea following antibiotic use.

Careful medical history is necessary because *C. difficile*–associated diarrhea has been reported to occur over 2 months after the administration of antibacterial agents.

If *C. difficile*–associated diarrhea is suspected or confirmed, ongoing antibiotic use not directed against *C. difficile* may need to be discontinued. Institute appropriate fluid and electrolyte management, protein supplementation, antibiotic treatment of *C. difficile*, and surgical evaluation as clinically indicated.

➤*Lactic acidosis:* Lactic acidosis has been reported with the use of linezolid. In reported cases, patients experienced repeated episodes of nausea and vomiting. Administer immediate medical evaluation to patients who develop recurrent nausea or vomiting, unexplained acidosis, or a low bicarbonate level while receiving linezolid.

➤*Serotonin syndrome:* Spontaneous reports of serotonin syndrome associated with the coadministration of linezolid and serotonergic agents, including antidepressants, such as selective serotonin reuptake inhibitors (SSRIs), have been reported.

Where administration of linezolid and concomitant serotonergic agents is clinically appropriate, closely observe patients for signs and symptoms of serotonin syndrome, such as cognitive dysfunction, hyperpyrexia, hyperreflexia, and incoordination. If signs or symptoms occur, consider discontinuation of either one or both agents. If the concomitant serotonergic agent is withdrawn, discontinuation symptoms can be observed.

➤*Peripheral and optic neuropathy:* Peripheral and optic neuropathy have been reported in patients treated with linezolid, primarily those patients treated for longer than the maximum recommended duration of 28 days. In cases of optic neuropathy that progressed to loss of vision, patients were treated for extended periods beyond the maximum recommended duration. Visual blurring has been reported in some patients treated with linezolid for less than 28 days.

If patients experience symptoms of visual impairment, such as changes in visual acuity, changes in color vision, blurred vision, or visual field defect, prompt ophthalmic evaluation is recommended. Monitor visual function in all patients taking linezolid for extended periods (at least 3 months) and in all patients reporting new visual symptoms, regardless of length of therapy with linezolid. If peripheral or optic neuropathy occurs, weigh the continued use of linezolid against the potential risks in these patients.

➤*Convulsions:* Convulsions have been reported in patients when treated with linezolid. In some of these cases, a history of seizures or risk factors for seizures was reported.

➤*Resistance:* Prescribing linezolid in the absence of a proven or strongly suspected bacterial infection or a prophylactic indication is unlikely to provide benefit to the patient and increases the risk of the development of drug-resistant bacteria.

➤*Duration of therapy:* The safety and efficacy of linezolid formulations given for longer than 28 days have not been evaluated in controlled clinical trials.

➤*Superinfection:* The use of antibiotics may promote the overgrowth of nonsusceptible organisms. If superinfection occurs during therapy, take appropriate measures.

➤*Pregnancy: Category C.* Linezolid was not teratogenic in mice or rats at exposure levels 6.5-fold (in mice) or equivalent to (in rats) the expected human exposure level, based on AUCs. However, embryo and fetal toxicities were seen (see following information). There are no adequate and well-controlled studies in pregnant women. It is not known if linezolid crosses the human placenta. The molecular weight (approximately 337) is low enough to

LINEZOLID — INJECTION

expect transfer to the fetus. Only use linezolid during pregnancy if the potential benefit justifies the potential risk to the fetus.

In mice, embryo and fetal toxicities were seen only at doses that caused maternal toxicity (clinical signs and reduced body weight gain). A dosage of 450 mg/kg/day (6.5-fold the estimated human exposure level based on AUCs) correlated with increased postimplantational embryo death, including total litter loss, decreased fetal body weights, and an increased incidence of costal cartilage fusion.

In rats, mild fetal toxicity was observed at 15 and 50 mg/kg/day (exposure levels 0.22-fold to approximately equivalent to the estimated human exposure, respectively, based on AUCs). The effects consisted of decreased fetal body weights and reduced ossification of sternebrae, a finding often seen in association with decreased fetal body weights. Slight maternal toxicity, in the form of reduced body weight gain, was seen at 50 mg/kg/day.

In rabbits, reduced fetal body weight occurred only in the presence of maternal toxicity (clinical signs, reduced body weight gain and food consumption) when administered at a dosage of 15 mg/kg/day (0.06-fold the estimated human exposure based on AUCs).

When female rats were treated with 50 mg/kg/day (approximately equivalent to the estimated human exposure based on AUCs) of linezolid during pregnancy and lactation, survival of pups was decreased on postnatal days 1 to 4. Male and female pups permitted to mature to reproductive age, when mated, showed an increase in preimplantation loss.

➤*Lactation:* Linezolid and its metabolites are excreted in the milk of lactating rats. Concentrations in milk were similar to those in maternal plasma. It is not known whether linezolid is excreted in human milk. The molecular weight (approximately 337) is low enough to expect excretion into breast milk. Because many drugs are excreted in human milk, exercise caution when linezolid is administered to a breast-feeding woman.

➤*Children:* See Administration and Dosage for more information.

➤*Monitoring:* Monitor complete blood cell counts weekly, particularly in those who receive linezolid for longer than 2 weeks, those with preexisting myelosuppression, those receiving concomitant drugs that produce bone marrow suppression, or those with a chronic infection who have received previous or concomitant antibiotic therapy.

Where administration of linezolid and concomitant serotonergic agents is clinically appropriate, closely observe patients for signs and symptoms of serotonin syndrome, such as cognitive dysfunction, hyperpyrexia, hyperreflexia, and incoordination.

Monitor visual function in all patients taking linezolid for extended periods (at least 3 months) and in all patients reporting new visual symptoms, regardless of length of therapy with linezolid.

Drug Interactions

Linezolid Drug Interactions

Precipitant drug	Object drug[a]		Description
Apraclonidine	Linezolid	↑	Linezolid is a reversible, nonselective MAOI[b]. Apraclonidine is contraindicated in patients receiving MAOIs. The risk of hypertension may be increased. Do not coadminister linezolid and apraclonidine within 14 days of each other.
Ginseng	Linezolid	↑	Use of linezolid with ginseng may produce unexpected toxic effects (eg, manic-like symptoms, headache). Avoid concomitant use.
MAOIs (eg, phenelzine)	Linezolid	↑	Linezolid is a reversible, nonselective MAOI; do not coadminister with any medicinal product that inhibits MAO A or B or within 2 weeks of use of such products.
Linezolid	MAOIs (eg, phenelzine)		
Rifamycins (eg, rifampin)	Linezolid	↓	Administration of linezolid 600 mg twice daily for 5 days with and without rifampin 600 mg once daily for 8 days decreased the linezolid maximum concentration and AUC 21% and 32%, respectively. Monitor the patient for a decreased response to linezolid. Be prepared to adjust therapy as needed.
Sibutramine	Linezolid	↑	The risk of serotonin syndrome may be increased. Serotonergic effects of these agents may be additive. MAOIs are contraindicated in patients receiving sibutramine.
Linezolid	Sibutramine		
Tetrabenazine	Linezolid	↑	The combination of linezolid and tetrabenazine may produce severe unexpected toxicity (eg, confusion, restlessness, behavioral changes). Coadministration of linezolid and tetrabenazine is contraindicated.
Tryptophan	Linezolid	↑	The risk of serotonin syndrome may be increased. Serotonergic effects of these agents may be additive. Carefully monitor patients for adverse reactions, including signs and symptoms of serotonin syndrome.
Linezolid	Tryptophan		
Linezolid	Atomoxetine	↑	Risk of serious or fatal reactions, including hyperthermia and rapid fluctuations in vital signs, may be increased. Coadministration of linezolid and atomoxetine within 14 days of each other is contraindicated.
Linezolid	Beta-2 agonists (eg, albuterol)	↑	Coadministration of linezolid and beta-2 agonists may result in adverse cardiovascular effects characterized by hypertension. Use caution with or within 14 days of coadministration of linezolid and beta-2 agonists. Monitor for potential increases in blood pressure with coadministration of these agents.
Linezolid	Bupropion	↑	The risk of hypertensive crisis is increased. Do not coadminister bupropion and linezolid within 14 days of each other.
Linezolid	Buspirone	↑	Unless patients are carefully observed for signs and symptoms of serotonin syndrome, do not coadminister linezolid with buspirone.
Linezolid	COMT[b] inhibitors (eg, entacapone)	↑	Coadministration of linezolid and COMT inhibitors may result in inhibition of the majority of pathways responsible for normal catecholamine metabolism. Excessive sympathetic stimulation may result. Use of linezolid with COMT inhibitors is not recommended.
Linezolid	Cyclobenzaprine	↑	The risk of hypertensive crisis, convulsions, and death is increased. Do not coadminister cyclobenzaprine and linezolid within 14 days of each other.
Linezolid	Dopaminergic agents (eg, dobutamine, dopamine)	↑	Unless patients are monitored for increases in blood pressure, do not coadminister linezolid with dopaminergic agents.
Linezolid	Levodopa	↑	Linezolid may increase the pharmacologic and toxic effects (flushing, headache, hypertension) of levodopa. Hypertensive crisis may occur. Avoid coadministration of levodopa and linezolid. If inadvertently given and hypertension occurs, give phentolamine.
Linezolid	Meperidine	↑	Unless patients are carefully observed for signs and symptoms of serotonin syndrome, do not coadminister linezolid with meperidine.
Linezolid	Methylphenidate	↑	The risk of hypertensive crisis is increased. Do not coadminister methylphenidate and linezolid within 14 days of each other.

LINEZOLID — INJECTION

Linezolid Drug Interactions

Precipitant drug	Object drug[a]		Description
Linezolid	Propoxyphene	⬆	A severe reaction potentially involving the respiratory, cardiac, and central nervous systems may occur shortly after administering propoxyphene to patients receiving linezolid. Use propoxyphene with caution in patients receiving linezolid.
Linezolid	Selective 5-HT_1 receptor agonists (eg, sumatriptan)	⬆	Unless patients are carefully observed for signs and symptoms of serotonin syndrome, do not coadminister linezolid with selective 5-HT_1 receptor agonists.
Linezolid	Serotonin reuptake inhibitors (eg, fluoxetine, paroxetine, sertraline, venlafaxine)	⬆	Linezolid has the potential for interaction with serotonergic agents. Unless patients are carefully observed for signs and symptoms of serotonin syndrome, do not coadminister linezolid with serotonin reuptake inhibitors.
Linezolid	Sympathomimetic agents (eg, pseudoephedrine)	⬆	Unless patients are monitored for increases in blood pressure, do not coadminister linezolid with sympathomimetic agents.
Linezolid	Tricyclic antidepressants (eg, amitriptyline)	⬆	Unless patients are carefully observed for signs and symptoms of serotonin syndrome, do not coadminister linezolid with tricyclic antidepressants.
Linezolid	Vasopressive agents (eg, epinephrine, norepinephrine)	⬆	Unless patients are monitored for increases in blood pressure, do not coadminister linezolid with vasopressive agents.

[a] ⬆ = object drug increased. ⬇ = object drug decreased.
[b] MAOI = monoamine oxidase inhibitor; COMT = catechol-O-methyl transferase.

➤*Drug/Food interactions:* Avoid large quantities of foods or beverages with high tyramine content while taking linezolid. Consume quantities of tyramine of less than 100 mg per meal.

Adverse Reactions

Adults –

Most common adverse reactions: The most common adverse reactions in patients treated with linezolid were diarrhea (incidence across studies is 2.8% to 11%), headache (incidence across studies is 0.5% to 11.3%), and nausea (incidence across studies is 3.4% to 9.6%).

Adverse reactions (2% or more):

Linezolid Adverse Reactions (≥ 2%)

Reaction	Linezolid (n = 2,046)	All comparators[a] (n = 2,001)
CNS		
Dizziness	2%	1.9%
Headache	6.5%	5.5%
Insomnia	2.5%	1.7%
GI		
Constipation	2.2%	2.1%
Diarrhea	8.3%	6.3%
Nausea	6.2%	4.6%
Vomiting	3.7%	2%
Miscellaneous		
Fever	1.6%	2.1%
Rash	2%	2.2%

[a] Comparators included cefpodoxime proxetil 200 mg orally every 12 hours; ceftriaxone 1 g IV every 12 hours; clarithromycin 250 mg orally every 12 hours; dicloxacillin 500 mg orally every 6 hours; oxacillin 2 g IV every 6 hours; vancomycin 1 g IV every 12 hours.

Other adverse reactions: Other adverse reactions reported in phase 2 and phase 3 studies included oral moniliasis, vaginal moniliasis, hypertension, dyspepsia, localized abdominal pain, pruritus, and tongue discoloration.

Adverse reactions by dose:

Linezolid Adverse Reactions (> 1%) by Dose

Adverse reactions	Uncomplicated skin and skin structure infections: Linezolid 400 mg orally every 12 h (n = 548)	Uncomplicated skin and skin structure infections: Clarithromycin 250 mg orally every 12 h (n = 537)	All other indications: Linezolid 600 mg every 12 h (n = 1,498)	All other indications: All other comparators[a] (n = 1,464)
Patients with 1 drug-related adverse reaction	25.4%	19.6%	20.4%	14.3%
Patients discontinuing because of drug-related adverse reactions[b]	3.5%	2.4%	2.1%	1.7%
CNS				
Dizziness	1.1%	1.5%	0.4%	0.3%
Headache	2.7%	2.2%	1.9%	1%
GI				
Diarrhea	5.3%	4.8%	4%	2.7%
Nausea	3.5%	3.5%	3.3%	1.8%
Oral moniliasis	0.4%	0%	1.1%	0.4%
Taste alteration	1.8%	2%	0.9%	0.2%
Tongue discoloration	1.1%	0%	0.2%	0%
Vomiting	0.9%	0.4%	1.2%	0.4%
Miscellaneous				
Abnormal liver function tests	0.4%	0%	1.3%	0.5%
Fungal infection	1.5%	0.2%	0.1%	< 0.1%
Vaginal moniliasis	1.6%	1.3%	1%	0.4%

[a] Comparators included cefpodoxime proxetil 200 mg orally every 12 hours; ceftriaxone 1 g IV every 12 hours; dicloxacillin 500 mg orally every 6 hours; oxacillin 2 g IV every 6 hours; vancomycin 1 g IV every 12 hours.
[b] The most commonly reported drug-related adverse reactions leading to discontinuation in patients treated with linezolid were nausea, headache, diarrhea, and vomiting.

➤*Children:*

Mortality – In the study of hospitalized children (birth through 11 years of age) with gram-positive infections who were randomized 2 to 1 (linezolid-:vancomycin), mortality was 6% in the linezolid arm and 3% in the vancomycin arm. However, given the severe underlying illness in the patient population, no causality could be established.

Adverse reactions (2% or more) –

Linezolid Adverse Reactions (≥ 2%) in Children

Reaction	Uncomplicated skin and skin structure infections[a]: Linezolid (n = 248)	Uncomplicated skin and skin structure infections[a]: Cefadroxil (n = 251)	All other indications[b]: Linezolid (n = 215)	All other indications[b]: Vancomycin (n = 101)
CNS				
Convulsion	0%	0%	2.8%	2%
Headache	6.5%	4%	0.9%	0%
Dermatologic				
Rash	1.6%	1.2%	7%	15.2%
Skin disorder	2%	0%	0.9%	1%
GI				
Diarrhea	7.8%	8%	10.8%	12.1%
Generalized abdominal pain	2.4%	2.8%	0.9%	2%
GI bleeding	0%	0%	2.3%	1%
Localized abdominal pain	2.4%	2.8%	0.9%	2%
Loose stools	1.6%	0.8%	2.3%	3%
Nausea	3.7%	3.2%	1.9%	0%
Vomiting	2.9%	6.4%	9.4%	9.1%
Hematologic				
Anemia	0%	0%	5.6%	7.1%
Thrombocythemia	0%	0%	2.8%	2%
Thrombocytopenia	0%	0%	4.7%	2%
Respiratory				
Apnea	0%	0%	2.3%	2%
Cough	2.4%	4%	0.9%	0%
Dyspnea	0%	0%	3.3%	1%
Pharyngitis	2.9%	1.6%	0.5%	1%
Pneumonia	0%	0%	2.8%	2%

LINEZOLID — INJECTION

Linezolid Adverse Reactions (≥ 2%) in Children				
	Uncomplicated skin and skin structure infections[a]		All other indications[b]	
Reaction	Linezolid (n = 248)	Cefadroxil (n = 251)	Linezolid (n = 215)	Vancomycin (n = 101)
Upper respiratory tract infection	3.7%	5.2%	4.2%	1%
Miscellaneous				
Fever	2.9%	3.6%	14.1%	14.1%
Generalized edema	0%	0%	2.3%	1%
Hypokalemia	0%	0%	2.8%	3%
Localized pain	2%	1.6%	0.9%	0%
Reaction at site of injection or of vascular catheter	0%	0%	3.3%	5.1%
Sepsis	0%	0%	8%	7.1%
Trauma	3.3%	4.8%	2.8%	2%

[a] Patients 5 through 11 years of age received linezolid 10 mg/kg orally every 12 hours or cefadroxil 15 mg/kg orally every 12 hours. Patients 12 years of age and older received linezolid 600 mg orally every 12 hours or cefadroxil 500 mg orally every 12 hours.
[b] Patients from birth through 11 years of age received linezolid 10 mg/kg IV/orally every 8 hours or vancomycin 10 to 15 mg/kg IV every 6 to 24 hours, depending on age and renal clearance.

Adverse reactions (more than 1%) –

Linezolid Adverse Reactions in Children (> 1% and > 1 Patient)				
	Uncomplicated skin and skin structure infections[a]		All other indications[b]	
Adverse reaction	Linezolid (n = 248)	Cefadroxil (n = 251)	Linezolid (n = 215)	Vancomycin (n = 101)
Patients with ≥ 1 drug-related adverse reaction	19.2%	14.1%	18.8%	34.3%
Patients discontinuing because of a drug-related adverse reaction	1.6%	2.4%	0.9%	6.1%
CNS				
Headache	2.4%	0.8%	0%	0%
Vertigo	1.2%	0.4%	0%	0%
Dermatologic				
Pruritus at nonapplication site	0.4%	0%	0%	2%
Rash	0.4%	1.2%	1.4%	7.1%
GI				
Diarrhea	5.7%	5.2%	3.8%	6.1%
Generalized abdominal pain	1.6%	1.2%	0%	0%
Localized abdominal pain	1.6%	1.2%	0%	0%
Loose stools	1.2%	0.8%	1.9%	0%
Nausea	3.3%	2%	1.4%	0%
Oral moniliasis	0%	0%	0.9%	4%
Vomiting	1.2%	2.4%	1.9%	1%
Hematologic				
Anemia	0%	0%	1.4%	1%
Eosinophilia	0.4%	0.4%	1.4%	0%
Thrombocytopenia	0%	0%	1.9%	0%
Miscellaneous				
Anaphylaxis	0%	0%	0%	10.1%[c]
Fever	0%	0%	0.5%	3%

[a] Patients 5 through 11 years of age received linezolid 10 mg/kg orally every 12 hours or cefadroxil 15 mg/kg orally every 12 hours. Patients 12 years of age and older received linezolid 600 mg orally every 12 hours or cefadroxil 500 mg orally every 12 hours.
[b] Patients from birth through 11 years of age received linezolid 10 mg/kg IV/orally every 8 hours or vancomycin 10 to 15 mg/kg IV every 6 to 24 hours, depending on age and renal clearance.
[c] These reports were of "red-man syndrome," which were coded as anaphylaxis.

➤*Thrombocytopenia:* Linezolid has been associated with thrombocytopenia when used in doses of up to and including 600 mg every 12 hours for up to 28 days. In phase 3, comparator-controlled trials, the percentage of adults who developed a substantially low platelet count (defined as less than 75% of lower limit of normal and/or baseline) was 2.4% (range among studies, 0.3% to 10%) with linezolid and 1.5% (range among studies, 0.4% to 7%) with a comparator. In a study of hospitalized children ranging from birth through 11 years of age, the percentage of patients who developed a substantially low platelet count (defined as less than 75% of lower limit of normal or baseline) was 12.9% with linezolid and 13.4% with vancomycin. In an outpatient study of children from 5 through 17 years of age, the percentage of patients who developed a substantially low platelet count was 0% with linezolid and 0.4% with cefadroxil. Thrombocytopenia associated with the use of linezolid appears to be dependent on duration of therapy (generally longer than 2 weeks of treatment). The platelet counts for most patients returned to the normal range/baseline during the follow-up period. No related clinical adverse reactions were identified in phase 3 clinical trials in patients developing thrombocytopenia. Bleeding reactions were identified in thrombocytopenic patients in a compassionate use program for linezolid; the role of linezolid in these reactions cannot be determined.

➤*Lab test abnormalities:*

Adults –

Linezolid Hematologic Adverse Reactions in Adults[a]				
	Uncomplicated skin and skin structure infections		All other indications	
Hematologic adverse reaction	Linezolid 400 mg every 12 h	Clarithromycin 250 mg every 12 h	Linezolid 600 mg every 12 h	All other comparators[b]
Hemoglobin (g/dL)	0.9%	0%	7.1%	6.6%
Platelet count (× 10³/mm³)	0.7%	0.8%	3%	1.8%
WBC[c] (× 10³/mm³)	0.2%	0.6%	2.2%	1.3%
Neutrophils (× 10³/mm³)	0%	0.2%	1.1%	1.2%

[a] Less than 75% (less than 50% for neutrophils) of lower limit of normal for values normal at baseline; less than 75% (less than 50% for neutrophils) of lower limit of normal and of baseline for values abnormal at baseline.
[b] Comparators included cefpodoxime proxetil 200 mg orally every 12 hours; ceftriaxone 1 g IV every 12 hours; dicloxacillin 500 mg orally every 6 hours; oxacillin 2 g IV every 6 hours; vancomycin 1 g IV every 12 hours.
[c] WBC = white blood cell count.

Linezolid Laboratory Abnormality in Adults[a]				
	Uncomplicated skin and skin structure infections		All other indications	
Laboratory abnormality	Linezolid 400 mg every 12 h	Clarithromycin 250 mg every 12 h	Linezolid 600 mg every 12 h	All other comparators[b]
AST (U/L)	1.7%	1.3%	5%	6.8%
ALT (U/L)	1.7%	1.7%	9.6%	9.3%
LDH[c] (U/L)	0.2%	0.2%	1.8%	1.5%
Alkaline phosphatase (U/L)	0.2%	0.2%	3.5%	3.1%
Lipase (U/L)	2.8%	2.6%	4.3%	4.2%
Amylase (U/L)	0.2%	0.2%	2.4%	2%
Total bilirubin (mg/dL)	0.2%	0%	0.9%	1.1%
BUN[c] (mg/dL)	0.2%	0%	2.1%	1.5%
Creatinine (mg/dL)	0.2%	0%	0.2%	0.6%

[a] Greater than 2 × ULN for values normal at baseline; greater than 2 × ULN and greater than 2 × baseline for values abnormal at baseline.
[b] Comparators included cefpodoxime proxetil 200 mg orally every 12 hours; ceftriaxone 1 g IV every 12 hours; dicloxacillin 500 mg orally every 6 hours; oxacillin 2 g IV every 6 hours; vancomycin 1 g IV every 12 hours.
[c] LDH = lactate dehydrogenase; BUN = serum urea nitrogen.

Children –

Linezolid Hematologic Abnormalities in Children[a]				
	Uncomplicated skin and skin structure infections[b]		All other indications[c]	
Hematologic abnormality	Linezolid	Cefadroxil	Linezolid	Vancomycin
Hemoglobin (g/dL)	0%	0%	15.7%	12.4%
Platelet count (× 10³/mm³)	0%	0.4%	12.9%	13.4%
WBC (× 10³/mm³)	0.8%	0.8%	12.4%	10.3%
Neutrophils (× 10³/mm³)	1.2%	0.8%	5.9%	4.3%

[a] Less than 75% (less than 50% for neutrophils) of lower limit of normal for values normal at baseline; less than 75% (less than 50% for neutrophils) of lower limit of normal and less than 75% (less than 50% for neutrophils, less than 90% for hemoglobin if baseline less than lower limit of normal) of baseline for values abnormal at baseline.
[b] Patients 5 through 11 years of age received linezolid 10 mg/kg orally every 12 hours or cefadroxil 15 mg/kg orally every 12 hours. Patients 12 years of age and older received linezolid 600 mg orally every 12 hours or cefadroxil 500 mg orally every 12 hours.
[c] Patients from birth through 11 years of age received linezolid 10 mg/kg IV/orally every 8 hours or vancomycin 10 to 15 mg/kg IV every 6 to 24 hours, depending on age and renal clearance.

LINEZOLID — INJECTION

Linezolid Laboratory Abnormality in Children[a]				
	Uncomplicated skin and skin structure infections[b]		All other indications[c]	
Laboratory abnormality	Linezolid	Cefadroxil	Linezolid	Vancomycin
ALT (U/L)	0%	0%	10.1%	12.5%
Lipase (U/L)	0.4%	1.2%		
Amylase (U/L)			0.6%	1.3%
Total bilirubin (mg/dL)			6.3%	5.2%
Creatinine (mg/dL)	0.4%	0%	2.4%	1%

[a] Greater than 2 times the ULN for values normal at baseline; greater than 2 times ULN and greater than 2 (greater than 1.5 for total bilirubin) times baseline for values abnormal at baseline.
[b] Patients 5 through 11 years of age received linezolid 10 mg/kg orally every 12 hours or cefadroxil 15 mg/kg orally every 12 hours. Patients 12 years of age and older received linezolid 600 mg orally every 12 hours or cefadroxil 500 mg orally every 12 hours.
[c] Patients from birth through 11 years of age received linezolid 10 mg/kg IV/orally every 8 hours or vancomycin 10 to 15 mg/kg IV every 6 to 24 hours, depending on age and renal clearance.

➤*Postmarketing:*

CNS – Convulsions, peripheral neuropathy, and optic neuropathy sometimes progressing to loss of vision. Serotonin syndrome has been reported in patients receiving concomitant serotonergic agents, including antidepressants, such as SSRIs, and linezolid.

Hematologic – Myelosuppression (including anemia, leukopenia, pancytopenia, and thrombocytopenia).

Miscellaneous – Anaphylaxis, angioedema, bullous skin disorders, such as those described as Stevens-Johnson syndrome, lactic acidosis, superficial tooth discoloration, and tongue discoloration

The tooth discoloration was removable with professional dental cleaning (manual descaling) in cases with known outcome.

Overdosage

➤*Treatment:* In the event of overdosage, supportive care is advised, with maintenance of glomerular filtration. Hemodialysis may facilitate more rapid elimination of linezolid. In a phase 1 clinical trial, approximately 30% of a dose of linezolid was removed during a 3-hour hemodialysis session beginning 3 hours after the dose of linezolid was administered. Data are not available for removal of linezolid with peritoneal dialysis or hemoperfusion.

Patient Information

Advise patients to inform their health care provider of any history of hypertension.

Advise patients to avoid large quantities of food or beverages with high tyramine content while taking linezolid. Instruct patients to consume quantities of tyramine less than 100 mg/meal. Foods high in tyramine content include those that may have undergone protein changes by aging, fermentation, pickling, or smoking to improve flavor, such as aged cheeses (tyramine 0 to 15 mg/ounce); fermented or air-dried meats (tyramine 0.1 to 8 mg/ounce); sauerkraut (tyramine 8 mg per 8 ounces); soy sauce (tyramine 5 mg/teaspoon); tap beers (tyramine 4 mg per 12 ounces); red wines (tyramine 0 to 6 mg per 8 ounces). The tyramine content of any protein-rich food may be increased if stored for long periods or improperly refrigerated.

Instruct patients to inform their health care provider if taking medications containing pseudoephedrine or phenylpropanolamine, such as cold remedies and decongestants, or if taking serotonin reuptake inhibitors or other antidepressants.

Instruct patients to inform their health care provider if experiencing changes in vision.

Instruct patients to inform their health care provider of any history of seizures.

Advise patient that diarrhea is a common problem caused by antibiotics that usually ends when the antibiotic is discontinued. Sometimes after starting treatment with antibiotics, patients can develop watery and bloody stools (with or without stomach cramps and fever), even as late as 2 or more months after having taken the last dose of the antibiotic. If this occurs, instruct patients to contact their health care provider as soon as possible.

Counsel patients to only use antibacterial drugs, including linezolid, to treat bacterial infections. They do not treat viral infections (eg, the common cold). When linezolid is prescribed to treat a bacterial infection, advise patients that although it is common to feel better early in the course of therapy, they must take the medication exactly as directed. Skipping doses or not completing the full course of therapy may decrease the effectiveness of the immediate treatment and increase the likelihood that bacteria will develop resistance and will not be treatable by linezolid or other antibacterial drugs in the future.

LINCOSAMIDES

WARNING

Pseudomembranous colitis has been reported with nearly all antibacterial agents, including lincosamides, and may range in severity from mild to life-threatening. Therefore, it is important to consider this diagnosis in patients who present with diarrhea subsequent to the administration of antibacterial agents.

Because lincosamide therapy has been associated with severe colitis, which may end fatally, it should be reserved for serious infections for which less toxic antimicrobial agents are inappropriate. It should not be used in patients with nonbacterial infections such as most upper respiratory tract infections. Treatment with antibacterial agents alters the normal flora of the colon and may permit overgrowth of clostridia. Studies indicate that a toxin produced by *Clostridium difficile* is one primary cause of antibiotic-associated colitis.

After the diagnosis of pseudomembranous colitis has been established, initiate therapeutic measures. Mild cases of pseudomembranous colitis usually respond to drug discontinuation alone. In moderate to severe cases, consider management with fluids and electrolytes, protein supplementation, and treatment with an antibacterial drug clinically effective against *C. difficile* colitis.

Diarrhea, colitis, and pseudomembranous colitis have begun up to several weeks following cessation of therapy with lincosamides.

Indications

➤*Serious infections:* For the treatment of serious infections caused by susceptible strains of streptococci, pneumococci, and staphylococci, and anaerobic bacteria. Its use should be reserved for penicillin-allergic patients or other patients for whom penicillin is inappropriate.

Because of the risk of antibiotic-associated pseudomembranous colitis, consider the nature of the infection and the suitability of less toxic alternatives (eg, erythromycin).

For specific indications, refer to individual monographs.

➤*Off-label uses:* Refer to individual monographs for further information.

Pelvic inflammatory disease –
Clindamycin: [1] = Good documentation.

Surgical prophylaxis –
Clindamycin: [2] = Fair documentation.

Toxoplasmosis –
Clindamycin: [1] = Good documentation.

Actions

➤*Pharmacology:* **Lincomycin** and **clindamycin**, collectively known as lincosamides, bind exclusively to the 50S subunit of bacterial ribosomes and suppress protein synthesis. Cross resistance has been demonstrated between these 2 agents.

➤*Pharmacokinetics:*

Pharmacokinetic Parameters						
	Bioavailability (%)	Mean peak serum level (mcg/mL)	Time to peak serum level (h)	Half-life (h)	Elimination in urine (%)	Elimination in feces (%)
Lincomycin						
IM[a]		11.6	1	4.4 to 6.4	17.3 (2 to 25)	
IV[b]		15.9	2		13.8 (5 to 30)	
Clindamycin						
Oral	90	2.5	0.75	2.4	10	3.6
IM		9 (adults) 6 (children)	3 (adults) 1 (children)			
IV		11.9 (adults) 10 (children)				

[a] IM = intramuscular.
[b] IV = intravenous.

Absorption – **Lincomycin** maintains therapeutic levels for 17 to 20 hours for most susceptible gram-positive organisms. **Clindamycin** is rapidly absorbed after oral administration.

Distribution – **Lincomycin** appears to diffuse into cerebrospinal fluid and the majority of body tissues. **Clindamycin** is widely distributed in body fluids and tissues (including bones).

Excretion – Tissue levels indicate that bile is an important route of excretion for **lincomycin**.

Special populations –

Elderly: After oral administration of **clindamycin**, elimination half-life is increased approximately 4 hours (range, 3.4 to 5.1 hours) in elderly patients compared with 3.2 hours (range, 2.1 to 4.2 hours) in younger adults.

Renal/Hepatic function impairment: The serum half-life of **lincomycin** may be prolonged in patients with severe renal function impairment compared with patients with healthy renal function. Serum half-life of **clindamycin** is increased slightly in patients with markedly reduced renal function. In patients with hepatic function impairment, **lincomycin** serum half-life may be 2-fold longer than in patients with healthy hepatic function.

➤*Microbiology:*

Lincosamide Microbiology Susceptibility		
	Lincomycin	Clindamycin
Gram-positive aerobes		
Corynebacterium diphtheriae	✓[a]	
Pneumococci	✓	✓
Staphylococcus aureus	✓[b]	✓[b,c]
Staphylococcus epidermidis		✓[a,b,c]
Streptococcus pneumoniae	✓	✓[d]
Streptococcus pyogenes	✓[a]	✓
Streptococcus agalactiae		✓[a]
Streptococcus anginosus		✓[a]
Streptococcus oralis		✓[a]
Streptococcus mitis		✓[a]
Viridans group streptococci	✓[a]	
Anerobes		
Actinomyces israelii		✓[a]
Bacteroides sp.		✓
Clostridium perfringens	✓[a]	✓
Clostridium clostridioforme		✓[a]
Clostridium tetani	✓[a]	
Eubacterium lentum		✓[a]
Fusobacterium necrophorum		✓
Fusobacterium nucleatum		✓
Microaerophilic streptococci		✓
Peptococcus sp.		✓
Peptostreptococcus anaerobius		✓
Peptostreptococcus micros		✓[a]
Peptostreptococcus magna		✓[a]
Prevotella melaninogenica		✓
Prevotella intermedia		✓[a]
Prevotella bivia		✓[a]
Propionibacterium acnes	✓[a]	✓[a]

[a] In vitro data only.
[b] Penicillinase- and nonpenicillinase-producing strains.
[c] Methicillin-susceptible strains.
[d] Penicillin-susceptible strains.

Contraindications

History of hypersensitivity to preparations containing clindamycin or lincomycin.

Warnings/Precautions

➤*Pseudomembranous colitis:* Pseudomembranous colitis has been reported with nearly all antibacterial agents, including lincosamides, and may range in severity from mild to life-threatening. Therefore, it is important to consider this diagnosis in patients who present with diarrhea subsequent to the administration of antibacterial agents (See Black Box Warning).

Treatment with antibacterial agents alters the normal flora of the colon and may permit overgrowth of clostridia. Studies indicate that a toxin produced by *C. difficile* is one primary cause of antibiotic-associated colitis.

After the diagnosis of pseudomembranous colitis has been established, initiate therapeutic measures. Mild cases of pseudomembranous colitis usually respond to drug discontinuation alone. In moderate to severe cases, consider management with fluids and electrolytes, protein supplementation, and treatment with an antibacterial drug clinically effective against *C. difficile* colitis.

Also consider other causes of colitis. Make a careful inquiry concerning previous sensitivities to drugs and other allergens.

➤*Meningitis:* **Clindamycin** does not diffuse adequately into cerebrospinal fluid; do not use for the treatment of meningitis. Although **lincomycin** does appear to diffuse into cerebrospinal fluid, levels may be inadequate for the treatment of meningitis.

➤*Administration:* Do not inject IV undiluted as a bolus; infuse over at least 10 to 60 minutes.

➤*Benzyl alcohol:* Some of these products contain benzyl alcohol, which has been associated with fatal "gasping syndrome" in premature infants.

➤*Drug resistant bacteria:* To reduce the development of drug-resistant bacteria and maintain the effectiveness of lincosamides and other antibacterial drugs, use lincosamides only to treat or prevent infections that are proven or strongly suspected to be caused by susceptible bacteria. When culture and susceptibility information are available, consider them in selecting or modifying antibacterial therapy. In the absence of such data, local epidemiology and susceptibility patterns may contribute to the empiric selection of therapy.

➤*Hypersensitivity reactions:* If hypersensitivity occurs, discontinue the drug and institute emergency treatment. Make a careful inquiry concerning previous sensitivities to drugs and other allergens. Serious anaphylactoid reactions require immediate emergency treatment with epinephrine. Administer oxygen and IV corticosteroids as indicated.

➤*Tartrazine sensitivity:* Some of the products contain tartrazine, which may cause allergic-type reactions (including bronchial asthma) in susceptible individuals. Although the incidence of tartrazine sensitivity in the general population is low, it is frequently seen in patients who also have aspirin sensitivity. Refer to the individual product listings.

➤*Renal/Hepatic function impairment:* Give cautiously to patients with severe renal or hepatic function impairment; monitor serum levels during high-dose therapy.

➤*Special risk:* Use with caution in patients with a history of asthma or significant allergies. Use with caution in atopic patients and in patients with GI disease, particularly colitis.

➤*Superinfection:* Use of antibiotics may result in bacterial or fungal overgrowth of nonsusceptible organisms, particularly yeasts. Such overgrowth may lead to a secondary infection. Take appropriate measures if superinfection occurs.

➤*Pregnancy: Category C* – **lincomycin** (per manufacturer prescribing information). *Category B* – **clindamycin**; **lincomycin** (per Briggs' *Drugs in Pregnancy and Lactation*). There are no adequate and well-controlled studies in pregnant women. Use these drugs during pregnancy only if clearly needed.

➤*Lactation:* **Clindamycin** appears in breast milk in ranges of 0.7 to 3.8 mcg/mL at doses of 150 mg orally to 600 mg IV. **Lincomycin** appears in breast milk in ranges of 0.5 to 2.4 mcg/mL. Because of the potential for serious adverse reactions in breast-feeding infants, decide whether to discontinue breast-feeding or the drug, taking into account the importance of the drug to the mother.

➤*Children:* Safety and effectiveness in children younger than 1 month of age have not been established for **lincomycin**. When **clindamycin** is administered to children (birth to 16 years of age), monitor organ system function. Each mL of **clindamycin** and **lincomycin** injection contains benzyl alcohol 9.45 mg.

➤*Elderly:* Older patients with associated severe illness may not tolerate diarrhea well; carefully monitor these patients for changes in bowel frequency.

➤*Monitoring:* For prolonged therapy, perform liver/kidney function tests and blood cell counts periodically. Monitor serum levels of lincosamides during high-dose therapy.

Drug Interactions

Lincosamide Drug Interactions			
Precipitant drug	Object drug[a]		Description
Erythromycin	Lincosamides	⬇	Antagonism has occurred in vitro between clindamycin and erythromycin. Because of possible clinical significance, do not coadminister the 2 drugs.
Kaolin-Pectin	Lincosamides	⬇	GI absorption is decreased for lincomycin and delayed for clindamycin when administered with kaolin-pectin antidiarrheals.
Lincosamides	Neuromuscular blockers (eg, pancuronium, tubocuraraine)	⬆	The actions of nondepolarizing neuromuscular blockers may be enhanced, possibly contributing to profound and severe respiratory depression.

[a] ⬆ = object drug increased; ⬇ = object drug decreased.

Adverse Reactions

Lincosamide Adverse Reactions		
Adverse reaction	Lincomycin	Clindamycin
Cardiovascular		
Cardiopulmonary arrest[a]	X[b]	X
Hypotension[a]	X	X
Dermatologic		
Dermatitis (exfoliative and vesiculobullous)	X	X
Pruritus		X
Skin rashes	X	X
Urticaria	X	X

Lincosamide Adverse Reactions		
Adverse reaction	Lincomycin	Clindamycin
GI		
Abdominal pain		X
Antibiotic associated diarrhea and colitis	X	X
Esophagitis		X
Glossitis	X	
Metallic taste[c]		X
Nausea	X	X
Pruritus ani	X	
Pseudomembranous colitis	X	X
Stomatitis	X	
Vomiting	X	X
GU		
Azotemia	X	X
Oliguria	X	X
Proteinuria	X	X
Vaginitis	X	X
Hematologic		
Agranulocytosis	X	X
Aplastic anemia	X	
Eosinophilia		X
Leukopenia	X	X
Neutropenia	X	X
Pancytopenia	X	
Thrombocytopenia		X
Thrombocytopenic purpura	X	
Hepatic		
Abnormal liver function tests	X	X
Jaundice	X	X
Local		
Abscess, sterile[d]		X
Induration[d]		X
Pain[d]	X	X
Thrombophlebitis[e]		X
Special senses		
Tinnitus	X	
Vertigo	X	
Miscellaneous		
Polyarthritis		X

[a] Reported following too rapid an IV administration.
[b] X = reported; no incidence given.
[c] Has been reported after IV administration of the higher doses of clindamycin phosphate.
[d] Reported after IV infusion.
[e] Reported after IM injection.

➤*Hypersensitivity:* Hypersensitivity reactions such as maculopapular rash, urticaria, angioneurotic edema, serum sickness, and anaphylaxis have been reported. Generalized mild to moderate morbilliform-like skin rashes are the most frequently reported of all adverse reactions. Rare instances of erythema multiforme, some resembling Stevens-Johnson syndrome, have been reported. A few cases of anaphylactoid reactions have been reported. If an allergic reaction occurs, discontinue the drug. Serious acute hypersensitivity reactions may require treatment with epinephrine and other emergency measures, including oxygen, IV fluids, IV antihistamines, corticosteroids, pressor amines, and airway management, as clinically indicated.

Overdosage

➤*Symptoms:* Significant mortality was observed in mice at an IV dose of **clindamycin** 855 mg/kg and in rats at an approximate oral or subcutaneous dose of **clindamycin** 2,618 mg/kg. In the mice, convulsions and depression were observed.

➤*Treatment:* Hemodialysis and peritoneal dialysis are not effective in removing **clindamycin** or **lincomycin** from the serum.

Patient Information

May cause diarrhea; advise patients to notify their health care provider immediately if this occurs. Advise patients not to treat diarrhea without notifying their health care provider.

Advise patient to take each dose of oral clindamycin with a full glass of water. Oral clindamycin may be taken without regard to meals.

Advise patient to complete the full course of therapy.

Advise patients these products may contain tartrazine dye.

Advise patient not to refrigerate clindamycin oral solution; when chilled, the solution may be difficult to pour. The oral solution is stable for 2 weeks at room temperature after reconstitution.

LINCOMYCIN

Rx	**Lincocin** (Upjohn)	**Injection, solution:** 300 mg/mL	As lincomycin hydrochloride. In 2 and 10 mL vials.[a]

[a] With benzyl alcohol 9.45 mg/mL.

LINCOMYCIN HYDROCHLORIDE — INJECTION

For complete and comparative prescribing information, refer to the Lincosamides group monograph.

WARNING

Pseudomembranous colitis has been reported with nearly all antibacterial agents, including lincomycin, and may range in severity from mild to life-threatening. Therefore, it is important to consider this diagnosis in patients who present with diarrhea subsequent to the administration of antibacterial agents.

Because lincomycin therapy has been associated with severe colitis, which may end fatally, reserve it for serious infections for which less toxic antimicrobial agents are inappropriate. Do not use it in patients with nonbacterial infections, such as most upper respiratory tract infections. Treatment with antibacterial agents alters the normal flora of the colon and may permit overgrowth of clostridia. Studies indicate that a toxin produced by *Clostridium difficile* is one primary cause of antibiotic-associated colitis.

After the diagnosis of pseudomembranous colitis has been established, initiate therapeutic measures. Mild cases of pseudomembranous colitis usually respond to drug discontinuation alone. In moderate to severe cases, consider management with fluids and electrolytes, protein supplementation, and treatment with an antibacterial drug clinically effective against *C. difficile* colitis.

Diarrhea, colitis, and pseudomembranous colitis may begin up to several weeks following cessation of therapy with lincomycin.

Indications

➤*Serious infections:* For the treatment of serious infections caused by susceptible strains of streptococci, pneumococci, and staphylococci. Its use should be reserved for penicillin-allergic patients or other patients for whom, in the judgment of the health care provider, a penicillin is inappropriate. Before selecting lincomycin and because of the risk of antibiotic-associated pseudomembranous colitis, consider the nature of the infection and the suitability of less toxic alternatives (eg, erythromycin).

Lincomycin has been demonstrated to be effective in the treatment of staphylococcal infections resistant to other antibiotics and susceptible to lincomycin. Staphylococcal strains resistant to lincomycin have been recovered; perform culture and susceptibility studies in conjunction with lincomycin therapy. In the case of macrolides, partial but not complete cross-resistance may occur. The drug may be administered concomitantly with other antimicrobial agents when indicated.

Administration and Dosage

➤*General dosing considerations:* Do not inject IV undiluted as a bolus; infuse over at least 60 minutes.

Severe cardiopulmonary reactions have occurred when this drug has been given at more than the recommended concentration and rate.

➤*Adults:*

Infections – For a list of infections, refer to Indications.

Serious infections: 600 mg (2 mL) IM every 24 hours, or 600 mg (2 mL) to 1 g by IV infusion (over at least 1 hour) every 8 to 12 hours.

More severe infections:

- *Usual dosage* – 600 mg (2 mL) IM every 12 hours or more often, or up to 8 g/day by IV infusion (over at least 1 hour).
- *Maximum dose* – 8 g/day by IV infusion.

Subconjunctival injection: 0.25 mL (75 mg) injected subconjunctivally will result in ocular fluid levels of antibiotic (lasting for at least 5 hours), with minimum inhibitory concentrations sufficient for most susceptible pathogens.

➤*Children:*

Infections – For a list of infections, refer to Indications.

Older than 1 month of age:

- *Intramuscular* –
  - *Serious infections:* 10 mg/kg IM every 24 hours.
  - *More severe infections:* 10 mg/kg IM every 12 hours or more often.
- *Intravenous* – 10 to 20 mg/kg/day by IV infusion (over at least 1 hour), depending on the severity of the infection, may be infused in divided doses as previously described for adults.

LINCOMYCIN HYDROCHLORIDE — INJECTION

➤*Renal function impairment:* When therapy with lincomycin is required in individuals with severe renal function impairment, an appropriate dose is 25% to 30% of that recommended for patients with normally functioning kidneys.

➤*Therapeutic drug monitoring:* Monitor serum lincomycin levels during high-dose therapy.

➤*Discontinuation of therapy:* If significant diarrhea occurs during therapy, this antibiotic should be discontinued.

➤*Preparation for administration:*

IV use – IV doses are given on the basis of lincomycin 1 g diluted in no less than 100 mL of appropriate solution.

➤*Administration:* Lincomycin may be given IV (infused over a period of no less than 1 hour), IM or subconjunctivally.

Lincomycin IV Infusion Rates

Dose	Volume diluent	Time
600 mg	100 mL	1 h
1 g	100 mL	1 h
2 g	200 mL	2 h
3 g	300 mL	3 h
4 g	400 mL	4 h

➤*Admixture compatibility:*

Compatibility –

Infusion solutions: Dextrose 5% injection, dextrose 10% injection, dextrose 5% and sodium chloride 0.9% injection, dextrose 10% and sodium chloride 0.9% injection, Ringer's injection, 1/6 M sodium lactate injection, Travert 10%-Electrolyte No. 1, and Dextran in Saline 6% w/v.

Vitamins in infusion solutions: B-complex and B-complex with ascorbic acid.

Antibiotics in infusion solutions: Penicillin G sodium (satisfactory for 4 hours), cephalothin, tetracycline, cephaloridine, colistimethate (satisfactory for 4 hours), ampicillin, methicillin, chloramphenicol, and polymyxin B sulfate.

Incompatibility – Novobiocin and kanamycin.

➤*Storage/Stability:* Store at 20° to 25°C (68° to 77°F). Diluted lincomycin in an appropriate solution is physically compatible for 24 hours at room temperature unless otherwise indicated.

CLINDAMYCIN

Rx	**Cleocin** (Pfizer)	**Capsules; oral:** 75 mg	As clindamycin hydrochloride. Tartrazine, lactose. (CLEOCIN 75 mg). Green. In 100s.
Rx	**Clindamycin Hydrochloride** (Various, eg, Ranbaxy, Teva)	**Capsules; oral:** 150 mg	As clindamycin hydrochloride. May contain lactose. In 100s.
Rx	**Cleocin** (Pfizer)		As clindamycin hydrochloride. Tartrazine, lactose. (CLEOCIN 150 mg). Light blue and green. In 100s and UD 100s.
Rx	**Clindamycin Hydrochloride** (Various, eg, Ranbaxy, Teva)	**Capsules; oral:** 300 mg	As clindamycin hydrochloride. May contain lactose. In 16s, 100s, and UD 100s.
Rx	**Cleocin** (Pfizer)		As clindamycin hydrochloride. Lactose. (CLEOCIN 300 mg). Light blue. In 100s and UD 100s.
Rx	**Clindamycin Palmitate Hydrochloride** (Various, eg, Greenstone, Paddock Laboratories)	**Granules for solution; oral:** 75 mg per 5 mL	As clindamycin palmitate hydrochloride. May contain cherry flavoring, dextrin, ethylparaben, sucrose. In 100 mL.
Rx	**Cleocin Pediatric** (Pfizer)		As clindamycin palmitate hydrochloride. Sucrose, ethylparaben. Cherry flavor. In 100 mL.
Rx	**Clindamycin Phosphate** (Various, eg, Abraxis)	**Injection, solution, concentrate:** 150 mg/mL	As clindamycin phosphate. May contain benzyl alcohol and disodium edetate. In 2, 4, and 6 mL vials and 2, 4, and 6 mL *ADD-Vantage* vials.
Rx	**Cleocin Phosphate** (Pharmacia & Upjohn)		As clindamycin phosphate. Benzyl alcohol, disodium edetate. In 2, 4, and 6 mL vials and 4 and 6 mL *ADD-Vantage* vials.
Rx	**Cleocin Phosphate IV** (Pharmacia & Upjohn)	**Injection:** 300 mg 600 mg 900 mg	As clindamycin phosphate. Disodium edetate. In 50 mL *Galaxy* plastic containers with dextrose 5%.

CLINDAMYCIN HYDROCHLORIDE — ORAL

For complete and comparative prescribing information, refer to the Lincosamides group monograph.

WARNING

Clostridium difficile–associated diarrhea (CDAD) has been reported with use of nearly all antibacterial agents, including clindamycin, and may range in severity from mild diarrhea to fatal colitis. Treatment with antibacterial agents alters the normal flora of the colon, leading to overgrowth of *C. difficile*.

Because clindamycin therapy has been associated with severe colitis, which may end fatally, reserve it for serious infections for which less toxic antimicrobial agents are inappropriate. Do not use clindamycin in patients with nonbacterial infections, such as most upper respiratory tract infections.

C. difficile produces toxins A and B, which contribute to the development of CDAD. Hypertoxin-producing strains of *C. difficile* cause increased morbidity and mortality, as these infections can be refractory to antimicrobial therapy and may require colectomy. CDAD must be considered in all patients who present with diarrhea following antibiotic use. Careful medical history is necessary because CDAD has been reported to occur more than 2 months after the administration of antibacterial agents.

If CDAD is suspected or confirmed, ongoing antibiotic use not directed against *C. difficile* may need to be discontinued. Institute appropriate fluid and electrolyte management, protein supplementation, antibiotic treatment of *C. difficile*, and surgical evaluation as clinically indicated.

Indications

➤*General information:* Clindamycin is indicated in the treatment of serious infections caused by susceptible anaerobic bacteria.

➤*Anaerobes:* Serious respiratory tract infections, such as empyema, anaerobic pneumonitis, and lung abscess; serious skin and soft tissue infections; septicemia; intra-abdominal infections, such as peritonitis and intra-abdominal abscess (typically resulting from anaerobic organisms resident in the normal GI tract); infections of the female pelvis and genital tract, such as endometritis, nongonococcal tubo-ovarian abscess, pelvic cellulitis, and postsurgical vaginal cuff infection.

➤*Pneumococci:* Serious respiratory tract infections.

➤*Serious infections:* Serious infections caused by susceptible strains of streptococci, pneumococci, and staphylococci. Reserve its use for patients allergic to penicillin or other patients for whom, in the judgment of the health care provider, a penicillin is inappropriate. Before selecting clindamycin, consider the nature of the infection and the suitability of less toxic alternatives (eg, erythromycin) because of the risk of colitis.

Streptococci/Staphylococci – Serious respiratory tract infections and serious skin and soft tissue infections.

➤*Off-label uses:*

Pelvic inflammatory disease – [1] = Good documentation. The Centers for Disease Control and Prevention (CDC) guidelines advise use of clindamycin, along with gentamicin, in treating pelvic inflammatory disease (PID).

Other possible off-label uses – Clindamycin 1,200 to 2,400 mg/day may be beneficial as an alternative to sulfonamides in combination with pyrimethamine in the acute treatment of CNS toxoplasmosis in AIDS patients.

Clindamycin is effective in the treatment of *Chlamydia trachomatis* infections in women.

Clindamycin 300 mg twice daily for 7 days is effective in treating bacterial vaginosis caused by *Gardnerella vaginalis* and may be an alternative to metronidazole.

Administration and Dosage

➤*General dosing considerations:* Serious infections caused by anaerobic bacteria are usually treated with clindamycin injection. However, in clinically appropriate circumstances, the health care provider may elect to initiate treatment or continue treatment with clindamycin capsules.

➤*Adults:*

Infections – For a list of infections, see Indications.

Serious infections: 150 to 300 mg every 6 hours.

More severe infections: 300 to 450 mg every 6 hours.

CLINDAMYCIN HYDROCHLORIDE — ORAL

Off-label dosing –

Pelvic inflammatory disease: [1] = Good documentation. 900 mg intravenously (IV) every 8 hours, given in conjunction with gentamicin. Clindamycin IV therapy should continue until 24 hours after clinical improvement is noted, at which time clindamycin oral therapy (450 mg orally 4 times daily) should be continued for a total of 14 days of treatment.

➤*Children:*

Infections – For a list of infections, see Indications.

Serious infections: 8 to 16 mg/kg/day (4 to 8 mg/lb/day) divided into 3 or 4 equal doses.

More severe infections: 16 to 20 mg/kg/day (8 to 10 mg/lb/day) divided into 3 or 4 equal doses.

Off-label dosing –

Infections: 10 to 30 mg/kg/day orally in divided doses every 6 to 8 hours.

Neonates (older than 7 days):
- *Weighing less than 1.2 kg* – 5 mg/kg/dose every 12 hours.
- *Weighing 1.2 to 2 kg* – 5 mg/kg/dose every 8 hours.
- *Weighing greater than 2 kg* – 5 to 7.5 mg/kg/dose every 6 hours.

Neonates (7 days and younger):
- *Weighing 2 kg or less* – 5 mg/kg/dose every 12 hours.
- *Weighing greater than 2 kg* – 5 mg/kg/dose every 8 hours.

Neonates:
- *Alternative dosage* – 5 to 7.5 mg/kg/dose using the dosing intervals that follow:

Clindamycin dosing intervals: PMA = postmenstrual age. Dose is based on gestational age plus postnatal age.
- *If PMA is 45 weeks or more* – For all postnatal ages, the dosing interval is 6 hours.
- *If PMA is 37 to 44 weeks* – For postnatal age more than 7 days, the dosing interval is 8 hours.

For postnatal age 0 to 7 days, the dosing interval is 12 hours.
- *If PMA is 30 to 36 weeks* – For postnatal age more than 14 days, the dosing interval is 8 hours.

For postnatal age 0 to 14 days, the dosing interval is 12 hours.
- *If PMA is 29 weeks or less* – For postnatal age 28 days or more, the dosing interval is 8 hours.

For postnatal age 0 to 28 days, the dosing interval is 12 hours.

Pelvic inflammatory disease: [1] = Good documentation.
- *Adolescents* – 900 mg IV every 8 hours, given in conjunction with gentamicin. Clindamycin IV therapy should continue until 24 hours after clinical improvement is noted, at which time clindamycin oral therapy (450 mg orally 4 times daily) should be continued for a total of 14 days of treatment.

Prevention of bacterial endocarditis:
- *Usual dose* – 20 mg/kg taken orally 1 hour before procedure.
- *Maximum dose* – 600 mg.

➤*Duration of therapy:* In cases of beta-hemolytic streptococcal infections, treatment should continue for at least 10 days.

➤*Discontinuation of therapy:* If significant diarrhea occurs during therapy, this antibiotic should be discontinued. (See Warning Box.)

➤*Administration:* To avoid the possibility of esophageal irritation, take clindamycin with a full glass of water.

➤*Storage/Stability:* Store at 20° to 25°C (68° to 77°F).

CLINDAMYCIN PALMITATE HYDROCHLORIDE — ORAL

For complete and comparative prescribing information, refer to the Lincosamides group monograph.

WARNING

Clostridium difficile–associated diarrhea (CDAD) has been reported with use of nearly all antibacterial agents, including clindamycin, and may range in severity from mild diarrhea to fatal colitis. Treatment with antibacterial agents alters the normal flora of the colon, leading to overgrowth of *C. difficile*.

Because clindamycin therapy has been associated with severe colitis, which may end fatally, reserve it for serious infections for which less toxic antimicrobial agents are inappropriate. Do not use clindamycin in patients with nonbacterial infections, such as most upper respiratory tract infections. *C. difficile* produces toxins A and B, which contribute to the development of CDAD. Hypertoxin-producing strains of *C. difficile* cause increased morbidity and mortality, as these infections can be refractory to antimicrobial therapy and may require colectomy. CDAD must be considered in all patients who present with diarrhea following antibiotic use. Careful medical history is necessary because CDAD has been reported to occur more than 2 months after the administration of antibacterial agents. If CDAD is suspected or confirmed, ongoing antibiotic use not directed against *C. difficile* may need to be discontinued. Institute appropriate fluid and electrolyte management, protein supplementation, antibiotic treatment of *C. difficile*, and surgical evaluation as clinically indicated.

Indications

➤*Anaerobes:* Serious respiratory tract infections such as empyema, anaerobic pneumonitis, and lung abscess; serious skin and soft tissue infections; septicemia; intra-abdominal infections, such as peritonitis and intra-abdominal abscess (typically resulting from anaerobic organisms resident in the normal GI tract); infections of the female pelvis and genital tract, such as endometritis, nongonococcal tubo-ovarian abscess, pelvic cellulitis, and postsurgical vaginal cuff infection.

➤*Pneumococci:* Serious respiratory tract infections.

➤*Serious infections:* Serious infections caused by strains of susceptible streptococci, pneumococci, and staphylococci. Reserve its use for penicillin-allergic patients or other patients for whom, in the judgment of the health care provider, a penicillin is inappropriate. Before selecting clindamycin, consider the nature of the infection and the suitability of less toxic alternatives (eg, erythromycin) because of the risk of colitis.

Streptococci/Staphylococci – Serious respiratory tract infections; serious skin and soft tissue infections.

Administration and Dosage

➤*Children:*

Anaerobic infections –

Usual dosage: In children weighing 10 kg or less, ½ teaspoon (37.5 mg) 3 times a day should be considered the minimum recommended dose.
- *Serious infections* – 8 to 12 mg/kg/day (4 to 6 mg/lb/day) divided into 3 or 4 equal doses.

Serious infections caused by anaerobic bacteria are usually treated with clindamycin injection. However, in clinically appropriate circumstances, the health care provider may elect to initiate treatment or continue treatment with clindamycin oral solution.
- *Severe infections* – 13 to 16 mg/kg/day (6.5 to 8 mg/lb/day) divided into 3 or 4 equal doses.
- *More severe infections* – 17 to 25 mg/kg/day (8.5 to 12.5 mg/lb/day) divided into 3 or 4 equal doses.

Off-label dosing –

Infections: 10 to 30 mg/kg/day orally in divided doses every 6 to 8 hours.

Prevention of bacterial endocarditis:
- *Usual dose* – 20 mg/kg taken orally 1 hour before the procedure.
- *Maximum dose* – 600 mg.

Neonates (older than 7 days):
- *Weighing less than 1.2 kg* – 5 mg/kg/dose every 12 hours.
- *Weighing 1.2 to 2 kg* – 5 mg/kg/dose every 8 hours.
- *Weighing greater than 2 kg* – 5 to 7.5 mg/kg/dose every 6 hours.

Neonates (7 days and younger):
- *Weighing 2 kg or less* – 5 mg/kg/dose every 12 hours.
- *Weighing greater than 2 kg* – 5 mg/kg/dose every 8 hours.

Neonates:
- *Alternative dosage* – 5 to 7.5 mg/kg/dose using the dosing intervals that follow:

Clindamycin dosing intervals: PMA = postmenstrual age. Dose is based on gestational age plus postnatal age.If PMA is 45 weeks or more For all postnatal ages, the dosing interval is 6 hours.If PMA is 37 to 44 weeks For postnatal age more than 7 days, the dosing interval is 8 hours.

For postnatal age 0 to 7 days, the dosing interval is 12 hours.If PMA is 30 to 36 weeks For postnatal age more than 14 days, the dosing interval is 8 hours.

For postnatal age 0 to 14 days, the dosing interval is 12 hours.If PMA is 29 weeks or less For postnatal age 28 days or more, the dosing interval is 8 hours.

For postnatal age 0 to 28 days, the dosing interval is 12 hours.

➤*Duration of therapy:* In cases of beta-hemolytic streptococcal infections, treatment should be continued for at least 10 days.

➤*Discontinuation of therapy:* If significant diarrhea occurs during therapy, discontinue this antibiotic. (See Warning Box.)

➤*Administration:* Coadministration of food does not adversely affect the absorption of clindamycin-flavored granules.

➤*Storage/Stability:* Store at 20° to 25°C (68° to 77°F).

Do not refrigerate the reconstituted solution; when chilled, the solution may thicken and be difficult to pour. The solution is stable for 2 weeks at room temperature.

CLINDAMYCIN PHOSPHATE — INJECTION

For complete and comparative prescribing information, refer to the Lincosamides group monograph.

WARNING

Clostridium difficile–associated diarrhea (CDAD) has been reported with use of nearly all antibacterial agents, including clindamycin, and may range in severity from mild diarrhea to fatal colitis. Treatment with antibacterial agents alters the normal flora of the colon, leading to overgrowth of *C. difficile*.

Because clindamycin therapy has been associated with severe colitis, which may end fatally, reserve it for serious infections for which less toxic antimicrobial agents are inappropriate. Do not use clindamycin in patients with nonbacterial infections, such as most upper respiratory tract infections. *C. difficile* produces toxins A and B, which contribute to the development of CDAD. Hypertoxin-producing strains of *C. difficile* cause increased morbidity and mortality, as these infections can be refractory to antimicrobial therapy and may require colectomy. CDAD must be considered in all patients who present with diarrhea following antibiotic use. Careful medical history is necessary because CDAD has been reported to occur more than 2 months after the administration of antibacterial agents.

If CDAD is suspected or confirmed, ongoing antibiotic use not directed against *C. difficile* may need to be discontinued. Institute appropriate fluid and electrolyte management, protein supplementation, antibiotic treatment of *C. difficile*, and surgical evaluation as clinically indicated.

Indications

➤*Bone and joint infections:* Acute hematogenous osteomyelitis caused by *Staphylococcus aureus* and as adjunctive therapy in the surgical treatment of chronic bone and joint infections caused by susceptible organisms.

➤*Gynecological infections:* Endometritis, nongonococcal tubo-ovarian abscess, pelvic cellulitis, and postsurgical vaginal cuff infection caused by susceptible anaerobes.

➤*Intra-abdominal infections:* Peritonitis and intra-abdominal abscess caused by susceptible anaerobic organisms.

➤*Lower respiratory tract infections:* Pneumonia, empyema, and lung abscess caused by anaerobes, *Streptococcus pneumoniae*, other streptococci (except *Enterococcus faecalis*), and *S. aureus*.

➤*Septicemia:* Caused by *S. aureus*, streptococci (except *E. faecalis*), and susceptible anaerobes.

➤*Serious infections:* For the treatment of serious infections caused by susceptible strains of streptococci, pneumococci, and staphylococci.

Reserve its use for penicillin-allergic patients or other patients for whom, in the judgment of the health care provider, a penicillin is inappropriate. Before selecting clindamycin, consider the nature of the infection and the suitability of less toxic alternatives (eg, erythromycin) because of the risk of antibiotic-associated pseudomembranous colitis.

➤*Skin and skin structure infections:* Caused by *Streptococcus pyogenes*, *S. aureus*, and anaerobes.

➤*Off-label uses:*

Pelvic inflammatory disease – [1] = Good documentation. The Centers for Disease Control and Prevention (CDC) guidelines advise use of clindamycin, along with gentamicin, in treating pelvic inflammatory disease (PID).

Surgical prophylaxis – [2] = Fair documentation. Evidence-based guidelines suggest that clindamycin may be used for surgical prophylaxis only in patients with a documented beta-lactam allergy requiring cardiothoracic, vascular, hip or knee arthroplasty, gynecologic, obstetric, or colorectal surgeries. The decision to use this agent should involve examination of local antibiotic resistance patterns.

Toxoplasmosis – [1] = Good documentation. According to New York State Department of Health (NYSDH) guidelines, clindamycin should be used as second-line therapy in combination with pyrimethamine and leucovorin for the treatment of toxoplasmic encephalitis and ocular toxoplasmosis, as well as for prevention of recurrent toxoplasmosis infections in immunocompromised men and nonpregnant women.

Administration and Dosage

➤*Adults:*

Serious infections caused by susceptible anaerobic bacteria –

Serious infections: 600 to 1,200 mg/day in 2, 3, or 4 equal doses administered intramuscularly (IM) or intravenously (IV) for infections caused by aerobic gram-positive cocci and the more susceptible anaerobes (not generally including *Bacteroides fragilis*, *Peptococcus* spp., and *Clostridium* spp. other than *Clostridium perfringens*.

More severe infections: 1,200 to 2,700 mg/day in 2, 3, or 4 equal doses administered IM or IV, in particular for infections caused by proven or suspected *B. fragilis*, *Peptococcus* spp., and *Clostridium* spp. other than *C. perfringens*.

Life-threatening situations: For more serious infections, these doses may have to be increased. In life-threatening situations caused by aerobes or anaerobes, these doses may be increased. Doses of as much as 4,800 mg daily have been given IV to adults.

Off-label dosing –

Pelvic inflammatory disease: [1] = Good documentation. 900 mg IV every 8 hours, given in conjunction with gentamicin. Clindamycin IV therapy should continue until 24 hours after clinical improvement is noted, at which time clindamycin oral therapy (450 mg orally 4 times daily) should be continued for a total of 14 days of treatment.

Surgical prophylaxis: [2] = Fair documentation. 600 to 900 mg IV infused over 10 to 60 minutes (do not exceed 30 mg/min) every 3 to 6 hours.

Toxoplasmosis: [1] = Good documentation. 600 to 1,200 mg IV every 12 hours for 4 to 6 weeks has been given as adjunctive therapy with pyrimethamine for the treatment of toxoplasmic encephalitis. Clindamycin dosing for ocular toxoplasmosis in immunocompromised, HIV-infected patients should be the same as for toxoplasmic encephalitis.

➤*Children:*

Serious infections caused by susceptible anaerobic bacteria –

1 month to 16 years of age:

- *Usual dosage* – 20 to 40 mg/kg/day in 3 or 4 equal doses administered IM or IV. Use the higher doses for more severe infections.
- *Alternative dosage* – Children may be dosed on a mg/m^2 basis for body surface area: 350 mg/m^2/day for serious infections and 450 mg/m^2/day for more severe infections.

Neonates (younger than 1 month of age): 15 to 20 mg/kg/day in 3 to 4 equal doses. The lower dose may be adequate for small premature infants.

Off-label dosing –

Infection:

- *Children older than 1 month of age* –
  - *Mild-to-moderate infection:* 15 to 25 mg/kg/day in divided doses every 6 to 8 hours administered IM or IV.
  - *Severe infection:* 25 to 40 mg/kg/day in divided doses every 6 to 8 hours administered IM or IV.
- *Neonates (older than 7 days of age)* –
  - *Weighing less than 1.2 kg:* 5 mg/kg/dose administered IM or IV every 12 hours.
  - *Weighing 1.2 to 2 kg:* 5 mg/kg/dose administered IM or IV every 8 hours.
  - *Weighing greater than 2 kg:* 5 to 7.5 mg/kg/dose administered IM or IV every 6 hours.
- *Neonates (7 days of age and younger)* –
  - *Weighing 2 kg or less:* 5 mg/kg/dose administered IM or IV every 12 hours.
  - *Weighing greater than 2 kg:* 5 mg/kg/dose administered IM or IV every 8 hours.
- *Neonates* –
  - *Alternative dosage:* 5 to 7.5 mg/kg/dose by IV infusion over 30 minutes using the dosing intervals that follow:

Clindamycin dosing intervals: PMA = postmenstrual age. Dose is based on gestational age plus postnatal age.

- *If PMA is 45 weeks or more* – For all postnatal ages, the dosing interval is 6 hours.
- *If PMA is 37 to 44 weeks* – For postnatal age more than 7 days, the dosing interval is 8 hours.

For postnatal age 0 to 7 days, the dosing interval is 12 hours.

- *If PMA is 30 to 36 weeks* – For postnatal age more than 14 days, the dosing interval is 8 hours.

For postnatal age 0 to 14 days, the dosing interval is 12 hours.

- *If PMA is 29 weeks or less* – For postnatal age 28 days or more, the dosing interval is 8 hours.

For postnatal age 0 to 28 days, the dosing interval is 12 hours.

Pelvic inflammatory disease: [1] = Good documentation.

- *Adolescents* – 900 mg IV every 8 hours, given in conjunction with gentamicin. Clindamycin IV therapy should continue until 24 hours after clinical improvement is noted, at which time clindamycin oral therapy (450 mg orally 4 times daily) should be continued for a total of 14 days of treatment.

Prevention of bacterial endocarditis:

- *Usual dose* – 20 mg/kg taken 20 to 30 minutes before procedure given IV.
- *Maximum dose* – 600 mg.

Surgical prophylaxis: [2] = Fair documentation. 10 mg/kg/dose administered IM or IV preoperatively.

- *Weight less than 10 kg* – Administer at least 37.5 mg every 3 to 6 hours.
- *Weight 10 kg or more* – Administer 3 to 6 mg/kg every 3 to 6 hours.

➤*Renal function impairment:*

Adults receiving continuous renal replacement therapy – One reference suggests a dosage of 150 to 450 mg IV every 6 hours.

Alternatively, a dosage of 600 to 900 mg IV every 8 hours is recommended for patients receiving continuous venovenous hemofiltration, continuous venovenous hemodialysis, or continuous venovenous hemodialfiltration. This recommendation assumes ultrafiltration and dialysis flow rates of 1 to 2 L/hr.

Adults receiving intermittent hemodialysis – 600 to 900 mg IV every 8 hours. This recommendation assumes the patient is receiving standard intermittent hemodialysis 3 times per week and completes the full dialysis sessions.

➤*Conversion from IV to oral:* Parenteral therapy may be changed to clindamycin for oral solution or clindamycin capsules when the condition warrants and at the discretion of the health care provider.

➤*Duration of therapy:* In cases of beta-hemolytic streptococcal infections, treatment should be continued for at least 10 days.

➤*Discontinuation of therapy:* If diarrhea occurs during therapy, this antibiotic should be discontinued. (See Warning Box.)

CLINDAMYCIN PHOSPHATE — INJECTION

➤*Preparation for administration:*

Galaxy plastic container – Premixed clindamycin IV solution is for IV administration using sterile equipment. Check for minute leaks prior to use by squeezing the bag firmly. If leaks are found, discard the solution because sterility may be impaired. Do not add supplementary medication.

Do not use unless solution is clear and seal is intact.

ADD-Vantage system –

For IV use only: Clindamycin 600 and 900 mg may be reconstituted in 50 or 100 mL, respectively, of dextrose 5% injection or sodium chloride 0.9% injection in the ADD diluent container. Refer to separate instructions for the *ADD-Vantage* system.

➤*Administration:* May be administered IM or IV. Single IM injections of more than 600 mg are not recommended. Administration of more than 1,200 mg in a single 1-hour infusion is not recommended.

Alternatively, the drug may be administered in the form of a single rapid infusion of the first dose, followed by continuous IV infusion as follows.

Clindamycin Injection Administration (Single Rapid Infusion)

To maintain serum clindamycin levels	Rapid infusion rate	Maintenance infusion rate
> 4 mcg/mL	10 mg/min for 30 min	0.75 mg/min
> 5 mcg/mL	15 mg/min for 30 min	1 mg/min
> 6 mcg/mL	20 mg/min for 30 min	1.25 mg/min

Dilution and infusion rates – Clindamycin must be diluted prior to IV administration. The concentration of clindamycin in diluent for infusion should not exceed 18 mg/mL. Infusion rates should not exceed 30 mg/min. The usual infusion dilutions and rates are as follows.

Clindamycin Injection Infusion Rates

Dose	Diluent	Time
300 mg	50 mL	10 min
600 mg	50 mL	20 min
900 mg	50 to 100 mL	30 min
1,200 mg	100 mL	40 min

➤*Admixture compatibility:*

Compatibility – Physical and biological compatibility studies monitored for 24 hours at room temperature have demonstrated no inactivation or incompatibility with the use of clindamycin in IV solutions containing sodium chloride, glucose, calcium or potassium, and solutions containing vitamin B complex in concentrations usually used clinically. No incompatibility has been demonstrated with the antibiotics cephalothin, kanamycin, gentamicin, penicillin, or carbenicillin.

Incompatibility – The following drugs are physically incompatible with clindamycin: ampicillin sodium, phenytoin sodium, barbiturates, aminophylline, calcium gluconate, and magnesium sulfate.

➤*Storage / Stability:* Store vials at a controlled room temperature, 20° to 25°C (68° to 77°F). Store *Galaxy* plastic containers at a room temperature, 25°C (77°F); avoid temperatures higher than 30°C (86°F).

Stability of diluted solutions –

Room temperature: The 6, 9, and 12 mg/mL (equivalent to clindamycin base) solutions in dextrose 5% injection, sodium chloride 0.9% injection, or Ringer's lactate injection in glass bottles or minibags demonstrated physical and chemical stability for at least 16 days at 25°C (77°F). Also, 18 mg/mL (equivalent to clindamycin base) in dextrose 5% injection in minibags demonstrated physical and chemical stability for at least 16 days at 25°C (77°F).

Refrigeration: The 6, 9, and 12 mg/mL (equivalent to clindamycin base) solutions in dextrose 5% injection, sodium chloride 0.9% injection, or Ringer's lactate injection in glass bottles or minibags demonstrated physical and chemical stability for at least 32 days at 4°C (39°F).

This chemical stability information in no way indicates that it would be acceptable practice to use this product well after the preparation time. Good professional practice suggests that compounded admixtures should be administered as soon after preparation as is feasible.

• *Frozen* – The 6, 9, and 12 mg/mL (equivalent to clindamycin base) solutions in dextrose 5% injection, sodium chloride 0.9% injection, or Ringer's lactate injection in minibags demonstrated physical and chemical stability for at least 8 weeks at −10°C (14°F). Frozen solutions should be thawed at room temperature and not refrozen.

AMINOGLYCOSIDES, PARENTERAL

WARNING

Toxicity – Aminoglycosides are associated with significant nephrotoxicity or ototoxicity. These agents are excreted primarily by glomerular filtration; thus, the serum half-life will be prolonged and significant accumulation will occur in patients with impaired renal function. Toxicity may develop even with conventional doses, particularly in patients with prerenal azotemia or impaired renal function.

Ototoxicity – Neurotoxicity, manifested as auditory (cochlear) and vestibular ototoxicity, can occur with any of these agents. Auditory changes are irreversible, usually bilateral and may be partial or total. Risk of hearing loss increases with the degree of exposure to high peak or high trough serum concentrations and continues to progress after drug withdrawal. The risk is higher in patients with renal function impairment and with preexisting hearing loss. High frequency deafness usually occurs first and can be detected by audiometric testing. When feasible, obtain serial audiograms. There may be no clinical symptoms to warn of developing cochlear damage. Tinnitus or vertigo may occur, and are evidence of vestibular injury. Other manifestations of neurotoxicity may include numbness, skin tingling, muscle twitching, and convulsions. Total or partial irreversible bilateral deafness may occur after drug discontinuation. Aminoglycoside-induced ototoxicity usually is irreversible. Vestibular toxicity is more predominant with gentamicin and streptomycin; auditory toxicity is more common with kanamycin and amikacin. Tobramycin affects both functions equally. Relative ototoxicity is streptomycin = kanamycin > amikacin = gentamicin = tobramycin. Kanamycin, amikacin, and streptomycin appear in this relative comparison based on high-dose (kanamycin, amikacin) and antituberculosis (streptomycin) therapy.

Renal toxicity – This may be characterized by decreased creatinine clearance (CrCl), cells or casts in the urine, decreased urine specific gravity, oliguria, proteinuria, or evidence of nitrogen retention (increasing blood urea nitrogen [BUN], nonprotein nitrogen [NPN], or serum creatinine). Renal damage usually is reversible. The relative nephrotoxicity of these agents is estimated to be kanamycin = amikacin = gentamicin > tobramycin > streptomycin.

Monitoring – Closely observe all patients treated with aminoglycosides. Monitoring renal and eighth cranial nerve function at onset of therapy is essential for patients with known or suspected renal function impairment and in those whose renal function initially is normal, but who develop signs of renal dysfunction. Evidence of renal function impairment or ototoxicity requires drug discontinuation or appropriate dosage adjustments. When feasible, monitor drug serum concentrations. Avoid concomitant use with other ototoxic, neurotoxic, or nephrotoxic drugs. Other factors that may increase risk of toxicity are dehydration and advanced age.

Indications

➤*General information:* The indications for specific agents are listed in individual drug monographs on the following pages. Reserve these drugs for treatment of infections caused by organisms not sensitive to less toxic agents. Safety for treatment periods longer than 14 days has not been established.

➤*Off-label uses:* Refer to individual monographs for further information.

Aerosolized –

Amikacin: [4] = Insufficient documentation.

Infective endocarditis (adults) –

Tobramycin: [1] = Good documentation.

Pelvic inflammatory disease –

Gentamicin: [1] = Good documentation.

Surgical prophylaxis –

Gentamicin: [1] = Good documentation.

Tuberculosis –

Amikacin: [1] = Good documentation.

Kanamycin: [1] = Good documentation.

Other possible off-label uses – In cystic fibrosis patients, the use of inhaled aminoglycosides may be beneficial in certain populations (eg, younger patients). Clinical outcome is not improved but deterioration of pulmonary function tests may be slowed or prevented.

Amikacin: Intrathecal/intraventricular administration has been suggested at 8 mg per 24 hours.

Amikacin 15 mg/day IV in divided doses every 8 to 12 hours may be used as a part of a multiple-drug regimen (generally 3 to 5 agents) for *Mycobacterium avium* complex, a common infection in AIDS patients.

Administration and Dosage

➤*Synergism:* In vitro studies indicate that aminoglycosides combined with penicillins or cephalosporins act synergistically against some strains of gram-negative organisms and enterococci (*Streptococcus faecalis*). Aminoglycosides may exhibit a synergistic effect when combined with carbenicillin or ticarcillin for *Pseudomonas* infections. Tests for antibiotic synergy are necessary. See also Admixture Incompatibility and Drug Interactions.

➤*Admixture incompatibility:* Beta-lactam antibiotics (eg, cephalosporins, penicillins) may inactivate aminoglycosides when admixed. Ticarcillin and carbenicillin are the worst β-lactam offenders; tobramycin and gentamicin are more susceptible than amikacin. This is most likely to occur: When the agents are mixed in the same container; during the aminoglycoside assay procedure; and in poor renal function. Concomitant cephalosporins also may falsely elevate creatinine determinations.

Ticarcillin and carbenicillin also may decrease aminoglycoside serum levels (see Overdosage).

Inactivation of tobramycin has not occurred in patients with normal renal function if they are given the drugs by separate routes. Kanamycin and methicillin inactivate each other in vitro, but this has not been seen in patients who receive them by different routes.

Guard against in vitro inactivation of aminoglycosides by β-lactam antibiotics in patients on combination therapy: 1) Place sample on ice immediately after drawing the specimen; test immediately. If testing is delayed, freeze serum as soon as possible; 2) draw the aminoglycoside level when the β-lactam antibiotic is at its trough level; 3) inactivation can still occur when the specimen is frozen (eg, ampicillin, kanamycin). If samples are to be frozen for a long period of time, inactivate the penicillin with penicillinase prior to freezing.

➤*Dosing interval:* Although further studies are needed, preliminary evidence indicates that aminoglycosides may be administered on a once daily basis without compromising efficacy and without increasing the potential for nephrotoxicity and ototoxicity. It is possible that the incidence of nephrotoxicity may be decreased.

Actions

➤*Pharmacology:* Aminoglycosides are bactericidal antibiotics used primarily in the treatment of gram-negative infections. They irreversibly bind to the 30S subunit of bacterial ribosomes, blocking the recognition step in protein synthesis and causing misreading of the genetic code. The ribosomes separate from messenger RNA; cell death ensues.

➤*Pharmacokinetics:* Because of the narrow range between therapeutic and toxic serum levels, careful attention to dosage calculations is essential, especially in patients with renal function impairment, women and elderly patients, those requiring high peak serum levels, patients on prolonged (longer than 10 days) therapy, patients with unstable renal function or those undergoing dialysis, those with abnormal extracellular fluid volume, or with prior exposure to ototoxic or nephrotoxic drugs. Age markedly affects peak concentration in children; generally, it is lower in young children and infants. Monitor drug serum levels. Peak levels indicate therapeutic levels. Trough serum level determinations (just before next dose) best indicate drug accumulation. Obtain serum levels within 48 hours of start of therapy and every 3 to 4 days assuming stable renal function; also, levels are indicated when dose is changed or in changing renal function. Generally, to measure peak levels, draw a serum sample about 30 minutes after IV infusion or 1 hour after an IM dose. For trough levels, obtain serum samples at 8 hours or just prior to the next dose.

Various Pharmacokinetic Parameters of the Aminoglycosides

Aminoglycoside	Half-life (h) Normal	Half-life (h) ESRD	Therapeutic serum levels (peak) (mcg/mL)	Toxic serum levels (mcg/mL) Peak[a]	Toxic serum levels (mcg/mL) Trough[b]	Dose (mg/kg/day) (normal CrCl)
Amikacin	2 to 3	24 to 60	16 to 32	> 35	> 10	15
Gentamicin	2	24 to 60	4 to 8	> 12	> 2	3 to 5
Kanamycin	2 to 3	24 to 60	15 to 40	> 35	> 10	15
Streptomycin	2.5	100	20 to 30	> 50	—	15
Tobramycin	2 to 2.5	24 to 60	4 to 8	> 12	> 2	3 to 5

[a] Measured 1 hour after IM administration.
[b] Measured immediately prior to next dose.

Absorption – Absorption from the GI tract is poor. Aminoglycosides are occasionally used orally for enteric infections (see Aminoglycosides, Oral monograph). Absorption from IM injection is rapid, with peak blood levels achieved within 1 hour.

Distribution – Aminoglycosides are widely distributed in extracellular fluids; peak serum concentrations may be lower than usual in patients whose extracellular fluid volume is expanded (eg, patients with edema or ascites). These drugs cross the placental barrier. Concentrations are found in bile, tissues, sputum, bronchial secretions and synovial, interstitial, peritoneal, abscess, and pleural fluids. Concentrations in renal cortex are several times higher than usual serum levels. Aminoglycosides exhibit low protein binding, except for streptomycin. They do not achieve significant cerebrospinal fluid (CSF) levels in healthy patients. Although penetration is enhanced in the presence of inflamed meninges, only low levels are achieved. When intrathecal gentamicin is given with systemic gentamicin, CSF levels are substantially increased, depending on location of injection. Peak CSF concentrations following intralumbar administration generally occur 1 to 6 hours after injection.

Newborn infants, postpartum women, and patients with ascites, spinal cord injury, and cystic fibrosis may have an enlarged apparent volume of distribution. Obesity will artificially contract the apparent volume of distribution because adipose tissue contains less water than lean body mass of equal weight.

Excretion – Done by glomerular filtration, largely as unchanged drug; thus, high urine levels are attained. Probenecid does not affect renal tubular transport. The serum half-lives of all the agents are between 2 to 3 hours in patients with normal renal function. Approximately 53% to 98% of a single IV dose is excreted in the urine in 24 hours. However, when renal function is impaired, significant accumulation and subsequent toxicity may occur rapidly if dosage is not adjusted. The serum half-life is longer in young infants, as the immature renal system is unable to excrete these drugs rapidly; during the first days of life, the half-life may exceed 5 to 6 hours. Prolonged half-life also may be noted in the elderly. In severely burned patients, the half-life may be significantly decreased and result in serum concentrations lower than anticipated. Febrile and anemic states may be associated with a shorter serum half-life; dosage adjustment is usually not necessary. Aminoglycosides are removed by hemodialysis (4 to 6 hours removes approximately 50%) and peritoneal dialysis (range, removal of 23% in 8 hours to only 4% in 22 hours).

➤*Microbiology:* The bactericidal activity of aminoglycosides is through inhibition of bacterial protein synthesis. One-way cross resistance is frequently noted. The following 3 mechanisms for the development of bacterial resistance to aminoglycosides have been identified: alteration of the drug target site (the bacterial ribosome); reduction or elimination of transport of the drug into the bacterial cell; inactivation of the drug by enzymatic modification (aminoglycoside inactivating enzymes; most significant).

Perform culture and sensitivity testing. Treat susceptible organisms with less toxic agents, especially if renal function is compromised. Resistance develops slowly, except with streptomycin. Development of streptomycin resistance may be a single-step process and may occur rapidly. Most streptococci species (particularly group D), including *S. pneumoniae*, anaerobic organisms (including *Bacteroides* sp. and *Clostridia* sp.), and anaerobic cocci are resistant to aminoglycosides.

Organisms Generally Susceptible to Aminoglycosides

	Organisms	Amikacin	Gentamicin	Kanamycin	Streptomycin	Tobramycin
Gram-positive	*Mycobacterium tuberculosis*	✓[a]			✓[b]	
	Staphylococci	✓[c]	✓[c]			✓
	S. aureus	✓	✓	✓[c]		✓
	S. epidermidis	✓		✓		
	Streptococci				✓[b]	
	S. faecalis		✓[b]		✓[b]	✓[b]
Gram-negative	*Acinetobacter* sp.	✓		✓		
	Brucella sp.				✓	
	Citrobacter sp.	✓	✓	✓	✓	✓
	Enterobacter sp.	✓	✓	✓	✓	✓
	Escherichia coli	✓	✓	✓	✓	✓
	Hemophilus influenzae	✓		✓	✓[b]	
	Hemophilus ducreyi				✓	
	Klebsiella sp.	✓	✓	✓	✓[b]	✓
	Morganella morganii					✓
	Neisseria sp.	✓		✓	✓	
	Proteus sp.	✓[d]	✓[d]	✓[d]	✓	✓[d]
	Providencia sp.	✓	✓	✓	✓	✓
	Pseudomonas sp.	✓				
	P. aeruginosa	✓	✓[b]		✓	✓
	Salmonella sp.	✓	✓	✓	✓	✓
	Serratia sp.	✓	✓	✓	✓	✓
	Shigella sp.	✓	✓	✓	✓	✓
	Yersinia (Pasteurella) pestis	✓	✓	✓	✓	✓

[a] ✓ = generally susceptible.
[b] Usually used concomitantly with other anti-infectives.
[c] Penicillinase-producing and nonpenicillinase-producing.
[d] Indole-positive and indole-negative.

Contraindications

Previous reactions to these agents. With the exception of the use of streptomycin in tuberculosis, these agents are generally not indicated in long-term therapy because of the ototoxic and nephrotoxic hazards of extended administration.

Warnings/Precautions

➤*Burn patients:* In patients with extensive burns, altered pharmacokinetics may result in reduced serum concentrations of aminoglycosides. In such patients, measurement of serum concentration is especially important for dosage determination.

➤*Hypomagnesemia:* This may occur in more than one third of patients whose oral diet is restricted or who are eating poorly.

➤*Neuromuscular blockade:* Neurotoxicity can occur after intrapleural and interperitoneal installation of large doses of an aminoglycoside; however, the reaction has followed IV, IM, and oral administration. Aminoglycosides may aggravate muscle weakness because of a potential curare-like effect on the neuromuscular junction. Use with caution in patients with neuromuscular disorders (eg, infant botulism, myasthenia gravis, parkinsonism).

Neuromuscular blockade resulting in respiratory paralysis has occurred with aminoglycosides, especially if given with or soon after anesthesia or muscle relaxants (see Drug Interactions).

During or following gentamicin therapy, paresthesias, tetany, positive Chvostek and Trousseau signs, and mental confusion have been described in patients with hypomagnesemia, hypocalcemia, and hypokalemia. When this occurred in infants, tetany and muscle weakness occurred. Adults and infants required appropriate corrective electrolyte therapy.

Use caution in newborns of mothers on magnesium sulfate; these hypermagnesemic infants may experience respiratory arrest after receiving aminoglycosides.

➤*Nephrotoxicity:* This may occur. Risk factors include the elderly, patients with a history of renal function impairment who are treated for longer periods or with higher doses than those recommended, a recent course of aminoglycosides (within 6 weeks), concurrent use of other nephrotoxic agents, frequent dosing, potassium depletion, and decreased intravascular volume. Adverse renal effects can occur in patients with initially normal renal function. Of patients receiving an aminoglycoside for several days or more, approximately 8% to 26% will develop mild renal function impairment that is generally reversible.

Because renal function may alter appreciably during therapy, test renal function daily or more frequently. Examine urine for increased excretion of protein and for presence of cells and casts, keeping in mind the effects of the primary illness on these tests. Obtain 1 or more of the following laboratory measurements at the onset of therapy, frequently during therapy and at, or shortly after, the end of therapy: CrCl rate (carefully measured or estimated from published nomograms or equations based on patient's age, sex, body weight, and serial creatinine concentrations; preferred over BUN); serum creatinine concentration (preferred over BUN); BUN. More frequent testing is desirable if renal function is changing. If signs of renal irritation appear, such as casts, white or red cells, and albumin, increase hydration; a dosage reduction may be desirable (see Administration and Dosage for individual agents). These signs usually disappear when treatment is completed. However, if azotemia or a progressive decrease of urine output occurs, stop treatment. Reduce dosage if other evidence of renal dysfunction occurs (decreased CrCl or urine-specific gravity, or increased BUN, creatinine, or oliguria).

The risk of toxic reactions is low in well-hydrated patients with normal renal function who do not receive **gentamicin** or **kanamycin** injections at higher doses or for longer periods of time than recommended.

Hydration – These drugs reach high concentrations in the renal system; keep patients well hydrated to minimize chemical irritation of tubules. Well-hydrated patients with normal renal function have low risk of nephrotoxic reactions if recommended dosage is not exceeded.

Streptomycin, given to patients with preexisting renal insufficiency, calls for extreme caution. In severely uremic patients, a single dose may produce high blood levels for several days, and the cumulative effect may produce ototoxic sequelae. Alkalinize the urine to minimize or prevent renal irritation.

➤*Intrathecal gentamicin:* A patient with multiple sclerosis for 7 years was given intra-lumbar gentamicin; disseminated microscopic brainstem lesions were found at autopsy. Tissue rarefaction and marked swelling of axis cylinders with occasional calcification, loss of oligodendroglia and astroglia, and poor inflammatory response were seen. Use of excessive (40 to 160 mg) doses of intrathecal gentamicin has produced neuromuscular disturbances (eg, ataxia, incontinence, paresis).

➤*Cross-allergenicity:* Occurrence among the aminoglycosides has been demonstrated and depends largely on inactivation by bacterial enzymes.

➤*Syphilis:* In the treatment of sexually transmitted disease, if concomitant syphilis is suspected, perform a darkfield examination before treatment is started. Perform monthly serologic tests for at least 4 months.

➤*Topical use:* Aminoglycosides are quickly and almost totally absorbed when applied topically in association with surgical procedures, except to the urinary bladder. Irreversible deafness, renal failure, and death because of neuromuscular blockade have occurred following irrigation of small and large surgical fields with an aminoglycoside preparation. Consider potential toxicity.

➤*Benzyl alcohol:* This is contained in some of these products as a preservative and has been associated with a fatal "gasping syndrome" in premature infants.

➤*Sulfite sensitivity:* Some products contain sulfites that may cause allergic-type reactions, including anaphylactic symptoms and life-threatening/less severe asthmatic episodes in susceptible people. Overall prevalence in general population is unknown and probably low. It is more frequent in asthmatics or atopic nonasthmatics.

➤*Superinfection:* Use of antibiotics (especially prolonged or repeated therapy) may result in bacterial or fungal overgrowth of nonsusceptible organisms. Such overgrowth may lead to a secondary infection. Take appropriate measures if this occurs.

➤*Pregnancy: Category D* – Amikacin, gentamicin (per manufacturer's prescribing information), kanamycin, tobramycin (per manufacturer's prescribing information). *Category C* (per Briggs' *Drugs in Pregnancy and Lactation*) – Gentamicin, paromomycin, tobramycin. Aminoglycosides can cause fetal harm when given to pregnant women. These agents cross the placenta. Fetal serum levels may reach 16% to 50% of maternal levels. There are reports of total irreversible bilateral congenital deafness in children whose mothers received **streptomycin** during pregnancy. Prolonged use of **gentamicin** during pregnancy may result in otological damage to the fetus. Serious side effects to the mother, fetus, or newborn have not been reported with other aminoglycosides, but the potential for harm exists. Although there is no clearly defined risk, such experience cannot exclude the possibility of infrequent or subtle damage to the fetus. If these drugs are used during pregnancy, or if the patient becomes pregnant while taking these drugs, apprise her of the potential hazards to the fetus.

➤*Lactation:* Small amounts of **amikacin**, **streptomycin** and **kanamycin** are excreted in breast milk. Decide whether to discontinue breastfeeding or discontinue the drug, taking into account the importance of the drug to the mother.

➤*Children:* Use with caution in premature infants and neonates because of their renal immaturity and the resulting prolongation of serum half-life of these drugs.

A syndrome of apparent CNS depression, characterized by stupor and flaccidity to coma and deep respiratory depression, has been reported in very young infants given **streptomycin** in doses higher than those recommended. Do not exceed recommended doses in infants.

➤*Elderly:* These patients may have reduced renal function that is not evident in the results of routine screening tests, such as BUN or serum creatinine. A CrCl determination may be more useful. Monitoring of renal function and drug levels during treatment is particularly important in such patients.

➤*Monitoring:* Collect urine specimens for examination during therapy (see Nephrotoxicity). Monitor peak and trough serum concentrations periodically to assure adequate levels and to avoid potentially toxic levels. Also monitor serum calcium, magnesium, and sodium (see Adverse Reactions).

Eighth cranial nerve function testing – Serial audiometric tests are suggested, particularly when renal function is impaired or prolonged aminoglycoside therapy is required; also repeat such tests periodically after treatment if there is evidence of a hearing deficit or vestibular abnormality before or during therapy, or when consecutive or concomitant use of other potentially ototoxic drugs is unavoidable. Discontinue therapy if tinnitus or subjective hearing loss develops, or if follow-up audiograms show loss of high frequency perception. Aminoglycoside-induced ototoxicity is usually irreversible.

Factors that may increase risk of aminoglycoside-induced ototoxicity include renal function impairment (especially if dialysis is required), excessive dosage, dehydration, coadministration of ethacrynic acid or furosemide, or previous use of other ototoxic drugs.

Cochlear damage usually is manifested initially by small changes in audiometric test results at the high frequencies and may not be associated with subjective hearing loss; vestibular dysfunction is usually manifested by nystagmus, vertigo, nausea, vomiting, or acute Meniere syndrome.

Drug Interactions

Aminoglycoside Drug Interactions

Precipitant drug	Object drug[a]		Description
Cephalosporins Enflurane Methoxyflurane Vancomycin	Aminoglycosides	↑	Risk of nephrotoxicity may increase above that with aminoglycoside alone. Monitor patients. With cephalosporins, bactericidal activity against certain pathogens may be enhanced (see Administration).
Indomethacin IV	Aminoglycosides		In preterm infants, the use of indomethacin for closure of patent ductus arteriosus resulted in aminoglycoside accumulation in 1 study.
Loop diuretics	Aminoglycosides	↑	Auditory toxicity appears to increase during concomitant use. Hearing loss of varying degrees may occur; it may be irreversible. Monitor patients.
Penicillins	Aminoglycosides	↑	Synergism of these agents is well documented; however, certain penicillins may inactivate certain aminoglycosides. The problem may be highest in vitro (see Administration).
Aminoglycosides	Neuromuscular blockers, depolarizing and nondepolarizing		The neuromuscular blocking effects are enhanced by aminoglycosides. Prolonged respiratory depression may occur.
Aminoglycosides	Polypeptide antibiotics	↑	Concurrent use of these agents may increase the risk of respiratory paralysis and renal dysfunction.

[a] ↑ = object drug increased.

Adverse Reactions

Aminoglycoside Adverse Reactions (%)

	Adverse reaction	Amikacin	Gentamicin	Kanamycin	Streptomycin	Tobramycin
CNS	Confusion		✓			✓
	Convulsions		✓			
	Disorientation					✓
	Dizziness		✓			✓
	Encephalopathy		✓			
	Fever		✓		✓	✓
	Headache	rare	✓[a]	rare		✓
	Lethargy		✓			✓
	Muscle twitching		✓			
	Myasthenia gravis-like syndrome		✓			
	Neuromuscular blockade[b]	✓		✓	✓	
	Numbness		✓			
	Paresthesia	rare		rare		
	Peripheral neuropathy		✓			
	Skin tingling		✓			
GI	Diarrhea			rare		✓
	Nausea	rare	✓	rare	✓	✓
	Vomiting	rare	✓	rare	✓	✓
Hematologic	Anemia	rare	✓			✓
	Eosinophilia	rare	✓		✓	✓
	Granulocytopenia		✓			✓
	Leukopenia		✓		✓	✓
	Thrombocytopenia		✓		✓	✓
Hypersensitivity	Anaphylaxis/Anaphylactoid reaction		✓		✓	
	Itching		✓			✓
	Rash	rare	✓	rare	✓	✓
	Urticaria		✓		✓	✓
Lab test abnormalities	Increased AST/ALT		✓			✓
	Increased bilirubin		✓			✓
	Increased serum LDH		✓			✓
Renal	Azotemia	✓		✓	✓	
	Casts	✓	✓			
	Decreasing CrCl			✓		
	Oliguria	✓	✓	✓		✓
	Proteinuria	✓	✓	✓		✓
	Red and white cells in urine	✓		✓		
	Rising BUN[b]		✓	✓		✓
	Rising NPN[b]		✓			✓
	Rising serum creatinine[b]	✓	✓	✓		✓
Special senses	Hearing loss/deafness	✓	✓	✓[c]	✓	✓
	Loss of balance	✓		✓[c]		
	Roaring in ears		✓			✓
	Tinnitus		✓			✓
	Vertigo		✓		✓	✓
	Visual disturbances/blurred vision		✓			
Miscellaneous	Acute muscular paralysis	✓		✓		
	Apnea	✓	✓	✓	✓	✓
	Decreased serum Ca, Na, K, Mg[b]		✓			✓
	Drug fever	rare		rare		
	Hypotension	rare	✓			
	Pain/Irritation at injection site		✓	✓		✓

[a] ✓ = Reported; no incidence given.
[b] See Warnings.
[c] Partially reversible to irreversible bilateral hearing loss.

➤*Renal:*

Renal function changes – These are usually reversible upon discontinuation. See Warnings.

➤*Amikacin:*

Miscellaneous – Arthralgia, tremor (rare).

➤*Gentamicin:*

CNS – Acute organic brain syndrome; depression; pseudotumor cerebri; respiratory depression.

GI – Decreased appetite; hypersalivation; stomatitis; weight loss.

Hematologic – Increased and decreased reticulocyte count; transient agranulocytosis.

Hypersensitivity – Generalized burning; laryngeal edema; purpura.

Miscellaneous – Alopecia; arachnoiditis or burning at injection site after intrathecal administration (see Warnings); Fanconi-like syndrome, with aminoaciduria and metabolic acidosis; hypertension; increased CSF protein; joint pain; leg cramps; pulmonary fibrosis; splenomegaly; subcutaneous atrophy or fat necrosis (rare); transient hepatomegaly.

➤*Kanamycin:*

Miscellaneous – Granular casts; "malabsorption syndrome" characterized by an increase in fecal fat, decrease in serum carotene, and fall in xylose absorption (prolonged therapy).

➤*Streptomycin:*

CNS – Facial, circumoral or peripheral paresthesia; muscular weakness.

Hypersensitivity – Angioneurotic edema; exfoliative dermatitis.

Miscellaneous – Amblyopia; hemolytic anemia; hepatic necrosis; myocarditis; pancytopenia; serum sickness; toxic epidermal necrolysis.

➤*Tobramycin:*

Miscellaneous – Cylindruria; delirium; leukocytosis.

Overdosage

➤*Symptoms:* The severity of the signs and symptoms following overdose are dependent on the dose administered, patient's renal function, state of hydration and age, and whether or not other medications with similar toxicities are being administered concurrently. Toxicity may occur in patients treated longer than 10 days or in patients with reduced renal function where dose has not been appropriately adjusted.

Nephrotoxicity following the parenteral administration of an aminoglycoside is most closely related to the area under the curve. Nephrotoxicity is more likely if trough concentrations fail to fall below the intended concentration. Patients who are elderly, have abnormal renal function, are receiving other nephrotoxic drugs, or are volume depleted are at higher risk for developing acute tubular necrosis. Auditory and vestibular toxicities have been associated with aminoglycoside overdose. These toxicities occur in patients treated longer than 10 days, in patients with abnormal renal function, in dehydrated patients, or in patients receiving medications with additive auditory toxicities. These patients may not have signs or symptoms, or may experience dizziness, tinnitus, vertigo, and a loss of high-tone acuity as ototoxicity progresses. Ototoxic signs and symptoms may not begin to occur until long after the drug has been discontinued.

Neuromuscular blockade or respiratory paralysis may occur following aminoglycoside administration. Neuromuscular blockade, respiratory failure, and prolonged respiratory paralysis may occur more commonly in patients with myasthenia gravis or Parkinson disease. Prolonged respiratory paralysis also may occur in patients receiving neuromuscular blockers. If neuromuscular blockade occurs, it may be reversed by the administration of calcium salts but mechanical assistance may be necessary.

If an aminoglycoside were ingested, toxicity would be less likely because they are poorly absorbed from an intact GI tract.

➤*Treatment:* The initial intervention is to establish an airway and ensure oxygenation and ventilation. Initiate resuscitative measures promptly if respiratory paralysis occurs. Adequately hydrate patients and carefully monitor fluid balance, CrCl, and plasma levels.

Peritoneal dialysis or hemodialysis will aid in removal from the blood. This is especially important if renal function is, or becomes, compromised. Hemodialysis is preferable because it is more efficient in reducing serum levels. Complexation with ticarcillin or carbenicillin (12 to 30 g/day) appears as effective as hemodialysis in lowering excessive aminoglycoside serum concentrations. In newborns, consider exchange transfusions.

Range of Aminoglycoside Half-Lives (Hours) During Dialysis[a]

Aminoglycosides	Interdialysis	Hemodialysis	Peritoneal dialysis
Kanamycin	40 to 96	5	12
Gentamicin	21 to 59	6 to 11	5 to 29
Tobramycin	27 to 70	3 to 10	10 to 37
Amikacin	28 to 87	4 to 7	18 to 29

[a] Patient renal function CrCl ≤ 5 mL/min.

STREPTOMYCIN SULFATE

Rx	**Streptomycin Sulfate** (Pfizer)	**Injection:** 400 mg/ml	In 2.5 mL amps.
Rx	**Streptomycin Sulfate** (Pharma-Tek)	**Lyophilized Cake/Powder for Injection:** 200 mg/ml	In 1 g vials.

STREPTOMYCIN SULFATE — INJECTION

For complete and comparative prescribing information, refer to the Aminoglycosides group monograph.

WARNING

The risk of severe neurotoxic reactions is sharply increased in patients with impaired renal function or prerenal azotemia. These include disturbances of vestibular and cochlear function, optic nerve dysfunction, peripheral neuritis, arachnoiditis, and encephalopathy. The incidence of clinically detectable, irreversible vestibular damage is particularly high in patients treated with streptomycin.

Renal function should be monitored carefully; patients with renal impairment and/or nitrogen retention should receive reduced doses. The peak serum concentration in individuals with kidney damage should not exceed 20 to 25 mcg/mL.

The concurrent or sequential use of other neurotoxic and/or nephrotoxic drugs with streptomycin sulfate, including neomycin, kanamycin, gentamicin, cephaloridine, paromomycin, viomycin, polymyxin B, colistin, tobramycin, and cyclosporine should be avoided.

The neurotoxicity of streptomycin can result in respiratory paralysis from neuromuscular blockage, especially when the drug is given soon after the use of anesthesia or muscle relaxants.

The administration of streptomycin in parenteral form should be reserved for patients where adequate laboratory and audiometric testing facilities are available during therapy.

Indications

➤*Mycobacterium tuberculosis:* The Advisory Council for the Elimination of Tuberculosis, the American Thoracic Society, and the Centers for Disease Control and Prevention recommend that either streptomycin or ethambutol be added as a fourth drug in a regimen containing isoniazid (INH), rifampin, and pyrazinamide for initial treatment of tuberculosis unless the likelihood of INH or rifampin resistance is very low. The need for a fourth drug should be reassessed when the results of susceptibility testing are known. In the past when the national rate of primary drug resistance to isoniazid was known to be < 4% and was either stable or declining, therapy with 2 and 3 drug regimens was considered adequate. If community rates of INH resistance are currently < 4%, an initial treatment regimen with

Streptomycin is also indicated for therapy of tuberculosis when one or more of the above drugs is contraindicated because of toxicity or intolerance. The management of tuberculosis has become more complex as a consequence of increasing rates of drug resistance and concomitant HIV infection. Additional consultation from experts in the treatment of tuberculosis may be desirable in those settings.

➤*Nontuberculosis infections:* The use of streptomycin should be limited to the treatment of infections caused by bacteria that have been shown to be susceptible to the antibacterial effects of streptomycin and that are not amenable to therapy with less potentially toxic agents. Organisms usually include sensitive *Pasteurella pestis* (plague); *Francisella tularensis* (tularemia); *Brucella*; *Calymmatobacterium granulomatis* (donovanosis, granuloma inguinale); *H. ducreyi* (chancroid); *H. influenzae* (in respiratory, endocardial, and meningeal infections, concomitantly with another antibacterial agent); *K. pneumoniae* pneumonia (concomitantly with another antibacterial agent); *E. coli*, *Proteus*, *A. aerogenes*, *K. pneumoniae*, and *Enterococcus faecalis* in urinary tract infections; *Streptococcus viridans*; *Enterococcus faecalis* (in endocardial infections, concomitantly with penicillin); gram-negative bacillary bacteremia (concomitantly with another antibacterial agent).

➤*Off-label uses:* Streptomycin 11 to 13 mg/kg/24 hrs IV or 15 mg/kg/day IM may be used as part of a multiple-drug regimen (generally 3 to 5 agents) for *Mycobacterium avium* complex, a common infection in AIDS patients.

Administration and Dosage

➤*General dosing considerations:* The standard regimen for the treatment of drug susceptible tuberculosis has been 2 months of isoniazid, rifampin, and pyrazinamide followed by 4 months of isoniazid and rifampin (patients with concomitant infection with tuberculosis and HIV may require treatment for a longer period). Streptomycin is added to this regimen because of suspected or proven drug resistance.

As higher doses or more prolonged therapy with streptomycin may be indicated for more severe or fulminating infections (endocarditis, meningitis), the physician should always take adequate measures to be immediately aware of any toxic signs or symptoms occurring in the patient as a result of streptomycin therapy.

➤*Adults:*

Bacterial endocarditis –

Enterococcal endocarditis: 1 g twice daily IM for 2 weeks and 500 mg twice daily IM for an additional 4 weeks in combination with penicillin. Ototoxicity may require termination of the streptomycin prior to completion of the 6-week course of treatment.

Streptococcal endocarditis: In penicillin-sensitive alpha and nonhemolytic *streptococcal endocarditis* (penicillin MIC less than or equal to 0.1 mcg/mL), streptomycin may be used for 2-week treatment concomitantly with penicillin. The streptomycin regimen is 1 g twice daily IM for the first week, and 500 mg twice daily IM for the second week.

Plague – 2 g/day IM in 2 divided doses for a minimum of 10 days.

Tuberculosis –

Streptomycin Adult Dosing in Tuberculosis			
	Daily	Twice daily	Thrice weekly
Adults	15 mg/kg	25 to 30 mg/kg	25 to 30 mg/kg
	Max 1 g	Max 1.5 g	Max 1.5 g

Streptomycin is usually administered daily as a single IM injection. A total dose of not more than 120 g over the course of therapy should be given unless there are no other therapeutic options. (see Warning Box).

The total period of drug treatment of tuberculosis is a minimum of 1 year; however, indications for terminating therapy with streptomycin may occur at any time as noted in Discontinuation of therapy. (See Discontinuation of Therapy).

Tularemia – 1 to 2 g daily in divided doses for 7 to 14 days until the patient is afebrile for 5 to 7 days.

Other infections – 1 to 2 g in divided doses every 6 to 12 hours for moderate to severe infections. Doses should generally not exceed 2 g/day. For use as concomitant therapy with other agents to which the infecting organism is also sensitive, streptomycin is considered a secondline agent for the treatment of gram-negative bacillary bacteremia, meningitis, and pneumonia; brucellosis; granuloma inguinale; chancroid, and urinary tract infection.

➤*Children:*

Tuberculosis –

Streptomycin Children's Dosing in Tuberculosis			
	Daily	Twice daily	Thrice weekly
Children	20 to 40 mg/kg	25 to 30 mg/kg	25 to 30 mg/kg
	Max 1 g	Max 1.5 g	Max 1.5 g

Streptomycin is usually administered daily as a single IM injection. A total dose of not more than 120 g over the course of therapy should be given unless there are no other therapeutic options. (see Warning Box).

The total period of drug treatment of tuberculosis is a minimum of 1 year; however, indications for terminating therapy with streptomycin may occur at any time as noted in Discontinuation of therapy. (See Discontinuation of Therapy).

Other infections – 20 to 40 mg/kg/day (8 to 20 mg/lb/day) in divided doses every 6 to 12 hours. Particular care should be taken to avoid excessive dosage in children. For use as concomitant therapy with other agents to which the infecting organism is also sensitive, streptomycin is considered a second-line agent for the treatment of gram-negative bacillary bacteremia, meningitis, and pneumonia; brucellosis; granuloma inguinale; chancroid, and urinary tract infection.

➤*Elderly:* In patients older than 60 years of age the drug should be used at a reduced dosage due to the risk of increased toxicity.

Bacterial endocarditis –

Streptococcal endocarditis: If the patient is older than 60 years of age, the dosage should be 500 mg twice daily for the entire 2-week period.

➤*Renal function impairment:* Renal function should be monitored carefully; patients with renal impairment and/or nitrogen retention should receive reduced doses. The peak serum concentration in individuals with kidney damage should not exceed 20 to 25 mcg/mL.

➤*Therapeutic drug monitoring:* The peak serum concentration in individuals with kidney damage should not exceed 20 to 25 mcg/mL. (See Warning Box).

➤*Discontinuation of therapy:* Therapy with streptomycin may be terminated when toxic symptoms have appeared, when impending toxicity is feared, when organisms become resistant, or when full treatment effect has been obtained.

➤*Preparation for administration:* The dry lyophilized cake is dissolved by adding water for injection in an amount to yield the desired concentration as indicated in the following table:

Concentration of Streptomycin	
Approximate concentration mg/mL	Volume (mL) of solvent
200	4.2
250	3.2
400	1.8

➤*Administration:* IM route only. Injection sites should be alternated.

Adults – The preferred site is the upper outer quadrant of the buttock (ie, gluteus maximus) or the mid-lateral thigh. The deltoid area should be used only if well developed such as in certain adults and older children, and then

STREPTOMYCIN SULFATE — INJECTION

only with caution to avoid radial nerve injury. IM injections should not be made into the lower and mid-third of the upper arm.

Children – It is recommended that IM injections be given preferably in the mid-lateral muscles of the thigh. In infants and small children the periphery of the upper outer quadrant of the gluteal region should be used only when necessary, such as in burn patients, in order to minimize the possibility of damage to the sciatic nerve.

➤*Storage/Stability:* Store dry powder at 15° to 30°C (59° to 86°F). Sterile reconstituted solutions should be protected from light and may be stored at room temperature for 1 week without significant loss of potency.

KANAMYCIN SULFATE

Rx	**Kanamycin Sulfate** (Various, eg, Smith & Nephew)	**Injection:** 500 mg	In 2 mL vials.[a]
Rx	**Kantrex** (Apothecon)		In 2 mL vials.[b]
Rx	**Kanamycin Sulfate** (Various, eg, Smith & Nephew)	**Injection:** 1 g	In 2 mL vials.[a]
Rx	**Kantrex** (Apothecon)		In 3 mL vials.[b]
Rx	**Kanamycin Sulfate** (Various, eg, Smith & Nephew)	**Pediatric Injection:** 75 mg	In 2 mL vials.[a]
Rx	**Kantrex** (Apothecon)		In 2 mL vials.[b]

[a] May contain sulfites.

[b] With sodium bisulfite.

KANAMYCIN SULFATE — INJECTION

For complete and comparative prescribing information, refer to the Aminoglycosides group monograph.

WARNING

Ototoxicity – Patients treated with aminoglycosides by any route should be under close clinical observation because of the potential toxicity associated with their use. As with other aminoglycosides, the major toxic effects of kanamycin sulfate are its action on the auditory and vestibular branches of the eighth nerve and the renal tubules. Neurotoxicity is manifested by bilateral auditory toxicity which often is permanent and, sometimes, by vestibular ototoxicity. Loss of high frequency perception usually occurs before there is noticeable clinical hearing loss and can be detected by audiometric testing. There may not be clinical symptoms to warn of developing cochlear damage. Vertigo may occur and may be evidence of vestibular injury. Other manifestations of neurotoxicity may include numbness, skin tingling, muscle twitching, and convulsions. The risk of hearing loss increases with the degree of exposure to either high peak or high trough serum concentrations and continues to progress after drug withdrawal.

Renal toxicity – Renal impairment may be characterized by decreased creatinine clearance, the presence of cells or casts, oliguria, proteinuria, decreased urine specific gravity, or evidence of increasing nitrogen retention (increasing serum urea nitrogen [BUN], nonprotein nitrogen [NPN], or serum creatinine).

The risks of severe ototoxic and nephrotoxic reactions are sharply increased in patients with impaired renal function and in those with normal renal function who receive high doses or prolonged therapy.

Monitoring – Renal and eighth nerve function should be closely monitored, especially in patients with known or suspected reduced renal function at the onset of therapy, and also in those whose renal function is initially normal but who develop signs of renal dysfunction during therapy. Serum concentrations of parenterally administered aminoglycosides should be monitored when feasible to assure adequate levels and to avoid potentially toxic levels. Urine should be examined for decreased specific gravity, increased excretion of protein, and the presence of cells or casts. BUN, serum creatinine, or creatinine clearance should be measured periodically. Serial audiograms should be obtained when feasible in patients old enough to be tested, particularly high risk patients. Evidence of ototoxicity (dizziness, vertigo, tinnitus, roaring in the ears, and hearing loss) or nephrotoxicity requires dosage adjustment or discontinuance of the drug.

Neuromuscular blockade – Neuromuscular blockade with respiratory paralysis may occur when kanamycin sulfate is instilled intraperitoneally concomitantly with anesthesia and muscle-relaxing drugs. Neuromuscular blockade has been reported following parenteral injection and the oral use of aminoglycosides. The possibility of the occurrence of neuromuscular blockade and respiratory paralysis should be considered if aminoglycosides are administered by any route, especially in patients receiving anesthetics, neuromuscular-blocking agents such as tubocurarine, succinylcholine, decamethonium, or in patients receiving massive transfusions of citrate-anticoagulated blood. If blockage occurs, calcium salts may reduce these phenomena but mechanical respiratory assistance may be necessary.

Concurrent therapy – The concurrent or sequential systemic, oral, or topical use of kanamycin and other potentially nephrotoxic, or neurotoxic drugs, particularly polymyxin B, bacitracin, colistin, amphotericin B, cisplatin, vancomycin, and all other aminoglycosides (including paromomycin) should be avoided because the toxicity may be additive. Other factors which may increase patient risk of toxicity are advanced age and dehydration.

Kanamycin sulfate should not be given concurrently with potent diuretics (ethacrynic acid, furosemide, meralluride sodium, sodium mercaptomerin, or mannitol). Some diuretics themselves cause ototoxicity, and IV administered diuretics may enhance aminoglycoside toxicity by altering antibiotic concentrations in serum and tissue.

Indications

➤*Initial therapy:*

Known pathogens – Kanamycin may be considered as initial therapy in the treatment of infections where one or more of the following are the known or suspected pathogens: *E. coli*, *Proteus* species (both indole-positive and indole-negative), *Enterobacter aerogenes*, *Klebsiella pneumoniae*, *Serratia marcescens*, *Acinetobacter* species. The decision to continue therapy with the drug should be based on results of the susceptibility tests, the response of the infection to therapy, and the important additional concepts contained in the Warning box.

Unknown pathogens – In serious infections when the causative organisms are unknown, kanamycin may be administered as initial therapy in conjunction with a penicillin- or cephalosporin-type drug before obtaining results of susceptibility testing. If anaerobic organisms are suspected, consideration should be given to using other suitable antimicrobial therapy in conjunction with kanamycin.

➤*Staphylococcal infections:* Although kanamycin is not the drug of choice for staphylococcal infections, it may be indicated under certain conditions for the treatment of known or suspected staphylococcal disease. These situations include the initial therapy of severe infections where the organism is thought to be either a gram-negative bacterium or a *Staphylococcus*, infections due to susceptible strains of staphylococci in patients allergic to other antibiotics, and mixed staphylococcal/gram-negative infections.

➤*Off-label uses:*

Tuberculosis – [1] = Good documentation. According to the American Thoracic Society, Centers for Disease Control and Prevention, and Infectious Diseases Society of America joint guidelines on the treatment of tuberculosis (TB), intravenous (IV) or intramuscular (IM) kanamycin can be used as second-line therapy for patients with drug-resistant TB whose isolate has demonstrated presumed susceptibility to kanamycin.

Other possible off-label uses – Kanamycin 11 to 13 mg/kg per 24 hours IV or 15 mg/kg/day IM may be used as part of a multiple-drug regimen (generally 3 to 5 agents) for *Mycobacterium avium* complex, a common infection in AIDS patients.

Administration and Dosage

➤*Maximum dose:* 15 mg/kg/day (IV) or 1.5 g/day (all routes of administration) according to the prescribing information.

➤*General dosing considerations:* The patient's pretreatment body weight should be obtained for calculation of the correct dosage. The dosage of an aminoglycoside in obese patients should be based on an estimate of the lean body mass.

Patients should be well hydrated before treatment to prevent irritation of the renal tubules.

Serum levels should be monitored carefully during treatment. (See Therapeutic Drug Monitoring.)

The status of renal function should be determined by measurement of serum creatinine concentration or calculation of the endogenous creatinine clearance (CrCl) rate. The BUN level is much less reliable for this purpose. Renal function should be reassessed frequently during therapy. (See Renal Function Impairment.)

➤*Adults:*

Infections – For a list of infections, refer to Indications.

Maximum dose: 15 mg/kg/day or 1.5 g/day (for heavier patients [ie, those weighing 100 kg or more]).

Aerosol: 250 mg 2 to 4 times a day by nebulization.

IM: 15 mg/kg/day IM in 2 equally divided dosages administered at equally divided intervals (ie, 7.5 mg/kg every 12 hours). If continuously high blood levels are desired, the daily dose of 15 mg/kg may be given in equally divided doses every 6 or 8 hours.

IV: The dose should not exceed 15 mg/kg/day IV and must be administered slowly. The total daily dose should be divided into 2 or 3 equally divided doses.

Intraperitoneal: Use following exploration for established peritonitis or after peritoneal contamination because of fecal spill during surgery. Kanamycin 500 mg diluted in 20 mL sterile distilled water may be instilled through a polyethylene catheter sutured into the wound at closure. If possible, installation should be postponed until the patient has fully recovered from the effects of anesthesia and muscle-relaxing drugs (see Warning Box).

Other routes of administration: Kanamycin in concentrations of 0.25% (2.5 mg/mL) has been used as an irrigating solution in abscess cavities, pleural space, and peritoneal and ventricular cavities. Possible absorption of kanamycin by such routes must be taken into account and dosage adjustments should be arranged so that a maximum total dose of 1.5 g/day by all routes of administration is not exceeded.

KANAMYCIN SULFATE — INJECTION

Off-label dosing –

Tuberculosis: [1] = Good documentation. Kanamycin 15 mg/kg/day (not to exceed 1 g/day) IV or IM, usually given as a single daily dose (5 to 7 days per week) initially, and then reduced to 2 or 3 times a week after the first 2 to 4 months or after culture conversion, depending on the efficacy of the other drugs in the regimen. For patients older than 59 years of age, the dosage should be reduced to 10 mg/kg/day. The dosing frequency should also be reduced in patients with renal insufficiency.

➤*Children:*

Infections – For a list of infections, refer to Indications.

Usual dosage: See Adults for dosing. Intraperitoneal administration is indicated only in adults.

Pediatric Dosing for Kanamycin Pediatric Injection, 75 mg per 2 mL (Amount per 24 Hours to be Given in Divided Doses)

Weight (lb)	Weight (kg)	Daily dosage (mg)	Daily dose (mL)
2.2	1	15	0.4
2.8	1.25	18.8	0.5
3.3	1.5	22.5	0.6
3.9	1.75	26.2	0.7
4.4	2	30	0.8
5	2.25	33.8	0.9
5.5	2.5	37.5	1
6	2.75	41.2	1.1
6.6	3	45	1.2
7.7	3.5	52.5	1.4
8.8	4	60	1.6
9.9	4.5	67.5	1.8
11	5	75	2

➤*Renal function impairment:* It is desirable to follow therapy by appropriate serum assays in patients with impaired renal function. If this is not feasible, a suggested method is to reduce the frequency of administration in patients with renal dysfunction. The interval between doses may be calculated with the following formula:

Serum creatinine (mg/100 mL) × 9 = dosage interval (in hours); eg, if the serum creatinine is 2 mg, the recommended dose (7.5 mg/kg) should be administered every 18 hours. Changes in creatinine concentration during therapy would, of course, necessitate changes in the dosage frequency.

➤*Therapeutic drug monitoring:* It is desirable to measure both peak and trough serum concentrations intermittently during therapy because both concentrations are used to determine the adequacy and safety of the dose and to adjust the dosage during treatment. Peak serum concentrations (30 to 90 minutes after injection) above 35 mcg/mL and trough concentrations (just prior to the next dose) higher than 10 mcg/mL should be avoided.

➤*Duration of therapy:* It is desirable to limit the duration of treatment with kanamycin to short term. At the recommended dosage level, uncomplicated infections caused by kanamycin-susceptible organisms should respond to therapy in 24 to 48 hours. The usual duration of treatment is 7 to 10 days. If longer therapy is required, measurement of kanamycin peak and trough serum concentrations is particularly important as a basis for determining the adequacy and safety of the dose. These patients should be carefully monitored for changes in renal, auditory, and vestibular function. Dosage should be adjusted as needed. The risks of toxicity multiply as the length of treatment increases.

➤*Discontinuation of therapy:* If definite clinical response does not occur within 3 to 5 days, therapy should be stopped and the antibiotic susceptibility pattern of the invading organism should be rechecked. Failure of the infection to respond may be caused by resistance of the organism or to the presence of septic foci requiring surgical drainage.

➤*Preparation for administration:*

Aerosol – Withdraw 250 mg (1 mL) from a 500 mg vial and dilute it with 3 mL of physiological saline and nebulize.

IV – For adults, the solution for IV use is prepared by adding the contents of a 500 mg vial to 100 to 200 mL of sterile diluent such as normal saline or dextrose 5% in water, or the contents of a 1 g vial to 200 to 400 mL of sterile diluent.

For children, the amount of diluent used should be sufficient to infuse the kanamycin over a 30- to 60-minute period.

Intraperitoneal – 500 mg diluted in 20 mL sterile distilled water.

➤*Administration:* May be given IM (deeply into the upper outer quadrant of the gluteal muscle) or IV over a 30- to 60-minute period. May also be given by other routes of administration. See Adults for more information.

➤*Admixture compatibility:* Kanamycin should not be physically mixed with other antibacterial agents, but each should be administered separately in accordance with its recommended route of administration and dosage schedule.

➤*Storage/Stability:* Store at 20° to 25° C (68° to 77°F). Occasionally, some vials may darken during the shelf-life of the product, but this does not indicate a loss of potency.

GENTAMICIN

Rx	**Gentamicin Sulfate** (Various, eg, Fujisawa, Major, Moore, Taylor)	**Injection:** 40 mg/mL (as sulfate)	In 2 and 20 mL vials and 1.5 and 2 mL cartridge-needle units.
Rx	**Gentamicin Sulfate** (Hospira)	**Injection:** 10 mg/mL (as sulfate)	In *ADD-Vantage* 60, 80, and 100 mg vials.
Rx	**Pediatric Gentamicin Sulfate** (Abraxis)		In 2 mL vials.
Rx	**Gentamicin Sulfate in 0.9% Sodium Chloride-** (Hospira)	**Injection:** 0.8 mg/mL (as gentamicin base)	In 100 mL single-dose flexible containers.
		0.9 mg/mL (as gentamicin base)	In 100 mL single-dose flexible containers.
		1 mg/mL (as gentamicin base)	In 100 mL single-dose flexible containers.
		1.2 mg/mL (as gentamicin base)	In 50 mL single-dose flexible containers.
		1.4 mg/mL (as gentamicin base)	In 50 mL single-dose flexible containers.
		1.6 mg/mL (as gentamicin base)	In 50 mL single-dose flexible containers.

GENTAMICIN SULFATE — INJECTION

For complete and comparative prescribing information, refer to the Aminoglycosides, Parenteral group monograph.

WARNING

Patients treated with aminoglycosides should be under close clinical observation because of the potential toxicity associated with their use.

As with other aminoglycosides, gentamicin sulfate injectable is potentially nephrotoxic. The risk of nephrotoxicity is greater in patients with impaired renal function and in those who receive high dosage or prolonged therapy.

Neurotoxicity manifested by ototoxicity, both vestibular and auditory, can occur in patients treated with gentamicin sulfate injectable, primarily in those with preexisting renal damage and in patients with healthy renal function treated with higher doses and/or for longer periods than recommended. Aminoglycoside-induced ototoxicity is usually irreversible. Other manifestations of neurotoxicity may include numbness, skin tingling, muscle twitching, and convulsions.

WARNING (cont.)

Renal and eighth cranial nerve functions should be closely monitored, especially in patients with known or suspected reduced renal function at onset of therapy, and also in those whose renal function is initially healthy but who develop signs of renal dysfunction during therapy. Urine should be examined for decreased specific gravity, increased excretion of protein, and the presence of cells or casts. Blood urea nitrogen, serum creatinine, or creatinine clearance should be determined periodically. When feasible, it is recommended that serial audiograms be obtained in patients old enough to be tested, particularly high-risk patients. Evidence of ototoxicity (dizziness, vertigo, ataxia, tinnitus, roaring in the ears, or hearing loss) or nephrotoxicity requires dosage adjustment or discontinuance of the drug. As with the other aminoglycosides, on rare occasions changes in renal and eighth cranial nerve function may not become manifest until soon after completion of therapy.

Serum concentrations of aminoglycosides should be monitored when feasible to ensure adequate levels and to avoid potentially toxic levels. When monitoring gentamicin peak concentrations, dosage should be adjusted so that prolonged levels above 12 mcg/mL are avoided. When monitoring gentamicin trough concentrations, dosage should be adjusted so that levels above 2 mcg/mL are avoided. Excessive peak or trough serum concentrations of aminoglycosides may increase the risk of renal and eighth cranial nerve toxicity. In the event of overdose or toxic reactions, hemodialysis may aid in the removal of gentamicin from the blood, especially if renal function is, or becomes, compromised. The rate of removal of gentamicin is considerably less by peritoneal dialysis than by hemodialysis.

GENTAMICIN SULFATE — INJECTION

WARNING (cont.)

Concurrent and/or sequential systemic or topical use of other potentially neurotoxic and/or nephrotoxic drugs, such as cisplatin, cephaloridine, kanamycin, amikacin, neomycin, polymyxin B, colistin, paromomycin, streptomycin, tobramycin, vancomycin, and viomycin, should be avoided. Other factors which may increase patient risk of toxicity are advanced age and dehydration.

The concurrent use of gentamicin with potent diuretics, such as ethacrynic acid or furosemide, should be avoided, because certain diuretics by themselves may cause ototoxicity. In addition, when administered intravenously, diuretics may enhance aminoglycoside toxicity by altering the antibiotic concentration in serum and tissue.

Indications

➤*Serious infections:* In the treatment of serious infections caused by susceptible strains of the following microorganisms: *Pseudomonas aeruginosa*, *Proteus* species (indole-positive and indole-negative), *Escherichia coli*, *Klebsiella-Enterobacter-Serratia* species, *Citrobacter* species, and *Staphylococcus* species (coagulase-positive and coagulase-negative).

Clinical studies have shown gentamicin sulfate injectable to be effective in bacterial neonatal sepsis; bacterial septicemia; and serious bacterial infections of the central nervous system (meningitis), urinary tract, respiratory tract, gastrointestinal tract (including peritonitis), skin, bone, and soft tissue (including burns). Aminoglycosides, including gentamicin, are not indicated in uncomplicated initial episodes of urinary tract infections unless the causative organisms are susceptible to these antibiotics and are not susceptible to antibiotics having less potential for toxicity.

Specimens for bacterial culture should be obtained to isolate and identify causative organisms and to determine their susceptibility to gentamicin.

➤*Gram-negative infections:* As initial therapy in suspected or confirmed gram-negative infections, and therapy may be instituted before obtaining results of susceptibility testing. The decision to continue therapy with this drug should be based on the results of susceptibility tests, the severity of the infection, and the important additional concepts contained in the warning box. If the causative organisms are resistant to gentamicin, other appropriate therapy should be instituted.

➤*Unknown pathogens:* In serious infections when the causative organisms are unknown, gentamicin sulfate injectable may be administered as initial therapy in conjunction with a penicillin-type or cephalosporin-type drug before obtaining results of susceptibility testing. If anaerobic organisms are suspected as etiologic agents, consideration should be given to using other suitable antimicrobial therapy in conjunction with gentamicin. Following identification of the organism and its susceptibility, appropriate antibiotic therapy should then be continued.

➤*Combination therapy:* In combination with carbenicillin for the treatment of life-threatening infections caused by *Pseudomonas aeruginosa*. It has also been found effective when used in conjunction with a penicillin-type drug for the treatment of endocarditis caused by group D streptococci.

➤*Staphylococcal infections:* Treatment of serious staphylococcal infections. While not the antibiotic of first choice, gentamicin sulfate injectable may be considered when penicillins or other less potentially toxic drugs are contraindicated and bacterial susceptibility tests and clinical judgment indicate its use. It may also be considered in mixed infections caused by susceptible strains of staphylococci and gram-negative organisms.

In the neonate with suspected bacterial sepsis or staphylococcal pneumonia, a penicillin-type drug is also usually indicated as concomitant therapy with gentamicin.

➤*Off-label uses:*

Pelvic inflammatory disease – [1] = Good documentation.

Surgical prophylaxis – [1] = Good documentation. Clinical guidelines recommend the use of gentamicin for surgical prophylaxis in patients with a documented beta-lactam allergy who are undergoing procedures with a high risk of infection from gram-negative bacteria, such as abdominal or vaginal hysterectomy or colorectal procedures.

Other possible off-label uses – An alternative regimen for pelvic inflammatory disease is gentamicin 2 mg/kg IV followed by 1.5 mg/kg 3 times daily (healthy renal function) plus clindamycin 600 mg IV 4 times daily. Continue for at least 4 days and at least 48 hours after patient improves; then continue clindamycin 450 mg orally 4 times daily for 10 to 14 days total therapy.

Administration and Dosage

➤*General dosing considerations:* The patient's pretreatment body weight should be obtained for calculation of correct dosage. The dosage of aminoglycosides in obese patients should be based on an estimate of the lean body mass. It is desirable to limit the duration of treatment with aminoglycosides to short term.

The following dosage schedules are not intended as rigid recommendations but are provided as guides to dosage when the measurement of gentamicin serum levels is not feasible.

In patients with extensive burns, altered pharmacokinetics may result in reduced serum concentrations of aminoglycosides. In such patients treated with gentamicin, measurement of serum concentrations is recommended as a basis for dosage adjustment.

Dosing interval – Although further studies are needed, preliminary evidence indicates that aminoglycosides may be administered on a once daily basis without compromising efficacy and without increasing the potential for nephrotoxicity and ototoxicity. It is possible that the incidence of nephrotoxicity may even be decreased.

➤*Adults:*

Infections – For a list of infections, refer to Indications.

Serious infections: 3 mg/kg/day IV or IM in 3 equal doses every 8 hours (see the following table).

Life-threatening infections: Up to 5 mg/kg/day IV or IM may be administered in 3 or 4 equal doses. This dosage should be reduced to 3 mg/kg/day as soon as clinically indicated (see the following table).

Gentamicin Dosing for Adults (Dosage at 8-Hour Intervals), 40 mg/mL

Patient's weight[a]		Serious infections 1 mg/kg every 8 hours (3 mg/kg/day)		Life-threatening infections (reduce as soon as clinically indicated) 1.7 mg/kg every 8 hours[b] (5 mg/kg/day)	
kg	lb	mg/dose	mL/dose	mg/dose	mL/dose
40	88	40	1	66	1.6
45	99	45	1.1	75	1.9
50	110	50	1.25	83	2.1
55	121	55	1.4	91	2.25
60	132	60	1.5	100	2.5
65	143	65	1.6	108	2.7
70	154	70	1.75	116	2.9
75	165	75	1.9	125	3.1
80	176	80	2	133	3.3
85	187	85	2.1	141	3.5
90	198	90	2.25	150	3.75
95	209	95	2.4	158	4
100	220	100	2.5	166	4.2

[a] The dosage of aminoglycosides in obese patients should be based on an estimate of lean body mass.
[b] For every-6-hour schedules, dosage should be recalculated.

Off-label dosing –

Pelvic inflammatory disease: [1] = Good documentation.

- *Loading dose* – 2 mg/kg IV or IM.
- *Maintenance dosage* – 1.5 mg/kg IV or IM every 8 hours. Single daily dosing may be substituted. Gentamicin is given in conjunction with clindamycin. Gentamicin therapy should continue until 24 hours after clinical improvement is noted; at this time, clindamycin oral therapy should be continued for a total of 14 days of treatment.

Surgical prophylaxis: [1] = Good documentation. 1.5 mg/kg IV over 30 to 60 minutes, 1 hour prior to incision. Redosing should be based on serum drug levels with discontinuation within 24 hours postoperation.

➤*Children:*

Infections – For a list of infections, refer to Indications.

Children: 6 to 7.5 mg/kg/day IV or IM (2 to 2.5 mg/kg every 8 hours).

Infants and neonates: 7.5 mg/kg/day IV or IM (2.5 mg/kg every 8 hours).

Premature or full-term neonates 1 week of age or younger: 5 mg/kg/day IV or IM (2.5 mg/kg every 12 hours).

Preterm infants younger than 32 weeks gestational age: A regimen of either 2.5 mg/kg every 18 hours or 3 mg/kg every 24 hours may also provide satisfactory peak and trough levels.

Off-label dosing –

Pelvic inflammatory disease: [1] = Good documentation.

- *Adolescents* –
  - *Loading dose:* 2 mg/kg IV or IM.
  - *Maintenance dosage:* 1.5 mg/kg IV or IM every 8 hours. Single daily dosing may be substituted. Gentamicin is given in conjunction with clindamycin. Gentamicin therapy should continue until 24 hours after clinical improvement is noted; at this time, clindamycin oral therapy should be continued for a total of 14 days of treatment.

➤*Renal function impairment:* Dosage must be adjusted in patients with impaired renal function to ensure therapeutically adequate, but not excessive, blood levels. Whenever possible, serum concentrations of gentamicin should be monitored. One method of dosage adjustment is to increase the interval between administrations of the usual doses. Because the serum creatinine concentration has a high correlation with the serum half-life of gentamicin, this laboratory test may provide guidance for adjustment of the interval between doses.

In adults, the interval between doses (in hours) may be approximated by multiplying the serum creatinine level (mg per 100 mL) by 8. For example, a patient weighing 60 kg with a serum creatinine level of 2 mg per 100 mL could be given 60 mg (1 mg/kg) every 16 hours (2 × 8). These guidelines may be considered when treating infants and children with serious renal impairment.

In patients with serious systemic infections and renal impairment, it may be desirable to administer the antibiotic more frequently but in reduced dosage. In such patients, serum concentrations of gentamicin should be measured so that adequate, but not excessive, levels result. A peak and trough concentration measured intermittently during therapy will provide optimal guidance for adjusting dosage. After the usual initial dose, a rough guide for determining reduced dosage at 8-hour intervals is to divide the normally recommended dose by the serum creatinine level (see the following table).

GENTAMICIN SULFATE — INJECTION

For example, after an initial dose of 60 mg (1 mg/kg), a patient weighing 60 kg with a serum creatinine level of 2 mg per 100 mL could be given 30 mg every 8 hours (60 divided by 2). After an initial dose of 20 mg (2 mg/kg), a child weighing 10 kg with a serum creatinine level of 2 mg per 100 mL could be given 10 mg every 8 hours (20 divided by 2). It should be noted that the status of renal function may be changing over the course of the infectious process.

It is important to recognize that deteriorating renal function may require a greater reduction in dosage than that specified in the previous guidelines for patients with stable renal impairment.

Gentamicin Dosing for Patients with Renal Impairment (Dosage at 8-Hour Intervals After the Usual Initial Dose)

Serum creatinine (mg/dL)	Approximate CrCl rate (mL/min per 1.73 m^2)	Percent of usual doses shown above
≤ 1	> 100	100%
1.1 to 1.3	70 to 100	80%
1.4 to 1.6	55 to 70	65%
1.7 to 1.9	45 to 55	55%
2 to 2.2	40 to 45	50%
2.3 to 2.5	35 to 40	40%
2.6 to 3	30 to 35	35%
3.1 to 3.5	25 to 30	30%
3.6 to 4	20 to 25	25%
4.1 to 5.1	15 to 20	20%
5.2 to 6.6	10 to 15	15%
6.7 to 8	< 10	10%

Alternative dosage – The following is an alternative dosage regimen for adults. Dosages are adjusted per pharmacy pharmacokinetic consult protocol.

CrCl of 30 to 80 mL/min: 2.5 to 4 mg/kg every 24 hours.
CrCl of 10 to 30 mL/min: 3 to 4 mg/kg every 48 hours.
CrCl of less than 10 mL/min: 2 mg/kg every 72 hours.

Hemodialysis –

Adults:

• *Continuous renal replacement therapy (CRRT)* – One reference suggests a dosage of 1.7 mg/kg IV every 12 to 48 hours with subsequent doses adjusted according to serum concentrations.

See the following table for alternative dosing recommendations. The recommendations assume ultrafiltration and dialysis flow rates of 1 to 2 L/h for patients receiving continuous venovenous hemofiltration (CVVH), continuous venovenous hemodialysis (CVVHD), or continuous venovenous hemodiafiltration (CVVHDF).

Consider performing first-dose pharmacokinetics for subsequent dosing. The volume of distribution and the elimination rate can be estimated based on the peak concentration and a 24-hour concentration. The 24-hour concentration should be performed in order to determine the dosing interval according to the patient's elimination rate.

• *Intermittent hemodialysis (IHD)* – The amount of gentamicin removed from the blood may vary depending on several factors, including the dialysis method used. An 8-hour hemodialysis may reduce serum concentrations of gentamicin by approximately 50%.

According to the prescribing information, the recommended dosage is 1 to 1.7 mg/kg (depending on the severity of infection) at the end of each dialysis period.

One reference suggests a dosage of 50% of the usual dosage administered after dialysis with subsequent doses adjusted according to serum concentrations.

The following table lists alternative dosing for patients receiving IHD and assumes the patient is receiving standard IHD 3 times per week and completes the full dialysis sessions.

Gentamicin Dosing for Adults Receiving Continuous Renal Replacement Therapy (CRRT) or Intermittent Hemodialysis (IHD)[b]

Indication	Loading dose	CRRT maintenance dose	IHD maintenance dose
Mild UTI or gram-positive cocci synergy (with beta-lactams or vancomycin) against	2 to 3 mg/kg	1 mg/kg IV every 24 to 36 hours[a] Redose when plasma concentration is less than 1 mg/L.	1 mg/kg IV every 48 to 72 hours after dialysis. Redose when pre-HD plasma concentration is less than 1 mg/L. Consider redosing when post-HD plasma concentration is less than 1 mg/L.
Moderate to severe UTI	2 to 3 mg/kg IV	1 to 1.5 mg/kg IV every 24 to 36 hours.[a] Redose when plasma concentration is less than 1.5 to 2 mg/L.	1 to 1.5 mg/kg IV every 48 to 72 hours after dialysis. Redose when pre-HD plasma concentration is less than 1.5 to 2 mg/L. Consider redosing when post-HD plasma concentration is less than 1 mg/L.
Systemic gram-negative rods infection	2 to 3 mg/kg IV	1.5 to 2.5 mg/kg IV every 24 to 48 hours.[a] Redose when plasma concentration is less than 3 to 5 mg/L.	1.5 to 2 mg/kg IV every 48 to 72 hours after dialysis. Redose when pre-HD plasma concentration is less than 3 to 5 mg/L. Consider redosing when post-HD plasma concentration is less than 2 mg/L.

[a] A standard dosage regimen may be started after achievement of target concentrations and the dialysis regimen is consistent. Periodically (eg, every 3 to 5 days) monitor gentamicin plasma concentrations.

[b] If IHD was started shortly after the loading dose, then consider administering the lower end of the maintenance dosage range for the second dose. If IHD was started more than a day after the administration of the loading dose, then consider using the higher end of the maintenance dosage range for the second dose.

Children: According to the prescribing information, the recommended dosage is 2 to 2.5 mg/kg (depending on the severity of infection) at the end of each dialysis period.

Continuous ambulatory peritoneal dialysis – For adults, 3 to 4 mg/L/day.

➤*Therapeutic drug monitoring:* It is desirable to measure periodically both peak and trough serum concentrations of gentamicin when feasible during therapy to ensure adequate, but not excessive, drug levels. For example, the peak concentration (at 30 to 60 minutes after IM injection) is expected to be in the range of 4 to 6 mcg/mL. When monitoring peak concentrations after IM or IV administration, dosage should be adjusted to avoid prolonged levels higher than 12 mcg/mL. When monitoring trough concentrations (just prior to the next dose), dosage should be adjusted to avoid levels higher than 2 mcg/mL. The susceptibility of the causative organism, severity of the infection, and status of the patient's host-defense mechanisms must be taken into consideration when determining the adequacy of a serum level for a particular patient.

➤*Duration of therapy:* The usual duration of treatment for all patients is 7 to 10 days. In difficult and complicated infections, a longer course of therapy may be necessary. In such cases, monitoring of renal, auditory, and vestibular functions is recommended because toxicity is more apt to occur with treatment extended for more than 10 days. Dosage should be reduced if clinically indicated.

➤*Preparation for administration:* For intermittent IV administration in adults, a single dose of gentamicin sulfate injectable may be diluted in 50 to 200 mL of sterile isotonic saline solution or in a sterile solution of dextrose 5% in water. For intermittent IV administration in children, a single dose of gentamicin sulfate pediatric injectable may be diluted in sterile isotonic saline solution or in a sterile solution of dextrose 5% in water.

➤*Administration:* May be given IM or IV. IV administration may be particularly useful for treating patients with bacterial septicemia or those in shock. It may also be the preferred route of administration for some patients with congestive heart failure, hematologic disorders, severe burns, or reduced muscle mass.

➤*Admixture compatibility:* Gentamicin should not be physically premixed with other drugs but should be administered separately in accordance with the recommended route of administration and dosage schedule.

➤*Storage/Stability:* Store at 15° to 30°C (59° to 86°F).

TOBRAMYCIN

Rx	**Tobramycin in 0.9% Sodium Chloride** (Hospira)	**Injection:** 0.8 mg/mL (as sulfate)	In 100 mL single-dose flexible containers.
		1.2 mg/mL (as sulfate)	In 50 mL single-dose flexible containers.
Rx	**Tobramycin Sulfate Pediatric** (Various, eg, Hospira, Apothecon)	**Solution for Injection:** 10 mg/ml	In 2 mL vials.
		40 mg/ml	In 1.5 and 2 mL syringes and 2 and 30 mL vials.
Rx	**Tobramycin Sulfate** (American Pharmaceutical Partners)	**Powder for injection:** 1.2 g (40 mg/mL after reconstitution)	Preservative free. In 50 mL pharmacy bulk package vial.
Rx	**TOBI** (Novartis)	**Solution; inhalation:** 300 mg per 5 mL	Preservative free. In 5 mL ampules.[a]

[a] With sodium chloride, sulfuric acid and sodium hydroxide.

TOBRAMYCIN — INJECTION

Information beginning in the Aminoglycoside group monograph must be considered when using these products.

WARNING

Keep patients treated with tobramycin injection and other aminoglycosides under close clinical observation because these drugs have an inherent potential for causing ototoxicity and nephrotoxicity.

Ototoxicity – Neurotoxicity, manifested as both auditory and vestibular ototoxicity, can occur. The auditory changes are irreversible, are usually bilateral, and may be partial or total. Eighth nerve impairment and nephrotoxicity may develop, primarily in patients having preexisting renal damage and in those with healthy renal function to whom aminoglycosides are administered for longer periods or in higher doses than those recommended. Other manifestations of neurotoxicity may include numbness, skin tingling, muscle twitching, and convulsions. The risk of aminoglycoside-induced hearing loss increases with the degree of exposure to either high peak or high trough serum concentrations. Patients who develop cochlear damage may not have symptoms during therapy to warn them of eighth-nerve toxicity, and partial or total irreversible bilateral deafness may continue to develop after the drug has been discontinued. Rarely, nephrotoxicity may not become apparent until the first few days after cessation of therapy. Aminoglycoside-induced nephrotoxicity usually is reversible.

Monitoring – Closely monitor renal and eighth nerve function in patients with known or suspected renal impairment and also in those whose renal function is initially normal but who develop signs of renal dysfunction during therapy. Periodically monitor peak and trough serum concentrations of aminoglycosides during therapy to assure adequate levels and to avoid potentially toxic levels. Prolonged serum concentrations above 12 mcg/mL should be avoided. Rising trough levels (above 2 mcg/mL) may indicate tissue accumulation. Such accumulation, excessive peak concentrations, advanced age, and cumulative dose may contribute to ototoxicity and nephrotoxicity. Examine urine for decreased specific gravity and increased excretion of protein, cells, and casts. Periodically measure serum urea nitrogen (BUN), serum creatinine, and creatinine clearance. When feasible, it is recommended that serial audiograms be obtained in patients old enough to be tested, particularly high-risk patients. Evidence of impairment of renal, vestibular, or auditory function requires discontinuation of the drug or dosage adjustment.

Use tobramycin injection with caution in premature and neonatal infants because of their renal immaturity and the resulting prolongation of serum half-life of the drug.

Concurrent therapy – Avoid concurrent and sequential use of other neurotoxic or nephrotoxic antibiotics, particularly other aminoglycosides (eg, amikacin, streptomycin, neomycin, kanamycin, gentamicin, paromomycin), cephaloridine, viomycin, polymyxin B, colistin, cisplatin, and vancomycin. Other factors that may increase patient risk are advanced age and dehydration.

Do not give aminoglycosides concurrently with potent diuretics, such as ethacrynic acid and furosemide. Some diuretics themselves cause ototoxicity, and intravenously (IV) administered diuretics enhance aminoglycoside toxicity by altering antibiotic concentrations in serum and tissue.

Pregnancy – Aminoglycosides can cause fetal harm when administered to a pregnant woman.

Indications

➤*Septicemia:* Septicemia in the pediatric patient and adult caused by *Pseudomonas aeruginosa*, *Escherichia coli*, and *Klebsiella* sp.

➤*Lower respiratory tract infections:* Lower respiratory tract infections caused by *P. aeruginosa*, *Klebsiella* sp., *Enterobacter* sp., *Serratia* sp., *E. coli*, and *Staphylococcus aureus* (penicillinase- and non-penicillinase-producing strains).

➤*Serious CNS infections (meningitis):* Serious CNS infections (meningitis) caused by susceptible organisms.

➤*Intra-abdominal infections:* Intra-abdominal infections, including peritonitis, caused by *E. coli*, *Klebsiella* sp., and *Enterobacter* sp.

➤*Skin, bone, and skin structure infections:* Skin, bone, and skin structure infections caused by *P. aeruginosa*, *Proteus* sp., *E. coli*, *Klebsiella* sp., *Enterobacter* sp., and *S. aureus*.

➤*Complicated and recurrent urinary tract infections:* Complicated and recurrent urinary tract infections caused by *P. aeruginosa*, *Proteus* sp. (indole-positive and indole-negative), *E. coli*, *Klebsiella* sp., *Enterobacter* sp., *Serratia* sp., *S. aureus*, *Providencia* sp., and *Citrobacter* sp.

Aminoglycosides, including tobramycin injection, are not indicated in uncomplicated initial episodes of urinary tract infections unless the causative organisms are not susceptible to antibiotics having less potential toxicity. Tobramycin injection may be considered in serious staphylococcal infections when penicillin or other potentially less toxic drugs are contraindicated, and when bacterial susceptibility testing and clinical judgment indicate its use.

➤*Off-label uses:*

Infective endocarditis (adults) – [1] = Good documentation. According to American Heart Association (AHA) guidelines, tobramycin, in combination with an extended-spectrum penicillin, ceftazidime, or cefepime, is a preferred therapy for infective endocarditis caused by *P. aeruginosa*.

Administration and Dosage

➤*General dosing considerations:* Tobramycin injection may be given intramuscularly (IM) or IV. Recommended dosages are the same for both routes. Obtain the patient's pretreatment body weight for calculation of correct dosage. (For obese patients, see Dosage in obese patients.) It is desirable to measure both peak and trough serum concentrations.

➤*Adults:*

Infections – For a list of infections, refer to Indications.

Serious infections: 3 mg/kg/day IV or IM divided in 3 equal doses every 8 hours.

Life-threatening infections: Up to 5 mg/kg/day IV or IM may be administered in 3 or 4 equal doses. The dosage should be reduced to 3 mg/kg/day as soon as clinically indicated. To prevent increased toxicity due to excessive blood levels, dosage should not exceed 5 mg/kg/day unless serum levels are monitored.

Off-label dosing –

Infective endocarditis (adults): [1] = Good documentation. 8 mg/kg IV or IM once daily with maintenance peak concentrations of 15 to 20 mcg/mL and trough concentrations no greater than 2 mcg/mL in combination with an extended-spectrum penicillin (eg, ticarcillin, piperacillin) or ceftazidime or cefepime in full doses for a minimum of 6 weeks for *P. aeruginosa*.

➤*Children:*

Septicemia caused by P. aeruginosa, E. coli, and Klebsiella species –

Older than 1 week of age: 6 to 7.5 mg/kg/day IV or IM in 3 or 4 equally divided doses (2 to 2.5 mg/kg every 8 hours or 1.5 to 1.89 mg/kg every 6 hours).

1 week of age or younger (premature or full-term neonates): Up to 4 mg/kg/day IV or IM may be administered in 2 equal doses every 12 hours.

➤*Renal function impairment:* Whenever possible, monitor serum tobramycin concentrations during therapy. (See Therapeutic Drug Monitoring.)

Following a loading dose of 1 mg/kg, subsequent dosage in these patients must be adjusted, either with reduced doses administered at 8-hour intervals or with normal doses given at prolonged intervals. Both of these methods are suggested as guides to be used when serum levels of tobramycin cannot be measured directly. They are based on either the creatinine clearance level or the serum creatinine level of the patient because these values correlate with the half-life of tobramycin. Use the dosage schedule derived from either method in conjunction with careful clinical and laboratory observations of the patient and modify as necessary. Do not use either method when dialysis is being performed.

Dosage adjustment based on CrCl –

30 to 80 mL/min: 2.5 to 4 mg/kg every 24 hours; adjust according to serum concentrations.

10 to 30 mL/min: 3 to 4 mg/kg every 48 hours; adjust according to serum concentrations.

Less than 10 mL/min: 2 mg/kg every 72 hours; adjust according to serum concentrations.

Reduced dosage at 8-hour intervals – A rough guide for determining reduced dosage at 8-hour intervals (for patients whose steady-state serum creatinine values are known) is to divide the normally recommended dose by the patient's serum creatinine.

Normal dosage at prolonged intervals – If the CrCl is not available, and the patient's condition is stable, a dosage frequency in hours can be determined by multiplying the patient's serum creatinine by 6.

Hemodialysis –

Continuous renal replacement therapy (CRRT): One reference suggests a dosage of 1.7 mg/kg IV every 24 to 48 hours with subsequent doses adjusted according to serum concentrations.

The following alternative recommendations are for gram-negative rod infections and assume ultrafiltration and dialysis flow rates of 1 to 2 L/h for patients receiving continuous venovenous hemofiltration (CVVH), continuous venovenous hemodialysis (CVVHD), or continuous venovenous hemodiafiltration (CVVHDF).

- *Loading dose* – 2 to 3 mg/kg IV.

TOBRAMYCIN — INJECTION

• *Maintenance dosage* – Consider performing first-dose pharmacokinetics for subsequent dosing. The volume of distribution and the elimination rate can be estimated based on the peak concentration and a 24-hour concentration. The 24-hour concentration should be performed in order to determine the dosing interval according to the patient's elimination rate.

One reference suggests a maintenance dosage of 1.5 to 2.5 mg/kg IV every 24 to 48 hours and to redose when the plasma concentration is less than 3 to 5 mg/L.

A standard dosage regimen may be started after the achievement of target concentrations and the dialysis regimen is consistent.

Periodically (eg, every 3 to 5 days) monitor tobramycin plasma concentrations.

Intermittent hemodialysis (IHD): A suggested dose is 50% of the normal dose as a supplement after dialysis and adjust according to serum concentrations.

Alternatively, administer a loading dose of 2 to 3 mg/kg IV. For systemic gram-negative rod infections, redose with 1 to 2 mg/kg (after dialysis) if the pre-IHD plasma concentration is approximately 3 to 5 mg/L. If IHD was started shortly after the loading dose, then consider administering the lower end of the maintenance dosage range for the second dose. If IHD was started more than a day after the administration of the loading dose, then consider using the higher end of the maintenance dosage range for the second dose. These recommendations assume the patient is receiving standard IHD 3 times per week and completes the full dialysis sessions.

Continuous ambulatory peritoneal dialysis – 3 to 4 mg/L/day.

➤*Cystic fibrosis patients:* In patients with cystic fibrosis, altered pharmacokinetics may result in reduced serum concentrations of aminoglycosides. Measurement of tobramycin serum concentration during treatment is especially important as a basis for determining appropriate dose. In patients with severe cystic fibrosis, an initial dosing regimen of 10 mg/kg/day in 4 equally divided doses is recommended. This dosing regimen is suggested only as a guide. Measure the serum levels of tobramycin directly during treatment due to wide interpatient variability.

➤*Dosage in obese patients:* The appropriate dose may be calculated by using the patient's estimated lean body weight plus 40% of the excess as the basic weight on which to figure mg/kg.

➤*Therapeutic drug monitoring:* Periodically measure tobramycin peak and trough serum levels during therapy. Avoid prolonged concentrations more than 12 mcg/mL. Rising trough levels (more than 2 mcg/mL) may indicate tissue accumulation. Such accumulation, advanced age, and cumulative dosage may contribute to ototoxicity and nephrotoxicity. It is particularly important to monitor serum levels closely in patients with known renal impairment.

A useful guideline would be to perform serum level assays after 2 or 3 doses, so that the dosage could be adjusted if necessary, and at 3- to 4-day intervals during therapy. In the event of changing renal function, obtain more frequent serum levels and adjust the dosage or dosage interval according to the guidelines.

In order to measure the peak level, a serum sample should be drawn about 30 minutes following IV infusion or 1 hour after an IM injection. Trough levels are measured by obtaining serum samples at 8 hours or just prior to the next dose of tobramycin injection. These suggested time intervals are intended only as guidelines and may vary according to institutional practices. It is important, however, that there be consistency within the individual patient program unless computerized pharmacokinetic dosing programs are available in the institution. These serum-level assays may be especially useful for monitoring the treatment of severely ill patients with changing renal function or of those infected with less susceptible organisms or those receiving maximum dosage.

➤*Duration of therapy:* It is desirable to limit treatment to short term. The usual duration of treatment is 7 to 10 days. A longer course of therapy may be necessary in difficult and complicated infections. In such cases, monitoring of renal, auditory, and vestibular functions is advised because neurotoxicity is more likely to occur when treatment is extended longer than 10 days.

➤*Preparation for administration:*

Directions for proper use of pharmacy bulk package – Not for direct infusion. The pharmacy bulk package is for use in the Hospital Pharmacy Admixture Service and only in a suitable work area, such as a laminar flow hood. Using aseptic technique, the closure may be penetrated only 1 time after reconstitution using a suitable sterile transfer device or dispensing set, which allows measured dispensing of the contents. Use of a syringe and needle is not recommended as it may cause leakage. After entry, entire contents of bulk vial should be dispensed within 24 hours.

The contents of the vial should be diluted with 30 mL of sterile water for injection to provide a solution containing tobramycin 40 mg/mL.

➤*Administration:*

IM administration – Tobramycin injection may be administered by withdrawing the appropriate dose directly from a vial or by using a prefilled syringe. The pharmacy bulk package and tobramycin in sodium chloride 0.9% is not intended for IM administration.

IV administration – For IV administration, the usual volume of diluent (sodium chloride 0.9% injection or dextrose 5% injection) is 50 to 100 mL for adult doses. For pediatric patients, the volume of diluent should be proportionately less than that for adults. The diluted solution usually should be infused over a period of 20 to 60 minutes. Infusion periods of less than 20 minutes are not recommended because peak serum levels may exceed 12 mcg/mL and should be avoided. Such accumulation, excessive peak concentrations, advanced age, and cumulative dose may contribute to ototoxicity and nephrotoxicity.

➤*Admixture compatibility:* Do not physically premix tobramycin injection with other drugs, but administer separately according to the recommended dose and route.

➤*Storage/Stability:* Store at controlled room temperature, 20° to 25°C (68° to 77°F).

Prior to reconstitution, store the pharmacy bulk package vial at controlled room temperature, 15° to 30°C (59° to 86°F). After reconstitution, keep the solution in a refrigerator and use within 96 hours. If kept at room temperature, the solution must be used within 24 hours.

TOBRAMYCIN SOLUTION FOR INHALATION

Information beginning in the Aminoglycoside group monograph must be considered when using these products.

Indications

➤*Cystic fibrosis:* For the management of cystic fibrosis patients with *Pseudomonas aeruginosa*.

Safety and efficacy have not been demonstrated in patients under the age of 6 years, patients with FEV_1 < 25% or greater than 75% predicted, or patients colonized with *Burkholderia cepacia*.

Administration and Dosage

➤*Adults:*

Cystic fibrosis patients with P. aeruginosa – 1 single-use ampule (300 mg) administered twice daily for 28 days. Dosage is not adjusted by weight. All patients should be administered 300 mg twice daily. The doses should be taken as close to 12 hours apart as possible; they should not be taken less than 6 hours apart.

Tobramycin is administered twice daily in alternating periods of 28 days. After 28 days of therapy, patients should stop tobramycin therapy for the next 28 days, and then resume therapy for the next "28 days on/28 days off" cycle.

➤*Children:* See Adults for dosing for children 6 years of age and older.

➤*Concurrent therapy:* During clinical studies, patients on multiple therapies were instructed to take them first, followed by tobramycin. The recommended order is as follows: Bronchodilator first, followed by chest physiotherapy, then other inhaled medications and, finally, tobramycin.

➤*Duration of therapy:* Tobramycin is administered twice daily in alternating periods of 28 days. After 28 days of therapy, patients should stop tobramycin therapy for the next 28 days, and then resume therapy for the next "28 days on/28 days off" cycle.

➤*Administration:* Tobramycin is administered by inhalation over a 10- to 15-minute period, using a handheld reusable nebulizer with a compressor (use only those supplied). Tobramycin solution for inhalation is not for subcutaneous, intravenous (IV), or intrathecal administration.

Tobramycin is inhaled while the patient is sitting or standing upright and breathing normally through the mouthpiece of the nebulizer. Nose clips may help the patient breathe through the mouth.

➤*Admixture compatibility:* Tobramycin should not be mixed with dornase alfa in the nebulizer.

➤*Storage/Stability:* Store refrigerated (2° to 8°C; 36° to 46°F). Upon removal from the refrigerator, or if refrigeration is unavailable, tobramycin solution for inhalation pouches (opened or unopened) may be stored at room temperature (up to 25°C; 77°F) for up to 28 days. Tobramycin should not be used beyond the expiration date stamped on the ampule when stored refrigerated (2° to 8°C; 36° to 46°F) or beyond 28 days when stored at room temperature (25°C; 77°F).

Tobramycin ampules should not be exposed to intense light. The solution in the ampule is slightly yellow, but may darken with age if not stored in the refrigerator; however, the color change does not indicate any change in the quality of the product as long as it is stored within the recommended storage conditions.

Tobramycin should not be used if it is cloudy, if there are particles in the solution, or if it has been stored at room temperature for longer than 28 days.

AMIKACIN SULFATE

Rx	**Amikacin** (Various, eg, Bedford Labs)	**Injection:** 250 mg/mL	In 2 and 4 mL vials.[a]
Rx	**Amikin** (Apothecon)		In 2 and 4 mL vials[b] and 2 mL disp syringes.[b]
	Amikacin (Various, eg, Gensia)	**Pediatric Injection:** 50 mg/mL	0.13% sodium metabisulfite, 0.5% sodium citrate dihydrate. In 2 and 4 mL vials.
Rx	**Amikin** (Apothecon)		In 2 mL vials.[b]

[a] May contain sodium metabisulfite, sodium citrate dihydrate or sulfuric acid.

[b] With sodium bisulfite and sulfuric acid.

AMIKACIN — INJECTION

Information beginning in the Aminoglycosides group monograph must be considered when using these products.

WARNING

Patients treated with parenteral aminoglycosides should be under close clinical observation because of the potential ototoxicity and nephrotoxicity associated with their use. Safety for treatment periods which are longer than 14 days has not been established.

Ototoxicity – Neurotoxicity, manifested as vestibular and permanent bilateral auditory ototoxicity, can occur in patients with preexisting renal damage and in patients with normal renal function treated at higher doses and/or periods longer than those recommended. The risk of aminoglycoside-induced ototoxicity is greater in patients with renal damage. High frequency deafness usually occurs first and can be detected only by audiometric testing. Vertigo may occur and may be evidence of vestibular injury. Other manifestations of neurotoxicity may include numbness, skin tingling, muscle twitching, and convulsions. The risk of hearing loss due to aminoglycosides increases with the degree of exposure to either high peak or high trough serum concentrations. Patients developing cochlear damage may not have symptoms during therapy to warn them of developing eighth-nerve toxicity, and total or partial irreversible bilateral deafness may occur after the drug has been discontinued. Aminoglycoside-induced ototoxicity is usually irreversible.

Nephrotoxicity – Aminoglycosides are potentially nephrotoxic. The risk of nephrotoxicity is greater in patients with impaired renal function and in those who receive high doses or prolonged therapy.

Neuromuscular blockade – Neuromuscular blockade and respiratory paralysis have been reported following parenteral injection, topical instillation (as in orthopedic and abdominal irrigation or in local treatment of empyema), and following oral use of aminoglycosides. The possibility of these phenomena should be considered if aminoglycosides are administered by any route, especially in patients receiving anesthetics, neuromuscular blocking agents such as tubocurarine, succinylcholine, decamethonium, or in patients receiving massive transfusions of citrate-anticoagulated blood. If blockage occurs, calcium salts may reverse these phenomena, but mechanical respiratory assistance may be necessary.

Monitoring – Renal and eighth-nerve function should be closely monitored especially in patients with known or suspected renal impairment at the onset of therapy and also in those whose renal function is initially normal but who develop signs of renal dysfunction during therapy. Serum concentrations of amikacin should be monitored when feasible to assure adequate levels and to avoid potentially toxic levels and prolonged peak concentrations above 35 mcg/mL. Urine should be examined for decreased specific gravity, increased excretion of proteins, and the presence of cells or casts. Blood urea nitrogen, serum creatinine, or creatinine clearance should be measured periodically. Serial audiograms should be obtained where feasible in patients old enough to be tested, particularly high-risk patients. Evidence of ototoxicity (dizziness, vertigo, tinnitus, roaring in the ears, and hearing loss) or nephrotoxicity requires discontinuation of the drug or dosage adjustment.

Concurrent therapy – Concurrent and/or sequential systemic, oral, or topical use of other neurotoxic or nephrotoxic products, particularly bacitracin, cisplatin, amphotericin B, cephaloridine, paromomycin, viomycin, polymyxin B, colistin, vancomycin, or other aminoglycosides should be avoided. Other factors that may increase risk of toxicity are advanced age and dehydration.

The concurrent use of amikacin with potent diuretics (ethacrynic acid, or furosemide) should be avoided because diuretics by themselves may cause ototoxicity. In addition, when administered intravenously, diuretics may enhance aminoglycoside toxicity by altering antibiotic concentrations in serum and tissue.

Indications

➤*Gram-negative infections:* In the short-term treatment of serious infections due to susceptible strains of gram-negative bacteria including *Pseudomonas* species, *Escherichia coli*, species of indole-positive and indole-negative *Proteus*, *Providencia* species, *Klebsiella-Enterobacter-Serratia* species, and *Acinetobacter* (Mima-Herellea) species.

➤*Serious infections:* Clinical studies have shown amikacin to be effective in bacterial septicemia (including neonatal sepsis); in serious infections of the respiratory tract, bones and joints, central nervous system (including meningitis) and skin and soft tissue; intra-abdominal infections (including peritonitis); and in burns and postoperative infections (including post-vascular surgery). Clinical studies have shown amikacin also to be effective in serious complicated and recurrent urinary tract infections due to these organisms. Aminoglycosides, including amikacin injectable, are not indicated in uncomplicated initial episodes of urinary tract infections unless the causative organisms are not susceptible to antibiotics having less potential toxicity.

➤*Suspected gram-negative infections:* Bacteriologic studies should be performed to identify causative organisms and their susceptibilities to amikacin. Amikacin may be considered as initial therapy in suspected gram-negative infections and therapy may be instituted before obtaining the results of susceptibility testing. Clinical trials demonstrated that amikacin was effective in infections caused by gentamicin and/or tobramycin-resistant strains of gram-negative organisms, particularly *Proteus rettgeri*, *Providencia stuartii*, *Serratia marcescens*, and *Pseudomonas aeruginosa*. The decision to continue therapy with the drug should be based on results of the susceptibility tests, the severity of the infection, the response of the patient and the important additional considerations contained in the Warning Box.

➤*Staphylococcal infections:* Amikacin has also been shown to be effective in staphylococcal infections and may be considered as initial therapy under certain conditions in the treatment of known or suspected staphylococcal disease such as, severe infections where the causative organism may be either a gram-negative bacterium or a staphylococcus, infections due to susceptible strains of staphylococci in patients allergic to other antibiotics, and in mixed staphylococcal/gram-negative infections. In certain severe infections such as neonatal sepsis, concomitant therapy with a penicillin-type drug may be indicated because of the possibility of infections due to gram-positive organisms such as streptococci or pneumococci.

➤*Off-label uses:*

Aerosolized – [4] = Insufficient documentation. Currently, there are limited available controlled data on the use of aerosolized amikacin in the treatment of pneumonia. Larger controlled trials are needed in patients with cystic fibrosis and those in nursing homes, 2 groups that could potentially benefit from effective antipseudomonal therapies.

Tuberculosis – [1] = Good documentation. According to the American Thoracic Society, Centers for Disease Control and Prevention, and Infectious Diseases Society of America joint guidelines on the treatment of tuberculosis (TB), intravenous (IV) or intramuscular (IM) amikacin can be used as second-line therapy for patients with drug-resistant TB whose isolate has demonstrated presumed susceptibility to amikacin.

Other possible off-label uses – Intrathecal/intraventricular administration has been suggested at 8 mg per 24 hours.

Amikacin 15 mg/day IV in divided doses every 8 to 12 hours may be used as a part of a multiple-drug regimen (generally 3 to 5 agents) for *Mycobacterium avium* complex, a common infection in AIDS patients.

In cystic fibrosis patients, the use of inhaled aminoglycosides may be beneficial in certain populations (eg, younger patients). Clinical outcome is not improved, but deterioration of pulmonary function tests may be slowed or prevented.

Administration and Dosage

➤*General dosing considerations:* The patient's pretreatment body weight should be obtained for calculation of correct dosage.

Because of the potential toxicity of aminoglycosides, "fixed dosage" recommendations that are not based on body weight are not advised. Rather, it is essential to calculate the dosage to fit the needs of each patient.

Whenever possible, serum amikacin concentrations should be monitored by appropriate assay procedures. (See Therapeutic drug monitoring.)

The status of renal function should be estimated by measurement of the serum creatinine concentration or calculation of the endogenous creatinine clearance (CrCl) rate. The serum urea nitrogen (BUN) is much less reliable for this purpose. Reassessment of renal function should be made periodically during therapy. (See Renal function impairment.)

➤*Adults:*

Infections – For a list of infections, refer to Indications.

Usual dosage: 15 mg/kg/day IM or IV, divided into 2 or 3 equal doses, administered at equally divided intervals (ie, 7.5 mg/kg every 12 hours or 5 mg/kg every 8 hours).

Amikacin Dosing for Adults and Children

Patient weight		Dosage	
lbs	kg	7.5 mg/kg every 12 hours	5 mg/kg every 8 hours
99 lbs	45 kg	337.5 mg	225 mg
110 lbs	50 kg	375 mg	250 mg
121 lbs	55 kg	412.5 mg	275 mg
132 lbs	60 kg	450 mg	300 mg
143 lbs	65 kg	487.5 mg	325 mg
154 lbs	70 kg	525 mg	350 mg
165 lbs	75 kg	562.5 mg	375 mg
176 lbs	80 kg	600 mg	400 mg
187 lbs	85 kg	637.5 mg	425 mg
198 lbs	90 kg	675 mg	450 mg
209 lbs	95 kg	712.5 mg	475 mg
220 lbs	100 kg	750 mg	500 mg

Maximum dose: 15 mg/kg/day or 1.5 g/day (for heavier patients).

Urinary tract infections (uncomplicated): 250 mg IM or IV twice daily may be used.

Off-label dosing –

Aerosolized: [4] = Insufficient documentation. 250 mg every 12 hours to 400 mg every 8 hours.

Tuberculosis: [1] = Good documentation. Amikacin 15 mg/kg/day (not to exceed 1 g/day) IV or IM, usually given as a single daily dose (5 to 7 days per week) initially, and then reduced to 2 or 3 times a week after the first 2 to 4 months or after culture conversion, depending on the efficacy of the other drugs in the regimen. For patients older than 59 years of age, the dosage should be reduced to 10 mg/kg/day. The dosing frequency should also be reduced in patients with renal insufficiency.

➤*Children:*

Infections – For a list of infections, refer to Indications.

AMIKACIN — INJECTION

See Adults for dosing for children and older infants.

Neonates:

- *Loading dose* – 10 mg/kg.
- *Maintenance dosage* – 7.5 mg/kg every 12 hours.

Off-label dosing –

Aerosolized: [4] = Insufficient documentation. 250 mg every 12 hours to 400 mg every 8 hours.

➤*Renal function impairment:* Doses may be adjusted in patients with impaired renal function either by administering normal doses at prolonged intervals or by administering reduced doses at a fixed interval. Both methods are based on the patient's CrCl or serum creatinine values because these have been found to correlate with aminoglycoside half-lives in patients with diminished renal function. These dosage schedules must be used in conjunction with careful clinical and laboratory observations of the patient and should be modified as necessary. Neither method should be used when dialysis is being performed.

These methods of dosage calculation may be misleading in patients who have undergone severe wasting and in elderly patients.

Normal dosage at prolonged intervals – If the CrCl rate is not available and the patient's condition is stable, a dosage interval in hours for the normal dose can be calculated by multiplying the patient's serum creatinine by 9 (eg, if the serum creatinine concentration is 2 mg per 100 mL) the recommended single dose (7.5 mg/kg) should be administered every 18 hours.

Reduced dosage at fixed time intervals – When renal function is impaired and it is desirable to administer amikacin at a fixed time interval, dosage must be reduced. In these patients, serum amikacin concentrations should be measured to ensure accurate administration of amikacin and to avoid concentrations above 35 mcg/mL.

First, initiate therapy by administering a normal dose, 7.5 mg/kg, as a loading dose. This loading dose is the same as the normally recommended dose, which would be calculated for a patient with normal renal function as previously described.

To determine the size of maintenance doses administered every 12 hours, the loading dose should be reduced in proportion to the reduction in the patient's CrCl rate:

Maintenance dose every 12 hours = observed CrCl (mL/min)/normal CrCl (mL/min) × calculated loading dose.

An alternate rough guide for determining reduced dosage at 12-hour intervals (for patients whose steady state serum creatinine values are known) is to divide the normally recommended dose by the patient's serum creatinine.

The previous dosage schedules are not intended to be rigid recommendations but are provided as guides to dosage when the measurement of amikacin serum levels is not feasible.

Alternative dosage – The following is an alternative dosage regimen for adults. Dosages are adjusted per pharmacy pharmacokinetic consult protocol.

CrCl 30 to 80 mL/min: 4 to 12 mg/kg every 24 hours.
CrCl 10 to 30 mL/min: 4 to 7.5 mg/kg every 48 hours.
CrCl less than 10 mL/min: 3 mg/kg every 72 hours.

Hemodialysis –

Adults receiving continuous renal replace therapy (CRRT): One reference suggests that 100% of a usual dosage be administered IV every 24 to 72 hours according to plasma concentrations.

The following alternative recommendations assume ultrafiltration and dialysis flow rates of 1 to 2 L/h.

- *Loading dose* – 10 mg/kg IV.
- *Maintenance dosage* – Consider performing first-dose pharmacokinetics for subsequent dosing. The volume of distribution and the elimination rate can be estimated based on the peak concentration and a 24-hour concentration. The 24-hour concentration should be performed in order to determine the dosing interval according to the patient's elimination rate.

Suggested maintenance dosage is 7.5 mg/kg IV every 24 to 48 hours for patients receiving continuous venovenous hemofiltration (CVVH), continuous venovenous hemodialysis (CVVHD), or continuous venovenous hemodialfiltration (CVVHDF). For patients with severe infections because of gram-negative rods, the target peak concentration should be 15 to 30 mg/L. When the plasma concentration declines to less than 10 mg/L, a dose should be administered.

Adults receiving intermittent hemodialysis (IHD): According to the prescribing information, approximately half the normal mg/kg dose can be given after hemodialysis.

An alternative dosage is 5 to 7.5 mg/kg IV every 48 to 72 hours administered after the dialysis session, and redose when the plasma concentration declines to less than 10 mg/L (prehemodialysis) or less than 6 to 8 mg/L (posthemodialysis). This recommendation assumes the patient is receiving standard IHD 3 times per week and completes the full dialysis sessions.

Peritoneal dialysis – A parenteral dose of 7.5 mg/kg is given, and amikacin is then instilled in peritoneal dialysate at a concentration desired in serum.

For continuous ambulatory peritoneal dialysis, give 15 to 20 mg/L/day.

➤*Therapeutic drug monitoring:* Whenever possible, amikacin concentrations in serum should be measured to ensure adequate but not excessive levels. It is desirable to measure both peak and trough serum concentrations intermittently during therapy. Peak concentrations (30 to 90 minutes after injection) above 35 mcg/mL and trough concentrations (just prior to the next dose) above 10 mcg per mL should be avoided. Dosage should be adjusted as indicated.

In adults, single doses of 500 mg (7.5 mg/kg) administered as an IV infusion over a period of 30 minutes produced a mean peak serum concentration over a period of 30 minutes, produced a mean peak serum concentration of 38 mcg/mL at the end of the infusion, and levels of 24, 18, and 0.75 mcg/mL at 30 minutes, 1 hour, and 10 hours postinfusion, respectively. Repeat infusions of 7.5 mg/kg every 12 hours were well tolerated and caused no drug accumulation.

➤*Duration of therapy:* The usual duration of treatment is 7 to 10 days. At the recommended dosage level, uncomplicated infections caused by amikacin-sensitive organisms should respond in 24 to 48 hours. It is desirable to limit the duration of treatment to short term whenever feasible. In difficult and complicated infections where treatment beyond 10 days is considered, the use of amikacin should be reevaluated. If continued, amikacin serum levels and renal, auditory, and vestibular functions should be monitored.

➤*Discontinuation of therapy:* If definite clinical response does not occur within 3 to 5 days, therapy should be stopped, and the antibiotic susceptibility pattern of the invading organism should be rechecked. Failure of the infection to respond may be due to resistance of the organism or to the presence of septic foci requiring surgical drainage.

➤*Preparation for administration:*

Adults – The solution for IV use is prepared by adding the contents of a 500 mg vial to 100 or 200 mL of sterile diluent such as sodium chloride 0.9% injection or dextrose 5% injection or any of the compatible solutions listed in Admixture compatibility. (See Admixture compatibility.)

Children – In children, the amount of fluid used will depend on the amount of amikacin ordered for the patient. It should be a sufficient amount to infuse the amikacin over a 30- to 60-minute period. Infants should receive a 1- to 2-hour infusion.

➤*Administration:* Amikacin may be given IM or IV (over a 30- to 60-minute period). Infants should receive a 1- to 2-hour infusion.

➤*Admixture compatibility:*

Compatibility – Amikacin is stable for 24 hours at room temperature at concentrations of 0.25 and 5 mg/mL in the following solutions:

- Dextrose 5% injection
- Dextrose 5% and Sodium chloride 0.2% injection
- Dextrose 5% and Sodium chloride 0.45% injection
- Sodium chloride 0.9% injection
- Ringer's lactate injection
- *Normosol M* in dextrose 5% injection (or *Plasma-Lyte 56* injection in dextrose 5% in water)
- *Normosol R* in dextrose 5% injection (or *Plasma-Lyte 148* injection in dextrose 5% in water)

Incompatibility – Aminoglycosides administered by any of the previous routes should not be physically premixed with other drugs; they should be administered separately.

➤*Storage/Stability:* Store at 15° to 30°C (59° to 86°F).

In the above solutions with amikacin concentrations of 0.25 and 5 mg/mL, solutions aged for 60 days at 4°C (39.2°F) and then stored at 25°C (77°F) had utility times of 24 hours. At the same concentrations, solutions frozen and aged for 30 days at −15°C (+5°F), thawed, and stored at 25°C (77°F) had utility times of 24 hours.

AMINOGLYCOSIDES, ORAL

For more complete information on aminoglycosides, refer to the Aminoglycosides, Parenteral group monograph. SPECIAL NOTE: See Warning Box in Aminoglycosides, Parenteral group monograph concerning toxicity.

Indications

➤*General information:* See individual monographs for specific information.

➤*Suppression of intestinal bacteria:* As adjunctive therapy for the suppression of intestinal bacteria.

➤*Hepatic coma:* As adjunctive therapy in the management of hepatic coma.

Actions

➤*Pharmacokinetics:* Oral aminoglycosides are poorly absorbed; therefore use only for suppression of GI bacterial flora. The small absorbed fraction is rapidly excreted with normal kidney function. The unabsorbed drug is eliminated unchanged in the feces. Most intestinal bacteria are rapidly eliminated with bacterial suppression persisting for 48 to 72 hours. Nonpathogenic yeasts and occasionally resistant strains of *Enterobacter aerogenes* replace the intestinal bacteria.

Contraindications

Presence of intestinal obstruction; hypersensitivity to aminoglycosides.

Warnings/Precautions

➤*Increased absorption:* Although negligible amounts are absorbed through intact mucosa, consider the possibility of increased absorption from ulcerated or denuded areas.

➤*Nephrotoxicity/Ototoxicity:* Because of reported cases of deafness and potential nephrotoxic effects, closely observe patients. Perform urine and blood examinations and audiometric tests prior to and during extended therapy, especially in those with hepatic or renal disease. If renal insufficiency develops, reduce dosage or discontinue the drug. Refer to the Warning Box in the Aminoglycosides, Parenteral monograph concerning aminoglycoside toxicity.

➤*Muscular disorders:* Use with caution in patients with muscular disorders such as myasthenia gravis or parkinsonism; these drugs may aggravate muscle weakness because of their potential curare-like effect on neuromuscular junction.

➤*GI effects:*

Neomycin – Orally administered neomycin increases fecal bile acid excretion and reduces intestinal lactase activity.

Paromomycin – Use with caution in individuals with ulcerative lesions of the bowel to avoid renal toxicity through inadvertent absorption.

➤*Superinfection:* Use of antibiotics (especially prolonged or repeated therapy) may result in bacterial or fungal overgrowth of nonsusceptible organisms. Such overgrowth may lead to a secondary infection. Take appropriate measures if superinfection occurs.

➤*Pregnancy: Category D* (**Neomycin**), (**Kanamycin** per Briggs's *Drugs in Pregnancy and Lactation*). Safety for use during pregnancy has not been established. Use only when clearly needed and when the potential benefits outweigh the potential hazards.

Neomycin – Aminoglycosides can cause fetal harm when administered to a pregnant woman. Aminoglycosides cross the placenta. Although serious side effects to fetus or newborn have not been reported in the treatment of pregnant women, the potential for harm exists. If neomycin is used during pregnancy, or if the patient becomes pregnant while taking this drug, apprise the patient of the potential hazard to the fetus.

➤*Lactation:* Neomycin is excreted in cow milk following a single IM injection. It is not known whether neomycin is excreted in human breast milk. Kanamycin is excreted in human breast milk. Other aminoglycosides are excreted in human breast milk. Because of the potential for serious adverse reactions from the aminoglycosides in nursing infants, decide whether to discontinue nursing or to discontinue the drug, taking into account the importance of the drug to the mother.

➤*Children:* The safety and efficacy of oral neomycin in patients < 18 years of age have not been established. If treatment is necessary, use with caution; do not exceed a treatment period of 3 weeks because of absorption from the GI tract.

Drug Interactions

Oral Aminoglycoside Drug Interactions

Precipitant drug	Object drug[a]		Description
Aminoglycosides	Anticoagulants	↑	A small rise in warfarin-induced hypoprothrombinemia may occur, possibly due to interference in absorption of dietary vitamin K by aminoglycosides.
Aminoglycosides	Digoxin	↓	Rate and extent of digoxin absorption may be reduced; however, in a small number of patients (< 10%), this may be offset by a reduction in digoxin's metabolism.
Aminoglycosides	Methotrexate	↓	Methotrexate's absorption and bioavailability may be decreased.
Aminoglycosides	Neuromuscular blockers - Depolarizing and nondepolarizing	↑	The actions of the neuromuscular blockers may be enhanced; prolonged respiratory depression may occur.
Aminoglycosides	Polypeptide antibiotics	↑	Concurrent use may increase the risk of respiratory paralysis and renal dysfunction.
Aminoglycosides	Vitamin A	↓	Serum retinol and plasma carotene levels may be decreased.

[a] ↑ = object drug increased; ↓ = object drug decreased.

Adverse Reactions

Nausea, vomiting and diarrhea are most common. The "malabsorption syndrome" characterized by increased fecal fat, decreased serum carotene and fall in xylose absorption has occurred with prolonged therapy. *Clostridium difficile*-associated colitis has occurred following neomycin therapy. Nephrotoxicity and ototoxicity have occurred following prolonged and high dosage therapy in hepatic coma.

Overdosage

Because of low absorption, it is unlikely that acute overdosage would occur with oral neomycin sulfate. However, prolonged administration could result in sufficient systemic drug levels to produce neurotoxicity, ototoxicity or nephrotoxicity. Hemodialysis will remove neomycin sulfate from the blood.

Patient Information

Complete full course of therapy; take until gone. May cause nausea, vomiting or diarrhea.

Notify physician if ringing in the ears, hearing impairment or rash, problems urinating or dizziness occurs.

Drink plenty of fluids.

➤*Neomycin:* Before administering the drug, inform patients or members of their families of possible toxic effects on the eighth cranial nerve. The possibility of acute toxicity increases in premature infants and neonates.

NEOMYCIN SULFATE

Rx	**Neomycin Sulfate** (Various, eg, Goldline)	**Tablets:** 500 mg	In 100s.
Rx	**Neo-fradin** (Pharma-Tek)	**Oral solution:** 125 mg per 5 mL	Parabens. In 480 mL.

NEOMYCIN SULFATE — ORAL

Refer to the general discussion of these products in the Aminoglycosides, Oral group monograph.

WARNING

Toxicity – Systemic absorption of neomycin occurs following oral administration, and toxic reactions may occur. Patients treated with neomycin should be under close clinical observation because of the potential toxicity associated with the use of neomycin. Neurotoxicity (including ototoxicity) and nephrotoxicity following the oral use of neomycin sulfate have been reported, even when used in recommended doses. The potential for nephrotoxicity, permanent bilateral auditory ototoxicity, and sometimes vestibular toxicity, is present in patients with healthy renal function when treated with higher doses of neomycin or for longer periods than recommended. Serial, vestibular and audiometric tests, as well as tests of renal function, should be performed (especially in high-risk patients). The risk of nephrotoxicity and ototoxicity is greater in patients with impaired renal function. Ototoxicity is often delayed in onset, and patients developing cochlear damage will not have symptoms during therapy to warn them of developing eighth nerve destruction, and total or partial deafness may occur long after neomycin has been discontinued.

Other factors which increase the risk of toxicity are advanced age and dehydration.

Neuromuscular blockage – Neuromuscular blockage and respiratory paralysis have been reported following the oral use of neomycin. The possibility of the occurrence of neuromuscular blockage and respiratory paralysis should be considered if neomycin is administered, especially to patients receiving anesthetics; neuromuscular-blocking agents such as tubocurarine, succinylcholine, decamethonium; or massive transfusions of citrate anticoagulated blood. If blockage occurs, calcium salts may reverse these phenomena, but mechanical respiratory assistance may be necessary.

WARNING (cont.)

Concurrent therapy – Concurrent or sequential systemic, oral or topical use of other aminoglycosides, including paromomycin and other potentially nephrotoxic or neurotoxic drugs such as bacitracin, cisplatin, vancomycin, amphotericin B, polymyxin B, colistin and viomycin, should be avoided because the toxicity may be additive.

The concurrent use of neomycin with potent diuretics such as ethacrynic acid or furosemide should be avoided, since certain diuretics by themselves may cause ototoxicity. In addition, when administered IV, diuretics may enhance neomycin toxicity by altering the antibiotic concentration in serum and tissue.

Indications

➤*Suppression of intestinal bacteria (tablets only):* Adjunctive therapy as part of a regimen for the suppression of the normal bacterial flora of the bowel (eg, preoperative preparation of the bowel). It is given concomitantly with erythromycin enteric-coated base (see Administration and Dosage).

➤*Hepatic coma (portal-systemic encephalopathy) (tablets and oral solution):* Neomycin sulfate oral preparations have been shown to be effective adjunctive therapy in hepatic coma by reduction of the ammonia-forming bacteria in the intestinal tract. The subsequent reduction in blood ammonia has resulted in neurologic improvement.

Administration and Dosage

➤*General dosing considerations:* The benefits to the patient should be weighed against the risks of nephrotoxicity, permanent ototoxicity, and neuromuscular blockade following the accumulation of neomycin in the tissues.

To minimize the risk of toxicity, use the lowest possible dose and the shortest possible treatment period to control the condition.

NEOMYCIN SULFATE — ORAL

➤*Adults:*

Hepatic coma – For use as an adjunct in the management of hepatic coma. Withdraw protein from diet. Avoid use of diuretic agents. Give supportive therapy, including blood products, as indicated.

Usual dosage: 4 to 12 g per day (8 to 24 tablets) in divided doses. Treatment should be continued over a period of 5 to 6 days, during which time protein should be returned incrementally to the diet.

If less potentially toxic drugs cannot be used for chronic hepatic insufficiency, neomycin in doses of up to 4 g daily (8 tablets/day) may be necessary.

Duration of therapy: 5 to 6 days; treatment for periods longer than 2 weeks is not recommended. The risk for the development of neomycin-induced toxicity progressively increases when treatment must be extended to preserve the life of a patient with hepatic encephalopathy who has failed to fully respond.

Monitoring: Frequent periodic monitoring of these patients to ascertain the presence of drug toxicity is mandatory. Also, neomycin serum concentrations should be monitored to avoid potentially toxic levels.

Suppression of intestinal bacteria – Neomycin tablets are indicated for the preoperative prophylaxis for elective colorectal surgery. Listed in the following sections is an example of a recommended bowel preparation regimen. A proposed surgery time of 8 am has been used.

Preoperative day 3: Minimum residue or clear liquid diet. Bisacodyl, 1 tablet orally at 6 pm.

Preoperative day 2: Minimum residue or clear liquid diet. Magnesium sulfate 30 mL, 50% solution (15 g) orally at 10 am, 2 pm, and 6 pm. Enema at 7 pm and 8 pm.

Preoperative day 1: Clear liquid diet. Supplemental (IV) fluids as needed. Magnesium sulfate 30 mL, 50% solution (15 g) orally at 10 am and 2 pm. Neomycin sulfate (1 g) and erythromycin base (1 g) orally at 1 pm, 2 pm and 11 pm. No enema.

Day of operation: Patient evacuates rectum at 6:30 am for scheduled operation at 8 am.

➤*Children:* The safety and efficacy of oral neomycin sulfate in patients younger than 18 years of age have not been established. If treatment of a patient younger than 18 years of age is necessary, neomycin should be used with caution, and the period of treatment should not exceed 2 weeks (tablets) or 3 weeks (oral solution) because of absorption from the GI tract.

➤*Renal function impairment:* Patients with renal insufficiency may develop toxic neomycin blood levels unless doses are properly regulated. If renal insufficiency develops during treatment, the dosage should be reduced or the antibiotic discontinued.

➤*Storage/Stability:* Store at 15° to 30°C (59° to 86°F). Dispense in tight containers.

PAROMOMYCIN

Rx	**Paromomycin Sulfate** (Caraco)	**Capsules; oral:** 250 mg paromomycin	As paromomycin sulfate. In 100s.
Rx	**Humatin** (Parke-Davis)		As paromomycin sulfate. In 16s.

PAROMOMYCIN SULFATE — ORAL

Refer to the general discussion of these products in the Aminoglycosides, Oral group monograph.

Indications

➤*Intestinal amebiasis:* Acute and chronic intestinal amebiasis.

It is not effective in extraintestinal amebiasis because it is not absorbed.

➤*Hepatic coma:* Management of hepatic coma as adjunctive therapy.

➤*Off-label uses:* Has been recommended for other parasitic infections, including *Dientamoeba fragilis* (25 to 30 mg/kg/day in 3 doses for 7 days); *Diphyllobothrium latum, Taenia saginata, T. solium, Dipylidium caninum* (for adults, 1 g every 15 minutes for 4 doses; for pediatric patients, 11 mg/kg every 15 minutes for 4 doses); *Hymenolepsis nana* (45 mg/kg/day for 5 to 7 days).

Administration and Dosage

➤*Adults:*

Hepatic coma – 4 g daily in divided doses, given at regular intervals for 5 to 6 days.

Intestinal amebiasis – 25 to 35 mg/kg daily, administered in 3 divided doses with meals, for 5 to 10 days.

➤*Children:* See Adults for dosing for intestinal amebiasis.

➤*Administration:* Give with meals.

➤*Storage/Stability:* Store at 15° to 30°C (59° to 86°F). Protect from moisture.

COLISTIMETHATE SODIUM

COLISTIMETHATE SODIUM

Rx	**Colistimethate Sodium** (Paddock)	**Injection, lyophilized cake:** 150 mg colistin base[a]	In vials.
Rx	**Coly-Mycin M** (JHP Pharmaceuticals)		In vials.

[a] As colistimethate sodium or pentasodium colistinmethane sulfonate.

COLISTIMETHATE SODIUM — INJECTION

Indications

➤*Gram-negative infections:* Treatment of acute or chronic infections due to sensitive strains of certain gram-negative bacilli. Particularly indicated when the infection is caused by sensitive strains of *P. aeruginosa*. Clinically effective in treatment of infections due to the following gram-negative organisms: *E. aerogenes, E. coli, K. pneumoniae* and *P. aeruginosa*. Pending results of bacteriologic cultures and sensitivity tests, colistimethate may be used to initiate therapy in serious infections that are suspected to be due to gram-negative organisms.

➤*Off-label uses:* Aerosolized colistin has been shown to be beneficial in the treatment of sensitive *Pseudomonas* infections in patients with cystic fibrosis. In addition, early aggressive use of the drug as adjunctive therapy may play a role in reducing chronic infections in this population.

Administration and Dosage

➤*Maximum dose:* 5 mg/kg/day according to the prescribing information.

➤*General dosing considerations:* In obese individuals, dosage should be based on ideal body weight.

➤*Adults:*

Infections – For a list of infections, refer to Indications.

Usual dosage: 2.5 to 5 mg/kg/day IV or IM in 2 to 4 divided doses, depending upon the severity of the infection.

Maximum dose: 5 mg/kg/day.

➤*Children:* See Adults for dosing.

➤*Renal function impairment:* Reduce the daily dose in the presence of any renal impairment.

Colistimethate Dosage Schedules for Adults with Impaired Renal Function

Renal function			Dosage			
Degree of impairment	Plasma creatinine (mg/dL)	Urea clearance % (of normal)	Dose[a] (mg)	Frequency (times per day)	Total daily dose (mg)	Approx. daily dose (mg/kg)
Normal	0.7 - 1.2	80 - 100	100 - 150	4 to 2	300	5
Mild	1.3 - 1.5	40 - 70	75 - 115	2	150 - 230	2.5 - 3.8
Moderate	1.6 - 2.5	25 - 40	66 - 150	2 or 1	133 - 150	2.5
Severe	2.6 - 4	10 - 25	100 - 150	q 36 h	100	1.5

[a] Suggested unit dose is 2.5 to 5 mg/kg; increase time interval between injections in presence of impaired renal function.

➤*Preparation for administration:* The 150 mg vial should be reconstituted with 2 mL sterile water for injection. During reconstitution swirl gently to avoid frothing. The reconstituted solution provides colistimethate sodium at a concentration equivalent to 75 mg/mL colistin base activity.

➤*Administration:* Colistimethate may be given IM or IV.

Direct intermittent administration – Inject one-half the total daily dose over a period of 3 to 5 minutes every 12 hours.

Continuous infusion – Slowly inject one-half the daily dose over 3 to 5 minutes. Add the remaining half of the total daily dose of colistimethate to one of the following: sodium chloride 0.9%; dextrose 5% in water; dextrose 5% with sodium chloride 0.9%; dextrose 5% with sodium chloride 0.45%; dextrose 5% with sodium chloride 0.225%; lactated Ringer's solution. Swirl gently to avoid frothing.

COLISTIMETHATE SODIUM — INJECTION

Administer by slow IV infusion starting 1 to 2 hours after the initial dose over the next 22 to 23 hours in the presence of normal renal function. In the presence of impaired renal function, reduce infusion rate. Choice of IV solution and volume to be employed are dictated by requirements of fluid and electrolyte management.

➤*Storage/Stability:* Store between 20° and 25°C (68° to 77°F). Store reconstituted solution in refrigerator (2° to 8°C; 36° to 46°F) or between 20° and 25°C (68° to 77°F) and use within 7 days.

Freshly prepare any infusion solution containing colistimethate and use for no longer than 24 hours.

Actions

➤*Pharmacokinetics:* Higher initial blood levels are obtained following IV administration. Blood levels peak at between 5 and 10 mcg/ml between 2 and 3 hours after IM administration. Serum half-life is 2 to 3 hours.

Average urinary levels range from about 270 mcg/ml at 2 hours to about 15 mcg/ml at 8 hours after IV administration and from about 200 to 25 mcg/ml during a similar period following IM administration.

➤*Microbiology:* Colistimethate has bactericidal activity against the following gram-negative bacilli: *Enterobacter aerogenes, Escherichia coli, Klebsiella pneumoniae* and *Pseudomonas aeruginosa*.

Contraindications

Hypersensitivity to colistimethate sodium; infections due to *Proteus* or *Neisseria* species.

Warnings/Precautions

➤*Maximum dosage:* Do not exceed 5 mg/kg/day in patients with normal renal function.

➤*Neurologic effects:* May occur transiently. These include circumoral paresthesia or numbness, tingling or formication of the extremities, generalized pruritus, vertigo, dizziness and slurring of speech. Warn patients not to drive vehicles or use hazardous machinery while on therapy. Dosage reduction may alleviate symptoms. Therapy need not be discontinued, but observe such patients carefully. Overdosage can result in renal insufficiency, muscle weakness and apnea.

➤*Respiratory effects:* Respiratory arrest has occurred following IM administration. Impaired renal function increases the possibility of apnea and neuromuscular blockade, generally because of failure to follow recommended guidelines, overdosage, failure to reduce dose commensurate with degree of renal impairment or concomitant use of other antibiotics or drugs with neuromuscular blocking potential. If apnea occurs, treat with assisted respiration, oxygen and calcium chloride injections.

➤*Nephrotoxicity:* A decrease in urine output or increase in BUN or serum creatinine can be signs of nephrotoxicity, which is probably a dose-dependent effect. These manifestations are reversible following discontinuation. Increases of BUN have occurred at dose levels of 1.6 to 5 mg/kg/day. Values returned to normal following cessation.

➤*Renal function impairment:* Since colistimethate is eliminated mainly by renal excretion, use with caution when the possibility of impaired renal function exists. Consider the decline in renal function with advanced age.

When actual renal impairment is present, use colistimethate with extreme caution; reduce the dosage in proportion to the extent of the impairment. Administration of amounts in excess of renal excretory capacity will lead to high serum levels. This can result in further impairment of renal function, initiating a cycle which, if not recognized, can lead to acute renal insufficiency, renal shutdown and further concentration of the antibiotic to toxic levels in the body. Interference with nerve transmission at neuromuscular junctions may occur and result in muscle weakness and apnea.

Signs indicating the development of impaired renal function are diminishing urine output and rising BUN or serum creatinine. If present, discontinue therapy immediately. If a life-threatening situation exists, reinstate therapy at a lower dosage after blood levels have fallen.

➤*Pregnancy: Category C.* Colistimethate sodium is transferred across the placental barrier, and blood levels of about 1 mcg/ml are obtained in the fetus following IV administration to the mother. Safety for use during pregnancy has not been established. Use only when clearly needed and when the potential benefits outweigh the potential hazards.

➤*Lactation:* Colistimethate is excreted into breast milk. The milk:plasma ratio is 0.17 to 0.18. Although this level is low, potential problems exist for the breast-feeding infant (eg, modification of bowel flora, direct effects on the infant, interference with the interpretation of culture results if a fever workup is required).

Drug Interactions

Colistimethate Drug Interactions

Precipitant drug	Object drug[a]		Description
Aminoglycosides	Colistimethate	↑	Concurrent use may increase the risk of respiratory paralysis and renal dysfunction.
Cephalothin	Colistimethate	↑	Concurrent use may increase the risk of renal dysfunction.
Colistimethate	Nondepolarizing muscle relaxants	↑	Neuromuscular blockade may be enhanced.

[a] ↑ = object drug increased.

Adverse Reactions

Respiratory arrest (see Warnings/Precautions); decreased urine output or increased BUN or serum creatinine (see Warnings/Precautions); paresthesia; tingling of the extremities or the tongue; generalized itching or urticaria; drug fever; GI upset; vertigo; slurring of speech. The subjective symptoms reported by the adult may not be manifest in infants or young children, thus requiring close attention to renal function.

POLYMYXIN B SULFATE

Rx	**Polymyxin B Sulfate** (Bedford)	**Injection:** 500,000 units	In vials.

POLYMYXIN B — INJECTION

WARNING

When this drug is given IM or intrathecally, it should be given only to hospitalized patients, so as to provide constant supervision by a physician.

Nephrotoxicity – Renal function should be carefully determined, and patients with renal damage and nitrogen retention should have reduced dosage. Patients with nephrotoxicity due to polymyxin B sulfate usually show albuminuria, cellular casts, and azotemia. Diminishing urine output and a rising blood urea nitrogen (BUN) are indications for discontinuing therapy with this drug.

Neurotoxicity – Neurotoxic reactions may be manifested by irritability, weakness, drowsiness, ataxia, perioral paresthesia, numbness of the extremities, and blurring of vision. These are usually associated with high serum levels found in patients with impaired renal function or nephrotoxicity.

Concurrent therapy – The concurrent or sequential use of other neurotoxic or nephrotoxic drugs with polymyxin B sulfate, particularly bacitracin, streptomycin, neomycin, kanamycin, gentamicin, tobramycin, amikacin, cephaloridine, paromomycin, viomycin, and colistin should be avoided.

Neuromuscular blockade – The neurotoxicity of polymyxin B sulfate can result in respiratory paralysis from neuromuscular blockade, especially when the drug is given soon after anesthesia or muscle relaxants.

Use in pregnancy – The safety of this drug in human pregnancy has not been established.

Indications

➤*Pseudomonal infections:* Polymyxin B sulfate is a drug of choice in the treatment of infections of the urinary tract, meninges, and bloodstream caused by susceptible strains of *Pseudomonas aeruginosa*.

➤*Serious infections:* It may be indicated in serious infections caused by susceptible strains of the following organisms, when less potentially toxic drugs are ineffective or contraindicated: *H. influenzae*, specifically meningeal infections; *Escherichia coli*, specifically urinary tract infections; *Aerobacter aerogenes*, specifically bacteremia; *Klebsiella pneumoniae*, specifically bacteremia.

In meningeal infections, polymyxin B sulfate should be administered only by the intrathecal route.

➤*Off-label uses:*

Hospital-acquired pneumonia – American Thoracic Society (ATS) and Infectious Diseases Society of America (IDSA) practice guidelines recommend polymyxin B in the treatment of hospital-acquired pneumonia, ventilator-associated pneumonia, and healthcare-associated pneumonia associated with multidrug-resistant (MDR) gram-negative bacteria, specifically cases associated with *P. aeruginosa* or *Acinetobacter* species that are resistant to systemic antibiotics. Data from a noncontrolled trial suggest that intravenous (IV) polymyxin B should be used only as a salvage monotherapy or adjunctive therapy. Data from a case series enrolling fewer than 20 patients suggest that aerosolized polymyxin B should be used as adjunctive salvage treatment in patients who have failed IV polymyxin B therapy. Larger randomized, controlled trials are needed to establish the role of polymyxin B in treating hospital-acquired pneumonia. The risk of nephrotoxicity and neurotoxicity may limit its use.

Hospital-acquired pneumonia (aerosolized): [3] = Safety concerns.
Hospital-acquired pneumonia (IV): [3] = Safety concerns.

Administration and Dosage

➤*Maximum dose:*

Adults and children – 25,000 units/kg/day (IV administration) according to the prescribing information.

POLYMYXIN B — INJECTION

Infants – Up to 40,000 units/kg/day IV or IM have been given to infants according to the prescribing information. Up to 45,000 units/kg/day IM have been given to premature and newborn infants according to the prescribing information.

➤*Adults:*

Infections – For a list of infections, refer to Indications.

IM use: 25,000 to 30,000 units/kg/day IM. The dosage may be divided and given at either 4- or 6-hour intervals.

Intrathecal use: 50,000 units once daily intrathecally for 3 to 4 days, then 50,000 units once every other day for at least 2 weeks after cultures of the cerebrospinal fluid are negative and sugar content has returned to normal.

IV use:

• *Usual dosage* – 15,000 to 25,000 units/kg/day IV. Infusions may be given every 12 hours; however, the total daily dose must not exceed 25,000 units/kg/day.

• *Maximum dose* – 25,000 units/kg/day.

Off-label dosing –

Hospital-acquired pneumonia (aerosolized): [3] = Safety concerns. 500,000 international units given by aerosolization twice daily (with aerosolized beta-2 agonist administered 20 minutes prior to prevent bronchospasm). Recommended duration is 14 to 16 days (range, 4 to 25 days). Used as adjunctive salvage therapy with IV antibiotics. The risk of nephrotoxicity and neurotoxicity has limited its use.

Hospital-acquired pneumonia (IV): [3] = Safety concerns.

• *Usual dose* – 15,000 to 25,000 units/kg/day IV divided every 12 hours used as salvage monotherapy or adjunctive therapy. It is possible to dose polymyxin B intramuscularly (IM); however, it is associated with severe pain at the injection site. Polymyxin B requires renal dosage adjustments when given IV or IM. The risk of nephrotoxicity and neurotoxicity has limited the use of IV polymyxin.

• *Maximum dose* – 25,000 units/kg/day.

• *Duration of therapy* – Recommended duration is 14 to 16 days (range, 4 to 34 days).

➤*Children:*

Infections – For a list of infections, refer to Indications.

IM use: See Adults for dosing for children.

• *Infants* – Infants with healthy renal function may receive up to 40,000 units/kg/day IM without adverse reactions.

Doses as high as 45,000 units/kg/day have been used in limited clinical studies in treating premature and newborn infants for sepsis caused by *Pseudomonas aeruginosa*.

Intrathecal use: See Adults for dosing for children 2 years of age and older.

• *Younger than 2 years of age* – 20,000 units once daily, intrathecally for 3 to 4 days or 25,000 units once every other day. Continue with a dose of 25,000 units once every other day for at least 2 weeks after cultures of the cerebrospinal fluid are negative and sugar content has returned to normal.

IV use: See Adults for dosing for children.

• *Infants* – Infants may receive up to 40,000 units/kg/day IV without adverse reactions.

➤*Renal function impairment:*

IM use – The dosage should be reduced in the presence of renal impairment.

IV use – The dosage should be reduced from 15,000 units/kg downward for adults and children with kidney impairment.

➤*Preparation for administration:*

IM – Dissolve 500,000 polymyxin B units in 2 mL of sterile water for injection or sodium chloride injection or procaine HCl injection 1%.

Intrathecal – Dissolve 500,000 polymyxin B units in 10 mL of sodium chloride injection for 50,000 units/mL dosage unit.

IV – Dissolve 500,000 polymyxin B units in 300 to 500 mL of parenteral dextrose injection 5% for continuous drip.

➤*Administration:* Polymyxin may be given IV, IM, or intrathecally. IM administration is not recommended routinely because of severe pain at injection sites, particularly in infants and children.

➤*Storage/Stability:*

Before reconstitution – Store at 15° to 30°C (59° to 86°F). Protect from light. Retain in carton until time of use.

After reconstitution – Product must be stored under refrigeration, between 2° and 8°C (36° and 46°F) and any unused portion should be discarded after 72 hours.

Actions

➤*Pharmacology:* Polymyxin B sulfate has a bactericidal action against almost all gram-negative bacilli except the *Proteus* group. Polymyxins increase the permeability of bacterial cell wall membranes.

➤*Pharmacokinetics:*

Absorption/Distribution – Polymyxin B sulfate is not absorbed from the normal alimentary tract. Since the drug loses 50% of its activity in the presence of serum, active blood levels are low. Repeated injections may give a cumulative effect. Levels tend to be higher in infants and children. Tissue diffusion is poor and the drug does not pass the blood-brain barrier into the cerebrospinal fluid.

Excretion – The drug is excreted slowly by the kidneys. In therapeutic dosage, polymyxin B sulfate causes some nephrotoxicity with tubule damage to a slight degree.

➤*Microbiology:* All gram-positive bacteria, fungi, and the gram-negative cocci, *N. gonorrhoeae* and *N. meningitidis*, are resistant.

Contraindications

Hypersensitivity reactions to polymyxins.

Warnings/Precautions

➤*Superinfection:* As with other antibiotics, use of this drug may result in overgrowth of nonsusceptible organisms, including fungi. If superinfection occurs, appropriate therapy should be instituted.

➤*Pregnancy: Category B* (per Briggs' *Drugs in Pregnancy and Lactation*). There is no information regarding the use of polymyxin B in pregnant women.

➤*Lactation:* There is no information regarding the use of polymyxin B in breast-feeding women.

➤*Monitoring:* Baseline renal function should be done prior to therapy, with frequent monitoring of renal function and blood levels of the drug during parenteral therapy. Renal function should be carefully determined, and patients with renal damage and nitrogen retention should have reduced dosage. Patients with nephrotoxicity due to polymyxin B sulfate usually show albuminuria, cellular casts, and azotemia. Diminishing urine output and a rising blood urea nitrogen (BUN) are indications for discontinuing therapy with this drug.

Drug Interactions

➤*Neurotoxic drugs:* Avoid concurrent use of a curariform muscle relaxant and other neurotoxic drugs (eg, ether, tubocurarine, succinylcholine, gallamine, decamethonium, sodium citrate) which may precipitate respiratory depression. If signs of respiratory paralysis appear, respiration should be assisted as required, and the drug discontinued.

Polymyxin B Drug Interactions

Precipitant drug	Object drug[a]		Description
Aminoglycosides	Polymyxin B	⬆	Concurrent use may increase the risk of respiratory paralysis and renal dysfunction.
Polymyxin B	Nondepolarizing muscle relaxants	⬆	Neuromuscular blockade may be enhanced.

[a] ⬆ = object drug increased.

Adverse Reactions

➤*CNS:*

Neurotoxic reactions – Facial flushing, dizziness progressing to ataxia, drowsiness, peripheral paresthesias (circumoral and stocking glove), apnea due to concurrent use of curariform muscle relaxants, other neurotoxic drugs or inadvertent overdosage, and signs of meningeal irritation with intrathecal administration (eg, fever, headache, stiff neck, increased cell count and protein cerebrospinal fluid).

➤*Renal:*

Nephrotoxic reactions – Albuminuria, cylinduria, azotemia, and rising blood levels without any increase in dosage.

➤*Miscellaneous:* Other reactions occasionally reported include the following: Drug fever, urticarial rash, pain (severe) at IM injection sites, and thrombophlebitis at IV injection sites.

BACITRACIN

Rx	**Bacitracin** (Various, eg, Upjohn)	**Injection, powder for solution:** 50,000 units	In vials.
Rx	**Baci-IM** (X-Gen Pharmaceuticals)		In vials.

BACITRACIN — INJECTION

WARNING

Nephrotoxicity – Bacitracin in parenteral (IM) therapy may cause renal failure due to tubular and glomerular necrosis. Its use should be restricted to infants with staphylococcal pneumonia and empyema when due to organisms shown to be susceptible to bacitracin. It should be used only where adequate laboratory facilities are available and when constant supervision of the patient is possible.

Renal function should be carefully determined prior to and daily during therapy. The recommended daily dose should not be exceeded, and fluid intake and urinary output should be maintained at proper levels to avoid kidney toxicity. If renal toxicity occurs the drug should be discontinued. The concurrent use of other nephrotoxic drugs, particularly streptomycin, kanamycin, polymyxin B, polymyxin E (colistin), and neomycin should be avoided.

Indications

➤*Pneumonia / Empyema:* The use of IM bacitracin is limited to the treatment of infants with pneumonia and empyema caused by staphylococci shown to be susceptible to the drug.

See the Warning box for more information.

➤*Off-label uses:* Oral use in antibiotic-associated colitis has been successful.

Administration and Dosage

➤*General dosing considerations:* Fluid intake and urinary output should be maintained at proper levels to avoid kidney toxicity.

➤*Children:*

Pneumonia and empyema caused by staphylococci –

Infants weighing more than 2,500 g: 1,000 units/kg/24 hours IM in 2 or 3 divided doses.

Infants weighing less than 2,500 g: 900 units/kg/24 hours IM in 2 or 3 divided doses.

➤*Preparation for administration:* Solutions should be dissolved in sodium chloride injection containing procaine HCl 2%. The concentration of the antibiotic in the solution should not be less than 5,000 units/mL or more than 10,000 units/mL.

Reconstitution of the 50,000 unit vial with 9.8 mL of diluent will result in a concentration of 5,000 units/mL.

➤*Administration:* This medication is to be administered IM only. IM injections of the solution should be given in the upper outer quadrant of the buttocks, alternating right and left and avoiding multiple injections in the same region because of the transient pain following injection.

➤*Admixture compatibility:* Diluents containing parabens should not be used to reconstitute bacitracin; cloudy solutions and precipitate formation have occurred.

➤*Storage / Stability:* Store the unreconstituted product in a refrigerator at 2° to 8°C (36° to 46°F).

Solutions are stable for 1 week when stored in a refrigerator at 2° to 8°C (36° to 46°F).

Actions

➤*Pharmacology:* Bacitracin exerts pronounced antibacterial action in vitro against a variety of gram-positive and a few gram-negative organisms. However, among systemic diseases, only staphylococcal infections qualify for consideration of bacitracin therapy. Bacitracin is assayed against a standard and its activity is expressed in units, 1 mg having a potency of not less than 50 units.

➤*Pharmacokinetics:*

Absorption – Absorption of bacitracin following IM injection is rapid and complete. A dose of 200 or 300 units/kg every 6 hours gives serum levels of 0.2 to 2 mcg/mL in individuals with healthy renal function.

Distribution – Bacitracin injection is widely distributed in all body organs and is demonstrable in ascitic and pleural fluids after IM injection.

Excretion – Bacitracin injection is excreted slowly by glomerular filtration.

Contraindications

Hypersensitivity or toxic reaction to the drug.

Warnings/Precautions

➤*Nephrotoxicity:* Bacitracin in parenteral (IM) therapy may cause renal failure due to tubular and glomerular necrosis. Its use should be restricted to infants with staphylococcal pneumonia and empyema when due to organisms shown to be susceptible to bacitracin. It should be used only where adequate laboratory facilities are available and when constant supervision of the patient is possible.

➤*Hydration:* Adequate fluid intake should be maintained orally, or if necessary, by parenteral method.

➤*Superinfection:* As with other antibiotics, use of this drug may result in overgrowth of nonsusceptible organisms, including fungi. If superinfection occurs, appropriate therapy should be instituted.

➤*Pregnancy:* *Category C* (per Briggs' *Drugs in Pregnancy and Lactation*). No reports linking the use of bacitracin with congenital defects have been located.

➤*Lactation:* No data are available on the use of bacitracin in breastfeeding women.

➤*Monitoring:* Renal function should be carefully determined prior to and daily during therapy. The recommended daily dose should not be exceeded, and fluid intake and urinary output should be maintained at proper levels to avoid kidney toxicity. If renal toxicity occurs, the drug should be discontinued.

Drug Interactions

Bacitracin Drug Interactions

Precipitant drug	Object drug[a]		Description
Aminoglycosides	Bacitracin	↑	Concurrent use may increase risk of respiratory paralysis and renal dysfunction.
Bacitracin	Nondepolarizing muscle relaxants	↑	Neuromuscular blockade may be enhanced.

[a] ↑ = object drug increased

➤*Other nephrotoxic drugs:* The concurrent use of other nephrotoxic drugs, particularly streptomycin, kanamycin, polymyxin B, polymyxin E (colistin), and neomycin should be avoided.

Adverse Reactions

➤*Dermatologic:* Skin rashes.

➤*GI:* Nausea and vomiting.

➤*Local:* Pain at site of injection.

➤*Renal:* Albuminuria, cylindruria, azotemia. Rising blood levels without any increase in dosage.

RIFAXIMIN

RIFAXIMIN

Rx	**Xifaxan** (Salix)	**Tablets; oral:** 200 mg	Disodium edetate. (Sx). Pink, round. Film-coated. In 30s, 100s, and UD 100s.
		550 mg	Disodium edetate. (rfx). Pink, oval. Film-coated. In 60s and UD 60s.

RIFAXIMIN — ORAL

Indications

➤*Hepatic encephalopathy (550 mg):* For reduction in risk of overt hepatic encephalopathy recurrence in patients 18 years of age and older.

Rifaximin has not been studied in patients with Model for End-Stage Liver Disease (MELD) scores greater than 25, and only 8.6% of patients in the controlled trial had MELD scores over 19. There is increased systemic exposure in patients with more severe hepatic dysfunction.

➤*Traveler's diarrhea (200 mg):* For the treatment of patients 12 years of age and older with traveler's diarrhea caused by noninvasive strains of *Escherichia coli*.

Do not use rifaximin tablets in patients with diarrhea complicated by fever or blood in the stool or diarrhea due to pathogens other than *E. coli*.

➤*Off-label uses:*

Irritable bowel syndrome – [2] = Fair documentation. Initial data from 2 controlled trials indicate that rifaximin may have a beneficial role in the management of irritable bowel syndrome (IBS) or symptoms of IBS in some patients. One trial was limited by the inclusion of patients with and without IBS. Larger trials with longer follow-up periods are needed that assess specific symptoms, including constipation.

Recurrent Clostridium difficile–associated diarrhea – [4] = Insufficient documentation. Initial data suggest that rifaximin may be an effective treatment option for recurrent *C. difficile*–associated diarrhea episodes that are unresponsive to first-line therapies. Long-term controlled trials are needed to further determine the efficacy and safety of this therapy.

Administration and Dosage

➤*Adults:*

Hepatic encephalopathy – 550 mg 2 times a day.

Traveler's diarrhea – 200 mg 3 times a day for 3 days.

Off-label dosing –

Irritable bowel syndrome: [2] = Fair documentation. 400 mg 2 or 3 times daily for 10 days.

RIFAXIMIN — ORAL

Recurrent C. difficile–associated diarrhea: [4] = Insufficient documentation. Ranges from 400 mg 3 times daily to 200 mg twice daily; most regimens were tapered.

➤*Children:*

Traveler's diarrhea –

12 years of age and older: 200 mg 3 times a day for 3 days.

➤*Administration:* Rifaximin tablets can be administered orally, with or without food.

➤*Storage/Stability:* Store at 20° to 25°C (68° to 77°F); excursions are permitted to 15° to 30°C (59° to 86°F).

Actions

➤*Pharmacology:* Rifaximin is a nonaminoglycoside semisynthetic antibacterial derived from rifamycin SV. Rifaximin acts by binding to the beta-subunit of bacterial DNA-dependent RNA polymerase, resulting in inhibition of bacterial RNA synthesis.

For hepatic encephalopathy, rifaximin is thought to have an effect on the GI flora.

➤*Pharmacokinetics:*

Absorption –

Hepatic encephalopathy: After a single dose and multiple doses of rifaximin 550 mg in healthy subjects, the mean time to reach peak plasma concentrations (T_{max}) was approximately 1 hour. The pharmacokinetic parameters were highly variable, and the accumulation ratio based on area under the curve (AUC) was 1.37.

The pharmacokinetics of rifaximin in patients with a history of hepatic encephalopathy were evaluated after administration of rifaximin 550 mg 2 times a day. The pharmacokinetic parameters were associated with a high variability, and mean rifaximin exposure (AUC_{tau}) in patients with a history of hepatic encephalopathy (147 ng•h/mL) was approximately 12-fold higher than that observed in healthy subjects following the same dosing regimen (12.3 ng•h/mL). When pharmacokinetic parameters were analyzed based on Child-Pugh class A, B, and C, the mean AUC_{tau} was 10-, 13-, and 20-fold higher, respectively, compared with healthy subjects.

Rifaximin Pharmacokinetic Parameters in Patients With a History of Hepatic Encephalopathy by Child-Pugh Class[a,b]

Parameter	Healthy subjects (n = 14)	Child-Pugh class A (n = 18)	B (n = 7)	C (n = 4)
AUC_{tau} (ng•h/mL)	12.3 ± 4.8	118 ± 67.8	161 ± 101	246 ± 120
C_{max}[c] (ng/mL)	3.4 ± 1.6	19.5 ± 11.4	25.1 ± 12.6	35.5 ± 12.5
T_{max}[d] (h)	0.8 (0.5 to 4)	1 (0.9 to 10)	1 (0.97 to 1)	1 (0 to 2)

[a] SD = standard deviation.
[b] Cross-study comparison with pharmacokinetic parameters in healthy subjects.
[c] C_{max} = maximum drug concentration.
[d] Median (range).

Traveler's diarrhea: Systemic absorption of rifaximin (200 mg 3 times daily) was evaluated in 13 subjects with shigellosis on days 1 and 3 of a 3-day course of treatment. Rifaximin plasma concentrations and exposures were low and variable. There was no evidence of accumulation of rifaximin following repeated administration for 3 days (9 doses). Rifaximin C_{max} after 3 and 9 consecutive doses ranged from 0.81 to 3.4 ng/mL on day 1 and 0.68 to 2.26 ng/mL on day 3. Similarly, the $AUC_{0\text{-last}}$ estimates were 6.95 ± 5.15 ng•h/mL on day 1 and 7.83 ± 4.94 ng•h/mL on day 3. Rifaximin is not suitable for treating systemic bacterial infections because of limited systemic exposure after oral administration.

Effect of food: A high-fat meal consumed 30 minutes prior to rifaximin dosing in healthy subjects delayed the mean T_{max} from 0.75 to 1.5 hours and increased the systemic exposure (AUC) of rifaximin by 2-fold.

Rifaximin 550 mg Single-Dose Pharmacokinetic Parameters Under Fasting and Fed Conditions (N = 12)

Parameter	Fasting	Fed
C_{max} (ng/mL)	4.1 ± 1.5	4.8 ± 4.3
T_{max}[a] (h)	0.8 (0.5 to 2.1)	1.5 (0.5 to 4.1)
Half-life (h)	1.8 ± 1.4	4.8 ± 1.3
AUC (ng•h/mL)	11.1 ± 4.2	22.5 ± 12

[a] Median (range).

Rifaximin can be administered with or without food.

Distribution – Rifaximin is moderately bound to human plasma proteins. In vivo, the mean protein-binding ratio was 67.5% in healthy subjects and 62% in patients with hepatic impairment when rifaximin 550 mg was administered.

Metabolism/Excretion – In a mass balance study, after administration of 400 mg ^{14}C-rifaximin orally to healthy volunteers, of the 96.94% total recovery, 96.62% of the administered radioactivity was recovered in feces almost exclusively as the unchanged drug and 0.32% was recovered in urine mostly as metabolites with 0.03% as the unchanged drug. Rifaximin accounted for 18% of radioactivity in plasma. This suggests that the absorbed rifaximin undergoes metabolism with minimal renal excretion of the unchanged drug. The enzymes responsible for metabolizing rifaximin are unknown.

In a separate study, rifaximin was detected in the bile after cholecystectomy in patients with intact GI mucosa, suggesting biliary excretion of rifaximin.

➤*Microbiology:* Rifaximin has been shown to be active against the following pathogen in clinical studies of infectious diarrhea: *E. coli* (enterotoxigenic and enteroaggregative strains).

Resistance – *E. coli* has been shown to develop resistance to rifaximin in vitro. However, the clinical significance of such an effect has not been studied.

Contraindications

Hypersensitivity to rifaximin, any of the rifamycin antimicrobial agents, or any of the components of rifaximin.

Warnings/Precautions

➤*Traveler's diarrhea not caused by E. coli:* Rifaximin tablets were not found to be effective in patients with diarrhea complicated by fever and/or blood in the stool or diarrhea due to pathogens other than *E. coli*. Rifaximin tablets are not effective in cases of traveler's diarrhea due to *Campylobacter jejuni*. The effectiveness of rifaximin tablets in traveler's diarrhea caused by *Shigella* spp. and *Salmonella* spp. has not been proven. Rifaximin tablets should not be used in patients where *C. jejuni*, *Shigella* spp., or *Salmonella* spp. may be suspected as causative pathogens.

Discontinue rifaximin tablets if diarrhea symptoms get worse or persist more than 24 to 48 hours, and consider alternative antibiotic therapy.

➤*Clostridium difficile–associated diarrhea:* *C. difficile*–associated diarrhea has been reported with use of nearly all antibacterial agents, including rifaximin, and may range in severity from mild diarrhea to fatal colitis. Treatment with antibacterial agents alters the normal flora of the colon, which may lead to overgrowth of *C. difficile*.

C. difficile produces toxins A and B, which contribute to the development of *Clostridium difficile*–associated diarrhea. Hypertoxin-producing strains of *C. difficile* cause increased morbidity and mortality, as these infections can be refractory to antimicrobial therapy and may require colectomy. *Clostridium difficile*–associated diarrhea must be considered in all patients who present with diarrhea following antibiotic use. Careful medical history is necessary because *Clostridium difficile*–associated diarrhea has been reported to occur more than 2 months after the administration of antibacterial agents.

If *Clostridium difficile*–associated diarrhea is suspected or confirmed, ongoing antibiotic use not directed against *C. difficile* may need to be discontinued. Institute appropriate fluid and electrolyte management, protein supplementation, antibiotic treatment of *C. difficile*, and surgical evaluation as clinically indicated.

➤*Resistance:* Prescribing rifaximin for traveler's diarrhea in the absence of a proven or strongly suspected bacterial infection or a prophylactic indication is unlikely to provide benefit to the patient and increases the risk of development of drug-resistant bacteria.

➤*Hypersensitivity reactions:* Hypersensitivity reactions have included exfoliative dermatitis, angioneurotic edema, and anaphylaxis.

➤*Hepatic function impairment:* Following administration of rifaximin 550 mg twice daily to patients with a history of hepatic encephalopathy, the systemic exposure (ie, AUC_{tau}) of rifaximin was about 10-, 13-, and 20-fold higher in those patients with mild (Child-Pugh class A), moderate (Child-Pugh class B), and severe (Child-Pugh class C) hepatic impairment, respectively, compared with that in healthy volunteers. Animal toxicity studies did not achieve systemic exposures that were seen in patients with severe hepatic impairment. The clinical trials were limited to patients with MELD scores less than 25. No dosage adjustment is recommended because rifaximin is presumably acting locally. Nonetheless, exercise caution when rifaximin is administered to patients with severe hepatic impairment.

➤*Pregnancy: Category C.* There are no adequate and well-controlled studies in pregnant women. Use during pregnancy only if the potential benefit outweighs the potential risk to the fetus.

In humans, the very small amounts absorbed systemically suggest that the embryo/fetal risk is low, if it exists at all. Although inadvertent exposure early in gestation appears to represent a low risk, the safest course, because of the animal data, is to avoid in the first trimester.

Rifaximin was teratogenic in rats at doses of 150 to 300 mg/kg (approximately 2.5 to 5 times the clinical dose for traveler's diarrhea [600 mg/day] and approximately 1.3 to 2.6 times the clinical dose for hepatic encephalopathy [1,100 mg/day], adjusted for body surface area). Rifaximin was teratogenic in rabbits at doses of 62.5 to 1,000 mg/kg (approximately 2 to 33 times the clinical dose for traveler's diarrhea [600 mg/day] and approximately 1.1 to 18 times the clinical dose for hepatic encephalopathy [1,100 mg/day], adjusted for body surface area). These effects include cleft palate, agnathia, jaw shortening, hemorrhage, eye partially open, small eyes, brachygnathia, incomplete ossification, and increased thoracolumbar vertebrae.

➤*Lactation:* It is not known whether rifaximin is excreted in human milk. The molecular weight (approximately 786) is low enough for excretion into breast milk, but only small amounts are absorbed into the systemic circulation. The effects of this exposure on a breast-feeding infant are unknown but appear to be negligible. Because many drugs are excreted in human milk and because of the potential for adverse reactions in breast-feeding infants from rifaximin, a decision should be made whether to discontinue breast-feeding or the drug, taking into account the importance of the drug to the mother.

➤*Children:* The safety and efficacy of rifaximin 200 mg in children with traveler's diarrhea younger than 12 years of age have not been established.

The safety and effectiveness of rifaximin 550 mg for hepatic encephalopathy have not been established in patients younger than 18 years of age.

RIFAXIMIN — ORAL

Drug Interactions

➤*Cytochrome 450 system:* In vitro studies have shown that rifaximin at concentrations ranging from 2 to 200 ng/mL does not inhibit CYP1A2, 2A6, 2B6, 2C9, 2C19, 2D6, 2E1, and CYP3A4. In an in vitro study, rifaximin was shown to induce CYP3A4 at the concentration of 0.2 mcM. However, in patients with healthy liver function, rifaximin at the recommended dosing regimen is not expected to induce CYP3A4. It is not known if rifaximin can affect the pharmacokinetics of concurrent CYP3A4 substrates in patients with decreased hepatic function who have elevated rifaximin concentrations.

➤*P-glycoprotein:* An in vivo study suggests that rifaximin is a substrate of P-glycoprotein (P-gp). In vitro, in the presence of the P-gp inhibitor verapamil, the efflux ratio of rifaximin was reduced more than 50%. The effect of P-gp inhibition on rifaximin was not evaluated in vivo. Therefore, it is not known if coadministration of drugs that inhibit P-gp can increase systemic exposure of rifaximin.

Adverse Reactions

➤*Hepatic encephalopathy:*

Adverse reactions (5% or more) – All adverse reactions that occurred at an incidence of 5% or more and at a higher incidence in rifaximin 550 mg–treated subjects than in the placebo group in the 6-month trial are provided in the following table. (These include adverse reactions that may be attributable to the underlying disease.)

Rifaximin Adverse Reactions in Patients With Hepatic Encephalopathy (≥ 5%)

Adverse reactions	Rifaximin 550 mg twice daily (n = 140)	Placebo (n = 159)
CNS		
Depression	7%	5%
Dizziness	13%	8%
Fatigue	12%	11%
Insomnia	7%	7%
Dermatologic		
Pruritus	9%	6%
Rash	5%	4%
GI		
Abdominal distension	8%	8%
Abdominal pain	9%	8%
Abdominal pain upper	6%	5%
Constipation	6%	6%
Nausea	14%	13%
Musculoskeletal		
Arthralgia	6%	5%
Back pain	6%	6%
Muscle spasms	9%	7%
Respiratory		
Cough	7%	7%
Dyspnea	6%	4%
Nasopharyngitis	7%	6%
Miscellaneous		
Anemia	8%	4%
Ascites	11%	9%
Edema peripheral	15%	8%
Pyrexia	6%	3%

Other adverse reactions –

CNS: Amnesia, confusional state, disturbance in attention, hypoesthesia, memory impairment, tremor.

GI: Abdominal pain lower, abdominal tenderness, anorexia, dry mouth, esophageal variceal bleed, stomach discomfort.

Metabolic/Nutritional: Dehydration, hyperglycemia, hyperkalemia, hypoglycemia, hyponatremia, weight increased.

Musculoskeletal: Myalgia, pain in extremity.

Respiratory: Epistaxis, pneumonia, rhinitis, upper respiratory tract infection not otherwise specified (NOS).

Miscellaneous: Cellulitis, chest pain, contusion, fall, generalized edema, hypotension, influenza-like illness, pain NOS, procedural pain, vertigo.

➤*Traveler's diarrhea:*

Discontinuation of therapy – Discontinuations due to adverse reactions occurred in 0.4% of patients. The adverse reactions leading to discontinuation were anorexia, dysentery, nasal passage irrigation, nausea, taste loss, and weight decrease.

Adverse reactions (2% or more) –

Rifaximin Adverse Reactions in Patients With Traveler's Diarrhea (≥ 2%)

	Number (%) of patients	
Adverse reactions	Rifaximin 600 mg/day (n = 320)	Placebo (n = 228)
GI		
Abdominal pain NOS	7%	10%
Constipation	4%	4%
Defecation urgency	6%	9%
Flatulence	11%	20%
Nausea	5%	8%
Rectal tenesmus	7%	9%
Vomiting NOS	2%	2%
Miscellaneous		
Headache	10%	9%
Pyrexia	3%	4%

Other adverse reactions –

Cardiovascular: Hot flashes NOS.

CNS: Abnormal dreams, dizziness, fatigue, insomnia, malaise, migraine NOS, syncope, weakness.

Dermatologic: Clamminess, increased sweating, rash NOS, sunburn.

GI: Abdominal distension, anorexia, blood in stool, diarrhea NOS, dry lips, dry throat, dysentery NOS, fecal abnormality NOS, gingival disorder NOS, inguinal hernia NOS, loss of taste, stomach discomfort.

GU: Blood in urine, choluria, dysuria, hematuria, polyuria, proteinuria, urinary frequency.

Hematologic/Lymphatic: Lymphocytosis, monocytosis, neutropenia.

Hepatic: Increased AST.

Metabolic/Nutritional: Decreased weight, dehydration.

Musculoskeletal: Arthralgia, muscle spasms, myalgia, neck pain.

Respiratory: Dyspnea NOS, nasal passage irritation, nasopharyngitis, pharyngitis, pharyngolaryngeal pain, respiratory tract infection NOS, rhinitis NOS, rhinorrhea, upper respiratory tract infection NOS.

Special senses: Ear pain, motion sickness, tinnitus.

Miscellaneous: Chest pain, pain NOS.

➤*Postmarketing:*

Hypersensitivity – Hypersensitivity reactions, including anaphylaxis, angioneurotic edema (swelling of face and tongue and difficulty swallowing), exfoliative dermatitis, flushing, rash, pruritus, and urticaria, have been reported. These events occurred as early as within 15 minutes of drug administration.

Miscellaneous – Cases of *C. difficile*–associated colitis have been reported.

Overdosage

➤*Symptoms:* No specific information is available on the treatment of overdosage with rifaximin. In clinical studies at doses higher than the recommended dosage (greater than 600 mg/day for traveler's diarrhea or more than 1,100 mg/day for hepatic encephalopathy), adverse reactions were similar to the recommended dosage (200 mg taken 3 times a day) and placebo.

➤*Treatment:* In the case of overdosage, discontinue rifaximin, treat symptomatically, and institute supportive measures as required.

Patient Information

Advise patients to contact their health care provider if diarrhea persists more than 24 to 48 hours or worsens. Advise the patient to seek medical care for fever and/or blood in the stool.

Advise patients to contact a health care provider as soon as possible if diarrhea occurs after therapy or does not improve or worsens during therapy.

Inform patients that rifaximin may be taken with our without food.

Counsel patients that antibacterial drugs, including rifaximin, should only be used to treat bacterial infections. They do not treat viral infections (eg, the common cold). When rifaximin is prescribed to treat a bacterial infection, inform patients that although it is common to feel better early in the course of therapy, the medication should be taken exactly as directed. Skipping doses or not completing the full course of therapy may decrease the effectiveness of the immediate treatment and increase the likelihood that bacteria will develop resistance and will not be treatable by rifaximin or other antibacterial drugs in the future.

METRONIDAZOLE

Rx	**Metronidazole** (Various, eg, Mutual, Teva, UDL)	**Tablets; oral:** 250 mg	In 25s, 100s, 250s, and 500s.
Rx	**Flagyl** (Pfizer)		(SEARLE 1831 FLAGYL 250). Blue. Film-coated. In 50s, 100s, and 2500s.
Rx	**Metronidazole** (Various, eg, Mutual, Teva, UDL)	**Tablets; oral:** 500 mg	In 25s, 50s, 100s, and 500s.
Rx	**Flagyl** (Pfizer)		(FLAGYL 500). Blue, oblong. Film-coated. In 50s, 100s, and 500s.
Rx	**Flagyl ER** (Pfizer)	**Tablets, extended-release; oral:** 750 mg	Lactose. (SEARLE 1961 FLAGYL ER). Blue, oval. Film-coated. In 30s.w
Rx	**Metronidazole** (Pliva)	**Capsules; oral:** 375 mg	(A 353). Yellow and grey. In 30s, 50s, 100s, 500s, and 1000s.
Rx	**Flagyl 375** (Pfizer)		(375 mg Flagyl). Iron gray/lt. green. In 50s and UD 100s.
Rx	**Metronidazole** (B. Braun)	**Injection, solution:** 5 mg/mL	In 100 mL vials.
Rx	**Metronidazole in Sodium Chloride** (Claris Lifesciences)		Sodium chloride 7.9 mg/mL. In 100 mL single-dose containers.

METRONIDAZOLE — ORAL

WARNING

Metronidazole has been shown to be carcinogenic in mice and rats. Unnecessary use of the drug should be avoided. Its use should be reserved for the conditions for which this drug is indicated.

Indications

➤*Tablets and capsules:*

Symptomatic trichomoniasis – For the treatment of symptomatic trichomoniasis in females and males when the presence of the trichomonad has been confirmed by appropriate laboratory procedures (wet smears or cultures).

Asymptomatic trichomoniasis – In the treatment of asymptomatic females when the organism is associated with endocervicitis, cervicitis, or cervical erosion. Since there is evidence that presence of the trichomonad can interfere with accurate assessment of abnormal cytological smears, additional smears should be performed after eradication of the parasite.

Treatment of asymptomatic consorts – *T. vaginalis* infection is a venereal disease. Therefore, asymptomatic sexual partners of treated patients should be treated simultaneously if the organism has been found to be present, in order to prevent reinfection of the partner. The decision as to whether to treat an asymptomatic male partner who has a negative culture or one for whom no culture has been attempted is an individual one. In making this decision, it should be noted that there is evidence that a woman may become reinfected if her partner is not treated. Also, since there can be considerable difficulty in isolating the organism from the asymptomatic male carrier, negative smears and cultures cannot be relied upon in this regard. In any event, the partner should be treated with metronidazole in cases of reinfection.

Amebiasis – In the treatment of acute intestinal amebiasis (amebic dysentery) and amebic liver abscess.

In amebic liver abscess, metronidazole therapy does not obviate the need for aspiration or drainage of pus.

Anaerobic bacterial infections – In the treatment of serious infections caused by susceptible anaerobic bacteria. Indicated surgical procedures should be performed in conjunction with metronidazole therapy. In a mixed aerobic and anaerobic infection, antimicrobials appropriate for the treatment of the aerobic infection should be used in addition to metronidazole.

Intra-abdominal infections – Peritonitis, intra-abdominal abscess, and liver abscess, caused by *Bacteroides* species including the *B. fragilis* group (*B. fragilis, B. distasonis, B. ovatus, B. thetaiotaomicron, B. vulgatus*), *Clostridium* species, *Eubacterium* species, *Peptococcus niger*, and *Peptostreptococcus* species.

Skin and skin structure infections – Caused by *Bacteroides* species including the *B. fragilis* group, *Clostridium* species, *Peptococcus niger*, *Peptostreptococcus* species, and *Fusobacterium* species.

Gynecologic infections – Including endometritis, endomyometritis, tubo-ovarian abscess, and postsurgical vaginal cuff infection, caused by *Bacteroides* species including the *B. fragilis* group, *Clostridium* species, *Peptococcus niger*, and *Peptostreptococcus* species.

Bacterial septicemia – Caused by *Bacteroides* species including the *B. fragilis* group, and *Clostridium* species.

Bone and joint infections – As adjunctive therapy, caused by *Bacteroides* species including the *B. fragilis* group.

CNS infections – Including meningitis and brain abscess, caused by *Bacteroides* species including the *B. fragilis* group.

Lower respiratory tract infections – Including pneumonia, empyema, and lung abscess, caused by *Bacteroides* species including the *B. fragilis* group.

Endocarditis – Caused by *Bacteroides* species including the *B. fragilis* group.

➤*Extended-release tablets:*

Bacterial vaginosis – In the treatment of women with bacterial vaginosis.

➤*Off-label uses:*

Pelvic inflammatory disease – [1] = Good documentation. The Centers for Disease Control and Prevention (CDC) guidelines advise use of metronidazole in treating pelvic inflammatory disease (PID) as part of a recommended regimen that includes a third-generation cephalosporin and doxycycline. If a parenteral cephalosporin is not feasible, the use of a fluoroquinolone with or without metronidazole may be considered.

Sinusitis – Evidence-based guidelines published by the American Academy of Allergy, Asthma and Immunology and the American College of Allergy, Asthma and Immunology suggest that metronidazole may be used in patients with sinusitis who fail initial therapy and when anaerobic bacteria is suspected as a cause.

Sinusitis (adults): [3] = Safety concerns.

Sinusitis (children/adolescents): [3] = Safety concerns.

Other possible off-label uses –

Bacterial vaginosis: Per CDC recommendations, metronidazole 500 mg twice/day for 7 days or 2 g orally in a single dose. *Flagyl ER* is approved for this use.

Crohn's disease: Metronidazole (250 mg 4 times/day) plus ciprofloxacin (500 mg twice/day) has been useful for patients with active acute-phase Crohn's disease.

Diarrhea associated with Clostridium difficile: Metronidazole (500 mg 3 times/day or 250 mg 4 times/day) has similar rates of efficacy compared with vancomycin.

Gardnerella vaginalis and giardiasis: The CDC has recommended the use of oral metronidazole for *Gardnerella vaginalis* (500 mg twice daily for 7 days) and for giardiasis (250 mg 3 times daily for 7 days).

Helicobacter pylori: Metronidazole is useful in eradicating *H. pylori* but should be used in combination therapy.

Hepatic encephalopathy: Metronidazole (800 mg/day) for 1 week has comparable efficacy to neomycin.

Prophylaxis after sexual assault: CDC guidelines recommend metronidazole 2 g orally in a single dose plus ceftriaxone and either azithromycin or doxycycline.

Recurrent and persistent urethritis: The CDC recommends metronidazole 2 g orally in a single dose plus erythromycin for 7 days.

Administration and Dosage

➤*General dosing considerations:* Pregnant patients should not be treated during the first trimester.

Alcoholic beverages should be avoided while taking metronidazole. (See Patient Information.)

➤*Adults:*

Amebiasis –

Acute intestinal amebiasis (acute amebic dysentery): 750 mg 3 times daily for 5 to 10 days.

Amebic liver abscess: 500 or 750 mg 3 times daily for 5 to 10 days.

Anaerobic bacteria – In the treatment of most serious anaerobic infections, metronidazole IV is usually administered initially.

Usual dosage: 7.5 mg/kg every 6 hours.

Maximum dose: 4 g daily.

Duration of therapy: 7 to 10 days; however, infections of the bone and joint, lower respiratory tract, and endocardium may require longer treatment.

Bacterial vaginosis –

Extended-release tablet: 750 mg once daily for 7 days.

Trichomoniasis –

Capsules: 375 mg twice daily for 7 days.

Tablets:

- *1-day treatment* – 2 g single dose or 1 g twice daily in the same day.
- *7-day treatment* – 250 mg 3 times daily for 7 days.

Re-treatment: When repeat courses of the drug are required, it is recommended that an interval of 4 to 6 weeks elapse between courses and that the presence of the trichomonad be reconfirmed by appropriate laboratory measures. Total and differential leukocyte counts should be made before and after re-treatment.

METRONIDAZOLE — ORAL

Off-label dosing –

Pelvic inflammatory disease: [1] = Good documentation. 500 mg orally twice daily for 14 days. Metronidazole can be given as adjunctive therapy with regimens consisting of a third-generation parenteral cephalosporin and doxycycline. If a parenteral cephalosporin is not feasible, the use of a fluoroquinolone with or without metronidazole may be considered.

Sinusitis (adults): [3] = Safety concerns. 7.5 mg/kg orally 4 times daily for 7 to 10 days. The maximum dose should not exceed 4 g in a 24-hour period.

➤*Children:*

Amebiasis – 35 to 50 mg/kg daily divided into 3 doses for 10 days.

Off-label dosing –

Infections:

Metronidazole Oral Off-Label Dosing in Children

Indication	Dosage
Anaerobic infection	
30 days and older	7.5 mg/kg every 6 hours. Maximum dose: 4 g daily.
7 to 29 days old and greater than 2 kg	15 mg/kg every 12 hours
7 to 29 days old and 1.2 to 2 kg	7.5 mg/kg every 12 hours
7 to 29 days old and less than 1.2 kg	7.5 mg/kg every 24 hours
Younger than 7 days old and greater than 2 kg	7.5 mg/kg every 12 hours
Younger than 7 days old and 1.2 to 2 kg	7.5 mg/kg every 24 hours
Younger than 7 days old and less than 1.2 kg	7.5 mg/kg/dose every 48 hours
Bacterial vaginosis (13 to 17 years of age)	500 mg twice daily for 7 days or 2 g single dose
Clostridium difficile	30 mg/kg daily divided every 6 hours for 10 days
Giardiasis	15 mg/kg daily divided 3 times daily for 5 days. Maximum dose: 750 mg daily
Helicobacter pylori	15 to 20 mg/kg daily divided twice daily for 4 weeks (use with amoxicillin and bismuth subsalicylate)
Other parasitic infections	15 to 30 mg/kg daily divided every 8 hours
Trichomoniasis	
13 years of age and older	**Capsules:** 375 mg twice daily for 7 days. **Tablets:** *1-day treatment:* 2 g single dose or 1 g twice daily in the same day. *7-day treatment:* 250 mg 3 times daily for 7 days. *Re-treatment:* When repeat courses of the drug are required, it is recommended that an interval of 4 to 6 weeks elapse between courses and that the presence of trichomonad be reconfirmed by appropriate laboratory measures. Total and differential leucocyte counts should be made before and after re-treatment.
Younger than 13 years of age	15 mg/kg daily divided 3 times daily for 7 days

Pelvic inflammatory disease: [1] = Good documentation.

• *Adolescents* – 500 mg orally twice daily for 14 days. Metronidazole can be given as adjunctive therapy with regimens consisting of a third-generation parenteral cephalosporin and doxycycline. If a parenteral cephalosporin is not feasible, the use of a fluoroquinolone with or without metronidazole may be considered.

Sinusitis (children/adolescents): [3] = Safety concerns. 7.5 mg/kg orally 3 times daily for 7 to 10 days. The maximum dose should not exceed 4 g in a 24-hour period.

➤*Hepatic function impairment:* Patients with severe hepatic disease metabolize metronidazole slowly, with resultant accumulation of metronidazole and its metabolites in the plasma. Cautiously administer doses below those usually recommended. Close monitoring of plasma metronidazole levels and toxicity is recommended.

➤*Pregnancy:* Pregnant patients should not be treated during the first trimester.

In pregnant patients in whom alternative treatment has been inadequate, the 1-day course of therapy should not be used, as it results in higher serum levels that can reach the fetal circulation.

➤*Administration:*

Extended-release tablet – Take under fasting conditions, at least 1 hour before or 2 hours after meals.

➤*Storage/Stability:*

Capsules – Store at 15° to 25°C (59° to 77°F).

Extended-release tablets – Store at 15° to 30°C (59° to 86°F) in a dry place. Protect from light.

Tablets – Store below 25°C (77°F) and protect from light.

Actions

➤*Pharmacology:* Metronidazole exerts an antimicrobial effect in an anaerobic environment by the following possible mechanism: Once metronidazole enters the organism, the drug is reduced by intracellular electron transport proteins. Because of this alteration to the metronidazole molecule, a concentration gradient is maintained, which promotes the drug's intracellular transport. Presumably, free radicals are formed, which in turn react with cellular components resulting in death of the microorganism.

➤*Pharmacokinetics:*

Absorption –

Tablets: Following oral administration, metronidazole is well absorbed with peak plasma concentrations occurring between 1 and 2 hours after administration. Plasma concentrations of metronidazole are proportional to the administered dose. Oral administration of 250, 500, or 2000 mg produced peak plasma concentrations of 6 mcg/mL, 12 mcg/mL, and 40 mcg/mL, respectively. Studies reveal no significant bioavailability differences between males and females; however, because of weight differences, the resulting plasma levels in males are generally lower.

Capsules: Metronidazole 375 mg capsules have been shown to have a rate and extent of absorption similar to metronidazole tablets and were bioequivalent at an equal single dose of 750 mg. In a study conducted with 23 adult, healthy, female volunteers, oral administration of two 375 mg metronidazole capsules under fasting conditions produced a mean (± 1 SD) peak plasma concentration (C_{max}) of 21.4 (± 2.8) mcg/mL with a mean t_{max} of 1.6 (± 0.7) hours and a mean area under the plasma concentration-time curve (AUC) of 223 (± 44) mcg•hr/mL. In the same study, three 250 mg metronidazole tablets produced a mean C_{max} of 20.4 (± 3.8) mcg/mL with a mean t_{max} of 1.4 (± 0.4) hours and a mean AUC of 218 (± 50) mcg•hr/mL.

Administration of metronidazole 375 mg capsules with food does not affect the extent of absorption of metronidazole; however, the presence of food results in a lower C_{max} and a delayed t_{max} compared to fasted conditions. In a study of 14 healthy, adult, female volunteers, administration of metronidazole 375 mg capsules under fasting conditions produced a mean C_{max} of 10.9 (± 1.5) mcg/mL, a mean t_{max} of 1.5 (± 1.4) hours, and a mean AUC of 110 (± 34) mcg•hr/mL compared to a mean C_{max} of 8.6 (± 1.6) mcg/mL, a mean t_{max} of 4.2 (± 1.7) hours, and a mean AUC of 99 (± 14) mcg•hr/mL under fed conditions.

Extended-release tablets: Relative to the fasting state, the rate of metronidazole absorption from the extended-release tablet is increased in the fed state resulting in alteration of the extended-release characteristics.

Distribution – Metronidazole appears in cerebrospinal fluid, saliva, and human milk in concentrations similar to those found in plasma. Bactericidal concentrations of metronidazole have also been detected in pus from hepatic abscesses.

Metabolism – Metronidazole is the major component appearing in the plasma, with lesser quantities of the 2-hydroxymethyl metabolite also being present. Less than 20% of the circulating metronidazole is bound to plasma proteins. Both the parent compound and the metabolite possess in vitro bactericidal activity against most strains of anaerobic bacteria and in vitro trichomonacidal activity.

Excretion – Disposition of metronidazole in the body is similar for both oral and IV dosage forms, with an average elimination half-life of 8 hours in healthy humans.

The major route of elimination of metronidazole and its metabolites is via the urine (60% to 80% of the dose), with fecal excretion accounting for 6% to 15% of the dose. The metabolites that appear in the urine result primarily from side-chain oxidation [1-(β-hydroxyethyl)-2-hydroxymethyl-5-nitroimidazole and 2-methyl-5-nitroimidazole-1-yl-acetic acid] and glucuronide conjugation, with unchanged metronidazole accounting for approximately 20% of the total. Renal clearance of metronidazole is approximately 10 mL/min/1.73 m^2.

Special populations –

Hepatic/Renal function impairment: Decreased renal function does not alter the single-dose pharmacokinetics of metronidazole. However, plasma clearance of metronidazole is decreased in patients with decreased liver function.

➤*Microbiology:*

Metronidazole has been shown to have in vitro and clinical activity against the following organisms –

Anaerobic gram-negative bacilli, including: Bacteroides species including the *Bacteroides fragilis* group (*B. fragilis, B. distasonis, B. ovatus, B. thetaiotaomicron, B. vulgatus*) and *Fusobacterium* species.

Anaerobic gram-positive bacilli: Clostridium species and susceptible strains of *Eubacterium*.

Anaerobic gram-positive cocci: Peptococcus niger and *Peptostreptococcus* species.

Protozoal parasites: Entamoeba histolytica and *Trichomonas vaginalis*.

Contraindications

A history of hypersensitivity to metronidazole or other nitroimidazole derivatives; during the first trimester of pregnancy.

METRONIDAZOLE — ORAL

Warnings/Precautions

➤*Neurologic effects:* Convulsive seizures and peripheral neuropathy, the latter characterized mainly by numbness or paresthesia of an extremity, have been reported in patients treated with metronidazole. The appearance of abnormal neurologic signs demands the prompt discontinuation of metronidazole therapy. Metronidazole should be administered with caution to patients with CNS diseases.

➤*Candidiasis:* Known or previously unrecognized candidiasis may present more prominent symptoms during therapy with metronidazole and requires treatment with a candidacidal agent.

➤*Hematologic effects:* Metronidazole is a nitroimidazole and should be used with caution in patients with evidence of or history of blood dyscrasia. A mild leukopenia has been observed during its administration; however, no persistent hematologic abnormalities attributable to metronidazole have been observed in clinical studies. Total and differential leukocyte counts are recommended before and after therapy for trichomoniasis and amebiasis, especially if a second course of therapy is necessary, and before and after therapy for anaerobic infections.

➤*Hepatic function impairment:* See Administration and Dosage for more information.

➤*Pregnancy: Category B.* Metronidazole crosses the placental barrier and enters the fetal circulation rapidly. Reproduction studies have been performed in rats at doses up to 5 times the human dose and have revealed no evidence of impaired fertility or harm to the fetus due to metronidazole. No fetotoxicity was observed when metronidazole was administered orally to pregnant mice at 20 mg/kg/day, approximately 1.5 times the most frequently recommended human dose (750 mg/day) based on mg/kg body weight. No fetotoxicity was observed when metronidazole was administered orally to pregnant mice at 60 mg/m^2/day, which is approximately 10% of the human dose when expressed as mg/m^2. However in a single small study where the drug was administered intraperitoneally, some intrauterine deaths were observed. The relationship of these findings to the drug is unknown. There are, however, no adequate and well-controlled studies in pregnant women. Because animal reproduction studies are not always predictive of human response, and because metronidazole is a carcinogen in rodents, this drug should be used during pregnancy only if clearly needed.

Use of metronidazole in the second and third trimesters of pregnancy or for trichomoniasis during pregnancy should be restricted to those in whom alternative treatment has been inadequate. Use of metronidazole in the first trimester or for trichomoniasis in pregnancy should be carefully evaluated because metronidazole crosses the placental barrier and its effects on the human fetal organogenesis are not known (see above).

➤*Lactation:* Because of the potential for tumorigenicity, shown for metronidazole in mouse and rat studies, a decision should be made whether to discontinue nursing or to discontinue the drug, taking into account the importance of the drug to the mother. Metronidazole is secreted in human milk in concentrations similar to those found in plasma.

➤*Children:* Safety and efficacy in children have not been established, except for the treatment of amebiasis (tablets and capsules only).

➤*Elderly:* No overall differences have been reported in safety and effectiveness between younger and older individuals, but greater sensitivity of some older individuals cannot be ruled out. Systemic exposure to the active metabolite, 2-hydroxymethyl metronidazole, is higher in the elderly. Metronidazole is known to be substantially excreted by the kidney, and the risk of toxic reactions to this drug may be greater in patients with impaired renal function. Although decreased renal function does not alter the single dose pharmacokinetics of metronidazole, because elderly patients are more likely to have decreased liver function, care should be taken in dose selection, and it may be useful to monitor renal function.

Plasma clearance of metronidazole is decreased in patients with decreased liver function. Therefore, in elderly patients, monitoring of serum levels may be necessary to adjust the metronidazole dosage accordingly.

➤*Monitoring:* Monitoring of serum levels in elderly patients may be necessary to adjust the metronidazole dosage accordingly.

Drug Interactions

Metronidazole Drug Interactions

Precipitant drug	Object drug[a]		Description
Barbiturates Phenytoin	Metronidazole	↓	Coadministration may accelerate the elimination of metronidazole, resulting in reduced plasma levels.
Cimetidine	Metronidazole	↑	Decreased metronidazole clearance and increased serum levels may occur; however, data conflict.
Metronidazole	Anticoagulants	↑	The anticoagulant effect of warfarin may be enhanced.
Metronidazole	Disulfiram	↑	Concurrent use may result in an acute psychosis or confusional state. Do not give metronidazole to patients who have taken disulfiram within the last 2 weeks.
Metronidazole	Ethanol	↑	A disulfiram-like reaction including symptoms of flushing, palpitations, tachycardia, nausea, vomiting, etc, may occur with concurrent use. Although the risk for most patients may be slight, caution is advised. Do not consume alcohol during therapy and for ≥ 1 to 3 days afterward.
Metronidazole	Hydantoins	↑	The total clearance of phenytoin may be decreased and its elimination half-life prolonged.
Metronidazole	Lithium	↑	In patients stabilized on relatively high lithium doses, short-term metronidazole has been associated with increased lithium levels and toxicity in some cases.

[a] ↑ = object drug increased; ↓ = object drug decreased.

➤*Drug/Lab test interactions:* Metronidazole may interfere with certain types of determinations of serum chemistry values, such AST, ALT, LDH, triglycerides, and hexokinase glucose. Values of zero may be observed. All of the assays in which interference has been reported involve enzymatic coupling of the assay to oxidation-reduction of nicotinamide adenine dinucleotide ($NAD^+ \rightleftarrows NADH$). Interference is due to the similarity in absorbance peaks of NADH (340 nm) and metronidazole (322 nm) at pH 7.

Adverse Reactions

➤*Extended-release tablets:* Most adverse events were described as being of mild or moderate severity. Among patients taking metronidazole extended-release who reported headaches, 10% considered them severe, and less than 2% of reported episodes of nausea were considered severe. Metallic taste was reported by 9% of patients taking metronidazole extended-release.

Adverse Reactions Irrespective of Treatment Causality (≥ 2%)

Adverse reaction	Metronidazole extended release tablets 7 days (n = 267)	Vaginal preparation (n = 285)
Headache	48 (18%)	44 (15%)
Vaginitis	39 (15%)	32 (12%)
Nausea	28 (10%)	8 (3%)
Taste perversion (metallic taste)	23 (9%)	1 (0%)
Infection bacterial	19 (7%)	17 (6%)
Influenza-like symptoms	17 (6%)	20 (7%)
Pruritus genital	14 (5%)	25 (9%)
Abdominal pain	10 (4%)	13 (5%)
Dizziness	11 (4%)	3 (1%)
Diarrhea	11 (4%)	3 (1%)
Upper respiratory tract infection	11 (4%)	10 (4%)
Rhinitis	12 (4%)	10 (4%)
Sinusitis	7 (3%)	6 (2%)
Urine abnormal	7 (3%)	4 (1%)
Pharyngitis	8 (3%)	4 (1%)
Dysmenorrhea	9 (3%)	7 (2%)
Moniliasis	9 (3%)	8 (3%)
Mouth dry	5 (2%)	2 (1%)
Urinary tract infection	6 (2%)	16 (6%)

➤*Adverse reactions reported during treatment with metronidazole:* The following reactions have also been reported during treatment with metronidazole:

Cardiovascular – Flattening of the T-wave may be seen in electrocardiographic tracings.

CNS – Two serious adverse reactions reported in patients treated with metronidazole have been convulsive seizures and peripheral neuropathy, the latter characterized mainly by numbness or paresthesia of an extremity. Since persistent peripheral neuropathy has been reported in some patients receiving prolonged administration of metronidazole, patients should be specifically warned about these reactions and should be told to stop the drug and report immediately to their physicians if any neurologic symptoms occur. In addition, patients have reported dizziness, vertigo, incoordination, ataxia, confusion, irritability, depression, weakness, and insomnia.

METRONIDAZOLE — ORAL

GI – The most common adverse reactions reported have been referable to the GI tract, particularly nausea reported by approximately 12% of patients, sometimes accompanied by headache, anorexia, and occasionally vomiting, diarrhea, epigastric distress, and abdominal cramping. Constipation has also been reported.

Hematologic – Reversible neutropenia (leukopenia); rarely, reversible thrombocytopenia.

Hypersensitivity – Urticaria, erythematous rash, flushing, nasal congestion, dryness of the mouth (or vagina or vulva), and fever.

Renal – Dysuria, cystitis, polyuria, incontinence, and a sense of pelvic pressure. Instances of darkened urine have been reported by approximately 1 patient in 100,000. Although the pigment, which is probably responsible for this phenomenon, has not been positively identified, it is almost certainly a metabolite of metronidazole and seems to have no clinical significance.

Special senses – A sharp, unpleasant metallic taste is not unusual. Furry tongue, glossitis, and stomatitis have occurred; these may be associated with a sudden overgrowth of *Candida*, which may occur during therapy.

Miscellaneous – Proliferation of *Candida* in the vagina, dyspareunia, decrease of libido, proctitis, and fleeting joint pains sometimes resembling "serum sickness." If patients receiving metronidazole drink alcoholic beverages, they may experience abdominal distress, nausea, vomiting, flushing, or headache. A modification of the taste of alcoholic beverages has also been reported. Rare cases of pancreatitis, which generally abated on withdrawal of the drug, have been reported.

Crohn disease – Crohn's disease patients are known to have an increased incidence of GI and certain extraintestinal cancers. There have been some reports in the medical literature of breast and colon cancer in Crohn's disease patients who have been treated with metronidazole at high doses for extended periods of time. A cause and effect relationship has not been established. Crohn's disease is not an approved indication for oral metronidazole.

Overdosage

➤*Symptoms:* Single oral doses of metronidazole up to 15 g have been reported in suicide attempts and accidental overdoses. Symptoms reported include nausea, vomiting, and ataxia.

Oral metronidazole has been studied as a radiation sensitizer in the treatment of malignant tumors. Neurotoxic effects, including seizures and peripheral neuropathy, have been reported after 5 to 7 days of doses of 6 to 10.4 g every other day.

➤*Treatment:* There is no specific antidote for metronidazole overdose; therefore, management of the patient should consist of symptomatic and supportive therapy.

Patient Information

Alcoholic beverages should be avoided while taking metronidazole and for at least 1 day (metronidazole tablets) or 3 days (metronidazole capsules and extended release tablets) after discontinuing.

METRONIDAZOLE — INJECTION

WARNING

Metronidazole has been shown to be carcinogenic in mice and rats. Its use, therefore, should be reserved for the conditions for which it is indicated.

Indications

➤*Anaerobic infections:* In the treatment of serious infections caused by susceptible anaerobic bacteria. Indicated surgical procedures should be performed in conjunction with metronidazole injection therapy. In a mixed aerobic and anaerobic infection, antibiotics appropriate for the treatment of the aerobic infection should be used in addition to metronidazole injection.

Effective in *Bacteroides fragilis* infections resistant to clindamycin, chloramphenicol, and penicillin.

Intra-abdominal infections – Intra-abdominal infections including peritonitis, intra-abdominal abscess, and liver abscess, caused by *Bacteroides* species including the *B. fragilis* group (*B. fragilis, B. distasonis, B. ovatus, B. thetaiotaomicron, B. vulgatus*), *Clostridium* species, *Eubacterium* species, *Peptococcus* species, and *Peptostreptococcus* species.

Skin and skin structure infections – Caused by *Bacteroides* species including the *B. fragilis* group, *Clostridium* species, *Peptococcus* species, *Peptostreptococcus* species, and *Fusobacterium* species.

Gynecologic infections – Including endometritis, endomyometritis, tubo-ovarian abscess, and postsurgical vaginal cuff infection, caused by *Bacteroides* species including the *B. fragilis* group, *Clostridium* species, *Peptococcus* species, and *Peptostreptococcus* species.

Bacterial septicemia – Caused by *Bacteroides* species including the *B. fragilis* group, and *Clostridium* species.

Bone and joint infections – As adjunctive therapy, caused by *Bacteroides* species including the *B. fragilis* group.

Central nervous system (CNS) infections – Including meningitis and brain abscess, caused by *Bacteroides* species including the *B. fragilis* group.

Lower respiratory tract infections – Including pneumonia, empyema, and lung abscess, caused by *Bacteroides* species including the *B. fragilis* group.

Endocarditis – Caused by *Bacteroides* species including the *B. fragilis* group.

➤*Prophylaxis:* The prophylactic administration of metronidazole injection preoperatively, intraoperatively, and postoperatively may reduce the incidence of postoperative infection in patients undergoing elective colorectal surgery which is classified as contaminated or potentially contaminated.

Prophylactic use of metronidazole injection should be discontinued within 12 hours after surgery. If there are signs of infection, specimens for cultures should be obtained for the identification of the causative organism(s) so that appropriate therapy may be given.

➤*Off-label uses:*

Pelvic inflammatory disease – As an alternative parenteral regimen, the CDC recommends metronidazole 500 mg IV every 8 hours combined with ofloxacin alone or ciprofloxacin plus doxycycline.

Administration and Dosage

➤*General dosing considerations:* Metronidazole injection is to be administered by slow intravenous (IV) drip infusion only (see Administration).

Alcoholic beverages should not be consumed during metronidazole therapy. (See Drug Interactions.)

➤*Adults:*

Anaerobic infections –

Maximum dose: 4 g daily.

Loading dose: 15 mg/kg IV over 1 hour.

Maintenance dosage: 7.5 mg/kg IV over 1 hour every 6 hours. The first maintenance dose should be instituted 6 hours following the initiation of the loading dose.

Duration of therapy: The usual duration of therapy is 7 to 10 days; however, infections of the bone and joint, lower respiratory tract, and endocardium may require longer treatment.

Conversion: IV therapy may be changed to oral when conditions warrant, based upon the severity of the disease and the response of the patient to metronidazole injection treatment. The usual adult oral dosage is 7.5 mg/kg every 6 hours.

Colorectal surgery prophylaxis – It is important that administration of the initial preoperative dose be completed approximately 1 hour before surgery so that adequate drug levels are present in the serum and tissues at the time of initial incision. Administer injection, if necessary, at 6-hour intervals to maintain effective drug levels.

Initial dosage: 15 mg/kg IV over 30 to 60 minutes and completed approximately 1 hour before surgery.

Maintenance dosage: 7.5 mg/kg IV over 30 to 60 minutes at 6 and 12 hours after the initial dose.

Duration of therapy: Limit to the day of surgery only.

➤*Children:*

Off-label dosing –

Infections:

Metronidazole Injection Off-Label Dosing in Children

Indication	Dosage
Anaerobic infection	
30 days and older	30 mg/kg daily IV over 1 hour divided every 6 hours. Maximum dose: 4 g daily
7 to 29 days old and greater than 2 kg	30 mg/kg daily IV over 1 hour divided every 12 hours
7 to 29 days old and 1.2 to 2 kg	15 mg/kg/day IV over 1 hour divided every 12 hours
7 to 29 days old and less than 1.2 kg	7.5 mg/kg/dose IV over 1 hour every 24 hours
Younger than 7 days old and greater than 2 kg	15 mg/kg daily IV over 1 hour divided every 12 hours
Younger than 7 days old and 1.2 to 2 kg	7.5 mg/kg/dose IV over 1 hour every 24 hours
Younger than 7 days old and less than 1.2 kg	7.5 mg/kg/dose IV over 1 hour every 48 hours
Clostridium difficile	30 mg/kg daily IV over 1 hour divided every 6 hours for 10 days. IV may be less efficacious than oral.
Surgical prophylaxis	Initial dosage: 15 mg/kg IV over 30 to 60 minutes 1 hour before surgery Maintenance dosage: 7.5 mg/kg IV at 6 and 12 hours after initial dose

➤*Renal function impairment:* For patients with a CrCl less than 10 mL/min, give 50% of the normal dose.

Adults receiving continuous renal replacement therapy (CRRT) – One reference suggests a dosage of 250 to 500 mg IV every 8 to 12 hours.

Alternatively, a dosage of 500 mg IV every 6 to 12 hours is recommended for patients receiving continuous venovenous hemofiltration (CVVH), continuous venovenous hemodialysis (CVVHD), or continuous venovenous hemodi-

METRONIDAZOLE — INJECTION

alfiltration (CVVHDF). This recommendation assumes ultrafiltration and dialysis flow rates of 1 to 2 L/hr.

Adults receiving intermittent hemodialysis (IHD): 500 mg IV every 8 to 12 hours. This recommendation assumes the patient is receiving standard IHD 3 times per week and completes the full dialysis sessions.

➤*Hepatic function impairment:* Patients with severe hepatic disease metabolize metronidazole slowly, with resultant accumulation of metronidazole and its metabolites in the plasma. Accordingly, for such patients, doses below those usually recommended should be administered with caution. Close monitoring of plasma metronidazole levels and toxicity is recommended.

➤*Nasogastric aspiration:* In patients receiving metronidazole injection in whom gastric secretions are continuously removed by nasogastric aspiration, sufficient metronidazole may be removed in the aspirate to cause a reduction in serum levels.

➤*Preparation for administration:*

Single-dose flexible containers – Ready-to-use isotonic solution. No dilution or buffering is required.

Single-dose lyophilized vials – Cannot be given by direct IV injection (IV bolus). Order of mixing is important.

Reconstitution: Add 4.4 mL of one of the compatible diluents and mix thoroughly. The resultant approximate withdrawal volume is 5 mL with an approximate concentration of 100 mg/mL.

The pH of the reconstituted product will be in the range of 0.5 to 2. Reconstituted metronidazole is clear, and pale yellow to yellow-green in color.

Dilution in IV solutions: Add reconstituted metronidazole to a glass or plastic IV container not to exceed a concentration of 8 mg/mL. Neutralization is required prior to administration.

Neutralization for IV infusion: Neutralize the IV solution containing metronidazole with approximately 5 mEq of sodium bicarbonate injection for each 500 mg of metronidazole used. Mix thoroughly. The pH of the neutralized IV solution will be approximately 6 to 7. Carbon dioxide gas will be generated with neutralization. It may be necessary to relieve gas pressure within the container.

When the contents of 1 vial (500 mg) are diluted and neutralized to 100 mL, the resultant concentration is 5 mg/mL. Do not exceed an 8 mg/mL concentration of metronidazole in the neutralized IV solution, since neutralization will decrease the aqueous solubility and precipitation may occur. Do not refrigerate neutralized solutions; otherwise, precipitation may occur.

➤*Administration:* Metronidazole injection is to be administered by slow IV drip infusion only either as a continuous or intermittent infusion. Avoid IV admixtures containing metronidazole and other drugs. Additives should not be introduced into this solution. If used with a primary IV fluid system, the primary solution should be discontinued during metronidazole infusion. Do not use equipment containing aluminum (eg, needles, cannulae) that would come in contact with the drug solution.

Single-dose flexible containers – Do not use in series connections. Such use could result in air embolism due to residual air being drawn from the primary container before administration of the fluid from the secondary container is complete.

Single-dose lyophilized vials – Metronidazole cannot be given by direct IV injection (IV bolus) because of the low pH (0.5 to 2) of the reconstituted product. Metronidazole must be further diluted and neutralized for IV infusion.

➤*Admixture compatibility:*

Reconstitution – Sterile water for injection, bacteriostatic water for injection, sodium chloride 0.9% injection, or bacteriostatic sodium chloride 0.9% injection.

Dilution in IV solutions – Sodium chloride 0.9% injection, dextrose 5% injection, or Ringer's lactate injection.

➤*Storage/Stability:*

Single-dose flexible containers – Store at 15° to 30°C (59° to 86°F) and protect from light during storage. Do not refrigerate.

Single-dose lyophilized vials – Reconstituted vials are chemically stable for 96 hours when stored below 30°C (86°F) in room light.

Use diluted and neutralized IV solutions containing metronidazole within 24 hours of mixing. Do not refrigerate neutralized solutions; otherwise, precipitation may occur.

Actions

➤*Pharmacology:* Metronidazole is a synthetic antibacterial compound. Disposition of metronidazole in the body is similar for both oral and IV dosage forms, with an average elimination half-life in healthy humans of 8 hours.

➤*Pharmacokinetics:*

Absorption/Distribution – Metronidazole appears in cerebrospinal fluid, saliva, and breast milk in concentrations similar to those found in plasma. Bactericidal concentrations of metronidazole have also been detected in pus from hepatic abscesses.

Plasma concentrations of metronidazole are proportional to the administered dose. An 8-hour IV infusion of 100 to 4000 mg of metronidazole in healthy subjects showed a linear relationship between dose and peak plasma concentration.

In patients treated with metronidazole, using a dosage regimen of 15 mg/kg loading dose followed 6 hours later by 7.5 mg/kg every 6 hours, peak steady-state plasma concentrations of metronidazole averaged 25 mcg/mL with trough (minimum) concentrations averaging 18 mcg/mL.

Metronidazole is the major component appearing in the plasma, with lesser quantities of the 2-hydroxymethyl metabolite also being present. Less than 20% of the circulating metronidazole is bound to plasma proteins. Both the parent compound and the metabolite possess in vitro bactericidal activity against most strains of anaerobic bacteria.

Metabolism/Excretion – The major route of elimination of metronidazole and its metabolites is via the urine (60% to 80% of the dose), with fecal excretion accounting for 6% to 15% of the dose. The metabolites that appear in the urine result primarily from side-chain oxidation [1-(β-hydroxyethyl)-2-hydroxymethyl-5-nitroimidazole and 2-methyl-5-nitroimidazole-1-yl-acetic acid] and glucuronide conjugation, with unchanged metronidazole accounting for approximately 20% of the total. Renal clearance of metronidazole is approximately 10 mL/min/1.73 m^2.

Special populations –

Hepatic function impairment: Decreased renal function does not alter the single-dose pharmacokinetics of metronidazole. However, plasma clearance of metronidazole is decreased in patients with decreased liver function.

Children: In 1 study, newborn infants appeared to demonstrate diminished capacity to eliminate metronidazole. The elimination half-life, measured during the first 3 days of life, was inversely related to gestational age. In infants whose gestational ages were between 28 and 40 weeks, the corresponding elimination half-lives ranged from 109 to 22.5 hours.

➤*Microbiology:* Metronidazole is active in vitro against most obligate anaerobes, but does not appear to possess any clinically relevant activity against facultative anaerobes or obligate aerobes. Against susceptible organisms, metronidazole is generally bactericidal at concentrations equal to or slightly higher than the minimal inhibitory concentrations. Metronidazole has been shown to have in vitro and clinical activity against the following organisms:

Anaerobic gram-negative bacilli, including *Bacteroides* species, including the *Bacteroides fragilis* group (*B. fragilis*, *B. distasonis*, *B. ovatus*, *B. thetaiotaomicron*, *B. vulgatus*) and *Fusobacterium* species.

Anaerobic gram-positive bacilli, including *Clostridium* species and susceptible strains of *Eubacterium*.

Anaerobic gram-positive cocci, including *Peptococcus* species and *Peptostreptococcus* species.

Contraindications

Hypersensitivity to metronidazole or other nitroimidazole derivatives.

Warnings/Precautions

➤*Neurologic effects:* Convulsive seizures and peripheral neuropathy, the latter characterized mainly by numbness or paresthesia of an extremity, have been reported in patients treated with metronidazole. The appearance of abnormal neurologic signs demands the prompt evaluation of the benefit/risk ratio of the continuation of therapy.

➤*Sodium content:* Administration of solutions containing sodium ions may result in sodium retention.

➤*Candidiasis:* Known or previously unrecognized candidiasis may present more prominent symptoms during therapy with metronidazole injection and requires treatment with a candidacidal agent.

➤*Hematologic effects:* Metronidazole is a nitroimidazole, and metronidazole injection should be used with care in patients with evidence of or history of blood dyscrasia. A mild leukopenia has been observed during its administration; however, no persistent hematologic abnormalities attributable to metronidazole have been observed in clinical studies. Total and differential leukocyte counts are recommended before and after therapy.

➤*Hepatic function impairment:* Patients with severe hepatic disease metabolize metronidazole slowly, with resultant accumulation of metronidazole and its metabolites in the plasma. Accordingly, for such patients, doses below those usually recommended should be administered cautiously.

➤*Special risk:* Care should be taken when administering metronidazole injection to patients receiving corticosteroids or to patients predisposed to edema.

➤*Pregnancy: Category B.* Metronidazole crosses the placental barrier and enters the fetal circulation rapidly. Reproduction studies have been performed in rats at doses up to 5 times the human dose and have revealed no evidence of impaired fertility or harm to the fetus due to metronidazole. Metronidazole administered intraperitoneally to pregnant mice at approximately the human dose caused fetotoxicity; administered orally to pregnant mice, no fetotoxicity was observed. There are, however, no adequate and well controlled studies in pregnant women. Because animal reproduction studies are not always predictive of human response, and because metronidazole is a carcinogen in rodents, these drugs should be used during pregnancy only if clearly needed.

➤*Lactation:* Because of the potential for tumorigenicity shown for metronidazole in mouse and rat studies, a decision should be made whether to discontinue nursing or to discontinue the drug, taking into account the importance of the drug to the mother. Metronidazole is secreted in breast milk in concentrations similar to those found in plasma.

➤*Children:* Safety and efficacy in children have not been established.

METRONIDAZOLE — INJECTION

Drug Interactions

Metronidazole Drug Interactions

Precipitant drug	Object drug[a]		Description
Barbiturates Phenytoin	Metronidazole	↓	Coadministration may accelerate the elimination of metronidazole, resulting in reduced plasma levels.
Cimetidine	Metronidazole	↑	Decreased metronidazole clearance and increased serum levels may occur; however, data conflict.
Metronidazole	Anticoagulants	↑	The anticoagulant effect of warfarin may be enhanced.
Metronidazole	Disulfiram	↑	Concurrent use may result in an acute psychosis or confusional state. Do not give metronidazole to patients who have taken disulfiram within the last 2 weeks.
Metronidazole	Ethanol	↑	A disulfiram-like reaction including symptoms of flushing, palpitations, tachycardia, nausea, vomiting, etc, may occur with concurrent use. Although the risk for most patients may be slight, caution is advised. Do not consume alcohol during therapy and for ≥ 1 to 3 days afterward.
Metronidazole	Hydantoins	↑	The total clearance of phenytoin may be decreased and its elimination half-life prolonged.
Metronidazole	Lithium	↑	In patients stabilized on relatively high lithium doses, short-term metronidazole has been associated with increased lithium levels and toxicity in some cases.

[a] ↑ = object drug increased; ↓ = object drug decreased.

➤*Drug/Lab test interactions:* Metronidazole may interfere with certain types of determinations of serum chemistry values, such as aspartate aminotransferase (AST), alanine aminotransferase (ALT), lactate dehydrogenase (LDH), triglycerides, and hexokinase glucose. Values of zero may be observed. All of the assays in which interference has been reported involve enzymatic coupling of the assay to oxidation-reduction of nicotine adenine dinucleotide ($NAD^+ \rightleftarrows NADH$). Interference is due to the similarity in absorbance peaks of NADH (340 nm) and metronidazole (322 nm) at pH 7.

Adverse Reactions

The 2 most serious adverse reactions reported in patients treated with metronidazole injection have been convulsive seizures and peripheral neuropathy, the latter characterized mainly by numbness or paresthesia of an extremity. Since persistent peripheral neuropathy has been reported in some patients receiving prolonged oral administration of metronidazole, patients should be observed carefully if neurologic symptoms occur and a prompt evaluation made of the benefit/risk ratio of the continuation of therapy.

The following reactions have also been reported during treatment with metronidazole injection:

➤*CNS:* Headache, dizziness, syncope, ataxia, and confusion.

➤*Dermatologic:* Erythematous rash and pruritus.

➤*GI:* Nausea, vomiting, abdominal discomfort, diarrhea, and an unpleasant metallic taste.

➤*Hematologic:* Reversible neutropenia (leukopenia).

➤*Local:* Thrombophlebitis after IV infusion. This reaction can be minimized or avoided by avoiding prolonged use of indwelling IV catheters.

➤*Miscellaneous:* Fever. Instances of a darkened urine have also been reported, and this manifestation has been the subject of a special investigation. Although the pigment which is probably responsible for this phenomenon has not been positively identified, it is almost certainly a metabolite of metronidazole and seems to have no clinical significance.

➤*Crohn disease:* Crohn's disease patients are known to have an increased incidence of GI and certain extraintestinal cancers. There have been some reports in the medical literature of breast and colon cancer in Crohn's disease patients who have been treated with metronidazole at high doses for extended periods of time. A cause-and-effect relationship has not been established. Crohn's disease is not an approved indication for metronidazole injection.

Overdosage

➤*Symptoms:* Use of dosages of metronidazole injection higher than those recommended has been reported. These include the use of 27 mg/kg 3 times a day for 20 days, and the use of 75 mg/kg as a single loading dose followed by 7.5 mg/kg maintenance doses. No adverse reactions were reported in either of the 2 cases. Single oral doses of metronidazole, up to 15 g, have been reported in suicide attempts and accidental overdoses. Symptoms reported include nausea, vomiting, and ataxia.

➤*Treatment:* There is no specific antidote for overdose; therefore, management of the patient should consist of symptomatic and supportive therapy.

SULFADIAZINE

Rx	**Sulfadiazine** (Sandoz)	**Tablets; oral:** 500 mg	(E 757). White, capsule shape. In 100s and 1,000s.

SULFADIAZINE — ORAL

For complete and comparative prescribing information, refer to the Sulfonamides group monograph.

Indications

➤*Chancroid:* For the treatment of chancroid.

➤*Conjunctivitis:* For the treatment of inclusion conjunctivitis.

➤*Malaria:* For the treatment of malaria caused by chloroquine-resistant strains of *Plasmodium falciparum* when used as adjunctive therapy.

➤*Meningitis:* For the prophylaxis of meningococcal meningitis when sulfonamide-sensitive group A strains are known to prevail in family groups or larger closed populations (the prophylactic usefulness of sulfonamides when group B or C infections are prevalent is not proved and may be harmful in closed population groups); for the treatment of meningococcal meningitis when the organism has been demonstrated to be susceptible; as an adjunct to therapy with parenteral streptomycin for the treatment of *Haemophilus influenzae* meningitis.

➤*Nocardiosis:* For the treatment of nocardiosis.

➤*Otitis media:* For the treatment of acute otitis media caused by *H. influenzae* when used concomitantly with adequate doses of penicillin.

➤*Rheumatic fever:* For prophylaxis against recurrences of rheumatic fever, as an alternative to penicillin.

➤*Toxoplasmosis encephalitis:* For the treatment of toxoplasmosis encephalitis in patients with and without AIDS, as adjunctive therapy with pyrimethamine.

➤*Trachoma:* For the treatment of trachoma.

➤*Urinary tract infections (UTIs):* For the treatment of UTIs (primarily pyelonephritis, pyelitis, and cystitis) in the absence of obstructive uropathy or foreign bodies, when these infections are caused by susceptible strains of the following organisms: *Escherichia coli*, *Klebsiella* species, *Enterobacter* species, *Staphylococcus aureus*, *Proteus mirabilis*, and *Proteus vulgaris*. Use sulfadiazine for urinary tract infections only after the use of more soluble sulfonamides has been unsuccessful.

Administration and Dosage

➤*General dosing considerations:* Adequate fluid intake must be maintained in order to prevent crystalluria and stone formation. (See Administration).

➤*Adults:*

Infections – For a list of infections, refer to Indications.

Initial dosage: 2 to 4 g.

Maintenance dosage: 2 to 4 g, divided into 3 to 6 doses, every 24 hours.

➤*Children:*

Infections – For a list of infections, refer to Indications.

2 months of age and older:

- *Maximum dose* – 6 g every 24 hours.
- *Initial dosage* – One half the 24-hour dose.
- *Maintenance dosage* – 150 mg/kg or 4 g/m², divided into 4 to 6 doses, every 24 hours.
- *Rheumatic fever prophylaxis* – Under 30 kg (66 lbs), 500 mg every 24 hours; over 30 kg (66 lbs), 1 g every 24 hours.

Younger than 2 months of age: Sulfadiazine is contraindicated in children younger than 2 months of age (except as adjunctive therapy with pyrimethamine in the treatment of congenital toxoplasmosis).

➤*Administration:* Administer each dose of sulfadiazine with 237 mL (8 ounces) of water and administer water at frequent intervals throughout the day.

➤*Storage/Stability:* Store at 20° to 25°C (68° to 77°F).

Actions

➤*Pharmacology:* The systemic sulfonamides are bacteriostatic agents with a similar spectrum of activity. Sulfonamides competitively inhibit bacterial synthesis of folic acid (pteroylglutamic acid) from aminobenzoic acid. Resistant strains are capable of utilizing folic acid precursors or preformed folic acid.

Sulfonamides exist in the blood in 3 forms: free, conjugated (acetylated and possibly others), and protein bound. The free form is considered to be therapeutically active.

SULFADIAZINE — ORAL

➤*Pharmacokinetics:*

Absorption – Sulfadiazine given orally is readily absorbed from the GI tract. After a single 2 g oral dose, a peak of 6.04 mg per 100 mL is reached in 4 hours; of this, 4.65 mg per 100 mL is free drug.

When a dose of 100 mg/kg of body weight is given initially and followed by 50 mg/kg every 6 hours, blood levels of free sulfadiazine are about 7 mg per 100 mL. Wide variations in blood levels may result with identical doses.

Distribution – Protein binding is 38% to 48%. Sulfadiazine diffuses into the cerebrospinal fluid; free drug reaches 32% to 65% of blood levels and total drug reaches 40% to 60%.

Excretion – Sulfadiazine is largely excreted in the urine, where concentrations are 10 to 25 times higher than serum levels. Approximately 10% of a single oral dose is excreted in the first 6 hours, 50% within 24 hours, and 60% to 85% in 48 to 72 hours. Of the amount excreted in the urine, 15% to 40% is in the acetyl form.

Contraindications

Hypersensitivity to sulfonamides; infants younger than 2 months of age (except as adjunctive therapy with pyrimethamine in the treatment of congenital toxoplasmosis); pregnancy at term and during the breast-feeding period because sulfonamides cross the placenta, are excreted in breast milk, and may cause kernicterus.

Warnings/Precautions

➤*Streptococcal infections:* Do not use sulfonamides for the treatment of group A beta-hemolytic streptococcal infections. In an established infection, they will not eradicate the streptococcus and, therefore, will not prevent sequelae, such as rheumatic fever and glomerulonephritis.

➤*Deaths:* Deaths associated with the administration of sulfonamides have been reported from hypersensitivity reactions, agranulocytosis, aplastic anemia, and other blood dyscrasias. The presence of such clinical signs as sore throat, fever, pallor, purpura, or jaundice may be early indications of serious blood disorders.

➤*Renal effects:* The frequency of renal complications is considerably lower in patients receiving more soluble sulfonamides.

➤*Asthma:* Give sulfonamides with caution to patients with bronchial asthma.

➤*Glucose-6-phosphate dehydrogenase (G6PD) deficiency:* Hemolysis may occur in individuals deficient in G6PD. This reaction is dose-related.

➤*Hydration:* Adequate fluid intake must be maintained in order to prevent crystalluria and stone formation.

➤*Hypersensitivity reactions:* Give sulfonamides with caution to patients with severe allergy.

➤*Renal/Hepatic function impairment:* Give sulfonamides with caution to patients with renal or hepatic function impairment.

➤*Pregnancy: Category C. Category D* if used near term (per Briggs' *Drugs in Pregnancy and Lactation*). Sulfadiazine is contraindicated for use in pregnancy at term because sulfonamides cross the placenta. The safe use of sulfonamides in pregnancy has not been established. The teratogenic potential of most sulfonamides has not been thoroughly investigated in animals or humans; however, a significant increase in the incidence of cleft palate and other bony abnormalities in offspring were observed when certain sulfonamides of the short-, intermediate-, and long-acting types were given to pregnant rats and mice in high oral doses (7 to 25 times the human therapeutic dose).

➤*Lactation:* Sulfadiazine is contraindicated for use in breast-feeding women because sulfonamides are excreted in breast milk and may cause kernicterus. Because of the potential for serious adverse reactions in breast-feeding infants from sulfadiazine, decide whether to discontinue breast-feeding or the drug, taking into account the importance of the drug to the mother.

➤*Children:* Sulfadiazine is contraindicated in infants younger than 2 months of age (except as adjunctive therapy with pyrimethamine in the treatment of congenital toxoplasmosis).

➤*Monitoring:* Frequently perform complete blood cell counts and urinalyses with careful microscopic examinations in patients receiving sulfonamides. Measure blood levels in patients receiving sulfonamides for serious infections. Free sulfonamide blood levels of 5 to 15 mg per 100 mL may be considered therapeutically effective for most infections, and blood levels of 12 to 15 mg per 100 mL may be considered optimal for serious infections. Because adverse reactions occur more frequently above this level, 20 mg per 100 mL should be the maximum total sulfonamide level.

Drug Interactions

Sulfadiazine Drug Interactions

Precipitant drug	Object drug[a]		Description
Indomethacin	Sulfadiazine	↑	Sulfadiazine may be displaced from plasma albumin, resulting in increased free-drug concentrations.
Probenecid	Sulfadiazine	↑	Sulfadiazine may be displaced from plasma albumin, resulting in increased free-drug concentrations.
Salicylates	Sulfadiazine	↑	Sulfadiazine may be displaced from plasma albumin, resulting in increased free-drug concentrations.
Sulfadiazine	Anticoagulants, oral (eg, warfarin)	↑	The anticoagulant action may be enhanced.
Sulfadiazine	Cyclosporine	↓	The action of cyclosporine may be reduced and the risk of nephrotoxicity is increased.
Sulfadiazine	Diuretics (eg, thiazide)	↑	Potentiation of the action of the thiazide diuretics may occur.
Sulfadiazine	Hydantoins (eg, phenytoin)	↑	Serum hydantoin levels may be increased, resulting in an increase in the pharmacologic and toxic effects of hydantoins.
Sulfadiazine	Methotrexate	↑	The risk of methotrexate-induced bone marrow suppression may be enhanced. Closely monitor patients for signs of hematologic toxicity.
Sulfadiazine	Sulfonylureas (eg, glipizide)	↑	Potentiation of the action of the sulfonylurea hypoglycemic agents may occur. Monitor blood glucose; the sulfonylurea dose may need to be decreased.
Sulfadiazine	Uricosuric agents	↑	Potentiations of the action of the uricosuric agents may occur.

[a] ↑ = object drug increased; ↓ = object drug decreased.

Adverse Reactions

➤*CNS:* Ataxia, convulsions, hallucinations, headache, insomnia, mental depression, peripheral neuritis, vertigo.

➤*Dermatologic:* Epidermal necrolysis, erythema multiforme (Stevens-Johnson syndrome), exfoliative dermatitis, generalized skin eruptions, photosensitization, pruritus, urticaria.

➤*Hematologic:* Agranulocytosis, aplastic anemia, hemolytic anemia, hypoprothrombinemia, leukopenia, methemoglobinemia, purpura, thrombocytopenia.

➤*Hypersensitivity:* Allergic myocarditis, anaphylactoid reactions.

➤*GI:* Abdominal pains, anorexia, diarrhea, emesis, hepatitis, nausea, pancreatitis, stomatitis.

➤*GU:* Crystalluria, stone formation, toxic nephrosis with oliguria and anuria; lupus erythematosus phenomenon and periarteritis nodosa have been noted.

➤*Special senses:* Conjunctival and scleral injection, periorbital edema, tinnitus.

➤*Miscellaneous:* Arthralgia, chills, drug fever, serum sickness. The sulfonamides bear certain chemical similarities to some goitrogens, diuretics (acetazolamide and the thiazides), and oral hypoglycemic agents. Goiter production, diuresis, and hypoglycemia have occurred rarely in patients receiving sulfonamides. Cross-sensitivity may exist with these agents.

Patient Information

Instruct patients to drink a 237 mL (8 ounces) glass of water with each dose of medication and at frequent intervals throughout the day.

Caution patients to promptly report the onset of sore throat, fever, pallor, purpura, or jaundice when taking this drug because these may be early indications of serious blood disorders.

NITROFURANTOIN

Rx	**Macrodantin** (Procter & Gamble)	**Capsules; oral:** 25 mg (as macrocrystals)	Lactose, talc. (MACRODANTIN 25 mg 0149-0007). White. In 100s.
Rx	**Nitrofurantoin** (Various, eg, Ivax, Mylan, Watson)	**Capsules; oral:** 50 mg (as macrocrystals)	In 100s, 500s, and 1,000s.
Rx	**Macrodantin** (Procter & Gamble)		Lactose, talc. (MACRODANTIN 50 mg 0149-0008). Yellow/White. In 100s and 1,000s.
Rx	**Nitrofurantoin** (Various, eg, Ivax, Mylan, Watson)	**Capsules; oral:** 100 mg (as macrocrystals)	In 100s, 500s, and 1,000s.
Rx	**Macrodantin** (Procter & Gamble)		Lactose, talc. (MACRODANTIN 100 mg 0149-0009). Yellow. In 100s and 1,000s.
Rx	**Nitrofurantoin** (Various, eg, Mylan, Watson)	**Capsules; oral:** 100 mg (as monohydrate/macrocrystals)	In 100s and 500s.
Rx	**Macrobid** (Procter & Gamble)		Lactose, talc. (Macrobid Norwich Eaton). Black/Yellow. In 100s.
Rx	**Furadantin** (Sciele Pharma, Inc.)	**Suspension; oral:** 25 mg per 5 mL	Parabens, saccharin, sorbitol. In 470 mL.

NITROFURANTOIN — ORAL

Indications

➤*Urinary tract infections (UTIs):* For the treatment of UTIs when caused by susceptible strains of *Escherichia coli*, enterococci, *Staphylococcus aureus*, and certain susceptible strains of *Klebsiella* and *Enterobacter* species.

Acute cystitis – Nitrofurantoin monohydrate/macrocrystals is indicated only for the treatment of acute uncomplicated UTIs (acute cystitis) caused by susceptible strains of *E. coli* or *Staphylococcus saprophyticus* in patients 12 years of age and older.

Nitrofurantoin is not indicated for the treatment of pyelonephritis or perinephric abscesses.

Administration and Dosage

➤*Adults:*

Urinary tract infections –

Macrocrystals and oral suspension:

• *Usual dosage* – 50 to 100 mg 4 times a day (the lower dosage level is recommended for uncomplicated UTIs).

• *Duration of therapy* – Continue therapy for 1 week or for at least 3 days after sterility of the urine is obtained. Continued infection indicates the need for reevaluation.

• *Prophylactic dosage* – For long-term suppressive therapy, a dosage reduction to 50 to 100 mg at bedtime may be adequate.

Monohydrate/Macrocrystals: 100 mg every 12 hours for 7 days.

➤*Children:*

Urinary tract infections –

Macrocrystals and oral suspension:

• *1 month of age and older* –

Usual dosage: 5 to 7 mg/kg of body weight per 24 hours, given in 4 divided doses.

Maximum dose: 400 mg/day for treatment and 100 mg/day for prophylaxis according to one reference.

Duration of therapy: Continue therapy for 1 week or for at least 3 days after sterility of the urine is obtained. Continued infection indicates the need for reevaluation.

Prophylactic dosage: For long-term suppressive therapy, doses as low as 1 mg/kg per 24 hours, given in a single dose or in 2 divided doses, may be adequate.

Oral suspension:

Nitrofurantoin Dosage in Children Based on Body Weight

Body weight		Dosage amount
Pounds	Kilograms	4 times daily
15 to 26	7 to 11	2.5 mL
27 to 46	12 to 21	5 mL
47 to 68	22 to 30	7.5 mL
69 to 91	31 to 41	10 mL

• *Younger than 1 month of age* – Use is contraindicated in children younger than 1 month of age.

Monohydrate/Macrocrystals:

• *12 years of age and older* – 100 mg every 12 hours for 7 days.

➤*Administration:* Give nitrofurantoin with food to improve drug absorption and, in some patients, tolerance.

➤*Storage/Stability:*

Oral suspension – Avoid exposure to strong light, which may darken the drug. It is stable when stored between 20° and 25°C (68° and 77°F). Protect from freezing. Dispense in glass amber bottles.

Capsules – Store at controlled room temperature, 15° to 30°C (59° to 86°F). Dispense in a tight container using a child-resistant closure.

Actions

➤*Pharmacology:* Nitrofurantoin is bactericidal in urine at therapeutic doses. The mechanism of the antimicrobial action of nitrofurantoin is unusual among antibacterials. Nitrofurantoin is reduced by bacterial flavoproteins to reactive intermediates that inactivate or alter bacterial ribosomal proteins and other macromolecules. As a result of such inactivations, the vital biochemical processes of protein synthesis, aerobic energy metabolism, DNA synthesis, RNA synthesis, and cell wall synthesis are inhibited. The broad-based nature of this mode of action may explain the lack of acquired bacterial resistance to nitrofurantoin, as the necessary multiple and simultaneous mutations of the target macromolecules would likely be lethal to the bacteria. Development of resistance to nitrofurantoin has not been a significant problem since its introduction in 1953. Cross-resistance with antibiotics and sulfonamides has not been observed, and transferable resistance is, at most, a very rare phenomenon.

➤*Pharmacokinetics:*

Absorption – Blood concentrations at therapeutic dosage are usually low.

Oral suspension: Oral nitrofurantoin is readily absorbed.

Macrocrystals: Nitrofurantoin macrocrystals are a larger, crystal form of nitrofurantoin. The absorption of nitrofurantoin macrocrystals is slower when compared with nitrofurantoin oral suspension.

Monohydrate/macrocrystals: Each monohydrate/macrocrystals capsule contains 2 forms of nitrofurantoin. Twenty-five percent is macrocrystalline nitrofurantoin, which has slower dissolution and absorption than nitrofurantoin monohydrate. The remaining 75% is nitrofurantoin monohydrate contained in the powder blend that, upon exposure to gastric and intestinal fluids, forms a gel matrix that releases nitrofurantoin over time.

Plasma nitrofurantoin concentrations after a single oral dose of the monohydrate/macrocrystals 100 mg capsule are low, with peak levels usually less than 1 mcg/mL.

Distribution – Unlike many drugs, the presence of food or agents delaying gastric emptying can increase the bioavailability of nitrofurantoin, presumably by allowing better dissolution in gastric juices.

When monohydrate/macrocrystals is administered with food, the bioavailability of nitrofurantoin is increased by approximately 40%.

Excretion – It is highly soluble in urine, to which it may impart a brown color.

Oral suspension: Nitrofurantoin oral suspension is rapidly excreted in urine. Following a dose regimen of 100 mg 4 times daily for 7 days, average urinary drug recoveries (0 to 24 hours) on day 1 and day 7 were 42.7% and 43.6%, respectively.

Macrocrystals: Excretion for nitrofurantoin macrocrystals is somewhat less when compared with nitrofurantoin oral suspension. Following a dose regimen of 100 mg 4 times daily for 7 days, average urinary drug recoveries (0 to 24 hours) on day 1 and day 7 were 37.9% and 35%, respectively.

Monohydrate/macrocrystals: Based on urinary pharmacokinetic data, the extent and rate of urinary excretion of nitrofurantoin from the monohydrate/macrocrystals 100 mg capsule are similar to those of the macrocrystals 50 or 100 mg capsule. Approximately 20% to 25% of a single dose of nitrofurantoin is recovered from the urine unchanged over 24 hours.

➤*Microbiology:* The minimal inhibitory concentration (MIC) in urine for most susceptible organisms is 32 mcg/mL or less. Resistant species generally have an MIC of at least 100 mcg/mL. Most gram-negative bacilli and gram-positive cocci associated with UTIs are susceptible, including: *E. coli*, *Klebsiella* and *Enterobacter* species, enterococci (eg, *Enterococcus faecalis*), *S. aureus*, and *S. saprophyticus*. Some strains of *Enterobacter* and *Klebsiella* species are resistant. Most strains of *Proteus* and *Serratia* species are resistant. It has no activity against *Pseudomonas* species. Susceptible bacteria do not readily develop resistance to nitrofurantoin during therapy. However, plasmid-mediated, transferable resistance has been demonstrated. Although in vitro susceptibility of *Salmonella*, *Shigella*, *Neisseria*, *Streptococcus pyogenes*, *S. pneumoniae*, *Corynebacterium*, and many anaerobes has been demonstrated, nitrofurantoin is of little clinical importance for infections caused by these organisms.

Contraindications

Anuria, oliguria, or significant impairment of renal function (creatinine clearance [Ccr] less than 60 mL/min or clinically significant elevated serum creatinine); hypersensitivity to nitrofurantoin.

Because of the possibility of hemolytic anemia caused by immature erythrocyte enzyme systems (glutathione instability), the drug is contraindicated in pregnant patients at term (38 to 42 weeks gestation), during labor and delivery, or when the onset of labor is imminent; also contraindicated in neonates younger than 1 month of age.

Warnings/Precautions

➤*Pulmonary reactions:* Acute, subacute, or chronic pulmonary reactions have been observed in patients treated with nitrofurantoin. If these reactions occur, discontinue nitrofurantoin and take appropriate measures. Reports have cited pulmonary reactions as a contributing cause of death.

NITROFURANTOIN — ORAL

Close monitoring of the pulmonary condition of patients receiving long-term therapy is warranted and requires that the benefits of therapy be weighed against potential risks.

Acute – Acute pulmonary reactions are commonly manifested by fever, chills, cough, chest pain, dyspnea, pulmonary infiltration with consolidation or pleural effusion on x-ray, and eosinophilia. Acute reactions usually occur within the first week of treatment and are reversible with cessation of therapy. Resolution often is dramatic.

Subacute – In subacute pulmonary reactions, fever and eosinophilia occur less often than in the acute form. Upon cessation of therapy, recovery may require several months. If the symptoms are not recognized as being drug-related and nitrofurantoin therapy is not stopped, the symptoms may become more severe.

Chronic – Chronic pulmonary reactions generally occur in patients who have received continuous treatment for 6 months or longer. Malaise, dyspnea on exertion, cough, and altered pulmonary function are common manifestations that can occur insidiously. Radiologic and histologic findings of diffuse interstitial pneumonitis or fibrosis, or both, also are common manifestations of the chronic pulmonary reaction. Fever is rarely prominent.

The severity of chronic pulmonary reactions and their degree of resolution appear to be related to the duration of therapy after the first clinical signs appear. Pulmonary function may be impaired permanently, even after cessation of therapy. The risk is greater when chronic pulmonary reactions are not recognized early.

➤*Peripheral neuropathy:* Peripheral neuropathy, which may become severe or irreversible, has occurred. Fatalities have been reported. Conditions such as renal impairment (Ccr less than 60 mL/min or clinically significant elevated serum creatinine), anemia, diabetes mellitus, electrolyte imbalance, vitamin B deficiency, and debilitating disease may enhance the occurrence of peripheral neuropathy. Periodically monitor patients receiving long-term therapy for changes in renal function.

➤*Optic neuritis:* Optic neuritis has been reported rarely in postmarketing experience with nitrofurantoin formulations.

➤*Hematologic effects:* Cases of hemolytic anemia of the primaquine-sensitivity type have been induced by nitrofurantoin. Hemolysis appears to be linked to a glucose-6-phosphate dehydrogenase deficiency in the red blood cells of the affected patients. This deficiency is found in 10% of black patients and a small percentage of ethnic groups of Mediterranean and Near-Eastern origin. Hemolysis is an indication for discontinuing nitrofurantoin; hemolysis ceases when the drug is withdrawn.

➤*Pseudomembranous colitis:* Pseudomembranous colitis has been reported with nearly all antibacterial agents, including nitrofurantoin, and may range from mild to life-threatening. Therefore, it is important to consider this diagnosis in patients with diarrhea subsequent to the administration of antibacterial agents.

Treatment with antibacterial agents alters the healthy flora of the colon and may permit overgrowth of clostridia. Studies indicate that a toxin produced by *Clostridium difficile* is one primary cause of antibiotic-associated colitis.

After the diagnosis of pseudomembranous colitis has been established, initiate appropriate therapeutic measures. Mild cases of pseudomembranous colitis usually respond to drug discontinuation alone. In moderate to severe cases, give consideration to management with fluids and electrolytes, protein supplementation, and treatment with an antibacterial drug clinically effective against *C. difficile* colitis.

➤*Hepatic reactions:* Hepatic reactions, including hepatitis, cholestatic jaundice, chronic active hepatitis, and hepatic necrosis, occur rarely. Fatalities have been reported. The onset of chronic active hepatitis may be insidious; periodically monitor patients for changes in biochemical tests that would indicate liver injury. If hepatitis occurs, withdraw the drug immediately and take appropriate measures.

➤*Drug resistance:* To reduce the development of drug-resistant bacteria and maintain the efficacy of nitrofurantoin and other antibacterial drugs, only use nitrofurantoin to treat or prevent infections that are proven or strongly suspected to be caused by bacteria. Prescribing nitrofurantoin in the absence of a proven or strongly suspected bacterial infection or a prophylactic indication is unlikely to provide benefit to the patient and increases the risk of the development of drug-resistant bacteria.

➤*Superinfection:* As with other antimicrobial agents, superinfections caused by resistant organisms (eg, *Pseudomonas* or *Candida* species) can occur. There are sporadic reports of *C. difficile* superinfections, or pseudomembranous colitis, with the use of nitrofurantoin.

➤*Pregnancy: Category B.* Because of the possibility of hemolytic anemia caused by immature erythrocyte enzyme systems (glutathione instability), the drug is contraindicated in pregnant patients at term (38 to 42 weeks gestation). In a single published study conducted in mice at 68 times the human dose (based on mg/kg administered to the dam), growth retardation and a low incidence of minor and common malformations were observed. However, at 25 times the human dose, fetal malformations were not observed; the relevance of these findings to humans is uncertain. There are, however, no adequate and well-controlled studies in pregnant women. Because animal reproduction studies are not always predictive of human response, use this drug during pregnancy only if clearly needed.

Nitrofurantoin has been shown in one published transplacental carcinogenicity study to induce lung papillary adenomas in the F1 generation mice at doses 19 times the human dose on a mg/kg basis. Because of the uncertainty regarding the human implications of these animal data, use this drug during pregnancy only if clearly needed.

Fertility impairment – Dosages of 10 mg/kg/day or greater in healthy men may, in certain unpredictable instances, produce a slight to moderate spermatogenic arrest with a decrease in sperm count.

Labor and delivery – Because of the possibility of hemolytic anemia caused by immature erythrocyte enzyme systems (glutathione instability), the drug is contraindicated in pregnant patients at term (38 to 42 weeks gestation), during labor and delivery, or when the onset of labor is imminent.

➤*Lactation:* Nitrofurantoin has been detected in human breast milk in trace amounts. Because of the potential for serious adverse reactions from nitrofurantoin in nursing infants younger than 1 month of age, decide whether to discontinue breast-feeding or to discontinue the drug, taking into account the importance of the drug to the mother.

➤*Children:* Nitrofurantoin is contraindicated in infants younger than 1 month of age.

Safety and efficacy of nitrofurantoin monohydrate/macrocrystals in pediatric patients younger than 12 years of age have not been established.

➤*Elderly:* Spontaneous reports suggest a higher proportion of pulmonary reactions, including fatalities, in elderly patients; these differences appear to be related to the higher proportion of elderly patients receiving long-term nitrofurantoin therapy. As in younger patients, chronic pulmonary reactions generally are observed in patients receiving therapy for 6 months or longer. Spontaneous reports also suggest an increased proportion of severe hepatic reactions, including fatalities, in elderly patients.

In general, consider the greater frequency of decreased hepatic, renal, or cardiac function, and of concomitant disease or other drug therapy when prescribing nitrofurantoin. This drug is known to be substantially excreted by the kidney, and the risk of toxic reactions to this drug may be greater in patients with impaired renal function. Anuria, oliguria, or significant impairment of renal function (Ccr less than 60 mL/min or clinically significant elevated serum creatinine) are contraindications. Because elderly patients are more likely to have decreased renal function, take care in dose selection; it may be useful to monitor renal function.

Per the Beers list, there is a potential for renal impairment with nitrofurantoin. Safer alternatives are available. Nitrofurantoin is also considered a high-risk medication for elderly patients according to the Centers of Medicare and Medicaid Services.

➤*Monitoring:* Periodically monitor patients receiving long-term therapy for changes in renal and pulmonary function.

Drug Interactions

Nitrofurantoin Drug Interactions			
Precipitant drug	Object drug[a]		Description
Anticholinergics	Nitrofurantoin	⬆	Anticholinergic drugs increase nitrofurantoin bioavailability by delaying gastric emptying and increasing absorption.
Magnesium salts	Nitrofurantoin	⬇	Magnesium salts may delay or decrease the absorption of nitrofurantoin.
Uricosurics	Nitrofurantoin	⬆	Administration of high doses of probenecid with nitrofurantoin decreases renal clearance and increases serum levels of nitrofurantoin. The result could be increased toxic effects.

[a] ⬆ = object drug increased; ⬇ = object drug decreased.

➤*Drug/Lab test interactions:* As a result of the presence of nitrofurantoin, a false-positive reaction for glucose in the urine may occur. This has been observed with Benedict and Fehling solutions but not with the glucose enzymatic test.

Adverse Reactions

➤*Cardiovascular:* Benign intracranial hypertension (pseudotumor cerebri) has been reported rarely. Bulging fontanels, as a sign of benign intracranial hypertension in infants, have been reported rarely. Changes in electrocardiogram (eg, nonspecific ST/T wave changes, bundle branch block) have been reported in association with pulmonary reactions.

➤*CNS:* Asthenia, confusion, depression, dizziness, drowsiness, headache, nystagmus, peripheral neuropathy (see Warnings), psychotic reactions, vertigo.

➤*Dermatologic:* Erythema multiforme (including Stevens-Johnson syndrome), exfoliative dermatitis (rare); transient alopecia.

➤*GI:* Abdominal pain, anorexia, diarrhea, emesis, nausea, pancreatitis, pseudomembranous colitis, sialadenitis.

➤*Hepatic:* Cholestatic jaundice, chronic active hepatitis, hepatic necrosis, hepatic reactions, hepatitis (rare).

➤*Hypersensitivity:* Anaphylaxis; angioedema; arthralgia; chills; drug fever; eczematous, erythematous, or maculopapular eruptions; lupus-like syndrome associated with pulmonary reactions; myalgia; pruritus; urticaria.

➤*Lab test abnormalities:* Agranulocytosis, decreased hemoglobin, eosinophilia, glucose-6-phosphate dehydrogenase deficiency anemia, granulocytopenia, hemolytic anemia, increased ALT, increased AST, increased serum phosphorus, leukopenia, megaloblastic anemia, thrombocytopenia. In most cases, these hematologic abnormalities resolved following cessation of therapy. Aplastic anemia (rare).

NITROFURANTOIN — ORAL

➤*Respiratory:* Chronic, subacute, or acute pulmonary hypersensitivity reactions may occur (see Warnings); cyanosis (rare).

➤*Miscellaneous:* Optic neuritis, superinfections caused by resistant organisms.

➤*Monohydrate/macrocrystals:* In clinical trials of monohydrate/macrocrystals, the most frequent adverse reactions that were reported as possibly or probably drug-related were nausea (8%), headache (6%), and flatulence (1.5%). Additional clinical adverse reactions reported as possibly or probably drug-related occurred in less than 1% of patients studied and are listed as the following.

CNS – Amblyopia, dizziness, drowsiness.

Dermatologic – Alopecia.

GI – Abdominal pain, constipation, diarrhea, dyspepsia, emesis.

Hypersensitivity – Pruritus, urticaria.

Respiratory – Acute pulmonary hypersensitivity reaction.

Miscellaneous – Chills, fever, malaise.

Overdosage

➤*Symptoms:* Occasional incidents of acute overdosage of nitrofurantoin have not resulted in any specific symptoms other than vomiting.

➤*Treatment:* There is no specific antidote, but a high fluid intake should be maintained to promote urinary excretion of the drug. It is dialyzable.

Patient Information

May cause brown discoloration of the urine.

Advise patients to take nitrofurantoin with food to further enhance tolerance and improve drug absorption. Instruct patients to complete the full course of therapy; however, advise them to contact their doctors if any unusual symptoms occur during therapy.

Many patients who cannot tolerate microcrystalline nitrofurantoin are able to take nitrofurantoin macrocrystals without nausea.

Advise patients not to use antacid preparations containing magnesium trisilicate while taking nitrofurantoin.

Counsel patients that antibacterial drugs, including nitrofurantoin, should only be used to treat bacterial infections. They do not treat viral infections (eg, the common cold). When nitrofurantoin is prescribed to treat a bacterial infection, tell patients that although it is common to feel better early in the course of therapy, the medication should be taken exactly as directed. Skipping doses or not completing the full course of therapy may (1) decrease the effectiveness of the immediate treatment, and (2) increase the likelihood that bacteria will develop resistance and will not be treatable by nitrofurantoin or other antibacterial drugs in the future.

METHENAMINES

Indications

➤*Urinary tract infections:* Prophylaxis or suppression/elimination of frequently recurring urinary tract infections when long-term therapy is considered necessary; for infected or residual urine sometimes accompanying neurologic disease (methenamine mandelate). Use only after eradication of the infection by other appropriate antimicrobial agents.

Actions

➤*Pharmacology:* In acid urine, methenamine is hydrolyzed to ammonia and formaldehyde, which is bactericidal. Methenamine does not liberate formaldehyde in the serum. The acid salts (mandelate and hippurate) help maintain a low urine pH.

➤*Pharmacokinetics:*

Absorption – Methenamine is readily absorbed following oral administration.

Distribution – Methenamine distributes widely into body fluids and is placentally transferred to the fetus during pregnancy.

Metabolism/Excretion – Generation of formaldehyde depends upon urinary pH, the concentration of methenamine and the duration that the urine is retained in the bladder. Peak concentrations of formaldehyde occur at a urine pH of 5.5 or less and are seen approximately 2 hours after a dose of methenamine hippurate and 3 to 8 hours after a dose of methenamine mandelate.

Excretion occurs via glomerular filtration and tubular secretion. Approximately 90% of the methenamine moiety is excreted in the urine within 24 hours.

Special populations –

Renal function impairment: Contraindicated in renal insufficiency.
Hepatic function impairment: Contraindicated in severe hepatic disease.

➤*Microbiology:* The nonspecific antibacterial action of formaldehyde is effective against gram-positive and gram-negative organisms and fungi. *Escherichia coli*, enterococci, and staphylococci are usually susceptible. *Enterobacter aerogenes* and *Proteus vulgaris* are generally resistant. Urea-splitting organisms (eg, *Proteus*, *Pseudomonas*) may be resistant because they raise the pH of the urine inhibiting the release of formaldehyde. An effective urine concentration of formaldehyde must persist for a minimum of 2 hours.

Methenamine is particularly suited for therapy of long-term infections because bacteria and fungi do not develop resistance to formaldehyde.

Contraindications

Renal insufficiency; severe dehydration; severe hepatic insufficiency; use alone for acute infections with parenchymal involvement causing systemic symptoms; hypersensitivity to the drug; concurrent sulfonamide therapy.

Warnings/Precautions

➤*Large doses:* Large doses of methenamine (8 g daily for 3 to 4 weeks) have caused bladder irritation, painful and frequent micturition, proteinuria, and gross hematuria.

➤*Acid urine:* Take care to maintain an acidic pH, especially when treating infections due to urea-splitting organisms, such as *Proteus* and strains of *Pseudomonas*. When acidification is contraindicated or unattainable (as with some urea-splitting bacteria) the drug is not recommended.

➤*Dysuria:* Dysuria may occur. This can be controlled by reducing the dosage and the acidification.

➤*Gout:* Methenamine salts may cause precipitation of urate crystals in the urine. Avoid use.

➤*Tartrazine sensitivity:* Some of these products contain tartrazine, which may cause allergic-type reactions (including bronchial asthma) in certain susceptible individuals. Although the overall incidence of tartrazine sensitivity in the general population is low, it is frequently seen in patients who also have aspirin hypersensitivity. Specific products containing tartrazine are identified in the product listings.

➤*Renal function impairment:* Contraindicated in renal insufficiency.

➤*Hepatic function impairment:* Contraindicated in severe hepatic disease. Patients with preexisting hepatic insufficiency may have adverse reactions from the small amounts of ammonia and formaldehyde that are produced.

➤*Pregnancy: Category C.* Safe use of methenamine in early pregnancy has not been established. Safety in the last trimester is suggested, but not proven. Methenamine passes into the fetus, but there is no evidence that methenamine salts cause fetal abnormalities. It is not known whether the drug can cause fetal harm when administered to a pregnant woman or can affect reproduction capacity. Give to pregnant women only if clearly needed.

➤*Lactation:* Methenamine passes into breast milk. No adverse effects on the breast-feeding infant have been reported. According to Briggs' *Drugs in Pregnancy and Lactation*, methenamine is probably compatible with breast-feeding.

➤*Children:* No data are available for children younger than 6 years of age.

➤*Monitoring:* Perform liver function studies periodically on patients receiving methenamine hippurate, especially those with liver dysfunction. Monitor urine pH.

Drug Interactions

Methenamine Drug Interactions

Precipitant drug	Object drug[a]		Description
Sulfonamides	Methenamine	⬇	An insoluble precipitate between the sulfonamide and formaldehyde may form in the urine. Concurrent use is contraindicated.
Urinary alkalinizers	Methenamine	⬇	Alkalinizing agents may decrease the efficacy of methenamine by inhibiting its conversion to formaldehyde.

[a] ⬇ = object drug decreased.

➤*Drug/Lab test interactions:* Methenamine may interfere with laboratory urine determinations of 17-hydroxycorticosteroids, **catecholamines**, and **vanillylmandelic acid** (false increases); and 5-hydroxyindoleacetic acid (false decrease).

Methenamine taken during pregnancy can interfere with laboratory tests of **urine estriol** (resulting in unmeasurably low values) when an acid hydrolysis procedure is used. This is due to the presence in the urine of methenamine or formaldehyde. Use enzymatic hydrolysis in place of acid hydrolysis.

Adverse Reactions

➤*Dermatologic:* Rash; pruritus (rare).

➤*GI:* Nausea, upset stomach, vomiting (3.5%).

➤*GU:* Dysuria (less than 3.5%); painful or difficult urination; microscopic and rarely gross hematuria.

Overdosage

➤*Treatment:* Immediately after ingestion of an overdose, further absorption of the drug may be minimized by gastric lavage, followed by administration of activated charcoal. Force fluids, either oral or parenteral, to tolerance.

Patient Information

Inform patient that it may be necessary to attempt to acidify the urine (eg, ascorbic acid, cranberry juice).

Advise patient to take with food to minimize GI upset.

Instruct patient to drink sufficient fluids to ensure adequate urine flow.

Advise patient to avoid excessive intake of alkalinizing foods (milk products) or medication (bicarbonate, carbonate).

Instruct patient to complete full course of therapy; take until gone.

Advise patient to notify health care provider if skin rash, painful urination, or intolerable GI upset occurs.

METHENAMINE

Rx	**Methenamine Mandelate** (Edenbridge Pharmaceuticals)	**Tablets; oral:** 500 mg	In 100s.
Rx	**Methenamine Mandelate** (Various, Edenbridge Pharmaceuticals, Seton Pharmaceuticals)	**Tablets; oral:** 1,000 mg	May contain PEG. In 100s.
Rx	**Methenamine Hippurate** (Various, CorePharma, County Line)	**Tablets; oral:** 1,000 mg	May contain saccharin. In 100s.
Rx	**Hiprex** (Sanofi-Aventis U.S.)		As methenamine hippurate. Tartrazine, saccharin. (Merrell 277). Yellow, capsule-shaped, scored. In 100s.
Rx	**Urex** (Vatring Pharmaceuticals)		As methenamine hippurate. Saccharin. (VP UREX). White, capsule-shaped, scored. In 100s.

METHENAMINE HIPPURATE — ORAL

For complete and comparative prescribing information refer to the Methenamines class monograph.

Indications

➤*Urinary tract infection:* For prophylactic or suppressive treatment of frequently recurring urinary tract infections when long-term therapy is considered necessary. Only use this drug after eradication of the infection by other appropriate antimicrobial agents.

Administration and Dosage

➤*General dosing considerations:* The antibacterial activity of methenamine hippurate is greater in acid urine. Therefore, restriction of alkalinizing foods and medications is desirable. If necessary, as indicated by urinary pH and clinical response, supplemental acidification of the urine may be instituted. The efficacy of therapy should be monitored by repeated urine cultures.

➤*Adults:*

Urinary tract infection – 1 g twice daily (morning and night).

➤*Children:*

Urinary tract infection –

13 years of age and older: See Adults for dosing.

6 to 12 years of age: 0.5 to 1 g twice daily (morning and night).

➤*Renal function impairment:* Contraindicated in patients with renal insufficiency.

➤*Administration:* Advise patients to take orally twice daily (morning and night).

➤*Storage/Stability:* Store at 15° to 30°C (59° to 86°F).

METHENAMINE MANDELATE — ORAL

For complete and comparative prescribing information, refer to the Methenamines class monograph.

Indications

➤*Urinary tract infection:* For the suppression or elimination of bacteriuria associated with pyelonephritis, cystitis, and other chronic urinary tract infections; for infected residual urine sometimes accompanying neurologic diseases.

Administration and Dosage

➤*General dosing considerations:* Because an acidic urine is essential for antibacterial activity, with maximum efficacy occurring at pH 5.5 or below, restriction of alkalinizing foods and medication is thus desirable. If testing of urine pH reveals the need, supplemental acidification should be given.

➤*Adults:*

Urinary tract infection – 4 g daily given as 1 g after each meal and at bedtime.

➤*Children:*

Urinary tract infection –

13 years of age and older: See Adults for dosing.

6 to 12 years of age: 2 g daily given as 500 mg after each meal and at bedtime.

5 years of age and younger: 250 mg for every 30 lb of body weight, 4 times daily.

➤*Renal function impairment:* Contraindicated in patients with renal insufficiency.

➤*Hepatic function impairment:* Contraindicated in patients with severe hepatic disease.

➤*Administration:* Advise patient to take after each meal and at bedtime.

➤*Storage/Stability:* Store at 15° and 30°C (59° and 86°F).

METHENAMINE COMBINATIONS

Rx	**Uretron D/S** (A. G. Marin)	**Tablets; oral:** 120 mg methenamine, 36.2 mg phenyl salicylate, 0.12 mg hyoscyamine sulfate, 10.8 mg methylene blue, 40.8 mg sodium biphosphate *Dose: Adults* - 1 tablet 4 times daily followed by liberal fluid intake; *older children* - individualize dosing	Parabens, sucrose. (URETRON D/S). Purple. Sugar-coated. In 100s.
Rx	**Urelle** (Pharmelle)	**Tablets; oral:** 81 mg methenamine, 32.4 mg phenyl salicylate, 10.8 mg methylene blue, 40.8 mg sodium phosphate monobasic, 0.12 mg hyoscyamine sulfate *Dose: Adults* - 1 tablet 4 times daily followed by liberal fluid intake; *older children* - individualize dosing	Sugar, mineral oil. (P-002). Blue. Sugar-coated. In 90s.
Rx	**Utrona-C** (Cypress Pharmaceutical)	**Tablets; oral:** 81.6 mg methenamine, 36.2 mg phenyl salicylate, 10.8 mg methylene blue, 40.8 mg sodium phosphate monobasic, 0.12 mg hyoscyamine sulfate *Dose: Adults* - 1 tablet 4 times daily followed by liberal fluid intake; *older children* - individualize dosing	Mineral oil, PEG, sugar. (HAW 513). Purple, oval. In 100s,
Rx	**Prosed/DS** (Ferring)	**Tablets; oral:** 81.6 mg methenamine, 36.2 mg phenyl salicylate, 10.8 mg methylene blue, 9 mg benzoic acid, 0.12 mg hyoscyamine sulfate *Dose:* 1 tablet 4 times daily	Sugar. (Prosed/DS). Dark blue, round. Sugar coated. In 100s.
Rx	**Uritact DS** (Cypress)	**Tablets; oral:** 81.6 mg methenamine, 36.2 mg phenyl salicylate, 10.8 mg methylene blue, 9 mg benzoic acid, 0.06 mg atropine sulfate, 0.06 mg hyoscyamine sulfate *Dose:* 1 tablet 4 times daily with liquid	Alcohol-free. (CYP 516). Light blue, capsule shape. In 100s.
Rx	**Uro Blue** (R. A. McNeil)	**Tablets; oral:** 120 mg methenamine, 40.8 mg sodium phosphate monobasic, 36.2 mg phenyl salicylate, 10.8 mg methylene blue, 0.12 mg hyoscyamine sulfate *Dose:* 1 tablet 4 times daily followed by liberal fluid intake	Sugar. (HMP). Purple. Sugar-coated. In 100s.
Rx	**Urogesic Blue** (Edwards)	**Tablets; oral:** 81.6 mg methenamine, 40.8 mg monobasic sodium phosphate, 10.8 mg methylene blue, 0.12 mg hyoscyamine sulfate *Dose:* 1 tablet 4 times daily followed by liberal fluid intake	Mannitol. (ED UB). Light blue to blue, oval, scored. In 100s.
Rx	**Urimax** (Xanodyne)	**Tablets, delayed release; oral:** 81.6 mg methenamine, 40.8 mg sodium biphosphate, 36.2 mg phenyl salicylate, 10.8 mg methylene blue, 0.12 mg hyoscyamine sulfate *Dose:* 1 tablet 4 times daily	(Urimax). Magenta. Film coated. In 100s.
Rx	**Urimar-T** (Marnel)	**Tablets; oral:** 120 mg methenamine, 40.8 mg sodium phosphate monobasic, 36.2 mg phenyl salicylate, 10.8 mg methylene blue, 0.12 mg hyoscyamine sulfate *Dose:* 1 tablet 4 times daily followed by liberal fluid intake; not recommended for children ≤ 6 years of age.	Sugar coated. (HMP). Purple. In 4s and 100s.

METHENAMINE COMBINATIONS

Rx	**Uroquid-Acid No. 2** (Beach)	**Tablets; oral:** 500 mg methenamine mandelate, 500 mg sodium acid phosphate monohydrate *Dose*: Initial - 2 tablets 4 times daily Maintenance - 2 to 4 tablets daily in divided doses	(Beach 1114). Yellow. Film coated. Capsule shape. In 100s.
RX	**Utac** (Breckenridge)	**Tablets; oral:** 500 mg methenamine mandelate, 500 mg sodium acid phosphate monobasic monohydrate *Dose*: Initial - 2 tablets 4 times daily Maintenance - 2 to 4 tablets daily in divided doses	(B 199). Yellow, oval. Film coated. In 100s
Rx	**Urisedamine** (PolyMedica)	**Tablets; oral:** 500 mg methenamine mandelate, 0.15 mg hyoscyamine *Dose*: 2 tablets 4 times daily Children (≥ 6 years) – Reduce dosage in proportion to age and weight	Sucrose. (W2210). Light blue. Capsule shape. In 100s.
Rx	**Atrosept** (Geneva)	**Tablets; oral:** 40.8 mg methenamine, 18.1 mg phenyl salicylate, 0.03 mg atropine sulfate, 0.03 mg hyoscyamine (as sulfate), 4.5 mg benzoic acid, 5.4 mg methylene blue *Dose*: Adults – 2 tablets 4 times daily Children (≥ 6 years) – Reduce dosage in proportion to age and weight	(220). Deep blue. Sugar coated. In 100s and 1000s.
Rx	**UAA** (Econo Med)		(UAA). Blue. Sugar coated. In 100s and 1000s.
Rx	**Urinary Antiseptic No. 2** (Various)		In 100s and 1000s.
Rx	**Uritin** (Various, eg, Gold-line)		In 1000s.
Rx	**MHP-A** (Cypress)	**Tablets; oral:** 40.8 mg methenamine, 18.1 mg phenyl salicylate, 0.03 mg atropine sulfate, 0.03 mg hyoscyamine sulfate, 4.5 mg benzoic acid, 5.4 mg methylene blue *Dose*: Adults – 2 tablets 4 times daily Children (≥ 6 years) – Dosage must be individualized by physician.	(CYP515). Green. In 100s.
Rx	**Uriseptic** (SDA Labs)	**Tablets; oral:** 40.8 mg methenamine, 18.1 mg phenyl salicylate, 0.03 mg atropine sulfate, 0.03 mg hyoscyamine sulfate, 4.5 mg benzoic acid, 5.4 mg methylene blue *Dose*: Adults – 2 tablets 4 times daily followed by liberal fluid intake Children (≥ 6 years) – Individualize dosage	Dk. blue. Film-coated. In 100s.
otc	**Cystex** (Numark)	**Tablets; oral:** 162 mg methenamine, 162.5 mg sodium salicylate, 32 mg benzoic acid *Dose*: Adults and children > 16 years old – 2 tablets 4 times daily with meals and at bedtime	In 40s and 100s.
Rx	**Ustell** (Biocomp Pharma)	**Capsules; oral:** 120 mg methenamine, 10 mg methylene blue, 36 mg phenyl salicylate, 40.8 mg sodium phosphate monobasic, 0.12 mg hyoscyamine sulfate *Dose*: Adults – 1 capsule 4 times per day followed by liberal fluid intake Older children – Individualize dosage	Ammonium hydroxide, propylene glycol. (S903). Blue. In 100s.
Rx	**Uticap** (Cypress)		(SJ 646). Blue. In 100s.

FOLATE ANTAGONISTS

TRIMETHOPRIM (TMP)

Rx	**Trimethoprim** (Various, eg, Biocraft, Moore, Parmed, Schein)	**Tablets:** 100 mg	In 14s, 30s, 100s and UD 100s.
Rx	**Proloprim** (GlaxoWellcome)		(Proloprim 09A). White, scored. In 100s.
Rx	**Trimethoprim** (Various, eg, Biocraft, Moore)	**Tablets:** 200 mg	In 100s.
Rx	**Proloprim** (GlaxoWellcome)		(Proloprim 200). Yellow, scored. In 100s.
Rx	**Primsol** (Ascent Pediatrics)	**Solution, oral:** 50 mg/5 ml	Parabens, sorbitol. Alcohol free. Bubble gum flavor. In 473 ml.

TRIMETHOPRIM — ORAL TABLETS

Indications

➤*Urinary tract infections:* For the treatment of initial episodes of uncomplicated urinary tract infections due to susceptible strains of the following organisms: *Escherichia coli*, *Proteus mirabilis*, *Klebsiella pneumoniae*, *Enterobacter* species and coagulase-negative *Staphylococcus* species, including *S. saprophyticus*.

Administration and Dosage

➤*Adults:*

Urinary tract infections – 100 mg every 12 hours or 200 mg every 24 hours, each for 10 days.

Off-label dosing –

Pneumocystis pneumonia treatment: 15 mg/kg in 3 divided doses with dapsone (see Dapsone for dosing).

➤*Children:*

Urinary tract infections – See Adults for dosing for children 12 years of age and older.

Off-label dosing –

Acute otitis media:

• *6 months of age and older* – 10 mg/kg/day divided twice daily for 10 days.

Pneumocystis carinii pneumonia, mild/moderate:

• *12 years of age and older* – 5 mg/kg orally 3 times daily for 21 days with dapsone 100 mg daily.

Urinary tract infections:

• *Younger than 12 years of age* – 4 to 6 mg/kg/day divided twice daily for 10 days.

➤*Renal function impairment:*

CrCl of 15 to 30 mL/min – 50 mg every 12 hours.

CrCl less than 15 mL/min – Use is not recommended.

➤*Storage/Stability:* Store at 15° to 25°C (59° to 77°F) in a dry place and protect from light.

Actions

➤*Pharmacokinetics:*

Absorption/Distribution – Trimethoprim is rapidly absorbed following oral administration. It exists in the blood as unbound, protein-bound and metabolized forms. The free form is considered to be the therapeutically active form. Approximately 44% of trimethoprim is bound to plasma proteins.

Mean peak serum concentrations of approximately 1 mcg/mL occur 1 to 4 hours after oral administration of a single 100 mg dose. A single 200 mg dose will result in serum levels approximately twice as high. The half-life of trimethoprim ranges from 8 to 10 hours. However, patients with severely impaired renal function exhibit an increase in the half-life of trimethoprim, which requires either dosage regimen adjustment or not using the drug in such patients. During a 13-week study of trimethoprim administered at a daily dosage of 200 mg (50 mg 4 times a day), the mean minimum steady-state concentration of the drug was 1.1 mcg/mL. Steady-state concentrations were achieved within 2 to 3 days of chronic administration and were maintained throughout the experimental period.

Since normal vaginal and fecal flora are the source of most pathogens causing urinary tract infections, it is relevant to consider the distribution of trimethoprim into these sites. Concentrations of trimethoprim in vaginal secretions are consistently greater than those found simultaneously in the serum, being typically 1.6 times the concentrations of simultaneously obtained serum samples. Sufficient trimethoprim is excreted in the feces to markedly reduce or eliminate trimethoprim-susceptible organisms from the fecal flora.

Trimethoprim also passes the placental barrier and is excreted in human milk.

Metabolism – Ten percent to 20% of trimethoprim is metabolized, primarily in the liver; the remainder is excreted unchanged in the urine. The principal metabolites of trimethoprim are the 1- and 3-oxides and the 3′- and 4′-hydroxy derivatives.

Excretion – Excretion of trimethoprim is primarily by the kidneys through glomerular filtration and tubular secretion. Urine concentrations of trimethoprim are considerably higher than are the concentrations in the blood. After a single oral dose of 100 mg, urine concentrations of trimethoprim ranged from 30 to 160 mcg/mL during the 0- to 4-hour period and declined to

TRIMETHOPRIM — ORAL TABLETS

approximately 18 to 91 mcg/mL during the 8- to 24-hour period. A 200 mg single oral dose will result in trimethoprim urine concentrations approximately twice as high. After oral administration, 50% to 60% of trimethoprim is excreted in urine within 24 hours, approximately 80% of this being unmetabolized trimethoprim.

➤*Microbiology:* Trimethoprim blocks the production of tetrahydrofolic acid from dihydrofolic acid by binding to and reversibly inhibiting the required enzyme, dihydrofolate reductase. This binding is very much stronger for the bacterial enzyme than for the corresponding mammalian enzyme. Thus, trimethoprim selectively interferes with bacterial biosynthesis of nucleic acids and proteins.

Trimethoprim has been shown to be active against most strains of the following microorganisms, both in vitro and in clinical infections.

Aerobic gram-positive microorganisms – *Staphylococcus* species (coagulase-negative strains, including *S. saprophyticus*).

Aerobic gram-negative microorganisms – *Enterobacter* species, *Escherichia coli, Klebsiella pneumoniae, Proteus mirabilis.*

Contraindications

Hypersensitivity to trimethoprim and in those with documented megaloblastic anemia due to folate deficiency.

Warnings/Precautions

➤*Hematologic effects:* Trimethoprim has been reported rarely to interfere with hematopoiesis, especially when administered in large doses or for prolonged periods.

The presence of clinical signs such as sore throat, fever, pallor or purpura may be early indications of serious blood disorders.

Obtain complete blood counts if any of these signs are noted in a patient receiving trimethoprim and discontinue the drug if a significant reduction in the count of any formed blood element is found.

➤*Folate deficiency:* Give trimethoprim with caution to patients with possible folate deficiency. Folates may be administered concomitantly without interfering with the antibacterial action of trimethoprim.

➤*Hypersensitivity reactions:* Serious hypersensitivity reactions have been reported rarely in patients on trimethoprim therapy.

➤*Renal/Hepatic function impairment:* Give trimethoprim with caution to patients with impaired renal or hepatic function.

➤*Pregnancy: Category C.* Trimethoprim has been shown to be teratogenic in the rat when given in doses 40 times the human dose. In some rabbit studies, the overall increase in fetal loss (dead and resorbed and malformed conceptuses) was associated with doses 6 times the human therapeutic dose.

While there are no large well-controlled studies on the use of trimethoprim in pregnant women, Brumfitt and Pursell (Brumfitt W., Pursell, R. Trimethoprim-sulfamethoxazole in the treatment of bacteriuria in women, *J Infect Dis*, 1973; 128 (suppl): S657 to S663) in a retrospective study, reported the outcome of 186 pregnancies during which the mother received either placebo or trimethoprim in combination with sulfamethoxazole. The incidence of congenital abnormalities was 4.5% (3 of 66) in those who received placebo and 3.3% (4 of 120) in those receiving trimethoprim plus sulfamethoxazole. There were no abnormalities in the 10 children whose mothers received the drug during the first trimester. In a separate survey, Brumfitt and Pursell also found no congenital abnormalities in 35 children whose mothers had received trimethoprim plus sulfamethoxazole at the time of conception or shortly thereafter.

Because trimethoprim may interfere with folic acid metabolism, use trimethoprim during pregnancy only if the potential benefit justifies the potential risk to the fetus.

➤*Lactation:* Trimethoprim is excreted in human milk. Because trimethoprim may interfere with folic acid metabolism, exercise caution when trimethoprim is administered to a nursing woman.

➤*Children:* Safety and efficacy in pediatric patients below the age of 2 months have not been established. The effectiveness of trimethoprim has not been established in pediatric patients under 12 years of age.

➤*Elderly:* Case reports of hyperkalemia in elderly patients receiving trimethoprim-sulfamethoxazole have been published. Trimethoprim is known to be substantially excreted by the kidney, and the risk of toxic reactions to this drug may be greater in patients with impaired renal function. Because elderly patients are more likely to have decreased renal function, care should be taken in dose selection, and it may be useful to monitor potassium concentrations and to monitor renal function by calculating creatinine clearance.

➤*Monitoring:* If any clinical signs of a blood disorder are noted in a patient receiving trimethoprim, obtain a complete blood count and discontinue the drug if a significant reduction in the count of any formed blood element is found.

Drug Interactions

➤*Phenytoin:* Trimethoprim may inhibit the hepatic metabolism of phenytoin. Trimethoprim, given at a common clinical dosage, increased the phenytoin half-life by 51% and decreased the phenytoin metabolic clearance rate by 30%. When administering these drugs concurrently, one should be alert for possible excessive phenytoin effect.

➤*Drug/Lab test interactions:* Trimethoprim can interfere with a serum methotrexate assay as determined by the competitive binding protein technique (CBPA) when a bacterial dihydrofolate reductase is used as the binding protein. No interference occurs, however, if methotrexate is measured by a radioimmunoassay (RIA).

The presence of trimethoprim may also interfere with the Jaffé alkaline picrate reaction assay for creatinine, resulting in overestimations of about 10% in the range of normal values.

Adverse Reactions

The adverse effects encountered most often with trimethoprim were rash and pruritus.

➤*CNS:* Aseptic meningitis has been rarely reported.

➤*Dermatologic:* Rash, pruritus and phototoxic skin eruptions. At the recommended dosage regimens of 100 mg twice daily or 200 mg daily, each for 10 days, the incidence of rash is 2.9% to 6.7%. In clinical studies which employed high doses of trimethoprim, an elevated incidence of rash was noted. These rashes were maculopapular, morbilliform, pruritic and generally mild to moderate, appearing 7 to 14 days after the initiation of therapy.

➤*GI:* Epigastric distress, glossitis, nausea, and vomiting.

➤*Hematologic:* Leukopenia, megaloblastic anemia, methemoglobinemia, neutropenia, and thrombocytopenia.

➤*Hepatic:* Cholestatic jaundice has been rarely reported. Elevation of serum transaminase and bilirubin has been noted, but the significance of this finding is unknown.

➤*Hypersensitivity:* Rare reports of anaphylaxis, erythema multiforme, exfoliative dermatitis, Stevens-Johnson syndrome, and toxic epidermal necrolysis (Lyell syndrome) have been received.

➤*Metabolic:* Hyperkalemia, hyponatremia.

➤*Miscellaneous:* Fever, increases in blood urea nitrogen (BUN) and serum creatinine levels.

Overdosage

➤*Acute:*

Symptoms – Signs of acute overdosage with trimethoprim may appear following ingestion of 1 g or more of the drug and include nausea, vomiting, dizziness, headaches, mental depression, confusion and bone marrow depression (see Chronic overdosage).

Treatment – Treatment consists of gastric lavage and general supportive measures. Acidification of the urine will increase renal elimination of trimethoprim. Peritoneal dialysis is not effective and hemodialysis is only moderately effective in eliminating the drug.

➤*Chronic:*

Symptoms – Use of trimethoprim at high doses or for extended periods of time may cause bone marrow depression manifested as thrombocytopenia, leukopenia or megaloblastic anemia.

Treatment – If signs of bone marrow depression occur, trimethoprim should be discontinued and the patient should be given leucovorin; 5 to 15 mg leucovorin daily has been recommended by some investigators.

TRIMETHOPRIM HYDROCHLORIDE — ORAL SOLUTION

Indications

➤*Adults:*

Urinary tract infections – For the treatment of initial episodes of uncomplicated urinary tract infections due to susceptible strains of the following organisms: *Escherichia coli, Proteus mirabilis, Klebsiella pneumoniae, Enterobacter* species and coagulase-negative *Staphylococcus* species, including *S. saprophyticus*.

➤*Children:*

Acute otitis media – For the treatment of acute otitis media due to susceptible strains of *Streptococcus pneumoniae* and *Haemophilus influenzae*. *Moraxella catarrhalis* isolates were found consistently resistant to trimethoprim in vitro. Therefore, when infection with *Moraxella catarrhalis* is suspected, consider the use of alternative antimicrobial agents. Trimethoprim is not indicated for prophylactic or prolonged administration in otitis media at any age.

Administration and Dosage

➤*Maximum dose:* There are no well-established maximum doses for the approved indications according to the prescribing information.

➤*Adults:*

Urinary tract infections – 100 mg (10 mL) every 12 hours or 200 mg (20 mL) every 24 hours, each for 10 days.

➤*Children:*

Acute otitis media –

6 months of age and older: 5 mg/kg every 12 hours for 10 days.

Trimethoprim Oral Solution Dosing for Children 6 Months of Age or Older

Weight		Dose (every 12 hours)	
lb	kg	tsp	mL
11	5	0.5	2.5
22	10	1	5

TRIMETHOPRIM HYDROCHLORIDE — ORAL SOLUTION

Trimethoprim Oral Solution Dosing for Children 6 Months of Age or Older			
Weight		Dose (every 12 hours)	
lb	kg	tsp	mL
33	15	1.5	7.5
44	20	2	10
55	25	2.5	12.5
66	30	3	15
77	35	3.5	17.5
≥ 88	≥ 40	4	20

Off-label dosing –
Acute otitis media:
Urinary tract infection:

• *12 years of age and older* – 100 mg every 12 hours or 200 mg every 24 hours for 10 days.
• *Infants and children younger than 12 years of age* – 4 to 6 mg/kg every 24 hours divided every 12 hours for 10 days.

Mild/moderate pneumocystis carinii pneumonia:
• *12 years of age and older* – 5 mg/kg 3 times daily with dapsone for 21 days. See Dapsone and www.aidsinfo.nih.gov/contentfiles/Pediatric_OI.pdf for more information.

➤*Renal function impairment:*

CrCl of 15 to 30 mL/min – Give half the dose recommended for patients of the same age with healthy renal function.

CrCl less than 15 mL/min – Use is not recommended.

➤*Storage/Stability:* Store between 15° and 25°C (59° and 77°F). Dispense in tight, light-resistant glass or PET plastic containers.

Actions

➤*Pharmacology:* Trimethoprim blocks the production of tetrahydrofolic acid from dihydrofolic acid by binding to and reversibly inhibiting the required enzyme, dihydrofolate reductase. This binding is very much stronger for the bacterial enzyme than for the corresponding mammalian enzyme. Thus, trimethoprim selectively interferes with bacterial biosynthesis of nucleic acids and proteins.

➤*Pharmacokinetics:*

Absorption/Distribution – Trimethoprim is rapidly absorbed following oral administration. It exists in the blood as unbound, protein-bound and metabolized forms. Approximately 44% of trimethoprim is bound to plasma proteins.

Mean peak plasma concentrations of approximately 1 mcg/mL occur 1 to 4 hours after oral administration of a single 100 mg dose. A single 200 mg dose will result in plasma concentrations approximately twice as high. The mean half-life of trimethoprim is approximately 9 hours (range, 8 to 10 hours). However, patients with severely impaired renal function exhibit an increase in the half-life of trimethoprim, which requires either dosage regimen adjustment or not using the drug in such patients. During a 13-week study of trimethoprim tablets administered at a dosage of 50 mg 4 times daily, the mean minimum steady-state concentration of the drug was 1.1 mcg/mL. Steady-state concentrations were achieved within 2 to 3 days of chronic administration and were maintained throughout the experimental period.

Trimethoprim also passes the placental barrier and is excreted in breast milk.

Since normal vaginal and fecal flora are the source of most pathogens causing urinary tract infections, it is relevant to consider the distribution of trimethoprim into these sites. Concentrations of trimethoprim in vaginal secretions are consistently greater than those found simultaneously in the serum, being typically 1.6 times the concentrations of simultaneously obtained serum samples. Sufficient trimethoprim is excreted in the feces to markedly reduce or eliminate trimethoprim-susceptible organisms from the fecal flora. The dominant non-Enterobacteriaceae fecal organisms, *Bacteroides* spp. and *Lactobacillus* spp, are not susceptible to trimethoprim concentrations obtained with the recommended dosage.

Trimethoprim also concentrates into middle ear fluid (MEF) very efficiently. In a study in children aged 1 to 12 years, administration of a single 4 mg/kg dose resulted in a mean peak MEF concentration of 2 mcg/mL.

Metabolism – Ten percent to 20% of trimethoprim is metabolized, primarily in the liver; the remainder is excreted unchanged in the urine. The principal metabolites of trimethoprim are the 1- and 3-oxides and the 3′- and 4′-hydroxy derivatives. The free form is considered to be the therapeutically active form.

Excretion – Excretion of trimethoprim is primarily by the kidneys through glomerular filtration and tubular secretion. Urine concentrations of trimethoprim are considerably higher than are the concentrations in the blood. After a single oral dose of 100 mg, urine concentrations of trimethoprim ranged from 30 to 160 mcg/mL during the 0- to 4-hour period and declined to approximately 18 to 91 mcg/mL during the 8- to 24-hour period. A 200 mg single oral dose will result in trimethoprim urine concentrations approximately twice as high. After oral administration, 50% to 60% of trimethoprim is excreted in the urine within 24 hours, approximately 80% of this being unmetabolized trimethoprim.

➤*Microbiology:* Trimethoprim has been shown to be active against most strains of the following microorganisms, both in vitro and in clinical infections.

Aerobic gram-positive microorganisms – *Staphylococcus* species (coagulase-negative strains, including *S. saprophyticus*), *Streptococcus pneumoniae* (penicillin-susceptible strains).

Aerobic gram-negative microorganisms – *Enterobacter* species, *Escherichia coli*, *Haemophilus influenzae* (excluding beta-lactamase-negative, ampicillin-resistant strains), *Klebsiella pneumoniae*, *Proteus mirabilis*.

Moraxella catarrhalis isolates were found consistently resistant to trimethoprim.

Contraindications

Hypersensitivity to trimethoprim and in those with documented megaloblastic anemia due to folate deficiency.

Warnings/Precautions

➤*Hematologic effects:* Experience with trimethoprim alone is limited, but it has been reported rarely to interfere with hematopoiesis, especially when administered in large doses or for prolonged periods.

If any clinical signs of a blood disorder are noted in a patient receiving trimethoprim, obtain a complete blood count and discontinue the drug if a significant reduction in the count of any formed blood element is found.

The presence of clinical signs such as sore throat, fever, pallor, or purpura may be early indications of serious blood disorders.

➤*Folate disorders:* Give with caution to patients with possible folate deficiency. Folates may be administered concomitantly without interfering with the antibacterial action of trimethoprim.

➤*Renal/Hepatic function impairment:* Give with caution to patients with impaired renal or hepatic function.

➤*Pregnancy: Category C.* Trimethoprim has been shown to be teratogenic in the rat when given in doses 40 times the human dose. In some rabbit studies, the overall increase in fetal loss (dead and resorbed and malformed conceptuses) was associated with doses 6 times the human therapeutic dose.

While there are no large well-controlled studies on the use of trimethoprim in pregnant women, Brumfitt and Pursell, in a retrospective study, reported the outcome of 186 pregnancies during which the mother received either placebo or trimethoprim in combination with sulfamethoxazole. The incidence of congenital abnormalities was 4.5% (3 of 66) in those who received placebo and 3.3% (4 of 120) in those receiving trimethoprim plus sulfamethoxazole. There were no abnormalities in the 10 children whose mothers received the drug during the first trimester. In a separate survey, Brumfitt and Pursell also found no congenital abnormalities in 35 children whose mothers had received trimethoprim plus sulfamethoxazole at the time of conception or shortly thereafter.

Because trimethoprim may interfere with folic acid metabolism, use during pregnancy only if the potential benefit justifies the potential risk to the fetus.

➤*Lactation:* Trimethoprim is excreted in human milk. Because trimethoprim may interfere with folic acid metabolism, exercise caution when trimethoprim is administered to a nursing woman.

➤*Children:* The safety of trimethoprim has not been established in pediatric patients below the age of 2 months.

The effectiveness of trimethoprim solution in the treatment of acute otitis media has not been established in patients below the age of 6 months.

Drug Interactions

➤*Phenytoin:* Trimethoprim oral solution may inhibit the hepatic metabolism of phenytoin. Trimethoprim, given at a common clinical dosage, increased the phenytoin half-life by 51% and decreased the phenytoin metabolic clearance rate by 30%. When administering these drugs concurrently, one should be alert for possible excessive phenytoin effect.

➤*Drug/Lab test interactions:* Trimethoprim can interfere with a serum methotrexate assay as determined by the competitive binding protein technique (CBPA) when a bacterial dihydrofolate reductase is used as the binding protein. No interference occurs, however, if methotrexate is measured by a radioimmunoassay (RIA).

The presence of trimethoprim may also interfere with the Jaffé alkaline picrate reaction assay for creatinine resulting in overestimations of about 10% in the range of normal values.

Adverse Reactions

➤*Children (oral solution):*

Trimethoprim vs Sulfamethoxazole/Trimethoprim Adverse Reactions in Children		
Adverse Event	Trimethoprim oral solution (n = 310)	Sulfamethoxazole + trimethoprim oral solution (n = 197)
Dermatologic		
Rash	1.3%	6.1%
GI		
Diarrhea	4.2%	4.6%

TRIMETHOPRIM HYDROCHLORIDE — ORAL SOLUTION

Trimethoprim vs Sulfamethoxazole/Trimethoprim Adverse Reactions in Children		
Adverse Event	Trimethoprim oral solution (n = 310)	Sulfamethoxazole + trimethoprim oral solution (n = 197)
Vomiting	1.6%	1.5%
Miscellaneous		
Abdominal pain	< 1%	2.5%

Hematologic – An increase in lymphocytes and eosinophils was noted in some pediatric patients following treatment with trimethoprim oral solution or sulfamethoxazole and trimethoprim oral suspension.

➤*Other adverse reactions reported for trimethoprim:* In addition to the adverse events listed above which have been observed in pediatric patients receiving trimethoprim oral solution, the following adverse reactions and altered laboratory tests have been previously reported for trimethoprim and, therefore, may occur with trimethoprim therapy:

Dermatologic – Pruritus and exfoliative dermatitis. At the recommended adult dosage regimens of 100 mg twice daily or 200 mg daily, each for 10 days, the incidence of rash is 2.9% to 6.7%. In clinical studies which employed high doses of trimethoprim in adults, an elevated incidence of rash was noted. These rashes were maculopapular, morbilliform, pruritic, and generally mild to moderate, appearing 7 to 14 days after the initiation of therapy.

GI – Epigastric distress, glossitis, and nausea.

Hematologic – Leukopenia, megaloblastic anemia, methemoglobinemia, neutropenia, and thrombocytopenia.

Metabolic – Hyperkalemia, hyponatremia.

Miscellaneous – Elevation of serum transaminase and bilirubin, fever, and increases in blood urea nitrogen (BUN) and serum creatinine levels.

Overdosage

➤*Acute:*

Symptoms – Signs of acute overdosage with trimethoprim may appear following ingestion of 1 g or more of the drug and include bone marrow depression, confusion, dizziness, headaches, mental depression, nausea, and vomiting.

Treatment – Treatment consists of gastric lavage and general supportive measures. Acidification of the urine will increase renal elimination of trimethoprim. Peritoneal dialysis is not effective, and hemodialysis is only moderately effective in eliminating the drug.

➤*Chronic:*

Symptoms – Use of trimethoprim at high doses or for extended periods of time may cause bone marrow depression manifested as thrombocytopenia, leukopenia or megaloblastic anemia.

Treatment – If signs of bone marrow depression occur, discontinue trimethoprim, and give the patient leucovorin, 3 to 6 mg IM daily for 3 days, or as required to restore normal hematopoiesis.

MISCELLANEOUS ANTI-INFECTIVES/ANTISEPTICS

METHYLENE BLUE

For complete and comparative prescribing information, see the Methylene blue oral monograph in the Endocrine and Metabolic Agents chapter.

FOSFOMYCIN TROMETHAMINE

Rx	**Monurol** (Forest)	Granules: 3 g	In single-dose packets.

FOSFOMYCIN TROMETHAMINE — ORAL

Indications

➤*Uncomplicated urinary tract infections:* For the treatment of uncomplicated urinary tract infections (acute cystitis) in women due to susceptible strains of *Escherichia coli* and *Enterococcus faecalis*. Fosfomycin tromethamine is not indicated for the treatment of pyelonephritis or perinephric abscess.

If persistence or reappearance of bacteriuria occurs after treatment with fosfomycin, other therapeutic agents should be selected.

Administration and Dosage

➤*General dosing considerations:* Fosfomycin should not be taken in its dry form. Always mix fosfomycin with water before ingesting. (See Preparation for administration.)

➤*Adults:*

Uncomplicated urinary tract infections –
Women: 3 g (1 sachet) as a single dose.

➤*Preparation for administration:* Pour the entire contents of a single-dose sachet of fosfomycin into 90 to 120 mL of water (½ cup) and stir to dissolve. Do not use hot water. Fosfomycin should be taken immediately after dissolving in water.

➤*Administration:* Fosfomycin should be taken orally. Fosfomycin may be taken with or without food.

➤*Storage/Stability:* Store at 15° to 30°C (59° to 86°F).

Actions

➤*Pharmacokinetics:*

Absorption – Fosfomycin tromethamine is rapidly absorbed following oral administration and converted to the free acid, fosfomycin. Absolute oral bioavailability under fasting conditions is 37%. After a single 3 g dose of fosfomycin tromethamine, the mean (± 1 SD) maximum serum concentration (C_{max}) achieved was 26.1 (± 9.1) mcg/mL within 2 hours. The oral bioavailability of fosfomycin is reduced to 30% under fed conditions. Following a single 3 g oral dose of fosfomycin tromethamine with a high-fat meal, the mean C_{max} achieved was 17.6 (± 4.4) mcg/mL within 4 hours. Cimetidine does not affect the pharmacokinetics of fosfomycin when coadministered with fosfomycin tromethamine. Metoclopramide lowers the serum concentrations and urinary excretion of fosfomycin when coadministered with fosfomycin.

Distribution – The mean apparent steady-state volume of distribution (Vss) is 136.1 (± 44.1) L following oral administration of fosfomycin tromethamine. Fosfomycin is not bound to plasma proteins. Fosfomycin is distributed to the kidneys, bladder wall, prostate, and seminal vesicles. Following a 50 mg/kg dose of fosfomycin to patients undergoing urological surgery for bladder carcinoma, the mean concentration of fosfomycin in the bladder, taken at a distance from the neoplastic site, was 18 mcg/g of tissue at 3 hours after dosing. Fosfomycin has been shown to cross the placental barrier in animals and man.

Excretion – Fosfomycin is excreted unchanged in both urine and feces. Following oral administration of fosfomycin tromethamine, the mean total body clearance (CL_{TB}) and mean renal clearance (CL_R) of fosfomycin were 16.9 (± 3.5) L/hr and 6.3 (± 1.7) L/hr, respectively. Approximately 38% of a 3 g dose of fosfomycin tromethamine is recovered from urine, and 18% is recovered from feces. Following intravenous administration, the mean CL_{TB} and mean CL_R of fosfomycin were 6.1 (± 1) L/hr and 5.5 (± 1.2) L/hr, respectively.

A mean urine fosfomycin concentration of 706 (± 466) mcg/mL was attained within 2 to 4 hours after a single oral 3 g dose of fosfomycin tromethamine under fasting conditions. The mean urinary concentration of fosfomycin was 10 mcg/mL in samples collected 72 to 84 hours following a single oral dose of fosfomycin tromethamine.

Following a 3 g dose of fosfomycin tromethamine administered with a high-fat meal, a mean urine fosfomycin concentration of 537 (± 252) mcg/mL was attained within 6 to 8 hours. Although the rate of urinary excretion of fosfomycin was reduced under fed conditions, the cumulative amount of fosfomycin excreted in the urine was the same, 1118 (± 201) mg (fed) vs 1140 (± 238) mg (fasting). Further, urinary concentrations greater than or equal to 100 mcg/mL were maintained for the same duration, 26 hours, indicating that fosfomycin tromethamine can be taken without regard to food.

Following oral administration of fosfomycin tromethamine, the mean half-life for elimination (t½) is 5.7 (± 2.8) hours.

Special populations –
Renal function impairment: In 5 anuric patients undergoing hemodialysis, the t½ of fosfomycin during hemodialysis was 40 hours. In patients with varying degrees of renal impairment (creatinine clearances varying from 54 mL/min to 7 mL/min), the t½ of fosfomycin increased from 11 hours to 50 hours. The percent of fosfomycin recovered in urine decreased from 32% to 11% indicating that renal impairment significantly decreases the excretion of fosfomycin.

➤*Microbiology:* Fosfomycin (the active component of fosfomycin tromethamine) has in vitro activity against a broad range of gram-positive and gram-negative aerobic microorganisms that are associated with uncomplicated urinary tract infections. Fosfomycin is bactericidal in urine at therapeutic doses. The bactericidal action of fosfomycin is due to its inactivation of the enzyme enolpyruvyl transferase, thereby irreversibly blocking the condensation of uridine diphosphate-N-acetylglucosamine with p-enolpyruvate, one of the first steps in bacterial cell wall synthesis. It also reduces adherence of bacteria to uroepithelial cells.

Fosfomycin has been shown to be active against most strains of the following microorganisms, both in vitro and in clinical infections.

Aerobic gram-positive microorganisms – *Enterococcus faecalis.*

Aerobic gram-negative microorganisms – *Escherichia coli.*

Contraindications

Hypersensitivity to the drug.

Warnings/Precautions

➤*Acute cystitis:* Do not use more than 1 single dose of fosfomycin tromethamine to treat a single episode of acute cystitis. Repeated daily doses of fosfomycin tromethamine did not improve the clinical success or

FOSFOMYCIN TROMETHAMINE — ORAL

microbiological eradication rates compared to single dose therapy, but did increase the incidence of adverse events.

➤*Pregnancy:* *Category B.* When administered intramuscularly as the sodium salt at a dose of 1 g to pregnant women, fosfomycin crosses the placental barrier. Fosfomycin crosses the placental barrier of rats; it does not produce teratogenic effects in pregnant rats at dosages as high as 1000 mg/kg/day (approximately 9 and 1.4 times the human dose based on body weight and mg/m^2, respectively). When administered to pregnant female rabbits at dosages as high as 1000 mg/kg/day (approximately 9 and 2.7 times the human dose based on body weight and mg/m^2, respectively), fetotoxicities were observed. However, these toxicities were seen at maternally toxic doses and were considered to be due to the sensitivity of the rabbit to changes in the intestinal microflora resulting from the antibiotic administration. There are, however, no adequate and well-controlled studies in pregnant women. Because animal reproduction studies are not always predictive of human response, this drug should be used during pregnancy only if clearly needed.

➤*Lactation:* It is not known whether fosfomycin tromethamine is excreted in human milk. Because many drugs are excreted in human milk and because of the potential for serious adverse reactions in nursing infants from fosfomycin, a decision should be made whether to discontinue nursing or the drug, taking into account the importance of the drug to the mother.

➤*Children:* Safety and efficacy in children age 12 years and under have not been established in adequate and well-controlled studies.

➤*Elderly:* In general, dose selection for an elderly patient should be cautious, starting at the low end of the dosing range, reflecting the greater frequency of decreased hepatic, renal, or cardiac function, and of concomitant disease or other drug therapy.

➤*Lab test abnormalities:* Significant laboratory changes reported in US clinical trials of fosfomycin tromethamine without regard to drug relationship include increased eosinophil count, increased or decreased WBC count, increased bilirubin, increased ALT, increased AST, increased alkaline phosphatase, decreased hematocrit, decreased hemoglobin, increased and decreased platelet count. The changes were generally transient and were not clinically significant.

➤*Monitoring:* Urine specimens for culture and susceptibility testing should be obtained before and after completion of therapy.

Drug Interactions

➤*Metoclopramide:* When coadministered with fosfomycin, metoclopramide, a drug that increases gastrointestinal motility, lowers the serum concentration and urinary excretion of fosfomycin. Other drugs that increase gastrointestinal motility may produce similar effects.

➤*Cimetidine:* Cimetidine does not affect the pharmacokinetics of fosfomycin when coadministered with fosfomycin tromethamine.

Adverse Reactions

➤*Adverse reactions from clinical trials:*

Drug-Related Adverse Reactions (%) In Fosfomycin and Comparator Populations (> 1%)				
Adverse reactions	Fosfomycin (n = 1233)	Nitrofurantoin (n = 374)	Trimethoprim/ sulfamethoxazole (n = 428)	Ciprofloxacin (n = 445)
Diarrhea	9%	6.4%	2.3%	3.1%
Vaginitis	5.5%	5.3%	4.7%	6.3%
Nausea	4.1%	7.2%	8.6%	3.4%
Headache	3.9%	5.9%	5.4%	3.4%
Dizziness	1.3%	1.9%	2.3%	2.2%
Asthenia	1.1%	0.3%	0.5%	0%
Dyspepsia	1.1%	2.1%	0.7%	1.1%

➤*Adverse events in the study population:* In clinical trials, the following adverse events occurring in the study population regardless of drug relationship:

CNS – Headache (10.3%); nervousness, somnolence, paresthesia, insomnia, migraine (less than 1%).

Dermatologic – Rash (1.4%); skin disorder, pruritus (less than 1%).

GI – Diarrhea (10.4%); nausea (5.2%); dyspepsia (1.8%); abnormal stools, dry mouth, flatulence, anorexia, constipation, vomiting (less than 1%).

GU – Vaginitis (7.6%); dysmenorrhea (2.6%); hematuria, menstrual disorder, dysuria (less than 1%).

Respiratory – Rhinitis (4.5%); pharyngitis (2.5%).

Miscellaneous – Back pain (3%); dizziness (2.3%); abdominal pain (2.2%); pain (2.2%); asthenia (1.7%); myalgia, ear disorder, fever, flu syndrome, infection, lymphadenopathy, AST increase (less than 1%). One patient developed unilateral optic neuritis, an event considered possibly related to fosfomycin therapy.

➤*Postmarketing:* Serious adverse events from the marketing experience with fosfomycin tromethamine outside of the United States have been rarely reported and include angioedema, aplastic anemia, asthma (exacerbation), cholestatic jaundice, hepatic necrosis, and toxic megacolon.

Overdosage

➤*Symptoms:* In acute toxicology studies, oral administration of high doses of fosfomycin tromethamine up to 5 g/kg were well-tolerated in mice and rats, produced transient and minor incidences of watery stool in rabbits, and produced diarrhea with anorexia in dogs occurring 2 to 3 days after single dose administration. These doses represent 50 to 125 times the human therapeutic dose.

➤*Treatment:* There have been no reported cases of overdosage. In the event of overdosage, treatment should be symptomatic and supportive.

Patient Information

Fosfomycin tromethamine can be taken with or without food. Symptoms should improve in 2 to 3 days after taking fosfomycin; if not improved, the patient should contact her healthcare provider.

ANTIBIOTIC COMBINATIONS

SULFAMETHOXAZOLE/TRIMETHOPRIM (Co-Trimoxazole; TMP-SMZ)

Rx	**Sulfamethoxazole/Trimethoprim** (Various, eg, Moore, Mutual)	**Tablets; oral:** sulfamethoxazole 400 mg and trimethoprim 80 mg	In 100s and 500s.
Rx	**Bactrim** (AR Scientific)		(Bactrim). White, round, scored. In 100s and 500s.
Rx	**Septra** (Monarch)		(M052). Pink, round, scored. In 100s.
Rx	**Sulfamethoxazole/Trimethoprim DS** (Various, eg, Geneva, Moore, Mutual)	**Tablets, double-strength; oral:** sulfamethoxazole 800 mg and trimethoprim 160 mg	In 100s and 500s.
Rx	**Bactrim DS** (AR Scientific)		(Bactrim DS). White, oval, scored. In 100s and 500s.
Rx	**Septra DS** (Monarch)		(M053). Pink, oval, scored. In 20s, 100s, and 500s.
Rx	**Sulfamethoxazole/Trimethoprim** (Hi Tech)	**Suspension; oral:** sulfamethoxazole 200 mg and trimethoprim 40 mg per 5 mL	Alcohol 0.26%, methylparaben, saccharin, sorbitol. Grape and cherry flavors. In 473 mL.
Rx	**Sulfatrim** (Activis MidAtlantic)		Alcohol < 0.5 %, parabens, saccharin, sucrose. Fruit-licorice and cherry flavors. In 473 mL.
Rx	**Trimethoprim/Sulfamethoxazole** (Various, eg, Teva)	**Injection, solution:** sulfamethoxazole 80 mg and trimethoprim 16 mg per mL	May contain alcohol, benzyl alcohol, and/or metabisulfite. In 5 mL single-use vials and 10 and 30 mL multiple-use vials.

SULFAMETHOXAZOLE/TRIMETHOPRIM — ORAL

Indications

Sulfamethoxazole and Trimethoprim Oral Indications[a]			
Indication	Adults	Children	Organism
FDA-approved uses			
Acute exacerbations of chronic bronchitis	X		*Haemophilus influenzae, Streptococcus pneumoniae*
Acute otitis media[b]		X	*H. influenzae, S. pneumoniae*
Enteritis	X	X	*Shigella flexneri, Shigella sonnei*
PCP prophylaxis[c]	X	X	*P. carinii*
PCP treatment	X	X	*P. carinii*
Traveler's diarrhea	X		Enterotoxigenic *Escherichia coli*
UTIs[d]	X	X	*E. coli, Klebsiella* and *Enterobacter* species, *Morganella morganii, Proteus mirabilis, Proteus vulgaris*
Off-label uses[e]			
Acute and chronic bacterial prostatitis	X		
Cholera and salmonella-type infections and nocardiosis	X		*Vibrio cholerae, Salmonella sp., Nocardia sp.*
Community-acquired pneumonia	X[f]		Methicillin-resistant *Staphylococcus aureus*
Prevention of recurrent UTIs in women	X		
Sinusitis	X[g]	X[g]	
Skin and soft-tissue infections	X	X	Methicillin-sensitive *S. aureus* or methicillin-resistant *S. aureus*

[a] FDA = Food and Drug Administration; PCP = *Pneumocystis carinii* pneumonia; UTI = urinary tract infection.
[b] Not indicated for prophylactic or prolonged administration in otitis media at any age.
[c] Prophylaxis against PCP in individuals who are immunosuppressed and considered to be at increased risk.
[d] Treat initial uncomplicated UTIs with a single antibacterial agent. Parenteral therapy is indicated in severe or complicated infections when oral therapy is not feasible.
[e] Low-dose sulfamethoxazole and trimethoprim has been studied in the prophylaxis of neutropenic patients with *P. carinii* infections or leukemia patients to reduce the incidence of gram-negative rod bacteremia. Prophylaxis with sulfamethoxazole 1,600 mg and trimethoprim 320 mg per day appears beneficial in reducing the incidence of bacterial infection following renal transplant and may provide protection against PCP.
[f] Good documentation.
[g] Fair documentation.

➤*Off-label uses:*

Community-acquired pneumonia – [1] = Good documentation. Infectious Diseases Society of America/American Thoracic Society guidelines on the management of community-acquired pneumonia (CAP) in adults recommend that sulfamethoxazole/trimethoprim may be useful in treating CAP suspected to be caused by methicillin-resistant *Staphylococcus aureus*. This medication could be chosen to reduce the risk of vancomycin resistance developing and because it is an inexpensive oral therapy.

Granuloma inguinale (donovanosis) – [1] = Good documentation. Centers for Disease Control and Prevention guidelines recommend sulfamethoxazole/trimethoprim as an alternative regimen in nonpregnant persons for treatment of granuloma inguinale when doxycycline is not appropriate. World Health Organization guidelines provide additional support for this recommendation.

Sinusitis – Evidence-based guidelines recommend that sulfamethoxazole/trimethoprim may be used as a first-line agent in the treatment of sinusitis in patients who are allergic to penicillin. Resistance to sulfamethoxazole/trimethoprim may be seen when treating sinusitis. For patients in whom resistance is likely, other treatments are recommended.

Sinusitis (adults): [2] = Fair documentation.

Sinusitis (children/adolescents): [2] = Fair documentation.

Administration and Dosage

➤*General dosing considerations:* Maintain adequate fluid intake to prevent crystalluria and stone formation.

Dosage adjustment required in patients with renal impairment (see Renal Function Impairment).

➤*Adults:*

Acute exacerbations of chronic bronchitis – Sulfamethoxazole 800 mg and trimethoprim 160 mg every 12 hours for 14 days.

Enteritis – Sulfamethoxazole 800 mg and trimethoprim 160 mg every 12 hours for 5 days.

P. carinii pneumonia –

Prophylactic dosage: Sulfamethoxazole 800 mg and trimethoprim 160 mg every 24 hours. (See also Off-Label Dosing.)

Treatment dosage: Sulfamethoxazole 75 to 100 mg/kg/day and trimethoprim 15 to 20 mg/kg in equally divided doses every 6 hours for 14 to 21 days.

Traveler's diarrhea – Sulfamethoxazole 800 mg and trimethoprim 160 mg every 12 hours for 5 days.

Urinary tract infections – Sulfamethoxazole 800 mg and trimethoprim 160 mg every 12 hours for 10 to 14 days.

Off-label dosing –

Acute and chronic bacterial prostatitis: Sulfamethoxazole 800 mg and trimethoprim 160 mg twice daily up to 12 weeks.

Community-acquired pneumonia: [1] = Good documentation. Empirically, sulfamethoxazole 800 mg and trimethoprim 160 mg twice daily for 10 to 14 days.

Granuloma inguinale (donovanosis): [1] = Good documentation. Trimethoprim 160 mg and sulfamethoxazole 800 mg (one double-strength tablet) orally twice a day for at least 3 weeks. Treatment should continue until all lesions have completely healed.

Nocardiosis: 15 mg/kg/day (based on trimethoprim) in 2 to 4 divided doses for 3 to 4 weeks, then decrease dosage to 10 mg/kg/day (based on trimethoprim) in 2 to 4 divided doses for 3 to 6 months.

P. carinii pneumonia:

• *Prophylactic dosage* – Sulfamethoxazole 400 mg and trimethoprim 80 mg orally every 24 hours or sulfamethoxazole 800 mg and trimethoprim 160 mg orally 3 times per week.

Prevention of recurrent urinary tract infections in women: Sulfamethoxazole 200 mg and trimethoprim 40 mg daily at bedtime, a minimum of 3 times weekly or postcoitally.

Sinusitis: [2] = Fair documentation. Sulfamethoxazole 800 mg and trimethoprim 160 mg twice daily for 3 to 14 days.

Skin and soft-tissue infections: Sulfamethoxazole 800 to 1,600 mg and trimethoprim 160 to 320 mg orally twice daily.

➤*Children:*

2 months of age and older –

Acute otitis media: Sulfamethoxazole 40 mg/kg and trimethoprim 8 mg/kg per day in 2 divided doses every 12 hours for 10 days.

Enteritis: Sulfamethoxazole 40 mg/kg and trimethoprim 8 mg/kg per day given in 2 divided doses every 12 hours for 5 days.

P. carinii pneumonia:

• *Prophylactic dosage* –

Usual dosage: Sulfamethoxazole 750 mg/m^2 with trimethoprim 150 mg/m^2 per day in equally divided doses twice a day, on 3 consecutive days per week. (See also Off-Label Dosing.)

Maximum dose: The total daily dose should not exceed sulfamethoxazole 1,600 mg and trimethoprim 320 mg.

Sulfamethoxazole and Trimethoprim Oral Prophylactic Dosage in Children With *P. carinii* Pneumonia		
	Dose every 12 hours	
Body surface area	Suspension	Tablets
0.26 m^2	2.5 mL	—
0.53 m^2	5 mL	½
1.06 m^2	10 mL	1

• *Treatment dosage* – Sulfamethoxazole 75 to 100 mg/kg and trimethoprim 15 to 20 mg/kg per day in divided doses every 6 hours for 14 to 21 days.

Sulfamethoxazole and Trimethoprim Oral Treatment Dosage in Children With *P. carinii* Pneumonia[a]		
	Dose every 6 hours	
Weight (kg)	Suspension	Tablets
8	5 mL	
16	10 mL	1
24	15 mL	1½
32	20 mL	2 or 1 double-strength tablet
40	25 mL	2½
48	30 mL	3 or 1½ double-strength tablet
64	40 mL	4 or 2 double-strength tablets
80	50 mL	5 or 2½ double-strength tablets

[a] Dosages are for the upper limit of the dosing range. For the lower limit, administer 75% of the dose.

Urinary tract infections: Sulfamethoxazole 40 mg/kg and trimethoprim 8 mg/kg per day given orally in 2 divided doses every 12 hours for 10 days.

Off-label dosing –

P. carinii pneumonia:

• *Prophylactic dosage* – Sulfamethoxazole 750 mg/m^2 and trimethoprim 150 mg/m^2 per day in a single daily dose for 3 consecutive days per week; sulfamethoxazole 750 mg/m^2 and trimethoprim 150 mg/m^2 per day in equally divided doses twice a day; or sulfamethoxazole 750 mg/m^2 and trimethoprim 150 mg/m^2 per day in equally divided doses twice a day 3 times per week on alternate days.

SULFAMETHOXAZOLE/TRIMETHOPRIM — ORAL

Prevention of urinary tract infection (based on trimethoprim): 2 to 4 mg/kg once daily.

Sinusitis: [2] = Fair documentation. Pediatric dosages outlined in recent guidelines for the management of sinusitis are substantially higher than dosages cited in other drug information sources. Standard pediatric references include the following dosing for children older than 2 months of age: For minor to moderate infections, 8 to 12 mg/kg/day (based on the trimethoprim component) given in 2 divided doses. For severe infections, 20 mg/kg daily given in divided doses every 6 to 8 hours.

Skin and soft-tissue infections: 8 to 12 mg/kg (based on the trimethoprim component) in equally divided doses every 12 hours.

➤*Elderly:* Make appropriate dosage adjustments for impaired kidney function (see Renal Function Impairment).

➤*Renal function impairment:*

Recommendations for dosage adjustment – According to the manufacturer's prescribing information for sulfamethoxazole and trimethoprim in patients with renal impairment, the dose should be adjusted based on the following recommendations:

Creatinine clearance 15 to 30 mL/min: ½ the usual regimen.

Creatinine clearance less than 15 mL/min: Not recommended.

Alternative dosing regimen –

Creatinine clearance 30 to 50 mL/min: Trimethoprim 5 to 7.5 mg/kg per dose every 8 hours.

Creatinine clearance 10 to 29 mL/min: Trimethoprim 5 to 10 mg/kg per dose every 12 hours.

Creatinine clearance less than 10 mL/min: Not recommended, but if used: trimethoprim 5 to 10 mg/kg per dose every 24 hours.

Hemodialysis: Not recommended, but if used: trimethoprim 5 to 10 mg/kg per dose every 24 hours.

Peritoneal dialysis: Not recommended, but if used: trimethoprim 5 to 10 mg/kg per dose every 24 hours.

Continuous renal replacement therapy: Trimethoprim 5 to 7.5 mg/kg per dose every 8 hours.

➤*Administration:* Instruct patient to take each oral dose with a full glass of water. Shake suspension well before using. Maintain adequate fluid intake.

Children – The following table is a guide for the dose of sulfamethoxazole and trimethoprim in the treatment of acute otitis media, enteritis, or UTI in children.

Sulfamethoxazole and Trimethoprim Oral Dosage Guidelines in Children 2 Months of Age and Older

Body weight (kg)	Dose every 12 hours: Suspension	Dose every 12 hours: Tablets
10	5 mL	—
20	10 mL	1
30	15 mL	1½
40	20 mL	2 (or 1 double-strength tablet)

➤*Storage/Stability:* Store at 15° to 25°C (59° to 77°F). Protect from light.

Actions

➤*Pharmacology:* Sulfamethoxazole inhibits bacterial synthesis of dihydrofolic acid by competing with para-aminobenzoic acid. Trimethoprim blocks the production of tetrahydrofolic acid from dihydrofolic acid by binding to and reversibly inhibiting the required enzyme, dihydrofolate reductase. Thus, sulfamethoxazole and trimethoprim block 2 consecutive steps in the biosynthesis of nucleic acids and proteins essential to many bacteria.

➤*Pharmacokinetics:*

Absorption – Sulfamethoxazole and trimethoprim is rapidly absorbed following oral administration. Peak blood levels for the individual components occur 1 to 4 hours after oral administration. Detectable amounts of sulfamethoxazole and trimethoprim are present in the blood 24 hours after drug administration. During administration of sulfamethoxazole 800 mg and trimethoprim 160 mg twice daily, the mean steady-state plasma concentration of trimethoprim was 1.72 mg/mL. The steady-state mean plasma levels of free and total sulfamethoxazole were 57.4 mg/mL and 68 mg/mL, respectively. These steady-state levels were achieved after 3 days of drug administration.

Distribution – Both sulfamethoxazole and trimethoprim exist in the blood as unbound, protein-bound, and metabolized forms; sulfamethoxazole also exists as the conjugated form. Approximately 70% of sulfamethoxazole and 44% of trimethoprim are bound to plasma proteins. The presence of sulfamethoxazole 10 mg percent in plasma decreases the protein binding of trimethoprim by an insignificant degree; trimethoprim does not influence the protein binding of sulfamethoxazole. Sulfamethoxazole and trimethoprim distribute to sputum, vaginal fluid, and middle ear fluid; trimethoprim also distributes to bronchial secretion, and both pass the placental barrier and are excreted in breast milk.

Metabolism – The metabolism of sulfamethoxazole occurs predominately by N_4-acetylation, although the glucuronide conjugate has been identified. The principal metabolites of trimethoprim are the 1- and 3-oxides and the 3′- and 4′-hydroxy derivatives. The free forms of sulfamethoxazole and trimethoprim are considered to be the therapeutically active forms.

Excretion – The mean serum half-lives of sulfamethoxazole and trimethoprim are 10 and 8 to 10 hours, respectively. Excretion of sulfamethoxazole and trimethoprim is primarily by the kidneys through glomerular filtration and tubular secretion. Urine concentrations of sulfamethoxazole and trimethoprim are considerably higher than are the concentrations in the blood. The average percentage of the dose recovered in urine from 0 to 72 hours after a single oral dose is 84.5% for total sulfonamide and 66.8% for free trimethoprim. Thirty percent of the total sulfonamide is excreted as free sulfamethoxazole, with the remaining as N_4-acetylated metabolite. When administered together, neither sulfamethoxazole nor trimethoprim affects the urinary excretion pattern of the other.

Special populations –

Renal function impairment: Patients with severely impaired renal function exhibit an increase in the half-lives of sulfamethoxazole and trimethoprim, requiring dosage regimen adjustment.

Elderly: After normalizing by body weight, the apparent total body clearance of trimethoprim was an average of 19% lower in elderly subjects compared with younger adult subjects.

➤*Microbiology:*

Resistance – In vitro studies have shown that bacterial resistance develops more slowly with sulfamethoxazole and trimethoprim than with either sulfamethoxazole or trimethoprim alone.

Susceptible organisms – In vitro serial dilution tests have shown that the spectrum of antibacterial activity of sulfamethoxazole and trimethoprim includes the common urinary tract pathogens with the exception of *Pseudomonas aeruginosa*. The following organisms are usually susceptible: *E. coli* (including susceptible enterotoxigenic strains implicated in traveler's diarrhea), *Klebsiella* species, *Enterobacter* species, *M. morganii*, *P. mirabilis*, and indole-positive *Proteus* species, including *P. vulgaris*.

The usual spectrum of antimicrobial activity of sulfamethoxazole and trimethoprim includes bacterial pathogens isolated from middle ear exudate and from bronchial secretions (*H. influenzae*, including ampicillin-resistant strains, and *S. pneumoniae*), and enterotoxigenic strains of *E. coli* causing bacterial gastroenteritis. *S. flexneri* and *S. sonnei* are also usually susceptible.

Sulfamethoxazole and trimethoprim have also been shown to be active against *P. carinii*.

Contraindications

Known hypersensitivity to trimethoprim or sulfonamides; documented megaloblastic anemia due to folate deficiency; pregnant patients; breastfeeding mothers; children younger than 2 months of age; marked hepatic damage; severe renal insufficiency when renal function status cannot be monitored.

Warnings/Precautions

➤*Severe reactions:* Fatalities associated with the administration of sulfonamides, although rare, have occurred because of severe reactions, including agranulocytosis, aplastic anemia, fulminant hepatic necrosis, Stevens-Johnson syndrome, toxic epidermal necrolysis, and other blood dyscrasias. Discontinue sulfamethoxazole and trimethoprim at the first appearance of skin rash or any sign of adverse reaction.

Clinical signs such as arthralgia, cough, fever, jaundice, pallor, purpura, rash, shortness of breath, or sore throat may be early indications of serious reactions. In rare instances, a skin rash may be followed by more severe reactions such as hepatic necrosis, serious blood disorder, Stevens- Johnson syndrome, or toxic epidermal necrolysis. Perform complete blood cell counts frequently in patients receiving sulfonamides.

➤*Respiratory effects:* Cough, pulmonary infiltrates, and shortness of breath are hypersensitivity reactions of the respiratory tract that have been reported in association with sulfonamide treatment.

➤*Group A beta-hemolytic streptococci:* Do not use sulfamethoxazole and trimethoprim for the treatment of group A beta-hemolytic streptococcal infections. In an established infection they will not eradicate the streptococcus and, therefore, will not prevent sequelae, such as rheumatic fever. Clinical studies have documented that patients with group A beta-hemolytic streptococcal tonsillopharyngitis have a greater incidence of bacteriologic failure when treated with this combination than do those patients treated with penicillin, as evidenced by failure to eradicate this organism from the tonsillopharyngeal area.

➤*Clostridium difficile–associated diarrhea: C. difficile*–associated diarrhea has been reported with use of nearly all antibacterial agents, including sulfamethoxazole and trimethoprim, and may range in severity from mild diarrhea to fatal colitis. Therefore, it is important to consider this diagnosis in patients who present with diarrhea subsequent to the administration of antibacterial agents. Treatment with antibacterial agents alters the healthy flora of the colon leading to overgrowth of *C. difficile*. Studies indicate that a toxin produced by *C. difficile* is one primary cause of antibiotic-associated colitis.

C. difficile produces toxins A and B, which contribute to the development of *C. difficile*–associated diarrhea. Hypertoxin-producing strains of *C. difficile* cause increased morbidity and mortality because these infections can be refractory to antimicrobial therapy and may require colectomy. *C. difficile*–associated diarrhea must be considered in all patients who present with diarrhea following antibiotic use.

Carefully obtaining a medical history is necessary because *C. difficile*–associated diarrhea has been reported to occur over 2 months after the use of antibacterial agents.

If *C. difficile*–associated diarrhea is suspected or confirmed, ongoing antibiotic use not directed against *C. difficile* may need to be discontinued. Institute appropriate fluid and electrolyte management, protein supplementation, antibiotic treatment of *C. difficile*, and surgical evaluation as clinically indicated.

SULFAMETHOXAZOLE/TRIMETHOPRIM — ORAL

➤*Administration:* During treatment, ensure adequate fluid intake and urinary output to prevent crystalluria. Patients who are "slow acetylators" may be more prone to idiosyncratic reactions to sulfonamides.

➤*Hematologic effects:* Hematologic changes indicative of folic acid deficiency may occur in elderly patients or in patients with preexisting folic acid deficiency or kidney failure. These effects are reversible by folinic acid therapy.

➤*Hyperkalemia:* A high dosage of trimethoprim, as used in patients with PCP, induces a progressive but reversible increase of serum potassium concentrations in a substantial number of patients. Even treatment with recommended doses may cause hyperkalemia when trimethoprim is administered to patients with underlying disorders of potassium metabolism, with renal insufficiency, or if drugs known to induce hyperkalemia are given concomitantly. Close monitoring of serum potassium is warranted in these patients.

➤*Hypoglycemia:* Cases of hypoglycemia in nondiabetic patients treated with sulfamethoxazole and trimethoprim are seen rarely, usually occurring after a few days of therapy. Patients with renal dysfunction, liver disease, malnutrition, or those receiving high doses of sulfamethoxazole and trimethoprim are particularly at risk.

➤*Phenylketonuria:* Trimethoprim has been noted to impair phenylalanine metabolism, but this is if no significance in phenylketonuric patients on appropriate dietary restriction.

➤*Drug-resistent bacteria:* Prescribing sulfamethoxazole and trimethoprim in the absence of a proven or strongly suspected bacterial infection or a prophylactic indication is unlikely to provide benefit to the patient and increases the risk of the development of drug-resistant bacteria.

➤*AIDS:* Patients with AIDS may not tolerate or respond to sulfamethoxazole and trimethoprim in the same manner as patients without AIDS. The incidence of adverse reactions, particularly rash, fever, leukopenia, and elevated aminotransferase (transaminase) values, with sulfamethoxazole and trimethoprim therapy in patients with AIDS who are being treated for PCP has been reported to be greatly increased compared with the incidence normally associated with the use of sulfamethoxazole and trimethoprim in patients without AIDS. The incidence of hyperkalemia and hyponatremia appears to be increased with patients with AIDS receiving sulfamethoxazole and trimethoprim. Adverse effects are generally less severe in patients receiving sulfamethoxazole and trimethoprim for prophylaxis. A history of mild intolerance to sulfamethoxazole and trimethoprim in patients with AIDS does not appear to predict intolerance of subsequent secondary prophylaxis. However, if a patient develops skin rash or any sign of adverse reaction, reevaluate therapy with sulfamethoxazole and trimethoprim.

The concomitant use of leucovorin with sulfamethoxazole and trimethoprim for the acute treatment of PCP in patients with HIV infection was associated with increased rates of treatment failure and morbidity in a placebo-controlled study.

➤*Renal function impairment:* Use with caution. Dosage adjustments are required (see Administration and Dosage). Contraindicated in severe renal insufficiency when renal function status cannot be monitored.

➤*Hepatic function impairment:* Use with caution. Contraindicated in marked hepatic damage.

➤*Special risk:* Give sulfamethoxazole and trimethoprim with caution to patients with possible folate deficiency (eg, elderly patients; chronic alcoholism; patients receiving anticonvulsant therapy; patients with malabsorption syndrome, porphyria, or thyroid dysfunction; patients in malnutrition states) and to those with severe allergies or bronchial asthma. In glucose-6-phosphate dehydrogenase deficient individuals, hemolysis may occur. This reaction is frequently dose-related.

➤*Pregnancy: Category C.* In rats, oral doses of sulfamethoxazole 533 mg/kg or trimethoprim 200 mg/kg produced teratological effects manifested mainly as cleft palates. The highest dose that did not cause cleft palates in rats was sulfamethoxazole 512 mg/kg or trimethoprim 192 mg/kg when administered separately. In 2 studies in rats, no teratology was observed when sulfamethoxazole 512 mg/kg was used in combination with trimethoprim 128 mg/kg. In 1 study, however, cleft palates were observed in 1 litter out of 9 when sulfamethoxazole 355 mg/kg was used in combination with trimethoprim 88 mg/kg.

In some rabbit studies, an overall increase in fetal loss (dead and resorbed and malformed conceptuses) was associated with doses of trimethoprim 6 times the human therapeutic dose.

While there are no large, well-controlled studies on the use of sulfamethoxazole and trimethoprim in pregnant women, a retrospective study reported the outcome of 186 pregnancies during which the mother received either placebo or sulfamethoxazole and trimethoprim. The incidence of congenital abnormalities was 4.5% in those who received placebo and 3.3% in those receiving sulfamethoxazole and trimethoprim. There were no abnormalities in the 10 children whose mothers received the drug during the first trimester. In a separate survey, there were no congenital abnormalities in 35 children whose mothers had received oral sulfamethoxazole and trimethoprim at the time of conception or shortly thereafter.

Trimethoprim (molecular weight approximately 290) crosses the placenta, producing similar levels in fetal and maternal serum and in amniotic fluid. Using an in vitro perfused human cotyledon, trimethoprim and sulfamethoxazole were shown to cross the placenta. Because sulfamethoxazole and trimethoprim may interfere with folic acid metabolism, use this product during pregnancy only if the potential benefit justifies the potential risk to the fetus.

➤*Lactation:* Sulfamethoxazole and trimethoprim is contraindicated in breast-feeding mothers because sulfonamides are excreted in breast milk and may cause kernicterus. Trimethoprim is excreted into breast milk in low concentrations. Following 160 mg twice daily for 5 days, milk concentrations varied between 1.2 and 2.4 mcg/mL (average, 1.8 mcg/mL) with peak levels occurring at 2 to 3 hours. No adverse effects were reported in the infants. The American Academy of Pediatrics classifies the combination of sulfamethoxazole and trimethoprim as compatible with breast-feeding.

➤*Children:* Contraindicated for use in children younger than 2 months of age.

➤*Elderly:* There may be an increased risk of severe adverse reactions in elderly patients, particularly when complicating conditions exist (eg, impaired kidney and/or liver function, or concomitant use of other drugs). Severe skin reactions, generalized bone marrow suppression, a specific decrease in platelets (with or without purpura), and hyperkalemia are the most frequently reported severe adverse reactions in elderly patients. In those concurrently receiving certain diuretics, primarily thiazides, an increased incidence of thrombocytopenia with purpura has been reported. Increased digoxin blood levels can occur with concomitant sulfamethoxazole and trimethoprim therapy, especially in elderly patients. Monitor serum digoxin levels. Hematological changes indicative of folic acid deficiency may occur in elderly patients. These effects are reversible by folinic acid therapy. Appropriately adjust the dosage for patients with impaired kidney function, and make the duration of use as short as possible to minimize risks of undesired reactions.

➤*Monitoring:* Perform complete blood cell counts frequently in patients receiving sulfamethoxazole and trimethoprim; if a significant reduction in the count of any formed blood element is noted, discontinue this drug product. Perform urinalysis with careful microscopic examination and renal function tests during therapy, particularly for those patients with impaired renal function. Monitor patient for signs and symptoms of skin rash or other adverse reactions.

Drug Interactions

➤*QT prolongation:* An additive effect of sulfamethoxazole and trimethoprim with other drugs that prolong the QT interval cannot be excluded. The following drugs may prolong the QT interval and increase the risk of life-threatening cardiac arrhythmias, including torsades de pointes: antiarrhythmic agents (eg, amiodarone, bretylium, disopyramide, dofetilide, procainamide, quinidine, sotalol), arsenic trioxide, chlorpromazine, cisapride, dolasetron, droperidol, mefloquine, mesoridazine, moxifloxacin, pentamidine, pimozide, tacrolimus, thioridazine, and ziprasidone. For a more complete list of drugs that may prolong the QT interval, see the appendix, Drug-Induced Prolongation of the QT Interval and Torsades de Pointes.

➤*Live vaccines:* The effectiveness of live vaccines may be decreased when sulfamethoxazole and trimethoprim is coadministered. Concurrent use is not recommended.

Sulfamethoxazole/Trimethoprim Drug Interactions

Precipitant drug	Object drug[a]		Description
ACE[b] inhibitors	Sulfamethoxazole/ Trimethoprim	↑	Hyperkalemia, possibly with cardiac arrhythmias or cardiac arrest, may occur with coadministration of sulfamethoxazole/trimethoprim and ACE inhibitors. Sulfamethoxazole/trimethoprim and ACE inhibitors may act additively to reduce aldosterone activity, resulting in hyperkalemia due to reduced potassium excretion. Monitor serum potassium concentrations.
Sulfamethoxazole/ Trimethoprim	ACE inhibitors		
Diuretics (primarily thiazides)	Sulfamethoxazole/ Trimethoprim	↑	The risk of thrombocytopenia with purpura may be increased. Monitor the platelet count. If an interaction is suspected, it may be necessary to discontinue one or both agents.
Sulfamethoxazole/ Trimethoprim	Diuretics (primarily thiazides)		
Indomethacin	Sulfamethoxazole/ Trimethoprim	↑	Sulfamethoxazole plasma concentrations may be elevated, increasing the pharmacologic effects and risk of adverse reactions. Observe the patient for sulfamethoxazole adverse reactions. If an interaction is suspected, adjust therapy as needed.
Methenamine	Sulfamethoxazole/ Trimethoprim	↑	Methenamine is contraindicated for use with sulfamethoxazole/trimethoprim because of the potential for formation of insoluble precipitates in the urine.
Sulfones (eg, dapsone)	Sulfamethoxazole/ Trimethoprim	↑	Plasma concentrations of trimethoprim and sulfones may be elevated, increasing the pharmacologic effects and toxicity of both agents. Measure plasma concentrations of both agents and closely monitor patients for sulfone toxicity (eg, methemoglobinemia). Adjust the doses or discontinue therapy as necessary.
Sulfamethoxazole/ Trimethoprim	Sulfones (eg, dapsone)		
Tretinoin	Sulfamethoxazole/ Trimethoprim	↑	Phototoxicity may be augmented if tretinoin and sulfamethoxazole are coadministered. Avoid coadministration.
Sulfamethoxazole/ Trimethoprim	Tretinoin		
Sulfamethoxazole/ Trimethoprim	Amantadine	↑	A single case of toxic delirium has been reported in a patient taking amantadine and sulfamethoxazole/trimethoprim concurrently. Monitor patients for CNS adverse reactions. If an interaction is suspected, it may be necessary to discontinue one or both drugs.

SULFAMETHOXAZOLE/TRIMETHOPRIM — ORAL

Sulfamethoxazole/Trimethoprim Drug Interactions			
Precipitant drug	Object drug[a]		Description
Sulfamethoxazole/ Trimethoprim	Cyclosporine	↓	Cyclosporine immunosuppressive effects may be decreased, while the risk of nephrotoxicity may be increased. If coadministration cannot be avoided, monitor cyclosporine blood or plasma concentration and serum creatinine concentrations. Monitor for clinical evidence of graft rejection. Adjust the dosage of cyclosporine accordingly or add additional immunosuppressive agents.
Sulfamethoxazole/ Trimethoprim	Ethanol (alcohol)	↑	Coadministration of alcohol and sulfamethoxazole/trimethoprim may produce an alcohol intolerance reaction. Advise patients receiving sulfamethoxazole/trimethoprim to avoid drinking alcohol and taking alcohol-containing medications.
Sulfamethoxazole/ Trimethoprim	Digoxin	↑	Digoxin plasma concentrations may be elevated, especially in elderly patients. Monitor digoxin concentrations and adjust the digoxin dose as needed.
Sulfamethoxazole/ Trimethoprim	Dofetilide	↑	Dofetilide plasma concentrations may be elevated, increasing the risk of ventricular arrhythmias, including torsades de pointes. Coadministration is contraindicated.
Sulfamethoxazole/ Trimethoprim	Hydantoins (eg, phenytoin)	↑	Phenytoin plasma concentrations may be elevated, and the half-life may be prolonged, increasing the pharmacologic effects and risk of toxicity. Monitor phenytoin concentrations and observe the patient for toxicity. If an interaction is suspected, adjust the phenytoin dose as needed.
Sulfamethoxazole/ Trimethoprim	Meglitinides (eg, repaglinide)	↑	Trimethoprim may elevate meglitinide plasma concentrations, increasing the risk of hypoglycemia. Closely monitor blood glucose after starting or stopping trimethoprim. Adjust the meglitinide dose as needed.
Sulfamethoxazole/ Trimethoprim	Methotrexate	↑	Sulfamethoxazole may displace methotrexate from its protein binding site. The pharmacologic effects and toxicity of methotrexate may be increased. In addition, trimethoprim may increase the risk of methotrexate-induced bone marrow suppression and megaloblastic anemia. Monitor hematologic status. A lower dose of methotrexate or higher leucovorin rescue dose may be needed during coadministration of sulfamethoxazole/trimethoprim. Methotrexate plasma concentrations may be helpful in making dosage adjustments. Discontinue both drugs if an interaction is suspected.
Sulfamethoxazole/ Trimethoprim	Procainamide	↑	Procainamide and N-acetylprocainamide (NAPA) plasma concentrations may be elevated, increasing the pharmacologic and toxic effects of procainamide. Monitor procainamide and NAPA plasma concentrations and cardiac function. Adjust the procainamide dose as needed.
Sulfamethoxazole/ Trimethoprim	Pyrimethamine	↑	The risk of megaloblastic anemia may be increased in patients receiving more than pyrimethamine 25 mg weekly. Assess the patient for hematologic and neurologic manifestations of megaloblastic anemia. If an interaction is suspected, administer corrective treatment (eg, folic acid if indicated). It may be necessary to discontinue one or both drugs.
Sulfamethoxazole/ Trimethoprim	Sulfonylureas (eg, glipizide)	↑	Sulfamethoxazole may increase the risk of hypoglycemia. Monitor blood glucose and adjust the sulfonylurea dose as needed.
Sulfamethoxazole/ Trimethoprim	Thiazolidinediones (eg, pioglitazone)	↑	Trimethoprim may elevate thiazolidinedione plasma concentrations, increasing the risk of hypoglycemia and other adverse reactions. Monitor blood glucose and for other adverse reactions. Adjust the thiazolidinedione dose as needed.
Sulfamethoxazole/ Trimethoprim	Tricyclic antidepressants (eg, amitriptyline)	↓	The effectiveness of tricyclic antidepressants may be decreased when sulfamethoxazole/trimethoprim is coadministered. Monitor the response of the patient and adjust the tricyclic antidepressant dose as needed.
Sulfamethoxazole/ Trimethoprim	Warfarin	↑	The anticoagulant effect of warfarin may be increased. Monitor coagulation parameters. Adjust the warfarin dose as needed.

[a] ↑ = object drug increased; ↓ = object drug decreased.
[b] ACE = angiotension-converting enzyme.

➤*Drug/Lab test interactions:* Trimethoprim can interfere with a serum methotrexate assay as determined by the competitive binding protein technique when a bacterial dihydrofolate reductase is used as the binding protein. No interference occurs, however, if methotrexate is measured by a radioimmunoassay. Sulfamethoxazole and trimethoprim may also interfere with the Jaffe alkaline pictate reaction assay for creatinine, resulting in overestimations of approximately 10% in the range of normal values.

Adverse Reactions

➤*Common adverse reactions:* The most common adverse reactions are GI disturbances (eg, anorexia, nausea, vomiting) and allergic skin reactions (eg, rash, urticaria).

➤*Severe adverse reactions:* Fatalities associated with the administration of sulfonamides, although rare, have occurred because of severe reactions, including agranulocytosis, aplastic anemia, fulminant hepatic necrosis, Stevens-Johnson syndrome, toxic epidermal necrolysis, and other blood dyscrasias.

➤*CNS:* Apathy, aseptic meningitis, ataxia, convulsions, depression, fatigue, hallucinations, headache, insomnia, nervousness, peripheral neuritis, tinnitus, vertigo.

➤*Dermatologic:* Erythema multiforme, exfoliative dermatitis, generalized skin eruptions, Henoch-Schönlein purpura, photosensitivity, pruritus, rash, Stevens-Johnson syndrome, toxic epidermal necrolysis, and urticaria.

➤*Endocrine:* The sulfonamides bear certain chemical similarities to some goitrogens, diuretics (acetazolamide and the thiazides), and oral hypoglycemic agents. Cross-sensitivity may exist with these agents. Diuresis and hypoglycemia have occurred rarely in patients receiving sulfonamides.

➤*GI:* Abdominal pain, anorexia, diarrhea, elevation of serum transaminase and bilirubin, emesis, glossitis, hepatitis (including cholestatic jaundice and hepatic necrosis), nausea, pancreatitis, pseudomembranous enterocolitis, stomatitis.

➤*GU:* Crystalluria, interstitial nephritis, nephrotoxicity in association with cyclosporine, renal failure, serum urea nitrogen and serum creatinine elevation, toxic nephrosis with oliguria and anuria.

➤*Hematologic:* Agranulocytosis, aplastic anemia, eosinophilia, hemolytic anemia, hypoprothrombinemia, leukopenia, megaloblastic anemia, methemoglobinemia, neutropenia, thrombocytopenia.

➤*Hypersensitivity:* Allergic myocarditis, anaphylaxis, angioedema, generalized allergic reactions.

➤*Metabolic:* Hyperkalemia, hyponatremia.

➤*Musculoskeletal:* Arthralgia, myalgia, rhabdomyolysis (mainly in patients with AIDS).

➤*Respiratory:* Cough, pulmonary infiltrates, shortness of breath.

➤*Miscellaneous:* Chills, conjunctival and scleral injection, drug fever, periarteritis nodosa, serum sickness–like syndrome, systemic lupus erythematosus, weakness.

Overdosage

➤*Symptoms:* Signs and symptoms of overdosage reported with sulfonamides include anorexia, colic, dizziness, drowsiness, headache, nausea, unconsciousness, and vomiting. Crystalluria, hematuria, and pyrexia may be noted. Blood dyscrasias and jaundice are potential late manifestations of overdosage. Signs of acute overdosage with trimethoprim include bone marrow depression, confusion, dizziness, headache, mental depression, nausea, and vomiting.

Use of sulfamethoxazole and trimethoprim at high doses and/or for extended periods of time may cause bone marrow depression manifested as leukopenia, megaloblastic anemia, and/or thrombocytopenia.

➤*Treatment:* General principles of treatment include the institution of gastric lavage, forcing oral fluids, and the administration of intravenous fluids if urine output is low and renal function is normal. Acidification of the urine will increase renal elimination of trimethoprim. Monitor the patient with blood cell counts and appropriate blood chemistries, including electrolytes. If a significant blood dyscrasia or jaundice occurs, institute specific therapy for these complications. Peritoneal dialysis is not effective and hemodialysis is only moderately effective in eliminating sulfamethoxazole and trimethoprim.

If signs of bone marrow depression occur, give the patient leucovorin 5 to 15 mg daily until normal hematopoiesis is restored.

Patient Information

Counsel patients that antibacterial drugs, including sulfamethoxazole and trimethoprim, should only be used to treat bacterial infections. They do not treat viral infections (eg, the common cold).

When sulfamethoxazole and trimethoprim is prescribed to treat a bacterial infection, tell patients that although it is common to feel better early in the course of therapy, the medication should be taken exactly as directed. Skipping doses or not completing the full course of therapy may decrease the effectiveness of the immediate treatment and increase the likelihood that bacteria will develop resistance and will not be treatable by sulfamethoxazole and trimethoprim or other antibacterial drugs in the future.

Sulfamethoxazole and trimethoprim tablets contain 1.8 mg (0.08 mEq) of sodium per tablet. Sulfamethoxazole and trimethoprim double-strength tablets contain 3.6 mg (0.16 mEq) of sodium per tablet.

Instruct patients to maintain an adequate fluid intake in order to prevent crystalluria and stone formation.

Instruct patients to report the following symptoms to a health care provider: fever, skin rash, sore throat, unusual bruising or bleeding.

Instruct patients to contact their health care provider immediately if they develop water and/or bloody stools, with or without stomach cramps and fever, even as late as 2 months after taking the last dose of medication.

Caution patients to avoid exposure to sunlight and to use sunscreen or wear protective clothing to avoid photosensitivity reaction.

SULFAMETHOXAZOLE/TRIMETHOPRIM — INJECTION

Indications

Sulfamethoxazole and Trimethoprim Injection Indications[a]	
Indication	Organism
FDA-approved	
Enteritis	*Shigella flexneri, Shigella sonnei*
PCP treatment	*P. carinii*
Severe or complicated urinary tract infections	*Escherichia coli, Klebsiella* and *Enterobacter* species, *Morganella morganii, Proteus* sp.[b]
Off-label	
Skin and soft-tissue infections in children	Methicillin-sensitive *Staphylococcus aureus*, methicillin-resistant *S. aureus*
Treatment of cholera and salmonella-type infections and nocardiosis	*Vibrio cholerae, Salmonella* sp., *Nocardia* sp.

[a] FDA = Food and Drug Administration; PCP = *Pneumocystis carinii* pneumonia.
[b] Parenteral therapy is indicated in severe or complicated infections when oral therapy is not feasible and when the organism is not susceptible to single agents effective in the urinary tract.

➤*Off-label uses:*

Catheter-related bloodstream infections – [2] = Fair documentation. Guidelines suggest that trimethoprim/sulfamethoxazole may be used for treatment of catheter-related bloodstream infections caused by *Stenotrophomonas maltophilia, Burkholderia cepacia*, and *Ochrobactrum anthropi*. Trimethoprim/sulfamethoxazole may be used as an alternative antimicrobial agent in resistant microorganisms if infection is caused by any of the following: methicillin-resistant *S. aureus*, coagulase-negative staphylococci, and *Chryseobacterium* species. This agent should not be used for empiric therapy. Further controlled trials defining the specific place for trimethoprim/sulfamethoxazole in therapy for catheter-related bloodstream infections are needed.

Administration and Dosage

➤*Maximum dose:*

Adults and children 2 months of age and older – 60 mL/day based on trimethoprim (may vary by indication).

➤*General dosing considerations:* Maintain adequate fluid intake to prevent crystalluria and stone formation.

Dosage adjustment required in patients with renal impairment (see Renal Function Impairment).

➤*Adults:*

Enteritis –

Usual dosage: 8 to 10 mg/kg/day (based on trimethoprim) in 2 to 4 divided doses every 6, 8, or 12 hours for 5 days by intravenous (IV) infusion.

Maximum dose: 60 mL/day (based on trimethoprim).

P. carinii pneumonia – 15 to 20 mg/kg/day (based on trimethoprim) in 3 or 4 equally divided doses every 6 to 8 hours for up to 14 days by IV infusion.

Severe or complicated urinary tract infections –

Usual dosage: 8 to 10 mg/kg/day (based on trimethoprim) in 2 to 4 divided doses every 6, 8, or 12 hours for up to 14 days by IV infusion.

Maximum dose: 60 mL/day (based on trimethoprim).

Off-label dosing –

Catheter-related bloodstream infections: [2] = Fair documentation. 3 to 5 mg/kg (based on trimethoprim) infused over 60 to 90 minutes, every 8 hours.

Nocardiosis: 15 mg/kg/day (based on trimethoprim) in 2 to 4 divided doses for 3 to 4 weeks, then decrease dosage to 10 mg/kg/day (based on trimethoprim) in 2 to 4 divided doses for 3 to 6 months.

➤*Children:*

2 months of age and older – See Adults for dosing.

Off-label dosing –

Catheter-related bloodstream infections: [2] = Fair documentation.

• *Infants 2 months of age and older and children* –

Mild to moderate infections: 6 to 12 mg/kg/day infused over 60 to 90 minutes in divided doses every 12 hours.

Serious infections: 15 to 20 mg/kg/day (based on trimethoprim) infused over 60 to 90 minutes in divided doses every 6 to 8 hours.

Skin and soft-tissue infections: 8 to 12 mg/kg (based on trimethoprim) in equally divided doses every 6 hours IV.

➤*Elderly:* Make appropriate dosage adjustments for impaired kidney function (see Renal Function Impairment).

➤*Renal function impairment:*

Recommendations for dosage adjustment – According to the manufacturer's prescribing information, the dose of sulfamethoxazole and trimethoprim in patients with renal impairment should be adjusted based on the following recommendations:

Creatinine clearance 15 to 30 mL/min: ½ the usual regimen.

Creatinine clearance less than 15 mL/min: Not recommended.

Alternative dosing regimen –

Creatinine clearance 30 to 50 mL/min: Trimethoprim 5 to 7.5 mg/kg per dose every 8 hours.

Creatinine clearance 10 to 29 mL/min: Trimethoprim 5 to 10 mg/kg per dose every 12 hours.

Creatinine clearance less than 10 mL/min: Not recommended, but if used: trimethoprim 5 to 10 mg/kg per dose every 24 hours.

Hemodialysis: Not recommended, but if used: trimethoprim 5 to 10 mg/kg per dose every 24 hours. Alternatively, 5 to 20 mg/kg IV 3 times per week in adults following dialysis. These recommendations assume the patient is receiving standard intermittent hemodialysis 3 times per week and completes the full dialysis sessions.

Peritoneal dialysis: Not recommended, but if used: trimethoprim 5 to 10 mg/kg per dose every 24 hours.

Continuous renal replacement therapy: Trimethoprim 5 to 7.5 mg/kg per dose every 8 hours.

• *Adults* – One reference suggests a dosage (based on trimethoprim) of 2.5 to 5 mg/kg IV every 12 hours for mild to moderate infections and 10 mg/kg every 12 hours for severe infections.

Alternatively, a dosage of 2.5 to 7.5 mg/kg (based on trimethoprim) IV every 12 hours is recommended for patients receiving continuous venovenous hemofiltration, continuous venovenous hemodialysis, or continuous venovenous hemodiafiltration. This recommendation assumes ultrafiltration and dialysis flow rates of 1 to 2 L/h.

For severely ill patients infected with *P. carinii* pneumonia who are receiving continuous venovenous hemodiafiltration, a dosage of up to 10 mg/kg IV every 12 hours may be necessary.

➤*Preparation for administration:* Injection solution must be diluted; add the contents of each 5 mL amp to 125 mL of dextrose 5% in water. Do not refrigerate and use within 6 hours. If a dilution of 5 mL per 100 mL of dextrose 5% in water is desired, use within 4 hours.

When fluid restriction is desirable, add each 5 mL amp to 75 mL of dextrose 5% in water. Mix solution just prior to use and administer within 2 hours.

➤*Administration:* Administer the injection by IV infusion over 60 to 90 minutes. Avoid rapid infusion or bolus injection. Do not give intramuscularly. The following infusion systems have been tested and found satisfactory: unit-dose glass containers, unit-dose polyvinyl chloride, and polyolefin containers.

➤*Admixture compatibility:* Do not mix the injection with other drugs or solutions.

➤*Storage/Stability:* Store vials at 15° to 30°C (59° to 86°F). Do not refrigerate. Protect from light. After initial entry into the multidose vials, use the remaining contents within 48 hours.

Actions

➤*Pharmacology:* Sulfamethoxazole inhibits bacterial synthesis of dihydrofolic acid by competing with para-aminobenzoic acid. Trimethoprim blocks the production of tetrahydrofolic acid from dihydrofolic acid by binding to and reversibly inhibiting the required enzyme, dihydrofolate reductase. Thus, this combination blocks 2 consecutive steps in the biosynthesis of nucleic acids and proteins essential to many bacteria.

➤*Pharmacokinetics:*

Absorption – Following a 1-hour IV infusion of a single dose of sulfamethoxazole 800 mg and trimethoprim 160 mg to 11 patients whose weight ranged from 105 to 165 lb (mean, 143 lb), the peak plasma concentrations of sulfamethoxazole and trimethoprim were 46.3 ± 2.7 mcg/mL and 3.4 ± 0.3 mcg/mL, respectively. Following repeated IV administration of the same dose at 8-hour intervals, the mean plasma concentrations just prior to and immediately after each infusion at steady state were 70.6 ± 7.3 mcg/mL and 105.6 ± 10.9 mcg/mL for sulfamethoxazole and 5.6 ± 0.6 mcg/mL and 8.8 ± 0.9 mcg/mL for trimethoprim. All of these 11 patients had healthy renal function, and their ages ranged from 17 to 78 years (median, 60 years).

Distribution – Sulfamethoxazole and trimethoprim exist in the blood as unbound, protein-bound, and metabolized forms; sulfamethoxazole also exists as the conjugated form. Approximately 70% of sulfamethoxazole and 44% of trimethoprim are bound to plasma proteins. The presence of sulfamethoxazole 10 mg percent in plasma decreases the protein binding of trimethoprim by an insignificant degree; trimethoprim does not influence the protein binding of sulfamethoxazole. Sulfamethoxazole and trimethoprim distribute to sputum and vaginal fluid; trimethoprim also distributes to bronchial secretions, and both pass the placental barrier and are excreted in breast milk.

Metabolism – The metabolism of sulfamethoxazole occurs predominately by N_4-acetylation, although the glucuronide conjugate has been identified. The principal metabolites of trimethoprim are the 1- and 3-oxides and the 3′- and 4′-hydroxy derivatives. The free forms of sulfamethoxazole and trimethoprim are considered to be the therapeutically active forms.

Excretion – The mean plasma half-life was 12.8 ± 1.8 hours for sulfamethoxazole and 11.3 ± 0.7 hours for trimethoprim. Excretion of sulfamethoxazole and trimethoprim is primarily by the kidneys through glomerular filtration and tubular secretion. Urine concentrations of sulfamethoxazole and trimethoprim are considerably higher than are the concentrations in the blood. The percent of dose excreted in urine over a 12-hour period following the IV administration of the first dose of sulfamethoxazole 1,200 mg and trimethoprim 240 mg on day 1 ranged from 7% to 12.7% as free sulfamethoxazole, 17% to 42.4% as free trimethoprim, and 36.7% to 56% as total (free plus the N_4-acetylated metabolite) sulfamethoxazole. When administered together, neither sulfamethoxazole nor trimethoprim affects the urinary excretion pattern of the other.

SULFAMETHOXAZOLE/TRIMETHOPRIM — INJECTION

Special populations –

Renal function impairment: Patients with severely impaired renal function exhibit an increase in the half-lives of both components, requiring dosage regimen adjustment.

➤*Microbiology:*

Resistance – In vitro studies have shown that bacterial resistance develops more slowly with this combination than with either sulfamethoxazole or trimethoprim alone.

Susceptible organisms – In vitro serial dilution tests have shown that the spectrum of antibacterial activity of sulfamethoxazole and trimethoprim includes common bacterial pathogens with the exception of *Pseudomonas aeruginosa*. The following organisms are usually susceptible: *E. coli*, *Klebsiella* species, *Enterobacter* species, *M. morganii*, *Proteus mirabilis*, indole-positive *Proteus* species including *Proteus vulgaris*, *Haemophilus influenzae* (including ampicillin-resistant strains), *Streptococcus pneumoniae*, *S. flexneri*, and *S. sonnei*. It should be noted, however, that there are little clinical data on the use of sulfamethoxazole and trimethoprim injection in serious systemic infections caused by *H. influenzae* and *S. pneumoniae*.

Contraindications

Known hypersensitivity to trimethoprim or sulfonamides; documented megaloblastic anemia caused by folate deficiency; pregnant patients; breast-feeding mothers; infants younger than 2 months of age.

Warnings/Precautions

➤*Severe reactions:* Fatalities associated with the administration of sulfonamides, although rare, have occurred because of severe reactions, including agranulocytosis, aplastic anemia, fulminant hepatic necrosis, Stevens-Johnson syndrome, toxic epidermal necrolysis, and other blood dyscrasias.

Discontinue sulfonamides, including sulfonamide-containing products, such as sulfamethoxazole and trimethoprim, at the first appearance skin rash or any sign of an adverse reaction. In rare instances, a skin rash may be followed by more severe reactions such as hepatic necrosis, serious blood disorders, Stevens-Johnson syndrome, and toxic epidermal necrolysis.

Clinical signs such as arthralgia, fever, jaundice, pallor, purpura, rash, or sore throat may be early indications of serious reactions.

➤*Respiratory effects:* Cough, pulmonary infiltrates, and shortness of breath are hypersensitivity reactions of the respiratory tract that have been reported in association with sulfonamide treatment.

➤*Group A beta-hemolytic streptococci:* Do not use the sulfonamides for the treatment of group A beta-hemolytic streptococcal infections. In an established infection, they will not eradicate the streptococcus and, therefore, will not prevent sequelae such as rheumatic fever.

➤*Clostridium difficile–associated diarrhea:* Pseudomembranous colitis has been reported with nearly all antibacterial agents, including sulfamethoxazole and trimethoprim, and may range in severity from mild to life-threatening. Therefore, it is important to consider this diagnosis in patients who present with diarrhea subsequent to the administration of antibacterial agents.

Treatment with antibacterial agents alters the normal flora of the colon and may permit overgrowth of clostridia. Studies indicate that a toxin produced by *C. difficile* is one primary cause of antibiotic-associated colitis.

After the diagnosis of pseudomembranous colitis has been established, initiate therapeutic measures. Mild cases of pseudomembranous colitis usually respond to drug discontinuation alone. In moderate to severe cases, consider management with fluids and electrolytes, protein supplementation, and treatment with an antibacterial drug effective against *C. difficile*.

➤*Local reactions:* Local irritation and inflammation due to extravascular infiltration of the infusion have been observed with sulfamethoxazole and trimethoprim. If these occur, discontinue the infusion and restart at another site.

➤*AIDS:* Patients with AIDS may not tolerate or respond to sulfamethoxazole and trimethoprim in the same manner as patients without AIDS. The incidence of adverse reactions, particularly elevated aminotransferase (transaminase) values, fever, leukopenia, and rash, with sulfamethoxazole and trimethoprim therapy in patients with AIDS who are being treated for PCP has been reported to be greatly increased compared with the incidence normally associated with the use of sulfamethoxazole and trimethoprim in patients without AIDS.

➤*Sulfite sensitivity:* Some formulations of sulfamethoxazole and trimethoprim may contain sodium metabisulfite, a sulfite that may cause allergic-type reactions, including anaphylactic symptoms and life-threatening or less severe asthmatic episodes in certain susceptible people. The overall prevalence of sulfite sensitivity in the general population is unknown and probably low. Sulfite sensitivity is seen more frequently in asthmatic than in nonasthmatic people.

➤*Renal function impairment:* Use with caution. Dosage adjustments required (see Administration and Dosage).

➤*Hepatic function impairment:* Use with caution.

➤*Special risk:* Give sulfamethoxazole and trimethoprim with caution to those with possible folate deficiency (eg, elderly patients, chronic alcoholism, patients receiving anticonvulsant therapy, patients with malabsorption syndrome, patients in malnutrition states) and to those with severe allergies or bronchial asthma. In glucose-6-phosphate dehydrogenase deficient individuals, hemolysis may occur. This reaction is frequently dose-related.

➤*Pregnancy:* Category *C*. In rats, oral doses of sulfamethoxazole 533 mg/kg or trimethoprim 200 mg/kg produced teratological effects manifested mainly as cleft palates.

The highest dose, which did not cause cleft palates in rats, was sulfamethoxazole 512 mg/kg or trimethoprim 192 mg/kg when administered separately. In 2 studies in rats, no teratology was observed when sulfamethoxazole 512 mg/kg was used in combination with trimethoprim 128 mg/kg. In 1 study, however, cleft palates were observed in 1 litter out of 9 when sulfamethoxazole 355 mg/kg was used in combination with trimethoprim 88 mg/kg.

In some rabbit studies, an overall increase in fetal loss (dead and resorbed and malformed conceptuses) was associated with doses of trimethoprim 6 times the human therapeutic dose.

While there are no large, well-controlled studies on the use of sulfamethoxazole and trimethoprim in pregnant women, a retrospective study reported the outcome of 186 pregnancies during which the mother received placebo or oral sulfamethoxazole and trimethoprim. The incidence of congenital abnormalities was 4.5% in those who received placebo and 3.3% in those receiving sulfamethoxazole and trimethoprim. There were no abnormalities in the 10 children whose mothers received the drug during the first trimester. In a separate survey, no congenital abnormalities were found in 35 children whose mothers had received oral sulfamethoxazole and trimethoprim at the time of conception or shortly thereafter.

Trimethoprim (molecular weight approximately 290) crosses the placenta, producing similar levels in fetal and maternal serum and in amniotic fluid. Using an in vitro perfused human cotyledon, sulfamethoxazole and trimethoprim were shown to cross the placenta. Because sulfamethoxazole and trimethoprim may interfere with folic acid metabolism, use sulfamethoxazole and trimethoprim during pregnancy only if the potential benefit justifies the potential risk to the fetus.

➤*Lactation:* Sulfamethoxazole and trimethoprim combination is contraindicated during breast-feeding because sulfonamides are excreted in the milk and may cause kernicterus. Trimethoprim is excreted into breast milk in low concentrations. Following 160 mg twice daily for 5 days, milk concentrations varied between 1.2 and 2.4 mcg/mL (average, 1.8 mcg/mL) with peak levels occurring at 2 to 3 hours. No adverse effects were reported in the infants. The American Academy of Pediatrics classifies the combination of sulfamethoxazole and trimethoprim as compatible with breast-feeding.

➤*Children:* Contraindicated for use in infants younger than 2 months of age. Some formulations may contain benzyl alcohol. In newborn infants, benzyl alcohol has been associated with an increased incidence of neurological and other complications that are sometimes fatal.

➤*Elderly:* There may be an increased risk of severe adverse reactions in elderly patients, particularly when complicating conditions exist (eg, impaired kidney and/or liver function, concomitant use of other drugs). Severe skin reactions, generalized bone marrow suppression, or a specific decrease in platelets (with or without purpura) are the most frequently reported severe adverse reactions in elderly patients. In those concurrently receiving certain diuretics, primarily thiazides, an increased incidence of thrombocytopenia with purpura has been reported. Make appropriate dosage adjustments for patients with impaired kidney function.

➤*Monitoring:* Perform appropriate culture and susceptibility studies before and throughout treatment. Perform complete blood cell counts frequently in patients receiving sulfamethoxazole and trimethoprim; if a significant reduction in the count of any formed blood element is noted, discontinue sulfamethoxazole and trimethoprim. Perform urinalyses with careful microscopic examination and renal function tests during therapy, particularly for those patients with impaired renal function. Monitor patient for signs and symptoms of skin rash or other adverse reactions.

Drug Interactions

➤*QT prolongation:* An additive effect of sulfamethoxazole and trimethoprim with other drugs that prolong the QT interval cannot be excluded. The following drugs may prolong the QT interval and increase the risk of life-threatening cardiac arrhythmias, including torsades de pointes: antiarrhythmic agents (eg, amiodarone, bretylium, disopyramide, dofetilide, procainamide, quinidine, sotalol), arsenic trioxide, chlorpromazine, cisapride, dolasetron, droperidol, mefloquine, mesoridazine, moxifloxacin, pentamidine, pimozide, tacrolimus, thioridazine, and ziprasidone. For a more complete list of drugs that may prolong the QT interval, see the appendix, Drug-Induced Prolongation of the QT Interval and Torsades de Pointes.

➤*Live vaccines:* The effectiveness of live vaccines may be decreased when sulfamethoxazole and trimethoprim is coadministered. Concurrent use is not recommended.

Sulfamethoxazole/Trimethoprim Drug Interactions

Precipitant drug	Object drug[a]		Description
ACE[b] inhibitors	Sulfamethoxazole/ Trimethoprim	⬆	Hyperkalemia, possibly with cardiac arrhythmias or cardiac arrest, may occur with coadministration of sulfamethoxazole/trimethoprim and ACE inhibitors. Sulfamethoxazole/trimethoprim and ACE inhibitors may act additively to reduce aldosterone activity, resulting in hyperkalemia due to reduced potassium excretion. Monitor serum potassium concentrations.
Sulfamethoxazole/ Trimethoprim	ACE inhibitors		
Diuretics (primarily thiazides)	Sulfamethoxazole/ Trimethoprim	⬆	The risk of thrombocytopenia with purpura may be increased. Monitor the platelet count. If an interaction is suspected, it may be necessary to discontinue one or both agents.
Sulfamethoxazole/ Trimethoprim	Diuretics (primarily thiazides)		

SULFAMETHOXAZOLE/TRIMETHOPRIM — INJECTION

Sulfamethoxazole/Trimethoprim Drug Interactions

Precipitant drug	Object drug[a]		Description
Indomethacin	Sulfamethoxazole/ Trimethoprim	↑	Sulfamethoxazole plasma concentrations may be elevated, increasing the pharmacologic effects and risk of adverse reactions. Observe the patient for sulfamethoxazole adverse reactions. If an interaction is suspected, adjust therapy as needed.
Methenamine	Sulfamethoxazole/ Trimethoprim	↑	Methenamine is contraindicated for use with sulfamethoxazole/trimethoprim because of the potential for formation of insoluble precipitates in the urine.
Sulfones (eg, dapsone)	Sulfamethoxazole/ Trimethoprim	↑	Plasma concentrations of trimethoprim and sulfones may be elevated, increasing the pharmacologic effects and toxicity of both agents. Measure plasma concentrations of both agents and closely monitor patients for sulfone toxicity (eg, methemoglobinemia). Adjust the doses or discontinue therapy as necessary.
Sulfamethoxazole/ Trimethoprim	Sulfones (eg, dapsone)		
Tretinoin	Sulfamethoxazole/ Trimethoprim	↑	Phototoxicity may be augmented if tretinoin and sulfamethoxazole are coadministered. Avoid coadministration.
Sulfamethoxazole/ Trimethoprim	Tretinoin		
Sulfamethoxazole/ Trimethoprim	Amantadine	↑	A single case of toxic delirium has been reported in a patient taking amantadine and sulfamethoxazole/trimethoprim concurrently. Monitor patients for CNS adverse reactions. If an interaction is suspected, it may be necessary to discontinue one or both drugs.
Sulfamethoxazole/ Trimethoprim	Cyclosporine	↓	Cyclosporine immunosuppressive effects may be decreased, while the risk of nephrotoxicity may be increased. If coadministration cannot be avoided, monitor cyclosporine blood or plasma concentration and serum creatinine concentrations. Monitor for clinical evidence of graft rejection. Adjust the dosage of cyclosporine accordingly or add additional immunosuppressive agents.
Sulfamethoxazole/ Trimethoprim	Ethanol (alcohol)	↑	Coadministration of alcohol and sulfamethoxazole/trimethoprim may produce an alcohol intolerance reaction. Advise patients receiving sulfamethoxazole/trimethoprim to avoid drinking alcohol or taking alcohol-containing medications.
Sulfamethoxazole/ Trimethoprim	Digoxin	↑	Digoxin plasma concentrations may be elevated, especially in elderly patients. Monitor digoxin concentrations and adjust the digoxin dose as needed.
Sulfamethoxazole/ Trimethoprim	Dofetilide	↑	Dofetilide plasma concentrations may be elevated, increasing the risk of ventricular arrhythmias, including torsades de pointes. Coadministration is contraindicated.
Sulfamethoxazole/ Trimethoprim	Hydantoins (eg, phenytoin)	↑	Phenytoin plasma concentrations may be elevated, and the half-life may be prolonged, increasing the pharmacologic effects and risk of toxicity. Monitor phenytoin concentrations and observe the patient for toxicity. If an interaction is suspected, adjust the phenytoin dose as needed.
Sulfamethoxazole/ Trimethoprim	Meglitinides (eg, repaglinide)	↑	Trimethoprim may elevate meglitinide plasma concentrations, increasing the risk of hypoglycemia. Closely monitor blood glucose after starting or stopping trimethoprim. Adjust the meglitinide dose as needed.
Sulfamethoxazole/ Trimethoprim	Methotrexate	↑	Sulfamethoxazole may displace methotrexate from its protein binding site. The pharmacologic effects and toxicity of methotrexate may be increased. In addition, trimethoprim may increase the risk of methotrexate-induced bone marrow suppression and megaloblastic anemia. Monitor hematologic status. A lower dose of methotrexate or higher leucovorin rescue dose may be needed during coadministration of sulfamethoxazole/trimethoprim. Methotrexate plasma concentrations may be helpful in making dosage adjustments. Discontinue both drugs if an interaction is suspected.
Sulfamethoxazole/ Trimethoprim	Procainamide	↑	Procainamide and N-acetylprocainamide (NAPA) plasma concentrations may be elevated, increasing the pharmacologic and toxic effects of procainamide. Monitor procainamide and NAPA plasma concentrations and cardiac function. Adjust the procainamide dose as needed.
Sulfamethoxazole/ Trimethoprim	Pyrimethamine	↑	The risk of megaloblastic anemia may be increased in patients receiving more than pyrimethamine 25 mg weekly. Assess the patient for hematologic and neurologic manifestations of megaloblastic anemia. If an interaction is suspected, administer corrective treatment (eg, folic acid if indicated). It may be necessary to discontinue one or both drugs.
Sulfamethoxazole/ Trimethoprim	Sulfonylureas (eg, glipizide)	↑	Sulfamethoxazole may increase the risk of hypoglycemia. Monitor blood glucose and adjust the sulfonylurea dose as needed.
Sulfamethoxazole/ Trimethoprim	Thiazolidinediones (eg, pioglitazone)	↑	Trimethoprim may elevate thiazolidinedione plasma concentrations, increasing the risk of hypoglycemia and other adverse reactions. Monitor blood glucose and for other adverse reactions. Adjust the thiazolidinedione dose as needed.
Sulfamethoxazole/ Trimethoprim	Tricyclic antidepressants (eg, amitriptyline)	↓	The effectiveness of tricyclic antidepressants may be decreased when sulfamethoxazole/trimethoprim is coadministered. Monitor the response of the patient and adjust the tricyclic antidepressant dose as needed.
Sulfamethoxazole/ Trimethoprim	Warfarin	↑	Anticoagulant effect of warfarin may be increased. Monitor coagulation parameters. Adjust the warfarin dose as needed.

[a] ↑ = object drug increased; ↓ = object drug decreased.
[b] ACE = angiotensin-converting enzyme.

➤*Drug/Lab test interactions:* Trimethoprim can interfere with a serum methotrexate assay as determined by the competitive binding protein technique when a bacterial dihydrofolate reductase is used as the binding protein. No interference occurs, however, if methotrexate is measured by a radioimmunoassay. Sulfamethoxazole and trimethoprim may also interfere with the Jaffe alkaline pictate reaction assay for creatinine, resulting in overestimations of approximately 10% in the range of normal values.

Adverse Reactions

➤*Common adverse reactions:* The most common adverse reactions are GI disturbances (eg, anorexia, nausea, vomiting) and allergic skin reactions (eg, rash, urticaria).

➤*Severe adverse reactions:* Fatalities associated with the administration of sulfonamides, although rare, have occurred because of severe reactions, including fulminant agranulocytosis, aplastic anemia, hepatic necrosis, Stevens-Johnson syndrome, toxic epidermal necrolysis, and other blood dyscrasias.

➤*CNS:* Apathy, aseptic meningitis, ataxia, convulsions, depression, fatigue, hallucinations, headache, insomnia, nervousness, peripheral neuritis, tinnitus, vertigo, weakness.

➤*Dermatologic:* Erythema multiforme, exfoliative dermatitis, generalized skin eruptions, Henoch-Schönlein purpura, photosensitivity, pruritus, rash, Stevens-Johnson syndrome, toxic epidermal necrolysis, and urticaria.

➤*Endocrine:* The sulfonamides bear certain chemical similarities to some goitrogens, diuretics (acetazolamide and the thiazides) and oral hypoglycemic agents. Cross-sensitivity may exist with these agents. Diuresis and hypoglycemia have occurred rarely in patients receiving sulfonamides.

➤*GI:* Abdominal pain, anorexia, diarrhea, elevation of serum transaminase and bilirubin, glossitis, emesis, hepatitis (including cholestatic jaundice and hepatic necrosis), nausea, pancreatitis, pseudomembranous enterocolitis, stomatitis.

➤*GU:* Crystalluria, interstitial nephritis, renal failure, serum urea nitrogen and serum creatinine elevation, toxic nephrosis with oliguria, and anuria.

➤*Hematologic:* Agranulocytosis, aplastic anemia, eosinophilia, hemolytic anemia, hypoprothrombinemia, leukopenia, megaloblastic anemia, methemoglobinemia, neutropenia, thrombocytopenia.

➤*Hypersensitivity:* Allergic myocarditis, anaphylaxis, angioedema, generalized allergic reactions.

➤*Local:* Local reaction and pain and slight irritation on IV administration are infrequent. Thrombophlebitis has rarely been observed.

➤*Musculoskeletal:* Arthralgia, myalgia.

➤*Miscellaneous:* Chills, conjunctival and scleral injection, drug fever, periarteritis nodosa, pulmonary infiltrates, serum sickness–like syndrome, systemic lupus erythematosus.

Overdosage

➤*Symptoms:* Signs and symptoms of overdosage reported with sulfonamides include anorexia, colic, dizziness, drowsiness, headache, nausea, unconsciousness, and vomiting. Crystalluria, hematuria, and pyrexia may be noted. Blood dyscrasias and jaundice are potential late manifestations of overdosage. Signs of acute overdosage with trimethoprim include bone marrow depression, confusion, dizziness, headache, mental depression, nausea, and vomiting.

SULFAMETHOXAZOLE/TRIMETHOPRIM — INJECTION

Use of sulfamethoxazole and trimethoprim at high doses and/or for extended periods of time may cause bone marrow depression manifested as leukopenia, megaloblastic anemia, and/or thrombocytopenia.

➤*Treatment:* General principles of treatment include the administration of IV fluids if urine output is low and renal function is healthy. Acidification of the urine will increase renal elimination of trimethoprim. Monitor the patient with blood cell counts and appropriate blood chemistries, including electrolytes. If a significant blood dyscrasia or jaundice occurs, institute specific therapy for these complications. Peritoneal dialysis is not effective, and hemodialysis is only moderately effective in eliminating trimethoprim and sulfamethoxazole.

If signs of bone marrow depression occur, give the patient leucovorin 5 to 15 mg daily until normal hematopoiesis is restored.

Patient Information

Encourage patients to maintain adequate fluid intake.

Educate patients and families to report any signs of super infection, such as fever, fatigue, vaginitis, and oral candidiasis.

Instruct patients to report the following symptoms to a health care provider: fever, skin rash, sore throat, unusual bruising or bleeding.

Instruct patients to contact their health care provider immediately if they develop watery and/or bloody stools, with or without stomach cramps and fever, even as late as 2 months after taking the last dose of medication.

Caution patients to avoid exposure to sunlight and to use sunscreen or wear protective clothing to avoid photosensitivity reaction.

ERYTHROMYCIN ETHYLSUCCINATE/SULFISOXAZOLE

Rx	**Erythromycin and Sulfisoxasole** (Various, eg, Barr, Goldline, Harber, Lederle, Moore, URL)	**Granules for Oral Suspension:** Erythromycin ethylsuccinate (equivalent to 200 mg erythromycin activity) and sulfisoxazole acetyl (equivalent to 600 mg sulfisoxazole) per 5 mL when reconstituted	In 100, 150 and 200 mL.

ERYTHROMYCIN ETHYLSUCCINATE/SULFISOXAZOLE — ORAL

For complete and comparative information on each of the components, refer to Erythromycin and Sulfisoxazole individual monographs.

Indications

➤*Acute otitis media in children:* Acute otitis media caused by susceptible strains of *Haemophilus influenzae*.

➤*Off-label uses:*

Sinusitis (children / adolescents) – [1] = Good documentation. Recently, guidelines published by the American Academy of Allergy, Asthma and Immunology and the American College of Allergy, Asthma and Immunology confirm erythromycin/sulfisoxazole as a therapeutic option for the treatment of sinusitis. It should be considered when first-line agents, such as amoxicillin, fail or as treatment alternative in areas with a high incidence of ampicillin-resistant *Haemophilus influenzae* and *Moraxella catarrhalis*. Patients should be treated for 10 to 14 days or until they are symptom free for 7 days.

Administration and Dosage

➤*Children:*

Acute otitis media –

2 months of age and older:

• *Usual dosage* – Erythromycin 50 mg/kg/day and sulfisoxazole 150 mg/kg/day (to a maximum of 6 g/day). Give in equally divided doses 4 times daily for 10 days.

Erythromycin/Sulfisoxazole Dosage Based on Weight

Weight		
kg	lb	Dose (every 6 hours)
< 8	< 18	Adjust dosage by body weight
8	18	2.5 mL
16	35	5 mL
24	53	7.5 mL
> 45	> 100	10 mL

• *Maximum dose* – Sulfisoxazole 6 g/day.

Off-label dosing –

Sinusitis (children / adolescents): [1] = Good documentation. Erythromycin 12.5 mg/kg and sulfisoxazole 37.5 mg/kg orally 4 times daily for 10 to 14 days, or until symptom free for 7 days.

➤*Administration:* Administer without regard to meals.

Warnings/Precautions

➤*Pregnancy: Category C.*

Teratogenic – At doses 7 times the human daily dose, sulfisoxazole was not teratogenic in either rats or rabbits. However, in 2 other teratogenicity studies, cleft palates developed in rats and mice after administration of 5 to 9 times the human therapeutic dose of sulfisoxazole.

There is no evidence of teratogenicity or any other adverse effects on reproduction in female rats fed erythromycin base (up to 0.25% of diet) prior to and during mating, during gestation, and through weaning of 2 successive litters. However, there are no adequate and well-controlled studies in pregnant women. Because animal reproduction studies are not always predictive of human response, use this drug during pregnancy only if clearly needed. Erythromycin has been reported to cross the placental barrier in humans, but fetal plasma levels are generally low.

There are no adequate or well-controlled studies of erythromycin ethylsuccinate and sulfisoxazole acetyl for oral suspension in either laboratory animals or pregnant women. It is not known whether erythromycin ethylsuccinate and sulfisoxazole acetyl for oral suspension can cause fetal harm when administered to a pregnant woman prior to term or can affect reproduction capacity. Use erythromycin ethylsuccinate and sulfisoxazole acetyl for oral suspension during pregnancy only if the potential benefit justifies the potential risk to the fetus.

Nonteratogenic – Kernicterus may occur in the newborn as a result of treatment of a pregnant woman at term with sulfonamides.

➤*Lactation:* Erythromycin and sulfisoxazole are excreted in human milk. Because of the potential for the development of kernicterus in neonates due to the displacement of bilirubin from plasma proteins by sulfisoxazole, a decision should be made whether to discontinue breast-feeding or the drug, taking into account the importance of the drug to the mother.

ANTIFUNGAL AGENTS

FLUCYTOSINE (5-FC; 5-Fluorocytosine)

Rx	**Ancobon** (ICN)	**Capsules:** 250 mg	Talc, lactose, and parabens. (Ancobon 250 ICN). Green and gray. In 100s.
		500 mg	Talc, lactose, and parabens. (Ancobon 500 ICN). White and gray. In 100s.

FLUCYTOSINE (5-FC; 5-Fluorocytosine) — ORAL

WARNING

Use with extreme caution in patients with renal impairment. Close monitoring of hematologic, renal, and hepatic status of all patients is essential.

Indications

➤*General information:* With the exception of urinary tract infection (UTI), use flucytosine in combination with amphotericin B for the treatment of systemic candidiasis and cryptococcosis because of rapid emergence of resistance to flucytosine in *Candida* and *Cryptococcus* isolates in patients receiving flucytosine alone.

➤*Candida:* Septicemia, endocarditis, and UTIs have been effectively treated. Limited trials in pulmonary infections justify the use of flucytosine.

➤*Cryptococcus:* For the treatment of meningitis and pulmonary infections. Good responses in septicemias and UTIs have occurred although studies are limited.

Administration and Dosage

➤*Adults:*

Infections – For a list of infections, refer to Indications.

Usual dosage: 50 to 150 mg/kg/day in divided doses at 6-hour intervals. To reduce or avoid nausea or vomiting, take capsules a few at a time over a 15-minute period.

➤*Renal function impairment:* Use a lower initial dose if BUN or serum creatinine is elevated or if there are other signs of renal impairment (see Warnings/Precautions). Adjust dosage to prevent progressive accumulation of the drug and to maintain the blood levels at less than 100 mcg/mL.

➤*Preparation for administration:* Flucytosine is considered a potential mutagen and teratogen. Follow safe handling procedures when preparing, administering, or dispensing flucytosine.

➤*Storage / Stability:* Store at 25°C (77°F); excursions permitted to 15° to 30°C (59° to 86°F).

Actions

➤*Pharmacology:* Flucytosine has in vitro and in vivo activity against *Candida* and *Cryptococcus*. Although the exact mechanism is unknown, it has been reported that flucytosine acts directly on fungal organisms by competi-

FLUCYTOSINE (5-FC; 5-Fluorocytosine) — ORAL

tive inhibition of purine and pyrimidine uptake and indirectly by intracellular metabolism to 5-fluorouracil. The 5-fluorouracil is extensively incorporated into fungal RNA and inhibits synthesis of DNA and RNA. The result is unbalanced growth and death of the fungal organism. It is rarely used alone; generally, it is used in combination with amphotericin B for synergistic antifungal activity (see Drug Interactions).

➤*Pharmacokinetics:*

Absorption/Distribution – Flucytosine is well absorbed after oral use with peak blood levels of 30 to 40 mcg/mL reached within 2 hours. After 5 days of continuous therapy, median peak levels in infants were 19.6, 27.7, and 83.9 mcg/mL at doses of 25, 50, and 100 mg/kg, respectively. Mean time to peak serum levels were approximately 2.5 hours, similar to that observed in adult patients. It is well distributed into aqueous humor and other body fluids and tissues; CSF concentrations are approximately 65% to 90% of serum levels. Bioavailability is 78% to 89%. Plasma protein binding is minimal. Toxicity occurs at blood levels higher than 100 mcg/mL.

Metabolism/Excretion – More than 90% of the dose is excreted unchanged in the urine by glomerular filtration; a small portion is found unchanged in the feces. Serum half-life is 2.4 and 4.8 hours in patients with normal renal function; half-life increases significantly, up to an average of 85 hours, in patients with renal failure. The median half-life observed in infants was 7.4 hours, approximately double that seen in adults. The drug is removed rapidly by hemodialysis.

➤*Microbiology:*

Fungal resistance –

Cryptococcus: Any isolate with an MIC greater than 12.5 mcg/mL is considered resistant. In vitro resistance has developed in originally susceptible strains during therapy. It is recommended that clinical cultures for susceptibility testing be taken initially and at weekly intervals during therapy. Reserve the initial culture as a reference in susceptibility testing of subsequent isolates.

Candida: As high as 40% to 50% of the pretreatment clinical isolates of *Candida* have been reported to be resistant to flucytosine. It is recommended that susceptibility studies be performed as early as possible and be repeated during therapy. An MIC value greater than 100 mcg/mL is considered resistant.

Contraindications

Hypersensitivity to flucytosine.

Warnings/Precautions

➤*Bone marrow depression:* Give with extreme caution to patients with bone marrow depression. Patients may be more prone to bone marrow depression if they have a hematologic disease, are being treated with radiation or marrow-suppressant drugs, or have a history of treatment with such drugs or radiation. Bone marrow toxicity can be irreversible and may lead to death in immunosuppressed patients. Frequently monitor hepatic function and the hematopoietic system during therapy.

➤*Renal function impairment:* Give with extreme caution; drug accumulation may occur. Monitor blood levels to determine the adequacy of renal excretion in such patients. Adjust dosage to prevent progressive accumulation of the drug and to maintain the blood levels at less than 100 mcg/mL.

➤*Pregnancy:* *Category C.* Flucytosine is teratogenic in rats at 40 mg/kg/day. At higher doses (700 mg/kg/day) cleft lip and palate and micrognathia were reported. There are no adequate and well-controlled studies in pregnant women. Use only if the potential benefit justifies the potential risk to the fetus.

➤*Lactation:* It is not known whether this drug is excreted in breast milk. Because of potential serious adverse reactions in nursing infants, decide whether to discontinue nursing or the drug, taking into account the importance of the drug to mother.

➤*Children:* Safety and efficacy in children have not been established. Hypokalemia and acidemia were reported in one patient who received flucytosine in combination with amphotericin B, and anemia was observed in a second patient who received flucytosine alone. Transient thrombocytopenia was noted in 2 additional patients, one of whom also received amphotericin B.

➤*Monitoring:* Before therapy is initiated, determine electrolytes and hematological and renal status of the patient (see Warnings/Precautions). Because renal impairment can cause accumulation of the drug, monitor blood concentrations and renal function during therapy. Monitor hematologic status (WBC and platelet count) and liver function (alkaline phosphatase, ALT, and AST) at frequent intervals during treatment.

Drug Interactions

Drugs that impair glomerular filtration may prolong the half-life of flucytosine.

➤*Amphotericin B:* Amphotericin B may increase the therapeutic action and toxicity of flucytosine.

➤*Cytosine:* Cytosine may inactivate the antifungal activity of flucytosine.

➤*Drug/Lab test interactions:* Determine measurement of serum creatinine levels by the Jaffe reaction, because flucytosine does not interfere with the determination of creatinine values by this method.

Adverse Reactions

➤*Cardiovascular:* Cardiac arrest; myocardial toxicity; ventricular dysfunction.

➤*CNS:* Ataxia; confusion; convulsions; fatigue; hallucinations; headache; hearing loss; paresthesia; parkinsonism; peripheral neuropathy; psychosis; pyrexia; sedation; vertigo; weakness.

➤*Dermatologic:* Photosensitivity; pruritus; rash; urticaria.

➤*GI:* Abdominal pain; anorexia; bilirubin elevation; diarrhea; dry mouth; duodenal ulcer; emesis; GI hemorrhage; hepatic dysfunction; elevation of hepatic enzymes; acute hepatic injury with possible fatal outcome in debilitated patients; jaundice; nausea; ulcerative colitis.

➤*GU:* Azotemia; creatinine and BUN elevation; crystalluria; renal failure.

➤*Hematologic:* Agranulocytosis; aplastic anemia; anemia; eosinophilia; leukopenia; pancytopenia; thrombocytopenia.

➤*Respiratory:* Chest pain; dyspnea; respiratory arrest.

➤*Miscellaneous:* Allergic reactions; hypoglycemia; hypokalemia; Lyell syndrome.

Overdosage

➤*Symptoms:* There is no experience with intentional overdosage. It is reasonable to expect pronounced manifestations of known clinical adverse reactions. Prolonged serum concentration in excess of 100 mcg/mL may be associated with an increased incidence of toxicity, especially GI (diarrhea, nausea, vomiting), hematologic (leukopenia, thrombocytopenia), and hepatic (hepatitis).

➤*Treatment:* Prompt gastric lavage or emetic use is recommended. Maintain adequate fluid intake by IV route if necessary, because flucytosine is excreted unchanged in the renal tract. Hemodialysis rapidly reduced serum concentrations in anuric patients. Monitor hematologic parameters frequently, and monitor liver and kidney function. If any abnormalities appear in any of these parameters, institute appropriate therapeutic measures. Refer to General Management of Acute Overdosage.

Patient Information

May cause GI upset (eg, nausea, vomiting, diarrhea). Inform patient that this can be reduced or avoided by taking capsules a few at a time over a 15-minute period. Instruct patient to notify physician if effects become intolerable.

Inform patients that lab tests will be required while taking this medication and to be sure to keep appointments.

Advise patients that this drug may cause photosensitivity (sensitivity to sunlight). Advise them to avoid prolonged exposure to the sun and other ultraviolet light (eg, tanning beds) and to use sunscreens and wear protective clothing until tolerance is determined.

Griseofulvin

Indications

➤*General information:* Griseofulvin is NOT effective in bacterial infections; candidiasis (moniliasis); histoplasmosis; actinomycosis; sporotrichosis; chromoblastomycosis; coccidioidomycosis; North American blastomycosis; cryptococcosis (torulosis); tinea versicolor; nocardiosis.

➤*Ringworm infections:* Treatment of ringworm infections of the skin, hair, and nails, namely the following: Tinea corporis, tinea pedis, tinea cruris, tinea barbae, tinea capitis, tinea unguium (onychomycosis) when caused by ≥ 1 of the following fungi: *Trichophyton rubrum, T. tonsurans, T. mentagrophytes, T. interdigitalis, T. verrucosum, T. megninii, T. gallinae, T. crateriform, T. sulphureum, T. schoenleinii, Microsporum audouinii, M. canis, M. gypseum,* and *Epidermophyton floccosum.*

➤*Note:* Prior to therapy, identify the types of fungi responsible for the infection. Use of this drug is not justified in minor or trivial infections that will respond to topical agents alone.

Administration and Dosage

Accurate diagnosis of the infecting organism is essential.

➤*Duration of therapy:* Continue medication until the infecting organism is completely eradicated, as indicated by appropriate clinical or laboratory examination. Representative treatment periods are as follows: Tinea capitis, 4 to 6 weeks; tinea corporis, 2 to 4 weeks; tinea pedis, 4 to 8 weeks; tinea unguium (depending on rate of growth) – fingernails, ≥ 4 months; toenails, ≥ 6 months.

➤*Hygiene:* Observe good hygiene to control sources of infection or reinfection. Concomitant use of appropriate topical agents is usually required, particularly in treatment of tinea pedis. In some forms of athlete's foot, yeasts and bacteria may be involved, as well as fungi. Griseofulvin will not eradicate the bacterial or monilial infection.

➤*Adults:*

Tinea corporis, tinea cruris, tinea capitis – A single or divided daily dose of 330 to 375 mg ultramicrosize will give a satisfactory response in most patients.

Tinea pedis, tinea unguium – 660 to 750 mg ultramicrosize per day in divided doses.

Griseofulvin

➤*Children:* Approximately 7.3 mg ultramicrosize/kg/day (3.3 mg/lb/day) is an effective dose for most children. The following dosage schedule is suggested:

Griseofulvin Dosage for Children Based on Weight		
Weight		Daily dose (mg)
lb	kg	ultramicrosize
30 to 50	13.6 to 22.6	82.5 to 165
> 50	> 22.6	165 to 330

Clinical experience indicates that a single daily dose is effective in children with tinea capitis.

Children (≤ 2 years of age) – Dosage not established.

➤*Storage/Stability:*

Tablets – Store between 2° and 30°C (36° and 86°F).

Capsules – Store at room temperature, ≈ 25°C (77°F). Dispense in a well-closed container.

Oral suspension – Store at room temperature in a tight, light-resistant container.

Actions

➤*Pharmacology:* Griseofulvin, an antibiotic derived from a species of *Penicillium*, is deposited in the keratin precursor cells, which are gradually exfoliated and replaced by noninfected tissue; it has a greater affinity for diseased tissue. The drug is tightly bound to the new keratin, which becomes highly resistant to fungal invasions.

➤*Pharmacokinetics:* The peak serum level found in fasting adults given 0.5 g griseofulvin microsize occurred at ≈ 4 hours and ranged between 0.5 to 1.5 mcg/ml. Some individuals are consistently "poor absorbers" and tend to attain lower blood levels at all times. The serum level may be increased by giving the drug with a high-fat meal. GI absorption varies considerably among individuals because of insolubility of the drug in aqueous media of the upper GI tract. The efficiency of GI absorption of the ultramicrocrystalline formulation is ≈ 1.5 times that of conventional microsized griseofulvin. This factor permits the oral intake of ⅔ as much ultramicrocrystalline griseofulvin as the microsized form; however, there is no evidence this confers any significant clinical differences in regard to safety and efficacy.

➤*Microbiology:* Griseofulvin is fungistatic with in vitro activity against species of *Microsporum*, *Epidermophyton*, and *Trichophyton*. It has no effect on bacteria or other fungi.

Contraindications

Hypersensitivity to griseofulvin; porphyria; hepatocellular failure.

Warnings/Precautions

➤*Prophylaxis:* Safety and efficacy for prophylaxis of fungal infections have not been established.

➤*Prolonged therapy:* Closely observe patients on prolonged therapy. Periodically monitor renal, hepatic, and hematopoietic function.

➤*Penicillin cross-sensitivity:* This is possible because griseofulvin is derived from species of *Penicillium*; however, known penicillin-sensitive patients have been treated without difficulty.

➤*Lupus erythematosus:* Lupus-like syndromes or exacerbation of lupus erythematosus have occurred in patients receiving griseofulvin.

➤*Hypersensitivity reactions:* Hypersensitivity reactions (eg, skin rashes, urticaria, angioneurotic edema, erythema multiforme-like reactions) may occur and necessitate withdrawal of therapy. Institute appropriate countermeasures; refer to Management of Acute Hypersensitivity Reactions.

➤*Photosensitivity:* Caution patients to take protective measures (eg, sunscreens, protective clothing) against exposure to ultraviolet light or sunlight. Photosensitivity reactions may aggravate lupus erythematosus.

➤*Pregnancy: Category C.* Griseofulvin was embryotoxic and teratogenic in rats. Rare cases of conjoined twins have been reported in patients taking griseofulvin during the first trimester of pregnancy. Do not give to pregnant women or women contemplating pregnancy.

Fertility impairment – Because griseofulvin has demonstrated harmful effects in vitro on the genotype bacteria, plants, and fungi, males should wait at least 6 months after completing therapy before fathering a child. Females should avoid risk of pregnancy while receiving griseofulvin.

Drug Interactions

Griseofulvin Drug Interactions			
Precipitant drug	Object drug[a]		Description
Griseofulvin	Anticoagulants	⬇	Griseofulvin may decrease the hypoprothrombinemic activity of warfarin; patients may require anticoagulant dosage adjustment.
Griseofulvin	Contraceptives, oral	⬇	Loss of contraceptive effectiveness may occur, possibly leading to breakthrough bleeding, amenorrhea, or unintended pregnancy.
Griseofulvin	Cyclosporine	⬇	Cyclosporine levels may be reduced, resulting in a decrease in pharmacologic effects.
Griseofulvin	Salicylates	⬇	Serum salicylate concentrations may be decreased.
Barbiturates	Griseofulvin	⬇	Serum griseofulvin levels may be decreased.

[a] ⬇ = object drug decreased.

Adverse Reactions

➤*Most common:* Hypersensitivity reactions such as skin rashes and urticaria (see Warnings).

➤*Occasional:* Oral thrush; nausea; vomiting; epigastric distress; diarrhea; headache; fatigue; dizziness; insomnia; mental confusion; impairment of performance of routine activities.

➤*Rare:* Angioneurotic edema and erythema multiforme-like drug reactions may occur.

Griseofulvin interferes with porphyrin metabolism. Proteinuria; nephrosis; leukopenia; hepatic toxicity; GI bleeding; menstrual irregularities; paresthesias of the hands and feet after extended therapy have occurred. Discontinue administration if granulocytopenia occurs.

Rarely, serious reactions occur with griseofulvin. They are usually associated with high dosages, long periods of therapy, or both.

Patient Information

Beneficial effects may not be noticeable for some time; continue taking medication for entire course of therapy.

Photosensitivity reactions may occur; avoid prolonged exposure to sunlight or sunlamps.

Notify physician if fever, sore throat, or skin rash occurs.

GRISEOFULVIN MICROSIZE

Rx	**Grifulvin V** (Ortho)	**Tablets:** 500 mg	(ORTHO 214). White, scored. In 100s and 500s.
Rx	**Griseofulvin Microsize** (Glades)	**Oral suspension:** 125 mL per 5 mL	Orange-cream flavors. In 120 mL.[a]

[a] With alcohol 0.2%, menthol, parabens, saccharin, sucrose.

GRISEOFULVIN MICROSIZE — ORAL

For complete and comparative prescribing information refer to the Griseofulvin group monograph.

GRISEOFULVIN ULTRAMICROSIZE

Rx	**Gris-PEG** (Pedinol)	**Tablets:** 125 mg	Lactose, parabens. (Gris-PEG 125). White, elliptical, scored. Film-coated. In 100s.
		250 mg	Parabens. (Gris-PEG 250). White, capsule shape, scored. Film-coated. In 100s and 500s.

GRISEOFULVIN ULTRAMICROSIZE — ORAL

For complete and comparative prescribing information refer to the Griseofulvin group monograph.

AMPHOTERICIN B

Rx	**Abelcet** (Enzon)	**Injection, suspension**: 5 mg/mL	As lipid complex. Preservative free. In 20 mL single-use vials with 5-micron filter needles.
Rx	**Amphotec** (Three Rivers Pharmaceuticals)	**Injection lyophilized, powder for solution**: 50 mg	As cholesteryl sulfate complex. Preservative free. Lactose 950 mg, edetate disodium 0.372 mg. In single-use vials.
		100 mg	As cholesteryl sulfate complex. Preservative free. Lactose 1,900 mg, edetate disodium 0.744 mg. In single-use vials.
Rx	**AmBisome** (Astellas)	**Injection, lyophilized, powder for suspension**: 50 mg	Sucrose 900 mg. In single-dose vials with 5-micron filter.
Rx	**Amphotericin B** (Pharma-Tek)	**Powder for Injection**: 50 mg (as desoxycholate)	In vials.

AMPHOTERICIN B CHOLESTERYL SULFATE COMPLEX

Indications

➤*Invasive aspergillosis:* For the treatment of *invasive aspergillosis* in patients in whom renal impairment or unacceptable toxicity precludes the use of amphotericin B deoxycholate in effective doses, and in patients with invasive aspergillosis in whom prior amphotericin B deoxycholate therapy has failed.

➤*Off-label uses:*

Other possible off-label uses – Prophylaxis of fungal infection in patients with bone marrow transplantation; for the treatment of primary amoebic meningoencephalitis caused by *Naegleria fowleri*; subconjunctival or intravitreal injection in ocular aspergillosis; as chemoprophylaxis by low-dose intravenous (IV), intranasal, or nebulized administration in immunocompromised patients at risk of aspergillosis; intra-articularly or intramuscularly for coccidioidal arthritis; treatment of *Aspergillus*, *Candida*, and *Cryptococcus* systemic fungal infections.

Administration and Dosage

➤*Adults:*

Aspergillosis, invasive – 3 to 4 mg/kg IV as required once a day.

➤*Children:*

Aspergillosis, invasive – See Adults for dosing.

Off-label dosing –

Fungal infections, systemic (eg, Aspergillus sp, Candida sp, Cryptococcus sp) in patients intolerant of or refractory to conventional amphotericin B:

- *Children and adolescents* –
  - *Usual dosage:* 3 to 6 mg/kg/day.
  - *Maximum dose:* 6 mg/kg/day. However, dosages as high as 7.5 mg/kg/day have been used.
- *Premature neonates* –
  - *Usual dosage:* 3 mg/kg/day on day 1, then 5 mg/kg/day thereafter.
  - *Maximum dose:* 6 mg/kg/day. However, dosages as high as 7.5 mg/kg/day have been used.

➤*Renal function impairment:* Use with caution in patients with reduced renal function.

Creatinine clearance of less than 10 mL/min – 3 to 6 mg/kg every 24 to 36 hours.

➤*Preparation for administration:*

Reconstitution – Do not filter or use an in-line filter. Reconstitute with sterile water for injection. Do not use saline or dextrose for reconstitution. Using a sterile syringe and a 20-gauge needle, rapidly add the following volumes to the vial to provide a liquid containing 5 mg/mL: for 50 mg/vial, add 10 mL of sterile water for injection; for 100 mg/vial, add 20 mL of sterile water for injection. Shake gently by hand, rotating the vial until all solids have dissolved. Note that the fluid may be opalescent or clear.

Dilution – For infusion, further dilute the reconstituted liquid to a final concentration of approximately 0.6 mg/mL (range, 0.16 to 0.83 mg/mL) with dextrose 5% for injection. The following table provides dilution recommendations.

Amphotericin B Cholesteryl Sulfate Complex Dilution Recommendations

Dose of amphotericin B cholesteryl sulfate complex	Volume of reconstituted amphotericin B cholesteryl sulfate complex	Infusion bag size for dextrose 5% injection
10 to 35 mg	2 to 7 mL	50 mL
35 to 70 mg	7 to 14 mL	100 mL
70 to 175 mg	14 to 35 mL	250 mL
175 to 350 mg	35 to 70 mL	500 mL
350 to 1,000 mg	70 to 200 mL	1,000 mL

➤*Administration:* Administer as an IV infusion at a rate of 1 mg/kg/h. Avoid rapid IV infusion.

If administered through an existing IV line, flush with dextrose 5% for injection prior to and following infusion; otherwise, administer via a separate line.

The infusion time may be shortened to a minimum of 2 hours for patients who show no evidence of intolerance or infusion-related reactions. If the patient experiences acute reactions or cannot tolerate the infusion volume, the infusion time may be extended.

Test dose – A test dose immediately preceding the first dose is advisable when commencing all new courses of treatment. A small amount of drug (eg, 10 mL of the final preparation containing between 1.6 and 8.3 mg) should be infused over 15 to 30 minutes and the patient carefully observed for the next 30 minutes.

Infusion reaction – Acute infusion-related reactions, including anorexia, chills, fever, headache, hypotension, hypoxia, nausea, and tachypnea, are common 1 to 3 hours after starting an IV infusion. These reactions are usually more severe or more frequent with the first few doses of amphotericin B and usually diminish with subsequent doses. Acute infusion-related reactions can be managed by pretreatment with antihistamines and corticosteroids and/or by reducing the rate of infusion and by prompt administration of antihistamines and corticosteroids. Avoid rapid IV infusion.

➤*Admixture compatibility:* Do not reconstitute with saline or dextrose solutions or mix with other drugs, saline, or electrolytes. The use of any solution other than those recommended or the presence of a bacteriostatic agent (eg, benzyl alcohol) may cause precipitation of amphotericin B cholesteryl sulfate.

➤*Storage/Stability:* Store unopened vials at 15° to 30°C (59° to 86°F). After reconstitution, refrigerate at 2° to 8°C (36° to 46°F) and use within 24 hours. Do not freeze. After further dilution with dextrose 5% for injection, refrigerate (2° to 8°C [36° to 46°F]) and use within 24 hours. Partially used vials should be discarded.

Actions

➤*Pharmacology:* Amphotericin B is a polyene antibiotic that acts by binding to sterols (primarily ergosterol) in cell membranes of sensitive fungi, with subsequent leakage of intracellular contents and cell death due to changes in membrane permeability. Amphotericin B also binds to the sterols (primarily cholesterol) in mammalian cell membranes, which is believed to account for its toxicity in animals and humans.

➤*Pharmacokinetics:*

Pharmacokinetic Parameters of Amphotericin B After Administration of Multiple Doses of Amphotericin B Cholesteryl Sulfate Complex[a,b]

	Amphotericin B cholesteryl sulfate complex	
Mean pharmacokinetic parameter	3 mg/kg/day	4 mg/kg/day
V_{ss} (L/kg)	3.8	4.1
Total plasma clearance (L/h/kg)	0.105	0.112
Distribution half-life (min)	3.5	3.5
Elimination half-life (h)	27.5	28.2
C_{max} (mcg/mL)	2.6	2.9
AUC_{ss} (mcg/mL·h)	29	36

[a] Data obtained using population modeling in 51 bone marrow transplant patients. The modeling assumes amphotericin B pharmacokinetics after administration of amphotericin B cholesteryl sulfate complex is best described by a 2-compartment model. Infusion rate = 1 mg/kg/h.
[b] V_{ss} = volume of distribution at steady state; C_{max} = maximum plasma concentration achieved at the end of an infusion; AUC_{ss} = area under the curve at steady state.

Absorption/Distribution – A population modeling approach was used to estimate pharmacokinetic parameters. The pharmacokinetics of amphotericin B, administered as amphotericin B cholesteryl sulfate complex, were best described by an open, 2-compartment structural model and were nonlinear. V_{ss} and total plasma clearance increased with escalating doses, resulting in less than proportional increases in plasma concentration over a dose range of 0.5 to 8 mg/kg/day. The increased volume of distribution probably reflected uptake by tissues. The covariates of body weight and dose level accounted for a substantial portion of the variability of the pharmacokinetic estimates between patients. The unexplained variability in clearance was 26%.

An analytical assay that is able to distinguish between amphotericin B in the amphotericin B cholesteryl sulfate complex and amphotericin B that is not complexed to cholesteryl sulfate was used to analyze samples from a study of 25 patients who were immunocompromised with aspergillosis or who were febrile and neutropenic. Following a 1 mg/kg/h infusion, 25 ± 18% (mean ± standard deviation [SD]) of the total amphotericin B concentration

AMPHOTERICIN B CHOLESTERYL SULFATE COMPLEX

measured in plasma was in the amphotericin B cholesteryl sulfate complex, dropping to 9.3 ± 7.9% at 1 hour and 7.5 ± 9.3% at 24 hours after the end of the infusion.

Special populations –

➤*Microbiology:*

Activity in vitro and in vivo – Amphotericin B cholesteryl sulfate complex is active in vitro against *Aspergillus* and *Candida* species. One hundred and twelve clinical isolates of 4 different *Aspergillus* species and 88 clinical isolates of 5 different *Candida* species were tested, with a majority of minimum inhibitory concentrations (MICs) less than 1 mcg/mL. Amphotericin B cholesteryl sulfate complex is also active in vitro against other fungi. In vitro, amphotericin B cholesteryl sulfate complex is fungistatic or fungicidal, depending upon the concentration of the drug and the susceptibility of the fungal organism. However, standardized techniques for susceptibility testing for antifungal agents have not been established, and results of susceptibility studies do not necessarily correlate with clinical outcome.

Amphotericin B cholesteryl sulfate complex is active in murine models against *Aspergillus fumigatus*, *Candida albicans*, *Coccidioides immitis*, and *Cryptococcus neoformans*, and in an immunosuppressed rabbit model of aspergillosis in which the end points were prolonged survival of infected animals and clearance of microorganisms from target organ(s). Amphotericin B cholesteryl sulfate complex was also active in a hamster model of visceral leishmaniasis, a disease caused by infection of macrophages of the mononuclear phagocytic system by a protozoal parasite of the genus *Leishmania*. In this hamster model, the end points were also prolonged survival of infected animals and clearance of microorganisms from target organ(s).

Drug resistance – Variants with reduced susceptibility to amphotericin B have been isolated from several fungal species after serial passage in cell culture media containing the drug and from some patients receiving prolonged therapy with amphotericin B deoxycholate. Although the relevance of drug resistance to clinical outcome has not been established, fungal organisms that are resistant to amphotericin B may also be resistant to amphotericin B cholesteryl sulfate complex.

Contraindications

Hypersensitivity to any of the product components, unless, in the opinion of the health care provider, the advantages of using amphotericin B cholesteryl sulfate complex outweigh the risks of hypersensitivity.

Warnings/Precautions

➤*Infusion reactions:* See Administration and Dosage for more information.

➤*Hypersensitivity reactions:* Anaphylaxis has been reported with amphotericin B deoxycholate and other amphotericin B–containing drugs. Immediate treatment of anaphylaxis or anaphylactoid reactions is required. Administer epinephrine, oxygen, IV steroids, and airway management as indicated. If severe respiratory distress occurs, immediately discontinue the infusion. The patient should not receive further infusions of amphotericin B cholesteryl sulfate complex.

➤*Pregnancy: Category B.* There are no reports of pregnant women having been treated with amphotericin B cholesteryl sulfate complex.

Reproductive studies with amphotericin B cholesteryl sulfate complex in rats at doses up to 0.4 times the recommended human dose and in rabbits at doses up to 1.1 times the recommended human dose have revealed no evidence of harm to the fetus due to treatment with amphotericin B cholesteryl sulfate complex.

Because animal reproduction studies are not always predictive of human response and because adequate and well-controlled studies have not been conducted in pregnant women, use amphotericin B cholesteryl sulfate complex during pregnancy only if the anticipated benefit to the patient outweighs the potential risk to the fetus.

➤*Lactation:* It is not known whether amphotericin B cholesteryl sulfate complex is excreted in milk. Because of the potential for serious adverse reactions in breast-feeding infants from amphotericin B, decide whether to discontinue breast-feeding or treatment with amphotericin B cholesteryl sulfate complex, taking into account the importance of the drug to the mother.

Because the drug is highly protein bound and has a large molecular weight, it is considered by most reviewers acceptable to use during breast-feeding.

➤*Children:* Ninety-seven children with systemic fungal infections have been treated with amphotericin B cholesteryl sulfate complex at daily doses (mg/kg) similar to those given to adults. No unexpected adverse reactions have been reported. In the same empiric, multicenter trial, children (younger than 16 years of age) treated with amphotericin B cholesteryl sulfate complex had significantly less renal toxicity than amphotericin B deoxycholate patients. Only 12% of children treated with amphotericin B cholesteryl sulfate complex developed nephrotoxicity compared with 52% of children receiving amphotericin B deoxycholate. Renal toxicity was defined as a doubling or increase of 1 mg/dL or more from baseline serum creatinine, or 50% or more decrease from baseline calculated creatinine clearance (CrCl).

➤*Elderly:* Sixty-eight patients at least 65 years of age have been treated with amphotericin B cholesteryl sulfate complex. No unexpected adverse reactions have been reported.

➤*Monitoring:* Monitor laboratory tests, particularly tests of renal and hepatic function, serum electrolytes, complete blood cell counts, and prothrombin time, as medically indicated.

Drug Interactions

Amphotericin B Drug Interactions

Precipitant drug	Object drug[a]		Description
Antineoplastic agents	Amphotericin B	↑	Coadministration may enhance the potential for renal toxicity, bronchospasm, and hypotension. Coadminister with caution.
Azole antifungals (eg, ketoconazole, miconazole)	Amphotericin B	↓	In vitro and in vivo animal studies suggest that imidazoles may induce fungal resistance to amphotericin B. Administer with caution, especially in immunocompromised patients.
Corticosteroids (eg, prednisone) and corticotropin	Amphotericin B	↑	Coadministration may potentiate hypokalemia and predispose patient to cardiac dysfunction. Do not give unless necessary to control adverse reactions. Closely monitor serum electrolytes and cardiac function.
Cyclosporine, tacrolimus	Amphotericin B	↑	Concomitant use of cyclosporine or tacrolimus and amphotericin B cholesteryl sulfate complex may increase the risk of nephrotoxicity. Also, the risk of cyclosporine neurotoxicity may be increased. Closely monitor patients and their renal function when coadministering cyclosporine and amphotericin B. If renal function declines or neurotoxicity occurs, decrease the dosage or stop one or both drugs.
Amphotericin B	Cyclosporine		
Foscarnet	Amphotericin B	↑	Because of additive or synergistic effects, the risk of renal toxicity may be increased. If the use of amphotericin B and foscarnet cannot be avoided, aggressive hydration and close clinical monitoring of renal function are indicated.
Amphotericin B	Foscarnet		
Leukocyte transfusions	Amphotericin B	↑	Acute pulmonary toxicity has been reported during simultaneous administration. Do not coadminister.
Nephrotoxic agents (eg, aminoglycosides, pentamidine)	Amphotericin B	↑	Coadministration may enhance the risk of drug-induced renal toxicity. Use caution when coadministering. Monitor renal function intensively.
Amphotericin B	Nephrotoxic agents (eg, aminoglycosides, pentamidine)		
Amphotericin B	Digitalis glycosides	↑	Coadministration may induce hypokalemia and may potentiate digitalis toxicity. Closely monitor serum potassium concentrations and promptly correct potassium deficits.
Amphotericin B	Flucytosine	↑	Flucytosine toxicity may be increased by increasing its cellular uptake and/or impairing renal excretion. Coadminister with caution.
Amphotericin B	Skeletal muscle relaxants (eg, tubocurarine)	↑	Amphotericin B–induced hypokalemia may enhance the curariform effect of skeletal muscle relaxants. Monitor serum potassium levels closely.

[a] ↑ = object drug increased; ↓ = object drug decreased.

Adverse Reactions

➤*Infusion-related adverse reactions:* Infusion-related adverse reactions (1 to 3 hours after starting IV infusion) occurred most frequently in association with the first infusion of amphotericin B cholesteryl sulfate complex; frequency and severity decreased with subsequent dosing. Based on the combined noncomparative studies, 35% of the patients reported chills or chills and fever, possibly or probably related to amphotericin B cholesteryl

AMPHOTERICIN B CHOLESTERYL SULFATE COMPLEX

sulfate complex, on the first day of dosing, compared with 14% by the seventh dose. In the comparative studies, a similar decreasing trend was noted for amphotericin B cholesteryl sulfate complex and amphotericin B deoxycholate.

➤*Adverse reactions (5% or more):*

Amphotericin B Cholesteryl Sulfate Complex Adverse Reactions (≥ 5%)				
	Noncomparative studies		Comparative studies[a]	
Adverse reaction	Amphotericin B cholesteryl sulfate complex (n = 572)	Amphotericin B cholesteryl sulfate complex aspergillosis patients (n = 161)	Amphotericin B cholesteryl sulfate complex (n = 150)	Amphotericin B deoxycholate (n = 146)
Cardiovascular				
Hypertension	7%	9%	7%	6%
Hypotension	10%	9%	12%	5%
Tachycardia	10%	12%	9%	5%
CNS				
Chills	50%	55%	77%	56%
Headache	5%	8%	4%	3%
GI				
Liver function test abnormal	4%	4%	11%	8%
Nausea	8%	12%	7%	7%
Nausea and vomiting	7%	11%	4%	7%
Vomiting	6%	8%	11%	8%
Metabolic/Nutritional				
Alkaline phosphatase increased	3%	3%	7%	8%
Creatinine increased[b]	12%	12%	21%	34%
Hyper-bilirubinemia	3%	2%	19%	17%
Hyper-glycemia	1%	1%	6%	9%
Hypokalemia	8%	7%	26%	29%
Hypomag-nesemia	4%	7%	6%	11%
Respiratory				
Dyspnea	5%	4%	9%	4%
Hypoxia	5%	6%	9%	5%
Miscellaneous				
Chills and fever	3%	3%	7%	2%
Fever	33%	34%	55%	47%
Thrombo-cytopenia	6%	7%	1%	1%

[a] From patients administered amphotericin B cholesteryl sulfate complex (4 or 6 mg/kg/day) and amphotericin B deoxycholate (0.8 or 1 mg/kg/day) in prospectively randomized, double-blinded studies of empiric treatment of febrile and neutropenic patients or treatment of first-line aspergillosis, respectively.
[b] Includes patients with kidney function abnormal that was associated with an increase in creatinine.

➤*Other adverse reactions (5% or more):*

Cardiovascular – Cardiovascular disorder, postural hypotension.

CNS – Abnormal thinking, confusion, dizziness, insomnia, somnolence, tremor.

Dermatologic – Maculopapular rash, pruritus, rash, sweating.

GI – Abdomen enlarged, abdominal pain, diarrhea, dry mouth, hematemesis, jaundice, stomatitis.

Hematologic/Lymphatic – Anemia, coagulation disorder, hemorrhage, prothrombin decreased.

Metabolic/Nutritional – Edema, generalized edema, hypocalcemia, hypophosphatemia, peripheral edema, weight gain.

Respiratory Apnea, asthma, epistaxis, hyperventilation, increased cough, lung disorder, rhinitis.

Miscellaneous – Back pain, chest pain, eye hemorrhage, face edema, hematuria, injection-site inflammation, mucous membrane disorder, pain, sepsis.

➤*Adverse reactions (1% to less than 5%):*

Cardiovascular – Arrhythmia, atrial fibrillation, bradycardia, congestive heart failure, heart arrest, phlebitis, shock, supraventricular tachycardia, syncope, vasodilatation, ventricular extrasystoles.

CNS – Agitation, anxiety, asthenia, convulsion, depression, hallucinations, hypertonia, hypothermia, nervousness, neuropathy, paresthesia, psychosis, speech disorder, stupor.

Dermatologic – Acne, alopecia, petechial rash, skin discoloration, skin disorder, skin nodule, skin ulcer, urticaria, vesiculobullous rash.

GI – Anorexia, bloody diarrhea, constipation, dyspepsia, fecal incontinence, gamma-glutamyl transpeptidase increased, GI disorder, GI hemorrhage, gingivitis, glossitis, hepatic failure, melena, mouth ulceration, oral moniliasis, rectal disorder.

GU – Albuminuria, dysuria, glycosuria, kidney failure, oliguria, urinary incontinence, urinary retention, urinary tract disorder.

Hematologic/Lymphatic – Ecchymosis, fibrinogen increased, hypochromic anemia, leukocytosis, leukopenia, petechia, thromboplastin decreased.

Hepatic – Veno-occlusive liver disease.

Local – Injection-site pain, injection-site reaction.

Metabolic/Nutritional – Acidosis, ALT increased, AST increased, dehydration, hyperkalemia, hyperlipemia, hypernatremia, hypervolemia, hypoglycemia, hyponatremia, hypoproteinemia, lactic dehydrogenase increased, serum urea nitrogen increased, weight loss.

Musculoskeletal – Arthralgia, myalgia, neck pain.

Respiratory – Hemoptysis, lung edema, pharyngitis, pleural effusion, respiratory disorder, sinusitis.

Special senses – Amblyopia, deafness, ear disorder, tinnitus.

Miscellaneous – Accidental injury, allergic reaction, death, immune system disorder, infection, injection-site reaction, local injection-site pain.

Overdosage

➤*Symptoms:* Amphotericin B deoxycholate overdose has been reported to result in cardiorespiratory arrest.

➤*Treatment:* Amphotericin B cholesteryl sulfate complex is not dialyzable.

Patient Information

Inform patients that this medication is administered by IV infusion and treatment may last for several weeks.

Advise patients to report to their health care provider any pain or swelling at the infusion site, difficulty breathing, chest pain, chills, nausea, swelling of the face or mouth, or any other infusion reactions.

AMPHOTERICIN B LIPID COMPLEX

Indications

➤*Fungal infections, systemic:* For the treatment of invasive fungal infections in patients who are refractory to or intolerant of conventional amphotericin B therapy.

➤*Off-label uses:* Prophylaxis of fungal infection in patients with bone marrow transplantation; for the treatment of primary amoebic meningoencephalitis caused by *Naegleria fowleri*; subconjunctival or intravitreal injection in ocular aspergillosis; as chemoprophylaxis by low-dose intravenous (IV), intranasal, or nebulized administration in immunocompromised patients at risk of aspergillosis; intra-articularly or intramuscularly (IM) for coccidioidal arthritis; empiric treatment of fungal infections; treatment of visceral leishmaniasis.

Administration and Dosage

➤*General dosing considerations:* As with any amphotericin B–containing product, during the initial dosing of amphotericin B lipid complex, administer the drug under close clinical observation by medically trained personnel.

Renal toxicity of amphotericin B lipid complex, as measured by serum creatinine levels, has been shown to be dose dependent. Decisions about dose adjustments should be made only after taking into account the overall clinical condition of the patient.

Amphotericin B lipid complex must be diluted prior to administration. (See Preparation for Administration.)

AMPHOTERICIN B LIPID COMPLEX

➤*Adults:*

Fungal infection, systemic – 5 mg/kg given as a single IV infusion daily.

➤*Children:* See Adults for dosing.

Off-label dosing –

Febrile neutropenia, empirical therapy:

- *Children 2 to 16 years of age* –
  Usual dosage: 5 mg/kg/day.
  Maximum dose: 5 mg/kg/day. However, dosages as high as 6.5 to 13 mg/kg/day have been given.

Fungal infections, systemic therapy (Aspergillus sp, Candida sp, Cryptococcus sp):

- *Infants and children 2 to 17 years of age* –
  Usual dosage: 2.5 to 5 mg/kg/day.
  Maximum dose: 5 mg/kg/day. However, dosages as high as 6.5 to 13 mg/kg/day have been given.
- *Neonates* –
  Usual dosage: 2.5 to 5 mg/kg/day. One study administered up to 6.5 mg/kg/day.
  Maximum dose: 5 mg/kg/day. However, dosages as high as 6.5 to 13 mg/kg/day have been given.

Visceral leishmaniasis (refractory or intolerant to conventional amphotericin B): 1 to 3 mg/kg/day for 5 days.

➤*Renal function impairment:* Use with caution in patients with reduced renal function.

Creatinine clearance of less than 10 mL/min – 5 mg/kg every 24 to 36 hours.

➤*Preparation for administration:* Shake the vial gently until there is no yellow sediment at the bottom. Withdraw the appropriate dose from the required number of vials into 1 or more sterile syringes using an 18-gauge needle. Remove the needle from each syringe filled with amphotericin B lipid complex and replace with a 5-micron filter needle supplied with each vial. Each filter needle may be used to filter the contents of up to four 100 mg vials. Insert the filter needle of the syringe into an IV bag containing dextrose 5% for injection and empty the contents of the syringe into the bag for a final concentration of 1 mg/mL (2 mg/mL for children and cardiovascular patients). Shake the bag until the contents are thoroughly mixed.

Do not use the admixture after dilution with dextrose 5% injection if there is any evidence of foreign matter. Vials are for single use. Unused materials should be discarded.

➤*Administration:* Before infusion, shake the bag until the contents are thoroughly mixed. Administer at a rate of 2.5 mg/kg/h. Do not use an in-line filter. If the infusion exceeds 2 hours, mix the contents by shaking the infusion bag every 2 hours.

An existing IV line should be flushed with dextrose 5% for injection before infusion of amphotericin B lipid complex, or a separate infusion line should be used.

Infusion reaction – Acute reactions, including fever and chills, may occur 1 to 2 hours after starting an IV infusion. These reactions are usually more common with the first few doses of amphotericin B lipid complex and usually diminish with subsequent doses. Infusion has been rarely associated with arrhythmias, bronchospasm, hypotension, and shock.

➤*Admixture compatibility:* Do not dilute with saline solutions or mix with other drugs or electrolytes because the compatibility of amphotericin B lipid complex with these materials has not been established. The use of any solution other than those recommended or the presence of a bacteriostatic agent (eg, benzyl alcohol) may cause precipitation of amphotericin B lipid complex.

➤*Storage/Stability:* Prior to admixture, store between 2° and 8°C (36° and 46°F). Protect from exposure to light. Do not freeze. Retain in the carton until time of use. The admixture may be stored for up to 48 hours between 2° and 8°C (36° and 46°F) and for an additional 6 hours at room temperature. Vials are for single use and any unused drug should be discarded.

Actions

➤*Pharmacology:* Amphotericin B is a polyene antifungal antibiotic that acts by binding to sterols in the cell membrane of susceptible fungi, with a resultant change in the permeability of the membrane. Mammalian cell membranes also contain sterols, and damage to human cells is believed to occur through the same mechanism of action.

➤*Pharmacokinetics:* The pharmacokinetics of amphotericin B after the administration of amphotericin B lipid complex are nonlinear. Volume of distribution (Vd) and clearance from blood increase with increasing dose of amphotericin B lipid complex, resulting in less than proportional increases in blood concentrations of amphotericin B over a dose range of 0.6 to 5 mg/kg/day.

Pharmacokinetic Parameters of Amphotericin B in Whole Blood in Patients Administered Multiple Doses of Amphotericin B Lipid Complex or Amphotericin B Desoxycholate[a]

Pharmacokinetic parameter	Amphotericin B lipid complex injection 5 mg/kg/day for 5 to 7 days mean ± SD	Amphotericin B 0.6 mg/kg/day for 42 days[b] mean ± SD
Peak concentration (mcg/mL)	1.7 ± 0.8 (n = 10)[c]	1.1 ± 0.2 (n = 5)
Concentration at end of dosing interval (mcg/mL)	0.6 ± 0.3 (n = 10)[c]	0.4 ± 0.2 (n = 5)
$AUC_{0\text{-}24h}$ (mcg•h/mL)	14 ± 7 (n = 14)[c,d]	17.1 ± 5 (n = 5)
Clearance (mL/h•kg)	436 ± 188.5 (n = 14)[c,d]	38 ± 15 (n = 5)
Apparent Vd_{area} (L/kg)	131 ± 57.7 (n = 8)[d]	5 ± 2.8 (n = 5)
Terminal elimination half-life (h)	173.4 ± 78 (n = 8)[d]	91.1 ± 40.9 (n = 5)
Amount excreted in urine over 24 hours after last dose (% of dose)[e]	0.9 ± 0.4 (n = 8)[d]	9.6 ± 2.5 (n = 8)

[a] SD = standard deviation; $AUC_{0\text{-}24h}$ = area under the curve.
[b] Data from patients with mucocutaneous leishmaniasis. Infusion rate was 0.25 mg/kg/h.
[c] Data from studies in patients with cytologically proven cancer being treated with chemotherapy or neutropenic patients with presumed or proven fungal infection. Infusion rate was 2.5 mg/kg/h.
[d] Data from patients with mucocutaneous leishmaniasis. Infusion rate was 4 mg/kg/h.
[e] Percentage of dose excreted in 24 hours after last dose.

Absorption – AUC of amphotericin B increased approximately 34% from day 1 after the administration of amphotericin B lipid complex 5 mg/kg/day for 7 days.

Distribution – The large Vd and high clearance from blood of amphotericin B after the administration of amphotericin B lipid complex probably reflect uptake by tissues.

Tissue concentrations of amphotericin B have been obtained at autopsy from 1 heart transplant patient who received 3 doses of amphotericin B lipid complex at 5.3 mg/kg/day.

Amphotericin B Concentration in Human Tissues after Administration of Amphotericin B Lipid Complex

Organ	Amphotericin B tissue concentration (mcg/g)
Spleen	290
Lung	222
Liver	196
Lymph node	7.6
Kidney	6.9
Heart	5
Brain	1.5

This pattern of distribution is consistent with that observed in preclinical studies in dogs in which greatest concentrations of amphotericin B after amphotericin B lipid complex administration were observed in the liver, spleen, and lung; however, the relationship of tissue concentrations of amphotericin B to its biological activity when administered as amphotericin B lipid complex is unknown.

Excretion – The long terminal elimination half-life probably reflects a slow redistribution from tissues. Although amphotericin B is excreted slowly, there is little accumulation in the blood after repeated dosing.

➤*Microbiology:*

Activity in vitro and in vivo – Amphotericin B lipid complex shows in vitro activity against *Aspergillus* sp (n = 3) and *Candida* sp (n = 10), with minimum inhibitory concentrations (MICs) generally less than 1 mcg/mL. Depending upon the species and strain of *Aspergillus* and *Candida* tested, significant in vitro differences in susceptibility to amphotericin B have been reported (MICs ranging from 0.1 to greater than 10 mcg/mL). However, standardized techniques for susceptibility testing for antifungal agents have not been established, and results of susceptibility studies do not necessarily correlate with clinical outcome.

Amphotericin B lipid complex is active in animal models against *Aspergillus fumigatus*; *Candida albicans*, *Candida guilliermondii*, *Candida stellatoidea*, and *Candida tropicalis*; *Cryptococcus* sp; *Coccidiomycoses* sp; *Histoplasma* sp; and *Blastomyces* sp in which end points were clearance of microorganisms from target organ(s) and/or prolonged survival of infected animals.

Drug resistance – Fungal species with decreased susceptibility to amphotericin B have been isolated after serial passage in culture media containing the drug and from some patients receiving prolonged therapy. Although the relevance of drug resistance to clinical outcome has not been established,

AMPHOTERICIN B LIPID COMPLEX

fungal species that are resistant to amphotericin B may also be resistant to amphotericin B lipid complex.

Contraindications

Hypersensitivity to amphotericin B or any other component in the formulation.

Warnings/Precautions

➤*Infusion reactions:* See Administration and Dosage for more information.

➤*Hypersensitivity reactions:* Anaphylaxis has been reported with amphotericin B desoxycholate and other amphotericin B–containing drugs. Anaphylaxis has been reported with amphotericin B lipid complex with an incidence rate of less than 0.1%. If severe respiratory distress occurs, immediately discontinue the infusion. The patient should not receive further infusions of amphotericin B lipid complex.

➤*Pregnancy: Category B.* There are no reports of pregnant women having been treated with amphotericin B lipid complex. Reproductive studies in rats and rabbits at doses of amphotericin B lipid complex up to 0.64 times the human dose revealed no harm to the fetus. Because animal reproductive studies are not always predictive of human response and adequate and well-controlled studies have not been conducted in pregnant women, use amphotericin B lipid complex during pregnancy only after taking into account the importance of the drug to the mother.

➤*Lactation:* It is not known whether amphotericin B lipid complex is excreted in human milk. Because many drugs are excreted in human milk and because of the potential for serious adverse reactions in breast-fed infants from amphotericin B lipid complex, decide whether to discontinue breast-feeding or the drug, taking into account the importance of the drug to the mother.

Because the drug is highly protein bound and has a large molecular weight, it is considered by most reviewers acceptable to use during breast-feeding.

➤*Children:* One-hundred eleven children (2 were enrolled twice and counted as separate patients) 16 years of age and younger, 11 of whom were younger than 1 year of age, have been treated with amphotericin B lipid complex at 5 mg/kg/day in 2 open-label studies and 1 small, prospective, single-arm study. In 1 single-center study, 5 children with hepatosplenic candidiasis were effectively treated with 2.5 mg/kg/day of amphotericin B lipid complex. No serious unexpected adverse reactions have been reported.

➤*Elderly:* Forty-nine elderly patients 65 years of age and older have been treated with amphotericin B lipid complex at 5 mg/kg/day in 2 open-label studies and 1 small, prospective, single-arm study. No serious unexpected adverse reactions have been reported.

➤*Monitoring:* Frequently monitor serum creatinine during amphotericin B lipid complex therapy. Regularly monitor liver function, serum electrolytes (particularly magnesium and potassium), and complete blood cell counts.

Drug Interactions

Amphotericin B Drug Interactions

Precipitant drug	Object drug[a]		Description
Antineoplastic agents	Amphotericin B	↑	Coadministration may enhance the potential for renal toxicity, bronchospasm, and hypotension. Coadminister with caution.
Azole antifungals (eg, ketoconazole, miconazole)	Amphotericin B	↓	In vitro and in vivo animal studies suggest that imidazoles may induce fungal resistance to amphotericin B. Administer with caution, especially in immunocompromised patients.
Corticosteroids (eg, prednisone) and corticotropin	Amphotericin B	↑	Coadministration may potentiate hypokalemia and predispose patient to cardiac dysfunction. Do not give unless necessary to control adverse reactions. Closely monitor serum electrolytes and cardiac function.
Cyclosporine	Amphotericin B	↑	Concomitant use of cyclosporine and amphotericin B lipid complex may increase the risk of nephrotoxicity. Also, the risk of cyclosporine neurotoxicity may be increased. Closely monitor patients and their renal function when coadministering cyclosporine and amphotericin B. If renal function declines or neurotoxicity occurs, decrease the dosage or stop one or both drugs.
Amphotericin B	Cyclosporine		
Foscarnet	Amphotericin B	↑	Because of additive or synergistic effects, the risk of renal toxicity may be increased. If the use of amphotericin B and foscarnet cannot be avoided, aggressive hydration and close clinical monitoring of renal function are indicated.
Amphotericin B	Foscarnet		
Leukocyte transfusions	Amphotericin B	↑	Acute pulmonary toxicity has been reported during simultaneous administration. Do not coadminister.
Nephrotoxic agents (eg, aminoglycosides, pentamidine)	Amphotericin B	↑	Coadministration may enhance risk of drug-induced renal toxicity. Use caution when administering concomitantly. Monitor renal function intensively.
Amphotericin B	Nephrotoxic agents (eg, aminoglycosides, pentamidine)		
Amphotericin B	Digitalis glycosides	↑	Coadministration may induce hypokalemia and may potentiate digitalis toxicity. Closely monitor serum potassium concentrations and promptly correct potassium deficits.
Amphotericin B	Flucytosine	↑	Flucytosine toxicity may be increased by increasing its cellular uptake and/or impairing renal excretion. Coadminister with caution.
Amphotericin B	Skeletal muscle relaxants (eg, tubocurarine)	↑	Amphotericin B–induced hypokalemia may enhance the curariform effect of skeletal muscle relaxants. Monitor serum potassium levels closely.

[a] ↑ = object drug increased; ↓ = object drug decreased.

Adverse Reactions

➤*Discontinuation of therapy:* Of the 556 patients treated with amphotericin B lipid complex, 9% discontinued treatment because of adverse reactions regardless of presumed relationship to study drug.

➤*Most common adverse reactions:* In general, the adverse reactions most commonly reported with amphotericin B lipid complex were transient chills and/or fever during infusion of the drug.

➤*Adverse reaction (3% or more):*

Amphotericin B Lipid Complex Adverse Reactions (≥ 3%)[a]

Adverse reaction	Amphotericin B lipid complex (n = 556)
Cardiovascular	
Heart arrest	6%
Hypertension	5%
Hypotension	8%
CNS	
Chills	18%
Headache	6%
GI	
Abdominal pain	4%
Diarrhea	6%
GI hemorrhage	4%
Nausea	9%
Nausea/Vomiting	3%
Vomiting	8%
Hematologic	
Anemia	4%
Leukopenia	4%
Thrombocytopenia	5%
Renal	
Increased serum creatinine	11%
Kidney failure	5%

AMPHOTERICIN B LIPID COMPLEX

Amphotericin B Lipid Complex Adverse Reactions (≥ 3%)[a]	
Adverse reaction	Amphotericin B lipid complex (n = 556)
Respiratory	
Dyspnea	7%
Respiratory disorder	4%
Respiratory failure	8%
Miscellaneous	
Bilirubinemia	4%
Chest pain	3%
Fever	14%
Hypokalemia	5%
Infection	5%
Multiple organ failure	11%
Pain	5%
Rash	4%
Sepsis	7%

[a] The causal association between these adverse reactions and amphotericin B lipid complex is uncertain.

➤*Other adverse reactions:*

Cardiovascular – Arrhythmias (including ventricular fibrillation), cardiac failure, cardiomyopathy, cerebral vascular accident, myocardial infarction, thrombophlebitis.

CNS – Convulsions, encephalopathy, extrapyramidal syndrome and other neurologic symptoms, malaise, peripheral neuropathy, transient vertigo.

Dermatologic – Erythema multiforme, exfoliative dermatitis, maculopapular rash, pruritus.

GI – Anorexia, cramping, diarrhea, dyspepsia, epigastric pain, melena.

GU – Anuria, dysuria, impotence, oliguria.

Hematologic – Blood dyscrasias (including eosinophilia), coagulation defects, leukocytosis.

Hepatic – Acute liver failure, cholangitis, cholecystitis, hepatomegaly, hepatitis, jaundice, veno-occlusive liver disease.

Hypersensitivity – Anaphylactoid and other allergic reactions, asthma, bronchospasm, wheezing.

Lab test abnormalities – Acidosis, hyperamylasemia, hypercalcemia, hyperglycemia, hyperkalemia, hyperuricemia, hypocalcemia, hypoglycemia, hypomagnesemia, hypophosphatemia, increased ALT, increased AST, increased alkaline phosphatase, increased serum urea nitrogen, increased lactate dehydrogenase.

Musculoskeletal – Myasthenia (including bone, muscle, and joint pain).

Renal – Decreased renal function, renal tubular acidosis.

Respiratory – Hemoptysis, pleural effusion, pulmonary edema, pulmonary embolus, tachypnea.

Special senses – Deafness, diplopia, hearing loss, tinnitus, visual impairment.

Miscellaneous – Injection-site reaction (including inflammation), shock, weight loss.

Overdosage

➤*Symptoms:* Amphotericin B desoxycholate overdose has been reported to result in cardiorespiratory arrest. Fifteen patients have been reported to have received 1 or more doses of amphotericin B lipid complex between 7 and 13 mg/kg. None of these patients had a serious acute reaction to amphotericin B lipid complex.

➤*Treatment:* If an overdose is suspected, discontinue therapy, monitor the patient's clinical status, and administer supportive therapy as required. Amphotericin B lipid complex is not hemodialyzable.

Patient Information

Instruct patients to report any symptoms of chills, fever, malaise, or any discomfort at injection site to their health care provider.

AMPHOTERICIN B LIPOSOME

Indications

➤*Cryptococcal meningitis in HIV:* Treatment of cryptococcal meningitis in HIV-infected patients.

➤*Fungal infections, empirical therapy:* For empirical treatment in febrile neutropenic patients with presumed fungal infection.

➤*Fungal infections, systemic therapy:* For use in patients refractory to conventional amphotericin B deoxycholate therapy or when renal impairment or unacceptable toxicity precludes the use of the deoxycholate formulation for the treatment of infections caused by *Aspergillus* sp, *Candida* sp, and/or *Cryptococcus* sp.

➤*Visceral leishmaniasis:* For treatment of visceral leishmaniasis.

➤*Off-label uses:*

Other possible off-label uses – Prophylaxis and treatment of fungal infection in patients with solid bone marrow transplantation; for the treatment of primary amoebic meningoencephalitis caused by *Naegleria fowleri*; subconjunctival or intravitreal injection in ocular aspergillosis; as chemoprophylaxis by low-dose intravenous (IV), intranasal, or nebulized administration in immunocompromised patients at risk of aspergillosis; intra-articularly or intramuscularly for coccidioidal arthritis.

Administration and Dosage

➤*General dosing considerations:* Dosing and rate of infusion should be individualized to the needs of the specific patient to ensure maximum efficacy while minimizing systemic toxicities or adverse reactions.

➤*Adults:*

Cryptococcal meningitis in HIV – 6 mg/kg/day.

Fungal infection, empirical – 3 mg/kg/day.

Fungal infection, systemic – 3 to 5 mg/kg/day.

Visceral leishmaniasis –

Immunocompetent patients: 3 mg/kg/day on days 1 through 5, 14, and 21; a repeat course of therapy may be useful if parasitic clearance is not achieved.

Immunocompromised patients: 4 mg/kg/day on days 1 through 5, 10, 17, 24, 31, and 38; seek expert advice regarding further therapy if parasitic clearance is not achieved or if relapse is experienced.

➤*Children:*

1 month of age and older – See Adults for dosing.

Off-label dosing –

Fungal infection, systemic:

- *Infants/Children/Adolescents* –
  Usual dosage: 3 to 5 mg/kg/day.
  Maximum dose: Dosages as high as 15 mg/kg/day have been used. Dosages as high as 10 mg/kg/day have been used in patients with *Aspergillus*.
- *Neonates (term and preterm)* – 3 to 5 mg/kg/day. Dosages as high as 7 mg/kg/day have been reported.

Solid bone marrow transplant, prophylaxis and treatment:

- *Children and adolescents* – 2 to 6 mg/kg/day IV over a mean of 25 days (range, 5 to 90 days). In hematopoietic stem cell transplant, 10 mg/kg/day once weekly may be useful for prophylaxis against fungal infections.

Visceral leishmaniasis:

- *Immunocompetent patients (children and adolescents)* – 4 mg/kg IV on days 1 to 5 and on day 10. Mediterranean visceral leishmaniasis has been treated with 20 mg/kg administered as 4 mg/kg for 5 days or 10 mg/kg for 2 days.

➤*Renal function impairment:* Use with caution in patients with reduced renal function.

Creatinine clearance less than 10 mL/min – 3 mg/kg every 24 hours.

Adults receiving continuous renal replacement therapy – A dosage of 3 to 5 mg/kg IV every 24 hours is recommended for patients receiving continuous venovenous hemofiltration (CVVH), continuous venovenous hemodialysis (CVVHD), or continuous venovenous hemodiafiltration (CVVHDF). This recommendation assumes ultrafiltration and dialysis flow rates of 1 to 2 L/h.

Adults receiving intermittent hemodialysis – 3 to 5 mg/kg IV every 24 hours administered after the dialysis session. This recommendation assumes the patient is receiving standard intermittent hemodialysis (IHD) 3 times per week and completes the full dialysis sessions.

➤*Preparation for administration:*

Reconstitution – Reconstitute using sterile water for injection (without a bacteriostatic agent). Add 12 mL of sterile water for injection to each vial to yield 4 mg/mL. Immediately shake the vial vigorously for 30 seconds to completely disperse the drug until a yellow, translucent suspension is formed. Visually inspect the vial for particulate matter and continue shaking until completely dispersed.

Dilution – Calculate the amount of reconstituted amphotericin B liposome (4 mg/mL) to be further diluted. Withdraw appropriate amount of reconstituted solution into sterile syringe, attach the 5-micron filter provided, and inject contents of syringe through filter needle into an appropriate amount of dextrose 5% (use only 1 filter needle per vial) to yield a final concentration of 1 to 2 mg/mL for administration. Lower concentrations of 0.2 to 0.5 mg/mL may be more appropriate for infants and small children. Discard partially used vials.

➤*Administration:* Administer using a controlled infusion device over approximately 120 minutes; infusion time may be reduced to 60 minutes if well tolerated or increased if patient experiences discomfort. An in-line membrane filter of at least 1 micron mean pore diameter may be used.

If administered through an existing IV line, flush with dextrose 5% for injection prior to and following infusion; otherwise, administer via a separate line.

Infusion reactions – Acute infusion-related reactions, including anorexia, chills, fever, headache, hypotension, nausea, and tachypnea, may occur 1 to 3 hours after starting an IV infusion. These reactions are usually

AMPHOTERICIN B LIPOSOME

more severe with the first few doses of amphotericin B and usually diminish with subsequent doses. Acute infusion-related reactions can be managed by pretreatment with antihistamines and corticosteroids or by reducing the rate of infusion and by prompt administration of antihistamines and corticosteroids.

➤*Admixture compatibility:* Do not reconstitute with saline solutions or mix with other drugs. The use of any solution other than those recommended or the presence of bacteriostatic agent (eg, benzyl alcohol) may cause precipitation of amphotericin B liposome.

➤*Storage/Stability:* Store unopened vials at 25°C (77°F). Store reconstituted product concentrate between 2° and 8°C (36° and 46°F) following reconstitution with sterile water for injection. Do not freeze. Use within 6 hours of dilution with dextrose 5%.

Actions

➤*Pharmacology:* Amphotericin B is a macrocyclic, polyene, antifungal antibiotic that acts by binding to the sterol component of a cell membrane, leading to alterations in cell permeability and cell death. While amphotericin B has a higher affinity for the ergosterol component of the fungal cell membrane, it can also bind to the cholesterol component of the mammalian cell, leading to cytotoxicity. Amphotericin B liposome, the liposomal preparation of amphotericin B, has been shown to penetrate the cell wall of both extracellular and intracellular forms of susceptible fungi.

➤*Pharmacokinetics:* The pharmacokinetics of amphotericin B after administration of amphotericin B liposome are nonlinear such that there is a greater than proportional increase in serum concentrations with an increase in dosage from 1 to 5 mg/kg/day.

Amphotericin B Liposome Pharmacokinetic Parameters[a]

Dose	1 mg/kg/day		2.5 mg/kg/day		5 mg/kg/day	
Day	1 (n = 8)	Last (n = 7)	1 (n = 7)	Last (n = 7)	1 (n = 12)	Last (n = 9)
Pharmacokinetic parameters						
C_{max} (mcg/mL)	7.3 ± 3.8	12.2 ± 4.9	17.2 ± 7.1	31.4 ± 17.8	57.6 ± 21	83 ± 35.2
AUC_{0-24} (mcg•h/mL)	27 ± 14	60 ± 20	65 ± 33	197 ± 183	269 ± 96	555 ± 311
Half-life (h)	10.7 ± 6.4	7 ± 2.1	8.1 ± 2.3	6.3 ± 2	6.4 ± 2.1	6.8 ± 2.1
V_{ss} (L/kg)	0.44 ± 0.27	0.14 ± 0.05	0.4 ± 0.37	0.16 ± 0.09	0.16 ± 0.1	0.1 ± 0.07
Clearance (mL/h/kg)	39 ± 22	17 ± 6	51 ± 44	22 ± 15	21 ± 14	11 ± 6

[a] C_{max} = maximum plasma concentration; AUC_{0-24} = area under the curve; V_{ss} = volume of distribution at steady state.

Absorption – Steady-state concentrations were generally achieved within 4 days of dosing.

Distribution – Although variable, mean trough concentrations of amphotericin B remained relatively constant with repeated administration of the same dose over the range of 1 to 5 mg/kg/day, indicating no significant drug accumulation in the serum.

Metabolism – The metabolic pathways of amphotericin B after administration of amphotericin B liposome are not known.

Excretion – Based on total amphotericin B concentrations measured within a dosing interval (24 hours) after administration of amphotericin B liposome, the mean half-life was 7 to 10 hours. However, based on total amphotericin B concentration measured up to 49 days after dosing of amphotericin B liposome, the mean half-life was 100 to 153 hours. The long terminal elimination half-life is probably a slow redistribution from tissues.

The mean clearance at steady state was independent of dose. The excretion of amphotericin B after administration of amphotericin B liposome has not been studied.

➤*Microbiology:*

Activity in vitro and in vivo – Amphotericin B liposome has shown in vitro activity comparable with amphotericin B against the following organisms: *Aspergillus* species (*Aspergillus fumigatus, Aspergillus flavus*), *Candida* species (*Candida albicans, Candida krusei, Candida lusitaniae, Candida parapsilosis, Candida tropicalis*), *Cryptococcus neoformans*, and *Blastomyces dermatitidis*. However, standardized techniques for susceptibility testing of antifungal agents have not been established and results of such studies do not necessarily correlate with clinical outcome.

Amphotericin B liposome is active in animal models against *A. fumigatus, C. albicans, C. krusei, C. lusitaniae, C. neoformans, B. dermatitidis, Coccidioides immitis, Histoplasma capsulatum, Paracoccidioides brasiliensis, Leishmania donovani*, and *Leishmania infantum*. The administration of amphotericin B liposome in these animal models demonstrated prolonged survival of infected animals, reduction of microorganisms from target organs, or a decrease in lung weight.

Drug resistance – Mutants with decreased susceptibility to amphotericin B have been isolated from several fungal species after serial passage in culture media containing the drug, and from some patients receiving prolonged therapy. Drug combination studies in vitro and in vivo suggest that imidazoles may induce resistance to amphotericin B. However, the clinical relevance of drug resistance has not been established.

Contraindications

Hypersensitivity to amphotericin B deoxycholate or any other constituents of the product.

Warnings/Precautions

➤*Administration:* As with any amphotericin B–containing product, medically trained personnel should administer the drug. During the initial dosing period, patients should be under close clinical observation. Amphotericin B liposome has been shown to be significantly less toxic than amphotericin B deoxycholate; however, adverse reactions may still occur.

➤*Infusion reactions:* See Administration and Dosage for more information.

➤*Hypersensitivity reactions:* Anaphylaxis has been reported with amphotericin B deoxycholate and other amphotericin B–containing drugs, including amphotericin B liposome. If a severe anaphylactic reaction occurs, immediately discontinue the infusion and do not administer further infusions of amphotericin B liposome.

➤*Pregnancy: Category B.* There have been no adequate and well-controlled studies of amphotericin B liposome in pregnant women. Systemic fungal infections have been successfully treated in pregnant women with amphotericin B deoxycholate, but the number of cases reported has been small. Only use amphotericin B liposome during pregnancy if the possible benefits to be derived outweigh the potential risks involved.

Segment II studies in rats and rabbits have concluded that amphotericin B liposome had no teratogenic potential in these species. In rats, the maternal nontoxic dose of amphotericin B liposome was estimated to be 5 mg/kg (equivalent to 0.16 to 0.8 times the recommended human clinical dose range of 1 to 5 mg/kg) and, in rabbits, 3 mg/kg (equivalent to 0.2 to 1 times the recommended human clinical dose range), based on body surface area correction. Rabbits receiving the higher doses (equivalent to 0.5 to 2 times the recommended human dose) of amphotericin B liposome experienced a higher rate of spontaneous abortions than the control groups.

➤*Lactation:* Many drugs are excreted in human milk. However, it is not known whether amphotericin B liposome is excreted in human milk. Because of the potential for serious adverse reactions in breast-fed infants, make a decision whether to discontinue breast-feeding or the drug, taking into account the importance of the drug to the mother.

Because the drug is highly protein bound and has a large molecular weight, it is considered by most reviewers acceptable to use during breast-feeding.

➤*Children:* Children 1 month to 16 years of age with presumed fungal infection (empirical therapy), confirmed systemic fungal infections, or visceral leishmaniasis have been successfully treated with amphotericin B liposome. In studies that included 302 children administered amphotericin B liposome, there was no evidence of any differences in efficacy or safety of amphotericin B liposome compared with adults. Because children have received amphotericin B liposome at doses comparable with those used in adults on a per kilogram body weight basis, no dosage adjustment is required in this population. Safety and effectiveness in children younger than 1 month of age have not been established.

➤*Elderly:* As with most other drugs, carefully monitor elderly patients receiving amphotericin B liposome.

➤*Monitoring:* Patient management should include laboratory evaluation of serum electrolytes (particularly magnesium and potassium) and renal, hepatic, and hematopoietic function.

Drug Interactions

Amphotericin B Liposome Drug Interactions

Precipitant drug	Object drug[a]		Description
Antineoplastic agents	Amphotericin B	⬆	Coadministration may enhance the potential for renal toxicity, bronchospasm, and hypotension. Coadminister with caution.
Azole antifungals (eg, ketoconazole, miconazole)	Amphotericin B	⬇	In vitro and in vivo animal studies suggest that imidazoles may induce fungal resistance to amphotericin B. Administer with caution, especially in immunocompromised patients.
Corticosteroids (eg, prednisone) and corticotropin	Amphotericin B	⬆	Coadministration may potentiate hypokalemia and predispose patient to cardiac dysfunction. Do not give unless necessary to control adverse reactions. Closely monitor serum electrolytes and cardiac function.

AMPHOTERICIN B LIPOSOME

Amphotericin B Liposome Drug Interactions			
Precipitant drug	Object drug[a]		Description
Cyclosporine	Amphotericin B	↑	Concomitant use of cyclosporine and amphotericin B may increase the risk of nephrotoxicity. Also, the risk of cyclosporine neurotoxicity may be increased. Closely monitor patients and their renal function when coadministering cyclosporine and amphotericin B. If renal function declines or neurotoxicity occurs, decrease the dosage or stop one or both drugs.
Amphotericin B	Cyclosporine		
Foscarnet	Amphotericin B liposome	↑	Because of additive or synergistic effects, the risk of renal toxicity may be increased. If the use of amphotericin B and foscarnet cannot be avoided, aggressive hydration and close clinical monitoring of renal function are indicated.
Amphotericin B liposome	Foscarnet		
Leukocyte transfusions	Amphotericin B	↑	Acute pulmonary toxicity has been reported during simultaneous administration. Do not coadminister.
Nephrotoxic agents (eg, aminoglycosides, pentamidine)	Amphotericin B	↑	Coadministration may enhance risk of drug-induced renal toxicity. Use caution when coadministering. Monitor renal function intensively.
Amphotericin B	Nephrotoxic agents (eg, aminoglycosides, pentamidine)		
Amphotericin B	Digitalis glycosides	↑	Coadministration may induce hypokalemia and may potentiate digitalis toxicity. Closely monitor serum potassium concentrations and promptly correct potassium deficits.
Amphotericin B	Flucytosine	↑	Flucytosine toxicity may be increased by increasing its cellular uptake and/or impairing renal excretion. Coadminister with caution.
Amphotericin B	Skeletal muscle relaxants (eg, tubocurarine)	↑	Amphotericin B–induced hypokalemia may enhance the curariform effect of skeletal muscle relaxants. Monitor serum potassium levels closely.

[a] ↑ = object drug increased; ↓ = object drug decreased.

Adverse Reactions

➤*Fungal infections, empiric therapy:*

Comparison with amphotericin B deoxycholate –

Adverse reaction	Amphotericin B liposome (n = 343)	Amphotericin B deoxycholate (n = 344)
Cardiovascular		
Chest pain	12%	11.6%
Hypertension	7.9%	16.3%
Hypotension	14.3%	21.5%
Tachycardia	13.4%	20.9%
CNS		
Anxiety	13.7%	11%
Asthenia	13.1%	10.8%
Chills	47.5%	75.9%
Confusion	11.4%	13.4%
Headache	19.8%	20.9%
Insomnia	17.2%	14.2%
Dermatologic		
Pruritus	10.8%	10.2%
Rash	24.8%	24.4%
Sweating	7%	10.8%
GI		
Abdominal pain	19.8%	21.8%
Diarrhea	30.3%	27.3%
GI hemorrhage	9.9%	11.3%
Nausea	39.7%	38.7%
Vomiting	31.8%	43.9%
Hepatic		
Alkaline phosphatase increased	22.2%	19.2%
ALT increased	14.6%	14%
AST increased	12.8%	12.8%
Bilirubinemia	18.1%	19.2%
Metabolic/Nutritional		
BUN[a] increased	21%	31.1%
Creatinine increased	22.4%	42.2%
Edema	14.3%	14.8%
Hyperglycemia	23%	27.9%
Hypernatremia	4.1%	11%
Hypervolemia	12.2%	15.4%
Hypocalcemia	18.4%	20.9%
Hypokalemia	42.9%	50.6%
Hypomagnesemia	20.4%	25.6%
Peripheral edema	14.6%	17.2%
Respiratory		
Cough increased	17.8%	21.8%
Dyspnea	23%	29.1%
Epistaxis	14.9%	20.1%
Hypoxia	7.6%	14.8%
Lung disorder	17.8%	17.4%
Pleural effusion	12.5%	9.6%
Rhinitis	11.1%	11%
Miscellaneous		
Back pain	12%	7.3%
Blood product transfusion reaction	18.4%	18.6%
Hematuria	14%	14%
Infection	11.1%	9.3%
Pain	14%	12.8%
Sepsis	14%	11.3%

[a] BUN = serum urea nitrogen.

Amphotericin B liposome was well tolerated. Amphotericin B liposome had a lower incidence of chills, hypokalemia, hypotension, hypoxia, hypertension, tachycardia, and various events related to decreased kidney function compared with amphotericin B deoxycholate.

In children 16 years of age or younger in this double-blind study, amphotericin B liposome compared with amphotericin B deoxycholate had a lower incidence of hypokalemia (37% vs 55%), chills (29% vs 68%), vomiting (27% vs 55%), and hypertension (10% vs 21%). Similar trends, although with a somewhat lower incidence, were observed in the open-label, randomized study 104-14 involving 205 febrile neutropenic children (141 treated with amphotericin B liposome and 64 treated with amphotericin B deoxycholate). Children appear to have more tolerance than older individuals for the nephrotoxic effects of amphotericin B deoxycholate.

Comparison with amphotericin B lipid complex –

Amphotericin B Liposome Empirical Therapy Adverse Reactions (> 10%)			
Adverse reaction	Amphotericin B liposome 3 mg/kg/day (n = 85)	Amphotericin B liposome 5 mg/kg/day (n = 81)	Amphotericin B lipid complex 5 mg/kg/day (n = 78)
Cardiovascular			
Chest pain	8.2%	11.1%	6.4%
Hypertension	10.6%	19.8%	23.1%
Hypotension	10.6%	7.4%	19.2%
Tachycardia	9.4%	18.5%	23.1%
CNS			
Anxiety	10.6%	7.4%	9%
Asthenia	8.2%	6.2%	11.5%
Chills/Rigors	40%	48.1%	89.7%

AMPHOTERICIN B LIPOSOME

Amphotericin B Liposome Empirical Therapy Adverse Reactions (> 10%)

Adverse reaction	Amphotericin B liposome 3 mg/kg/day (n = 85)	Amphotericin B liposome 5 mg/kg/day (n = 81)	Amphotericin B lipid complex 5 mg/kg/day (n = 78)
Confusion	12.9%	8.6%	3.8%
Headache	9.4%	17.3 %	10.3%
GI			
Abdominal pain	12.9%	9.9%	11.5%
Diarrhea	15.3%	17.3%	14.1%
Nausea	25.9%	29.6%	37.2%
Vomiting	22.4%	25.9%	30.8%
Hepatic			
Alkaline phosphatase increased	7.1%	8.6%	12.8%
Bilirubinemia	16.5%	11.1%	11.5%
Liver function tests abnormal	10.6%	7.4%	11.5%
Metabolic/Nutritional			
BUN increased	20%	18.5%	28.2%
Creatinine increased	20%	18.5%	48.7%
Edema	12.9%	12.3%	12.8%
Hyperglycemia	8.2%	8.6%	14.1%
Hypervolemia	8.2%	11.1%	14.1%
Hypocalcemia	10.6%	4.9%	5.1%
Hypokalemia	37.6%	43.2%	39.7%
Hypomagnesemia	15.3%	25.9%	15.4%
Respiratory			
Dyspnea	17.6%	22.2%	23.1%
Epistaxis	10.6%	8.6%	14.1%
Hypoxia	7.1%	6.2%	20.5%
Lung disorder	14.1%	13.6%	15.4%
Miscellaneous			
Rash	23.5%	22.2%	14.1%
Sepsis	12.9%	7.4%	11.5%
Transfusion reaction	10.6%	8.6%	5.1%

➤*Cryptococcal meningitis in HIV: Adverse reactions (more than 10%)* –

Amphotericin B Liposome Cryptococcal Meningitis Adverse Reactions (> 10%)

Adverse reactions	Amphotericin B liposome 3 mg/kg/day (n = 86)	Amphotericin B liposome 6 mg/kg/day (n = 94)	Amphotericin B 0.7 mg/kg/day (n = 87)
CNS			
Dizziness	7%	8.5%	10.3%
Insomnia	22.1%	17%	20.7%
GI			
Abdominal pain	7%	7.4%	10.3%
Anorexia	14%	9.6%	11.5%
Constipation	15.1%	14.9%	20.7%
Diarrhea	10.5%	16%	10.3%
Nausea	16.3%	21.3%	25.3%
Vomiting	10.5%	21.3%	20.7%
Hematologic/Lymphatic			
Anemia	26.7%	47.9%	43.7%
Leukopenia	15.1%	17%	17.2%
Thrombocytopenia	5.8%	12.8%	6.9%
Metabolic/Nutritional			
Bilirubinemia	0%	8.5%	12.6%
BUN increased	9.3%	7.4%	10.3%
Creatinine increased	18.6%	39.4%	43.7%
Hyperglycemia	9.3%	12.8%	17.2%
Hypocalcemia	12.8%	17%	13.8%
Hypokalemia	31.4%	51.1%	48.3%
Hypomagnesemia	29.1%	48.9%	40.2%
Hyponatremia	11.6%	8.5%	9.2%
Liver function tests abnormal	12.8%	4.3%	9.2%
Miscellaneous			
Cough increased	8.1%	2.1%	10.3%
Infection	12.8%	11.7%	6.9%
Phlebitis	9.3%	10.6%	25.3%
Procedural complication	8.1%	9.6%	10.3%
Rash	4.7%	11.7%	4.6%

➤*Infusion-related reactions:* Amphotericin B liposome–treated patients had a lower incidence of infusion-related fever (17% vs 44%), chills/rigors (18% vs 54%) and vomiting (6% vs 8%) on day 1 as compared with amphotericin B deoxycholate–treated patients.

Amphotericin B Liposome Day 1 Infusion-Related Reactions

	Children (≤ 16 years of age)		Adults (> 16 years of age)	
	Amphotericin B liposome	Amphotericin B	Amphotericin B liposome	Amphotericin B
Total number of patients receiving at least 1 dose of study drug	n = 48	n = 47	n = 295	n = 297
Patients with fever[a] increase ≥ 1°C	13%	47%	18%	43%
Patients with chills/rigors	8%	47%	20%	56%
Patients with nausea	8%	9%	13%	10%
Patients with vomiting	4%	15%	6%	7%
Patients with other reactions	21%	28%	16%	23%

[a] Increased above the temperature taken within 1 hour prior to infusion (preinfusion temperature) or above the lowest infusion value (no preinfusion temperature recorded).

Cardiorespiratory reactions, except for vasodilatation (flushing), during all study drug infusions were more frequent in amphotericin B–treated patients.

Amphotericin B Liposome Infusion-Related Cardiorespiratory Reactions

Adverse reaction	Amphotericin liposome (n = 343)	Amphotericin B (n = 344)
Dyspnea	4.7%	7.3%
Hypotension	3.5%	8.1%
Hypoxia	0.3%	6.4%
Hypertension	2.3%	11.3%
Hyperventilation	1.2%	4.9%
Tachycardia	2.3%	12.5%
Vasodilatation	5.2%	0.6%

The percentage of patients who received drugs either for the treatment or prevention of infusion-related reactions (eg, acetaminophen, diphenhydramine, hydrocortisone, meperidine) was lower in amphotericin B liposome–treated patients compared with amphotericin B deoxycholate–treated patients.

In the empirical therapy study 97-0-034, on day 1, where no premedication was administered, the overall incidence of infusion-related events of chills/rigors was significantly lower for patients administered amphotericin B liposome compared with amphotericin B lipid complex. Fever, chills/rigors, and hypoxia were significantly lower for each amphotericin B liposome group compared with the amphotericin B lipid complex group. The infusion-related event hypoxia was reported for 11.5% of amphotericin B lipid complex–treated patients compared with 0% of patients administered amphotericin B liposome 3 mg/kg/day and 1.2% of patients treated with amphotericin B liposome 5 mg/kg/day.

AMPHOTERICIN B LIPOSOME

Amphotericin B Liposome Day 1 Infusion-Related Reactions: Empirical Therapy

	Amphotericin B liposome			Amphotericin B lipid complex
	3 mg/kg/day n = 85	5 mg/kg/day n = 81	Both n = 166	5 mg/kg/day n = 78
Chills/Rigors (day 1)	18.8%	23.5%	21.1%	79.5%
Dyspnea	4.7%	9.9%	7.2%	10.3%
Fever[a] (≥ 1°C increase in temperature)	23.5%	19.8%	21.7%	57.7%
Hypertension	4.7%	8.6%	6.6%	15.4%
Hypoxia	0%	1.2%	< 1%	11.5%
Nausea	10.6%	8.6%	9.6%	11.5%
Tachycardia	2.4%	9.9%	6%	17.9%
Vomiting	5.9%	6.2%	6%	14.1%

[a] Day 1 body temperature increased above the temperature taken within 1 hour prior to infusion (preinfusion temperature) or above the lowest infusion value (no preinfusion temperature recorded).

Patients were not administered premedications to prevent infusion-related reactions prior to the day 1 study drug infusion.

In study 94-0-013, a randomized, double-blind multicenter trial comparing amphotericin B liposome with amphotericin B deoxycholate as initial therapy for cryptococcal meningitis, premedications to prevent infusion-related reactions were permitted. Amphotericin B liposome–treated patients had a lower incidence of chill/rigors, fever, and respiratory adverse reactions.

Amphotericin B Liposome Infusion-Related Reactions in Cryptococcal Meningitis Patients

	Amphotericin B liposome 3 mg/kg	Amphotericin B liposome 6 mg/kg	Amphotericin B
Total number of patients receiving at least 1 dose of study drug	n = 86	n = 94	n = 87
Fever increase of > 1°C	7%	9%	28%
Chills/Rigors	6%	9%	48%
Nausea	13%	14%	20%
Vomiting	16%	14%	18%
Respiratory adverse reactions	0%	1%	9%

There have been a few reports of flushing, back pain with or without chest tightness, and chest pain associated with amphotericin B liposome administration; on occasion, this has been severe. Where these symptoms were noted, the reaction developed within a few minutes after the start of infusion and disappeared rapidly when the infusion was stopped. The symptoms do not occur with every dose and usually do not recur on subsequent administrations when the infusion rate is slowed.

➤*Toxicity and discontinuation of dosing:* In study 94-0-002, a significantly lower incidence of grade 3 or 4 toxicity was observed in the amphotericin B liposome group compared with the amphotericin B group. In addition, nearly 3 times as many patients who were administered amphotericin B required a reduction in dose because of toxicity or discontinued the study drug because of an infusion-related reaction compared with those administered amphotericin B liposome.

In empirical therapy study 97-0-034, a greater proportion of patients in the amphotericin B lipid complex group discontinued the study drug because of an adverse reaction than in the amphotericin B liposome groups.

➤*Other adverse reactions (2% to 10%):*

Cardiovascular – Arrhythmia, atrial fibrillation, bradycardia, cardiac arrest, cardiomegaly, hemorrhage, postural hypotension, valvular heart disease, vascular disorder, vasodilatation (flushing).

CNS – Agitation, coma, convulsion, cough, depression, dysesthesia, dizziness, hallucinations, malaise, nervousness, paresthesia, somnolence, thinking abnormality, tremor.

Dermatologic – Alopecia, dry skin, herpes simplex, injection-site inflammation, maculopapular rash, purpura, skin discoloration, skin disorder, skin ulcer, urticaria, vesiculobullous rash.

GI – Abdomen enlarged, anorexia, constipation, dry mouth/nose, dyspepsia, dysphagia, eructation, fecal incontinence, flatulence, hemorrhoids, gum/oral hemorrhage, hematemesis, hepatocellular damage, hepatomegaly, liver function test abnormal, ileus, mucositis, rectal disorder, stomatitis, venoocclusive liver disease, ulcerative stomatitis.

GU – Abnormal renal function, acute kidney failure, acute renal failure, dysuria, kidney failure, toxic nephropathy, urinary incontinence, vaginal hemorrhage.

Hematologic/Lymphatic – Anemia, coagulation disorder, ecchymosis, fluid overload, petechia, prothrombin decreased, prothrombin increased, thrombocytopenia.

Metabolic/Nutritional – Acidosis, amylase increased, hyperchloremia, hyperkalemia, hypermagnesemia, hyperphosphatemia, hyponatremia, hypophosphatemia, hypoproteinemia, lactate dehydrogenase increased, nonprotein nitrogen increased, respiratory alkalosis.

Musculoskeletal – Arthralgia, bone pain, dystonia, myalgia, neck pain, rigors.

Respiratory – Asthma, atelectasis, hemoptysis, hiccup, hyperventilation, influenza-like symptoms, lung edema, pharyngitis, pneumonia, respiratory insufficiency, respiratory failure, sinusitis.

Special senses – Conjunctivitis, dry eyes, eye hemorrhage.

Miscellaneous – Allergic reaction, cellulitis, cell-mediated immunological reaction, face edema, graft versus host disease, procedural complication.

➤*Laboratory test abnormalities:* The effect of amphotericin B liposome on renal and hepatic function and on serum electrolytes was assessed from laboratory values measured repeatedly in study 94-0-002. The frequency and magnitude of hepatic test abnormalities were similar in the amphotericin B liposome and amphotericin B groups. Nephrotoxicity was defined as creatinine values increasing 100% or more over pretreatment levels in children, and creatinine values increasing 100% or more over pretreatment levels in adult patients provided the peak creatinine concentration was more than 1.2 mg/dL. Hypokalemia was defined as potassium levels of 2.5 mmol/L or lower any time during treatment.

Nephrotoxicity – Incidence of nephrotoxicity, mean peak serum creatinine concentration, mean change from baseline in serum creatinine, and incidence of hypokalemia in the double-blind randomized study were lower in the amphotericin B liposome group as summarized in the following table:

Amphotericin B Liposome Laboratory Evidence of Nephrotoxicity

	Amphotericin B liposome	Amphotericin B
Total number of patients receiving at least 1 dose of study drug	n = 343	n = 344
Nephrotoxicity	18.7%	33.7%
Mean peak creatinine	1.24 mg/dL	1.52 mg/dL
Mean change from baseline in creatinine	0.48 mg/dL	0.77 mg/dL
Hypokalemia	6.7%	11.6%

In empirical therapy study 97-0-034, the incidence of nephrotoxicity as measured by increases of serum creatinine from baseline was significantly lower for patients administered amphotericin B liposome (individual dose groups and combined) compared with amphotericin B lipid complex.

Amphotericin B Liposome Incidence of Nephrotoxicity: Empirical Therapy

	Amphotericin B liposome			Amphotericin B lipid complex
	3 mg/kg/day n = 85	5 mg/kg/day n = 81	Both n = 166	5 mg/kg/day n = 78
Number with nephrotoxicity				
1.5 × baseline serum creatinine value	29.4%	25.9%	27.7%	62.8%
2 × baseline serum creatinine value	14.1%	14.8%	14.5%	42.3%

The incidence of nephrotoxicity in study 94-0-013, comparative trial in cryptococcal meningitis was lower in the amphotericin B liposome groups.

Amphotericin B Liposome Laboratory Evidence of Nephrotoxicity in Cryptococcal Meningitis

	Amphotericin B liposome 3 mg/kg	Amphotericin B liposome 6 mg/kg	Amphotericin B
Total number of patients receiving at least 1 dose of study drug	n = 86	n = 94	n = 87
Number with nephrotoxicity			
1.5 × baseline serum creatinine	35%	47%	60%
2 × baseline serum creatinine	14%	21%	33%

➤*Postmarketing:* The following infrequent adverse experiences have been reported in postmarketing surveillance, in addition to those mentioned previously: agranulocytosis, angioedema, bronchospasm, cyanosis/hypoventilation, erythema, hemorrhagic cystitis, pulmonary edema, urticaria.

AMPHOTERICIN B LIPOSOME

Overdosage

➤*Symptoms:* The toxicity of amphotericin B liposome due to overdose has not been defined. Repeated daily doses up to 10 mg/kg in children and 15 mg/kg in adult patients have been administered in clinical trials with no reported dose-related toxicity.

➤*Treatment:* If overdosage occurs, cease administration immediately. Institute symptomatic supportive measures. Give particular attention to monitoring renal function. Hemodialysis or peritoneal dialysis do not appear to significantly affect the elimination of amphotericin B liposome.

Patient Information

Inform patients that this medication is administered by IV infusion and treatment may last for several weeks.

Advise patients to report to their health care provider any pain or swelling at infusion site, difficulty breathing or chest pain, chills, nausea, swelling of the face or mouth, or any other infusion reactions.

AMPHOTERICIN B DESOXYCHOLATE — INJECTION

WARNING

This drug should be used primarily for treatment of patients with progressive and potentially life-threatening fungal infections; it should not be used to treat noninvasive forms of fungal disease such as oral thrush, vaginal candidiasis, and esophageal candidiasis in patients with normal neutrophil counts.

Exercise caution to prevent inadvertent overdose with amphotericin B. Verify the product name and dosage if dose exceeds 1.5 mg/kg.

Indications

➤*Life-threatening fungal infections:* Amphotericin B for injection, USP should be administered primarily to patients with progressive, potentially life-threatening fungal infections. This potent drug should not be used to treat noninvasive fungal infections, such as oral thrush, vaginal candidiasis and esophageal candidiasis in patients with normal neutrophil counts.

Amphotericin B for injection is specifically intended to treat potentially life-threatening fungal infections: Aspergillosis, cryptococcosis (torulosis), North American blastomycosis, systemic candidiasis, coccidioidomycosis, histoplasmosis, zygomycosis including mucormycosis due to susceptible species of the genera *Absidia*, *Mucor* and *Rhizopus*, and infections due to related susceptible species of *Conidiobolus* and *Basidiobolus*, and sporotrichosis.

➤*Leishmaniasis:* Amphotericin B may be useful in the treatment of American mucocutaneous leishmaniasis, but it is not the drug of choice as primary therapy.

➤*Off-label uses:*

Bladder irrigation for candidal cystitis – [4] = Insufficient documentation. Studies have shown that amphotericin B given by bladder irrigation may quickly resolve candidal cystitis, but recurrence is common. Guidelines suggest that amphotericin B is rarely indicated for candidal cystitis, except for use as a diagnostic test. Treatment recommendations for candidal cystitis involve intravenous (IV) amphotericin B, oral or IV fluconazole, or oral flucytosine.

Ocular aspergillosis – [1] = Good documentation. Although topical administration of amphotericin B drops may be adequate in cases of aspergillus keratitis, more advanced ophthalmic infections may require more invasive techniques for delivering the drug to the deeper layers of the eye. Some debate exists among ophthalmologists about whether amphotericin B should be administered into the vitreous humor (intravitreal injection) or into the aqueous humor (intracameral injection), for the treatment of aspergillus endophthalmitis. IDSA guidelines recommend intravitreal injection for endophthalmitis and intracameral injection for refractory keratitis that does not respond to topical therapy.

Other possible off-label uses – Prophylaxis of fungal infection in patients with bone marrow transplantation (0.1 mg/kg/day); for the treatment of primary amoebic meningoencephalitis caused by *Naegleria fowleri*; as chemoprophylaxis by low-dose IV, intranasal, or nebulized administration in immunocompromised patients at risk of *aspergillosis*; intrathecally for patients with severe meningitis unresponsive to IV therapy; intra-articularly or IM for coccidioidal arthritis.

Administration and Dosage

➤*General dosing considerations:* Because patient tolerance varies greatly, the dosage of amphotericin B must be individualized and adjusted according to the patient's clinical status (eg, site and severity of infection, etiologic agent, cardio-renal function).

A test dose is recommended prior to administration. (See Test dose).

Infusion reactions – Acute reactions, including fever, shaking, chills, hypotension, anorexia, nausea, vomiting, headache, and tachypnea, are common 1 to 3 hours after starting an IV infusion. These reactions are usually more severe with the first few doses of amphotericin B and usually diminish with subsequent doses.

Rapid IV infusion has been associated with hypotension, hypokalemia, arrhythmias, and shock and should, therefore, be avoided. (See also Administration.)

➤*Adults:*

Life-threatening fungal infections –

Maximum dose: 1.5 mg/kg per day. Amphotericin B overdoses can result in cardiorespiratory arrest.

Test dose: A single IV test dose (1 mg in 20 mL of dextrose 5% solution) administered over 20 to 30 minutes may be preferred. The patient's temperature, pulse, respiration, and blood pressure should be recorded every 30 minutes for 2 to 4 hours.

Initial dosage: In patients with good cardio-renal function and a well-tolerated test dose, therapy is usually initiated with a daily dose of 0.25 mg/kg of body weight. However, in those patients having severe and rapidly progressive fungal infection, therapy may be initiated with a daily dose of 0.3 mg/kg of body weight. In patients with impaired cardio-renal function or a severe reaction to the test dose, therapy should be initiated with smaller daily doses (ie, 5 to 10 mg).

Maintenance dosage: Depending on the patient's cardio-renal status, doses may gradually be increased by 5 to 10 mg/day to final daily dosage of 0.5 to 0.7 mg/kg.

There are insufficient data presently available to define total dosage requirements and duration of treatment necessary for eradication of specific mycoses. The optimal dose is unknown. Total daily dosage may range up to 1 mg/kg/day or up to 1.5 mg/kg when given on alternate days.

Therapy interruption: Whenever medication is interrupted for a period of more than 7 days, therapy should be resumed by starting with the lowest dosage level (eg, 0.25 mg/kg of body weight) and increased gradually.

Aspergillosis: Aspergillosis has been treated with amphotericin B intravenously for a period up to 11 months with a total dose up to 3.6 g.

Rhinocerebral phycomycosis: A cumulative dose of at least 3 g of amphotericin B is recommended. Although a total dose of 3 to 4 g will infrequently cause lasting renal impairment, this would seem a reasonable minimum where there is clinical evidence of invasion of deep tissue.

Sporotrichosis: Therapy with IV amphotericin B for sporotrichosis has ranged up to 9 months with a total dose up to 2.5 g.

Off-label dosing –

Bladder irrigation for candidal cystitis: [4] = Insufficient documentation.

- *Continuous irrigation* – Concentrations of 10 and 50 mg/L administered into the bladder continuously over 24 to 48 hours in patients with indwelling catheters. In one study, amphotericin B was administered into the bladder at a rate of 42 mL/h.
- *Intermittent irrigation* – Doses of 20 to 40 mg or 5 to 200 mg/L administered into the bladder (and retained there for 90 minutes) every 8 hours for 3 days have been used.

Ocular aspergillosis: [1] = Good documentation.

- *Intraocular* – 5 to 10 mcg per injection administered intaviterally or intracamerally, repeated in cases of ongoing infection at intervals of approximately 1 week after resolution of any local inflammatory response from the previous injection. The recommended volume for each injection is 0.1 mL.
- *Topical* – Amphotericin B 0.15% to 0.2% drops applied topically every 30 to 60 minutes until symptoms resolve. Therapy usually continues for days to weeks.

➤*Renal function impairment:* In some patients, hydration and sodium repletion prior to amphotericin B administration may reduce the risk of developing nephrotoxicity.

For patients with creatinine clearance of less than 10 mL/min, the dosage should be 0.5 to 0.7 mg/kg every 24 to 48 hours.

Adults receiving continuous renal replacement therapy (CRRT) – A dosage of 0.5 to 1 mg/kg IV every 24 hours is recommended for patients receiving continuous venovenous hemofiltration (CVVH), continuous venovenous hemodialysis (CVVHD), or continuous venovenous hemodialfiltration (CVVHDF). This recommendation assumes ultrafiltration and dialysis flow rates of 1 to 2 L/h.

Adults receiving intermittent hemodialysis (IHD) – 0.5 to 1 mg/kg IV every 24 hours administered after the dialysis session. This recommendation assumes the patient is receiving standard IHD 3 times per week and completes the full dialysis sessions.

➤*Preparation for administration:* Reconstitute as follows: See also Admixture compatibility. An initial concentrate of 5 mg amphotericin B per mL is first prepared by rapidly expressing 10 mL of sterile water for injection without a bacteriostatic agent directly into the lyophilized cake, using a sterile needle (minimum diameter, 20 gauge) and syringe. Shake the vial immediately until the colloidal solution is clear. The infusion solution, providing amphotericin B 0.1 mg per mL, is then obtained by further dilution (1:50) with dextrose 5% injection of pH greater than 4.2. The pH of each container of dextrose injection should be ascertained before use. Commercial dextrose injection usually has a pH greater than 4.2; however, if it is less than 4.2, then 1 or 2 mL of buffer should be added to the dextrose injection before it is used to dilute the concentrated solution of amphotericin B. The recommended buffer has the following composition:

- Dibasic sodium phosphate (anhydrous) equals 1.59 g
- Monobasic sodium phosphate (anhydrous) equals 0.96 g
- Water for injection equals quantity sufficient 100 mL
- The buffer should be sterilized before it is added to the dextrose injection, either by filtration through a bacterial retentive stone, mat, or membrane, or by autoclaving for 30 minutes at 15 lbs pressure (approximately 121°C; 249.8°F).

Aseptic technique must be strictly observed in all handling, because no preservative or bacteriostatic agent is present in the antibiotic or in the materials used to prepare it for administration. All entries into the vial or into the diluents must be made with a sterile needle.

AMPHOTERICIN B DESOXYCHOLATE — INJECTION

Do not use the initial concentrate or the infusion solution if there is any evidence of precipitation or foreign matter in either one.

➤*Administration:* Avoid rapid IV infusion because it has been associated with hypotension, hypokalemia, arrhythmias, and shock. Administer by slow IV infusion. IV infusion should be given over a period of approximately 2 to 6 hours (depending on the dose) observing the usual precautions for IV therapy. The recommended concentration for IV infusion is 0.1 mg per mL (1 mg per 10 mL).

An inline membrane filter may be used for IV infusion of amphotericin B; however, the mean pore diameter of the filter should not be less than 1 micron in order to ensure passage of the antibiotic dispersion.

➤*Admixture compatibility:* Do not reconstitute with saline solutions. The use of any diluent other than the ones recommended or the presence of bacteriostatic agent (eg, benzyl alcohol) in the diluent may cause precipitation of the antibiotic.

➤*Storage/Stability:* Prior to reconstitution, amphotericin B for injection should be stored in the refrigerator, protected against exposure to light. The concentrate (amphotericin B 5 mg per mL after reconstitution with sterile water for injection 10 mL) may be stored in the dark, at room temperature for 24 hours, or at refrigerator temperatures for 1 week with minimal loss of potency and clarity. Any unused material should then be discarded. Solutions prepared for IV infusion (less than or equal to amphotericin B 0.1 mg per mL) should be used promptly after preparation and should be protected from light during administration.

Actions

➤*Pharmacology:* Amphotericin B is fungistatic or fungicidal depending on the concentration obtained in body fluids and the susceptibility of the fungus. The drug acts by binding to sterols in the cell membrane of susceptible fungi with a resultant change in membrane permeability allowing leakage of intracellular components. Mammalian cell membranes also contain sterols and it has been suggested that the damage to human cells and fungal cells may share common mechanisms.

➤*Pharmacokinetics:* An initial IV infusion of 1 to 5 mg of amphotericin B per day, gradually increased to 0.4 to 0.6 mg/kg/day, produces peak plasma concentrations ranging from ≈ 0.5 to 2 mcg/mL. Following a rapid initial fall, plasma concentrations plateau at ≈ 0.5 mcg/mL. An elimination half-life of ≈ 15 days follows an initial plasma half-life of ≈ 24 hours. Amphotericin B circulating in plasma is highly bound (> 90%) to plasma proteins and is poorly dialyzable. Approximately two-thirds of concurrent plasma concentrations have been detected in fluids from inflamed pleura, peritoneum, synovium, and aqueous humor. Concentrations in the cerebrospinal fluid seldom exceed 2.5% of those in the plasma. Little amphotericin B penetrates into vitreous humor or normal amniotic fluid. Complete details of tissue distribution are not known.

Amphotericin B is excreted very slowly (over weeks to months) by the kidneys with 2% to 5% of a given dose being excreted in the biologically active form. Details of possible metabolic pathways are not known. After treatment is discontinued, the drug can be detected in the urine for at least 7 weeks due to the slow disappearance of the drug. The cumulative urinary output over a 7-day period amounts to ≈ 40% of the amount of drug infused.

➤*Microbiology:* Amphotericin B shows a high order of in vitro activity against many species of fungi. *Histoplasma capsulatum, Coccidioides immitis, Candida* species, *Blastomyces dermatitidis, Rhodotorula, Cryptococcus neoformans, Sporothrix schenckii, Mucor mucedo,* and *Aspergillus fumigatus* are all inhibited by concentrations of amphotericin B ranging from 0.03 to 1 mcg/mL in vitro. While *Candida albicans* is generally quite susceptible to amphotericin B, non*albicans* species may be less susceptible. *Pseudallescheria boydii* and *Fusarium* sp. are often resistant to amphotericin B. The antibiotic is without effect on bacteria, rickettsiae, and viruses.

Contraindications

This product is contraindicated in patients who have shown hypersensitivity to amphotericin B or any other component in the formulation unless, in the opinion of the physician, the condition requiring treatment is life-threatening and amenable only to amphotericin B therapy.

Warnings/Precautions

➤*Life-threatening fungal disease:* Amphotericin B is frequently the only effective treatment available for potentially life-threatening fungal disease. In each case, its possible lifesaving benefit must be balanced against its untoward and dangerous side effects.

➤*Administration:* Administer IV under close clinical observation by medically trained personnel. It should be reserved for treatment of patients with progressive, potentially life-threatening fungal infections due to susceptible organisms (see Indications).

➤*Infusion reactions:* Acute reactions including fever, shaking chills, hypotension, anorexia, nausea, vomiting, headache, and tachypnea are common 1 to 3 hours after starting an IV infusion. These reactions are usually more severe with the first few doses of amphotericin B and usually diminish with subsequent doses.

Rapid IV infusion has been associated with hypotension, hypokalemia, arrhythmias, and shock and should, therefore, be avoided (see Administration and Dosage).

➤*Leukocyte transfusions:* Since acute pulmonary reactions have been reported in patients given amphotericin B during or shortly after leukocyte transfusions, it is advisable to temporarily separate these infusions as far as possible and to monitor pulmonary function (see Drug Interactions).

➤*Leukoencephalopathy:* Leukoencephalopathy has been reported following use of amphotericin B. Literature reports have suggested that total body irradiation may be a predisposition.

➤*Therapy interruption:* Whenever medication is interrupted for a period of > 7 days, therapy should be resumed by starting with the lowest dosage level (eg, 0.25 mg/kg of body weight) and increased gradually as outlined under Administration and Dosage.

➤*Renal function impairment:* Amphotericin B should be used with care in patients with reduced renal function; frequent monitoring of renal function is recommended (see Precautions and Adverse Reactions). In some patients, hydration and sodium repletion prior to amphotericin B administration may reduce the risk of developing nephrotoxicity. Supplemental alkali medication may decrease renal tubular acidosis complications.

➤*Pregnancy: Category B.* Reproduction studies in animals have revealed no evidence of harm to the fetus due to amphotericin B for injection. Systemic fungal infections have been successfully treated in pregnant women with amphotericin B for injection without obvious effects to the fetus, but the number of cases reported has been small. Because animal reproduction studies are not always predictive of human response, and adequate and well-controlled studies have not been conducted in pregnant women, this drug should be used during pregnancy only if clearly indicated.

➤*Lactation:* It is not known whether amphotericin B is excreted in human milk. Because many drugs are excreted in human milk and considering the potential toxicity of amphotericin B, it is prudent to advise a nursing mother to discontinue nursing.

➤*Children:* Safety and efficacy in children have not been established through adequate and well-controlled studies. Systemic fungal infections have been successfully treated in children without reports of unusual side effects. Amphotericin B for injection, when administered to children, should be limited to the smallest dose compatible with an effective therapeutic regimen.

➤*Lab test abnormalities:* Serum electrolytes, liver function tests, renal function tests, and other test abnormalities have been reported including the following: Hypomagnesemia, hypo- and hyperkalemia, hypocalcemia; elevations of AST, ALT, GGT, bilirubin, and alkaline phosphatase; elevations of BUN and serum creatinine.

➤*Monitoring:* Renal function should be monitored frequently during amphotericin B therapy (see Warnings and Adverse Reactions). It is also advisable to monitor on a regular basis liver function, serum electrolytes (particularly magnesium and potassium), blood counts, and hemoglobin concentrations. Laboratory test results should be used as a guide to subsequent dosage adjustments.

Drug Interactions

Amphotericin B Desoxycholate Drug Interactions

Precipitant drug	Object drug[a]		Description
Antineoplastic agents	Amphotericin B	↑	Concurrent administration may enhance the potential for renal toxicity, bronchospasm, and hypotension.
Azole antifungals	Amphotericin B	↓	In vitro animal studies suggest that imidazoles may induce fungal resistance to amphotericin B. Administer with caution, especially in immunocompromised patients.
Corticosteroids and corticotropin	Amphotericin B	↑	Concurrent administration may potentiate hypokalemia and predispose patients to cardiac dysfunction. Do not give unless necessary to control adverse reactions.
Zidovudine	Amphotericin B	↑	Increases in myelotoxicity and nephrotoxicity were observed in dogs administered zidovudine concomitantly with amphotericin B desoxycholate.
Amphotericin B	Cyclosporine	↑	The risk of renal toxicity is increased with concomitant administration. Severe muscle tremors were reported in 1 patient.
Cyclosporine	Amphotericin B		
Amphotericin B	Digitalis glycosides	↑	Concurrent administration may induce hypokalemia and may potentiate digitalis toxicity.
Amphotericin B	Flucytosine	↑	A synergistic relationship with amphotericin B has been reported. Flucytosine toxicity may be increased by increasing its cellular uptake or impairing renal excretion.

AMPHOTERICIN B DESOXYCHOLATE — INJECTION

Amphotericin B Desoxycholate Drug Interactions

Precipitant drug	Object drug[a]		Description
Amphotericin B	Nephrotoxic agents	⬆	Concomitant administration may enhance risk of drug-induced renal toxicity. Use caution when administering concomitantly. Monitor renal function intensively.
Nephrotoxic agents	Amphotericin B		
Amphotericin B	Skeletal muscle relaxants	⬆	Amphotericin B-induced hypokalemia may enhance the curariform effect of skeletal muscle relaxants. Monitor serum potassium levels closely.
Amphotericin B	Thiazides	⬆	Electrolyte depletion may be intensified, particularly hypokalemia. Monitor potassium levels.

[a] ⬆ = object drug increased; ⬇ = object drug decreased.

Adverse Reactions

➤*Prevention of adverse reactions:* Although some patients may tolerate full IV doses of amphotericin B without difficulty, most will exhibit some intolerance, often at less than the full therapeutic dose.

Tolerance may be improved by treatment with aspirin, antipyretics (eg, acetaminophen), antihistamines, or antiemetics. Meperidine (25 to 50 mg IV) has been shown in some patients to decrease the duration of shaking chills, and fever that may accompany the infusion of amphotericin B.

Administration of amphotericin B on alternate days may decrease anorexia and phlebitis.

IV administration of small doses of adrenal corticosteroids just prior to or during the amphotericin B infusion may help decrease febrile reactions. Dosage and duration of such corticosteroid therapy should be kept to a minimum (see Drug Interactions).

Addition of heparin (1000 units per infusion) and the use of pediatric scalp-vein needle may lessen the incidence of thrombophlebitis. Extravasation may cause chemical irritation.

➤*Most common adverse reactions:*

CNS – Headache.

GI – Anorexia; nausea; vomiting; diarrhea; dyspepsia; cramping; epigastric pain.

Hematologic – Normochromic anemia; normocytic anemia.

Local – Pain at the injection site with or without phlebitis or thrombophlebitis.

Musculoskeletal – Generalized pain, including muscle and joint pains.

Pulmonary – Hypotension; tachypnea.

Renal – Decreased renal function and renal function abnormalities including azotemia, hypokalemia, hyposthenuria, renal tubular acidosis, and nephrocalcinosis. These usually improve with interruption of therapy. However, some permanent impairment often occurs, especially in those patients receiving large amounts (greater than 5 g) of amphotericin B or receiving other nephrotoxic agents. In some patients hydration and sodium repletion prior to amphotericin B administration may reduce the risk of developing nephrotoxicity. Supplemental alkali medication may decrease renal tubular acidosis.

Miscellaneous – Fever (sometimes accompanied by shaking chills usually occurring within 15 to 20 minutes after initiation of treatment); malaise; weight loss.

➤*Other adverse reactions:*

Allergic – Anaphylactoid and other allergic reactions; bronchospasm; wheezing.

CNS – Convulsions; hearing loss; tinnitus; transient vertigo; visual impairment; diplopia; peripheral neuropathy; encephalopathy (see Precautions); other neurologic symptoms.

Dermatologic – Rash, in particular maculopapular; pruritus.

GI – Acute liver failure; hepatitis; jaundice; hemorrhagic gastroenteritis; melena.

Hematologic – Agranulocytosis; coagulation defects; thrombocytopenia; leukopenia; eosinophilia; leukocytosis.

Lab test abnormalities –

Serum electrolytes: Hypomagnesemia; hypo- and hyperkalemia; hypocalcemia.

Liver function tests: Elevations of AST, ALT, GGT, bilirubin, and alkaline phosphatase.

Renal function tests: Elevations of BUN and serum creatinine.

Cardiopulmonary – Cardiac arrest; shock; cardiac failure; pulmonary edema; hypersensitivity pneumonitis; arrhythmias, including ventricular fibrillation; dyspnea; hypertension.

Renal – Acute renal failure; anuria; oliguria.

Miscellaneous – Flushing.

Overdosage

➤*Symptoms:* Amphotericin B overdoses can result in cardiorespiratory arrest.

➤*Treatment:* If an overdose is suspected, discontinue therapy and monitor the patient's clinical status (eg, cardiorespiratory, renal, and liver function, hematologic status, serum electrolytes) and administer supportive therapy, as required. Amphotericin B is not hemodialyzable.

Prior to reinstituting therapy, the patient's condition should be stabilized (including correction of electrolyte deficiencies).

NYSTATIN

Rx	**Nystatin** (Various, eg, Major, Teva)	**Tablets**: 500,000 units	In 100s.
Rx	**Mycostatin** (Bristol-Myers Squibb)		Lactose. (Squibb 580). Light brown, biconvex. Film-coated. In 100s.
Rx	**Nystatin** (Various, eg, Geneva, NMC, Parmed)	**Oral suspension**: 100,000 units/mL	In 5, 60 and 480 mL.
Rx	**Nilstat** (Lederle)		Cherry flavor. In 60 and 473 mL.
Rx	**Nystatin** (Paddock)	**Bulk Powder**: 50 million units	
Rx	**Nilstat** (Lederle)	**Bulk Powder**: 150 million units	
Rx	**Nystatin** (Paddock)		
Rx	**Nystatin** (Paddock)	**Bulk Powder**: 500 million units	
Rx	**Nilstat** (Lederle)	**Bulk Powder**: 1 billion units	
Rx	**Nystatin** (Paddock)		
Rx	**Nilstat** (Lederle)	**Bulk Powder**: 2 billion units	
Rx	**Nystatin** (Paddock)		
Rx	**Nystatin** (Paddock)	**Bulk Powder**: 5 billion units	

NYSTATIN — ORAL

Indications

➤*Tablets:* Nystatin tablets are intended for the treatment of nonesophageal mucous membrane GI candidiasis.

➤*Oral suspension:* For the treatment of candidiasis in the oral cavity.

➤*Powder for extemporaneous preparation of oral suspension:* Nystatin powder for oral suspension is indicated for the treatment of intestinal and oral cavity infections caused by *Candida (Monilia) albicans*.

Administration and Dosage

➤*Adults:*

Oral suspension –

Oral cavity infections caused by Candida (Monilia) albicans: 400,000 to 600,000 units 4 times daily (one-half of dose in each side of mouth, retaining the drug as long as possible before swallowing).

Powder for extemporaneous preparation of oral suspension –

Intestinal Candidiasis (moniliasis): 500,000 to 1 million units (approximately ⅛ to ¼ teaspoonful) 3 times daily.

Oral cavity infections caused by Candida (Monilia) albicans: 400,000 to 600,000 units 4 times daily (one-half of dose in each side of mouth, retaining the drug as long as possible before swallowing).

Tablets –

Nonesophageal mucous membrane GI Candidiasis: 1 to 2 tablets (500,000 to 1 million units) 3 times daily.

➤*Children:*

Oral suspension –

Oral cavity infections caused by Candida (Monilia) albicans:

• *1 year of age and older* – 400,000 to 600,000 units 4 times daily (one-half of dose in each side of mouth, retaining the drug as long as possible before swallowing).

NYSTATIN — ORAL

• *Younger than 1 year of age* – 200,000 units 4 times daily (100,000 units in each side of the mouth).

• *Premature and low birth weight infants* – Limited clinical studies indicate that 100,000 units (50,000 units in each side of the mouth) 4 times daily is effective.

Powder for extemporaneous preparation of oral suspension –

Intestinal Candidiasis (moniliasis): 500,000 to 1 million units (approximately ⅛ to ¼ teaspoonful) 3 times daily.

Oral cavity infections caused by Candida (Monilia) albicans:

• *1 year of age and older* – 400,000 to 600,000 units 4 times daily (one-half of dose in each side of mouth, retaining the drug as long as possible before swallowing).

• *Younger than 1 year of age* – 200,000 units (100,000 units in each side of the mouth) 4 times daily.

• *Premature and low birth weight infants* – Limited clinical studies indicate that 100,000 units (50,000 units in each side of the mouth) 4 times daily is effective.

➤*Duration of therapy:* Treatment should generally be continued for at least 48 hours after clinical cure to prevent relapse.

➤*Preparation for administration:*

Powder for extemporaneous preparation of oral suspension – For adults and older children, add ⅛ teaspoonful (approximately 500,000 units) of nystatin to about ½ cup of water and stir well. One-eighth teaspoonful of nystatin is equivalent to the recommended dose for adults and children of nystatin oral suspension (4 to 6 mL, or 400,000 to 600,000 units). This product contains no preservatives. Therefore, use immediately after mixing and do not store. It is designed for extemporaneous preparation of a single dose at a time.

➤*Administration:*

Oral suspension – Retain the drug in the mouth as long as possible before swallowing.

➤*Storage/Stability:*

Tablets – Store at controlled room temperature, 15° to 30°C (59° to 86°F). Dispense in a tight, light-resistant container.

Powder for extemporaneous preparation of oral suspension – Store in a refrigerator, 2° to 8°C (36° to 46°F). Protect from light. Dispense in a tight, light-resistant container. Use immediately after mixing and do not store.

Note: The potency of this product cannot be ensured for longer than 90 days after the container is first opened.

Actions

➤*Pharmacology:* Nystatin acts by binding to sterols in the cell membrane of susceptible fungi, with a resultant change in membrane permeability, allowing leakage of intracellular components. Nystatin exhibits no appreciable activity against bacteria, protozoa, or viruses.

➤*Pharmacokinetics:*

Absorption – GI absorption of nystatin is insignificant. Most oral nystatin is passed unchanged in the stool. In patients with renal insufficiency receiving oral therapy with conventional dosage forms, significant plasma concentrations of nystatin may occasionally occur.

➤*Microbiology:* Nystatin is both fungistatic and fungicidal in vitro against a wide variety of yeasts and yeast-like fungi. *Candida albicans* demonstrates no significant resistance to nystatin in vitro on repeated subculture in increasing levels of nystatin; other *Candida* species become quite resistant. Generally, resistance does not develop in vivo.

Contraindications

Nystatin tablets and oral suspension are contraindicated in patients with histories of hypersensitivity to any of the components.

Warnings/Precautions

➤*Systemic mycoses:* Do not use these medications for the treatment of systemic mycoses. Discontinue treatment if sensitization or irritation is reported during use.

➤*Hypersensitivity reactions:* If irritation or hypersensitivity develops with nystatin, discontinue treatment and institute appropriate therapy.

➤*Pregnancy: Category C.*

Teratogenic – Animal reproduction studies have not been conducted with nystatin. It is also not known whether nystatin can cause fetal harm when administered to a pregnant woman or can affect reproduction capacity. Give nystatin to a pregnant woman only if clearly needed.

➤*Lactation:* It is not known whether nystatin is excreted in human milk. Although GI absorption is insignificant, because many drugs are excreted in human milk, exercise caution when nystatin is administered to a nursing woman.

➤*Lab test abnormalities:*

Lack of therapeutic response – If there is a lack of therapeutic response, repeat appropriate microbiological studies (eg, KOH smears or cultures) to confirm the diagnosis of candidiasis and rule out other pathogens before instituting another course of therapy.

Adverse Reactions

Nystatin is generally well tolerated, even with prolonged therapy. Oral irritation and sensitization have been reported. Nausea has been reported occasionally during therapy.

➤*Dermatologic:* Rash, including urticaria, has been reported rarely. Stevens-Johnson syndrome has been reported very rarely.

➤*GI:* Diarrhea (including 1 case of bloody diarrhea), nausea, vomiting, GI upset disturbances.

Large oral doses of nystatin have occasionally produced irritation of the stomach that may result in nausea and vomiting.

➤*Miscellaneous:* Tachycardia, bronchospasm, facial swelling, and nonspecific myalgia have also been rarely reported.

Overdosage

➤*Symptoms:* Oral doses of nystatin in excess of 5 million units daily have caused nausea and GI upset. There have been no reports of serious toxic effects or superinfections.

Patient Information

Retain the drug in the mouth as long as possible. Continue use at least 2 days after symptoms have subsided.

Imidazole Antifungal

KETOCONAZOLE

Rx	**Ketoconazole** (Various, eg, Mutual, Mylan, Novopharm, Taro, Teva)	**Tablets:** 200 mg	In 30s, 50s, 100s, 250s, 500s, 1000s, blister packs of 10, and UD 30s, 50s, and 100s.

KETOCONAZOLE — ORAL

WARNING

Hepatotoxicity – When used orally, ketoconazole has been associated with hepatic toxicity, including some fatalities. Patients receiving this drug should be informed by the physician of the risk and should be closely monitored (see Warnings/Precautions).

Drug interactions –

Terfenadine: Coadministration of terfenadine with ketoconazole tablets is contraindicated. Rare cases of serious cardiovascular adverse events, including death, ventricular tachycardia and torsades de pointes have been observed in patients taking ketoconazole tablets concomitantly with terfenadine, due to increased terfenadine concentrations induced by ketoconazole tablets (see Contraindications, Warnings/Precautions, and Drug Interactions).

Astemizole: Pharmacokinetic data indicate that oral ketoconazole inhibits the metabolism of astemizole, resulting in elevated plasma levels of astemizole and its active metabolite desmethylastemizole which may prolong QT intervals. Coadministration of astemizole with ketoconazole tablets is therefore contraindicated (see Contraindications, Warnings/Precautions, and Drug Interactions).

Cisapride: Coadministration of cisapride with ketoconazole is contraindicated. Serious cardiovascular adverse events including ventricular tachycardia, ventricular fibrillation and torsades de pointes have occurred in patients taking ketoconazole concomitantly with cisapride (see Contraindications, Warnings/Precautions, and Drug Interactions).

Indications

➤*Fungal infections:* Treatment of the following systemic fungal infections: Candidiasis, chronic mucocutaneous candidiasis, oral thrush, candiduria, blastomycosis, coccidioidomycosis, histoplasmosis, chromomycosis, and paracoccidioidomycosis. Ketoconazole should not be used for fungal meningitis because it penetrates poorly into the cerebrospinal fluid.

➤*Severe recalcitrant cutaneous dermatophyte infections:* Treatment of patients with severe recalcitrant cutaneous dermatophyte infections who have not responded to topical therapy or oral griseofulvin, or who are unable to take griseofulvin.

➤*Off-label uses:*

Cushing syndrome – [3] = Safety concerns. Ketoconazole appears to be effective for lowering cortisol levels in patients with Cushing syndrome. It can be used prior to or after surgical therapy, or it can be used to medically manage cortisol levels. Although ketoconazole was well tolerated in clinical studies and case reports, the risk of liver toxicity and drug interactions may limit its use.

Depression – [3] = Safety concerns. Most of the studies included patients with refractory depression with a psychotic or nonpsychotic component. Initial data from 2 small trials suggest that nonpsychotic patients may be better candidates for successful response, but larger studies will be needed to verify this initial hypothesis. If psychotic patients are slower to respond, treatment longer than 8 weeks may be necessary to document response. It is not clear if patients with nonrefractory depression may respond differently. Although this initial information suggests that ketoconazole may be a pos-

KETOCONAZOLE — ORAL

sible alternative for patients with hypercortisolemia-related refractory depression, further controlled studies are needed in this area.

Onychomycosis – [3] = Safety concerns. The necessity for long-term treatment of onychomycosis limits the use of ketoconazole because of its adverse effects and drug interactions. Because of a lack of clinical data demonstrating efficacy over newer systemic therapies and significant safety concerns, oral ketoconazole should not be used as a first-line treatment for onychomycosis.

Tinea capitis – [5] = Poor documentation. Because of the lack of clinical data demonstrating efficacy over griseofulvin and significant safety concerns, oral ketoconazole is not recommended for treatment of tinea capitis.

Tinea cruris – [4] = Insufficient documentation. Guidelines include oral ketoconazole as a treatment option for severe tinea cruris; however, the availability of more favorable agents and the risk of liver toxicity and drug interactions limit its use to patients who have severe or chronic infections or who have been unresponsive to topical therapies.

Tinea versicolor – [3] = Safety concerns. Oral ketoconazole is effective in the treatment of tinea versicolor. Cure rates vary depending on the severity of the infection and the dose and duration of treatment. Patients with more extensive infection may require a higher dose or longer duration of therapy. In clinical trials, adverse events were minimal; however, the risk of hepatotoxicity and availability of antifungal agents with improved safety and efficacy may limit its use.

Other possible off-label uses – Ketoconazole has been used successfully in the treatment of tinea pedis, corporis, and vaginal candidiasis.

High-dose (800 to 1,200 mg/day) ketoconazole has shown some success in treating CNS fungal infections.

Ketoconazole in dosages of 400 mg every 8 hours has been used in the treatment of advanced prostate cancer (see Warnings/Precautions).

Administration and Dosage

➤*Adults:*

Fungal infections – For a list of infections, see Indications.

Initial dosage: 200 mg once daily.

Dosage adjustment: In very serious infections or if clinical responsiveness is insufficient within the expected time, the dose may be increased to 400 mg once daily.

Off-label dosing –

Cushing syndrome: [3] = Safety concerns. 200 to 1,200 mg/day administered in divided doses twice daily. Most patients require at least 600 mg/day.

Depression: [3] = Safety concerns. Doses have ranged from 200 to 1,200 mg/day in most noncontrolled and controlled trials for 3 to 8 weeks. Two trials used lower dosages initially, with titration to higher doses. Titration schedules were 200 mg/day, increased by 200 mg every 3 to 4 days for 6 weeks (mean dose, 900 mg/day). Another titration schedule was 200 mg 3 times a day, increased by 200 mg every 4 to 7 days to a maximum of 1,200 mg/day for 8 weeks. In 2 patients, ketoconazole was used for longer periods, ranging from 15 to 24 months.

To avoid acute adrenal insufficiency and prevent rebound morning corticotropin surge, nighttime doses of cortisol or equivalents (20 mg) were administered in some reports. It is unclear what effect this had on results because this was not compared with control groups.

Onychomycosis: [3] = Safety concerns. 200 mg daily for 4 months or 400 mg once weekly for up to 48 weeks.

Tinea cruris: [4] = Insufficient documentation. 200 mg orally daily for up to 8 weeks.

Tinea versicolor: [3] = Safety concerns. 200 mg/day for up to 5 weeks or 400 mg/wk for 2 weeks results in a greater than 70% mycological cure rate.

In 1 study, a single dose of ketoconazole 400 mg was as effective as a 10-day course of 200 mg/day, demonstrating a 42% and 51% mycological cure rate 1 month after therapy, respectively.

In another study, a single dose of ketoconazole 400 mg followed by 400 mg every 2 weeks for 3 months demonstrated greater cure rates and lower rates of relapse in patients with more extensive infection than in a single 400 mg dose in patients with mild infection (97.2% vs 70.1% cure and 5.7% vs 47.7% relapse, respectively). Additionally, a dosage of 400 mg daily for 2 days cured 81.7% of moderately infected patients and had a 29.9% relapse rate.

➤*Children:*

Fungal infections – For a list of infections, see Indications.

Two years of age and older: 3.3 to 6.6 mg/kg once daily.

➤*Duration of therapy:* Treatment should be continued until tests indicate that active fungal infection has subsided. Inadequate periods of treatment may yield poor response and lead to early recurrence of clinical symptoms. Minimum treatment for candidiasis is 1 or 2 weeks. Patients with chronic mucocutaneous candidiasis usually require maintenance therapy. Minimum treatment for the other indicated systemic mycoses is 6 months.

Minimum treatment for recalcitrant dermatophyte infections is 4 weeks in cases involving glabrous skin. Palmar and plantar infections may respond more slowly. Apparent cures may subsequently recur after discontinuation of therapy in some cases.

➤*Administration:* Patients should not take ketoconazole with antacids; this may cause dizziness.

➤*Storage/Stability:* Store at 15° to 25°C (59° to 77°F). Protect from moisture.

Actions

➤*Pharmacology:* In vitro studies suggest that ketoconazole impairs the synthesis of ergosterol, which is a vital component of fungal cell membranes. This allows impaired permeability and leakage of cellular components.

➤*Pharmacokinetics:*

Absorption/Distribution – Mean peak plasma levels of ≈ 3.5 mcg/mL are reached within 1 to 2 hours, following oral administration of a single 200 mg dose taken with a meal. In vitro, the plasma protein binding is ≈ 99% mainly to the albumin fraction. Only a negligible proportion of ketoconazole reaches the cerebrospinal fluid. Ketoconazole is a weak dibasic agent and thus requires acidity for dissolution and absorption.

Metabolism – Following absorption from the GI tract, ketoconazole is converted into several inactive metabolites. The major identified metabolic pathways are oxidation and degradation of the imidazole and piperazine rings, oxidative O-dealkylation and aromatic hydroxylation.

Excretion – About 13% of the dose is excreted in the urine, of which 2% to 4% is unchanged drug. The major route of excretion is through the bile into the intestinal tract.

Plasma elimination is biphasic with a half-life of 2 hours during the first 10 hours and 8 hours thereafter.

➤*Microbiology:* Ketoconazole is active against clinical infections with *Blastomyces dermatitidis*, *Candida* sp, *Coccidioides immitis*, *Histoplasma capsulatum*, *Paracoccidioides brasiliensis*, and *Phialophora*sp. Ketoconazole is also active against *Trichophyton* sp, *Epidermophyton* sp, and *Microsporum* sp. Ketoconazole is also active in vitro against a variety of fungi and yeast. In animal models, activity has been demonstrated against *Candida* sp, *Blastomyces dermatitidis*, *Histoplasma capsulatum*, *Malassezia furfur*, *Coccidioides immitis*, and *Cryptococcus neoformans*.

Contraindications

Coadministration with terfenadine, astemizole, cisapride, or oral triazolam (see Warning Box, Warnings, and Drug Interactions); hypersensitivity to the drug.

Warnings/Precautions

➤*Cardiac dysrhythmias:* See the Warning box for more information.

➤*Prostate cancer:* In European clinical trials involving 350 patients with metastatic prostatic cancer, 11 deaths were reported within 2 weeks of starting treatment with high doses of ketoconazole tablets (1200 mg/day). It is not possible to ascertain from the information available whether death was related to ketoconazole therapy in these patients with serious underlying disease. However, high doses of ketoconazole are known to suppress adrenal corticosteroid secretion.

➤*Hepatotoxicity:* Hepatotoxicity, primarily of the hepatocellular type, has been associated with the use of ketoconazole, including rare fatalities. The reported incidence of hepatotoxicity has been about 1:10,000 exposed patients, but this probably represents some degree of underreporting, as is the case for most reported adverse reactions to drugs. The median duration of ketoconazole therapy in patients who developed symptomatic hepatotoxicity was ≈ 28 days, although the range extended to as low as 3 days. The hepatic injury has usually, but not always, been reversible upon discontinuation of ketoconazole treatment. Several cases of hepatitis have been reported in children.

Prompt recognition of liver injury is essential. Liver function tests (such as alkaline phosphatase, ALT, AST and bilirubin) should be measured before starting treatment and at frequent intervals during treatment. Patients receiving ketoconazole concurrently with other potentially hepatotoxic drugs should be carefully monitored, particularly those patients requiring prolonged therapy or those who have had a history of liver disease.

Most of the reported cases of hepatic toxicity have to date been in patients treated for onychomycosis. Of 180 patients worldwide developing idiosyncratic liver dysfunction during ketoconazole therapy, 61.3% had onychomycosis and 16.8% had chronic recalcitrant dermatophytoses.

Transient minor elevations in liver enzymes have occurred during treatment with ketoconazole. The drug should be discontinued if these persist, if the abnormalities worsen, or if the abnormalities become accompanied by symptoms of possible liver injury.

➤*Hormone levels:* Ketoconazole has been demonstrated to lower serum testosterone. Once therapy with ketoconazole has been discontinued, serum testosterone levels return to baseline values. Testosterone levels are impaired with doses of 800 mg/day and abolished by 1600 mg per day. Ketoconazole also decrease ACTH-induced corticosteroid serum levels at similar high doses. The recommended dose of 200 mg to 400 mg daily should be followed closely.

➤*Gastric acidity:* In 4 subjects with drug-induced achlorhydria, a marked reduction in ketoconazole absorption was observed. Ketoconazole requires acidity for dissolution. If concomitant antacids, anticholinergics, and H_2-blockers are needed, they should be given at least 2 hours after administration of ketoconazole. In cases of achlorhydria, the patients should be instructed to dissolve each tablet in 4 mL aqueous solution of 0.2 N HCl. For ingesting the resulting mixture, they should use a drinking straw so as to avoid contact with the teeth. This administration should be followed with a cup of tap water.

➤*Hypersensitivity reactions:* In rare cases anaphylaxis has been reported after the first dose. Several cases of hypersensitivity reactions including urticaria have also been reported.

KETOCONAZOLE — ORAL

➤*Pregnancy: Category C.* Ketoconazole has been shown to be teratogenic (syndactylia and oligodactylia) in the rat when given in the diet at 80 mg/kg/day (10 times the maximum recommended human dose). However, these effects may be related to maternal toxicity, evidence of which also was seen at this and higher dose levels.

There are no adequate and well-controlled studies in pregnant women. Ketoconazole tablets should be used during pregnancy only if the potential benefit justifies the potential risk to the fetus.

➤*Lactation:* Since ketoconazole is probably excreted in the milk, mothers who are under treatment should not breastfeed.

➤*Children:* Ketoconazole have not been systematically studied in children of any age, and essentially no information is available on children younger than 2 years. Ketoconazole should not be used in pediatric patients unless the potential benefit outweighs the risks.

Drug Interactions

➤*QT prolongation:* An additive effect of ketoconazole with other drugs that prolong the QT interval cannot be excluded. The following drugs may prolong the QT interval and increase the risk of life-threatening cardiac arrhythmias, including torsade de pointes: Antiarrhythmic agents (eg, amiodarone, bretylium, disopyramide, dofetilide, procainamide, quinidine, and sotalol), arsenic trioxide, chlorpromazine, cisapride, dolasetron, droperidol, mefloquine, mesoridazine, moxifloxacin, pentamidine, pimozide, tacrolimus, thioridazine, and ziprasidone. For a more complete list of drugs that may prolong the QT interval, see the appendix, Drug-Induced Prolongation of the QT Interval and Torsade de Pointes.

Ketoconazole Drug Interactions

Precipitant drug	Object drug[a]		Description
Antacids	Ketoconazole	⬇	Increased gastric pH may inhibit ketoconazole absorption. Consider giving antacids ≥ 2 hours after ketoconazole.
Didanosine	Ketoconazole	⬇	The therapeutic effects of ketoconazole may be decreased. The buffers in didanosine chewable tablets decrease the absorption of ketoconazole.
Ketoconazole	Protease inhibitors Indinavir Ritonavir Saquinavir	⬆	Plasma protease inhibitors concentrations may be elevated, increasing the risk of toxicity. Ketoconazole may inhibit the hepatic metabolism of protease inhibitors.
Ketoconazole	Tricyclic antidepressants	⬆	Serum tricyclic antidepressant concentrations may be elevated, resulting in an increase in therapeutic and adverse effects.
Ketoconazole	Carbamazepine	⬆	Plasma concentrations of carbamazepine may be elevated, increasing clinical and adverse effects. Ketoconazole may inhibit the metabolism of carbamazepine.
Sucralfate	Ketoconazole	⬇	The therapeutic effects of ketoconazole may be reduced. The mechanism of action is unknown but likely because of a decrease in ketoconazole bioavailability. When clinical situation permits, administer ketoconazole ≥ 2 hours before sucralfate.
Proton pump inhibitors	Ketoconazole	⬇	The effects of ketoconazole may be decreased. The bioavailability of ketoconazole may be decreased because of a possible reduction in tablet dissolution in the presence of a high gastric pH.
Ketoconazole	Quinidine	⬆	Serum quinidine levels may be elevated, increasing therapeutic and toxic effects. Ketoconazole may inhibit quinidine metabolism.
Ketoconazole	Sulfonylureas	⬆	Serum sulfonylurea concentrations may be elevated increasing the hypoglycemic effect.
Ketoconazole	Benzodiazepines	⬆	Increased and prolonged serum levels, CNS depression, and psychomotor impairment with certain benzodiazepines are possible for several days after stopping ketoconazole. Concomitant administration of ketoconazole with oral triazolam is contraindicated.
Ketoconazole	Buspirone	⬆	Plasma buspirone concentrations may be elevated, increasing pharmacologic and adverse effects.
Ketoconazole	Contraceptives, oral	⟷	The therapeutic efficacy of oral contraceptives may be reduced. In addition, elevated ethinyl estradiol blood levels may occur. The mechanism of action is unknown. Inform women of the possible increased risk of oral contraceptive failure. Consider an alternative method of contraception.
Ketoconazole	Donepezil	⬆	Donepezil plasma concentration and side effects may be increased.
Ketoconazole	HMG-CoA Reductase Inhibitors	⬆	Increased plasma levels and side effects of HMG-CoA reductase inhibitors may occur. Rhabdomyolysis has been reported. If concurrent administration cannot be avoided, consider reducing the HMG-CoA reductase inhibitor dose.
Ketoconazole	Nisoldipine	⬆	Nisoldipine concentrations may be elevated, increasing pharmacologic and adverse effects.
Ketoconazole	Tacrolimus	⬆	Plasma concentrations may be elevated, increasing the risk of toxicity because of inhibition of tacrolimus gut metabolism.
Ketoconazole	Vinca alkaloids	⬆	Increased risk of vinca alkaloid toxicity has occurred because of inhibition of vinca alkaloid metabolism (CYP3A4) by ketoconazole.
Ketoconazole	Zolpidem	⬆	Plasma concentrations and the therapeutic effects of zolpidem may be increased.
Histamine H_2 antagonists	Ketoconazole	⬇	Increased gastric pH may inhibit ketoconazole absorption.
Isoniazid	Ketoconazole	⬇	Bioavailability of ketoconazole may be decreased.
Rifampin	Ketoconazole	⬇	Decreased serum levels of either drug may occur. Avoid concurrent use if possible.
Ketoconazole	Warfarin	⬆	The anticoagulant response may be enhanced secondary to inhibition of warfarin metabolism.
Ketoconazole	Corticosteroids	⬆	Corticosteroid bioavailability may be increased and clearance may be decreased, possibly resulting in toxicity.
Ketoconazole	Cyclosporine	⬆	Increased cyclosporine concentrations may occur because of inhibition of metabolism, resulting in toxicity. Because the effect on cyclosporine levels is consistent and predictable, this interaction has been used beneficially to decrease cyclosporine dosage in some patients.
Ketoconazole	Theophyllines	⬇	Decreased absorption of theophylline may occur, resulting in decreased theophylline serum levels.

[a] ⬆ = object drug increased; ⬇ = object drug decreased; ⟷ = undetermined clinical effect.

➤*Cytochrome P-450 3A4:* Ketoconazole is a potent inhibitor of the cytochrome P-450 3A4 enzyme system. Coadministration of ketoconazole and drugs primarily metabolized by the cytochrome P-450 3A4 enzyme system may result in increased plasma concentrations of the drugs that could increase or prolong both therapeutic and adverse effects. Therefore, unless otherwise specified, appropriate dosage adjustments may be necessary. The following drug interactions have been identified involving ketoconazole and other drugs metabolized by the cytochrome P-450 3A4 enzyme system:

➤*Cyclosporine, tacrolimus, methylprednisolone:* Ketoconazole may alter the metabolism of cyclosporine, tacrolimus, and methylprednisolone, resulting in elevated plasma concentrations of the latter drugs. Dosage adjustment may be required if cyclosporine, tacrolimus, or methylprednisolone are given concomitantly with ketoconazole.

➤*Midazolam, triazolam:* Coadministration of ketoconazole with midazolam or triazolam has resulted in elevated plasma concentrations of the latter 2 drugs. This may potentiate and prolong hypnotic and sedative effects, especially with repeated dosing or chronic administration of these agents. These agents should not be used in patients treated with ketoconazole. If midazolam is administered parenterally, special precaution is required since the sedative effect may be prolonged.

➤*Digoxin:* Rare cases of elevated plasma concentrations of digoxin have been reported. It is not clear whether this was due to the combination of therapy. It is, therefore, advisable to monitor digoxin concentrations in patients receiving ketoconazole.

➤*Hypoglycemic agents:* Because severe hypoglycemia has been reported in patients concomitantly receiving oral miconazole (an imidazole) and oral hypoglycemic agents, such a potential interaction involving the latter agents when used concomitantly with ketoconazole tablets (an imidazole) can not be ruled out.

➤*Phenytoin:* Concomitant administration of ketoconazole with phenytoin may alter the metabolism of one or both of the drugs. It is suggested to monitor both ketoconazole and phenytoin.

➤*Loratadine:* After the coadministration of 200 mg oral ketoconazole twice daily and one 20 mg dose of loratadine to 11 subjects, the AUC and C_{max} of loratadine averaged 302% (± 142 S.D.) and 251% (± 68 S.D.), respectively, of those obtained after cotreatment with placebo. The AUC and C_{max} of descarboethoxyloratadine, an active metabolite, averaged 155% (± 27 S.D.) and 141% (± 35 S.D.), respectively. However, no related changes were noted in the QTc on ECG taken at 2, 6, and 24 hours after the coadministration. Also, there were no clinically significant differences in adverse events when loratadine was administered with or without ketoconazole.

➤*Alcohol:* Rare cases of a disulfiram-like reaction to alcohol have been reported. These experiences have been characterized by flushing, rash, peripheral edema, nausea, and headache. Symptoms resolved within a few hours.

KETOCONAZOLE — ORAL

Adverse Reactions

In rare cases, anaphylaxis has been reported after the first dose. Several cases of hypersensitivity reactions including urticaria have also been reported. However, the most frequent adverse reactions were nausea or vomiting in ≈ 3%, abdominal pain in 1.2%, pruritus in 1.5%, and the following in less than 1% of the patients: Headache, dizziness, somnolence, fever and chills, photophobia, diarrhea, gynecomastia, impotence, thrombocytopenia, leukopenia, hemolytic anemia, and bulging fontanelles. Oligospermia has been reported in investigational studies with the drug at dosages above those currently approved. Oligospermia has not been reported at dosages up to 400 mg daily; however, sperm counts have been obtained infrequently in patients treated with these dosages. Most of these reactions were mild and transient and rarely required discontinuation of ketoconazole. In contrast, the rare occurrences of hepatic dysfunction require special attention (see Warnings/Precautions).

In worldwide postmarketing experience with ketoconazole there have been rare reports of alopecia, paresthesia, and signs of increased intracranial pressure including bulging fontanelles and papilledema. Hypertriglyceridemia has also been reported but a causal association with ketoconazole is uncertain.

➤*Cardiovascular:* Ventricular dysrhythmias (prolonged QT intervals) have occurred with the concomitant use of terfenadine with ketoconazole tablets (see Warning Box, Contraindications, and Warnings). Data suggest that coadministration of ketoconazole tablets and cisapride can result in prolongation of the QT interval and has rarely been associated with ventricular arrhythmias (see Contraindications, Warnings, and Drug Interactions).

➤*Psychiatric:* Neuropsychiatric disturbances, including suicidal tendencies and severe depression, have occurred rarely in patients using ketoconazole tablets.

Overdosage

➤*Treatment:* In the event of accidental overdosage, supportive measures, including gastric lavage with sodium bicarbonate, should be employed.

Patient Information

Patients should not take ketoconazole with antacids; this may cause dizziness.

Patients should be instructed to report any signs and symptoms which may suggest liver dysfunction so that appropriate biochemical testing can be done. Such signs and symptoms may include unusual fatigue, anorexia, nausea or vomiting, jaundice, dark urine or pale stools (see Warnings/Precautions).

MICONAZOLE

Rx	**Oravig** (Strativa Pharmaceuticals)	**Tablet; buccal**: 50 mg	Lactose, milk protein concentrate. L. Off-white, round. In 14s.

MICONAZOLE — BUCCAL

Indications

➤*Oropharyngeal candidiasis:* For the local treatment of oropharyngeal candidiasis in adults.

Administration and Dosage

➤*Adults:*

Oropharyngeal candidiasis –

Usual dosage: 50 mg (1 tablet) to the upper gum region (canine fossa) once daily.

Duration of therapy: Fourteen consecutive days.

➤*Children:*

Oropharyngeal candidiasis –

16 years of age and older: See Adults for dosing.

➤*Administration:* Apply typically to the gum in the morning with dry hands, after brushing the teeth. Do not crush, chew, or swallow the tablet. The rounded side surface of the tablet should be placed against the upper gum just above the incisor tooth (canine fossa) and held in place with slight pressure over the upper lip for 30 seconds to ensure adhesion. The tablet is round on one side for comfort, but either side of the tablet can be applied to the gum. Food and drink can be taken normally when the tablet is in place, but chewing gum should be avoided.

Once applied, the tablet stays in position and gradually dissolves. Subsequent applications should be made to alternate sides of the mouth. Before applying the next tablet, the patient should clear away any remaining tablet material.

If the tablet does not adhere or falls off within the first 6 hours, the same tablet should be repositioned immediately. If the tablet still does not adhere, a new tablet should be placed.

If the tablet is swallowed within the first 6 hours, the patient should drink a glass of water and a new tablet should be applied only once.

If the tablet falls off or is swallowed after it was in place for 6 hours or more, a new tablet should not be applied until the next regularly scheduled dose.

➤*Storage/Stability:* Store at 20° to 25°C (68° and 77°F); excursions are permitted between 15° and 30°C (59° and 86°F). Protect from moisture.

Actions

➤*Pharmacology:* Miconazole is an antifungal drug and inhibits the enzyme cytochrome P450 14-alpha-demethylase, which leads to inhibition of ergosterol synthesis, an essential component of the fungal cell membrane. Miconazole also affects the synthesis of triglycerides and fatty acids and inhibits oxidative and peroxidative enzymes, increasing the amount of reactive oxygen species within the cell.

➤*Pharmacokinetics:*

Absorption/Distribution –

Salivary:

Miconazole Pharmacokinetic Parameters in Saliva (N = 18)[a]	
Salivary pharmacokinetic parameters	Mean ± SD (min to max)
AUC_{0-24h} (mcg•h/mL)	55.2 ± 35.1 (0.5 to 128.3)
C_{max} (mcg/mL)	15.1 ± 16.2 (0.5 to 64.8)
T_{max} (hour)	7[b] (2 to 24.1)

[a] SD = standard deviation; AUC = area under the curve; C_{max} = maximum plasma concentration; T_{max} = time to C_{max}.
[b] Median.

In healthy volunteers, the duration of buccal adhesion was on average 15 hours following a single dose application.

Plasma: Plasma concentrations of miconazole were below the lower limit of quantification (0.4 mcg/mL) in 97% of samples from healthy volunteers following single-dose application. Measurable plasma concentrations ranged from 0.5 to 0.83 mcg/mL.

Plasma concentrations of miconazole evaluated after 7 days of treatment in 40 patients with HIV were all below the limit of quantification (0.1 mcg/mL).

Metabolism/Excretion – Most of the absorbed miconazole is metabolized by the liver, with less than 1% of the administered dose found unchanged in urine. In healthy volunteers, the terminal half-life is 24 hours following systemic administration. There are no active metabolites of miconazole.

Contraindications

Known hypersensitivity (eg, anaphylaxis) to miconazole, milk protein concentrate, or any other component of the product.

Warnings/Precautions

➤*Hypersensitivity reactions:* Allergic reactions, including anaphylactic reactions and hypersensitivity, have been reported with the administration of miconazole products, including the buccal tablets. Discontinue miconazole immediately at the first sign of hypersensitivity.

There is no information regarding cross-hypersensitivity between miconazole and other azole antifungal agents. Monitor patients with a history of hypersensitivity to azoles.

➤*Hepatic function impairment:* While miconazole systemic exposure is minimal following the application of miconazole, administer miconazole with caution in patients with hepatic impairment.

➤*Pregnancy: Category C.* There are no adequate and well-controlled clinical trials of miconazole in pregnant women. Do not use miconazole during pregnancy unless the potential benefit to the mother outweighs the potential risk to the fetus.

Miconazole nitrate administered orally at dosages of 80 mg/kg/day or higher to pregnant rats or rabbits crossed the placenta and resulted in embryo- and fetotoxicity, including increased fetal resorptions. These doses also resulted in prolonged gestation and dystocia in rats, but not in rabbits.

➤*Lactation:* It is not known whether this drug is excreted in human milk. Because many drugs are excreted in human milk, exercise caution when miconazole is administered to a breast-feeding woman. Miconazole is classified as probably compatible with breast-feeding.

➤*Children:* Safety and effectiveness of miconazole in children younger than 16 years of age have not been established. The ability of children to comply with the application instructions has not been evaluated. Use in younger children is not recommended because of the potential risk of choking.

➤*Monitoring:* Monitor patients with a history of hypersensitivity to azoles.

MICONAZOLE — BUCCAL

Drug Interactions

Miconazole Drug Interactions			
Precipitant drug	Object drug[a]		Description
Miconazole	CYP2C9 and CYP3A4 substrates (eg, ergot derivatives [eg, ergotamine], hydantoins [eg, phenytoin], oral hypoglycemic agents [eg, glyburide])	↔	Because miconazole is a known inhibitor of CYP2C9 and CYP3A4, the potential for interaction with these substrates cannot be ruled out.
Miconazole	Warfarin	↑	While miconazole buccal tablets may not produce high systemic levels, systemic miconazole therapy has been associated with enhanced anticoagulant effects when used with warfarin. Cases of bleeding have been reported following concomitant use of warfarin and miconazole. Patients requiring miconazole therapy while using warfarin should have their prothrombin time and international normalized ratio monitored closely and should be instructed to report any bleeding. Adjust the warfarin dose as needed.

[a] ↑ = object drug increased; ↔ = undetermined clinical effect.

Adverse Reactions

➤*Discontinuation:* Discontinuation of miconazole because of adverse drug reactions occurred in 0.6% of patients overall.

➤*Patients with HIV:*

Miconazole Adverse Reactions in Patients With HIV (≥ 2%)		
Adverse reaction	Miconazole (n = 290)	Clotrimazole troches (n = 287)
Any adverse reaction	54.5%	50.9%
CNS	13.1%	8.4%
Ageusia	2.4%	0.3%
Fatigue	2.8%	2.1%
Headache	7.6%	6.6%
GI	25.9%	23.7%
Abdominal pain upper	1.7%	2.8%
Diarrhea	9%	8%
Dry mouth	2.8%	1.7%
Gastroenteritis	1.4%	2.8%
Nausea	6.6%	7.7%
Vomiting	3.8%	3.1%
Hematologic	6.9%	8.4%
Anemia	2.8%	1.7%
Lymphopenia	1.7%	2.1%
Neutropenia	0.7%	2.1%
Lab test abnormalities	5.5%	6.3%
Increased GGT[a]	1%	2.8%
Respiratory	5.2%	7.7%
Cough	2.8%	1.7%
Pharyngeal pain	0.7%	2.4%
Upper respiratory infection	2.1%	2.4%
Miscellaneous		
General disorders and administration-site conditions	6.6%	8%
Infections and infestations	15.9%	17.1%
Pain	1%	2.8%

[a] GGT = gamma-glutamyl transferase.

Local – Overall local adverse reactions, including altered taste, application-site pain or discomfort, dry mouth, gingival pain, gingival pruritis, gingival swelling, glossodynia, loss of taste, mouth ulceration, oral burning, oral discomfort, oral pain, tongue ulceration, and toothache, were reported by 12.1% of patients who received miconazole buccal tablets compared with 9.4% of patients who received clotrimazole troches.

➤*Head and neck cancer patients:*

Miconazole Adverse Reactions in Head and Neck Cancer Patients (≥ 2%)		
Adverse reaction	Miconazole buccal tablets (n = 147)	Miconazole gel (n = 147)
At least 1 adverse reaction	20.4%	21.8%
CNS	5.4%	1.4%
Dysgeusia	4.1%	0%
Dermatologic	3.4%	0.7%
Pruritus	2%	0.7%
GI	8.8%	13.6%
Abdominal pain upper	1.4%	2%
Glossodynia	0%	2%
Nausea	0.7%	2.7%
Oral discomfort	2.7%	2.7%
Vomiting	0.7%	2%

Local – Overall local adverse reactions, including altered taste, application-site discomfort or pain, dry mouth, glossodynia, loss of taste, mouth ulceration, oral discomfort, oral pain, tongue ulceration, and tooth disorder, were experienced by 9.5% of patients who used miconazole buccal tablets compared with 0.9% of patients who used miconazole gel.

➤*Adverse reactions (2% or more):*

Miconazole Adverse Reactions (≥ 2%)	
Adverse reaction	Miconazole (n = 480)
At least 1 adverse reaction	43.5%
CNS	10.6%
Dysgeusia	2.9%
Headache	5%
GI	20.6%
Abdominal pain upper	2.5%
Diarrhea	6%
Nausea	4.6%
Vomiting	2.5%
Miscellaneous	—
Infections and infestations	11.9%

Overdosage

➤*Treatment:* Symptomatic and supportive care is the basis for management.

Patient Information

Advise patient to use the tablet immediately after removal from the bottle.

Instruct patients not to crush, chew, or swallow the tablet.

Inform patients to apply the rounded side of the tablet to the upper gum above the incisor tooth in the morning, after brushing the teeth.

Advise patients to hold the tablet in place for 30 seconds with slight pressure of the finger over the upper lip to make the tablet stick to the gum. The tablet may be used if it sticks to the cheek, inside of the lip, or the gum. If the tablet does not adhere, it should be repositioned. As the miconazole tablet absorbs moisture from the mouth, it will slowly dissolve over time and should be left in place; there is no need to remove the tablet. Subsequent applications of miconazole should be made to alternate sides of the gum.

Inform patients that if miconazole does not stick or falls off within the first 6 hours, to reposition the same tablet immediately. If the tablet does not adhere, place a new tablet. If miconazole is swallowed within the first 6 hours, the patient should drink a glass of water and a new tablet should be applied only once. If miconazole falls off or is swallowed after it was in place for 6 hours or more, a new tablet should not be applied until the next regularly scheduled dose.

Advise patients to avoid situations that could interfere with the sticking of the tablet, including touching or pressing the tablet after placement, wearing upper denture, chewing gum, hitting tablet when brushing teeth, and rinsing mouth too vigorously.

Inform patients that if they develop hives, skin rash, or other symptoms of an allergic reaction, or swelling or pain at the tablet application site, to stop using miconazole and contact a health care provider. Patients may experience other adverse reactions, including diarrhea, headache, nausea, and change in taste.

VORICONAZOLE

Rx	**Voriconazole** (Various, eg, Greenstone, Mylan)	**Tablets; oral:** 50	May include lactose. In 30s.
Rx	**Vfend** (Roerig)	**Tablets; oral:** 50 mg	Lactose. (Pfizer VOR50). White, round. Film-coated. In 30s.
	Voriconazole (Various, eg, Greenstone, Mylan)	**Tablets; oral:** 200 mg	May include lactose. In 30s.
	Vfend (Roerig)	**Tablets; oral:** 200 mg	Lactose. (Pfizer VOR200). White, capsule shape. Film-coated. In 30s.
Rx	**Vfend** (Roerig)	**Powder for suspension; oral:** 40 mg/mL (after reconstitution)	Sucrose, sodium benzoate. Orange flavoring. In 100 mL with a 5 mL oral dispenser.
Rx	**Vfend** (Roerig)	**Injection, lyophilized powder for solution**[a]: 200 mg	Preservative free. In single-use vials.

[a] Contains intravenous (IV) vehicle of 3,200 mg of sulfobutyl ether beta-cyclodextrin sodium (SBECD).

VORICONAZOLE — ORAL

Indications

➤*Candidemia:* For the treatment of Candidemia in nonneutropenic patients and the following *Candida* infections: disseminated infections in skin and infections in abdomen, bladder wall, kidney, and wounds.

➤*Esophageal candidiasis:* For the treatment of esophageal candidiasis.

➤*Invasive aspergillosis:* For the treatment of invasive aspergillosis. In clinical trials, the majority of isolates recovered were *Aspergillus fumigatus*. There was a small number of cases of culture-proven disease caused by species of *Aspergillus* other than *A. fumigatus*.

➤*Serious fungal infections:* For the treatment of serious fungal infections caused by *Scedosporium apiospermum* (asexual form of *Pseudallescheria boydii*) and *Fusarium* spp., including *Fusarium solani*, in patients intolerant of, or refractory to, other therapy.

Administration and Dosage

➤*Adults:*

Infections –

Usual dosage:

Voriconazole Recommended Adult Dosing Regimen			
	Loading dosage	Maintenance dosage	
Infection	IV[a]	IV	Oral[b]
Candidemia in nonneutropenic patients and other deep tissue *Candida* infections	6 mg/kg every 12 hours for the first 24 hours	3 to 4 mg/kg every 12 hours[c]	200 mg every 12 hours
Esophageal candidiasis	[d]	[d]	200 mg every 12 hours
Invasive aspergillosis	6 mg/kg every 12 hours for the first 24 hours	4 mg/kg every 12 hours	200 mg every 12 hours
Scedosporiosis and fusariosis	6 mg/kg every 12 hours for the first 24 hours	4 mg/kg every 12 hours	200 mg every 12 hours

[a] IV = intravenous.
[b] Patients who weigh ≥ 40 kg should receive an oral maintenance dosage of voriconazole 200 mg every 12 hours. Patients who weigh
[c] In clinical trials, patients with candidemia received 3 mg/kg every 12 hours as primary therapy, while patients with other deep tissue *Candida* infections received 4 mg/kg as salvage therapy. Base appropriate dose on the severity and nature of the infection.
[d] Not evaluated in patients with esophageal candidiasis.

Dosage adjustment: If patient response is inadequate, the oral maintenance dosage may be increased from 200 mg every 12 hours to 300 mg every 12 hours. For patients weighing less than 40 kg, the oral maintenance dosage may be increased from 100 mg every 12 hours to 150 mg every 12 hours.

If patients are unable to tolerate 300 mg orally every 12 hours, reduce the oral maintenance dosage by 50 mg steps to a minimum of 200 mg every 12 hours (or to 100 mg every 12 hours for adults weighing 40 kg or less).

➤*Children:* See Adults for dosing for children 12 years of age and older.

➤*Renal function impairment:*

Oral – No adjustment is necessary for oral dosing in patients with mild to severe renal impairment.

IV – In patients with moderate or severe renal impairment (creatinine clearance [CrCl] less than 50 mL/min), accumulation of the IV vehicle SBECD occurs. Oral voriconazole should be administered to these patients, unless an assessment of the benefit/risk to the patient justifies the use of IV voriconazole.

Hemodialysis – Voriconazole is hemodialyzed with clearance of 121 mL/min.

Adults receiving continuous renal replacement therapy – The following recommendations assume ultrafiltration and dialysis flow rates of 1 to 2 L/h.

Loading dose: 400 mg orally every 12 hours for 2 doses.

Maintenance dosage: A dosage of 200 mg orally every 12 hours is recommended for patients receiving continuous venovenous hemofiltration, continuous venovenous hemodialysis, or continuous venovenous hemodialfiltration. This recommendation assumes ultrafiltration and dialysis flow rates of 1 to 2 L/h.

Adults receiving intermittent hemodialysis – 200 mg orally every 12 hours. This recommendation assumes the patient is receiving standard intermittent hemodialysis 3 times per week and completes the full dialysis sessions.

➤*Hepatic function impairment:*

Mild to moderate hepatic impairment – It is recommended that the standard loading-dose regimens be used, but that the maintenance dose be halved in patients with mild to moderate hepatic cirrhosis (Child-Pugh class A and B).

➤*Duration of therapy:*

Candidemia in nonneutropenic patients and other deep tissue Candida infections – Patients should be treated for a minimum of 14 days after resolution of symptoms, or following last positive culture, whichever is longer.

Esophageal candidiasis – Patients should be treated for a minimum of 14 days and for at least 7 days following resolution of symptoms.

➤*Administration:* Should be taken orally at least 1 hour before or 1 hour after a meal.

➤*Admixture compatibility:* Voriconazole suspension should not be mixed with any other medication or additional flavoring agent, and the suspension should not be diluted further with water or other vehicles.

➤*Storage/Stability:*

Tablets – Store at 15° to 30°C (59° to 86°F).

Suspension – Store in a refrigerator at 2° to 8°C (36° to 46°F) before reconstitution. Store the reconstituted suspension at 15° to 30°C (59° to 86°F). Do not refrigerate or freeze. Keep the container tightly closed. Discard any remaining suspension 14 days after reconstitution.

Actions

➤*Pharmacology:* Voriconazole is a triazole antifungal agent. The primary mode of action of voriconazole is the inhibition of fungal cytochrome P 450 (CYP-450)–mediated 14 alpha-lanosterol demethylation, an essential step in fungal ergosterol biosynthesis. The accumulation of 14 alpha-methyl sterols correlates with the subsequent loss of ergosterol in the fungal cell wall and may be responsible for the antifungal activity of voriconazole. Voriconazole has been shown to be more selective for fungal CYP-450 enzymes than for various mammalian CYP-450 enzyme systems.

➤*Pharmacokinetics:*

Absorption – Based on a population pharmacokinetic analysis of pooled data in healthy subjects (n = 207), the oral bioavailability of voriconazole is estimated to be 96% (coefficient of variation [CV] 13%). Maximum plasma concentration (C_{max}) is achieved 1 to 2 hours after dosing.

Greater than proportional increase in exposure is observed with increasing dose. It is estimated that, on average, increasing the oral dosage in healthy subjects from 200 mg every 12 hours to 300 mg every 12 hours leads to a 2.5-fold increase in exposure (AUC_{tau}).

Voriconazole Oral Pharmacokinetic Parameters		
Pharmacokinetic parameter	200 mg orally every 12 h	300 mg orally every 12 h
AUC_{tau}[a] (mcg•h/mL) (CV%)	19.86 (94%)	50.32 (74%)

[a] Mean AUC_{tau} are predicted values from population pharmacokinetic analysis of data from 236 volunteers.

When the recommended oral loading dose regimen is administered to healthy subjects, peak plasma concentrations close to steady state are achieved within the first 24 hours of dosing. Without the loading dose, accumulation occurs during twice-daily multiple dosing, with steady-state voriconazole C_{max} achieved by day 6 in the majority of subjects.

VORICONAZOLE — ORAL

Voriconazole Oral Pharmacokinetic Parameters from Loading Dose and Maintenance Dose Regimens		
	400 mg every 12 h on day 1, 200 mg every 12 h on days 2 to 10 (n = 17)	
Pharmacokinetic parameter	Day 1, first dose	Day 10
AUC_{tau}[a] (mcg•h/mL) (CV%)	9.31 (38%)	11.13 (103%)
C_{max} (mcg/mL) (CV%)	2.3 (19%)	2.08 (62%)

[a] AUC_{tau} values are calculated over a 12-hour dosing interval. Pharmacokinetic parameters for loading and maintenance doses summarized for same cohort of volunteers.

Steady-state trough plasma concentrations with voriconazole are achieved after approximately 5 days of oral dosing without a loading dose regimen.

Effect of food: When multiple doses of voriconazole are administered with high-fat meals, the mean C_{max} and AUC_{tau} are reduced by 34% and 24%, respectively, when administered as a tablet, and by 58% and 37%, respectively, when administered as the suspension.

Distribution – The volume of distribution at steady state for voriconazole is estimated to be 4.6 L/kg, suggesting extensive distribution into tissues. Plasma protein binding is estimated to be 58% and was shown to be independent of plasma concentrations achieved after single and multiple oral doses of 200 or 300 mg (approximate range is 0.9 to 15 mcg/mL). Varying degrees of hepatic and renal impairment do not affect the protein binding of voriconazole.

Metabolism – In vitro studies showed that voriconazole is metabolized by the human hepatic CYP-450 enzymes, CYP2C19, CYP2C9, and CYP3A4. The major metabolite of voriconazole is the N-oxide, which accounts for 72% of the circulating radiolabeled metabolites in plasma. Because this metabolite has minimal antifungal activity, it does not contribute to the overall efficacy of voriconazole.

Excretion – Voriconazole is eliminated via hepatic metabolism, with less than 2% of the dose excreted unchanged in the urine. After administration of a single radiolabeled dose of voriconazole, preceded by multiple dosing, approximately 80% to 83% of the radioactivity is recovered in the urine. The majority (more than 94%) of the total radioactivity is excreted in the first 96 hours after dosing.

As a result of nonlinear pharmacokinetics, the terminal half-life of voriconazole is dose dependent and, therefore, not useful in predicting the accumulation or elimination of voriconazole.

Special populations –

Renal function impairment:

Hepatic function impairment: After a single oral dose of voriconazole 200 mg in 8 subjects with mild (Child-Pugh class A) and 4 patients with moderate (Child-Pugh class B) hepatic impairment, the mean AUC was 3.2-fold higher than in age- and weight-matched controls with healthy hepatic function. There was no difference in mean C_{max} between the groups. When only the patients with mild (Child-Pugh class A) hepatic impairment were compared with controls, there still was a 2.3-fold increase in the mean AUC in the group with hepatic impairment compared with controls.

In an oral multiple-dose study, AUC_{tau} was similar in 6 subjects with moderate hepatic impairment (Child-Pugh class B) given a lower maintenance dosage of 100 mg twice daily compared with 6 subjects with healthy hepatic function given the standard 200 mg twice-daily maintenance dose. The mean C_{max} was 20% lower in the hepatically impaired group.

See Administration and Dosage for more information.

Gender: In an oral multiple-dose study, the mean C_{max} and AUC_{tau} for healthy younger women were 83% and 113% higher, respectively, than in healthy younger men (18 to 45 years of age) after tablet dosing. In the same study, no significant differences in the mean C_{max} and AUC_{tau} were observed between healthy elderly men and healthy elderly women (65 years of age and older). In a similar study, after dosing with the oral suspension, the mean AUC for healthy younger women was 45% higher than in healthy younger men, whereas the mean C_{max} was comparable between genders. The steady-state trough voriconazole concentrations (C_{min}) in women were 100% and 91% higher than in men receiving the tablet and the suspension, respectively.

➤*Microbiology:*

Activity in vitro – Voriconazole has been shown to be active against most strains of the following microorganisms, both in vitro and in clinical infections: *A. fumigatus, Aspergillus flavus, Aspergillus niger, Aspergillus terreus, Candida albicans, Candida glabrata* (in clinical studies, the voriconazole minimum inhibitory concentration [MIC_{90}] was 4 mcg/mL), *Candida krusei, Candida parapsilosis, Candida tropicalis, Fusarium* spp. including *Fusarium solani*, and *S. apiospermum*. In clinical studies, voriconazole MIC_{90} for *C. glabrata* baseline isolates was 4 mcg/mL; 26% of *C. glabrata* baseline isolates were resistant (MIC at least 4 mcg/mL) to voriconazole. However, based on 1,054 isolates tested in surveillance studies, the MIC_{90} was 1 mcg/mL.

Voriconazole exhibits in vitro MICs of 1 mcg/mL or less against most (at least 90%) isolates of the following microorganisms; however, the safety and effectiveness of voriconazole in treating clinical infections due to these *Candida* species have not been established in adequate and well-controlled clinical trials: *Candida lusitaniae* and *Candida guilliermondii*.

Contraindications

Hypersensitivity to voriconazole or its excipients; coadministration with CYP3A4 substrates (terfenadine, astemizole, cisapride, pimozide, quinidine), sirolimus, rifampin, carbamazepine, long-acting barbiturates, ritonavir (400 mg every 12 hours), rifabutin, ergot alkaloids (ergotamine and dihydroergotamine), and St. John's wort.

Warnings/Precautions

➤*Ophthalmic effects:* The effect of voriconazole on visual function is not known if treatment continues beyond 28 days. There have been postmarketing reports of prolonged visual adverse reactions, including optic neuritis and papilledema. If treatment continues beyond 28 days, monitor visual function, including visual acuity, visual field, and color perception.

➤*Hepatic toxicity:* In clinical trials, there have been uncommon cases of serious hepatic reactions during treatment with voriconazole (including clinical hepatitis, cholestasis, and fulminant hepatic failure, including fatalities). Instances of hepatic reactions were noted to occur primarily in patients with serious underlying medical conditions (predominantly hematological malignancy). Hepatic reactions, including hepatitis and jaundice, have occurred among patients with no other identifiable risk factors. Liver dysfunction usually has been reversible on discontinuation of therapy.

Evaluate liver function tests (LFTs) at the start of and during the course of voriconazole therapy. Monitor patients who develop abnormal LFTs during voriconazole therapy for the development of more severe hepatic injury. Patient management should include laboratory evaluation of hepatic function (particularly LFTs and bilirubin). Consider discontinuation of voriconazole if clinical signs and symptoms consistent with liver disease develop that may be attributable to voriconazole.

➤*Galactose intolerance:* Voriconazole tablets contain lactose; do not give to patients with rare hereditary problems of galactose intolerance, Lapp lactase deficiency, or glucose-galactose malabsorption.

➤*Cardiovascular effects:* Some azoles, including voriconazole, have been associated with prolongation of the QT interval on the ECG. During clinical development and postmarketing surveillance, there have been rare cases of arrhythmias (including ventricular arrhythmias, such as torsades de pointes), cardiac arrests, and sudden deaths in patients taking voriconazole. These cases usually involved seriously ill patients with multiple confounding risk factors, such as histories of cardiotoxic chemotherapy, cardiomyopathy, hypokalemia, and concomitant medications, that may have been contributory.

Administer voriconazole with caution to patients with these potentially proarrhythmic conditions.

➤*Renal toxicity:* Acute renal failure has been observed in severely ill patients undergoing treatment with voriconazole. Patients being treated with voriconazole are likely to be treated concomitantly with nephrotoxic medications and have concurrent conditions that may result in decreased renal function.

➤*Dermatological reactions:* See Adverse Reactions for more information.

➤*Hypersensitivity reactions:* There is no information regarding cross-sensitivity between voriconazole and other azole antifungal agents. Use caution when prescribing voriconazole to patients with hypersensitivity to other azoles.

➤*Renal function impairment:* See Administration and Dosage for more information.

➤*Hepatic function impairment:* See Administration and Dosage for more information.

➤*Hazardous tasks:* Advise patients to avoid potentially hazardous tasks, such as driving or operating machinery, if they perceive any change in vision.

➤*Photosensitivity:* See Administration and Dosage for more information.

➤*Pregnancy: Category D.* Voriconazole can cause fetal harm when administered to a pregnant woman. It is not known if voriconazole crosses the placenta to the fetus; however, the molecular weight (approximately 349) is low enough that exposure of the embryo and/or fetus should be expected.

If this drug is used during pregnancy, or if the patient becomes pregnant while taking this drug, apprise the patient of the potential hazard to the fetus.

Voriconazole was teratogenic in rats (cleft palates, hydronephrosis/hydroureter) from 10 mg/kg (0.3 times the recommended maintenance dose on a mg/m^2 basis) and embryotoxic in rabbits at 100 mg/kg (6 times the recommended maintenance dose). Other effects in rats included reduced ossification of sacral and caudal vertebrae, skull, pubic and hyoid bone, supernumerary ribs, anomalies of the sternebrae, and dilatation of the ureter/renal pelvis. Plasma estradiol in pregnant rats was reduced at all dose levels. Voriconazole treatment in rats produced increased gestational length and dystocia, which were associated with increased perinatal pup mortality at the 10 mg/kg dose. The effects seen in rabbits were an increased embryomortality; reduced fetal weight; and increased incidences of skeletal variations, cervical ribs, and extrasternebral ossification sites.

Instruct women of childbearing potential to use effective contraception during treatment.

➤*Lactation:* The excretion of voriconazole in breast milk has not been investigated. The molecular weight (approximately 349) suggests that voriconazole will be excreted in breast milk. There is potential for toxicity in breast-feeding infants, especially during the neonatal period when hepatic function is immature. Do not use voriconazole in breast-feeding mothers unless the benefit clearly outweighs the risk.

➤*Children:* Safety and efficacy in children younger than 12 years of age have not been established.

VORICONAZOLE — ORAL

There have been postmarketing reports of pancreatitis in children.

➤*Monitoring:* Monitor patients with risk factors for acute pancreatitis (eg, recent chemotherapy, hematopoietic stem cell transplantation) for the development of pancreatitis.

Correct electrolyte disturbances, such as hypocalcemia, hypokalemia, and hypomagnesemia, prior to initiation of therapy.

Monitor patients for the development of abnormal renal function. This includes laboratory evaluation, particularly serum creatinine.

Evaluate LFTs and bilirubin at the start of and during the course of voriconazole therapy. Monitor patients who develop abnormal LFTs during voriconazole therapy for the development of more severe hepatic injury. Patients with hepatic insufficiency must be carefully monitored for drug toxicity.

If treatment continues beyond 28 days, monitor visual function, including visual acuity, visual field, and color perception.

Drug Interactions

➤*QT prolongation:* An additive effect of voriconazole with other drugs that prolong the QT interval cannot be excluded. The following drugs may prolong the QT interval and increase the risk of life-threatening cardiac arrhythmias, including torsades de pointes: antiarrhythmic agents (eg, amiodarone, bretylium, disopyramide, dofetilide, procainamide, quinidine, sotalol), arsenic trioxide, chlorpromazine, cisapride, dolasetron, droperidol, mefloquine, mesoridazine, moxifloxacin, pentamidine, pimozide, tacrolimus, thioridazine, and ziprasidone. For a more complete list of drugs that may prolong the QT interval, see the appendix Drug-Induced Prolongation of the QT Interval and Torsades de Pointes.

Voriconazole Drug Interactions

Precipitant drug	Object drug[a]		Description
Barbiturates, long acting (eg, mephobarbital, phenobarbital), carbamazepine	Voriconazole	↓	Coadministration may decrease voriconazole plasma concentrations. Coadministration is contraindicated.
Cimetidine	Voriconazole	↑	Cimetidine increased voriconazole C_{max} and AUC by an average of 18% and 23%, respectively. No dosage adjustment is required.
Contraceptives, hormonal (eg, containing ethinyl estradiol and norethindrone)	Voriconazole		Voriconazole administration to healthy women receiving oral contraceptives increased ethinyl estradiol C_{max} and AUC by an average of 36% and 61%, respectively, and norethindrone C_{max} and AUC by an average of 15% and 53%, respectively. Voriconazole C_{max} and AUC increased by an average of 14% and 46%, respectively. Monitor for adverse reactions related to the contraceptive agent as well as voriconazole.
Voriconazole	Contraceptives, hormonal (eg, containing ethinyl estradiol and norethindrone)	↑	
Fluconazole	Voriconazole	↑	Fluconazole increased voriconazole C_{max} and AUC by an average of 57% and 79%, respectively. Coadministration is not recommended. Close clinical monitoring is recommended if voriconazole is given sequentially after fluconazole, especially within 24 hours of the last fluconazole dose.
NNRTIs[b] (eg, delavirdine, nevirapine)	Voriconazole	↑↓	Coadministration may induce or inhibit the metabolism of voriconazole. Monitor for toxicity and effectiveness of voriconazole. Voriconazole also may inhibit the metabolism of an NNRTI. Monitor for drug toxicity. Coadministration of efavirenz and voriconazole decreases voriconazole plasma concentrations. When voriconazole is coadministered with efavirenz, increase the voriconazole maintenance dosage to 400 mg every 12 hours and decrease the efavirenz dosage to 300 mg every 24 hours. When voriconazole is discontinued, restore the initial dosage of efavirenz.
Voriconazole	NNRTIs (eg, delavirdine, efavirenz)	↑	

Voriconazole Drug Interactions

Precipitant drug	Object drug[a]		Description
Phenytoin	Voriconazole	↓	Phenytoin may decrease the C_{max} and AUC of voriconazole by 50% and 70%, respectively. Voriconazole may increase the C_{max} and AUC of phenytoin up to 2 times. Monitor for phenytoin adverse reactions and phenytoin plasma concentrations. If phenytoin is administered with voriconazole, increase the voriconazole dosage from 200 to 400 mg every 12 hours (100 to 200 mg every 12 hours in adults weighing less than 40 kg).
Voriconazole	Phenytoin	↑	
Protease inhibitors (eg, amprenavir, ritonavir, saquinavir)	Voriconazole	↑↓	Voriconazole may inhibit the metabolism of certain protease inhibitors, and the metabolism of voriconazole may be inhibited or induced by certain protease inhibitors. Monitor closely for toxicity. Coadministration with indinavir showed no significant effects on voriconazole or indinavir exposure.
Voriconazole	Protease inhibitors (eg, amprenavir, nelfinavir, ritonavir, saquinavir)	↑	Ritonavir (400 mg every 12 hours) decreased voriconazole AUC and C_{max} by approximately 82% and 66%, respectively. Coadministration with ritonavir (400 mg every 12 hours) is contraindicated. Avoid coadministration with ritonavir 100 mg every 12 hours unless assessment of benefit/risk justifies the use of voriconazole.
Proton pump inhibitors (eg, omeprazole)	Voriconazole	↑	Omeprazole may increase the C_{max} and AUC of voriconazole by an average of 15% and 40%, respectively. No dosage adjustment of voriconazole is recommended. Voriconazole may increase the C_{max} and AUC of omeprazole by an average of 2 and 4 times, respectively. When initiating voriconazole in patients already receiving omeprazole doses of 40 mg or more, reduce the dose of omeprazole by 50%. Voriconazole also may inhibit the metabolism of other proton pump inhibitors that are CYP2C19 substrates.
Voriconazole	Proton pump inhibitors (eg, omeprazole)		
Rifampin, rifabutin	Voriconazole	↓	Voriconazole plasma concentrations are significantly reduced during coadministration. In healthy subjects, rifampin 600 mg once daily decreased the steady-state C_{max} and AUC of voriconazole (200 mg every 12 hours for 7 days) by an average of 93% and 96%, respectively. Voriconazole may increase the C_{max} and AUC of rifabutin by an average of 3 and 4 times, respectively. Coadministration is contraindicated.
Voriconazole	Rifabutin	↑	
St. John's wort	Voriconazole	↓	Multiple oral doses of St. John's wort followed by a single dose of voriconazole decreased the voriconazole AUC by 59%. In contrast, coadministration of single oral doses of St. John's wort and voriconazole had no effect on voriconazole AUC. Coadministration is contraindicated.
Voriconazole	Anticoagulants (eg, warfarin)	↑	Coadministration may significantly increase PT by approximately 2 times. Closely monitor coagulation tests and adjust warfarin dose accordingly.

VORICONAZOLE — ORAL

Voriconazole Drug Interactions

Precipitant drug	Object drug[a]		Description
Voriconazole	Aripiprazole	↑	Aripiprazole plasma concentrations may be elevated, increasing the pharmacologic effects and risks of adverse reactions. Monitor the clinical response and adjust the aripiprazole dose as needed.
Voriconazole	Benzodiazepines (eg, alprazolam, midazolam, triazolam)	↑	Voriconazole may increase the plasma concentrations of benzodiazepines that are metabolized by CYP3A4. Frequent monitoring for benzodiazepine adverse events and toxicity is warranted. Adjust benzodiazepine dose if needed.
Voriconazole	Cabazitaxel	↑	Cabazitaxel plasma concentrations may be elevated, increasing the pharmacologic effects and risk of adverse reactions. Avoid coadministration.
Voriconazole	Calcium channel blockers (eg, felodipine)	↑	Voriconazole may increase plasma concentrations of calcium channel blockers that are metabolized by CYP3A4 (eg, felodipine). Frequent monitoring for calcium channel adverse events and toxicity is warranted. Adjust calcium channel blocker dose if needed.
Voriconazole	Cisapride, pimozide, quinidine	↑	Voriconazole may inhibit the metabolism of these drugs. Increased plasma concentration may lead to QT prolongation and rare occurrences of torsades de pointes. Coadministration is contraindicated.
Voriconazole	Clopidogrel	↓	Coadministration may decrease clopidogrel plasma concentrations, decreasing the pharmacologic effects. Avoid coadministration.
Voriconazole	Cyclosporine	↑	Coadministration of oral voriconazole increased cyclosporine C_{max} and AUC an average of 1.1 and 1.7 times, respectively. When initiating voriconazole therapy in patients already receiving cyclosporine, reduce the dose of cyclosporine to 50% of the original dose. Frequently monitor cyclosporine levels during coadministration and when voriconazole is discontinued.
Voriconazole	Docetaxel	↑	Docetaxel plasma concentrations may be elevated, increasing the pharmacologic effects and risk of toxicity. Avoid coadministration. If coadministration cannot be avoided, consider reducing the docetaxel dose by 50% with close clinical and laboratory monitoring.
Voriconazole	Dronedarone	↑	Dronedarone plasma concentrations may be elevated, increasing the pharmacologic effects and risk of toxicity, including life-threatening cardiotoxicity. Coadministration is contraindicated.
Voriconazole	Ergot alkaloids (eg, dihydroergotamine, ergotamine)	↑	Voriconazole may increase the plasma concentrations of ergot alkaloids and lead to ergotism. Coadministration is contraindicated.
Voriconazole	Erlotinib	↑	Erlotinib plasma concentrations may be elevated, increasing the risk of adverse reactions. Frequent monitoring for erlotinib adverse events and toxicity is warranted. Erlotinib dose reduction may be needed.

Voriconazole Drug Interactions

Precipitant drug	Object drug[a]		Description
Voriconazole	Erythromycin	↑	Erythromycin plasma concentrations may be elevated, increasing the risk of adverse reactions, including sudden death due to cardiac causes. Avoid coadministration.
Voriconazole	HMG-CoA reductase inhibitors (eg, lovastatin)	↑	Voriconazole has been shown to inhibit lovastatin metabolism. Voriconazole may increase the plasma concentrations of statins that are metabolized by CYP3A4. The risk of adverse reactions, including rhabdomyolysis, may be increased. Frequent monitoring for adverse events and toxicity to statins is warranted. Consider dosage adjustment of the statin during coadministration.
Voriconazole	Ixabepilone	↑	Ixabepilone plasma concentrations may be elevated, increasing the pharmacologic effects and risk of adverse reactions. Avoid coadministration. If coadministration cannot be avoided, an ixabepilone dose reduction may be needed.
Voriconazole	Maraviroc	↑	Maraviroc plasma concentrations may be elevated, increasing the pharmacologic effects and risk of adverse reactions. A maraviroc dose reduction may be needed. Coadministration is contraindicated in patients with severe renal impairment (CrCl ≤ 30 mL/min).
Voriconazole	mTOR[c] inhibitors (eg, everolimus, temsirolimus)	↑	The mTOR inhibitor's plasma concentrations may be elevated, increasing the pharmacologic effects and risk of adverse reactions. Avoid coadministration. If coadministration cannot be avoided, frequent monitoring for mTOR inhibitor–related adverse events is warranted. A reduction in the mTOR inhibitor dose may be needed.
Voriconazole	Nilotinib	↑	Nilotinib plasma concentrations may be elevated, increasing the pharmacologic effects and risk of adverse reactions. Avoid coadministration. If coadministration cannot be avoided, it is recommended that nilotinib therapy be interrupted.
Voriconazole	NSAIDs (eg, diclofenac, ibuprofen)	↑	NSAID plasma concentrations may be increased. Frequent monitoring for NSAID-related adverse events and toxicity is warranted. NSAID dose reduction may be needed.
Voriconazole	Opioid analgesics (eg, alfentanil, fentanyl, methadone, oxycodone)	↑	Opioid analgesic plasma concentrations may be increased. Extended and frequent monitoring for respiratory depression and other adverse events is warranted. Increased concentrations of methadone may cause QT prolongation. Reduce the opioid dose if needed.
Voriconazole	Prednisolone	↑	Voriconazole may increase the C_{max} and AUC of prednisolone by an average 11% and 34%, respectively. No dosage adjustment is recommended.

VORICONAZOLE — ORAL

Voriconazole Drug Interactions			
Precipitant drug	Object drug[a]		Description
Voriconazole	Romidepsin	↑	Romidepsin plasma concentrations may be elevated, increasing the pharmacologic effects and risk of adverse reactions, including QT prolongation. Avoid coadministration. If coadministration cannot be avoided, frequent monitoring for romidepsin-related adverse events is warranted. Romidepsin dose reduction may be needed.
Voriconazole	Sirolimus	↑	Voriconazole can significantly increase the C_{max} and AUC of sirolimus an average of 7- and 11-fold, respectively. Coadministration is contraindicated.
Voriconazole	Sulfonylureas	↑	Voriconazole may increase plasma concentrations of sulfonylureas. Monitor for hypoglycemia. Dose adjustment of the sulfonylurea is recommended.
Voriconazole	Tacrolimus	↑	Voriconazole can significantly increase the C_{max} and AUC of tacrolimus by an average of 2- and 3-fold, respectively. When initiating voriconazole therapy in patients already receiving tacrolimus, reduce the dose of tacrolimus to 33% of the original dose. Frequently monitor tacrolimus levels during coadministration and when voriconazole is discontinued.
Voriconazole	Tyrosine kinase receptor inhibitors (eg, dasatinib, lapatinib, pazopanib, sunitinib)	↑	Tyrosine kinase receptor inhibitor plasma concentrations may be elevated, increasing the pharmacologic effects and risk of adverse reactions. Avoid coadministration. If coadministration cannot be avoided, frequent monitoring for tyrosine kinase receptor inhibitor–related adverse events is warranted. A reduction in the tyrosine kinase receptor inhibitor dose may be needed.
Voriconazole	Vinca alkaloids (eg, vinblastine, vincristine)	↑	Coadministration may increase the plasma concentrations of the vinca alkaloids and lead to neurotoxicity. Consider adjusting the dose of the vinca alkaloid and monitor for toxicity (eg, neurotoxicty).
Voriconazole	Zolpidem	↑	Zolpidem plasma concentrations may be elevated, increasing the pharmacologic effects and risk of adverse reactions. Frequent monitoring for zolpidem-related adverse events is warranted. A reduction in the zolpidem dose may be needed.

[a] ↓ = object drug decreased; ↑ = object drug increased; ↑↓ = object drug is both increased and decreased.
[b] NNRTIs = nonnucleoside reverse transcriptase inhibitors.
[c] mTOR = mammalian target of rapamycin.

➤*Drug/Food interactions:* When multiple doses of voriconazole are administered with high-fat meals, the mean C_{max} and AUC are reduced 34% and 24%, respectively, when administered as a tablet and by 58% and 37%, respectively, when administered as the oral suspension.

Adverse Reactions

➤*Most frequent adverse reactions:* The most frequently reported adverse reactions (all causalities) in the therapeutic trials were abdominal pain, diarrhea, fever, headache, nausea, peripheral edema, rash, respiratory disorder, sepsis, visual disturbances, and vomiting.

➤*Discontinuation:* The treatment-related adverse reactions that most often led to discontinuation of voriconazole therapy were elevated LFTs, rash, and visual disturbances.

➤*Adverse reactions (2% or more):*

Voriconazole All Therapeutic Studies Population Adverse Reactions (≥ 2%)						
	All therapeutic studies	Studies 307/602[a] and 608[b] (IV/oral therapy)			Study 305[c] oral therapy	
Adverse reactions	Voriconazole (n = 1,655)	Voriconazole (n = 468)	Amphotericin B[d] (n = 185)	Amphotericin B followed by fluconazole (n = 131)	Voriconazole (n = 200)	Fluconazole (n = 191)
CNS						
Hallucinations	2.4%	2.8%	0.5%	0%	0%	0%
Headache	3%	1.9%	4.3%	0.8%	0%	0.5%
GI						
Nausea	5.4%	3.8%	15.7%	1.5%	1%	1.6%
Vomiting	4.4%	3.2%	9.7%	0.8%	1%	0.5%
Hepatic						
ALT increased	1.8%	1.9%	0.5%	1.5%	3%	1%
AST increased	1.9%	1.9%	0%	0.8%	4%	1%
Bilirubinemia	0.9%	1.1%	1.6%	1.5%	0.5%	0%
Cholestatic jaundice	1%	1.7%	0%	0.8%	1.5%	0%
Hepatic enzymes increased	1.8%	2.4%	2.7%	0.8%	1.5%	0%
LFTs abnormal	2.7%	3.2%	2.2%	0.8%	3%	1%
Metabolic/Nutritional						
Alkaline phosphatase increased	3.6%	4.1%	2.2%	2.3%	5%	1.6%
Hypokalemia	1.6%	0.6%	19.5%	12.2%	0%	0%
Renal						
Acute kidney failure	0.4%	0.4%	5.9%	5.3%	0%	0%
Creatinine increased	0.2%	0%	31.9%	7.6%	0.5%	0%
Kidney function abnormal	0.6%	1.3%	21.6%	6.9%	0.5%	0.5%
Special senses						
Abnormal vision	18.7%	13.5%	0.5%	0%	15.5%	4.2%
Chromatopsia	1.2%	0.4%	0%	0%	1%	0%
Photophobia	2.2%	1.7%	0%	0%	2.5%	1%
Miscellaneous						
Chills	3.7%	0.2%	19.5%	6.1%	0.5%	0%
Fever	5.7%	1.7%	13.5%	3.8%	0%	0%
Rash	5.3%	4.3%	3.8%	0.8%	1.5%	0.5%
Tachycardia	2.4%	1.3%	2.7%	0%	0%	0%

[a] In study 307/602, 381 patients (196 on voriconazole, 185 on amphotericin B) were treated to compare voriconazole with amphotericin B followed by other licensed antifungal therapy in the primary treatment of patients with acute invasive aspergillosis.
[b] In study 608, 403 patients with candidemia were treated to compare voriconazole (272 patients) with the regimen of amphotericin B followed by fluconazole (131 patients).
[c] Study 305 evaluated the effects of voriconazole oral (200 patients) and fluconazole oral (191 patients) in the treatment of esophageal candidiasis.
[d] Amphotericin B followed by other licensed antifungal therapy.

Dermatologic – Dermatological reactions were common in patients treated with voriconazole. The mechanism underlying these dermatologic adverse reactions remains unknown. In clinical trials, rashes considered related to therapy were reported by 7% of voriconazole-treated patients. The majority of rashes were of mild to moderate severity. Patients have rarely developed serious cutaneous reactions, including Stevens-Johnson syndrome, toxic epidermal necrolysis, and erythema multiforme during treatment with voriconazole. If patients develop an exfoliative cutaneous reaction, discontinue voriconazole. In addition, voriconazole has been associated with photosensitivity skin reactions. It is recommended that patients avoid strong, direct sunlight during voriconazole therapy. In patients with photosensitivity skin reactions, squamous cell carcinoma of the skin and melanoma have been reported during long-term therapy. If a patient develops a skin lesion consistent with squamous cell carcinoma or melanoma, discontinue voriconazole.

VORICONAZOLE — ORAL

Ophthalmic – Voriconazole treatment-related visual disturbances are common. In therapeutic trials, approximately 21% of patients experienced abnormal vision, color vision change, and/or photophobia. The visual disturbances were generally mild and rarely resulted in discontinuation. Visual disturbances may be associated with higher plasma concentrations and/or doses. There have been postmarketing reports of prolonged visual adverse events, including optic neuritis and papilledema.

The mechanism of action of the visual disturbance is unknown, although the site of action is most likely within the retina. In a study in healthy volunteers investigating the effect of 28-day treatment with voriconazole on retinal function, voriconazole caused a decrease in the electroretinogram (ERG) waveform amplitude, a decrease in the visual field, and an alteration in color perception. The ERG measures electrical currents in the retina. The effects were noted early in administration of voriconazole and continued through the course of study drug dosing. Fourteen days after end of dosing, ERG, visual fields, and color perception returned to normal.

➤*Adverse reactions (less than 2%):*

Cardiovascular – Atrial arrhythmia, atrial fibrillation, atrioventricular block complete, bigeminy, bradycardia, bundle branch block, cardiomegaly, cardiomyopathy, cerebral hemorrhage, cerebral ischemia, cerebrovascular accident, congestive heart failure, deep thrombophlebitis, endocarditis, extrasystoles, heart arrest, hypertension, hypotension, myocardial infarction, nodal arrhythmia, palpitation, phlebitis, postural hypotension, pulmonary embolus, QT interval prolonged, supraventricular extrasystoles, supraventricular tachycardia, syncope, thrombophlebitis, vasodilatation, ventricular arrhythmia, ventricular fibrillation, ventricular tachycardia (including torsades de pointes).

CNS – Abnormal dreams, acute brain syndrome, agitation, akathisia, amnesia, anxiety, asthenia, ataxia, brain edema, coma, confusion, convulsion, delirium, dementia, depersonalization, depression, diplopia, dizziness, encephalitis, encephalopathy, euphoria, extrapyramidal syndrome, grand mal convulsion, Guillain-Barré syndrome, hypertonia, hypesthesia, insomnia, intracranial hypertension, libido decreased, neuralgia, neuropathy, nystagmus, oculogyric crisis, paresthesia, psychosis, somnolence, suicidal ideation, tremor, vertigo.

Dermatologic – Alopecia, angioedema, contact dermatitis, discoid lupus erythematosis, eczema, erythema multiforme, exfoliative dermatitis, fixed drug eruption, furunculosis, herpes simplex, maculopapular rash, melanosis, melanoma, photosensitivity, pruritus, psoriasis, pseudoporphyria, skin discoloration, skin disorder, skin dry, skin reaction, squamous cell carcinoma, Stevens-Johnson syndrome, sweating, toxic epidermal necrolysis, urticaria.

Endocrine – Adrenal cortex insufficiency, diabetes insipidus, hyperthyroidism, hypothyroidism.

GI – Abdomen enlarged, abdominal pain, anorexia, cheilitis, cholecystitis, cholelithiasis, constipation, diarrhea, duodenal ulcer perforation, duodenitis, dyspepsia, dysphagia, dry mouth, enlarged liver, esophageal ulcer, esophagitis, flatulence, gastroenteritis, gamma-glutamyl transferase (GGT)/lactic dehydrogenase (LDH) elevated, GI hemorrhage, gingivitis, glossitis, gum hemorrhage, gum hyperplasia, hematemesis, hepatic coma, hepatic failure, hepatitis, intestinal perforation, intestinal ulcer, jaundice, melena, mouth ulceration, pancreatitis, parotid gland enlargement, periodontitis, proctitis, pseudomembranous colitis, rectal disorder, rectal hemorrhage, stomach ulcer, stomatitis, tongue edema.

GU – Anuria, blighted ovum, CrCl decreased, dysmenorrhea, dysuria, epididymitis, glycosuria, hemorrhagic cystitis, hematuria, hydronephrosis, impotence, kidney pain, kidney tubular necrosis, metrorrhagia, nephritis, nephrosis, oliguria, scrotal edema, urinary incontinence, urinary retention, urinary tract infection, uterine hemorrhage, vaginal hemorrhage.

Hematologic/Lymphatic – Agranulocytosis, anemia (macrocytic, megaloblastic, microcytic, normocytic), aplastic anemia, bleeding time increased, cyanosis, disseminated intravascular coagulation, ecchymosis, enlarged spleen, eosinophilia, hemolytic anemia, hypervolemia, leukopenia, lymphadenopathy, lymphangitis, marrow depression, pancytopenia, petechia, purpura, thrombocytopenia, thrombotic thrombocytopenic purpura.

Metabolic/Nutritional – Albuminuria, creatine phosphokinase increased, edema, glucose tolerance decreased, hypercalcemia, hypercholesteremia, hyperglycemia, hyperkalemia, hypermagnesemia, hypernatremia, hyperuricemia, hypocalcemia, hypoglycemia, hypomagnesemia, hyponatremia, hypophosphatemia, peripheral edema, serum urea nitrogen increased, uremia.

Musculoskeletal – Arthralgia, arthritis, back pain, bone necrosis, bone pain, leg cramps, myalgia, myasthenia, myopathy, osteomalacia, osteoporosis.

Respiratory – Cough increased, dyspnea, epistaxis, hemoptysis, hypoxia, lung edema, pharyngitis, pleural effusion, pneumonia, respiratory disorder, respiratory distress syndrome, respiratory tract infection, rhinitis, sinusitis, voice alteration.

Special senses – Abnormality of accommodation, blepharitis, color blindness, conjunctivitis, corneal opacity, deafness, dry eyes, ear pain, eye hemorrhage, eye pain, hypoacusis, keratitis, keratoconjunctivitis, mydriasis, night blindness, optic atrophy, optic neuritis, otitis externa, papilledema, retinal hemorrhage, retinitis, scleritis, taste loss, taste perversion, tinnitus, uveitis, visual field defect.

Miscellaneous – Allergic reaction, anaphylactoid reaction, ascites, bacterial infection, cellulitis, chest pain, edema, face edema, flank pain, flu syndrome, fungal infection, graft versus host reaction, granuloma, infection, mucous membrane disorder, multiorgan failure, pain, pelvic pain, peritonitis, sepsis, substernal chest pain.

➤*Lab test abnormalities:* The overall incidence of clinically significant transaminase abnormalities in all therapeutic studies was 12.4% of patients treated with voriconazole. Increased incidence of LFT abnormalities may be associated with higher plasma concentrations and/or doses. The majority of abnormal LFTs resolved during treatment without dose adjustment or after dose adjustment, including discontinuation of therapy.

Voriconazole Lab Test Abnormalities in Patients With Esophageal Candidiasis (Study 305)

Laboratory abnormality	Criteria[a]	Voriconazole	Fluconazole
Total bilirubin	> 1.5 × ULN[b]	4.3%	3.8%
AST	> 3 × ULN	20.3%	8.1%
ALT	> 3 × ULN	10.7%	6.5%
Alkaline phosphatase	> 3 × ULN	10.2%	7.5%

[a] Without regard to baseline value.
[b] ULN = upper limit of normal.

Voriconazole Lab Test Abnormalities in Patients With Invasive Aspergillosis (Study 307/602)

Laboratory abnormality	Criteria[a]	Voriconazole	Amphotericin B[b]
Total bilirubin	> 1.5 × ULN	19.4%	26.6%
AST	> 3 × ULN	11.7%	10.3%
ALT	> 3 × ULN	18.9%	23.1%
Alkaline phosphatase	> 3 × ULN	16%	22%
Creatinine	> 1.3× ULN	21.4%	57.6%
Potassium	< 0.9 × LLN[c]	16.6%	39.3%

[a] Without regard to baseline value.
[b] Amphotericin B followed by other licensed antifungal therapy.
[c] LLN = lower limit of normal.

Voriconazole Lab Test Abnormalities in Patients With Candidemia (Study 608)

Lab test abnormality	Criteria[a]	Voriconazole	Amphotericin B followed by fluconazole
Total bilirubin	> 1.5 × ULN	19.2%	27%
AST	> 3 × ULN	15.3%	13.8%
ALT	> 3 × ULN	8.4%	12.9%
Alkaline phosphatase	> 3 × ULN	22.6%	22.6%
Creatinine	> 1.3 × ULN	15%	27.1%
Potassium	< 0.9 × LLN	16.7%	29.7%

[a] Without regard to baseline value.

Overdosage

➤*Symptoms:* In clinical trials, there were 3 cases of accidental overdose. All occurred in children who received up to 5 times the recommended IV dose of voriconazole. A single adverse reaction of photophobia of 10 minutes' duration was reported.

➤*Treatment:* There is no known antidote to voriconazole.

Voriconazole is hemodialyzed with clearance of 121 mL/min. In an overdose, hemodialysis may assist in the removal of voriconazole from the body.

Patient Information

Advise patients to take voriconazole at least 1 hour before or 1 hour after a meal.

Advise patients not to drive at night while taking voriconazole. Voriconazole may cause changes to vision, including blurring and/or photophobia.

Advise patients to avoid potentially hazardous tasks, such as driving or operating machinery, if they perceive any change in vision.

Advise patients to avoid strong, direct sunlight during voriconazole therapy.

Advise women of childbearing potential to use effective contraception during treatment.

Voriconazole suspension contains sucrose and is not recommended for patients with rare hereditary problems of fructose intolerance, sucrase-isomaltase deficiency, or glucose-galactose malabsorption.

VORICONAZOLE — INJECTION

Indications

➤*Candidemia:* For the treatment of candidemia in nonneutropenic patients and the following *Candida* infections: disseminated infections in skin and infections in abdomen, kidney, bladder wall, and wounds.

➤*Esophageal candidiasis:* For the treatment of esophageal candidiasis.

➤*Invasive aspergillosis:* For the treatment of invasive aspergillosis. In clinical trials, the majority of isolates recovered were *Aspergillus fumigatus*. There was a small number of cases of culture-proven disease caused by species of *Aspergillus* other than *A. fumigatus*.

➤*Serious fungal infections:* For the treatment of serious fungal infections caused by *Scedosporium apiospermum* (asexual form of *Pseudallescheria boydii*) and *Fusarium* spp., including *Fusarium solani*, in patients intolerant of, or refractory to, other therapy.

➤*Off-label uses:*

Catheter-related bloodstream infections (children) – [2] = Fair documentation. Guidelines suggest that voriconazole may be used as an alternative treatment option to amphotericin B for the treatment of catheter-related bloodstream infections caused by *Malassezia furfur*. There are currently no randomized controlled trials for the use of voriconazole in children with catheter-related bloodstream infections.

Administration and Dosage

➤*Adults:*

Infections –

Usual dosage:

Voriconazole Recommended Adult Dosing Regimen

Infection	Loading dosage	Maintenance dosage	
	IV[a]	IV	Oral[b]
Candidemia in nonneutropenic patients and other deep tissue *Candida* infections	6 mg/kg every 12 h for the first 24 h	3 to 4 mg/kg every 12 h[c]	200 mg every 12 h
Esophageal candidiasis	[d]	[d]	200 mg every 12 h
Invasive aspergillosis	6 mg/kg every 12 h for the first 24 h	4 mg/kg every 12 h	200 mg every 12 h
Scedosporiosis and fusariosis	6 mg/kg every 12 h for the first 24 h	4 mg/kg every 12 h	200 mg every 12 h

[a] IV = intravenous.
[b] Patients who weigh ≥ 40 kg should receive an oral maintenance dosage of voriconazole 200 mg every 12 hours. Patients who weigh
[c] In clinical trials, patients with candidemia received 3 mg/kg every 12 hours as primary therapy, while patients with other deep tissue *Candida* infections received 4 mg/kg as salvage therapy. Base appropriate dosage on the severity and nature of the infection.
[d] Not evaluated in patients with esophageal candidiasis.

Dosage adjustment: If patients are unable to tolerate 4 mg/kg IV, reduce the IV maintenance dosage to 3 mg/kg every 12 hours.

➤*Children:* See Adults for dosing for children 12 years and older.

Off-label dosing –

Catheter-related bloodstream infections (children): [2] = Fair documentation.

• *2 years and older* – 6 mg/kg administered IV every 12 hours for 2 doses on day 1 (loading dose), followed by 4 mg/kg administered IV every 12 hours.

Infection:

• *Children 12 months and older –*
Loading dose: 6 to 8 mg/kg IV every 12 hours for 2 doses.
Maintenance dosage: 4 to 7 mg/kg IV every 12 hours.

• *Neonates and infants –*
Loading dose: 3 to 8 mg/kg IV every 12 hours for 2 doses.
Maintenance dosage: 2 to 6 mg/kg IV every 12 hours.

➤*Renal function impairment:*

Moderate to severe renal impairment – In patients with moderate or severe renal impairment (creatinine clearance [CrCl] less than 50 mL/min), accumulation of the IV vehicle sulfobutylether 7-beta-cyclodextrin (SBECD) occurs. Oral voriconazole should be administered to these patients, unless an assessment of the benefit/risk to the patient justifies the use of IV voriconazole. Serum creatinine levels should be monitored closely in these patients, and, if increases occur, consideration should be given to changing to oral voriconazole therapy.

Hemodialysis – According to the prescribing information, voriconazole is hemodialyzed with clearance of 121 mL/min. The IV vehicle SBECD is hemodialyzed with clearance of 55 mL/min. A 4-hour hemodialysis session does not remove a sufficient amount of voriconazole to warrant dose adjustment.

Adults receiving continuous renal replacement therapy: The oral doseform of voriconazole is recommended because of the IV vehicle. The following recommendations assume ultrafiltration and dialysis flow rates of 1 to 2 L/h.

• *Loading dose* – 400 mg orally every 12 hours for 2 doses.

• *Maintenance dosage* – A dosage of 200 mg orally every 12 hours is recommended for patients receiving continuous venovenous hemofiltration, continuous venovenous hemodialysis, or continuous venovenous hemodialfiltration. This recommendation assumes ultrafiltration and dialysis flow rates of 1 to 2 L/h.

Adults receiving intermittent hemodialysis: 200 mg orally every 12 hours. This recommendation assumes the patient is receiving standard intermittent hemodialysis 3 times per week and completes the full dialysis sessions.

➤*Hepatic function impairment:*

Mild to moderate hepatic impairment – It is recommended that the standard loading-dose regimens be used but that the maintenance dose be halved in patients with mild to moderate hepatic cirrhosis (Child-Pugh class A and B, respectively).

➤*Concomitant therapy:*

Phenytoin – Phenytoin may be coadministered with voriconazole if the IV maintenance dosage of voriconazole is increased to 5 mg/kg every 12 hours.

Efavirenz – When voriconazole is coadministered with efavirenz, the voriconazole maintenance dosage should be increased to 400 mg every 12 hours and the efavirenz dose should be decreased to 300 mg every 24 hours. When treatment with voriconazole is stopped, the initial dosage of efavirenz should be restored.

➤*Duration of therapy:*

Candidemia in nonneutropenic patients and other deep tissue Candida infections – Patients should be treated for at least 14 days following resolution of symptoms or following last positive culture, whichever is longer.

Esophageal candidiasis – Patients should be treated for a minimum of 14 days and for at least 7 days following resolution of symptoms.

➤*Preparation for administration:*

Reconstitution – The powder is reconstituted with 19 mL of water for injection to obtain an extractable volume of 20 mL of clear concentrate containing voriconazole 10 mg/mL. It is recommended that a standard 20 mL (nonautomated) syringe be used to ensure that the exact amount (19 mL) of water for injection is dispensed. Discard the vial if a vacuum does not pull the diluent into the vial. Shake the vial until all the powder is dissolved.

Dilution – See Admixture Compatibility for a list of compatible solutions. The required volume of the voriconazole 10 mg/mL concentrate should be further diluted as follows. Calculate the volume of voriconazole 10 mg/mL concentrate required based on the patient's weight. In order to allow the required volume of voriconazole concentrate to be added, withdraw and discard at least an equal volume of diluent from the infusion bag or bottle to be used. The volume of diluent remaining in the bag or bottle should be such that when the voriconazole 10 mg/mL concentrate is added, the final concentration is not less than 0.5 mg/mL nor greater than 5 mg/mL. Using a suitable size syringe and aseptic technique, withdraw the required volume of voriconazole concentrate from the appropriate number of vials and add to the infusion bag or bottle. Discard partially used vials.

Voriconazole Injection Required Volumes of 10 mg/mL Concentrate

Body weight (kg)	Volume of voriconazole concentrate (10 mg/mL) required for:		
	3 mg/kg dose	4 mg/kg dose	6 mg/kg dose
30	9 mL (1 vial)	12 mL (1 vial)	18 mL (1 vial)
35	10.5 mL (1 vial)	14 mL (1 vial)	21 mL (2 vials)
40	12 mL (1 vial)	16 mL (1 vial)	24 mL (2 vials)
45	13.5 mL (1 vial)	18 mL (1 vial)	27 mL (2 vial)
50	15 mL (1 vial)	20 mL (1 vial)	30 mL (2 vials)
55	16.5 mL (1 vial)	22 mL (2 vials)	33 mL (2 vials)
60	18 mL (1 vial)	24 mL (2 vials)	36 mL (2 vials)
65	19.5 mL (1 vial)	26 mL (2 vials)	39 mL (2 vials)
70	21 mL (2 vials)	28 mL (2 vials)	42 mL (3 vials)
75	22.5 mL (2 vials)	30 mL (2 vials)	45 mL (3 vials)
80	24 mL (2 vials)	32 mL (2 vials)	48 mL (3 vials)
85	25.5 mL (2 vials)	34 mL (2 vials)	51 mL (3 vials)
90	27 mL (2 vials)	36 mL (2 vials)	54 mL (3 vials)
95	28.5 mL (2 vials)	38 mL (2 vials)	57 mL (3 vials)
100	30 mL (2 vials)	40 mL (2 vials)	60 mL (3 vials)

➤*Administration:* Not for IV bolus injection. Voriconazole must be infused at a maximum rate of 3 mg/kg/h over 1 to 2 hours at a concentration of 5 mg/mL or less.

Infusion reactions – During infusion, anaphylactoid-type reactions, including flushing, fever, sweating, tachycardia, chest tightness, dyspnea, faintness, nausea, pruritus, and rash, have occurred uncommonly. Symptoms appeared immediately upon initiating the infusion. Consideration should be given to stopping the infusion should these reactions occur.

➤*Admixture compatibility:*

Compatibility – The reconstituted solution can be diluted with the following: sodium chloride 9 mg/mL (0.9%); Ringer's lactate; dextrose 5% and Ringer's lactate; dextrose 5% and sodium chloride 0.45% dextrose; dextrose 5%; dextrose 5% and potassium chloride 20 mEq; sodium chloride 0.45%; dextrose 5% and sodium chloride 0.9%.

VORICONAZOLE — INJECTION

Voriconazole can be infused at the same time as other IV solutions containing (nonconcentrated) electrolytes but must be infused through a separate line.

Voriconazole can be infused at the same time as total parenteral nutrition (TPN), but must be infused in a separate line. If infused through a multiple-lumen catheter, TPN needs to be administered using a different port from the one used for voriconazole.

Incompatibility – Voriconazole must not be diluted with sodium bicarbonate 4.2% infusion. The mildly alkaline nature of this diluent caused slight degradation of voriconazole after 24-hours storage at room temperature. Although refrigerated storage is recommended following reconstitution, use of this diluent is not recommended as a precautionary measure. Compatibility with other concentrations is unknown.

Voriconazole must not be infused concomitantly with any blood product or short-term infusion of concentrated electrolytes, even if the 2 infusions are running in separate IV lines (or cannulas).

➤*Storage/Stability:* Store unreconstituted vials at 15° to 30°C (59° to 86°F). Following reconstitution, use the solution immediately. If not used immediately, may be stored for no longer than 24 hours at 2° to 8°C (36° to 46°F). The injection solution is unpreserved and is for single use only; discard any unused solution.

Actions

➤*Pharmacology:* Voriconazole is a triazole antifungal agent. The primary mode of action of voriconazole is the inhibition of fungal cytochrome P450 (CYP-450)–mediated 14 alpha-lanosterol demethylation, an essential step in fungal ergosterol biosynthesis. The accumulation of 14 alpha-methyl sterols correlates with the subsequent loss of ergosterol in the fungal cell wall and may be responsible for the antifungal activity of voriconazole. Voriconazole has been shown to be more selective for fungal CYP-450 enzymes than for various mammalian CYP-450 enzyme systems.

➤*Pharmacokinetics:*

Absorption – Maximum plasma concentrations (C_{max}) are achieved 1 to 2 hours after dosing.

Greater than proportional increase in exposure is observed with increasing dose. It is estimated that, on average, increasing the IV dosage from 3 mg/kg every 12 hours to 4 mg/kg every 12 hours produces a 2.3-fold increase in exposure (AUC_{tau}).

Voriconazole IV Pharmacokinetic Parameters		
Pharmacokinetic parameter	3 mg/kg IV every 12 h	4 mg/kg IV every 12 h
AUC_{tau}[a] (mcg•h/mL) (CV%[b])	21.81 (100%)	50.4 (83%)

[a] Mean AUC_{tau} are predicted values from population pharmacokinetic analysis of data from 236 volunteers.
[b] Percent coefficient of variation.

When the recommended IV loading-dose regimen is administered to healthy subjects, peak plasma concentrations close to steady state are achieved within the first 24 hours of dosing. Without the loading dose, accumulation occurs during twice-daily multiple dosing, with steady-state voriconazole C_{max} being achieved by day 6 in the majority of subjects.

Voriconazole IV Pharmacokinetic Parameters from Loading Dose and Maintenance Dose Regimens		
	6 mg/kg IV[a] every 12 h on day 1, 3 mg/kg IV every 12 h on days 2 to 10 (n = 9)	
Pharmacokinetic parameter	Day 1, first dose	Day 10
AUC_{tau}[b] (mcg•h/mL) (CV%)	13.22 (22%)	13.25 (58%)
C_{max} (mcg/mL) (CV%)	4.7 (22%)	3.06 (31%)

[a] IV infusion over 60 minutes.
[b] AUC_{tau} values are calculated over a dosing interval of 12 hours. Pharmacokinetic parameters for loading and maintenance doses summarized for same cohort of volunteers.

Steady-state trough plasma concentrations with voriconazole are achieved after approximately 5 days of IV dosing without a loading dose regimen. However, when an IV loading dose regimen is used, steady-state trough plasma concentrations are achieved within 1 day.

Distribution – The volume of distribution at steady state for voriconazole is estimated to be 4.6 L/kg, suggesting extensive distribution into tissues. Plasma protein binding is estimated to be 58%. Varying degrees of hepatic and renal impairment do not affect the protein binding of voriconazole.

Metabolism – In vitro studies showed that voriconazole is metabolized by the human hepatic CYP-450 enzymes CYP2C19, CYP2C9, and CYP3A4. The major metabolite of voriconazole is the N-oxide, which accounts for 72% of the circulating radiolabeled metabolites in plasma. Because this metabolite has minimal antifungal activity, it does not contribute to the overall efficacy of voriconazole.

Excretion – Voriconazole is eliminated via hepatic metabolism with less than 2% of the dose excreted unchanged in the urine. After administration of a single radiolabeled dose of IV voriconazole, preceded by multiple dosing, approximately 80% to 83% of the radioactivity is recovered in the urine. The majority (greater than 94%) of the total radioactivity is excreted in the first 96 hours after IV dosing.

As a result of nonlinear pharmacokinetics, the terminal half-life of voriconazole is dose dependent and, therefore, not useful in predicting the accumulation or elimination of voriconazole.

Special populations –

Renal function impairment: In patients with moderate renal dysfunction (CrCl 30 to 50 mL/min), accumulation of the IV vehicle SBECD occurs. The AUC and C_{max} of SBECD were increased by 4-fold and almost 50%, respectively, in the moderately impaired group compared with the healthy control group.

Avoid IV voriconazole in patients with moderate or severe renal impairment (CrCl less than 50 mL/min), unless an assessment of the benefit/risk to the patient justifies the use of IV voriconazole.

Hepatic function impairment: See Administration and Dosage for more information.

Elderly: In the clinical program, no dosage adjustment was made on the basis of age. An analysis of pharmacokinetic data obtained from 552 patients from 10 voriconazole clinical trials showed that the median voriconazole plasma concentrations in the elderly patients (65 years and older) were approximately 80% to 90% higher than those in the younger patients (65 years and younger) after administration. However, the safety profile of voriconazole in younger and elderly subjects was similar and, therefore, no dosage adjustment is necessary for elderly patients.

➤*Microbiology:*

Activity in vitro – Voriconazole has been shown to be active against most strains of the following microorganisms, both in vitro and in clinical infection: *A. fumigatus*, *Aspergillus flavus*, *Aspergillus niger*, *Aspergillus terreus*, *Candida albicans*, *Candida glabrata* (in clinical studies, the voriconazole minimum inhibitory concentration [MIC_{90}] was 4 mcg/mL), *Candida krusei*, *Candida parapsilosis*, *Candida tropicalis*, and *Fusarium* spp. including *F. solani*, and *S. apiospermum*. In clinical studies, voriconazole MIC_{90} for *C. glabrata* baseline isolates was 4 mcg/mL; 26% of *C. glabrata* baseline isolates were resistant (MIC at least 4 mcg/mL) to voriconazole. However, based on 1,054 isolates tested in surveillance studies, the MIC_{90} was 1 mcg/mL.

Voriconazole exhibits in vitro MICs of 1 mcg/mL or less against most (at least 90%) isolates of the following microorganisms; however, the safety and effectiveness of voriconazole in treating clinical infections due to these *Candida* species have not been established in adequate and well-controlled clinical trials: *Candida lusitaniae* and *Candida guilliermondii*.

Contraindications

Hypersensitivity to voriconazole or its excipients; coadministration with CYP3A4 substrates (terfenadine, astemizole, cisapride, pimozide, quinidine), sirolimus, rifampin, carbamazepine, long-acting barbiturates, ritonavir (400 mg every 12 hours), rifabutin, ergot alkaloids (ergotamine and dihydroergotamine), and St. John's wort.

Warnings/Precautions

➤*Ophthalmic effects:* The effect of voriconazole on visual function is not known if treatment continues beyond 28 days. There have been postmarketing reports of prolonged visual adverse reactions, including optic neuritis and papilledema. If treatment continues beyond 28 days, monitor visual function, including visual acuity, visual field, and color perception.

➤*Hepatic toxicity:* In clinical trials, there have been uncommon cases of serious hepatic reactions during treatment with voriconazole (including clinical hepatitis, cholestasis, and fulminant hepatic failure, including fatalities). Instances of hepatic reactions were noted to occur primarily in patients with serious underlying medical conditions (predominantly hematological malignancy). Hepatic reactions, including hepatitis and jaundice, have occurred among patients with no other identifiable risk factors. Liver dysfunction has usually been reversible on discontinuation of therapy.

Evaluate liver function tests (LFTs) at the start of and during the course of voriconazole therapy. Monitor patients who develop abnormal LFTs during voriconazole therapy for the development of more severe hepatic injury. Patient management should include laboratory evaluation of hepatic function (particularly LFTs and bilirubin). Consider discontinuation of voriconazole if clinical signs and symptoms consistent with liver disease develop that may be attributable to voriconazole.

➤*Cardiovascular effects:* Some azoles, including voriconazole, have been associated with prolongation of the QT interval on the electrocardiogram. During clinical development and postmarketing surveillance, there have been rare cases of arrhythmias (including ventricular arrhythmias, such as torsades de pointes), cardiac arrests, and sudden deaths in patients taking voriconazole. These cases usually involved seriously ill patients with multiple confounding risk factors, such as histories of cardiotoxic chemotherapy, cardiomyopathy, hypokalemia, and concomitant medications, that may have been contributory.

Administer voriconazole with caution to patients with these potentially proarrhythmic conditions.

➤*Infusion-related reactions:* During infusion of the IV formulation of voriconazole in healthy subjects, anaphylactoid-type reactions, including flushing, fever, sweating, tachycardia, chest tightness, dyspnea, faintness, nausea, pruritus, and rash, have occurred uncommonly. Symptoms appeared immediately on initiating the infusion. Consider stopping the infusion if these reactions occur.

➤*Renal toxicity:* Acute renal failure has been observed in severely ill patients undergoing treatment with voriconazole. Patients being treated with voriconazole are likely to be treated concomitantly with nephrotoxic medications and have concurrent conditions that may result in decreased renal function.

VORICONAZOLE — INJECTION

➤*Dermatological reactions:* Patients have rarely developed serious exfoliative cutaneous reactions (eg, Stevens-Johnson syndrome) during treatment with voriconazole. If a patient develops an exfoliative cutaneous reaction, discontinue voriconazole.

➤*Hypersensitivity reactions:* There is no information regarding cross-sensitivity between voriconazole and other azole antifungal agents. Use caution when prescribing voriconazole to patients with hypersensitivity to other azoles.

➤*Renal function impairment:* See Administration and Dosage for more information.

➤*Hepatic function impairment:* See Administration and Dosage for more information.

➤*Hazardous tasks:* Advise patients to avoid potentially hazardous tasks, such as driving or operating machinery, if they perceive any change in vision.

➤*Photosensitivity:* See Adverse Reactions for more information.

➤*Pregnancy: Category D.* Voriconazole can cause fetal harm when administered to a pregnant woman. It is not known if voriconazole crosses the placenta to the fetus; however, the molecular weight (approximately 349) is low enough to expect exposure of the embryo and/or fetus.

If this drug is used during pregnancy or if the patient becomes pregnant while taking this drug, apprise the patient of the potential hazard to the fetus.

Voriconazole was teratogenic in rats (cleft palates, hydronephrosis/hydroureter) from 10 mg/kg (0.3 times the recommended maintenance dose on a mg/m^2 basis) and embryotoxic in rabbits at 100 mg/kg (6 times the recommended maintenance dose). Other effects in rats included reduced ossification of sacral and caudal vertebrae, skull, pubic and hyoid bone, supernumerary ribs, anomalies of the sternebrae, and dilatation of the ureter/renal pelvis. Plasma estradiol in pregnant rats was reduced at all dose levels. Voriconazole treatment in rats produced increased gestational length and dystocia, which were associated with increased perinatal pup mortality at the 10 mg/kg dose. The effects seen in rabbits were an increased embryomortality, reduced fetal weight, and increased incidences of skeletal variations, cervical ribs, and extrasternebral ossification sites.

Instruct women of childbearing potential to use effective contraception during treatment.

➤*Lactation:* The excretion of voriconazole in breast milk has not been investigated. The molecular weight (approximately 349) suggests that voriconazole will be excreted into breast milk. There is potential for toxicity in breast-feeding infants, especially during the neonatal period when hepatic function is immature. Instruct breast-feeding mothers to not use voriconazole unless the benefit clearly outweighs the risk.

➤*Children:* Safety and efficacy in children younger than 12 years have not been established.

There have been postmarketing reports of pancreatitis in children.

➤*Monitoring:* Monitor patients with risk factors for acute pancreatitis (eg, recent chemotherapy, hematopoietic stem cell transplantations) for the development of pancreatitis.

Correct electrolyte disturbances, such as hypokalemia, hypomagnesemia, and hypocalcemia, prior to initiation of voriconazole therapy.

Monitor patients for the development of abnormal renal function. This includes laboratory evaluation, particularly serum creatinine.

Evaluate LFTs and bilirubin at the start of and during the course of voriconazole therapy. Monitor patients who develop abnormal LFTs during voriconazole therapy for the development of more severe hepatic injury. Patients with hepatic insufficiency must be carefully monitored for drug toxicity.

If treatment continues beyond 28 days, monitor visual function, including visual acuity, visual field, and color perception.

Drug Interactions

➤*QT prolongation:* An additive effect of voriconazole with other drugs that prolong the QT interval cannot be excluded. The following drugs may prolong the QT interval and increase the risk of life-threatening cardiac arrhythmias, including torsades de pointes: antiarrhythmic agents (eg, amiodarone, bretylium, disopyramide, dofetilide, procainamide, quinidine, sotalol), arsenic trioxide, chlorpromazine, cisapride, dolasetron, droperidol, mefloquine, mesoridazine, moxifloxacin, pentamidine, pimozide, tacrolimus, thioridazine, and ziprasidone. For a more complete list of drugs that may prolong the QT interval, see the appendix Drug-Induced Prolongation of the QT Interval and Torsades de Pointes.

Voriconazole Drug Interactions

Precipitant drug	Object drug[a]		Description
Barbiturates, long acting (eg, mephobarbital, phenobarbital), carbamazepine	Voriconazole	↓	Coadministration may decrease voriconazole plasma concentrations. Coadministration is contraindicated.
Cimetidine	Voriconazole	↑	Cimetidine increased voriconazole C_{max} and AUC by an average of 18% and 23%, respectively. No dosage adjustment is required.
Contraceptives, hormonal (eg, containing ethinyl estradiol and norethindrone)	Voriconazole	↑	Voriconazole administration to healthy women receiving oral contraceptives increased ethinyl estradiol C_{max} and AUC by an average of 36% and 61%, respectively, and norethindrone C_{max} and AUC by an average of 15% and 53%, respectively. Voriconazole C_{max} and AUC increased by an average of 14% and 46%, respectively. Monitor for adverse reactions related to the contraceptive agent, as well as voriconazole.
Voriconazole	Contraceptives, hormonal (eg, containing ethinyl estradiol and norethindrone)	↑	
Fluconazole	Voriconazole	↑	Fluconazole increased voriconazole C_{max} and AUC by an average of 57% and 79%, respectively. Coadministration is not recommended. Close clinical monitoring is recommended if voriconazole is given sequentially after fluconazole, especially within 24 hours of the last fluconazole dose.
NNRTIs[b] (eg, delavirdine, nevirapine)	Voriconazole	↑↓	Coadministration may induce or inhibit the metabolism of voriconazole. Monitor for toxicity and effectiveness of voriconazole. Voriconazole also may inhibit the metabolism of an NNRTI. Monitor for drug toxicity. Coadministration of efavirenz and voriconazole decreases voriconazole plasma concentrations. When voriconazole is coadministered with efavirenz, increase voriconazole maintenance dosage to 400 mg every 12 hours and decrease the efavirenz dosage to 300 mg every 24 hours. When voriconazole is discontinued, restore initial dosage of efavirenz.
Voriconazole	NNRTIs (eg, delavirdine, efavirenz)	↑	
Phenytoin	Voriconazole	↓	Phenytoin may decrease the C_{max} and AUC of voriconazole by 50% and 70%, respectively. Voriconazole may increase the C_{max} and AUC of phenytoin up to 2 times. Monitor for phenytoin adverse reactions and phenytoin plasma concentrations. If phenytoin is administered with voriconazole, increase the voriconazole dosage 5 mg/kg every 12 hours.
Voriconazole	Phenytoin	↑	
Protease inhibitors (eg, amprenavir, ritonavir, saquinavir)	Voriconazole	↑↓	Voriconazole may inhibit the metabolism of certain protease inhibitors, and the metabolism of voriconazole may be inhibited or induced by certain protease inhibitors. Monitor closely for toxicity. Coadministration with indinavir showed no significant effects on voriconazole or indinavir exposure. Ritonavir (400 mg every 12 hours) decreased voriconazole AUC and C_{max} by approximately 82% and 66%, respectively. Coadministration with ritonavir (400 mg every 12 hours) is contraindicated. Avoid coadministration with ritonavir 100 mg every 12 hours unless assessment of benefit/risk justifies the use of voriconazole.
Voriconazole	Protease inhibitors (eg, amprenavir, nelfinavir, ritonavir, saquinavir)	↑	

VORICONAZOLE — INJECTION

Voriconazole Drug Interactions

Precipitant drug	Object drug[a]		Description
Proton pump inhibitors (eg, omeprazole)	Voriconazole	↑	Omeprazole may increase the C_{max} and AUC of voriconazole by an average of 15% and 40%, respectively. No dosage adjustment of voriconazole is recommended. Voriconazole may increase the C_{max} and AUC of omeprazole by an average of 2 and 4 times, respectively. When initiating voriconazole in patients already receiving omeprazole doses of 40 mg or more, reduce the dose of omeprazole by 50%. Voriconazole also may inhibit the metabolism of other proton pump inhibitors that are CYP2C19 substrates.
Voriconazole	Proton pump inhibitors (eg, omeprazole)		
Rifampin, rifabutin	Voriconazole	↓	Voriconazole plasma concentrations are significantly reduced during coadministration. In healthy subjects, rifampin 600 mg once daily decreased the steady-state C_{max} and AUC of voriconazole (200 mg every 12 hours for 7 days) by an average of 93% and 96%, respectively. Voriconazole may increase the C_{max} and AUC of rifabutin by an average of 3 and 4 times, respectively. Coadministration is contraindicated.
Voriconazole	Rifabutin	↑	
St. John's wort	Voriconazole	↓	Multiple oral doses of St. John's wort followed by a single dose of voriconazole decreased the voriconazole AUC by 59%. In contrast, coadministration of single oral doses of St. John's wort and voriconazole had no effect on voriconazole AUC. Coadministration is contraindicated.
Voriconazole	Anticoagulants (eg, warfarin)	↑	Coadministration may significantly increase prothrombin time by approximately 2 times. Closely monitor coagulation tests and adjust warfarin dose accordingly.
Voriconazole	Aripiprazole	↑	Aripiprazole plasma concentrations may be elevated, increasing the pharmacologic effects and risks of adverse reactions. Monitor the clinical response and adjust the aripiprazole dose as needed.
Voriconazole	Benzodiazepines (eg, alprazolam, midazolam, triazolam)	↑	Voriconazole may increase the plasma concentrations of benzodiazepines that are metabolized by CYP3A4. Frequent monitoring for benzodiazepine adverse events and toxicity is warranted. Adjust benzodiazepine dose if needed.
Voriconazole	Cabazitaxel	↑	Cabazitaxel plasma concentrations may be elevated, increasing the pharmacologic effects and risk of adverse reactions. Avoid coadministration.
Voriconazole	Calcium channel blockers	↑	Voriconazole may increase plasma concentrations of calcium channel blockers that are metabolized by CYP3A4 (eg, felodipine). Frequent monitoring for calcium channel adverse events and toxicity is warranted. Adjust calcium channel blocker dose if needed.
Voriconazole	Cisapride, pimozide, quinidine	↑	Voriconazole may inhibit the metabolism of these drugs. Increased plasma concentration may lead to QT prolongation and rare occurrences of torsades de pointes. Coadministration is contraindicated.

Voriconazole Drug Interactions

Precipitant drug	Object drug[a]		Description
Voriconazole	Clopidogrel	↓	Coadministration may decrease clopidogrel plasma concentrations, decreasing the pharmacologic effects. Avoid coadministration.
Voriconazole	Cyclosporine	↑	Coadministration of oral voriconazole increased cyclosporine C_{max} and AUC an average of 1.1 and 1.7 times, respectively. When initiating voriconazole therapy in patients already receiving cyclosporine, reduce the dose of cyclosporine to 50% of the original dose. Frequently monitor cyclosporine levels during coadministration and when voriconazole is discontinued.
Voriconazole	Docetaxel	↑	Docetaxel plasma concentrations may be elevated, increasing the pharmacologic effects and risk of toxicity. Avoid coadministration. If coadministration cannot be avoided, consider reducing the docetaxel dose by 50% with close clinical and laboratory monitoring.
Voriconazole	Dronedarone	↑	Dronedarone plasma concentrations may be elevated, increasing the pharmacologic effects and risk of toxicity, including life-threatening cardiotoxicity. Coadministration is contraindicated.
Voriconazole	Ergot alkaloids (eg, dihydroergotamine, ergotamine)	↑	Voriconazole may increase the plasma concentrations of ergot alkaloids and lead to ergotism. Coadministration is contraindicated.
Voriconazole	Erlotinib	↑	Erlotinib plasma concentrations may be elevated, increasing the risk of adverse reactions. Frequent monitoring for erlotinib adverse events and toxicity is warranted. Erlotinib dose reduction may be needed.
Voriconazole	Erythromycin	↑	Erythromycin plasma concentrations may be elevated, increasing the risk of adverse reactions, including sudden death due to cardiac causes. Avoid coadministration.
Voriconazole	HMG-CoA reductase inhibitors (eg, lovastatin)	↑	Voriconazole has been shown to inhibit lovastatin metabolism. Voriconazole may increase the plasma concentrations of statins that are metabolized by CYP3A4. The risk of adverse reactions, including rhabdomyolysis, may be increased. Frequent monitoring for adverse events and toxicity to statins is warranted. Consider dosage adjustment of the statin during coadministration.
Voriconazole	Ixabepilone	↑	Ixabepilone plasma concentrations may be elevated, increasing the pharmacologic effects and risk of adverse reactions. Avoid coadministration. If coadministration cannot be avoided, an ixabepilone dose reduction may be needed.
Voriconazole	Maraviroc	↑	Maraviroc plasma concentrations may be elevated, increasing the pharmacologic effects and risk of adverse reactions. A maraviroc dose reduction may be needed. Coadministration is contraindicated in patients with severe renal impairment (CrCl ≤ 30 mL/min).

VORICONAZOLE — INJECTION

Voriconazole Drug Interactions			
Precipitant drug	Object drug[a]		Description
Voriconazole	mTOR[c] inhibitors (eg, everolimus, temsirolimus)	↑	The mTOR inhibitor's plasma concentrations may be elevated, increasing the pharmacologic effects and risk of adverse reactions. Avoid coadministration. If coadministration cannot be avoided, frequent monitoring for mTOR inhibitor–related adverse events is warranted. A reduction in the mTOR inhibitor dose may be needed.
Voriconazole	Nilotinib	↑	Nilotinib plasma concentrations may be elevated, increasing the pharmacologic effects and risk of adverse reactions. Avoid coadministration. If coadministration cannot be avoided, it is recommended that nilotinib therapy be interrupted.
Voriconazole	NSAIDs (eg, diclofenac, ibuprofen)	↑	NSAID plasma concentrations may be increased. Frequent monitoring for NSAID-related adverse events and toxicity is warranted. NSAID dose reduction may be needed.
Voriconazole	Opioid analgesics (eg, alfentanil, fentanyl, methadone, oxycodone)	↑	Opioid analgesic plasma concentrations may be increased. Extended and frequent monitoring for respiratory depression and other adverse events is warranted. Increased concentrations of methadone may cause QT prolongation. Reduce the opioid dose if needed.
Voriconazole	Prednisolone	↑	Voriconazole may increase the C_{max} and AUC of prednisolone by an average of 11% and 34%, respectively. No dosage adjustment is recommended.
Voriconazole	Romidepsin	↑	Romidepsin plasma concentrations may be elevated, increasing the pharmacologic effects and risk of adverse reactions, including QT prolongation. Avoid coadministration. If coadministration cannot be avoided, frequent monitoring for romidepsin-related adverse events is warranted. Romidepsin dose reduction may be needed.
Voriconazole	Sirolimus	↑	Voriconazole can significantly increase the C_{max} and AUC of sirolimus an average of 7- and 11-fold, respectively. Coadministration is contraindicated.
Voriconazole	Sulfonylureas	↑	Voriconazole may increase plasma concentrations of sulfonylureas. Monitor for hypoglycemia. Dose adjustment of the sulfonylurea is recommended.
Voriconazole	Tacrolimus	↑	Voriconazole can significantly increase the C_{max} and AUC of tacrolimus by an average of 2- and 3-fold, respectively. When initiating voriconazole therapy in patients already receiving tacrolimus, reduce the dose of tacrolimus to 33% of the original dose. Frequently monitor tacrolimus levels during coadministration and when voriconazole is discontinued.
Voriconazole	Tyrosine kinase receptor inhibitors (eg, dasatinib, lapatinib, pazopanib, sunitinib)	↑	Tyrosine kinase receptor inhibitor plasma concentrations may be elevated, increasing the pharmacologic effects and risk of adverse reactions. Avoid coadministration. If coadministration cannot be avoided, frequent monitoring for tyrosine kinase receptor inhibitor–related adverse events is warranted. A reduction in the tyrosine kinase receptor inhibitor dose may be needed.
Voriconazole	Vinca alkaloids (eg, vinblastine, vincristine)	↑	Coadministration may increase the plasma concentrations of the vinca alkaloids and lead to neurotoxicity. Consider adjusting the dose of the vinca alkaloid and monitor for toxicity (eg, neurotoxicity).
Voriconazole	Zolpidem	↑	Zolpidem plasma concentrations may be elevated, increasing the pharmacologic effects and risk of adverse reactions. Frequent monitoring for zolpidem-related adverse events is warranted. A reduction in the zolpidem dose may be needed.

[a] ↓ = object drug decreased; ↑ = object drug increased; ↑↓ = object drug is both increased and decreased.
[b] NNRTI = nonnucleoside reverse transcriptase inhibitor.
[c] mTOR = mammalian target of rapamycin.

Adverse Reactions

➤*Most frequent adverse reactions:* The most frequently reported adverse reactions (all causalities) in the therapeutic trials were abdominal pain, diarrhea, fever, headache, nausea, peripheral edema, rash, respiratory disorder, sepsis, visual disturbances, and vomiting.

➤*Discontinuation:* The treatment-related adverse reactions that most often led to discontinuation of voriconazole therapy were elevated LFTs, rash, and visual disturbances.

➤*Adverse reactions (2% or more):*

Voriconazole All Therapeutic Studies Population Adverse Reactions (≥ 2%)						
	All therapeutic studies	Studies 307/602[a] and 608[b] (IV/oral therapy)			Study 305[c] (oral therapy)	
Adverse reactions	Voriconazole (n = 1,655)	Voriconazole (n = 468)	Amphotericin B[d] (n = 185)	Amphotericin B followed by fluconazole (n = 131)	Voriconazole (n = 200)	Fluconazole (n = 191)
CNS						
Hallucinations	2.4%	2.8%	0.5%	0%	0%	0%
Headache	3%	1.9%	4.3%	0.8%	0%	0.5%
GI						
Nausea	5.4%	3.8%	15.7%	1.5%	1%	1.6%
Vomiting	4.4%	3.2%	9.7%	0.8%	1%	0.5%
Hepatic						
ALT increased	1.8%	1.9%	0.5%	1.5%	3%	1%
AST increased	1.9%	1.9%	0%	0.8%	4%	1%
Bilirubinemia	0.9%	1.1%	1.6%	1.5%	0.5%	0%
Cholestatic jaundice	1%	1.7%	0%	0.8%	1.5%	0%
Hepatic enzymes increased	1.8%	2.4%	2.7%	0.8%	1.5%	0%
LFTs abnormal	2.7%	3.2%	2.2%	0.8%	3%	1%
Metabolic/Nutritional						
Alkaline phosphatase increased	3.6%	4.1%	2.2%	2.3%	5%	1.6%
Hypokalemia	1.6%	0.6%	19.5%	12.2%	0%	0%

VORICONAZOLE — INJECTION

Voriconazole All Therapeutic Studies Population Adverse Reactions (≥ 2%)						
	All therapeutic studies	Studies 307/602[a] and 608[b] (IV/oral therapy)			Study 305[c] (oral therapy)	
Adverse reactions	Voriconazole (n = 1,655)	Voriconazole (n = 468)	Amphotericin B[d] (n = 185)	Amphotericin B followed by fluconazole (n = 131)	Voriconazole (n = 200)	Fluconazole (n = 191)
Renal						
Acute kidney failure	0.4%	0.4%	5.9%	5.3%	0%	0%
Creatinine increased	0.2%	0%	31.9%	7.6%	0.5%	0%
Kidney function abnormal	0.6%	1.3%	21.6%	6.9%	0.5%	0.5%
Special senses						
Abnormal vision	18.7%	13.5%	0.5%	0%	15.5%	4.2%
Chromatopsia	1.2%	0.4%	0%	0%	1%	0%
Photophobia	2.2%	1.7%	0%	0%	2.5%	1%
Miscellaneous						
Chills	3.7%	0.2%	19.5%	6.1%	0.5%	0%
Fever	5.7%	1.7%	13.5%	3.8%	0%	0%
Rash	5.3%	4.3%	3.8%	0.8%	1.5%	0.5%
Tachycardia	2.4%	1.3%	2.7%	0%	0%	0%

[a] In study 307/602, 381 patients (196 taking voriconazole, 185 taking amphotericin B) were treated to compare voriconazole with amphotericin B followed by other licensed antifungal therapy in the primary treatment of patients with acute invasive aspergillosis.
[b] In study 608, 403 patients with candidemia were treated to compare voriconazole (272 patients) to the regimen of amphotericin B followed by fluconazole (131 patients).
[c] Study 305 evaluated the effects of oral voriconazole (200 patients) and oral fluconazole (191 patients) in the treatment of esophageal candidiasis.
[d] Amphotericin B followed by other licensed antifungal therapy.

Dermatologic – Dermatological reactions were common in the patients treated with voriconazole. The mechanism underlying these dermatologic adverse reactions remains unknown. In clinical trials, rashes considered related to therapy were reported by 7% of voriconazole-treated patients. The majority of rashes were of mild to moderate severity. Patients have rarely developed serious cutaneous reactions, including Stevens-Johnson syndrome, toxic epidermal necrolysis, and erythema multiforme during treatment with voriconazole. Discontinue voriconazole if a patient develops an exfoliative cutaneous reaction. In addition, voriconazole has been associated with photosensitivity skin reactions. It is recommended that patients avoid strong, direct sunlight during voriconazole therapy. In patients with photosensitivity skin reactions, squamous cell carcinoma of the skin and melanoma have been reported during long-term therapy. If a patient develops a skin lesion consistent with squamous cell carcinoma or melanoma, discontinue voriconazole.

Ophthalmic – Voriconazole treatment-related visual disturbances are common. In therapeutic trials, approximately 21% of patients experienced abnormal vision, color vision change, and/or photophobia. The visual disturbances were generally mild and rarely resulted in discontinuation. Visual disturbances may be associated with higher plasma concentrations and/or doses. There have been postmarketing reports of prolonged visual adverse reactions, including optic neuritis and papilledema.

The mechanism of action of the visual disturbance is unknown, although the site of action is most likely to be within the retina. In a study in healthy volunteers investigating the effect of 28-day treatment with voriconazole on retinal function, voriconazole caused a decrease in the electroretinogram (ERG) waveform amplitude, a decrease in the visual field, and an alteration in color perception. The ERG measures electrical currents in the retina. The effects were noted early in administration of voriconazole and continued through the course of study drug dosing.

Fourteen days after end of dosing, ERG, visual fields, and color perception returned to normal.

➤*Adverse reactions (less than 2%):*

Cardiovascular – Atrial arrhythmia, atrial fibrillation, atrioventricular block complete, bigeminy, bradycardia, bundle branch block, cardiomegaly, cardiomyopathy, cerebral hemorrhage, cerebral ischemia, cerebrovascular accident, congestive heart failure, deep thrombophlebitis, endocarditis, extrasystoles, heart arrest, hypertension, hypotension, myocardial infarction, nodal arrhythmia, palpitation, phlebitis, postural hypotension, pulmonary embolus, QT interval prolonged, supraventricular extrasystoles, supraventricular tachycardia, syncope, thrombophlebitis, vasodilatation, ventricular arrhythmia, ventricular fibrillation, ventricular tachycardia (including torsades de pointes).

CNS – Abnormal dreams, acute brain syndrome, agitation, akathisia, amnesia, anxiety, asthenia, ataxia, brain edema, coma, confusion, convulsion, delirium, dementia, depersonalization, depression, diplopia, dizziness, encephalitis, encephalopathy, euphoria, extrapyramidal syndrome, grand mal convulsion, Guillain-Barré syndrome, hypertonia, hypesthesia, insomnia, intracranial hypertension, libido decreased, neuralgia, neuropathy, nystagmus, oculogyric crisis, paresthesia, psychosis, somnolence, suicidal ideation, tremor, vertigo.

Dermatologic – Alopecia, angioedema, contact dermatitis, discoid lupus erythematosis, eczema, erythema multiforme, exfoliative dermatitis, fixed drug eruption, furunculosis, herpes simplex, maculopapular rash, melanoma, melanosis, photosensitivity skin reaction, pruritus, pseudoporphyria, psoriasis, skin discoloration, skin disorder, skin dry, Stevens-Johnson syndrome, squamous cell carcinoma, sweating, toxic epidermal necrolysis, urticaria.

Endocrine – Adrenal cortex insufficiency, diabetes insipidus, hyperthyroidism, hypothyroidism.

GI – Abdomen enlarged, abdominal pain, anorexia, cheilitis, cholecystitis, cholelithiasis, constipation, diarrhea, dry mouth, duodenal ulcer perforation, duodenitis, dyspepsia, dysphagia, enlarged liver, esophageal ulcer, esophagitis, flatulence, gastroenteritis, gamma-glutamyl transferase/lactic dehydrogenase elevated, GI hemorrhage, gingivitis, glossitis, gum hemorrhage, gum hyperplasia, hematemesis, hepatic coma, hepatic failure, hepatitis, intestinal perforation, intestinal ulcer, jaundice, melena, mouth ulceration, pancreatitis, parotid gland enlargement, periodontitis, proctitis, pseudomembranous colitis, rectal disorder, rectal hemorrhage, stomach ulcer, stomatitis, tongue edema.

GU – Anuria, blighted ovum, CrCl decreased, dysmenorrhea, dysuria, epididymitis, glycosuria, hematuria, hemorrhagic cystitis, hydronephrosis, impotence, kidney pain, kidney tubular necrosis, metrorrhagia, nephritis, nephrosis, oliguria, scrotal edema, urinary incontinence, urinary retention, urinary tract infection, uterine hemorrhage, vaginal hemorrhage.

Hematologic/Lymphatic – Agranulocytosis, anemia (macrocytic, megaloblastic, microcytic, normocytic), aplastic anemia, hemolytic anemia, bleeding time increased, cyanosis, disseminated intravascular coagulation, ecchymosis, enlarged spleen, eosinophilia, hypervolemia, leukopenia, lymphadenopathy, lymphangitis, marrow depression, pancytopenia, petechia, purpura, thrombocytopenia, thrombotic thrombocytopenic purpura.

Metabolic/Nutritional – Albuminuria, creatine phosphokinase increased, edema, glucose tolerance decreased, hypercalcemia, hypercholesteremia, hyperglycemia, hyperkalemia, hypermagnesemia, hypernatremia, hyperuricemia, hypocalcemia, hypoglycemia, hypomagnesemia, hyponatremia, hypophosphatemia, peripheral edema, serum urea nitrogen increased, uremia.

Musculoskeletal – Arthralgia, arthritis, back pain, bone necrosis, bone pain, leg cramps, myalgia, myasthenia, myopathy, osteomalacia, osteoporosis.

Respiratory – Cough increased, dyspnea, epistaxis, hemoptysis, hypoxia, lung edema, pharyngitis, pleural effusion, pneumonia, respiratory disorder, respiratory distress syndrome, respiratory tract infection, rhinitis, sinusitis, voice alteration.

Special senses – Abnormality of accommodation, blepharitis, color blindness, conjunctivitis, corneal opacity, deafness, dry eyes, ear pain, eye hemorrhage, eye pain, hypoacusis, keratitis, keratoconjunctivitis, mydriasis, night blindness, optic atrophy, optic neuritis, otitis externa, papilledema, retinal hemorrhage, retinitis, scleritis, taste loss, taste perversion, tinnitus, uveitis, visual field defect.

Miscellaneous – Allergic reaction, anaphylactoid reaction, ascites, bacterial infection, cellulitis, chest pain, edema, face edema, flank pain, flu syndrome, fungal infection, graft versus host reaction, granuloma, infection, injection-site infection/inflammation, injection-site pain, mucous membrane disorder, multiorgan failure, pain, pelvic pain, peritonitis, sepsis, substernal chest pain.

➤*Lab test abnormalities:* The overall incidence of clinically significant transaminase abnormalities in all therapeutic studies was 12.4% (206/1,655) of patients treated with voriconazole. Increased incidence of LFT abnormalities may be associated with higher plasma concentrations and/or doses. The majority of abnormal LFTs either resolved during treatment without dosage adjustment or following dose adjustment, including discontinuation of therapy.

Voriconazole Lab Test Abnormalities in Patients With Esophageal Candidiasis (Study 305)			
Laboratory abnormality	Criteria[a]	Voriconazole	Fluconazole
Total bilirubin	> 1.5 × ULN[b]	4.3%	3.8%
AST	> 3 × ULN	20.3%	8.1%
ALT	> 3 × ULN	10.7%	6.5%
Alkaline phosphatase	> 3 × ULN	10.2%	7.5%

[a] Without regard to baseline value.
[b] ULN = upper limit of normal.

Voriconazole Lab Test Abnormalities in Patients With Invasive Aspergillosis (Study 307/602)			
Laboratory abnormality	Criteria[a]	Voriconazole	Amphotericin B[b]
Total bilirubin	> 1.5 × ULN	19.4%	26.6%
AST	> 3 × ULN	11.7%	10.3%
ALT	> 3 × ULN	18.9%	23.1%
Alkaline phosphatase	> 3 × ULN	16%	22%

VORICONAZOLE — INJECTION

Voriconazole Lab Test Abnormalities in Patients With Invasive Aspergillosis (Study 307/602)			
Laboratory abnormality	Criteria[a]	Voriconazole	Amphotericin B[b]
Creatinine	> 1.3 × ULN	21.4%	57.6%
Potassium	< 0.9 × LLN[c]	16.6%	39.3%

[a] Without regard to baseline value.
[b] Amphotericin B followed by other licensed antifungal therapy.
[c] LLN = lower limit of normal.

Voriconazole Lab Test Abnormalities in Patients With Candidemia (Study 608)			
Laboratory abnormality	Criteria[a]	Voriconazole	Amphotericin B followed by fluconazole
Total bilirubin	> 1.5 × ULN	19.2%	27%
AST	> 3 × ULN	15.3%	13.8%
ALT	> 3 × ULN	8.4%	12.9%
Alkaline phosphatase	> 3 × ULN	22.6%	22.6%

Voriconazole Lab Test Abnormalities in Patients With Candidemia (Study 608)			
Laboratory abnormality	Criteria[a]	Voriconazole	Amphotericin B followed by fluconazole
Creatinine	> 1.3 × ULN	15%	27.1%
Potassium	< 0.9 × LLN	16.7%	29.7%

[a] Without regard to baseline value.

Overdosage

➤*Symptoms:* In clinical trials, there were 3 cases of accidental overdose. All occurred in children who received up to 5 times the recommended IV dose of voriconazole. A single adverse reaction of photophobia of 10 minutes' duration was reported.

➤*Treatment:* There is no known antidote to voriconazole.

Voriconazole is hemodialyzed, with clearance of 121 mL/min. The IV vehicle, SBECD, is hemodialyzed, with clearance of 55 mL/min. In an overdose, hemodialysis may assist in the removal of voriconazole and SBECD from the body.

Patient Information

Advise patients not to drive at night while taking voriconazole. Voriconazole may cause changes to vision, including blurring and/or photophobia.

Advise patients to avoid potentially hazardous tasks, such as driving or operating machinery, if they perceive any change in vision.

Advise patients to avoid strong, direct sunlight during voriconazole therapy.

Advise women of childbearing potential to use effective contraception during treatment.

POSACONAZOLE

Rx	**Noxafil** (Schering Corporation)	**Suspension, oral:** 40 mg/mL	Polysorbate 80, simethicone, sodium benzoate, xanthan gum, glucose. Cherry flavored. In 105 mL with calibrated dosing spoon.

POSACONAZOLE — ORAL

Indications

➤*Oropharyngeal candidiasis:* For the treatment of oropharyngeal candidiasis, including oropharyngeal candidiasis refractory to itraconazole and/or fluconazole.

➤*Prophylaxis of invasive fungal infection:* Prophylaxis of invasive *Aspergillus* and *Candida* infections in patients 13 years of age and older who are at high risk of developing these infections because of being severely immunocompromised, such as hematopoietic stem cell transplant (HSCT) recipients with graft versus host disease (GVHD) or patients with hematologic malignancies with prolonged neutropenia from chemotherapy.

Administration and Dosage

➤*Adults:*

Oropharyngeal candidiasis –

Loading dose: 100 mg (2.5 mL) twice daily on the first day.

Maintenance dosage: 100 mg (2.5 mL) once daily for 13 days.

Oropharyngeal candidiasis refractory to itraconazole and/or fluconazole –

Usual dosage: 400 mg (10 mL) twice daily.

Duration of therapy: Duration of therapy should be based on the severity of the patient's underlying disease and clinical response.

Prophylaxis of invasive fungal infections –

Usual dosage: 200 mg (5 mL) 3 times daily.

Duration of therapy: The duration of therapy is based on recovery from neutropenia or immunosuppression.

➤*Children:* See Adults for dosing for children 13 years of age and older.

➤*Preparation for administration:* Shake posaconazole oral suspension well before use.

➤*Administration:* Each dose of posaconazole oral suspension should be administered with a full meal or liquid nutritional supplement. For patients who cannot eat a full meal or tolerate an oral nutritional supplement, alternative antifungal therapy should be considered or patients should be monitored closely for breakthrough fungal infections.

➤*Storage/Stability:* Store at 25°C (77°F); excursions are permitted to 15° to 30°C (59° to 86°F). Do not freeze.

Actions

➤*Pharmacology:* Posaconazole is a triazole antifungal agent. As a triazole antifungal agent, posaconazole blocks the synthesis of ergosterol, a key component of the fungal cell membrane, through the inhibition of the enzyme lanosterol 14α-demethylase and accumulation of methylated sterol precursors.

➤*Pharmacokinetics:*

Summary of pharmacokinetic parameters –

Mean (% CV) (Min, Max) Posaconazole Steady-State Pharmacokinetic Parameters[a]					
Dosage[b]	Steady-state plasma concentrations[c] (ng/mL)	AUC[d] (ng•h/mL)	CL/F (L/h)	V/F (L)	$t_{1/2}$ (h)
200 mg 3 times daily[e] (n = 252)	1,103 (67) [21.5 to 3,650]	ND	ND	ND	ND
200 mg 3 times daily[f] (n = 215)	583 (65) [89.7 to 2,200]	15,900 (62) [4,100 to 56,100]	51.2 (54) [10.7 to 146]	2,425 (39) [828 to 5,702]	37.2 (39) [19.1 to 148]
400 mg twice daily[g] (n = 23)	723 (86) [6.7 to 2,256]	9,093 (80) [1,564 to 26,794]	76.1 (78) [14.9 to 256]	3,088 (84) [407 to 13,140]	31.7 (42) [12.4 to 67.3]

[a] V/F = apparent volume of distribution; ND = not done.
[b] Oral suspension administration.
[c] Steady-state plasma concentrations based on observed data; other pharmacokinetic parameters based on estimates from population pharmacokinetic analyses.
[d] $AUC_{(0-24\ h)}$ for 200 mg 3 times daily and $AUC_{(0-12\ h)}$ for 400 mg twice daily.
[e] Allogenic HSCT recipients with GVHD.
[f] Neutropenic patients who were receiving cytotoxic chemotherapy for acute myelogenous leukemia or myelodysplastic syndromes.
[g] Febrile neutropenic patients or patients with refractory invasive fungal infections, steady-state plasma concentrations (n = 24).

Absorption – Posaconazole is absorbed with a medium time to reach maximum drug concentration (T_{max}) of approximately 3 to 5 hours. Dose-proportional increases in plasma exposure (area under the curve [AUC]) to posaconazole were observed following single oral doses from 50 to 800 mg and following multiple-dose administration from 50 to 400 mg twice daily. No further increases in exposure were observed when the dose was increased from 400 to 600 mg twice daily in febrile neutropenic patients or those with refractory invasive fungal infections. Steady-state plasma concentrations are attained at 7 to 10 days following multiple-dose administration.

Food effects: Following single-dose administration of posaconazole 200 mg, the mean AUC and maximal drug concentration (C_{max}) are approximately 3 times higher when administered with a nonfat meal and approximately 4 times higher when administered with a high-fat meal (approximately 50 g of fat), relative to the fasted state. Following single-dose administration of posaconazole 400 mg, the mean AUC and C_{max} are approximately 3 times higher when administered with a liquid nutritional supplement (14 g of fat), relative to the fasted state (see the following table). In order to ensure attainment of adequate plasma concentrations, administering posaconazole with food or a nutritional supplement is recommended.

POSACONAZOLE — ORAL

Posaconazole Pharmacokinetic Parameters Under Fed and Fasted Conditions[a]

Dose (mg)	C_{max} (ng/mL)	T_{max} [b] (h)	AUC(I) (ng•h/mL)	CL/F (L/h)	t½ (h)
200 mg fasted (n = 20)[c]	132 (50) [45 to 267]	3.5 [1.5 to 36][d]	4,179 (31) [2,705 to 7,269]	51 (25) [28 to 74]	23.5 (25) [15.3 to 33.7]
200 mg nonfat (n = 20)[c]	378 (43) [131 to 834]	4 [3 to 5]	10,753 (35) [4,579 to 17,092]	21 (39) [12 to 44]	22.2 (18) [17.4 to 28.7]
200 mg high-fat (54 g of fat) (n = 20)[c]	512 (34) [241 to 1,106]	5 [4 to 5]	15,059 (26) [10,341 to 24,476]	14 (24) [8.2 to 19]	23 (19) [17.2 to 33.4]
400 mg fasted (n = 23)[e]	121 (75) [27 to 366]	4 [2 to 12]	5,258 (48) [2,834 to 9,567]	91 (40) [42 to 141]	27.3 (26) [16.8 to 38.9]
400 mg with liquid nutritional supplement (14 g of fat) (n = 23)[e]	355 (43) [145 to 720]	5 [4 to 8]	11,295 (40) [3,865 to 20,592]	43 (56) [19 to 103]	26 (19) [18.2 to 35]

[a] CL/F = total body clearance; t½ = mean half-life.
[b] Median (min, max).
[c] n = 15 for AUC(I), CL/F, and t½.
[d] The subject with T_{max} of 36 hours had relatively constant plasma levels over 36 hours (1.7 ng/mL difference between 4 and 36 hours).
[e] n = 10 for AUC(I), CL/F, and t½.

Distribution – Posaconazole has an apparent volume of distribution of 1,774 L, suggesting extensive extravascular distribution and penetration into the body tissues. Posaconazole is highly protein bound (greater than 98%), predominantly to albumin.

Metabolism – Posaconazole primarily circulates as the parent compound in plasma. Of the circulating metabolites, the majority are glucuronide conjugates formed via uridine diphosphate (UDP) glucuronidation (phase 2 enzymes). Posaconazole does not have any major circulating oxidative (CYP-450–mediated) metabolites. The excreted metabolites in urine and feces account for approximately 17% of the administered radiolabeled dose.

Excretion – Posaconazole is eliminated with a mean half-life of 35 hours (range, 20 to 66 hours) and a CL/F of 32 L/h. Posaconazole is predominantly eliminated in the feces (71% of the radiolabeled dose up to 120 hours), with the major component eliminated as parent drug (66% of the radiolabeled dose). Renal clearance is a minor elimination pathway, with 13% of the radiolabeled dose excreted in urine up to 120 hours (less than 0.2% of the radiolabeled dose is parent drug).

The variability in average plasma posaconazole concentrations in patients was relatively higher than that in healthy subjects.

Special populations –

Renal function impairment: In subjects with severe renal function impairment (Ccr less than 20 mL/min/1.73 m^2), the mean plasma exposure (AUC) was similar to that in patients with healthy renal function (Ccr greater than 80 mL/min/1.73 m^2). However, the range of the AUC estimates was highly variable (CV = 96%) in those subjects with severe renal function impairment, as compared with that in the other renal function impairment groups (CV less than 40%). Because of the variability in exposure, closely monitor patients with severe renal function impairment for breakthrough fungal infections.

Hepatic function impairment: The pharmacokinetic data in subjects with hepatic function impairment was not sufficient to determine if dose adjustment is necessary. It is recommended that posaconazole be used with caution in patients with hepatic function impairment.

➤*Microbiology:*

Activity in vitro and in vivo – Posaconazole has shown in vitro activity against *Aspergillus fumigatus* and *Candida albicans*, including *C. albicans* isolates from patients refractory to itraconazole or fluconazole or both drugs.

In immunocompetent and/or immunocompromised mice and rabbits with pulmonary or disseminated infection with *A. fumigatus*, posaconazole administered prophylactically was effective in prolonging survival and reducing mycological burden. Prophylactic posaconazole also prolonged survival of immunocompetent mice challenged with *C. albicans* or *Aspergillus flavus*.

Drug resistance – Clinical isolates of *C. albicans* and *Candida glabrata* with decreases in posaconazole susceptibility were observed in oral swish samples taken during prophylaxis with posaconazole and fluconazole, suggesting a potential for development of resistance. These isolates also showed reduced susceptibility to other azoles, suggesting cross-resistance between azoles. The clinical significance of this finding is not known.

Contraindications

Hypersensitivity to the active substance or to any of the excipients; coadministration with ergot alkaloids; coadministration with the CYP3A4 substrates terfenadine, astemizole, cisapride, pimozide, halofantrine, or quinidine because this may result in increased plasma concentrations of the drugs, leading to QTc prolongation and rare occurrence of torsades de pointes.

Warnings/Precautions

➤*Hepatic toxicity:* In clinical trials, there were infrequent cases of hepatic reactions (eg, mild to moderate elevations in ALT, AST, alkaline phosphatase, total bilirubin, and/or clinical hepatitis). The elevations in liver function tests were generally reversible upon discontinuation of therapy and, in some instances, these tests normalized without drug interruption and rarely required drug discontinuation. Rarely, more severe hepatic reactions, including cholestasis or hepatic failure including fatalities, were reported in patients with serious underlying medical conditions (eg, hematologic malignancy) during treatment with posaconazole. These severe hepatic reactions were seen primarily in subjects receiving posaconazole 800 mg daily (400 mg twice daily or 200 mg 4 times daily) in another indication.

Evaluate liver function tests at the start of and during the course of posaconazole therapy. Monitor patients who develop abnormal liver function tests during posaconazole therapy for the development of more severe hepatic injury. Patient management includes laboratory evaluation of hepatic function (particularly liver function tests and bilirubin). Consider discontinuation of posaconazole if the patient demonstrates clinical signs and symptoms consistent with liver disease that may be attributable to the drug.

➤*Cardiac effects:* Administer posaconazole with caution to patients with potentially proarrhythmic conditions; do not administer with drugs that are known to prolong the QTc interval and are metabolized through CYP3A4. Make rigorous attempts to correct potassium, magnesium, and calcium before starting posaconazole.

Some azoles, including posaconazole, have been associated with prolongation of the QT interval on the electrocardiogram. Results from a multiple, time-matched electrocardiogram analysis in healthy volunteers did not show any increase in the mean of the QTc interval. During clinical development, there was 1 case of torsades de pointes in a patient taking posaconazole. This patient was seriously ill, with multiple confounding risk factors including a history of cardiotoxic chemotherapy, hypokalemia, and concomitant medications, which may have been contributory.

➤*Hypersensitivity reactions:* There is no information regarding cross-sensitivity between posaconazole and other azole antifungal agents. Use caution when prescribing posaconazole to patients with hypersensitivity to other azoles.

➤*Pregnancy: Category C.* Posaconazole has been shown to cause skeletal malformations (cranial malformations and missing ribs) in rats when given in doses of 27 mg/kg or more (at least 1.4 times the 400 mg twice-daily regimen based on steady-state plasma concentrations of drug in healthy volunteers). The no-effect dose for malformations in rats was 9 mg/kg, which is 0.7 times the exposure achieved with the 400 mg twice-daily regimen. No malformations were seen in rabbits at doses up to 80 mg/kg. In the rabbit, the no-effect dose was 20 mg/kg, while high doses of 40 and 80 mg/kg (2.9 or 5.2 times the exposure achieved with the 400 mg twice-daily regimen) caused an increase in resorption. In rabbits dosed at 80 mg/kg, a reduction in the body weight gain of females and a reduction in litter size were seen. There are no adequate and well-controlled studies in pregnant women. Use posaconazole in pregnancy only if the potential benefit justifies the potential risk to the fetus.

➤*Lactation:* Posaconazole is excreted in the milk of lactating rats. The excretion of posaconazole in human breast milk has not been investigated. Do not prescribe posaconazole to breast-feeding mothers unless the benefit clearly outweighs the potential risk to the infant.

➤*Children:* Safety and efficacy of posaconazole in children younger than 13 years of age have not been established.

➤*Monitoring:* Evaluate liver function tests at the start of and during the course of posaconazole therapy. Monitor for the development of more severe hepatic injury in patients who develop abnormal liver function tests during posaconazole therapy.

Closely monitor for breakthrough fungal infections in patients who have severe diarrhea or vomiting.

Make rigorous attempts to correct potassium, magnesium, and calcium before starting posaconazole therapy.

Closely monitor patients with severe renal function impairment for breakthrough invasive fungal infection.

Generally avoid coadministration of drugs that can decrease the plasma concentrations of posaconazole unless the benefit outweighs the risk. If such drugs are necessary, closely monitor patients for breakthrough fungal infections.

Drug Interactions

Posaconazole Drug Interactions

Precipitant drug	Object drug[a]		Description
Cimetidine	Posaconazole	⬇	Coadministration resulted in a 39% decrease in both posaconazole C_{max} and AUC. Avoid concomitant use unless the benefit outweighs the risk.

POSACONAZOLE — ORAL

Posaconazole Drug Interactions			
Precipitant drug	Object drug[a]		Description
Phenytoin	Posaconazole	⬇	Coadministration resulted in a 41% and 50% decrease in posaconazole C_{max} and AUC, respectively, and a 16% increase in both phenytoin C_{max} and AUC. Avoid concomitant use unless the benefit outweighs the risk. Perform frequent monitoring of phenytoin concentrations and consider dose reduction of phenytoin during coadministration.
Posaconazole	Phenytoin	⬆	
Rifabutin	Posaconazole	⬇	Coadministration resulted in a 43% and 49% decrease in posaconazole C_{max} and AUC, respectively, and a 31% and 72% increase in rifabutin C_{max} and AUC, respectively. Avoid concomitant use unless the benefit outweighs the risk. If coadministration is required, frequent monitoring of complete blood cell counts and adverse reactions due to increased rifabutin levels (eg, leukopenia, uveitis) is recommended.
Posaconazole	Rifabutin	⬆	
Posaconazole	Benzodiazepines metabolized by CYP3A4 (eg, midazolam)	⬆	Coadministration resulted in an 83% increase in midazolam AUC. Perform frequent monitoring for adverse reactions and consider dose reduction of these benzodiazepines during coadministration.
Posaconazole	Calcium channel blockers metabolized through CYP3A4 (eg, felodipine)	⬆	Frequent monitoring for adverse reactions and toxicity related to calcium channel blockers is recommended during coadministration. Dose reduction of the calcium channel blocker may be needed.
Posaconazole	CYP3A4 substrates (eg, astemizole, cisapride, halofantrine, pimozide, quinidine, terfenadine)	⬆	Increased plasma concentrations of these drugs can lead to QT prolongation with rare occurrences of torsades de pointes. Coadministration is contraindicated.
Posaconazole	Ergot alkaloids (eg, ergotamine, dihydroergotamine)	⬆	Posaconazole may increase the plasma concentrations of ergot alkaloids, which may lead to ergotism. Coadministration is contraindicated.
Posaconazole	HMG-CoA reductase inhibitors metabolized through CYP3A4 (eg, atorvastatin)	⬆	It is recommended that dose reduction of statins be considered during coadministration. Increased statin concentrations in plasma can be associated with rhabdomyolysis.
Posaconazole	Immunosuppressants (eg, cyclosporine, sirolimus, tacrolimus)	⬆	Cases of elevated cyclosporine levels resulting in rare but serious adverse reactions, including nephrotoxicity, leukoencephalopathy, and death, have been reported. Reduce the dose of cyclosporine and tacrolimus by three fourths and one third of the original dose, respectively. Perform frequent clinical monitoring of cyclosporine, tacrolimus, and sirolimus whole blood concentrations when posaconazole therapy is initiated and discontinued.
Posaconazole	Vinca alkaloids (eg, vincristine, vinblastine)	⬆	Posaconazole may increase the plasma concentrations of vinca alkaloids, which may lead to neurotoxicity. Consider dosage adjustment of the vinca alkaloid.

[a] ⬇ = object drug decreased; ⬆ = object drug increased.

➤*Drug/Food interactions:* Following single-dose administration of posaconazole 200 mg, the mean AUC and C_{max} of posaconazole are approximately 3 times higher when administered with a nonfat meal and approximately 4 times higher when administered with a high-fat meal (approximately 50 g of fat), relative to the fasted state. Following single-dose administration of 400 mg, the mean C_{max} and AUC of posaconazole are approximately 3 times higher when administered with a liquid nutritional supplement (14 g of fat), relative to the fasted state. In order to ensure attainment of adequate plasma concentrations, it is recommended to administer posaconazole with food or a nutritional supplement.

Adverse Reactions

➤*Prophylaxis of Aspergillus and Candida:*

Posaconazole Adverse Reactions in Prophylaxis Studies (> 10%)			
Adverse reaction	Posaconazole (n = 605)	Fluconazole (n = 539)	Itraconazole (n = 58)
Subjects reporting any adverse reaction	98%	99%	100%
Cardiovascular			
Hypertension	18%	16%	5%
Hypotension	14%	15%	17%
Tachycardia	12%	14%	5%
CNS			
Anxiety	9%	11%	16%
Dizziness	11%	10%	9%
Fatigue	17%	18%	9%
Headache	28%	26%	40%
Insomnia	17%	17%	19%
Weakness	8%	10%	3%
Dermatologic			
Pruritus	11%	12%	19%
Rash	19%	18%	43%
GI			
Abdominal pain	27%	27%	36%
Anorexia	15%	17%	28%
Constipation	21%	17%	17%
Diarrhea	42%	39%	60%
Dyspepsia	10%	9%	10%
Mucositis NOS[a]	17%	13%	26%
Nausea	38%	37%	52%
Vomiting	29%	32%	41%
GU			
Vaginal hemorrhage[b]	10%	9%	12%
Hematologic/Lymphatic			
Anemia	25%	23%	28%
Febrile neutropenia	20%	16%	40%
Neutropenia	23%	23%	40%
Petechiae	11%	10%	16%
Thrombocytopenia	29%	27%	34%
Hepatic			
Bilirubinemia	10%	9%	19%
Metabolic/Nutritional			
Hyperglycemia	11%	14%	3%
Hypocalcemia	9%	10%	9%
Hypokalemia	30%	26%	52%
Hypomagnesemia	18%	16%	19%
Musculoskeletal			
Arthralgia	11%	12%	9%
Back pain	10%	12%	7%
Musculoskeletal pain	16%	15%	16%
Rigors	20%	16%	29%
Respiratory			
Coughing	24%	24%	24%
Dyspnea	20%	22%	26%
Epistaxis	14%	14%	21%
Pharyngitis	12%	11%	21%
Upper respiratory tract infection	7%	10%	9%
Miscellaneous			
Bacteremia	18%	18%	28%
Cytomegalovirus infection	14%	13%	0%
Edema	9%	13%	14%

POSACONAZOLE — ORAL

Posaconazole Adverse Reactions in Prophylaxis Studies (> 10%)			
Adverse reaction	Posaconazole (n = 605)	Fluconazole (n = 539)	Itraconazole (n = 58)
Edema, legs	15%	12%	19%
Fever	45%	47%	55%
Herpes simplex	15%	11%	17%

[a] NOS = not otherwise specified.
[b] Percentages of sex-specific adverse reactions are based on the number of male/female patients.

The 2 following tables present treatment-related adverse reactions observed at an incidence of 2% or more in posaconazole prophylaxis studies.

Posaconazole Adverse Reactions (Study 1) (≥ 2%)		
Adverse reaction	Posaconazole (n = 301)	Fluconazole (n = 299)
Subjects reporting any adverse reaction	36%	38%
Cardiovascular		
Hypertension	1%	2%
CNS		
Dizziness	1%	2%
Fatigue	1%	2%
Headache	1%	3%
Tremor	1%	2%
Weakness	1%	2%
GI		
Abdominal pain	1%	2%
Anorexia	1%	2%
Constipation	< 1%	2%
Diarrhea	3%	4%
Dyspepsia	1%	2%
Nausea	7%	9%
Vomiting	4%	5%
Hepatic		
ALT increased	3%	1%
AST increased	3%	1%
Bilirubinemia	3%	2%
GGT[a] increased	3%	2%
Hepatic enzymes increased	3%	2%
Metabolic/Nutritional		
Phosphatase alkaline increased	2%	2%
Renal		
Blood creatinine increased	2%	2%
Special senses		
Taste perversion	1%	2%
Vision blurred	1%	2%
Miscellaneous		
Drug level altered	2%	1%

[a] GGT = gamma-glutamyl transferase.

Posaconazole Adverse Reactions (Study 2) (≥ 2%)				
Adverse reaction	Posaconazole (n = 304)	Fluconazole/ Itraconazole (n = 298)	Fluconazole (n = 240)	Itraconazole (n = 58)
Subjects reporting any adverse reaction	34%	34%	30%	52%
Cardiovascular				
QT/QTc prolongation	4%	3%	2%	7%
CNS				
Headache	2%	< 1%	0%	2%
Dermatologic				
Rash	3%	4%	4%	2%
GI				
Abdominal pain	3%	3%	3%	2%
Constipation	1%	2%	3%	0%
Diarrhea	7%	7%	5%	16%
Dyspepsia	2%	1%	1%	0%
Mucositis NOS	2%	0%	0%	0%
Nausea	7%	8%	7%	14%
Vomiting	5%	7%	6%	10%
Hepatic				
ALT increased	2%	2%	2%	2%
AST increased	2%	2%	2%	2%
Bilirubinemia	2%	3%	2%	5%
GGT increased	2%	1%	< 1%	2%
Hepatic enzymes increased	2%	1%	1%	0%
Metabolic/Nutritional				
Hypokalemia	3%	2%	2%	2%

➤*Most common adverse reactions (1%):* The most common treatment-related serious adverse reactions (1% each) in the combined prophylaxis studies were the following:

GI – Nausea, vomiting.

Hepatic – Bilirubinemia, hepatocellular damage, increased hepatic enzymes.

➤*Adverse reactions in HIV-infected subjects with oropharyngeal candidiasis:*

Posaconazole Adverse Reactions in Oropharyngeal Candidiasis Studies (%)			
	Controlled oropharyngeal candidiasis pool		Refractory oropharyngeal candidiasis pool
Adverse reaction	Posaconazole (n = 557)	Fluconazole (n = 262)	Posaconazole (n = 239)
Subjects reporting any adverse reaction[a]	64%	67%	92%
CNS			
Asthenia	2%	2%	13%
Fatigue	3%	5%	13%
Headache	8%	9%	20%
Insomnia	1%	1%	16%
Dermatologic			
Rash	3%	4%	15%
Sweating increased	2%	2%	10%
GI			
Abdominal pain	5%	6%	18%
Anorexia	2%	2%	19%
Diarrhea	10%	13%	29%
Nausea	9%	11%	29%
Vomiting	7%	7%	28%
GU			
Acute renal failure	0%	0%	3%
Hematologic/Lymphatic			
Anemia	2%	2%	14%
Neutropenia	4%	3%	16%
Neutropenia aggravated	0%	0%	2%
Thrombocytopenia	1%	< 1%	5%
Hepatic			
ALT increased	1%	2%	3%
AST increased	1%	2%	3%
Bilirubinemia	1%	1%	3%
Hepatic enzymes increased	< 1%	< 1%	3%
Hepatic function abnormal	1%	2%	0%
Hepatitis	1%	0%	2%
Hepatomegaly	0%	0%	3%
Jaundice	0%	0%	2%
Metabolic/Nutritional			
Dehydration	1%	3%	11%
Hypokalemia	1%	1%	6%
Weight decrease	1%	1%	14%

POSACONAZOLE — ORAL

Posaconazole Adverse Reactions in Oropharyngeal Candidiasis Studies (%)			
	Controlled oropharyngeal candidiasis pool		Refractory oropharyngeal candidiasis pool
Adverse reaction	Posaconazole (n = 557)	Fluconazole (n = 262)	Posaconazole (n = 239)
Respiratory			
Coughing	3%	4%	25%
Dyspnea	1%	3%	12%
Miscellaneous			
Candidiasis, oral	1%	< 1%	12%
Fever	6%	8%	34%
Herpes simplex	3%	3%	11%
Pain	1%	1%	11%
Pneumonia	3%	2%	10%
Rigors	< 1%	2%	12%

[a] Number of subjects reporting treatment-emergent adverse reactions at least once during the study, without regard to relationship to treatment. Subjects may have reported more than 1 reaction.

Posaconazole Oropharyngeal Candidiasis Adverse Reactions (Any Grade; ≥ 2%)			
	Controlled oropharyngeal candidiasis pool		Refractory oropharyngeal candidiasis pool
Adverse reaction	Posaconazole (n = 557)	Fluconazole (n = 262)	Posaconazole (n = 239)
Subjects reporting any adverse reaction[a]	27%	27%	56%
CNS			
Asthenia	1%	1%	3%
Dizziness	2%	2%	3%
Fatigue	1%	2%	3%
Headache	3%	2%	8%
Insomnia	1%	0%	3%
Somnolence	1%	2%	1%
Dermatologic			
Pruritus	1%	1%	2%
Rash	1%	2%	4%
GI			
Abdominal pain	2%	3%	5%
Anorexia	1%	< 1%	3%
Diarrhea	3%	5%	11%
Flatulence	1%	0%	5%
Mouth dry	1%	2%	2%
Nausea	5%	7%	8%
Vomiting	4%	2%	7%
Hematologic/Lymphatic			
Anemia	< 1%	0%	3%
Neutropenia	2%	2%	8%
Thrombocytopenia	1%	0%	2%
Hepatic			
Hepatic enzymes increased	< 1%	0%	2%
Hepatic function abnormal	1%	2%	0%
Metabolic/Nutritional			
Phosphatase alkaline increased	1%	1%	2%
Musculoskeletal			
Myalgia	< 1%	0%	2%
Miscellaneous			
Fever	2%	< 1%	3%

[a] Number of subjects reporting treatment-related adverse reactions at least once during the study, without regard to relationship to treatment. Subjects may have reported more than 1 reaction.

Adverse reactions were reported more frequently in the pool of patients with refractory oropharyngeal candidiasis. Among these highly immunocompromised patients with advanced HIV disease, serious adverse reactions were reported in 55% (132/239). The most commonly reported serious adverse reactions were fever (13%) and neutropenia (10%).

Treatment-related serious adverse reactions were reported for 14% (34/239) of these patients and included neutropenia (5%) and abdominal pain (2%). Posaconazole was discontinued in 2 patients who developed neutropenia that was considered serious and treatment-related. All other reported treatment-related serious adverse reactions occurred in up to 1% of subjects on posaconazole.

➤*Other adverse reactions:* Uncommon and rare treatment-related serious or medically significant adverse reactions reported during clinical trials in prophylaxis, oropharyngeal candidiasis/refractory oropharyngeal candidiasis, or other indications with posaconazole include adrenal insufficiency and allergic and/or hypersensitivity reactions.

Rare cases of hemolytic uremic syndrome, thrombotic thrombocytopenic purpura, and pulmonary embolus have been reported primarily among patients who had been receiving concomitant cyclosporine or tacrolimus for management of transplant rejection or GVHD.

During clinical development there was a single case of torsades de pointes in a patient taking posaconazole. This report involved a seriously ill patient with multiple confounding, potentially contributory risk factors, such as a history of palpitations, recent cardiotoxic chemotherapy, hypokalemia, and hypomagnesemia.

➤*Lab test abnormalities:* In healthy volunteers and patients, elevation of liver function test values did not appear to be associated with higher plasma concentrations of posaconazole. The majority of abnormal liver function tests were minor, transient, and did not lead to discontinuation of therapy.

For the prophylaxis studies, the number of patients with changes in liver function tests from Common Toxicity Criteria grade 0, 1, or 2 at baseline to grade 3 or 4 during the study is presented in the following table.

Posaconazole Lab Test Abnormalities[a]				
	Study 1		Study 2	
Laboratory parameter	Posaconazole (n = 301)	Fluconazole (n = 299)	Posaconazole (n = 304)	Fluconazole/ Itraconazole (n = 298)
Alkaline phosphatase	9/271 (3%)	8/271 (3%)	4/281 (1%)	1/276 (< 1%)
ALT	47/271 (17%)	39/272 (14%)	18/289 (6%)	13/284 (5%)
AST	11/266 (4%)	13/266 (5%)	9/286 (3%)	5/280 (2%)
Bilirubin	24/271 (9%)	20/275 (7%)	20/290 (7%)	25/285 (9%)

[a] Change from grade 0 to 2 at baseline to grade 3 or 4 during the study. These data are presented in the form X/Y, where X represents the number of patients who met the criterion as indicated, and Y represents the number of patients who had a baseline observation and at least 1 postbaseline observation.

The number of patients treated for oropharyngeal candidiasis with clinically significant liver function test abnormalities at any time during the studies is provided in the following table (liver function test abnormalities were present in some of these patients prior to initiation of the study drug).

Clinically Significant Laboratory Test Abnormalities Without Regard to Baseline Value			
	Controlled		Refractory
Laboratory test	Posaconazole (n = 557)	Fluconazole (n = 262)	Posaconazole (n = 239)
ALT > 3 × ULN[a]	16/537 (3%)	13/254 (5%)	25/226 (11%)
AST > 3 × ULN	33/537 (6%)	26/254 (10%)	39/223 (17%)
Total bilirubin > 1.5 × ULN	15/536 (3%)	5/254 (2%)	9/197 (5%)
Alkaline phosphatase > 3 × ULN	17/535 (3%)	15/253 (6%)	24/190 (13%)

[a] ULN = upper limit of normal.

Overdosage

During the clinical trials, some patients received posaconazole up to 1,600 mg/day with no adverse reactions noted that were different from the lower doses. In addition, accidental overdose was noted in 1 patient who took 1,200 mg twice daily for 3 days. No related adverse reactions were noted by the investigator. Posaconazole is not removed by hemodialysis.

Patient Information

Advise patients to take each dose of posaconazole oral suspension with a full meal or liquid nutritional supplement in order to enhance absorption; inform their health care provider if they develop severe diarrhea or vomiting because these conditions may change blood levels of posaconazole and inform their health care provider if they are taking or planning to take other drugs because certain drugs can change blood levels.

FLUCONAZOLE

Rx	**Fluconazole** (Various, eg, Greenstone, Ivax, Ranbaxy, Sandoz, Teva)	**Tablets:** 50 mg	May contain lactose. In 30s, 100s, 500s, and UD 100s.
Rx	**Diflucan** (Pfizer)		Lactose. (Diflucan 50 Roerig). Pink, trapezoid shape. In 30s.
Rx	**Fluconazole** (Various, eg, Greenstone, Ivax, Ranbaxy, Sandoz, Teva)	**Tablets:** 100 mg	May contain lactose. In 30s, 100s, 500s, and UD 100s.
Rx	**Diflucan** (Pfizer)		Lactose. (Diflucan 100 Roerig). Pink, trapezoid shape. In 30s and UD 100s.
Rx	**Fluconazole** (Various, eg, Greenstone, Ivax, Ranbaxy, Sandoz, Teva)	**Tablets:** 150 mg	May contain lactose. In UD 1s and 12s.
Rx	**Diflucan** (Pfizer)		Lactose. (Diflucan 150 Roerig). Pink, oval. In UD 1s.
Rx	**Fluconazole** (Various, eg, Greenstone, Ivax, Ranbaxy, Sandoz, Teva)	**Tablets:** 200 mg	May contain lactose. In 30s, 100s, 500s, and UD 100s.
Rx	**Diflucan** (Pfizer)		Lactose. (Diflucan 200 Roerig). Pink, trapezoid shape. In 30s and UD 100s.
Rx	**Fluconazole** (Various, eg, Greenstone, Ranbaxy)	**Powder for oral suspension:** 10 mg/mL when reconstituted	May contain sucrose. In 35 mL.
Rx	**Diflucan** (Pfizer)		Sucrose. Orange flavor. In 35 mL.
Rx	**Fluconazole** (Various, eg, Greenstone, Ranbaxy)	**Powder for oral suspension:** 40 mg/mL when reconstituted	May contain sucrose. In 35 mL.
Rx	**Diflucan** (Pfizer)		Sucrose. Orange flavor. In 35 mL.
Rx	**Fluconazole** (Various, eg, Greenstone, Hospira, Mayne, West-Ward Pharmaceutical Corp.)	**Injection:** 2 mg/mL	In 100 and 200 mL.

[a] Contains 9 mg/mL NaCl.

[b] Contains 56 mg/mL dextrose, hydrous.

FLUCONAZOLE — ORAL

Indications

➤*Vaginal candidiasis:* Vaginal yeast infections caused by *Candida*.

➤*Oropharyngeal and esophageal candidiasis:* In open, noncomparative studies of relatively small numbers of patients, fluconazole was also effective for the treatment of *Candida* urinary tract infections, peritonitis, and systemic *Candida* infections including candidemia, disseminated candidiasis, and pneumonia.

➤*Cryptococcal meningitis:* Treatment of cryptococcal meningitis.

➤*Prophylaxis:* Fluconazole is also indicated to decrease the incidence of candidiasis in patients undergoing bone marrow transplantation who receive cytotoxic chemotherapy or radiation therapy.

Administration and Dosage

➤*Maximum dose:*

Children – The following maximum doses are according to the prescribing information:

Cryptococcal meningitis, esophageal candidiasis, oropharyngeal candidiasis, systemic Candida infections: 600 mg/day.

➤*General dosing considerations:* Because oral absorption is rapid and almost complete, the daily dose of fluconazole is the same for oral (tablets and suspension) and intravenous (IV) administration. In general, a loading dose of twice the daily dose is recommended on the first day of therapy to result in plasma concentrations close to steady state by the second day of therapy.

The daily dose of fluconazole for the treatment of infections other than vaginal candidiasis should be based on the infecting organism and the patient's response to therapy. Treatment should be continued until clinical parameters or laboratory tests indicate that active fungal infection has subsided. An inadequate period of treatment may lead to recurrence of active infection. Patients with AIDS and cryptococcal meningitis or recurrent oropharyngeal candidiasis usually require maintenance therapy to prevent relapse.

➤*Adults:*

Cryptococcal meningitis –

Usual dosage: 400 mg on the first day, followed by 200 mg once daily. A dosage of 400 mg once daily may be used based on medical judgment of the patient's response to therapy.

Duration of therapy: 10 to 12 weeks after the cerebrospinal fluid becomes culture negative.

Suppression of relapse in patients with AIDS: 200 mg once daily.

Esophageal candidiasis –

Usual dosage: 200 mg on the first day, followed by 100 mg once daily. Doses of up to 400 mg/day may be used based on medical judgment of the patient's response to therapy.

Duration of therapy: A minimum of 3 weeks and for at least 2 weeks following resolution of symptoms.

Oropharyngeal candidiasis –

Usual dosage: 200 mg on the first day, followed by 100 mg once daily.

Duration of therapy: Clinical evidence of oropharyngeal candidiasis generally resolves within several days, but treatment should be continued for at least 2 weeks to decrease the likelihood of relapse.

Peritonitis – Doses of 50 to 200 mg/day have been used in open, noncomparative studies of small numbers of patients.

Prophylaxis in patients undergoing bone marrow transplantation –

Usual dosage: 400 mg once daily.

Duration of therapy: Patients who are anticipated to have severe granulocytopenia (less than 500 neutrophils/mm^3) should start fluconazole prophylaxis several days before the anticipated onset of neutropenia and continue for 7 days after the neutrophil count rises above 1,000 cells/mm^3.

Systemic Candida infections – Doses of up to 400 mg daily have been used in open, noncomparative studies of small numbers of patients. For systemic *Candida* infections, including candidemia, disseminated candidiasis, and pneumonia, optimal therapeutic dosage and duration of therapy have not been established.

Urinary tract infections – Doses of 50 to 200 mg/day have been used in open, noncomparative studies of small numbers of patients.

Vaginal candidiasis – 150 mg as a single dose.

➤*Children:*

Equivalent Fluconazole Dosage in Children vs Adults	
Children	Adults
3 mg/kg	100 mg
6 mg/kg	200 mg
12 mg/kg[a]	400 mg

[a] Some older children may have clearances similar to those of older adults. Absolute doses exceeding 600 mg/day are not recommended.

Experience with fluconazole in neonates is limited to pharmacokinetic studies in premature newborns (see Pharmacokinetics). Based on the prolonged half-life seen in premature newborns (gestational age, 26 to 29 weeks), in the first 2 weeks of life these children should receive the same dosage (mg/kg) as older children, but it should be administered every 72 hours. After the first 2 weeks, these children should be dosed once daily. No information regarding fluconazole pharmacokinetics in full-term newborns is available.

Cryptococcal meningitis –

Usual dosage: 12 mg/kg on the first day, followed by 6 mg/kg once daily. A dosage of 12 mg/kg once daily may be used based on medical judgment of the patient's response to therapy.

Duration of therapy: The recommended duration of treatment for initial therapy is 10 to 12 weeks after the cerebrospinal fluid becomes culture negative.

Suppression of relapse in patients with AIDS: 6 mg/kg once daily.

FLUCONAZOLE — ORAL

Esophageal candidiasis –

Usual dosage: 6 mg/kg on the first day, followed by 3 mg/kg once daily. Doses of up to 12 mg/kg/day may be used based on medical judgment of the patient's response to therapy.

Duration of therapy: Patients should be treated for a minimum of 3 weeks and for at least 2 weeks following the resolution of symptoms.

Oropharyngeal candidiasis –

Usual dosage: 6 mg/kg on the first day, followed by 3 mg/kg once daily.

Duration of therapy: Treatment should be administered for at least 2 weeks to decrease the likelihood of relapse.

Systemic Candida infections –

Usual dosage: Daily doses of 6 to 12 mg/kg/day have been used in an open, noncomparative study of a small number of children for the treatment of candidemia and disseminated *Candida* infections.

Premature neonates (gestational age, 26 to 29 weeks) – For the first 2 weeks of life, these children should receive the same dosage as older children, but it should be administered every 72 hours. After the first 2 weeks of life, these children should be dosed once daily.

➤*Renal function impairment:*

Adults – Fluconazole is cleared primarily by renal excretion as unchanged drug. There is no need to adjust single dose therapy for vaginal candidiasis because of renal function impairment. In patients with renal function impairment who will receive multiple doses of fluconazole, an initial loading dose of 50 to 400 mg should be given. After the loading dose, the daily dose (according to indication) should be based on the following table.

These are suggested dose adjustments based on pharmacokinetics following administration of multiple doses. Further adjustment may be needed depending on clinical condition.

Fluconazole Dose in Patients with Renal Impairment

CrCl[a] (mL/min)	Percent of recommended dose
> 50	100%
≤ 50 (no dialysis)	50%
Regular dialysis	100% after each dialysis

[a] CrCl = creatinine clearance.

$$\text{Males: } \frac{\text{Weight (kg)} \times (140 - \text{age})}{72 \times \text{serum creatinine (mg/dL)}} = \text{CrCl}$$

Females: $0.85 \times$ male value

➤*Storage/Stability:* Store tablets and powder for oral suspension below 30°C (86°F). Store reconstituted suspension between 5° and 30°C (41° and 86°F) and discard unused portion after 2 weeks. Protect from freezing.

Actions

➤*Pharmacology:* Fluconazole is a highly selective inhibitor of fungal cytochrome P-450 sterol C-14 alpha-demethylation. Mammalian cell demethylation is much less sensitive to fluconazole inhibition. The subsequent loss of normal sterols correlates with the accumulation of 14 alpha-methyl sterols in fungi and may be responsible for the fungistatic activity of fluconazole.

➤*Pharmacokinetics:*

Absorption/Distribution – The pharmacokinetic properties of fluconazole are similar following administration by the intravenous or oral routes. In healthy volunteers, the bioavailability of orally administered fluconazole is greater than 90% compared with intravenous administration. Bioequivalence was established between the 100 mg tablet and both suspension strengths when administered as a single 200 mg dose.

Peak plasma concentrations (C_{max}) in fasted healthy volunteers occur between 1 and 2 hours. In fasted healthy volunteers, administration of a single oral 400 mg dose of fluconazole leads to a mean C_{max} of 6.72 mcg/mL (range, 4.12 to 8.08 mcg/mL) and after single oral doses of 50 to 400 mg, fluconazole plasma concentrations and AUC (area under the plasma concentration-time curve) are dose proportional.

Administration of a single oral 150 mg tablet of fluconazole to 10 lactating women resulted in a mean C_{max} of 2.61 mcg/mL (range, 1.57 to 3.65 mcg/mL).

Steady state concentrations are reached within 5 to 10 days following oral doses of 50 to 400 mg given once daily. Administration of a loading dose (on day 1) of twice the usual daily dose results in plasma concentrations close to steady-state by the second day. The apparent volume of distribution of fluconazole approximates that of total body water. Plasma protein binding is low (11% to 12%). Following either single- or multiple-oral doses for up to 14 days, fluconazole penetrates into all body fluids studied. In healthy volunteers, saliva concentrations of fluconazole were equal to or slightly greater than plasma concentrations regardless of dose, route, or duration of dosing. In patients with bronchiectasis, sputum concentrations of fluconazole following a single 150 mg oral dose were equal to plasma concentrations at both 4 and 24 hours post dose. In patients with fungal meningitis, fluconazole concentrations in the CSF are approximately 80% of the corresponding plasma concentrations.

Metabolism/Excretion – In healthy volunteers, fluconazole is cleared primarily by renal excretion, with approximately 80% of the administered dose appearing in the urine as unchanged drug. About 11% of the dose is excreted in the urine as metabolites.

Clearance corrected for body weight was not affected by age in these studies. Mean body clearance in adults is reported to be 0.23 (17%) mL/min/kg.

Fluconazole has a terminal plasma elimination half-life of approximately 30 hours (range, 20 to 50 hours) after oral administration.

Special populations –

Renal function impairment: The pharmacokinetics of fluconazole are markedly affected by reduction in renal function. There is an inverse relationship between the elimination half-life and creatinine clearance. The dose of fluconazole may need to be reduced in patients with impaired renal function. A 3-hour hemodialysis session decreases plasma concentrations by approximately 50%.

Premature newborns: In premature newborns (gestational age 26 to 29 weeks), the mean (% cv) clearance within 36 hours of birth was 0.18 (35%, n = 7) mL/min/kg, which increased with time to a mean of 0.218 (31%, n = 9) mL/min/kg 6 days later and 0.333 (56%, n = 4) mL/min/kg 12 days later. Similarly, the half-life was 73.6 hours, which decreased with time to a mean of 53.2 hours 6 days later and 46.6 hours 12 days later.

➤*Microbiology:* Fluconazole exhibits in vitro activity against *Cryptococcus neoformans* and *Candida* spp. Fungistatic activity has also been demonstrated in normal and immunocompromised animal models for systemic and intracranial fungal infections due to *Cryptococcus neoformans* and for systemic infections due to *Candida albicans*.

In common with other azole antifungal agents, most fungi show a higher apparent sensitivity to fluconazole in vivo than in vitro. Fluconazole administered orally or intravenously was active in a variety of animal models of fungal infection using standard laboratory strains of fungi. Activity has been demonstrated against fungal infections caused by *Aspergillus flavus*and *Aspergillus fumigatus* in normal mice. Fluconazole has also been shown to be active in animal models of endemic mycoses, including one model of *Blastomyces dermatitidis* pulmonary infections in normal mice; one model of *Coccidioides immitis* intracranial infections in normal mice; and several models of *Histoplasma capsulatum* pulmonary infection in normal and immunosuppressed mice. The clinical significance of results obtained in these studies is unknown.

Contraindications

Hypersensitivity to fluconazole or to any of its excipients. There is no information regarding cross-hypersensitivity between fluconazole and other azole antifungal agents. Caution should be used in prescribing fluconazole to patients with hypersensitivity to other azoles. Coadministration with terfenadine or cisapride (see Drug Interactions).

Warnings/Precautions

➤*Hepatic injury:* Fluconazole has been associated with rare cases of serious hepatic toxicity, including fatalities primarily in patients with serious underlying medical conditions. In cases of fluconazole-associated hepatotoxicity, no obvious relationship to total daily dose, duration of therapy, sex or age of the patient has been observed. Fluconazole hepatotoxicity has usually, but not always, been reversible on discontinuation of therapy. Patients who develop abnormal liver function tests during fluconazole therapy should be monitored for the development of more severe hepatic injury. Fluconazole should be discontinued if clinical signs and symptoms consistent with liver disease develop that may be attributable to fluconazole.

➤*Dermatologic disorders:* Patients have rarely developed exfoliative skin disorders during treatment with fluconazole. In patients with serious underlying diseases (predominantly AIDS and malignancy), these have rarely resulted in a fatal outcome. Patients who develop rashes during treatment with fluconazole should be monitored closely and the drug discontinued if lesions progress.

➤*Vaginal candidiasis:* The convenience and efficacy of the single dose oral tablet of fluconazole regimen for the treatment of vaginal yeast infections should be weighed against the acceptability of a higher incidence of drug-related adverse events with fluconazole (26%) versus intravaginal agents (16%) in US comparative clinical studies (see Drug interactions, and Adverse reactions).

➤*Hypersensitivity reactions:* In rare cases, anaphylaxis has been reported.

➤*Pregnancy: Category C.* Fluconazole was administered orally to pregnant rabbits during organogenesis in 2 studies, at 5, 10, and 20 mg/kg and at 5, 25, and 75 mg/kg, respectively. Maternal weight gain was impaired at all dose levels, and abortions occurred at 75 mg/kg (≈ 20 to 60 times the recommended human dose); no adverse fetal effects were detected. In several studies in which pregnant rats were treated orally with fluconazole during organogenesis, maternal weight gain was impaired and placental weights were increased at 25 mg/kg. There were no fetal effects at 5 or 10 mg/kg; increases in fetal anatomical variants (supernumerary ribs, renal pelvis dilation) and delays in ossification were observed at 25 and 50 mg/kg and higher doses. At doses ranging from 80 mg/kg (≈ 20 to 60 times the recommended human dose) to 320 mg/kg embryolethality in rats was increased and fetal abnormalities included wavy ribs, cleft palate, and abnormal cranio-facial ossification. These effects are consistent with the inhibition of estrogen synthesis in rats and may be a result of known effects of lowered estrogen on pregnancy, organogenesis, and parturition.

There are no adequate and well-controlled studies in pregnant women. There have been reports of multiple congenital abnormalities in infants whose mothers were being treated for 3 or more months with high dose (400 to 800 mg/day) fluconazole therapy for coccidioidomycosis (an unindicated use). The relationship between fluconazole use and these events is unclear. Fluconazole should be used in pregnancy only if the potential benefit justifies the possible risk to the fetus.

➤*Lactation:* Fluconazole is secreted in human milk at concentrations similar to plasma. Therefore, the use of fluconazole in nursing mothers is not recommended.

FLUCONAZOLE — ORAL

➤*Children:* An open-label, randomized, controlled trial has shown fluconazole to be effective in the treatment of oropharyngeal candidiasis in children 6 months to 13 years of age.

The use of fluconazole in children with cryptococcal meningitis, *Candida* esophagitis, or systemic *Candida* infections is supported by the efficacy shown for these indications in adults and by the results from several small noncomparative pediatric clinical studies. In addition, pharmacokinetic studies in children (see Pharmacokinetics) have established a dose proportionality between children and adults (see Administration and Dosage).

Efficacy of fluconazole has not been established in infants younger than 6 months of age. A small number of patients (29) ranging in age from 1 day to 6 months have been treated safely with fluconazole.

Drug Interactions

➤*QT prolongation:* An additive effect of fluconazole with other drugs that prolong the QT interval cannot be excluded. The following drugs may prolong the QT interval and increase the risk of life-threatening cardiac arrhythmias, including torsade de pointes: Antiarrhythmic agents (eg, amiodarone, bretylium, disopyramide, dofetilide, procainamide, quinidine, and sotalol), arsenic trioxide, chlorpromazine, cisapride, dolasetron, droperidol, mefloquine, mesoridazine, moxifloxacin, pentamidine, pimozide, tacrolimus, thioridazine, and ziprasidone. For a more complete list of drugs that may prolong the QT interval, see the appendix, Drug-Induced Prolongation of the QT Interval and Torsade de Pointes.

Fluconazole Drug Interactions

Precipitant drug	Object drug[a]		Description
Cimetidine	Fluconazole	↓	Cimetidine resulted in a reduction in fluconazole AUC and C_{max}.
Hydrochlorothiazide	Fluconazole	↑	Concomitant use resulted in a significant increase in fluconazole C_{max} and AUC, which can be attributed to reduced renal clearance.
Rifampin	Fluconazole	↓	Rifampin enhances the metabolism of concurrently administered fluconazole. Depending on the clinical circumstances, give consideration when increasing the dose of fluconazole when administered with rifampin.
Fluconazole	Alfentanil	↑	The pharmacologic and adverse effects of alfentanil may be increased. Possible inhibition of alfentanil metabolism (CYP3A4) by fluconazole may occur. Monitor for prolonged or recurrent respiratory depression. It may be necessary to administer a lower dose of alfentanil.
Fluconazole	Benzodiazepines	↑	Increased and prolonged serum levels, CNS depression, and psychomotor impairment with certain benzodiazepines may occur, possibly lasting for several days after stopping fluconazole.
Fluconazole	Buspirone	↑	Plasma buspirone concentrations may be elevated because of inhibition of buspirone metabolism. The pharmacologic and adverse effects of buspirone may be increased. Adjust the dose of buspirone as needed.
Fluconazole	Carbamazepine	↑	Plasma concentrations of carbamazepine may be elevated, increasing clinical and adverse effects because of possible inhibition of carbamazepine metabolism (CYP3A4) by fluconazole. Monitor carbamazepine concentrations.
Fluconazole	Cisapride	↑	Concurrent use may increase cisapride concentrations and cardiotoxicity may occur. Coadministration is contraindicated.

Fluconazole Drug Interactions

Precipitant drug	Object drug[a]		Description
Fluconazole	Contraceptives, oral	↔	Concurrent use with an OC containing ethinyl estradiol/levonorgestrel produced an overall mean increase in the levels of the OC components; however, in some cases there were decreases ≤ 47% and 33% of ethinyl estradiol and levonorgestrel levels, respectively.
Fluconazole	Corticosteroids	↑	The effects of corticosteroids may be enhanced, resulting in increased toxicity because of inhibition of corticosteroid metabolism. Adjust corticosteroid dose as needed.
Fluconazole	Cyclosporine	↑	Significant increases in cyclosporine C_{max}, C_{min}, and AUC values and a significant decrease in oral clearance occurred following fluconazole use.
Fluconazole	Haloperidol	↑	Concurrent use may increase haloperidol plasma concentrations, increasing the risk of side effects. Adjust haloperidol dose as needed.
Fluconazole	HMG-CoA reductase inhibitors	↑	Coadministration causes increased plasma levels of the HMG-CoA reductase inhibitors. Rhabdomyolysis has been reported. If concurrent use can not be avoided, consider reducing the dose of the HMG-CoA reductase inhibitor. Pravastatin levels appear to be the least affected by concurrent use.
Fluconazole	Losartan	↑	The antihypertensive and adverse effects of losartan may be increased because of possible inhibition of metabolism (CYP2D9) of losartan by fluconazole. Monitor blood pressure.
Fluconazole	Nisoldipine	↑	Serum nisoldipine concentrations may be elevated, increasing pharmacologic and adverse effects. Fluconazole, especially > 200 mg/day, may inhibit CYP3A4.
Fluconazole	Phenytoin	↑	Coadministration resulted in an increase of phenytoin AUC values. Monitor phenytoin levels and adjust dose as needed.
Fluconazole	Protease inhibitors	↑	Concurrent use may elevate protease inhibitor levels, increasing the risk of toxicity. Adjust protease inhibitor dose as needed.
Fluconazole	Rifabutin	↑	Coadministration may increase rifabutin levels. Cases of uveitis have been reported in patients receiving both drugs. Monitor closely.
Fluconazole	Sirolimus	↑	Plasma sirolimus concentrations may be elevated because of an inhibition of sirolimus gut metabolism.
Fluconazole	Sulfonylureas	↑	Fluconazole reduces the metabolism of sulfonylureas and increases the plasma concentrations of these agents. Carefully monitor blood glucose concentrations and adjust the sulfonylurea dose as necessary when these agents are coadministered.
Fluconazole	Tacrolimus	↑	There have been reports of nephrotoxicity in patients when these agents were coadministered. Carefully monitor.
Fluconazole	Theophylline	↑	Theophylline AUC, C_{max}, and half-life were significantly increased, and clearance was decreased.

FLUCONAZOLE — ORAL

Fluconazole Drug Interactions			
Precipitant drug	Object drug[a]		Description
Fluconazole	Tolterodine	⬆	Concurrent use may increase tolterodine plasma levels. Adjust tolterodine dose as needed. Do not give more than 1 mg of tolterodine twice daily when coadministered with azole antifungals.
Fluconazole	Tricyclic antidepressants (ie, amitriptyline, nortriptyline)	⬆	Serum tricyclic antidepressant (TCA) concentrations may be elevated, resulting in an increase in therapeutic and adverse effects including cardiac arrhythmia. Inhibition of TCA metabolism is suspected (CYP2C9 by fluconazole). Adjust the TCA dose as needed.
Fluconazole	Vinca alkaloids (eg, vincristine)	⬆	The risk of vinca alkaloid toxicity (eg, constipation, myalgia, neutropenia) may be increased. Avoid coadministration of these agents whenever possible.
Fluconazole	Warfarin	⬆	The anticoagulant effect of warfarin may be increased. A single warfarin dose after 14 days of fluconazole resulted in an increase in the PT response. Monitor PT and INR frequently.
Fluconazole	Zidovudine	⬆	There was a significant increase in zidovudine AUC following fluconazole administration.
Fluconazole	Zolpidem	⬆	Plasma concentrations and therapeutic effects of zolpidem may be increased. The dose of zolpidem may need to be decreased during coadministration of azole antifungal agents.

[a] ⬆ = object drug increased; ⬇ = object drug decreased; ⬌ = undetermined clinical effect.

Adverse Reactions

➤*Patients receiving multiple doses for other infections:* Sixteen percent of over 4000 patients treated with fluconazole in clinical trials of 7 days or more experienced adverse reactions. Treatment was discontinued in 1.5% of patients due to adverse clinical events and in 1.3% of patients due to laboratory test abnormalities.

Clinical adverse events were reported more frequently in HIV infected patients (21%) than in non-HIV infected patients (13%); however, the patterns in HIV infected and non-HIV infected patients were similar. The proportions of patients discontinuing therapy due to clinical adverse events were similar in the 2 groups (1.5%).

The following treatment-related clinical adverse events occurred at an incidence of 1% or greater in 4048 patients receiving fluconazole for 7 or more days in clinical trials: Nausea 3.7%, headache 1.9%, skin rash 1.8%, vomiting 1.7%, abdominal pain 1.7%, diarrhea 1.5%.

The following adverse events have occurred under conditions where a causal association is probable.

Allergic – In rare cases, anaphylaxis has been reported.

Hepatic – In combined clinical trials and marketing experience, there have been rare cases of serious hepatic reactions during treatment with fluconazole (see Warnings). The spectrum of these hepatic reactions has ranged from mild transient elevations in transaminases to clinical hepatitis, cholestasis, and fulminant hepatic failure, including fatalities. Instances of fatal hepatic reactions were noted to occur primarily in patients with serious underlying medical conditions (predominantly AIDS or malignancy) and often while taking multiple concomitant medications. Transient hepatic reactions, including hepatitis and jaundice, have occurred among patients with no other identifiable risk factors. In each of these cases, liver function returned to baseline on discontinuation of fluconazole.

➤*Adverse reactions with an unknown relationship to fluconazole:* The following adverse events have occurred under conditions where a causal association is uncertain.

CNS – Seizures.

Dermatologic – Exfoliative skin disorders including Stevens-Johnson syndrome and toxic epidermal necrolysis (see Warnings), alopecia.

Hematologic/Lymphatic – Leukopenia, including neutropenia and agranulocytosis, thrombocytopenia.

Metabolic – Hypercholesterolemia, hypertriglyceridemia, hypokalemia.

➤*Children:* In Phase II/III clinical trials conducted in the United States and in Europe, 577 pediatric patients, ages 1 day to 17 years were treated with fluconazole at doses up to 15 mg/kg/day for up to 1616 days. Thirteen percent of children experienced treatment related adverse events. The most commonly reported events were vomiting (5%), abdominal pain (3%), nausea (2%), and diarrhea (2%). Treatment was discontinued in 2.3% of patients due to adverse clinical events and in 1.4% of patients due to laboratory test abnormalities. The majority of treatment-related laboratory abnormalities were elevations of transaminases or alkaline phosphatase.

Fluconazole Adverse Reactions in Children		
Adverse reaction	Percentage of patients with treatment-related side effects fluconazole (n = 577)	Comparative agents (n = 451)
With any side effect	13%	9.3%
Vomiting	5.4%	5.1%
Abdominal pain	2.8%	1.6%
Nausea	2.3%	1.6%
Diarrhea	2.1%	2.2%

Overdosage

➤*Symptoms:* There has been 1 reported case of overdosage with fluconazole. A 42-year-old patient infected with human immunodeficiency virus developed hallucinations and exhibited paranoid behavior after reportedly ingesting 8200 mg of fluconazole. The patient was admitted to the hospital, and his condition resolved within 48 hours.

➤*Treatment:* In the event of overdose, symptomatic treatment (with supportive measures and gastric lavage if clinically indicated) should be instituted.

Fluconazole is largely excreted in urine. A 3-hour hemodialysis session decreases plasma levels by ≈ 50%.

In mice and rats receiving very high doses of fluconazole, clinical effects in both species included decreased motility and respiration, ptosis, lacrimation, salivation, urinary incontinence, loss of righting reflex, and cyanosis; death was sometimes preceded by clonic convulsions.

FLUCONAZOLE — INJECTION

Indications

➤*Vaginal candidiasis:* Vaginal yeast infections caused by *Candida*.

➤*Oropharyngeal and esophageal candidiasis:* In open noncomparative studies of relatively small numbers of patients, fluconazole was also effective for the treatment of *Candida* urinary tract infections, peritonitis, and systemic *Candida* infections including candidemia, disseminated candidiasis, and pneumonia.

➤*Cryptococcal meningitis:* Treatment of cryptococcal meningitis.

➤*Prophylaxis:* Fluconazole is also indicated to decrease the incidence of candidiasis in patients undergoing bone marrow transplantation who receive cytotoxic chemotherapy or radiation therapy.

Administration and Dosage

➤*Maximum dose:*

Children – The following maximum doses are according to the prescribing information:

Cryptococcal meningitis, esophageal candidiasis, oropharyngeal candidiasis, systemic Candidainfections: 600 mg/day.

➤*General dosing considerations:* Because oral absorption is rapid and almost complete, the daily dose of fluconazole is the same for oral (tablets and suspension) and intravenous (IV) administration. In general, a loading dose of twice the daily dose is recommended on the first day of therapy to result in plasma concentrations close to steady-state by the second day of therapy.

The daily dose of fluconazole should be based on the infecting organism and the patient's response to therapy. Treatment should be continued until clinical parameters or laboratory tests indicate that active fungal infection has subsided. An inadequate period of treatment may lead to recurrence of active infection. Patients with AIDS and cryptococcal meningitis or recurrent oropharyngeal candidiasis usually require maintenance therapy to prevent relapse.

➤*Adults:*

Cryptococcal meningitis –

Usual dosage: 400 mg IV on the first day, followed by 200 mg IV once daily. A dosage of 400 mg IV once daily may be used based on medical judgment of the patient's response to therapy.

Duration of therapy: 10 to 12 weeks after the cerebrospinal fluid becomes culture negative.

Suppression of relapse in patients with AIDS: 200 mg IV once daily.

Esophageal candidiasis –

Usual dosage: 200 mg IV on the first day, followed by 100 mg IV once daily. Doses of up to 400 mg/day may be used based on medical judgment of the patient's response to therapy.

Duration of therapy: Patients should be treated for a minimum of 3 weeks and for at least 2 weeks following resolution of symptoms.

FLUCONAZOLE — INJECTION

Oropharyngeal candidiasis –

Usual dosage: 200 mg IV on the first day, followed by 100 mg IV once daily.

Duration of therapy: Clinical evidence of oropharyngeal candidiasis generally resolves within several days, but treatment should be continued for at least 2 weeks to decrease the likelihood of relapse.

Peritonitis – Doses of 50 to 200 mg/day IV have been used in open, noncomparative studies of small numbers of patients.

Prophylaxis in patients undergoing bone marrow transplantation –

Usual dosage: 400 mg IV once daily.

Duration of therapy: Patients who are anticipated to have severe granulocytopenia (less than 500 neutrophils/mm^3) should start fluconazole prophylaxis several days before the anticipated onset of neutropenia and continue for 7 days after the neutrophil count rises above 1,000 cells/mm^3.

Systemic Candida infections – Doses of up to 400 mg IV daily have been used in open, noncomparative studies of small numbers of patients. For systemic *Candida* infections, including candidemia, disseminated candidiasis, and pneumonia, optimal therapeutic dosage and duration of therapy have not been established.

Urinary tract infections – Doses of 50 to 200 mg/day IV have been used in open, noncomparative studies of small numbers of patients.

➤*Children:*

Equivalent Fluconazole Dosage in Children vs Adults

Children	Adults
3 mg/kg	100 mg
6 mg/kg	200 mg
12 mg/kg[a]	400 mg

[a] Some older children may have clearances similar to those of older adults. Absolute doses exceeding 600 mg/day are not recommended.

Cryptococcal meningitis –

Usual dosage: 12 mg/kg IV on the first day, followed by 6 mg/kg IV once daily. A dosage of 12 mg/kg IV once daily may be used based on medical judgment of the patient's response to therapy.

Duration of therapy: The recommended duration of treatment for initial therapy is 10 to 12 weeks after the cerebrospinal fluid becomes culture negative.

Suppression of relapse in patients with AIDS: 6 mg/kg IV once daily.

Esophageal candidiasis –

Usual dosage: 6 mg/kg IV on the first day, followed by 3 mg/kg IV once daily. Doses of up to 12 mg/kg/day may be used based on medical judgment of the patient's response to therapy.

Duration of therapy: Patients should be treated for a minimum of 3 weeks and for at least 2 weeks following the resolution of symptoms.

Oropharyngeal candidiasis –

Usual dosage: 6 mg/kg IV on the first day, followed by 3 mg/kg IV once daily.

Duration of therapy: Treatment should be administered for at least 2 weeks to decrease the likelihood of relapse.

Systemic Candida infections –

Usual dosage: 6 to 12 mg/kg/day IV has been used in an open, noncomparative study of a small number of children.

Premature neonates (gestational age, 26 to 29 weeks) – For the first 2 weeks of life, these children should receive the same dosage (mg/kg) as older children, but it should be administered every 72 hours. After the first 2 weeks, these children should be dosed once daily.

➤*Renal function impairment:*

Adults – Fluconazole is cleared primarily by renal excretion as unchanged drug. There is no need to adjust single-dose therapy for vaginal candidiasis because of impaired renal function. In patients with impaired renal function who will receive multiple doses of fluconazole, an initial loading dose of 50 to 400 mg should be given. After the loading dose, the daily dose (according to indication) should be based on the following table.

These are suggested dose adjustments based on pharmacokinetics following administration of multiple doses. Further adjustment may be needed, depending on clinical condition.

Fluconazole Dose in Patients with Renal Impairment

CrCl[a] (mL/min)	Percent of recommended dose
> 50	100%
≤ 50 (no dialysis)	50%
Regular dialysis	100% after each dialysis

[a] CrCl = creatinine clearance.

Continuous renal replacement therapy (CRRT): One reference suggests a dosage of 200 to 400 mg IV every 24 hours.

The following alternative recommendations assume ultrafiltration and dialysis flow rates of 1 to 2 L/h.

- *Loading dose* – 400 to 800 mg IV.
- *Maintenance dosage* –
  - *Continuous venovenous hemofiltration (CVVH):* 200 to 400 mg IV every 24 hours.
  - *Continuous venovenous hemodialysis (CVVHD):* 400 to 800 mg IV every 24 hours.
  - *Continuous venovenous hemodialfiltration (CVVHDF):* 800 mg IV every 24 hours. An alternative dosage is 500 to 600 mg IV every 12 hours.

Intermittent hemodialysis (IHD): As an alternative dosage to the dosage listed in the previous table, administer 200 to 400 mg IV every 48 to 72 hours or 100 to 200 mg IV every 24 hours. Doses should be administered after the dialysis session. These recommendations assume the patient is receiving standard IHD 3 times per week and completes the full dialysis sessions.

Continuous ambulatory peritoneal dialysis: Give 50% of the usual dose.

Children – Although the pharmacokinetics of fluconazole have not been studied in children with renal insufficiency, dosage reduction in children with renal insufficiency should parallel that recommended for adults. The following formula may be used to estimate CrCl in children (where K = 0.55 for children older than 1 year of age and 0.45 for infants):

$$\text{CrCl (mL/min/1.73 m}^2) = K \times \frac{\text{body length or height (cm)}}{\text{serum creatinine (mg/dL)}}$$

➤*Administration:* Fluconazole injection has been used safely for up to 14 days of IV therapy. The IV infusion of fluconazole should be administered at a maximum rate of approximately 200 mg/h, given as a continuous infusion.

Fluconazole injections in glass and *Viaflex Plus* plastic containers are only intended for IV administration using sterile equipment.

Do not use if the solution is cloudy or precipitated or if the seal is not intact.

➤*Storage/Stability:* Store fluconazole injections in glass bottles between 5° and 30°C (41° and 86°F). Protect from freezing.

Store fluconazole injections in *Viaflex Plus* plastic containers between 5° and 25°C (41° and 77°F). Brief exposure of up to 40°C (104°F) does not adversely affect the product. Protect from freezing.

Actions

➤*Pharmacology:* Fluconazole is a highly selective inhibitor of fungal cytochrome P-450 sterol C-14 alpha-demethylation. Mammalian cell demethylation is much less sensitive to fluconazole inhibition. The subsequent loss of normal sterols correlates with the accumulation of 14 alpha-methyl sterols in fungi and may be responsible for the fungistatic activity of fluconazole.

➤*Pharmacokinetics:*

Absorption/Distribution – The pharmacokinetic properties of fluconazole are similar following administration by the intravenous or oral routes. In healthy volunteers, the bioavailability of orally administered fluconazole is greater than 90% compared with intravenous administration. Bioequivalence was established between the 100 mg tablet and both suspension strengths when administered as a single 200 mg dose.

Peak plasma concentrations (C_{max}) in fasted healthy volunteers occur between 1 and 2 hours with a terminal plasma elimination half-life of approximately 30 hours (range, 20 to 50 hours) after oral administration. In fasted healthy volunteers, administration of a single oral 400 mg dose of fluconazole leads to a mean C_{max} of 6.72 mcg/mL (range, 4.12 to 8.08 mcg/mL) and after single oral doses of 50 to 400 mg, fluconazole plasma concentrations and AUC (area under the plasma concentration-time curve) are dose proportional.

Administration of a single oral 150 mg tablet of fluconazole to 10 lactating women resulted in a mean C_{max} of 2.61 mcg/mL (range, 1.57 to 3.65 mcg/mL).

Steady state concentrations are reached within 5 to 10 days following oral doses of 50 to 400 mg given once daily. Administration of a loading dose (on day 1) of twice the usual daily dose results in plasma concentrations close to steady-state by the second day. The apparent volume of distribution of fluconazole approximates that of total body water. Plasma protein binding is low (11% to 12%). Following either single- or multiple-oral doses for up to 14 days, fluconazole penetrates into all body fluids studied. In healthy volunteers, saliva concentrations of fluconazole were equal to or slightly greater than plasma concentrations regardless of dose, route, or duration of dosing. In patients with bronchiectasis, sputum concentrations of fluconazole following a single 150 mg oral dose were equal to plasma concentrations at both 4 and 24 hours post dose. In patients with fungal meningitis, fluconazole concentrations in the CSF are approximately 80% of the corresponding plasma concentrations.

Metabolism/Excretion – In healthy volunteers, fluconazole is cleared primarily by renal excretion, with approximately 80% of the administered dose appearing in the urine as unchanged drug. About 11% of the dose is excreted in the urine as metabolites.

Clearance corrected for body weight was not affected by age in these studies. Mean body clearance in adults is reported to be 0.23 (17%) mL/min/kg.

Special populations –

Renal function impairment: The pharmacokinetics of fluconazole are markedly affected by reduction in renal function. There is an inverse relationship between the elimination half-life and creatinine clearance. The dose of fluconazole may need to be reduced in patients with renal function impairment. A 3-hour hemodialysis session decreases plasma concentrations by approximately 50%.

Premature newborns: In premature newborns (gestational age 26 to 29 weeks), the mean (% cv) clearance within 36 hours of birth was 0.18 (35%, n = 7) mL/min/kg, which increased with time to a mean of 0.218 (31%, n = 9) mL/min/kg 6 days later and 0.333 (56%, n = 4) mL/min/kg 12 days later. Similarly, the half-life was 73.6 hours, which decreased with time to a mean of 53.2 hours 6 days later and 46.6 hours 12 days later.

FLUCONAZOLE — INJECTION

➤*Microbiology:* Fluconazole exhibits in vitro activity against *Cryptococcus neoformans* and *Candida* spp. Fungistatic activity has also been demonstrated in normal and immunocompromised animal models for systemic and intracranial fungal infections due to *Cryptococcus neoformans* and for systemic infections due to *Candida albicans*.

In common with other azole antifungal agents, most fungi show a higher apparent sensitivity to fluconazole in vivo than in vitro. Fluconazole administered orally or intravenously was active in a variety of animal models of fungal infection using standard laboratory strains of fungi. Activity has been demonstrated against fungal infections caused by *Aspergillus flavus* and *Aspergillus fumigatus* in normal mice. Fluconazole has also been shown to be active in animal models of endemic mycoses, including one model of *Blastomyces dermatitidis* pulmonary infections in normal mice; one model of *Coccidioides immitis* intracranial infections in normal mice; and several models of *Histoplasma capsulatum* pulmonary infection in normal and immunosuppressed mice. The clinical significance of results obtained in these studies is unknown.

Contraindications

Fluconazole is contraindicated in patients who have shown hypersensitivity to fluconazole or to any of its excipients. There is no information regarding cross-hypersensitivity between fluconazole and other azole antifungal agents. Caution should be used in prescribing fluconazole to patients with hypersensitivity to other azoles. Coadministration of terfenadine is contraindicated in patients receiving fluconazole at multiple doses of 400 mg or higher based upon results of a multiple dose interaction study. Coadministration of cisapride is contraindicated in patients receiving fluconazole (see Drug Interactions).

Warnings/Precautions

➤*Hepatic injury:* Fluconazole has been associated with rare cases of serious hepatic toxicity, including fatalities primarily in patients with serious underlying medical conditions. In cases of fluconazole-associated hepatotoxicity, no obvious relationship to total daily dose, duration of therapy, sex or age of the patient has been observed. Fluconazole hepatotoxicity has usually, but not always, been reversible on discontinuation of therapy. Patients who develop abnormal liver function tests during fluconazole therapy should be monitored for the development of more severe hepatic injury. Fluconazole should be discontinued if clinical signs and symptoms consistent with liver disease develop that may be attributable to fluconazole.

➤*Dermatologic:* Patients have rarely developed exfoliative skin disorders during treatment with fluconazole. In patients with serious underlying diseases (predominantly AIDS and malignancy), these have rarely resulted in a fatal outcome. Patients who develop rashes during treatment with fluconazole should be monitored closely and the drug discontinued if lesions progress.

➤*Hypersensitivity reactions:* In rare cases, anaphylaxis has been reported.

➤*Pregnancy: Category C.* Fluconazole was administered orally to pregnant rabbits during organogenesis in 2 studies, at 5, 10, and 20 mg/kg and at 5, 25, and 75 mg/kg, respectively. Maternal weight gain was impaired at all dose levels, and abortions occurred at 75 mg/kg (≈ 20 to 60 times the recommended human dose); no adverse fetal effects were detected. In several studies in which pregnant rats were treated orally with fluconazole during organogenesis, maternal weight gain was impaired and placental weights were increased at 25 mg/kg. There were no fetal effects at 5 or 10 mg/kg; increases in fetal anatomical variants (supernumerary ribs, renal pelvis dilation) and delays in ossification were observed at 25 and 50 mg/kg and higher doses. At doses ranging from 80 mg/kg (≈ 20 to 60 times the recommended human dose) to 320 mg/kg embryolethality in rats was increased and fetal abnormalities included wavy ribs, cleft palate, and abnormal cranio-facial ossification. These effects are consistent with the inhibition of estrogen synthesis in rats and may be a result of known effects of lowered estrogen on pregnancy, organogenesis, and parturition.

There are no adequate and well-controlled studies in pregnant women. There have been reports of multiple congenital abnormalities in infants whose mothers were being treated for 3 or more months with high dose (400 to 800 mg/day) fluconazole therapy for coccidioidomycosis (an unindicated use). The relationship between fluconazole use and these events is unclear. Fluconazole should be used in pregnancy only if the potential benefit justifies the possible risk to the fetus.

➤*Lactation:* Fluconazole is secreted in human milk at concentrations similar to plasma. Therefore, the use of fluconazole in nursing mothers is not recommended.

➤*Children:* An open-label, randomized, controlled trial has shown fluconazole to be effective in the treatment of oropharyngeal candidiasis in children 6 months to 13 years of age.

The use of fluconazole in children with cryptococcal meningitis, *Candida* esophagitis, or systemic *Candida* infections is supported by the efficacy shown for these indications in adults and by the results from several small noncomparative pediatric clinical studies. In addition, pharmacokinetic studies in children (see Pharmacokinetics) have established a dose proportionality between children and adults (see Administration and Dosage).

Efficacy of fluconazole has not been established in infants younger than 6 months of age. A small number of patients (29) ranging in age from 1 day to 6 months have been treated safely with fluconazole.

Drug Interactions

➤*QT prolongation:* An additive effect of fluconazole with other drugs that prolong the QT interval cannot be excluded. The following drugs may prolong the QT interval and increase the risk of life-threatening cardiac arrhythmias, including torsade de pointes: Antiarrhythmic agents (eg, amiodarone, bretylium, disopyramide, dofetilide, procainamide, quinidine, and sotalol), arsenic trioxide, chlorpromazine, cisapride, dolasetron, droperidol, mefloquine, mesoridazine, moxifloxacin, pentamidine, pimozide, tacrolimus, thioridazine, and ziprasidone. For a more complete list of drugs that may prolong the QT interval, see the appendix, Drug-Induced Prolongation of the QT Interval and Torsade de Pointes.

Fluconazole Drug Interactions

Precipitant drug	Object drug[a]		Description
Cimetidine	Fluconazole	⬇	Cimetidine resulted in a reduction in fluconazole AUC and C_{max}.
Hydrochlorothiazide	Fluconazole	⬆	Concomitant use resulted in a significant increase in fluconazole C_{max} and AUC, which can be attributed to reduced renal clearance.
Rifampin	Fluconazole	⬇	Rifampin enhances the metabolism of concurrently administered fluconazole. Depending on the clinical circumstances, give consideration when increasing the dose of fluconazole when administered with rifampin.
Fluconazole	Alfentanil	⬆	The pharmacologic and adverse effects of alfentanil may be increased. Possible inhibition of alfentanil metabolism (CYP3A4) by fluconazole may occur. Monitor for prolonged or recurrent respiratory depression. It may be necessary to administer a lower dose of alfentanil.
Fluconazole	Benzodiazepines	⬆	Increased and prolonged serum levels, CNS depression, and psychomotor impairment with certain benzodiazepines may occur, possibly lasting for several days after stopping fluconazole.
Fluconazole	Buspirone	⬆	Plasma buspirone concentrations may be elevated because of inhibition of buspirone metabolism. The pharmacologic and adverse effects of buspirone may be increased. Adjust the dose of buspirone as needed.
Fluconazole	Carbamazepine	⬆	Plasma concentrations of carbamazepine may be elevated, increasing clinical and adverse effects because of possible inhibition of carbamazepine metabolism (CYP3A4) by fluconazole. Monitor carbamazepine concentrations.
Fluconazole	Cisapride	⬆	Concurrent use may increase cisapride concentrations and cardiotoxicity may occur. Coadministration is contraindicated.
Fluconazole	Contraceptives, oral	⬌	Concurrent use with an OC containing ethinyl estradiol/ levonorgestrel produced an overall mean increase in the levels of the OC components; however, in some cases there were decreases ≤ 47% and 33% of ethinyl estradiol and levonorgestrel levels, respectively.
Fluconazole	Corticosteroids	⬆	The effects of corticosteroids may be enhanced, resulting in increased toxicity because of inhibition of corticosteroid metabolism. Adjust corticosteroid dose as needed.
Fluconazole	Cyclosporine	⬆	Significant increases in cyclosporine C_{max}, C_{min}, and AUC values and a significant decrease in oral clearance occurred following fluconazole use.

FLUCONAZOLE — INJECTION

Fluconazole Drug Interactions			
Precipitant drug	Object drug[a]		Description
Fluconazole	Haloperidol	↑	Concurrent use may increase haloperidol plasma concentrations, increasing the risk of side effects. Adjust haloperidol dose as needed.
Fluconazole	HMG-CoA reductase inhibitors	↑	Coadministration causes increased plasma levels of the HMG-CoA reductase inhibitors. Rhabdomyolysis has been reported. If concurrent use can not be avoided, consider reducing the dose of the HMG-CoA reductase inhibitor. Pravastatin levels appear to be the least affected by concurrent use.
Fluconazole	Losartan	↑	The antihypertensive and adverse effects of losartan may be increased because of possible inhibition of metabolism (CYP2D9) of losartan by fluconazole. Monitor blood pressure.
Fluconazole	Nisoldipine	↑	Serum nisoldipine concentrations may be elevated, increasing pharmacologic and adverse effects. Fluconazole, especially > 200 mg/day, may inhibit CYP3A4.
Fluconazole	Phenytoin	↑	Coadministration resulted in an increase of phenytoin AUC values. Monitor phenytoin levels and adjust dose as needed.
Fluconazole	Protease inhibitors	↑	Concurrent use may elevate protease inhibitor levels, increasing the risk of toxicity. Adjust protease inhibitor dose as needed.
Fluconazole	Rifabutin	↑	Coadministration may increase rifabutin levels. Cases of uveitis have been reported in patients receiving both drugs. Monitor closely.
Fluconazole	Sirolimus	↑	Plasma sirolimus concentrations may be elevated because of an inhibition of sirolimus gut metabolism.
Fluconazole	Sulfonylureas	↑	Fluconazole reduces the metabolism of sulfonylureas and increases the plasma concentrations of these agents. Carefully monitor blood glucose concentrations and adjust the sulfonylurea dose as necessary when these agents are coadministered.
Fluconazole	Tacrolimus	↑	There have been reports of nephrotoxicity in patients when these agents were coadministered. Carefully monitor.
Fluconazole	Theophylline	↑	Theophylline AUC, C_{max}, and half-life were significantly increased, and clearance was decreased.
Fluconazole	Tolterodine	↑	Concurrent use may increase tolterodine plasma levels. Adjust tolterodine dose as needed. Do not give more than 1 mg of tolterodine twice daily when coadministered with azole antifungals.
Fluconazole	Tricyclic antidepressants (ie, amitriptyline, nortriptyline)	↑	Serum tricyclic antidepressant (TCA) concentrations may be elevated, resulting in an increase in therapeutic and adverse effects including cardiac arrhythmia. Inhibition of TCA metabolism is suspected (CYP2C9 by fluconazole). Adjust the TCA dose as needed.
Fluconazole	Vinca alkaloids (eg, vincristine)	↑	The risk of vinca alkaloid toxicity (eg, constipation, myalgia, neutropenia) may be increased. Avoid coadministration of these agents whenever possible.
Fluconazole	Warfarin	↑	The anticoagulant effect of warfarin may be increased. A single warfarin dose after 14 days of fluconazole resulted in an increase in the PT response. Monitor PT and INR frequently.
Fluconazole	Zidovudine	↑	There was a significant increase in zidovudine AUC following fluconazole administration.
Fluconazole	Zolpidem	↑	Plasma concentrations and therapeutic effects of zolpidem may be increased. The dose of zolpidem may need to be decreased during coadministration of azole antifungal agents.

[a] ↑ = object drug increased; ↓ = object drug decreased; ↔ = undetermined clinical effect.

Adverse Reactions

➤*Patients receiving multiple doses for other infections:* Sixteen percent of over 4000 patients treated with fluconazole in clinical trials of 7 days or more experienced adverse events. Treatment was discontinued in 1.5% of patients due to adverse clinical events and in 1.3% of patients due to laboratory test abnormalities.

Clinical adverse events were reported more frequently in HIV infected patients (21%) than in non-HIV infected patients (13%); however, the patterns in HIV infected and non-HIV infected patients were similar. The proportions of patients discontinuing therapy due to clinical adverse events were similar in the 2 groups (1.5%).

The following treatment-related clinical adverse events occurred at an incidence of 1% or greater in 4048 patients receiving fluconazole for 7 or more days in clinical trials: Nausea (3.7%), headache (1.9%), skin rash (1.8%), vomiting (1.7%), abdominal pain (1.7%), diarrhea (1.5%).

The following adverse events have occurred under conditions where a causal association is probable.

Allergic – In rare cases, anaphylaxis has been reported.

Hepatic – In combined clinical trials and marketing experience, there have been rare cases of serious hepatic reactions during treatment with fluconazole (see Warnings). The spectrum of these hepatic reactions has ranged from mild transient elevations in transaminases to clinical hepatitis, cholestasis, and fulminant hepatic failure, including fatalities. Instances of fatal hepatic reactions were noted to occur primarily in patients with serious underlying medical conditions (predominantly AIDS or malignancy) and often while taking multiple concomitant medications. Transient hepatic reactions, including hepatitis and jaundice, have occurred among patients with no other identifiable risk factors. In each of these cases, liver function returned to baseline on discontinuation of fluconazole.

➤*Adverse reactions of uncertain causal association with fluconazole:* The following adverse reactions have occurred under conditions where a causal association is uncertain.

CNS – Seizures.

Dermatologic – Exfoliative skin disorders including Stevens-Johnson syndrome and toxic epidermal necrolysis (see Warnings), alopecia.

Hematologic/Lymphatic – Leukopenia, including neutropenia and agranulocytosis, thrombocytopenia.

Metabolic – Hypercholesterolemia, hypertriglyceridemia, hypokalemia.

➤*Children:* In Phase II/III clinical trials conducted in the United States and in Europe, 577 pediatric patients, ages 1 day to 17 years were treated with fluconazole at doses up to 15 mg/kg/day for up to 1616 days.

Fluconazole Adverse Reactions in Children		
Adverse reactions	Percentage of patients with treatment-related side effects fluconazole (n = 577)	Comparative agents (n = 451)
With any side effect	13%	9.3%
Vomiting	5.4%	5.1%
Abdominal pain	2.8%	1.6%
Nausea	2.3%	1.6%
Diarrhea	2.1%	2.2%

Overdosage

➤*Symptoms:* There has been 1 reported case of overdosage with fluconazole. A 42-year-old patient infected with human immunodeficiency virus developed hallucinations and exhibited paranoid behavior after reportedly

FLUCONAZOLE — INJECTION

ingesting 8200 mg of fluconazole. The patient was admitted to the hospital, and his condition resolved within 48 hours.

➤*Treatment:* In the event of overdose, symptomatic treatment (with supportive measures and gastric lavage if clinically indicated) should be instituted.

Fluconazole is largely excreted in urine. A 3-hour hemodialysis session decreases plasma levels by approximately 50%.

Animal toxicology – In mice and rats receiving very high doses of fluconazole, clinical effects in both species included decreased motility and respiration, ptosis, lacrimation, salivation, urinary incontinence, loss of righting reflex, and cyanosis; death was sometimes preceded by clonic convulsions.

ITRACONAZOLE

Rx	**Itraconazole** (Various, eg, Eon)	**Capsules:** 100 mg	In 28s, 30s, 100s, 500s, and UD 28s and 30s.
Rx	**Sporanox** (Janssen)		Sucrose, sugar. (Janssen Sporanox 100). Blue/pink. In 30s, UD 30s, and *PulsePak* 28s.
Rx	**Sporanox** (Ortho Biotech)	**Oral solution:** 10 mg/mL	Saccharin, sorbitol. Cherry/caramel flavor. In 150 mL.

ITRACONAZOLE — ORAL

WARNING

Congestive heart failure (CHF) – If signs or symptoms of CHF occur during administration of itraconazole, reassess continued itraconazole use.

Do not administer itraconazole capsules for the treatment of onychomycosis in patients with evidence of ventricular dysfunction such as CHF or a history of CHF. If signs or symptoms of CHF occur during administration of itraconazole capsules, discontinue administration. When itraconazole was administered intravenously (IV) to dogs and healthy human volunteers, negative inotropic effects were seen.

Drug interactions – Coadministration of cisapride, pimozide, quinidine, or dofetilide with itraconazole is contraindicated. Itraconazole, a potent cytochrome P450 3A4 isoenzyme system (CYP3A4) inhibitor, may increase plasma concentrations of drugs metabolized by this pathway. Serious cardiovascular events, including QT prolongation, torsades de pointes, ventricular tachycardia, cardiac arrest, and/or sudden death have occurred in patients using cisapride, pimozide, or quinidine concomitantly with itraconazole and/or other CYP3A4 inhibitors.

Indications

➤*Aspergillosis (capsules):* Treatment of pulmonary and extrapulmonary aspergillosis in immunocompromised and nonimmunocompromised patients who are intolerant of or who are refractory to amphotericin B therapy.

➤*Blastomycosis (capsules):* Treatment of pulmonary and extrapulmonary blastomycosis in immunocompromised and nonimmunocompromised patients.

➤*Febrile neutropenia, empiric (oral solution):* For empiric therapy of febrile neutropenic patients with suspected fungal infections. Note: In a comparative trial, the overall response rate for itraconazole-treated subjects was higher than for amphotericin B-treated subjects. However, compared with amphotericin B-treated subjects, a larger number of itraconazole-treated subjects discontinued treatment because of persistent fever and a change in antifungal medication because of fever. Whereas a larger number of amphotericin B-treated subjects discontinued because of drug intolerance.

➤*Histoplasmosis (capsules):* Treatment of histoplasmosis, including chronic cavitary pulmonary disease and disseminated, nonmeningeal histoplasmosis in immunocompromised and nonimmunocompromised patients.

➤*Onychomycosis (capsules):* Treatment of onychomycosis of the toenail, with or without fingernail involvement, caused by dermatophytes (*tinea unguium*) and onychomycosis of the fingernail caused by dermatophytes (*tinea unguium*) in nonimmunocompromised patients.

Prior to initiating treatment, obtain appropriate nail specimens for laboratory testing (potassium hydroxide [KOH] preparation, fungal culture, or nail biopsy) to confirm the diagnosis of onychomycosis.

➤*Oropharyngeal/esophageal candidiasis (oral solution):* Treatment of oropharyngeal and esophageal candidiasis.

➤*Off-label uses:* Itraconazole solution (200 mg/day) is recommended as an alternative to fluconazole as secondary prevention of oropharyngeal, vaginal, or esophageal candidiasis in HIV-infected patients who have severe or frequent recurrences; itraconazole capsules (200 mg/day) have been used as an alternative to fluconazole for primary prevention of cryptococcosis in adults with advanced HIV disease (CD4 counts less than 50 cells/mcL) and are recommended as an alternate to fluconazole for lifelong secondary prevention of cryptococcal disease in HIV-infected adults; itraconazole capsules (200 mg/day) are recommended as first-line agent in the primary prevention of histoplasmosis in adults with advanced HIV disease (CD4 counts less than 100 cells/mcL) and live in endemic areas (rate greater than or equal to 10 cases per 100 patient-years) and also as first-line agent for lifelong secondary prophylaxis (200 mg twice daily); itraconazole capsules (200 mg twice daily) are recommended as an alternate agent to fluconazole for lifelong secondary prevention of coccidioidomycosis in HIV-infected adults; oral itraconazole also is recommended for secondary prevention of histoplasmosis (first line; 2 to 5 mg/kg every 12 to 48 hours), cryptococcal disease (alternate therapy; 2 to 5 mg/kg every 12 to 24 hours), and coccidioidomycosis (alternate therapy; 2 to 5 mg/kg every 12 to 48 hours) in children with HIV; oral itraconazole (2 to 5 mg/kg every 12 to 24 hours) is recommended for primary prevention of histoplasmosis (first-line agent) and cryptococcal disease (alternate therapy) in children with HIV, severe immunosuppression, and live in endemic areas (histoplasmosis).

Administration and Dosage

➤*General dosing considerations:* The itraconazole capsule is a different preparation than itraconazole oral solution, and the 2 doseforms should not be used interchangeably; drug exposure is greater with the oral solution than with the capsules when the same dose of drug is given. In addition, the topical effects of mucosal exposure may be different between the 2 formulations. Only the oral solution has been demonstrated to be effective for oral and/or esophageal candidiasis.

➤*Adults:*

Capsules –

Aspergillosis: 200 to 400 mg/day.

Blastomycosis:

- *Usual dosage* – 200 mg once daily.
- *Maximum dose* – 400 mg/day.
- *Dosage adjustment* – If there is no obvious improvement, or if there is evidence of progressive fungal disease, increase the dose in 100 mg increments to a maximum of 400 mg daily. Give doses above 200 mg/day in 2 divided doses.

Histoplasmosis:

- *Usual dosage* – 200 mg once daily.
- *Maximum dose* – 400 mg/day.
- *Dosage adjustment* – If there is no obvious improvement, or if there is evidence of progressive fungal disease, increase the dose in 100 mg increments to a maximum of 400 mg daily. Give doses above 200 mg/day in 2 divided doses.

Life-threatening situations: In life-threatening situations, use a loading dose. Although clinical studies did not provide for a loading dose, it is recommended, based on pharmacokinetic data, that a loading dose of 200 mg (2 capsules) 3 times daily (600 mg/day) be given for the first 3 days of treatment.

Continue treatment for a minimum of 3 months and until clinical parameters and laboratory tests indicate that the active fungal infection has subsided. An inadequate period of treatment may lead to recurrence of active infection.

Onychomycosis:

- *Fingernails only* – 2 treatment pulses, each consisting of 200 mg twice daily (400 mg/day) for 1 week. The pulses are separated by a 3-week period without itraconazole.
- *Toenails with or without fingernail involvement* – 200 mg once daily for 12 consecutive weeks.

Oral solution –

Esophageal candidiasis: 100 mg (10 mL) daily for a minimum of 3 weeks. Vigorously swish the solution in the mouth (10 mL at a time) for several seconds and swallow. Continue treatment for 2 weeks following resolution of symptoms. Doses up to 200 mg (20 mL) per day may be used, based on medical judgement of the patient's response to therapy.

Febrile neutropenia, empiric: 200 mg IV twice daily for 4 doses, followed by 200 mg once daily for up to 14 days. Continue treatment with itraconazole oral solution 200 mg (20 mL) twice daily until resolution of clinically significant neutropenia occurs. The safety and efficacy of itraconazole use exceeding 28 days in empiric therapy of febrile neutropenia is not known.

Oropharyngeal candidiasis: 200 mg (20 mL) daily for 1 to 2 weeks. Vigorously swish the solution in the mouth (10 mL at a time) for several seconds and swallow. Clinical signs and symptoms of oropharyngeal candidiasis generally resolve within several days.

For patients with oropharyngeal candidiasis unresponsive/refractory to treatment with fluconazole tablets, the recommended dose is 100 mg (10 mL) twice daily. For patients responding to therapy, clinical response will be seen in 2 to 4 weeks. Patients may relapse shortly after discontinuing therapy. Limited data on the safety of long-term use (more than 6 months) of itraconazole oral solution are available at this time.

➤*Children:* A small number of patients 3 to 16 years of age have been treated with itraconazole capsules 100 mg/day for systemic fungal infections, and no serious unexpected adverse events have been reported.

A pharmacokinetic study was conducted with itraconazole oral solution in 26 pediatric patients 6 months to 12 years of age who required systemic antifungal treatment. Itraconazole was dosed at 5 mg/kg once daily for 2 weeks, and no serious unexpected adverse events were reported.

➤*Renal function impairment:*

Adults receiving continuous renal replacement therapy – A dosage of 200 mg IV every 12 hours for 4 doses followed by 200 mg IV every

ITRACONAZOLE — ORAL

24 hours is recommended for patients receiving continuous venovenous hemofiltration, continuous venovenous hemodialysis, or continuous venovenous hemodiafiltration. This recommendation assumes ultrafiltration and dialysis flow rates of 1 to 2 L/h.

Adults receiving intermittent hemodialysis (IHD) – 200 mg IV every 12 hours for 4 doses followed by 200 mg IV every 24 hours. This recommendation assumes the patient is receiving standard IHD 3 times per week and completes the full dialysis sessions.

➤*Hepatic function impairment:* Carefully monitor patients with hepatic function impairment. If clinical signs or symptoms develop that are consistent with liver disease, discontinue treatment.

➤*Administration:*

Capsules – Itraconazole capsules should be taken with a full meal to ensure maximal absorption.

Oral solution – Itraconazole oral solution should be taken without food, if possible.

➤*Storage/Stability:*

Capsules – Store at controlled room temperature 15° to 25°C (59° to 77°F). Protect from light and moisture.

Oral solution – Store at or below 25°C (77°F). Do not freeze.

Actions

➤*Pharmacology:* Itraconazole is a systemic triazole antifungal agent. In vitro, itraconazole inhibits the cytochrome P450-dependent synthesis of ergosterol, which is a vital component of fungal membranes.

➤*Pharmacokinetics:*

Absorption/Distribution –

The plasma protein binding of itraconazole is 99.8% and that of hydroxyitraconazole is 99.5%. Following IV administration, the volume of distribution of itraconazole averaged 796 ± 185 L.

The pharmacokinetics of itraconazole after IV administration and its absolute oral bioavailability from an oral solution were studied in a randomized crossover study in 6 healthy men. The observed absolute oral bioavailability of itraconazole was 55%.

Capsules: The oral bioavailability of itraconazole is maximal when itraconazole capsules are taken with a full meal. The pharmacokinetics of itraconazole were studied in 6 healthy men who received, in a crossover design, single doses of itraconazole 100 mg as a polyethylene glycol capsule, with or without a full meal. The same 6 volunteers also received 50 or 200 mg with a full meal in a crossover design. In this study, only itraconazole plasma concentrations were measured.

Pharmacokinetics of Various Dosages of Itraconazole Capsules (N = 6)

	50 mg (fed)	100 mg (fed)	100 mg (fasted)	200 mg (fed)
C_{max} (ng/mL)	45 ± 16[a]	132 ± 67	38 ± 20	289 ± 100
t_{max} (hours)	3.2 ± 1.3	4 ± 1.1	3.3 ± 1	4.7 ± 1.4
$AUC_{0-\infty}$ (ng•h/mL)	567 ± 264	1899 ± 838	722 ± 289	5211 ± 2116

[a] Mean ± standard deviation.

Doubling the itraconazole dose results in approximately a 3-fold increase in the itraconazole plasma concentrations.

Values given in the following table represent data from a crossover pharmacokinetics study in which 27 healthy male volunteers each took a single dose of itraconazole capsules 200 mg with or without a full meal:

Pharmacokinetics of a Single Itraconazole Capsule 200 mg (N = 27)

	Itraconazole		Hydroxyitraconazole	
	Fed	Fasted	Fed	Fasted
C_{max} (ng/mL)	239 ± 85[a]	140 ± 65	397 ± 103	286 ± 101
t_{max} (hours)	4.5 ± 1.1	3.9 ± 1	5.1 ± 1.6	4.5 ± 1.1
$AUC_{0-\infty}$ (ng•h/mL)	3423 ± 1154	2094 ± 905	7978 ± 2648	5191 ± 2489
t½ (hours)	21 ± 5	21 ± 7	12 ± 3	12 ± 3

[a] Mean ± standard deviation.

Absorption of itraconazole under fasted conditions in individuals with relative or absolute achlorhydria, such as patients with AIDS or volunteers taking gastric acid secretion suppressors (eg, H_2 receptor antagonists), was increased when itraconazole capsules were administered with a cola beverage. Eighteen men with AIDS received single doses of itraconazole capsules 200 mg under fasted conditions with 240 mL of water or 240 mL of a cola beverage in a crossover design. The absorption of itraconazole was increased when itraconazole capsules were coadministered with a cola beverage, with AUC_{0-24} and C_{max} increasing 75% ± 121% and 95% ± 128%, respectively.

Steady-state concentrations were reached within 15 days following oral doses of 50 to 400 mg daily. Values given in the information below are data at steady-state from a pharmacokinetics study in which 27 healthy male volunteers took itraconazole capsules 200 mg twice daily (with a full meal) for 15 days:

Steady-State Pharmacokinetics of Itraconazole Capsules

	Itraconazole	Hydroxyitraconazole
C_{max} (ng/mL)	2282 ± 514[a]	3488 ± 742
C_{min} (ng/mL)	1855 ± 535	3349 ± 761
t_{max} (hours)	4.6 ± 1.8	3.4 ± 3.4
$AUC_{0-12\ hr}$ (ng•h/mL)	22569 ± 5375	38572 ± 8450
t½ (hours)	64 ± 32	56 ± 24

[a] Mean ± standard deviation.

Oral solution: The absolute bioavailability of itraconazole administered as a nonmarketed solution formulation under fed conditions was 55% in 6 healthy men. However, the bioavailability of itraconazole oral solution is increased under fasted conditions reaching higher maximum plasma concentrations (C_{max}) in a shorter period of time. In 27 healthy men, the steady-state area under the plasma concentration versus time curve (AUC_{0-24hr}) of itraconazole (itraconazole oral solution, 200 mg daily for 15 days) under fasted conditions was 131 ± 30% of that obtained under fed conditions. Therefore, unlike itraconazole capsules, it is recommended that itraconazole oral solution be administered without food. Presented in the table below are the steady-state (day 15) pharmacokinetic parameters for itraconazole and hydroxyitraconazole (itraconazole oral solution) under fasted and fed conditions:

Steady-State Pharmacokinetic Parameters for Itraconazole Oral Solution

	Itraconazole		Hydroxy-itraconazole	
	Fasted	Fed	Fasted	Fed
C_{max} (ng/mL)	1963 ± 601[a]	1435 ± 477	2055 ± 487	1781 ± 397
t_{max} (hours)	2.5 ± 0.8	4.4 ± 0.7	5.3 ± 4.3	4.3 ± 1.2
$AUC_{0-24\ h}$ (ng•h/mL)	29271 ± 10285	22815 ± 7098	45184 ± 10981	38823 ± 8907
t½ (hours)	39.7 ± 13	37.4 ± 13	27.3 ± 13	26.1 ± 10

[a] Mean ± standard deviation.

The bioavailability of itraconazole oral solution relative to itraconazole capsules was studied in 30 healthy men who received itraconazole 200 mg as the oral solution and capsules under fed conditions. The $AUC_{0-\infty}$ from itraconazole oral solution was 149 ± 68% of that obtained from itraconazole capsules; a similar increase was observed for hydroxyitraconazole. In addition, a cross study comparison of itraconazole and hydroxyitraconazole pharmacokinetics following the administration of single doses of itraconazole oral solution 200 mg (under fasted conditions) or itraconazole capsules (under fed conditions) indicates that when these 2 formulations are administered under conditions which optimize their systemic absorption, the bioavailability of the solution relative to capsules is expected to be increased further. Therefore, it is recommended that itraconazole oral solution and itraconazole capsules not be used interchangeably. The following table contains pharmacokinetic parameters for itraconazole and hydroxyitraconazole following single doses of itraconazole oral solution 200 mg (n = 27) or itraconazole capsules (n = 30) administered to healthy men under fasted and fed conditions, respectively:

Pharmacokinetic Parameters for Itraconazole Capsules (N = 30) vs Oral Solution (N = 27)

	Itraconazole		Hydroxy-itraconazole	
	Oral solution fasted	Capsules fed	Oral solution fasted	Capsules fed
C_{max} (ng/mL)	544 ± 213[a]	302 ± 119	622 ± 116	504 ± 132
t_{max} (hours)	2.2 ± 0.8	5 ± 0.8	3.5 ± 1.2	5 ± 1
$AUC_{0-24\ hr}$ (ng•h/mL)	4505 ± 1670	2682 ± 1084	9552 ± 1835	7293 ± 2144

[a] Mean ± standard deviation.

Metabolism/Excretion – Itraconazole is metabolized predominately by the cytochrome P450 3A4 isoenzyme system (CYP3A4), resulting in the formation of several metabolites, including hydroxyitraconazole, the major metabolite. Results of a pharmacokinetics study suggest that itraconazole may undergo saturable metabolism with multiple dosing. Fecal excretion of the parent drug varies between 3% to 18% of the dose. Renal excretion of the parent drug is less than 0.03% of the dose. About 40% of the dose is excreted as inactive metabolites in the urine. No single excreted metabolite represents more than 5% of a dose. Itraconazole total plasma clearance averaged 381 ± 95 mL/minute following IV administration.

Special populations –

Renal function impairment: A pharmacokinetic study using a single dose of itraconazole 200 mg (four 50 mg capsules) was conducted in 3 groups of patients with renal function impairment (uremia [n = 7]; hemodialysis [n = 7]; and continuous ambulatory peritoneal dialysis [n = 5]). In uremic subjects with a mean creatinine clearance of 13 mL/min × 1.73 m^2, the bioavailability was slightly reduced compared with healthy population parameters. This study did not demonstrate any significant effect of hemodialysis or continuous ambulatory peritoneal dialysis on the pharmacokinetics of itraconazole (t_{max}, C_{max}, and AUC_{0-8}). Plasma concentration-versus-time profiles showed wide intersubject variation in all 3 groups.

Hepatic function impairment: Carefully monitor patients with hepatic function impairment when taking itraconazole. Consider the prolonged

ITRACONAZOLE — ORAL

elimination half-life of itraconazole observed in cirrhotic patients when deciding to initiate therapy with other medications metabolized by CYP3A4, such as lovastatin, simvastatin, cisapride, pimozide, quinidine, dofetilide, triazolam, and oral midazolam. Itraconazole has been associated with rare cases of hepatotoxicity, including liver failure and death. If clinical signs or symptoms develop that are consistent with liver disease, discontinue treatment.

• *Capsules* – A pharmacokinetic study using a single dose of itraconazole 100 mg (one 100 mg capsule) was conducted in 6 healthy and 12 cirrhotic subjects. No statistically significant differences in AUC were seen between these 2 groups. A statistically significant reduction in mean C_{max} (47%) and a 2-fold increase in the elimination half-life (37 ± 17 hours) of itraconazole were noted in cirrhotic subjects compared with healthy subjects.

Children:

• *Oral solution* – The pharmacokinetics of itraconazole oral solution were studied in 26 pediatric patients requiring systemic antifungal therapy. Patients were stratified by age: 6 months to 2 years of age (n = 8), 2 to 5 years of age (n = 7) and 5 to 12 years of age (n = 11), and received itraconazole oral solution 5 mg/kg once daily for 14 days. Pharmacokinetic parameters at steady-state (day 14) were not significantly different among the age strata and are summarized in the table below for all 26 patients:

Pharmacokinetics of Itraconazole Oral Solution in Pediatric Patients (N = 26)

	Itraconazole	Hydroxyitraconazole
C_{max} (ng/mL)	582.5 ± 382.4[a]	692.4 ± 355
C_{min} (ng/mL)	187.5 ± 161.4	403.8 ± 336.1
$AUC_{0-24\ h}$ (ng•h/mL)	7706.7 ± 5245.2	13356.4 ± 8942.4
t½ (hours)	35.8 ± 35.6	17.7 ± 13

[a] Mean ± standard deviation.

Decreased cardiac contractility: When itraconazole was administered IV to anesthetized dogs, a dose-related negative inotropic effect was documented. In a healthy volunteer study of itraconazole injection (IV infusion), transient, asymptomatic decreases in left ventricular ejection fraction were observed using gated SPECT imaging; these resolved before the next infusion, 12 hours later.

• *CHF* –

Capsules: If signs or symptoms of CHF appear during administration of itraconazole capsules, discontinue itraconazole.

Oral solution: If signs or symptoms of CHF appear during administration of itraconazole oral solution, monitor carefully and consider other treatment alternatives which may include discontinuation of itraconazole oral solution administration.

Cystic fibrosis: Seventeen cystic fibrosis patients, 7 to 28 years of age, were administered itraconazole oral solution 2.5 mg/kg twice daily for 14 days in a pharmacokinetic study. Sixteen patients completed the study. Steady state trough concentrations more than 250 ng/mL were achieved in 6 out of 11 patients 16 years of age and older, but none of the 5 patients younger than 16 years of age. Large variability was observed in the pharmacokinetic data (%CV for trough concentrations = 98% and 70% for 16 years of age and older and less than 16 years of age, respectively; %CV for AUC = 75% and 58% for 16 years of age and older and less than 16 years of age, respectively). If a patient with cystic fibrosis does not respond to itraconazole oral solution, consider switching to alternative therapy.

➤*Microbiology:* In vitro studies have demonstrated that itraconazole inhibits the cytochrome P-450–dependent synthesis of ergosterol, which is a vital component of fungal cell membranes.

Activity in vitro and in vivo – Itraconazole exhibits in vitro activity against *Blastomyces dermatitidis*, *Histoplasma capsulatum*, *Histoplasma duboisii*, *Aspergillus flavus*, *Aspergillus fumigatus*, *Candida albicans*, and *Cryptococcus neoformans*. Itraconazole also exhibits varying in vitro activity against *Sporothrix schenckii*, *Trichophyton* species, *Candida krusei*, and other *Candida* species. The bioactive metabolite, hydroxyitraconazole, has not been evaluated against *Histoplasma capsulatum* and *Blastomyces dermatitidis*. Correlation between minimum inhibitory concentration (MIC) results in vitro and clinical outcome has yet to be established for azole antifungal agents.

Resistance –

Several in vitro studies have reported that some fungal clinical isolates, including *Candida* species, with reduced susceptibility to 1 azole antifungal agent may also be less susceptible to other azole derivatives. The finding of cross-resistance is dependent on a number of factors, including the species evaluated, its clinical history, the particular azole compounds compared, and the type of susceptibility test that is performed. The relevance of these in vitro susceptibility data to clinical outcome remains to be elucidated.

Contraindications

Do not administer itraconazole capsules for the treatment of onychomycosis in patients with evidence of ventricular dysfunction such as CHF or a history of CHF.

Coadministration with certain drugs metabolized by the cytochrome P-450 3A4 isoenzyme system (CYP3A4), cisapride, oral midazolam, pimozide, quinidine, dofetilide, triazolam, HMG-CoA reductase inhibitors metabolized by CYP3A4, such as lovastatin and simvastatin, and ergot alkaloids metabolized by CYP3A4, such as dihydroergotamine, ergotamine, ergonovine, and methylergonovine (see Drug interactions).

Itraconazole is contraindicated for patients who have shown hypersensitivity to itraconazole or its excipients. There is no information regarding cross-hypersensitivity between itraconazole and other azole antifungal agents. Use caution when prescribing itraconazole to patients with hypersensitivity to other azoles.

Warnings/Precautions

➤*Interchangeability:* Do not use itraconazole capsules and itraconazole oral solution interchangeably. This is because drug exposure is greater with the oral solution than with the capsules when the same dose of drug is given. In addition, the topical effects of mucosal exposure may be different between the 2 formulations. Only the oral solution has been demonstrated effective for oral and/or esophageal candidiasis.

➤*Cardiac dysrhythmias:* Life-threatening cardiac dysrhythmias and/or sudden death have occurred in patients using cisapride, pimozide, or quinidine concomitantly with itraconazole and/or other CYP3A4 inhibitors. Coadministration of these drugs with itraconazole is contraindicated.

➤*Cardiac disease:* For patients with risk factors for CHF, carefully review the risks and benefits of itraconazole therapy. These risk factors include cardiac disease such as ischemic and valvular disease; significant pulmonary disease such as chronic obstructive pulmonary disease; and renal failure and other edematous disorders. Inform such patients of the signs and symptoms of CHF, treat with caution, and monitor for signs and symptoms of CHF during treatment. If signs or symptoms of CHF appear during administration of itraconazole capsules, discontinue administration.

See Actions for more information.

Cases of CHF, peripheral edema, and pulmonary edema have been reported in the postmarketing period among patients being treated for onychomycosis and/or systemic fungal infections.

Capsules – Do not administer itraconazole capsules for the treatment of onychomycosis in patients with evidence of ventricular dysfunction such as CHF or a history of CHF. Do not use itraconazole capsules for other indications in patients with evidence of ventricular dysfunction unless the benefit clearly outweighs the risk.

Oral solution – Do not use itraconazole oral solution in patients with evidence of ventricular dysfunction unless the benefit clearly outweighs the risk. If signs or symptoms of CHF appear during administration of itraconazole oral solution, monitor carefully and consider other treatment alternatives which may include discontinuation of itraconazole oral solution administration.

➤*Cystic fibrosis:* If a patient with cystic fibrosis does not respond to itraconazole oral solution, consider switching to alternative therapy.

➤*Severely neutropenic patients:* Itraconazole oral solution as treatment for oropharyngeal and/or esophageal candidiasis was not investigated in severely neutropenic patients. Because of its pharmacokinetic properties, itraconazole oral solution is not recommended for initiation of treatment in patients at immediate risk of systemic candidiasis.

➤*Hepatotoxicity:* Itraconazole has been associated with rare cases of serious hepatotoxicity, including liver failure and death. Some of these cases had neither preexisting liver disease nor a serious underlying medical condition and some of these cases developed within the first week of treatment. If clinical signs or symptoms develop that are consistent with liver disease, discontinue treatment and perform liver function testing. Continued itraconazole use or reinstitution of treatment with itraconazole is strongly discouraged unless there is a serious or life-threatening situation where the expected benefit exceeds the risk.

In patients with elevated or abnormal liver enzymes or active liver disease, or who have experienced liver toxicity with other drugs, treatment with itraconazole is strongly discouraged unless there is a serious or life-threatening situation where the expected benefit exceeds the risk.

➤*Neuropathy:* If neuropathy occurs that may be attributable to itraconazole, discontinue the treatment.

➤*Decreased gastric acidity:*

Capsules – Administer itraconazole capsules after a full meal. The oral bioavailability of itraconazole is maximal when itraconazole capsules are taken with a full meal.

Under fasted conditions, itraconazole absorption was decreased in the presence of decreased gastric acidity. The absorption of itraconazole may be decreased with the concomitant administration of antacids or gastric acid secretion suppressors. Studies conducted under fasted conditions demonstrated that administration with 240 mL of a cola beverage resulted in increased absorption of itraconazole in AIDS patients with relative or absolute achlorhydria. This increase relative to the effects of a full meal is unknown.

Because hypochlorhydria has been reported in HIV-infected individuals, the absorption of itraconazole in these patients may be decreased.

➤*Pregnancy: Category C.* There are no studies in pregnant women. Use itraconazole for the treatment of systemic fungal infections in pregnancy only if the benefit outweighs the potential risk. Do not administer itraconazole for the treatment of onychomycosis to pregnant patients or to women contemplating pregnancy.

Itraconazole was found to cause a dose-related increase in maternal toxicity, embryotoxicity, and teratogenicity in rats at dosage levels of approximately 40 to 160 mg/kg/day (5 to 20 times MRHD), and in mice at dosage levels of approximately 80 mg/kg/day (10 times MRHD). In rats, the teratogenicity consisted of major skeletal defects; in mice, it consisted of encephaloceles and/or macroglossia.

During postmarketing experience, cases of congenital abnormalities have been reported.

ITRACONAZOLE — ORAL

Women of childbearing potential – Do not administer itraconazole to women of childbearing potential for the treatment of onychomycosis unless they are using effective measures to prevent pregnancy and they begin therapy on the second or third day following the onset of menses. Continue effective contraception throughout itraconazole therapy and for 2 months following the end of treatment.

➤*Lactation:* Itraconazole is excreted in human milk; therefore, weigh the expected benefits of itraconazole therapy for the mother against the potential risk from exposure of itraconazole to the infant. The US Public Health Service Centers for Disease Control and Prevention advises HIV-infected women not to breast-feed to avoid potential transmission of HIV to uninfected infants.

➤*Children:* The efficacy and safety of itraconazole have not been established in pediatric patients.

The long-term effects of itraconazole on bone growth in children are unknown. In 3 toxicology studies using rats, itraconazole induced bone defects at dosage levels as low as 20 mg/kg/day (2.5 times MRHD). The induced defects included reduced bone plate activity, thinning of the zona compacta of the large bones, and increased bone fragility. At a dosage level of 80 mg/kg/day (10 times MRHD) over 1 year or 160 mg/kg/day (20 times MRHD) for 6 months, itraconazole induced small tooth pulp with hypocellular appearance in some rats. No such bone toxicity has been reported in adult patients.

➤*Monitoring:* Monitor liver function in patients with preexisting hepatic function abnormalities or those who have experienced liver toxicity with other medications, and consider monitoring liver function in all patients receiving itraconazole. Stop treatment immediately and conduct liver function testing in patients who develop signs and symptoms suggestive of liver dysfunction.

Drug Interactions

➤*Cytochrome P450 system:* Concomitant administration of itraconazole and certain drugs metabolized by the cytochrome P450 3A4 isoenzyme system (CYP3A4) may result in increased plasma concentrations of those drugs, leading to potentially serious and/or life-threatening adverse events. Cisapride, oral midazolam, pimozide, quinidine, dofetilide, and triazolam are contraindicated with itraconazole. HMG-CoA reductase inhibitors metabolized by CYP3A4, such as lovastatin and simvastatin, are also contraindicated with itraconazole. Ergot alkaloids metabolized by CYP3A4 such as dihydroergotamine, ergonovine, and methylergonovine are contraindicated with itraconazole. Use cilostazol and eletriptan (CYP3A4 metabolized drugs) with caution when coadministered with itraconazole.

Itraconazole and its major metabolite, hydroxyitraconazole, are inhibitors of CYP3A4.

Itraconazole may decrease the elimination of drugs metabolized by CYP3A4, resulting in increased plasma concentrations of these drugs when they are administered with itraconazole. These elevated plasma concentrations may increase or prolong both therapeutic and adverse effects of these drugs. Whenever possible, monitor plasma concentrations of these drugs, and make dosage adjustments after concomitant itraconazole therapy is initiated. When appropriate, clinical monitoring for signs or symptoms of increased or prolonged pharmacologic effects is advised. Upon discontinuation, depending on the dose and duration of treatment, itraconazole plasma concentrations decline gradually (especially in patients with hepatic cirrhosis or in those receiving CYP3A4 inhibitors). This is particularly important when initiating therapy with drugs whose metabolism is affected by itraconazole.

Inducers of CYP3A4 may decrease the plasma concentrations of itraconazole. Itraconazole may not be effective in patients concomitantly taking itraconazole and 1 of these drugs. Therefore, administration of these drugs with itraconazole is not recommended.

Other inhibitors of CYP3A4 may increase the plasma concentrations of itraconazole. Monitor patients who must take itraconazole concomitantly with 1 of these drugs for signs or symptoms of increased or prolonged pharmacologic effects of itraconazole.

➤*QT prolongation:* An additive effect of itraconazole with other drugs that prolong the QT interval cannot be excluded. The following drugs may prolong the QT interval and increase the risk of life-threatening cardiac arrhythmias, including torsade de pointes: Antiarrhythmic agents (eg, amiodarone, bretylium, disopyramide, dofetilide, procainamide, quinidine, and sotalol), arsenic trioxide, chlorpromazine, cisapride, dolasetron, droperidol, mefloquine, mesoridazine, moxifloxacin, pentamidine, pimozide, tacrolimus, thioridazine, and ziprasidone. For a more complete list of drugs that may prolong the QT interval, see the appendix, Drug-Induced Prolongation of the QT Interval and Torsade de Pointes.

Itraconazole Drug Interactions

Precipitant drug	Object drug[a]		Description
Antacids Proton pump inhibitors H_2-antagonists	Itraconazole	⬇	Absorption of itraconazole capsules is impaired when gastric acidity is decreased. Administer at least 1 hour before or 2 hours after itraconazole capsules. Administer itraconazole with a cola beverage when coadministering with H_2-antagonists or other gastric acid suppressors.
Didanosine (buffered formulation only)	Itraconazole	⬇	The therapeutic effects of itraconazole may be decreased. Administer itraconazole ≥ 2 hours before didanosine (buffered formulation only).
Macrolide antibiotics Erythromycin Clarithromycin	Itraconazole	⬆	Macrolide antibiotics may increase plasma itraconazole concentrations through inhibition of CYP3A4.
Nevirapine	Itraconazole	⬇	Coadministration may lead to decreased itraconazole plasma levels and, therefore, is not recommended.
Phenobarbital	Itraconazole	⬇	The plasma concentration of itraconazole may be decreased.
Itraconazole	Alfentanil	⬆	Pharmacologic and adverse effects may be increased. Use caution when administering concurrently. Lower the alfentanil dose as needed.
Itraconazole	Amphotericin B	⬇	Studies suggest that amphotericin B activity may be suppressed by prior azole antifungal therapy. Clinical significance is unknown.
Itraconazole	Aripiprazole	⬆	Aripiprazole plasma concentrations may be elevated, increasing the pharmacologic and adverse effects. Reduce the aripiprazole dose 50% of the normal dose when coadministering with itraconazole.
Itraconazole	Benzodiazepines Triazolam Midazolam Alprazolam Diazepam	⬆	Increased and prolonged serum levels, CNS depression, and psychomotor impairment with certain benzodiazepines may occur, possibly several days after stopping itraconazole. Concurrent use of triazolam and oral midazolam is contraindicated.
Itraconazole	Buspirone	⬆	Plasma buspirone concentrations may be elevated, increasing the pharmacologic and adverse effects. In patients receiving itraconazole when buspirone is started, it may be prudent to start with a conservative dose. Monitor closely when an antifungal agent is stopped, started, or changed in dose in patients on buspirone therapy. Adjust the dose of buspirone as needed.
Itraconazole	Busulfan	⬆	Itraconazole may elevate busulfan plasma levels, increasing the risk of toxicity (eg, pancytopenia). Monitor patients for increased toxicity and adjust the busulfan dose as needed.
Itraconazole	Calcium channel blockers	⬆	Concomitant administration may increase negative inotropic effects. Edema has also been reported with concomitant therapy. Itraconazole may inhibit the metabolism of calcium channel blockers such as dihydropyridines (eg, felodipine, nisoldipine, nifedipine) and verapamil. Coadminister with caution and adjust the dose of calcium channel blockers accordingly.
Itraconazole	Carbamazepine	⬆	Plasma concentrations of carbamazepine may be elevated, increasing clinical and adverse effects. Monitor serum levels.
Carbamazepine	Itraconazole	⬇	Decreased itraconazole plasma concentrations may occur with coadministration.

ITRACONAZOLE — ORAL

Itraconazole Drug Interactions

Precipitant drug	Object drug[a]		Description
Itraconazole	Cilostazol	↑	Cilostazol plasma concentrations may be elevated, increasing the pharmacologic and adverse effects. Use caution with coadministration.
Itraconazole	Cisapride	↑	Increased cisapride concentrations with cardiotoxicity may occur. Itraconazole is contraindicated in patients receiving cisapride.
Itraconazole	Corticosteroids Budesonide Dexamethasone Methylprednisolone	↑	Itraconazole may inhibit the metabolism of certain corticosteroids, enhancing the effects and possibly resulting in increased toxicity. Monitor patients for adverse effects and adjust corticosteroids dose accordingly.
Itraconazole	Cyclosporine	↑	Increased cyclosporine levels may occur. Monitor cyclosporine levels and serum creatinine when itraconazole is added or discontinued.
Itraconazole	Digoxin	↑	Serum digoxin concentrations may be increased, enhancing its pharmacologic and adverse effects. Monitor plasma digoxin concentrations and observe the patient for signs of digoxin toxicity. Adjust digoxin dose accordingly.
Itraconazole	Disopyramide	↑	Serum disopyramide concentrations may be elevated. A high plasma concentration has the potential to increase the QT interval.
Itraconazole	Docetaxel	↑	Itraconazole may inhibit docetaxel metabolism.
Itraconazole	Dofetilide	↑	Elevated dofetilide plasma concentrations may occur with increased risk of ventricular arrhythmias, including torsades de pointes. Administration with itraconazole is contraindicated.
Itraconazole	Eletriptan Almotriptan	↑	Plasma concentrations of eletriptan may be elevated, increasing the pharmacologic and adverse effects. Eletriptan should not be taken within 72 hours of itraconazole.
Itraconazole	Eplerenone	↑	Elevated eplerenone plasma concentrations may occur, increasing the risk of hyperkalemia and associated serious arrhythmias. Coadministration is contraindicated.
Itraconazole	Ergot alkaloids Dihydroergotamine Ergonovine Ergotamine Methylergonovine	↑	The risk of ergot toxicity (eg, peripheral vasospasm, ischemia of the extremities and/or cerebral ischemia) may be increased. Concomitant administration is contraindicated.
Itraconazole	Halofantrine	↑	Halofantrine plasma concentrations may be elevated, increasing the potential of prolonging the QT interval. Use caution with coadministration.
Itraconazole	Haloperidol	↑	Haloperidol concentrations may be elevated, increasing the risk of side effects. Adjust dose as needed.

Itraconazole Drug Interactions

Precipitant drug	Object drug[a]		Description
Itraconazole	HMG-CoA reductase inhibitors Atorvastatin Simvastatin Lovastatin	↑	Increased plasma levels and side effects of certain HMG-CoA reductase inhibitors may occur. If concurrent administration of these agents cannot be avoided, consider reducing the HMG-CoA reductase inhibitor dose. Coadministration with lovastatin and simvastatin is contraindicated.
Itraconazole	Hydantoins (eg, phenytoin)	↑	The plasma concentrations and pharmacologic effects of itraconazole may be decreased while those of hydantoins may be increased. Avoid concomitant use if possible.
Hydantoins (eg, phenytoin)	Itraconazole	↓	
Itraconazole	Oral hypoglycemic agents		Severe hypoglycemia has been reported in those receiving concomitant therapy. Monitor blood glucose levels carefully.
Itraconazole	Phosphodiesterase Type 5 Inhibitors Sildenafil Tadalafil Vardenafil		Phosphodiesterase Type 5 (PDE5) inhibitor plasma levels may be elevated, increasing the risk of side effects. Give PDE5 inhibitors with caution and in reduced doses to patients.
Itraconazole	Pimozide	↑	Concomitant use may increase pimozide plasma concentrations, resulting in serious cardiac effects. Administration with itraconazole is contraindicated.
Itraconazole	Protease inhibitors	↑	Plasma concentrations of protease inhibitors metabolized by CYP3A4 (eg, indinavir, ritonavir, saquinavir) may be elevated, increasing the risk of toxicity. Consider reducing the dose of the protease inhibitor during concurrent administration with itraconazole. Plasma concentrations of itraconazole may be increased by indinavir and ritonavir.
Protease inhibitors Indinavir Ritonavir	Itraconazole		
Itraconazole	Quinidine	↑	Quinidine concentrations may be elevated, increasing the risk of serious cardiovascular events. Coadministration is contraindicated.
Itraconazole	Rifamycins Rifabutin Rifampin Rifapentine Isoniazid	↑	Itraconazole levels may be decreased. Itraconazole may increase rifabutin plasma levels and toxicity. Anticipate similar effects with isoniazid. Coadministration is not recommended. If coadministration cannot be avoided, monitor antimicrobial activity and adjust dosage.
Rifamycins Rifabutin Rifampin Rifapentine Isoniazid	Itraconazole	↓	
Itraconazole	Sirolimus	↑	Coadministration may lead to increased sirolimus plasma levels. Monitor sirolimus plasma concentrations and observe patient for toxicity when starting or stopping itraconazole. Adjust sirolimus dose accordingly.
Itraconazole	Tacrolimus	↑	Tacrolimus concentrations may be elevated, increasing the toxicity risk.
Itraconazole	Tolterodine	↑	Tolterodine plasma concentrations may be elevated, increasing the pharmacologic and adverse effects. Patients receiving itraconazole should not receive more than 1 mg tolterodine twice daily.
Itraconazole	Trimetrexate	↑	Itraconazole may inhibit trimetrexate metabolism.
Itraconazole	Vinca alkaloids Vincristine Vinblastine	↑	Vinca alkaloid toxicity (constipation, myalgia, neutropenia) may be increased. Avoid concurrent administration of these agents if possible.

ITRACONAZOLE — ORAL

Itraconazole Drug Interactions			
Precipitant drug	Object drug[a]		Description
Itraconazole	Warfarin	↑	The anticoagulant effect of warfarin may be increased. Monitor prothrombin time (PT) and international normalized ratio (INR) values frequently when adding or discontinuing itraconazole. Adjust warfarin dose accordingly.
Itraconazole	Zolpidem	↑	Plasma concentrations and therapeutic effects of zolpidem may be increased. Monitor the clinical response of the patient. The dose of zolpidem may need to be decreased.

[a] ↑ = object drug increased; ↓ = object drug decreased.

➤*Drug/Food interactions:* The oral bioavailability of itraconazole is maximal when itraconazole capsules are taken with a full meal. The absorption of itraconazole was increased when itraconazole capsules were coadministered with a cola beverage. The bioavailability of itraconazole oral solution is increased under fasted conditions reaching higher maximum plasma concentrations (C_{max}) in a shorter period of time. Therefore, unlike itraconazole capsules, it is recommended that itraconazole oral solution be administered without food.

Adverse Reactions

Itraconazole has been associated with rare cases of serious hepatotoxicity, including liver failure and death. Some of these cases had neither preexisting liver disease nor a serious underlying medical condition. If clinical signs or symptoms develop that are consistent with liver disease, discontinue treatment and perform liver function testing. Reassess the risks and benefits of itraconazole use.

➤*Capsules:*

Adverse events in the treatment of systemic fungal infections – Adverse event data were derived from 602 patients treated for systemic fungal disease in US clinical trials who were immunocompromised or receiving multiple concomitant medications. Treatment was discontinued in 10.5% of patients because of adverse events. The median duration before discontinuation of therapy was 81 days (range, 2 to 776 days).

Itraconazole Capsules Adverse Events During Clinical Trials of Systemic Fungal Infections ≥ 1%	
Adverse reaction	Incidence (%) (n = 602)
CNS	
Dizziness	2%
Fatigue	3%
Headache	4%
Libido decreased	1%
Malaise	1%
Somnolence	1%
Dermatologic	
Pruritus	3%
Rash[a]	9%
GI	
Abdominal pain	2%
Anorexia	1%
Diarrhea	3%
Nausea	11%
Vomiting	5%
Miscellaneous	
Albuminuria	1%
Edema	4%
Fever	3%
Hepatic function abnormal	3%
Hypertension	3%
Hypokalemia	2%
Impotence	1%

[a] Rash tends to occur more frequently in immunocompromised patients receiving immunosuppressive medications.

Adverse events infrequently reported in all studies included adrenal insufficiency, constipation, depression, gastritis, gynecomastia, insomnia, male breast pain, menstrual disorder, and tinnitus.

Adverse events reported in toenail onychomycosis clinical trials – Patients in these trials were on a continuous dosing regimen of 200 mg once daily for 12 consecutive weeks.

Patients Temporarily or Permanently Discontinuing Itraconazole Treatment of Onychomycosis of the Toenail Because of Adverse Events (%)	
Adverse reaction	Itraconazole (n = 112)
Elevated liver enzymes (greater than twice the upper limit of normal)	4%
GI disorders	4%
Headache	1%
Hypertension	2%
Malaise	1%
Myalgia	1%
Orthostatic hypotension	1%
Rash	3%
Vasculitis	1%
Vertigo	1%

The following adverse events occurred with an incidence of greater than or equal to 1% (n = 112): headache (10%); rhinitis (9%); upper respiratory tract infection (8%); injury, sinusitis (7%); abdominal pain, diarrhea, dizziness, dyspepsia, flatulence, rash (4%); cystitis, liver function abnormality, myalgia, nausea, urinary tract infection (3%); abnormal dreaming, appetite increased, asthenia, constipation, fever, gastritis, gastroenteritis, herpes zoster, pain, pharyngitis, tremor (2%).

Adverse events reported in fingernail onychomycosis clinical trials – Patients in these trials were on a pulse regimen consisting of two 1-week treatment periods of 200 mg twice daily, separated by a 3-week period without drug.

Patients Temporarily or Permanently Discontinuing Itraconazole Treatment of Onychomycosis of the Fingernail Because of Adverse Events (%)	
Adverse reaction	Itraconazole (n = 37)
Hypertriglyceridemia	3%
Rash/pruritus	3%

The following adverse events occurred with an incidence of greater than or equal to 1% (n = 37): headache (8%); nausea, pruritus, rhinitis (5%); abdominal pain, anxiety, bursitis, constipation, depression, dyspepsia, fatigue, gingivitis, hypertriglyceridemia, injury, malaise, pain, rash, sinusitis, ulcerative stomatitis (3%).

Itraconazole Capsules Adverse Events in Clinical Trials of Onychomycosis of the Toenail (≥ 1%)	
Adverse reaction	Incidence (n = 112)
CNS	
Abnormal dreaming	2%
Asthenia	4%
Dizziness	2%
Headache	10%
Tremor	2%
GI	
Abdominal pain	4%
Appetite increased	2%
Constipation	2%
Diarrhea	4%
Dyspepsia	4%
Flatulence	4%
Gastritis	2%
Gastroenteritis	2%
Nausea	3%
GU	
Cystitis	3%
Urinary tract infection	3%
Respiratory	
Pharyngitis	2%
Rhinitis	9%
Sinusitis	7%
Upper respiratory tract infection	8%
Miscellaneous	
Fever	2%
Herpes zoster	2%
Injury	7%
Liver function abnormality	3%
Myalgia	3%
Pain	2%
Rash	4%

ITRACONAZOLE — ORAL

Itraconazole Capsules Adverse Events in Clinical Trials of Onychomycosis of the Fingernail (≥ 1%)

Adverse reaction	Incidence (n = 37)
CNS	
Anxiety	3%
Depression	3%
Fatigue	3%
Headache	8%
Malaise	3%
Dermatologic	
Pruritus	5%
Rash	3%
GI	
Abdominal pain	3%
Constipation	3%
Dyspepsia	3%
Gingivitis	3%
Nausea	5%
Ulcerative stomatitis	3%
Respiratory	
Rhinitis	5%
Sinusitis	3%
Miscellaneous	
Bursitis	3%
Hypertriglyceridemia	3%
Injury	3%
Pain	3%

➤*Oral solution:*

Adverse events reported in empiric therapy in febrile neutropenic (ETFN) patients – Adverse events considered at least possibly drug related in a clinical trial of empiric therapy in 384 febrile, neutropenic patients (192 treated with itraconazole and 192 with amphotericin B) with suspected fungal infections are listed in the table below. Patients received a regimen of itraconazole injection followed by itraconazole oral solution. The dose of itraconazole injection was 200 mg twice daily for the first 2 days followed by a single daily dose of 200 mg for the remainder of the intravenous treatment period. The majority of patients received between 7 and 14 days of itraconazole injection. The dose of itraconazole oral solution was 200 mg (20 mL) twice daily for the remainder of therapy.

Itraconazole Oral Solution Adverse Events in a Clinical Trial of Empiric Therapy in Febrile Neutropenic Patients (≥ 2%)

Adverse reaction	Itraconazole (n = 192)	Amphotericin B (n = 192)
Cardiovascular		
Hypertension	0%	2%
Hypotension	1%	3%
Tachycardia	1%	3%
Dermatologic		
Rash	5%	3%
Sweating increased	2%	1%
GI		
Abdominal pain	3%	3%
Diarrhea	10%	9%
Nausea	11%	15%
Vomiting	7%	10%
Hepatic		
ALT increased	3%	1%
AST increased	2%	1%
Bilirubinemia	6%	3%
Hepatic function abnormal	3%	2%
Jaundice	2%	1%
Metabolic		
Alkaline phosphatase increased	2%	2%
Blood urea nitrogen increased	1%	6%
Fluid overload	1%	3%
Hypocalcemia	1%	2%
Hypokalemia	9%	28%
Hypomagnesemia	2%	4%
LDH increased	2%	0%
Serum creatinine increased	3%	25%
Miscellaneous		
Dyspnea	1%	3%
Edema	2%	2%
Fever	0%	7%
Headache	2%	2 %
Renal function abnormal	1%	12%
Rigors	1%	34%

The following additional adverse events considered at least possibly related occurred in between 1% and 2% of patients who received itraconazole injection and oral solution: constipation, dizziness, erythematous rash, GGT increased, hypophosphatemia, pruritus, pulmonary infiltration, and tremor.

Adverse events reported in oropharyngeal or esophageal candidiasis trials – US adverse experience data are derived from 350 immunocompromised patients (332 HIV seropositive/AIDS) treated for oropharyngeal or esophageal candidiasis. The table below lists adverse events reported by at least 2% of patients treated with itraconazole oral solution in US clinical trials. Data on patients receiving comparator agents in these trials are included for comparison.

Itraconazole Oral Solution Adverse Events in Clinical Trials of Oropharyngeal Candidiasis (≥ 2%)

	Itraconazole			
Adverse reaction	Total (n = 350[a])	All controlled studies (n = 272)	Fluconazole (n = 125[b])	Clotrimazole (n = 81[c])
CNS				
Depression	2%	1%	0%	1%
Dizziness	2%	2%	4%	1%
Headache	4%	4%	6%	6%
Dermatologic				
Increased sweating	3%	4%	6%	1%
Rash	4%	5%	4%	6%
Skin disorder, unspecified	2%	2%	2%	1%
GI				
Abdominal pain	6%	4%	7%	7%
Constipation	2%	2%	1%	0%
Diarrhea	11%	10%	10%	4%
Nausea	11%	10%	11%	5%
Vomiting	7%	6%	8%	1%
Respiratory				
Coughing	4%	4%	10%	0%
Dyspnea	2%	3%	5%	1%
Pneumonia	2%	2%	0%	0%
Sinusitis	2%	2%	4%	0%
Sputum increased	2%	3%	3%	1%
Miscellaneous				
Chest pain	3%	3%	2%	0%
Fatigue	2%	1%	2%	0%
Fever	7%	6%	8%	5%
Pain	2%	2%	4%	0%
Pneumocystis carinii infection	2%	2%	2%	0%

[a] Of the 350 patients, 209 were treated for oropharyngeal candidiasis in controlled studies, 63 were treated for esophageal candidiasis in controlled studies and 78 were treated for oropharyngeal candidiasis in an open study.
[b] Of the 125 patients, 62 were treated for oropharyngeal candidiasis and 63 were treated for esophageal candidiasis.
[c] All 81 patients were treated for oropharyngeal candidiasis.

Adverse events reported by less than 2% of patients in US clinical trials with itraconazole included: adrenal insufficiency, asthenia, back pain, dehydration, dyspepsia, dysphagia, flatulence, gynecomastia, hematuria, hemor-

ITRACONAZOLE — ORAL

rhoids, hot flushes, implantation complication, infection unspecified, injury, insomnia, male breast pain, myalgia, pharyngitis, pruritus, rhinitis, rigors, stomatitis ulcerative, taste perversion, tinnitus, upper respiratory tract infection, vision abnormal, and weight decrease. Edema, hypokalemia, and menstrual disorders have been reported in clinical trials with itraconazole capsules.

➤*Postmarketing:* Worldwide postmarketing experiences with the use of itraconazole include adverse events of GI origin, such as abdominal pain, constipation, diarrhea, dyspepsia, nausea, and vomiting. Other reported adverse events include allergic reactions (eg, pruritus, rash, urticaria, angioedema, anaphylaxis), alopecia, anaphylactic, anaphylactoid, and allergic reaction, CHF and pulmonary edema, dizziness, headache, hepatitis, hypertriglyceridemia, hypokalemia, liver failure, menstrual disorders, neutropenia, peripheral edema, peripheral neuropathy, photosensitivity, reversible increases in hepatic enzymes, and Stevens-Johnson syndrome.

Congenital abnormalities – There is limited information on the use of itraconazole during pregnancy. Cases of congenital abnormalities, including skeletal, genitourinary tract, cardiovascular, and ophthalmic malformations, as well as chromosomal and multiple malformations have been reported during postmarketing experience. A causal relationship with itraconazole has not been established.

Overdosage

➤*Symptoms:* Limited data exist on the outcomes of patients ingesting high doses of itraconazole. In patients taking either itraconazole oral solution 1,000 mg or itraconazole capsules up to 3,000 mg, the adverse event profile was similar to that observed at recommended doses.

➤*Treatment:* Itraconazole is not removed by dialysis. In the event of accidental overdosage, employ supportive measures, including gastric lavage with sodium bicarbonate.

Patient Information

➤*Capsules:* The topical effects of mucosal exposure may be different between the itraconazole capsules and oral solution. Only the oral solution has been demonstrated effective for oral and/or esophageal candidiasis. Do not use itraconazole capsules interchangeably with itraconazole oral solution.

Instruct patients to take itraconazole capsules with a full meal.

Instruct patients about the signs and symptoms of CHF, and if these signs or symptoms occur during itraconazole administration, to discontinue itraconazole and contact their healthcare provider immediately.

Instruct patients to stop itraconazole treatment immediately and contact their healthcare provider if any signs and symptoms suggestive of liver dysfunction develop. Such signs and symptoms may include unusual anorexia, dark urine, fatigue, jaundice, nausea and/or vomiting, or pale stools.

Instruct patients to contact their physician before taking any concomitant medications with itraconazole to ensure there are no potential drug interactions.

➤*Oral solution:* Only itraconazole oral solution has been demonstrated effective for oral and/or esophageal candidiasis. Itraconazole oral solution contains the excipient hydroxypropyl-β-cyclodextrin which produced pancreatic adenocarcinomas in a rat carcinogenicity study. These findings were not observed in a similar mouse carcinogenicity study. The clinical relevance of these findings is unknown.

Taking itraconazole oral solution under fasted conditions improves the systemic availability of itraconazole. Instruct patients to take itraconazole oral solution without food, if possible.

Do not use itraconazole oral solution interchangeably with itraconazole capsules.

Patients taking itraconazole oral solution for the treatment of oropharyngeal and esophageal candidiasis should be instructed to vigorously swish in the mouth (10 mL at a time) for several seconds and swallowed.

TERBINAFINE

Rx	**Terbinafine Hydrochloride** (Various, eg, Aurobindo, Blu,[a] Teva, Sandoz)	**Tablet; oral:** 250 mg	As terbinafine hydrochloride. In 30s, 90s, 100s, 500s.
Rx	**Lamisil** (Novartis)		As terbinafine hydrochloride. (Lamisil 250). White to yellow-tinged white, biconvex. In 30s and 100s.
Rx	**Terbinex** (JSJ Pharmaceuticals)		As terbinafine hydrochloride. (IG 209). White, round. In kits with 42 tablets and 12 mL topical Eco Formula.
Rx	**Lamisil** (Novartis)	**Granules; oral:** 125 mg/packet	As terbinafine hydrochloride. PEG. Off-white to yellowish, biconvex. Film-coated. In cartons containing 14 or 42 packets.
		187.5 mg/packet	As terbinafine hydrochloride. PEG. Off-white to yellowish, biconvex. Film-coated. In cartons containing 14 or 42 packets.

[a] Blu Pharmaceuticals, 301 Robey St., Franklin, KY 42134; 1-877-264-0258; http://www.blurx.us.

TERBINAFINE HYDROCHLORIDE — ORAL

For complete and comparative prescribing information, refer to the Terbinafine Topical monograph.

Indications

➤*Onychomycosis (tablets):* For the treatment of onychomycosis of the toenail or fingernail caused by dermatophytes (tinea unguium).

Prior to initiating treatment, obtain appropriate nail specimens for laboratory testing (potassium hydroxide [KOH] preparation, fungal culture, or nail biopsy) to confirm the diagnosis of onychomycosis.

➤*Tinea capitis (oral granules):* For the treatment of tinea capitis in patients 4 years of age and older.

Administration and Dosage

➤*General dosing considerations:* The optimal clinical effect for the treatment of onychomycosis is seen some months after mycological cure and cessation of treatment. This is related to the period required for outgrowth of healthy nail.

➤*Adults:*

Onychomycosis of the fingernail – One 250 mg tablet once daily for 6 weeks.

Onychomycosis of the toenail – One 250 mg tablet once daily for 12 weeks.

Tinea capitis – 250 mg once daily for 6 weeks (oral granules only).

➤*Children:*

Tinea capitis –

4 years of age and older:

Terbinafine Oral Granules Dosage by Body Weight	
Body weight	Dosage
< 25 kg	125 mg once daily for 6 weeks
25 to 35 kg	187.5 mg once daily for 6 weeks
> 35 kg	250 mg once daily for 6 weeks

• *Duration of therapy* – 2 to 4 weeks of *Trichophyton* species or 2 to 8 weeks for *Microsporum* species.

Off-label dosing –

Onychomycosis:

Terbinafine Oral Tablets Dosage by Body Weight	
Body weight	Dosage
Standard dose	
10 to 20 kg	62.5 mg daily
20 to 40 kg	125 mg daily
> 40 kg	250 mg daily
High dose	
10 to 15 kg	125 mg daily
16 to 25 kg	187.5 mg daily
> 25 kg	250 mg daily

• *Duration of therapy* – 6 to 12 weeks for onchomycosis (12 weeks for toenail, 6 for fingernail).

TERBINAFINE HYDROCHLORIDE — ORAL

➤*Renal function impairment:* In patients with renal function impairment (CrCl of 50 mL/min or less), the use of terbinafine has not been adequately studied and, therefore, is not recommended.

➤*Hepatic function impairment:* Terbinafine is not recommended for patients with chronic or active liver disease.

➤*Administration:*

Oral granules – Sprinkle the contents of each packet on a spoonful of pudding or other soft, nonacidic food, such as mashed potatoes, and swallow the entire spoonful (without chewing); do not use applesauce or fruit-based foods. Take with food. If 2 packets (250 mg) are required with each dose, the content of both packets may be sprinkled on 1 spoonful, or the contents of both packets may be sprinkled on 2 spoonfuls of nonacidic food as previously directed.

➤*Storage/Stability:*

Oral granules – Store at 25°C (77°F); excursions are permitted to 15° to 30°C (59° to 86°F).

Tablets – Store below 25°C (77°F) in a tightly closed container. Protect from light.

Actions

➤*Pharmacology:* Terbinafine is a synthetic allylamine derivative. Terbinafine is hypothesized to act by inhibiting squalene epoxidase, thus blocking the biosynthesis of ergosterol, an essential component of fungal cell membranes. In vitro, mammalian squalene epoxidase is only inhibited at higher (4,000-fold) concentrations than is needed for inhibition of the dermatophyte enzyme. Depending on the concentration of the drug and the fungal species test in vitro, terbinafine may be fungicidal. However, the clinical significance of in vitro data is unknown.

➤*Pharmacokinetics:*

Absorption/Distribution –

Tablets: Following oral administration, terbinafine is well absorbed (more than 70%), and the bioavailability as a result of first-pass metabolism is approximately 40%. Peak plasma concentrations (C_{max}) of 1 mcg/mL appear within 2 hours after a single 250 mg dose; the area under the curve (AUC) is approximately 4.56 mcg•h/mL. In plasma, terbinafine is more than 99% bound to plasma proteins and there are no specific binding sites. At steady state, in comparison with a single dose, the C_{max} of terbinafine is 25% higher, and plasma AUC increases by a factor of 2.5; the increase in plasma AUC is consistent with an effective half-life of approximately 36 hours. Terbinafine is distributed to the sebum and skin.

• *Food effects* – An increase in the AUC of terbinafine of less than 20% is observed when terbinafine is administered with food.

Oral granules: The pharmacokinetics in children 4 to 8 years of age with tinea capitis were investigated in a pharmacokinetic study after single and repeated (for 42 days) oral administration of terbinafine oral granules (N = 16) once daily using the body weight groups and doses. The systemic exposure C_{max} and AUC_{0-24} of terbinafine in children had a relatively high inter-individual variability (ranging from 36% to 64%). At steady state, the AUC_{0-24} increased by a mean factor of 1.9 to 2.1 across doses. In plasma, terbinafine is more than 99% bound to plasma proteins.

Metabolism/Excretion –

Tablets: Prior to excretion, terbinafine is extensively metabolized. No metabolites have been identified that have antifungal activity similar to terbinafine. Approximately 70% of the administered dose is eliminated in the urine. A terminal half-life of 200 to 400 hours may represent the slow elimination of terbinafine from tissues such as skin and adipose.

Oral granules: Prior to excretion, terbinafine is rapidly and extensively metabolized by at least 7 cytochrome P450 (CYP-450) isoenzymes, with major contributions from CYP2C9, CYP1A2, CYP3A4, CYP2C8, and CYPC19. No metabolites have been identified that have antifungal activity similar to terbinafine. The mean standard deviation effective half-life obtained from the observed accumulation was 26.7 (13.8) hours and 30.5 (9.3) hours for the 125 and 187.5 mg doses, respectively. Approximately 70% of the administered dose is eliminated in the urine.

Systemic exposure to terbinafine in the children did not exceed the highest values of the systemic exposure in adults receiving repeated once daily doses of terbinafine 250 mg tablets. A population pharmacokinetic evaluation of oral terbinafine that included children 4 to 12 years of age and adults 18 to 45 years of age (N = 113) found that clearance (CL/F) of terbinafine is dependent on body weight in a nonlinear manner. For a typical child of 25 kg, CL/F was predicted to be 19 L/h, and for a typical adult of 70 kg body weight, it was predicted to be 27 L/h. Over the weight range for children included in the analysis (14.1 to 68 kg), the predicted CL/F ranged between 15.6 and 26.7 L/h.

Special populations –

Renal and hepatic function impairment: In patients with renal function impairment (creatinine clearance [CrCl] 50 mL/min or less) or hepatic cirrhosis, the clearance of terbinafine is decreased by approximately 50% compared with healthy volunteers.

➤*Microbiology:* Terbinafine has been shown to be active against most strains of the following microorganisms both in vitro and in clinical infections: *Trichophyton mentagrophytes* and *Trichophyton rubrum*.

The following in vitro data are available, but their clinical significance is unknown. In vitro, terbinafine exhibits satisfactory minimum inhibitory concentrations against most strains of the following microorganisms; however, the safety and efficacy of terbinafine in treating clinical infections caused by these microorganisms have not been established in adequate and well-controlled clinical trials: *Candida albicans, Epidermophyton floccosum*, and *Scopulariopsis brevicaulis*.

Contraindications

Hypersensitivity to terbinafine or to any other ingredients of the formulation.

Warnings/Precautions

➤*Hepatic effects:* Cases of liver failure, some leading to death or liver transplant, have occurred with the use of terbinafine for the treatment of onychomycosis in patients with and without preexisting liver disease.

In the majority of liver cases reported in association with terbinafine use, the patients had serious underlying systemic conditions and an uncertain causal association with terbinafine. The severity of hepatic events and/or their outcomes may be worse in patients with active or chronic liver disease. Discontinue treatment with terbinafine tablets if biochemical or clinical evidence of liver injury develops.

➤*Dermatologic effects:* There have been isolated reports of serious skin reactions (eg, Stevens-Johnson syndrome, toxic epidermal necrolysis). If progressive skin rash occurs, discontinue treatment with terbinafine.

➤*Systemic lupus erythematosus:* During postmarketing experience, precipitation and exacerbation of cutaneous and systemic lupus erythematosus have been reported infrequently in patients taking terbinafine. Discontinue terbinafine therapy in patients with clinical signs and symptoms suggestive of lupus erythematosus.

➤*Ophthalmic effects:* Changes in the ocular lens and retina have been reported following the use of terbinafine tablets in controlled trials. The clinical significance of these changes is unknown.

➤*Hematologic effects:*

Absolute lymphocyte counts – Transient decreases in absolute lymphocyte counts (ALCs) have been observed in controlled clinical trials. In placebo-controlled trials, 8 of 465 (1.7%) terbinafine-treated patients and 3 of 137 (2.2%) placebo-treated patients had decreases in ALC to less than 1,000/mm^3 on 2 or more occasions. The clinical significance of this observation is unknown. However, in patients with known or suspected immunodeficiency, consider monitoring complete blood cell counts (CBCs) if terbinafine therapy will exceed 6 weeks.

Neutropenia – Isolated cases of severe neutropenia have been reported. These were reversible upon discontinuation of terbinafine, with or without supportive therapy. If clinical signs and symptoms suggestive of secondary infection occur, obtain a CBC. If the neutrophil count is 1,000 cells/mm^3 or less, discontinue terbinafine and start supportive management.

➤*Renal function impairment:* In patients with renal function impairment (CrCl of 50 mL/min or less), the use of terbinafine has not been adequately studied and, therefore, is not recommended.

➤*Hepatic function impairment:* Terbinafine is not recommended for patients with chronic or active liver disease. Before prescribing terbinafine, assess preexisting liver disease. Hepatotoxicity may occur in patients with and without preexisting liver disease. Pretreatment serum transaminase (ALT and AST) tests are advised for all patients before taking terbinafine. Warn patients prescribed terbinafine to report immediately to their health care provider any symptoms of anorexia, dark urine or pale stools, fatigue, persistent nausea, right upper abdominal pain or jaundice, or vomiting. Advise patients with these symptoms to discontinue taking oral terbinafine, and immediately evaluate the patient's liver function.

➤*Pregnancy: Category B.* There are no adequate and well-controlled studies in pregnant women. Because animal reproduction studies are not always predictive of human response, and because treatment of onychomycosis can be postponed until after pregnancy is completed, it is recommended that terbinafine not be initiated during pregnancy.

➤*Lactation:* After oral administration, terbinafine is present in the breast milk of breast-feeding mothers. The ratio of terbinafine in milk to plasma is 7:1. Treatment with terbinafine is not recommended in breast-feeding mothers.

➤*Children:*

Tablets – The safety and efficacy of terbinafine have not been established in children.

Oral granules – Terbinafine oral granules were studied in 2 randomized, active-controlled trials in which 1,021 subjects with a clinical diagnosis of tinea capitis confirmed by KOH microscopy were treated with terbinafine at the labeled dose for up to 6 weeks. The most common adverse reactions were cough, headache, nasopharyngitis, pyrexia, upper respiratory tract infection, and vomiting.

➤*Monitoring:* In patients with known or suspected immunodeficiency, consider monitoring CBCs in patients using terbinafine therapy for more than 6 weeks.

Pretreatment serum transaminase (ALT and AST) tests are advised for all patients before taking terbinafine.

Drug Interactions

➤*CYP-450 system:* In vivo studies have shown that terbinafine is an inhibitor of the CYP-450 2D6 isozyme. Carefully monitor drugs predominantly metabolized by the CYP-450 2D6 isozyme; a reduction in a dose of the 2D6-metabolized drug may be required.

TERBINAFINE HYDROCHLORIDE — ORAL

Terbinafine Drug Interactions[a]

Precipitant drug	Object drug[b]		Description
Cimetidine	Terbinafine	↑	Terbinafine clearance is decreased 33% by cimetidine.
Fluconazole	Terbinafine	↑	Coadministration of a single dose of fluconazole (100 mg) with a single dose of terbinafine resulted in a 52% and 69% increase in terbinafine C_{max} and AUC, respectively.
Rifampin	Terbinafine	↓	Terbinafine clearance is increased 100% by rifampin.
Terbinafine	Antiarrhythmics class type 1C (eg, flecainide, propafenone)	↑	Terbinafine is an inhibitor of the CYP2D6 isozyme; therefore, drugs predominantly metabolized by this isozyme, such as antiarrhythmics type 1C, should be done with careful monitoring and may require a dose reduction.
Terbinafine	Beta-blockers	↑	Terbinafine is an inhibitor of the CYP2D6 isozyme; therefore, drugs predominantly metabolized by this isozyme, such as beta-blockers, should be done with careful monitoring and may require a dose reduction.
Terbinafine	Caffeine	↑	Terbinafine decreases the clearance of caffeine by 19%.
Terbinafine	Cyclosporine	↓	Terbinafine increases the clearance of cyclosporine by 15%.
Terbinafine	Dextromethorphan	↑	Plasma dextromethorphan concentrations may be elevated, increasing the pharmacologic and adverse reactions. Reduce the dose of dextromethorphan as needed.
Terbinafine	MAOIs type B (eg, rasagiline, selegiline)	↑	Terbinafine is an inhibitor of the CYP2D6 isozyme; therefore, drugs predominantly metabolized by this isozyme, such as MAOIs type B, should be done with careful monitoring and may require a dose reduction.
Terbinafine	SRIs (eg, paroxetine, venlafaxine)	↑	SRI plasma concentrations may be elevated, increasing the pharmacologic effects and adverse reactions. Adjust the SRI dose as needed.
Terbinafine	Tricyclic antidepressants (eg, amitriptyline, desipramine, nortriptyline)	↑	The pharmacologic and toxic effects of tricyclic antidepressants may be increased. Monitor for signs of tricyclic antidepressant toxicity and adjust the dose as needed.
Terbinafine	Warfarin	↑↓	Spontaneous reports of increase or decrease in prothrombin times in patients concomitantly taking terbinafine and warfarin have been reported; however, a casual relationship has not been established.

[a] MAOI = monoamine oxidase inhibitor; SRI = serotonin reuptake inhibitor.
[b] ↑ = object drug increased; ↓ = object drug decreased; ↑↓ = object drug both increased and decreased.

➤*Drug/Food interactions:*

Tablets – An increase in the AUC of terbinafine tablets of less than 20% is observed when terbinafine is administered with food.

Adverse Reactions

➤*Onychomycosis (tablets):*

Terbinafine (Tablets) Adverse Reactions

	Adverse reaction		Discontinuation	
Adverse reactions	Terbinafine (n = 465)	Placebo (n = 137)	Terbinafine (n = 465)	Placebo (n = 137)
CNS				
Headache	12.9%	9.5%	0.2%	0%
Dermatologic				
Pruritus	2.8%	1.5%	0.2%	0%
Rash	5.6%	2.2%	0.9%	0.7%
Urticaria	1.1%	0%	0%	0%
GI				
Abdominal pain	2.4%	1.5%	0.4%	0%
Diarrhea	5.6%	2.9%	0.6%	0%
Dyspepsia	4.3%	2.9%	0.4%	0%
Flatulence	2.2%	2.2%	0%	0%
Nausea	2.6%	2.9%	0.2%	0%
Hepatic				
Liver enzyme abnormalities[a]	3.3%	1.4%	0.2%	0%
Special senses				
Taste disturbance	2.8%	0.7%	0.2%	0%
Visual disturbance	1.1%	1.5%	0.9%	0%

[a] Liver enzyme abnormalities 2 or more times the upper limit of normal range.

➤*Other adverse reactions:* Adverse reactions, based on worldwide experience with terbinafine tablets use, include the following:

Dermatologic – Acute generalized exanthematous pustulosis, precipitation and exacerbation of cutaneous and systemic lupus erythematosus, psoriasiform eruptions or exacerbation of psoriasis, and serious skin reactions (eg, Stevens-Johnson syndrome and toxic epidermal necrolysis) have been reported in patients taking terbinafine.

Hematologic – Severe neutropenia, thrombocytopenia.

Hepatic – Idiosyncratic and symptomatic hepatic injury and, more rarely, cases of liver failure, some leading to death or liver transplant.

Hypersensitivity – Allergic reactions (including anaphylaxis), angioedema.

Musculoskeletal – Arthralgia, myalgia.

Special senses – Terbinafine may cause taste disturbance (including taste loss), which usually recovers within several weeks after discontinuation of the drug. There have been isolated reports of prolonged (more than 1 year) taste disturbances. Rarely, taste disturbances associated with oral terbinafine have been reported to be severe enough to result in decreased food intake leading to significant and unwanted weight loss.

Miscellaneous – Fatigue, hair loss, malaise, vomiting.

➤*Tinea capitis (oral granules):*

Terbinafine (Oral Granules) Adverse Reactions (≥ 1%)

Adverse reactions	Terbinafine oral granules (n = 1,042)	Griseofulvin oral suspension (n = 507)
CNS		
Headache	7%	8%
Dermatologic		
Pruritus	1%	1%
Rash	2%	2%
GI		
Abdominal pain	2%	1%
Diarrhea	3%	4%
Nausea	2%	2%
Toothache	1%	1%
Upper abdominal pain	4%	4%
Vomiting	5%	5%
Respiratory		
Cough	6%	5%
Nasal congestion	2%	1%
Nasopharyngitis	10%	11%
Pharyngolaryngeal pain	2%	2%
Rhinorrhea	2%	0%
Upper respiratory tract infection	5%	5%

Allylamine Antifungal

TERBINAFINE HYDROCHLORIDE — ORAL

Terbinafine (Oral Granules) Adverse Reactions (≥ 1%)		
Adverse reactions	Terbinafine oral granules (n = 1,042)	Griseofulvin oral suspension (n = 507)
Miscellaneous		
Pyrexia	7%	6%
Influenza	2%	1%

Adverse reactions leading to discontinuation – In the pooled pivotal trials, 2% (17/1,042) of subjects in the terbinafine group and 25% (6/507) in the griseofulvin group experienced discontinuation of study drug because of adverse reactions. The most common categories of adverse reactions causing discontinuation in those exposed to terbinafine included GI disorders, skin and subcutaneous disorders, and infections and infestations.

Ophthalmic – For visual acuity, 1% (11/837) of subjects treated with terbinafine and 2% (7/426) of subjects treated with griseofulvin showed a doubling of visual angle after 6 weeks of treatment, while 2% (15/837) treated with terbinafine and 3% (12/426) treated with griseofulvin showed a halving of the visual angle after 6 weeks of treatment. Of subjects who completed yellow-blue color vision assessment for acquired defects, 5% (13/262) of subjects treated with terbinafine and 6% (8/129) of subjects treated with griseofulvin had color confusion on more than 1 symbol at week 6 than at baseline, while 13% (33/262) of subjects treated with terbinafine and 13% (17/129) of subjects treated with griseofulvin identified more symbols correctly at week 6 than at baseline.

➤*Postmarketing:* Altered prothrombin time (prolongation and reduction) in patients concomitantly treated with warfarin and terbinafine, agranulocytosis (rare), and precipitation and exacerbation of cutaneous and systemic lupus erythematosus have been reported infrequently.

Overdosage

➤*Oral granules:* In a 52-week toxicology study conducted in juvenile maturing dogs, increased heart and liver weights were noted in males and signs of CNS disturbance, including 3 cases of single episodes of seizures, were noted in females at the highest dosage tested, 100 mg/kg/day (19 times [males] and 10 times [females] the maximum recommended human dose (MRHD) based on AUC comparisons of the parent terbinafine). No treatment-related findings were noted at 30 mg/kg/day (1.6 times [males] and 1.9 times [females]) the MRHD based on AUC comparisons of the parent terbinafine) in this study.

➤*Symptoms:* Clinical experience regarding overdose with terbinafine is limited. Doses of up to 5 g in adults (20 times the therapeutic daily dose) have been taken without inducing serious adverse reactions. The symptoms of overdose included abdominal pain, dizziness, frequent urination, headache, nausea, rash, and vomiting.

Patient Information

Warn patients prescribed terbinafine to report immediately to their health care provider any symptoms of anorexia, dark urine, fatigue, pale stools, persistent nausea, right upper abdominal pain or jaundice, or vomiting. Instruct patients with these symptoms to discontinue taking oral terbinafine, and immediately evaluate the patient's liver function.

Echinocandins

CASPOFUNGIN ACETATE

Rx	**Cancidas** (Merck)	**Injection, lyophilized powder for solution:** 50 mg	Sucrose 39 mg, mannitol 26 mg. In single-use vials.
		70 mg	Sucrose 54 mg, mannitol 36 mg. In single-use vials.

CASPOFUNGIN ACETATE — INJECTION

Indications

➤*Candidemia and other Candida infections:* For the treatment of candidemia and the following *Candida* infections in patients 3 months of age and older: intra-abdominal abscesses, peritonitis, and pleural space infections.

➤*Esophageal candidiasis:* For the treatment of esophageal candidiasis in patients 3 months of age and older.

➤*Fungal infections, empirical therapy:* For empirical therapy for presumed fungal infections in febrile, neutropenic patients 3 months of age and older.

➤*Invasive aspergillosis:* For the treatment of invasive aspergillosis in patients 3 months of age and older who are refractory to or intolerant of other therapies (eg, amphotericin B, lipid formulations of amphotericin B, itraconazole).

Administration and Dosage

➤*Adults:*

Usual dosage – A single 70 mg loading dose followed by 50 mg once daily thereafter. The safety and efficacy of a dosage of 150 mg daily (range, 1 to 51 days; median, 14 days) has been studied in 100 adult patients with candidemia and other *Candida* infections. The efficacy of caspofungin at this higher dosage was not significantly better than the efficacy of the 50 mg daily dosage of caspofungin. The efficacy of dosages higher than 50 mg daily in the other adult patients for whom caspofungin is indicated is not known.

Candidemia and other Candida infections –

Loading dose: A single 70 mg intravenous (IV) infusion on day 1.

Maintenance dosage: Follow the loading dose with 50 mg IV once daily.

Duration of therapy: The patient's clinical and microbiological response should dictate duration of treatment. In general, continue antifungal therapy for at least 14 days after the last positive culture. Patients who remain persistently neutropenic may warrant a longer course of therapy pending resolution of neutropenia.

Esophageal candidiasis –

Usual dosage: 50 mg IV once daily. A 70 mg loading dose has not been studied with this indication.

Duration of therapy: Continue therapy for 7 to 14 days after symptom resolution. Because of the risk of relapse of oropharyngeal candidiasis in patients with HIV infection, suppressive oral therapy may be considered.

Fungal infections, empirical therapy –

Loading dose: A single 70 mg IV infusion over 1 hour on day 1.

Maintenance dosage: Follow the loading dose with 50 mg IV once daily.

Dosage adjustment: If the 50 mg dose is well tolerated but does not provide an adequate clinical response, the daily dose can be increased to 70 mg.

Duration of therapy: Base duration of treatment on the patient's clinical response. Continue empirical therapy until resolution of neutropenia. Treat patients found to have a fungal infection for a minimum of 14 days; continue treatment for at least 7 days after neutropenia and clinical symptoms are resolved.

Invasive aspergillosis –

Loading dose: A single 70 mg IV infusion on day 1.

Maintenance dosage: Follow the loading dose with 50 mg IV once daily.

Duration of therapy: Base duration of treatment on the severity of the patient's underlying disease, recovery from immunosuppression, and clinical response.

➤*Children:*

Fungal infections – For a list of infections, refer to Indications.

3 months to 17 years of age:

• *Maximum dose* – The maximum loading dose and the daily maintenance dose should not exceed 70 mg, regardless of the patient's calculated dose.

• *Loading dose* – A single 70 mg/m² IV infusion on day 1.

• *Maintenance dosage* – Follow the loading dose with 50 mg/m² IV once daily.

• *Dosage adjustment* – If the 50 mg/m² daily dose is well tolerated but does not provide an adequate clinical response, the daily dose can be increased to 70 mg/m² daily (not to exceed 70 mg).

• *Duration of therapy* – Duration of treatment should be individualized to the indication, as described for each indication in adults. (See Adults.)

Off-label dosing –

Neonates and infants younger than 3 months of age:

• *Usual dose* – 1 mg/kg/day IV for 2 days, followed by 2 mg/kg/day. Dosage was administered by slow IV infusion (over approximately 1 hour).

• *Alternative dosage* – Other reported dosage regimens include 5 mg/kg/day (50 mg/m²) IV for 3 days, followed by 2.5 mg/kg/day (25 mg/m²) or 1.5 to 8 mg/kg/day IV on day 1, followed by 1 to 6 mg/kg/day.

➤*Hepatic function impairment:*

Adults –

Moderate hepatic impairment (Child-Pugh score, 7 to 9): 35 mg IV once daily. When recommended, a 70 mg loading dose should still be administered on day 1.

Severe hepatic impairment (Child-Pugh score, greater than 9): There is no clinical experience.

➤*Concomitant therapy:*

Adults – Adult patients on rifampin should receive an IV infusion of caspofungin 70 mg once daily. Patients on nevirapine, efavirenz, carbamazepine, dexamethasone, or phenytoin may require an increase in dosage to caspofungin 70 mg once daily.

Children – When caspofungin is coadministered with inducers of drug clearance to children, such as rifampin, efavirenz, nevirapine, phenytoin, dexamethasone, or carbamazepine, consider a caspofungin dosage of 70 mg/m² IV infusion once daily (not to exceed 70 mg).

➤*Preparation for administration:*

Reconstitution – Equilibrate the refrigerated vial of caspofungin to room temperature. Aseptically add 10.8 mL of sodium chloride 0.9% injection, sterile water for injection, bacteriostatic water for injection with methylparaben and propylparaben, or bacteriostatic water for injection with benzyl alcohol 0.9% to the vial. Each vial of caspofungin contains an intentional overfill of caspofungin. Thus, the drug concentration of the resulting solution is listed in the following table.

CASPOFUNGIN ACETATE — INJECTION

Caspofungin Acetate Injection Reconstitution			
Caspofungin vial	Total drug content (including overfill)	Reconstitution volume to be added	Resulting concentration following reconstitution
50 mg	54.6 mg	10.8 mL	5 mg/mL
70 mg	75.6 mg	10.8 mL	7 mg/mL

The white to off-white cake will dissolve completely. Mix gently until a clear solution is obtained.

Dilution – Aseptically transfer the appropriate volume (mL) of reconstituted caspofungin to an IV bag (or bottle) containing 250 mL of sodium chloride 0.9%, 0.45%, or 0.225% injection or Ringer's lactate injection. Alternatively, the volume (mL) of reconstituted caspofungin can be added to a reduced volume of sodium chloride 0.9%, 0.45%, or 0.225% injection or Ringer's lactate injection, not to exceed a final concentration of 0.5 mg/mL.

Special considerations for children older than 3 months of age – Follow the reconstitution procedures using either the 70 or 50 mg vial to create the reconstituted solution. From the reconstituted solution in the vial, remove the volume of drug equal to the calculated loading dose or calculated maintenance dose based on a concentration of 7 mg/mL (if reconstituted from the 70 mg vial) or a concentration of 5 mg/mL (if reconstituted from the 50 mg vial).

The choice of vial should be based on total milligram dose of drug to be administered to the child. If available, it is recommended to use 50 mg vials (with a concentration of 5 mg/mL) for pediatric doses less than 50 mg to help ensure accurate dosing. The 70 mg vial should be reserved for children requiring doses greater than 50 mg.

➤*Administration:* Administer by slow IV infusion over approximately 1 hour. Caspofungin should not be administered by IV bolus administration.

➤*Admixture compatibility:* Do not mix or coinfuse caspofungin with other medications because there are no data available on the compatibility of caspofungin with other IV substances, additives, or medications. Do not use diluents containing dextrose (alpha-d-glucose) because caspofungin is not stable in diluents containing dextrose.

➤*Storage/Stability:* Store the lyophilized vials refrigerated at 2° to 8°C (36° to 46°F). Reconstituted caspofungin in the vial may be stored at 25°C or below (77°F or below) for 1 hour prior to the preparation of the patient infusion solution. Caspofungin vials are for single use only; discard any remaining solutions. The final infusion solution in the IV bag or bottle can be stored at 25°C or below (77°F or below) for 24 hours or at 2° to 8°C (36° to 46°F) for 48 hours.

Actions

➤*Pharmacology:* Caspofungin is an echinocandin antifungal drug that inhibits the synthesis of beta (1,3)-D-glucan, an essential component of the cell wall of susceptible *Aspergillus* and *Candida* species. Beta (1,3)-D-glucan is not present in mammalian cells. Caspofungin has shown activity against *Candida* species and in regions of active cell growth of the hyphae of *Aspergillus fumigatus*.

➤*Pharmacokinetics:*

Caspofungin Pharmacokinetic Parameters in Children 3 Months to 17 Years of Age and Adults[a]							
			Pharmacokinetic parameters (mean ± SD)				
Population	n	Daily dose	AUC_{0-24h} (mcg•h/mL)	C_{1h} (mcg/mL)	C_{24h} (mcg/mL)	Half-life (h)[b]	Clearance (mL/min)
Children							
Adolescents 12 to 17 years of age	8	50 mg/m²	124.9 ± 50.4	14 ± 6.9	2.4 ± 1	11.2 ± 1.7	12.6 ±5.5
Children 2 to 11 years of age	9	50 mg/m²	120 ± 33.4	16.1 ± 4.2	1.7 ± 0.8	8.2 ± 2.4	6.4 ± 2.6
Young children 3 to 23 months of age	8	50 mg/m²	131.2 ± 17.7	17.6 ± 3.9	1.7 ± 0.7	8.8 ± 2.1	3.2 ± 0.4
Adult patients							
Adults with esophageal candidiasis	6[c]	50 mg	87.3 ± 30	8.7 ± 2.1	1.7 ± 0.7	13 ± 1.9	10.6 ± 3.8
Adults receiving empirical therapy	119[d]	50 mg[e]		8 ± 3.4	1.6 ± 0.7		

[a] SD = standard deviation; AUC = area under the curve.
[b] Harmonic mean ± jackknife standard deviation.
[c] n = 5 for $C_{1\,h}$ and AUC $_{0\text{-}24\,h}$; n = 6 for $C_{24\,h}$.
[d] n = 117 for $C_{24\,h}$; n =119 for $C_{1\,h}$.
[e] Following an initial 70 mg loading dose on day 1.

Distribution – Plasma concentrations of caspofungin decline in a polyphasic manner following single 1-hour IV infusions. A short alpha phase occurs immediately postinfusion, followed by a beta phase (half-life, 9 to 11 hours) that characterizes much of the profile and exhibits clear log-linear behavior from 6 to 48 hours postdose, during which the plasma concentration decreases 10-fold. An additional, longer half-life phase, gamma phase (half-life, 40 to 50 hours), also occurs. There is little excretion or biotransformation of caspofungin during the first 30 hours after administration.

Distribution, rather than excretion or biotransformation, is the dominant mechanism influencing plasma clearance. Caspofungin is bound extensively to albumin (approximately 97%), and distribution into red blood cells is minimal. Mass balance results showed that approximately 92% of the administered radioactivity was distributed to tissues by 36 to 48 hours after a single dose of [^{3}H] caspofungin 70 mg.

Metabolism – Caspofungin is metabolized slowly by hydrolysis and N-acetylation. Caspofungin also undergoes spontaneous chemical degradation to an open-ring peptide compound, L-747969. At later time points (at least 5 days postdose), there is a low level (7 picomoles/mg protein or less, or 1.3% or less of administered dose) of covalent binding of radiolabel in plasma following single-dose administration of [^{3}H] caspofungin, which may be caused by 2 reactive intermediates formed during the chemical degradation of caspofungin to L-747969. Additional metabolism involves hydrolysis into constitutive amino acids and their degradates, including dihydroxyhomotyrosine and N-acetyl-dihydroxyhomotyrosine. These 2 tyrosine derivatives are found only in urine, suggesting rapid clearance by the kidneys.

Excretion – Two single-dose pharmacokinetic studies were conducted with radiolabeled caspofungin. In 1 study, plasma, urine, and feces were collected over 27 days, and in the second study, plasma was collected over 6 months. Plasma concentrations of radioactivity and of caspofungin were similar during the first 24 to 48 hours postdose; thereafter, drug levels fell more rapidly. In plasma, caspofungin concentrations fell below the limit of quantitation after 6 to 8 days postdose, while radiolabel fell below the limit of quantitation at 22.3 weeks postdose. After single IV administration of [^{3}H] caspofungin, excretion of caspofungin and its metabolites in humans was 35% of the dose in feces and 41% of the dose in urine. A small amount of caspofungin is excreted unchanged in urine (approximately 1.4% of the dose). Renal clearance of the parent drug is low (approximately 0.15 mL/min), and total clearance of caspofungin is 12 mL/min.

Special populations –

Hepatic function impairment: Adult patients with moderate hepatic impairment (Child-Pugh score, 7 to 9) who received a single dose of caspofungin 70 mg had an average plasma caspofungin increase of 76% in the AUC compared with healthy subjects. A dosage reduction is recommended for adults with moderate hepatic impairment based on this pharmacokinetic data. There is no clinical experience in adults with severe hepatic impairment (Child-Pugh score, greater than 9) or in children with any degree of hepatic impairment.

Gender: After 13 daily 50 mg doses, caspofungin plasma concentrations in women were elevated slightly (approximately 22% in AUC) relative to men. No dosage adjustment is necessary based on gender.

➤*Microbiology:*

Activity in vitro – Caspofungin has been shown to be active in in vitro and clinical infections against most strains of the following microorganisms: *A. fumigatus*, *Aspergillus flavus*, *Aspergillus terreus* and *Candida albicans*, *Candida glabrata*, *Candida guilliermondii*, *Candida krusei*, *Candida parapsilosis*, and *Candida tropicalis*.

Drug resistance – A caspofungin minimum inhibitory concentration of 2 mcg/mL or less (susceptible) indicates that the *Candida* isolate is likely to be inhibited if caspofungin therapeutic concentrations are achieved; there is insufficient treatment outcome information on isolates with reduced caspofungin susceptibility to define categories other than susceptible. Breakthrough infections with *Candida* isolates requiring caspofungin concentrations greater than 2 mcg/mL for growth inhibition have developed in a mouse model of *C. albicans* infection and in some patients with *Candida* infections. Some of these isolates had mutations in the FKS1 gene. The incidence of drug resistance by various clinical isolates of *Candida* and *Aspergillus* species is unknown.

Contraindications

Hypersensitivity (eg, anaphylaxis) to any component of this product.

Warnings/Precautions

➤*Concomitant use with cyclosporine:* Limit concomitant use of caspofungin with cyclosporine to patients for whom the potential benefit outweighs the potential risk. In one clinical study, 3 of 4 healthy adult subjects who received caspofungin 70 mg on days 1 through 10, and also received two 3 mg/kg doses of cyclosporine 12 hours apart on day 10, developed transient elevations of ALT on day 11 that were 2 to 3 times the upper limit of normal (ULN). In a separate panel of adult subjects in the same study, 2 of 8 who received caspofungin 35 mg daily for 3 days and cyclosporine (two 3 mg/kg doses administered 12 hours apart) on day 1 had small increases in ALT (slightly above the ULN) on day 2. In both groups, elevations in AST paralleled ALT elevations, but were of lesser magnitude. In another clinical study, 2 of 8 healthy men developed transient ALT elevations of less than 2 times the ULN. In this study, cyclosporine 4 mg/kg was administered on days 1 and 12, and caspofungin 70 mg was administered daily on days 3 through 13. In 1 subject, the ALT elevation occurred on days 7 and 9 and, in the other subject, the ALT elevation occurred on day 19. These elevations returned to normal by day 27. In all groups, elevations in AST paralleled ALT elevations but were of lesser magnitude. In these clinical studies, cyclosporine (4 mg/kg dose or two 3 mg/kg doses) increased the AUC of caspofungin by approximately 35%.

CASPOFUNGIN ACETATE — INJECTION

Given the limitations of these data, only use caspofungin and cyclosporine concomitantly in those patients for whom the potential benefit outweighs the potential risk. Monitor patients who develop abnormal liver function tests during concomitant therapy and evaluate the risks/benefits of continuing therapy.

➤*Hepatic effects:* Laboratory abnormalities in liver function tests have been seen in healthy volunteers and in adults and children treated with caspofungin. In some patients with serious underlying conditions who were receiving multiple concomitant medications along with caspofungin, isolated cases of clinically significant hepatic dysfunction, hepatitis, or worsening hepatic failure have been reported; a causal relationship to caspofungin has not been established. Monitor patients who develop abnormal liver function tests during caspofungin therapy for evidence of worsening hepatic function and evaluate them for the risks/benefits of continuing caspofungin therapy.

➤*Hepatic function impairment:* See Administration and Dosage for more information.

➤*Pregnancy: Category C.* There are no adequate and well-controlled studies with the use of caspofungin in pregnant women. It is unknown if caspofungin crosses the human placenta, but it does cross the placenta in rats and rabbits. If indicated, avoid maternal treatment in the first trimester, if possible. Use caspofungin during pregnancy only if the potential benefit justifies the potential risk to the fetus.

In animal studies, caspofungin caused embryofetal toxicity, including increased resorptions, increased peri-implantation loss, and incomplete ossification at multiple fetal sites. In offspring born to pregnant rats treated with caspofungin at doses comparable with the human dose based on body surface area (BSA) comparisons, there was incomplete ossification of the skull and torso and increased incidences of cervical rib. There was also an increase in resorptions and peri-implantation losses. In pregnant rabbits treated with caspofungin at doses comparable with 2 times the human dose based on BSA comparisons, there was an increased incidence of incomplete ossification of the talus/calcaneus in offspring and increases in fetal resorptions. Caspofungin crosses the placenta in rats and rabbits and was detectable in fetal plasma. Animal data suggest human risk, especially if exposure occurs in the first trimester.

➤*Lactation:* Caspofungin was found in the milk of lactating, drug-treated rats. It is not known whether caspofungin is present in human milk. Because many drugs are excreted in human milk, exercise caution when caspofungin is administered to a breast-feeding woman. The high molecular weight (approximately 1,213) and extensive plasma protein binding (approximately 97%) should limit the amount of drug excreted in breast milk, but the long gamma-phase half-life may allow for some drug in the milk. Breast-feeding appears to be compatible, and the risk of harm appears to be low. Monitor infants for symptoms of histamine release (eg, facial swelling, rash) and GI symptoms.

➤*Children:* The efficacy and safety of caspofungin has not been adequately studied in prospective clinical trials involving neonates and infants younger than 3 months of age. Although limited pharmacokinetic data were collected in neonates and infants younger than 3 months of age, these data are insufficient to establish a safe and effective dose of caspofungin in the treatment of neonatal candidiasis. Invasive candidiasis in neonates has a higher rate of CNS and multiorgan involvement than in older patients; the ability of caspofungin to penetrate the blood-brain barrier and to treat patients with meningitis and endocarditis is unknown.

Caspofungin has not been studied in children with endocarditis, osteomyelitis, and meningitis caused by *Candida*. Caspofungin has also not been studied as initial therapy for invasive aspergillosis in children.

In clinical trials, 171 children (0 months to 17 years of age), including 18 patients who were younger than 3 months of age, were given IV caspofungin. Pharmacokinetic studies enrolled a total of 66 children, and an additional 105 children received caspofungin in safety and efficacy studies. The majority of the children received caspofungin at a once-daily maintenance dose of 50 mg/m² for a mean duration of 12 days (median, 9 days; range, 1 to 87 days). In all studies, safety was assessed by the investigator throughout study therapy and for 14 days following cessation of study therapy. The most common adverse reactions in children treated with caspofungin were pyrexia (29%), blood potassium decreased (15%), diarrhea (14%), increased AST (12%), rash (12%), increased ALT (11%), hypotension (11%), and chills (11%).

Postmarketing hepatobiliary adverse reactions have been reported in children with serious underlying medical conditions.

➤*Elderly:* Plasma concentrations of caspofungin in healthy elderly men and women (65 years of age and older) were increased slightly (approximately 28% in AUC) compared with young healthy men. A similar effect of age on pharmacokinetics was seen in patients with candidemia or other *Candida* infections (intra-abdominal abscesses, peritonitis, or pleural space infections). No dose adjustment is recommended for elderly patients; however, greater sensitivity of some older individuals cannot be ruled out.

➤*Monitoring:* Monitor patients who develop abnormal liver function tests during caspofungin therapy for evidence of worsening hepatic function and for development of abnormal liver function tests during concomitant therapy with cyclosporine, and evaluate them for the risks/benefits of continuing caspofungin therapy.

Drug Interactions

Caspofungin Drug Interactions			
Precipitant drug	Object drug[a]		Description
Cyclosporine	Caspofungin	⬆	Cyclosporine increased the AUC of caspofungin ≈ 35%. Concurrent use also produced transient elevations (≤ 5 times the ULN) in ALT and AST. Use concomitantly only if the potential benefit outweighs the potential risk. Monitor liver function closely. See Warnings/Precautions for more information.
Inducers of drug clearance or mixed inducer/inhibitors (eg, carbamazepine, dexamethasone, efavirenz, nevirapine, phenytoin, rifampin)	Caspofungin	⬇	Coadministration may result in clinically meaningful reductions in caspofungin concentrations. Rifampin decreased caspofungin trough concentrations 30%. Give patients receiving rifampin caspofungin 70 mg daily. When coadministering caspofungin with the other drugs listed, consider an increase in the daily dose of caspofungin to 70 mg in adults who are not clinically responding or to 70 mg/m² (not to exceed 70 mg daily) in children.
Caspofungin	Tacrolimus	⬇	Coadministration produced a decrease in the AUC of tacrolimus ≈ 20%, C_{max}[b] by 16%, and 12-hour blood concentration by 26%. Monitor tacrolimus blood concentrations and adjust the dose accordingly.

[a] ⬆ = object drug increased; ⬇ = object drug decreased.
[b] C_{max} = maximum plasma concentration.

Adverse Reactions

➤*Hypersensitivity:* Possible histamine-mediated symptoms have been reported, including reports of rash, facial swelling, pruritus, sensation of warmth, or bronchospasm. Anaphylaxis has been reported during administration of caspofungin.

➤*Adults:*

Empirical therapy –

In this study, clinical or laboratory hepatic adverse reactions were reported in 39% and 45% of patients in the caspofungin and amphotericin B liposome groups, respectively. Also reported was an isolated, serious adverse reaction of hyperbilirubinemia considered possibly related to caspofungin.

Caspofungin Adverse Reactions Among Adults With Persistent Fever and Neutropenia (≥ 7.5%)[a,b]		
Adverse reactions	Caspofungin[c] (n = 564)	Amphotericin B liposome injection[d] (n = 547)
All systems, any adverse reaction	95%	97%
Cardiovascular, NOS[e]	16%	19%
Hypotension	6%	10%
Tachycardia	7%	9%
Vascular disorders, NOS	20%	23%
CNS, NOS	25%	27%
Headache	11%	12%
Dermatologic, NOS	42%	37%
Rash	16%	14%
GI, NOS	50%	55%
Abdominal pain	9%	11%
Diarrhea	20%	16%
Nausea	11%	20%
Vomiting	9%	17%
Lab test abnormalities, NOS	58%	63%
ALT increased	18%	20%
AST increased	14%	17%
Bilirubin conjugated increased	5%	9%
Blood albumin decreased	7%	8%
Blood alkaline phosphatase increased	15%	23%
Blood bilirubin increased	10%	14%

CASPOFUNGIN ACETATE — INJECTION

Caspofungin Adverse Reactions Among Adults With Persistent Fever and Neutropenia (≥ 7.5%)[a,b]

Adverse reactions	Caspofungin[c] (n = 564)	Amphotericin B liposome injection[d] (n = 547)
Blood creatinine increased	3%	11%
Blood glucose increased	6%	9%
Blood magnesium decreased	7%	9%
Blood potassium decreased	15%	23%
Blood urea increased	4%	8%
Metabolic/Nutritional, NOS	21%	24%
Hypokalemia	6%	8%
Peripheral edema	11%	12%
Respiratory, NOS	47%	49%
Cough	11%	10%
Dyspnea	9%	10%
Pneumonia	11%	10%
Rales	7%	8%
Miscellaneous		
Chills	23%	31%
General disorders and administration-site conditions, NOS	57%	63%
Infections and infestations, NOS	45%	42%
Mucosal inflammation	6%	8%
Pyrexia	27%	29%

[a] Within any system organ class, individuals may experience > 1 adverse reaction.
[b] Regardless of causality.
[c] 70 mg on day 1, then 50 mg once daily for the remainder of treatment; the daily dose was increased to 70 mg for 73 patients.
[d] 3 mg/kg/day; dosage was increased to 5 mg/kg/day for 74 patients.
[e] NOS = not otherwise specified.

Infusion-related adverse reactions: The proportion of patients who experienced an infusion-related adverse reaction was significantly lower in the group treated with caspofungin (35%) than in the group treated with amphotericin B liposome (52%). An infusion-related adverse reaction was defined as a systemic event, such as anaphylaxis, chills, dyspnea, flushing, hypertension, hypotension, pyrexia, rash, tachycardia, or tachypnea, that developed during the study therapy infusion and 1 hour following infusion.

Renal: Among patients whose baseline CrCl was greater than 30 mL/min, the incidence of nephrotoxicity was significantly lower in the group treated with caspofungin (3%) than in the group treated with amphotericin B liposome (12%). Clinical renal events, regardless of causality, were similar between caspofungin (13%) and amphotericin B liposome (16%).

Candidemia and other Candida infections –

Caspofungin Adverse Reactions Among Adults With Candidemia or Other *Candida* Infections (≥ 10%)[a,b,c]

Adverse reactions	Caspofungin 50 mg[d] (n = 114)	Amphotericin B (n = 125)
All systems, any adverse reaction	96%	99%
Cardiovascular, NOS	26%	34%
Hypotension	10%	16%
Tachycardia	8%	12%
Vascular disorders, NOS	25%	38%
Dermatologic, NOS	25%	28%
Rash	4%	10%
GI, NOS	49%	53%
Diarrhea	14%	10%
Nausea	9%	17%
Vomiting	17%	16%
Hematologic/Lymphatic, NOS	15%	13%
Anemia	11%	9%
Lab test abnormalities, NOS	67%	82%
ALT increased	16%	15%
AST increased	16%	14%
Bilirubin conjugated increased	8%	14%
Blood alkaline phosphatase increased	21%	32%
Blood bilirubin increased	13%	17%
Blood creatinine increased	11%	28%
Blood potassium decreased	23%	32%
Blood urea increased	9%	23%
Hematocrit decreased	13%	18%
Hemoglobin decreased	18%	23%
Red blood cells urine positive	10%	10%
Respiratory, NOS	40%	54%
Pleural effusion	9%	14%
Pneumonia	4%	10%
Respiratory failure	11%	12%
Tachypnea	1%	11%
Miscellaneous		
Chills	9%	30%
General disorders and administration-site conditions, NOS	47%	63%
Infections and infestations, NOS	48%	54%
Peripheral edema	11%	12%
Pyrexia	13%	33%
Septic shock	11%	9%

[a] Within any system organ class, individuals may experience > 1 adverse reaction.
[b] Intra-abdominal abscesses, peritonitis, and pleural space infections.
[c] Regardless of causality.
[d] Patients received caspofungin 70 mg on day 1 then 50 mg daily for the remainder of their treatment.

Infusion-related adverse reactions: The proportion of patients who experienced an infusion-related adverse reaction was significantly lower in the group treated with caspofungin (20%) than in the group treated with amphotericin B (49%). An infusion-related adverse reaction was defined as a systemic event, such as anaphylaxis, chills, dyspnea, flushing, hypertension, hypotension, pyrexia, rash, tachycardia, or tachypnea that developed during the study therapy infusion and 1 hour following infusion.

Renal: In a subgroup of patients whose baseline CrCl was greater than 30 mL/min, the incidence of nephrotoxicity was significantly lower in the group treated with caspofungin than in the group treated with amphotericin B.

High-dose caspofungin:

Caspofungin Adverse Reactions Among Patients With Candidemia or Other *Candida* Infections (≥ 5%)[a,b,c]

Adverse reactions	Caspofungin 50 mg[d] (n = 104)	Caspofungin 150 mg (n = 100)
All systems, any adverse reaction	83%	83%
Cardiovascular		
Hypertension	5%	6%
Hypotension	7%	3%
Vascular disorders, NOS	19%	18%
Dermatologic, NOS	15%	15%
Decubitus ulcer	3%	5%
GI, NOS	30%	33%
Diarrhea	6%	7%
Nausea	5%	7%
Vomiting	11%	6%
Lab test abnormalities, NOS	28%	35%
Alkaline phosphatase increased	12%	9%
ALT increased	4%	7%
AST increased	6%	9%
Blood potassium decreased	6%	8%
Respiratory, NOS	23%	26%
Pneumonia	5%	7%
Respiratory failure	6%	2%
Miscellaneous		
General disorders and administration-site conditions, NOS	33%	27%
Infections and infestations, NOS	44%	43%
Pyrexia	6%	6%

CASPOFUNGIN ACETATE — INJECTION

Caspofungin Adverse Reactions Among Patients With Candidemia or Other *Candida* Infections (≥ 5%)[a,b,c]		
Adverse reactions	Caspofungin 50 mg[d] (n = 104)	Caspofungin 150 mg (n = 100)
Sepsis	5%	7%
Septic shock	13%	14%

[a] Within any system organ class, individuals may experience > 1 adverse reaction.
[b] Regardless of causality.
[c] Intra-abdominal abscesses, peritonitis, and pleural space infections.
[d] Patients received caspofungin 70 mg on day 1, then 50 mg once daily for the remainder of their treatment.

Esophageal candidiasis and oropharyngeal candidiasis –

Caspofungin Adverse Reactions Among Adults With Esophageal and/or Oropharyngeal Candidiasis (≥ 10%)[a,b]		
Adverse reactions	Caspofungin 50 mg[c] (n = 83)	Fluconazole IV 200 mg[c] (n = 94)
All systems, any adverse reaction	90%	93%
Cardiovascular		
Phlebitis	18%	11%
Vascular disorders, NOS	19%	15%
CNS, NOS	18%	17%
Headache	15%	9%
GI, NOS	58%	50%
Diarrhea	27%	18%
Nausea	15%	15%
Lab test abnormalities, NOS	53%	61%
ALT increased	12%	17%
AST increased	13%	19%
Blood alkaline phosphatase increased	13%	17%
Hematocrit decreased	18%	16%
Hemoglobin decreased	21%	16%
White blood cell count decreased	12%	19%
Miscellaneous		
General disorders and administration-site conditions, NOS	31%	36%
Pyrexia	21%	21%

[a] Within any system organ class, individuals may experience > 1 adverse reaction.
[b] Regardless of causality.
[c] Derived from a comparator-controlled clinical study.

Invasive aspergillosis – In the open-label, noncomparative aspergillosis study, in which 69 patients received caspofungin (70 mg loading dose on day 1 followed by 50 mg daily), the following treatment-emergent adverse reactions were observed with an incidence of at least 12.5%: blood alkaline phosphatase increased (22%); hypotension, respiratory failure (20%); pyrexia (17%); diarrhea, nausea, headache (15%); rash, aspergillosis, ALT increased, AST increased, blood bilirubin increased, blood potassium decreased (13%). Also reported infrequently in this patient population were pulmonary edema, adult respiratory distress syndrome, and radiographic infiltrates.

➤*Children:*

Serious adverse reactions – One (0.6%) patient receiving caspofungin and 3 (12%) patients receiving amphotericin B liposome developed a serious drug-related adverse reaction.

Discontinuation of therapy – Two (1%) patients were discontinued from caspofungin and 3 (12%) patients were discontinued from amphotericin B liposome because of a drug-related adverse reaction.

Infusion-related adverse reactions – The proportion of patients who experienced an infusion-related adverse reaction was 22% in the group treated with caspofungin and 35% in the group treated with amphotericin B liposome. An infusion-related adverse reaction was defined as a systemic event, such as anaphylaxis, chills, dyspnea, flushing, hypertension, hypotension, pyrexia, rash, tachycardia, or tachypnea that developed during the study therapy infusion and 1 hour following infusion.

Adverse reactions (7.5% or more) –

Caspofungin Adverse Reactions Among Children (0 Months to 17 Years of Age) (≥ 7.5%)[a,b]			
	Noncomparative clinical studies	Comparator-controlled clinical study of empirical therapy	
Adverse reactions	Caspofungin any dose (n = 115)	Caspofungin 50 mg/m^2[c] (n = 56)	Amphotericin B liposome 3 mg/kg (n = 26)
All systems, any adverse reaction	95%	96%	89%
Cardiovascular, NOS	17%	13%	19%
Hypertension	10%	9%	4%
Hypotension	12%	9%	8%
Tachycardia	4%	11%	19%
Vascular disorders, NOS	24%	21%	19%
CNS, NOS	13%	16%	8%
Headache	5%	9%	4%
Dermatologic, NOS	33%	41%	39%
Erythema	4%	9%	0%
Pruritus	7%	6%	8%
Rash	6%	23%	8%
Hematologic/Lymphatic, NOS	10%	2%	15%
Anemia	2%	0%	8%
GI, NOS	42%	41%	35%
Abdominal pain	7%	4%	12%
Diarrhea	17%	7%	15%
Nausea	4%	4%	8%
Vomiting	8%	11%	12%
Lab test abnormalities, NOS	55%	41%	50%
ALT increased	14%	5%	12%
AST increased	17%	2%	12%
Blood potassium decreased	18%	9%	27%
Blood potassium increased	3%	0%	8%
Protein total decreased	0%	0%	8%
Metabolic/Nutritional, NOS	22%	11%	23%
Edema	3%	4%	8%
Hypokalemia	8%	5%	4%
Musculoskeletal, NOS	11%	14%	12%
Back pain	4%	0%	8%
Respiratory, NOS	43%	32%	27%
Cough	6%	9%	8%
Respiratory distress	8%	0%	4%
Miscellaneous			
Central line infection	1%	9%	0%
Chills	10%	13%	8%
General disorders and administration-site conditions, NOS	47%	59%	42%
Graft versus host disease	1%	4%	8%
Immune system disorders, NOS	7%	7%	12%
Infections and infestations, NOS	40%	30%	35%
Mucosal inflammation	10%	4%	4%
Pyrexia	29%	30%	23%

[a] Within any system organ class, individuals may experience > 1 adverse reaction.
[b] Regardless of causality.
[c] 70 mg/m^2 on day 1, then 50 mg/m^2 once daily for the remainder of the treatment.

CASPOFUNGIN ACETATE — INJECTION

➤*Other adverse reactions (adults and children):*

Caspofungin Treatment-Emergent[a] Adverse Reactions in Adults and Children From 34 Clinical Studies (≥ 5%)[b]	
Adverse reactions[c]	Caspofungin (n = 1,951)
All systems, any adverse reaction	85%
Cardiovascular	
Hypotension	6%
Vascular disorders, NOS	18%
CNS, NOS	21%
Headache	10%
Dermatologic, NOS	27%
Erythema	5%
Rash	8%
GI, NOS	39%
Abdominal pain	6%
Diarrhea	14%
Nausea	9%
Vomiting	8%
Lab test abnormalities, NOS	46%
ALT increased	13%
AST increased	12%
Blood alkaline phosphatase increased	12%
Blood bilirubin increased	6%
Blood potassium decreased	11%
Respiratory, NOS	31%
Cough	6%
Pneumonia	6%
Miscellaneous	43%
Chills	10%
General disorders and administration-site conditions, NOS	43%
Infections and infestations, NOS	37%
Peripheral edema	6%
Pyrexia	20%

[a] Defined as an adverse reaction, regardless of causality, while receiving caspofungin or during the 14-day post-caspofungin follow-up period.
[b] Incidence for each preferred term is ≥ 5% among individuals who received ≥ 1 dose of caspofungin.
[c] Within any system organ class, individuals may experience > 1 adverse reaction.

Adverse reactions (less than 5%) – Clinically significant adverse reactions, regardless of causality or incidence that occurred in these trials are as follows.

Cardiovascular – Arrhythmia, atrial fibrillation, bradycardia, cardiac arrest, flushing, hypertension, myocardial infarction, phlebitis, tachycardia.

CNS – Anxiety, asthenia, confusional state, convulsion, depression, dizziness, fatigue, insomnia, somnolence, tremor.

Dermatologic – Erythema, petechiae, skin lesion, urticaria.

GI – Abdominal distension, anorexia, constipation, dyspepsia, upper abdominal pain.

GU – Hematuria, renal failure, urinary tract infection.

Hematologic/Lymphatic – Anemia, coagulopathy, febrile neutropenia, neutropenia, thrombocytopenia.

Hepatic – Hepatic failure, hepatomegaly, hepatotoxicity, hyperbilirubinemia, jaundice.

Metabolic/Nutritional – Decreased appetite, edema, fluid overload, hypercalcemia, hyperglycemia, hypokalemia, hypomagnesemia.

Musculoskeletal – Arthralgia, back pain, pain in extremity.

Respiratory – Dyspnea, epistaxis, hypoxia, tachypnea.

Miscellaneous – Bacteremia, infusion-site pain/pruritus/swelling, mucosal inflammation, sepsis.

➤*Postmarketing:*

Dermatologic – Erythema multiforme, skin exfoliation, Stevens-Johnson syndrome.

Miscellaneous – Clinically significant renal dysfunction, hepatic necrosis, pancreatitis, swelling and peripheral edema.

Overdosage

➤*Symptoms:* In 6 healthy subjects who received a single 210 mg dose, no significant adverse reactions were reported. Multiple doses above 150 mg daily have not been studied.

In clinical trials, 1 child 16 years of age unintentionally received a single dose of caspofungin 113 mg (on day 1), followed by 80 mg daily for an additional 7 days. No clinically significant adverse reactions were reported.

➤*Treatment:* Caspofungin is not dialyzable.

Patient Information

Inform patients that there have been isolated reports of serious hepatic effects from caspofungin therapy and that their health care provider will assess the risk/benefit of continuing caspofungin therapy if abnormal liver function tests occur during treatment.

Inform patients that caspofungin can cause hypersensitivity reactions, including rash, facial swelling, pruritus, sensation of warmth, or bronchospasm.

MICAFUNGIN SODIUM

Rx	**Mycamine** (Astellas)	**Injection, lyophilized, powder for solution:** 50 mg	Preservative free. Lactose 200 mg. In single-use vials.
		100 mg	Preservative free. Lactose 200 mg. In single-use vials.

MICAFUNGIN SODIUM — INJECTION

Indications

➤*Candidemia, acute disseminated candidiasis, Candida peritonitis, and abscesses:* For the treatment of patients with candidemia, acute disseminated candidiasis, *Candida* peritonitis, and abscesses.

➤*Esophageal candidiasis:* For the treatment of patients with esophageal candidiasis.

➤*Prophylaxis of Candida infections:* For prophylaxis of *Candida* infections in patients undergoing hematopoietic stem cell transplantation (HSCT).

Administration and Dosage

➤*Adults:*

Abscesses – 100 mg/day IV. The mean duration of treatment was 15 days (range, 10 to 47 days).

Acute disseminated candidiasis – 100 mg/day administered by IV infusion over 1 hour. The mean duration of treatment was 15 days (range, 10 to 47 days).

Candida peritonitis – 100 mg/day administered by IV infusion over 1 hour. The mean duration of treatment was 15 days (range, 10 to 47 days).

Candidemia – 100 mg/day administered by IV infusion over 1 hour. The mean duration of treatment was 15 days (range, 10 to 47 days).

Esophageal candidiasis – 150 mg/day administered by IV infusion over 1 hour. The mean duration of treatment was 15 days (range, 10 to 30 days).

Prophylaxis of Candida infections – 50 mg/day administered by IV infusion over 1 hour. In HSCT recipients who experienced success of prophylactic therapy, the mean duration of prophylaxis was 19 days (range, 6 to 51 days).

➤*Preparation for administration:* The diluent to be used for reconstitution and dilution is sodium chloride 0.9% injection (without a bacteriostatic agent). Alternatively, dextrose 5% injection may be used for reconstitution and dilution of micafungin.

Reconstitution – Aseptically add 5 mL of sodium chloride 0.9% injection (without a bacteriostatic agent) to each 50 mg vial to yield a preparation containing approximately 10 mg/mL of micafungin.

Aseptically add 5 mL of sodium chloride 0.9% injection (without a bacteriostatic agent) to each 100 mg vial to yield a preparation containing approximately 20 mg/mL of micafungin.

To minimize excessive foaming, gently dissolve the micafungin powder by swirling the vial. Do not vigorously shake the vial.

Dilution – Diluted solution should be protected from light. It is not necessary to cover the infusion drip chamber or the tubing.

Candidemia, acute disseminated candidiasis, Candida peritonitis, and abscesses: Add reconstituted micafungin 100 mg into 100 mL of sodium chloride 0.9% injection or 100 mL of dextrose 5% injection.

Prophylaxis of Candida infections: Add reconstituted micafungin 50 mg into 100 mL of sodium chloride 0.9% injection or 100 mL of dextrose 5% injection.

Esophageal candidiasis: Add micafungin 150 mg reconstituted into 100 mL of sodium chloride 0.9% injection or 100 mL of dextrose 5% injection.

➤*Administration:* Micafungin should be administered by IV infusion over 1 hour. More rapid infusions may result in more frequent histamine-

MICAFUNGIN SODIUM — INJECTION

mediated reactions. An existing IV line should be flushed with sodium chloride 0.9% injection prior to infusion of micafungin.

➤*Admixture compatibility:* Do not mix or coinfuse micafungin with other medications. Micafungin has been shown to precipitate when mixed directly with other commonly used medications.

➤*Storage/Stability:* Unopened vials of lyophilized material must be stored at 25°C (77°F); excursions are permitted to 15° to 30°C (59° to 86°F). The reconstituted product may be stored in the original vial for up to 24 hours at 25°C (77°F). Protect the diluted infusion from light. It may be stored for up to 24 hours at 25°C (77°F). Discard partially used vials.

Actions

➤*Pharmacology:* Micafungin, a member of the echinocandin class of antifungal agents, inhibits the synthesis of 1,3-β-D-glucan, an essential component of fungal cell walls, which is not present in mammalian cells.

➤*Pharmacokinetics:* Steady-state pharmacokinetic parameters in relevant patient populations after repeated daily administration are presented in the following table.

Micafungin Pharmacokinetic Parameters

			Pharmacokinetic parameters (mean ± SD[a])			
Population	n	Dose	C_{max}[b] (mcg/mL)	$AUC_{0\text{-}24}$[c] (mcg•h/mL)	t½[d] (h)	Clearance (mL/min/kg)
Patients with candidemia or other *Candida* infections						
Day 1	20	100 mg	5.7 ± 2.2	83 ± 51	14.5 ± 7	0.359 ± 0.179
Steady state	20	100 mg	10.1 ± 4.4	97 ± 29	13.4 ± 2	0.298 ± 0.115
HIV-positive patients with esophageal candidiasis						
Day 1	20	50 mg	4.1 ± 1.4	36 ± 9	14.9 ± 4.3	0.321 ± 0.098
	20	100 mg	8 ± 2.4	108 ± 31	13.8 ± 3	0.327 ± 0.093
	14	150 mg	11.6 ± 3.1	151 ± 45	14.1 ± 2.6	0.34 ± 0.092
Day 14 or 21	20	50 mg	5.1 ± 1	54 ± 13	15.6 ± 2.8	0.3 ± 0.063
	20	100 mg	10.1 ± 2.6	115 ± 25	16.9 ± 4.4	0.301 ± 0.086
	14	150 mg	16.4 ± 6.5	167 ± 40	15.2 ± 2.2	0.297 ± 0.081
HSCT recipients						
Day 7	8	3 mg/kg	21.1 ± 2.84	234 ± 34	14 ± 1.4	0.214 ± 0.031
	10	4 mg/kg	29.2 ± 6.2	339 ± 72	14.2 ± 3.2	0.204 ± 0.036
	8	6 mg/kg	38.4 ± 6.9	479 ± 157	14.9 ± 2.6	0.224 ± 0.064
	8	8 mg/kg	60.8 ± 26.9	663 ± 212	17.2 ± 2.3	0.223 ± 0.081

[a] SD = standard deviation.
[b] C_{max} = peak plasma concentration.
[c] AUC = area under the curve; $AUC_{0\text{-infinity}}$ is presented for day 1; $AUC_{0\text{-}24}$ is presented for steady state.
[d] t½ = half-life.

Absorption – The relationship of AUC to micafungin dose was linear over the daily dose range of 50 to 150 mg and 3 to 8 mg/kg body weight. Typically, 85% of the steady-state concentration is achieved after 3 daily micafungin doses.

Distribution – The mean ± SD volume of distribution of micafungin at terminal phase was 0.39 ± 0.11 L/kg body weight when determined in adult patients with esophageal candidiasis at the dose range of 50 to 150 mg.

Micafungin is highly (more than 99%) protein bound in vitro, independent of plasma concentrations over the range of 10 to 100 mcg/mL. The primary binding protein is albumin; however, micafungin at therapeutically relevant concentrations does not competitively displace bilirubin binding to albumin. Micafungin also binds to a lesser extent to alpha-1 acid glycoprotein.

Metabolism – Micafungin is metabolized to M-1 (catechol form) by arylsulfatase, with further metabolism to M-2 (methoxy form) by catechol-O-methyltransferase. M-5 is formed by hydroxylation at the side chain (ω-1 position) of micafungin catalyzed by CYP-450 isozymes. Even though micafungin is a substrate for, and a weak inhibitor of, CYP3A in vitro, hydroxylation by CYP3A is not a major pathway for micafungin metabolism in vivo. Micafungin is neither a P-glycoprotein substrate nor inhibitor in vitro.

In 4 healthy volunteer studies, the ratio of metabolite to parent exposure (AUC) at a dose of 150 mg/day was 6% for M-1, 1% for M-2, and 6% for M-5. In patients with esophageal candidiasis, the ratio of metabolite to parent exposure (AUC) at a dose of 150 mg/day was 11% for M-1, 2% for M-2, and 12% for M-5.

Excretion – The excretion of radioactivity following a single IV dose of ^{14}C-micafungin for injection (25 mg) was evaluated in healthy volunteers. At 28 days after administration, mean urinary and fecal recovery of total radioactivity accounted for 82.5% (76.4% to 87.9%) of the administered dose. Fecal excretion is the major route of elimination (total radioactivity 28 days after administration was 71% of the administered dose).

Special populations –

Hepatic function impairment: A single 1-hour infusion of micafungin 100 mg was administered to 8 subjects with moderate hepatic function impairment (Child-Pugh score, 7 to 9) and 8 age-, gender-, and weight-matched subjects with healthy hepatic function. The C_{max} and AUC values of micafungin were lower by approximately 22% in subjects with moderate hepatic function impairment. This difference in micafungin exposure does not require dose adjustment of micafungin in patients with moderate hepatic function impairment. The pharmacokinetics of micafungin have not been studied in patients with severe hepatic function impairment.

➤*Microbiology:*

Activity in vitro – Micafungin exhibited in vitro activity against *Candida albicans*, *Candida glabrata*, *Candida guilliermondii*, *Candida krusei*, *Candida parapsilosis*, and *Candida tropicalis*.

Contraindications

Hypersensitivity to micafungin, to any component of the product, or to other echinocandins.

Warnings/Precautions

➤*Hematological effects:* Acute intravascular hemolysis and hemoglobinuria was seen in a healthy volunteer during infusion of micafungin (200 mg) and oral prednisolone (20 mg). This event was transient, and the subject did not develop significant anemia. Isolated cases of significant hemolysis and hemolytic anemia have also been reported in patients treated with micafungin. Closely monitor patients who develop clinical or laboratory evidence of hemolysis or hemolytic anemia during micafungin therapy for evidence of worsening of these conditions, and evaluate them for the risk/benefit of continuing micafungin therapy.

➤*Hepatic effects:* Laboratory abnormalities in liver function tests have been seen in healthy volunteers and patients treated with micafungin. In some patients with serious underlying conditions who were receiving micafungin along with multiple concomitant medications, clinical hepatic abnormalities have occurred, and isolated cases of significant hepatic function impairment, hepatitis, and hepatic failure have been reported. Monitor patients who develop abnormal liver function tests during micafungin therapy for evidence of worsening hepatic function, and evaluate them for the risk/benefit of continuing micafungin therapy.

➤*Renal effects:* Elevations in serum urea nitrogen (BUN) and creatinine and isolated cases of significant renal function impairment or acute renal failure have been reported in patients who received micafungin. In controlled trials, the incidence of drug-related renal adverse reactions was 0.4% for micafungin-treated patients and 0.5% for fluconazole-treated patients. Monitor patients who develop abnormal renal function tests during micafungin therapy for evidence of worsening renal function.

➤*Hypersensitivity reactions:* Isolated cases of serious hypersensitivity (anaphylaxis and anaphylactoid) reactions, including shock, have been reported in patients receiving micafungin. If these reactions occur, discontinue micafungin infusion and administer appropriate treatment.

➤*Pregnancy: Category C.* Micafungin administration to pregnant rabbits (IV dosing on days 6 to 18 of gestation) resulted in visceral abnormalities and abortion at 32 mg/kg, a dose equivalent to about 4 times the recommended dose based on BSA comparisons. Visceral abnormalities included abnormal lobation of the lung, levocardia, retrocaval ureter, anomalous right subclavian artery, and dilatation of the ureter. There are no adequate and well-controlled studies of micafungin in pregnant women. Animal reproduction studies in rabbits showed visceral abnormalities and increased abortion at 4 times the recommended human dose. However, animal studies are not always predictive of human response. Use micafungin during pregnancy only if the potential benefit justifies the potential risk to the fetus.

➤*Lactation:* Micafungin was found in the milk of lactating, drug-treated rats. It is not known whether micafungin is excreted in human milk. Exercise caution when micafungin is administered to a breast-feeding woman.

➤*Children:* The safety and efficacy of micafungin in children has not been established.

➤*Elderly:* No overall differences in safety or efficacy were observed between these subjects and younger subjects. Other reported clinical experience has not identified differences in responses between the elderly and younger patients, but greater sensitivity of some older individuals cannot be ruled out.

➤*Monitoring:* Closely monitor patients who develop clinical or laboratory evidence of hemolysis or hemolytic anemia during micafungin therapy for evidence of worsening of these conditions, and evaluate them for the risk/benefit of continuing micafungin therapy. Monitor patients who develop abnormal liver function tests during micafungin therapy for evidence of worsening hepatic function, and evaluate them for the risk/benefit of continuing micafungin therapy. Monitor patients who develop abnormal renal function tests during micafungin therapy for evidence of worsening renal function.

MICAFUNGIN SODIUM — INJECTION

Drug Interactions

Micafungin Drug Interactions			
Precipitant drug	Object drug[a]		Description
Micafungin	Cyclosporine	↑	Cyclosporine whole-blood concentrations may be elevated, increasing the pharmacologic effects and adverse reactions. Monitor cyclosporine whole-blood concentrations and adjust the dose as needed.
Micafungin	Itraconazole	↑	Coadministration resulted in itraconazole AUC and C_{max} increases of 22% and 11%, respectively. Monitor for itraconazole toxicity and reduce the dose as necessary.
Micafungin	Nifedipine	↑	Nifedipine AUC and C_{max} were increased 18% and 42%, respectively, in the presence of steady-state micafungin. Monitor for nifedipine toxicity and reduce the dose as needed.
Micafungin	Sirolimus	↑	Sirolimus AUC was increased by 21% in the presence of steady-state micafungin. Monitor for sirolimus toxicity and reduce the dose as needed.

[a] ↑ = object drug increased.

Adverse Reactions

➤*Hypersensitivity:* Possible histamine-mediated symptoms have been reported with micafungin, including rash, pruritus, facial swelling, and vasodilatation.

➤*Local:* Injection site reactions, including phlebitis and thrombophlebitis, have been reported at micafungin doses of 50 to 150 mg/day. These reactions tended to occur more often in patients receiving micafungin via peripheral IV administration.

➤*Candidemia and other Candida infections:*

Micafungin Adverse Reactions in Patients With Candidemia and Other *Candida* Infections (≥ 5%)[a,b]			
Adverse reaction[c]	Micafungin 100 mg (n = 200)	Micafungin 150 mg (n = 202)	Caspofungin[d] (n = 193)
All systems, any adverse reaction	91.5%	92.6%	88.6%
Cardiovascular			
Atrial fibrillation	2.5%	5%	0%
Bradycardia, NOS[e]	2.5%	5%	4.1%
Cardiac disorders	17.5%	23.8%	18.7%
Hypertension, NOS	3%	5%	6.2%
Hypotension, NOS	10%	5.9%	7.8%
Tachycardia, NOS	3%	3.5%	6.7%
Vascular disorders	21.5%	23.3%	18.7%
CNS			
Headache, NOS	2%	5%	5.7%
Insomnia	5.5%	4%	8.3%
Nervous system disorders	10.5%	20.8%	16.6%
Psychiatric disorders	15.5%	13.4%	17.1%
Dermatologic			
Decubitus ulcer	4.5%	5.9%	4.7%
Skin/Subcutaneous tissue disorders	13%	16.8%	17.1%
GI			
Abdominal pain, NOS	2.5%	2%	5.2%
Diarrhea, NOS	7.5%	12.9%	7.3%
GI disorders	40.5%	44.1%	39.4%
Nausea	9.5%	7.4%	10.4%
Vomiting, NOS	9%	7.4%	8.3%
Hematologic/Lymphatic			
Anemia, NOS	2.5%	3%	6.7%
Anemia aggravated, NOS	2%	5%	2.6%
Blood/Lymphatic system disorders	19%	22.3%	19.2%
Thrombocytopenia	4%	4%	5.7%
Metabolic/Nutritional			
Hyperkalemia	5%	4%	2.6%
Hypernatremia	4%	6.4%	4.1%
Hypoglycemia, NOS	6%	6.9%	4.7%
Hypokalemia	14%	16.8%	14.5%
Hypomagnesaemia	5.5%	8.4%	7.3%
Metabolism and nutrition disorders	38.5%	41.1%	37.8%
Miscellaneous			
Bacteremia	5%	8.9%	5.7%
Blood alkaline phosphatase increased, NOS	5.5%	7.9%	4.1%
Edema peripheral	5.5%	5.9%	7.3%
Infections and infestations	33.5%	40.1%	30.6%
General disorders/administration site conditions	29.5%	27.7%	26.4%
Pneumonia, NOS	1.5%	5.4%	2.1%
Pyrexia	7%	10.9%	7.8%
Sepsis, NOS	5.5%	5%	5.7%
Septic shock	7.5%	4.5%	4.7%

[a] Patient base: all randomized patients who received at least 1 dose of trial drug.
[b] During IV treatment + 3 days.
[c] Within a system organ class, patients may experience more than 1 adverse reaction.
[d] 70 mg loading dose on day 1 followed by 50 mg/day thereafter (caspofungin).
[e] NOS = not otherwise specified.

In a second supportive, randomized, double-blind study for treatment of candidemia and other *Candida* infections, treatment-emergent adverse reactions occurred in 245 of 264 (92.8%) and 250 of 265 (94.3%) patients in the micafungin (100 mg/day) and lipid based amphotericin B (3 mg/kg/day) treatment groups, respectively. The most common treatment-emergent adverse reactions occurring in 5% or more of the micafungin-treated patients at least 16 years of age were pyrexia (15.2% vs 17%), hypokalemia (16.7% vs 20.8%), nausea (9.5% vs 8.3%), diarrhea (10.6% vs 11.3%), and vomiting (12.9% vs 9.4%) in the micafungin and lipid based amphotericin B treatment groups, respectively. Other important treatment-emergent adverse reactions that occurred at less than 5% frequency were abnormal liver function tests (4.2% vs 3%), increased aspartate aminotransferase (2.7% vs 1.9%), and increased blood alkaline phosphatase (3% vs 2.3%) in the micafungin and lipid based amphotericin B treatment groups, respectively.

➤*Esophageal candidiasis:*

Micafungin Adverse Reactions in Patients With Esophageal Candidiasis (≥ 5%)[a,b]		
Adverse reaction[c]	Micafungin 150 mg/day (n = 260)	Fluconazole 200 mg/day (n = 258)
All systems, any adverse reaction	77.7%	72.1%
Cardiovascular		
Phlebitis, NOS	18.8%	5%
Vascular disorders	20.8%	8.1%
CNS		
Headache, NOS	8.5%	7.8%
Insomnia	3.5%	5%
Nervous system disorders	16.2%	15.5%
Psychiatric disorders	7.7%	8.1%
Dermatologic		
Rash, NOS	5.4%	2.3%
Skin and subcutaneous tissue disorders	13.8%	10.1%
GI		
Abdominal pain, NOS	3.8%	5.8%
Diarrhea, NOS	10.4%	11.2%
GI disorders	32.3%	36%
Nausea	7.7%	8.9%
Vomiting, NOS	6.5%	6.6%
Hematologic/Lymphatic		
Anemia, NOS	3.1%	6.2%
Blood/Lymphatic system disorders	14.6%	16.7%

MICAFUNGIN SODIUM — INJECTION

Micafungin Adverse Reactions in Patients With Esophageal Candidiasis (≥ 5%)[a,b]		
Adverse reaction[c]	Micafungin 150 mg/day (n = 260)	Fluconazole 200 mg/day (n = 258)
Miscellaneous		
General disorders/administration site conditions	20%	17.4%
Pyrexia	13.1%	8.1%

[a] Patient base: all randomized patients who received at least 1 dose of trial drug.
[b] During treatment + 3 days.
[c] Within a system organ class, patients may experience more than 1 adverse reaction.

➤*Prophylaxis of Candida infections in HSCT recipients:*

Micafungin Adverse Reactions During Prophylaxis of *Candida* Infection in HSCT Recipients (≥ 15%)[a,b]		
Adverse reaction[c]	Micafungin 50 mg/day (n = 425)	Fluconazole 400 mg/day (n = 457)
All systems, any adverse reactions	100%	100%
Cardiovascular		
Cardiac disorders	34.6%	35.4%
Flushing	11.1%	15.3%
Hypertension, NOS	21.4%	24.7%
Hypotension, NOS	18.6%	19.5%
Tachycardia, NOS	24.7%	22.3%
Vascular disorders	52.7%	58.4%
CNS		
Anxiety	22.4%	20.1%
Dizziness	12.9%	18.2%
Fatigue	29.6%	31.7%
Headache, NOS	42.1%	36.1%
Insomnia	35.8%	31.9%
Nervous system disorders	61.4%	58.6%
Psychiatric disorders	60.5%	54.5%
Rigors	26.4%	25.8%
Dermatologic		
Erythema	11.3%	15.5%
Pruritus, NOS	17.6%	19%
Rash, NOS	25.9%	22.3%
Skin and subcutaneous tissue disorders	68.2%	69.1%
GI		
Abdominal pain, NOS	27.1%	23.4%
Anorexia	27.3%	26.5%
Appetite decreased, NOS	20.5%	20.4%
Constipation	30.4%	31.3%
Diarrhea, NOS	71.1%	76.1%
Dyspepsia	24.5%	26.7%
GI disorders	99.1%	98.2%
Nausea	69.6%	67.6%
Vomiting, NOS	66.1%	67.2%
Hematologic/Lymphatic		
Anemia, NOS	35.5%	37.9%
Blood and lymphatic system disorders	96%	93.9%
Febrile neutropenia	36.5%	36.3%
Neutropenia	75.3%	71.6%
Thrombocytopenia	72.2%	66.5%
Metabolic/Nutritional		
Edema peripheral	20.7%	21.9%
Fluid overload	17.4%	21%
Fluid retention	16.2%	14.4%
Hyperglycemia, NOS	16%	20.1%
Hypocalcemia	16.9%	17.9%
Hypokalemia	49.2%	50.8%
Hypomagnesaemia	50.4%	56%
Metabolism and nutrition disorders	90.6%	93.7%

Micafungin Adverse Reactions During Prophylaxis of *Candida* Infection in HSCT Recipients (≥ 15%)[a,b]		
Adverse reaction[c]	Micafungin 50 mg/day (n = 425)	Fluconazole 400 mg/day (n = 457)
Respiratory		
Cough	23.1%	24.5%
Dyspnea, NOS	12.7%	14%
Epistaxis	11.5%	18.4%
Respiratory, thoracic, and mediastinal disorders	68.5%	73.5%
Miscellaneous		
Bacteremia	15.5%	18.8%
General disorders/administration site conditions	96.5%	96.3%
Infections and infestations	41.9%	45.5%
Mucosal inflammation, NOS	75.8%	78.8%
Pyrexia	44.9%	47.7%

[a] Patient base: all randomized patients who received at least 1 dose of trial drug.
[b] During treatment + 3 days.
[c] Within a system organ class, patients may experience more than 1 adverse reaction.

➤*Overall safety experience:*

Micafungin Adverse Reactions (≥ 5%)[a,b]	
Adverse reactions[c]	Micafungin (N = 3,083)
All systems, any adverse reaction	91.1%
Cardiovascular	
Cardiac disorders	18.3%
Hypertension, NOS	6.9%
Hypotension, NOS	9.1%
Phlebitis, NOS	5.6%
Tachycardia, NOS	7.5%
Vascular disorders	28.1%
CNS	
Anxiety	6.4%
Fatigue	6.4%
Headache, NOS	15.9%
Insomnia	9.8%
Nervous system disorders	28.8%
Psychiatric disorders	23.6
Rigors	9.1%
Dermatologic	
Pruritus, NOS	6.1%
Rash, NOS	8.7%
Skin and subcutaneous tissue disorders	30.5%
GI	
Abdominal pain	9.7%
Anorexia	6.2%
Constipation	11.1%
Diarrhea, NOS	23.3%
Dyspepsia	5.7%
GI disorders	57.2%
Nausea	22%
Vomiting, NOS	21.7%
Hematologic/Lymphatic	
ALT increased	5.4%
Anemia, NOS	9.8%
AST increased	5.6%
Blood alkaline phosphatase increased, NOS	5.4%
Blood and lymphatic system disorders	34%
Neutropenia	14.1%
Thrombocytopenia	15.4%
Metabolic/Nutritional	
Edema peripheral	6.8%
Fluid overload	5%
Hyperglycemia, NOS	5.6%

MICAFUNGIN SODIUM — INJECTION

Micafungin Adverse Reactions (≥ 5%)[a,b]	
Adverse reactions[c]	Micafungin (N = 3,083)
Hypocalcemia	6.5%
Hypokalemia	18%
Hypomagnesemia	13.3%
Metabolism and nutrition disorders	42.7%
Respiratory	
Cough	8.1%
Dyspnea, NOS	5.9%
Epistaxis	5.6%
Respiratory, thoracic, and mediastinal disorders	39.5%
Miscellaneous	
Back pain	5.4%
Bacteremia	6%
Febrile neutropenia	6.1%
General disorders/administration site conditions	45.6%
Infections and infestations	39.8%
Mucosal inflammation, NOS	14.2%
Musculoskeletal disorders	18.8%
Pyrexia	20%
Sepsis, NOS	5.1%

[a] Patient base: all randomized patients who received at least 1 dose of trial drug.
[b] During treatment + 3 days.
[c] Within a system organ class, patients may experience more than 1 adverse reaction.

➤*Other adverse reactions:*

Cardiovascular – Arrhythmia, atrial fibrillation, cardiac arrest, cyanosis, deep venous thrombosis, hypertension, hypotension, myocardial infarction, tachycardia.

CNS – Convulsions, delirium, encephalopathy, intracranial hemorrhage.

Dermatologic – Erythema multiforme, skin necrosis, urticaria.

GI – Abdominal pain upper, dyspepsia

Hematologic/Lymphatic – Coagulopathy, febrile neutropenia, hemolysis, hemolytic anemia, pancytopenia, thrombotic thrombocytopenic purpura.

Hepatic – Hepatic failure, hepatocellular damage, hepatomegaly, jaundice.

Metabolic/Nutritional – Acidosis, anorexia, hyponatremia.

Renal – Anuria, hemoglobinuria, oliguria, renal failure acute, renal tubular necrosis.

Respiratory – Apnea, dyspnea, hypoxia, pneumonia, pulmonary embolism.

Miscellaneous – Arthralgia, infection, injection-site thrombosis, sepsis.

➤*Postmarketing:*

CNS – Shock.

Hematologic/Lymphatic – Hemolytic anemia, white blood cell count decreased.

Hepatic – Hepatic disorder, hepatic function abnormal, hepatocellular damage, hyperbilirubinemia.

Renal – Acute renal failure and renal function impairment.

Overdosage

➤*Symptoms:* No cases of micafungin overdosage have been reported. Repeated daily doses of up to 8 mg/kg (maximum total dose, 896 mg) in adult patients have been administered in clinical trials with no reported dose-limiting toxicity.

➤*Treatment:* Micafungin is highly protein bound and, therefore, is not dialyzable.

Patient Information

Advise patients of the potential benefits and risks of micafungin. Inform patients about the common adverse reactions of micafungin, including hypersensitivity reactions (anaphylaxis and anaphylactoid reactions, including shock), hematological effects (acute intravascular hemolysis, hemolytic anemia, and hemoglobinuria), hepatic effects (abnormal liver function tests, hepatic function impairment, hepatitis, or worsening hepatic failure), and renal effects (elevations in BUN and creatinine, renal function impairment, or acute renal failure).

Instruct patients to inform their health care provider if they develop any unusual symptom, or if any known symptom persists or worsens.

Instruct patients to inform their health care provider of any other medications they are currently taking with micafungin, including nonprescription medications.

ANIDULAFUNGIN

Rx	**Eraxis** (Roerig)	**Injection, lyophilized, powder for solution:** 50 mg	Preservative free. In single-use vial with diluent.
		100 mg	Preservative free. In single-use vial with diluent.

ANIDULAFUNGIN — INJECTION

Indications

➤*Candidemia and other Candida infections:* For the treatment of candidemia and other forms of *Candida* infections (intra-abdominal abscess and peritonitis). Anidulafungin has not been studied in endocarditis, osteomyelitis, and meningitis caused by *Candida*, and it has not been studied in sufficient numbers of neutropenic patients to determine efficacy in this group.

➤*Esophageal candidiasis:* For the treatment of esophageal candidiasis.

➤*Off-label uses:*

Catheter-related bloodstream infections (children/adolescents) – [2] = Fair documentation. Guidelines suggest that anidulafungin may be used as a first-line treatment option for catheter-related bloodstream infections caused by *Candida* species. There are currently no randomized controlled trials evaluating the use of anidulafungin in pediatric patients with catheter-related bloodstream infections.

Administration and Dosage

➤*Adults:*

Candidemia and other Candida infections –

Loading dose: On day 1, administer a single 200 mg IV infusion (at a rate not to exceed 1.1 mg/min).

Maintenance dosage: Follow loading dose with 100 mg/day as an IV infusion given at a rate not to exceed 1.1 mg/min.

Duration of therapy: The duration of treatment should be based on the patient's clinical response. In general, antifungal therapy should be continued for at least 14 days after the last positive culture.

Esophageal candidiasis –

Loading dose: On day 1, administer a single 100 mg IV infusion (at a rate not to exceed 1.1 mg/min).

Maintenance dosage: Follow loading dose with 50 mg/day as an IV infusion given at a rate not to exceed 1.1 mg/min.

Duration of therapy: Patients should be treated for a minimum of 14 days and for at least 7 days following resolution of symptoms. The duration of treatment should be based on the patient's clinical response. Because of the risk of relapse of esophageal candidiasis in patients with HIV infection, suppressive antifungal therapy may be considered after a course of treatment.

➤*Children:*

Off-label dosing –

Catheter-related bloodstream infections (children/adolescents): [2] = Fair documentation.

• *2 years of age and older* – 1.5 mg/kg/day IV, with a maximum daily dosage of 100 mg.

➤*Preparation for administration:* Anidulafungin must be reconstituted with the companion diluent (dehydrated alcohol 20% [w/w] in water for injection) and subsequently diluted with only dextrose 5% injection or sodium chloride 0.9% injection.

Reconstitution –

50 mg vial: Aseptically reconstitute each 50 mg vial with 15 mL of the companion diluent (dehydrated alcohol 20% [w/w] in water for injection) to provide a concentration of 3.33 mg/mL. The reconstituted solution must be further diluted and administered within 24 hours.

100 mg vial: Aseptically reconstitute each 100 mg vial with 30 mL of the companion diluent (dehydrated alcohol 20% [w/w] in water for injection) to provide a concentration of 3.33 mg/mL. The reconstituted solution must be further diluted and administered within 24 hours.

Dilution – Aseptically transfer the contents of the reconstituted vials into the appropriately sized IV bag (or bottle) containing dextrose 5% injection or sodium chloride 0.9% injection. The following table provides the number of unit packs (anidulafungin vial and companion diluent vial), volumes, and infusion solution concentration for each dose.

Dilution Requirements for Anidulafungin Administration					
Dose	Number of unit packs required	Total reconstituted volume required	Infusion volume[a]	Total infusion volume	Infusion solution concentration
50 mg	One 50 mg	15 mL	100 mL	115 mL	0.43 mg/mL
100 mg	Two 50 mg or one 100 mg	30 mL	250 mL	280 mL	0.36 mg/mL

ANIDULAFUNGIN — INJECTION

Dilution Requirements for Anidulafungin Administration					
Dose	Number of unit packs required	Total reconstituted volume required	Infusion volume[a]	Total infusion volume	Infusion solution concentration
200 mg	Four 50 mg or two 100 mg	60 mL	500 mL	560 mL	0.36 mg/mL

[a] Either dextrose 5% injection or sodium chloride 0.9% injection.

➤*Administration:* The rate of IV infusion should not exceed 1.1 mg/min.

➤*Admixture compatibility:* The compatibility of reconstituted anidulafungin with IV substances, additives, or medications other than dextrose 5% injection or sodium chloride 0.9% injection has not been established.

➤*Storage/Stability:* Unreconstituted vials, reconstituted vials, and diluted product should be stored at 25°C (77°F); excursions are permitted to 15° to 30°C (59° to 86°F). Do not refrigerate or freeze. The reconstituted vials must be further diluted and administered within 24 hours.

Actions

➤*Pharmacology:* Anidulafungin is a semisynthetic echinocandin with antifungal activity. Anidulafungin inhibits glucan synthase, an enzyme present in fungal but not mammalian cells. This results in inhibition of the formation of 1,3-β-D-glucan, an essential component of the fungal cell wall.

➤*Pharmacokinetics:*

Absorption – Systemic exposures of anidulafungin are dose proportional and have low intersubject variability (coefficient of variation [CV] less than 25%) (see the following table). Steady state was achieved on the first day after a loading dose (twice the daily maintenance dose), and the estimated plasma accumulation factor at steady state is approximately 2.

Anidulafungin Mean (% CV) Pharmacokinetic Parameters in Adults			
	Anidulafungin IV dosing regimen (LD/MD, mg)[a]		
Pharmacokinetic parameter[b]	70/35[c,d] (n = 6)	200/100 (n = 10)	260/130[d,e] (n = 10)
$C_{max, ss}$[f] (mg/L)	3.55 (13.2)	8.6 (16.2)	10.9 (11.7)
AUC_{ss}[g] (mg•h/L)	42.3 (14.5)	111.8 (24.9)	168.9 (10.8)
Clearance (L/h)	0.84 (13.5)	0.94 (24)	0.78 (11.3)
Half-life (h)	43.2 (17.7)	52 (11.7)	50.3 (9.7)

[a] LD/MD = loading dose/maintenance dose once daily for 10 days.
[b] Parameters were obtained from separate studies.
[c] Data were collected on day 7.
[d] Safety and efficacy of these doses have not been established.
[e] See Overdosage section.
[f] $C_{max, ss}$ = the steady-state peak concentration.
[g] AUC_{ss} = the steady-state area under the concentration-time curve.

Distribution – The pharmacokinetics of anidulafungin following IV administration are characterized by a short distribution half-life (0.5 to 1 hour) and a volume of distribution of 30 to 50 L that is similar to total body fluid volume. Anidulafungin is extensively bound (more than 99%) to human plasma proteins.

Metabolism – Anidulafungin undergoes slow chemical degradation at physiologic temperature and pH to a ring-opened peptide that lacks antifungal activity. The in vitro degradation half-life of anidulafungin under physiologic conditions is about 24 hours. In vivo, the ring-opened product is subsequently converted to peptidic degradants and eliminated.

Excretion – The clearance of anidulafungin is about 1 L/h, and anidulafungin has a terminal elimination half-life of 40 to 50 hours.

In a single-dose clinical study, radiolabeled (^{14}C) anidulafungin was administered to healthy subjects. Approximately 30% of the administered radioactive dose was eliminated in the feces over 9 days, of which less than 10% was intact drug. Less than 1% of the administered radioactive dose was excreted in the urine. Anidulafungin concentrations fell below the lower limits of quantitation 6 days postdose. Negligible amounts of drug-derived radioactivity were recovered in blood, urine, and feces 8 weeks postdose.

➤*Microbiology:*

Activity in vitro – Anidulafungin is active in vitro against *Candida albicans, Candida glabrata, Candida parapsilosis,* and *Candida tropicalis*.

Minimum inhibitory concentrations were determined according to the Clinical and Laboratory Standards Institute-approved standard reference method M27 for susceptibility testing of yeasts. However, no correlation between in vitro activity as determined by this method and clinical outcome has been established.

Activity in vivo – Parenterally administered anidulafungin was effective against *C. albicans* in immunocompetent and immunosuppressed mice and rabbits with disseminated infection as measured by prolonged survival and reduction in mycological burden. Anidulafungin also reduced the mycological burden of fluconazole-resistant *C. albicans* in an oropharyngeal/esophageal infection model in immunosuppressed rabbits.

Contraindications

Known hypersensitivity to anidulafungin, to any of its components, or to other echinocandins.

Warnings/Precautions

➤*Hepatic effects:* Laboratory abnormalities in liver function tests have been seen in healthy volunteers and patients treated with anidulafungin. In some patients with serious underlying medical conditions who were receiving multiple concomitant medications along with anidulafungin, clinically significant hepatic abnormalities have occurred. Isolated cases of significant hepatic function impairment, hepatitis, or worsening hepatic failure have been reported in patients; a causal relationship to anidulafungin has not been established. Monitor patients who develop abnormal liver function tests during anidulafungin therapy for evidence of worsening hepatic function and evaluate for risk/benefit of continuing anidulafungin therapy.

➤*Pregnancy: Category C.* Embryofetal development studies were conducted with doses of up to 20 mg/kg/day in rats and rabbits (equivalent to 2 and 4 times, respectively, the proposed therapeutic maintenance dose of 100 mg/day on the basis of relative body surface area). Anidulafungin administration resulted in skeletal changes in rat fetuses, including incomplete ossification of various bones and wavy, misaligned, or misshapen ribs. These changes were not dose-related and were within the range of the laboratory's historical control database. Developmental effects observed in rabbits (slightly reduced fetal weights) occurred in the high-dose group, a dose that also produced maternal toxicity. Anidulafungin crossed the placental barrier in rats and was detected in fetal plasma.

There are no adequate and well-controlled studies in pregnant women. Because animal reproduction studies are not always predictive of human response, use anidulafungin during pregnancy only if the potential benefit justifies the risk to the fetus.

➤*Lactation:* Administer to breast-feeding mothers only if the potential benefit justifies the risk. Anidulafungin was found in the milk of lactating rats. It is not known whether anidulafungin is excreted in human milk.

➤*Children:* Safety and effectiveness of anidulafungin in children have not been established.

➤*Monitoring:* Monitor patients who develop abnormal liver function tests during anidulafungin therapy for evidence of worsening hepatic failure.

Drug Interactions

➤*Cyclosporine:* Coadministration with cyclosporine slightly increased the steady-state AUC of anidulafungin by 22%.

Adverse Reactions

➤*Hypersensitivity:* Possible histamine-mediated symptoms have been reported with anidulafungin, including dyspnea, flushing, hypotension, pruritus, rash, and urticaria. These reactions are infrequent when the rate of anidulafungin infusion does not exceed 1.1 mg/min.

➤*Candidemia/Other Candida infections:*

Anidulafungin Adverse Reactions[a] in Patients With Candidemia/Other *Candida* Infections (≥ 2%)		
Adverse reaction	Anidulafungin 100 mg[b] (n = 131)	Fluconazole 400 mg[b] (n = 125)
Subjects with ≥ 1 treatment-related adverse reaction	24.4%	26.4%
Hepatic		
Alkaline phosphatase increased	1.5%	4%
ALT increased	2.3%	3.2%
AST increased	0.8%	2.4%
Hepatic enzyme increased	1.5%	7.2%
Miscellaneous		
Deep vein thrombosis	0.8%	2.4%
Diarrhea	3.1%	1.6%
Hypokalemia	3.1%	2.4%

[a] Treatment-related adverse reactions are defined as those that are possibly or probably related to study treatment, as determined by the investigator.
[b] Maintenance dose.

➤*Esophageal candidiasis:*

Anidulafungin Adverse Reactions[a] in Patients With Esophageal Candidiasis (≥ 1%)		
Adverse reaction	Anidulafungin 50 mg[b] (n = 300)	Fluconazole 100 mg[b] (n = 301)
Subjects with ≥ 1 treatment-related adverse reaction	14.3%	16.6%
GI		
Dyspepsia aggravated	0.3%	1%
Nausea	1%	1%
Vomiting	0.7%	1%
Hematologic		
Leukopenia	0.7%	1.3%

ANIDULAFUNGIN — INJECTION

Anidulafungin Adverse Reactions[a] in Patients With Esophageal Candidiasis (≥ 1%)

Adverse reaction	Anidulafungin 50 mg[b] (n = 300)	Fluconazole 100 mg[b] (n = 301)
Neutropenia	1%	—
Hepatic		
ALT increased	—	1%
AST increased	0.3%	2.3%
Gamma-glutamyl transferase increased	1.3%	1.3%
Miscellaneous		
Headache	1.3%	1%
Phlebitis	0.7%	1.3%
Pyrexia	0.7%	1%
Rash	1%	0.7%

[a] Treatment-related adverse reactions include those that are of possible, probable, or unknown relationship to study treatment, as determined by the investigator.
[b] Maintenance dose.

The following reactions occurred in less than 2% of patients treated for candidemia/other *Candida* infections or in less than 1% of patients treated for esophageal candidiasis and were judged by investigators to be at least possibly related to anidulafungin.

➤*Cardiovascular:* Atrial fibrillation, bundle branch block (right), electrocardiogram early transition, electrocardiogram QT prolonged, flushing, hot flushes, hypertension, hypotension, sinus arrhythmia, thrombophlebitis superficial, ventricular extrasystoles.

➤*CNS:* Convulsion, dizziness, headache.

➤*Dermatologic:* Angioneurotic edema, erythema, pruritus, pruritus generalized, sweating increased, urticaria.

➤*GI:* Abdominal pain upper, constipation, diarrhea, dyspepsia, fecal incontinence, nausea, vomiting.

➤*Hematologic/Lymphatic:* Coagulopathy, thrombocytopenia.

➤*Hepatic:* Abnormal liver function tests, cholestasis, hepatic necrosis.

➤*Lab test abnormalities:* Amylase increased, bilirubin increased, creatine phosphokinase increased, creatinine increased, gamma-glutamyl transferase increased, lipase increased, magnesium decreased, platelet count decreased, platelet count increased, potassium decreased, prothrombin time prolonged, urea increased.

➤*Metabolic/Nutritional:* Hypercalcemia, hyperglycemia, hyperkalemia, hypernatremia, hypomagnesemia.

➤*Musculoskeletal:* Back pain, rigors.

➤*Ophthalmic:* Eye pain, vision blurred, visual disturbance.

➤*Miscellaneous:* Candidiasis, clostridial infection, cough, fungemia, infusion-related reaction, oral candidiasis, peripheral edema.

Overdosage

➤*Symptoms:* During clinical trials, a single dose of anidulafungin 400 mg was inadvertently administered as a loading dose. No clinical adverse reactions were reported. In a study of 10 healthy subjects administered a loading dose of 260 mg followed by 130 mg daily, anidulafungin was generally well tolerated; 3 of the 10 subjects experienced transient, asymptomatic transaminase elevations (up to 3 times the upper limit of normal).

Patient Information

Advise patients that this medicine only works against fungus; it does not treat viral infections (eg, the common cold).

Be sure to tell patients to use this medicine for the full course of treatment. If they do not, the medicine may not clear up the infection completely.

Instruct patients to notify their health care provider if any of the following most common adverse reactions persist or become bothersome: diarrhea; headache; pain, swelling, or redness at the injection site.

Instruct patients to seek medical attention right away if any of the following severe adverse reactions occur: severe allergic reactions (rash; hives; itching; difficulty breathing; tightness in the chest; swelling of the mouth, face, lips, or tongue; unusual hoarseness); dark urine; fever, chills, or persistent sore throat; irregular heartbeat; leg redness, swelling, or pain; pale stools; seizures; severe or persistent stomach pain; shortness of breath; unusual bruising or bleeding; yellowing of the skin or eyes.

ANTIMALARIAL PREPARATIONS

Cinchona Alkaloid

QUININE SULFATE

Rx	**Qualaquin** (AR Scientific)	**Capsules; oral:** 324 mg	(AR 102). In 30s, 100s, 500s, and 1,000s.

QUININE SULFATE — ORAL

Indications

➤*Malaria:* Only for treatment of uncomplicated *Plasmodium falciparum* malaria. Quinine has been shown to be effective in geographical regions where resistance to chloroquine has been documented.

➤*Off-label uses:* Nocturnal recumbency leg cramps, prevention, and treatment. Dose: 260 to 300 mg at bedtime.

Administration and Dosage

➤*Adults:*

Malaria – 648 mg (2 capsules) every 8 h for 7 days.

➤*Children:*

Malaria –

16 years of age and older: 648 mg (2 capsules) every 8 h for 7 days.

Off-label dosing –

Malaria caused by P. falciparum or species unknown: 8.3 mg base/kg (= 10 mg salt/kg) 3 times daily for 3 to 7 days plus one of the following: clindamycin 20 mg base/kg/day 3 times daily for 7 days or doxycycline 2.2 mg/kg every 12 h for 7 days or tetracycline 25 mg/kg/day 4 times daily for 7 days.

Malaria caused by Plasmodium vivax: 8.3 mg base/kg (= 10 mg salt/kg) 3 times daily for 3 to 7 days and primaquine 0.5 mg base/kg/day for 14 days plus one of the following: doxycycline 2.2 mg/kg every 12 h for 7 days or tetracycline 25 mg/kg/day 4 times daily for 7 days.

➤*Renal function impairment:*

Severe chronic renal failure – Loading dose of 648 mg followed 12 h later by maintenance doses of 324 mg every 12 h.

➤*Administration:* Take with food to minimize stomach upset.

➤*Storage/Stability:* Store at 25° to 30°C (77° to 86°F).

Actions

➤*Pharmacology:* Quinine inhibits nucleic acid synthesis, protein synthesis, and glycolysis in *P. falciparum* and can bind with hemazoin in parasitized erythrocytes. However, the precise mechanism of the antimalarial activity of quinine is not completely understood.

➤*Pharmacokinetics:*

Absorption – The oral bioavailability of quinine is 76% to 88% in healthy adults. Quinine exposure is higher in patients with malaria than in healthy subjects. After a single oral dose of quinine, the mean quinine time to reach maximum concentration (T_{max}) was longer, and mean area under the curve (AUC) and maximum plasma concentration (C_{max}) were higher in patients with uncomplicated *P. falciparum* malaria than in healthy subjects.

Quinine Pharmacokinetic Parameters after a Single Dose[a] of Quinine Capsules

Pharmacokinetic parameter	Healthy subjects (n = 23) mean ± SD	Uncomplicated *P. falciparum* malaria patients (n = 15) mean ± SD
Dose (mg/kg)[a]	8.7	10
T_{max} (h)	2.8 ± 0.8	5.9 ± 4.7
C_{max} (mcg/mL)	3.2 ± 0.7	8.4
$AUC_{0\ to\ 12}$(mcg•h/mL)	28	73

[a] Quinine dose was 648 mg (approximately 8.7 mg/kg) in healthy subjects, and 10 mg/kg in patients with malaria.

Effects of food: Quinine capsules may be administered without regard to meals. Take with food to minimize possible GI irritation. When a single oral 324 mg capsule of quinine was administered to healthy volunteers (n = 26) with a standardized high-fat breakfast, the mean T_{max} of quinine was prolonged to about 4 hours, but the mean C_{max} and $AUC_{0\text{-}24h}$ were similar to those achieved when quinine was given under fasted conditions.

Distribution – In patients with malaria, the volume of distribution (Vd/f) decreases in proportion to the severity of the infection. In published studies with healthy subjects who received a single oral 600 mg dose of quinine, the mean Vd/f ranged from 2.5 to 7.1 L/kg.

Quinine is moderately protein-bound in blood in healthy subjects, ranging from 69% to 92%. During active malarial infection, protein binding of quinine is increased to 78% to 95%, corresponding to the increase in alpha-1 acid glycoprotein that occurs with malaria infection.

Intra-erythrocytic levels of quinine are approximately 30% to 50% of the plasma concentration. Quinine penetrates relatively poorly into the cerebrospinal fluid (CSF) in patients with cerebral malaria, with CSF concentration approximately 2% to 7% of plasma concentration.

In one study, quinine concentrations in placental cord blood and breast milk were approximately 32% and 31%, respectively, of quinine concentrations in

QUININE SULFATE — ORAL

maternal plasma. The estimated total dose of quinine secreted into breast milk was less than 2 to 3 mg per day.

Metabolism – Quinine is metabolized almost exclusively via hepatic oxidative cytochrome P450 (CYP-450) pathways, resulting in 4 primary metabolites, 3-hydroxyquinine, 2'-quinone, O-desmethylquinine, and 10,11-dihydroxydihydroquinine. Six secondary metabolites result from further biotransformation of the primary metabolites. The major metabolite, 3-hydroxyquinine, is less active than the parent drug. In vitro studies using human liver microsomes and recombinant P-450 enzymes have shown that quinine is metabolized mainly by CYP3A4. Depending on the in vitro experimental conditions, other enzymes, including CYP1A2, CYP2C8, CYP2C9, CYP2C19, CYP2D6, and CYP2E1, were shown to have some role in the metabolism of quinine.

Excretion – Quinine is eliminated primarily via hepatic biotransformation. Approximately 20% of quinine is excreted unchanged in urine. Because quinine is reabsorbed when the urine is alkaline, renal excretion of the drug is twice as rapid when the urine is acidic than when it is alkaline.

In various published studies, healthy subjects who received a single oral 600 mg dose of quinine exhibited a mean plasma clearance ranging from 0.08 to 0.47 L/h/kg (median value, 0.17 L/h/kg) with a mean plasma elimination half-life of 9.7 to 12.5 hours.

In 15 patients with uncomplicated malaria who received a 10 mg/kg oral dose of quinine, the mean total clearance of quinine was slower (approximately 0.09 L/h/kg) during the acute phase of the infection, and faster (approximately 0.16 L/h/kg) during the recovery or convalescent phase.

Special populations –

Renal function impairment: Following a single oral 600 mg dose of quinine in otherwise healthy subjects with severe chronic renal failure not receiving any form of dialysis (mean serum creatinine, 9.6 mg/dL), the median AUC was higher by 195% and the median C_{max} was higher by 79% than in subjects with healthy renal function (mean serum creatinine, 1 mg/dL). The mean plasma half-life in subjects with severe chronic renal impairment was prolonged to 26 hours compared with 9.7 hours in the healthy controls. Computer-assisted modeling and simulation indicates that in patients with malaria and severe chronic renal failure, a dosage regimen consisting of 1 loading dose of 648 mg quinine followed 12 hours later by a maintenance dosing regimen of 324 mg every 12 hours will provide adequate systemic exposure to quinine. The effects of mild and moderate renal impairment on the pharmacokinetics and safety of quinine are not known. Negligible to minimal amounts of circulating quinine in the blood are removed by hemodialysis or hemofiltration. In subjects with chronic renal failure (CRF) on hemodialysis, only about 6.5% of quinine is removed in 1 hour. Plasma quinine concentrations do not change during or shortly after hemofiltration in subjects with CRF.

Hepatic function impairment: In otherwise healthy subjects with moderate hepatic impairment (Child-Pugh B; n = 9) who received a single oral 600 mg dose of quinine, the mean AUC increased 55% without a significant change in mean C_{max}, as compared with healthy volunteer controls (n = 6). In subjects with hepatitis, the absorption of quinine was prolonged, the elimination half-life was increased, the apparent volume of distribution was higher, but there was no significant difference in weight-adjusted clearance. Therefore, in patients with mild to moderate hepatic impairment, dosage adjustment is not needed, but closely monitor patients for adverse reactions of quinine. No pharmacokinetic data are available for patients with severe hepatic impairment (Child-Pugh C).

Elderly: Following a single oral dose of quinine 600 mg, the mean AUC was about 38% higher in 8 healthy elderly subjects (65 to 78 years of age) than in 12 younger subjects (20 to 35 years of age). The mean T_{max} and C_{max} were similar in elderly and younger subjects after a single oral dose of quinine 600 mg. The mean oral clearance of quinine was significantly decreased, and the mean elimination half-life was significantly increased in elderly subjects compared with younger subjects (0.06 vs 0.08 L/h/kg, and 18.4 vs 10.5 hours, respectively). Although there was no significant difference in the renal clearance of quinine between the 2 age groups, elderly subjects excreted a larger proportion of the dose in urine as unchanged drug than younger subjects (16.6% vs 11.2%). Despite these pharmacokinetic changes, an alteration in the quinine dosage regimen in elderly patients is not needed.

Cigarette smoking (CYP1A2 inducer): In healthy male heavy smokers, the mean quinine AUC following a single 600 mg dose was 44% lower, the mean C_{max} was 18% lower, and the elimination half-life was shorter (7.5 vs 12 hours) than in their nonsmoking counterparts. However, in malaria patients who received the full 7-day course of quinine therapy, cigarette smoking produced only a 25% decrease in median quinine AUC and a 16.5% decrease in median C_{max}, suggesting that the already reduced clearance of quinine in acute malaria could have diminished the metabolic induction effect of smoking. Because smoking did not appear to influence the therapeutic outcome in malaria patients, it is not necessary to increase the dose of quinine in the treatment of acute malaria in heavy cigarette smokers.

➤*Microbiology:*

Activity in vitro and in vivo – Quinine acts primarily on the blood schizont form of *P. falciparum*; it is not gametocidal and has little effect on the sporozoite or pre-erythrocytic forms.

Drug resistance – Strains of *P. falciparum* with decreased susceptibility to quinine can be selected in vivo. *P. falciparum* malaria that is clinically resistant to quinine has been reported in some areas of South America, Southeast Asia, and Bangladesh.

Contraindications

In patients with a prolonged QT interval; glucose-6-phosphate dehydrogenase (G-6-PD) deficiency; myasthenia gravis; optic neuritis; known hypersensitivity to quinine, mefloquine, or quinidine; history of potential hypersensitivity reactions associated with previous quinine use (ie, thrombotic thrombocytopenic purpura [TTP] or hemolytic uremic syndrome [HUS]); thrombocytopenia, blackwater fever [acute intravascular hemolysis, hemoglobinuria, and hemoglobinemia]).

Warnings/Precautions

➤*Nocturnal leg cramps:* Quinine may cause unpredictable serious and life-threatening hypersensitivity reactions, QT prolongation, serious cardiac arrhythmias, including torsades de pointes, and other serious adverse reactions requiring medical intervention and hospitalization. Fatalities have also been reported. The risk associated with the use of quinine in the absence of evidence of its effectiveness for treatment or prevention of nocturnal leg cramps outweighs any potential benefit in treating and/or preventing this benign, self-limiting condition. Because 157 adverse drug reactions attributed to quinine were reported from 1969 to 1992, the Food and Drug Administration (FDA) concluded that quinine was not safe for use in this condition. In 1994, the FDA prohibited the marketing of quinine for nocturnal leg cramps and discontinued its availability and the labeling of products for this use in prescription and nonprescription form.[3]

➤*QT prolongation and ventricular arrhythmias:* QT interval prolongation has been a consistent finding in studies which evaluated electrocardiographic changes with oral or parenteral quinine administration, regardless of age, clinical status, or severity of disease. The maximum increase in QT interval has been shown to correspond with peak quinine plasma concentration. Quinine sulfate has been rarely associated with potentially fatal cardiac arrhythmias, including torsades de pointes and ventricular fibrillation.

Quinine should also be avoided in patients with known prolongation of QT interval, in elderly patients, and in patients with clinical conditions known to prolong the QT interval, such as uncorrected hypokalemia, bradycardia, and certain cardiac conditions.

➤*Glucose-6-phosphate dehydrogenase deficiency:* Hemolysis and hemolytic anemia can occur in patients with G-6-PD deficiency who receive quinine. Stop quinine immediately upon the appearance of evidence of hemolysis.

➤*Myasthenia gravis:* Quinine has neuromuscular blocking activity, and may exacerbate muscle weakness in patients with myasthenia gravis.

➤*Atrial fibrillation and flutter:* Use quinine with caution in patients with atrial fibrillation or atrial flutter. A paradoxical increase in ventricular response rate may occur with quinine, similar to that observed with quinidine. If digoxin is used to prevent a rapid ventricular response, closely monitor serum digoxin levels, because digoxin levels may be increased with use of quinine.

➤*Hypoglycemia:* Quinine stimulates release of insulin from the pancreas, and patients, especially pregnant women, may experience clinically significant hypoglycemia.

➤*Hypersensitivity reactions:* Serious hypersensitivity reactions reported with quinine include anaphylactic shock, anaphylactoid reactions, urticaria, serious skin rashes, including Stevens-Johnson syndrome and toxic epidermal necrolysis, angioedema, facial edema, bronchospasm, and pruritus. A number of other serious adverse reactions reported with quinine, including TTP and HUS, thrombocytopenia, immune thrombocytopenic purpura, blackwater fever, disseminated intravascular coagulation, leukopenia, neutropenia, granulomatous hepatitis, and acute interstitial nephritis, may also be due to hypersensitivity reactions. Discontinue quinine in case of any signs or symptoms of hypersensitivity.

➤*Pregnancy: Category C* (per manufacturer's prescribing information). *Category D* (per Briggs' *Drugs in Pregnancy and Lactation*). There are no adequate and well-controlled studies in pregnant women.

Hypoglycemia, due to increased pancreatic secretion of insulin, has been associated with quinine use, particularly in pregnant women. Quinine crosses the placenta and gives measurable blood concentrations in the fetus. In 8 women who delivered live infants 1 to 6 days after starting quinine therapy, placental cord plasma quinine concentrations were between 1 and 4.6 mg/L (mean, 2.4 mg/L) and the mean (± SD) ratio of cord plasma to maternal plasma quinine concentrations was 0.32 ± 0.14.

Quinine levels in the fetus may not be therapeutic. If congenital malaria is suspected after delivery, evaluate the infant and treat appropriately.

Rare and isolated case reports describe deafness and optic nerve hypoplasia in children exposed in utero because of maternal ingestion of high doses of quinine.

P. falciparum malaria carries a higher risk of morbidity and mortality in pregnant women than in the general population. Pregnant women with *P. falciparum* malaria have an increased incidence of fetal loss (including spontaneous abortion and stillbirth), preterm labor and delivery, intrauterine growth retardation, low birth weight, and maternal death. Therefore, treatment of malaria in pregnancy is important. Use quinine during pregnancy only if the potential benefit justifies the potential risk to the fetus. Consider the risks and benefits of alternative treatment. If quinine is used during pregnancy, or if the patient becomes pregnant while taking this drug, apprise the patient of the potential hazards to the fetus.

Teratogenic effects have been demonstrated in some animal species but not in others when quinine was given by the subcutaneous or intramuscular route at dose levels in the same range as the maximum recommended human dose. Teratogenic effects were observed in rabbits (death in utero, degenerated auditory nerve and spiral ganglion, and CNS anomalies, such as anencephaly and microcephaly), dogs (death in utero), guinea pigs (hemorrhage and mitochondrial change in cochlea), and chinchillas (death and

QUININE SULFATE — ORAL

growth suppression in utero and CNS anomalies, such as anencephaly and microcephaly). There were no teratogenic findings in mice, rats, and monkeys.

Labor and delivery – There is no evidence that quinine causes uterine contractions at the doses recommended for the treatment of malaria. In doses several times higher than those used to treat malaria, quinine may stimulate the pregnant uterus.

➤*Lactation:* Quinine is excreted into breast milk. Although quinine is generally considered compatible with breast-feeding, the risks and benefits to infant and mother should be assessed. The American Academy of Pediatrics classifies quinine as compatible with breast-feeding.

If malaria is suspected in the infant, appropriate evaluation and treatment should be provided. Plasma quinine levels may not be therapeutic in infants of breast-feeding mothers receiving quinine.

➤*Children:* The safety and efficacy of quinine in children younger than 16 years of age have not been established.

➤*Lab test abnormalities:* Quinine may produce an elevated value for urinary 17-ketogenic steroids when the Zimmerman method is used.

Drug Interactions

➤*Cytochrome P450 system:* Since quinine is metabolized mainly by the CYP3A enzyme systems, substances known to inhibit these enzymes may decrease metabolism or increase bioavailability of quinine, as indicated by increased whole blood or plasma concentrations. Drugs known to induce these enzyme systems may result in an increased metabolism of quinine or decreased bioavailability, as indicated by decreased whole blood or plasma concentrations. Monitoring of blood concentrations and appropriate dosage adjustments are essential when such drugs are used concomitantly.

➤*QT prolongation:* An additive effect of quinine with other drugs that prolong the QT interval cannot be excluded. The following drugs may prolong the QT interval and increase the risk of life-threatening cardiac arrhythmias, including torsade de pointes: antiarrhythmic agents (eg, amiodarone, bretylium, disopyramide, dofetilide, procainamide, quinidine, sotalol), arsenic trioxide, astemizole (this drug is no longer marketed in the United States), chlorpromazine, cisapride (available from the manufacturer on a limited-access protocol), dolasetron, droperidol, halofantrine, mefloquine, mesoridazine, moxifloxacin, pentamidine, pimozide, tacrolimus, terfenadine (this drug is no longer marketed in the United States), thioridazine, and ziprasidone. Coadministration of these agents with quinine is not recommended.

Quinine Drug Interactions

Precipitant drug	Object drug[a]		Description
Antacids (eg, aluminum and/or magnesium)	Quinine	⬇	Concurrent use may delay or decrease absorption of quinine. Avoid coadministration.
Anticonvulsants (eg, carbamazepine, phenobarbital, phenytoin)	Quinine	⬇	Quinine plasma concentrations may be decreased with concurrent use. Coadministration also increased the C_{max} and AUC of carbamazepine and phenobarbital. If concomitant use cannot be avoided, frequently monitor anticonvulsant drug concentration. Also, observe the clinical response of the patient and adjust the quinine dose as needed.
Quinine	Anticonvulsants (eg, carbamazepine, phenobarbital)	⬆	
Cigarette smoking	Quinine	⬇	Quinine AUC and C_{max} may be reduced and the $t_{1/2}$ shortened. However, dosage adjustment does not appear to be necessary in treating acute malaria.
CYP-450 inhibitors (eg, cimetidine, erythromycin, ketoconazole, ranitidine, ritonavir)	Quinine	⬆	Concurrent use may increase quinine plasma levels and the risk of adverse reactions. Closely monitor for quinine adverse reactions and adjust the quinine dose as needed. Avoid concomitant use with erythromycin.
Rifamycins (eg, rifampin)	Quinine	⬇	Avoid concurrent use due to decreased plasma concentrations of quinine; treatment failures may result.
Tetracycline	Quinine	⬆	Plasma quinine concentrations are about 2-fold higher with coadministration. Monitor patient for adverse reactions associated with quinine and adjust treatment as needed.
Urinary alkalinizers (eg, acetazolamide, sodium bicarbonate)	Quinine	⬆	Urinary alkalinizing agents may increase plasma quinine concentrations. Monitor the clinical response of the patient. If an interaction is suspected, adjust the quinine dose as needed.

Quinine Drug Interactions

Precipitant drug	Object drug[a]		Description
Xanthine derivatives (eg, aminophylline, theophylline)	Quinine	⬆	Quinine plasma concentrations may be elevated, increasing the risk of adverse reactions. Closely monitor for quinine adverse reactions and adjust treatment as needed. While theophylline plasma concentrations may be decreased, possibly reducing the effect. Plasma theophylline concentrations should be monitored frequently during concurrent therapy and the theophylline dose adjusted as needed.
Quinine	Xanthine derivatives (eg, aminophylline, theophylline)	⬇	
Quinine	Anticholinesterases (eg, neostigmine)	⬇	Beneficial effects of anticholinesterases in the treatment of myasthenia gravis may be reversed by quinine. Avoid coadministration in patients receiving anticholinesterases for myasthenia gravis.
Quinine	Anticoagulants (eg, heparin, warfarin)	⬆	Quinine may depress hepatic enzyme synthesis of vitamin-K dependent coagulation pathway proteins and may enhance the action of anticoagulants. Monitor prothrombin time, partial thromboplastin time, and international normalization ratio closely during coadministration. Adjust the anticoagulant dose as needed.
Quinine	CYP2D6 substrates (eg, debrisoquine, desipramine, dextromethorphan, flecainide, metoprolol, paroxetine)	⬆	Quinine may inhibit the metabolism of drugs that are CYP2D6 substrates, elevating plasma concentrations and increasing the pharmacologic effect and risk of adverse reactions. Monitor patient for adverse reactions and adjust treatment as needed.
Quinine	Digoxin	⬆	Digoxin levels may be increased with concurrent use. Monitor serum digoxin levels closely and adjust the digoxin dose as needed.
Quinine	HMG-CoA[b] reductase inhibitors (eg, atorvastatin, lovastatin, simvastatin)	⬆	Quinine may increase plasma concentration of HMG-CoA reductase inhibitors, thereby increasing the risk of myopathy or rhabdomyolysis. Consider lower starting and maintenance doses of the HMG-CoA reductase inhibitors. Closely monitor patients for signs or symptoms of muscle pain, tenderness, or weakness. If symptoms occur in conjunction with elevated creatine phosphokinase, the HMG-CoAb reductase inhibitor should be discontinued.
Quinine	Neuromuscular blocking agents (eg, pancuronium, succinylcholine, tubocurarine)	⬆	Quinine may potentiate neuromuscular blockade, resulting in respiratory depression and apnea. Avoid use of quinine during administration of and for several hours after recovery from non-depolarizing muscle relaxants. If this combination is required, closely monitor neuromuscular function, titrate the dose of neuromuscular blocking agent, and provide mechanical respiratory support as needed.

[a] ⬆ = object drug increased; ⬇ = object drug decreased.
[b] HMG-CoA = 3-hydroxy-3-methylglutanyl coenzyme A.

➤*Drug/Lab test interactions:* An elevated value for urinary 17-ketogenic steroids measured by the Zimmerman method may occur.1

➤*Drug/Food interactions:* See Actions for more information.

Adverse Reactions

➤*Common adverse reactions:* Quinine can adversely affect almost every body system. The most common adverse reactions associated with quinine use are a cluster of symptoms called cinchonism, which occurs to some degree in almost all patients taking quinine. Symptoms of mild cinchonism include headache, vasodilation and sweating, nausea, tinnitus, hearing impairment, vertigo or dizziness, blurred vision, and disturbance in color perception. More severe symptoms of cinchonism are vomiting, diarrhea, abdominal pain, deafness, blindness, and disturbances in cardiac rhythm or conduction. Most symptoms of cinchonism are reversible and resolve with discontinuation of quinine.

➤*Cardiovascular:* Atrial fibrillation, atrioventricular block, bradycardia, cardiac arrest, chest pain, hypotension, irregular rhythm, palpitations, postural hypotension, nodal escape beats, QT prolongation, syncope, tachycardia, torsades de pointes, unifocal premature ventricular contractions, U waves, vasodilatation, ventricular fibrillation, and ventricular tachycardia.

➤*CNS:* Acute dystonic reaction, altered mental status, aphasia, ataxia, coma, confusion, diplopia, disorientation, headache, restlessness, seizures, suicide, and tremors.

QUININE SULFATE — ORAL

➤*Dermatologic:* Cutaneous rashes, including urticarial, papular, or scarlatinal rashes, acral necrosis, allergic contact dermatitis, bullous dermatitis, cutaneous vasculitis, erythema multiforme, exfoliative dermatitis, fixed drug eruption, photosensitivity reactions, pruritus, Stevens-Johnson syndrome, and toxic epidermal necrolysis.

➤*GI:* Abdominal pain, diarrhea, esophagitis, gastric irritation, nausea, and vomiting.

➤*Hematologic:* Agranulocytosis, aplastic anemia, blackwater fever, coagulopathy, disseminated intravascular coagulation, ecchymosis, hemolytic anemia, hemolytic uremic syndrome, hemorrhage, hypoprothrombinemia, idiopathic thrombocytopenic purpura, leukopenia, lupus anticoagulant, neutropenia, pancytopenia, petechiae, thrombocytopenia, and thrombotic thrombocytopenic purpura.

➤*Hepatic:* Abnormal liver function tests, granulomatous hepatitis, hepatitis, and jaundice.

➤*Metabolic/Nutritional:* Anorexia and hypoglycemia.

➤*Musculoskeletal:* Muscle weakness and myalgias.

➤*Renal:* Acute interstitial nephritis, hemoglobinuria, renal failure, and renal impairment.

➤*Respiratory:* Asthma, dyspnea, pulmonary edema.

➤*Special senses:* Visual disturbances, including blindness, blurred vision with scotomata, diminished visual fields, diplopia, fixed pupillary dilatation, disturbed color vision, night blindness, optic neuritis, photophobia, sudden loss of vision; vertigo, including tinnitus, hearing impairment, and deafness.

➤*Miscellaneous:* Asthenia, chills, fever, flushing, hypersensitivity reactions, lupus-like syndrome, and sweating.

Overdosage

➤*Symptoms:* Quinine overdose can be associated with serious complications, including visual impairment, hypoglycemia, cardiac arrhythmias, and death. Visual impairment can range from blurred vision and defective color perception to visual field constriction and permanent blindness. Cinchonism occurs in virtually all patients with quinine overdose. Symptoms range from headache, nausea, vomiting, abdominal pain, diarrhea, tinnitus, vertigo, hearing impairment, sweating, flushing, and blurred vision to deafness, blindness, serious cardiac arrhythmias, hypotension, and circulatory collapse. CNS toxicity (drowsiness, disturbances of consciousness, ataxia, convulsions, respiratory depression, and coma) has also been reported with quinine overdose, as well as pulmonary edema and adult respiratory distress syndrome.

Most toxic reactions are dose-related; however, some reactions may be idiosyncratic because of the variable sensitivity of patients to the toxic effects of quinine. A lethal dose of quinine has not been clearly defined, but fatalities have been reported after the ingestion of 2 to 8 g in adults.

Quinine, like quinidine, has class I antiarrhythmic properties. The cardiotoxicity of quinine is due to its negative inotropic action, and to its effect on cardiac conduction, resulting in decreased rates of depolarization and conduction, and increased action potential and effective refractory period. Electrocardiogram (ECG) changes observed with quinine overdose include sinus tachycardia, PR prolongation, T-wave inversion, bundle branch block, an increased QT interval, and a widening of the QRS complex. Quinines alpha-blocking properties may result in hypotension and further exacerbate myocardial depression by decreasing coronary perfusion. Quinine overdose has also been associated with hypotension, cardiogenic shock, and circulatory collapse, ventricular arrhythmias, including ventricular tachycardia, ventricular fibrillation, idioventricular rhythm, and torsades de pointes, as well as bradycardia, and atrioventricular block.

➤*Treatment:* Quinine is rapidly absorbed, and attempts to remove residual quinine from the stomach by gastric lavage may not be effective. Multiple-dose activated charcoal has been shown to decrease plasma quinine concentrations. Forced acid diuresis, hemodialysis, charcoal column hemoperfusion, and plasma exchange were not found to be effective in significantly increasing quinine elimination in a series of 16 patients.

Administration of multiple-dose activated charcoal (50 g administered 4 hours after quinine dosing followed by 3 further doses over the next 12 hours) decreased the mean quinine elimination half-life from 8.2 to 4.6 hours, and increased the mean quinine clearance by 56% (from 11.8 to 18.4 L/h) in 7 healthy adult volunteers who received a single oral 600 mg dose of quinine. Likewise, in 5 symptomatic patients with acute quinine poisoning who received multiple-dose activated charcoal (50 g every 4 hours), the mean quinine elimination half-life was shortened to 8.1 hours in comparison with a half-life of approximately 26 hours in patients who did not receive activated charcoal.

In 6 patients with quinine poisoning, forced acid diuresis did not change the half-life of quinine elimination (25.1 ± 4.6 hours vs 26.5 ± 5.8 hours), or the amount of unchanged quinine recovered in the urine, in comparison with 8 patients not treated in this manner.

Patient Information

Advise patients to take all of the medication as directed.

Advise patients to take no more of the medication than the amount prescribed.

Advise patients to take with food to minimize possible GI irritation.

If a dose is missed, instruct patients not to double the next dose. If more than 4 hours has elapsed since the missed dose, instruct the patient to wait and take the next dose as previously scheduled.

Quinine may cause diarrhea, nausea, stomach cramps or pain, vomiting, or ringing in the ears; advise patient to notify their health care provider if these become pronounced.

Quinine may produce blurred vision, vertigo, restlessness, confusion, or dizziness; advise patients to observe caution while driving or performing other tasks requiring alertness.

Advise patients to stop the drug if there is any evidence of allergy, such as flushing, itching, rash, fever, stomach pain, difficult breathing, ringing in the ears, or vision problems.

ANTIMALARIAL PREPARATIONS

MEFLOQUINE HYDROCHLORIDE

Rx	**Mefloquine HCl** (Geneva)	**Tablets**: 250 mg	(GP 118). White, scored. In 25s.

MEFLOQUINE HYDROCHLORIDE — ORAL

Indications

➤*Acute malaria infections:* For the treatment of mild-to-moderate acute malaria caused by mefloquine-susceptible strains of *P. falciparum* (both chloroquine-susceptible and resistant strains) or by *Plasmodium vivax*. There are insufficient clinical data to document the effect of mefloquine in malaria caused by *P. ovale* or *P. malariae*.

➤*Prevention of malaria:* For the prophylaxis of *P. falciparum* and *P. vivax* malaria infections, including prophylaxis of chloroquine-resistant strains of *P. falciparum*.

Administration and Dosage

➤*General dosing considerations:* If a full treatment course with mefloquine does not lead to improvement within 48 to 72 hours, mefloquine should not be used for retreatment. An alternative treatment should be used. Similarly, if previous prophylaxis with mefloquine has failed, mefloquine should not be used for curative treatment.

Patients with acute *P. vivax* malaria, treated with mefloquine, are at high risk of relapse because mefloquine does not eliminate exoerythrocytic (hepatic-phase) parasites. To avoid relapse after initial treatment of the acute infection with mefloquine, patients should subsequently be treated with an 8-aminoquinoline (eg, primaquine).

➤*Adults:*

Malaria prevention –

Usual dosage: 250 mg once weekly beginning 1 week before arrival in an endemic area. Subsequent weekly doses should be taken regularly, always on the same day of each week preferably after the main meal.

Duration of therapy: To reduce the risk of malaria after leaving an endemic area, prophylaxis must be continued for 4 additional weeks to ensure suppressive blood levels of the drug when merozoites emerge from the liver.

Malaria treatment (mild-to-moderate) – 1,250 mg (5 tablets) given as a single oral dose.

➤*Children:*

Malaria prevention –

Usual dosage: 5 mg/kg body weight once weekly.

- *Over 45 kg* – 250 mg (1 tablet) once weekly.
- *31 to 45 kg* – 187.5 mg (3/4 tablet) once weekly.
- *21 to 30 kg* – 125 mg (1/2 tablet) once weekly.
- *11 to 20 kg* – 62.5 mg (1/4 tablet) once weekly.
- *5 to 10 kg* – 31.25 mg (1/8 tablet; approximate tablet fraction based on a dosage of 5 mg/kg body weight. Exact doses for children weighing less than 10 kg may best be prepared and dispensed by pharmacists.)

Malaria treatment (mild-to-moderate) –

6 months of age and older:

- *Usual dosage* – 20 to 25 mg/kg. Splitting the total therapeutic dose into 2 doses taken 6 to 8 hours apart may reduce the occurrence or severity of adverse reactions. (See Administration.)
- *Repeating dose due to vomiting* – In children, the administration of mefloquine for the treatment of malaria has been associated with early vomiting. In some cases, early vomiting has been cited as a possible cause of treatment failure. If a significant loss of drug product is observed or suspected because of vomiting, a second full dose of mefloquine should be administered to patients who vomit less than 30 minutes after receiving the drug. If vomiting occurs 30 to 60 minutes after a dose, an additional half-dose should be given. If vomiting recurs, the patient should be monitored closely and alternative malaria treatment considered if improvement is not observed within a reasonable period of time.

➤*Concomitant therapy:* In certain cases (eg, when a traveler is taking other medication), it may be desirable to start prophylaxis 2 to 3 weeks prior to departure, in order to ensure that the combination of drugs is well tolerated (see Drug Interactions).

MEFLOQUINE HYDROCHLORIDE — ORAL

➤*Administration:*

Adults – The drug should not be taken on an empty stomach and should be administered with at least 240 mL of water.

Children – The drug should not be taken on an empty stomach and should be administered with ample water. For very young patients, the dose may be crushed and suspended in a small amount of water, milk or other beverage for administration to small children and other persons unable to swallow them whole.

➤*Storage/Stability:* Tablets should be stored at 25°C (77°F); excursions permitted to 15° to 30°C (59° to 86°F).

Actions

➤*Pharmacology:* Mefloquine HCl is an antimalarial agent which acts as a blood schizonticide. Its exact mechanism of action is not known.

➤*Pharmacokinetics:*

Absorption – The absolute oral bioavailability of mefloquine has not been determined since an intravenous formulation is not available. The bioavailability of the tablet formation compared with an oral solution was over 85%. The presence of food significantly enhances the rate and extent of absorption, leading to about a 40% increase in bioavailability. In healthy volunteers, plasma concentrations peak 6 to 24 hours (median, about 17 hours) after a single dose of mefloquine HCl. In a similar group of volunteers, maximum plasma concentrations in mcg/L are roughly equivalent to the dose in milligrams (for example, a single 1000 mg dose produces a maximum concentration of about 1000 mcg/L).

In healthy volunteers, a dose of 250 mg once weekly, produces maximum steady-state plasma concentrations of 1000 to 2000 mcg/L, which are reached after 7 to 10 weeks.

Distribution – In healthy adults, the apparent volume of distribution, approximately 20 L/kg, indicates extensive tissue distribution. Mefloquine HCl may accumulate in parasitized erythrocytes. Experiments conducted in vitro with human blood using concentrations between 50 and 1000 mg/mL showed a relatively constant erythrocyte-to-plasma concentration ratio of about 2 to 1. The equilibrium reached in less than 30 minutes, was found to be reversible. Protein binding is about 98%.

Mefloquine crosses the placenta. Excretion into breast milk appears to be minimal (see Warnings).

Metabolism – Two metabolites have been identified in humans. The main metabolite, 2,8-bis-trifluoromethyl-4-quinoline carboxylic acid, is inactive in Plasmodium falciparum. In a study in healthy volunteers, the carboxylic acid metabolite appeared in plasma 2 to 4 hours after a single oral dose. Maximum plasma concentrations, which were about 50% higher than those of mefloquine, were reached after 2 weeks. Thereafter, plasma levels of the main metabolite and mefloquine declined at a similar rate. The area under the plasma concentration-time curve (AUC) of the main metabolite was 3 to 5 times larger than that of the parent drug. The other metabolite, an alcohol, was present in minute quantities only.

Excretion – In several studies in healthy adults, the mean elimination half-life of mefloquine varied between 2 and 4 weeks, with an average of about 3 weeks. The total clearance of the drug, which is essentially all hepatic, is approximately 30 mL/min. There is evidence that mefloquine is excreted mainly in the bile and feces. In volunteers, urinary excretion of unchanged mefloquine and its main metabolite under steady-state condition accounted for about 9% and 4% of the dose, respectively. Concentrations of other metabolites could not be measured in the urine.

➤*Microbiology:*

Activity in vitro and in vivo – Mefloquine is active against the erythrocytic stages of *Plasmodium* species (see Indications). However, the drug has no effect against the exoerythrocytic (hepatic) stages of the parasite. Mefloquine is effective against malaria parasites resistant to chloroquine (see Indications).

Drug resistance – Strains of *P. falciparum* with decreased susceptibility to mefloquine can be selected in vitro or in vivo. Resistance of *P. falciparum* to mefloquine have been reported in areas of multi-drug resistance in South East Asia. Increased incidences of resistance have also been reported in other parts of the world.

Contraindications

Hypersensitivity to mefloquine or related compounds (eg, quinine, quinidine) or to any of the excipients contained in the formulation. Mefloquine HCl should not be prescribed for prophylaxis in patients with active depression, generalized anxiety disorder, a recent history of depression, psychosis, or schizophrenia or other major psychiatric disorders, or with a history of convulsions.

Warnings/Precautions

➤*Life-threatening P. falciparum infections:* In case of life-threatening, serious or overwhelming malaria infections due to *P. falciparum*, patients should be treated with an IV antimalarial drug. Following completion of IV treatment, mefloquine HCl may be given to complete the course of therapy.

➤*Psychiatric disturbances:* Mefloquine HCl may cause psychiatric symptoms in a number of patients, ranging from anxiety, paranoia, and depression to hallucinations and psychotic behavior. On occasions, these symptoms have been reported to continue long after mefloquine has been stopped. Rare cases of suicidal ideation and suicide have been reported; though no relationship to drug administration has been confirmed. To minimize the chances of these adverse events, mefloquine should not be taken for prophylaxis in patients with active depression or with a recent history of depression, generalized anxiety disorder, psychosis, or schizophrenia or other major psychiatric disorders. Mefloquine HCl should be used with caution in patients with a history of depression.

During prophylactic use, if psychiatric symptoms such as acute anxiety, depression, restlessness or confusion occur, these may be considered prodromal to a more serious event. In these cases, the drug must be discontinued, and an alternative medication should be substituted.

➤*Ocular lesions:* Although retinal abnormalities seen in humans with long-term chloroquine use have not been observed with mefloquine use, long-term feeding of mefloquine to rats resulted in dose-related ocular lesions. All surviving rats given 30 mg/kg/day had ocular lesions in both eyes characterized by retinal degeneration, opacity of the lens, and retinal edema. Similar but less severe lesions were observed in 80% of female and 22% of male rats fed 12.5 mg/kg/day for 2 years. At doses of 5 mg/kg/day, only corneal lesions were observed. They occurred in 9% of rats studied. Therefore, periodic ophthalmic examinations are recommended.

➤*Cardiac effects:* Parenteral studies in animals show that mefloquine, a myocardial depressant, possesses 20% of the antifibrillatory action of quinidine and produces 50% of the increase in the PR interval reported with quinine. The effect of mefloquine on the compromised cardiovascular system has not been evaluated. However, transitory and clinically silent ECG alterations have been reported during the use of mefloquine. Alterations included sinus bradycardia, sinus arrhythmia, first-degree AV block, prolongation of the QTc interval and abnormal T-waves. The benefits of mefloquine HCl therapy should be weighed against the possibility of adverse effects in patients with cardiac disease.

➤*Epilepsy:* In patients with epilepsy, mefloquine HCl may increase the risk of convulsions. The drug should therefore be prescribed only for curative treatment in such patients and only if there are compelling medical reasons for its use.

➤*Hypersensitivity reactions:* Hypersensitivity reactions ranging from mild cutaneous events to anaphylaxis cannot be predicted.

➤*Hepatic function impairment:* In patients with impaired liver function, the elimination of mefloquine may be prolonged, leading to higher plasma levels.

➤*Special risk:* Mefloquine HCl should be used with caution in patients with psychiatric disturbances because mefloquine use has been associated with emotional disturbances.

➤*Hazardous tasks:* Caution should be exercised with regard to activities requiring alertness and fine motor coordination such as driving, piloting aircraft and operating machinery, and deep-sea diving, as dizziness, a loss of balance, or other disorders of the central or peripheral nervous system have been reported during and following the use of mefloquine HCl. These effects may occur after therapy is discontinued due to the long half-life of the drug.

➤*Pregnancy:* *Category C.*

Teratogenic – Mefloquine has been demonstrated to be teratogenic in rats and mice at a dose of 100 mg/kg/day. In rabbits, a high dose of 160 mg/kg/day was embryotoxic and teratogenic, and a dose of 80 mg/kg/day was teratogenic but not embryotoxic. There are no adequate and well-controlled studies in pregnant women. However, clinical experience with mefloquine HCl has not revealed an embryotoxic or teratogenic effect. Mefloquine should be used during pregnancy only if the potential benefit justifies the potential risk to the fetus. Women of childbearing potential who are traveling to areas where malaria is endemic should be warned against becoming pregnant. Women of childbearing potential should also be advised to practice contraception during malaria prophylaxis with mefloquine HCl and for up to 3 months thereafter. However, in the case of unplanned pregnancy, malaria chemoprophylaxis with mefloquine HCl is not considered an indication for pregnancy termination.

➤*Lactation:* Mefloquine is excreted in human milk in small amounts, the activity of which is unknown. Based on a study in a few subjects, low concentrations (3% to 4%) of mefloquine were excreted in human milk following a dose equivalent to 250 mg of the free base. Because of the potential for serious adverse reactions in nursing infants from mefloquine, a decision should be made whether to discontinue the drug, taking into account the importance of the drug to the mother.

➤*Children:* Use of mefloquine HCl to treat acute, uncomplicated *P. falciparum* malaria in pediatric patients is supported by evidence from adequate and well-controlled studies of mefloquine HCl in adults with additional data from published open-label and comparative trials using mefloquine HCl to treat malaria caused by *P. falciparum* in patients younger than 16 years of age. The safety and efficacy of mefloquine HCl for the treatment of malaria in pediatric patients below the age of 6 months have not been established.

Early vomiting – See Administration and Dosage for more information.

➤*Monitoring:* This drug has been administered for greater than 1 year. If the drug is to be administered for a prolonged period, periodic evaluations, including liver function tests, should be performed.

Drug Interactions

➤*QT prolongation:* An additive effect of mefloquine with other drugs that prolong the QT interval cannot be excluded. The following drugs may prolong the QT interval and increase the risk of life-threatening cardiac arrhythmias, including torsade de pointes: Antiarrhythmic agents (eg, amiodarone, bretylium, disopyramide, dofetilide, procainamide, quinidine, and sotalol), arsenic trioxide, chlorpromazine, cisapride, dolasetron, droperidol, mesoridazine, moxifloxacin, pentamidine, pimozide, tacrolimus, thioridazine, and ziprasidone. For a more complete list of drugs that may prolong the QT interval, see the appendix, Drug-Induced Prolongation of the QT Interval and Torsade de Pointes.

MEFLOQUINE HYDROCHLORIDE — ORAL

Mefloquine Drug Interactions			
Precipitant drug	Object drug[a]		Description
Beta-adrenergic blockers (propranolol)	Mefloquine	↑	There is one report of cardiopulmonary arrest with full recovery in a patient taking propranolol.
Chloroquine	Mefloquine	↑	The risk of convulsions may be increased with concomitant mefloquine.
Halofantrine	Mefloquine	↑	Do not give halofantrine with or subsequently to mefloquine because of the danger of a potentially fatal prolongation of the QT_c interval.
Mefloquine	Bacterial vaccines, live attenuated (ie, oral live typhoid vaccines)	↓	When mefloquine is taken concurrently with oral live typhoid vaccines, attenuation of immunization cannot be excluded. Vaccinations with attenuated live bacteria should therefore be completed at least 3 days before the first dose of mefloquine.
Mefloquine	Quinine or Quinidine	↑	Coadministration may produce ECG abnormalities. If these agents are to be used in the initial treatment of severe malaria, delay mefloquine administration at least 12 hours after the last dose of quinine or quinidine. The risk of convulsions also may be increased with concurrent mefloquine and quinine.
Mefloquine	Anticonvulsants (eg, valproic acid, carbamazepine, phenobarbital, phenytoin)	↓	Monitor anticonvulsant blood levels and adjust the dosage as necessary. Coadministration may reduce seizure control by lowering the plasma levels of the anticonvulsant.

[a] ↑ = object drug increased; ↓ = object drug decreased.

Adverse Reactions

At the doses used for treatment of acute malaria infections, the symptoms possibly attributable to drug administration cannot be distinguished from those symptoms usually attributable to the disease itself.

➤*Prophylaxis of malaria:* Among subjects who received mefloquine for prophylaxis of malaria, the most frequently observed adverse experience was vomiting (3%). Dizziness, syncope, extrasystoles and other complaints affecting less than 1% were also reported.

➤*Treatment of malaria:* Among subjects who received mefloquine for treatment, the most frequently observed adverse experiences included the following: Dizziness, myalgia, nausea, fever, headache, vomiting, chills, diarrhea, skin rash, abdominal pain, fatigue, loss of appetite, and tinnitus. Those side effects occurring in less than 1% included bradycardia, hair loss, emotional problems, pruritus, asthenia, transient emotional disturbances and telogen effluvium (loss of resting hair). Seizures have also been reported.

Two serious adverse reactions were cardiopulmonary arrest in 1 patient shortly after ingesting a single prophylactic dose of mefloquine while concomitantly using propranolol (see Precautions), and encephalopathy of unknown etiology during prophylactic mefloquine administration. The relationship of encephalopathy to drug administration could not be clearly established.

➤*Postmarketing:* Postmarketing surveillance indicates that the same adverse experiences are reported during prophylaxis, as well as acute treatment.

The most frequently reported adverse events are nausea, vomiting, loose stools or diarrhea, abdominal pain, dizziness or vertigo, loss of balance, and neuropsychiatric events such as headache, somnolence, and sleep disorders (insomnia, abnormal dreams). These are usually mild and may decrease despite continued use.

Psychiatric – Occasionally, more severe neuropsychiatric disorders have been reported such as the following: Sensory and motor neuropathies (including paresthesia, tremor and ataxia), convulsions, agitation or restlessness, anxiety, depression, mood changes, panic attacks, forgetfulness, confusion, hallucinations, aggression, psychotic or paranoid reactions and encephalopathy. Rare cases of suicidal ideation and suicide have been reported, though no relationship to drug administration has been confirmed.

Other infrequent adverse reactions include:

Cardiovascular – Circulatory disturbances (hypotension, hypertension, flushing, syncope), chest pain, tachycardia or palpitation, bradycardia, irregular pulse, extrasystoles, AV block and other transient cardiac conduction alterations.

Dermatologic – Rash, exanthema, erythema, urticaria, pruritus, hair loss, erythema multiforme and Stevens-Johnson syndrome.

Lab test abnormalities – The most frequently observed laboratory alterations which could be possibly attributable to drug administration were decreased hematocrit, transient elevation of transaminases, leukopenia and thrombocytopenia. These alterations were observed in patients with acute malaria who received treatment doses of the drug and were attributed to the disease itself.

During prophylactic administration of mefloquine to indigenous populations in malaria-endemic areas, the following occasional alterations in laboratory values were observed: Transient elevation of transaminases, leukocytosis or thrombocytopenia.

Because of the long half-life of mefloquine, adverse reactions to mefloquine HCl may occur or persist up to several weeks after the last dose.

Musculoskeletal – Muscle weakness, muscle cramps, myalgia, arthralgia.

Miscellaneous – Visual disturbances, vestibular disorders (including tinnitus and hearing impairment), dyspnea, asthenia, malaise, fatigue, fever, sweating, chills, dyspepsia, and loss of appetite.

Overdosage

➤*Symptoms:* In cases of overdosage with mefloquine HCl, the adverse reactions may be more pronounced.

➤*Treatment:* The following procedure is recommended in case of overdosage: Induce vomiting or perform gastric lavage, as appropriate. Monitor cardiac function (if possible by ECG) and neurologic and psychiatric status for at least 24 hours. Provide symptomatic and intensive supportive treatment as required, particularly for cardiovascular disturbances. Treat vomiting or diarrhea with standard fluid therapy.

Patient Information

As required by law, a mefloquine HCl medication guide is supplied to patients when mefloquine HCl is dispensed. Patients should be instructed to read the *MedGuide* when mefloquine HCl is received.

Malaria can be a life-threatening infection in the traveler.

In a small percentage of cases, patients are unable to take this medication because of side effects, and it may be necessary to change medications.

When used as prophylaxis, the first dose of mefloquine HCl should be taken 1 week prior to arrival in an endemic area

If the patients experience psychiatric symptoms such as acute anxiety, depression, restlessness or confusion, these may be considered prodromal to a more serious event. In these cases, the drug must be discontinued, and an alternative medication should be substituted.

No chemoprophylactic regimen is 100% effective, and protective clothing, insect repellents, and bednets are important components of malaria prophylaxis.

Seek medical attention for any febrile illness that occurs after return from a malarious area and inform their physician that they may have been exposed to malaria.

DOXYCYCLINE

For complete prescribing information, refer to the Doxycycline monograph in the Tetracyclines section of the Systemic Anti-Infectives chapter.

HYDROXYCHLOROQUINE

For hydroxychloroquine prescribing information, see the Hydroxychloroquine Sulfate monograph in the Antirheumatic Agents section of the Biological and Immunologic Agents chapter.

CHLOROQUINE PHOSPHATE

Rx	**Chloroquine Phosphate** (Various, eg, Gallipot)	**Tablets:** 250 mg (equiv. to 150 mg base)	In 100s and 1000s.
Rx	**Aralen Phosphate** (Sanofi Synthelabo)	**Tablets:** 500 mg (equiv. to 300 mg base)	(W/A77). Pink. Film coated. In 25s.

CHLOROQUINE PHOSPHATE — ORAL

WARNING

Physicians should completely familiarize themselves with the complete contents of this monograph before prescribing chloroquine phosphate.

Indications

➤*Malaria:* For the suppressive treatment and for acute attacks of malaria due to *P. vivax*, *P. malariae P. ovale*, and susceptible strains of *P. falciparum*.

➤*Extraintestinal amebiasis:* For the treatment of extraintestinal amebiasis.

Administration and Dosage

➤*General dosing considerations:* The dosage of chloroquine phosphate is often expressed or calculated in terms of equivalent chloroquine base. Each 250 mg tablet of chloroquine phosphate is equivalent to 150 mg base and each 500 mg tablet of chloroquine phosphate is equivalent to 300 mg base. In infants and children, the dosage is preferably calculated on the body weight.

For radical cure of vivax and malariae malaria, concomitant therapy with an 8-aminoquinoline compound is necessary.

➤*Adults:*

Extraintestinal amebiasis – One gram (600 mg base) daily for 2 days, followed by 500 mg (300 mg base) daily for at least 2 to 3 weeks. Treatment is usually combined with an effective intestinal amebicide.

Malaria suppression –

Usual dosage: 500 mg (300 mg base) on exactly the same day of each week. If circumstances permit, suppressive therapy should begin 2 weeks prior to exposure. However, failing this in adults, an initial double (loading) dose of 1 g (600 mg base) may be taken in 2 divided doses, 6 hours apart.

Duration of therapy: The suppressive therapy should be continued for 8 weeks after leaving the endemic area.

Malaria treatment –

Usual dosage: 2.5 g chloroquine phosphate (1.5 g base) in 3 days, as follows:

- *First dose* – 1 g (600 mg base) on day 1.
- *Second dose* – 500 mg (300 mg base) 6 to 8 hours after the first dose.
- *Third and fourth doses* – 500 mg (300 mg base) on each of 2 consecutive days.

Alternative dosage: The dosage for adults of low body weight should be calculated on the basis of body weight. A total dose representing 25 mg of base per kg of body weight administered in 3 days, as follows:

- *First dose* – 10 mg (base) per kg (but not exceeding a single dose of 600 mg base).
- *Second dose* – 5 mg (base) per kg (but not exceeding a single dose of 300 mg base) 6 hours after first dose.
- *Third dose* – 5 mg (base) per kg 18 hours after second dose.
- *Fourth dose* – 5 mg (base) per kg 24 hours after third dose.

➤*Children:*

Malaria suppression –

Usual dosage: 5 mg/kg weekly (calculated as base), but should not exceed the adult dose regardless of weight. If circumstances permit, suppressive therapy should begin 2 weeks prior to exposure. However, failing this in children, 10 mg base/kg may be taken in 2 divided doses, 6 hours apart.

Maximum dose: 500 mg (300 mg base).

Duration of therapy: The suppressive therapy should be continued for 8 weeks after leaving the endemic area.

Malaria treatment – A total dose representing 25 mg of base per kg of body weight administered in 3 days, as follows:

First dose: 10 mg (base) per kg (but not exceeding a single dose of 600 mg base).

Second dose: 5 mg (base) per kg (but not exceeding a single dose of 300 mg base) 6 hours after first dose.

Third dose: 5 mg (base) per kg 18 hours after second dose.

Fourth dose: 5 mg (base) per kg 24 hours after third dose.

➤*CDC recommended schedule for chloroquine as an alternative to mefloquine:* Travelers to areas of risk where chloroquine-resistant *P. falciparum* is endemic and for whom mefloquine is contraindicated may elect to use an alternative regimen. Chloroquine alone taken weekly is recommended for travelers who cannot use mefloquine or doxycycline, especially pregnant women and children less than 15 kg. In addition, give these travelers a single treatment dose of sulfadoxine/pyrimethamine to keep during travel and to take promptly in the event of a febrile illness during their travel when professional medical care is not readily available. Continue weekly chloroquine prophylaxis after presumptive treatment with sulfadoxine/pyrimethamine.

➤*Storage/Stability:* Store at 15° to 30°C (59° to 86°F). Protect from light and moisture. Dispense in a tight, light-resistant container using a child-resistant closure.

Actions

➤*Pharmacology:* Chloroquine phosphate has been found to be active against the erythrocytic forms of *Plasmodium vivax* and *Plasmodium malariae* and most strains of *Plasmodium falciparum* (but not the gametocytes of *P. falciparum*).

The mechanism of plasmodicidal action of chloroquine is not completely certain. While the drug can inhibit certain enzymes, its effect is believed to result, at least in part, from its interaction with DNA.

➤*Pharmacokinetics:*

Absorption/Distribution – Chloroquine is rapidly and almost completely absorbed from the GI tract, and only a small proportion of the administered dose is found in the stools. Approximately 55% of the drug in the plasma is bound to nondiffusible plasma constituents. Chloroquine is deposited in the tissues in considerable amounts. In animals, from 200 to 700 times the plasma concentration may be found in the liver, spleen, kidney, and lung; leukocytes also concentrate the drug. The brain and spinal cord, in contrast, contain only 10 to 30 times the amount present in plasma.

Metabolism/Excretion – Chloroquine undergoes appreciable degradation in the body. The main metabolite is desethylchloroquine, which accounts for one-fourth of the total material appearing in the urine; bisdesethylchloroquine, a carboxylic acid derivative, and other metabolic products as yet uncharacterized are found in small amounts. Slightly more than half of the urinary drug products can be accounted for as unchanged chloroquine. Excretion of chloroquine is quite slow, but is increased by acidification of the urine.

➤*Microbiology:* Chloroquine phosphate has been found to be highly active against the erythrocytic forms of *Plasmodium vivax* and malariae and most strains of *Plasmodium falciparum* (but not the gametocytes of *P. falciparum*). The precise mechanism of action of the drug is not known.

In vitro studies with trophozoites of *Entamoeba histolytica* have demonstrated that chloroquine phosphate also possesses amebicidal activity comparable to that of emetine.

Contraindications

Use of this drug is contraindicated in the presence of retinal or visual field changes either attributable to 4-aminoquinoline compounds or to any other etiology, and in patients with known hypersensitivity to 4-aminoquinoline compounds. However, in the treatment of acute attacks of malaria caused by susceptible strains of plasmodia, the physician may elect to use this drug after carefully weighing the possible benefits and risks to the patient.

Warnings/Precautions

➤*Resistance:* In recent years it has been found that certain strains of *P. falciparum* have become resistant to 4-aminoquinoline compounds (including chloroquine and hydroxychloroquine) as shown by the fact that normally adequate doses have failed to prevent or cure clinical malaria or parasitemia. Treatment with quinine or other specific forms of therapy is therefore advised for patients infected with a resistant strain of parasites.

➤*Retinopathy:* Irreversible retinal damage has been observed in some patients who had received long-term or high-dosage 4-aminoquinoline therapy. Retinopathy has been reported to be dose related.

When prolonged therapy with any antimalarial compound is contemplated, initial (baseline) and periodic ophthalmologic examinations (including visual acuity, expert slit-lamp, funduscopic, and visual-field tests) should be performed.

If there is any indication (past or present) of abnormality in the visual acuity, visual field, or retinal macular areas (such as pigmentary changes, loss of foveal reflex), or any visual symptoms (such as light flashes and streaks) which are not fully explainable by difficulties of accommodation or corneal opacities, the drug should be discontinued immediately and the patient closely observed for possible progression. Retinal changes (and visual disturbances) may progress even after cessation of therapy.

➤*Muscular weakness:* All patients on long-term therapy with this preparation should be questioned and examined periodically, including testing knee and ankle reflexes, to detect any evidence of muscular weakness. If weakness occurs, discontinue the drug.

➤*Psoriases/Porphyria:* Use of chloroquine phosphate in patients with psoriasis may precipitate a severe attack of psoriasis. When used in patients with porphyria the condition may be exacerbated. The drug should not be used in these conditions unless in the judgment of the physician the benefit to the patient outweighs the possible hazard.

➤*Hematologic effects:* If any severe blood disorder appears which is not attributable to the disease under treatment, discontinuance of the drug should be considered.

4-Aminoquinoline Compounds

CHLOROQUINE PHOSPHATE — ORAL

➤*Glucose-6 phosphate dehydrogenase:* The drug should be administered with caution to patients having G-6-PD (glucose-6 phosphate dehydrogenase) deficiency.

➤*Hepatic function impairment:* Since this drug is known to concentrate in the liver, it should be used with caution in patients with hepatic disease or alcoholism or in conjunction with known hepatotoxic drugs.

➤*Pregnancy: Category C* (per Briggs' *Drugs in Pregnancy and Lactation*). Chloroquine crosses the placenta to the fetus with fetal concentrations approximating those in the mother. Chloroquine is not a major teratogen, but small increases in birth defects cannot be excluded.

➤*Lactation:* Chloroquine is excreted into breast milk. Although the amounts of chloroquine excreted into milk are not considered to be harmful to a breast-feeding infant, they are insufficient to provide adequate protection against malaria. The American Academy of Pediatrics classifies chloroquine as compatible with breast-feeding. Because of the potential for serious adverse reactions in breast-feeding infants from chloroquine, a decision should be made whether to discontinue breast-feeding or to discontinue the drug, taking into account the importance of the drug to the mother.

➤*Children:* A number of fatalities have been reported following the accidental ingestion of chloroquine, sometimes in relatively small doses (0.75 g or 1 g chloroquine phosphate in one 3-year-old child). Patients should be strongly warned to keep this drug out of the reach of children because they are especially sensitive to the 4-aminoquinoline compounds.

Malaria suppression – See Administration and Dosage for more information.

Treatment of acute attack – See Administration and Dosage for more information.

➤*Monitoring:* Complete blood cell counts should be made periodically if patients are given prolonged therapy.

Adverse Reactions

➤*Cardiovascular:* Rarely, hypotension, electrocardiographic change.

➤*CNS:* Convulsive seizures; mild and transient headache; psychic stimulation.

➤*Dermatologic:* Pleomorphic skin eruptions, skin and mucosal pigmentary changes; lichen planus-like eruptions, pruritus, and hair loss.

➤*GI:* Anorexia, nausea, vomiting, diarrhea, abdominal cramps.

➤*Ophthalmic:* Irreversible retinal damage in patients receiving long-term or high-dosage 4-aminoquinoline therapy; visual disturbances (blurring of vision and difficulty of focusing or accommodation); nyctalopia; scotomatous vision with field defects of paracentral, pericentral ring types, and typically temporal scotomas (eg, difficulty in reading with words tending to disappear, seeing half an object, misty vision, and fog before the eyes).

➤*Special senses:* Nerve-type deafness; tinnitus; reduced hearing in patients with preexisting auditory damage.

Overdosage

➤*Symptoms:* Chloroquine is very rapidly and completely absorbed after ingestion. Toxic doses of chloroquine can be fatal. As little as 1 g may be fatal in children. Toxic symptoms can occur within minutes. These consist of headache, drowsiness, visual disturbances, nausea and vomiting, cardiovascular collapse, and convulsions followed by sudden and early respiratory and cardiac arrest. The electrocardiogram may reveal atrial standstill, nodal rhythm, prolonged intraventricular conduction time, and progressive bradycardia leading to ventricular fibrillation or arrest.

➤*Treatment:* Treatment is symptomatic and must be prompt with immediate evacuation of the stomach by emesis (at home, before transportation to the hospital) or gastric lavage until the stomach is completely emptied. If finely powdered, activated charcoal is introduced by stomach tube, after lavage, and within 30 minutes after ingestion of the antimalarial, it may inhibit further intestinal absorption of the drug. To be effective, the dose of activated charcoal should be at least 5 times the estimated dose of chloroquine ingested.

Convulsions, if present, should be controlled before attempting gastric lavage. If due to cerebral stimulation, cautious administration of an ultra short-acting barbiturate may be tried but, if due to anoxia, it should be corrected by oxygen administration and artificial respiration. In shock with hypotension, a potent vasopressor should be administered. Because of the importance of supporting respiration, tracheal intubation or tracheostomy, followed by gastric lavage, may also be necessary. Peritoneal dialysis and exchange transfusions have also been suggested to reduce the level of the drug in the blood.

A patient who survives the acute phase and is asymptomatic should be closely observed for at least 6 hours. Fluids may be forced, and sufficient ammonium chloride (8 g daily in divided doses for adults) may be administered for a few days to acidify the urine to help promote urinary excretion in cases of both overdosage or sensitivity.

8–Aminoquinoline Compound

PRIMAQUINE

Rx	Primaquine Phosphate (Sanofi Winthrop)	Tablets; oral: 26.3 mg	Equiv. to 15 mg primaquine base. Lactose. (W P97). Pink. Film-coated. In 100s.

PRIMAQUINE PHOSPHATE — ORAL

WARNING

Health care providers should completely familiarize themselves with the complete contents of this monograph before prescribing primaquine phosphate.

Indications

➤*Vivax malaria:* For the radical cure (prevention of relapse) of vivax malaria.

Recommended only for the radical cure of vivax malaria, the prevention of relapse in vivax malaria, or following the termination of chloroquine phosphate suppressive therapy in an area where vivax malaria is endemic.

Administration and Dosage

➤*Adults:*

Vivax malaria – 26.3 mg (equivalent to 15 mg base; 1 tablet) daily for 14 days.

➤*Concomitant therapy:* Patients suffering from an attack of vivax malaria or having parasitized red blood cells should receive a course of chloroquine phosphate, which quickly destroys the erythrocytic parasites and terminates the paroxysm. Primaquine phosphate should be administered concurrently in order to eradicate the exoerythrocytic parasites.

➤*Administration:* May be taken with or without food. If stomach upset occurs, instruct patients to take with food to reduce stomach irritation. Caution patients to avoid grapefruit products while taking primaquine. Advise patients to take primaquine with a liquid other than grapefruit juice.

➤*Storage/Stability:* Store at 25°C (77°F); excursions are permitted to 15° to 30°C (59° to 86°F).

Actions

➤*Pharmacology:* Primaquine phosphate is an 8-amino-quinoline compound that eliminates tissue (exoerythrocytic) infection. Thereby, it prevents the development of the blood (erythrocytic) forms of the parasite, which are responsible for relapses in vivax malaria. Primaquine phosphate is also active against gametocytes of *Plasmodium falciparum*.

Contraindications

In acutely ill patients suffering from systemic disease manifested by tendency to granulocytopenia, such as rheumatoid arthritis and lupus erythematosus; in patients concurrently receiving other potentially hemolytic drugs or depressants of myeloid elements of the bone marrow; coadministration with quinacrine.

Warnings/Precautions

➤*Hemolytic anemia:* Discontinue the use of primaquine phosphate promptly if signs suggestive of hemolytic anemia occur (eg, darkening of the urine, marked fall of hemoglobin or erythrocytic count).

Hemolytic reactions (moderate to severe) may occur in glucose-6-phosphate dehydrogenase (G-6-PD) deficient white patients (particularly in Sardinians and in persons with a family or personal history of favism). Dark-skinned persons have a great tendency to develop hemolytic anemia (due to congenital deficiency of erythrocytic G-6-PD) while receiving primaquine and related drugs.

If primaquine phosphate is prescribed for a patient who has shown a previous idiosyncrasy to primaquine phosphate (as manifested by hemolytic anemia, leukopenia, and methemoglobinemia), a patient with a family or personal history of favism, or a patient with erythrocytic G-6-PD deficiency or nicotinamide adenine dinucleotide (NADH) methemoglobin reductase deficiency, observe the patient closely for tolerance. Discontinue the drug immediately if marked darkening of the urine or a sudden decrease in hemoglobin concentration or leukocyte count occurs.

➤*Pregnancy: Category C.* Safe use of this preparation in pregnancy has not been established. Therefore, avoid its use during pregnancy except when, in the judgment of the health care provider, the benefit outweighs the possible hazard.

➤*Lactation:* There are no data regarding primaquine in breast-feeding women.

➤*Elderly:* In general, be cautious about dose selection for elderly patients, usually starting at the low end of the dosing range, reflecting the greater frequency of decreased cardiac, hepatic, or renal function, and of concomitant disease or other drug therapy.

➤*Monitoring:* Since anemia, methemoglobinemia, and leukopenia have been observed following administration of large doses of primaquine, do not exceed the adult dosage of 1 tablet (equivalent to 15 mg base) daily for

8–Aminoquinoline Compound

PRIMAQUINE PHOSPHATE — ORAL

14 days. It is also advisable to make routine blood examinations (particularly blood cell counts and hemoglobin determinations) during therapy.

Drug Interactions

➤*Quinacrine:* Because quinacrine hydrochloride appears to potentiate the toxicity of antimalarial compounds that are structurally related to primaquine, the use of quinacrine in patients receiving primaquine is contraindicated. Similarly, do not administer primaquine to patients who have received quinacrine recently because toxicity is increased.

➤*Drug/Food interactions:* Grapefruit juice increased the maximum concentration and area under the curve of primaquine 23% and 19%, respectively, compared with fasting state values. Primaquine plasma concentrations may be elevated, increasing the toxic effects. Advise patients taking primaquine to avoid ingestion of grapefruit juice.

Adverse Reactions

➤*GI:* Abdominal cramps, epigastric distress, nausea, vomiting.

➤*Hematologic:* Hemolytic anemia in G-6-PD deficient persons, leukopenia, and methemoglobinemia in NADH methemoglobin reductase–deficient persons.

Overdosage

➤*Symptoms:* Symptoms of overdosage of primaquine phosphate are similar to those seen after overdosage of pamaquine. They include the following: abdominal cramps, anemia, burning epigastric distress, CNS and cardiovascular disturbances, cyanosis, methemoglobinemia, moderate leukocytosis or leukopenia, and vomiting. The most striking symptoms are granulocytopenia and acute hemolytic anemia in sensitive persons. Acute hemolysis occurs, but patients recover completely if the dosage is discontinued.

Patient Information

- Caution patients to avoid grapefruit products while taking primaquine. Advise patients to take primaquine with a liquid other than grapefruit juice.
- This medicine may be taken with or without food. If stomach upset occurs, instruct patients to take with food to reduce stomach irritation.
- Instruct patients that if a dose of this medicine is missed, to take it as soon as possible. If it is almost time for your next dose, tell patient to skip the missed dose and go back to their regular dosing schedule. Two doses should not be taken at once.

Folic Acid Antagonist

PYRIMETHAMINE

Rx	**Daraprim** (Amedra Pharmaceuticals)	**Tablets; oral:** 25 mg	Lactose. (Daraprim A3A). White, scored. In 100s.

PYRIMETHAMINE — ORAL

Indications

➤*Chemoprophylaxis of malaria:* In susceptible strains of plasmodia only. It is not suitable as a prophylactic agent for travelers to most areas because of prevalent resistance worldwide.

➤*Toxoplasmosis:* Use with a sulfonamide; synergism exists with this combination.

➤*Acute malaria:* In conjunction with a sulfonamide (eg, sulfadoxine) to initiate transmission control and suppression for susceptible strains of plasmodia. Fast-acting schizonticides (chloroquine, quinine) are preferable for the treatment of acute malaria.

Administration and Dosage

➤*General dosing considerations:* Pyrimethamine is not recommended for use alone to treat acute malaria. Fast-acting schizonticides (chloroquine, quinine) are indicated for treatment of acute malaria.

For the treatment of toxoplasmosis, at the dosage required there is marked variation in tolerance. Young patients may tolerate higher doses than older patients. Coadministration of folinic acid (leucovorin) is strongly recommended in all patients. The dosage of pyrimethamine required for the treatment of toxoplasmosis is 10 to 20 times the recommended antimalaria dosage and approaches the toxic level (see Warnings/Precautions).

➤*Adults:*

Malaria prophylaxis –

Usual dosage: 25 mg once weekly.

Maximum dose: 25 mg once weekly.

Malaria treatment –

Initial dosage: 25 mg/day for 2 days with a sulfonamide.

Maintenance dosage: Clinical cure should be followed with 25 mg once weekly. Extend regimens, which include suppression through any characteristic periods of early recrudescence and late relapse (ie, for at least 10 weeks in each case).

Alternative dosage: If pyrimethamine must be used alone in semi-immune people, the dose is 50 mg/day for 2 days followed by the maintenance dosage as discussed previously.

Concomitant therapy: Concomitant use with a sulfonamide will initiate transmission control and suppression of nonfalciparum malaria.

Toxoplasmosis –

Initial dosage: Pyrimethamine 50 to 75 mg/day with 1 to 4 g of a sulfonamide of the sulfapyrimidine type (eg, sulfadoxine). Continue for 1 to 3 weeks, depending on response and tolerance.

Maintenance dosage: Dosage for each drug may be reduced by one-half and continued for an additional 4 or 5 weeks.

Concomitant therapy: Administer with a sulfonamide of the sulfapyrimidine type (eg, sulfadoxine). (See the previous information). Also, coadministration of folinic acid (leucovorin) is strongly recommended in all patients.

Patients with convulsive disorders: Use lower initial dose to avoid potential CNS toxicity.

➤*Children:*

Malaria prophylaxis – See Adults for dosing for children 10 years of age and older.

4 to 10 years of age:
- *Usual dosage* – 12.5 mg once weekly.
- *Maximum dose* – 12.5 mg once weekly.

Younger than 4 years of age:
- *Usual dosage* – 6.25 mg once weekly.
- *Maximum dose* – 6.25 mg once weekly.

Malaria treatment – See Adults for dosing for children 10 years of age and older.

4 to 10 years of age:
- *Initial dosage* – 25 mg/day for 2 days.
- *Maintenance dosage* – Follow with 12.5 mg once weekly. Extend regimens that include suppression through any characteristic periods of early recrudescence and late relapse (ie, for at least 10 weeks in each case).
- *Concomitant therapy* – Concomitant use with a sulfonamide will initiate transmission control and suppression of nonfalciparum malaria.

Toxoplasmosis –

Initial dosage: 1 mg/kg/day divided into 2 equal daily doses for 2 to 4 days given in conjunction with a sulfonamide (given at the usual pediatric dosage).

Maintenance dosage: After the initial dosage, reduce to 0.5 mg/kg/day divided into 2 equal daily doses and continue for approximately 1 month.

Concomitant therapy: Administer with a sulfonamide (given at the usual pediatric dosage). Also, coadministration of folinic acid (leucovorin) is strongly recommended in all patients.

Patients with convulsive disorders: Use lower initial dose to avoid potential CNS toxicity.

➤*Administration:* Administer with food to minimize vomiting.

➤*Storage/Stability:* Store at 15° to 25°C (59° to 77°F) in a dry place and protect from light.

Actions

➤*Pharmacology:* Pyrimethamine is a folic acid antagonist; its therapeutic action is based on differential requirement between host and parasite for nucleic acid precursors involved in growth as it selectively inhibits plasmodial dihydrofolate reductase. Pyrimethamine inhibits the enzyme dihydrofolate reductase, which catalyzes the reduction of dihydrofolate to tetrahydrofolate. This activity is highly selective against plasmodia and *Toxoplasma gondii*. It does not destroy gametocytes but arrests sporogony in the mosquito. Pyrimethamine possesses blood schizonticidal and some tissue schizonticidal activity against human malaria parasites. The action of pyrimethamine against *T. gondii* is greatly enhanced when used in conjunction with sulfonamides.

➤*Pharmacokinetics:* Pyrimethamine is well absorbed after oral use. Peak plasma concentrations occur in 2 to 6 hours. Plasma half-life is approximately 4 days; suppressive concentrations are maintained for approximately 2 weeks (but lower in malaria patients). It is approximately 87% plasma protein-bound. Several metabolites appear in the urine.

Contraindications

Hypersensitivity to the drug or any components of the formulation; megaloblastic anemia caused by folate deficiency.

Warnings/Precautions

➤*Folic acid deficiency:* The dosage of pyrimethamine required for the treatment of toxoplasmosis is 10 to 20 times the recommended antimalaria dosage and approaches the toxic level. If signs of folate deficiency develop, reduce dosage or discontinue drug according to patient response. Folinic acid (leucovorin) may be given in a dosage of 5 to 15 mg/day (oral, IM, or IV) until normal hematopoiesis is restored. Use with caution in possible folate deficiency (eg, malabsorption syndrome, alcoholism, pregnancy, phenytoin usage).

➤*Accidental ingestion:* Keep pyrimethamine out of the reach of infants and children as they are extremely susceptible to adverse effects from an overdose. Deaths in pediatric patients have been reported after accidental ingestion.

➤*G-6-PD:* Large doses of pyrimethamine may precipitate hemolytic anemia in patients with glucose-6-phosphate dehydrogenase deficiency.

Folic Acid Antagonist

PYRIMETHAMINE — ORAL

➤*Hypersensitivity reactions:* Occasionally severe hypersensitivity reactions (eg, Stevens-Johnson syndrome, toxic epidermal necrolysis, erythema multiforme, and anaphylaxis) have occurred, particularly if given with a sulfonamide (see Adverse Reactions). Refer to Management of Acute Hypersensitivity Reactions.

➤*Renal/Hepatic function impairment:* Use with caution.

➤*Pregnancy: Category C.* Pyrimethamine has been shown to be teratogenic in rats when given in oral doses 7 times the human dose for chemoprophylaxis of malaria or 2.5 times the human dose for treatment of toxoplasmosis. At these doses in rats, there was a significant increase in abnormalities such as cleft palate, brachygnathia, oligodactyly, and microphthalmia. Pyrimethamine also has been shown to produce terata such as meningocele in hamsters and cleft palate in miniature pigs when given in oral doses 170 and 5 times the human dose, respectively, for chemoprophylaxis of malaria or for treatment of toxoplasmosis. There are no adequate and well-controlled studies in pregnant women. Use pyrimethamine during pregnancy only if the potential benefit justifies the potential risk to the fetus. Coadministration of folinic acid is strongly recommended when treating toxoplasmosis during pregnancy.

➤*Lactation:* Pyrimethamine is excreted in breast milk. Because of the potential for serious adverse reactions in nursing infants from pyrimethamine and from concurrent use of a sulfonamide with pyrimethamine for treatment of some patients with toxoplasmosis, decide whether to discontinue nursing or discontinue the drug, taking into account the importance of the drug to the mother.

➤*Children:* See Administration and Dosage.

➤*Elderly:* Dose selection for an elderly patient should be cautious, usually starting at the low end of the dosing range, reflecting the greater frequency of decreased hepatic, renal, or cardiac function, and of concomitant disease or other drug therapy.

➤*Monitoring:* For toxoplasmosis, perform semiweekly blood counts, including platelet counts. Because of the long half-life of pyrimethamine, daily monitoring of peripheral blood counts is recommended for up to several weeks after an overdose until normal hematological values are restored.

Drug Interactions

➤*Antifolate drugs or agents associated with myelosuppression (eg, proguanil, zidovudine, cytostatic agents [eg, methotrexate], sulfonamides, trimethoprim-sulfamethoxazole):* Concurrent use of antifolic acids and pyrimethamine may increase the risk of bone marrow suppression. Discontinue pyrimethamine if signs of folate deficiency develop. Administer folinic acid (leucovorin) until normal hematopoiesis is restored (see Warnings).

➤*Lorazepam:* Mild hepatotoxicity has been reported when lorazepam and pyrimethamine were coadministered.

Adverse Reactions

➤*GI:* Anorexia, vomiting (large doses); atrophic glossitis. Vomiting may be minimized by giving with meals; it usually disappears promptly upon dosage reduction.

➤*Hematologic:* Megaloblastic anemia, leukopenia, thrombocytopenia, pancytopenia, hematuria.

➤*Hypersensitivity:* Hypersensitivity reactions, occasionally severe (eg, Stevens-Johnson syndrome, toxic epidermal necrolysis, erythema multiforme, anaphylaxis), and hyperphenylalaninemia have occurred particularly when coadministered with a sulfonamide.

➤*Miscellaneous:* Rhythm disorders; pulmonary eosinophilia (rare).

Overdosage

➤*Symptoms:* Following the ingestion of 300 mg or more of pyrimethamine, GI and/or CNS signs may be present, including convulsions. Initial GI symptoms include abdominal pain, nausea, and severe and repeated vomiting possibly including hematemesis. CNS toxicity is manifested by initial excitability; generalized and prolonged convulsions, which may be followed by respiratory depression; circulatory collapse; and death within a few hours. Neurological symptoms appear rapidly (30 minutes to 2 hours after drug ingestion), suggesting that in gross overdosage, pyrimethamine has a direct toxic effect on the CNS.

Fatal dose is variable; the smallest reported fatal single dose is 375 mg. There are reports of children who have recovered after taking 375 to 625 mg.

➤*Treatment:* There is no specific antidote for pyrimethamine. Gastric lavage is effective. Use parenteral diazepam to control convulsions. Administer folinic acid (leucovorin) within 2 hours of ingestion to counteract effects on the hematopoietic system. Because of the long half-life of pyrimethamine, daily monitoring of peripheral blood counts is recommended for up to several weeks after the overdose until normal hematological values are restored. Treatment includes usual supportive measures. Refer to General Management of Acute Overdosage.

Patient Information

May cause anorexia or vomiting; inform patients to take with food or meals.

At first appearance of a skin rash, inform patients to discontinue the drug and immediately seek medical attention.

Warn patients that the appearance of sore throat, pallor, purpura, or glossitis may be early indications of serious disorders that require seeking medical treatment.

Warn women of childbearing potential against becoming pregnant.

Advise patients to keep medication out of the reach of children.

Advise patients not to exceed recommended doses.

Coadministration of folinic acid (leucovorin) is strongly recommended in all patients when used for the treatment of toxoplasmosis.

ANTIMALARIAL PREPARATIONS

ARTEMETHER/LUMEFANTRINE

Rx	**Coartem** (Novartis)	**Tablets; oral:** artemether 20 mg/lumefantrine 120 mg N/C CG. Yellow, round. Scored. In 24s.

ARTEMETHER/LUMEFANTRINE — ORAL

Indications

➤*Malaria:* For the treatment of acute, uncomplicated malaria infections due to *Plasmodium falciparum* in patients weighing 5 kg or more.

Administration and Dosage

➤*Adults:*

Malaria – A 3-day treatment schedule with a total of 6 doses is recommended for adult patients weighing 35 kg or more:

Four tablets as a single initial dose, 4 tablets again after 8 hours, and then 4 tablets twice daily (morning and evening) for the following 2 days (total course of 24 tablets).

For patients weighing less than 35 kg, see Children for dosing.

➤*Children:*

Malaria –

16 years of age or younger or weighing less than 35 kg: A 3-day treatment schedule with a total of 6 doses is recommended as the following:

- *Weighing 35 kg or more* – See Adults for dosing.
- *Weighing 25 kg to less than 35 kg* – Three tablets as an initial dose, 3 tablets again after 8 hours, and then 3 tablets twice daily (morning and evening) for the following 2 days (total course of 18 tablets).
- *Weighing 15 kg to less than 25 kg* – Two tablets as an initial dose, 2 tablets again after 8 hours, and then 2 tablets twice daily (morning and evening) for the following 2 days (total course of 12 tablets).
- *Weighing 5 kg to less than 15 kg* – One tablet as an initial dose, 1 tablet again after 8 hours, and then 1 tablet twice daily (morning and evening) for the following 2 days (total course of 6 tablets).

➤*Hepatic function impairment:* Exercise caution when administering artemether/lumefantrine tablets in patients with severe hepatic impairment.

No specific pharmacokinetic studies have been carried out in patients with hepatic impairment. Most patients with acute malaria present with some degree of related hepatic impairment. In clinical studies, the adverse reaction profile did not differ in patients with mild or moderate hepatic impairment compared with patients with normal hepatic function. No specific dose adjustments are needed for patients with mild or moderate hepatic impairment.

➤*Administration:* Artemether/lumefantrine tablets should be taken with food. Patients with acute malaria are frequently averse to food. Patients should be encouraged to resume normal eating as soon as food can be tolerated because this improves absorption of artemether and lumefantrine.

For patients who are unable to swallow the tablets, such as infants and children, artemether/lumefantrine tablets may be crushed and mixed with a small amount of water (1 to 2 teaspoons) in a clean container for administration immediately prior to use. The container can be rinsed with more water and the contents swallowed by the patient. The crushed tablet preparation should be followed whenever possible by food/drink (eg, milk, formula, pudding, broth, porridge).

In the event of vomiting within 1 to 2 hours of administration, a repeat dose should be taken. If the repeat dose is vomited, the patient should be given an alternative antimalarial for treatment.

➤*Storage/Stability:* Store at 25°C (77°F); excursions are permitted to 15° to 30°C (59° to 86°F).

ARTEMETHER/LUMEFANTRINE — ORAL

Actions

➤*Pharmacology:* Artemether/lumefantrine tablets, a fixed dose combination of artemether and lumefantrine in the ratio of 1:6, is an antimalarial agent. Both components are blood schizontocides.

Artemether is rapidly metabolized into an active metabolite dihydroartemisinin. The antimalarial activity of artemether and dihydroartemisinin has been attributed to endoperoxide moiety. The exact mechanism by which lumefantrine exerts its antimalarial effect is not well defined. Available data suggest lumefantrine inhibits the formation of beta-hematin by forming a complex with hemin. Both artemether and lumefantrine were shown to inhibit nucleic acid and protein synthesis.

Pharmacodynamics –

Electrocardiogram: In a healthy adult volunteer parallel group study including a placebo and moxifloxacin control group (n = 42 per group), the administration of the 6-dose regimen of artemether/lumefantrine tablets was associated with prolongation of QTcF (Fridericia). Following administration of a 6-dose regimen of artemether/lumefantrine tablets consisting of 4 tablets per dose (total of 4 tablets of artemether 80 mg/lumefantrine 480 mg) taken with food, the maximum mean change from baseline and placebo adjusted QTcF was 7.5 msec (1-sided 95%, upper confidence interval [CI], 11 msec). There was a concentration-dependent increase in QTcF for lumefantrine.

In clinical trials conducted in children, no patient had QTcF greater than 500 msec. Over 5% of patients had an increase in QTcF of over 60 msec.

In clinical trials conducted in adults, QTcF prolongation of greater than 500 msec was reported in 3 (0.3%) of patients. Over 6% of adults had a QTcF increase of over 60 msec from baseline.

➤*Pharmacokinetics:*

Absorption – Following administration of artemether/lumefantrine tablets to healthy volunteers and patients with malaria, artemether is absorbed with peak plasma concentrations (C_{max}) about 2 hours after dosing. Absorption of lumefantrine, a highly lipophilic compound, starts after a lag-time of up to 2 hours, with peak plasma concentrations about 6 to 8 hours after administration. The single dose (4 tablets) pharmacokinetic parameters for artemether, dihydroartemisinin, an active antimalarial metabolite of artemether, and lumefantrine in adult white healthy volunteers are given in the following table. Multiple dose data after the 6-dose regimen of artemether/lumefantrine tablets in adult malaria patients are given in the table following the one below.

Artemether, Dihydroartemisinin, and Lumefantrine Pharmacokinetics[a] Under Fed Conditions[b]

	Study 2102 (n = 50)	Study 2104 (n = 48)
Artemether		
C_{max} (ng/mL)	60.0 ± 32.5	83.8 ± 59.7
T_{max} (h)	1.5	2
AUC_{last} (ng•h/mL)	146 ± 72.2	259 ± 150
t½ (h)	1.6 ± 0.7	2.2 ± 1.9
Dihydroartemisinin		
C_{max} (ng/mL)	104 ± 35.3	90.4 ± 48.9
T_{max} (h)	1.76	2
AUC_{last} (ng•h/mL)	284 ± 83.8	285 ± 98
t½ (h)	1.6 ± 0.6	2.2 ± 1.5
Lumefantrine		
C_{max} (mcg/mL)	7.38 ± 3.19	9.80 ± 4.2
T_{max} (h)	6.01	8
AUC_{last} (mcg•h/mL)	158 ± 70.1	243 ± 117
t½ (h)	101 ± 35.6	119 ± 51

[a] Mean ± standard deviation (SD) C_{max}, AUC_{last}, t½ and Median T_{max}.
[b] T_{max} = time to C_{max}; AUC = area under the curve; t½ = terminal half-life.

Effect of food: Food enhances the absorption of both artemether and lumefantrine. In healthy volunteers, the relative bioavailability of artemether was increased between 2- to 3-fold, and that of lumefantrine 16-fold when artemether/lumefantrine tablets were taken after a high-fat meal compared with under fasted conditions. Encourage patients to take artemether/lumefantrine tablets with a meal as soon as food can be tolerated.

Distribution – Artemether and lumefantrine are both highly bound to human serum proteins in vitro (95.4% and 99.7%, respectively). Dihydroartemisinin is also bound to human serum proteins (47% to 76%). Protein binding to human plasma proteins is linear.

Metabolism – In human liver microsomes and recombinant cytochrome P450 (CYP-450) enzymes, the metabolism of artemether was catalyzed predominantly by CYP3A4/5. Dihydroartemisinin is an active metabolite of artemether. The metabolism of artemether was also catalyzed to a lesser extent by CYP2B6, CYP2C9, and CYP2C19. In vitro studies with artemether at therapeutic concentrations revealed no significant inhibition of the metabolic activities of CYP1A2, CYP2A6, CYP2C9, CYP2C19, CYP2D6, CYP2E1, CYP3A4/5, and CYP4A9/11.

During repeated administration of artemether/lumefantrine tablets, systemic exposure of artemether decreased significantly, while concentrations of dihydroartemisinin increased, although not to a statistically significant degree. The artemether/dihydroartemisinin AUC ratio is 1.2 after a single dose and 0.3 after 6 doses given over 3 days. This suggests that there was induction of CYP3A4/5 responsible for the metabolism of artemether.

In human liver microsomes and in recombinant CYP-450 enzymes, lumefantrine was metabolized mainly by CYP3A4 to desbutyl-lumefantrine. The systemic exposure to the metabolite desbutyl-lumefantrine was less than 1% of the exposure to the parent compound. In vitro, lumefantrine significantly inhibits the activity of CYP2D6 at therapeutic plasma concentrations.

Excretion – Artemether and dihydroartemisinin are cleared from plasma with an elimination half-life of about 2 hours. Lumefantrine is eliminated more slowly, with a terminal half-life of 3 to 6 days in healthy volunteers and in patients with *falciparum* malaria.

No urinary excretion data are available for humans. In animal studies, artemether metabolites were largely excreted in the urine. However, urinary excretion of artemether, lumefantrine, and lumefantrine metabolites was negligible. While animal data are informative, they do not always predict human results.

Special populations –

➤*Microbiology:*

Activity in vitro and in vivo – Artemether and lumefantrine are active against the erythrocytic stages of *Plasmodium falciparum*.

Drug resistance – Strains of *P. falciparum* with a moderate decrease in susceptibility to artemether or lumefantrine alone can be selected in vitro or in vivo, but not maintained in the case of artemether. The clinical relevance of such an effect is not known.

Contraindications

Patients hypersensitive to artemether, lumefantrine, or to any of the excipients of artemether/lumefantrine tablets.

Warnings/Precautions

➤*Prolongation of the QT interval:* Some antimalarials (eg, halofantrine, quinine, quinidine) including artemether/lumefantrine tablets have been associated with prolongation of the QT interval on the electrocardiogram.

Artemether/lumefantrine tablets should be avoided in patients with the following:

- congenital prolongation of the QT interval (eg, long QT syndrome) or any other clinical condition known to prolong the QTc interval, such as patients with a history of symptomatic cardiac arrhythmias, with clinically relevant bradycardia, or with severe cardiac disease;
- a family history of congenital prolongation of the QT interval or sudden death;
- known disturbances of electrolyte balance (eg, hypokalemia, hypomagnesemia);
- administration of other medications that prolong the QT interval, such as class IA (eg, quinidine, procainamide, disopyramide) or class III (eg, amiodarone, sotalol) antiarrhythmic agents; antipsychotics (eg, pimozide, ziprasidone); antidepressants; certain antibiotics (eg, macrolide antibiotics, fluoroquinolone antibiotics, imidazole, triazole antifungal agents); certain nonsedating antihistamines (eg, terfenadine, astemizole), or cisapride;
- administration of medications that are metabolized by the cytochrome enzyme CYP2D6 that also have cardiac effects (eg, flecainide, imipramine, amitriptyline, clomipramine).

➤*Recrudescence:* Food enhances absorption of artemether and lumefantrine following administration of artemether/lumefantrine tablets. Closely monitored patients who remain averse to food during treatment, because the risk of recrudescence may be greater.

In the event of recrudescent *P. falciparum* infection after treatment with artemether/lumefantrine tablets, patients should be treated with a different antimalarial drug.

➤*Plasmodium vivax* Infection: Artemether/lumefantrine tablets have been shown in limited data (43 patients) to be effective in treating the erythrocytic stage of *P. vivax* infection. However, relapsing malaria caused by *P. vivax* requires additional treatment with other antimalarial agents to achieve radical cure (ie, eradication of any hypnozoite forms that may remain dormant in the liver).

➤*Renal/Hepatic function impairment:* Artemether/lumefantrine have not been studied for efficacy and safety in patients with severe hepatic and/or renal impairment. No dosage adjustment is necessary in patients with mild to moderate hepatic and/or renal impairment.

➤*Pregnancy: Category C.* Artemether/lumefantrine tablets should be used during pregnancy only if the potential benefit justifies the potential risk to the fetus. Safety data from an observational pregnancy study of approximately 500 pregnant women who were exposed to artemether/lumefantrine tablets (including a third of patients who were exposed in the first trimester), and published data of over 1,000 pregnant patients who were exposed to artemisinin derivatives, did not show an increase in adverse pregnancy outcomes or teratogenic effects over background rate.

The efficacy of artemether/lumefantrine tablets in the treatment of acute, uncomplicated malaria in pregnant women has not been established.

Pregnant rats dosed during the period of organogenesis at or higher than a dose of about half the highest clinical dose of artemether/lumefantrine 1,120 mg per day (based on body surface area comparisons) showed increases in fetal loss, early resorptions, and postimplantation loss. No adverse effects were observed in animals dosed at about one-third the highest clinical dose. Similarly, dosing in pregnant rabbits at about 3 times the clinical dose (based on body surface area comparisons) resulted in abortions,

ARTEMETHER/LUMEFANTRINE — ORAL

preimplantation loss, postimplantation loss, and decreases in the number of live fetuses. No adverse reproductive effects were detected in rabbits at 2 times the clinical dose. Embryo-fetal loss is a significant reproductive toxicity. Other artemisinins are known to be embryotoxic in animals. However, because metabolic profiles in animals and humans are dissimilar, artemether exposures in animals may not be predictive of human exposures. These data cannot rule out an increased risk for early pregnancy loss or fetal defects in humans.

➤*Lactation:* It is not known whether artemether or lumefantrine is excreted in human milk. Because many drugs are excreted in human milk, exercise caution when artemether/lumefantrine tablets are administered to a nursing woman. Animal data suggest both artemether and lumefantrine are excreted into breast milk. Weigh the benefits of breastfeeding to mother and infant against potential risk from infant exposure to artemether and lumefantrine through breast milk.

➤*Children:* The safety and effectiveness of artemether/lumefantrine tablets have been established for the treatment of acute, uncomplicated malaria in studies involving children weighing 5 kg or more. The safety and efficacy have not been established in children weighing less than 5 kg. Children from nonendemic countries were not included in clinical trials.

➤*Elderly:* Clinical studies of artemether/lumefantrine tablets did not include sufficient numbers of subjects 65 years of age and older to determine if they respond differently than younger subjects. In general, consider the greater frequency of decreased hepatic, renal, or cardiac function, and of concomitant disease or other drug therapy in elderly patients when prescribing artemether/lumefantrine tablets.

Drug Interactions

An additive effect of artemether/lumefantrine with other drugs that prolong the QT interval cannot be excluded. The following drugs may prolong the QT interval and increase the risk of life-threatening cardiac arrhythmias, including torsade de pointes: Antiarrhythmic agents (eg, amiodarone, bretylium, disopyramide, dofetilide, procainamide, quinidine, sotalol), arsenic trioxide, chlorpromazine, cisapride, dolasetron, droperidol, mefloquine, mesoridazine, moxifloxacin, pentamidine, pimozide, tacrolimus, thioridazine, and ziprasidone. For a more complete list of drugs that may prolong the QT interval, see the appendix Drug-Induced Prolongation of the QT Interval and Torsade de Pointes.

Artemether/Lumefantrine Drug Interactions

Precipitant drug	Object drug[a]		Description
Antibiotics (eg, macrolides, fluoroquinolones, imidazole, triazole antifungals)	Artemether/lumefantrine	↑	Potential for additive effects on the QT interval. Avoid coadministration.
Artemether/lumefantrine	Antibiotics (eg, macrolides, fluoroquinolones, imidazole, triazole antifungals)		
Antidepressants	Artemether/lumefantrine	↑	Potential for additive effects on the QT interval. Avoid coadministration.
Artemether/lumefantrine	Antidepressants		
Antimalarials (eg, quinine, quinidine)	Artemether/lumefantrine	↑	Potential for additive effects on the QT interval. Avoid coadministration.
Artemether/lumefantrine	Antimalarials (eg, quinine, quinidine)		
Antipsychotics (eg, pimozide, ziprasidone)	Artemether/lumefantrine	↑	Potential for additive effects on the QT interval. Avoid coadministration.
Artemether/lumefantrine	Antipsychotics (eg, pimozide, ziprasidone)		
Antiretroviral drugs (eg, nonnucleoside reverse transcriptase inhibitors, protease inhibitors)	Artemether/lumefantrine	↑	May result in increased lumefantrine concentrations causing QT prolongation, decreased concentration of antiretroviral resulting in loss of efficacy, or decrease in artemether/lumefantrine concentrations resulting in loss of efficacy.
Artemether/lumefantrine	Antiretroviral drugs (eg, nonnucleoside reverse transcriptase inhibitors, protease inhibitors)	↓	
Cisapride	Artemether/lumefantrine	↑	Potential for additive effects on the QT interval. Avoid coadministration.
Artemether/lumefantrine	Cisapride		
Class IA antiarrhythmic agents (eg, disopyramide, procainamide, quinidine)	Artemether/lumefantrine	↑	Potential for additive effects on the QT interval. Avoid coadministration.
Artemether/lumefantrine	Class IA antiarrhythmic agents (eg, disopyramide, procainamide, quinidine)		
Class III antiarrhythmic agents (eg, amiodarone, sotalol)	Artemether/lumefantrine	↑	Potential for additive effects on the QT interval. Avoid coadministration.
Artemether/lumefantrine	Class III antiarrhythmic agents (eg, amiodarone, sotalol)		
CYP3A4 inducers	Artemether/lumefantrine	↓	May result in decreased concentrations of artemether/lumefantrine and loss of antimalarial efficacy.
CYP3A4 inhibitors (eg, grapefruit juice, ketoconazole)	Artemether/lumefantrine	↑	May result in increased concentrations of artemether/lumefantrine and potentiate QT prolongation.
Halofantrine	Artemether/lumefantrine	↑	Potential for additive effects on the QT interval. Avoid coadministration.
Artemether/lumefantrine	Halofantrine		
Mefloquine	Artemether/lumefantrine	↓	If mefloquine is administered immediately prior to artemether/lumefantrine, there may be decreased exposure to lumefantrine. Monitor patients for decreased efficacy and encourage food consumption.
Artemether/lumefantrine	Contraceptives, hormonal	↓	May reduce the effectiveness of hormonal contraceptives. Advise patients to use an additional nonhormonal method of birth control.
Nonsedating antihistamines (eg, astemizole, terfenadine)	Artemether/lumefantrine	↑	Potential for additive effects on the QT interval. Avoid coadministration.
Artemether/lumefantrine	Nonsedating antihistamines (eg, astemizole, terfenadine)		
Artemether/lumefantrine	CYP2D6 metabolized drugs (eg, amitriptyline, clomipramine, flecainide, imipramine)	↑	Coadministration may significantly increase plasma concentrations and increase the risk for adverse effects, including QT interval prolongation.
Artemether/lumefantrine	CYP3A4 substrates	↓	May result in decreased concentrations of the substrate and potential loss of substrate efficacy.

[a] ↑ = object drug increased; ↓ = object drug decreased.

Adverse Reactions

The data described below reflect exposure to a 6-dose regimen of artemether/lumefantrine tablets in 1,979 patients including 647 adults (older than 16 years of age) and 1,332 children (16 years of age and younger). For the 6-dose regimen, artemether/lumefantrine tablets was studied in active-controlled (366 patients) and noncontrolled, open-label trials (1,613 patients). The 6-dose artemether/lumefantrine tablets population was patients with malaria between 2 months and 71 years of age: 67% (1,332) were 16 years of age and younger and 33% (647) were older than 16 years of age. Males represented 73% and 53% of the adult and pediatric populations, respectively. The majority of adult patients were enrolled in studies in Thailand, while the majority of pediatric patients were enrolled in Africa.

In adults, the most frequently reported adverse reactions were anorexia, asthenia, dizziness, and headache. In children, the adverse reactions were anorexia, cough, headache, pyrexia, and vomiting. Most adverse reactions were mild, did not lead to discontinuation of study medication, and resolved.

ARTEMETHER/LUMEFANTRINE — ORAL

The discontinuation rate of artemether/lumefantrine tablets due to adverse drug reactions occurring in 1.1% of patients treated with the 6-dose regimen overall was 0.2% (1/647) in adults and 1.6% (21/1,332) in children.

Artemether/Lumefantrine 6-Dose Regimen Adverse Reactions (≥ 3%) in Adults

Adverse reactions	Adults[a] N = 647 (%)
CNS	
Asthenia	38%
Dizziness	39%
Fatigue	17%
Headache	56%
Insomnia	5%
Malaise	3%
Sleep disorder	22%
Vertigo	3%
Dermatologic	
Pruritus	4%
Rash	3%
GI	
Abdominal pain	17%
Anorexia	40%
Diarrhea	7%
Nausea	26%
Vomiting	17%
Hematologic/Lymphatic	
Anemia	4%
Splenomegaly	9%
Musculoskeletal	
Arthralgia	34%
Myalgia	32%
Respiratory	
Cough	6%
Nasopharyngitis	3%
Miscellaneous	
Chills	23%
Hepatomegaly	9%
Malaria	3%
Palpitations	18%
Pyrexia	25%

[a] Adult patients defined as > 16 years of age.

Artemether/Lumefantrine 6-Dose Regimen Adverse Reactions (≥ 3%) in Children

Adverse reactions	Children[a] N = 1,332 (%)
CNS	
Asthenia	5%
Dizziness	4%
Fatigue	3%
Headache	13%
GI	
Abdominal pain	8%
Anorexia	13%
Diarrhea	8%
Nausea	5%
Vomiting	18%
P. falciparum infection	17%
Hematologic/Lymphatic	
Anemia	9%
Splenomegaly	9%
Hepatic	
AST increased	4%
Hepatomegaly	6%
Musculoskeletal	
Arthralgia	3%
Myalgia	3%
Respiratory	
Cough	23%
Rhinitis	4%
Miscellaneous	
Chills	5%
Pyrexia	29%
Rash	3%

[a] Children defined as patients ≤ 16 years of age.

➤*Other adverse reactions (less than 3%):* Clinically significant adverse reactions reported in adults and/or children treated with the 6-dose regimen of artemether/lumefantrine tablets that occurred in clinical studies at less than 3% regardless of causality are the following:

CNS – Agitation, ataxia, clonus, fine motor delay, hyperreflexia, hypesthesia, mood swings, nystagmus, tremor.

Dermatologic – Impetigo, urticaria.

GI – Constipation, dyspepsia, dysphagia, gastroenteritis, peptic ulcer.

GU – Hematuria, proteinuria, urinary tract infection.

Hematologic / Lymphatic – Eosinophilia, hematocrit decreased, lymphocyte morphology abnormal, platelet count decreased, platelet count increased, white blood cell count decreased, white blood cell count increased.

Hepatic – ALT increased, AST increased.

Respiratory – Asthma, bronchitis, lower respiratory tract infection, nasopharyngitis, pharyngolaryngeal pain, pneumonia, respiratory tract infection, upper respiratory tract infection.

Special senses – Conjunctivitis, tinnitus.

Miscellaneous – Abscess, acrodermatitis, back pain, ear infection, gait disturbance, helminthic infection, hookworm infection, hypokalemia, influenza, malaria, oral herpes, subcutaneous abscess.

➤*Postmarketing:* Hypersensitivity including urticaria and angioedema; serious skin reactions (bullous eruption) have been rarely reported.

Overdosage

➤*Symptoms:* There is no information on overdoses of artemether/lumefantrine tablets higher than the doses recommended for treatment.

➤*Treatment:* In cases of suspected overdosage, give symptomatic and supportive therapy, which would include electrocardiogram and blood electrolyte monitoring, as appropriate.

Patient Information

Instruct patients to take artemether/lumefantrine tablets with food. Patients who do not have an adequate intake of food are at risk for recrudescence of malaria.

Patients hypersensitive to artemether, lumefantrine, or to any of the excipients should not receive artemether/lumefantrine tablets.

Instruct patients to inform their health care provider of any personal or family history of QT prolongation or proarrhythmic conditions, such as hypokalemia, bradycardia, or recent myocardial ischemia.

Instruct patients to inform their health care provider if they are taking any other medications that prolong the QT interval, such as class IA (eg, disopyramide, procainamide, quinidine) or class III (eg, amiodarone, sotalol) antiarrhythmic agents; antipsychotics (eg, pimozide, ziprasidone); antidepressants; certain antibiotics (eg, fluoroquinolone antibiotics, imidazole, macrolide antibiotics, triazole antifungal agents); certain nonsedating antihistamines (eg, terfenadine, astemizole) or cisapride.

Instruct patients to notify their health care provider if they have any symptoms of prolongation of the QT interval, including prolonged heart palpitations or a loss of consciousness.

Instruct patients to avoid medications that are metabolized by the cytochrome enzyme CYP2D6 while receiving artemether/lumefantrine tablets, because these drugs also have cardiac effects (eg, amitriptyline, clomipramine, flecainide, imipramine).

Inform patients that based on animal data, artemether/lumefantrine tablets administered during pregnancy may result in fetal loss. Fetal defects have been reported when artemisinins are administered to animals.

Halofantrine and artemether/lumefantrine tablets should not be administered within 1 month of each other because of potential additive effects on the QT interval.

Antimalarials should not be given concomitantly with artemether/lumefantrine tablets, unless there is no other treatment option, because of limited safety data.

QT prolonging drugs, including quinine and quinidine, should be used cautiously following artemether/lumefantrine tablets due to the long elimination half-life of lumefantrine and the potential for additive effects on the QT interval.

Closely monitor food intake in patients who received mefloquine immediately prior to treatment with artemether/lumefantrine tablets.

ARTEMETHER/LUMEFANTRINE — ORAL

Use artemether/lumefantrine tablets cautiously in patients receiving other drugs that are substrates, inhibitors, or inducers of CYP3A4, including grapefruit juice, especially those that prolong the QT interval or are antiretroviral drugs.

Artemether/lumefantrine tablets may reduce the effectiveness of hormonal contraceptives. Therefore, advise patients using oral, transdermal patch, or other systemic hormonal contraceptives to use an additional nonhormonal method of birth control.

Inform patients that artemether/lumefantrine tablets can cause hypersensitivity reactions. Instruct patients to discontinue the drug at the first sign of a skin rash, hives, or other skin reactions; a rapid heartbeat; difficulty swallowing or breathing; any swelling suggesting angioedema (eg, swelling of the lips, tongue, face, tightness of the throat, hoarseness); or other symptoms of an allergic reaction.

ATOVAQUONE/PROGUANIL HYDROCHLORIDE

Rx	**Malarone** (GlaxoSmithKline)	**Tablets**: atovaquone 250 mg/ proguanil hydrochloride 100 mg	(GX CM3). Pink, biconvex. Film-coated. In 100s and UD 24s.
Rx	**Malarone Pediatric** (GlaxoSmithKline)	**Tablets**: atovaquone 62.5 mg/ proguanil hydrochloride 25 mg	(GX CG7). Pink, biconvex. Film-coated. In 100s.

ATOVAQUONE/PROGUANIL HYDROCHLORIDE — ORAL

Indications

➤*Malaria prevention:* Prophylaxis of *Plasmodium falciparum* malaria, including areas where chloroquine resistance has been reported.

➤*Malaria treatment:* Treatment of acute, uncomplicated *P. falciparum* malaria. Atovaquone and proguanil have been shown to be effective in regions where the drugs chloroquine, halofantrine, mefloquine, and amodiaquine may have unacceptable failure rates, presumably because of drug resistance.

Administration and Dosage

➤*Adults:*

Malaria prevention – 1 tablet (atovaquone 250 mg/proguanil 100 mg) per day. Start prophylactic treatment 1 or 2 days before entering a malaria-endemic area and continue daily during the stay and for 7 days after return.

Malaria treatment – 4 tablets (total daily dose, atovaquone 1 g/proguanil 400 mg) as a single daily dose for 3 consecutive days.

➤*Children:*

Malaria prevention –

Children weighing 11 kg or more: Start prophylactic treatment 1 or 2 days before entering a malaria-endemic area and continue daily during the stay and for 7 days after return.

Dosage of Atovaquone/Proguanil for Prevention of Malaria in Children

Weight (kg)	Atovaquone/ Proguanil total daily dose	Dosage regimen
more than 40	250 mg/100 mg	1 tablet (adult strength) as a single daily dose
31 to 40	187.5 mg/75 mg	3 tablets (pediatric strength) as a single daily dose
21 to 30	125 mg/50 mg	2 tablets (pediatric strength) as a single daily dose
11 to 20	62.5 mg/25 mg	1 tablet (pediatric strength) daily

Malaria treatment –

Children weighing 5 kg or more:

Atovaquone/Proguanil for Treatment of Acute Malaria in Children

Weight (kg)	Atovaquone/ Proguanil total daily dose	Dosage regimen
more than 40	1 g/400 mg	4 tablets (adult strength) as a single daily dose for 3 consecutive days
31 to 40	750 mg/300 mg	3 tablets (adult strength) as a single daily dose for 3 consecutive days
21 to 30	500 mg/200 mg	2 tablets (adult strength) as a single daily dose for 3 consecutive days
11 to 20	250 mg/100 mg	1 tablet (adult strength) daily for 3 consecutive days
9 to 10	187.5 mg/75 mg	3 tablets (pediatric strength) daily for 3 consecutive days
5 to 8	125 mg/50 mg	2 tablets (pediatric strength) daily for 3 consecutive days

Off-label dosing –

Malaria prevention: Begin treatment 1 to 2 days before travel and continue throughout stay and for 1 week after leaving.

- *Children 9 to 10 kg* – ¾ tablet (pediatric strength) daily.
- *Children 5 to 8 kg* – ½ tablet (pediatric strength) daily.

➤*Renal function impairment:* Do not use for malaria prophylaxis in patients with severe renal impairment (CrCl less than 30 mL/min). Use with caution for the treatment of malaria in patients with severe renal impairment (CrCl less than 30 mL/min) only if the benefits of the 3-day treatment regimen outweigh the potential risks associated with increased drug exposure. Administer with caution to patients with severe pre-existing renal failure because proguanil is eliminated by renal excretion.

➤*Administration:* Take the daily dose at the same time each day with food or milk. In the event of vomiting within 1 hour after dosing, instruct patient to repeat dose. Tablets may be crushed and mixed with condensed milk just prior to administration for children who may have difficulty swallowing tablets.

➤*Storage/Stability:* Store at 25°C (77°F); excursions permitted between 15° and 30°C (59° and 86°F).

Actions

➤*Pharmacology:* Atovaquone/proguanil is a fixed-dose combination. The constituents of the combination interfere with 2 different pathways involved in the biosynthesis of pyrimidines required for nucleic acid replication. Atovaquone is a selective inhibitor of parasite mitochondrial electron transport. Proguanil primarily exerts its effect by means of the metabolite cycloguanil, a dihydrofolate reductase inhibitor. Inhibition of dihydrofolate reductase in the malaria parasite disrupts deoxythymidylate synthesis.

Atovaquone and cycloguanil (an active metabolite of proguanil) are active against the erythrocytic and exoerythrocytic stages of *Plasmodium* spp. Enhanced efficacy of the combination compared with either atovaquone or proguanil alone was demonstrated in clinical studies in immune and nonimmune patients.

Drug resistance – Strains of *P. falciparum* with decreased susceptibility to atovaquone or proguanil/cycloguanil alone can be selected in vitro or in vivo. The combination of atovaquone and proguanil may not be effective for treatment of recrudescent malaria that develops after prior therapy with the combination.

➤*Pharmacokinetics:*

Absorption – Atovaquone is a highly lipophilic compound with low aqueous solubility. The bioavailability of atovaquone shows considerable interindividual variability.

See Drug Interactions for more information.

Distribution – Atovaquone is highly protein bound (more than 99%) over the concentration range of 1 to 90 mcg/mL. The apparent volume of distribution of atovaquone in adults and children after oral administration is approximately 8.8 L/kg.

Proguanil is 75% protein bound. The apparent volume of distribution of proguanil in adults and children older than 15 years of age with body weights from 31 to 110 kg ranged from 1,617 to 2,502 L. In children 15 years of age and younger with body weights from 11 to 56 kg, the apparent volume of distribution of proguanil ranged from 462 to 966 L. In human plasma, the binding of atovaquone and proguanil was unaffected by the presence of the other.

Metabolism – There is indirect evidence that atovaquone may undergo limited metabolism; however, a specific metabolite has not been identified. Proguanil is metabolized to cycloguanil (primarily via CYP2C19) and 4-chlorophenylbiguanide. The main routes of elimination are hepatic biotransformation and renal excretion.

Excretion – In a study where atovaquone was administered to healthy volunteers, greater than 94% of the dose was recovered unchanged in the feces over 21 days. There was little or no excretion of atovaquone in the urine (less than 0.6%). Between 40% to 60% of proguanil is excreted by the kidneys. The elimination half-life of atovaquone is approximately 2 to 3 days in adult patients. The mean oral clearance of proguanil is 3.22 L/h/kg. The elimination half-life of proguanil is 12 to 21 hours in adult and pediatric patients but may be longer in individuals who are slow metabolizers.

Special populations –

Renal function impairment: In patients with moderate renal impairment (Ccr 30 to 50 mL/min), mean oral clearance for proguanil was reduced by approximately 35% compared with patients with normal renal function (Ccr greater than 80 mL/min) and the oral clearance of atovaquone was comparable between patients with normal renal function and mild renal impairment. In patients with severe renal impairment (Ccr less than 30 mL/min), atovaquone C_{max} and AUC are reduced, but the elimination half-lives for proguanil and cycloguanil are prolonged, with corresponding increases in AUC, resulting in the potential of drug accumulation and toxicity with repeated dosing.

Hepatic function impairment: In patients with moderate hepatic impairment, the elimination half-life of atovaquone was increased (point estimate = 1.28, 90% CI = 1 to 1.63). Proguanil AUC, C_{max}, and half-life increased in subjects with mild hepatic impairment when compared with healthy subjects. The proguanil AUC and half-life increased in patients with moderate hepatic

ATOVAQUONE/PROGUANIL HYDROCHLORIDE — ORAL

impairment when compared with healthy subjects. Consistent with the increase in proguanil AUC, there were marked decreases in the systemic exposure of cycloguanil (C_{max} and AUC) and an increase in its elimination half-life in subjects with mild hepatic impairment when compared with healthy volunteers.

Elderly: In elderly subjects, the extent of systemic exposure (AUC) of cycloguanil was increased (point estimate = 2.36, CI = 1.7, 3.28). T_{max} was longer in elderly subjects (median, 8 hours) compared with younger subjects (median, 4 hours) and average elimination half-life was longer in elderly subjects (mean, 14.9 hours) compared with younger subjects (mean, 8.3 hours).

Children: The pharmacokinetics of proguanil and cycloguanil are similar in adult and pediatric patients. However, the elimination half-life of atovaquone is shorter in pediatric patients (1 to 2 days) than in adult patients (2 to 3 days).

Contraindications

Hypersensitivity to atovaquone, proguanil, or any component of the formulation.

For prophylaxis of *P. falciparum* malaria in patients with severe renal impairment (Ccr less than 30 mL/min).

Warnings/Precautions

➤*Cerebral malaria:* Atovaquone/proguanil combination has not been evaluated for the treatment of cerebral malaria or other severe manifestations of complicated malaria, including hyperparasitemia, pulmonary edema, or renal failure. Patients with severe malaria are not candidates for oral therapy.

➤*Diarrhea/vomiting:* Absorption of atovaquone may be reduced in patients with diarrhea or vomiting. If atovaquone/proguanil combination is used in patients who are vomiting (see Administration and Dosage), closely monitor parasitemia and consider the use of an antiemetic. Vomiting occurred in 19% or less of pediatric patients given treatment doses. In controlled clinical trials, 15.3% of adults who were treated with atovaquone/proguanil received an antiemetic. Of these patients, 98.3% were successfully treated. In patients with severe or persistent diarrhea or vomiting, alternative antimalarial therapy may be required.

➤*Relapse:* Parasite relapse occurred commonly when *Plasmodium vivax* malaria was treated with atovaquone/proguanil alone. In the event of recrudescent *P. falciparum* infections after treatment with or failure of chemoprophylaxis with atovaquone/proguanil, treat patients with a different blood schizonticide.

➤*Renal function impairment:* Do not use for malaria prophylaxis in patients with severe renal impairment (Ccr less than 30 mL/min). Use with caution for the treatment of malaria in patients with severe renal impairment (Ccr less than 30 mL/min) only if the benefits of the 3-day treatment regimen outweigh the potential risks associated with increased drug exposure. Administer with caution to patients with severe pre-existing renal failure because proguanil is eliminated by renal excretion.

➤*Pregnancy: Category C.* Falciparum malaria carries a higher risk of morbidity and mortality in pregnant women than in the general population. Maternal death and fetal loss are known complications of falciparum malaria in pregnancy. In pregnant women who must travel to malaria-endemic areas, personal protection against mosquito bites should always be employed (see Patient Information) in addition to antimalarials.

In rabbits, atovaquone caused maternal toxicity at plasma concentrations that were approximately 0.6 to 1.3 times the estimated human exposure during treatment of malaria. Adverse fetal effects in rabbits, including decreased fetal body lengths and increased early resorption and postimplantation losses, were observed only in the presence of maternal toxicity. Concentrations of atovaquone in rabbit fetuses averaged 30% of the concurrent maternal plasma concentrations.

While there are no adequate and well-controlled studies of atovaquone or proguanil in pregnant women; the combination may be used if the potential benefit justifies the potential risk to the fetus. The proguanil component acts by inhibiting the parasitic dihydrofolate reductase (see Pharmacology). However, there are no clinical data indicating that folate supplementation diminishes drug efficacy, and for women of childbearing age receiving folate supplements to prevent neural tube birth defects, such supplements may be continued while taking the atovaquone/proguanil combination.

➤*Lactation:* It is not known whether atovaquone is excreted in breast milk. In a rat study, atovaquone concentrations in the milk were 30% of the concurrent atovaquone concentrations in the maternal plasma. Proguanil is excreted in breast milk in small quantities. Exercise caution when the atovaquone/proguanil combination is administered to a nursing woman.

➤*Children:* The safety and efficacy of atovaquone/proguanil for the treatment of malaria have been established in controlled studies involving pediatric patients weighing 5 kg or more. Safety and efficacy have not been established in pediatric patients who weigh less than 5 kg.

The safety and efficacy of atovaquone/proguanil have been established for the prophylaxis of malaria in controlled studies involving children weighing 11 kg or more. Safety and efficacy have not been established in children who weigh less than 11 kg.

Drug Interactions

Atovaquone is highly protein bound (more than 99%) but does not displace other highly protein-bound drugs in vitro. Proguanil is metabolized primarily by CYP2C19. Potential pharmacokinetic interactions with other substrates or inhibitors of this pathway are unknown.

Atovaquone/Proguanil Drug Interactions			
Precipitant drug	Object drug[a]		Description
Metoclopramide	Atovaquone	⬇	Concomitant treatment with metoclopramide has been associated with decreased bioavailability of atovaquone. Use only if other antiemetics are not available.
Rifampin Rifabutin	Atovaquone	⬇	Concomitant administration of rifampin or rifabutin is known to reduce atovaquone levels by approximately 50% and 34% respectively. The concomitant administration of these agents is not recommended. The mechanism of this interaction is unknown.
Tetracycline	Atovaquone	⬇	Concomitant treatment with tetracycline has been associated with ≈ 40% reduction in plasma concentrations of atovaquone. Closely monitor parasitemia in patients receiving tetracycline.
Atovaquone	Zidovudine	⬆	Zidovudine concentrations may be elevated, increasing the risk of zidovudine toxicity.

[a] ⬇ = object drug decreased; ⬆ = object drug increased.

➤*Drug/Food interactions:* Dietary fat taken with atovaquone increases the rate and extent of absorption, increasing AUC 2 to 3 times and C_{max} 5 times over fasting. The absolute bioavailability of the tablet formulation of atovaquone when taken with food is 23%. Atovaquone/proguanil tablets should be taken with food or a milky drink. Proguanil is extensively absorbed regardless of food intake.

Adverse Reactions

➤*Malaria prevention:* Among subjects who received atovaquone/proguanil for prophylaxis of malaria, adverse reactions occurred in similar proportions of subjects receiving the combination or placebo. The most commonly reported adverse experiences possibly attributable to atovaquone/proguanil or placebo were headache and abdominal pain. Prophylaxis was discontinued prematurely because of treatment-related adverse experiences in 3 of 381 adults and 0 of 125 pediatric patients.

In an additional placebo-controlled study of malaria prophylaxis with atovaquone/proguanil involving 330 pediatric patients, the most common treatment-emergent adverse events with atovaquone/proguanil were abdominal pain and headache (13%) and cough (10%). Abdominal pain (13% vs 8%) and vomiting (5% vs 3%) were reported more often with atovaquone/proguanil than with placebo, while fever (5% vs 12%) and diarrhea (1% vs 5%) were more common with placebo.

➤*Malaria treatment:* Among adults who received atovaquone/proguanil for malaria treatment, attributable adverse experiences that occurred in 5% or more of patients were abdominal pain (17%); nausea, vomiting (12%); headache (10%); diarrhea, asthenia (8%); anorexia, dizziness (5%). Treatment was discontinued prematurely because of an adverse experience in 4 of 436 adults.

Among children (weighing 11 to 40 kg) who received atovaquone/proguanil for malaria treatment, attributable adverse experiences that occurred in 5% or more of patients were vomiting (10%) and pruritus (6%). Vomiting occurred in 43 of 319 (13%) pediatric patients who did not have symptomatic malaria but were given treatment doses of atovaquone/proguanil for 3 days in a clinical trial. The design of this clinical trial required that any patient who vomited be withdrawn from the trial. Among pediatric patients with symptomatic malaria treated with the combination, treatment was discontinued prematurely because of an adverse experience in 1 of 116 (0.9%).

In a study of 100 pediatric patients (5 to less than 11 kg body weight) who received atovaquone/proguanil for the treatment of uncomplicated *P. falciparum* malaria, only diarrhea (6%) occurred in 5% or more of patients as an adverse experience attributable to atovaquone/proguanil. In 3 patients (3%), treatment was discontinued prematurely because of an adverse experience.

➤*Lab test abnormalities:* Abnormalities in laboratory tests reported in clinical trials were limited to elevations of transaminases in malaria patients being treated with atovaquone/proguanil. The frequency of these abnormalities varied substantially across studies of treatment and were not observed in the randomized portions of the prophylaxis trials.

In one phase 3 trial of malaria treatment in Thai adults, early elevations of AST and ALT were observed to occur more frequently in patients treated with atovaquone/proguanil compared with patients treated with an active control drug. Rates for patients who had normal baseline levels of these clinical laboratory parameters were: day 7 – ALT 26.7% vs 15.6%; AST 16.9% vs 8.6%. By day 14 of this 28-day study, the frequency of transaminase elevations equalized across the 2 groups.

In this and other studies in which transaminase elevations occurred, they were noted to persist for 4 weeks or less following treatment with atovaquone/proguanil for malaria. None were associated with untoward clinical events.

ATOVAQUONE/PROGUANIL HYDROCHLORIDE — ORAL

Adverse Reactions of Atovaquone/Proguanil Combination for Prophylaxis of Malaria (%)

Adverse reaction	Adults			Children and adolescents	
	Placebo (n = 206)	Atovaquone/ Proguanil[a] (n = 206)	Atovaquone/ Proguanil[b] (n = 381)	Placebo (n = 140)	Atovaquone/ Proguanil (n = 125)
Any adverse event	32%	17%	17%	41%	42%
GI					
Abdominal pain	5%	4%	3%	29	31%
Diarrhea	3%	2%	1%	1%	0%
Dyspepsia	4%	2%	1%	0%	0%
Gastritis	2%	3%	2%	0%	0%
Vomiting	< 1%	< 1%	< 1%	6%	7%
Respiratory					
Cough	< 1%	< 1%	1%	0%	0%
Upper respiratory tract infection	0%	0%	0%	0%	0%
Miscellaneous					
Back pain	0%	0%	0%	0%	0%
Fever	1%	0%	0%	< 1%	0%
Flu syndrome	0%	0%	0%	0%	0%
Headache	7%	3%	5%	14%	14%
Myalgia	0%	0%	0%	0%	0%

[a] Subjects receiving the recommended dose of atovaquone and proguanil in placebo-controlled trials.
[b] Subjects receiving the recommended dose of atovaquone and proguanil in any trial.

➤*Postmarketing:*

CNS – Rare cases of seizures and psychotic events (eg, hallucinations); however, a causal relationship has not been established.

Dermatologic – Cutaneous reactions ranging from rash, photosensitivity, and urticaria to rare cases of erythema multiforme and Stevens-Johnson syndrome.

Overdosage

There have been no reports of overdosage of atovaquone/proguanil combination tablets substantially higher than the doses recommended for treatment.

➤*Symptoms:*

Atovaquone – Overdoses with 31,500 mg or less of atovaquone have been reported. In one such patient who also took an unspecified dose of dapsone, methemoglobinemia occurred. Rash also has been reported after overdose.

Proguanil – Overdoses of proguanil as large as 1,500 mg have been followed by complete recovery, and doses as high as 700 mg twice daily have been taken for more than 2 weeks without serious toxicity. Adverse events occasionally associated with proguanil doses of 100 to 200 mg/day, such as epigastric discomfort and vomiting, would be likely to occur with overdose. There also are reports of reversible hair loss and scaling of the skin on the palms or soles, reversible aphthous ulceration, and hematologic side effects.

➤*Treatment:*

Atovaquone – There is no known antidote for atovaquone, and it is currently unknown if atovaquone is dialyzable. The median lethal dose is higher than the maximum oral dose tested in mice and rats (1,825 mg/kg/day).

Patient Information

Instruct patients to do the following:

- Take atovaquone/proguanil combination tablets at the same time each day with food or a milky drink.
- Take a repeat dose of the combination if vomiting occurs within 1 hour after dosing.
- Consult a health care professional regarding alternative forms of prophylaxis if prophylaxis with atovaquone/proguanil is prematurely discontinued for any reason.
- Include protective clothing, insect repellants, and bed nets as important components of malaria prophylaxis.
- No chemoprophylactic regimen is 100% effective; therefore, patients should seek medical attention for any febrile illness that occurs during or after return from a malaria-endemic area and inform their health care professional that they may have been exposed to malaria.
- *Falciparum* malaria carries a higher risk of death and serious complications in pregnant women than in the general population. Pregnant women anticipating travel to malarious areas should discuss the risks and benefits of such travel with their physicians (see Pregnancy section).
- If a dose is missed, take it as soon as possible, then return to the normal schedule. If a dose is skipped, do not double the next dose.

ANTITUBERCULOSIS AGENTS

Antituberculosis drugs have been described in terms of the following 3 areas of activity: Bactericidal activity, sterilizing activity, and drug resistance prevention. Isoniazid is the most potent bactericidal antituberculosis agent, although rifampin and streptomycin have some bactericidal activity. Rifampin and pyrazinamide are the most potent sterilizing drugs for tuberculosis. Drugs that eliminate all bacterial populations and do not allow the emergence of resistant organisms prevent drug resistance.

Standard treatment regimens are divided into the following 2 phases: An initial phase, during which agents are used to kill rapidly multiplying populations of *Mycobacterium tuberculosis* and to prevent the emergence of drug resistance, followed by a continuation phase, during which sterilizing drugs kill the intermittently dividing populations.

The initial phase of the regimen must contain ≥ 3 of the following drugs: Isoniazid, rifampin, and pyrazinamide, along with either ethambutol or streptomycin if the local resistance pattern to isoniazid is not documented or is more than 4%.

➤*Directly observed therapy (DOT):* Adherence to the treatment regimen can be achieved by DOT, the "gold standard." The health care provider watches the patient swallow each dose of medication. This allows for monitoring the number of doses that an individual has taken.

DOT may be given intermittently (2 to 3 times/week) or daily. Intermittent therapy was introduced when it was shown in controlled clinical trials that therapeutic serum levels of the various antituberculosis drugs were maintained even when medications were given only 2 or 3 times/week. Intermittent regimens do not have more toxic effects than daily regimens; allow drug administration to be adapted to local conditions. All intermittent regimens must involve DOT.

Recommended Drugs for the Treatment of Tuberculosis in Children and Adults[a]

Drug	Daily dose[b]		Maximum daily dose in children and adults	Twice weekly dose		3 times/week dose	
	Children	Adults		Children	Adults	Children	Adults
Initial treatment							
Isoniazid	10 to 20 mg/kg PO or IM	5 mg/kg PO or IM	300 mg	20 to 40 mg/kg max 900 mg	15 mg/kg max 900 mg	20 to 40 mg/kg max 900 mg	15 mg/kg max 900 mg
Rifampin	10 to 20 mg/kg PO	10 mg/kg PO	600 mg	10 to 20 mg/kg max 600 mg	10 mg/kg max 600 mg	10 to 20 mg/kg max 600 mg	10 mg/kg max 600 mg
Pyrazinamide	15 to 30 mg/kg PO	15 to 30 mg/kg PO	2 g	50 to 70 mg/kg max 4 g	50 to 70 mg/kg max 4 g	50 to 70 mg/kg max 3 g	50 to 70 mg/kg max 3 g
Streptomycin	20 to 40 mg/kg IM	15 mg/kg IM	1 g[c]	25 to 30 mg/kg IM max 1.5 g	25 to 30 mg/kg IM max 1.5 g	25 to 30 mg/kg max 1.5 g	25 to 30 mg/kg max 1.5 g
Ethambutol	15 to 25 mg/kg PO	15 to 25 mg/kg PO	—	50 mg/kg	50 mg/kg	25 to 30 mg/kg	25 to 30 mg/kg
Rifapentine	—	—	—	—	600 mg PO	—	—
Second-line treatment							
Cycloserine	15 to 20 mg/kg PO	15 to 20 mg/kg PO	1 g				

Recommended Drugs for the Treatment of Tuberculosis in Children and Adults[a]

Drug	Daily dose[b]		Maximum daily dose in children and adults	Twice weekly dose		3 times/week dose	
	Children	Adults		Children	Adults	Children	Adults
Ethionamide	15 to 20 mg/kg PO	15 to 20 mg/kg PO	1 g	—	—	—	—
Capreomycin	15 to 30 mg/kg IM	15 to 30 mg/kg IM	1 g	—	—	—	—
Kanamycin	15 to 30 mg/kg IM or IV	15 to 30 mg/kg IM or IV	1 g	—	—	—	—
Ciprofloxacin	—	1000 to 1500 mg PO	1500 mg	—	—	—	—
Ofloxacin	—	800 mg PO	800 mg	—	—	—	—
Levofloxacin	—	500 to 750 mg PO	750 mg	—	—	—	—
Sparfloxacin	—	200 mg PO	200 mg	—	—	—	—
P-aminosalicylic acid	150 mg/kg PO	150 mg/kg PO	12 g	—	—	—	—
Rifabutin	—	300 to 450 mg PO	—	—	—	—	—

[a] For detailed dosing information and frequency, see individual monographs.
[b] Doses based on weight. Adjust as weight changes.
[c] In people ≥ 60 years of age, limit the daily dose of streptomycin to 0.5 g IM.

➤*Treatment regimens:* Treatment for tuberculosis is a long-term process. Begin treatment as soon as possible after diagnosis. Combination therapy is required. The CDC recommends at least a 3-drug regimen with rifampin, isoniazid, and pyrazinamide for a minimum of 2 months, followed by rifampin and isoniazid for 4 months in areas with a low incidence of tuberculosis. Administer streptomycin or ethambutol for the first 2 months in areas with a high incidence of tuberculosis.

➤*Retreatment:* Retreatment is necessary when treatment fails because of noncompliance or inadequate drug treatment. Retreatment regimens include ≥ 4 drugs; however, depending on disease progression and the bacteriostatic or bactericidal activity of the drug, ≤ 7 drugs can be used. Retreatment drug regimens most commonly include the second-line agents of ethionamide, aminosalicylic acid, cycloserine, and capreomycin, as well as ofloxacin and ciprofloxacin.

Therapy includes 2 or 3 agents not given previously when current susceptibility data are unavailable. Add to the initial 4-drug regimen of isoniazid, rifampin, pyrazinamide, and ethambutol or streptomycin, ≥ 2 drugs to which the organism is susceptible on the basis of local resistance patterns. The ineffective agents may be discontinued once susceptibility test results are available.

Individualize treatment on the basis of the susceptibility pattern of the infecting organism when re-treating patients known to be infected with drug-resistant isolates. Include in this regimen ≥ 3 new drugs to which the organism is susceptible. Continue therapy until sputum cultures convert to negative and then continue therapy for an additional 12 months with 2 drugs. Treatment may be continued for 24 months after sputum culture conversion.

➤*HIV:* The initial phase of a 6-month tuberculosis regimen consists of isoniazid, rifabutin, pyrazinamide, and ethambutol for patients receiving therapy with protease inhibitors or nonnucleoside reverse transcriptase inhibitors. These drugs are administered a) daily for at least the first 2 weeks, followed by twice weekly dosing for 6 weeks or b) daily for 8 weeks to complete the 2-month induction phase. The second phase of treatment consists of rifabutin and isoniazid administered twice weekly or daily for 4 months.

Patients for whom the use of rifamycins is limited or contraindicated for any reason (eg, patient/clinician decision not to combine antiretroviral therapy with rifabutin, intolerance to rifamycins), the initial phase of a 9-month tuberculosis regimen consists of isoniazid, streptomycin, pyrazinamide, and ethambutol administered a) daily for at least the first 2 weeks, followed by twice weekly dosing for 6 weeks or b) daily for 8 weeks to complete the 2-month induction phase. The second phase of treatment consists of isoniazid, streptomycin, and pyrazinamide administered 2 to 3 times/week for 7 months.

The preferred option for patients who are not candidates for antiretroviral therapy or for whom a decision is made not to combine the initiation of tuberculosis therapy with antiretroviral therapy is to administer a 6-month regimen of isoniazid, rifampin, pyrazinamide, and ethambutol or streptomycin. These drugs are administered a) daily for at least the first 2 weeks, followed by 2 or 3 times/week dosing for 6 weeks or b) daily for 8 weeks to complete the 2-month induction phase. The second phase of treatment consists of isoniazid and rifampin administered daily or 2 to 3 times/week for 4 months. Isoniazid, rifampin, pyrazinamide, and ethambutol or streptomycin can be administered 3 times/week for 6 months.

Do not use tuberculosis regimens consisting of isoniazid, ethambutol, and pyrazinamide (ie, 3-drug regimens that do not contain a rifamycin, an aminoglycoside [eg, streptomycin, amikacin, kanamycin], or capreomycin) for the treatment of patients with HIV-related tuberculosis. The minimum duration of therapy is 18 months (or 12 months after documented culture conversion) if these regimens are used for the treatment of tuberculosis.

Administer pyridoxine (vitamin B_6) 25 to 50 mg daily or 50 to 100 mg twice weekly to all HIV-infected patients who are undergoing tuberculosis treatment with isoniazid to reduce the occurrence of isoniazid-induced side effects in the central and peripheral nervous system.

Because the MMWR's most recent recommendations for the use of antiretroviral therapy strongly advise against interruptions of therapy, and because alternative tuberculosis treatments that do not contain rifampin are available, previous antituberculosis therapy options that involved stopping protease inhibitor therapy to allow the use of rifampin are no longer recommended.

➤*Pregnancy:* Do not delay treatment for suspected or confirmed tuberculosis during pregnancy. The best therapeutic choices with the least danger to the fetus appear to be combinations of isoniazid, ethambutol, and rifampin. Pyrazinamide and streptomycin are not recommended during pregnancy because of possible teratogenic effects. Administer pyridoxine to all pregnant women receiving tuberculosis treatment to prevent peripheral neuropathy as a result of taking isoniazid. In pregnant women, delay prophylaxis until after delivery.

➤*Multidrug resistance:* The most recent cultures should undergo susceptibility testing to all antituberculosis drugs if cultures remain positive after 3 to 4 months of treatment. The patient may continue to receive the most recent treatment regimen, if his or her condition is clinically stable, while awaiting results of drug susceptibility testing. Alternatively, add ≥ 2 new drugs to the original medications if the patient is acutely ill. Administer an aminoglycoside or capreomycin as one of the medications, because these drugs lead to earlier sputum conversion.

➤*Chemoprophylaxis:* Administer isoniazid to adults in a daily dose of 300 mg for 1 year. Administer 10 mg/kg to a maximum daily dose of 300 mg for 1 year to children. Consider prophylactic therapy for the following: Those exposed to tuberculosis but who have no evidence of infection; those with infection (positive tuberculin test: greater than 5 mm [HIV infected] or 10 mm [not immunocompromised] of induration to 5 units purified protein derivative [PPD]) and no apparent disease; those with a history of tuberculosis but in whom the disease is presently "inactive;" and anergic people from populations at risk for tuberculosis. Prophylaxis with isoniazid is contraindicated for patients who have had reactions to the drug or have active hepatic disease. There are insufficient data on the advisability of prophylaxis with alternative drugs such as rifampin.

ISONIAZID (Isonicotinic acid hydrazide; INH)

Rx	**Isoniazid** (Various, eg, Barr, Eon, Paddock, UDL)	**Tablets; oral:** 100 mg	In 30s, 100s, and 1000s.
Rx	**Isoniazid** (Various, eg, Barr, Eon, Major, UDL)	**Tablets; oral:** 300 mg	In 30s, 60s, 100s, 200s, and 1000s.
Rx	**Isoniazid** (Carolina Medical)	**Syrup; oral:** 50 mg/5 ml	Sorbitol. Orange flavor. In pt.
Rx	**Isoniazid** (Sandoz)	**Injection solution:** 100 mg/ml	In 10 mL vials.[a]
Rx	**Nydrazid** (Apothecon)		In 10 ml vials.[a]

[a] With 0.25% chlorobutanol.

ISONIAZID — ORAL

WARNING

Hepatitis – Severe and sometimes fatal hepatitis associated with isoniazid therapy has been reported and may occur or may develop even after many months of treatment. The risk of developing hepatitis is age related. Approximate case rates by age are as follows: less than 1/1,000 for persons younger than 20 years of age, 3/1,000 for persons in the 20- to 34-years of age group, 12/1,000 for persons in the 35- to 49-years of age group, 23/1,000 for persons in the 50- to 64-years of age group, and 8/1,000 for persons older than 65 years of age. The risk of hepatitis is increased with daily consumption of alcohol. Precise data to provide a fatality rate for isoniazid-related hepatitis is not available; however, in a US public health service surveillance study of 13,838 persons taking isoniazid, there were 8 deaths among 174 cases of hepatitis.

Therefore, carefully monitor patients given isoniazid and interview patients at monthly intervals. For persons older than 35 years of age, in addition to monthly symptom reviews, measure hepatic enzymes (specifically, AST and ALT) prior to starting isoniazid therapy and periodically throughout treatment. Isoniazid-associated hepatitis usually occurs during the first 3 months of treatment. Usually, enzyme levels return to normal despite continuance of drug, but, in some cases, progressive liver dysfunction occurs. Other factors associated with an increased risk of hepatitis include daily use of alcohol, chronic liver disease, and injection drug use. A recent report suggests an increased risk of fatal hepatitis associated with isoniazid among women, particularly black and Hispanic women. The risk may also be increased during the postpartum period. Consider more careful monitoring in these groups, possibly including more frequent laboratory monitoring. If abnormalities of liver function exceed 3 to 5 times the upper limit of normal (ULN), strongly consider discontinuation of isoniazid. Liver function tests are not a substitute for a clinical evaluation at monthly intervals or for the prompt assessment of signs or symptoms of adverse reactions occurring between regularly scheduled evaluations. Instruct patients to immediately report signs or symptoms consistent with liver damage or other adverse reactions. These include any of the following: unexplained anorexia, nausea, vomiting, dark urine, icterus, rash, persistent paresthesias of the hands and feet, persistent fatigue, weakness or fever of greater than 3-day duration or abdominal tenderness, especially right-upper-quadrant discomfort. If these symptoms appear or if signs suggestive of hepatic damage are detected, promptly discontinue isoniazid, because continued use of the drug in these cases has been reported to cause a more severe form of liver damage.

Give patients with tuberculosis who have hepatitis attributed to isoniazid appropriate treatment with alternative drugs. If isoniazid must be reinstituted, do so only after symptoms and laboratory abnormalities have cleared. Restart the drug in very small and gradually increasing doses and withdraw immediately if there is any indication of recurrent liver involvement.

Defer preventive treatment in persons with acute hepatic diseases.

Indications

➤*General information:* The risk of hepatitis must be weighed against the risk of tuberculosis in positive tuberculin reactors older than 35 of age. However, the use of isoniazid is for those with the additional risk factors listed above and on an individual basis in situations where there is likelihood of serious consequences to contacts who may become infected.

➤*Tuberculosis treatment:* For all forms of tuberculosis in which organisms are susceptible. However, active tuberculosis must be treated with multiple, concomitant antituberculosis medications to prevent the emergence of drug resistance. Single-drug treatment of active tuberculosis with isoniazid, or any other medication, is inadequate therapy.

➤*Prophylaxis:* Isoniazid is recommended as preventive therapy for the following groups, regardless of age. (Note: The criterion for a positive reaction to a skin test [in millimeters (mm) of induration] for each group is given in parenthesis).

HIV – Persons with HIV infection (greater than or equal to 5 mm) and persons with risk factors for HIV infection whose HIV infection status is unknown but who are suspected of having HIV infection. Preventive therapy may be considered for HIV-infected persons who are tuberculin negative but belong to groups in which the prevalence of tuberculosis is high. Candidates for preventive therapy who have HIV infection should have a minimum of 12 months of therapy.

Close contacts of people with infectious tuberculosis – Close contacts of persons with newly diagnosed infectious tuberculosis (greater than or equal to 5 mm). In addition, tuberculin-negative (less than 5 mm) children and adolescents who have been close contacts of infectious persons within the past 3 months are candidates for preventive therapy until a repeat tuberculin skin test is done 12 weeks after the infectious source. If the repeat skin test is positive (greater than 5 mm), continue therapy.

Recent converters – Recent converters, as indicated by a tuberculin skin test (greater than or equal to 10 mm increase within a 2-year period for those younger than 35 years old; greater than or equal to 15 mm increase for those 35 years of age and older). All infants and children younger than 4 years of age with a greater than 10 mm skin test are included in this category.

Abnormal chest radiographs – Persons with abnormal chest radiographs that show fibrotic lesions likely to represent old healed tuberculosis (greater than or equal to 5 mm). Candidates for preventive therapy who have fibrotic pulmonary lesions consistent with healed tuberculosis or who have pulmonary silicosis should have 12 months of isoniazid or 4 months of rifampin, concomitantly.

IV drug users – Intravenous (IV) drug users known to be HIV-seronegative (greater than 10 mm).

Increased risk of tuberculosis – Persons with the following medical conditions that have been reported to increase the risk of tuberculosis (greater than or equal to 10 mm); silicosis; diabetes mellitus; prolonged therapy with adrenocorticosteroids; immunosuppressive therapy; some hematologic and reticuloendothelial diseases, such as leukemia or Hodgkin disease; end-stage renal disease; clinical situations associated with substantial rapid weight loss or chronic undernutrition (including the following: intestinal bypass surgery for obesity, the postgastrectomy state with or without weight loss, chronic peptic ulcer disease, chronic malabsorption syndromes, and carcinomas of the oropharynx and upper GI tract that prevent adequate nutritional intake). Candidates for preventive therapy who have fibrotic pulmonary lesions consistent with healed tuberculosis pulmonary silicosis should have 12 months of isoniazid or 4 months of isoniazid and rifampin, concomitantly.

Adults younger than 35 years of age with tuberculin skin test reaction of greater than or equal to 10 mm – Additionally, in the absence of any of the above risk factors, persons younger than 35 years of age with a tuberculin skin test reaction of greater than or equal to 10 mm are also appropriate candidates for preventive therapy if they are a member of any of the following high-incidence groups.

- Foreign-born persons from high-prevalence countries who never received BCG vaccine.
- Medically underserved low-income populations, including high-risk racial or ethnic minority populations, especially blacks, Hispanics, and Native Americans.
- Residents of facilities for long-term care (eg, correctional institutions, nursing homes, mental institutions).

Children younger than 4 years of age – Children who are younger than 4 years old are candidates for isoniazid-preventive therapy if they have greater than 10 mm induration from a purified protein derivative (PPD) Mantoux tuberculin skin test.

Adults younger than 35 years of age with tuberculin skin test reaction of greater than or equal to 15 mm – Finally, persons younger than 35 years of age who: have none of the above risk factors, belong to none of the high-incidence groups, and have tuberculin skin test reactions of 15 mm or more, are appropriate candidates for preventive therapy.

➤*Off-label uses:*

Tuberculosis (once-weekly dosing) – [1] = Good documentation. According to the official joint statement of the American Thoracic Society, Centers for Disease Control and Prevention (CDC), and Infectious Diseases Society of America for the treatment of tuberculosis, oral isoniazid is given in combination with rifampin, pyrazinamide, and ethambutol for a 2-month initial phase and a 4- to 7-month continuation phase. The Food and Drug Administration (FDA) has approved oral isoniazid 5 mg/kg daily, or 15 mg/kg 2 or 3 times weekly. The guidelines also recommend oral isoniazid 15 mg/kg once per week (not to exceed 900 mg).

Administration and Dosage

➤*General dosing considerations:* Before isoniazid preventive therapy is initiated, bacteriologically positive or radiographically progressive tuberculosis must be excluded. Perform appropriate evaluations if extrapulmonary tuberculosis is suspected.

Continuous administration of isoniazid for a sufficient period is an essential part of the regimen because relapse rates are higher if chemotherapy is stopped prematurely. In the treatment of tuberculosis, resistant organisms may multiply and the emergence of resistant organisms during the treatment may necessitate a change in the regimen.

Isoniazid is used in conjunction with other effective antituberculosis agents. Perform drug susceptibility testing on the organisms initially isolated from all patients with newly diagnosed tuberculosis. If the bacilli becomes resistant, therapy must be changed to agents which the bacilli are susceptible.

➤*Adults:*

Tuberculosis prophylaxis – 300 mg in a single daily dose for adults weighing more than 30 kg.

Tuberculosis treatment –

Usual dosage: 5 mg/kg (up to 300 mg) in a single daily dose, or 15 mg/kg (up to 900 mg) given 2 or 3 times per week.

Maximum dose: 300 mg/day (daily regimen); 900 mg (2- or 3-times-per-week regimen).

Off-label dosing –

Tuberculosis (once-weekly dosing): [1] = Good documentation. Oral isoniazid 15 mg/kg once per week (not to exceed 900 mg/day).

➤*Children:*

Tuberculosis prophylaxis –

Usual dosage: 10 mg/kg (up to 300 mg daily) in a single daily dose.

Maximum dose: 300 mg/day (daily regimen); 900 mg (twice weekly regimen).

Alternative dosage: In situations where adherence with daily preventive therapy cannot be assured, 20 to 30 mg/kg IM (not to exceed 900 mg) twice weekly under the direct observation of a health care worker at the time of administration is recommended.

ISONIAZID — ORAL

Tuberculosis treatment –

Usual dosage: 10 to 15 mg/kg (up to 300 mg) in a single daily dose, or 20 to 40 mg/kg (up to 900 mg) given 2 or 3 times per week.

Maximum dose: 300 mg/day (daily regimen); 900 mg (2- or 3-times-weekly regimen).

Alternative dosage: The Centers for Disease Control and Prevention recommends a dose of 20 to 30 mg/kg (up to 900 mg) given 2 times/week as an alternative to the previously described daily regimen.

➤*Hepatic function impairment:* Give patients with tuberculosis who have hepatitis attributed to isoniazid appropriate treatment with alternative drugs. Defer preventive treatment in people with acute hepatic diseases. (See Warning Box.)

➤*Directly observed therapy:* A major cause of drug-resistant tuberculosis is patient noncompliance with treatment. The use of directly observed therapy can help ensure patient compliance with drug therapy. Directly observed therapy is the observation of the patient by a health care provider or other responsible person as the patient ingests antituberculosis medications. Directly observed therapy can be achieved with daily, twice-weekly, or thrice-weekly regimens and is recommended for all patients.

➤*Concomitant pyridoxine therapy:* Coadministration of pyridoxine (B_6) is recommended in malnourished and in those predisposed to neuropathy (eg, alcoholics, diabetics).

➤*Pulmonary tuberculosis without HIV infection:* There are 3 regimen options for the initial treatment of tuberculosis:

Option 1 – Daily isoniazid, rifampin, and pyrazinamide for 8 weeks followed by 16 weeks of isoniazid and rifampin daily or 2 to 3 times weekly. Add ethambutol or streptomycin to the initial regimen until sensitivity to isoniazid and rifampin is demonstrated. The addition of a fourth drug is optional if the relative prevalence of isoniazid-resistant *Mycobacterium tuberculosis* isolates in the community is less than or equal to 4%.

Option 2 – Daily isoniazid, rifampin, pyrazinamide, and streptomycin or ethambutol for 2 weeks followed by twice-weekly administration of the same drugs for 6 weeks; subsequently, twice-weekly isoniazid and rifampin for 16 weeks.

Option 3 – Three times weekly with isoniazid, rifampin, pyrazinamide, and ethambutol or streptomycin for 6 months.

Administer all regimens given twice weekly or 3 times weekly by directly observed therapy. (See Directly Observed Therapy.)

The above treatment guidelines apply only when the disease is caused by organisms that are susceptible to the standard antituberculous agents. Because of the impact of resistance to isoniazid and rifampin on the response to therapy, it is essential that health care providers initiating therapy for tuberculosis be familiar with the prevalence of drug resistance in their communities. It is suggested that ethambutol not be used in children whose visual acuity cannot be monitored.

➤*Pulmonary tuberculosis and HIV infection:* The response of the immunologically impaired host to treatment may not be as satisfactory as that of a person with normal host responsiveness. For this reason, therapeutic decisions for the impaired host must be individualized. Since patients coinfected with HIV may have problems with malabsorption, screening of antimycobacterial drug levels, especially in patients with advanced HIV disease, may be necessary to prevent the emergence of multidrug-resistant tuberculosis (MDRTB).

➤*Extrapulmonary tuberculosis:* The basic principles that underlie the treatment of pulmonary tuberculosis also apply to extrapulmonary forms of the disease. Although there have not been the same kinds of carefully conducted controlled trials of treatment of extrapulmonary tuberculosis as for pulmonary disease, increasing clinical experience indicates that a 6- to 9-month short-course regimen is effective. Because of the insufficient data, military tuberculosis, bone/joint tuberculosis, and tuberculous meningitis in infants and children should receive 12-month therapy.

Bacteriologic evaluation of extrapulmonary tuberculosis may be limited by the relative inaccessibility of the sites of disease. Thus, response to treatment often must be judged on the basis of clinical and radiographic findings.

The use of adjunctive therapies such as surgery and corticosteroids is more commonly required in extrapulmonary tuberculosis than in pulmonary disease. Surgery may be necessary to obtain specimens for diagnosis and to treat such processes as constrictive pericarditis and spinal cord compression from Pott disease. Corticosteroids have been shown to be of benefit in preventing cardiac constriction from tuberculous pericarditis and in decreasing the neurologic sequelae of all stages of tuberculosis meningitis, especially when administered early in the course of the disease.

➤*Pregnant women with tuberculosis:* The treatment options previously listed must be adjusted for the pregnant patient. Streptomycin interferes with in utero development of the ear and may cause congenital deafness. Routine use of pyrazinamide is also not recommended in pregnancy because of inadequate teratogenicity data. The initial treatment regimen should consist of isoniazid and rifampin. Include ethambutol unless primary isoniazid resistance is unlikely (isoniazid resistance rate documented to be less than 4%).

➤*Multiple-drug resistant tuberculosis:* MDRTB (ie, resistance to at least isoniazid and rifampin) presents difficult treatment problems. Treatment must be individualized and based on susceptibility studies. In such cases, consultation with an expert in tuberculosis is recommended.

➤*Therapeutic drug monitoring:* The Potts-Cozart test, a simple colorimetric method of checking for isoniazid in the urine is a useful tool for ensuring patient compliance, which is essential for effective tuberculosis control. Additionally, isoniazid test strips are also available to check patient compliance.

➤*Administration:* Do not administer isoniazid with food. Studies have shown that the bioavailability of isoniazid is reduced significantly when administered with food.

➤*Storage/Stability:* Store at 15° to 30°C (59° to 86°F). Protect from moisture and light. Dispense in a well-closed and light-resistant container with a child-resistant closure.

Actions

➤*Pharmacology:* Isoniazid inhibits the synthesis of mycoloic acids, an essential component of the bacterial cell wall. At therapeutic levels isoniazid is bacteriocidal against activity growing intracellular and extracellular *M. tuberculosis* organisms.

Isoniazid-resistant *Mycobacterium tuberculosis* bacilli develop rapidly when isoniazid monotherapy is administered.

➤*Pharmacokinetics:*

Absorption/Distribution – Within 1 to 2 hours after oral administration, isoniazid produces peak blood levels that decline to 50% or less within 6 hours. It diffuses readily into all body fluids (cerebrospinal, pleural, and ascitic fluids), tissues, organs, and excreta (saliva, sputum, and feces). The drug also passes through the placental barrier and into milk in concentrations comparable with those in the plasma.

Metabolism – Isoniazid is metabolized primarily by acetylation and dehydrazination. The rate of acetylation is genetically determined. Approximately 50% of black patients and white patients are "slow inactivators" and the rest are "rapid inactivators"; the majority of Eskimo and Asian patients are "rapid inactivators."

The rate of acetylation does not significantly alter the efficacy of isoniazid. However, slow acetylation may lead to higher blood levels of the drug and, thus, to an increase in toxic reactions.

Pyridoxine (vitamin B_6) deficiency is sometimes observed in adults with high doses of isoniazid and is considered probably due to its competition with pyridoxal phosphate for the enzyme apotryptophanase.

Excretion – From 50% to 70% of a dose of isoniazid is excreted in the urine within 24 hours.

Contraindications

Severe hypersensitivity reactions, including drug-induced hepatitis; previous isoniazid-associated severe adverse reactions to isoniazid such as drug fever, chills, or arthritis; and acute liver disease of any etiology.

Warnings/Precautions

➤*Hepatitis:* See the Warning box for more information.

➤*Hypersensitivity reactions:* All drugs should be stopped and an evaluation made at the first sign of a hypersensitivity reaction. If isoniazid therapy must be reinstituted, give the drug only after symptoms have cleared. Restart the drug in very small and gradually increasing doses and withdraw immediately if there is any indication of a recurrent hypersensitivity reaction.

➤*Special risk:* Because there is a higher frequency of isoniazid-associated hepatitis among certain patient groups, including those older than 35 years of age, daily users of alcohol, chronic liver disease, drug use, and women belonging to minority groups, particularly in the postpartum period, obtain transaminase measurements prior to starting and monthly during preventive therapy, or more frequently as needed. If any of the values exceed 3 to 5 times the ULN, temporarily discontinue isoniazid and consider restarting therapy.

➤*Pregnancy: Category C.* Isoniazid has been shown to have an embryocidal effect in rats and rabbits when given orally during pregnancy. Isoniazid was not teratogenic in reproduction studies in mice, rats and rabbits. There are no adequate and well-controlled studies in pregnant women. Use isoniazid as a treatment for active tuberculosis during pregnancy because the benefit justifies the potential risk to the fetus. Weigh the benefit of preventive therapy against a possible risk to the fetus. Generally, start preventive therapy after delivery to prevent putting the fetus at risk of exposure; the low levels of isoniazid in breast milk do not threaten the neonate. Since isoniazid is known to cross the placental barrier, carefully observe neonates of isoniazid-treated mothers for any evidence of adverse effects.

➤*Lactation:* The small concentrations of isoniazid in breast milk do not produce toxicity in the breast-feeding newborn; therefore, do not discourage breast-feeding. However, because levels of isoniazid are so low in breast milk, they can not be relied upon for prophylaxis or therapy of breast-feeding infants.

➤*Monitoring:* Carefully monitor use of isoniazid in the following: Daily users of alcohol (daily ingestion of alcohol may be associated with a higher incidence of isoniazid hepatitis); patients with active chronic liver disease or severe renal dysfunction; older than 35 years of age; concurrent use of any chronically administered medication; history of previous discontinuation of isoniazid; existence of peripheral neuropathy or conditions predisposing to neuropathy; pregnancy; injection drug use; women belonging to minority groups, particularly in the postpartum period; HIV-seropositive patients.

Drug Interactions

Isoniazid Drug Interactions			
Precipitant drug	Object drug[a]		Description
Rifampin	Isoniazid	↑	Hepatotoxicity may occur at a rate higher than either agent alone. If alterations in liver function tests occur, consider discontinuation of one or both of these agents.
Isoniazid	Acetaminophen	↑	Hepatotoxicity has been reported due to inhibition of acetaminophen metabolism. Monitor patient for acetaminophen toxicity.
Isoniazid	Carbamazepine	↑	Isoniazid hepatotoxicity may result due to carbamazepine increasing isoniazid degradation to hepatotoxic metabolites. Carbamazepine toxicity may result due to inhibition of carbamazepine metabolism by isoniazid. Monitor serum carbamazepine concentrations, monitor liver function, and adjust doses as necessary.
Carbamazepine	Isoniazid	↑	
Isoniazid	Chlorzoxazone	↑	Plasma concentrations of chlorzoxazone may be elevated, increasing therapeutic and adverse effects. Adjust the dose of chlorzoxazone as appropriate.
Isoniazid	Disulfiram	↑	The coadministration of disulfiram and isoniazid may result in acute behavioral and coordination changes. The mechanism is unknown; possible excess dopaminergic activity may occur. If acute behavioral or coordination changes develop during concurrent administration of disulfiram and isoniazid, the disulfiram dose may need to be decreased or the drug discontinued.
Isoniazid	Enflurane	↑	In rapid isoniazid acetylators, high output renal failure may occur due to nephrotoxic concentrations of inorganic fluoride. Monitor renal function in patients receiving this combination, particularly those who are rapid acetylators.
Isoniazid	Hydantoins (eg, phenytoin)	↑	Serum hydantoin levels may be increased, producing an increase in the pharmacologic and toxic effects of hydantoins. In usual therapeutic doses, phenytoin toxicity appears to be most significant in patients who are slow acetylators of isoniazid. Monitor serum hydantoin levels and observe for toxicity.
Isoniazid	Ketoconazole	↓	The therapeutic benefit of ketoconazole may be attenuated. Avoid concomitant use if possible. Monitoring of ketoconazole serum levels or antifungal activity may be necessary.
Isoniazid	Valproate	↑	A recent case study has shown a possible increase in the plasma level of valproate when coadministered with isoniazid. Monitor plasma valproate concentration when isoniazid and valproate are coadministered and make appropriate dosage adjustments of valproate.
Isoniazid	Theophylline	↑	Isoniazid may increase theophylline plasma levels. Also a slight decrease in isoniazid elimination has been noted. Monitor and adjust the dose as necessary.
Theophylline	Isoniazid	↑	

[a] ↑ = object drug increased; ↓ = object drug decreased.

➤*Drug/Food interactions:* Do not administer isoniazid with food. Studies have shown that the bioavailability of isoniazid is reduced significantly when administered with food.

Adverse Reactions

The most frequent reactions are those affecting the nervous system and the liver.

➤*CNS:* Peripheral neuropathy is the most common toxic effect. It is dose related, occurs most often in the malnourished and in those predisposed to neuritis (eg, alcoholics, diabetics), and is usually preceded by paresthesias of the feet and hands. The incidence is higher in "slow inactivators".

Other neurotoxic effects, which are uncommon with conventional doses, are convulsions, toxic encephalopathy, optic neuritis and atrophy, memory impairment, and toxic psychosis.

➤*GI:* Nausea, vomiting, epigastric distress.

➤*Hematologic:* Agranulocytosis; hemolytic, sideroblastic, or aplastic anemia; thrombocytopenia; eosinophilia.

➤*Hepatic:* Elevated serum transaminase (AST, ALT), bilirubinemia, bilirubinuria, jaundice, and occasionally severe and sometimes fatal hepatitis. The common prodromal symptoms of hepatitis are anorexia, nausea, vomiting, fatigue, malaise, and weakness. Mild hepatic dysfunction, evidenced by mild and transient elevation of serum transaminase levels occurs in 10% to 20% of patients taking isoniazid.

See the Warning box for more information.

➤*Hypersensitivity:* Fever, skin eruptions (morbilliform, maculopapular, purpuric, or exfoliative), lymphadenopathy, vasculitis.

➤*Metabolic/Nutritional:* Pyridoxine deficiency, pellagra, hyperglycemia, metabolic acidosis, gynecomastia.

➤*Miscellaneous:* Rheumatic syndrome, systemic lupus erythematosus-like syndrome.

Overdosage

➤*Symptoms:* Isoniazid overdosage produces signs and symptoms within 30 minutes to 3 hours after ingestion. Nausea, vomiting, dizziness, slurring of speech, blurring of vision, and visual hallucinations (including bright colors and strange designs) are among the early manifestations. With marked overdosage, respiratory distress and CNS depression, progressing rapidly from stupor to profound coma, are to be expected, along with severe, intractable seizures. Severe metabolic acidosis, acetonuria, and hyperglycemia are typical laboratory findings.

➤*Treatment:*

For the asymptomatic patient – Absorption of drugs from the GI tract may be decreased by giving activated charcoal. Employ gastric emptying in the asymptomatic patient. Safeguard the patient's airway when employing these procedures. Patients who acutely ingest greater than 80 mg/kg should be treated with pyridoxine IV on a gram per gram (g) basis equal to the isoniazid dose. If an unknown amount of isoniazid is ingested, consider an initial dose of 5 g of pyridoxine given over 30 to 60 minutes in adults, 80 mg/kg of pyridoxine in children.

For the symptomatic patient – Ensure adequate ventilation, support cardiac output, and protect the airway while treating seizures and attempting to limit absorption. If the dose of isoniazid is known, initially treat the patient with a slow IV bolus of pyridoxine, over 3 to 5 minutes, on a gram per gram basis, equal to the isoniazid dose. If the quantity of isoniazid ingestion is unknown, then consider an initial IV bolus of pyridoxine of 5 g in the adult or 80 mg/kg in the child. If seizures continue, the dosage of pyridoxine may be repeated. It would be rare that greater than 10 g of pyridoxine would need to be given. The maximum safe dose for pyridoxine in isoniazid intoxication is not known. If the patient does not respond to pyridoxine, diazepam may be administered. Use phenytoin cautiously because isoniazid interferes with the metabolism of phenytoin.

General – Obtain blood samples for immediate determination of gases, electrolytes, serum urea nitrogen (BUN), glucose; type and cross-match blood in preparation for possible hemodialysis.

Rapid control of metabolic acidosis – Patients with this degree of isoniazid intoxication are likely to have hypoventilation. The administration of sodium bicarbonate under these circumstances can cause exacerbation of hypercarbia. Ventilation must be monitored carefully, by measuring blood carbon dioxide levels, and supported mechanically, if there is respiratory impairment.

Dialysis – Both peritoneal and hemodialysis have been used in the management of isoniazid overdosage. These procedures are probably not required if control of seizures and acidosis is achieved with pyridoxine, diazepam, and bicarbonate.

Along with measures based on initial and repeated determination of blood gases and other laboratory tests as needed, utilize meticulous respiratory and other intensive care to protect against hypoxia, hypotension, aspiration, and pneumonitis.

ISONIAZID — INJECTION

WARNING

Hepatitis – Severe and sometimes fatal hepatitis associated with isoniazid therapy has been reported and may occur or may develop even after many months of treatment. The risk of developing hepatitis is age related. Approximate case rates by age are as follows: Less than $1/1000$ for persons younger than 20 years of age, $3/1000$ for persons in the 20- to 34-year age group, $12/1000$ for persons in the 35- to 49-year age group, $23/1000$ for persons in the 50- to 64-year age group, and $8/1000$ for persons older than 65 years of age. The risk of hepatitis is increased with daily consumption of alcohol. Precise data to provide a fatality rate for isoniazid-related hepatitis are not available; however, in a US Public Health Service surveillance study of 13,838 persons taking isoniazid, there were 8 deaths among 174 cases of hepatitis.

Therefore, patients given isoniazid should be carefully monitored and interviewed at monthly intervals. For persons 35 years of age and older, in addition to monthly symptom reviews, hepatic enzymes (specifically, AST and ALT) should be measured prior to starting isoniazid therapy and periodically throughout treatment. Isoniazid-associated hepatitis usually occurs during the first 3 months of treatment. Usually, enzyme levels return to normal despite continuance of drug, but in some cases progressive liver dysfunction occurs. Other factors associated with an increased risk of hepatitis include daily use of alcohol, chronic liver disease and injection drug use. A report suggests an increased risk of fatal hepatitis associated with isoniazid among women, particularly black and Hispanic women. The risk may also be increased during the postpartum period. More careful monitoring should be considered in these groups, possibly including more frequent laboratory monitoring. If abnormalities of liver function exceed 3 to 5 times the upper limit of normal, discontinuation of isoniazid should be strongly considered. Liver function tests are not a substitute for a clinical evaluation at monthly intervals or for the prompt assessment of signs or symptoms of adverse reactions occurring between regularly scheduled evaluations. Patients should be instructed to immediately report signs or symptoms consistent with liver damage or other adverse effects. These include any of the following: Unexplained anorexia, nausea, vomiting, dark urine, icterus, rash, persistent paresthesias of the hands and feet, persistent fatigue, weakness or fever of more than 3-day duration or abdominal tenderness, especially right upper quadrant discomfort. If these symptoms appear, or if signs suggestive of hepatic damage are detected, isoniazid should be discontinued promptly, since continued use of the drug in these cases has been reported to cause a more severe form of liver damage.

Patients with tuberculosis who have hepatitis attributed to isoniazid should be given appropriate treatment with alternative drugs. If isoniazid must be reinstituted, it should be reinstituted only after symptoms and laboratory abnormalities have cleared. The drug should be restarted in very small and gradually increasing doses and should be withdrawn immediately if there is any indication of recurrent liver involvement.

Preventive treatment should be deferred in persons with acute hepatic diseases.

Indications

➤*General information:* The risk of hepatitis must be weighed against the risk of tuberculosis in positive tuberculin reactors older than 35 years of age. However, the use of isoniazid is recommended for those with the additional risk factors listed above and on an individual basis in situations where there is likelihood of serious consequences to contacts who may become infected.

➤*Tuberculosis treatment:* For all forms of tuberculosis in which organisms are susceptible.

However, active tuberculosis must be treated with multiple concomitant antituberculosis medications to prevent the emergence of drug resistance. Single-drug treatment of active tuberculosis with isoniazid, or any other medication, is inadequate therapy.

➤*Preventive therapy:* Isoniazid is recommended as preventive therapy for the following groups, regardless of age (the criterion for a positive reaction to a skin test [in mm of induration] for each group is given in parenthesis).

HIV – Persons with human immunodeficiency virus (HIV) infection (greater than or equal to 5 mm) and persons with risk factors for HIV infection whose HIV infection status is unknown but who are suspected of having HIV infection. Preventive therapy may be considered for HIV-infected persons who are tuberculin-negative but belong to groups in which the prevalence of tuberculosis infection is high. Candidates for preventive therapy who have HIV infection should have a minimum of 12 months of therapy.

Close contacts of people with infectious tuberculosis – Close contacts of persons with newly diagnosed infectious tuberculosis (greater than or equal to 5 mm). In addition, tuberculin-negative (less than 5 mm) children, and adolescents who have been close contacts of infectious persons within the past 3 months, are candidates for preventive therapy until a repeat tuberculin skin test is done 12 weeks after contact with the infectious source. If the repeat skin test is positive (greater than 5 mm), therapy should be continued.

Recent converters – Recent converters, as indicated by a tuberculin skin test (greater than or equal to 10 mm increase within a 2-year period for those younger than 35 years old; greater than or equal to 15 mm increase for those 35 years of age and older). All infants and children younger than 4 years of age with a greater than 10 mm skin test are included in this category.

Abnormal chest radiographs – Persons with abnormal chest radiographs that show fibrotic lesions likely to represent old healed tuberculosis (greater than or equal to 5 mm). Candidates for preventive therapy who have fibrotic pulmonary lesions consistent with healed tuberculosis or who have pulmonary silicosis should have 12 months of isoniazid or 4 months of isoniazid and rifampin, concomitantly.

IV drug users – IV drug users known to be HIV-seronegative (greater than 10 mm).

Increased risk of tuberculosis – Persons with the following medical conditions that have been reported to increase the risk of tuberculosis (greater than or equal to 10 mm): Silicosis; diabetes mellitus; prolonged therapy with adrenocorticosteroids; immunosuppressive therapy; some hematologic and reticuloendothelial diseases such as leukemia or Hodgkin's disease; end-stage renal disease; clinical situations associated with substantial rapid weight loss or chronic undernutrition (eg, intestinal bypass surgery for obesity, the postgastrectomy state with or without weight loss, chronic peptic ulcer disease, chronic malabsorption syndromes, and carcinomas of the oropharynx and upper GI tract that prevent adequate nutritional intake). Candidates for preventive therapy who have fibrotic pulmonary lesions consistent with healed tuberculosis or who have pulmonary silicosis should have 12 months of isoniazid or 4 months of isoniazid and rifampin, concomitantly.

Adults younger than 35 years of age with tuberculin skin test reaction of greater than or equal to 10 mm – Additionally, in the absence of any of the above risk factors, persons younger than 35 years of age with a tuberculin skin test reaction of greater than or equal to 10 mm are also appropriate candidates for preventive therapy if they are a member of any of the following high-incidence groups: Foreign-born persons from high-prevalence countries who never received BCG vaccine; medically underserved low-income populations, including high-risk racial or ethnic minority populations, especially black patients, Hispanic patients, and Native Americans; residents of facilities for long-term care (eg, correctional institutions, nursing homes, and mental institutions).

Children less than 4 years of age – Children who are younger than 4 years old are candidates for isoniazid preventive therapy if they have greater than 10 mm induration from a PPD Mantoux tuberculin skin test.

Adults less than 35 years of age – Persons younger than 35 years of age who have none of the above risk factors, belong to none of the high-incidence groups, and have a tuberculin skin test reaction of greater than or equal to 15 mm, are appropriate candidates for preventive therapy.

Administration and Dosage

➤*General dosing considerations:* Isoniazid is used in conjunction with other effective antituberculous agents. There are 3 regimen options for the initial treatment of tuberculosis in children and adults. (See also Pulmonary Tuberculosis Without HIV Infection.)

Before isoniazid preventive therapy is initiated, bacteriologically positive or radiographically progressive tuberculosis must be excluded. Perform appropriate evaluations if extrapulmonary tuberculosis is suspected.

Continuous administration of isoniazid for a sufficient period of time is an essential part of the regimen because relapse rates are higher if chemotherapy is stopped prematurely. In the treatment of tuberculosis, resistant organisms may multiply and the emergence during the treatment may necessitate a change in the regimen.

Drug susceptibility testing should be performed on the organism initially isolated from all patients with newly diagnosed tuberculosis. If the bacilli becomes resistant, therapy must be changed to agents to which the bacilli are susceptible.

Dosage adjustment required for patients with renal function impairment. (See Renal Function Impairment.)

➤*Adults:*

Tuberculosis prophylaxis – 300 mg intramuscularly (IM) in a single daily dose for adults weighing more than 30 kg.

Tuberculosis treatment –

Usual dosage: 5 mg/kg IM (up to 300 mg) in a single daily dose, or 15 mg/kg IM (up to 900 mg) given 2 or 3 times per week.

Maximum dose: 300 mg/day (daily regimen); 900 mg (2 or 3 times/week regimen).

Off-label dosing –

Tuberculosis (once-weekly dosing): [1] = Good documentation. Oral isoniazid 15 mg/kg once per week (not to exceed 900 mg/day).

➤*Children:*

Tuberculosis prophylaxis –

Usual dosage: 10 mg/kg (up to 300 mg daily) IM in a single daily dose.

Maximum dose: 300 mg/day (daily regimen); 900 mg (twice-weekly regimen).

Alternative dosage: In situations where adherence with daily preventive therapy cannot be assured, 20 to 30 mg/kg (not to exceed 900 mg) twice weekly under the direct observation of a health care worker at the time of administration is recommended.

Tuberculosis treatment –

Usual dosage: 10 to 15 mg/kg IM (up to 300 mg) in a single daily dose, or 20 to 40 mg/kg IM (up to 900 mg) given 2 or 3 times per week.

Maximum dose: 300 mg/day (daily regimen); 900 mg (2- or 3-times-weekly regimen).

Alternative dosage: The Centers for Disease Control and Prevention recommends a dose of 20 to 30 mg/kg (up to 900 mg) given 2 times per week as an alternative to the previously described daily regimen.

➤*Renal function impairment:*

Creatinine clearance less than 10 mL/min – 50% of usual dose.

ISONIAZID — INJECTION

Hemodialysis – Dose after dialysis.

Continuous ambulatory peritoneal dialysis – 50% of usual dose given every 24 hours.

➤*Directly observed therapy:* A major cause of drug-resistant tuberculosis is patient noncompliance with treatment. The use of DOT can help ensure patient compliance with drug therapy. DOT is the observation of the patient by a health care provider or other responsible person as the patient ingests antituberculosis medications. DOT can be achieved with daily, twice-weekly or 3-times-per-week regimens, and is recommended for all patients.

➤*Concomitant pyridoxine therapy:* Coadministration of pyridoxine (B_6) is recommended in the malnourished and in those predisposed to neuropathy (eg, alcoholics, diabetics).

➤*Pulmonary tuberculosis without HIV infection:* There are 3 regimen options for the initial treatment of tuberculosis:

Option 1 – Daily isoniazid, rifampin, and pyrazinamide for 8 weeks followed by 16 weeks of isoniazid and rifampin daily or 2 to 3 times weekly. Ethambutol or streptomycin should be added to the initial regimen until sensitivity to isoniazid and rifampin is demonstrated. The addition of a fourth drug is optional if the relative prevalence of isoniazid-resistant *Mycobacterium tuberculosis* isolates in the community is less than or equal to 4%.

Option 2 – Daily isoniazid, rifampin, pyrazinamide, and streptomycin or ethambutol for 2 weeks, followed by twice-weekly administration of the same drugs for 6 weeks, subsequently twice-weekly administration of isoniazid and rifampin for 16 weeks.

Option 3 – Three times weekly with isoniazid, rifampin, pyrazinamide, and ethambutol or streptomycin for 6 months.

All regimens given twice weekly or 3 times weekly should be administered by directly observed therapy. (See Directly Observed Therapy.)

The above treatment guidelines apply only when the disease is caused by organisms that are susceptible to the standard antituberculous agents. Because of the impact of resistance to isoniazid and rifampin on the response to therapy, it is essential that health care providers initiating therapy for tuberculosis be familiar with the prevalence of drug resistance in their communities. It is suggested that ethambutol not be used in children whose vital acuity cannot be monitored.

➤*Pulmonary tuberculosis and HIV infection:* The response of the immunologically impaired host to treatment may not be satisfactory as that of a person with healthy host responsiveness. For this reason, therapeutic decisions for the impaired host must be individualized. Because patients coinfected with HIV may have problems with malabsorption, screening of antimycobacterial drug levels, especially in patients with advanced HIV disease, may be necessary to prevent the emergence of multidrug-resistant tuberculosis (MDRTB).

➤*Extrapulmonary tuberculosis:* The basic principles that underlie the treatment of pulmonary tuberculosis also apply to extrapulmonary forms of the disease. Although there have not been the same kinds of carefully conducted controlled trials of treatment of extrapulmonary tuberculosis as for pulmonary disease, increasing clinical experience indicates that 6- to 9-month short-course regimens are effective. Because of the insufficient data, miliary tuberculosis, bone/joint tuberculosis, and tuberculosis meningitis in infants and children should receive 12-month therapy.

Bacteriologic evaluation of extra pulmonary tuberculosis may be limited by the relative inaccessibility of the sites of disease. Thus, response to treatment often must be judged on the basis of clinical and radiographic findings.

The use of adjunctive therapies such as surgery and corticosteroids is more commonly required in extrapulmonary tuberculosis than in pulmonary disease. Surgery may be necessary to obtain specimens for diagnosis and to treat such processes as constrictive pericarditis and spinal cord compression from Pott disease. Corticosteroids have been shown to be of benefit in preventing cardiac constriction from tuberculous pericarditis and in decreasing the neurologic sequelae of all stages of tuberculosis meningitis, especially when administered early in the course of the disease.

➤*Pregnant women with tuberculosis:* The options previously listed must be adjusted for the pregnant patient. Streptomycin interferes with in utero development of the ear and may cause congenital deafness. Routine use of pyrazinamide is also not recommended in pregnancy because of inadequate teratogenicity data. The initial treatment regimen should consist of isoniazid and rifampin. Include ethambutol unless primary isoniazid resistance is unlikely (isoniazid resistance rate documented to be less than 4%).

➤*Multiple-drug resistant tuberculosis:* MDRTB (ie, resistance to at least isoniazid and rifampin) presents difficult treatment problems. Treatment must be individualized and based on susceptibility studies. In such cases, consultation with an expert in tuberculosis is recommended.

➤*Therapeutic drug monitoring:* The Potts-Cozart test, a simple colorimetric method of checking for isoniazid in the urine, is a useful tool for assuring patient compliance, which is essential for effective tuberculosis control. Additionally, isoniazid test strips are also available to check patient compliance.

➤*Administration:* For IM injection.

Parenteral drug products should be inspected for particulate matter and discoloration prior to administration, whenever solution and container permit.

➤*Storage/Stability:* Store at 15° to 30°C (59° to 86°F). Protect from light. Isoniazid injection may crystallize at low temperatures. If this occurs, warm the vial to room temperature before use to redissolve the crystals.

Actions

➤*Pharmacology:* Pyridoxine (B_6) deficiency is sometimes observed in adults with high doses of isoniazid and is considered probably due to its competition with pyridoxal phosphate for the enzyme apotryptophanase.

Isoniazid inhibits the synthesis of mycoloic acids, an essential component of the bacterial cell wall. At therapeutic levels isoniazid is bactericidal against actively growing intracellular and extracellular *Mycobacterium tuberculosis* organisms.

➤*Pharmacokinetics:*

Absorption/Distribution – Within 1 to 2 hours after oral administration, isoniazid produces peak blood levels which decline to ≤ 50% within 6 hours. The medicine diffuses readily into all body fluids (cerebrospinal, pleural, and ascitic), tissues, organs, and excreta (saliva, sputum, and feces). The drug also passes through the placental barrier and into milk in concentrations comparable to those in the plasma.

Metabolism – Isoniazid is metabolized primarily by acetylation and dehydrazination. The rate of acetylation is genetically determined. Approximately 50% of black patients and white patients are "slow acetylators" and the rest are "rapid acetylators"; the majority of Eskimos and Asian patients are "rapid acetylators."

The rate of acetylation does not significantly alter the effectiveness of isoniazid therapy when dosage is administered daily. However, slow acetylation may lead to higher blood levels of the drug and thus an increase in toxic reactions.

Excretion – From 50% to 70% of a dose of isoniazid is excreted in the urine in 24 hours.

➤*Microbiology:* Isoniazid-resistant *Mycobacterium tuberculosis* bacilli develop rapidly when isoniazid monotherapy is administered.

Contraindications

Severe hypersensitivity reactions, including the following: Drug-induced hepatitis; previous isoniazid-associated hepatic injury; severe adverse reactions to isoniazid such as drug fever, chills, arthritis; acute liver disease of any etiology.

Warnings/Precautions

➤*Hepatitis:* See Warning Box.

➤*Hypersensitivity reactions:* All drugs should be stopped and an evaluation made at the first sign of a hypersensitivity reaction. If isoniazid therapy must be reinstituted, the drug should be given only after symptoms have cleared. The drug should be restarted in very small and gradually increasing doses and should be withdrawn immediately if there is any indication of recurrent hypersensitivity reaction.

➤*Special risk:* Use of isoniazid should be carefully monitored in the following: Daily users of alcohol (daily ingestion of alcohol may be associated with a higher incidence of + isoniazid hepatitis); patients with active chronic liver disease or severe renal dysfunction; patients older than 35 years of age; patients with concurrent use of any chronically administered medication; patients with a history of previous discontinuation of isoniazid; patients with the existence of peripheral neuropathy or conditions predisposing to neuropathy; pregnant patients; patients with injection drug use; women belonging to minority groups, particularly in the postpartum period; HIV-seropositive patients.

➤*Pregnancy: Category C.* Isoniazid has been shown to have an embryocidal effect in rats and rabbits when given orally during pregnancy. There are no adequate and well-controlled studies in pregnant women. Isoniazid should be used as a treatment for active tuberculosis during pregnancy because the benefit justifies the potential risk to the fetus. The benefit of preventive therapy also should be weighed against a possible risk to the fetus. Preventive therapy generally should be started after delivery to prevent putting the fetus at risk of exposure; the low levels of isoniazid in breast milk do not threaten the neonate.

Since isoniazid is known to cross the placental barrier, neonates of isoniazid-treated mothers should be carefully observed for any evidence of adverse effects.

➤*Lactation:* The small concentrations of isoniazid in breast milk do not produce toxicity in the nursing newborn; therefore, breastfeeding should not be discouraged. However, because levels of isoniazid are so low in breast milk, they can not be relied upon for prophylaxis or therapy of nursing infants.

➤*Monitoring:* Periodic ophthalmologic examinations during isoniazid therapy are recommended when visual symptoms occur.

Because there is a higher frequency of isoniazid-associated hepatitis among certain patient groups, including those older than 35 years of age, daily users of alcohol, those with chronic liver disease, patients with injection drug use and women belonging to minority groups (particularly in the postpartum period), transaminase measurements should be obtained prior to starting, and monthly during, preventive therapy, or more frequently as needed. If any of the values exceed 3 to 5 times the upper limit of normal, isoniazid should be temporarily discontinued and consideration given to restarting therapy.

Drug Interactions

Isoniazid Drug Interactions

Precipitant drug	Object drug[a]		Description
Rifampin	Isoniazid	↑	Hepatotoxicity may occur at a rate higher than either agent alone. If alterations in liver function tests occur, consider discontinuation of one or both of these agents.
Isoniazid	Acetaminophen	↑	Hepatotoxicity has been reported due to inhibition of acetaminophen metabolism. Monitor patient for acetaminophen toxicity.
Isoniazid	Carbamazepine	↑	Isoniazid hepatotoxicity may result due to carbamazepine increasing isoniazid degradation to hepatotoxic metabolites. Carbamazepine toxicity may result due to inhibition of carbamazepine metabolism by isoniazid. Monitor serum carbamazepine concentrations, monitor liver function, and adjust doses as necessary.
Carbamazepine	Isoniazid	↑	
Isoniazid	Chlorzoxazone	↑	Plasma concentrations of chlorzoxazone may be elevated, increasing therapeutic and adverse effects. Adjust the dose of chlorzoxazone as appropriate.
Isoniazid	Disulfiram	↑	The coadministration of disulfiram and isoniazid may result in acute behavioral and coordination changes. The mechanism is unknown; possible excess dopaminergic activity may occur. If acute behavioral or coordination changes develop during concurrent administration of disulfiram and isoniazid, the disulfiram dose may need to be decreased or the drug discontinued.
Isoniazid	Enflurane	↑	In rapid isoniazid acetylators, high output renal failure may occur due to nephrotoxic concentrations of inorganic fluoride. Monitor renal function in patients receiving this combination, particularly those who are rapid acetylators.
Isoniazid	Hydantoins (eg, phenytoin)	↑	Serum hydantoin levels may be increased, producing an increase in the pharmacologic and toxic effects of hydantoins. In usual therapeutic doses, phenytoin toxicity appears to be most significant in patients who are slow acetylators of isoniazid. Monitor serum hydantoin levels and observe for toxicity.
Isoniazid	Ketoconazole	↓	The therapeutic benefit of ketoconazole may be attenuated. Avoid concomitant use if possible. Monitoring of ketoconazole serum levels or antifungal activity may be necessary.
Isoniazid	Valproate	↑	A recent case study has shown a possible increase in the plasma level of valproate when coadministered with isoniazid. Plasma valproate concentration should be monitored when isoniazid and valproate are coadministered, and appropriate dosage adjustments of valproate should be made.
Isoniazid	Theophylline	↑	Isoniazid may increase theophylline plasma levels. Also a slight decrease in isoniazid elimination has been noted. Monitor and adjust the dose as necessary.
Theophylline	Isoniazid	↑	

[a] ↑ = object drug increased; ↓ = object drug decreased.

Adverse Reactions

The most frequent reactions are those affecting the nervous system and the liver.

➤*CNS:* Peripheral neuropathy is the most common toxic effect. It is dose related, occurs most often in the malnourished and in those predisposed to neuritis (eg, alcoholics, diabetics), and is usually preceded by paresthesias of the feet and hands. The incidence is higher in "slow acetylators."

Other neurotoxic effects which are uncommon with conventional doses are convulsions, toxic encephalopathy, optic neuritis and atrophy, memory impairment, and toxic psychosis.

➤*GI:* Nausea, vomiting, and epigastric distress.

➤*Hematologic:* Agranulocytosis; hemolytic, sideroblastic, or aplastic anemia; thrombocytopenia; eosinophilia.

➤*Hepatic:* See Warning Box. Elevated serum transaminases (AST; ALT), bilirubinemia, bilirubinuria, jaundice, and occasionally severe and sometimes fatal hepatitis. The common prodromal symptoms of hepatitis are anorexia, nausea, vomiting, fatigue, malaise, and weakness. Mild hepatic dysfunction, evidenced by mild and transient elevation of serum transaminase levels occurs in 10% to 20% of patients taking isoniazid.

See the Warning box for more information.

➤*Hypersensitivity:* Fever, skin eruptions (morbilliform, maculopapular, purpuric, or exfoliative), lymphadenopathy, and vasculitis.

➤*Local:* Local irritation has been observed at the site of IM injection.

➤*Metabolic/Nutritional:* Pyridoxine deficiency, pellagra, hyperglycemia, metabolic acidosis, and gynecomastia.

➤*Miscellaneous:* Rheumatic syndrome and systemic lupus erythematosus-like syndrome.

Overdosage

➤*Symptoms:* Isoniazid overdosage produces signs and symptoms within 30 minutes to 3 hours after ingestion. Nausea, vomiting, dizziness, slurring of speech, blurring of vision, and visual hallucinations (including bright colors and strange designs) are among the early manifestations. With marked overdosage, respiratory distress and CNS depression, progressing rapidly from stupor to profound coma, are to be expected, along with severe, intractable seizures. Severe metabolic acidosis, acetonuria, and hyperglycemia are typical laboratory findings.

➤*Treatment:* Untreated or inadequately treated cases of gross isoniazid overdosage, 80 mg/kg to 150 mg/kg, can cause neurotoxicity and terminate fatally, but good response has been reported in most patients brought under adequate treatment within the first few hours after drug ingestion.

For the asymptomatic patient – Absorption of drugs from the GI tract may be decreased by giving activated charcoal. Gastric emptying should also be employed in the asymptomatic patient. Safeguard the patient's airway when employing these procedures. Patients who acutely ingest more than 80 mg/kg should be treated with IV pyridoxine on a gram per gram basis equal to the isoniazid dose. If an unknown amount if isoniazid is ingested, consider an initial dose of 5 g of pyridoxine given over 30 to 60 minutes in adults, or 80 mg/kg of pyridoxine in children.

For the symptomatic patient – Ensure adequate ventilation, support cardiac output, and protect the airway while treating seizures and attempting to limit absorption. If the dose of isoniazid is known, the patient should be treated initially with a slow IV bolus of pyridoxine, over 3 to 5 minutes, on a gram per gram basis, equal to the isoniazid dose. If the quantity of isoniazid ingestion is unknown, then consider an initial IV bolus of pyridoxine of 5 g in the adult or 80 mg/kg in the child. If seizures continue, the dosage of pyridoxine may be repeated. It would be rare that more than 10 g of pyridoxine would need to be given. The maximum safe dose of pyridoxine in isoniazid intoxication is not known. If the patient does not respond to pyridoxine, diazepam may be administered. Phenytoin should be used cautiously, because isoniazid interferes with the metabolism of phenytoin.

Obtain blood samples for immediate determination of gases, electrolytes, BUN, glucose; type and cross-match blood in preparation for possible hemodialysis.

Rapid control of metabolic acidosis – Patients with this degree of INH intoxication are likely to have hypoventilation. The administration of sodium bicarbonate under these circumstances can cause exacerbation of hypercarbia. Ventilation must be monitored carefully, by measuring blood carbon dioxide levels, and supported mechanically, if there is respiratory insufficiency.

Dialysis – Both peritoneal and hemodialysis have been used in the management of isoniazid overdosage. These procedures are probably not required if control of seizures and acidosis is achieved with pyridoxine, diazepam and bicarbonate.

Patient Information

Use as directed. Do not discontinue except on the advice of a physician.

Avoid certain foods (eg, fish [skipjack, tuna], and perhaps tyramine-containing products).

Notify physician of weakness, fatigue, loss of appetite, nausea and vomiting, yellowing of skin or eyes, darkening of urine, or numbness or tingling in hands and feet.

ISONIAZID COMBINATIONS

Rx	**Rifater** (Aventis)	**Tablets:** 120 mg rifampin, 50 mg isoniazid, 300 mg pyrazinamide	(Rifater). Sugar-coated. Light beige. In 60s.
Rx	**IsonaRif** (VersaPharm)	**Capsules:** 300 mg rifampin and 150 mg isoniazid	Lactose. (West-ward 3238). Scarlet opaque. In 60s.
Rx	**Rifamate** (Aventis)		(RIFAMATE). Red. In 60s.

ISONIAZID COMBINATIONS — ORAL

Refer to the general discussion in the Antituberculosal Agents Introduction.

Indications

➤*ISONIAZID:* Bacteriocidal against *Mycobacterium tuberculosis.* See individual monograph.

➤*PYRAZINAMIDE:* Acts against *M. tuberculosis.* See individual monograph.

➤*RIFAMPIN:* Bactericidal against *M. tuberculosis.* See individual monograph.

Warnings/Precautions

➤*Pregnancy: Category C.* Although rifampin has been reported to cross the placental barrier and appear in cord blood, the effect of rifampin, alone or in combination with other antituberculosis drugs, on the human fetus is not known. An increase in congenital malformations, primarily spina bifida and cleft palate, has been reported in the offspring of rodents given oral doses of rifampin 150 to 250 mg/kg/day during pregnancy. The possible teratogenic potential in women capable of bearing children should be carefully weighed against the benefits of therapy.

In rats and rabbits, it has been reported that isoniazid may exert an embryocidal effect when administered orally during pregnancy, although no isoniazid-related congenital anomalies have been found in reproduction studies in mammalian species (mice, rats, and rabbits). These drugs should be prescribed during pregnancy only when therapeutically necessary. The benefit of preventive therapy should be weighed against a possible risk to the fetus. Preventive treatment generally should be started after delivery because of the increased risk of tuberculosis for new mothers.

➤*Lactation:* Because rifampin, isoniazid, and pyrazinamide are known to pass into maternal breast milk, a decision should be made whether to discontinue nursing or to discontinue rifampin, isoniazid, and pyrazinamide, taking into account the importance of the drug to the mother.

RIFAMPIN (Rifampicin)

Rx	**Rifampin** (Various, eg, Eon)	**Capsules; oral:** 150 mg	In 30s and 100s.
Rx	**Rifadin** (Sanofi-Aventis)		(Rifadin 150). Maroon and scarlet. In 30s.
Rx	**Rifampin** (Various, eg, Eon, UDL)	**Capsules; oral:** 300 mg	In 30s, 60s, 100s, and 500s.
Rx	**Rifadin** (Sanofi-Aventis)		(Rifadin 300). Maroon and scarlet. In 60s and 100s.
Rx	**Rimactane** (Novartis)		(Ciba 154). Scarlet and caramel. In 30s, 60s, and 100s.
Rx	**Rifampin** (Akorn Strides)	**Injection, lyophilized powder for solution:** 600 mg	In vials.
Rx	**Rifadin** (Sanofi-Aventis)		In vials.

RIFAMPIN — ORAL AND INJECTION

Refer to the general discussion in the Antituberculosis Agents Introduction.

Indications

➤*Neisseria meningitidis carriers:* For treatment of asymptomatic carriers of *N. meningitidis* to eliminate meningococci from the nasopharynx. Rifampin is not indicated for the treatment of meningococcal infection because of the possibility of the rapid emergence of resistant organisms.

➤*Tuberculosis:*

Oral – For the treatment of all forms of tuberculosis. A 3-drug regimen consisting of rifampin, isoniazid, and pyrazinamide is recommended in the initial phase of short-course therapy that is usually continued for 2 months. The Advisory Council for the Elimination of Tuberculosis (ACET), the American Thoracic Society (ATS), and Centers for Disease Control and Prevention (CDC) recommend that either streptomycin or ethambutol be added as a fourth drug in a regimen containing isoniazid, rifampin, and pyrazinamide for initial treatment of tuberculosis unless the likelihood of isoniazid resistance is very low. Reassess the need for a fourth drug when the results of susceptibility testing are known. If community rates of isoniazid resistance are currently less than 4%, an initial treatment regimen with fewer than 4 drugs may be considered.

Intravenous – For initial treatment and retreatment of tuberculosis when the drug cannot be taken by mouth.

➤*Off-label uses:*

Catheter-related bloodstream infections (adults) – [2] = Fair documentation. The use of rifampin in catheter-related bloodstream infections may be appropriate when added to vancomycin when the infection is caused by methicillin-resistant *Staphylococcus aureus*.

Cholestatic pruritus (adults) – [1] = Good documentation. The American Association for the Study of Liver Diseases practice guideline for the management of primary biliary cirrhosis recommends cholestyramine as the first-line drug for the treatment of pruritus associated with liver disease. In patients who are intolerant of or who fail therapy with cholestyramine, rifampin is recommended as a second-line agent.

Tuberculosis (intermittent dosing) – [1] = Good documentation. According to the ATS, CDC, and Infectious Diseases Society of America joint guidelines on the treatment of tuberculosis, oral or intravenous (IV) rifampin should be given as initial treatment in combination with isoniazid, pyrazinamide, and ethambutol for 2 months, followed by a 4- to 7-month continuation phase. The Food and Drug Administration has approved oral or IV rifampin 10 mg/kg daily, not to exceed 600 mg/day. The guidelines also recommended oral or IV rifampin 10 mg 2 or 3 times weekly.

Other possible off-label uses – Rifampin has a broad antibacterial spectrum. Use in monotherapy is limited to *Haemophilus influenzae* type B. Rifampin, in combination with other effective agents, has been used in combination for the following: To clear pharyngeal carriage of group A beta-hemolytic streptococcus; eradicate pharyngeal carriage of group b streptococci (GBS) in infants who have had recurrent GBS sepsis; treat manifestations of cat scratch disease caused by *Bartonella henselae*; treat resistant *Streptococcus pneumoniae meningitis*; treat severe staphylococcal bone and joint infections; treat prosthetic valve endocarditis due to coagulase-negative staphylococci; treat *Aspergillus*; treat Leprosy. Rifampin, in combination with other agents, has also shown activity against *S. pneumoniae, S. aureus, Staphylococcus epidermidis, Corynebacterium jeikeium, Listeria monocytogenes, Neisseria gonorrhoeae, Moraxella catarrhalis, Francisella tularensis, Brucella* sp, *N. meningitides*, and *Chlamydia trachomatis*. Rifampin has been used for prophylaxis in high-risk, close contacts of patients infected with *Neisseria meningitidis*. Dosage in adults is 600 mg every 12 hours for 2 days; dosage in children older than 1 month is 10 mg/kg (maximum dose 600 mg) every 12 hours for 2 days; dosage in infants ≤ 1 month is 5 mg/kg every 12 hours for 2 days.

Administration and Dosage

➤*General dosing considerations:* IV doses are the same as oral doses.

Use with at least one other antituberculous agent.

➤*Adults:*

N. meningitidis carriers – 600 mg every 12 hours for 2 days.

Tuberculosis –

Usual dosage: 10 mg/kg in a single daily administration not to exceed 600 mg once daily.

Maximum dose: 600 mg/day.

Duration of therapy: Following the initial phase, continue treatment with rifampin and isoniazid for at least 4 months. Continue treatment for longer if the patient is still sputum- or culture-positive, if resistant organisms are present, or if the patient is HIV positive.

Concomitant therapy: A 3-drug regimen consisting of rifampin, isoniazid, and pyrazinamide is recommended in the initial phase of short-course therapy that is usually continued for 2 months. The ACET, the ATS, and CDC recommend that either streptomycin or ethambutol be added as a fourth drug in a regimen containing isoniazid, rifampin, and pyrazinamide for initial treatment of tuberculosis unless the likelihood of isoniazid resistance is very low. Reassess the need for a fourth drug when the results of susceptibility testing are known. If community rates of isoniazid resistance are currently less than 4%, an initial treatment regimen with fewer than 4 drugs may be considered.

Off-label dosing –

Catheter-related bloodstream infections (adults): [2] = Fair documentation. 10 mg/kg, in a single daily administration, not to exceed 600 mg/day, orally or IV.

Cholestatic pruritus: [1] = Good documentation. 150 mg/day orally if bilirubin is less than 3 mg/dL or 150 mg twice daily if bilirubin is 3 mg/dL or higher.

Tuberculosis (intermittent dosing): [1] = Good documentation. 10 mg/kg orally or IV twice weekly or 3 times weekly, not to exceed 600 mg/day.

➤*Children:*

N. meningitidis carriers –

1 month of age or older:

- *Usual dosage* – 10 mg/kg (up to 600 mg/dose) every 12 hours for 2 days.
- *Maximum dose* – 600 mg/dose.

Younger than 1 month of age: 5 mg/kg every 12 hours for 2 days.

Tuberculosis –

Usual dosage: 10 to 20 mg/kg (up to 600 mg/day).

Maximum dose: 600 mg/day.

RIFAMPIN — ORAL AND INJECTION

Duration of therapy: Following the initial phase, continue treatment with rifampin and isoniazid for at least 4 months. Continue treatment for longer if the patient is still sputum- or culture-positive, if resistant organisms are present, or if the patient is HIV positive.

Concomitant therapy: A 3-drug regimen consisting of rifampin, isoniazid, and pyrazinamide is recommended in the initial phase of short-course therapy that is usually continued for 2 months. The Advisory Council for the Elimination of Tuberculosis, the American Thoracic Society (ATS), and Centers for Disease Control and Prevention (CDC) recommend that either streptomycin or ethambutol be added as a fourth drug in a regimen containing isoniazid, rifampin, and pyrazinamide for initial treatment of tuberculosis unless the likelihood of isoniazid resistance is very low. Reassess the need for a fourth drug when the results of susceptibility testing are known. If community rates of isoniazid resistance are currently less than 4%, an initial treatment regimen with fewer than 4 drugs may be considered.

➤*Renal function impairment:* For patients with creatinine clearance less than 50 mL/min or for patients receiving hemodialysis or continuous ambulatory peritoneal dialysis, administer 50% to 100% of the usual dose. No supplemental dose is required after dialysis.

For patients receiving continuous renal replacement therapy, one reference suggests 300 to 600 mg IV every 12 to 24 hours. The appropriate dosing regimen is highly dependent on the clinical indication.

➤*Preparation for administration:*

Extemporaneous oral suspension – Preparation of suspension (to contain rifampin 10 mg/mL). Empty the contents of 4 rifampin 300 mg (or 8 rifampin 150 mg) capsules onto a piece of weighing paper. If necessary, gently crush the capsule contents with a spatula to produce a fine powder. Transfer the powder into a 4 oz amber glass or plastic (high density polyethylene [HDPE], polypropylene, or polycarbonate) prescription bottle. Rinse the paper and spatula with 20 mL of simple syrup (*Syrup NF*, Humco Laboratories), *Syrpalta syrup* (Emerson Laboratories), or raspberry syrup (Humco Laboratories), and add the rinse to the bottle. Shake vigorously. Add 100 mL of syrup to the bottle. Shake vigorously.

Shake well prior to administration.

Solution for IV infusion – Reconstitute the lyophilized powder by transferring 10 mL of sterile water for injection to a vial containing 600 mg of rifampin. Swirl vial gently to completely dissolve the antibiotic. The resultant solution contains rifampin 60 mg/mL and is stable at room temperature for 24 hours. Withdraw a volume equivalent to the amount of rifampin calculated to be administered and add to 500 mL of infusion medium. Mix well and infuse at a rate allowing for complete infusion in 3 hours. Alternatively, the amount of rifampin calculated to be administered may be added to 100 mL of infusion medium and infused in 30 minutes.

➤*Administration:* Rifampin can be administered by the oral route or by IV infusion.

Oral administration – It is recommended that oral rifampin be administered once daily, either 1 hour before or 2 hours after a meal, with a full glass of water. For patients in whom capsule swallowing is difficult or when lower doses are needed, a rifampin suspension can be prepared (see Preparation for Administration).

IV administration – Add rifampin calculated to be administered to 500 mL of infusion medium and infuse at a rate allowing for complete infusion in 3 hours. Alternatively, the amount of rifampin calculated to be administered may be added to 100 mL of infusion medium and infused in 30 minutes. Rifampin must not be administered by IM or subcutaneous route.

➤*Extravasation:* Avoid extravasation during injection; local irritation and inflammation because of extravascular infiltration of the infusion have been observed. If these occur, discontinue the infusion and restart at another site.

➤*Admixture compatibility:* Physical incompatibility (precipitate) was observed with undiluted (5 mg/mL) and diluted (1 mg/mL in normal saline) diltiazem and rifampin (6 mg/mL in normal saline) during simulated Y-site administration.

➤*Storage/Stability:*

Capsules – Store in a dry place and avoid excessive heat.

Extemporaneous oral suspension – The extemporaneously prepared oral suspension is stable for 4 weeks when stored at room temperature or in a refrigerator (2° to 8°C [36° to 46°F]).

Solutions for IV infusion – Reconstitutions with sterile water for injection are stable at room temperature for 24 hours. Dilutions in dextrose 5% for injection are stable at room temperature for up to 4 hours and should be prepared and used within this time. Precipitation of rifampin from the infusion solution may occur beyond this time. Dilutions in normal saline are stable at room temperature for up to 24 hours and should be prepared and used within this time. Other infusion solutions are not recommended.

Actions

➤*Pharmacology:* Rifampin inhibits DNA-dependent RNA polymerase activity in susceptible cells. Specifically, it interacts with bacterial RNA polymerase but does not inhibit the mammalian enzyme. Cross-resistance has only been shown with other rifamycins. Rifampin at therapeutic levels has demonstrated bactericidal activity against intracellular and extracellular *Mycobacterium tuberculosis* organisms.

➤*Pharmacokinetics:*

Absorption/Distribution – Rifampin, 600 mg administered orally, is almost completely absorbed and achieves mean peak plasma levels within 1 to 4 hours. The peak level averages at 7 mcg/mL but may vary from 4 to 32 mcg/mL. In children, mean peak serum levels range from 3.5 to 15 mcg/mL. Absorption of rifampin is reduced by approximately 30% when the drug is ingested with food.

Following administration of a 300 or 600 mg IV dose in 12 volunteers, mean peak plasma concentrations were 9 and 17 mcg/mL, respectively. The average plasma concentrations remained detectable for 8 and 12 hours, respectively. Volumes of distribution at steady state were approximately 0.66 and approximately 0.64 L/kg for the 300 and 600 mg IV doses, respectively. After repeated once daily infusions of 600 mg in 5 patients for 7 days, concentrations decreased from 5.8 mcg/mL 8 hours after the infusion on day 1 to 2.6 mcg/mL 8 hours after the infusion on day 7.

Metabolism – Rifampin is metabolized in the liver by deacetylation; the metabolite is still active against *M. tuberculosis*. It undergoes enterohepatic circulation; however, the deacetylated metabolite is poorly absorbed. The half-life is approximately 3 hours after a 600 mg oral dose, up to 5.1 hours after a 900 mg oral dose. With repeated administration, the half-life decreases and averages approximately 2 to 3 hours.

Excretion – Elimination occurs mainly through the bile and, to a much lesser extent, the urine. Dosage adjustment is not necessary in renal failure, but is with hepatic dysfunction. Rifampin is not significantly removed by hemodialysis. The elimination of the larger dose was not as rapid.

Special populations –

Children:

• *Oral* – In 1 study, pediatric patients 6 to 58 months of age were given rifampin suspended in simple syrup or as dry powder mixed with applesauce at a dose of 10 mg/kg body weight. Peak serum concentrations of approximately 10.7 and approximately 11.5 mcg/mL were obtained 1 hour after preprandial ingestion of the drug suspension and the applesauce mixture, respectively. After the administration of either preparation, the half-life of rifampin averaged 2.9 hours. It should be noted that in other studies in pediatric populations, at doses of 10 mg/kg body weight, mean peak serum concentrations of 3.5 to 15 mcg/mL have been reported.

• *IV* – In children 0.25 to 12.8 years of age (n = 12), the mean peak serum concentration was 26 mcg/mL following a 300 mg/m² infusion, 11.7 to 41.5 mcg/mL 1 to 4 days after initiation of therapy, and 13.6 to 37.4 mcg/mL 5 to 14 days after initiation of therapy. The half-life was 1.17 to 3.19 hours.

Contraindications

Hypersensitivity to any rifamycin; patients who are also receiving ritonavir-boosted saquinavir due to an increased risk of severe hepatocellular toxicity; patients who are also receiving atazanavir, darunavir, fosamprenavir, saquinavir, or tipranavir due to the potential of rifampin to substantially decrease plasma concentrations of these antiviral drugs, which may result in loss of antiviral efficacy and/or development of viral resistance.

Warnings/Precautions

➤*Hepatotoxicity:* There have been fatalities associated with jaundice in patients with liver disease or patients receiving rifampin concomitantly with other hepatotoxic agents. Since an increased risk may exist for individuals with liver disease, weigh benefits against risk of further liver damage. Carefully monitor liver function, especially AST and ALT, prior to therapy and then every 2 to 4 weeks during therapy. Withdraw rifampin if signs of hepatocellular damage occur.

➤*Hyperbilirubinemia:* This results from competition between rifampin and bilirubin for excretory pathways of the liver at the cell level can occur in the early days of treatment. An isolated report showing a moderate rise in bilirubin or transaminase level is not in itself an indication to interrupt treatment. Make the decision based on repeat tests and the patient's clinical condition.

➤*Porphyria:* Isolated reports have associated porphyria exacerbation with rifampin administration.

➤*Meningococci resistance:* The possibility of rapid emergence of resistant meningococci restricts use to short-term treatment of asymptomatic carrier state. Rifampin is not to be used for treatment of meningococcal disease.

➤*Intermittent therapy:* May be used if the patient cannot or will not self-administer drugs on a daily basis. Closely monitor patients on intermittent therapy for compliance, and caution against intentional or accidental interruption of prescribed therapy because of increased risk of serious adverse reactions.

➤*Red discoloration of body fluids:* Urine, sputum, sweat, and tears may be red-orange colored. Soft contact lenses may be permanently stained. Advise patients of these possibilities.

➤*Thrombocytopenia:* This reaction has occurred, primarily with high dose intermittent therapy, but has also been noted after resumption of interrupted treatment. It rarely occurs during well-supervised daily therapy. This effect is reversible if the drug is discontinued as soon as purpura occurs. Cerebral hemorrhage and fatalities have occurred when rifampin administration has continued or resumed after appearance of purpura.

➤*Hypersensitivity reactions:* These reactions have occurred during intermittent therapy or when treatment was resumed following accidental or intentional interruption and were reversible with rifampin discontinuation and appropriate therapy. Refer to Management of Acute Hypersensitivity Reactions (see Adverse Reactions).

➤*Pregnancy: Category C.* The effect of rifampin (alone or in combination with other antituberculous drugs) on the human fetus is not known. Rifampin crosses the placental barrier and appears in cord blood. It is teratogenic in rodents given oral doses of 15 to 25 times the human dose. An increase in congenital malformations, primarily spina bifida and cleft palate, has occurred in the offspring of rodents given oral doses of 150 to 250 mg/kg/day. Imperfect osteogenesis and embryotoxicity occurred in rabbits given doses

RIFAMPIN — ORAL AND INJECTION

up to 20 times the usual human daily dose. When administered during the last few weeks of pregnancy, rifampin can cause postnatal hemorrhages in the mother and infant for which treatment with vitamin K may be indicated. Carefully weigh possible teratogenic potential in women capable of bearing children against benefits of therapy (also see Antituberculosal Drugs introduction).

Carefully observe neonates of rifampin-treated mothers for any adverse effects.

➤*Lactation:* Rifampin is excreted in breast milk. Decide whether to discontinue nursing or discontinue the drug, taking into account the importance of the drug to the mother.

➤*Children:* Safety and efficacy in pediatric patients have not been established.

➤*Monitoring:* Perform baseline measurements of hepatic enzymes, bilirubin, serum creatinine, a complete blood count, and a platelet count (or estimate) in adults treated for tuberculosis with rifampin. Baseline tests are unnecessary in pediatric patients unless a complicating condition is known or clinically suspected.

Drug Interactions

Rifampin Drug Interactions

Precipitant drug	Object drug[a]		Description
Aminosalicylic acid, oral	Rifampin	↓	Aminosalicylic acid decreases the effect of rifampin. Give the combination of these 2 agents at an interval of 8 to 12 hours apart.
Halothane	Rifampin	↑	Hepatotoxicity and hepatic encephalopathy have been reported.
Rifampin	Antiarrhythmics (eg, amiodarone, disopyramide, mexiletine, propafenone, quinidine, tocainide)	↓	Serum concentrations of antiarrhythmics may be decreased because of CYP3A4 induction by rifampin. Closely monitor serum concentrations when starting or stopping rifampin.
Rifampin	ACE inhibitors (eg, enalapril)	↓	The pharmacologic effects of enalapril may be decreased, resulting in a decrease in antihypertensive control. The mechanism by which this occurs is unknown. Monitor the patient's blood pressure; consider an alternative antihypertensive if blood pressure remains uncontrolled.
Rifampin	Anticoagulants	↓	Rifampin decreases the anticoagulation activity of warfarin because of increased hepatic microsomal enzyme metabolism. Increased dosage of anticoagulants may be needed. Monitor coagulation parameters closely when rifampin is discontinued.
Rifampin	Azole antifungals (eg, fluconazole, itraconazole, ketoconazole)	↓	Rifampin may induce the metabolism of azole antifungal agents. Ketoconazole may interfere with rifampin absorption decreasing serum rifampin levels. If concurrent use cannot be avoided, monitor and adjust the dosages as needed.
Azole antifungals (eg, fluconazole, itraconazole, ketoconazole)	Rifampin	↓	
Rifampin	Barbiturates	↓	Rifampin may stimulate liver microsomal enzymes resulting in more rapid degradation of barbiturates. When rifampin is added to the regimen of a patient receiving a barbiturate, monitor the patient for changes in clinical status and plasma barbiturate levels. The barbiturate dosage may need to be raised.
Rifampin	Benzodiazepines (eg, diazepam, midazolam, triazolam)	↓	The pharmacologic effects of diazepam, midazolam, and triazolam may be decreased because of increased metabolism of benzodiazepines. Monitor the clinical response to the benzodiazepine when starting or stopping rifampin.
Rifampin	Beta blockers (eg, bisoprolol, metoprolol, propranolol)	↓	The pharmacologic effects of certain beta blockers (eg, bisoprolol, metoprolol, propranolol) may be reduced possibly because of increased hepatic metabolism from enzyme induction by rifampin. A 3- to 4-week washout period may be necessary for the enzyme induction effect to diminish. Close monitoring of therapeutic response is essential.
Rifampin	Buspirone	↓	Buspirone plasma concentrations and pharmacologic effects may be decreased because of induction of first-pass metabolism (CYP3A4) by rifampin. Escalation of buspirone dose may be necessary.
Rifampin	Chloramphenicol	↓	Chloramphenicol metabolism may be increased because of induction of hepatic microsomal enzymes by rifampin.
Rifampin	Contraceptives, oral	↓	Reduced oral contraceptive efficacy and an increased incidence of menstrual abnormalities may occur. Advise patients to use an additional form of birth control while receiving rifampin therapy.
Rifampin	Corticosteroids	↓	The pharmacologic effects of corticosteroids may be decreased. Lack of effect may occur within a few days of adding rifampin and reverse 2 to 3 weeks following discontinuation. Avoid coadministration.
Rifampin	Cyclosporine	↓	The immunosuppressive effects of cyclosporine may be reduced 2 days following the initiation of rifampin and persist for 1 to 3 weeks after discontinuation. Cyclosporine bioavailability is decreased because of induction of intestinal cytochrome P450 enzymes. Increased doses may be necessary; avoid this combination if possible.
Rifampin	Delavirdine	↓	Rifampin may increase the metabolism of delavirdine by enzyme induction thereby decreasing the plasma concentrations. Avoid concurrent use.
Rifampin	Digoxin	↓	Rifampin coadministration may decrease the serum concentration of digoxin. An increased digoxin dosage may be necessary.
Rifampin	Doxycycline	↓	Rifampin may decrease the serum concentration and half-life of doxycycline, possibly reducing the therapeutic effect. Monitor the clinical response.
Rifampin	Estrogens	↓	Rifampin may impair the effectiveness of estrogens by inducing drug metabolism, decreasing AUC, and half-life. Consider alternate methods of contraception.
Rifampin	Fluoroquinolones	↓	Rifampin may accelerate the metabolism of fluoroquinolones. It may be necessary to adjust the dosage of a fluoroquinolone.
Rifampin	Haloperidol	↓	Rifampin may decrease the plasma concentration and clinical effectiveness of haloperidol. When adding or discontinuing rifamycin therapy, carefully monitor the clinical response of the patient. Adjust the haloperidol dose as indicated.
Rifampin	Hydantoins	↓	Serum hydantoin levels may be decreased because of rifampin increasing hepatic enzyme metabolism. Monitor serum hydantoin levels and observe the patient.
Rifampin	Isoniazid	↑	Hepatotoxicity may occur at a rate higher than with either agent alone. If alterations in liver function tests occur, consider discontinuation of one or both agents.
Isoniazid	Rifampin	↑	

RIFAMPIN — ORAL AND INJECTION

Rifampin Drug Interactions			
Precipitant drug	Object drug[a]		Description
Rifampin	Losartan	⬇	Rifampin may increase the metabolism of losartan. Observe the clinical response of the patient when starting or stopping rifampin.
Rifamycins	Macrolide antibiotics (eg, clarithromycin)	⬇	The metabolism of rifampin may be inhibited, while the metabolism of the macrolide antibiotic may be increased. Monitor for increased side effects and a decrease in the response to the macrolide antibiotic.
Macrolide antibiotics (eg, clarithromycin)	Rifamycins	⬆	
Rifampin	Narcotic analgesics (eg, methadone, morphine)	⬇	Patients may experience withdrawal symptoms. Rifampin primarily appears to stimulate the hepatic metabolism of methadone. A higher dose of narcotic analgesics may be required during concurrent administration of rifampin.
Rifampin	Nifedipine	⬇	The therapeutic effects of nifedipine may be reduced. Monitor blood pressure and angina symptoms. Adjust the nifedipine dose accordingly or consider a different antihypertensive medication.
Rifampin	Ondansetron	⬇	Plasma concentrations of ondansetron may be reduced. Consider use of an alternative antiemetic.
Rifampin	Progestins	⬇	Rifampin may increase the elimination rate of progestin-containing oral contraceptives. Avoid coadministration.
Rifampin	Protease inhibitors (eg, indinavir, nelfinavir, ritonavir)	⬇	Rifampin may increase the metabolism of protease inhibitors while protease inhibitors may decrease rifampin metabolism. Avoid concomitant use.
Protease inhibitors (eg, indinavir, nelfinavir, ritonavir)	Rifampin	⬆	
Rifampin	Quinine derivatives	⬇	Rifampin increases the hepatic clearance of quinine derivatives. Enzyme induction can persist for several days following discontinuation of rifampin. Addition of rifampin to stable quinine derivative regimens may require increased doses of quinine derivatives to maintain the desired therapeutic effect. Withdrawal of rifampin may result in quinine derivative dose-related toxicity. Monitor quinine derivative serum levels and the ECG.
Rifampin	Sulfapyridine	⬇	Plasma concentrations of sulfapyridine may be reduced following the concomitant administration of sulfasalazine and rifampin. This finding may be the result of alteration in the colonic bacteria responsible for the reduction of sulfasalazine to sulfapyridine and mesalamine.
Rifampin	Sulfones	⬇	The pharmacologic effect of dapsone may be decreased because of increased metabolism of dapsone. Higher doses of dapsone may be necessary.
Rifampin	Sulfonylureas	⬇	Rifampin may decrease the half-life and serum levels while increasing the clearance of tolbutamide and chlorpropamide, possibly resulting in hyperglycemia. Closely monitor blood glucose and possibly increase the sulfonylurea dose.
Rifampin	Tacrolimus	⬇	The immunosuppressive effects of tacrolimus may be reduced as early as 2 days following the initiation of rifampin. Closely monitor tacrolimus whole blood concentrations when starting or stopping rifampin.
Rifampin	Theophylline	⬇	The addition of rifampin may result in decreased theophylline levels and exacerbation of pulmonary symptoms. Monitor theophylline levels.
Rifampin	Thyroid hormones	⬇	Thyroid stimulating hormone (TSH) levels may be increased, resulting in hypothyroidism. Monitor thyroid status in patients receiving both drugs.
Rifampin	Tricyclic antidepressants (TCAs)	⬇	TCA levels may decrease because of increased hepatic metabolism of TCAs. Consider monitoring TCA concentrations when starting, stopping, or altering the rifampin dose.
Rifampin	Verapamil	⬇	There is an increase in first-pass hepatic metabolism resulting in a lowered bioavailability of oral verapamil. Use IV verapamil or substitute another agent for either verapamil or rifampin.
Rifampin	Zidovudine	⬇	The pharmacologic effects of zidovudine may be decreased possibly because of increased hepatic metabolism.
Rifampin	Zolpidem	⬇	Plasma concentrations and therapeutic effects of zolpidem may be reduced. Monitor the clinical response of the patient.

[a] ⬇ = object drug decreased; ⬆ = object drug increased.

➤*Cytochrome P450:* Rifampin is known to induce certain cytochrome P450 enzymes. Administration of rifampin with drugs that undergo biotransformation through these metabolic pathways may accelerate elimination of coadministered drugs. To maintain optimum therapeutic blood levels, dosages of drugs metabolized by these enzymes may require adjustment when starting or stopping concomitantly administered rifampin.

➤*Drug/Lab test interactions:* Therapeutic levels of rifampin inhibit standard assays for serum folate and vitamin B_{12}. Consider alternative methods when determining folate and vitamin B_{12} concentrations in the presence of rifampin.

Hepatitis or shock-like syndrome with hepatic involvement and abnormal liver function tests have been reported.

Transient abnormalities in liver function tests (eg, elevation in serum bilirubin, alkaline phosphatase, and serum transaminases), and reduced biliary excretion of contrast media used for visualization of the gallbladder have also been observed. Therefore, perform these tests before the morning dose of rifampin.

➤*Drug/Food interactions:* Food interferes with the absorption of rifampin, possibly resulting in increased peak plasma concentrations. Take on an empty stomach, either 1 hour before or 2 hours after a meal, with a full glass of water.

Adverse Reactions

High doses of rifampin (more than 600 mg) given once or twice weekly have resulted in a high incidence of adverse reactions including: The "flu-like" syndrome (eg, fever, chills, malaise); hematopoietic reactions (eg, leukopenia, thrombocytopenia, acute hemolytic anemia); cutaneous, GI and hepatic reactions; shortness of breath; shock; renal failure. Recent studies indicate that regimens using twice-weekly doses of rifampin 600 mg plus isoniazid 15 mg/kg are much better tolerated.

➤*CNS:* Headache; ataxia; drowsiness; fatigue; dizziness; inability to concentrate; mental confusion; psychoses; generalized numbness; behavioral changes (rare).

➤*Dermatologic:* Rash; flushing; itching (with or without rash).

➤*GI:* Heartburn; epigastric distress; anorexia; nausea; vomiting; gas; cramps; diarrhea; jaundice; pseudomembranous colitis.

➤*Hematologic:* Transient leukopenia; hemolytic anemia; decreased hemoglobin; hemolysis; disseminated intravascular coagulation; thrombocytopenia (see Precautions).

➤*Hepatic:* Hepatitis or shock-like syndrome with hepatic involvement (rare); abnormal liver function tests; transient abnormalities in liver function tests (elevations in serum bilirubin, BSP, alkaline phosphatase, serum transaminases). Perform BSP test prior to the morning dose of rifampin to avoid false-positive results.

➤*Hypersensitivity:* Pruritus; urticaria; pemphigoid reaction; erythema multiforme including Stevens-Johnson syndrome; toxic epidermal necrolysis; vasculitis; eosinophilia; sore mouth; sore tongue; conjunctivitis. Rarely hemolysis, hemoglobinuria, hematuria, renal insufficiency, or acute renal failure have occurred.

➤*Musculoskeletal:* Ataxia; muscular weakness; pain in extremities; myopathy.

➤*Renal:* Interstitial nephritis; acute tubular necrosis.

RIFAMPIN — ORAL AND INJECTION

➤*Miscellaneous:* Visual disturbances; menstrual disturbances; fever; elevations in BUN and serum uric acid; adrenal insufficiency in patients with compromised adrenal function; edema of face and extremities; shortness of breath; wheezing; decrease in blood pressure; shock; flu syndrome (eg, fever, chills, headache, dizziness, bone pain).

Overdosage

➤*Symptoms:* The minimum acute lethal or toxic dose is not well established. However, nonfatal acute overdoses in adults have been reported with doses ranging from 9 to 12 g rifampin. Fatal acute overdoses in adults have been reported with doses ranging from 14 to 60 g. Alcohol or a history of alcohol abuse was involved in some of the fatal and nonfatal reports. Nonfatal overdoses in pediatric patients ages 1 to 4 years of age or 100 mg/kg for 1 to 2 doses has been reported.

Nausea, vomiting, abdominal pain, pruritus, headache, and increasing lethargy will probably occur shortly after ingestion; unconsciousness may occur with severe hepatic disease. Transient increases in liver enzymes or bilirubin may occur. Brownish-red or orange discoloration of skin, urine, sweat, saliva, tears, and feces is proportional to amount ingested. Facial or periorbital edema has also been reported in pediatric patients. Hypotension, sinus tachycardia, ventricular arrhythmias, seizures, and cardiac arrest were reported in some fatal cases. Liver enlargement, possibly with tenderness, can develop within a few hours after severe overdosage, and jaundice may develop rapidly. Hepatic involvement may be more marked in patients with prior impairment of hepatic function. Other physical findings remain essentially normal.

Direct and total bilirubin levels may increase rapidly with severe overdosage; hepatic enzyme levels may be affected, especially with prior impairment of hepatic function. A direct effect on the hematopoietic system, electrolyte levels, or acid-base balance is unlikely.

➤*Treatment:* Nausea and vomiting are likely to be present. Gastric lavage is probably preferable to inducing emesis. Instill activated charcoal slurry into stomach after evacuation of gastric contents to help absorb any remaining drug in GI tract. Antiemetic medication may be required to control severe nausea or vomiting.

Forced diuresis (with measured intake and output) will promote excretion of the drug. Hemodialysis may be of value in some patients. Bile drainage may be indicated in the presence of serious impairment of hepatic function lasting more than 24 to 48 hours; extracorporeal hemodialysis may be required. In patients with previously adequate hepatic function, reversal of liver enlargement, and impaired hepatic excretory function probably will be noted within 72 hours, with rapid return toward normal thereafter.

Patient Information

Take on an empty stomach, greater than or equal to 1 hour before or 2 hours after meals, with a full glass of water.

Take medication on a regular basis; avoid missing doses. Do not discontinue therapy except on advice of physician.

Advise patient that the reliability of oral or other systemic hormonal contraceptive may be affected; give consideration to using alternative contraceptive measures.

Medication may cause a reddish-orange discoloration of urine, stools, saliva, tears, sweat, and sputum. This is to be expected and is not harmful. It may also permanently discolor soft contact lenses.

Notify physician if fever, loss of appetite, malaise, nausea, vomiting, darkened urine, or yellowish discoloration of skin or eyes occurs.

RIFABUTIN

Rx	**Mycobutin** (Pharmacia & Upjohn)	**Capsules:** 150 mg	(MYCOBUTIN/PHARMACIA & UPJOHN). Red/brown. In 100s.

RIFABUTIN — ORAL

Refer to the general discussion in the Antituberculosis Agents Introduction.

Indications

➤*Mycobacterium avium complex:* For the prevention of disseminated *Mycobacterium avium* complex (MAC) disease in patients with advanced human immunodeficiency virus (HIV) infection.

➤*Off-label uses:*

Tuberculosis – [1] = Good documentation. The American Thoracic Society, Centers for Disease Control and Prevention (CDC), and Infectious Diseases Society of America joint guidelines on the treatment of tuberculosis recommend rifabutin as a substitute for rifampin in patients who are concurrently receiving medications that have unacceptable interactions with rifampin or who have intolerance to rifampin.

Administration and Dosage

➤*Adults:*

Mycobacterium avium complex prevention –

Usual dosage: 300 mg once daily. For those patients with propensity to nausea, vomiting, or other GI upset, administration of rifabutin at doses of 150 mg twice daily taken with food may be useful.

Concomitant therapy: Reduction of the dose of rifabutin may also be needed for patients receiving concomitant treatment with certain other drugs (see Drug Interactions).

Off-label dosing –

Tuberculosis: [1] = Good documentation. 5 mg/kg orally daily, 2 or 3 times weekly, not to exceed 300 mg/day.

➤*Renal function impairment:* For patients with severe renal impairment (creatinine clearance less than 30 mL/min), the dose of rifabutin should be reduced by 50%.

➤*Administration:* Administration with food may be useful for those patients with propensity to nausea, vomiting, or other GI upset.

➤*Storage/Stability:* Store at 25°C (77°F); excursions permitted to 15° to 30°C (59° to 86°F) Keep tightly closed and dispense in a tight container.

Actions

➤*Pharmacology:* Rifabutin inhibits DNA-dependent RNA polymerase in susceptible strains of *Escherichia coli* and *Bacillus subtilis* but not in mammalian cells. In resistant strains of *E. coli*, rifabutin, like rifampin, did not inhibit this enzyme. It is not known whether rifabutin inhibits DNA-dependent RNA polymerase in *Mycobacterium avium* or in *M. intracellulare* which comprise *M. avium* complex (MAC).

➤*Pharmacokinetics:*

Absorption – Following a single oral dose of 300 mg to nine healthy adult volunteers, rifabutin was readily absorbed from the gastrointestinal tract with mean (± SD) peak plasma levels (C_{max}) of 375 (± 267) ng/mL (range: 141 to 1033 ng/mL) attained in 3.3 (± 0.9) hours (T_{max} range: 2 to 4 hours). Absolute bioavailability assessed in 5 HIV-positive patients, who received both oral and intravenous doses, averaged 20%. Total recovery of radioactivity in the urine indicates that at least 53% of the orally administered rifabutin dose is absorbed from the gastrointestinal tract. The bioavailability of rifabutin from the capsule dosage form, relative to an oral solution, was 85% in 12 healthy adult volunteers. High-fat meals slow the rate without influencing the extent of absorption from the capsule dosage form. Plasma concentrations post-C_{max} declined in an apparent biphasic manner. Pharmacokinetic dose-proportionality was established over the 300 to 600 mg dose range in 9 healthy adult volunteers (crossover design) and in 16 early symptomatic HIV-positive patients over a 300 to 900 mg dose range.

Distribution – Due to its high lipophilicity, rifabutin demonstrates a high propensity for distribution and intracellular tissue uptake. Following intravenous dosing, estimates of apparent steady-state distribution volume (9.3 ± 1.5 L/kg) In 5 HIV-positive patients exceeded total body water by approximately 15-fold. Substantially higher intracellular tissue levels than those seen in plasma have been observed in both rat and man. The lung-to-plasma concentration ratio, obtained at 12 hours, was approximately 6.5 in 4 surgical patients who received an oral dose. Mean rifabutin steady-state trough levels ($C_{p,min}{}^{ss}$; 24-hour post-dose) ranged from 50 to 65 ng/mL in HIV-positive patients and in healthy adult volunteers. About 85% of the drug is bound in a concentration-independent manner to plasma proteins over a concentration range of 0.05 to 1 mcg/mL. Binding does not appear to be influenced by renal or hepatic dysfunction. Rifabutin was slowly eliminated from plasma in 7 healthy adult volunteers, presumably because of distribution-limited elimination, with a mean terminal half-life of 45 (±17) hours (range: 16 to 69 hours). Although the systemic levels of rifabutin following multiple dosing decreased by 38%. Its terminal half-life remained unchanged.

Metabolism – Of the 5 metabolites that have been identified, 25-O-desacetyl and 31-hydroxy are the most predominant, and show a plasma metabolite: Parent area under the curve ratio of 0.1 and 0.07, respectively. The former has an activity equal to the parent drug and contributes up to 10% to the total antimicrobial activity.

Excretion – A mass-balance study in 3 healthy adult volunteers with ^{14}C-labeled rifabutin showed that 53% of the oral dose was excreted in the urine, primarily as metabolites. About 30% of the dose is excreted in the feces. Mean systemic clearance (CL_s/F) in healthy adult volunteers following a single oral dose was 0.69 (± 0.32) L/hr/kg (range: 0.46 to 1.34 L/hr/kg). Renal and biliary clearance of unchanged drug each contribute approximately 5% to CL_s/F.

Special populations –

Renal function impairment: The disposition of rifabutin (300 mg) was studied in 18 patients with varying degrees of renal function. Area under plasma concentration time curve (AUC) increased by about 71% in patients with severe renal insufficiency (creatinine clearance below 30 mL/min) compared to patients with creatinine clearance (CrCl) between 61 to 74 mL/min. In patients with mild to moderate renal insufficiency (CrCl between 30 to 61 mL/min), the AUC increased by about 41%. A reduction in the dosage of rifabutin is recommended for patients with CrCl less than 30 mL/min (see Administration and Dosage).

Contraindications

Clinically significant hypersensitivity to rifabutin or to any other rifamycins.

Warnings/Precautions

➤*Active tuberculosis:* Rifabutin capsules must not be administered for MAC prophylaxis to patients with active tuberculosis. Tuberculosis in HIV-positive patients is common and may present with atypical or extrapulmonary findings. Patients are likely to have a nonreactive purified protein derivative (PPD) despite active disease. In addition to chest X-ray and sputum culture, the following studies may be useful in the diagnosis of tuberculosis in the HIV-positive patient: Blood culture, urine culture, or biopsy of a suspicious lymph node.

RIFABUTIN — ORAL

Patients who develop complaints consistent with active tuberculosis while on prophylaxis with rifabutin should be evaluated immediately, so that those with active disease may be given an effective combination regimen of antituberculosis medications. Administration of rifabutin as a single agent to patients with active tuberculosis is likely to lead to the development of tuberculosis that is resistant both to rifabutin and to rifampin.

There is no evidence that rifabutin is effective prophylaxis against *M. tuberculosis*. Patients requiring prophylaxis against both *M. tuberculosis* and *Mycobacterium avium* complex may be given isoniazid and rifabutin concurrently.

➤*Pregnancy: Category B.* In rats, given 200 mg/kg/day, there was a decrease in fetal viability. In rats, at 40 mg/kg/day (8 times the recommended human daily dose), rifabutin caused an increase in fetal skeletal variants. In rabbits, at 80 mg/kg/day (16 times the recommended human daily dose), rifabutin caused maternotoxicity and increase in fetal skeletal anomalies. There are no adequate and well-controlled studies in pregnant women. Because animal reproduction studies are not always predictive of human response, rifabutin should be used in pregnant women only if the potential benefit justifies the potential risk to the fetus.

➤*Lactation:* It is not known whether rifabutin is excreted in human milk. Because many drugs are excreted in human milk and because of the potential for serious adverse reactions in nursing infants, a decision should be made whether to discontinue nursing or discontinue the drug, taking into account the importance of the drug to the mother.

➤*Children:* Safety and effectiveness of rifabutin for prophylaxis of MAC in children have not been established. Limited safety data are available from treatment use in 22 HIV-positive children with MAC who received rifabutin in combination with at least two other antimycobacterials for periods from 1 to 183 weeks. Mean doses (mg/kg) for these children were: 18.5 (range 15 to 25) for infants 1 year of age; 8.6 (range 4.4 to 18.8) for children 2 to 10 years of age; and 4 (range 2.8 to 5.4) for adolescents 14 to 16 years of age. There is no evidence that doses greater than 5 mg/kg daily are useful. Adverse experiences were similar to those observed in the adult population, and included leukopenia, neutropenia and rash. In addition, corneal deposits have been observed in some patients during routine ophthalmologic surveillance of HIV-positive pediatric patients receiving rifabutin as part of a multiple-drug regimen for MAC prophylaxis. These are tiny, almost transparent, asymptomatic peripheral and central corneal deposits which do not impair vision. Doses of rifabutin may be administered mixed with foods such as applesauce.

➤*Monitoring:* Because treatment with rifabutin capsules may be associated with neutropenia, and more rarely thrombocytopenia, physicians should consider obtaining hematologic studies periodically in patients receiving prophylaxis with rifabutin.

Drug Interactions

Rifabutin Drug Interactions

Precipitant drug	Object drug[a]		Description
Rifamycins	Anticoagulants	↓	Rifampin decreases the anticoagulation action of warfarin. Increased doses of anticoagulants may be needed when rifamycins are administered concomitantly.
Rifamycins	Azole antifungal agents (eg, ketoconazole, itraconazole, fluconazole)	↓	Plasma levels of azole antifungal agents may be decreased, reducing antifungal activity. Ketoconazole may decrease serum rifamycin levels. Itraconazole may increase rifabutin plasma levels and toxicity. If concurrent use cannot be avoided, monitor antimicrobial activity, and adjust doses as needed.
Azole antifungal agents (eg, ketoconazole, itraconazole)	Rifamycins	↔	
Rifamycins	Benzodiazepines	↓	The pharmacologic effects of certain benzodiazepines may be decreased. Monitor the clinical response to the benzodiazepines when starting or stopping the rifamycin.
Rifamycins	Beta blockers	↓	The pharmacologic effects of certain beta blockers may be reduced by rifampin. May need a 3- to 4-week wash-out period for the enzyme induction effect to disappear. Closely monitor therapeutic response (eg, blood pressure).
Rifamycins	Buspirone	↓	Buspirone plasma concentrations and pharmacologic effects may be decreased. Escalation of buspirone dose may be necessary. Buspirone concentrations may increase following discontinuation of concomitantly administered rifamycins.
Rifamycins	Corticosteroids	↓	The pharmacologic effects of corticosteroids may be markedly decreased with initiation of rifampin therapy. This appears to occur within a few days of adding rifampin and to reverse 2 to 3 weeks following its administration. Double corticosteroid dosage after the addition of rifampin 300 mg/day.
Rifamycins	Cyclosporine	↓	Immunosuppressive effects of cyclosporine may be reduced as early as 2 days following rifamycin initiation. Avoid this combination if possible; otherwise, frequently monitor.
Rifamycins	Dapsone	↓	Rifabutin (300 mg/day) decreased the AUC of dapsone (50 mg/day) in HIV-infected patients (n = 16) by about 27% to 40%.
Rifamycins	Delavirdine	↓	Rifamycins decrease delavirdine plasma concentrations. Avoid concurrent use if possible.
Rifamycins	Didanosine	↔	In 12 HIV-infected patients, coadministration of rifabutin (300 or 600 mg/day) and didanosine (167 to 375 mg twice daily) did not alter the pharmacokinetics of either drug.
Rifamycins	Doxycycline	↓	Rifamycins may decrease the serum concentration of doxycycline. Monitor the clinical response. Streptomycin does not appear to decrease doxycycline concentrations.
Rifamycins	Hydantoins	↓	Serum hydantoin levels may be decreased, resulting in a decreased pharmacologic hydantoin effect. Monitor hydantoin levels.
Rifamycins	Indinavir	↓	Rifamycins may decrease indinavir serum concentrations. In addition, indinavir may elevate serum rifabutin concentrations, increasing the risk of rifabutin toxicity. It is recommended to reduce the rifabutin dose by 50% when administered with indinavir.
Indinavir	Rifamycins	↑	
Rifamycins	Losartan	↓	Losartan plasma concentrations may be reduced, decreasing antihypertensive effects. Observe the clinical response when rifamycin is started or stopped and adjust therapy as needed.
Rifamycins	Macrolide antibiotics (eg, clarithromycin, erythromycin)	↓	The antimicrobial effects of macrolide antibiotics may be decreased. The frequency of GI adverse reactions may be increased.
Rifamycins	Methadone	↓	The actions of methadone may be reduced, requiring higher doses of methadone during rifampin administration. Patients receiving methadone treatment may experience withdrawal symptoms.
Rifamycins	Morphine	↓	The analgesic effects of morphine may be decreased.
Rifamycins	Nelfinavir	↓	Rifamycins may decrease nelfinavir serum concentrations, decreasing the pharmacologic effects. Avoid concomitant rifampin and nelfinavir administration.
Rifamycins	Oral contraceptives	↓	In 22 healthy female volunteers receiving an oral contraceptive (35 mcg ethinyl estradiol (EE) and 1 mg norethindrone (NE) daily for 21 days, rifabutin decreased EE (AUC) and C_{max} by 35% and 20%, respectively, and NE AUC by 46%.
Rifamycins	Quinine, Quinidine	↓	Addition of rifamycins to stable quinine derivative regimens may require increased doses of quinine derivative to maintain the desired therapeutic effect. Monitor quinine derivative serum levels and the ECG.
Rifamycins	Saquinavir	↓	In 12 HIV-infected patients, rifabutin (300 mg/day) decreased the AUC of saquinavir (600 mg 3 times daily) by about 40%.

RIFABUTIN — ORAL

Rifabutin Drug Interactions

Precipitant drug	Object drug[a]		Description
Rifamycins	Sulfamethoxazole-trimethoprim	⬇	Coadministration of rifabutin (300 mg/day) and sulfamethoxazole-trimethoprim (double strength) in 12 HIV-infected patients decreased the AUC of sulfamethoxazole-trimethoprim by about 15% to 20%. When trimethoprim was given alone, the AUC of trimethoprim was decreased by 14% and the C_{max} by 6%. Sulfamethoxazole-trimethoprim did not alter the pharmacokinetics of rifabutin.
Rifamycins	Theophylline, Aminophylline	⬇	The addition of rifamycin may cause decreased theophylline levels and exacerbation of pulmonary symptoms. Monitor theophylline levels and the patient's response.
Rifamycins	Tricyclic antidepressants	⬇	Tricyclic antidepressant (TCA) levels may be decreased, resulting in a decrease in pharmacologic effects. Consider monitoring the TCA concentrations when starting, discontinuing, or altering the rifamycin dose.
Rifamycins	Zidovudine	⬇	In 16 HIV-infected patients on zidovudine (100 or 200 mg every 4 hours), rifabutin (300 or 450 mg/day) lowered the C_{max} and AUC of zidovudine by about 48% and 32%, respectively. However, zidovudine levels remained within the therapeutic range during coadministration of rifabutin. Zidovudine did not affect the pharmacokinetics of rifabutin.
Rifamycins	Zolpidem	⬇	Plasma concentrations and therapeutic effects of zolpidem may be reduced. Monitor the clinical response, possibly increasing the dose of zolpidem during concomitant administration of rifamycins.
Ritonavir	Rifabutin	⬆	Coadministration of ritonavir (500 mg every 12 hours) and rifabutin (150 mg/day) increased the AUC and C_{max} of rifabutin by more than 400% and 250%, respectively.

[a] ⬇ = object drug decreased; ⬆ = object drug increased; ⬌ = undetermined clinical effect.

➤*Cytochrome P450 system:* Rifabutin induces the enzymes of the cytochrome P450 3A subfamily (CYP3A) and therefore may reduce the plasma concentrations of drugs that are principally metabolized by those enzymes. Rifabutin is also metabolized by CYP3A. Thus, some drugs that inhibit CYP3A may significantly increase plasma concentrations of rifabutin.

Adverse Reactions

Rifabutin capsules were generally well tolerated in the controlled clinical trials. Discontinuation of therapy due to an adverse event was required in 16% of patients receiving rifabutin compared to 8% of patients receiving placebo in these trials. Primary reasons for discontinuation of rifabutin were rash (4% of treated patients), gastrointestinal intolerance (3%), and neutropenia (2%).

The following table enumerates adverse experiences that occurred at a frequency of 1% or greater, among the patients treated with rifabutin in studies 023 and 027.

Clinical Adverse Reactions Reported With Rifabutin (≥ 1%)

Adverse reaction	Rifabutin (n = 566)	Placebo (n = 580)
CNS		
Insomnia	1%	1%
Dermatologic		
Rash	11%	8%
GI		
Anorexia	2%	2%
Diarrhea	3%	3%
Dyspepsia	3%	1%
Eructation	3%	1%
Flatulence	2%	1%
Nausea	6%	5%
Nausea and vomiting	3%	2%
Vomiting	1%	1%
GU		
Discolored urine	30%	6%
Musculoskeletal		
Myalgia	2%	1%
Special senses		
Taste perversion	3%	1%
Miscellaneous		
Abdominal pain	4%	3%
Asthenia	1%	1%
Chest pain	1%	1%
Fever	2%	1%
Headache	3%	5%
Pain	1%	2 %

➤*Additional (less than 1%):* Considering data from the 023 and 027 pivotal trials, and from other clinical studies, rifabutin appears to be a likely cause of the following adverse events which occurred in less than 1% of treated patients: Flu-like syndrome, hepatitis, hemolysis, arthralgia, myositis, chest pressure or pain with dyspnea, and skin discoloration.

The following adverse events have occurred in more than one patient receiving rifabutin, but an etiologic role has not been established: Seizure, paresthesia, aphasia, confusion, and nonspecific T wave changes on electrocardiogram.

When rifabutin was administered at doses from 1050 mg/day to 2400 mg/day, generalized arthralgia and uveitis were reported. These adverse experiences abated when rifabutin was discontinued.

➤*Lab test abnormalities:* The following table enumerates the changes in laboratory values that were considered as laboratory abnormalities in studies 023 and 027.

Laboratory Abnormalities In Rifabutin Use

Laboratory abnormalities	Rifabutin (n = 566)	Placebo (n = 580)
Chemistry		
Increased alkaline phosphatase[a]	less than 1%	3%
Increased AST[b]	7%	12%
Increased ALT[b]	9%	11%
Hematology		
Anemia[c]	6%	7%
Eosinophilia	1%	1%
Leukopenia[d]	17%	16%
Neutropenia[e]	25%	20%
Thrombocytopenia[f]	5%	4%

[a] Includes grade 3 or 4 toxicities as specified: 1 all values greater than 450 U/L
[b] 2 all values greater than 150 U/L
[c] 3 all hemoglobin values less than 8 g/dL
[d] 4 all WBC values less than 1500/mm³
[e] 5 all ANC values less than 750/mm³
[f] 6 all platelet count values less than 50,000/mm³

➤*Neutropenia:* The incidence of neutropenia in patients treated with rifabutin was significantly greater than in patients treated with placebo ($P = 0.03$). Although thrombocytopenia was not significantly more common among patients treated with rifabutin in these trials, rifabutin has been clearly linked to thrombocytopenia in rare cases. One patient in study 023 developed thrombotic thrombocytopenic purpura, which was attributed to rifabutin.

➤*Uveitis:* Uveitis is rare when rifabutin is used as a single agent at 300 mg/day for prophylaxis of MAC in HIV-infected persons, even with the concomitant use of fluconazole and/or macrolide antibiotics. However, if higher doses of rifabutin are administered in combination with these agents, the incidence of uveitis is higher.

Patients who developed uveitis had mild to severe symptoms that resolved after treatment with corticosteroids and/or mydriatic eye drops; in some severe cases, however, resolution of symptoms occurred after several weeks.

When uveitis occurs, temporary discontinuance of rifabutin and ophthalmologic evaluation are recommended. In most mild cases, rifabutin may be restarted; however, if signs or symptoms recur, use of rifabutin should be discontinued.

Overdosage

➤*Treatment:* While there is no experience in the treatment of overdose with rifabutin, clinical experience with rifamycins suggest that gastric lavage to evacuate gastric contents (within a few hours of overdose), followed by instillation of an activated charcoal slurry into the stomach, may help absorb any remaining drug from the gastrointestinal tract.

Rifabutin is 85% protein bound and distributed extensively into tissues (V_{ss}: 8 to 9 L/kg). It is not primarily excreted via the urinary route (less than 10% as unchanged drug), therefore, neither hemodialysis nor forced diuresis is

RIFABUTIN — ORAL

expected to enhance the systemic elimination of unchanged rifabutin from the body in a patient with an overdose of rifabutin.

Patient Information

Patients should be advised of the signs and symptoms of both MAC and tuberculosis, and should be instructed to consult their physicians if they develop new complaints consistent with either of these diseases. In addition, since rifabutin may rarely be associated with myositis and uveitis, patients should be advised to notify their physicians if they develop signs or symptoms suggesting either of these disorders.

Urine, feces, saliva, sputum, perspiration, tears, and skin may be colored brown-orange with rifabutin and some of its metabolites. Soft contact lenses may be permanently stained. Patients to be treated with rifabutin should be made aware of these possibilities.

Advise patients using oral contraceptives to consider changing to nonhormonal methods of birth control because rifabutin, like rifampin, may decrease their efficacy.

ETHAMBUTOL HYDROCHLORIDE

Rx	**Ethambutol Hydrochloride** (Heritage)	**Tablets; oral:** 100 mg	Sorbitol, sucrose. (E 6). Film-coated. In 100s.
Rx	**Myambutol** (X-Gen)		(M6). White. Film coated. In 100s.
Rx	**Ethambutol Hydrochloride** (Heritage)	**Tablets; oral:** 400 mg	Sorbitol, sucrose. (E 7). Scored. Film-coated. In 100s.
Rx	**Myambutol** (X-Gen)		(M7). White, scored. Film coated. In 100s, 1000s, and UD 10s.

ETHAMBUTOL HYDROCHLORIDE — ORAL

Refer to the general discussion in the Antituberculosal Agents Introduction.

Indications

➤*Pulmonary tuberculosis:* For the treatment of pulmonary tuberculosis. It should not be used as the sole antituberculous drug, but should be used in conjunction with at least one other antituberculous drug. Selection of the companion drug should be based on clinical experience, considerations of comparative safety and appropriate in vitro susceptibility studies. In patients who have not received previous antituberculous therapy (ie, initial treatment) the most frequently used regimens have been ethambutol plus isoniazid and ethambutol plus isoniazid plus streptomycin.

In patients who have received previous antituberculous therapy, mycobacterial resistance to other drugs used in initial therapy is frequent. Consequently, in such retreatment patients, combine ethambutol with at least 1 of the second line drugs not previously administered to the patient and to which bacterial susceptibility has been indicated by appropriate in vitro studies. Antituberculous drugs used with ethambutol have included cycloserine, ethionamide, pyrazinamide, viomycin, and other drugs. Isoniazid, aminosalicylic acid, and streptomycin have also been used in multiple drug regimens. Alternating drug regimens have also been utilized.

Administration and Dosage

➤*General dosing considerations:* Ethambutol should not be used alone in initial treatment or in re-treatment. Please consult the CDC for the most current recommendations regarding treatment of tuberculosis. In general, continue therapy until bacteriological conversion has become permanent and maximal clinical improvement has occurred.

During the period when a patient is on a daily dose of 25 mg/kg, monthly eye examinations are advised.

➤*Adults:*

Pulmonary tuberculosis –

Therapy-naive patients:

• *Usual dosage* – 15 mg/kg (7 mg/lb), as a single oral dose once every 24 hours in patients who have not received previous antituberculous therapy. See the following table.

• *Concomitant therapy* – In the more recent studies, isoniazid has been administered concurrently in a single, daily, oral dose.

Therapy-experienced patients:

• *Usual dosage* – 25 mg/kg (11 mg/lb), as a single oral dose once every 24 hours in patients who have received previous antituberculous therapy. After 60 days of ethambutol administration, decrease the dose to 15 mg/kg (7 mg/lb) of body weight, and administer as a single oral dose once every 24 hours. See the following table.

• *Concomitant therapy* – Coadminister at least 1 other antituberculous drug that the organisms have been demonstrated to be susceptible by appropriate in vitro tests. Suitable drugs usually consist of those not previously used in the treatment of the patient.

Ethambutol Weight-Dose Table

Weight range		Daily dose
Pounds	Kilograms	In mg
15 mg/kg (7 mg/lb) schedule		
Under 85 lbs	Under 37 kg	500
85 to 94.5	37 to 43	600
95 to 109.5	43 to 50	700
110 to 124.5	50 to 57	800
125 to 139.5	57 to 64	900
140 to 154.5	64 to 71	1,000
155 to 169.5	71 to 79	1,100
170 to 184.5	79 to 84	1,200
185 to 199.5	84 to 90	1,300
200 to 214.5	90 to 97	1,400
215 and over	Over 97	1,500

Ethambutol Weight-Dose Table

Weight range		Daily dose
Pounds	Kilograms	In mg
25 mg/kg (11 mg/lb) schedule		
less than 85 lbs	less than 38 kg	900
85 to 92.5	38 to 42	1,000
93 to 101.5	42 to 45.5	1,100
102 to 109.5	45.5 to 50	1,200
110 to 118.5	50 to 54	1,300
119 to 128.5	54 to 58	1,400
129 to 136.5	58 to 62	1,500
137 to 146.5	62 to 67	1,600
147 to 155.5	67 to 71	1,700
156 to 164.5	71 to 75	1,800
165 to 173.5	75 to 79	1,900
174 to 182.5	79 to 83	2,000
183 to 191.5	83 to 87	2,100
192 to 199.5	87 to 91	2,200
200 to 209.5	91 to 95	2,300
210 to 218.5	95 to 99	2,400
≥ 219	over 99	2,500

➤*Children:*

Pulmonary tuberculosis –

13 years of age and older: See Adults for dosing for children 13 years of age and older.

➤*Renal function impairment:* Patients with decreased renal function need the dosage reduced, as determined by serum levels of ethambutol, because the main path of excretion of this drug is by the kidneys.

➤*Administration:* Administer ethambutol on a once every 24-hour basis only. Absorption is not significantly altered by administration with food.

➤*Storage/Stability:* Store at 20° to 25°C (68° to 77°F).

Actions

➤*Pharmacology:* Ethambutol diffuses into actively growing mycobacterium cells such as tubercle bacilli. Ethambutol appears to inhibit the synthesis of 1 or more metabolites, thus causing impairment of cell metabolism, arrest of multiplication, and cell death. No cross-resistance with other available antimycobacterial agents has been demonstrated.

➤*Pharmacokinetics:*

Absorption/Distribution – Ethambutol following a single oral dose of 25 mg/kg of body weight, attains a peak of 2 to 5 mcg/mL in serum 2 to 4 hours after administration. When the drug is administered daily for longer periods of time at this dose, serum levels are similar. The serum level of ethambutol falls to undetectable levels by 24 hours after the last dose except in some patients with abnormal renal function. The intracellular concentrations of erythrocytes reach peak values approximately twice those of plasma and maintain this ratio throughout the 24 hours.

Metabolism/Excretion – During the 24-hour period following oral administration of ethambutol, approximately 50% of the initial dose is excreted unchanged in the urine, while an additional 8% to 15% appears in the form of metabolites. The main path of metabolism appears to be an initial oxidation of the alcohol to an aldehydic intermediate, followed by conversion to a dicarboxylic acid. From 20% to 22% of the initial dose is excreted in the feces as unchanged drug. No drug accumulation has been observed with consecutive single daily doses of 25 mg/kg in patients with healthy kidney function, although marked accumulation has been demonstrated in patients with renal insufficiency.

ETHAMBUTOL HYDROCHLORIDE — ORAL

Contraindications

Hypersensitive to ethambutol; optic neuritis unless clinical judgement determines that it may be used; in patients who are unable to appreciate and report visual side effects or changes in vision (eg, young children, unconscious patients).

Warnings/Precautions

➤*Visual disturbances:* See Adverse Reactions for more information.

➤*Hepatic effects:* Liver toxicities including fatalities have been reported.

➤*Renal function impairment:* Patients with decreased renal function need the dosage reduced as determined by serum levels of ethambutol, since the main path of excretion of this drug is by the kidneys.

➤*Pregnancy: Category C.* There are no adequate and well-controlled studies in pregnant women. There are reports of ophthalmic abnormalities occurring in infants born to women on antituberculous therapy that included ethambutol. Use ethambutol during pregnancy only if the benefit justifies the potential risk to the fetus.

Ethambutol has been shown to be teratogenic in pregnant mice and rabbits when given in high doses. When pregnant mice or rabbits were treated with high doses of ethambutol, fetal mortality was slightly but not significantly (P greater than 0.05) increased. Female rats treated with ethambutol displayed slight but insignificant (P greater than 0.05) decreases in fertility and litter size.

In fetuses born of mice treated with high doses of ethambutol during pregnancy, a low incidence of cleft palate, exencephaly, and abnormality of the vertebral column were observed. Minor abnormalities of the cervical vertebra were seen in the newborn of rats treated with high doses of ethambutol during pregnancy. Rabbits receiving high doses of ethambutol during pregnancy gave birth to 2 fetuses with monophthalmia, 1 with a shortened right forearm accompanied by bilateral wrist-joint contracture, and 1 with hare lip and cleft palate.

➤*Lactation:* Ethambutol is excreted into breast milk. Consider the use of ethambutol only if the expected benefit to the mother outweighs the potential risk to the infant.

➤*Children:* See Administration and Dosage for more information.

➤*Monitoring:* As with any potent drug, perform baseline and periodic assessments of organ system functions, including renal, hepatic, and hematopoietic.

Because this drug may have adverse effects on vision, physical examination should include ophthalmoscopy, finger perimetry, and testing of color discrimination. In patients with visual defects such as cataracts, recurrent inflammatory conditions of the eye, optic neuritis, and diabetic retinopathy, the evaluation of changes in visual acuity is more difficult. Take care to be sure the variations in vision are not due to the underlying disease conditions. In such patients, give consideration to the relationship between benefits expected and possible visual deterioration because evaluation of visual changes is difficult.

Drug Interactions

➤*Aluminum-containing antacids:* The results of a study of coadministration of ethambutol (50 mg/kg) with an aluminum hydroxide containing antacid to 13 patients with tuberculosis showed a reduction of mean serum concentrations and urinary excretion of ethambutol of approximately 20% and 13%, respectively, suggesting that the oral absorption of ethambutol may be reduced by these antacid products. It is recommended to avoid concurrent administration of ethambutol with aluminum hydroxide containing antacids for at least 4 hours following ethambutol administration.

Adverse Reactions

➤*Ophthalmic:* Ethambutol may produce decreases in visual acuity, including irreversible blindness, which appear to be due to optic neuritis. Optic neuropathy including optic neuritis or retrobulbar neuritis occurring in association with ethambutol therapy may be characterized by 1 or more of the following events: decreased visual acuity, scotoma, color blindness, and/or visual defect. These events have also been reported in the absence of a diagnosis of optic or retrobulbar neuritis.

Advise patients to report promptly to their physicians any change of visual acuity.

Recovery of visual acuity generally occurs over a period of weeks to months after the drug has been discontinued. Patients have then received ethambutol again without recurrence of loss of visual acuity.

➤*Hypersensitivity:* Hypersensitivity syndrome consisting of cutaneous reaction (such as rash or exfoliative dermatitis), eosinophilia, and 1 or more of the following: Hepatitis, pneumonitis, nephritis, myocarditis, pericarditis. Fever and lymphadenopathy may be present.

➤*Miscellaneous:* Other adverse reactions reported include hypersensitivity, anaphylactoid reactions, dermatitis, pruritus and joint pain, anorexia, nausea, vomiting, gastrointestinal upset, abdominal pain, fever, malaise, headache, and dizziness, mental confusion, disorientation and possible hallucinations, thrombocytopenia, leukopenia, and neutropenia. Numbness and tingling of the extremities due to peripheral neuritis have been reported infrequently.

Elevated serum uric acid levels occur and precipitation of acute gout has been reported. Pulmonary infiltrates and eosinophilia also have been reported during ethambutol therapy. Liver toxicities, including fatalities, have been reported. Since ethambutol is recommended for therapy in conjunction with one or more other antituberculous drugs, these changes may be related to the concurrent therapy.

PYRAZINAMIDE

Rx	**Pyrazinamide** (Various, eg, Allscripts, Pharmpak, VersaPharm)	**Tablets; oral:** 500 mg	In 60s, 90s, 100s, 500s, and UD 100s.

PYRAZINAMIDE — ORAL

Refer to the general discussion in the Antituberculosal Agents Introduction.

Indications

➤*Tuberculosis:*

Drug-susceptible disease – Initial treatment of active tuberculosis in adults and children when combined with other antituberculous agents.

The current recommendation of the Centers for Disease Control and Prevention (CDC) for drug-susceptible disease is to use a 6-month regimen for initial treatment of active tuberculosis, consisting of isoniazid, pyrazinamide, and rifampin given for 2 months, followed by isoniazid and rifampin for 4 months.

Drug-resistant disease – Treat patients with a drug-resistant disease with regimens individualized to their situation. Pyrazinamide frequently will be an important component of such therapy.

Treatment failure – Pyrazinamide is also indicated after treatment failure with other primary drugs in any form of active tuberculosis.

Administration and Dosage

➤*General dosing considerations:* Pyrazinamide should always be administered with other effective antituberculous drugs. It is administered for the initial 2 months of a 6-month or longer treatment regimen for drug-susceptible patients. Patients who are known or suspected to have drug-resistant disease should be treated with regimens individualized to their situation.

➤*Adults:*

Tuberculosis –

Usual dosage: 15 to 30 mg/kg once daily. (See the following table). Older regimens employed 3 or 4 divided doses daily, but the most current recommendations are for once-daily administration.

Maximum dose: 3 g/day for once-daily administration. The CDC recommendations do not exceed 2 g/day when given as a daily regimen.

Alternative dosage: 50 to 70 mg/kg twice weekly based on lean body weight. (See the following table). This dosing has been developed to promote patient compliance with a regimen on an outpatient basis. In studies evaluating the twice-weekly regimen, dosages of pyrazinamide in excess of 3 g twice weekly have been administered. This exceeds the recommended maximum 3 g daily dose. However, an increased incidence of adverse reactions has not been reported.

Dosing table –

Recommended Drugs for Initial and Twice-Weekly Treatment of Tuberculosis in Adults

Drug	Daily dose[a]	Twice-weekly dose
Isoniazid	5 mg/kg orally or IM[b] (max, 300 mg)	15 mg/kg (max, 900 mg)
Rifampin	10 mg/kg orally (max, 600 mg)	10 mg/kg (max, 600 mg)
Pyrazinamide	15 to 30 mg/kg orally (max, 2 g)	50 to 70 mg/kg
Streptomycin	15 mg/kg[c] IM (max, 1 g[c])	25 to 30 mg/kg IM
Ethambutol	15 to 25 mg/kg orally (max, 2.5 g)	50 mg/kg

[a] Doses based on weight should be adjusted as weight changes.
[b] IM = intramuscularly.
[c] In individuals older than 60 years of age, the daily dose of streptomycin should be limited to 10 mg/kg, with a maximal dose of 750 mg.

➤*Children:*

Tuberculosis – See Adults and the following table for dosing information.

Dosing table –

Recommended Drugs for Initial and Twice-Weekly Treatment of Tuberculosis in Children

Drug	Daily dose[a]	Twice-weekly dose
Isoniazid	10 to 20 mg/kg orally or IM[b] (max, 300 mg)	20 to 40 mg/kg (max, 900 mg)

PYRAZINAMIDE — ORAL

Recommended Drugs for Initial and Twice-Weekly Treatment of Tuberculosis in Children

Drug	Daily dose[a]	Twice-weekly dose
Rifampin	10 to 20 mg/kg orally (max, 600 mg)	10 to 20 mg/kg (max, 600 mg)
Pyrazinamide	15 to 30 mg/kg orally (max, 2 g)	50 to 70 mg/kg
Streptomycin	20 to 40 mg/kg IM (max, 1 g)	25 to 30 mg/kg IM
Ethambutol	15 to 25 mg/kg orally (max, 2.5 g)	50 mg/kg

[a] Doses based on weight should be adjusted as weight changes.
[b] IM = intramuscularly.

➤*HIV infection:* Patients with concomitant HIV infection may require longer courses of therapy. Be alert to any revised recommendations from the CDC for this group of patients.

➤*Storage/Stability:* Store in a well-closed container at 15° to 30°C (59° to 86°F). Dispense in a well-closed container with a child-resistant closure.

Actions

➤*Pharmacology:* Pyrazinamide, the pyrazine analog of nicotinamide, is an antituberculous agent. Pyrazinamide may be bacteriostatic or bactericidal against *Mycobacterium tuberculosis*, depending on the concentration of the drug attained at the site of infection. The mechanism of action is unknown. The drug is active only at a slightly acidic pH in vitro and in vivo.

➤*Pharmacokinetics:*

Absorption/Distribution – Pyrazinamide is well absorbed from the GI tract and attains peak plasma concentrations within 2 hours. Plasma concentrations generally range from 30 to 50 mcg/mL with doses of 20 to 25 mg/kg. Pyrazinamide is widely distributed in body tissues and fluids, including the liver, lungs, and cerebrospinal fluid (CSF). The CSF concentration is approximately equal to concurrent steady-state plasma concentrations in patients with inflamed meninges. Pyrazinamide is approximately 10% bound to plasma proteins.

Metabolism/Excretion – The half-life of pyrazinamide is 9 to 10 hours in patients with healthy renal and hepatic function. The plasma half-life may be prolonged in patients with renal or hepatic function impairment. Pyrazinamide is hydrolyzed in the liver to its major active metabolite, pyrazinoic acid. Pyrazinoic acid is hydroxylated to the main excretory product, 5-hydroxypyrazinoic acid.

Approximately 70% of an oral dose is excreted in urine, mainly by glomerular filtration, within 24 hours. Pyrazinamide is dialyzable.

Contraindications

Hypersensitivity to the drug; severe hepatic damage; acute gout.

Warnings/Precautions

➤*Combination therapy:* Use pyrazinamide only in conjunction with other effective antituberculous agents. Individualize regimens to treat patients with drug-resistant disease. Pyrazinamide frequently will be an important component of such therapy.

➤*HIV infection:* In patients with concomitant HIV infection, be aware of current CDC recommendations. It is possible these patients may require a longer course of treatment.

➤*Hyperuricemia:* Pyrazinamide inhibits renal excretion of urates, frequently resulting in hyperuricemia, which is usually asymptomatic. Determine baseline serum acid for patients started on pyrazinamide. Discontinue pyrazinamide if hyperuricemia is accompanied by acute gouty arthritis.

➤*Diabetes mellitus:* Use with caution in patients with a history of diabetes mellitus because management may be more difficult.

➤*Drug-resistant disease:* Primary resistance of *M. tuberculosis* to pyrazinamide is uncommon. In cases with known or suspected drug resistance, perform in vitro susceptibility tests with recent cultures of *M. tuberculosis* against pyrazinamide and the usual primary drugs. There are few reliable in vitro tests for pyrazinamide resistance. A reference laboratory capable of performing these studies must be employed.

➤*Renal function impairment:* It may be prudent to select doses at the low end of the dosing range.

➤*Hepatic function impairment:* Closely follow patients with preexisting liver disease or those at increased risk for drug-related hepatitis (eg, alcohol abusers). Discontinue pyrazinamide and do not resume if signs of hepatocellular damage appear.

➤*Pregnancy: Category C.* Animal reproduction studies have not been conducted with pyrazinamide. It is not known whether pyrazinamide can cause fetal harm when administered to a pregnant woman or if it can affect reproduction capacity. Give pyrazinamide to a pregnant woman only if clearly needed.

➤*Lactation:* Pyrazinamide has been found in small amounts in breast milk. Therefore, use pyrazinamide with caution in breast-feeding mothers, taking into account the risk-benefit of this therapy.

➤*Children:* Pyrazinamide regimens employed in adults are probably equally effective in children. Pyrazinamide appears to be well tolerated in children.

➤*Elderly:* In general, dose selection for an elderly patient should be cautious, usually starting at the low end of the dosing range, reflecting the greater frequency of decreased hepatic or renal function, and of concomitant disease or other drug therapy.

➤*Monitoring:* Determine baseline liver function studies (especially ALT and AST) and uric acid levels prior to therapy. Perform appropriate laboratory testing at periodic intervals and if any clinical signs or symptoms occur during therapy.

Drug Interactions

➤*Drug/Lab test interactions:* Pyrazinamide has been reported to interfere with *Acetest* and *Ketostix* urine tests to produce a pink-brown color.

Adverse Reactions

➤*GI:* Anorexia, nausea, vomiting.

➤*Hematologic:* Increased serum iron concentration, thrombocytopenia and sideroblastic anemia with erythroid hyperplasia, and vacuolation of erythrocytes have occurred rarely with this drug. Adverse reactions on blood-clotting mechanisms have also been rarely reported.

➤*Hepatic:* The principal adverse reaction is a hepatic reaction. Hepatotoxicity appears to be dose related and may appear at any time during therapy.

➤*Metabolic:* Gout.

➤*Miscellaneous:* Mild arthralgia and myalgia have been reported frequently. Hypersensitivity reactions, including pruritus, rashes, and urticaria, have been reported. Acne, dysuria, fever, interstitial nephritis, photosensitivity, and porphyria have been reported rarely.

Overdosage

➤*Symptoms:* Overdosage experience is limited. In one case report of overdose, abnormal liver function tests developed. These spontaneously reverted to normal when the drug was stopped.

➤*Treatment:* Employ clinical monitoring and supportive therapy. Pyrazinamide is dialyzable.

Patient Information

Instruct patients to notify their health care provider promptly if they experience any of the following: darkened urine, fever, loss of appetite, malaise, nausea and vomiting, pain or swelling of the joints, yellowish discoloration of the skin and eyes.

Emphasize compliance with the full course of therapy; stress the importance of not missing any doses.

ETHIONAMIDE

Rx	**Trecator** (Wyeth)	**Tablets; oral:** 250 mg	(W 4177). Orange. Film-coated. In 100s.

ETHIONAMIDE — ORAL

Refer to the general discussion in the Antituberculosal Agents Introduction.

Indications

➤*Tuberculosis:* Ethionamide is primarily indicated for the treatment of active tuberculosis in patients with *Mycobacterium tuberculosis* resistant to isoniazid or rifampin, or when there is intolerance on the part of the patient to other drugs. Its use alone in the treatment of tuberculosis results in the rapid development of resistance. It is essential, therefore, to give a suitable companion drug or drugs, the choice being based on the results of susceptibility tests. If the susceptibility tests indicate that the patient's organism is resistant to one of the first-line antituberculosis drugs (ie, isoniazid or rifampin) yet susceptible to ethionamide, ethionamide should be accompanied by at least one drug to which the *M. tuberculosis* isolate is known to be susceptible. If the tuberculosis is resistant to both isoniazid and rifampin, yet susceptible to ethionamide, ethionamide should be accompanied by at least two other drugs to which the *M. tuberculosis* isolate is known to be susceptible.

Drugs which have been used as companion agents are rifampin, ethambutol, pyrazinamide, cycloserine, kanamycin, streptomycin, and isoniazid. The usual warnings, precautions, and dosage regimens for these companion drugs should be observed.

Administration and Dosage

➤*General dosing considerations:* In the treatment of tuberculosis, a major cause of the emergence of drug-resistant organisms and, thus, treatment failure, is patient nonadherence to prescribed treatment. Treatment failure and drug-resistant organisms can be life-threatening and may result in other serious health risks. It is, therefore, important that patients adhere to the drug regimen for the full duration of treatment. Directly observed therapy is recommended when patients are receiving treatment for tuberculosis. Consultation with an expert in the treatment of drug-resistant tuberculosis is advised for patients in whom drug-resistant tuberculosis is suspected or likely.

ETHIONAMIDE — ORAL

In patients with concomitant tuberculosis and HIV infection, malabsorption syndrome may be present. Drug malabsorption should be suspected in patients who adhere to therapy, but who fail to respond appropriately. In such cases, consideration should be given to therapeutic drug monitoring.

➤*Adults:*

Tuberculosis –

Maximum dose: 1 g/day.

Initial dosage: 250 mg daily, with gradual titration to optimal doses as tolerated by the patient. A regimen of 250 mg daily for 1 or 2 days, followed by 250 mg twice daily for 1 or 2 days with a subsequent increase to 1 g in 3 or 4 divided doses has been reported.

Maintenance dosage: 15 to 20 mg/kg/day, administered once daily or, if patient exhibits poor GI tolerance, in divided doses. Thus far, there is insufficient evidence to indicate the lowest effective dosage levels. Therefore, in order to minimize the risk of resistance developing to the drug or to the companion drug, the principle of giving the highest tolerated dose (based on GI intolerance) has been followed. In adult patients, this would seem to be between 0.5 and 1 g daily, with an average of 0.75 g daily.

➤*Children:*

Tuberculosis – 10 to 20 mg/kg daily in 2 or 3 divided doses given after meals or 15 mg/kg as a single daily dose have been recommended. The optimum dosage for pediatric patients has not been established.

➤*Concomitant therapy:* Coadministration of pyridoxine is recommended. Ethionamide should be administered with at least 1, sometimes 2, other drugs to which the organism is known to be susceptible (see Indications).

➤*Duration of therapy:* Duration of treatment should be based on individual clinical response. In general, continue therapy until bacteriological conversion has become permanent and maximal clinical improvement has occurred.

➤*Administration:* May be administered without regard to timing of meals. The best times of administration are those that the individual patient finds most suitable in order to avoid or minimize GI intolerance, which is usually at mealtimes. Every effort should be made to encourage patients to persevere with treatment when GI side effects appear, because they may diminish in severity as treatment proceeds.

➤*Storage/Stability:* Store at approximately 25°C (77°F). Dispense in a tight container.

Actions

➤*Pharmacology:* Ethionamide may be bacteriostatic or bactericidal in action, depending on the concentration of the drug attained at the site of infection and the susceptibility of the infecting organism. The exact mechanism of action of ethionamide has not been fully elucidated, but the drug appears to inhibit peptide synthesis in susceptible organisms.

➤*Pharmacokinetics:*

Absorption/Distribution – Ethionamide is essentially completely absorbed following oral administration and is not subjected to any appreciable first pass metabolism. Following a single 250 mg oral dose of ethionamide in healthy volunteers, peak plasma concentrations of about 2 mcg/mL were attained at 2 hours in most cases. Normal serum concentrations of 1 to 5 mcg/mL are usually seen 2 hours following doses of 250 mg to 500 mg. These concentrations approximate the therapeutic range for this drug when the therapeutic range is defined by those serum concentrations associated with a high probability of success and a low probability of dose-related toxicity. The drug is ≈ 30% bound to plasma proteins. Ethionamide is rapidly and widely distributed into body tissues and fluids, with concentrations in plasma and various organs being approximately equal. Significant concentrations also are present in cerebrospinal fluid.

Metabolism/Excretion – Ethionamide is extensively metabolized to active and inactive metabolites with less than 1% excreted as the free form in urine. Metabolism is presumed to occur in the liver and thus far 6 metabolites have been isolated: 2-ethylisonicotinamide, carbamoyldihydropyridine, thiocarbamoyl-dihydropyridine, S-oxocarbamoyl dihydropyridine, 2-ethylthioiso-nicotinamide, and ethionamide sulphoxide. The sulphoxide metabolite has been demonstrated to have antimicrobial activity against *Mycobacterium tuberculosis*. Ethionamide has a plasma elimination half-life of ≈ 2 hours after oral dosing.

Contraindications

In patients with severe hepatic impairment and in patients who are hypersensitive to the drug.

Warnings/Precautions

➤*Resistance:* The use of ethionamide alone in the treatment of tuberculosis results in rapid development of resistance. It is essential, therefore, to give a suitable companion drug or drugs, the choice being based on the results of susceptibility testing.

However, therapy may be initiated prior to receiving the results of susceptibility tests as deemed appropriate by the physician. Ethionamide should be administered with at least one, sometimes two, other drugs to which the organism is known to be susceptible (see Indications).

➤*Compliance:* Patient compliance is essential to the success of the antituberculosis therapy and to prevent the emergence of drug-resistant organisms. Therefore, patients should adhere to the drug regimen for the full duration of treatment. It is recommended that directly observed therapy be practiced when patients are receiving antituberculous medication. Additional consultation from experts in the treatment of drug-resistant tuberculosis is recommended when patients develop drug-resistant organisms.

➤*Pregnancy: Category C.* Animal studies conducted with ethionamide indicate that the drug has teratogenic potential in rabbits and rats. The doses used in these studies on a mg/kg basis were considerably in excess of those recommended in humans. There are no adequate and well-controlled studies in pregnant women. Because of these animal studies, however, it must be recommended that ethionamide be withheld from women who are pregnant, or who are likely to become pregnant while under therapy, unless the prescribing physician considers it to be an essential part of the treatment.

➤*Lactation:* Because no information is available on the excretion of ethionamide in human milk, ethionamide should be administered to nursing mothers only if the benefits outweigh the risks. Newborns who are breastfed by mothers who are taking ethionamide should be monitored for adverse effects.

➤*Children:* Due to the fact that pulmonary tuberculosis resistant to primary therapy is rarely found in neonates, infants, and children, investigations have been limited in these age groups. At present, the drug should not be used in pediatric patients under 12 years of age except when the organisms are definitely resistant to primary therapy and systemic dissemination of the disease, or other life-threatening complications of tuberculosis, is judged to be imminent.

➤*Monitoring:* Determination of serum transaminases (AST/ALT) should be made prior to initiation of therapy and should be monitored monthly. If serum transaminases become elevated during therapy, ethionamide and the companion antituberculosis drug or drugs may be discontinued temporarily until the laboratory abnormalities have resolved. Ethionamide and the companion antituberculosis medication(s) then should be reintroduced sequentially to determine which drug (or drugs) is (are) responsible for the hepatotoxicity.

Blood glucose determinations should be made prior to and periodically throughout therapy with ethionamide. Diabetic patients should be particularly alert for episodes of hypoglycemia.

Periodic monitoring of thyroid function tests is recommended as hypothyroidism, with or without goiter, has been reported with ethionamide therapy.

Ophthalmologic examinations (including ophthalmoscopy) should be performed before and periodically during therapy with ethionamide.

Drug Interactions

➤*Antituberculous agents:* Ethionamide has been found to temporarily raise serum concentrations of isoniazid. Ethionamide may potentiate the adverse effects of other antituberculous drugs administered concomitantly. In particular, convulsions have been reported when ethionamide is administered with cycloserine and special care should be taken when the treatment regimen includes both of these drugs.

➤*Ethanol:* Excessive ethanol ingestion should be avoided because a psychotic reaction has been reported.

Adverse Reactions

➤*CNS:* Psychotic disturbances (including mental depression), drowsiness, dizziness, restlessness, headache, and postural hypotension have been reported with ethionamide. Rare reports of peripheral neuritis, optic neuritis, diplopia, blurred vision, and a pellagra-like syndrome also have been reported. Concurrent administration of pyridoxine has been recommended to prevent or relieve neurotoxic effects.

➤*GI:* The most common side effects of ethionamide are gastrointestinal disturbances including nausea, vomiting, diarrhea, abdominal pain, excessive salivation, metallic taste, stomatitis, anorexia and weight loss. Adverse gastrointestinal effects appear to be dose related, with ≈ 50% of patients unable to tolerate 1 g as a single dose. Gastrointestinal effects may be minimized by decreasing dosage, by changing the time of drug administration, or by the concurrent administration of an antiemetic agent.

➤*Hepatic:* Transient increases in serum bilirubin, AST, ALT; hepatitis (with or without jaundice).

➤*Hypersensitivity:* Hypersensitivity reactions including rash, photosensitivity, thrombocytopenia and purpura have been reported rarely.

➤*Miscellaneous:* Hypoglycemia, gynecomastia, impotence, and acne also have occurred. The management of patients with diabetes mellitus may become more difficult in those receiving ethionamide.

Overdosage

➤*Treatment:* No specific information is available on the treatment of overdosage with ethionamide. If it should occur, standard procedures to evacuate gastric contents and to support vital functions should be employed.

Patient Information

Patients should be advised to consult their physician should blurred vision or any loss of vision, with or without eye pain, occur during treatment.

Excessive ethanol ingestion should be avoided because a psychotic reaction has been reported.

AMINOSALICYLIC ACID (p-aminosalicylic acid; 4-aminosalicylic acid)

Rx	**Paser** (Jacobus Pharm)	**Granules, delayed-release:** 4 g	In packets.

AMINOSALICYLIC ACID — ORAL

Refer to the general discussion in the Antituberculosal Agents Introduction.

Indications

➤*Tuberculosis:* For the treatment of tuberculosis in combination with other active agents. It is most commonly used in patients with multi-drug resistant TB (MDR-TB) or in situations when therapy with isoniazid and rifampin is not possible due to a combination of resistance or intolerance. When aminosalicylic acid is added to the treatment regimen in patients with proven or suspected drug resistance, it should be accompanied by at least 1 and preferably 2 other new agents to which the patient's organism is known or expected to be susceptible.

Administration and Dosage

➤*General dosing considerations:* Aminosalicylic acid granules should be administered with other drugs to which the organism is known or expected to be susceptible. It is most commonly administered to patients with MDR-TB or in other situations in which therapy with isoniazid or rifampin is not possible because of a combination of resistance or intolerance.

➤*Adults:*

Tuberculosis – 4 g (1 packet) 3 times per day. See Administration.

➤*Children:*

Tuberculosis – Correspondingly smaller doses than the adult dosage should be given. See Administration.

➤*Renal function impairment:* Patients with end stage renal disease should not receive aminosalicylic acid.

➤*Administration:* The contents of the packet may be sprinkled on apple sauce or yogurt or by swirling in a glass to suspend the granules in an acidic drink such as tomato or orange juice.

Do not use if packet is swollen or the granules have lost their tan color and turned dark brown or purple.

➤*Storage/Stability:* Store below 15°C (59°F) (in a refrigerator or freezer). Patients are urged to store aminosalicylic acid in a refrigerator or freezer. Aminosalicylic acid packets may be stored at room temperature for short periods of time. Avoid excessive heat. Do not use if packet is swollen or the granules have lost their tan color, turning dark brown or purple.

Actions

➤*Pharmacology:* Aminosalicylic acid is bacteriostatic against *Mycobacterium tuberculosis*. It inhibits the onset of bacterial resistance to streptomycin and isoniazid. The mechanism of action has been postulated to be inhibition of folic acid synthesis (but without potentiation with antifolic compounds) or inhibition of synthesis of the cell wall component, mycobactin, thus reducing iron uptake by *M. tuberculosis*.

Enteric coating – After 2 hours in simulated gastric fluid, 10% of unprotected aminosalicylic acid is decarboxylated to form meta-aminophenol, a known hepatotoxin. The acid-resistant coating of the aminosalicylic acid granules protects against degradation in the stomach.

The small granules are designed to escape the usual restriction on gastric emptying of large particles. Under neutral conditions such as are found in the small intestine or in neutral foods, the acid-resistant coating is dissolved within 1 minute. Care must be taken in the administration of these granules to protect the acid-resistant coating by maintaining the granules in an acidic food during dosage administration. Patients who have neutralized gastric acid with antacids will not need to protect the acid resistant coating with an acidic food since no acid is present to spoil the drug. Antacids may influence the absorption of other medications and are not necessary for aminosalicylic acid consumed with an acidic food.

Because aminosalicylic acid granules are protected by an enteric coating, absorption does not commence until they leave the stomach. The soft skeletons of the granules remain and may be seen in the stool.

➤*Pharmacokinetics:*

Absorption/Distribution – In a single 4 g pharmacokinetic study with food in healthy volunteers the initial time to a 2 mcg/mL serum level of aminosalicylic acid was 2 hours with a range of 45 minutes to 24 hours; the median time to peak was 6 hours with a range of 1.5 to 24 hours. The mean peak level was 20 mcg/mL with a range of 9 to 35 mcg/mL; a level of 2 mcg/mL was maintained for an average of 7.9 hours with a range of 5 to 9; a level of 1 mcg/mL was maintained for an average of 8.8 hours with a range of 6 to 11.5 hours. The recommended schedule is 4 g every 8 hours.

Penetration into the cerebrospinal fluid occurs only if the meninges are inflamed.

Approximately 50% to 60% of aminosalicylic acid is protein bound; binding is reported to be reduced 50% in kwashiorkor.

Excretion – Eighty percent (80%) of aminosalicylic acid is excreted in the urine, with 50% or more of the dosage excreted in acetylated form. The acetylation process is not genetically determined as is the case for isoniazid. Aminosalicylic acid is excreted by glomerular filtration; although previously reported otherwise, probenecid, a tubular blocking agent, does not enhance plasma concentration. In a 1954 study thyroxine synthesis but not iodide uptake was reported reduced about 40% when the sodium salt (not aminosalicylic acid granules) of aminosalicylic acid was administered 1 hour before radioiodine; the sodium salt typically produces a serum level over 120 mcg/mL at 1 hour lasting 1 hour. Occasional goiter development can be prevented by the administration of thyroxine but not iodide.

Contraindications

Hypersensitivity to any component of this medication; severe renal disease.

Warnings/Precautions

➤*Hepatitis:* In 1 retrospective study of 7492 patients on rapidly absorbed aminosalicylic acid preparations, drug-induced hepatitis occurred in 38 patients (0.5%): In these 38, the first symptom usually appeared within 3 months of the start of therapy with a rash as the most common event followed by fever and much less frequently by GI disturbances of anorexia, nausea or diarrhea. Only 1 patient was diagnosed on routine biochemistry.

➤*Malabsorption syndrome:* A malabsorption syndrome can develop in patients on aminosalicylic acid but is usually not complete. The complete syndrome includes steatorrhea, an abnormal small bowel pattern on x-ray, villus atrophy, depressed cholesterol, reduced D-xylose, and iron absorption. Triglyceride absorption always is normal.

➤*Hypersensitivity reactions:* All drugs should be stopped at the first sign suggesting a hypersensitivity reaction. They may be restarted one at a time in very small but gradually increasing doses to determine whether the manifestations are drug-induced and, if so, which drug is responsible.

Desensitization has been accomplished successfully in 15 of 17 patients starting with 10 mg aminosalicylic acid given as a single dose. The dosage is doubled every 2 days until reaching a total of 1 g after which the dosage is divided to follow the regular schedule of administration. If a mild temperature rise or skin reaction develops, the increment is to be dropped back 1 level or the progression held for 1 cycle.

Reactions are rare after a total dosage of 1.5 g.

➤*Renal function impairment:* Patients with severe renal disease will accumulate aminosalicylic acid and its acetyl metabolite but will continue to acetylate, thus leading exclusively to the inactive acetylated form; deacetylation, if any, is not significant.

➤*Pregnancy:* *Category C.* Aminosalicylic acid has been reported to produce occipital malformations in rats when given at doses within the human dose range. Although there probably is a dose response, the frequency of abnormalities was comparable to controls at the highest level tested (2 times the human dosage). When administered to rabbits at 5 mg/kg, throughout all 3 trimesters, no teratologic or embryocidal effects were seen. Literature reports on aminosalicylic acid in pregnant women always report coadministration of other medications. Because there are no adequate and well controlled studies of aminosalicylic acid in humans, aminosalicylic acid granules should be given to a pregnant woman only if clearly needed.

➤*Lactation:* After administration of a different preparation of aminosalicylic acid to 1 patient, the maximum concentration in the milk was 1 mcg/mL at 3 hours with a half-life of 2.5 hours; the maximum maternal plasma concentration was 70 mcg/mL at 2 hours.

Drug Interactions

Aminosalicylic Acid Drug Interactions

Precipitant	Object drug[a]		Description
Aminosalicylic acid	Isoniazid	⬆	Aminosalicylic acid at a dose of 12 g in a rapidly available form has been reported to produce a 20% decrease in the acetylation of INH, especially in fast acetylators. The effect is dose related and, while it has not been studied with the current delayed-release formulation, the lower serum levels with this preparation will result in a reduced effect on the acetylation of INH. Special precautions are not deemed necessary.
Aminosalicylic acid	Digoxin	⬇	Oral absorption of digoxin may be reduced when given concomitantly with aminosalicylic acid. Monitor serum digoxin levels.
Aminosalicylic acid	Vitamin B_{12}	⬇	Aminosalicylic acid impairs the absorption of vitamin B_{12}. Consider vitamin B_{12} therapy for patients on aminosalicylic acid therapy more than 1 month.

[a] ⬆ = object drug increased; ⬇ = object drug decreased.

➤*Drug/Lab test interactions:* Aminosalicylic acid has been reported to interfere technically with the serum determinations of albumin by dye-binding, AST by the azoene dye method and with qualitative urine tests for ketones, bilirubin, urobilinogen, or porphobilinogen.

Adverse Reactions

➤*GI:* The most common side effect is gastrointestinal intolerance manifested by nausea, vomiting, diarrhea, and abdominal pain.

➤*Miscellaneous:* Fever, skin eruptions of various types, including exfoliative dermatitis, infectious mononucleosis-like, or lymphoma-like syndrome,

AMINOSALICYLIC ACID — ORAL

leukopenia, agranulocytosis, thrombocytopenia, Coombs' positive hemolytic anemia, jaundice, hepatitis, pericarditis, hypoglycemia, optic neuritis, encephalopathy, Leoffler's syndrome, vasculitis, and a reduction in prothrombin.

Crystalluria may be prevented by the maintenance of urine at a neutral or an alkaline pH.

Patient Information

The patient should be advised that the first signs of hypersensitivity include a rash, often followed by fever, and much less frequently, GI disturbances of anorexia, nausea, or diarrhea. If such symptoms develop, the patient should immediately cease taking the medication and arrange for a prompt clinical visit.

Patients should be advised that poor compliance in taking anti-TB medication often leads to treatment failure, and, not infrequently, to the development of resistance of the organisms in the individual patient.

Patients should be advised that the skeleton of the granules may be seen in the stool.

The coating to protect the aminosalicylic acid granules dissolves promptly under neutral conditions; the granules therefore should be administered by sprinkling on acidic foods such as apple sauce or yogurt or by suspension in a fruit drink which will protect the coating, but the granules sink and will have to be swirled. The coating will last at least 2 hours in either system. All juices tested to date have been satisfactory; tested are: Tomato, orange, grapefruit, grape, cranberry, apple, "fruit punch".

Patients should be advised to store aminosalicylic acid in a refrigerator or freezer. Aminosalicylic acid packets may be stored at room temperature for short periods of time.

Patients should be advised not to use if the packets are swollen or the granules have lost their tan color and are dark brown or purple. The patient should inform the pharmacist or physician immediately and return the medication.

CYCLOSERINE

Rx	**Seromycin Pulvules** (Eli Lilly and Co.)	**Capsules:** 250 mg	(51479 019). Red/gray. In 40s.

CYCLOSERINE — ORAL

Refer to the general discussion in the Antituberculosal Agents Introduction.

Indications

➤*Active pulmonary and extrapulmonary tuberculosis:* Treatment of active pulmonary and extrapulmonary tuberculosis (including renal disease) when the causative organisms are susceptible to this drug and when treatment with the primary medications (streptomycin, isoniazid, rifampin, and ethambutol) has proved inadequate. Like all antituberculosis drugs, cycloserine should be administered in conjunction with other effective chemotherapy and not as the sole therapeutic agent.

➤*Acute urinary tract infections:* Treatment of acute urinary tract infections caused by susceptible strains of gram-positive and gram-negative bacteria, especially *Enterobacter* sp. and *Escherichia coli*. It is generally no more and is usually less effective than other antimicrobial agents in the treatment of urinary tract infections caused by bacteria other than mycobacteria. Use of cycloserine in these infections should be considered only when more conventional therapy has failed and when the organism has been demonstrated to be susceptible to the drug.

Administration and Dosage

➤*Adults:*

Tuberculosis (active pulmonary and extrapulmonary) –

Maximum dose: 1 g/day.

Initial dosage: 250 mg twice daily at 12-hour intervals for the first 2 weeks.

Maintenance dosage: 500 mg to 1 g daily in divided doses monitored by blood levels.

Urinary tract infections (acute) –

Maximum dose: 1 g/day.

Initial dosage: 250 mg twice daily at 12-hour intervals for the first 2 weeks.

Maintenance dosage: 500 mg to 1 g daily in divided doses monitored by blood levels.

➤*Renal function impairment:* Contraindicated in patients with severe renal insufficiency.

➤*Storage/Stability:* Store at 15° to 30°C (59° to 86°F).

Actions

➤*Pharmacology:* Cycloserine inhibits cell-wall synthesis in susceptible strains of gram-positive and gram-negative bacteria and in *Mycobacterium* tuberculosis.

➤*Pharmacokinetics:*

Absorption – After oral administration, cycloserine is readily absorbed from the GI tract, with peak blood levels occurring in 4 to 8 hours.

Distribution – Blood levels of 25 to 30 mcg/mL can generally be maintained with the usual dosage of 250 mg twice a day, although the relationship of plasma levels to dosage is not always consistent. Concentrations in the cerebrospinal fluid, pleural fluid, fetal blood, and mother's milk approach those found in the serum. Detectable amounts are found in ascitic fluid, bile, sputum, amniotic fluid, and lung and lymph tissues.

Metabolism/Excretion – The remaining 35% is apparently metabolized to unknown substances.

Approximately 65% of a single dose of cycloserine can be recovered in the urine within 72 hours after oral administration. The maximum excretion rate occurs 2 to 6 hours after administration, with 50% of the drug eliminated in 12 hours.

Contraindications

Hypersensitivity to cycloserine; epilepsy; depression, severe anxiety, or psychosis; severe renal insufficiency; excessive concurrent use of alcohol.

Warnings/Precautions

➤*CNS toxicity:* Administration of cycloserine should be discontinued or the dosage reduced if the patient develops symptoms of CNS toxicity, such as convulsions, psychosis, somnolence, depression, confusion, hyperreflexia, headache, tremor, vertigo, paresis, or dysarthria.

The risk of convulsions is increased in chronic alcoholics.

➤*Allergic dermatitis:* Administration should be discontinued or the dosage reduced if the patient develops allergic dermatitis.

➤*Toxicity:* The toxicity of cycloserine is closely related to excessive blood levels (above 30 mcg/mL), as determined by high dosage or inadequate renal clearance. The ratio of toxic dose to effective dose in tuberculosis is small.

➤*Anticonvulsants or sedatives:* Anticonvulsant drugs or sedatives may be effective in controlling symptoms of CNS toxicity, such as convulsions, anxiety, and tremor. Patients receiving more than 500 mg of cycloserine daily should be closely observed for such symptoms. The value of pyridoxine in preventing CNS toxicity from cycloserine has not been proved.

➤*Anemia:* Administration of cycloserine and other antituberculosis drugs has been associated in a few instances with vitamin B_{12} or folic-acid deficiency, megaloblastic anemia, and sideroblastic anemia. If evidence of anemia develops during treatment, appropriate studies and therapy should be instituted.

➤*Pregnancy: Category C.* It is not known whether cycloserine can cause fetal harm when administered to a pregnant woman or can affect reproduction capacity. Cycloserine should be given to a pregnant woman only if clearly needed.

➤*Lactation:* Because of the potential for serious adverse reactions in nursing infants from cycloserine, a decision should be made whether to discontinue nursing or to discontinue the drug, taking into account the importance of the drug to the mother.

➤*Children:* Safety and effectiveness in pediatric patients have not been established.

➤*Monitoring:* Patients should be monitored by hematologic, renal excretion, blood level, and liver function studies.

Blood levels should be determined at least weekly for patients with reduced renal function, for individuals receiving a daily dosage of more than 500 mg, and for those showing signs and symptoms suggestive of toxicity. The dosage should be adjusted to keep the blood level below 30 mcg/mL.

Drug Interactions

➤*Ethionamide:* Concurrent administration of ethionamide has been reported to potentiate neurotoxic side effects.

➤*Alcohol:* Alcohol and cycloserine are incompatible, especially during a regimen calling for large doses of the latter. Alcohol increases the possibility and risk of epileptic episodes.

➤*Isoniazid:* Concurrent administration of isoniazid may result in increased incidence of CNS effects, such as dizziness or drowsiness. Dosage adjustments may be necessary and patients should be monitored closely for signs of CNS toxicity.

Adverse Reactions

Most adverse reactions occurring during therapy with cycloserine involve the nervous system or are manifestations of drug hypersensitivity. The following side effects have been observed in patients receiving cycloserine:

➤*Allergic:* Allergy apparently not related to dosage.

➤*Cardiovascular:* Sudden development of congestive heart failure in patients receiving 1 to 1.5 g of cycloserine daily has been reported.

➤*CNS:* Nervous system symptoms that appear to be related to higher dosages of the drug, ie, greater than 500 mg daily, are convulsions, drowsiness and somnolence, headache, tremor, dysarthria, vertigo, confusion and disorientation with loss of memory, psychoses, possibly with suicidal tendencies, character changes, hyperirritability, aggression, paresis, hyperreflexia, paresthesia, major and minor (localized) clonic seizures, coma.

➤*Dermatologic:* Skin rash.

➤*Miscellaneous:* Elevated serum transaminase, especially in patients with preexisting liver disease.

Overdosage

➤*Symptoms:* Acute toxicity from cycloserine can occur if more than 1 g is ingested by an adult. Chronic toxicity from cycloserine is dose related and can occur if more than 500 mg is administered daily. Patients with renal

CYCLOSERINE — ORAL

impairment will accumulate cycloserine and may develop toxicity if the dosing regimen is not modified. Patients with severe renal impairment should not receive the drug. The central nervous system is the most common organ system involved with toxicity. Toxic effects may include headache, vertigo, confusion, drowsiness, hyperirritability, paresthesias, dysarthria, and psychosis. Following larger ingestions, paresis, convulsions, and coma often occur. Ethyl alcohol may increase the risk of seizures in patients receiving cycloserine.

The oral median lethal dose in mice is 5290 mg/kg.

➤*Treatment:* Overdoses of cycloserine have been reported rarely. The following is provided to serve as a guide should such an overdose be encountered.

Protect the patient's airway and support ventilation and perfusion. Meticulously monitor and maintain, within acceptable limits, the patient's vital signs, blood gases, serum electrolytes, etc. Absorption of drugs from the GI tract may be decreased by giving activated charcoal, which, in many cases, is more effective than emesis or lavage; consider charcoal instead of or in addition to gastric emptying. Repeated doses of charcoal over time may hasten elimination of some drugs that have been absorbed. Safeguard the patient's airway when employing gastric emptying or charcoal.

In adults, many of the neurotoxic effects of cycloserine can be both treated and prevented with the administration of 200 to 300 mg of pyridoxine daily.

The use of hemodialysis has been shown to remove cycloserine from the bloodstream. This procedure should be reserved for patients with life-threatening toxicity that is unresponsive to less invasive therapy.

STREPTOMYCIN SULFATE

For complete prescribing information, refer to the Streptomycin Sulfate monograph in the Parenteral Aminoglycosides section.

CAPREOMYCIN

Rx	**Capastat Sulfate** (Akorn)	**Injection, powder for solution:** 1 g	As capreomycin sulfate. In 10 mL vials.

CAPREOMYCIN — INJECTION

Refer to the general discussion in the Antituberculosal Agents Introduction.

WARNING

The use of capreomycin for injection, USP in patients with renal insufficiency or preexisting auditory impairment must be undertaken with great caution, and the risk of additional cranial nerve VIII impairment or renal injury should be weighed against the benefits derived from therapy.

Since other parenteral antituberculosis agents (streptomycin, viomycin) also have similar and sometimes irreversible toxic effect, particularly on cranial nerve VIII and renal function, simultaneous administration of these agents with capreomycin is not recommended. Use with nonantituberculosis drugs (polymyxin A sulfate, colistin sulfate, amikacin, gentamicin, tobramycin, vancomycin, kanamycin, and neomycin) having ototoxic or nephrotoxic potential should be undertaken only with great caution.

Pregnancy – The safety of the use capreomycin in pregnancy has not been determined.

Children – Safety and effectiveness in pediatric patients have not been established.

Indications

➤*Tuberculosis:* Pulmonary infections caused by capreomycin-susceptible strains of *M. tuberculosis* when the primary agents (isoniazid, rifampin, ethambutol, aminosalicylic acid, and streptomycin) have been ineffective or cannot be used because of toxicity or the presence of resistant tubercle bacilli.

Susceptibility studies should be performed to determine the presence of a capreomycin-susceptible strain of *M. tuberculosis*.

Administration and Dosage

➤*General dosing considerations:* Capreomycin is always administered in combination with at least 1 other antituberculosis agent to which the patient's strain of tubercle bacilli is susceptible.

If facilities for administering injectable medication are not available, a change to appropriate oral therapy is indicated on the patient's release from the hospital.

➤*Adults:*

Tuberculosis –

Maximum dose: 20 mg/kg/day.

Initial dosage: 1 g daily (not to exceed 20 mg/kg/day), given IM or by IV infusion for 60 to 120 days.

Maintenance dosage: 1 g IM or by IV infusion 2 or 3 times weekly.

Duration of therapy: Therapy for tuberculosis should be maintained for 12 to 24 months.

➤*Renal function impairment:* Patients with reduced renal function should have dosage reduction based on creatinine clearance (CrCl) using the following guidelines. These dosages are designed to achieve a mean steady-state capreomycin level of 10 mcg/mL.

Estimated Dosages to Attain Mean Steady-State Serum Capreomycin Concentration of 10 mcg/mL (Based on CrCl)

CrCl (mL/min)	Capreomycin clearance (L/gr × 10^{-2})	Half-life (hours)	Dose[a] (mg/kg) for the following dosing intervals: 24 hours	48 hours	72 hours
0	0.54	55.5	1.29	2.58	3.87
10	1.01	29.4	2.43	4.87	7.3
20	1.49	20	3.58	7.16	10.7
30	1.97	15.1	4.72	9.45	14.2
40	2.45	12.2	5.87	11.7	
50	2.92	10.2	7.01	14	
60	3.4	8.8	8.16		
80	4.35	6.8	10.4[b]		
100	5.31	5.6	12.7[b]		
110	5.78	5.2	13.9[b]		

[a] For patients with renal impairment, initial maintenance dose estimates are given for optional dosing intervals; longer dosing intervals are expected to provide greater peak and lower trough serum capreomycin levels than shorter dosing intervals.
[b] The usual dosage for patients with healthy renal function is 1 g daily, not to exceed 20 mg/kg/day, for 60 to 120 days, then 1 g 2 to 3 times weekly.

➤*Preparation for administration:* Reconstitution is achieved by dissolving the vial contents (1 g) in 2 mL of sodium chloride 0.9% injection or sterile water for injection. Two to 3 minutes should be allowed for complete dissolution.

IM use – For administration of a 1 g dose, the entire contents of the vial should be given. For doses lower than 1 g, the following dilution table may be used.

Capreomycin Dilution Table

Diluent added to 1 g (10 mL) vial	Volume of capreomycin for injection solution	Concentration (approximate)
2.15 mL	2.85 mL	350 mg[a]/mL
2.63 mL	3.33 mL	300 mg[a]/mL
3.3 mL	4 mL	250 mg[a]/mL
4.3 mL	5 mL	200 mg[a]/mL

[a] Equivalent to capreomycin activity.

IV use – Reconstituted capreomycin should be diluted in 100 mL of sodium chloride 0.9% injection.

➤*Administration:* Capreomycin may be administered IM or by IV infusion following reconstitution.

IM use – Give by deep IM injection into a large muscle mass because superficial injection may be associated with increased pain and the development of sterile abscesses.

IV use – Administer over 60 minutes.

➤*Storage/Stability:* Store at 15° to 30°C (59° to 86°F) prior to reconstitution. The solution may acquire a pale straw color and darken with time, but this is not associated with loss of potency or the development of toxicity. After reconstitution, all solutions of capreomycin may be stored for up to 24 hours under refrigeration.

Actions

➤*Pharmacology:* Capreomycin is a polypeptide antibiotic isolated from *Streptomyces capreolus*.

➤*Pharmacokinetics:* Capreomycin is not absorbed in significant quantities from the gastrointestinal tract and must be administered parenterally. In 2 studies of 10 patients each, peak serum concentrations following 1 g of capreomycin given intramuscularly were achieved 1 to 2 hours after administration, and average peak levels reached were 28 and 32 mcg/mL respectively (range, 20 to 47 mcg/mL). Low serum concentrations were present at 24 hours. However, 1 g of capreomycin daily for 30 days or more produced no significant accumulation in subjects with healthy renal function. Two patients with marked reduction of renal function had high serum concentrations 24 hours after administration of the drug. When a 1 g dose of capreomycin was given intramuscularly to healthy volunteers, 52% was excreted in the urine within 12 hours.

Lehmann, et al, examined the pharmacokinetics of single dose capreomycin (1 g) administered intramuscularly and by intravenous infusion (1 hour) in 6 healthy volunteers. The area under the serum concentration vs. time curve

CAPREOMYCIN — INJECTION

was similar for the 2 routes of administration. Capreomycin peak concentrations after intravenous infusion were 30 ± 47% higher than after intramuscular administration.

Paper chromatographic studies indicated that capreomycin is excreted essentially unaltered. Urine concentrations averaged 1.68 mcg/mL (average urine volume, 228 mL) during the 6 hours following a 1 g dose.

Contraindications

Hypersensitivity to capreomycin.

Warnings/Precautions

➤*Hypokalemia:* Since hypokalemia may occur during therapy, serum potassium levels should be determined frequently.

➤*Ototoxicity:* Audiometric measurements and assessment of vestibular function should be performed prior to initiation of therapy with capreomycin and at regular intervals during treatment.

➤*Nephrotoxicity:* Renal injury, with tubular necrosis, elevation of the blood urea nitrogen (BUN) or serum creatinine, and abnormal urinary sediment, has been noted. Slight elevation of the BUN and serum creatinine has been observed in a significant number of patients receiving prolonged therapy. The appearance of casts, red cells, and white cells in the urine has been noted in a high percentage of these cases. Elevation of the BUN above 30 mg/100 mL or any other evidence of decreasing renal function with or without a rise in BUN levels calls for careful evaluation of the patient, and the dosage should be reduced or the drug completely withdrawn. The clinical significance of abnormal urine sediment and slight elevation in the BUN (or serum creatinine) observed during long-term therapy with capreomycin has not been established.

➤*Neuromuscular blockade:* The peripheral neuromuscular blocking action that has been attributed to other polypeptide antibiotics (colistin sulfate, polymyxin A sulfate, paromomycin, and viomycin) and to aminoglycoside antibiotics (streptomycin, dihydrostreptomycin, neomycin, and kanamycin) has been studied with capreomycin. A partial neuromuscular blockade was demonstrated after large intravenous doses of capreomycin. This action was enhanced by ether anesthesia (as has been reported for neomycin) and was antagonized by neostigmine.

➤*Hypersensitivity reactions:* Caution should be exercised in the administration of antibiotics, including capreomycin, to any patient who has demonstrated some form of allergy, particularly to drugs.

➤*Renal function impairment:* Regular tests of renal function should be made throughout the period of treatment, and reduced dosage should be employed in patients with known or suspected renal impairment.

➤*Pregnancy: Category C.* Capreomycin has been shown to be teratogenic in rats when given in doses 3 ½ times the human dose. There are no adequate and well-controlled studies in pregnant women. Capreomycin should be used during pregnancy only if the potential benefit justifies the potential risk to the fetus (see Warning Box and Animal Pharmacology).

➤*Lactation:* It is not known whether this drug is excreted in human milk. Because many drugs are excreted in human milk, caution should be exercised when capreomycin is administered to a nursing woman.

➤*Children:* Safety and effectiveness in pediatric patients have not been established (see Warning Box).

➤*Monitoring:* Renal function studies should be made both before therapy with capreomycin is started and on a weekly basis during treatment.

Drug Interactions

For neuromuscular blocking action of this drug, see Precautions.

Adverse Reactions

➤*Hematologic:* Leukocytosis and leukopenia have been observed. The majority of patients treated have had eosinophilia exceeding 5% while receiving daily injections of capreomycin. This has subsided with reduction of the capreomycin dosage to 2 or 3 g weekly.

Pain and induration at the injection site have been observed. Excessive bleeding at the injection site has been reported. Sterile abscesses have been noted. Rare cases of thrombocytopenia have been reported.

➤*Hepatic:* Serial tests of liver function have demonstrated a decrease in BSP excretion without change in SGOT or SGPT in the presence of preexisting liver disease. Abnormal results in liver function tests have occurred in many persons receiving capreomycin in combination with other antituberculosis agents that also are known to cause changes in hepatic function. The role of capreomycin in producing these abnormalities is not clear; however, periodic determinations of liver function are recommended.

➤*Hypersensitivity:* Urticaria and maculopapular skin rashes associated in some cases with febrile reactions have been reported when capreomycin and other antituberculosis drugs were given concomitantly.

➤*Renal:* In 36% of 722 patients treated with capreomycin, elevation of the BUN above 20 mg/100 mL has been observed. In many instances, there was also depression of PSP excretion and abnormal urine sediment. In 10% of this series, the BUN elevation exceeded 30 mg/100 mL.

Toxic nephritis was reported in 1 patient with tuberculosis and portal cirrhosis who was treated with capreomycin (1 g) and aminosalicylic acid daily for 1 month. This patient developed renal insufficiency and oliguria and died. Autopsy showed subsiding acute tubular necrosis.

Electrolyte disturbances resembling Bartter's syndrome have been reported in 1 patient.

➤*Special senses:* Subclinical auditory loss was noted in ≈ 11% of 722 patients undergoing treatment with capreomycin. This was a 5- to 10-decibel loss in the 4000- to 8000-CPS range. Clinically apparent hearing loss occurred in 3% of the 722 subjects. Some audiometric changes were reversible. Other cases with permanent loss were not progressive following withdrawal of capreomycin.

Tinnitus and vertigo have occurred.

Overdosage

➤*Symptoms:* Nephrotoxicity following the parenteral administration of capreomycin is most closely related to the area under the curve of the serum concentration vs time graph. The elderly patient, patients with abnormal renal function or dehydration, and patients receiving other nephrotoxic drugs are at much greater risk for developing acute tubular necrosis.

Damage to the auditory and vestibular divisions of cranial nerve VIII has been associated with capreomycin given to patients with abnormal renal function or dehydration and in those receiving medications with additive auditory toxicities. These patients often experience dizziness, tinnitus, vertigo, and a loss of high-tone acuity.

Neuromuscular blockage or respiratory paralysis may occur following rapid intravenous infusion.

If capreomycin is ingested, toxicity would be unlikely because it is poorly absorbed (less than 1%) from an intact gastrointestinal system.

Hypokalemia, hypocalcemia, hypomagnesemia, and an electrolyte disturbance resembling Bartter's syndrome have been reported to occur in patients with capreomycin toxicity.

The subcutaneous median lethal dose in mice was 514 mg/kg.

➤*Treatment:* Protect the patient's airway and support ventilation and perfusion. Meticulously monitor and maintain, within acceptable limits, the patient's vital signs, blood gases, serum electrolytes, etc. Absorption of drugs from the gastrointestinal tract may be decreased by giving activated charcoal, which, in many cases, is more effective than emesis or lavage; consider charcoal instead of or in addition to gastric emptying. Repeated doses of charcoal over time may hasten elimination of some drugs that have been absorbed. Safeguard the patient's airway when employing gastric emptying or charcoal.

Patients who have received an overdose of capreomycin and have normal renal function should be carefully hydrated to maintain a urine output of 3 to 5 mL/kg/hr. Fluid balance, electrolytes, and creatinine clearance should be carefully monitored.

Hemodialysis may be effectively used to remove capreomycin in patients with significant renal disease.

RIFAPENTINE

Rx	**Priftin** (Aventis)	**Tablets:** 150 mg	EDTA, polyethylene glycol. (Priftin 150). Dark pink. Film coated. In 32s.

RIFAPENTINE — ORAL

Refer to the general discussion in the Antituberculosis Agents Introduction.

Indications

➤*Pulmonary tuberculosis:* For the treatment of pulmonary tuberculosis. Rifapentine oral must always be used in conjunction with at least one other antituberculosis drug to which the isolate is susceptible. In the intensive phase of the short-course treatment of pulmonary tuberculosis, rifapentine oral should be administered twice weekly for 2 months, with an interval of no less than 3 days (72 hours) between doses, as part of an appropriate regimen which includes daily companion drugs. It may also be necessary to add either streptomycin or ethambutol until the results of susceptibility testing are known. Compliance with all drugs in the intensive phase (ie, rifapentine oral, isoniazid, pyrazinamide, ethambutol or streptomycin) is imperative to ensure early sputum conversion and protection against relapse. Following the intensive phase, continuation phase treatment should be continued with rifapentine oral for 4 months. During this phase, rifapentine oral should be administered on a once-weekly basis in combination with an appropriate antituberculous agent for susceptible organisms.

Administration and Dosage

➤*General dosing considerations:* Rifapentine should not be used alone, in initial treatment or in retreatment of pulmonary tuberculosis.

The following recommendations apply to patients with drug-susceptible organisms. Patients with drug-resistant organisms may require longer duration treatment with other drug regimens.

➤*Adults:*

Pulmonary tuberculosis –

Intensive phase:

- *Usual dosage* – 600 mg (four 150 mg tablets) twice weekly with an interval of not less than 3 days (72 hours) between doses.
- *Duration of therapy* – 2 months for short-course therapy.

RIFAPENTINE — ORAL

• *Concomitant therapy* – In the intensive phase, rifapentine must be administered in combination as part of an appropriate regimen that includes daily companion drugs. Compliance with all drugs (ie, rifapentine, isoniazid, pyrazinamide, ethambutol, or streptomycin), especially on days when rifapentine is not administered, is imperative to assure early sputum conversion and protection against relapse. The Advisory Council for the Elimination of Tuberculosis, the American Thoracic Society (ATS), and the Centers for Disease Control and Prevention (CDC) also recommend that either streptomycin or ethambutol be added to the regimen unless the likelihood of isoniazid resistance is very low. The need for streptomycin or ethambutol should be reassessed when the results of susceptibility testing are known. An initial treatment regimen with less than 4 drugs may be considered if there is little possibility of drug resistance (that is, less than 4% primary resistance to isoniazid in the community, and the patient has had no previous treatment with antituberculosis medications, is not from a country with a high prevalence of drug resistance, and has no known exposure to a drug-resistant case).

Continuation phase: Following the intensive phase, continue treatment with rifapentine once weekly for 4 months in combination with isoniazid or an appropriate agent for susceptible organisms. If the patient is still sputum smear positive or culture positive, if resistant organisms are present, or if the patient is HIV positive, follow the ATS/CDC treatment guidelines.

➤*Children:*

Pulmonary tuberculosis –

12 years of age and older: See Adults for dosing for children 12 years of age and older.

➤*Concomitant pyridoxine therapy:* Concomitant administration of pyridoxine (vitamin B_6) is recommended in patients who are malnourished, in those predisposed to neuropathy (eg, alcoholics, diabetics), and in adolescents.

➤*Administration:* For those patients with propensity to nausea, vomiting or GI upset, administration of rifapentine with food may be useful.

➤*Storage/Stability:* Store at 25°C (77°F); excursions are permitted 15° to 30°C (59° to 86°F). Protect from excessive heat and humidity.

Actions

➤*Pharmacology:* Rifapentine, a cyclopentyl rifamycin, inhibits DNA-dependent RNA polymerase in susceptible strains of *Mycobacterium tuberculosis* but not in mammalian cells. At therapeutic levels, rifapentine exhibits bactericidal activity against both intracellular and extracellular *M. tuberculosis* organisms. Both rifapentine and the 25-desacetyl metabolite accumulate in human monocyte-derived macrophages with intracellular/extracellular ratios of approximately 24 to 1 and 7 to 1, respectively.

➤*Pharmacokinetics:*

Absorption – The absolute bioavailability of rifapentine has not been determined. The relative bioavailability (with an oral solution as a reference) of rifapentine after a single 600 mg dose to healthy adult volunteers was 70%. The maximum concentrations were achieved from 5 to 6 hours after administration of the 600 mg rifapentine dose. Food (850 total calories: 33 g protein, 55 g fat and 58 g carbohydrate) increased $AUC_{(0-\infty)}$ and C_{max} by 43% and 44%, respectively, over that observed when administered under fasting conditions. When oral doses of rifapentine were administered once daily or once every 72 hours to healthy volunteers for 10 days, single dose $AUC_{(0-\infty)}$ value of rifapentine was similar to its steady-state $AUC_{SS\ (0\text{-}24\ hr)}$ or $AUC_{SS\ (0\text{-}72\ hr)}$ values, suggesting no significant auto-induction effect on steady-state pharmacokinetics of rifapentine. Steady-state conditions were achieved by day 10 following daily administration of rifapentine 600 mg. The pharmacokinetic characteristics of rifapentine and 25-desacetyl rifapentine (active metabolite) on day 10 following oral administration of 600 mg rifapentine every 72 hours to healthy volunteers are discussed below.

Select Pharmacokinetic Parameters of Rifapentine

Pharmacokinetic parameter	Rifapentine[a] (n = 12)	25-desacetyl rifapentine[a] (n = 12)
C_{max} (mcg/ml)	≈ 15.05	≈ 6.26
AUC (0-72 hr) (mcg•hr/ml)	≈ 319.54	≈ 215.88
t½ (hr)	≈ 13.19	≈ 13.35
T_{max} (hr)	≈ 4.83	≈ 11.25
Cl_{po} (L/hr)	≈ 2.03	–

[a] Mean values, day 10.

Distribution – In a population pharmacokinetic analysis in 351 tuberculosis patients who received 600 mg rifapentine in combination with isoniazid, pyrazinamide and ethambutol, the estimated apparent volume of distribution was 70.2 ± 9.1 L. In healthy volunteers, rifapentine and 25-desacetyl rifapentine were 97.7% and 93.2% bound to plasma proteins, respectively. Rifapentine was mainly bound to albumin. Similar extent of protein binding was observed in healthy volunteers, asymptomatic HIV-infected subjects and hepatically impaired subjects.

Metabolism/Excretion – Following a single 600 mg oral dose of radiolabelled rifapentine to healthy volunteers (n = 4), 87% of the total ^{14}C rifapentine was recovered in the urine (17%) and feces (70%). Greater than 80% of the total ^{14}C rifapentine dose was excreted from the body within 7 days. Rifapentine was hydrolyzed by an esterase enzyme to form a microbiologically active 25-desacetyl rifapentine. Rifapentine and 25-desacetyl rifapentine accounted for 99% of the total radioactivity in plasma. Plasma $AUC_{(0-\infty)}$ and C_{max} values of the 25-desacetyl rifapentine metabolite were one-half and one-third those of the rifapentine, respectively. Based upon relative in vitro activities and $AUC_{(0-\infty)}$ values, rifapentine and 25-desacetyl rifapentine potentially contributes 62% and 38% to the clinical activities against *M. tuberculosis*, respectively.

Special populations –

Asymptomatic HIV-infected volunteers: Following oral administration of a single 600 mg dose of rifapentine to asymptomatic HIV-infected volunteers (n = 15) under fasting conditions, mean C_{max} and $AUC_{(0-\infty)}$ of rifapentine were lower (20 to 32%) than that observed in other studies in healthy volunteers (n = 55). In a cross-study comparison, mean C_{max} and AUC values of the 25-desacetyl metabolite of rifapentine, when compared to healthy volunteers were higher (6 to 21%) in one study (n = 20), but lower (15 to 16%) in a different study (n = 40). The clinical significance of this observation is not known. Food (850 total calories: 33 g protein, 55 g fat, and 58 g carbohydrate) increases the mean AUC and C_{max} of rifapentine observed under fasting conditions in asymptomatic HIV-infected volunteers by about 51% and 53%, respectively.

Contraindications

Hypersensitivity to any of the rifamycins (eg, rifampin, rifabutin).

Warnings/Precautions

➤*Compliance:* Poor compliance with the dosage regimen, particularly the daily administered non-rifamycin drugs in the Intensive Phase, was associated with late sputum conversion and a high relapse rate in the rifapentine arm of Clinical Study 008. Therefore, compliance with the full course of therapy must be emphasized, and the importance of not missing any doses must be stressed.

➤*Hyperbilirubinemia:* Hyperbilirubinemia resulting from competition for excretory pathways between rifapentine and bilirubin cannot be excluded since competition between the related drug rifampin and bilirubin can occur. An isolated report showing a moderate rise in bilirubin and/or transaminase level is not in itself an indication for interrupting treatment; rather, the decision should be made after repeating the tests, noting trends in the levels and considering them in conjunction with the patient's clinical condition.

➤*Pseudomembranous colitis:* Pseudomembranous colitis has been reported to occur with various antibiotics, including other rifamycins. Diarrhea, particularly if severe and/or persistent, occurring during treatment or in the initial weeks following treatment may be symptomatic of *Clostridium difficile*-associated disease, the most severe form of which is pseudomembranous colitis. If pseudomembranous colitis is suspected, rifapentine should be stopped immediately and the patient should be treated with supportive and specific treatment without delay (eg, oral vancomycin). Products inhibiting peristalsis are contraindicated in this clinical situation.

➤*HIV-infected patients:* Experience in HIV-infected patients is limited. In an ongoing CDC TB trial, 5 out of 30 HIV-infected patients randomized to once weekly rifapentine (plus INH) in the Continuation Phase who completed treatment, relapsed. Four of these patients developed rifampin monoresistant (RMR) TB. Each RMR patient had late-stage HIV infection, low CD4 counts and extrapulmonary disease, and documented coadministration of antifungal azoles. These findings are consistent with the literature in which an emergence of RMR TB in HIV-infected TB patients has been reported in recent years. Further study in this sub-population is warranted. As with other antituberculous treatments, when rifapentine is used in HIV-infected patients, a more aggressive regimen should be employed (eg, more frequent dosing). Based on results to date of the CDC trial (see above), once weekly dosing during the continuation phase of treatment is not recommended at this time.

➤*Red discoloration of body fluids:* Rifapentine may produce a predominately red-orange discoloration of body tissues and/or fluids (eg, skin, teeth, tongue, urine, feces, saliva, sputum, tears, sweat, and cerebrospinal fluid).

Contact lenses or dentures may become permanently stained.

➤*Porphyria:* Rifapentine should not be used in patients with porphyria. Rifampin has enzyme-inducing properties, including induction of delta amino levulinic acid synthetase. Isolated reports have associated porphyria exacerbation with rifampin administration. Based on these isolated reports with rifampin, it may be assumed that rifapentine has a similar effect.

➤*Hepatic function impairment:* Since antituberculous multidrug treatments, including the rifamycin class, are associated with serious hepatic events, patients with abnormal liver tests and/or liver disease should only be given rifapentine in cases of necessity and then with caution and under strict medical supervision. In these patients, careful monitoring of liver tests (especially serum transaminases) should be carried out prior to therapy and then every 2 to 4 weeks during therapy. If signs of liver disease occur or worsen, rifapentine should be discontinued. Hepatotoxicity of other antituberculosis drugs (eg, isoniazid, pyrazinamide) used in combination with rifapentine should also be taken into account.

➤*Pregnancy: Category C.* Rifapentine has been shown to be teratogenic in rats and rabbits. In rats, when given in doses 0.6 times the human dose (based on body surface area comparisons) during the period of organogenesis, pups showed cleft palates, right aortic arch and increased incidence of delayed ossification and increased number of ribs. Rabbits treated with drug at doses between 0.3 and 1.3 times the human dose (based on body surface area comparison) displayed major malformations including ovarian agenesis, pes varus, arhinia, microphthalmia and irregularities of the ossified facial tissues (4 of 321 examined fetuses).

In rats, rifapentine administration was associated with increased resorption rate and post implantation loss, decreased mean fetus weight, increased number of stillborn pups and slightly increased mortality during lactation. Rabbits given 1.3 times the human dose (based on body surface area comparisons) showed higher postimplantation losses and an increased incidence of stillborn pups.

RIFAPENTINE — ORAL

When rifapentine was administered at 0.3 times the human dose (based on body surface area comparisons) to mated female rats late in gestation (from day 15 of gestation to day 21 postpartum), pup weights and gestational survival (live pups born/pups born) were reduced compared to controls.

There are no adequate and well-controlled studies in pregnant women. In Clinical Study 008, 6 patients randomized to rifapentine became pregnant; 2 had normal deliveries; 2 had first trimester spontaneous abortions, 1 had an elective abortion and 1 patient was lost to follow-up. Of the 2 patients who spontaneously aborted, co-morbid conditions of ethanol abuse in 1 and HIV infection in the other were noted.

When administered during the last few weeks of pregnancy, rifampin can cause postnatal hemorrhages in the mother and infant for which treatment with vitamin K may be indicated.

Thus, patients and infants who receive rifapentine during the last few weeks of pregnancy should have appropriate clotting parameters evaluated.

Rifapentine should be used during pregnancy only if the potential benefit justifies the potential risk to the fetus.

➤*Lactation:* It is not known whether rifapentine is excreted in human milk. Because many drugs are excreted in human milk and because of the potential for serious adverse reactions in nursing infants, a decision should be made whether to discontinue nursing or discontinue the drug, taking into account the importance of the drug to the mother. Since rifapentine may produce a red-orange discoloration of body fluids, there is a potential for discoloration of breast milk.

➤*Children:* The safety and effectiveness of rifapentine in pediatric patients under the age of 12 have not been established. A pharmacokinetic study was conducted in 12- to 15-year-old healthy volunteers. The pharmacokinetics of rifapentine were similar to those observed in healthy adults.

➤*Elderly:* In general, dose selection for an elderly patient should be cautious, usually starting at the low end of the dosing range, reflecting the greater frequency of decreased hepatic, renal, or cardiac function and of concomitant disease or other drug therapy.

➤*Monitoring:* Adults treated for tuberculosis with rifapentine should have baseline measurements of hepatic enzymes, bilirubin, a complete blood count, and a platelet count (or estimate).

Patients should be seen at least monthly during therapy and should be specifically questioned concerning symptoms associated with adverse reactions. All patients with abnormalities should have follow-up, including laboratory testing, if necessary. Routine laboratory monitoring for toxicity in people with normal baseline measurements is generally not necessary.

Drug Interactions

➤*Indinavir:* In a study in which 600 mg rifapentine was administered twice weekly for 14 days followed by rifapentine twice weekly plus 800 mg indinavir 3 times a day for an additional 14 days, indinavir C_{max} decreased by 55% while AUC reduced by 70%. Clearance of indinavir increased by 3-fold in the presence of rifapentine while half-life did not change. But when indinavir was administered for 14 days followed by coadministration with rifapentine for an additional 14 days, indinavir did not affect the pharmacokinetics of rifapentine. Rifapentine should be used with extreme caution, if at all, in patients who are also taking protease inhibitors.

➤*Cytochrome P450 system:* Rifapentine is an inducer of cytochromes P450 3A4 and P450 2C8/9. Therefore, rifapentine may increase the metabolism of other coadministered drugs that are metabolized by these enzymes. Induction of enzyme activities by rifapentine occurred within 4 days after the first dose. Enzyme activities returned to baseline levels 14 days after discontinuing rifapentine. In addition, the magnitude of enzyme induction by rifapentine was dose and dosing frequency dependent; less enzyme induction occurred when 600 mg oral doses of rifapentine were given once every 72 hours versus daily. In vitro and in vivo enzyme induction studies have suggested rifapentine induction potential may be less than rifampin but more potent than rifabutin. Rifampin has been reported to accelerate the metabolism and may reduce the activity of the following drugs; hence, rifapentine may also increase the metabolism and decrease the activity of these drugs.

Dosage adjustments of the following drugs or of drugs metabolized by cytochrome P450 3A4 or P450 2C8/9 may be necessary if they are given concurrently with rifapentine. Patients using oral or other systemic hormonal contraceptives should be advised to change to nonhormonal methods of birth control.

Drugs That May Require Dosage Adjustment When Given Concurrently with Rifapentine	
Anticonvulsants (eg, phenytoin)	Haloperidol
Antiarrhythmics (eg, disopyramide, mexiletine, quinidine, tocainide	HIV protease inhibitors (eg, indinavir, ritonavir, nelfinavir, saquinavir; see indinavir interaction above)
Antibiotics (eg, chloramphenicol, clarithromycin, dapsone, doxycycline, fluoroquinolones such as ciprofloxacin)	Oral hypoglycemic agents (eg, sulfonylureas).
Anticoagulants, oral (eg, warfarin)	Immunosuppressants (eg, cyclosporine, tacrolimus)
Antifungals (eg, fluconazole, itraconazole, ketoconazole)	Levothyroxine
Barbiturates	Narcotic analgesics (eg, methadone)
Benzodiazepines (eg, diazepam)	Progestins
Beta blockers, calcium channel blockers (eg, diltiazem, nifedipine, verapamil)	Quinine
Corticosteroids	Reverse transcriptase inhibitors (eg, delavirdine, zidovudine)
Cardiac glycoside preparations	Sildenafil
Clofibrate	Theophylline
Oral or other systemic hormonal contraceptives	Tricyclic antidepressants (eg, amitriptyline, nortriptyline)

Esterase enzyme – The conversion of rifapentine to 25-desacetyl rifapentine is mediated by an esterase enzyme. There is minimal potential for rifapentine metabolism to be inhibited or induced by another drug, or for rifapentine to inhibit the metabolism of another drug based upon the characteristics of the esterase enzymes. Rifapentine does not induce its own metabolism. Since rifapentine is highly bound to albumin, drug displacement interactions may also occur.

Antacids – In Clinical study 008, patients were advised to take rifapentine at least 1 hour before or 2 hours after ingestion of antacids.

➤*Drug/Lab test interactions:* Therapeutic concentrations of rifampin have been shown to inhibit standard microbiological assays for serum folate and Vitamin B_{12}. Similar drug-laboratory interactions should be considered for rifapentine; thus, alternative assay methods should be considered.

Adverse Reactions

A patient may have experienced the same adverse event more than once during the course of the study, therefore, patient counts across the columns may not equal the patient counts in the total column. "Greater than or equal to 1%" refers to rifapentine in the total column.

Rifapentine Treatment-Related Adverse Events Occurring in ≥ 1% of the Patients in Study 008

Preferred term	Intensive phase[a]		Continuation phase[b]		Total	
	Rifapentine combination (n = 361) n (%)	Rifampin combination (n = 361) n (%)	Rifapentine combination (n = 321) n (%)	Rifampin combination (n = 307) n (%)	Rifapentine combination (n = 361) n (%)	Rifampin combination (n = 361) n (%)
Hyperuricemia	78 (21.6%)	55 (15.2%)	0	0	78 (21.6%)	55 (15.%2)
ALT increased	12 (3.3%)	17 (4.7%)	6 (1.9%)	7 (2.3%)	18 (5%)	24 (6.6%)
AST increased	11 (3%)	16 (4.4%)	5 (1.6%)	7 (2.3%)	15 (4.2%)	23 (6.4%)
Neutropenia	7 (1.9%)	9 (2.5%)	12 (3.7%)	9 (2.9%)	18 (5%)	18 (5%)
Pyuria	11 (3%)	10 (2.8%)	6 (1.9%)	3 (1%)	14 (3.9%)	12 (3.3%)
Proteinuria	15 (4.2%)	10 (2.8%)	2 (0.6%)	1 (0.3%)	17 (4.7%)	11 (3%)
Hematuria	10 (2.8%)	12 (3.3%)	4 (1.2%)	4 (1.3%)	13 (3.6%)	15 (4.2%)
Lymphopenia	14 (3.9%)	13 (3.6%)	3 (0.9%)	1 (0.3%)	16 (4.4%)	14 (3.9%)
Urinary casts	11 (3%)	3 (0.8%)	4 (1.2%)	0	14 (3.9%)	3 (0.8%)
Rash	9 (2.5%)	19 (5.3%)	4 (1.2%)	3 (1%)	13 (3.6%)	21 (5.8%)
Pruritus	8 (2.2%)	15 (4.2%)	1 (0.3%)	1 (0.3%)	9 (2.5%)	16 (4.4%)
Acne	5 (1.4%)	3 (0.8%)	2 (0.6%)	1 (0.3%)	7 (1.9%)	4 (1.1%)
Anorexia	6 (1.7%)	8 (2.2%)	3 (0.9%)	4 (1.3%)	8 (2.2%)	10 (2.8%)
Anemia	7 (1.9%)	9 (2.5%)	2 (0.6%)	1 (0.%3)	9 (2.5%)	10 (2.8%)
Leukopenia	4 (1.1%)	4 (1.1%)	3 (0.9%)	5 (1.6%)	7 (1.9%)	8 (2.2%)
Arthralgia	9 (2.5%)	7 (1.9%)	0	0	9 (2.5%)	7 (1.9%)
Pain	7 (1.9%)	5 (1.4%)	0	1 (0.3%)	7 (1.9%)	6 (1.7%)
Nausea	7 (1.9%)	2 (0.6%)	0	1 (0.3%)	7 (1.9%)	3 (0.8%)
Vomiting	4 (1.1%)	6 (1.7%)	1 (0.3%)	1 (0.3%)	5 (1.4%)	7 (1.9%)
Headache	3 (0.8%)	4 (1.1%)	1 (0.3%)	3 (1%)	4 (1.1%)	7 (1.9%)
Dyspepsia	3 (0.8%)	5 (1.4%)	2 (0.6%)	3 (1%)	4 (1.1%)	8 (2.2%)
Hypertension	3 (0.8%)	0 (0.0%)	1 (0.3%)	1 (0.3%)	4 (1.1%)	1 (0.3%)
Dizziness	4 (1.1%)	0	0	1 (0.3%)	4 (1.1%)	1 (0.3%)
Thrombocytosis	4 (1.1%)	2 (0.6%)	0	0	4 (1.1%)	2 (0.6%)
Diarrhea	4 (1.1%)	0	0	0	4 (1.1%)	0
Rash maculopapular	4 (1.1%)	3 (0.8%)	0	0	4 (1.1%)	3 (0.8%)
Hemoptysis	2 (0.6%)	0	2 (0.6%)	0	4 (1.1%)	0

[a] Intensive phase consisted of therapy with either rifapentine or rifampin combined with isoniazid, pyrazinamide, and ethambutol administered daily (rifapentine twice weekly) for 60 days.

[b] Continuation phase consisted of therapy with either rifapentine or rifampin combined with isoniazid for 120 days. Rifapentine patients were dosed once weekly; rifampin patients were dosed twice weekly. Events recorded in this phase includes those reported up to 3 months after continuation phase therapy was completed.

Treatment-related adverse events of moderate or severe intensity in less than 1% of the rifapentine combination therapy patients in Study 008 are presented below.

➤*Dermatologic:* Urticaria, skin discoloration.

RIFAPENTINE — ORAL

➤*GI:* Constipation, esophagitis, gastritis, pancreatitis.

➤*Hematologic:* Thrombocytopenia, neutrophilia, leukocytosis, purpura, hematoma.

➤*Hepatic:* Bilirubinemia, hepatitis.

➤*Metabolic/Nutritional:* Hyperkalemia, hypovolemia, alkaline phosphatase increased, LDH increased.

➤*Musculoskeletal:* Gout, arthrosis.

➤*Miscellaneous:* Aggressive reaction, peripheral edema, fatigue. Three (3) patients (2 rifampin combination therapy patients and 1 rifapentine combination therapy patient) were discontinued in the Intensive Phase as a result of hepatitis with increased liver function tests (ALT, AST, LDH, and bilirubin). Concomitant medications for all 3 patients included isoniazid, pyrazinamide, ethambutol, and pyridoxine. The 2 rifampin patients and 1 rifapentine patient recovered without sequelae.

Twenty-two (22) deaths occurred in Study 008 (11 in the rifampin combination therapy group and 11 in the rifapentine combination therapy group). None of the deaths were attributed to study medication. In the study, 18/361 (5%) rifampin combination therapy patients discontinued the study due to an adverse event compared to 11/361 (3%) rifapentine combination therapy patients.

The overall occurrence rate of treatment-related adverse events was higher in males with the rifapentine combination regimen (50%) versus the rifampin combination regimen (43%), while in females the overall rate was greater in the rifampin combination group (68%) compared to the rifapentine combination group (59%). However, there were higher frequencies of treatment-related hematuria and ALT increases for female patients in both treatment groups compared to those for male patients.

Adverse events associated with rifampin may occur with rifapentine: Effects of enzyme induction to increase metabolism resulting in decreased concentration of endogenous substrates, including adrenal hormones, thyroid hormones, and vitamin D.

Overdosage

There is no experience with the treatment of acute overdose with rifapentine at doses exceeding 1200 mg per dose. In a pharmacokinetic study involving healthy volunteers (n = 9), single oral doses up to 1200 mg have been administered without serious adverse reactions. The only adverse reactions reported with the 1200 mg dose were heartburn (3/8), headache (2/8) and increased urinary frequency (1/8). In clinical trials, tuberculosis patients ranging in age from 20 to 74 years accidentally received continuous daily doses of rifapentine 600 mg. Some patients received continuous daily dosing for up to 20 days without evidence of serious adverse effects. One patient experienced a transient elevation in AST and glucose (the latter attributed to pre-existing diabetes); a second patient experienced slight pruritus. While there is no experience with the treatment of acute overdose with rifapentine, clinical experience with rifamycins suggests that gastric lavage to evacuate gastric contents (within a few hours of overdose), followed by instillation of an activated charcoal slurry into the stomach, may help absorb any remaining drug from the gastrointestinal tract.

Rifapentine and 25-desacetyl rifapentine are 97.7% and 93.2% plasma protein bound, respectively. Rifapentine and related compounds excreted in urine account for only 17% of the administered dose; therefore, neither hemodialysis nor forced diuresis is expected to enhance the systemic elimination of unchanged rifapentine from the body of a patient with a rifapentine overdose.

Patient Information

The patient should be told that rifapentine may produce a reddish coloration of the urine, sweat, sputum, tears, and breast milk and the patient should be forewarned that contact lenses or dentures may be permanently stained. The patient should be advised that the reliability of oral or other systemic hormonal contraceptives may be affected; consideration should be given to using alternative contraceptive measures. For those patients with a propensity to nausea, vomiting, or gastrointestinal upset, administration of rifapentine with food may be useful. Patients should be instructed to notify their physician promptly if they experience any of the following: Fever, loss of appetite, malaise, nausea and vomiting, darkened urine, yellowish discoloration of the skin and eyes, and pain or swelling of the joints.

Compliance with the full course of therapy must be emphasized, and the importance of not missing any doses of the daily administered companion medications in the intensive phase must be stressed.

AMEBICIDES

PAROMOMYCIN

For complete prescribing information, refer to the Paromomycin Sulfate monograph in the Oral Aminoglycosides section.

IODOQUINOL (Diiodohydroxyquin)

Rx	Yodoxin (Glenwood)	Tablets: 210 mg	In 100s and 1,000s.
		650 mg	In 100s and 1,000s.
		Powder	In 25 g.

IODOQUINOL — ORAL

Indications

➤*Intestinal amebiasis:* Treatment of intestinal amebiasis.

Administration and Dosage

➤*Adults:*

Intestinal amebiasis – 650 mg 3 times per day after meals for 20 days.

➤*Children:*

Intestinal amebiasis – 10 to 13.3 mg/kg 3 times per day (not to exceed 1.95 g in 24 hours) for 20 days.

➤*Administration:* Take after meals.

➤*Storage/Stability:* Store at 15° to 30°C (59° to 86°F).

Actions

➤*Pharmacology:* Iodoquinol is amebicidal against *Entamoeba histolytica* and is considered effective against the trophozoite and cyst forms.

Contraindications

Hypersensitivity to iodine and 8-hydroxyquinolines; hepatic damage.

Warnings/Precautions

➤*CNS and ophthalmic effects:* Optic neuritis, optic atrophy, and peripheral neuropathy have been reported following prolonged high dosage therapy with halogenated 8-hydroxyquinolines.

➤*Thyroid disease:* Use iodoquinol with caution in patients with thyroid disease.

➤*Pregnancy: Category C.* Safety for use during pregnancy has not been established.

➤*Lactation:* Safety for use during lactation has not been established.

Drug Interactions

➤*Drug/Lab test interactions:* Protein-bound serum iodine levels may be increased during treatment with iodoquinol and therefore interfere with certain thyroid function tests. These effects may persist for as long as 6 months after discontinuation of therapy.

Adverse Reactions

➤*CNS:* Chills, headache, vertigo; peripheral neuropathy (associated with prolonged high-dosage 8-hydroxyquinoline therapy).

➤*Dermatologic:* Various forms of skin eruptions (acneiform papular and pustular bullae; vegetating or tuberous iododerma), urticaria, pruritus.

➤*GI:* Abdominal cramps, diarrhea, nausea, pruritus ani, and vomiting.

➤*Ophthalmic:* Optic neuritis and optic atrophy (associated with prolonged high-dosage 8-hydroxyquinoline therapy).

➤*Miscellaneous:* Fever, enlargement of thyroid.

CHLOROQUINE PHOSPHATE

For complete prescribing information, refer to the Chloroquine Phosphate monograph in the Antimalarial section.

CHLOROQUINE HYDROCHLORIDE

For chlorquine prescribing information, refer to the Chloroquine Phosphate monograph in the Antimalarial section.

FOSCARNET SODIUM (Phosphonoformic acid; PFA)

Rx	**Foscarnet Sodium** (Hospira)	**Injection:** 24 mg/mL	Preservative-free. In 250 and 500 mL.

FOSCARNET SODIUM — INJECTION

WARNING

Renal impairment is the major toxicity of foscarnet sodium. Frequent monitoring of serum creatinine, with dose adjustment for changes in renal function, and adequate hydration with administration of foscarnet sodium, is imperative (see Administration and Dosage, Hydration).

Seizures, related to alterations in plasma minerals and electrolytes, have been associated with foscarnet sodium treatment. Therefore, patients must be carefully monitored for such changes and their potential sequelae. Mineral and electrolyte supplementation may be required.

Foscarnet sodium is indicated for use only in immunocompromised patients with cytomegalovirus (CMV) retinitis and mucocutaneous acyclovir-resistant herpes simplex virus (HSV) infections (see Indications).

Indications

➤*CMV retinitis:* For the treatment of CMV retinitis in patients with acquired immunodeficiency syndrome (AIDS). Combination therapy with foscarnet sodium and ganciclovir is indicated for patients who have relapsed after monotherapy with either drug. Safety and efficacy of foscarnet sodium have not been established for treatment of other CMV infections (eg, pneumonitis, gastroenteritis); congenital or neonatal CMV disease; or nonimmunocompromised individuals.

➤*Mucocutaneous acyclovir-resistant HSV infections:* For the treatment of acyclovir-resistant mucocutaneous HSV infections in immunocompromised patients. Safety and efficacy of foscarnet sodium have not been established for treatment of other HSV infections (eg, retinitis, encephalitis); congenital or neonatal HSV disease; or HSV in nonimmunocompromised individuals.

Administration and Dosage

➤*General dosing considerations:* The recommended dosage, frequency, or infusion rates should not be exceeded.

All doses must be individualized for patient's renal function. To reduce the risk of nephrotoxicity, creatinine clearance (CrCl) (mL/min/kg) should be calculated even if serum creatinine is within the healthy range, and doses should be adjusted accordingly. (See Renal Function Impairment.)

An infusion pump must be used to control the rate of infusion. (See Administration.)

Adequate hydration is recommended to establish a diuresis (see Hydration for recommendation), both prior to and during treatment to minimize renal toxicity (see Warnings), provided there are no clinical contraindications.

➤*Adults:*

CMV retinitis –

Initial dosage: Either 90 mg/kg (1½- to 2-hour infusion) every 12 hours or 60 mg/kg (minimum 1-hour infusion) every 8 hours over 2 to 3 weeks depending on clinical response.

Maintenance dosage: 90 to 120 mg/kg/day (individualized for renal function) given as a single daily IV infusion over 2 hours. Because the superiority of the 120 mg/kg/day has not been established in controlled trials, and given the likely relationship of higher plasma foscarnet levels to toxicity, it is recommended that most patients be started on maintenance treatment with a dose of 90 mg/kg/day. Escalation to 120 mg/kg/day may be considered should early reinduction be required because of retinitis progression. Some patients who show excellent tolerance to foscarnet may benefit from initiation of maintenance treatment at 120 mg/kg/day earlier in their treatment.

Progression of retinitis: Patients who experience progression of retinitis while receiving foscarnet maintenance therapy may be retreated with the induction and maintenance regimens given above or with a combination of foscarnet and ganciclovir.

Because of physical incompatibility, foscarnet and ganciclovir must not be mixed.

Mucocutaneous acyclovir-resistant HSV infections – The initial dosage is 40 mg/kg (minimum 1-hour infusion) either every 8 or 12 hours for 2 to 3 weeks or until healed.

➤*Renal function impairment:* Foscarnet should be used with caution in patients with abnormal renal function because reduced plasma clearance of foscarnet will result in elevated plasma levels (see Pharmacokinetics). In addition, foscarnet has the potential to further impair renal function (see Warnings). Safety and efficacy data for patients with baseline serum creatinine levels more than 2.8 mg/dL or measured 24-hour creatinine clearances less than 50 mL/min are limited.

Renal function must be monitored carefully at baseline and during induction and maintenance therapy with appropriate dose adjustments for foscarnet as outlined in the following table. During foscarnet therapy if creatinine clearance falls below the limits of the dosing nomograms (0.4 mL/min/kg), foscarnet should be discontinued, the patient hydrated, and the patient monitored daily until resolution of renal impairment is ensured.

Foscarnet dosing must be individualized according to the patient's renal function status. Refer below for recommended doses and adjust the dose as indicated. Even patients with serum creatinine in the healthy range may require dose adjustment; therefore, the dose should be calculated at baseline and frequently thereafter.

To use this dosing guide, actual 24-hour creatinine clearance (mL/min) must be divided by body weight (kg), or the estimated creatinine clearance in mL/min/kg can be calculated from serum creatinine (mg/dL) using the following formula (modified Cockcroft and Gault equation):

$$\text{Males: } \frac{\text{Weight (kg)} \times (140 - \text{age})}{72 \times \text{serum creatinine (mg/dL)}} = \text{CrCl}$$

$$\text{Females: } 0.85 \times \text{male value}$$

Foscarnet Dosing Based on CrCl for Induction

CrCl (mL/min/kg)	HSV dosage equivalent to: 80 mg/kg/day total (40 mg/kg every 12 hours)	HSV dosage equivalent to: 120 mg/kg/day total (40 mg/kg every 8 hours)	CMV dosage equivalent to: 180 mg/kg/day total (60 mg/kg every 8 hours)	CMV dosage equivalent to: 180 mg/kg/day total (90 mg/kg every 12 hours)
> 1.4	40 mg/kg every 12 hours	40 mg/kg every 8 hours	60 mg/kg every 8 hours	90 mg/kg every 12 hours
> 1 to 1.4	30 mg/kg every 12 hours	30 mg/kg every 8 hours	45 mg/kg every 8 hours	70 mg/kg every 12 hours
> 0.8 to 1	20 mg/kg every 12 hours	35 mg/kg every 12 hours	50 mg/kg every 12 hours	50 mg/kg every 12 hours
> 0.6 to 0.8	35 mg/kg every 24 hours	25 mg/kg every 12 hours	40 mg/kg every 12 hours	80 mg/kg every 24 hours
> 0.5 to 0.6	25 mg/kg every 24 hours	40 mg/kg every 24 hours	60 mg/kg every 24 hours	60 mg/kg every 24 hours
≥ 0.4 to 0.5	20 mg/kg every 24 hours	35 mg/kg every 24 hours	50 mg/kg every 24 hours	50 mg/kg every 24 hours
< 0.4	Not recommended	Not recommended	Not recommended	Not recommended

Foscarnet Dosing Based on CrCl for Maintenance

CrCl (mL/min/kg)	CMV: equivalent to 90 mg/kg/day (once daily)	CMV: equivalent to 120 mg/kg/day (once daily)
> 1.4	90 mg/kg every 24 hours	120 mg/kg every 24 hours
> 1 to 1.4	70 mg/kg every 24 hours	90 mg/kg every 24 hours
> 0.8 to 1	50 mg/kg every 24 hours	65 mg/kg every 24 hours
> 0.6 to 0.8	80 mg/kg every 48 hours	105 mg/kg every 48 hours
> 0.5 to 0.6	60 mg/kg every 48 hours	80 mg/kg every 48 hours
≥ 0.4 to 0.5	50 mg/kg every 48 hours	65 mg/kg every 48 hours
< 0.4	Not recommended	Not recommended

➤*Hydration:* Hydration may reduce the risk of nephrotoxicity. It is recommended that 750 to 1,000 mL of normal saline or 5% dextrose solution should be given prior to the first infusion of foscarnet to establish diuresis. With subsequent infusions, 750 to 1,000 mL of hydration fluid should be given with 90 to 120 mg/kg of foscarnet, and 500 mL with 40 to 60 mg/kg of foscarnet. Hydration fluid may need to be decreased if clinically warranted.

After the first dose, the hydration fluid should be administered concurrently with each infusion of foscarnet.

➤*Accidental exposure:* Accidental skin and eye contact with foscarnet solution may cause local irritation and burning sensation. If accidental contact occurs, the exposed area should be flushed with water.

➤*Preparation for administration:* When a peripheral vein catheter is used, the 24 mg/mL must be diluted to 12 mg/mL with dextrose 5% in water or with a normal saline solution prior to administration to avoid local irritation of peripheral veins.

➤*Administration:* Do not administer foscarnet by rapid or bolus IV injection. The toxicity of foscarnet may be increased as a result of excessive plasma levels. Care should be taken to avoid unintentional overdose by carefully controlling the rate of infusion. Therefore, an infusion pump must be used. In spite of the use of an infusion pump, overdoses have occurred.

Foscarnet is administered by controlled IV infusion, either by using a central venous line or by using a peripheral vein. The standard 24 mg/mL solution may be used with or without dilution when using a central venous catheter for infusion. When a peripheral vein catheter is used, the 24 mg/mL must be diluted to 12 mg/mL with 5% dextrose in water or with a normal saline solution prior to administration to avoid local irritation of peripheral veins.

Since the dose of foscarnet is calculated on the basis of body weight, it may be desirable to remove and discard any unneeded quantity from the bottle before starting with the infusion to avoid overdosage. Solutions thus prepared should be used within 24 hours of first entry into a sealed bottle.

FOSCARNET SODIUM — INJECTION

➤*Admixture compatibility:*

Compatibility – Other drugs and supplements can be administered to a patient receiving foscarnet. However, care must be taken to ensure the foscarnet is only administered with normal saline or dextrose 5% solution and that no other drug or supplement is administered concurrently via the same catheter.

Incompatibility – Foscarnet has been reported to be chemically incompatible with dextrose 30%, amphotericin B, and solutions containing calcium such as Ringer's lactate and TPN. Physical incompatibility with other IV drugs has also been reported including acyclovir sodium, ganciclovir, trimetrexate glucuronate, pentamidine isethionate, vancomycin, trimethoprim/sulfamethoxazole, diazepam, midazolam, digoxin, phenytoin, leucovorin, and prochlorperazine. Because of foscarnet's chelating properties, a precipitate can potentially occur when divalent cautions are administered concurrently in the same catheter.

➤*Storage/Stability:* Store at 15° to 30°C (59° to 86°F), and protect from excessive heat (above 40°C; 104°F) and from freezing. Foscarnet should be used only if the bottle and seal are intact, a vacuum is present, and the solution is clear and colorless.

Actions

➤*Pharmacology:* Foscarnet sodium is an organic analogue of inorganic pyrophosphate that inhibits replication of herpes viruses in vitro including CMV and HSV types 1 and 2 (HSV-1 and HSV-2).

Foscarnet sodium exerts its antiviral activity by a selective inhibition at the pyrophosphate binding site on virus-specific DNA polymerases at concentrations that do not affect cellular DNA polymerases. Foscarnet sodium does not require activation (phosphorylation) by thymidine kinase or other kinases and therefore is active in vitro against HSV TK deficient mutants and CMV UL97 mutants. Thus, HSV strains resistant to acyclovir or CMV strains resistant to ganciclovir may be sensitive to foscarnet sodium. However, acyclovir— or ganciclovir—resistant mutants with alterations in the viral DNA polymerase may be resistant to foscarnet sodium and may not respond to therapy with foscarnet sodium. The combination of foscarnet sodium and ganciclovir has been shown to have enhanced activity in vitro.

➤*Pharmacokinetics:*

Absorption/Distribution – In vitro studies have shown that 14% to 17% of foscarnet is protein bound at plasma drug concentrations of 1 to 1000 mcM.

The pharmacokinetics of foscarnet have been determined after administration as an intermittent intravenous infusion during induction therapy in AIDS patients with CMV retinitis. Observed plasma foscarnet concentrations in 4 studies (FOS-01, ACTG-015, FP48PK, FP49PK) are summarized in the following table:

Foscarnet Sodium Pharmacokinetic Characteristics[a]

Parameter	60 mg/kg every 8 hours	90 mg/kg every 12 hours
C_{max} at steady state (mcM)	589 ± 192 (24)	623 ± 132 (19)
C_{trough} at steady state (mcM)	114 ± 91 (24)	63 ± 57 (17)
Volume of distribution (L/kg)	0.41 ± 0.13 (12)	0.52 ± 0.2 (18)
Plasma half-life (hours)	4 ± 2 (n = 24)	3.3 ± 1.4 (18)
Systemic clearance (L/hr)	6.2 ± 2.1 (24)	7.1 ± 2.7 (18)
Renal clearance (L/hr)	5.6 ± 1.9 (5)	6.4 ± 2.5 (13)
CSF:plasma ratio	0.69 ± 0.19 (9)[b]	0.66 ± 0.11 (5)[c]

[a] Values expressed as mean ± SD (number of subjects studied) for each parameter.
[b] 50 mg/kg every 8 hours for 28 days, samples taken 3 hours after end of 1 hour infusion (Astra Report 815–04 AC025–1).
[c] 90 mg/kg every 12 hours for 28 days, samples taken 1 hour after end of 2-hour infusion.

Metabolism/Excretion – The foscarnet terminal half-life determined by urinary excretion was 87.5 ± 41.8 hours, possibly due to release of foscarnet from bone. Postmortem data on several patients in European clinical trials provide evidence that foscarnet does accumulate in bone in humans; however, the extent to which this occurs has not been determined. In animal studies (mice), 40% of an intravenous dose of foscarnet sodium was deposited in bone in young animals and 7% was deposited in adult animals.

Special populations –

Renal function impairment: The pharmacokinetic properties of foscarnet have been determined in a small group of adult subjects with healthy and impaired renal function, as summarized in the following table:

Pharmacokinetic Parameters (Mean ± SD) After a Single 60 mg/kg Dose of Foscarnet Sodium in 4 Groups[a] of Adults with Varying Degrees of Renal Function

Parameter	Group 1 (n = 6)	Group 2 (n = 6)	Group 3 (n = 6)	Group 4 (n = 4)
Creatinine clearance (mL/min)	108 ± 16	68 ± 8	34 ± 9	20 ± 4
Foscarnet CL (mL/min/kg)	2.13 ± 0.71	1.33 ± 0.43	0.46 ± 0.14	0.43 ± 0.26
Foscarnet half-life (hours)	1.93 ± 0.12	3.35 ± 0.87	13 ± 4.05	25.3 ± 18.7

[a] Group 1 patients had healthy renal function defined as a creatinine clearance (C_{cr} of greater than 80 mL/min. Group 2 C_{cr} was 50 to 80 mL min. Group 3 C_{cr} was 25 to 49 mL/min and Group 4 C_{cr} was 10 to 24 mL/min.

Total systemic clearance of foscarnet decreased and half-life increased with diminishing renal function (as expressed by creatinine clearance). Based on these observations, it is necessary to modify the dosage of foscarnet in patients with renal impairment (see Administration and Dosage).

Contraindications

Clinically significant hypersensitivity to foscarnet sodium.

Warnings/Precautions

➤*Mineral and electrolyte abnormalities:* Foscarnet sodium has been associated with changes in serum electrolytes including hypocalcemia, hypophosphatemia, hyperphosphatemia, hypomagnesemia, and hypokalemia (see Adverse Reactions). Foscarnet sodium may also be associated with a dose-related decrease in ionized serum calcium which may not be reflected in total serum calcium. This effect is likely to be related to chelation of divalent metal ions such as calcium by foscarnet. Patients should be advised to report symptoms of low ionized calcium such as perioral tingling, numbness in the extremities and paresthesias. Particular caution and careful management of serum electrolytes is advised in patients with altered calcium or other electrolyte levels before treatment and especially in those with neurologic or cardiac abnormalities and those receiving other drugs known to influence minerals and electrolytes (see Administration and Dosage, Patient monitoring and Drug Interactions). Physicians should be prepared to treat these abnormalities and their sequelae such as tetany, seizures or cardiac disturbances. The rate of foscarnet sodium infusion may also affect the decrease in ionized calcium. Therefore, an infusion pump must be used for administration to prevent rapid intravenous infusion (see Administration and Dosage). Slowing the infusion rate may decrease or prevent symptoms.

➤*Seizures:* Seizures related to mineral and electrolyte abnormalities have been associated with foscarnet sodium treatment (see Warnings; Mineral and electrolyte abnormalities). Several cases of seizures were associated with death. Risk factors associated with seizures included impaired baseline renal function, low total serum calcium, and underlying CNS conditions.

➤*Nephrotoxicity:* The major toxicity of foscarnet sodium is renal impairment (see Adverse Reactions). Renal impairment is most likely to become clinically evident during the second week of induction therapy, but may occur at any time during foscarnet sodium treatment. Renal function should be monitored carefully during both induction and maintenance therapy (see Administration and Dosage, Patient monitoring). Elevations in serum creatinine are usually, but not always, reversible following discontinuation or dose adjustment of foscarnet sodium. Safety and efficacy data for patients with baseline serum creatinine levels > 2.8 mg/dL or measured 24-hour creatinine clearances < 50 mL/min are limited.

Because of foscarnet sodium's potential to cause renal impairment, dose adjustment based on serum creatinine is necessary.

➤*Hydration:* See Administration and Dosage for more information.

➤*Local irritation:* Care must be taken to infuse solutions containing foscarnet sodium only into veins with adequate blood flow to permit rapid dilution and distribution to avoid local irritation (see Administration and Dosage). Local irritation and ulcerations of penile epithelium have been reported in male patients receiving foscarnet sodium, possibly related to the presence of drug in the urine. One case of vulvovaginal ulcerations in a female receiving foscarnet sodium has been reported. Adequate hydration with close attention to personal hygiene may minimize the occurrence of such events.

➤*Hemopoietic system:* Anemia has been reported in 33% of patients receiving foscarnet sodium in controlled studies. Granulocytopenia has been reported in 17% of patients receiving foscarnet sodium in controlled studies; however, only 1% (2/189) were terminated from these studies because of neutropenia.

➤*Pregnancy: Category C.* Daily subcutaneous doses up to 75 mg/kg administered to female rats prior to and during mating, during gestation, and 21 days post-partum caused a slight increase (

These studies are inadequate to define the potential teratogenicity at levels to which women will be exposed. There are no adequate and well-controlled studies in pregnant women. Because animal reproductive studies are not always predictive of human response, foscarnet sodium should be used during pregnancy only if clearly needed.

➤*Lactation:* It is not known whether foscarnet sodium is excreted in human milk; however, in lactating rats administered 75 mg/kg, foscarnet sodium was excreted in maternal milk at concentrations three times higher than peak maternal blood concentrations.

➤*Children:* The safety and effectiveness of foscarnet sodium in pediatric patients have not been established. Foscarnet sodium is deposited in teeth and bone and deposition is greater in young and growing animals. Foscarnet sodium has been demonstrated to adversely affect development of tooth enamel in mice and rats. The effects of this deposition on skeletal development have not been studied. Since deposition in human bone has also been shown to occur, it is likely that it does so to a greater degree in developing bone in pediatric patients. Administration to pediatric patients should be

FOSCARNET SODIUM — INJECTION

undertaken only after careful evaluation and only if the potential benefits for treatment outweigh the risks.

➤*Elderly:* No studies of the efficacy or safety of foscarnet sodium in persons over age 65 have been conducted. Since these individuals frequently have reduced glomerular filtration, particular attention should be paid to assessing renal function before and during foscarnet sodium administration (see Administration and Dosage).

➤*Monitoring:* The majority of patients will experience some decrease in renal function due to foscarnet sodium administration. Therefore it is recommended that creatinine clearance, either measured or estimated using the modified Cockcroft and Gault equation based on serum creatinine, be determined at baseline, 2 to 3 times per week during induction therapy and at least every 1 to 2 weeks during maintenance therapy, with foscarnet sodium dose adjusted accordingly (see Dose Adjustment). More frequent monitoring may be required for some patients. It is also recommended that a 24-hour creatinine clearance be determined at baseline and periodically thereafter to ensure correct dosing (assuming verification of an adequate collection using creatinine index). Foscarnet sodium should be discontinued if creatinine clearance drops below 0.4 mL/min/kg.

Due to foscarnet sodium's propensity to chelate divalent metal ions and alter levels of serum electrolytes, patients must be monitored closely for such changes. It is recommended that a schedule similar to that recommended for serum creatinine (see above) be used to monitor serum calcium, magnesium, potassium and phosphorus. Particular caution is advised in patients with decreased total serum calcium or other electrolyte levels before treatment, as well as in patients with neurologic or cardiac abnormalities, and in patients receiving other drugs known to influence serum calcium levels. Any clinically significant metabolic changes should be corrected. Also, patients who experience mild (eg, perioral numbness or paresthesias) or severe (eg, seizures) symptoms of electrolyte abnormalities should have serum electrolyte and mineral levels assessed as close in time to the event as possible.

Careful monitoring and appropriate management of electrolytes, calcium, magnesium, and creatinine are of particular importance in patients with conditions that may predispose them to seizures (see Warnings).

Drug Interactions

➤*QT prolongation:* An additive effect of foscarnet with other drugs that prolong the QT interval cannot be excluded. The following drugs may prolong the QT interval and increase the risk of life-threatening cardiac arrhythmias, including torsade de pointes: Antiarrhythmic agents (eg, amiodarone, bretylium, disopyramide, dofetilide, procainamide, quinidine, and sotalol), arsenic trioxide, chlorpromazine, cisapride, dolasetron, droperidol, mefloquine, mesoridazine, moxifloxacin, pentamidine, pimozide, tacrolimus, thioridazine, and ziprasidone. For a more complete list of drugs that may prolong the QT interval, see the appendix, Drug-Induced Prolongation of the QT Interval and Torsade de Pointes.

Foscarnet Drug Interactions

Precipitant drug	Object drug[a]		Description
Nephrotoxic drugs (eg, aminoglycosides, amphotericin B, IV pentamidine)	Foscarnet	↑	Because of foscarnet's tendency to cause renal impairment, avoid the use of foscarnet in combination with potentially nephrotoxic drugs unless the potential benefits outweigh the risks to the patient.
Ritonavir/ Saquinavir	Foscarnet	↑	Abnormal renal function has occurred with concomitant use.
Foscarnet	Calcium	↓	Foscarnet decreases serum concentrations of ionized calcium. Avoid concurrent use.
Foscarnet	Pentamidine	↑	Concomitant treatment of four patients with foscarnet and IV pentamidine may have caused hypocalcemia; one patient died with severe hypocalcemia. Toxicity associated with concomitant use of aerosolized pentamidine has not been reported.

[a] ↑ = object drug increased; ↓ = object drug decreased.

Adverse Reactions

➤*Electrolyte disturbance:* Foscarnet sodium has been associated with changes in serum electrolytes including hypocalcemia (15% to 30%), hypophosphatemia (8% to 26%) and hyperphosphatemia (6%), hypomagnesemia (15% to 30%), and hypokalemia (16% to 48%) (see Warnings). The higher percentages were derived from those patients receiving hydration.

➤*Renal:* The major toxicity of foscarnet sodium is renal impairment (see Warnings). Approximately 33% of 189 patients with AIDS and CMV retinitis who received foscarnet sodium (60 mg/kg 3 times daily), without adequate hydration, developed significant impairment of renal function (serum creatinine ≥ 2 mg/dL). The incidence of renal impairment in subsequent clinical trials in which 1,000 mL of normal saline or 5% dextrose solution was given with each infusion of foscarnet sodium was 12% (34/280).

➤*Seizures:* Foscarnet sodium treatment was associated with seizures in 18/189 (10%) AIDS patients in the initial 5 controlled studies (see Warnings). Risk factors associated with seizures included impaired baseline renal function, low total serum calcium, and underlying CNS conditions predisposing the patient to seizures. The rate of seizures did not increase with duration of treatment. Three cases were associated with overdoses of foscarnet sodium (see Overdosage). In five controlled US clinical trials the most frequently reported adverse events in patients with AIDS and CMV retinitis are shown in the following table. These figures were calculated without reference to drug relationship or severity.

Foscarnet Adverse Reactions Reported in US Clinical Trials

Adverse reaction	n = 189
Fever	65%
Nausea	47%
Anemia	33%
Diarrhea	30%
Abnormal renal function	27%
Vomiting	26%
Headache	26%
Seizures	10%

From these same controlled trials, adverse events categorized by investigator as "severe" are shown in the following table. Although death was specifically attributed to foscarnet in only 1 case, other complications of foscarnet (ie, renal impairment, electrolyte abnormalities, and seizures) may have contributed to patient deaths (see Warnings).

Severe Foscarnet Adverse Reactions

Adverse reaction	n = 189
Death	14%
Abnormal renal function	14%
Marrow suppression	10%
Anemia	9%
Seizures	7%

➤*Incidence ≥ 5%:* From the 5 initial US controlled trials of foscarnet sodium, the following list of adverse events has been compiled regardless of causal relationship to foscarnet sodium. Evaluation of these reports was difficult because of the diverse manifestations of the underlying disease and because most patients received numerous concomitant medications.

CNS – Headache, paresthesia, dizziness, involuntary muscle contractions, hypoesthesia, neuropathy, seizures including grand mal seizures (see Warnings).

Dermatologic – Rash, increased sweating.

GI – Anorexia, nausea, diarrhea, vomiting, abdominal pain.

GU – Alterations in renal function included increased serum creatinine, decreased creatinine clearance, and abnormal renal function (see Warnings).

Hematologic – Anemia, granulocytopenia, leukopenia (see Precautions).

Metabolic/Nutritional – Mineral and electrolyte imbalances (see Warnings) including hypokalemia, hypocalcemia, hypomagnesemia, hypophosphatemia, hyperphosphatemia.

Psychiatric – Depression, confusion, anxiety.

Respiratory – Coughing, dyspnea.

Special senses – Vision abnormalities.

Miscellaneous – Fever, fatigue, rigors, asthenia, malaise, pain, infection, sepsis, death.

➤*Incidence 1% to < 5%:*

Cardiovascular – Hypertension, palpitations, ECG abnormalities including sinus tachycardia, first degree AV block and non-specific ST-T segment changes, hypotension, flushing, cerebrovascular disorder (see Warnings).

CNS – Tremor, ataxia, dementia, stupor, generalized spasms, sensory disturbances, meningitis, aphasia, abnormal coordination, leg cramps, EEG abnormalities (see Warnings).

Dermatologic – Pruritus, skin ulceration, seborrhea, erythematous rash, maculopapular rash, skin discoloration.

GI – Constipation, dysphagia, dyspepsia, rectal hemorrhage, dry mouth, melena, flatulence, ulcerative stomatitis, pancreatitis.

GU – Albuminuria, dysuria, polyuria, urethral disorder, urinary retention, urinary tract infections, acute renal failure, nocturia, facial edema.

Hematologic – Thrombocytopenia, platelet abnormalities, thrombosis, white blood cell abnormalities, lymphadenopathy.

Hepatic – Abnormal A-G ratio, abnormal hepatic function, increased ALT, increased AST.

Metabolic/Nutritional – Hyponatremia, decreased weight, increased alkaline phosphatase, increased LDH, increased BUN, acidosis, cachexia, thirst, hypercalcemia (see Warnings).

Musculoskeletal – Arthralgia, myalgia.

Psychiatric – Insomnia, somnolence, nervousness, amnesia, agitation, aggressive reaction, hallucination.

Respiratory – Pneumonia, sinusitis, pharyngitis, rhinitis, respiratory disorders, respiratory insufficiency, pulmonary infiltration, stridor, pneumothorax, hemoptysis, bronchospasm.

Special senses – Taste perversions, eye abnormalities, eye pain, conjunctivitis.

FOSCARNET SODIUM — INJECTION

Miscellaneous – Back pain, chest pain, edema, influenza-like symptoms, bacterial infections, moniliasis, fungal infections, abscess.

Application Site: Injection site pain, injection site inflammation.

Neoplasms: Lymphoma-like disorder, sarcoma.

➤*Incidence < 1%:* Selected adverse events occurring at a rate of less than 1% in the five initial US controlled clinical trials of foscarnet sodium include: syndrome of inappropriate antidiuretic hormone secretion, pancytopenia, hematuria, dehydration, hypoproteinemia, increases in amylase and creatine phosphokinase, cardiac arrest, coma, and other cardiovascular and neurologic complications. Selected adverse event data from the Foscarnet vs Ganciclovir CMV Retinitis Trial (FGCRT), performed by the Studies of the Ocular Complications of AIDS (SOCA) Research Group are shown in the following table.

Foscarnet vs Ganciclovir CMV Retinitis Trial: Selected Adverse Reactions[a]

	Ganciclovir			Foscarnet		
Adverse reaction	No. of events	No. of patients	Rates[b]	No. of events	No. of patients	Rates[b]
Absolute neutrophil count decreasing < 0.50•10⁹ per liter	63	41	1.3	31	17	0.72
Serum creatinine increasing to > 260 mcmol per liter (> 2.9 mg/dL)	6	4	0.12	13	9	0.3
Seizure[c]	21	13	0.37	19	13	0.37
Catheterization-related infection	49	27	1.26	51	28	1.46
Hospitalization	209	91	4.74	202	75	5.03

[a] Values for the treatment groups refer only to patients who completed at least 1 follow-up visit (ie, 113 to 119 patients in the ganciclovir group and 93 to 100 in the foscarnet group. "Events" denotes all events observed and "patients" the number of patients with 1 or more of the indicated events.
[b] Per person-year at risk.
[c] Final frozen SOCA 1 database dated October 1991.

Selected adverse events from ACTG Study 228 (CRRT) comparing combination therapy with foscarnet sodium or ganciclovir monotherapy are shown in the following table. The most common reason for a treatment change in patients assigned to either foscarnet sodium or ganciclovir was retinitis progression. The most frequent reason for a treatment change in the combination treatment group was toxicity.

Foscarnet CMV Retinitis Retreatment Trial: Selected Adverse Reactions

	Foscarnet (n = 88)			Ganciclovir (n = 93)			Combination (n = 93)		
Adverse reaction	No. events	No. patients[a]	Rate[b]	No. events	No. patients[a]	Rate[b]	No. events	No. patients[a]	Rate[b]
Anemia (Hgb < 70 g/L)	11	7	0.20	9	7	0.14	19	15	0.33
Neutropenia[c]									
ANC $0.75 \cdot 10^9$ cells/L	86	32	1.53	95	41	1.51	107	51	1.91
ANC $0.50 \cdot 10^9$ cells/L	50	25	0.91	49	28	0.8	50	28	0.85
Thrombocytopenia									
Platelets $50 \cdot 10^9$/L	28	14	0.5	19	8	0.43	40	15	0.56
Platelets $20 \cdot 10^9$/L	1	1	0.01	6	2	0.05	7	6	0.18

Foscarnet CMV Retinitis Retreatment Trial: Selected Adverse Reactions

	Foscarnet (n = 88)			Ganciclovir (n = 93)			Combination (n = 93)		
Adverse reaction	No. events	No. patients[a]	Rate[b]	No. events	No. patients[a]	Rate[b]	No. events	No. patients[a]	Rate[b]
Nephrotoxicity									
Creatinine > 260 mcmol/L (> 2.9 mg/dL)	9	7	0.15	10	7	0.17	11	10	0.2
Seizures	6	6	0.17	7	6	0.15	10	5	0.18
Hospitalizations	86	53	1.86	111	59	2.36	118	64	2.36

[a] Patients with event.
[b] Rate = events/person/year.
[c] ANC = absolute neutrophil count.

Postmarketing – Adverse events that have been reported in postmarketing surveillance include: Ventricular arrhythmia, prolongation of QT interval, diabetes insipidus (usually nephrogenic), renal calculus, and muscle disorders including myopathy, myositis, muscle weakness and rare cases of rhabdomyolysis. Cases of vesiculobullous eruptions including erythema multiforme, toxic epidermal necrolysis, and Stevens-Johnson syndrome have been reported. In most cases, patients were taking other medications that have been associated with toxic epidermal necrolysis or Stevens-Johnson syndrome.

Overdosage

➤*Symptoms:* In controlled clinical trials performed in the United States, overdosage with foscarnet sodium was reported in 10 out of 189 patients. All 10 patients experienced adverse events and all except 1 made a complete recovery. One patient died after receiving a total daily dose of 12.5 g for 3 days instead of the intended 10.9 g. The patient suffered a grand mal seizure and became comatose. Three days later the patient expired with the cause of death listed as respiratory/cardiac arrest. The other 9 patients received doses ranging from 1.14 times to 8 times their recommended doses with an average of 4 times their recommended doses. Overall, 3 patients had seizures, 3 patients had renal function impairment, 4 patients had paresthesias either in limbs or periorally, and 5 patients had documented electrolyte disturbances primarily involving calcium and phosphate.

➤*Treatment:* There is no specific antidote for foscarnet sodium overdose. Hemodialysis and hydration may be of benefit in reducing drug plasma levels in patients who receive an overdosage of foscarnet sodium, but the effectiveness of these interventions has not been evaluated. The patient should be observed for signs and symptoms of renal impairment and electrolyte imbalance. Medical treatment should be instituted if clinically warranted.

Patient Information

➤*CMV retinitis:* Patients should be advised that foscarnet sodium is not a cure for CMV retinitis, and that they may continue to experience progression of retinitis during or following treatment. They should be advised to have regular ophthalmologic examinations.

➤*Mucocutaneous acyclovir-resistant HSV infections:* Patients should be advised that foscarnet sodium is not a cure for HSV infections. While complete healing is possible, relapse occurs in most patients. Because relapse may be due to acyclovir-sensitive HSV, sensitivity testing of the viral isolate is advised. In addition, repeated treatment with foscarnet sodium has led to the development of resistance associated with poorer response. In the case of poor therapeutic response, sensitivity testing of the viral isolate also is advised.

➤*General:* Patients should be informed that the major toxicities of foscarnet are renal impairment, electrolyte disturbances, and seizures, and that dose modifications and possibly discontinuation may be required. The importance of close monitoring while on therapy must be emphasized. Patients should be advised of the importance of reporting to their physicians symptoms of perioral tingling, numbness in the extremities or paresthesias during or after infusion as possible symptoms of electrolyte abnormalities. Should such symptoms occur, the infusion of foscarnet sodium should be stopped, appropriate laboratory samples for assessment of electrolyte concentrations obtained, and a physician consulted before resuming treatment. The rate of infusion must be no more than 1 mg/kg/minute. The potential for renal impairment may be minimized by accompanying foscarnet sodium administration with hydration adequate to establish and maintain a diuresis during dosing.

GANCICLOVIR (DHPG)

Rx	**Ganciclovir** (Ranbaxy)	**Capsules:** 250 mg	(RX 636). Green. In 180s.
Rx	**Ganciclovir** (Ranbaxy)	**Capsules:** 500 mg	(RX 637). Yellow/Green. In 180s.
Rx	**Ganciclovir** (APP Pharmaceuticals)	**Injection, lyophilized powder for solution:** 500 mg	As ganciclovir sodium. Sodium 46 mg. In 10 mL vials.
Rx	**Cytovene** (Roche)		As ganciclovir sodium. Sodium 46 mg. In 10 mL vials.

GANCICLOVIR SODIUM — ORAL

WARNING

The clinical toxicity of ganciclovir includes granulocytopenia, anemia and thrombocytopenia. In animal studies ganciclovir was carcinogenic, teratogenic and caused aspermatogenesis.

Ganciclovir capsules are indicated only for prevention of cytomegalovirus (CMV) disease in patients with advanced HIV infection at risk for CMV disease, for maintenance treatment of CMV retinitis in immunocompromised patients, and for prevention of CMV disease in solid organ transplant recipients.

Because ganciclovir capsules are associated with a risk of more rapid rate of CMV retinitis progression, they should be used as maintenance treatment only in those patients for whom this risk is balanced by the benefit associated with avoiding daily intravenous infusions.

Indications

➤*CMV disease:* For the prevention of cytomegalovirus (CMV) disease in solid organ transplant recipients and in individuals with advanced HIV infection at risk for developing CMV disease.

➤*CMV retinitis:* An alternative to the intravenous formulation for maintenance treatment of CMV retinitis in immunocompromised patients, including patients with AIDS, in whom retinitis is stable following appropriate induction therapy and for whom the risk of more rapid progression is balanced by the benefit associated with avoiding daily IV infusions.

Safety and efficacy of ganciclovir has not been established for congenital or neonatal CMV disease; nor for the treatment of established CMV disease other than retinitis; nor for use in nonimmunocompromised individuals. The safety and efficacy of ganciclovir capsules have not been established for treating any manifestation of CMV disease other than maintenance treatment of CMV retinitis.

Administration and Dosage

➤*Adults:*

Cytomegalovirus disease (prophylaxis) –

Usual dosage: 1,000 mg 3 times a day with food.

Duration of therapy: The duration of treatment in transplant recipients is dependent upon the duration and degree of immunosuppression. In a controlled clinical trial of liver allograft recipients, treatment with ganciclovir was continued through week 14 posttransplantation.

Cytomegalovirus retinitis – For patients who experience progression of CMV retinitis while receiving maintenance treatment with either formulation of ganciclovir, reinduction treatment is recommended.

Maintenance dosage: 1,000 mg 3 times a day with food. This maintenance dosage follows induction treatment with ganciclovir injection. Ganciclovir capsules should not be used for induction treatment.

Alternative dosage: 500 mg 6 times daily every 3 hours with food during waking hours.

➤*Children:* Ganciclovir capsules have not been studied in pediatric patients younger than 13 years of age.

See Adults for dosing for children 13 years of age and older.

➤*Elderly:* Dosage reduction may be required in elderly patients with underlying renal function impairment. (See Renal Function Impairment.)

➤*Renal function impairment:*

Ganciclovir Oral Dosing in Renal Function Impairment

Creatinine clearance[a] (mL/min)	Ganciclovir capsule doses
≥ 70	1,000 mg 3 times daily or 500 mg every 3 hours, 6 times daily
50 to 69	1,500 mg once daily or 500 mg 3 times daily
25 to 49	1,000 mg once daily or 500 mg twice daily
10 to 24	500 mg once daily
< 10	500 mg 3 times per week following hemodialysis

[a] Creatinine clearance can be related to serum creatinine by the following formulas:

Creatinine clearance for males = (140 − age in years) (body weight in kg)/(72) (serum creatinine in mg/dL).

Creatinine clearance for females = 0.85 × male value.

➤*Patients with hematologic abnormalities:* Consider dosage reductions for patients with neutropenia, anemia, and/or thrombocytopenia. Ganciclovir should not be administered in patients with severe neutropenia (absolute neutrophil count [ANC] less than 500/mcL) or severe thrombocytopenia (platelets less than 25,000/mcL). (See also Warnings/Precautions.)

➤*Preparation for administration:* Ganciclovir is an immunosuppressant agent and is also considered a mutagen and potential teratogen. Follow safe handling procedures when preparing, administering, or dispensing ganciclovir.

Caution should be exercised in the handling of ganciclovir capsules. Avoid direct contact with the skin or mucous membranes of the powder contained in ganciclovir capsules. If such contact occurs, wash thoroughly with soap and water; rinse eyes thoroughly with plain water.

➤*Administration:* Take capsules with food. Capsules should not be opened or crushed.

➤*Storage/Stability:* Store at controlled room temperature, 20° to 25°C (68° to 77°F); excursions are permitted between 15° and 30°C (59° and 86°F).

Actions

➤*Pharmacology:* Ganciclovir is an acyclic nucleoside analogue of 2′-deoxyguanosine that inhibits replication of herpes viruses. Ganciclovir has been shown to be active against cytomegalovirus (CMV) and herpes simplex virus (HSV) in human clinical studies.

To achieve anti-CMV activity, ganciclovir is phosphorylated first to the monophosphate form by a CMV-encoded (UL97 gene) protein kinase homologue, then to the di- and triphosphate forms by cellular kinases. Ganciclovir triphosphate concentrations may be 100-fold greater in CMV-infected than in uninfected cells, indicating preferential phosphorylation in infected cells. Ganciclovir triphosphate, once formed, persists for days in the CMV-infected cell. Ganciclovir triphosphate is believed to inhibit viral DNA synthesis by competitive inhibition of viral DNA polymerases; and incorporation into viral DNA, resulting in eventual termination of viral DNA elongation.

➤*Pharmacokinetics:*

Absorption – The absolute bioavailability of oral ganciclovir under fasting conditions was approximately 5% (n = 6) and following food was 6% to 9% (n = 32). When ganciclovir was administered orally with food at a total daily dosage of 3 g/day (500 mg every 3 hours, 6 times daily and 1000 mg 3 times a day), the steady-state absorption as measured by area under the serum concentration vs time curve (AUC) over 24 hours and maximum serum concentrations (C_{max}) were similar following both regimens with an AUC_{0-24} of 15.9 ± 4.2 (mean ± SD) and 15.4 ± 4.3 mcg•hr/mL and C_{max} of 1.02 ± 0.24 and 1.18 ± 0.36 mcg/mL, respectively (n = 16).

When ganciclovir capsules were given with a meal containing 602 calories and 46.5% fat at a dosage of 1000 mg every 8 hours to 20 HIV-positive subjects, the steady-state AUC increased by 22% ± 22% (range, −6% to 68%) and there was a significant prolongation of time to peak serum concentrations (t_{max}) from 1.8 ± 0.8 to 3 ± 0.6 hours and a higher C_{max} (0.85 ± 0.25 vs 0.96 ± 0.27 mcg/mL) (n = 20).

Distribution – For ganciclovir capsules, no correlation was observed between AUC and reciprocal weight (range, 55 to 128 kg); oral dosing according to weight is not required. Binding to plasma proteins was 1% to 2% over ganciclovir concentrations of 0.5 and 51 mcg/mL.

Metabolism – Following oral administration of a single 1000 mg dose of ^{14}C-labeled ganciclovir, 86% ± 3% of the administered dose was recovered in the feces and 5% ± 1% was recovered in the urine (n = 4). No metabolite accounted for more than 1% to 2% of the radioactivity recovered in urine or feces.

Excretion – When administered orally, it exhibits linear kinetics up to a total daily dose of 4 g/day. Renal excretion of unchanged drug by glomerular filtration and active tubular secretion is the major route of elimination of ganciclovir. After oral administration of ganciclovir, steady-state is achieved within 24 hours. Renal clearance following oral administration was 3.1 ± 1.2 mL/min/kg (n = 22). Half-life was 4.8 ± 0.9 hours (n = 39) following oral administration.

Special populations –

Renal function impairment: The pharmacokinetics of ganciclovir following oral administration of ganciclovir capsules were evaluated in 44 patients, who were either solid organ transplant recipients or HIV positive. Apparent oral clearance of ganciclovir decreased and $AUC_{0-24\,hr}$ increased with diminishing renal function (as expressed by creatinine clearance). Based on these observations, it is necessary to modify the dosage of ganciclovir in patients with renal impairment.

Hemodialysis: See Administration and Dosage for more information.

Contraindications

Hypersensitivity to ganciclovir or acyclovir.

Warnings/Precautions

➤*Hematologic:* Ganciclovir should not be administered if the absolute neutrophil count is less than 500 cells/mcL or the platelet count is less than 25,000 cells/mcL. Granulocytopenia (neutropenia), anemia and thrombocytopenia have been observed in patients treated with ganciclovir. The frequency and severity of these events vary widely in different patient populations.

Ganciclovir should, therefore, be used with caution in patients with preexisting cytopenias or with a history of cytopenic reactions to other drugs, chemicals or irradiation. Granulocytopenia usually occurs during the first or second week of treatment but may occur at any time during treatment. Cell counts usually begin to recover within 3 to 7 days of discontinuing drug.

➤*Renal function impairment:* Ganciclovir should be used with caution in patients with impaired renal function because the half-life and plasma/serum concentrations of ganciclovir will be increased due to reduced renal clearance.

Hemodialysis has been shown to reduce plasma levels of ganciclovir by approximately 50%.

Since ganciclovir is excreted by the kidneys, normal clearance depends on adequate renal function. If renal function is impaired, dosage adjustments are required for ganciclovir IV and should be considered for ganciclovir capsules. Such adjustments should be based on measured or estimated creatinine clearance values.

➤*Pregnancy: Category C.* Because of the mutagenic and teratogenic potential of ganciclovir, women of childbearing potential should be advised to use

GANCICLOVIR SODIUM — ORAL

effective contraception during treatment. Similarly, men should be advised to practice barrier contraception during and for at least 90 days following treatment with ganciclovir.

Ganciclovir has been shown to be embryotoxic in rabbits and mice following intravenous administration and teratogenic in rabbits. Fetal resorptions were present in at least 85% of rabbits and mice administered 60 mg/kg/day and 108 mg/kg/day (2× the human exposure based on AUC comparisons), respectively. Effects observed in rabbits included fetal growth retardation, embryolethality, teratogenicity or maternal toxicity. Teratogenic changes included cleft palate, anophthalmia/microphthalmia, aplastic organs (kidney and pancreas), hydrocephaly, and brachygnathia. In mice, effects observed were maternal/fetal toxicity and embryolethality.

Ganciclovir may be teratogenic or embryotoxic at dose levels recommended for human use. There are no adequate and well-controlled studies in pregnant women. Ganciclovir should be used during pregnancy only if the potential benefits justify the potential risk to the fetus.

Fertility impairment – Although data in humans have not been obtained, it is considered probable that ganciclovir at the recommended doses causes temporary or permanent inhibition of spermatogenesis. Animal data also indicate that suppression of fertility in females may occur.

➤*Lactation:* It is not known whether ganciclovir is excreted in human milk. However, many drugs are excreted in human milk and, because carcinogenic and teratogenic effects occurred in animals treated with ganciclovir, the possibility of serious adverse reactions from ganciclovir in nursing infants is considered likely. Mothers should be instructed to discontinue nursing if they are receiving ganciclovir. The minimum interval before nursing can safely be resumed after the last dose of ganciclovir is unknown.

➤*Children:* Ganciclovir capsules have not been studied in pediatric patients under age 13 years.

Safety and efficacy of ganciclovir in pediatric patients have not been established. The use of ganciclovir in the pediatric population warrants extreme caution due to the probability of long-term carcinogenicity and reproductive toxicity. Administration to pediatric patients should be undertaken only after careful evaluation and only if the potential benefits of treatment outweigh the risks.

➤*Elderly:* Clinical studies of ganciclovir did not include sufficient numbers of subjects aged 65 years and over to determine whether they respond differently from younger subjects. In general, dose selection for an elderly patient should be cautious, reflecting the greater frequency of decreased hepatic, renal, or cardiac function, and of concomitant disease or other drug therapy. Ganciclovir capsules are known to be substantially excreted by the kidney, and the risk of toxic reactions to this drug may be greater in patients with impaired renal function. Because elderly patients are more likely to have decreased renal function, care should be taken in dose selection. In addition, renal function should be monitored and dosage adjustments should be made accordingly.

➤*Monitoring:* Due to the frequency of neutropenia, anemia, and thrombocytopenia in patients receiving ganciclovir, it is recommended that complete blood counts and platelet counts be performed frequently, especially in patients in whom ganciclovir or other nucleoside analogues have previously resulted in leukopenia, or in whom neutrophil counts are less than 1000 cells/mcL at the beginning of treatment. Increased serum creatinine levels have been observed in trials evaluating both ganciclovir. Patients should have serum creatinine or creatinine clearance values monitored carefully to allow for dosage adjustments in renally impaired patients.

HIV-positive patients with CMV retinitis – Ganciclovir is not a cure for CMV retinitis, and immunocompromised patients may continue to experience progression of retinitis during or following treatment. Patients should be advised to have ophthalmologic follow-up examinations at a minimum of every 4 to 6 weeks while being treated with ganciclovir capsules. Some patients will require more frequent follow-up.

Drug Interactions

Ganciclovir Drug Interactions

Precipitant drug	Object drug[a]		Description
Ganciclovir	Cytotoxic drugs	↑	Cytotoxic drugs that inhibit replication of rapidly dividing cell populations such as bone marrow, spermatogonia, and germinal layers of skin and GI mucosa may have additive toxicity when administered concomitantly with ganciclovir. Therefore, consider the concomitant use of drugs such as dapsone, pentamidine, flucytosine, vincristine, vinblastine, adriamycin, amphotericin B, trimethoprim/sulfamethoxazole combinations, or other nucleoside analogs only if potential benefits outweigh the risks.
Imipenem-cilastatin	Ganciclovir	↑	Generalized seizures occurred in patients who received ganciclovir and imipenem-cilastatin. Do not use these drugs concomitantly unless the potential benefits outweigh the risks.
Nephrotoxic drugs	Ganciclovir	↑	Increases in serum creatinine were observed following concurrent use of ganciclovir and either cyclosporine or amphotericin B.
Probenecid	Ganciclovir	↑	Ganciclovir AUC increased 53% (range, -14% to 299%) in the presence of probenecid. Renal clearance of ganciclovir decreased 22% (range, -54% to -4%), which is consistent with an interaction involving competition for renal tubular secretion.
Ganciclovir	Didanosine	↑	Steady-state didanosine AUC increased 111% (range, 10% to 493%) when didanosine was administered either 2 hours prior to or simultaneously with ganciclovir. A decrease in steady-state ganciclovir AUC of 21% (range, -44% to 5%) was observed when didanosine was administered 2 hours prior to administration of ganciclovir, but ganciclovir AUC was not affected by the presence of didanosine when the 2 drugs were administered simultaneously.
Didanosine	Ganciclovir	↓	
Ganciclovir	Zidovudine	↑	Mean steady-state ganciclovir AUC decreased 17% (range, -52% to 23%) in the presence of zidovudine (100 mg every 4 hours [n = 12]). Steady-state zidovudine AUC increased 19% (range, -11% to 74%) in the presence of ganciclovir. Because both drugs can cause neutropenia and anemia, some patients will not tolerate combination therapy at full dosage.
Zidovudine	Ganciclovir	↓	

[a] ↑ = object drug increased; ↓ = object drug decreased.

Adverse Reactions

Adverse events that occurred during clinical trials of ganciclovir capsules are summarized below, according to the participating study subject population.

➤*AIDS patients:* Three controlled, randomized, phase 3 trials comparing ganciclovir IV and ganciclovir capsules for maintenance treatment of CMV retinitis have been completed. During these trials, ganciclovir IV or ganciclovir capsules were prematurely discontinued in 9% of subjects because of adverse events. In a placebo-controlled, randomized, phase 3 trial of ganciclovir capsules for prevention of CMV disease in AIDS, treatment was prematurely discontinued because of adverse events, new or worsening intercurrent illness, or laboratory abnormalities in 19.5% of subjects treated with ganciclovir capsules and 16% of subjects receiving placebo.

➤*Lab test abnormalities:* Laboratory data and adverse events reported during the conduct of these controlled trials are summarized below.

Selected Ganciclovir Laboratory Abnormalities in Trials For Treatment of CMV Retinitis and Prevention of CMV Disease

	CMV retinitis treatment[a]		CMV disease preventions[b]	
Treatment	Ganciclovir capsules[c] 3000 mg/day	Ganciclovir IV[d] 5 mg/kg/day	Ganciclovir capsules[e] 3000 mg/day	Placebo[f]
Subjects, number	320	175	478	234
Neutropenia				
< 500 ANC/mcL	18%	25%	10%	6%
500 to < 749 ANC/mcL	17%	14%	16%	7%
750 to < 1000 ANC/mcL	19%	26%	22%	16%
Anemia				
Hemoglobin				
< 6.5 g/dL	2%	5%	1%	< 1%
6.5 to < 8 g/dL	10%	16%	5%	3%
8 to < 9.5 g/dL	25%	26%	15%	16%

GANCICLOVIR SODIUM — ORAL

Selected Ganciclovir Laboratory Abnormalities in Trials For Treatment of CMV Retinitis and Prevention of CMV Disease				
	CMV retinitis treatment[a]		CMV disease preventions[b]	
Treatment	Ganciclovir capsules[c] 3000 mg/day	Ganciclovir IV[d] 5 mg/kg/day	Ganciclovir capsules[e] 3000 mg/day	Placebo[f]
Maximum serum creatinine				
≥ 2.5 mg/dL	1%	2%	1%	2%
≥ 1.5 to < 2.5 mg/dL	12%	14%	19%	11%

[a] Pooled data from treatment studies, ICM 1653, study ICM 1774, and study AVI 034.
[b] Data from prevention study, ICM 1654.
[c] Mean time on therapy = 91 days, including allowed reinduction treatment periods.
[d] Mean time on therapy = 103 days, including allowed reinduction treatment periods.
[e] Mean time on ganciclovir = 269 days.
[f] Mean time on placebo = 240 days.

➤*Adverse events reported in 5% or more of the subjects:*

Adverse Reactions in 3 Randomized Phase 3 Studies of Ganciclovir Capsules vs Ganciclovir IV Solution for Maintenance Treatment of CMV Retinitis and In 1 Phase 3 Randomized Study of Ganciclovir Capsules vs Placebo for CMV Disease Prevention (≥ 5%)					
		Maintenance treatment		Prevention study	
Body system	Adverse reaction	Capsules (n = 326)	IV (n = 179)	Capsules (n = 478)	Placebo (n = 234)
Miscellaneous	Fever	38%	48%	35%	33%
	Sweating	11%	12%	14%	12%
	Pruritus	6%	5%	10%	9%
	Infection	9%	13%	8%	4%
	Chills	7%	10%	7%	4%
	Sepsis	4%	15%	3%	2%
GI	Diarrhea	41%	44%	48%	42%
	Anorexia	15%	14%	19%	16%
	Vomiting	13%	13%	14%	11%
Hemic/lymphatic	Leukopenia	29%	41%	17%	9%
	Anemia	19%	25%	9%	7%
	Thrombocytopenia	6%	6%	3%	1%
CNS	Neuropathy	8%	9%	21%	15%
Catheter related[a]	Total catheter events	6%	22%	-	-
	Catheter infection	4%	9%	-	-
	Catheter sepsis	1%	8%	-	-

[a] Some of these events also appear under other body systems.

➤*The following events were frequently observed in clinical trials but occurred with equal or greater frequency in placebo-treated subjects:* Abdominal pain, nausea, flatulence, pneumonia, paresthesia, rash.

➤*Retinal detachment:* Retinal detachment has been observed in subjects with CMV retinitis both before and after initiation of therapy with ganciclovir. Its relationship to therapy with ganciclovir is unknown.

Retinal detachment occurred in 11% of patients treated with ganciclovir IV solution and in 8% of patients treated with ganciclovir capsules. Patients with CMV retinitis should have frequent ophthalmologic evaluations to monitor the status of their retinitis and to detect any other retinal pathology.

➤*Transplant recipients:* There has been 1 controlled clinical trial of ganciclovir capsules for the prevention of CMV disease in transplant recipients. Laboratory data and adverse events reported during this trial is summarized below.

Laboratory data – The following table shows the frequency of granulocytopenia (neutropenia) and thrombocytopenia observed:

Neutropenia and Thrombocytopenia with Ganciclovir Capsules in Liver Allograft[a]		
	Ganciclovir capsules (n = 150)	Placebo (n = 154)
Neutropenia		
Minimum ANC < 500/mcL	3%	1%
Minimum ANC 500 to 1000/mcL	3%	2%
Total ANC ≤ 1000/mcL	6%	3%
Thrombocytopenia		
Platelet count < 25,000/mcL	0%	3%
Platelet count 25,000 to 50,000/mcL	5%	3%
Total platelet ≤ 50,000/mcL	5%	6%

[a] Study GAN040. Mean duration of ganciclovir treatment = 82 days.

The following table shows the frequency of elevated serum creatinine values in these controlled clinical trials.

Elevated Serum Creatinine with Ganciclovir Capsules in Liver Allograft (Study 040)		
Maximum serum creatinine levels	Ganciclovir capsules (n = 150)	Placebo (n = 154)
Serum creatinine ≥ 2.5 mg/dL	16%	10%
Serum creatinine ≥ 1.5 to < 2.5 mg/dL	39%	42%

In 3 out of 4 trials, patients receiving either ganciclovir IV solution or ganciclovir capsules had elevated serum creatinine levels when compared to those receiving placebo. Most patients in these studies also received cyclosporine. The mechanism of impairment of renal function is not known. However, careful monitoring of renal function during therapy with ganciclovir capsules is essential, especially for those patients receiving concomitant agents that may cause nephrotoxicity.

➤*"Probably" or "possibly" related to ganciclovir IV solution or ganciclovir capsules:* Other adverse events that were thought to be in controlled clinical studies in either subjects with AIDS or transplant recipients are listed below. These events all occurred in at least 3 subjects.

Cardiovascular – Hypertension, phlebitis, vasodilatation.

CNS – Abnormal dreams, anxiety, confusion, depression, dizziness, dry mouth, insomnia, seizures, somnolence, thinking abnormal, tremor.

Dermatologic – Alopecia, dry skin.

GI – Abnormal liver function test, aphthous stomatitis, constipation, dyspepsia, eructation.

GU – Creatinine clearance decreased, kidney failure, kidney function abnormal, urinary frequency.

Hematologic/Lymphatic – Pancytopenia.

Metabolic/Nutritional – Creatinine increased, AST increased, ALT increased, weight loss.

Musculoskeletal – Arthralgia, leg cramps, myalgia, myasthenia.

Respiratory – Cough increased, dyspnea.

Special senses – Abnormal vision, taste perversion, tinnitus, vitreous disorder.

Miscellaneous – Abdomen enlarged, asthenia, chest pain, edema, headache, injection site inflammation, malaise, pain.

Fatal adverse events – The following adverse events reported in patients receiving ganciclovir may be potentially fatal: Gastrointestinal perforation, multiple organ failure, pancreatitis and sepsis.

➤*Postmarketing:* The following events have been identified during post-approval use of the drug. Because they are reported voluntarily from a population of unknown size, estimates of frequency cannot be made. These events have been chosen for inclusion due to either the seriousness, frequency of reporting, the apparent causal connection or a combination of these factors:

Acidosis, allergic reaction, anaphylactic reaction, arthritis, bronchospasm, cardiac arrest, cardiac conduction abnormality, cataracts, cholelithiasis, cholestasis, congenital anomaly, dry eyes, dysesthesia, dysphagia, elevated triglyceride levels, encephalopathy, exfoliative dermatitis, extrapyramidal reaction, facial palsy, hallucinations, hemolytic anemia, hemolytic uremic syndrome, hepatic failure, hepatitis, hypercalcemia, hyponatremia, inappropriate serum ADH, infertility, intestinal ulceration, intracranial hypertension, irritability, loss of memory, loss of sense of smell, myelopathy, oculomotor nerve paralysis, peripheral ischemia, pulmonary fibrosis, renal tubular disorder, rhabdomyolysis, Stevens-Johnson syndrome, stroke, testicular hypotrophy, torsades de pointes, vasculitis, and ventricular tachycardia.

Overdosage

➤*Symptoms:* There have been no reports of overdosage with ganciclovir capsules. Doses as high as 6000 mg/day, given either as 1000 mg 6 times daily or as 2000 mg 3 times a day, did not result in overt toxicity other than transient neutropenia. Daily doses of more than 6000 mg have not been studied.

➤*Treatment:* Since ganciclovir is dialyzable, dialysis may be useful in reducing serum concentrations. Adequate hydration should be maintained. The use of hematopoietic growth factors should be considered.

Patient Information

All patients should be informed that the major toxicities of ganciclovir are granulocytopenia (neutropenia), anemia, and thrombocytopenia and that dose modifications may be required, including discontinuation. The importance of close monitoring of blood counts while on therapy should be emphasized. Patients should be informed that ganciclovir has been associated with elevations in serum creatinine.

Patients should be instructed to take ganciclovir capsules with food to maximize bioavailability.

Patients should be advised that ganciclovir has caused decreased sperm production in animals and may cause infertility in humans. Women of childbearing potential should be advised that ganciclovir causes birth defects in animals and should not be used during pregnancy and to use effective contraception during treatment with ganciclovir capsules. Similarly, men should be advised to practice barrier contraception during and for at least 90 days following treatment with ganciclovir capsules.

GANCICLOVIR SODIUM — ORAL

Patients should be advised that ganciclovir causes tumors in animals. Although there is no information from human studies, ganciclovir should be considered a potential carcinogen.

➤*All HIV-positive patients:* These patients may be receiving zidovudine. Patients should be counseled that treatment with both ganciclovir and zidovudine simultaneously may not be tolerated by some patients and may result in severe granulocytopenia (neutropenia). Patients with AIDS may be receiving didanosine. Patients should be counseled that concomitant treatment with both ganciclovir and didanosine can cause didanosine serum concentrations to be significantly increased.

➤*HIV-positive patients with CMV retinitis:* Ganciclovir is not a cure for CMV retinitis, and immunocompromised patients may continue to experience progression of retinitis during or following treatment. Patients should be advised to have ophthalmologic follow-up examinations at a minimum of every 4 to 6 weeks while being treated with ganciclovir capsules. Some patients will require more frequent follow-up.

GANCICLOVIR SODIUM — INJECTION

WARNING

The clinical toxicity of ganciclovir IV includes granulocytopenia, anemia and thrombocytopenia. In animal studies ganciclovir was carcinogenic, teratogenic and caused aspermatogenesis.

Ganciclovir IV is indicated for use only in the treatment of cytomegalovirus (CMV) retinitis in immunocompromised patients and for the prevention of CMV disease in transplant patients at risk for CMV disease.

Indications

➤*CMV retinitis:* Treatment of CMV retinitis in immunocompromised patients, including patients with acquired immunodeficiency syndrome (AIDS).

➤*CMV disease prevention:* Prevention of CMV disease in transplant recipients at risk for CMV disease.

Safety and efficacy of ganciclovir IV has not been established for congenital or neonatal CMV disease; nor for the treatment of established CMV disease other than retinitis; nor for use in non-immunocompromised individuals.

➤*Off-label uses:* Ganciclovir may be beneficial in CMV pneumonia in organ transplant patients.

Administration and Dosage

➤*Adults:*

Cytomegalovirus disease (prophylaxis) –

Maximum dose: The following doses should not be exceeded.

Initial dosage: 5 mg/kg given IV at a constant rate over 1 hour every 12 hours for 7 to 14 days.

Maintenance dosage: 5 mg/kg once daily 7 days per week, or 6 mg/kg once daily 5 days per week. Dose is given IV at a constant rate over 1 hour.

Duration of therapy: The duration of treatment in transplant recipients is dependent upon the duration and degree of immunosuppression. In controlled clinical trials in bone marrow allograft recipients, treatment with ganciclovir IV was continued until day 100 to 120 posttransplantation. CMV disease occurred in several patients who discontinued treatment with ganciclovir IV prematurely. In heart allograft recipients, the onset of newly diagnosed CMV disease occurred after treatment with ganciclovir IV was stopped at day 28 posttransplant, suggesting that continued dosing may be necessary to prevent late occurrence of CMV disease in this patient population. In a controlled clinical trial of liver allograft recipients, treatment with ganciclovir capsules was continued through week 14 posttransplantation.

Cytomegalovirus retinitis – For patients who experience progression of CMV retinitis while receiving maintenance treatment with either formulation of ganciclovir, reinduction treatment is recommended.

Maximum dose: The following doses should not be exceeded.

Initial dosage: 5 mg/kg given IV at a constant rate over 1 hour every 12 hours for 14 to 21 days. Capsules should not be used for induction.

Maintenance dosage: 5 mg/kg once daily 7 days per week, or 6 mg/kg once daily 5 days per week. Dose is given IV at a constant rate over 1 hour.

➤*Elderly:* Dosage reduction may be required in elderly patients with underlying renal function impairment. (See Renal function impairment.)

➤*Renal function impairment:*

Ganciclovir IV Dosing in Renal Function Impairment

Creatinine clearance[a] (mL/min)	Induction		Maintenance	
	IV induction dose (mg/kg)	Dosing interval (hours)	IV maintenance dose (mg/kg)	Dosing interval (hours)
≥ 70	5	12	5	24
50 to 69	2.5	12	2.5	24
25 to 49	2.5	24	1.25	24
10 to 24	1.25	24	0.625	24
< 10	1.25	3 times per week following hemodialysis	0.625	3 times per week following hemodialysis

[a] Creatinine clearance can be related to serum creatinine by the following formulas:

Creatinine clearance for males = (140 − age in years) (body weight in kg)/(72) (serum creatinine in mg/dL).

Creatinine clearance for females = 0.85 × male value.

Adults receiving continuous renal replacement therapy (CRRT) – One reference suggests an induction dose of 2.5 mg/kg IV every 24 hours followed by a maintenance dosage of 1.25 mg/kg IV every 24 hours.

The following alternative recommendations assume ultrafiltration and dialysis flow rates of 1 to 2 L/h. The following recommendations are for CMV infection.

Continuous venovenous hemofiltration (CVVH): 2.5 mg/kg IV every 24 hours (induction dose); 1.25 mg/kg IV every 24 hours (maintenance dosage).

Continuous venovenous hemodialysis (CVVHD) or continuous venovenous hemodialfiltration (CVVHDF): 2.5 mg/kg IV every 12 hours (induction dose); 2.5 mg/kg IV every 24 hours (maintenance dosage).

Adults receiving intermittent hemodialysis (IHD) – According to the prescribing information, dosing for patients undergoing hemodialysis should not exceed 1.25 mg/kg 3 times per week following each hemodialysis session. Ganciclovir IV should be given shortly after completion of the hemodialysis session because hemodialysis has been shown to reduce plasma levels by approximately 50%.

An alternative dosing regimen for CMV infection is 1.25 mg/kg IV every 48 to 72 hours as the induction dose and 0.625 mg/kg IV every 48 to 72 hours as the maintenance dose. Doses are to be administered after the dialysis session. These recommendations assume the patient is receiving standard IHD 3 times per week and completes the full dialysis sessions.

➤*Patients with hematologic abnormalities:* Consider dosage reductions for patients with neutropenia, anemia, and/or thrombocytopenia. Ganciclovir should not be administered in patients with severe neutropenia (absolute neutrophil count [ANC] less than 500/mcL) or severe thrombocytopenia (platelets less than 25,000/mcL). (See also Warnings/Precautions.)

➤*Preparation for administration:* Ganciclovir is an immunosuppressant agent and is also considered a mutagen and potential teratogen. Follow safe handling procedures when preparing, administering, or dispensing ganciclovir.

Caution should be exercised in the handling and preparation of solutions of ganciclovir IV. Solutions of ganciclovir IV are alkaline (pH 11). Avoid direct contact with the skin or mucous membranes of the powder contained in ganciclovir capsules or of ganciclovir IV solutions. If such contact occurs, wash thoroughly with soap and water; rinse eyes thoroughly with plain water.

Reconstitution –

1.) Reconstitute lyophilized ganciclovir IV by injecting 10 mL of sterile water for injection into the vial.
2.) Shake the vial to dissolve the drug.
3.) Visually inspect the reconstituted solution for particulate matter and discoloration prior to proceeding with infusion solution. Discard the vial if particulate matter or discoloration is observed.

Infusion solution – Based on patient weight, the appropriate volume of the reconstituted solution (ganciclovir concentration 50 mg/mL) should be removed from the vial and added to an acceptable infusion fluid (typically 100 mL) for delivery over the course of 1 hour. Infusion concentrations greater than 10 mg/mL are not recommended. (See Admixture compatibility.)

➤*Administration:* Administer IV at a constant rate over 1 hour. Do not administer ganciclovir IV solution by rapid or bolus IV injection. The toxicity of ganciclovir IV may be increased as a result of excessive plasma levels.

Intramuscular or subcutaneous injection or reconstituted ganciclovir IV solution may result in severe tissue irritation because of the high pH of 11.

➤*Admixture compatibility:*

Compatibilities – Sodium chloride 0.9%, dextrose 5%, Ringer's Injection and Ringer's Lactate Injection.

Incompatibilities – Do not use bacteriostatic water for injection containing parabens. It is incompatible with ganciclovir IV and may cause precipitation.

➤*Storage/Stability:* Store vials at temperatures below 40°C (104°F).

Reconstituted solution – Reconstituted solution in the vial is stable at room temperature for 12 hours. It should not be refrigerated.

Ganciclovir IV, when reconstituted with sterile water for injection, further diluted with 0.9% sodium chloride injection, and stored refrigerated at 5°C (41°F) in polyvinyl chloride (PVC) bags, remains physically and chemically stable for 14 days.

However, because ganciclovir IV is reconstituted with nonbacteriostatic sterile water, it is recommended that the infusion solution be used within 24 hours of dilution to reduce the risk of bacterial contamination. The infusion should be refrigerated. Freezing is not recommended.

Actions

➤*Pharmacology:* Ganciclovir is an acyclic nucleoside analogue of 2′-deoxyguanosine that inhibits replication of herpes viruses. Ganciclovir has been shown to be active against cytomegalovirus (CMV) and herpes simplex virus (HSV) in human clinical studies.

To achieve anti-CMV activity, ganciclovir is phosphorylated first to the monophosphate form by a CMV-encoded (UL97 gene) protein kinase homologue, then to the di- and triphosphate forms by cellular kinases. Ganciclovir

GANCICLOVIR SODIUM — INJECTION

triphosphate concentrations may be 100-fold greater in CMV-infected than in uninfected cells, indicating preferential phosphorylation in infected cells. Ganciclovir triphosphate, once formed, persists for days in the CMV-infected cell. Ganciclovir triphosphate is believed to inhibit viral DNA synthesis by competitive inhibition of viral DNA polymerases; and incorporation into viral DNA, resulting in eventual termination of viral DNA elongation.

➤*Pharmacokinetics:*

Absorption – The absolute bioavailability of oral ganciclovir under fasting conditions was approximately 5% (n = 6) and following food was 6% to 9% (n = 32). When ganciclovir was administered orally with food at a total daily dosage of 3 g/day (500 mg every 3 hours, 6 times daily and 1000 mg 3 times a day), the steady-state absorption as measured by area under the serum concentration vs time curve (AUC) over 24 hours and maximum serum concentrations (C_{max}) were similar following both regimens with an AUC_{0-24} of 15.9 ± 4.2 (mean ± SD) and 15.4 ± 4.3 mcg•hr/mL and C_{max} of 1.02 ± 0.24 and 1.18 ± 0.36 mcg/mL, respectively (n = 16).

When ganciclovir capsules were given with a meal containing 602 calories and 46.5% fat at a dosage of 1000 mg every 8 hours to 20 HIV-positive subjects, the steady-state AUC increased by 22 ± 22% (range, −6% to 68%) and there was a significant prolongation of time to peak serum concentrations (T_{max}) from 1.8 ± 0.8 to 3 ± 0.6 hours and a higher C_{max} (0.85 ± 0.25 vs 0.96 ± 0.27 mcg/mL) (n = 20).

Distribution – The steady-state volume of distribution of ganciclovir after intravenous administration was 0.74 ± 0.15 L/kg (n = 98). For ganciclovir capsules, no correlation was observed between AUC and reciprocal weight (range, 55 to 128 kg); oral dosing according to weight is not required. Cerebrospinal fluid concentrations obtained 0.25 to 5.67 hours postdose in 3 patients who received 2.5 mg/kg ganciclovir intravenously every 8 hours or every 12 hours ranged from 0.31 to 0.68 mcg/mL representing 24% to 70% of the respective plasma concentrations. Binding to plasma proteins was 1% to 2% over ganciclovir concentrations of 0.5 and 51 mcg/mL.

Metabolism – Following oral administration of a single 1000 mg dose of ^{14}C-labeled ganciclovir, 86% ± 3% of the administered dose was recovered in the feces and 5% ± 1% was recovered in the urine (n = 4). No metabolite accounted for more than 1% to 2% of the radioactivity recovered in urine or feces.

Excretion – When administered intravenously, ganciclovir exhibits linear pharmacokinetics over the range of 1.6 to 5 mg/kg and when administered orally, it exhibits linear kinetics up to a total daily dose of 4 g/day. Renal excretion of unchanged drug by glomerular filtration and active tubular secretion is the major route of elimination of ganciclovir. In patients with healthy renal function, 91.3% ± 5% (n = 4) of intravenously administered ganciclovir was recovered unmetabolized in the urine. Systemic clearance of intravenously administered ganciclovir was 3.52 ± 0.8 mL/min/kg (n = 98) while renal clearance was 3.20 ± 0.8 mL/min/kg (n = 47), accounting for 91% ± 11% of the systemic clearance (n = 47). After oral administration of ganciclovir, steady-state is achieved within 24 hours. Renal clearance following oral administration was 3.1 ± 1.2 mL/min/kg (n = 22). Half-life was 3.5 ± 0.9 hours (n = 98) following IV administration and 4.8 ± 0.9 hours (n = 39) following oral administration.

Special populations –

Renal function impairment: The pharmacokinetics following intravenous administration of ganciclovir IV solution were evaluated in 10 immunocompromised patients with renal impairment who received doses ranging from 1.25 to 5 mg/kg.

Ganciclovir Injection Pharmacokinetics in Renal Impairment

Estimated creatinine clearance (mL/min)	n	Dose	Clearance (mL/min) Mean ± SD	Half-life (hours) Mean ± SD
50 to 79	4	3.2 to 5 mg/kg	128 ± 63	4.6 ± 1.4
25 to 49	3	3 to 5 mg/kg	57 ± 8	4.4 ± 0.4
< 25	3	1.25 to 5 mg/kg	30 ± 13	10.7 ± 5.7

• *Hemodialysis* – See Administration and Dosage for more information.

Contraindications

Hypersensitivity to ganciclovir or acyclovir.

Warnings/Precautions

➤*Hematologic:* Ganciclovir IV should not be administered if the absolute neutrophil count is less than 500 cells/mcL or the platelet count is less than 25,000 cells/mcL. Granulocytopenia (neutropenia), anemia and thrombocytopenia have been observed in patients treated with ganciclovir IV and ganciclovir. The frequency and severity of these events vary widely in different patient populations (see Adverse Reactions).

Ganciclovir IV should, therefore, be used with caution in patients with preexisting cytopenias or with a history of cytopenic reactions to other drugs, chemicals or irradiation. Granulocytopenia usually occurs during the first or second week of treatment but may occur at any time during treatment. Cell counts usually begin to recover within 3 to 7 days of discontinuing drug. Colony-stimulating factors have been shown to increase neutrophil and white blood cell counts in patients receiving ganciclovir IV solution for treatment of CMV retinitis.

➤*Large doses/Rapid infusion:* In clinical studies with ganciclovir IV, the maximum single dose administered was 6 mg/kg by intravenous infusion over 1 hour. Larger doses have resulted in increased toxicity. It is likely that more rapid infusions would also result in increased toxicity (see Overdosage). Administration of ganciclovir IV solution should be accompanied by adequate hydration.

➤*Phlebitis/Pain at injection site:* Initially reconstituted solutions of ganciclovir IV have a high pH (pH 11). Despite further dilution in intravenous fluids, phlebitis or pain may occur at the site of intravenous infusion. Care must be taken to infuse solutions containing ganciclovir IV only into veins with adequate blood flow to permit rapid dilution and distribution (see Administration and Dosage).

➤*Renal function impairment:* Ganciclovir IV should be used with caution in patients with impaired renal function because the half-life and plasma/serum concentrations of ganciclovir will be increased due to reduced renal clearance (see Administration and Dosage and Adverse Reactions, Renal).

Hemodialysis has been shown to reduce plasma levels of ganciclovir by approximately 50%.

Since ganciclovir is excreted by the kidneys, normal clearance depends on adequate renal function. If renal function is impaired, dosage adjustments are required for ganciclovir IV. Such adjustments should be based on measured or estimated creatinine clearance values (see Administration and Dosage).

➤*Pregnancy: Category C.* Dose comparisons are based on the human AUC following administration of a single 5 mg/kg intravenous infusion of ganciclovir IV as used during the maintenance phase of treatment. Compared with the single 5 mg/kg intravenous infusion, human exposure is doubled during the intravenous induction phase (5 mg/kg 2 times a day) and approximately halved during maintenance treatment with ganciclovir capsules (1000 mg 3 times a day). The cross-species dose comparisons should be divided by 2 for intravenous induction treatment with ganciclovir IV.

Ganciclovir has been shown to be embryotoxic in rabbits and mice following intravenous administration and teratogenic in rabbits. Fetal resorptions were present in at least 85% of rabbits and mice administered 60 mg/kg/day and 108 mg/kg/day (2× the human exposure based on AUC comparisons), respectively. Effects observed in rabbits included fetal growth retardation, embryolethality, teratogenicity or maternal toxicity. Teratogenic changes included cleft palate, anophthalmia/microphthalmia, aplastic organs (kidney and pancreas), hydrocephaly and brachygnathia. In mice, effects observed were maternal/fetal toxicity and embryolethality.

Ganciclovir may be teratogenic or embryotoxic at dose levels recommended for human use. There are no adequate and well-controlled studies in pregnant women. Ganciclovir IV should be used during pregnancy only if the potential benefits justify the potential risk to the fetus.

Because of the mutagenic and teratogenic potential of ganciclovir, women of childbearing potential should be advised to use effective contraception during treatment. Similarly, men should be advised to practice barrier contraception during and for at least 90 days following treatment with ganciclovir IV.

Fertility impairment – Although data in humans have not been obtained, it is considered probable that ganciclovir at the recommended doses causes temporary or permanent inhibition of spermatogenesis. Animal data also indicate that suppression of fertility in females may occur.

➤*Lactation:* It is not known whether ganciclovir is excreted in human milk. However, many drugs are excreted in human milk and, because carcinogenic and teratogenic effects occurred in animals treated with ganciclovir, the possibility of serious adverse reactions from ganciclovir in nursing infants is considered likely (see Pregnancy). Mothers should be instructed to discontinue nursing if they are receiving ganciclovir IV. The minimum interval before nursing can safely be resumed after the last dose of ganciclovir IV is unknown.

➤*Children:* Safety and efficacy of ganciclovir IV in pediatric patients have not been established. The use of ganciclovir IV in the pediatric population warrants extreme caution due to the probability of long-term carcinogenicity and reproductive toxicity. Administration to pediatric patients should be undertaken only after careful evaluation and only if the potential benefits of treatment outweigh the risks.

The spectrum of adverse events reported in 120 immunocompromised pediatric clinical trial participants with serious CMV infections receiving ganciclovir IV solution were similar to those reported in adults. Granulocytopenia (17%) and thrombocytopenia (10%) were the most common adverse events reported.

➤*Elderly:* Clinical studies of ganciclovir IV did not include sufficient numbers of subjects aged 65 and over to determine whether they respond differently from younger subjects. In general, dose selection for an elderly patient should be cautious, reflecting the greater frequency of decreased hepatic, renal, or cardiac function, and of concomitant disease or other drug therapy. Ganciclovir IV is known to be substantially excreted by the kidney, and the risk of toxic reactions to this drug may be greater in patients with impaired renal function. Because elderly patients are more likely to have decreased renal function, care should be taken in dose selection. In addition, renal function should be monitored and dosage adjustments should be made accordingly (see Warnings, Renal impairment and Administration and Dosage).

➤*Monitoring:* Due to the frequency of neutropenia, anemia, and thrombocytopenia in patients receiving ganciclovir IV (see Adverse Events), it is recommended that complete blood counts and platelet counts be performed frequently, especially in patients in whom ganciclovir or other nucleoside analogues have previously resulted in leukopenia, or in whom neutrophil counts are less than 1000 cells/mcL at the beginning of treatment. Increased serum creatinine levels have been observed in trials evaluating ganciclovir IV. Patients should have serum creatinine or creatinine clearance values monitored carefully to allow for dosage adjustments in renally impaired patients (see Administration and Dosage).

GANCICLOVIR SODIUM — INJECTION

Drug Interactions

Ganciclovir Drug Interactions			
Precipitant drug	Object drug[a]		Description
Ganciclovir	Cytotoxic drugs	↑	Cytotoxic drugs that inhibit replication of rapidly dividing cell populations such as bone marrow, spermatogonia, and germinal layers of skin and GI mucosa may have additive toxicity when administered concomitantly with ganciclovir. Therefore, consider the concomitant use of drugs such as dapsone, pentamidine, flucytosine, vincristine, vinblastine, adriamycin, amphotericin B, trimethoprim/sulfamethoxazole combinations, or other nucleoside analogs only if potential benefits outweigh the risks.
Imipenem-cilastatin	Ganciclovir	↑	Generalized seizures occurred in patients who received ganciclovir and imipenem-cilastatin. Do not use these drugs concomitantly unless the potential benefits outweigh the risks.
Nephrotoxic drugs	Ganciclovir	↑	Increases in serum creatinine were observed following concurrent use of ganciclovir and either cyclosporine or amphotericin B.
Probenecid	Ganciclovir	↑	Ganciclovir AUC increased 53% (range, -14% to 299%) in the presence of probenecid. Renal clearance of ganciclovir decreased 22% (range, -54% to -4%), which is consistent with an interaction involving competition for renal tubular secretion.
Ganciclovir	Didanosine	↑	Steady-state didanosine AUC increased 111% (range, 10% to 493%) when didanosine was administered either 2 hours prior to or simultaneously with ganciclovir. A decrease in steady-state ganciclovir AUC of 21% (range, -44% to 5%) was observed when didanosine was administered 2 hours prior to administration of ganciclovir, but ganciclovir AUC was not affected by the presence of didanosine when the 2 drugs were administered simultaneously.
Didanosine	Ganciclovir	↓	
Ganciclovir	Zidovudine	↑	Mean steady-state ganciclovir AUC decreased 17% (range, -52% to 23%) in the presence of zidovudine (100 mg every 4 hours [n = 12]). Steady-state zidovudine AUC increased 19% (range, -11% to 74%) in the presence of ganciclovir. Because both drugs can cause neutropenia and anemia, some patients will not tolerate combination therapy at full dosage.
Zidovudine	Ganciclovir	↓	

[a] ↑ = object drug increased; ↓ = object drug decreased.

Adverse Reactions

Adverse events that occurred during clinical trials of ganciclovir IV solution and ganciclovir capsules are summarized below, according to the participating study subject population.

➤*AIDS patients:* Three controlled, randomized, phase 3 trials comparing ganciclovir IV and ganciclovir capsules for maintenance treatment of CMV retinitis have been completed. During these trials, ganciclovir IV or ganciclovir capsules were prematurely discontinued in 9% of subjects because of adverse events. In a placebo-controlled, randomized, phase 3 trial of ganciclovir capsules for prevention of CMV disease in AIDS, treatment was prematurely discontinued because of adverse events, new or worsening intercurrent illness, or laboratory abnormalities in 19.5% of subjects treated with ganciclovir capsules and 16% of subjects receiving placebo. Laboratory data and adverse events reported during the conduct of these controlled trials are summarized below.

➤*Lab test abnormalities:*

Selected Ganciclovir Laboratory Abnormalities in Trials For Treatment of CMV Retinitis and Prevention of CMV Disease				
	CMV retinitis treatment[a]		CMV disease prevention[b]	
Lab test abnormality	Ganciclovir capsules 3000 mg/day[c]	Ganciclovir IV 5 mg/kg/day[d]	Ganciclovir capsules 3000 mg/day[e]	Placebo[f]
Subjects, number	320	175	478	234
Neutropenia:				
< 500 ANC/mcL	18%	25%	10%	6%
500 to < 749 ANC/mcL	17%	14%	16%	7%
750 to < 1000 ANC/mcL	19%	26%	22%	16%
Anemia: *Hemoglobin*:				
< 6.5 g/dL	2%	5%	1%	< 1%
6.5 to < 8 g/dL	10%	16%	5%	3%
8 to < 9.5 g/dL	25%	26%	15%	16%
Maximum serum creatinine:				
≥ 2.5 mg/dL	1%	2%	1%	2%
≥ 1.5 to < 2.5 mg/dL	12%	14%	19%	11%

[a] Pooled data from treatment studies, ICM 1653, study ICM 1774, and study AVI 034.
[b] Data from prevention study, ICM 1654.
[c] Mean time on therapy = 91 days, including allowed reinduction treatment periods.
[d] Mean time on therapy = 103 days, including allowed reinduction treatment periods.
[e] Mean time on ganciclovir = 269 days.
[f] Mean time on placebo = 240 days.

➤*Adverse events reported in 5% or more of the subjects:*

Adverse Reactions in 3 Randomized Phase 3 Studies of Ganciclovir Capsules vs Ganciclovir IV Solution for Maintenance Treatment of CMV Retinitis and in 1 Phase 3 Randomized Study of Ganciclovir Capsules vs Placebo for CMV Disease Prevention (≥ 5%)					
		Maintenance treatment studies		Prevention study	
Body system	Adverse reaction	Capsules (n = 326)	IV (n = 179)	Capsules (n = 478)	Placebo (n = 234)
Miscellaneous	Fever	38%	48%	35%	33%
	Sweating	11%	12%	14%	12%
	Pruritus	6%	5%	10%	9%
	Infection	9%	13%	8%	4%
	Chills	7%	10%	7%	4%
	Sepsis	4%	15%	3%	2%
GI	Diarrhea	41%	44%	48%	42%
	Anorexia	15%	14%	19%	16%
	Vomiting	13%	13%	14%	11%
Hemic/lymphatic	Leukopenia	29%	41%	17%	9%
	Anemia	19%	25%	9%	7%
	Thrombocytopenia	6%	6%	3%	1%
CNS	Neuropathy	8%	9%	21%	15%
Catheter related[a]	Total catheter events	6%	22%		
	Catheter infection	4%	9%		
	Catheter sepsis	1%	8%		

[a] Some of these events also appear under other body systems.

➤*The following events were frequently observed in clinical trials but occurred with equal or greater frequency in placebo-treated subjects:* Abdominal pain, nausea, flatulence, pneumonia, paresthesia, rash.

➤*Retinal detachment:* Retinal detachment has been observed in subjects with CMV retinitis both before and after initiation of therapy with ganciclovir. Its relationship to therapy with ganciclovir is unknown.

Ophthalmic – Retinal detachment occurred in 11% of patients treated with ganciclovir IV solution and in 8% of patients treated with ganciclovir capsules. Patients with CMV retinitis should have frequent ophthalmologic evaluations to monitor the status of their retinitis and to detect any other retinal pathology.

➤*Transplant recipients:* There have been 3 controlled clinical trials of ganciclovir IV solution and 1 controlled clinical trial of ganciclovir capsules for the prevention of CMV disease in transplant recipients. Laboratory data and adverse events reported during these trials are summarized below.

Laboratory data – The following table shows the frequency of granulocytopenia (neutropenia) and thrombocytopenia observed.

GANCICLOVIR SODIUM — INJECTION

Adverse Reactions in Controlled Trials for Ganciclovir in Transplant Recipients						
	Ganciclovir IV				Ganciclovir capsules	
	Heart allograft[a]		Bone marrow allograft[b]		Liver allograft[c]	
Adverse reaction	Ganciclovir IV (n = 76)	Placebo (n = 73)	Ganciclovir IV (n = 57)	Control (n = 55)	Ganciclovir capsules (n = 150)	Placebo (n = 154)
Neutropenia						
Minimum ANC < 500/mcL	4%	3%	12%	6%	3%	1%
Minimum ANC 500 to 1000/mcL	3%	8%	29%	17%	3%	2%
Total ANC ≤ 1000/mcL	7%	11%	41%	23%	6%	3%
Thrombocytopenia						
Platelet count < 25,000/mcL	3%	1%	32%	28%	0%	3%
Platelet count 25,000 to 50,000/mcL	5%	3%	25%	37%	5%	3%
Total platelet ≤ 50,000/mcL	8%	4%	57%	65%	5%	6%

[a] Study ICM 1496. Mean duration of treatment = 28 days.
[b] Study ICM 1570 and ICM 1689. Mean duration of treatment = 45 days.
[c] Study GAN040. Mean duration of ganciclovir treatment = 82 days.

Frequency of elevated serum creatinine values in clinical trials – The following table shows the frequency of elevated serum creatinine values in these controlled clinical trials.

Elevated Serum Creatinine in Controlled Trials for Ganciclovir in Transplant Recipients								
	Ganciclovir IV						Ganciclovir capsules	
	Heart allograft ICM 1496		Bone marrow allograft ICM 1570		Bone marrow allograft ICM 1689		Liver allograft study 040	
Maximum serum creatinine levels	Ganciclovir IV (n = 76)	Placebo (n = 73)	Ganciclovir IV (n = 20)	Control (n = 20)	Ganciclovir IV (n = 37)	Placebo (n = 35)	Ganciclovir capsules (n = 150)	Placebo (n = 154)
Serum creatinine ≥ 2.5 mg/dL	18%	4%	20%	0%	0%	0%	16%	10%
Serum creatinine ≥ 1.5 to	58%	69%	50%	35%	43%	44%	39%	42%

In 3 out of 4 trials, patients receiving either ganciclovir IV solution or ganciclovir capsules had elevated serum creatinine levels when compared to those receiving placebo. Most patients in these studies also received cyclosporine. The mechanism of impairment of renal function is not known. However, careful monitoring of renal function during therapy with ganciclovir IV solution or ganciclovir capsules is essential, especially for those patients receiving concomitant agents that may cause nephrotoxicity.

➤*Other adverse events:* Other adverse events that were thought to be "probably" or "possibly" related to ganciclovir IV solution or ganciclovir capsules in controlled clinical studies in either subjects with AIDS or transplant recipients are listed below. These events all occurred in at least 3 subjects.

Cardiovascular – Hypertension, phlebitis, vasodilatation.

CNS – Abnormal dreams, anxiety, confusion, depression, dizziness, dry mouth, insomnia, seizures, somnolence, thinking abnormal, tremor.

Dermatologic – Alopecia, dry skin.

GI – Abnormal liver function test, aphthous stomatitis, constipation, dyspepsia, eructation.

GU – Creatinine clearance decreased, kidney failure, kidney function abnormal, urinary frequency.

Hematologic/Lymphatic – Pancytopenia.

Metabolic/Nutritional – Creatinine increased, SGOT increased, SGPT increased, weight loss.

Musculoskeletal – Arthralgia, leg cramps, myalgia, myasthenia.

Respiratory – Cough increased, dyspnea.

Special senses – Abnormal vision, taste perversion, tinnitus, vitreous disorder.

Miscellaneous – Abdomen enlarged, asthenia, chest pain, edema, headache, injection site inflammation, malaise, pain.

Fatal adverse events: The following adverse events reported in patients receiving ganciclovir may be potentially fatal: Gastrointestinal perforation, multiple organ failure, pancreatitis and sepsis.

➤*Postmarketing:* The following events have been identified during postapproval use of the drug. Because they are reported voluntarily from a population of unknown size, estimates of frequency cannot be made. These events have been chosen for inclusion due to either the seriousness, frequency of reporting, the apparent causal connection or a combination of these factors:

Miscellaneous – Acidosis, allergic reaction, anaphylactic reaction, arthritis, bronchospasm, cardiac arrest, cardiac conduction abnormality, cataracts, cholelithiasis, cholestasis, congenital anomaly, dry eyes, dysesthesia, dysphasia, elevated triglyceride levels, encephalopathy, exfoliative dermatitis, extrapyramidal reaction, facial palsy, hallucinations, hemolytic anemia, hemolytic uremic syndrome, hepatic failure, hepatitis, hypercalcemia, hyponatremia, inappropriate serum ADH, infertility, intestinal ulceration, intracranial hypertension, irritability, loss of memory, loss of sense of smell, myelopathy, oculomotor nerve paralysis, peripheral ischemia, pulmonary fibrosis, renal tubular disorder, rhabdomyolysis, Stevens-Johnson syndrome, stroke, testicular hypotrophy, torsades de pointes, vasculitis, ventricular tachycardia.

Overdosage

➤*Symptoms:* Overdosage with ganciclovir IV has been reported in 17 patients (13 adults and 4 children under 2 years of age). Five patients experienced no adverse events following overdosage at the following doses: 7 doses of 11 mg/kg over a 3-day period (adult), single dose of 3500 mg (adult), single dose of 500 mg (72.5 mg/kg) followed by 48 hours of peritoneal dialysis (4-month-old), single dose of ≈ 60 mg/kg followed by exchange transfusion (18-month-old), 2 doses of 500 mg instead of 31 mg (21-month-old).

Irreversible pancytopenia developed in 1 adult with AIDS and CMV colitis after receiving 3000 mg of ganciclovir IV solution on each of 2 consecutive days. He experienced worsening GI symptoms and acute renal failure that required short-term dialysis. Pancytopenia developed and persisted until his death from a malignancy several months later. Other adverse events reported following overdosage included: persistent bone marrow suppression (1 adult with neutropenia and thrombocytopenia after a single dose of 6000 mg), reversible neutropenia or granulocytopenia (4 adults, overdoses ranging from 8 mg/kg daily for 4 days to a single dose of 25 mg/kg), hepatitis (1 adult receiving 10 mg/kg daily, and one 2 kg infant after a single 40 mg dose), renal toxicity (1 adult with transient worsening of hematuria after a single 500 mg dose, and 1 adult with elevated creatinine (5.2 mg/dL) after a single 5000 to 7000 mg dose), and seizure (1 adult with known seizure disorder after 3 days of 9 mg/kg). In addition, 1 adult received 0.4 mL (instead of 0.1 mL) ganciclovir IV solution by intravitreal injection, and experienced temporary loss of vision and central retinal artery occlusion secondary to increased intraocular pressure related to the injected fluid volume.

➤*Treatment:* Since ganciclovir is dialyzable, dialysis may be useful in reducing serum concentrations. Adequate hydration should be maintained. The use of hematopoietic growth factors should be considered.

Patient Information

All patients should be informed that the major toxicities of ganciclovir are granulocytopenia (neutropenia), anemia and thrombocytopenia and that dose modifications may be required, including discontinuation. The importance of close monitoring of blood counts while on therapy should be emphasized. Patients should be informed that ganciclovir has been associated with elevations in serum creatinine.

Patients should be advised that ganciclovir has caused decreased sperm production in animals and may cause infertility in humans. Women of childbearing potential should be advised that ganciclovir causes birth defects in animals and should not be used during pregnancy and to use effective contraception during treatment with ganciclovir IV. Similarly, men should be advised to practice barrier contraception during and for at least 90 days following treatment with ganciclovir IV.

Patients should be advised that ganciclovir causes tumors in animals. Although there is no information from human studies, ganciclovir should be considered a potential carcinogen.

➤*All HIV positive patients:* These patients may be receiving zidovudine. Patients should be counseled that treatment with both ganciclovir and zidovudine simultaneously may not be tolerated by some patients and may result in severe granulocytopenia (neutropenia). Patients with AIDS may be receiving didanosine. Patients should be counseled that concomitant treatment with both ganciclovir and didanosine can cause didanosine serum concentrations to be significantly increased.

➤*HIV positive patients with CMV retinitis:* Ganciclovir is not a cure for CMV retinitis, and immunocompromised patients may continue to experience progression of retinitis during or following treatment. Patients should be advised to have ophthalmologic follow-up examinations at a minimum of every 4 to 6 weeks while being treated with ganciclovir IV. Some patients will require more frequent follow-up.

➤*Transplant recipients:* Transplant recipients should be counseled regarding the high frequency of impaired renal function in transplant recipients who received ganciclovir IV solution in controlled clinical trials, particularly in patients receiving concomitant administration of nephrotoxic agents such as cyclosporine and amphotericin B. Although the specific mechanism of this toxicity, which in most cases was reversible, has not been determined, the higher rate of renal impairment in patients receiving ganciclovir IV solution compared with those who received placebo in the same trials may indicate that ganciclovir IV played a significant role.

VALGANCICLOVIR

Rx	Valcyte (Roche)	Tablets; oral: 450 mg	Equiv. to valganciclovir hydrochloride 496.3 mg. (VGC 450). Pink, oval. Film-coated. In 60s.
		Powder for solution; oral: 50 mg/mL	Mannitol, saccharin. Tutti-frutti flavor. In 100 mL glass bottles with bottle adapter and 2 oral dispensers.

VALGANCICLOVIR HYDROCHLORIDE — ORAL

WARNING

The clinical toxicity of valganciclovir, which is metabolized to ganciclovir, includes granulocytopenia, anemia, and thrombocytopenia. In animal studies, ganciclovir was carcinogenic and teratogenic and caused aspermatogenesis.

Indications

➤*Cytomegalovirus disease:* For the prevention of CMV disease in kidney, heart, and kidney-pancreas transplant adult patients at high risk (donor CMV seropositive/recipient CMV seronegative [D+/R−]); for the prevention of CMV disease in kidney and heart transplant pediatric patients (4 months to 16 years of age) at high risk.

➤*Cytomegalovirus retinitis:* For the treatment of cytomegalovirus (CMV) retinitis in adults with AIDS.

Administration and Dosage

➤*General dosing considerations:* The bioavailability of ganciclovir from valganciclovir is significantly higher than from ganciclovir capsules. Therefore, valganciclovir tablets cannot be substituted for ganciclovir capsules on a 1-to-1 basis.

➤*Adults:*

Cytomegalovirus retinitis –

Active disease:

• *Initial dosage* – 900 mg twice a day for 21 days.

• *Maintenance dosage* – 900 mg once daily following initial dosage.

Inactive disease: 900 mg once daily.

Cytomegalovirus disease prevention – 900 mg once daily starting within 10 days of transplantation until 100 days posttransplantation.

➤*Children:*

Cytomegalovirus disease prevention kidney and heart transplantation –

4 months to 16 years of age:

• *Usual dosage* – Dose is administered once daily starting within 10 days of transplantation until 100 days posttransplantation and is calculated using the following equation (BSA = body surface area; CrCl = creatinine clearance):

Dose (mg) = 7 × BSA × CrCl (calculated using a modified Schwartz formula) where

$$BSA\ (m^2) = \sqrt{\frac{ht\ (cm) \times wt\ (kg)}{3600}}$$

$$CrCl\ (mL/min/1.73\ m^2) = K \times \frac{\text{body length or height (cm)}}{\text{serum creatinine (mg/dL)}}$$

Where K = 0.45 for patients younger than 1 year of age; K = 0.45 for patients 1 to younger than 2 years of age (note: K value is 0.45 instead of the typical value of 0.55); K = 0.55 for boys 2 to younger than 13 years of age and for girls 2 to 16 years of age; and K = 0.7 for boys 13 to 16 years of age.

All calculated doses should be rounded to the nearest 25 mg increment for the actual deliverable dose. If the calculated dose exceeds 900 mg, a maximum dose of 900 mg should be administered.

• *Maximum dose* – 900 mg once daily.

Off-label dosing –

Cytomegalovirus disease prevention in liver transplantation:

• *Children 1 year of age and older* – A dosage of 15 to 18 mg/kg daily for 100 days following transplantation was used in a small study.

Cytomegalovirus retinitis:

• *Children 12 years of age and older –*

Induction therapy: 900 mg twice daily for 21 days.

Maintenance therapy: 900 mg daily.

➤*Renal function impairment:*

Adults –

Valganciclovir Dose Modifications in Adults With Impaired Renal Function

CrCl (mL/min)	Initial dosage	Maintenance/Prevention dosage
≥ 60	900 mg twice daily	900 mg once daily
40 to 59	450 mg twice daily	450 mg once daily
25 to 39	450 mg once daily	450 mg every 2 days
10 to 24	450 mg every 2 days	450 mg twice weekly
< 10 (on hemodialysis[a])	Not recommended	Not recommended

[a] For patients on hemodialysis, it is recommended that ganciclovir be used (in accordance with the dose-reduction algorithm cited in the Ganciclovir Injection and Ganciclovir Oral monographs in Administration and Dosage) rather than valganciclovir.

Children – Dosing in children with renal impairment can be done using the recommended equations because CrCl is a component in the calculation.

➤*Preparation for administration:*

Oral solution –

Measure 91 mL of purified water in a graduated cylinder. Shake the valganciclovir bottle to loosen the powder. Remove the child-resistant bottle cap and add approximately half the total amount of water for constitution to the bottle and shake the closed bottle well for approximately 1 minute. Add the remainder of water and shake the closed bottle well for approximately 1 minute. This prepared solution contains 50 mg of valganciclovir free base per 1 mL. Remove the child-resistant bottle cap and push the bottle adapter into the neck of the bottle. Close bottle with child-resistant bottle cap tightly. This will ensure the proper seating of the bottle adapter in the bottle and child-resistant status of the cap. Write the date of expiration of the constituted solution on the bottle label.

➤*Administration:* Instruct patients to take with food. Tablets should not be broken or crushed.

Adults should use valganciclovir tablets, not valganciclovir oral solution.

Children – Valganciclovir for oral solution is the preferred formulation because it provides the ability to administer a dose calculated according to the previous formula; however, valganciclovir tablets may be used if the calculated doses are within 10% of the available tablet strength (450 mg). For example, if the calculated dose is between 405 and 495 mg, one 450 mg tablet may be taken.

➤*Storage / Stability:* Store at 25°C (77°F); excursions are permitted to 15° to 30°C (59° to 86°F). Store constituted solution under refrigeration at 2° to 8°C (36° to 46°F) for no longer than 49 days. Do not freeze.

Handling and disposal – Caution should be exercised in the handling of valganciclovir. Because valganciclovir is considered a potential teratogen and carcinogen in humans, caution should be observed in handling broken tablets, the powder for oral solution, and the constituted oral solution. Avoid direct contact of broken or crushed tablets, the powder for oral solution, and the constituted oral solution with skin or mucous membranes. If such contact occurs, wash thoroughly with soap and water, and rinse eyes thoroughly with plain water.

Actions

➤*Pharmacology:* Valganciclovir is an L-valyl ester (prodrug) of ganciclovir that exists as a mixture of 2 diastereomers. After oral administration, both diastereomers are rapidly converted to ganciclovir by intestinal and hepatic esterases. Ganciclovir is a synthetic analog of 2′-deoxyguanosine, which inhibits replication of human CMV in cell culture and in vivo.

In CMV-infected cells, ganciclovir is initially phosphorylated to ganciclovir monophosphate by the viral protein kinase, pUL97. Further phosphorylation occurs by cellular kinases to produce ganciclovir triphosphate, which is then slowly metabolized intracellularly (half-life, 18 hours). As the phosphorylation is largely dependent on the viral kinase, phosphorylation of ganciclovir occurs preferentially in virus-infected cells. The virustatic activity of ganciclovir is due to inhibition of viral DNA synthesis by ganciclovir triphosphate.

➤*Pharmacokinetics:* The pharmacokinetics of valganciclovir and ganciclovir after administration of valganciclovir tablets have been evaluated in HIV- and CMV-seropositive patients, patients with AIDS and CMV retinitis, and in solid organ transplant patients.

Mean Ganciclovir Pharmacokinetic[a] Measures in Healthy Volunteers and HIV-Positive/CMV-Positive Adults at Maintenance Dosage[b]

Formulation	Valganciclovir 900 mg tablets once daily with food	Ganciclovir 5 mg/kg IV once daily	Ganciclovir 1,000 mg capsules 3 times daily with food
$AUC_{0\text{-}24h}$ (mcg•h/mL)	29.1 ± 9.7 (n = 57)	26.5 ± 5.9 (n = 68)	Range of means 12.3 to 19.2 (n = 94)
C_{max} (mcg/mL)	5.61 ± 1.52 (n = 58)	9.46 ± 2.02 (n = 68)	Range of means 0.955 to 1.4 (n = 94)

VALGANCICLOVIR HYDROCHLORIDE — ORAL

Mean Ganciclovir Pharmacokinetic[a] Measures in Healthy Volunteers and HIV-Positive/CMV-Positive Adults at Maintenance Dosage[b]

Formulation	Valganciclovir 900 mg tablets once daily with food	Ganciclovir 5 mg/kg IV once daily	Ganciclovir 1,000 mg capsules 3 times daily with food
Absolute oral bioavailability (%)	59.4 ± 6.1 (n = 32)	Not applicable	Range of means 6.22 ± 1.29 to 8.53 ± 1.53 (n = 32)
Elimination half-life (h)	4.08 ± 0.76 (n = 73)	3.81 ± 0.71 (n = 69)	Range of means 3.86 to 5.03 (n = 61)
Renal clearance (mL/min/kg)	3.21 ± 0.75 (n = 20)	2.99 ± 0.67 (n = 16)	Range of means 2.67 to 3.98 (n = 30)

[a] Data were obtained from single- and multiple-dose studies in healthy volunteers, HIV-positive patients, and HIV-positive/CMV-positive patients with and without retinitis. Patients with CMV retinitis tended to have higher ganciclovir plasma concentrations than patients without CMV retinitis.
[b] IV = intravenously; AUC = area under the curve; C_{max} = maximal drug concentration.

In solid organ transplant recipients, the mean systemic exposure to ganciclovir was 1.7 times higher following administration of valganciclovir 900 mg tablets once daily versus ganciclovir 1,000 mg capsules 3 times daily, when both drugs were administered according to their renal function dosing algorithms. The systemic ganciclovir exposures attained were comparable across kidney, heart, and liver transplant recipients based on a population pharmacokinetics evaluation.

Mean Ganciclovir Pharmacokinetic Measures by Organ Transplant Type (Study PV16000)

Parameter	Ganciclovir 1,000 mg capsules 3 times daily with food	Valganciclovir 900 mg tablets once daily with food
Heart transplant recipients	(n = 13)	(n = 17)
AUC_{0-24h} (mcg•h/mL)	26.6 ± 11.6	40.2 ± 11.8
C_{max} (mcg/mL)	1.4 ± 0.5	4.9 ± 1.1
Elimination half-life (h)	8.47 ± 2.84	6.58 ± 1.5
Liver transplant recipients	(n = 33)	(n = 75)
AUC_{0-24h} (mcg•h/mL)	24.9 ± 10.2	46 ± 16.1
C_{max} (mcg/mL)	1.3 ± 0.4	5.4 ± 1.5
Elimination half-life (h)	7.68 ± 2.74	6.18 ± 1.42
Kidney transplant recipients[a]	(n = 36)	(n = 68)
AUC_{0-24h} (mcg•h/mL)	31.3 ± 10.3	48.2 ± 14.6
C_{max} (mcg/mL)	1.5 ± 0.5	5.3 ± 1.5
Elimination half-life (h)	9.44 ± 4.37	6.77 ± 1.25

[a] Includes kidney-pancreas.

Absorption – Valganciclovir is well absorbed from the GI tract and rapidly metabolized in the intestinal wall and liver to ganciclovir. The absolute bioavailability of ganciclovir from valganciclovir tablets following administration with food was approximately 60% (3 studies: n = 18, n = 16, n = 28). Ganciclovir median time to peak plasma concentration (T_{max}) following administration of valganciclovir 450 to 2,625 mg tablets ranged from 1 to 3 hours. Dose proportionality with respect to ganciclovir AUC following administration of valganciclovir tablets was demonstrated only under fed conditions. Systemic exposure to the prodrug valganciclovir is transient and low, and the AUC_{24} and C_{max} values are approximately 1% and 3% of those of ganciclovir, respectively.

Food effect: When valganciclovir tablets were administered with a high-fat meal containing approximately 600 total calories (31.1 g of fat, 51.6 g of carbohydrates, and 22.2 g of protein) at a dose of 875 mg once daily to 16 HIV-positive subjects, the steady-state ganciclovir AUC increased by 30% (95% confidence interval [CI], 12% to 51%), and the C_{max} increased by 14% (95% CI, −5% to 36%), without any prolongation in T_{max}. Administer valganciclovir tablets with food.

Distribution – Because of the rapid conversion of valganciclovir to ganciclovir, plasma protein binding of valganciclovir was not determined. Plasma protein binding of ganciclovir is 1% to 2% over concentrations of 0.5 and 51 mcg/mL. When ganciclovir was administered IV, the steady-state volume of distribution of ganciclovir was 0.703 ± 0.134 L/kg (n = 69).

Metabolism – Valganciclovir is rapidly hydrolyzed to ganciclovir; no other metabolites have been detected. No metabolite of orally administered radiolabeled ganciclovir (1,000 mg single dose) accounted for more than 1% to 2% of the radioactivity recovered in the feces or urine.

Excretion – The major route of elimination of valganciclovir is by renal excretion as ganciclovir through glomerular filtration and active tubular secretion. Systemic clearance of IV administered ganciclovir was 3.07 ± 0.64 mL/min/kg (n = 68), while renal clearance was 2.99 ± 0.67 mL/min/kg (n = 16).

The terminal half-life ($t_{½}$) of ganciclovir following oral administration of valganciclovir tablets to either healthy or HIV-positive/CMV-positive subjects was 4.08 ± 0.76 hours (n = 73), and following administration of IV ganciclovir was 3.81 ± 0.71 hours (n = 69). In heart, kidney, kidney-pancreas, and liver transplant patients, the terminal elimination half-life of ganciclovir following oral administration of valganciclovir was 6.48 ± 1.38 hours, and following oral administration of ganciclovir was 8.56 ± 3.62 hours.

Special populations –

Renal function impairment:

Pharmacokinetics of Ganciclovir From a Single Oral Dose of Valganciclovir 900 mg Tablets

Estimated CrCl (mL/min)	N	Apparent clearance (mL/min) Mean ± SD[a]	AUC_{last} (mcg•h/mL) Mean ± SD	Half-life (h) Mean ± SD
51 to 70	6	249 ± 99	49.5 ± 22.4	4.85 ± 1.4
21 to 50	6	136 ± 64	91.9 ± 43.9	10.2 ± 4.4
11 to 20	6	45 ± 11	223 ± 46	21.8 ± 5.2
≤ 10	6	12.8 ± 8	366 ± 66	67.5 ± 34

[a] SD = standard deviation.

Decreased renal function results in decreased clearance of ganciclovir from valganciclovir and a corresponding increase in terminal half-life. Therefore, dosage adjustment is required for patients with impaired renal function.

• *Hemodialysis* – Hemodialysis reduces plasma concentrations of ganciclovir by approximately 50% following valganciclovir administration. Adult patients receiving hemodialysis (CrCl less than 10 mL/min) cannot use valganciclovir hydrochloride tablets because the daily dose of valganciclovir hydrochloride tablets required for these patients is less than 450 mg.

Children: The pharmacokinetics of ganciclovir were evaluated following the administration of valganciclovir in 63 pediatric solid organ transplant patients 4 months to 16 years of age. In this study, patients received oral doses of valganciclovir (either tablets or oral solution) to produce exposure equivalent to an adult 900 mg dose.

The pharmacokinetics of ganciclovir were similar across organ types and age ranges. Population pharmacokinetic modeling suggested that bioavailability was approximately 60%. Clearance was positively influenced by body surface area and renal function. The mean total clearance was 5.3 L/h (88.3 mL/min) for a patient with CrCl of 70.4 mL/min.

Mean (SD) Pharmacokinetics of Ganciclovir by Age in Pediatric Solid Organ Transplant Patients

	Pharmacokinetic parameter	Age group ≤ 2 y (n = 2)	> 2 to < 12 y (n = 10)[a,b]	≥ 12 y (n = 19)
Kidney (n = 31)	AUC_{0-24h} (mcg•h/mL)	67.6 (13)	55.9 (12.1)	47.8 (12.4)
	C_{max} (mcg/mL)	10.4 (0.4)	8.7 (2.1)	7.7 (2.1)
	$t_{½}$ (h)	4.5 (1.5)	4.8 (1)	6 (1.3)
		≤ 2 (n = 9)	> 2 to < 12 (n = 6)	≥ 12 (n = 2)
Liver (n = 17)	AUC_{0-24h} (mcg•h/mL)	69.9 (37)	59.4 (8.1)	35.4 (2.8)
	C_{max} (mcg/mL)	11.9 (3.7)	9.5 (2.3)	5.5 (1.1)
	$t_{½}$ (h)	2.8 (1.5)	3.8 (0.7)	4.4 (0.2)
		≤ 2 (n = 6)	> 2 to < 12 (n = 2)	≥ 12 (n = 4)
Heart (n = 12)	AUC_{0-24h} (mcg•h/mL)	55.4 (22.8)	59.6 (21)	60.6 (25)
	C_{max} (mcg/mL)	8.2 (2.5)	12.5 (1.2)	9.5 (3.3)
	$t_{½}$ (h)	3.8 (1.7)	2.8 (0.9)	4.9 (0.8)

[a] There was 1 subject in this age group who received both a kidney and liver transplant. The pharmacokinetic profile for this subject has not been included in this table because it is not possible to determine whether the effects observed are from the kidney/liver transplant or neither.
[b] The pharmacokinetic profiles for 2 subjects in this age group who received kidney transplants have not been included in this table because the data were determined to be nonevaluable.

➤*Microbiology:*

Viral resistance – Viruses resistant to ganciclovir can arise after prolonged treatment with valganciclovir by selection of mutations in either the viral protein kinase gene (UL97) responsible for ganciclovir monophosphorylation and/or in the viral polymerase gene (UL54). A virus with mutations in the UL97 gene is resistant to ganciclovir alone, whereas a virus with mutations in the UL54 gene may show cross-resistance to other antivirals that target the same sites on viral DNA polymerase.

The current working definition of CMV resistance to ganciclovir in cell culture assays is EC_{50} of 1.5 mcg/mL or higher (6 mcM or more). CMV resistance to ganciclovir has been observed in individuals (immunocompromised and neonates) receiving prolonged treatment with ganciclovir or valganci-

VALGANCICLOVIR HYDROCHLORIDE — ORAL

clovir. Consider the possibility of viral resistance in patients who show poor clinical response or experience persistent viral excretion during therapy.

Contraindications

Hypersensitivity (eg, anaphylaxis) to valganciclovir, ganciclovir, or any component of the formulation.

Warnings/Precautions

➤*Hematologic effects:* Do not administer valganciclovir if the absolute neutrophil count is less than 500 cells/mcL, the platelet count is less than 25,000/mcL, or the hemoglobin is less than 8 g/dL.

Severe leukopenia, neutropenia, anemia, thrombocytopenia, pancytopenia, bone marrow aplasia, and aplastic anemia have been reported in patients treated with valganciclovir tablets (and ganciclovir).

Use valganciclovir with caution in patients with preexisting cytopenias, or who have received or are receiving myelosuppressive drugs or irradiation. Cytopenia may occur at any time during treatment and may worsen with continued dosing. Cell counts usually begin to recover within 3 to 7 days of discontinuing the drug.

➤*Acute renal failure:* Acute renal failure may occur in elderly patients with or without reduced renal function, patients receiving potential nephrotoxic drugs, and patients without adequate hydration. Exercise caution when administering valganciclovir to elderly patients and patients receiving potential nephrotoxic drugs. A dosage reduction is recommended for patients with renal impairment. Maintain adequate hydration for all patients.

➤*Renal function impairment:* Dose reduction is recommended when administering valganciclovir to patients with renal impairment. See Administration and Dosage for more information.

For adult patients on hemodialysis (CrCl less than 10 mL/min), it is recommended that ganciclovir be used (in accordance with the dose-reduction algorithm cited in the Ganciclovir Injection and Ganciclovir Oral monographs in Administration and Dosage) rather than valganciclovir tablets.

➤*Pregnancy: Category C.* Valganciclovir is converted to ganciclovir and therefore is expected to have reproductive toxicity effects similar to ganciclovir. There are no adequate and well-controlled studies of valganciclovir or ganciclovir use in pregnant women. In animal studies of ganciclovir, embryofetal toxicity and structural malformations occurred. Use valganciclovir during pregnancy only if the potential benefit justifies the potential risk to the fetus.

In animal studies, pregnant mice and rabbits received ganciclovir at doses that produced 2 times the human exposure (based on AUC comparison). Treated rabbits had increased rates of fetal resorption, fetal growth retardation, embryolethality, maternal toxicity, cleft palate, anophthalmia/microphthalmia, aplastic organs (kidney and pancreas), hydrocephaly, and brachygnathia. In mice, increased fetal resorptions and embryolethality occurred in the presence of maternal/fetal toxicity.

Daily IV doses of approximately 1.7 times the human exposure (based on AUC) administered to female mice prior to mating, during gestation, and during lactation caused hypoplasia of the testes and seminal vesicles in month-old male offspring, as well as pathologic changes in the nonglandular region of the stomach.

Data from an ex vivo human placental model showed that ganciclovir crosses the human placenta. The transfer occurred by passive diffusion and was not saturable over a concentration range of 1 to 10 mg/mL.

In animal studies, ganciclovir was found to be teratogenic, mutagenic, and carcinogenic. Therefore, consider valganciclovir to have the potential to cause birth defects and cancers in humans.

Because of the mutagenic and teratogenic potential of ganciclovir, advise women of childbearing potential to use effective contraception during treatment and for at least 30 days following treatment with valganciclovir. Similarly, advise men to practice barrier contraception during, and for at least 90 days following, treatment with valganciclovir.

Fertility impairment – In men, valganciclovir at the recommended doses may cause temporary or permanent inhibition of spermatogenesis. Animal data also indicate that suppression of fertility in females may occur.

➤*Lactation:* It is not known whether ganciclovir (active drug) or valganciclovir (prodrug) is excreted in human milk. Because valganciclovir caused granulocytopenia, anemia, and thrombocytopenia in clinical trials and ganciclovir was mutagenic and carcinogenic in animal studies, serious adverse events may occur from ganciclovir exposure in breast-feeding infants. Because of the potential for serious adverse events in breast-feeding infants, decide whether to discontinue breast-feeding or the drug, taking into consideration the importance of the drug to the mother. The Centers for Disease Control and Prevention recommend that HIV-infected mothers not breastfeed their infants to avoid risking postnatal transmission of HIV.

➤*Children:* The use of valganciclovir for the prevention of CMV disease in children 4 months to 16 years of age with kidney or heart transplant is based on pharmacokinetic, safety, and efficacy data from an open-label trial with oral valganciclovir (oral solution or tablets) in pediatric solid organ transplant recipients at risk for developing CMV disease. The results of this study were supported by previous demonstration of efficacy in adults.

The safety and efficacy of valganciclovir for oral solution and tablets have not been established in children for prevention of CMV disease in liver transplant patients, solid organ transplants other than those indicated, pediatric solid organ transplant patients younger than 4 months of age, or for treatment of congenital CMV disease

➤*Elderly:* No studies of valganciclovir have been conducted in adults older than 65 years of age. Clinical studies of valganciclovir did not include sufficient numbers of subjects 65 years of age and older to determine whether they respond differently from younger subjects. In general, dose selection for an elderly patient should be cautious, usually starting at the low end of the dosing range, reflecting the greater frequency of decreased hepatic, renal, or cardiac function, and of concomitant disease or other drug therapy. Valganciclovir hydrochloride is known to be substantially excreted by the kidneys, and the risk of toxic reactions to this drug may be greater in patients with impaired renal function. Because elderly patients are more likely to have decreased renal function, care should be taken in dose selection. In addition, monitor renal function and make dosage adjustments accordingly.

➤*Monitoring:* Due to the frequency of neutropenia, anemia, and thrombocytopenia in patients receiving valganciclovir, it is recommended that complete blood counts with differential and platelet counts be performed frequently, especially in patients in whom ganciclovir or other nucleoside analogs have previously resulted in leukopenia, or in whom neutrophil counts are less than 1,000 cells/mcL at the beginning of treatment. Increased monitoring for cytopenias may be warranted if therapy with oral ganciclovir is changed to valganciclovir because of increased plasma concentrations of ganciclovir after valganciclovir administration.

Increased serum creatinine levels have been observed in trials evaluating valganciclovir tablets. Monitor serum creatinine or creatinine clearance values carefully to allow for dosage adjustments in renally impaired patients. The mechanism of impairment of renal function is not known.

Drug Interactions

No in vivo drug-drug interaction studies were conducted with valganciclovir. However, because valganciclovir is rapidly and extensively converted to ganciclovir, interactions associated with ganciclovir are expected for valganciclovir.

Ganciclovir Drug Interactions

Precipitant drug	Object drug[a]		Description
Didanosine	Ganciclovir	↑↓	Steady-state didanosine AUC increased 111% when didanosine was administered either 2 hours prior to or simultaneously with ganciclovir. Closely monitor for didanosine toxicity. A decrease in steady-state ganciclovir AUC of 21% was observed when didanosine was administered 2 hours prior to administration of ganciclovir, but ganciclovir AUC was not affected by the presence of didanosine when the 2 drugs were administered simultaneously. Didanosine dosage adjustment may be needed.
Ganciclovir	Didanosine		
Mycophenolate mofetil	Ganciclovir	↔	In patients with healthy renal function, no pharmacokinetic interaction was observed. However, closely monitor patients with renal function impairment because concentrations of ganciclovir and mycophenolate metabolites may be increased.
Ganciclovir	Mycophenolate mofetil		
Myelosuppressive drugs or irradiation	Ganciclovir	↑	Risk of cytopenia may be increased. Use with caution.
Ganciclovir	Myelosuppressive drugs or irradiation		
Nephrotoxic drugs	Ganciclovir	↑	Risk of renal failure may be increased. Use with caution.
Probenecid	Ganciclovir	↑	Ganciclovir AUC increased 53% and renal clearance of ganciclovir decreased 22%, which is consistent with an interaction involving competition for renal tubular secretion. Monitor for ganciclovir toxicity. Probenecid dosage adjustment may be needed.
Trimethoprim	Ganciclovir	↑	Coadministration resulted in decreased ganciclovir renal clearance and increased $t_{1/2}$.
Zidovudine	Ganciclovir	↑↓	Mean steady-state ganciclovir AUC decreased 17% in the presence of zidovudine. Zidovudine AUC increased 19% in the presence of ganciclovir. Because both drugs can cause neutropenia and anemia, many patients will not tolerate combination therapy at full dosage.
Ganciclovir	Zidovudine		

[a] ↑ = object drug increased; ↑↓ = object drug both increased and decreased; ↔ = undetermined clinical effect.

➤*Drug/Food interactions:* When valganciclovir tablets were administered with a high-fat meal containing approximately 600 total calories

VALGANCICLOVIR HYDROCHLORIDE — ORAL

(31.1 g of fat, 51.6 g of carbohydrates, and 22.2 g of protein) at a dose of 875 mg once daily to 16 HIV-positive subjects, the steady-state ganciclovir AUC increased by 30% (95% CI, 12% to 51%), and the C_{max} increased by 14% (95% CI, −5% to 36%), without any prolongation in T_{max}. Administer valganciclovir tablets with food.

Adverse Reactions

Valganciclovir, a prodrug of ganciclovir, is rapidly converted to ganciclovir after oral administration. Adverse reactions known to be associated with ganciclovir usage can therefore be expected to occur with valganciclovir.

➤*Most common adverse reactions:* The most common adverse reactions and laboratory abnormalities reported in at least 1 indication by 20% or more of adults treated with valganciclovir are anemia, diarrhea, graft rejection, nausea, neutropenia, pyrexia, thrombocytopenia, tremor, and vomiting. The most common reported adverse reactions and laboratory abnormalities reported in more than 10% of pediatric solid organ transplant recipients treated with valganciclovir for oral solution or tablets are anemia, constipation, cough, diarrhea, hypertension, nausea, neutropenia, pyrexia, upper respiratory tract infection, and vomiting.

➤*Treatment of cytomegalovirus retinitis in AIDS patients:*

Valganciclovir Adverse Events in Patients With Cytomegalovirus Retinitis (≥ 5%)

Adverse reactions	Valganciclovir tablets (n = 370)
CNS	
Headache	22%
Insomnia	16%
Paresthesia	8%
Peripheral neuropathy	9%
GI	
Abdominal pain	15%
Diarrhea	41%
Nausea	30%
Vomiting	21%
Miscellaneous	
Pyrexia	31%
Retinal detachment	15%

Lab test abnormalities –

Valganciclovir Laboratory Abnormalities in Patients With Cytomegalovirus Retinitis

Laboratory abnormalities	Valganciclovir tablets (n = 370)
Neutropenia: ANC/mcL	
< 500	19%
500 to < 750	17%
750 to < 1,000	17%
Anemia: hemoglobin g/dL	
< 6.5	7%
6.5 to < 8	13%
8 to < 9.5	16%
Thrombocytopenia: platelets/mcL	
< 25,000	4%
25,000 to < 50,000	6%
50,000 to < 100,000	22%
Serum creatinine: mg/dL	
> 2.5	3%
> 1.5 to 2.5	12%

➤*Prevention of cytomegalovirus disease in selected solid organ transplantation:* The following table shows selected adverse reactions regardless of severity and drug relationship with an incidence of 5% or more from a clinical trial (up to 28 days after study treatment) in which heart, kidney, kidney-pancreas, and liver transplant patients received valganciclovir tablets (n = 244) or oral ganciclovir (n = 126). The majority of the adverse reactions were of mild or moderate intensity.

Valganciclovir Grades 1 to 4 Adverse Reactions in Selected Solid Organ Transplant Patients (≥ 5%)

Adverse reactions	Valganciclovir (n = 244)	Oral ganciclovir (n = 126)
CNS		
Headache	22%	27%
Insomnia	20%	16%
Tremors	28%	25%
GI		
Diarrhea	30%	29%
Nausea	23%	23%
Vomiting	16%	14%
Miscellaneous		
Graft rejection	24%	30%
Hypertension	18%	15%
Pyrexia	13%	14%

Lab test abnormalities –

Valganciclovir Laboratory Abnormalities in Solid Organ Transplant Patients[a]

Laboratory abnormalities	Valganciclovir (n = 244)	Oral ganciclovir (n = 126)
Neutropenia: ANC/mcL		
< 500	5%	3%
500 to < 750	3%	2%
750 to < 1,000	5%	2%
Anemia: hemoglobin g/dL		
< 6.5	1%	2%
6.5 to < 8	5%	7%
8 to < 9.5	31%	25%
Thrombocytopenia: platelets/mcL		
< 25,000	0%	2%
25,000 to < 50,000	1%	3%
50,000 to < 100,000	18%	21%
Serum creatinine: mg/dL		
> 2.5	14%	21%
> 1.5 to 2.5	45%	47%

[a] Laboratory abnormalities are those reported by investigators.

➤*Other adverse reactions (5% or more):* Adverse reactions not included in the previous table that occurred at a frequency of 5% or more in a clinical study with solid organ transplant patients or were selected serious adverse reactions reported in studies with patients with CMV retinitis or in studies with solid organ transplant patients with a frequency of less than 5% are listed in the following sections.

Cardiovascular – Hypotension.

CNS – Agitation, confusion, convulsion, depression, dizziness (excluding vertigo), fatigue, hallucinations, paresthesia, psychosis, weakness.

Dermatologic – Acne, dermatitis, pruritus.

GI – Abdominal distention, abdominal pain, ascites, constipation, dyspepsia.

GU – Decreased creatinine clearance, dysuria, renal impairment, urinary tract infection.

Hematologic – Anemia, aplastic anemia, bone marrow depression, neutropenia, pancytopenia, potentially life-threatening bleeding associated with thrombocytopenia, thrombocytopenia.

Hepatic – Abnormal hepatic function.

Hypersensitivity – Valganciclovir hypersensitivity.

Metabolic/Nutritional – Appetite decreased, dehydration, edema, hyperglycemia, hyperkalemia, hypocalcemia, hypokalemia, hypomagnesemia, hypophosphatemia, peripheral edema.

Musculoskeletal – Arthralgia, back pain, limb pain, muscle cramps.

Respiratory – Cough, dyspnea, pharyngitis/nasopharyngitis, pleural effusion, rhinorrhea, upper respiratory tract infection.

Miscellaneous – Increased wound drainage, local and systemic infections and sepsis, pain, postoperative complications, postoperative pain, postoperative wound infection, wound dehiscence.

➤*Children:* Valganciclovir for oral solution and tablets have been studied in 109 pediatric (4 months to 16 years of age) solid organ transplant patients who were at risk for developing CMV disease and in 24 neonates (8 to 34 days of age) with symptomatic congenital CMV disease, with duration of ganciclovir exposure ranging from 2 to 100 days. The overall safety profile was similar in children compared with adults. However, the rates of certain adverse reactions and laboratory abnormalities, such as anemia, nasopharyngitis, neutropenia, pyrexia, and upper respiratory tract infection, were reported more frequently in children than in adults.

Overdosage

➤*Symptoms:*

Overdose with valganciclovir – One adult developed fatal bone marrow depression (medullary aplasia) after several days of dosing that was at least 10-fold greater than recommended for the patient's estimated degree of renal impairment.

VALGANCICLOVIR HYDROCHLORIDE — ORAL

An overdose of valganciclovir could also possibly result in increased renal toxicity.

Overdose with IV ganciclovir – Reports of overdoses with IV ganciclovir have been received from clinical trials and during postmarketing experience. The majority of patients experienced one or more of the following adverse events.

Hematological toxicity: Pancytopenia, bone marrow depression, medullary aplasia, leukopenia, neutropenia, granulocytopenia.

Hepatotoxicity: Hepatitis, liver function disorder.

Renal toxicity: Worsening of hematuria in a patient with preexisting renal impairment, acute renal failure, elevated creatinine.

GI toxicity: Abdominal pain, diarrhea, vomiting.

Neurotoxicity: Generalized tremor, convulsion.

➤*Treatment:* Because ganciclovir is dialyzable, dialysis may be useful in reducing serum concentrations in patients who have received an overdose of valganciclovir. Maintain adequate hydration. Consider the use of hematopoietic growth factors.

Patient Information

Advise patients that valganciclovir tablets cannot be substituted for ganciclovir capsules on a 1-to-1 basis. Advise patients switching from ganciclovir capsules of the risk of overdosage if they take more than the prescribed number of valganciclovir tablets.

Instruct patients that adults should use valganciclovir tablets, not valganciclovir for oral solution.

Valganciclovir is changed to ganciclovir once it is absorbed into the body. Inform all patients that the major toxicities of ganciclovir include granulocytopenia (neutropenia), anemia, and thrombocytopenia and that dose modifications may be required, including discontinuation. Emphasize the importance of close monitoring of blood counts while on therapy. Inform patients that ganciclovir has been associated with elevations in serum creatinine.

Instruct patients to take valganciclovir with food to maximize bioavailability.

Advise patients that ganciclovir causes decreased sperm production in animals and may cause decreased fertility in humans. Advise women of childbearing potential that ganciclovir causes birth defects in animals and should not be used during pregnancy. Because of the potential for serious adverse events in breast-feeding infants, instruct mothers not to breast-feed if they are receiving valganciclovir. Advise women of childbearing potential to use effective contraception during and for at least 30 days following treatment with valganciclovir tablets. Similarly, advise men to practice barrier contraception during and for at least 90 days following treatment with valganciclovir.

Although there is no information from human studies, advise patients that ganciclovir should be considered a potential carcinogen.

Advise patients that convulsions, sedation, dizziness, ataxia, or confusion have been reported with the use of valganciclovir or ganciclovir. If they occur, such effects may affect tasks requiring alertness, including the patient's ability to drive and operate machinery.

Advise patients that ganciclovir is not a cure for CMV retinitis, and that they may continue to experience progression of retinitis during or following treatment. Advise patients to have ophthalmologic follow-up examinations at a minimum of every 4 to 6 weeks while being treated with valganciclovir tablets. Some patients will require more frequent follow-up.

Antiherpes Virus Agents

ACYCLOVIR (Acycloguanosine)

Rx	**Acyclovir** (Various, eg, Mylan, PAR, Purepac, Teva, Zenith-Goldline)	**Tablets:** 400 mg	In 100s, 500s, and 1000s.
Rx	**Zovirax** (GlaxoSmithKline)		(Zovirax). White, shield shape. In 100s.
Rx	**Acyclovir** (Various, eg, Mylan, PAR, Purepac, Teva, Zenith-Goldline)	**Tablets:** 800 mg	In 100s and 500s.
Rx	**Zovirax** (GlaxoSmithKline)		(Zovirax 800 mg). Blue, oval. In 100s and UD 100s.
Rx	**Acyclovir** (Various, eg, Mylan, PAR, Purepac, Teva, Zenith-Goldline)	**Capsules:** 200 mg	In 100s.
Rx	**Zovirax** (GlaxoSmithKline)		Lactose. (Wellcome Zovirax 200). Blue. In 100s.[a]
Rx	**Acyclovir** (Various, eg, Alpharma, Xactdose)	**Suspension:** 200 mg/5 mL	In 473 mL.
Rx	**Zovirax** (GlaxoSmithKline)		Banana flavor. In 473 mL.[b]
Rx	**Acyclovir** (Various, eg, Bertek, APP)	**Injection:** 50 mg/mL (as sodium)	In cartons of 10.
Rx	**Acyclovir** (Various, eg, Abbott, Bedford, Gensia Sicor, Novaplus)	**Powder for injection:** 500 mg/vial (as sodium)[c]	In 10 mL vials.
		1000 mg/vial (as sodium)	In 20 mL vials.

[a] May contain parabens.
[b] With 0.1% methylparaben, 0.02% propylparaben, and sorbitol.
[c] Contains 49 mg of sodium.

ACYCLOVIR — ORAL

Indications

➤*Herpes zoster infections:* Acyclovir is indicated for the acute treatment of herpes zoster (shingles).

➤*Genital herpes:* Acyclovir is indicated for the treatment of initial episodes and the management of recurrent episodes of genital herpes.

➤*Chickenpox:* Acyclovir is indicated for the treatment of chickenpox (varicella).

➤*Off-label uses:*

Prevention of recurrent ocular herpes infection – [2] = Fair documentation. Published data evaluating safety and efficacy of acyclovir for the prevention of recurrent ocular herpes simplex virus (HSV) infection are limited to 1 controlled trial in immunocompetent patients and 1 open-label pilot study. While results from these trials are promising, the patient population who would most benefit from therapy is not yet defined. (See Administration and Dosage.)

Other possible off-label uses – Cytomegalovirus and HSV infection following bone marrow or renal transplantation; disseminated primary eczema herpeticum; herpes simplex-associated erythema multiforme; herpes simplex labialis; varicella pneumonia; herpes simplex proctitis; herpes simplex whitlow; herpes zoster encephalitis; infectious mononucleosis.

Administration and Dosage

➤*General dosing considerations:*

Bioequivalence – Acyclovir suspension was shown to be bioequivalent to acyclovir capsules (n = 20), and 1 acyclovir 800 mg tablet was shown to be bioequivalent to 4 acyclovir 200 mg capsules (n = 24).

➤*Adults:*

Chickenpox – 800 mg 4 times daily for 5 days.

Genital herpes (initial episodes) – 200 mg every 4 hours, 5 times daily for 10 days.

Genital herpes (recurrent episodes) – 200 mg every 4 hours, 5 times daily for 5 days. Therapy should be initiated at the earliest sign or symptom (prodrome) of recurrence.

Genital herpes (chronic suppressive therapy) –

Usual dosage: 400 mg 2 times daily for up to 12 months, followed by re-evaluation.

Alternative dosage: Alternative regimens have included doses ranging from 200 mg 3 times daily to 200 mg 5 times daily.

Herpes zoster – 800 mg every 4 hours orally, 5 times daily for 7 to 10 days.

Off-label dosing –

Prevention of recurrent ocular herpes infection: [2] = Fair documentation. 600 to 800 mg daily was administered for 8 to 12 months.

➤*Children:*

Chickenpox –

2 years of age and older: 20 mg/kg per dose orally 4 times daily (80 mg/kg per day) for 5 days.

Over 40 kg: 800 mg 4 times daily for 5 days.

Off-label dosing –

Cytomegalovirus prophylaxis:

- *Usual dose* – 800 to 3,200 mg/day divided every 6 to 24 hours during risk period.
- *Maximum dose* – 80 mg/kg/day.

Genital herpes (first episode):

- *12 years of age and older* –
  Usual dosage: 1,000 to 1,200 mg/day in 3 to 5 divided doses for 7 to 10 days.
  Maximum dose: 80 mg/kg/day divided every 6 to 8 hours in children.

Genital herpes (recurrence):

- *12 years of age and older* –
  Usual dosage: 1,000 mg/day in 5 divided doses. 1,200 mg/day in 3 divided doses, or 1,600 mg/day in 2 divided doses for 5 days.
  Maximum dose: 80 mg/kg/day divided every 6 to 8 hours in children.
  Alternative dosage: 2,400 mg/day in 3 divided doses for 2 days.

Genital and/or ocular herpes chronic suppressive therapy:

- *12 years of age and older* –
  Usual dosage: 800 to 1,000 mg/day in 2 to 5 divided doses for up to 12 months.

ACYCLOVIR — ORAL

Maximum dose: 80 mg/kg/day divided every 6 to 8 hours in children.

Herpes simplex virus infection prophylaxis (immunocompromised):

• *2 years of age and older* – 600 to 1,000 mg daily in 3 to 5 divided doses during risk period.

Herpes simplex virus infection treatment (immunocompromised):

• *2 years of age and older* – 1,000 mg daily in 3 to 5 divided doses for 7 to 14 days.

Varicella (immunocompetent):

• *2 years of age and older* –

Usual dosage: 80 mg/kg/day in 4 divided doses for 5 days.

Maximum dose: 3,200 mg/day.

Varicella or zoster (immunocompromised): 250 to 600 mg/m² per dose 4 to 5 times per day.

Zoster (immunocompetent):

• *12 years of age and older* – 4,000 mg daily in 5 divided doses for 5 to 7 days.

➤*Elderly:* Dosage reduction may be required in elderly patients with underlying renal impairment. (See Renal Function Impairment.)

➤*Renal function impairment:*

Acyclovir Oral Dosage Modification in Adults with Renal Impairment

Normal dosage regimen	Creatinine clearance (mL/min/1.73 m²)	Adjusted dosage regimen: Dose (mg)	Adjusted dosage regimen: Dosing interval
200 mg every 4 hours	> 10	200	every 4 hours, 5 times daily
	0 to 10	200	every 12 hours
400 mg every 12 hours	> 10	400	every 12 hours
	0 to 10	200	every 12 hours
800 mg every 4 hours	> 25	800	every 4 hours, 5 times daily
	10 to 25	800	every 8 hours
	0 to 10	800	every 12 hours

Hemodialysis –

The patient's dosing schedule should be adjusted so that an additional dose is administered after each dialysis.

➤*Administration:* Administer with or without food.

➤*Storage/Stability:* Store at 15° to 25°C (59° to 77°F) and protect from moisture.

Actions

➤*Pharmacology:* Acyclovir is a synthetic purine nucleoside analogue with in vitro and in vivo inhibitory activity against herpes simplex virus types 1 (HSV-1), 2 (HSV-2), and varicella-zoster virus (VZV). In cell culture, acyclovir's highest antiviral activity is against HSV-1, followed in decreasing order of potency against HSV-2 and VZV.

The inhibitory activity of acyclovir is highly selective due to its affinity for the enzyme thymidine kinase (TK) encoded by HSV and VZV. This viral enzyme converts acyclovir into acyclovir monophosphate, a nucleotide analogue. The monophosphate is further converted into diphosphate by cellular guanylate kinase and into triphosphate by a number of cellular enzymes. In vitro, acyclovir triphosphate stops replication of herpes viral DNA. This is accomplished in three ways: Competitive inhibition of viral DNA polymerase; incorporation into and termination of the growing viral DNA chain; and inactivation of the viral DNA polymerase. The greater antiviral activity of acyclovir against HSV compared to VZV is due to its more efficient phosphorylation by the viral TK.

➤*Pharmacokinetics:*

Absorption/Distribution – The pharmacokinetics of acyclovir after oral administration have been evaluated in healthy volunteers and in immunocompromised patients with herpes simplex or varicella-zoster virus infection. Acyclovir pharmacokinetic parameters are summarized in the following table.

Acyclovir Oral Pharmacokinetic Characteristics (Range)

Parameter	Range
Plasma protein binding	9% to 33%
Plasma elimination half-life	2.5 to 3.3 hours
Average oral bioavailability	10% to 20%[a]

[a] Bioavailability decreases with increasing dose.

In one multiple-dose, cross-over study in healthy subjects (n = 23), it was shown that increases in plasma acyclovir concentrations were less than dose proportional with increasing dose, as shown in the following table. The decrease in bioavailability is a function of the dose and not the dosage form.

Acyclovir Oral Peak and Trough Concentrations at Steady State

Parameter	200 mg	400 mg	800 mg
Css_{max}	0.83 mcg/mL	1.21 mcg/mL	1.61 mcg/mL
Css_{trough}	0.46 mcg/mL	0.63 mcg/mL	0.83 mcg/mL

There was no effect of food on the absorption of acyclovir (n = 6); therefore, acyclovir capsules, tablets, and suspension may be administered with or without food.

Metabolism – The only known urinary metabolite is 9-]guanine.

Special populations –

Renal function impairment: The half-life and total body clearance of acyclovir are dependent on renal function. A dosage adjustment is recommended for patients with reduced renal function.

Elderly: Acyclovir plasma concentrations are higher in geriatric patients compared to younger adults, in part due to age-related changes in renal function. Dosage reduction may be required in geriatric patients with underlying renal impairment.

Contraindications

Hypersensitivity to acyclovir or valacyclovir.

Warnings/Precautions

➤*Oral use:* Acyclovir capsules, tablets, and suspension are intended for oral ingestion only.

➤*Thrombotic thrombocytopenic purpura/hemolytic uremic syndrome (TTP/HUS):* TTP/HUS, which has resulted in death, has occurred in immunocompromised patients receiving acyclovir therapy.

➤*Renal effects:* Renal failure, in some cases resulting in death, has been observed with acyclovir therapy.

➤*Herpes zoster:* There are no data on treatment initiated more than 72 hours after onset of the zoster rash. Patients should be advised to initiate treatment as soon as possible after a diagnosis of herpes zoster.

➤*Genital herpes infections:* Patients should be informed that acyclovir is not a cure for genital herpes. There are no data evaluating whether acyclovir will prevent transmission of infection to others. Because genital herpes is a sexually transmitted disease, patients should avoid contact with lesions or intercourse when lesions and/or symptoms are present to avoid infecting partners. Genital herpes can also be transmitted in the absence of symptoms through asymptomatic viral shedding. If medical management of a genital herpes recurrence is indicated, patients should be advised to initiate therapy at the first sign or symptom of an episode.

➤*Chickenpox:* Chickenpox in otherwise healthy children is usually a self-limited disease of mild to moderate severity. Adolescents and adults tend to have more severe disease. Treatment was initiated within 24 hours of the typical chickenpox rash in the controlled studies, and there is no information regarding the effects of treatment begun later in the disease course.

➤*Renal function impairment:* Dosage adjustment is recommended when administering acyclovir to patients with renal impairment. Caution should also be exercised when administering acyclovir to patients receiving potentially nephrotoxic agents since this may increase the risk of renal dysfunction and/or the risk of reversible central nervous system symptoms such as those that have been reported in patients treated with intravenous acyclovir.

➤*Pregnancy: Category B.* There are no adequate and well-controlled studies in pregnant women. A prospective epidemiologic registry of acyclovir use during pregnancy was established in 1984 and completed in April 1999. There were 749 pregnancies followed in women exposed to systemic acyclovir during the first trimester of pregnancy resulting in 756 outcomes. The occurrence rate of birth defects approximates that found in the general population. However, the small size of the registry is insufficient to evaluate the risk for less common defects or to permit reliable or definitive conclusions regarding the safety of acyclovir in pregnant women and their developing fetuses. In a population-based historical cohort study, 2% of 1,561 infants exposed to acyclovir during the first trimester were diagnosed with a major birth defect compared to 2.4% of the 19,920 infants that were not exposed to antivirals. The authors of the study concluded that exposure to acyclovir during the first trimester of pregnancy was not associated with an increased risk of major birth defects. Acyclovir should be used during pregnancy only if the potential benefit justifies the potential risk to the fetus.

➤*Lactation:* Acyclovir concentrations have been documented in breast milk in 2 women following oral administration of acyclovir and ranged from 0.6 to 4.1 times corresponding plasma levels. These concentrations would potentially expose the nursing infant to a dose of acyclovir as high as 0.3 mg/kg/day. Acyclovir should be administered to a nursing mother with caution and only when indicated.

➤*Children:* Safety and effectiveness in pediatric patients younger than 2 years of age have not been established.

➤*Elderly:* Of 376 subjects who received acyclovir in a clinical study of herpes zoster treatment in immunocompetent subjects 50 years of age and older, 244 were 65 years of age and older while 111 were 75 years of age and older. No overall differences in effectiveness for time to cessation of new lesion formation or time to healing were reported between geriatric subjects and younger adult subjects. The duration of pain after healing was longer in patients 65 years of age and older. Nausea, vomiting, and dizziness were reported more frequently in elderly subjects. Elderly patients are more likely to have reduced renal function and require dose reduction. Elderly patients are also more likely to have renal or CNS adverse events. With respect to CNS adverse events observed during clinical practice, somnolence, hallucinations, confusion, and coma were reported more frequently in elderly patients.

ACYCLOVIR — ORAL

Drug Interactions

Acyclovir Drug Interactions			
Precipitant drug	Object drug[a]		Description
Probenecid	Acyclovir	⬆	Acyclovir bioavailability and terminal plasma half-life may be increased, and renal clearance may be decreased.
Acyclovir	Theophyllines	⬆	Coadministration may result in increased theophylline plasma concentrations; monitor plasma levels and side effects. Adjust theophylline dose as necessary.
Acyclovir	Hydantoins Valproic acid	⬇	Plasma levels of hydantoins and valproic acid may be decreased with coadministration of acyclovir.

[a] ⬆ = object drug increased; ⬇ = object drug decreased.

Adverse Reactions

Herpes simplex –

Short-term administration: The most frequent adverse events reported during clinical trials of treatment of genital herpes with acyclovir 200 mg administered orally 5 times daily every 4 hours for 10 days were nausea or vomiting in 8 of 298 patient treatments (2.7%). Nausea or vomiting occurred in 2 of 287 (0.7%) patients who received placebo.

Long-term administration: The most frequent adverse events reported in a clinical trial for the prevention of recurrences with continuous administration of 400 mg (two 200 mg capsules) 2 times daily for 1 year in 586 patients treated with acyclovir were nausea (4.8%) and diarrhea (2.4%).

The 589 control patients receiving intermittent treatment of recurrences with acyclovir for 1 year reported diarrhea (2.7%), nausea (2.4%), and headache (2.2%).

Herpes zoster – The most frequent adverse event reported during 3 clinical trials of treatment of herpes zoster (shingles) with 800 mg of oral acyclovir 5 times daily for 7 to 10 days in 323 patients was malaise (11.5%). The 323 placebo recipients reported malaise (11.1%).

Chickenpox – The most frequent adverse event reported during 3 clinical trials of treatment of chickenpox with oral acyclovir at doses of 10 to 20 mg/kg 4 times daily for 5 to 7 days or 800 mg 4 times daily for 5 days in 495 patients was diarrhea (3.2%). The 498 patients receiving placebo reported diarrhea (2.2%).

➤*Postmarketing:* In addition to adverse events reported from clinical trials, the following events have been identified during postapproval use of acyclovir. Because they are reported voluntarily from a population of unknown size, estimates of frequency cannot be made. These events have been chosen for inclusion due to a combination of their seriousness, frequency of reporting, or potential causal connection to acyclovir, or a combination of these factors.

CNS – Aggressive behavior, agitation, ataxia, coma, confusion, decreased consciousness, delirium, dizziness, dysarthria, encephalopathy, hallucinations, paresthesia, psychosis, seizure, somnolence, tremors. These symptoms may be marked, particularly in older adults or in patients with renal impairment.

Dermatologic – Alopecia, erythema multiforme, photosensitive rash, pruritus, rash, Stevens-Johnson syndrome, toxic epidermal necrolysis, urticaria.

GI – Diarrhea; gastrointestinal distress; nausea.

GU – Renal failure, elevated blood urea nitrogen, elevated creatinine, hematuria.

Hematologic/Lymphatic – Anemia, leukocytoclastic vasculitis, leukopenia, lymphadenopathy, thrombocytopenia.

Hepatic – Elevated liver function tests, hepatitis, hyperbilirubinemia, jaundice.

Musculoskeletal – Myalgia.

Special senses – Visual abnormalities.

Miscellaneous – Anaphylaxis, fever, angioedema, headache, pain, peripheral edema.

Overdosage

➤*Symptoms:* Overdoses involving ingestion of up to 100 capsules (20 g) have been reported. Adverse events that have been reported in association with overdosage include agitation, coma, seizures, and lethargy. Precipitation of acyclovir in renal tubules may occur when the solubility (2.5 mg/mL) is exceeded in the intratubular fluid. Overdosage has been reported following bolus injections or inappropriately high doses and in patients whose fluid and electrolyte balance were not properly monitored. This has resulted in elevated BUN and serum creatinine and subsequent renal failure.

➤*Treatment:* In the event of acute renal failure and anuria, the patient may benefit from hemodialysis until renal function is restored.

Patient Information

Patients are instructed to consult with their physicians if they experience severe or troublesome adverse reactions, they become pregnant or intend to become pregnant, they intend to breastfeed while taking orally administered acyclovir, or they have any other questions.

There are no data on treatment initiated more than 72 hours after onset of the zoster rash. Patients should be advised to initiate treatment as soon as possible after a diagnosis of herpes zoster.

Patients should be informed that acyclovir is not a cure for genital herpes. There are no data evaluating whether acyclovir will prevent transmission of infection to others. Because genital herpes is a sexually transmitted disease, patients should avoid contact with lesions or intercourse when lesions and/or symptoms are present to avoid infecting partners. Genital herpes can also be transmitted in the absence of symptoms through asymptomatic viral shedding. If medical management of a genital herpes recurrence is indicated, patients should be advised to initiate therapy at the first sign or symptom of an episode.

Chickenpox in otherwise healthy children is usually a self-limited disease of mild to moderate severity. Adolescents and adults tend to have more severe disease. Treatment was initiated within 24 hours of the typical chickenpox rash in the controlled studies, and there is no information regarding the effects of treatment begun later in the disease course.

ACYCLOVIR — INJECTION

Indications

➤*Herpes simplex infections in immunocompromised patients:* Acyclovir for injection is indicated for the treatment of initial and recurrent mucosal and cutaneous herpes simplex (HSV-1 and HSV-2) in immunocompromised patients.

➤*Initial episodes of herpes genitalis:* Treatment of severe initial clinical episodes of herpes genitalis in immunocompetent patients.

➤*Herpes simplex encephalitis:* Treatment of herpes simplex encephalitis.

➤*Neonatal herpes simplex virus infection:* Treatment of neonatal herpes infections.

➤*Varicella-zoster infections in immunocompromised patients:* Treatment of varicella-zoster (shingles) infections in immunocompromised patients.

➤*Off-label uses:* Prophylaxis of mucocutaneous HSV infection in immunosuppressed HSV-seropositive patients (oral and IV); high-dose IV acyclovir may reduce the risk of CMV infection in CMV-seropositive patients undergoing bone-marrow transplantation.

Administration and Dosage

➤*Adults:* For obese patients, administer the recommended adult dose using ideal body weight.

Herpes genitalis (severe initial episodes) – 5 mg/kg infused at a constant rate over 1 hour, every 8 hours for 5 days.

Herpes simplex encephalitis – 10 mg/kg infused at a constant rate over 1 hour, every 8 hours for 10 days.

Herpes simplex infections (mucosal and cutaneous herpes simplex [HSV-1 and HSV-2] infections) in immunocompromised patients – 5 mg/kg infused at a constant rate over 1 hour, every 8 hours for 7 days.

Varicella-zoster infections in immunocompromised patients – 10 mg/kg infused at a constant rate over 1 hour, every 8 hours for 7 days.

➤*Children:*

Herpes genitalis (severe initial episodes) –

12 years of age and older: See Adults.

Herpes simplex encephalitis –

12 years of age and older: 10 mg/kg infused at a constant rate over 1 hour, every 8 hours for 10 days. One reference suggests a treatment duration of 14 to 21 days.

3 months to 12 years of age: 20 mg/kg infused at a constant rate over 1 hour, every 8 hours for 10 days. One reference suggests a treatment duration of 14 to 21 days.

Herpes simplex infections (mucosal and cutaneous herpes simplex [HSV-1 and HSV-2] infections) in immunocompromised patients – See also Off-label Dosing for additional dosing recommendations.

12 years of age and older: See Adults.

Younger than 12 years of age: 10 mg/kg infused at a constant rate over 1 hour, every 8 hours for 7 days.

Neonatal herpes simplex virus infection –

Birth to 3 months of age: 10 mg/kg infused at a constant rate over 1 hour, every 8 hours for 10 days. In neonatal herpes simplex infections, doses of 15 mg/kg or 20 mg/kg (infused at a constant rate over 1 hour every 8 hours) have been used; the safety and efficacy of these doses are not known. See also Off-label Dosing for additional dosing recommendations.

Varicella-zoster infections in immunocompromised patients –See also Off-label Dosing for additional dosing recommendations.

12 years of age and older: See Adults.

Younger than 12 years of age: 20 mg/kg infused at a constant rate over 1 hour, every 8 hours for 7 days.

ACYCLOVIR — INJECTION

Off-label dosing –

Cytomegalovirus prophylaxis: 1,500 mg/m²/day divided every 8 hours during risk period.

Herpes simplex virus encephalitis:

• *3 months to 12 years of age* – 45 to 60 mg/kg per day divided every 8 hours for 14 to 21 days.

Herpes simplex virus prophylaxis: 750 mg/m²/day in 3 divided doses during risk period.

Herpes simplex virus treatment (immunocompromised): 15 mg/kg/day or 750 to 1,500 mg/m²/day divided every 8 hours for 7 to 14 days.

Neonatal herpes simplex virus: 60 mg/kg per day divided every 8 hours for 14 to 21 days. Another reference suggests 40 mg/kg per day divided every 12 hours for 14 to 21 days for neonates less than 35 weeks postconceptional age.

Varicella (immunocompetent):

• *2 years of age and older* – 30 mg/kg/day or 1,500 mg/m²/day in 3 divided doses for 7 to 10 days.

Varicella (immunocompromised):

• *1 year of age and older* – 30 mg/kg/day or 1,500 mg/m²/day in 3 divided doses for 7 to 10 days.

• *Younger than 1 year of age* – 30 mg/kg/day in 3 divided doses for 7 to 10 days.

Zoster (immunocompetent): 30 mg/kg/day or 1,500 mg/m²/day in 3 divided doses for 7 to 10 days.

Zoster (immunocompromised): 30 mg/kg/day in 3 divided doses for 7 to 10 days.

➤*Elderly:* Dosage reduction may be required in elderly patients with underlying renal impairment. (See Renal Function Impairment.)

➤*Renal function impairment:* See the recommended doses, and adjust the dosing interval as indicated in the following table.

Acyclovir Injection Dosage Adjustments in Renal Impairment

Creatinine clearance (mL/min per 1.73 m²)	Percent of recommended dose	Dosing interval (hours)
> 50	100%	8
25 to 50	100%	12
10 to 25	100%	24
0 to 10	50%	24

Hemodialysis –

The patient's dosing schedule should be adjusted so that an additional dose is administered after each dialysis.

Adults receiving continuous renal replacement therapy (CRRT): One reference suggests a dosage of 5 to 10 mg/kg IV every 24 hours.

The following alternative recommendations assume ultrafiltration and dialysis flow rates of 1 to 2 L/h. A higher dosage is recommended when treating viral meningoencephalitis and varicella-zoster virus infections.

• *Continuous venovenous hemofiltration (CVVH)* – 5 to 10 mg/kg IV every 24 hours.

• *Continuous venovenous hemodialysis (CVVHD) or continuous venovenous hemodialfiltration (CVVHDF)* – 5 to 10 mg/kg IV every 12 to 24 hours.

Adults receiving intermittent hemodialysis (IHD): 2.5 to 5 mg/kg IV every 24 hours administered after the dialysis session. This recommendation assumes the patient is receiving standard IHD 3 times per week and completes the full dialysis sessions. Patients receiving extended daily dialysis may require increased doses. A higher dosage is recommended when treating viral meningoencephalitis and varicella-zoster virus infections.

➤*Preparation for administration:*

Reconstitution – The contents of the vial should be dissolved in sterile water for injection as follows:

Acyclovir Injection Reconstitution

Contents of vial	Amount of diluent
500 mg	10 mL
1,000 mg	20 mL

The resulting solution in each case contains acyclovir 50 mg/mL (pH approximately 11). Shake the vial well to ensure complete dissolution before measuring and transferring each individual dose.

Dilution – Remove and add the calculated dose to any appropriate intravenous (IV) solution at a volume selected for administration during each 1-hour infusion. Infusion concentrations of approximately 7 mg/mL or lower are recommended. In clinical studies, the average 70 kg adult received between 60 and 150 mL of fluid per dose. Higher concentrations (eg, 10 mg/mL) may produce phlebitis or inflammation at the injection site upon inadvertent extravasation.

Once diluted for administration, use each dose within 24 hours.

➤*Administration:* Administer by constant infusion over 1 hour. Rapid or bolus IV injection must be avoided. Intramuscular (IM) or subcutaneous injection must also be avoided.

➤*Extravasation:* Extravasation may occur during administration of acyclovir. If signs or symptoms of extravasation occur, stop the infusion immediately. If possible, withdraw 3 to 5 mL of blood to remove some of the drug. Remove the infusion needle. Delineate the infiltrated area on the patient's skin with a felt-tip marker. Hyaluronidase is an effective antidote for hyperosmolar drug infiltrations; administer promptly within the first few minutes to 1 hour after extravasation. Higher doses (150 units) have primarily been used in adults while lower doses (15 units) have been used in children. Administer hyaluronidase according to the following steps. Dilute hyaluronidase to desired concentration, depending on the dose and product used. (Note: Some products do not require dilution.) For example, if the total dose is 15 units, make 15 units/mL dilution. If the total dose is 150 units, make 150 units/mL dilution. Cleanse area with povidone-iodine. Inject hyaluronidase locally, subcutaneously or intradermally, using a 25-gauge needle or smaller. The dose is given as five 0.2 mL injections at the leading edge of the extravasation site. Change needle after each injection. Elevate for 48 hours above heart level using a sling or stockinette dressing with an observation window cut in the dressing. Avoid pressure or friction. Do not rub area. Observe for signs of increased erythema, pain, or skin necrosis. If increased symptoms occur, consult a plastic surgeon. Ensure that no medication is given distally to extravasation site. After 48 hours, encourage the patient to use the extremity normally to promote full range of motion.

➤*Admixture compatibility:* When reconstituting the contents of the vial, do not use bacteriostatic water for injection containing benzyl alcohol or parabens.

Standard, commercially available electrolyte and glucose solutions are suitable for IV administration; biologic or colloidal fluids (eg, blood products, protein solutions) are not recommended.

➤*Storage/Stability:* Store at 15° to 25°C (59° to 77°F).

The reconstituted solution should be used within 12 hours. Refrigeration of reconstituted solution may result in the formation of a precipitate that will redissolve at room temperature.

Actions

➤*Pharmacology:* Acyclovir is a synthetic purine nucleoside analogue with in vitro and in vivo inhibitory activity against HSV-1, HSV-2, and varicella-zoster virus (VZV). In cell culture, acyclovir's highest antiviral activity is against HSV-1, followed in decreasing order of potency against HSV-2 and VZV.

The inhibitory activity of acyclovir is highly selective due to its affinity for the enzyme thymidine kinase (TK) encoded by HSV and VZV. This viral enzyme converts acyclovir into acyclovir monophosphate, a nucleoside analogue. The monophosphate is further converted into diphosphate by cellular guanylate kinase and into triphosphate by a number of cellular enzymes. In vitro, acyclovir triphosphate stops replication of herpes viral DNA. This is accomplished in three ways: Competitive inhibition of viral DNA polymerase, incorporation into and termination of the growing viral DNA chain, and inactivation of the viral DNA polymerase. The greater antiviral activity of acyclovir against HSV compared with VZV is due to its more efficient phosphorylation by the viral TK.

➤*Pharmacokinetics:*

Absorption/Distribution – The pharmacokinetics of acyclovir after IV administration have been evaluated in adult patients with normal renal function during Phase 1 and 2 studies after single doses ranging from 0.5 to 15 mg/kg and after multiple doses ranging from 2.5 to 15 mg/kg every 8 hours. Proportionality between dose and plasma levels is seen after single doses or at steady-state after multiple dosing.

Average steady-state peak and trough concentrations from 1-hour infusions administered every 8 hours are given in the following table.

Acyclovir Injection Peak and Trough Concentrations at Steady-State

Dosage regimen	Css_{max}	Css_{trough}
5 mg/kg every 8 hours (n = 8)	9.8 mcg/mL	0.7 mcg/mL
	range: 5.5 to 13.8	range: 0.2 to 1
10 mg/kg every 8 hours (n = 7)	22.9 mcg/mL	1.9 mcg/mL
	range: 14.1 to 44.1	range: 0.5 to 2.9

Concentrations achieved in the cerebrospinal fluid are approximately 50% of plasma values. Plasma protein binding is relatively low (9% to 33%) and drug interactions involving binding site displacement are not anticipated.

Metabolism/Excretion – Renal excretion of unchanged drug is the major route of acyclovir elimination accounting for 62% to 91% of the dose. The only major urinary metabolite detected is 9-carboxymethoxymethylguanine, accounting for up to 14.1% of the dose in patients with healthy renal function.

The half-life and total body clearance of acyclovir are dependent on renal function as shown in the following table.

Acyclovir Injection Half-Life and Total Body Clearance

Creatinine clearance (mL/min per 1.73 m²)	Half-life (h)	Total body clearance (mL/min per 1.73 m²)	Total body clearance (mL/min/kg)
> 80	2.5	327	5.1
50 to 80	3	248	3.9
15 to 50	3.5	190	3.4
0 (anuric)	19.5	29	0.5

Special populations –

Renal function impairment: Acyclovir was administered at a dose of 2.5 mg/kg to 6 adult patients with severe renal failure. The peak and trough plasma levels during the 47 hours preceding hemodialysis were 8.5 mcg/mL and 0.7 mcg/mL, respectively.

ACYCLOVIR — INJECTION

Elderly: Acyclovir plasma concentrations are higher in geriatric patients compared with younger adults, in part due to age-related changes in renal function. Dosage reduction may be required in geriatric patients with underlying renal impairment.

Contraindications

Hypersensitivity to acyclovir or valacyclovir.

Warnings/Precautions

➤*Administration:* Reconstituted acyclovir IV has a pH of approximately 11 and should not be administered by mouth.

Acyclovir for injection is intended for IV infusion only; do not administer topically, IM, orally, subcutaneously, or in the eye. IV infusions must be given over a period of at least 1 hour to reduce the risk of renal tubular damage.

➤*Thrombotic thrombocytopenic purpura/hemolytic uremic syndrome (TTP/HUS):* TTP/HUS, which has resulted in death, has occurred in immunocompromised patients receiving acyclovir therapy.

➤*Aseptic conditions:* Acyclovir IV contains no antimicrobial preservative. Reconstitution and dilution should be carried out under full aseptic conditions immediately before use and any unused solution discarded. Do not refrigerate the reconstituted or diluted solutions.

➤*Renal effects:* Precipitation of acyclovir crystals in renal tubules can occur if the maximum solubility of free acyclovir (2.5 mg/mL at 37°C [98.6°F] in water) is exceeded or if the drug is administered by bolus injection. Ensuing renal tubular damage can produce acute renal failure.

Abnormal renal function (decreased creatinine clearance) can occur as a result of acyclovir administration and depends on the state of the patient's hydration, other treatments, and the rate of drug administration. Concomitant use of other nephrotoxic drugs, preexisting renal disease, and dehydration make further renal impairment with acyclovir more likely.

When dosage adjustments are required, they should be based on estimated creatinine clearance.

➤*Hydration:* Administration of acyclovir by IV infusion must be accompanied by adequate hydration.

➤*Encephalopathic changes:* Approximately 1% of patients receiving IV acyclovir have manifested encephalopathic changes characterized by either lethargy, obtundation, tremors, confusion, hallucinations, agitation, seizures, or coma. Use acyclovir with caution in those patients who have underlying neurologic abnormalities and those with serious renal, hepatic, or electrolyte abnormalities, or significant hypoxia.

➤*Extravasation:* See Administration and Dosage for more information.

➤*Renal function impairment:* The dose of acyclovir must be adjusted in patients with impaired renal function in order to avoid accumulation of acyclovir in the body.

In patients receiving acyclovir at higher doses, (eg, for herpes encephalitis), take specific care regarding renal function, particularly when patients are dehydrated or have any renal impairment.

Renal failure, in some cases resulting in death, has been observed with acyclovir therapy.

➤*Pregnancy: Category B.* There are no adequate and well-controlled studies in pregnant women. A prospective epidemiologic registry of acyclovir use during pregnancy was established in 1984 and completed in April 1999. There were 749 pregnancies followed in women exposed to systemic acyclovir during the first trimester of pregnancy resulting in 756 outcomes. The occurrence rate of birth defects approximates that found in the general population. However, the small size of the registry is insufficient to evaluate the risk for less common defects or to permit reliable or definitive conclusions regarding the safety of acyclovir in pregnant women and their developing fetuses. Use acyclovir during pregnancy only if the potential benefit justifies the potential risk to the fetus.

➤*Lactation:* Acyclovir concentrations have been documented in breast milk in 2 women following oral administration of acyclovir and ranged from 0.6 to 4.1 times corresponding plasma levels. These concentrations would potentially expose the nursing infant to a dose of acyclovir up to 0.3 mg/kg/day. Administer acyclovir to a breast-feeding mother with caution and only when indicated.

➤*Elderly:* Clinical studies of acyclovir for injection did not include sufficient numbers of patients 65 years of age and older to determine whether they respond differently from younger patients. Other reported clinical experience has identified differences in the severity of CNS adverse reactions between elderly and younger patients. In general, dose selection for an elderly patient should be cautious, reflecting the greater frequency of decreased renal function, and of concomitant disease or other drug therapy. This drug is known to be substantially excreted by the kidney, and the risk of toxic reactions to this drug may be greater in patients with impaired renal function. Because elderly patients are more likely to have decreased renal function, take care in dose selection, and it may be useful to monitor renal function.

Drug Interactions

Acyclovir Drug Interactions			
Precipitant drug	Object drug[a]		Description
Probenecid	Acyclovir	↑	Acyclovir bioavailability and terminal plasma half-life may be increased, and renal clearance may be decreased.
Acyclovir	Theophyllines	↑	Coadministration may result in increased theophylline plasma concentrations; monitor plasma levels and side effects. Adjust theophylline dose as necessary.
Acyclovir	Hydantoins Valproic acid	↓	Plasma levels of hydantoins and valproic acid may be decreased with coadministration of acyclovir.

[a] ↑ = object drug increased; ↓ = object drug decreased.

Adverse Reactions

The most frequent adverse reactions reported during administration of acyclovir were inflammation or phlebitis at the injection site in approximately 9% of the patients, and transient elevations of serum creatinine or blood urea nitrogen in 5% to 10% (the higher incidence occurred usually following rapid [less than 10 minutes] IV infusion). Nausea or vomiting occurred in approximately 7% of the patients (the majority occurring in nonhospitalized patients who received 10 mg/kg). Itching, rash, or hives occurred in approximately 2% of patients. Elevation of transaminases occurred in 1% to 2% of patients.

The following hematologic abnormalities occurred at a frequency of less than 1%: Anemia, neutropenia, thrombocytopenia, thrombocytosis, leukocytosis, and neutrophilia. In addition, anorexia and hematuria were observed.

➤*Postmarketing:* In addition to adverse reactions reported from clinical trials, the following reactions have been identified during post-approval use of acyclovir for injection in clinical practice. Because they are reported voluntarily from a population of unknown size, estimates of frequency cannot be made. These reactions have been chosen for inclusion due to either their seriousness, frequency of reporting, potential causal connection to acyclovir, or a combination of these factors.

Cardiovascular – Hypotension.

CNS – Aggressive behavior, agitation, ataxia, coma, confusion, delirium, dizziness, dysarthria, encephalopathy, hallucinations, obtundation, paresthesia, psychosis, seizure, somnolence, tremor. These symptoms may be marked, particularly in older adults.

Dermatologic – Alopecia, erythema multiforme, photosensitive rash, pruritus, rash, Stevens-Johnson syndrome, toxic epidermal necrolysis, urticaria. Severe local inflammatory reactions, including tissue necrosis, have occurred following infusion of acyclovir into extravascular tissues.

GI – Abdominal pain, diarrhea, GI distress, nausea.

GU – Renal failure, elevated blood urea nitrogen, elevated creatinine.

Hematologic/Lymphatic – Disseminated intravascular coagulation, hemolysis, leukocytoclastic vasculitis, leukopenia, lymphadenopathy.

Hepatic – Elevated liver function tests, hepatitis, hyperbilirubinemia, jaundice.

Musculoskeletal – Myalgia.

Special senses – Visual abnormalities.

Miscellaneous – Anaphylaxis, angioedema, fatigue, fever, headache, pain, peripheral edema.

Overdosage

➤*Symptoms:* Overdoses involving ingestions of up to 20 g have been reported. Adverse reactions that have been reported in association with overdosage include agitation, coma, seizures, and lethargy. Precipitation of acyclovir in renal tubules may occur when the solubility (2.5 mg/mL) is exceeded in the intratubular fluid. Overdosage has been reported following bolus injections or inappropriately high doses, and in patients whose fluid and electrolyte balance were not properly monitored. This has resulted in elevated blood urea nitrogen and serum creatinine, and subsequent renal failure.

➤*Treatment:* In the event of acute renal failure and anuria, the patient may benefit from hemodialysis until renal function is restored.

FAMCICLOVIR

Rx	**Famciclovir** (Teva Pharmaceuticals)	**Tablets; oral:** 125 mg	Polydextrose. (8117 93). White. Film-coated. In 30s.
Rx	**Famvir** (Novartis)		Lactose. (Famvir 125). White, round. Film-coated. In 30s.
Rx	**Famciclovir** (Teva Pharmaceuticals)	**Tablets; oral:** 250 mg	Polydextrose. (8118 93). White. Film-coated. In 30s.
Rx	**Famvir** (Novartis)		(Famvir 250). White, round. Film-coated. In 30s.

FAMCICLOVIR

Rx	**Famciclovir** (Teva Pharmaceuticals)	**Tablets; oral:** 500 mg	Polydextrose. (8119 93). Capsule shape. Film-coated. In 30s.
Rx	**Famvir** (Novartis)		Lactose. (Famvir 500). White, oval. Film-coated. In 30s and UD 50s.

FAMCICLOVIR — ORAL

Indications

➤*Genital herpes infections:*

Recurrent episodes – For the treatment of recurrent episodes of genital herpes in immunocompetent patients.

Suppressive therapy – For long-term suppressive therapy of recurrent episodes of genital herpes in immunocompetent patients.

➤*Herpes labialis (cold sores):* For the treatment of recurrent herpes labialis (cold sores) in immunocompetent patients.

➤*Herpes zoster (shingles):* For the treatment of herpes zoster in immunocompetent patients.

➤*Recurrent orolabial or genital herpes:* For the treatment of recurrent episodes of orolabial or genital herpes in HIV-infected adults.

➤*Limitations of use:* The efficacy and safety of famciclovir have not been established for patients younger than 18 years of age, patients with first episode of genital herpes, patients with ophthalmic zoster, immunocompromised patients other than for the treatment of recurrent orolabial or genital herpes in HIV-1–infected patients, or black and African American patients with recurrent genital herpes.

➤*Off-label uses:* Management of initial episodes of herpes genitalis (250 mg 3 times/day for 5 days).

Administration and Dosage

➤*Adults:*

Genital herpes –

Recurrent episodes: 1,000 mg twice daily for 1 day.

Suppressive episodes: 250 mg twice daily.

Herpes labialis (cold sores) – 1,500 mg as a single dose.

Herpes zoster (shingles) – 500 mg every 8 hours for 7 days.

Recurrent orolabial or genital herpes – 500 mg twice daily for 7 days in HIV-infected patients.

➤*Renal function impairment:*

Famciclovir Dosage in Renal Function Impairment

Indication and normal dosage regimen	CrCl[a] (mL/min)	Adjusted dosage regimen dose (mg)	Dosing interval
Single-day dosing regimens			
Recurrent genital herpes			
1,000 mg every 12 hours for 1 day	≥ 60	1,000	every 12 hours for 1 day
	40 to 59	500	every 12 hours for 1 day
	20 to 39	500	single dose
	< 20	250	single dose
	HD[b]	250	single dose following dialysis
Recurrent herpes labialis			
1,500 mg single dose	≥ 60	1,500	single dose
	40 to 59	750	single dose
	20 to 39	500	single dose
	< 20	250	single dose
	HD[b]	250	single dose following dialysis
Multiple-day dosing regimens			
Herpes zoster			
500 mg every 8 hours	≥ 60	500	every 8 hours
	40 to 59	500	every 12 hours
	20 to 39	500	every 24 hours
	< 20	250	every 24 hours
	HD[b]	250	following each dialysis

Famciclovir Dosage in Renal Function Impairment

Indication and normal dosage regimen	CrCl[a] (mL/min)	Adjusted dosage regimen dose (mg)	Dosing interval
Suppression of recurrent genital herpes			
250 mg every 12 hours	≥ 40	250	every 12 hours
	20 to 39	125	every 12 hours
	< 20	125	every 24 hours
	HD[b]	125	following each dialysis
Recurrent orolabial and genital herpes simplex infection in HIV-infected patients			
500 mg every 12 hours	≥ 40	500	every 12 hours
	20 to 39	500	every 24 hours
	< 20	250	every 24 hours
	HD[b]	250	following each dialysis

[a] CrCl = creatinine clearance.
[b] HD = hemodialysis.

➤*Administration:* May be taken without regard to meals.

➤*Storage/Stability:* Store at 25°C (77°F); excursions are permitted to 15° to 30°C (59° to 86°F).

Actions

➤*Pharmacology:* Famciclovir undergoes rapid biotransformation to the active antiviral compound penciclovir, which has inhibitory activity against herpes simplex virus types 1 (HSV-1) and 2 (HSV-2) and varicella zoster virus (VZV). In cells infected with HSV-1, HSV-2, or VZV, the viral thymidine kinase phosphorylates penciclovir to a monophosphate form that, in turn, is converted to penciclovir triphosphate by cellular kinases. In vitro studies demonstrate that penciclovir triphosphate inhibits HSV-2 DNA polymerase competitively with deoxyguanosine triphosphate. Consequently, herpes viral DNA synthesis and, therefore, replication are selectively inhibited.

➤*Pharmacokinetics:*

Absorption – Famciclovir is the diacetyl 6-deoxy analog of the active antiviral compound penciclovir. Following oral administration, little or no famciclovir is detected in plasma or urine.

The absolute bioavailability of famciclovir is 77% ± 8% as determined following the administration of a famciclovir 500 mg oral dose and a penciclovir 400 mg intravenous (IV) dose to 12 healthy male subjects.

Penciclovir concentrations increased in proportion to dose over a famciclovir dose range of 125 to 1,000 mg administered as a single dose. Single oral-dose administration of famciclovir 125, 250, 500, or 1,000 mg to healthy male volunteers across 17 studies gave the following pharmacokinetic parameters.

Famciclovir Pharmacokinetic Parameters

Dose	$AUC_{(0-\infty)}$[a] (mcg h/mL)	C_{max}[b] (mcg/mL)	T_{max}[c] (h)
125 mg	2.24	0.8	0.9
250 mg	4.48	1.6	0.9
500 mg	8.95	3.3	0.9
1,000 mg	17.9	6.6	0.9

[a] $AUC_{(0-\infty)}$ = area under the plasma concentration-time profile extrapolated to infinity.
[b] C_{max} = maximum observed plasma concentration.
[c] T_{max} = time to C_{max}.

Following single oral-dose administration of famciclovir 500 mg to 7 patients with herpes zoster, the mean ± standard deviation (SD) AUC, C_{max}, and T_{max} were 12.1 ± 1.7 mcg h/mL, 4 ± 0.7 mcg/mL, and 0.7 ± 0.2 hours, respectively. The AUC of penciclovir was approximately 35% greater in patients with herpes zoster as compared with healthy volunteers. Some of this difference may be due to differences in renal function between the 2 groups.

There is no accumulation of penciclovir after the administration of famciclovir 500 mg 3 times a day for 7 days.

Food effects: Penciclovir C_{max} decreased approximately 50%, and T_{max} was delayed by 1.5 hours when a capsule formulation of famciclovir was administered with food (nutritional content was approximately 910 kcal and 26% fat). There was no effect on the extent of availability (AUC) of penciclovir. There was an 18% decrease in C_{max} and a delay in T_{max} of about 1 hour when famciclovir was given 2 hours after a meal as compared with its administration 2 hours before a meal. Because there was no effect on the

FAMCICLOVIR — ORAL

extent of systemic availability of penciclovir, it appears that famciclovir can be taken without regard to meals.

Distribution – The volume of distribution ($Vd_β$) was 1.08 ± 0.17 L/kg in 12 healthy male subjects following a single IV dose of penciclovir at 400 mg administered as a 1-hour IV infusion.

Penciclovir is less than 20% bound to plasma proteins over the concentration range of 0.1 to 20 mcg/mL. The blood/plasma ratio of penciclovir is approximately 1.

Metabolism – Following oral administration, famciclovir is deacetylated and oxidized to form penciclovir. Metabolites that are inactive include 6-deoxy penciclovir, monoacetylated penciclovir, and 6-deoxy monoacetylated penciclovir (5%, less than 0.5%, and less than 0.5% of the dose in the urine, respectively). Little or no famciclovir is detected in plasma or urine.

An in vitro study using human liver microsomes demonstrated that CYP-450 does not play an important role in famciclovir metabolism. The conversion of 6-deoxy penciclovir to penciclovir is catalyzed by aldehyde oxidase.

Excretion – Approximately 94% of administered radioactivity was recovered in urine over 24 hours (83% of the dose was excreted in the first 6 hours) after the administration of 5 mg/kg radiolabeled penciclovir as a 1-hour infusion to 3 healthy male volunteers. Penciclovir accounted for 91% of the radioactivity excreted in the urine.

Following the oral administration of a single 500 mg dose of radiolabeled famciclovir to 3 healthy male volunteers, 73% and 27% of administered radioactivity were recovered in urine and feces over 72 hours, respectively. Penciclovir accounted for 82%, and 6-deoxy penciclovir accounted for 7% of the radioactivity excreted in the urine. Approximately 60% of the administered radiolabeled dose was collected in urine in the first 6 hours.

After IV administration of penciclovir in 48 healthy male volunteers, mean ± SD total plasma clearance of penciclovir was 36.6 ± 6.3 L/h (0.48 ± 0.09 L/h/kg). Penciclovir renal clearance accounted for 74.5 ± 8.8% of total plasma clearance.

Renal clearance of penciclovir following the oral administration of a single 500 mg dose of famciclovir to 109 healthy male volunteers was 27.7 ± 7.6 L/h.

The plasma elimination half-life of penciclovir was 2 ± 0.3 hours after IV administration of penciclovir to 48 healthy male volunteers and 2.3 ± 0.4 hours after oral administration of famciclovir 500 mg to 124 healthy male volunteers. The half-life in 17 patients with herpes zoster was 2.8 ± 1 hours and 2.7 ± 1 hours after single and repeated doses, respectively.

Special populations –

Renal function impairment:

Famciclovir Pharmacokinetic Parameters in Patients With Renal Function Impairment

Parameter (mean ± SD)	CrCl ≥ 60 (mL/min) (n = 15)	CrCl 40 to 59 (mL/min) (n = 5)	CrCl 20 to 39 (mL/min) (n = 4)	CrCl < 20 (mL/min) (n = 3)
CrCl (mL/min)	88.1 ± 20.6	49.3 ± 5.9	26.5 ± 5.3	12.7 ± 5.9
CL_R (L/h)	30.1 ± 10.6	13 ± 1.3[a]	4.2 ± 0.9	1.6 ± 1
CL/F[b] (L/h)	66.9 ± 27.5	27.3 ± 2.8	12.8 ± 1.3	5.8 ± 2.8
Half-life (hours)	2.3 ± 0.5	3.4 ± 0.7	6.2 ± 1.6	13.4 ± 10.2

[a] n = 4.
[b] CL/F consists of bioavailability factor and famciclovir to penciclovir conversion factor.

A dosage adjustment is recommended for patients with renal function impairment.

Hepatic function impairment: Well-compensated chronic liver disease (chronic hepatitis [n = 6], chronic ethanol abuse [n = 8], or primary biliary cirrhosis [n = 1]) had no effect on the extent of availability (AUC) of penciclovir following a single dose of famciclovir 500 mg. However, there was a 44% decrease in penciclovir mean C_{max}, and T_{max} was increased by 0.75 hours in patients with hepatic function impairment, compared with healthy volunteers. No dosage adjustment is recommended for patients with well-compensated hepatic function impairment. The pharmacokinetics of penciclovir have not been evaluated in patients with severe uncompensated hepatic function impairment.

Elderly: Based on cross-study comparisons, mean penciclovir AUC was 40% larger, and penciclovir renal clearance was 22% lower after the oral administration of famciclovir in elderly volunteers (n = 18, 65 to 79 years of age), compared with younger volunteers. Some of this difference may be due to differences in renal function between the 2 groups.

Contraindications

Hypersensitivity to the product, its components, or penciclovir cream.

Warnings/Precautions

➤*Initial episodes/immunocompromised patients:* The efficacy of famciclovir has not been established for initial episode genital herpes infection, ophthalmic zoster, disseminated zoster, or in immunocompromised patients with herpes zoster.

➤*Lactose intolerance:* Famciclovir 125, 250, and 500 mg tablets contain lactose (26.9, 53.7, and 107.4 mg, respectively). Patients with rare hereditary problems of galactose intolerance, a severe lactase deficiency, or glucose-galactose malabsorption should not take famciclovir 125, 250, and 500 mg tablets.

➤*Renal function impairment:* Dosage adjustment is recommended when administering famciclovir to patients with CrCl values less than 60 mL/min. In patients with underlying renal disease who have received inappropriately high doses of famciclovir for their level of renal function, acute renal failure has been reported.

➤*Pregnancy: Category B.* There are no adequate and well-controlled studies in pregnant women. Because animal reproduction studies are not always predictive of human response, use famciclovir during pregnancy only if the benefit to the patient clearly exceeds the potential risk to the fetus.

Pregnancy registry – To monitor maternal fetal outcomes of pregnant women exposed to famciclovir, the manufacturer Novartis Pharmaceutical Corporation maintains a famciclovir pregnancy registry. Health care providers are encouraged to register their patients by calling 1-888-669-6682.

➤*Lactation:* Following oral administration of famciclovir to lactating rats, penciclovir was excreted in breast milk at concentrations higher than those seen in the plasma. It is not known whether it is excreted in human milk. There are no data on the safety of famciclovir in infants.

➤*Children:* Safety and efficacy in children younger than 18 years of age have not been established.

➤*Elderly:* In general, exercise appropriate caution in the administration and monitoring of famciclovir in elderly patients, reflecting the greater frequency of decreased hepatic, renal, or cardiac function, and of concomitant disease or other drug therapy.

Drug Interactions

➤*Aldehyde oxidase:* The conversion of 6-deoxy penciclovir to penciclovir is catalyzed by aldehyde oxidase. Interactions with other drugs metabolized by this enzyme could potentially occur.

➤*Probenecid:* Concurrent use with probenecid or other drugs significantly eliminated by active renal tubular secretion may result in increased plasma concentrations of penciclovir.

➤*Drug/Food interactions:* See Administration and Dosage for more information.

Adverse Reactions

➤*Immunocompetent patients:*

Famciclovir Adverse Reactions[a]

	Incidence							
	Herpes zoster[b]		Recurrent genital herpes[c]		Genital herpes-suppression[d]		Herpes labialis[c]	
Adverse reaction	Famciclovir 500 mg 3 times daily (n = 273)	Placebo (n = 146)	Famciclovir 1 gm twice daily (n = 163)	Placebo (n = 166)	Famciclovir 250 mg twice daily (n = 458)	Placebo (n = 63)	Famciclovir 1,500 mg single dose (n = 227)	Placebo (n = 254)
CNS								
Fatigue	4.4%	3.4%	0.6%	0%	4.8%	3.2%	1.3%	0.4%
Headache	22.7%	17.8%	13.5%	5.4%	39.3%	42.9%	9.7%	6.7%
Migraine	0.7%	0.7%	0.6%	0.6%	3.1%	0%	0%	0%
Paresthesia	2.6%	0%	0%	0%	0.9%	0%	0%	0%
Dermatologic								
Pruritus	3.7%	2.7%	0%	0.6%	2.2%	0%	0%	0%
Rash	0.4%	0.7%	0%	0%	3.3%	1.6%	0%	0%
GI								
Abdominal pain	1.1%	3.4%	0%	1.2%	7.9%	7.9%	0%	0.4%
Diarrhea	7.7%	4.8%	4.9%	1.2%	9%	9.5%	1.8%	0.8%
Flatulence	1.5%	0.7%	0.6%	0%	4.8%	1.6%	0%	0%
Nausea	12.5%	11.6%	2.5%	3.6%	7.2%	9.5%	2.2%	3.9%
Vomiting	4.8%	3.4%	1.2%	0.6%	3.1%	1.6%	0%	0%
GU								
Dysmenorrhea	0%	0.7%	1.8%	0.6%	7.6%	6.3%	0.9%	0%

[a] Patients may have entered into more than 1 clinical trial.
[b] 7 days of treatment.
[c] 1 day of treatment.
[d] Daily treatment.

➤*Lab test abnormalities:*

Famciclovir Laboratory Abnormalities[a]

Lab test abnormality	Famciclovir (n = 660)[b]	Placebo (n = 210)[b]
Anemia (< 0.8 X MR:[c])	0.1%	0%
Leukopenia (< 0.75 X NRL)	1.3%	0.9%
Neutropenia (< 0.8 X NRL)	3.2%	1.5%
AST (> 2 × NRH[d])	2.3%	1.2%

FAMCICLOVIR — ORAL

Famciclovir Laboratory Abnormalities[a]		
Lab test abnormality	Famciclovir (n = 660)[b]	Placebo (n = 210)[b]
ALT (> 2 × NRH)	3.2%	1.5%
Total bilirubin (> 1.5 × NRH)	1.9%	1.2%
Serum creatinine (> 1.5 × NRH)	0.2%	0.3%
Amylase (> 1.5 × NRH)	1.5%	1.9%
Lipase (> 1.5 × NRH)	4.9%	4.7%

[a] Percentage of patients with laboratory abnormalities that were increased or decreased from baseline and were outside of specified ranges.
[b] n values represent the minimum number of patients assessed for each laboratory parameter.
[c] NRL = normal range low.
[d] NRH = normal range high.

➤*HIV-infected patients:* In HIV-infected patients, the most frequently reported adverse reactions for famciclovir (500 mg twice daily; n = 150) and acyclovir (400 mg, 5 times a day; n = 143), respectively, were headache (16% versus 15.4%), nausea (10.7% versus 12.6%), diarrhea (6.7% versus 10.5%), vomiting (4.7% versus 3.5%), fatigue (4% versus 2.1%), and abdominal pain (3.3% versus 5.6%).

➤*Postmarketing:* The following adverse reactions have been reported during postapproval use of famciclovir: urticaria, serious skin reactions (eg, erythema multiforme), jaundice, thrombocytopenia, hallucinations, and confusion (including delirium, disorientation, and confusional state, occurring predominantly in the elderly). Because these adverse reactions are reported voluntarily from a population of unknown size, estimates of frequency cannot be made.

Overdosage

➤*Treatment:* Give appropriate symptomatic and supportive therapy. Penciclovir is removed by hemodialysis.

Patient Information

Inform patients that famciclovir is not a cure for genital herpes. There are no data evaluating whether famciclovir will prevent transmission of infection to others. As genital herpes is a sexually transmitted disease, patients should avoid contact with lesions or intercourse when lesions or symptoms are present to avoid infecting partners. Genital herpes can also be transmitted in the absence of symptoms through asymptomatic viral shedding. If medical management of recurrent episodes is indicated, advise patients to initiate therapy at the first sign or symptom.

There is no evidence that famciclovir will affect the ability of a patient to drive or to use machines. However, patients who experience dizziness, somnolence, confusion, or other CNS disturbances while taking famciclovir should refrain from driving or operating machinery.

VALACYCLOVIR HYDROCHLORIDE

Rx	**Valacyclovir Hydrochloride** (Ranbaxy)	**Tablets; oral:** 500 mg	PEG 400, PEG 6000. (RX 904). Blue, capsule shape. Film-coated. In 10s, 30s, and 500s.
Rx	**Valtrex** (GlaxoSmithKline)		(VALTREX 500 mg). Blue, capsule shape. Film-coated. In 30s, 90s, and UD 100s.
Rx	**Valacyclovir Hydrochloride** (Ranbaxy)	**Tablets; oral:** 1 g	PEG 400, PEG 6000. (RX 905). Blue, capsule shape, scored. Film-coated. In 10s, 30s, and 500s.
Rx	**Valtrex** (GlaxoSmithKline)		(VALTREX 1 gram). Blue, capsule shape. Film-coated. In 30s and 90s.

VALACYCLOVIR HYDROCHLORIDE — ORAL

Indications

➤*Adults:*

Cold sores (herpes labialis) – For the treatment of cold sores (herpes labialis).

The efficacy of valacyclovir initiated after the development of clinical signs of a cold sore (eg, papule, vesicle, or ulcer) has not been established.

Genital herpes –

Initial episode: For the treatment of the initial episode of genital herpes in immunocompetent adults.

The efficacy of treatment of valacyclovir when initiated more than 72 hours after the onset of signs and symptoms has not been established.

Recurrent episodes: For treatment of recurrent episodes of genital herpes in immunocompetent adults.

The efficacy of treatment with valacyclovir when initiated more than 24 hours after the onset of signs and symptoms has not been established.

Suppressive therapy: For chronic suppressive therapy of recurrent episodes of genital herpes in immunocompetent and in HIV-infected adults.

The efficacy and safety of valacyclovir for the suppression of genital herpes beyond 1 year in immunocompetent patients and beyond 6 months in HIV-infected patients have not been established.

Reduction of transmission: For the reduction of transmission of genital herpes in immunocompetent adults. The efficacy of valacyclovir for the reduction of transmission of genital herpes beyond 8 months in discordant couples has not been established.

The efficacy of valacyclovir for the reduction of transmission of genital herpes in individuals with multiple partners and non heterosexual couples has not been established. Safer sex practices should be used with suppressive therapy (see current Centers for Disease Control and Prevention [CDC] *Sexually Transmitted Diseases Treatment Guidelines*).

Herpes zoster – For the treatment of herpes zoster (shingles) in immunocompetent adults.

The efficacy of valacyclovir when initiated more than 72 hours after the onset of rash and the efficacy and safety of valacyclovir for treatment of disseminated herpes zoster have not been established.

➤*Children:*

Chickenpox – For the treatment of chickenpox in immunocompetent pediatric patients 2 to younger than 18 years of age. Based on efficacy data from clinical studies with oral valacyclovir, treatment with valacyclovir should be initiated within 24 hours after the onset of rash.

Cold sores (herpes labialis) – For the treatment of cold sores (herpes labialis) in pediatric patients 12 years of age and older.

The efficacy of valacyclovir initiated after the development of clinical signs of a cold sore (eg, papule, vesicle, or ulcer) has not been established.

➤*Limitations of use:* The efficacy and safety of valacyclovir have not been established in:

- immunocompromised patients other than for the suppression of genital herpes in HIV-infected patients with a CD4+ cell count of 100 cells/mm^3 or higher.
- patients younger 12 years of age with cold sores (herpes labialis).
- patients younger 2 years of age or older than 18 years of age with chickenpox.
- patients younger 18 years of age with genital herpes.
- patients younger 18 years of age with herpes zoster.
- neonates and infants as suppressive therapy following neonatal herpes simplex virus (HSV) infection.

Administration and Dosage

➤*Adults:*

Cold sores (herpes labialis) – 2 g twice daily for 1 day, taken about 12 hours apart. Therapy should be initiated at the earliest symptom of a cold sore (eg, tingling, itching, burning).

Genital herpes (initial episode) – 1 g twice daily for 10 days. Therapy was most effective when administered within 48 hours of the onset of signs and symptoms.

Genital herpes (recurrent episodes) – 500 mg twice daily for 3 days. Initiate treatment at the first sign or symptom of an episode.

Genital herpes (chronic suppressive therapy) –

Usual dosage: 1 g once daily in patients with healthy immune function.

Alternative dosage: 500 mg once daily in patients with a history of 9 or fewer recurrences per year.

HIV-infected patients: In HIV-infected patients with a CD4+ cell count of at least 100 cells/mm^3, the recommended dose of valacyclovir for chronic suppressive therapy of recurrent genital herpes is 500 mg twice daily.

Genital herpes (reduction of transmission) – 500 mg once daily for the source partner with a history of 9 or fewer recurrences per year.

Herpes zoster – 1 g orally 3 times daily for 7 days. Therapy should be initiated at the earliest sign or symptom of herpes zoster and is most effective when started within 48 hours of the onset of zoster rash.

➤*Children:*

Chickenpox –

Children 2 to 18 years of age:

- *Usual dosage* – 20 mg/kg administered 3 times daily for 5 days. Therapy should be initiated at the earliest sign or symptom.
- *Maximum dose* – 1 g 3 times daily.

Cold sores (herpes labialis) –

Children 12 years of age and older: 2 g twice daily for 1 day taken 12 hours apart. Therapy should be initiated at the earliest symptoms of a cold sore (eg, tingling, itching, burning).

Off-label dosing –

Chickenpox:

- *Children 2 to 18 years of age* –
  Alternative dosing by weight6 to 19 kg: 250 mg 3 times daily.20 to 31 kg 500 mg 3 times daily.More than 32 kg 750 mg 3 times daily.

Genital herpes:

- *Children 12 years of age or older* –
  Initial episode: 1 g twice a day for 10 days.
  Recurrent episodes: 500 mg twice a day for 3 days.
  Suppressive therapy: 500 to 1,000 mg once daily for 1 year, then reassess for recurrences.

VALACYCLOVIR HYDROCHLORIDE — ORAL

Patients with less than 9 recurrences per year: 500 mg once daily for 1 year.

➤*Renal function impairment:*

Valacyclovir Dosage Adjustments for Adults with Renal Function Impairment

Indications	Normal dosage regimen (CrCl[a] ≥ 50 mL/min)	CrCl (mL/min) 30 to 49	10 to 29	< 10
Cold Sores (herpes labialis) (Do not exceed 1 day of treatment)	Two 2 g doses taken 12 h apart	Two 1 g doses taken 12 h apart	Two 500 mg doses taken 12 h apart	500 mg single dose
Genital herpes: Initial episode	1 g every 12 h	No reduction	1 g every 24 h	500 mg every 24 h
Genital herpes: Recurrent episodes	500 mg every 12 h	No reduction	500 mg every 24 h	500 mg every 24 h
Genital herpes: Suppressive therapy Immunocompetent patients	1 g every 24 h	No reduction	500 mg every 24 h	500 mg every 24 h
Suppressive therapy Alternate dose for immunocompetent patients with ≤ 9 recurrences/year	500 mg every 24 h	No reduction	500 mg every 48 h	500 mg every 48 h
Suppressive therapy in HIV-infected patients	500 mg every 12 h	No reduction	500 mg every 24 h	500 mg every 24 h
Herpes zoster	1 g every 8 h	1 g every 12 h	1 g every 24 h	500 mg every 24 h

[a] CrCl = creatinine clearance.

Hemodialysis – Patients requiring hemodialysis should receive the recommended dose of valacyclovir after hemodialysis.

Peritoneal dialysis – Supplemental doses of valacyclovir should not be required following chronic ambulatory peritoneal dialysis (CAPD) or continuous arteriovenous hemofiltration/dialysis (CAVHD).

➤*Preparation for administration:*

Extemporaneous preparation of oral suspension – Valacyclovir oral suspension (25 or 50 mg/mL) may be prepared extemporaneously from valacyclovir 500 mg tablets for use in children for whom a solid doseform is not appropriate. Ingredients required include the following: Valacyclovir tablets 500 mg, cherry flavor, and Suspension Structured Vehicle USP-NF (SSV). Valacyclovir oral suspension (25 or 50 mg/mL) should be prepared in lots of 100 mL.

➤*Administration:* Valacyclovir may be given without regard to meals.

➤*Storage/Stability:* Store at 15° to 25°C (59° to 77°F).

Actions

➤*Pharmacology:* Valacyclovir is rapidly converted to acyclovir, which has demonstrated antiviral activity against herpes simplex virus types 1 (HSV-1) and 2 (HSV-2) and varicella-zoster virus (VZV) both in vitro and in vivo.

The inhibitory activity of acyclovir is highly selective because of its affinity for the enzyme thymidine kinase (TK) encoded by HSV and VZV. This viral enzyme converts acyclovir into acyclovir monophosphate, a nucleotide analogue. The monophosphate is further converted into diphosphate by cellular guanylate kinase and into triphosphate by a number of cellular enzymes. In vitro, acyclovir triphosphate stops replication of herpes viral deoxyribonucleic acid (DNA). This is accomplished in the following 3 ways: competitive inhibition of viral DNA polymerase, incorporation and termination of the growing viral DNA chain, and inactivation of the viral DNA polymerase. The greater antiviral activity of acyclovir against HSV compared with VZV is due to its more efficient phosphorylation by the viral TK.

➤*Pharmacokinetics:*

Absorption – The pharmacokinetics of valacyclovir and acyclovir after oral administration of valacyclovir have been investigated in 14 volunteer studies involving 283 adults. The absolute bioavailability of acyclovir after administration of valacyclovir is 54.5% ± 9.1%, as determined following an oral dose of valacyclovir 1 g and an intravenous (IV) dose of acyclovir 350 mg to 12 healthy volunteers. Acyclovir bioavailability from the administration of valacyclovir is not altered by administration with food (30 minutes after an 873 kcal breakfast, which included 51 g of fat).

There was a lack of dose proportionality in acyclovir maximum concentration (C_{max}) and area under the acyclovir concentration-time curve (AUC) after single-dose administration of 100 mg, 250 mg, 500 mg, 750 mg, and 1 g of valacyclovir to 8 healthy volunteers. The mean C_{max} (± standard deviation [SD]) was 0.83 (± 0.14), 2.15 (± 0.5), 3.28 (± 0.83), 4.17 (± 1.14), and 5.65 (± 2.37) mcg/mL, respectively, and the mean AUC (± SD) was 2.28 (± 0.4), 5.76 (± 0.6), 11.59 (± 1.79), 14.11 (± 3.54), and 19.52 (± 6.04) mcg•h/mL, respectively.

There was also a lack of dose proportionality in acyclovir C_{max} and AUC after the multiple-dose administration of 250 mg, 500 mg, and 1 g of valacyclovir administered 4 times daily for 11 days in parallel groups of 8 healthy volunteers. The mean C_{max} (± SD) was 2.11 (± 0.33), 3.69 (± 0.87), and 4.96 (± 0.64) mcg/mL, respectively, and the mean AUC (±SD) was 5.66 (± 1.09), 9.88 (± 2.01), and 15.7 (± 2.27) mcg/mL•h, respectively.

There is no accumulation of acyclovir after the administration of valacyclovir at the recommended dosage regimens to healthy volunteers with healthy renal function.

Distribution – The binding of valacyclovir to human plasma proteins ranged from 13.5% to 17.9%.

Metabolism – After oral administration, valacyclovir is rapidly absorbed from the GI tract. Valacyclovir is converted to acyclovir and L-valine by first-pass intestinal and/or hepatic metabolism. Acyclovir is converted to a small extent to inactive metabolites by aldehyde oxidase and by alcohol and aldehyde dehydrogenase. Neither valacyclovir nor acyclovir is metabolized by cytochrome P-450 enzymes. Plasma concentrations of unconverted valacyclovir are low and transient, generally becoming nonquantifiable by 3 hours after administration. Peak plasma valacyclovir concentrations are generally less than 0.5 mcg/mL at all doses. After single-dose administration of valacyclovir 1 g, average plasma valacyclovir concentrations observed were 0.5, 0.4, and 0.8 mcg/mL in patients with hepatic function impairment, those with renal function impairment, and in healthy volunteers who received concomitant cimetidine and probenecid, respectively.

Excretion – The pharmacokinetic disposition of acyclovir delivered by valacyclovir is consistent with previous experience from IV and oral acyclovir. Following the oral administration of a single 1 g dose of radiolabeled valacyclovir to 4 healthy subjects, 45.6% and 47.12% of administered radioactivity was recovered in urine and feces over 96 hours, respectively. Acyclovir accounted for 88.6% of the radioactivity excreted in the urine. Renal clearance of acyclovir following the administration of a single 1 g dose of valacyclovir to 12 healthy volunteers was approximately 255 ± 86 mL/min, which represents 41.9% of total acyclovir apparent plasma clearance.

The plasma elimination half-life of acyclovir typically averaged 2.5 to 3.3 hours in all studies of valacyclovir in volunteers with healthy renal function.

Special populations –

Renal function impairment: Following administration of valacyclovir to volunteers with ESRD, the average acyclovir half-life is approximately 14 hours. During hemodialysis, the acyclovir half-life is approximately 4 hours. Approximately one-third of acyclovir in the body is removed by dialysis during a 4-hour hemodialysis session. Apparent plasma clearance of acyclovir in dialysis patients was 86.3 ± 21.3 mL/min/1.73 m^2, compared with 679.16 ± 162.76 mL/min/1.73 m^2 in healthy volunteers.

Reduction in dosage is recommended in patients with renal function impairment.

Hepatic function impairment: Administration of valacyclovir to patients with moderate (biopsy-proven cirrhosis) or severe (with and without ascites and biopsy-proven cirrhosis) liver disease indicated that the rate but not the extent of conversion of valacyclovir to acyclovir is reduced, and the acyclovir half-life is not affected. Dosage modification is not recommended for patients with cirrhosis.

Elderly: After single-dose administration of valacyclovir 1 g in healthy elderly volunteers, the half-life of acyclovir was 3.11 ± 0.51 hours, compared with 2.91 ± 0.63 hours in healthy volunteers. The pharmacokinetics of acyclovir after a single dose of valacyclovir 1 g was unchanged by coadministration of digoxin (2 doses of 0.75 mg). The pharmacokinetics of acyclovir following single- and multiple-dose oral administration of valacyclovir in elderly volunteers varied with renal function. Dose reduction may be required in elderly patients, depending on the underlying renal status of the patient.

➤*Microbiology:*

Antiviral activities – The quantitative relationship between the in vitro susceptibility of herpes viruses to antivirals and the clinical response to therapy has not been established in humans, and virus-sensitivity testing has not been standardized. Sensitivity testing results, expressed as the concentration of drug required to inhibit by 50% the growth of virus in cell culture (inhibitory concentration [IC_{50}]), vary greatly depending upon a number of factors. Using plaque-reduction assays, the IC_{50} against HSV isolates ranges from 0.02 to 13.5 mcg/mL for HSV-1 and from 0.01 to 9.9 mcg/mL for HSV-2. The IC_{50} for acyclovir against most laboratory strains and clinical isolates of VZV ranges from 0.12 to 10.8 mcg/mL. Acyclovir also demonstrates activity against the Oka vaccine strain of VZV with a mean IC_{50} of 1.35 mcg/mL.

Drug resistance – Resistance of HSV and VZV to acyclovir can result from qualitative or quantitative changes in the viral TK and/or DNA polymerase. Clinical isolates of VZV with reduced susceptibility to acyclovir have been recovered from patients with AIDS. In these cases, TK-deficient mutants of VZV have been recovered.

Resistance of HSV and VZV to acyclovir occurs by the same mechanisms. While most of the acyclovir-resistant mutants isolated thus far from immunocompromised patients have been found to be TK-deficient mutants, other mutants involving the viral TK gene (TK partial and TK altered) and DNA polymerase have also been isolated. TK-negative mutants may cause severe disease in immunocompromised patients. Consider the possibility of viral resistance to valacyclovir (and, therefore, to acyclovir) in patients who show poor clinical response during therapy.

Contraindications

Known hypersensitivity or intolerance to valacyclovir, acyclovir, or any component of the formulation.

VALACYCLOVIR HYDROCHLORIDE — ORAL

Warnings/Precautions

➤*Thrombotic thrombocytopenic purpura/hemolytic uremic syndrome (TTP/HUS):* TTP/HUS, in some cases resulting in death, has occurred in patients with advanced HIV disease and also in allogeneic bone marrow transplant– and renal transplant–recipients participating in clinical trials of valacyclovir at doses of 8 g/day.

➤*Immunocompromised patients:* The safety and efficacy of valacyclovir have not been established in immunocompromised patients, other than for the suppression of genital herpes in HIV-infected patients. The safety and efficacy of valacyclovir for suppression of recurrent genital herpes in patients with advanced HIV disease (CD4 cell count less than 100 cells/mm^3) have not been established. The efficacy of valacyclovir for the treatment of genital herpes in HIV-infected patients has not been established. The safety and efficacy of valacyclovir have not been established for the treatment of disseminated herpes zoster.

➤*Transmission of genital herpes:* The efficacy of valacyclovir for reducing transmission of genital herpes has not been established in individuals with multiple partners and nonheterosexual couples.

➤*Cold sore treatment:* Given the dosage recommendations for treatment of cold sores, pay special attention when prescribing valacyclovir for cold sores in patients who are elderly or who have impaired renal function. Treatment should not exceed 1 day (2 doses of 2 g in 24 hours). Therapy beyond 1 day does not provide additional clinical benefit.

➤*Renal function impairment:* Dose reduction is recommended when administering valacyclovir to patients with renal function impairment. Acute renal failure and CNS symptoms (agitation, hallucinations, confusion, delirium, and encephalopathy) have been reported in patients with underlying renal disease who have received inappropriately high doses of valacyclovir for their level of renal function. Exercise similar caution when administering valacyclovir to elderly patients and patients receiving potentially nephrotoxic agents.

Precipitation of acyclovir in renal tubules may occur when the solubility (2.5 mg/mL) is exceeded in the intratubular fluid. Maintain adequate hydration. In the event of acute renal failure and anuria, the patient may benefit from hemodialysis until renal function is restored.

➤*Pregnancy: Category B.*

Teratogenic – There are no adequate and well-controlled studies of valacyclovir or acyclovir in pregnant women. A prospective epidemiologic registry of acyclovir use during pregnancy was established in 1984 and completed in April 1999. There were 749 pregnancies followed in women exposed to systemic acyclovir during the first trimester of pregnancy, resulting in 756 outcomes. The occurrence rate of birth defects approximates that found in the general population. However, the small size of the registry is insufficient to evaluate the risk for less common defects or to permit reliable or definitive conclusions regarding the safety of acyclovir in pregnant women and their developing fetuses. In a population-based historical cohort study, 3.1% of 229 infants exposed to valacyclovir during the first trimester were diagnosed with a major birth defect compared to 2.4% of the 19,920 infants that were not exposed to antivirals. The authors of the study concluded that exposure to valacyclovir during the first trimester of pregnancy was not associated with an increased risk of major birth defects. Use valacyclovir during pregnancy only if the potential benefit justifies the potential risk to the fetus.

➤*Lactation:* Following oral administration of a dose of valacyclovir 500 mg to 5 breast-feeding mothers, peak acyclovir concentrations (C_{max}) in breast milk ranged from 0.5 to 2.3 times (median, 1.4) the corresponding maternal acyclovir serum concentrations. The acyclovir breast milk AUC ranged from 1.4 to 2.6 (median, 2.2) maternal serum AUC. A maternal dosage of valacyclovir 500 mg twice daily would provide a breast-feeding infant with an oral acyclovir dosage of approximately 0.6 mg/kg/day. This would result in less than 2% of the exposure obtained after administration of a standard neonatal dose of 30 mg/kg/day of IV acyclovir to the breast-feeding infant. Unchanged valacyclovir was not detected in maternal serum, breast milk, or infant urine. Administer valacyclovir to a breast-feeding mother with caution and only when indicated.

➤*Children:* Safety and efficacy of valacyclovir in prepubertal children have not been established.

➤*Elderly:* Of the total number of patients included in clinical studies of valacyclovir, 906 were 65 years of age or older, and 352 were 75 years of age or older. In a clinical study of herpes zoster, the duration of pain after healing (postherpetic neuralgia) was longer in patients 65 years of age and older, compared with younger adults. Elderly patients are more likely to have reduced renal function and to require dose reduction. Elderly patients are more likely to have renal or CNS adverse reactions. With respect to CNS adverse reactions observed during clinical practice, agitation, hallucinations, confusion, delirium, and encephalopathy were reported more frequently in elderly patients.

Adverse Reactions

Frequently reported adverse reactions in clinical trials of valacyclovir in healthy patients are listed in the following table:

Valacyclovir Adverse Reactions

Adverse reaction	Herpes zoster: Valacyclovir 1 g 3 times daily (n = 967)	Herpes zoster: Placebo (n = 195)	Genital herpes treatment: Valacyclovir 1 g twice daily (n = 1,194)	Genital herpes treatment: Valacyclovir 500 mg twice daily (n = 1,159)	Genital herpes treatment: Placebo (n = 439)	Genital herpes suppression: Valacyclovir 1 g once daily (n = 269)	Genital herpes suppression: Valacyclovir 500 mg once daily (n = 266)	Genital herpes suppression: Placebo (n = 134)
CNS								
Depression	NA[a]	NA	1%	0%	< 1%	7%	5%	5%
Dizziness	3%	2%	3%	2%	3%	4%	2%	1%
Headache	14%	12%	16%	15%	14%	35%	38%	34%
GI								
Abdominal pain	3%	2%	2%	1%	3%	11%	9%	6%
Nausea	15%	8%	6%	5%	8%	11%	11%	8%
Vomiting	6%	3%	1%	< 1%	< 1%	3%	3%	2%
Lab test abnormalities								
AST (2 × ULN[b])	1%	0%	1%	—[c]	0.5%	4.1%	3.8%	3%
Hemoglobin (< 0.8 X LLN[d])	0.8%	0%	0.3%	0.2%	0%	0%	0.8%	0.8%
Platelet count (< 100,000/mm^3)	1%	1.2%	0.3%	0.1%	0.7%	0.4%	1.1%	1.5%
Serum creatinine (> 1.5 × ULN)	0.2%	0%	0.7%	0%	0%	0%	0%	0%
White blood cells (< 0.75 X LLN)	1.3%	0.6%	0.7%	0.6%	0.2%	0.7%	0.8%	1.5%
Miscellaneous								
Arthralgia	NA	NA	< 1%	< 1%	< 1%	6%	5%	4%
Dysmenorrhea	NA	NA	< 1%	< 1%	1%	8%	5%	4%

[a] NA = not applicable.
[b] ULN = upper limit of normal.
[c] Data were not collected prospectively.
[d] LLN = lower limit of normal.

➤*Suppression of genital herpes in HIV-infected patients:* In HIV-infected patients, frequently reported adverse reactions for valacyclovir (500 mg twice daily; n = 194; median days on therapy, 172) and placebo (n = 99; median days on therapy, 59) included headache (13% vs 8%, respectively), fatigue (8% vs 5%, respectively), and rash (8% vs 1%, respectively). Post randomization laboratory abnormalities that were reported more frequently in valacyclovir subjects vs placebo included elevated alkaline phosphatase (4% vs 2%), elevated ALT (14% vs 10%), elevated AST (16% vs 11%), decreased neutrophil counts (18% vs 10%), and decreased platelet counts (3% vs 0%).

➤*Reduction of transmission:* In a clinical study for the reduction of transmission of genital herpes, the adverse reactions reported by patients receiving valacyclovir 500 mg once daily (n = 743) or placebo once daily (n = 741) included headache (valacyclovir, 29%; placebo, 26%), nasopharyngitis

VALACYCLOVIR HYDROCHLORIDE — ORAL

(valacyclovir, 16%; placebo, 15%), and upper respiratory tract infection (valacyclovir, 9%; placebo, 10%). In this 8-month study, there were no clinically significant changes from baseline laboratory parameters in subjects receiving valacyclovir compared with placebo.

➤*Cold sores (herpes labialis):* In clinical studies for the treatment of cold sores, the adverse reactions reported by patients receiving valacyclovir (n = 609) or placebo (n = 609) included headache (valacyclovir, 14%; placebo, 10%) and dizziness (valacyclovir, 2%; placebo, 1%). The frequencies of abnormal ALT (greater than 2 times the ULN) were 1.8% for patients receiving valacyclovir, compared with 0.8% for placebo. Other laboratory abnormalities (hemoglobin, white blood cells, alkaline phosphatase, and serum creatinine) occurred with similar frequencies in the 2 groups.

➤*Postmarketing:* The following events have been identified during postapproval use of valacyclovir in clinical practice. Because they are reported voluntarily from a population of unknown size, estimates of frequency cannot be made. These events have been chosen for inclusion because of their seriousness, frequency of reporting, or causal connection to valacyclovir, or a combination of these factors.

Cardiovascular – Hypertension, tachycardia.

CNS – Aggressive behavior; agitation; ataxia; coma; confusion; decreased consciousness; dysarthria; encephalopathy; mania; psychosis, including auditory and visual hallucinations; seizures; tremors.

Dermatologic – Alopecia; erythema multiforme; rashes, including photosensitivity.

GI – Diarrhea.

Hematologic – Aplastic anemia, leukocytoclastic vasculitis, thrombocytopenia, TTP/HUS.

Hepatic – Hepatitis, liver enzyme abnormalities.

Hypersensitivity – Acute hypersensitivity reactions, including anaphylaxis, angioedema, dyspnea, pruritus, rash, and urticaria.

Ophthalmic – Visual abnormalities.

Renal – Elevated creatinine, renal failure.

Renal failure and CNS symptoms have been reported in patients with renal function impairment who received valacyclovir or acyclovir at greater than the recommended dose. Dosage reduction is recommended in this patient population.

Miscellaneous – Facial edema.

Overdosage

Exercise caution to prevent inadvertent overdose.

➤*Symptoms:* Precipitation of acyclovir in renal tubules may occur when the solubility (2.5 mg/mL) is exceeded in the intratubular fluid.

➤*Treatment:* In the event of acute renal failure and anuria, the patient may benefit from hemodialysis until renal function is restored.

Patient Information

Advise patients to maintain adequate hydration.

➤*Herpes zoster:* There are no data on treatment initiated greater than 72 hours after onset of the zoster rash. Advise patients to initiate treatment as soon as possible after a diagnosis of herpes zoster.

➤*Genital herpes:* Inform patients that valacyclovir is not a cure for genital herpes. Because genital herpes is a sexually transmitted disease, patients should avoid contact with lesions or intercourse when lesions and/or symptoms are present to avoid infecting partners. Genital herpes is frequently transmitted in the absence of symptoms through asymptomatic viral shedding. Therefore, counsel patients to use safer sex practices in combination with suppressive therapy with valacyclovir. Advise sex partners of infected persons that they might be infected even if they have no symptoms. Type-specific serologic testing of asymptomatic partners of persons with genital herpes can determine whether risk of HSV-2 acquisition exists.

Valacyclovir has not been shown to reduce transmission of sexually transmitted infections other than HSV-2.

If medical management of a genital herpes recurrence is indicated, advise patients to initiate therapy at the first sign or symptom of an episode.

There are no data on the efficacy of treatment initiated greater than 72 hours after the onset of signs and symptoms of a first episode of genital herpes or more than 24 hours after the onset of signs and symptoms of a recurrent episode.

There are no data on the safety or efficacy of chronic suppressive therapy of greater than 1 year's duration in otherwise healthy patients. There are no data on the safety or efficacy of chronic suppressive therapy of more than 6 months' duration in HIV-infected patients.

➤*Cold sores (herpes labialis):* Advise patients to initiate treatment at the earliest symptom of a cold sore (eg, tingling, itching, burning). There are no data on the efficacy of treatment initiated after the development of clinical signs of a cold sore (eg, papule, vesicle, ulcer). Instruct patients that treatment for cold sores should not exceed 1 day (2 doses) and that their doses should be taken about 12 hours apart. Inform patients that valacyclovir is not a cure for cold sores.

AMANTADINE HYDROCHLORIDE

Rx	**Amantadine Hydrochloride** (Upsher-Smith)	**Tablets:** 100 mg	(832 AMT). Peach. In 100s and 500s.
Rx	**Symmetrel** (Endo)		(SYMMETREL). Orange, triangular. In 100s and 500s.
Rx	**Amantadine HCl** (Various, eg, Banner, Geneva, Major, Martec, UDL, URL)	**Capsules:** 100 mg	In 100s, 500s, and UD 100s.
Rx	**Amantadine HCl** (Various, eg, Alpharma, Endo, Morton Grove)	**Syrup:** 50 mg per 5 mL	May contain sorbitol and parabens. In 480 mL.
Rx	**Symmetrel** (Endo)		Sorbitol and parabens. In 480 mL.

AMANTADINE HYDROCHLORIDE — ORAL

Indications

➤*Influenza A prophylaxis:* For chemoprophylaxis against signs and symptoms of influenza A virus infection when early vaccination is not feasible or when the vaccine is contraindicated or not available. In the prophylaxis of influenza, early vaccination on an annual basis as recommended by the Centers for Disease Control's Immunization Practices Advisory Committee is the method of choice. Because amantadine hydrochloride does not completely prevent the host immune response to influenza A infection, individuals who take this drug may still develop immune responses to natural disease or vaccination and may be protected when later exposed to antigenically related viruses. Following vaccination during an influenza A outbreak, amantadine hydrochloride prophylaxis should be considered for the 2- to 4-week time period required to develop an antibody response.

➤*Influenza A treatment:* Treatment of uncomplicated respiratory tract illness caused by influenza A virus strains especially when administered early in the course of illness. There are no well-controlled clinical studies demonstrating that treatment with amantadine hydrochloride will avoid the development of influenza A virus pneumonitis or other complications in high-risk patients.

➤*Parkinson disease:* Treatment of idiopathic Parkinson's disease (paralysis agitans), postencephalitic parkinsonism, and symptomatic parkinsonism which may follow injury to the nervous system by carbon monoxide intoxication. It is indicated in those elderly patients believed to develop parkinsonism in association with cerebral arteriosclerosis. In the treatment of Parkinson's disease, amantadine hydrochloride is less effective than levodopa, (-)-3-(3,4-dihydroxyphenyl)-L-alanine, and its efficacy in comparison with the anticholinergic antiparkinson drugs has not yet been established.

➤*Drug-induced extrapyramidal reactions:* In the treatment of drug-induced extrapyramidal reactions. Although anticholinergic-type side effects have been noted with amantadine hydrochloride when used in patients with drug-induced extrapyramidal reactions, there is a lower incidence of these side effects than that observed with the anticholinergic antiparkinson drugs.

➤*Off-label uses:*

Attention deficit hyperactivity disorder – [4] = Insufficient documentation. Initial data from case reports and noncontrolled studies suggest that amantadine may have some benefit as adjunctive therapy in the management of attention deficit hyperactivity disorder (ADHD), but results are conflicting.

Multiple sclerosis–related fatigue – [5] = Poor documentation. Although limited benefit may be seen, National Institute for Clinical Excellence guidelines suggest the evidence does not support the use of amantadine for the treatment of multiple sclerosis (MS)–associated fatigue at this time. Further quality studies are needed to determine if true benefits exist.

Postpoliomyelitis syndrome–related fatigue – [5] = Poor documentation. Evidence from a limited number of controlled and noncontrolled studies evaluating amantadine in the treatment of postpoliomyelitis syndrome–related fatigue has demonstrated conflicting results. International guidelines state that this agent is not effective in the management of postpoliomyelitis syndrome–related fatigue.

Restless legs syndrome – [4] = Insufficient documentation. The use of amantadine for the treatment of restless legs syndrome (RLS) has been limited to a noncontrolled investigation in fewer than 30 patients. Although this study suggested some benefit in the management of RLS, there were several limitations to the design and patient population. This drug is not routinely recommended for the treatment of RLS.

Tardive dyskinesia – [4] = Insufficient documentation. Data supporting amantadine's use in tardive dyskinesia management are minimal.

AMANTADINE HYDROCHLORIDE — ORAL

Other possible off-label uses –

H1N1 influenza A (swine flu): Per the Centers for Disease Control and Prevention (CDC) recommendations for treatment and chemoprophylaxis of H1N1 influenza A (swine flu) virus infection, refer to the Oseltamivir and Zanamivir monographs. The H1N1 virus is resistant to the antiviral medication amantadine. http://www.cdc.gov/h1n1flu/recommendations.htm

Administration and Dosage

➤*Adults:*

Drug-induced extrapyramidal reactions – 100 mg twice a day. Occasionally, patients whose responses are not optimal with 200 mg daily may benefit from an increase up to 300 mg daily in divided doses.

Influenza A virus infection –

Usual dosage: For prophylaxis or treatment of influenza A virus infection, the dosage is 200 mg as a single daily dose. The daily dosage may be split into 100 mg twice a day. If CNS effects develop during once-a-day dosing, a split dosage schedule may reduce such complaints.

Prophylactic dosing should be started in anticipation of an influenza A outbreak and before or after contact with individuals with influenza A virus respiratory tract illness.

Treatment of influenza A virus illness should be started as soon as possible, preferably within 24 to 48 hours after onset of signs and symptoms.

Alternative dosage: A 100 mg daily dose has also been shown in experimental challenge studies to be effective as prophylaxis in healthy adults who are not at high risk for influenza-related complications. However, it has not been demonstrated that a 100 mg daily dose is as effective as a 200 mg daily dose for prophylaxis, nor has the 100 mg daily dose been studied in the treatment of acute influenza illness. In recent clinical trials, the incidence of CNS adverse effects associated with the 100 mg daily dose was at or near the level of placebo. The 100 mg dose is recommended for persons who have demonstrated intolerance to amantadine 200 mg/day because of CNS adverse effects or other toxicities.

Duration of therapy:

- *Prophylaxis* – Amantadine should be continued daily for at least 10 days following a known exposure. If used chemoprophylactically in conjunction with inactivated influenza A virus vaccine until protective antibody responses develop, then it should be administered for 2 to 4 weeks after the vaccine has been given. When inactivated influenza A virus vaccine is unavailable or contraindicated, amantadine should be administered for the duration of known influenza A in the community because of repeated and unknown exposure.
- *Treatment* – Continue for 24 to 48 hours after the disappearance of signs and symptoms.

Parkinsonism –

Usual dosage: 100 mg twice a day when used alone. Amantadine has an onset of action usually within 48 hours.

Initial dosage: 100 mg daily for patients with serious associated medical illnesses or who are receiving high doses of other antiparkinson drugs.

Dosage titration: After one to several weeks at 100 mg once daily, the dose may be increased to 100 mg twice daily, if necessary. Occasionally, patients whose responses are not optimal with amantadine 200 mg daily may benefit from an increase up to 400 mg daily in divided doses. However, such patients should be supervised closely by their health care providers.

Concomitant therapy: Some patients who do not respond to anticholinergic antiparkinson drugs may respond to amantadine.

When amantadine or anticholinergic antiparkinson drugs are each used with marginal benefit, concomitant use may produce additional benefit. When amantadine and levodopa are initiated concurrently, the patient can exhibit rapid therapeutic benefits. Amantadine should be held constant at 100 mg daily or twice daily while the daily dose of levodopa is gradually increased to optimal benefit.

When amantadine is added to optimal well-tolerated doses of levodopa, additional benefit may result, including smoothing out the fluctuations in improvement, which sometimes occur in patients on levodopa alone. Patients who require a reduction in their usual doses of levodopa because of development of adverse effects may possibly regain lost benefit with the addition of amantadine.

Loss of effectiveness: Patients initially deriving benefit from amantadine not uncommonly experience a fall-off of effectiveness after a few months. Benefit may be regained by increasing the dose to 300 mg daily. Alternatively, temporary discontinuation of amantadine for several weeks, followed by reinitiation of the drug, may result in regaining benefit in some patients. A decision to use other antiparkinson drugs may be necessary.

Off-label dosing –

Restless legs syndrome: [4] = Insufficient documentation. For patients with symptoms primarily at bedtime, amantadine was administered before bedtime. Patients with symptoms earlier in the evening were administered a dose 1 to 2 hours prior to the usual time of onset of symptoms and, if necessary, redosed before sleep. For patients with daytime symptoms, amantadine was administered 1 to 2 hours prior to the usual time of onset of symptoms, then 1 to 2 doses were administered later during the day or night as needed.

- *Maximum dose* – 300 mg/day.
- *Initial dosage* – 100 mg/day.
- *Dosage titration* – Increase by 100 mg every 3 to 5 days, up to a maximum dosage of 300 mg/day until significant relief of symptoms or tolerance.
- *Duration of therapy* – Duration of treatment was not clearly stated, but duration of response was reported as at least 2 to 13 months in responders.

Tardive dyskinesia: [4] = Insufficient documentation. 100 to 300 mg daily. The studied duration of therapy was 7 weeks, and it is unclear at which time benefits occurred.

➤*Children:*

Influenza A virus infection –

Usual dosage: The following dosage recommendations are for prophylaxis or treatment of influenza A virus infection.

- *9 to 12 years of age* – 100 mg twice a day (200 mg/day).
- *1 to 9 years of age* – 4.4 to 8.8 mg/kg/day, not to exceed 150 mg/day.

Maximum dose: 150 mg/day for children 1 to 9 years of age.

Duration of therapy: See Adults for more information.

Off-label dosing –

Attention deficit hyperactivity disorder: [4] = Insufficient documentation. Children and adolescents 5 to 13 years of age with ADHD who were stimulant- and ADHD treatment–naive were treated with 150 to 200 mg/day, initiated at 50 mg/day and titrated up over approximately 1 week. Studies have evaluated amantadine treatment for up to 6 weeks.

Influenza A virus infection (prophylaxis and treatment): The following dosing recommendations are according to the CDC.

- *1 to 9 years of age –*
  Usual dosage: 5 mg/kg/day given in 2 divided doses.
  Maximum dose: 150 mg/day.
- *10 years of age and older –*
  Weighing at least 40 kg: 100 mg twice daily.
  Weighing less than 40 kg: 5 mg/kg/day given in 2 divided doses up to 150 mg/day.

➤*Elderly:* The dose of amantadine should be reduced in patients who are 65 years of age and older. For the prophylaxis and treatment of influenza A virus infection, the recommended dosage is 100 mg daily.

➤*Renal function impairment:*

Amantadine Dosage in Renal Function Impairment	
CrCl (mL/min/1.73 m^2)	Dosage
30 to 50	200 mg first day; 100 mg each day thereafter
15 to 29	200 mg first day followed by 100 mg on alternate days
< 15	200 mg every 7 days

Hemodialysis – 200 mg every 7 days.

➤*Congestive heart failure, peripheral edema, or orthostatic hypotension:* The dose of amantadine may need reduction in patients with congestive heart failure, peripheral edema, or orthostatic hypotension.

➤*Storage/Stability:* Store at controlled room temperature 25°C (77°F), excursions permitted to 15° to 30°C (59° to 86°F).

Dispense in a tight container as defined in the USP, with a child-resistant closure (as required). Protect from moisture.

Actions

➤*Pharmacology:*

Parkinson's disease – The mechanism of action of amantadine in the treatment of Parkinson's disease and drug-induced extrapyramidal reactions is not known. Data from animal studies have either shown or suggested amantadine hydrochloride to enhance extracellular concentrations of dopamine by increasing dopamine release or decreasing reuptake of dopamine into presynaptic neurons; to stimulate the dopamine receptor itself; or drive the postsynaptic dopaminergic system to a more dopamine sensitive status.

However, doses employed in the animal studies were often of a magnitude greater than the clinically therapeutic doses. More recent work using doses in the low clinically therapeutic range (low mcM) showed amantadine to inhibit the N-methyl-D-aspartic acid (NMDA) receptor-mediated stimulation of acetylcholine release from rat stratum, most likely at the MK-801 site. Although amantadine does not possess anticholinergic activity in dogs at doses of 31.5 mg/kg, equivalent to an approximate human dose of 15.8 mg/kg (based on body surface area conversions), clinically, it exhibits anticholinergic-like side effects such as dry mouth, urinary retention, and constipation.

Antiviral – The mechanism by which amantadine exerts its antiviral activity is not clearly understood. It appears to mainly prevent the release of infectious viral nucleic acid into the host cell by interfering with the function of the transmembrane domain of the viral M2 protein. In certain cases, amantadine is also known to prevent virus assembly during virus replication. It does not appear to interfere with the immunogenicity of inactivated influenza A virus vaccine.

➤*Pharmacokinetics:* Amantadine hydrochloride is well absorbed orally. Maximum plasma concentrations are directly related to dose for doses up to 200 mg/day. Doses above 200 mg/day may result in a greater than proportional increase in maximum plasma concentrations. It is primarily excreted unchanged in the urine by glomerular filtration and tubular secretion. Eight metabolites of amantadine have been identified in human urine. One metabolite, an N-acetylated compound, was quantified in human urine and accounted for 5% to 15% of the administered dose. Plasma acetylamantadine accounted for up to 80% of the concurrent amantadine plasma concentration in 5 of 12 healthy volunteers following the ingestion of a 200 mg dose of amantadine. Acetylamantadine was not detected in the plasma of the remaining 7 volunteers. The contribution of this metabolite to efficacy or toxicity is not known.

Amantadine pharmacokinetics were determined in 24 healthy adult male volunteers after the oral administration of a single amantadine hydrochloride 100 mg capsule. The mean ± SD maximum plasma concentration was 0.22 ± 0.03 mcg/mL (range, 0.18 to 0.32 mcg/mL). The time to peak concen-

AMANTADINE HYDROCHLORIDE — ORAL

tration was 3.3 ± 1.5 hours (range, 1.5 to 8 hours). The apparent oral clearance was 0.28 ± 0.11 L/hr/kg (range, 0.14 to 0.62 L/hr/kg). The half-life was 17 ± 4 hours (range, 10 to 25 hours). Across other studies, amantadine plasma half-life has averaged 16 ± 6 hours (range, 9 to 31 hours) in 19 healthy volunteers.

Plasma amantadine clearance ranged from 0.2 to 0.3 L/kg/hr after the administration of 5 mg to 25 mg intravenous doses of amantadine to 15 healthy volunteers.

In 6 healthy volunteers, the ratio of amantadine renal clearance to apparent oral plasma clearance was 0.79 ± 0.17 (mean ± SD).

The volume of distribution determined after the intravenous administration of amantadine to 15 healthy subjects was 3 to 8 L/kg, suggesting tissue binding. Amantadine, after single oral 200 mg doses to 6 healthy young subjects and to 6 healthy elderly subjects has been found in nasal mucus at mean ± SD concentrations of 0.15 ± 0.16, 0.28 ± 0.26, and 0.39 ± 0.34 mcg/g at 1, 4, and 8 hours after dosing, respectively. These concentrations represented 31 ± 33%, 59 ± 61%, and 95 ± 86% of the corresponding plasma amantadine concentrations. Amantadine is approximately 67% bound to plasma proteins over a concentration range of 0.1 to 2 mcg/mL. Following the administration of amantadine 100 mg as a single dose, the mean ± SD red blood cell to plasma ratio ranged from 2.7 ± 0.5 in 6 healthy subjects to 1.4 ± 0.2 in 8 patients with renal insufficiency.

Special populations –

Renal function impairment: Compared with otherwise healthy adult individuals, the clearance of amantadine is significantly reduced in adult patients with renal insufficiency. The elimination half-life increases 2- to 3-fold or greater when creatinine clearance is less than 40 mL/min/1.73 m^2 and averages 8 days in patients on chronic maintenance hemodialysis. Amantadine is removed in negligible amounts by hemodialysis.

Elderly: The apparent oral plasma clearance of amantadine is reduced and the plasma half-life and plasma concentrations are increased in healthy elderly individuals age 60 and older. After single dose administration of 25 to 75 mg to 7 healthy, elderly male volunteers, the apparent plasma clearance of amantadine was 0.1 ± 0.04 L/hr/kg (range 0.06 to 0.17 L/hr/kg) and the half-life was 29 ± 7 hours (range 20 to 41 hours). Whether these changes are due to decline in renal function or other age related factors is not known.

Drug interactions – The pH of the urine has been reported to influence the excretion rate of amantadine hydrochloride. Since the excretion rate of amantadine hydrochloride increases rapidly when the urine is acidic, the administration of urine acidifying drugs may increase the elimination of the drug from the body.

Contraindications

Hypersensitivity to amantadine hydrochloride.

Warnings/Precautions

➤*Deaths:* Deaths have been reported from overdose with amantadine hydrochloride. The lowest reported acute lethal dose was 1 g. Acute toxicity may be attributable to the anticholinergic effects of amantadine. Drug overdose has resulted in cardiac, respiratory, renal or central nervous system toxicity. Cardiac dysfunction includes arrhythmia, tachycardia and hypertension (see Overdosage).

➤*Suicide attempts:* Suicide attempts, some of which have been fatal, have been reported in patients treated with amantadine hydrochloride, many of whom received short courses for influenza treatment or prophylaxis. The incidence of suicide attempts is not known and the pathophysiologic mechanism is not understood. Suicide attempts and suicidal ideation have been reported in patients with and without history of psychiatric illness. Amantadine hydrochloride can exacerbate mental problems in patients with a history of psychiatric disorders or substance abuse. Patients who attempt suicide may exhibit abnormal mental states which include disorientation, confusion, depression, personality changes, agitation, aggressive behavior, hallucinations, paranoia, other psychotic reactions, and somnolence or insomnia. Because of the possibility of serious adverse effects, caution should be observed when prescribing amantadine hydrochloride to patients being treated with drugs having CNS effects, or for whom the potential risks outweigh the benefit of treatment. Because some patients have attempted suicide by overdosing with amantadine, prescriptions should be written for the smallest quantity consistent with good patient management.

➤*CNS effects:* Patients with a history of epilepsy or other "seizures" should be observed closely for possible increased seizure activity.

Patients receiving amantadine hydrochloride who note central nervous system effects or blurring of vision should be cautioned against driving or working in situations where alertness and adequate motor coordination are important.

➤*CHF or peripheral edema:* Patients with a history of congestive heart failure or peripheral edema should be followed closely as there are patients who developed congestive heart failure while receiving amantadine hydrochloride.

Because amantadine hydrochloride has anticholinergic effects and may cause mydriasis, it should not be given to patients with untreated angle closure glaucoma.

➤*Parkinson disease:* Patients with Parkinson's disease improving on amantadine hydrochloride should resume normal activities gradually and cautiously, consistent with other medical considerations, such as the presence of osteoporosis or phlebothrombosis.

➤*Abrupt withdrawal:* Amantadine hydrochloride should not be discontinued abruptly in patients with Parkinson's disease since a few patients have experienced a parkinsonian crisis (ie, a sudden marked clinical deterioration) when this medication was suddenly stopped. The dose of anticholinergic drugs or of amantadine hydrochloride should be reduced if atropine-like effects appear when these drugs are used concurrently. Abrupt discontinuation may also precipitate delirium, agitation, delusions, hallucinations, paranoid reaction, stupor, anxiety, depression and slurred speech.

➤*Neuroleptic malignant syndrome (NMS):* Sporadic cases of possible neuroleptic malignant syndrome (NMS) have been reported in association with dose reduction or withdrawal of amantadine hydrochloride therapy. Therefore, patients should be observed carefully when the dosage of amantadine hydrochloride is reduced abruptly or discontinued, especially if the patient is receiving neuroleptics.

➤*Bacterial infections:* Serious bacterial infections may begin with influenza-like symptoms or may coexist with or occur as complications during the course of influenza. Amantadine hydrochloride has not been shown to prevent such complications.

➤*Renal function impairment:* Because amantadine hydrochloride is mainly excreted in the urine, it accumulates in the plasma and in the body when renal function declines. Thus, the dose of amantadine hydrochloride should be reduced in patients with renal impairment and in individuals who are greater than or equal to 65 years of age. Hemodialysis does not remove significant amounts of amantadine hydrochloride; in patients with renal failure, a 4-hour hemodialysis removed 7 to 15 mg after a single 300 mg oral dose.

➤*Hepatic function impairment:* Care should be exercised when administering amantadine hydrochloride to patients with liver disease. Rare instances of reversible elevation of liver enzymes have been reported in patients receiving amantadine hydrochloride, though a specific relationship between the drug and such changes has not been established.

➤*Special risk:* The dose of amantadine hydrochloride may need careful adjustment in patients with congestive heart failure, peripheral edema, or orthostatic hypotension. Care should be exercised when administering amantadine hydrochloride to patients with a history of recurrent eczematoid rash, or to patients with psychosis or severe psychoneurosis not controlled by chemotherapeutic agents.

➤*Hazardous tasks:* See Warnings/Precautions for more information.

➤*Pregnancy: Category C.* Amantadine hydrochloride has been shown to be teratogenic in rats at 50 mg/kg/day and embryotoxic at 100 mg/kg/day (estimated human equivalent dose of 7.1 mg/kg/day and 14.2 mg/kg/day, respectively, based on body surface area conversion). There are no adequate and well-controlled studies in pregnant women. Human data regarding teratogenicity after maternal use of amantadine is scarce. Teratology of Fallot and tibial hemimelia (normal karyotype) occurred in an infant exposed to amantadine during the first trimester of pregnancy (100 mg by mouth for 7 days during the sixth and seventh week of gestation). Cardiovascular maldevelopment (single ventricle with pulmonary atresia) was associated with maternal exposure to amantadine (100 mg/day) administered during the first 2 weeks of pregnancy. Amantadine hydrochloride should be used during pregnancy only if the potential benefit justifies the potential risk to the embryo or fetus.

Fertility impairment – Failed fertility has been reported during human in vitro fertilization (IVF) when the sperm donor ingested amantadine 2 weeks prior to, and during the IVF cycle.

➤*Lactation:* Amantadine hydrochloride is excreted in human milk. Use is not recommended in nursing mothers.

➤*Children:* The safety and efficacy of amantadine hydrochloride in newborn infants and infants below the age of 1 year have not been established.

➤*Elderly:* Because amantadine hydrochloride is primarily excreted in the urine, it accumulates in the plasma and in the body when renal function declines. Thus, the dose of amantadine hydrochloride should be reduced in patients with renal impairment and in individuals who are greater than or equal to 65 years of age. The dose of amantadine hydrochloride may need reduction in patients with congestive heart failure, peripheral edema, or orthostatic hypotension.

Drug Interactions

➤*QT prolongation:* An additive effect of amantadine with other drugs that prolong the QT interval cannot be excluded. The following drugs may prolong the QT interval and increase the risk of life-threatening cardiac arrhythmias, including torsade de pointes: Antiarrhythmic agents (eg, amiodarone, bretylium, disopyramide, dofetilide, procainamide, quinidine, and sotalol), arsenic trioxide, chlorpromazine, cisapride, dolasetron, droperidol, mefloquine, mesoridazine, moxifloxacin, pentamidine, pimozide, tacrolimus, thioridazine, and ziprasidone. For a more complete list of drugs that may prolong the QT interval, see the appendix, Drug-Induced Prolongation of the QT Interval and Torsade de Pointes.

Amantadine Drug Interactions

Precipitant drug	Object drug[a]		Description
Anticholinergic agents	Amantadine	↑	Concurrent administration may potentiate the anticholinergic-like side effects of amantadine. Consider reducing the dose of the anticholinergic agent if atropine-like effects appear.
Quinidine Quinine	Amantadine	↑	Coadministration was shown to reduce renal clearance of amantadine.

AMANTADINE HYDROCHLORIDE — ORAL

Amantadine Drug Interactions

Precipitant drug	Object drug[a]		Description
Triamterene Thiazide diuretics	Amantadine	↑	Coadministration resulted in a higher plasma amantadine concentration.
Trimethoprim/ sulfamethoxazole	Amantadine	↑	Coadministration may impair renal clearance of amantadine, resulting in higher plasma concentrations.
Amantadine	CNS stimulants	↑	Careful observation is required during concomitant administration.
Thioridazine	Amantadine	↑	Coadministration of thioridazine has been reported to worsen the tremor in elderly patients with Parkinson's disease; however, it is not known if other phenothiazines produce a similar response.

[a] ↑ = object drug increased.

Adverse Reactions

The adverse reactions reported most frequently at the recommended dose of amantadine hydrochloride (5% to 10%) are nausea, dizziness (lightheadedness), and insomnia.

Less frequently (1% to 5%) reported adverse reactions are the following: Depression, anxiety and irritability, hallucinations, confusion, anorexia, dry mouth, constipation, ataxia, livedo reticularis, peripheral edema, orthostatic hypotension, headache, somnolence, nervousness, dream abnormality, agitation, dry nose, diarrhea, and fatigue.

Infrequently (0.1% to 1%) occurring adverse reactions are as follows: Congestive heart failure, psychosis, urinary retention, dyspnea, fatigue, skin rash, vomiting, weakness, slurred speech, euphoria, confusion, thinking abnormality, amnesia, hyperkinesia, hypertension, decreased libido, and visual disturbance, including punctate subepithelial or other corneal opacity, corneal edema, decreased visual acuity, sensitivity to light, and optic nerve palsy.

Rare (less than 0.1%) occurring adverse reactions are the following: Instances of convulsion, leukopenia, neutropenia, eczematoid dermatitis, oculogyric episodes, suicidal attempt, suicide, and suicidal ideation.

➤*Postmarketing:*

Cardiovascular – Cardiac arrest, arrhythmias including malignant arrhythmias, hypotension, and tachycardia.

CNS – Coma, stupor, delirium, hypokinesia, hypertonia, delusions, aggressive behavior, paranoid reaction, manic reaction, involuntary muscle contractions, gait abnormalities, paresthesia, EEG changes, and tremor. Abrupt discontinuation may also precipitate delirium, agitation, delusions, hallucinations, paranoid reaction, stupor, anxiety, depression and slurred speech.

Dermatologic – Pruritus and diaphoresis.

GI – Dysphagia.

Hematologic – Leukocytosis.

Lab test abnormalities – Elevated CPK, BUN, serum creatine, alkaline phosphatase, LDH, bilirubin, GGT, AST, and ALT.

Respiratory – Acute respiratory failure, pulmonary edema, and tachypnea.

Special senses – Keratitis and mydriasis.

Miscellaneous – Neuroleptic malignant syndrome (see Warnings), allergic reactions including anaphylactic reactions, edema, and fever.

Overdosage

➤*Symptoms:* Deaths have been reported from overdose with amantadine hydrochloride. The lowest reported acute lethal dose was 1 g. Because some patients have attempted suicide by overdosing with amantadine, prescriptions should be written for the smallest quantity consistent with good patient management.

Acute toxicity may be attributable to the anticholinergic effects of amantadine. Drug overdose has resulted in cardiac, respiratory, renal or central nervous system toxicity. Cardiac dysfunction includes arrhythmia, tachycardia and hypertension. Pulmonary edema and respiratory distress (including adult respiratory distress syndrome [ARDS]) have been reported; renal dysfunction including increased BUN, decreased creatinine clearance and renal insufficiency can occur. Central nervous system effects that have been reported include insomnia, anxiety, aggressive behavior, hypertonia, hyperkinesia, tremor, confusion, disorientation, depersonalization, fear, delirium, hallucinations, psychotic reactions, lethargy, somnolence and coma. Seizures may be exacerbated in patients with history of seizure disorders. Hyperthermia has also been observed in cases where a drug overdose has occurred.

➤*Treatment:* There is no specific antidote for an overdose of amantadine hydrochloride. However, slowly administered intravenous physostigmine in 1 and 2 mg doses in an adult at 1- to 2-hour intervals and 0.5 mg doses in a child at 5- to 10-minute intervals up to a maximum of 2 mg/hr have been reported to be effective in the control of central nervous system toxicity caused by amantadine hydrochloride. For acute overdosing, general supportive measures should be employed along with immediate gastric lavage or induction of emesis. Fluids should be forced, and if necessary, given intravenously. Hemodialysis does not remove significant amounts of amantadine hydrochloride; in patients with renal failure, a 4-hour hemodialysis removed 7 to 15 mg after a single 300 mg oral dose. The pH of the urine has been reported to influence the excretion rate of amantadine hydrochloride. Since the excretion rate of amantadine hydrochloride increases rapidly when the urine is acidic, the administration of urine acidifying drugs may increase the elimination of the drug from the body. The blood pressure, pulse, respiration and temperature should be monitored. The patient should be observed for hyperactivity and convulsions; if required, sedation, and anticonvulsant therapy should be administered. The patient should be observed for the possible development of arrhythmias and hypotension; if required, appropriate antiarrhythmic and antihypotensive therapy should be given. The blood electrolytes, urine pH and urinary output should be monitored. If there is no record of recent voiding, catheterization should be done.

Care should be exercised when administering adrenergic agents, such as isoproterenol, to patients with a amantadine hydrochloride overdose, since the dopaminergic activity of amantadine hydrochloride has been reported to induce malignant arrhythmias.

Patient Information

Patients should be advised of the following information:

Blurry vision and/or impaired mental acuity may occur.

Gradually increase physical activity as the symptoms of Parkinson's disease improve.

Avoid excessive alcohol usage, because it may increase the potential for CNS effects such as dizziness, confusion, lightheadedness, and orthostatic hypotension.

Avoid getting up suddenly from a sitting or lying position. If dizziness or lightheadedness occurs, notify physician.

Notify physician if mood/mental changes, swelling of extremities, difficulty urinating, or shortness of breath occurs.

Do not take more medication than prescribed because of the risk of overdose. If there is no improvement in a few days, or if medication appears less effective after a few weeks, discuss with a physician.

Consult physician before discontinuing medication.

Seek medical attention immediately if it is suspected that an overdose of medication has been taken.

CIDOFOVIR

Rx	**Vistide** (Gilead Sciences)	**Injection:** 75 mg/mL	Preservative free. In 5 mL single-use vials.

CIDOFOVIR — INJECTION

WARNING

Renal impairment is the major toxicity of cidofovir. Cases of acute renal failure resulting in dialysis or contributing to death have occurred with as few as 1 or 2 doses of cidofovir. To reduce possible nephrotoxicity, IV prehydration with normal saline and administration of probenecid must be used with each cidofovir infusion. Renal function (serum creatinine and urine protein) must be monitored within 48 hours prior to each dose of cidofovir and the dose of cidofovir modified for changes in renal function as appropriate (see Administration and Dosage). Cidofovir is contraindicated in patients who are receiving other nephrotoxic agents.

Neutropenia has been observed in association with cidofovir treatment. Therefore, neutrophil counts should be monitored during cidofovir therapy.

Cidofovir is indicated only for the treatment of cytomegalovirus (CMV) retinitis in patients with acquired immunodeficiency syndrome (AIDS).

In animal studies, cidofovir was carcinogenic, teratogenic and caused hypospermia (see Warnings, Carcinogenesis, Mutagenesis, and Fertility impairment).

Indications

➤*CMV retinitis:* Treatment of cytomegalovirus (CMV) retinitis in patients with AIDS. The safety and efficacy of cidofovir have not been established for treatment of other CMV infections (such as pneumonitis or gastroenteritis), congenital or neonatal CMV disease, or CMV disease in non-HIV-infected individuals.

Administration and Dosage

➤*General dosing considerations:* To minimize potential nephrotoxicity, probenecid, and IV saline prehydration must be administered with each cidofovir infusion.

➤*Adults:*

Cytomegalovirus retinitis –

Maximum dose: 5 mg/kg.

Initial dosage: 5 mg/kg body weight (given as an IV infusion at a constant rate over 1 hour) administered once weekly for 2 consecutive weeks for patients with a serum creatinine of 1.5 mg/dL or less, a calculated creatinine clearance greater than 55 mL/min, and a urine protein less than 100 mg/dL (equivalent to less than 2+ proteinuria).

CIDOFOVIR — INJECTION

Maintenance dosage: 5 mg/kg body weight (given as an IV infusion at a constant rate over 1 hour), administered once every 2 weeks.

Concomitant therapy:

• *Probenecid* – 2 g of probenecid must be administered 3 hours prior to each cidofovir dose and 1 g administered at 2 hours and again at 8 hours after completion of the 1 hour cidofovir infusion (for a total of 4 g). Ingestion of food prior to each dose of probenecid may reduce drug-related nausea and vomiting. Administration of an antiemetic may reduce the potential for nausea associated with probenecid ingestion. In patients who develop allergic or hypersensitivity symptoms to probenecid, the use of an appropriate prophylactic or therapeutic antihistamine or acetaminophen should be considered.

• *Hydration* – Patients must receive at least 1 L of 0.9% (normal) saline solution IV with each infusion of cidofovir. The saline solution should be infused over a 1- to 2-hour period immediately before the cidofovir infusion. Patients who can tolerate the additional fluid load should receive a second liter. If administered, the second liter of saline should be initiated either at the start of the cidofovir infusion or immediately afterward, and infused over a 1- to 3-hour period.

➤*Renal function impairment:* Cidofovir is contraindicated in patients with a serum creatinine concentration greater than 1.5 mg/dL, a calculated creatinine clearance 55 mL/min or less, or a urine protein 100 mg/dL or greater (equivalent to at least 2+ proteinuria).

Because serum creatinine in patients with advanced AIDS and CMV retinitis may not provide a complete picture of the patient's underlying renal status, it is important to utilize the Cockcroft-Gault formula to more precisely estimate creatinine clearance (CrCl). As creatinine clearance is dependent on serum creatinine and patient weight, it is necessary to calculate clearance prior to initiation of cidofovir. CrCl (mL/min) should be calculated according to the following formula:

$$\text{CrCl}_{\text{males}} = \frac{[140 - \text{age (in years)}] \times [\text{body weight (in kg)}]}{72 \times [\text{serum creatinine (mg/dL)}]}$$

$$\text{CrCl}_{\text{females}} = \frac{0.85 \times [140 - \text{age (in years)}] \times [\text{body weight (in kg)}]}{72 \times [\text{serum creatinine (mg/dL)}]}$$

Dosage adjustment – The maintenance dose of cidofovir must be reduced from 5 mg/kg to 3 mg/kg for an increase in serum creatinine of 0.3 to 0.4 mg/dL above baseline. Cidofovir therapy must be discontinued for an increase in serum creatinine of 0.5 mg/dL or greater above baseline or development of at least 3+ proteinuria.

➤*Preparation for administration:* Cidofovir is considered a potential teratogen and mutagen. Follow safe handling procedures when preparing, administering, or dispensing cidofovir.

With a syringe, extract the appropriate volume of cidofovir from the vial and transfer the dose to an infusion bag containing 100 mL 0.9% (normal) saline solution.

Handling and disposal – Due to the mutagenic properties of cidofovir, adequate precautions including the use of appropriate safety equipment are recommended for the preparation, administration, and disposal of cidofovir. The National Institutes of Health presently recommends that such agents be prepared in a class II laminar flow biological safety cabinet and that personnel preparing drugs of this class wear surgical gloves and a closed front surgical-type gown with knit cuffs. If cidofovir contacts the skin, wash membranes, and flush thoroughly with water. Excess cidofovir and all other materials used in the admixture preparation and administration should be placed in a leak-proof, puncture-proof container. The recommended method of disposal is high temperature incineration.

➤*Administration:* Cidofovir must not be administered by intraocular injection. Infuse the entire volume IV into the patient at a constant rate over a 1-hour period. Use of a standard infusion pump for administration is recommended.

➤*Admixture compatibility:* The chemical stability of cidofovir admixtures was demonstrated in polyvinyl chloride composition and ethylene/propylene copolymer composition commercial infusion bags and in glass bottles.

➤*Storage/Stability:* Cidofovir should be stored at controlled room temperature (20° to 25°C; 68° to 77°F).

It is recommended that cidofovir infusion admixtures be administered within 24 hours of preparation and that refrigerator or freezer storage not be used to extend this 24-hour limit.

If admixtures are not intended for immediate use, they may be stored under refrigeration (2° to 8°C; 35.6° to 46.4°F) for no more than 24 hours. Refrigerated admixtures should be allowed to equilibrate to room temperature prior to use.

Cidofovir is supplied in single-use vials. Partially used vials should be discarded.

Actions

➤*Pharmacokinetics:*

Absorption/Distribution – Cidofovir must be administered with probenecid. The pharmacokinetics of cidofovir, administered both without and with probenecid, are described below.

In vitro, cidofovir was < 6% bound to plasma or serum proteins over the cidofovir concentration range 0.25 to 25 mcg/mL. Cerebrospinal fluid (CSF) concentrations of cidofovir following IV infusion of cidofovir 5 mg/kg with concomitant probenecid and IV hydration were undetectable (< 0.1 mcg/mL, assay detection threshold) at 15 minutes after the end of a 1-hour infusion in one patient whose corresponding serum concentration was 8.7 mcg/mL.

The pharmacokinetics of cidofovir without probenecid were evaluated in 27 HIV-infected patients with or without asymptomatic CMV infection. Dose-independent pharmacokinetics were demonstrated after 1-hour infusions of 1 (n = 5), 3 (n = 10), 5 (n = 2) and 10 (n = 8) mg/kg. There was no evidence of cidofovir accumulation after 4 weeks of repeated administration of 3 mg/kg/week (n = 5) without probenecid. In patients with healthy renal function, ≈ 80% to 100% of the cidofovir dose was recovered unchanged in urine within 24 hours (n = 27). The renal clearance of cidofovir was greater than creatinine clearance, indicating renal tubular secretion contributes to the elimination of cidofovir.

Cidofovir Pharmacokinetic Parameters Following 3 and 5 mg/kg Infusions Without and With Probenecid[a]

Parameters	Cidofovir injection administered without probenecid		Cidofovir for injection administered with probenecid	
	3 mg/kg (n = 10)	5 mg/kg (n = 2)	3 mg/kg (n = 12)	5 mg/kg (n = 6)
AUC (mcg•hr/mL)	20 ± 2.3	28.3	25.7 ± 8.5	40.8 ± 9
C_{max} (end of infusion) (mcg/mL)	7.3 ± 1.4	11.5	9.8 ± 3.7	19.6 ± 7.2
V_{dss} (mL/kg)	537 ± 126 (n = 12)		410 ± 102 (n = 18)	
Clearance (mL/min/1.73 m²)	179 ± 23.1 (n = 12)		148 ± 38.8 (n = 18)	
Renal clearance (mL/min/1.73 m²)	150 ± 26.9 (n = 12)		98.6 ± 27.9 (n = 11)	

[a] See Administration and Dosage.

Special populations –

Renal function impairment: Pharmacokinetic data collected from subjects with creatinine clearance values as low as 11 mL/min indicate that cidofovir clearance decreases proportionally with creatinine clearance.

High-flux hemodialysis has been shown to reduce the serum levels of cidofovir by ≈ 75%.

Initiation of therapy with cidofovir is contraindicated in patients with serum creatinine > 1.5 mg/dL, a calculated creatinine clearance ≤ 55 mL/min, or a urine protein ≥ 100 mg/dL (equivalent to ≥ 2+ proteinuria) (see Contraindications).

Contraindications

Initiation of therapy in patients with a serum creatinine > 1.5 mg/dL, a calculated creatinine clearance ≤ 55 mL/min, or a urine protein ≥ 100 mg/dL (equivalent to ≥ 2+ proteinuria); in patients receiving agents with nephrotoxic potential (such agents must be discontinued at least 7 days prior to starting therapy with cidofovir); hypersensitivity to cidofovir or a history of clinically severe hypersensitivity to probenecid or other sulfa-containing medications; direct intraocular injection; direct injection of cidofovir has been associated with iritis, ocular hypotony, and permanent impairment of vision.

Warnings/Precautions

➤*Hematological toxicity:* Neutropenia may occur during cidofovir therapy. Neutrophil count should be monitored while receiving cidofovir therapy.

➤*Decreased IOP/ocular hypotony:* Decreased intraocular pressure (IOP) may occur during cidofovir therapy, and in some instances has been associated with decreased visual acuity. IOP should be monitored during cidofovir therapy. Among the subset of patients monitored for intraocular pressure changes, a ≥ 50% decrease from baseline intraocular pressure was reported in 17 of 70 (24%) patients at the 5 mg/kg maintenance dose. Severe hypotony (intraocular pressure of 0 to 1 mm Hg) has been reported in 3 patients. Risk of ocular hypotony may be increased in patients with preexisting diabetes mellitus.

➤*Metabolic acidosis:* Decreased serum bicarbonate associated with proximal tubule injury and renal wasting syndrome (including Fanconi's syndrome) have been reported in patients receiving cidofovir (see Adverse Reactions). Mucormycosis, aspergillus, disseminated mycobacterial infection, cases of metabolic acidosis in association with liver dysfunction and pancreatitis resulting in death have been reported in patients receiving cidofovir.

➤*Nephrotoxicity:* Dose-dependent nephrotoxicity is the major dose-limiting toxicity related to cidofovir administration. Cases of acute renal failure resulting in dialysis or contributing to death have occurred with as few as 1 or 2 doses of cidofovir. Renal function (serum creatinine and urine protein) must be monitored within 48 hours prior to each dose of cidofovir. Dose adjustment or discontinuation is required for changes in renal function (serum creatinine or urine protein) while on therapy. Proteinuria, as measured by urinalysis in a clinical laboratory, may be an early indicator of cidofovir-related nephrotoxicity. Continued administration of cidofovir may lead to additional proximal tubular cell injury, which may result in glycosuria, decreases in serum phosphate, uric acid, and bicarbonate, elevations in serum creatinine, or acute renal failure, in some cases, resulting in the need for dialysis. Patients with these adverse events occurring concurrently and meeting a criteria of Fanconi's syndrome have been reported. Renal function that did not return to baseline after drug discontinuation has been observed in clinical studies of cidofovir.

➤*IV infusion only:* Cidofovir is formulated for IV infusion only and must not be administered by intraocular injection. Administration of cidofovir by infusion must be accompanied by oral probenecid and IV saline prehydration (see Administration and Dosage).

CIDOFOVIR — INJECTION

➤*Uveitis/iritis:* Uveitis or iritis was reported in clinical trials and during postmarketing in patients receiving cidofovir therapy. Treatment with topical corticosteroids with or without topical cycloplegic agents should be considered. Patients should be monitored for signs and symptoms of uveitis/iritis during cidofovir therapy.

➤*Renal function impairment:* See Administration and Dosage for more information.

➤*Pregnancy: Category C.* Cidofovir was embryotoxic (reduced fetal body weights) in rats at 1.5 mg/kg/day and in rabbits at 1 mg/kg/day, doses which were also maternally toxic, following daily IV dosing during the period of organogenesis. The no-observable-effect levels for embryotoxicity in rats (0.5 mg/kg/day) and in rabbits (0.25 mg/kg/day) were ≈ 0.04 and 0.05 times the clinical dose (5 mg/kg every other week) based on AUC, respectively. An increased incidence of fetal external, soft tissue, and skeletal anomalies (meningocele, short snout, and short maxillary bones) occurred in rabbits at the high dose (1 mg/kg/day) which was also maternally toxic. There are no adequate and well-controlled studies in pregnant women. Cidofovir should be used during pregnancy only if the potential benefit justifies the potential risk to the fetus.

➤*Lactation:* It is not known whether cidofovir is excreted in human milk. Since many drugs are excreted in human milk and because of the potential for adverse reactions as well as the potential for tumorigenicity shown for cidofovir in animal studies, cidofovir should not be administered to nursing mothers. The US Public Health Service Centers for Disease Control and Prevention advises HIV-infected women not to breastfeed to avoid postnatal transmission of HIV to a child who may not yet be infected.

➤*Children:* Safety and efficacy in children have not been studied. The use of cidofovir in children with AIDS warrants extreme caution due to the risk of long-term carcinogenicity and reproductive toxicity. Administration of cidofovir to children should be undertaken only after careful evaluation and only if the potential benefits of treatment outweigh the risks.

➤*Elderly:* No studies of the safety or efficacy of cidofovir in patients over the age of 60 have been conducted. Since elderly individuals frequently have reduced glomerular filtration, particular attention should be paid to assessing renal function before and during cidofovir administration (see Administration and Dosage).

➤*Monitoring:* Serum creatinine and urine protein must be monitored within 48 hours prior to each dose. White blood cell counts with differential should be monitored prior to each dose. In patients with proteinuria, IV hydration should be administered and the test repeated. Intraocular pressure, visual acuity, and ocular symptoms should be monitored periodically.

Drug Interactions

➤*Nephrotoxic agents:* Concomitant administration of cidofovir and agents with nephrotoxic potential (eg, IV aminoglycosides [eg, tobramycin, gentamicin, and amikacin], amphotericin B, foscarnet, IV pentamidine, vancomycin, and nonsteroidal anti-inflammatory agents) is contraindicated. Such agents must be discontinued at least 7 days prior to starting therapy with cidofovir.

Adverse Reactions

➤*Nephrotoxicity:* Renal toxicity, as manifested by ≥ 2+ proteinuria, serum creatinine elevations of ≥ 0.4 mg/dL, or decreased creatinine clearance ≤ 55 mL/min, occurred in 79 of 135 (59%) patients receiving cidofovir at a maintenance dose of 5 mg/kg every other week. Maintenance dose reductions from 5 mg/kg to 3 mg/kg due to proteinuria or serum creatinine elevations were made in 12 of 41 (29%) patients who had not received prior therapy for CMV retinitis (Study 106) and in 19 of 74 (26%) patients who had received prior therapy for CMV retinitis (Study 107). Prior foscarnet use has been associated with an increased risk of nephrotoxicity; therefore, such patients must be monitored closely (see Contraindications, Warnings, Administration and Dosage).

➤*Neutropenia:* In clinical trials, at the 5 mg/kg maintenance dose, a decrease in absolute neutrophil count to ≤ 500 cells/mm³ occurred in 24% of patients. Granulocyte colony-stimulating factor (G-CSF) was used in 39% of patients.

➤*Decreased IOP/ocular hypotony:* Among the subset of patients monitored for IOP changes, a ≥ 50% decrease from baseline IOP was reported in 17 of 70 (24%) patients at the 5 mg/kg maintenance dose. Severe hypotony (intraocular pressure of 0 to 1 mmHg) has been reported in 3 patients. Risk of ocular hypotony may be increased in patients with preexisting diabetes mellitus.

➤*Anterior uveitis/iritis:* Uveitis or iritis has been reported in clinical trials and during postmarketing in patients receiving cidofovir therapy. Uveitis or iritis was reported in 15 of 135 (11%) patients receiving 5 mg/kg maintenance dosing. Treatment with topical corticosteroids with or without topical cycloplegic agents may be considered. Patients should be monitored for signs and symptoms of uveitis/iritis during cidofovir therapy.

➤*Metabolic acidosis:* A diagnosis of Fanconi's syndrome, as manifested by multiple abnormalities of proximal renal tubular function, was reported in 1% of patients. Decreases in serum bicarbonate to ≤ 16 mEq/L occurred in 16% of cidofovir-treated patients. Cases of metabolic acidosis in association with liver dysfunction and pancreatitis resulting in death have been reported in patients receiving cidofovir.

Lab test abnormalities – In clinical trials, cidofovir was withdrawn due to adverse events in 39% of patients treated with 5 mg/kg every other week as maintenance therapy.

The incidence of adverse reactions reported as serious in 3 controlled clinical studies in patients with CMV retinitis, regardless of presumed relationship to drug, is listed in the following table.

Cidofovir Serious Clinical Adverse Reactions or Laboratory Abnormalities (> 5%)

Laboratory abnormality/Adverse reaction	Frequency (n = 135)[a]
Proteinuria (≥ 100 mg/dL)	68 (50%)
Neutropenia (≤ 500 cells/mm³)	33 (24%)
Decreased intraocular pressure [b]	17 (24%)
Decreased serum bicarbonate (≤ 16 mEq/L)	21 (16%)
Fever	19 (14%)
Infection	16 (12%)
Creatinine elevation (≥ 2 mg/dL)	16 (12%)
Pneumonia	12 (9%)
Dyspnea	11 (8%)
Nausea/vomiting	10 (7%)

[a] Patients receiving 5 mg/kg maintenance regimen in studies 105, 106 and 107.
[b] Defined as decreased IOP to ≤ 50% that at baseline. Based on 70 patients receiving 5 mg/kg maintenance dosing (studies 105, 106 and 107) for whom baseline and follow-up IOP determinations were recorded.

➤*Observed adverse reactions/intercurrent illnesses in clinical trials (causal relationship unknown):* The following adverse reactions/intercurrent illnesses have been observed in clinical studies of cidofovir and are listed below regardless of causal relationship to cidofovir. Evaluation of these reports was difficult because of the diverse manifestations of the underlying disease and because most patients received numerous concomitant medicines.

Cardiovascular – Cardiomyopathy, cardiovascular disorder, congestive heart failure, hypertension, hypotension, migraine, pallor, peripheral vascular disorder, phlebitis, postural hypotension, shock, syncope, tachycardia, vascular disorder, and edema.

CNS – Abnormal dreams, abnormal gait, acute brain syndrome, agitation, amnesia, anxiety, ataxia, cerebrovascular disorder, confusion, convulsion, delirium, dementia, depression, dizziness, drug dependence, dry mouth, encephalopathy, facial paralysis, hallucinations, headache, hemiplegia, hyperesthesia, hypertonia, hypotony, incoordination, increased libido, insomnia, myoclonus, nervousness, neuropathy, paresthesia, personality disorder, somnolence, speech disorder, tremor, twitching, vasodilatation, and vertigo.

Dermatologic – Acne, alopecia, angioedema, dry skin, eczema, exfoliative dermatitis, furunculosis, herpes simplex, nail disorder, pruritus, rash, seborrhea, skin discoloration, skin disorder, skin hypertrophy, skin ulcer, sweating, and urticaria.

Endocrine – Adrenal cortex insufficiency.

GI – Anorexia, abdominal pain, cholangitis, colitis, constipation, esophagitis, diarrhea, dry mouth, dyspepsia, dysphagia, fecal incontinence, flatulence, gastritis, GI hemorrhage, gingivitis, hepatitis, hepatomegaly, hepatosplenomegaly, jaundice, abnormal liver function, liver damage, liver necrosis, melena, oral candidiasis, pancreatitis, proctitis, rectal disorder, stomatitis, aphthous stomatitis, tongue discoloration, mouth ulceration, and tooth caries.

GU – Decreased creatinine clearance, dysuria, glycosuria, hematuria, kidney stone, mastitis, metorrhagia, nocturia, polyuria, prostatic disorder, toxic nephrophathy, urethritis, urinary casts, urinary incontinence, urinary retention, and urinary tract infection.

Hematologic/Lymphatic – Hypochromic anemia, leukocytosis, leukopenia, lymphadenopathy, lymphoma like reaction, pancytopenia, splenic disorder, splenomegaly, thrombocytopenia, and thrombocytopenic purpura.

Metabolic/Nutritional – Cachexia, dehydration, edema, hypercalcemia, hyperglycemia, hyperkalemia, hyperlipemia, hypocalcemia, hypoglycemia, hypoglycemic reaction, hypokalemia, hypomagnesemia, hyponatremia, hypophosphatemia, hypoproteinemia, increased alkaline phosphatase, increased BUN, increased lactic dehydrogenase, increased AST, increased ALT, peripheral edema, respiratory alkalosis, thirst, weight loss, and weight gain.

Musculoskeletal – Arthralgia, arthrosis, bone necrosis, bone pain, joint disorder, leg cramps, myalgia, myasthenia, and pathological fracture.

Respiratory – Asthma, bronchitis, coughing, epistaxis, hemoptysis, hiccup, hyperventilation, hypoxia, increased sputum, larynx edema, lung disorder, pharyngitis, pneumothorax, rhinitis, and sinusitis.

Special senses – Abnormal vision, amblyopia, blindness, cataract, conjunctivitis, corneal lesion, corneal opacity, diplopia, dry eyes, ear disorder, ear pain, eye disorder, eye pain, hypotony, hyperacusis, iritis, keratitis, miosis, otitis externa, otitis media, refraction disorder, retinal detachment, retinal disorder, taste perversion, tinnitus, uveitis, visual field defect, and hearing loss.

Miscellaneous – Abdominal pain, accidental injury, AIDS, allergic reaction, back pain, catheter blocked, cellulitis, chest pain, chills and fever, cryptococcosis, cyst, death, face edema, flu-like syndrome, hypothermia, injection site reaction, malaise, mucous membrane disorder, neck pain, overdose, photosensitivity reaction, sarcoma, and sepsis.

CIDOFOVIR — INJECTION

➤*Most frequently reported adverse reactions, regardless of relationship to study drugs or severity:* The most frequently reported adverse events regardless of relationship to study drugs (cidofovir or probenecid) or severity are shown in the table below.

Adverse Reactions, Laboratory Abnormalities or Intercurrent Illnesses Regardless of Severity Occurring with Cidofovir (> 15%)

Adverse reaction	Frequency (n = 115)[a]
Any adverse reaction	115 (100%)
Proteinuria (≥ 30 mg/dL)	101 (88%)
Nausea with or without vomiting	79 (69%)
Fever	67 (58%)
Neutropenia (< 750 cells/mm³)	50 (43%)
Asthenia	50 (43%)
Headache	34 (30%)
Rash	34 (30%)
Infection	32 (28%)
Alopecia	31 (27%)
Diarrhea	30 (26%)
Pain	29 (25%)
Creatinine elevation (> 1.5 mg/dL)	28 (24%)
Anemia	28 (24%)
Anorexia	26 (23%)
Dyspnea	26 (23%)
Chills	25 (22%)
Increased cough	22 (19%)
Oral moniliasis	21 (18%)

[a] Patients receiving 5 mg/kg maintenance regimen in studies 106 and 107.

➤*Reporting of adverse reactions:* Malignancies or serious adverse reactions that occur in patients who have received cidofovir should be reported to patients' healthcare providers.

Overdosage

➤*Symptoms:* Two cases of cidofovir overdose have been reported. These patients received single doses of cidofovir at 16.3 mg/kg and 17.4 mg/kg, respectively, with concomitant oral probenecid and IV hydration. Significant changes in renal function were not observed in either patient.

➤*Treatment:* In both cases, the patients were hospitalized and received oral probenecid (1 g 3 times daily) and vigorous IV hydration with normal saline for 3 to 5 days.

Patient Information

Patients should be advised that cidofovir is not a cure for CMV retinitis, and that they may continue to experience progression of retinitis during and following treatment. Patients receiving cidofovir should be advised to have regular follow-up ophthalmologic examinations. Patients may also experience other manifestations of CMV disease despite cidofovir therapy.

HIV-infected patients may continue taking antiretroviral therapy, but those taking zidovudine should be advised to temporarily discontinue zidovudine administration or decrease their zidovudine dose by 50%, on days of cidofovir administration only, because probenecid reduces metabolic clearance of zidovudine.

Patients should be informed of the major toxicity of cidofovir, namely renal impairment, and that dose modification, including reduction, interruption, and possibly discontinuation, may be required. Close monitoring of renal function (routine urinalysis and serum creatinine) while on therapy should be emphasized.

The importance of completing a full course of probenecid with each cidofovir dose should be emphasized. Patients should be warned of potential adverse events caused by probenecid (eg, headache, nausea, vomiting, hypersensitivity reactions). Hypersensitivity/allergic reactions may include rash, fever, chills, and anaphylaxis. Administration of probenecid after a meal or use of antiemetics may decrease the nausea. Prophylactic or therapeutic antihistamines or acetaminophen can be used to ameliorate hypersensitivity reactions.

Patients should be advised that cidofovir causes tumors, primarily mammary adenocarcinomas, in rats. Cidofovir should be considered a potential carcinogen in humans (see Warnings). Women should be advised of the limited enrollment of women in clinical trials of cidofovir.

Patients should be advised that cidofovir caused reduced testes weight and hypospermia in animals. Such changes may occur in humans and cause infertility. Women of childbearing potential should be advised that cidofovir is embryotoxic in animals and should not be used during pregnancy. Women of childbearing potential should be advised to use effective contraception during and for 1 month following treatment with cidofovir. Men should be advised to practice barrier contraceptive methods during and for 3 months after treatment with cidofovir.

RIBAVIRIN

Rx	**Ribavirin** (Various, eg, Sandoz, Teva, Zydus)	**Tablets; oral:** 200 mg	In 168s, 180s, 1,000s, and UD 100s.
Rx	**Copegus** (Genentech)		(RIB 200 ROCHE). Lt. pink to pink, oval. Film-coated. In 168s.
Rx	**Ribasphere** (Three Rivers)		Lactose. (200 3RP). Lt. blue, capsule shape. Film-coated. In 168s and 500s.
Rx	**Ribasphere** (Three Rivers)	**Tablets; oral:** 400 mg	Lactose. (400 3RP). Medium blue, capsule shape. Film-coated. In 56s, 500s, and **RibaPak** 800 and 1,000 dose packs.[a]
Rx	**Ribasphere** (Three Rivers)	**Tablets; oral:** 600 mg	Lactose. (600 3RP). Dark blue, capsule shape. Film-coated. In 56s, 250s, and **RibaPak** 1,000 and 1,200 dose packs.[a]
Rx	**Ribavirin** (Various, eg, Sandoz, Teva, Zydus)	**Capsules; oral:** 200 mg	In 42s, 56s, 70s, 84s, 140s, 168s, 180s, 1,000s, and UD 100s.
Rx	**Rebetol** (Schering)		Lactose. (REBETOL 200 mg). White/Opaque. In 42s, 56s, 70s, and 84s.
Rx	**Ribasphere** (Three Rivers)		Lactose. Pellet-filled. (riba 200). White/opaque. In 42s, 56s, 70s, 84s, 140s, 168s, and 180s.
Rx	**Rebetol** (Schering)	**Solution; oral:** 40 mg/mL	Glycerin, propylene glycol, sodium benzoate, sorbitol, sucrose. Bubble gum flavor. In 100 mL.
Rx	**Virazole** (Valent)	**Lyophilized powder for solution; inhalation:** 6 g	In vials.

[a] Each *RibaPak* 800 dose pack contains 14 ribavirin 400 mg tablets. Each *RibaPak* 1,000 dose pack contains 7 ribavirin 400 mg tablets and 7 ribavirin 600 mg tablets. Each *RibaPak* 1,200 dose pack contains 14 ribavirin 600 mg tablets.

RIBAVIRIN — ORAL

WARNING

Ribavirin monotherapy is not effective for the treatment of chronic hepatitis C virus (HCV) infection and should not be used alone for this indication.

The primary clinical toxicity of ribavirin is hemolytic anemia, which may result in worsening of cardiac disease and lead to fatal and nonfatal myocardial infarctions (MIs). Do not treat patients with a history of significant or unstable cardiac disease with ribavirin.

Significant teratogenic and/or embryocidal effects have been demonstrated in all animal species exposed to ribavirin. In addition, ribavirin has a multiple-dose half-life of 12 days, and it may persist in nonplasma compartments for as long as 6 months. Therefore, ribavirin therapy is contraindicated in women who are pregnant and in the male partners of women who are pregnant. Extreme care must be taken to avoid pregnancy during therapy and for 6 months after completion of treatment in women receiving ribavirin therapy and female partners of men who are taking ribavirin therapy. At least 2 reliable forms of effective contraception must be used during treatment and during the 6-month posttreatment follow-up period.

Indications

➤*Chronic hepatitis C virus:*

Tablets – In combination with peginterferon alfa-2a for the treatment of adults with chronic HCV infection who have compensated liver disease and have not previously been treated with interferon alpha.

Patients in whom efficacy was demonstrated included patients with compensated liver disease and histological evidence of cirrhosis (Child-Pugh class A). Efficacy of *Copegus* was also demonstrated in patients with HIV disease that is clinically stable (eg, antiretroviral therapy not required or receiving stable antiretroviral therapy).

Capsules / Solution –

Ribasphere: In combination with interferon alfa-2b for the treatment of chronic HCV in patients 18 years of age and older with compensated liver disease previously untreated with alpha interferon and in patients 18 years of age and older who have relapsed following alpha interferon therapy; in combination with peginterferon alfa-2b for the treatment of chronic HCV in patients with compensated liver disease who have not previously been treated with interferon alpha and are at least 18 years of age.

Rebetol: In combination with interferon alfa-2b (pegylated and nonpegylated) for the treatment of chronic HCV in patients 3 years of age and older with compensated liver disease.

➤*Off-label uses:* Treatment of viral hemorrhagic fevers, such as Crimean-Congo hemorrhagic fever.

Administration and Dosage

➤*Adults:*

Chronic hepatic C virus infection –

Copegus or *Ribasphere* tablets/peginterferon alfa-2a: 800 to 1,200 mg administered orally in 2 divided doses. Individualize the dose to the patient, depending on baseline disease characteristics (eg, genotype), response to therapy, and tolerability of the regimen.

Copegus or Ribasphere Tablets/Peginterferon Alfa-2a Dosing Recommendations

Genotype[a]	Peginterferon alfa-2a dose	Ribavirin tablet dose[b]	Duration
Genotype 1, 4	180 mcg	< 75 kg = 1,000 mg	48 weeks
		≥ 75 kg = 1,200 mg	48 weeks
Genotype 2, 3	180 mcg	800 mg	24 weeks

[a] Non-1 genotypes showed no increased response to treatment beyond 24 weeks. Data on genotypes 5 and 6 are insufficient for dosing recommendations.
[b] Administer in 2 divided doses.

• *Duration of therapy* – 24 to 48 weeks for patients previously untreated with ribavirin and interferon.

Rebetol or *Ribasphere* capsules/interferon alfa-2b:

• *Usual dosage* –

76 kg or more: 600 mg in the morning and 600 mg in the evening with interferon alfa-2b 3 million units 3 times weekly subcutaneously.

75 kg or less: 400 mg in the morning and 600 mg in the evening with interferon alfa-2b 3 million units 3 times weekly subcutaneously.

• *Duration of therapy* – 24 to 48 weeks for patients previously untreated with interferon; 24 weeks for patients who relapsed following nonpegylated interferon monotherapy.

Ribasphere capsules/peginterferon alfa-2b: *Ribasphere* 800 mg/day in 2 divided doses (400 mg in the morning and 400 mg in the evening).

Rebetol/Peginterferon alfa-2b:

• *Usual dosage* –

Rebetol/Peginterferon Alfa-2b Dosing Recommendations in Adults

Body weight	Peginterferon alfa-2b strength	Amount of peginterferon alfa-2b to administer	Volume[a] of peginterferon alfa-2b to administer	*Rebetol* daily dose	Number of *Rebetol* capsules
< 40 kg	50 mcg per 0.5 mL	50 mcg	0.5 mL	800 mg/day	2 × 200 mg capsules in the morning 2 × 200 mg capsules in the evening
40 to 50 kg	80 mcg per 0.5 mL	64 mcg	0.4 mL	800 mg/day	2 × 200 mg capsules in the morning 2 × 200 mg capsules in the evening
51 to 60 kg		80 mcg	0.5 mL	800 mg/day	2 × 200 mg capsules in the morning 2 × 200 mg capsules in the evening
61 to 65 kg	120 mcg per 0.5 mL	96 mcg	0.4 mL	800 mg/day	2 × 200 mg capsules in the morning 2 × 200 mg capsules in the evening
66 to 75 kg		96 mcg	0.4 mL	1,000 mg/day	2 × 200 mg capsules in the morning 3 × 200 mg capsules in the evening
76 to 80 kg		120 mcg	0.5 mL	1,000 mg/day	2 × 200 mg capsules in the morning 3 × 200 mg capsules in the evening
81 to 85 kg				1,200 mg/day	3 × 200 mg capsules in the morning 3 × 200 mg capsules in the evening
86 to 105 kg	150 mcg per 0.5 mL	150 mcg	0.5 mL	1,200 mg/day	3 × 200 mg capsules in the morning 3 × 200 mg capsules in the evening
> 105 kg	†[b]	†[b]	†[b]	1,400 mg/day	3 × 200 mg capsules in the morning 4 × 200 mg capsules in the evening

[a] When reconstituted as directed.
[b] For patients weighing > 105 kg, the peginterferon alfa-2b dosage of 1.5 mcg/kg/wk should be calculated based on the individual patient's weight. Two vials of peginterferon alfa-2b may be necessary to provide the dose.

• *Duration of therapy* –

Interferon alpha–naive patients: 48 weeks for patients with genotype 1; 24 weeks for patients with genotypes 2 and 3.

Re-treatment with peginterferon alfa-2b of prior treatment failures: 48 weeks, regardless of HCV genotype.

Chronic hepatic C virus with HIV coinfection –

Copegus/Peginterferon alfa-2a:

• *Usual dosage* – *Copegus* 800 mg/day and peginterferon alfa-2a 180 mcg subcutaneously once weekly.

• *Duration of therapy* – 48 weeks regardless of genotype.

➤*Children:* See also Off-Label Uses.

Chronic hepatic C virus infection –

Rebetol/Interferon alfa-2b:

• *Usual dosage* –

76 kg or more: 600 mg in the morning and 600 mg in the evening with interferon alfa-2b 3 million units 3 times weekly subcutaneously.

62 to 75 kg: 400 mg in the morning and 600 mg in the evening with interferon alfa-2b 3 million units 3 times weekly subcutaneously.

25 to 61 kg: 15 mg/kg/day (divided dose in the morning and in the evening) with interferon alfa-2b 3 million units/m^2 3 times weekly subcutaneously.

• *Duration of therapy* – 48 weeks for children with genotype 1; 24 weeks for children with genotype 2 and 3.

RIBAVIRIN — ORAL

Rebetol/Peginterferon alfa-2b combination:

• *3 to 17 years of age* –

Usual dosage:

Ribavirin[a] Dosing Guidelines in Children		
Body weight	Ribavirin daily dose	Number of ribavirin capsules
< 47 kg	15 mg/kg/day	Use oral solution[b]
47 to 59 kg	800 mg/day	2 × 200 mg capsules in the morning 2 × 200 mg capsules in the evening
60 to 73 kg	1,000 mg/day	2 × 200 mg capsules in the morning 3 × 200 mg capsules in the evening
> 73 kg	1,200 mg/day	3 × 200 mg capsules in the morning 3 × 200 mg capsules in the evening

[a] Ribavirin to be used in combination with peginterferon alfa-2b 60 mcg/m² weekly. Patients who reach their 18th birthday while receiving these medications should remain on the pediatric dosing regimen.
[b] Ribavirin solution may be used for any patient regardless of body weight.

Duration of therapy: 48 weeks for patients with genotype 1; 24 weeks for patients with genotypes 2 and 3.

Off-label dosing –

Hepatitis C:

• *3 years of age and older* –

Capsule or solution in combination with interferon alfa-2b 3 million units 3 times weekly subcutaneously50 to 61 kg: 400 mg twice daily.37 to 49 kg 200 mg in the morning and 400 mg in the evening.25 to 36 kg 200 mg twice daily.

➤*Renal function impairment:* Do not use in patients with creatinine clearance (CrCl) less than 50 mL/min.

Rebetol –

Dose Modification and Discontinuation of *Rebetol* Combination Therapy in Adults and Children					
	Adults	Children		Adults	Children
Laboratory values	Peginterferon alfa-2b/ interferon alfa-2b	Peginterferon alfa-2b	Interferon alfa-2b	*Rebetol*	
Hb < 10 g/dL	For patients with cardiac disease, reduce by 50%[a]	See footnote[a]	See footnote[a]	Adjust dose[b]	1st reduction to 12 mg/kg/day 2nd reduction to 8 mg/kg/day
WBC[c] < 1.5 × 10⁹/L	Adjust dose[d]	1st reduction to 40 mcg/m²/wk 2nd reduction to 20 mcg/m²/wk	Reduce by 50%	No dose change	No dose change
Neutrophils < 0.75 × 10⁹/L					
Platelets < 50 × 10⁹/L (adults) < 70 × 10⁹/L (children)					
Hb < 8.5 g/dL	Permanently discontinue	Permanently discontinue	Permanently discontinue	Permanently discontinue	Permanently discontinue
WBC < 1 × 10⁹/L					
Neutrophils < 0.5 × 10⁹/L					
Creatinine > 2 mg/dL (children)					
Platelets < 25 × 10⁹/L (adults) < 50 × 10⁹/L (children)					

[a] For adults with a history of stable cardiac disease receiving peginterferon alfa-2b or interferon alfa-2b in combination with ribavirin, the peginterferon alfa-2b or interferon alfa-2b dose should be reduced by half and the ribavirin dose by 200 mg/day if a > 2 g/dL decrease in Hb is observed during any 4-week period. Both peginterferon alfa-2b and ribavirin or interferon alfa-2b and ribavirin should be permanently discontinued if patients have Hb levels < 12 g/dL after this ribavirin dose reduction. Children who have preexisting cardiac conditions and experience a Hb decrease ≥ 2 g/dL during any 4-week period during treatment should have weekly evaluations and hematology testing.
[b] First dose reduction of ribavirin is by 200 mg/day, except in patients receiving the 1,400 mg dose it is by 400 mg/day; second dose reduction of ribavirin (if needed) is by an additional 200 mg/day.
[c] WBC = white blood cell count.
[d] For patients on ribavirin/peginterferon alfa-2b combination therapy: first dose reduction of peginterferon alfa-2b is to 1 mcg/kg/wk, second dose reduction (if needed) of peginterferon alfa-2b is to 0.5 mcg/kg/wk. For patients receiving ribavirin/interferon alfa-2b combination therapy, reduce interferon alfa-2b dose by 50%.

➤*Discontinuation of therapy:*

Ribavirin/Interferon alfa-2b – Treatment discontinuation should be considered in any patient who has not achieved an HCV-RNA below the limit of detection of the assay by 24 weeks.

Ribavirin/Peginterferon alfa-2a – Consider discontinuation in patients who do not achieve at least a 2 log_{10} drop from baseline in HCV-RNA at 12 weeks, or undetectable HCV-RNA levels after 24 weeks of therapy. Retreated patients who fail to achieve undetectable HCV-RNA at week 12 of therapy, or whose HCV-RNA remains detectable after 24 weeks of therapy, are highly unlikely to achieve sustained virologic response, and discontinuation of therapy should be considered. Discontinue ribavirin tablets in patients who develop hepatic decompensation during treatment.

➤*Preparation for administration:* Ribavirin is considered a teratogen. Follow safe handling procedures when preparing, administering, or dispensing ribavirin.

➤*Administration:* Administer *Copegus*, *Rebetol*, and *Ribasphere* tablets with food. Do not open, crush, or break the capsules.

Ribasphere capsules may be administered without regard to food but should be administered in a consistent manner with respect to food intake.

➤*Storage/Stability:*

Capsules/Tablets – Store at 25°C (77°F); excursions are permitted between 15° and 30°C (59° and 86°F).

➤*Hepatic function impairment:* Discontinue therapy in patients who develop hepatic decompensation during treatment.

➤*Dose modifications:* If severe adverse reactions or laboratory abnormalities develop during combination therapy, modify or discontinue the dose, if appropriate, until the adverse reactions abate or decrease in severity. If intolerance persists after dose adjustment, discontinue combination therapy.

Ribavirin –

Adults:

Ribavirin Dosage Modification and Discontinuation Guidelines		
Hb[a]	Reduce ribavirin dose to 600 mg/day[b] if:	Discontinue ribavirin tablets if:
Patients with no cardiac disease	Hb < 10 g/dL	Hb < 8.5 g/dL
Patients with history of stable cardiac disease	≥ 2 g/dL decrease in Hb during any 4-week treatment period	Hb < 12 g/dL despite 4 weeks at reduced dose

[a] Hb = hemoglobin.
[b] One 200 mg tablet in the morning and two 200 mg tablets in the evening.

• *Tablets* – Once ribavirin has been withheld because of a laboratory abnormality or clinical manifestation, an attempt may be made to restart ribavirin at 600 mg/day and further increase the dosage to 800 mg/day. However, it is not recommended that ribavirin be increased to the original assigned dose (1,000 to 1,200 mg).

Children: Modify the recommended dose from the original starting dosages of 15 mg/kg daily in a 2-step process to 12 mg/kg/day, then to 8 mg/kg/day if needed.

Solution – Store at 2° to 8°C (36° to 46°F) or at 25°C (77°F); excursions are permitted between 15° and 30°C (59° and 86°F).

Actions

➤*Pharmacology:* Ribavirin is a synthetic nucleoside analog (purine analog) with antiviral activity. The mechanism by which the combination of ribavirin and an interferon product exerts its effect against HCV has not been fully established. Ribavirin has direct antiviral activity in tissue culture against many RNA viruses. Ribavirin increases the mutation frequency in the genomes of several viruses, and ribavirin triphosphate inhibits HCV polymerase in a biochemical reaction.

➤*Pharmacokinetics:*

Ribavirin Capsules/Solution Mean (% CV) Pharmacokinetic Parameters in Adults[a]			
Pharmacokinetic parameter	Single-dose ribavirin 600 mg solution (n = 14)	Single-dose ribavirin 600 mg capsules (n = 12)	Multiple-dose ribavirin 600 mg twice daily capsules (n = 12)
T_{max} (h)	1 (34%)	1.7 (46%)[b]	3 (60%)
C_{max} (ng/mL)	872 (42%)	782 (37%)	3,680 (85%)
AUC_{tf} (ng•h/mL)	14,098 (38%)	13,400 (48%)	228,000 (25%)

RIBAVIRIN — ORAL

Ribavirin Capsules/Solution Mean (% CV) Pharmacokinetic Parameters in Adults[a]			
Pharmacokinetic parameter	Single-dose ribavirin 600 mg solution (n = 14)	Single-dose ribavirin 600 mg capsules (n = 12)	Multiple-dose ribavirin 600 mg twice daily capsules (n = 12)
Half-life (h)		43.6 (47%)	298 (30%)
Apparent volume of distribution (L)	—	2,825 (9%)[c]	—
Apparent clearance (L/h)	—	38.2 (40%)	—
Absolute bioavailability	—	64% (44%)[d]	—

[a] CV = coefficient of variation; T_{max} = time to maximal drug concentration; C_{max} = maximal drug concentration; AUC = area under the curve.
[b] n = 11.
[c] Data obtained from a single-dose pharmacokinetic study using ^{14}C-labeled ribavirin; n = 5.
[d] n = 6.

Absorption –

Tablets: Multiple-dose ribavirin pharmacokinetic data are available for patients with HCV who received ribavirin in combination with peginterferon alfa-2a. Following administration of 1,200 mg/day with food for a mean of 12 weeks ± standard deviation (SD) (n = 39; body weight more than 75 kg), the AUC_{0-12h} was 25,361 ± 7,110 ng•h/mL and C_{max} was 2,748 ± 818 ng/mL. The average T_{max} was 2 hours. There is extensive accumulation after multiple dosing (twice daily), such that the C_{max} at steady state was 4-fold higher than that of a single dose.

Trough ribavirin plasma concentrations following 12 weeks of dosing with food were 1,662 ± 545 ng/mL in patients with HCV infection who received 800 mg/day (n = 89) and 2,112 ± 810 ng/mL in patients who received 1,200 mg/day (n = 75; body weight more than 75 kg).

Capsules / Solution: Ribavirin was rapidly and extensively absorbed following oral administration. However, because of first-pass metabolism, the absolute bioavailability averaged 64% (44%). There was a linear relationship between dose and AUC from time zero to last measurable concentration (AUC_{tf}) following single doses of ribavirin 200 to 1,200 mg. The relationship between dose and C_{max} was curvilinear, tending to asymptote above single doses of 400 to 600 mg.

Upon multiple oral dosing, based on AUC_{12h}, a 6-fold accumulation of ribavirin was observed in plasma. Following oral dosing with 600 mg twice daily, steady state was reached by approximately 4 weeks, with mean steady-state plasma concentrations of 2,200 ng/mL (37%).

Effect of food: For ribavirin tablets, bioavailability of a single oral dose of ribavirin was increased by coadministration with a high-fat meal. The absorption was slowed (T_{max} was doubled), and the AUC_{0-192h} and C_{max} increased 42% and 66%, respectively, when taken with a high-fat meal compared with fasting conditions. Both AUC_{tf} and C_{max} increased 70% when ribavirin capsules were administered with a high-fat meal (841 kcal, 53.8 g of fat, 31.6 g of protein, and 57.4 g of carbohydrates) in a single-dose pharmacokinetic study.

Distribution –

Capsules / Solution: Ribavirin transport into nonplasma compartment has been most extensively studied in red blood cells, and has been identified to be primarily via an e_s-type equilibrative nucleoside transporter. This type of transporter is present on virtually all cell types and may account for the extensive volume of distribution. Ribavirin does not bind to plasma proteins.

Metabolism –

Tablets: The contribution of renal and hepatic pathways to ribavirin elimination after administration is not known. In vitro studies indicate that ribavirin is not a substrate of cytochrome P450 (CYP-450) enzymes.

Capsules / Solution: Ribavirin has 2 pathways of metabolism: a reversible phosphorylation pathway in nucleated cells and a degradative pathway involving deribosylation and amide hydrolysis to yield a triazole carboxylic acid metabolite.

Excretion –

Tablets: The terminal half-life following single-dose administration is approximately 120 to 170 hours. The total apparent clearance is approximately 26 L/h.

Capsules / Solution: Ribavirin and its triazole carboxamide and triazole carboxylic acid metabolites are excreted renally. After oral administration of ^{14}C-ribavirin 600 mg, approximately 61% and 12% of the radioactivity was eliminated in the urine and feces, respectively, in 336 hours. Unchanged ribavirin accounted for 17% of the administered dose. Upon discontinuation of dosing, the mean half-life was 298 (30%) hours, which probably reflects slow elimination from nonplasma compartments.

Special populations –

Renal function impairment:

• *Tablets* – The pharmacokinetics of ribavirin following administration in patients with renal impairment have not been studied, and there are limited data from clinical trials on administration of ribavirin in patients with CrCl less than 50 mL/min. Do not administer ribavirin to patients with CrCl less than 50 mL/min.

• *Capsules / Solution* – The pharmacokinetics of ribavirin were assessed after administration of a single oral dose of ribavirin 400 mg to non–HCV-infected subjects with varying degrees of renal dysfunction. The mean AUC_{tf} value was 3-fold greater in subjects with CrCl values between 10 and 30 mL/min compared with control subjects (CrCl more than 90 mL/min). In subjects with CrCl values between 30 and 60 mL/min, AUC_{tf} was 2-fold greater compared with control subjects. The increased AUC_{tf} appears to be due to reduction of renal and nonrenal clearance in these patients. Phase 3 efficacy trials included subjects with CrCl values of more than 50 mL/min. The multiple-dose pharmacokinetics of ribavirin cannot be accurately predicted in patients with renal impairment. Ribavirin is not effectively removed by hemodialysis. Do not treat patients with CrCl less than 50 mL/min with ribavirin.

Hepatic function impairment:

• *Capsules / Solution* – The effect of hepatic dysfunction was assessed after a single oral dose of ribavirin 600 mg. The mean AUC_{tf} values were not significantly different in subjects with mild, moderate, or severe hepatic dysfunction (Child-Pugh class A, B, or C) compared with control subjects. However, the mean C_{max} values increased with severity of hepatic dysfunction and were 2-fold greater in subjects with severe hepatic impairment compared with control subjects.

Children:

• *Capsules / Solution* –

Ribavirin Capsule Mean (% CV) Multiple-Dose Pharmacokinetic Parameters in Children		
Pharmacokinetic parameters	Ribavirin capsules 15 mg/kg/day as 2 divided doses (n = 17)	Interferon alfa-2b 3 million units/m² 3 times weekly (n = 54)
T_{max} (h)	1.9 (83%)	5.9 (36%)
C_{max} (ng/mL)	3,275 (25%)	51 (48%)
AUC[a]	29,774 (26%)	622 (48%)
Apparent clearance (L/h/kg)	0.27 (27%)	ND[b]

[a] AUC_{12} (ng•h/mL) for ribavirin; AUC_{0-24} (units•h/mL) for interferon alfa-2b.
[b] ND = not done.

Contraindications

Patients with hemoglobinopathies (eg, thalassemia major, sickle-cell anemia); women who are or who may become pregnant or in men whose female partners are pregnant because ribavirin may cause fetal harm when administered to a pregnant woman; autoimmune hepatitis; in cirrhotic chronic HCV monoinfected patients with hepatic decompensation (Child-Pugh score of more than 6; class B and C) before or during treatment, and in cirrhotic chronic HCV patients coinfected with HIV who have hepatic decompensation with a Child-Pugh score of 6 or more before or during treatment (in combination with peginterferon alfa-2a); known hypersensitivity reactions, such as Stevens-Johnson syndrome, toxic epidermal necrolysis, and erythema multiforme, to ribavirin or any component of the product; CrCl less than 50 mL/min; coadministration with didanosine.

Warnings/Precautions

➤*Monotherapy:* See the Warning box for more information.

➤*Combination therapy adverse reactions:* There are significant adverse reactions caused by ribavirin tablets/peginterferon alfa-2a therapy and by ribavirin capsules/interferon alfa-2b or peginterferon alfa-2b therapy, including severe depression and suicidal ideation, hemolytic anemia, suppression of bone marrow function, autoimmune and infectious disorders, pulmonary dysfunction, pancreatitis, and diabetes. Review the respective interferon alfa-2b, peginterferon alfa-2b, or peginterferon alfa-2a monographs and Medication Guides in their entirety for additional safety information prior to initiation of combination treatment.

➤*Suicidal ideation:* Suicidal ideation or suicide attempts occurred more frequently among children, primarily adolescents, compared with adults (2.4% vs 1%) during treatment and off-therapy follow-up.

➤*Hemolytic anemia:* The primary toxicity of ribavirin is hemolytic anemia (Hb less than 10 g/dL), which was observed in approximately 13% of ribavirin/peginterferon alfa-2a–treated patients and approximately 10% of ribavirin/interferon alfa-2b–treated patients in clinical trials. The anemia associated with ribavirin occurs within 1 to 2 weeks of initiation of therapy. Because the initial drop in Hb may be significant, it is advised that Hb or hematocrit be obtained pretreatment and at weeks 2 and 4 of therapy, or more frequently if clinically indicated. Then follow patients as clinically appropriate.

➤*Cardiovascular effects:* Fatal and nonfatal MIs have been reported in patients with anemia caused by ribavirin. Assess patients for underlying cardiac disease before initiation of ribavirin therapy. Before treatment, administer electrocardiograms (ECGs) to patients with preexisting disease, and monitor these patients appropriately during therapy. If there is any deterioration of cardiovascular status, suspend or discontinue therapy. Because cardiac disease may be worsened by drug-induced anemia, patients with a history of significant or unstable cardiac disease should not use ribavirin.

➤*Pulmonary effects:* Pulmonary symptoms, including dyspnea, pneumonia, pneumonitis, and pulmonary infiltrates, have been reported during therapy with ribavirin and alpha interferon. Occasional cases of fatal pneumonia have occurred. In addition, sarcoidosis or exacerbation of sarcoidosis has been reported. If there is evidence of pulmonary infiltrates or pulmonary impairment, closely monitor the patient and, if appropriate, discontinue treatment.

➤*Ophthalmologic disorders:* Ribavirin is used in combination therapy with alpha interferons. Decrease or loss of vision; retinopathy, including macular edema, retinal artery or vein, thrombosis, retinal hemorrhages, and cotton wool spots; optic neuritis; papilledema; and serous retinal detach-

RIBAVIRIN — ORAL

ment are induced or aggravated by treatment with alpha interferons. Give all patients an eye examination at baseline. Give patients with preexisting ophthalmologic disorders (eg, diabetic or hypertensive retinopathy) periodic ophthalmologic exams during combination therapy with alpha interferon treatment. Perform a prompt and complete eye examination in any patient who develops ocular symptoms. Discontinue combination therapy with alpha interferons in patients who develop new or worsening ophthalmologic disorders.

➤*Dental and periodontal disorders:* Dental and periodontal disorders have been reported in patients receiving ribavirin and interferon or peginterferon combination therapy. In addition, dry mouth could have a damaging effect on teeth and mucous membranes of the mouth during long-term treatment with the combination of ribavirin and interferon alfa-2b or pegylated interferon alfa-2b. Instruct patients to brush their teeth thoroughly twice daily and to have regular dental examinations. Advise patient that if vomiting occurs, to rinse out their mouth thoroughly afterwards.

➤*Pancreatitis:* Suspend ribavirin and interferon alfa-2b, peginterferon alfa-2b, or peginterferon alfa-2a therapy in patients with signs and symptoms of pancreatitis, and discontinue in patients with confirmed pancreatitis.

➤*Organ transplant recipients:* Safety and efficacy of interferon alfa-2b and peginterferon alfa-2b alone or in combination with ribavirin for the treatment of HCV in liver or other organ transplant recipients have not been established. In a small (N = 16), single-center, uncontrolled case experience, renal failure in renal allograft recipients receiving interferon alpha and ribavirin combination therapy was more frequent than expected from the center's previous experience with renal allograft recipients not receiving combination therapy. The relationship of the renal failure to renal allograft rejection is not clear.

➤*HIV or hepatitis B virus coinfection:* The safety and efficacy of peginterferon alfa-2b/ribavirin and interferon alfa-2b/ribavirin for the treatment of patients with HCV coinfected with hepatitis B virus or HIV and a CD4+ cell count less than 100 cells/mcL have not been established.

➤*Other infections and conditions:* The safety and efficacy of ribavirin with peginterferon alfa-2a, interferon alfa-2b, or peginterferon alfa-2b combination therapy for the treatment of HIV infection, adenovirus, respiratory syncytial virus, parainfluenza, or influenza infections have not been established. Do not use oral ribavirin for these indications. Consult the ribavirin inhalation monograph if ribavirin inhalation therapy is being considered.

The safety and efficacy of ribavirin and interferon alfa-2b or peginterferon alfa-2a combination therapy have not been established in patients with decompensated liver disease due to HCV infection or in patients who are nonresponders to interferon therapy.

➤*Hepatic effects:* Chronic HCV patients with cirrhosis may be at risk of hepatic decompensation and death when treated with alpha interferons. Cirrhotic chronic HCV patients coinfected with HIV receiving highly active antiretroviral therapy (HAART) and interferon alfa-2a, with or without ribavirin, appear to be at an increased risk for the development of hepatic decompensation compared with patients not receiving HAART. In study NR15961, among 129 chronic HCV/HIV cirrhotic patients receiving HAART, 11% of these patients across all treatment arms developed hepatic decompensation, which resulted in 6 deaths. All 14 patients were on nucleoside reverse transcriptase inhibitors (NRTIs), including abacavir, didanosine, lamivudine, stavudine, and zidovudine. These small numbers of patients do not permit discrimination between specific NRTIs or the associated risk. During treatment, closely monitor patients' clinical status and hepatic function, and discontinue peginterferon alfa-2a treatment immediately if decomposition (Child-Pugh score of 6 or more) is observed.

Discontinue ribavirin and peginterferon alfa-2a in patients who develop evidence of hepatic decompensation during treatment.

➤*Hypersensitivity reactions:* Severe acute hypersensitivity reactions (eg, urticaria, angioedema, bronchoconstriction, anaphylaxis) have been observed rarely during alpha interferon and ribavirin therapy. If such reactions occur, discontinue therapy and immediately institute appropriate medical therapy. Serious skin reactions, including vesiculobullous eruptions, reactions in the spectrum of Stevens-Johnson syndrome (erythema multiforme major) with varying degrees of skin and mucosal involvement, and exfoliative dermatitis (erythroderma), have been rarely reported in patients receiving peginterferon alfa-2a with and without ribavirin. Patients developing signs or symptoms of severe skin reactions must discontinue therapy.

Transient rashes do not necessitate interruption of treatment.

➤*Renal function impairment:* See Administration and Dosage for more information.

➤*Pregnancy: Category X.* Ribavirin has produced significant teratogenic effects (eg, malformation of skull, palate, eye, jaw, limbs, skeleton, GI tract) and/or embryocidal effects in all animal species in which adequate studies have been conducted. These effects occurred at doses as low as one-twentieth of the recommended human dose of ribavirin. The incidence and severity of teratogenic effects increased with escalation of the drug dose. Survival of fetuses and offspring was reduced.

Ribavirin may cause birth defects and/or death of the exposed fetus. Extreme care must be taken to avoid pregnancy in female patients and in female partners of male patients. Do not start ribavirin therapy until a report of a negative pregnancy test has been obtained immediately prior to planned initiation of therapy. Instruct male and female patients to use at least 2 forms of effective contraception during treatment and during the 6-month period after treatment has been stopped based on a multiple-dose half-life of ribavirin of 12 days. Perform pregnancy testing monthly during ribavirin therapy and for 6 months after therapy has stopped.

In conventional embryotoxicity/teratogenicity studies in rats and rabbits, observed no-effects dosage levels were well below those for proposed clinical use (0.3 mg/kg/day for rats and rabbits; approximately 0.06 times the recommended human 24-hour dose of ribavirin). No maternal toxicity or effects on offspring were observed in a perinatal/postnatal toxicity study in rats dosed orally at up to 1 mg/kg/day (estimated human equivalent dose of 0.17 mg/kg based on body surface area (BSA) adjustment for a 60 kg adult; approximately 0.01 times the maximum recommended human 24-hour dose of ribavirin).

Ribavirin is known to accumulate in intracellular components, where it is cleared very slowly. It is not known whether ribavirin contained in sperm will exert a potential teratogenic effect upon fertilization of the ova. In a study in rats, it was concluded that dominant lethality was not induced by ribavirin at doses of up to 200 mg/kg for 5 days (estimated human equivalent doses of 7.14 to 28.6 mg/kg based on BSA adjustment for a 60 kg adult; up to 1.7 times the maximum recommended human dose of ribavirin). However, because of the potential human teratogenic effects of ribavirin, advise male patients to take every precaution to avoid the risk of pregnancy in their female partners.

Pregnancy registry – A ribavirin pregnancy registry has been established to monitor maternal-fetal outcomes of pregnancies of female patients and female partners of male patients exposed to ribavirin during treatment and for 6 months following cessation of treatment. Health care providers and patients are encouraged to report such cases by calling 1-800-593-2214.

➤*Lactation:* It is not known if ribavirin is excreted in human milk. The molecular weight (approximately 244) and prolonged plasma elimination half-life (12 days) suggest that the drug will be excreted into breast milk. The effects of this exposure on a breast-feeding infant are unknown, but the drug causes toxicity in lactating animals and their offspring. Because many drugs are excreted in human milk and to avoid any potential for serious adverse reactions in breast-feeding infants from ribavirin, decide whether to discontinue breast-feeding or to delay or discontinue ribavirin, taking into consideration the importance of therapy to the mother.

➤*Children:*

Tablets – Safety and efficacy of ribavirin tablets have not been established in children younger than 18 years of age.

Capsules / Solution – During a 48-week course of therapy, there was a decrease in the rate of linear growth (mean percentile assignment decrease of 9%) and a decrease in the rate of weight gain (mean percentile assignment decrease of 13%). A general reversal of these trends was noted during the 24-week posttreatment period.

Suicidal ideation or suicide attempts occurred more frequently among children, primarily adolescents, compared with adult patients (2.4% vs 1%) during treatment and off-therapy follow-up. As in adult patients, children experienced anemia, neutropenia, and other psychiatric adverse reactions (eg, depression, emotional lability, somnolence).

Safety and effectiveness of *Rebetol*/peginterferon alfa-2b has not been established in children younger than 3 years of age. Safety and effectiveness of *Ribasphere*/peginterferon alfa-2b have not been established in children. For treatment with ribavirin/interferon alfa-2b, evidence of disease progression, such as hepatic inflammation and fibrosis, as well as prognostic factors for response, consider HCV genotype and viral load when deciding to treat a child. Weigh the benefits of treatment against the safety findings observed.

➤*Elderly:*

Tablets – The risk of toxic reactions to this drug may be greater in patients with impaired renal function. Do not administer ribavirin to patients with CrCl less than 50 mL/min.

Capsules / Solution – In clinical trials, elderly subjects had a higher frequency of anemia (67%) than younger patients.

In general, cautiously administer ribavirin to elderly patients, starting at the lower end of the dosing range, reflecting the greater frequency of decreased hepatic or cardiac function, and of concomitant disease or other drug therapy.

Ribavirin is known to be substantially excreted by the kidney, and the risk of toxic reactions to this drug may be greater in patients with renal impairment. Take care in dose selection because elderly patients often have decreased renal function. Monitor renal function and make dosage adjustments accordingly. Do not use ribavirin in elderly patients with CrCl less than 50 mL/min.

➤*Lab test abnormalities:* Peginterferon alfa-2b in combination with ribavirin may cause severe decreases in neutrophil and platelet counts, and hematologic, endocrine (eg, thyroid-stimulating hormone [TSH]), and hepatic abnormalities.

➤*Monitoring:* Assess patients for underlying cardiac disease before initiation of ribavirin therapy and appropriately monitor them during therapy. Measure HCV-RNA periodically during treatment.

Tablets – Before beginning ribavirin therapy, standard hematological and biochemical laboratory tests must be conducted for all patients. Pregnancy screening for women of childbearing potential must be done.

After initiation of therapy, perform hematological tests at 2 and 4 weeks and biochemical tests at 4 weeks. Perform additional testing periodically during therapy. Perform monthly pregnancy testing during combination therapy and for 6 months after discontinuing therapy.

RIBAVIRIN — ORAL

The following entrance criteria used for the clinical studies of ribavirin and peginterferon alfa-2a combination therapy may be considered as a guideline to acceptable baseline values for initiation of treatment:

- platelet count of 90,000 cells/mm^3 or more (as low as 75,000 cells/mm^3 in patients with cirrhosis)
- for *Copegus*, a platelet count as low as 70,000 cells/mm^3 in patients with chronic HCV and HIV
- absolute neutrophil count of 1,500 cells/mm^3 or more
- TSH and thyroxine (T_4) within normal limits or adequately controlled thyroid function
- ECG
- CD4+ cell count of 200 cells/mcL or more or CD4+ cell count of at least 100 cells/mcL but less than 200 cells/mcL and HIV-1 RNA less than 5,000 copies/mL in patients coinfected with HIV (*Copegus* only)
- Hb 12 g/dL or more for women and 13 g/dL or more for men in chronic HCV monoinfected patients
- Hb 11 g/dL or more for women and 12 g/dL or more for men in patients with chronic HCV and HIV (*Copegus* only)

The maximum drop in Hb usually occurred during the first 8 weeks of ribavirin therapy. Because of this initial acute drop in Hb, it is advised that a complete blood cell count (CBC) be obtained pretreatment and at weeks 2 and 4 of therapy, or more frequently if clinically indicated. Perform additional testing periodically during therapy. Follow patients as clinically appropriate.

Capsules / Oral solution – The following laboratory tests are recommended for all patients treated with ribavirin prior to beginning treatment and periodically thereafter:

- standard hematologic tests, including Hb (pretreatment, week 2, and week 4 of therapy, and as clinically appropriate), CBC and differential WBC counts, and platelet count
- liver function tests and TSH
- pregnancy, including monthly monitoring for women of childbearing potential and for 6 months after discontinuing therapy
- ECG

In the adult clinical trial, CBC (including Hb, neutrophil, and platelet counts) and chemistries (including AST, ALT, bilirubin, and uric acid) were measured during the treatment period at weeks 2, 4, 8, 12, and then at 6-week intervals or more frequently if abnormalities developed. In children, the same laboratory parameters were evaluated, with additional assessment of Hb at treatment week 6. TSH levels were measured every 12 weeks during the treatment period.

Drug Interactions

Ribavirin Drug Interactions

Precipitant drug	Object drug[a]		Description
Ribavirin/ Peginterferon alfa-2a	NRTIs (eg, didanosine, lamivudine, stavudine, zidovudine)	↑↓	Coadministration of ribavirin and didanosine is contraindicated. Fatal hepatic failure, peripheral neuropathy, pancreatitis, and symptomatic hyperlactatemia/ lactic acidosis have been reported. Ribavirin may antagonize the in vitro antiviral activity of lamivudine, stavudine, and zidovudine against HIV. Combination therapy with zidovudine, ribavirin, and peginterferon alfa-2a resulted in severe neutropenia and severe anemia. Use with caution. Monitor closely for treatment-associated toxicities. Consider dose reduction or discontinuation of ribavirin, peginterferon alfa-2a, or both if worsening toxicities occur.
Ribavirin	Thiopurines (eg, azathioprine, mercaptopurine)	↑	The risk of thiopurine-related myelosuppression (eg, pancytopenia) may be increased. If coadministration cannot be avoided, closely monitor for myelosuppression. Be prepared to discontinue one or both agents.
Ribavirin	Warfarin	↓	The anticoagulant action of warfarin may be decreased. Monitor international normalized ratio closely during the first 4 weeks of combination therapy and upon discontinuation.

[a] ↑ = object drug increased; ↓ = object drug decreased; ↑↓ = object drug both increased and decreased.

Adverse Reactions

➤*Tablets:*

Ribavirin / peginterferon alfa-2a –

Most common adverse reactions: The most common life-threatening or fatal reactions induced or aggravated by ribavirin/peginterferon alfa-2a were bacterial infections, depression, relapse of drug abuse/overdose, and suicide; each occurred at a frequency of less than 1%. Hepatic decompensation occurred in 2% of chronic HCV/HIV patients.

Nearly all patients in clinical trials experienced 1 or more adverse reaction. The most commonly reported adverse reactions were psychiatric reactions (including anxiety, depression, insomnia, and irritability) and flu-like symptoms (such as fatigue, headache, myalgia, pyrexia, and rigors). Other common reactions were alopecia, anorexia, arthralgia, diarrhea, injection-site reactions, nausea and vomiting, and pruritus.

Discontinuation of therapy: Ten percent of chronic HCV monoinfected patients receiving 48 weeks of therapy with peginterferon alfa-2a in combination with ribavirin discontinued therapy; 16% of chronic HCV/HIV coinfected patients discontinued therapy. The most common reasons for discontinuation of therapy were dermatologic and GI disorders, flu-like syndrome (eg, fatigue, headache, lethargy), laboratory abnormalities (anemia, neutropenia, and thrombocytopenia), and psychiatric reactions.

Dosage modification: Overall, 39% of patients with chronic HCV or chronic HCV/HIV required modification of peginterferon alfa-2a and/or ribavirin therapy.

The most common reason for dose modification of ribavirin in chronic HCV and chronic HCV/HIV patients was anemia (22% and 16%, respectively). The ribavirin dose was reduced in 21% of patients receiving 1,000 to 1,200 mg for 48 weeks and 12% in patients receiving 800 mg for 24 weeks.

The most common reason for dose modification of peginterferon alfa-2a in chronic HCV and chronic HCV/HIV patients was laboratory abnormalities, neutropenia (20% and 27%, respectively), and thrombocytopenia (4% and 6%, respectively). The peginterferon alfa-2a dose was reduced in 12% of patients receiving ribavirin 1,000 to 1,200 mg tablets for 48 weeks and in 7% of patients receiving ribavirin 800 mg tablets for 24 weeks.

24- vs 48-week therapy duration: Chronic HCV monoinfected patients treated for 24 weeks with peginterferon alfa-2a and ribavirin 800 mg were observed to have a lower incidence of the following: serious adverse reactions (3% vs 10%), Hb less than 10 g/dL (3% vs 15%), dose modification of peginterferon alfa-2a (30% vs 36%) and ribavirin (19% vs 38%), and withdrawal from treatment (5% vs 15%), compared with patients treated for 48 weeks with peginterferon alfa-2a and ribavirin 1,000 or 1,200 mg. On the other hand, the overall incidence of adverse reactions appeared to be similar in the 2 treatment groups.

Adverse reactions (5% or more):

Ribavirin Tablet Adverse Reactions (≥ 5%)

Adverse reactions	Peginterferon alfa-2a 180 mcg + ribavirin 1,000 or 1,200 mg tablets 48 weeks (n = 451)	Interferon alfa-2b + ribavirin 1,000 or 1,200 mg capsules 48 weeks (n = 443)
CNS		
Anxiety/ Irritability/ Nervousness	33%	38%
Asthenia/Fatigue	65%	68%
Depression	20%	28%
Dizziness (excluding vertigo)	14%	14%
Headache	43%	49%
Impaired concentration	10%	13%
Insomnia	30%	37%
Memory impairment	6%	5%
Mood alteration	5%	6%
Rigors	25%	37%
Dermatologic		
Alopecia	28%	33%
Dermatitis	16%	13%
Dry skin	10%	13%
Eczema	5%	4%
Injection-site reaction	23%	16%
Pruritus	19%	18%
Rash	8%	5%
Sweating increased	6%	5%
GI		
Abdominal pain	8%	9%
Anorexia	24%	26%
Diarrhea	11%	10%
Dry mouth	4%	7%
Dyspepsia	6%	5%
Nausea/Vomiting	25%	29%
Weight decrease	10%	10%

RIBAVIRIN — ORAL

Ribavirin Tablet Adverse Reactions (≥ 5%)		
Adverse reactions	Peginterferon alfa-2a 180 mcg + ribavirin 1,000 or 1,200 mg tablets 48 weeks (n = 451)	Interferon alfa-2b + ribavirin 1,000 or 1,200 mg capsules 48 weeks (n = 443)
Hematologic[a]		
Anemia	11%	11%
Lymphopenia	14%	12%
Neutropenia	27%	8%
Thrombocytopenia	5%	< 1%
Musculoskeletal		
Arthralgia	22%	23%
Back pain	5%	5%
Myalgia	40%	49%
Respiratory		
Cough	10%	7%
Dyspnea	13%	14%
Dyspnea, exertional	4%	7%
Miscellaneous		
Hypothyroidism	4%	5%
Overall resistance mechanism disorders	12%	10%
Pain	10%	9%
Pyrexia	41%	55%
Vision blurred	5%	2%

[a] Severe hematologic abnormalities (lymphocyte < 0.5×10^9/L; Hb < 10 g/dL; neutrophil < 0.75×10^9/L; platelet < 50×10^9/L).

Serious adverse reactions: In all studies, 1 or more serious adverse reaction occurred in 10% of chronic HCV monoinfected patients and in 19% of chronic HCV/HIV patients receiving peginterferon alfa-2a alone or in combination with ribavirin. The most common serious adverse reaction (3% in chronic HCV; 5% in chronic HCV/HIV) was bacterial infection (eg, endocarditis, osteomyelitis, pneumonia, pyelonephritis, sepsis). Other serious adverse reactions that occurred at a frequency of less than 1% included the following: aggression, angina, anxiety, aplastic anemia, arrhythmia, autoimmune phenomena (eg, hyperthyroidism, hypothyroidism, sarcoidosis, rheumatoid arthritis, systemic lupus erythematous), cerebral hemorrhage, cholangitis, colitis, coma, corneal ulcer, diabetes mellitus, drug abuse and drug overdose, fatty liver, GI bleeding, hallucination, hepatic dysfunction, myositis, pancreatitis, peptic ulcer, peripheral neuropathy, psychosis, psychotic disorder, pulmonary embolism, suicidal ideation, suicide, and thrombotic thrombocytopenic purpura.

Chronic hepatitis C virus with HIV coinfection – The adverse reaction profile of coinfected patients treated with peginterferon alfa-2a and ribavirin in study NR15961 was generally similar to that shown for monoinfected patients. Reactions occurring more frequently in coinfected patients were neutropenia (40%), weight decrease (16%), anemia (14%), mood alteration (9%), and thrombocytopenia (8%).

➤*Capsules/Solution:*

Common adverse reactions – More than 96% of all subjects in clinical trials experienced one or more adverse reactions. The most commonly reported adverse reactions in adult subjects receiving peginterferon alfa-2b or interferon alfa-2b in combination with ribavirin were anxiety/emotional lability/irritability, fatigue/asthenia, fever, headache, injection-site inflammation/reaction, myalgia, nausea, and rigors. The most common adverse reactions in children 3 years of age and older receiving ribavirin in combination with peginterferon alfa-2b or interferon alfa-2b were anorexia, fatigue, headache, injection-site erythema, neutropenia, pyrexia, and vomiting.

Serious adverse reactions – Serious adverse reactions have occurred in approximately 12% of subjects in clinical trials with peginterferon alfa-2b with or without ribavirin. The most common serious reactions occurring in subjects treated with peginterferon alfa-2b and ribavirin were depression and suicidal ideation, each occurring at a frequency of less than 1%. Suicidal ideation or attempts occurred more frequently among children, primarily adolescents, compared with adults (2.4% vs 1%) during treatment and off-therapy follow-up. The most common fatal reactions occurring in subjects treated with peginterferon alfa-2b and ribavirin was cardiac arrest, suicide ideation, and suicide attempt, all occurring in less than 1% of subjects.

Anemia – The primary toxicity of ribavirin is hemolytic anemia. Reductions in Hb levels occurred within the first 1 to 2 weeks of oral therapy. Cardiac and pulmonary reactions associated with anemia occurred in approximately 10% of patients.

Ribavirin/Peginterferon alfa-2b –

Adults: Overall, in clinical trials, 14% of patients receiving ribavirin/peginterferon alfa-2b combination therapy discontinued therapy compared with 13% of patients treated with ribavirin/interferon alfa-2b. The most common reasons for discontinuation of therapy were related to psychiatric, systemic (eg, fatigue, headache), or GI adverse reactions.

Ribavirin Combination Therapy Adverse Reactions in Adults (> 5%)		
Adverse reactions[a]	Peginterferon alfa-2b 1.5 mcg/kg + ribavirin (n = 511)	Interferon alfa-2b + ribavirin (n = 505)
CNS		
Agitation	8%	5%
Anxiety/Emotional lability/Irritability	47%	47%
Asthenia/Fatigue	66%	63%
Depression	31%	34%
Dizziness	21%	17%
Headache	62%	58%
Impaired concentration	17%	21%
Insomnia	40%	41%
Malaise	4%	6%
Nervousness	6%	6%
Rigors	48%	41%
Dermatologic		
Alopecia	36%	32%
Flushing	4%	3%
Injection-site inflammation	25%	18%
Injection-site reaction	58%	36%
Pruritus	29%	28%
Rash	24%	23%
Skin dry	24%	23%
Sweating increased	11%	7%
GI		
Abdominal pain	13%	13%
Anorexia	32%	27%
Constipation	5%	5%
Diarrhea	22%	17%
Dry mouth	12%	8%
Dyspepsia	9%	8%
Nausea	43%	33%
Right upper quadrant pain	12%	6%
Vomiting	14%	12%
Weight decrease	29%	20%
Hematologic		
Anemia	12%	17%
Leukopenia	6%	5%
Neutropenia	26%	14%
Thrombocytopenia	5%	2%
Musculoskeletal		
Arthralgia	34%	28%
Musculoskeletal pain	21%	19%
Myalgia	56%	50%
Respiratory		
Coughing	23%	16%
Dyspnea	26%	24%
Pharyngitis	12%	13%
Rhinitis	8%	6%
Sinusitis	6%	5%
Special senses		
Conjunctivitis	4%	5%
Taste perversion	9%	4%
Vision blurred	5%	6%
Miscellaneous		
Chest pain	8%	7%
Fever	46%	33%
Hepatomegaly	4%	4%
Hypothyroidism	5%	4%
Infection, fungal	6%	1%

RIBAVIRIN — ORAL

Ribavirin Combination Therapy Adverse Reactions in Adults (> 5%)		
Adverse reactions[a]	Peginterferon alfa-2b 1.5 mcg/kg + ribavirin (n = 511)	Interferon alfa-2b + ribavirin (n = 505)
Infection, viral	12%	12%
Menstrual disorder	7%	6%

[a] A patient may have reported > 1 adverse reaction within a body system/organ class category.

Ribavirin Combination Therapy Treatment-Related Adverse Reactions (≥ 10%)			
Adverse reactions	Peginterferon alfa-2b 1.5 mcg/kg with ribavirin capsules (n = 1,019)	Peginterferon alfa-2b 1 mcg/kg with ribavirin capsules (n = 1,016)	Peginterferon alfa-2a 180 mcg with ribavirin tablets (n = 1,035)
CNS			
Anxiety	11%	11%	10%
Depression	25%	19%	20%
Dizziness	16%	14%	13%
Fatigue	67%	68%	64%
Headache	50%	47%	41%
Insomnia	38%	37%	41%
Irritability	25%	25%	25%
Dermatologic			
Alopecia	23%	20%	17%
Dry skin	11%	11%	12%
Pruritus	18%	15%	19%
Rash	29%	25%	34%
GI			
Abdominal pain	10%	10%	10%
Anorexia	29%	25%	21%
Diarrhea	15%	16%	14%
Nausea	40%	35%	34%
Vomiting	12%	10%	9%
Weight decreased	13%	10%	10%
Hematologic/Lymphatic			
Anemia	35%	30%	34%
Leukopenia	9%	7%	10%
Neutropenia	26%	19%	31%
Musculoskeletal			
Arthralgia	21%	22%	22%
Myalgia	27%	26%	22%
Respiratory			
Cough	15%	16%	17%
Dyspnea	21%	20%	22%
Miscellaneous			
Chills	39%	36%	23%
Influenza-like illness	16%	15%	15%
Injection-site reactions	34%	35%	23%
Pyrexia	35%	32%	21%
Unspecified pain	12%	13%	9%

• *Serious adverse reactions* – The incidence of serious adverse reactions was comparable in all studies. In study 3, there was a similar incidence of serious adverse reactions reported for the weight-based ribavirin group (12%) and with the flat-dose ribavirin regimen. In study 2, the incidence of serious adverse reactions was 17% in the peginterferon alfa-2b/ribavirin groups compared with 14% in the interferon alfa-2b/ribavirin group.

In many, but not all cases, adverse reactions resolved after dose reduction or discontinuation of therapy. Some subjects experienced ongoing or new serious adverse reactions during the 6-month follow-up period. In study 2, many subjects continued to experience adverse reactions several months after discontinuation of therapy. By the end of the 6-month follow-up period, the incidence of ongoing adverse reactions by body class in the peginterferon alfa-2b 1.5 mcg/ribavirin group was 33% (psychiatric), 20% (musculoskeletal), and 10% (endocrine and for GI). In approximately 10% to 15% of subjects, fatigue, headache, and weight loss had not resolved.

There have been 31 subject deaths that occurred during treatment or during follow-up in these clinical trials. In study 1, there was 1 suicide in a subject receiving peginterferon alfa-2b monotherapy and 2 deaths among subjects receiving interferon alfa-2b monotherapy (1 murder/suicide and 1 sudden death). In study 2, there was 1 suicide in a subject receiving peginterferon alfa-2b/ribavirin and 1 subject death in the interferon alfa-2b/ribavirin group (motor vehicle accident). There were 31 deaths that occurred during treatment or during follow-up in the 3 clinical trials. In study 3, there were 14 deaths, 2 of which were probable suicides, and 1 was an unexplained death in a person with a relevant medical history of depression. In study 4, there were 12 deaths, 6 of which occurred in subjects who received peginterferon alfa-2b/ribavirin, 5 in the peginterferon alfa-2b 1.5 mcg/ribavirin arm (n = 1,019) and 1 in the peginterferon alfa-2b 1 mcg/ribavirin arm (n = 1,016), and 6 of which occurred in subjects receiving peginterferon alfa-2a/ribavirin tablets (n = 1,035). There were 3 suicides that occurred during the off-treatment follow-up period in subjects who received peginterferon alfa-2b (1.5 mcg/kg)/ribavirin.

• *Discontinuation of therapy* – In studies 1 and 2, 10% to 14% of subjects receiving peginterferon alfa-2b alone or in combination with ribavirin discontinued therapy compared with 6% treated with interferon alfa-2b alone and 13% treated with interferon alfa-2b in combination with ribavirin. Similarly, in study 3, 15% of subjects receiving peginterferon alfa-2b in combination with weight-based ribavirin and 14% of subjects receiving peginterferon alfa-2b and flat-dose ribavirin discontinued therapy because of an adverse reaction. The most common reasons for discontinuation of therapy were related to known interferon effects of psychiatric, systemic (eg, fatigue, headache), or GI adverse reactions. In study 4, 13% of subjects in the peginterferon alfa-2b 1.5 mcg/ribavirin arm, 10% in the peginterferon alfa-2b 1 mcg/ribavirin arm, and 13% in the peginterferon alfa-2a 180 mcg/ribavirin tablet arm discontinued because of adverse reactions.

• *Dosage reduction* – In study 2, dose reductions because of adverse reactions occurred in 42% of subjects receiving peginterferon alfa-2b (1.5 mcg/kg)/ribavirin and in 34% of those receiving interferon alfa-2b/ribavirin. The majority (57%) of subjects weighing 60 kg or less receiving peginterferon alfa-2b (1.5 mcg/kg)/ribavirin required dose reduction. Reductions of interferon were dose related (peginterferon alfa-2b 1.5 mcg/kg more than peginterferon alfa-2b 0.5 mcg/kg or interferon alfa-2b), 40%, 27%, and 28%, respectively. Dose reductions for ribavirin were similar across all 3 groups (33% to 35%). The most common reasons for dose modifications were neutropenia (18%) or anemia (9%). Other common reasons included depression, fatigue, nausea, and thrombocytopenia. In study 3, dose modifications because of adverse reactions occurred more frequently with weight-based dosing compared with flat dosing (29% and 23%, respectively). In study 4, 16% of subjects had a dose reduction of peginterferon alfa-2b to 1 mcg/kg in combination with ribavirin, with an additional 4% requiring a second dose reduction of peginterferon alfa-2b to 0.5 mcg/kg because of adverse reactions, compared with 15% of subjects in the peginterferon alfa-2a/ribavirin tablet arm who required a dosage reduction to 135 mcg/wk with peginterferon alfa-2a, with an additional 7% in the peginterferon alfa-2a/ribavirin tablet arm requiring a second dosage reduction to 90 mcg/wk with peginterferon alfa-2a.

• *Most common adverse reactions* – In the peginterferon alfa-2b/ribavirin combination trials, the most common adverse reactions were psychiatric and occurred among 77% of subjects in study 2 and 68% to 69% of subjects in study 3. These psychiatric adverse reactions most commonly included depression, insomnia, and irritability, each reported by approximately 30% to 40% of subjects in all treatment groups. Suicidal behavior (ideation, attempts, and suicides) occurred in 2% of all subjects during treatment or during follow-up after treatment cessation. In study 4, psychiatric adverse reactions occurred in 58% of subjects in the peginterferon alfa-2b 1.5 mcg/ribavirin arm, 55% of subjects in the peginterferon alfa-2b 1 mcg/ribavirin arm, and 57% of subjects in the peginterferon alfa-2a 180 mcg/ribavirin tablet arm.

Peginterferon alfa-2b induced fatigue or headache in approximately two-thirds of subjects, with fever or rigors in approximately half of the subjects. The severity of some of these systemic symptoms (eg, fever, headache) tends to decrease as treatment continues. In studies 1 and 2, application-site inflammation and reaction (eg, bruise, irritation, itchiness) occurred at approximately twice the incidence with peginterferon alfa-2b therapies (in up to 75% of subjects) compared with interferon alfa-2b. However, injection-site pain was infrequent (2% to 3%) in all groups. In study 3, there was a 23% to 24% incidence overall for injection-site reactions or inflammation.

Children:

• *Most common adverse reactions* – In the pediatric study, the most prevalent adverse reactions in all subjects were pyrexia (80%), headache (62%), neutropenia (33%), fatigue (30%), anorexia (29%), injection-site erythema (29%), and vomiting (27%). The majority of adverse reactions reported in the study were mild or moderate in severity.

• *Severe/important adverse reactions* – Severe adverse reactions were reported in 7% of all subjects and included pyrexia (4%), headache (1%), injection-site pain (1%), neutropenia (1%), and pain in extremity (1%). Important adverse reactions that occurred in this subject population were nervousness (7%), aggression (3%), anger (2%), and depression (1%). Five subjects received levothyroxine treatment, 3 with clinical hypothyroidism and 2 with asymptomatic TSH elevations.

• *Dosage modifications* – Dose modifications of peginterferon alfa-2b and/or ribavirin were required in 25% of subjects because of treatment-related adverse reactions, most commonly for anemia, neutropenia, and weight loss.

• *Discontinuation of therapy* – Two (2%) subjects discontinued therapy as a result of an adverse reaction.

Ribavirin Combination Therapy Adverse Reactions (≥ 10%) in Children	
Adverse reactions	Peginterferon alfa-2b + ribavirin (N = 107)
CNS	
Asthenia	15%

RIBAVIRIN — ORAL

Ribavirin Combination Therapy Adverse Reactions (≥ 10%) in Children	
Adverse reactions	Peginterferon alfa-2b + ribavirin (N = 107)
Dizziness	14%
Fatigue	30%
Headache	62%
GI	
Abdominal pain	21%
Anorexia	29%
Decreased appetite	22%
Nausea	18%
Upper abdominal pain	12%
Vomiting	27%
Hematologic	
Anemia	11%
Leukopenia	10%
Neutropenia	33%
Musculoskeletal	
Arthralgia	17%
Myalgia	17%
Miscellaneous	
Alopecia	17%
Chills	21%
Injection-site erythema	29%
Irritability	14%
Pyrexia	80%
Weight loss	19%

Data on the effects of peginterferon alfa-2b plus ribavirin on growth come from an open-label study in subjects 3 to 17 years of age, and weight and height changes are compared with US normative population data. In general, the weight and height gain of children treated with peginterferon alfa-2b plus ribavirin lags behind that predicted by normative population data for the entire length of treatment. Approximately 6 months posttreatment (follow-up week 24), subjects had weight gain rebounds and regained their weight to the 53rd percentile, above the average of the normative population and similar to that predicted by their average baseline weight (57th percentile). Approximately 6 months posttreatment, height gain stabilized and subjects treated with peginterferon alfa-2b plus ribavirin had an average height in the 44th percentile, which was less than the average of the normative population and less than their average baseline height (51st percentile). Severely inhibited growth velocity (below the 3rd percentile) was observed in 70% of the subjects while on treatment. Of the subjects experiencing severely inhibited growth, 20% had continued inhibited growth velocity (below the 3rd percentile) after 6 months of follow-up.

Among the boys studied, the age groups of 3 to 11 years and 12 to 17 years had similar height percentile decreases of approximately 5 percentiles after 6 months posttreatment; weight gain continued to be similar to their average baseline percentile. Girls 3 to 11 years of age treated for 48 weeks had the largest average drop in height and weight percentiles (13th percentiles and 7th percentiles, respectively), whereas girls 12 to 17 years of age continued along their average baseline height and weight percentiles after 6 months posttreatment.

Ribavirin/Interferon alfa-2b –

Adults: In clinical trials, 19% and 6% of previously untreated and relapse patients, respectively, discontinued therapy because of adverse reactions in the combination arms compared with 13% and 3% in the interferon arms.

Children: In clinical trials of 118 children 3 to 16 years of age, 6% discontinued therapy because of adverse reactions. Dose modifications were required in 30% of patients, most commonly for anemia and neutropenia. Anorexia, emotional lability, fever, injection-site disorders, and vomiting occurred more frequently in children compared with adults. Conversely, children experienced less arthralgia, dyspepsia, dyspnea, fatigue, impaired concentration, insomnia, irritability, and pruritus compared with adults.

Ribavirin Adverse Reactions: Previously Untreated and Relapse Patients							
	Previously untreated adults				Relapsed adults		Previously untreated children
	24 weeks of treatment		48 weeks of treatment		24 weeks of treatment		48 weeks of treatment
Adverse reactions[a]	Interferon alfa-2b + ribavirin (n = 228)	Interferon alfa-2b + placebo (n = 231)	Interferon alfa-2b + ribavirin (n = 228)	Interferon alfa-2b + placebo (n = 225)	Interferon alfa-2b + ribavirin (n = 77)	Interferon alfa-2b + placebo (n = 76)	Interferon alfa-2b + ribavirin (n = 118)
CNS							
Asthenia	9%	4%	9%	9%	10%	4%	5%
Depression	32%	25%	36%	37%	23%	14%	13%
Dizziness	17%	15%	23%	19%	26%	21%	20%
Emotional lability	7%	6%	11%	8%	12%	8%	16%
Fatigue	68%	62%	70%	72%	60%	53%	58%
Headache	63%	63%	66%	67%	66%	68%	69%
Impaired concentration	11%	14%	14%	14%	10%	12%	5%
Insomnia	39%	27%	39%	30%	26%	25%	14%
Irritability	23%	19%	32%	27%	25%	20%	10%
Nervousness	4%	2%	4%	4%	5%	4%	3%
Rigors	40%	32%	42%	39%	43%	37%	25%
Dermatologic							
Alopecia	28%	27%	32%	28%	27%	26%	23%
Injection-site inflammation	13%	10%	12%	14%	6%	8%	14%
Injection-site reaction	7%	9%	8%	9%	5%	3%	19%
Pruritus	21%	9%	19%	8%	13%	4%	12%
Rash	20%	9%	28%	8%	21%	5%	17%
GI							
Anorexia	27%	16%	25%	19%	21%	14%	51%
Dyspepsia	14%	6%	16%	9%	16%	9%	< 1%
Nausea	38%	35%	46%	33%	47%	33%	33%
Vomiting	11%	10%	9%	13%	12%	8%	42%
Musculoskeletal							
Arthralgia	30%	27%	33%	36%	29%	29%	15%
Musculoskeletal pain	20%	26%	28%	32%	22%	28%	21%
Myalgia	61%	57%	64%	63%	61%	58%	32%
Respiratory							
Dyspnea	19%	9%	18%	10%	17%	12%	5%
Sinusitis	9%	7%	10%	14%	12%	7%	< 1%
Miscellaneous							
Chest pain	5%	4%	9%	8%	6%	7%	5%
Fever	37%	35%	41%	40%	32%	36%	61%
Influenza-like symptoms	14%	18%	18%	20%	13%	13%	31%
Taste perversion	7%	4%	8%	4%	6%	5%	< 1%

[a] Patients reporting ≥ 1 adverse reaction. A patient may have reported > 1 adverse reaction within a body system/organ class category.

Lab test abnormalities –

Tablets:

- *Hemoglobin* – Anemia (Hb less than 10 g/dL) due to hemolysis is the most significant toxicity of ribavirin therapy. Hb less than 10 g/dL was observed in 13% of ribavirin/peginterferon alfa-2a patients in clinical trials. The maximum drop in Hb occurred during the first 8 weeks of initiation of ribavirin therapy.

Capsules:

- *Ribavirin/Interferon alfa-2b –*

  Hemoglobin: Hb decreases among patients receiving ribavirin therapy began at week 1, with stabilization by week 4. In previously untreated patients who were treated for 48 weeks, the mean maximum decrease from baseline was 3.1 g/dL in the US study and 2.9 g/dL in the international study. In relapse patients, the mean maximum decrease from baseline was 2.8 g/dL in the US study and 2.6 g/dL in the international study. Hb values returned to pretreatment levels within 4 to 8 weeks of cessation of therapy in most patients.

  Bilirubin and uric acid: Increases in bilirubin and uric acid associated with hemolysis were noted in clinical trials. Most were moderate biochemical changes and were reversed within 4 weeks after treatment discontinuation. This observation occurs most frequently in patients with a previous diagnosis of Gilbert syndrome. This has not been associated with hepatic impairment or clinical morbidity.

RIBAVIRIN — ORAL

Ribavirin/Interferon Alfa-2b Laboratory Abnormalities

Laboratory parameter	Previously untreated adults, 24 weeks of treatment: Interferon alfa-2b + ribavirin (n = 228)	Previously untreated adults, 24 weeks of treatment: Interferon alfa-2b + placebo (n = 231)	Previously untreated adults, 48 weeks of treatment: Interferon alfa-2b + ribavirin (n = 228)	Previously untreated adults, 48 weeks of treatment: Interferon alfa-2b + placebo (n = 225)	Relapsed adults, 24 weeks of treatment: Interferon alfa-2b + ribavirin (n = 77)	Relapsed adults, 24 weeks of treatment: Interferon alfa-2b + placebo (n = 76)	Previously untreated children, 48 weeks of treatment: Interferon alfa-2b + ribavirin (n = 118)
Hemoglobin (g/dL)							
9.5 to 10.9	24%	1%	32%	1%	21%	3%	24%
8 to 9.4	5%	0%	4%	0%	4%	0%	3%
6.5 to 7.9	0%	0%	0%	0.4%	0%	0%	0%
< 6.5	0%	0%	0%	0%	0%	0%	0%
Leukocytes (× 10^9/L)							
2 to 2.9	40%	20%	38%	23%	45%	26%	35%
1.5 to 1.9	4%	1%	9%	2%	5%	3%	8%
1 to 1.4	0.9%	0%	2%	0%	0%	0%	0%
< 1	0%	0%	0%	0%	0%	0%	0%
Neutrophils (× 10^9/L)							
1 to 1.49	30%	32%	31%	44%	42%	34%	37%
0.75 to 0.99	14%	15%	14%	11%	16%	18%	15%
0.5 to 0.74	9%	9%	14%	7%	8%	4%	16%
< 0.5	11%	8%	11%	5%	5%	8%	3%
Platelets (× 10^9/L)							
70 to 99	9%	11%	11%	14%	6%	12%	0.8%
50 to 69	2%	3%	2%	3%	0%	5%	2%
30 to 49	0%	0.4%	0%	0.4%	0%	0%	0%
< 30	0.9%	0%	1%	0.9%	0%	0%	0%
Total bilirubin (mg/dL)							
1.5 to 3	27%	13%	32%	13%	21%	7%	2%
3.1 to 6	0.9%	0.4%	2%	0%	3%	0%	0%
6.1 to 12	0%	0%	0.4%	0%	0%	0%	0%
> 12	0%	0%	0%	0%	0%	0%	0%

• *Ribavirin/Peginterferon alfa-2b* –

Ribavirin/Peginterferon Alfa-2b Laboratory Abnormalities

Laboratory parameter	Adults: Ribavirin/ peginterferon alfa-2b (n = 511)	Adults: Ribavirin/ interferon alfa-2b (n = 505)	Children: Ribavirin/ peginterferon alfa-2b (n = 107)[a]
ALT			
2 × baseline	0.6%	0.2%	1%
2.1 to 5 × baseline	3%	1%	5%
5.1 to 10 × baseline	0%	0%	3%
> 10 × baseline	0%	0%	—
Hemoglobin (g/dL)			
9.5 to < 11	26%	27%	30%
8 to < 9.5	3%	3%	2%
6.5 to 7.9	0.2%	0.2%	
Leukocytes (× 10^9/L)			
2 to 2.9	46%	41%	39%
1.5 to < 2	24%	8%	3%
1 to 1.4	5%	1%	
Neutrophils (× 10^9/L)			
1 to 1.5	33%	37%	35%
0.75 to < 1	25%	13%	26%
0.5 to 0.75	18%	7%	13%
< 0.5	4%	2%	3%
Platelets (× 10^9/L)			
70 to 100	15%	5%	1%
50 to < 70	3%	0.8%	
30 to 49	0.2%	0.2%	
25 to < 50	—	—	1%
Total bilirubin (mg/dL)			
1.5 to 3	10%	13%	—
1.26 to 2.59 × ULN[b]	—	—	7%
3.1 to 6	0.6%	0.2%	
6.1 to 12	0%	0.2%	

[a] The table summarizes the worst category observed within the period per subject per laboratory test. Only subjects with ≥ 1 treatment value for a given laboratory test are included.
[b] ULN = upper limit of normal.

Hemoglobin: Hb levels decreased to less than 11 g/dL in approximately 30% of subjects in study 2. In study 3, 47% of subjects receiving weight-based dosing of ribavirin and 33% receiving flat-dose ribavirin had decreases in Hb levels of less than 11 g/dL. Reductions in Hb to less than 9 g/dL occurred more frequently in subjects receiving weight-based dosing compared with flat dosing (4% and 2%, respectively). In study 2, dose modification was required in 9% and 13% of subjects in the peginterferon alfa-2b/ribavirin and interferon alfa-2b/ribavirin groups. In study 4, patients receiving peginterferon alfa-2b (1.5 mcg/kg)/ribavirin had decreases in Hb levels to between 8.5 and less than 10 g/dL (28%) and to less than 8.5 g/dL (3%), whereas in patients receiving peginterferon alfa-2a 180 mcg/ribavirin tablets, these decreases occurred in 26% and 4% of subjects, respectively. On average, Hb levels become stable by treatment weeks 4 to 6. The typical pattern observed was a decrease in Hb levels by treatment week 4, followed by stabilization and a plateau, which was maintained to the end of treatment. In the peginterferon alfa-2b monotherapy trial, Hb decreases were generally mild, and dose modifications were rarely necessary.

Neutrophils: Decreases in neutrophil counts were observed in a majority (85%) of adults treated with combination therapy with ribavirin in study 2 and interferon alfa-2b/ribavirin (60%). Severe, potentially life-threatening neutropenia (less than 0.5 × 10^9/L) occurred in 2% of subjects treated with interferon alfa-2b/ribavirin and in approximately 4% of subjects treated with peginterferon alfa-2b/ribavirin in study 2. Subjects receiving peginterferon alfa-2b/ribavirin (18%) in study 2 required modification of interferon dosage. Few subjects (less than 1%) required permanent discontinuation of treatment. Neutrophil counts generally return to pretreatment levels 4 weeks after cessation of therapy.

RIBAVIRIN — ORAL

Platelets: Platelet counts decreased to less than 100,000/mm^3 in approximately 20% of subjects treated with peginterferon alfa-2b alone or with ribavirin and in 6% of adult subjects treated with interferon alfa-2b/ribavirin. Severe decreases in platelet counts (less than 50,000/mm^3) occur in less than 4% of adult subjects. Subjects may require discontinuation or dose modification as a result of platelet decreases. In study 2, 1% or 3% of subjects required dose modification of interferon alfa-2b or peginterferon alfa-2b, respectively. Platelet counts generally returned to pretreatment levels 4 weeks after the cessation of therapy.

Thyroid function: Development of TSH abnormalities, with and without clinical manifestations, are associated with interferon therapies. In study 2, clinically apparent thyroid disorders occur among subjects treated with either interferon alfa-2b or peginterferon alfa-2b (with or without ribavirin) at a similar incidence (5% for hypothyroidism and 3% for hyperthyroidism). Subjects developed new-onset TSH abnormalities while on treatment and during the follow-up period. At the end of the follow-up period, 7% of subjects still had abnormal TSH values.

Bilirubin and uric acid: In study 2, 10% to 14% of subjects developed hyperbilirubinemia and 33% to 38% developed hyperuricemia in association with hemolysis. Six subjects developed mild to moderate gout.

➤*Postmarketing:*

Hematologic/Lymphatic – Aplastic anemia, pure red cell aplasia.

Special senses – Hearing disorder, hearing loss, serous retinal detachment, vertigo.

Miscellaneous – Dehydration, diabetes, pulmonary hypertension, serious skin reactions.

Overdosage

➤*Symptoms:*

Tablets – No cases of overdose have been reported in clinical trials. Hypocalcemia and hypomagnesemia have been observed in persons administered more than the recommended dosage of ribavirin. In most of these cases, ribavirin was administered intravenously at dosages up to and, in some cases, exceeding 4 times the recommended maximum oral daily dose.

Capsules/Solution – There is limited experience with overdosage. Acute ingestion of ribavirin up to 20 g, ingestion of interferon alfa-2b up to 120 million units, and subcutaneous doses of interferon alfa-2b up to 10 times the recommended dose have been reported. The primary effects observed were increased severity of adverse reactions related to the therapeutic use of interferon alfa-2b and ribavirin. However, hepatic enzyme abnormalities, renal failure, hemorrhage, and MI have been reported with administration of single subcutaneous doses of interferon alfa-2b that exceed dosing recommendations.

➤*Treatment:* There is no known specific antidote for interferon alfa-2b and ribavirin overdose, nor are hemodialysis or peritoneal dialysis effective.

Patient Information

Inform patients that ribavirin may cause birth defects and/or death of the exposed fetus. Ribavirin must not be used by women who are pregnant or by men whose female partners are pregnant. Extreme care must be taken to avoid pregnancy in these individuals. Do not initiate ribavirin until a report of a negative pregnancy test has been obtained immediately prior to initiation of therapy. Inform patients that they must perform a pregnancy test monthly during therapy and for 6 months posttherapy. Counsel women of childbearing potential about the use of effective contraception (2 reliable forms) prior to initiating therapy. Advise patients (men and women) of the teratogenic/embryocidal risks and instruct them to practice effective contraception during ribavirin and for 6 month posttherapy. Advise patients to immediately notify their health care provider in the event of pregnancy.

If pregnancy does occur during treatment or during 6 months posttherapy, advise the patient of the teratogenic/embryocidal risks of ribavirin therapy to the fetus. Instruct patients or partners of patients to immediately report any pregnancy that occurs during treatment or within 6 months after treatment cessation to their health care provider. Health care providers should report such cases by calling 1-800-593-2214.

Inform patients receiving ribavirin of the benefits and risks associated with treatment, and direct patients in its appropriate use.

Inform patients that the effect of treatment of HCV infection on transmission is not known and to take appropriate precautions to prevent transmission of HCV.

Inform patients that the most common adverse reaction associated with ribavirin is anemia, which may be severe. Advise patients that laboratory evaluations are required prior to starting therapy and periodically thereafter.

Advise patients to be well hydrated, especially during the initial stages of treatment.

Caution patients who develop dizziness, confusion, somnolence, and fatigue to avoid driving or operating machinery.

Advise patients to take *Copegus*, *Rebetol*, and *Ribasphere* tablets with food. *Ribasphere* capsules may be administered without regard to food, but should be administered in a consistent manner with respect to food intake. Instruct patients not to open, crush, or break capsules.

Inform patients about what to do if they miss a dose of ribavirin. The missed dose should be taken as soon as possible during the same day. Instruct patients not to double the next dose. Advise patients to contact their health care provider if they have questions.

RIBAVIRIN — INHALATION

WARNING

Use of ribavirin in patients requiring mechanical ventilator assistance should be undertaken only by health care providers and support staff familiar with this mode of administration and the specific ventilator being used. Strict attention must be paid to procedures that have been shown to minimize the accumulation of drug precipitate, which can result in mechanical ventilator dysfunction and associated increases in pulmonary pressures.

Sudden deterioration of respiratory function has been associated with the initiation of ribavirin use in infants. Carefully monitor respiratory function during treatment. If the initiation of ribavirin treatment appears to produce sudden deterioration of respiratory function, stop treatment and reinstitute only with extreme caution, continuous monitoring, and consideration of coadministration of bronchodilators.

Aerosolized ribavirin is not indicated for use in adults. Be aware that ribavirin has been shown to produce testicular lesions in rodents and to be teratogenic in all animal species in which adequate studies have been conducted (rodents and rabbits).

Indications

➤*Severe respiratory syncytial virus infection:* For the treatment of hospitalized infants and young children with severe lower respiratory tract infection due to severe respiratory syncytial virus (RSV). Treatment early in the course of severe lower respiratory tract infection may be necessary to achieve efficacy.

Diagnosis – Document RSV infection by a rapid diagnostic method, such as demonstration of viral antigen in respiratory tract secretions by immunofluorescence or an enzyme-linked immunoabsorbent assay, before or during the first 24 hours of treatment. Treatment may be initiated while awaiting rapid diagnostic test results. However, do not continue treatment without documentation of RSV infection. Nonculture antigen detection techniques may have false positive or false negative results. Assessment of the clinical situation, the time of year, and other parameters may warrant reevaluation of the laboratory diagnosis.

➤*Off-label uses:* Aerosol ribavirin has shown some success against influenza A and B viruses and herpes simplex virus.

Administration and Dosage

➤*Children:*

Severe respiratory syncytial virus infection –

Infants and young children:

• *Usual dosage* – 20 mg/mL as the starting solution in the drug reservoir of the small-particle aerosol generator (SPAG-2) unit, with continuous aerosol administration for 12 to 18 hours per day.

• *Duration of therapy* – 3 to 7 days.

➤*Preparation for administration:* Ribavirin is considered a teratogen. Follow safe handling procedures when preparing, administering, or dispensing ribavirin.

Using sterile technique, reconstitute the drug with a minimum of 75 mL of sterile water for injection or inhalation in the original 100 mL glass vial. Shake well. Transfer to the clean, sterilized 500 mL SPAG-2 reservoir and further dilute to a final volume of 300 mL with sterile water for injection or inhalation. The final concentration should be 20 mg/mL. Solutions in the SPAG-2 unit should be discarded at least every 24 hours and when the liquid level is low before adding newly reconstituted solution.

➤*Administration:* For aerosol administration only with Valeant SPAG-2 (see SPAG-2 manual). Aerosolized ribavirin should not be administered with any other aerosol-generating device.

Nonmechanically ventilated infants – Deliver ribavirin to an infant oxygen hood from the SPAG-2 aerosol generator. Administration by face mask or oxygen tent may be necessary if a hood cannot be employed (see SPAG-2 manual). However, the volume and condensation area are larger in a tent, which may alter delivery dynamics of the drug.

Mechanically ventilated infants – The recommended dose and administration schedule for infants who require mechanical ventilation is the same as for those who do not. Either a pressure or volume cycle ventilator may be used in conjunction with the SPAG-2. In either case, patients should have their endotracheal tubes suctioned every 1 to 2 hours and their pulmonary pressures monitored frequently (every 2 to 4 hours). For pressure and volume ventilators, heated wire connective tubing and bacteria filters in series in the expiratory limb of the system (which must be changed frequently [ie, every 4 hours]) must be used to minimize the risk of ribavirin precipitation in the system and the subsequent risk of ventilator dysfunction. Water column pressure release valves should be used in the ventilator circuit for pressure-cycled ventilators and may be utilized with volume-cycled ventilators (see SPAG-2 manual).

RIBAVIRIN — INHALATION

➤*Admixture compatibility:* Ribavirin should not be administered in a mixture for combined aerosolization or simultaneously with other aerosolized medications. The sterile water for injection or inhalation should not have had any antimicrobial agent or other substance added.

➤*Storage/Stability:* Store vials in a dry place at 25°C (77°F); excursions are permitted between 15° and 30°C (59° and 86°F). Reconstituted solutions may be stored under sterile conditions between 20° and 30°C (68° and 86°F) for 24 hours. Discard solutions that have been placed in the SPAG-2 unit at least every 24 hours.

Actions

➤*Pharmacology:* Ribavirin is a synthetic nucleoside with antiviral activity. In cell cultures, the inhibitory activity of ribavirin for RSV is selective. The mechanism of action is unknown. The reversal of the in vitro antiviral activity by guanosine or xanthosine suggests ribavirin may act as an analog of these cellular metabolites. In addition, ribavirin has been shown to have in vitro activity against influenza A and B viruses and herpes simplex virus, but the clinical significance of these data is unknown.

➤*Pharmacokinetics:*

Absorption/Distribution – Ribavirin, when administered by aerosol, is absorbed systemically. Four children inhaling ribavirin aerosol administered by face mask for 2.5 hours each day for 3 days had plasma concentrations ranging from 0.44 to 1.55 mcM, with a mean concentration of 0.76 mcM. Three children inhaling aerosolized ribavirin administered by face mask or mist tent for 20 hours each day for 5 days had plasma concentrations ranging from 1.5 to 14.3 mcM, with a mean concentration of 6.8 mcM.

The bioavailability of aerosolized ribavirin is unknown and may depend on the mode of aerosol delivery. After aerosol treatment, peak plasma concentrations of ribavirin are 85% to 98% less than the concentration that reduced RSV plaque formation in tissue culture. After aerosol treatment, respiratory tract secretions are likely to contain ribavirin in concentrations many-fold higher than those required to reduce plaque formation. However, RSV is an intracellular virus, and it is unknown whether plasma concentrations or respiratory secretion concentrations of the drug better reflect intracellular concentrations in the respiratory tract.

In humans, rats, and rhesus monkeys, accumulation of ribavirin and/or metabolites in red blood cells has been noted, plateauing in red cells in humans in approximately 4 days and gradually declining, with an apparent half-life of 40 days (the half-life of erythrocytes). The extent of accumulation of ribavirin following inhalation therapy is not well defined.

Metabolism/Excretion – The plasma half-life was reported to be 9.5 hours.

Assay for ribavirin in human materials is by radioimmunoassay, which detects ribavirin and at least 1 metabolite.

Contraindications

Hypersensitivity to the drug or its components; women who are or may become pregnant during exposure to the drug.

Warnings/Precautions

➤*Deterioration of respiratory function:* See Warnings/Precautions for more information.

➤*Use with mechanical ventilators:* Use of ribavirin in patients requiring mechanical ventilator assistance should be undertaken only by health care providers and support staff familiar with this mode of administration and the specific ventilator being used. Strict attention must be paid to procedures that have been shown to minimize the accumulation of drug precipitate, which can result in mechanical ventilator dysfunction and associated increases in pulmonary pressure. These procedures include the use of bacteria filters in series in the expiratory limb of the ventilator circuit with frequent changes (every 4 hours), water column pressure release valves to indicate elevated ventilator pressure, frequent monitoring of these devices, verification that ribavirin crystals have not accumulated within the ventilator circuitry, and frequent suctioning and monitoring of the patient.

➤*Health care personnel information:* Be aware that ribavirin has been shown to be teratogenic in all animal species in which adequate studies have been conducted (rodents and rabbits). Although no reports of teratogenesis in the offspring of mothers who were exposed to aerosolized ribavirin during pregnancy have been confirmed, no controlled studies have been conducted in pregnant women. Studies of environmental exposure in treatment settings have shown that the drug can disperse into the immediate bedside area during routine patient-care activities, with highest ambient levels closest to the patient and extremely low levels outside of the immediate bedside area. Adverse reactions resulting from actual occupational exposure in adults are described in the following paragraph. Some studies have documented ambient drug concentrations at the bedside that could potentially lead to systemic exposures above those considered safe for exposure during pregnancy (1/1,000 of the no observable teratogenic effects level dose in the most sensitive animal species).

A 1992 study conducted by the National Institute of Occupational Safety and Health (NIOSH) demonstrated measurable urine levels of ribavirin in health workers exposed to aerosol in the course of direct patient care. Levels were lowest in workers caring for infants receiving ribavirin with mechanical ventilation and highest in those caring for patients being administered the drug via an oxygen tent or hood. This study employed a more sensitive assay to evaluate ribavirin levels in urine than was available for several previous studies of environmental exposure that failed to detect measurable ribavirin levels in exposed workers. Creatinine-adjusted urine levels in the NIOSH study ranged from less than 0.001 to 0.14 mcM of ribavirin per gram of creatinine in exposed workers. However, the relationship between urinary ribavirin levels in exposed workers, plasma levels in animal studies, and the specific risk of teratogenesis in exposed pregnant women is unknown.

It is good practice to avoid unnecessary occupational exposure to chemicals wherever possible. Hospitals are encouraged to conduct training programs to minimize potential occupational exposure to ribavirin. Instruct pregnant health care workers to consider avoiding direct care of patients receiving aerosolized ribavirin. If close patient contact cannot be avoided, take precautions to limit exposure. These include administration of ribavirin in negative-pressure rooms, adequate room ventilation (at least 6 air exchanges per hour), using ribavirin aerosol scavenging devices, turning off the SPAG-2 device for 5 to 10 minutes prior to prolonged patient contact, and wearing appropriately fitted respirator masks. Surgical masks do not provide adequate filtration of ribavirin particles. Further information is available from NIOSH's Hazard Evaluation and Technical Assistance Branch, and additional recommendations have been published in an Aerosol Consensus Statement by the American Respiratory Care Foundation and the American Association for Respiratory Care.

➤*Pregnancy:* *Category X.* Ribavirin has demonstrated significant teratogenic and/or embryocidal potential in all animal species in which adequate studies have been conducted.

Teratogenic effects were evident after single oral doses of 2.5 mg/kg or more in hamsters, and after daily oral doses of 0.3 and 1 mg/kg in rabbits and rats, respectively (estimated human equivalent doses of 0.12 and 0.14 mg/kg, based on body surface area [BSA] adjustment for an adult). Malformations of the skull, palate, eye, jaw, limbs, skeleton, and GI tract were noted. The incidence and severity of teratogenic effects increased with escalation of the drug dose. Survival of fetuses and offspring was reduced. Ribavirin caused embryolethality in rabbits at daily oral dose levels as low as 1 mg/kg. No teratogenic effects were evident in rabbits and rats administered daily oral doses of 0.1 and 0.3 mg/kg, respectively (estimated human equivalent doses of 0.01 and 0.04 mg/kg, based on BSA adjustment). These doses are considered to define the no observable teratogenic effects level for ribavirin in rabbits and rats.

Following oral administration of ribavirin in pregnant rats (1 mg/kg) and rabbits (0.3 mg/kg), mean plasma levels of the drug ranged from 0.1 to 0.2 mcM (0.024 to 0.049 g/mL) at 1 hour after dosing to undetectable levels at 24 hours. At 1 hour following the administration of 0.3 or 0.1 mg/kg in rats and rabbits (no observable teratogenic effects level), respectively, mean plasma levels of the drug in both species were near or below the limit of detection (0.05 mcM).

Although clinical studies have not been performed, ribavirin may cause fetal harm in humans. As noted previously, ribavirin is concentrated in red blood cells and persists for the life of the cell. Thus, the terminal half-life for the systemic elimination of ribavirin is essentially that of the half-life of circulating erythrocytes. The minimum interval following exposure to ribavirin before pregnancy may be safely initiated is unknown.

➤*Lactation:* It is not known if ribavirin is excreted in human milk. The molecular weight (approximately 244) and prolonged plasma elimination half-life (12 days) suggest that the drug will be excreted into breast milk. The effects of this exposure on a breast-feeding infant are unknown, but the drug causes toxicity in lactating animals and their offspring.

➤*Monitoring:* Patients with severe lower respiratory tract infections due to RSV require optimum monitoring and attention to respiratory and fluid status.

Drug Interactions

None well documented.

Adverse Reactions

➤*Deaths:* Deaths during or shortly after treatment with ribavirin have been reported in 20 cases of patients treated with ribavirin (12 of these patients were being treated for RSV infection). Several cases have been characterized as possibly related to ribavirin by the treating health care provider; these were in infants who experienced worsening respiratory status related to bronchospasm while being treated with the drug. Several other cases have been attributed to mechanical ventilator malfunction in which ribavirin precipitation within the ventilator apparatus led to excessively high pulmonary pressures and diminished oxygenation. In these cases, the monitoring procedures described in the current package insert were not employed.

➤*Adverse reactions:*

Cardiovascular – Bradycardia, cardiac arrest, digitalis toxicity, hypotension. Bigeminy, bradycardia, and tachycardia have been described in patients with underlying congenital heart disease.

Pulmonary – Apnea, atelectasis, bacterial pneumonia, bronchospasm, cyanosis, dyspnea, hypoventilation, pneumothorax, pulmonary edema, ventilator dependence, worsening of respiratory status.

Pulmonary function significantly deteriorated during ribavirin treatment in 6 of 6 adults with chronic obstructive lung disease and in 4 of 6 asthmatic adults. Dyspnea and chest soreness were also reported in the latter group. Minor abnormalities in pulmonary function were also seen in healthy adult volunteers. In the original study population of approximately 200 infants who received ribavirin, several serious adverse reactions occurred in severely ill infants with life-threatening underlying diseases, many of whom required assisted ventilation. The role of ribavirin in these reactions is indeterminate. Since the drug's approval in 1986, additional reports of similar serious, although nonfatal, reactions have been filed infrequently.

Hematologic – Although anemia was not reported with the use of aerosolized ribavirin in controlled clinical trials, most infants treated with the aerosol have not been evaluated 1 to 2 weeks posttreatment, when anemia is likely to occur. Anemia has been shown to occur frequently with experimental oral and intravenous (IV) ribavirin in humans. Also, cases of anemia

RIBAVIRIN — INHALATION

(type unspecified), reticulocytosis, and hemolytic anemia associated with aerosolized ribavirin use have been reported through postmarketing reporting systems. All have been reversible with discontinuation of the drug.

➤*Additional adverse reactions:* Some subjects requiring assisted ventilation experienced serious difficulties because of inadequate ventilation and gas exchange. Precipitation of drug within the ventilatory apparatus, including the endotracheal tube, has resulted in increased positive end expiratory pressure and increased positive inspiratory pressure. Accumulation of fluid in tubing (ie, rain out) has also been noted. Carefully follow measures to avoid these complications.

Conjunctivitis and rash and have been associated with the use of aerosolized ribavirin. These usually resolve within hours of discontinuing therapy. Asthenia and seizures associated with experimental IV ribavirin therapy have also been reported.

➤*Adverse reactions in health care workers:* Studies of environmental exposure to aerosolized ribavirin in health care workers administering care to patients receiving aerosolized ribavirin have not detected adverse signs or symptoms related to exposure. However, 152 health care workers have reported experiencing adverse reactions through postmarketing surveillance. Nearly all were in individuals providing direct care to infants receiving aerosolized ribavirin. Of 358 reactions from these 152 individual health care worker reports, the most common signs and symptoms were headache (51% of reports); conjunctivitis (32%); and dizziness, lacrimation, nausea, pharyngitis, rash, or rhinitis (10% to 20% each). Several cases of bronchospasm and/or chest pain were also reported, usually in individuals with known underlying reactive airway disease. Several case reports of damage to contact lenses after prolonged close exposure to aerosolized ribavirin have also been reported. Most signs and symptoms reported as having occurred in exposed health care workers resolved within minutes to hours of discontinuing close exposure to aerosolized ribavirin.

Overdosage

➤*Symptoms:* No overdosage with ribavirin by aerosol administration has been reported in humans.

Patient Information

Advise the patient's family or caregiver that ribavirin will be prepared and administered by health care providers in a hospital setting.

RIMANTADINE HYDROCHLORIDE

Rx	**Rimantadine Hydrochloride** (Various, eg, Global, Sandoz)	**Tablets; oral:** 100 mg	In 100s and 1,000s.
Rx	**Flumadine** (Caraco)		(FLUMADINE 100 FOREST). Orange, oval. Film-coated. In 100s.

RIMANTADINE HYDROCHLORIDE — ORAL

Indications

➤*Influenza A virus:* For the prophylaxis and treatment of illness caused by various strains of influenza A virus in adults and for prophylaxis against influenza A virus in children.

General considerations – Consider the following points before initiating treatment or prophylaxis with rimantadine:

- Rimantadine is not a substitute for early vaccination on an annual basis, as recommended by the Centers for Disease Control and Prevention (CDC) Advisory Committee on Immunization Practices.
- Influenza viruses change over time. Emergence of resistance mutations could decrease drug effectiveness. Other factors (eg, changes in viral virulence) might also diminish clinical benefit of antiviral drugs. Consider available information on influenza drug susceptibility patterns and treatment effects when deciding whether to use rimantadine.

➤*Off-label uses:*

H1N1 influenza A (swine flu) – Per the CDC recommendations for treatment and chemoprophylaxis of H1N1 influenza A (swine flu) virus infection, refer to the oseltamivir and zanamivir monographs. The H1N1 virus is resistant to the antiviral medication rimantadine. For more information, seehttp://www.cdc.gov/h1n1flu/recommendations.htm.

Other possible off-label uses – Treatment of influenza A virus in children.

Administration and Dosage

➤*Adults:*

Prophylaxis of influenza A virus –

Usual dosage: 100 mg twice daily.

Treatment of influenza A virus –

Usual dosage: 100 mg twice daily. Initiate therapy as soon as possible, preferably within 48 hours after onset of signs and symptoms of influenza A infection.

Duration of therapy: Therapy should be continued for approximately 7 days from the initial onset of symptoms.

➤*Children:*

Prophylaxis of influenza A virus – See also Off-Label dosing.

10 years of age and older:

- *Usual dosage* – 100 mg twice daily.

1 to 9 years of age:

- *Usual dosage* – 5 mg/kg once daily.
- *Maximum dose* – 150 mg.

Off-label dosing –

Prophylaxis of influenza A virus:

- *10 years of age and older and less than 40 kg* –
  Usual dosage: 5 mg/kg/day in 1 or 2 divided doses.
  Maximum dose: 150 mg/day.
- *Treatment of influenza A virus* –
  10 years of age and older40 kg or more: 100 mg twice daily; initiate within 48 hours of onset of illness. 5 to 7 days.Less than 40 kg 5 mg/kg/day in 1 or 2 divided doses; initiate within 48 hours of onset of illness. 150 mg/day. 5 to 7 days.
  1 to 9 years of age: 5 mg/kg once daily; initiate within 48 hours of onset of illness. 150 mg/day. 5 to 7 days.

➤*Elderly:* In elderly nursing home patients, a dosage reduction to 100 mg daily is recommended.

➤*Renal function impairment:*

Severe renal impairment (creatinine clearance 5 to 29 mL/min) or renal failure (creatinine clearance 10 mL/min or less) – 100 mg daily is recommended.

➤*Hepatic function impairment:*

Severe hepatic dysfunction – 100 mg daily is recommended.

➤*Preparation for administration:*

Compounding of oral suspension – Calculate the amount of rimantadine in milligrams needed for the duration of therapy: daily dose × number of days = rimantadine (milligrams); for example, 75 mg/day × 10 days = 750 mg. Round up the milligrams of rimantadine amount to the next 100 mg designation; for example, round 750 mg up to 800 mg. Calculate the number of 100 mg tablets that are required for the compounded oral suspension: rounded milligrams of rimantadine divided by 100 mg/tablet = number of tablets; for example, 800 mg divided by 100 mg/tablet = 8 tablets. Calculate the total volume of compounded oral suspension (10 mg/mL): rounded milligrams of rimantadine divided by 10 mg/mL = total volume; for example, 800 mg divided by 10 mg/mL = 80 mL.

Place the required number of 100 mg tablets into a clean mortar of sufficient size to contain the tablets and volume of vehicle, *Ora-Sweet*. Grind the tablets and triturate to a fine powder using a pestle. Powder on the sides of the mortar or pestle should be removed using a spatula and incorporated into the trituration throughout the process. Slowly add approximately one-third of the total volume of vehicle to the mortar while triturating until a uniform suspension is achieved. Transfer the suspension to an amber glass or PET plastic bottle. Other types of bottles, such as non-PET plastic or uncolored bottles, have not been evaluated and should not be used. A funnel may be used to eliminate any spillage. Slowly add the second one-third of the total volume of vehicle to the mortar, rinse the pestle and mortar by a triturating motion, and transfer the contents into the bottle. Repeat the rinsing with the remaining one-third of the vehicle, transferring the remaining contents to the fullest extent possible. Verify that the suspension is at the desired total volume or add additional vehicle if needed. Close the bottle and shake well to ensure a homogenous suspension.

➤*Administration:* For oral use only. Shake the compounded suspension gently before each use.

➤*Storage/Stability:* Store at 25°C (77°F); excursions are permitted between 15° and 30°C (59° and 86°F).

Compounded suspension – Stable for 14 days when stored in ambient room temperature conditions.

Actions

➤*Pharmacology:* The mechanism of action of rimantadine is not fully understood. Rimantadine appears to exert its inhibitory effect early in the viral replicative cycle, possibly inhibiting the uncoating of the virus. Genetic studies suggest that a virus protein specified by the virion M2 gene plays an important role in the susceptibility of influenza A virus to inhibition by rimantadine.

➤*Pharmacokinetics:*

Absorption/Distribution – Rimantadine is absorbed after oral administration. The mean ± standard deviation peak plasma concentration after a single rimantadine 100 mg dose was 74 ± 22 mg/mL (range, 45 to 138 mg/mL). The time to peak concentration was 6 ± 1 hour in healthy adults (20 to 44 years of age).

After the administration of rimantadine 100 mg twice daily to healthy volunteers (18 to 70 years of age) for 10 days, area under the curve (AUC) values were approximately 30% higher than predicted from a single dose. Plasma trough levels (C_{min}) at steady state ranged between 118 and 468 mg/mL. In these patients, no age-related differences in pharmacokinetics were detected.

The in vitro human plasma protein binding of rimantadine is approximately 40% over typical plasma concentrations. Albumin is the major binding protein.

Metabolism – Following oral administration, rimantadine is extensively metabolized in the liver, with less than 25% of the dose excreted in the urine as unchanged drug. Three hydroxylated metabolites have been found in

RIMANTADINE HYDROCHLORIDE — ORAL

plasma. These metabolites, an additional conjugated metabolite, and parent drug account for 74% ± 10% (n = 4) of a single rimantadine 200 mg dose excreted in urine over 72 hours.

Excretion – The single-dose elimination half-life in healthy adults (20 to 44 years of age) was 25.4 ± 6.3 hours (range, 13 to 65 hours). The single-dose elimination half-life in a group of healthy patients 71 to 79 years of age was 32 ± 16 hours (range, 20 to 65 hours).

Special populations –

Renal function impairment: In subjects with severe renal impairment, rimantadine maximal drug concentration, C_{min}, and $AUC_{0\text{-tau}}$ on day 14 increased by 75%, 82%, and 81%, respectively, compared with healthy subjects. The rimantadine elimination half-life was slightly prolonged (increase of 18% or less) in subjects with mild and moderate renal impairment but increased by 49% in subjects with severe renal impairment compared with healthy subjects.

• *Hemodialysis* – After a single rimantadine 200 mg oral dose was given to 8 hemodialysis patients (creatinine clearance 0 to 10 mL/min), there was a 1.6-fold increase in the elimination half-life and a 40% decrease in apparent clearance compared with age-matched healthy subjects. Hemodialysis did not contribute to the clearance of rimantadine.

Hepatic function impairment: After administration of a single rimantadine 200 mg dose to patients (n = 10) with severe hepatic dysfunction, AUC was approximately 3-fold larger, elimination half-life was approximately 2-fold longer, and apparent clearance was approximately 50% lower compared with historic data from healthy subjects.

Elderly: In a comparison of 3 groups of healthy older subjects (50 to 60, 61 to 70, and 71 to 79 years of age), the 71 to 79 years of age group had average AUC values, peak concentrations, and elimination half-life values at steady state that were 20% to 30% higher than the other 2 groups. Steady-state concentrations in elderly nursing home patients (68 to 102 years of age) were 2- to 4-fold higher than those seen in healthy younger and elderly adults.

Contraindications

Hypersensitivity to drugs of the adamantane class, including rimantadine and amantadine.

Warnings/Precautions

➤*Seizures:* An increased incidence of seizures has been reported in patients with a history of epilepsy who received the related drug amantadine. In clinical trials of rimantadine, the occurrence of seizure-like activity was observed in a small number of patients with a history of seizures who were not receiving anticonvulsant medication while taking rimantadine. If seizures develop, discontinue rimantadine.

➤*Resistant strains:* Consider transmission of rimantadine-resistant virus when treating patients whose contacts are at high risk of influenza A illness. Influenza A virus strains resistant to rimantadine can emerge during treatment, and such resistant strains have been shown to be transmissible and to cause typical influenza illness. Although the frequency, rapidity, and clinical significance of the emergence of drug-resistant virus are not yet established, several small studies have demonstrated that 10% to 30% of patients with initially sensitive virus, upon treatment with rimantadine, shed rimantadine-resistant virus.

➤*Bacterial infections:* Serious bacterial infections may begin with influenza-like symptoms or may coexist with or occur as complications during the course of influenza. Rimantadine has not been shown to prevent these complications.

➤*Live vaccines:* The concurrent use of rimantadine with live, attenuated intranasal influenza vaccine has not been evaluated. However, because of the potential interference between these products, do not administer the live, attenuated intranasal influenza vaccine until 48 hours after cessation of rimantadine, and do not administer rimantadine until 2 weeks after the administration of live, attenuated intranasal influenza vaccine unless medically indicated. The concern about potential interferences arises principally from the potential for antiviral drugs to inhibit replication of the live vaccine virus.

➤*Renal function impairment:* Because of the potential for increased accumulation of rimantadine metabolites in renally-impaired patients, exercise caution when these patients are treated with rimantadine.

See Actions for more information.

➤*Hepatic function impairment:* Because of the potential for accumulation of rimantadine and its metabolites in plasma, exercise caution when patients with hepatic insufficiency are treated with rimantadine.

See Actions for more information.

➤*Pregnancy: Category C.* There are no adequate and well-controlled studies in pregnant women. It is unknown whether rimantadine crosses the human placenta to the fetus, but the relatively low molecular weight (approximately 216) probably ensures that transfer occurs. Use rimantadine during pregnancy only if the potential benefit justifies the risk to the fetus.

Rimantadine is reported to cross the placenta in mice. Rimantadine has been shown to be embryotoxic in rats when given at a dosage of 200 mg/kg/day (11 times the recommended human dose based on mg/m^2). At this dose, the embryotoxic effect consisted of increased fetal resorption in rats; this dose also produced a variety of maternal effects, including ataxia, tremors, convulsions, and significantly reduced weight gain. No embryotoxicity was observed when rabbits were given dosages of up to 50 mg/kg/day (approximately 0.1 times the maximum recommended human dose [MRHD] based on AUC). However, there was evidence of a developmental abnormality in the form of a change in the ratio of fetuses with 12 or 13 ribs. This ratio is normally approximately 50:50 in a litter but was 80:20 after rimantadine treatment. However, in a repeat embryofetal toxicity study in rabbits at dosages of up to 50 mg/kg/day (approximately 0.1 times the MRHD based on AUC), this abnormality was not observed.

Rimantadine was administered to pregnant rats in a peri- and postnatal reproduction toxicity study at dosages of 30, 60, and 120 mg/kg/day (1.7, 3.4, and 6.8 times the recommended human dose based on mg/m^2). Maternal toxicity during gestation was noted at the 2 higher doses of rimantadine. At the highest dosage, 120 mg/kg/day, there was an increase in pup mortality during the first 2 to 4 days postpartum. Decreased fertility of the F1 generation was also noted for the 2 higher doses.

➤*Lactation:* Do not administer rimantadine to breast-feeding mothers because of the adverse effects noted in offspring of rats treated with rimantadine during the breast-feeding period. Rimantadine is concentrated in rat milk in a dose-related manner: 2 to 3 hours following administration of rimantadine, rat breast milk levels were approximately twice those observed in the serum. There are no reports describing the use of rimantadine during human lactation, but anticipate passage of the drug into human milk because of its low molecular weight (approximately 216).

➤*Children:* The safety and effectiveness of rimantadine in the treatment of symptomatic influenza infection in children 1 to 16 years of age have not been established. Prophylaxis studies with rimantadine have not been performed in children younger than 1 year of age.

➤*Monitoring:* Monitor patients with any degree of renal or hepatic insufficiency for adverse reactions and adjust the dose as needed.

Drug Interactions

➤*Live vaccines:* See Warnings/Precautions for more information.

Rimantadine Drug Interactions

Precipitant drug	Object drug[a]		Description
Acetaminophen	Rimantadine	⬇	Coadministration with acetaminophen reduced the peak concentration and AUC values for rimantadine by approximately 11%. Based on the magnitude of the interaction, a clinically important consequence is unlikely.
Aspirin	Rimantadine	⬇	The peak plasma concentration and AUC of rimantadine were reduced approximately 10% when coadministered with aspirin. Based on the magnitude of the interaction, a clinically important consequence is unlikely.
Cimetidine	Rimantadine	⬆	When a single rimantadine 100 mg dose was administered 1 hour after cimetidine (300 mg 4 times/day) in healthy adults, the AUC increased 20% and the apparent total rimantadine clearance decreased 18%. Based on the magnitude of the interaction, a clinically important consequence is unlikely.

[a] ⬆ = object drug increased; ⬇ = object drug decreased.

Adverse Reactions

➤*Most frequent adverse reactions (1% to 3%):*

Rimantadine Adverse Reactions (> 1%)

Adverse reactions	Rimantadine (n = 1,027)	Control (n = 986)
CNS		
Asthenia	1.4%	0.5%
Dizziness	1.9%	1.1%
Fatigue	1%	0.9%
Headache	1.4%	1.3%
Insomnia	2.1%	0.9%
Nervousness	1.3%	0.6%
GI		
Abdominal pain	1.4%	0.8%
Anorexia	1.6%	0.8%
Dry mouth	1.5%	0.6%
Nausea	2.8%	1.6%
Vomiting	1.7%	0.6%

➤*Less frequent adverse reactions (0.3% to 1%):*

CNS – Agitation, ataxia, depression, impairment of concentration, somnolence.

GI – Diarrhea, dyspepsia.

Miscellaneous – Dyspnea, rash, tinnitus.

RIMANTADINE HYDROCHLORIDE — ORAL

➤*Additional adverse reactions (less than 0.3%):*

Cardiovascular – Cardiac failure, cerebrovascular disorder, heart block, hypertension, pallor, palpitation, pedal edema, syncope, tachycardia.

CNS – Confusion, convulsions, euphoria, gait abnormality, hallucination, hyperkinesia, tremor.

Respiratory – Bronchospasm, cough.

Special senses – Parosmia, taste loss/change.

Miscellaneous – Nonpuerperal lactation.

➤*High dosage:*

CNS – Agitation, hypesthesia, rigors.

GI – Constipation, dysphagia, stomatitis.

Special senses – Eye pain, increased lacrimation.

Miscellaneous – Diaphoresis, fever, increased micturition frequency.

➤*Elderly:* Elderly patients who received rimantadine 200 or 400 mg daily for 1 to 50 days experienced considerably more CNS and GI adverse reactions than comparable elderly patients receiving placebo. CNS reactions, including anxiety, asthenia, dizziness, fatigue, and headache, occurred up to 2 times more often in patients treated with rimantadine than in those treated with placebo. GI symptoms, particularly abdominal pain, nausea, and vomiting, occurred at least twice as frequently in subjects receiving rimantadine than in those receiving placebo. The GI symptoms appeared to be dose related.

See Administration and Dosage for more information.

Overdosage

➤*Symptoms:* Overdoses of a related drug, amantadine, have been reported, with adverse reactions consisting of agitation, cardiac arrhythmia, death, and hallucinations.

➤*Treatment:* The administration of intravenous physostigmine (a cholinergic agent) at doses of 1 to 2 mg in adults and 0.5 mg in children, repeated as needed as long as the dose did not exceed 2 mg/h, has been reported anecdotally to be beneficial in patients with CNS effects from overdoses of amantadine. As with any overdose, administer supportive therapy as indicated.

Patient Information

Advise patients to use this medication for the full course of treatment.

Inform patients that this medication only works on certain types of flu and that it does not treat other viral infections (eg, common cold).

Advise patients not to take this medication until 2 weeks after they receive a live nasal flu vaccine and not to receive a live nasal flu vaccine within 48 hours after they stop taking this medication.

Advise patients using the compounded suspension to shake well prior to administration.

ZANAMIVIR

Rx	**Relenza** (GlaxoSmithKline)	**Powder; inhalation:** 5 mg	Lactose. In 4 blisters with 5 *Rotadisks* and 1 *Diskhaler.*

ZANAMIVIR — INHALATION

Indications

➤*Influenza:*

Prophylaxis – For the prophylaxis of influenza in adults and children 5 years of age and older.

Treatment – For the treatment of uncomplicated acute illness caused by influenza A and B virus in adults and children 7 years of age and older who have been symptomatic for no more than 2 days.

➤*Off-label uses:*

H1N1 influenza A (swine flu) – For treatment and chemoprophylaxis of H1N1 influenza A (swine flu) virus infection. This includes patients with confirmed, probable or suspected H1N1 influenza A (swine flu) virus infection and their close contacts. For more information, refer to the CDC guidelines at http://www.cdc.gov/h1n1flu/recommendations.htm. (See Administration and Dosage for Adults and Children.)

Administration and Dosage

➤*Adults:*

Influenza prophylaxis –

Household setting:

• *Usual dosage* – 10 mg inhaled once daily for 10 days. The dose should be administered at approximately the same time each day. There are no data on the effectiveness of prophylaxis with zanamivir in a household setting when initiated more than 1.5 days after the onset of signs or symptoms in the index case.

• *Duration of therapy* – 10 days.

Community outbreaks:

• *Usual dosage* – 10 mg inhaled once daily for 28 days. The dose should be administered at approximately the same time each day. There are no data on the effectiveness of prophylaxis with zanamivir in a community outbreak when initiated more than 5 days after the outbreak was identified in the community.

• *Duration of therapy* – 28 days. The safety and effectiveness of prophylaxis with zanamivir have not been evaluated for longer than 28 days' duration.

Influenza treatment –

Usual dosage: 10 mg inhaled twice daily (approximately 12 hours apart) for 5 days. Two doses should be taken on the first day of treatment whenever possible, provided there are at least 2 hours between doses. On subsequent days, doses should be about 12 hours apart (eg, morning and evening) at approximately the same time each day.

Duration of therapy: 5 days. The safety and efficacy of repeated treatment courses have not been studied.

➤*Children:*

Influenza prophylaxis –

Household setting:

• *5 years of age and older* – See Adults for dosing.

Community outbreaks:

• *Adolescents 12 to 16 years of age* – See Adults for dosing.

Influenza treatment –

7 years of age and older: See Adults for dosing.

➤*Administration:* Zanamivir is for administration to the respiratory tract by oral inhalation only, using the *Diskhaler* device provided. The 10 mg dose is provided by 2 inhalations (one 5 mg blister per inhalation). Patients should be instructed in the use of the delivery system. Instructions should include a demonstration whenever possible. If zanamivir is prescribed for children, it should be used only under adult supervision and instruction, and the supervising adult should first be instructed by a health care provider.

Patients scheduled to use an inhaled bronchodilator at the same time as zanamivir should use their bronchodilator before taking zanamivir.

➤*Storage/Stability:* Store at 25°C (77°F); excursions are permitted between 15° and 30°C (59° and 86°F). Keep out of the reach of children. Do not puncture any zanamivir *Rotadisk* blister until taking a dose using the *Diskhaler*.

Actions

➤*Pharmacology:* Zanamivir is an antiviral drug and is an inhibitor of influenza virus neuraminidase, affecting release of viral particles.

➤*Pharmacokinetics:*

Absorption/Distribution – Pharmacokinetic studies of orally inhaled zanamivir indicate that approximately 4% to 17% of the inhaled dose is systemically absorbed. The peak serum concentrations ranged from 17 to 142 ng/mL within 1 to 2 hours following a 10 mg dose. The area under the curve (AUC_∞) ranged from 111 to 1,364 ng•h/mL.

Zanamivir has limited plasma protein binding (less than 10%).

Metabolism/Excretion – Zanamivir is renally excreted as unchanged drug. No metabolites have been detected in humans.

The serum half-life of zanamivir following administration by oral inhalation ranges from 2.5 to 5.1 hours. It is excreted unchanged in the urine, with excretion of a single dose completed within 24 hours. Total clearance ranges from 2.5 to 10.9 L/h. Unabsorbed drug is excreted in the feces.

Special populations –

Renal function impairment: After a single intravenous (IV) dose of zanamivir 4 or 2 mg in volunteers with mild to moderate or severe renal function impairment, respectively, significant decreases in renal clearance (and hence, total clearance: normal 5.3 L/h, mild to moderate 2.7 L/h, and severe 0.8 L/h; median values) and significant increases in half-life (normal 3.1 hours, mild to moderate 4.7 hours, and severe 18.5 hours; median values) and systemic exposure were observed. Safety and efficacy have not been documented in the presence of severe renal function impairment. Because of the low systemic bioavailability of zanamivir following oral inhalation, no dosage adjustments are necessary in patients with renal function impairment; however, consider the potential for drug accumulation.

Children: The pharmacokinetics of zanamivir were evaluated in children with signs and symptoms of respiratory illness. Sixteen patients 6 to 12 years of age received a single dose of zanamivir 10 mg dry powder via the *Diskhaler*. Five patients had undetectable zanamivir serum concentrations or low drug concentrations (8.32 to 10.38 ng/mL) that were not detectable after 1.5 hours. Eleven patients had maximum effective plasma concentration (C_{max}) median values of 43 ng/mL (range, 15 to 74 ng/mL) and AUC_∞ median values of 167 ng•h/mL (range, 58 to 279 ng/mL). Low or undetectable serum concentrations were related to lack of measurable peak inspiratory flow rates (PIFRs) in individual patients.

Contraindications

History of allergic reaction to any ingredient of zanamivir including lactose (which contains milk proteins).

Warnings/Precautions

➤*Bronchospasm:* Zanamivir is not recommended for the treatment or prophylaxis of influenza in individuals with underlying airway disease (eg, asthma, chronic obstructive pulmonary disease [COPD]).

Serious cases of bronchospasm, including fatalities, have been reported during treatment with zanamivir in patients with and without underlying air-

ZANAMIVIR — INHALATION

way disease. Many of these cases were reported during postmarketing and causality was difficult to assess.

Discontinue zanamivir in any patient who develops bronchospasm or declines in respiratory function; immediate treatment and hospitalization may be required. Some patients without prior pulmonary disease may also have respiratory abnormalities from acute respiratory infection that could resemble adverse drug reactions or increase patient vulnerability to adverse drug reactions.

If treatment with zanamivir is considered for a patient with underlying airway disease, carefully weigh the potential risks and benefits. If a decision is made to prescribe zanamivir for such a patient, do this only under conditions of careful monitoring of respiratory function, close observation, and appropriate supportive care, including availability of fast-acting bronchodilators.

➤*Neuropsychiatric effects:* Influenza can be associated with a variety of neurologic and behavioral symptoms, which can include reactions such as seizures, hallucinations, delirium, and abnormal behavior, in some cases resulting in fatal outcomes. These reactions may occur in the setting of encephalitis or encephalopathy but can occur without obvious severe disease.

There have been postmarketing reports (mostly from Japan) of delirium and abnormal behavior leading to injury in patients with influenza who were receiving neuraminidase inhibitors, including zanamivir. Because these reactions were reported voluntarily during clinical practice, estimates of frequency cannot be made, but they appear to be uncommon based on usage data for zanamivir. These reactions were reported primarily among pediatric patients and often had an abrupt onset and rapid resolution. The contribution of zanamivir to these reactions has not been established. Closely monitor patients with influenza for signs of abnormal behavior. If neuropsychiatric symptoms occur, the risks and benefits of continuing treatment should be evaluated for each patient.

➤*Bacterial infections:* Serious bacterial infections may begin with influenza-like symptoms or may coexist with or occur as complications during the course of influenza. Zanamivir has not been shown to prevent such complications.

➤*Proper use of Diskhaler:* See Administration and Dosage for more information.

➤*Influenza vaccination:* Use of zanamivir should not affect the evaluation of individuals for annual influenza vaccination and is not a substitute for early vaccination on an annual basis in accordance with guidelines of the Centers for Disease Control and Prevention Advisory Committee on Immunization Practices.

➤*Other viral illness:* There is no evidence for the efficacy of zanamivir in any illness caused by agents other than influenza viruses A and B.

➤*Vaccines:* See Drug Interactions for more information.

➤*Hypersensitivity reactions:* Allergic-like reactions, including oropharyngeal edema, serious skin rashes, and anaphylaxis, have been reported in postmarketing experience with zanamivir. Stop zanamivir and institute appropriate treatment if an allergic reaction occurs or is suspected.

➤*Pregnancy: Category C.* There are no adequate and well-controlled studies of zanamivir in pregnant women. Use zanamivir during pregnancy only if the potential benefit justifies the potential risk to the fetus.

Per the CDC recommendations for the treatment of H1N1 influenza A (swine flu), oseltamivir is the preferred choice because of its systemic activity. The drug of choice for prophylaxis is less clear. Zanamivir may be preferable because of its limited systemic absorption; however, respiratory complications that may be associated with zanamivir because of its inhaled route of administration need to be considered, especially in women at risk for respiratory problems. For more information, refer to the CDC guidelines at http://www.cdc.gov/h1n1flu/recommendations.htm.

In a subchronic study in rats at the 90 mg/kg/day IV dose, the AUC values were more than 300 times the human exposure at the proposed clinical dose.

An additional embryo/fetal study, in a different strain of rat, was conducted using subcutaneous administration of zanamivir 3 times daily at doses of 1, 9, or 80 mg/kg during days 7 to 17 of pregnancy. There was an increase in the incidence rates of a variety of minor skeleton alterations and variants in the exposed offspring in this study. Based on AUC measurements, the 80 mg/kg dose produced an exposure more than 1,000 times the human exposure at the proposed clinical dose. However, the individual incidence rate of each skeletal alteration or variant, in most instances, remained within the background rates of the historical occurrence in the strain studied.

Zanamivir has been shown to cross the placenta in rats and rabbits. In these animals, fetal blood concentrations of zanamivir were significantly lower than zanamivir concentrations in the maternal blood.

There are no adequate and well-controlled studies of zanamivir in pregnant women. Use zanamivir during pregnancy only if the potential benefit justifies the potential risk to the fetus.

➤*Lactation:* Studies in rats have demonstrated that zanamivir is excreted in milk. It has been suggested that zanamivir may cross the human placenta due to the molecular weight (about 332), along with the lack of metabolism and plasma protein binding, and the moderately long elimination half-life. Exercise caution when zanamivir is administered to a breast-feeding woman.

➤*Children:* Safety and efficacy of zanamivir have not been established for the treatment of influenza in children younger than 7 years of age and for the prophylaxis of influenza in children younger than 5 years of age.

➤*Elderly:* No overall differences in safety or efficacy were observed between these subjects and younger patients, and other reported clinical experience has not identified differences in responses between elderly and younger patients; however, greater sensitivity of some older individuals cannot be ruled out. Elderly subjects may need assistance with use of the device.

➤*Monitoring:* Closely monitor patients with influenza for signs of abnormal behavior. If neuropsychiatric symptoms occur, evaluate the risks and benefits of continuing treatment for each patient.

Drug Interactions

➤*Vaccines:* Because of the potential interference between live attenuated influenza vaccine and zanamivir, do not administer live attenuated influenza vaccine within 2 weeks before or 48 hours after administration of zanamivir, unless medically indicated. The concern about possible interference arises from the potential for antiviral drugs to inhibit replication of live vaccine virus.

Trivalent inactivated influenza vaccine can be administered at any time relative to use of zanamivir.

Adverse Reactions

See Warnings and Precautions for more information about risk of serious adverse reactions such as bronchospasm, allergic-like reactions, and for safety information in patients with underlying airways disease.

➤*Influenza treatment:*

Adults and adolescents –

Zanamivir Adverse Reactions in Adults and Adolescents (≥ 12 Years of Age) (≥ 1.5%)			
Adverse reactions	Zanamivir 10 mg inhaled twice daily (n = 1,132)	All zanamivir dosing regimens[a] (n = 2,289)	Placebo (lactose vehicle) (n = 1,520)
CNS			
Dizziness	2%	1%	< 1%
Headaches	2%	2%	3%
GI			
Diarrhea	3%	3%	4%
Nausea	3%	3%	3%
Vomiting	1%	1%	2%
Respiratory			
Bronchitis	2%	2%	3%
Cough	2%	2%	3%
Ear, nose, and throat infections	2%	1%	2%
Nasal signs and symptoms	2%	3%	3%
Sinusitis	3%	2%	2%

[a] Includes studies in which zanamivir was administered intranasally (6.4 mg 2 to 4 times daily in addition to inhaled preparation) and/or inhaled more frequently (4 times daily) than the currently recommended dose.

Other adverse reactions (less than 1.5%) – Abdominal pain, arthralgia, fatigue, fever, malaise, myalgia, urticaria.

Lab test abnormalities – The most frequent laboratory abnormalities in phase 3 treatment studies included elevations of liver enzymes and creatine phosphokinase, lymphopenia, and neutropenia. These were reported in similar proportions of zanamivir and lactose-vehicle placebo recipients with acute influenza-like illness.

Children –

Zanamivir Adverse Reactions in Children (≥ 1.5%)[a]		
Adverse reactions	Zanamivir 10 mg inhaled twice daily (n = 291)	Placebo (lactose vehicle) (n = 318)
GI		
Diarrhea	2%	2%
Nausea	< 1%	2%
Vomiting	2%	3%
Respiratory		
Asthma	< 1%	2%
Cough	< 1%	2%
Ear, nose, and throat hemorrhage	< 1%	2%
Ear, nose, and throat infections	5%	5%

[a] Includes a subset of patients receiving zanamivir for treatment of influenza in a prophylaxis study.

In 1 of the 2 studies described in the previous table, some additional information is available from children 5 to 12 years of age without acute influenza-like illness who received an investigational prophylaxis regimen of zanamivir; 132 children received zanamivir and 145 children received placebo. Among these children, nasal signs and symptoms (zanamivir, 20%; placebo, 9%), cough (zanamivir, 16%; placebo, 8%), and throat/tonsil discomfort and pain (zanamivir, 11%; placebo, 6%) were reported more frequently with zanamivir than placebo. In a subset with chronic pulmonary disease, lower respiratory tract adverse reactions (described as asthma, cough, or viral res-

ZANAMIVIR — INHALATION

piratory infections that could include influenza-like symptoms) were reported in 7 of 7 zanamivir recipients and 5 of 12 placebo recipients.

➤*Influenza prophylaxis:*

Family / Household prophylaxis –

Zanamivir Adverse Reactions Incidence During 10-Day Prophylaxis Studies in Adults, Adolescents, and Children ≥ 5 Years of Age (≥ 1.5%)[a]		
Adverse reactions	Zanamivir (n = 1,068)	Placebo (n = 1,059)
CNS		
Fatigue/Malaise	5%	5%
Headaches	13%	14%
GI		
Anorexia/Decreased or increased appetite	2%	2%
Nausea/Vomiting	1%	2%
Respiratory		
Cough	7%	9%
Nasal inflammation	1%	2%
Nasal signs and symptoms	12%	12%
Throat/Tonsil discomfort and pain	8%	9%
Viral respiratory infections	13%	19%
Miscellaneous		
Chills/Fever	5%	4%
Muscle pain	3%	3%

[a] In prophylaxis studies, symptoms associated with influenza-like illness were captured as adverse reactions. Subjects were enrolled during a winter respiratory season; any symptoms that occurred were captured as adverse reactions.

Community prophylaxis –

Zanamivir Adverse Reactions During 28-Day Prophylaxis in Adults, Adolescents, and Children ≥ 5 Years of Age (≥ 1.5%)[a]		
Adverse reactions	Zanamivir (n = 2,231)	Placebo (n = 2,239)
CNS		
Fatigue/Malaise	8%	8%
Headaches	24%	26%
GI		
Anorexia/Decreased or increased appetite	4%	4%
Diarrhea	2%	2%
Nausea/Vomiting	2%	3%
Musculoskeletal		
Arthralgia/Articular rheumatism	2%	< 1%
Muscle pain	8%	8%
Musculoskeletal pain	6%	6%
Respiratory		
Cough	17%	18%
Ear, nose, and throat infections	2%	2%
Nasal signs and symptoms	12%	13%
Throat/Tonsil discomfort and pain	19%	20%
Viral respiratory infections	3%	4%
Miscellaneous		
Chills and/or fever	9%	10%

[a] In prophylaxis studies, symptoms associated with influenza-like illness were captured as adverse reactions. Subjects were enrolled during a winter respiratory season; any symptoms that occurred were captured as adverse reactions.

➤*Postmarketing:*

Cardiovascular – Arrhythmias, syncope.

CNS – Delirium, including symptoms such as abnormal behavior, agitation, altered level of consciousness, anxiety, confusion, delusions, hallucinations, nightmares, seizures.

Dermatologic – Facial edema; rash, including serious cutaneous reactions; urticaria.

Hypersensitivity – Allergic or allergic-like reaction, including oropharyngeal edema.

Respiratory – Bronchospasm, dyspnea.

Overdosage

There have been no reports of overdosage from administration of zanamivir.

Patient Information

Instruct patients in the use of the delivery system. Include a demonstration with the instructions whenever possible.

Advise patients that the use of zanamivir for treatment of influenza has not been shown to reduce the risk of transmission of influenza to others.

Advise patients of the risk of bronchospasm, especially in the setting of underlying airway disease, and to stop zanamivir and contact their health care provider if they experience increased respiratory symptoms during treatment, such as worsening wheezing, shortness of breath, or other signs or symptoms of bronchospasm. If a decision is made to prescribe zanamivir for a patient with asthma or COPD, make the patient aware of the risks and advise them to have a fast-acting bronchodilator available. Advise patients scheduled to take inhaled bronchodilators at the same time as zanamivir to use their bronchodilators before taking zanamivir.

Inform patients with influenza (the flu), particularly children and adolescents, may be at an increased risk of seizures, confusion, or abnormal behavior early in their illness. These reactions may occur after beginning zanamivir or may occur when flu is not treated. These reactions are uncommon but may result in accidental injury to the patient. Therefore, observe patients for signs of unusual behavior and contact a health care provider immediately if the patient shows any signs of unusual behavior.

If zanamivir is prescribed for children, it should be used only under adult supervision and instruction, and only after the supervising adult receives instruction by a health care provider.

OSELTAMIVIR

Rx	**Tamiflu** (Genentech USA)	**Capsules; oral:** 30 mg	As oseltamivir phosphate. (ROCHE 30 mg). Lt. yellow. In UD 10s.
		45 mg	As oseltamivir phosphate. (ROCHE 45 mg). Gray. In UD 10s.
		75 mg	As oseltamivir phosphate. (ROCHE 75 mg). Gray/Lt. yellow. In UD 10s.
		Powder for suspension; oral: 12 mg/mL (after reconstitution)	As oseltamivir phosphate. Saccharin, sorbitol. Tutti-frutti flavor. In 25 mL glass bottle with bottle adapter and oral dispenser.

OSELTAMIVIR PHOSPHATE — ORAL

Indications

➤*Prophylaxis of influenza:* For the prophylaxis of influenza in patients 1 year of age and older.

Influenza viruses change over time. Emergence of resistance mutations could decrease drug effectiveness. Other factors (eg, changes in viral virulence) might also diminish clinical benefit of antiviral drugs. Health care providers should consider available information on influenza drug susceptibility patterns and treatment effects when deciding whether to use oseltamivir.

➤*Treatment of influenza:* For the treatment of uncomplicated acute illness caused by influenza infection in patients 1 year of age and older who have been symptomatic for no more than 2 days.

➤*Off-label uses:*

H1N1 influenza A (swine flu) – For treatment and chemoprophylaxis of H1N1 influenza A (swine flu) virus infection. This includes patients with confirmed, probable, or suspected H1N1 influenza A (swine flu) virus infection and their close contacts. For more information, refer to the CDC guidelines at http://www.cdc.gov/h1n1flu/recommendations.htm.

Administration and Dosage

➤*Adults:*

Prophylaxis of influenza –

Usual dosage: 75 mg once daily for at least 10 days following close contact with an infected individual. Therapy should begin within 2 days of exposure. The recommended dosage for prophylaxis during a community outbreak of influenza is 75 mg once daily.

Duration of therapy: For a community outbreak, safety and efficacy have been demonstrated for up to 6 weeks. The duration of protection lasts for as long as dosing is continued.

Treatment of influenza – 75 mg twice daily for 5 days. Treatment should begin within 2 days of onset of influenza symptoms.

➤*Children:*

Prophylaxis of influenza –

13 years of age and older: See Adults for dosing.

1 to 12 years of age:

• *Usual dosage* – Therapy should begin within 2 days of exposure.

OSELTAMIVIR PHOSPHATE — ORAL

Oseltamivir Dosing for the Prophylaxis of Influenza in Children				
Body weight (kg)	Body weight (lbs)	Recommended dosage for 10 days	Number of bottles of oral suspension needed to obtain the recommended dose for a 10-day regimen	Number of capsules needed to obtain the recommended dose for a 10-day regimen
≤ 15 kg	≤ 33 lbs	30 mg once daily	1	10 (30 mg)
> 15 to 23 kg	> 33 to 51 lbs	45 mg once daily	2	10 (45 mg)
> 23 to 40 kg	> 51 to 88 lbs	60 mg once daily	2	20 (30 mg)
> 40 kg	> 88 lbs	75 mg once daily	3	10 (75 mg)

• *Duration of therapy* – Prophylaxis in children following close contact with an infected individual is recommended for 10 days. Prophylaxis in patients 1 to 12 years of age has not been evaluated for longer than 10 days' duration.

Treatment of influenza –
13 years of age and older: See Adults for dosing.
1 to 12 years of age:
• *Usual dosage* – Treatment should begin within 2 days of onset of influenza symptoms.

Oseltamivir Dosing for the Treatment of Influenza in Children (1 to 12 years of age)				
Body weight (kg)	Body weight (lbs)	Recommended dosage for 5 days	Number of bottles of oral suspension needed to obtain the recommended dose for a 5-day regimen	Number of capsules needed to obtain the recommended dose for a 5-day regimen
≤ 15 kg	≤ 33 lbs	30 mg twice daily	1	10 (30 mg)
> 15 to 23 kg	> 33 to 51 lbs	45 mg twice daily	2	10 (45 mg)
> 23 to 40 kg	> 51 to 88 lbs	60 mg twice daily	2	20 (30 mg)
> 40 kg	> 88 lbs	75 mg twice daily	3	10 (75 mg)

➤*Renal function impairment:*

Prophylaxis of influenza – For patients with creatinine clearance (CrCl) between 10 and 30 mL/min, reduce dosage to 75 mg every other day or 30 mg every day.

Treatment of influenza – For patients with CrCl between 10 and 30 mL/min, reduce dosage to 75 mg once daily for 5 days.

➤*Emergency pharmacy-compounded suspension from oseltamivir 75 mg capsules:* The compounding procedure results in a 15 mg/mL suspension, which is different from the commercially available oseltamivir for oral suspension (12 mg/mL). (See also Preparation for Administration.)

Dosing for Emergency Pharmacy-Compounded Suspension (15 mg/mL) From Oseltamivir 75 mg Capsules[a]					
Body weight (kg)	Body weight (lbs)	Dose (mg)	Volume per dose 15 mg/mL	Treatment dosage (for 5 days)	Prophylaxis dosage (for 10 days)
≤ 15 kg	≤ 33 lbs	30 mg	2 mL	2 mL twice daily	2 mL once daily
16 to 23 kg	34 to 51 lbs	45 mg	3 mL	3 mL twice daily	3 mL once daily
24 to 40 kg	52 to 88 lbs	60 mg	4 mL	4 mL twice daily	4 mL once daily
≥ 41 kg	≥ 89 lbs	75 mg	5 mL	5 mL twice daily	5 mL once daily

[a] 1 teaspoon = 5 mL.

➤*Preparation for administration:*

Powder for oral suspension

1.) Tap the closed bottle several times to loosen the powder.
2.) Measure 23 mL of water in a graduated cylinder.
3.) Add the total amount of water for reconstitution to the bottle and shake the closed bottle well for 15 seconds.
4.) Remove the child-resistant cap and push the bottle adapter into the neck of the bottle.
5.) Tightly close the bottle with the child-resistant cap. This will ensure the proper seating of the bottle adapter in the bottle and child-resistant status of the cap.

Emergency compounding of an oral suspension from oseltamivir capsules (final concentration of 15 mg/mL) – The following directions are provided for use only during emergency situations. These directions are not intended to be used if the FDA-approved, commercially manufactured oseltamivir oral suspension is readily available from wholesalers or the manufacturer.

Compounding an oral suspension with this procedure will provide 1 patient with enough medication for a 5-day course of treatment or a 10-day course of prophylaxis.

Commercially manufactured oseltamivir oral suspension (12 mg/mL) is the preferred product for children and adult patients who have difficulty swallowing capsules or when lower doses are needed. In the event that oseltamivir oral suspension is not available, the pharmacist may compound a suspension (15 mg/mL) from oseltamivir 75 mg capsules using either of 2 vehicles: cherry syrup (*Humco*) or *Ora-Sweet SF* (sugar-free). Other vehicles have not been studied. This compounded suspension should not be used for convenience or when the FDA-approved oseltamivir oral suspension is commercially available.

First, calculate the total volume of an oral suspension needed to be compounded and dispensed for each patient. The total volume required is determined by the weight of each patient.

Volume of Oseltamivir Oral Suspension (15 mg/mL) Needed to be Compounded Based Upon the Patient's Weight		
Body weight (kg)	Body weight (lbs)	Total volume to compound per patient (mL)
≤ 15 kg	≤ 33 lbs	30 mL
16 to 23 kg	34 to 51 lbs	40 mL
24 to 40 kg	52 to 88 lbs	50 mL
≥ 41 kg	≥ 89 lbs	60 mL

Second, determine the number of capsules and the amount of vehicle (cherry syrup or *Ora-Sweet SF*) that is needed to prepare the total volume (calculated from the previous table: 30, 40, 50, or 60 mL) of compounded oral suspension (15 mg/mL).

Number of Oseltamivir 75 mg Capsules and Amount of Vehicle Needed to Prepare the Total Volume of a Compounded Oral Suspension (15 mg/mL)		
Total volume of compounded oral suspension needed to be prepared	Required number of oseltamivir 75 mg capsules	Required volume of vehicle
30 mL	6 capsules (450 mg)	29 mL
40 mL	8 capsules (600 mg)	38.5 mL
50 mL	10 capsules (750 mg)	48 mL
60 mL	12 capsules (900 mg)	57 mL

Third, refer to the following procedure for compounding the oral suspension (15 mg/mL) from oseltamivir 75 mg capsules.

1.) Carefully separate the capsule body and cap and transfer the contents of the required number of oseltamivir 75 mg capsules into a clean mortar.
2.) Triturate the granules to a fine powder.
3.) Add one-third of the specified amount of vehicle and triturate the powder until a uniform suspension is achieved.
4.) Transfer the suspension to an amber glass or amber polyethylene terephthalate bottle. A funnel may be used to eliminate any spillage.
5.) Add another one-third of the vehicle to the mortar, rinse the pestle and mortar with a triturating motion, and transfer the vehicle into the bottle.
6.) Repeat the rinsing (step 5) with the remainder of the vehicle.
7.) Close the bottle using a child-resistant cap.
8.) Shake well to completely dissolve the active drug and to ensure homogeneous distribution of the dissolved drug in the resulting suspension. (Note: The active drug, oseltamivir, readily dissolves in the specified vehicles. The suspension is caused by some of the inert ingredients of oseltamivir capsules, which are insoluble in these vehicles.)
9.) Put an ancillary label on the bottle indicating "Shake gently before use" (this compounded suspension should be shaken gently prior to administration to minimize the tendency for air entrapment, particularly with the *Ora-Sweet SF* preparation).
10.) Instruct the parent or guardian that any remaining material following completion of therapy must be discarded by either affixing an ancillary label to the bottle or adding a statement to the pharmacy label instructions.
11.) Place an appropriate expiration date label according to storage condition.

Consider dispensing the suspension with a graduated oral syringe for measuring small amounts of suspension. If possible, mark or highlight the graduation corresponding to the appropriate dose (2, 3, 4, or 5 mL) on the oral syringe for each patient. The dosing device dispensed with the commercially available oseltamivir for oral suspension should not be used with the compounded suspension because they have different concentrations.

➤*Administration:* May take with or without food. Tolerability may be enhanced if taken with food. Shake the oral suspension well before each use.

An oral dosing dispenser with 30, 45, and 60 mg graduations is provided with the oral suspension; the 75 mg dose can be measured using a combination of 30 and 45 mg. It is recommended that patients use this dispenser. In the event that the dispenser provided is lost or damaged, another dosing syringe or other device may be used to deliver the following volumes: 2.5 mL (½ teaspoon) for children weighing 15 kg or less; 3.8 mL (¾ teaspoon) for

OSELTAMIVIR PHOSPHATE — ORAL

children weighing 15 to 23 kg; 5 mL (1 teaspoon) for children weighing 23 to 40 kg; and 6.2 mL (1¼ teaspoon) for children weighing more than 40 kg.

Oseltamivir oral suspension may also be used by patients who cannot swallow a capsule. For children who cannot swallow capsules, oseltamivir oral suspension is the preferred formulation.

If the oral suspension is not available, oseltamivir capsules may be opened and mixed with sweetened liquids such as regular or sugar-free chocolate syrup.

➤*Storage/Stability:*

Dry powder for suspension/capsules – Store at 25°C (77°F); excursions are permitted between 15° and 30°C (59° and 86°F).

Reconstituted suspension – Store under refrigeration between 2° and 8°C (36° and 46°F). Do not freeze. Patients should use the reconstituted oral suspension within 10 days of preparation.

Pharmacy-compounded suspension –
Refrigeration: Stable for 5 weeks (35 days) when stored in a refrigerator between 2° and 8°C (36° and 46°F).
Room temperature: Stable for 5 days when stored at room temperature, 25°C (77°F).

Actions

➤*Pharmacology:* Oseltamivir is an ethyl ester prodrug requiring ester hydrolysis for conversion to the active form, oseltamivir carboxylate. Oseltamivir carboxylate is an inhibitor of influenza virus neuraminidase affecting release of viral particles.

➤*Pharmacokinetics:*

Absorption – Oseltamivir is readily absorbed from the GI tract after oral administration and is extensively converted, predominantly by hepatic esterases, to oseltamivir carboxylate. At least 75% of an oral dose reaches the systemic circulation as oseltamivir carboxylate. Exposure to oseltamivir is less than 5% of the total exposure after oral dosing. See the following table.

Oseltamivir and Oseltamivir Carboxylate Mean (% CV[a]) Pharmacokinetic Parameters After a Multiple 75 mg Capsule Twice-Daily Oral Dosage		
Parameter	Oseltamivir (n = 20)	Oseltamivir carboxylate (n = 20)
C_{max}[b] (ng/mL)	65.2 (26%)	348 (18%)
$AUC_{0\text{-}12h}$[c] (ng•h/mL)	112 (25%)	2,719 (20%)

[a] CV = coefficient of variation.
[b] C_{max} = maximal drug concentration.
[c] $AUC_{0\text{-}12h}$ = area under the curve from 0 to 12 hours.

Plasma concentrations of oseltamivir carboxylate are proportional to doses of up to 500 mg given twice daily.

Distribution – The volume of distribution of oseltamivir carboxylate, following intravenous administration in 24 subjects, ranged between 23 and 26 L.

The binding of oseltamivir carboxylate to human plasma protein is low (3%). The binding of oseltamivir to human plasma protein is 42%, which is insufficient to cause significant displacement-based drug interactions.

Metabolism – Oseltamivir is extensively converted to oseltamivir carboxylate by esterases located predominantly in the liver. Neither oseltamivir nor oseltamivir carboxylate is a substrate for, or inhibitor of, CYP-450 isoforms.

Excretion – Absorbed oseltamivir is primarily (more than 90%) eliminated by conversion to oseltamivir carboxylate. Plasma concentrations of oseltamivir declined with a half-life of 1 to 3 hours in most subjects after oral administration. Oseltamivir carboxylate is not further metabolized and is eliminated in the urine. Plasma concentrations of oseltamivir carboxylate declined, with a half-life of 6 to 10 hours in most subjects after oral administration. Oseltamivir carboxylate is eliminated entirely (more than 99%) by renal excretion. Renal clearance (18.8 L/h) exceeds glomerular filtration rate (7.5 L/h), indicating that tubular secretion occurs in addition to glomerular filtration. Less than 20% of an oral radiolabeled dose is eliminated in feces.

Special populations –
Renal function impairment: Administration of oseltamivir 100 mg twice daily for 5 days to patients with various degrees of renal impairment showed that exposure to oseltamivir carboxylate is inversely proportional to declining renal function. Oseltamivir carboxylate exposures in patients with healthy and unhealthy renal function administered various dose regimens of oseltamivir are described in the following table.

Oseltamivir Carboxylate Exposures in Patients With Healthy and Reduced Serum CrCl								
	Healthy renal function			Renal function impairment				
				CrCl < 10 mL/min		CrCl > 10 and < 30 mL/min		
				CAPD[a]	Hemodialysis			
Parameter	75 mg once daily	75 mg twice daily	150 mg twice daily	30 mg weekly	30 mg alternate hemodialysis cycle	75 mg daily	75 mg alternate days	30 mg daily
C_{max}	259[b]	348[b]	705[b]	766	850	1,638	1,175	655
C_{min}[c]	39[b]	138[b]	288[b]	62	48	864	209	346
AUC_{48}[d]	7,476[b]	10,876[b]	21,864[b]	17,381	12,429	62,636	21,999	25,054

[a] CAPD = continuous ambulatory peritoneal dialysis.
[b] Observed values. All other values are predicted.
[c] C_{min} = minimum drug concentration.
[d] AUC normalized to 48 hours.

Elderly: Exposure to oseltamivir carboxylate at steady state was 25% to 35% higher in elderly patients (range, 65 to 78 years of age) than in young adults given comparable doses of oseltamivir. Based on drug exposure and tolerability, dosage adjustments are not required for elderly patients for either treatment or prophylaxis.

Children: Younger children cleared the prodrug and active metabolite faster than adult patients, resulting in a lower exposure for a given mg/kg dose. For oseltamivir carboxylate, apparent total clearance decreases linearly with increasing age (up to 12 years of age). The pharmacokinetics of oseltamivir in children older than 12 years of age are similar to those in adult patients.

Contraindications

Hypersensitivity to any of the components of the product.

Warnings/Precautions

➤*Treatment initiation:* Efficacy of oseltamivir in patients who begin treatment after 40 hours of symptoms has not been established.

➤*Repeated courses:* Safety and efficacy of repeated treatment or prophylaxis courses have not been studied.

➤*Bacterial infections:* Serious bacterial infections may begin with influenza-like symptoms or may coexist with or occur as complications during the course of influenza. Oseltamivir has not been shown to prevent such complications.

➤*Neuropsychiatric reactions:* Influenza can be associated with a variety of neurologic and behavioral symptoms, which can include events such as hallucinations, delirium, and abnormal behavior, in some cases resulting in fatal outcomes. These events may occur in the setting of encephalitis or encephalopathy but can occur without obvious severe disease.

There have been postmarketing reports (mostly from Japan) of delirium and abnormal behavior leading to injury, sometimes resulting in fatal outcomes, in patients with influenza who were receiving oseltamivir. Because these events were voluntarily reported during clinical practice, estimates of frequency cannot be made, but they appear to be uncommon based on oseltamivir usage data. These events were primarily reported among children and often had an abrupt onset and rapid resolution. The contribution of oseltamivir to these events has not been established. Closely monitor patients with influenza for signs of abnormal behavior. If neuropsychiatric symptoms occur, evaluate the risks and benefits of continuing treatment for each patient.

➤*Hypersensitivity reactions:* Rare cases of anaphylaxis and serious skin reactions, including erythema multiforme, Stevens-Johnson syndrome, and toxic epidermal necrolysis (TEN), have been reported in postmarketing experience with oseltamivir. Stop oseltamivir and institute appropriate treatment if an allergic-like reaction occurs or is suspected.

Live vaccines – The concurrent use of oseltamivir with intranasal live attenuated influenza vaccine has not been evaluated; however, because of the potential for interference between these products, do not administer live attenuated influenza vaccine within 2 weeks before or 48 hours after administration of oseltamivir, unless medically indicated. The concern about possible interference arises from the potential for antiviral drugs to inhibit replication of live vaccine virus. Trivalent inactivated influenza vaccine can be administered at any time relative to oseltamivir use.

➤*Renal function impairment:* Dosage adjustment is recommended for patients with a CrCl of less than 30 mL/min.

➤*Pregnancy: Category C.* Because animal reproductive studies may not be predictive of human response and there are no adequate and well-controlled studies in pregnant women, use oseltamivir during pregnancy only if the potential benefit justifies the potential risk to the fetus. It is not known if oseltamivir or oseltamivir carboxylate cross the placenta to the human fetus. The molecular weight (about 312 for the free base of oseltamivir) is low enough that transfer to the fetus should be expected.

Per the CDC recommendations for the treatment of H1N1 influenza A (swine flu), oseltamivir is the preferred choice because of its systemic activity. The drug of choice for prophylaxis is less clear. Zanamivir may be preferable because of its limited systemic absorption; however, respiratory

OSELTAMIVIR PHOSPHATE — ORAL

complications that may be associated with zanamivir because of its inhaled route of administration need to be considered, especially in women at risk for respiratory problems. For more information, refer to the CDC guidelines at http://www.cdc.gov/h1n1flu/recommendations.htm.

Pharmacokinetic studies indicated that fetal exposure was seen in both rats and rabbits. In the rat study, minimal maternal toxicity was reported in the 1,500 mg/kg/day group. In the rabbit study, slight and marked maternal toxicities were observed in the 150 and 500 mg/kg/day groups, respectively. There was a dose-dependent increase in the incidence rates of a variety of minor skeletal abnormalities and variants in the exposed offspring in these studies; however, the individual incidence rate of each skeletal abnormality or variant remained within the background rates of occurrence in the species studied.

Because animal reproductive studies may not be predictive of human response and there are no adequate and well-controlled studies in pregnant women, use oseltamivir during pregnancy only if the potential benefit justifies the potential risk to the fetus.

➤*Lactation:* In lactating rats, oseltamivir and oseltamivir carboxylate are excreted in the milk. Because the molecular weight of oseltamivir (about 312 for the free base) is low enough, excretion into breast milk should be expected. It is not known whether oseltamivir or oseltamivir carboxylate is excreted in human milk. Only use oseltamivir if the potential benefit for the breast-feeding mother justifies the potential risk to the infant.

➤*Children:* The safety and efficacy of oseltamivir in children younger than 1 year of age have not been studied. Oseltamivir is not indicated for treatment or prophylaxis of influenza in children younger than 1 year of age because of uncertainties regarding the rate of development of the human blood-brain barrier and the unknown clinical significance of nonclinical animal toxicology data for human infants.

➤*Monitoring:* Closely monitor patients with influenza for signs of unhealthy behavior throughout the treatment period.

Drug Interactions

➤*Live vaccines:* See Warnings/Precautions for more information.

➤*Probenecid:* Coadministration of probenecid results in an approximate 2-fold increase in exposure to oseltamivir carboxylate because of a decrease in active anionic tubular secretion in the kidney. However, because of the safety margin of oseltamivir carboxylate, no dosage adjustments are required with probenecid coadministration.

Adverse Reactions

➤*Adults and adolescents (13 years of age and older): Treatment and prophylaxis of influenza –*

Oseltamivir Treatment and Prophylaxis of Influenza Adverse Reactions in Patients 13 Years of Age and Older (≥ 1%)

	Influenza treatment		Influenza prophylaxis	
Adverse reaction	Placebo (n = 716)	Oseltamivir 75 mg twice daily (n = 724)	Placebo/ no prophylaxis[a] (n = 1,688)	Oseltamivir 75 mg daily (n = 1,790)
CNS				
Dizziness	3%	2%	1%	1%
Fatigue	1%	1%	10%	8%
Headache	2%	2%	18%	18%
Insomnia	1%	1%	1%	1%
Vertigo	1%	1%	< 1%	< 1%
GI				
Abdominal pain	2%	2%	1%	2%
Diarrhea	10%	7%	2%	3%
Nausea (without vomiting)	6%	10%	3%	7%
Vomiting	3%	9%	1%	2%
Respiratory				
Bronchitis	2%	2%	1%	1%
Cough	2%	1%	7%	5%

[a] The majority of subjects received placebo; 254 subjects from a randomized, open-label, postexposure prophylaxis study in households did not receive placebo or prophylaxis therapy.

Other adverse reactions (less than 1%) – Anemia, humerus fracture, peritonsillar abscess, pneumonia, pseudomembranous colitis, pyrexia, unstable angina.

➤*Children (1 to 12 years of age): Treatment and prophylaxis of influenza –*

Oseltamivir Treatment and Prophylaxis of Influenza Adverse Reactions in Children (≥ 1%)

	Influenza treatment trials[a]		Household influenza prophylaxis trial[b]	
Adverse reaction	Placebo (n = 517)	Oseltamivir 2 mg/kg twice daily (n = 515)	No prophylaxis[c] (n = 87)	Prophylaxis with oseltamivir daily[c] (n = 99)
GI				
Abdominal pain	4%	5%	—	3%
Diarrhea	11%	10%	—	1%
Nausea	4%	3%	1%	4%
Vomiting	9%	15%	2%	10%
Respiratory				
Asthma (including aggravated)	4%	3%	1%	1%
Bronchitis	2%	2%	2%	—
Epistaxis	3%	3%	—	1%
Pneumonia	3%	2%	2%	—
Sinusitis	3%	2%	—	—
Special senses				
Conjunctivitis	< 1%	1%	—	—
Ear disorder	1%	2%	—	—
Otitis media	11%	9%	2%	2%
Tympanic membrane disorder	1%	1%	—	—
Miscellaneous				
Dermatitis	2%	1%	—	—
Lymphadenopathy	2%	1%	—	—

[a] Pooled data from phase 3 trials of oseltamivir treatment of naturally acquired influenza.
[b] A randomized, open-label study of household transmission in which household contacts received either prophylaxis or no prophylaxis but treatment if they became ill. Only contacts who received prophylaxis or who remained on no prophylaxis are included in this table.
[c] Unit dose = age-based dosing: 1 to 2 years of age received prophylaxis (10 days) 30 mg once daily; 3 to 5 years of age received prophylaxis (10 days) 45 mg once daily; 6 to 12 years of age received prophylaxis (10 days) 60 mg once daily.

➤*Postmarketing:*

CNS – Abnormal behavior, agitation, anxiety, confusion, delirium (including symptoms such as altered level of consciousness), delusions, hallucinations, nightmares, seizure.

Dermatologic – Dermatitis, eczema, erythema multiforme, rash, Stevens-Johnson syndrome, TEN, urticaria.

GI – GI bleeding, hemorrhagic colitis.

Hepatic – Abnormal liver function tests, hepatitis.

Hypersensitivity – Allergy, anaphylactic/anaphylactoid reactions, swelling of the face or tongue.

Miscellaneous – Aggravation of diabetes; arrhythmia.

Overdosage

➤*Symptoms:* At present, there has been no experience with overdose. Single doses of up to 1,000 mg have been associated with nausea and/or vomiting.

Patient Information

Instruct patients to begin treatment with oseltamivir as soon as possible after the first appearance of flu symptoms. Similarly, prevention should begin as soon as possible after exposure, at the recommendation of a health care provider.

Instruct patients to take any missed doses as soon as they remember, unless it is near the time of the next scheduled dose (within 2 hours), and then to continue to take oseltamivir at the usual times.

Oseltamivir is not a substitute for a flu vaccination. Instruct patients to continue receiving an annual flu shot according to guidelines on immunization practices.

A bottle of oseltamivir 13 g for oral suspension contains approximately 11 g of sorbitol. One dose of 75 mg oseltamivir for oral suspension delivers sorbitol 2 g. For patients with hereditary fructose intolerance, this is above the daily maximum limit of sorbitol and may cause dyspepsia and diarrhea.

PERAMIVIR (INVESTIGATIONAL)

Rx	**Peramivir**[a] (BioCryst)	**Injection, solution:** 200 mg per 20 mL (10 mg/mL)	Preservative free. In single-dose vials.

[a] Peramivir is an investigational agent. It is for use under an emergency use authorization (EUA) for treatment of certain patients with 2009 H1N1 influenza.

PERAMIVIR — INJECTION

Indications

➤*H1N1 influenza A (swine flu) emergency treatment:* Peramivir is an intravenous (IV) investigational drug authorized for emergency use for the treatment of certain hospitalized patients with known or suspected 2009 H1N1 influenza.

➤*Authorized use:* Peramivir is authorized for use under an EUA for treatment of certain patients with suspected or laboratory-confirmed 2009 H1N1 infection or infection caused by nonsubtypable influenza A virus suspected to be 2009 H1N1, based on community epidemiology. Specifically, peramivir is authorized only for the following patients who are admitted to a hospital and for whom an IV agent is clinically appropriate based upon one of the following reasons:

Adults –

1.) Patient is not responding to either oral or inhaled antiviral therapy, or
2.) drug delivery by a route other than IV (eg, enteral oseltamivir or inhaled zanamivir) is not expected to be dependable or is not feasible, or
3.) the health care provider judges IV therapy to be appropriate because of other circumstances.

Children –

1.) Patient is not responding to either oral or inhaled antiviral therapy, or
2.) drug delivery by a route other than IV (eg, enteral oseltamivir or inhaled zanamivir) is not expected to be dependable or is not feasible.

Only the United States' Centers for Disease Control and Prevention (CDC) is authorized to distribute peramivir to a hospital at the request of the licensed treating clinician. A peramivir IV request must be submitted electronically to the CDC to obtain peramivir via the CDC's Peramivir IV Electronic Request System.

Administration and Dosage

➤*General dosing considerations:* Peramivir is an investigational drug. Maintain adequate records showing receipt, use, and disposition of peramivir. For unused intact vials, maintain adequate records showing use and disposition of peramivir.

All patients with known or suspected renal insufficiency must have creatinine clearance (CrCl) determined and dosing of peramivir adjusted accordingly. (See also Renal Function Impairment.)

➤*Adults:* 600 mg given IV over 30 minutes once daily for 5 to 10 days.

➤*Children:*

Usual dosage –

Peramivir Dose Recommendations in Children[a]

Age	Dosage
Birth through 30 days	6 mg/kg IV over 60 minutes once daily for 5 to 10 days
31 through 90 days	8 mg/kg IV over 60 minutes once daily for 5 to 10 days
91 through 180 days	10 mg/kg IV over 60 minutes once daily for 5 to 10 days
181 days through 5 years	12 mg/kg IV over 60 minutes once daily for 5 to 10 days
6 through 17 years	10 mg/kg IV over 60 minutes once daily for 5 to 10 days

[a] Maximum daily dose is 600 mg IV.

Maximum dose – 600 mg/day once daily for 5 to 10 days.

➤*Renal function impairment:*

Adults –

Peramivir Dosage Recommendations in Adults With Renal Function Impairment

CrCl[a] or estimated clearance (CL_{CRRT}[b] + residual renal clearance)	Daily dose (IV)
Mild renal impairment (CrCl 50 to 80 mL/min)	600 mg
Moderate renal impairment (CrCl 31 to 49 mL/min)	150 mg
Severe renal impairment (CrCl 10 to 30 mL/min)	100 mg
CrCl < 10 mL/min who are not on dialysis or renal replacement therapy	100 mg on day 1 of dosing, followed by 15 mg once daily thereafter
ESRD[c] on intermittent hemodialysis	100 mg on day 1, then 100 mg given 2 h after each hemodialysis session on dialysis days only

[a] Calculated using Cockcroft and Gault equation, when serum creatinine represents a steady state of renal function.
[b] Calculated using equation applicable to type of continuous renal replacement therapy (CRRT). See equations in Calculation of CRRT Clearance for Various Types of CRRT table.
[c] ESRD = end-stage renal disease.

Continuous venovenous hemofiltration or other CRRT: Very limited data available for peramivir in the setting of continuous venovenous hemofiltration (CVVH) and continuous venovenous hemodialysis (CVVHD) indicate peramivir is efficiently cleared by CRRT. Ultrafiltrate concentrations from a single adult patient on CVVH revealed a high sieving coefficient (approximately 80%), consistent with peramivir's low protein binding (less than 30%).

For renally impaired patients receiving CRRT, the peramivir dose should be selected according to the previous table, but using the CRRT clearance (CL_{CRRT}, as outlined below) instead of calculated CrCl determined with the Cockcroft and Gault equation. If the patient has any residual renal function while on CRRT, an estimate of the patient's renal clearance should be added to CL_{CRRT} in order to estimate total clearance before using the previous table.

The following equations were derived from previously published recommendations for drug dosing in the setting of CRRT and are based on several assumptions about peramivir, including low or negligible protein binding (f_u = 1) and a high sieving coefficient (SC = 100%). These assumptions may result in overestimation of clearance depending on actual protein binding or sieving coefficient. For CRRT methods with a diffusive component (CVVHD and continuous arteriovenous hemodialysis [CAVHD]), the following equation does not account for dialysate saturation, which may result in a higher CL_{CRRT} estimate than is actually observed.

Dose modifications should be made, as appropriate, for changes in patient renal function, changes to ultrafiltrate or dialysate flow rate, or initiation, discontinuation, or changes to CRRT.

Peramivir Calculation of CRRT Clearance for Various Types of CRRT[a]

Type of CRRT	Equation for calculation of CRRT clearance[b]
For SCUF or CAVH or CVVH	$CL_{CRRT} = Q_f$
For CAVHD or CVVHD	$CL_{CRRT} = Q_d$
For CAVHDF and CVVHDF	$CL_{CRRT} = Q_f + Q_d$

[a] SCUF = slow continuous ultrafiltration; CAVH = continuous arteriovenous hemofiltration; CAVHDF = continuous arteriovenous hemodiafiltration; CVVHDF = continuous venovenous hemodiafiltration.
[b] Q_f = ultrafiltration rate (mL/min); Q_d = dialysate flow rate (mL/min)

Children –

Peramivir Dosage Recommendations in Children With Renal Function Impairment

Age	CrCl[a] or estimated clearance (CL_{CRRT}[b] + residual renal CL): 50 to 80 mL/min per 1.73 m²	31 to 49 mL/min per 1.73 m²	10 to 30 mL/min per 1.73 m²	< 10 mL/min per 1.73 m² and not on intermittent hemodialysis or CRRT	ESRD (< 10 mL/min per 1.73 m²) on intermittent hemodialysis
Birth through 30 days	6 mg/kg once daily	1.5 mg/kg once daily	1 mg/kg once daily	1 mg/kg on day 1, then 0.15 mg/kg once daily	1 mg/kg on day 1, then 1 mg/kg given 2 h after each hemodialysis session on dialysis days only

PERAMIVIR — INJECTION

Peramivir Dosage Recommendations in Children With Renal Function Impairment					
	CrCl[a] or estimated clearance (CL_{CRRT}[b] + residual renal CL)				
Age	50 to 80 mL/min per 1.73 m²	31 to 49 mL/min per 1.73 m²	10 to 30 mL/min per 1.73 m²	< 10 mL/min per 1.73 m² and not on intermittent hemodialysis or CRRT	ESRD (< 10 mL/min per 1.73 m²) on intermittent hemodialysis
31 through 90 days	8 mg/kg once daily	2 mg/kg once daily	1.3 mg/kg once daily	1.3 mg/kg on day 1, then 0.2 mg/kg once daily	1.3 mg/kg on day 1, then 1.3 mg/kg given 2 h after each hemodialysis session on dialysis days only
91 through 180 days	10 mg/kg once daily	2.5 mg/kg once daily	1.6 mg/kg once daily	1.6 mg/kg on day 1, then 0.25 mg/kg once daily	1.6 mg/kg on day 1, then 1.6 mg/kg given 2 h after each hemodialysis session on dialysis days only
181 days through 5 years	12 mg/kg once daily	3 mg/kg once daily	1.9 mg/kg once daily	1.9 mg/kg on day 1, then 0.3 mg/kg once daily	1.9 mg/kg on day 1, then 1.9 mg/kg given 2 h after each hemodialysis session on dialysis days only
6 through 17 years	10 mg/kg once daily	2.5 mg/kg once daily	1.6 mg/kg once daily	1.6 mg/kg on day 1, then 0.25 mg/kg once daily	1.6 mg/kg on day 1, then 1.6 mg/kg given 2 h after each hemodialysis session on dialysis days only

[a] Calculated using Schwartz equation when serum creatinine represents a steady state of renal function.

[b] Calculated using equation applicable to type of continuous renal replacement therapy. See equations in Adults in Calculation of CRRT Clearance for Various Types of CRRT table.

CVVH or other CRRT: For renally impaired children receiving CRRT, the peramivir dose should be selected according to the previous table, but using the CRRT clearance (CL_{CRRT}) instead of calculated CrCl determined with the Schwartz equation. If the patient has any residual renal function while on CRRT, an estimate of the patient's renal clearance should be added to CL_{CRRT} in order to estimate total clearance before using the previous table. See the equations in Adults in Calculation of CRRT Clearance for Various Types of CRRT table.

➤*Duration of therapy:* Initial treatment courses are for 5 to 10 days' duration. For adults, treatment beyond 10 days is permitted depending on clinical presentation, such as critical illness (eg, respiratory failure or intensive care unit admission), continued viral shedding, or unresolved clinical influenza illness.

➤*Preparation for administration:* Peramivir must be diluted in sodium chloride 0.9% or 0.45% injection that does not contain dextrose or other electrolytes.

Adults – Transfer 600 mg (60 mL, or appropriate volume based on recommended dose for patients with renal impairment) of peramivir to an empty sterile container for IV use. Add 40 mL (or appropriate volume to reach a total of 100 mL based on the adjusted renal dose) of sodium chloride 0.9% or 0.45% injection to the container. The total volume of diluted solution should be 100 mL, with a maximum final concentration of 6 mg/mL.

Children – Calculate the recommended age-based dose according to the previous tables. Dilute the calculated dose using sodium chloride 0.9% or 0.45% injection in an empty sterile container for IV use. The final concentration of the diluted solution should not exceed 6 mg/mL. The diluted solution should be administered IV over 60 minutes, or an undiluted dose must be administered using an infusion device (eg, piggyback system, timed syringe system, pump) that allows infusion into an open IV line with sodium chloride injection over 60 minutes.

➤*Administration:* Infusion rates should not exceed 40 mg per minute. To the extent possible, a separate IV line or separate IV lumen in a multilumen catheter is recommended for infusion of peramivir. Do not administer as an intramuscular (IM) injection.

Administer over 30 minutes in adults and over 60 minutes in children.

Any unused portion of a single-use peramivir injection vial should be discarded after a diluted solution is prepared.

➤*Admixture compatibility:* The prepared diluted solution should not be administered simultaneously with any other medication. The compatibility of peramivir injection with IV solutions and medications other than sodium chloride injection is not known.

Heparin lock – Before infusion of peramivir via a heparin lock, the port should be flushed with 3 to 5 mL of sterile saline. After the infusion of peramivir is complete, the port should be flushed again with sterile saline and then heparin can be added to maintain patency of this catheter.

Single or multilumen catheter – If other medications are also administered via a single lumen catheter or a single lumen of a multilumen catheter, at least 10 mL of sterile saline should be administered between the infusion of any other medication and the administration of peramivir to ensure that all medication is flushed from the catheter tubing before peramivir is administered.

Peramivir may be piggybacked into an existing saline infusion line. When possible, the saline infusion rate should be reduced to ensure that peramivir IV is infused over 30 minutes for adults and over 60 minutes for pediatric patients.

➤*Storage/Stability:* Peramivir is authorized for use under an EUA.

Vials of peramivir should be stored at ambient temperature (15° to 30°C [59° to 86°F]). However, temperature extremes encountered during shipment and storage (including freezing) would likely not adversely affect the quality of this product. Once a diluted solution has been prepared, it should be administered immediately or stored under refrigerated conditions (2° to 8°C [36° to 46°F]). If refrigerated, the refrigerated diluted solution should be allowed to reach room temperature prior to administration. The diluted solution should be administered within 24 hours following preparation. Any unused diluted solution must be discarded after 24 hours.

Actions

➤*Pharmacology:* Peramivir is a cyclopentane analog that binds to the active site of influenza virus neuraminidase. It has inhibitory activity against human influenza A and influenza B viruses.

➤*Pharmacokinetics:*

Excretion – The half-life of peramivir following administration of 0.5 to 8 mg/kg as a single dose or 4 mg/kg twice daily for 1 day ranged from 7.7 to 20.8 hours. The major route of elimination of peramivir is via the kidney. Renal clearance of unchanged peramivir accounts for approximately 90% of total clearance.

Special populations –

Renal function impairment:

• *Mild renal impairment (CrCl 50 to 80 mL/min)* – The mean systemic exposures in patients with mild renal impairment are expected to be approximately 24% higher than the systemic exposures in patients with healthy renal function. These higher exposures in patients with mild renal impairment are not expected to be clinically relevant. Therefore, no dose adjustments are needed for patients with mild renal impairment.

• *Moderate renal impairment (CrCl 30 to 49 mL/min)* – The mean systemic exposures in patients with moderate renal impairment are expected to be approximately 3.4-fold higher than the exposures in patients with healthy renal function. Therefore, the dose of peramivir is reduced to 150 mg in order to achieve exposures similar to those in patients with healthy renal function after administration of a single 600 mg IV dose.

• *Severe renal impairment (CrCl 10 to 30 mL/min)* – The mean systemic exposures in patients with severe renal impairment are expected to be approximately 6-fold higher than the exposures in patients with healthy renal function. Therefore, the dose of peramivir is reduced to 100 mg in order to achieve exposures similar to those in patients with healthy renal function after administration of a single 600 mg IV dose.

PERAMIVIR — INJECTION

• *Patients with end-stage renal disease on intermittent hemodialysis –*

Predicted Peramivir Pharmacokinetic Parameters in Patients With End-Stage Renal Disease on Intermittent Hemodialysis[a]

	Healthy renal function (600 mg once daily)	Intermittent hemodialysis (100 mg on day 1, then 100 mg given 2 hours after each hemodialysis session)
AUC_{0-24} (average[b]) (ng•h/mL)	107,000	98,000
C_{max} (ng/mL)[c]	34,100	13,100
C_{min} (ng/mL)[c]	56	370

[a] Simulations were performed assuming a 4-hour hemodialysis session every 48 hours. Simulations were performed for a 7-day dosing duration.
[b] Average area under the curve (AUC_{0-24}) is the average of all AUC_{0-24} values predicted for the 7-day treatment duration.
[c] Maximal drug concentration (C_{max}) is the highest predicted C_{max}, and minimum plasma drug concentration (C_{min}) is the lowest predicted C_{min} for the simulated dosing period.

• *Patients with CrCl less than 10 mL/min who are not receiving intermittent hemodialysis or CRRT –*

Predicted Peramivir Pharmacokinetic Parameters in Patients With CrCl[a]

	Healthy renal function	CrCl < 10 mL/min and not receiving intermittent hemodialysis or CRRT
	600 mg once daily	100 mg on day 1, followed by 15 mg once daily
AUC_{0-24} (average)[b] (ng•h/mL)	107,000	122,000
AUC_{0-24} (day 1) (ng•h/mL)	106,000	142,000
C_{max}[c] (ng/mL)	34,100	10,300
C_{min}[c] (ng/mL)	56	4,060

[a] Simulations were performed assuming a 7-day dosing duration.
[b] Average AUC_{0-24} is the average of all AUC_{0-24} values predicted for the 7-day treatment duration.
[c] C_{max} is the highest predicted C_{max}, and C_{min} is the lowest predicted C_{min} for the simulated dosing period.

• *Patients undergoing CVVH or other CRRT* – Very limited data are available from patients on CVVH or CVVHD who received peramivir IV under emergency IND procedures. The pharmacokinetic sampling from these patients was sparse (2 to 4 samples per patient), timing of samples with respect to dose or CRRT is not well documented, and no information is provided regarding filter type, flow rate, or duration of renal replacement therapy. Ultrafiltrate concentrations from a single adult patient on CVVH revealed a high sieving coefficient (approximately 80%), consistent with peramivir's low protein binding (less than 30%).

Elderly: Comparisons of the pharmacokinetics of peramivir administered IV in healthy young volunteers with data from healthy volunteers (65 years of age and older) suggest patients in the 65 years of age and older group had approximately a 46% increase in dose-normalized AUC and, on average, approximately 26% lower clearance of peramivir primarily because of a decrease in kidney function. Peramivir C_{max} was independent of age and dose adjustment is not currently recommended for patients 65 years of age and older.

Contraindications

History of severe allergic reaction to any other neuraminidase inhibitors (zanamivir or oseltamivir) or any ingredient of peramivir.

Warnings/Precautions

➤*GI effects:* Monitor patients for development of diarrhea and administer appropriate evaluation and/or treatment, as indicated, including evaluation for other causes of diarrhea as clinically warranted.

All GI events, regardless of causality, were seen in 12.4% of patients receiving peramivir IV 600 mg compared with 18% of patients receiving oseltamivir. In the phase 3 trial, the incidence of diarrhea was similar between peramivir 600 mg IV and oseltamivir.

➤*Bacterial infections:* Serious bacterial infections may begin with influenza-like symptoms or may coexist with or develop as complications during the course of influenza illness. Monitor, evaluate, and treat patients for suspected bacterial infections as clinically warranted while administering peramivir.

➤*Neuropsychiatric events:* Influenza infection itself can be associated with a variety of neurologic and behavioral symptoms that can include events such as seizures, hallucinations, delirium, and abnormal behavior, in some cases resulting in fatal outcomes. These events may occur in the setting of encephalitis or encephalopathy but can occur without clinically apparent severe disease.

There have been postmarketing reports (mostly from Japan) of delirium and abnormal behavior leading to injury in patients with influenza who were receiving the approved neuraminidase inhibitors zanamivir or oseltamivir. These events appear to be uncommon based on usage data, have been reported primarily among children, and often had an abrupt onset and rapid resolution. Because peramivir is also a neuraminidase inhibitor and based on limited data from clinical trials, it is possible that these types of reactions or other types of neurologic and behavioral events could occur in patients receiving peramivir. Closely monitor patients with influenza for signs of abnormal behavior. If neuropsychiatric symptoms occur, evaluate the risks and benefits of continuing treatment for each patient.

➤*Hypersensitivity reactions:* Serious allergic-like reactions have not been reported in clinical trials in patients receiving peramivir to date. However, allergic-like reactions, including oropharyngeal edema, serious skin rashes, and anaphylaxis, have been reported with use of neuraminidase inhibitors, including zanamivir and oseltamivir. Discontinue peramivir and institute appropriate treatment if an allergic reaction occurs or is suspected.

➤*Pregnancy:* No adequate and well-controlled studies of peramivir use in pregnant women have been conducted. Use peramivir during pregnancy only if the potential benefit justifies the potential risk for the mother and fetus. No teratogenicity was detected in fertility and developmental studies conducted in rats and rabbits. Peramivir administered IV at 200 mg/kg caused severe maternal toxicity (dose-limiting nephrosis) in pregnant rabbits and an increased incidence of abortion and embryotoxicity, considered to be related to the maternal toxicity. Peramivir did not produce significant maternal toxicity or embryotoxicity (up to 600 mg/kg) in pregnant rats.

➤*Lactation:* Peramivir has not been studied in breast-feeding mothers. Studies in rats demonstrated peramivir is excreted in milk. Lactating rats excreted peramivir into the milk at levels below the mother's plasma drug concentrations. However, inform breast-feeding mothers that it is not known whether peramivir is excreted in human milk.

➤*Children:* Peramivir has not been administered to any children (younger than 18 years of age) in clinical trials. However, limited use of peramivir in adults and children has been allowed for peramivir under emergency IND procedures.

➤*Elderly:* Clinical studies of peramivir do not include sufficient numbers of patients 65 year of age and older to determine whether they respond differently from younger patients. In general, appropriate caution should be exercised in the administration of peramivir IV and monitoring of elderly patients, reflecting the greater frequency of decreased hepatic, renal, or cardiac function, and of concomitant disease or other drug therapy.

➤*Monitoring:*

Peramivir Recommended Monitoring

Assessment	Laboratory parameter	Timing
Complete blood cell count with differential and a basic metabolic profile	Glucose, calcium, sodium, potassium, chloride, serum bicarbonate, creatinine, and blood urea nitrogen	Upon initiation, day 3 of therapy, and end of therapy.
Liver-associated tests	ALT, AST, alkaline phosphatase, and total and direct bilirubin	Upon initiation and conclusion of therapy and during therapy, if clinically indicated.
Urinalysis[a]		Upon initiation and conclusion of therapy and during therapy, if clinically indicated. If significant proteinuria develops while on therapy, consider appropriate further evaluation, including laboratory testing, 24-hour urine collection, and possible nephrology consultation.
Assessment of renal function	Serum creatinine (at a minimum)	Completed prior to initiation of dosing and followed carefully throughout dosing, as clinically appropriate.
Vital signs	Body temperature, noninvasive blood pressure, heart rate, respiratory rate, and oxygen saturation	Daily (at a minimum).

[a] Because renal abnormalities were observed in animal studies, renal parameters, including proteinuria, were closely monitored in phase 1 and 2 studies. Based on the limited data, no dose-related proteinuria or other renal abnormalities possibly related to peramivir were observed; however, monitoring is recommended.

Monitor, evaluate, and treat patients for suspected bacterial infections as clinically warranted while administering peramivir. Closely monitor patients with influenza for signs of abnormal behavior.

It is especially important for patients in whom abnormal laboratory values are noted at the time peramivir treatment is initiated to be monitored through the duration of therapy for worsening.

Continually assess patients with significant or serious metabolic abnormalities with regard to the risks and potential benefits of continued peramivir therapy.

Perform careful follow-up and, at a minimum, repeat assessment within 1 to 2 weeks of the conclusion of therapy to assess normalization in patients with abnormal laboratory parameters.

PERAMIVIR — INJECTION

Monitor patients for development of diarrhea and administer appropriate evaluation and/or treatment, as indicated, including evaluation for other causes of diarrhea as clinically warranted.

Drug Interactions

➤*Renally eliminated drugs:* Peramivir is primarily eliminated by the kidneys; coadministration of peramivir with drugs that reduce renal function or compete for active tubular secretion may increase plasma concentrations of peramivir and/or increase the concentrations of other renally eliminated drugs. Use caution with medications that are eliminated by the kidneys and monitor the patient's renal function as appropriate.

Adverse Reactions

➤*Common adverse reactions:*

GI – Diarrhea, nausea, vomiting.

Miscellaneous – Neutrophil count decreased.

➤*Less common adverse reactions:*

Cardiovascular – Electrocardiogram abnormalities (prolonged QTc interval observed in 1 patient in a phase 1 trial), elevated blood pressure.

CNS – Depression, dizziness, feeling agitated, headache, insomnia, nervousness, nightmares, somnolence.

GU – Cystitis, hematuria, proteinuria.

Miscellaneous – Anorexia, hyperbilirubinemia, hyperglycemia.

Overdosage

➤*Treatment:* Treatment of overdose with peramivir should consist of general supportive measures, including monitoring of vital signs and observation of the clinical status of the patient. There is no specific antidote for overdose with peramivir.

Peramivir IV is cleared by hemodialysis.

Patient Information

Advise patients that peramivir is an unapproved product. The Food and Drug Administration (FDA) has authorized the emergency use of peramivir under an EUA.

Peramivir is not for the treatment of seasonal influenza A or B virus infections, for outpatients with acute uncomplicated 2009 H1N1 virus infection, or for pre- or postexposure chemoprophylaxis (prevention) of influenza.

ADEFOVIR DIPIVOXIL

Rx	Hepsera (Gilead Sciences)	Tablets; oral: 10 mg	Lactose. (10 GILEAD). White. In 30s.

ADEFOVIR DIPIVOXIL — ORAL

WARNING

Severe acute exacerbations of hepatitis have been reported in patients who have discontinued anti–hepatitis B therapy, including adefovir. Closely monitor hepatic function with both clinical and laboratory follow-up for at least several months in patients who discontinue anti–hepatitis B therapy. If appropriate, resumption of anti–hepatitis B therapy may be warranted.

In patients at risk of or having underlying renal dysfunction, chronic administration of adefovir may result in nephrotoxicity. Closely monitor renal function in these patients; they may require dose adjustment.

HIV resistance may emerge in chronic hepatitis B patients with unrecognized or untreated HIV infection treated with anti–hepatitis B therapies that may have activity against HIV (eg, adefovir).

Lactic acidosis and severe hepatomegaly with steatosis, including fatal cases, have been reported with the use of nucleoside analogs alone or in combination with other antiretrovirals.

Indications

➤*Chronic hepatitis B:* For the treatment of chronic hepatitis B virus (HBV) in patients 12 years of age and older with evidence of active viral replication and either evidence of persistent elevations in serum aminotransferases (ALT or AST) or histologically active disease.

Administration and Dosage

➤*Adults:*

Chronic hepatitis B –

Usual dosage: 10 mg once daily taken without regard to food.

➤*Children:*

Chronic hepatitis B – See Adults for dosing for children 12 years of age and older.

➤*Renal function impairment:*

Adefovir Dosing Interval Adjustment in Adults With Renal Function Impairment

	CrCl (mL/min)[a]			
	≥ 50	30 to 49	10 to 29	Hemodialysis patients
Recommended dosage and dosing interval	10 mg every 24 hours	10 mg every 48 hours	10 mg every 72 hours	10 mg every 7 days following dialysis

[a] CrCl calculated by Cockroft-Gault method using lean or ideal body weight.

➤*Administration:* May be taken with or without food.

➤*Storage/Stability:* Store in original container at 25°C (77°F); excursions are permitted between 15° and 30°C (59° and 86°F).

Actions

➤*Pharmacology:* Adefovir, an antiviral drug, is an acyclic nucleotide analog of adenosine monophosphate, which is phosphorylated to the active metabolite adefovir diphosphate by cellular kinases. Adefovir diphosphate inhibits hepatitis B virus (HBV) DNA polymerase (reverse transcriptase) by competing with the natural substrate deoxyadenosine triphosphate and by causing DNA chain termination after its incorporation into viral DNA. The inhibition constant (K_i) for adefovir diphosphate for HBV DNA polymerase was 0.1 mcM. Adefovir diphosphate is a weak inhibitor of human DNA polymerases α and γ with K_i values of 1.18 and 0.97 mcM, respectively.

➤*Pharmacokinetics:*

Absorption – Adefovir is a diester prodrug of the active moiety adefovir. Based on a cross study comparison, the approximate oral bioavailability of adefovir from adefovir is 59%.

Following oral administration of a 10 mg single dose of adefovir to chronic hepatitis B patients (n = 14), the peak adefovir plasma concentration (C_{max}) was 18.4 ± 6.26 ng/mL (mean ± standard deviation [SD]) and occurred between 0.58 and 4 hours (median, 1.75 hours) postdose. The adefovir area under the plasma concentration-time curve ($AUC_{0-\infty}$) was 220 ± 70 ng•h/mL. Plasma adefovir concentrations declined in a biexponential manner.

Distribution – In vitro binding of adefovir to human plasma or human serum proteins is 4% or less over the adefovir concentration range of 0.1 to 25 mcg/mL. The volume of distribution at steady state following intravenous (IV) administration of 1 or 3 mg/kg/day is 392 ± 75 and 352 ± 9 mL/kg, respectively.

Metabolism/Excretion – Following oral administration, adefovir is rapidly converted to adefovir. Forty-five percent of the dose is recovered as adefovir in the urine over 24 hours at steady state following oral doses of adefovir 10 mg. Adefovir is renally excreted by a combination of glomerular filtration and active tubular secretion. Terminal elimination half-life ($t_{1/2}$) is 7.48 ± 1.65 hours.

Special populations –

Renal function impairment:

Adefovir Pharmacokinetic Parameters (Mean ± SD) in Patients With Varying Degrees of Renal Function

Pharmacokinetic parameter	Renal function group and baseline CrCl (mL/min): Unimpaired > 80 (n = 7)	Mild 50 to 80 (n = 8)	Moderate 30 to 49 (n = 7)	Severe 10 to 29 (n = 10)
C_{max} (ng/mL)	17.8 ± 3.22	22.4 ± 4.04	28.5 ± 8.57	51.6 ± 10.3
$AUC_{0\ to\ \infty}$ (ng•h/mL)	201 ± 40.8	266 ± 55.7	455 ± 176	1,240 ± 629
CL/F[a] (mL/min)	469 ± 99	356 ± 85.6	237 ± 118	91.7 ± 51.3
CL_{renal} (mL/min)	231 ± 48.9	148 ± 39.3	83.9 ± 27.5	37 ± 18.4

[a] CL/F = apparent total clearance.

A 4-hour period of hemodialysis removed approximately 35% of the adefovir dose. The effect of peritoneal dialysis on adefovir removal has not been evaluated.

Contraindications

Previously demonstrated hypersensitivity to any of the components of the product.

Warnings/Precautions

➤*Exacerbations of hepatitis after discontinuation of treatment:* In clinical trials of adefovir, exacerbations of hepatitis (ALT elevations 10 times the upper limit of normal or greater) occurred in up to 25% of patients after discontinuation of adefovir. These reactions were identified in studies GS-98-437 and GS-98-438 (n = 492). Most of these reactions occurred within 12 weeks of drug discontinuation. These exacerbations generally occurred in the absence of HBeAg seroconversion, and presented as serum ALT elevations in addition to reemergence of viral replication. In the HBeAg-positive and HBeAg-negative studies in patients with compensated liver function, the exacerbations were not generally accompanied by hepatic decompensation. However, patients with advanced liver disease or cirrhosis may be at higher risk for hepatic decompensation. Although most reactions appear to have been self-limited or resolved with reinitiation of treatment, severe hepatitis exacerbations, including fatalities, have been reported; therefore, closely monitor patients after stopping treatment.

See the Warning box for more information.

➤*Nephrotoxicity:* It is important to monitor renal function for all patients during treatment with adefovir, particularly for those with preexisting or other risks for renal function impairment. Patients with renal function impairment at baseline or during treatment may require dose adjustment. Carefully evaluate the risks and benefits of adefovir treatment prior to discontinuing adefovir in a patient with treatment-emergent nephrotoxicity.

ADEFOVIR DIPIVOXIL — ORAL

Nephrotoxicity characterized by a delayed onset of gradual increases in serum creatinine and decreases in serum phosphorus was historically shown to be the treatment-limiting toxicity of adefovir therapy at substantially higher doses in HIV-infected patients (60 and 120 mg daily) and in chronic hepatitis B patients (30 mg daily). Chronic administration of adefovir (10 mg once daily) may result in nephrotoxicity. The overall risk of nephrotoxicity in patients with adequate renal function is low. However, this is of special importance in patients at risk of or that have underlying renal function impairment and patients taking concomitant nephrotoxic agents such as cyclosporine, tacrolimus, aminoglycosides, vancomycin, and nonsteroidal anti-inflammatory drugs.

➤*HIV resistance:* Prior to initiating adefovir therapy, offer HIV antibody testing to all patients. Treatment with anti–hepatitis B therapies, such as adefovir, that have activity against HIV in a chronic hepatitis B patient with unrecognized or untreated HIV infection may result in emergence of HIV resistance. Adefovir has not been shown to suppress HIV RNA in patients; however, there are limited data on the use of adefovir to treat patients with chronic hepatitis B coinfected with HIV.

➤*Lactic acidosis/severe hepatomegaly with steatosis:* Lactic acidosis and severe hepatomegaly with steatosis, including fatal cases, have been reported with the use of nucleoside analogs alone or in combination with antiretrovirals.

➤*Clinical resistance:* Resistance to adefovir can result in viral load rebound, which may result in exacerbation of hepatitis B and, in the setting of diminished hepatic function, lead to liver decompensation and possible fatal outcome.

In order to reduce the risk of resistance in patients with lamivudine resistant HBV, adefovir should be used in combination with lamivudine and not as adefovir monotherapy.

In order to reduce the risk of resistance in all patients receiving adefovir monotherapy, a modification of treatment should be considered if serum HBV DNA remains above 1,000 copies/mL with continued treatment.

Long-term (144 weeks) data from study 438 (n = 124) show that patients with HBV DNA levels greater than 1,000 copies/mL at week 48 of treatment with adefovir were at greater risk of developing resistance than patients with serum HBV DNA levels below 1,000 copies/mL at week 48 of therapy.

➤*Renal function impairment:* It is recommended that the dosing interval for adefovir be modified in adult patients with baseline CrCl less than 50 mL/min. The pharmacokinetics of adefovir have not been evaluated in nonhemodialysis patients with CrCl of less than 10 mL/min or in adolescent patients with renal function impairment; therefore, no dosing recommendations are available for these patients.

The efficacy and safety of adefovir have not been studied in patients younger than 18 years of age with different degrees of renal function impairment and no data are available to make dosage recommendations in these patients. Exercise caution when prescribing adefovir to adolescents with underlying renal function impairment, and closely monitor renal function in these patients.

➤*Pregnancy: Category C.* There are no adequate, well-controlled studies of adefovir in pregnant women. Chronic hepatitis B is a serious condition that requires treatment. Use adefovir during pregnancy only if the potential benefit to the mother justifies the potential risk to the fetus.

Embryotoxicity and an increased incidence of fetal malformations (anasarca, depressed eye bulge, umbilical hernia, and kinked tail) occurred when adefovir was administered IV to pregnant rats at 38 times the human therapeutic exposure. These adverse reproductive effects did not occur following an IV dose where exposure was 12 times the human therapeutic exposure.

Because animal reproductive studies are not always predictive of human response, use adefovir during pregnant only if clearly needed and after careful consideration of the risks and benefits.

Adefovir should not be withheld because of pregnancy if indicated for hepatitis B because chronic hepatitis B has significant morbidity and mortality.

Pregnancy registry – To monitor fetal outcomes of pregnant women exposed to adefovir, a pregnancy registry has been established. Health care providers are encouraged to register patients by calling 1-800-258-4263.

Labor and delivery – There are no studies in pregnant women and no data on the effect of adefovir on the transmission of HBV from mother to infant. Therefore, use appropriate infant immunizations to prevent neonatal acquisition of HBV.

➤*Lactation:* It is not known whether adefovir is excreted in human milk.

The relative lack of protein binding, moderately long terminal $t_{1/2}$, and molecular weight (approximately 501) of the prodrug adefovir dipivoxil suggest that adefovir will be excreted into human milk.

Because many drugs are excreted into human milk and because of the potential for serous adverse reactions in breast-feeding infants from adefovir, decide whether to discontinue adefovir or breast-feeding, taking into account the importance of the drug to the mother.

If adefovir is used during breast-feeding for the treatment of maternal infection, there is a potential risk of toxicity for the breast-fed infant, such as nephrotoxicity seen in adults.

➤*Children:*

Children (2 to younger than 12 years of age) – Adefovir is not recommended for use in children younger than 12 years of age.

➤*Elderly:* Clinical studies of adefovir did not include sufficient numbers of patients 65 years of age and older to determine whether they respond differently from younger patients. In general, exercise caution when prescribing to elderly patients because they have greater frequency of decreased renal or cardiac function caused by concomitant disease or other drug therapy.

➤*Monitoring:* Closely monitor hepatic function at repeated intervals with both clinical and laboratory follow-up for at least several months in patients who discontinue anti–hepatitis B therapy.

Closely monitor patients for adverse reactions when adefovir is coadministered with drugs that are renally excreted or with other drugs known to affect renal function.

Closely monitor renal function in all patients during therapy, especially patients at risk of having underlying renal function impairment or patients who develop renal function impairment during therapy with adefovir.

Drug Interactions

➤*Renally eliminated drugs:* Adefovir is eliminated by the kidney; coadministration of adefovir with drugs that reduce renal function or compete for active tubular secretion may increase serum concentrations of either adefovir and/or these coadministered drugs.

Adverse Reactions

The following adverse reactions have been discussed in previous sections:

1.) Severe acute exacerbations of hepatitis (see the Black Box Warning and Warnings/Precautions).
2.) Nephrotoxicity (see the Black Box Warning and Warnings/Precautions).

➤*Clinical trials:* Because clinical trials are conducted under widely varying conditions, adverse reaction rates observed in the clinical trials of a drug cannot be directly compared with rates in the clinical trials of another drug and may not reflect the rates observed in practice.

Placebo-controlled and open-label studies –

Adefovir Adverse Reactions (Grade 1 to 4) (≥ 3%)[a]

Adverse reactions	Adefovir 10 mg (n = 294)	Placebo (n = 228)
CNS		
Asthenia	13%	14%
Headache	9%	10%
GI		
Abdominal pain	9%	11%
Diarrhea	3%	4%
Dyspepsia	3%	2%
Flatulence	4%	4%
Nausea	5%	8%

[a] In these studies, the overall incidence of adverse reactions with adefovir was similar to that reported with placebo. The incidence of adverse reactions is derived from treatment events as identified by the study evaluations.

No patients treated with adefovir developed a confirmed serum creatinine increase of 0.5 mg/dL or more or confirmed phosphorus decrease of 2 mg/dL or less from baseline by week 48. By week 96, 2% of adefovir-treated patients, by Kaplan-Meier estimate, had increases in serum creatinine of 0.5 or more mg/dL from baseline (no placebo-controlled results were available for comparison beyond week 48). For patients who chose to continue adefovir for up to 240 weeks in study 438, 4 of 125 (3%) patients had a confirmed increase of 0.5 mg/dL from baseline. The creatinine elevation resolved in one patient who permanently discontinued treatment and remained stable in 3 patients who continued treatment. For 65 patients who chose to continue adefovir for up to 240 weeks in study 437, 6 had a confirmed increase in serum creatinine of greater than or equal to 0.5 mg/dL from baseline with 2 patients discontinuing from the study because of the elevated serum creatinine concentration.

➤*Pre– and post–liver transplantation patients:* Additional adverse reactions observed from an open-label (study 435) in pre– and post–liver transplantation patients with chronic hepatitis B and lamivudine-resistant hepatitis B administered adefovir once daily for up to 203 weeks include abnormal renal function, pruritis, rash, renal failure, and vomiting.

Changes in renal function occurred in pre– and post–liver transplantation patients with risk factors for renal function impairment, including concomitant use of cyclosporine and tacrolimus, renal function impairment at baseline, hypertension, diabetes, and on-study transplantation. Therefore, the contributory role of adefovir to these changes in renal function is difficult to assess.

Increase in serum creatinine of 0.3 mg/dL or more from baseline were observed in 37% and 53% of pre–liver transplantation patients by weeks 48 and 96, respectively, by Kaplan-Meier estimates. Increases in serum creatinine of 0.3 or more mg/dL from baseline were observed in 32% and 51% of post–liver transplantation patients by weeks 48 and 96, respectively, by Kaplan-Meier estimates. Serum phosphorous values of less than 2 mg/dL were observed in 3 of 226 (1.3%) pre–liver transplantation patients and in 6 of 241 (2.5%) post–liver transplantation patients by last study visit. Four percent (19/467) of patients discontinued treatment with adefovir because of renal adverse reactions.

➤*Children:* Assessment of adverse reactions is based on a placebo-controlled study (study 518) in which 173 children 2 to younger than 18 years of age with chronic hepatitis B and compensated liver disease received double-blind treatment with adefovir (n = 115), or placebo (n = 58) for 48 weeks.

ADEFOVIR DIPIVOXIL — ORAL

The safety profile of adefovir in patients older than 12 and younger than 18 years of age (n = 56) was similar to that observed in adults. No children treated with adefovir developed a confirmed serum creatinine increase of 0.5 mg/dL or more or confirmed phosphorous decrease 2 mg/dL or less from baseline by week 48.

➤*Postmarketing:*

GU – Fanconi syndrome, proximal renal tubulopathy, renal failure.

Metabolic/Nutritional – Hypophosphatemia.

Musculoskeletal – Myopathy, osteomalacia (both associated with proximal renal tubulopathy).

Overdosage

➤*Symptoms:* Doses of adefovir 500 mg/day for 2 weeks and 250 mg/day for 12 weeks have been associated with GI adverse reactions.

➤*Treatment:* If overdose occurs, monitor the patient for evidence of toxicity and apply standard supportive treatment as necessary. Following a single dose of adefovir 10 mg, a 4-hour hemodialysis session removed approximately 35% of the adefovir dose.

Patient Information

Inform patients of the potential risks and benefits of adefovir and of alternative modes of therapy.

Instruct patients to read the patient package insert before starting adefovir therapy; follow a regular dosing schedule to avoid missing doses; immediately report any severe abdominal pain, muscle pain, yellowing of the eyes, dark urine, pale stools, and/or loss of appetite; and inform their health care provider or pharmacist if they develop any unusual symptoms or if any known symptom persists or worsens.

Patients should remain under the care of a health care provider when using adefovir.

Advise patients that the optimal duration of adefovir treatment and the relationship between treatment response and long-term outcomes such as hepatocellular carcinoma or decompensated cirrhosis are not known; they should not discontinue adefovir without first informing their health care provider; routine laboratory monitoring and follow-up with a health care provider is important; obtaining HIV antibody testing prior to starting adefovir is important; lamivudine-resistant patients should use adefovir in combination with lamivudine and not as adefovir monotherapy.

Inform women of childbearing age about the risks associated with exposure to adefovir during pregnancy.

Patients should inform their health care provider if they become pregnant while using adefovir.

Inform pregnant patients using adefovir about the adefovir pregnancy registry and offer them the opportunity to enroll.

Inform patients that it is not known whether adefovir is excreted into human milk or if it can harm a breast-feeding infant. Therefore, a decision should be made whether to discontinue breast-feeding or the drug.

ENTECAVIR

Rx	Baraclude (Bristol-Myers Squibb)	Tablets; oral: 0.5 mg	Lactose. (BMS 1611). White to off-white, triangular. Film-coated. In 30s and 90s.
		1 mg	Lactose. (BMS 1612). Pink, triangular. Film-coated. In 30s.
		Solution; oral: 0.05 mg/mL	Maltitol, parabens. Orange flavor. In 210 mL.

ENTECAVIR — ORAL

WARNING

Severe acute exacerbations of hepatitis B – Severe acute exacerbations of hepatitis B have been reported in patients who have discontinued anti–hepatitis B therapy, including entecavir. Closely monitor hepatic function with clinical and laboratory follow-up for at least several months in patients who discontinue anti–hepatitis B therapy. If appropriate, initiation of anti–hepatitis B therapy may be warranted.

Patients co-infected with HIV and chronic hepatitis B virus – Limited clinical experience suggests there is a potential for the development of resistance to HIV nucleoside reverse transcriptase inhibitors if entecavir is used to treat chronic hepatitis B virus (HBV) infection in patients with HIV infection not being treated. Therapy with entecavir is not recommended for HIV/HBV co-infected patients who are not also receiving highly active antiretroviral therapy.

Lactic acidosis and severe hepatomegaly – Lactic acidosis and severe hepatomegaly with steatosis, including fatal cases, have been reported with the use of nucleoside analogues alone or in combination with antiretrovirals.

Indications

➤*Chronic hepatitis B:* For the treatment of chronic HBV infection in adults with evidence of active viral replication and either evidence of persistent elevations in serum aminotransferases (ALT or AST) or histologically active disease.

Administration and Dosage

➤*Adults:*

Chronic hepatitis B –

Compensated liver disease:

- *Nucleoside-treatment naive* –
  Usual dosage: 0.5 mg once daily.
- *History of hepatitis B viremia while receiving lamivudine or with known lamivudine- or telbivudine-resistance mutations (rtM204I/V with or without rtL180M, rtL80I/V, or rtV173L)* –
  Usual dosage: 1 mg once daily.

Decompensated liver disease: 1 mg once daily.

➤*Children:*

Chronic hepatitis B –

16 years of age and older: See Adults for dosing.

➤*Renal function impairment:* The once-daily dosing regimens are preferred.

Entecavir Dosage for Patients With Renal Impairment[a]

CrCl (mL/min)	Usual dosage (0.5 mg)	Lamivudine-refractory or decompensated liver disease (1 mg)
≥ 50	0.5 mg once daily	1 mg once daily
30 to < 50	0.25 mg once daily[b] or 0.5 mg every 48 h	0.5 mg once daily or 1 mg every 48 h
10 to < 30	0.15 mg once daily[b] or 0.5 mg every 72 h	0.3 mg once daily[b] or 1 mg every 72 h
< 10 Hemodialysis[c] or CAPD	0.05 mg once daily[b] or 0.5 mg every 7 days	0.1 mg once daily[b] or 1 mg every 7 days

[a] CrCl = creatinine clearance; CAPD = continuous ambulatory peritoneal dialysis.
[b] For doses less than 0.5 mg, entecavir oral solution is recommended.
[c] If administered on a hemodialysis day, administer after the hemodialysis session.

➤*Administration:* Administer entecavir on an empty stomach (at least 2 hours after a meal and 2 hours before the next meal).

➤*Storage/Stability:* Store tablets in a tightly closed container and oral solution in the outer carton at 25°C (77°F); excursions are permitted between 15° and 30°C (59° and 86°F). Protect oral solution from light.

Actions

➤*Pharmacology:* Entecavir, an antiviral drug, is a guanosine nucleoside analog with activity against HBV reverse transcriptase and is efficiently phosphorylated to the active triphosphate form, which has an intracellular half-life of 15 hours. By competing with the natural substrate deoxyguanosine triphosphate, entecavir triphosphate functionally inhibits all 3 activities of the HBV reverse transcriptase: base priming, reverse transcription of the negative strand from the pregenomic messenger RNA, and synthesis of the positive strand of HBV DNA. Entecavir triphosphate is a weak inhibitor of cellular DNA polymerases alpha, beta, and delta and mitochondrial DNA polymerase gamma, with K_i values ranging from 18 to more than 160 mcM.

➤*Pharmacokinetics:*

Absorption – Following oral administration in healthy subjects, entecavir peak plasma concentrations (C_{max}) occurred between 0.5 and 1.5 hours. Following multiple daily doses ranging from 0.1 to 1 mg, C_{max} and area under the curve (AUC) at steady state increased in proportion to dose. Steady state was achieved after 6 to 10 days of once-daily administration, with approximately 2-fold accumulation. For a 0.5 mg oral dose, C_{max} at steady state was 4.2 ng/mL, and trough plasma concentration (C_{trough}) was 0.3 ng/mL. For a 1 mg oral dose, C_{max} was 8.2 ng/mL, and C_{trough} was 0.5 ng/mL.

Bioequivalence: In healthy subjects, the bioavailability of the tablet was 100% relative to the oral solution. The oral solution and tablet may be used interchangeably.

Food effects: Oral administration of entecavir 0.5 mg with a standard high-fat meal (945 kcal, 54.6 g fat) or a light meal (379 kcal, 8.2 g fat) resulted in a delay in absorption (1 to 1.5 hours fed vs 0.75 hours fasted), a decrease in C_{max} of 44% to 46%, and a decrease in AUC of 18% to 20%.

Distribution – Based on the pharmacokinetic profile of entecavir after oral dosing, the estimated apparent volume of distribution is in excess of total body water, suggesting that entecavir is extensively distributed into tissues.

Binding of entecavir to human serum proteins in vitro was approximately 13%.

ENTECAVIR — ORAL

Metabolism/Excretion – Following administration of ^{14}C-entecavir in humans and rats, no oxidative or acetylated metabolites were observed. Minor amounts of phase 2 metabolites (glucuronide and sulfate conjugates) were observed.

After reaching C_{max}, entecavir plasma concentrations decreased in a biexponential manner, with a terminal elimination half-life of approximately 128 to 149 hours. The observed drug accumulation index is approximately 2-fold with once-daily dosing, suggesting an effective accumulation half-life of approximately 24 hours.

Entecavir is predominantly eliminated by the kidney, with urinary recovery of unchanged drug at steady state ranging from 62% to 73% of the administered dose. Renal clearance is independent of dose and ranges from 360 to 471 mL/min, suggesting that entecavir undergoes both glomerular filtration and net tubular secretion.

Special populations –

Renal function impairment:

Entecavir Pharmacokinetic Parameters in Subjects With Selected Degrees of Renal Impairment[a]

	Baseline CrCl					
Parameters	Unimpaired > 80 mL/min (n = 6)	Mild > 50 to ≤ 80 mL/min (n = 6)	Moderate 30 to 50 mL/min (n = 6)	Severe < 30 mL/min (n = 6)	Severe managed with hemodialysis (n = 6)[b]	Severe managed with CAPD (n = 4)
C_{max} (ng/mL) (CV%)	8.1 (30.7)	10.4 (37.2)	10.5 (22.7)	15.3 (33.8)	15.4 (56.4)	16.6 (29.7)
$AUC_{(0\ to\ T)}$ (ng•h/mL) (CV)	27.9 (25.6)	51.5 (22.8)	69.5 (22.7)	145.7 (31.5)	233.9 (28.4)	221.8 (11.6)
CLR (mL/min) (SD)	383.2 (101.8)	197.9 (78.1)	135.6 (31.6)	40.3 (10.1)	NA	NA
CLT/F (mL/min) (SD)	588.1 (153.7)	309.2 (62.6)	226.3 (60.1)	100.6 (29.1)	50.6 (16.5)	35.7 (19.6)

[a] CV = coefficient of variation; CLR = renal clearance; NA = not available; SD = standard deviation; CLT/F = apparent oral clearance.
[b] Dosed immediately following hemodialysis.

• *Dialysis* – Following a single dose of entecavir 1 mg administered 2 hours before the hemodialysis session, hemodialysis removed approximately 13% of the entecavir dose over 4 hours. CAPD removed approximately 0.3% of the dose during 7 days. Administer entecavir after hemodialysis.

Elderly: The effect of age on the pharmacokinetics of entecavir was evaluated following administration of a single 1 mg oral dose in healthy younger and elderly volunteers. Entecavir AUC was 29.3% higher in elderly subjects compared with younger subjects. The disparity in exposure between elderly and younger subjects most likely was attributable to differences in renal function. Base dosage adjustment of entecavir on the patient's renal function rather than age.

Liver transplant: The safety and efficacy of entecavir in liver transplant recipients are unknown. However, in a small pilot study of entecavir use in HBV-infected liver transplant recipients on a stable dose of cyclosporine A (n = 5) or tacrolimus (n = 4), entecavir exposure was approximately 2-fold the exposure in healthy subjects with healthy renal function. Altered renal function contributed to the increase in entecavir exposure in these patients. The potential for pharmacokinetic interactions between entecavir and cyclosporine A or tacrolimus was not formally evaluated.

Contraindications

None well documented.

Warnings/Precautions

➤*Severe acute exacerbations of hepatitis B:* See the Warning box for more information.

➤*HIV/HBV co-infection:* Entecavir has not been evaluated in HIV/HBV co-infected patients who were not simultaneously receiving effective HIV treatment. Before initiating entecavir therapy, offer HIV antibody testing to all patients. Entecavir has not been studied as a treatment for HIV infection and is not recommended for this use.

See the Warning box for more information.

➤*Lactic acidosis/severe hepatomegaly with steatosis:* See the Warning box for more information.

The majority of these cases have been in women. Obesity and prolonged nucleoside exposure may be risk factors. Exercise particular caution when administering nucleoside analogues to any patient with known risk factors for liver disease; however, cases have also been reported in patients with no known risk factors. Suspend treatment with entecavir in any patient who develops clinical or laboratory findings suggestive of lactic acidosis or pronounced hepatotoxicity (which may include hepatomegaly and steatosis even in the absence of marked transaminase elevations).

➤*Liver transplant recipients:* The safety and efficacy of entecavir in liver transplant recipients are unknown. If entecavir treatment is necessary for a liver transplant recipient who has received or is receiving an immunosuppressant that may affect renal function, such as cyclosporine or tacrolimus, renal function must be carefully monitored before and during treatment with entecavir.

➤*Renal function impairment:* See Administration and Dosage for more information.

➤*Pregnancy: Category C.* There are no adequate and well-controlled studies in pregnant women. Because animal reproduction studies are not always predictive of human response, only use entecavir during pregnancy if clearly needed and after careful consideration of the risks and benefits.

In rats, maternal toxicity, embryofetal toxicity (resorptions), lower fetal body weights, tail and vertebral malformations, reduced ossification (vertebrae, sternebrae, and phalanges), and extra lumbar vertebrae and ribs were observed at exposures 3,100 times those in humans. In rabbits, embryofetal toxicity (resorptions), reduced ossification (hyoid), and an increased incidence of 13th rib were observed at exposures 883 times those in humans.

Pregnancy registry – To monitor fetal outcomes of pregnant women exposed to entecavir, a pregnancy registry has been established. Health care providers are encouraged to register patients by calling 1-800-258-4263.

Labor and delivery – There are no studies in pregnant women and no data on the effect of entecavir on transmission of HBV from mother to infant. Therefore, use appropriate interventions to prevent neonatal acquisition of HBV.

➤*Lactation:* Entecavir is excreted in the milk of rats. It is not known whether this drug is excreted in human milk. However, the molecular weight (approximately 277), long elimination half-life (128 to 149 hours), and minimal metabolism suggest that the drug will be excreted into breast milk.Because many drugs are excreted into human milk and because of the potential for serious adverse reactions in breast-feeding infants from entecavir, decide whether to discontinue breast-feeding or entecavir, taking into consideration the importance of continued hepatitis B therapy to the mother and the known benefits of breast-feeding.

➤*Children:* The safety and efficacy of entecavir in children younger than 16 years of age have not been established.

➤*Elderly:* Entecavir is substantially excreted by the kidney, and the risk of toxic reactions to this drug may be greater in patients with renal impairment. Because elderly patients are more likely to have decreased renal function, take care in dose selection and monitor renal function.

➤*Monitoring:* Periodic monitoring of hepatic function is recommended during treatment and for at least several months after treatment in patients who discontinue antihepatitis B therapy. Monitor patients closely for adverse reactions when entecavir is coadministered with drugs that are renally eliminated or known to affect renal function. Monitor patients for signs/symptoms of lactic acidosis/hepatomegaly.

Drug Interactions

➤*Drugs affected by renal impairment:* Because entecavir is primarily eliminated by the kidneys, coadministration of entecavir with drugs that reduce renal function or compete for active tubular secretion may increase serum concentrations of entecavir or the coadministered drug. Monitor patients closely for adverse reactions when entecavir is coadministered with such drugs.

➤*Drug/Food interactions:* See Actions for more information.

Adverse Reactions

➤*Compensated liver disease:*

Most common adverse reactions – The most common adverse reactions of any severity (at least 3%) with at least a possible relation to study drug for entecavir-treated patients were dizziness, fatigue, headache, and nausea. The most common adverse reactions among lamivudine-treated patients were dizziness, fatigue, and headache.

Discontinuation of treatment – One percent of entecavir-treated patients in these 4 studies compared with 4% of lamivudine-treated patients discontinued for adverse reactions or abnormal laboratory test results.

Adverse reactions (Grade 2 to 4) –

Entecavir Adverse Reactions Over 2 Years[a] (Moderate to Severe Intensity) (Grades 2 to 4)

	Nucleoside-naive[b]		Lamivudine-refractory[c]	
Adverse reactions	Entecavir 0.5 mg (n = 679)	Lamivudine 100 mg (n = 668)	Entecavir 1 mg (n = 183)	Lamivudine 100 mg (n = 190)
Any grade 2 to 4 adverse reaction[a]	15%	18%	22%	23%
CNS				
Dizziness	< 1%	< 1%	0%	1%
Fatigue	1%	1%	3%	3%
Headache	2%	2%	4%	1%
Insomnia	< 1%	< 1%	0%	< 1%
Somnolence	< 1%	< 1%	0%	0%
GI				
Diarrhea	< 1%	0%	1%	0%
Dyspepsia	< 1%	< 1%	1%	0%
Nausea	< 1%	< 1%	< 1%	2%
Vomiting	< 1%	< 1%	< 1%	0%

[a] Includes reactions of possible, probable, certain, or unknown relationship to treatment regimen.
[b] Studies AI463022 and AI463027.
[c] Includes study AI463026 and the entecavir 1 mg and lamivudine treatment arms of study AI463014, a phase 2, multinational, randomized, double-blind study of 3 doses of entecavir (0.1, 0.5, and 1 mg) once daily versus continued lamivudine 100 mg once daily for up to 52 weeks in patients who experienced recurrent viremia on lamivudine therapy.

ENTECAVIR — ORAL

Lab test abnormalities –

Entecavir Laboratory Test Abnormalities[a,b]				
	Nucleoside-naive[c]		Lamivudine-refractory[d]	
Lab test	Entecavir 0.5 mg (n = 679)	Lamivudine 100 mg (n = 668)	Entecavir 1 mg (n = 183)	Lamivudine 100 mg (n = 190)
Any grade 3 to 4 laboratory abnormality[e]	35%	36%	37%	45%
ALT > 10 × ULN and 2 × baseline	2%	4%	2%	11%
ALT > 5 × ULN	11%	16%	12%	24%
Albumin < 2.5 g/dL	< 1%	< 1%	0%	2%
Total bilirubin > 2.5 × ULN	2%	2%	3%	2%
Lipase ≥ 2.1 × ULN	7%	6%	7%	7%
Creatinine > 3 × ULN	0%	0%	0%	0%
Confirmed creatinine increase ≥ 0.5 mg/dL	1%	1%	2%	1%
Hyperglycemia, fasting 250 mg/dL	2%	1%	3%	1%
Glycosuria[f]	4%	3%	4%	6%
Hematuria[g]	9%	10%	9%	6%
Platelet count < 50,000/mm^3	< 1%	< 1%	< 1%	< 1%

[a] ULN = upper limit of normal.
[b] On-treatment value worsened from baseline to grade 3 or 4 for all parameters except albumin (any on-treatment value < 2.5 g/dL), confirmed creatinine increase ≥ 0.5 mg/dL, and ALT > 10 × ULN and > 2 × baseline.
[c] Studies AI463022 and AI463027.
[d] Includes study AI463026 and the entecavir 1 mg and lamivudine treatment arms of study AI463014, a phase 2, multinational, randomized, double-blind study of 3 doses of entecavir (0.1, 0.5, and 1 mg) once daily versus continued lamivudine 100 mg once daily for up to 52 weeks in patients who experienced recurrent viremia on lamivudine therapy.
[e] Includes hematology, routine chemistries, renal and liver function tests, pancreatic enzymes, and urinalysis.
[f] Grade 3 = 3+, large, ≥ 500 mg/dL; grade 4 = 4+, marked, severe.
[g] Grade 3 = 3+, large; grade 4 = ≥ 4+, marked, severe, many.

Among entecavir-treated patients in these studies, on-treatment ALT elevations of more than 10 times the ULN and more than 2 times baseline generally resolved with continued treatment. A majority of these exacerbations were associated with at least a 2 $\log_{10}$/mL reduction in viral load that preceded or coincided with the ALT elevation. Periodic monitoring of hepatic function is recommended during treatment.

Exacerbations of hepatitis or ALT elevations after discontinuation of treatment – An exacerbation of hepatitis or ALT flare was defined as ALT of more than 10 times the ULN and more than 2 times the patient's reference level (minimum of the baseline or last measurement at end of dosing). In these studies, a subset of patients was allowed to discontinue treatment at or after 52 weeks if they achieved a protocol-defined response to therapy. If entecavir is discontinued without regard to treatment response, the rate of posttreatment flares could be higher.

Entecavir Exacerbations of Hepatitis During Off-Treatment Follow-up, Subjects in Studies AI463022, AI463027, and AI463026				
	Patients with ALT elevations > 10 × ULN and > 2 × reference[a]			
	n	Entecavir	n	Lamivudine
Nucleoside-naive				
HBeAg-positive	174	2%	147	9%
HBeAg-negative	302	8%	270	11%
Lamivudine-refractory	52	12%	16	0%

[a] Reference is the minimum of the baseline or last measurement at end of dosing. Median time to off-treatment exacerbation was 23 weeks for entecavir-treated patients and 10 weeks for lamivudine-treated patients.

➤*Decompensated liver disease:* Among the 102 subjects receiving entecavir, the most common treatment-emergent adverse events of any severity, regardless of causality, occurring through week 48 were peripheral edema (16%), ascites (15%), pyrexia (14%), hepatic encephalopathy (10%), and upper respiratory infection (10%). Clinical adverse reactions not listed in the previous tables that were observed through week 48 include blood bicarbonate decreased (2%) and renal failure (less than 1%).

Eighteen percent of subjects treated with entecavir and 20% of subjects treated with adefovir dipivoxil died during the first 48 weeks of therapy. The majority (11 in the entecavir group and 16 in the adefovir dipivoxil group) of deaths were due to liver-related causes, such as hepatic failure, hepatic encephalopathy, hepatorenal syndrome, and upper GI hemorrhage. The rate of hepatocellular carcinoma through week 48 was 6% for subjects treated with entecavir and 8% for subjects treated with adefovir dipivoxil. Five percent of subjects in either treatment arm discontinued therapy due to an adverse event through week 48.

No subject in either treatment arm experienced an on-treatment hepatic flare (ALT more than 2 × baseline and more than 10 × ULN) through week 48. 11% of subjects treated with entecavir and 13% of subjects treated with adefovir dipivoxil had a confirmed increase in serum creatinine of 0.5 mg/dL through week 48.

Overdosage

➤*Symptoms:* There is limited experience of entecavir overdosage reported in patients. Healthy subjects who received single entecavir doses of up to 40 mg or multiple doses of up to 20 mg/day for up to 14 days had no increase in or unexpected adverse reactions.

➤*Treatment:* If overdose occurs, the patient must be monitored for evidence of toxicity and standard supportive treatment applied as necessary. Following a single dose of entecavir 1 mg, a 4-hour hemodialysis session removed approximately 13% of the entecavir dose.

Patient Information

Advise patients to remain in the care of a health care provider while taking entecavir, and advise them to discuss any new symptoms or concurrent medications with their health care provider.

Advise patients to take entecavir on an empty stomach (at least 2 hours after a meal and 2 hours before the next meal).

Advise patients to take a missed dose as soon as remembered unless it is almost time for the next dose. Instruct patients not to take 2 doses at the same time.

Inform patients that deterioration of liver disease may occur in some cases if treatment is discontinued, and tell them to discuss any change in regimen with their health care provider.

Advise patients that treatment with entecavir will not cure HBV and has not been shown to reduce the risk of transmission of HBV to others through sexual contact or blood contamination.

Instruct patients using the oral solution to hold the dosing spoon in a vertical position and fill it gradually to the mark corresponding to the prescribed dose. Recommend rinsing of the spoon with water after each daily dose.

Offer HIV antibody testing to all patients before starting entecavir therapy. Inform patients that if they have HIV infection and are not receiving effective HIV treatment, entecavir may increase the chance of HIV resistance to HIV medication.

ANTIRETROVIRAL AGENTS

Protease Inhibitors

SAQUINAVIR

Rx	**Invirase** (Genentech)	**Tablets; oral:** 500 mg	As saquinavir mesylate. Lactose. (ROCHE SQV 500). Lt. orange to grayish or brownish orange, oval cylindrical. Film-coated. In 120s.
		Capsules; oral: 200 mg	As saquinavir mesylate. Lactose. (ROCHE 0245). Lt. brown/green, opaque. In 270s.

SAQUINAVIR MESYLATE — ORAL

Indications

➤*HIV infection:* For the treatment of HIV-1 infectionin adults (older than 16 years of age) in combination with ritonavir and other antiretroviral agents.

Administration and Dosage

➤*General dosing considerations:* Saquinavir must be used in combination with ritonavir because it significantly inhibits saquinavir's metabolism to provide increased plasma saquinavir levels.

➤*Adults:*

HIV infection –

Usual dosage: 1,000 mg twice daily with ritonavir 100 mg twice daily.

SAQUINAVIR MESYLATE — ORAL

Dosage adjustment: For serious or severe toxicities that occur with saquinavir, saquinavir should be interrupted until etiology of the event is identified or the toxicity resolves.

Concomitant therapy: Must be administered with ritonavir (100 mg twice daily) at the same time as saquinavir.

When administered with lopinavir 400 mg/ritonavir 100 mg twice daily, the appropriate dosage of saquinavir is 1,000 mg twice daily (with no additional ritonavir).

➤*Children:*

HIV infection –

16 years of age and older: See Adults for dosing.

➤*Hepatic function impairment:* Saquinavir in combination with ritonavir is contraindicated in patients with severe hepatic impairment.

➤*Administration:* Take within 2 hours after a meal.

➤*Storage/Stability:* Store at 25°C (77°F); excursions are permitted between 15° and 30°C (59° and 86°F).

Actions

➤*Pharmacology:* Saquinavir is an inhibitor of HIV-1 protease. HIV-1 protease is an enzyme required for the proteolytic cleavage of viral polyprotein precursors into individual functional proteins found in HIV-1 particles. Saquinavir is a peptide-like substrate analog that binds to the protease active site and inhibits the activity of the enzyme. Saquinavir inhibition prevents cleavage of the viral polyproteins, resulting in the formation of immature noninfectious virus particles.

➤*Pharmacokinetics:*

Absorption – Absolute bioavailability of saquinavir averaged 4% (coefficient of variation [CV], 73%; range, 1% to 9%) in 8 healthy volunteers who received a single 600 mg dose (3 × 200 mg) of saquinavir following a high-fat breakfast (48 g protein, 60 g carbohydrate, 57 g fat; 1,006 kcal). The low bioavailability is thought to be due to a combination of incomplete absorption and extensive first-pass metabolism.

Saquinavir Pharmacokinetic Parameters[a]

Dosing regimen	AUC_{Tau}[b] (ng•h/mL)	AUC_{24h} (ng•h/mL)	C_{min} (ng/mL)
Saquinavir 600 mg 3 times daily (arithmetic mean, % CV) (n = 10)	866 (62)	2,598	79
Saquinavir soft gel capsules 1,200 mg 3 times daily (arithmetic mean) (n = 31)	7,249	21,747	216
Saquinavir 1,000 mg twice daily + ritonavir 100 mg twice daily (geometric mean and 95% CI) (n = 24)	14,607 (10,218 to 20,882)	29,214	371 (245 to 561)
Saquinavir soft gel capsules 1,000 mg twice daily + ritonavir 100 mg twice daily (geometric mean and 95% CI) (n = 24)	19,085 (13,943 to 26,124)	38,170	433 (301 to 622)

[a] AUC = area under the curve; C_{min} = minimum plasma concentration; CI = confidence interval.
[b] Tau is the dosing interval (ie, 8 hours if 3 times daily and 12 hours if twice daily).

Effect of food: The mean 24-hour AUC after a single 600 mg oral dose (6 × 100 mg) in healthy volunteers (n = 6) was increased from 24 ng•h/mL (CV 33%) under fasting conditions to 161 ng•h/mL (CV 35%) when saquinavir was given following a high-fat breakfast (48 g protein, 60 g carbohydrate, 57 g fat; 1,006 kcal). Saquinavir 24-hour AUC and maximal plasma concentration (C_{max}) following the administration of a higher-calorie meal (943 kcal, 54 g fat) were on average 2 times higher than after a lower-calorie, lower-fat meal (355 kcal, 8 g fat). The effect of food has been shown to persist for up to 2 hours. Take saquinavir/ritonavir within 2 hours after a meal.

Distribution – The mean steady-state volume of distribution following intravenous (IV) administration of a 12 mg dose of saquinavir was 700 L (CV 39%), suggesting saquinavir partitions into tissues. Saquinavir was approximately 98% bound to plasma proteins over a concentration range of 15 to 700 ng/mL. In 2 patients receiving saquinavir 600 mg 3 times daily, cerebrospinal fluid concentrations were negligible when compared with concentrations from matching plasma samples.

Metabolism/Excretion – In vitro studies using human liver microsomes have shown that the metabolism of saquinavir is cytochrome P450 (CYP-450)–mediated, with the specific isoenzyme CYP3A4 responsible for more than 90% of the hepatic metabolism. Based on in vitro studies, saquinavir is rapidly metabolized to a range of mono- and di-hydroxylated inactive compounds. In a mass balance study using 600 mg of ^{14}C-saquinavir, 88% and 1% of the oral radioactivity was recovered in feces and urine, respectively, within 5 days of dosing. In an additional 4 subjects administered 10.5 mg of ^{14}C-saquinavir IV, 81% and 3% of the IV radioactivity was recovered in feces and urine, respectively, within 5 days of dosing. In mass balance studies, 13% of circulating radioactivity in plasma was attributed to unchanged drug after oral administration and the remainder attributed to saquinavir metabolites. Following IV administration, 66% of circulating radioactivity was attributed to unchanged drug and the remainder to saquinavir metabolites, suggesting that saquinavir undergoes extensive first-pass metabolism.

Systemic clearance of saquinavir was rapid, 1.14 L/h/kg (CV 12%) after IV doses of 6, 36, and 72 mg. The mean residence time of saquinavir was 7 hours.

Special populations –

Renal function impairment: Patients with severe renal impairment or end-stage renal disease have not been studied; and concentrations of saquinavir may be elevated in these populations.

Hepatic function impairment: The mean (% CV in parentheses) values for saquinavir AUC_{0-12h} and C_{max} were 24.3 (102%) mcg•h/mL and 3.6 (83%) µg•/mL, respectively, for HIV-1–infected patients with moderate hepatic impairment. The corresponding values in the control group were 28.5 (71%) mcg•h/mL and 4.3 (68%) mcg/mL. The geometric mean ratio (90% CI) was 0.7 (0.3 to 1.6) for both AUC_{0-12} and C_{max}, which suggests approximately 30% reduction in saquinavir exposure in patients with moderate hepatic impairment.

Gender: A gender difference was observed, with women showing higher saquinavir exposure than men (mean AUC 56% higher, mean C_{max} 26% higher) in the relative bioavailability study comparing saquinavir 500 mg tablets with the saquinavir 200 mg capsules in combination with ritonavir. There was no evidence that age and body weight explained the gender difference in this study.

Contraindications

Congenital long QT syndrome; refractory hypokalemia or hypomagnesemia; complete atrioventricular (AV) block without implanted pacemakers, or patients who are at high risk of complete AV block; hypersensitivity (eg, anaphylactic reaction, Stevens-Johnson syndrome) to saquinavir, saquinavir mesylate, or any of the components contained in the capsule or tablet, or to ritonavir; severe hepatic impairment when coadministered with ritonavir; coadministration with drugs that both increase saquinavir plasma concentrations and prolong the QT interval; coadministration with CYP3A substrates (alfuzosin, amiodarone, bepridil, cisapride, dihydroergotamine, dofetilide, ergonovine, ergotamine, flecainide, lidocaine [systemic], lovastatin, methylergonavine, midazolam [orally administered], pimozide, propafenone, quinidine, rifampin, sildenafil [for the treatment of pulmonary arterial hypertension], simvastatin, trazodone, or triazolam). (See Drug Interactions.)

Warnings/Precautions

➤*Concomitant therapy:* Saquinavir must be used in combination with ritonavir.

➤*Toxicity:* If a serious or severe toxicity occurs during treatment with saquinavir, interrupt saquinavir until the etiology of the event is identified or the toxicity resolves. At that time, resumption of treatment with full-dose saquinavir may be considered.

➤*Cardiovascular effects:*

PR interval prolongation – Saquinavir/ritonavir prolongs the PR interval in a dose-dependent fashion. Cases of second- or third-degree AV block have been reported rarely. Patients with underlying structural heart disease, pre-existing conduction system abnormalities, cardiomyopathies, and ischemic heart disease may be at increased risk for developing cardiac conduction abnormalities.

See Drug Interactions for more information.

➤*QT interval prolongation:* Saquinavir/ritonavir causes dose-dependent QT prolongation. Torsades de pointes has been reported rarely postmarketing. Avoid saquinavir/ritonavir in patients with long QT syndrome. Electrocardiogram (ECG) monitoring is recommended if therapy is initiated in patients with congestive heart failure, bradyarrhythmias, hepatic impairment, or electrolyte abnormalities. Correct hypokalemia or hypomagnesemia prior to initiating saquinavir/ritonavir and monitor these electrolytes periodically during therapy. Do not use in combination with drugs that both increase saquinavir plasma concentrations and prolong the QT interval.

Perform an ECG prior to initiation of treatment. Ensure that patients with a QT interval more than 450 msec do not receive ritonavir-boosted saquinavir. For patients with a QT interval less than 450 msec, an on-treatment ECG is suggested after approximately 3 to 4 days of therapy; discontinue ritonavir-boosted saquinavir in patients with a QT interval more than 480 msec or prolongation over pretreatment by more than 20 msec.

Only use medications with the potential to increase the QT interval and concomitant ritonavir boosted saquinavir when no alternative therapy is available and the potential benefits outweigh the potential risks. Perform an ECG prior to initiation of the concomitant therapy, and do not initiate the concomitant therapy in patients with a QT interval more than 450 msec. If baseline QT interval is less than 450 msec, perform an on-treatment ECG after 3 to 4 days of therapy. For patients demonstrating a subsequent increase in QT interval to more than 480 msec or increase by more than 20 msec after commencing concomitant therapy, use best clinical judgment to discontinue either ritonavir-boosted saquinavir or the concomitant therapy or both.

➤*Diabetes mellitus and hyperglycemia:* New-onset diabetes mellitus, exacerbation of preexisting diabetes mellitus, and hyperglycemia have been reported during postmarketing surveillance in patients infected with HIV receiving protease inhibitor therapy. Some patients required either initiation or dose adjustments of insulin or oral hypoglycemic agents for the treatment of these events. In some cases, diabetic ketoacidosis has occurred. In those patients who discontinued protease inhibitor therapy, hyperglycemia persisted in some cases.

SAQUINAVIR MESYLATE — ORAL

➤*Hemophilia:* There have been reports of spontaneous bleeding in patients with hemophilia A and B treated with protease inhibitors. In some patients, additional factor VIII was required. In the majority of reported cases, treatment with protease inhibitors was continued or restarted.

➤*Hyperlipidemia:* Elevated cholesterol and/or triglyceride levels have been observed in some patients taking saquinavir in combination with ritonavir. Marked elevation in triglyceride levels is a risk factor for development of pancreatitis. Monitor cholesterol and triglyceride levels prior to initiating combination dosing regimen of saquinavir with ritonavir and at periodic intervals while on such therapy.

➤*Fat redistribution:* Redistribution or accumulation of body fat, including breast enlargement, central obesity, "cushingoid appearance," dorsocervical fat enlargement (buffalo hump), facial wasting, and peripheral wasting, has been observed in patients receiving antiretroviral therapy.

➤*Immune reconstitution syndrome:* Immune reconstitution syndrome has been reported in patients treated with combination antiretroviral therapy, including saquinavir. During the initial phase of combination antiretroviral treatment, patients whose immune systems respond may develop an inflammatory response to indolent or residual opportunistic infections (eg, *Mycobacterium avium* infection, cytomegalovirus, *Pneumocystis jiroveci* pneumonia, tuberculosis) that may necessitate further evaluation and treatment.

➤*Renal function impairment:* Patients with severe renal impairment or end-stage renal disease have not been studied; exercise caution when prescribing saquinavir in this population.

➤*Hepatic function impairment:* In patients with underlying hepatitis B or C, cirrhosis, chronic alcoholism, and/or other underlying liver abnormalities, there have been reports of worsening liver disease.

See Contraindications for more information.

➤*Pregnancy:* *Category B.* Clinical experience in pregnant women is limited. Use saquinavir during pregnancy only if the potential benefit justifies the potential risk to the fetus.

It is not known if saquinavir crosses the human placenta. The molecular weight of the free base (approximately 671) is low enough that some degree of transfer should be anticipated.

In 2006, the updated US Department of Health and Human Services guidelines for the use of antiretroviral agents in patients infected with HIV-1 continued the recommendation that therapy, with the exception of efavirenz, be continued during pregnancy. Therefore, If indicated, do not withhold protease inhibitors, including saquinavir, in pregnancy because the expected benefit to the mother who is HIV-positive outweighs the unknown risk to the fetus.

Antiretroviral pregnancy registry – To monitor maternal-fetal outcomes of pregnant women exposed to antiretroviral medications, including saquinavir, an antiretroviral pregnancy registry has been established. Health care providers are encouraged to register patients by calling 1-800-258-4263.

➤*Lactation:* The Centers for Disease Control and Prevention recommend that mothers infected with HIV not breast-feed their infants to avoid risking postnatal transmission of HIV. It is not known whether saquinavir is excreted in human milk. The molecular weight of the free base (approximately 671) is low enough that excretion into breast milk should be expected. Because of the potential for HIV transmission and the potential for serious adverse reactions in breast-feeding infants, instruct mothers not to breast-feed if they are receiving saquinavir.

➤*Children:* The safety and efficacy of saquinavir in children younger than 16 years of age have not been established.

➤*Monitoring:* Perform clinical chemistry tests, viral load, and CD_4 count prior to initiating saquinavir therapy and at appropriate intervals thereafter. Monitor cholesterol and triglyceride levels prior to initiating the combination dosing regimen and at periodic intervals during therapy. Monitor potassium and magnesium prior to starting therapy and periodically thereafter. Monitor ECG prior to initiation of treatment. Perform ECG monitoring in patients with CHF, bradyarrhythmias, hepatic impairment, structural heart disease, electrolyte abnormalities, pre-existing conduction abnormalities, cardiomyopathies, and/or ischemic heart disease.

Drug Interactions

➤*Cytochrome P450 system:* Because saquinavir is metabolized mainly by the CYP3A enzyme systems, substances known to inhibit these enzymes may decrease metabolism or increase bioavailability of saquinavir, as indicated by increased whole blood or plasma concentrations. Drugs known to induce these enzyme systems may result in an increased metabolism or saquinavir or decreased bioavailability, as indicated by decreased whole blood or plasma concentrations. Monitoring of blood concentrations and appropriate dosage adjustments are essential when such drugs are used concomitantly.

➤*P-glycoprotein:* Saquinavir is a substrate for p-glycoprotein. Drugs that affect p-glycoprotein may alter the pharmacokinetics of saquinavir. Also, saquinavir may alter the pharmacokinetics of drugs that are substrates for p-glycoprotein.

➤*QT prolongation:* An additive effect of saquinavir with other drugs that prolong the QT interval cannot be excluded. The following drugs may prolong the QT interval and increase the risk of life-threatening cardiac arrhythmias, including torsade de pointes: antiarrhythmic agents (eg, amiodarone, bretylium, disopyramide, dofetilide, procainamide, quinidine, sotalol), arsenic trioxide, chlorpromazine, cisapride, dolasetron, droperidol, gatifloxacin, halofantrine, levomethadyl, mefloquine, mesoridazine, moxifloxacin, pentamidine, pimozide, probucol, sparfloxacin, tacrolimus, thioridazine, ziprasidone. For a more complete list of drugs that prolong the QT interval, see the appendix Drug-Induced Prolongation of the QT Interval and Torsades De Pointes.

Saquinavir Drug Interactions[a]

Precipitant drug	Object drug[b]		Description
Anticonvulsants (eg, carbamazepine, phenobarbital, phenytoin)	Saquinavir	↓	Saquinavir may be less effective because of decreased plasma concentrations. Use with caution.
Saquinavir	Anticonvulsants (eg, carbamazepine)	↑	Carbamazepine plasma concentrations may be elevated, increasing the risk of toxicity (eg, neurotoxicity). Closely monitor carbamazepine plasma concentrations when starting, stopping, or changing the saquinavir dose. Adjust carbamazepine dose as needed or consider alternative treatment.
Antimycobacterials (eg, rifampin)	Saquinavir	↓	Coadministration of rifampin and saquinavir is contraindicated. Rifamycins may decrease saquinavir serum concentrations. Do not administer rifampin in patients taking ritonavir-boosted saquinavir as part of an antiretroviral therapy regimen because of the risk of severe hepatocellular toxicity. In addition, saquinavir was shown to increase serum rifabutin concentrations. Rifabutin dosage reduction of ≥ 75% of the usual dosage of 300 mg/day is recommended (ie, a maximum dosage of 150 mg every other day or 3 times per week). Increased monitoring for adverse reactions is warranted. Consider monitoring rifabutin concentrations to ensure adequate exposure.
Saquinavir	Antimycobacterials (eg, rifabutin)	↑	
Atazanavir	Saquinavir	↑	May result in increased saquinavir plasma concentrations.
Azole antifungals (eg, itraconazole, ketoconazole)	Saquinavir	↑	Azole antifungals may inhibit the metabolism of saquinavir, resulting in an increase in plasma concentrations. Azole antifungal agent plasma concentrations may be elevated. Monitor the patient for toxicity and adjust the dose of either agent as needed. Dosages of ketoconazole or itraconazole > 200 mg/day are not recommended.
Saquinavir	Azole antifungals (eg, itraconazole, ketoconazole)		
Clarithromycin	Saquinavir	↑	Concurrent use increased saquinavir and clarithromycin concentrations but decreased concentrations of the active metabolite 14-OH clarithromycin. For patients with CrCl 30 to 60 mL/min, the clarithromycin dose should be reduced 50%. For patients with CrCl < 30 mL/min, the clarithromycin dose should be decreased 75%.
Saquinavir	Clarithromycin	↑↓	
Delavirdine	Saquinavir	↑	Delavirdine may increase saquinavir plasma concentrations and pharmacologic effects, while saquinavir may decrease delavirdine plasma concentrations and pharmacologic effects. Monitor the patient. Saquinavir dosage reduction and delavirdine dosage increase may be needed.
Saquinavir	Delavirdine		
Dexamethasone	Saquinavir	↓	Dexamethasone may decrease saquinavir levels and efficacy. Use with caution.
Efavirenz	Saquinavir	↓	Coadministration may decrease saquinavir and/or efavirenz plasma levels.
Saquinavir	Efavirenz	↓	

SAQUINAVIR MESYLATE — ORAL

Saquinavir Drug Interactions[a]

Precipitant drug	Object drug[b]		Description
Garlic	Saquinavir	↓	Coadministration is not recommended because of the risk of decreased and possibly subtherapeutic saquinavir plasma concentrations.
Indinavir	Saquinavir	↑	Saquinavir concentrations increased when given with indinavir. Effect on indinavir is not established.
Loperamide	Saquinavir	↓	Saquinavir plasma concentrations and clinical effect may be decreased, while loperamide concentrations may be elevated, increasing the pharmacologic effects and risk of adverse reactions. If coadministration cannot be avoided, closely monitor the patient for a decrease in antiretroviral activity.
Saquinavir	Loperamide	↑	
Lopinavir/ritonavir	Saquinavir	↔	Ritonavir levels may be decreased. Coadminister with caution. Additive effects of QT and/or PR interval prolongation may occur with saquinavir. The recommended dosage with this combination is saquinavir 1,000 mg plus lopinavir 400 mg/ritonavir 100 mg twice daily.
Nevirapine	Saquinavir	↓	Saquinavir plasma levels and clinical efficacy may be reduced. Appropriate doses for the coadministration of nevirapine and saquinavir/ritonavir have not been established.
Proton pump inhibitors (eg, omeprazole)	Saquinavir	↑	Saquinavir plasma concentrations may be elevated and proton pump inhibitor plasma concentrations may be decreased. Use with caution. Monitor for saquinavir toxicity (eg, GI symptoms, increased triglycerides, deep vein thrombosis, QT prolongation). Adjust the saquinavir dose as needed.
Saquinavir	Proton pump inhibitors (eg, omeprazole)	↓	
QT prolonging agents (eg, halofantrine, ibutilide, neuroleptic agents [eg, clozapine, haloperidol, mesoridazine, phenothiazines, thioridazine, ziprasidone], pentamidine, sotalol)	Saquinavir	↑	Coadminister with caution. Additive effects on QT and/or PR interval prolongation may occur.
Saquinavir	QT prolonging agents (eg, halofantrine, ibutilide, neuroleptic agents [eg, clozapine, haloperidol, mesoridazine, phenothiazines, thioridazine, ziprasidone], pentamidine, sotalol)	↑	
St. John's wort	Saquinavir	↓	Coadministration may lead to loss of virologic response and possible resistance to saquinavir or to the class of protease inhibitors. Concomitant use is not recommended.

Saquinavir Drug Interactions[a]

Precipitant drug	Object drug[b]		Description
Tipranavir/Ritonavir	Saquinavir	↓	Saquinavir plasma concentrations may be decreased. Coadministration of saquinavir with tipranavir/ritonavir is not recommended.
Saquinavir	Antiarrhythmics (eg, amiodarone, bepridil, dofetilide, dronedarone, flecainide, lidocaine [systemic], propafenone, quinidine)	↑	Coadministration is contraindicated because of the potential for serious and/or life-threatening reactions.
Saquinavir	Antipsychotic agents (eg, aripiprazole, quetiapine, risperidone)	↑	Plasma concentrations and pharmacologic effects of these antipsychotics may be increased. Avoid coadministration with risperidone. Consider reducing the aripiprazole dose 50% when given with saquinavir.
Saquinavir	Benzodiazepines (eg, alprazolam, clorazepate, diazepam, flurazepam, midazolam, triazolam)	↑	Saquinavir may inhibit the CYP3A4 metabolism of certain benzodiazepines; a decrease in benzodiazepine dose may be needed. Oral midazolam and triazolam are contraindicated with saquinavir because of the potential for serious and/or life-threatening reactions, such as prolonged or increased sedation or respiratory depression. If midazolam IV is given with saquinavir, closely monitor for respiratory depression and/or prolonged sedation and adjust the midazolam dose as needed.
Saquinavir	Bosentan	↑	Bosentan plasma concentrations may be elevated. In patients receiving saquinavir/ritonavir for at least 10 days when bosentan is started, start bosentan at 62.5 mg once daily or every other day based on tolerability. In patients receiving bosentan, discontinue bosentan at least 36 hours before starting saquinavir/ritonavir. At least 10 days after initiation of saquinavir/ritonavir, resume bosentan at 62.5 mg once daily or every other day based on tolerability.
Saquinavir	Buspirone	↑	Buspirone plasma concentrations may be elevated, increasing the pharmacologic effects and risks of adverse reactions. Closely monitor the clinical response of the patient when starting, stopping, or changing the dose of saquinavir. Adjust the buspirone dose as needed.
Saquinavir	Calcium channel blockers (eg, amlodipine, diltiazem, felodipine, isradipine, nicardipine, nifedipine, nimodipine, nisoldipine, verapamil)	↑	Calcium channel blocker concentration may be increased when given with saquinavir. Use with caution and monitor closely. Adjust calcium channel blocker dose as needed.
Saquinavir	Cabazitaxel	↑	Cabazitaxel plasma concentrations may be elevated, increasing the pharmacologic effects and risk of adverse reactions. Avoid concurrent use.
Saquinavir	Cisapride[c]	↑	Coadministration is contraindicated because of the potential for serious and/or life-threatening reactions, such as cardiac arrhythmias.

SAQUINAVIR MESYLATE — ORAL

Saquinavir Drug Interactions[a]

Precipitant drug	Object drug[b]		Description
Saquinavir	Colchicine	↑	Do not coadminister to patients with hepatic or renal impairment. For treatment of gout flares, coadminister colchicine 0.6 mg followed by 0.3 mg 1 hour later. Dose to be repeated no earlier than 3 days. For prophylaxis of gout flares, if the original colchicine regimen was colchicine 0.6 mg twice daily, adjust the dose to 0.3 mg once a day. If the original colchicine dosage was 0.6 mg once daily, adjust the regimen to colchicine 0.3 mg every other day. For treatment of familial Mediterranean fever, coadminister colchicine at a maximum of 0.3 mg twice a day.
Saquinavir	Digoxin	↑	Digoxin plasma concentrations may be elevated, increasing the risk of toxicity. Use with caution. Monitor digoxin concentrations when starting or stopping saquinavir. Adjust the digoxin dose as needed.
Saquinavir	Docetaxel	↑	Docetaxel plasma concentrations may be elevated, increasing the pharmacologic effects and risk of toxicity. Avoid concurrent use. If coadministration cannot be avoided, consider reducing the docetaxel dose by 50% with close clinical and laboratory monitoring.
Saquinavir	Eplerenone	↑	Saquinavir may increase plasma concentrations and pharmacologic or toxic effects of eplerenone. Close clinical monitoring is indicated with coadministration.
Saquinavir	Ergot derivatives (eg, dihydroergotamine, ergonovine, ergotamine, methylergonovine)	↑	Coadministration is contraindicated because of the potential for serious and/or life-threatening reactions, such as acute ergot toxicity, characterized by peripheral vasospasm and ischemia of the extremities and other tissues.
Saquinavir	Erlotinib	↑	Plasma concentrations of erlotinib may be elevated, increasing the risk of erlotinib adverse reactions. If an interaction is suspected, reduce the erlotinib dose.
Saquinavir	Erythromycin	↑	Plasma concentration of erythromycin may be increased by concurrent use of saquinavir. Additive effects on the QT and/or PR interval prolongation may occur. Avoid coadministration.
Erythromycin	Saquinavir		
Saquinavir	Eszopiclone	↑	Plasma concentrations of eszopiclone may be elevated, increasing the pharmacologic effects and risk of adverse reactions. Reduce the eszopiclone dose when saquinavir is coadministered.
Saquinavir	Fluoxetine	↑	Fluoxetine and saquinavir plasma concentrations may be elevated, increasing the risk of adverse reactions to both drugs. Serotonin syndrome has been reported.
Fluoxetine	Saquinavir		
Saquinavir	Fluticasone (inhaled/nasal)	↑	Concomitant use may increase plasma concentrations of fluticasone, resulting in significantly reduced serum cortisol concentrations. Coadministration is not recommended unless the potential benefit outweighs the risk of systemic corticosteroid adverse reactions.
Saquinavir	HMG-CoA reductase inhibitors (eg, atorvastatin, lovastatin, rosuvastatin, simvastatin)	↑↓	Concentrations of certain HMG-CoA reductase inhibitors may be elevated, increasing the risk of adverse reactions, such as myopathy, including rhabdomyolysis. In addition, pravastatin levels may be reduced. Coadministration of saquinavir with lovastatin or simvastatin is contraindicated. Use the lowest dose of atorvastatin or rosuvastatin with careful monitoring or consider the use of fluvastatin.
Saquinavir	Contraceptives, oral (eg, ethinyl estradiol)		Concurrent use may decrease ethinyl estradiol concentrations. Use alternative or additional contraceptive measures when estrogen-based oral contraceptives are taken with saquinavir.
Saquinavir	Iloperidone	↑	Plasma concentrations and pharmacologic effects of iloperidone may be increased by saquinavir. Reduce the dose of iloperidone by one-half when coadministered with saquinavir. If saquinavir is discontinued, increase the dose of iloperidone to the original dose.
Saquinavir	Immunosuppressants (eg, cyclosporine, rapamycin, tacrolimus)	↑	Immunosuppressant concentrations may be increased. Saquinavir plasma concentrations may increase with concomitant cyclosporin use. Monitor immunosuppressant levels and adjust the dose as needed.
Immunosuppressants (eg, cyclosporine, rapamycin, tacrolimus)	Saquinavir		
Saquinavir	Ixabepilone	↑	Ixabepilone plasma concentrations may be elevated, increasing the risk of toxicity. Avoid coadministration. If concomitant use cannot be avoided, consider reducing the ixabepilone dose.
Saquinavir	Maraviroc	↑	Maraviroc plasma concentrations may be increased. The maraviroc dosage should be 150 mg twice daily when administered with saquinavir/ritonavir.
Saquinavir	Methadone	↓	Methadone levels may decrease. Monitor the response of the patient. Adjust methadone dose as needed when starting or stopping saquinavir. Use with caution. Additive effects on QT and/or PR interval prolongation may occur with saquinavir/ritonavir.
Saquinavir	mTOR inhibitors (eg, everolimus, temsirolimus)	↑	mTOR plasma concentrations may be elevated, increasing the pharmacologic effects and risk of adverse reactions. Avoid coadministration. If coadministration of saquinavir is necessary, monitor the clinical response of the patient and adjust the mTOR dose as needed.
Saquinavir	Muscarinic receptor antagonists (eg, darifenacin, fesoterodine, solifenacin, tolterodine)	↑	Muscarinic receptor antagonist plasma concentrations may be increased by saquinavir. When saquinavir is coadministered, the dosage of darifenacin should not exceed 7.5 mg daily, the dosage of fesoterodine should not exceed 4 mg daily, the dosage of solifenacin should not exceed 5 mg daily, and the dosage of tolterodine should not exceed 2 mg daily.

SAQUINAVIR MESYLATE — ORAL

Saquinavir Drug Interactions[a]			
Precipitant drug	Object drug[b]		Description
Saquinavir	Nilotinib	↑	Nilotinib plasma concentrations may be elevated. Avoid coadministration. If concurrent use cannot be avoided, closely monitor for adverse reactions, including QT prolongation. Nilotinib dosage adjustments may be needed when saquinavir is started or stopped.
Saquinavir	Opioid analgesics (eg, buprenorphine, fentanyl, oxycodone)	↑	Concurrent use may increase opioid analgesic plasma concentrations and prolong the half-life, increasing the risk of adverse reactions (eg, respiratory depression). Closely monitor respiratory function during coadministration, and for a longer period than usual after stopping the opioid analgesic. If the opioid analgesic is administered continuously, reduce the opioid analgesic dose as needed.
Saquinavir	PDE5 inhibitors (eg, sildenafil, tadalafil, vardenafil)	↑	Concurrent use may increase the PDE5 inhibitor concentration, resulting in severe and potentially fatal hypotension. For treatment of erectile dysfunction: Reduce the dose and increase the dosing interval of the PDE5 inhibitor. Use with caution and increase monitoring of adverse reactions. Do not exceed sildenafil 25 mg every 48 hours, tadalafil 10 mg every 72 hours, or vardenafil 2.5 mg every 72 hours. For treatment of pulmonary arterial hypertension: Coadministration of sildenafil and saquinavir/ritonavir is contraindicated. In patients receiving saquinavir/ritonavir for at least 1 week, start tadalafil at 20 mg once daily. Increase to 40 mg once daily based on tolerability. Avoid tadalafil during initiation of saquinavir/ritonavir. Stop tadalafil at least 24 hours prior to starting saquinavir/ritonavir. After at least one week following the initiation of saquinavir/ritonavir, resume tadalafil at 20 mg once daily. Increase the dosage to 40 mg once daily based on tolerability.
Saquinavir	Pimozide	↑	Coadministration is contraindicated because of the potential for serious and/or life-threatening reactions.
Saquinavir	Quinazolines (eg, alfuzosin, silodosin, tamsulosin)	↑	Plasma concentrations of these agents may be increased by saquinavir. Avoid concurrent use. Coadministration of alfuzosin and saquinavir is contraindicated.
Saquinavir	Ranolazine	↑	Ranolazine plasma concentrations may be elevated, increasing the risk of dose-related prolongation in the QTc interval, torsades de pointes–type arrhythmias, and sudden death. Coadministration is contraindicated.
Saquinavir	Romidepsin	↑	Romidepsin plasma concentrations may be elevated, increasing the pharmacologic effects and risk of adverse reactions, including QT prolongation. Avoid coadministration. If alternatives to saquinavir are not acceptable, careful clinical, laboratory, and ECG monitoring are indicated. Adjust the romidepsin dose as needed.
Saquinavir	Salmeterol	↑	Salmeterol plasma concentrations may be elevated, increasing the risk of cardiovascular adverse reactions associated with salmeterol, including QT prolongation, palpitations, and sinus tachycardia. Coadministration is not recommended.
Saquinavir	Selective 5-HT_1 receptor agonists (eg, eletriptan)	↑	Saquinavir may increase plasma concentrations and pharmacologic effects of these agents. It is recommended that triptans not be given within 72 hours of ritonavir.
Saquinavir	Thyroid hormones (eg, levothyroxine)	↑↓	Thyroxine serum concentrations may be increased or decreased, resulting in hyperthyroidism or hypothyroidism. Closely monitor thyroid function status when saquinavir is started or stopped. Adjust the thyroid hormone dosage as needed.
Saquinavir	Trazodone	↑	Trazodone concentrations may be elevated, increasing the risk of adverse reactions. Coadministration is contraindicated.
Saquinavir	Tricyclic antidepressants (eg, amitriptyline, imipramine)	↑	Tricyclic antidepressant concentrations may be increased. Monitor tricyclic antidepressant plasma concentrations and the response of the patient, and adjust the dose as needed.
Saquinavir	Tyrosine kinase inhibitors (eg, dasatinib, lapatinib)	↑	Tyrosine kinase inhibitor plasma concentrations may be increased, increasing the pharmacologic effects and risk of adverse reactions. Closely monitor the clinical response of the patient and adjust the tyrosine kinase inhibitor dose as needed.
Saquinavir	Vasopressin receptor antagonists (eg, conivaptan, tolvaptan)	↑	Plasma concentrations and pharmacologic effects of vasopressin receptor antagonists may be increased. Coadministration is contraindicated.
Saquinavir	Warfarin	↑↓	Concentrations of warfarin may be affected. Monitor patient's international normalized ratio. Adjust warfarin dose as needed.

[a] CrCl = creatinine clearance; HMG-CoA = beta-hydroxy-beta-methylglutaryl-CoA; mTOR = mammalian target of rapamycin; PDE5 = phosphodiesterase type 5.
[b] ↑ = object drug increased; ↓ = object drug decreased; ↔ = undetermined clinical effect; ↑↓ = object drug is both increased and decreased.
[c] Available from the manufacturer on a limited-access protocol.

➤*Drug/Food interactions:* See Actions for more information.

Grapefruit – Saquinavir plasma levels may be elevated, increasing the pharmacologic and adverse reactions. Avoid coadministration of saquinavir and grapefruit products. Caution patients to take saquinavir with a liquid other than grapefruit juice.

Adverse Reactions

➤*Adverse reactions (2% or more):*

Saquinavir Adverse Reactions (≥ 2%)[a]	
Adverse reactions	Saquinavir plus ritonavir (N = 148)
Dermatologic	
Dry lips/skin	2%
Eczema	2%
Pruritus	3.4%
Rash	3.4%
GI	
Abdominal pain	6.1%
Constipation	2%
Diarrhea	8.1%
Nausea	10.8%
Vomiting	7.4%

SAQUINAVIR MESYLATE — ORAL

Saquinavir Adverse Reactions (≥ 2%)[a]	
Adverse reactions	Saquinavir plus ritonavir (N = 148)
Metabolic	
Diabetes mellitus/ hyperglycemia	2.7%
Lipodystrophy	5.4%
Respiratory	
Bronchitis	2.7%
Influenza	2.7%
Pneumonia	5.4%
Sinusitis	2.7%
Miscellaneous	
Back pain	2%
Fatigue	6.1%
Fever	3.4%

[a] Includes reactions with an unknown relationship to study drug.

Hepatic – In a study investigating the drug-drug interaction of rifampin 600 mg/day daily and saquinavir 1,000 mg/ritonavir 100 mg twice daily (ritonavir-boosted saquinavir) involving 28 healthy volunteers, 65% of healthy volunteers exposed concomitantly to rifampin and ritonavir-boosted saquinavir developed severe hepatocellular toxicity that presented as increased hepatic transaminases. In some subjects, transaminases increased up to more than 20-fold the upper limit of normal and were associated with GI symptoms, including abdominal pain, gastritis, nausea, and vomiting. Following discontinuation of all 3 drugs, clinical symptoms abated and the increased hepatic transaminases normalized.

➤*Other adverse reactions:*

Cardiovascular – Heart murmur, hypertension, hypotension, peripheral vasoconstriction, syncope, thrombophlebitis.

CNS – Abnormal coordination, anxiety, asthenia, confusion, convulsions, depression, dizziness, dysgeusia, headache, hypoaesthesia, insomnia, intracranial hemorrhage leading to death, lethargy, libido disorder, loss of consciousness, paresthesia, peripheral neuropathy, psychotic disorder, sleep disorder, somnolence, suicide attempt, tremor, unconsciousness.

Dermatologic – Acne, alopecia, bullous dermatitis, drug eruption, erythema, papillomatosis, severe cutaneous reaction associated with increased liver function tests, Stevens-Johnson syndrome, sweating increased, urticaria.

GI – Abdominal discomfort, anorexia, ascites, mucosa ulceration, dry mouth, dyspepsia, dysphagia, eructation, flatulence, gastritis, GI hemorrhage, intestinal obstruction, pancreatitis.

GU – Nephrolithiasis.

Hematologic – Acute myeloid leukemia, anemia, hemolytic anemia, leukopenia, neutropenia, pancytopenia, thrombocytopenia.

Hepatic – Chronic active hepatitis, hepatitis, hepatomegaly, hyperbilirubinemia, jaundice, portal hypertension.

Lab test abnormalities – ALT increase, AST increase, increased alkaline phosphatase, increased creatinine phosphokinase, increased gamma-glutamyltransferase, raised amylase, raised lactate dehydrogenase.

Metabolic – Appetite decrease, appetite increase, dehydration, hypertriglyceridemia, weight increase.

Musculoskeletal – Arthralgia, muscle spasm, myalgia, polyarthritis.

Respiratory Cough, dyspnea.

Special senses – Tinnitus, visual impairment.

Miscellaneous – Allergic reaction, chest pain, edema, lymphadenopathy, wasting syndrome.

Overdosage

➤*Treatment:* Treatment of overdose with saquinavir should consist of general supportive measures including monitoring of vital signs and ECG and observations of the patient's clinical status. Because saquinavir is highly protein bound, dialysis is unlikely to be beneficial in significant removal of the active substance.

Patient Information

Inform patients that saquinavir is not a cure for HIV-1 infection and that they may continue to acquire illnesses associated with advanced HIV-1 infection, including opportunistic infections. Advise patients that saquinavir may be used only if it is combined with ritonavir, which significantly inhibits saquinavir's metabolism to provide increased plasma saquinavir levels.

Advise patients to report to their health care providers the use of any other prescription medication, nonprescription medication, or herbal products, particularly St. John's wort.

Inform patients that saquinavir may produce changes in the ECG (PR interval or QT interval prolongation). Instruct patients to consult their health care provider if they are experiencing symptoms such as dizziness, lightheadedness, or palpitations.

Inform patients that redistribution or accumulation of body fat may occur in patients receiving protease inhibitors and that the cause and long-term health effects of these conditions are not known at this time.

Inform patients that saquinavir must be used in combination with ritonavir, which significantly inhibits saquinavir's metabolism to provide increased plasma saquinavir levels.

Inform them that saquinavir therapy has not been shown to reduce the risk of transmitting HIV to others through sexual contact or blood contamination.

Advise patients to take saquinavir administered with ritonavir within 2 hours after a full meal. When saquinavir is taken without food, concentrations of saquinavir in the blood are substantially reduced and may result in no antiviral activity. Advise patients of the importance of taking their medication every day, as prescribed, to achieve maximum benefit, and tell them not to alter the dose or discontinue therapy without consulting their health care provider. If a dose is missed, advise patients to take the next dose as soon as possible. However, tell patients not to double the next dose.

RITONAVIR

Rx	**Norvir** (Abbott)	**Tablets; oral:** 100 mg	Sorbitan. (NK). White, oval. Film-coated. In 30s.
		Capsules, softgel; oral: 100 mg	Ethanol, polyoxyl 35 castor oil. (100 DS). White. In 30s.
		Solution; oral: 80 mg/mL	Saccharin, ethanol, polyoxyl 35 castor oil. Peppermint and caramel flavor. In 240 mL.

RITONAVIR — ORAL

When coadministering ritonavir with other protease inhibitors, see the full prescribing information for that protease inhibitor.

WARNING

Coadministration of ritonavir with sedative hypnotics, antiarrhythmics, or ergot alkaloid preparations may result in potentially serious and/or life-threatening adverse reactions due to possible effects of ritonavir on the hepatic metabolism of certain drugs. See Contraindications and Drug Interactions for more information.

Indications

➤*HIV infection:* In combination with other antiretroviral agents for the treatment of HIV infection.

Administration and Dosage

➤*General dosing considerations:* Patients should be aware that frequently observed adverse reactions, such as mild to moderate GI disturbances and paresthesias, may diminish as capsule therapy is continued. In addition, patients initiating combination regimens with ritonavir and reverse transcriptase inhibitors may improve GI tolerance by initiating ritonavir alone and subsequently adding the reverse transcriptase inhibitors before completing 2 weeks of ritonavir monotherapy.

➤*Adults:*

HIV infection –

Maximum dose: 600 mg twice daily.

Initial dosage: 300 mg twice daily; increase at 2- to 3-day intervals by 100 mg twice daily.

Maintenance dosage: 600 mg twice daily.

➤*Children:*

HIV infection –

Older than 1 month of age:

- *Maximum dose* – 600 mg twice daily.
- *Initial dosage* – 250 mg/m², 2 times per day; increase at 2- to 3-day intervals by 50 mg/m² twice daily.
- *Maintenance dosage* – 350 to 400 mg/m² twice daily. If patients do not tolerate 400 mg/m² twice daily because of adverse reactions, the highest tolerated dose may be used for maintenance therapy in combination with other antiretroviral agents; however, consider alternative therapy.

Ritonavir Dosage Guidelines in Children				
BSA[a] (m²)	Twice-daily dose 250 mg/m²	Twice-daily dose 300 mg/m²	Twice-daily dose 350 mg/m²	Twice-daily dose 400 mg/m²
0.2	0.6 mL (50 mg)	0.75 mL (60 mg)	0.9 mL (70 mg)	1 mL (80 mg)

RITONAVIR — ORAL

Ritonavir Dosage Guidelines in Children				
BSA[a] (m^2)	Twice-daily dose 250 mg/m^2	Twice-daily dose 300 mg/m^2	Twice-daily dose 350 mg/m^2	Twice-daily dose 400 mg/m^2
0.25	0.8 mL (62.5 mg)	0.9 mL (75 mg)	1.1 mL (87.5 mg)	1.25 mL (100 mg)
0.5	1.6 mL (125 mg)	1.9 mL (150 mg)	2.2 mL (175 mg)	2.5 mL (200 mg)
0.75	2.3 mL (187.5 mg)	2.8 mL (225 mg)	3.3 mL (262.5 mg)	3.75 mL (300 mg)
1	3.1 mL (250 mg)	3.75 mL (300 mg)	4.4 mL (350 mg)	5 mL (400 mg)
1.25	3.9 mL (312.5 mg)	4.7 mL (375 mg)	5.5 mL (437.5 mg)	6.25 mL (500 mg)
1.5	4.7 mL (375 mg)	5.6 mL (450 mg)	6.6 mL (525 mg)	7.5 mL (600 mg)

[a] Body surface area (BSA; m^2) can be calculated with the following equation:

$$BSA\ (m^2) = \sqrt{\frac{ht\ (cm) \times wt\ (kg)}{3600}}$$

Off-label dosing –

Infants younger than 1 months of age: 450 mg/m^2 BSA twice daily.

➤*Hepatic function impairment:* Not recommended for use in severe hepatic impairment.

➤*Concomitant therapy with other protease inhibitors:* Dose reduction of ritonavir is necessary when used with other protease inhibitors (eg, amprenavir, atazanavir, darunavir, fosamprenavir, saquinavir, tipranavir).

Conversion – Patients who take ritonavir capsules may experience more GI adverse reactions, such as nausea, vomiting, abdominal pain, or diarrhea, when switching from the capsule to the tablet because of greater maximum plasma concentration (C_{max}) achieved with the tablet formulation relative to the capsule. Patients should also be aware that these adverse reactions (GI or paresthesias) may diminish as therapy is continued.

➤*Administration:* Ritonavir is administered orally and should be taken with meals.

Tablets – Ritonavir tablets should be swallowed whole, and not chewed, broken, or crushed.

Solution – Shake well before each use. When possible, administer the dose using a calibrated dosing syringe. Patients may improve the taste of the solution by mixing with chocolate milk or enteral nutritional therapy liquids (eg, *Advera, Ensure*) within 1 hour of dosing.

➤*Storage/Stability:*

Tablets – Store at 20° to 25°C (68° to 77°F); excursions are permitted between 15° and 30°C (59° and 86°F). Dispense in original container or equivalent tight container (60 mL or less). Exposure of this product to high humidity outside the original or equivalent tight container for longer than 2 weeks is not recommended.

Capsules – Store at 2° to 8°C (36° to 46°F) until dispensed. Refrigeration of capsules by the patient is recommended, but not required if used within 30 days and stored below 25°C (77°F). Protect from light. Avoid exposure to excessive heat.

Solution – Store at 20° to 25°C (68° to 77°F). Do not refrigerate. Store and dispense in the original container. Avoid exposure to excessive heat.

Actions

➤*Pharmacology:* Ritonavir, an antiviral drug, is a peptidomimetic inhibitor of the HIV-1 and HIV-2 proteases. Inhibition of HIV protease renders the enzyme incapable of processing the gag-pol polyprotein precursor that leads to production of noninfectious immature HIV particles.

Electrophysiology – QTcF interval was evaluated in a randomized, placebo- and active- (moxifloxacin 400 mg once daily) controlled crossover study in 45 healthy adults, with 10 measurements over 12 hours on day 3. The maximum mean (95% upper confidence bound) time-matched difference in QTcF from placebo after baseline correction was 5.5 (7.6) msec for ritonavir 400 mg twice daily. Ritonavir 400 mg twice daily resulted in day 3 ritonavir exposure that was approximately 1.5-fold higher than observed with the ritonavir 600 mg twice-daily dosage at steady state.

PR interval prolongation also was noted in subjects receiving ritonavir in the same study on day 3. The maximum mean (95% confidence interval [CI]) difference from placebo in the PR interval after baseline correction was 22 (25) msec for ritonavir 400 mg twice daily.

➤*Pharmacokinetics:* Ritonavir tablets are not bioequivalent to ritonavir capsules.

Ritonavir Pharmacokinetic Characteristics[a]		
Parameter	n	Values (mean ± SD)
C_{max} SS[b]	10	11.2 ± 3.6 mcg/mL
C_{trough} SS[b]	10	3.7 ± 2.6 mcg/mL
V_{beta}/F[c]	91	0.41 ± 0.25 L/kg
t½		3 to 5 h
CL/F, SS[b]	10	8.8 ± 3.2 L/h
CL/F[c]	91	4.6 ± 1.6 L/h
CL_R	62	< 0.1 L/h
RBC/Plasma ratio		0.14
Percent bound[d]		98% to 99%

[a] SD = standard deviation; C_{max} SS = maximal steady-state drug concentration; C_{trough} SS = trough drug concentration at steady-state; V_{beta}/F = apparent volume of distribution; t½ = half-life; CL/F = apparent oral clearance; CL/F SS = apparent steady state oral clearance; CL_R = renal clearance; RBC = red blood cell.
[b] Patients taking ritonavir 600 mg every 12 hours.
[c] Single ritonavir 600 mg dose.
[d] Primarily bound to human serum albumin and alpha-1 acid glycoprotein over the ritonavir concentration range of 0.01 to 30 mcg/mL.

Absorption – The absolute bioavailability of ritonavir has not been determined. After a 600 mg dose of oral solution, peak concentrations of ritonavir were achieved approximately 2 and 4 hours after dosing under fasting and nonfasting (514 kcal; 9% fat, 12% protein, and 79% carbohydrate) conditions, respectively.

Effect of food: When the oral solution was given under nonfasting conditions, peak ritonavir concentrations decreased 23%, and the extent of absorption decreased 7% relative to fasting conditions. Relative to fasting conditions, the extent of absorption of ritonavir from the capsule was 13% higher when administered with a meal (615 kcal; 14.5% fat, 9% protein, and 76% carbohydrate).

A food effect is observed for ritonavir tablets. Food decreased the bioavailability of the ritonavir tablets when a single 100 mg dose of ritonavir was administered. Under high-fat conditions (907 kcal; 52% fat, 15% protein, and 33% carbohydrates), a 23% decrease in mean area under the curve ($AUC_{0-\infty}$) (90% CI, −30% to −15%), and a 23% decrease in mean C_{max} (90% CI, −34% to −11%) was observed relative to fasting conditions. Under moderate-fat conditions, a 21% decrease in mean $AUC_{0-\infty}$ (90% CI, −28% to −13%) and a 22% decrease in mean C_{max} (90% CI, −33% to −9%) was observed relative to fasting conditions. However, the type of meal administered did not change ritonavir tablet bioavailability when high-fat meals were compared with moderate-fat meals.

Metabolism – Nearly all of the plasma radioactivity after a single oral dose of ^{14}C-ritonavir 600 mg oral solution (n = 5) was attributed to unchanged ritonavir. Five ritonavir metabolites have been identified in human urine and feces. The isopropylthiazole oxidation metabolite (M-2) is the major metabolite and has antiviral activity similar to that of parent drug; however, the concentrations of this metabolite in plasma are low. In vitro studies utilizing human liver microsomes have demonstrated that CYP3A is the major isoform involved in ritonavir metabolism, although CYP2D6 also contributes to the formation of M-2.

Excretion – In a study of 5 subjects receiving a dose of ^{14}C-ritonavir 600 mg oral solution, 11.3% ± 2.8% of the dose was excreted into the urine, with 3.5% ± 1.8% of the dose excreted as unchanged parent drug. In that study, 86.4% ± 2.9% of the dose was excreted in the feces, with 33.8% ± 10.8% of the dose excreted as unchanged parent drug. Upon multiple dosing, ritonavir accumulation is less than predicted from a single dose, possibly because of a time- and dose-related increase in clearance.

Special populations –

Hepatic function impairment: Dose-normalized steady-state ritonavir exposures in subjects with moderate hepatic impairment (400 mg twice daily; n = 6) were about 40% lower than those in subjects with healthy hepatic function (500 mg twice daily; n = 6).

No dosage adjustment is recommended in patients with mild or moderate hepatic impairment. However, be aware of the potential for lower ritonavir concentrations in patients with moderate hepatic impairment; monitor patient response carefully. Ritonavir has not been studied in patients with severe hepatic impairment.

Children: Steady-state pharmacokinetics were evaluated in 37 patients 2 to 14 years of age who were HIV-infected and receiving dosages ranging from 250 to 400 mg/m^2 twice daily in study 310, and in 41 patients 1 month to 2 years of age who were HIV-infected at dosages of 350 and 450 mg/m^2 twice daily in study 345. Across dose groups, ritonavir steady-state oral clearance (CL/F/m^2) was approximately 1.5 to 1.7 times faster in children than in adults.

The following observations were seen regarding ritonavir concentrations after administration with 350 or 450 mg/m^2 twice daily in children younger than 2 years of age. Higher ritonavir exposures were not evident with 450 mg/m^2 twice daily compared with the 350 mg/m^2 twice daily. Ritonavir trough concentrations were somewhat lower than those obtained in adults receiving 600 mg twice daily. The AUC and trough concentrations obtained after administration with 350 or 450 mg/m^2 twice daily in children younger than 2 years of age were approximately 16% and 60% lower, respectively, than those obtained in adults receiving 600 mg twice daily.

Contraindications

Coadministration with alfuzosin, amiodarone, bepridil, cisapride, dihydroergotamine, ergonovine, ergotamine, flecainide, lovastatin, methylergonovine, oral midazolam, pimozide, propafenone, quinidine, St. John's wort (*Hypericum perforatum*), sildenafil (*Revatio*; only when used for the treatment of pulmonary arterial hypertension [PAH]), simvastatin, triazolam, voriconazole; hypersensitivity to ritonavir or any of its ingredients.

RITONAVIR — ORAL

Warnings/Precautions

➤*Hepatic effects:* Hepatic transaminase elevations exceeding 5 times the upper limit of normal, clinical hepatitis, and jaundice have occurred in patients receiving ritonavir alone or in combination with other antiretroviral drugs. There may be an increased risk of transaminase elevations in patients with underlying hepatitis B or C. Therefore, exercise caution when administering ritonavir to patients with preexisting liver diseases, liver enzyme abnormalities, or hepatitis. Consider increased AST/ALT monitoring in these patients, especially during the first 3 months of ritonavir treatment.

There have been postmarketing reports of hepatic impairment, including some fatalities. These have generally occurred in patients taking multiple concomitant medications and/or in patients with advanced AIDS.

➤*Pancreatitis:* Pancreatitis has been observed in patients receiving ritonavir therapy, including those who developed hypertriglyceridemia. In some cases, fatalities have been observed. Patients with advanced HIV disease may be at increased risk of elevated triglycerides and pancreatitis.

Consider pancreatitis if clinical symptoms (eg, abdominal pain, nausea, vomiting) or abnormalities in laboratory values (eg, increased serum lipase or amylase values) suggestive of pancreatitis occur. Evaluate patients who exhibit these signs or symptoms and discontinue ritonavir therapy if a diagnosis of pancreatitis is made.

➤*Diabetes mellitus/hyperglycemia:* New-onset diabetes mellitus, exacerbation of preexisting diabetes mellitus, and hyperglycemia have been reported during postmarketing surveillance in patients who are infected with HIV receiving protease inhibitor therapy. Some patients required initiation or dosage adjustments of insulin or oral hypoglycemic agents for treatment of these events. In some cases, diabetic ketoacidosis has occurred. In those patients who discontinued protease inhibitor therapy, hyperglycemia persisted in some cases. Because these events have been reported voluntarily during clinical practice, estimates of frequency cannot be made and a causal relationship between protease inhibitor therapy and these events has not been established.

➤*Resistance/Cross resistance:* Varying degrees of cross resistance among protease inhibitors have been observed. Continued administration of ritonavir therapy following loss of viral suppression may increase the likelihood of cross resistance to other protease inhibitors.

➤*Hemophilia:* There have been reports of increased bleeding, including spontaneous skin hematomas and hemarthrosis, in patients with hemophilia type A and B treated with protease inhibitors. In some patients, additional factor VIII was given. In more than half of the reported cases, treatment with protease inhibitors was continued or reintroduced. A causal relationship between protease inhibitor therapy and these events has not been established.

➤*PR interval prolongation:* Ritonavir prolongs the PR interval in some patients. Postmarketing cases of second- or third-degree atrioventricular (AV) block have been reported in patients. Use ritonavir with caution in patients with underlying structural heart disease, preexisting conduction system abnormalities, ischemic heart disease, and cardiomyopathies, as these patients may be at increased risk for developing cardiac conduction abnormalities. The impact on the PR interval of coadministration of ritonavir with other drugs that prolong the PR interval (including calcium channel blockers, beta-adrenergic blockers, digoxin, and atazanavir) has not been evaluated. As a result, undertake caution with coadministration of ritonavir with these drugs, particularly with those drugs metabolized by CYP3A. Clinical monitoring is recommended.

➤*Fat redistribution:* Redistribution/accumulation of body fat, including central obesity, dorsocervical fat enlargement ("buffalo hump"), peripheral wasting, facial wasting, breast enlargement, and "cushingoid appearance" have been observed in patients receiving antiretroviral therapy. The mechanism and long-term consequences of these events are currently unknown. A causal relationship has not been established.

➤*Lipid disorders:* Treatment with ritonavir therapy alone or in combination with saquinavir has resulted in substantial increases in the concentration of total triglycerides and cholesterol. Perform triglyceride and cholesterol testing prior to initiating ritonavir therapy and at periodic intervals during therapy. Manage lipid disorders as clinically appropriate taking into account any potential drug-drug interactions with ritonavir and HMG-CoA reductase inhibitors.

➤*Immune reconstitution syndrome:* Immune reconstitution syndrome has been reported in patients infected with HIV treated with combination antiretroviral therapy, including ritonavir. During the initial phase of combination antiretroviral treatment, patients whose immune system responds may develop an inflammatory response to indolent or residual opportunistic infections (such as *Mycobacterium avium* infection, cytomegalovirus, *Pneumocystis jiroveci* pneumonia, or tuberculosis), which may necessitate further evaluation and treatment.

➤*Hypersensitivity reactions:* Allergic reactions (eg, urticaria, mild skin eruptions, bronchospasm, angioedema) have been reported. Rare cases of anaphylaxis and Stevens-Johnson syndrome also have been reported. Discontinue treatment if severe reactions develop.

➤*Hepatic function impairment:* Ritonavir is principally metabolized by the liver. Therefore, exercise caution when administering this drug to patients with impaired hepatic function.

See Administration and Dosage for more information.

➤*Pregnancy: Category B.* There are no adequate and well-controlled studies in pregnant women. Because animal reproduction studies are not always predictive of human response, only use this drug during pregnancy if clearly needed.

Developmental toxicity observed in rats (early resorptions, decreased fetal body weight and ossification delays, and developmental variations) occurred at a maternally toxic dosage at an exposure equivalent to approximately 30% of that achieved with the proposed therapeutic dose. A slight increase in the incidence of cryptorchidism was also noted in rats at an exposure approximately 22% of that achieved with the proposed therapeutic dose. Developmental toxicity observed in rabbits (resorptions, decreased litter size, and decreased fetal weights) also occurred at a maternally toxic dosage equivalent to 1.8 times the proposed therapeutic dose based on a BSA conversion factor.

In 2006, the updated US Department of Health and Human Services guidelines for the use of antiretroviral agents in patients with HIV-1 infection continued the recommendation that therapy, with the exception of efavirenz, should be continued during pregnancy. Therefore, if indicated, protease inhibitors, including ritonavir, should not be withheld in pregnancy because the expected benefit to the mother who is HIV positive outweighs the unknown risk to the fetus.

Antiretroviral pregnancy registry – To monitor maternal-fetal outcomes of pregnant women exposed to ritonavir, an antiretroviral pregnancy registry has been established. Health care providers are encouraged to register patients by calling 1-800-258-4263.

➤*Lactation:* The Centers for Disease Control and Prevention recommend that mothers who are HIV-infected do not breast-feed their infants to avoid risking postnatal transmission of HIV. It is not known whether ritonavir is secreted in human breast milk. The molecular weight (about 721) is low enough that excretion into breast milk should be expected. Because of the potential for HIV transmission and the potential for serious adverse reactions in breast-feeding infants, instruct mothers not to breast-feed if they are receiving ritonavir.

➤*Elderly:* Make dose selection for an elderly patient with caution, usually starting at the low end of the dosing range, reflecting the greater frequency of decreased hepatic, renal, or cardiac function, and of concomitant disease or other drug therapy.

➤*Monitoring:* Consider increased AST/ALT monitoring in patients with hepatitis B or C, especially during the first 3 months of ritonavir treatment.

Ritonavir has been shown to increase triglycerides, cholesterol, AST, ALT, gamma-glutamyltransferase (GGT), creatine phosphokinase (CPK), and uric acid. Perform appropriate laboratory testing prior to initiating ritonavir therapy and at periodic intervals or if any clinical signs or symptoms occur during therapy. Monitor blood glucose closely.

Drug Interactions

➤*Cytochrome P450 system:* Because ritonavir is metabolized mainly by the CYP3A enzyme systems, substances known to inhibit these enzymes may decrease metabolism or increase bioavailability of ritonavir, as indicated by increased plasma concentrations. Drugs known to induce these enzyme systems may result in an increased metabolism of ritonavir or decreased bioavailability, as indicated by decreased plasma concentrations. Monitoring of plasma concentrations and appropriate dosage adjustments are essential when such drugs are used concomitantly.

Ritonavir Drug Interactions

Precipitant drug	Object drug[a]		Description
Aldesleukin	Ritonavir	↑	Ritonavir concentrations may be elevated. Adjust ritonavir dose as needed.
Anticonvulsants (eg, carbamazepine)	Ritonavir	↑↓	Carbamazepine may decrease ritonavir levels, resulting in treatment failure. Ritonavir may increase plasma concentrations of carbamazepine and ethosuximide. Divalproex, lamotrigine, and phenytoin levels may be decreased; therefore, a dose increase may be needed when coadministered with ritonavir. Close clinical monitoring is indicated if concomitant use cannot be avoided. Closely monitor carbamazepine plasma concentrations when starting, stopping, or changing the dose of ritonavir. Observe the clinical response during coadministration of carbamazepine. Adjust the dose of one or both drugs as needed.
Ritonavir	Anticonvulsants (eg, carbamazepine, divalproex, ethosuximide, lamotrigine, phenytoin)		

RITONAVIR — ORAL

Ritonavir Drug Interactions

Precipitant drug	Object drug[a]		Description
Azole antifungals (fluconazole, itraconazole, ketoconazole)	Ritonavir	↑↓	Ritonavir plasma concentrations may be elevated. Ketoconazole AUC increased 3.4-fold and the C_{max} increased by 55%. High doses of ketoconazole or itraconazole (> 200 mg/day) are not recommended. Itraconazole and ketoconazole levels may be increased. Voriconazole levels may be decreased when coadministered with ritonavir and may lead to loss of antifungal response. Therefore, coadministration of voriconazole and ritonavir 400 mg every 12 hours or greater is contraindicated. Coadministration of voriconazole and ritonavir 100 mg should be avoided.
Ritonavir	Azole antifungals (itraconazole, ketoconazole, voriconazole)		
Clarithromycin	Ritonavir	↑	Concurrent use may increase ritonavir and clarithromycin levels. Dosage adjustment is not needed in patients with healthy renal function. For patients with CrCl[b] 30 to 60 mL/min, decrease clarithromycin dose by 50%. For patients with CrCl < 30 mL/min, decrease clarithromycin dose by 75%.
Ritonavir	Clarithromycin		
Immunosuppressants (eg, cyclosporine)	Ritonavir	↑	Plasma concentrations and pharmacologic effects of both drugs may increase when immunosuppressants and ritonavir are coadministered. Increased concentrations of these agents may occur within 3 days of concurrent therapy. Additional plasma concentrations and clinical monitoring are indicated. Adjust the dose accordingly.
Ritonavir	Immunosuppressants (eg, cyclosporine, rapamycin, sirolimus, tacrolimus)		
Mefloquine	Ritonavir	↓	Plasma concentrations of ritonavir may be reduced. Monitor the clinical response of the patient for a possible decrease in efficacy. Adjust the ritonavir dose as needed.
NNRTIs[b] (eg, delavirdine, efavirenz, nevirapine)	Ritonavir	↑↓	Ritonavir plasma levels and clinical efficacy may be reduced when coadministered with efavirenz and nevirapine. Delavirdine may increase ritonavir AUC and C_{max}. Appropriate doses of this combination have not been established. The combination of atazanavir/ritonavir, fosamprenavir/ritonavir, or tipranavir/ritonavir should not be coadministered with NNRTIs.
Rifamycins (eg, rifampin)	Ritonavir	↓	Coadministration of ritonavir with rifampin may lead to loss of virologic response to ritonavir. Consider alternate antimycobacterial agents (eg, rifabutin). Do not coadminister saquinavir/ritonavir with rifampin because of the risk of severe hepatotoxicity if the 3 drugs are given together. Coadministration of ritonavir with rifabutin may increase rifabutin (and its metabolite) concentrations. Reduce rifabutin dose by at least 75% (eg, 150 mg every other day or 3 times weekly). Further dosage reduction may be necessary.
Ritonavir	Rifamycins (eg, rifabutin, rifampin)	↑	
St. John's wort (*Hypericum perforatum*)	Ritonavir	↓	Coadministration may lead to loss of virologic response and possible resistance to ritonavir. Coadministration is contraindicated.

Ritonavir Drug Interactions

Precipitant drug	Object drug[a]		Description
Ritonavir	Alfuzosin	↑	Alfuzosin blood concentrations may be elevated, increasing the pharmacologic effects and adverse reactions, such as hypotension. Coadministration is contraindicated.
Ritonavir	Antiarrhythmic agents (eg, amiodarone, bepridil, disopyramide, flecainide, lidocaine, mexiletine, propafenone, quinidine)	↑	Coadministration of ritonavir with amiodarone, bepridil, flecainide, propafenone, or quinidine is contraindicated because of the potential for serious and/or life-threatening cardiac arrhythmias secondary to increases in plasma concentrations of antiarrhythmics. Coadministration of ritonavir with other antiarrhythmics (eg, disopyramide, lidocaine, mexiletine) may also cause an increase in the antiarrhythmic concentration. Use with caution and monitor the therapeutic concentration of the antiarrhythmics.
Ritonavir	Antidepressants (eg, bupropion, desipramine, nefazodone, SSRIs[b], trazodone, tricyclics)	↑↓	A dosage decrease may be needed when these antidepressants are coadministered with ritonavir. Concurrent use increased desipramine AUC by 145% and C_{max} by 22%; dosage reduction and concentration monitoring is recommended. Fluoxetine may increase ritonavir levels. Bupropion plasma concentrations may be reduced, decreasing the efficacy. Monitor the clinical response and adjust the bupropion dose as needed.
SSRIs (eg, fluoxetine)	Ritonavir	↑	
Ritonavir	Antineoplastic agents (eg, vinblastine, vincristine)	↑	Vinblastine and vincristine plasma concentrations may be elevated. Consider either temporarily withholding ritonavir-containing regimens in patients who develop severe adverse reactions or using alternative treatment with an antiretroviral agent that does not inhibit CYP3A of P-glycoprotein.
Ritonavir	Antipsychotics (eg, aripiprazole, olanzapine, perphenazine, pimozide, quetiapine, risperidone, thioridazine)	↑↓	Coadministration with pimozide is contraindicated because of the potential for cardiac arrhythmias. Aripiprazole, quetiapine, perphenazine, risperidone, and thioridazine levels may be increased; olanzapine levels may be decreased. Adjust dose as needed.
Ritonavir	Atovaquone	↓	Atovaquone levels may be decreased. A dosage increase may be needed.
Ritonavir	Benzodiazepines (eg, alprazolam, clonazepam, clorazepate, diazepam, estazolam, flurazepam, midazolam, triazolam)	↑↓	Coadministration of ritonavir with oral midazolam or triazolam is contraindicated because of the risk of prolonged or increased sedation or respiratory depression. Plasma levels of the other benzodiazepines, including parenteral midazolam, may be increased; therefore, a decrease in the benzodiazepine dose may be needed. Alprazolam plasma concentrations may be decreased. Coadminister parenteral midazolam in a setting that ensures close medical monitoring and appropriate medical management in case of respiratory depression and/or prolonged sedation.
Ritonavir	Beta-blockers (eg, metoprolol, timolol)	↑	Metoprolol and timolol concentrations may be increased. Use with caution and monitor patients. A dosage decrease of the beta-blocker may be needed.

RITONAVIR — ORAL

Ritonavir Drug Interactions

Precipitant drug	Object drug[a]		Description
Ritonavir	Bosentan	↑	Bosentan concentrations may be elevated, increasing the risk of adverse reactions. Coadministration is contraindicated.
Ritonavir	Buspirone	↑	Increased serum buspirone levels may occur; therefore, a dosage decrease may be needed with coadministration.
Ritonavir	Calcium channel blockers (eg, amlodipine, diltiazem, nifedipine, verapamil)	↑	Calcium channel blocker levels may be increased. Use with caution and monitor patients. A decrease in the calcium channel blocker dose may be needed.
Ritonavir	Cisapride	↑	Coadministration is contraindicated because of the risk of cardiac arrhythmias.
Ritonavir	Colchicine	↑	Colchicine plasma concentrations may be elevated, increasing the risk of toxicity. Coadministration is contraindicated in patients with hepatic or renal impairment. In patients with healthy renal and hepatic function, coadminister ritonavir and colchicine with caution, using a maximum colchicine dosage of 0.3 mg twice daily.
Ritonavir	Conivaptan	↑	Coadministration is contraindicated because of the increased risk of adverse reactions.
Ritonavir	Corticosteroids (eg, dexamethasone, fluticasone, prednisone)	↑	Steroid levels may be increased. A decrease in dose may be needed for these drugs. Coadministration of ritonavir with fluticasone (nasal spray) increased fluticasone AUC by 350-fold and C_{max} by 25-fold and caused a significant decrease (86%) in plasma cortisol AUC. Coadministration of ritonavir with fluticasone is not recommended. Consider using a less systemically available steroid such as beclomethasone or budesonide.
Ritonavir	Contraceptives, hormonal	↓	Coadministration decreased the ethinyl estradiol AUC by 40% and the C_{max} by 32%. Consider alternate nonhormonal contraceptive measures.
Ritonavir	Deferasirox	↓	Plasma concentrations and pharmacologic effects of deferasirox may be decreased by ritonavir; avoid coadministration. If concurrent use cannot be avoided, consider a starting dose of deferasirox 30 mg/kg/day. Adjust the deferasirox dose further according to serum ferritin concentrations and clinical response.
Ritonavir	Didanosine	↓	Coadministration for 4 days decreased the didanosine AUC by 13% and the C_{max} by 16%. These changes are not likely to be clinically important.
Ritonavir	Digoxin	↑	Digoxin levels may be elevated, increasing the risk of toxicity. Monitor digoxin levels closely and adjust dosage as needed.
Ritonavir	Disulfiram Metronidazole	↑	Ritonavir formulations contain alcohol, which can produce disulfiram-like reactions when coadministered with disulfiram or other drugs that produce this reaction (eg, metronidazole).
Ritonavir	Dronabinol	↑	Dronabinol levels may be increased. A decrease in dosage of dronabinol may be needed.
Ritonavir	Dronedarone	↑	Dronedarone plasma concentrations may be elevated, increasing the pharmacologic effects and risk of adverse reactions. Coadministration is contraindicated.
Ritonavir	Eplerenone	↑	Eplerenone levels may be elevated, increasing the risk for hyperkalemia and associated serious arrhythmias. Coadministration is contraindicated.
Ritonavir	Ergot derivatives (eg, dihydroergotamine, ergonovine, ergotamine, methylergonovine)	↑	The risk of ergot toxicity (eg, vasospasm and ischemia of the extremities and other tissues including the CNS) may be increased. Coadministration is contraindicated.
Ritonavir	Eszopiclone	↑	Eszopiclone concentrations may be elevated, increasing the pharmacologic effects and risk for adverse reactions. Monitor for increased pharmacologic effects. Consider eszopiclone dosage reduction during coadministration of ritonavir.
Ritonavir	HMG-CoA reductase inhibitors (eg, atorvastatin, lovastatin, pravastatin, rosuvastatin, simvastatin)	↑↓	Concurrent use increases the risk of myopathy, including rhabdomyolysis. Coadministration with lovastatin or simvastatin is contraindicated. If using atorvastatin or rosuvastatin, start with the lowest possible dose and monitor carefully or consider pravastatin or fluvastatin. However, pravastatin plasma levels may be reduced, decreasing the efficacy.
Ritonavir	Iloperidone	↑	Plasma concentrations and pharmacologic effects of iloperidone may be increased by ritonavir. Reduce the dose of iloperidone by one-half when coadministered with ritonavir. If ritonavir is discontinued, increase the dose of iloperidone to the original dose.
Ritonavir	Ixabepilone	↑	Ixabepilone plasma concentrations may be elevated, increasing the pharmacologic effects and risk of adverse reactions. Avoid coadministration.
Ritonavir	Levothyroxine	↑↓	Thyroxine serum concentrations may be increased or decreased. Monitor patients when starting or stopping ritonavir. Adjust the levothyroxine dose as needed.
Ritonavir	Maraviroc	↑	Maraviroc plasma concentrations may be increased. When coadministered with ritonavir, maraviroc dosage adjustments may be necessary.
Ritonavir	Methamphetamine	↑	Methamphetamine levels may be increased; therefore, a dose decrease of methamphetamine may be needed.
Ritonavir	Muscarinic receptor antagonists (eg, darifenacin, fesoterodine, solifenacin, tolterodine)	↑	Muscarinic receptor antagonist plasma concentrations may be increased by ritonavir. When ritonavir is coadministered, the dose of darifenacin should not exceed 7.5 mg daily, the dose of solifenacin should not exceed 5 mg daily, the dose of tolterodine should not exceed 2 mg daily, and the dose of fesoterodine should not exceed 4 mg daily.

RITONAVIR — ORAL

Ritonavir Drug Interactions			
Precipitant drug	Object drug[a]		Description
Ritonavir	Nilotinib	↑	Nilotinib plasma concentrations may be elevated, increasing the pharmacologic effects and risk of adverse reactions. Avoid coadministration of ritonavir and nilotinib.
Ritonavir	Opioid analgesics (eg, fentanyl, meperidine, methadone, propoxyphene, tramadol)	↑↓	Plasma concentrations of alfentanil, buprenorphine, fentanyl, propoxyphene, sufentanil, and tramadol may be increased, possibly causing toxicity. A dose decrease may be needed for these drugs when coadministered with ritonavir. Methadone concentration may be decreased; therefore, consider dosage increase of methadone. Meperidine levels may decrease, possibly decreasing efficacy. However, the levels of the metabolite normeperidine may be increased, possibly leading to increased neurologic toxicity (eg, seizures). Dosage increase and long-term use of meperidine with ritonavir are not recommended.
Ritonavir	PDE5[b] inhibitors (eg, sildenafil, tadalafil, vardenafil)	↑	Coadministration with sildenafil, when used for the treatment of PAH, is contraindicated. Use concomitantly with caution and with increased monitoring for adverse reactions; the PDE5 inhibitor dose should not exceed the following: sildenafil 25 mg within 48 hours; tadalafil 10 mg every 72 hours; vardenafil 2.5 mg every 72 hours.
Ritonavir	Protease inhibitors (eg, atazanavir, darunavir, fosamprenavir, indinavir, saquinavir, tipranavir)	↑	Ritonavir may increase the AUC and C_{max} of other coadministered protease inhibitors. Coadministration of tipranavir and ritonavir has been associated with hepatitis and fatal hepatic decompensation. Use with caution in patients with chronic hepatitis B or hepatitis C coinfection. Adjust the dose of one or both agents as needed.
Ritonavir	Quinine	↑	Quinine levels may be increased. A decrease of the quinine dose may be needed.
Ritonavir	Ranolazine	↑	Coadministration is contraindicated. Increased ranolazine concentrations may increase the risk of QT prolongation, torsades de pointes, and sudden death.
Ritonavir	Salmeterol	↑	Pharmacologic effects of salmeterol may be increased by ritonavir, increasing the risk of cardiovascular toxicity (eg, QT prolongation, palpitations, sinus tachycardia). Coadministration is not recommended.
Ritonavir	Selective 5-HT_1 receptor agonists (eg, eletriptan)	↑	Ritonavir may increase plasma concentrations and pharmacologic effects of these agents. It is recommended that eletriptan not be given within 72 hours of ritonavir.
Ritonavir	Sulfamethoxazole	↓	Coadministration of ritonavir with sulfamethoxazole/trimethoprim decreased sulfamethoxazole AUC by 20%. This decrease is not likely to be clinically important.
Ritonavir	Theophylline	↓	Coadministration decreased the theophylline AUC 43% and the C_{max} 32%. Consider monitoring of theophylline levels; increased dosage may be needed.
Ritonavir	Trimethoprim	↑	Coadministration of ritonavir with sulfamethoxazole/trimethoprim increased trimethoprim AUC 20%. This increase is not likely to be clinically important.
Ritonavir	Tyrosine kinase receptor inhibitors (eg, dasatinib)	↑	Ritonavir may elevate plasma concentrations, increasing the pharmacologic effects and risk of adverse reactions of these agents. Closely monitor the clinical response of the patient. Adjust the dose of tyrosine kinase receptor inhibitor as needed.
Ritonavir	Warfarin	↑↓	Initial frequent monitoring of international normalized ratio is indicated. Adjust the warfarin dose as needed.
Ritonavir	Zidovudine	↓	Coadministration decreased zidovudine AUC 25% and C_{max} 27%. Observe the clinical response of the patient. If an interaction is suspected, adjust the zidovudine dose as needed.
Ritonavir	Zolpidem	↑	Zolpidem levels may be increased, resulting in possible severe sedation and respiratory depression. Closely monitor the patient and adjust the zolpidem dose as needed.

[a] ↑ = object drug increased; ↓ = object drug decreased; ↑↓ = object drug both increased and decreased.
[b] NNRTI = nonnucleoside reverse transcriptase inhibitors; SSRIs = selective serotonin reuptake inhibitors; PDE5 = phosphodiesterase type 5; CrCl = creatinine clearance.

➤*Drug/Food interactions:* See Actions for more information.

Grapefruit juice may increase the plasma concentrations and pharmacologic effects of ritonavir. If grapefruit juice cannot be avoided, close clinical monitoring is indicated. Adjust the ritonavir dose accordingly.

Adverse Reactions

➤*Adults:*

Ritonavir Adverse Reactions in Adults[a] (≥ 2%)						
	Study 245 naive patients[b]			Study 247 advanced patients[c]		Study 462 protease inhibitor–naive patients[d]
Adverse reactions	Ritonavir + zidovudine (n = 116)	Ritonavir (n = 117)	Zidovudine (n = 119)	Ritonavir (n = 541)	Placebo (n = 545)	Ritonavir + saquinavir (n = 141)
Cardiovascular						
Syncope	0.9%	1.7%	0.8%	0.6%	0%	2.1%
Vasodilation	3.4%	1.7%	0.8%	1.7%	0%	3.5%
CNS						
Abnormal thinking	2.6%	0%	0.8%	0.9%	0.4%	0.7%
Anxiety	0.9%	0%	0.8%	1.7%	0.9%	2.1%
Asthenia	28.4%	10.3%	11.8%	15.3%	6.4%	16.3%
Circumoral paresthesia	5.2%	3.4%	0%	6.7%	0.4%	6.4%
Confusion	0%	0.9%	0%	0.6%	0.6%	2.1%
Depression	1.7%	1.7%	2.5%	1.7%	0.7%	7.1%
Dizziness	5.2%	2.6%	3.4%	3.9%	1.1%	8.5%
Headache	7.8%	6%	6.7%	6.5%	5.7%	4.3%
Insomnia	3.4%	2.6%	0.8%	2%	1.8%	2.8%
Malaise	5.2%	1.7%	3.4%	0.7%	0.2%	2.8%
Paresthesia	5.2%	2.6%	0%	3%	0.4%	2.1%
Peripheral paresthesia	0%	6%	0.8%	5%	1.1%	5.7%
Somnolence	2.6%	2.6%	0%	2.4%	0.2%	0%
Dermatologic						
Rash	0.9%	0%	0.8%	3.5%	1.5%	0.7%
Sweating	3.4%	2.6%	1.7%	1.7%	1.1%	2.8%

RITONAVIR — ORAL

Ritonavir Adverse Reactions in Adults[a] (≥ 2%)						
	Study 245 naive patients[b]			Study 247 advanced patients[c]		Study 462 protease inhibitor–naive patients[d]
Adverse reactions	Ritonavir + zidovudine (n = 116)	Ritonavir (n = 117)	Zidovudine (n = 119)	Ritonavir (n = 541)	Placebo (n = 545)	Ritonavir + saquinavir (n = 141)
GI						
Abdominal pain	5.2%	6%	5.9%	8.3%	5.1%	2.1%
Anorexia	8.6%	1.7%	4.2%	7.8%	4.2%	4.3%
Constipation	3.4%	0%	0.8%	0.2%	0.4%	1.4%
Diarrhea	25%	15.4%	2.5%	23.3%	7.9%	22.7%
Dyspepsia	2.6%	0%	1.7%	5.9%	1.5%	0.7%
Fecal incontinence	0%	0%	0%	0%	0%	2.8%
Flatulence	2.6%	0.9%	1.7%	1.7%	0.7%	3.5%
Local throat irritation	0.9%	1.7%	0.8%	2.8%	0.4%	1.4%
Nausea	46.6%	25.6%	26.1%	29.8%	8.4%	18.4%
Taste perversion	17.2%	11.1%	8.4%	7%	2.2%	5%
Vomiting	23.3%	13.7%	12.6%	17.4%	4.4%	7.1%
Weight loss	0%	0%	0%	2.4%	1.7%	0%
Musculoskeletal						
Arthralgia	0%	0%	0%	1.7%	0.7%	2.1%
Myalgia	1.7%	1.7%	0.8%	2.4%	1.1%	2.1%
Miscellaneous						
Fever	1.7%	0.9%	1.7%	5%	2.4%	0.7%
Nocturia	0%	0%	0%	0.2%	0%	2.8%
Pain (unspecified)	0.9%	1.7%	0.8%	2.2%	1.8%	4.3%
Pharyngitis	0.9%	2.6%	0%	0.4%	0.4%	1.4%

[a] Includes those adverse reactions at least possibly related to study drug or of unknown relationship and excludes concurrent HIV conditions.
[b] The median duration of treatment for patients randomized to regimens containing ritonavir in study 245 was 9.1 months.
[c] The median duration of treatment for patients randomized to regimens containing ritonavir in study 247 was 9.4 months.
[d] The median duration of treatment for patients in ongoing study 462 was 48 weeks.

Other adverse reactions –

Cardiovascular: Cardiovascular disorder, cerebral ischemia, cerebral venous thrombosis, hypertension, hypotension, myocardial infarction, palpitation, peripheral vascular disorder, phlebitis, postural hypotension, tachycardia, vasospasm (less than 2%).

CNS: Abnormal dreams, abnormal gait, agitation, amnesia, aphasia, ataxia, coma, convulsion, dementia, depersonalization, emotional lability, euphoria, generalized tonic-clonic seizure, hallucinations, hyperesthesia, hyperkinesia, hypesthesia, incoordination, libido decreased, manic reaction, migraine, nervousness, neuralgia, neuropathy, paralysis, peripheral neuropathic pain, peripheral neuropathy, peripheral sensory neuropathy, personality disorder, sleep disorder, speech disorder, stupor, subdural hematoma, tremor, vertigo, vestibular disorder (less than 2%).

Dermatologic: Acne, contact dermatitis, dry skin, eczema, erythema multiforme, exfoliative dermatitis, folliculitis, fungal dermatitis, furunculosis, maculopapular rash, molluscum contagiosum, onychomycosis, pruritus, psoriasis, pustular rash, seborrhea, skin discoloration, skin disorder, skin hypertrophy, skin melanoma, urticaria, vesiculobullous rash (less than 2%).

Endocrine: Adrenal cortex insufficiency, diabetes mellitus (less than 2%).

GI: Abnormal stools, bloody diarrhea, cheilitis, colitis, dry mouth, dysphagia, enlarged abdomen, eructation, esophageal ulcer, esophagitis, gastritis, gastroenteritis, GI disorder, GI hemorrhage, gingivitis, ileus, melena, mouth ulcer, pancreatitis, pseudomembranous colitis, rectal disorder, rectal hemorrhage, sialadenitis, stomatitis, tenesmus, thirst, tongue edema, ulcerative colitis (less than 2%).

GU: Acute kidney failure, breast pain, cystitis, dysuria, hematuria, impotence, kidney calculus, kidney failure, kidney function abnormal, kidney pain, menorrhagia, pelvic pain, penis disorder, polyuria, urethritis, urinary frequency, urinary retention, urinary tract infection, vaginitis (less than 2%).

Hematologic/Lymphatic: Acute myeloblastic leukemia, anemia, ecchymosis, leukopenia, lymphadenopathy, lymphocytosis, myeloproliferative disorder, thrombocytopenia (less than 2%).

Hepatic: Cholestatic jaundice, hepatic coma, hepatitis, hepatomegaly, hepatosplenomegaly, liver damage (less than 2%).

Metabolic/Nutritional: Albuminuria, alcohol intolerance, avitaminosis, cachexia, dehydration, edema, enzymatic abnormality, facial edema, glycosuria, gout, hormone level altered, hypercholesteremia, peripheral edema, serum urea nitrogen increased, xanthomatosis (less than 2%).

Musculoskeletal: Arthritis, arthrosis, back pain, bone disorder, bone pain, joint disorder, leg cramps, muscle cramps, muscle weakness, myositis, neck pain, neck rigidity, twitching (less than 2%).

Respiratory: Asthma, bronchitis, dyspnea, epistaxis, hiccup, hypoventilation, increased cough, interstitial pneumonia, larynx edema, lung disorder, rhinitis, sinusitis (less than 2%).

Special senses: Abnormal electro-oculogram, abnormal electroretinogram, abnormal vision, amblyopia/blurred vision, blepharitis, conjunctivitis, diplopia, ear pain, extraocular palsy, eye disorder, eye pain, hearing impairment, increased cerumen, iritis, parosmia, photophobia, taste loss, tinnitus, uveitis, visual field defect, vitreous disorder (less than 2%).

Miscellaneous: Accidental injury, allergic reaction, chest pain, chills, facial pain, flu syndrome, hypothermia, photosensitivity reaction, substernal chest pain (less than 2%).

➤*Children:* Vomiting, diarrhea, and skin rash/allergy were the only drug-related clinical adverse reactions of moderate to severe intensity observed in 2% or more children enrolled in ritonavir clinical trials.

➤*Lab test abnormalities:*

Adults –

Ritonavir Laboratory Abnormalities in Adults (> 3%)							
		Study 245 naive patients			Study 247 advanced patients		Study 462 protease inhibitor–naive patients
Variable	Limit	Ritonavir + zidovudine	Ritonavir	Zidovudine	Ritonavir	Placebo	Ritonavir + saquinavir
Chemistry values	High						
Cholesterol	> 240 mg/dL	30.7%	44.8%	9.3%	36.5%	8%	65.2%
CPK	> 1,000 units/L	9.6%	12.1%	11%	9.1%	6.3%	9.9%
GGT	> 300 units/L	1.8%	5.2%	1.7%	19.6%	11.3%	9.2%
AST	> 180 units/L	5.3%	9.5%	2.5%	6.4%	7%	7.8%
ALT	> 215 units/L	5.3%	7.8%	3.4%	8.5%	4.4%	9.2%
Triglycerides	> 800 mg/dL	9.6%	17.2%	3.4%	33.6%	9.4%	23.4%
Triglycerides	> 1,500 mg/dL	1.8%	2.6%	—[a]	12.6%	0.4%	11.3%
Triglycerides fasting	> 1,500 mg/dL	1.5%	1.3%	—[a]	9.9%	0.3%	—[a]
Uric acid	> 12 mg/dL	—[a]	—[a]	—[a]	3.8%	0.2%	1.4%
Hematology values	Low						
Hematocrit	< 30%	2.6%	—[a]	0.8%	17.3%	22%	0.7%
Hemoglobin	< 8 g/dL	0.9%	—[a]	—[a]	3.8%	3.9%	—[a]
Neutrophils	$\leq 0.5 \times 10^9$/L	—[a]	—[a]	—[a]	6%	8.3%	—[a]
RBC	$< 3 \times 10^{12}$/L	1.8%	—[a]	5.9%	18.6%	24.4%	—[a]
WBC[b] count	$< 2.5 \times 10^9$/L	—[a]	0.9%	6.8%	36.9%	59.4%	3.5%

[a] Indicates no reactions reported.
[b] WBC = white blood cell.

Children – The following grade 3 to 4 laboratory abnormalities occurred in at least 3% of children who received treatment with ritonavir either alone or in combination with reverse transcriptase inhibitors: neutropenia (9%), hyperamylasemia (7%), thrombocytopenia (5%), anemia (4%), and elevated AST (3%).

➤*Postmarketing:*

Cardiovascular – First-degree AV block, second-degree AV block, third-degree AV block, right bundle branch block.

Endocrine – Cushing syndrome and adrenal suppression (when coadministered with fluticasone).

Miscellaneous – Dehydration, usually associated with GI symptoms, and sometimes resulting in hypotension, syncope, or renal insufficiency has been reported; syncope, orthostatic hypotension, and renal insufficiency also have been reported without known dehydration; redistribution/accumulation of body fat; seizure; increased bleeding in patients with hemophilia A or B.

Overdosage

➤*Symptoms:* Human experience of acute overdose with ritonavir is limited. One patient in clinical trials took ritonavir 1,500 mg/day for 2 days. The patient reported paresthesias that resolved after the dosage was decreased. A postmarketing case of renal failure with eosinophilia has been reported with ritonavir overdose.

Ritonavir oral solution contains 43% alcohol by volume. Accidental ingestion of the product by a young child could result in significant alcohol-related toxicity and could approach the potential lethal dose of alcohol.

RITONAVIR — ORAL

➤*Treatment:* Treatment of overdose with ritonavir consists of general supportive measures, including monitoring of vital signs and observation of the clinical status of the patient. There is no specific antidote for overdose with ritonavir. If indicated, achieve elimination of unabsorbed drug by gastric lavage; observe usual precautions to maintain the airway. Administration of activated charcoal also may be used to aid in removal of unabsorbed drug. Because ritonavir is extensively metabolized by the liver and is highly protein bound, dialysis is unlikely to be beneficial in significant removal of the drug. Consult a certified poison control center for up-to-date information on the management of overdose with ritonavir.

Patient Information

Instruct patients to read the patient package insert before starting ritonavir therapy and to reread it each time the prescription is refilled.

Inform patients that ritonavir is not a cure for HIV infection and that they may continue to acquire illnesses associated with advanced HIV infection, including opportunistic infections.

Tell patients that the long-term effects of ritonavir are unknown at this time. Inform them that ritonavir therapy has not been shown to reduce the risk of transmitting HIV to others through sexual contact or blood contamination. For their health and the health of others, it is important that they always practice safer sex by using a latex or polyurethane condom or other barrier method to lower the chance of sexual contact with any body fluids such as semen, vaginal secretions, or blood. They should also be advised to never re-use or share needles.

Advise patients to take ritonavir with food, if possible.

Instruct patients to take ritonavir and other concomitant antiretroviral therapy every day as prescribed. Ritonavir must always be used in combination with other antiretroviral drugs. Instruct patients not to alter the dose or discontinue ritonavir without consulting their health care provider. If a dose is missed, instruct patients to take the next dose as soon as possible. However, if a dose is skipped, advise the patient not to double the next dose.

Inform patients that redistribution or accumulation of body fat may occur in patients receiving antiretroviral therapy and that the cause and long-term health effects of these conditions are not known at this time.

Ritonavir may interact with some drugs; therefore, advise patients to report to their health care provider the use of any other prescription or nonprescription medications or herbal products, particularly St. John's wort.

Advise patients receiving PDE5 inhibitors for erectile dysfunction (eg, sildenafil, tadalafil, vardenafil) that they may be at an increased risk of associated adverse reactions, including hypotension, visual changes, and sustained erection, and to promptly report any symptoms to their health care provider. Concomitant use of sildenafil with ritonavir is contraindicated in patients with PAH.

Advise patients that their liver function tests will need to be monitored closely, especially during the first several months of ritonavir treatment, and to notify their health care provider if they develop the signs and symptoms of worsening liver disease, including loss of appetite, abdominal pain, jaundice, and itchy skin.

Advise patients to inform their health care provider of signs and symptoms (nausea, vomiting, and abdominal pain) that might be suggestive of pancreatitis.

Advise patients to contact their health care provider if they develop a rash while taking ritonavir. The health care provider will determine if treatment should be continued or if an alternative antiretroviral regimen should be used.

Instruct patients receiving estrogen-based hormonal contraceptives to use additional or alternate contraceptive measures during therapy with ritonavir.

Inform patients that ritonavir may produce changes in the electrocardiogram (eg, PR prolongation). Advise patient to consult their health care provider if experiencing symptoms such as dizziness, light-headedness, abnormal heart rhythm, or loss of consciousness.

Advise patients that treatment with ritonavir therapy can result in substantial increases in the concentration of total cholesterol and triglycerides.

Advise patients to notify their health care provider if they develop the signs and symptoms of diabetes mellitus, including frequent urination, excessive thirst, extreme hunger, unusual weight loss, and/or increased blood sugar, while taking ritonavir as they may require a change in their diabetes treatment or new treatment.

Advise patients that immune reconstitution syndrome has been reported in HIV-infected patients treated with combination antiretroviral therapy, including ritonavir.

Advise patients with hemophilia that they may experience increased bleeding when treated with protease inhibitors such as ritonavir.

INDINAVIR

Rx	**Crixivan** (Merck)	**Capsules; oral:** 100 mg	Equivalent to indinavir sulfate 125 mg. Lactose. (CRIXIVAN 100 mg). White. In 180s.
		200 mg	Equivalent to indinavir sulfate 250 mg. Lactose. (CRIXIVAN 200 mg). White. In 360s.
		400 mg	Equivalent to indinavir sulfate 500 mg. Lactose. (CRIXIVAN 400 mg). White. In 18s, 90s, 120s, 180s, and UD 42s.

INDINAVIR SULFATE — ORAL

Indications

➤*HIV infection:* For the treatment of HIV infection in combination with other antiretroviral agents.

Administration and Dosage

➤*Adults:*

HIV infection – 800 mg (usually two 400 mg capsules) orally every 8 hours.

Concomitant therapy –

Delavirdine: Dosage reduction of indinavir to 600 mg every 8 hours should be considered when administering delavirdine 400 mg 3 times a day.

Didanosine: If indinavir and didanosine are coadministered, they should be administered at least 1 hour apart on an empty stomach.

Itraconazole: Dosage reduction of indinavir to 600 mg every 8 hours is recommended when coadministering itraconazole 200 mg twice daily.

Ketoconazole: Dosage reduction of indinavir to 600 mg every 8 hours is recommended when coadministering ketoconazole.

Rifabutin: Dose reduction of rifabutin to half the standard dose and a dosage increase of indinavir to 1,000 mg every 8 hours are recommended when rifabutin and indinavir are coadministered.

➤*Children:*

Off-label dosing –

HIV infection: 500 mg/m^2 (maximum, 800 mg/dose) every 8 hours has been studied in uncontrolled studies of 70 children 3 to 18 years of age. The optimal dosing regimen for use of indinavir in children has not been established.

➤*Hepatic function impairment:* Reduce dosage to 600 mg every 8 hours in patients with mild to moderate hepatic insufficiency caused by cirrhosis.

➤*Nephrolithiasis/Urolithiasis:* In addition to adequate hydration, medical management in patients who experience nephrolithiasis/urolithiasis may include temporary interruption (eg, 1 to 3 days) or discontinuation of therapy.

➤*Administration:* Indinavir must be taken at intervals of 8 hours. To ensure adequate hydration, it is recommended that the patient drink at least 1.5 L (approximately 48 ounces) of liquids during the course of 24 hours. For optimal absorption, indinavir should be administered without food but with water 1 hour before or 2 hours after a meal. Alternatively, indinavir may be administered with other liquids, such as skim milk, juice, coffee, or tea, or with a light meal (eg, dry toast with jelly, juice, and coffee with skim milk and sugar; or corn flakes, skim milk, and sugar).

➤*Storage/Stability:* Store in a tightly closed container at 15° to 30°C (59° to 86°F).

Indinavir capsules are sensitive to moisture; protect from moisture. Dispense and store indinavir in the original container. The desiccant should remain in the original bottle.

Actions

➤*Pharmacology:* HIV-1 protease is an enzyme required for the proteolytic cleavage of the viral polyprotein precursors into the individual functional proteins found in infectious HIV-1. Indinavir binds to the protease active site and inhibits the activity of the enzyme. This inhibition prevents cleavage of the viral polyproteins, resulting in the formation of immature noninfectious viral particles.

➤*Pharmacokinetics:*

Absorption – Indinavir was rapidly absorbed in the fasted state with a time to peak plasma concentration (T_{max}) of 0.8 ± 0.3 hours (mean ± standard deviation) (n = 11). A greater than dose-proportional increase in indinavir plasma concentrations was observed over the 200 to 1,000 mg dose range. At a dosing regimen of 800 mg every 8 hours, steady-state area under the curve (AUC) was 30,691 ± 11,407 nM•h (n = 16), the peak plasma concentration (C_{max}) was 12,617 ± 4,037 nM (n = 16), and the plasma concentration 8 hours postdose (trough) was 251 ± 178 nM (n = 16).

Effect of food: Administration of indinavir with a meal high in calories, fat, and protein (784 kcal, fat 48.6 g, protein 31.3 g) resulted in a 77% ± 8% reduction in AUC and an 84% ± 7% reduction in C_{max} (n = 10). Administration with lighter meals (eg, a meal of dry toast with jelly, apple juice, and coffee with skim milk and sugar; or a meal of corn flakes, skim milk, and sugar) resulted in little or no change in AUC, C_{max}, or trough concentration.

Distribution – Indinavir was approximately 60% bound to human plasma proteins over a concentration range of 81 to 16,300 nM.

Metabolism – Following a dose of ^{14}C-indinavir 400 mg, 83 ± 1% (n = 4) and 19 ± 3% (n = 6) of the total radioactivity was recovered in feces and urine, respectively; radioactivity caused by parent drug in feces and urine was 19.1% and 9.4%, respectively. Seven metabolites have been identified,

INDINAVIR SULFATE — ORAL

1 glucuronide conjugate and 6 oxidative metabolites. In vitro studies indicate that CYP3A4 is the major enzyme responsible for formation of the oxidative metabolites.

Excretion – Less than 20% of indinavir is excreted unchanged in the urine. Mean urinary excretion of unchanged drug was 10.4 ± 4.9% (n = 10) and 12 ± 4.9% (n = 10) following a single 700 and 1,000 mg dose, respectively. Indinavir was rapidly eliminated with a half-life of 1.8 ± 0.4 hours (n = 10). Significant accumulation was not observed after multiple dosing at 800 mg every 8 hours.

Special populations –

Hepatic function impairment: Patients with mild to moderate hepatic insufficiency and clinical evidence of cirrhosis had evidence of decreased metabolism of indinavir, resulting in an approximately 60% higher mean AUC following a single 400 mg dose (n = 12). The half-life of indinavir increased to 2.8 ± 0.5 hours. Indinavir pharmacokinetics have not been studied in patients with severe hepatic insufficiency. See Administration and Dosage for more information.

Children: The optimal dosing regimen for use of indinavir in children has not been established. In children 4 to 15 years of age infected with HIV, a dosage regimen of indinavir 500 mg/m^2 capsules every 8 hours produced $AUC_{0\text{-}8h}$ of 38,742 ± 24,098 nM•h (n = 34), C_{max} of 17,181 ± 9,809 nM (n = 34), and trough concentrations of 134 ± 91 nM (n = 28). The pharmacokinetic profiles of indinavir in children were not comparable with profiles previously observed in adults infected with HIV who where receiving the recommended dosage of 800 mg every 8 hours. The AUC and C_{max} values were slightly higher and the trough concentrations were considerably lower in children. Approximately 50% of the children had trough values below 100 nM; however, approximately 10% of adult patients had trough levels below 100 nM. The relationship between specific trough values and inhibition of HIV replication has not been established.

Pregnancy: The optimal dosing regimen for use of indinavir in pregnant patients has not been established. An indinavir dosage of 800 mg every 8 hours (with zidovudine 200 mg every 8 hours and lamivudine 150 mg twice daily) has been studied in 16 pregnant patients infected with HIV who were at 14 to 28 weeks of gestation at enrollment (study PACTG 358). The mean indinavir plasma $AUC_{0\text{-}8h}$ at weeks 30 to 32 of gestation (n = 11) was 9,231 nM•h, which is 74% (95% confidence interval [CI], 50% to 86%) lower than that observed 6 weeks postpartum. Six of these 11 (55%) patients had mean indinavir plasma concentrations 8 hours postdose (minimum plasma concentration) below assay threshold of reliable quantification. The pharmacokinetics of indinavir in these 11 patients at 6 weeks postpartum were generally similar to those observed in nonpregnant patients in another study.

➤*Microbiology:*

Drug resistance – Isolates of HIV-1 with reduced susceptibility to the drug have been recovered from some patients treated with indinavir. Viral resistance was correlated with the accumulation of mutations that resulted in the expression of amino acid substitutions in the viral protease. Eleven amino acid residue positions (L10I/V/R, K20I/M/R, L24I, M46I/L, I54A/V, L63P, I64V, A71T/V, V82A/F/T, I84V, and L90M), at which substitutions are associated with resistance, have been identified. Resistance was mediated by the coexpression of multiple and variable substitutions at these positions. No single substitution was either necessary or sufficient for measurable resistance (at least 4-fold increase in inhibitory concentration [IC_{95}]). In general, higher levels of resistance were associated with the coexpression of greater numbers of substitutions, although their individual effects varied and were not additive. At least 3 amino acid substitutions must be present for phenotypic resistance to indinavir to reach measurable levels. In addition, mutations in the p7/p1 and p1/p6 gag cleavage sites were observed in some indinavir-resistant HIV-1 isolates.

Cross-resistance – Varying degrees of HIV-1 cross-resistance have been observed between indinavir and other HIV-1 protease inhibitors. In studies with ritonavir, saquinavir, and amprenavir, the extent and spectrum of cross-resistance varied with the specific mutational patterns observed. In general, the degree of cross-resistance increased with the accumulation of resistance-associated amino acid substitutions. Within a panel of 29 viral isolates from indinavir-treated patients that exhibited measurable (at least 4-fold) phenotypic resistance to indinavir, all were resistant to ritonavir. Of the indinavir resistant HIV-1 isolates, 63% showed resistance to saquinavir and 81% to amprenavir.

Contraindications

Hypersensitivity to any of the components of indinavir; coadministration with alfuzosin, amiodarone, dihydroergotamine, ergonovine, ergotamine, methylergonovine, cisapride, pimozide, oral midazolam, triazolam, alprazolam, and sildenafil (when used for the treatment of pulmonary arterial hypertension).

Warnings/Precautions

➤*Nephrolithiasis/Urolithiasis:* Nephrolithiasis/urolithiasis has occurred with indinavir therapy. The cumulative frequency of nephrolithiasis is substantially higher in children (29%) than in adult patients (12.4%; range across individual trials, 4.7% to 34.4%). The cumulative frequency of nephrolithiasis events increases with increasing exposure to indinavir; however, the risk over time remains relatively constant. In some cases, nephrolithiasis/urolithiasis has been associated with renal insufficiency or acute renal failure, and/or pyelonephritis with or without bacteremia. If signs or symptoms of nephrolithiasis/urolithiasis (including flank pain, with or without hematuria or microscopic hematuria) occur, consider temporary interruption (eg, 1 to 3 days) or discontinuation of therapy. Adequate hydration is recommended in all patients treated with indinavir.

➤*Hemolytic anemia:* Acute hemolytic anemia, including cases resulting in death, has been reported in patients treated with indinavir. Once a diagnosis is apparent, institute appropriate measures for the treatment of hemolytic anemia, including discontinuation of indinavir.

➤*Hepatitis:* Hepatitis, including cases resulting in hepatic failure and death, has been reported in patients treated with indinavir. Because the majority of these patients had confounding medical conditions and/or were receiving concomitant therapy(ies), a causal relationship between indinavir and these events has not been established.

➤*Hyperglycemia:* New-onset diabetes mellitus, exacerbation of preexisting diabetes mellitus, and hyperglycemia have been reported during postmarketing surveillance in patients infected with HIV receiving protease inhibitor therapy. Some patients required either initiation or dose adjustments of insulin or oral hypoglycemic agents for treatment of these events. In some cases, diabetic ketoacidosis has occurred. In those patients who discontinued protease inhibitor therapy, hyperglycemia persisted in some cases. Because these events have been reported voluntarily during clinical practice, estimates of frequency cannot be made, and a causal relationship between protease inhibitor therapy and these events has not been established.

➤*Hyperbilirubinemia:* Indirect hyperbilirubinemia has occurred frequently during treatment with indinavir and has infrequently been associated with increases in serum transaminases. It is not known whether indinavir will exacerbate the physiologic hyperbilirubinemia seen in neonates.

➤*Tubulointerstitial nephritis:* Reports of tubulointerstitial nephritis with medullary calcification and cortical atrophy have been observed in patients with asymptomatic severe leukocyturia (more than 100 cells per high-power field). Closely follow patients with asymptomatic severe leukocyturia, and frequently monitor with urinalysis. Further diagnostic evaluation may be warranted; consider discontinuation of indinavir in all patients with severe leukocyturia.

➤*Immune reconstitution syndrome:* Immune reconstitution syndrome has been reported in patients treated with combination antiretroviral therapy, including indinavir. During the initial phase of treatment, patients responding to antiretroviral therapy whose immune system responds to combination antiretroviral therapy may develop an inflammatory response to indolent or residual opportunistic infections (eg, *Mycobacterium avium*, cytomegalovirus, *Pneumocystis carinii* pneumonia, tuberculosis), which may necessitate further evaluation and treatment.

➤*Hemophilia:* There have been reports of spontaneous bleeding in patients with hemophilia A and B treated with protease inhibitors. In some patients, additional factor VIII was required. In many of the reported cases, treatment with protease inhibitors was continued or restarted. A causal relationship between protease inhibitor therapy and these episodes has not been established.

➤*Fat redistribution:* Redistribution/accumulation of body fat, including central obesity, dorsocervical fat enlargement (buffalo hump), peripheral wasting, facial wasting, breast enlargement, and cushingoid appearance, have been observed in patients receiving antiretroviral therapy. The mechanism and long-term consequences of these events are currently unknown. A causal relationship has not been established.

➤*Hepatic function impairment:* In patients with hepatic insufficiency caused by cirrhosis, lower the dosage of indinavir because of decreased metabolism of indinavir (see Administration and Dosage for more information).

➤*Pregnancy:* *Category C.* Developmental toxicity studies were performed in rabbits (at dosages of up to 240 mg/kg/day), dogs (at dosages of up to 80 mg/kg/day), and rats (at dosages of up to 640 mg/kg/day). Treatment-related increases over controls in the incidence of supernumerary ribs (at exposures at or below those in humans) and of cervical ribs (at exposures comparable with or slightly greater than those in humans) were seen in rats. In all 3 species, no treatment-related effects on embryonic/fetal survival or fetal weights were observed.

Indinavir was administered to rhesus monkeys during the third trimester of pregnancy (at dosages of up to 160 mg/kg twice daily) and to neonatal rhesus monkeys (at dosages of up to 160 mg/kg twice daily). When administered to neonates, indinavir caused an exacerbation of the transient physiologic hyperbilirubinemia seen in this species after birth; serum bilirubin values were approximately 4-fold above controls at 160 mg/kg twice daily.

There are no adequate and well-controlled studies in pregnant women. Use during pregnancy only if the potential benefit justifies the potential risk to the fetus.

A dosage of indinavir 800 mg every 8 hours with zidovudine 200 mg every 8 hours and lamivudine 150 mg twice daily has been studied in 16 pregnant patients infected with HIV at 14 to 28 weeks of gestation at enrollment (study PACTG 358). Given the substantially lower antepartum exposures observed and the limited data in this patient population, indinavir use is not recommended in pregnant patients infected with HIV.

Antiviral pregnancy registry – To monitor maternal-fetal outcomes of pregnant women exposed to indinavir, an antiretroviral pregnancy registry has been established. Health care providers are encouraged to register patients by calling 1-800-258-4263.

Hyperbilirubinemia – Hyperbilirubinemia has occurred during treatment with indinavir. It is unknown whether indinavir administered to the mother in the perinatal period will exacerbate physiologic hyperbilirubinemia in neonates.

INDINAVIR SULFATE — ORAL

➤*Lactation:* Studies in lactating rats have demonstrated that indinavir is excreted in milk. Although it is not known whether indinavir is excreted in human milk, there exists the potential for adverse reactions from indinavir in breast-feeding infants. The molecular weight of indinavir (approximately 712) is low enough that excretion into breast milk should be expected. Instruct mothers to discontinue breast-feeding if they are receiving indinavir. This is consistent with the recommendation by the US Public Health Service Centers for Disease Control and Prevention that mothers infected with HIV not breast-feed their infants to avoid risking postnatal transmission of HIV.

➤*Children:* The optimal dosing regimen for use of indinavir in children has not been established. A dosage of 500 mg/m^2 every 8 hours has been studied in uncontrolled studies of 70 children 3 to 18 years of age. The pharmacokinetic profiles of indinavir at this dose were not comparable with profiles previously observed in adults receiving the recommended dose. Although viral suppression was observed in some of the 32 children who were followed on this regimen through 24 weeks, a substantially higher rate of nephrolithiasis was reported when compared with adult historical data. Health care providers considering the use of indinavir in children without other protease inhibitor options should be aware of the limited data available in this population and the increased risk of nephrolithiasis.

➤*Elderly:* In general, exercise caution in dose selection for an elderly patient, reflecting the greater frequency of decreased hepatic, renal, or cardiac function, and of concomitant disease or other drug therapy.

➤*Monitoring:* Monitor patients for signs or symptoms of nephrolithiasis/urolithiasis (including flank pain, with or without hematuria or microscopic hematuria); if signs or symptoms occur, consider temporary interruption (eg, 1 to 3 days) or discontinuation of therapy.

Monitor blood glucose levels closely; new-onset diabetes or exacerbation of preexisting diabetes has been associated with protease inhibitor therapy.

Closely follow patients with asymptomatic severe leukocyturia and frequently monitor with urinalysis.

Drug Interactions

➤*Cytochrome P450 system:* Indinavir is an inhibitor of the cytochrome P450 isoform CYP3A4. Coadministration of indinavir and drugs primarily metabolized by CYP3A4 may result in increased plasma concentrations of the other drug, which could increase or prolong its therapeutic and adverse effects.

Indinavir is metabolized by CYP3A4. Drugs that induce CYP3A4 activity are expected to increase the clearance of indinavir, resulting in lowered plasma concentrations of indinavir. Coadministration of indinavir and other drugs that inhibit CYP3A4 may decrease the clearance of indinavir and may result in increased plasma concentrations of indinavir.

Indinavir Drug Interactions

Precipitant drug	Object drug[a]		Description
Anticonvulsants (eg, carbamazepine, phenobarbital, phenytoin)	Indinavir	↓	Indinavir may not be effective because of decreased indinavir concentrations in patients taking these agents concomitantly. Use with caution.
Azole antifungals (itraconazole, ketoconazole)	Indinavir	↑	Plasma indinavir concentrations may be elevated, increasing the toxicity. Dosage reduction of indinavir to 600 mg every 8 hours is recommended.
Clarithromycin	Indinavir	↑	Concentrations of clarithromycin and indinavir may be elevated, increasing the pharmacologic effects and adverse reactions. The appropriate dose with respect to safety and efficacy for this combination has not been established.
Indinavir	Clarithromycin		
Didanosine	Indinavir	↓	The therapeutic effect of indinavir may be decreased by the buffered formulation of didanosine. Administer indinavir and buffered didanosine formulations at least 1 hour apart on an empty stomach.
Fluoxetine	Indinavir	↑	Indinavir may increase plasma concentrations of fluoxetine. Similarly, fluoxetine may increase plasma concentrations of indinavir. Closely monitor the patient for adverse reactions, including serotonin syndrome. Dosage reduction of fluoxetine and/or indinavir may be needed during coadministration of these agents.
Indinavir	Fluoxetine		
Interleukins (eg, aldesleukin)	Indinavir	↑	Indinavir concentrations may be elevated, increasing the risk of toxicity. Adjust dose of indinavir as needed when interleukins are started or stopped.
Nonnucleoside reverse transcriptase inhibitors (eg, delavirdine, efavirenz, nevirapine)	Indinavir	↑↓	Coadministration of delavirdine may increase plasma concentrations of indinavir, increasing the pharmacologic effects and adverse reactions. Reduce dosage of indinavir to 600 mg every 8 hours when administering delavirdine 400 mg 3 times daily. Coadministration of efavirenz and/or nevirapine with indinavir may decrease indinavir plasma concentrations. The optimal dose of indinavir, when given in combination with efavirenz, is not known. Increasing the indinavir dosage to 1,000 mg every 8 hours does not compensate for the increased indinavir metabolism caused by efavirenz.
Protease inhibitors (eg, atazanavir, nelfinavir, ritonavir)	Indinavir	↑	Coadministration of indinavir with other protease inhibitors is expected to increase exposure to other protease inhibitors. Both indinavir and atazanavir are associated with indirect (unconjugated) hyperbilirubinemia. Combinations of these drugs have not been studied and coadministration of indinavir and atazanavir is not recommended. Nelfinavir and ritonavir may increase indinavir concentrations. The appropriate dose for combined use of indinavir and nelfinavir, ritonavir, or saquinavir has not been established. The incidence of nephrolithiasis is higher in patients receiving indinavir in combination with ritonavir compared with patients receiving indinavir 800 mg every 8 hours.
Indinavir	Protease inhibitors (eg, atazanavir, ritonavir, saquinavir)		
Proton pump inhibitors (eg, esomeprazole, lansoprazole, omeprazole, pantoprazole)	Indinavir	↓	Coadministration may reduce the antiviral activity of indinavir. Monitor the clinical response of the patient and adjust the indinavir dose as needed.
Rifamycins (eg, rifabutin, rifampin)	Indinavir	↓↑	Rifamycins may decrease indinavir serum concentrations, which may lead to loss of virologic response and possible resistance to indinavir or to the class of protease inhibitors. Coadministration is not recommended. Indinavir may elevate serum rifabutin and rifampin concentrations, increasing the risk of toxicity. Dose reduction of rifabutin to half the standard dose and a dosage increase of indinavir to 1,000 mg (three 333 mg capsules) every 8 hours are recommended when rifabutin and indinavir are coadministered.
Indinavir	Rifamycins (eg, rifabutin, rifampin)		
St. John's wort (*Hypericum perforatum*)	Indinavir	↓	Coadministration substantially decreases indinavir concentrations, which may lead to loss of virologic response and possible resistance to indinavir or to the class of protease inhibitors. Coadministration is not recommended.

INDINAVIR SULFATE — ORAL

Indinavir Drug Interactions			
Precipitant drug	Object drug[a]		Description
Venlafaxine	Indinavir	⬇	In a study of 9 healthy volunteers, venlafaxine administered under steady-state conditions at 150 mg/day resulted in a 28% decrease in the AUC of a single oral dose of indinavir 800 mg and a 36% decrease in indinavir C_{max}. Indinavir did not affect the pharmacokinetics of venlafaxine and its active metabolite. The clinical significance of this finding is unknown.
Indinavir	Alfuzosin	⬆	Alfuzosin plasma concentrations may be elevated, increasing the risk of hypotension. Coadministration is contraindicated.
Indinavir	Amiodarone	⬆	Increases in serum amiodarone concentrations may occur, increasing the risk of serious and/or life-threatening reactions, such as cardiac arrhythmias. Coadministration is contraindicated.
Indinavir	Antiarrhythmics (eg, bepridil, lidocaine [systemic], quinidine)	⬆	Caution is warranted and monitoring of therapeutic concentration is recommended for antiarrhythmics when coadministered with indinavir.
Indinavir	Aripiprazole	⬆	Aripiprazole plasma concentrations may be elevated, increasing the pharmacologic effects and risk of adverse reactions. Monitor the patient and adjust the aripiprazole dose as needed when indinavir is started or stopped.
Indinavir	Benzodiazepines (eg, alprazolam, midazolam, triazolam)	⬆	Serum concentrations of benzodiazepines may be elevated, resulting in prolonged or increased sedation or respiratory depression. Alprazolam, oral midazolam, and triazolam are contraindicated in patients taking indinavir. If parenteral midazolam is coadministered, use with caution. Closely monitor for respiratory depression and/or prolonged sedation. Adjust the midazolam dose as needed.
Indinavir	Bosentan	⬆	Start at or adjust bosentan to 62.5 mg daily or every other day based upon individual tolerability. Monitor the clinical response of the patient.
Indinavir	Buspirone	⬆	Plasma concentrations and pharmacologic effects of buspirone may be increased by indinavir. Closely monitor the patient for signs of new-onset parkinsonian symptoms (eg, ataxia, shuffling gait, cogwheel rigidity, resting tremor, sad affect, masked facies) when buspirone and indinavir are coadministered.
Indinavir	Calcium channel blockers (eg, felodipine, nicardipine, nifedipine)	⬆	Caution is warranted and clinical monitoring of patients is recommended.
Indinavir	Cisapride[b]	⬆	Increased cisapride plasma concentrations may occur, increasing the risk for serious and/or life-threatening reactions, such as cardiac arrhythmias. Coadministration is contraindicated.
Indinavir	Colchicine	⬆	Colchicine and indinavir should not be coadministered to patients with hepatic or renal impairment. For treatment of gout flares, coadminister colchicine 0.6 mg followed by 0.3 mg 1 hour later. Dose to be repeated no earlier than 3 days. For prophylaxis of gout flares, if the original colchicine regimen was colchicine 0.6 mg twice daily, adjust the dosage to 0.3 mg once daily. If the original colchicine dosage was 0.6 mg once daily, adjust the regimen to colchicine 0.3 mg once every other day. For treatment of familial Mediterranean fever, coadminister colchicine at a maximum daily dosage of 0.3 mg twice daily.
Indinavir	Corticosteroids, inhaled/nasal (eg, fluticasone)	⬆	Corticosteroid plasma concentrations may be increased. Monitor for signs of adrenal insufficiency. Consider alternatives to fluticasone for long-term use.
Indinavir	Dronedarone	⬆	Dronedarone plasma concentrations may be elevated, increasing the pharmacologic effects and risk of toxicity. Avoid coadministration.
Indinavir	Eletriptan	⬆	Eletriptan plasma concentrations may be elevated by indinavir, increasing the pharmacologic effects and risk of adverse reactions. Eletriptan should not be used within 72 hours of indinavir.
Indinavir	Eplerenone	⬆	Eplerenone plasma concentrations may be elevated, increasing the pharmacologic effects and risk of toxicity. Close clinical monitoring is indicated when eplerenone is coadministered with indinavir. Adjust the eplerenone dose as needed.
Indinavir	Ergot derivatives (eg, dihydroergotamine, ergonovine, ergotamine, methylergonovine)	⬆	The risk of ergot toxicity (peripheral vasospasm, ischemia of the extremities) may be increased. Coadministration is contraindicated.
Indinavir	Erlotinib	⬆	Plasma concentration of erlotinib may be elevated, increasing the pharmacologic effects and risk of adverse reactions. Monitor the patient for clinical response and adverse reactions. Adjust the erlotinib dose as needed.
Indinavir	Erythromycin	⬆	Plasma concentration of erythromycin may be elevated, increasing the risk of sudden death from cardiac causes. Avoid concurrent use.
Indinavir	Eszopiclone	⬆	Eszopiclone plasma concentrations may be elevated, increasing the pharmacologic effects and risk of adverse reactions. Close monitoring is indicated. Consider reducing the eszopiclone dose when coadministered with indinavir.

INDINAVIR SULFATE — ORAL

Indinavir Drug Interactions

Precipitant drug	Object drug[a]		Description
Indinavir	HMG-CoA reductase inhibitors (atorvastatin, lovastatin, rosuvastatin, simvastatin)	↑	Coadministration of indinavir may result in elevated plasma levels of these agents, increasing the risk of myopathy, including rhabdomyolysis. Lovastatin, rosuvastatin, and simvastatin are not recommended for concomitant use with indinavir. Use the lowest possible dose of atorvastatin or rosuvastatin and monitor for adverse reactions. The interaction of indinavir with fluvastatin or pravastatin is not known.
Indinavir	Iloperidone	↑	Iloperidone plasma concentrations and pharmacologic effects may be increased. A modification of the iloperidone dosage is recommended. The dose of iloperidone should be reduced by one-half when coadministered with indinavir. If therapy with indinavir is discontinued, the dose of iloperidone should be increased to the original dose.
Indinavir	Immunosuppressant agents (eg, cyclosporine, sirolimus, tacrolimus)	↑	Plasma concentrations of immunosuppressants may be increased by indinavir. Monitor the clinical response of the patient and immunosuppressant concentrations. Adjust the immunosuppressant dose as needed.
Indinavir	Ixabepilone	↑	Ixabepilone plasma concentrations may be elevated, increasing the risk of ixabepilone toxicity. Avoid coadministration or consider a dose reduction of ixabepilone.
Indinavir	Maraviroc	↑	Maraviroc plasma concentrations may be elevated, increasing the pharmacologic effects and risk of adverse reactions. Monitor the response of the patient and adjust the maraviroc dose as needed.
Indinavir	mTOR[c] inhibitors (eg, everolimus, temsirolimus)	↑	Plasma concentrations of mTOR inhibitors may be elevated, increasing the pharmacologic effects and risk of adverse reactions. If coadministration cannot be avoided, monitor the clinical response of the patient and adjust the mTOR inhibitor dose as needed.
Indinavir	Muscarinic receptor antagonists (eg, darifenacin, fesoterodine solifenacin, tolterodine)	↑	Muscarinic receptor antagonist plasma concentrations may be increased by indinavir. When indinavir is coadministered, the dosage of darifenacin should not exceed 7.5 mg daily, the dosage of fesoterodine should not exceed 4 mg daily, the dosage of solifenacin should not exceed 5 mg daily, and the dosage of tolterodine should not exceed 2 mg daily.
Indinavir	Nilotinib	↑	Plasma concentrations and pharmacologic effects of nilotinib may be increased by indinavir. Avoid coadministration. If indinavir must be given, consider interrupting nilotinib therapy. If indinavir must be coadministered with nilotinib, consult official package labeling for specific recommendations.

Indinavir Drug Interactions

Precipitant drug	Object drug[a]		Description
Indinavir	Opioid analgesics (eg, buprenorphine, fentanyl, oxycodone)	↑	Indinavir may increase plasma concentrations and pharmacologic effects of opioid analgesics. Severe respiratory depression may occur. Closely monitor the clinical status of the patient, including respiratory function. Adjust the opioid analgesic dose as needed.
Indinavir	Phosphodiesterase type 5 inhibitors (eg, sildenafil, tadalafil, vardenafil)	↑	Coadministration of sildenafil and indinavir is contraindicated for the treatment of pulmonary arterial hypertension. Elevated plasma concentrations of sildenafil, tadalafil, and vardenafil may occur, resulting in an increase in adverse reactions, including hypotension, visual changes, and priapism. A safe and effective dose has not been established when used with indinavir. For treatment of pulmonary arterial hypertension in patients receiving indinavir, start or adjust the tadalafil dosage to 20 mg once daily. Increase to 40 mg once daily based upon individual tolerability. For the treatment of erectile dysfunction in patients receiving indinavir, the sildenafil dose should not exceed a maximum of 25 mg in a 48-hour period, the tadalafil dose should not exceed a maximum of 10 mg in a 72-hour period, and the vardenafil dose should not exceed a maximum of 2.5 mg in a 24-hour period.
Indinavir	Pimozide	↑	Inhibition of CYP3A4 by indinavir can result in elevated plasma concentrations of pimozide, potentially causing serious and/or life-threatening reactions. Coadministration is contraindicated.
Indinavir	Quetiapine	↑	Quetiapine plasma concentrations may be elevated, increasing the pharmacologic effects and risk of adverse reactions. Administer with caution and closely monitor the clinical response. Adjust the quetiapine dose as needed.
Indinavir	Ranolazine	↑	Ranolazine plasma concentrations may be elevated, increasing the risk of dose-related prolongation in the QTc interval, torsades de pointes–type arrythmias, and sudden death. Coadministration is contraindicated.
Indinavir	Risperidone	↑	Risperidone plasma concentrations may be elevated, increasing the pharmacologic effects and risk of adverse reactions. Closely monitor the clinical response of the patient. Adjust the risperidone dose as needed.
Indinavir	Romidepsin	↑	Romidepsin plasma concentrations may be elevated, increasing the pharmacologic effects and risk of adverse reactions, including QT prolongation. If coadministration cannot be avoided, close clinical, laboratory, and electrocardiograph monitoring are indicated. Adjust the dosage of romidepsin accordingly.
Indinavir	Salmeterol	↑	The risk of cardiovascular adverse events associated with salmeterol, including QT prolongation, palpitation, and sinus tachycardia, may be increased. Coadministration is not recommended.

INDINAVIR SULFATE — ORAL

Indinavir Drug Interactions			
Precipitant drug	Object drug[a]		Description
Indinavir	Thyroid hormones (eg, levothyroxine)	↑↓	Thyroxine serum concentrations may be increased or decreased, resulting in hyper- or hypothyroidism. Closely monitor thyroid function when indinavir is started or stopped. Adjust the thyroid hormone dose as needed.
Indinavir	Trazodone	↑	Trazodone plasma concentrations may be elevated, increasing the pharmacologic effects and adverse reactions (eg, dizziness, hypotension, syncope). Use with caution. Monitor the patient and adjust the dose of trazodone as needed.
Indinavir	Tyrosine kinase inhibitors (ie, dasatinib, lapatinib, pazopanib, sorafenib, sunitinib)	↑	Protein-tyrosine kinase inhibitor plasma concentrations may be elevated, increasing the pharmacologic effects and risk of adverse reactions. If coadministration cannot be avoided, closely monitor the response of the patient and adjust the protein-tyrosine kinase inhibitor dose as needed.
Indinavir	Vasopressin receptor antagonists (eg, conivaptan, tolvaptan)	↑	Vasopressin receptor antagonist plasma concentrations may be elevated, increasing the pharmacologic effects and risk of adverse reactions. Coadministration is contraindicated.
Indinavir	Warfarin	↓	The anticoagulant effect of warfarin may be decreased. Monitor coagulation parameters when indinavir is started or stopped. Adjust the warfarin dose as needed.

[a] ↑ = object drug increased; ↓ = object drug decreased; ↑↓ = object drug both increased and decreased.
[b] Available from the manufacturer on a limited-access protocol.
[c] mTOR = mammalian target of rapamycin.

➤*Drug/Food interactions:* See Actions for more information.

Garlic may reduce indinavir plasma concentrations, decreasing the pharmacologic effects. Avoid garlic ingestion.

Grapefruit – Administering indinavir with grapefruit may delay the time to reach indinavir peak plasma concentrations.

Adverse Reactions

➤*Adverse reactions (2% or more):*

Indinavir Adverse Reactions (≥ 2%)					
Adverse reactions	Indinavir (n = 332)	Indinavir + zidovudine (n = 332)	Zidovudine (n = 332)	Indinavir + zidovudine + lamivudine (n = 571)	Zidovudine + lamivudine (n = 575)
CNS					
Asthenia/Fatigue	2.1%	4.2%	3.6%	2.4%	4.5%
Dizziness	3%	3.9%	0.9%	0.5%	0.7%
Headache	5.4%	9.6%	6%	2.4%	2.8%
Malaise	2.1%	2.7%	1.8%	0%	0%
Somnolence	2.4%	3.3%	3.3%	0%	0%
Dermatologic					
Pruritus	4.2%	2.4%	1.8%	0.5%	0%
Rash	1.2%	0.6%	2.4%	1.1%	0.5%
GI					
Abdominal pain	16.6%	16%	12%	1.9%	0.7%
Acid regurgitation	2.7%	5.4%	1.8%	0.4%	0%
Anorexia	2.7%	5.4%	3%	0.5%	0.2%
Appetite increase	2.1%	1.5%	1.2%	0%	0%
Diarrhea	3.3%	3%	2.4%	0.9%	1.2%
Dyspepsia	1.5%	2.7%	0.9%	0%	0%
Jaundice	1.5%	2.1%	0.3%	0%	0%
Nausea	11.7%	31.9%	19.6%	2.8%	1.4%
Taste perversion	2.7%	8.4%	1.2%	0.2%	0%
Vomiting	8.4%	17.8%	9%	1.4%	1.4%
GU					
Dysuria	1.5%	2.4%	0.3%	0.4%	0.2%
Nephrolithiasis/Urolithiasis[a]	8.7%	7.8%	2.1%	2.6%	0.3%
Respiratory					
Cough	1.5%	0.3%	0.6%	1.6%	1%
Difficulty breathing/dyspnea/shortness of breath	0%	0.6%	0.3%	1.8%	1%
Miscellaneous					
Anemia	0.6%	1.2%	2.1%	2.4%	3.5%
Back pain	8.4%	4.5%	1.5%	0.9%	0.7%
Fever	1.5%	1.5%	2.1%	3.8%	3%

[a] Including renal colic, and flank pain with and without hematuria.

➤*Hyperbilirubinemia:* Asymptomatic hyperbilirubinemia (total bilirubin at least 2.5 mg/dL), reported predominantly as elevated indirect bilirubin, has occurred in approximately 14% of patients treated with indinavir. In less than 1%, this was associated with elevations in ALT or AST.

Hyperbilirubinemia occurred more frequently at dosages exceeding 2.4 g/day compared with dosages less than or equal to 2.4 g/day.

➤*Nephrolithiasis/Urolithiasis:* Nephrolithiasis/urolithiasis, including flank pain with or without hematuria (including microscopic hematuria), has been reported in approximately 12.4% (range across individual trials, 4.7% to 34.4%) of patients receiving indinavir at the recommended dosage in clinical trials with a median follow-up of 47 weeks (range, 1 day to 242 weeks; 2,238 patient-years follow-up). The cumulative frequency of nephrolithiasis events increases with duration of exposure to indinavir; however, the risk over time remains relatively constant. Of the patients treated with indinavir who developed nephrolithiasis/urolithiasis in clinical trials during the double-blind phase, 2.8% were reported to develop hydronephrosis and 4.5% underwent stent placement. Following the acute episode, 4.9% of patients discontinued therapy.

Nephrolithiasis/urolithiasis occurred more frequently at dosages exceeding 2.4 g/day compared with dosages less than or equal to 2.4 g/day.

➤*Other adverse reactions:* In phase 1 and 2 controlled trials, the following adverse reactions were reported significantly more frequently by those randomized to the arms containing indinavir than by those randomized to nucleoside analogs: dry skin, pharyngitis, rash, taste perversion, upper respiratory tract infection.

➤*Lab test abnormalities:*

Indinavir Selected Laboratory Abnormalities					
Lab test abnormalities	Indinavir (n = 329)	Indinavir + zidovudine (n = 320)	Zidovudine (n = 330)	Indinavir + zidovudine + lamivudine (n = 571)	Zidovudine + lamivudine (n = 575)
Blood chemistry					
Increased ALT > 500% ULN[a]	4.9%	4.1%	3%	2.6%	2.6%
Increased AST > 500% ULN	3.7%	2.8%	2.7%	3.3%	2.8%
Total serum bilirubin > 250% ULN	11.9%	9.7%	0.6%	6.1%	1.4%
Increased serum amylase > 200% ULN	2.1%	1.9%	1.8%	0.9%	0.3%
Increased glucose > 250 mg/dL	0.9%	0.9%	0.6%	1.6%	1.9%
Increased creatinine > 300% ULN	0%	0%	0.6%	0.2%	0%
Hematology					
Decreased hemoglobin < 7 g/dL	0.6%	0.9%	3.3%	2.4%	3.5%
Decreased platelet count < 50,000/mm³	0.9%	0.9%	1.8%	0.2%	0.9%
Decreased neutrophils < 750/mm³	2.4%	2.2%	6.7%	5.1%	14.6%

[a] ULN = upper limit of the normal range.

➤*Postmarketing:*

Cardiovascular – Cardiovascular disorders (including myocardial infarction and angina pectoris), cerebrovascular disorder.

CNS – Depression, oral paresthesia.

Dermatologic – Alopecia, hyperpigmentation, ingrown toenails and/or paronychia, pruritus, rash (including erythema multiforme and Stevens-Johnson syndrome).

INDINAVIR SULFATE — ORAL

Endocrine – Exacerbation of preexisting diabetes mellitus, hyperglycemia, new-onset diabetes mellitus.

GI – Abdominal distention, dyspepsia, pancreatitis.

GU – Crystalluria; dysuria; interstitial nephritis, sometimes with indinavir crystal deposits (in some patients, the interstitial nephritis did not resolve following discontinuation of indinavir); leukocyturia; nephrolithiasis/urolithiasis, in some cases resulting in renal insufficiency or acute renal failure; pyelonephritis with or without bacteremia; renal failure; renal insufficiency.

Hematologic – Acute hemolytic anemia, increased spontaneous bleeding in patients with hemophilia.

Hepatic – Hepatitis (including reports of hepatic failure), jaundice, liver function abnormalities.

Hypersensitivity – Anaphylactoid reactions, urticaria, vasculitis.

Lab test abnormalities – Increased serum cholesterol, increased serum triglycerides.

Miscellaneous – Arthralgia, redistribution/accumulation of body fat.

Overdosage

➤*Symptoms:* There have been more than 60 reports of acute or chronic human overdosage (up to 23 times the recommended total daily dose of 2,400 mg) with indinavir. The most commonly reported symptoms were renal (eg, flank pain, hematuria, nephrolithiasis/urolithiasis) and GI (eg, diarrhea, nausea, vomiting).

Patient Information

Indinavir is not a cure for HIV infection. Advise patients that they may continue to develop opportunistic infections and other complications associated with HIV disease. The long-term effects of indinavir are unknown at this time. Advise patients that indinavir has not been shown to reduce the risk of transmission of HIV to others through sexual contact or blood contamination.

Advise patients to remain under the care of a health care provider when using indinavir and not to modify or discontinue treatment without first consulting their health care provider. Therefore, if a dose is missed, advise patients to take the next dose at the regularly scheduled time and to not double this dose. Initiate and maintain therapy with indinavir at the recommended dosage.

Indinavir may interact with some drugs; therefore, advise patients to report the use of any other prescription medication, nonprescription medication, or herbal products, particularly St. John's wort, to their health care provider.

For optimal absorption, administer indinavir without food but with water 1 hour before or 2 hours after a meal. Alternatively, indinavir may be administered with other liquids such as skim milk, juice, coffee, or tea, or with a light meal (eg, dry toast with jelly, juice, and coffee with skim milk and sugar; or corn flakes, skim milk, and sugar). Ingestion of indinavir with a meal high in calories, fat, and protein reduces the absorption of indinavir.

Advise patients receiving a phosphodiesterase type 5 (PDE5) inhibitor (sildenafil, tadalafil, vardenafil) that they may be at an increased risk of PDE5-associated adverse reactions (including hypotension, priapism, visual changes) and to promptly report any symptoms to their health care provider.

Inform patients that redistribution or accumulation of body fat may occur in patients receiving antiretroviral therapy and that the cause and long-term health effects of these conditions are not known at this time.

Indinavir capsules are sensitive to moisture. Inform patients to store and use indinavir in the original container and to leave the desiccant in the bottle.

TIPRANAVIR

Rx	Aptivus (Boehringer Ingelheim)	Capsules; oral: 250 mg	Dehydrated alcohol 7% w/w, polyoxyl 35 castor oil. (TPV 250). Pink, oblong. In 120s.
		Solution; oral: 100 mg/mL	PEG 400, vitamin E polyethylene glycol succinate,[a] propylene glycol. Buttermint-butter toffee flavor. In 95 mL with 5 mL oral dispensing syringe.

[a] Each mL of oral solution contains vitamin E 116 units.

TIPRANAVIR — ORAL

WARNING

Hepatotoxicity – Clinical hepatitis and hepatic decompensation, including some fatalities, have been reported. Extra vigilance is warranted in patients with chronic hepatitis B or hepatitis C coinfection, as these patients have an increased risk of hepatotoxicity.

Intracranial hemorrhage – Both fatal and nonfatal intracranial hemorrhage have been reported.

Indications

➤*HIV infection:* Tipranavir, coadministered with ritonavir, is indicated for combination antiretroviral treatment of patients infected with HIV-1 who are treatment experienced and infected with HIV-1 strains resistant to more than 1 protease inhibitor (PI).

Administration and Dosage

➤*General dosing considerations:* Tipranavir must be coadministered with ritonavir to exert its therapeutic effect. Failure to correctly coadminister tipranavir with ritonavir will result in plasma levels of tipranavir that will be insufficient to achieve the desired antiviral effect and will alter some drug interactions.

Tipranavir may be administered as capsules or oral solution to adults and children 2 years of age and older.

Health care providers should pay special attention to accurate calculation of the dose of tipranavir, transcription of the medication order, dispensing information, and dosing instruction to minimize risk for medication errors, overdose, and underdose.

➤*Adults:*

HIV infection – Tipranavir 500 mg (two 250 mg capsules or 5 mL oral solution) coadministered with ritonavir 200 mg twice daily.

➤*Children:*

2 to 18 years of age –

HIV-1 infection:

• *Usual dosage* – Tipranavir 14 mg/kg with ritonavir 6 mg/kg twice daily. Alternatively, tipranavir 375 mg/m² coadministered with ritonavir 150 mg/m² twice daily.

• *Maximum dose* – Tipranavir 500 mg coadministered with ritonavir 200 mg twice daily.

• *Dosage adjustment* – For children who develop intolerance or toxicity and cannot continue with tipranavir 14 mg/kg with ritonavir 6 mg/kg, health care providers may consider decreasing the dose to tipranavir 12 mg/kg with ritonavir 5 mg/kg (or tipranavir 290 mg/m² coadministered with ritonavir 115 mg/m²) taken twice daily, provided their virus is not resistant to multiple PIs.

➤*Hepatic function impairment:* Tipranavir/ritonavir is contraindicated in patients with moderate or severe (Child-Pugh class B and C, respectively) hepatic impairment.

➤*Administration:* Tipranavir coadministered with ritonavir capsules or solution can be taken with or without food.

Tipranavir coadministered with ritonavir tablets must only be taken with meals.

Before prescribing tipranavir capsules, children should be assessed for the ability to swallow capsules. If a child is unable to reliably swallow a tipranavir capsule, the tipranavir oral solution formulation should be prescribed.

➤*Storage/Stability:*

Capsules – Store in a refrigerator, 2° to 8°C (36° to 46°F), prior to opening the bottle. After opening the bottle, the capsules may be stored at 25°C (77°F); excursions are permitted to 15° to 30°C (59° to 86°F). Medication must be used within 60 days after first opening the bottle.

Oral solution – Store at 25°C (77°F); excursions are permitted between 15° and 30°C (59° and 86°F). Do not refrigerate or freeze. The solution must be used within 60 days after first opening the bottle.

Actions

➤*Pharmacology:* Tipranavir is an HIV-1 PI that inhibits the virus-specific processing of the viral Gag and Gag-Pol polyproteins in HIV-1–infected cells, thus preventing formation of mature virions.

➤*Pharmacokinetics:* In order to achieve effective tipranavir plasma concentrations and a twice-daily dosing regimen, coadministration of tipranavir with ritonavir is essential. Ritonavir inhibits hepatic CYP3A, the intestinal P-glycoprotein (P-gp) efflux pump, and, possibly, intestinal CYP3A. In a dose-ranging evaluation in 113 HIV-1–negative male and female volunteers, there was a 29-fold increase in the geometric mean morning steady-state trough plasma concentrations of tipranavir following tipranavir coadministered with low-dose ritonavir (tipranavir 500 mg/ritonavir 200 mg twice daily), compared with tipranavir 500 mg twice daily without ritonavir. In adults, the mean systemic ritonavir concentration when ritonavir 200 mg was given with tipranavir 500 mg was similar to the concentrations observed when 100 mg was given with the other PIs.

Absorption – Absorption of tipranavir in humans is limited, although no absolute quantification of absorption is available. Tipranavir is a P-gp substrate, a weak P-gp inhibitor, and appears to be a potent P-gp inducer as well. In vivo data suggest that tipranavir/ritonavir, at the dose of tipranavir 500 mg/ritonavir 200 mg, is a P-gp inhibitor after the first dose and that induction of P-gp occurs over time. Tipranavir trough concentrations at steady state are approximately 70% lower than those on day 1, presumably because of intestinal P-gp induction. Steady state is attained in most subjects after 7 to 10 days of dosing.

TIPRANAVIR — ORAL

Dosing with tipranavir 500 mg concomitant with ritonavir 200 mg twice daily for more than 2 weeks and without meal restriction produced the following pharmacokinetic parameters for female and male HIV-1–positive patients.

Pharmacokinetic Parameters[a] of Tipranavir 500 mg/Ritonavir 200 mg for HIV-1–Positive Patients by Gender[b]

Parameter	Women (n = 14)	Men (n = 106)
Cp_{trough} (mcM)	41.6 ± 24.3	35.6 ± 16.7
C_{max} (mcM)	94.8 ± 22.8	77.6 ± 16.6
T_{max} (h)	2.9	3
AUC_{0-12h} (mcM•h)	851 ± 309	710 ± 207
CL (L/h)	1.15	1.27
Vd (L)	7.7	10.2
t½ (h)	5.5	6

[a] Population pharmacokinetic parameters reported as mean ± standard deviation.
[b] Cp_{trough} = trough plasma concentration; C_{max} = maximum drug concentration; T_{max} = time to maximum concentration; AUC_{0-12h} = area under the curve from 0 to 12 hours; CL = clearance; Vd = volume of distribution; t½ = elimination half-life.

Food effects: For tipranavir capsules or oral solution coadministered with ritonavir at steady state, no clinically significant changes in C_{max}, Cp12h, and AUC were observed under fed conditions (500 to 682 Kcal, 23% to 25% calories from fat) compared with fasted conditions. Tipranavir coadministered with ritonavir may be taken with or without food.

Distribution – Tipranavir is extensively bound to plasma proteins (more than 99.9%). It binds to both human serum albumin and alpha-1 acid glycoprotein. The mean fraction of tipranavir (dosed without ritonavir) unbound in plasma was similar in clinical samples from healthy volunteers and HIV-1–positive patients. Total plasma tipranavir concentrations for these samples ranged from 9 to 82 mcM. The unbound fraction of tipranavir appeared to be independent of total drug concentration over this concentration range.

Metabolism – In vitro metabolism studies with human liver microsomes indicated that CYP3A4 is the predominant CYP enzyme involved in tipranavir metabolism.

The oral clearance of tipranavir decreased after the addition of ritonavir, which may represent diminished first-pass clearance of the drug at the GI tract as well as the liver.

The metabolism of tipranavir in the presence of ritonavir 200 mg is minimal. Administration of ^{14}C-tipranavir to subjects who received tipranavir 500 mg/ritonavir 200 mg dosed to steady state demonstrated that unchanged tipranavir accounted for 98.4% or more of the total plasma radioactivity circulating at 3, 8, or 12 hours after dosing. Only a few metabolites were found in plasma, and all were at trace levels (0.2% or less of the plasma radioactivity). In feces, unchanged tipranavir represented the majority of fecal radioactivity (79.9% of fecal radioactivity). The most abundant fecal metabolite, at 4.9% of fecal radioactivity (3.2% of the dose), was a hydroxyl metabolite of tipranavir. In urine, unchanged tipranavir was found in trace amounts (0.5% of urine radioactivity). The most abundant urinary metabolite, at 11% of urine radioactivity (0.5% of the dose), was a glucuronide conjugate of tipranavir.

Excretion – Administration of ^{14}C-tipranavir to subjects (n = 8) who received tipranavir 500 mg/ritonavir 200 mg dosed to steady state demonstrated that most radioactivity (median, 82.3%) was excreted in feces, while only a median of 4.4% of the radioactive dose administered was recovered in urine. In addition, most (56%) radioactivity was excreted between 24 and 96 hours after dosing. The effective mean elimination half-life of tipranavir/ritonavir in healthy volunteers (n = 67) and HIV-1–infected adult patients (n = 120) was approximately 4.8 and 6 hours, respectively, at steady state following a dosage of tipranavir 500 mg/ritonavir 200 mg twice daily with a light meal.

Special populations –
Gender: Evaluation of steady-state plasma tipranavir trough concentrations at 10 to 14 hours after dosing from the controlled clinical trials 1182.12 and 1182.48 demonstrated that women generally had higher tipranavir concentrations than men. After 4 weeks of tipranavir 500 mg/ritonavir 200 mg twice daily, the median plasma trough concentration of tipranavir was 43.9 mcM for women and 31.1 mcM for men. The difference in concentrations does not warrant a dose adjustment.

➤*Microbiology:* Tipranavir inhibits the replication of laboratory strains of HIV-1 and clinical isolates in acute models of T-cell infection, with 50% effective concentrations (EC_{50}) ranging from 0.03 to 0.07 mcM (18 to 42 ng/mL). Tipranavir demonstrates antiviral activity in cell culture against a broad panel of HIV-1 group M nonclade B isolates (A, C, D, F, G, H, CRF01 AE, CRF02 AG, CRF12 BF). Group O and HIV-2 isolates have reduced susceptibility in cell culture to tipranavir, with EC_{50} values ranging from 0.164 to 1 mcM and 0.233 to 0.522 mcM, respectively. When used with other antiretroviral agents in cell culture, the combination of tipranavir was additive to antagonistic with other PIs (amprenavir, atazanavir, indinavir, lopinavir, nelfinavir, ritonavir, and saquinavir) and generally additive with the nonnucleoside reverse transcriptase inhibitors (NNRTIs) (delavirdine, efavirenz, and nevirapine) and the nucleoside reverse transcriptase inhibitors (NRTIs) (abacavir, didanosine, emtricitabine, lamivudine, stavudine, tenofovir, and zidovudine). Tipranavir was synergistic with the HIV-1 fusion inhibitor enfuvirtide. There was no antagonism of the in cell culture combinations of tipranavir with either adefovir or ribavirin, used in the treatment of viral hepatitis.

Resistance –
Treatment-experienced patients: In controlled clinical trials 1182.12 and 1182.48, multiple PI-resistant HIV-1 isolates from 59 treatment-experienced adult patients who received tipranavir/ritonavir and experienced virologic rebound developed amino acid substitutions that were associated with resistance to tipranavir. The most common amino acid substitutions that developed on tipranavir 500 mg/ritonavir 200 mg in more than 20% of tipranavir/ritonavir virologic failure isolates were L33V/I/F, V82T, and I84V. Other substitutions that developed in 10% to 20% of tipranavir/ritonavir virologic failure isolates included L10V/I/S, I13V, E35D/G/N, I47V, 154V/A/M, K55R, V82L, and L89V/M. Evolution at protease Gag polyprotein cleavage sites was also observed. Among 28 children in clinical trial 1182.14 who experienced virologic failure or nonresponse, the emergent protease amino acid codon substitutions were similar to those observed in adult virologic failure isolates.

In clinical trials 1182.12 and 1182.48, tipranavir resistance was detected at virologic rebound after an average of 38 weeks of tipranavir/ritonavir treatment, with a median 14-fold decrease in tipranavir susceptibility. Similarly reduced tipranavir susceptibility was associated with emergent mutations in pediatric patient isolates.

Cross-resistance – Cross-resistance among PIs has been observed. Tipranavir had a less than 4-fold decreased susceptibility against 90% (94/105) of HIV-1 clinical isolates resistant to amprenavir, atazanavir, indinavir, lopinavir, nelfinavir, ritonavir, or saquinavir. Tipranavir-resistant viruses that emerged in cell culture from wild-type HIV-1 had decreased susceptibility to the PIs amprenavir, atazanavir, indinavir, lopinavir, nelfinavir, and ritonavir, but remained sensitive to saquinavir.

Contraindications

Moderate or severe (Child-Pugh class B or C, respectively) hepatic impairment; coadministration of tipranavir/ritonavir with the following drugs that are highly dependent on CYP3A for clearance or are potent CYP3A inducers: alfuzosin, amiodarone, bepridil, cisapride, dihydroergotamine, ergonovine, ergotamine, flecainide, lovastatin, methylergonovine, midazolam (oral), pimozide, propafenone, quinidine, rifampin, sildenafil (*Revatio* [for the treatment of pulmonary arterial hypertension]), simvastatin, St. John's wort (*Hypericum perforatum*), and triazolam.

Because of the need for coadministration of tipranavir with ritonavir, refer to the Ritonavir monograph for a description of ritonavir contraindications.

Warnings/Precautions

➤*Coadministration with ritonavir:* Tipranavir must be coadministered with ritonavir 200 mg to exert its therapeutic effect. Failure to correctly coadminister tipranavir with ritonavir will result in reduced plasma levels of tipranavir that will be insufficient to achieve the desired antiviral effect and will alter some drug interactions (effect of tipranavir and ritonavir on other drugs).

Refer to the Ritonavir monograph for additional information on precautionary measures.

➤*Hepatic toxicity:* Tipranavir coadministered with ritonavir 200 mg has been associated with reports of clinical hepatitis and hepatic decompensation, including some fatalities. These have generally occurred in patients with advanced HIV-1 disease taking multiple concomitant medications. A causal relationship to tipranavir/ritonavir could not be established. Closely follow all patients with clinical and laboratory monitoring, especially those with chronic hepatitis B or C coinfection because these patients have an increased risk of hepatotoxicity. Perform liver function tests prior to initiating therapy with tipranavir/ritonavir and frequently throughout the duration of treatment.

Treatment-experienced patients with chronic hepatitis B or C coinfection or elevations in transaminases are at an approximately 2-fold risk for developing grade 3 or 4 transaminase elevations or hepatic decompensation. In 2 large, randomized, open-label, controlled clinical trials with an active comparator (1182.12 and 1182.48) of treatment-experienced patients, grade 3 and 4 increases in hepatic transaminases were observed in 10.3% (10.9/100 PEY) receiving tipranavir/ritonavir through week 48. In a study of treatment-naive patients, 20.3% (21/100 PEY) experienced grade 3 or 4 hepatic transaminase elevations while receiving tipranavir 500 mg/ritonavir 200 mg through week 48.

Health care providers and patients should be vigilant for the appearance of signs or symptoms of hepatitis, such as fatigue, malaise, anorexia, nausea, jaundice, bilirubinuria, acholic stools, liver tenderness, or hepatomegaly. Instruct patients with signs or symptoms of clinical hepatitis to discontinue tipranavir/ritonavir treatment and seek medical evaluation.

If asymptomatic elevations in AST or ALT greater than 10 times the upper limit of normal occur, tipranavir/ritonavir therapy should be discontinued. If asymptomatic elevations in AST or ALT between 5 and 10 times the upper limit of normal (ULN) and increases in total bilirubin greater than 2.5 times the ULN occur, discontinue the tipranavir/ritonavir therapy.

➤*Intracranial hemorrhage:* Tipranavir, coadministered with ritonavir 200 mg, has been associated with reports of both fatal and nonfatal intracranial hemorrhage. Many of these patients had other medical conditions or were receiving concomitant medications that may have caused or contributed to these events. No pattern of abnormal coagulation parameters has been observed in patients in general, or preceding the development of intracranial hemorrhage. Therefore, routine measurement of coagulation parameters is not currently indicated in the management of patients on tipranavir.

TIPRANAVIR — ORAL

➤*Platelet aggregation and coagulation:* In in vitro experiments, tipranavir was observed to inhibit human platelet aggregation at levels consistent with exposures observed in patients receiving tipranavir/ritonavir.

Use tipranavir/ritonavir with caution in patients who may be at risk of increased bleeding from trauma, surgery, or other medical conditions, or who are receiving medications known to increase the risk of bleeding, such as antiplatelet agents and anticoagulants, or who are taking supplemental high doses of vitamin E.

In rats, tipranavir treatment alone induced dose-dependent changes in coagulation parameters, bleeding events and death. Coadministration with vitamin E significantly increased these effects. However, analyses of stored plasma from adult patients treated with tipranavir capsules and children treated with tipranavir oral solution (which contains a vitamin E derivative) showed no effect of tipranavir/ritonavir on vitamin K–dependent coagulation factors (factor II and VII), factor V, or on prothrombin or activated partial thromboplastin times.

➤*Vitamin E:* Advise patients taking tipranavir oral solution not to take supplemental vitamin E greater than a standard multivitamin because tipranavir oral solution contains vitamin E 116 units/mL, which is higher than the reference daily intake (adults, 30 units; children, approximately 10 units).

➤*Rash:* Rash, including urticarial rash, maculopapular rash, and possible photosensitivity, has been reported in subjects receiving tipranavir/ritonavir. In some cases, rash was accompanied by joint pain or stiffness, throat tightness, or generalized pruritus. In controlled adult clinical trials, rash (all grades, all causality) was observed in 10% of women and in 8% of men receiving tipranavir/ritonavir through 48 weeks of treatment. The median time to onset of rash was 53 days, and the median duration of rash was 22 days. The discontinuation rate for rash in clinical trials was 0.5%. In an uncontrolled compassionate use program (n = 3,920), cases of rash, some of which were severe, accompanied by myalgia, fever, erythema, desquamation, and mucosal erosions, were reported. In the pediatric clinical trial, the frequency of rash (all grades, all causality) through 48 weeks of treatment was 21%. Overall, most of the children had mild rash and 5 (5%) had moderate rash. Overall, 3% of children interrupted tipranavir treatment because of rash, and the discontinuation rate for rash in children was 0.9%. Discontinue and initiate appropriate treatment if severe skin rash develops.

➤*Diabetes mellitus / Hyperglycemia:* New-onset diabetes mellitus, exacerbation of preexisting diabetes mellitus, and hyperglycemia have been reported during postmarketing surveillance in HIV-1–infected patients receiving PI therapy. Some patients required either initiation or dose adjustments of insulin or oral hypoglycemic agents for treatment of these events. In some cases, diabetic ketoacidosis has occurred. In those patients who discontinued PI therapy, hyperglycemia persisted in some cases. Because these events have been reported voluntarily during clinical practice, estimates of frequency cannot be made, and a causal relationship between PI therapy and these events has not been established.

➤*Immune reconstitution syndrome:* Immune reconstitution syndrome has been reported in patients treated with combination antiretroviral therapy, including tipranavir. During the initial phase of combination antiretroviral treatment, patients whose immune system responds may develop an inflammatory response to indolent or residual opportunistic infections (eg, *Mycobacterium avium* infection, cytomegalovirus, *Pneumocystis jiroveci* pneumonia, tuberculosis, reactivation of herpes simplex and herpes zoster), which may necessitate further evaluation and treatment.

➤*Fat redistribution:* Redistribution/accumulation of body fat, including central obesity, dorsocervical fat enlargement (buffalo hump), peripheral wasting, facial wasting, breast enlargement, and "cushingoid appearance," have been observed in patients receiving antiretroviral therapy. The mechanism and long-term consequences of these reactions are currently unknown. A causal relationship has not been established.

➤*Lipid elevations:* Treatment with tipranavir coadministered with ritonavir 200 mg has resulted in large increases in the concentration of total cholesterol and triglycerides. Perform triglyceride and cholesterol testing prior to initiating tipranavir/ritonavir therapy and at periodic intervals during therapy. Manage lipid disorders as clinically appropriate, taking into account any potential drug-drug interactions.

➤*Hemophilia:* There have been reports of increased bleeding, including spontaneous skin hematomas and hemarthrosis in patients with hemophilia type A and B treated with PIs. In some patients, additional factor VIII was given. In more than half of the reported cases, treatment with PIs was continued or reintroduced if treatment had been discontinued. A causal relationship between PIs and these reactions has not been established.

➤*Resistance / Cross-resistance:* Because the potential for HIV-1 cross-resistance among PIs has not been fully explored in tipranavir/ritonavir-treated patients, it is unknown what effect therapy with tipranavir will have on the activity of subsequently administered PIs.

➤*Hypersensitivity reactions:* Use tipranavir with caution in patients with a known sulfonamide allergy. Tipranavir contains a sulfonamide moiety. The potential for cross-sensitivity between drugs in the sulfonamide class and tipranavir is unknown.

➤*Hepatic function impairment:* Tipranavir is principally metabolized by the liver. Therefore, exercise caution when administering tipranavir/ritonavir to patients with mild hepatic impairment (Child-Pugh class A) because tipranavir concentrations may be increased. Tipranavir is contraindicated in patients with moderate or severe (Child-Pugh class B or C, respectively) hepatic impairment.

➤*Pregnancy: Category C.* There are no adequate and well-controlled studies in pregnant women for the treatment of HIV-1 infection. Use tipranavir during pregnancy only if the potential benefit justifies the potential risk to the fetus.

At 400 mg/kg/day and above in rats, fetal toxicity (decreased sternebrae ossification and body weights) was observed, corresponding to an AUC of 1,310 mcM•h or approximately 0.8-fold human exposure at the recommended dose.

In pre- and postdevelopment studies in rats, tipranavir showed no adverse effects at 40 mg/kg/day (approximately 0.2-fold human exposure), but caused growth inhibition in pups and maternal toxicity at dose levels of 400 mg/kg/day (approximately 0.8-fold human exposure). No postweaning functions were affected at any dose level.

Antiretroviral pregnancy registry – To monitor maternal-fetal outcomes of pregnant women exposed to tipranavir, an antiretroviral pregnancy registry has been established. Health care providers are encouraged to register patients by calling 1-800-258-4263.

➤*Lactation:* The Centers for Disease Control and Prevention recommend that HIV-infected mothers not breast-feed their infants to avoid risking postnatal transmission of HIV-1. Because of the potential for HIV-1 transmission and possible adverse effects of tipranavir, instruct mothers not to breast-feed if they are receiving tipranavir.

The molecular weight (approximately 603), minimal metabolism, and elimination half-life (6 hours) suggest that the drug will be excreted in breast milk.

➤*Children:* The safety, pharmacokinetic profile, and virologic and immunologic responses of tipranavir oral solution and capsules were evaluated in HIV-1 infected children 2 to 18 years of age.

The most frequent adverse reactions (grades 2 to 4) were similar to those described in adults. However, rash was reported more frequently in children than in adults.

The risk-benefit has not been established in children younger than 2 years of age.

➤*Elderly:* In general, exercise caution in the administration and monitoring of tipranavir in elderly patients, reflecting the greater frequency of decreased hepatic, renal, or cardiac function, and of concomitant disease or other drug therapy.

➤*Monitoring:* Perform liver function tests prior to initiating therapy with tipranavir/ritonavir and frequently throughout the duration of treatment.

Perform triglyceride and cholesterol testing prior to initiating tipranavir/ritonavir therapy and at periodic intervals during therapy. Manage lipid disorders as clinically appropriate.

Monitor patients for signs or symptoms of hepatitis (eg, acholic stools, anorexia, bilirubinuria, fatigue, hepatomegaly, jaundice, liver tenderness, malaise, nausea).

Drug Interactions

➤*Cytochrome P450 system:* Tipranavir coadministered with ritonavir 200 mg at the recommended dosage is a net inhibitor of CYP3A and may increase plasma concentrations of agents that are primarily metabolized by CYP3A. Thus, coadministration of tipranavir/ritonavir with drugs highly dependent on CYP3A for clearance, and for which elevated plasma concentrations are associated with serious and/or life-threatening reactions, is contraindicated. Coadministration with other CYP3A substrates may require a dose adjustment or additional monitoring.

Tipranavir is a CYP3A substrate and a P-gp substrate. Coadministration of tipranavir/ritonavir and drugs that induce CYP3A and/or P-gp may decrease tipranavir plasma concentrations. Coadministration of tipranavir/ritonavir and drugs that inhibit P-gp may increase tipranavir plasma concentrations.

Coadministration of tipranavir/ritonavir with drugs that inhibit CYP3A may not further increase tipranavir plasma concentrations because the level of metabolites is low following steady-state administration of tipranavir 500 mg/ritonavir 200 mg twice daily.

Tipranavir Drug Interactions

Precipitant drug	Object drug[a]		Description
Aluminum- and magnesium-based antacids	Tipranavir	⬇	Aluminum- and magnesium-based antacids may decrease tipranavir absorption. Consider separating tipranavir/ritonavir dosing from antacid administration.
Anticonvulsants (eg, carbamazepine, phenobarbital, phenytoin)	Tipranavir	⬇	Tipranavir plasma concentrations may be reduced, decreasing the efficacy. Use with caution.
Tipranavir	Anticonvulsants (eg, valproic acid)		Valproic acid plasma concentrations may be reduced, decreasing the efficacy. Use with caution.

TIPRANAVIR — ORAL

Tipranavir Drug Interactions

Precipitant drug	Object drug[a]		Description
Azole antifungals (eg, fluconazole)	Tipranavir	↑	Fluconazole may increase tipranavir concentrations. Dosage adjustment is not needed. High doses (> 200 mg) of fluconazole, itraconazole, and ketoconazole are not recommended. Studies have not been done with itraconazole, ketoconazole, or voriconazole.
Tipranavir	Azole antifungals (eg, fluconazole, itraconazole, ketoconazole, voriconazole)	↔	
Buprenorphine	Tipranavir	↓	Tipranavir concentrations may be decreased. However, dose adjustments cannot be recommended.
Clarithromycin	Tipranavir	↑	Concurrent use may increase tipranavir and clarithromycin levels. Dosage adjustment is not needed in patients with healthy renal function. For patients with CrCl[b] 30 to 60 mL/min, decrease clarithromycin dose 50%. For patients with CrCl < 30 mL/min, decrease the clarithromycin dose 75%.
Tipranavir	Clarithromycin		
Delavirdine	Tipranavir	↑	Delavirdine may increase plasma concentrations and pharmacologic effects of tipranavir. Tipranavir may decrease plasma concentrations and pharmacologic effects of delavirdine. Dosage reduction of tipranavir may be needed during coadministration of delavirdine. Dosage increases may be required for delavirdine when coadministered with tipranavir.
Tipranavir	Delavirdine	↓	
Efavirenz	Tipranavir	↓	Efavirenz coadministered with tipranavir 500 mg/ritonavir 100 mg twice daily may cause tipranavir concentrations to decrease. Higher doses of tipranavir/ritonavir did not cause changes in tipranavir pharmacokinetics. Monitor tipranavir concentrations and the clinical response of the patient. If an interaction is suspected, it may be necessary to increase the tipranavir dose.
Enfuvirtide	Tipranavir	↑	Tipranavir concentrations may be increased. However, dose adjustments are not recommended.
Etravirine	Tipranavir	↑	Tipranavir concentrations may be increased. Tipranavir/ritonavir have been reported to decrease etravirine concentrations while atazanavir/ritonavir have been reported to increase etravirine concentrations. High-dose ritonavir (600 mg twice daily) has been reported to decrease etravirine concentrations. Coadministration of tipranavir/ritonavir with etravirine is not recommended.
Tipranavir	Etravirine	↓↑	
Nevirapine	Tipranavir	↓	Tipranavir plasma concentrations may be reduced, decreasing the efficacy. Monitor tipranavir concentrations and the clinical response of the patient when nevirapine is started or stopped. Adjust the tipranavir dose as needed.
Protease inhibitors (eg, atazanavir)	Tipranavir	↑	Atazanavir may increase tipranavir concentrations. Tipranavir may decrease protease inhibitor concentrations. Coadministration is not recommended.
Tipranavir	Protease inhibitors (eg, atazanavir, fosamprenavir, lopinavir, saquinavir)	↓	
Rifamycins (eg, rifampin)	Tipranavir	↓	Coadministration of tipranavir with rifampin may lead to loss of virologic response and possible resistance to tipranavir. Coadministration is contraindicated. Coadministration of tipranavir with rifabutin may increase concentrations of rifabutin and its metabolite. Reduce rifabutin dose 75% (eg, 150 mg every other day) and increase monitoring.
Tipranavir	Rifamycins (eg, rifabutin)	↑	
St. John's wort	Tipranavir	↓	Coadministration may lead to loss of virologic response and possible resistance to tipranavir. Coadministration is contraindicated.
Tenofovir	Tipranavir	↓	Coadministration may decrease the concentrations of both tipranavir and tenofovir. Monitor tenofovir and tipranavir concentrations and the response of the patient. If an interaction is suspected, adjust therapy as indicated.
Tipranavir	Tenofovir		
Tipranavir	Alfuzosin	↑	Alfuzosin plasma concentrations may be elevated, increasing the risk of hypotension. Coadministration is contraindicated.
Tipranavir	Antiarrhythmic agents (eg, amiodarone, bepridil, flecainide, propafenone, quinidine)	↑	Coadministration is contraindicated because of the potential for serious and/or life-threatening reactions, such as cardiac arrhythmias secondary to increases in plasma concentrations of antiarrhythmics.
Tipranavir	Anticholinergic agents (eg, darifenacin, fesoterodine, solifenacin, tolterodine)	↑	Plasma concentrations of the anticholinergic agent may be elevated, increasing the pharmacologic effects and risk of adverse reactions. When coadministered with tipranavir, the daily dose of darifenacin should not exceed 7.5 mg, the daily dose of fesoterodine should not exceed 4 mg, the daily dose of solifenacin should not exceed 5 mg, and the daily dose of tolterodine should not exceed 2 mg.
Tipranavir	Aripiprazole	↑	Aripiprazole plasma concentrations may be elevated, increasing the pharmacologic effects and risk of adverse reactions. Monitor the patient and adjust the aripiprazole dose as needed.
Tipranavir	Benzodiazepines (eg, midazolam, triazolam)	↑	Coadministration of tipranavir and triazolam or oral midazolam is contraindicated because of the risk of prolonged or increased sedation or respiratory depression. If parenteral midazolam is coadministered, closely monitor for respiratory depression and/or prolonged sedation. Adjust the midazolam dose as needed.
Tipranavir	Bosentan	↑	In patients taking bosentan, discontinue use of bosentan at least 36 hours before starting tipranavir/ritonavir. At least 10 days after starting tipranavir/ritonavir, resume bosentan 62.5 mg once daily or every other day based on individual tolerability. In patients on tipranavir/ritonavir for at least 10 days, start bosentan at 62.5 mg once daily or every other day based on individual tolerability.

TIPRANAVIR — ORAL

Tipranavir Drug Interactions

Precipitant drug	Object drug[a]		Description
Tipranavir	Calcium channel blockers (eg, diltiazem, felodipine, nicardipine, nisoldipine, verapamil)	↔	Although not studied, caution is warranted and clinical monitoring is recommended.
Tipranavir	Cisapride	↑	Coadministration is contraindicated because of the risk of cardiac arrhythmias.
Tipranavir	Colchicine	↑	Colchicine plasma concentrations may be increased. Life-threatening and fatal colchicine toxicity may occur. Avoid coadministration in patients with hepatic or renal impairment. In patients with healthy renal and hepatic function, coadministration of tipranavir and colchicine should be undertaken using a maximum dosage of colchicine 0.3 mg twice daily with careful monitoring for colchicine-related adverse effects.
Tipranavir	Contraceptives, hormonal (estrogen-containing)	↓	Concurrent use may decrease ethinyl estradiol 50%. Use alternative methods of nonhormonal contraception. Monitor patients taking estrogen-based hormone replacement therapy for signs of estrogen deficiency. Patients also may have an increased risk of rash.
Tipranavir	Desipramine	↑	Although not studied, increased desipramine levels are expected. Dosage reduction and concentration monitoring of desipramine are recommended.
Tipranavir	Digoxin	↑	Tipranavir may increase plasma concentrations and pharmacologic effects of digoxin. Closely monitor for clinical and laboratory signs of digoxin toxicity when tipranavir is added to a stable digoxin regimen. Digoxin dose reductions may be necessary.
Tipranavir	Disulfiram, metronidazole	↑	Tipranavir capsules contain alcohol that can produce disulfiram-like reactions when coadministered with disulfiram or other drugs that can produce this reaction (eg, metronidazole). Inform patients of this risk.
Tipranavir	Dronedarone	↑	Dronedarone plasma concentrations may be elevated, increasing the pharmacologic effects and risk of toxicity. Avoid coadministration.
Tipranavir	Eletriptan	↑	Eletriptan plasma concentrations may be elevated by tipranavir/ritonavir, increasing the pharmacologic effects and risk of adverse reactions. Eletriptan should not be used within 72 hours of tipranavir/ritonavir.
Tipranavir	Eplerenone	↑	Eplerenone plasma concentrations may be elevated, increasing the pharmacologic effects and risk of toxicity. Close clinical monitoring is indicated when eplerenone is coadministered with tipranavir. Adjust the eplerenone dose as needed.

Tipranavir Drug Interactions

Precipitant drug	Object drug[a]		Description
Tipranavir	Ergot derivatives (eg, dihydroergotamine, ergonovine, ergotamine, methylergonovine)	↑	The risk of ergot toxicity (peripheral vasospasms and ischemia of the extremities and other tissues) is increased. Coadministration is contraindicated.
Tipranavir	Erlotinib	↑	Erlotinib plasma concentrations may be elevated, increasing the pharmacologic effects and risk of adverse reactions. In patients receiving erlotinib, monitor for erlotinib adverse reactions when tipranavir is started. Adjust the erlotinib dose as needed.
Tipranavir	Erythromycin	↑	Plasma concentration of erythromycin may be elevated, increasing the risk of sudden death from cardiac causes. Concurrent use should be avoided.
Tipranavir	Eszopiclone	↑	Eszopiclone plasma concentrations may be elevated, increasing the pharmacologic effects and risk of adverse reactions. Close monitoring is indicated when eszopiclone is coadministered with tipranavir. Consider reducing the eszopiclone dose when coadministered with tipranavir.
Tipranavir	Fluticasone	↑	Concomitant use of fluticasone and tipranavir/ritonavir may increase plasma concentrations of fluticasone, resulting in reduced serum cortisol concentrations. This combination is not recommended unless the potential benefit outweighs the risk of systemic corticosteroid adverse reactions.
Tipranavir	HMG-CoA reductase inhibitors (eg, atorvastatin, lovastatin, rosuvastatin, simvastatin)	↑	Concurrent use increases the risk of myopathy, including rhabdomyolysis. Concurrent use of tipranavir with lovastatin or simvastatin is contraindicated. If using atorvastatin or rosuvastatin, start with the lowest possible dose with careful monitoring. Consider using fluvastatin or pravastatin as alternative therapy when tipranavir is used concomitantly with ritonavir 200 mg.
Tipranavir	Hypoglycemic agents (eg, glimepiride, glipizide, glyburide, pioglitazone, repaglinide, tolbutamide)	↔	Although not studied, careful glucose monitoring is recommended.
Tipranavir	Iloperidone	↑	Iloperidone plasma concentrations and pharmacologic effects may be increased. A modification of the iloperidone dosage is recommended. The dose of iloperidone should be reduced by one-half when coadministered with tipranavir. If therapy with tipranavir is discontinued, the dose of iloperidone should be increased to the original dose.
Tipranavir	Immunosuppressants (eg, cyclosporine, sirolimus, tacrolimus)	↔	Although not studied, careful drug concentration monitoring is recommended.
Tipranavir	Maraviroc	↑	Maraviroc plasma concentrations may be elevated, increasing the pharmacologic effects and risk of adverse reactions. Monitor the response of the patient and adjust the maraviroc dose as needed.

TIPRANAVIR — ORAL

Tipranavir Drug Interactions

Precipitant drug	Object drug[a]		Description
Tipranavir	NRTIs (eg, abacavir, didanosine, zidovudine)	↓	Plasma concentrations of NRTIs may be decreased. The clinical relevance is unknown. Separate didanosine dosing from tipranavir/ritonavir by at least 2 hours.
Tipranavir	Omeprazole	↓	Omeprazole dosage may need to be increased when coadministered with tipranavir and ritonavir.
Tipranavir	Opioid analgesics (eg, meperidine, methadone)	↑↓	Although not studied, the levels of meperidine and methadone may be decreased. However, the levels of the metabolite normeperidine may be increased and thus increase the risk for seizures. Increased dosage and long-term use of meperidine are not recommended. Methadone dosage may need to be increased.
Tipranavir	PDE5[b] inhibitors (eg, sildenafil, tadalafil, vardenafil)	↑	Sildenafil, for the treatment of pulmonary arterial hypertension, is contraindicated in patients receiving tipranavir/ritonavir. In patients with pulmonary arterial hypertension who have received tipranavir/ritonavir for at least 1 week, start tadalafil at 20 mg once daily. The tadalafil dosage may be increased to 40 mg once daily based upon individual tolerability. In patients already on tadalafil, stop tadalafil at least 24 hours prior to starting tipranavir/ritonavir. After at least 1 week following the start of tipranavir/ritonavir, resume tadalafil at 20 mg once daily. The tadalafil dosage may be increased to 40 mg once daily based upon individual tolerability. Coadminister with caution for the treatment of erectile dysfunction and do not exceed the following doses: sildenafil 25 mg within 48 hours, tadalafil 10 mg every 72 hours, vardenafil 2.5 mg every 72 hours.
Tipranavir	Pimozide	↑	Coadministration is contraindicated because of the potential for cardiac arrhythmias.
Tipranavir	Propoxyphene	↑	Propoxyphene plasma concentrations may be increased by tipranavir/ritonavir. Clinical monitoring for signs of adverse effects due to propoxyphene is indicated. Propoxyphene dosage reduction may be required.
Tipranavir	Protein-tyrosine kinase inhibitors (eg, dasatinib, lapatinib, pazopanib, sorafenib, sunitinib)	↑	Protein-tyrosine kinase inhibitor plasma concentrations may be elevated, increasing the pharmacologic effects and risk of adverse reactions. Monitor the response of the patient and adjust the protein-tyrosine kinase inhibitor dose as needed.
Tipranavir	Quetiapine	↑	Quetiapine plasma concentrations may be elevated, increasing the pharmacologic effects and risk of adverse reactions. Monitor the response of the patient and adjust the quetiapine dose as needed.
Tipranavir	Ranolazine	↑	Ranolazine plasma concentrations may be elevated, increasing the risk of dose-related prolongation of the QTc interval, torsades de pointes–type arrhythmias, and sudden death. Coadministration of ranolazine and other potent or moderate CYP3A4 inhibitors such as tipranavir/ritonavir is contraindicated.
Tipranavir	Risperidone	↑	Risperidone plasma concentrations may be elevated, increasing the pharmacologic effects and risk of adverse reactions. Closely monitor the clinical response when tipranavir/ritonavir therapy is started or stopped. Adjust the risperidone dose as needed.
Tipranavir	Salmeterol	↑	Salmeterol plasma concentrations may be elevated, increasing the risk of cardiovascular adverse events (eg, QT prolongation, palpitations, sinus tachycardia). Coadministration is not recommended.
Tipranavir	SSRIs[b] (eg, fluoxetine, paroxetine, sertraline)	↑	Although not studied, SSRI dose may need to be adjusted upon initiation of tipranavir/ritonavir.
Tipranavir	Trazodone	↑	Concomitant use of trazodone and tipranavir/ritonavir may increase plasma concentrations of trazodone. If trazodone is used with CYP3A4 inhibitors such as tipranavir/ritonavir, use the combination with caution and consider a lower dose of trazodone.
Tipranavir	Vasopressin receptor antagonists (eg, conivaptan, tolvaptan)	↑	Vasopressin receptor antagonist plasma concentrations may be elevated, increasing the pharmacologic effects and risk of adverse reactions. Avoid coadministration.
Tipranavir	Warfarin	↔	Monitor the international normalized ratio frequently upon initiation of tipranavir/ritonavir.
Tipranavir	Zolpidem	↑	Zolpidem concentrations may be increased, resulting in possible severe sedation and respiratory depression. Closely monitor the patient for signs of zolpidem adverse reactions. Zolpidem dosage adjustments may be needed when tipranavir/ritonavir is started or stopped.

[a] ↑ = object drug increased; ↓ = object drug decreased; ↑↓ = object drug both increased and decreased; ↔ = undetermined clinical effect.
[b] CrCl = creatinine clearance; PDE5 = phosphodiesterase type 5; SSRIs = selective serotonin reuptake inhibitors.

➤*Drug/Food interactions:* See Actions for more information. Garlic may reduce tipranavir plasma concentrations, decreasing the pharmacologic effects. Avoid garlic ingestion.

Adverse Reactions

Because of the need for coadministration of tipranavir with ritonavir, refer to the Ritonavir monograph for ritonavir-associated adverse reactions.

➤*Adults:*

Discontinuation of therapy – The 48-week Kaplan-Meier rates of adverse reactions leading to discontinuation were 13.3% for tipranavir/ritonavir-treated patients and 10.8% for the comparator arm patients.

Most common adverse reactions – In 1182.12 and 1182.48 in the tipranavir/ritonavir arm, the most frequent adverse reactions were abdominal pain, diarrhea, fatigue, headache, nausea, pyrexia, and vomiting.

TIPRANAVIR — ORAL

Adverse reactions (2% or more) –

Tipranavir Adverse Reactions (Grades 2 to 4) (≥ 2%)[a,b]

Adverse reactions	Percentage of patients (rate per 100 patient-exposure years)	
	Tipranavir 500 mg/ ritonavir 200 mg twice daily + OBR (757.4 patient-exposure years) (n = 749)	Comparator PI/ritonavir[c] + OBR (503.9 patient-exposure years (n = 737)
CNS		
Fatigue	5.7% (5.9)	5.6% (8.4)
Headache	5.2% (5.3)	4.2% (6.3)
Insomnia	1.7% (1.7)	3.7% (5.5)
Peripheral neuropathy	1.5% (1.5)	2% (3)
GI		
Abdominal pain	4.4% (4.5)	3.4% (5.1)
Abdominal pain, upper	1.5% (1.5)	2.3% (3.4)
Diarrhea	15% (16.5)	13.4% (21.6)
Nausea	8.5% (9)	6.4% (9.7)
Vomiting	5.9% (6)	4.1% (6.1)
Weight decreased	3.1% (3.1)	2.2% (3.2)
Hematologic		
Anemia	3.3% (3.4)	2.3% (3.4)
Neutropenia	2% (2)	1% (1.4)
Metabolic/Nutritional		
Dehydration	2.1% (2.1)	1.1% (1.6)
Hyperlipidemia	2.5% (2.6)	0.8% (1.2)
Hypertriglyceridemia	3.9% (4)	2% (3)
Miscellaneous		
ALT increased	2% (2)	0.5% (0.8)
GGT increased	2% (2)	0.4% (0.6)
Dyspnea	2.1% (2.1)	1% (1.4)
Myalgia	2.3% (2.3)	1.8% (2.6)
Pyrexia	7.5% (7.7)	5.4% (8.2)
Rash	3.1% (3.1)	3.8% (5.7)

[a] Excludes laboratory abnormalities that were adverse reactions.
[b] OBR = optimized background regimen; GGT = gamma-glutamyl transferase.
[c] Comparator PI/ritonavir: lopinavir 400 mg/ritonavir 100 mg twice daily, indinavir 800 mg/ritonavir 100 mg twice daily, saquinavir 1,000 mg/ritonavir 100 mg twice daily, amprenavir 600 mg/ritonavir 100 mg twice daily.

Other adverse reactions (less than 2%) – The following are other adverse reactions reported in less than 2% of adults (n = 1,474) treated with tipranavir 500 mg/ritonavir 200 mg in phase 2 and 3 clinical trials.

CNS – Dizziness, sleep disorder, somnolence.

Dermatologic – Acquired lipodystrophy, exanthem, lipoatrophy, lipohypertrophy, pruritus.

GI – Abdominal distension, anorexia, dyspepsia, flatulence, gastroesophageal reflux disease, pancreatitis.

Hepatic – Cytolytic hepatitis, hepatic failure, hepatic steatosis, hepatitis, hyperbilirubinemia, toxic hepatitis.

Lab test abnormalities – Hepatic enzymes increased, lipase increased, liver function test abnormal.

Metabolic/Nutritional – Decreased appetite, diabetes mellitus, facial wasting, hyperamylasemia, hypercholesterolemia, hyperglycemia, mitochondrial toxicity.

Musculoskeletal – Malaise, muscle cramp.

Miscellaneous – Hypersensitivity, influenza-like illness, intracranial hemorrhage, renal insufficiency, thrombocytopenia.

➤*Children:* Tipranavir coadministered with ritonavir has been studied as combination therapy in 135 children 2 through 18 years of age who where infected with HIV-1. This study enrolled HIV-1–infected, treatment-experienced children (with the exception of 3 treatment-naive patients), with baseline HIV-1 RNA of at least 1,500 copies/mL. One hundred ten patients were enrolled in a randomized, open-label, 48-week clinical trial (study 1182.14), and 25 patients were enrolled in other clinical studies including Expanded Access and Emergency Use Programs.

The adverse reactions profile seen in study 1182.14 was similar to adults. Pyrexia (6.4%), cough (5.5%), rash (5.5%), vomiting (5.5%), nausea (4.5%), and diarrhea (3.6%) were the most frequently reported adverse reactions (grade 2 to 4, all causes) in children. Rash was reported more frequently in children than in adults.

The most common grade 3 to 4 laboratory abnormalities were increase in creatine phosphokinase (11%), ALT (6.5%), and amylase (7.5%).

Because of previous reports of both fatal and nonfatal intracranial hemorrhage, an analysis of bleeding events was performed. At 48 weeks of treatment, the frequency of children with any bleeding adverse reactions was 7.5%. No drug-related serious bleeding adverse reaction was reported. The most frequent bleeding adverse reaction was epistaxis (3.7%). No other bleeding adverse reaction was reported in frequency of more than 1%. Additional trial follow-up through 100 weeks showed a cumulative 12% frequency of any bleeding adverse reaction.

➤*Lab test abnormalities:*

Tipranavir Treatment-Emergent Laboratory Abnormalities Reported in Adults (≥ 2%)

Lab test abnormality	Limit	Percentage of patients (rate per 100 patient-exposure years)	
		Tipranavir 500 mg/ ritonavir 200 mg twice daily + OBR (n = 738)	Comparator PI/ritonavir + OBR[a] (n = 724)
Hematology			
White blood cell count decrease			
Grade 3	< 2 × 10³/mcL	5.4% (5.6)	4.8% (7.7)
Grade 4	< 1 × 10³/mcL	0.3% (0.3)	1.1% (1.7)
Chemistry			
Amylase			
Grade 3	> 2.5 × ULN	5.7% (5.9)	6.4% (10.4)
Grade 4	> 5 × ULN	0.3% (0.3)	0.7% (1.1)
ALT			
Grade 2	> 2.5 to 5 × ULN	14.9% (16.5)	7.5% (12.4)
Grade 3	> 5 to 10 × ULN	5.6% (5.7)	1.7% (2.6)
Grade 4	> 10 × ULN	4.1% (4.1)	0.4% (0.7)
AST			
Grade 2	> 2.5 to 5 × ULN	9.9% (10.5)	8% (13.3)
Grade 3	> 5 to 10 × ULN	4.5% (4.6)	1.4% (2.2)
Grade 4	> 10 × ULN	1.6% (1.6)	0.4% (0.6)
ALT and/or AST			
Grades 2 to 4	> 2.5 × ULN	26% (31.5)	13.7% (23.8)
Cholesterol			
Grade 2	> 300 to 400 mg/dL	15.6% (17.7)	6.4% (10.5)
Grade 3	> 400 to 500 mg/dL	3.3% (3.3)	0.3% (0.4)
Grade 4	> 500 mg/dL	0.9% (1)	0.1% (0.2)
Triglycerides			
Grade 2	400 to 750 mg/dL	35.9% (49.9)	26.8% (51)
Grade 3	> 750 to 1,200 mg/dL	16.9% (19.4)	8.7% (14.6)
Grade 4	> 1,200 mg/dL	8% (8.4)	4.3% (7)

[a] Comparator PI/ritonavir: lopinavir 400 mg/ritonavir 100 mg twice daily, indinavir 800 mg/ritonavir 100 mg twice daily, saquinavir 1,000 mg/ritonavir 100 mg twice daily, amprenavir 600 mg/ritonavir 100 mg twice daily.

In controlled clinical trials 1182.12 and 1182.48 extending up to 96 weeks, the proportion of patients who developed grade 2 to 4 ALT and/or AST elevations increased from 26% at week 48 to 32.1% at week 96 with tipranavir/ritonavir. The risk of developing transaminase elevations is greater during the first year of therapy.

Overdosage

➤*Treatment:* There is no known antidote for tipranavir overdose. Treatment of overdose should consist of general supportive measures, including monitoring of vital signs and observation of the patient's clinical status. If indicated, achieve elimination of unabsorbed tipranavir by gastric lavage. Administration of activated charcoal also may be used to aid in removal of unabsorbed drug. Because tipranavir is highly protein bound, dialysis is unlikely to provide significant removal of this medicine.

Patient Information

Inform patients that tipranavir coadministered with ritonavir 200 mg has been associated with severe liver disease, including some deaths. Instruct patients with signs or symptoms of clinical hepatitis to discontinue tipranavir/ritonavir treatment and seek medical evaluation. Symptoms of hepatitis include fatigue, malaise, anorexia, nausea, jaundice, bilirubinuria, acholic stools, liver tenderness, or hepatomegaly. Extra vigilance is needed for patients with chronic hepatitis B or C coinfection because these patients have an increased risk of hepatotoxicity.

Advise patients that liver function tests will be performed prior to initiating therapy with tipranavir and ritonavir 200 mg and frequently throughout the duration of treatment. Patients with chronic hepatitis B or C coinfection or elevations in liver enzymes prior to treatment are at increased risk (approxi-

TIPRANAVIR — ORAL

mately 2-fold) for developing further liver enzyme elevations or severe liver disease. Exercise caution when administering tipranavir/ritonavir to patients with liver enzyme abnormalities or history of chronic liver disease. Increased liver function testing is warranted in these patients. Do not give tipranavir to patients with moderate to severe hepatic impairment.

Inform patients that tipranavir coadministered with ritonavir 200 mg has been associated with reports of both fatal and nonfatal intracranial hemorrhage. Instruct patients to report any unusual or unexplained bleeding to their health care provider.

Tipranavir may interact with some drugs; therefore, advise patients to report to their health care provider the use of any other prescription or nonprescription medications or herbal products, particularly St. John's wort.

Advise patients taking tipranavir oral solution not to take more supplemental vitamin E than is in a standard multivitamin because tipranavir oral solution contains 116 units/mL of vitamin E and, when taken at the recommended maximum dose of tipranavir 500 mg/ritonavir 200 mg twice daily, results in a daily dose of 1,160 units. This intake is higher than the reference daily intake (adults, 30 units; children, approximately 10 units).

Inform patients that rash, including flat or raised rashes or sensitivity to the sun, has been reported in approximately 10% of subjects receiving tipranavir. Some patients who developed rash also had 1 or more of the following symptoms: joint pain or stiffness, throat tightness, generalized itching, muscle aches, fever, redness, blisters, or peeling of the skin. Women taking birth control pills may get a skin rash. Tell patients to discontinue use of tipranavir and call their health care provider right away if any of these symptoms develop.

Tell patients to report any history of sulfonamide allergy to their health care provider.

Instruct women receiving estrogen-based hormonal contraceptives to use additional or alternative contraceptive measures during therapy with tipranavir/ritonavir. There may be an increased risk of rash when tipranavir is given with hormonal contraceptives.

Inform patients that redistribution or accumulation of body fat may occur in patients receiving antiretroviral therapy, and that the cause and long-term health effects of these conditions are not known at this time.

Inform patients that tipranavir must be coadministered with ritonavir to ensure its therapeutic effect. Failure to correctly coadminister tipranavir with ritonavir will result in reduced plasma levels of tipranavir that may be insufficient to achieve the desired antiviral effect.

Tell patients that sustained decreases in plasma HIV-1 RNA have been associated with a reduced risk of progression to AIDS and death. Instruct patients to remain under the care of a health care provider while using tipranavir. Advise patients to take tipranavir and other concomitant antiretroviral therapy every day as prescribed. Tipranavir coadministered with ritonavir must be given in combination with other antiretroviral drugs. Instruct patients not to alter the dose or discontinue therapy without consulting their health care provider. If a dose of tipranavir is missed, instruct patients to take the dose as soon as possible and then return to their normal schedule. However, if a dose is skipped, advise patients not to double the next dose.

Inform patients that tipranavir is not a cure for HIV-1 infection and that they may continue to develop opportunistic infections and other complications associated with HIV-1 disease. The long-term effects of tipranavir are unknown at this time. Tell patients that there are currently no data demonstrating that therapy with tipranavir can reduce the risk of transmitting HIV-1 to others through sexual contact.

Advise patients that tipranavir can be taken with or without food.

DARUNAVIR

Rx	**Prezista** (Tibotec Therapeutics[a])	**Tablets; oral:** 75 mg	As darunavir ethanolate. (75 TMC). White, capsule shape. Film-coated. In 480s.
		150 mg	As darunavir ethanolate. (150 TMC). White, oval. Film-coated. In 240s.
		400 mg	As darunavir ethanolate. (400 TMC). Light orange, oval. Film-coated. In 60s.
		600 mg	As darunavir ethanolate. (600 TMC). Orange, oval. Film-coated. In 60s.

[a] Tibotec Therapeutics, 1020 Stony Hill Rd, Ste. 300, Yardley, PA 19067; 1-609-730-7500; http://www.tibotectherapeutics.com

DARUNAVIR ETHANOLATE — ORAL

Indications

➤*HIV-1 infection:* For the treatment of HIV-1 infection, coadministered with ritonavir and other antiretroviral agents in adults and children 6 years of age and older.

Administration and Dosage

➤*General dosing considerations:* Darunavir must be coadministered with ritonavir and food to exert its therapeutic effect. Failure to correctly coadminister darunavir with ritonavir will result in plasma levels of darunavir that will be insufficient to achieve the desired antiviral effect and will alter some drug interactions.

➤*Adults:*

HIV-1 infection –

Treatment-naive: 800 mg taken with ritonavir 100 mg once daily and food.

Treatment–experienced:

Darunavir Dosing for Treatment–Experienced Adults

With no darunavir resistance-associated substitutions[a]	With ≥ 1 darunavir resistance-associated substitution[a]
800 mg darunavir once daily with ritonavir 100 mg once daily and food	600 mg darunavir twice daily with ritonavir 100 mg twice daily and food

[a] V11I, V32I, L33F, I47V, I50V, I54L, I54M, T74P, L76V, I84V, and L89V.

For antiretroviral treatment–experienced patients genotypic testing is recommended. However, when genotypic testing is not feasible, darunavir 600 mg with ritonavir 100 mg twice-daily dosing is recommended.

➤*Children:*

HIV-1 infection –

6 to younger than 18 years of age and weighing at least 20 kg:

• *Usual dosage –*

Darunavir Recommended Dosage for Children

Body weight	Dosage
≥ 20 kg to < 30 kg	Darunavir 375 mg with ritonavir 50 mg twice daily and food
≥ 30 kg to < 40 kg	Darunavir 450 mg with ritonavir 60 mg twice daily and food
≥ 40 kg	Darunavir 600 mg with ritonavir 100 mg twice daily and food

• *Maximum dose –* Darunavir 600 mg with ritonavir 100 mg twice daily.

➤*Hepatic function impairment:* Darunavir/ritonavir is not recommended for use in patients with severe hepatic impairment.

➤*Missed dose:* In patients taking darunavir once daily, if the patient misses a dose of darunavir or ritonavir by more than 12 hours, instruct the patient to wait and then take the next dose of darunavir and ritonavir at the regularly scheduled time. If the patient misses a dose of darunavir or ritonavir by less than 12 hours, instruct the patient to take darunavir and ritonavir immediately, and then take the next dose of darunavir and ritonavir at the regularly scheduled time. If a dose of darunavir or ritonavir is skipped, advise the patient not to double the next dose. Inform the patient not to take more or less than the prescribed dose of darunavir or ritonavir.

In patients taking darunavir twice daily, if the patient misses a dose of darunavir or ritonavir by more than 6 hours, instruct the patient to wait and then take the next dose of darunavir and ritonavir at the regularly scheduled time. If the patient misses a dose of darunavir or ritonavir by less than 6 hours, instruct the patient to take darunavir and ritonavir immediately, and then take the next dose of darunavir and ritonavir at the regularly scheduled time. If a dose of darunavir or ritonavir is skipped, instruct the patient not to double the next dose. Instruct the patient not to take more or less than the prescribed dose of darunavir or ritonavir.

➤*Administration:* Administer with food. Before prescribing darunavir, children should be assessed for the ability to swallow tablets. If a child is unable to reliably swallow a tablet, the use of darunavir may not be appropriate. Do not use once-daily dosing in children.

➤*Storage/Stability:* Store at 25°C (77°F); excursions are permitted between 15° and 30°C (59° and 86°F).

Actions

➤*Pharmacology:* Darunavir, an HIV antiviral drug, is an inhibitor of the HIV protease. It selectively inhibits the cleavage of HIV-encoded Gag-Pol polyproteins in infected cells, thereby preventing the formation of mature virus particles.

➤*Pharmacokinetics:*

Absorption – Darunavir, coadministered with ritonavir 100 mg twice daily, was absorbed following oral administration with a time to maximum concentration of approximately 2.5 to 4 hours. The absolute oral bioavailability of a single dose of darunavir 600 mg alone and after coadministration with ritonavir 100 mg twice daily was 37% and 82%, respectively.

Darunavir is primarily metabolized by CYP3A. Ritonavir inhibits CYP3A, thereby increasing the plasma concentrations of darunavir. When a single dose of darunavir 600 mg was given orally in combination with ritonavir 100 mg twice daily, there was an approximate 14-fold increase in the systemic exposure of darunavir. Therefore, only use darunavir in combination with ritonavir 100 mg to achieve sufficient exposures of darunavir.

Effect of food: When administered with food, the maximum effective plasma concentration and area under the curve (AUC) of darunavir coadministered with ritonavir is approximately 30% higher relative to the fasting state. Therefore, always take darunavir tablets coadministered with ritonavir with food.

Distribution – Darunavir is approximately 95% bound to plasma proteins. Darunavir binds primarily to plasma alpha-1 acid glycoprotein.

DARUNAVIR ETHANOLATE — ORAL

Metabolism – In vitro experiments with human liver microsomes indicate that darunavir primarily undergoes oxidative metabolism. Darunavir is extensively metabolized by CYP enzymes, primarily by CYP3A. A mass-balance study in healthy volunteers showed that after a single-dose administration of ^{14}C-darunavir 400 mg coadministered with ritonavir 100 mg, the majority of the radioactivity in the plasma was caused by darunavir. At least 3 oxidative metabolites of darunavir have been identified in humans; all showed activity that was at least 90% less than the activity of darunavir against wild-type HIV.

In vivo data suggest that darunavir/ritonavir is an inhibitor of the P-glycoprotein transporters.

Excretion – A mass-balance study in healthy volunteers showed that after single-dose administration of ^{14}C-darunavir 400 mg coadministered with ritonavir 100 mg, approximately 79.5% and 13.9% of the administered dose of ^{14}C-darunavir was recovered in the feces and urine, respectively. Unchanged darunavir accounted for approximately 41.2% and 7.7% of the administered dose in feces and urine, respectively. The terminal elimination half-life of darunavir was approximately 15 hours when combined with ritonavir. After intravenous administration, the clearance of darunavir, administered alone and coadministered with twice-daily ritonavir 100 mg, was 32.8 L/h and 5.9 L/h, respectively.

Special populations –

Gender: Population pharmacokinetic analysis showed higher mean darunavir exposure in HIV-infected women compared with men. This difference is not clinically relevant.

Contraindications

Coadministration with drugs that are highly dependent on CYP3A for clearance and drugs for which elevated plasma concentrations are associated with serious and/or life-threatening events (narrow therapeutic index) (eg, alfuzosin, ergot derivatives [dihydroergotamine, ergonovine, ergotamine, methylergonovine]; cisapride; pimozide; orally administered midazolam; triazolam; St. John's wort; lovastatin; simvastatin; rifampin).

Phosphodiesterase type 5 (PDE5) inhibitors (eg, sildenafil for treatment of pulmonary arterial hypertension) are contraindicated. A safe and effective dose for the treatment of pulmonary arterial hypertension has not been established. There is an increased potential for sildenafil-associated adverse events, which include visual disturbances, hypotension, prolonged erection, and syncope.

Warnings/Precautions

➤*Administration:* See Administration and Dosage for more information.

➤*Hepatotoxicity:* Drug-induced hepatitis (eg, acute hepatitis, cytolytic hepatitis) has been reported with darunavir/ritonavir. During the clinical development program, hepatitis was reported in 0.5% of patients receiving combination therapy with darunavir/ritonavir. Patients with preexisting hepatic impairment, including chronic active hepatitis B or C, have an increased risk for hepatic function abnormalities, including severe hepatic adverse reactions.

Postmarketing cases of liver injury, including some fatalities, have been reported. These have generally occurred in patients with advanced HIV-1 disease taking multiple concomitant medications, having comorbidities (eg, hepatitis B or C coinfection), and/or developing immune reconstitution syndrome. A causal relationship with darunavir/ritonavir therapy has not been established.

Conduct appropriate laboratory testing prior to initiating therapy with darunavir/ritonavir, and monitor patients during treatment. Consider increased AST/ALT monitoring in patients with underlying chronic hepatitis or cirrhosis or in patients who have pretreatment elevations of transaminases, especially during the first several months of darunavir/ritonavir treatment.

If there is evidence of new or worsening liver dysfunction (including clinically significant elevations of liver enzymes and/or symptoms such as anorexia, dark urine, fatigue, hepatomegaly, jaundice, liver tenderness, nausea) in patients on darunavir/ritonavir, interruption or discontinuation of treatment must be considered.

➤*Dermatologic effects:* During the clinical development program, severe skin reactions, accompanied by fever and/or elevations of transaminases in some cases, have been reported in 0.4% of subjects. Stevens-Johnson syndrome was rarely (less than 0.1%) reported during the clinical development program. During postmarketing experience, toxic epidermal necrolysis has been reported. Discontinue darunavir/ritonavir immediately if signs or symptoms of severe skin reactions develop. These can include, but are not limited to, severe rash or rash accompanied with fever, general malaise, fatigue, muscle or joint aches, blisters, oral lesions, conjunctivitis, hepatitis, and/or eosinophilia.

Rash (all grades, regardless of causality) occurred in 10.3% of subjects treated with darunavir. Rash was mostly mild to moderate, often occurring within the first 4 weeks of treatment and resolving with continued dosing. The discontinuation rate because of rash in subjects using darunavir/ritonavir was 0.5%.

➤*Sulfa allergy:* Darunavir contains a sulfonamide moiety. Use darunavir with caution in patients with known sulfonamide allergy. In clinical studies with darunavir/ritonavir, the incidence and severity of rash was similar in subjects with or without a history of sulfonamide allergy.

➤*Diabetes mellitus/hyperglycemia:* New-onset diabetes mellitus, exacerbation of preexisting diabetes mellitus, and hyperglycemia have been reported during postmarketing surveillance in HIV-infected patients receiving protease inhibitor therapy. Some patients required initiation or dosage adjustments of insulin or oral hypoglycemic agents for treatment of these reactions. In some cases, diabetic ketoacidosis has occurred. In those patients who discontinued protease inhibitor therapy, hyperglycemia persisted in some cases. Because these reactions have been reported voluntarily during clinical practice, estimates of frequency cannot be made, and causal relationships between protease inhibitor therapy and these reactions have not been established.

➤*Fat redistribution:* Redistribution/accumulation of body fat, including central obesity, dorsocervical fat enlargement (buffalo hump), peripheral wasting, facial wasting, breast enlargement, and "cushingoid appearance" have been observed in patients receiving antiretroviral therapy. The mechanism and long-term consequences of these reactions are currently unknown. A causal relationship has not been established.

➤*Immune reconstitution syndrome:* During the initial phase of treatment, patients responding to antiretroviral therapy may develop an inflammatory response to indolent or residual opportunistic infections (eg, cytomegalovirus, *Mycobacterium avium* complex, *Pneumocystis jeroveci* pneumonia, tuberculosis), which may necessitate further evaluation and treatment.

➤*Hemophilia:* There have been reports of increased bleeding, including spontaneous skin hematomas and hemarthrosis, in patients with hemophilia type A and B treated with protease inhibitors. In some patients, additional factor VIII was given. In more than half of the reported cases, treatment with protease inhibitors was continued or reintroduced if treatment had been discontinued. A causal relationship between protease inhibitor therapy and these episodes has not been established.

➤*Resistance/Cross-resistance:* Because the potential for HIV cross-resistance among protease inhibitors has not been fully explored in darunavir/ritonavir–treated patients; it is unknown what effect therapy with darunavir will have on the activity of subsequently administered protease inhibitors.

➤*Hepatic function impairment:* Darunavir/ritonavir is not recommended for use in patients with severe hepatic impairment.

➤*Pregnancy:* *Category C* (per manufacturer's prescribing information); *Category B* (per Briggs' *Drugs in Pregnancy and Lactation*).

No adequate and well-controlled studies have been conducted in pregnant women. It is not known if darunavir crosses the human placenta. The molecular weight (about 594) and prolonged elimination half-life suggest that the drug will cross to the embryo and fetus. Use darunavir during pregnancy only if the potential benefit justifies the potential risk.

In the rat pre-and postnatal development study, a reduction in pup body weight gain was observed with darunavir alone or in combination with ritonavir during lactation. This was because of exposure of pups to drug substances via the milk.

In the juvenile toxicity study where rats were directly dosed with darunavir, deaths occurred from postnatal day 5 through day 11 at plasma exposure levels ranging from 0.1 to 1 of the human exposure levels.

In 2006, the updated US Department of Health and Human Services guidelines for the use of antiretroviral agents in HIV-1–infected patients continued the recommendation that therapy, with the exception of efavirenz, should be continued during pregnancy. Therefore, if indicated, protease inhibitors, including darunavir, should not be withheld in pregnancy because the expected benefit to the HIV-positive mother outweighs the unknown risk to the fetus.

Antiretroviral pregnancy registry – To monitor maternal-fetal outcomes of pregnant women exposed to darunavir, an antiretroviral pregnancy registry has been established. Patients can be registered by calling 1-800-258-4263.

➤*Lactation:* The Centers for Disease Control and Prevention recommend that HIV-infected mothers not breast-feed their infants in order to avoid risking postnatal transmission of HIV. Although it is not known whether darunavir is secreted in human milk, darunavir is secreted into the milk of lactating rats. The molecular weight (about 594) and prolonged elimination half-life (about 15 hours) suggest that the drug will be excreted into breast milk. The effects on a breast-feeding infant are not known. Because of the potential for HIV transmission and the potential for serious adverse reactions in breast-feeding infants, instruct mothers not to breast-feed if they are receiving darunavir.

➤*Children:* Do not administer darunavir/ritonavir in children younger than 3 years of age, in view of toxicity and mortality observed in juvenile rats dosed with darunavir (from 20 mg/kg to 1,000 mg/kg) up to days 23 to 26 of age. The safety, pharmacokinetics, tolerability, and efficacy of darunavir/ritonavir in children 3 to younger than 6 years of age have not been established.

Do not administer darunavir/ritonavir once daily in children.

➤*Elderly:* In general, exercise caution in administration and monitoring of darunavir in elderly patients, reflecting the greater frequency of decreased hepatic function and of concomitant disease or other drug therapy.

➤*Monitoring:* Conduct appropriate laboratory testing prior to initiating therapy with darunavir/ritonavir, and monitor patients during treatment. Consider increased AST/ALT monitoring in patients with underlying chronic hepatitis, cirrhosis, or in patients who have pretreatment elevations of transaminases, especially during the first several months of darunavir/ritonavir treatment. Monitor pregnant women taking protease inhibitors for hyperglycemia.

DARUNAVIR ETHANOLATE — ORAL

Drug Interactions

➤*Protease inhibitors:*

Cytochrome P450 system – Darunavir and ritonavir are inhibitors of CYP3A and CYP2D6. Coadministration of darunavir and ritonavir with drugs that are primarily metabolized by CYP3A and CYP2D6 may result in increased plasma concentrations of such drugs, which could increase or prolong their therapeutic effect and adverse reactions. Darunavir and ritonavir are metabolized by CYP3A. Drugs that induce CYP3A activity would be expected to increase the clearance of darunavir and ritonavir, resulting in lowered plasma concentrations of darunavir and ritonavir. Coadministration of darunavir and ritonavir and other drugs that inhibit CYP3A may decrease the clearance of darunavir and ritonavir and may result in increased plasma concentrations of darunavir and ritonavir.

Darunavir Drug Interactions

Precipitant drug	Object drug[a]		Description
Alpha-1 adrenoreceptor antagonists (eg, alfuzosin)	Darunavir	↑	There is a potential for serious and/or life-threatening reactions, such as hypotension if coadministered. Coadministration is contraindicated.
Anticonvulsants (eg, phenobarbital, phenytoin)	Darunavir	↓	Coadministration may cause a significant decrease in darunavir or anticonvulsant plasma concentrations and may result in loss of therapeutic effect. If this coadministration cannot be avoided, monitor phenytoin and phenobarbital concentrations and adjust the dose as needed.
Darunavir	Anticonvulsants (eg, phenobarbital, phenytoin)	↓	
Azole antifungals (eg, itraconazole, ketoconazole)	Darunavir	↑	Concomitant systemic use of ketoconazole or itraconazole may increase plasma concentrations of darunavir. Plasma concentrations of ketoconazole or itraconazole may be increased in the presence of darunavir/ritonavir. When coadministration is required, do not exceed a daily dose of ketoconazole or itraconazole 200 mg. Do not administer voriconazole to patients receiving darunavir/ritonavir unless an assessment of the benefit/risk ratio justifies the use.
Darunavir	Azole antifungals (eg, itraconazole, ketoconazole, voriconazole)	↑	
Carbamazepine	Darunavir	↓	Carbamazepine may decrease plasma concentrations and pharmacologic effects of darunavir. Darunavir may increase carbamazepine plasma concentrations. Close clinical monitoring is indicated if concomitant use cannot be avoided. Consider drugs other than carbamazepine as an alternative. Amitriptyline, gabapentin, or tramadol may be alternatives for postherpetic neuralgia; valproic acid or lamotrigine may be alternatives for seizures.
Darunavir	Carbamazepine	↑	
Corticosteroids (eg, dexamethasone)	Darunavir	↓	Systemic dexamethasone induces CYP3A and can thereby decrease darunavir plasma concentrations, resulting in loss of darunavir therapeutic effect. Use with caution. Concomitant use of inhaled fluticasone and darunavir/ritonavir may increase plasma concentrations of fluticasone. Consider an alternative to fluticasone, especially for long-term use.
Darunavir	Corticosteroids (eg, inhaled fluticasone, propionate)	↑	
Indinavir	Darunavir	↑	The appropriate dose of indinavir in combination with darunavir/ritonavir has not been established.
Darunavir	Indinavir		
Lopinavir/Ritonavir	Darunavir	↓	Coadministration may decrease plasma concentrations of darunavir and may increase plasma concentrations of lopinavir. Appropriate doses of this combination have not been established. It is not recommended to coadminister lopinavir/ritonavir and darunavir with or without ritonavir.
Darunavir	Lopinavir/Ritonavir	↑	
NNRT inhibitors[b] (eg, efavirenz, nevirapine)	Darunavir	↓	Coadministration may decrease darunavir plasma levels and clinical efficacy may be reduced. Efavirenz and nevirapine concentrations may be increased while etravirine concentrations may be decreased. Use with caution. Monitor the response of the patient and adjust treatment as needed.
Darunavir	NNRT inhibitors (eg, efavirenz, nevirapine)	↑↓	
Rifamycins (eg, rifabutin, rifampin)	Darunavir	↑↓	Coadministration is contraindicated; rifampin may cause significant decreases in darunavir plasma concentrations, resulting in loss of therapeutic effect. Concomitant use of rifabutin and darunavir in the presence of ritonavir is expected to increase rifabutin plasma concentrations and decrease darunavir plasma concentrations. Administer rifabutin 150 mg once every other day when coadministered with darunavir/ritonavir. Increase monitoring for adverse reactions. Further rifabutin dose reductions may be necessary.
Darunavir	Rifamycins (eg, rifabutin)	↑	
Saquinavir	Darunavir	↓	Darunavir AUC may decrease by approximately 26%. It is not recommended to coadminister saquinavir and darunavir, with or without ritonavir.
St. John's wort	Darunavir	↓	St. John's wort may cause significant decreases in darunavir plasma concentrations, which may result in loss of therapeutic effect. Coadministration is contraindicated.
Darunavir	Antiarrhythmic agents (eg, amiodarone, bepridil, flecainide, lidocaine, propafenone, quinidine)	↑	Coadministration may increase the concentrations of these antiarrhythmics. Use with caution and monitor therapeutic concentrations.
Darunavir	Antipsychotics (eg, risperidone, thioridazine)	↑	A dose decrease may be needed for these drugs when coadministered with darunavir/ritonavir. Monitor the clinical response of the patient.
Darunavir	Benzodiazepines (eg, midazolam, triazolam)	↑	Coadministration is contraindicated with triazolam and orally administered midazolam because of the risk of potential life-threatening reactions, such as prolonged or increased sedation or respiratory depression. Concomitant use of IV midazolam and darunavir/ritonavir may increase plasma concentrations of midazolam. Closely monitor for respiratory function and prolonged sedation. Consider midazolam dose reduction, especially if more than a single IV midazolam dose is administered.

DARUNAVIR ETHANOLATE — ORAL

Darunavir Drug Interactions

Precipitant drug	Object drug[a]		Description
Darunavir	Beta-blockers (eg, metoprolol, timolol)	↑	Use with caution. A dosage decrease may be needed for these beta-blockers when coadministered with darunavir/ritonavir.
Darunavir	Calcium channel blockers (eg, felodipine, nicardipine, nifedipine)	↑	Plasma concentrations of felodipine, nicardipine, and nifedipine may increase when administered with darunavir/ritonavir. Administer with caution and monitor patients.
Darunavir	Cisapride[c]	↑	Coadministration is contraindicated because of the potential for serious and/or life-threatening reactions, such as cardiac arrhythmias.
Darunavir	Clarithromycin	↑	Concurrent use may increase clarithromycin levels. Dosage adjustment is not needed in patients with healthy renal function. For patients with a CrCl 30 to 60 mL/min, decrease clarithromycin dose by 50%. For patients with a CrCl less than 30 mL/min, decrease clarithromycin dose 75%.
Darunavir	Colchicine	↑	Colchicine plasma concentrations may be elevated, increasing the risk of life-threatening and fatal colchicine toxicity. Coadministration of darunavir and colchicine is contraindicated in patients with renal or hepatic impairment. In patients with normal renal and hepatic function, undertake coadministration of darunavir and colchicine using a maximum colchicine dose of 0.3 mg twice daily, with close monitoring for colchicine-related adverse reactions.
Darunavir	Contraceptives, hormonal (eg, ethinyl estradiol, norethindrone)	↓	Concurrent use may decrease plasma concentrations of ethinyl estradiol because of induction of metabolism by ritonavir. Use alternative or additional contraceptive measures when estrogen-containing contraceptives are coadministered.
Darunavir	Desipramine	↑	Concomitant use may increase plasma concentrations of desipramine. Use with caution and consider a lower dose of desipramine.
Darunavir	Dextromethorphan	↑	Plasma concentrations of dextromethorphan may be increased. Monitor the patient for dextromethorphan-induced adverse reactions. If an interaction is suspected, adjust the dextromethorphan dose as needed.
Darunavir	Didanosine	↔	It is recommended that didanosine be administered on an empty stomach. Therefore, administer didanosine 1 hour before or 2 hours after darunavir/ritonavir (which are administered with food).
Didanosine	Darunavir		
Darunavir	Digoxin	↑	Concomitant use of darunavir/ritonavir with digoxin results in a significant increase in serum concentrations of digoxin. Monitor digoxin levels closely and use the lowest possible dose. Use digoxin serum concentrations to gauge digoxin dose titration.
Darunavir	Dronedarone	↑	Plasma concentrations and pharmacologic effects of dronedarone may be increased by darunavir. Coadministration of dronedarone and darunavir/ritonavir is contraindicated.
Darunavir	Ergot derivatives (eg, dihydroergotamine, ergonovine)	↑	Concomitant use may increase the potential for serious and/or life-threatening reactions (eg, acute ergot toxicity characterized by peripheral vasospasm and ischemia of the extremities and other tissues). Coadministration is contraindicated.
Darunavir	HMG-CoA reductase inhibitors (eg, atorvastatin, lovastatin, pravastatin, rosuvastatin, simvastatin)	↑	Coadministration may increase the risk for serious reactions, such as myopathy, including rhabdomyolysis. It is recommended to start with the lowest possible dose of atorvastatin, pravastatin, or rosuvastatin with careful monitoring, or consider using fluvastatin. Concurrent use increased pravastatin AUC by 81%. Coadministration with lovastatin and simvastatin is contraindicated.
Darunavir	Immunosuppressants (eg, cyclosporine, sirolimus, tacrolimus)	↑	Coadministration may increase plasma concentrations of cyclosporine, sirolimus, or tacrolimus. Therapeutic concentration monitoring of the immunosuppressive agent is recommended.
Darunavir	Iloperidone	↑	Plasma concentrations and pharmacologic effects of iloperidone may be increased by darunavir. Reduce the dose of iloperidone by one-half when coadministered with darunavir. If therapy with darunavir is discontinued, increase the dose of iloperidone to the original dose.
Darunavir	Maraviroc	↑	Concomitant use may increase plasma concentrations of maraviroc. When used in combination, the maraviroc dose should be 150 mg twice daily.
Darunavir	Methadone	↓	During concurrent use, monitor patients for opiate-abstinence syndrome. Methadone dosage may need to be increased.
Darunavir	Omeprazole	↓	Plasma concentrations of omeprazole may be decreased, reducing the efficacy. Monitor the patient. If an interaction is suspected, it may be necessary to increase the omeprazole dose.
Darunavir	Opioid analgesics (eg, buprenorphine, fentanyl)	↑	Opioid analgesic plasma concentrations may be increased and the half-life prolonged, increasing the risk of adverse reactions (eg, respiratory depression). Closely monitor respiratory function.
Darunavir	PDE5 inhibitors	↑	Use concomitantly with caution. The PDE5 inhibitor dose should not exceed the following when coadministered with darunavir/ritonavir: sildenafil 25 mg within 48 hours; tadalafil 10 mg within 72 hours; or vardenafil 2.5 mg within 72 hours. Coadministration with sildenafil is contraindicated when used for the treatment of pulmonary arterial hypertension. (See Contraindications.)
Darunavir	Pimozide	↑	Coadministration is contraindicated because of the potential for life-threatening reactions, such as cardiac arrhythmias.

DARUNAVIR ETHANOLATE — ORAL

Darunavir Drug Interactions

Precipitant drug	Object drug[a]		Description
Darunavir	Quetiapine	↑	Quetiapine plasma concentrations may be elevated, increasing the pharmacologic effects and risk of adverse reactions. Use with caution and closely monitor the patient. Adjust the quetiapine dose as needed.
Darunavir	SSRIs[b] (eg, paroxetine, sertraline)	↓	The SSRI dose may need to be carefully titrated based on antidepressant response.
Darunavir	Tenofovir	↑	Darunavir/ritonavir increased the AUC of tenofovir by 22%. This change is not considered clinically important.
Darunavir	Trazodone	↑	Concomitant use may increase plasma concentrations of trazodone. Use with caution and consider a lower dose of trazodone.
Darunavir	Warfarin	↓	Warfarin concentrations may be decreased during coadministration. Monitor the international normalized ratio frequently upon initiation of darunavir/ritonavir.

[a] ↑ = object drug increased; ↓ = object drug decreased; ↑↓ = object drug both increased and decreased; ↔ = undetermined clinical effect.
[b] NNRT = nonnucleoside reverse transcriptase; SSRI = selective serotonin reuptake inhibitor.
[c] Available from the manufacturer on a limited-access protocol.

Because of the need for darunavir to be coadministered with ritonavir, refer to the ritonavir monograph for additional drug interactions.

➤*Drug/Food interactions:* See Actions for more information.

Adverse Reactions

➤*Treatment-naive adults:*

Common adverse reactions – The most common adverse reactions from darunavir 800 mg/ritonavir 100 mg once daily (at least 5%) of at least moderate intensity (at least grade 2) were abdominal pain, diarrhea, headache, and rash.

Discontinuation – 2.3% of subjects in the darunavir arm discontinued treatment because of adverse reactions.

Adverse reactions (at least 2%) –

Darunavir Adverse Reactions [a] (≥ Grade 2) in Treatment-Naive Adults (≥ 2%)

Adverse reactions	Darunavir 800 mg/ritonavir 100 mg once daily + tenofovir disoproxil fumarate/emtricitabine (n = 343)	Lopinavir 800 mg/ritonavir 200 mg per day + tenofovir disoproxil fumarate/emtricitabine (n = 346)
CNS		
Fatigue	< 1%	3%
Headache	6%	5%
Dermatologic		
Rash	5%	6%
GI		
Abdominal pain	5%	6%
Anorexia	2%	< 1%
Diarrhea	8%	15%
Nausea	3%	4%
Vomiting	2%	3%

[a] Excluding laboratory abnormalities reported as adverse drug reactions.

Adverse reactions (less than 2%) –

CNS: Abnormal dreams, asthenia.
Dermatologic: Angioedema, pruritus, Stevens-Johnson syndrome, urticaria.
GI: Acute pancreatitis, dyspepsia, flatulence.
Hepatic: Acute hepatitis (eg, cytolytic hepatitis, hepatotoxicity).
Miscellaneous: Diabetes mellitus, hypersensitivity, myalgia.

Laboratory abnormalities –

Darunavir Grade 2 to 4 Laboratory Abnormalities in Treatment-Naive Adults[a]

Laboratory abnormality	Limit	Darunavir 800 mg/ritonavir 100 mg once daily + tenofovir disoproxil fumarate/emtricitabine (n = 343)	Lopinavir 800 mg/ritonavir 200 mg per day + tenofovir disoproxil fumarate/emtricitabine (n = 346)
ALT			
Grade 2	> 2.5 to ≤ 5 × ULN[b]	7%	6%
Grade 3	> 5 to ≤ 10 × ULN	3%	3%
Grade 4	> 10 × ULN	< 1%	3%
AST			
Grade 2	> 2.5 to ≤ 5 × ULN	6%	6%
Grade 3	> 5 to ≤ 10 × ULN	4%	2%
Grade 4	> 10 × ULN	1%	2%
Alkaline phosphatase			
Grade 2	> 2.5 to ≤ 5 × ULN	2%	1%
Grade 3	> 5 to ≤ 10 × ULN	0%	< 1%
Grade 4	> 10 × ULN	0%	0%
Hyperbilirubinemia			
Grade 2	> 1.5 to ≤ 2.5 × ULN	< 1%	4%
Grade 3	> 2.5 to ≤ 5 × ULN	< 1%	< 1%
Grade 4	> 5 × ULN	0%	0%
Triglycerides			
Grade 2	5.65 to 8.48 mmol/L 500 to 750 mg/dL	3%	8%
Grade 3	8.49 to 13.56 mmol/L 751 to 1,200 mg/dL	1%	5%
Grade 4	> 13.56 mmol/L > 1,200 mg/dL	< 1%	< 1%
Total cholesterol			
Grade 2	6.2 to 7.77 mmol/L 240 to 300 mg/dL	16%	23%
Grade 3	> 7.77 mmol/L > 300 mg/dL	1%	5%
LDL[c] cholesterol			
Grade 2	4.13 to 4.9 mmol/L 160 to 190 mg/dL	14%	10%
Grade 3	≥ 4.91 mmol/L ≥ 191 mg/dL	5%	5%
Elevated glucose levels			
Grade 2	6.95 to 13.88 mmol/L 126 to 250 mg/dL	7%	8%
Grade 3	13.89 to 27.75 mmol/L 251 to 500 mg/dL	< 1%	0%
Grade 4	> 27.75 mmol/L > 500 mg/dL	0%	0%
Pancreatic lipase			
Grade 2	> 1.5 to ≤ 3 × ULN	2%	1%
Grade 3	> 3 to ≤ 5 × ULN	< 1%	< 1%
Grade 4	> 5 × ULN	0%	< 1%
Pancreatic amylase			
Grade 2	> 1.5 to ≤ 2 × ULN	5%	2%
Grade 3	> 2 to ≤ 5 × ULN	3%	3%
Grade 4	> 5 × ULN	0%	< 1%

[a] Grade 4 data not applicable in Division of AIDS grading scale.
[b] ULN = upper limit of normal.
[c] LDL = low-density lipoprotein.

➤*Treatment-experienced adults:*

Common adverse reactions – The most common adverse reactions to darunavir 600 mg/ritonavir 100 mg twice daily (at least 5%) of at least moderate intensity (at least grade 2) were abdominal pain, diarrhea, nausea, rash, and vomiting.

Discontinuation – 4.7% of subjects in the darunavir/ritonavir arm discontinued treatment because of adverse reactions.

DARUNAVIR ETHANOLATE — ORAL

Adverse reactions (2% or more) –

Darunavir Adverse Reactions (≥ Grade 2) in Treatment-Experienced Adults (≥ 2%)[a]

Adverse reactions	Darunavir 600 mg/ ritonavir 100 mg twice daily + OBR[b] (n = 298)	Lopinavir 400 mg/ ritonavir 100 mg twice daily + OBR (n = 297)
CNS		
Asthenia	3%	1%
Fatigue	2%	1%
Headache	3%	3%
GI		
Abdominal distension	2%	< 1%
Abdominal pain	6%	3%
Anorexia	2%	2%
Diarrhea	14%	20%
Dyspepsia	2%	1%
Nausea	7%	6%
Vomiting	5%	3%
Miscellaneous		
Diabetes mellitus	2%	< 1%
Rash	7%	3%

[a] Excluding laboratory abnormalities reported as adverse drug reactions.
[b] OBR = optimized background regimen.

Adverse reactions (less than 2%) –

Dermatologic: Pruritus, urticaria.
GI: Acute pancreatitis, flatulence.
Miscellaneous: Abnormal dreams, myalgia.

Laboratory abnormalities –

Darunavir Grade 2 to 4 Laboratory Abnormalities in Treatment-Experienced Adults[a]

Laboratory abnormality	Limit	Darunavir 600 mg/ ritonavir 100 mg twice daily + OBR[b] (n = 298)	Lopinavir 400 mg/ ritonavir 100 mg twice daily + OBR (n = 297)
ALT			
Grade 2	> 2.5 to ≤ 5 × ULN	7%	5%
Grade 3	> 5 to ≤ 10 × ULN	2%	2%
Grade 4	> 10 × ULN	1%	2%
AST			
Grade 2	> 2.5 to ≤ 5 × ULN	6%	6%
Grade 3	> 5 to ≤ 10 × ULN	2%	2%
Grade 4	> 10 × ULN	< 1%	2%
Alkaline phosphatase			
Grade 2	> 2.5 to ≤ 5 × ULN	< 1%	0%
Grade 3	> 5 to ≤ 10 × ULN	< 1%	< 1%
Grade 4	> 10 × ULN	0%	0%
Hyperbilirubinemia			
Grade 2	> 1.5 to ≤ 2.5 × ULN	< 1%	2%
Grade 3	> 2.5 to ≤ 5 × ULN	< 1%	< 1%
Grade 4	> 5 × ULN	< 1%	0%
Triglycerides			
Grade 2	5.65 to 8.48 mmol/L 500 to 750 mg/dL	10%	11%
Grade 3	8.49 to 13.56 mmol/L 751 to 1,200 mg/dL	7%	10%
Grade 4	> 13.56 mmol/L > 1,200 mg/dL	3%	6%
Total cholesterol			
Grade 2	6.2 to 7.77 mmol/L 240 to 300 mg/dL	25%	23%
Grade 3	> 7.77 mmol/L > 300 mg/dL	10%	14%
LDL cholesterol			
Grade 2	4.13 to 4.9 mmol/L 160 to 190 mg/dL	14%	14%
Grade 3	≥ 4.91 mmol/L ≥ 191 mg/dL	8%	9%
Elevated glucose levels			
Grade 2	6.95 to 13.88 mmol/L 126 to 250 mg/dL	10%	11%
Grade 3	13.89 to 27.75 mmol/L 251 to 500 mg/dL	1%	< 1%
Grade 4	> 27.75 mmol/L > 500 mg/dL	< 1%	0%
Pancreatic lipase			
Grade 2	> 1.5 to ≤ 3 × ULN	3%	4%
Grade 3	> 3 to ≤ 5 × ULN	2%	< 1%
Grade 4	> 5 × ULN	< 1%	0%
Pancreatic amylase			
Grade 2	> 1.5 to ≤ 2 × ULN	6%	7%
Grade 3	> 2 to ≤ 5 × ULN	7%	3%
Grade 4	> 5 × ULN	0%	0%

[a] Grade 4 data not applicable in Division of AIDS grading scale.
[b] OBR = optimized background regimen.

➤*Serious adverse reactions (at least grade 2):*

CNS – Asthenia, fatigue, headache.

Dermatologic – Rash, Stevens-Johnson syndrome.

Endocrine – Diabetes mellitus, hypercholesterolemia, hyperglycemia, hypertriglyceridemia.

GI – Abdominal pain, acute hepatitis, acute pancreatitis, anorexia, diarrhea, hepatic enzyme increased, nausea, pancreatic enzyme increased, vomiting.

Miscellaneous – Immune reconstitution syndrome, LDL increased; osteonecrosis (identified from other clinical trials).

➤*Children:* Adverse reactions from darunavir/ritonavir (all grades, at least 3%), excluding laboratory abnormalities reported as adverse reactions, were vomiting (13%), diarrhea (11%), abdominal pain (10%), headache (9%), rash (5%), nausea (4%), and fatigue (3%).

Grade 3 or 4 laboratory abnormalities were ALT increased (grade 3, 3%; grade 4, 1%), AST increased (grade 3, 1%), pancreatic amylase increased (grade 3, 4%, grade 4, 1%), pancreatic lipase increased (grade 3, 1%), total cholesterol increased (grade 3, 1%), and LDL increased (grade 3, 3%).

➤*Postmarketing:*

Dermatologic – Toxic epidermal necrolysis.

Miscellaneous – Redistribution of body fat, rhabdomyolysis (associated with coadministration with HMG-CoA reductase inhibitors and darunavir/ritonavir).

Overdosage

➤*Treatment:* There is no specific antidote for overdose with darunavir. Treatment of overdose with darunavir consists of general supportive measures, including monitoring of vital signs and observation of the clinical status of the patient. If indicated, elimination of unabsorbed active substance is to be achieved by gastric lavage. Administration of activated charcoal may also be used to aid in removal of unabsorbed active substance. Because darunavir is highly protein bound, dialysis is unlikely to be beneficial in significant removal of the active substance.

Patient Information

Inform patients that darunavir is not a cure for HIV infection and that they may continue to develop opportunistic infections and other complications associated with HIV disease. Inform patients that there are currently no data demonstrating that therapy with darunavir can reduce the risk of transmitting HIV to others.

Inform patients that sustained decreases in plasma HIV RNA have been associated with a reduced risk of progression to AIDS and death. Instruct patients to remain under the care of a health care provider while using darunavir.

Advise patients to take darunavir and ritonavir with food every day as prescribed. Instruct patients to swallow the tablets whole with a drink, such as water or milk. Darunavir must always be used with ritonavir 100 mg in combination with other antiretroviral drugs. Instruct patients not to alter

DARUNAVIR ETHANOLATE — ORAL

the dose of darunavir or ritonavir, discontinue ritonavir, or discontinue therapy with darunavir without consulting their health care provider.

In patients taking darunavir once daily, if the patient misses a dose of darunavir or ritonavir by more than 12 hours, instruct the patient to wait and then take the next dose of darunavir and ritonavir at the regularly scheduled time. If the patient misses a dose of darunavir or ritonavir by less than 12 hours, instruct the patient to take darunavir and ritonavir immediately, and then take the next dose of darunavir and ritonavir at the regularly scheduled time. If a dose of darunavir or ritonavir is skipped, advise the patient not to double the next dose. Inform the patient not to take more or less than the prescribed dose of darunavir or ritonavir.

In patients taking darunavir twice daily, if the patient misses a dose of darunavir or ritonavir by more than 6 hours, instruct the patient to wait and then take the next dose of darunavir and ritonavir at the regularly scheduled time. If the patient misses a dose of darunavir or ritonavir by less than 6 hours, instruct the patient to take darunavir and ritonavir immediately, and then take the next dose of darunavir and ritonavir at the regularly scheduled time. If a dose of darunavir or ritonavir is skipped, instruct the patient not to double the next dose. Instruct the patient not to take more or less than the prescribed dose of darunavir or ritonavir at any one time.

Darunavir/ritonavir may interact with many drugs; therefore, advise patients to report to their health care provider the use of any other prescription or nonprescription medication or herbal products, including St. John's wort.

Instruct patients receiving estrogen-based contraceptives to use alternate contraceptive measures during therapy with darunavir/ritonavir because hormonal levels may decrease.

Inform patients that redistribution or accumulation of body fat may occur in patients receiving antiretroviral therapy, including darunavir/ritonavir, and that the cause and long-term health effects of these conditions are not known at this time.

NELFINAVIR MESYLATE

Rx	**Viracept** (Pfizer U.S.)	**Tablets; oral:** 250 mg (as base)	(Viracept 250 mg). Lt. blue, capsule shape. In 270s and 300s.
		625 mg (as base)	(V 625). White, oval. In 120s.
		Powder; oral: 50 mg/g (as base)	Aspartame, phenylalanine 11.2 mg/g, sucrose. In multiple-dose bottles containing 144 g powder with 1 g scoop.

NELFINAVIR MESYLATE — ORAL

Indications

➤*HIV infection:* In combination with other antiretroviral agents, for the treatment of HIV infection.

➤*Off-label uses:* Used as part of a 3-drug regimen for occupational HIV postexposure prophylaxis in cases where there is an increased risk for transmission; for HIV infection in neonates; twice daily dosing for HIV infection in children older than 6 years of age.

Administration and Dosage

➤*General dosing considerations:* For children unable to take tablets, nelfinavir oral powder may be administered. Assess appropriate formulation and dosage for each patient. Crushed 250 mg tablets can be used in lieu of powder.

➤*Adults:*

HIV infection – 1,250 mg twice daily or 750 mg 3 times daily.

➤*Children:*

HIV infection –

2 to 13 years of age:

• *Maximum dose* – 2,500 mg/day (twice daily dosing) or 2,250 mg/day (3 times daily dosing).

• *Maintenance dosage* – 45 to 55 mg/kg twice daily or 25 to 35 mg/kg 3 times daily.

Nelfinavir Tablets: Dosing for Children ≥ 2 Years of Age

Body weight		Twice daily 45 to 55 mg/kg (No. of 250 mg tablets)	3 times daily 25 to 35 mg/kg (No. of 250 mg tablets)
Kg	Lbs		
≥ 21	≥ 46.2	4 to 5[a]	3[b]
19 to 20	41.8 to 44	4	2
13 to 18	28.6 to 39.6	3	2
10 to 12	22 to 26.4	2	1

[a] For twice-daily dosing, the maximum dose per day is 5 tablets twice daily.
[b] For 3-times-daily dosing, the maximum dose per day is 3 tablets 3 times a day.

Nelfinavir Oral Powder: Dosing for Children ≥ 2 Years of Age

Body weight		Twice daily 45 to 55 mg/kg		3 times daily 25 to 35 mg/kg	
Kg	Lbs	Scoops of powder (50 mg/g)	Teaspoons[a] of powder	Scoops of powder (50 mg/g)	Teaspoons[a] of powder
≥ 23	≥ 50.5	Not recommended[b]	Not recommended[b]	15	3 ¾
18 to < 23	39.5 to < 50.5	Not recommended[b]	Not recommended[b]	12	3
16 to < 18	35 to < 39.5	Not recommended[b]	Not recommended[b]	10	2½
14 to < 16	31 to < 35	15	3¾	9	2¼
12 to < 14	26.5 to < 31	13	3¼	8	2
10.5 to < 12	23 to < 26.5	11	2¾	7	1¾
9 to < 10.5	20 to < 23	10	2½	6	1½

[a] If a teaspoon is used to measure nelfinavir oral powder, 1 level teaspoon contains nelfinavir 200 mg (4 level scoops equals 1 level teaspoon).
[b] Use nelfinavir 250 mg tablet.

➤*Administration:* Take with a meal.

Tablets – Patients unable to swallow the 250 or 625 mg tablets may dissolve the tablets in a small amount of water. Once dissolved, mix the cloudy liquid well and consume it immediately. Rinse the glass with water and swallow the rinse to ensure the entire dose is consumed.

Oral powder – The oral powder may be mixed with a small amount of water, milk, formula, soy formula, soy milk, or dietary supplements; once mixed, consume the entire contents in order to obtain the full dose. If the mixture is not consumed immediately, store it under refrigeration, but storage must not exceed 6 hours. Acidic food or juice (eg, orange juice, apple juice, applesauce) are not recommended to be used in combination with nelfinavir because the combination may result in a bitter taste. Do not reconstitute oral powder with water in its original container.

➤*Storage/Stability:* Store at 15° to 30°C (59° to 86°F). Keep container tightly closed. Dispense in original container.

Actions

➤*Pharmacology:* Nelfinavir is an inhibitor of the HIV-1 protease. Inhibition of the viral protease prevents cleavage of the gag and gag-pol polyprotein resulting in the production of immature, noninfectious virus.

➤*Pharmacokinetics:*

Absorption – The pharmacokinetic properties of nelfinavir were evaluated in healthy volunteers and HIV-infected patients; no substantial differences were observed between the 2 groups.

Summary of a Pharmacokinetic Study in HIV-Positive Patients with Multiple Dosing of Nelfinavir 1,250 mg Twice a Day for 28 Days and 750 mg 3 Times a Day for 28 Days

Regimen	AUC_{24} mg•hr/L	C_{max} mg/L	C_{trough} morning mg/L	C_{trough} afternoon or evening mg/L
1,250 mg twice a day	52.8 ± 15.7	4 ± 0.8	2.2 ± 1.3	0.7 ± 0.4
750 mg 3 times a day	43.6 ± 17.8	3 ± 1.6	1.4 ± 0.6	1 ± 0.5

Data are mean ± SD.

The difference between morning and afternoon or evening trough concentrations for the 3-times-a-day and 2-times-a-day regimens was also observed in healthy volunteers who were dosed at precisely 8- or 12-hour intervals.

In healthy volunteers receiving a single 1,250 mg dose, the 625 mg tablet was not bioequivalent to the 250 mg tablet formulation. Under fasted conditions (n = 27), the AUC and C_{max} were 34% and 24% higher, respectively, for the 625 mg tablets. In a relative bioavailability assessment under fed conditions (n = 28), the AUC was 24% higher for the 625 mg tablet; the C_{max} was comparable for both formulations.

NELFINAVIR MESYLATE — ORAL

Food increases nelfinavir exposure and decreases nelfinavir pharmacokinetic variability relative to the fasted state. In one study, healthy volunteers received a single dose of 1,250 mg of nelfinavir 250 mg tablets (5 tablets) under fasted or fed conditions (3 different meals). In a second study, healthy volunteers received single doses of 1,250 mg nelfinavir (5 × 250 mg tablets) under fasted or fed conditions (2 different fat content meals).

Increase in AUC, C_{max} and t_{max} for Nelfinavir in Fed State Relative to Fasted State Following 1,250 mg Nelfinavir (5 × 250 mg Tablets)

Number of Kcal	% fat	Number of subjects	AUC fold increase	C_{max} fold increase	Increase in t_{max} (hr)
125	20	n = 21	2.2	2	1
500	20	n = 22	3.1	2.3	2
1,000	50	n = 23	5.2	3.3	2

Increase in Nelfinavir AUC, C_{max} and t_{max} in Fed Low-Fat (20%) vs High-Fat (50%) State Relative to Fasted State Following 1,250 mg Nelfinavir (5 × 250 mg Tablets)

Number of Kcal	% fat	Number of subjects	AUC fold increase	C_{max} fold increase	Increase in t_{max} (hr)
500	20	n = 22	3.1	2.5	1.8
500	50	n = 22	5.1	3.8	2.1

Nelfinavir exposure can be increased by increasing the calorie or fat content in meals taken with nelfinavir.

Distribution – The apparent volume of distribution following oral administration of nelfinavir was 2 to 7 L/kg. Nelfinavir in serum is extensively protein bound (greater than 98%).

Metabolism – Unchanged nelfinavir comprised 82% to 86% of the total plasma radioactivity after a single oral 750 mg dose of ^{14}C-nelfinavir. In vitro, multiple cytochrome P450 enzymes including CYP3A and CYP2C19 are responsible for metabolism of nelfinavir. One major and several minor oxidative metabolites were found in plasma. The major oxidative metabolite has in vitro antiviral activity comparable to the parent drug.

Excretion – The terminal half-life in plasma was typically 3.5 to 5 hours. The majority (87%) of an oral 750 mg dose containing ^{14}C-nelfinavir was recovered in the feces; fecal radioactivity consisted of numerous oxidative metabolites (78%) and unchanged nelfinavir (22%). Only 1% to 2% of the dose was recovered in urine, of which unchanged nelfinavir was the major component.

Special populations –

Children: The pharmacokinetics of nelfinavir have been investigated in 5 studies in pediatric patients from birth to 13 years of age either receiving nelfinavir 3 times or twice daily.

Summary of Steady-State AUC_{24} of Nelfinavir in Pediatric Studies

Protocol no.	Dosing regimen[a]	N[b]	Age	AUC_{24} (mg•hr/L) arithmetic mean ± SD
AG1343-524	20 (19 to 28) mg/kg 3 times daily	14	2 to 13 years	56.1 ± 29.8
PACTG 725	55 (48 to 60) mg/kg twice daily	6	3 to 11 years	101.8 ± 56.1
PENTA 7	40 (34 to 43) mg/kg 3 times daily	4	2 to 9 months	33.8 ± 8.9
PENTA 7	75 (55 to 83) mg/kg twice daily	12	2 to 9 months	37.2 ± 19.2
PACTG 353	40 (14 to 56) mg/kg twice daily	10	6 weeks	44.1 ± 27.4
			1 week	45.8 ± 32.1

[a] Protocol specified dose (actual dose range).
[b] N: Number of subjects with evaluable pharmacokinetic results C_{trough} values are not presented in the table because they are not available for all studies.

Overall, use of nelfinavir in the pediatric population is associated with highly variable drug exposure. The high variability may be due to inconsistent food intake in pediatric patients.

➤*Microbiology:*

Antiviral activity in vitro – The antiviral activity of nelfinavir in vitro has been demonstrated in both acute or chronic HIV infections in lymphoblastoid cell lines, peripheral blood lymphocytes, and monocytes/macrophages. Nelfinavir was found to be active against several laboratory strains of HIV-1 and several clinical isolates of HIV-1 and the HIV-2 strain ROD. The EC_{95} (95% effective concentration) of nelfinavir ranged from 7 to 196 nM. Drug combination studies with protease inhibitors showed nelfinavir had antagonistic interactions with indinavir, additive interactions with ritonavir or saquinavir, and synergistic interactions with amprenavir and lopinavir. Minimal to no cellular cytotoxicity was observed with any of these protease inhibitors alone or in combination with nelfinavir. In combination with reverse transcriptase inhibitors, nelfinavir demonstrated additive (didanosine or stavudine) to synergistic (abacavir, delavirdine, efavirenz, lamivudine, nevirapine, tenofovir, zalcitabine, or zidovudine) antiviral activity in vitro without enhanced cytotoxicity.

Drug resistance – HIV-1 isolates with reduced susceptibility to nelfinavir have been selected in vitro. HIV isolates from selected patients treated with nelfinavir alone or in combination with reverse transcriptase inhibitors were monitored for phenotypic (n = 19) and genotypic (n = 195, 157 of which were evaluable) changes in clinical trials over a period of 2 to 82 weeks. One or more virus protease mutations at amino acid positions 30, 35, 36, 46, 71, 77, and 88 were detected in the HIV-1 of greater than 10% of patients with evaluable isolates. The overall incidence of the D30N mutation in the virus protease of evaluable patients (n = 157) receiving nelfinavir monotherapy or nelfinavir in combination with zidovudine and lamivudine or stavudine was 54.8%. The overall incidence of other mutations associated with primary protease inhibitor resistance was 9.6% for the L90M substitution whereas substitutions at 48, 82, or 84 were not observed. Of 19 clinical isolates for which both phenotypic and genotypic analyses were performed on clinical isolates, 9 showed reduced susceptibility (5- to 93-fold) to nelfinavir in vitro. All 9 patients possessed 1 or more mutations in the virus protease gene. Amino acid position 30 appeared to be the most frequent mutation site.

Cross-resistance –

Nonclinical studies: Patient-derived recombinant HIV isolates containing the D30N mutation (n = 4) and demonstrating high-level (greater than 10-fold) NFV-resistance remained susceptible (less than 2.5-fold resistance) to amprenavir, indinavir, lopinavir, and saquinavir, in vitro. Patient-derived recombinant HIV isolates containing the L90M mutation (n = 8) demonstrated moderate-to high-level resistance to NFV and had varying levels of susceptibility to amprenavir, indinavir, lopinavir, and saquinavir, in vitro. Most patient-derived recombinant isolates with phenotypic and genotypic evidence of reduced susceptibility (greater than 2.5-fold) to amprenavir, indinavir, lopinavir, or saquinavir demonstrated high-level cross-resistance to nelfinavir, in vitro. Mutations associated with resistance to other PIs (eg, G48V, V82A/F/T, I84V, L90M) appeared to confer high-level cross-resistance to NFV Following ritonavir therapy, 6 of 7 clinical isolates with decreased ritonavir susceptibility (8- to 113-fold) in vitro compared to baseline also exhibited decreased susceptibility to nelfinavir in vitro (5- to 40-fold). Cross-resistance between nelfinavir and reverse transcriptase inhibitors is unlikely because different enzyme targets are involved. Clinical isolates (n = 5) with decreased susceptibility to zidovudine, lamivudine, or nevirapine remain fully susceptible to nelfinavir in vitro.

Contraindications

Hypersensitivity to any of its components.

Coadministration of nelfinavir is contraindicated with drugs that are highly dependent on CYP3A for clearance and for which elevated plasma concentrations are associated with serious or life-threatening events.

Drugs That are Contraindicated with Nelfinavir

Drug class	Drugs within class that are contraindicated with nelfinavir
Antiarrhythmics	Amiodarone, quinidine
Ergot derivatives	Dihydroergotamine, ergonovine, ergotamine, methylergonovine
Neuroleptic	Pimozide
Sedative/hypnotics	Midazolam, triazolam

Warnings/Precautions

➤*Phenylketonurics:* Nelfinavir mesylate oral powder contains 11.2 mg phenylalanine per g of powder.

➤*Diabetes mellitus/hyperglycemia:* New onset diabetes mellitus, exacerbation of preexisting diabetes mellitus, and hyperglycemia have been reported during postmarketing surveillance in HIV-infected patients receiving protease inhibitor therapy. Some patients required either initiation or dose adjustments of insulin or oral hypoglycemic agents for treatment of these events. In some cases, diabetic ketoacidosis has occurred. In those patients who discontinued protease inhibitor therapy, hyperglycemia persisted in some cases. Because these events have been reported voluntarily during clinical practice, estimates of frequency cannot be made and a causal relationship between protease inhibitor therapy and these events has not been established.

➤*Resistance/cross-resistance:* HIV cross-resistance between protease inhibitors has been observed.

➤*Hemophilia:* There have been reports of increased bleeding, including spontaneous skin hematomas and hemarthrosis, in patients with hemophilia type A and B treated with protease inhibitors. In some patients, additional Factor VIII was given. In more than half of the reported cases, treatment with protease inhibitors was continued or reintroduced. A causal relationship has not been established.

➤*Redistribution/accumulation of body fat:* Redistribution/accumulation of body fat including central obesity, dorsocervical fat enlargement (buffalo hump), peripheral wasting, breast enlargement, and "cushingoid appearance" have been observed in patients receiving antiretroviral therapy. The mechanism and long-term consequences of these events are currently unknown. A causal relationship has not been established.

➤*Hepatic function impairment:* Nelfinavir is principally metabolized by the liver. Therefore, exercise caution when administering this drug to patients with hepatic impairment.

➤*Pregnancy: Category B.* There are no adequate and well-controlled studies in pregnant women. Because animal reproduction studies are not always predictive of human response, use nelfinavir mesylate during pregnancy only if clearly needed.

Antiretroviral pregnancy registry (APR) – To monitor maternal-fetal outcomes of pregnant women exposed to nelfinavir mesylate and other anti-

NELFINAVIR MESYLATE — ORAL

retroviral agents, an Antiretroviral Pregnancy Registry has been established. Register patients by calling (800) 258-4263.

➤*Lactation:* The Centers for Disease Control and Prevention advises HIV-infected women not to breastfeed to avoid postnatal transmission of HIV to a child who may not yet be infected. Studies in lactating rats have demonstrated that nelfinavir is excreted in milk. Because of both the potential for HIV transmission and the potential for serious adverse reactions in nursing infants, instruct mothers not to breastfeed if they are receiving nelfinavir.

➤*Children:* The safety and effectiveness of nelfinavir have been established in patients from 2 to 13 years of age. The use of nelfinavir in these age groups is supported by evidence from adequate and well-controlled studies of nelfinavir in adults and pharmacokinetic studies and studies supporting activity in pediatric patients. In patients less than 2 years of age, nelfinavir was found to be safe at the doses studied but a reliably effective dose could not be established.

Drug Interactions

CYP3A and CYP2C19 appear to be the predominant enzymes that metabolize nelfinavir in humans. The potential ability of nelfinavir to inhibit the major human cytochrome P450 isoforms (CYP3A, CYP2C19, CYP2D6, CYP2C9, CYP1A2 and CYP2E1) has been investigated in vitro. Only CYP3A was inhibited at concentrations in the therapeutic range.

Nelfinavir Drug Interactions

Precipitant drug	Object drug[a]		Description
Anticonvulsants (ie, carbamazepine, phenobarbital)	Nelfinavir	↓	Concurrent use may decrease nelfinavir plasma concentrations.
Azithromycin	Nelfinavir	↓	Coadministration resulted in a decrease in the AUC and C_{max} of nelfinavir by 15% and 10%, respectively.
Nelfinavir	Azithromycin	↑	Coadministration resulted in an increase in the AUC of 112% and C_{max} of 136% of azithromycin. Dose adjustment is not recommended; closely monitor for liver enzyme abnormalities and hearing impairment.
Azole antifungals	Nelfinavir	↑	May inhibit the metabolism of protease inhibitors. Ketoconazole increased nelfinavir AUC and C_{max} by 35% and 25%, respectively. Monitor for protease inhibitor toxicity and adjust dose as needed.
Efavirenz Delavirdine	Nelfinavir	↑	Coadministration resulted in an increase in the AUC and C_{max} of nelfinavir, 107% and 88% with delavirdine, and 20% and 21% with efavirenz, respectively.
Nelfinavir	Efavirenz Delavirdine	↓	Coadministration caused a decrease in the AUC and C_{max} of efavirenz of 12% and 12%, respectively, and delavirdine of 31% and 27%, respectively.
Indinavir	Nelfinavir	↑	Coadministration resulted in an 83% increase in nelfinavir AUC and a 51% increase in indinavir AUC.
Nelfinavir	Indinavir		
Interleukins	Nelfinavir	↑	May inhibit protease inhibitor metabolism. May be necessary to adjust protease inhibitor dose.
Nevirapine	Nelfinavir	↓	Increased hepatic metabolism of the protease inhibitor is suspected. Monitor protease inhibitor blood levels and adjust dose as necessary.
Rifabutin	Nelfinavir	↓	Coadministration resulted in a 32% decrease in nelfinavir AUC and a 207% increase in rifabutin AUC. It is recommended that the dose of rifabutin be reduced to one half the usual dose when administered with nelfinavir.
Nelfinavir	Rifabutin	↑	
Rifampin	Nelfinavir	↓	Coadministration resulted in an 83% decrease in nelfinavir AUC. Do not coadminister nelfinavir with rifampin.

Nelfinavir Drug Interactions

Precipitant drug	Object drug[a]		Description
Ritonavir	Nelfinavir	↑	Coadministration resulted in a 152% increase in nelfinavir AUC and very little change in ritonavir AUC.
Saquinavir	Nelfinavir	↑	Coadministration resulted in an 18% increase in nelfinavir AUC and a 392% increase in saquinavir AUC. If used in combination, no dose adjustments are needed.
Nelfinavir	Saquinavir		
St. John's wort	Nelfinavir	↓	Increased metabolism of the protease inhibitor is suspected and may lead to loss of virologic response and possible resistance to nelfinavir. Avoid coadministration.
Nelfinavir	Didanosine	↔	It is recommended that didanosine be administered on an empty stomach; administer nelfinavir (with food) 1 hour after or > 2 hours before didanosine.
Nelfinavir	HMG-CoA reductase inhibitors (atorvastatin, lovastatin, simvastatin)	↑	Coadministration resulted in an increase in the C_{max} and AUC of simvastatin (517% and 505%) and atorvastatin (122% and 74%). Concomitant administration with nelfinavir is contraindicated due to potential for serious reactions such as risk of myopathy including rhabdomyolysis.
Nelfinavir	Lamivudine	↑	Coadministration resulted in an increase in lamivudine's AUC and C_{max} by 10% and 31%, respectively.
Nelfinavir	Oral contraceptives	↓	Coadministration resulted in a 47% decrease in ethinyl estradiol and an 18% decrease in norethindrone plasma levels. Use alternate or additional contraceptive measures during nelfinavir therapy.
Nelfinavir	Phenytoin	↓	Coadministration resulted in a decrease in the AUC and C_{max} of phenytoin, 29% and 21%, respectively. Monitor phenytoin plasma levels and adjust dose as necessary.
Nelfinavir	Pimozide	↑	Coadministration is contraindicated due to potential for serious or life-threatening reactions such as cardiac arrhythmias.
Nelfinavir	Zidovudine	↓	Coadministration of zidovudine with nelfinavir resulted in a 35% decrease in zidovudine AUC.
Nelfinavir	Antiarrhythmics (amiodarone, quinidine)	↑	Protease inhibitors may inhibit the metabolism via cytochrome P450 3A4 isoenzyme. Coadministration with nelfinavir is contraindicated.
Nelfinavir	Benzodiazepines	↑	Possibly severe sedation and respiratory depression caused by the inhibition of the metabolism of benzodiazepines that undergo oxidation. Midazolam and triazolam are contraindicated in patients receiving nelfinavir.
Nelfinavir	Cisapride	↑	Protease inhibitors may inhibit the metabolism of cisapride via cytochrome P450 3A4 isoenzyme.
Nelfinavir	Ergot alkaloids	↑	Protease inhibitors may inhibit the metabolism of ergot alkaloids via cytochrome P450 3A4 isoenzyme. Coadministration with nelfinavir is contraindicated due to potential for serious or life-threatening reactions, such as acute ergot toxicity characterized by peripheral vasospasm and ischemia of the extremities and other tissues.

NELFINAVIR MESYLATE — ORAL

Nelfinavir Drug Interactions			
Precipitant drug	Object drug[a]		Description
Nelfinavir	Fentanyl	↑	Possible inhibition of metabolism of fentanyl. Closely monitor respiratory function if coadministered. A reduction in the fentanyl dose may be necessary.
Nelfinavir	Methadone	↓	Increased metabolism of methadone is suspected. Coadministration resulted in a decrease of the AUC and C_{max} of methadone, 47% and 46%, respectively. Monitor for withdrawal symptoms and adjust dose as necessary.
Nelfinavir	Sildenafil	↑	Inhibition of sildenafil metabolism. Coadminister with extreme caution; sildenafil should not exceed a maximum single dose of 25 mg/48 hours when used concomitantly.
Nelfinavir	Tacrolimus Sirolimus	↑	Plasma concentrations of the immunosuppressants may be increased with concomitant administration. Carefully monitor renal function and immunosuppressant concentrations when starting, stopping, or changing the dose of a protease inhibitor and adjust the dose of the immunosuppressant as necessary.

[a] ↑ = object drug increased; ↓ = object drug decreased; ↔ = undetermined clinical effect.

Nelfinavir is an inhibitor of CYP3A enzyme. Coadministration of nelfinavir mesylate and drugs primarily metabolized by CYP3A (eg, dihydropyridine calcium channel blockers, HMG-CoA reductase inhibitors, immunosuppressants, sildenafil) may result in increased plasma concentrations of the other drug that could increase or prolong both its therapeutic and adverse effects. Exercise caution when inhibitors of CYP3A, including nelfinavir, are coadministered with drugs that are metabolized by CYP3A and that prolong the QT interval. Nelfinavir is metabolized by CYP3A and CYP2C19. Coadministration of nelfinavir mesylate and drugs that induce CYP3A or CYP2C19, such as rifampin, may decrease nelfinavir plasma concentrations and reduce its therapeutic effect. Coadministration of nelfinavir mesylate and drugs that inhibit CYP3A or CYP2C19 may increase nelfinavir plasma concentrations.

Adverse Reactions

The safety of nelfinavir mesylate was studied in over 5,000 patients who received drug either alone or in combination with nucleoside analogues. The majority of adverse events were of mild intensity. The most frequently reported adverse event among patients receiving nelfinavir mesylate was diarrhea, which was generally of mild to moderate intensity. The frequency of nelfinavir-associated diarrhea may be increased in patients receiving the 625 mg tablet because of the increased bioavailability of this formulation.

Nelfinavir Percentage of Patients with Treatment-Emergent[a] Adverse Reactions of Moderate or Severe Intensity Reported in ≥ 2% of Patients

Adverse events	Study 511; 24 weeks			Study 542; 48 weeks	
	Placebo + zidovudine/ lamivudine (n = 101)	500 mg 3 times daily nelfinavir mesylate + zidovudine/ lamivudine (n = 97)	750 mg 3 times daily nelfinavir mesylate + zidovudine/ lamivudine (n = 100)	1,250 mg twice daily nelfinavir mesylate + stavudine/ lamivudine (n = 344)	750 mg 3 times daily nelfinavir mesylate + stavudine/ lamivudine (n = 210)
Dermatologic					
Rash	1%	1%	3%	2%	1%
GI					
Diarrhea	3%	14%	20%	20%	15%
Flatulence	0%	5%	2%	1%	1%
Nausea	4%	3%	7%	3%	3%

[a] Includes those adverse events at least possibly related to study drug or of unknown relationship and excludes concurrent HIV conditions.

Adverse events occurring in less than 2% of patients receiving nelfinavir mesylate in all phase 2/3 clinical trials and considered at least possibly related or of unknown relationship to treatment and of at least moderate severity are listed below.

➤*CNS:* Anxiety, depression, dizziness, emotional lability, hyperkinesia, insomnia, migraine, paresthesia, seizures, sleep disorder, somnolence, and suicidal ideation.

➤*Dermatologic:* Dermatitis, folliculitis, fungal dermatitis, maculopapular rash, pruritus, sweating, and urticaria.

➤*GI:* Anorexia, dyspepsia, epigastric pain, GI bleeding, hepatitis, mouth ulceration, pancreatitis, vomiting, and abdominal pain.

➤*GU:* Kidney calculus, sexual dysfunction, and urine abnormality.

➤*Hematologic/Lymphatic:* Anemia, leukopenia, and thrombocytopenia.

➤*Metabolic/Nutritional:* Increases in alkaline phosphate, amylase, creatine phosphokinase, lactic dehydrogenase, ALT, AST and gamma glutamyl transpeptidase; hyperlipemia, hyperuricemia, hyperglycemia, hypoglycemia, dehydration, and abnormal liver function tests.

➤*Musculoskeletal:* Arthralgia, arthritis, cramps, myalgia, myasthenia, and myopathy.

➤*Respiratory:* Dyspnea, pharyngitis, rhinitis, and sinusitis.

➤*Special senses:* Acute iritis and eye disorder.

➤*Miscellaneous:* Accidental injury, allergic reaction, back pain, fever, headache, malaise, pain and redistribution/accumulation of body fat including central obesity, dorsocervical fat enlargement (buffalo hump), peripheral wasting, breast enlargement, and "cushingoid appearance".

➤*Postmarketing:* The following additional adverse experiences have been reported from postmarketing surveillance as at least possibly related or of unknown relationship to nelfinavir mesylate:

Cardiovascular – QTc prolongation, torsades de pointes.

GI – Jaundice.

Metabolic/Nutritional – Bilirubinemia, metabolic acidosis.

Miscellaneous – Hypersensitivity reactions (including bronchospasm, moderate to severe rash, fever, and edema).

➤*Lab test abnormalities:* The percentage of patients with marked laboratory abnormalities in studies 542 and 511 are presented below. Marked laboratory abnormalities are defined as a Grade 3 or 4 abnormality in a patient with a normal baseline value or a Grade 4 abnormality in a patient with a Grade 1 abnormality at baseline.

Nelfinavir Marked Laboratory Abnormalities (> 2%)

Lab abnormality	Study 511			Study 542	
	Placebo + zidovudine/ lamivudine (n = 101)	500 mg 3 times daily nelfinavir mesylate + zidovudine/ lamivudine (n = 97)	750 mg 3 times daily nelfinavir mesylate + zidovudine/ lamivudine (n = 100)	1,250 mg twice daily nelfinavir mesylate + stavudine/ lamivudine (n = 344)	750 mg 3 times daily nelfinavir mesylate + stavudine/ lamivudine (n = 210)
Chemistry					
ALT	6%	1%	1%	2%	1%
AST	4%	1%	0%	2%	1%
Creatine kinase	7%	2%	2%	N/A	N/A
Hematology					
Hemoglobin	6%	3%	2%	0%	0%
Lymphocytes	1%	6%	1%	1%	0%
Neutrophils	4%	3%	5%	2%	1%

[a] Marked laboratory abnormalities are defined as a shift from Grade 0 at baseline to at least Grade 3 or from Grade 1 to Grade 4.

Children – The most commonly reported drug-related, treatment-emergent adverse events reported in the pediatric studies included diarrhea, leukopenia/neutropenia, rash, anorexia, and abdominal pain. Diarrhea, regardless of assigned relationship to study drug, was reported in 39% to 47% of pediatric patients receiving nelfinavir in 2 of the larger treatment trials. Leukopenia/neutropenia was the laboratory abnormality most commonly reported as a significant event across the pediatric studies.

Overdosage

➤*Treatment:* Human experience of acute overdose with nelfinavir mesylate is limited. There is no specific antidote for overdose with nelfinavir mesylate. If indicated, achieve elimination of unabsorbed drug by emesis or gastric lavage. Administration of activated charcoal may also be used to aid removal of unabsorbed drug. Since nelfinavir is highly protein bound, dialysis is unlikely to significantly remove drug from blood.

Patient Information

For optimal absorption, advise patients to take nelfinavir mesylate with food. Maximum plasma concentrations and area under the plasma concentration-time curve (AUC) were 2 – to 3-fold higher under fed conditions compared to fasting. The effect of food on nelfinavir absorption was evaluated in 2 studies (n = 14, total). The meals evaluated contained 517 to 759 Kcal, with 153 to 313 Kcal derived from fat.

NELFINAVIR MESYLATE — ORAL

Inform patients that nelfinavir mesylate is not a cure for HIV infection and that they may continue to acquire illnesses associated with advanced HIV infection, including opportunistic infections.

Tell patients that there is currently no data demonstrating that nelfinavir mesylate therapy can reduce the risk of transmitting HIV to others through sexual contact or blood contamination.

Tell patients that sustained decreases in plasma HIV RNA have been associated with a reduced risk of progression to AIDS and death. Advise patients to take nelfinavir mesylate and other concomitant antiretroviral therapy every day as prescribed. Patients should not alter the dose or discontinue therapy without consulting with their doctor. If a dose of nelfinavir mesylate is missed, patients should take the dose as soon as possible and then return to their normal schedule. However, if a dose is skipped, the patient should not double the next dose.

Inform patients that nelfinavir tablets are film-coated and that this film-coating is intended to make the tablets easier to swallow.

The most frequent adverse event associated with nelfinavir mesylate is diarrhea, which can usually be controlled with nonprescription drugs, such as loperamide, which slow GI motility.

Inform patients that redistribution or accumulation of body fat may occur in patients receiving antiretroviral therapy including protease inhibitors and that the cause and long-term health effects of these conditions are not known at this time.

Nelfinavir may interact with some drugs; therefore, advise patients to report to their doctor the use of any other prescription, nonprescription medication, or herbal products, particularly St. John's wort.

Instruct patients receiving oral contraceptives to use alternate or additional contraceptive measures during therapy with nelfinavir mesylate.

Advise patients receiving sildenafil and nelfinavir that they may be at an increased risk of sildenafil-associated adverse events including hypotension, visual changes, and prolonged penile erection, and should promptly report any symptoms to their doctor.

FOSAMPRENAVIR

Rx	Lexiva (GlaxoSmithKline)	Tablets; oral: 700 mg	As fosamprenavir calcium.[a] (GX LL7). Pink, capsule shape. Film-coated. In 60s.
		Suspension; oral: 50 mg/mL	As fosamprenavir calcium.[a] Parabens, sucralose. Grape/bubble gum/peppermint flavor. In 225 mL.

[a] Fosamprenavir calcium is a prodrug of amprenavir. For the tablets, fosamprenavir 700 mg is equivalent to ≈ 600 mg of amprenavir. For the oral suspension, fosamprenavir 50 mg/mL is equivalent to ≈ 43 mg/mL of amprenavir.

FOSAMPRENAVIR CALCIUM — ORAL

Indications

➤*HIV infection:* In combination with other antiretroviral agents for the treatment of HIV-1 infection.

Administration and Dosage

➤*General dosing considerations:* Higher than approved dose combinations of fosamprenavir plus ritonavir are not recommended because of an increased risk of transaminase elevations.

➤*Adults:*

HIV infection –

Protease inhibitor (PI)-experienced patients: 700 mg twice daily plus ritonavir 100 mg twice daily.

Therapy-naive patients: 1,400 mg twice daily (without ritonavir), 1,400 mg once daily plus ritonavir 200 mg once daily, 1,400 mg once daily plus ritonavir 100 mg once daily, or 700 mg twice daily plus ritonavir 100 mg twice daily.

➤*Children:*

HIV infection –

When administered without ritonavir, the adult regimen of fosamprenavir 1,400 mg tablets twice daily may be used for children weighing at least 47 kg.

When administered in combination with ritonavir, fosamprenavir tablets may be used for children weighing at least 39 kg; ritonavir capsules may be used for children weighing at least 33 kg.

Therapy-experienced patients:

- *6 years of age and older* –
  - *Usual dosage:* 18 mg/kg twice daily (suspension) plus ritonavir 3 mg/kg twice daily.
  - *Maximum dose:* 700 mg twice daily plus ritonavir 100 mg twice daily.

Therapy-naive patients:

- *6 years of age and older* –
  - *Usual dosage:* 30 mg/kg twice daily (suspension), or 18 mg/kg twice daily (suspension) plus ritonavir 3 mg/kg twice daily.
  - *Maximum dose:* 1,400 mg twice daily, or 700 mg twice daily plus ritonavir 100 mg twice daily.
- *2 to 5 years of age* –
  - *Usual dosage:* 30 mg/kg twice daily (suspension).
  - *Maximum dose:* 1,400 mg twice daily.

➤*Hepatic function impairment:*

Mild hepatic impairment (Child-Pugh score 5 to 6) – 700 mg twice daily without ritonavir (therapy-naive patients), or 700 mg twice daily plus ritonavir 100 mg once daily (therapy-naive or PI–experienced patients).

Moderate hepatic impairment (Child-Pugh score 7 to 9) – 700 mg twice daily without ritonavir (therapy-naive patients), or 450 mg twice daily plus ritonavir 100 mg once daily (therapy-naive or PI–experienced patients).

Severe hepatic impairment (Child-Pugh score 10 to 15) – 350 mg twice daily without ritonavir (therapy-naive patients) or 300 mg twice daily plus ritonavir 100 mg once daily (therapy-naive or PI–experienced patients).

➤*Preparation for administration:* Instruct patients to shake the bottle vigorously before each use. Inform patients that refrigeration may improve the taste.

➤*Administration:*

Tablets – May be taken with or without food.

Suspension – Adults should take the suspension without food. Children should take the suspension with food. If emesis occurs within 30 minutes after dosing, redose fosamprenavir.

➤*Storage/Stability:* Store tablets at 25°C (77°F); excursions are permitted between 15° and 30°C (59° and 86°F). Keep the container tightly closed.

Store suspension between 5° and 30°C (41° and 86°F). Shake vigorously before using. Do not freeze.

Actions

➤*Pharmacology:* Fosamprenavir is an antiviral agent and a prodrug that is rapidly hydrolyzed to amprenavir by cellular phosphatases in the gut epithelium as it is absorbed. Amprenavir is an inhibitor of HIV-1 protease. Amprenavir binds to the active site of HIV-1 protease and thereby prevents the processing of viral Gag and Gag-Pol polyprotein precursors, resulting in the formation of immature, noninfectious viral particles.

➤*Pharmacokinetics:*

Absorption – After administration of a single dose of fosamprenavir to HIV-1–infected patients, the time to peak amprenavir concentration (T_{max}) occurred between 1.5 and 4 hours (median, 2.5 hours). The absolute oral bioavailability of amprenavir after administration of fosamprenavir in humans has not been established.

Steady-State Plasma Amprenavir Pharmacokinetic Parameters in Adults[a]

Regimen	C_{max} (mcg/mL)	T_{max} (h)[b]	AUC_{24} (mcg•h/mL)	C_{min} (mcg/mL)
Fosamprenavir 1,400 mg twice daily	4.82 (4.06 to 5.72)	1.3 (0.8 to 4)	33 (27.6 to 39.2)	0.35 (0.27 to 0.46)
Fosamprenavir 1,400 mg once daily plus ritonavir 200 mg once daily	7.24 (6.32 to 8.28)	2.1 (0.8 to 5)	69.4 (59.7 to 80.8)	1.45 (1.16 to 1.81)
Fosamprenavir 1,400 mg once daily plus ritonavir 100 mg once daily	7.93 (7.25 to 8.68)	1.5 (0.75 to 5)	66.4 (61.1 to 72.1)	0.86 (0.74 to 1.01)
Fosamprenavir 700 mg twice daily plus ritonavir 100 mg twice daily	6.08 (5.38 to 6.86)	1.5 (0.75 to 5)	79.2 (69 to 90.6)	2.12 (1.77 to 2.54)

[a] C_{max} = maximal drug concentration; AUC = area under the curve; C_{mm} = trough drug concentration.
[b] Data shown are median (range).

Food effect: After administration of a single 1,400 mg dose in the fasted state, fosamprenavir 50 mg/mL oral suspension and fosamprenavir 700 mg tablets provided similar amprenavir exposures (AUC); however, the C_{max} of amprenavir after administration of the suspension formulation was 14.5% higher compared with the tablet.

Fosamprenavir tablets may be taken with or without food. Administration of a single 1,400 mg dose of fosamprenavir tablets in the fed state (standardized high-fat meal: 967 kcal, 67 g of fat, 33 g of protein, 58 g of carbohydrate) compared with the fasted state was associated with no significant changes in amprenavir C_{max}, T_{max}, or $AUC_{0-\infty}$.

For adults, fosamprenavir oral suspension should be taken without food. However, children should take the oral suspension with food. Administration of a single 1,400 mg dose of fosamprenavir oral suspension in the fed state (standardized high-fat meal: 967 kcal, 67 g of fat, 33 g of protein, 58 g of carbohydrate) compared with the fasted state was associated with a 46% reduction in C_{max}, a 0.72 hour delay in T_{max}, and a 28% reduction in amprenavir $AUC_{0-\infty}$.

Distribution – In vitro, amprenavir is approximately 90% bound to plasma proteins, primarily to alpha-1 acid glycoprotein. In vitro,

FOSAMPRENAVIR CALCIUM — ORAL

concentration-dependent binding was observed over the concentration range of 1 to 10 mcg/mL, with decreased binding at higher concentrations. The partitioning of amprenavir into erythrocytes is low, but increases as amprenavir concentrations increase, reflecting the higher amount of unbound drug at higher concentrations.

Metabolism – After oral administration, fosamprenavir is rapidly and almost completely hydrolyzed to amprenavir and inorganic phosphate prior to reaching the systemic circulation. This occurs in the gut epithelium during absorption. Amprenavir is metabolized in the liver by the CYP3A4 enzyme system. The 2 major metabolites result from oxidation of the tetrahydrofuran and aniline moieties. Glucuronide conjugates of oxidized metabolites have been identified as minor metabolites in the urine and feces.

Excretion – Excretion of unchanged amprenavir in the urine and feces is minimal. Unchanged amprenavir in the urine accounts for approximately 1% of the dose; unchanged amprenavir was not detectable in the feces. Approximately 14% and 75% of an administered single dose of ^{14}C-amprenavir can be accounted for as metabolites in the urine and feces, respectively. Two metabolites accounted for more than 90% of the radiocarbon in fecal samples. The plasma elimination half-life of amprenavir is approximately 7.7 hours.

Special populations –

Hepatic function impairment: The pharmacokinetics of amprenavir have been studied after the administration of fosamprenavir in combination with ritonavir to adult HIV-1–infected patients with mild, moderate, and severe hepatic impairment. Following 2 weeks of dosing with fosamprenavir plus ritonavir, the AUC of amprenavir was increased by approximately 22% in patients with mild hepatic impairment, by approximately 70% in patients with moderate hepatic impairment, and by approximately 80% in patients with severe hepatic impairment compared with HIV-1–infected patients with healthy hepatic function. Protein binding of amprenavir was decreased in patients with hepatic impairment. The unbound fraction at 2 hours (approximate C_{max}) ranged between a decrease of −7% to an increase of 57%, while the unbound fraction at the end of the dosing interval (C_{min}) increased from 50% to 102%.

Children:

Geometric Mean (95% CI[a]) Steady-State Plasma Amprenavir Pharmacokinetic Parameters in Children Receiving Fosamprenavir

Parameter	Children 2 to 5 years of age: n	Fosamprenavir 30 mg/kg twice daily
$AUC_{(24)}$ (mcg•h/mL)	8	31.4 (13.7 to 72.4)
C_{max} (mcg/mL)	8	5 (1.95 to 12.8)
C_{min} (mcg/mL)	17	0.454 (0.342 to 0.604)

[a] CI = confidence interval.

Geometric Mean (95% CI) Steady-State Plasma Amprenavir Pharmacokinetic Parameters in Children Receiving Fosamprenavir Plus Ritonavir Twice Daily

	Children 6 to 11 years of age		Children 12 to 18 years of age	
Parameter	n	Fosamprenavir 18 mg/kg plus ritonavir 3 mg/kg twice daily	n	Fosamprenavir 700 mg plus ritonavir 100 mg twice daily
$AUC_{(0-24)}$ (mcg•h/mL)	9	93.4 (67.8 to 129)	8	58.8 (38.8 to 89)
C_{max} (mcg/mL)	9	6.07 (4.4 to 8.38)	8	4.33 (2.82 to 6.65)
C_{min} (mcg/mL)	17	2.69 (2.15 to 3.36)	24	1.61 (1.21 to 2.15)

➤*Microbiology:*

Antiviral activity – Fosamprenavir has little or no antiviral activity in vitro.

The in vitro antiviral activity of amprenavir was evaluated against HIV-1 IIIB in both acutely and chronically infected lymphoblastic cell lines (MT-4, CEM-CCRF, H9) and in peripheral blood lymphocytes. The 50% effective concentration (EC_{50}) of amprenavir ranged from 0.012 to 0.08 mcM in acutely infected cells and was 0.41 mcM in chronically infected cells (1 mcM = 0.5 mcg/mL). The median EC_{50} value of amprenavir against HIV-1 isolates from clades A to G was 0.00095 mcM in peripheral blood mononuclear cells. Similarly, the EC_{50} values for amprenavir against monocytes/macrophage tropic HIV-1 isolates (clade B) ranged from 0.003 to 0.075 mcM in monocyte/macrophage cultures. The EC_{50} values of amprenavir against HIV-2 isolates grown in peripheral blood mononuclear cells were higher than those for HIV-1 isolates and ranged from 0.003 to 0.11 mcM. Amprenavir exhibited synergistic anti–HIV-1 activity in combination with the nucleoside reverse transcriptase inhibitors (NRTIs) abacavir, didanosine, lamivudine, stavudine, tenofovir, and zidovudine; the nonnucleoside reverse transcriptase inhibitors (NNRTIs) delavirdine and efavirenz; and the PIs atazanavir and saquinavir. Amprenavir exhibited additive anti–HIV-1 activity in combination with the (NNRTI) nevirapine; the PIs indinavir, lopinavir, nelfinavir, and ritonavir; and the fusion inhibitor enfuvirtide. These drug combinations have not been adequately studied in humans.

Resistance – HIV-1 isolates with a decreased susceptibility to amprenavir have been selected in vitro and obtained from patients treated with fosamprenavir. Genotypic analysis of isolates from treatment-naive patients failing amprenavir-containing regimens showed mutations in the HIV-1 protease gene, resulting in amino acid substitutions primarily at positions V32I, M46I/L, I47V, I50V, I54L/M, and I84V, as well as mutations in the p7/p1 and p1/p6 Gag and Gag-Pol polyprotein precursor cleavage sites. Some of these amprenavir resistance-associated mutations also have been detected in HIV-1 isolates from antiretroviral-naive patients treated with fosamprenavir. Of the 488 antiretroviral-naive patients treated with fosamprenavir 1,400 mg twice daily or fosamprenavir 1,400 mg plus ritonavir 200 mg once daily in studies APV 30001 and APV 30002, respectively, 61 patients (29 receiving fosamprenavir and 32 receiving fosamprenavir plus ritonavir) with virological failure (plasma HIV-1 RNA more than 1,000 copies/mL on 2 occasions on or after week 12) were genotyped. Five of the 29 (17%) antiretroviral-naive patients receiving fosamprenavir without ritonavir in study APV 30001 had evidence of genotypic resistance to amprenavir: I54L/M (n = 2), I54L + L33F (n = 1), V32I + I47V (n = 1), and M46I + I47V (n = 1). No amprenavir resistance-associated mutations were detected in antiretroviral-naive patients treated with fosamprenavir plus ritonavir for 48 weeks in study APV 30002. However, the M46I and I50V mutations were detected in isolates from 1 virologically failed patient receiving fosamprenavir plus ritonavir once daily at week 160 (HIV-1 RNA more than 500 copies/mL). Upon retrospective analysis of stored samples using an ultrasensitive assay, these resistant mutants were traced back to week 84 (76 weeks prior to clinical virologic failure).

Cross-resistance – Varying degrees of cross-resistance among HIV-1 PIs have been observed. An association between virologic response at 48 weeks (HIV-1 RNA level less than 400 copies/mL) and PI-resistance mutations detected in baseline HIV-1 isolates from PI-experienced patients receiving fosamprenavir plus ritonavir twice daily (n = 88) or lopinavir plus ritonavir twice daily (n = 85) in study APV 30003 is shown in the following table. The majority of subjects had previously received 1 (47%) or 2 (36%) PIs, most commonly nelfinavir (57%) and indinavir (53%). Out of the 102 subjects with baseline phenotypes receiving twice-daily fosamprenavir plus ritonavir, 54% (n = 55) had resistance to at least 1 PI, with 98% (n = 54) of those having resistance to nelfinavir. Out of the 97 subjects with baseline phenotypes in the lopinavir plus ritonavir arm, 60% (n = 58) had resistance to at least 1 PI, with 97% (n = 56) of those having resistance to nelfinavir.

Fosamprenavir Plus Ritonavir Responders at Study Week 48 by Presence of Baseline PI Resistance-Associated Mutations[a]

PI mutations[b]	Fosamprenavir + ritonavir twice daily (n = 88)	Lopinavir + ritonavir twice daily (n = 85)
D30N	21/22 (95%)	17/19 (89%)
N88D/S	20/22 (91%)	12/12 (100%)
L90M	16/31 (52%)	17/29 (59%)
M46I/L	11/22 (50%)	12/24 (50%)
V82A/F/T/S	2/9 (22%)	6/17 (35%)
I54V	2/11 (18%)	6/11 (55%)
I84V	1/6 (17%)	2/5 (40%)

[a] Interpret results with caution because the subgroups were small.
[b] Most patients had a > 1 PI resistance-associated mutation at baseline.

The virologic response based upon baseline phenotype was assessed. Baseline isolates from PI-experienced patients responding to fosamprenavir plus ritonavir twice daily had a median shift in susceptibility to amprenavir relative to a standard wild-type reference strain of 0.7 (range, 0.1 to 5.4; n = 62), and baseline isolates from individuals failing therapy had a median shift in susceptibility of 1.9 (range, 0.2 to 14; n = 29). Because this was a select patient population, these data do not constitute definitive clinical susceptibility break points. Additional data are needed to determine clinically relevant break points for fosamprenavir.

Isolates from 15 of the 20 patients receiving twice-daily fosamprenavir plus ritonavir up to week 48 and experiencing virologic failure/ongoing replication were subjected to genotypic analysis. The following amprenavir resistance-associated mutations were found either alone or in combination: V32I, M46I/L, I47V, I50V, I54L/M, and I84V. Isolates from 4 of the 16 patients continuing to receive fosamprenavir plus ritonavir twice daily up to week 96 who experienced virologic failure underwent genotypic analysis. Isolates from 2 patients contained amprenavir resistance-associated mutations: V32I, M46I, and I47V in 1 isolate and I84V in the other.

Contraindications

Previously demonstrated clinically significant hypersensitivity (eg, Stevens-Johnson syndrome) to any of the components of this product or to amprenavir; coadministration with cisapride, delavirdine, dihydroergotamine, ergonovine, ergotamine, lovastatin, methylergonovine, midazolam, pimozide, rifampin, simvastatin, St. John's wort, and triazolam. If fosamprenavir is coadministered with ritonavir, the antiarrhythmic agents flecainide and propafenone also are contraindicated; refer to the full prescribing information for ritonavir for additional contraindications (see also Drug Interactions).

Warnings/Precautions

➤*Skin reactions:* Severe and life-threatening skin reactions, including 1 case of Stevens-Johnson syndrome among 700 patients treated with fosam-

FOSAMPRENAVIR CALCIUM — ORAL

prenavir were reported in clinical studies. Discontinue treatment with fosamprenavir for severe or life-threatening rashes and for moderate rashes accompanied by systemic symptoms.

➤*Hepatic toxicity:* Use of fosamprenavir with ritonavir at higher-than-recommended dosages may result in transaminase elevations and should not be used. Patients with underlying hepatitis B or C or marked elevations in transaminases prior to treatment may be at increased risk for developing or worsening of transaminase elevations. Conduct appropriate laboratory testing prior to initiating therapy with fosamprenavir and closely monitor patients during treatment.

➤*Diabetes mellitus/hyperglycemia:* New-onset diabetes mellitus, exacerbation of preexisting diabetes mellitus, and hyperglycemia have been reported during postmarketing surveillance in HIV-infected patients receiving PI therapy. Some patients required initiation or dosage adjustments of insulin or oral hypoglycemic agents for treatment of these events. In some cases, diabetic ketoacidosis has occurred. In those patients who discontinued PI therapy, hyperglycemia persisted in some cases. Because these events have been reported voluntarily during clinical practice, estimates of frequency cannot be made, and causal relationships between PI therapy and these events have not been established.

➤*Immune reconstitution syndrome:* Immune reconstitution syndrome has been reported in patients treated with combination antiretroviral therapy, including fosamprenavir. During the initial phase of combination antiretroviral treatment, a patient whose immune system responds may develop an inflammatory response to indolent or residual opportunistic infections (ie, *Mycobacterium avium* infection, cytomegalovirus, *Pneumocystis jirovecii* pneumonia, tuberculosis), which may necessitate further evaluation and treatment.

➤*Fat redistribution:* Redistribution/accumulation of body fat, including breast enlargement, central obesity, cushingoid appearance, dorsocervical fat enlargement (buffalo hump), facial wasting, and peripheral wasting, have been observed in patients receiving antiretroviral therapy, including fosamprenavir. The mechanism and long-term consequences of these reactions are currently unknown. A causal relationship has not been established.

➤*Lipid elevations:* Treatment with fosamprenavir plus ritonavir has resulted in increases in the concentration of triglycerides and cholesterol. Perform triglyceride and cholesterol testing prior to initiating therapy with fosamprenavir and at periodic intervals during therapy. Manage lipid disorders as clinically appropriate.

➤*Hemolytic anemia:* Acute hemolytic anemia has been reported in a patient treated with amprenavir.

➤*Hemophilia:* There have been reports of spontaneous bleeding in patients with hemophilia A and B treated with PIs. In some patients, additional factor VIII was required. In many of the reported cases, treatment with PIs was continued or restarted. A causal relationship between PI therapy and these episodes has not been established.

➤*Nephrolithiasis:* Cases of nephrolithiasis were reported during postmarketing surveillance in HIV-infected patients receiving fosamprenavir. Because these events were reported voluntarily during clinical practice, estimates of frequency cannot be made. If signs or symptoms of nephrolithiasis occur, temporary interruption or discontinuation of therapy may be considered.

➤*Resistance/Cross-resistance:* Because the potential for HIV cross-resistance among PIs has not been fully explored, it is unknown what effect therapy with fosamprenavir will have on the activity of subsequently administered PIs. Fosamprenavir has been studied in patients who have experienced treatment failure with PIs.

➤*Hypersensitivity reactions:* Use fosamprenavir with caution in patients with a known sulfonamide allergy. Fosamprenavir contains a sulfonamide moiety. The potential for cross-sensitivity between drugs in the sulfonamide class and fosamprenavir is unknown. In a clinical study of fosamprenavir used as the sole PI, rash occurred in 2 of 10 (20%) patients with a history of sulfonamide allergy, compared with 42 of 126 (33%) patients with no history of sulfonamide allergy. In 2 clinical studies of fosamprenavir plus low-dose ritonavir, rash occurred in 8 of 50 (16%) patients with a history of sulfonamide allergy, compared with 50 of 412 (12%) patients with no history of sulfonamide allergy.

➤*Hepatic function impairment:* Amprenavir is principally metabolized by the liver; therefore, exercise caution when administering fosamprenavir to patients with hepatic impairment because amprenavir concentrations may be increased. Patients with impaired hepatic function receiving fosamprenavir with or without concurrent ritonavir require dose reduction.

➤*Pregnancy: Category C.* Although the limited human data do not allow a prediction as to the safety of fosamprenavir during pregnancy, the animal data indicate that the drug may represent a low risk to the developing fetus. PIs should not be withheld in pregnancy because the expected benefit to the HIV-positive mother outweighs the unknown risk to the fetus. Monitor pregnant women taking PIs for hyperglycemia. Advise women receiving antiretroviral therapy during pregnancy to continue therapy, but, regardless of the regimen, zidovudine administration is recommended during the intrapartum period to prevent vertical transmission of HIV to the newborn.

Embryofetal development studies were conducted in rats (dosed from day 6 to 17 of gestation) and rabbits (dosed from day 7 to 20 of gestation). Administration of fosamprenavir to pregnant rats and rabbits produced no major effects on embryofetal development; however, the incidence of abortion was increased in rabbits that were administered fosamprenavir. Systemic exposures ($AUC_{0\text{-}24\ h}$) to amprenavir at these dosages were 0.8 (rabbits) to 2 (rats) times the exposures in humans following administration of the maximum recommended human dose (MRHD) of fosamprenavir alone or 0.3 (rabbits) to 0.7 (rats) times the exposures in humans following administration of the MRHD of fosamprenavir in combination with ritonavir. In contrast, administration of amprenavir was associated with abortions and an increased incidence of minor skeletal variations resulting from deficient ossification of the femur, humerus, and trochlea in pregnant rabbits at the tested dosage, approximately 5% of the exposure seen at the recommended human dosage.

The mating and fertility of the F_1 generation born to female rats given fosamprenavir was not different from control animals; however, fosamprenavir did cause a reduction in pup survival and body weights. Surviving F_1 female rats showed an increased time to successful mating, an increased length of gestation, a reduced number of uterine implantation sites per litter, and reduced gestational body weights compared with control animals. Systemic exposure ($AUC_{0\text{-}24\ h}$) to amprenavir in the F_0 pregnant rats was approximately 2 times higher than exposures in humans following administration of the MRHD of fosamprenavir alone or approximately the same as those seen in humans following administration of the MRHD of fosamprenavir in combination with ritonavir.

There are no adequate and well-controlled studies in pregnant women. Use fosamprenavir during pregnancy only if the potential benefit justifies the potential risk to the fetus.

Antiretroviral pregnancy registry – To monitor maternal-fetal outcomes of pregnant women exposed to fosamprenavir, an antiretroviral pregnancy registry has been established. Health care providers are encouraged to register patients by calling 1-800-258-4263.

➤*Lactation:* The Centers for Disease Control and Prevention recommend that HIV-infected mothers not breast-feed their infants to avoid risking postnatal transmission of HIV. Although it is not known if amprenavir is excreted in human milk, amprenavir is secreted into the milk of lactating rats. The molecular weight of amprenavir (approximately 506) is low enough that excretion into human breast milk should be expected. Because of the potential for HIV transmission and serious adverse reactions in breast-feeding infants, instruct mothers not to breast-feed if they are receiving fosamprenavir.

➤*Children:* The safety, pharmacokinetic profile, and virologic response of fosamprenavir oral suspension and tablets were evaluated in children 2 to 18 years of age in 2 open-label studies. No data are available for children younger than 2 years of age.

The adverse reaction profile seen in children was similar to that seen in adults. Vomiting regardless of causality was more frequent in children than in adults.

➤*Monitoring:* Perform triglyceride and cholesterol testing prior to initiating therapy with fosamprenavir and at periodic intervals during therapy. Monitor liver function tests prior to initiating therapy and periodically thereafter.

Drug Interactions

➤*Cytochrome P450 system:* Amprenavir, the active metabolite of fosamprenavir, is an inhibitor of CYP3A4 metabolism; therefore, do not coadminister with medications with narrow therapeutic windows that are substrates of CYP3A4. Data also suggest that amprenavir induces CYP3A4. Use caution when coadministering medications that are substrates, inhibitors, or inducers of CYP3A4, or potentially toxic medications that are metabolized by CYP3A4. Amprenavir does not inhibit CYP2D6, CYP1A2, CYP2C9, CYP2C19, CYP2E1, or uridine glucuronosyltransferase.

Fosamprenavir Drug Interactions

Precipitant drug	Object drug[a]		Description
Anticonvulsants (eg, carbamazepine, phenobarbital, phenytoin)	Fosamprenavir	⬇	Fosamprenavir may be less effective because of decreased amprenavir plasma concentrations with coadministration. Use with caution.
Azole antifungals (eg, itraconazole, ketoconazole)	Fosamprenavir	⬆	Coadministration may lead to an increase in ketoconazole or itraconazole adverse reactions. Dosage reduction of ketoconazole or itraconazole may be needed in patients receiving more than 400 mg/day of ketoconazole or itraconazole. Increase monitoring for adverse reactions. Coadministration of fosamprenavir plus ritonavir: High doses of ketoconazole or itraconazole (more than 200 mg/day) are not recommended. Plasma concentrations of amprenavir may be elevated, increasing the risk of toxicity. Monitor patients for amprenavir toxicity and adjust dosage as needed.
Fosamprenavir	Azole antifungals (eg, itraconazole, ketoconazole)		

FOSAMPRENAVIR CALCIUM — ORAL

Fosamprenavir Drug Interactions

Precipitant drug	Object drug[a]		Description
Contraceptives, hormonal (eg, ethinyl estradiol/ norethindrone)	Fosamprenavir	↓	Coadministration may decrease amprenavir AUC, and may lead to loss of virologic response. Coadministration of fosamprenavir with ethinyl estradiol/ norethindrone may alter hormone levels. Alternative methods of nonhormonal contraception are recommended.
Fosamprenavir	Contraceptives, hormonal (eg, ethinyl estradiol/ norethindrone)	↑↓	
CYP3A4 inhibitors (eg, clarithromycin)	Fosamprenavir	↑	Use with caution. Coadministering medications that are inhibitors of CYP3A4 may lead to increased amprenavir plasma concentrations.
Delavirdine	Fosamprenavir	↑	Coadministration may increase amprenavir concentrations. Coadministration may lead to loss of virologic response and possible resistance to delavirdine. Coadministration is contraindicated.
Fosamprenavir	Delavirdine	↓	
Dexamethasone	Fosamprenavir	↓	Fosamprenavir may be less effective because of decreased amprenavir plasma concentrations in patients taking these agents concomitantly. Use with caution.
Efavirenz	Fosamprenavir	↓	Coadministration led to decreases in amprenavir concentrations. An additional 100 mg/day (300 mg total) of ritonavir is recommended when efavirenz is administered with fosamprenavir plus ritonavir once daily. No change in the ritonavir dosage is required when efavirenz is administered with fosamprenavir plus ritonavir twice daily.
Efavirenz/ Ritonavir	Fosamprenavir	↑	Coadministration of efavirenz/ ritonavir with fosamprenavir plus ritonavir led to increases in amprenavir C_{max} and AUC by 18% and 11%, respectively.
Histamine H_2-receptor antagonists (eg, cimetidine, famotidine, nizatidine, ranitidine)	Fosamprenavir	↓	Fosamprenavir may be less effective because of decreased amprenavir plasma concentrations in patients taking these agents concomitantly. Use with caution.
HMG-CoA[b] reductase inhibitors (eg, atorvastatin, lovastatin, rosuvastatin, simvastatin)	Fosamprenavir	↓	Coadministration may increase the risk of myopathy, including rhabdomyolysis. Coadministration of fosamprenavir with lovastatin or simvastatin is contraindicated. Use the lowest possible dose of atorvastatin or rosuvastatin. Carefully monitor the patient. Consider use of fluvastatin or pravastatin as an alternative agent.
Fosamprenavir	HMG-CoA reductase inhibitors (eg, atorvastatin, lovastatin, rosuvastatin, simvastatin)	↑	
Indinavir	Fosamprenavir	↑	Coadministration has led to increases in amprenavir concentrations. Appropriate dosages of the combinations have not been established. Coadministration may decrease indinavir concentrations.
Fosamprenavir	Indinavir	↓	

Fosamprenavir Drug Interactions

Precipitant drug	Object drug[a]		Description
Lopinavir plus ritonavir	Fosamprenavir	↓	Coadministration of lopinavir plus ritonavir with fosamprenavir decreased amprenavir C_{max} and AUC. Coadministration increased lopinavir plus ritonavir C_{max} and AUC. An increased rate of adverse reactions has been observed with coadministration of these agents. Appropriate dosages of the combinations with respect to safety and efficacy have not been established.
Fosamprenavir	Lopinavir plus ritonavir	↑	
Methadone	Fosamprenavir	↓	Coadministration of amprenavir and methadone compared with a nonmatched historical control resulted in a 30%, 27%, and 25% decrease in serum amprenavir AUC, C_{max}, and C_{min}, respectively. Methadone concentrations may be decreased. The dose of methadone may need to be increased when coadministered with fosamprenavir. Monitor for opioid withdrawal symptoms.
Fosamprenavir	Methadone		
Nevirapine	Fosamprenavir	↓	Coadministration of nevirapine and fosamprenavir without ritonavir is not recommended. Coadministration has led to decreases in amprenavir levels and may increase nevirapine plasma concentrations. No dosage adjustment is required when nevirapine is administered with fosamprenavir/ritonavir twice daily.
Fosamprenavir	Nevirapine	↑	
Rifabutin	Fosamprenavir	↑	When coadministered with fosamprenavir, a dosage reduction of rifabutin by ≥ 50% of the recommended dose is required. When coadministered with fosamprenavir and ritonavir, a dosage reduction of rifabutin by ≥ 75% of the usual dosage is recommended (maximum dosage of 150 mg every other day or 3 times/wk). Monitor for neutropenia weekly when coadministered. Coadministration may also increase amprenavir AUC and C_{max} 35% and 36%, respectively.
Fosamprenavir	Rifabutin		
Rifampin	Fosamprenavir	↓	Rifampin reduces plasma concentrations of amprenavir by 82%, which may lead to loss of virologic response and possible resistance to fosamprenavir or to the class of PIs. Coadministration is contraindicated.
Saquinavir	Fosamprenavir	↓	Coadministration has led to decreases in amprenavir levels. Appropriate dosages have not been established.
St. John's wort	Fosamprenavir	↓	Coadministration may substantially decrease amprenavir concentrations, leading to the loss of virologic response and possible resistance to fosamprenavir or to the class of PIs. Coadministration is contraindicated.
Zidovudine	Fosamprenavir	↑	Coadministration may increase amprenavir AUC. Coadministration may increase zidovudine exposure. Monitor the patient for adverse reactions and adjust the zidovudine dose as needed.
Fosamprenavir	Zidovudine		

FOSAMPRENAVIR CALCIUM — ORAL

Fosamprenavir Drug Interactions

Precipitant drug	Object drug[a]		Description
Fosamprenavir	Antiarrhythmics (eg, amiodarone, bepridil, flecainide, lidocaine [systemic], propafenone, quinidine)	↑	Coadministration of fosamprenavir plus ritonavir with antiarrhythmics may increase the plasma concentrations of the antiarrhythmic agent, causing serious and/or life-threatening reactions such as cardiac arrhythmias. Coadministration of flecainide or propafenone is contraindicated if fosamprenavir is given with ritonavir. Use other antiarrhythmic agents with caution. Monitor antiarrhythmic concentrations.
Fosamprenavir	Anticholinergic agents (eg, darifenacin, fesoterodine, solifenacin, tolterodine)	↑	Plasma concentrations of the anticholinergic agent may be elevated, increasing the pharmacologic effects and risk adverse reactions. When coadministered with fosamprenavir, the daily dose of darifenacin should not exceed 7.5 mg, the daily dose of solifenacin should not exceed 5 mg, the daily dose of tolterodine should not exceed 2 mg and the daily dose of fesoterodine should not exceed 4 mg.
Fosamprenavir	Aripiprazole	↑	Aripiprazole plasma concentrations may be elevated, increasing the pharmacologic effects and risk of adverse reactions. Monitor the patient and adjust the aripiprazole dose as needed.
Fosamprenavir plus ritonavir	Atazanavir	↓	Fosamprenavir plus ritonavir may decrease atazanavir concentrations. Appropriate doses of the combinations with respect to safety and efficacy have not been established.
Fosamprenavir	Benzodiazepines (eg, alprazolam, clorazepate, diazepam, flurazepam, midazolam, triazolam)	↑	Coadministration with midazolam or triazolam is contraindicated because of the potential for serious and/or life-threatening reactions such as prolonged or increased sedation or respiratory depression. Alprazolam, clorazepate, diazepam, and flurazepam serum concentrations may be elevated, resulting in increased pharmacologic effects; a lower dosage may be needed.
Fosamprenavir	Calcium channel blockers (eg, amlodipine, diltiazem, felodipine, isradipine, nicardipine, nifedipine, nimodipine, nisoldipine, verapamil)	↑	The concentrations of calcium channel blockers may be increased when given with fosamprenavir. Monitor patients and use with caution.
Fosamprenavir	Carbamazepine	↑	Carbamazepine levels may be elevated, increasing the risk of toxicity.
Fosamprenavir	Cisapride	↑	Coadministration is contraindicated because of the potential for serious and/or life-threatening reactions such as cardiac arrhythmias.

Fosamprenavir Drug Interactions

Precipitant drug	Object drug[a]		Description
Fosamprenavir	Colchicine	↑	Colchicine plasma concentrations may be increased. Life-threatening and fatal colchicine toxicity may occur. Avoid coadministration in patients with hepatic or renal impairment. In patients with healthy renal and hepatic function, coadministration of fosamprenavir and colchicine should be undertaken using a maximum dose of colchicine 0.3 mg twice daily, with careful monitoring for colchicine-related adverse effects.
Fosamprenavir	Corticosteroids (eg, nasal fluticasone, oral prednisone)	↑	Corticosteroid metabolism (CYP3A4) may be inhibited, increasing the risk for toxicity. Coadministration of fluticasone and fosamprenavir plus ritonavir is not recommended unless the potential benefit to the patient outweighs the risk of systemic corticosteroid adverse reactions.
Fosamprenavir	Dronedarone	↑	Dronedarone plasma concentrations may be elevated, increasing the pharmacologic effects and risk of toxicity. Avoid coadministration.
Fosamprenavir	Eplerenone	↑	Eplerenone plasma concentrations may be elevated, increasing the pharmacologic effects and risk of toxicity. Close clinical monitoring is indicated when eplerenone is coadministered with fosamprenavir. Adjust the eplerenone dose as needed.
Fosamprenavir	Ergot derivatives (eg, dihydroergotamine, ergonovine, ergotamine, methylergonovine)	↑	Contraindicated because of the potential for serious and/or life-threatening reactions such as acute ergot toxicity (peripheral vasospasm and ischemia of the extremities and other tissues).
Fosamprenavir	Erythromycin	↑	Erythromycin plasma concentrations may be elevated, increasing the pharmacologic effects and risk of adverse reactions such as cardiac arrhythmias. Avoid coadministration.
Fosamprenavir	Esomeprazole	↑	Esomeprazole exposure may be increased. Monitor for adverse reactions and adjust the esomeprazole dose as needed.
Fosamprenavir	Eszopiclone	↑	Eszopiclone plasma concentrations may be elevated, increasing the pharmacologic effects and risk of adverse reactions. Close clinical monitoring is indicated when eszopiclone is coadministered with fosamprenavir. Adjust the eszopiclone dose as needed.
Fosamprenavir	Immunosuppressants (eg, cyclosporine, rapamycin, tacrolimus)	↑	Immunosuppressant concentrations may be increased. Therapeutic concentration monitoring of immunosuppressants is recommended. Toxicity may occur. Adjust the immunosuppressant dose as needed.
Fosamprenavir	Ixabepilone	↑	Ixabepilone plasma concentrations may be elevated, increasing the pharmacologic effects and risk of adverse reactions. Avoid coadministration. If fosamprenavir must be given with ixabepilone, ixabepilone dosage adjustment may be needed.

FOSAMPRENAVIR CALCIUM — ORAL

Fosamprenavir Drug Interactions

Precipitant drug	Object drug[a]		Description
Fosamprenavir	Maraviroc	↑	Maraviroc plasma concentrations may be elevated, increasing the pharmacologic effects and risk of adverse reactions. Monitor the response of the patient and adjust the maraviroc dose as needed.
Fosamprenavir	mTOR[c] inhibitors (eg, everolimus, temsirolimus)	↑	mTOR plasma concentrations may be elevated, increasing the pharmacologic effects and risk of adverse reactions. Avoid coadministration. If coadministration of fosamprenavir is necessary, monitor the clinical response of the patient and adjust the mTOR dose as needed.
Fosamprenavir	Nilotinib	↑	Nilotinib plasma concentrations may be elevated, increasing the pharmacologic effects and risk of adverse reactions such as cardiac arrhythmias. Avoid coadministration. If coadministration of fosamprenavir is necessary, it is recommended that therapy with nilotinib be interrupted. If fosamprenavir must be given with nilontinib, nilotinib dosage adjustment may be needed.
Fosamprenavir	Opioid analgesics (eg, alfentanil, buprenorphine, fentanyl, sufentanil)	↑	Opioid analgesic plasma concentrations may be increased and the half-life prolonged, increasing the risk of adverse reactions. Monitor respiratory function and adjust the opioid dose as needed.
Fosamprenavir	PDE5[d] inhibitors (eg, sildenafil, tadalafil, vardenafil)	↑	Coadministration substantially elevates the PDE5 inhibitor concentrations, resulting in an increase in adverse reactions (eg, hypotension, priapism, and visual changes). Use sildenafil with caution at reduced dosages of 25 mg every 48 hours. Use tadalafil with caution at reduced dosages of no more than 10 mg every 72 hours. Use vardenafil with caution at reduced dosages of no more than 2.5 mg every 24 hours. When coadministering vardenafil with fosamprenavir plus ritonavir, reduce dosage to no more than 2.5 mg every 72 hours. Increase monitoring for adverse reactions.
Fosamprenavir plus ritonavir	Paroxetine	↓	Coadministration of fosamprenavir and ritonavir with paroxetine decreased plasma levels of paroxetine. Adjust paroxetine dose based on clinical effect (tolerability and efficacy).
Fosamprenavir plus ritonavir	Phenytoin	↓	Fosamprenavir plus ritonavir may decrease phenytoin concentrations. Monitor phenytoin concentrations and increase phenytoin dose as appropriate.
Fosamprenavir	Pimozide	↑	Coadministration is contraindicated because of the potential for serious and/or life-threatening reactions such as cardiac arrhythmias.
Fosamprenavir	Protein-tyrosine kinase inhibitors (eg, dasatinib, suitinib, sorafenib)	↑	Protein-tyrosine kinase inhibitor plasma concentrations may be elevated, increasing the pharmacologic effects and risk of adverse reactions. Monitor the response of the patient and adjust the protein-tyrosine kinase inhibitor dose as needed.
Fosamprenavir	Quetiapine	↑	Quetipine plasma concentrations may be elevated, increasing the pharmacologic effects and risk of adverse reactions. Monitor the response of the patient and adjust the quetiapine dose as needed.
Fosamprenavir	Ranolazine	↑	Ranolazine plasma concentrations may be elevated, increasing the risk of dose-related prolongation of the QTc interval, torsades de pointes–type arrythmias, and sudden death. Coadministration of ranolazine and certain PIs is contraindicated.
Fosamprenavir	Trazodone	↑	Coadministration with fosamprenavir with or without ritonavir may elevate plasma concentrations of trazodone, increasing the pharmacologic and adverse reactions. Use the combination with caution and consider a lower dosage of trazodone.
Fosamprenavir	Tricyclic antidepressants (eg, amitriptyline, imipramine)	↑	Serious and/or life-threatening reactions could occur. Consider monitoring tricyclic antidepressant concentration with coadministration.
Fosamprenavir	Vasopressin receptor antagonists (eg, conivaptan, tolvaptan)	↑	Vasopressin receptor antagonist plasma concentrations may be elevated, increasing the pharmacologic effects and risk of adverse reactions. Avoid coadministration.
Fosamprenavir	Warfarin	↔	Concentrations of warfarin may be affected. Monitor international normalized ratio.

[a] ↑ = object drug increased; ↓ = object drug decreased; ↑↓ = object drug both increased and decreased; ↔ = undetermined clinical effect.
[b] HMG-CoA = 3–hydroxy-3–methylglutaryl coenzyme A.
[c] mTOR = mammalian target of rapamycin inhibitors.
[d] PDE5 = phosphodiesterase 5.

➤*Drug/Food interactions:* Administration of a single dose of fosamprenavir 1,400 mg oral suspension in the fed state (standardized high-fat meal: 967 kcal, 67 g of fat, 33 g of protein, 58 g of carbohydrate) compared with the fasted state was associated with a 46% reduction in C_{max}, a 0.72-hour delay in T_{max}, and a 28% reduction in amprenavir $AUC_{0-\infty}$. Grapefruit juice may increase plasma concentrations of amprenavir. If grapefruit juice cannot be avoided, closely monitor the patient and adjust the fosamprenavir dose as needed.Garlic ingestion may reduce amprenavir plasma concentrations, decreasing the pharmacologic effects. Avoid garlic ingestion.

Adverse Reactions

➤*Most common adverse reactions:* The most common moderate to severe adverse reactions in clinical studies of fosamprenavir were diarrhea, rash, nausea, vomiting, and headache.

➤*Discontinuation of therapy:* Treatment discontinuation because of adverse reactions occurred in 6.4% of patients receiving fosamprenavir and in 5.9% of patients receiving comparator treatments. The most common adverse reactions leading to discontinuation of fosamprenavir (incidence of 1% or less) included diarrhea, nausea, vomiting, AST increased, ALT increased, and rash.

➤*Adults:* The data for the 3 active-controlled clinical trials described in the following sectionreflect exposure of 700 HIV-1 infected patients to fosamprenavir tablets, including 599 patients exposed to fosamprenavir for longer than 24 weeks and 409 patients exposed for longer than 48 weeks. The population age ranged from 17 to 72 years. Of these patients, 26% were female, 51% were white patients, 31% were black, 16% were American Hispanic, and 70% were antiretroviral-naive. Sixty-one percent received fosamprenavir 1,400 mg once daily plus ritonavir 200 mg once daily, 24% received fosamprenavir 1,400 mg twice daily, and 15% received fosamprenavir 700 mg twice daily plus ritonavir 100 mg twice daily.

➤*Skin reactions:* See Warnings/Precautions for more information.

Skin rash (without regard to causality) occurred in approximately 19% of patients treated with fosamprenavir in the pivotal efficacy studies. Rashes were usually maculopapular and of mild or moderate intensity, some with pruritus. Rash had a median onset of 11 days after initiation of fosamprenavir and a median duration of 13 days. Skin rash led to discontinuation of fosamprenavir in less than 1% of patients. In some patients with mild or moderate rash, dosing with fosamprenavir often was continued without interruption; if interrupted, reintroduction of fosamprenavir generally did not result in rash recurrence.

FOSAMPRENAVIR CALCIUM — ORAL

➤*Antiretroviral-naive patients:*

Fosamprenavir Moderate to Severe Adverse Reactions in Antiretroviral-Naive Adult Patients (≥ 2%)[a]				
Adverse reactions	Fosamprenavir 1,400 mg twice daily (n = 166)	Nelfinavir 1,250 mg twice daily (n = 83)	Fosamprenavir 1,400 mg once daily/ ritonavir 200 mg once daily (n = 322)	Nelfinavir 1,250 mg twice daily (n = 327)
CNS				
Fatigue	2%	1%	4%	2%
Headache	2%	4%	3%	3%
Dermatologic				
Rash	8%	2%	3%	2%
GI				
Abdominal pain	1%	0%	2%	2%
Diarrhea	5%	18%	10%	18%
Nausea	7%	4%	7%	5%
Vomiting	2%	4%	6%	4%

[a] All patients also received abacavir and lamivudine twice daily.

PI-experienced patients –

Fosamprenavir Moderate to Severe Adverse Reactions in PI-Experienced Adult Patients (≥ 2%)		
Adverse reactions	Fosamprenavir 700 mg twice daily/ ritonavir 100 mg twice daily[a] (n = 106)	Lopinavir 400 mg twice daily/ ritonavir 100 mg twice daily[a] (n = 103)
GI		
Abdominal pain	< 1%	2%
Diarrhea	13%	11%
Nausea	3%	9%
Vomiting	3%	5%
Miscellaneous		
Headache	4%	2%
Rash	3%	0%

[a] All patients also received 2 reverse transcriptase inhibitors.

➤*Lab test abnormalities:*

Fosamprenavir Grade 3/4 Laboratory Abnormalities in Antiretroviral-Naive Adults (≥ 2%)[a]				
Laboratory abnormality	Fosamprenavir 1,400 mg twice daily (n = 166)	Nelfinavir 1,250 mg twice daily (n = 83)	Fosamprenavir 1,400 mg once daily/ ritonavir 200 mg once daily (n = 322)	Nelfinavir 1,250 mg twice daily (n = 327)
ALT (> 5 × ULN[b])	6%	5%	8%	8%
AST (> 5 × ULN)	6%	6%	6%	7%
Neutrophil count, absolute (< 750 cells/mm^3)	3%	6%	3%	4%
Serum lipase (> 2 × ULN)	8%	4%	6%	4%
Triglycerides[c] (> 750 mg/dL)	0%	1%	6%	2%

[a] All patients also received abacavir and lamivudine twice daily.
[b] ULN = upper limit of normal.
[c] Fasting specimens.

The incidence of grade 3 or 4 hyperglycemia in antiretroviral-naive patients who received fosamprenavir in the pivotal studies was less than 1%.

Fosamprenavir Grade 3/4 Laboratory Abnormalities in PI-Experienced Adults (≥ 2%)		
Laboratory abnormality	Fosamprenavir 700 mg twice daily/ ritonavir 100 mg twice daily[a] (n = 104)	Lopinavir 400 mg twice daily/ ritonavir 100 mg twice daily[a] (n = 103)
ALT (> 5 × ULN)	4%	4%
AST (> 5 × ULN)	4%	2%
Glucose (> 251 mg/dL)	2%[b]	2%[b]
Serum lipase (> 2 × ULN)	5%	12%
Triglycerides[c] (> 750 mg/dL)	11%[b]	6%[b]

[a] All patients also received 2 reverse transcriptase inhibitors.
[b] n = 100 for fosamprenavir plus ritonavir; n = 98 for lopinavir plus ritonavir.
[c] Fasting specimens.

➤*Children:* Fosamprenavir, with and without ritonavir, was studied in 144 children 2 to 18 years of age in 2 open-label studies. Safety information from 75 children receiving fosamprenavir twice daily, with or without ritonavir, is as follows.

All adverse reactions regardless of causality, all drug-related adverse reactions, and all laboratory reactions occurred with similar frequency in children compared with adults, with the exception of vomiting. Vomiting, regardless of causality, occurred more frequently among children receiving fosamprenavir twice daily with ritonavir (30%, all between 2 and 18 years of age) and without ritonavir (56%, all between 2 and 5 years of age), compared with adults receiving fosamprenavir twice daily with ritonavir (10%) and without ritonavir (16%). The median duration of drug-related vomiting episodes was 1 day (range, 1 to 62 days). Vomiting required temporary dose interruptions in 4 children and was treatment limiting in 1 child, all of whom were receiving fosamprenavir twice daily with ritonavir.

➤*Postmarketing:* Angioedema, hypercholesterolemia, myocardial infarction, nephrolithiasis, and oral paresthesia.

Overdosage

➤*Symptoms:* In a healthy volunteer repeat-dose pharmacokinetic study evaluating high-dose combinations of fosamprenavir plus ritonavir, an increased frequency of grade 2/3 ALT elevations (more than 2.5 times the ULN) was observed with fosamprenavir 1,400 mg twice daily plus ritonavir 200 mg twice daily (4/25 subjects). Concurrent grade 1/2 elevations in AST (more than 1.25 times the ULN) were noted in 3 of these 4 subjects. These transaminase elevations resolved following discontinuation of dosing.

➤*Treatment:* There is no known antidote for fosamprenavir. It is not known whether amprenavir can be removed by peritoneal dialysis or hemodialysis. If overdosage occurs, monitor the patient for evidence of toxicity and apply standard supportive treatment as necessary.

Patient Information

Inform patients that fosamprenavir is not a cure for HIV infection and that they may continue to develop opportunistic infections and other complications associated with HIV disease. The long-term effects of fosamprenavir are unknown at this time. Tell patients that there currently are no data demonstrating that therapy with fosamprenavir can reduce the risk of transmitting HIV to others.

Inform patients that sustained decreases in plasma HIV-1 RNA have been associated with a reduced risk of progression to AIDS and death. Advise patients to remain under the care of a health care provider while using fosamprenavir.

Advise patients to take fosamprenavir every day as prescribed. Fosamprenavir must always be used in combination with other antiretroviral drugs. Advise patients not to alter the dosage or discontinue therapy without consulting their health care provider. If a dose is missed by less than 4 hours, instruct patients to take the dose as soon as possible and then return to their normal schedule. However, if a dose is skipped, instruct the patient not to double the next dose.

Instruct patients to inform their health care provider if they have a sulfa allergy. The potential for cross-sensitivity between drugs in the sulfonamide class and fosamprenavir is unknown.

Fosamprenavir may interact with many drugs; therefore, advise patients to report to their health care provider the use of any other prescription or nonprescription medication or herbal products, particularly St. John's wort.

Advise patients receiving PDE5 inhibitors that they may be at an increased risk of PDE5 inhibitor–associated adverse reactions, including hypotension, priapism, and visual changes, and instruct them to promptly report any symptoms to their health care provider.

Instruct patients receiving hormonal contraceptives to use alternate contraceptive measures during therapy with fosamprenavir because hormonal levels may be altered, and, if used in combination with fosamprenavir and ritonavir, liver enzyme elevations may occur.

Inform patients that redistribution or accumulation of body fat may occur in patients receiving antiretroviral therapy, including fosamprenavir, and that the cause and long-term health effects of these conditions are not known at this time.

Tell patients to take fosamprenavir tablets with or without food.

➤*Oral suspension:* Instruct patients to shake the bottle vigorously before each use. Inform patients that refrigeration of the oral suspension may improve the taste.

Tell adults to take fosamprenavir oral suspension without food. Children should take fosamprenavir oral suspension with food. If vomiting occurs within 30 minutes of dosing, repeat the dose.

ATAZANAVIR

Rx	**Reyataz** (Bristol-Myers Squibb)	**Capsules; oral:** 100 mg	As atazanavir sulfate. Lactose. (BMS 100 mg 3623). Blue/White. In 60s.
		150 mg	As atazanavir sulfate. Lactose. (BMS 150 mg 3624). Blue/Powder blue. In 60s.
		200 mg	As atazanavir sulfate. Lactose. (BMS 200 mg 3631). Blue. In 60s.
		300 mg	As atazanavir sulfate. Lactose. (BMS 300 mg 3622). Red/Blue. In 30s.

ATAZANAVIR SULFATE — ORAL

Indications

➤*HIV infection:* In combination with other antiretroviral agents for the treatment of HIV-1 infection.

Administration and Dosage

➤*General dosing considerations:* The recommended oral dosage of atazanavir depends on the treatment history of the patient and use of other coadministered drugs. When coadministered with H_2-receptor antagonists or proton pump inhibitors, dose separation may be required.

Safety and efficacy of atazanavir with ritonavir in dosages greater than 100 mg once daily have not been established. The use of higher ritonavir doses might alter the safety profile of atazanavir (eg, cardiac effects, hyperbilirubinemia) and, therefore, is not recommended. Consult the complete monograph for ritonavir when using this agent.

➤*Adults:*

HIV infection, therapy-naive patients –

Usual dosage: Atazanavir 300 mg with ritonavir 100 mg once daily all as a single dose with food. For patients who are unable to tolerate ritonavir, the recommended dosage is atazanavir 400 mg (without ritonavir) once daily taken with food.

Concomitant therapy:

• *Didanosine* – When coadministered with didanosine buffered or enteric-coated formulations, atazanavir should be given with food 2 hours before or 1 hour after didanosine.

• *Tenofovir* – Atazanavir 300 mg with ritonavir 100 mg once daily (all as a single dose with food) with tenofovir.

• *H_2-receptor antagonist* – The H_2-receptor antagonist dosage should not exceed a dosage comparable with famotidine 40 mg twice daily. Atazanavir 300 mg and ritonavir 100 mg should be administered simultaneously with, and/or at least 10 hours after, the dose of the H_2-receptor antagonist. For patients unable to tolerate ritonavir, atazanavir 400 mg once daily with food should be administered at least 2 hours before and at least 10 hours after the H_2-receptor antagonist. For these patients, no single dose of the H_2-receptor antagonist should exceed a dose comparable with famotidine 20 mg, and the total daily dose should not exceed a dose comparable with famotidine 40 mg.

• *Proton pump inhibitors* – The proton pump inhibitor dose should not exceed a dose comparable with omeprazole 20 mg and must be taken approximately 12 hours prior to the atazanavir 300 mg and ritonavir 100 mg doses.

• *Efavirenz* – If atazanavir is combined with efavirenz, atazanavir 400 mg (two 200 mg capsules) with ritonavir 100 mg should be administered once daily all as a single dose with food, and efavirenz should be administered on an empty stomach, preferably at bedtime.

HIV infection, therapy-experienced patients – Atazanavir without ritonavir is not recommended for treatment-experienced patients with prior virologic failure.

Usual dosage: Atazanavir 300 mg with ritonavir 100 mg once daily (all as a single dose with food).

Concomitant therapy:

• *Didanosine* – When coadministered with didanosine buffered or enteric-coated formulations, atazanavir should be given (with food) 2 hours before or 1 hour after didanosine.

• *Efavirenz* – Do not coadminister atazanavir with efavirenz in treatment-experienced patients because of decreased atazanavir exposure.

• *H_2-receptor antagonist* – Whenever an H_2-receptor antagonist is given to a patient receiving atazanavir with ritonavir, the H_2-receptor antagonist dosage should not exceed a dosage comparable with famotidine 20 mg twice daily, and the atazanavir and ritonavir doses should be administered simultaneously with, and/or at least 10 hours after, the dose of the H_2-receptor antagonist.

Atazanavir 300 mg with ritonavir 100 mg once daily should be given all as a single dose with food if taken with an H_2-receptor antagonist.

Atazanavir 400 mg (two 200 mg capsules) with ritonavir 100 mg once daily should be given all as a single dose with food if taken with both tenofovir and an H_2-receptor antagonist.

• *Proton pump inhibitors* – Proton pump inhibitors should not be used in treatment-experienced patients receiving atazanavir.

➤*Children:* The recommended dosage of atazanavir for children 6 to younger than 18 years of age is based on body weight and should not exceed the recommended adult dosage.

HIV infection, therapy-naive patients –

Treatment without ritonavir:

• *13 years of age and older (weighing at least 39 kg)* – For treatment-naive patients 13 years of age and older weighing at least 39 kg who are unable to tolerate ritonavir, the recommended dosage is atazanavir 400 mg (without ritonavir) once daily with food.

Treatment with ritonavir:

• *6 to younger than 18 years of age –*

Usual dosage:

Atazanavir Dosage for Treatment-Naive Children 6 to Younger Than 18 Years of Age

Body weight (kg)	Atazanavir dose[a,b]	Ritonavir dose[b]
15 to < 25	150 mg	80 mg[c]
25 to < 32	200 mg	100 mg[d]
32 to < 39	250 mg	100 mg[d]
≥ 39	300 mg	100 mg[d]

[a] The recommended dosage of atazanavir can be achieved using a combination of commercially available capsule strengths.
[b] The dosage of atazanavir and ritonavir was calculated as follows:
• 15 kg to < 20 kg: atazanavir 8.5 mg/kg with ritonavir 4 mg/kg once daily with food.
• ≥ 20 kg: atazanavir 7 mg/kg with ritonavir 4 mg/kg once daily with food, not to exceed atazanavir 300 mg and ritonavir 100 mg.
[c] Ritonavir liquid.
[d] Ritonavir capsule or liquid.

Maximum dose: Atazanavir 300 mg/ritonavir 100 mg.

HIV infection, therapy-experienced patients –

6 to younger than 18 years of age:

• *Usual dosage* – The data are insufficient to recommend dosing of treatment-experienced children weighing less than 25 kg.

Atazanavir Dosage for Treatment-Experienced Children 6 to Younger Than 18 Years of Age

Body weight (kg)	Atazanavir dose[a,b]	Ritonavir dose[b]
25 to < 32	200 mg	100 mg[c]
32 to < 39	250 mg	100 mg[c]
≥ 39	300 mg	100 mg[c]

[a] The recommended dosage of atazanavir can be achieved using a combination of commercially available capsule strengths.
[b] The dosage was calculated as atazanavir 7 mg/kg with ritonavir 4 mg/kg once daily with food, not to exceed atazanavir 300 mg and ritonavir 100 mg.
[c] Ritonavir capsule or liquid.

• *Maximum dose* – Atazanavir 300 mg/ritonavir 100 mg.

➤*Renal function impairment:*

Hemodialysis – Treatment-naive patients with end-stage renal disease managed with hemodialysis should receive atazanavir 300 mg with ritonavir 100 mg. Atazanavir should not be administered to HIV-treatment–experienced patients with end-stage renal disease managed with hemodialysis.

➤*Hepatic function impairment:* Atazanavir should be used with caution in patients with mild to moderate hepatic impairment. For patients with moderate hepatic impairment (Child-Pugh class B) who have not experienced prior virologic failure, a dosage reduction to 300 mg once daily should be considered. Atazanavir should not be used in patients with severe hepatic impairment (Child-Pugh class C). Atazanavir/ritonavir has not been studied in subjects with hepatic impairment and is not recommended.

➤*Administration:* Atazanavir must be taken with food.

➤*Storage/Stability:* Store at 25°C (77°F); excursions are permitted between 15° and 30°C (59° and 86°F).

Actions

➤*Pharmacology:* Atazanavir, an antiviral drug, is an azapeptide HIV-1 protease inhibitor. The compound selectively inhibits the virus-specific processing of viral Gag and Gag-Pol polyproteins in HIV-1 infected cells, thus preventing formation of mature virions.

➤*Pharmacokinetics:*

Atazanavir With Ritonavir Steady-State Pharmacokinetics in Adults[a]

Pharmacokinetic parameter	Atazanavir 400 mg once daily: Healthy subjects (n = 14)	Atazanavir 400 mg once daily: HIV-infected patients (n = 13)	Atazanavir 300 mg with ritonavir 100 mg once daily: Healthy subjects (n = 28)	Atazanavir 300 mg with ritonavir 100 mg once daily: HIV-infected patients (n = 10)
C_{max} (ng/mL)				
Geometric mean (CV %)	5,199 (26%)	2,298 (71%)	6,129 (31%)	4,422 (58%)
Mean (SD)	5,358 (1,371)	3,152 (2,231)	6,450 (2,031)	5,233 (3,033)

ATAZANAVIR SULFATE — ORAL

Atazanavir With Ritonavir Steady-State Pharmacokinetics in Adults[a]				
	Atazanavir 400 mg once daily		Atazanavir 300 mg with ritonavir 100 mg once daily	
Pharmacokinetic parameter	Healthy subjects (n = 14)	HIV-infected patients (n = 13)	Healthy subjects (n = 28)	HIV-infected patients (n = 10)
T_{max} (h)				
Median	2.5	2	2.7	3
AUC (ng•h/mL)				
Geometric mean (CV%)	28,132 (28%)	14,874 (91%)	57,039 (37%)	46,073 (66%)
Mean (SD)	29,303 (8,263)	22,262 (20,159)	61,435 (22,911)	53,761 (35,294)
Half-life (h)				
Mean (SD)	7.9 (2.9)	6.5 (2.6)	18.1 (6.2)[b]	8.6 (2.3)
C_{min} (ng/mL)				
Geometric mean (CV%)	159 (88%)	120 (109%)	1,227 (53%)	636 (97%)
Mean (SD)	218 (191)	273 (298)[c]	1,441 (757)	862 (838)

[a] C_{max} = maximum plasma concentration; CV = coefficient of variation; SD = standard deviation; T_{max} = time to reach C_{max}; AUC = area under the curve; C_{min} = minimum plasma concentration.
[b] n = 26.
[c] n = 12.

Absorption – Atazanavir is rapidly absorbed, with a T_{max} of approximately 2.5 hours. Atazanavir demonstrates nonlinear pharmacokinetics with greater than dose-proportional increases in AUC and C_{max} values over the dosage range of 200 to 800 mg once daily. Steady state is achieved between days 4 and 8, with an accumulation of approximately 2.3-fold.

Effect of food: Administration of atazanavir with food enhances bioavailability and reduces pharmacokinetic variability. Administration of a single atazanavir 400 mg dose with a light meal (357 kcal, fat 8.2 g, protein 10.6 g) resulted in a 70% increase in AUC and 57% increase in C_{max} relative to the fasting state. Administration of a single atazanavir 400 mg dose with a high-fat meal (721 kcal, fat 37.3 g, protein 29.4 g) resulted in a mean increase in AUC of 35%, with no change in C_{max} relative to the fasting state. Administration of atazanavir with a light meal or high-fat meal decreased the CV of AUC and C_{max} by approximately one-half compared with the fasting state.

Coadministration of a single dose of atazanavir 300 mg and a dose of ritonavir 100 mg with a light meal (336 kcal, fat 5.1 g, protein 9.3 g) resulted in a 33% increase in the AUC and a 40% increase in both the C_{max} and the 24-hour concentration of atazanavir relative to the fasting state. Coadministration with a high-fat meal (951 kcal, fat 54.7 g, protein 35.9 g) did not affect the AUC of atazanavir relative to fasting conditions, and the C_{max} was within 11% of fasting values. The 24-hour concentration following a high-fat meal was increased by approximately 33% because of the delayed absorption; the median T_{max} increased from 2 to 5 hours. Coadministration of atazanavir with ritonavir with a light or a high-fat meal decreased the CV of AUC and C_{max} by approximately 25% compared with the fasting state.

Distribution – Atazanavir is 86% bound to human serum proteins, and protein binding is independent of concentration. Atazanavir binds to both alpha-1 acid glycoprotein and albumin to a similar extent (89% and 86%, respectively). In a multiple-dose study in HIV-infected patients dosed with atazanavir 400 mg once daily with a light meal for 12 weeks, atazanavir was detected in the cerebrospinal fluid and semen. The cerebrospinal fluid/plasma ratio for atazanavir (n = 4) ranged between 0.0021 and 0.0226, and the seminal fluid/plasma ratio (n = 5) ranged between 0.11 and 4.42.

Metabolism – Atazanavir is extensively metabolized in humans. The major biotransformation pathways of atazanavir in humans consisted of monooxygenation and dioxygenation. Other minor biotransformation pathways for atazanavir or its metabolites consisted of glucuronidation, N-dealkylation, hydrolysis, and oxygenation with dehydrogenation. Two minor metabolites of atazanavir in plasma have been characterized. Neither metabolite demonstrated in vitro antiviral activity. In vitro studies using human liver microsomes suggested that atazanavir is metabolized by CYP3A.

Excretion – Following a single dose of ^{14}C-atazanavir 400 mg, 79% and 13% of the total radioactivity was recovered in the feces and urine, respectively. Unchanged drug accounted for approximately 20% and 7% of the administered dose in the feces and urine, respectively. The mean elimination half-life of atazanavir in healthy volunteers (n = 214) and HIV-infected adults (n = 13) was approximately 7 hours at steady state following a dose of 400 mg daily with a light meal.

Special populations –

Renal function impairment: In healthy subjects, the renal elimination of unchanged atazanavir was approximately 7% of the administered dose. Atazanavir has been studied in adults with severe renal impairment (n = 20), including those on hemodialysis, at multiple doses of 400 mg once daily. The mean atazanavir C_{max} was 9% lower, AUC was 19% higher, and C_{min} was 96% higher in subjects with severe renal impairment not undergoing hemodialysis (n = 10) than in age-, weight-, and gender-matched subjects with healthy renal function. Atazanavir was not appreciably cleared during hemodialysis. In a 4-hour dialysis session, 2.1% of the administered dose was removed. When atazanavir was administered prior to or following hemodialysis (n = 10), the geometric means for C_{max}, AUC, and C_{min} were approximately 25% to 43% lower compared with subjects with healthy renal function. The mechanism of this decrease is unknown. Do not administer atazanavir to HIV-treatment–experienced patients with end-stage renal disease managed with hemodialysis.

Hepatic function impairment: Atazanavir is metabolized and eliminated primarily by the liver. Atazanavir has been studied in adults with moderate to severe hepatic impairment (14 Child-Pugh class B and 2 Child-Pugh class C subjects) after a single 400 mg dose. The mean $AUC_{(0-\infty)}$ was 42% greater in subjects with hepatic impairment than in healthy volunteers. The mean half-life of atazanavir in subjects with hepatic impairment was 12.1 hours compared with 6.4 hours in healthy volunteers. Increased concentrations of atazanavir are expected in patients with moderate or severe hepatic impairment. The pharmacokinetics of atazanavir in combination with ritonavir have not been studied in subjects with hepatic impairment. Do not administer atazanavir to patients with severe hepatic impairment. Atazanavir/ritonavir is not recommended for use in patients with hepatic impairment.

Children:

Atazanavir Steady-State Pharmacokinetics in Children 6 to < 18 Years of Age in the Fed State		
	Atazanavir 205 mg/m² with ritonavir 100 mg/m² once daily	
	≥ 6 to 13 years of age (n = 17)	≥ 13 to 18 years of age (n = 10)
Dose (mg)		
Median	200	400
(min-max)	(150 to 400)	(250 to 500)
C_{max} ng/mL		
Geometric mean (CV%)	4,451 (33%)	3,711 (46%)
AUC ng•h/mL		
Geometric mean (CV%)	42,503 (36%)	44,970 (34%)
C_{min} ng/mL		
Geometric mean (CV%)	535 (62%)	1,090 (60%)

➤*Microbiology:*

Antiviral activity in cell culture – Atazanavir exhibits anti–HIV-1 activity, with a mean 50% effective concentration (EC_{50}) in the absence of human serum of 2 to 5 nM against a variety of laboratory and clinical HIV-1 isolates grown in peripheral blood mononuclear cells, macrophages, CEM-SS cells, and MT-2 cells. Atazanavir has activity against HIV-1 group M subtype viruses A, B, C, D, AE, AG, F, G, and J isolates in cell culture. Atazanavir has variable activity against HIV-2 isolates (1.9 to 32 nM), with EC_{50} values above the EC_{50} values of failure isolates. Two-drug combination antiviral activity studies with atazanavir showed no antagonism in cell culture with nonnucleoside reverse transcriptase inhibitors (NNRTIs) (eg, delavirdine, efavirenz, nevirapine), protease inhibitors (eg, amprenavir, indinavir, lopinavir, nelfinavir, ritonavir, saquinavir), nucleoside reverse transcriptase inhibitors (NRTIs) (eg, abacavir, didanosine, emtricitabine, lamivudine, stavudine, tenofovir, zalcitabine, zidovudine), the HIV-1 fusion inhibitor enfuvirtide, and 2 compounds used in the treatment of viral hepatitis (adefovir and ribavirin) without enhanced cytotoxicity.

Resistance –

Cell culture: HIV-1 isolates with a decreased susceptibility to atazanavir have been selected in cell culture and obtained from patients treated with atazanavir or atazanavir/ritonavir. HIV-1 isolates that had 93- to 183-fold reduced susceptibility to atazanavir from 3 different viral strains were selected in cell culture by 5 months. The substitutions in these HIV-1 viruses that contributed to atazanavir resistance included I50L, N88S, I84V, A71V, and M46I. Changes were also observed at the protease cleavage sites following drug selection. Recombinant viruses containing the I50L substitution without other major protease inhibitor substitutions were growth impaired and displayed increases in cell culture susceptibility to other protease inhibitors (eg, amprenavir, indinavir, lopinavir, nelfinavir, ritonavir, saquinavir). The I50L and I50V substitutions yielded selective resistance to atazanavir and amprenavir, respectively, and did not appear to be cross-resistant.

Cross-resistance – Cross-resistance among protease inhibitors has been observed. Baseline phenotypic and genotypic analyses of clinical isolates from atazanavir clinical trials of protease inhibitor–experienced patients showed that isolates cross-resistant to multiple protease inhibitors were cross-resistant to atazanavir. More than 90% of the isolates with substitutions that included I84V or G48V were resistant to atazanavir. More than 60% of isolates containing L90M, G73S/T/C, A71V/T, I54V, M46I/L, or a change at V82 were resistant to atazanavir, and 38% of isolates containing a D30N substitution in addition to other changes were resistant to atazanavir. Isolates resistant to atazanavir were also cross-resistant to other protease inhibitors, with more than 90% of the isolates resistant to indinavir, lopinavir, nelfinavir, ritonavir, and saquinavir, and 80% resistant to amprenavir. In treatment-experienced patients, protease inhibitor–resistant viral isolates that developed the I50L substitution in addition to other protease inhibitor resistance-associated substitution were also cross-resistant to other protease inhibitors.

Contraindications

Previously demonstrated clinically significant hypersensitivity (eg, Stevens-Johnson syndrome, erythema multiforme, toxic skin eruptions) to any of the

ATAZANAVIR SULFATE — ORAL

components of the product; coadministration with the following drugs that are highly dependent on CYP3A or UGT1A1 for clearance and for which elevated plasma concentrations are associated with serious and/or life-threatening events: alfuzosin, cisapride, dihydroergotamine, ergonovine, ergotamine, indinavir, irinotecan, lovastatin, methylergonovine, midazolam (orally administered), pimozide, rifampin, sildenafil when dosed as *Revatio* for the treatment of pulmonary arterial hypertension, St. John's wort (*Hypericum perforatum*), simvastatin, and triazolam.

Warnings/Precautions

➤*Cardiac conduction abnormalities:* Atazanavir prolonged the PR interval of the electrocardiogram (ECG) in some patients. In healthy volunteers and in patients, abnormalities in atrioventricular (AV) conduction were asymptomatic and generally limited to first-degree AV block. There have been rare reports of second-degree AV block and other conduction abnormalities. Because of limited clinical experience, use atazanavir with caution in patients with preexisting conduction system disease (eg, marked first-degree AV block or second- or third-degree AV block).

➤*Dermatologic effects:* In controlled clinical trials, rash (all grades, regardless of causality) occurred in approximately 20% of patients treated with atazanavir. The median time to onset of rash in clinical studies was 7.3 weeks, and the median duration of rash was 1.4 weeks. Rashes were generally mild to moderate maculopapular skin eruptions. Treatment-emergent adverse reactions of moderate or severe rash (occurring at a rate of 2% or more) are presented for the individual clinical studies. Dosing with atazanavir was often continued without interruption in patients who developed rash. The discontinuation rate for rash in clinical trials was less than 1%. Discontinue atazanavir if severe rash develops. Cases of Stevens-Johnson syndrome, erythema multiforme, and toxic skin eruptions have been reported in patients receiving atazanavir.

➤*Hyperbilirubinemia:* Most patients taking atazanavir experience asymptomatic elevations in indirect (unconjugated) bilirubin related to inhibition of uridine disphosphoglucuronosyl transferase. This hyperbilirubinemia is reversible upon discontinuation of atazanavir. Evaluate hepatic transaminase elevations that occur with hyperbilirubinemia for alternative causes. No long-term safety data are available for patients experiencing persistent elevations in total bilirubin more than 5 times the upper limit of normal (ULN). Consider alternative antiretroviral therapy to atazanavir if jaundice or scleral icterus associated with bilirubin elevations presents cosmetic concerns for patients. Dose reduction of atazanavir is not recommended because long-term efficacy of reduced doses has not been established.

➤*Nephrolithiasis:* Cases of nephrolithiasis were reported during postmarketing surveillance in HIV-infected patients receiving atazanavir therapy. Because these events were reported voluntarily during clinical practice, estimates of frequency cannot be made. If signs and symptoms of nephrolithiasis occur, consider temporary interruption or discontinuation of therapy.

➤*Diabetes mellitus / hyperglycemia:* New-onset diabetes mellitus, exacerbation of preexisting diabetes mellitus, and hyperglycemia have been reported during postmarketing surveillance in HIV-infected patients receiving protease inhibitor therapy. Some patients required initiation or dose adjustments of insulin or oral hypoglycemic agents for treatment of these reactions. In some cases, diabetic ketoacidosis occurred. In patients who discontinued protease inhibitor therapy, hyperglycemia persisted in some cases. Because these reactions have been reported voluntarily during clinical practice, estimates of frequency cannot be made, and a causal relationship between protease inhibitor therapy and these reactions has not been established.

➤*Immune reconstitution syndrome:* Immune reconstitution syndrome has been reported in patients treated with combination antiretroviral therapy, including atazanavir. During the initial phase of combination antiretroviral treatment, patients whose immune systems responds may develop an inflammatory response to indolent or residual opportunistic infections (such as *Mycobacterium avium* infection, cytomegalovirus, *Pneumocystis jiroveci* pneumonia, or tuberculosis), which may necessitate further evaluation and treatment.

➤*Fat redistribution:* Redistribution/accumulation of body fat, including central obesity, dorsocervical fat enlargement (buffalo hump), peripheral wasting, facial wasting, breast enlargement, and cushingoid appearance, has been observed in patients receiving antiretroviral therapy. The mechanism and long-term consequences of these events are currently unknown. A causal relationship has not been established.

➤*Hemophilia:* There have been reports of increased bleeding, including spontaneous skin hematomas and hemarthrosis, in patients with hemophilia type A and B treated with protease inhibitors. In some patients, additional factor VIII was given. In more than half of the reported cases, treatment with protease inhibitors was continued or reintroduced. A causal relationship between protease inhibitor therapy and these reactions has not been established.

➤*Resistance / Cross-resistance:* Various degrees of cross-resistance among protease inhibitors have been observed. Resistance to atazanavir may not preclude the subsequent use of other protease inhibitors.

➤*Hepatic function impairment:* Exercise caution when administering this drug to patients with hepatic impairment because atazanavir concentrations may be increased. Patients with underlying hepatitis B or C viral infections or marked elevations in transaminases before treatment may be at increased risk of developing further transaminase elevations or hepatic decompensation. Conduct appropriate laboratory testing prior to initiation of therapy with atazanavir and monitor patients during treatment.

➤*Pregnancy:* *Category B.* There are no adequate and well-controlled studies of atazanavir use during pregnancy. Cases of lactic acidosis syndrome and symptomatic hyperlactatemia have occurred in pregnant women receiving atazanavir in combination with nucleoside analogs. In animal reproduction and pre- and postnatal development studies, there was no evidence of adverse fetal effects or teratogenicity. Because animal reproduction studies are not always predictive of human response, use atazanavir during pregnancy only if clearly needed.

Cases of lactic acidosis syndrome, sometimes fatal, and symptomatic hyperlactatemia have been reported in patients (including pregnant women) receiving atazanavir in combination with nucleoside analogs. Nucleoside analogs are associated with an increased risk of lactic acidosis syndrome. In addition, hyperbilirubinemia occurred frequently during treatment with atazanavir. It is not known whether atazanavir administered to the mother during pregnancy will exacerbate physiological hyperbilirubinemia or increase the risk of kernicterus in neonates and young infants. In the prepartum period, consider additional monitoring and alternative therapy to atazanavir.

Antiretroviral pregnancy registry – To monitor maternal-fetal outcomes of pregnant women exposed to atazanavir, an antiretroviral pregnancy registry has been established. Register patients by calling 1-800-258-4263.

➤*Lactation:* The Centers for Disease Control and Prevention recommends that HIV-infected mothers not breast-feed their infants to avoid risking postnatal transmission of HIV. It is not known whether atazanavir is present in human breast milk. However, the molecular weight (approximately 705 for the free base) and the moderately long elimination half-life (approximately 7 hours) suggest that the drug will be excreted into human breast milk. Because of both the potential for HIV transmission and the potential for serious adverse reactions in breast-feeding infants, instruct mothers not to breast-feed if they are receiving atazanavir.

➤*Children:* Do not administer atazanavir to children younger than 3 months of age because of the risk of kernicterus.

The safety, activity, and pharmacokinetic profiles of atazanavir in children 3 months to younger than 6 years of age have not been established.

➤*Elderly:* In general, exercise appropriate caution in the administration and monitoring of atazanavir in elderly patients, reflecting the greater frequency of decreased hepatic, renal, or cardiac function, and of concomitant disease or other drug therapy.

➤*Monitoring:* Monitor ECG at baseline and periodically during treatment. Monitor glucose, lipids, and liver function tests. Monitor CD4+ cell count and HIV RNA load. Monitor patients for signs and symptoms of lactic acidosis.

Drug Interactions

➤*Cytochrome P450 system:* Coadministration of atazanavir and drugs primarily metabolized by cytochrome P450 (CYP) 3A, CYP2C8, or UGT1A1 may result in increased plasma concentrations of the other drug that could increase or prolong its therapeutic effects and adverse reactions.

Coadministration of atazanavir and drugs that induce CYP3A may decrease atazanavir plasma concentrations and reduce its therapeutic effect. Coadministration of atazanavir and drugs that inhibit CYP3A may increase atazanavir plasma concentrations.

➤*Drugs that prolong the PR interval:* Pharmacokinetic studies between atazanavir and other drugs that prolong the PR interval, including beta-blockers (other than atenolol), verapamil, and digoxin, have not been performed. An additive effect of atazanavir and these drugs cannot be excluded; therefore, exercise caution when giving atazanavir concurrently with these drugs, especially drugs that are metabolized by CYP3A (eg, verapamil).

Atazanavir Drug Interactions

Precipitant drug	Object drug[a]		Description
Antacids and buffered medications	Atazanavir	⬇	Reduced plasma concentrations of atazanavir are expected with coadministration. Administer atazanavir 2 hours before or 1 hour after these medications.
Antifungals (eg, itraconazole, ketoconazole, voriconazole)	Atazanavir	⬆	Plasma atazanavir and azole antifungal agent levels may be elevated, increasing the risk of toxicity. Coadministration of ketoconazole with atazanavir without ritonavir resulted in a negligible increase in atazanavir AUC and C_{max}. Coadministration of voriconazole with atazanavir may increase atazanavir concentrations. Use caution when high doses of ketoconazole or itraconazole are coadministered with atazanavir/ritonavir. Coadministration of voriconazole with atazanavir/ritonavir is not recommended.
Atazanavir	Antifungals (eg, itraconazole, ketoconazole, voriconazole)		

ATAZANAVIR SULFATE — ORAL

Atazanavir Drug Interactions

Precipitant drug	Object drug[a]		Description
Bosentan	Atazanavir	↓	Atazanavir plasma concentrations may be decreased when bosentan is administered without ritonavir. Coadministration of atazanavir and bosentan without ritonavir is not recommended. Bosentan plasma concentrations may be elevated, increasing the pharmacologic effect and risk of adverse reactions. For patients who have been receiving atazanavir/ritonavir for at least 10 days, start bosentan at 62.5 mg once daily or every other day based on individual tolerability. In patients on bosentan, discontinue bosentan at least 36 hours before starting atazanavir/ritonavir. At least 10 days after starting atazanavir/ritonavir, resume bosentan at 62.5 mg once daily or every other day based on individual tolerability.
Atazanavir	Bosentan	↑	
Carbamazepine	Atazanavir	↓	Carbamazepine levels may be elevated, increasing the risk of toxicity, while atazanavir levels may decrease, resulting in antiretroviral treatment failure. If coadministration cannot be avoided, close clinical monitoring is indicated. Consider alternative therapy for carbamazepine.
Atazanavir	Carbamazepine	↑	
Cat's claw (*Uncaria tomentosa*)	Atazanavir	↑	Atazanavir concentrations may be elevated, increasing the risk of toxicity. Patients receiving atazanavir should avoid use of the herbal product cat's claw.
Clarithromycin	Atazanavir	↑	Increased concentrations of clarithromycin may cause QTc prolongations; therefore, reduce the dose of clarithromycin by 50%. Concentrations of the active metabolite 14-OH clarithromycin are significantly reduced; consider alternative therapy for indications other than *Mycobacterium avium* complex. Coadministration of atazanavir/ritonavir with clarithromycin has not been studied.
Atazanavir	Clarithromycin	↑↓	
Delavirdine	Atazanavir	↑	Delavirdine may increase plasma concentrations and pharmacologic effects of atazanavir, while atazanavir may decrease plasma concentrations and pharmacologic effects of delavirdine. Dosage reduction of atazanavir may be needed during coadministration of delavirdine. Dosage increases may be required for delavirdine when coadministered with atazanavir. Closely monitor the patient and adjust therapy as needed.
Atazanavir	Delavirdine	↓	
Didanosine (buffered)	Atazanavir	↓	Coadministration of atazanavir and buffered didanosine may decrease atazanavir concentrations. Take atazanavir 2 hours before or 1 hour after the buffered formulation of didanosine. Coadministration of didanosine enteric-coated capsules and atazanavir decreased didanosine exposure. Administer atazanavir and didanosine at different times.
Atazanavir	Didanosine (enteric-coated)		
Digoxin	Atazanavir	↑	An additive effect of atazanavir and digoxin on PR interval prolongation cannot be excluded; therefore, use with caution.
Atazanavir	Digoxin		

Atazanavir Drug Interactions

Precipitant drug	Object drug[a]		Description
Fluoxetine	Atazanavir	↑	Atazanavir may increase plasma concentrations of fluoxetine resulting in possible fluoxetine toxicity. Similarly, fluoxetine may increase plasma concentrations of atazanavir. Closely monitor the patient for adverse reactions, including serotonin syndrome. Dosage reduction of fluoxetine and/or atazanavir may be needed during coadministration of these agents.
Atazanavir	Fluoxetine		
H_2-receptor antagonists (eg, famotidine)	Atazanavir	↓	Plasma concentrations of atazanavir were substantially decreased when administered simultaneously with famotidine, which may result in loss of therapeutic effect and development of resistance (see Administration and Dosage).
NNRTIs (eg, efavirenz, nevirapine)	Atazanavir	↓	Atazanavir plasma levels and clinical efficacy may be reduced. In treatment-naive patients, administer atazanavir 400 mg and ritonavir 100 mg with efavirenz 600 mg. Do not coadminister atazanavir with efavirenz in treatment-experienced patients. Nevirapine may decrease atazanavir exposure and coadministration may increase nevirapine exposure. Coadministration is not recommended (see Administration and Dosage).
Atazanavir	NNRTIs (eg, nevirapine)	↑	
Protease inhibitors (eg, amprenavir, darunavir, fosamprenavir, indinavir, nelfinavir, ritonavir, saquinavir, tipranavir)	Atazanavir	↑	If atazanavir is coadministered with ritonavir, decrease the dose of atazanavir to 300 mg once daily with ritonavir 100 mg once daily. The coadministration of atazanavir with other protease inhibitors is expected to increase exposure to the other protease inhibitor. Coadministration is not recommended. Coadministration of atazanavir and indinavir is contraindicated because both drugs are associated with indirect (unconjugated) hyperbilirubinemia. Saquinavir 1,200 mg coadministered with atazanavir 400 mg and tenofovir 300 mg plus NRTIs did not provide adequate efficacy.
Atazanavir	Protease inhibitors (eg, indinavir, ritonavir)		
Proton pump inhibitors (eg, omeprazole)	Atazanavir	↓	Plasma concentrations of atazanavir were substantially decreased when administered with omeprazole, which may result in loss of therapeutic effect and development of resistance. In treatment-naive patients, administer proton pump inhibitors 12 hours prior to the atazanavir dose (see Administration and Dosage).
Rifampin	Atazanavir	↓	Rifampin may decrease plasma concentrations of atazanavir, which may result in loss of therapeutic effect and development of resistance. Coadministration is contraindicated.
St. John's wort	Atazanavir	↓	Atazanavir plasma concentrations and clinical efficacy may be decreased. Coadministration is contraindicated.

ATAZANAVIR SULFATE — ORAL

Atazanavir Drug Interactions

Precipitant drug	Object drug[a]		Description
Tenofovir	Atazanavir	↓	Tenofovir may decrease the AUC and C_{min} of atazanavir. Atazanavir without ritonavir should not be coadministered with tenofovir. Dose as atazanavir 300 mg, ritonavir 100 mg, and tenofovir 300 mg. Atazanavir increases tenofovir concentrations. Monitor for tenofovir-associated adverse reactions.
Atazanavir	Tenofovir	↑	
Tetracyclines (eg, minocycline)	Atazanavir	↓	Tetracyclines may reduce atazanavir plasma concentrations, which may decrease the therapeutic effect. Closely monitor atazanavir concentrations and the clinical response of the patient. Adjust the atazanavir dose as needed.
Atazanavir	Alfuzosin	↑	Alfuzosin plasma concentrations may be elevated, increasing the risk of hypotension. Coadministration is contraindicated.
Atazanavir	Antiarrhythmics (eg, amiodarone, bepridil, systemic lidocaine, quinidine)	↑	Concurrent use has the potential to produce serious and/or life-threatening adverse reactions. Use with caution. Monitoring the therapeutic concentration of the antiarrhythmic agent is recommended.
Atazanavir	Anticoagulants (eg, warfarin)	↑	Coadministration has the potential to produce serious and/or life-threatening bleeding. Monitor INR.[b]
Atazanavir	Aripiprazole	↑	Aripiprazole plasma concentrations may be elevated, increasing the pharmacologic effects and risk of adverse reactions. Monitor the patient and adjust the aripiprazole dose as needed when atazanavir is started or stopped.
Atazanavir	Benzodiazepines (eg, midazolam, triazolam)	↑	Oral midazolam and triazolam are contraindicated because of the potential for serious and/or life-threatening events, such as prolonged or increased sedation or respiratory depression. Use intravenous midazolam with caution.
Atazanavir	Calcium channel blockers (eg, amlodipine, diltiazem, felodipine, nicardipine, nifedipine, verapamil)	↑	Atazanavir has the potential to prolong the PR interval in some patients. Caution is warranted. Consider a dose reduction of diltiazem by 50% and dose titration of other calcium channel blockers. Monitor ECG.
Atazanavir	Cisapride	↑	Contraindicated because of the potential for serious and/or life-threatening reactions such as cardiac arrhythmias.
Atazanavir	Colchicine	↑	Colchicine and atazanavir should not be coadministered to patients with hepatic or renal impairment. For treatment of gout flares, coadminister colchicine 0.6 mg followed by 0.3 mg 1 hour later. Repeat dose no earlier than 3 days. For prophylaxis of gout flares, if the original colchicine regimen was colchicine 0.6 mg twice daily, adjust the dose to 0.3 mg once a day. If the original colchicine dose was 0.6 mg once daily, adjust the regimen to colchicine 0.3 mg every other day. For treatment of familial Mediterranean fever, coadminister colchicine at a maximum daily dose of 0.3 mg twice a day.

Atazanavir Drug Interactions

Precipitant drug	Object drug[a]		Description
Atazanavir	Contraceptives, hormonal (eg, ethinyl estradiol, norethindrone, norgestimate)	↑	Because contraceptive steroid concentrations may be altered, alternative methods of nonhormonal contraception are recommended.
Atazanavir	Corticosteroids (eg, fluticasone, prednisone)	↑	Corticosteroid plasma concentrations may be increased. Monitor for signs of adrenal insufficiency. Consider alternatives to fluticasone for long-term use.
Atazanavir	Dronedarone	↑	Dronedarone plasma concentrations may be elevated, increasing the pharmacologic effects and risk of toxicity. Avoid coadministration.
Atazanavir	Eletriptan	↑	Eletriptan plasma concentrations may be elevated by atazanavir, increasing the pharmacologic effects and risk of adverse reactions. Eletriptan should not be used within 72 hours of atazanavir.
Atazanavir	Eplerenone	↑	Eplerenone plasma concentrations may be elevated, increasing the pharmacologic effects and risk of toxicity. Close clinical monitoring is indicated when eplerenone is coadministered with atazanavir. Adjust the eplerenone dose as needed.
Atazanavir	Ergot derivatives (eg, dihydroergotamine, ergonovine, ergotamine, methylergonovine)	↑	Contraindicated because of the potential for serious and/or life-threatening events such as acute ergot toxicity (peripheral vasospasm, ischemia of the extremities).
Atazanavir	Erlotinib	↑	Plasma concentration of erlotinib may be elevated, increasing the pharmacologic effects and risk of adverse reactions. Monitor the clinical response of the patient and for adverse reactions. Adjust the erlotinib dose as needed.
Atazanavir	Erythromycin	↑	Plasma concentration of erythromycin may be elevated, increasing the risk of sudden death from cardiac causes. Avoid concurrent use.
Atazanavir	Eszopiclone	↑	Eszopiclone plasma concentrations may be elevated, increasing the pharmacologic effects and risk of adverse reactions. Close monitoring is indicated. Consider reducing the eszopiclone dose when coadministered with atazanavir.
Atazanavir	HMG-CoA reductase inhibitors (eg, atorvastatin, lovastatin, rosuvastatin, simvastatin)	↑	Atazanavir may increase serum concentrations of HMG-CoA reductase inhibitors, which could increase their toxicity, including rhabdomyolysis. Coadministration with simvastatin or lovastatin is contraindicated. If using atorvastatin or rosuvastatin, start with the lowest possible dose with careful monitoring. Consider pravastatin or fluvastatin in combination with atazanavir.
Atazanavir	Iloperidone	↑	Iloperidone plasma concentrations and pharmacologic effects may be increased. A modification of the iloperidone dosage is recommended. Reduce the dose of iloperidone by one-half when coadministered with atazanavir. If therapy with atazanavir is discontinued, increase the dose of iloperidone to the original dose.

ATAZANAVIR SULFATE — ORAL

Atazanavir Drug Interactions

Precipitant drug	Object drug[a]		Description
Atazanavir	Immunosuppressants (eg, cyclosporine, sirolimus, tacrolimus)	↑	Immunosuppressant levels may increase. Therapeutic concentration monitoring is recommended for immunosuppressant agents when coadministered with atazanavir.
Atazanavir	Irinotecan	↑	Atazanavir may interfere with the metabolism of irinotecan, resulting in increased toxicity. Coadministration is contraindicated.
Atazanavir	Ixabepilone	↑	Ixabepilone plasma concentrations may be elevated. Avoid coadministration.
Atazanavir	Maraviroc	↑	Maraviroc plasma concentrations may be elevated, increasing the pharmacologic effects and risk of adverse reactions. Monitor the response of the patient and adjust the maraviroc dose as needed.
Atazanavir	mTOR[b] inhibitors (eg, everolimus, temsirolimus)	↑	mTOR inhibitor plasma concentrations may be elevated, increasing the pharmacologic effects and risk of adverse reactions. If coadministration cannot be avoided, monitor the clinical response of the patient and adjust the mTOR inhibitor dose as needed.
Atazanavir	Muscarinic receptor antagonists (eg, darifenacin, fesoterodine solifenacin, tolterodine)	↑	Muscarinic receptor antagonist plasma concentrations may be increased by atazanavir. When atazanavir is coadministered, do not exceed the following doses: darifenacin 7.5 mg daily, fesoterodine 4 mg daily; solifenacin 5 mg daily, and tolterodine 2 mg daily.
Atazanavir	Nilotinib	↑	Plasma concentrations and pharmacologic effects of nilotinib may be increased. Avoid coadministration. If atazanavir must be given, consider interrupting nilotinib therapy. If atazanavir must be coadministered with nilotinib, consult official package labeling for specific recommendations.
Atazanavir	Opioid analgesics (eg, buprenorphine, fentanyl, oxycodone, sufentanil)	↑	Reduced dose of opioid may be necessary. Plasma concentrations and half-life of opioid may be increased. Closely monitor respiratory function during opioid administration and for a longer period than usual after stopping the opioid. Atazanavir without ritonavir should not be administered with buprenorphine.
Atazanavir	PDE5[b] inhibitors (eg, sildenafil, tadalafil, vardenafil)	↑	Coadministration of atazanavir and sildenafil for the treatment of pulmonary arterial hypertension is contraindicated. Coadministration may result in an increase in PDE5 inhibitor–associated adverse reactions, including hypotension, visual changes, and priapism. In patients with pulmonary arterial hypertension, who have received atazanavir for at least 1 week, start tadalafil at 20 mg once daily. The tadalafil dose may be increased to 40 mg once daily based on individual tolerability. In patients with pulmonary hypertension already taking tadalafil, avoid tadalafil during initiation of atazanavir. Stop tadalafil at least 24 hours prior to starting atazanavir. After at least 1 week following the start of atazanavir, resume tadalafil at 20 mg once daily. The tadalafil dose may be increased to 40 mg once daily based on individual tolerability. For the treatment of erectile dysfunction, use with caution at reduced dosages and increase monitoring for adverse events. Limit dosage of sildenafil to 25 mg every 48 hours, tadalafil to 10 mg every 72 hours, or vardenafil to no more than 2.5 mg every 24 hours. Use vardenafil with atazanavir/ritonavir with caution at reduced doses of no more than 2.5 mg every 72 hours.
Atazanavir	Pimozide	↑	Contraindicated because of the potential for serious and/or life-threatening reactions such as cardiac arrhythmias.
Atazanavir	Quetiapine	↑	Quetiapine plasma concentrations may be elevated, increasing the pharmacologic effects and risk of adverse reactions. Administer with caution and closely monitor the clinical response. Adjust the quetiapine dose as needed.
Atazanavir	Raltegravir	↑	Plasma concentrations and pharmacologic effects of raltegravir may be increased by atazanavir. Closely monitor the clinical response of the patient and adjust the raltegravir dose as needed.
Atazanavir	Ranolazine	↑	Increased risk of dose-related prolongation in the QTc interval, torsades de pointes–type arrhythmias, and sudden death. Coadministration with potent CYP3A inhibitors, such as atazanavir, is contraindicated.
Atazanavir	Rifabutin	↑	A rifabutin dosage reduction of up to 75% (eg, 150 mg every other day or 3 times a week) is recommended.
Atazanavir	Risperidone	↑	Risperidone plasma concentrations may be elevated, increasing the pharmacologic effects and risk of adverse reactions. Closely monitor the clinical response of the patient. Adjust the risperidone dose as needed.

ATAZANAVIR SULFATE — ORAL

Atazanavir Drug Interactions			
Precipitant drug	Object drug[a]		Description
Atazanavir	Romidepsin	↑	Romidepsin plasma concentrations may be elevated, increasing the pharmacologic effects and risk of adverse reactions, including QT prolongation. If coadministration cannot be avoided, close clinical, laboratory, and ECG monitoring are indicated. Adjust the dosage of romidepsin accordingly.
Atazanavir	Salmeterol	↑	Salmeterol concentrations may be elevated, increasing the risk of cardiovascular events, including QT prolongation, palpitations, and sinus tachycardia. Coadministration is not recommended.
Atazanavir	Trazodone	↑	Increased plasma concentrations of trazodone may lead to an increase in adverse reactions. Use with caution and reduce the dose of trazodone.
Atazanavir	Tricyclic antidepressants (eg, amitriptyline)	↑	Coadministration has the potential to produce serious and/or life-threatening adverse reactions. Monitor the concentration of the tricyclic antidepressant.
Atazanavir	Tyrosine kinase inhibitors (ie, dasatinib, lapatinib, pazopanib, sorafenib, sunitinib)	↑	Protein-tyrosine kinase inhibitor plasma concentrations may be elevated, increasing the pharmacologic effects and risk of adverse reactions. If coadministration cannot be avoided, closely monitor the response of the patient and adjust the protein-tyrosine kinase inhibitor dose as needed.
Atazanavir	Vasopressin receptor antagonists (eg, conivaptan, tolvaptan)	↑	Vasopressin receptor antagonist plasma concentrations may be elevated, increasing the pharmacologic effects and risk of adverse reactions. Coadministration is contraindicated.

[a] ↑ = object drug increased; ↓ = object drug decreased; ↑↓ = object drug both increased and decreased.
[b] INR = international normalized ratio; mTOR = mammalian target of rapamycin; PDE5 = phosphodiesterase type 5.

➤*Drug/Food interactions:* See Actions for more information.

Garlic may reduce atazanavir plasma concentrations, decreasing the pharmacologic effects. Avoid garlic ingestion.

Grapefruit juice may increase the atazanavir plasma concentrations and pharmacologic effects. If grapefruit juice cannot be avoided, closely monitor the clinical response of the patient and adjust the atazanavir dose as needed.

Adverse Reactions

➤*Treatment-naive adults:*

Most common adverse reactions – The most common adverse reactions are nausea, jaundice/scleral icterus, and rash.

Adverse reactions of 2% or more –

Atazanavir Adverse Reactions[a] of Moderate or Severe Intensity Reported in Adult Treatment-Naive Patients (≥ 2%): 96 weeks		
	96 weeks[b]	
Adverse reactions	Atazanavir 300 mg with ritonavir 100 mg (once daily) and tenofovir with emtricitabine[c] (n = 441)	Lopinavir 400 mg with ritonavir 100 mg (twice daily) and tenofovir with emtricitabine[c] (n = 437)
Dermatologic		
Rash	3%	2%
GI		
Diarrhea	2%	12%
Jaundice/scleral icterus	5%	–[d]
Nausea	4%	8%

[a] Includes reactions of possible, probable, certain, or unknown relationship to treatment regimen.
[b] Median time on therapy.
[c] As a fixed-dose combination: tenofovir 300 mg, emtricitabine 200 mg once daily.
[d] None reported in this treatment arm.

Atazanavir Adverse Reactions[a] of Moderate or Severe Intensity Reported in Adult Treatment-Naive Patients (≥ 2%)[b]: 64 weeks, 73 weeks, and 120 weeks				
	Study AI424-034		Studies AI424-007, -008	
	64 weeks[c]	64 weeks[c]	120 weeks[c,d]	73 weeks[c,d]
Adverse reactions	Atazanavir 400 mg once daily + lamivudine + zidovudine[e] (n = 404)	Efavirenz 600 mg once daily + lamivudine + zidovudine[e] (n = 401)	Atazanavir 400 mg once daily + stavudine + lamivudine or didanosine (n = 279)	Nelfinavir 750 mg 3 times daily or 1,250 mg twice daily + stavudine + lamivudine or didanosine (n = 191)
CNS				
Dizziness	2%	7%	< 1%	–
Headache	6%	6%	1%	2%
Insomnia	3%	3%	< 1%	–
Peripheral neurologic symptoms	< 1%	1%	4%	3%
Dermatologic				
Rash	7%	10%	5%	1%
GI				
Abdominal pain	4%	4%	4%	2%
Diarrhea	1%	2%	3%	16%
Jaundice/Scleral icterus	7%	–	7%	–
Nausea	14%	12%	6%	4%
Vomiting	4%	7%	3%	3%

[a] Includes reactions of possible, probable, certain, or unknown relationship to treatment regimen.
[b] Based on regimens containing atazanavir.
[c] Median time on therapy.
[d] Includes long-term follow-up.
[e] As a fixed-dose combination: lamivudine 150 mg and zidovudine 300 mg twice daily.

➤*Treatment-experienced adults:*

Most common adverse reactions – The most common reactions are jaundice/scleral icterus and myalgia.

Adverse reactions (2% or more) –

Atazanavir Adverse Reactions[a] of Moderate or Severe Intensity Reported in Adult Treatment-Experienced Patients[b] (≥ 2%)		
	48 weeks[c]	48 weeks[c]
Adverse reactions	Atazanavir 300 mg/ ritonavir 100 mg once daily + tenofovir + NRTI (n = 119)	Lopinavir 400 mg/ ritonavir 100 mg twice daily[d] + tenofovir + NRTI (n = 118)
GI		
Diarrhea	3%	11%
Jaundice/Scleral icterus	9%	–
Nausea	3%	2%
Miscellaneous		
Depression	2%	< 1%
Fever	2%	–
Myalgia	4%	–

[a] Includes reactions of possible, probable, certain, or unknown relationship to treatment regimen.
[b] Based on the regimen containing atazanavir.
[c] Median time on therapy.
[d] As a fixed-dose combination.

➤*Children:*

Most common adverse reactions – The most common grade 2 to 4 adverse reactions (5% or more, regardless of causality) reported in children were cough (21%), fever (19%), rash (14%), jaundice/scleral icterus (13%), diarrhea, vomiting (8%), headache (7%), and rhinorrhea (6%). Asymptomatic second-degree AV block was reported in 2% of patients.

ATAZANAVIR SULFATE — ORAL

➤*Lab test abnormalities:*

Treatment-naive adults –

Atazanavir Grade 3 to 4 Laboratory Abnormalities in Adult Treatment-Naive Patients[a] (≥ 2%): 96 weeks

Laboratory abnormality	ULN	Study AI424-138 96 weeks[b]: Atazanavir 300 mg with ritonavir 100 mg (once daily) and tenofovir with emtricitabine[c] (n = 441)	Study AI424-138 96 weeks[b]: Lopinavir 400 mg with ritonavir 100 mg (twice daily) and tenofovir with emtricitabine[c] (n = 437)
Chemistry		High	
AST	≥ 5.1 × ULN	3%	1%
ALT	≥ 5.1 × ULN	3%	2%
Total bilirubin	≥ 2.6 × ULN	44%	< 1%
Lipase	≥ 2.1 × ULN	2%	2%
Creatine kinase	≥ 5.1 × ULN	8%	7%
Total cholesterol	≥ 240 mg/dL	11%	25%
Hematology		Low	
Neutrophils	< 750 cells/mm³	5%	2%

[a] Based on the regimen containing atazanavir.
[b] Median time on therapy.
[c] As a fixed-dose combination: tenofovir 300 mg, emtricitabine 200 mg once daily.

Atazanavir Grade 3 to 4 Laboratory Abnormalities in Adult Treatment-Naive Patients[a] (≥ 2%): 64 weeks, 73 weeks, and 120 weeks

Laboratory abnormality	ULN	Study AI424-034, 64 weeks[b]: Atazanavir 400 mg once daily + lamivudine + zidovudine[d] (n = 404)	Study AI424-034, 64 weeks[b]: Efavirenz 600 mg once daily + lamivudine + zidovudine[d] (n = 401)	Studies AI424-007, -008, 120 weeks[b,c]: Atazanavir 400 mg once daily + stavudine + lamivudine or + stavudine + didanosine (n = 279)	Studies AI424-007, -008, 73 weeks[b,c]: Nelfinavir 750 mg 3 times daily or 1,250 mg twice daily + stavudine + lamivudine or + stavudine + didanosine (n = 191)
Chemistry	High				
ALT	≥ 5.1 × ULN	4%	3%	9%	7%
Amylase	≥ 2.1 × ULN	—	—	14%	10%
AST	≥ 5.1 × ULN	2%	2%	7%	5%
Creatine kinase	≥ 5.1 × ULN	6%	6%	11%	9%
Lipase	≥ 2.1 × ULN	< 1%	1%	4%	5%
Total bilirubin	≥ 2.6 × ULN	35%	< 1%	47%	3%
Total cholesterol	≥ 240 mg/dL	6%	24%	19%	48%
Triglycerides	≥ 751 mg/dL	< 1%	3%	4%	2%
Hematology	Low				
Hemoglobin	< 8 g/dL	5%	3%	< 1%	4%
Neutrophils	< 750 cells/mm³	7%	9%	3%	7%

[a] Based on regimen(s) containing atazanavir.
[b] Median time on therapy.
[c] Includes long-term follow-up.
[d] As a fixed-dose combination: lamivudine 150 mg and zidovudine 300 mg twice daily.

Lipids:

Atazanavir Lipid Values, Mean Change From Baseline, Study AI424-138

Lipid	Atazanavir/Ritonavir[a,b] Baseline mg/dL (n = 428[d])	Week 48 mg/dL (n = 372[d])	Week 48 Change[e] (n = 372[d])	Week 96 mg/dL (n = 342[d])	Week 96 Change[e] (n = 342[d])	Lopinavir/Ritonavir[b,c] Baseline mg/dL (n = 424[d])	Week 48 mg/dL (n = 335[d])	Week 48 Change[e] (n = 335[d])	Week 96 mg/dL (n = 291[d])	Week 96 Change[e] (n = 291[d])
LDL-C[f]	92	105	+ 14%	105	+14%	93	111	+ 19%	110	+17%
HDL-C[f]	37	46	+ 29%	44	+21%	36	48	+ 37%	46	+29%
Total cholesterol[f]	149	169	+ 13%	169	+13%	150	187	+ 25%	186	+25%
Triglycerides[f]	126	145	+ 15%	140	+13%	129	194	+ 52%	184	+50%

[a] Atazanavir 300 mg with ritonavir 100 mg once daily with the fixed-dose combination: tenofovir 300 mg, emtricitabine 200 mg once daily.
[b] Values obtained after initiation of serum lipid-reducing agents were not included in these analyses. At baseline, serum lipid-reducing agents were used in 1% in the lopinavir/ritonavir treatment arm and 1% in the atazanavir/ritonavir arm. Through week 48, serum lipid-reducing agents were used in 8% in the lopinavir/ritonavir treatment arm and 2% in the atazanavir/ritonavir arm. Through week 96, serum lipid-reducing agents were used in 10% in the lopinavir/ritonavir treatment arm and 3% in the atazanavir/ritonavir arm.
[c] Lopinavir 400 mg with ritonavir 100 mg twice daily with the fixed-dose combination tenofovir 300 mg, emtricitabine 200 mg once daily.
[d] Number of patients with LDL-C measured.
[e] The change from baseline is the mean of within-patient changes from baseline for patients with both baseline and week 48 or week 96 values and is not a simple difference of the baseline and week 48 or week 96 mean values, respectively.
[f] Fasting. LDL-C = low-density lipoprotein cholesterol; HDL-C = high-density lipoprotein cholesterol.

ATAZANAVIR SULFATE — ORAL

Atazanavir Lipid Values, Mean Change from Baseline, Study AI424-034

Lipid	Atazanavir[a,b]			Efavirenz[b,c]		
	Baseline	Week 48		Baseline	Week 48	
	mg/dL (n = 383[e])	mg/dL (n = 283[e])	Change[d] (n = 272[e])	mg/dL (n = 378[e])	mg/dL (n = 264[e])	Change[d] (n = 253[e])
HDL-C	39	43	+13%	38	46	+24%
LDL-C[f]	98	98	+1%	98	114	+18%
Total cholesterol	164	168	+2%	162	195	+21%
Triglycerides[f]	138	124	−9%	129	168	+23%

[a] Atazanavir 400 mg once daily with the following fixed-dose combination: lamivudine 150 mg and zidovudine 300 mg twice daily.
[b] Values obtained after initiation of serum lipid-reducing agents were not included in these analyses. At baseline, serum lipid-reducing agents were used in 0% in the efavirenz treatment arm and < 1% in the atazanavir arm. Through week 48, serum lipid-reducing agents were used in the efavirenz treatment arm (3%) and atazanavir arm (1%).
[c] Efavirenz 600 mg once daily with the following fixed-dose combination: lamivudine 150 mg and zidovudine 300 mg twice daily.
[d] The change from baseline is the mean of within-patient changes from baseline for patients with both baseline and week 48 values and is not a simple difference of the baseline and week 48 mean values.
[e] Number of patients with LDL-C measured.
[f] Fasting.

Treatment-experienced patients –

Atazanavir Grade 3 to 4 Laboratory Abnormalities in Adult Treatment-Experienced Patients, Study AI424-045[a] (≥ 2%)

Laboratory abnormality	ULN	48 weeks[b] Atazanavir 300 mg/ritonavir 100 mg once daily + tenofovir + NRTI (n = 119)	Lopinavir 400 mg/ritonavir 100 mg twice daily[c] + tenofovir + NRTI (n = 118)
Chemistry		High	
ALT	≥ 5.1 × ULN	4%	3%
AST	≥ 5.1 × ULN	3%	3%
Creatine kinase	≥ 5.1 × ULN	8%	8%
Glucose	≥ 251 mg/dL	5%	< 1%
Lipase	≥ 2.1 × ULN	5%	6%
Total bilirubin	≥ 2.6 × ULN	49%	< 1%
Total cholesterol	≥ 240 mg/dL	25%	26%
Triglycerides	≥ 751 mg/dL	8%	12%
Hematology		Low	
Platelets	< 50,000 cells/mm^3	2%	3%
Neutrophils	< 750 cells/mm^3	7%	8%

[a] Based on regimen(s) containing atazanavir.
[b] Median time on therapy.
[c] As a fixed-dose combination.

Lipids:

Atazanavir Lipid Values, Mean Change from Baseline, Study AI424-045

Lipid	Atazanavir/Ritonavir[a,b]			Lopinavir/Ritonavir[b,c]		
	Baseline	Week 48		Baseline	Week 48	
	mg/dL (n = 111[d])	mg/dL (n = 75[d])	Change[e] (n = 74[d])	mg/dL (n = 108[d])	mg/dL (n = 76[d])	Change[e] (n = 73[d])
LDL-C[f]	108	98	−10%	104	103	+1%
HDL-C	40	39	−7%	39	41	+2%
Total cholesterol	188	170	−8%	181	187	+6%
Triglycerides[f]	215	161	−4%	196	224	+30%

[a] Atazanavir 300 mg once daily plus ritonavir plus tenofovir plus 1 NRTI.
[b] Values obtained after initiation of serum lipid-reducing agents were not included in these analyses. At baseline, serum lipid-reducing agents were used in 4% in the lopinavir/ritonavir treatment arm and 4% in the atazanavir/ritonavir arm. Through week 48, serum lipid-reducing agents were used in the lopinavir/ritonavir treatment arm (19%) and the atazanavir/ritonavir arm (8%).
[c] Lopinavir 400 mg/ritonavir 100 mg twice daily plus tenofovir plus 1 NRTI.
[d] Number of patients with LDL-C measured.
[e] The change from baseline is the mean of within-patient changes from baseline for patients with both baseline and week 48 values and is not a simple difference of the baseline and week 48 mean values.
[f] Fasting.

Children – The most common grade 3 to 4 laboratory abnormality was elevation of total bilirubin (3.2 mg/dL or more), which occurred in 49% of children. All other grade 3 to 4 laboratory abnormalities occurred with a frequency of less than 3%.

Hepatitis B and/or hepatitis C virus coinfection – Monitor liver function tests in patients with a history of hepatitis B or C. In study AI424-138, 60 patients treated with atazanavir 300 mg/ritonavir 100 mg once daily and 51 patients treated with lopinavir 400 mg/ritonavir 100 mg twice daily, each with fixed-dose tenofovir/emtricitabine, were seropositive for hepatitis B and/or C at study entry. ALT levels more than 5 times the ULN developed in 10% of the atazanavir/ritonavir-treated patients and 8% of the lopinavir/ritonavir-treated patients. AST levels more than 5 times the ULN developed in 10% of the atazanavir/ritonavir-treated patients and none of the lopinavir/ritonavir-treated patients.

In studies AI424-008 and AI424-034, 74 patients treated with atazanavir 400 mg once daily (58 of whom received efavirenz), and 12 patients who received nelfinavir were seropositive for hepatitis B and/or C at study entry. ALT levels higher than 5 times the ULN developed in 15% of the atazanavir-treated patients, 14% of the efavirenz-treated patients, and 17% of the nelfinavir-treated patients. AST levels higher than 5 times the ULN developed in 9% of the atazanavir-treated patients, 5% of the efavirenz-treated patients, and 17% of the nelfinavir-treated patients. Within atazanavir and control regimens, no difference in frequency of bilirubin elevations was noted between seropositive and seronegative patients.

In study AI424-045, 20 patients treated with atazanavir 300 mg/ritonavir 100 mg once daily and 18 patients treated with lopinavir 400 mg/ritonavir 100 mg twice daily were seropositive for hepatitis B and/or C at study entry. ALT levels greater than 5 times the ULN developed in 25% of the atazanavir/ritonavir-treated patients and 6% of the lopinavir/ritonavir-treated patients. AST levels greater than 5 times the ULN developed in 10% of the atazanavir/ritonavir-treated patients and 6% of the lopinavir/ritonavir-treated patients.

➤*Postmarketing:*

Cardiovascular – Left bundle branch block, QTc prolongation, second-degree AV block, third-degree AV block.

Dermatologic – Alopecia, maculopapular rash, pruritus.

Hepatic – Cholecystitis, cholelithiasis, cholestasis, hepatic function abnormalities.

Metabolic/Nutritional – Diabetes mellitus, hyperglycemia.

Miscellaneous – Arthralgia, edema, nephrolithiasis, pancreatitis.

Overdosage

➤*Symptoms:* A single self-administered overdose of atazanavir 29.2 g in an HIV-infected patient (73 times the 400 mg recommended dose) was associated with asymptomatic bifascicular block and PR interval prolongation. These events resolved spontaneously. At high doses that lead to high drug exposures, jaundice due to indirect (unconjugated) hyperbilirubinemia (without associated liver function test changes) or PR interval prolongation may be observed.

➤*Treatment:* Treatment of overdosage with atazanavir should consist of general supportive measures, including monitoring of vital signs and ECG, and observations of the patient's clinical status. If indicated, achieve elimination of unabsorbed atazanavir by gastric lavage. Administration of activated charcoal may also be used to aid removal of unabsorbed drug. There is no specific antidote for overdose with atazanavir. Because atazanavir is extensively metabolized by the liver and is highly protein bound, dialysis is unlikely to be beneficial in significant removal of this medicine.

Patient Information

Inform patients to take atazanavir with food to enhance absorption.

Inform patients that sustained decreases in plasma HIV RNA have been associated with a reduced risk of progression to AIDS and death. Patients should remain under the care of a health care provider while using atazanavir. Advise patients to take atazanavir with food every day and take other concomitant antiretroviral therapy as prescribed. Atazanavir must always be used in combination with other antiretroviral drugs. Advise patients not to alter the dose or discontinue therapy without consulting their health care provider. If a dose of atazanavir is missed, advise patients to take the dose as soon as possible and then return to their normal schedule. If a dose is skipped, tell the patient not to double the next dose.

Inform patients that atazanavir is not a cure for HIV infection and that they may continue to develop opportunistic infections and other complications associated with HIV disease. Inform patients that there are currently no data demonstrating that therapy with atazanavir can reduce the risk of transmitting HIV to others through sexual contact.

Atazanavir may interact with some drugs; therefore, advise patients to report to their health care providers the use of any other prescription or nonprescription medication, or herbal products, particularly St. John's wort.

Advise patients receiving a PDE5 inhibitor and atazanavir that they may be at an increased risk of PDE5 inhibitor–associated adverse reactions, including hypotension, syncope, visual disturbances, and prolonged penile erection, and that they should promptly report any symptoms to their health care providers.

Inform patients that sildenafil (ie, *Revatio*) (used to treat pulmonary arterial hypertension) is contraindicated with atazanavir and that dose adjustments are necessary when atazanavir is used with tadalafil (eg, *Cialis*), vardenafil (*Levitra*), or sildenafil (eg, *Viagra*) (used to treat erectile dysfunction), or tadalafil (eg, *Adcirca*) (used to treat pulmonary arterial hypertension).

ATAZANAVIR SULFATE — ORAL

Inform patients that atazanavir may produce changes in the ECG (PR prolongation). Patients should consult their health care provider if they are experiencing symptoms such as dizziness or light-headedness.

Inform patients that mild rashes without other symptoms have been reported with atazanavir use. These rashes go away within 2 weeks with no change in treatment. However, there have been a few reports of severe skin reactions (eg, Stevens-Johnson syndrome, erythema multiforme, toxic skin eruptions) with atazanavir use. Patients developing signs or symptoms of severe skin reactions or hypersensitivity reactions (including, but not limited to, severe rash or rash accompanied by 1 or more of the following: fever, general malaise, muscle or joint aches, blisters, oral lesions, conjunctivitis, facial edema, hepatitis, eosinophilia, granulocytopenia, lymphadenopathy, and renal dysfunction) must discontinue atazanavir and seek medical evaluation immediately.

Inform patients that asymptomatic elevations in indirect bilirubin have occurred in patients receiving atazanavir. These elevations may be accompanied by yellowing of the skin or whites of the eyes; consider alternative antiretroviral therapy if the patient has cosmetic concerns.

Inform patients that redistribution or accumulation of body fat may occur in patients receiving antiretroviral therapy, including protease inhibitors, and that the cause and long-term health effects of these conditions are not known at this time. It is unknown whether long-term use of atazanavir will result in a lower incidence of lipodystrophy than with other protease inhibitors.

LOPINAVIR/RITONAVIR

Rx	**Kaletra** (Abbott)	**Tablets; oral**: lopinavir 100 mg/ritonavir 25 mg	Sorbitan. (KC, "A" logo). Pale yellow, oval. Film-coated. In 60s.
		lopinavir 200 mg/ritonavir 50 mg	Sorbitan. (KA, "A" logo). Yellow, oval. Film-coated. In 120s.
		Solution; oral: lopinavir 80 mg/ritonavir 20 mg per mL	Light yellow to orange. Acesulfame K, alcohol 42.4%, castor oils, corn syrup, cotton candy flavoring, glycerin, *Magnasweet*, menthol, peppermint oil, propylene glycol, saccharin, vanilla flavoring. In 160 mL with dosing cup.

LOPINAVIR/RITONAVIR — ORAL

Indications

➤*HIV infection:* In combination with other antiretroviral agents for the treatment of HIV-1 infection.

Administration and Dosage

➤*General dosing considerations:* Dosage adjustments are required when lopinavir/ritonavir is used concomitantly with efavirenz, nevirapine, (fos)amprenavir, or nelfinavir. (See Concomitant Therapy.)

Based on weight – Patient's weight (kg) × prescribed lopinavir dose (mg/kg) = administered lopinavir dose (mg).

Based on body surface area – Patient's body surface area (BSA) (m^2) × prescribed lopinavir dose (mg/m^2) = administered lopinavir dose (mg).

➤*Adults:*

HIV infection –

Usual dosage: Lopinavir 400 mg/ritonavir 100 mg twice daily or lopinavir 800 mg/ritonavir 200 mg once daily in patients with less than 3 lopinavir resistance–associated substitutions.

Concomitant therapy:

• *Anticonvulsants* – Lopinavir/ritonavir should not be administered once daily in combination with carbamazepine, phenobarbital, or phenytoin.

• *Antiretrovirals* – Lopinavir/ritonavir should not be administered as a once-daily regimen in combination with efavirenz, nevirapine, (fos)amprenavir, or nelfinavir.

Tablets: Lopinavir 500 mg/ritonavir 125 mg twice daily when used in combination with efavirenz, nevirapine, (fos)amprenavir, or nelfinavir.

Oral solution: Lopinavir 533 mg/ritonavir 133 mg (6.5 mL) twice daily taken with food when used in combination with efavirenz, nevirapine, (fos)amprenavir, or nelfinavir.

➤*Children:* Lopinavir/ritonavir should not be administered once daily to children.

HIV infection –

6 months to 18 years of age:

• *Without concomitant efavirenz, (fos)amprenavir, nelfinavir, or nevirapine* –

Usual dosage:

Solution – Lopinavir 230 mg/ritonavir 57.5 mg/m^2 twice daily with food. If dosing by body weight, lopinavir 12 mg/ritonavir 3 mg per kg for patients less than 15 kg, or lopinavir 10 mg/ritonavir 2.5 mg per kg for patients 15 to 40 kg, given twice daily with food.

Tablets –

Lopinavir/Ritonavir Tablet Dosing for Children 6 Months to 18 Years of Age Without Concomitant Efavirenz, Nevirapine, (Fos)amprenavir, or Nelfinavir

Body weight (kg)	BSA (m^2)[a]	Recommended number of lopinavir 100 mg/ritonavir 25 mg tablets twice daily
15 to 25	≥ 0.6 to < 0.9	2
> 25 to 35	≥ 0.9 to < 1.4	3
> 35	≥ 1.4	4 (or two lopinavir 200 mg/ritonavir 50 mg tablets)

[a] Lopinavir/ritonavir oral solution is available for children with a BSA [2] or those who are unable to reliably swallow a tablet.

Maximum dose: Lopinavir 400 mg/ritonavir 100 mg twice daily.

• *With concomitant efavirenz, (fos)amprenavir, nelfinavir, or nevirapine* –

Usual dosage:

Solution – Lopinavir 300 mg/ritonavir 75 mg/m^2 twice daily (both treatment-naive and treatment-experienced). If dosing by body weight, lopinavir 13 mg/ritonavir 3.25 mg per kg given twice daily for patients weighing less than 15 kg and lopinavir 11 mg/ritonavir 2.75 mg per kg given twice daily for patients weighing 15 to 45 kg.

Tablets –

Lopinavir/Ritonavir Tablet Dosing for Children 6 Months to 18 Years of Age With Concomitant Efavirenz,[a] Nevirapine, (Fos)amprenavir,[a] or Nelfinavir[a]

Body weight (kg)	BSA (m^2)[b]	Recommended number of lopinavir 100 mg/ritonavir 25 mg tablets twice daily
15 to 20	≥ 0.6 to < 0.8	2
> 20 to 30	≥ 0.8 to < 1.2	3
> 30 to 45	≥ 1.2 to < 1.7	4 (or two lopinavir 200 mg/ritonavir 50 mg tablets)
> 45	≥ 1.7	5 (or two lopinavir 200 mg/ritonavir 50 mg tablets and one lopinavir 100 mg/ritonavir 25 mg tablets)

[a] Refer to the individual product labels for appropriate dosing in children.
[b] Lopinavir/ritonavir oral solution is available for children with a BSA [2] or those who are unable to reliably swallow a tablet.

Maximum dose: Lopinavir 533 mg/ritonavir 133 mg (oral solution) or lopinavir 500 mg/ritonavir 125 mg (tablets) twice daily.

14 days to 6 months of age:

• *Usual dosage* – Lopinavir 16 mg/ritonavir 4 mg per kg or lopinavir 300 mg/ritonavir 75 mg per m^2 twice daily.

➤*Preparation for administration:*

Oral solution – If lopinavir/ritonavir oral solution is used, the volume (mL) of lopinavir/ritonavir solution can be determined as follows:

Volume of lopinavir/ritonavir solution (mL) = administered lopinavir dose (mg) ÷ 80 (mg/mL)

➤*Administration:*

Tablets – May be taken with or without food. Tablets should be swallowed whole and not chewed, broken, or crushed.

Oral solution – Must be taken with food. The dose of the oral solution should be administered using a calibrated syringe.

➤*Storage/Stability:*

Tablets – Store at 20° to 25°C (68° to 77°F); excursions are permitted to 15° to 30°C (59° to 86°F). Dispense in original container. Exposure to high humidity outside the container for longer than 2 weeks is not recommended.

Oral solution – Store in a refrigerator at 2° to 8°C (36° to 46°F) until dispensed. Avoid exposure to excessive heat. Under refrigeration, the solution remains stable until the expiration date printed on the label. If stored at room temperature up to 25°C (77°F), use within 2 months.

LOPINAVIR/RITONAVIR — ORAL

Actions

➤*Pharmacology:* Lopinavir, an HIV-1 protease inhibitor, prevents cleavage of the Gag-Pol polyprotein, resulting in the production of immature, noninfectious viral particles. Ritonavir inhibits the CYP3A-mediated metabolism of lopinavir, thereby providing increased plasma levels of lopinavir.

➤*Pharmacokinetics:*

Absorption – In a pharmacokinetic study in subjects who were positive for HIV-1 (N = 19), multiple dosing with lopinavir 400 mg/ritonavir 100 mg twice daily with food for 3 weeks produced a mean ± standard deviation (SD) lopinavir peak plasma concentration (C_{max}) of 9.8 ± 3.7 mcg/mL, occurring approximately 4 hours after administration. The mean steady-state trough concentration prior to the morning dose was 7.1 ± 2.9 mcg/mL and minimum concentration within a dosing interval was 5.5 ± 2.7 mcg/mL. Lopinavir area under the curve (AUC) over a 12-hour dosing interval averaged 92.6 ± 36.7 mcg•h/mL. The absolute bioavailability of lopinavir coformulated with ritonavir in humans has not been established. Under nonfasting conditions (500 kcal, 25% from fat), lopinavir concentrations were similar following administration of lopinavir/ritonavir coformulated capsules and liquid. When administered under fasting conditions, the mean AUC and C_{max} of lopinavir were 22% lower for the lopinavir/ritonavir liquid relative to the capsule formulation.

Once-daily dosing: Multiple dosing of lopinavir 800 mg/ritonavir 200 mg once daily for 4 weeks with food (n = 24) produced a mean ± SD lopinavir C_{max} of 11.8 ± 3.7 mcg/mL, occurring approximately 6 hours after administration. The mean steady-state trough concentration prior to the morning dose was 3.2 ± 2.1 mcg/mL, and minimum concentration within a dosing interval was 1.7 ± 1.6 mcg/mL. Lopinavir AUC over a 24-hour dosing interval averaged 154.1 ± 61.4 mcg•h/mL.

Effect of food:

• *Oral solution* – Relative to fasting, administration of oral solution with a moderate-fat meal (500 to 682 kcal, 23% to 25% calories from fat) increased lopinavir AUC and C_{max} by 80% and 54%, respectively. Relative to fasting, administration of oral solution with a high-fat meal (872 kcal, 56% calories from fat) increased lopinavir AUC and C_{max} by 130% and 56%, respectively. To enhance bioavailability and minimize pharmacokinetic variability, instruct patients to take the oral solution with food.

Distribution – At steady state, lopinavir is approximately 98% to 99% bound to plasma proteins. Lopinavir binds to both alpha-1-acid glycoprotein (AAG) and albumin, but has a higher affinity for AAG. At steady state, lopinavir protein binding remains constant over the range of observed concentrations after lopinavir 400 mg/ritonavir 100 mg twice daily and is similar between healthy volunteers and patients who are HIV-1–positive.

Metabolism – In vitro experiments with human hepatic microsomes indicate that lopinavir primarily undergoes oxidative metabolism. Lopinavir is extensively metabolized by the hepatic cytochrome P450 (CYP-450) system, almost exclusively by the CYP3A isozyme. Ritonavir is a potent CYP3A inhibitor that inhibits the metabolism of lopinavir and, therefore, increases plasma levels of lopinavir. A ^{14}C-lopinavir study in humans showed that 89% of the plasma radioactivity after a single lopinavir 400 mg/ritonavir 100 mg dose was due to the parent drug. At least 13 lopinavir oxidative metabolites have been identified in humans. Ritonavir has been shown to induce metabolic enzymes, resulting in the induction of its own metabolism. Predose lopinavir concentrations decline with time during multiple dosing, stabilizing after approximately 10 to 16 days.

Excretion – Following a ^{14}C-lopinavir 400 mg/ritonavir 100 mg dose, approximately 10.4% ± 2.3% and approximately 82.6% ± 2.5% of an administered dose of ^{14}C-lopinavir can be accounted for in urine and feces, respectively, after 8 days. Unchanged lopinavir accounted for approximately 2.2% and 19.8% of the administered dose in urine and feces, respectively. After multiple dosing, less than 3% of the lopinavir dose is excreted unchanged in the urine. The apparent oral clearance of lopinavir is 5.98 ± 5.75 L/h (mean ± SD, n = 19).

Special populations –

Hepatic function impairment: Multiple dosing of lopinavir 400 mg/ritonavir 100 mg twice daily to patients coinfected with HIV-1 and hepatitis C virus with mild to moderate hepatic impairment (n = 12) resulted in a 30% increase in lopinavir AUC and a 20% increase in C_{max} compared with patients infected with HIV-1 with healthy hepatic function (n = 12). Additionally, the plasma protein binding of lopinavir was statistically significantly lower in both mild and moderate hepatic impairment compared with controls (99.09% vs 99.31%, respectively). Exercise caution when administering lopinavir/ritonavir to subjects with hepatic impairment. Lopinavir/ritonavir has not been studied in patients with severe hepatic impairment.

Children: The mean steady-state lopinavir AUC, C_{max}, and minimum concentration (C_{min}) were 72.6 ± 31.1 mcg•h/mL, 8.2 ± 2.9 mcg/mL, and 3.4 ± 2.1 mcg/mL, respectively, after lopinavir oral solution 230 mg/ritonavir 57 mg per m^2 twice daily without nevirapine (n = 12), and were 85.8 ± 36.9 mcg•h/mL, 10 ± 3.3 mcg/mL and 3.6 ± 3.5 mcg/mL, respectively, after lopinavir 300 mg/ritonavir 75 mg per m^2 twice daily with nevirapine (n = 12). The nevirapine regimen was 7 mg/kg twice daily (6 months to 8 years of age) or 4 mg/kg twice daily (older than 8 years of age).

The pharmacokinetics of approximately lopinavir oral solution 300 mg/ritonavir 75 mg per m^2 twice-daily also have been evaluated in infants at approximately 6 weeks of age (n = 9) and between 6 weeks and 6 months of age (n = 18) in study 1030. The mean steady-state lopinavir AUC_{12}, C_{max}, and C_{12} were 43.4 ± 14.8 mcg• h/mL, 5.2 ± 1.8 mcg/mL, and 1.9 ± 1.1 mcg/mL, respectively, in infants at approximately 6 weeks of age, and 74.5 ± 37.9 mcg•h/mL, 9.4 ± 4.9, and 3.1 ± 1.8 mcg/mL, respectively, in infants between 6 weeks and 6 months of age after lopinavir/ritonavir oral solution was administered at approximately lopinavir 300 mg/ritonavir 75 mg per m^2 twice daily without concomitant nonnucleoside reverse transcriptase inhibitor (NNRTI) therapy.

Contraindications

Hypersensitivity (eg, toxic epidermal necrolysis, Stevens-Johnson syndrome, erythema multiforme) to any of the ingredients, including ritonavir; coadministration with drugs that are highly dependent on CYP3A for clearance and for which elevated plasma concentrations are associated with serious and/or life-threatening reactions; coadministration with potent CYP3A inducers where significantly reduced lopinavir plasma concentrations may be associated with the potential for loss of virologic response and possible resistance and cross-resistance; coadministration with alfuzosin, cisapride, dihydroergotamine, ergonovine, ergotamine, lovastatin, methylergonovine, oral midazolam, pimozide, rifampin, sildenafil when used to treat pulmonary arterial hypertension, simvastatin, St. John's wort, and triazolam.

Warnings/Precautions

➤*Pancreatitis:* Pancreatitis has been observed in patients receiving lopinavir/ritonavir therapy, including those who developed marked triglyceride elevations. In some cases, fatalities have occurred. Although a causal relationship to lopinavir/ritonavir has not been established, marked triglyceride elevations is a risk factor for development of pancreatitis. Patients with advanced HIV-1 disease may be at increased risk of elevated triglycerides and pancreatitis, and patients with a history of pancreatitis may be at increased risk for recurrence during lopinavir/ritonavir therapy.

Consider pancreatitis if clinical symptoms (eg, abdominal pain, nausea, vomiting) or abnormalities in laboratory values (eg, increased serum lipase or amylase values) suggestive of pancreatitis occur. Evaluate patients who exhibit these signs or symptoms and suspend lopinavir/ritonavir and/or other antiretroviral therapy as clinically appropriate.

➤*Hepatotoxicity:* Patients with underlying hepatitis B or C or marked elevations in transaminase prior to treatment may be at increased risk for developing or worsening of transaminase elevations or hepatic decompensation with use of lopinavir/ritonavir.

There have been postmarketing reports of hepatic dysfunction, including some fatalities. These have generally occurred in patients with advanced HIV-1 disease taking multiple concomitant medications in the setting of underlying chronic hepatitis or cirrhosis. A causal relationship with lopinavir/ritonavir therapy has not been established.

Elevated transaminases with or without elevated bilirubin levels have been reported in HIV-1 mono-infected and uninfected patients as early as 7 days after the initiation of lopinavir/ritonavir in conjunction with other antiretroviral agents. In some cases, the hepatic dysfunction was serious; however, a definitive causal relationship with lopinavir/ritonavir therapy has not been established.

Conduct appropriate laboratory testing prior to initiating therapy with lopinavir/ritonavir and closely monitor patients during treatment. Consider increasing AST and ALT monitoring in patients with underlying chronic hepatitis or cirrhosis, especially during the first several months of ritonavir/lopinavir treatment.

➤*Diabetes mellitus/hyperglycemia:* New-onset diabetes mellitus, exacerbation of preexisting diabetes mellitus, and hyperglycemia have been reported during postmarketing surveillance in patients infected with HIV-1 receiving protease inhibitor therapy. Some patients required either initiation or dose adjustments of insulin or oral hypoglycemic agents for treatment of these reactions. In some cases, diabetic ketoacidosis has occurred. In those patients who discontinued protease inhibitor therapy, hyperglycemia persisted in some cases. Because these reactions have been reported voluntarily during clinical practice, estimates of frequency cannot be made and a causal relationship between protease inhibitor therapy and these reactions has not been established.

➤*Cardiovascular effects:*

PR interval prolongation – Lopinavir/ritonavir prolongs the PR interval in some patients. Cases of second or third degree atrioventricular block have been reported. Use lopinavir/ritonavir with caution in patients with underlying structural heart disease, preexisting conduction system abnormalities, ischemic heart disease, or cardiomyopathies, because these patients may be at increased risk for developing cardiac conduction abnormalities.

The impact on the PR interval of coadministered lopinavir/ritonavir with other drugs that prolong the PR interval (including calcium channel blockers, beta-adrenergic blockers, digoxin, and atazanavir) has not been evaluated. As a result, undertake coadministration of lopinavir/ritonavir with these drugs with caution, particularly with those drugs metabolized by CYP3A. Clinical monitoring is recommended.

QT interval prolongation – Postmarketing cases of QT interval prolongation and torsade de pointes have been reported, although causality of lopinavir/ritonavir could not be established. Avoid use in patients with congenital long QT syndrome, those with hypokalemia, and with other drugs that prolong the QT interval.

➤*Immune reconstitution syndrome:* Immune reconstitution syndrome has been reported in patients treated with combination antiretroviral therapy, including lopinavir/ritonavir. During the initial phase of combination antiretroviral treatment, patients whose immune system responds may develop an inflammatory response to indolent or residual opportunistic infections (eg, *Mycobacterium avium* infection, cytomegalovirus, *Pneumocystis jirovecii* pneumonia, tuberculosis), which may necessitate further evaluation and treatment.

LOPINAVIR/RITONAVIR — ORAL

➤*Fat redistribution:* Redistribution/accumulation of body fat, including central obesity, dorsocervical fat enlargement (buffalo hump), peripheral wasting, facial wasting, breast enlargement, and cushingoid appearance, have been observed in patients receiving antiretroviral therapy. The mechanism and long-term consequences of these reactions are currently unknown. A causal relationship has not been established.

➤*Lipid elevations:* Treatment with lopinavir/ritonavir has resulted in large increases in the concentration of total cholesterol and triglycerides. Perform triglyceride and cholesterol testing prior to initiating therapy and at periodic intervals during therapy. Manage lipid disorders as clinically appropriate, taking into account any potential drug-drug interactions with lopinavir/ritonavir and hydroxymethylglutaryl coenzyme A (HMG-CoA) reductase inhibitors.

➤*Hemophilia:* There have been reports of increased bleeding, including spontaneous skin hematomas and hemarthrosis, in patients with hemophilia types A and B treated with protease inhibitors. In some patients, additional factor VIII was given. In more than 50% of the reported cases, treatment with protease inhibitors was continued or reintroduced. A causal relationship between protease inhibitor therapy and these reactions has not been established.

➤*Hepatic function impairment:* Lopinavir/ritonavir is principally metabolized by the liver; therefore, exercise caution when administering this drug to patients with hepatic impairment because lopinavir concentrations may be increased.

➤*Pregnancy: Category C.* There are no adequate and well-controlled studies in pregnant women. Consistent with the molecular weight (approximately 629) and lipid solubility, lopinavir crosses the human placenta. An in vitro experiment using term perfused human placentas demonstrated that the placental transfer of ritonavir was concentration dependent and that the clearance index, at both maternal trough and peak concentrations, was very low. The investigators attributed the low transfer to the molecular weight (approximately 721) and solubility characteristics of ritonavir. However, experience in human pregnancies suggest that embryo/fetal risk is low. According to the US Department of Health and Human Services guidelines for the use of antiretroviral agents in patients infected with HIV, lopinavir/ritonavir is a recommended protease inhibitor. Use lopinavir/ritonavir during pregnancy only if the potential benefit justifies the potential risk to the fetus.

Embryonic and fetal developmental toxicities (early resorption, decreased fetal viability, decreased fetal body weight, increased incidence of skeletal variations, and skeletal ossification delays) occurred in rats at a maternally toxic dosage. Based on AUC measurements, the drug exposures in rats at the toxic doses were approximately 0.7-fold for lopinavir and 1.8-fold for ritonavir that of the exposures in humans at the recommended therapeutic dosage (lopinavir 400 mg/ritonavir 100 mg twice daily) for males and females. In a perinatal and postnatal study in rats, a developmental toxicity (a decrease in survival in pups between birth and postnatal day 21) occurred.

Antiretroviral pregnancy registry – To monitor maternal-fetal outcomes of pregnant women exposed to lopinavir/ritonavir, an antiretroviral pregnancy registry has been established. Health care providers are encouraged to register patients by calling 1-800-258-4263.

➤*Lactation:* The Centers for Disease Control and Prevention recommend that mothers infected with HIV-1 not breast-feed their infants to avoid risking postnatal transmission of HIV-1. Studies in rats have demonstrated that lopinavir is secreted in breast milk. The molecular weights of lopinavir (approximately 629) and ritonavir (approximately 721) combined with their lipid solubility suggest that the drugs will be excreted into human breast milk, although the extensive plasma protein binding (98% to 99%) should limit this excretion. Because of both the potential for HIV-1 transmission and the potential for serious adverse reactions in breast-feeding infants, instruct mothers not to breast-feed if they are receiving lopinavir/ritonavir.

➤*Children:* The safety, efficacy, and pharmacokinetic profiles of lopinavir/ritonavir in children younger than 14 days of age have not been established. Lopinavir/ritonavir once daily has not been evaluated in children.

➤*Elderly:* Exercise appropriate caution in the administration and monitoring of lopinavir/ritonavir in elderly patients, reflecting the greater frequency of decreased hepatic, renal, or cardiac function and of concomitant disease or other drug therapy.

➤*Monitoring:* Monitor patients for hepatic dysfunction prior to initiating treatment and closely during treatment. There may be an increased risk for further transaminase elevations in patients with underlying hepatitis B or C or marked transaminase elevations. Consider increased AST/ALT monitoring in these patients, especially during the first several months of therapy.

Perform triglyceride and cholesterol testing prior to initiating lopinavir/ritonavir therapy and at periodic intervals during therapy.

Monitor blood glucose levels closely. New-onset diabetes mellitus or exacerbation of preexisting diabetes mellitus has been associated with protease inhibitor therapy.

Drug Interactions

➤*Contraindicated drugs:* See Contraindications for more information.

Lopinavir/Ritonavir Drug Interactions

Precipitant drug	Object drug[a]		Description
Aldesleukin (IL-2)	Lopinavir/Ritonavir	↑	Protease inhibitor concentrations may be elevated, increasing the risk of toxicity. Monitor the clinical response of the patient when aldesleukin is started or stopped. Adjust the lopinavir/ritonavir dose as needed.
Anticonvulsants (eg, carbamazepine, phenobarbital, phenytoin)	Lopinavir/Ritonavir	↓	Carbamazepine levels may be increased; a dosage decrease may be needed when coadministered with ritonavir. Divalproex, lamotrigine, and phenytoin levels may be decreased; therefore, a dose increase may be needed when coadministered with ritonavir. Monitor therapeutic concentrations. Lopinavir/ritonavir may be less effective because of decreased lopinavir plasma concentrations in patients taking carbamazepine, phenobarbital, and phenytoin. Do not administer lopinavir/ritonavir once daily with this combination.
Lopinavir/Ritonavir	Anticonvulsants (eg, carbamazepine, divalproex, lamotrigine, phenytoin)	↑↓	
Azole antifungals (eg, itraconazole, ketoconazole, voriconazole)	Lopinavir/Ritonavir	↑↓	Ketoconazole and itraconazole levels may be increased. High doses of ketoconazole or itraconazole (> 200 mg/day) are not recommended. Voriconazole levels may be decreased when coadministered with ritonavir; therefore, voriconazole coadministered with ritonavir is contraindicated. Plasma ritonavir concentrations may be elevated, increasing the risk of toxicity. Consider using an alternative antifungal agent.
Lopinavir/Ritonavir	Azole antifungals (eg, itraconazole, ketoconazole, voriconazole)		
Cat's claw (*Uncaria tomentosa*)	Lopinavir/Ritonavir	↓	Ritonavir plasma concentrations may be elevated, increasing the risk of toxicity. Avoid coadministration.
Clarithromycin	Lopinavir/Ritonavir	↑	Ritonavir and clarithromycin plasma levels may be increased. For patients with CrCl[b] 30 to 60 mL/min, reduce the dose of clarithromycin 50%; for patients with CrCl < 30 mL/min, reduce the dose of clarithromycin 75%.
Lopinavir/Ritonavir	Clarithromycin		
Corticosteroids (eg, dexamethasone)	Lopinavir/Ritonavir	↑↓	Lopinavir/ritonavir may be less effective when coadministered with corticosteroids because of decreased lopinavir plasma concentrations. Corticosteroid plasma concentrations may be elevated, increasing the pharmacologic and toxic effects (ie, Cushing syndrome with secondary adrenal insufficiency). Coadministration of inhaled fluticasone and lopinavir/ritonavir is not recommended unless the potential benefit outweighs the risk of adverse reactions. Use the lowest effective dose of triamcinolone when coadministered with lopinavir/ritonavir. Close clinical monitoring for signs and symptoms of adrenal suppression and Cushing Syndrome is recommended.
Lopinavir/Ritonavir	Corticosteroids (eg, fluticasone propionate [inhaled], prednisone, triamcinolone)		
Darunavir	Lopinavir/Ritonavir	↑↓	Darunavir plasma concentrations may be reduced, decreasing the pharmacologic effects. Lopinavir/ritonavir plasma concentrations may be elevated, increasing the pharmacologic effects and risk of adverse reactions. Coadministration is not recommended.
Lopinavir/Ritonavir	Darunavir		
Evening primrose	Lopinavir/Ritonavir	↓	Ritonavir plasma concentrations may be elevated, increasing the risk of toxicity. Avoid coadministration.

LOPINAVIR/RITONAVIR — ORAL

Lopinavir/Ritonavir Drug Interactions			
Precipitant drug	Object drug[a]		Description
Fosamprenavir	Lopinavir/Ritonavir	↓	Plasma concentrations and pharmacologic effects of lopinavir/ritonavir may be decreased by fosamprenavir and plasma concentrations and pharmacologic effects of fosamprenavir may be decreased by lopinavir/ritonavir. An increase in lopinavir/ritonavir dosage using a twice-daily regimen is recommended.
Lopinavir/Ritonavir	Fosamprenavir		
Nelfinavir	Lopinavir/Ritonavir	↓	Lopinavir concentrations may be reduced, decreasing the efficacy. Consider a dosage increase of lopinavir/ritonavir in treatment-experienced patients when decreased susceptibility to lopinavir is clinically suspected. Nelfinavir concentrations may be increased. Do not administer lopinavir/ritonavir once daily in combination with nelfinavir (see Administration and Dosage).
Lopinavir/Ritonavir	Nelfinavir	↑	
NNRTIs (eg, delavirdine, efavirenz, nevirapine)	Lopinavir/Ritonavir	↑↓	Lopinavir and ritonavir plasma levels and clinical efficacy may be reduced when coadministered with efavirenz and nevirapine. Consider a dosage increase of lopinavir/ritonavir when used in combination with efavirenz or nevirapine (see Administration and Dosage). Delavirdine may increase lopinavir and ritonavir concentrations. Appropriate doses of this combination have not been established.
Rifamycins (eg, rifabutin, rifampin, rifapentine)	Lopinavir/Ritonavir	↓↑	Coadministration may lead to loss of virologic response and possible resistance to lopinavir/ritonavir or to the class of protease inhibitors or other coadministered antiretroviral agents when administered with rifampin. Coadministration with rifampin is contraindicated. Ritonavir may elevate serum rifabutin levels; therefore, dosage reduction of rifabutin by $\geq$ 75% of the usual dose of 300 mg/day is recommended (ie, a maximum dosage of 150 mg every other day or 3 times per week). Monitor for adverse reactions.
Lopinavir/Ritonavir	Rifamycins (ie, rifabutin)		
SSRIs[b] (eg, fluoxetine)	Lopinavir/Ritonavir	↑↓	The AUC of ritonavir may be increased. SSRI levels may be increased. Serotonin syndrome may occur; closely monitor for adverse reactions. A dose decrease may be needed. Lopinavir/ritonavir significantly decreased plasma levels of paroxetine with coadministration. Any dose adjustment should be guided by clinical effect.
Lopinavir/Ritonavir	Selective serotonin reuptake inhibitors (SSRIs) (eg, fluoxetine, paroxetine)		
St. John's wort (*H. perforatum*)	Lopinavir/Ritonavir	↓	Concomitant use is contraindicated. Coadministration of protease inhibitors with St. John's wort, is expected to substantially decrease protease inhibitor concentrations and may result in suboptimal levels of lopinavir and lead to loss of virologic response and possible resistance to lopinavir or to the protease inhibitors class.
Tipranavir	Lopinavir/Ritonavir	↓	Coadministration may decrease lopinavir AUC and C_{min}. Avoid coadministration.
Lopinavir/Ritonavir	Antiarrhythmics (eg, amiodarone, bepridil[c], lidocaine [systemic], quinidine)	↑	Caution is warranted and therapeutic concentration monitoring (if available) is recommended for antiarrhythmics with coadministration.
Lopinavir/Ritonavir	Antihistamines (ie, astemizole,[c] terfenadine[c])	↑	Coadministration is contraindicated because of the potential for serious and/or life-threatening reactions, such as cardiac arrhythmias.
Lopinavir/Ritonavir	Aripiprazole	↑	Aripiprazole plasma concentrations may be elevated, increasing the pharmacologic effects and risk of adverse reactions. Consider reducing the aripiprazole by 50% when used in combination with lopinavir/ritonavir.
Lopinavir/Ritonavir	Atovaquone	↓	Clinical significance is unknown; however, increase of atovaquone doses may be needed.
Lopinavir/Ritonavir	Benzodiazepines (eg, midazolam, triazolam)	↑	Midazolam (oral) and triazolam are contraindicated because of potential serious and/or life-threatening reactions, such as prolonged or increased sedation or respiratory depression. Plasma levels of other benzodiazepines, including parenteral midazolam, may be increased. Closely monitor for respiratory depression and prolonged sedation. Adjust the benzodiazepine dose as needed.
Lopinavir/Ritonavir	Beta-blockers (eg, metoprolol, timolol)	↑	Metoprolol and timolol concentrations may be increased. Use with caution and monitor patient. A dose decrease of the beta-blocker may be needed.
Lopinavir/Ritonavir	Bosentan	↑	Bosentan plasma concentrations may be elevated, increasing the pharmacologic effect and risk of adverse reactions. Discontinue bosentan at least 36 hours prior to starting lopinavir/ritonavir therapy. Bosentan 62.5 mg once daily or every other day can be resumed at least 10 days after starting lopinavir/ritonavir.
Lopinavir/Ritonavir	Bupropion	↓	Decreased serum bupropion concentrations may occur, decreasing the therapeutic effects. Monitor the clinical response of the patient to bupropion and adjust the dose as needed.
Lopinavir/Ritonavir	Buspirone	↑	Buspirone plasma concentration may be elevated, increasing the pharmacologic effects and risk of adverse reactions. Closely monitor the patient for signs of new-onset parkinsonian symptoms (eg, ataxia, shuffling gait, cogwheel rigidity, resting tremor) with coadministration.
Lopinavir/Ritonavir	Calcium channel blockers, (eg, amlodipine, diltiazem, felodipine, nicardipine, nifedipine)	↑	Caution is warranted and clinical monitoring of patients is recommended. A decrease in calcium channel blocker dose may be needed.
Lopinavir/Ritonavir	Cisapride[d]	↑	Contraindicated because of potential for serious and/or life-threatening reactions, such as cardiac arrhythmias.
Lopinavir/Ritonavir	Colchicine	↑	Colchicine plasma concentrations may be elevated, increasing the risk of toxicity. Coadministration is contraindicated in patients with hepatic or renal impairment. For the treatment of gout flares, give colchicine 0.6 mg once, followed by 0.3 mg 1 hour later. Repeat no earlier than 3 days. For the prophylaxis of gout flares, if the original colchicine regimen was 0.6 mg twice daily, adjust dose to 0.3 mg once daily. If the original regimen was 0.6 mg once daily, adjust dose to 0.3 mg once every other day. In patients with Mediterranean fever and healthy renal and hepatic function, coadminister lopinavir/ritonavir and colchicine with caution, using a maximum colchicine dosage of 0.3 mg twice daily. Carefully monitor for colchicine-related adverse reactions.
Lopinavir/Ritonavir	Conivaptan	↑	Conivaptan plasma concentrations may be elevated, increasing the risk of adverse reactions. Coadministration is contraindicated.
Lopinavir/Ritonavir	Contraceptives, hormonal (eg, ethinyl estradiol)	↓	Loss of hormonal contraceptive effectiveness, possibly leading to unintended pregnancy. Use alternative or additional nonhormonal contraceptive measures with coadministration.
Lopinavir/Ritonavir	Deferasirox	↓	Deferasirox plasma concentrations may be reduced, decreasing the pharmacologic effect. If coadministration cannot be avoided, consider an initial dose of deferasirox 30 mg/kg/day. Adjust the deferasirox dosages according to serum ferritin concentrations and clinical response.

LOPINAVIR/RITONAVIR — ORAL

Lopinavir/Ritonavir Drug Interactions

Precipitant drug	Object drug[a]		Description
Lopinavir/Ritonavir	Didanosine	⬇	Ritonavir may decrease didanosine concentrations. Lopinavir/ritonavir tablets may be administered simultaneously with didanosine without food. Because it is recommended that didanosine be administered on an empty stomach, give didanosine 1 hour before or 2 hours after lopinavir/ritonavir oral solution (give with food).
Lopinavir/Ritonavir	Digoxin	⬆	Ritonavir may increase digoxin plasma concentrations. Monitor digoxin plasma concentrations and adjust dose as needed.
Lopinavir/Ritonavir	Disulfiram/Metronidazole	⬆	Lopinavir/ritonavir oral solution contains alcohol, which can produce disulfiram-like reactions when coadministered with disulfiram or other drugs that produce this reaction (eg, metronidazole). Avoid lopinavir/ritonavir solution in patients taking disulfiram or metronidazole.
Lopinavir/Ritonavir	Docetaxel	⬆	Plasma concentrations and pharmacologic effects of docetaxel may be increased. Use of lopinavir/ritonavir with docetaxel may increase the risk of neutropenia. If coadministration cannot be avoided, close clinical and laboratory monitoring are indicated. A docetaxel dosage reduction may be needed.
Lopinavir/Ritonavir	Dronabinol	⬆	Dronabinol levels may be increased. A decrease in dose of dronabinol may be needed.
Lopinavir/Ritonavir	Dronedarone	⬆	Plasma concentrations and pharmacologic effects of dronedarone may be increased. Coadministration of lopinavir/ritonavir with dronedarone is contraindicated.
Lopinavir/Ritonavir	Eletriptan	⬆	Plasma concentrations and pharmacologic effects of eletriptan may be increased by lopinavir/ritonavir. Eletriptan should not be used within 72 hours of lopinavir/ritonavir.
Lopinavir/Ritonavir	Eplerenone	⬆	Ritonavir inhibits the metabolism of eplerenone, which may increase risk of hyperkalemia and arrhythmias. Coadministration is contraindicated.
Lopinavir/Ritonavir	Ergot derivatives (eg, dihydroergotamine, ergonovine,[c] ergotamine, methylergonovine[c])	⬆	Contraindicated because of the potential for serious and/or life-threatening reactions, such as acute ergot toxicity characterized by peripheral vasospasm and ischemia of the extremities and other tissues.
Lopinavir/Ritonavir	Erlotinib	⬆	Erlotinib plasma concentration may be elevated, increasing the pharmacologic effects and risk of adverse reactions. If an interaction is suspected (eg, severe adverse reactions) erlotinib dosage reduction may be needed.
Lopinavir/Ritonavir	Erythromycin	⬆	Erythromycin plasma concentration may be elevated, increasing the risk of sudden death from cardiac causes. Avoid concurrent use.
Lopinavir/Ritonavir	Eszopiclone	⬆	Eszopiclone plasma concentration may be elevated, increasing the pharmacologic effects and risk of adverse reactions. Reduce the dose of eszopiclone when coadministered with lopinavir/ritonavir. Closely monitor the patient for signs of excessive effects.
Lopinavir/Ritonavir	HMG-CoA reductase inhibitors (eg, atorvastatin, lovastatin, rosuvastatin, simvastatin)	⬆	Use the lowest possible dose of atorvastatin or rosuvastatin with careful monitoring, or consider other HMG-CoA reductase inhibitors, such as pravastatin or fluvastatin, in combination with lopinavir/ritonavir. Coadministration with simvastatin or lovastatin is contraindicated because of the potential for serious reactions such as the risk of myopathy, including rhabdomyolysis.
Lopinavir/Ritonavir	Iloperidone	⬆	Iloperidone plasma concentrations and pharmacologic effects may be increased. A modification of the iloperidone dosage is recommended. Reduce the dose of iloperidone by one-half when coadministered with lopinavir/ritonavir. If therapy with lopinavir/ritonavir is discontinued, increase the dose of iloperidone to the original dose.
Lopinavir/Ritonavir	Immunosuppressants (ie, cyclosporine, rapamycin, tacrolimus)	⬆	Therapeutic concentration monitoring is recommended for immunosuppressant agents when coadministered with lopinavir/ritonavir.
Lopinavir/Ritonavir	Indinavir	⬆	Indinavir plasma levels may be elevated, increasing the pharmacologic and adverse reactions. Decrease indinavir dosage to 600 mg twice daily when coadministered with lopinavir 400 mg/ritonavir 100 mg twice daily.
Lopinavir/Ritonavir	Irinotecan	⬆	Irinotecan plasma levels may be elevated, increasing the pharmacologic and risk of toxicity (eg, diarrhea, neutropenia). Closely monitor for irinotecan toxicity.
Lopinavir/Ritonavir	Ixabepilone	⬆	Ixabepilone plasma levels may be elevated, increasing the pharmacologic and adverse reactions. If coadministration cannot be avoided, consider a reduction in ixabepilone dose. Consult the package labeling for ixabepilone for the specific recommendations.
Lopinavir/Ritonavir	Levothyroxine	⬆⬇	Thyroxine serum concentrations may be increased or decreased. Monitor thyroid function status when lopinavir/ritonavir is started or stopped. Adjust the levothyroxine dose as needed.
Lopinavir/Ritonavir	Maraviroc	⬆	Maraviroc plasma concentrations may be increased. When coadministered, patients should receive maraviroc 150 mg twice daily.
Lopinavir/Ritonavir	Methamphetamine	⬆	Methamphetamine levels may be increased; therefore, a dose decrease may be needed with coadministration. Use with caution.
Lopinavir/Ritonavir	mTOR[b] inhibitors (eg, everolimus, temsirolimus)	⬆	mTOR plasma concentrations may be elevated[b], increasing the pharmacologic effects and risk of adverse reactions. Avoid coadministration. If coadministration of lopinavir/ritonavir is necessary, monitor the clinical response of the patient and adjust the mTOR dose as needed.
Lopinavir/Ritonavir	Muscarinic receptor antagonists (eg, darifenacin, fesoterodine solifenacin, tolterodine)	⬆	Muscarinic receptor antagonist plasma concentrations may be increased by lopinavir/ritonavir. When lopinavir/ritonavir is coadministered, the dose of darifenacin should not exceed 7.5 mg daily, the dose of fesoterodine should not exceed 4 mg daily; the dose of solifenacin should not exceed 5 mg daily, and the dose of tolterodine should not exceed 2 mg daily.
Lopinavir/Ritonavir	Nefazodone	⬆	Nefazodone levels may be increased. A decrease in nefazodone dose may be needed.
Lopinavir/Ritonavir	Nilotinib	⬆	Plasma concentrations and pharmacologic effects of nilotinib may be increased, including life-threatening cardiac arrhythmias. If coadministration cannot be avoided, closely monitor for adverse reactions, including QT prolongation. Nilotinib dosage adjustments may be needed when lopinavir/ritonavir is started or stopped.
Lopinavir/Ritonavir	NRTIs[b] (eg, abacavir, tenofovir, zidovudine)	⬆⬇	Lopinavir/ritonavir increases tenofovir concentrations; monitor for adverse reactions. Lopinavir/ritonavir induces glucuronidation; therefore, it has the potential to reduce abacavir and zidovudine plasma concentrations. The clinical significance is unknown.
Lopinavir/Ritonavir	Olanzapine	⬇	Olanzapine plasma concentrations may be reduced. Adjust the olanzapine dose as needed.

LOPINAVIR/RITONAVIR — ORAL

Lopinavir/Ritonavir Drug Interactions

Precipitant drug	Object drug[a]		Description
Lopinavir/Ritonavir	Opioid analgesics (eg, buprenorphine, fentanyl, meperidine, methadone, propoxyphene)	↓↑	Dosage of methadone may need to be increased when coadministered with lopinavir/ritonavir. Plasma concentrations of buprenorphine and fentanyl may be increased, possibly causing toxicity. Monitor respiratory function and adjust the dose as needed. Meperidine levels may decrease, possibly decreasing efficacy, but the normeperidine serum levels may increase, increasing neurologic toxicity. Concurrent use of propoxyphene or meperidine is contraindicated with ritonavir.
Lopinavir/Ritonavir	Phenothiazines (eg, perphenazine, thioridazine)	↑	Phenothiazine levels may be increased by ritonavir; therefore, a phenothiazine dosage decrease may be needed.
Lopinavir/Ritnavir	PDE5[b] inhibitors (eg, sildenafil, tadalafil, vardenafil)	↑	Coadministration with sildenafil is contraindicated when used for the treatment of pulmonary arterial hypertension. Use caution when coadministering, with increased monitoring for adverse reactions. The PDE5 dosage should not exceed the following: sildenafil 25 mg every 48 hours, tadalafil 10 mg every 72 hours, or vardenafil 2.5 mg every 72 hours.
Lopinavir/Ritonavir	Pimozide	↑	Contraindicated because of potential serious and/or life-threatening reactions (eg, cardiac arrhythmias).
Lopinavir/Ritonavir	Quetiapine	↑	Quetiapine plasma concentrations may be elevated, increasing the pharmacologic effects and risk of adverse reactions. Coadminister with caution and closely monitor the clinical response. Adjust the quetiapine dose as needed.
Lopinavir/Ritonavir	Quinazolines (eg, alfuzosin, silodosin, tamsulosin)	↑	Quinazoline plasma concentrations may be elevated. Coadministration of alfuzosin or silodosin and ritonavir is contraindicated. Similarly, do not coadminister tamsulosin with lopinavir/ritonavir.
Lopinavir/Ritonavir	Quinine	↑	Quinine levels may be increased, increasing the pharmacologic effects and risk of adverse reactions; therefore, a dose decrease may be needed.
Lopinavir/Ritonavir	Ranolazine	↑	Ranolazine plasma concentrations may be elevated, increasing the risk of dose-related prolongation of the QTc interval, torsades de pointes–type arrhythmias, and sudden death. Coadministration is contraindicated.
Lopinavir/Ritonavir	Risperidone	↑	Risperidone plasma concentrations may be elevated. increasing the pharmacologic effects and risk of adverse reactions. Closely monitor the clinical response when risperidone therapy is started or stopped. Adjust dose as needed.
Lopinavir/Ritonavir	Romidepsin	↑	Romidepsin plasma concentrations may be elevated, increasing the pharmacologic effects and risk of adverse reactions (including QT prolongation). If coadministration cannot be avoided, close, clinical, laboratory, and ECG[b] monitoring are indicated. Adjust the romidepsin dose as needed.
Lopinavir/Ritonavir	Salmeterol	↑	The risk of cardiovascular adverse reactions associated with salmeterol, including QT prolongation, palpitation, and sinus tachycardia may be increased. Coadministration is not recommended.
Lopinavir/Ritonavir	Saquinavir	↑	Saquinavir plasma concentrations may be elevated. Saquinavir dosage is 1,000 mg twice daily when coadministered with lopinavir 400 mg/ritonavir 100 mg twice daily.
Lopinavir/Ritonavir	Theophylline	↓	Coadministration may decrease theophylline concentrations. Monitor theophylline levels; adjust dosage as needed.
Lopinavir/Ritonavir	Trazodone	↑	Trazodone plasma concentrations may be elevated, increasing the risk of adverse reactions (eg, hypotension, syncope). Use with caution. Consider a lower dose of trazodone.
Lopinavir/Ritonavir	Tricyclic antidepressants (eg, desipramine)	↑	Concurrent use increased the desipramine AUC 145% and the C_{max} 22%. Dosage reduction and concentration monitoring of desipramine is recommended.
Lopinavir/Ritonavir	Tyrosine kinase receptor inhibitors (eg, dasatinib, lapatinib, sorafenib, sunitinib)	↑	Lopinavir/ritonavir may increase plasma concentrations of these agents, increasing the pharmacologic effects and risk of adverse reactions. Closely monitor the clinical response of the patient and adjust the tyrosine kinase receptor inhibitor dose as needed (eg, lapatinib 500 mg daily is recommended if used concurrently).
Lopinavir/Ritonavir	Vasopressin receptor antagonists (eg, conivaptan, tolvaptan)	↑	Vasopressin receptor antagonist plasma concentrations may be elevated, increasing the risk of adverse reactions. Coadministration is contraindicated.
Lopinavir/Ritonavir	Vinblastine, vincristine	↑	Vinblastine or vincristine concentrations may be elevated, increasing the risk of adverse reactions. Consider temporarily withholding lopinavir/ritonavir in patients who develop hematologic or GI side effects. If lopinavir/ritonavir must be withheld for a prolonged period, consider initiating a revised regimen that does not include a CYP3A or P-glycoprotein inhibitor.
Lopinavir/Ritonavir	Warfarin	↑↓	The anticoagulant effect of warfarin may be affected. Carefully monitor the international normalized ratio when starting or stopping a protease inhibitor. Adjust the warfarin dose as needed.
Lopinavir/Ritonavir	Zolpidem	↑	Zolpidem levels may be increased, resulting in possible severe sedation and respiratory depression. Closely monitor the patient for signs of zolpidem adverse reactions. Zolpidem dosage adjustments may be needed when lopinavir/ritonavir is started or stopped.

[a] ↑ = object drug increased; ↓ = object drug decreased; ↑↓ = object drug both increased and decreased.
[b] CrCl = creatinine clearance; SSRIs = selective serotonin reuptake inhibitors; mTOR = mammalian target of rapamycin inhibitors; NRTIs = nucleoside reverse transcriptase inhibitors; PDE5 = phosphodiesterase type 5; ECG = electrocardiogram.
[c] No longer marketed in the United States.
[d] Available from the manufacturer on a limited-access protocol.

➤*Drug/Food interactions:* See Actions for more information.

Grapefruit juice may increase the plasma concentrations of lopinavir/ritonavir. If grapefruit juice cannot be avoided, closely monitor the clinical response of the patient and adjust the lopinavir/ritonavir dose as needed. Garlic may reduce lopinavir/ritonavir plasma concentrations, decreasing the pharmacologic effects. Avoid garlic ingestion.

Adverse Reactions

➤*Adults:*

Most common adverse reaction – The most common adverse reaction was diarrhea, which was generally of mild to moderate severity. In study 730, the incidence of diarrhea of any severity during 48 weeks of therapy was 60% in patients receiving lopinavir/ritonavir once daily compared with 57% in patients receiving lopinavir/ritonavir twice daily. More patients receiving lopinavir/ritonavir once daily (4.2%) had ongoing diarrhea at the time of discontinuation as compared with patients receiving lopinavir/ritonavir twice daily (1.8%). In study 802, the incidence of diarrhea of any severity during 48 weeks of therapy was 50% in patients receiving lopinavir/ritonavir once daily compared with 39% in patients receiving lopinavir/ritonavir twice daily. Moderate or severe drug-related diarrhea occurred in 14% of patients receiving lopinavir/ritonavir once daily compared with 11% in patients receiving lopinavir/ritonavir twice daily. At the time of discontinuation, 6.3% of patients receiving lopinavir/ritonavir once daily had ongoing diarrhea, compared with 3.7% of patients receiving lopinavir/ritonavir twice daily.

Discontinuation of therapy – In study 730, discontinuations because of any adverse reaction were 4.8% in patients receiving lopinavir/ritonavir once daily compared with 3% in patients receiving lopinavir/ritonavir twice daily. Discontinuations because of any adverse reaction occurred in 4.3% of patients receiving lopinavir/ritonavir once daily compared with 7% in patients receiving lopinavir/ritonavir twice daily in study 802. Rates of dis-

LOPINAVIR/RITONAVIR — ORAL

continuation of randomized therapy caused by adverse reactions were 3.4% in lopinavir/ritonavir-treated patients and 3.7% in nelfinavir-treated patients in study 863.

Adverse reactions (2% or more) –

Lopinavir/Ritonavir Adverse Reactions in Adult Antiretroviral-Naive Patients (≥ 2%)[a]

Adverse reactions	Study 863 (48 wk): Lopinavir 400 mg/ ritonavir 100 mg twice daily + stavudine and lamivudine (n = 326)	Study 863 (48 wk): Nelfinavir 750 mg 3 times daily + stavudine and lamivudine (n = 327)	Study 730 (48 weeks): Lopinavir 800 mg/ ritonavir 200 mg daily + tenofovir and emtricitabine (n = 333)	Study 730 (48 weeks): Lopinavir 400 mg/ ritonavir 100 mg twice daily + tenofovir and emtricitabine (n = 331)	Study 720 (360 wk): Lopinavir/ Ritonavir twice daily[b] + stavudine and lamivudine (n = 100)
CNS					
Asthenia	4%	3%	< 1%	< 1%	9%
Depression	1%	2%	0%	0%	0%
Headache	2%	2%	2%	2%	6%
Insomnia	2%	1%	1%	0%	3%
Libido decreased	< 1%	< 1%	0%	< 1%	2%
Paresthesia	1%	1%	0%	0%	2%
GI					
Abdominal pain	4%	3%	1%	1%	11%
Anorexia	1%	< 1%	< 1%	1%	2%
Diarrhea	16%	17%	17%	15%	28%
Dyspepsia	2%	< 1%	0%	0%	6%
Flatulence	2%	1%	1%	0%	4%
Nausea	7%	5%	7%	1%	16%
Vomiting	2%	2%	3%	5%	6%
Miscellaneous					
Bronchitis	0%	0%	0%	< 1	2%
Hypogonadism	0%	0%	0%	0%	2%
Myalgia	1%	1%	0%	0%	2%
Rash	1%	2%	< 1%	1%	5%
Vasodilation	0%	0%	0%	0%	3%
Weight decreased	1%	< 1%	0%	< 1	2%

[a] Includes adverse reactions of possible or probable relationship to study drug.
[b] Includes adverse reaction data from dosage group 1 (lopinavir 200 mg/ritonavir 100 mg twice daily only [n = 16] and lopinavir 400 mg/ritonavir 100 mg twice daily [n = 16]) and dosage group 2 (lopinavir 400 mg/ritonavir 100 mg twice daily [n = 35] and lopinavir 400 mg/ritonavir 200 mg twice daily [n = 33]). Within dosing groups, moderate to severe nausea of probable/possible relationship to lopinavir/ritonavir occurred at a higher rate in the lopinavir 400 mg/ritonavir 200 mg dosage arm compared with the lopinavir 400 mg/ritonavir 100 mg dosage arm in group 2.

Adverse Reactions in Adult Protease Inhibitor–Experienced Patients (≥ 2%)[a]

Adverse reactions	Study 888 (48 wk): Lopinavir 400 mg/ ritonavir 100 mg twice daily + nevirapine and NRTIs (n = 148)	Study 888 (48 wk): Investigator-selected protease inhibitor(s) + nevirapine and NRTIs (n = 140)	Study 957[b] and study 765[c] (84 to 144 wk): Lopinavir/ Ritonavir twice daily + NNRTI and NRTIs (n = 127)	Study 802 (48 weeks): Lopinavir 800 mg/ ritonavir 200 mg once daily + NRTIs (n = 300)	Study 802 (48 weeks): Lopinavir 400 mg/ ritonavir 100 mg twice daily + NRTIs (n = 299)
CNS					
Asthenia	3%	6%	9%	< 1%	< 1%
Depression	1%	2%	3%	< 1%	0%
Headache	2%	3%	2%	< 1%	0%
Insomnia	0%	2%	2%	0%	< 1%
Paresthesia	0%	1%	2%	0%	0%
GI					
Abdominal pain	2%	2%	4%	2%	< 1%
Abdominal pain upper	NA[d]	NA	NA	1%	2%
Anorexia	1%	3%	0%	0%	1%
Diarrhea	7%	9%	23%	14%	11%
Dyspepsia	1%	1%	2%	1%	< 1%
Dysphagia	2%	1%	0%	0%	0%
Flatulence	1%	2%	2%	1%	1%
Nausea	7%	16%	5%	3%	7%
Vomiting	4%	12%	2%	2%	3%
Miscellaneous					
Chills	2%	0%	0%	0%	0%
Pyrexia	2%	1%	2%	0%	< 1%
Hypertension	0%	0%	2%	0%	0%

LOPINAVIR/RITONAVIR — ORAL

Adverse Reactions in Adult Protease Inhibitor–Experienced Patients (≥ 2%)[a]					
	Study 888 (48 wk)		Study 957[b] and study 765[c] (84 to 144 wk)	Study 802 (48 weeks)	
Adverse reactions	Lopinavir 400 mg/ ritonavir 100 mg twice daily + nevirapine and NRTIs (n = 148)	Investigator-selected protease inhibitor(s) + nevirapine and NRTIs (n = 140)	Lopinavir/ Ritonavir twice daily + NNRTI and NRTIs (n = 127)	Lopinavir 800 mg/ ritonavir 200 mg once daily + NRTIs (n = 300)	Lopinavir 400 mg/ ritonavir 100 mg twice daily + NRTIs (n = 299)
Myalgia	1%	1%	2%	0%	0%
Rash	2%	1%	2%	0%	0%
Weight decreased	0%	1%	3%	< 1%	< 1%

[a] Includes adverse reactions of possible or probable relationship to study drug.
[b] Includes adverse reaction data from patients receiving lopinavir 400 mg/ritonavir 100 mg twice daily (n = 29) or lopinavir 533 mg/ritonavir 133 mg twice daily (n = 28) for 84 weeks. Patients received lopinavir/ritonavir in combination with NRTIs and efavirenz.
[c] Includes adverse reaction data from patients receiving lopinavir 400 mg/ritonavir 100 mg twice daily (n = 36) or lopinavir 400 mg/ritonavir 200 mg twice daily (n = 34) for 144 weeks. Patients received lopinavir/ritonavir in combination with NRTIs and nevirapine.
[d] NA = not available.

Other adverse reactions – Less than 2%:

Cardiovascular – Angina pectoris, atrial fibrillation, atrioventricular (AV) block, cerebral infarction, deep vein thrombosis, myocardial infarction, orthostatic hypotension, palpitation, thrombophlebitis, tricuspid valve incompetence, varicose veins, vasculitis.

CNS – Ageusia, abnormal dreams, abnormal thinking, affect lability, agitation, amnesia, anxiety, apathy, ataxia, balance disorder, confusion, convulsion, dizziness, disorientation, dysgeusia, dyskinesia, encephalopathy, extrapyramidal disorder, facial palsy, fatigue, hypertonia, malaise, migraine, mood swings, nervousness, neuropathy, peripheral neuropathy, somnolence, tremor, vertigo.

Dermatologic – Acne, alopecia, benign neoplasm of the skin, dry skin, cellulitis, dermatitis acneiform, dermatitis allergic, eczema, exfoliative dermatitis, face swelling, folliculitis, furuncle, generalized rash, hyperhidrosis, idiopathic capillaritis, maculopapular rash, nail disorder, pruritus, seborrhea, skin discoloration, skin hypertrophy, skin striae, skin ulcer.

Endocrine – Cushing syndrome, diabetes mellitus, hypothyroidism.

GI – Abdominal discomfort, abdominal distention, abdomen pain lower, cholangitis, cholecystitis, constipation, decreased appetite, dry mouth, duodenitis, enteritis, enterocolitis, eructation, esophagitis, fecal incontinence, gastric disorder, gastric ulcer, gastritis, gastroenteritis, gastroesophageal reflux disease, hemorrhagic enterocolitis, hemorrhoids, increased appetite, mouth ulceration, pancreatitis, periodontitis, rectal hemorrhage, sialadenitis, stomach discomfort, stomatitis.

GU – Breast enlargement, ejaculation disorder, erectile dysfunction, gynecomastia, hematuria, menorrhagia, nephritis, nephrolithiasis, perineal abscess, renal disorder, urine abnormality, urine odor abnormal.

Hematologic/Lymphatic – Anemia, leukopenia, lymphadenopathy, neutropenia, splenomegaly.

Hepatic – Cytolytic hepatitis, hepatic steatosis, hepatitis, hepatomegaly, jaundice, liver tenderness.

Hypersensitivity – Drug hypersensitivity, hypersensitivity.

Metabolic/Nutritional – Decreased glucose tolerance, dehydration, edema, hypovitaminosis, lactic acidosis, lipomatosis, obesity, peripheral edema, weight increased.

Musculoskeletal – Arthralgia, arthropathy, back pain, muscular weakness, osteoarthritis, osteonecrosis, pain in extremity.

Respiratory – Asthma, bronchopneumonia, cough, dyspnea, pharyngitis, pulmonary edema, rhinitis, sinusitis.

Special senses – Eye disorder, hyperacusis, otitis media, tinnitus, visual disturbance.

Miscellaneous – Bacterial infection, chest pain, cyst, drug interaction, drug level increased, face edema, hypertrophy, immune reconstitution syndrome, influenza, lipoma, neoplasm, viral infection.

➤*Children:* Lopinavir/ritonavir oral solution dosed at lopinavir 300 mg/ ritonavir 75 mg per m^2 has been studied in 31 children 14 days to 6 months of age. The adverse reaction profile in study 1030 was similar to that observed in older children and adults. No adverse reaction was reported in more than 10% of subjects. Adverse drug reactions of moderate to severe intensity occurring in 2 or more subjects included decreased neutrophil count (n = 3), anemia (n = 2), high potassium (n = 2), and low sodium (n = 2).

Lopinavir/ritonavir oral solution and soft gelatin capsules dosed at higher than recommended doses including lopinavir 400 mg/ritonavir 100 mg per m^2 (without concomitant NNRTI) and lopinavir 480 mg/ritonavir 120 mg per m^2 (with concomitant NNRTI) have been studied in 26 children 7 to 18 years of age in study 1038. Patients also had saquinavir added to their regimen at week 4. Abnormal blood cholesterol (12%), abnormal blood triglycerides (12%), and rash (12%) were the only adverse reactions reported in more than 10% of subjects. Adverse drug reactions of moderate to severe intensity occurring in 2 or more subjects included rash (n = 3), abnormal blood triglycerides (n = 3), and ECG QT prolonged (n = 2). Both subjects with QT prolongation had additional predisposing conditions such as electrolyte abnormalities, concomitant medications, or preexisting cardiac abnormalities.

Lopinavir/ritonavir oral solution dosed up to 300 mg/75 mg/m^2 has been studied in 100 children 6 months to 12 years of age. The adverse reaction profile seen during study 940 was similar to that for adults. Dysgeusia (22%), vomiting (21%), and diarrhea (12%) were the most common adverse reactions of any severity reported in children treated with combination therapy for up to 48 weeks in study 940. Eight children experienced moderate or severe adverse reactions. The adverse reactions meeting these criteria and reported for the 8 subjects include hypersensitivity (characterized by fever, jaundice, and rash), ALT increased, constipation, dry skin, dysgeusia, hepatomegaly, pancreatitis, pyrexia, rash, viral infection, and vomiting. Rash was the only reaction of those listed that occurred in 2 or more subjects (n = 3).

➤*Lab test abnormalities:*

Adults –

Lopinavir/Ritonavir Grade 3 to 4 Laboratory Test Abnormalities in Adult Antiretroviral-Naive Patients (≥ 2%)[a]						
		Study 863 (48 wk)		Study 720 (360 wk)	Study 730 (48 wk)	
Variable	Limit	Lopinavir 400 mg/ ritonavir 100 mg twice daily + stavudine and lamivudine (n = 326)	Nelfinavir 750 mg 3 times daily + stavudine and lamivudine (n = 327)	Lopinavir/ Ritonavir twice daily + stavudine and lamivudine (n = 100)	Lopinavir/ Ritonavir once daily + tenofovir and emtricitabine (n = 333)	Lopinavir/ Ritonavir twice daily + tenofovir and emtricitabine (n = 331)
Chemistry high						
Glucose	> 250 mg/dL	2%	2%	4%	0%	< 1%
Uric acid	> 12 mg/dL	2%	2%	5%	< 1%	1%
AST[b]	> 180 units/L	2%	4%	10%	1%	2%
ALT[b]	> 215 units/L	4%	4%	11%	1%	1%
GGT	> 300 units/L	NA	NA	10%	NA	NA
Total cholesterol	> 300 mg/dL	9%	5%	27%	4%	3%
Triglycerides	> 750 mg/dL	9%	1%	29%	3%	6%
Amylase	> 2 × ULN	3%	2%	4%	NA	NA

LOPINAVIR/RITONAVIR — ORAL

Lopinavir/Ritonavir Grade 3 to 4 Laboratory Test Abnormalities in Adult Antiretroviral-Naive Patients (≥ 2%)[a]

		Study 863 (48 wk)		Study 720 (360 wk)	Study 730 (48 wk)	
Variable	Limit	Lopinavir 400 mg/ ritonavir 100 mg twice daily + stavudine and lamivudine (n = 326)	Nelfinavir 750 mg 3 times daily + stavudine and lamivudine (n = 327)	Lopinavir/ Ritonavir twice daily + stavudine and lamivudine (n = 100)	Lopinavir/ Ritonavir once daily + tenofovir and emtricitabine (n = 333)	Lopinavir/ Ritonavir twice daily + tenofovir and emtricitabine (n = 331)
Lipase	> 2 × ULN	NA	NA	NA	3%	5%
Chemistry low						
Calculated CrCl	< 50 mL/min	NA	NA	NA	2%	2%
Hematology low						
Neutrophils	< 0.75 × 10^9/L	1%	3%	5%	2%	1%

[a] GGT = gamma-glutamyltransferase; ULN = upper limit of normal.

[b] Criterion for study 730 was > 5 × ULN (AST/ALT).

Lopinavir/Ritonavir Grade 3 to 4 Laboratory Test Abnormalities in Adult Protease Inhibitor–Experienced Patients (≥ 2%)

		Study 888 (48 wk)		Study 957[a] and study 765[b] (84 to 144 wk)	Study 802 (48 wk)	
Variable	Limit	Lopinavir 400 mg/ ritonavir 100 mg twice daily + nevirapine and NRTIs (n = 148)	Investigator-selected protease inhibitor(s) + nevirapine and NRTIs (n = 140)	Lopinavir/ Ritonavir twice daily + NNRTI and NRTIs (n = 127)	Lopinavir 800 mg/ ritonavir 200 mg once daily + NRTIs (n = 300)	Lopinavir 400 mg/ ritonavir 100 mg twice daily + NRTIs (n = 299)
Chemistry high						
Glucose	> 250 mg/dL	1%	2%	5%	2%	2%
Total bilirubin	> 3.48 mg/dL	1%	3%	1%	1%	1%
AST[c]	> 180 units/L	5%	11%	8%	3%	2%
ALT[c]	> 215 units/L	6%	13%	10%	2%	2%
GGT	> 300 units/L	NA	NA	29%	NA	NA
Total cholesterol	> 300 mg/dL	20%	21%	39%	6%	7%
Triglycerides	> 750 mg/dL	25%	21%	36%	5%	6%
Amylase	> 2 × ULN	4%	8%	8%	4%	4%
Lipase	> 2 × ULN	NA	NA	NA	4%	1%
Creatine phosphokinase	> 4 × ULN	NA	NA	NA	4%	5%
Chemistry low						
Calculated CrCl	< 50 mL/min	NA	NA		3%	3%
Inorganic phosphorus	< 1.5 mg/dL	1%	0%	2%	1%	< 1%
Hematology low						
Neutrophils	< 0.75 × 10^9/L	1%	2%	4%	3%	4%
Hemoglobin	< 80 g/L	1%	1%	1%	1%	2%

[a] Includes clinical laboratory data from patients receiving lopinavir 400 mg/ritonavir 100 mg twice daily (n = 29) or lopinavir 533 mg/ritonavir 133 mg twice daily (n = 28) for 84 weeks. Patients received lopinavir/ritonavir in combination with NRTIs and efavirenz.

[b] Includes clinical laboratory data from patients receiving lopinavir 400 mg/ritonavir 100 mg twice daily (n = 36) or lopinavir 400 mg/ritonavir 200 mg twice daily (n = 34) for 144 weeks. Patients received lopinavir/ritonavir in combination with NRTIs and nevirapine.

[c] Criterion for study 802 was > 5 × ULN (AST/ALT).

Children –

Lopinavir/Ritonavir Grade 3 to 4 Laboratory Test Abnormalities in Children (≥ 2%)

Variable	Limit	Lopinavir/Ritonavir twice daily + RTIs[a] (N = 100)
Chemistry high		
Sodium	> 149 mEq/L	3%
Total bilirubin	≥ 3 × ULN	3%
AST	> 180 units/L	8%
ALT	> 215 units/L	7%
Total cholesterol	> 300 mg/dL	3%
Amylase	> 2.5 × ULN	7%[b]
Chemistry low		
Sodium	< 130 mEq/L	3%
Hematology low		
Platelet count	< 50 × 10^9/L	4%
Neutrophils	< 0.4 × 10^9/L	2%

[a] RTIs = reverse transcriptase inhibitors.

[b] Subjects with grade 3 to 4 amylase confirmed by elevations in pancreatic amylase.

➤*Postmarketing:*

Cardiovascular – Bradyarrhythmias, first-degree AV block, QTc interval prolongation, second-degree AV block, third-degree AV block, torsades de pointes.

Dermatologic – Erythema multiforme, Stevens-Johnson syndrome

Miscellaneous – Redistribution/accumulation of body fat.

Overdosage

➤*Symptoms:* Overdoses with lopinavir/ritonavir oral solution have been reported. One of these reports described fatal cardiogenic shock in a 2.1 kg infant who received a single dose of lopinavir/ritonavir 6.5 mL oral solution 9 days prior. However, a causal relationship between the overdose and the outcome could not be established. Be aware that lopinavir/ritonavir oral solution is highly concentrated and, therefore, pay special attention to accurate calculation of the dose of lopinavir/ritonavir, transcription of the medication order, dispensing information, and dosing instructions to minimize the risk for medication errors and overdose. This is especially important for infants and young children.

Lopinavir/ritonavir oral solution contains 42.4% alcohol (v/v). Accidental ingestion of the product by a young child could result in significant alcohol-related toxicity and could approach the potential lethal dose of alcohol.

➤*Treatment:* Human experience of acute overdosage with lopinavir/ritonavir is limited. Treatment of overdose with lopinavir/ritonavir should consist of general supportive measures, including monitoring of vital signs and observation of the clinical status of the patient. There is no specific antidote for overdose with lopinavir/ritonavir. If indicated, achieve elimination

Protease Inhibitor Combinations

LOPINAVIR/RITONAVIR — ORAL

of unabsorbed drug by gastric lavage. Administration of activated charcoal also may be used to aid in removal of unabsorbed drug. Because lopinavir/ritonavir is highly protein bound, dialysis is unlikely to be beneficial in significant removal of the drug.

Patient Information

Advise patients and/or their health care providers to pay special attention to accurate administration of their dose to minimize the risk of accidental overdose or underdose of lopinavir/ritonavir.

Instruct patients to inform their health care provider if their children's weight changes to ensure that the child's lopinavir/ritonavir dose is correct.

Instruct patients to take the prescribed dose of lopinavir/ritonavir as directed and to set up a daily routine in order to do so.

Inform patients that sustained decreases in plasma HIV-1 RNA have been associated with a reduced risk of progression to AIDS and death. Instruct patients to remain under the care of a health care provider while using lopinavir/ritonavir.

Advise patients to take lopinavir/ritonavir and other concomitant antiretroviral therapy every day as prescribed; lopinavir/ritonavir must always be used in combination with other antiretroviral drugs. Instruct patients not to alter the dose or discontinue therapy without consulting their health care provider. If a dose is missed, instruct the patient to take the dose as soon as possible and then return to their normal schedule. However, if a dose is skipped, instruct the patient not to double the next dose.

Inform patients that lopinavir/ritonavir is not a cure for HIV-1 infection and that they may continue to develop opportunistic infections and other complications associated with HIV-1 disease. The long-term effects of lopinavir/ritonavir are unknown at this time. There are currently no data demonstrating that therapy with lopinavir/ritonavir can reduce the risk of transmitting HIV-1 to others through sexual contact, sharing needles, or being exposed to blood. For their health and the health of others, it is important that they always practice safer sex by using a latex or polyurethane condom or other barrier method to lower the chance of sexual contact with any body fluids, such as semen, vaginal secretions, or blood. Advise patients never to reuse or share needles.

Lopinavir/ritonavir may interact with some drugs; therefore, advise patients to report to their health care provider the use of any other prescription or nonprescription medication or herbal product, particularly St. John's wort.

Lopinavir/ritonavir tablets can be taken at the same time as didanosine without food. Instruct patients taking didanosine to take didanosine 1 hour before or 2 hours after lopinavir/ritonavir oral solution.

Advise patients receiving sildenafil, tadalafil, or vardenafil that they may be at an increased risk of associated adverse reactions, including hypotension, visual changes, and sustained erection, and to promptly report any symptoms to their health care provider.

Instruct patients receiving estrogen-based hormonal contraceptives to use additional or alternate contraceptive measures during therapy.

If they are taking or before they begin using salmeterol and lopinavir/ritonavir, instruct them to talk to their doctor about problems these medications may cause when taken together. Their health care provider may choose not to keep someone on salmeterol.

Advise patients to contact their health care provider if they develop a rash while taking lopinavir/ritonavir.

Advise patients that appropriate liver function testing will be conducted prior to initiating and during therapy with lopinavir/ritonavir. Advise patients that their liver function tests will need to be monitored closely, especially during the first several months of lopinavir/ritonavir treatment; instruct patients to notify their health care provider if they develop the signs and symptoms of worsening liver disease, including loss of appetite, abdominal pain, jaundice, and itchy skin.

Advise patients to notify their health care provider if they develop the signs and symptoms of diabetes mellitus, including frequent urination, excessive thirst, extreme hunger, unusual weight loss, and/or an increased blood sugar, while taking lopinavir/ritonavir, because they may require a change in their diabetes treatment or new treatment.

Instruct patients to consult their health care provider if they experience symptoms such as dizziness, light-headedness, abnormal heart rhythm, or loss of consciousness.

Instruct patients to seek medical assistance immediately if they develop a sustained penile erection lasting more than 4 hours while taking lopinavir/ritonavir and a PDE5 inhibitor, such as *Viagra*, *Cialis*, or *Levitra*.

Take lopinavir/ritonavir tablets with or without food. Take lopinavir/ritonavir oral solution with food to enhance absorption.

Inform patients that redistribution or accumulation of body fat may occur in patients receiving antiretroviral therapy, including protease inhibitors, and that the cause and long-term health effects of these conditions are not known at this time.

Inform patients that there may be a greater chance of developing diarrhea with the once-daily regimen compared with the twice-daily regimen.

Nucleotide Analog Reverse Transcriptase Inhibitor

TENOFOVIR DISOPROXIL FUMARATE

Rx	**Viread** (Gilead Sciences)	**Tablets; oral:** 300 mg	Equiv. to tenofovir disoproxil 245 mg. Lactose. (GILEAD 4331 300). Lt. blue, almond shape. Film-coated. In 30s.

TENOFOVIR DISOPROXIL FUMARATE — ORAL

WARNING

Lactic acidosis/severe hepatomegaly with steatosis – Lactic acidosis and severe hepatomegaly with steatosis, including fatal cases, have been reported with the use of nucleoside analogs, including tenofovir, in combination with other antiretrovirals.

Posttreatment exacerbation of hepatitis – Severe acute exacerbations of hepatitis have been reported in hepatitis B virus (HBV)–infected patients who have discontinued anti–hepatitis B therapy, including tenofovir. Monitor hepatic function closely with clinical and laboratory follow-up for at least several months in patients who discontinue anti–hepatitis B therapy, including tenofovir. If appropriate, resumption of anti–hepatitis B therapy may be warranted.

Indications

➤*Chronic hepatitis B:* For the treatment of chronic hepatitis B in adults.

➤*HIV infection:* In combination with other antiretroviral agents for the treatment of HIV-1 infection in adults and children 12 years of age and older.

Administration and Dosage

➤*Adults:*

Chronic hepatitis B –

Usual dosage: 300 mg once daily.

HIV infection – 300 mg once daily.

➤*Children:*

HIV infection –

12 years of age and older and 35 kg or more: 300 mg once daily.

➤*Renal function impairment:*

Adults –

Creatinine clearance 30 to 49 mL/min: 300 mg every 48 hours.

Creatinine clearance 10 to 29 mL/min: 300 mg every 72 to 96 hours.

Creatinine clearance less than 10 mL/min:

• *Hemodialysis* – 300 mg every 7 days or after a total of approximately 12 hours of dialysis. Generally once weekly, assuming 3 hemodialysis sessions a week of approximately 4 hours' duration. Administer following completion of dialysis.

➤*Storage/Stability:* Store at 25°C (77°F); excursions are permitted between 15° and 30°C (59° and 86°F).

Actions

➤*Pharmacology:* Tenofovir disoproxil fumarate (a prodrug of tenofovir) is a nucleotide analog reverse transcriptase inhibitor antiviral drug. Tenofovir is an acyclic nucleoside phosphonate diester analog of adenosine monophosphate. Tenofovir disoproxil fumarate requires initial diester hydrolysis for conversion to tenofovir and subsequent phosphorylations by cellular enzymes to form tenofovir diphosphate, an obligate chain terminator. Tenofovir diphosphate inhibits the activity of HIV-1 reverse transcriptase and HBV polymerase by competing with the natural substrate deoxyadenosine 5′-triphosphate and, after incorporation into DNA, by DNA chain termination. Tenofovir diphosphate is a weak inhibitor of mammalian DNA polymerases alpha, beta, and mitochondrial DNA polymerase gamma.

➤*Pharmacokinetics:*

Absorption – Tenofovir disoproxil fumarate is a water-soluble diester prodrug of the active ingredient tenofovir. The oral bioavailability of tenofovir from tenofovir disoproxil fumarate in fasted patients is approximately 25%. Following oral administration of a single dose of tenofovir 300 mg to HIV-1–infected patients in the fasted state, maximum serum concentrations (C_{max}) are achieved in 1 ± 0.4 hours. C_{max} and area under the curve (AUC) values are 0.3 ± 0.09 mcg/mL and 2.29 ± 0.69 mcg•h/mL, respectively.

Effect of food: Administration of tenofovir following a high-fat meal (approximately 700 to 1,000 kcal containing 40% to 50% fat) increases the oral bioavailability, with an increase in tenofovir $AUC_{0-\infty}$ of approximately 40% and an increase in C_{max} of approximately 14%. However, administration of tenofovir with a light meal did not have a significant effect on the pharmacokinetics of tenofovir compared with fasted administration of the drug. Food delays the time to tenofovir C_{max} by approximately 1 hour. C_{max} and AUC of tenofovir were 0.33 ± 0.12 mcg/mL and 3.32 ± 1.37 mcg•h/mL, respectively, following multiple doses of tenofovir 300 mg once daily in the fed state when meal content was not controlled.

TENOFOVIR DISOPROXIL FUMARATE — ORAL

Distribution – In vitro binding of tenofovir to human plasma or serum proteins is less than 0.7% and 7.2%, respectively, over the tenofovir concentration range of 0.01 to 25 mcg/mL. The volume of distribution at steady state is 1.3 ± 0.6 L/kg and 1.2 ± 0.4 L/kg following intravenous (IV) administration of tenofovir 1 and 3 mg/kg.

Metabolism/Excretion – Following IV administration of tenofovir, approximately 70% to 80% of the dose is recovered in the urine as unchanged tenofovir within 72 hours of dosing. Following single-dose oral administration of tenofovir, the terminal elimination half-life of tenofovir is approximately 17 hours. After multiple oral doses of tenofovir 300 mg once daily (under fed conditions), 32% ± 10% of the administered dose is recovered in the urine over 24 hours.

Tenofovir is eliminated by a combination of glomerular filtration and active tubular secretion. There may be competition for elimination with other compounds that are also renally eliminated.

Special populations –

Renal function impairment: See Administration and Dosage for more information.

Tenofovir Pharmacokinetic Parameters (Mean ± SD)[a] in Patients With Renal Impairment[b]

Pharmacokinetic parameter	CrCl > 80 mL/min (n = 3)	CrCl 50 to 80 mL/min (n = 10)	CrCl 30 to 49 mL/min (n = 8)	CrCl 12 to 29 mL/min (n = 11)
C_{max} (mcg/mL)	0.34 ± 0.03	0.33 ± 0.06	0.37 ± 0.16	0.6 ± 0.19
$AUC_{0-\infty}$ (mcg•h/mL)	2.18 ± 0.26	3.06 ± 0.93	6.01 ± 2.5	15.98 ± 7.22
CL/F (mL/min)	1,043.7 ± 115.4	807.7 ± 279.2	444.4 ± 209.8	177 ± 97.1
CL_{renal} (mL/min)	243.5 ± 33.3	168.6 ± 27.5	100.6 ± 27.5	43 ± 31.2

[a] Single dose of tenofovir 300 mg.
[b] CrCl = creatinine clearance; SD = standard deviation; CL/F = apparent oral clearance; CL_{renal} = renal clearance.

• *Hemodialysis* – Tenofovir is removed efficiently by hemodialysis with an extraction coefficient of approximately 54%. Following a single dose of tenofovir 300 mg, a 4-hour hemodialysis session removed approximately 10% of the administered tenofovir dose.

Contraindications

None well documented.

Warnings/Precautions

➤*Lactic acidosis/severe hepatomegaly with steatosis:* Lactic acidosis and severe hepatomegaly with steatosis, including fatal cases, have been reported with the use of nucleoside analogs, including tenofovir, in combination with other antiretrovirals.

A majority of these cases have been in women. Obesity and prolonged nucleoside exposure may be risk factors. Exercise particular caution when administering nucleoside analogs to any patient with known risk factors for liver disease; however, cases have also been reported in patients with no known risk factors. Suspend treatment with tenofovir in any patient who develops clinical or laboratory findings suggestive of lactic acidosis or pronounced hepatotoxicity (which may include hepatomegaly and steatosis even in the absence of marked transaminase elevations).

➤*Exacerbation of hepatitis:* See the Warning box for more information.

➤*Renal effects:* Renal impairment, including cases of acute renal failure and Fanconi syndrome (renal tubular injury with severe hypophosphatemia), has been reported with the use of tenofovir.

➤*HIV and hepatitis B virus coinfection:* Because of the risk of development of HIV-1 resistance, only use tenofovir in HIV-1 and HBV coinfected patients as part of an appropriate antiretroviral combination regimen.

Offer HIV-1 antibody testing to all HBV-infected patients before initiating therapy with tenofovir. It is recommended that all patients with HIV be tested for the presence of chronic HBV before initiating tenofovir.

➤*Bone effects:* Consider assessment of bone mineral density (BMD) for adults and children 12 years of age and older who have a history of pathologic bone fracture or other risk factors for osteoporosis or bone loss. Although the effect of supplementation with calcium and vitamin D was not studied, such supplementation may be beneficial for all patients. If bone abnormalities are suspected, then obtain appropriate consultation.

Cases of osteomalacia (associated with proximal renal tubulopathy and may contribute to fractures) have been reported in association with the use of tenofovir.

➤*Fat redistribution:* Redistribution/accumulation of body fat, including breast enlargement, central obesity, cushingoid appearance, dorsocervical fat enlargement (buffalo hump), facial wasting, and peripheral wasting, have been observed in patients receiving combination antiretroviral therapy.

➤*Immune reconstitution syndrome:* Immune reconstruction syndrome has been reported in HIV-infected patients treated with combination antiretroviral therapy, including tenofovir. During the initial phase of combination antiretroviral treatment, a patient whose immune system responds may develop an inflammatory response to indolent or residual opportunistic infections (eg, cytomegalovirus, *Mycobacterium avium* infection, *Pneumocystis jirovecii* pneumonia, tuberculosis), which may necessitate further evaluation and treatment.

➤*Early virologic failure:* Clinical studies in HIV-infected subjects have demonstrated that certain regimens that only contain 3 nucleoside reverse transcriptase inhibitors (NRTIs) are generally less effective than triple-drug regimens containing 2 NRTIs in combination with a nonnucleoside reverse transcriptase inhibitor (NNRTI) or an HIV-1 protease inhibitor. In particular, early virologic failure and high rates of resistance substitutions have been reported. Therefore, use triple nucleoside regimens with caution. Carefully monitor and consider for treatment modification patients on a therapy utilizing a triple nucleoside–only regimen.

➤*Renal function impairment:* Tenofovir is principally eliminated by the kidney. Dosing interval adjustment and close monitoring of renal function are recommended in all patients with CrCl less than 50 mL/min or in patients with end-stage renal disease who require dialysis. No safety or efficacy data are available in patients with renal impairment who received tenofovir using these dosing guidelines; therefore, assess the potential benefit of tenofovir therapy against the potential risk of renal toxicity. (See Administration and Dosage.)

➤*Pregnancy: Category B.* There are no adequate and well-controlled studies in pregnant women. Reproduction studies have been performed in rats and rabbits at doses of up to 14 and 19 times the human dose based on body surface are (BSA) comparisons and revealed no evidence of impaired fertility or harm to the fetus caused by tenofovir. The molecular weight (approximately 636 for the prodrug) and low plasma and serum protein binding, combined with the data from monkeys, suggest that the drug will cross to the human embryo and fetus. Because animal reproduction studies are not always predictive of human response, use tenofovir during pregnancy only if clearly needed.

The US Department of Health and Human Services recommends that the current antiretroviral agents, with the exception of efavirenz, be continued during pregnancy in HIV-1 infected patients. If indicated, do not withhold tenofovir in pregnancy because the expected benefit to the HIV-positive mother outweighs the unknown risk to the fetus. Updated guidelines for the use of antiretroviral drugs to reduce perinatal HIV-1 transmission also were released in 2006. Advise women receiving antiretroviral therapy during pregnancy to continue the therapy but, regardless of the regimen, zidovudine administration is recommended during the intrapartum period to prevent vertical transmission of HIV to the newborn.

Antiretroviral pregnancy registry – To monitor fetal outcomes of pregnant women exposed to tenofovir, an antiretroviral pregnancy registry has been established. Health care providers are encouraged to register patients by calling 1-800-258-4263.

➤*Lactation:* The Centers for Disease Control and Prevention (CDC) recommends that HIV-1–infected mothers not breast-feed their infants to avoid risking postnatal transmission of HIV-1. Studies in rats have demonstrated that tenofovir is secreted in milk. It is not known whether tenofovir is excreted in human milk. The molecular weight (approximately 636 for the prodrug) and low plasma (approximately 1%) and serum (approximately 7%) protein binding suggest that the drug will be excreted into human breast milk. Because HIV-1 is transmitted in milk, and because of the potential for HIV-1 transmission and serious adverse reactions in breast-feeding infants, instruct mothers not to breast-feed if they are receiving tenofovir.

➤*Children:* The safety and effectiveness in children younger than 12 years of age have not been established.

➤*Elderly:* Use caution during dose selection for elderly patients, keeping in mind the greater frequency of decreased hepatic, renal, or cardiac function, and of concomitant disease or other drug therapy.

➤*Monitoring:* Consider BMD monitoring for HIV-infected patients who have a history of pathologic bone fractures or are at risk for osteopenia. Monitor patients for signs and symptoms of lactic acidosis. Monitor hepatic function closely with both clinical and laboratory follow-up for at least several months in patients who discontinue tenofovir and are coinfected with HIV and HBV.

Calculate CrCl and serum phosphorus in all patients prior to initiating therapy and as clinically appropriate during therapy, especially patients at risk for renal impairment or with CrCl less than 50 mL/min or in patients with end-stage renal disease (ESRD) who require dialysis. Monitor patients at risk for, or with a history of, renal impairment and patients receiving concomitant nephrotoxic agents for changes in serum creatinine and phosphorus.

Drug Interactions

Tenofovir Drug Interactions

Precipitant drug	Object drug[a]		Description
Atazanavir	Tenofovir	⬆	Concurrent use increased tenofovir AUC by 24% and C_{max} by 14%. Monitor closely. Coadministration of tenofovir and atazanavir resulted in decreased atazanavir AUC by 25% and C_{max} by 21%. Do not administer atazanavir without ritonavir in patients receiving tenofovir
Tenofovir	Atazanavir	⬇	

TENOFOVIR DISOPROXIL FUMARATE — ORAL

Tenofovir Drug Interactions			
Precipitant drug	Object drug[a]		Description
Indinavir	Tenofovir	↑	Coadministration increased tenofovir C_{max} ≈ 14%, but AUC remained unchanged. The C_{max} of indinavir decreased ≈ 11%, but AUC remained unchanged.
Tenofovir	Indinavir	↓	
Lopinavir/ Ritonavir	Tenofovir	↑	Concurrent use increased tenofovir AUC by 32%. Monitor closely.
Nephrotoxic agents	Tenofovir	↑	Risk of nephrotoxicity may be increased. Avoid tenofovir in patients who are currently or recently have been treated with a nephrotoxic agent.
NSAIDs[b] (eg, ibuprofen)	Tenofovir	↑	NSAIDs may increase the pharmacologic and toxic effects (eg, nephrotoxicity) of tenofovir. Coadminister with caution.
Tacrolimus	Tenofovir	↑	Coadministration increased C_{max} of tenofovir by 13%. Monitor closely.
Tenofovir	Abacavir	↑	Concurrent use increased abacavir C_{max} by 12%, but AUC remained unchanged.
Tenofovir	Acyclovir, adefovir dipivoxil, cidofovir, ganciclovir, valacyclovir, valganciclovir	↑	Coadministration of tenofovir with drugs that reduce renal function or compete for active tubular secretion may increase serum concentrations of tenofovir and/or increase the concentrations of other renally eliminated drugs. Avoid coadministration with adefovir dipivoxil.
Acyclovir, adefovir dipivoxil, cidofovir, ganciclovir, valacyclovir, valganciclovir	Tenofovir		
Tenofovir	Didanosine (buffered formulation or enteric-coated)	↑	The C_{max} and AUC of didanosine increased significantly when given with tenofovir. Increases in didanosine concentrations could potentiate adverse reactions, including pancreatitis, lactic acidosis, and neuropathy. In adults weighing > 60 kg, reduce the didanosine dose to 250 mg when administered with tenofovir. Monitor patients closely for adverse reactions and use with caution. Discontinue didanosine in patients who develop adverse reactions. Give under fasting conditions.
Tenofovir	Entecavir	↑	Coadministration increased entecavir AUC by 13%.
Tenofovir	Lamivudine	↓	Concurrent use decreased lamivudine C_{max} by 24%, but AUC remained unchanged.
Tenofovir	Saquinavir/ Ritonavir	↑	Concurrent use increased saquinavir AUC by 29% and C_{max} by 22%. These changes are not expected to be clinically relevant.

[a] ↑ = object drug increased; ↓ = object drug decreased.
[b] NSAIDs = nonsteroidal anti-inflammatory drugs.

➤*Drug/Food interactions:* Administration of tenofovir following a high-fat meal (approximately 700 to 1,000 kcal containing 40% to 50% fat) increases the oral bioavailability, with an increase in tenofovir $AUC_{0-\infty}$ of approximately 40% and an increase in C_{max} of approximately 14%. Food delays the time to tenofovir C_{max} by approximately 1 hour.

Adverse Reactions

➤*Chronic hepatitis B:*

Adverse reactions (more than 5%) – In controlled clinical trials in patients with chronic hepatitis B, more patients treated with tenofovir experienced nausea (9% with tenofovir vs 2% with adefovir). Other treatment-emergent adverse reactions reported in more than 5% of patients treated with tenofovir include abdominal pain, back pain, diarrhea, dizziness, fatigue, headache, nasopharyngitis, and skin rash.

Most frequent adverse reactions – The most frequently reported treatment-emergent adverse reactions of any severity were abdominal pain (22%), nausea (20%), insomnia (18%), pruritus (16%), vomiting (13%), dizziness (13%), and pyrexia (11%).

Mortality – Four percent of subjects died through week 48 of the study because of progression of liver disease.

Discontinuation – Seven percent of subjects discontinued treatment because of an adverse event.

Renal – Nine percent of subjects experienced a confirmed increase in serum creatinine of 0.5 mg/dL (1 subject also had a confirmed serum phosphorus less than 2 mg/dL through week 48). Three of these subjects (each of whom had a Child-Pugh score of at least 10 and Mayo End-Stage Liver Disease (MELD) score of at least 14 at entry) developed renal failure. Because tenofovir and decompensated liver disease may have an impact on renal function, the contribution of tenofovir to renal impairment in this population is difficult to ascertain.

Hepatic – One of 45 subjects experienced an on-treatment hepatic flare during the 48-week study.

➤*HIV infection:*

Most common adverse reactions – The most common adverse reactions (incidence of 10% or more, grades 2 to 4) identified from any of the 3 large controlled clinical trials include asthenia, depression, diarrhea, headache, nausea, pain, and rash.

Treatment-naive adults –

Most common adverse reactions:

Tenofovir Adverse Reactions (Grade 2 to 4)[a] in HIV-Treatment–Naive Adults (≥ 5%)		
Adverse reactions	Tenofovir + lamivudine + efavirenz (n = 299)	Stavudine + lamivudine + efavirenz (n = 301)
CNS		
Anxiety	6%	6%
Asthenia	6%	7%
Depression	11%	10%
Dizziness	3%	6%
Headache	14%	17%
Insomnia	5%	8%
Peripheral neuropathy[b]	1%	5%
GI		
Abdominal pain	7%	12%
Diarrhea	11%	13%
Dyspepsia	4%	5%
Nausea	8%	9%
Vomiting	5%	9%
Musculoskeletal		
Arthralgia	5%	7%
Back pain	9%	8%
Myalgia	3%	5%
Miscellaneous		
Fever	8%	7%
Lipodystrophy[c]	1%	8%
Pain	13%	12%
Pneumonia	5%	5%
Rash[d]	18%	12%

[a] Frequencies of adverse reactions are based on all treatment-emergent adverse reactions, regardless of relationship to study drug.
[b] Peripheral neuropathy includes peripheral neuritis and neuropathy.
[c] Lipodystrophy represents a variety of investigator-described adverse reactions, not a protocol-defined syndrome.
[d] Includes maculopapular rash, pruritus, pustular rash, rash, urticaria, and vesiculobullous rash.

Tenofovir Adverse Reactions[a] (Grades 2 to 4) in HIV-Treatment–Naive Adults (≥ 5%)		
Adverse reactions	Tenofovir[b] + emtricitabine + efavirenz (n = 257)	Zidovudine/ Lamivudine + efavirenz (n = 254)
CNS		
Depression	9%	7%
Dizziness	8%	7%
Fatigue	9%	8%
Headache	6%	5%
Insomnia	5%	7%

TENOFOVIR DISOPROXIL FUMARATE — ORAL

Tenofovir Adverse Reactions[a] (Grades 2 to 4) in HIV-Treatment–Naive Adults (≥ 5%)		
Adverse reactions	Tenofovir[b] + emtricitabine + efavirenz (n = 257)	Zidovudine/ Lamivudine + efavirenz (n = 254)
Dermatologic		
Rash[c]	7%	9%
GI		
Diarrhea	9%	5%
Nausea	9%	7%
Vomiting	2%	5%
Respiratory		
Nasopharyngitis	5%	3%
Sinusitis	8%	4%
Upper respiratory tract infections	8%	5%

[a] Frequencies of adverse reactions are based on all treatment-emergent adverse reactions, regardless of relationship to study drug.
[b] From weeks 96 to 144 of the study, patients received emtricitabine/tenofovir with efavirenz in place of tenofovir + emtricitabine with efavirenz.
[c] Includes rash, exfoliative rash, rash generalized, rash macular, rash maculopapular, rash pruritic, and rash vesicular.

Treatment-experienced adults:

Tenofovir Adverse Reactions[a] (Grades 2 to 4) in HIV-Treatment–Experienced Adults (≥ 3%)				
Adverse reactions	Tenofovir (n = 368) (weeks 0 to 24)	Placebo (n = 182) (weeks 0 to 24)	Tenofovir (n = 368) (weeks 0 to 48)	Placebo crossover to tenofovir (n = 170) (weeks 24 to 48)
CNS				
Asthenia	7%	6%	11%	1%
Depression	4%	3%	8%	4%
Dizziness	1%	3%	3%	1%
Headache	5%	5%	8%	2%
Insomnia	3%	2%	4%	4%
Peripheral neuropathy[b]	3%	3%	5%	2%
Dermatologic				
Rash[c]	5%	4%	7%	1%
Sweating	3%	2%	3%	1%
GI				
Abdominal pain	4%	3%	7%	6%
Anorexia	3%	2%	4%	1%
Diarrhea	11%	10%	16%	11%
Dyspepsia	3%	2%	4%	2%
Flatulence	3%	1%	4%	1%
Nausea	8%	5%	11%	7%
Vomiting	4%	1%	7%	5%
Musculoskeletal				
Back pain	3%	3%	4%	2%
Myalgia	3%	3%	4%	1%
Miscellaneous				
Chest pain	3%	1%	3%	2%
Fever	2%	2%	4%	2%
Pain	7%	7%	12%	4%
Pneumonia	2%	0%	3%	2%
Weight loss	2%	1%	4%	2%

[a] Frequencies of adverse reactions are based on all treatment-emergent adverse reactions, regardless of relationship to study drug.
[b] Includes peripheral neuritis and neuropathy.
[c] Includes maculopapular rash, pruritus, pustular rash, rash, urticaria, and vesiculobullous rash.

➤*Lab test abnormalities:*
Chronic hepatitis B –

Tenofovir Laboratory Abnormalities Grade 3/4 in Chronic Hepatitis B (≥ 1%)		
Laboratory abnormality	Tenofovir (n = 426)	Adefovir (n = 215)
Any ≥ grade 3 laboratory abnormality	19%	13%
AST (Men: > 180 units/L) (Women: > 170 units/L)	4%	4%
ALT (Men: > 215 units/L) (Women: > 170 units/L)	10%	6%
Creatine kinase (Men: > 990 units/L) (Women: > 845 units/L)	2%	3%
Glycosuria (≥ 3+)	3%	< 1%
Serum amylase (> 175 units/L)	4%	1%

The overall incidence of on-treatment ALT elevations (defined as serum ALT more than 2 times baseline and more than 10 times the upper limit of normal, with or without associated symptoms) was similar between tenofovir (2.6%) and adefovir (2%). ALT elevations generally occurred within the first 4 to 8 weeks of treatment and were accompanied by decreases in HBV DNA levels. No patient had evidence of decompensation. ALT flares typically resolved within 4 to 8 weeks without changes in study medication.

HIV infection –
Treatment-naive adults:

Tenofovir Laboratory Abnormalities (Grade 3 and 4) in HIV-Treatment–Naive Adults (≥ 1%)		
Laboratory abnormality	Tenofovir + lamivudine + efavirenz (n = 299)	Stavudine + lamivudine + efavirenz (n = 301)
Any ≥ grade 3 laboratory abnormality	36%	42%
ALT (Men: > 215 units/L) (Women: > 170 units/L)	4%	5%
AST (Men: > 180 units/L) (Women: > 170 units/L)	5%	7%
Creatine kinase (Men: > 990 units/L) (Women: > 845 units/L)	12%	12%
Fasting cholesterol (> 240 mg/dL)	19%	40%
Fasting triglyceride (> 750 mg/dL)	1%	9%
Hematuria (> 100 red blood cells per high-power field)	7%	7%
Neutrophils (< 750/mm^3)	3%	1%
Serum amylase (> 175 units/L)	9%	8%

Tenofovir Significant Laboratory Abnormalities in HIV-Treatment–Naive Adults (≥ 1%)		
Laboratory abnormality	Tenofovir[a] + emtricitabine + efavirenz (n = 257)	Zidovudine/ Lamivudine + efavirenz (n = 254)
Any ≥ grade 3 laboratory abnormality	30%	26%
Alkaline phosphatase (> 550 units/L)	1%	0%
ALT (Men: > 215 units/L) (Women: > 170 units/L)	2%	3%
AST (Men: > 180 units/L) (Women: > 170 units/L)	3%	3%
Creatine kinase (Men: > 990 units/L) (Women: > 845 units/L)	9%	7%

TENOFOVIR DISOPROXIL FUMARATE — ORAL

Tenofovir Significant Laboratory Abnormalities in HIV-Treatment–Naive Adults (≥ 1%)		
Laboratory abnormality	Tenofovir[a] + emtricitabine + efavirenz (n = 257)	Zidovudine/ Lamivudine + efavirenz (n = 254)
Fasting cholesterol (> 240 mg/dL)	22%	24%
Fasting triglycerides (> 750 mg/dL)	4%	2%
Glycosuria (≥ 3+)	< 1%	1%
Hematuria (> 75 red blood cells per high-power field)	3%	2%
Hemoglobin (< 8 mg/dl)	0%	4%
Hyperglycemia (> 250 mg/dL)	2%	1%
Neutrophils (< 750/mm^3)	3%	5%
Serum amylase (> 175 units/L)	8%	4%

[a] From weeks 96 to 144 of the study, patients received emtricitabine/tenofovir with efavirenz in place of tenofovir + emtricitabine with efavirenz.

Treatment-experienced adults:

Tenofovir Laboratory Abnormalities Grade 3/4 in HIV-Treatment–Experienced Adults (≥ 1%)				
Laboratory abnormality	Tenofovir (n = 368) (weeks 0 to 24)	Placebo (n = 182) (weeks 0 to 24)	Tenofovir (n = 368) (weeks 0 to 48)	Placebo crossover to tenofovir (n = 170) (weeks 24 to 48)
Any ≥ grade 3 laboratory abnormality	25%	38%	35%	34%
ALT (Men: > 215 units/L) (Women: > 170 units/L)	2%	2%	4%	5%
AST (Men: > 180 units/L) (Women: > 170 units/L)	3%	3%	4%	5%
Creatine kinase (Men: > 990 units/L) (Women: > 845 units/L)	7%	14%	12%	12%
Glycosuria (≥ 3+)	3%	3%	3%	2%
Neutrophils (< 750 mg/mm^3)	1%	1%	2%	1%
Serum amylase (> 175 units/L)	6%	7%	7%	6%
Serum glucose (> 250 units/L)	2%	4%	3%	3%
Triglycerides (> 750 mg/dL)	8%	13%	11%	9%

➤*Postmarketing:*

GI – Abdominal pain, increased amylase, pancreatitis.

GU – Acute renal failure, acute tubular necrosis, Fanconi syndrome, increased creatinine, interstitial nephritis (including acute cases), nephrogenic diabetes insipidus, polyuria, proteinuria, proximal tubulopathy, renal failure, renal insufficiency.

Hepatic – Hepatic steatosis, hepatitis, increased liver enzymes (most commonly AST, ALT, gamma-glutamyl transpeptidase).

Metabolic/Nutritional – Hypokalemia, hypophosphatemia (may occur as a consequence of proximal renal tubulopathy). lactic acidosis.

Musculoskeletal – Muscular weakness, myopathy, osteomalacia (manifested as bone pain and may contribute to fractures), rhabdomyolysis (may occur as a consequence of proximal renal tubulopathy).

Miscellaneous – Allergic reaction (including angioedema), asthenia, dyspnea, rash.

Overdosage

➤*Treatment:* If overdose occurs, monitor the patient for evidence of toxicity, and apply standard supportive treatment as necessary.

Tenofovir is efficiently removed by hemodialysis with an extraction coefficient of approximately 54%. Following a single dose of tenofovir 300 mg, a 4-hour hemodialysis session removed approximately 10% of the administered tenofovir dose.

Patient Information

Inform patients that tenofovir is not a cure for HIV-1 infection and patients may continue to experience illnesses associated with HIV-1 infection, including opportunistic infections. Patients should remain under the care of a health care provider when using tenofovir.

Inform patients that the use of tenofovir has not been shown to reduce the risk of transmission of HIV-1 or HBV to others through sexual contact or blood contamination. Advise patients to continue to practice safe sex and to use latex or polyurethane condoms to lower the chance of sexual contact with any body fluids such as semen, vaginal secretions, or blood. Advise patients never to reuse or share needles.

Inform patients that the long-term effects of tenofovir are unknown.

Advise patients not to discontinue tenofovir without first informing their health care provider.

Inform patients with HIV-1 infection, with or without HBV coinfection, that it is important to take tenofovir with combination therapy.

Advise patients that it is important to take tenofovir on a regular dosing schedule and to avoid missing doses.

Inform patients that lactic acidosis and severe hepatomegaly with steatosis, including fatal cases, have been reported. Suspend treatment with tenofovir in any patient who develops clinical symptoms suggestive of lactic acidosis or pronounced hepatotoxicity (including nausea, vomiting, unusual or unexpected stomach discomfort, and weakness).

Advise patients with HIV-1 to be tested for HBV before initiating antiretroviral therapy.

Inform patients with chronic hepatitis B to obtain HIV antibody testing prior to initiating therapy with tenofovir.

Inform patients that severe acute exacerbations of hepatitis have been reported in patients who are infected with HBV or coinfected with HBV and HIV-1 and who have discontinued tenofovir.

Inform patients that renal impairment, including cases of acute renal failure and Fanconi syndrome, has been reported. Tenofovir should be avoided with concurrent or recent use of a nephrotoxic agent. The dosing interval of tenofovir may need adjustment in patients with renal impairment.

Do not coadminister tenofovir with the fixed-dose combination products emtricitabine/tenofovir and efavirenz/emtricitabine/tenofovir because it is a component of these products.

Do not administer tenofovir in combination with adefovir.

Inform patients that decreases in BMD have been observed with the use of tenofovir in patients with HIV. Consider BMD monitoring in patients who have a history of pathologic bone fracture or who are at risk for osteopenia.

Inform patients that in the treatment of chronic hepatitis B, the optimal duration of treatment is unknown. The relationship between response and long-term prevention of outcomes such as hepatocellular carcinoma is not known.

Advise HIV-infected mothers not to breast-feed to prevent infecting infant with HIV.

DIDANOSINE (ddI; dideoxyinosine)

Rx	**Didanosine** (Various, eg, Aurobindo, Mylan)	**Capsules, delayed-release; oral:** 125 mg	In 30s, 500s, and UD 140s.
Rx	**Videx EC**[a] (Bristol-Myers Squibb)		(BMS 125 mg 6671). Tan. In 30s.
Rx	**Didanosine**[a] (Various, eg, Aurobindo, Mylan)	**Capsules, delayed-release; oral:** 200 mg	In 30s, 500s, and UD 100s.
Rx	**Videx EC**[a] (Bristol-Myers Squibb)		(BMS 200 mg 6672). Green. In 30s.
Rx	**Didanosine**[a] (Various, eg, Aurobindo, Mylan)	**Capsules, delayed-release; oral:** 250 mg	In 30s, 500s, and UD 100s.
Rx	**Videx EC**[a] (Bristol-Myers Squibb)		(BMS 250 mg 6673). Blue. In 30s.
Rx	**Didanosine**[a] (Various, eg, Aurobindo, Mylan)	**Capsules, delayed-release; oral:** 400 mg	In 30s, 500s, and UD 100s.
Rx	**Videx EC**[a] (Bristol-Myers Squibb)		(BMS 400 mg 6674). Red. In 30s.
Rx	**Videx** (Bristol-Myers Squibb)	**Powder for solution; oral:** 2 g	In 4 oz bottles.
		4 g	In 8 oz bottles.

[a] Capsule contains enteric-coated beadlets.

DIDANOSINE – ORAL

WARNING

Pancreatitis – Fatal and nonfatal pancreatitis has occurred during therapy with didanosine used alone or in combination regimens in both treatment-naive and treatment-experienced patients, regardless of the degree of immunosuppression. Suspend didanosine in patients with suspected pancreatitis; discontinue didanosine in patients with confirmed pancreatitis.

Lactic acidosis/severe hepatomegaly – Lactic acidosis and severe hepatomegaly with steatosis, including fatal cases, have been reported with the use of nucleoside analogs alone or in combination, including didanosine and other antiretrovirals. Fatal lactic acidosis has been reported in pregnant women who received the combination of didanosine and stavudine with other antiretroviral agents. Use the combination of didanosine and stavudine with caution during pregnancy; the combination is recommended only if the potential benefit clearly outweighs the potential risk.

Indications

➤*HIV infection:* For the treatment of HIV-1 infection in combination with other antiretroviral agents.

Administration and Dosage

➤*Adults:*

HIV infection –

Delayed-release capsule:

- *60 kg or greater* – 400 mg once daily.
- *25 kg to less than 60 kg* – 250 mg once daily.
- *20 kg to less than 25 kg* – 200 mg once daily.

Powder for oral solution:

- *60 kg or greater* – 200 mg twice daily (preferred) or 400 mg once daily.
- *Less than 60 kg* – 125 mg twice daily (preferred) or 250 mg once daily.

➤*Children:*

HIV infection –

Delayed-release capsule: See Adults for dosing.

Powder for oral solution:

- *Older than 8 months* – 120 mg/m² twice daily, not to exceed the adult dosing recommendation.
- *2 weeks to 8 months of age* – 100 mg/m² twice daily, not to exceed the adult dosing recommendation.

Off-label dosing –

Treatment naive (3 to 21 years of age): 240 mg/m² daily.

Older than 8 months:

- *Alternative dosing* – 90 to 150 mg/m² twice daily.

Neonates/infants (2 weeks to younger than 3 months): 50 mg/m² twice daily.

➤*Renal function impairment:*

Recommended Didanosine Dosage in Adults With Renal Impairment[a]

CrCl[b] (mL/min)	Patient weight ≥ 60 kg: Delayed-release capsule	Patient weight ≥ 60 kg: Powder for oral suspension	Patient weight < 60 kg: Delayed-release capsule	Patient weight < 60 kg: Powder for oral suspension
≥ 60	400 mg once daily	200 mg twice daily[c]	250 mg once daily	125 mg twice daily[c]
30 to 59	200 mg once daily	200 mg once daily or 100 mg twice daily	125 mg once daily	150 mg once daily or 75 mg twice daily
10 to 29	125 mg once daily	150 mg once daily	125 mg once daily	100 mg once daily
< 10	125 mg once daily	100 mg once daily	[d]	75 mg once daily

[a] Based on studies using a buffered formulation of didanosine.
[b] CrCl = creatinine clearance.
[c] 400 mg once daily (≥ 60 kg) or 250 mg once daily (< 60 kg) for patients whose management requires once-daily frequency of administration.
[d] Not suitable for use in patients weighing < 60 kg with CrCl

Children – Urinary excretion is also a major route of elimination of didanosine in children; therefore, the clearance of didanosine may be altered in children with renal impairment. Although there are insufficient data to recommend a specific dose adjustment of didanosine in this patient population, a reduction in the dose should be considered.

Hemodialysis/Continuous ambulatory peritoneal dialysis – For patients requiring continuous ambulatory peritoneal dialysis (CAPD) or hemodialysis, follow dosing recommendations for patients with CrCl of less than 10 mL/min. It is not necessary to administer a supplemental dose of didanosine following hemodialysis.

➤*Concomitant therapy:*

Tenofovir – In patients who are also taking tenofovir, a dose reduction of didanosine to 250 mg (adults weighing at least 60 kg with CrCl of at least 60 mL/min) or 200 mg (adults weighing less than 60 kg with CrCl of at least 60 mL/min) once daily taken together with tenofovir is recommended. The appropriate dose of didanosine coadministered with tenofovir in patients with CrCl of less than 60 mL/min has not been established.

➤*Preparation for administration:*

Powder for oral solution – Prior to dispensing, the pharmacist must constitute dry powder with purified water to an initial concentration of 20 mg/mL and immediately mix the resulting solution with antacid to a final concentration of 10 mg/mL as follows:

20 mg/mL initial solution: Reconstitute the product to 20 mg/mL by adding 100 or 200 mL of purified water to the didanosine 2 or 4 g powder, respectively, in the product bottle.

10 mg/mL final admixture: Immediately mix 1 part of the 20 mg/mL initial solution with 1 part of *Maximum Strength Mylanta* liquid (aluminum hydroxide/magnesium hydroxide/simethicone) for a final dispensing concentration of didanosine 10 mg/mL. For patient home use, the admixture should be dispensed in appropriately sized, flint-glass or plastic (HDPE, PET, or PETG) bottles with child-resistant closures.

➤*Administration:* Administer on an empty stomach, at least 30 minutes before or 2 hours after eating.

Delayed-release capsule – May take didanosine and tenofovir together with a light meal (400 kcal or less, 20% fat or less) or in the fasted state.

The capsules should be administered once daily and swallowed intact.

Powder for oral solution – May take didanosine and tenofovir together in the fasted state. Alternatively, if tenofovir is taken with food, didanosine should be taken on an empty stomach (at least 30 minutes before or 2 hours after food).

The preferred dosing frequency is twice daily because there is more evidence to support the effectiveness of this dosing regimen. Once-daily dosing should be considered only for adult patients whose management requires once-daily dosing of didanosine. Shake well prior to use.

➤*Storage/Stability:*

Delayed-release capsules – Store in a tightly closed container at 25°C (77°F). Excursions are permitted between 15° and 30°C (59° and 86°F).

Powder for oral solution – Store the bottles of powder at 15° to 30°C (59° to 86°F). The didanosine admixture may be stored up to 30 days in a refrigerator between 2° and 8°C (36° and 46°F). Discard any unused portion after 30 days.

Actions

➤*Pharmacology:* Didanosine, an antiviral agent, is a synthetic nucleoside analog of the naturally occurring nucleoside deoxyadenosine, in which the 3′-hydroxyl group is replaced by hydrogen. Intracellularly, didanosine is converted by cellular enzymes to the active metabolite, dideoxyadenosine 5′-triphosphate. Dideoxyadenosine 5′-triphosphate inhibits the activity of HIV-1 reverse transcriptase by competing with the natural substrate deoxyadenosine 5′-triphosphate, and by its incorporation into viral DNA, causing termination of viral DNA chain elongation.

DIDANOSINE — ORAL

➤*Pharmacokinetics:*

Mean ± Standard Deviation Pharmacokinetic Parameters for Didanosine Powder for Oral Solution in Adults and Children

Parameter	Adults[a]	n	Children[b] 8 mo to 19 y	n	2 wk to 4 mo	n
Oral bioavailability (%)	42 ± 12	6	25 ± 20	46	ND[c]	
Apparent volume of distribution[d] (L/m²)	43.7 ± 8.9	6	28 ± 15	49	ND	
CSF[e]-plasma ratio[f]	21 ± 0.03%[g]	5	46% (range, 12% to 85%)	7	ND	
Systemic clearance[d] (mL/min/m²)	526 ± 64.7	6	516 ± 184	49	ND	
Renal clearance[h] (mL/min/m²)	223 ± 85	6	240 ± 90	15	ND	
Apparent oral clearance[i] (mL/min/m²)	1,252 ± 154	6	2,064 ± 736	48	1,353 ± 759	41
Elimination half-life[h] (h)	1.5 ± 0.4	6	0.8 ± 0.3	60	1.2 ± 0.3	21
Urinary recovery of didanosine[h] (%)	18 ± 8	6	18 ± 10	15	ND	

[a] Parameter units for adults were converted to the same units in children to facilitate comparisons among populations: mean adult body weight = 70 kg and mean adult body surface area = 1.73 m².
[b] In 1-day old infants (n = 10), the mean ± standard deviation (SD) apparent oral clearance was 1,523 ± 1,176 mL/min/m², and half-life was 2 ± 0.7 h.
[c] ND = not determined.
[d] Following intravenous (IV) administration.
[e] CSF = cerebrospinal fluid.
[f] Following IV administration in adults and IV or oral administration in children.
[g] Mean ± standard error.
[h] Following oral administration.
[i] Apparent oral clearance estimate was determined as the ratio of the mean systemic clearance and the mean oral bioavailability estimate.

Pharmacokinetic Parameters for Didanosine Delayed-Release Capsules in Patients Infected With HIV

Parameter[a]	Children 20 to < 25 kg (n = 10)	25 to < 60 kg (n = 17)	≥ 60 kg (n = 7)	Adults ≥ 60 kg (n = 44)
Apparent clearance (L/h)	89.5 ± 21.6	116.2 ± 38.6	196 ± 55.8	174.5 ± 69.7
Apparent volume of distribution (L)	98.1 ± 30.2	154.7 ± 55	363 ± 137.7	308.3 ± 164.3
Elimination half-life (h)	0.75 ± 0.13	0.92 ± 0.09	1.26 ± 0.19	1.19 ± 0.21
Steady-state AUC[b] (mg•h/L)	2.38 ± 0.66	2.36 ± 0.7	2.25 ± 0.89	2.65 ± 1.07

[a] The pharmacokinetic parameters (mean ± SD) of didanosine were determined by a population pharmacokinetic model based on combined clinical studies.
[b] AUC = area under the curve.

Absorption/Distribution – Didanosine is rapidly absorbed, with peak plasma concentrations generally observed from 0.25 to 1.5 hours following oral dosing with a buffered formulation. Increases in plasma didanosine concentrations were dose proportional over the range of 50 to 400 mg. In adults, the mean (± SD) oral bioavailability following single oral dosing with a buffered formulation is 42 (± 12)%. The CSF-plasma ratio following IV administration is 21 (± 0.03)%. Steady-state pharmacokinetic parameters did not differ significantly from values obtained after a single dose. Binding of didanosine to plasma proteins in vitro was low (less than 5%).

Comparison of formulations: In the delayed-release capsules, didanosine is protected against stomach acid degradation by the use of an enteric coating on the beadlets in the capsule. The enteric coating dissolves when the beadlets empty into the small intestine, the site of drug absorption. With buffered formulations of didanosine, administration with antacid provides protection from degradation by stomach acid.

In healthy volunteers, as well as subjects infected with HIV, the AUC is equivalent for didanosine administered as the delayed-release capsule formulation relative to a buffered tablet formulation. The peak plasma concentration (C_{max}) of didanosine, administered as delayed-release capsules, is reduced approximately 40% relative to didanosine buffered tablets. The time to peak concentration (T_{max}) increased from approximately 0.67 hours for didanosine buffered tablets to 2 hours for didanosine delayed-release capsules.

Effect of food: Didanosine C_{max} and AUC were decreased by approximately 55% when didanosine tablets were administered up to 2 hours after a meal. Administration of didanosine tablets up to 30 minutes before a meal did not result in any significant changes in bioavailability. In the presence of food, the C_{max} and AUC for didanosine delayed-release capsules were reduced by approximately 46% and 19%, respectively, compared with the fasting state. Instruct patients to take didanosine on an empty stomach.

Metabolism/Excretion – Based on data from in vitro and animal studies, it is presumed that the metabolism of didanosine in humans occurs by the same pathways responsible for the elimination of endogenous purines. After oral administration, the urinary recovery of didanosine is approximately 18 (± 8)% of the dose.

Special populations –

Renal function impairment: Data from 2 studies indicated that the apparent oral clearance of didanosine decreased and the terminal elimination half-life increased as creatinine clearance decreased. Following oral administration, didanosine was not detectable in peritoneal dialysate fluid (n = 6); recovery in hemodialysate (n = 5) ranged from 0.6% to 7.4% of the dose over a 3- to 4-hour dialysis period. The absolute bioavailability of didanosine was not affected in patients requiring dialysis.

Mean ± SD Pharmacokinetic Parameters for Didanosine Buffered Formulation (Single Dose) in Patients With Renal Function Impairment[a]

Parameter	CrCl (mL/min) ≥ 90 (n = 12)	60 to 90 (n = 6)	30 to 59 (n = 6)	10 to 29 (n = 3)	Dialysis patients (n = 11)
CrCl (mL/min)	112 ± 22	68 ± 8	46 ± 8	13 ± 5	ND
CL/F (mL/min)	2,164 ± 638	1,566 ± 833	1,023 ± 378	628 ± 104	543 ± 174
CL_R (mL/min)	458 ± 164	247 ± 153	100 ± 44	20 ± 8	< 10
Half-life (h)	1.42 ± 0.33	1.59 ± 0.13	1.75 ± 0.43	2 ± 0.3	4.1 ± 1.2

[a] ND = not determined due to anuria; CL/F = apparent oral clearance; CL_R = renal clearance.

Hepatic function impairment: The pharmacokinetics of didanosine have been studied in 12 subjects not infected with HIV with moderate (n = 8) to severe (n = 4) hepatic impairment (Child-Pugh class B or C). Mean AUC and C_{max} values following a single didanosine 400 mg dose were approximately 13% and 19% higher, respectively, in patients with hepatic impairment compared with matched healthy subjects. No dose adjustment is needed because a similar range and distribution of AUC and C_{max} values were observed for subjects with hepatic impairment and matched healthy controls.

Children: The pharmacokinetics of didanosine have been evaluated in HIV-exposed and HIV-infected children from birth to adulthood. Overall, the pharmacokinetics of didanosine in children are similar to those of didanosine in adults. Didanosine plasma concentrations increased in proportion to oral doses ranging from 25 to 120 mg/m² in children younger than 5 months and from 80 to 180 mg/m² in children older than 8 months.

➤*Microbiology:*

Resistance – HIV-1 isolates with reduced sensitivity to didanosine have been selected in cell culture and were also obtained from patients treated with didanosine. Genetic analysis of isolates from didanosine-treated patients showed mutations in the reverse transcriptase gene that resulted in the amino acid substitutions K65R, L74V, and M184V. The L74V mutation was most frequently observed in clinical isolates. Phenotypic analysis of HIV-1 isolates from 60 patients (some with prior zidovudine treatment) receiving 6 to 24 months of didanosine monotherapy showed that isolates from 10 of 60 patients exhibited an average of a 10-fold decrease in susceptibility to didanosine in vitro compared with baseline isolates. Clinical isolates that exhibited a decrease in didanosine susceptibility harbored 1 or more didanosine resistance-associated substitutions.

Cross-resistance – HIV-1 isolates from 2 of 39 patients receiving combination therapy for up to 2 years with zidovudine and didanosine exhibited decreased susceptibility to zidovudine, didanosine, zalcitabine, stavudine, and lamivudine in cell culture. These isolates harbored 5 substitutions (A62V, V751, F77L, F116Y, and Q151M) in the reverse transcriptase gene. In data from clinical studies, the presence of thymidine analog mutations (M41L, D67N, L210W, T215Y, K219Q) has been shown to decrease the response to didanosine.

Contraindications

Coadministration with allopurinol or ribavirin.

Warnings/Precautions

➤*Pancreatitis:* See the Warning box for more information.

When treatment with life-sustaining drugs known to cause pancreatic toxicity is required, suspension of didanosine therapy is recommended. In patients with risk factors for pancreatitis, administer didanosine with extreme caution and only if clearly indicated. Patients with advanced HIV infection, especially elderly patients, are at increased risk of pancreatitis; follow these patients closely. Patients with renal impairment may be at greater risk for pancreatitis if treated without dose adjustment. Patients treated with didanosine in combination with stavudine, with or without hydroxyurea, may be at increased risk for pancreatitis.

The frequency of pancreatitis is dose related.

➤*Lactic acidosis/severe hepatomegaly with steatosis:* See the Warning box for more information.

Suspend treatment with didanosine in any patient who develops clinical signs or symptoms with or without laboratory findings suggestive of symptomatic hyperlactatemia, lactic acidosis, or pronounced hepatotoxicity (which may include hepatomegaly and steatosis even in the absence of marked transaminase elevations). See also Pregnancy for additional details.

➤*Hepatotoxicity:* Hepatotoxicity and hepatic failure resulting in death were reported during postmarketing surveillance in HIV-infected patients treated with hydroxyurea and other antiretroviral agents. Fatal hepatic

DIDANOSINE — ORAL

events were reported most often in patients treated with the combination of hydroxyurea, didanosine, and stavudine. Avoid this combination.

➤*Noncirrhotic portal hypertension:* Postmarketing cases of noncirrhotic portal hypertension have been reported, including cases leading to liver transplantation or death. Cases of didanosine-associated noncirrhotic portal hypertension were confirmed by liver biopsy in patients with no evidence of viral hepatitis. Onset of signs and symptoms ranged from months to years after the start of didanosine therapy. Common presenting features included elevated liver enzymes, esophageal varices, hematemesis, ascites, and splenomegaly.

Monitor patients receiving didanosine for early signs of portal hypertension (eg, thrombocytopenia and splenomegaly) during routine medical visits. Consider appropriate laboratory testing, including liver enzymes, serum bilirubin, albumin, complete blood count, and international normalized ratio and ultrasonography. Discontinue didanosine in patients with evidence of noncirrhotic portal hypertension.

➤*Peripheral neuropathy:* Peripheral neuropathy, manifested by numbness, tingling, or pain in the hands or feet, has been reported in patients receiving didanosine therapy. Peripheral neuropathy has occurred more frequently in patients with advanced HIV, in patients with a history of neuropathy, or in patients being treated with neurotoxic drug therapy, including stavudine. Consider discontinuation of didanosine in patients who develop peripheral neuropathy.

➤*Ophthalmic effects:* Retinal changes and optic neuritis have been reported in adults and children. Consider periodic retinal examinations for patients receiving didanosine.

➤*Fat redistribution:* Redistribution/accumulation of body fat, including central obesity, dorsocervical fat enlargement ("buffalo hump"), peripheral wasting, facial wasting, breast enlargement, and "cushingoid appearance," have been observed in patients receiving antiretroviral therapy. The mechanism and long-term consequences of these events are currently unknown. A causal relationship has not been established.

➤*Immune reconstitution syndrome:* Immune reconstitution syndrome has been reported in patients treated with combination antiretroviral therapy, including didanosine. During the initial phase of combination antiretroviral treatment, patients whose immune systems respond may develop an inflammatory response to indolent or residual opportunistic infections, such as *Mycobacterium avium* infection, cytomegalovirus, *Pneumocystis jiroveci* pneumonia (PCP), or tuberculosis, which may necessitate further evaluation and treatment.

➤*Renal function impairment:* Patients with renal impairment (CrCl less than 60 mL/min) may be at greater risk of toxicity from didanosine because of decreased drug clearance. A dose reduction is recommended in these patients.

➤*Hepatic function impairment:* The safety and efficacy of didanosine have not been established in HIV-infected patients with significant underlying liver disease. During combination antiretroviral therapy, patients with preexisting liver dysfunction, including long-term, active hepatitis, have an increased frequency of liver abnormalities, including severe and potentially fatal hepatic adverse events; monitor according to standard practice. If there is evidence of worsening liver disease in such patients, interruption or discontinuation of treatment must be considered.

➤*Pregnancy: Category B.* There are no adequate and well-controlled studies in pregnant women. Because animal reproduction studies are not always predictive of human response, use this drug during pregnancy only if the benefit justifies the potential risk.

In 2006, the updated US Department of Health and Human Services guidelines for the use of antiretroviral agents in HIV-1–infected patients continued the recommendations that therapy, with the exception of efavirenz, should be continued during pregnancy. If indicated, didanosine should not be withheld in pregnancy because the expected benefit to the HIV-positive mother outweighs the unknown risk to the fetus.

Fatal lactic acidosis has been reported in pregnant women who received the combination of didanosine and stavudine with other antiretroviral agents. It is unclear if pregnancy augments the risk of lactic acidosis/hepatic steatosis syndrome reported in nonpregnant individuals receiving nucleoside analogs. Use the combination of didanosine and stavudine with caution during pregnancy; this combination is recommended only if the potential benefit clearly outweighs the potential risk. Be alert for early diagnosis of lactic acidosis/hepatic steatosis syndrome when caring for HIV-infected pregnant women receiving didanosine.

At approximately 12 times the estimated human exposure, didanosine was slightly toxic to female rats and their pups during mid and late lactation. These rats showed reduced food intake and body weight gains, but the physical and functional development of the offspring was not impaired, and there were no major changes in the F2 generation. A study in rats showed that didanosine and/or its metabolites are transferred to the fetus through the placenta.

Antiretroviral pregnancy registry – To monitor maternal-fetal outcomes of pregnant women exposed to didanosine and other antiretroviral agents, an Antiretroviral Pregnancy Registry has been established. Register patients by calling 1-800-258-4263.

➤*Lactation:* The Centers for Disease Control and Prevention recommend that HIV-infected mothers not breast-feed their infants to avoid risking postnatal transmission of HIV. A study in rats showed that, following oral administration, didanosine and/or its metabolites were excreted into the milk of lactating rats. It is not known if didanosine is excreted in human milk. The molecular weight (approximately 236) is low enough that excretion into milk should be expected. Because of both the potential for HIV transmission and the potential for serious adverse reactions in breast-feeding infants, instruct mothers not to breast-feed if they are receiving didanosine.

➤*Children:* Use of didanosine in children from 2 weeks of age through adolescence is supported by evidence from adequate and well-controlled studies of didanosine in adults and children.

Powder for oral solution – Dosing recommendations for didanosine in patients younger than 2 weeks cannot be made because the pharmacokinetics of didanosine in these children are too variable to determine an appropriate dose.

Delayed-release capsules – Additional pharmacokinetic studies in children support use in children who weigh at least 20 kg.

➤*Elderly:* In an Expanded Access Program using a buffered formulation of didanosine for patients with advanced HIV infection, patients 65 years and older had a higher frequency of pancreatitis (10%) than younger patients (5%). Didanosine is known to be substantially excreted by the kidney, and the risk of toxic reactions to this drug may be greater in patients with impaired renal function. Because elderly patients are more likely to have decreased renal function, take care in dose selection. In addition, monitor renal function and make dosage adjustments accordingly.

➤*Monitoring:* Monitor patients receiving didanosine for early signs of portal hypertension (eg, thrombocytopenia and splenomegaly) during routine medical visits. Consider appropriate laboratory testing, including liver enzymes, serum bilirubin, albumin, complete blood count, and international normalized ratio and ultrasonography.

Patients with advanced HIV infection, especially elderly patients, are at increased risk of pancreatitis; follow these patients closely. Consider periodic retinal examinations for patients receiving didanosine. During combination antiretroviral therapy, patients with preexisting liver dysfunction, including long-term, active hepatitis, have an increased frequency of liver abnormalities, including severe and potentially fatal hepatic adverse events; monitor according to standard practice. If there is evidence of worsening liver disease in such patients, interruption or discontinuation of treatment must be considered.

Drug Interactions

Coadministration of didanosine with drugs that are known to cause pancreatitis may increase the risk of this toxicity. Because didanosine formulations either contain buffers or are mixed with antacids before administration, interactions may be anticipated with drugs whose absorption can be affected by the level of acidity in the stomach and with drugs that have been demonstrated to interact with antacids containing magnesium, calcium, or aluminum. Predicted drug interactions with didanosine are listed in the following table.

Didanosine Drug Interactions

Precipitant drug	Object drug[a]		Description
Allopurinol	Didanosine	↑	The AUC of didanosine was increased ≈ 4-fold when allopurinol 300 mg/day was coadministered with a single dose of didanosine 200 mg to 2 patients with renal impairment. Coadministration of these 2 drugs is contraindicated.
Ganciclovir	Didanosine	↑	Administration of didanosine 2 hours prior to or concurrent with oral ganciclovir was associated with an increase in the steady-state AUC of didanosine. A decrease in the steady-state AUC of ganciclovir was observed when didanosine was administered 2 hours prior to ganciclovir but not when the 2 drugs were administered simultaneously. Monitor the clinical response and for didanosine toxicity. Adjust the didanosine dose as needed.
Didanosine	Ganciclovir	↓	
Methadone	Didanosine	↓	Administration of a single dose of didanosine 200 mg with long-term methadone dosing decreased the AUC and C_{max} of didanosine by 57% and 66%, respectively. Do not administer methadone with didanosine powder for oral solution due to decreases in didanosine concentrations. If coadministration of methadone and didanosine is necessary, the didanosine delayed-release capsule formulation is recommended. Monitor the clinical response and adjust the didanosine dose as needed.

DIDANOSINE — ORAL

Didanosine Drug Interactions

Precipitant drug	Object drug[a]		Description
Neurotoxic drugs	Didanosine	↑	The risk of neuropathy may be increased. Use with caution. If coadministration cannot be avoided, suspension of didanosine therapy is recommended.
Didanosine	Neurotoxic drugs		
Ribavirin	Didanosine	↑	Exposure to the active metabolite of didanosine is increased when it is coadministered with ribavirin. Fatal hepatic failure, as well as peripheral neuropathy, pancreatitis, and symptomatic hyperlactatemia/lactic acidosis have been reported in patients receiving didanosine and ribavirin. Coadministration is contraindicated.
Tenofovir	Didanosine	↑	Didanosine plasma levels may be elevated, increasing the risk of life-threatening adverse reactions (eg, lactic acidosis, pancreatitis). A dose reduction of didanosine to 250 mg (≥ 60 kg with CrCl ≥ 60 mL/min) or 200 mg (
Didanosine	Antacids	↑	Coadministration of antacids containing magnesium or aluminum with didanosine powder for oral solution may potentiate adverse reactions associated with the antacid components. Use powder for oral solution with caution.
Didanosine	Azole antifungal agents (eg, ketoconazole, itraconazole)	↓	The therapeutic effects of azole antifungal agents may be decreased. The buffers in didanosine appear to decrease the absorption of azole antifungal agents. Administer the azole antifungal drugs ≥ 2 hours before the buffered didanosine formulation.
Didanosine	Delavirdine, indinavir	↓	Significant decreases in the AUC of delavirdine and indinavir occurred following simultaneous administration of these agents with didanosine. To avoid this interaction, give delavirdine or indinavir 1 hour prior to dosing with didanosine.
Didanosine	Fluoroquinolones (eg, ciprofloxacin)	↓	Plasma concentrations of some fluoroquinolone antibiotics are decreased when administered with antacids containing magnesium, calcium, or aluminum as well as the buffers present in didanosine tablets. Therefore, if concurrent use cannot be avoided, give the fluoroquinolone ≥ 2 hours before or 6 hours after buffered didanosine formulations.
Didanosine	Hydroxyurea	↑	Patients treated with didanosine in combination with stavudine, with or without hydroxyurea, may be at increased risk for pancreatitis and hepatotoxicity, which may be fatal, and severe peripheral neuropathy. The combination of didanosine and hydroxyurea should be avoided.
Didanosine	Nelfinavir	↑	Nelfinavir concentrations may be increased. However, the pharmacokinetics of nelfinavir are not altered to a clinically significant degree when it is administered with a light meal 1 hour after didanosine.
Didanosine	Stavudine	↑	Combination therapy of didanosine, stavudine, and other antiretrovirals has caused fatal lactic acidosis in women. The risk of fatal lactic acidosis may be increased in pregnant women. Peripheral neuropathy has occurred more frequently in patients treated with neurotoxic drugs, including stavudine. Close clinical monitoring is recommended.
Didanosine	Tetracyclines	↓	Plasma concentrations of tetracycline antibiotics are decreased when administered with antacids containing magnesium, calcium, or aluminum as well as the buffers present in didanosine tablets. Therefore, if concurrent use cannot be avoided, separate the administration times of tetracyclines and buffered didanosine formulations by 3 to 4 hours.

[a] ↑ = object drug increased; ↓ = object drug decreased.

➤*Drug/Food interactions:* See Actions for more information.

Adverse Reactions

When didanosine is used in combination with other agents with similar toxicities, the incidence of these toxicities may be higher than when didanosine is used alone. Thus, patients treated with didanosine in combination with stavudine, with or without hydroxyurea, may be at increased risk for pancreatitis and hepatotoxicity, which may be fatal. Patients treated with didanosine in combination with stavudine may also be at increased risk for peripheral neuropathy.

➤*Adults:*

Delayed-release capsules –

Didanosine Delayed-Release Adverse Reactions[a]

Adverse reactions	Didanosine delayed-release + stavudine + nelfinavir[b,c] (n = 258)	Zidovudine/Lamivudine[d] + nelfinavir[b,c] (n = 253)
CNS		
Headache	22%	17%
Peripheral neurologic symptoms/neuropathy	25%	11%
Dermatologic		
Rash	14%	12%
GI		
Diarrhea	57%	58%
Nausea	24%	36%
Pancreatitis	< 1%	[e]
Vomiting	14%	19%

[a] Median duration of treatment was 62 wk in the didanosine + stavudine + nelfinavir group and 61 wk in the zidovudine/lamivudine + nelfinavir group.
[b] Percentages based on treated patients.
[c] The incidences reported included all severity grades and all reactions regardless of causality.
[d] Zidovudine/lamivudine combination tablet.
[e] This event was not observed in this study arm.

Powder for oral solution –

Didanosine Powder for Oral Solution Adverse Reactions From Monotherapy Studies[a]

Adverse reactions	ACTG 116A		ACTG 116B/117	
	Didanosine (n = 197)	Zidovudine (n = 212)	Didanosine (n = 298)	Zidovudine (n = 304)
GI				
Abdominal pain	13%	8%	7%	8%
Diarrhea	19%	15%	28%	21%
Pancreatitis	7%	3%	6%	2%
Miscellaneous				
Peripheral neurologic symptoms/neuropathy	17%	14%	20%	12%
Rash/Pruritus	7%	8%	9%	5%

[a] The incidences reported included all severity grades and all reactions regardless of causality.

DIDANOSINE — ORAL

Didanosine Powder for Oral Solution Adverse Reactions From Combination Studies[a,b]

Adverse reactions	AI454-148[c]		START 2[c]	
	Didanosine + stavudine + nelfinavir (n = 482)	Zidovudine + lamivudine + nelfinavir (n = 248)	Didanosine + stavudine + indinavir (n = 102)	Zidovudine + lamivudine + indinavir (n = 103)
CNS				
Headache	21%	30%	46%	37%
Peripheral neurologic symptoms/neuropathy	26%	6%	21%	10%
GI				
Diarrhea	70%	60%	45%	39%
Nausea	28%	40%	53%	67%
Vomiting	12%	14%	30%	35%
Miscellaneous				
Pancreatitis	1%	[d]	< 1%	[d]
Rash	13%	16%	30%	18%

[a] Percentages based on treated subjects.
[b] The incidences reported included all severity grades and all reactions regardless of causality.
[c] Median duration of treatment 48 wk.
[d] This reaction was not observed in this study arm.

➤*Children:* In pediatric phase 1 studies, pancreatitis occurred in 3% of patients treated at entry doses lower than 300 mg/m^2/day and in 13% of patients treated at higher doses. In study ACTG 152, pancreatitis occurred in none of the 281 children who received didanosine 120 mg/m^2 every 12 hours and in less than 1% of the 274 children who received didanosine 90 mg/m^2 every 12 hours in combination with zidovudine.

Retinal changes and optic neuritis have been reported in children.

➤*Pancreatitis:* The frequency of pancreatitis is dose related. In phase 3 studies, incidence ranged from 1% to 10% with doses higher than are currently recommended and 1% to 7% with the recommended dose.

Pancreatitis resulting in death was observed in 1 patient who received didanosine plus stavudine plus nelfinavir in study AI454-148 and in 1 patient who received didanosine plus stavudine plus indinavir in the START 2 study. In addition, pancreatitis resulting in death was observed in 2 of 68 patients who received didanosine plus stavudine plus indinavir plus hydroxyurea in an ACTG clinical trial. In an early access program, pancreatitis resulting in death was observed in 1 patient who received didanosine delayed-release plus stavudine plus hydroxyurea plus ritonavir plus indinavir plus efavirenz.

Delayed-release capsules –

Didanosine Delayed-Release Lab Test Abnormalities[a,b]

Parameter	Didanosine delayed-release + stavudine + nelfinavir (n = 258)		Zidovudine/Lamivudine[c] + nelfinavir (n = 253)	
	Grades 3 to 4[d]	All grades	Grades 3 to 4[d]	All grades
AST	5%	46%	5%	19%
ALT	6%	44%	5%	22%
Lipase	5%	23%	2%	13%
Bilirubin	< 1%	9%	< 1%	3%

[a] Median duration of treatment was 62 wk in the didanosine + stavudine + nelfinavir group and 61 wk in the zidovudine/lamivudine + nelfinavir group.
[b] Percentages based on treated patients.
[c] Zidovudine/lamivudine combination tablet.
[d] Greater than 5 × upper limit of normal (ULN) for AST and ALT, ≥ 2.1 × ULN for lipase, and ≥ 2.6 × ULN for bilirubin.

Powder for oral solution –

Didanosine Powder for Oral Solution Lab Test Abnormalities From Monotherapy Studies

Parameter	ACTG 116A		ACTG 116B/117	
	Didanosine (n = 197)	Zidovudine (n = 212)	Didanosine (n = 298)	Zidovudine (n = 304)
AST (> 5 × ULN)	9%	4%	7%	6%
ALT (> 5 × ULN)	9%	6%	6%	6%
Alkaline phosphatase (> 5 × ULN)	4%	1%	1%	1%
Amylase (≥ 1.4 × ULN)	17%	12%	15%	5%
Uric acid (> 12 mg/dL)	3%	1%	2%	1%

Didanosine Powder for Oral Solution Lab Test Abnormalities From Combination Studies (Grades 3 to 4)[a,b]

Parameter	AI454-148[c]		START 2[c]	
	Didanosine + stavudine + nelfinavir (n = 482)	Zidovudine + lamivudine + nelfinavir (n = 248)	Didanosine + stavudine + indinavir (n = 102)	Zidovudine + lamivudine + indinavir (n = 103)
Bilirubin (> 2.6 × ULN)	< 1%	< 1%	16%	8%
AST (> 5 × ULN)	3%	2%	7%	7%
ALT (> 5 × ULN)	3%	3%	8%	5%
GGT[d] > 5 × ULN)	NC	NC	5%	2%
Lipase (> 2 × ULN)	7%	2%	5%	5%
Amylase (> 2 × ULN)	NC	NC	8%	2%

[a] NC = not collected.
[b] Percentages based on treated subjects.
[c] Median duration of treatment 48 weeks.
[d] GGT = gamma-glutamyl transpeptidase.

Didanosine Powder for Oral Solution Lab Test Abnormalities From Combination Studies (All Grades)[a]

Parameter	AI454-148[b]		START 2[b]	
	Didanosine + stavudine + nelfinavir (n = 482)	Zidovudine + lamivudine + nelfinavir (n = 248)	Didanosine + stavudine + indinavir (n = 102)	Zidovudine + lamivudine + indinavir (n = 103)
Bilirubin	7%	3%	68%	55%
AST	42%	23%	53%	20%
ALT	37%	24%	50%	18%
GGT	NC	NC	28%	12%
Lipase	17%	11%	26%	19%
Amylase	NC	NC	31%	17%

[a] Percentages based on treatment subjects.
[b] Median duration of treatment 48 weeks.

➤*Postmarketing:*

CNS – Asthenia, chills/fever.

GI – Abdominal pain, alopecia, anorexia, dry mouth, dyspepsia, flatulence, pancreatitis (including fatal cases), parotid gland enlargement, sialoadenitis.

Hematologic – Anemia, leukopenia, thrombocytopenia.

Hepatic – Symptomatic hyperlactatemia/lactic acidosis and hepatic steatosis; hepatitis and liver failure; noncirrhotic portal hypertension.

Metabolic – Diabetes mellitus, elevated serum alkaline phosphatase level, elevated serum amylase level, elevated serum GGT level, elevated serum uric acid level, hypoglycemia, hyperglycemia.

Musculoskeletal – Myalgia (with or without increases in creatine kinase), rhabdomyolysis, including acute renal failure and hemodialysis, arthralgia, myopathy.

Ophthalmic – Dry eyes, optic neuritis, retinal depigmentation.

Miscellaneous – Anaphylactoid reaction, pain, redistribution/accumulation of body fat.

Overdosage

➤*Symptoms:* In phase 1 studies, in which didanosine was initially administered at doses 10 times the currently recommended dose, toxicities included pancreatitis, peripheral neuropathy, diarrhea, hyperuricemia, and hepatic dysfunction.

➤*Treatment:* There is no known antidote for didanosine overdosage. Didanosine is not dialyzable by peritoneal dialysis, although there is some clearance by hemodialysis.

Patient Information

Inform patients that pancreatitis, a serious toxicity of didanosine when used alone and in combination regimens, has been fatal.

Advise patients that peripheral neuropathy, manifested by numbness, tingling, or pain in the hands or feet, may develop during therapy with didanosine. Counsel patients that peripheral neuropathy occurs with greatest frequency in patients with advanced HIV disease or a history of peripheral neuropathy, and that discontinuation of didanosine may be required if toxicity develops.

Inform patients that lactic acidosis and severe hepatomegaly with steatosis, including fatal cases, have been reported with the use of nucleoside analogues alone or in combination, including didanosine and other antiretrovirals.

Inform patients that hepatotoxicity, including fatal hepatic adverse events, were reported in patients with preexisting liver dysfunction. The safety and

DIDANOSINE — ORAL

efficacy of didanosine have not been established in HIV-infected patients with significant underlying liver disease.

Inform patients that noncirrhotic portal hypertension has been reported in patients taking didanosine, including cases leading to liver transplantation or death.

Inform patients that retinal changes and optic neuritis have been reported in adults and children.

Inform patients that when didanosine is used in combination with other agents with similar toxicities, the incidence of adverse events may be higher than when didanosine is used alone.

Caution patients about the use of medications or other substances, including alcohol, that may exacerbate didanosine toxicities.

Inform patients that didanosine is not a cure for HIV infection, and patients may continue to develop HIV-associated illnesses, including opportunistic infections. Therefore, instruct patients to remain under the care of a health care provider when using didanosine. Advise patients that didanosine therapy has not been shown to reduce the risk of HIV transmission to others through sexual contact or blood contamination. Advise patients to continue to practice safe sex and take precautions to prevent others from coming in contact with infected blood and other body fluids.

Inform patients that the preferred dosing frequency of didanosine powder for oral solution is twice daily because there is more evidence to support the effectiveness of this dosing frequency. Consider once-daily dosing only for adult patients whose management requires once-daily dosing of didanosine.

Instruct patients to swallow didanosine delayed-release capsules whole and to not open the capsules.

Instruct patients not to miss a dose but that if they do, that they should take didanosine as soon as possible. Tell patients that if it is almost time for the next dose, they should skip the missed dose and continue with the regular dosing schedule.

Inform patients that redistribution or accumulation of body fat may occur in patients receiving antiretroviral therapy and that the cause and long-term health effects of these conditions are not known at this time.

TELBIVUDINE

Rx	**Tyzeka** (Novartis)	**Tablets; oral:** 600 mg	(LDT). White/Slightly yellowish, ovaloid. Film-coated. In 30s.
		Solution; oral: 100 mg per 5 mL	Benzoic acid, saccharin, sodium 47 mg per 30 mL. Passion fruit flavor. In 300 mL bottles.

TELBIVUDINE — ORAL

WARNING

Lactic acidosis and severe hepatomegaly with steatosis, including fatal cases, have been reported with the use of nucleoside analogs alone or in combination with antiretrovirals.

Severe, acute exacerbations of hepatitis B have been reported in patients who have discontinued anti–hepatitis B therapy, including telbivudine. Closely monitor hepatic function with clinical and laboratory follow-up for at least several months in patients who discontinue anti–hepatitis B therapy. If appropriate, resumption of anti–hepatitis B therapy may be warranted.

Indications

➤*Chronic hepatitis B:* For treatment of chronic hepatitis B in adult patients with evidence of viral replication and evidence of persistent elevations in serum aminotransferases (ALT or AST) or histologically active disease.

Administration and Dosage

➤*Adults:*

Chronic hepatitis B – 600 mg once daily.

➤*Children:*

Chronic hepatitis B –

16 years of age and older: 600 mg once daily.

➤*Renal function impairment:*

Telbivudine Dosage Adjustment in Patients With Renal Impairment[a]

CrCl (mL/min)	Telbivudine solution	Telbivudine tablet
≥ 50 mL/min	30 mL once daily	1 tablet every 24 h
30 to 49 mL/min	20 mL once daily	1 tablet every 48 h
< 30 mL/min (not requiring dialysis)	10 mL once daily	1 tablet every 72 h
ESRD	—[b]	1 tablet every 96 h[c]

[a] CrCl = creatinine clearance; ESRD = end-stage renal disease.
[b] Dosing recommendations for telbivudine solution in patients with ESRD have not been established.
[c] When administered on hemodialysis days, telbivudine should be administered after hemodialysis.

➤*Administration:* Take orally with or without food. Telbivudine solution may be considered for patients who have difficulty swallowing tablets.

➤*Storage/Stability:* Store in the original container at 25°C (77°F); excursions are permitted between 15° and 30°C (59° and 86°F). Use solution within 2 months after opening the bottle. Do not freeze.

Actions

➤*Pharmacology:* Telbivudine, an antiviral drug, is a synthetic thymidine nucleoside analog with activity against HBV DNA polymerase. It is phosphorylated by cellular kinases to the active triphosphate form, which has an intracellular half-life of 14 hours. Telbivudine 5′-triphosphate inhibits HBV DNA polymerase (reverse transcriptase) by competing with the natural substrate, thymidine 5′-triphosphate. Incorporation of telbivudine 5′-triphosphate into viral DNA causes DNA chain termination. Telbivudine is an inhibitor of HBV first strand (median effective concentration [EC_{50}] value, 1.3 ± 1.6 mcM) and second strand synthesis (EC_{50} value, 0.2 ± 0.2 mcM).

➤*Pharmacokinetics:*

Absorption – Following oral administration of telbivudine 600 mg once daily in healthy subjects (n = 12), steady-state peak plasma concentration (C_{max}) was 3.69 ± 1.25 mcg/mL (mean ± standard deviation [SD]), which occurred between 1 and 4 hours (median, 2 hours); area under the curve (AUC) was 26.1 ± 7.2 mcg•h/mL (mean ± SD); and trough plasma concentrations were approximately 0.2 to 0.3 mcg/mL. Steady state was achieved after approximately 5 to 7 days of once-daily administration with approximately 1.5-fold accumulation, suggesting an effective half-life of approximately 15 hours.

Distribution – In vitro binding of telbivudine to human plasma proteins is low (3.3%). After oral dosing, the estimated apparent volume of distribution is in excess of total body water, suggesting that telbivudine is widely distributed into tissues. Telbivudine was equally partitioned between plasma and blood cells.

Metabolism/Excretion –

After reaching the peak concentration, plasma concentrations of telbivudine declined in a biexponential manner with a terminal elimination half-life of 40 to 49 hours. Telbivudine is eliminated primarily by urinary excretion of unchanged drug. The renal clearance of telbivudine approaches normal glomerular filtration rate, suggesting that passive diffusion is the main mechanism of excretion. Approximately 42% of the dose is recovered in the urine over 7 days following a single oral dose of telbivudine 600 mg.

Special populations –

Renal function impairment: See Administration and Dosage for more information.

Telbivudine Pharmacokinetic Parameters (Mean ± SD) in Renal Impairment

	Normal CrCl (> 80 mL/min) (n = 8) 600 mg	Mild CrCl (50 to 80 mL/min) (n = 8) 600 mg	Moderate CrCl (30 to 49 mL/min) (n = 8) 400 mg	Severe CrCl (< 30 mL/min) (n = 6) 200 mg	ESRD/ Hemodialysis (n = 6) 200 mg
C_{max} (mcg/mL)	3.4 ± 0.9 mL/min	3.2 ± 0.9 mL/min	2.8 ± 1.3 mL/min	1.6 ± 0.8 mL/min	2.1 ± 0.9 mL/min
$AUC_{0-\infty}$ (mcg•h/mL)	28.5 ± 9.6 mL/min	32.5 ± 10.1 mL/min	36 ± 13.2 mL/min	32.5 ± 13.2 mL/min	67.4 ± 36.9 mL/min
Renal clearance (L/h)	7.6 ± 2.9 mL/min	5 ± 1.2 mL/min	2.6 ± 1.2 mL/min	0.7 ± 0.4 mL/min	

• *Hemodialysis* – Hemodialysis (up to 4 hours) reduces systemic telbivudine exposure by approximately 23%. Following dose regimen adjustment for CrCl, no additional dose modification is necessary during routine hemodialysis. Administer telbivudine after hemodialysis.

Contraindications

None well documented.

Warnings/Precautions

➤*Lactic acidosis:* Lactic acidosis and severe hepatomegaly with steatosis, including fatal cases, have been reported with the use of nucleoside analogs alone or in combination with antiretrovirals. Female gender, obesity, and prolonged nucleoside exposure may be risk factors. Exercise particular caution when administering HBV nucleoside analog reverse transcriptase inhibitors to patients with known risk factors for liver disease; however, cases have also been reported in patients with no known risk factors. Suspend treatment with telbivudine in any patient who develops clinical or laboratory findings suggestive of lactic acidosis or pronounced hepatotoxicity (which may include hepatomegaly and steatosis, even in the absence of marked transaminase elevations).

➤*Exacerbations of hepatitis:* See the Warning box for more information.

➤*Myopathy:* Cases of myopathy/myositis have been reported with telbivudine use several weeks to months after starting therapy. Myopathy also has been reported with some other drugs in this class. Rhabdomyolysis has been reported during postmarketing use of telbivudine.

TELBIVUDINE — ORAL

Uncomplicated myalgia has been reported in telbivudine-treated patients. Consider myopathy, defined as persistent unexplained muscle aches and/or muscle weakness in conjunction with increases in creatine kinase (CK) values, in any patient with diffuse myalgias, muscle tenderness, or muscle weakness. Among patients with telbivudine-associated myopathy, no pattern with regard to the degree or timing of CK elevations has been observed. In addition, the predisposing factors for the development of myopathy among telbivudine recipients are unknown. Advise patients to promptly report unexplained muscle aches, pain, tenderness, or weakness. Interrupt telbivudine therapy if myopathy is suspected, and discontinue if myopathy is confirmed. It is not known if the risk of myopathy during treatment with drugs in this class is increased with coadministration of other drugs associated with myopathy, including, but not limited to, certain azole antifungals, certain beta-hydroxy-beta-methylglutaryl-CoA (HMG-CoA) reductase inhibitors, chloroquine, corticosteroids, cyclosporine, erythromycin, fibric acid derivatives, hydroxychloroquine, niacin, penicillamine, and/or zidovudine. When initiating concomitant treatment with any drug associated with myopathy, monitor patients closely for any signs or symptoms of unexplained muscle pain, tenderness, or weakness.

➤*Peripheral neuropathy:* Peripheral neuropathy has been reported with telbivudine alone or in combination with pegylated interferon alfa-2a and other interferons. In 1 clinical trial, an increased risk and severity of peripheral neuropathy was observed with the combination use of telbivudine with pegylated interferon alfa-2a compared with telbivudine alone. The safety and efficacy of telbivudine in combination with pegylated interferons or other interferons for the treatment of chronic hepatitis B has not been demonstrated. Advise patients to report any burning sensations, numbness, and/or tingling in the arms and/or legs, with or without gait disturbance. Interrupt telbivudine therapy if peripheral neuropathy is suspected and discontinue if peripheral neuropathy is confirmed.

➤*Renal function impairment:* See Administration and Dosage for more information.

➤*Pregnancy: Category B.* There are no adequate and well-controlled studies of telbivudine in pregnant women. Studies in pregnant rats and rabbits showed that telbivudine crosses the placenta. Because animal reproductive toxicity studies are not always predictive of human response, use telbivudine during pregnancy only if potential benefits outweigh the risks.

Theoretically, exposure to agents in this class at the time of implantation could impair fertility as a result of embryonic cytotoxicity. Avoiding treatment during pregnancy is the safest course, but if a pregnant woman requires this agent it should not be withheld. However, avoiding treatment during organogenesis (20 to 55 days postconception or 34 to 69 days after the first day of the last menstrual period) should be considered.

Pregnancy registry – To monitor fetal outcomes of pregnant women exposed to telbivudine, health care providers are encouraged to register these patients in the antiretroviral pregnancy registry by calling 1-800-258-4263.

➤*Lactation:* Telbivudine is excreted in the milk of rats. It is not known whether telbivudine is excreted in human milk. Instruct mothers not to breast-feed if they are receiving telbivudine.

The low molecular weight (about 242) and plasma protein binding (3%), and long elimination half-life (40-49 hours), suggest that telbivudine will be excreted into breast milk. If the mother elects to breastfeed, the infant should be monitored closely for the most common telbivudine-induced toxicities observed in adults, such as upper respiratory infection, fatigue, malaise, abdominal pain, cough, fever, insomnia, rash, nausea, vomiting, diarrhea, and loose stools.

➤*Children:* Safety and effectiveness in children younger than 16 years of age have not been established.

➤*Elderly:* In general, exercise caution when prescribing telbivudine to elderly patients, considering the greater frequency of decreased renal function because of concomitant disease or other drug therapy. Monitor renal function in elderly patients and make dosage adjustments accordingly.

➤*Monitoring:* Periodically monitor hepatic function. Closely monitor hepatic function with clinical and laboratory follow-up for at least several months in patients who discontinue anti–hepatitis B therapy. Monitor patients for any signs or symptoms of unexplained muscle pain, tenderness, or weakness, particularly during periods of upward dosage titration. Monitor renal function in elderly patients and in patients taking drugs that may alter renal function (eg, cyclosporine, tacrolimus).

Drug Interactions

Telbivudine Drug Interactions

Precipitant drug	Object drug[a]		Description
Drugs associated with myopathy (eg, azole antifungals [eg, ketoconazole], chloroquine, corticosteroids, cyclosporine, erythromycin, fibric acid derivatives [eg, gemfibrozil], HMG-CoA reductase inhibitors [eg, simvastatin], hydroxychloroquine, niacin, penicillamine, zidovudine)	Telbivudine	↔	Myopathy has been reported during postmarketing experience with telbivudine. It is unknown if the risk of myopathy increases with coadministration of telbivudine and other drugs associated with myopathy. Closely monitor patients for signs and symptoms of unexplained muscle pain, tenderness, or weakness if telbivudine is coadministered with another drug associated with myopathy. Interrupt telbivudine treatment if myopathy is suspected and discontinue if confirmed.
Drugs that alter renal function (eg, cyclosporine, tacrolimus)	Telbivudine	↔	Because telbivudine is eliminated primarily by renal excretion, coadministration of telbivudine with drugs that alter renal function (eg, cyclosporine, tacrolimus) may alter plasma concentrations of tacrolimus. Monitor renal function and adjust the telbivudine dose as needed.
Interferons (eg, pegylated interferon alfa-2a)	Telbivudine	↑	A clinical trial investigating the combination of telbivudine 600 mg daily with pegylated interferon alfa-2a 180 mcg once weekly by subcutaneous administration indicates that this combination may be associated with an increased risk of peripheral neuropathy occurrence and severity, in comparison with telbivudine alone. Closely monitor patients. Interrupt telbivudine treatment if peripheral neuropathy is suspected and discontinue if confirmed.

[a] ↑ = object drug increased; ↔ = undetermined clinical effect.

Adverse Reactions

Telbivudine Adverse Reactions (≥ 3%)

Adverse reactions	Telbivudine (n = 847)	Lamivudine (n = 852)
CNS		
Dizziness	4%	5%
Fatigue	13%	11%
Headache	10%	11%
Insomnia	3%	3%
Dermatologic		
Pruritus	2%	3%
Rash	4%	3%
GI		
Abdominal distension	3%	2%
Abdominal pain	3%	4%
Abdominal pain, upper	6%	6%
Diarrhea	6%	5%
Dyspepsia	3%	5%
Nausea	5%	5%
Musculoskeletal		
Arthralgia	4%	5%
Back pain	4%	4%
Myalgia	3%	2%
Respiratory		
Cough	6%	5%
Pharyngolaryngeal pain	5%	4%

TELBIVUDINE — ORAL

Telbivudine Adverse Reactions (≥ 3%)		
Adverse reactions	Telbivudine (n = 847)	Lamivudine (n = 852)
Miscellaneous		
ALT increased	3%	4%
CK increased	11%	6%
Hepatitis B exacerbation	2%	4%
Pyrexia	4%	3%

➤*Moderate to severe adverse reactions:* Moderate to severe (grade 2 to 4) adverse reactions were reported in 28% of telbivudine recipients and 27% of lamivudine recipients. The profile of adverse reactions of moderate to severe intensity was similar in both treatment groups and no individual adverse reaction was reported in more than 2% of subjects in either treatment group.

➤*Discontinuation:* Discontinuations because of adverse reactions were reported in 4% of telbivudine recipients and 4% of lamivudine recipients. The most common adverse reactions resulting in telbivudine discontinuation included diarrhea, fatigue, increased CK, myalgia, myopathy, and nausea.

➤*Peripheral neuropathy:* Peripheral neuropathy was reported as an adverse reaction in less than 1% of patients receiving telbivudine monotherapy.

➤*Myopathy/Myositis:* Of telbivudine-treated patients, less than 1% were diagnosed with myopathy/myositis (presenting with muscular weakness).

➤*Exacerbations of hepatitis:* In the subset of patients who discontinued treatment prematurely for reasons other than efficacy or who elected not to continue telbivudine in another clinical trial, 6% of telbivudine-treated and 6% of lamivudine-treated patients experienced an exacerbation of hepatitis (ALT elevation of more than 2 × baseline and more than 10 × upper limit of normal [ULN]) in the 4-month posttreatment period.

➤*Lab test abnormalities:*

Telbivudine Grade 3 to 4 Laboratory Abnormalities[a]		
Laboratory abnormality	Telbivudine 600 mg (n = 847)	Lamivudine 100 mg (n = 852)
CK > 7 × ULN	13%	4%
ALT > 10 × ULN and 2 × baseline[b]	5%	8%
ALT > 3 × baseline	7%	13%
AST > 3 × baseline	6%	10%
Lipase > 2.5 × ULN	2%	4%
Amylase > 3 × ULN	< 1%	< 1%
Total bilirubin > 5 × ULN	< 1%	< 1%
Neutropenia (ANC[c] ≤ 749/mm³)	2%	2%
Thrombocytopenia (platelets ≤ 49,999/mm³)	< 1%	< 1%

[a] On-treatment value worsened from baseline to grade 3 or 4 during therapy.
[b] American Association for the Study of Liver Disease definition of acute hepatitis flare.
[c] ANC = absolute neutrophil count.

Creatine kinase elevations – Among telbivudine-treated patients with grade 1 to 4 CK elevations, 10% developed a musculoskeletal adverse reaction compared with 5% of lamivudine-treated patients. A total of 2% of telbivudine-treated subjects interrupted or discontinued study drug because of CK elevation or musculoskeletal adverse reactions (includes preferred terms: back pain, chest discomfort, chest wall pain, flank pain, muscle cramp, muscular weakness, musculoskeletal pain, musculoskeletal chest pain, musculoskeletal discomfort, musculoskeletal stiffness, myalgia, myofascial pain syndrome, myopathy, myositis, neck pain, noncardiac chest pain, and pain in extremity).

ALT flares – The incidence of ALT flares, defined as ALT more than 10 × ULN and more than 2 × baseline, was similar in the 2 treatment arms (3%) in the first 6 months. After week 24, ALT flares were reported less frequently in the telbivudine arm (2%) compared with the lamivudine arm (5%). Periodic monitoring of hepatic function is recommended during long-term hepatitis B treatment.

➤*Postmarketing:*

CNS – Hypesthesia, paresthesia.

Musculoskeletal – Lactic acidosis, rhabdomyolysis.

Overdosage

➤*Treatment:* In the event of an overdose, discontinue telbivudine. The patient must be monitored for evidence of toxicity, and appropriate general supportive treatment applied as necessary.

In case of overdosage, hemodialysis may be considered. Within 2 hours, following a single dose of telbivudine 200 mg, a 4-hour hemodialysis session removed approximately 23% of the telbivudine dose.

Patient Information

Advise patients to remain under the care of a health care provider while taking telbivudine. Tell them to discuss any new symptoms or concurrent medications with their health care provider.

Advise patients to promptly report unexplained muscle pain, tenderness, or weakness.

Advise patients to promptly report any burning sensations, numbness, and/or tingling in the arms and/or legs, with or without difficulty walking.

Advise patients that telbivudine is not a cure for hepatitis B, and that the long-term treatment benefits of telbivudine are unknown at this time. In particular, the relationship of initial treatment response to outcomes such as hepatocellular carcinoma and decompensated cirrhosis is unknown.

Inform patients that deterioration of liver disease may occur in some cases if treatment is discontinued and tell them to discuss any change in regimen with their health care provider.

Advise patients that treatment with telbivudine has not been shown to reduce the risk of transmission of HBV to others through sexual contact or blood contamination. Discuss HBV prevention strategies with patients, including safe sexual practices and avoidance of needle sharing or sharing any personal items that may contain residual blood or body fluids, such as razor blades or toothbrushes. Additionally, a vaccine is available for prevention of hepatitis B infection in susceptible individuals.

Advise patients on a low-sodium diet that telbivudine solution contains approximately 47 mg of sodium per 600 mg (30 mL) dose.

LAMIVUDINE (3TC)

Rx	**Epivir-HBV** (GlaxoSmithKline)	**Tablets; oral:** 100 mg	(GX CG5). Butterscotch color, capsule shape. Film-coated. In 60s.
Rx	**Epivir** (GlaxoSmithKline)	**Tablets; oral:** 150 mg	PEG. (GX CJ7). White, diamond shape, scored. Film-coated. In 60s.
		300 mg	PEG. (GX EJ7). Gray, diamond shape. Film-coated. In 30s.
Rx	**Epivir-HBV** (GlaxoSmithKline)	**Solution; oral:** 5 mg/mL	Parabens, sucrose 200 mg/mL. Strawberry-banana flavor. In 240 mL.
Rx	**Epivir** (GlaxoSmithKline)	**Solution; oral:** 10 mg/mL	Parabens, sucrose 200 mg/mL. Strawberry-banana flavor. In 240 mL.

LAMIVUDINE — ORAL

WARNING

Lactic acidosis and severe hepatomegaly with steatosis, including fatal cases, have been reported with the use of nucleoside analogs alone or in combination, including lamivudine and other antiretrovirals. Suspend treatment with lamivudine in any patient who develops clinical or laboratory findings suggestive of lactic acidosis or pronounced hepatotoxicity.

Lamivudine tablets and oral solution (used to treat HIV) contain a higher dose of the active ingredient (lamivudine) than lamivudine-HBV tablets and oral solution (used to treat chronic hepatitis B). Patients with HIV should receive only dosing forms appropriate for treatment of HIV. The formulation and dosage of lamivudine-HBV are not appropriate for patients dually infected with hepatitis B virus (HBV) and HIV (see Warnings/Precautions).

WARNING (cont.)

Offer HIV counseling and testing to all patients before beginning lamivudine-HBV and periodically during treatment, because lamivudine-HBV contains a lower dose of the same active ingredient as lamivudine tablets and oral solution used to treat HIV. If treatment with lamivudine-HBV is prescribed for chronic hepatitis B for a patient with unrecognized or untreated HIV infection, rapid emergence of HIV resistance is likely because of the subtherapeutic dose and inappropriate monotherapy.

Severe acute exacerbations of hepatitis B have been reported in patients who have discontinued anti–hepatitis B therapy (including lamivudine-HBV) or are coinfected with HBV and HIV and have discontinued lamivudine. Monitor hepatic function closely with both clinical and laboratory follow-up for at least several months in patients who discontinue anti–hepatitis B therapy or who discontinue lamivudine and are coinfected with HIV and HBV. If appropriate, initiation of anti–hepatitis B therapy may be warranted.

LAMIVUDINE — ORAL

Indications

➤*Chronic hepatitis B (lamivudine-HBV):* For the treatment of chronic hepatitis B associated with evidence of hepatitis B viral replication and active liver inflammation.

➤*HIV infection (lamivudine):* In combination with other antiretroviral agents for the treatment of HIV.

Administration and Dosage

➤*General dosing considerations:* If lamivudine is administered to a patient dually infected with HIV and HBV, the dosage indicated for HIV therapy should be used as part of an appropriate combination regimen. The formulation and dosage of lamivudine-HBV are not appropriate for patients dually infected with HBV and HIV.

➤*Adults:*

Chronic hepatitis B –

Usual dosage: 100 mg once daily.

HIV infection – 300 mg daily, administered as 150 mg twice daily or 300 mg once daily, in combination with other antiretroviral agents.

➤*Children:*

Chronic hepatitis B –

2 to 17 years of age:

• *Usual dosage* – 3 mg/kg once daily.

• *Maximum dose* – 100 mg daily.

• *Duration of therapy* – Safety and efficacy of treatment beyond 1 year have not been established, and the optimum duration of treatment is not known.

HIV –

Lamivudine oral solution:

• *3 months to 16 years of age –*

Usual dosage: 4 mg/kg twice daily administered in combination with other antiretroviral agents.

Maximum dose: 150 mg twice a day in combination with other antiretroviral agents.

Lamivudine scored tablets: Lamivudine is also available as a scored tablet for HIV-infected children who weigh at least 14 kg and for whom a solid dosage form is appropriate. Before prescribing lamivudine tablets, children should be assessed for the ability to swallow tablets. If a child is unable to reliably swallow lamivudine tablets, the oral solution formulation should be prescribed.

Dosing Recommendations for Lamivudine Tablets in Children

Weight (kg)	Dosage regimen using scored 150 mg tablets: AM dose	PM dose	Total daily dose
14 to 21	½ tablet (75 mg)	½ tablet (75 mg)	150 mg
> 21 to < 30	½ tablet (75 mg)	1 tablet (150 mg)	225 mg
≥ 30	1 tablet (150 mg)	1 tablet (150 mg)	300 mg

Off-label dosing –

Prevention of maternal-fetal HIV transmission:

• *Neonates 35 weeks of age and older* – 2 mg/kg twice daily for 7 days in combination with zidovudine 2 mg/kg orally every 6 hours starting within 12 hours after birth and continuing through 6 weeks of age.

• *Neonates younger than 35 weeks of age but older than 30 weeks of age* – 2 mg/kg twice daily for 7 days in combination with zidovudine 2 mg/kg orally every 12 hours, advanced to every 8 hours at 2 weeks of age and continued through 6 weeks of age.

• *Neonates younger than 30 weeks of age* – 2 mg/kg every 12 hours for 7 days in combination with zidovudine 2 mg/kg orally every 12 hours, advanced to every 8 hours at 4 weeks of age and continued through 6 weeks of age.

➤*Renal function impairment:*

Adults –

Chronic hepatitis B:

Lamivudine-HBV Dosage Adjustment in Adults According to CrCl[a]

CrCl (mL/min)	Recommended dosage
≥ 50	100 mg once daily
30 to 49	100 mg first dose, then 50 mg once daily
15 to 29	100 mg first dose, then 25 mg once daily
5 to 14	35 mg first dose, then 15 mg once daily
< 5	35 mg first dose, then 10 mg once daily

[a] CrCl = creatinine clearance.

HIV: Dosing of lamivudine is adjusted in accordance with renal function.

Lamivudine Dosage Adjustment in Adults According to CrCl[a]

CrCl (mL/min)	Recommended dosage
≥ 50	150 mg twice daily or 300 mg once daily
30 to 49	150 mg once daily
15 to 29	150 mg first dose, then 100 mg once daily
5 to 14	150 mg first dose, then 50 mg daily
< 5	50 mg first dose, then 25 mg once daily

[a] CrCl = creatinine clearance.

Children –

Chronic hepatitis B: Although there are insufficient data to recommend a specific dose adjustment of lamivudine-HBV or lamivudine in children with renal function impairment, a dose reduction should be considered.

HIV: Although there are insufficient data to recommend a specific dose adjustment of lamivudine in children with renal function impairment, a reduction in the dose and/or an increase in the dosing interval should be considered.

For renal dosing in adolescents, see Renal function impairment, Adults for more information.

➤*Storage/Stability:* Store tablets at 25°C (77°F); excursions are permitted to 15° to 30°C (59° to 86°F). Store lamivudine solution in tightly closed bottles at 25°C (77°F). Store lamivudine-HBV solution at a controlled room temperature of 20° to 25°C (68° to 77°F) in tightly closed bottles.

Actions

➤*Pharmacology:* Lamivudine is a synthetic nucleoside analog. Intracellularly, lamivudine is phosphorylated to its active 5-triphosphate metabolite, lamivudine triphosphate (3TC-TP). The principal mode of action of 3TC-TP is the inhibition of HIV-1 reverse transcriptase (RT) via DNA chain termination after incorporation of the nucleotide analog into viral DNA. Incorporation of the monophosphate form into viral DNA by HBV polymerase results in DNA chain termination. 3TC-TP is a weak inhibitor of mammalian DNA polymerases alpha, beta, and gamma.

➤*Pharmacokinetics:*

Absorption –

Lamivudine: Lamivudine was rapidly absorbed after oral administration in HIV-infected patients. Absolute bioavailability in 12 adult patients was 86% ± 16% (mean ± standard deviation [SD]) for the 150 mg tablet and 87% ± 13% for the 10 mg/mL oral solution. After oral administration of 2 mg/kg twice daily to 9 adults with HIV, the peak serum lamivudine concentration (C_{max}) was 1.5 ± 0.5 mcg/mL (mean ± SD). The area under the curve (AUC) and C_{max} increased in proportion to oral dose over the range from 0.25 to 10 mg/kg.

• *Food effects* – An investigational lamivudine 25 mg dosage form was administered orally to 12 asymptomatic, HIV-infected patients on 2 occasions, once in the fasted state and once with food (1,099 kcal; 75 g fat, 34 g protein, 72 g carbohydrate). Absorption of lamivudine was slower in the fed state (time to C_{max} [T_{max}], 3.2 ± 1.3 hours) compared with the fasted state (T_{max}, 0.9 ± 0.3 hours); C_{max} in the fed state was 40% ± 23% (mean ± SD) lower than in the fasted state. There was no significant difference in AUC_{∞} in the fed and fasted states; therefore, lamivudine tablets and oral solution may be administered with or without food.

Lamivudine-HBV: Lamivudine was rapidly absorbed after oral administration in HBV-infected patients and healthy subjects. Following single oral doses of 100 mg, the C_{max} in HBV-infected patients (steady state) and healthy subjects (single dose) was 1.28 ± 0.56 mcg/mL and 1.05 ± 0.32 mcg/mL (mean ± SD), respectively, which occurred between 0.5 and 2 hours after administration. The AUC_{0-24h} following lamivudine 100 mg oral single and repeated daily doses to steady state was 4.3 ± 1.4 (mean ± SD) and 4.7 ± 1.7 mcg•h/mL, respectively. The relative bioavailability of the tablet and solution was then demonstrated in healthy subjects. Although the solution demonstrated a slightly higher C_{max}, there was no significant difference in AUC_{∞} between the solution and the tablet. Therefore, the solution and the tablet may be used interchangeably.

After oral administration of lamivudine once daily to HBV-infected adults, the AUC and C_{max} increased in proportion to dose over a range of 5 to 600 mg once daily.

• *Food effects* – The 100 mg tablet was administered orally to 24 healthy subjects on 2 occasions, once in the fasted state and once with food (standard meal: 967 kcal; 67 g fat, 33 g protein, 58 g carbohydrate). There was no significant difference in AUC_{∞} in the fed and fasted states; therefore, lamivudine-HBV tablets and oral solution may be administered with or without food.

Distribution – The apparent volume of distribution after intravenous (IV) administration of lamivudine to 20 asymptomatic, HIV-infected patients was 1.3 ± 0.4 L/kg, suggesting that lamivudine distributes into extravascular spaces. Volume of distribution was independent of dose and did not correlate with body weight.

Distribution of lamivudine into cerebrospinal fluid (CSF) was assessed in 38 children after multiple oral dosing with lamivudine. CSF samples were collected between 2 and 4 hours postdose. At the dosage of 8 mg/kg/day, CSF lamivudine concentrations in 8 patients ranged from 5.6% to 30.9% (mean ± SD of 14.2% ± 7.9%) of the concentration in a simultaneous serum sample, with CSF lamivudine concentrations ranging from 0.04 to 0.3 mcg/mL.

LAMIVUDINE — ORAL

Binding of lamivudine to human plasma proteins is low (less than 36%) and independent of dose. In vitro studies showed that, over a concentration range of 0.1 to 100 mcg/mL, the amount of lamivudine associated with erythrocytes ranged from 53% to 57% and was independent of concentration.

Metabolism – Metabolism of lamivudine is a minor route of elimination. In humans, the only known metabolite of lamivudine is the trans-sulfoxide metabolite.

Lamivudine: Within 12 hours after a single oral dose of lamivudine in 6 HIV-infected adults, 5.2% ± 1.4% (mean ± SD) of the dose was excreted as the trans-sulfoxide metabolite in the urine. Serum concentrations of the trans-sulfoxide metabolite have not been determined.

Lamivudine-HBV: In 9 healthy subjects receiving lamivudine 300 mg as single oral doses, a total of 4.2% (range, 1.5% to 7.5%) of the dose was excreted as the trans-sulfoxide metabolite in the urine, the majority of which was excreted in the first 12 hours. Serum concentrations of the trans-sulfoxide metabolite have not been determined.

Excretion – The majority of lamivudine is eliminated unchanged in urine by active organic cationic secretion. In 9 healthy subjects given a single oral dose of lamivudine 300 mg, renal clearance was 199.7 ± 56.9 mL/min (mean ± SD). In 20 HIV-infected patients given a single IV dose, renal clearance was 280.4 ± 75.2 mL/min (mean ± SD), representing 71% ± 16% (mean ± SD) of total clearance of lamivudine.

In most single-dose studies in HIV-infected patients, HBV-infected patients, or healthy subjects with serum sampling for 24 hours after dosing, the observed mean elimination half-life ranged from 5 to 7 hours. In HIV-infected patients, total clearance was 398.5 ± 69.1 mL/min (mean ± SD). Oral clearance and elimination half-life were independent of dose and body weight over an oral dosing range from 0.25 to 10 mg/kg.

Special populations –

Renal function impairment: AUC_∞, C_{max}, and half-life increased with diminishing renal function (as expressed by CrCl). Apparent total oral clearance (Cl/F) of lamivudine decreased as CrCl decreased. T_{max} was not significantly affected by renal function. Based on these observations, it is recommended that the dosage of lamivudine be modified in patients with renal function impairment.

• *Lamivudine* –

Pharmacokinetic Parameters (Mean ± SD) After a Single Oral Dose of Lamivudine 300 mg in Adults With Varying Degrees of Renal Function

	CrCl		
Parameter	> 60 mL/min (n = 6)	10 to 30 mL/min (n = 4)	< 10 mL/min (n = 6)
CrCl (mL/min)	111 ± 14	28 ± 8	6 ± 2
C_{max} (mcg/mL)	2.6 ± 0.5	3.6 ± 0.8	5.8 ± 1.2
AUC_∞ (mcg•h/mL)	11 ± 1.7	48 ± 19	157 ± 74
Cl/F (mL/min)	464 ± 76	114 ± 34	36 ± 11

• *Lamivudine-HBV* –

Pharmacokinetic Parameters (Mean ± SD) Dose-Normalized to a Single Oral Dose of Lamivudine-HBV 100 mg in Subjects With Varying Degrees of Renal Function

	CrCl		
Parameter	≥ 80 mL/min (n = 9)	20 to 59 mL/min (n = 8)	< 20 mL/min (n = 6)
CrCl (mL/min)	97 (range, 82 to 117)	39 (range, 25 to 49)	15 (range, 13 to 19)
C_{max} (mcg/mL)	1.31 ± 0.35	1.85 ± 0.4	1.55 ± 0.31
AUC_∞ (mcg•h/mL)	5.28 ± 1.01	14.67 ± 3.74	27.33 ± 6.56
Cl/F (mL/min)	326.4 ± 63.8	120.1 ± 29.5	64.5 ± 18.3

Children:

• *Lamivudine* – Systemic clearance decreased with increasing age in children.

After oral administration of lamivudine 4 mg/kg twice daily to 11 children ranging from 4 months to 14 years of age, C_{max} was 1.1 ± 0.6 mcg/mL, and half-life was 2 ± 0.6 hours. In adults with similar blood sampling, the half-life was 3.7 ± 1 hours. Total exposure to lamivudine, as reflected by mean AUC values, was comparable between children receiving an 8 mg/kg/day dose and adults receiving a 4 mg/kg/day dose.

• *Lamivudine-HBV* –

Limited, uncontrolled pharmacokinetic and safety data are available from administration of lamivudine (and zidovudine) in 36 infants up to 1 week of age in 2 studies in South Africa. In these studies, lamivudine clearance was substantially reduced in neonates 1 week of age relative to children (older than 3 months of age) studied previously. There is insufficient information to establish the time course of changes in clearance between the immediate neonatal period and the age ranges older than 3 months.

➤*Microbiology:*

Antiviral activity in vitro –

Lamivudine: In HIV-1–infected MT-4 cells, lamivudine in combination with zidovudine at various ratios exhibited synergistic antiretroviral activity.

Drug resistance –

Lamivudine: Lamivudine-resistant variants of HIV-1 have been selected in cell culture. Genotypic analysis showed that the resistance was because of a specific amino acid substitution in the HIV-1 reverse transcriptase at codon 184, changing the methionine residue to isoleucine or valine (M184V/I).

HIV-1 strains resistant to lamivudine and zidovudine have been isolated from patients. Susceptibility of clinical isolates to lamivudine and zidovudine was monitored in controlled clinical trials. In patients receiving lamivudine monotherapy or combination therapy with lamivudine plus zidovudine, HIV-1 isolates from most patients became phenotypically and genotypically resistant to lamivudine within 12 weeks. In some patients harboring zidovudine-resistant virus at baseline, phenotypic sensitivity to zidovudine was restored by 12 weeks of treatment with lamivudine and zidovudine. Combination therapy with lamivudine plus zidovudine delayed the emergence of mutations conferring resistance to zidovudine.

Lamivudine-resistant HBV isolates develop substitutions (rtM204V/I) in the YMDD motif of the catalytic domain of the viral reverse transcriptase. rtM204V/I substitutions are frequently accompanied by other substitutions (rtV173L, rtL180M) that enhance the level of lamivudine resistance or act as compensatory mutations improving replication efficiency. Other substitutions detected in lamivudine-resistant HBV isolates include rtL80I and rtA181T. Similar HBV mutants have been reported in HIV-1–infected patients who received lamivudine-containing antiretroviral regimens in the presence of concurrent infections with HBV.

Lamivudine-HBV: In a controlled study, treatment-naive patients with HBeAg-positive chronic hepatitis B were treated with lamivudine or lamivudine plus adefovir dipivoxil combination therapy. Following 104 weeks of therapy, YMDD-mutant HBV was detected in 7 of 40 (18%) patients receiving combination therapy compared with 15 of 35 (43%) patients receiving lamivudine-only therapy. In another controlled study, combination therapy was evaluated in adult patients with HBeAg-positive chronic hepatitis B who had YMDD-mutant HBV and diminished clinical and virologic response to lamivudine. Following 52 weeks of lamivudine plus adefovir dipivoxil combination therapy (n = 46) or lamivudine-only therapy (n = 49), YMDD-mutant HBV was detected less frequently in patients receiving combination therapy, 62% vs 96%.

A published study suggested that the rates of lamivudine resistance in patients treated for HBeAg-negative chronic hepatitis B appear to be more variable (0% to 27% at 1 year and 10% to 56% at 2 years).

Cross-resistance –

Lamivudine: Lamivudine-resistant HIV-1 mutants were cross-resistant to didanosine and zalcitabine. In some patients treated with zidovudine plus didanosine or zalcitabine, isolates resistant to multiple RT inhibitors, including lamivudine, have emerged.

Lamivudine-HBV: HBV containing lamivudine resistance-associated substitutions (rtL180M, rtM204I, rtM204V, rtL180M + rtM204V, rtV173L + L180M + rtM204V) retain susceptibility to adefovir dipivoxil but have reduced susceptibility to entecavir (30-fold) and telbivudine (more than 100-fold). The lamivudine resistance-associated substitution rtA181T results in diminished response to adefovir and telbivudine. Similarly, HBV with entecavir resistance-associated substitutions (I169T/M250V and T184G/S202I) have more than 1,000-fold reductions in susceptibility to lamivudine.

In studies of HIV-1 infected patients who received lamivudine monotherapy or combination therapy with lamivudine plus zidovudine for at least 12 weeks, HIV-1 isolates with reduced in vitro susceptibility to lamivudine were detected in most patients.

Contraindications

Previously demonstrated clinically significant hypersensitivity to any of the components of the products.

Warnings/Precautions

➤*Lactic acidosis/severe hepatomegaly with steatosis:* Lactic acidosis and severe hepatomegaly with steatosis, including fatal cases, have been reported with the use of nucleoside analogs alone or in combination, including lamivudine and other antiretrovirals. A majority of these cases have been in women. Obesity and prolonged nucleoside exposure may be risk factors. Most of these reports have described patients receiving nucleoside analogs for treatment of HIV infection, but there have been reports of lactic acidosis in patients receiving lamivudine for hepatitis B. Exercise particular caution when administering lamivudine to any patient with known risk factors for liver disease; however, cases have also been reported in patients with no known risk factors. Suspend treatment with lamivudine or lamivudine HBV in any patient who develops clinical or laboratory findings suggestive of lactic acidosis or pronounced hepatotoxicity (which may include hepatomegaly and steatosis, even in the absence of marked transaminase elevations).

➤*Differences among lamivudine-containing products:* Lamivudine-HBV tablets and oral solution contain a lower dose of lamivudine than lamivudine tablets and oral solution, lamivudine/zidovudine combination tablets, and abacavir/lamivudine/zidovudine combination tablets used to treat HIV infection. The formulation and dosage of lamivudine in lamivudine-HBV are not appropriate for patients dually infected with HBV and HIV. Lamivudine has not been adequately studied for treatment of chronic hepatitis B in patients dually infected with HIV and HBV.

➤*Coinfection with HIV and chronic hepatitis B:* If treatment with lamivudine-HBV is prescribed for chronic hepatitis B for a patient with unrecognized or untreated HIV infection, rapid emergence of HIV resistance is likely to result because of the subtherapeutic dose and the inappropriateness of monotherapy HIV treatment. If a decision is made to administer lamivudine to patients dually infected with HIV and HBV, use lamivudine tablets, lamivudine oral solution, lamivudine/zidovudine tablets, or abacavir and lamivudine tablets as part of an appropriate combination regimen. Do not coadminister a fixed-dose combination tablet of lamivudine/zidovudine with lamivudine, lamivudine-HBV, abacavir/lamivudine, zidovudine, or

LAMIVUDINE — ORAL

abacavir/lamivudine/zidovudine, or with emtricitabine-containing products, including efavirenz/emtricitabine/tenofovir, emtricitabine, or emtricitabine/tenofovir.

The safety and efficacy of lamivudine have not been established for treatment of chronic hepatitis B in patients dually infected with HIV and HBV. In non-HIV-infected patients treated with lamivudine for chronic hepatitis B, emergence of lamivudine-resistant HBV has been detected and has been associated with diminished treatment response. Emergence of HBV variants associated with resistance to lamivudine has also been reported in HIV-infected patients who have received lamivudine-containing antiretroviral regimens in the presence of concurrent infection with HBV. Posttreatment exacerbations of hepatitis have also been reported.

➤*Posttreatment exacerbations of hepatitis:* In clinical trials in non–HIV-infected patients treated with lamivudine for chronic hepatitis B, clinical and laboratory evidence of exacerbations of hepatitis have occurred after discontinuation of lamivudine-HBV. These exacerbations have been detected primarily by serum ALT elevations, in addition to the reemergence of HBV DNA commonly observed after stopping treatment. Although most reactions appear to have been self-limited, fatalities have been reported in some cases. Similar reactions have been reported from postmarketing experience after changes from lamivudine-containing HIV treatment regimens to non–lamivudine-containing regimens in patients infected with both HIV and HBV. The causal relationship to discontinuation of lamivudine treatment is unknown. Closely monitor patients with clinical and laboratory follow-up for at least several months after stopping treatment. There is insufficient evidence to determine whether reinitiation of lamivudine alters the course of posttreatment exacerbations of hepatitis.

➤*Pancreatitis:* Pancreatitis has been reported in patients receiving lamivudine, particularly in HIV-infected children with prior nucleoside exposure.

In children with a history of antiretroviral nucleoside exposure, a history of pancreatitis, or other significant risk factors for the development of pancreatitis, use lamivudine with caution. Stop treatment with lamivudine immediately if clinical signs, symptoms, or laboratory abnormalities suggestive of pancreatitis occur.

➤*Use with interferon- and ribavirin-based regimens:* In vitro studies have shown ribavirin can reduce the phosphorylation of pyrimidine nucleoside analogs, such as lamivudine. Although no evidence of a pharmacokinetic or pharmacodynamic interaction (eg, loss of HIV/hepatitis C virus [HCV] virologic suppression) was seen when ribavirin was coadministered with lamivudine in HIV/HCV coinfected patients, hepatic decompensation (some fatal) has occurred in HIV/HCV coinfected patients receiving combination antiretroviral therapy for HIV and interferon alfa, with or without ribavirin. Closely monitor patients receiving interferon alfa, with or without ribavirin, and lamivudine for treatment-associated toxicities, especially hepatic decompensation. Consider discontinuation of lamivudine as medically appropriate. Also consider dose reduction or discontinuation of interferon alfa, ribavirin, or both if worsening clinical toxicities are observed, including hepatic decompensation (eg, Child-Pugh more than 6).

➤*Immune reconstitution syndrome:* Immune reconstitution syndrome has been reported in patients treated with combination antiretroviral therapy, including lamivudine. During the initial phase of combination antiretroviral treatment, patients whose immune systems respond may develop an inflammatory response to indolent or residual opportunistic infections (such as *Mycobacterium avium* infection, cytomegalovirus, *Pneumocystis jirovecii* pneumonia, or tuberculosis), which may necessitate further evaluation and treatment.

➤*Differences between dosing regimens:* Trough levels of lamivudine in plasma and intracellular lamivudine triphosphate were lower with once-daily dosing than with twice-daily dosing. The clinical significance of this observation is not known.

➤*Fat redistribution:* Redistribution/accumulation of body fat, including central obesity, dorsocervical fat enlargement (buffalo hump), peripheral wasting, facial wasting, breast enlargement, and "cushingoid appearance," has been observed in patients receiving antiretroviral therapy. The mechanism and long-term consequences of these events are currently unknown. A causal relationship has not been established.

➤*Emergence of resistance-associated HBV mutations:* In controlled clinical trials, YMDD-mutant HBV was detected in patients with on-lamivudine reappearance of HBV DNA after an initial decline to less than the solution hybridization assay limit. These mutations can be detected by a research assay and have been associated with reduced susceptibility to lamivudine in vitro.

See Actions for more information.

➤*Renal function impairment:* Reduction of the dose of lamivudine or lamivudine-HBV is recommended for patients with renal function impairment. See Administration and Dosage for more information.

➤*Special risk:* The safety and efficacy of lamivudine-HBV have not been established in patients with decompensated liver disease or organ transplants; children younger than 2 years of age; patients dually infected with HBV and HCV, hepatitis delta, or HIV; or other populations not included in the principal phase 3 controlled studies. There are no studies in pregnant women and no data regarding effect on vertical transmission; use appropriate infant immunizations to prevent neonatal acquisition of HBV.

➤*Pregnancy: Category C.* There are no adequate and well-controlled studies in pregnant women. Because animal reproductive toxicity studies are not always predictive of human response, use lamivudine during pregnancy only if the potential benefits outweigh the risks.

The US Department of Health and Human Services Guidelines recommend that the current antiretroviral agents in HIV-1–infected patients continue their therapy, with the exception of efavirenz, during pregnancy. If indicated, do not withhold lamivudine in pregnancy because the expected benefit to the mother outweighs the unknown risk to the fetus.

For lamivudine, sufficient numbers of first trimester exposures have been monitored to detect at least a 1.5-fold increase in risk of overall birth defects; no such increases have been detected to date.

In a subset of subjects from whom amniotic fluid specimens were obtained following natural rupture of membranes, amniotic fluid concentrations of lamivudine ranged from 1.2 to 2.5 mcg/mL (150 mg twice daily) and 2.1 to 5.2 mcg/mL (300 mg twice daily) and were typically more than 2 times the maternal serum levels. Use lamivudine during pregnancy only if the potential benefits outweigh the risks.

It is not known whether the risks of adverse reactions associated with lamivudine are altered in pregnant women compared with other HIV-1–infected patients.

Lamivudine-HBV – Lamivudine has not been shown to affect the transmission of HBV from mother to infant; use appropriate infant immunizations to prevent neonatal acquisition of HBV.

Antiretroviral pregnancy registry – To monitor maternal-fetal outcomes of pregnant women exposed to lamivudine, a pregnancy registry has been established. Health care providers are encouraged to register patients by calling 1-800-258-4263.

➤*Lactation:* The CDC recommends that HIV-infected mothers do not breast-feed their infants to avoid risking postnatal transmission of HIV.

In developing countries, extended antiretroviral prophylaxis in breast-fed infants with antiretroviral drugs appears to reduce the rate of HIV transmission during breast-feeding by about half, but the optimal regimen and duration of prophylaxis has not yet been defined. In this setting, lamivudine is often used as part of a regimen that decreases mother-to-child transmission of HIV and is generally well tolerated by the infant. Lamivudine has not been studied in HIV-negative breast-feeding mothers being treated for hepatitis B infection, but the low doses used would not be expected to cause any serious adverse effects in breast-feeding infants.

A study in lactating rats administered lamivudine 45 mg/kg showed that lamivudine concentrations in milk were slightly higher than those in plasma. Lamivudine is also excreted in human milk. Samples of breast milk obtained from 20 mothers receiving lamivudine monotherapy (300 mg twice daily) or combination therapy (lamivudine 150 mg twice daily and zidovudine 300 mg twice daily) had measurable concentrations of lamivudine.

Because of the potential for serious adverse reactions in breast-feeding infants, instruct mothers not to breast-feed if they are receiving lamivudine or lamivudine-HBV.

➤*Children:*

Lamivudine – The safety and efficacy of twice-daily lamivudine in combination with other antiretroviral agents have been established in children 3 months of age and older.

Lamivudine-HBV – The safety and efficacy in children younger than 2 years of age have not been established. The safety and efficacy of lamivudine for treatment of chronic hepatitis B in children have been studied in children from 2 to 17 years of age in a controlled clinical trial.

➤*Elderly:* Because lamivudine is substantially excreted by the kidney and elderly patients are more likely to have decreased renal function, monitor renal function and make dose adjustments accordingly.

➤*Monitoring:* Monitor patients regularly during treatment by a health care provider experienced in the management of chronic hepatitis B. The safety and efficacy of treatment with lamivudine-HBV beyond 1 year have not been established. During treatment, combinations of events such as return of persistently elevated ALT, increasing levels of HBV DNA over time after an initial decline less than assay limit, progression of clinical signs or symptoms of hepatic disease, and/or worsening of hepatic necroinflammatory findings may be considered as potentially reflecting loss of therapeutic response. Take such observations into consideration when determining the advisability of continuing therapy with lamivudine-HBV. Closely monitor patients receiving interferon alfa, with or without ribavirin, and lamivudine for treatment-associated toxicities, especially hepatic decompensation.

The optimal duration of treatment, the durability of HBeAg seroconversions occurring during treatment, and the relationship between treatment response and long-term outcomes, such as hepatocellular carcinoma or decompensated cirrhosis, are not known.

Drug Interactions

Lamivudine is predominantly eliminated in the urine by active organic cationic secretion. Consider the possibility of interactions with other coadministered drugs, particularly when their main route of elimination is active renal secretion via the organic cationic transport system (eg, trimethoprim).

LAMIVUDINE — ORAL

Lamivudine Drug Interactions

Precipitant drug	Object drug[a]		Description
Interferon alfa	Lamivudine	↑	Hepatic decompensation (some fatal) has occurred in HIV/HCV coinfected patients receiving antiretroviral therapy for HIV and interferon alfa, with or without ribavirin. Monitor closely for treatment-associated toxicities, especially hepatic decompensation. Consider discontinuation of lamivudine as medically appropriate. Also consider dose reduction or discontinuation of interferon alfa, ribavirin, or both if worsening clinical toxicities are observed.
Ribavirin	Lamivudine	↓	Ribavirin may reduce the phosphorylation of lamivudine.
Trimethoprim/Sulfamethoxazole	Lamivudine	↑	Coadministration of lamivudine with trimethoprim 160 mg and sulfamethoxazole 800 mg has been shown to increase lamivudine AUC 44%. Dosage adjustments are not needed.
Zalcitabine	Lamivudine	↓	Lamivudine and zalcitabine may inhibit the intracellular phosphorylation of one another. Coadministration is not recommended.
Lamivudine	Zalcitabine		
Lamivudine	Zidovudine	↑	Coadministration resulted in an increase of approximately 39% in the C_{max} of zidovudine.

[a] ↑ = object drug increased; ↓ = object drug decreased.

Adverse Reactions

The following adverse reactions are discussed in greater detail in the Warnings/Precautions section: lactic acidosis and severe hepatomegaly with steatosis, severe acute exacerbations of hepatitis B, hepatic decompensation in patients coinfected with HIV-1 and hepatitis C, and pancreatitis.

➤*HIV infection (lamivudine):*

Adults – The most common adverse reactions in both treatment groups were dizziness, dreams, fatigue and/or malaise, headache, insomnia and other sleep disorders, nasal signs and symptoms, diarrhea, cough, nausea, and skin rash.

Lamivudine Adverse Reactions in HIV Clinical Trials (≥ 5%)

Adverse reactions	Lamivudine 150 mg twice daily plus zidovudine (n = 251)	Zidovudine[a] (n = 230)
CNS		
Depressive disorders	9%	4%
Dizziness	10%	4%
Headache	35%	27%
Insomnia and other sleep disorders	11%	7%
Malaise/fatigue	27%	23%
Neuropathy	12%	10%
GI		
Abdominal cramps	6%	3%
Abdominal pain	9%	11%
Anorexia or decreased appetite	10%	7%
Diarrhea	18%	22%
Dyspepsia	5%	5%
Nausea	33%	29%
Nausea/vomiting	13%	12%
Musculoskeletal		
Arthralgia	5%	5%
Musculoskeletal pain	12%	10%
Myalgia	8%	6%
Respiratory		
Cough	18%	13%
Nasal signs/symptoms	20%	11%
Miscellaneous		
Fever or chills	10%	12%
Skin rashes	9%	6%

[a] Either zidovudine monotherapy or zidovudine in combination with zalcitabine.

The types and frequencies of clinical adverse reactions reported in patients receiving lamivudine 300 mg once daily or lamivudine 150 mg twice daily (in 3-drug combination regimens in EPV20001 and EPV40001) for 48 weeks were similar.

Pancreatitis: Pancreatitis was observed in 9 of 2,613 (0.3%) adult patients who received lamivudine in the controlled clinical trials EPV20001, NUCA3001, NUCB3001, NUCA3002, NUCB3002, and NUCB3007.

Lab test abnormalities:

Lamivudine Laboratory Abnormalities in Adults With HIV[a]

Test (threshold level)	24-week surrogate end point studies[b]		Clinical end point study[b]	
	Lamivudine plus zidovudine	Zidovudine[c]	Lamivudine plus current therapy	Placebo plus current therapy[d]
ANC (³)	7.2%	5.4%	15%	13%
Hemoglobin (< 8 g/dL)	2.9%	1.8%	2.2%	3.4%
Platelets (< 50,000/mm³)	0.4%	1.3%	2.8%	3.8%
ALT (> 5 × ULN)	3.7%	3.6%	3.8%	1.9%
AST (> 5 × ULN)	1.7%	1.8%	4%	2.1%
Bilirubin (> 2.5 × ULN)	0.8%	0.4%	ND	ND
Amylase (> 2 × ULN)	4.2%	1.5%	2.2%	1.1%

[a] ANC = absolute neutrophil count; ULN = upper limit of normal; ND = not done.
[b] The median duration on study was 12 months.
[c] Zidovudine monotherapy or zidovudine in combination with zalcitabine.
[d] Current therapy was zidovudine, zidovudine plus didanosine, or zidovudine plus zalcitabine.

Children –

Lamivudine Adverse Reactions in Children With HIV (≥ 5%)

Adverse reactions	Lamivudine plus zidovudine (n = 236)	Didanosine (n = 235)
GI		
Diarrhea	8%	6%
Hepatomegaly	11%	11%
Nausea/vomiting	8%	7%
Splenomegaly	5%	8%
Stomatitis	6%	12%
Respiratory		
Abnormal breath sounds/wheezing	7%	9%
Cough	15%	18%
Nasal discharge or congestion	8%	11%
Miscellaneous		
Fever	25%	32%
Lymphadenopathy	9%	11%
Signs or symptoms of ears[a]	7%	6%
Skin rashes	12%	14%

[a] Includes pain, discharge, erythema, or swelling of an ear.

Pancreatitis: Pancreatitis, which has been fatal in some cases, has been observed in antiretroviral nucleoside-experienced children receiving lamivudine alone or in combination with other antiretroviral agents. In an open-label, dose-escalation study (NUCA2002), 14 (14%) patients developed pancreatitis while receiving monotherapy with lamivudine. Three of these patients died of complications of pancreatitis. In a second open-label study (NUCA2005), 12 (18%) patients developed pancreatitis. In study ACTG300, pancreatitis was not observed in 236 patients randomized to lamivudine plus zidovudine. Pancreatitis was observed in 1 patient in this study who received open-label lamivudine in combination with zidovudine and ritonavir following discontinuation of didanosine monotherapy.

CNS: Paresthesias and peripheral neuropathies were reported in 15 (15%) patients in study NUCA2002, 6 (9%) patients in study NUCA2005, and 2 (less than 1%) patients in study ACTG300.

Lab test abnormalities:

Lamivudine Laboratory Abnormalities in Children With HIV

Test (threshold level)	Lamivudine plus zidovudine	Didanosine
ANC (³)	8%	3%
Hemoglobin (< 7 g/dL)	4%	2%
Platelets (< 50,000/mm³)	1%	3%
ALT (> 10 × ULN)	1%	3%
AST (> 10 × ULN)	2%	4%

LAMIVUDINE — ORAL

Lamivudine Laboratory Abnormalities in Children With HIV

Test (threshold level)	Lamivudine plus zidovudine	Didanosine
Lipase (> 2.5 × ULN)	3%	3%
Total amylase (> 2.5 × ULN)	3%	3%

Neonates – Limited short-term safety information is available from 2 small, uncontrolled studies in South Africa in neonates receiving lamivudine, with or without zidovudine, for the first week of life following maternal treatment starting at week 38 or 36 of gestation. Adverse reactions reported in these neonates included anemia, diarrhea, electrolyte disturbances, hypoglycemia, increased liver function tests, jaundice and hepatomegaly, rash, respiratory infections, and sepsis; 3 neonates died (1 from gastroenteritis with acidosis and convulsions, 1 from traumatic injury, and 1 from unknown causes). Two other nonfatal gastroenteritis or diarrhea cases were reported, including 1 with convulsions; 1 infant had transient renal insufficiency associated with dehydration. The absence of control groups further limits assessments of causality, but assume that perinatally exposed infants may be at risk for adverse reactions comparable with those reported in HIV-infected children and adults treated with lamivudine-containing combination regimens. Long-term effects of in utero and infant lamivudine exposure are not known.

➤*HBV (lamivudine-HBV):* Several serious adverse reactions reported with lamivudine (lactic acidosis and severe hepatomegaly with steatosis, posttreatment exacerbations of hepatitis B, pancreatitis, and emergence of viral mutants associated with reduced drug susceptibility and diminished treatment response) have occurred (see Warnings/Precautions).

Adults –

Lamivudine Adverse Reactions in Patients With Chronic HBV[a] (≥ 5%)

Adverse reactions	Lamivudine-HBV (n = 332)	Placebo (n = 200)
CNS		
Headache	21%	21%
Malaise and fatigue	24%	28%
Dermatologic		
Skin rashes	5%	5%
GI		
Abdominal discomfort and pain	16%	17%
Diarrhea	14%	12%
Nausea/vomiting	15%	17%
Musculoskeletal		
Arthralgia	7%	5%
Myalgia	14%	17%
Miscellaneous		
Ear, nose, and throat infections	25%	21%
Fever or chills	7%	9%
Sore throat	13%	8%

[a] Includes patients treated for 52 to 68 weeks.

Lab test abnormalities:

Lamivudine Laboratory Abnormalities in Adults With HBV[a]

Test (abnormal level)	Patients with abnormality/ patients with observations[a] Lamivudine-HBV	Placebo
ALT (> 3 × baseline[b])	11%	13%
Albumin (< 2.5 g/dL)	0%	1%
Amylase (> 3 × baseline)	< 1%	2%
Serum lipase (≥ 2.5 × the ULN[c])	10%	7%
Creatine kinase (≥ 7 × baseline)	9%	5%
Neutrophils (< 750/mm^3)	0%	< 1%
Platelets (< 50,000/mm^3)	4%	3%

[a] Includes patients treated for 52 to 68 weeks.
[b] See the posttreatment ALT values table.
[c] Includes observations during and after treatment in the 2 placebo-controlled trials that collected this information.

Lamivudine Posttreatment ALT Elevations in Adults

Abnormal value	Patients with ALT elevation/ patients with observations[a] Lamivudine-HBV	Placebo
ALT ≥ 2 × baseline value	27%	19%
ALT ≥ 3 × baseline value[b]	21%	8%

Lamivudine Posttreatment ALT Elevations in Adults

Abnormal value	Patients with ALT elevation/ patients with observations[a] Lamivudine-HBV	Placebo
ALT ≥ 2 × baseline value and absolute ALT > 500 units/L	15%	7%
ALT ≥ 2 × baseline value and bilirubin > 2 × ULN and ≥ 2 × baseline value	0.7%	0.9%

[a] Each patient may be represented in 1 or more category.
[b] Comparable to a grade 3 toxicity in accordance with modified World Health Organization criteria.

Children with hepatitis B – The most commonly observed adverse reactions in the pediatric trials were similar to those in adult trials; in addition, respiratory symptoms (eg, cough, bronchitis, viral respiratory tract infections) were reported in both lamivudine and placebo recipients. Posttreatment transaminase elevations were observed in some patients after cessation of lamivudine.

Children with HIV infection – In early, open-label studies of lamivudine in children with HIV, peripheral neuropathy and neutropenia were reported, and pancreatitis was observed in 14% to 15% of patients.

➤*Lamivudine (HIV) versus lamivudine-HBV:* In HIV-infected patients, safety information reflects a higher dose of lamivudine (150 mg twice daily) than the dose used to treat chronic hepatitis B in HIV-negative patients. In clinical trials using lamivudine as part of a combination regimen for the treatment of HIV infection, several clinical adverse reactions occurred more often in lamivudine-containing treatment arms than in comparator arms. These included nasal signs and symptoms (20% vs 11%), dizziness (10% vs 4%), and depressive disorders (9% vs 4%). Pancreatitis was observed in 9 of 2,613 (less than 0.5%) adult patients who received lamivudine in controlled clinical trials. Laboratory abnormalities reported more often in lamivudine-containing arms included neutropenia and elevations of liver function tests (also more frequent in lamivudine-containing arms for a retrospective analysis of HIV/HBV dually infected patients in 1 study), and amylase elevations.

➤*Postmarketing:*

CNS – Paresthesia, peripheral neuropathy, weakness.

Dermatologic – Alopecia, pruritus, rash.

Endocrine – Hyperglycemia.

GI – Stomatitis.

Hematologic/Lymphatic – Anemia (including pure red cell aplasia and severe anemias progressing on therapy), lymphadenopathy, splenomegaly.

Hepatic – Lactic acidosis and hepatic steatosis, pancreatitis, posttreatment exacerbation of hepatitis B.

Hypersensitivity – Anaphylaxis, urticaria.

Musculoskeletal – Creatine kinase elevation, muscle weakness, rhabdomyolysis.

Respiratory – Abnormal breath sounds, wheezing.

Miscellaneous – Redistribution/accumulation of body fat.

Overdosage

➤*Symptoms:* One case of an adult ingesting lamivudine 6 g was reported; there were no clinical signs or symptoms noted, and hematologic tests remained normal. Two cases of overdose in children were reported in ACTG300. One case was a single dose of lamivudine 7 mg/kg; the second case involved use of lamivudine 5 mg/kg twice daily for 30 days. There were no clinical signs or symptoms noted in either case.

➤*Treatment:* There is no known antidote for lamivudine. It is not known whether lamivudine can be removed by peritoneal dialysis or hemodialysis. Because a negligible amount of lamivudine was removed via (4-hour) hemodialysis, continuous ambulatory peritoneal dialysis, and automated peritoneal dialysis, it is not known if continuous hemodialysis would provide clinical benefit in a lamivudine overdose event. If overdose occurs, monitor the patient, and apply standard supportive treatment as required.

Patient Information

➤*Lamivudine:* Advise patients that lamivudine is not a cure for HIV infection and they may continue to experience illnesses associated with HIV infection, including opportunistic infections. Patients should remain under the care of a health care provider when using lamivudine. Advise patients that the use of lamivudine has not been shown to reduce the risk of transmission of HIV to others through sexual contact or blood contamination.

Advise patients that lamivudine tablets and oral solution contain a higher dose of the same active ingredient (lamivudine) as lamivudine-HBV tablets and oral solution. If a decision is made to include lamivudine in the HIV treatment regimen of a patient dually infected with HIV and HBV, use the formulation and dosage of lamivudine in *Epivir* (not *Epivir-HBV*).

Inform patients coinfected with HIV and HBV that deterioration of liver disease has occurred in some cases when treatment with lamivudine was discontinued. Advise patients to discuss any changes in regimen with their health care provider.

LAMIVUDINE — ORAL

Advise patients that the long-term effects of lamivudine are unknown at this time.

Advise patients of the importance of taking lamivudine with combination therapy on a regular dosing schedule and to avoid missing doses.

Advise patients of the importance of taking lamivudine exactly as it is prescribed.

Advise patients to not take lamivudine with drugs containing lamivudine or emtricitabine, including lamivudine/zidovudine, abacavir/lamivudine, abacavir/lamivudine/zidovudine, efavirenz/emtricitabine/tenofovir, emtricitabine, or emtricitabine/tenofovir.

Advise parents or guardians to monitor children for signs and symptoms of pancreatitis.

Inform patients that redistribution or accumulation of body fat may occur in patients receiving antiretroviral therapy and that the cause and long-term effects of these conditions are not known at this time.

Advise diabetic patients that each 15 mL dose of lamivudine oral solution contains 3 g of sucrose.

➤*Lamivudine-HBV:* Patients should remain under the care of a health care provider while taking lamivudine-HBV. Advise patients to discuss any new symptoms or concurrent medications with their health care provider.

Advise patients that lamivudine-HBV is not a cure for hepatitis B, that the long-term treatment benefits of lamivudine-HBV are unknown at this time, and, in particular, that the relationship of initial treatment response to outcomes, such as hepatocellular carcinoma and decompensated cirrhosis, is unknown. Inform patients that deterioration of liver disease has occurred in some cases if treatment was discontinued, and advise them to discuss any change in regimen with their health care provider. Inform patients that emergence of resistant HBV and worsening of disease can occur during treatment, and advise them to promptly report any new symptoms to their health care provider.

Counsel patients on the importance of testing for HIV to avoid inappropriate therapy and development of resistant HIV; offer HIV counseling and testing before starting lamivudine-HBV and periodically during therapy. Advise patients that lamivudine-HBV tablets and lamivudine-HBV oral solution contain a lower dose of the same active ingredient (lamivudine) as lamivudine tablets, lamivudine oral solution, lamivudine/zidovudine tablets, and abacavir/lamivudine/zidovudine tablets. Do not take lamivudine-HBV concurrently with lamivudine, lamivudine/zidovudine, or abacavir/lamivudine/zidovudine. Patients infected with both HBV and HIV who are planning to change their HIV treatment regimen to a regimen that does not include lamivudine, lamivudine/zidovudine, or abacavir/lamivudine/zidovudine should discuss continued therapy for hepatitis B with their health care provider.

Advise patients that treatment with lamivudine-HBV has not been shown to reduce the risk of transmission of HBV to others through sexual contact or blood contamination.

Advise diabetic patients that each 20 mL dose of lamivudine-HBV oral solution contains 4 g of sucrose.

STAVUDINE (d4T)

Rx	**Stavudine** (Mylan)	**Capsules; oral:** 15 mg	May contain lactose. In 60s, 100s, and 500s.
Rx	**Zerit** (Bristol-Myers Squibb)		Lactose. (BMS 1964 15). Lt. yellow/dark red. In 60s.
Rx	**Stavudine** (Mylan)	**Capsules; oral:** 20 mg	May contain lactose. In 60s, 100s, and 500s.
Rx	**Zerit** (Bristol-Myers Squibb)		Lactose. (BMS 1965 20). Lt. brown. In 60s.
Rx	**Stavudine** (Mylan)	**Capsules; oral:** 30 mg	May contain lactose. In 60s, 100s, and 500s.
Rx	**Zerit** (Bristol-Myers Squibb)		Lactose. (BMS 1966 30). Lt. orange/dark orange. In 60s.
Rx	**Stavudine** (Mylan)	**Capsules; oral:** 40 mg	May contain lactose. In 60s, 100s, and 500s.
Rx	**Zerit** (Bristol-Myers Squibb)		Lactose. (BMS 1967 40). Dark orange. In 60s.
Rx	**Zerit** (Bristol-Myers Squibb)	**Powder for solution; oral:** 1 mg/mL when reconstituted	Sucrose, parabens. Dye free. Fruit flavor. In 200 mL.

STAVUDINE — ORAL

WARNING

Lactic acidosis and hepatomegaly with steatosis – Lactic acidosis and severe hepatomegaly with steatosis, including fatal cases, have been reported with the use of nucleoside analogues alone or in combination, including stavudine and other antiretrovirals. Fatal lactic acidosis has been reported in pregnant women who received the combination of stavudine and didanosine with other antiretroviral agents. Use the combination of stavudine and didanosine with caution during pregnancy and only if the potential benefit clearly outweighs the potential risk.

Pancreatitis – Fatal and nonfatal pancreatitis have occurred during therapy when stavudine was part of a combination regimen that included didanosine in both treatment-naive and treatment-experienced patients, regardless of degree of immunosuppression.

Indications

➤*HIV infection:* For the treatment of HIV-1 infection in combination with other antiretroviral agents.

Administration and Dosage

➤*Adults:*

HIV infection –

Patients weighing 60 kg or more: 40 mg every 12 hours.

Patients weighing less than 60 kg: 30 mg every 12 hours.

➤*Children:*

HIV infection –

14 days of age and older:

- *Patients weighing 60 kg or more* – 40 mg every 12 hours.
- *Patients weighing 30 to less than 60 kg* – 30 mg every 12 hours.
- *Patients weighing less than 30 kg* – 1 mg/kg every 12 hours.

Birth to 13 days of age: 0.5 mg/kg every 12 hours.

➤*Renal function impairment:*

Adults –

Stavudine Dosage Adjustment for Renal Impairment

CrCl[a] (mL/min)	Recommended dose: Patient weight ≥ 60 kg	Recommended dose: Patient weight < 60 kg
> 50	40 mg every 12 hours	30 mg every 12 hours
26 to 50	20 mg every 12 hours	15 mg every 12 hours
10 to 25	20 mg every 24 hours	15 mg every 24 hours

[a] CrCl = creatinine clearance.

Hemodialysis: 20 mg every 24 hours for patients weighing at least 60 kg, or 15 mg every 24 hours for patients weighing less than 60 kg, administered after the completion of hemodialysis on dialysis days and at the same time of day on nondialysis days.

➤*Administration:* Stavudine may be taken without regard to meals.

The interval between doses should be 12 hours.

➤*Storage / Stability:*

Capsules – Store in tightly closed containers at 25°C (77°F); excursions are permitted between 15° and 30°C (59° and 86°F).

Oral solution – Protect from excessive moisture and store in tightly closed containers at 25°C (77°F). Excursions are permitted between 15° and 30°C (59° and 86°F). After constitution, store tightly closed containers in a refrigerator, 2° to 8°C (36° to 46°F). Discard any unused portion after 30 days.

Actions

➤*Pharmacology:* Stavudine, a nucleoside analogue of thymidine, is phosphorylated by cellular kinases to the active metabolite stavudine triphosphate. Stavudine triphosphate inhibits the activity of HIV-1 reverse transcriptase (RT) by competing with the natural substrate thymidine triphosphate (K_i = 0.0083 to 0.032 mcM) and by causing DNA chain termination following its incorporation into viral DNA. Stavudine triphosphate inhibits cellular DNA polymerases beta and gamma, and markedly reduces the synthesis of mitochondrial DNA.

➤*Pharmacokinetics:* The pharmacokinetics of stavudine have been evaluated in HIV-1–infected adults and children.

Pharmacokinetic Parameters of Stavudine in HIV-1–Infected Adults

Parameter	Mean ± SD[a]
Oral bioavailability (n = 25)	86.4 ± 18.2%
Volume of distribution (n = 44)[b]	46 ± 21 L
Total body clearance[b] (n = 44)	594 ± 164 mL/min
Apparent oral clearance[c] (n = 113)	560 ± 182[d] mL/min
Renal clearance[b] (n = 39)	237 ± 98 mL/min
Elimination half-life, IV dose[b] (n = 44)	1.15 ± 0.35 h

STAVUDINE — ORAL

Pharmacokinetic Parameters of Stavudine in HIV-1–Infected Adults	
Parameter	Mean ± SD[a]
Elimination half-life, oral dose[c] (n = 8)	1.6 ± 0.23 h
Urinary recovery of stavudine (% of dose)[b,e] (n = 39)	42 ± 14%

[a] SD = standard deviation.
[b] Following 1-hour intravenous (IV) infusion.
[c] Following single oral dose.
[d] Assuming a body weight of 70 kg.
[e] Over 12 to 24 hours.

Absorption – Following oral administration, stavudine is rapidly absorbed, with peak plasma concentrations (C_{max}) occurring within 1 hour after dosing. The systemic exposure to stavudine is the same following administration as capsules or solution.

C_{max} and area under the curve (AUC) increased in proportion to dose after single and multiple doses ranging from 0.03 to 4 mg/kg. There was no significant accumulation of stavudine with repeated administration every 6, 8, or 12 hours.

Steady-State Pharmacokinetic Parameters of Stavudine in HIV-1–Infected Adults	
Parameter	Stavudine 40 mg twice daily Mean ± SD (n = 8)
AUC_{0-24}	2,568 ± 454 ng•h/mL
C_{max}	536 ± 146 ng/mL
C_{min}[a]	8 ± 9 ng/mL

[a] C_{min} = trough or minimum plasma concentration.

Distribution – Binding of stavudine to serum proteins was negligible over the concentration range of 0.01 to 11.4 mcg/mL. Stavudine distributes equally between red blood cells and plasma.

Metabolism – Metabolism plays a limited role in the clearance of stavudine. Unchanged stavudine was the major drug-related component circulating in plasma after an 80 mg dose of ^{14}C-stavudine, while metabolites constituted minor components of the circulating radioactivity. Minor metabolites include oxidized stavudine, glucuronide conjugates of stavudine and its oxidized metabolite, and an *N*-acetylcysteine conjugate of the ribose after glycosidic cleavage, suggesting that thymine is also a metabolite of stavudine.

Excretion – Following an 80 mg dose of ^{14}C-stavudine to healthy subjects, approximately 95% and 3% of the total radioactivity was recovered in urine and feces, respectively. Radioactivity due to parent drug in urine and feces was 73.7% and 62%, respectively. The mean terminal elimination half-life is approximately 2.3 hours following single oral doses. Mean renal clearance of the parent compound is approximately 272 mL/min, accounting for approximately 67% of the apparent oral clearance.

In HIV-1–infected patients, renal elimination accounted for approximately 40% of the overall clearance regardless of the route of administration.

The mean renal clearance is about twice the average endogenous CrCl, indicating active tubular secretion in addition to glomerular filtration.

Special populations –

Renal function impairment: Data from 2 studies in adults indicated that the apparent oral clearance of stavudine decreased and the terminal elimination half-life increased as CrCl decreased. C_{max} and time to maximum concentration (T_{max}) were not significantly altered by renal insufficiency. The mean ± SD hemodialysis clearance value of stavudine was 120 ± 18 mL/min (n = 12); the mean ± SD percentage of the stavudine dose recovered in the dialysate, timed to occur between 2 to 6 hours postdose, was 31 ± 5%. Based on these observations, it is recommended that stavudine dosage be modified in patients with reduced CrCl and in patients receiving maintenance hemodialysis.

Mean ± SD Pharmacokinetic Parameter Values of Stavudine[a] in Adults With Varying Degrees of Renal Function[b]				
	CrCl			
Parameter	> 50 mL/min (n = 10)	26 to 50 mL/min (n = 5)	9 to 25 mL/min (n = 5)	Hemodialysis patients[c] (n = 11)
CrCl (mL/min)	104 ± 28	41 ± 5	17 ± 3	NA
CL/F (mL/min)	335 ± 57	191 ± 39	116 ± 25	105 ± 17
CL_R (mL/min)	167 ± 65	73 ± 18	17 ± 3	NA
t½ (h)	1.7 ± 0.4	3.5 ± 2.5	4.6 ± 0.9	5.4 ± 1.4

[a] Single 40 mg oral dose.
[b] CL/F = apparent oral clearance; CL_R = renal clearance; t½ = terminal elimination half-life; NA = not applicable.
[c] Determined while patients were off dialysis.

Children:

Pharmacokinetic Parameters (Mean ± SD) of Stavudine in HIV-1–Exposed or HIV-1–Infected Children						
Parameter	Ages 5 weeks to 15 years	n	Ages 14 to 28 days	n	Day of birth	n
Oral bioavailability	76.9% ± 31.7%	20	ND[a]		ND	
Volume of distribution[b]	0.73 ± 0.32 L/kg	21	ND		ND	
Ratio of CSF:plasma concentrations[c]	59% ± 35%	8	ND		ND	
Total body clearance[b]	9.75 ± 3.76 mL/min/kg	21	ND		ND	
Apparent oral clearance[d]	13.75 ± 4.29 mL/min/kg	20	11.52 ± 5.93 mL/min/kg	30	5.08 ± 2.8 mL/min/kg	17
Elimination half-life, IV dose[b]	1.11 ± 0.28 h	21	ND		ND	
Elimination half-life oral dose[d]	0.96 ± 0.26 h	20	1.59 ± 0.29 h	30	5.27 ± 2.01 h	17
Urinary recovery of stavudine (% of dose)[d,e]	34% ± 16%	19	ND		ND	

[a] ND = not determined.
[b] Following 1-hour IV infusion.
[c] CSF = cerebrospinal fluid. At median time of 2.5 hours (range, 2 to 3 hours) following multiple oral doses.
[d] Following single oral doses.
[e] Over 8 hours.

➤*Microbiology:*

Antiviral activity – The cell culture antiviral activity of stavudine was measured in peripheral blood mononuclear cells, monocytic cells, and lymphoblastoid cell lines. The concentration of drug necessary to inhibit HIV-1 replication by 50% (median effective concentration [EC_{50}]) ranged from 0.009 to 4 mcM against laboratory and clinical isolates of HIV-1. In cell culture, stavudine exhibited additive to antagonistic activity in combination with zidovudine. Stavudine in combination with either abacavir, didanosine, tenofovir, or zalcitabine exhibited additive to synergistic anti–HIV-1 activity. Ribavirin, at the 9 to 45 mcM concentrations tested, reduced the anti–HIV-1 activity of stavudine by 2.5- to 5-fold. The relationship between cell culture susceptibility of HIV-1 to stavudine and the inhibition of HIV-1 replication in humans has not been established.

Drug resistance – HIV isolates with reduced susceptibility to stavudine have been selected in cell culture (strain-specific) and were also obtained from patients treated with stavudine. Phenotypic analysis of HIV-1 isolates from 61 patients receiving prolonged (6 to 29 months) stavudine monotherapy showed that posttherapy isolates from 4 patients exhibited EC_{50} values more than 4-fold (range, 7- to 16-fold) higher than the average pretreatment susceptibility of baseline isolates. Of these, HIV-1 isolates from 1 patient contained the zidovudine-resistance–associated substitutions T215Y and K219E, and isolates from another patient contained the multiple-nucleoside-resistance–associated substitution Q151M. Mutations in the RT gene of HIV-1 isolates from the other 2 patients were not detected. The genetic basis for stavudine susceptibility changes has not been identified.

Cross-resistance – Cross-resistance among HIV-1 reverse transcriptase inhibitors has been observed. Several studies have demonstrated that prolonged stavudine treatment can select and/or maintain thymidine analogue mutations (TAMS) (M41L, D67N, K70R, L210W, T215Y/F, K219Q/E) associated with zidovudine resistance. HIV-1 isolates with 1 or more TAMs exhibited reduced susceptibility to stavudine in cell culture. These TAMs are seen at a similar frequency with stavudine and zidovudine in virological treatment. The clinical relevance of these findings suggests that stavudine should be avoided in the presence of thymidine analogue mutations.

Contraindications

Clinically significant hypersensitivity to stavudine or to any of the components contained in the formulation.

Warnings/Precautions

➤*Lactic acidosis/severe hepatomegaly with steatosis:* Lactic acidosis and severe hepatomegaly with steatosis, including fatal cases, have been reported with the use of nucleoside analogues alone or in combination, including stavudine and other antiretrovirals. Although relative rates of lactic acidosis have not been assessed in prospective well-controlled trials, longitudinal cohort and retrospective studies suggest that this infrequent event may be more often associated with antiretroviral combinations containing stavudine. Female gender, obesity, and prolonged nucleoside exposure may be risk factors.

See the Warning box for more information.

Exercise particular caution when administering stavudine to any patient with known risk factors for liver disease; however, cases of lactic acidosis have also been reported in patients with no known risk factors. Generalized fatigue; digestive symptoms (nausea, vomiting, abdominal pain, and unexplained weight loss); respiratory symptoms (tachypnea and dyspnea); or

STAVUDINE — ORAL

neurologic symptoms, including motor weakness (see Neurologic Symptoms), might be indicative of lactic acidosis syndrome or the development of symptomatic hyperlactatemia.

Suspend treatment with stavudine in any patient who develops clinical or laboratory findings suggestive of symptomatic hyperlactatemia, lactic acidosis, or pronounced hepatotoxicity, which may include hepatomegaly and steatosis even in the absence of marked transaminase elevations. Consider permanent discontinuation of stavudine for patients with confirmed lactic acidosis.

➤*Hepatic toxicity:* The safety and efficacy of stavudine have not been established in HIV-infected patients with significant underlying liver disease. During combination antiretroviral therapy, patients with preexisting liver dysfunction, including chronic active hepatitis, have an increased frequency of liver function abnormalities, including severe and potentially fatal hepatic adverse events, and should be monitored according to standard practice. If there is evidence of worsening liver disease in such patients, interruption or discontinuation of treatment must be considered.

Hepatotoxicity and hepatic failure resulting in death were reported during postmarketing surveillance in HIV-infected patients treated with hydroxyurea and other antiretroviral agents. Fatal hepatic events were reported most often in patients treated with the combination of hydroxyurea, didanosine, and stavudine. Avoid this combination.

➤*Neurologic symptoms:* Motor weakness has been reported rarely in patients receiving combination antiretroviral therapy including stavudine. Most of these cases occurred in the setting of lactic acidosis. The evolution of motor weakness may mimic the clinical presentation of Guillain-Barré syndrome, including respiratory failure. If motor weakness develops, discontinue stavudine. Symptoms may continue or worsen following discontinuation of therapy.

Peripheral sensory neuropathy, manifested by numbness, tingling, or pain in the hands or feet, has been reported in patients receiving stavudine therapy. Peripheral neuropathy, which can be severe, is dose related and occurs more frequently in patients with advanced HIV-1 disease or a history of peripheral neuropathy, or in patients receiving other drugs that have been associated with neuropathy, including didanosine.

Stavudine-related peripheral neuropathy may resolve if therapy is withdrawn promptly. If peripheral neuropathy develops, consider permanent discontinuation of stavudine. In some cases, symptoms may worsen temporarily following discontinuation of therapy.

➤*Pancreatitis:* See the Warning box for more information.

The combination of stavudine and didanosine and any other agents that are toxic to the pancreas should be suspended in patients with suspected pancreatitis. Reinstitution of stavudine after a confirmed diagnosis of pancreatitis should be undertaken with particular caution and close patient monitoring; avoid use in combination with didanosine.

➤*Fat redistribution:* Redistribution/accumulation of body fat, including central obesity, dorsocervical fat enlargement (buffalo hump), peripheral wasting, facial wasting, breast enlargement, and "cushingoid appearance," have been observed in patients receiving antiretroviral therapy.

In randomized controlled trials of treatment-naive patients, clinical lipoatrophy or lipodystropy developed in a higher proportion of patients treated with stavudine compared with other nucleosides (tenofovir or abacavir). Dual-energy x-ray absorptiometry (DEXA) scans demonstrated overall limb fat loss in stavudine-treated patients compared with limb fat gain or no gain in patients treated with other nucleosides (abacavir, tenofovir, or zidovudine). The incidence and severity of lipoatrophy or lipodystrophy are cumulative over time with stavudine-containing regimens. In clinical trials, switching from stavudine to other nucleosides (tenofovir or abacavir) resulted in increases in limb fat with modest to no improvements in clinical lipoatrophy. Monitor patients receiving stavudine for symptoms or signs of lipoatrophy or lipodystrophy and question them about body changes related to lipoatrophy or lipodystrophy. Given the potential risks of using stavudine including lipoatrophy or lipodystrophy, make a benefit-risk assessment for each patient and consider an alternative antiretroviral.

➤*Immune reconstitution syndrome:* Immune reconstitution syndrome has been reported in patients treated with combination antiretroviral therapy, including stavudine. During the initial phase of combination antiretroviral treatment, patients whose immune systems respond may develop an inflammatory response to indolent or residual opportunistic infections (such as *Mycobacteriam avium* infection, cytomegalovirus, *Pneumocystis jiroveci* pneumonia [PCP], or tuberculosis), which may necessitate further evaluation and treatment.

➤*Renal function impairment:* See Actions for more information. See Administration and Dosage for more information.

➤*Pregnancy: Category C.* There are no adequate and well-controlled studies of stavudine in pregnant women. Use stavudine during pregnancy only if the potential benefit justifies the potential risk.

Fatal lactic acidosis has been reported in pregnant women who received the combination of stavudine and didanosine with other antiretroviral agents. It is unclear if pregnancy augments the risk of lactic acidosis/hepatic steatosis syndrome reported in nonpregnant individuals receiving nucleoside analogues. Use the combination of stavudine and didanosine with caution during pregnancy and only if the potential benefit clearly outweighs the potential risk. Health care providers caring for HIV-infected pregnant women receiving stavudine should be alert for early diagnosis of lactic acidosis/hepatic steatosis syndrome.

Reproduction studies have been performed in rats and rabbits with exposures (based on C_{max}) up to 399 and 183 times, respectively, of that seen at a clinical dosage of 1 mg/kg/day and have revealed no evidence of teratogenicity. The incidence in fetuses of a common skeletal variation, unossified or incomplete ossification of sternebra, was increased in rats at 399 times human exposure, while no effect was observed at 216 times human exposure. A slight postimplantation loss was noted at 216 times the human exposure with no effect noted at approximately 135 times the human exposure. An increase in early rat neonatal mortality (birth to 4 days of age) occurred at 399 times the human exposure, while survival of neonates was unaffected at approximately 135 times the human exposure. A study in rats showed that stavudine is transferred to the fetus through the placenta. The concentration in fetal tissue was approximately one-half the concentration in maternal plasma. Animal reproduction studies are not always predictive of human response.

Antiretroviral pregnancy registry – To monitor maternal-fetal outcomes of pregnant women exposed to stavudine and other antiretroviral agents, an antiretroviral pregnancy registry has been established. Health care providers are encouraged to register patients by calling 1-800-258-4263.

➤*Lactation:* The Centers for Disease Control and Prevention (CDC) recommend that HIV-infected mothers not breast-feed their infants to avoid risking postnatal transmission of HIV. Studies in lactating rats demonstrated that stavudine is excreted in milk. The molecular weight (about 224) suggests that stavudine will be excreted in breast milk. Although it is not known whether stavudine is excreted in human breast milk, there exists the potential for adverse effects from stavudine in breast-feeding infants. Because of the potential for HIV transmission and the potential for serious adverse reactions in breast-feeding infants, instruct mothers not to breast-feed if they are receiving stavudine.

➤*Children:* Use of stavudine in children from birth through adolescence is supported by evidence from adequate and well-controlled studies of stavudine in adults with additional pharmacokinetic and safety data in children.

➤*Elderly:* In a monotherapy expanded access program for patients with advanced HIV-1 infection, peripheral neuropathy or peripheral neuropathic symptoms were observed in 38% of elderly patients receiving 40 mg twice daily and 16% of elderly patients receiving 20 mg twice daily. Of the approximately 12,000 patients enrolled in the expanded access program, peripheral neuropathy or peripheral neuropathic symptoms developed in 30% of patients receiving 40 mg twice daily and 25% of patients receiving 20 mg twice daily. Closely monitor elderly patients for signs and symptoms of peripheral neuropathy.

Stavudine is known to be substantially excreted by the kidney, and the risk of toxic reactions to this drug may be greater in patients with impaired renal function. Because elderly patients are more likely to have decreased renal function, it may be useful to monitor renal function. Dose adjustment is recommended for patients with renal impairment.

➤*Monitoring:* Monitor patients for the development of peripheral neuropathy and pancreatitis.

Monitor patients with preexisting liver dysfunction for liver function abnormalities according to standard practice.

Monitor patients for development of lactic acidosis and for severe hepatomegaly with steatosis.

Drug Interactions

Stavudine Drug Interactions

Precipitant drug	Object drug[a]		Description
Didanosine	Stavudine	↑	Coadministration may increase the risk for lactic acidosis, hepatotoxicity, pancreatitis, or peripheral neuropathy (see Warnings/Precautions). Use stavudine in combination with didanosine with caution during pregnancy.
Doxorubicin	Stavudine	↓	Phosphorylation of stavudine is inhibited at relevant concentrations by doxorubicin. Coadminister with caution. Closely monitor for treatment-associated toxicities, especially hepatic decompensation.
Hydroxyurea	Stavudine	↑	Coadministration may increase the risk for lactic acidosis, hepatotoxicity, pancreatitis, or peripheral neuropathy (see Warnings/Precautions). Avoid combined administration of stavudine and hydroxyurea with or without didanosine.

STAVUDINE — ORAL

Stavudine Drug Interactions

Precipitant drug	Object drug[a]		Description
Methadone	Stavudine	⬇	Coadministration produced a 23% decrease in AUC and a 44% decrease in peak drug concentration of stavudine. Close clinical and laboratory monitoring is warranted when methadone is started or stopped. Adjust the stavudine dose as needed.
Ribavirin	Stavudine	⬇	Phosphorylation of stavudine is inhibited at relevant concentrations by ribavirin. Coadminister with caution. Closely monitor for treatment-associated toxicities, especially hepatic decompensation.
Zidovudine	Stavudine	⬇	Zidovudine may competitively inhibit the intracellular phosphorylation of stavudine. Coadministration is not recommended.

[a] ⬆ = object drug increased; ⬇ = object drug decreased.

Drug interaction studies have demonstrated that there are no clinically significant pharmacokinetic interactions between stavudine and the following: didanosine, lamivudine, or nelfinavir.

Adverse Reactions

➤*Adults:*

Stavudine Adverse Reactions in Study AI455-019[a] (Monotherapy)

Adverse reactions	Stavudine[b] (40 mg twice daily) (n = 412)	Zidovudine (200 mg 3 times daily) (n = 402)
CNS		
Headache	54%	49%
Peripheral neurologic symptoms/neuropathy	52%	39%
Dermatologic		
Rash	40%	35%
GI		
Diarrhea	50%	44%
Nausea/Vomiting	39%	44%

[a] The incidences reported included all severity grades and all reactions regardless of causality.
[b] Median duration of stavudine therapy = 79 weeks; median duration of zidovudine therapy = 53 weeks.

Pancreatitis was observed in 3 of the 412 adults who received stavudine in study AI455-019.

Stavudine Adverse Reactions[a] in START 1 and START 2[b] Studies (Combination Therapy)

	START 1		START 2[b]	
Adverse reactions	Stavudine + lamivudine + indinavir (n = 100)[c]	Zidovudine + lamivudine + indinavir (n = 102)	Stavudine + didanosine + indinavir (n = 102)[c]	Zidovudine + lamivudine + indinavir (n = 103)
CNS				
Headache	25%	26%	46%	37%
Peripheral neurologic symptoms/ neuropathy	8%	7%	21%	10%
Dermatologic				
Rash	18%	13%	30%	18%
GI				
Diarrhea	34%	16%	45%	39%
Nausea	43%	63%	53%	67%
Vomiting	18%	33%	30%	35%

[a] The incidences reported included all severity grades and all reactions regardless of causality.
[b] START 2 compared 2 triple-combination regimens in 205 treatment-naive patients. Patients received either stavudine (40 mg twice daily) plus didanosine plus indinavir or zidovudine plus lamivudine plus indinavir.
[c] Duration of stavudine therapy = 48 weeks.

Lab test abnormalities –

Stavudine Laboratory Abnormalities in Study AI455-019[a,b]

Parameter	Stavudine (40 mg twice daily) (n = 412)	Zidovudine (200 mg 3 times daily) (n = 402)
AST (> 5 × ULN[c])	11%	10%
ALT (> 5 × ULN)	13%	11%
Amylase (≥ 1.4 × ULN)	14%	13%

[a] Data presented for patients for whom laboratory evaluations were performed.
[b] Median duration of stavudine therapy = 79 weeks; median duration of zidovudine therapy = 53 weeks.
[c] ULN = upper limit of normal.

Stavudine Laboratory Test Abnormalities in START 1 and START 2 (Grades 3 to 4)[a]

	START 1		START 2	
Parameter	Stavudine + lamivudine + indinavir (n = 100)	Zidovudine + lamivudine + indinavir (n = 102)	Stavudine + didanosine + indinavir (n = 102)	Zidovudine + lamivudine + indinavir (n = 103)
Bilirubin (> 2.6 × ULN)	7%	6%	16%	8%
AST (> 5 × ULN)	5%	2%	7%	7%
ALT (> 5 × ULN)	6%	2%	8%	5%
GGT (> 5 × ULN)	2%	2%	5%	2%
Lipase (> 2 × ULN)	6%	3%	5%	5%
Amylase (> 2 × ULN)	4%	< 1%	8%	2%

[a] GGT = gamma-glutamyltransferase.

Stavudine Laboratory Test Abnormalities in START 1 and START 2 Studies (All Grades)

	START 1		START 2	
Parameter	Stavudine + lamivudine + indinavir (n = 100)	Zidovudine + lamivudine + indinavir (n = 102)	Stavudine + didanosine + indinavir (n = 102)	Zidovudine + lamivudine + indinavir (n = 103)
Total bilirubin	65%	60%	68%	55%
AST	42%	20%	53%	20%
ALT	40%	20%	50%	18%
GGT	15%	8%	28%	12%
Lipase	27%	12%	26%	19%
Amylase	21%	19%	31%	17%

➤*Children:* Adverse reactions and serious laboratory abnormalities in children from birth through adolescence were similar in type and frequency to those seen in adults.

➤*Postmarketing:*

CNS – Insomnia, severe motor weakness (most often reported in the setting of lactic acidosis.

GI – Abdominal pain, anorexia, pancreatitis (including fatal cases).

Hematologic – Anemia, leukopenia, macrocytosis, neutropenia, thrombocytopenia.

Hepatic – Symptomatic hyperlactatemia/lactic acidosis and hepatic steatosis, hepatitis and liver failure.

Metabolic/Nutritional – Diabetes mellitus, hyperglycemia, lipoatrophy, lipodystrophy.

Miscellaneous – Allergic reaction, chills/fever, myalgia, redistribution/accumulation of body fat.

Use with didanosine- and hydroxyurea-based regimens – When stavudine is used in combination with other agents with similar toxicities, the incidence of these toxicities may be higher than when stavudine is used alone. Therefore, patients treated with stavudine in combination with didanosine, with or without hydroxyurea, may be at increased risk for pancreatitis and hepatotoxicity, which may be fatal, and severe peripheral neuropathy. Avoid the combination of stavudine and hydroxyurea, with or without didanosine.

Overdosage

➤*Symptoms:* Experience with adults treated with 12 to 24 times the recommended daily dosage revealed no acute toxicity. Complications of chronic overdosage include peripheral neuropathy and hepatic toxicity.

➤*Treatment:* Stavudine can be removed by hemodialysis; the mean ± SD hemodialysis clearance of stavudine is 120 ± 18 mL/min. Whether stavudine is eliminated by peritoneal dialysis has not been studied.

Patient Information

Inform patients of the importance of early recognition of symptoms of symptomatic hyperlactatemia or lactic acidosis syndrome, which include unexplained weight loss, abdominal discomfort, nausea, vomiting, fatigue,

STAVUDINE — ORAL

dyspnea, and motor weakness. Inform patients in whom these symptoms develop to seek medical attention immediately. Discontinuation of stavudine therapy may be required.

Inform patients that an important toxicity of stavudine is peripheral neuropathy. Advise patients that peripheral neuropathy is manifested by numbness, tingling, or pain in the hands or feet, and to report these symptoms to their health care providers. Counsel patients that peripheral neuropathy occurs with greatest frequency in patients who have advanced HIV disease or a history of peripheral neuropathy, and that discontinuation of stavudine may be required if toxicity develops. Instruct caregivers of young children receiving stavudine therapy regarding detection and reporting of peripheral neuropathy.

Inform patients that an increased risk of pancreatitis, which may be fatal, may occur in patients treated with the combination of stavudine and didanosine. Inform patients that they will be closely monitored for symptoms of pancreatitis.

Inform patients that an increased risk of hepatotoxicity, which may be fatal, may occur in patients treated with stavudine in combination with didanosine and hydroxyurea.

Inform patients that stavudine is not a cure for HIV-1 infection, and that they may continue to acquire illnesses associated with HIV infection, including opportunistic infections. Advise patients to remain under the care of a health care provider when using stavudine, and the importance of adherence to any antiretroviral regimen, including those that contain stavudine. Advise them that stavudine therapy has not been shown to reduce the risk of transmission of HIV-1 to others through sexual contact or blood contamination. Inform patients that when stavudine is used in combination with other agents with similar toxicities, the incidence of adverse reactions may be higher than when stavudine is used alone.

Instruct patients that if they miss a dose to take it as soon as possible. If it is almost time for the next dose, skip the missed dose and continue the regular dosing schedule.

Instruct patients that if they take too much stavudine they should contact a poison control center or emergency department right away.

Advise patients with diabetes that stavudine for oral solution contains 50 mg of sucrose (sugar) per mL.

Inform patients that the CDC recommends that HIV-infected mothers not breast-feed infants to reduce the risk of postnatal transmission of HIV infection.

Inform patients that redistribution or accumulation of body fat may occur in patients receiving antiretroviral therapy, including stavudine.

Instruct patients to avoid alcohol while taking stavudine. Alcohol may increase the patient's risk of pancreatitis or liver damage.

ZIDOVUDINE (Azidothymidine; AZT; Compound S)

Rx	**Zidovudine** (Various, eg, Aurobindo, Ranbaxy, Roxane)	**Tablets; oral:** 300 mg	In 60s.
Rx	**Retrovir** (GlaxoSmithKline)		(GX CW3 300). White, round. Film-coated. In 60s.
Rx	**Zidovudine** (Aurobindo Pharma)	**Capsules; oral:** 100 mg	(D 01). In 100s and UD 100s.
Rx	**Retrovir** (GlaxoSmithKline)		(Wellcome Y9C 100). White. In 100s and UD 100s.
Rx	**Zidovudine** (Aurobindo)	**Syrup; oral:** 50 mg per 5 mL	Sucrose. Strawberry flavor. In 240 mL.
Rx	**Retrovir** (GlaxoSmithKline)		Sodium benzoate 0.2% sucrose. Strawberry flavor. In 240 mL.
Rx	**Retrovir** (GlaxoSmithKline)	**Injection, solution:** 10 mg/mL	In 20 mL single-use vial.

ZIDOVUDINE — ORAL

WARNING

Hematologic toxicity – Zidovudine has been associated with hematologic toxicity, including neutropenia and severe anemia, particularly in patients with advanced HIV disease.

Myopathy – Prolonged use of zidovudine has been associated with symptomatic myopathy.

Lactic acidosis severe hepatomegaly – Lactic acidosis and severe hepatomegaly with steatosis, including fatal cases, have been reported with the use of nucleoside analogues alone or in combination, including zidovudine and other antiretrovirals. Suspend treatment if clinical or laboratory findings suggestive of lactic acidosis or pronounced hepatotoxicity occur.

Indications

➤*HIV infection:* For the treatment of HIV-1 infection in combination with other antiretroviral agents.

➤*Maternal-fetal HIV transmission:* For the prevention of maternal-fetal HIV-1 transmission. The indication is based on a dosing regimen that included 3 components: antepartum therapy of HIV-1 infected mothers, intrapartum therapy of HIV-1 infected mothers, and postpartum therapy of HIV-1 exposed neonate. Points to consider prior to initiating zidovudine in pregnant women for the prevention of maternal-fetal HIV-1 transmission include:

- In most cases, zidovudine for prevention of maternal-fetal HIV-1 transmission should be given in combination with other antiretroviral drugs.
- Prevention of HIV-1 transmission in women who have received zidovudine for a prolonged period before pregnancy has not been evaluated.
- Because the fetus is most susceptible to the potential teratogenic effects of drugs during the first 10 weeks of gestation and the risks of therapy with zidovudine during that period are not fully known, women in the first trimester of pregnancy who do not require immediate initiation of antiretroviral therapy for their own health may consider delaying use; this indication is based on use after 14 weeks' gestation.

Administration and Dosage

➤*Adults:*

HIV infection – 600 mg/day in divided doses in combination with other antiretroviral agents.

Prevention of maternal-fetal HIV transmission – 100 mg orally 5 times/day until labor starts. During labor and delivery, zidovudine IV should be administered at 2 mg/kg (total body weight) over 1 hour, followed by a continuous IV infusion of 1 mg/kg/h (total body weight) until clamping of the umbilical cord occurs.

➤*Children:* Zidovudine syrup should be used to provide accurate dosage when whole tablets or capsules are not appropriate.

HIV infection –

4 weeks to younger than 18 years of age:

Zidovudine Pediatric Dosage (≥4 Weeks of Age)			
Body weight (kg)	Total daily dose	Dosage regimen and dose	
		Twice daily	3 times daily
4 to < 9	24 mg/kg/day	12 mg/kg	8 mg/kg
≥ 9 to < 30	18 mg/kg/day	9 mg/kg	6 mg/kg
≥ 30	600 mg/day	300 mg	200 mg

Alternatively, dosing of zidovudine can be based on body surface area (BSA) for each child. The recommended oral dose of zidovudine is 480 mg/m^2/day in divided doses (240 mg/m^2 twice daily or 160 mg/m^2 3 times daily). In some cases, the dose calculated by mg/kg will not be the same as that calculated by BSA.

Prevention of maternal-fetal HIV transmission – The recommended dosage regimens for administration to pregnant women (greater than 14 weeks of pregnancy) and their neonates are as follows.

Maternal: 100 mg orally 5 times per day until the start of labor. During labor and delivery, intravenous zidovudine should be administered at 2 mg/kg (total body weight) over 1 hour followed by a continuous intravenous infusion of 1 mg/kg/hour (total body weight) until clamping of the umbilical cord.

Neonates: 2 mg/kg orally every 6 hours starting within 12 hours of birth and continuing through 6 weeks of age. Neonates unable to receive oral dosing may be administered zidovudine IV at 1.5 mg/kg infused over 30 minutes every 6 hours.

➤*Renal function impairment:* In patients with severe renal function impairment (creatinine clearance [CrCl] less than 15 mL/min), dosage reduction is recommended. In patients maintained on hemodialysis or peritoneal dialysis, the recommended dosing is 100 mg every 6 to 8 hours.

➤*Patients with hematologic abnormalities:* Significant anemia (hemoglobin level of less than 7.5 g/dL or reduction of greater than 25% of baseline) and/or significant neutropenia (granulocyte count of less than 750 cells/mm^3 or reduction of greater than 50% from baseline) may require a dose interruption until evidence of marrow recovery is observed. In patients who develop significant anemia, dose interruption does not necessarily eliminate the need for transfusion. If marrow recovery occurs following dose interruption, resumption of dose may be appropriate using adjunctive measures such as epoetin alfa at recommended doses, depending on hematologic indices such as serum erythropoietin level and patient tolerance.

➤*Preparation for administration:* Zidovudine is considered a potential teratogen. Follow safe handling procedures when preparing, administering, or dispensing zidovudine.

➤*Administration:* May be administered with or without food.

➤*Storage/Stability:* Store at 15° to 25°C (59° to 77°F). Protect capsules from moisture.

ZIDOVUDINE — ORAL

Actions

➤*Pharmacology:* Zidovudine (formally called azidothymidine [AZT]) is a pyrimidine nucleoside analog active against HIV. Intracellularly, zidovudine is phosphorylated to its active 5″-triphosphate metabolite, zidovudine triphosphate (ZDV-TP). The principal mode of action of ZDV-TP is inhibition of reverse transcriptase (RT) via DNA chain termination after incorporation of the nucleotide analogue. ZDV-TP is a weak inhibitor of the cellular DNA polymerases α and γ and has been reported to be incorporated into the DNA of cells in culture.

➤*Pharmacokinetics:*

Absorption/Distribution – Following oral administration, zidovudine is rapidly absorbed and extensively distributed, with peak serum concentrations occurring within 0.5 to 1.5 hours. Binding to plasma protein is low.

Food effects: Zidovudine may be administered with or without food. The extent of zidovudine absorption (area under the curve [AUC]) was similar when a single dose of zidovudine was administered with food.

Bioequivalence: The extent of absorption (AUC) was equivalent when zidovudine was administered as zidovudine tablets or syrup compared with zidovudine capsules.

Zidovudine Pharmacokinetic Parameters in Fasting Adult Patients

Parameter	Mean ± SD[a] (except where noted)
Oral bioavailability (%)	64 ± 10 (n = 5)
Apparent volume of distribution (L/kg)	1.6 ± 0.6 (n = 8)
Plasma protein binding (%)	< 38
CSF[b]:plasma ratio[c]	0.6 [0.04 to 2.62] (n = 39)
Systemic clearance (L/h/kg)	1.6 ± 0.6 (n = 6)
Renal clearance (L/h/kg)	0.34 ± 0.05 (n = 9)
Elimination half-life (h)[d]	0.5 to 3 (n = 19)

[a] SD = standard deviation.
[b] CSF = cerebrospinal fluid.
[c] Median [range].
[d] Approximate range.

Metabolism/Excretion – Zidovudine is primarily eliminated by hepatic metabolism. The major metabolite of zidovudine is 3'-azido-3'-deoxy-5'-O-β-D-glucopyranuronosylthymidine (GZDV). GZDV AUC is about 3-fold greater than the zidovudine AUC. Urinary recovery of zidovudine and GZDV accounts for 14% and 74%, respectively, of the dose following oral administration. Pharmacokinetics of zidovudine were dose independent at oral dosing regimens ranging from 2 mg/kg every 8 hours to 10 mg/kg every 4 hours.

Special populations –

Renal function impairment: Zidovudine clearance was decreased, resulting in increased zidovudine and GZDV half-life and AUC in patients with impaired renal function (n = 14) following a single 200 mg oral dose (see the following table). Plasma concentrations of 3'-amino-3'-deoxythymidine (AMT) were not determined. A dose adjustment should not be necessary for patients with creatinine clearance (Ccr) of 15 mL/min or greater.

Zidovudine Pharmacokinetic Parameters in Patients With Severe Renal Function Impairment[a]

Parameter	Control subjects (healthy renal function) (n = 6)	Patients with renal function impairment (n = 14)
Ccr (mL/min)	120 ± 8	18 ± 2
Zidovudine AUC (ng•h/mL)	1,400 ± 200	3,100 ± 300
Zidovudine half-life (h)	1 ± 0.2	1.4 ± 0.1

[a] Data are expressed as mean ± SD.

The pharmacokinetics and tolerance of zidovudine were evaluated in a multiple-dose study in patients undergoing hemodialysis (n = 5) or peritoneal dialysis (n = 6) receiving escalating doses up to 200 mg 5 times daily for 8 weeks. Daily doses of 500 mg or less were well tolerated despite significantly elevated GZDV plasma concentrations. Apparent zidovudine oral clearance was approximately 50% of that reported in patients with healthy renal function. Hemodialysis and peritoneal dialysis appeared to have a negligible effect on the removal of zidovudine, whereas GZDV elimination was enhanced. A dosage adjustment is recommended for patients undergoing hemodialysis or peritoneal dialysis.

Hepatic function impairment: Data describing the effect of hepatic function impairment on the pharmacokinetics of zidovudine are limited. However, because zidovudine is eliminated primarily by hepatic metabolism, it is expected that zidovudine clearance would be decreased and plasma concentrations would be increased following administration of the recommended adult doses to patients with hepatic function impairment.

Children:

Zidovudine Pharmacokinetic Parameters in Children[a]

Parameter	Birth to 14 days of age	14 days to 3 months of age	3 months to 12 years of age
Oral bioavailability (%)	89 ± 19 (n = 15)	61 ± 19 (n = 17)	65 ± 24 (n = 18)
CSF:plasma ratio	no data	no data	0.68 [0.03 to 3.25][b] (n = 38)
Clearance (L/h/kg)	0.65 ± 0.29 (n = 18)	1.14 ± 0.24 (n = 16)	1.85 ± 0.47 (n = 20)
Elimination half-life (h)	3.1 ± 1.2 (n = 21)	1.9 ± 0.7 (n = 18)	1.5 ± 0.7 (n = 21)

[a] Data presented as mean ± SD except where noted.
[b] Median (range).

➤*Microbiology:*

Antiviral activity – The antiviral activity of zidovudine against HIV-1 was assessed in a number of cell lines (including monocytes and fresh human peripheral blood lymphocytes). The median effective concentration (EC_{50}) and EC_{90} values for zidovudine were 0.01 to 0.49 mcM (1 mcM = 0.27 mcg/mL) and 0.1 to 9 mcM, respectively. HIV from therapy-naive subjects with no mutations associated with resistance gave median EC_{50} values of 0.011 mcM (range, 0.005 to 0.11 mcM) from Virco (n = 93 baseline samples from COLA40263) and 0.02 mcM (0.01 to 0.03 mcM) from Monogram Biosciences (n = 135 baseline samples from ESS30009). The EC_{50} values of zidovudine against different HIV-1 clades (A-G) ranged from 0.00018 to 0.02 mcM, and against HIV-2 isolates from 0.00049 to 0.004 mcM. In cell culture drug combination studies, zidovudine demonstrates synergistic activity with the nucleoside reverse transcriptase inhibitors (NRTIs) abacavir, didanosine, lamivudine, and zalcitabine; the nonnucleoside reverse transcriptase inhibitors (NNRTIs) delavirdine and nevirapine; and the protease inhibitors indinavir, nelfinavir, ritonavir, and saquinavir; and additive activity with interferon alfa. Ribavirin has been found to inhibit the phosphorylation of zidovudine in cell culture.

Resistance – Genotypic analyses of the isolates selected in cell culture and recovered from zidovudine-treated patients showed mutations in the HIV-1 RT gene resulting in 6 amino acid substitutions (M41L, D67N, K70R, L210W, T215Y or F, and K219Q) that confer zidovudine resistance. In general, higher levels of resistance were associated with a greater number of mutations. In some patients harboring zidovudine-resistant virus at baseline, phenotypic sensitivity to zidovudine was restored by 12 weeks of treatment with lamivudine and zidovudine. Combination therapy with lamivudine plus zidovudine delayed the emergence of mutations conferring resistance to zidovudine.

Cross-resistance – In a study of 167 HIV-infected patients, isolates (n = 2) with multidrug resistance to didanosine, lamivudine, stavudine, zalcitabine, and zidovudine were recovered from patients treated for 1 year or more with zidovudine plus didanosine or zidovudine plus zalcitabine. The pattern of resistance-associated mutations with such combination therapies was different (A62V, V75I, F77L, F116Y, Q151M) from the pattern with zidovudine monotherapy, with the Q151M mutation being most commonly associated with multidrug resistance. The mutation at codon 151 in combination with mutations at 62, 75, 77, and 116 results in a virus with reduced susceptibility to didanosine, lamivudine, stavudine, zalcitabine, and zidovudine. Thymidine analogue mutations are selected by zidovudine and confer cross-resistance to abacavir, didanosine, stavudine, tenofovir, and zalcitabine.

Contraindications

Potentially life-threatening allergic reactions to any of the components of the formulations.

Warnings/Precautions

➤*Combination products:* Lamivudine plus zidovudine (*Combivir*) and abacavir plus lamivudine plus zidovudine (*Trizivir*) are combination product tablets that contain zidovudine as one of their components. Do not coadminister zidovudine with these combinations.

➤*Bone marrow suppression:* Use zidovudine with caution in patients who have bone marrow compromise evidenced by granulocyte count less than 1,000 cells/mm^3 or hemoglobin less than 9.5 g/dL. In patients with advanced symptomatic HIV disease, anemia and neutropenia were the most significant adverse reactions observed. There have been reports of pancytopenia associated with the use of zidovudine, which was reversible in most instances after discontinuance of the drug. However, significant anemia, in many cases requiring dose adjustment, discontinuation of zidovudine, and/or blood transfusions has occurred during treatment with zidovudine alone or in combination with other antiretrovirals.

Frequent blood counts are strongly recommended in patients with advanced HIV disease who are treated with zidovudine. For HIV-infected persons and patients with asymptomatic or early HIV disease, periodic blood cell counts are recommended. If anemia or neutropenia develops, dosage adjustments may be necessary.

➤*Myopathy:* Myopathy and myositis with pathological changes, similar to that produced by HIV disease, have been associated with prolonged use of zidovudine.

➤*Lactic acidosis/severe hepatomegaly with steatosis:* Lactic acidosis and severe hepatomegaly with steatosis, including fatal cases, have been reported with the use of nucleoside analogues alone or in combination, including zidovudine and other antiretrovirals. A majority of these cases

ZIDOVUDINE — ORAL

have been in women. Obesity and prolonged exposure to antiretroviral nucleoside analogues may be risk factors. Exercise particular caution when administering zidovudine to any patient with known risk factors for liver disease; however, cases have also been reported in patients with no known risk factors. Suspend treatment with zidovudine in any patient who develops clinical or laboratory findings suggestive of lactic acidosis or pronounced hepatotoxicity (which may include hepatomegaly and steatosis even in the absence of marked transaminase elevations).

➤*Immune reconstitution syndrome:* Immune reconstitution syndrome has been reported in patients treated with combination antiretroviral therapy including zidovudine. During the initial phase of combination antiretroviral treatment, patients whose immune system responds may develop an inflammatory response to indolent or residual opportunistic infections (such as *Mycobacterium avium* infection, cytomegalovirus, *Pneumocystis jirovecii* pneumonia [PCP], or tuberculosis), which may necessitate further evaluation and treatment.

➤*Fat redistribution:* Redistribution/accumulation of body fat, including central obesity, dorsocervical fat enlargement (buffalo hump), peripheral wasting, facial wasting, breast enlargement, and "cushingoid appearance," have been observed in patients receiving antiretroviral therapy. The mechanism and long-term consequences of these events are currently unknown. A causal relationship has not been established.

➤*Renal/Hepatic function impairment:* Zidovudine is eliminated from the body primarily by renal excretion following metabolism in the liver (glucuronidation). In patients with severe renal function impairment (Ccr less than 15 mL/min), dosage reduction is recommended. Although the data are limited, zidovudine concentrations appear to be increased in patients with severe hepatic function impairment that may increase the risk of hematologic toxicity.

➤*Pregnancy: Category C.* Oral teratology studies in the rat and in the rabbit at doses up to 500 mg/kg/day revealed no evidence of teratogenicity with zidovudine. Zidovudine treatment resulted in embryo/fetal toxicity as evidenced by an increase in the incidence of fetal resorptions in rats given 150 or 450 mg/kg/day and rabbits given 500 mg/kg/day. The doses used in the teratology studies resulted in peak zidovudine plasma concentrations (after one half of the daily dose) in rats 66 to 226 times, and in rabbits 12 to 87 times, mean steady-state peak human plasma concentrations (after one sixth of the daily dose) achieved with the recommended daily dosage (100 mg every 4 hours). In an in vitro experiment with fertilized mouse oocytes, zidovudine exposure resulted in a dose-dependent reduction in blastocyst formation. In an additional teratology study in rats, a dose of 3,000 mg/kg/day (very near the oral median lethal dose in rats of 3,683 mg/kg) caused marked maternal toxicity and an increase in the incidence of fetal malformations. This dose resulted in peak zidovudine plasma concentrations 350 times peak human plasma concentrations. (Estimated AUC in rats at this dose level was 300 times the daily AUC in humans given 600 mg/day.) No evidence of teratogenicity was seen in this experiment at doses of 600 mg/kg/day or less.

A randomized, double-blind, placebo-controlled trial was conducted in HIV-infected pregnant women to determine the utility of zidovudine for the prevention of maternal-fetal HIV-transmission. Congenital abnormalities occurred with similar frequency between neonates born to mothers who received zidovudine and neonates born to mothers who received placebo. Abnormalities were either problems in embryogenesis (prior to 14 weeks) or were recognized on ultrasound before or immediately after initiation of study drug.

Antiretroviral pregnancy registry – To monitor maternal-fetal outcomes of pregnant women exposed to zidovudine, an antiretroviral pregnancy registry has been established. Health care providers are encouraged to register patients by calling 1-800-258-4263.

➤*Lactation:* The Centers for Disease Control and Prevention (CDC) recommend that HIV-infected mothers not breast-feed their infants to avoid risking postnatal transmission of HIV. Zidovudine is excreted in human milk. Because of both the potential for HIV transmission and the potential for serious adverse reactions in breast-feeding infants, instruct mothers not to breast-feed if they are receiving zidovudine.

➤*Children:* Zidovudine has been studied in HIV-infected children older than 3 months of age who had HIV-related symptoms or who were asymptomatic with abnormal laboratory values indicating significant HIV-related immunosuppression. Zidovudine has also been studied in neonates perinatally exposed to HIV.

➤*Elderly:* In general, dose selection for an elderly patient should be cautious, reflecting the greater frequency of decreased hepatic, renal, or cardiac function, and of concomitant disease or other drug therapy.

➤*Monitoring:* The incidence of adverse reactions appears to increase with disease progression; monitor patients carefully, especially as disease progression occurs.

Hematologic toxicities appear to be related to pretreatment bone marrow reserve and to dose and duration of therapy. In patients with poor bone marrow reserve, particularly in patients with advanced symptomatic HIV disease, frequent monitoring of hematologic indices is recommended to detect serious anemia or neutropenia. In patients who experience hematologic toxicity, reduction in hemoglobin may occur as early as 2 to 4 weeks, and neutropenia usually occurs after 6 to 8 weeks.

Drug Interactions

Zidovudine Drug Interactions

Precipitant drug	Object drug[a]		Description
Atovaquone	Zidovudine	↑	Atovaquone appears to inhibit glucuronidation of zidovudine, thus increasing zidovudine concentrations and increasing the risk of zidovudine toxicity.
Doxorubicin	Zidovudine	↓	Avoid coadministration. An antagonistic relationship has been demonstrated.
Fluconazole	Zidovudine	↑	Concurrent use may increase the zidovudine AUC. Consider zidovudine dose reduction in patients experiencing pronounced anemia or other severe zidovudine-associated reactions.
Ganciclovir	Zidovudine	↑	Concomitant use may increase zidovudine plasma levels and AUC, thus increasing risk of life-threatening hematologic toxicities. Avoid coadministration.
Methadone	Zidovudine	↑	Zidovudine serum concentrations and AUC may be elevated, increasing the risk of side effects.
Nelfinavir/ Ritonavir	Zidovudine	↓	Zidovudine AUC is decreased.
Probenecid	Zidovudine	↑	Probenecid may increase zidovudine AUC by inhibiting glucuronidation or reducing renal excretion. Some patients have developed symptoms consisting of myalgia, malaise or fever, and maculopapular rash.
Ribavirin	Zidovudine	↑	Ribavirin can reduce phosphorylation of zidovudine. Cases of hepatic decompensation (some fatal) have occurred in HIV/hepatitis C virus coinfected patients receiving this combination.
Rifamycins	Zidovudine	↓	The AUC of zidovudine may be decreased.
Stavudine, ribavirin	Zidovudine	↓	Avoid concomitant use because some nucleoside analogs affect viral replication and may antagonize antiviral activity of zidovudine against HIV.
Valproic acid	Zidovudine	↑	Concurrent use may inhibit glucuronide metabolism, thus increasing zidovudine AUC. Consider zidovudine dose reduction in patients experiencing pronounced anemia or other severe zidovudine-associated reactions.
Zidovudine	Phenytoin	↔	Phenytoin levels have been reported to increase, decrease, or not change with concurrent use. In addition, zidovudine clearance was decreased by phenytoin.
Phenytoin	Zidovudine	↑	

[a] ↑ = object drug increased; ↓ = object drug decreased; ↔ = undetermined clinical effect.

➤*Drug/Food interactions:* The extent of zidovudine absorption (AUC) was similar when a single dose of zidovudine was administered with food.

Adverse Reactions

➤*Adults:* The frequency and severity of adverse reactions associated with the use of zidovudine are greater in patients with more advanced infection at the time of initiation of therapy. The following table summarizes reactions reported at a statistically significant greater incidence for patients receiving zidovudine in a monotherapy study.

Zidovudine Adverse Reactions (≥ 5%)

Adverse reaction	Zidovudine 500 mg/day (n = 453)	Placebo (n = 428)
GI		
Anorexia	20.1%	10.5%
Constipation	6.4%[a]	3.5%
Nausea	51.4%	29.9%

ZIDOVUDINE — ORAL

Zidovudine Adverse Reactions (≥ 5%)		
Adverse reaction	Zidovudine 500 mg/day (n = 453)	Placebo (n = 428)
Vomiting	17.2%	9.8%
Miscellaneous		
Asthenia	8.6%[a]	5.8%
Headache	62.5%	52.6%
Malaise	53.2%	44.9%

[a] Not statistically significant versus placebo.

Selected laboratory abnormalities observed during a clinical study of monotherapy with zidovudine are shown in the following table.

Zidovudine Laboratory Abnormalities		
Adverse reaction	Zidovudine 500 mg/day (n = 453)	Placebo (n = 428)
Anemia (Hgb[a] < 8 g/dL)	1.1%	0.2%
Granulocytopenia (< 750 cells/mm³)	1.8%	1.6%
Thrombocytopenia (platelets < 50,000/mm³)	0%	0.5%
ALT (> 5 × ULN[b])	3.1%	2.6%
AST (> 5 × ULN)	0.9%	1.6%
Alkaline phosphatase (> 5 × ULN)	0%	0%

[a] Hgb = hemoglobin.
[b] ULN = upper limit of normal.

➤*Other adverse reactions:*

CNS – Fatigue, insomnia.

GI – Abdominal cramps, abdominal pain, dyspepsia.

Musculoskeletal – Arthralgia, musculoskeletal pain, myalgia.

Miscellaneous – Chills, hyperbilirubinemia, neuropathy.

➤*Children:* Selected clinical adverse reactions and physical findings with a frequency of at least 5% during therapy with lamivudine 4 mg/kg twice daily plus zidovudine 160 mg/m² 3 times daily compared with didanosine in therapy-naive (56 or fewer days of antiretroviral therapy) children are listed in the following table.

Zidovudine Adverse Reactions (≥ 5%) in Children		
Adverse reaction	Lamivudine plus zidovudine (n = 236)	Didanosine (n = 235)
GI		
Diarrhea	8%	6%
Hepatomegaly	11%	11%
Nausea/Vomiting	8%	7%
Splenomegaly	5%	8%
Stomatitis	6%	12%
Respiratory		
Abnormal breath sounds/wheezing	7%	9%
Cough	15%	18%
Special senses		
Nasal discharge or congestion	8%	11%
Signs or symptoms of ears[a]	7%	6%
Miscellaneous		
Fever	25%	32%
Lymphadenopathy	9%	11%
Skin rashes	12%	14%

[a] Includes discharge, erythema, pain, or swelling of an ear.

Lab test abnormalities – Selected laboratory abnormalities experienced by therapy-naive (56 or fewer days of antiretroviral therapy) children are listed in the following table.

Zidovudine Laboratory Abnormalities in Children		
Adverse reaction	Lamivudine plus zidovudine	Didanosine
Neutropenia (ANC[a] < 400 cells/mm³)	8%	3%
Anemia (Hgb < 7 g/dL)	4%	2%
Thrombocytopenia (platelets < 50,000/mm³)	1%	3%
ALT (> 10 × ULN)	1%	3%
AST (> 10 × ULN)	2%	4%
Lipase (> 2.5 × ULN)	3%	3%
Total amylase (> 2.5 × ULN)	3%	3%

[a] ANC = absolute neutrophil count.

➤*Other adverse reactions:*

Cardiovascular – Congestive heart failure, electrocardiogram abnormality, left ventricular dilation.

CNS – Decreased reflexes, nervousness/irritability.

GU – Hematuria.

Hematologic – Macrocytosis.

Miscellaneous – Edema, weight loss. The clinical adverse reactions reported among adult recipients of zidovudine may also occur in children.

➤*Maternal-fetal transmission of HIV:* In a randomized, double-blind, placebo-controlled trial in HIV-infected women and their neonates conducted to determine the utility of zidovudine for the prevention of maternal-fetal HIV transmission, zidovudine 2 mg/kg syrup was administered every 6 hours for 6 weeks to neonates beginning within 12 hours following birth. The most commonly reported adverse reactions were anemia (hemoglobin less than 9 g/dL) and neutropenia (less than 1,000 cells/mm³). Anemia occurred in 22% of the neonates who received zidovudine and in 12% of the neonates who received placebo. The mean difference in hemoglobin values was less than 1 g/dL for neonates receiving zidovudine compared with neonates receiving placebo. No neonates with anemia required transfusion and all hemoglobin values spontaneously returned to normal within 6 weeks after completion of therapy with zidovudine. Neutropenia was reported with similar frequency in the group that received zidovudine (21%) and in the group that received placebo (27%). The long-term consequences of in utero and infant exposure to zidovudine are unknown.

➤*Postmarketing:*

Cardiovascular – Cardiomyopathy, syncope.

CNS – Anxiety, confusion, depression, dizziness, loss of mental acuity, mania, paresthesia, seizures, somnolence, vertigo.

Dermatologic – Changes in skin and nail pigmentation, pruritus, rash, Stevens-Johnson syndrome, sweat, toxic epidermal necrolysis, urticaria.

Endocrine – Gynecomastia.

GI – Constipation, dysphagia, flatulence, mouth ulcer, oral mucosa pigmentation.

GU – Urinary frequency, urinary hesitancy.

Hematologic/Lymphatic – Aplastic anemia, hemolytic anemia, leukopenia, lymphadenopathy, pancytopenia with marrow hypoplasia, pure red cell aplasia.

Hepatic – Hepatitis, hepatomegaly with steatosis, jaundice, lactic acidosis, pancreatitis.

Lab test abnormalities – Increased creatine phosphokinase, increased lactate dehydrogenase.

Musculoskeletal – Back pain, muscle spasm, myopathy and myositis with pathological changes (similar to that produced by HIV disease), rhabdomyolysis, tremor.

Respiratory – Cough, dyspnea, rhinitis, sinusitis.

Special senses – Amblyopia, hearing loss, macular edema, photophobia, taste perversion.

Miscellaneous – Breast enlargement, chest pain, flu-like syndrome, generalized pain, sensitization reactions including anaphylaxis and angioedema, vasculitis. Redistribution/accumulation of body fat, including central obesity, dorsocervical fat enlargement (buffalo hump), facial wasting, peripheral wasting, and "cushingoid appearance," have been observed in patients receiving antiretroviral therapy.

Overdosage

➤*Symptoms:* Acute overdoses of zidovudine have been reported in children and adults. These involved exposures up to 50 g. No specific symptoms or signs have been identified following acute overdosage with zidovudine apart from those listed as adverse reactions (eg, fatigue, headache, vomiting, occasional reports of hematological disturbances). All patients recovered without permanent sequelae.

➤*Treatment:* Hemodialysis and peritoneal dialysis appear to have a negligible effect on the removal of zidovudine while elimination of its primary metabolite, GZDV, is enhanced.

Patient Information

Zidovudine is not a cure for HIV infection, and patients may continue to acquire illnesses associated with HIV infection, including opportunistic infections. Therefore, advise patients to seek medical care for any significant change in their health status.

The safety and efficacy of zidovudine in women, IV drug users, and racial minorities is not significantly different than that observed in white men.

ZIDOVUDINE — ORAL

Inform patients that the major toxicities of zidovudine are neutropenia and/or anemia. The frequency and severity of these toxicities are greater in patients with more advanced disease and in those who initiate therapy later in the course of their infection. They should be told that if toxicity develops, they may require transfusions or dose modifications, including possible drug discontinuation. They should be told of the extreme importance of having their blood cell counts followed closely while on therapy, especially for patients with advanced symptomatic HIV disease. Caution them about the use of other medications, including ganciclovir and interferon alpha, that may exacerbate the toxicity of zidovudine. Inform patients that other adverse reactions of zidovudine include nausea and vomiting. Also encourage patients to contact their health care provider if they experience muscle weakness, shortness of breath, symptoms of hepatitis or pancreatitis, or any other unexpected adverse reactions while being treated with zidovudine.

Zidovudine tablets, capsules, and syrup are for oral ingestion only. Tell patients of the importance of taking zidovudine exactly as prescribed. Tell them not to share medication and not to exceed the recommended dose. Tell patients that the long-term effects of zidovudine are unknown at this time.

Advise pregnant women considering the use of zidovudine during pregnancy for prevention of HIV-transmission to their infants that transmission may still occur in some cases despite therapy. The long-term consequences of in utero and infant exposure to zidovudine are unknown, including the possible risk of cancer.

Advise HIV-infected pregnant women not to breast-feed to avoid postnatal transmission of HIV to a child who may not yet be infected.

Advise patients that therapy with zidovudine has not been shown to reduce the risk of transmission of HIV to others through sexual contact or blood contamination.

Inform patients that redistribution or accumulation of body fat may occur in patients receiving antiretroviral therapy and that the cause and long-term health effects of these conditions are not known at this time.

ZIDOVUDINE — INJECTION

WARNING

Zidovudine has been associated with hematologic toxicity, including neutropenia and severe anemia, particularly in patients with advanced HIV disease. Prolonged use of zidovudine has been associated with symptomatic myopathy.

Lactic acidosis and severe hepatomegaly with steatosis, including fatal cases, have been reported with the use of nucleoside analogues alone or in combination, including zidovudine and other antiretrovirals.

Indications

➤*HIV infection:* For the treatment of HIV infection in combination with other antiretroviral agents.

➤*Maternal-fetal HIV transmission:* For the prevention of maternal-fetal HIV transmission as part of a regimen that includes oral zidovudine beginning between 14 and 34 weeks of gestation, zidovudine intravenous (IV) during labor, and administration of zidovudine syrup to the neonate after birth. The efficacy of this regimen for preventing HIV transmission in women who have received zidovudine for a prolonged period before pregnancy has not been evaluated. The safety of zidovudine for the mother or fetus during the first trimester of pregnancy has not been assessed.

Administration and Dosage

➤*General dosing considerations:* Patients should receive zidovudine IV infusion only until oral therapy can be administered. The IV dosing regimen equivalent to the oral administration of 100 mg every 4 hours is approximately 1 mg/kg IV every 4 hours.

➤*Adults:*

HIV infection – 1 mg/kg infused over 1 hour. This dose should be administered 5 to 6 times daily (5 to 6 mg/kg daily).

Prevention of maternal-fetal HIV transmission – 100 mg orally 5 times/day until labor starts. During labor and delivery, IV zidovudine should be administered at 2 mg/kg (total body weight) over 1 hour, followed by a continuous IV infusion of 1 mg/kg/h (total body weight) until clamping of the umbilical cord occurs.

➤*Children:*

Prevention of maternal-fetal HIV transmission – The recommended dosage regimens for administration to pregnant women (greater than 14 weeks of pregnancy) and their neonates are as follows.

Maternal: 100 mg orally 5 times per day until the start of labor. During labor and delivery, intravenous zidovudine should be administered at 2 mg/kg (total body weight) over 1 hour followed by a continuous intravenous infusion of 1 mg/kg/hour (total body weight) until clamping of the umbilical cord.

Neonates: 2 mg/kg orally every 6 hours, starting within 12 hours of birth and continuing through 6 weeks of age. Neonates unable to receive oral dosing may be administered zidovudine IV at 1.5 mg/kg, infused over 30 minutes, every 6 hours.

➤*Renal function impairment:* In patients maintained on hemodialysis or peritoneal dialysis (creatinine clearance [CrCl] less than 15 mL/min), recommended dosing is 1 mg/kg every 6 to 8 hours.

➤*Hepatic function impairment:* There are insufficient data to recommend dose adjustment of zidovudine in patients with mild to moderate impaired hepatic function or liver cirrhosis. Because zidovudine is eliminated primarily by hepatic metabolism, a reduction in the daily dose may be necessary in these patients. Frequent monitoring of hematologic toxicities is advised.

➤*Patients with hematologic abnormalities:* Significant anemia (hemoglobin less than 7.5 g/dL or reduction of more than 25% from baseline) and/or significant neutropenia (granulocyte count less than 750 cells/mm^3 or reduction of more than 50% from baseline) may require a dose interruption until evidence of marrow recovery is observed. In patients who develop significant anemia, dose interruption does not necessarily eliminate the need for transfusion. If marrow recovery occurs following dose interruption, resumption of dose may be appropriate, using adjunctive measures such as epoetin alfa at recommended doses, depending on hematologic indices such as serum erythropoietin level and patient tolerance.

For patients experiencing pronounced anemia while receiving chronic coadministration of zidovudine and some of the drugs (eg, fluconazole, valproic acid) listed in drug interactions, zidovudine dose reduction may be considered.

➤*Preparation for administration:* Zidovudine is considered a potential mutagen. Follow safe handling procedures when preparing, administering, or dispensing zidovudine.

Zidovudine IV infusion must be diluted prior to administration. The calculated dose should be removed from the 20 mL vial and added to dextrose 5% injection solution in order to achieve a concentration of no more than 4 mg/mL.

If particulate matter or discoloration is observed, the solution should be discarded, and a fresh solution should be prepared.

➤*Administration:* Zidovudine IV infusion is administered IV at a constant rate over 1 hour. Rapid infusion or bolus injection should be avoided. Zidovudine IV infusion should not be given intramuscularly.

➤*Admixture compatibility:*

Compatibility – Zidovudine is compatible with dextrose 5% injection.

Incompatibility – Admixture in biologic or colloidal fluids (eg, blood products, protein solutions) is not recommended.

To screen for specific compatibilities, see *Trissel's IV-Chek*.

➤*Storage/Stability:* Store vials at 15° to 25°C (59° to 77°F) and protect from light.

After dilution, the solution is physically and chemically stable for 24 hours at room temperature and 48 hours if refrigerated at 2° to 8°C (36° to 46°F). Care should be taken during admixture to prevent inadvertent contamination. As an additional precaution, the diluted solution should be administered within 8 hours if stored at 25°C (77°F) or 24 hours if refrigerated at 2° to 8°C (36° to 46°F) to minimize potential administration of a microbially contaminated solution.

Actions

➤*Pharmacology:* Zidovudine is a synthetic nucleoside analogue. Intracellularly, zidovudine is phosphorylated to its active 5'-triphosphate metabolite, zidovudine triphosphate (ZDV-TP). The principal mode of action of ZDV-TP is inhibition of reverse transcriptase via DNA chain termination after incorporation of the nucleotide analogue. ZDV-TP is a weak inhibitor of the cellular DNA polymerases α and γ and has been reported to be incorporated into the DNA of cells in culture.

➤*Pharmacokinetics:*

Absorption/Distribution – The pharmacokinetics of zidovudine have been evaluated in 22 adult HIV-infected patients in a phase 1 dose-escalation study. Following IV dosing, dose-independent kinetics was observed over the range of 1 to 5 mg/kg.

The mean steady-state peak and trough concentrations of zidovudine at 2.5 mg/kg every 4 hours were 1.06 and 0.12 mcg/mL, respectively.

The zidovudine cerebrospinal fluid (CSF)/plasma concentration ratio was determined in 39 patients receiving chronic therapy with zidovudine. The median ratio measured in 50 paired samples drawn 1 to 8 hours after the last dose of zidovudine was 0.6.

Zidovudine Pharmacokinetic Parameters Following IV Administration in HIV-Infected Patients

Parameter	Mean ± SD[a] (except where noted)
Apparent volume of distribution (L/kg)	1.6 ± 0.6 (n = 11)
Plasma protein binding (%)	< 38
CSF:plasma ratio[b]	0.6 [0.04 to 2.62] (n = 39)
Systemic clearance (L/h/kg)	1.6 (0.8 to 2.7) (n = 18)
Renal clearance (L/h/kg)	0.34 ± 0.05 (n = 16)
Elimination half-life (h)[c]	1.1 (0.5 to 2.9) (n = 19)

[a] SD = standard deviation.
[b] Median [range].
[c] Approximate range.

ZIDOVUDINE — INJECTION

Metabolism/Excretion – The major metabolite of zidovudine is 3'-azido-3'-deoxy-5'-O-β-D-glucopyranuronosylthymidine (GZDV). GZDV area under the curve (AUC) is about 3-fold greater than the zidovudine AUC. Urinary recovery of zidovudine and GZDV accounts for 18% and 60%, respectively, following IV dosing. A second metabolite, 3'-amino-3'-deoxythymidine (AMT), has been identified in the plasma following single-dose IV administration of zidovudine. The AMT AUC was one fifth of the zidovudine AUC.

Special populations –

Renal function impairment: Zidovudine clearance was decreased, resulting in increased zidovudine and GZDV half-life and AUC in patients with renal function impairment (n = 14) following a single 200 mg oral dose (see the following table). Plasma concentrations of AMT were not determined. A dose adjustment should not be necessary for patients with Ccr 15 mL/min or more.

Zidovudine Pharmacokinetic Parameters in Patients With Severe Renal Function Impairment[a]

Parameter	Control subjects (healthy renal function) (n = 6)	Patients with renal function impairment (n = 14)
Ccr (mL/min)	120 ± 8	18 ± 2
Zidovudine AUC (ng•h/mL)	1,400 ± 200	3,100 ± 300
Zidovudine half-life (h)	1 ± 0.2	1.4 ± 0.1

[a] Data are expressed as mean ± SD.

Hepatic function impairment: Data describing the effect of hepatic function impairment on the pharmacokinetics of zidovudine are limited. However, because zidovudine is eliminated primarily by hepatic metabolism, it is expected that zidovudine clearance would be decreased and plasma concentrations would be increased following administration of the recommended adult doses to patients with hepatic function impairment.

Children:

• *Patients younger than 3 months of age* – Zidovudine pharmacokinetics have been evaluated in children from birth to 3 months of age. Zidovudine elimination was determined immediately following birth in 8 neonates who were exposed to zidovudine in utero. The half-life was 13 ± 5.8 hours. In neonates 14 days old or younger, bioavailability was greater, total body clearance was slower, and half-life was longer than in children older than 14 days.

Zidovudine Pharmacokinetic Parameters in Children[a]

Parameter	Birth to 14 days of age	14 days to 3 months of age	3 months to 12 years of age
Oral bioavailability (%)	89 ± 19 (n = 15)	61 ± 19 (n = 17)	65 ± 24 (n = 18)
CSF:plasma ratio	no data	no data	0.26 ± 0.17[b] (n = 28)
CL (L/h/kg)	0.65 ± 0.29 (n = 18)	1.14 ± 0.24 (n = 16)	1.85 ± 0.47 (n = 20)
Elimination half-life (h)	3.1 ± 1.2 (n = 21)	1.9 ± 0.7 (n = 18)	1.5 ± 0.7 (n = 21)

[a] Data presented as mean ± SD except where noted.
[b] CSF ratio determined at steady state on constant IV infusion.

Contraindications

Potentially life-threatening allergic reactions to any component of the formulation.

Warnings/Precautions

➤*Combination products:* Lamivudine/zidovudine tablets and abacavir/lamivudine/zidovudine tablets are combination products that contain zidovudine as one of their components. Do not administer zidovudine concomitantly with lamivudine/zidovudine tablets or abacavir sulfate/lamivudine/zidovudine tablets.

➤*Bone marrow suppression:* Use zidovudine with caution in patients who have bone marrow compromise evidenced by a granulocyte count less than 1,000 cells/mm^3 or hemoglobin less than 9.5 g/dL. In patients with advanced symptomatic HIV disease, anemia and neutropenia were the most significant adverse reactions observed. There have been reports of pancytopenia associated with the use of zidovudine, which was reversible in most instances, after discontinuance of the drug. However, significant anemia, in many cases requiring dose adjustment, discontinuation of zidovudine, and/or blood transfusions, has occurred during treatment with zidovudine alone or in combination with other antiretrovirals.

Hematologic toxicities appear to be related to pretreatment bone marrow reserve and to dose and duration of therapy. In patients with poor bone marrow reserve, particularly in patients with advanced symptomatic HIV disease, frequent monitoring of hematologic indices is recommended to detect serious anemia or neutropenia. In patients who experience hematologic toxicity, reduction in hemoglobin may occur as early as 2 to 4 weeks, and neutropenia usually occurs after 6 to 8 weeks.

➤*Myopathy:* Myopathy and myositis with pathological changes, similar to that produced by HIV disease, have been associated with prolonged use of zidovudine.

➤*Lactic acidosis/severe hepatomegaly with steatosis:* Lactic acidosis and severe hepatomegaly with steatosis, including fatal cases, have been reported with the use of nucleoside analogues alone or in combination, including zidovudine and other antiretrovirals. A majority of these cases have been in women. Obesity and prolonged exposure to antiretroviral nucleoside analogues may be risk factors. Exercise particular caution when administering zidovudine to any patient with known risk factors for liver disease; however, cases have also been reported in patients with no known risk factors. Suspend treatment with zidovudine in any patient who develops clinical or laboratory findings suggestive of lactic acidosis or pronounced hepatotoxicity (which may include hepatomegaly and steatosis even in the absence of marked transaminase elevations).

➤*Immune reconstitution syndrome:* Immune reconstitution syndrome has been reported in patients treated with combination antiretroviral therapy, including zidovudine. During the initial phase of combination antiretroviral treatment, patients whose immune system responds may develop an inflammatory response to indolent or residual opportunistic infections (such as *Mycobacterium avium* infection, cytomegalovirus, *Pneumocystis jirovecii* pneumonia [PCP], or tuberculosis), which may necessitate further evaluation and treatment.

➤*Renal/Hepatic function impairment:* Zidovudine is eliminated from the body primarily by renal excretion following metabolism in the liver (glucuronidation).

See Administration and Dosage for more information.

➤*Pregnancy: Category C.* Oral teratology studies in the rat and in the rabbit at doses up to 500 mg/kg/day revealed no evidence of teratogenicity with zidovudine. Zidovudine treatment resulted in embryo/fetal toxicity as evidenced by an increase in the incidence of fetal resorptions in rats given 150 or 450 mg/kg/day and rabbits given 500 mg/kg/day. The doses used in the teratology studies resulted in peak zidovudine plasma concentrations (after one half of the daily dose) in rats 66 to 226 times, and in rabbits 12 to 87 times, mean steady-state peak human plasma concentrations (after one sixth of the daily dose) achieved with the recommended daily dose (100 mg every 4 hours). In an in vitro experiment with fertilized mouse oocytes, zidovudine exposure resulted in a dose-dependent reduction in blastocyst formation. In an additional teratology study in rats, a dose of 3,000 mg/kg/day (very near the oral median lethal dose in rats of 3,683 mg/kg) caused marked maternal toxicity and an increase in the incidence of fetal malformations. This dose resulted in peak zidovudine plasma concentrations 350 times peak human plasma concentrations. (Estimated AUC in rats at this dose level was 300 times the daily AUC in humans given 600 mg per day.) No evidence of teratogenicity was seen in this experiment at doses of 600 mg/kg/day or less.

A randomized, double-blind, placebo-controlled trial was conducted in HIV-infected pregnant women to determine the utility of zidovudine for the prevention of maternal-fetal HIV transmission. Congenital abnormalities occurred with similar frequency between neonates born to mothers who received zidovudine and neonates born to mothers who received placebo. Abnormalities were either problems in embryogenesis (prior to 14 weeks) or were recognized on ultrasound before or immediately after initiation of study drug.

Antiretroviral pregnancy registry – To monitor maternal-fetal outcomes of pregnant women exposed to zidovudine, an antiretroviral pregnancy registry has been established. Health care providers are encouraged to register patients by calling 1-800-258-4263.

➤*Lactation:* The Centers for Disease Control and Prevention recommend that HIV-infected mothers not breast-feed their infants to avoid risking postnatal transmission of HIV.

Zidovudine is excreted in human milk. Because of both the potential for HIV transmission and the potential for serious adverse reactions in breast-feeding infants, instruct mothers not to breast-feed if they are receiving zidovudine.

➤*Elderly:* In general, dose selection for an elderly patient should be cautious, reflecting the greater frequency of decreased hepatic, renal, or cardiac function, and of concomitant disease or other drug therapy.

➤*Monitoring:* Frequent blood counts are strongly recommended in patients with advanced HIV disease who are treated with zidovudine. For HIV-infected individuals and patients with asymptomatic or early HIV disease, periodic blood counts are recommended. Significant anemia (hemoglobin less than 7.5 g/dL or reduction of more than 25% of baseline) and/or significant neutropenia (granulocyte count less than 750 cells/mm^3 or reduction of more than 50% from baseline) may require a dose interruption until evidence of marrow recovery is observed.

Closely monitor patients receiving interferon alfa with or without ribavirin and zidovudine for treatment-associated toxicities, especially hepatic decompensation, neutropenia, and anemia. Consider discontinuation of zidovudine medically appropriate. Also consider dose reduction or discontinuation of interferon alfa, ribavirin, or both if worsening clinical toxicities are observed, including hepatic decompensation (eg, Childs-Pugh more than 6).

The incidence of adverse reactions appears to increase with disease progression; monitor patients carefully, especially as disease progression occurs.

Drug Interactions

➤*Interferon- and ribavirin-based regimens:* In vitro studies have shown ribavirin can reduce the phosphorylation of pyrimidine nucleoside analogues such as zidovudine. Although no evidence of a pharmacokinetic or pharmacodynamic interaction (eg, loss of HIV/hepatitis C virus [HCV] virologic suppression) was seen when ribavirin was coadministered with zidovudine in HIV/HCV co-infected patients, hepatic decompensation (some fatal)

ZIDOVUDINE — INJECTION

has occurred in HIV/HCV coinfected patients receiving combination antiretroviral therapy for HIV and interferon alfa with or without ribavirin.

Zidovudine Drug Interactions

Precipitant drug	Object drug[a]		Description
Atovaquone	Zidovudine	↑	Atovaquone appears to inhibit glucuronidation of zidovudine, thus increasing zidovudine concentrations and decreasing clearance.
Bone marrow suppressive/ cytotoxic agents (eg, interferon-alpha, interferon-beta-1b)	Zidovudine	↑	Coadministration may increase the hematologic toxicity of zidovudine.
Doxorubicin	Zidovudine	↓	Avoid coadministration. An antagonistic relationship has been demonstrated.
Fluconazole	Zidovudine	↑	Concurrent use may increase the zidovudine AUC. Zidovudine dose reduction may be considered.
Ganciclovir	Zidovudine	↑	Concomitant use may increase zidovudine plasma levels and AUC, thus increasing risk of life-threatening hematologic toxicities.
Methadone	Zidovudine	↑	Zidovudine serum concentrations and AUC may be elevated, increasing the risk of adverse reactions.
Nelfinavir/ Ritonavir	Zidovudine	↓	Zidovudine AUC is decreased.
Probenecid	Zidovudine	↑	Probenecid may increase zidovudine AUC by inhibiting glucuronidation or reducing renal excretion. Some patients have developed symptoms consisting of myalgia, malaise or fever, and maculopapular rash.
Rifamycins	Zidovudine	↓	The AUC of zidovudine may be decreased.
Stavudine, ribavirin	Zidovudine	↓	Avoid concomitant use because some nucleoside analogs affect viral replication and may antagonize antiviral activity of zidovudine against HIV.
Valproic acid	Zidovudine	↑	Concurrent use may inhibit glucuronide metabolism, thus increasing zidovudine AUC. Zidovudine dose reduction may be considered.
Zidovudine	Phenytoin	↔	Phenytoin levels have been reported to increase, decrease, or not change with concurrent use.
Phenytoin	Zidovudine	↑	In addition, zidovudine clearance was decreased by phenytoin.

[a] ↑ = object drug increased; ↓ = object drug decreased; ↔ = undetermined clinical effect.

➤*Drug/Food interactions:* The rate and extent of zidovudine absorption may be decreased by fatty meals. Administer zidovudine at least 1 hour before meals.

Adverse Reactions

The adverse reactions reported during administration of zidovudine IV infusion are similar to those reported with oral administration; neutropenia and anemia were reported most frequently. Long-term IV administration beyond 2 to 4 weeks has not been studied in adults and may enhance hematologic adverse reactions. Local reaction, pain, and slight irritation during IV administration occur infrequently.

➤*Adults:*

Zidovudine Adverse Reactions (≥ 5%)

Adverse reaction	Zidovudine (n = 453)	Placebo (n = 428)
CNS		
Asthenia	8.6%[a]	5.8%
Headache	62.5%	52.6%
Malaise	53.2%	44.9%
GI		
Anorexia	20.1%	10.5%
Constipation	6.4%[a]	3.5%
Nausea	51.4%	29.9%
Vomiting	17.2%	9.8%

[a] Not statistically significant vs placebo.

➤*Other adverse reactions:* In addition to the adverse reactions listed in the previous table, the following other adverse reactions were observed in clinical studies.

CNS – Fatigue, insomnia, neuropathy.

GI – Abdominal cramps, abdominal pain, dyspepsia.

Musculoskeletal – Arthralgia, musculoskeletal pain, myalgia.

Miscellaneous – Chills, hyperbilirubinemia.

Lab test abnormalities –

Zidovudine Laboratory Abnormalities (Grade 3/4)[a]

Adverse reaction	Zidovudine (n = 453)	Placebo (n = 428)
Anemia (Hb < 8 g/dL)	1.1%	0.2%
Granulocytopenia (< 750 cells/mm^3)	1.8%	1.6%
Thrombocytopenia (platelets < 50,000/mm^3)	0%	0.5%
ALT (> 5 × ULN)[a]	3.1%	2.6%
AST (> 5 × ULN)[a]	0.9%	1.6%
Alkaline phosphate (> 5 × ULN)	0%	0%

[a] Hb = hemoglobin; ULN = upper limit of normal.

➤*Children:*

Zidovudine Adverse Reactions in Children (≥ 5%)

Adverse reaction	Lamivudine plus zidovudine (n = 236)	Didanosine (n = 235)
Dermatologic		
Skin rashes	12%	14%
GI		
Diarrhea	8%	6%
Nausea and vomiting	8%	7%
Stomatitis	6%	12%
Respiratory		
Abnormal breathing sounds/ wheezing	7%	9%
Cough	15%	18%
Nasal discharge or congestion	8%	11%
Miscellaneous		
Fever	25%	32%
Hepatomegaly	11%	11%
Lymphadenopathy	9%	11%
Signs or symptoms of ears[a]	7%	6%
Splenomegaly	5%	8%

[a] Includes pain, discharge, erythema, or swelling of an ear.

Lab test abnormalities –

Zidovudine Laboratory Abnormalities (Grade 3/4) in Children

Adverse reaction	Lamivudine plus zidovudine	Didanosine
Neutropenia (ANC < 400 cells/mm^3)[a]	8%	3%
Anemia (Hb < 7.0 g/dL)	4%	2%
Thrombocytopenia (platelets < 50,000/mm^3)	1%	3%
ALT (> 10 × ULN)[b]	1%	3%
AST (> 10 × ULN)[b]	2%	4%
Lipase (> 2.5 × ULN)[b]	3%	3%
Total amylase (> 2.5 × ULN)[b]	3%	3%

[a] ANC = absolute neutrophil count
[b] ULN = upper limit of normal

ZIDOVUDINE — INJECTION

➤*Other adverse reactions:* Additional adverse reactions were reported in open-label studies in children receiving zidovudine 180 mg/m^2 every 6 hours.

Cardiovascular – Congestive heart failure, electrocardiogram abnormality, left ventricular dilation.

CNS – Decreased reflexes, nervousness/irritability.

Miscellaneous – Edema, hematuria, macrocytosis, weight loss.

➤*Zidovudine use for the prevention of maternal-fetal transmission of HIV:* In a randomized, double-blind, placebo-controlled trial in HIV-infected women and their neonates conducted to determine the utility of zidovudine for the prevention of maternal-fetal HIV transmission, zidovudine syrup at 2 mg/kg was administered every 6 hours for 6 weeks to neonates beginning within 12 hours following birth. The most commonly reported adverse reactions were anemia (hemoglobin less than 9 g/dL) and neutropenia (less than 1,000 cells/mm^3). Anemia occurred in 22% of the neonates who received zidovudine and in 12% of the neonates who received placebo. The mean difference in hemoglobin values was less than 1 g/dL for neonates receiving zidovudine compared with neonates receiving placebo. No neonates with anemia required transfusion and all hemoglobin values spontaneously returned to normal within 6 weeks after completion of therapy with zidovudine. Neutropenia was reported with similar frequency in the group that received zidovudine (21%) and in the group that received placebo (27%). The long-term consequences of in utero and infant exposure to zidovudine are unknown.

➤*Postmarketing:*

Cardiovascular – Cardiomyopathy, syncope.

CNS – Anxiety, confusion, depression, dizziness, loss of mental acuity, mania, paresthesia, seizures, somnolence, vertigo.

Dermatologic – Changes in skin and nail pigmentation, pruritus, rash, Stevens-Johnson syndrome, sweat, toxic epidermal necrolysis, urticaria.

Endocrine – Gynecomastia.

GI – Constipation, dysphagia, flatulence, mouth ulcer, oral mucosal pigmentation.

GU – Urinary frequency, urinary hesitancy.

Hematologic / Lymphatic – Aplastic anemia, hemolytic anemia, leukopenia, lymphadenopathy, pancytopenia with marrow hypoplasia, pure red cell aplasia.

Hepatic – Hepatitis, hepatomegaly with steatosis, jaundice, lactic acidosis, pancreatitis.

Hypersensitivity – Sensitization reactions including anaphylaxis and angioedema.

Musculoskeletal – Increased creatine phosphokinase, increased lactate dehydrogenase, muscle spasm, myopathy and myositis with pathological changes (similar to that produced by HIV disease), rhabdomyolysis, tremor.

Respiratory – Cough, dyspnea, rhinitis, sinusitis.

Special senses – Amblyopia, hearing loss, macular edema, photophobia, taste perversion.

Miscellaneous – Back pain, chest pain, flu-like syndrome, generalized pain, vasculitis.

Overdosage

➤*Symptoms:* No specific symptoms or signs have been identified following acute overdosage with zidovudine apart from those listed as adverse reactions such as fatigue, headache, vomiting, and occasional reports of hematological disturbances. All patients recovered without permanent sequelae.

➤*Treatment:* Hemodialysis and peritoneal dialysis appear to have a negligible effect on the removal of zidovudine, while elimination of its primary metabolite, GZDV, is enhanced.

Patient Information

Zidovudine is not a cure for HIV infection, and patients may continue to acquire illnesses associated with HIV infection, including opportunistic infections. Therefore, advise patients to seek medical care for any significant change in their health status.

The safety and efficacy of zidovudine in treating women, IV drug users, and racial minorities is not significantly different than that observed in white men.

Inform patients that the major toxicities of zidovudine are neutropenia and/or anemia. The frequency and severity of these toxicities are greater in patients with more advanced disease and in those who initiate therapy later in the course of their infection. Tell patients that if toxicity develops, they may require transfusions or drug discontinuation. Tell patients of the extreme importance of having their blood counts followed closely while on therapy, especially for patients with advanced symptomatic HIV disease. Caution them about the use of other medications, including ganciclovir and interferon alfa, which may exacerbate the toxicity of zidovudine. Inform patients that other adverse reactions of zidovudine include nausea and vomiting. Encourage patients to contact their health care providers if they experience muscle weakness, shortness of breath, symptoms of hepatitis or pancreatitis, or any other unexpected adverse reactions while being treated with zidovudine.

Advise pregnant women considering the use of zidovudine during pregnancy for prevention of HIV transmission to their infants that transmission may still occur in some cases despite therapy. The long-term consequences of in utero and neonatal exposure to zidovudine are unknown, including the possible risk of cancer.

Advise HIV-infected pregnant women not to breast-feed to avoid postnatal transmission of HIV to a child who may not yet be infected.

Advise patients that therapy with zidovudine has not been shown to reduce the risk of transmission of HIV to others through sexual contact or blood contamination.

ABACAVIR

Rx	**Ziagen** (ViiV Healthcare)	**Tablets; oral:** 300 mg	As abacavir sulfate. (GX 623). Yellow, capsule shape. Film-coated. In 60s and UD 60s.
		Solution; oral: 20 mg/mL	As abacavir sulfate. Parabens, saccharin, sorbitol. Strawberry-banana flavor. In 240 mL.

ABACAVIR SULFATE — ORAL

WARNING

Hypersensitivity reactions – Serious and sometimes fatal hypersensitivity reactions have been associated with abacavir therapy. Hypersensitivity to abacavir is a multiorgan clinical syndrome usually characterized by a sign or symptom in 2 or more of the following groups:

- constitutional, including achiness, fatigue, or generalized malaise;
- fever;
- GI, including abdominal pain, diarrhea, nausea, or vomiting;
- rash;
- respiratory, including cough, dyspnea, or pharyngitis.

Discontinue abacavir as soon as a hypersensitivity reaction is suspected.

Patients who carry the HLA-B*5701 allele are at high risk for experiencing a hypersensitivity reaction to abacavir. Prior to initiating therapy with abacavir, screening for the HLA-B*5701 allele is recommended; this approach has been found to decrease the risk of hypersensitivity reaction. Screening is also recommended prior to reinitiation of abacavir in patients of unknown HLA-B*5701 status who have previously tolerated abacavir. HLA-B*5701–negative patients may develop a suspected hypersensitivity reaction to abacavir; however, this occurs significantly less frequently than in HLA-B*5701–positive patients.

Regardless of HLA-B*5701 status, permanently discontinue abacavir if hypersensitivity cannot be ruled out, even when other diagnoses are possible.

Following a hypersensitivity reaction to abacavir, never restart abacavir or any abacavir-containing product because more severe symptoms can occur within hours and may include life-threatening hypotension and death.

WARNING (cont.)

Reintroduction of abacavir or any other abacavir-containing product, even in patients who have no identified history or unrecognized symptoms of hypersensitivity to abacavir therapy, can result in serious or fatal hypersensitivity reactions. Such reactions can occur within hours.

Lactic acidosis and severe hepatomegaly – Lactic acidosis and severe hepatomegaly with steatosis, including fatal cases, have been reported with the use of nucleoside analogs alone or in combination, including abacavir and other antiretrovirals.

Indications

➤*HIV infection:* For the treatment of HIV-1 infection, in combination with other antiretroviral agents.

Administration and Dosage

➤*General dosing considerations:* Abacavir should always be used in combination with other antiretroviral agents.

Dispense a Medication Guide and warning card that provide information about recognition of hypersensitivity reactions with each new prescription and refill. To facilitate reporting of hypersensitivity reactions and collection of information on each case, an abacavir hypersensitivity registry has been established. Health care providers should register patients by calling 1-800-270-0425.

➤*Adults:*

HIV infection – 600 mg daily, administered as 300 mg twice daily or 600 mg once daily, in combination with other antiretroviral agents.

ABACAVIR SULFATE — ORAL

➤*Children:*

HIV infection –

3 months to 16 years of age:

• *Usual dosage* – 8 mg/kg twice daily (up to a maximum of 300 mg twice daily) in combination with other antiretroviral agents.

• *Maximum dose* – 300 mg twice daily.

➤*Hepatic function impairment:*

Mild hepatic function impairment (Child-Pugh score 5 to 6) – 200 mg twice daily. To enable dose reduction, use abacavir oral solution (10 mL twice daily) for the treatment of these patients.

Moderate or severe hepatic function impairment – The safety, efficacy, and pharmacokinetic properties of abacavir have not been established in patients with moderate or severe hepatic function impairment; therefore, abacavir is contraindicated in these patients.

➤*Administration:* Abacavir may be taken with or without food.

➤*Storage/Stability:* Store tablets and oral solution at 20° to 25°C (68° to 77°F). Oral solution may be refrigerated; do not freeze.

Actions

➤*Pharmacology:* Abacavir is an antiviral agent classified as a carbocyclic synthetic nucleoside analog. Abacavir is converted by cellular enzymes to the active metabolite carbovir triphosphate, an analog of deoxyguanosine 5′-triphosphate (dGTP). Carbovir triphosphate inhibits the activity of HIV-1 reverse transcriptase (RT) by competing with the natural substrate dGTP and by its incorporation into viral DNA. The lack of a 3′-OH group in the incorporated nucleoside analog prevents the formation of the 5′ to 3′ phosphodiester linkage essential for DNA chain elongation and, therefore, the viral DNA growth is terminated. Abacavir is a weak inhibitor of cellular DNA polymerases alpha, beta, and gamma.

➤*Pharmacokinetics:*

Absorption –

Abacavir was rapidly and extensively absorbed after oral administration. The geometric mean absolute bioavailability of the tablet was 83%. After oral administration of 300 mg twice daily in 20 patients, the steady-state peak serum abacavir concentration (C_{max}) was 3 ± 0.89 mcg/mL (mean ± standard deviation [SD]) and area under the curve ($AUC_{0\text{-}12h}$) was 6.02 ± 1.73 mcg•h/mL. After oral administration of a single dose of abacavir 600 mg in 20 patients, C_{max} was 4.26 ± 1.19 mcg/mL (mean ± SD) and AUC_{∞} was 11.95 ± 2.51 mcg•h/mL.

Systemic exposure to abacavir was comparable after administration of abacavir oral solution and tablets. Therefore, these products may be used interchangeably.

Distribution – The apparent volume of distribution after intravenous (IV) administration of abacavir was 0.86 ± 0.15 L/kg, suggesting that abacavir distributes into extravascular space. In 3 subjects, the cerebrospinal fluid $AUC_{0\text{-}6h}$ to plasma abacavir $AUC_{0\text{-}6h}$ ratio ranged from 27% to 33%.

Binding of abacavir to human plasma proteins is approximately 50%. Binding of abacavir to plasma proteins was independent of concentration. Total blood and plasma drug-related radioactivity concentrations are identical, demonstrating that abacavir readily distributes into erythrocytes.

Metabolism – In humans, abacavir is not significantly metabolized by CYP-450 enzymes. The primary routes of elimination of abacavir are metabolism by alcohol dehydrogenase (to form the 5′-carboxylic acid) and glucuronyl transferase (to form the 5′-glucuronide). The metabolites do not have antiviral activity. In vitro experiments reveal that abacavir does not inhibit human CYP3A4, CYP2D6, or CYP2C9 activity at clinically relevant concentrations.

Excretion – Elimination of abacavir was quantified in a mass-balance study following administration of a ^{14}C-abacavir 600 mg dose as follows: 99% of the radioactivity was recovered; 1.2% was excreted in the urine as abacavir, 30% as the 5′-carboxylic acid metabolite, 36% as the 5′-glucuronide metabolite, and 15% as unidentified minor metabolites in the urine. Fecal elimination accounted for 16% of the dose.

In single-dose studies, the observed elimination half-life) was 1.54 ± 0.63 hours. After IV administration, total clearance was 0.8 ±0.24 L/h/kg (mean ± SD).

Special populations –

Hepatic function impairment: The pharmacokinetics of abacavir have been studied in patients with mild hepatic impairment (Child-Pugh score 5 to 6). Results show that there was a mean increase of 89% in the abacavir AUC, and an increase of 58% in the half-life of abacavir after a single dose of abacavir 600 mg. The AUCs of the metabolites were not modified by mild liver disease; however, the rates of formation and elimination of the metabolites were decreased. A dose of 200 mg (provided by 10 mL of abacavir oral solution) administered twice daily is recommended for patients with mild liver disease. The safety, efficacy, and pharmacokinetics of abacavir have not been studied in patients with moderate or severe hepatic impairment; therefore, abacavir is contraindicated in these patients.

Children: The pharmacokinetics of abacavir have been studied after single or repeat doses of abacavir in 68 children. Following multiple-dose administration of abacavir 8 mg/kg twice daily, steady-state $AUC_{0\text{-}12h}$ and C_{max} were 9.8 ± 4.56 mcg•h/mL and 3.71 ± 1.36 mcg/mL (mean ± SD), respectively. The safety and efficacy of abacavir have been established in children 3 months to 13 years of age.

Contraindications

Hypersensitivity to abacavir or any other component of the products; moderate or severe hepatic impairment. See the Warning box for more information.

Warnings/Precautions

➤*Lactic acidosis/severe hepatomegaly with steatosis:* Lactic acidosis and severe hepatomegaly with steatosis, including fatal cases, have been reported with the use of nucleoside analogs alone or in combination, including abacavir and other antiretrovirals. A majority of these cases have been in women. Obesity and prolonged nucleoside exposure may be risk factors. Exercise particular caution when administering abacavir to any patient with known risk factors for liver disease; however, cases also have been reported in patients with no known risk factors. Suspend treatment with abacavir in any patient who develops clinical or laboratory findings suggestive of lactic acidosis or pronounced hepatotoxicity (which may include hepatomegaly and steatosis even in the absence of marked transaminase elevations).

➤*Immune reconstitution syndrome:* Immune reconstitution syndrome has been reported in patients treated with combination antiretroviral therapy, including abacavir. During the initial phase of combination antiretroviral treatment, patients whose immune systems respond may develop an inflammatory response to indolent or residual opportunistic infections (such as *Mycobacterium avium* infection, cytomegalovirus, *Pneumocystis jirovecii* pneumonia, or tuberculosis), which may necessitate further evaluation and treatment.

➤*Fat redistribution:* See Adverse Reactions for more information.

➤*Myocardial infarction:* As a precaution, consider the underlying risk of coronary heart disease when prescribing antiretroviral therapies (including abacavir) and taking action to minimize all modifiable risk factors (eg, hypertension, hyperlipidemia, diabetes mellitus, smoking).

➤*Hypersensitivity reactions:* Serious and sometimes fatal hypersensitivity reactions have been associated with abacavir and other abacavir-containing products. Patients who carry the HLA-B*5701 allele are at high risk for experiencing a hypersensitivity reaction to abacavir. Prior to initiating therapy with abacavir, screening for the HLA-B*5701 allele is recommended; this approach has been found to decrease the risk of a hypersensitivity reaction. Screening is also recommended prior to reinitiation of abacavir in patients of unknown HLA-B*5701 status who have previously tolerated abacavir. For HLA-B*5701–positive patients, treatment with an abacavir-containing regimen is not recommended and should be considered only with close medical supervision and under exceptional circumstances when the potential benefit outweighs the risk.

HLA-B*5701–negative patients may develop a hypersensitivity reaction to abacavir; however, this occurs significantly less frequently than in HLA-B*5701–positive patients. Regardless of HLA-B*5701 status, permanently discontinue abacavir if hypersensitivity cannot be ruled out, even when other diagnoses are possible.

See the Warning box for more information.

Other less common signs and symptoms of hypersensitivity include abnormal chest x-ray findings (predominantly infiltrates, which can be localized), edema, lethargy, myolysis, and paresthesia. Adult respiratory distress syndrome, anaphylaxis, death, hypotension, liver failure, renal failure, and respiratory failure have occurred in association with hypersensitivity reactions. In one study, 4 patients (11%) receiving abacavir 600 mg once daily experienced hypotension with a hypersensitivity reaction compared with 0 patients receiving abacavir 300 mg twice daily.

Physical findings associated with hypersensitivity to abacavir in some patients include lymphadenopathy, mucous membrane lesions (conjunctivitis and mouth ulcerations), and rash. The rash usually appears as maculopapular or urticarial, but may be variable in appearance. There have been reports of erythema multiforme. Hypersensitivity reactions have occurred without rash.

Laboratory abnormalities associated with hypersensitivity to abacavir in some patients include elevated liver function tests, elevated creatinine phosphokinase, elevated creatinine, and lymphopenia.

Hypersensitivity reaction registry – An abacavir hypersensitivity registry has been established to facilitate reporting of hypersensitivity reactions and collection of information on each case. Health care providers should register patients by calling 1-800-270-0425.

➤*Hepatic function impairment:* See Contraindications for more information.

➤*Pregnancy: Category C.* There are no adequate and well-controlled studies in pregnant women. Abacavir does cross the human placenta. Use abacavir during pregnancy only if the potential benefits outweigh the risk.

Updated guidelines were released in 2006 for the use of antiretroviral drugs to reduce the perinatal transmission of HIV-1. According to Public Health Service task force recommendations, women receiving antiretroviral therapy during pregnancy should continue the therapy, and zidovudine administration is recommended during the intrapartum period to prevent vertical HIV transmission to the newborn.

Antiretroviral pregnancy registry – To monitor maternal-fetal outcomes of pregnant women exposed to abacavir, an antiretroviral pregnancy registry has been established. Health care providers are encouraged to register patients by calling 1-800-258-4263.

ABACAVIR SULFATE — ORAL

➤*Lactation:* The Centers for Disease Control and Prevention recommends that HIV-infected mothers not breast-feed their infants to avoid risking postnatal transmission of HIV infection.

Although it is not known if abacavir is excreted in human milk, abacavir is secreted into the milk of lactating rats. The molecular weight (approximately 671) suggests abacavir will be excreted into human breast milk. Instruct mothers not to breast-feed if they are receiving abacavir because of the potential for HIV transmission and for serious adverse reactions in breast-fed infants.

➤*Elderly:* In general, use caution in dose selection for an elderly patient, reflecting the greater frequency of decreased hepatic, renal, or cardiac function, and of concomitant disease or other drug therapy.

Drug Interactions

➤*Ethanol:* Coadministration of ethanol and abacavir resulted in a 41% increase in abacavir AUC_∞ and a 26% increase in abacavir half-life.

➤*Methadone:* Oral methadone clearance increased 22% (90% confidence interval [CI], 6% to 42%) with abacavir coadministration. This alteration will not result in a methadone dose modification in the majority of patients; however, an increased methadone dose may be required in a small number of patients.

Adverse Reactions

Serious and sometimes fatal hypersensitivity reactions have been associated with abacavir. In 1 study, once-daily dosing of abacavir was associated with more severe hypersensitivity reactions (see Warnings and Precautions).

➤*Clinical trials experience:*

Adults –

Therapy-naive adults:

• *Study CNA30024 –*

Abacavir Adverse Reactions in Therapy-Naive Adults (CNA30024) (≥ 5%)[a]

Adverse reactions	Abacavir + lamivudine + efavirenz (n = 324)	Zidovudine + lamivudine + efavirenz (n = 325)
CNS		
Depressive disorders	6%	6%
Dizziness	6%	6%
Dreams/Sleep disorders	10%	10%
Fatigue/Malaise	7%	10%
Headaches/Migraine	7%	11%
GI		
Abdominal pain/gastritis/ GI signs and symptoms	6%	8%
Diarrhea	7%	6%
Nausea	7%	11%
Vomiting	2%	9%
Miscellaneous		
Bronchitis	4%	5%
Drug hypersensitivity	9%	< 1%[b]
Musculoskeletal pain	6%	5%
Rash	6%	12%

[a] This study used double-blind ascertainment of suspected hypersensitivity reactions. During the blinded portion of the study, suspected hypersensitivity to abacavir was reported by investigators in 9% of 324 patients in the abacavir group and 3% of 325 patients in the zidovudine group.

[b] Ten (3%) cases of suspected drug hypersensitivity were reclassified as not being caused by abacavir following unblinding.

• *Study CNA3005 –*

Abacavir Adverse Reactions in Therapy-Naive Adults (CNA3005) (≥ 5%)

Adverse reactions	Abacavir + lamivudine/zidovudine (n = 262)	Indinavir + lamivudine/zidovudine (n = 264)
CNS		
Anxiety	5%	3%
Depressive disorders	6%	4%
Headache	13%	9%
Malaise and fatigue	12%	12%
GI		
Diarrhea	7%	5%
Nausea	19%	17%
Nausea and vomiting	10%	10%
Miscellaneous		
Ear/Nose/Throat infections	5%	4%
Fever and/or chills	6%	3%
Hypersensitivity reaction	8%	2%
Musculoskeletal pain	5%	7%
Pain (non–site-specific)	< 1%	5%
Renal signs/symptoms	< 1%	5%
Skin rash	5%	4%
Viral respiratory infections	5%	5%

Five patients receiving abacavir in study CNA3005 experienced worsening of preexisting depression compared with none in the indinavir arm. The background rates of preexisting depression were similar in the 2 treatment arms.

Children –

Therapy-experienced children:

Abacavir Adverse Reactions in Therapy-Experienced Children (CNA3006) (≥ 5%)

Adverse reactions	Abacavir + lamivudine + zidovudine (n = 102)	Lamivudine + zidovudine (n = 103)
Ear/Nose/Throat infections	5%	1%
Fever and/or chills	9%	7%
Headache	1%	5%
Nausea and vomiting	9%	2%
Pneumonia	4%	5%
Skin rash	7%	1%

➤*Miscellaneous:* Another adverse reaction observed in the expanded access program was pancreatitis.

➤*Lab test abnormalities:*

Adults –

Abacavir Laboratory Abnormalities in Therapy-Naive Adults (CNA30024)[a]

Grade 3/4 laboratory abnormalities	Abacavir + lamivudine + efavirenz (n = 324)	Zidovudine + lamivudine + efavirenz (n = 325)
Elevated CPK (> 4 × ULN)	8%	8%
Elevated ALT (> 5 × ULN)	6%	6%
Elevated AST (> 5 × ULN)	6%	5%
Hypertriglyceridemia (> 750 mg/dL)	6%	5%
Hyperamylasemia (> 2 × ULN)	4%	5%
Neutropenia (ANC < 750/mm³)	2%	4%
Anemia (hemoglobin ≤ 6.9 g/dL)	< 1%	2%
Thrombocytopenia (platelets < 50,000/mm³)	1%	< 1%
Leukopenia (WBC ≤ 1,500/mm³)	< 1%	2%

[a] CPK = creatine phosphokinase; ULN = upper limit of normal; ANC = absolute neutrophil count; WBC = white blood cell.

ABACAVIR SULFATE — ORAL

Study CNA3005 –

Abacavir Treatment-Emergent Laboratory Abnormalities (Grades 3/4) in Therapy-Naive Adults (CNA3005)		
	Number of subjects by treatment group	
Grade 3/4 laboratory abnormalities	Abacavir + lamivudine/zidovudine (n = 262)	Indinavir + lamivudine/zidovudine (n = 264)
Elevated CPK (> 4 × ULN)	7%	7%
ALT (> 5 × ULN)	6%	6%
Neutropenia (< 750/mm^3)	5%	5%
Hypertriglyceridemia (> 750 mg/dL)	2%	1%
Hyperamylasemia (> 2 × ULN)	2%	< 1%
Hyperglycemia (> 13.9 mmol/L)	< 1%	< 1%
Anemia (hemoglobin ≤ 6.9 g/dL)	0%	1%

Children –

Study CNA3006: In study CNA3006, laboratory abnormalities (eg, anemia, CPK elevations, liver function test abnormalities, neutropenia) were observed with similar frequencies as in a study of therapy-naive adults (CNA30024). Mild elevations of blood glucose were more frequent in children receiving abacavir (CNA3006) compared with adult patients (CNA30024). Another laboratory abnormality observed in the expanded access program was increased gamma-glutamyltransferase.

➤*Postmarketing:*

Cardiovascular – Myocardial infarction.

Dermatologic – Suspected Stevens-Johnson syndrome and toxic epidermal necrolysis have been reported in patients receiving abacavir primarily in combination with medications known to be associated with suspected Stevens-Johnson syndrome and toxic epidermal necrolysis, respectively. Because of the overlap of clinical signs and symptoms between hypersensitivity to abacavir and suspected Stevens-Johnson syndrome and toxic epidermal necrolysis, and the possibility of multiple-drug sensitivities in some patients, discontinue abacavir and do not restart in such cases. There also have been reports of erythema multiforme.

Hepatic – Hepatic steatosis, lactic acidosis.

Miscellaneous – Redistribution/accumulation of body fat, including breast enlargement, central obesity, cushingoid appearance, dorsocervical fat enlargement (buffalo hump), facial wasting, and peripheral wasting have been observed in patients receiving antiretroviral therapy. The mechanism and long-term consequences of these reactions are currently unknown. A causal relationship has not been established.

Patient Information

Inform patients that some HIV medicines, including abacavir, may cause a rare but serious condition called lactic acidosis with liver enlargement (hepatomegaly).

Abacavir is not a cure for HIV infection, and patients may continue to experience illnesses associated with HIV infection, including opportunistic infections. Patients should remain under the care of a health care provider when using abacavir. Advise patients that the use of abacavir has not been shown to reduce the risk of transmission of HIV to others through sexual contact or blood contamination.

Inform patients that redistribution or accumulation of body fat may occur in patients receiving antiretroviral therapy, and the cause and long-term health effects of these conditions are not known at this time.

Advise patients of the importance of taking HIV medications exactly as prescribed.

EMTRICITABINE

Rx	**Emtriva** (Gilead Sciences)	**Capsules; oral:** 200 mg	(200 mg GILEAD). Blue/White. In 30s.
		Solution; oral: 10 mg/mL	Edetate disodium, xylitol, parabens. Cotton candy flavor. In 170 mL with dosing cup.

EMTRICITABINE — ORAL

WARNING

Lactic acidosis and severe hepatomegaly with steatosis, including fatal cases, have been reported with the use of nucleoside analogs alone or in combination with other antiretrovirals.

Emtricitabine is not approved for the treatment of chronic hepatitis B virus (HBV) infection, and the safety and efficacy of emtricitabine have not been established in patients coinfected with HBV and HIV-1. Severe acute exacerbations of hepatitis B have been reported in patients who have discontinued emtricitabine. Closely monitor hepatic function with clinical and laboratory follow-up for at least several months in patients who discontinue emtricitabine and are coinfected with HIV-1 and HBV. If appropriate, initiation of anti-HBV therapy may be warranted.

Indications

➤*HIV infection:* For the treatment of HIV-1 infection in combination with other antiretroviral agents.

Administration and Dosage

➤*Adults:*

HIV infection –

Capsules: 200 mg once daily.
Solution: 240 mg (24 mL) once daily.

➤*Children:*

HIV infection –

3 months to 17 years of age weighing more than 33 kg:
- *Capsules* – 200 mg once daily.
- *Solution –*
  Usual dosage: 6 mg/kg once daily.
  Maximum dose: 240 mg (24 mL) once daily.

0 to 3 months of age:
- *Solution* – 3 mg/kg once daily.

➤*Renal function impairment:*

Adults –

Emtricitabine Dosage Adjustment in Adult Patients With Renal Impairment				
	CrCl			
Formulation	≥ 50 mL/min	30 to 49 mL/min	15 to 29 mL/min	< 15 mL/min or on hemodialysis[a]
Capsule	200 mg every 24 h	200 mg every 48 h	200 mg every 72 h	200 mg every 96 h

Emtricitabine Dosage Adjustment in Adult Patients With Renal Impairment				
	CrCl			
Formulation	≥ 50 mL/min	30 to 49 mL/min	15 to 29 mL/min	< 15 mL/min or on hemodialysis[a]
Solution	240 mg every 24 h (24 mL)	120 mg every 24 h (12 mL)	80 mg every 24 h (8 mL)	60 mg every 24 h (6 mL)

[a] Hemodialysis patients: If dosing on day of dialysis, administer after dialysis.

Children – Although there are insufficient data to recommend a specific dose adjustment of emtricitabine in children with renal impairment, a dose reduction and/or an increase in the dosing interval similar to adjustments for adults should be considered.

➤*Administration:* May be taken without regard to food.

➤*Storage/Stability:* Store capsules at 25°C (77°F); excursions are permitted to 15° to 30°C (59° to 86°F). Refrigerate solution at 2° to 8°C (36° to 46°F). Use solution within 3 months if stored at 25°C (77°F); excursions are permitted to 15° to 30°C (59° to 86°F).

Actions

➤*Pharmacology:* Emtricitabine, a synthetic nucleoside analog of cytosine, is phosphorylated by cellular enzymes to form emtricitabine 5′-triphosphate. Emtricitabine 5′-triphosphate inhibits the activity of the HIV-1 reverse transcriptase by competing with the natural substrate deoxycytidine 5′-triphosphate and by being incorporated into nascent viral DNA, which results in chain termination. Emtricitabine 5′-triphosphate is a weak inhibitor of mammalian DNA polymerase α, β, ε, and mitochondrial DNA polymerase γ.

➤*Pharmacokinetics:*

Absorption – Emtricitabine is rapidly and extensively absorbed following oral administration with peak plasma concentrations occurring at 1 to 2 hours postdose. Following multiple-dose oral administration of emtricitabine capsules to 20 HIV-1–infected subjects, the (mean ± standard deviation [SD]) steady-state plasma emtricitabine peak concentration (C_{max}) was 1.8 ± 0.7 mcg/mL and the area under the curve (AUC) over a 24-hour dosing interval was 10 ± 3.1 mcg•h/mL. The mean steady-state plasma trough concentration at 24 hours postdose was 0.09 mcg/mL. The mean absolute bioavailability of emtricitabine capsules was 93%, while the mean absolute bioavailability of emtricitabine oral solution was 75%. The relative bioavailability of emtricitabine oral solution was approximately 80% of emtricitabine capsules.

The multiple-dose pharmacokinetics of emtricitabine are dose proportional over a dose range of 25 to 200 mg.

EMTRICITABINE — ORAL

Effect of food: Emtricitabine capsules and oral solution may be taken with or without food. Emtricitabine AUC was unaffected, while C_{max} decreased by 29% when emtricitabine capsules were administered with food (an approximately 1,000 kcal high-fat meal).

Distribution – In vitro binding of emtricitabine to human plasma proteins was less than 4% and independent of concentration over the range of 0.02 to 200 mcg/mL. At peak plasma concentration, the mean plasma to blood drug concentration ratio was approximately 1, and the mean semen to plasma drug concentration ratio was approximately 4.

Metabolism – In vitro studies indicate that emtricitabine is not an inhibitor of human cytochrome P450 enzymes. Following administration of ^{14}C-emtricitabine, complete recovery of the dose was achieved in urine (approximately 86%) and feces (approximately 14%). Thirteen percent of the dose was recovered in urine as 3 putative metabolites. The biotransformation of emtricitabine includes oxidation of the thiol moiety to form the 3′-sulfoxide diastereomers (approximately 9% of the dose) and conjugation with glucuronic acid to form 2′-O-glucuronide (approximately 4% of the dose). No other metabolites were identifiable.

Excretion – The plasma emtricitabine half-life is approximately 10 hours. The renal clearance of emtricitabine is greater than the estimated CrCl, suggesting elimination by glomerular filtration and active tubular secretion. There may be competition for elimination with other compounds that also are renally eliminated.

Special populations –

Renal function impairment: See Administration and Dosage for more information.

Emtricitabine Mean ± SD Pharmacokinetic Parameters in Adults With Renal Impairment[a]

CrCl (mL/min)	> 80 (n = 6)	50 to 80 (n = 6)	30 to 49 (n = 6)	< 30 (n = 5)	ESRD[b] < 30 (n = 5)
Baseline CrCl (mL/min)	107 ± 21	59.8 ± 6.5	40.9 ± 5.1	22.9 ± 5.3	8.8 ± 1.4
C_{max} (mcg/mL)	2.2 ± 0.6	3.8 ± 0.9	3.2 ± 0.6	2.8 ± 0.7	2.8 ± 0.5
AUC (mcg•h/mL)	11.8 ± 2.9	19.9 ± 1.2	25.1 ± 5.7	33.7 ± 2.1	53.2 ± 9.9
CL/F (mL/min)	302 ± 94	168 ± 10	138 ± 28	99 ± 6	64 ± 12
CLr (mL/min)	213 ± 89	121 ± 39	69 ± 32	30 ± 11	NA[c]

[a] ESRD = end-stage renal disease; CL/F = apparent oral clearance; CLr = apparent renal clearance.
[b] Patients with ESRD requiring dialysis
[c] NA = not applicable.

• *Hemodialysis* – Hemodialysis treatment removes approximately 30% of the emtricitabine dose over a 3-hour dialysis period starting within 1.5 hours of emtricitabine dosing (blood flow rate of 400 mL/min and a dialysate flow rate of 600 mL/min). It is not known whether emtricitabine can be removed by peritoneal dialysis.

Children:

Emtricitabine Mean ± SD Pharmacokinetic Parameters in Children

	HIV-1–exposed neonates	HIV-1–infected children			
Age	0 to 3 mo (n = 20)[a]	3 to 24 mo (n = 14)	25 mo to 6 y (n = 19)	7 to 12 y (n = 17)	13 to 17 y (n = 27)
Formulation					
Capsules	n = 0	n = 0	n = 0	n = 10	n = 26
Solution	n = 20	n = 14	n = 19	n = 7	n = 1
Dose (mg/kg)[b]	3.1 (2.9 to 3.4)	6.1 (5.5 to 6.8)	6.1 (5.6 to 6.7)	5.6 (3.1 to 6.6)	4.4 (1.8 to 7)
C_{max} (mcg/mL)	1.6 ± 0.6	1.9 ± 0.6	1.9 ± 0.7	2.7 ± 0.8	2.7 ± 0.9
AUC (mcg•h/mL)	11 ± 4.2	8.7 ± 3.2	9 ± 3	12.6 ± 3.5	12.6 ± 5.4
$t_{½}$[c] (h)	12.1 ± 3.1	8.9 ± 3.2	11.3 ± 6.4	8.2 ± 3.2	8.9 ± 3.3

[a] Two pharmacokinetic evaluations were conducted in 20 neonates over the first 3 months of life. Median (range) age of infant on day of pharmacokinetic evaluation was 26 (5 to 81) days.
[b] Mean (range).
[c] $t_{½}$ = terminal half-life.

Contraindications

Previously demonstrated hypersensitivity to any of the components of the products.

Warnings/Precautions

➤*Lactic acidosis/severe hepatomegaly with steatosis:* Lactic acidosis and severe hepatomegaly with steatosis, including fatal cases, have been reported with the use of nucleoside analogs alone or in combination, including emtricitabine and other antiretrovirals. A majority of these cases have been in women. Obesity and prolonged nucleoside exposure may be risk factors. Exercise particular caution when administering nucleoside analogs to any patient with known risk factors for liver disease; however, cases have also been reported in patients with no known risk factors. Suspend treatment with emtricitabine in any patient who develops clinical or laboratory findings suggestive of lactic acidosis or pronounced hepatotoxicity (which may include hepatomegaly and steatosis even in the absence of marked transaminase elevations).

➤*HIV-1 and hepatitis B virus coinfection:* It is recommended that all patients with HIV-1 be tested for the presence of chronic HBV before initiating antiretroviral therapy.

See the Warning box for more information.

➤*Fat redistribution:* Redistribution/accumulation of body fat, including central obesity, dorsocervical fat enlargement ("buffalo hump"), peripheral wasting, facial wasting, breast enlargement, and "cushingoid appearance," have been observed in patients receiving antiretroviral therapy. The mechanism and long-term consequences of these events are currently unknown. A causal relationship has not been established.

➤*Immune reconstitution syndrome:* Immune reconstitution syndrome has been reported in patients treated with combination antiretroviral therapy, including emtricitabine. During the initial phase of combination antiretroviral treatment, patients whose immune system responds may develop an inflammatory response to indolent or residual opportunistic infections (eg, *Mycobacterium avium* infection, cytomegalovirus, *Pneumocystis jirovecii* pneumonia, tuberculosis), which may necessitate further evaluation and treatment.

➤*Renal function impairment:* Emtricitabine is principally eliminated by the kidney. It is recommended that the dose or dosing interval for emtricitabine be modified in patients with CrCl less than 50 mL/min or in patients who require dialysis (see Administration and Dosage).

➤*Pregnancy: Category B.* There are no adequate and well-controlled studies in pregnant women. The relatively low molecular weight (approximately 247), low plasma protein binding, and long elimination half-life suggest that emtricitabine will cross the human placenta. Because animal reproduction studies are not always predictive of human response, use emtricitabine during pregnancy only if clearly needed.

Antiretroviral pregnancy registry – To monitor fetal outcomes of pregnant women exposed to emtricitabine, an antiretroviral pregnancy registry has been established. Health care providers are encouraged to register patients by calling 1-800-258-4263.

➤*Lactation:* The Centers for Disease Control and Prevention recommends that HIV-1–infected mothers not breast-feed their infants to avoid risking postnatal transmission of HIV-1. It is not known whether emtricitabine is secreted into human milk. Emtricitabine's low molecular weight, low plasma protein binding, and long plasma elimination half-life suggest that it will be excreted in human milk. Because of the potential for HIV-1 transmission and for serious adverse reactions in breast-feeding infants, instruct mothers not to breast-feed if they are receiving emtricitabine.

➤*Elderly:* In general, exercise caution in dose selection for elderly patients, keeping in mind the greater frequency of decreased hepatic, renal, or cardiac function, and of concomitant disease or other drug therapy.

➤*Monitoring:* Monitor patient for signs of lactic acidosis. Closely monitor hepatic function with clinical and laboratory follow-up for at least several months in patients who discontinue emtricitabine and are coinfected with HIV-1 and HBV. HBV testing is recommended prior to initiation of therapy. Closely monitor clinical response to treatment and renal function in patients with baseline CrCl less than 50 mL/min.

Drug Interactions

➤*Coadministration with other drugs containing emtricitabine:* Emtricitabine is a component of *Truvada* (a fixed-dose combination of emtricitabine and tenofovir disoproxil fumarate) and *Atripla* (a fixed-dose combination of efavirenz, emtricitabine, and tenofovir disproxil fumarate). Do not coadminister emtricitabine with *Truvada* or *Atripla*. Because of similarities between emtricitabine and lamivudine, do not coadminister emtricitabine with other drugs containing lamivudine, including lamivudine/zidovudine, abacavir/lamivudine, or abacavir/lamivudine/zidovudine.

➤*Drug/Food interactions:* See Actions for more information.

Adverse Reactions

➤*Adults:* The most common adverse reactions (incidence of at least 10%, any severity) identified from any of the 3 large controlled trials included abdominal pain, abnormal dreams, asthenia, depression, diarrhea, dizziness, fatigue, headache, increased cough, insomnia, nausea, rash, and rhinitis. The most common adverse reactions that occurred in patients receiving emtricitabine with other antiretroviral agents in clinical trials were headache, diarrhea, nausea, and rash, which were generally of mild to moderate severity. Approximately 1% of patients discontinued participation in the clinical studies because of these reactions. All adverse reactions were reported with similar frequency in emtricitabine and control treatment groups, with the exception of skin discoloration, which was reported with higher frequency in the emtricitabine-treated group.

Skin discoloration, manifested by hyperpigmentation on the palms and/or soles, was generally mild and asymptomatic. The mechanism and clinical significance are unknown.

EMTRICITABINE — ORAL

Study 301A/303:

Emtricitabine Adverse Reactions (≥ 3%)				
	Study 303		Study 301A	
Adverse reaction	Emtricitabine + zidovudine or stavudine + NNRTI/PI[a] (n = 294)	Lamivudine + zidovudine or stavudine + NNRTI/PI (n = 146)	Emtricitabine + didanosine + efavirenz (n = 286)	Stavudine + didanosine + efavirenz (n = 285)
CNS				
Abnormal dreams	2%	< 1%	11%	19%
Asthenia	16%	10%	12%	17%
Depressive disorders	6%	10%	9%	13%
Dizziness	4%	5%	25%	26%
Headache	13%	6%	22%	25%
Insomnia	7%	3%	16%	21%
Neuropathy/ Peripheral neuritis	4%	3%	4%	13%
Paresthesia	5%	7%	6%	12%
Dermatologic				
Rash event[b]	17%	14%	30%	33%
GI				
Abdominal pain	8%	11%	14%	17%
Diarrhea	23%	18%	23%	32%
Dyspepsia	4%	5%	8%	12%
Nausea	18%	12%	13%	23%
Vomiting	9%	7%	9%	12%
Musculoskeletal				
Arthralgia	3%	4%	5%	6%
Myalgia	4%	4%	6%	3%
Respiratory				
Increased cough	14%	11%	14%	8%
Rhinitis	18%	12%	12%	10%

[a] PI = protease inhibitor; NNRTI = nonnucleoside reverse transcriptase inhibitor.
[b] Rash event includes allergic reaction, maculopapular rash, pruritus, pustular rash, rash, urticaria, and vesiculobullous rash.

Study 934:

Emtricitabine Adverse Reactions (Grades 2 to 4) (≥ 5%)[a]		
Adverse reaction	Tenofovir disproxil fumarate[b] + emtricitabine + efavirenz (n = 257)	Zidovudine/Lamivudine + efavirenz (n = 254)
CNS		
Depression	9%	7%
Dizziness	8%	7%
Fatigue	9%	8%
Headache	6%	5%
Insomnia	5%	7%
Dermatologic		
Rash event[c]	7%	9%
GI		
Diarrhea	9%	5%
Nausea	9%	7%
Vomiting	2%	5%
Respiratory		
Nasopharyngitis	5%	3%
Sinusitis	8%	4%
Upper respiratory tract infections	8%	5%

[a] Frequencies of adverse reactions are based on all treatment-emergent adverse reactions, regardless of relationship to study drug.
[b] From weeks 96 to 144 of the study, patients received tenofovir disproxil fumarate/emtricitabine with efavirenz in place of tenofovir disproxil fumarate + emtricitabine with efavirenz.
[c] Rash event includes rash, exfoliative rash, generalized rash, macular rash, maculopapular rash, pruritic rash, and vesicular rash.

➤*Children:* Selected treatment-emergent adverse reactions, regardless of causality, reported in children during 48 weeks of treatment were the following: infection (44%), hyperpigmentation (32%), increased cough (28%), vomiting (23%), otitis media (23%), rash (21%), rhinitis (20%), diarrhea (20%), fever (18%), pneumonia (15%), gastroenteritis (11%), abdominal pain (10%), and anemia (7%).

➤*Lab test abnormalities:*

Adults –

Study 301A/303:

Emtricitabine Grade 3/4 Laboratory Abnormalities (≥ 1%)				
	Study 303		Study 301A	
	Emtricitabine + zidovudine or stavudine + NNRTI/PI (n = 294)	Lamivudine + zidovudine or stavudine + NNRTI/PI (n = 146)	Emtricitabine + didanosine + efavirenz (n = 286)	Stavudine + didanosine + efavirenz (n = 285)
Percentage with grade 3 or 4 laboratory abnormality	31%	28%	34%	38%
ALT (> 5 × ULN[a])	2%	1%	5%	6%
AST (> 5 × ULN)	3%	< 1%	6%	9%
Bilirubin (> 2.5 × ULN)	1%	2%	< 1%	< 1%
Creatine kinase (> 4 × ULN)	11%	14%	12%	11%
Neutrophils (< 750 mm^3)	5%	3%	5%	7%
Pancreatic amylase (> 2 × ULN)	2%	2%	< 1%	1%
Serum amylase (> 2 × ULN)	2%	2%	5%	10%
Serum glucose (< 40 or > 250 mg/dL)	3%	3%	2%	3%
Serum lipase (> 2 × ULN)	< 1%	< 1%	1%	2%
Triglycerides (> 750 mg/dL)	10%	8%	9%	6%

[a] ULN = upper limit of normal.

Study 934:

Emtricitabine Laboratory Abnormalities (≥ 1%)		
	Tenofovir disproxil fumarate[a] + emtricitabine + efavirenz (n = 257)	Zidovudine/lamivudine + efavirenz (n = 254)
Any ≥ grade 3 laboratory abnormality	30%	26%
Alkaline phosphatase (> 550 units/L)	1%	0%
ALT (M: > 215 units/L) (F: > 170 units/L)	2%	3%
AST (M: > 180 units/L) (F: > 170 units/L)	3%	3%
Creatine kinase (M: > 990 units/L) (F: > 845 units/L)	9%	7%
Fasting cholesterol (>240 mg/dL)	22%	24%
Fasting triglycerides (> 750 mg/dL)	4%	2%
Glycosuria (3+)	< 1%	1%
Hematuria (> 75 red blood cells per high-power field)	3%	2%
Hemoglobin (< 8 mg/dL)	0%	4%
Hyperglycemia (> 250 mg/dL)	2%	1%
Neutrophils (< 750/mm^3)	3%	5%
Serum amylase (> 175 units/L)	8%	4%

[a] From weeks 96 to 144 of the study, patients received emtricitabine/tenofovir disproxil fumarate with efavirenz in place of tenofovir disproxil fumarate + emtricitabine with efavirenz.

EMTRICITABINE — ORAL

Children – Treatment-emergent grade 3/4 laboratory abnormalities in study 203 were experienced by 9% of children, including amylase greater than 2 × ULN (n = 4), neutrophils less than 750/mm³ (n = 3), ALT greater than 5 × ULN (n = 2), elevated creatine phosphokinase (greater than 4 × ULN) (n = 2), and 1 patient each with elevated bilirubin (greater than 3 × ULN), elevated gamma-glutamyltransferase (greater than 10 × ULN), elevated lipase (greater than 2.5 × ULN), decreased hemoglobin (less than 7 g/dL), and decreased glucose (less than 40 g/dL).

Overdosage

➤*Treatment:* There is no known antidote for emtricitabine. If overdose occurs, monitor the patient for signs of toxicity and apply standard supportive treatment as necessary.

Hemodialysis treatment removes approximately 30% of the emtricitabine dose over a 3-hour dialysis period, starting within 1.5 hours of emtricitabine dosing (blood flow rate of 400 mL/min and a dialysate flow rate of 600 mL/min). It is not known whether emtricitabine can be removed by peritoneal dialysis.

Patient Information

Inform patients that emtricitabine is not a cure for HIV-1 infection and patients may continue to experience illnesses associated with HIV-1 infection, including opportunistic infections. Advise patients to remain under the care of a health care provider when using this medicine.

Advise patients that the use of emtricitabine has not been shown to reduce the risk of transmission of HIV-1 to others through sexual contact or blood contamination. The long-term effects of emtricitabine are unknown.

Advise patients that emtricitabine capsules and solution are for oral ingestion only.

Advise patients that it is important to take emtricitabine with combination therapy on a regular dosing schedule to avoid missing doses.

Inform patients that lactic acidosis and severe hepatomegaly with steatosis, including fatal cases, have been reported. Suspend treatment with emtricitabine in any patient who develops clinical symptoms suggestive of lactic acidosis or pronounced hepatotoxicity (including nausea, vomiting, unusual or unexpected stomach discomfort, and weakness).

Inform patients that severe acute exacerbation of hepatitis B has been reported in patients who are coinfected with HBV and HIV-1 and have discontinued emtricitabine.

Advise patients that emtricitabine should not be coadministered with other drugs containing lamivudine, including lamivudine/zidovudine, lamivudine, abacavir/lamivudine, or abacavir/lamivudine/zidovudine.

Advise patients with HIV-1 to be tested for HBV before initiating antiretroviral therapy.

Inform patients that redistribution or accumulation of body fat may occur in patients receiving antiretroviral therapy and the cause and long-term health effects of these conditions are not known.

Nucleoside Analog Reverse Transcriptase Inhibitor Combinations

LAMIVUDINE/ZIDOVUDINE (3TC/ZDV, 3TC/AZT)

Rx	**Combivir** (GlaxoSmithKline)	**Tablets; oral:** lamivudine 150 mg/zidovudine 300 mg	(PEG GXFC3). White, capsule shape. Scored. Film-coated. In 60s and UD 120s.

LAMIVUDINE/ZIDOVUDINE — ORAL

Consult the complete prescribing information for each agent, lamivudine and zidovudine, prior to administration of lamivudine/zidovudine combination tablets.

WARNING

Zidovudine, one of the 2 active ingredients in lamivudine/zidovudine, has been associated with hematologic toxicity, including neutropenia and anemia, particularly in patients with advanced HIV-1 disease. Prolonged use of zidovudine has been associated with symptomatic myopathy.

Lactic acidosis and hepatomegaly with steatosis, including fatal cases, have been reported with use of nucleoside analogs alone or in combination, including lamivudine, zidovudine, and other antiretrovirals. Suspend treatment if clinical or laboratory findings suggestive of lactic acidosis or pronounced hepatotoxicity occur.

Acute exacerbations of hepatitis B have been reported in patients who are coinfected with hepatitis B virus (HBV) and HIV-1 and have discontinued lamivudine, which is 1 component of lamivudine/zidovudine. Monitor hepatic function closely with both clinical and laboratory follow-up for at least several months in patients who discontinue lamivudine/zidovudine and are coinfected with HIV-1 and HBV. If appropriate, initiation of hepatitis B therapy may be warranted.

Indications

➤*HIV infection:* For the treatment of HIV-1 infection in combination with other antiretrovirals.

Administration and Dosage

➤*Adults:*

HIV infection – Lamivudine 150 mg/zidovudine 300 mg orally twice daily.

➤*Children:*

HIV infection – See Adults for dosing in children weighing more than 30 kg.

➤*Elderly:* In general, use caution in dose selection for an elderly patient, reflecting the greater frequency of decreased hepatic, renal, or cardiac function, and of concomitant disease or other drug therapy.

➤*Renal function impairment:*

Creatinine clearance less than 50 mL/min – Not recommended.

➤*Hepatic function impairment:* Because lamivudine/zidovudine is a fixed-dose combination that cannot be adjusted for patients with impaired hepatic function or liver cirrhosis, it is not recommended.

➤*Storage/Stability:* Store between 2° and 30°C (36° and 86°F).

Actions

➤*Pharmacology:* Lamivudine/zidovudine is an antiviral agent.

Lamivudine – Intracellularly, lamivudine is phosphorylated to its active 5′-triphosphate metabolite, lamivudine triphosphate (3TC-TP). The principal mode of action of 3TC-TP is inhibition of reverse transcriptase (RT) via DNA chain termination after incorporation of the nucleotide analog. 3TC-TP is a weak inhibitor of cellular DNA polymerases alpha, beta, and gamma.

Zidovudine – Intracellularly, zidovudine is phosphorylated to its active 5′-triphosphate metabolite, zidovudine triphosphate (ZDV-TP). The principal mode of action of ZDV-TP is inhibition of RT via DNA chain termination after incorporation of the nucleotide analog. ZDV-TP is a weak inhibitor of the cellular DNA polymerases alpha and gamma, and has been reported to be incorporated into the DNA of cells in culture.

➤*Pharmacokinetics:*

Lamivudine and Zidovudine Pharmacokinetic Parameters[a] in Fasting Adults

Pharmacokinetic parameter	Lamivudine	Zidovudine
Oral bioavailability (%)	86 ± 16	64 ± 10
Apparent volume of distribution (L/kg)	1.3 ± 0.4	1.6 ± 0.6
Plasma protein binding	< 36%	< 38%
CSF:plasma ratio[b]	0.12 (0.04 to 0.47)	0.6 (0.04 to 2.62)
Systemic clearance (L/h/kg)	0.33 ± 0.06	1.6 ± 0.6
Renal clearance (L/h/kg)	0.22 ± 0.06	0.34 ± 0.05
Elimination half-life[c]	5 to 7 h	0.5 to 3 h

[a] Data presented as mean ± standard deviation except where noted.
[b] Median (range).
[c] Approximate range.

Absorption/Distribution – Following oral administration, lamivudine and zidovudine are rapidly absorbed and extensively distributed. Binding to plasma protein is low.

Effect of food: Lamivudine/zidovudine may be administered with or without food. The extent of lamivudine and zidovudine absorption (area under the curve [AUC]) following administration of lamivudine/zidovudine with food was similar when compared with fasting healthy subjects (n = 24).

Metabolism/Excretion –

Lamivudine: Approximately 70% of an intravenous dose of lamivudine is recovered as unchanged drug in the urine. Metabolism of lamivudine is a minor route of elimination. In humans, the only known metabolite is the trans-sulfoxide metabolite (approximately 5% of an oral dose after 12 hours).

Zidovudine: Zidovudine is eliminated primarily by hepatic metabolism. The major metabolite of zidovudine is 3′-azido-3′-deoxy-5′-*O*-β-*D*- glucopyranuronosylthymidine (GZDV). GZDV AUC is about 3-fold greater than the zidovudine AUC. Urinary recovery of zidovudine and GZDV accounts for 14% and 74%, respectively, of the dose following oral administration. A second metabolite, 3′-amino- 3′-deoxythymidine (AMT), has been identified in plasma. The AMT AUC was ⅕ of the zidovudine AUC.

Special populations –

Children: See Administration and Dosage for more information.

Contraindications

Previously demonstrated clinically significant hypersensitivity (eg, anaphylaxis, Stevens-Johnson syndrome) to any of the components of this product.

Warnings/Precautions

➤*Bone marrow suppression:* Zidovudine, a component of lamivudine/zidovudine, has been associated with hematologic toxicity including neutropenia and anemia, particularly in patients with advanced HIV-1 disease. Use lamivudine/zidovudine with caution in patients who have bone marrow compromise evidenced by granulocyte count less than 1,000 cells/mm^3 or hemoglobin less than 9.5 g/dL. Frequent blood cell counts are strongly recommended in patients with advanced HIV-1 disease who are treated with lamivudine/zidovudine. For other HIV-1-infected patients, periodic blood cell counts are recommended. If anemia or neutropenia develops, dosage interruption may be needed.

➤*Myopathy:* Myopathy and myositis, with pathological changes similar to that produced by HIV-1 disease, have been associated with prolonged use of zidovudine and, therefore, may occur with lamivudine/zidovudine therapy.

➤*Lactic acidosis/hepatomegaly with steatosis:* Lactic acidosis and hepatomegaly with steatosis, including fatal cases, have been reported with the use of nucleoside analogs alone or in combination, including lamivudine, zidovudine, and other antiretrovirals. A majority of these cases have been in women. Obesity and prolonged nucleoside exposure may be risk factors. Exercise particular caution when administering lamivudine/zidovudine to any patient with known risk factors for liver disease; however, cases have also been reported in patients with no known risk factors. Suspend treatment with lamivudine/zidovudine in any patient who develops clinical or laboratory findings suggestive of lactic acidosis or pronounced hepatotoxicity (which may include hepatomegaly and steatosis even in the absence of marked transaminase elevations).

➤*HIV-1 and hepatitis B virus coinfection:*

Posttreatment exacerbations of hepatitis – In clinical trials in non-HIV-1–infected patients treated with lamivudine for chronic HBV, clinical and laboratory evidence of exacerbations of hepatitis have occurred after discontinuation of lamivudine. These exacerbations have been detected primarily by serum ALT elevations in addition to reemergence of HBV DNA. Although most events appear to have been self-limited, fatalities have been reported in some cases. Similar events have been reported from postmarketing experience after changes from lamivudine-containing HIV-1 treatment regimens to non-lamivudine–containing regimens in patients infected with both HIV-1 and HBV. The causal relationship to discontinuation of lamivudine treatment is unknown. Closely monitor patients with both clinical and laboratory follow-up for at least several months after stopping treatment. There is insufficient evidence to determine whether reinitiation of lamivudine alters the course of posttreatment exacerbations of hepatitis.

➤*Lamivudine-resistant hepatitis B virus:* In non-HIV-1–infected patients treated with lamivudine for chronic hepatitis B, emergence of lamivudine-resistant HBV has been detected and associated with diminished treatment response. Emergence of HBV variants associated with resistance to lamivudine has also been reported in HIV-1–infected patients who have received lamivudine-containing antiretroviral regimens in the presence of concurrent infection with HBV.

➤*Pancreatitis:* Use lamivudine/zidovudine with caution in patients with a history of pancreatitis or other significant risk factors for the development of pancreatitis. Stop treatment with lamivudine/zidovudine immediately if clinical signs, symptoms, or laboratory abnormalities suggestive of pancreatitis occur.

➤*Immune reconstitution syndrome:* Immune reconstitution syndrome has been reported in patients treated with combination antiretroviral therapy, including lamivudine/zidovudine. During the initial phase of combination antiretroviral treatment, patients whose immune systems respond may develop an inflammatory response to indolent or residual opportunistic infections (eg, *Mycobacterium avium* infection, cytomegalovirus, *Pneumocystis jirovecii* pneumonia, tuberculosis), which may necessitate further evaluation and treatment.

➤*Fat redistribution:* Redistribution/accumulation of body fat, including central obesity, dorsocervical fat enlargement (buffalo hump), peripheral wasting, facial wasting, breast enlargement, and cushingoid appearance, has been observed in patients receiving antiretroviral therapy. The mechanism and long-term consequences of these events are currently unknown. A causal relationship has not been established.

➤*Renal function impairment:* See Administration and Dosage for more information.

➤*Hepatic function impairment:* See Administration and Dosage for more information.

➤*Pregnancy: Category C.*

Lamivudine/Zidovudine – There are no adequate and well-controlled studies of lamivudine/zidovudine in pregnant women. Treatment of HIV during pregnancy optimizes the health of mother and fetus. Clinical trial data reviewed by the FDA demonstrate that maternal zidovudine treatment significantly reduces vertical transmission of HIV-1 infection to the fetus. Published data suggest that combination antiretroviral regimens may reduce the rate of vertical transmission even further. Only use lamivudine/zidovudine during pregnancy if the potential benefits outweigh the potential risk to the fetus.

Antiretroviral pregnancy registry – To monitor maternal-fetal outcomes of pregnant women exposed to lamivudine/zidovudine and other antiretroviral agents, an antiretroviral pregnancy registry has been established. Register patients by calling 1-800-258-4263.

➤*Lactation:* The Centers for Disease Control and Prevention recommend that HIV-1-infected mothers in the United States not breast-feed their infants to avoid risking postnatal transmission of HIV-1 infection. Because of both the potential for HIV-1 transmission and the potential for serious adverse reactions in breast-feeding infants, instruct mothers not to breast-feed if they are receiving lamivudine/zidovudine.

Although no studies of lamivudine/zidovudine excretion in breast milk have been performed, lactation studies performed with lamivudine and zidovudine show that both drugs are excreted in human breast milk. Samples of breast milk obtained from 20 mothers receiving lamivudine monotherapy (300 mg twice daily) or combination therapy (lamivudine 150 mg twice daily and zidovudine 300 mg twice daily) had measurable concentrations of lamivudine. In another study, after administration of a single dose of zidovudine 200 mg to 13 HIV-1-infected women, the mean concentration of zidovudine was similar in human milk and serum.

➤*Children:* See Administration and Dosage for more information.

➤*Elderly:* See Administration and Dosage for more information.

➤*Monitoring:* Blood cell count monitoring is recommended frequently for patients with advanced HIV-1 disease and periodically for patients with asymptomatic or early HIV-1 disease.

Monitor hepatic function closely with clinical and laboratory follow-up for at least several months in patients who discontinue lamivudine/zidovudine and are coinfected with HIV-1 and HBV.

Drug Interactions

➤*Use with other lamivudine-, zidovudine-, and/or emtricitabine-containing products:* Lamivudine/zidovudine is a fixed-dose combination of lamivudine and zidovudine. Lamivudine/zidovudine should not be administered concomitantly with other lamivudine- or zidovudine-containing products including lamivudine tablets and oral solution; lamivudine-HBV tablets and oral solution; zidovudine tablets, capsules, syrup, and IV infusion; abacavir and lamivudine tablets; abacavir, lamivudine, and zidovudine tablets; or emtricitabine-containing products, including efavirenz, emtricitabine, and tenofovir; emtricitabine; or emtricitabine and tenofovir.

➤*Ribavirin:* Hepatic decompensation (some fatal) has occurred in HIV-1/hepatitis C virus (HCV) coinfected patients receiving combination antiretroviral therapy for HIV-1 and interferon alfa with or without ribavirin. Closely monitor patients receiving coadministration for treatment-associated toxicities, especially hepatic decompensation, neutropenia, and anemia. Consider discontinuation of lamivudine/zidovudine as medically appropriate. Consider dose reduction or discontinuation of interferon alfa, ribavirin, or both if worsening clinical toxicities are observed, including hepatic decompensation (eg, Child-Pugh more than 6).

Exacerbation of anemia has been reported in HIV-1/HCV coinfected patients receiving ribavirin and zidovudine. Coadministration of ribavirin and zidovudine is not advised.

Lamivudine/Zidovudine Drug Interactions			
Precipitant drug	Object drug[a]		Description
Acetaminophen	Zidovudine	↓	Acetaminophen may decrease the AUC of zidovudine.
Atovaquone	Zidovudine	↑	Atovaquone appears to inhibit glucuronidation of zidovudine, thus increasing zidovudine concentrations and decreasing clearance.
Bone marrow suppressive/ cytotoxic agents (eg, ganciclovir, interferon alfa)	Zidovudine	↑	Coadministration may increase the hematologic toxicity of zidovudine. Avoid coadministration of ganciclovir and zidovudine.
Clarithromycin	Zidovudine	↑↓	Peak serum zidovudine concentrations may be increased or decreased.
Doxorubicin	Zidovudine	↓	Avoid coadministration. An antagonistic relationship has been demonstrated.
Fluconazole	Zidovudine	↑	Concurrent use may increase the zidovudine AUC.
Methadone	Zidovudine	↑	Zidovudine serum concentrations and AUC may be elevated, increasing the risk of adverse reactions.
Nelfinavir Ritonavir	Zidovudine	↓	Zidovudine AUC is decreased.
Nelfinavir	Lamivudine	↑	Lamivudine AUC is increased.
Probenecid	Zidovudine	↑	Probenecid may increase zidovudine AUC by inhibiting glucuronidation or reducing renal excretion. Some patients have developed symptoms consisting of myalgia, malaise, fever, and maculopapular rash.

LAMIVUDINE/ZIDOVUDINE — ORAL

Lamivudine/Zidovudine Drug Interactions			
Precipitant drug	Object drug[a]		Description
Ribavirin/ Interferon	Zidovudine	↑	Coadministration of zidovudine in combination with pegylated interferon and ribavirin, may increase the hematologic and hepatic toxicity of zidovudine. Closely monitor patients receiving coadministration for treatment-associated toxicities, especially hepatic decompensation, neutropenia, and anemia. Coadministration of ribavirin and zidovudine is not advised.
Rifamycins	Zidovudine	↓	The AUC of zidovudine may be decreased.
Stavudine	Zidovudine	↓	Avoid coadministration. An antagonistic relationship has been demonstrated.
Trimethoprim Trimethoprim/ Sulfamethoxazole	Lamivudine/ Zidovudine	↑	Plasma lamivudine concentrations may be increased. Trimethoprim appears to inhibit the renal secretion of lamivudine. Serum levels of zidovudine and its metabolite may be increased, especially in patients with impaired hepatic glucuronidation from liver disease or drug inhibition.
Valproic acid	Zidovudine	↑	Concurrent use may inhibit glucuronide metabolism, thus increasing zidovudine AUC.
Zalcitabine	Lamivudine	↓	Lamivudine and zalcitabine may inhibit the intracellular phosphorylation of one another. Severe pancreatitis may occur. Coadministration is not recommended.
Lamivudine	Zalcitabine		
Zidovudine	Didanosine	↓	The AUC of didanosine may be decreased, while the plasma concentration of zidovudine may be increased.
Didanosine	Zidovudine	↑	

[a] ↑ = object drug increased; ↓ = object drug decreased; ↑↓ = object drug both increased and decreased.

Adverse Reactions

➤*Lamivudine plus zidovudine:*

Lamivudine and Zidovudine Adverse Reactions (≥ 5%)	
Adverse reactions	Lamivudine 300 mg/day Plus Zidovudine 600 mg/day (n = 251)
CNS	
Depressive disorders	9%
Dizziness	10%
Headache	35%
Insomnia and other sleep disorders	11%
Malaise and fatigue	27%
Neuropathy	12%
GI	
Abdominal cramps	6%
Abdominal pain	9%
Anorexia and/or decreased appetite	10%
Diarrhea	18%
Dyspepsia	5%
Nausea	33%
Nausea and vomiting	13%
Musculoskeletal	
Arthralgia	5%
Musculoskeletal pain	12%
Myalgia	8%
Miscellaneous	
Cough	18%
Fever or chills	10%
Nasal signs and symptoms	20%
Skin rashes	9%

Pancreatitis was observed in 9 of the 2,613 adult patients (0.3%) who received lamivudine in controlled clinical trials.

Lamivudine Plus Zidovudine Laboratory Abnormalities[a,b]	
Laboratory abnormality	Lamivudine 300 mg/day plus zidovudine 600 mg/day
ALT (> 5 × ULN)	3.7%
Amylase (> 2 × ULN)	4.2%
Anemia (hemoglobin	2.9%
AST (> 5 × ULN)	1.7%
Bilirubin (> 2.5 × ULN)	0.8%
Neutropenia (ANC < 750/mm^3)	7.2%
Thrombocytopenia (platelets < 50,000/mm^3)	0.4%

[a] Frequencies of these laboratory abnormalities were higher in patients with mild laboratory abnormalities at baseline.
[b] ANC = absolute neutrophil count; ULN = upper limit of normal.

➤*Postmarketing:*

CNS – Paresthesia, peripheral neuropathy, seizures, weakness.

Dermatologic – Alopecia, erythema multiforme, Stevens-Johnson syndrome.

GI – Oral mucosal pigmentation, stomatitis.

Hematologic/Lymphatic – Anemia (including pure red cell aplasia and anemias progressing on therapy), lymphadenopathy, splenomegaly.

Hepatic – Lactic acidosis and hepatic steatosis, pancreatitis, posttreatment exacerbation of hepatitis B.

Hypersensitivity – Sensitization reactions (including anaphylaxis), urticaria.

Metabolic – Gynecomastia, hyperglycemia.

Musculoskeletal – Creatine phosphokinase elevation, muscle weakness, rhabdomyolysis.

Respiratory –

Miscellaneous – Abnormal breath sounds/wheezing, cardiomyopathy, redistribution/accumulation of body fat, vasculitis.

Overdosage

➤*Symptoms:* One case of an adult ingesting 6 g of lamivudine was reported; there were no clinical signs or symptoms noted and hematologic tests remained normal.

Acute overdoses of zidovudine have been reported in children and adults. These involved exposures up to 50 g. The only consistent findings were nausea and vomiting. Other reported occurrences included headache, dizziness, drowsiness, lethargy, confusion, and 1 report of a grand mal seizure. Hematologic changes were transient. All patients recovered.

➤*Treatment:* There is no known antidote for lamivudine/zidovudine. Because a negligible amount of lamivudine was removed via hemodialysis (4 hours), continuous ambulatory peritoneal dialysis, and automated peritoneal dialysis, it is not known if continuous hemodialysis would provide clinical benefit in a lamivudine overdose event. Hemodialysis and peritoneal dialysis appear to have a negligible effect on the removal of zidovudine, while elimination of its primary metabolite, GZDV, is enhanced.

Patient Information

Lamivudine/zidovudine is not a cure for HIV-1 infection and patients may continue to experience illnesses associated with HIV-1 infection, including opportunistic infections. Advise patients that the use of lamivudine/zidovudine has not been shown to reduce the risk of transmission of HIV-1 to others through sexual contact or blood contamination. Advise patients of the importance of taking lamivudine/zidovudine exactly as it is prescribed.

Inform patients that redistribution or accumulation of body fat may occur in patients receiving antiretroviral therapy and that the cause and long-term health effects of these conditions are not known at this time.

Caution patients about the use of other medications, including ganciclovir, interferon alfa, and ribavirin, which may exacerbate the toxicity of zidovudine.

Lamivudine/zidovudine should not be coadministered with drugs containing lamivudine, zidovudine, or emtricitabine, including *Epivir* (lamivudine), *Epvir-HBV* (lamivudine-HBV), *Retrovir* (zidovudine), *Epzicom* (abacavir sulfate and lamivudine), *Trizivir* (abacavir sulfate, lamivudine, and zidovudine), *Atripla* (efavirenz, emtricitabine, and tenofovir), *Emtriva* (emtricitabine), or *Truvada* (emtricitabine and tenofovir).

Inform patients coinfected with HIV-1 and HBV that deterioration of liver disease has occurred in some cases when treatment with lamivudine was discontinued. Advise patients to discuss any changes in regimen with their health care provider.

Inform patients that the important toxicities associated with zidovudine are neutropenia and/or anemia. Tell patients about the importance of having their blood cell counts followed closely while on therapy, especially patients with advanced HIV-1 disease.

ABACAVIR SULFATE/LAMIVUDINE/ZIDOVUDINE

Rx	**Trizivir** (ViiV Healthcare)	**Tablets; oral:** abacavir sulfate 300 mg/lamivudine 150 mg/zidovudine 300 mg	(GX LL1). Blue-green, capsule shape. Film-coated. In 60s.

ABACAVIR SULFATE/LAMIVUDINE/ZIDOVUDINE — ORAL

Consult the complete prescribing information for each agent (ie, abacavir, lamivudine, zidovudine) prior to administration of abacavir/lamivudine/zidovudine combination tablets.

WARNING

This product contains 3 nucleoside analogs (ie, abacavir sulfate, lamivudine, zidovudine) and is intended only for patients whose regimen would otherwise include these 3 components.

Hypersensitivity reactions – Serious and sometimes fatal hypersensitivity reactions have been associated with abacavir sulfate, a component of abacavir/lamivudine/zidovudine. Hypersensitivity to abacavir is a multi-organ clinical syndrome usually characterized by a sign or symptom in 2 or more of the following groups: fever; rash; GI (eg, abdominal pain, diarrhea, nausea, vomiting); constitutional (eg, achiness, fatigue, generalized malaise); respiratory (eg, cough, dyspnea, pharyngitis).

Discontinue abacavir/lamivudine/zidovudine as soon as a hypersensitivity reaction is suspected.

Patients who carry the HLA-B*5701 allele are at high risk for experiencing a hypersensitivity reaction to abacavir. Prior to initiating therapy with abacavir, screening for HLA-B*5701 allele is recommended; this approach has been found to decrease the risk of hypersensitivity reaction. Screening is also recommended prior to reinitiation of abacavir in patients of unknown HLA-B*5701 status who have previously tolerated abacavir. HLA-B*5701–negative patients may develop a suspected hypersensitivity reaction to abacavir; however, this occurs significantly less frequently than in HLA-B*5701–positive patients.

Regardless of HLA-B*5701 status, permanently discontinue abacavir/lamivudine/zidovudine if hypersensitivity cannot be ruled out, even when other diagnoses are possible.

Following a hypersensitivity reaction to abacavir, never restart abacavir/lamivudine/zidovudine or any other abacavir-containing product because more severe symptoms can occur within hours and may include life-threatening hypotension and death.

Reintroduction of abacavir/lamivudine/zidovudine or any other abacavir-containing product, even in patients who have no identified history or unrecognized symptoms of hypersensitivity to abacavir therapy, can result in serious or fatal hypersensitivity reactions. Such reactions can occur within hours (see Warnings/Precautions).

Hematologic toxicity – Zidovudine has been associated with hematologic toxicity, including neutropenia and severe anemia, particularly in patients with advanced HIV-1 disease. Prolonged use of zidovudine has been associated with symptomatic myopathy.

Lactic acidosis and severe hepatomegaly – Lactic acidosis and severe hepatomegaly with steatosis, including fatal cases, have been reported with the use of nucleoside analogs alone or in combination, including abacavir, lamivudine, zidovudine, and other antiretrovirals.

Exacerbations of hepatitis B – Severe acute exacerbations of hepatitis B have been reported in patients who are coinfected with hepatitis B virus (HBV) and HIV-1 and have discontinued lamivudine, which is one component of abacavir/lamivudine/zidovudine. Monitor hepatic function closely with both clinical and laboratory follow-up for at least several months in patients who discontinue abacavir/lamivudine/zidovudine and are coinfected with HIV-1 and HBV. If appropriate, initiation of anti-HBV therapy may be warranted.

Indications

➤*HIV infection:* In combination with other antiretroviral agents or alone for the treatment of HIV-1 infection in patients weighing more than 40 kg.

Administration and Dosage

➤*Adults:*

HIV –

Usual dosage:

- *Weighing 40 kg or more* – 1 tablet twice daily.
- *Weighing less than 40 kg* – Abacavir/lamivudine/zidovudine is not recommended in adolescents who weigh less than 40 kg because it is a fixed-dose tablet.

Dosage adjustment: Because it is a fixed-dose tablet, abacavir/lamivudine/zidovudine should not be prescribed for patients requiring dosage adjustment or patients experiencing dose-limiting adverse reactions.

➤*Children:*

HIV –

Usual dosage:

- *Adolescents weighing 40 kg or more* – See Adults for dosing.
- *Children and adolescents weighing less than 40 kg* – Abacavir/lamivudine/zidovudine is not intended for use in children weighing less than 40 kg.

➤*Renal function impairment:* Because abacavir/lamivudine/zidovudine is a fixed-dose tablet and the dosage of the individual components cannot be altered, patients with creatinine clearance (CrCl) less than 50 mL/min should not receive abacavir/lamivudine/zidovudine.

➤*Hepatic function impairment:* Because abacavir/lamivudine/zidovudine is a fixed-dose combination that cannot be adjusted for this patient population, abacavir/lamivudine/zidovudine is contraindicated in patients with hepatic function impairment.

➤*Storage/Stability:* Store at 25°C (77°F); excursions are permitted to 15° to 30°C (59° to 86°F).

Actions

➤*Pharmacology:*

Abacavir – Abacavir is a carbocyclic synthetic nucleoside analog. Abacavir is converted by cellular enzymes to the active metabolite carbovir triphosphate (CBV-TP), an analog of deoxyguanosine-5′-triphosphate (dGTP). CBV-TP inhibits the activity of HIV-1 reverse transcriptase (RT) by competing with the natural substrate dGTP and by its incorporation into viral DNA. The lack of a 3′-OH group in the incorporated nucleotide analog prevents the formation of the 5′ to 3′ phosphodiester linkage essential for DNA chain elongation, and, therefore, the viral DNA growth is terminated. CBV-TP is a weak inhibitor of cellular DNA polymerases alpha, beta, and gamma.

Lamivudine – Lamivudine is a synthetic nucleoside analog. Intracellularly, lamivudine is phosphorylated to its active 5′-triphosphate metabolite, lamivudine triphosphate (3TC-TP). The principal mode of action of 3TC-TP is inhibition of RT via DNA chain termination after incorporation of the nucleotide analog. 3TC-TP is a weak inhibitor of cellular DNA polymerases alpha, beta, and gamma.

Zidovudine – Zidovudine is a synthetic nucleoside analog. Intracellularly, zidovudine is phosphorylated to its active 5′-triphosphate metabolite, zidovudine triphosphate (ZDV-TP). The principal mode of action of ZDV-TP is inhibition of RT via DNA chain termination after incorporation of the nucleotide analog. ZDV-TP is a weak inhibitor of the cellular DNA polymerases alpha and gamma and has been reported to be incorporated into the DNA of cells in culture.

➤*Pharmacokinetics:*

Pharmacokinetic Parameters for Abacavir, Lamivudine, and Zidovudine in Adults[a]

Parameter	Abacavir	Lamivudine	Zidovudine
Oral bioavailability (%)	86 ± 2.5	86 ± 16	64 ± 10
Apparent volume of distribution (L/kg)	0.86 ± 0.15	1.3 ± 0.4	1.6 ± 0.6
Systemic clearance (L/h/kg)	0.8 ± 0.24	0.33 ± 0.06	1.6 ± 0.6
Renal clearance (L/h/kg)	0.007 ± 0.008	0.22 ± 0.06	0.34 ± 0.05
Elimination half-life (h)[b]	1.45 ± 0.32	5 to 7	0.5 to 3

[a] Data presented as mean ± standard deviation except where noted.
[b] Approximate range.

Absorption/Distribution – In a single-dose, 3-way, crossover bioavailability study of 1 abacavir/lamivudine/zidovudine tablet versus 1 abacavir 300 mg tablet, 1 lamivudine 150 mg tablet, plus 1 zidovudine 300 mg tablet administered simultaneously in healthy subjects (n = 24), there was no difference in the extent of absorption, as measured by the area under the curve (AUC) and maximal peak concentration (C_{max}) of all 3 components.

Abacavir: Following oral administration, abacavir is rapidly absorbed and extensively distributed. Binding of abacavir to human plasma proteins is approximately 50%. Binding of abacavir to plasma proteins was independent of concentration. Total blood and plasma drug-related radioactivity concentrations are identical, demonstrating that abacavir readily distributes into erythrocytes.

Lamivudine/zidovudine: Following oral administration, lamivudine and zidovudine are rapidly absorbed and extensively distributed. Binding to plasma protein is low.

Bioequivalence: One abacavir/lamivudine/zidovudine tablet was bioequivalent to one abacavir 300 mg tablet, one lamivudine 150 mg tablet, plus one zidovudine 300 mg tablet following single-dose administration to fasting healthy subjects (n = 24).

Food effects: Abacavir/lamivudine/zidovudine may be administered with or without food. Administration with food in a single-dose bioavailability study resulted in lower C_{max}, similar to results observed previously for the reference formulations. The average (90% confidence interval [CI]) decrease in abacavir, lamivudine, and zidovudine C_{max} was 32% (24% to 38%), 18% (10% to 25%), and 28% (13% to 40%), respectively, when administered with a high-fat meal, compared with administration under fasted conditions. Administration of abacavir/lamivudine/zidovudine with food did not alter the extent of abacavir, lamivudine, and zidovudine absorption (AUC), compared with administration under fasted conditions (n = 24).

Metabolism/Excretion –

Abacavir: The primary routes of elimination of abacavir are metabolism by alcohol dehydrogenase to form the 5′-carboxylic acid and glucuronyl transferase to form the 5′-glucuronide.

Lamivudine: Approximately 70% of an intravenous (IV) dose of lamivudine is recovered as unchanged drug in the urine. Metabolism of lamivudine

ABACAVIR SULFATE/LAMIVUDINE/ZIDOVUDINE — ORAL

is a minor route of elimination. In humans, the only known metabolite is the trans-sulfoxide metabolite (approximately 5% of an oral dose after 12 hours).

Zidovudine: Zidovudine is eliminated primarily by hepatic metabolism. The major metabolite of zidovudine is 3′-azido-3′-deoxy-5′-*O*-β-*D*-glucopyranuronosylthymidine. AUC of 3′-azido-3′-deoxy-5′-*O*-β-*D*-glucopyranuronosylthymidine is about 3-fold greater than the zidovudine AUC. Urinary recovery of zidovudine and 3′-azido-3′-deoxy-5′-*O*-β-*D*-glucopyranuronosylthymidine accounts for 14% and 74% of the dose following oral administration, respectively. A second metabolite, 3′-amino-3′-deoxythymidine, has been identified in plasma. The 3′-amino-3′-deoxythymidine AUC was one-fifth of the zidovudine AUC.

Special populations –

Renal function impairment: Because lamivudine and zidovudine require dose adjustment in the presence of renal insufficiency, abacavir/lamivudine/zidovudine is not recommended for use in patients with CrCl less than 50 mL/min.

Hepatic function impairment: A reduction in the daily dose of zidovudine may be necessary in patients with mild to moderate hepatic function impairment or liver cirrhosis. Abacavir is contraindicated in patients with moderate to severe hepatic impairment, and dose reduction is required in patients with mild hepatic impairment. Because abacavir/lamivudine/zidovudine is a fixed-dose combination that cannot be adjusted for this patient population, abacavir/lamivudine/zidovudine is contraindicated for patients with hepatic function impairment.

Children: Abacavir/lamivudine/zidovudine is not intended for use in children. Do not administer abacavir/lamivudine/zidovudine to adolescents who weigh less than 40 kg because it is a fixed-dose tablet that cannot be dose adjusted for this patient population.

Contraindications

Hypersensitivity to abacavir or any other component of the product (see Black Box Warning for more information); hepatic impairment.

Warnings/Precautions

➤*Hypersensitivity reactions:* Serious and sometimes fatal hypersensitivity reactions have been associated with abacavir/lamivudine/zidovudine and other abacavir-containing products.

Patients who carry the HLA-B*5701 allele are at high risk for experiencing a hypersensitivity reaction to abacavir. Prior to initiating therapy with abacavir, screening for the HLA-B*5701 allele is recommended; this approach has been found to decrease the risk of a hypersensitivity reaction. Screening is also recommended prior to reinitiation of abacavir in patients of unknown HLA-B*5701 status who have previously tolerated abacavir. For HLA-B*5701–positive patients, treatment with an abacavir-containing regimen is not recommended; consider only with close medical supervision and under exceptional circumstances when the potential benefit outweighs the risk.

HLA-B*5701–negative patients may develop a hypersensitivity reaction to abacavir; however, this occurs significantly less frequently than in HLA-B*5701–positive patients. Regardless of HLA-B*5701 status, permanently discontinue abacavir/lamivudine/zidovudine if hypersensitivity cannot be ruled out, even when other diagnoses are possible.

Abacavir hypersensitivity reaction registry – To facilitate reporting of hypersensitivity reactions and collection of information on each case, an abacavir hypersensitivity registry has been established. Register patients by calling 1-800-270-0425.

➤*Lactic acidosis/severe hepatomegaly with steatosis:* Lactic acidosis and severe hepatomegaly with steatosis, including fatal cases, have been reported with the use of nucleoside analogs alone or in combination, including abacavir, lamivudine, zidovudine, and other antiretrovirals. A majority of these cases have been in women. Obesity and prolonged nucleoside exposure may be risk factors. Exercise particular caution when administering abacavir/lamivudine/zidovudine to any patient with known risk factors for liver disease; however, cases have also been reported in patients with no known risk factors. Suspend treatment in any patient who develops clinical or laboratory findings suggestive of lactic acidosis or pronounced hepatotoxicity (which may include hepatomegaly and steatosis, even in the absence of marked transaminase elevations).

➤*Bone marrow suppression:* Because abacavir/lamivudine/zidovudine contains zidovudine, use abacavir/lamivudine/zidovudine with caution in patients who have bone marrow compromise evidenced by a granulocyte count less than 1,000 cells/mm^3 or hemoglobin less than 9.5 g/dL. Frequent blood cells counts are strongly recommended in patients with advanced HIV-1 disease who are treated with abacavir/lamivudine/zidovudine. For HIV-1–infected individuals and patients with asymptomatic or early HIV-1 disease, periodic blood cell counts are recommended.

➤*Myopathy:* Myopathy and myositis, with pathological changes similar to those produced by HIV-1 disease, have been associated with prolonged use of zidovudine, and, therefore, may occur with therapy with abacavir/lamivudine/zidovudine.

➤*Posttreatment exacerbations of hepatitis:* In clinical trials in non–HIV-1-infected patients treated with lamivudine for chronic HBV, clinical and laboratory evidence of exacerbations of hepatitis have occurred after discontinuation of lamivudine. These exacerbations have been detected primarily by serum ALT elevations in addition to reemergence of HBV DNA. Although most events appear to have been self-limited, fatalities have been reported in some cases. Similar events have been reported from postmarketing experience after changes from lamivudine-containing HIV-1 treatment regimens to non–lamivudine-containing regimens in patients infected with both HIV-1 and HBV. The causal relationship to discontinuation of lamivudine treatment is unknown. Closely monitor patients with clinical and laboratory follow-up for at least several months after stopping treatment. There is insufficient evidence to determine whether reinitiation of lamivudine alters the course of posttreatment exacerbations of hepatitis.

➤*Fixed-dose combination:* Abacavir/lamivudine/zidovudine contains fixed doses of 3 nucleoside analogs: abacavir, lamivudine, and zidovudine; do not coadminister with abacavir, lamivudine, emtricitabine, or zidovudine. Do not coadminister abacavir/lamivudine/zidovudine with the fixed-dose combination drugs: lamivudine/zidovudine, abacavir and lamivudine, or emtricitabine and tenofovir.

Because abacavir/lamivudine/zidovudine is a fixed-dose tablet, do not prescribe it for adolescents who weigh less than 40 kg or other patients requiring dosage adjustment.

➤*Therapy-experienced patients:* In clinical trials, patients with prolonged prior NRTI exposure or who had HIV-1 isolates that contained multiple mutations conferring resistance to NRTIs had limited response to abacavir. Consider the potential for cross-resistance between abacavir and other NRTIs when choosing new therapeutic regimens in therapy-experienced patients.

➤*HIV and HBV coinfection:* Safety and efficacy of lamivudine have not been established for treatment of chronic hepatitis B in patients dually infected with HIV-1 and HBV. In non–HIV-1-infected patients treated with lamivudine for chronic hepatitis B, emergence of lamivudine-resistant HBV has been detected and has been associated with diminished treatment response. Emergence of HBV variants associated with resistance to lamivudine has also been reported in HIV-1–infected patients who have received lamivudine-containing antiretroviral regimens in the presence of concurrent infection with HBV.

➤*Immune reconstitution syndrome:* Immune reconstitution syndrome has been reported in patients treated with combination antiretroviral therapy, including abacavir/lamivudine/zidovudine. During the initial phase of combination antiretroviral treatment, patients whose immune systems respond may develop an inflammatory response to indolent or residual opportunistic infections (eg, *Mycobacterium avium* infection, cytomegalovirus, *Pneumocystis jirovecii* pneumonia [PCP], tuberculosis), which may necessitate further evaluation and treatment.

➤*Fat redistribution:* Redistribution/accumulation of body fat, including central obesity, dorsocervical fat enlargement (buffalo hump), peripheral wasting, facial wasting, breast enlargement, and cushingoid appearance, have been observed in patients receiving antiretroviral therapy. The mechanism and long-term consequences of these events are currently unknown. A causal relationship has not been established.

➤*Myocardial infarction:* In a published prospective, observational, epidemiological study designed to investigate the rate of myocardial infarction (MI) in patients on combination antiretroviral therapy, the use of abacavir within the previous 6 months was correlated with an increased risk of MI. In a sponsor-conducted pooled analysis of clinical trials, no excess risk of MI was observed in abacavir-treated patients compared with control subjects. In totality, the available data from the observational cohort and from clinical trials are inconclusive.

As a precaution, consider the underlying risk of coronary heart disease when prescribing antiretroviral therapies, including abacavir, and take action to minimize all modifiable risk factors (eg, diabetes mellitus, hyperlipidemia, hypertension, smoking).

➤*Renal function impairment:* Because abacavir/lamivudine/zidovudine is a fixed-dose tablet and the dosage of the individual components cannot be altered, patients with CrCl less than 50 mL/min should not receive abacavir/lamivudine/zidovudine.

➤*Hepatic function impairment:* Abacavir/lamivudine/zidovudine is contraindicated in patients with hepatic impairment because it is a fixed-dose tablet and the dosage of the individual components cannot be altered.

➤*Pregnancy:* *Category C.* There are no adequate and well-controlled studies of abacavir/lamivudine/zidovudine in pregnant women. Use abacavir/lamivudine/zidovudine during pregnancy only if the potential benefits outweigh the risks.

Abacavir – Studies in pregnant rats showed that abacavir is transferred to the fetus through the placenta. Fetal malformations (increased incidences of fetal anasarca and skeletal malformations) and developmental toxicity (depressed fetal body weight and reduced crown-rump length) were observed in rats at a dose that produced 35 times the human exposure, based on AUC. Embryonic and fetal toxicities (increased resorptions, decreased fetal body weights) and toxicities to the offspring (increased incidence of stillbirth and lower body weights) occurred at half of the above-mentioned dose in separate fertility studies conducted in rats.

Lamivudine – Studies in pregnant rats and rabbits showed that lamivudine is transferred to the fetus through the placenta. Reproduction studies with orally administered lamivudine have been performed in rats and rabbits at dosages up to 4,000 mg/kg/day and 1,000 mg/kg/day, respectively, producing plasma levels up to approximately 35 times that for the adult HIV dose. No evidence of teratogenicity caused by lamivudine was observed. Evidence of early embryolethality was seen in the rabbit at exposure levels similar to those observed in humans, but there was no indication of this effect in the rat at exposure levels up to 35 times that in humans.

Zidovudine – Zidovudine treatment resulted in embryo/fetal toxicity, as evidenced by an increase in the incidence of fetal resorptions in rats given 150 or 450 mg/kg/day and rabbits given 500 mg/kg/day. The doses used in the teratology studies resulted in peak zidovudine plasma concentrations

ABACAVIR SULFATE/LAMIVUDINE/ZIDOVUDINE — ORAL

(after one-half of the daily dose) in rats 66 to 226 times, and in rabbits 12 to 87 times, mean steady-state peak human plasma concentrations (after one-sixth of the daily dose) achieved with the recommended daily dosage (100 mg every 4 hours). In an additional teratology study in rats, a dosage of 3,000 mg/kg/day (very near the oral median lethal dose in rats of approximately 3,700 mg/kg) caused marked maternal toxicity and an increase in the incidence of fetal malformations. This dose resulted in peak zidovudine plasma concentrations 350 times peak human plasma concentrations. No evidence of teratogenicity was seen in this experiment at dosages of 600 mg/kg/day or less.

Antiretroviral pregnancy registry – To monitor maternal-fetal outcomes of pregnant women exposed to abacavir/lamivudine/zidovudine or other antiretroviral agents, an antiretroviral pregnancy registry has been established. Register patients by calling 1-800-258-4263.

➤*Lactation:* The CDC recommends that HIV-1–infected mothers not breast-feed their infants to avoid risking postnatal transmission of HIV-1 infection.

Lamivudine and zidovudine are excreted in human breast milk; abacavir and lamivudine are secreted into the milk of lactating rats.

Because of both the potential for HIV transmission and the potential for serious adverse reactions in breast-feeding infants, instruct mothers not to breast-feed if they are receiving abacavir/lamivudine/zidovudine.

➤*Children:* Abacavir/lamivudine/zidovudine is not intended for use in children. Do not administer abacavir/lamivudine/zidovudine to adolescents who weigh less than 40 kg because it is a fixed-dose tablet that cannot be adjusted for this patient population.

Therapy-experienced children – A randomized, double-blind study, CNA3006, compared abacavir plus lamivudine and zidovudine with lamivudine and zidovudine in children, most of whom were extensively pretreated with nucleoside analog antiretroviral agents. Patients in this study had a limited response to abacavir.

➤*Elderly:* In general, use caution in dose selection for an elderly patient, reflecting the greater frequency of decreased hepatic, renal, or cardiac function, and of concomitant disease or other drug therapy. Abacavir/lamivudine/zidovudine is not recommended for patients with impaired renal function (ie, CrCl less than 50 mL/min).

➤*Monitoring:* Monitor patients with coinfection with HBV and HIV for posttreatment exacerbations of hepatitis B for several months after stopping treatment. Frequent blood cell counts are strongly recommended in patients with advanced HIV-1 disease who are being treated with abacavir/lamivudine/zidovudine. For HIV-1–infected individuals and patients with asymptomatic or early HIV-1 disease, periodic blood cell counts are recommended.

Drug Interactions

Abacavir/Lamivudine/Zidovudine Drug Interactions

Precipitant drug	Object drug[a]		Description
Acetaminophen	Abacavir/ Lamivudine/ Zidovudine	↓	Acetaminophen may decrease the AUC of zidovudine.
Atovaquone	Abacavir/ Lamivudine/ Zidovudine	↑	Atovaquone appears to inhibit glucuronidation of zidovudine, thus increasing zidovudine concentrations and decreasing clearance.
Bone marrow suppressive/ cytotoxic agents (eg, interferon alpha, interferon beta-1b, ganciclovir)	Abacavir/ Lamivudine/ Zidovudine	↑	Coadministration may increase the hematologic toxicity of zidovudine.
Clarithromycin	Abacavir/ Lamivudine/ Zidovudine	↑↓	Peak serum zidovudine concentrations may be increased or decreased.
Doxorubicin	Abacavir/ Lamivudine/ Zidovudine	↓	Avoid coadministration. An antagonistic relationship has been demonstrated.
Ethanol	Abacavir/ Lamivudine/ Zidovudine	↑	Coadministration of ethanol and abacavir resulted in a 41% increase in abacavir AUC and a 26% increase in abacavir half-life.
Fluconazole	Abacavir/ Lamivudine/ Zidovudine	↔	Concurrent use may increase the zidovudine AUC. Clinical significance is not known.
Ganciclovir	Abacavir/ Lamivudine/ Zidovudine	↑	Concomitant use may increase zidovudine plasma levels and AUC, thus increasing risk of life-threatening hematologic toxicities.
Nelfinavir Ritonavir	Abacavir/ Lamivudine/ Zidovudine	↓	Zidovudine AUC is decreased, decreasing the pharmacologic effects.
Probenecid	Abacavir/ Lamivudine/ Zidovudine	↑	Probenecid may increase zidovudine AUC by inhibiting glucuronidation or reducing renal excretion. Some patients have developed symptoms consisting of maculopapular rash, myalgia, and malaise or fever.
Ribavirin	Abacavir/ Lamivudine/ Zidovudine	↓	Ribavirin may inhibit the phosphorylation of lamivudine and zidovudine, thus reducing therapeutic effectiveness.
Ribavirin/ Interferon	Abacavir/ Lamivudine/ Zidovudine	↑	Coadministration of zidovudine in combination with pegylated interferon/ribavirin may increase the hematologic and hepatic toxicity of zidovudine. Closely monitor patients receiving this combination for treatment-associated toxicities, especially anemia, hepatic decompensation, and neutropenia.
Rifamycins (eg, rifabutin, rifampin)	Abacavir/ Lamivudine/ Zidovudine	↓	The AUC of zidovudine may be decreased.
Stavudine Ribavirin	Abacavir/ Lamivudine/ Zidovudine	↓	Avoid concomitant use because some nucleoside analogs affect viral replication and may antagonize antiviral activity of zidovudine against HIV.
Trimethoprim/ Sulfamethoxazole	Abacavir/ Lamivudine/ Zidovudine	↑	Plasma concentrations of lamivudine and zidovudine may be increased.
Valproic acid	Abacavir/ Lamivudine/ Zidovudine	↑	Concurrent use may inhibit glucuronide metabolism, thus increasing zidovudine AUC.
Abacavir/ Lamivudine/ Zidovudine	Methadone	↓↑	Abacavir increased oral methadone clearance by 22%. This alteration will not result in a methadone dose modification in the majority of patients; however, an increased methadone dose may be required in a small number of patients. Zidovudine serum concentrations and AUC may be elevated, increasing the risk of adverse reactions.
Methadone	Abacavir/ Lamivudine/ Zidovudine		
Abacavir/ lamivudine/ zidovudine	Phenytoin	↔	Phenytoin levels have been reported to increase, decrease, or not change with concurrent use. In addition, zidovudine clearance was decreased by phenytoin.
Phenytoin	Abacavir/ Lamivudine/ Zidovudine	↑	

[a] ↑ = object drug increased; ↓ = object drug decreased; ↔ = undetermined clinical effect.

Adverse Reactions

➤*Hypersensitivity:* Serious and sometimes fatal hypersensitivity reactions have been associated with abacavir sulfate, a component of abacavir/lamivudine/zidovudine (see Black Box Warning and Warnings/Precautions for more information).

➤*Treatment-emergent adverse reactions:* Treatment-emergent clinical adverse reactions (rated by the investigator as moderate or severe) with a 5% or more frequency during therapy with abacavir 300 mg twice daily, lamivudine 150 mg twice daily, and zidovudine 300 mg twice daily compared with indinavir 800 mg 3 times daily, lamivudine 150 mg twice daily, and zidovudine 300 mg twice daily from CNA3005 are listed in the following table.

Abacavir/Lamivudine/Zidovudine Adverse Reactions in Therapy-Naive Adults (≥ 5%)

Adverse reaction	Abacavir plus lamivudine/zidovudine (n = 262)	Indinavir plus lamivudine/zidovudine (n = 264)
CNS		
Anxiety	5%	3%
Depressive disorders	6%	4%

ABACAVIR SULFATE/LAMIVUDINE/ZIDOVUDINE — ORAL

Abacavir/Lamivudine/Zidovudine Adverse Reactions in Therapy-Naive Adults (≥ 5%)

Adverse reaction	Abacavir plus lamivudine/zidovudine (n = 262)	Indinavir plus lamivudine/zidovudine (n = 264)
Headache	13%	9%
Malaise and fatigue	12%	12%
GI		
Diarrhea	7%	5%
Nausea	19%	17%
Nausea and vomiting	10%	10%
Hypersensitivity		
Hypersensitivity reaction	8%	2%
Skin rashes	5%	4%
Miscellaneous		
Ear/Nose/Throat infections	5%	4%
Fever and/or chills	6%	3%
Musculoskeletal pain	5%	7%
Pain (non-site-specific)	< 1%	5%
Renal sign/symptoms	< 1%	5%
Viral respiratory infections	5%	5%

Five patients receiving abacavir in study CNA3005 experienced worsening of preexisting depression compared with none in the indinavir arm. The background rates of preexisting depression were similar in the 2 treatment arms.

➤*Other adverse reactions:* In addition, other adverse reactions observed in the expanded access program for abacavir were pancreatitis and increased gamma-glutamyltransferase.

➤*Lab test abnormalities:*

Abacavir Plus Lamivudine/Zidovudine Treatment-Emergent Laboratory Abnormalities (Grades 3 to 4) in Study CNA3005[a]

Grade 3/4 laboratory abnormalities	Abacavir plus lamivudine/zidovudine (n = 262)	Indinavir plus lamivudine/zidovudine (n = 264)
Elevated CPK (> 4 × ULN)	7%	7%
ALT (> 5 × ULN)	6%	6%
Neutropenia (< 750/mm^3)	5%	5%
Hypertriglyceridemia (> 750 mg/dL)	2%	1%
Hyperamylasemia (> 2 × ULN)	2%	< 1%
Hyperglycemia (> 13.9 mmol/L)	< 1%	< 1%
Anemia (Hgb ≤ 6.9 g/dL)	0%	1%

[a] CPK = creatine phosphokinase; ULN = upper limit of normal; Hgb = hemoglobin.

➤*Abacavir:*

Cardiovascular – MI.

Dermatologic – Suspected Stevens-Johnson syndrome and toxic epidermal necrolysis (TEN) have been reported in patients receiving abacavir primarily in combination with medications known to be associated with Stevens-Johnson syndrome and TEN, respectively. Because of the overlap of clinical signs and symptoms between hypersensitivity to abacavir and SJS and TEN, and the possibility of multiple drug sensitivities in some patients, discontinue abacavir and do not restart it in such cases.

There have also been reports of erythema multiforme with abacavir use.

➤*Abacavir, lamivudine, and/or zidovudine:*

CNS – Dizziness, insomnia and other sleep disorders, paresthesia, peripheral neuropathy, seizures, weakness.

Dermatologic – Alopecia, erythema multiforme, Stevens-Johnson syndrome.

Endocrine – Gynecomastia, hyperglycemia.

GI – Anorexia and/or decreased appetite, abdominal pain, dyspepsia, oral mucosal pigmentation, stomatitis.

Hematologic/Lymphatic – Aplastic anemia, anemia (including pure red cell aplasia and severe anemias progressing on therapy), lymphadenopathy, splenomegaly, thrombocytopenia.

Hepatic – Hepatic steatosis and lactic acidosis, elevated bilirubin, elevated transaminases, pancreatitis, posttreatment exacerbation of hepatitis B.

Hypersensitivity – Sensitization reactions (including anaphylaxis), urticaria.

Musculoskeletal – Arthralgia, CPK elevation, myalgia, muscle weakness, rhabdomyolysis.

Respiratory – Abnormal breath sounds/wheezing.

Miscellaneous – Cardiomyopathy, redistribution/accumulation of body fat, vasculitis.

Overdosage

➤*Abacavir:* There is no known antidote for abacavir. It is not known whether abacavir can be removed by peritoneal dialysis or hemodialysis.

➤*Lamivudine:* One case of an adult ingesting lamivudine 6 g was reported; there were no clinical signs or symptoms noted and hematologic tests remained normal. Because a negligible amount of lamivudine was removed via (4-hour) hemodialysis, continuous ambulatory peritoneal dialysis, and automated peritoneal dialysis, it is not known if continuous hemodialysis would provide clinical benefit in a lamivudine overdose event.

➤*Zidovudine:* Acute overdoses of zidovudine have been reported in children and adults. These involved exposures of up to 50 g. The only consistent findings were nausea and vomiting. Other reported occurrences included headache, dizziness, drowsiness, lethargy, and confusion. Hematologic changes were transient. All patients recovered. Hemodialysis and peritoneal dialysis appear to have a negligible effect on the removal of zidovudine, while elimination of its primary metabolite, 3′-azido-3′-deoxy-5′-*O*-β-*D*-glucopyranuronosylthymidine, is enhanced.

Patient Information

➤*Abacavir hypersensitivity reaction:* Inform patients of the following:

- a *Medication Guide* and warning card summarizing the symptoms of the abacavir hypersensitivity reaction and other product information will be dispensed by the pharmacist with each new prescription and refill of abacavir/lamivudine/zidovudine. Encourage the patient to read the *Medication Guide* and warning card every time to obtain any new information that may be present about abacavir/lamivudine/zidovudine.
- to carry the warning card with them.
- how to identify a hypersensitivity reaction (see Warnings and *Medication Guide*). If they develop symptoms consistent with a hypersensitivity reaction, they should call their health care provider right away to determine if they should stop taking abacavir/lamivudine/zidovudine.
- that a hypersensitivity reaction can worsen and lead to hospitalization or death if abacavir/lamivudine/zidovudine is not immediately discontinued.
- to not restart abacavir/lamivudine/zidovudine or any other abacavir-containing product following a hypersensitivity reaction because more severe symptoms can occur within hours and may include life-threatening hypotension and death.
- that a hypersensitivity reaction is usually reversible if it is detected promptly and abacavir/lamivudine/zidovudine is stopped right away.
- that if they have interrupted abacavir/lamivudine/zidovudine for reasons other than symptoms of hypersensitivity (ie, those who have an interruption in drug supply), a serious or fatal hypersensitivity reaction may occur with reintroduction of abacavir.
- to not restart abacavir/lamivudine/zidovudine or any other abacavir-containing product without medical consultation and that restarting abacavir needs to be undertaken only if medical care can be readily accessed by the patient or others.
- abacavir/lamivudine/zidovudine should not be coadministered with lamivudine/zidovudine combination, emtricitabine, lamivudine, abacavir/lamivudine combination, zidovudine, emtricitabine/tenofovir combination, or abacavir.

➤*Lamivudine:* Inform patients coinfected with HIV and HBV that deterioration of liver disease has occurred in some cases when treatment with lamivudine was discontinued. Advise patients to discuss any changes in regimen with their health care provider.

➤*Zidovudine:* Inform patients that the important toxicities associated with zidovudine are neutropenia and/or anemia. Inform them of the extreme importance of having their blood cell counts followed closely while on therapy, especially for patients with advanced HIV disease.

➤*Abacavir/Lamivudine/Zidovudine:* Inform patients that some HIV-1 medicines, including abacavir/lamivudine/zidovudine, can cause a rare, but serious condition called lactic acidosis with liver enlargement (hepatomegaly).

Abacavir/lamivudine/zidovudine is not a cure for HIV-1 infection, and patients may continue to experience illnesses associated with HIV-1 infection, including opportunistic infections. Patients should remain under the care of a health care provider when using abacavir/lamivudine/zidovudine. Advise patients that the use of abacavir/lamivudine/zidovudine has not been shown to reduce the risk of transmission of HIV-1 to others through sexual contact or blood contamination.

Inform patients that redistribution or accumulation of body fat may occur in patients receiving antiretroviral therapy and that the cause and long-term health effects of these conditions are not known at this time.

Abacavir/lamivudine/zidovudine tablets are for oral ingestion only.

Advise patients of the importance of taking abacavir/lamivudine/zidovudine exactly as prescribed.

EMTRICITABINE/TENOFOVIR DISOPROXIL FUMARATE

Rx	Truvada (Gilead Sciences)	**Tablets; oral:** emtricitabine 200 mg/tenofovir disoproxil fumarate 300 mg	Equiv. to tenofovir disoproxil 245 mg. Lactose. Gluten free. (GILEAD 701). Blue, capsule shape. Film-coated. In 30s.

EMTRICITABINE/TENOFOVIR DISOPROXIL FUMARATE — ORAL

Consult the Emtricitabine and Tenofovir Disoproxil Fumarate individual monographs prior to administration of emtricitabine/tenofovir combination tablets.

WARNING

Lactic acidosis and severe hepatomegaly with steatosis, including fatal cases, have been reported with the use of nucleoside analogs, including tenofovir (a component of emtricitabine/tenofovir), in combination with other antiretrovirals.

Emtricitabine/tenofovir is not approved for the treatment of chronic hepatitis B virus (HBV) infection, and the safety and efficacy of emtricitabine/tenofovir have not been established in patients coinfected with HBV and HIV-1. Severe, acute exacerbations of hepatitis B have been reported in patients who are coinfected with HBV and HIV-1 and have discontinued emtricitabine/tenofovir. Closely monitor hepatic function with clinical and laboratory follow-up for at least several months in patients who discontinue emtricitabine/tenofovir and are coinfected with HIV-1 and HBV. If appropriate, initiation of anti–hepatitis B therapy may be warranted.

Indications

➤*HIV infection:* For the treatment of HIV-1 infection in adults in combination with other antiretroviral agents (eg, nonnucleoside reverse transcriptase inhibitors [NNRTIs], protease inhibitors).

Administration and Dosage

➤*Adults:*
HIV infection – One tablet (emtricitabine 200 mg/tenofovir 300 mg) once daily.

➤*Renal function impairment:*

Emtricitabine/Tenofovir Dosage Adjustment for Patients With Altered CrCl[a]

	CrCl (mL/min)[b]		
	≥ 50	30 to 49	< 30[c]
Recommended dosing interval	Every 24 h	Every 48 h	Do not administer

[a] CrCl = creatinine clearance.
[b] Calculated using ideal (lean) body weight.
[c] Including patients requiring hemodialysis.

➤*Administration:* Administer with or without food.

➤*Storage/Stability:* Store at 25°C (77°F); excursions are permitted between 15° and 30°C (59° and 86°F). Dispense only in the original container.

Actions

➤*Pharmacology:*
Emtricitabine – Emtricitabine, a synthetic nucleoside analog of cytidine, is phosphorylated by cellular enzymes to form emtricitabine 5′-triphosphate. Emtricitabine 5′-triphosphate inhibits the activity of the HIV-1 reverse transcriptase by competing with the natural substrate deoxycytidine 5′-triphosphate and by being incorporated into nascent viral DNA, which results in chain termination. Emtricitabine 5′-triphosphate is a weak inhibitor of mammalian DNA polymerase alpha, beta, epsilon, and mitochondrial DNA polymerase gamma.

Tenofovir – Tenofovir is an acyclic nucleoside phosphonate diester analog of adenosine monophosphate. Tenofovir requires initial diester hydrolysis for conversion to tenofovir and subsequent phosphorylations by cellular enzymes to form tenofovir diphosphate. Tenofovir diphosphate inhibits the activity of HIV-1 reverse transcriptase by competing with the natural substrate deoxyadenosine 5′-triphosphate and, after incorporation into DNA, by DNA chain termination. Tenofovir diphosphate is a weak inhibitor of mammalian DNA polymerases alpha, beta, and mitochondrial DNA polymerase gamma.

➤*Pharmacokinetics:*

Emtricitabine and Tenofovir Single-Dose Pharmacokinetic Parameters in Adults

Pharmacokinetic parameter	Emtricitabine	Tenofovir
Fasted oral bioavailability[a]	92% (83.1% to 106.4%)	25% (NC[b] to 45%)
Plasma terminal elimination half-life[a] (h)	10 (7.4 to 18)	17 (12 to 25.7)
C_{max}[c,d] (mcg/mL)	1.8 ± 0.72[e]	0.3 ± 0.09
AUC[c,f] (mcg•h/mL)	10 ± 3.12[e]	2.29 ± 0.69
CL/F[c,g] (mL/min)	302 ± 94	1,043 ± 115
CL_{renal}[c,h] (mL/min)	213 ± 89	243 ± 33

[a] Median (range).
[b] NC = not calculated.
[c] Mean (± standard deviation).
[d] C_{max} = maximal drug concentration.
[e] Data presented as steady-state values.
[f] AUC = area under the curve.
[g] CL/F = apparent total clearance.
[h] CL_{renal} = renal clearance.

Absorption/Distribution –
Emtricitabine: Following oral administration, emtricitabine is rapidly absorbed, with C_{max} occurring at 1 to 2 hours postdose. In vitro binding of emtricitabine to human plasma proteins is less than 4% and is independent of concentration over the range of 0.02 to 200 mcg/mL.

Tenofovir: Following oral administration of tenofovir, maximum tenofovir serum concentrations are achieved in 1 ± 0.4 hours. In vitro binding of tenofovir to human plasma proteins is less than 0.7% and is independent of concentration over the range of 0.01 to 25 mcg/mL.

Effect of food: Emtricitabine/tenofovir may be administered with or without food. Administration of emtricitabine/tenofovir following a high-fat meal (784 kcal; 49 g of fat) or light meal (373 kcal; 8 g of fat) delayed the time of tenofovir C_{max} approximately 45 minutes. The mean increases in tenofovir AUC and C_{max} were approximately 35% and 15%, respectively, when administered with a high-fat or light meal, compared with administration in the fasted state. In previous safety and efficacy studies, tenofovir was taken under fed conditions. Emtricitabine systemic exposures (AUC and C_{max}) were unaffected when emtricitabine/tenofovir was administered with a high-fat or light meal.

Metabolism/Excretion –
Emtricitabine: Following administration of radiolabeled emtricitabine, approximately 86% is recovered in the urine and 13% is recovered as metabolites. The metabolites of emtricitabine include 3′-sulfoxide diastereomers and their glucuronic acid conjugate. Emtricitabine is eliminated by a combination of glomerular filtration and active tubular secretion. Following a single oral dose of emtricitabine, the plasma emtricitabine half-life is approximately 10 hours.

Tenofovir: Approximately 70% to 80% of the intravenous (IV) dose of tenofovir is recovered as unchanged drug in the urine. Tenofovir is eliminated by a combination of glomerular filtration and active tubular secretion. Following a single oral dose of tenofovir, the terminal elimination half-life of tenofovir is approximately 17 hours.

Special populations –
Renal function impairment: The pharmacokinetics of emtricitabine and tenofovir are altered in patients with renal impairment. In patients with CrCl of less than 50 mL/min, C_{max} and $AUC_{(0-\infty)}$ of emtricitabine and tenofovir were increased. It is recommended that the dosing interval for emtricitabine/tenofovir be modified in patients with a CrCl of 30 to 49 mL/min. Do not use emtricitabine/tenofovir in patients with a CrCl of less than 30 mL/min or in patients with end-stage renal disease requiring dialysis.

Contraindications

None well documented.

Warnings/Precautions

➤*Lactic acidosis/severe hepatomegaly with steatosis:* A majority of cases of lactic acidosis and severe hepatomegaly with steatosis have been in women. Obesity and prolonged nucleoside exposure may be risk factors. Exercise particular caution when administering nucleoside analogs to any patient with known risk factors for liver disease; however, cases also have been reported in patients with no known risk factors. Suspend treatment with emtricitabine/tenofovir in any patient who develops clinical or laboratory findings suggestive of lactic acidosis or pronounced hepatotoxicity, which may include hepatomegaly and steatosis, even in the absence of marked transaminase elevations.

➤*HIV-1 and hepatitis B coinfection:* It is recommended that all patients with HIV-1 be tested for the presence of chronic HBV before initiating antiretroviral therapy.

See the Warning box for more information.

➤*Renal effects:* Renal function, including cases of acute renal failure and Fanconi syndrome (renal tubular injury with severe hypophosphatemia), has been reported in association with the use of tenofovir.

➤*Bone effects:* Consider bone mineral density (BMD) monitoring for HIV-1–infected patients who have a history of pathologic bone fracture or are at risk for osteopenia. Although the effect of supplementation with calcium and vitamin D was not studied, such supplementation may be beneficial for all patients. If bone abnormalities are suspected, obtain appropriate consultation.

EMTRICITABINE/TENOFOVIR DISOPROXIL FUMARATE — ORAL

In a 144-week study of treatment-naive patients, decreases in BMD were seen at the lumbar spine and hip in both arms of the study. At week 144, there was a significantly greater mean percentage decrease from baseline in BMD at the lumbar spine in patients receiving tenofovir plus lamivudine plus efavirenz compared with patients receiving stavudine plus lamivudine plus efavirenz. Changes in BMD at the hip were similar between the 2 treatment groups. In both groups, the majority of the reduction in BMD occurred in the first 24 to 48 weeks of the study, and this reduction was sustained through 144 weeks. Twenty-eight percent of tenofovir-treated patients versus 21% of the comparator patients lost at least 5% of BMD at the spine or 7% of BMD at the hip. Clinically relevant fractures (excluding fingers and toes) were reported in 4 patients in the tenofovir group and 6 patients in the comparator group. Tenofovir was associated with significant increases in biochemical markers of bone metabolism (serum bone-specific alkaline phosphatase, serum osteocalcin, serum C-telopeptide, and urinary N-telopeptide), suggesting increased bone turnover. Serum parathyroid hormone levels and 1,25 vitamin D levels were also higher in patients receiving tenofovir. The effects of tenofovir-associated changes in BMD and biochemical markers on long-term bone health and future fracture risk are unknown. For additional information, consult the tenofovir monograph.

Cases of osteomalacia associated with proximal renal tubulopathy, which may contribute to fractures, have been reported in association with the use of tenofovir.

➤*Fat redistribution:* Redistribution/accumulation of body fat, including central obesity, dorsocervical fat enlargement (buffalo hump), peripheral wasting, facial wasting, breast enlargement, and "cushingoid appearance," have been observed in patients receiving antiretroviral therapy. The mechanism and long-term consequences of these events are currently unknown. A causal relationship has not been established.

➤*Immune reconstitution syndrome:* Immune reconstitution syndrome has been reported in patients treated with combination antiretroviral therapy, including emtricitabine/tenofovir. During the initial phase of combination antiretroviral treatment, patients whose immune system responds may develop an inflammatory response to indolent or residual opportunistic infections (eg, *Mycobacterium avium* infection, cytomegalovirus, *Pneumocystis jirovecii* pneumonia, or tuberculosis), which may necessitate further evaluation and treatment.

➤*Early virologic failure:* Clinical studies in HIV-infected patients have demonstrated that certain regimens that only contain 3 nucleoside reverse transcriptase inhibitors (NRTIs) are generally less effective than triple drug regimens containing 2 NRTIs in combination with either a NNRTI or an HIV-1 protease inhibitor. In particular, early virological failure and high rates of resistance substitutions have been reported. Triple nucleoside regimens should therefore be used with caution. Carefully monitor patients on a therapy utilizing a triple nucleoside-only regimen and consider them for treatment modification.

➤*Renal function impairment:* See Administration and Dosage for more information.

➤*Pregnancy: Category B.* There are no adequate and well-controlled studies in pregnant women. Because animal reproduction studies are not always predictive of human response, use emtricitabine/tenofovir during pregnancy only if clearly needed. In 2006, the updated guidelines for the use of antiretroviral agents in HIV-1–infected patients recommended continuing therapy during pregnancy.

Antiretroviral pregnancy registry – To monitor fetal outcomes of pregnant women exposed to emtricitabine/tenofovir, an antiretroviral pregnancy registry has been established. Health care providers are encouraged to register patients by calling 1-800-258-4263.

➤*Lactation:* The Centers for Disease Control and Prevention recommends that HIV-infected mothers not breast-feed their infants to avoid risking postnatal transmission of HIV-1. Studies in rats have demonstrated that tenofovir is secreted in milk. The low molecular weight (approximately 247), low plasma protein binding (less than 4%), and long plasma elimination half-life (approximately 10 hours) suggest that emtricitabine will be excreted into human breast milk. It is not known whether emtricitabine is excreted in human milk. Because of the potential for HIV transmission and the potential for serious adverse reactions in breast-feeding infants, instruct mothers not to breast-feed if they are receiving emtricitabine/tenofovir.

➤*Children:* Emtricitabine/tenofovir is not recommended for patients younger than 18 years of age because it is a fixed-dose combination tablet containing tenofovir, for which safety and efficacy have not been established in this age group.

➤*Elderly:* In general, use caution when selecting dosages for elderly patients, keeping in mind the greater frequency of decreased hepatic, renal, or cardiac function, and of concomitant disease or other drug therapy.

➤*Monitoring:* Monitor for signs of lactic acidosis. For at least several months, closely monitor hepatic function with clinical and laboratory follow-up in patients who discontinue emtricitabine/tenofovir and who are coinfected with HIV and HBV.

Calculate CrCl in all patients prior to initiating therapy and as clinically appropriate during therapy with emtricitabine/tenofovir. Routinely monitor calculated CrCl and serum phosphorus in patients at risk for renal impairment. Consider BMD monitoring for patients who have a history of pathologic bone fracture or are at risk for osteopenia.

Carefully monitor patients on a therapy utilizing a triple nucleoside-only regimen, and consider them for treatment modification.

Drug Interactions

➤*Fixed-dose combination:* Emtricitabine/tenofovir is a fixed-dose combination of emtricitabine and tenofovir. Do not administer emtricitabine/tenofovir with efavirenz/emtricitabine/tenofovir, emtricitabine, or tenofovir.

Emtricitabine/Tenofovir Drug Interactions

Precipitant drug	Object drug[a]		Description
Acyclovir, adefovir dipivoxil, cidofovir, ganciclovir, valacyclovir, valganciclovir	Emtricitabine/ Tenofovir	↑	Coadministration of tenofovir with drugs that reduce renal function or compete for active tubular secretion may increase serum concentrations of tenofovir and/or increase the concentrations of other renally eliminated drugs. Do not administer emtricitabine/ tenofovir with adefovir.
Emtricitabine/ Tenofovir	Acyclovir, adefovir dipivoxil, cidofovir, ganciclovir, valacyclovir, valganciclovir		
Atazanavir	Emtricitabine/ Tenofovir	↑	Concurrent use increased tenofovir AUC by 24% and C_{max} by 14%. Monitor closely. Coadministration of tenofovir and atazanavir resulted in decreased atazanavir AUC by 25% and C_{max} by 21%. Do not coadminister without the addition of ritonavir.
Tenofovir	Atazanavir	↓	
Indinavir	Emtricitabine/ Tenofovir	↑	Coadministration increased tenofovir C_{max} by approximately 14%, but AUC remained unchanged. The C_{max} of indinavir decreased by approximately 11%, but AUC remained unchanged. The magnitude of these changes is not likely to be clinically important.
Emtricitabine/ Tenofovir	Indinavir	↓	
Lopinavir/ Ritonavir	Emtricitabine/ Tenofovir	↑	Concurrent use increased tenofovir AUC by 32%. Monitor closely for emtricitabine/tenofovir-associated adverse reactions. Discontinue in patients who develop adverse reactions.
Nephrotoxic agents	Emtricitabine/ Tenofovir	↑	The risk of nephrotoxicity may be increased. Avoid emtricitabine/ tenofovir with concurrent or recent use of a nephrotoxic agent.
Emtricitabine/ Tenofovir	Nephrotoxic agents		
Tacrolimus	Emtricitabine/ Tenofovir	↑	Concurrent use increased tenofovir C_{max} by 13%, but AUC remained unchanged. The magnitude of this change is not likely to be clinically important.
Emtricitabine/ Tenofovir	Abacavir	↑	Concurrent use increased abacavir C_{max} by 12%, but AUC remained unchanged. The magnitude of this change is not likely to be clinically important.
Emtricitabine/ Tenofovir	Didanosine (buffered formulation or enteric-coated)	↑	The C_{max} and AUC of didanosine (buffered formulation or enteric-coated) increased when given with tenofovir. Increases in didanosine concentrations could potentiate adverse reactions, including pancreatitis, lactic acidosis, and neuropathy. In adults weighing > 60 kg, reduce the didanosine dose to 250 mg. Monitor patients closely and administer under fasting conditions or with a light meal (ie, less than 400 kcal, 20% fat).
Emtricitabine/ Tenofovir	Entecavir	↑	Concurrent uses increased entecavir AUC by 13% The magnitude of this change is not likely to be clinically important.

EMTRICITABINE/TENOFOVIR DISOPROXIL FUMARATE — ORAL

Emtricitabine/Tenofovir Drug Interactions			
Precipitant drug	Object drug[a]		Description
Emtricitabine/ Tenofovir	Lamivudine	↓	Concurrent use decreased lamivudine C_{max} by 24%, but AUC remained unchanged. Do not coadminister emtricitabine/ tenofovir with lamivudine or lamivudine-containing products, including lamivudine/zidovudine, abacavir/lamivudine, or abacavir/ lamivudine/zidovudine.
Emtricitabine/ Tenofovir	Saquinavir/ Ritonavir	↑	Concurrent use increased saquinavir AUC by 29% and C_{max} by 22%. These changes are not expected to be clinically relevant.
Emtricitabine/ Tenofovir	Zidovudine	↑	Concurrent use increased zidovudine C_{max} by 17% and AUC by 13%. The magnitude of these changes is not likely to be clinically important.

[a] ↑ = object drug increased; ↓ = object drug decreased.

➤*Drug/Food interactions:* See Actions for more information.

Adverse Reactions

➤*Common adverse reactions (10% or more):* The most common adverse reactions (incidence of at least 10%, any severity) occurring in study 934, an active-controlled clinical study of efavirenz, emtricitabine, and tenofovir, included abnormal dreams, depression, diarrhea, dizziness, fatigue, headache, insomnia, nausea, and rash. Skin discoloration, manifested by hyperpigmentation on the palms and/or soles, was generally mild and asymptomatic. The mechanism and clinical significance are unknown.

➤*Adverse reactions (5% or more):*

Emtricitabine/Tenofovir Adverse Reactions[a] (Grades 2 to 4) (≥ 5%)		
Adverse reaction	Emtricitabine + tenofovir + efavirenz[b] (n = 257)	Zidovudine/ lamivudine + efavirenz (n = 254)
CNS		
Depression	9%	7%
Dizziness	8%	7%
Fatigue	9%	8%
Headache	6%	5%
Insomnia	5%	7%
Dermatologic		
Rash[c]	7%	9%
GI		
Diarrhea	9%	5%
Nausea	9%	7%
Vomiting	2%	5%
Respiratory		
Nasopharyngitis	5%	3%
Sinusitis	8%	4%
Upper respiratory tract infection	8%	5%

[a] Frequencies of adverse reactions are based on all treatment-emergent adverse reactions, regardless of relationship to study drug.
[b] From weeks 96 to 144 of the study, patients received emtricitabine/tenofovir with efavirenz in place of tenofovir plus emtricitabine with efavirenz.
[c] Rash reaction includes rash, exfoliative rash, rash generalized, rash macular, rash maculopapular, rash pruritic, and rash vesicular.

➤*Other adverse reactions (5% or more):*

CNS – Anxiety, paresthesia, peripheral neuropathy (including peripheral neuritis and neuropathy).

GI – Abdominal pain, dyspepsia.

Musculoskeletal – Arthralgia, back pain, myalgia.

Respiratory – Cough increased, pneumonia, and rhinitis.

Miscellaneous – Fever, pain.

➤*Lab test abnormalities:*

Emtricitabine/Tenofovir Laboratory Abnormalities (≥ 1%)		
	Emtricitabine + tenofovir + efavirenz[a] (n = 257)	Zidovudine/ lamivudine + efavirenz (n = 254)
Any ≥ grade 3 laboratory abnormality	30%	26%
Fasting cholesterol (> 240 mg/dL)	22%	24%
Creatine kinase (M[b]: > 990 units/L) (F[b]: > 845 units/L)	9%	7%
Serum amylase (> 175 units/L)	8%	4%
Alkaline phosphatase (> 550 units/L)	1%	0%
AST (M: > 180 units/L) (F: > 170 units/L)	3%	3%
ALT (M: > 215 units/L) (F: > 170 units/L)	2%	3%
Hemoglobin (< 8 mg/dL)	0%	4%
Hyperglycemia (> 250 mg/dL)	2%	1%
Hematuria (> 75 RBC/HPF[c])	3%	2%
Glycosuria (≥ 3+)	< 1%	1%
Neutrophils (< 750/mm^3)	3%	5%
Fasting triglycerides (> 750 mg/dL)	4%	2%

[a] From weeks 96 to 144 of the study, patients received emtricitabine/tenofovir with efavirenz in place of tenofovir plus emtricitabine with efavirenz.
[b] M = male; F = female.
[c] RBC/HPF = red blood cells per high-power field.

Additional lab test abnormalities – In addition to the laboratory abnormalities described previously for study 934, grade 3/4 elevations of bilirubin (more than 2.5 times upper limit of normal [ULN]), pancreatic amylase (more than 2 times the ULN), serum glucose (less than 40 or more than 250 mg/dL), and serum lipase (more than 2 times the ULN) occurred in up to 3% of patients treated with emtricitabine or tenofovir with other antiretroviral agents in clinical trials.

➤*Postmarketing:*

Tenofovir –

GI: Abdominal pain, increased amylase, pancreatitis.

GU: Acute renal failure, acute tubular necrosis, Fanconi syndrome, increased creatinine, interstitial nephritis (including acute cases), nephrogenic diabetes insipidus, polyuria, proteinuria, proximal tubulopathy, renal failure, renal insufficiency.

Hepatic: Hepatic steatosis, hepatitis, increased liver enzymes (most commonly AST, ALT, gamma-glutamyltransferase).

Metabolic/Nutritional: Hypokalemia, hypophosphatemia, lactic acidosis.

Musculoskeletal: Muscular weakness, myopathy, osteomalacia (manifested as bone pain and which may contribute to fractures), rhabdomyolysis.

Miscellaneous: Allergic reaction, angioedema, asthenia, dyspnea, rash. The following adverse reactions may occur as a consequence of proximal renal tubulopathy: hypokalemia, hypophosphatemia, muscular weakness, myopathy, osteomalacia, rhabdomyolysis.

Overdosage

➤*Treatment:* If overdose occurs, monitor the patient for evidence of toxicity and apply standard supportive treatment as necessary.

Emtricitabine – Hemodialysis treatment removes approximately 30% of the emtricitabine dose over a 3-hour dialysis period, starting within 1.5 hours of emtricitabine dosing (blood flow rate of 400 mL/min and a dialysate flow rate of 600 mL/min). It is not known whether emtricitabine can be removed by peritoneal dialysis.

Tenofovir – Tenofovir is efficiently removed by hemodialysis, with an extraction coefficient of approximately 54%. Following a single dose of tenofovir 300 mg, a 4-hour hemodialysis session removed approximately 10% of the administered tenofovir dose.

Patient Information

Inform patients that emtricitabine/tenofovir is not a cure for HIV-1 infection, and they may continue to experience illnesses associated with HIV-1 infection, including opportunistic infections. Advise patients to remain under the care of their health care provider when using emtricitabine/ tenofovir.

EMTRICITABINE/TENOFOVIR DISOPROXIL FUMARATE — ORAL

Inform patients that the use of emtricitabine/tenofovir has not been shown to reduce the risk of transmission of HIV-1 to others through sexual contact or blood contamination.

Advise patients to continue to practice safer sex and to use latex or polyurethane condoms to lower the chance of sexual contact with any body fluids such as semen, vaginal secretions, or blood. Patients should be advised never to re-use or share needles.

Inform patients that the long-term effects of emtricitabine/tenofovir are unknown.

Advise patients that emtricitabine/tenofovir tablets are for oral ingestion only.

Inform patients that it is important to take emtricitabine/tenofovir with combination therapy on a regular dosing schedule to avoid missing doses.

Inform patients that redistribution or accumulation of body fat may occur in patients receiving antiretroviral therapy, and the cause and long-term effects of these conditions are not known.

Inform patients that lactic acidosis and severe hepatomegaly with steatosis, including fatal cases, have been reported. Treatment with emtricitabine/tenofovir should be suspended in any patients who develop clinical symptoms suggestive of lactic acidosis or pronounced hepatotoxicity (including nausea, vomiting, unusual or unexpected stomach discomfort, and weakness).

Advise all patients with HIV-1 to be tested for HBV before initiating antiretroviral therapy.

Inform patients that severe acute exacerbations of hepatitis B have been reported in patients who are coinfected with HBV and HIV-1 and have discontinued emtricitabine/tenofovir.

Inform patients that renal impairment, including cases of acute renal failure and Fanconi syndrome, has been reported in association with the use of tenofovir. Emtricitabine/tenofovir should be avoided with concurrent or recent use of a nephrotoxic agent. The dosing interval of emtricitabine/tenofovir may need adjustment in patients with renal impairment.

Inform patients that emtricitabine/tenofovir should not be coadministered with efavirenz/emtricitabine/tenofovir, emtricitabine, or tenofovir, or with drugs containing lamivudine, including lamivudine/zidovudine, lamivudine, abacavir/lamivudine, or abacavir/lamivudine/zidovudine.

Inform patients that emtricitabine/tenofovir should not be administered with adefovir dipivoxil.

Inform patients that decreases in BMD have been observed with the use of tenofovir. Consider bone monitoring in patients who have a history of pathologic bone fracture or who are at risk for osteopenia.

ABACAVIR/LAMIVUDINE

Rx	**Epzicom** (GlaxoSmithKline)	**Tablets; oral:** abacavir 600 mg/lamivudine 300 mg	As abacavir sulfate. (GS FC2). Orange, capsule-shaped. Film-coated. In 30s.

ABACAVIR SULFATE/LAMIVUDINE — ORAL

Consult the Abacavir Sulfate and Lamivudine individual monographs prior to administration of abacavir/lamivudine combination tablets.

WARNING

This product contains 2 nucleoside analogs (abacavir and lamivudine) and is intended only for patients whose regimen would otherwise include these 2 components.

Hypersensitivity reactions – Serious and sometimes fatal hypersensitivity reactions have been associated with abacavir. Hypersensitivity to abacavir is a multiorgan clinical syndrome usually characterized by a sign or symptom in 2 or more of the following groups: fever, rash, GI (eg, nausea, vomiting, diarrhea, abdominal pain), constitutional (eg, generalized malaise, fatigue, achiness), and respiratory (eg, dyspnea, cough, pharyngitis). Discontinue abacavir/lamivudine as soon as a hypersensitivity reaction is suspected.

Patients who carry the HLA-B*5701 allele are at high risk for experiencing a hypersensitivity reaction to abacavir. Prior to initiating therapy with abacavir, screening for the HLA-B*5701 allele is recommended; this approach has been found to decrease the risk of hypersensitivity reaction. Screening is also recommended prior to reinitiation of abacavir in patients of unknown HLA-B*5701 status who have previously tolerated abacavir. HLA-B*5701–negative patients may develop a suspected hypersensitivity reaction to abacavir; however, this occurs significantly less frequently than in HLA-B*5701–positive patients.

Regardless of HLA-B*5701 status, permanently discontinue abacavir/lamivudine if hypersensitivity cannot be ruled out, even when other diagnoses are possible.

Following a hypersensitivity reaction to abacavir, never restart abacavir/lamivudine or any other abacavir-containing product because more severe symptoms can occur within hours and may include life-threatening hypotension and death.

Reintroduction of abacavir/lamivudine or any other abacavir-containing product, even in patients who have no identified history or unrecognized symptoms of hypersensitivity to abacavir therapy, can result in serious or fatal hypersensitivity reactions. Such reactions can occur within hours.

Lactic acidosis and severe hepatomegaly – Lactic acidosis and severe hepatomegaly with steatosis, including fatal cases, have been reported with the use of nucleoside analogs alone or in combination, including abacavir, lamivudine, and other antiretrovirals.

Exacerbations of hepatitis B – Severe acute exacerbations of hepatitis B have been reported in patients who are coinfected with hepatitis B virus (HBV) and HIV-1 and have discontinued lamivudine, which is one component of abacavir/lamivudine. Closely monitor hepatic function with clinical and laboratory follow-up for at least several months in patients who discontinue abacavir/lamivudine and are coinfected with HIV-1 and HBV. If appropriate, initiation of anti–hepatitis B therapy may be warranted.

Indications

➤*HIV infection:* For use in combination with other antiretroviral agents for the treatment of HIV-1 infection.

Administration and Dosage

➤*General dosing considerations:* Because it is a fixed-dose tablet, abacavir/lamivudine should not be prescribed to patients requiring dosage adjustment, such as those with a creatinine clearance (CrCl) of less than 50 mL/min, those with hepatic impairment, or those experiencing dose-limiting adverse reactions. Use of lamivudine oral solution and abacavir oral solution may be considered.

➤*Adults:*

HIV infection – 1 tablet daily, in combination with other antiretroviral agents.

➤*Elderly:* Dose selection for an elderly patient should be made with caution, reflecting the greater frequency of decreased hepatic, renal, or cardiac function, and of concomitant disease or other drug therapy.

➤*Renal function impairment:* Abacavir/lamivudine is not recommended for use in patients with CrCl less than 50 mL/min.

➤*Hepatic function impairment:* Abacavir/lamivudine is contraindicated in patients with hepatic impairment.

➤*Administration:* May be taken with or without food.

➤*Storage/Stability:* Store at 25°C (77°F); excursions are permitted to 15° to 30°C (59° to 86°F).

Actions

➤*Pharmacology:* Abacavir/lamivudine contains 2 synthetic nucleoside analogs with inhibitory activity against HIV.

Abacavir is a carbocyclic synthetic nucleoside analog. Abacavir is converted by cellular enzymes to the active metabolite, carbovir triphosphate (CBV-TP), an analog of deoxyguanosine-5′-triphosphate (dGTP). CBV-TP inhibits the activity of HIV-1 reverse transcriptase by competing with the natural substrate dGTP and by its incorporation into viral DNA. The lack of a 3′-OH group in the incorporated nucleotide analog prevents the formation of the 5′ to 3′ phosphodiester linkage essential for DNA chain elongation and, therefore, the viral DNA growth is terminated. CBV-TP is a weak inhibitor of cellular DNA polymerases alpha, beta, and gamma.

Lamivudine is a synthetic nucleoside analog. Intracellularly, lamivudine is phosphorylated to its active 5′-triphosphate metabolite, lamivudine triphosphate (3TC-TP). The principal mode of action of 3TC-TP is inhibition of reverse transcriptase via DNA chain termination after incorporation of the nucleotide analog. CBV-TP and 3TC-TP are weak inhibitors of cellular DNA polymerases alpha, beta, and gamma.

➤*Pharmacokinetics:*

Absorption/Distribution –

Abacavir: Following oral administration, abacavir is rapidly absorbed and extensively distributed. After oral administration of a single dose of abacavir 600 mg in 20 patients, C_{max} was 4.26 ± 1.19 mcg/mL (mean ± standard deviation [SD]) and AUC_{∞} was 11.95 ± 2.51 mcg•h/mL. Binding of abacavir to human plasma proteins is approximately 50% and was independent of concentration. Total blood and plasma drug-related radioactivity concentrations are identical, demonstrating that abacavir readily distributes into erythrocytes.

Lamivudine: Following oral administration, lamivudine is rapidly absorbed and extensively distributed. After multiple-dose oral administration of lamivudine 300 mg once daily for 7 days to 60 healthy volunteers, steady-state C_{max} ($C_{max,ss}$) was 2.04 ± 0.54 mcg/mL (mean ± SD) and the 24-hour steady-state AUC ($AUC_{24,ss}$) was 8.87 ± 1.83 mcg•h/mL. Binding to plasma protein is low.

The steady-state pharmacokinetic properties of the lamivudine 300 mg tablet once daily for 7 days compared with the lamivudine 150 mg tablet twice daily for 7 days were assessed in a crossover study in 60 healthy volunteers. Lamivudine 300 mg once daily resulted in lamivudine exposures that were

ABACAVIR SULFATE/LAMIVUDINE — ORAL

similar to lamivudine 150 mg twice daily with respect to plasma $AUC_{24,ss}$; however, $C_{max,ss}$ was 66% higher and the trough value was 53% lower compared with the 150 mg twice-daily regimen. Intracellular lamivudine triphosphate exposures in peripheral blood mononuclear cells were also similar with respect to $AUC_{24,ss}$ and $C_{max24,ss}$; however, trough values were lower compared with the 150 mg twice-daily regimen. Intersubject variability was greater for intracellular lamivudine triphosphate concentrations versus lamivudine plasma trough concentrations. The clinical significance of observed differences for both plasma lamivudine concentrations and intracellular lamivudine triphosphate concentrations is not known.

Effect of food: Abacavir/lamivudine may be administered with or without food. Administration with a high-fat meal in a single-dose bioavailability study resulted in no change in AUC_{last}, AUC_{∞}, and C_{max} for lamivudine. Food did not alter the extent of systemic exposure to abacavir (AUC_{∞}), but the rate of absorption (C_{max}) was decreased approximately 24% compared with fasted conditions (n = 25). These results are similar to those from previous studies of the effect of food on abacavir and lamivudine tablets administered separately.

Metabolism / Excretion – The primary routes of elimination of abacavir are metabolism by alcohol dehydrogenase to form the 5′-carboxylic acid and glucuronyl transferase to form the 5′-glucuronide.

Approximately 70% of an intravenous dose of lamivudine is recovered as unchanged drug in the urine. Metabolism of lamivudine is a minor route of elimination. In humans, the only known metabolite is the trans-sulfoxide metabolite (approximately 5% of an oral dose after 12 hours).

In humans, abacavir and lamivudine are not significantly metabolized by cytochrome P450 enzymes.

Abacavir and Lamivudine Pharmacokinetic Parameters[a]

Parameter	Abacavir		Lamivudine	
Oral bioavailability (%)	86 ± 25	n = 6	86 ± 16	n = 12
Apparent volume of distribution (L/kg)	0.86 ± 0.15	n = 6	1.3 ± 0.4	n = 20
Systemic clearance (L/h/kg)	0.8 ±0.24	n = 6	0.33 ± 0.06	n = 20
Renal clearance (L/h/kg)	0.007 ± 0.008	n = 6	0.22 ± 0.06	n = 20
Elimination half-life (h)	1.45 ± 0.32	n = 20	5 to 7[b]	

[a] Data presented as mean ± SD except where noted.
[b] Approximate range.

Special populations –

Renal function impairment: Lamivudine requires dose adjustment in the presence of renal insufficiency; abacavir/lamivudine is not recommended for use in patients with CrCl less than 50 mL/min.

Hepatic function impairment: Abacavir is contraindicated in patients with moderate to severe hepatic impairment, and dose reduction is required in patients with mild hepatic impairment. Because abacavir/lamivudine is a fixed-dose combination and cannot be dose adjusted, abacavir/lamivudine is contraindicated for patients with hepatic impairment.

➤*Microbiology:*

Antiviral activity –

Abacavir: The antiviral activity of abacavir against HIV-1 was evaluated against a T-cell tropic laboratory strain $HIV\text{-}1_{IIIB}$ in lymphoblastic cell lines, a monocyte/macrophage tropic laboratory strain $HIV\text{-}1_{BaL}$ in primary monocytes/macrophages, and clinical isolates in peripheral blood mononuclear cells. The concentration of drug necessary to effect viral replication by 50 percent (EC_{50}) ranged from 3.7 to 5.8 mcM (1 mcM = 0.28 mcg/mL) and 0.07 to 1 mcM against $HIV\text{-}1_{IIIB}$ and $HIV\text{-}1_{BaL}$, respectively, and was 0.26 ± 0.18 mcM against 8 clinical isolates. The EC_{50} values of abacavir against different HIV-1 clades (A-G) ranged from 0.0015 to 1.05 mcM, and against HIV-2 isolates, from 0.024 to 0.49 mcM. Ribavirin (50 mcM) had no effect on the anti–HIV-1 activity of abacavir in cell culture.

Lamivudine: The antiviral activity of lamivudine against HIV-1 was assessed in a number of cell lines (including monocytes and fresh human peripheral blood lymphocytes) using standard susceptibility assays. EC_{50} values were in the range of 0.003 to 15 mcM (1 mcM = 0.23 mcg/mL). HIV-1 from therapy-naive subjects with no amino acid substitutions associated with resistance gave median EC_{50} values of 0.429 mcM (range, 0.2 to 2.007 mcM) from Virco (n = 92 baseline samples from COLA40263) and 2.35 mcM (1.37 to 3.68 mcM) from Monogram Biosciences (n = 135 baseline samples from ESS30009). The EC_{50} values of lamivudine against different HIV-1 clades (A-G) ranged from 0.001 to 0.12 mcM, and against HIV-2 isolates from 0.003 to 0.12 mcM in peripheral blood mononuclear cells. Ribavirin (50 mcM) decreased the anti–HIV-1 activity of lamivudine by 3.5-fold in MT-4 cells.

The combination of abacavir and lamivudine has demonstrated antiviral activity in cell culture against non-subtype B isolates and HIV-2 isolates with equivalent antiviral activity as for subtype B isolates. Abacavir/lamivudine had additive to synergistic activity in cell culture in combination with the nucleoside reverse transcriptase inhibitors (NRTIs) emtricitabine, stavudine, tenofovir, zalcitabine, and zidovudine; the nonnucleoside reverse transcriptase inhibitors (NNRTIs) delavirdine, efavirenz, and nevirapine; the protease inhibitors (PIs) amprenavir, indinavir, lopinavir, nelfinavir, ritonavir, and saquinavir; or the fusion inhibitor enfuvirtide. Ribavirin, used in combination with interferon for the treatment of hepatitis C virus (HCV) infection, decreased the anti–HIV-1 potency of abacavir/lamivudine reproducible by 2- to 6-fold in cell culture.

Resistance – HIV-1 isolates with reduced susceptibility to the combination of abacavir and lamivudine have been selected in cell culture and have also been obtained from patients failing abacavir/lamivudine-containing regimens. Genotypic characterization of abacavir/lamivudine-resistant viruses selected in cell culture identified amino acid substitutions M184V/I, K65R, L74V, and Y115F in HIV-1 reverse transcriptase.

Genotypic analysis of isolates selected in cell culture and recovered from abacavir-treated patients demonstrated that amino acid substitutions K65R, L74V, Y115F, and M184V/I in HIV-1 reverse transcriptase contributed to abacavir resistance. Genotypic analysis of isolates selected in cell culture and recovered from lamivudine-treated patients showed that the resistance was due to a specific amino acid substitution in HIV-1 reverse transcriptase at codon 184 changing the methionine to either isoleucine or valine (M184V/I). In a study of therapy-naive adults receiving abacavir 600 mg once daily (n = 384) or 300 mg twice daily (n = 386) in a background regimen of lamivudine 300 mg and efavirenz 600 mg once daily (study CNA30021), the incidence of virologic failure at 48 weeks was similar between the 2 groups (11% in both arms). Genotypic (n = 38) and phenotypic analyses (n = 35) of virologic failure isolates from this study showed that the reverse transcriptase substitutions that emerged during abacavir/lamivudine once-daily and twice-daily therapy were K65R, L74V, Y115F, and M184V/I. The abacavir- and lamivudine-associated resistance substitution M184V/I was the most commonly observed substitution in virologic failure isolates from patients receiving abacavir/lamivudine once daily (56%) and twice daily (40%).

Thirty-nine percent of the isolates from patients who experienced virologic failure in the abacavir once-daily arm had a more than 2.5-fold decrease in abacavir susceptibility, with a median-fold decrease of 1.3 (range, 0.5 to 11), compared with 29% of the failure isolates in the twice-daily arm, with a median-fold decrease of 0.92 (range, 0.7 to 13). Fifty-six percent of the virologic failure isolates in the once-daily abacavir group compared with 41% of the failure isolates in the twice-daily abacavir group had a more than 2.5-fold decrease in lamivudine susceptibility, with median-fold changes of 81 (range, 0.79 to more than 116) and 1.1 (range, 0.68 to more than 116) in the once-daily and twice-daily abacavir arms, respectively.

Cross-resistance – Cross-resistance has been observed among NRTIs. Viruses containing abacavir and lamivudine resistance-associated amino acid substitutions, namely, K65R, L74V, M184V, and Y115F, exhibit cross-resistance to didanosine, emtricitabine, lamivudine, tenofovir, and zalcitabine in cell culture and in patients. The K65R substitution can confer resistance to abacavir, didanosine, emtricitabine, lamivudine, stavudine, tenofovir, and zalcitabine; the L74V substitution can confer resistance to abacavir, didanosine, and zalcitabine; and the M184V substitution can confer resistance to abacavir, didanosine, emtricitabine, lamivudine, and zalcitabine.

The combination of abacavir/lamivudine has demonstrated decreased susceptibility to viruses with the substitutions K65R with or without the M184V/I substitution, viruses with L74V plus the M184V/I substitution, and viruses with thymidine analog mutations (M41L, D67N, K70R, L210W, T215Y/F, K219 E/R/H/Q/N) plus M184V. An increasing number of thymidine analog mutations is associated with a progressive reduction in abacavir susceptibility.

Contraindications

Hepatic impairment or a previously demonstrated hypersensitivity to abacavir or to any other component of the product.

Warnings/Precautions

➤*Serious and sometimes fatal hypersensitivity reactions:* Serious and sometimes fatal hypersensitivity reactions have been associated with abacavir/lamivudine and other abacavir-containing products. Patients who carry the HLA-B*5701 allele are at high risk for experiencing a hypersensitivity reaction to abacavir. Prior to initiating therapy with abacavir, screening for the HLA-B*5701 allele is recommended; this approach has been found to decrease the risk of a hypersensitivity reaction. Screening is also recommended prior to reinitiation of abacavir in patients of unknown HLA-B*5701 status who have previously tolerated abacavir. For patients who are HLA-B*5701–positive, treatment with an abacavir-containing regimen is not recommended and should be considered only with close medical supervision and under exceptional circumstances when the potential benefit outweighs the risk.

See the Warning box for more information.

Signs and symptoms of hypersensitivity – Hypersensitivity to abacavir is a multiorgan clinical syndrome usually characterized by a sign or symptom in 2 or more of the following groups: fever, rash, GI (including abdominal pain, diarrhea, nausea, or vomiting), constitutional (including achiness, generalized malaise, or fatigue), respiratory (including cough, dyspnea, or pharyngitis).

Hypersensitivity to abacavir following the presentation of a single sign or symptom has been reported infrequently.

Hypersensitivity to abacavir was reported in approximately 8% of 2,670 patients (n = 206) in 9 clinical trials (range, 2% to 9%) from November 1999 to February 2002. Data on time to onset and symptoms of suspected hypersensitivity were collected on a detailed data collection module. Symptoms usually appeared within the first 6 weeks of treatment with abacavir, although the reaction may occur at any time during therapy. Median time to onset was 9 days; 89% appeared within the first 6 weeks; 95% of patients reported symptoms from 2 or more of the 5 groups listed previously.

Other less common signs and symptoms of hypersensitivity include lethargy, myolysis, edema, abnormal chest x-ray findings (predominantly infiltrates, which can be localized), and paresthesia.

Anaphylaxis, liver failure, renal failure, hypotension, adult respiratory distress syndrome, respiratory failure, and death have occurred in association

ABACAVIR SULFATE/LAMIVUDINE — ORAL

with hypersensitivity reactions. In 1 study, 4 (11%) patients receiving abacavir 600 mg once daily experienced hypotension with a hypersensitivity reaction compared with 0 patients receiving abacavir 300 mg twice daily.

Physical findings associated with hypersensitivity to abacavir in some patients include lymphadenopathy, mucous membrane lesions (conjunctivitis and mouth ulcerations), and rash. The rash usually appears maculopapular or urticarial but may be variable in appearance. There have been reports of erythema multiforme. Hypersensitivity reactions have occurred without rash.

Laboratory abnormalities associated with hypersensitivity to abacavir in some patients include elevated liver function tests, elevated creatine phosphokinase, elevated creatinine, and lymphopenia.

Clinical management of hypersensitivity – Discontinue abacavir/lamivudine as soon as a hypersensitivity reaction is suspected. To minimize the risk of a life-threatening hypersensitivity reaction, permanently discontinue abacavir/lamivudine if hypersensitivity cannot be ruled out, even when other diagnoses are possible (eg, acute-onset respiratory diseases, such as pneumonia, bronchitis, pharyngitis, or influenza; gastroenteritis; or reactions to other medications).

Following a hypersensitivity reaction to abacavir, never restart abacavir/lamivudine or any other abacavir-containing product because more severe symptoms can occur within hours and may include life-threatening hypotension and death.

When therapy with abacavir/lamivudine has been discontinued for reasons other than symptoms of a hypersensitivity reaction, and if reinitiation of abacavir/lamivudine or any other abacavir-containing product is under consideration, carefully evaluate the reason for discontinuation of abacavir/lamivudine to ensure that the patient did not have symptoms of a hypersensitivity reaction. If the patient is of unknown HLA-B*5701 status, screening for the allele is recommended prior to reinitiation of abacavir/lamivudine.

If hypersensitivity cannot be ruled out, do not reintroduce abacavir/lamivudine or any other abacavir-containing product. Even in the absence of the HLA-B*5701 allele, it is important to permanently discontinue abacavir and not rechallenge with abacavir if a hypersensitivity reaction cannot be ruled out on clinical grounds because the potential for a severe or even fatal reaction.

If symptoms consistent with hypersensitivity are not identified, reintroduction can be undertaken with continued monitoring for symptoms of a hypersensitivity reaction. Make patients aware that a hypersensitivity reaction can occur with reintroduction of abacavir/lamivudine or any other abacavir-containing product and that reintroduction of abacavir/lamivudine or introduction of any other abacavir-containing product needs to be undertaken only if medical care can be readily accessed by the patient or others.

*HLA-B*5701 allele risk factor* – Studies have shown that carriage of the HLA-B*5701 allele is associated with a significantly increased risk of a hypersensitivity reaction to abacavir.

CNA106030 (PREDICT-1), a randomized, double-blind study, evaluated the clinical utility of prospective HLA-B*5701 screening on the incidence of abacavir hypersensitivity reaction in adults who are abacavir-naive and HIV-1–infected (n = 1,650). In this study, use of pretherapy screening for the HLA-B*5701 allele and exclusion of subjects with this allele reduced the incidence of clinically suspected abacavir hypersensitivity reactions from 7.8% to 3.4%. Based on this study, it is estimated that 61% of patients with the HLA-B*5701 allele will develop a clinically suspected hypersensitivity reaction during the course of abacavir treatment compared with 4% of patients who do not have the HLA-B*5701 allele.

Screening for carriage of the HLA-B*5701 allele is recommended prior to initiating treatment with abacavir. Screening is also recommended prior to reinitiation of abacavir in patients of unknown HLA-B*5701 status who have previously tolerated abacavir. For HLA-B*5701–positive patients, initiating or reinitiating treatment with an abacavir-containing regimen is not recommended and should be considered only with close medical supervision and under exceptional circumstances for which potential benefit outweighs the risk.

Skin patch testing is used as a research tool and should not be used to aid in the clinical diagnosis of abacavir hypersensitivity.

In any patient treated with abacavir, the clinical diagnosis of hypersensitivity reaction must remain the basis of clinical decision-making. Even in the absence of the HLA-B*5701 allele, it is important to permanently discontinue abacavir and not rechallenge with abacavir if a hypersensitivity reaction cannot be ruled out on clinical grounds because of to the potential for a severe or even fatal reaction.

Abacavir hypersensitivity reaction registry – An abacavir hypersensitivity registry has been established to facilitate reporting of hypersensitivity reactions and collection of information on each case. Health care providers should register patients by calling 1-800-270-0425.

➤*Lactic acidosis/severe hepatomegaly with steatosis:* Lactic acidosis and severe hepatomegaly with steatosis, including fatal cases, have been reported with the use of nucleoside analogs alone or in combination, including abacavir and lamivudine and other antiretrovirals. A majority of these cases have been in women. Obesity and prolonged nucleoside exposure may be risk factors. Exercise particular caution when administering abacavir/lamivudine to any patient with known risk factors for liver disease; however, cases also have been reported in patients with no known risk factors. Suspend abacavir/lamivudine treatment in any patient who develops clinical or laboratory findings suggestive of lactic acidosis or pronounced hepatotoxicity (which may include hepatomegaly and steatosis even in the absence of marked transaminase elevations).

➤*Exacerbations of hepatitis:* In clinical trials in non-HIV–infected patients treated with lamivudine for chronic HBV, clinical and laboratory evidence of exacerbations of hepatitis have occurred after discontinuation of lamivudine. These exacerbations have been detected primarily by serum ALT elevations in addition to re-emergence of HBV DNA. Although most events appear to have been self-limited, fatalities have been reported in some cases. Similar events have been reported from postmarketing experience after changes from lamivudine-containing HIV-1 treatment regimens to non-lamivudine–containing regimens in patients infected with both HIV-1 and HBV. The causal relationship to discontinuation of lamivudine treatment is unknown. Closely monitor patients with clinical and laboratory follow-up for at least several months after stopping treatment. There is insufficient evidence to determine whether reinitiation of lamivudine alters the course of posttreatment exacerbations of hepatitis.

➤*Fixed-dose combination:* Abacavir/lamivudine contains fixed doses of 2 nucleoside analogs, abacavir and lamivudine, and should not be coadministered with other abacavir-containing and/or lamivudine-containing products. Consult the individual monographs for all agents being considered for use with abacavir/lamivudine before initiating combination therapy with abacavir/lamivudine.

➤*Therapy-experienced patients:* In clinical trials, patients with prolonged prior NRTI exposure or who had HIV-1 isolates that contained multiple mutations conferring resistance to NRTIs had limited response to abacavir. Consider the potential for cross-resistance between abacavir and other NRTIs when choosing new therapeutic regimens in therapy-experienced patients.

➤*HIV-1 and hepatitis B virus coinfection:* Safety and efficacy of lamivudine have not been established for treatment of chronic hepatitis B in patients dually infected with HIV-1 and HBV. In non-HIV-1–infected patients treated with lamivudine for chronic hepatitis B, emergence of lamivudine-resistant HBV has been detected and has been associated with diminished treatment response. Emergence of hepatitis B virus variants associated with resistance to lamivudine has also been reported in HIV-1–infected patients who have received lamivudine-containing antiretroviral regimens in the presence of concurrent infection with hepatitis B virus.

➤*Immune reconstitution syndrome:* Immune reconstitution syndrome has been reported in patients treated with combination antiretroviral therapy, including abacavir/lamivudine. During the initial phase of combination antiretroviral treatment, patients whose immune system responds may develop an inflammatory response to indolent or residual opportunistic infections (such as *Mycobacterium avium* infection, cytomegalovirus, *Pneumocystis jirovecii* pneumonia, or tuberculosis), which may necessitate further evaluation and treatment.

➤*Fat redistribution:* Redistribution/accumulation of body fat, including central obesity, dorsocervical fat enlargement (buffalo hump), peripheral wasting, facial wasting, breast enlargement, and cushingoid appearance, have been observed in patients receiving antiretroviral therapy. The mechanism and long-term consequences of these events are currently unknown. A causal relationship has not been established.

➤*Myocardial infarction:* In a published prospective, observational, epidemiological study designed to investigate the rate of myocardial infarction (MI) in patients on combination antiretroviral therapy, the use of abacavir within the previous 6 months was correlated with an increased risk of MI. In a sponsor-conducted pooled analysis of clinical trials, no excess risk of MI was observed in abacavir-treated subjects as compared with control subjects. In totality, the available data from the observational cohort and from clinical trials are inconclusive.

As a precaution, consider the underlying risk of coronary heart disease when prescribing antiretroviral therapies, including abacavir, and take action to minimize all modifiable risk factors (eg, hypertension, hyperlipidemia, diabetes mellitus, smoking).

➤*Hypersensitivity reactions:* See Serious and Sometimes Fatal Hypersensitivity Reactions and Black Box Warning for more information.

➤*Renal function impairment:* Because abacavir/lamivudine is a fixed-dose tablet and the dosage of the individual components cannot be altered, patients with CrCl less than 50 mL/min should not receive abacavir/lamivudine.

➤*Hepatic function impairment:* Abacavir/lamivudine is contraindicated in patients with hepatic impairment because it is a fixed-dose tablet, and the dosage of the individual components cannot be altered.

➤*Pregnancy: Category C.* There are no adequate and well-controlled studies of abacavir/lamivudine in pregnant women. Use abacavir/lamivudine during pregnancy only if the potential benefits outweigh the risks.

In 2006, the updated US Department of Health and Human Services guidelines for the use of antiretroviral agents in HIV-1–infected patients continued the recommendation that therapy, with the exception of efavirenz, should be continued during pregnancy. If indicated, abacavir should not be withheld in pregnancy because the expected benefit to the HIV-positive mother outweighs the unknown risk to the fetus. Women receiving antiretroviral therapy during pregnancy should continue the therapy, but regardless of the regimen, zidovudine administration is recommended during the intrapartum period to prevent vertical transmission of HIV to the newborn.

Abacavir – Studies in pregnant rats showed that abacavir is transferred to the fetus through the placenta. Abacavir crosses the human placenta. Fetal malformations (increased incidences of fetal anasarca and skeletal

ABACAVIR SULFATE/LAMIVUDINE — ORAL

malformations) and developmental toxicity (depressed fetal body weight and reduced crown-rump length) were observed in rats at a dose that produced 35 times the human exposure, based on AUC. Embryonic and fetal toxicities (increased resorptions, decreased fetal body weights) and toxicities to the offspring (increased incidence of stillbirth and lower body weights) occurred at half of the above-mentioned dose in separate fertility studies conducted in rats.

Lamivudine – Studies in pregnant rats showed that lamivudine is transferred to the fetus through the placenta. The low molecular weight (about 229) of lamivudine suggests that it will cross the placenta. Evidence of early embryolethality was seen in rabbits at exposure levels similar to those observed in humans, but there was no indication of this effect in rats at exposure levels up to 35 times those in humans.

Antiretroviral pregnancy registry – To monitor maternal-fetal outcomes of pregnant women exposed to abacavir/lamivudine or other antiretroviral agents, an Antiretroviral Pregnancy Registry has been established. Health care providers are encouraged to register patients by calling 1-800-258-4263.

➤*Lactation:* The Centers for Disease Control and Prevention recommend that HIV-1–infected mothers not breast-feed their infants to avoid risking postnatal transmission of HIV-1 infection. Abacavir is secreted into the milk of lactating rats. The molecular weight (about 67) suggests that the drug will be excreted in human breast milk. Lamivudine is excreted in human breast milk and into the milk of lactating rats. Samples of breast milk obtained from 20 mothers receiving lamivudine monotherapy (300 mg twice daily) or combination therapy (lamivudine 150 mg twice daily and zidovudine 300 mg twice daily) had measurable concentrations of lamivudine. Because of the potential for HIV-1 transmission and the potential for serious adverse reactions in breast-fed infants, instruct mothers not to breast-feed if they are receiving abacavir/lamivudine.

➤*Children:* Safety and effectiveness of abacavir/lamivudine in children have not been established.

➤*Elderly:* In general, dose selection for an elderly patient should be made with caution, reflecting the greater frequency of decreased hepatic, renal, or cardiac function, and of concomitant disease or other drug therapy. Abacavir/lamivudine is not recommended for patients with impaired renal function or impaired hepatic function.

➤*Monitoring:* Screening for carriage of the HLA-B*5701 allele is recommended prior to initiating treatment with abacavir.

Monitor patients for signs and symptoms of a hypersensitivity reaction. Closely monitor chronic HBV patients with both clinical and laboratory follow-up for at least several months after stopping treatment.

Closely monitor patients receiving interferon alfa with or without ribavirin and abacavir/lamivudine for treatment-associated toxicities, especially hepatic decompensation. Consider discontinuation of abacavir/lamivudine as medically appropriate. Also consider dose reduction or discontinuation of interferon alfa, ribavirin, or both if worsening clinical toxicities are observed, including hepatic decompensation (eg, Child-Pugh score greater than 6) (see the individual monographs for interferon and ribavirin).

Drug Interactions

Abacavir/Lamivudine Drug Interactions

Precipitant drug	Object drug[a]		Description
Ethanol	Abacavir/ lamivudine	↑	Ethanol decreases the elimination of abacavir, causing an increase in overall exposure. Dosage adjustments are not needed.
Interferon alfa	Abacavir/ lamivudine	↑	Hepatic decompensation (some fatal) has occurred in HIV-1/HCV coinfected patients receiving combination antiretroviral therapy for HIV-1 and interferon alfa with or without ribavirin. Closely monitor patients for treatment-associated toxicities during coadministration.
Ribavirin	Abacavir/ lamivudine	↓	Ribavirin may reduce the phosphorylation of lamivudine.
Trimethoprim/ Sulfamethoxazole	Abacavir/ lamivudine	↑	Coadministration of lamivudine with trimethoprim 160 mg/ sulfamethoxazole 800 mg increased lamivudine AUC 43%. Dosage adjustments are not needed.
Zalcitabine	Abacavir/ lamivudine	↓	Lamivudine and zalcitabine may inhibit the intracellular phosphorylation of one another. Coadministration is not recommended.
Abacavir/ lamivudine	Zalcitabine		
Abacavir/ lamivudine	Methadone	↓	Methadone clearance increased 22% during coadministration. In the majority of patients, this alteration will not result in a methadone dose modification. In addition, methadone may delay the absorption of abacavir/ lamivudine, resulting in a decrease in bioavailability.
Methadone	Abacavir/lamivudine		

[a] ↑ = object drug increased; ↓ = object drug decreased.

➤*Drug/Food interactions:* Food did not alter the extent of systemic exposure to abacavir (AUC_{∞}), but the rate of absorption (C_{max}) was decreased approximately 24% compared with a fasted condition. Abacavir/ lamivudine may be administered with or without food.

Adverse Reactions

➤*Therapy-naive adults:*

Abacavir + Lamivudine + Efavirenz Treatment-Emergent Adverse Reactions (Grades 2 to 4) Through 48 Weeks of Treatment (≥ 5%)

Adverse reactions	Abacavir 600 mg once daily + lamivudine + efavirenz (n = 384)	Abacavir 300 mg twice daily + lamivudine + efavirenz (n = 386)
CNS		
Abnormal dreams	4%	5%
Anxiety	3%	5%
Depression/Depressed mood	7%	7%
Dizziness/Vertigo	6%	6%
Fatigue/Malaise	6%	8%
Headache/Migraine	7%	6%
Insomnia	7%	9%
GI		
Abdominal pain/gastritis	4%	5%
Diarrhea[a]	5%	6%
Nausea	5%	6%
Miscellaneous		
Drug hypersensitivity[ab]	9%	7%
Pyrexia	5%	3%
Rash	5%	5%

[a] Patients receiving abacavir 600 mg once daily experienced a significantly higher incidence of severe drug hypersensitivity reactions and severe diarrhea compared with patients who received abacavir 300 mg twice daily. Five percent of patients receiving abacavir 600 mg once daily had severe drug hypersensitivity reactions compared with 2% of patients receiving abacavir 300 mg twice daily. Two percent of patients receiving abacavir 600 mg once daily had severe diarrhea, while none of the patients receiving abacavir 300 mg twice daily had this reaction.

[b] Study CNA30024 was a multicenter, double-blind, controlled study in which 649 HIV-1–infected, therapy-naive adults were randomized and received abacavir (300 mg twice daily), lamivudine (150 mg twice daily), and efavirenz (600 mg once daily) or zidovudine (300 mg twice daily), lamivudine (150 mg twice daily), and efavirenz (600 mg once daily). CNA30024 used double-blind ascertainment of suspected hypersensitivity reactions. During the blinded portion of the study, suspected hypersensitivity to abacavir was reported by investigators in 9% of 324 patients in the abacavir group and 3% of 325 patients in the zidovudine group.

➤*Hypersensitivity:* See the Warning box for more information. See Warnings/Precautions for more information.

➤*Lab test abnormalities:* Laboratory abnormalities observed in clinical studies of abacavir were anemia, neutropenia, liver function test abnormalities, and elevations of creatine phosphokinase (CPK), blood glucose, and triglycerides. Additional laboratory abnormalities observed in clinical studies of lamivudine were thrombocytopenia and elevated levels of bilirubin, amylase, and lipase.

➤*Miscellaneous:* In addition to adverse reactions listed previously, other adverse reactions observed in the expanded access program for abacavir were pancreatitis and increased gamma-glutamyl transferase.

➤*Postmarketing:*

Cardiovascular – MI (abacavir).

CNS – Paresthesia, peripheral neuropathy, seizures (abacavir/lamivudine).

Dermatologic – Suspected Stevens-Johnson syndrome and toxic epidermal necrolysis (TEN) have been reported in patients receiving abacavir primarily in combination with medications known to be associated with Stevens-Johnson syndrome and TEN, respectively. Because of the overlap of clinical signs and symptoms between hypersensitivity to abacavir and Stevens-Johnson syndrome and TEN, as well as the possibility of multiple drug sensitivities in some patients, discontinue abacavir and do not restart it in such cases.

ABACAVIR SULFATE/LAMIVUDINE — ORAL

There also have been reports of erythema multiforme (abacavir); alopecia, erythema multiforme, and Stevens-Johnson syndrome (abacavir/lamivudine).

GI – Pancreatitis, stomatitis (abacavir/lamivudine).

Hematologic/Lymphatic – Anemia (including pure red cell aplasia and severe anemias progressing upon therapy), aplastic anemia, lymphadenopathy, splenomegaly (abacavir/lamivudine).

Hepatic – Lactic acidosis and hepatic steatosis, posttreatment exacerbation of hepatitis B (abacavir/lamivudine).

Hypersensitivity – Sensitization reactions (including anaphylaxis), urticaria (abacavir/lamivudine).

Musculoskeletal – CPK elevation, muscle weakness, rhabdomyolysis (abacavir/lamivudine).

Respiratory – Abnormal breath sounds/wheezing (abacavir/lamivudine).

Miscellaneous – Hyperglycemia, redistribution/accumulation of body fat, weakness (abacavir/lamivudine).

Overdosage

➤*Symptoms:* One case of an adult ingesting lamivudine 6 g was reported; there were no clinical signs or symptoms noted and hematologic tests remained normal.

➤*Treatment:* There is no known antidote for abacavir. It is not known whether abacavir or lamivudine can be removed by peritoneal dialysis or hemodialysis.

Patient Information

Advise patients to carry the Warning Card with them.

Inform patients how to identify a hypersensitivity reaction.

Inform patients that if they develop symptoms consistent with a hypersensitivity reaction they should call their health care provider right away to determine if they should stop taking abacavir/lamivudine.

Inform patients that a hypersensitivity reaction can worsen and lead to hospitalization or death if abacavir/lamivudine is not immediately discontinued.

Advise patients not to restart abacavir/lamivudine or any other abacavir-containing product following a hypersensitivity reaction because more severe symptoms can occur within hours and may include life-threatening hypotension and death.

Inform patients that a hypersensitivity reaction is usually reversible if it is detected promptly and abacavir/lamivudine is stopped right away.

Inform patients that if they have interrupted abacavir/lamivudine for reasons other than symptoms of hypersensitivity (eg, those who have an interruption in drug supply), a serious or fatal hypersensitivity reaction may occur with reintroduction of abacavir.

Inform patients that in one study, more severe hypersensitivity reactions were seen when abacavir was dosed at 600 mg once daily.

Inform patients not to restart abacavir/lamivudine or any other abacavir-containing product without medical consultation and that restarting abacavir needs to be undertaken only if medical care can be readily accessed by the patient or others.

Inform patients coinfected with HIV-1 and HBV that deterioration of liver disease has occurred in some cases when treatment with lamivudine was discontinued. Advise patients to discuss any changes in regimen with their health care provider.

Inform patients that some HIV-1 medicines, including abacavir/lamivudine, can cause a rare but serious condition called lactic acidosis with liver enlargement (hepatomegaly).

Abacavir/lamivudine is not a cure for HIV-1 infection, and patients may continue to experience illnesses associated with HIV-1 infection, including opportunistic infections. Patients should remain under the care of a health care provider when using abacavir/lamivudine. Advise patients that the use of abacavir/lamivudine has not been shown to reduce the risk of transmission of HIV-1 to others through sexual contact or blood contamination.

Inform patients that redistribution or accumulation of body fat may occur in patients receiving antiretroviral therapy and that the cause and long-term health effects of these conditions are not known at this time.

Advise patients that abacavir/lamivudine tablets are for oral ingestion only.

Advise patients of the importance of taking abacavir/lamivudine exactly as it is prescribed.

ETRAVIRINE

Rx	**Intelence** (Tibotec Therapeutics)	**Tablets; oral:** 100 mg	Lactose. (TMC125 100). White to off-white, oval. In 120s.
		200 mg	(T200). White to off-white, oblong. In 60s.

ETRAVIRINE — ORAL

Indications

➤*HIV infection:* In combination with other antiretroviral agents for the treatment of HIV-1 infection in antiretroviral treatment–experienced adult patients who have evidence of viral replication and HIV-1 strains resistant to nonnucleoside reverse transcriptase inhibitors (NNRTIs) and other antiretroviral agents.

Treatment history and, when available, resistance testing should guide the use of etravirine. The use of other active antiretroviral agents with etravirine is associated with an increased likelihood of treatment response. In patients who have experienced virologic failure on an NNRTI-containing regimen, do not use etravirine in combination with only nucleotide reverse transcriptase inhibitors (NtRTIs). The risks and benefits of etravirine have not been established in children or in treatment-naive adult patients.

Administration and Dosage

➤*Adults:*

HIV infection – 200 mg (one 200 mg tablet or two 100 mg tablets) taken twice daily following a meal.

➤*Administration:* Etravirine should be taken following a meal twice daily. The type of food does not affect the exposure to etravirine. Tablets should be swallowed whole with a liquid such as water.

Patients who are unable to swallow etravirine tablets whole may disperse the tablets in a glass of water. Once dispersed, patients should stir the dispersion well and drink it immediately. The glass should be rinsed with water several times and each rinse completely swallowed to ensure that the entire dose is consumed.

➤*Storage/Stability:* Store at 25°C (77°F); excursions are permitted between 15° and 30°C (59° and 86°F). Store in the original bottle. Keep the bottle tightly closed to protect from moisture. Do not remove the desiccant pouches.

Actions

➤*Pharmacology:* Etravirine is an antiviral drug and an NNRTI of HIV-1.

Etravirine binds directly to reverse transcriptase and blocks the RNA- and DNA-dependent DNA polymerase activities by causing a disruption of the enzyme's catalytic site. Etravirine does not inhibit the human DNA polymerases alpha, beta, and gamma.

➤*Pharmacokinetics:*

Absorption – Following oral administration, etravirine was absorbed with a time to maximum plasma concentration (T_{max}) of approximately 2.5 to 4 hours. The absolute oral bioavailability of etravirine is unknown.

The pharmacokinetic properties of etravirine were determined in healthy adults and in treatment-experienced HIV-1–infected adults. The systemic exposures (area under the curve [AUC]) to etravirine were lower in HIV-1–infected subjects than in healthy subjects.

Etravirine Population Pharmacokinetic Estimates of HIV-1–Infected Subjects (Integrated Data From Phase 3 Trials at Week 48)[a]

Parameter	Etravirine 200 mg twice daily (N = 575)
$AUC_{12\ h}$ (ng•h/mL)	
Geometric mean ± SD[b]	4,522 ± 4,710
Median (range)	4,380 (458 to 59,084)
C_{0h}[c] (ng/mL)	
Geometric mean ± SD	297 ± 391
Median (range)	298 (2 to 4,852)

[a] All HIV-1–infected subjects enrolled in phase 3 clinical trials received darunavir 600 mg/ritonavir 100 mg twice daily as part of their background regimen. Therefore, the pharmacokinetic parameter estimates shown in this table account for reductions in the pharmacokinetic parameters of etravirine caused by the coadministration of etravirine and darunavir/ritonavir. Note: the median protein binding adjusted median effective concentration (EC_{50}) for MT4 cells infected with HIV-1/IIIB in vitro is 4 ng/mL.
[b] SD = standard deviation.
[c] C_{0h} = predose concentration.

Effect of food: The systemic exposure (AUC) to etravirine was decreased by approximately 50% when etravirine was administered under fasting conditions, compared with etravirine administration following a meal; therefore, etravirine should always be taken following a meal. Within the range of meals studied, the systemic exposures to etravirine were similar. The total caloric content of the various meals evaluated ranged from 345 kcal (17 g fat) to 1,160 kcal (70 g fat).

Distribution – Etravirine is approximately 99.9% bound to plasma proteins, primarily to albumin (99.6%) and alpha-1 acid glycoprotein (97.66% to 99.02%) in vitro. The distribution of etravirine into compartments other than plasma (eg, cerebrospinal fluid, genital tract secretions) has not been evaluated in humans.

Metabolism – In vitro experiments with human liver microsomes indicate that etravirine primarily undergoes metabolism by CYP3A4, CYP2C9, and CYP2C19 enzymes. The major metabolites, formed by methyl hydroxylation of the dimethylbenzonitrile moiety, were at least 90% less active than etravirine against wild-type HIV in cell culture.

ETRAVIRINE — ORAL

Excretion – After single-dose oral administration of ^{14}C-etravirine 800 mg, 93.7% and 1.2% of the administered dose of ^{14}C-etravirine was recovered in feces and urine, respectively. Unchanged etravirine accounted for 81.2% to 86.4% of the administered dose in feces. Unchanged etravirine was not detected in urine. The mean (±SD) terminal elimination half-life of etravirine was approximately 41 (±20) hours.

Special populations –

Hepatic function impairment:

• *Hepatitis B and/or hepatitis C virus coinfection* – Population pharmacokinetic analysis of the TMC125-C206 and TMC125-C216 trials showed reduced clearance for etravirine in HIV-1–infected subjects with hepatitis B and/or C virus (HBV and/or HCV) coinfection. Based on the safety profile, no dosage adjustment is necessary in patients coinfected with HBV and/or HCV.

➤*Microbiology:*

Resistance –

Treatment-experienced subjects: In the phase 3 trials TMC125-C206 and TMC125-C216, substitutions that developed most commonly in subjects with virologic failure at week 48 to the etravirine–containing regimen were V179F, V179I, and Y181C, which usually emerged in a background of multiple other NNRTI resistance–associated substitutions. In all of the trials conducted with etravirine in HIV-1–infected subjects, the following substitutions emerged most commonly: L100I, E138G, V179F, V179I, Y181C, and H221Y. Other NNRTI resistance–associated substitutions that emerged on etravirine treatment in less than 10% of the virologic failure isolates included K101E H/P, K103N/R, V106I/M, V108I, Y181I, Y188L, V189I, G190S/C, N348I and R356K. The emergence of NNRTI substitutions on etravirine treatment contributed to decreased susceptibility to etravirine with a median fold-change in etravirine susceptibility of 40-fold from reference and a median fold-change of 6-fold from baseline.

Cross-resistance –

Site-directed nonnucleoside reverse transcriptase inhibitors mutant virus: Etravirine showed antiviral activity against 55 of 65 (85%) HIV-1 strains with single amino acid substitutions at reverse transcriptase positions associated with NNRTI resistance, including the most commonly found K103N. The single amino acid substitutions associated with an etravirine reduction in susceptibility more than 3-fold were K101A, K101P, K101Q, E138G, E138Q, Y181C, Y181I, Y181T, Y181V, and M230L, and of these, the greatest reductions were Y181I (13 fold-change in EC_{50} value) and Y181V (17 fold-change in EC_{50} value). Mutant strains containing a single NNRTI resistance–associated substitution (K101P, K101Q, E138Q, or M230L) had cross-resistance between etravirine and efavirenz. The majority (64%) of the NNRTI mutant viruses with 2 or 3 amino acid substitutions associated with NNRTI resistance had decreased susceptibility to etravirine (fold-change of more than 3). The highest levels of resistance to etravirine were observed for HIV-1 harboring a combination of substitutions V179F + Y181C (187 fold-change), V179F + Y181I (123 fold-change), or V179F + Y181C + F227C (888 fold-change).

Contraindications

None well documented.

Warnings/Precautions

➤*Skin reactions:* Severe and potentially life-threatening and fatal skin reactions have been reported. These include Stevens-Johnson syndrome, toxic epidermal necrolysis, and erythema multiforme. Hypersensitivity reactions have also been reported and were characterized by constitutional findings, rash, and sometimes organ dysfunction, including hepatic failure. In phase 3 clinical trials, grade 3 and 4 rashes were reported in 1.3% of subjects receiving etravirine compared with 0.2% of placebo subjects. A total of 2.2% of HIV-1–infected subjects receiving etravirine discontinued from phase 3 trials because of rash. Rash occurred most commonly during the first 6 weeks of therapy.

Discontinue etravirine immediately if signs or symptoms of severe skin reactions or hypersensitivity reactions develop, including, but not limited to, severe rash or rash accompanied by angioedema, blisters, conjunctivitis, eosinophilia, facial edema, fatigue, fever, general malaise, hepatitis, muscle or joint aches, or oral lesions. Monitor clinical status, including liver transaminases, and initiate appropriate therapy. Delay in stopping etravirine treatment after the onset of severe rash may result in a life-threatening reaction.

➤*Fat redistribution:* Redistribution/accumulation of body fat, including breast enlargement, central obesity, cushingoid appearance, dorsocervical fat enlargement (buffalo hump), facial wasting, and peripheral wasting have been observed in patients receiving antiretroviral therapy. The mechanism and long-term consequences of these reactions are currently unknown. A causal relationship has not been established.

➤*Immune reconstitution syndrome:* Immune reconstitution syndrome has been reported in patients treated with combination antiretroviral therapy, including etravirine. During the initial phase of combination antiretroviral treatment, patients whose immune system responds may develop an inflammatory response to indolent or residual opportunistic infections, such as *Mycobacterium avium* complex, cytomegalovirus, *Pneumocystis jiroveci* pneumonia, and tuberculosis, which may necessitate further evaluation and treatment.

➤*Renal function impairment:* Because the renal clearance of etravirine is negligible (less than 1.2%), a decrease in total body clearance is not expected in patients with renal impairment. No dose adjustments are required in patients with renal impairment. Because etravirine is highly bound to plasma proteins, it is unlikely that it will be significantly removed by hemodialysis or peritoneal dialysis.

➤*Hepatic function impairment:* No dosage adjustment is required in patients with mild (Child-Pugh class A) or moderate (Child-Pugh class B) hepatic impairment. The pharmacokinetics of etravirine have not been evaluated in patients with severe hepatic impairment (Child-Pugh class C).

➤*Pregnancy:* Category B. No adequate and well-controlled studies of etravirine use in pregnant women have been conducted. Use etravirine during pregnancy only if the potential benefit justifies the potential risk to the fetus. In addition, no pharmacokinetic studies have been conducted in pregnant patients.

Antiretroviral pregnancy registry – To monitor maternal-fetal outcomes of pregnant women exposed to etravirine, an antiretroviral pregnancy registry has been established. Health care providers are encouraged to register patients by calling 1-800-258-4263.

➤*Lactation:* The Centers for Disease Control and Prevention recommends that mothers infected with HIV not breast-feed their infants to avoid risking postnatal transmission of HIV. It is not known whether etravirine is secreted in human milk. Because of the potential for HIV transmission and the potential for adverse reactions in breast-feeding infants, advise mothers not to breast-feed if they are receiving etravirine.

➤*Children:* Safety and effectiveness in children have not been established.

➤*Elderly:* Make dose selection for an elderly patient with caution, reflecting the greater frequency of decreased hepatic, renal, or cardiac function, and of concomitant disease or other drug therapy.

➤*Monitoring:* Monitor clinical status, including liver transaminases, in patients who develop signs and symptoms of severe skin reactions (eg, Stevens-Johnson syndrome, toxic epidermal necrosis) or hypersensitivity reactions.

Drug Interactions

➤*Cytochrome P450 system:* Etravirine is a substrate of CYP3A4, CYP2C9, and CYP2C19; therefore, coadministration of etravirine with drugs that induce or inhibit CYP3A4, CYP2C9, and CYP2C19 may alter the therapeutic effect or adverse reaction profile of etravirine. Etravirine is an inducer of CYP3A4 and inhibitor of CYP2C9 and CYP2C19; therefore, coadministration of drugs that are substrates of CYP3A4, CYP2C9, and CYP2C19 with etravirine may alter the therapeutic effect or adverse reaction profile of the coadministered drug(s).

Etravirine Drug Interactions

Precipitant drug	Object drug[a]		Description
Anticonvulsants (eg, carbamazepine, phenobarbital, phenytoin)	Etravirine	↓	Carbamazepine, phenobarbital, and phenytoin are inducers of CYP-450[b] enzymes and when coadministered with etravirine may cause a significant decrease in etravirine plasma concentrations and loss of therapeutic effect of etravirine. Avoid coadministration.
Antifungals (eg, fluconazole, itraconazole, ketoconazole, posaconazole, voriconazole)	Etravirine	↑	Coadministration of fluconazole, itraconazole, ketoconazole, and posaconazole with etravirine may increase plasma concentrations of etravirine. Plasma concentrations of itraconazole or ketoconazole may be decreased by etravirine. Concomitant use of voriconazole and etravirine may increase plasma concentration of voriconazole and etravirine. Use with caution. Dose adjustments for itraconazole, ketoconazole, or posaconazole may be necessary.
Etravirine	Antifungals (eg, itraconazole, ketoconazole, voriconazole)	↑↓	
Atazanavir/Ritonavir	Etravirine	↑	The AUC of etravirine after coadministration of atazanavir/ritonavir with etravirine is anticipated to be approximately 100% higher. Concomitant use of etravirine with atazanavir/ritonavir may cause a significant decrease in atazanavir minimum plasma concentration by approximately 38% and a loss of therapeutic effect of atazanavir. Avoid coadministration.
Etravirine	Atazanavir	↓	
Charcoal	Etravirine	↓	Charcoal can decrease the absorption of etravirine, reducing its effectiveness or toxicity.
Darunavir/Ritonavir	Etravirine	↓	The AUC of etravirine was reduced by approximately 37% when etravirine was coadministered with darunavir/ritonavir. May be coadministered without adjustments.

ETRAVIRINE — ORAL

Etravirine Drug Interactions

Precipitant drug	Object drug[a]		Description
Dexamethasone (systemic)	Etravirine	↓	Systemic dexamethasone can decrease etravirine plasma concentrations, resulting in loss of therapeutic effect. Use with caution or consider an alternative corticosteroid, particularly if used long-term.
Lopinavir/Ritonavir	Etravirine	↓	The AUC of etravirine was reduced after coadministration of lopinavir/ritonavir. Because the AUC reduction is similar to the reduction in the presence of darunavir/ritonavir, etravirine can be coadministered with lopinavir/ritonavir without dose adjustments.
NNRTIs (eg, delavirdine, efavirenz, nevirapine)	Etravirine	↑↓	Concomitant use of etravirine with efavirenz or nevirapine may cause a significant decrease in the plasma concentrations of etravirine and loss of therapeutic effect. Etravirine plasma concentrations may be increased when coadministered with delavirdine. Avoid coadministration.
Rifabutin	Etravirine	↓	If etravirine is not coadministered with a protease inhibitor/ritonavir, the recommended rifabutin dose is 300 mg daily. If etravirine is administered with darunavir/ritonavir or saquinavir/ritonavir, do not coadminister rifabutin because of the potential for reductions in etravirine exposure.
Rifampin, rifapentine	Etravirine	↓	Do not use etravirine with rifampin or rifapentine because coadministration may cause significant decreases in etravirine plasma concentrations and loss of therapeutic effect.
Ritonavir	Etravirine	↓	Concomitant use of etravirine with ritonavir 600 mg twice daily may cause a significant decrease in the plasma concentration of etravirine and loss of therapeutic effect. Do not coadminister.
Saquinavir/Ritonavir	Etravirine	↓	The AUC of etravirine was reduced by approximately 33% when coadministered with saquinavir/ritonavir. No dose adjustment is necessary.
St. John's wort (*Hypericum perforatum*)	Etravirine	↓	Concomitant use of etravirine with products containing St. John's wort may cause a significant decrease in etravirine plasma concentrations and loss of therapeutic effect. Avoid coadministration.
Tipranavir/Ritonavir	Etravirine	↓	Concomitant use of etravirine with tipranavir/ritonavir may cause a significant decrease in the plasma concentrations of etravirine and loss of therapeutic effect. Avoid coadministration.
Etravirine	Antiarrhythmic agents (eg, amiodarone, bepridil, disopyramide, flecainide, lidocaine [systemic], mexiletine, propafenone, quinidine)	↓	Concentrations of these antiarrhythmics may be decreased when coadministered with etravirine. Use with caution and monitor drug concentrations if available.

Etravirine Drug Interactions

Precipitant drug	Object drug[a]		Description
Etravirine	Clarithromycin	↑↓	Clarithromycin exposure was decreased by etravirine; however, concentrations of the active metabolite (14-hydroxy-clarithromycin) were increased. Consider alternatives such as azithromycin.
Etravirine	Clopidogrel	↓	Conversion of clopidogrel to its active metabolite may be decreased. Consider alternatives to clopidogrel treatment.
Etravirine	Diazepam	↑	Concomitant use may increase plasma concentrations of diazepam. A decrease in the diazepam dose may be necessary.
Etravirine	Digoxin	↑	When initiating treatment with etravirine and digoxin, start with the lowest dose of digoxin. When initiating etravirine treatment in a patient on a stable digoxin regimen, no dose adjustment in either etravirine or digoxin is needed. Monitor digoxin concentrations and adjust the dose as needed.
Etravirine	Fosamprenavir/Ritonavir	↑	Because of significant increase in the systemic exposure of amprenavir, the appropriate dose of the combination of etravirine and fosamprenavir/ritonavir has not been established. Avoid coadministration.
Etravirine	HMG-CoA reductase inhibitors[b] (eg, atorvastatin, fluvastatin, lovastatin, simvastatin)	↑↓	Coadministration may reduce lovastatin and simvastatin plasma levels and increase fluvastatin levels. Dose adjustments may be necessary. The combination of atorvastatin and etravirine may be given without dose adjustments; however, the dose of atorvastatin may need to be altered based on clinical response.
Etravirine	Immunosuppressants (eg, cyclosporine, sirolimus, tacrolimus)	↓	Coadminister etravirine and systemic immunosuppressants with caution because plasma concentrations of cyclosporine, sirolimus, and tacrolimus may be affected.
Etravirine	Maraviroc	↑↓	Maraviroc plasma concentrations may be reduced when etravirine is administered with maraviroc in the absence of a potent CYP3A inhibitor (eg, ritonavir boosted protease inhibitor). In this instance, the recommended maraviroc dose is 600 mg twice daily.
			Maraviroc plasma concentrations may be increased when etravirine is administered with maraviroc in the presence of a potent CYP3A inhibitor. In this instance, the recommended maraviroc dose is 150 mg twice daily.
Etravirine	Methadone	↔	Etravirine and methadone can be coadministered without dose adjustments; however, clinical monitoring for withdrawal symptoms is recommended because methadone maintenance therapy may need to be adjusted in some patients.
Etravirine	PDE5[b] inhibitors (eg, sildenafil, tadalafil, vardenafil)	↓	Etravirine and sildenafil may be coadministered without dose adjustments; however, the dose of sildenafil may need to be altered based on clinical effect.

ETRAVIRINE — ORAL

Etravirine Drug Interactions			
Precipitant drug	Object drug[a]		Description
Etravirine	Protease inhibitors (eg, atazanavir, fosamprenavir, indinavir, nelfinavir)	↑↓	Concomitant use of etravirine with protease inhibitors without coadministration of low-dose ritonavir may cause a significant alteration in the plasma concentrations of the protease inhibitor. Do not coadminister etravirine with protease inhibitors without low-dose ritonavir.
Etravirine	Warfarin	↑	Warfarin concentrations may be increased when coadministered with etravirine. Monitor INR[b] when warfarin is combined with etravirine.

[a] ↑ = object drug increased; ↓ = object drug decreased; ↑↓ = object drug both increased and decreased; ↔ = undetermined clinical effect.
[b] CYP-450 = cytochrome P450; HMG-CoA = 3-hydroxy-3-methylglutaryl coenzyme A; PDE5 = phosphodiesterase type 5; INR = international normalized ratio.

➤*Drug/Food interactions:* Etravirine systemic exposure is reduced approximately 50% when administered under fasting conditions, compared with being given after a meal. Instruct patients to always take etravirine following a meal.

Adverse Reactions

➤*Dermatologic:* The most frequently reported adverse reaction at least grade 2 in severity was rash (10%). Stevens-Johnson syndrome, drug hypersensitivity reaction, and erythema multiforme were reported in less than 0.1% of subjects during clinical development with etravirine. A total of 2.2% of HIV-1–infected subjects in phase 3 trials receiving etravirine discontinued because of rash. In general, in clinical trials, rash was mild to moderate, occurred primarily in the second week of therapy, and was infrequent after week 4. Rash generally resolved within 1 to 2 weeks on continued therapy. The incidence of rash was higher in women compared with men in the etravirine arm in the phase 3 trials. Patients with a history of NNRTI-related rash did not appear to be at increased risk of the development of etravirine-related rash compared with patients without a history of NNRTI-related rash.

➤*Common adverse reactions (2% or more):*

Etravirine Adverse Reactions (≥ 2%)[a,b]		
	Pooled TMC 125-C206 and TMC 125-C216 trials	
Adverse reactions	Etravirine + BR[c] (n = 599)	Placebo + BR (n = 604)
CNS		
Peripheral neuropathy	4%	2%
Dermatologic		
Rash	10%	3%

[a] Includes adverse reactions at least possibly, probably, or very likely related to the drug.
[b] Intensities are defined as follows: moderate (discomfort enough to cause interference with usual activity); severe (incapacitating with inability to work or do usual activity).
[c] BR = background regimen

➤*Less common adverse reactions (less than 2%):*

Cardiovascular – Angina pectoris, atrial fibrillation, myocardial infarction.

CNS – Abnormal dreams, anxiety, confused state, disorientation, disturbance in attention, hypersomnia, hypesthesia, insomnia, nervousness, nightmares, paresthesia, sleep disorders, sluggishness, somnolence, tremor.

Dermatologic – Dry skin, hyperhidrosis, lipohypertrophy, night sweats, prurigo, swelling face.

GI – Abdominal distension, anorexia, constipation, dry mouth, flatulence, gastritis, gastroesophageal reflux disease, hematemesis, pancreatitis, retching, stomatitis.

GU – Acute renal failure, gynecomastia.

Hematologic – Anemia, hemolytic anemia.

Hepatic – Cytolytic hepatitis, hepatic failure, hepatic steatosis, hepatitis, hepatomegaly.

Metabolic/Nutritional – Diabetes mellitus, dyslipidemia.

Respiratory – Bronchospasm, exertional dyspnea.

Special senses – Blurred vision, vertigo.

Miscellaneous – Drug hypersensitivity, immune reconstitution syndrome.

➤*Other adverse reactions (0.5% or less):* Additional adverse reactions of at least moderate intensity observed in other trials were acquired lipodystrophy, angioneurotic edema, erythema multiforme, and hemorrhagic stroke.

➤*Lab test abnormalities:*

Etravirine Laboratory Abnormalities (Grade 2 to 4)			
		Pooled TMC125-C206 and TMC125-C216 trials	
Laboratory parameter	Division of AIDS toxicity range	Etravirine + BR[a] (n = 599)	Placebo + BR (n = 604)
Pancreatic amylase			
Grade 2	> 1.5 to 2 × ULN[a]	7%	8%
Grade 3	> 2 to 5 × ULN	7%	8%
Grade 4	> 5 × ULN	2%	1%
Lipase			
Grade 2	> 1.5 to 3 × ULN	4%	6%
Grade 3	> 3 to 5 × ULN	2%	2%
Grade 4	> 5 × ULN	1%	< 1%
Creatinine			
Grade 2	> 1.4 to 1.8 × ULN	6%	5%
Grade 3	> 1.9 to 3.4 × ULN	2%	1%
Grade 4	> 3.4 × ULN	0%	< 1%
Hemoglobin decreased			
Grade 2	90 to 99 g/L	2%	4%
Grade 3	70 to 89 g/L	< 1%	< 1%
Grade 4	< 70 g/L	< 1%	< 1%
White blood cell count			
Grade 2	1,500 to 1,999/mm³	2%	3%
Grade 3	1,000 to 1,499/mm³	1%	4%
Grade 4	< 1,000/mm³	1%	< 1%
Neutrophils			
Grade 2	750 to 999 mm³	5%	6%
Grade 3	500 to 749 mm³	4%	4%
Grade 4	< 500 mm³	2%	3%
Platelet count			
Grade 2	50,000 to 99,999 mm³	3%	5%
Grade 3	25,000 to 49,999 mm³	1%	1%
Grade 4	< 25,000 mm³	< 1%	< 1%
Total cholesterol			
Grade 2	> 6.2 to 7.77 mmol/L 240 to 300 mg/dL	20%	17%
Grade 3	> 7.77 mmol/L > 300 mg/dL	8%	5%
Low-density lipoprotein			
Grade 2	4.13 to 4.9 mmol/L 160 to 190 mg/dL	13%	12%
Grade 3	> 4.9 mmol/L > 190 mg/dL	7%	7%
Triglycerides			
Grade 2	5.65 to 8.48 mmol/L 500 to 750 mg/dL	9%	7%
Grade 3	8.49 to 13.56 mmol/L 751 to 1,200 mg/dL	6%	4%
Grade 4	> 13.56 mmol/L > 1,200 mg/dL	4%	2%
Glucose levels elevated			
Grade 2	6.95 to 13.88 mmol/L 161 to 250 mg/dL	15%	13%
Grade 3	13.89 to 27.75 mmol/L 251 to 500 mg/dL	4%	2%
Grade 4	> 27.75 mmol/L > 500 mg/dL	0%	< 1%

ETRAVIRINE — ORAL

Etravirine Laboratory Abnormalities (Grade 2 to 4)			
		Pooled TMC125-C206 and TMC125-C216 trials	
Laboratory parameter	Division of AIDS toxicity range	Etravirine + BR[a] (n = 599)	Placebo + BR (n = 604)
ALT			
Grade 2	2.6 to 5 × ULN	6%	5%
Grade 3	5.1 to 10 × ULN	3%	2%
Grade 4	> 10 × ULN	1%	< 1%
AST			
Grade 2	2.6 to 5 × ULN	6%	8%
Grade 3	5.1 to 10 × ULN	3%	2%
Grade 4	> 10 × ULN	< 1%	< 1%

[a] BR = background regimen; ULN = upper limit of normal.

Patients coinfected with hepatitis B and hepatitis C virus – In phase 3 trials TMC125-C206 and TMC125-C216, 139 (12.3%) subjects with chronic HBV and/or HCV coinfection (out of 1,129 subjects) were permitted to enroll. AST and ALT abnormalities occurred more frequently in HBV and/or HCV coinfected subjects for both treatment groups. Grade 2 or higher laboratory abnormalities that represent a worsening from baseline of AST, ALT, or total bilirubin occurred in 27.8% , 25%, and 7.1%, respectively, of coinfected etravirine-treated subjects, compared with 6.7%, 7.5%, and 1.8% of noncoinfected etravirine-treated subjects. In general, adverse reactions reported by etravirine-treated subjects with HBV and/or HCV coinfection were similar to etravirine-treated subjects without HBV and/or HCV coinfection.

➤*Postmarketing:* Fatal cases of toxic epidermal necrolysis have been reported. Severe hypersensitivity reactions, including cases of hepatic failure, have been reported.

Overdosage

➤*Treatment:* There is no specific antidote for overdose with etravirine. Human experience of overdose with etravirine is limited. The highest dosage studied in healthy volunteers was 400 mg once daily. Treatment of overdose with etravirine consists of general supportive measures, including monitoring of vital signs and observation of the clinical status of the patient. If indicated, elimination of an unabsorbed active substance is to be achieved by gastric lavage. Administration of activated charcoal also may be used to aid in the removal of the unabsorbed active substances. Because etravirine is highly protein bound, dialysis is unlikely to result in significant removal of the active substance.

Patient Information

A statement to patients and health care providers is included on the product's bottle label: Alert: Find out about medicines that should not be taken with etravirine from your health care provider. A patient package insert for etravirine is available for patient information.

Inform patients that etravirine is not a cure for HIV infection and that they may continue to develop opportunistic infections and other complications associated with HIV disease. Inform patients that etravirine does not reduce the risk of passing HIV to others through sexual contact, sharing needles, or exposure to blood. Advise patients to continue to practice safer sex and to use latex or polyurethane condoms to lower the chance of sexual contact with any body fluids, such as semen, vaginal secretions, or blood. Advise patients to never reuse or share needles. Tell patients that sustained decreases in plasma HIV RNA have been associated with a reduced risk of progression to AIDS and death. Advise patients to remain under the care of a health care provider while using etravirine.

Advise patients to take etravirine following a meal twice daily as prescribed. The type of food does not affect the exposure to etravirine. Instruct patients to swallow the tablets whole with a liquid such as water. Advise patients who are unable to swallow the etravirine tablets whole that they may disperse the tablets in a glass of water. Once dispersed, instruct patients to stir the dispersion well, and drink it immediately. The glass must be rinsed with water several times and each rinse completely swallowed to ensure the entire dose is consumed.

Always use etravirine in combination with other antiretroviral drugs. Advise patients not to alter the etravirine dose or discontinue etravirine therapy without consulting their health care provider. If the patient misses a dose of etravirine within 6 hours of the time it is usually taken, tell the patient to take etravirine following a meal as soon as possible, and then take the next dose of etravirine at the regularly scheduled time. If a patient misses a dose of etravirine by more than 6 hours of the time it is usually taken, tell the patient not to take the missed dose and simply resume the usual dosing schedule. Inform the patient not to take more or less than the prescribed dose of etravirine at any one time.

Etravirine may interact with many drugs. Advise patients to report the use of any other prescription or nonprescription medication or herbal products, including St. John's wort, to their health care provider.

Inform patients that severe and potentially life-threatening rash has been reported with etravirine. Rash has been reported most commonly in the first 6 weeks of therapy. Advise patients to immediately contact their health care provider if they develop rash. Instruct patients to immediately stop taking etravirine and seek medical attention if they develop a rash associated with any of the following symptoms as it may be a sign of a more serious reaction, such as Stevens-Johnson syndrome, toxic epidermal necrolysis, or severe hypersensitivity: blisters, extreme tiredness, eye inflammation, facial swelling, fever, generally ill feeling, muscle or joint aches, oral lesions; swelling of the eyes, lips, or mouth; breathing difficulty; and/or signs and symptoms of liver problems (eg, dark or tea-colored urine, loss of appetite, nausea, pale-colored stools/bowel movements, vomiting, yellowing of the skin or whites of the eyes, or pain, aching, or sensitivity on the right side below your ribs). Explain to patients that if severe rash occurs, they will be closely monitored, laboratory tests will be ordered, and appropriate therapy will be initiated.

Inform patients that redistribution or accumulation of body fat may occur in patients receiving antiretroviral therapy, including etravirine, and that the cause and long-term health effects of these conditions are not known at this time.

NEVIRAPINE

Rx	**Viramune** (Boehringer Ingelheim)	**Tablets; oral:** 200 mg	Lactose. (54 193). White, oval. In 60s.
		Suspension; oral: 50 mg per 5 mL	As nevirapine hemihydrate. Parabens, polysorbate 80, sorbitol, sucrose. In 240 mL.
Rx	**Viramune XR** (Boehringer Ingelheim)	**Tablets, extended-release; oral:** 400 mg	Lactose. (V04). Yellow, oval. In 30s.

NEVIRAPINE — ORAL

WARNING

Hepatotoxicity – Severe, life-threatening, and, in some cases, fatal hepatotoxicity, particularly in the first 18 weeks, has been reported in patients treated with nevirapine. In some cases, patients presented with nonspecific prodromal signs or symptoms of hepatitis and progressed to hepatic failure. These events are often associated with rash. Women and patients with higher CD4+ cell counts at initiation of therapy are at increased risk. Women with CD4+ cell counts higher than 250 cells/mm^3, including pregnant women receiving nevirapine in combination with other antiretrovirals for treatment of HIV-1 infection, are at the greatest risk. However, hepatotoxicity associated with nevirapine use can occur in both genders, at all CD4+ cell counts, and at any time during treatment. Hepatic failure has also been reported in patients without HIV taking nevirapine for post-exposure prophylaxis. Use of nevirapine for occupational and nonoccupational postexposure prophylaxis is contraindicated. Patients with signs or symptoms of hepatitis, or with increased transaminases combined with rash or other systemic symptoms, must discontinue nevirapine and seek medical evaluation immediately.

WARNING (cont.)

Skin reactions – Severe, life-threatening skin reactions, including fatal cases, have occurred in patients treated with nevirapine. These have included cases of Stevens-Johnson syndrome, toxic epidermal necrolysis, and hypersensitivity reactions characterized by rash, constitutional findings, and organ dysfunction. Patients developing signs or symptoms of severe skin reactions or hypersensitivity reactions must discontinue nevirapine and seek medical evaluation immediately. Check transaminase levels immediately for all patients who develop a rash in the first 18 weeks of treatment. The 14-day lead-in period with immediate-release nevirapine 200 mg daily dosing has been observed to decrease the incidence of rash and must be followed.

Monitoring – It is essential that patients be monitored intensively during the first 18 weeks of therapy with nevirapine to detect potentially life-threatening hepatotoxicity or skin reactions. Extra vigilance is warranted during the first 6 weeks of therapy, which is the period of greatest risk of these reactions. Do not restart nevirapine following clinical hepatitis, or transaminase elevations combined with rash or other systemic symptoms, or following severe skin rash or hypersensitivity reactions. In some cases, hepatic injury has progressed despite discontinuation of treatment.

NEVIRAPINE — ORAL

Indications

➤*HIV infection:* For use in combination with other antiretroviral agents for the treatment of HIV-1 infection in adults.

Administration and Dosage

➤*General dosing considerations:* A patient experiencing mild to moderate rash without constitutional symptoms during the 14-day lead-in period should not have their nevirapine dose increased until the rash has resolved. The total duration of the once-daily lead-in dosing period should not exceed 28 days, at which point an alternative regimen should be sought.

➤*Adults:*

HIV infection –

Maximum dose: 400 mg daily.

Initial dosage: 200 mg immediate release daily for the first 14 days.

Maintenance dosage: 200 mg immediate release twice daily or 400 mg extended release (ER) daily.

Missed doses: Patients who interrupt nevirapine dosing for more than 7 days should restart using one 200 mg immediate-release tablet daily for the first 14 days (lead-in) followed by one 200 mg immediate-release tablet twice daily or 400 mg ER tablet daily.

Conversion: Patients already on a regimen of nevirapine immediate release twice daily in combination with other antiretroviral agents can be switched to nevirapine ER 400 mg once daily in combination with other antiretroviral agents without the 14-day lead-in period.

➤*Children:*

HIV infection –

15 days and older (immediate release only):

- *Maximum dose* – 400 mg daily; 200 mg per dose.
- *Initial dosage* – 150 mg/m² once daily for 14 days.
- *Maintenance dosage* – 150 mg/m² twice daily.

Nevirapine Suspension for Dosing in Children Based on a Dose of 150 mg/m² of BSA[a]

BSA range	Volume
0.06 to 0.12 m²	1.25 mL
0.12 to 0.25 m²	2.5 mL
0.25 to 0.42 m²	5 mL
0.42 to 0.58 m²	7.5 mL
0.58 to 0.75 m²	10 mL
0.75 to 0.92 m²	12.5 mL
0.92 to 1.08 m²	15 mL
1.08 to 1.25 m²	17.5 mL
> 1.25 m²	20 mL

[a] BSA = body surface area.

- *Missed doses* – Patients who interrupt nevirapine dosing for more than 7 days should restart using 150 mg/m² per day for the first 14 days (lead-in) followed by 150 mg/m² twice daily.

14 days and younger: See Off-Label Dosing.

ER formulation – The safety and efficacy of nevirapine ER in children have not been established.

Off-label dosing –

HIV infection:

- *Birth to 2 months of age* –
  Initial dosage: 5 mg/kg or 120 mg/m² daily for 14 days.
  Dosage titration: 120 mg/m² every 12 hours for 14 days.
  Maintenance dosage: 200 mg/m² every 12 hours.

Prevention of maternal-fetal HIV transmission:

- *Neonates 35 weeks gestational age and older* – 2 mg/kg given as a single dose between birth and 72 hours of age in combination with zidovudine 2 mg/kg orally every 6 hours starting within 12 hours after birth and continuing through 6 weeks of age and lamivudine 2 mg/kg twice daily for 7 days.
- *Neonates younger than 35 weeks gestational age but older than 30 weeks of age* – 2 mg/kg given as a single dose between birth and 72 hours of age in combination with zidovudine 2 mg/kg orally every 12 hours, advanced to every 8 hours at 2 weeks of age continuing through 6 weeks of age, and lamivudine 2 mg/kg twice daily for 7 days.
- *Neonates younger than 30 weeks gestational age* – 2 mg/kg given as a single dose between birth and 72 hours of age in combination with zidovudine 2 mg/kg orally every 12 hours, advanced to every 8 hours at 4 weeks of age continuing through 6 weeks of age, and lamivudine 2 mg/kg twice daily for 7 days.

➤*Elderly:* Use caution with dose selection, reflecting the greater frequency of decreased hepatic, renal, or cardiac function, and of concomitant disease or other drug therapy.

➤*Renal function impairment:*

Dialysis – An additional nevirapine 200 mg immediate-release dose following each dialysis treatment is indicated in patients requiring dialysis. Nevirapine metabolites may accumulate in patients receiving dialysis; however, the clinical significance of this accumulation is not known.

➤*Hepatic function impairment:* Contraindicated in patients with moderate or severe (Child-Pugh class B or C, respectively) hepatic impairment.

➤*Discontinuation of therapy:* Nevirapine should be discontinued if patients experience severe rash or any rash accompanied by constitutional findings. If a clinical (symptomatic) hepatic event occurs, nevirapine should be permanently discontinued and not restarted after recovery.

➤*Administration:* Administer with or without food.

Suspension – Shake the suspension gently prior to administration. It is important to administer the entire measured dose of the suspension by using an oral dosing syringe or dosing cup. An oral dosing syringe is recommended, particularly for volumes of 5 mL or less. If a dosing cup is used, it should be thoroughly rinsed with water, and the rinse should also be administered to the patient.

➤*Storage/Stability:* Store at 25°C (77°F); excursions are permitted between 15° and 30°C (59° and 86°F).

Actions

➤*Pharmacology:* Nevirapine, an antiviral drug, is a nonnucleoside reverse transcriptase inhibitor (NNRTI) of HIV-1. Nevirapine binds directly to reverse transcriptase (RT) and blocks the RNA- and DNA-dependent DNA polymerase activities by causing a disruption of the enzyme's catalytic site. The activity of nevirapine does not compete with template or nucleoside triphosphates. HIV-2 RT and eukaryotic DNA polymerases (such as human DNA polymerases alpha, beta, gamma, or delta) are not inhibited by nevirapine.

➤*Pharmacokinetics:*

Absorption – Nevirapine is readily absorbed (more than 90%) after oral administration in healthy volunteers and in adults with HIV-1 infection. Absolute bioavailability in 12 healthy adults following single-dose administration was 93% ± 9% (mean ± standard deviation [SD]) for a 50 mg tablet and 91% ± 8% for an oral solution. Peak plasma nevirapine concentrations of 2 ± 0.4 mcg/mL (7.5 mcM) were attained by 4 hours following a single 200 mg dose. After multiple doses, nevirapine peak concentrations appear to increase linearly in the dose range of 200 to 400 mg/day. Steady-state trough nevirapine concentrations of 4.5 ± 1.9 mcg/mL (17 ± 7 mcM) (n = 242) were attained at 400 mg/day. Nevirapine tablets and suspension have been shown to be comparably bioavailable and interchangeable at doses of up to 200 mg.

Distribution – Nevirapine is highly lipophilic and is essentially nonionized at physiologic pH. Following intravenous administration to healthy adults, the apparent volume of distribution of nevirapine was 1.21 ± 0.09 L/kg, suggesting that nevirapine is widely distributed in humans. Nevirapine readily crosses the placenta and is found in breast milk. Nevirapine is approximately 60% bound to plasma proteins in the plasma concentration range of 1 to 10 mcg/mL. Nevirapine concentrations in human cerebrospinal fluid (n = 6) were 45% (± 5%) of the concentrations in plasma; this ratio is approximately equal to the fraction not bound to plasma protein.

Metabolism/Excretion – In vivo studies in humans and in vitro studies with human liver microsomes have shown that nevirapine is extensively biotransformed via the cytochrome P450 (CYP-450) (oxidative) metabolism to several hydroxylated metabolites. In vitro studies with human liver microsomes suggest that oxidative metabolism of nevirapine is mediated primarily by CYP-450 isozymes from the CYP3A and CYP2B6 families, although other isozymes may have a secondary role. In a mass balance/excretion study in 8 healthy male volunteers dosed to steady state with nevirapine 200 mg given twice daily followed by a single ^{14}C-nevirapine 50 mg dose, approximately 91.4% ± 10.5% of the radiolabeled dose was recovered, with urine (81.3% ± 11.1%) representing the primary route of excretion, compared with feces (10.1% ± 1.5%). More than 80% of the radioactivity in urine was made up of glucuronide conjugates of hydroxylated metabolites; therefore, CYP-450 metabolism, glucuronide conjugation, and urinary excretion of glucuronidated metabolites represent the primary route of nevirapine biotransformation and elimination in humans. Only a small fraction (less than 5%) of the radioactivity in urine (representing less than 3% of the total dose) was made up of the parent compound; therefore, renal excretion plays a minor role in elimination of the parent compound.

Nevirapine is an inducer of hepatic CYP-450 metabolic enzymes 3A and 2B6. Nevirapine induces CYP3A and CYP2B6 by approximately 20% to 25%, as indicated by erythromycin breath test results and urine metabolites. Autoinduction of CYP3A- and CYP2B6-mediated metabolism leads to an approximately 1.5- to 2-fold increase in the apparent oral clearance of nevirapine as treatment continues from a single dose to 2 to 4 weeks of dosing with 200 to 400 mg/day. Autoinduction also results in a corresponding decrease in the terminal phase half-life of nevirapine in plasma from approximately 45 hours (single dose) to approximately 25 to 30 hours following multiple dosing with 200 to 400 mg/day.

Special populations –

Renal function impairment: Subjects requiring dialysis exhibited a 44% reduction in nevirapine area under the curve (AUC) over a 1-week exposure period. There was also evidence of accumulation of nevirapine hydroxy-metabolites in plasma in subjects requiring dialysis. An additional 200 mg dose following each dialysis treatment is indicated.

Hepatic function impairment: In a pharmacokinetic study in which HIV-1–negative cirrhotic patients with mild (Child-Pugh class A; n = 6) or moderate (Child-Pugh class B; n = 4) hepatic impairment received a single nevirapine 200 mg dose, a significant increase in the AUC of nevirapine was observed in 1 patient with Child-Pugh class B and ascites suggesting that patients with worsening hepatic function and ascites may be at risk of accumulating nevirapine in the systemic circulation. Because nevirapine induces its own metabolism with multiple dosing, a single-dose study may not reflect the impact of hepatic impairment on multiple-dose pharmacokinetics.

NEVIRAPINE — ORAL

See Contraindications for more information.

Gender: Women showed a 13.8% lower clearance of nevirapine than men. Because neither body weight nor body mass index (BMI) had an influence on the clearance of nevirapine, the effect of gender cannot solely be explained by body size.

Contraindications

Moderate or severe (Child-Pugh class B or C, respectively) hepatic impairment; for use as part of occupational and nonoccupational postexposure prophylaxis regimens.

Warnings/Precautions

➤*Hepatotoxicity:* Severe, life-threatening, and, in some cases, fatal hepatotoxicity, including fulminant and cholestatic hepatitis, hepatic necrosis, and hepatic failure, have been reported in patients treated with nevirapine. In controlled clinical trials, symptomatic hepatic reactions (regardless of severity) occurred in 4% (range, 0% to 11%) of patients who received nevirapine and 1.2% of patients in control groups.

The risk of symptomatic hepatic reactions regardless of severity was greatest in the first 6 weeks of therapy. The risk continued to be greater in the nevirapine groups compared with controls through 18 weeks of treatment. However, hepatic events may occur at any time during treatment. In some cases, patients presented with nonspecific, prodromal signs or symptoms of anorexia, fatigue, hepatomegaly, jaundice, liver tenderness, malaise, or nausea, with or without initially abnormal serum transaminase levels. Rash was observed in approximately half of the patients with symptomatic hepatic adverse reactions. Fever and flu-like symptoms accompanied some of these hepatic events. Some events, particularly those with rash and other symptoms, have progressed to hepatic failure with transaminase elevation, with or without hyperbilirubinemia, eosinophilia, hepatic encephalopathy, or prolonged partial thromboplastin time. Rhabdomyolysis has been observed in some patients experiencing skin and/or liver reactions associated with nevirapine use. Advise patients with signs or symptoms of hepatitis to discontinue nevirapine and immediately seek medical evaluation, including liver function tests.

If clinical hepatitis or transaminase elevations combined with rash or other systemic symptoms occur, permanently discontinue nevirapine. Do not restart nevirapine after recovery. In some cases, hepatic injury progresses despite discontinuation of treatment.

The patients at greatest risk of hepatic events, including potentially fatal events, are women with high CD4+ cell counts. In general, during the first 6 weeks of therapy, women have a 3-fold higher risk than men for symptomatic, often rash-associated, hepatic events (5.8% vs 2.2%), and patients with higher CD4+ cell counts at initiation of nevirapine therapy are at higher risk for symptomatic hepatic events with nevirapine. In a retrospective review, women with CD4+ cell counts higher than 250 cells/mm^3 had a 12-fold higher risk of symptomatic hepatic adverse events compared with women with CD4+ cell counts lower than 250 cells/mm^3 (11% vs 0.9%). An increased risk was observed in men with CD4+ cell counts higher than 400 cells/mm^3 (6.3% vs 1.2% for men with CD4+ cell counts lower than 400 cells/mm^3). However, monitor all patients regardless of gender, CD4+ cell count, or antiretroviral treatment history for hepatotoxicity because symptomatic hepatic adverse events have been reported at all CD4+ cell counts. Coinfection with hepatitis B or C and/or increased transaminase elevations at the start of therapy with nevirapine are associated with a greater risk of later symptomatic events (6 weeks or more after starting nevirapine) and asymptomatic increases in AST or ALT.

See Contraindications for more information.

➤*Skin reactions:* Severe and life-threatening skin reactions, including fatal cases, have been reported, occurring most frequently during the first 6 weeks of therapy. These have included cases of Stevens-Johnson syndrome, toxic epidermal necrolysis, and hypersensitivity reactions characterized by rash, constitutional findings, and organ dysfunction. Rhabdomyolysis has been observed in some patients experiencing skin and/or liver reactions associated with nevirapine use. In controlled clinical trials, grade 3 and 4 rashes were reported during the first 6 weeks in 1.5% of nevirapine recipients, compared with 0.1% of placebo subjects.

Patients developing signs or symptoms of severe skin reactions or hypersensitivity reactions (including, but not limited to, severe rash or rash accompanied by fever, general malaise, fatigue, muscle or joint aches, blisters, oral lesions, conjunctivitis, facial edema, and/or hepatitis, eosinophilia, granulocytopenia, lymphadenopathy, and renal dysfunction) must permanently discontinue nevirapine and seek medical evaluation immediately. Do not restart nevirapine following severe skin rash, skin rash combined with increased transaminases or other symptoms, or hypersensitivity reaction.

If patients present with a suspected nevirapine-associated rash, measure transaminases immediately. Permanently discontinue nevirapine in patients with rash-associated transaminase elevations.

Therapy with nevirapine must be initiated with a 14-day lead-in period of 200 mg/day (150 mg/m^2/day in children), which has been shown to reduce the frequency of rash. Discontinue nevirapine if a patient experiences severe rash or any rash accompanied by constitutional findings. A patient experiencing a mild to moderate rash without constitutional symptoms during the 14-day lead-in period of 200 mg/day (150 mg/m^2/day in children) should not have their nevirapine dose increased until the rash has resolved. The total duration of the once-daily lead-in dosing period should not exceed 28 days, at which point an alternative regimen should be sought. Closely monitor patients if isolated rash of any severity occurs. Delay in stopping nevirapine treatment after the onset of rash may result in a more serious reaction. Women appear to be at higher risk than men of developing rash with nevirapine.

➤*Resistance:* Do not use nevirapine as a single agent to treat HIV-1 or added on as a sole agent to a failing regimen. Resistant viruses emerge rapidly when nevirapine is administered as monotherapy. The choice of new antiretroviral agents to be used in combination with nevirapine should take into consideration the potential for cross-resistance. When discontinuing an antiretroviral regimen containing nevirapine, take the long half-life of nevirapine into account; if antiretrovirals with shorter half-lives than nevirapine are stopped concurrently, low plasma concentrations of nevirapine alone may persist for a week or longer, and virus resistance may subsequently develop.

➤*Immune reconstitution syndrome:* Immune reconstitution syndrome has been reported in patients treated with combination antiretroviral therapy, including nevirapine. During the initial phase of combination antiretroviral treatment, patients whose immune system responds may develop an inflammatory response to indolent or residual opportunistic infections (eg, *Mycobacterium avium* infection, cytomegalovirus, *Pneumocystis jirovecii* pneumonia, tuberculosis), which may necessitate further evaluation and treatment.

➤*Fat redistribution:* Redistribution/accumulation of body fat, including breast enlargement, cushingoid appearance, central obesity, dorsocervical fat enlargement (buffalo hump), facial wasting, and peripheral wasting, have been observed in patients receiving antiretroviral therapy. The mechanism and long-term consequences of these events are currently unknown. A causal relationship has not been established.

➤*Renal function impairment:* See Administration and Dosage for more information.

➤*Hepatic function impairment:* See Contraindications for more information.

➤*Pregnancy: Category B.* according to the manufacturer; *Category C* per Briggs' *Drugs in Pregnancy and Lactation.* Nevirapine readily crosses the placenta. However, there are no adequate and well-controlled studies in pregnant women. The antiretroviral pregnancy registry, which has been surveying pregnancy outcomes since January 1989, has not found an increased risk of birth defects following first trimester exposures to nevirapine. The prevalence of birth defects after any trimester exposure to nevirapine is comparable with the prevalence observed in the general population. Use nevirapine during pregnancy only if the potential benefit justifies the potential risk to the fetus.

No observable teratogenicity was detected in reproductive studies performed in pregnant rats and rabbits. The maternal and developmental no-observable-effect level dosages produced systemic exposures approximately equivalent to or approximately 50% higher in rats and rabbits, respectively, than those seen at the recommended daily human dose, based on AUC. In rats, decreased fetal body weights were observed because of administration of a maternally toxic dose (exposures approximately 50% higher than that seen at the recommended human clinical dose).

Severe hepatic events, including fatalities, have been reported in pregnant women receiving long-term nevirapine therapy as part of combination treatment of HIV-1 infection. Regardless of pregnancy status, do not initiate nevirapine in women with CD4+ cell counts greater than 250 cells/mm^3 unless the benefit outweighs the risk. It is unclear if pregnancy augments the risk observed in nonpregnant women.

In 2006, the updated US Department of Health and Human Services guidelines for the use of antiretroviral agents in HIV-1–infected patients continued the recommendation that therapy, with the exception of efavirenz, should be continued during pregnancy. If indicated, nevirapine should not be withheld in pregnancy because the expected benefit to the HIV-positive mother outweighs the unknown risk to the fetus. Updated guidelines for the use of antiretroviral drugs to reduce perinatal HIV-1 transmission also were released in 2006. Women receiving antiretroviral therapy during pregnancy should continue the therapy, but regardless of the regimen, zidovudine administration is recommended during the intrapartum period to prevent vertical transmission of HIV to the newborn.

Antiretroviral pregnancy registry – To monitor maternal-fetal outcomes of pregnant women exposed to nevirapine, an antiretroviral pregnancy registry has been established. Register patients by calling 1-800-258-4263.

➤*Lactation:* The CDC recommends that HIV-1–infected mothers not breast-feed their infants to avoid risking postnatal transmission of HIV-1. Nevirapine is excreted in breast milk with a median milk:maternal plasma ratio of 60.5% (range, 25.3% to 122.2%). Because of both the potential for HIV-1 transmission and the potential for serious adverse reactions in breast-feeding infants, instruct mothers not to breast-feed if they are receiving nevirapine. In developing countries, breast-feeding is undertaken despite the risk because there are no affordable milk substitutes available. Zidovudine, zidovudine plus lamivudine, and nevirapine have all been shown to reduce, but not eliminate, the risk of HIV-1 transmission during breast-feeding.

➤*Children:* See Administration and Dosage for more information.

See Adverse Reactions for more information.

➤*Elderly:* Use caution in dose selection for an elderly patient; dosing should reflect the greater frequency of decreased hepatic, renal, or cardiac function, and of concomitant disease or other drug therapy.

➤*Monitoring:* The first 18 weeks of therapy with nevirapine are a critical period during which intensive clinical and laboratory monitoring of patients is required to detect potentially life-threatening hepatic events and skin

NEVIRAPINE — ORAL

reactions. The optimal frequency of monitoring during this time period has not been established. Some experts recommend clinical and laboratory monitoring more often than once per month, and in particular, would include monitoring of liver enzyme test at baseline, prior to dose escalation, and at 2 weeks postdose escalation. After the initial 18-week period, continue frequent clinical and laboratory monitoring throughout nevirapine treatment. In some cases, hepatic injury has progressed despite discontinuation of treatment.

Perform liver function tests immediately if a patient experiences signs or symptoms suggestive of hepatitis and/or hypersensitivity reaction. Obtain liver function tests immediately for all patients who develop a rash in the first 18 weeks of treatment. Carefully monitor patients with hepatic fibrosis or cirrhosis for evidence of drug-induced toxicity.

Drug Interactions

➤*CYP-450 system:* Nevirapine is principally metabolized by the liver via the CYP-450 isoenzymes, 3A4 and 2B6. Nevirapine is known to be an inducer of these enzymes. As a result, drugs that are metabolized by these enzyme systems may have lower than expected plasma levels when coadministered with nevirapine.

Nevirapine Drug Interactions

Precipitant drug	Object drug[a]		Description
Fluconazole	Nevirapine	↑	Nevirapine concentrations may be increased. Use with caution and monitor for nevirapine-induced adverse reactions.
Rifamycins (eg, rifampin)	Nevirapine	↓	Nevirapine plasma concentrations may be reduced; therefore, do not use with rifampin. When treating tuberculosis, use rifabutin instead.
Nevirapine	Rifamycins (eg, rifampin, rifabutin)	↑	Rifabutin and its metabolite concentrations are moderately increased when coadministered with nevirapine. Use this combination with caution. Rifampin AUC also may increase slightly.
St. John's wort	Nevirapine	↓	Nevirapine concentrations may be substantially reduced because of increased hepatic metabolism, possibly leading to loss of virologic response to nevirapine and to the class of NNRTIs. Coadministration is not recommended.
Nevirapine	Antiarrhythmics (eg, amiodarone, disopyramide, lidocaine)	↓	Plasma concentrations of these antiarrhythmics may be decreased. Use with caution.
Nevirapine	Anticonvulsants (eg, carbamazepine, clonazepam, ethosuximide)	↓	Plasma concentrations of these anticonvulsants may be decreased. Use with caution.
Nevirapine	Cabazitaxel	↓	Cabazitaxel plasma concentrations may be decreased, reducing the pharmacologic effect. Avoid concurrent use.
Nevirapine	Calcium channel blockers (eg, diltiazem, nifedipine, verapamil)	↓	Plasma levels of these calcium channel blockers may be decreased. Use with caution.
Nevirapine	Cisapride[b]	↓	Plasma levels of cisapride may be decreased. Coadminister with caution.
Nevirapine	Clarithromycin	↑↓	Clarithromycin exposure may be decreased; however, the active metabolite's (14-OH clarithromycin) concentration may be increased. Consider an alternative to clarithromycin, such as azithromycin.
Nevirapine	Contraceptives, hormonal	↓	Estrogen and progestogen concentrations may be decreased. Reduced contraceptive efficacy may occur. An alternative nonhormonal or additional method of contraception is recommended.
Nevirapine	Cyclophosphamide	↓	Coadminister with caution. Plasma levels of cyclophosphamide may be decreased.
Nevirapine	Efavirenz	↓	Efavirenz plasma concentration may be decreased. In addition, coadministration has been associated with an increase in adverse reactions and no improvement in efficacy. Appropriate dose for this combination has not been established. Concurrent use is not recommended.
Nevirapine	Ergot alkaloids (eg, ergotamine)	↓	Plasma levels of the ergot alkaloids may be decreased. Coadminister with caution.
Nevirapine	Exemestane	↓	Exemestane plasma concentrations may be decreased, reducing the pharmacologic effect. Monitor the clinical response when nevirapine is started or stopped, and adjust the exemestane dose as needed.
Nevirapine	Immunosuppressants (eg, cyclosporine, sirolimus, tacrolimus)	↓	Plasma levels of immunosuppressants may be decreased. Coadminister with caution.
Nevirapine	Itraconazole, ketoconazole	↓	Itraconazole and ketoconazole plasma concentrations may be decreased, reducing the pharmacologic effect. Do not coadminister.
Nevirapine	Maraviroc	↑	Coadministration may increase plasma concentrations of maraviroc. Monitor the clinical response and adjust the dose of maraviroc as needed.
Nevirapine	Opioid analgesics (eg, fentanyl, methadone)	↓	Fentanyl and methadone levels may be decreased. Narcotic withdrawal syndrome has been reported. Monitor methadone-maintained patients for evidence of withdrawal when nevirapine is started, and adjust the methadone dose as needed.
Nevirapine	Protease inhibitors (eg, atazanavir, darunavir, fosamprenavir, indinavir, lopinavir, nelfinavir, ritonavir, saquinavir)	↑↓	Nevirapine may decrease plasma levels and clinical efficacy of protease inhibitors. An increase in indinavir and saquinavir dose may be required. See the lopinavir/ritonavir monograph for dosing recommendations when used with nevirapine. Do not coadminister nevirapine and atazanavir because atazanavir exposure is substantially decreased. Coadministration of nevirapine and fosamprenavir without ritonavir is not recommended. When combined with nevirapine, the appropriate doses of indinavir, nelfinavir, and saquinavir/ritonavir have not been established. An increase in the dosage of indinavir may be required. Coadministration with darunavir/ritonavir may increase plasma concentrations of darunavir/ritonavir.
Nevirapine	Tyrosine kinase receptor inhibitors (eg, lapatinib, nilotinib, pazopanib)	↓	Tyrosine kinase receptor inhibitor plasma concentrations may be decreased, reducing the pharmacologic effect. Avoid concurrent use.
Nevirapine	Warfarin	↑↓	Warfarin plasma concentrations may be increased or decreased with coadministration. Monitor coagulation parameters when starting or stopping nevirapine. Adjust the warfarin dose as needed.

NEVIRAPINE — ORAL

Nevirapine Drug Interactions			
Precipitant drug	Object drug[a]		Description
Nevirapine	Zidovudine	↓	Coadministration decreased zidovudine AUC and C_{max}[c] 28% and 30%, respectively. Monitor the clinical response and adjust the zidovudine dose as needed.

[a] ↑ = object drug increased; ↓ = object drug decreased; ↑↓ = object drug both increased and decreased.
[b] Available from the manufacturer on a limited-access protocol.
[c] C_{max} = maximal plasma concentration.

Adverse Reactions

➤*Serious adverse reactions:* The most serious adverse reactions associated with nevirapine are hepatitis/hepatic failure, hypersensitivity reactions, Stevens-Johnson syndrome, and toxic epidermal necrolysis. Hepatitis/hepatic failure may be isolated or associated with signs of hypersensitivity, which can include severe rash or rash accompanied by blisters, conjunctivitis, eosinophilia, facial edema, fatigue, fever, general malaise, granulocytopenia, lymphadenopathy, muscle or joint aches, oral lesions, or renal dysfunction.

➤*Adults:*

Dermatologic – The most common clinical toxicity of nevirapine is rash, which can be severe or life-threatening. Rash occurs most frequently within the first 6 weeks of therapy. Rashes are usually mild to moderate maculopapular erythematous cutaneous eruptions, with or without pruritus, located on the trunk, face, and extremities. In controlled clinical trials (trials 1037, 1038, 1046, and 1090), grade 1 and 2 rashes were reported in 13.3% of patients receiving nevirapine compared with 5.8% receiving placebo during the first 6 weeks of therapy. Grade 3 or 4 rashes were reported in 1.5% of nevirapine recipients compared with 0.1% of subjects receiving placebo. Women tend to be at higher risk for development of nevirapine-associated rash.

Hepatic – In controlled clinical trials, symptomatic hepatic events, regardless of severity, occurred in 4% (range, 0% to 11%) of patients who received nevirapine and 1.2% of patients in control groups. Female gender and higher CD4+ cell counts (higher than 250 cells/mm^3 in women and higher than 400 cells/mm^3 in men) place patients at increased risk of these events.

Asymptomatic transaminase elevations (ALT or AST greater than 5 times the upper limit of normal) were observed in 5.8% (range, 0% to 9.2%) of patients who received nevirapine and 5.5% of patients in control groups. Coinfection with hepatitis B or C and/or increased transaminase elevations at the start of therapy with nevirapine are associated with a greater risk of later symptomatic events (6 weeks or more after starting nevirapine) and asymptomatic increases in AST or ALT.

Adverse reactions (more than 2%) –

Nevirapine Moderate or Severe Adverse Reactions (> 2%)				
	Trial 1090[a]		Trials 1037, 1038, 1046[b]	
Adverse reaction	Nevirapine (n = 1121)	Placebo (n = 1128)	Nevirapine (n = 253)	Placebo (n = 203)
Median exposure	58 weeks	52 weeks	28 weeks	28 weeks
Any adverse reaction	14.5%	11.1%	31.6%	13.3%
CNS				
Fatigue	0.2%	0.3%	4.7%	3.9%
Headache	0.7%	0.4%	3.6%	0.5%
GI				
Abdominal pain	0.1%	0.4%	2%	0%
Diarrhea	0.2%	0.8%	2%	0.5%
Nausea	0.5%	1.1%	8.7%	3.9%
Lab test abnormalities				
ALT > 250 units/L	5.3%	4.4%	14%	4%
AST > 250 units/L	3.7%	2.5%	7.6%	1.5%
Bilirubin > 2.5 mg/dL	1.7%	2.2%	1.7%	1.5%
Hemoglobin < 8 g/dL	3.2%	4.1%	0%	0%
Platelets < 50,000/mm^3	1.3%	1%	0.4%	1.5%
Neutrophils < 750/mm^3	13.3%	13.5%	3.6%	1%
Miscellaneous				
Granulocytopenia	1.8%	2.8%	0.4%	0%
Myalgia	0.2%	0%	1.2%	2%
Rash	5.1%	1.8%	6.7%	1.5%

[a] Background therapy included lamivudine for all patients and combinations of NRTIs and protease inhibitors. Patients had CD4+ cell counts < 200 cells/mm^3.
[b] Background therapy included zidovudine and zidovudine plus didanosine; nevirapine monotherapy was administered in some patients. Patients had CD4+ cell counts of ≥ 200 cells/mm^3.

Lab test abnormalities – Liver function test abnormalities (AST, ALT, gamma-glutamyltransferase [GGT]) were observed more frequently in patients receiving nevirapine than in controls. Asymptomatic elevations in GGT occur frequently but are not a contraindication to continue nevirapine therapy in the absence of elevations in other liver function tests. Other laboratory abnormalities (eg, anemia, bilirubin, neutropenia, thrombocytopenia) were observed with similar frequencies in clinical trials comparing nevirapine and control regimens.

➤*Children:* The most frequently reported adverse reactions related to nevirapine in children were similar to those observed in adults, with the exception of granulocytopenia, which was more commonly observed in children receiving both zidovudine and nevirapine. Cases of allergic reaction, including 1 case of anaphylaxis, were also reported.

Rash (all causality) was reported in 21% of the patients, 3% of whom discontinued the drug because of rash. All 4 patients experienced the rash early in the course of therapy (less than 4 weeks) and resolved upon nevirapine discontinuation. Other clinically important adverse reactions (all causality) include neutropenia (8.9%), anemia (7.3%), and hepatotoxicity (2.4%).

➤*Postmarketing:*

CNS – Paresthesia, somnolence.

Hematologic – Anemia, eosinophilia, neutropenia. Anemia has been more commonly observed in children, although development of anemia due to concomitant medication cannot be ruled out.

Hepatic – Fulminant and cholestatic hepatitis, hepatic failure, hepatic necrosis, jaundice.

Hypersensitivity – Allergic reactions, including anaphylaxis, angioedema, bullous eruptions, ulcerative stomatitis, and urticaria; hypersensitivity syndrome and hypersensitivity reactions with rash associated with constitutional findings, such as blistering, conjunctivitis, facial edema, fatigue, fever, general malaise, muscle or joint aches, oral lesions, or significant hepatic abnormalities plus 1 or more of the following: eosinophilia, granulocytopenia, hepatitis, lymphadenopathy, and/or renal dysfunction.

Musculoskeletal – Arthralgia, rhabdomyolysis associated with skin and/or liver reactions.

Miscellaneous – Drug withdrawal, fever, redistribution/accumulation of body fat, vomiting.

Overdosage

➤*Symptoms:* Cases of nevirapine overdose at dosages ranging from 800 to 1,800 mg/day for up to 15 days have been reported. Patients have experienced reactions including edema, erythema nodosum, fatigue, fever, headache, insomnia, nausea, pulmonary infiltrates, rash, vertigo, vomiting, and weight decrease.

Patient Information

Inform patients of the possibility of severe liver disease or skin reactions associated with nevirapine that may result in death. Instruct patients developing signs or symptoms of liver disease or severe skin reactions to discontinue nevirapine and seek medical attention immediately, including laboratory monitoring. Symptoms of liver disease include acholic stools, anorexia, fatigue, hepatomegaly, jaundice, liver tenderness, malaise, or nausea. Symptoms of severe skin or hypersensitivity reactions include rash accompanied by blisters, conjunctivitis, facial edema, fatigue, fever, general malaise, hepatitis, muscle or joint aches, and/or oral lesions.

Intensive clinical and laboratory monitoring, including liver enzymes, is essential during the first 18 weeks of therapy with nevirapine to detect potentially life-threatening hepatotoxicity and skin reactions. However, liver disease can occur after this period; therefore, continue monitoring at frequent intervals throughout nevirapine treatment. Extra vigilance is warranted during the first 6 weeks of therapy, which is the period of greatest risk of hepatic and skin reactions. Advise patients with signs and symptoms of hepatitis to discontinue nevirapine and seek medical evaluation immediately. If nevirapine is discontinued because of hepatotoxicity, do not restart it. Patients, particularly women, with increased CD4+ cell counts at initiation of nevirapine therapy (higher than 250 cells/mm^3 in women and higher than 400 cells/mm^3 in men) are at substantially higher risk for development of symptomatic hepatic events, often associated with rash. Advise patients that coinfection with hepatitis B or C and/or increased transaminases at the start of antiretroviral therapy are associated with a greater risk of later symptomatic events (6 weeks or more after starting nevirapine) and asymptomatic increases in AST or ALT.

The majority of rashes associated with nevirapine occur within the first 6 weeks of initiation of therapy. If any rash occurs during the 2-week lead-in period, do not escalate the nevirapine dose until the rash resolves. The total duration of the once-daily lead-in dosing period should not exceed 28 days, at which point an alternative regimen may need to be started. Instruct any patient experiencing a rash to have their liver enzymes (AST, ALT) evaluated immediately. Advise any patient experiencing severe rash or hypersensitivity reactions to discontinue nevirapine immediately and consult a health care provider. Do not restart nevirapine following severe skin rash or hypersensitivity reaction. Women tend to be at higher risk for development of nevirapine-associated rash.

Instruct women not to use hormonal methods of birth control, other than depot medroxyprogesterone acetate (DMPA), as their sole method of contraception because nevirapine may lower the plasma levels of these medications. Additionally, when oral contraceptives are used for hormonal regulation during nevirapine therapy, monitor the therapeutic effect of the hormonal therapy.

NEVIRAPINE — ORAL

Inform patients that nevirapine therapy has not been shown to reduce the risk of transmission of HIV-1 to others through sexual contact or blood contamination. The long-term effects of nevirapine are unknown at this time.

Nevirapine is not a cure for HIV-1 infection; patients may continue to experience illnesses associated with advanced HIV-1 infection, including opportunistic infections. Advise patients to remain under the care of their health care provider when using nevirapine.

Instruct patients to take nevirapine every day as prescribed. Instruct patients to not alter the dose without consulting their health care provider.

If a dose is missed, advise patients to take the next dose as soon as possible. However, if a dose is skipped, instruct patients not to double the next dose. Advise patients to report to their health care provider the use of any other medications.

Nevirapine may interact with some drugs; therefore, advise patients to report to their health care provider the use of any other prescription or nonprescription medication or herbal products, particularly St. John's wort.

Inform patients that redistribution or accumulation of body fat may occur in patients receiving antiretroviral therapy and that the cause and long-term health effects of these conditions are not known at this time.

DELAVIRDINE MESYLATE

Rx	**Rescriptor** (Agouron)	**Tablets:** 100 mg	Lactose. (U 3761). White, capsule shape. In 360s.
		200 mg	Lactose. (RESCRIPTOR 200 mg). White, capsule shape. In 180s.

DELAVIRDINE MESYLATE — ORAL

WARNING

Delavirdine tablets are indicated for the treatment of HIV-1 infection in combination with appropriate antiretroviral agents when therapy is warranted. This indication is based on surrogate marker changes in clinical studies. Clinical benefit was not demonstrated for delavirdine based on survival or incidence of AIDS-defining clinical events in a completed trial comparing delavirdine plus didanosine with didanosine monotherapy.

Resistant virus emerges rapidly when delavirdine is administered as monotherapy. Therefore, always administer delavirdine in combination with appropriate antiretroviral therapy.

Indications

➤*HIV infection:* For the treatment of HIV-1 (human immunodeficiency virus type 1infection) in combination with at least 2 other active antiretroviral agents when therapy is warranted.

Administration and Dosage

➤*Adults:*

HIV infection – 400 mg 3 times daily.

➤*Children:*

HIV infection –

16 years of age and older: 400 mg 3 times daily.

➤*Concomitant therapy:* Patients taking both delavirdine and antacids should be advised to take them at least 1 hour apart.

➤*Administration:* Delavirdine tablets may be administered with or without food. Patients with achlorhydria should take delavirdine with an acidic beverage (eg, orange or cranberry juice). However, the effect of an acidic beverage on the absorption of delavirdine in patients with achlorhydria has not been investigated.

The delavirdine 100 mg tablets may be dispersed in water prior to consumption. To prepare a dispersion, add 4 delavirdine 100 mg tablets to at least 3 ounces of water; allow the dispersion to stand for a few minutes and then stir until a uniform dispersion occurs. The dispersion should be consumed promptly. The glass should be rinsed with water and the rinse swallowed to ensure the entire dose is consumed. The 200 mg tablets should be taken as intact tablets because they are not readily dispersed in water. Note: The 200 mg tablets are approximately one-third smaller in size than the 100 mg tablets.

➤*Storage/Stability:* Store at 20° to 25°C (68° to 77°F). Keep container tightly closed. Protect from high humidity.

Actions

➤*Pharmacokinetics:*

Absorption – Delavirdine is rapidly absorbed following oral administration, with peak plasma concentrations occurring at approximately 1 hour. Following administration of delavirdine 400 mg 3 times a day (n = 67, HIV-1-infected patients), the mean ± SD steady-state peak plasma concentration (C_{max}) was 35 ± 20 mcM (range, 2 to 100 mcM), systemic exposure (AUC) was 180 ± 100 mcM•hr (range, 5 to 515 mcM•hr) and trough concentration (C_{min}) was 15 ± 10 mcM (range, 0.1 to 45 mcM). The single-dose bioavailability of delavirdine tablets relative to an oral solution was 85 ± 25% (n = 16, non-HIV-infected subjects). The single-dose bioavailability of delavirdine tablets (100 mg strength) was increased by approximately 20% when a slurry of drug was prepared by allowing delavirdine tablets to disintegrate in water before administration (n = 16, non-HIV-infected subjects). The bioavailability of the 200 mg strength delavirdine tablets has not been evaluated when administered as a slurry, because they are not readily dispersed in water (see Administration and Dosage).

Effect of food: Delavirdine may be administered with or without food. In a multiple-dose study, delavirdine was administered every 8 hours with food or every 8 hours, 1 hour before or 2 hours after a meal (n = 13, HIV-1-infected patients). Patients remained on their typical diet throughout the study; meal content was not standardized. When multiple doses of delavirdine were administered with food, mean C_{max} was reduced by 22% but AUC and C_{min} were not altered.

Distribution – Delavirdine is extensively bound (approximately 98%) to plasma proteins, primarily albumin. The percentage of delavirdine that is protein bound is constant over a delavirdine concentration range of 0.5 to 196 mcM. In 5 HIV-1-infected patients whose total daily dose of delavirdine ranged from 600 to 1200 mg, cerebrospinal fluid concentrations of delavirdine averaged 0.4% ± 0.07% of the corresponding plasma delavirdine concentrations; this represents about 20% of the fraction not bound to plasma proteins. Steady-state delavirdine concentrations in saliva (n = 5, HIV-1-infected patients who received delavirdine 400 mg 3 times a day) and semen (n = 5 healthy volunteers who received delavirdine 300 mg 3 times a day) were about 6% and 2%, respectively, of the corresponding plasma delavirdine concentrations collected at the end of a dosing interval.

Metabolism/Excretion – Delavirdine is extensively converted to several inactive metabolites. Delavirdine is primarily metabolized by cytochrome P450 3A (CYP3A), but in vitro data suggest that delavirdine may also be metabolized by CYP2D6. The major metabolic pathways for delavirdine are N-desalkylation and pyridine hydroxylation. Delavirdine exhibits nonlinear steady-state elimination pharmacokinetics, with apparent oral clearance decreasing by about 22-fold as the total daily dose of delavirdine increases from 60 to 1200 mg/day. In a study of ^{14}C-delavirdine in 6 healthy volunteers who received multiple doses of delavirdine tablets 300 mg 3 times a day, approximately 44% of the radiolabeled dose was recovered in feces, and approximately 51% of the dose was excreted in urine. Less than 5% of the dose was recovered unchanged in urine. The apparent plasma half-life of delavirdine increases with dose; mean half-life following 400 mg 3 times a day is 5.8 hours, with a range of 2 to 11 hours.

In vitro and in vivo studies have shown that delavirdine reduces CYP3A activity and inhibits its own metabolism. In vitro studies have also shown that delavirdine reduces CYP2C9, CYP2D6, and CYP2C19 activity. Inhibition of CYP3A by delavirdine is reversible within 1 week after discontinuation of drug.

➤*Microbiology:* Delavirdine is a non-nucleoside reverse transcriptase inhibitor (NNRTI) of HIV-1. Delavirdine binds directly to reverse transcriptase (RT) and blocks RNA-dependent and DNA-dependent DNA polymerase activities. Delavirdine does not compete with template: primer or deoxynucleoside triphosphates. HIV-2 RT and human cellular DNA polymerases α, γ, or δ are not inhibited by delavirdine. In addition, HIV-1 group O, a group of highly divergent strains that are uncommon in North America, may not be inhibited by delavirdine.

In vitro HIV-1 susceptibility – In vitro anti-HIV-1 activity of delavirdine was assessed by infecting cell lines of lymphoblastic and monocytic origin and peripheral blood lymphocytes with laboratory and clinical isolates of HIV-1. IC_{50} and IC_{90} values (50% and 90% inhibitory concentrations) for laboratory isolates (n = 5) ranged from 0.005 to 0.03 mcM and 0.04 to 0.1 mcM, respectively. Mean IC_{50} of clinical isolates (n = 74) was 0.038 mcM (range, 0.001 to 0.69 mcM); 73 of 74 clinical isolates had an $IC_{50} \le 0.18$ mcM. The IC_{90} of 24 of these clinical isolates ranged from 0.05 to 0.1 mcM. In drug combination studies of delavirdine with zidovudine, didanosine, zalcitabine, lamivudine, interferon-α, and protease inhibitors, additive to synergistic anti-HIV-1 activity was observed in cell culture. The relationship between the in vitro susceptibility of HIV-1 RT inhibitors and the inhibition of HIV replication in humans has not been established.

Drug resistance – Phenotypic analyses of isolates from patients treated with delavirdine as monotherapy showed a 50-fold to 500-fold reduction in sensitivity in 14 of 15 patients by week 8 of therapy. Genotypic analyses of HIV-1 isolates from patients receiving delavirdine plus zidovudine combination therapy (n = 79) showed resistance conferring mutations in all isolates by week 24 of therapy. In delavirdine treated patients the mutations in RT occurred predominantly at amino acid positions 103 and less frequently at positions 181 and 236. In a separate study, an average 86-fold increase in the zidovudine susceptibility of patient isolates (n = 24) was observed after 24 weeks on delavirdine and zidovudine combination therapy. The clinical relevance of the phenotypic and the genotypic changes associated with delavirdine therapy has not been determined.

Cross-resistance – Delavirdine may confer cross-resistance to other NNRTIs when used alone or in combination. Mutations at positions 103 or 181 has been found in resistant virus during treatment with delavirdine and other NNRTIs. These mutations have been associated with cross-resistance among NNRTIs in vitro.

Contraindications

Hypersensitivity to delavirdine or any of its ingredients. Coadministration of delavirdine mesylate is contraindicated with drugs that are highly dependent on CYP3A for clearance and for which elevated plasma concentrations are associated with serious or life-threatening events.

DELAVIRDINE MESYLATE — ORAL

Drugs That are Contraindicated With Delavirdine Mesylate	
Drug class	Drugs within class that are contraindicated with delavirdine mesylate
Antihistamines	Astemizole, terfenadine
Ergot derivatives	Dihydroergotamine, ergonovine, ergotamine, methylergonovine
GI motility agent	Cisapride
Neuroleptic	Pimozide
Sedative/hypnotics	Alprazolam, midazolam, triazolam

Warnings/Precautions

➤*Cytochrome P-450 inhibition:* Coadministration of delavirdine mesylate with certain nonsedating antihistamines, sedative hypnotics, antiarrhythmics, calcium channel blockers, ergot alkaloid preparations, amphetamines, cisapride, and sildenafil, may result in potentially serious or life-threatening adverse events due to possible effects of delavirdine mesylate on the hepatic metabolism of certain drugs (see Drug Interactions).

➤*Resistance/cross-resistance:* Non-nucleoside reverse transcriptase inhibitors, when used alone or in combination, may confer cross-resistance to other nonnucleoside reverse transcriptase inhibitors.

➤*Fat redistribution:* Redistribution/accumulation of body fat including central obesity, dorsocervical fat enlargement (buffalo hump), peripheral wasting, facial wasting, breast enlargement, and "cushingoid appearance" have been observed in patients receiving antiretroviral therapy. The mechanism and long-term consequences of these events are currently unknown. A causal relationship has not been established.

➤*Skin rash:* Severe rash including rare cases of erythema multiforme and Stevens-Johnson syndrome have been reported in patients receiving delavirdine mesylate. Erythema multiforme and Stevens-Johnson syndrome were rarely seen in clinical trials and resolved after withdrawal of delavirdine mesylate. Any patient experiencing severe rash or rash accompanied by symptoms such as fever, blistering, oral lesions, conjunctivitis, swelling, muscle or joint aches should discontinue delavirdine mesylate and consult a physician. Two cases of Stevens-Johnsons syndrome have been reported through postmarketing surveillance out of a total of 339 surveillance reports.

In studies 21 part II and 13C, rash (including maculopapular rash) was reported in more patients who were treated with delavirdine mesylate 400 mg 3 times a day (35% and 32%, respectively) than in those who were not treated with delavirdine mesylate (21% and 16%, respectively). The highest intensity of rash reported in these studies was severe (grade 3), which was observed in approximately 4% of patients treated with delavirdine in each study and in none of the patients who were not treated with delavirdine mesylate. Also in studies 21 part II and 13C, discontinuations due to rash were reported in more patients who received delavirdine mesylate 400 mg 3 times a day (3% and 4%, respectively) than in those who did not receive delavirdine mesylate (0% and 1%, respectively).

In most cases, the duration of the rash was less than 2 weeks and did not require dose reduction or discontinuation of delavirdine mesylate. Most patients were able to resume therapy after rechallenge with delavirdine mesylate following a treatment interruption due to rash. The distribution of the rash was mainly on the upper body and proximal arms, with decreasing intensity of the lesions on the neck and face, and progressively less on the rest of the trunk and limbs. Occurrence of a delavirdine-associated rash after 1 month is uncommon. Symptomatic relief has been obtained using diphenhydramine hydrochloride, hydroxyzine hydrochloride, or topical corticosteroids.

➤*Hepatic function impairment:* Delavirdine is metabolized primarily by the liver. Therefore, caution should be exercised when administering delavirdine mesylate tablets to patients with impaired hepatic function.

➤*Pregnancy: Category C.* Delavirdine has been shown to be teratogenic in rats. Delavirdine caused ventricular septal defects in rats at doses of 50, 100, and 200 mg/kg/day when administered during the period of organogenesis. The lowest dose of delavirdine that caused malformations produced systemic exposures in pregnant rats equal to or lower than the expected human exposure to delavirdine mesylate (C_{min} 15 mcM) at the recommended dose. Exposure in rats approximately 5-fold higher than the expected human exposure resulted in marked maternal toxicity, embryotoxicity, fetal developmental delay, and reduced pup survival. Additionally, reduced pup survival on postpartum day 0 occurred at an exposure (mean C_{min}) approximately equal to the expected human exposure.

Delavirdine at doses of 200 and 400 mg/kg/day administered during the period of organogenesis caused maternal toxicity, embryotoxicity, and abortions in rabbits. The lowest dose of delavirdine that resulted in these toxic effects produced systemic exposures in pregnant rabbits approximately 6-fold higher than the expected human exposure to delavirdine mesylate (C_{min} 15 mcM) at the recommended dose. The no-observed-adverse-effect dose in the pregnant rabbit was 100 mg/kg/day. Various malformations were observed at this dose, but the incidence of such malformations was not statistically significantly different from those observed in the control group. Systemic exposures in pregnant rabbits at a dose of 100 mg/kg/day were lower than those expected in humans at the recommended clinical dose. Malformations were not apparent at 200 and 400 mg/kg/day; however, only a limited number of fetuses were available for examination as a result of maternal and embryo death.

No adequate and well-controlled studies in pregnant women have been conducted. Delavirdine mesylate should be used during pregnancy only if the potential benefit justifies the potential risk to the fetus. Of 9 pregnancies reported in premarketing clinical studies and postmarketing experience, a total of 10 infants were born (including 1 set of twins). Eight of the infants were born healthy. One infant was born HIV-positive but was otherwise healthy and with no congenital abnormalities detected, and 1 infant was born prematurely (34 to 35 weeks) with a small muscular ventricular septal defect that spontaneously resolved. The patient received approximately 6 weeks of treatment with delavirdine and zidovudine early in the course of the pregnancy.

Antiretroviral pregnancy registry – To monitor maternal-fetal outcomes of pregnant women exposed to delavirdine and other antiretroviral agents, an Antiretroviral Pregnancy Registry has been established. Physicians are encouraged to register patients by calling (800) 258–4263.

➤*Lactation:* Delavirdine was excreted in the milk of lactating rats at a concentration 3 to 5 times that of rat plasma.

The US public health services Centers for Disease Control and Prevention advises HIV-infected women not to breastfeed to avoid postnatal transmission of HIV. Because of both the potential for HIV transmission and any possible adverse reactions in nursing infants, mothers should be instructed not to breastfeed if they are receiving delavirdine.

➤*Children:* Safety and effectiveness of delavirdine in combination with other antiretroviral agents have not been established in HIV-1-infected individuals younger than 16 years of age.

➤*Elderly:* Clinical studies of delavirdine did not include sufficient numbers of subjects aged 65 and older to determine whether they respond differently from younger subjects. In general, caution should be taken when dosing delavirdine in elderly patients due to the greater frequency of decreased hepatic, renal or cardiac function and of concomitant disease or other drug therapy.

Drug Interactions

➤*Serious drug interactions:* Because delavirdine may inhibit the metabolism of many different drugs (eg, antiarrhythmics, calcium channel blockers, sedative hypnotics and others), serious or life-threatening drug interactions could result from inappropriate coadministration of some drugs with delavirdine. In addition, some drugs may markedly reduce delavirdine plasma concentrations, resulting suboptimal antiviral activity and subsequent emergence of drug resistance. All prescribers should become familiar with the data available in this section and in Contraindications, Warnings, and Pharmacokinetics.

➤*Cytochrome P-450 system:* Delavirdine is an inhibitor of CYP3A isoform and other CYP isoforms to a lesser extent including CYP2C9, CYP2D6, and CYP2C19. Coadministration of delavirdine and drugs primarily metabolized by CYP3A (eg, HMG-CoA reductase inhibitors and sildenafil) may result in increased plasma concentrations of the coadministered drug that could increase or prolong both its therapeutic or adverse effects.

Delavirdine is metabolized primarily by CYP3A, but in vitro data suggest that delavirdine may also be metabolized by CYP2D6. Coadministration of delavirdine and drugs that induce CYP3A, such as rifampin, may decrease delavirdine plasma concentrations and reduce its therapeutic effect. Coadministration of delavirdine and drugs that inhibit CYP3A may increase delavirdine plasma concentrations. See the following table:

Drugs That Should Not be Coadministered With Delavirdine Mesylate	
Drug class: drug name	Clinical comment
Anticonvulsant agents: phenytoin, phenobarbital, and carbamazepine	May lead to loss of virologic response and possible resistance to delavirdine or to the class of nonnucleoside reverse transcriptase inhibitors.
Antihistamines: astemizole and terfenadine	Contraindicated due to potential for serious or life-threatening reactions such as cardiac arrhythmias.
Antimycobacterials: rifabutin[a], rifampin[a]	May lead to loss of virologic response and possible resistance to delavirdine mesylate or to the class of nonnucleoside reverse transcriptase inhibitors or other coadministered antiviral agents.
Ergot derivatives: dihydroergotamine, ergonovine, ergotamine, methylergonovine	Contraindicated due to potential for serious or life-threatening reactions such as acute ergot toxicity characterized by peripheral vasospasm and ischemia of the extremities and other tissues.
GI motility agent: cisapride	Contraindicated due to potential for serious or life-threatening reactions such as cardiac arrhythmias.

DELAVIRDINE MESYLATE — ORAL

Drugs That Should Not be Coadministered With Delavirdine Mesylate

Drug class: drug name	Clinical comment
Herbal products: St. John's wort (*hypericum perforatum*)	May lead to loss of virologic response and possible resistance to delavirdine mesylate or to the class of nonnucleoside reverse transcriptase inhibitors.
HMG-CoA reductase inhibitors: lovastatin, simvastatin	Potential for serious reactions such as risk of myopathy including rhabdomyolysis.
Neuroleptic: pimozide	Contraindicated due to potential for serious or life-threatening reactions such as cardiac arrhythmias.
Sedative/hypnotics: alprazolam, midazolam, triazolam	Contraindicated due to potential for serious or life-threatening reactions such as prolonged or increased sedation or respiratory depression.

[a] See Pharmacokinetics for magnitude of interactions.

Delavirdine Drug Interactions

Precipitant drug	Object drug[a]		Description
Antacids	Delavirdine	↓	Separate administration by ≥ 1 hour because antacids may reduce absorption of delavirdine.
Anticonvulsants (eg, phenytoin, phenobarbital, carbamazepine)	Delavirdine	↓	Coadministration not recommended because anticonvulsants may decrease plasma delavirdine concentrations.
Clarithromycin	Delavirdine	↑	Clarithromycin may increase plasma delavirdine concentrations.
Didanosine	Delavirdine	↓	Coadministration reduces AUC of both drugs by 20%. Separate administration times by ≥ 1 hour.
Delavirdine	Didanosine		
Fluoxetine, ketoconazole	Delavirdine	↑	These drugs may increase trough plasma delavirdine concentrations by ≈ 50%.
H_2 receptor antagonists	Delavirdine	↓	H_2 antagonists increase gastric pH and may decrease absorption of delavirdine. Although the effect on delavirdine absorption is unknown, chronic use is not recommended.
Rifabutin, rifampin	Delavirdine	↓	Coadministration not recommended because plasma delavirdine concentrations may be decreased.
Saquinavir	Delavirdine	↓	Coadministration with saquinavir may decrease delavirdine AUC. Monitor ALT/AST closely when coadministering.
Delavirdine	Amprenavir	↑	Plasma concentrations of amprenavir may be increased.
Delavirdine	Benzodiazepines (eg, alprazolam, midazolam, triazolam)	↑	Alprazolam, midazolam, and triazolam plasma concentrations may be increased.
Delavirdine	Cisapride	↑	Plasma concentrations of cisapride may be increased.
Delavirdine	Clarithromycin, dapsone, rifabutin	↑	Rifabutin, clarithromycin, or dapsone plasma concentrations of may be increased.
Delavirdine	Dihydropyridine calcium channel blockers	↑	Delavirdine may increase plasma concentrations of nifedipine and other dihydropyridine calcium channel blockers.
Delavirdine	Ergot derivatives	↑	Coadministration is not recommended because of increased risk for ergot toxicity.
Delavirdine	Indinavir	↑	Delavirdine inhibits metabolism of indinavir. When coadministered, reduce indinavir dose to 600 mg 3 times daily.
Delavirdine	Quinidine	↑	Plasma concentrations of quinidine may be increased.
Delavirdine	Saquinavir	↑	Saquinavir AUC increased 5-fold when coadministered with delavirdine. Monitor ALT/AST closely when coadministered.
Delavirdine	Sildenafil	↑	Delavirdine may increase sildenafil plasma concentration. Do not exceed a single 25 mg dose of sildenafil in a 48-hour period.
Delavirdine	Warfarin	↑	Plasma concentrations of warfarin may be increased.

[a] ↑ = object drug increased; ↓ = object drug decreased. See Pharmacokinetics for magnitude of interaction.

Adverse Reactions

Patients with Treatment-Emergent Rash in Pivotal Trials (Studies 21 Part II and 13C)[a]

	Description of rash grade[b]	Delavirdine mesylate 400 mg 3 times a day (n = 412)	Control group patients (n = 295)
Grade 1 rash	Erythema, pruritus	69 (16.7%)	35 (11.9%)
Grade 2 rash	Diffuse maculopapular rash, dry desquamation	59 (14.3%)	17 (5.8%)
Grade 3 rash	Vesiculation, moist desquamation, ulceration	18 (4.4%)	0 (0%)
Grade 4 rash	Erythema multiforme, Stevens-Johnson syndrome, toxic epidermal necrolysis, necrosis requiring surgery, exfoliative dermatitis	0 (0%)	0 (0%)
Rash of any grade		146 (35.4%)	52 (17.6%)
Treatment discontinuation as a result of rash		13 (3.2%)	1 (0.3%)

[a] Includes events reported regardless of causality.
[b] ACTG toxicity grading system, includes events reported as "rash", "maculopapular rash", and "urticaria".

➤*Adverse events of moderate to severe intensity:*

Treatment-Emergent Events (Regardless of Causality) of Moderate to Severe or Life-Threatening Intensity Reported by Evaluable[a] Patients in Any Treatment Group (≥ 5%)

	Study 21 part II			Study 13C	
Adverse reactions	ZDV + 3TC (n = 123)	400 mg 3 times a day delavirdine mesylate + ZDV (n = 123)	400 mg 3 times a day delavirdine mesylate + ZDV + 3TC (n = 119)	ZDV + ddI, ddC or 3TC (n = 172)	400 mg 3 times a day delavirdine mesylate + ZDV + ddI, ddC or 3TC (n = 170)
CNS					
Anxiety	1.6% (2)	2.4% (3)	6.7% (8)	4.1% (7)	3.5% (6)
Depressive symptoms	6.5% (8)	4.9% (6)	12.6% (15)	3.5% (6)	5.9% (10)
Insomnia	4.9% (6)	4.9% (6)	5% (6)	2.9% (5)	1.2% (2)
Dermatologic					
Rashes	3.3% (4)	19.5% (24)	13.4% (16)	7.6% (13)	18.8% (32)
GI					
Diarrhea	8.1% (10)	2.4% (3)	4.2% (5)	8.1% (14)	5.9% (10)
Nausea	17.1% (21)	20.3% (25)	16.8% (20)	9.3% (16)	14.7% (25)
Vomiting	8.9% (11)	4.9% (6)	2.5% (3)	4.1% (7)	6.5% (11)
Respiratory					
Bronchitis	4.1% (5)	6.5% (8)	6.7% (8)	3.5% (6)	3.5% (6)
Cough	9.8% (12)	4.1% (5)	5% (6)	5.2% (9)	3.5% (6)
Pharyngitis	6.5% (8)	1.6% (2)	5% (6)	4.1% (7)	3.5% (6)
Sinusitis	8.9% (11)	7.3% (9)	5% (6)	2.3% (4)	1.2% (2)
Upper respiratory tract infection	11.4% (14)	6.5% (8)	7.6% (9)	8.7% (15)	4.7% (8)
Miscellaneous					
Abdominal pain generalized	2.4% (3)	3.3% (4)	5% (6)	1.7% (3)	2.4% (4)
Asthenia/fatigue	16.3% (20)	15.4 %(19)	16% (19)	8.1% (14)	5.3% (9)

DELAVIRDINE MESYLATE — ORAL

Treatment-Emergent Events (Regardless of Causality) of Moderate to Severe or Life-Threatening Intensity Reported by Evaluable[a] Patients in Any Treatment Group (≥ 5%)					
	Study 21 part II			Study 13C	
Adverse reactions	ZDV + 3TC (n = 123)	400 mg 3 times a day delavirdine mesylate + ZDV (n = 123)	400 mg 3 times a day delavirdine mesylate + ZDV + 3TC (n = 119)	ZDV + ddI, ddC or 3TC (n = 172)	400 mg 3 times a day delavirdine mesylate + ZDV + ddI, ddC or 3TC (n = 170)
Fever	2.4% (3)	1.6% (2)	3.4% (4)	6.4 %(11)	7.1% (12)
Flu syndrome	4.9% (6)	7.3% (9)	5% (6)	5.2% (9)	2.4% (4)
Headache	14.6% (18)	12.2% (15)	16.8% (20)	12.8% (22)	11.2% (19)
Localized pain	4.9% (6)	5.7% (7)	5% (6)	2.9% (5)	1.8% (3)

[a] Evaluable patients in Study 21 part II were those who received at least 1 dose of study medication and returned for at least 1 clinic visit. Evaluable patients in Study 13C were those who received at least 1 dose of study medication.

➤*Other adverse events:*

Cardiovascular – Abnormal cardiac rate and rhythm, cardiac insufficiency, cardiomyopathy, hypertension, migraine, pallor, peripheral vascular disorder, and postural hypotension.

CNS – Abnormal coordination, agitation, amnesia, change in dreams, cognitive impairment, confusion, decreased libido, disorientation, dizziness, emotional lability, euphoria, hallucination, hyperesthesia, hyperreflexia, hypertonia, hypesthesia, impaired concentration, manic symptoms, muscle cramp, nervousness, neuropathy, nystagmus, paralysis, paranoid symptoms, restlessness, sleep cycle disorder, somnolence, tingling, tremor, vertigo, and weakness.

Dermatologic – Angioedema, dermal leukocytoclastic vasculitis, dermatitis, desquamation, diaphoresis, discolored skin, dry skin, erythema, erythema multiforme, folliculitis, fungal dermatitis, hair loss, herpes zoster or simplex, nail disorder, petechiae, pruritus non-application site, seborrhea, skin hypertrophy, skin disorder, skin nodule, Stevens-Johnson syndrome, urticaria, vesiculobullous rash, and wart.

GI – Anorexia, bloody stool, colitis, constipation, decreased appetite, diarrhea (*Clostridium difficile*), diverticulitis, dry mouth, dyspepsia, dysphagia, enteritis at all levels, eructation, fecal incontinence, flatulence, gagging, gastroenteritis, gastroesophageal reflux, gastrointestinal bleeding, gastrointestinal disorder, gingivitis, gum hemorrhage, hepatomegaly, increased appetite, increased saliva, increased thirst, jaundice, mouth or tongue inflammation or ulcers, nonspecific hepatitis, oral/enteric moniliasis, pancreatitis, rectal disorder, sialadenitis, tooth abscess, and toothache.

GU – Amenorrhea, breast enlargement, calculi of the kidney, chromaturia, epididymitis, hematuria, hemospermia, urinary tract infection, impaired urination, impotence, kidney pain, metrorrhagia, nocturia, polyuria, proteinuria, testicular pain, and vaginal moniliasis.

Hematologic / Lymphatic – Adenopathy, bruising, eosinophilia, granulocytosis, leukopenia, pancytopenia, purpura, spleen disorder, and thrombocytopenia, and prolonged prothrombin time.

Metabolic / Nutritional – Alcohol intolerance, amylase increased, bilirubinemia, hyperglycemia, hyperkalemia, hypertriglyceridemia, hyperuricemia, hypocalcemia, hyponatremia, hypophosphatemia, increased AST, increased gamma glutamyl transpeptidase, increased lipase, increased serum alkaline phosphatase; increased serum creatine, and weight increase or decrease.

Musculoskeletal – Arthralgia or arthritis of single and multiple joints, bone disorder, bone pain, myalgia, tendon disorder, tenosynovitis, tetany, and vertigo.

Ophthalmic – Blepharitis, blurred vision, conjunctivitis, diplopia, dry eyes, and photophobia.

Respiratory – Chest congestion, dyspnea, epistaxis, hiccups, laryngismus, pneumonia, and rhinitis.

Special senses – Ear pain, parosmia, otitis media, taste perversion, and tinnitus.

Miscellaneous – Abdominal cramps, abdominal distention, abdominal pain (localized), abscess, allergic reaction, chills, edema (generalized or localized), epidermal cyst, fever, infection, infection viral, lip edema, malaise, *Mycobacterium tuberculosis* infection, neck rigidity, redistribution/accumulation of body fat (see Precautions, Fat redistribution, and sebaceous cyst.

➤*Postmarketing:*

Hepatic – Hepatic failure.

Hematologic / Lymphatic – Hemolytic anemia.

Musculoskeletal – Rhabdomyolysis.

Renal – Acute kidney failure.

➤*Lab test abnormalities:*

Marked Laboratory Abnormalities (≥ 2%)						
		Study 21 part II			Study 13C	
Lab abnormality	Toxicity limit	ZDV + 3TC (n = 123)	400 mg 3 times a day delavirdine mesylate + ZDV (n = 123)	400 mg 3 times a day delavirdine mesylate + ZDV + 3TC (n = 119)	ZDV + ddI, ddC or 3TC (n = 172)	400 mg 3 times a day delavirdine mesylate + ZDV + ddI, ddC or 3TC (n = 170)
Hematology						
Hemoglobin	< 7 mg/dL	4.1%	2.5%	0.9%	1.7%	2.9%
Neutrophils	< 750/mm³	5.7%	4.9%	3.4%	10.4%	7.6%
PT[a]	> 1.5 × ULN	0%	0%	1.7%	2.9%	2.4%
APTT[b]	> 2.33 × ULN	0%	0.8%	0%	5.8%	2.4%
Chemistry						
ALT[c]	> 5 × ULN	2.5%	4.1%	5.1%	3.5%	4.1%
Amylase	> 2 × ULN	0.8%	2.5%	2.6%	3.5%	2.9%
AST[d]	> 5 × ULN	1.6%	2.5%	3.4%	3.5%	2.3%
Bilirubin	> 2.5 × ULN	0.8%	2.5%	1.7%	1.2%	0%
GGT[e]	> 5 × ULN	N/A	N/A	N/A	4.1%	1.8%
Glucose[f]	< 40 mg/dL > 250 mg/dL	4.1%	0.8%	1.7%	1.2%	0%

[a] Prothrombin time.
[b] Activated partial thromboplastin.
[c] Alananine aminotransferase.
[d] Aspartate aminotransferase.
[e] Gamma glutamyl transferase.
[f] Hypo/hyperglycemia.
N/A = Not applicable because no predose values were obtained for patients.

Overdosage

➤*Treatment:* Human experience of acute overdose with delavirdine mesylate is limited.

Treatment of overdosage with delavirdine mesylate should consist of general supportive measures, including monitoring of vital signs and observation of the patient's clinical status. There is no specific antidote for overdosage with delavirdine mesylate. If indicated, elimination of unabsorbed drug should be achieved by emesis or gastric lavage. Since delavirdine is extensively metabolized by the liver and is highly protein bound, dialysis is unlikely to result in significant removal of the drug.

Patient Information

Patients should be informed that delavirdine mesylate is not a cure for HIV-1 infection and that they may continue to acquire illnesses associated with HIV-1 infection, including opportunistic infections. Treatment with delavirdine mesylate has not been shown to reduce the incidence or frequency of such illnesses, and patients should be advised to remain under the care of a physician when using delavirdine mesylate.

Patients should be advised that the use of delavirdine mesylate has not been shown to reduce the risk of transmission of HIV-1.

Patients should be instructed that the major toxicity of delavirdine mesylate is rash and should be advised to promptly notify their physician should rash occur. The majority of rashes associated with delavirdine mesylate occur within 1 to 3 weeks after initiating treatment with delavirdine mesylate. The rash normally resolves in 3 to 14 days and may be treated symptomatically while therapy with delavirdine mesylate is continued. Any patient experiencing severe rash or rash accompanied by symptoms such as fever, blistering, oral lesions, conjunctivitis, swelling, muscle or joint aches should discontinue medication and consult a physician.

Patients should be informed that redistribution or accumulation of body fat may occur in patients receiving antiretroviral therapy and that the cause and long-term health effects of these conditions are not known at this time.

Patients should be informed to take delavirdine mesylate every day as prescribed. Patients should not alter the dose of delavirdine mesylate without consulting their doctor. If a dose is missed, patients should take the next dose as soon as possible. However, if a dose is skipped, the patient should not double the next dose.

Patients with achlorhydria should take delavirdine mesylate with an acidic beverage (eg, orange or cranberry juice). However, the effect of an acidic beverage on the absorption of delavirdine in patients with achlorhydria has not been investigated.

Patients taking both delavirdine mesylate and antacids should be advised to take them at least 1 hour apart.

DELAVIRDINE MESYLATE — ORAL

Because delavirdine mesylate may interact with certain drugs, patients should be advised to report to their doctor the use of any prescription, nonprescription medication or herbal products, particularly St. John's wort.

Patients receiving sildenafil and delavirdine mesylate should be advised that they may be at an increased risk of sildenafil-associated adverse events, including hypotension, visual changes, and prolonged penile erection, and should promptly report any symptoms to their doctor.

EFAVIRENZ

Rx	**Sustiva** (Bristol-Myers Squibb)	**Capsules; oral:** 50 mg	Lactose. (SUSTIVA 50 mg). Gold/white. In 30s.
		200 mg	Lactose. (SUSTIVA 200 mg). Gold. In 90s.
		Tablets; oral: 600 mg	Lactose. (SUSTIVA). Yellow, capsule shape. Film-coated. In 30s.

EFAVIRENZ — ORAL

Indications

➤*HIV infection:* In combination with other antiretroviral agents for the treatment of HIV-1 infection.

Administration and Dosage

➤*Adults:*

HIV infection –

Usual dosage: 600 mg once daily at bedtime.

Concomitant therapy: If efavirenz is coadministered with voriconazole, the voriconazole maintenance dosage should be increased to 400 mg every 12 hours, and the efavirenz dosage should be decreased to 300 mg once daily using the capsule formulation (one 200 mg and two 50 mg capsules or six 50 mg capsules). Give in combination with a protease inhibitor and/or nucleoside analog reverse transcriptase inhibitors (NRTIs).

➤*Children:*

HIV infection –

3 years of age and older:

Efavirenz Dosing in Children 3 Years of Age and Older	
Body weight	Dosage
≥ 40 kg	600 mg at bedtime
32.5 to < 40 kg	400 mg at bedtime
25 to < 32.5 kg	350 mg at bedtime
20 to < 25 kg	300 mg at bedtime
15 to < 20 kg	250 mg at bedtime
10 to < 15 kg	200 mg at bedtime

Concomitant therapy – Give in combination with a protease inhibitor and/or NRTIs. Consider prophylaxis with antihistamines prior to initiating therapy to prevent rash.

➤*Administration:* Take on an empty stomach, preferably at bedtime. The increased efavirenz concentrations observed following administration of efavirenz with food may lead to an increase in the frequency of adverse reactions. Dosing at bedtime may improve the tolerability of nervous system symptoms.

Efavirenz tablets should not be broken.

➤*Storage/Stability:* Store at 25°C (77°F); excursions are permitted between 15° and 30°C (59° and 86°F).

Actions

➤*Pharmacology:* Efavirenz, an antiviral drug, is a non-NRTI (NNRTI) of HIV-1. Efavirenz activity is mediated predominantly by noncompetitive inhibition of HIV-1 reverse transcriptase (RT).

➤*Pharmacokinetics:*

Absorption – Peak efavirenz plasma concentrations of 1.6 to 9.1 mcM were attained by 5 hours following single oral doses of 100 to 1,600 mg administered to uninfected volunteers. Dose-related increases in maximal drug concentration (C_{max}) and area under the curve (AUC) were seen for doses of up to 1,600 mg; the increases were less than proportional, suggesting diminished absorption at higher doses.

In HIV-infected patients at steady state, mean C_{max}, mean minimal drug concentration (C_{min}), and mean AUC were dose-proportional following 200, 400, and 600 mg daily doses. Time-to-peak plasma concentrations were approximately 3 to 5 hours, and steady-state plasma concentrations were reached in 6 to 10 days. In 35 patients receiving efavirenz 600 mg once daily, steady-state C_{max} was 12.9 ± 3.7 mcM (mean ± standard deviation [SD]), steady-state C_{min} was 5.6 ± 3.2 mcM, and AUC was 184 ± 73 mcM•h.

Effect of food:

• *Capsules –* Administration of a single efavirenz 600 mg dose with a high-fat/high-caloric meal (894 kcal, 54 g of fat, 54% calories from fat) or a reduced-fat/normal-caloric meal (440 kcal, 2 g of fat, 4% calories from fat) was associated with a mean increase of 22% and 17% in efavirenz AUC_∞ and a mean increase of 39% and 51% in efavirenz C_{max}, respectively, relative to the exposures achieved when given under fasted conditions.

• *Tablets –* Administration of a single efavirenz 600 mg tablet with a high-fat/high-caloric meal (approximately 1,000 kcal, 500 to 600 kcal from fat) was associated with a 28% increase in mean AUC_∞ of efavirenz and a 79% increase in mean C_{max} of efavirenz relative to the exposures achieved under fasted conditions.

Distribution – Efavirenz is highly protein bound (approximately 99.5% to 99.75%) to human plasma proteins, predominantly albumin. In HIV-1–infected patients (n = 9) who received efavirenz 200 to 600 mg once daily for at least 1 month, cerebrospinal fluid concentrations ranged from 0.26% to 1.19% (mean, 0.69%) of the corresponding plasma concentration. This proportion is approximately 3-fold higher than the nonprotein-bound (free) fraction of efavirenz in plasma.

Metabolism – Studies in humans and in vitro studies using human liver microsomes have demonstrated that efavirenz is principally metabolized by the cytochrome P450 (CYP-450) system to hydroxylated metabolites, with subsequent glucuronidation of these hydroxylated metabolites. These metabolites are essentially inactive against HIV-1. The in vitro studies suggest that CYP3A4 and CYP2B6 are the major isozymes responsible for efavirenz metabolism.

Efavirenz has been shown to induce CYP-450 enzymes, resulting in the induction of its own metabolism. Multiple doses of 200 to 400 mg/day for 10 days resulted in a lower-than-predicted extent of accumulation (22% to 42% lower).

Excretion – Efavirenz has a terminal half-life of 52 to 76 hours after single doses and 40 to 55 hours after multiple doses. A 1-month mass balance/excretion study was conducted using 400 mg/day with a ^{14}C-labeled dose administered on day 8. Approximately 14% to 34% of the radiolabel was recovered in the urine, and 16% to 61% was recovered in the feces. Nearly all of the urinary excretion of the radiolabeled drug was in the form of metabolites. Efavirenz accounted for the majority of the total radioactivity measured in the feces.

Special populations –

➤*Microbiology:*

Antiviral activity in cell culture – The concentration of efavirenz inhibiting replication of wild-type laboratory-adapted strains and clinical isolates in cell culture by 90% to 95% (effective concentration $[EC]_{90-95}$) ranged from 1.7 to 25 nM in lymphoblastoid cell lines, peripheral blood mononuclear cells (PBMCs), and macrophage/monocyte cultures. Efavirenz demonstrated antiviral activity against most nonclade B isolates (subtypes A, AE, AG, C, D, F, G, J, N), but had reduced antiviral activity against group O viruses. Efavirenz demonstrated additive antiviral activity without cytotoxicity against HIV-1 in cell culture when combined with the NNRTIs delavirdine and nevirapine; NRTIs abacavir, didanosine, emtricitabine, lamivudine, stavudine, tenofovir, zalcitabine, and zidovudine; protease inhibitors amprenavir, indinavir, lopinavir, nelfinavir, ritonavir, and saquinavir; and the fusion inhibitor enfuvirtide. Efavirenz demonstrated additive to antagonistic antiviral activity in cell culture with atazanavir. Efavirenz was not antagonistic with adefovir, used for the treatment of hepatitis B virus (HBV) infection, or ribavirin, used in combination with interferon for the treatment of hepatitis C virus infection.

Contraindications

Coadministration with bepridil, cisapride, midazolam, pimozide, St. John's wort (*Hypericum perforatum*), triazolam, or ergot derivatives (eg, dihydroergotamine, ergonovine, ergotamine, methylergonovine); hypersensitivity (eg, Stevens-Johnson syndrome, erythema multiforme, or toxic skin eruptions) to efavirenz or any of its components.

Warnings/Precautions

➤*Resistance:* Efavirenz must not be used as a single agent to treat HIV-1 infection or added on as a sole agent to a failing regimen. Resistant virus emerges rapidly when efavirenz is administered as monotherapy. Consider the potential for viral cross-resistance when choosing new antiretroviral agents to be used in combination with efavirenz.

➤*Psychiatric effects:* Serious psychiatric adverse reactions have been reported in patients treated with efavirenz. In controlled trials of 1,008 patients treated with regimens containing efavirenz for a mean of 2.1 years and 635 patients treated with control regimens for a mean of 1.5 years, the frequency (regardless of causality) of specific serious psychiatric reactions among patients who received efavirenz or control regimens, respectively, were as follows: severe depression (2.4%, 0.9%), suicidal ideation (0.7%, 0.3%), nonfatal suicide attempts (0.5%, 0%), aggressive behavior (0.4%, 0.5%), paranoid reactions (0.4%, 0.3%), and manic reactions (0.2%, 0.3%). When psychiatric symptoms similar to those previously noted were combined and evaluated as a group in a multifactorial analysis of data from study 006, treatment with efavirenz was associated with an increase in the occurrence of these selected psychiatric symptoms. Other factors associated with an increase in the occurrence of these psychiatric symptoms were history of injection drug use, psychiatric history, and receipt of psychiatric medication at study entry; similar associations were observed in both the efavirenz and control treatment groups. In study 006, onset of new serious psychiatric symptoms occurred throughout the study for efavirenz- and control-treated patients. One percent of efavirenz-treated patients discontinued or interrupted treatment because of one or more of these selected psychiatric symptoms. There have also been occasional postmarketing reports of death by suicide, delusions, and psychosis-like behavior, although a causal relationship to the use of efavirenz cannot be determined from these reports. Urge patients with serious psychiatric adverse reactions to

EFAVIRENZ — ORAL

seek immediate medical evaluation to assess the possibility that the symptoms may be related to the use of efavirenz, and, if so, to determine whether the risks of continued therapy outweigh the benefits.

➤*CNS effects:* Fifty-three percent of patients receiving efavirenz in controlled trials reported CNS symptoms (any grade, regardless of causality) compared with 25% of patients receiving control regimens. These symptoms included, but were not limited to, dizziness (28.1%), insomnia (16.3%), impaired concentration (8.3%), somnolence (7%), abnormal dreams (6.2%), and hallucinations (1.2%). These symptoms were severe in 2% of patients, and 2.1% of patients discontinued therapy as a result. These symptoms usually begin during the first or second day of therapy and generally resolve after the first 2 to 4 weeks of therapy. After 4 weeks of therapy, the prevalence of nervous system symptoms of at least moderate severity ranged from 5% to 9% in patients treated with regimens containing efavirenz and from 3% to 5% in patients treated with a control regimen. Inform patients that these common symptoms were likely to improve with continued therapy and were not predictive of subsequent onset of the less frequent psychiatric symptoms. Dosing at bedtime may improve the tolerability of these nervous system symptoms.

Analysis of long-term data from study 006 (median follow-up, 180 weeks, 102 weeks, and 76 weeks for patients treated with efavirenz plus zidovudine plus lamivudine, efavirenz plus indinavir, and indinavir plus zidovudine plus lamivudine, respectively) showed that, beyond 24 weeks of therapy, the incidences of new-onset nervous system symptoms among efavirenz-treated patients were generally similar to those in the indinavir-containing control arm.

See Drug Interactions for more information.

➤*Dermatologic effects:* In controlled clinical trials, 26% of patients treated with efavirenz 600 mg experienced new-onset skin rash, compared with 17% of patients treated in control groups. Rash associated with blistering, moist desquamation, or ulceration occurred in 0.9% of patients treated with efavirenz. The incidence of grade 4 rash (eg, erythema multiforme, Stevens-Johnson syndrome) in patients treated with efavirenz in all studies and expanded access was 0.1%. Rashes are usually mild-to-moderate maculopapular skin eruptions that occur within the first 2 weeks of initiating therapy with efavirenz (the median time to onset of rash in adults was 11 days) and, in most patients continuing therapy with efavirenz, rash resolves within 1 month (median duration, 16 days). The discontinuation rate for rash in clinical trials was 1.7%. Efavirenz can be reinitiated in patients interrupting therapy because of rash. Discontinue efavirenz in patients developing severe rash associated with blistering, desquamation, mucosal involvement, or fever. Appropriate antihistamines and/or corticosteroids may improve the tolerability and hasten the resolution of rash.

Rash was reported in 46% of 57 children treated with efavirenz capsules. One child experienced grade 3 rash (confluent rash with fever), and 2 patients had grade 4 rash (erythema multiforme). The median time to onset of rash in children was 8 days. Consider prophylaxis with appropriate antihistamines prior to initiating therapy with efavirenz in children.

➤*Hepatotoxicity:* A few of the postmarketing reports of hepatic failure occurred in patients with no preexisting hepatic disease or other identifiable risk factors.

In patients with persistent elevations of serum transaminases to more than 5 times the upper limit of normal (ULN) range, the benefit of continued therapy with efavirenz needs to be weighed against the unknown risks of significant liver toxicity.

➤*Convulsions:* Convulsions have been observed in patients receiving efavirenz, generally in the presence of known medical history of seizures. Caution must be taken in any patient with a history of seizures. Patients who are receiving concomitant anticonvulsant medications primarily metabolized by the liver, such as phenytoin and phenobarbital, may require periodic monitoring of plasma levels.

➤*Lipid effects:* Treatment with efavirenz has resulted in increases in the concentration of total cholesterol and triglycerides.

➤*Immune reconstitution syndrome:* Immune reconstitution syndrome has been reported in patients treated with combination antiretroviral therapy, including efavirenz. During the initial phase of combination antiretroviral treatment, patients whose immune systems respond may develop an inflammatory response to indolent or residual opportunistic infections (eg, *Mycobacterium avium* infection, cytomegalovirus, *Pneumocystis jiroveci* pneumonia, tuberculosis), which may necessitate further evaluation and treatment.

➤*Fat redistribution:* Redistribution/accumulation of body fat, including central obesity, dorsocervical fat enlargement (buffalo hump), peripheral wasting, facial wasting, breast enlargement, and "cushingoid appearance," have been observed in patients receiving antiretroviral therapy. The mechanism and long-term consequences of these events are currently unknown. A causal relationship has not been established.

➤*Hepatic function impairment:* Because of the extensive CYP-450–mediated metabolism of efavirenz and limited clinical experience in patients with hepatic function impairment, exercise caution in administering efavirenz to these patients.

➤*Hazardous tasks:* Advise patients who experience CNS symptoms, such as dizziness, impaired concentration, and/or drowsiness, to avoid potentially hazardous tasks, such as driving or operating machinery.

➤*Pregnancy: Category D* (per manufacturer's prescribing information); *Category C* (per Briggs' *Drugs in Pregnancy and Lactation*). Efavirenz may cause fetal harm when administered during the first trimester to a pregnant woman. Advise women receiving efavirenz to avoid pregnancy. Advise patients to always use barrier contraception in combination with other methods of contraception (eg, oral, other hormonal contraceptives). Because of the long half-life of efavirenz, use of adequate contraceptive measures for 12 weeks after discontinuation of efavirenz is recommended. Ensure women of childbearing potential undergo pregnancy testing prior to initiation of efavirenz. If this drug is used during the first trimester of pregnancy, or if the patient becomes pregnant while taking this drug, apprise the patient of the potential harm to the fetus.

There are no adequate and well-controlled studies in pregnant women. It is not known if efavirenz crosses the human placenta to the fetus. The relatively low molecular weight (approximately 316) suggests that the drug is transferred to the fetus. Use efavirenz during pregnancy only if the potential benefit justifies the potential risk to the fetus, such as in pregnant women without other therapeutic options. As of July 2009, the Antiretroviral Pregnancy Registry has received prospective reports of 661 pregnancies exposed to efavirenz-containing regimens, nearly all of which were first-trimester exposures (606 pregnancies). Birth defects occurred in 14 of 501 live births (first-trimester exposure) and 2 of 55 live births (second/third-trimester exposure). One of these prospectively reported defects with first-trimester exposure was a neural tube defect. A single case of anophthalmia with first-trimester exposure to efavirenz has also been prospectively reported; however, this case included severe oblique facial clefts and amniotic banding, a known association with anophthalmia. There have been 6 retrospective reports of findings consistent with neural tube defects, including meningomyelocele. All mothers were exposed to efavirenz-containing regimens in the first trimester. Although a causal relationship of these events to the use of efavirenz has not been established, similar defects have been observed in preclinical studies of efavirenz.

Malformations have been observed in 3 of 20 fetuses/infants from efavirenz-treated cynomolgus monkeys (versus 0 of 20 concomitant controls) in a developmental toxicity study. The pregnant monkeys were dosed throughout pregnancy (postcoital days 20 to 150) with efavirenz 60 mg/kg daily, a dosage that resulted in plasma drug concentrations similar to those in humans given efavirenz 600 mg/day. Anencephaly and unilateral anophthalmia were observed in 1 fetus, micro-ophthalmia was observed in another fetus, and cleft palate was observed in a third fetus. Efavirenz crosses the placenta in cynomolgus monkeys and produces fetal blood concentrations similar to maternal blood concentrations.

Efavirenz crosses the placenta in rats and rabbits and produces fetal blood concentrations of efavirenz similar to maternal concentrations. An increase in fetal resorptions was observed in rats at efavirenz doses that produced peak plasma concentrations and AUC values in female rats equivalent to or lower than those achieved in humans given efavirenz 600 mg once daily.

Antiretroviral pregnancy registry – To monitor fetal outcomes of pregnant women exposed to efavirenz, an Antiretroviral Pregnancy Registry has been established. Health care providers are encouraged to register patients by calling 1-800-258-4263. The US Department of Health and Human Services guidelines for the use of antiretroviral agents in HIV-1–infected patients recommend continuation of therapy, with the exception of efavirenz, during pregnancy.

➤*Lactation:* The Centers for Disease Control and Prevention recommend that HIV-infected mothers not breast-feed their infants to avoid risking postnatal transmission of HIV. Although it is not known if efavirenz is secreted in human milk, efavirenz is secreted into the milk of lactating rats. The molecular weight of efavirenz (approximately 316) is low enough that excretion into breast milk should be expected. Because of the potential for HIV transmission and the potential for serious adverse reactions in breast-feeding infants, instruct mothers not to breast-feed if they are receiving efavirenz.

➤*Children:* ACTG 382 is an ongoing, open-label study in 57 NRTI-experienced children to characterize the safety, pharmacokinetics, and antiviral activity of efavirenz in combination with nelfinavir 20 to 30 mg/kg 3 times a day and NRTIs. Mean age was 8 years (range, 3 to 16 years).

➤*Elderly:* In general, use caution in dose selection for an elderly patient, reflecting the greater frequency of decreased hepatic, renal, or cardiac function, and of concomitant disease or other therapy.

➤*Monitoring:* Monitoring of liver enzymes before and during treatment is recommended for patients with underlying hepatic disease, including hepatitis B or C infection; patients with marked transaminase elevations; and patients treated with other medications associated with liver toxicity.

Consider monitoring liver enzymes for patients without preexisting hepatic dysfunction or other risk factors.

Perform cholesterol and triglyceride testing before initiating efavirenz therapy and at periodic intervals during therapy.

Drug Interactions

➤*CYP-450 system:* Efavirenz has been shown in vivo to induce CYP3A4. Other compounds that are substrates of CYP3A4 may have decreased plasma concentrations when coadministered with efavirenz. In vitro studies have demonstrated that efavirenz inhibits CYP2C9, CYP2C19, and CYP3A4 isozymes in the range of observed efavirenz plasma concentrations. Coadministration of efavirenz with drugs primarily metabolized by these isozymes may result in altered plasma concentrations of the coadministered drug. Therefore, appropriate dose adjustments may be necessary for these drugs. Drugs that induce CYP3A4 activity (eg, phenobarbital, rifampin, rifabutin) would be expected to increase the clearance of efavirenz, resulting in lowered plasma concentrations.

Non-Nucleoside Reverse Transcriptase Inhibitors

EFAVIRENZ — ORAL

Efavirenz Drug Interactions			
Precipitant drug	Object drug[a]		Description
Anticonvulsants (carbamazepine, phenobarbital, phenytoin)	Efavirenz	⬇	Potential for reduction in anticonvulsant and/or efavirenz plasma levels; periodically monitor anticonvulsant plasma levels and adjust the anticonvulsant dose as needed or administer an alternative anticonvulsant.
Efavirenz	Anticonvulsants (carbamazepine, phenobarbital, phenytoin)		
Azole antifungals (ie, voriconazole)	Efavirenz	⬆	Voriconazole may elevate efavirenz plasma concentrations, increasing the pharmacologic effects and risk of adverse reactions. Efavirenz has the potential to decrease plasma concentrations of azole antifungal agents. Coadministration of efavirenz and voriconazole is contraindicated at standard doses. Efavirenz significantly decreases voriconazole plasma concentrations and may decrease therapeutic effectiveness. Consider use of an alternative antifungal agent. If efavirenz is coadministered with voriconazole, the voriconazole maintenance dosage should be increased to 400 mg every 12 hours, and the efavirenz dosage should be decreased to 300 mg once daily using the capsule formulation.
Efavirenz	Azole antifungals (ie, itraconazole, ketoconazole, posaconazole, voriconazole)	⬇	
Nevirapine	Efavirenz	⬇⬆	Efavirenz plasma concentrations and clinical efficacy may be reduced. However, the risk of adverse reactions may be increased. Coadministration is not recommended.
Rifabutin Rifampin	Efavirenz	⬇	Rifabutin and rifampin would be expected to increase the clearance of efavirenz caused by CYP3A4 induction. Coadministration also may decrease rifabutin concentration. Increase daily dose of rifabutin by 50%. Consider doubling the rifabutin dose when rifabutin is given 2 to 3 times per week.
Efavirenz	Rifabutin Rifampin		
Ritonavir	Efavirenz	⬆	With concurrent use, the concentration for each drug was increased. This combination was associated with a higher frequency of adverse reactions (eg, dizziness, nausea, paresthesia) and laboratory abnormalities (elevated liver enzymes). Monitoring of liver enzymes is recommended.
Efavirenz	Ritonavir		
St. John's wort (*Hypericum perforatum*)	Efavirenz	⬇	Concomitant use may lead to loss of efavirenz virologic response and possible resistance to efavirenz or the class of NNRTIs. Coadministration is not recommended.
Efavirenz	Amprenavir,[b] fosamprenavir	⬇	Efavirenz has the potential to decrease serum concentrations of amprenavir. Appropriate doses of unboosted fosamprenavir and efavirenz with respect to safety and efficacy have not been established. Add 100 mg (300 mg total) of ritonavir with coadministration of fosamprenavir/ritonavir once daily. No additional dose required with twice daily regimen.
Efavirenz	Atazanavir	⬇	Atazanavir plasma concentrations and clinical efficacy may be reduced. When coadministered with efavirenz in treatment-naive patients, the recommended dosage of atazanavir is 400 mg with ritonavir 100 mg once daily and efavirenz 600 mg once daily. In treatment-experienced patients, coadministration of efavirenz and atazanavir is not recommended.
Efavirenz	Cabazitaxel	⬇	Cabazitaxel plasma concentrations and clinical efficacy may be reduced. Avoid concurrent use.
Efavirenz	Calcium channel blockers (eg, diltiazem, felodipine, nicardipine, nifedipine, verapamil)	⬇	Coadministration may reduce diltiazem plasma concentrations. The potential exists for reduction in plasma concentrations for other calcium channel blockers. Guide dose adjustments by clinical response.
Efavirenz	Clarithromycin	⬌	Clarithromycin plasma levels decreased while clarithromycin hydroxymetabolite levels increased. The clinical significance of these changes is unknown. No dose adjustment of efavirenz is recommended. Consider alternatives to clarithromycin, such as azithromycin. Other macrolide antibiotics have not been studied.
Efavirenz	CYP-450 3A4 inhibitors (eg, astemizole, bepridil, cisapride[c], dihydroergotamine, ergonovine, ergotamine, ergot derivatives, methylergotamine, midazolam, pimozide, triazolam)	⬆	Contraindicated; do not coadminister. Competition for CYP3A4 by efavirenz could result in serious or life-threatening adverse reactions (eg, acute ergot toxicity, cardiac arrhythmias, prolonged or increased sedation, respiratory depression).
Efavirenz	HMG-CoA reductase inhibitors (eg, atorvastatin, pravastatin, simvastatin)	⬇	Coadministration decreased plasma concentrations of atorvastatin, pravastatin, and simvastatin. Monitor LDL[d] concentrations after starting efavirenz.
Efavirenz	Hormonal contraceptives (eg, etonogestrel, levonorgestrel, norgestimate)	⬇	Efavirenz does not affect ethinyl estradiol concentrations, but progestin concentrations are markedly decreased. A reliable method of barrier contraception must be used in addition to hormonal contraception.
Efavirenz	Immunosuppressants (eg, cyclosporine, sirolimus, tacrolimus)	⬇	Decreased exposure of immunosuppressants metabolized by CYP3A4 may be expected. Closely monitor immunosuppressant concentrations for at least 2 weeks when starting or stopping efavirenz.
Efavirenz	Indinavir	⬇	Indinavir plasma concentrations and clinical efficacy may be decreased. The optimal dose of indinavir when administered in combination with efavirenz is not known.
Efavirenz	Ixabepilone	⬇	Ixabepilone plasma concentrations and clinical efficacy may be reduced. Avoid concurrent use.

EFAVIRENZ — ORAL

Efavirenz Drug Interactions			
Precipitant drug	Object drug[a]		Description
Efavirenz	Lopinavir	↓	Lopinavir plasma concentrations and clinical efficacy may be decreased. Lopinavir/ritonavir should not be administered once daily with efavirenz. A dose increase in lopinavir/ritonavir may be considered when used concurrently with efavirenz in treatment experienced patients.
Efavirenz	Maraviroc	↓	Maraviroc plasma concentrations and clinical efficacy may be decreased. A dosage adjustment of maraviroc may be required if maraviroc is coadministered with efavirenz. Consult full maraviroc prescribing information. Coadministration of maraviroc and efavirenz is contraindicated in patients with severe renal impairment (CrCl 30 mL/min).
Efavirenz	Methadone	↓	Coadministration decreased methadone AUC and C_{max}. Monitor for withdrawal symptoms and increase methadone dose as needed.
Efavirenz	Saquinavir	↓	Saquinavir plasma concentrations and clinical efficacy may be decreased. Saquinavir should not be used as the sole protease inhibitor in combination with efavirenz.
Efavirenz	Sertraline	↓	The AUC and C_{max} of sertraline may be decreased. Guide an increase in sertraline dose by clinical response.
Efavirenz	Warfarin	↑↓	Plasma concentrations and effects potentially increased or decreased by efavirenz. Monitor coagulation parameters and adjust the warfarin dose as needed.

[a] ↑ = object drug increased; ↓ = object drug decreased; ↔ = undetermined clinical effect; ↑↓ = object drug both increased and decreased.
[b] Not currently marketed in the United States.
[c] Available from the manufacturer on a limited-access protocol.
[d] LDL = low-density lipoprotein.

➤*Drug/Lab test interactions:* Efavirenz does not bind to cannabinoid receptors. False-positive urine cannabinoid test results have been observed in non–HIV-infected volunteers receiving efavirenz when the Microgenics *Cedia* DAU Multi-Level THC assay was used for screening. Negative results were obtained when more specific confirmatory testing was performed with gas chromatography/mass spectrometry.

➤*Drug/Food interactions:* Food increases efavirenz concentrations and may increase the frequency of adverse reactions. Efavirenz should be taken on an empty stomach.

Adverse Reactions

➤*Significant adverse reactions:* Adverse reactions observed in patients treated with efavirenz are nervous system symptoms, psychiatric symptoms, and rash.

➤*Most common adverse reactions (more than 5%):* The most common (greater than 5% in either efavirenz treatment group) adverse reactions of at least moderate severity among patients in study 006 treated with efavirenz in combination with zidovudine/lamivudine or indinavir were rash, dizziness, nausea, headache, fatigue, insomnia, and vomiting.

➤*Adults:*

Efavirenz Adverse Reactions in Adults (≥ 2%)[a]						
	Study 006 lamivudine-, NNRTI-, and protease inhibitor–naive patients			Study ACTG 364 NRTI-experienced, NNRTI-naive, and protease inhibitor–naive patients		
Adverse reactions	Efavirenz[b] + zidovudine + lamivudine (n = 412) 180 weeks[c]	Efavirenz[b] + indinavir (n = 415) 102 weeks[c]	Indinavir + zidovudine + lamivudine (n = 401) 76 weeks[c]	Efavirenz[b] + nelfinavir + NRTIs (n = 64) 71.1 weeks[c]	Efavirenz[b] + NRTIs (n = 65) 70.9 weeks[c]	Nelfinavir + NRTIs (n = 66) 62.7 weeks[c]
CNS						
Abnormal dreams	3%	1%	0%	—[d]	—	—
Anxiety	2%	4%	< 1%	—	—	—
Concentration impaired	5%	3%	< 1%	0%	0%	0%
Depression	5%	4%	< 1%	3%	0%	5%
Dizziness	9%	9%	2%	2%	6%	6%
Fatigue	8%	5%	9%	0%	2%	3%
Headache	8%	5%	3%	5%	2%	3%
Insomnia	7%	7%	2%	0%	0%	2%
Nervousness	2%	2%	0%	2%	0%	2%
Somnolence	2%	2%	< 1%	0%	0%	0%
Dermatologic						
Pruritus	< 1%	1%	1%	9%	5%	9%
Rash[d]	11%	16%	5%	9%	5%	9%
GI						
Abdominal pain	2%	2%	5%	3%	3%	3%
Anorexia	1%	< 1%	< 1%	0%	2%	2%
Diarrhea	3%	5%	6%	14%	3%	9%
Dyspepsia	4%	4%	6%	0%	0%	2%
Nausea	10%	6%	24%	3%	2%	2%
Vomiting	6%	3%	14%	—	—	—
Miscellaneous						
Pain	1%	2%	8%	13%	6%	17%

[a] Includes adverse reactions at least possibly related to study drug or of unknown relationship for study 006. Includes all adverse reactions regardless of relationship to study drug for study ACTG 364.
[b] Efavirenz provided as 600 mg once daily.
[c] Median duration of treatment.
[d] — = not specified.
[e] Includes erythema multiforme, rash, rash erythematous, rash follicular, rash maculopapular, rash petechial, rash pustular, and urticaria for study 006 and macules, papules, rash, erythema, redness, inflammation, allergic rash, urticaria, welts, hives, itchy, and pruritus for ACTG 3564.

EFAVIRENZ — ORAL

Pancreatitis – Pancreatitis has been reported, although a causal relationship with efavirenz has not been established. Asymptomatic increases in serum amylase levels were observed in a significantly higher number of patients treated with efavirenz 600 mg than in control patients.

CNS adverse reactions –

Efavirenz Nervous System Adverse Reactions[a,b]

Symptom description	Efavirenz 600 mg once daily (n = 1,008)	Control groups (n = 635)
Symptoms of any severity	52.7%	24.6%
Mild symptoms[c]	33.3%	15.6%
Moderate symptoms[d]	17.4%	7.7%
Severe symptoms[e]	2%	1.3%
Treatment discontinuation as a result of symptoms	2.1%	1.1%

[a] Includes reactions reported regardless of causality. Reactions include: abnormal dreaming, abnormal thinking, agitation, amnesia, confusion, depersonalization, dizziness, euphoria, hallucinations, impaired concentration, insomnia, somnolence, and stupor.
[b] Data from study 006 and 3 phase 2/3 studies.
[c] "Mild" = symptoms that do not interfere with patients' daily activities.
[d] "Moderate" = symptoms that may interfere with daily activities.
[e] "Severe" = events that interrupt patients' usual daily activities.

Serious psychiatric adverse reactions (3% or more) – Serious psychiatric adverse reactions have been reported in patients treated with efavirenz. In controlled trials, psychiatric symptoms observed at a frequency of greater than 2% among patients treated with efavirenz or control regimens, respectively, were depression (19%, 16%), anxiety (13%, 9%), and nervousness (7%, 2%).

Dermatologic adverse reactions –

Efavirenz Dermatologic Adverse Reactions[a,b]

	Description of rash	Efavirenz 600 mg once daily adults (n = 1,008)	Efavirenz children (n = 57)	Control groups adults (n = 635)
Rash, any grade	—	26.3%	45.6%	17.5%
Grade 1 rash	Erythema, pruritus	10.7%	8.8%	9.8%
Grade 2 rash	Diffuse maculopapular rash, dry desquamation	14.7%	31.6%	7.4%
Grade 3 rash	Vesiculation, moist desquamation, ulceration	0.8%	1.8%	0.3%
Grade 4 rash	Erythema multiforme, Stevens-Johnson syndrome, toxic epidermal necrolysis, necrosis requiring surgery, exfoliative dermatitis	0.1%	3.5%	0%
Treatment discontinuation because of rash	—	1.7%	8.8%	0.3%

[a] Includes reactions reported regardless of causality.
[b] Data from study 006 and 3 phase 2/3 studies.

Discontinuation due to rash – Experience with efavirenz in patients who discontinued other antiretroviral agents of the NNRTI class is limited. Nineteen patients who discontinued nevirapine because of rash have been treated with efavirenz. Nine of these patients developed mild to moderate rash while receiving therapy with efavirenz, and 2 of these patients discontinued because of rash.

➤*Children:*

CNS – Dizziness/light-headedness/fainting (16%), headache (11%), nervous system symptoms was (18%).

Dermatologic – Rash (46%); discontinued because of rash (9%), grade 3 rash, grade 4 rash.

GI – Diarrhea/loose stools (39%), nausea/vomiting (12%).

Miscellaneous – Ache/pain/discomfort (14%), cough (16%), fever (21%).

➤*Adults:*

Efavirenz Grade 3 to 4 Laboratory Abnormalities in Adults (≥ 2%)

		Study 006 lamivudine-, NNRTI-, and protease inhibitor–naive patients			Study ACTG 364 NRTI-experienced, NNRTI- and protease inhibitor–naive patients		
Laboratory abnormality	Limit	Efavirenz[a] + zidovudine lamivudine (n = 412) 180 weeks[b]	Efavirenz[a] + indinavir (n = 415) 102 weeks[b]	Indinavir + zidovudine + lamivudine (n = 401) 76 weeks[b]	Efavirenz[a] + nelfinavir + NRTIs (n = 64) 71.1 weeks[b]	Efavirenz[a] + NRTIs (n = 65) 70.9 weeks[b]	Nelfinavir + NRTIs (n = 66) 62.7 weeks[b]
ALT	> 5 × ULN	5%	8%	5%	2%	6%	3%
AST	> 5 × ULN	5%	6%	5%	6%	8%	8%
GGT[c]	> 5 × ULN	8%	7%	3%	5%	0%	5%
Amylase	> 2 × ULN	4%	4%	1%	0%	6%	2%
Glucose	> 250 mg/dL	3%	3%	3%	5%	2%	3%
Triglycerides[d]	≥ 751 mg/dL	9%	6%	6%	11%	8%	17%
Neutrophils	< 750/mm[3]	10%	3%	5%	2%	3%	2%

[a] Efavirenz provided as 600 mg once daily.
[b] Median duration of treatment.
[c] GGT = gamma-glutamyltransferase. Isolated elevations of GGT in patients receiving efavirenz may reflect enzyme induction not associated with liver toxicity.
[d] Nonfasting.

Hepatitis B or C coinfection – Monitor liver function tests in patients with a history of hepatitis B and/or C. In the long-term data set from study 006, 137 patients treated with efavirenz-containing regimens (median duration of therapy, 68 weeks) and 84 treated with a control regimen (median duration, 56 weeks) were seropositive at screening for hepatitis B (surface antigen positive) and/or C (hepatitis C antibody positive). Among these coinfected patients, elevations in AST to more than 5 times the ULN developed in 13% of patients in the efavirenz arms and 7% of those in the control arm, and elevations in ALT to greater than 5 times ULN developed in 20% of patients in the efavirenz arms and 7% patients in the control arm. Among coinfected patients, 3% of those treated with efavirenz-containing regimens and 2% in the control arm discontinued from the study because of liver or biliary system disorders.

Lipids – Increases from baseline in total cholesterol of 10% to 20% have been observed in some uninfected volunteers receiving efavirenz. In patients treated with efavirenz plus zidovudine plus lamivudine, increases from baseline in nonfasting total cholesterol and high-density lipoprotein (HDL) of approximately 20% and 25%, respectively, were observed. In patients treated with efavirenz plus indinavir, increases from baseline in nonfasting cholesterol and HDL of approximately 40% and 35%, respectively, were observed. Nonfasting total cholesterol levels of 240 mg/dL or more and 300 mg/dL or more were reported in 34% and 9%, respectively, of patients treated with efavirenz plus zidovudine plus lamivudine; 54% and 20%, respectively, of patients treated with efavirenz plus indinavir; and 28% and 4%, respectively, of patients treated with indinavir plus zidovudine plus lamivudine. The effects of efavirenz on triglycerides and LDL were not well

EFAVIRENZ — ORAL

characterized because samples were taken from nonfasting patients. The clinical significance of these findings is unknown.

➤*Postmarketing:*

CNS – Abnormal coordination, aggressive reactions, agitation, asthenia, ataxia, cerebellar coordination and balance disturbances, convulsions, delusions, emotional lability, hypesthesia, mania, neuropathy, neurosis, paranoia, paresthesia, psychosis, suicide, tremor.

Dermatologic – Erythema multiforme, flushing, photoallergic dermatitis, Stevens-Johnson syndrome.

GI – Constipation, malabsorption.

Hepatic – Hepatic enzyme increase, hepatic failure, hepatitis. A few of the postmarketing reports of hepatic failure, including cases in patients with no preexisting hepatic disease or other identifiable risk factors, were characterized by a fulminant course, progressing in some cases to transplantation or death.

Metabolic/Nutritional – Hypercholesterolemia, hypertriglyceridemia.

Musculoskeletal – Arthralgia, myalgia, myopathy.

Special senses – Abnormal vision, tinnitus.

Miscellaneous – Allergic reactions, dyspnea, gynecomastia, palpitations, redistribution/accumulation of body fat.

Overdosage

➤*Symptoms:* Some patients accidentally taking 600 mg twice daily have reported increased nervous system symptoms. One patient experienced involuntary muscle contractions.

➤*Treatment:* Treatment of overdose with efavirenz should consist of general supportive measures, including monitoring of vital signs and observation of the patient's clinical status. Administration of activated charcoal may be used to aid removal of unabsorbed drug. There is no specific antidote for overdose with efavirenz. Because efavirenz is highly protein bound, dialysis is unlikely to significantly remove the drug from blood.

Patient Information

Inform patients that efavirenz is not a cure for HIV-1 infection and that they may continue to experience illnesses associated with HIV-1 infection, including opportunistic infections. Tell patients that the use of efavirenz has not been shown to reduce the risk of transmitting HIV-1 to others through sexual contact or blood contamination.

Advise patients to take efavirenz every day as prescribed. Efavirenz must always be used in combination with other antiretroviral drugs. Advise patients to take efavirenz on an empty stomach, preferably at bedtime. Taking efavirenz with food increases efavirenz concentrations and may increase the frequency of adverse reactions. Dosing at bedtime may improve the tolerability of nervous system symptoms. Advise patients to remain under the care of a health care provider while taking efavirenz.

Inform patients that CNS symptoms, including abnormal dreams, dizziness, drowsiness, impaired concentration, and insomnia, are commonly reported during the first weeks of therapy with efavirenz. Dosing at bedtime may improve the tolerability of these symptoms, and these symptoms are likely to improve with continued therapy.

Alert patients to the potential for additive CNS effects when efavirenz is used concomitantly with alcohol or psychoactive drugs. Instruct patients who experience these symptoms to avoid potentially hazardous tasks such as driving or operating machinery.

Inform patients that serious psychiatric symptoms, including severe depression, suicide attempts, aggressive behavior, delusions, paranoia, and psychosis-like symptoms, have also been reported in patients receiving efavirenz. Inform patients that if they experience severe psychiatric adverse reactions they should seek immediate medical evaluation. Advise patients to inform their health care provider of any history of mental illness or substance abuse.

Inform patients that another common adverse reaction is rash. These rashes usually go away without any change in treatment. However, because rash may be serious, advise patients to contact their health care provider promptly if rash occurs.

Instruct women receiving efavirenz to avoid pregnancy. Advise women to always use a reliable form of barrier contraception in combination with other methods of contraception, including oral or other hormonal contraception. Because of the long half-life of efavirenz, use of adequate contraceptive measures for 12 weeks after discontinuation of efavirenz is recommended. Advise women to notify their health care provider if they become pregnant while taking efavirenz. If this drug is used during the first trimester of pregnancy, or if the patient becomes pregnant while taking this drug, apprise her of the potential harm to the fetus.

Efavirenz may interact with some drugs; therefore, advise patients to report to their health care provider the use of any other prescriptions, nonprescription medications, or herbal products, particularly St. John's wort.

Inform patients that redistribution or accumulation of body fat may occur in patients receiving antiretroviral therapy and that the cause and long-term health effects of these conditions are not known.

EFAVIRENZ/EMTRICITABINE/TENOFOVIR DISOPROXIL FUMARATE

Rx	**Atripla** (Bristol-Myers Squibb/Gilead Sciences)	**Tablets; oral:** efavirenz 600 mg/emtricitabine 200 mg/tenofovir disoproxil fumarate 300 mg	Equiv. to tenofovir disoproxil 245 mg. (123). Pink, capsule shape. Film-coated. In 30s.

EFAVIRENZ/EMTRICITABINE/TENOFOVIR DISOPROXIL FUMARATE — ORAL

Consult the complete prescribing information for each agent (ie, efavirenz, emtricitabine, tenofovir) prior to administration of efavirenz/emtricitabine/tenofovir combination tablet.

WARNING

Lactic acidosis/severe hepatomegaly – Lactic acidosis and severe hepatomegaly with steatosis, including fatal cases, have been reported with the use of nucleoside analogs in combination with other antiretrovirals.

Hepatitis B coinfection – Efavirenz/emtricitabine/tenofovir is not approved for the treatment of chronic hepatitis B virus (HBV) infection, and the safety and efficacy of efavirenz/emtricitabine/tenofovir has not been established in patients coinfected with HBV and HIV. Severe acute exacerbations of hepatitis B have been reported in patients who have discontinued emtricitabine or tenofovir. Closely monitor hepatic function with both clinical and laboratory follow-up for at least several months in patients who discontinue efavirenz/emtricitabine/tenofovir and are coinfected with HIV and HBV. If appropriate, initiation of anti–hepatitis B therapy may be warranted.

Indications

➤*HIV infection:* For use alone as a complete regimen or in combination with other antiretroviral agents for the treatment of HIV-1 infection in adults.

Administration and Dosage

➤*Adults:*

HIV infection – One tablet once daily taken on an empty stomach. Dosing at bedtime may improve the tolerability of nervous system symptoms.

➤*Renal function impairment:* Because efavirenz/emtricitabine/tenofovir is a fixed-dose combination, it should not be prescribed for patients requiring dosage adjustment, such as those with moderate or severe renal impairment (creatinine clearance [CrCl] less than 50 mL/min).

➤*Administration:* Take on an empty stomach.

➤*Storage/Stability:* Store at 25°C (77°F); excursions are permitted between 15° and 30°C (59° and 86°F). Keep the container tightly closed, dispense only in the original container, and do not use if the seal over the bottle opening is broken or missing.

Actions

➤*Pharmacology:*

Efavirenz – Efavirenz is a nonnucleoside reverse transcriptase inhibitor of HIV-1. Efavirenz activity is mediated predominantly by noncompetitive inhibition of HIV-1 reverse transcriptase. HIV-2 reverse transcriptase and human cellular DNA polymerases alpha, beta, gamma, and delta are not inhibited by efavirenz.

Emtricitabine – Emtricitabine, a synthetic nucleoside analog of cytidine, is phosphorylated by cellular enzymes to form emtricitabine 5′-triphosphate. Emtricitabine 5′-triphosphate inhibits the activity of the HIV-1 reverse transcriptase by competing with the natural substrate deoxycytidine 5′-triphosphate and by being incorporated into nascent viral DNA, which results in chain termination. Emtricitabine 5′-triphosphate is a weak inhibitor of mammalian DNA polymerases alpha, beta, and epsilon and mitochondrial DNA polymerase gamma.

Tenofovir – Tenofovir is an acyclic nucleoside phosphonate diester analog of adenosine monophosphate. Tenofovir disoproxil fumarate requires initial diester hydrolysis for conversion to tenofovir and subsequent phosphorylations by cellular enzymes to form tenofovir diphosphate. Tenofovir diphosphate inhibits the activity of HIV-1 reverse transcriptase by competing with the natural substrate deoxyadenosine 5′-triphosphate and, after incorporation into DNA, by DNA chain termination. Tenofovir diphosphate is a weak inhibitor of mammalian DNA polymerases alpha and beta and mitochondrial DNA polymerase gamma.

➤*Pharmacokinetics:*

Absorption/Distribution –

Efavirenz: In HIV-infected patients, time to peak plasma concentrations (C_{max}) was approximately 3 to 5 hours, and steady-state plasma concentrations were reached in 6 to 10 days. In 35 HIV-1–infected patients receiving efavirenz 600 mg once daily, the steady-state C_{max} was 12.9 ± 3.7 mcM (mean ± standard deviation [SD]), the minimum serum concentration was 5.6 ± 3.2 mcM, and the area under the curve (AUC) was 184 ± 73 mcM•h. Efavirenz is highly bound (approximately 99.5% to 99.75%) to human plasma proteins, predominantly albumin.

Emtricitabine: Following oral administration, emtricitabine is rapidly absorbed, with C_{max} occurring at 1 to 2 hours postdose. Following multiple-dose oral administration of emtricitabine to 20 patients infected with HIV, the steady-state emtricitabine C_{max} was 1.8 ± 0.7 mcg/mL (mean ± SD), and the AUC over a 24-hour dosing interval was 10 ± 3.1 mcg•h/mL. The

EFAVIRENZ/EMTRICITABINE/TENOFOVIR DISOPROXIL FUMARATE — ORAL

mean steady-state plasma trough concentration at 24 hours postdose was 0.09 mcg/mL. The mean absolute bioavailability of emtricitabine was 93%. In vitro binding of emtricitabine to human plasma proteins is less than 4% and is independent of concentration over the range of 0.02 to 200 mcg/mL.

Tenofovir: Following oral administration of a single dose of tenofovir 300 mg to patients infected with HIV-1 in the fasted state, C_{max} was achieved in 1 ± 0.4 hours (mean ± SD), and C_{max} and AUC values were 296 ± 90 ng/mL and 2,287 ± 685 ng•h/mL, respectively. The oral bioavailability of tenofovir from tenofovir disoproxil fumarate in fasted patients is approximately 25%. In vitro binding of tenofovir to human plasma proteins is less than 0.7% and is independent of concentration over the range of 0.01 to 25 mcg/mL.

Effect of food: Efavirenz/emtricitabine/tenofovir has not been evaluated in the presence of food. Administration of efavirenz with a high-fat meal increased the mean AUC and C_{max} of efavirenz 28% and 79%, respectively, compared with administration in the fasted state. Compared with fasted administration, dosing of tenofovir and emtricitabine in combination with either a high-fat or light meal increased the mean AUC and C_{max} of tenofovir 35% and 15%, respectively, without affecting emtricitabine exposures.

Metabolism/Excretion –

Efavirenz: Following administration of ^{14}C-labeled efavirenz, 14% to 34% of the dose was recovered in the urine (mostly as metabolites), and 16% to 61% was recovered in the feces (mostly as parent drug). In vitro studies suggest that CYP3A4 and CYP2B6 are the major isozymes responsible for efavirenz metabolism. Efavirenz has been shown to induce cytochrome P450 (CYP-450) enzymes, resulting in induction of its own metabolism. Efavirenz has a terminal half-life of 52 to 76 hours after single doses and 40 to 55 hours after multiple doses.

Emtricitabine: Following administration of radiolabeled emtricitabine, approximately 86% is recovered in the urine and 13% is recovered as metabolites. The metabolites of emtricitabine include 3′-sulfoxide diastereomers and their glucuronic acid conjugates. Emtricitabine is eliminated by a combination of glomerular filtration and active tubular secretion, with a renal clearance in adults with healthy renal function of 213 ± 89 mL/min (mean ± SD). Following a single oral dose, the plasma emtricitabine half-life is approximately 10 hours.

Tenofovir: Approximately 70% to 80% of an intravenous dose of tenofovir is recovered as unchanged drug in the urine. Tenofovir is eliminated by a combination of glomerular filtration and active tubular secretion, with a renal clearance in adults with healthy renal function of 243 ± 33 mL/min (mean ± SD). Following a single oral dose, the terminal elimination half-life of tenofovir is approximately 17 hours.

Special populations –

Renal function impairment:

• *Emtricitabine/Tenofovir* – The pharmacokinetics of emtricitabine and tenofovir are altered in patients with renal impairment. In patients with CrCl less than 50 mL/min, the C_{max} and $AUC_{(0-\infty)}$ of emtricitabine and tenofovir were increased.

Contraindications

Previously demonstrated hypersensitivity (eg, Stevens-Johnson syndrome, erythema multiforme, toxic skin eruptions) to efavirenz; coadministration with bepridil, cisapride, ergot derivatives (eg, dihydroergotamine, ergotamine), midazolam, pimozide, St. John's wort, triazolam, or voriconazole. (See also Drug Interactions.)

Warnings/Precautions

➤*Lactic acidosis/severe hepatomegaly with steatosis:* Lactic acidosis and severe hepatomegaly with steatosis, including fatal cases, have been reported with the use of nucleoside analogs in combination with other antiretrovirals. A majority of these cases has been in women. Obesity and prolonged nucleoside exposure may be risk factors. Exercise particular caution when administering nucleoside analogs to any patient with known risk factors of liver disease; however, cases have also been reported in patients with no known risk factors. Discontinue treatment with efavirenz/emtricitabine/tenofovir in any patient who develops clinical or laboratory findings suggestive of lactic acidosis or pronounced hepatotoxicity, which may include hepatomegaly and steatosis, even in the absence of marked transaminase elevations.

➤*Patients with HIV and HBV coinfection:* See the Warning box for more information.

➤*Psychiatric symptoms:* Serious psychiatric adverse reactions have been reported in patients treated with efavirenz. In controlled trials of 1,008 patients treated with regimens containing efavirenz for a mean of 2.1 years and 635 patients treated with control regimens for a mean of 1.5 years, the frequency (regardless of causality) of specific serious psychiatric reactions among patients who received efavirenz or control regimens, respectively, were severe depression (2.4%, 0.9%), suicidal ideation (0.7%, 0.3%), nonfatal suicide attempts (0.5%, 0%), aggressive behavior (0.4%, 0.5%), paranoid reactions (0.4%, 0.3%), and manic reactions (0.2%, 0.3%). When psychiatric symptoms similar to those previously noted were combined and evaluated as a group in a multifactorial analysis of data from study AI266006 (006), treatment with efavirenz was associated with an increase in the occurrence of these selected psychiatric symptoms. Other factors associated with an increase in the occurrence of these psychiatric symptoms were history of injection drug use, psychiatric history, and receipt of psychiatric medication at study entry; similar associations were observed in both the efavirenz and control treatment groups. In study 006, onset of new serious psychiatric symptoms occurred throughout the study for both efavirenz- and control-treated patients. Of efavirenz-treated patients, 1% discontinued or interrupted treatment because of 1 or more of these selected psychiatric symptoms. There also have been occasional postmarketing reports of death by suicide, delusions, and psychosis-like behavior, although a causal relationship between these reactions and the use of efavirenz cannot be determined from these reports. Instruct patients with serious psychiatric adverse reactions to seek immediate medical evaluation in order to assess the possibility that the symptoms may be related to the use of efavirenz, and, if so, to determine whether the risks of continued therapy outweigh the benefits.

➤*CNS effects:* In controlled trials, 53% of patients receiving efavirenz reported CNS symptoms (any grade, regardless of causality) compared with 25% of patients receiving control regimens. These symptoms included dizziness (28.1%), insomnia (16.3%), impaired concentration (8.3%), somnolence (7%), abnormal dreams (6.2%), and hallucinations (1.2%). Other reported symptoms were abnormal thinking, agitation, amnesia, confusion, depersonalization, euphoria, and stupor. The majority of these symptoms were mild to moderate (50.7%); symptoms were severe in 2% of patients. Overall, 2.1% of patients discontinued therapy as a result. These symptoms usually began during the first or second day of therapy and generally resolved after the first 2 to 4 weeks of therapy. After 4 weeks of therapy, the prevalence of nervous system symptoms of at least moderate severity ranged from 5% to 9% in patients treated with regimens containing efavirenz and from 3% to 5% in patients treated with a control regimen. Inform patients that these common symptoms are likely to improve with continued therapy and are not predictive of subsequent onset of the less frequent psychiatric symptoms. Dosing at bedtime may improve the tolerability of these nervous system symptoms.

Alert patients receiving efavirenz/emtricitabine/tenofovir to the potential for additive CNS reactions when used concomitantly with alcohol or psychoactive drugs.

➤*Skin rash:* In controlled clinical trials, 26% of patients treated with efavirenz 600 mg experienced new-onset skin rash compared with 17% of patients treated in control groups. Rash associated with blistering, moist desquamation, or ulceration occurred in 0.9% of patients treated with efavirenz. The incidence of grade 4 rash (eg, erythema multiforme, Stevens-Johnson syndrome) in patients treated with efavirenz in all studies and expanded access was 0.1%. Rashes were usually mild to moderate maculopapular skin eruptions that occurred within the first 2 weeks of efavirenz therapy initiation (median time to onset of rash in adults was 11 days), and in most patients continuing therapy with efavirenz, the rash resolved within 1 month (median duration, 16 days). The discontinuation rate for rash in clinical trials was 1.7%. Efavirenz/emtricitabine/tenofovir can be reinitiated in patients interrupting therapy because of rash.

Discontinue efavirenz/emtricitabine/tenofovir in patients developing severe rash associated with blistering, desquamation, fever, or mucosal involvement. Appropriate antihistamines and/or corticosteroids may improve tolerability and hasten the resolution of rash.

Experience with efavirenz in patients who discontinued nucleoside reverse transcriptase inhibitors is limited. Nineteen patients who discontinued nevirapine because of rash have been treated with efavirenz. Nine of these patients developed mild to moderate rash while receiving therapy with efavirenz, and 2 of these patients discontinued because of rash.

➤*Bone effects:*

Bone mineral density – Consider bone mineral density (BMD) monitoring for HIV-infected patients who have a history of pathologic bone fracture or are at risk of osteopenia. Although the effect of supplementation with calcium and vitamin D was not studied, such supplementation may be beneficial for all patients. If bone abnormalities are suspected, obtain appropriate consultation.

In a 144-week study of treatment-naive patients receiving tenofovir, decreases in BMD were seen at the lumbar spine and hip in both arms of the study. At week 144, there was a significantly greater mean percentage decrease from baseline in BMD at the lumbar spine in patients receiving tenofovir plus lamivudine plus efavirenz compared with patients receiving stavudine plus lamivudine plus efavirenz. Changes in BMD at the hip were similar between the treatment groups. In both groups, the majority of the reduction in BMD occurred in the first 24 to 48 weeks of the study, and this reduction was sustained through 144 weeks. Of tenofovir-treated patients, 28% versus 21% of the comparator patients lost at least 5% of BMD at the spine or 7% of BMD at the hip. Clinically relevant fractures (excluding fingers and toes) were reported in 4 patients in the tenofovir group and 6 patients in the comparator group.

Tenofovir was associated with significant increases in biochemical markers of bone metabolism (eg, serum bone-specific alkaline phosphatase, serum osteocalcin, serum C-telopeptide, urinary N-telopeptide), suggesting increased bone turnover. Serum parathyroid hormone levels and 1,25-vitamin D levels were also higher in patients receiving tenofovir. The effects of tenofovir-associated changes in BMD and biochemical markers on long-term bone health and future fracture risk are unknown.

Osteomalacia – Cases of osteomalacia (associated with proximal renal tubulopathy (and which may contribute to fractures) have been reported in association with the use of tenofovir.

➤*Convulsions:* Convulsions have been observed in patients receiving efavirenz, generally in those with a known medical history of seizures. Exercise caution in any patient with a history of seizures.

Patients who are receiving concomitant anticonvulsant medications primarily metabolized by the liver, such as phenytoin and phenobarbital, may require periodic monitoring of plasma levels.

➤*Immune reconstitution syndrome:* Immune reconstitution syndrome has been reported in patients treated with combination antiretroviral therapy, including efavirenz/emtricitabine/tenofovir. During the initial phase of combination antiretroviral treatment, patients whose immune systems respond may develop an inflammatory response to indolent or residual

EFAVIRENZ/EMTRICITABINE/TENOFOVIR DISOPROXIL FUMARATE — ORAL

opportunistic infections (eg, *Mycobacterium avium* infection, cytomegalovirus, *Pneumocystis jiroveci* pneumonia [PCP], tuberculosis), which may necessitate further evaluation and treatment.

➤*Fat redistribution:* Redistribution/accumulation of body fat, including breast enlargement, central obesity, "cushingoid appearance," dorsocervical fat enlargement (buffalo hump), facial wasting, and peripheral wasting have been observed in patients receiving antiretroviral therapy. The mechanism and long-term consequences of these reactions are currently unknown. A causal relationship has not been established.

➤*Renal function impairment:* See Administration and Dosage for more information.

Renal function impairment, including cases of acute renal failure and Fanconi syndrome (renal tubular injury with severe hypophosphatemia), has been reported in association with the use of tenofovir.

It is recommended that CrCl be calculated in all patients prior to initiating therapy and as clinically appropriate during therapy with efavirenz/emtricitabine/tenofovir. Perform routine monitoring of calculated CrCl and serum phosphorus in patients at risk of renal impairment, including patients who have previously experienced renal events while receiving adefovir.

Avoid efavirenz/emtricitabine/tenofovir in the case of concurrent or recent use of a nephrotoxic agent.

➤*Hepatic function impairment:* Monitoring of liver enzymes before and during treatment is recommended for patients with underlying hepatic disease (including hepatitis B or C infection), patients with marked transaminase elevations, and patients treated with other medications associated with liver toxicity. A few of the postmarketing reports of hepatic failure occurred in patients with no preexisting hepatic disease or other identifiable risk factors. Also consider liver enzyme monitoring for patients without preexisting hepatic dysfunction or other risk factors. In patients with persistent elevations of serum transaminases to greater than 5 times the upper limit of the normal (ULN), weigh the benefits of continued therapy with efavirenz/emtricitabine/tenofovir against the unknown risks of significant liver toxicity.

Because of the extensive CYP-450–mediated metabolism of efavirenz and limited clinical experience in patients with hepatic function impairment, exercise caution when administering efavirenz/emtricitabine/tenofovir to these patients.

➤*Hazardous tasks:* Advise patients who experience CNS symptoms, such as dizziness, drowsiness, and/or impaired concentration, to avoid potentially hazardous tasks, such as driving or operating machinery.

➤*Pregnancy:* *Category D.* Efavirenz may cause fetal harm when administered during the first trimester to a pregnant woman. Instruct women receiving efavirenz/emtricitabine/tenofovir to avoid pregnancy. Advise women of childbearing potential to always use barrier contraception in combination with other methods of contraception (eg, oral or other hormonal contraceptives). Because of the long half-life of efavirenz, use of adequate contraceptive measures for 12 weeks after discontinuation of efavirenz/emtricitabine/tenofovir is recommended. Perform pregnancy testing in women of childbearing potential before initiating efavirenz/emtricitabine/tenofovir. If this drug is used during the first trimester of pregnancy or if the patient becomes pregnant while taking this drug, inform the patient of the potential harm to the fetus.

There are no adequate and well-controlled studies of efavirenz/emtricitabine/tenofovir in pregnant women. Only use efavirenz/emtricitabine/tenofovir during pregnancy if the potential benefit justifies the potential risk to the fetus, such as in pregnant women without other therapeutic options.

Antiretroviral pregnancy registry – To monitor fetal outcomes of pregnant women, an antiretroviral pregnancy registry has been established. Health care providers are encouraged to register patients who become pregnant by calling 1-800-258-4263.

➤*Lactation:* The Centers for Disease Control and Prevention (CDC) recommend that women infected with HIV not breast-feed their infants in order to avoid risking postnatal transmission of HIV. Studies in rats have demonstrated that efavirenz and tenofovir are secreted in milk. It is not known whether efavirenz, emtricitabine, or tenofovir are excreted in human milk. Because of the relatively low molecular weight of efavirenz (approximately 316), emtricitabine (approximately 247), and tenofovir (approximately 636 for the prodrug), excretion into breast milk should be expected. The effect on a breast-feeding infant is unknown. Because of the potential for HIV transmission and serious adverse reactions in breast-feeding infants, instruct women not to breast-feed if they are receiving efavirenz/emtricitabine/tenofovir.

➤*Children:* Efavirenz/emtricitabine/tenofovir is not recommended for patients younger than 18 years because it is a fixed-dose combination tablet containing the component tenofovir, for which safety and effectiveness have not been established in this age group.

➤*Elderly:* In general, use caution during dose selection for elderly patients, keeping in mind the greater frequency of decreased hepatic, renal, or cardiac function, and of concomitant disease or other drug therapy.

➤*Monitoring:* It is recommended that all patients with HIV be tested for the presence of chronic HBV before initiating antiretroviral therapy. Closely monitor hepatic function with clinical and laboratory follow-up for at least several months in patients who discontinue efavirenz/emtricitabine/tenofovir and are coinfected with HIV and HBV. If appropriate, initiation of anti–hepatitis B therapy may be warranted.

Perform pregnancy testing in women of childbearing potential before initiating efavirenz/emtricitabine/tenofovir.

It is recommended that CrCl be calculated in all patients prior to initiating therapy and as clinically appropriate during therapy with efavirenz/emtricitabine/tenofovir. Perform routine monitoring of calculated CrCl and serum phosphorus in patients at risk of renal impairment.

Monitor liver enzymes before and during treatment in patients with underlying hepatic disease, including hepatitis B or C infection and in patients treated with other medications associated with liver toxicity. In patients with persistent elevations of serum transaminases and in patients with marked transaminase elevations to greater than 5 times the ULN, weigh the benefits of continued therapy with efavirenz/emtricitabine/tenofovir against the unknown risks of significant liver toxicity.

Consider BMD monitoring for HIV-infected patients who have a history of pathologic bone fracture or are at risk of osteopenia. Although the effect of supplementation with calcium and vitamin D was not studied, such supplementation may be beneficial for all patients. If bone abnormalities are suspected, obtain appropriate consultation.

Patients who are receiving concomitant anticonvulsant medications primarily metabolized by the liver, such as phenytoin and phenobarbital, may require periodic monitoring of plasma levels.

Drug Interactions

➤*Coadministration with related drugs:* Related drugs not for coadministration with efavirenz/emtricitabine/tenofovir include emtricitabine, tenofovir, emtricitabine/tenofovir, and efavirenz, which contain the same active components as efavirenz/emtricitabine/tenofovir. Because of similarities between emtricitabine and lamivudine, do not coadminister efavirenz/emtricitabine/tenofovir with drugs containing lamivudine, including lamivudine/zidovudine, lamivudine, lamivudine-HBV, abacavir/lamivudine, or abacavir/lamivudine/zidovudine.

➤*Cytochrome P450 system:* Efavirenz plasma concentrations may be altered by substrates, inhibitors, or inducers of CYP3A. Similarly, efavirenz may alter plasma concentrations of drugs metabolized by CYP3A. In vitro studies demonstrate that efavirenz inhibits CYP2C9, 2C19, and 3A4 isozymes in the range of observed efavirenz plasma concentrations. Concomitant use of efavirenz with drugs primarily metabolized by these isozymes may result in altered plasma concentrations of the coadministered drug. Therefore, appropriate dose adjustments may be necessary for these drugs.

➤*Drugs eliminated by kidneys:* Because emtricitabine and tenofovir are primarily eliminated by the kidneys, coadministration of efavirenz/emtricitabine/tenofovir with drugs that reduce renal function or compete for active tubular secretion may increase serum concentrations of emtricitabine, tenofovir, and/or other renally eliminated drugs. Some examples include, but are not limited to, acyclovir, adefovir dipivoxil, cidofovir, ganciclovir, valacyclovir, and valganciclovir.

Efavirenz/Emtricitabine/Tenofovir Drug Interactions

Precipitant drug	Object drug[a]		Description
Anticonvulsants (eg, carbamazepine, phenobarbital, phenytoin)	Efavirenz/Emtricitabine/Tenofovir	↓	There is potential for reduction in anticonvulsant and/or efavirenz plasma levels. Conduct periodic monitoring of phenytoin or phenobarbital plasma levels. Use anticonvulsant therapy other than carbamazepine.
Efavirenz/Emtricitabine/Tenofovir	Anticonvulsants (eg, carbamazepine, phenobarbital, phenytoin)		
Atazanavir	Efavirenz/Emtricitabine/Tenofovir	↑↓	Atazanavir has the potential to increase serum concentrations of tenofovir. Closely monitor for tenofovir-associated adverse reactions. Plasma concentrations of atazanavir may be decreased by both efavirenz and tenofovir. Coadministration is not recommended.
Efavirenz/Emtricitabine/Tenofovir	Atazanavir		
Azole antifungals (eg, itraconazole, ketoconazole, posaconazole, voriconazole)	Efavirenz/Emtricitabine/Tenofovir	↓↑	Efavirenz has the potential to decrease plasma concentrations of itraconazole, ketoconazole, and posaconazole. Avoid concomitant use unless the benefit outweighs the risks. Coadministration of efavirenz and voriconazole is contraindicated. Voriconazole increases efavirenz plasma concentrations, which may increase the risk of efavirenz-associated adverse reactions. Efavirenz significantly decreases voriconazole plasma concentrations, which may decrease voriconazole efficacy.
Efavirenz/Emtricitabine/Tenofovir	Azole antifungals (eg, voriconazole)		

EFAVIRENZ/EMTRICITABINE/TENOFOVIR DISOPROXIL FUMARATE — ORAL

Efavirenz/Emtricitabine/Tenofovir Drug Interactions

Precipitant drug	Object drug[a]		Description
Ginkgo biloba	Efavirenz/ Emtricitabine/ Tenofovir	↓	Efavirenz plasma concentrations may be reduced, decreasing the efficacy. Avoid efavirenz in patients taking *Ginkgo biloba*.
Lopinavir/ Ritonavir	Efavirenz/ Emtricitabine/ Tenofovir	↑↓	Lopinavir/ritonavir has the potential to increase serum concentrations of tenofovir. Closely monitor for tenofovir-associated adverse reactions. Efavirenz/emtricitabine/ tenofovir may decrease plasma concentrations of lopinavir. A dosage increase of lopinavir/ritonavir to 600 mg/150 mg twice daily may be considered when decreased susceptibility to lopinavir is clinically suspected.
Efavirenz/ Emtricitabine/ Tenofovir	Lopinavir/ Ritonavir		
Nevirapine	Efavirenz/ Emtricitabine/ Tenofovir	↓	Efavirenz plasma concentrations may be reduced; however, the risk of adverse reactions may be increased. Coadministration is not recommended.
Rifabutin Rifampin	Efavirenz/ Emtricitabine/ Tenofovir	↓	Rifabutin and rifampin would be expected to increase the clearance of efavirenz caused by CYP3A4 induction. Coadministration may also decrease rifabutin concentration. Increase daily dose of rifabutin by 50%. Consider doubling the rifabutin dose when rifabutin is given 2 to 3 times a week.
Efavirenz/ Emtricitabine/ Tenofovir	Rifabutin Rifampin		
Ritonavir	Efavirenz/ Emtricitabine/ Tenofovir	↑	With concurrent use, the concentration of efavirenz and ritonavir was increased. The combination was associated with a higher frequency of adverse reactions (eg, dizziness, nausea, paresthesia) and elevated liver enzymes. Monitor liver enzymes.
Efavirenz/ Emtricitabine/ Tenofovir	Ritonavir		
St. John's wort	Efavirenz/ Emtricitabine/ Tenofovir	↓	Concomitant use is contraindicated. St. John's wort is expected to substantially decrease plasma levels of efavirenz and lead to a loss of virologic response and possible resistance to efavirenz.
Efavirenz/ Emtricitabine/ Tenofovir	Amprenavir, fosamprenavir	↓	Efavirenz has the potential to decrease serum concentrations of amprenavir (fosamprenavir active metabolite). An additional 100 mg/day (300 mg total) is recommended when efavirenz/ emtricitabine/tenofovir is administered with fosamprenavir/ ritonavir once daily.
Efavirenz/ Emtricitabine/ Tenofovir	Benzodiazepines (eg, midazolam, triazolam)	↑	Concomitant use is contraindicated because of the potential for serious and/or life-threatening adverse reactions, such as increased sedation or respiratory depression.
Efavirenz/ Emtricitabine/ Tenofovir	Bepridil	↑	Concomitant use is contraindicated because of the potential for serious and/or life-threatening reactions, such as cardiac arrhythmias.
Efavirenz/ Emtricitabine/ Tenofovir	Calcium channel blockers (eg, diltiazem, felodipine, nicardipine, nifedipine, verapamil)	↓	There is a potential for reduction in calcium channel blocker plasma levels. Guide dose adjustments by clinical response.
Efavirenz/ Emtricitabine/ Tenofovir	Cisapride[c]	↑	Concomitant use is contraindicated because of the potential for serious and/or life-threatening reactions, such as cardiac arrhythmias.

Efavirenz/Emtricitabine/Tenofovir Drug Interactions

Precipitant drug	Object drug[a]		Description
Efavirenz/ Emtricitabine/ Tenofovir	Clarithromycin	↔	Clarithromycin plasma levels may decrease, while clarithromycin hydroxy metabolite levels increase with coadministration. In uninfected volunteers, 46% developed a rash while receiving efavirenz/emtricitabine/tenofovir and clarithromycin. The clinical significance of this is unknown. Consider alternatives (eg, azithromycin) to clarithromycin.
Efavirenz/ Emtricitabine/ Tenofovir	Contraceptives, hormonal (eg, ethinyl estradiol)	↔	Clinical significance is unknown. Because the potential interaction of efavirenz with oral contraceptives has not been fully characterized, use a reliable barrier contraceptive in addition to oral contraceptives.
Efavirenz/ Emtricitabine/ Tenofovir	Didanosine	↑	Tenofovir has the potential to increase didanosine concentrations and could potentiate didanosine-associated adverse reactions, including pancreatitis and neuropathy. In adults weighing > 60 kg, reduce the didanosine dose to 250 mg with coadministration. When coadministered, efavirenz/emtricitabine/tenofovir and didanosine enteric-coated tablets may be taken under fasted conditions or with a light meal (< 400 kcal, 20% fat). Coadminister didanosine buffered formulation with efavirenz/emtricitabine/ tenofovir under fasted conditions. Use with caution and monitor patients closely.
Efavirenz/ Emtricitabine/ Tenofovir	Ergot derivatives (eg, dihydroergotamine, ergonovine, ergotamine)	↑	Concomitant use is contraindicated because of the potential for serious and/or life-threatening reactions, such as acute ergot toxicity characterized by peripheral vasospasm and ischemia of the extremities and other tissues.
Efavirenz/ Emtricitabine/ Tenofovir	Etravirine	↓	Plasma concentrations and pharmacologic effects of etravirine may be decreased. Larger dosages of etravirine may be needed. Clinical and laboratory monitoring for therapeutic efficacy is warranted.
Efavirenz/ Emtricitabine/ Tenofovir	HMG-CoA[d] reductase inhibitors (eg, atorvastatin, pravastatin, simvastatin)	↓	Plasma concentrations of atorvastatin, pravastatin, and simvastatin may be decreased with efavirenz administration. Close clinical monitoring of LDL[d] levels after starting or stopping efavirenz is warranted during coadministration with HMG-CoA reductase inhibitors.
Efavirenz/ Emtricitabine/ Tenofovir	Immunosuppressants (eg, cyclosporine, sirolimus, tacrolimus)	↓	Immunosuppressant concentrations may be reduced. Immunosuppressant dosage adjustment may be needed. Closely monitor immunosuppressant concentrations for at least 2 weeks (until stable concentrations are reached) when starting or stopping efavirenz/emtricitabine/tenofovir treatment.
Efavirenz/ Emtricitabine/ Tenofovir	Indinavir	↓	Efavirenz may increase the metabolism of indinavir. Increasing the indinavir dosage does not compensate for the increased indinavir metabolism.

EFAVIRENZ/EMTRICITABINE/TENOFOVIR DISOPROXIL FUMARATE — ORAL

Efavirenz/Emtricitabine/Tenofovir Drug Interactions			
Precipitant drug	Object drug[a]		Description
Efavirenz/ Emtricitabine/ Tenofovir	Maraviroc	↓	Efavirenz may decrease maraviroc plasma concentrations. A dosage adjustment of maraviroc may be required. Consult official package labeling. Coadministration is contraindicated in patients with severe renal impairment (CrCl 30 mL/min).
Efavirenz/ Emtricitabine/ Tenofovir	Methadone	↓	Coadministration in HIV-infected patients with a history of injection drug use resulted in decreased plasma levels of methadone and signs of opiate withdrawal. Monitor patients for signs of withdrawal and increase their methadone dose as required in order to alleviate withdrawal symptoms.
Efavirenz/ Emtricitabine/ Tenofovir	Pimozide	↑	Concomitant use is contraindicated because of the potential for serious and/or life-threatening reactions, such as cardiac arrhythmias.
Efavirenz/ Emtricitabine/ Tenofovir	Progestins (eg, norethindrone)	↓	The efficacy of norethindrone may be reduced. A higher dose of progestin may be needed. If the progestin is being used for contraception, instruct the patient to always use a barrier method of contraception in addition to hormonal contraception.
Efavirenz/ Emtricitabine/ Tenofovir	Protease inhibitors (eg, atazanavir, fosamprenavir, indinavir, nelfinavir, ritonavir, saquinavir)	↑↓	Protease inhibitor plasma levels and clinical efficacy may be reduced. Nelfinavir concentrations may be increased.
Efavirenz/ Emtricitabine/ Tenofovir	Saquinavir	↓	Do not use saquinavir with efavirenz/emtricitabine/tenofovir as the sole protease inhibitor because of decreased AUC and C_{max} of saquinavir.
Efavirenz/ Emtricitabine/ Tenofovir	Sertraline	↓	Efavirenz/emtricitabine/tenofovir has the potential to decrease serum concentrations of sertraline. Guide increases in sertraline dose by clinical response.
Efavirenz/ Emtricitabine/ Tenofovir	Warfarin	↑↓	Plasma concentrations and effects of warfarin may be potentially increased or decreased by efavirenz. Monitor coagulation parameters and adjust the warfarin dose as needed.

[a] ↑ = object drug increased; ↓ = object drug decreased; ↔ = undetermined clinical effect; ↑↓ = object drug both increased and decreased.
[b] This drug is no longer marketed in the United States.
[c] Available from the manufacturer on a limited-access protocol.
[d] HMG-CoA = 3-hydroxy-3-methylglutaryl coenzyme A; LDL = low-density lipoprotein.

➤*Drug/Lab test interactions:*

Cannabinoid test interaction – Efavirenz does not bind to cannabinoid receptors. False-positive urine cannabinoid test results have been observed in volunteers not infected with HIV receiving efavirenz when the Microgenics *CEDIA* DAU multilevel tetrahydrocannabinol assay was used for screening. Negative results were obtained when more specific confirmatory testing was performed with gas chromatography/mass spectrometry. For more information, see the Efavirenz monograph.

➤*Drug/Food interactions:* Administration of efavirenz with a high-fat meal increased the mean AUC and C_{max} of efavirenz by 28% and 79%, respectively, compared with administration in the fasted state. Compared with fasted administration, dosing of tenofovir and emtricitabine in combination with a high-fat or light meal increased the mean AUC and C_{max} of tenofovir by 35% and 15%, respectively, without affecting emtricitabine exposures. Administer efavirenz/emtricitabine/tenofovir on an empty stomach.

Minimally or noninteracting drugs – Drug interaction studies were performed with efavirenz and other drugs likely to be coadministered. There were no clinically important interactions between efavirenz and azithromycin, cetirizine, fluconazole, lamivudine, lorazepam, paroxetine, or zidovudine. Single doses of famotidine or an aluminum and magnesium antacid with simethicone had no effect of efavirenz exposure.

Adverse Reactions

For more information on lactic acidosis, severe hepatomegaly with steatosis, psychiatric and other CNS symptoms, convulsions, renal impairment, hepatoxicity, rash, BMD decreases, osteomalacia, immune reconstitution syndrome, and fat redistribution, refer to Warnings/Precautions.

➤*Efavirenz/Emtricitabine/Tenofovir:* The most common adverse reactions (incidence 10% or more, any severity) occurring in study 934 include abnormal dreams, depression, diarrhea, dizziness, fatigue, headache, insomnia, nausea, and rash. Adverse reactions observed in study 934 were generally consistent with those seen in previous studies of the individual components.

Efavirenz/Emtricitabine/Tenofovir Adverse Reactions[a] (Grades 2 to 4) (≥ 5%)		
Adverse reactions	Emtricitabine + tenofovir + efavirenz[b] (n = 257)	Zidovudine/Lamivudine + efavirenz (n = 254)
CNS		
Anxiety	5%	4%
Depression	9%	7%
Dizziness	8%	7%
Fatigue	9%	8%
Headache	6%	5%
Insomnia	5%	7%
GI		
Diarrhea	9%	5%
Nausea	9%	7%
Vomiting	2%	5%
Respiratory		
Nasopharyngitis	5%	3%
Sinusitis	8%	4%
Upper respiratory tract infections	8%	5%
Miscellaneous		
Rash event[c]	7%	9%

[a] Frequencies of adverse reactions are based on all treatment-emergent adverse events, regardless of relationship to study drug.
[b] From weeks 96 to 144 of the study, subjects received emtricitabine/tenofovir coadministered with efavirenz in place of emtricitabine plus tenofovir with efavirenz.
[c] Rash event includes rash, exfoliative rash, rash generalized, rash macular, rash maculopapular, rash pruritic, and rash vesicular.

In study 073, subjects with stable, virologic suppression on antiretroviral therapy and no history of virologic failure were randomized to receive efavirenz/emtricitabine/tenofovir or stay on their baseline regimen. The adverse reactions observed in study 073 were generally consistent with those seen in study 934 and those seen with the individual components of efavirenz/emtricitabine/tenofovir when each was administered in combination with other antiretroviral agents.

➤*Emtricitabine and tenofovir:* Adverse reactions that occurred in at least 5% of patients receiving emtricitabine or tenofovir with other antiretroviral agents in clinical trials include abdominal pain, anxiety, arthralgia, back pain, dyspepsia, fever, increased cough, myalgia, pain, paresthesia, peripheral neuropathy (including peripheral neuritis and neuropathy), pneumonia, rash event (including allergic reaction, maculopapular rash, pruritus, pustular rash, rash, urticaria, and vesiculobullous rash), and rhinitis.

Skin discoloration has been reported with higher frequency among emtricitabine-treated patients. Skin discoloration, manifested by hyperpigmentation on the palms and/or soles, was generally mild and asymptomatic. The mechanism and clinical significance are unknown.

➤*Efavirenz:* The most significant adverse reactions observed in patients treated with efavirenz are CNS symptoms, psychiatric symptoms, and rash. See Warnings/Precautions for more information.

Selected adverse reactions of moderate or severe intensity observed in at least 2% of efavirenz-treated patients in 2 controlled clinical trials included abdominal pain, abnormal dreams,anorexia, dyspepsia, impaired concentration, nervousness, pain, pruritus, and somnolence.

Pancreatitis has been reported, although a causal relationship with efavirenz has not been established. Asymptomatic increases in serum amylase levels were observed in a significantly higher number of patients treated with efavirenz 600 mg than in control patients.

EFAVIRENZ/EMTRICITABINE/TENOFOVIR DISOPROXIL FUMARATE — ORAL

➤*Lab test abnormalities:*

Efavirenz/Emtricitabine/Tenofovir Significant Laboratory Abnormalities (≥ 1%)		
Lab abnormality	Emtricitabine + tenofovir + efavirenz [a] (n = 257)	Zidovudine/ lamivudine + efavirenz (n = 254)
Any ≥ grade 3 laboratory abnormality	30%	26%
Alkaline phosphatase (> 550 units/L)	1%	0%
ALT (women: > 170 units/L) (men: > 215 units/L)	2%	3%
AST (women: > 170 units/L) (men: > 180 units/L)	3%	3%
Creatine kinase (women: > 845 units/L) (men: > 990 units/L)	9%	7%
Fasting cholesterol (> 240 mg/mL)	22%	24%
Fasting triglyceride (> 750 mg/dL)	4%	2%
Glycosuria (≥3t)		1%
Hematuria (> 75 RBC/hpf[b])	3%	2%
Hemoglobin (< 8 mg/dL)	0%	4%
Hyperglycemia (> 250 mg/dL)	2%	1%
Neutrophils (< 750/mm^3)	3%	5%
Serum amylase (> 175 units/L)	8%	4%

[a] From weeks 96 to 144 of the study, subjects received emtricitabine/tenofovir coadministered with efavirenz in place of emtricitabine plus tenofovir with efavirenz.
[b] RBC/hpf = red blood cells per high power field.

Hepatic events – In study 934, 19 subjects treated with efavirenz, emtricitabine, and tenofovir and 20 subjects treated with efavirenz and fixed-dose zidovudine/lamivudine were hepatitis B surface antigen or hepatitis C antibody–positive. Among these coinfected subjects, 1 subject (1/19) in the efavirenz, emtricitabine, and tenofovir arm had elevations in transaminases to more then 5 times the ULN through 144 weeks. In the fixed-dose zidovudine/lamivudine arm, 2 subjects (2/20) had elevations in transaminases to more than 5 times ULN through 144 weeks. No HBV and/or hepatitis C virus coinfected subject discontinued from the study due to hepatobiliary disorders.

➤*Postmarketing:*

CNS – Abnormal coordination, aggressive reactions, agitation, asthenia, ataxia, cerebellar coordination and balance disturbances, convulsions, delusions, emotional lability, hypoesthesia, mania, neuropathy, neurosis, paranoia, paresthesia, psychosis, suicide, tremor (efavirenz); asthenia (tenofovir).

Dermatologic – Erythema multiforme, flushing, photoallergic dermatitis, Stevens-Johnson syndrome (efavirenz); rash (tenofovir).

GI – Constipation, malabsorption (efavirenz); abdominal pain, increased amylase, pancreatitis (tenofovir).

Hepatic – Hepatic enzyme increase, hepatic failure, hepatitis. A few of the postmarketing reports of hepatic failure, including cases in patients with no preexisting hepatic disease or other identifiable risk factors, were characterized by a fulminant course, progressing in some cases to transplantation or death (efavirenz); hepatic steatosis, hepatitis, increased liver enzymes (most commonly AST, ALT, gamma-glutamyl transferase) (tenofovir).

Metabolic/Nutritional – Hypercholesterolemia, hypertriglyceridemia, redistribution/accumulation of body fat (efavirenz); hypokalemia, hypophosphatemia, lactic acidosis (tenofovir).

Musculoskeletal – Arthralgia, myalgia, myopathy (efavirenz); muscular weakness, myopathy, osteomalacia (manifested as bone pain and may contribute to fractures), rhabdomyolysis (tenofovir).

Renal – Acute renal failure, acute tubular necrosis, Fanconi syndrome, increased creatinine, interstitial nephritis (including acute cases), nephrogenic diabetes insipidus, polyuria, proteinuria, proximal renal tubulopathy, renal failure, renal impairment (tenofovir).

Special senses – Abnormal vision, tinnitus (efavirenz).

Miscellaneous – Allergic reaction, dyspnea, gynecomastia, palpitations (efavirenz); allergic reaction including angioedema, dyspnea (tenofovir).

The following adverse reactions, listed under the previous body system headings, may occur as a consequence of proximal renal tubulopathy: hypokalemia, hypophosphatemia, muscular weakness, myopathy, osteomalacia, and rhabdomyolysis.

Overdosage

➤*Symptoms:*

Efavirenz – Some patients accidentally taking efavirenz 600 mg twice daily have reported increased nervous system symptoms. One patient experienced involuntary muscle contractions.

➤*Treatment:*

Efavirenz/Emtricitabine/Tenofovir – If overdosage occurs, monitor the patient for evidence of toxicity, including monitoring of vital signs and observation of the patient's clinical status. Then apply standard supportive treatment as necessary. Administration of activated charcoal may be used to aid removal of unabsorbed efavirenz. Hemodialysis can remove both emtricitabine and tenofovir, but it is unlikely to significantly remove efavirenz from the blood.

Emtricitabine – Hemodialysis treatment removes approximately 30% of the emtricitabine dose over a 3-hour dialysis period starting within 1.5 hours of emtricitabine dosing (blood flow rate of 400 mL/min and a dialysate flow rate of 600 mL/min). It is not known whether emtricitabine can be removed by peritoneal dialysis.

Tenofovir – Tenofovir is efficiently removed by hemodialysis, with an extraction coefficient of approximately 54%. Following a single dose of tenofovir 300 mg, a 4-hour hemodialysis session removed approximately 10% of the administered tenofovir dose.

Patient Information

Advise patients to take efavirenz/emtricitabine/tenofovir on an empty stomach and that it is important to take efavirenz/emtricitabine/tenofovir on a regular dosing schedule to avoid missing doses.

Advise patients that efavirenz/emtricitabine/tenofovir is not a cure for HIV infection, and patients may continue to experience illnesses associated with HIV infection, including opportunistic infections. Instruct patients to remain under the care of a health care provider when using efavirenz/emtricitabine/tenofovir.

Advise patients that the use of efavirenz/emtricitabine/tenofovir has not been shown to reduce the risk of transmission of HIV to others through sexual contact or blood contamination. Advise patients to continue to practice safer sex and to use latex or polyurethane condoms to lower the chance of sexual contact with body fluids, such as semen, vaginal secretions, or blood. Advise patients to never re-use or share needles.

Advise patients that the long-term effects of efavirenz/emtricitabine/tenofovir are unknown.

Advise patients that redistribution or accumulation of body fat may occur in patients receiving antiretroviral therapy and that the cause and long-term health effects of this are unknown.

Instruct patients not to coadminister efavirenz/emtricitabine/tenofovir with efavirenz; emtricitabine; tenofovir; emtricitabine/tenofovir; drugs containing lamivudine, including lamivudine/zidovudine, abacavir/lamivudine, or abacavir/lamivudine/zidovudine; or adefovir.

Inform patients that lactic acidosis and severe hepatomegaly with steatosis, including fatal cases, have been reported. Inform patients that treatment will be suspended in any patients who develop clinical symptoms suggestive of lactic acidosis or pronounced hepatotoxicity (including nausea, vomiting, unusual or unexpected stomach discomfort, and weakness).

Instruct patients with HIV that they will be tested for HBV before initiating antiretroviral therapy.

Advise patients that severe acute exacerbations of hepatitis B have been reported in patients who are coinfected with HBV and HIV and have discontinued emtricitabine or tenofovir, which are components of efavirenz/emtricitabine/tenofovir.

Advise patients that renal impairment, including cases of acute renal failure and Fanconi syndrome, has been reported. Advise patients to avoid efavirenz/emtricitabine/tenofovir with concurrent or recent use of a nephrotoxic agent.

Inform patients that decreases in BMD have been observed with the use of tenofovir. Inform patients that BMD monitoring may be performed in patients who have a history of pathologic bone fracture or are at risk of osteopenia.

Inform patients that CNS symptoms, including abnormal dreams, dizziness, drowsiness, impaired concentration, and insomnia, are commonly reported during the first weeks of therapy with efavirenz. Advise patients that dosing at bedtime may improve the tolerability of these symptoms, and these symptoms are likely to improve with continued therapy. Alert patients to the potential for additive CNS effects when efavirenz/emtricitabine/tenofovir is used concomitantly with alcohol or psychoactive drugs. Inform patients to avoid potentially hazardous tasks, such as driving or operating machinery, if they experience these symptoms.

Inform patients that serious psychiatric symptoms, including aggressive behavior, delusions, paranoia, psychosis-like symptoms, severe depression, and suicide attempts, have also been reported in patients receiving efavirenz. Inform patients to seek immediate medical evaluation if they experience severe psychiatric adverse reactions.

Inform patients that another common adverse reaction is rash. These rashes usually go away without any change in treatment. However, because rash

EFAVIRENZ/EMTRICITABINE/TENOFOVIR DISOPROXIL FUMARATE — ORAL

may be serious, advise patients to contact their health care provider promptly if they develop a rash.

Instruct women receiving efavirenz/emtricitabine/tenofovir to avoid pregnancy and to always use a reliable form of barrier contraception in combination with other methods of contraception, including oral or other hormonal contraception. Advise patients that the use of adequate contraceptive measures for 12 weeks after discontinuation efavirenz/emtricitabine/tenofovir is recommended. Advise women to notify their health care provider if they become pregnant or plan to become pregnant while taking efavirenz/emtricitabine/tenofovir. If this drug is used during the first trimester of pregnancy or if the patient becomes pregnant while taking this drug, inform her of the potential harm to the fetus.

Efavirenz/emtricitabine/tenofovir may interact with some drugs; therefore, advise patients to report the use of any other prescription and nonprescription medication or herbal products (particularly St. John's wort) to their health care provider.

Cellular Chemokine Receptor (CCR5) Antagonist

MARAVIROC

Rx	Selzentry (Pfizer)	Tablets; oral: 150 mg	(Pfizer MVC 150). Blue, oval. Film-coated. In 60s.
		300 mg	(Pfizer MVC 300). Blue, oval. Film-coated. In 60s.

MARAVIROC — ORAL

WARNING

Hepatotoxicity has been reported with maraviroc use. Evidence of a systemic allergic reaction (eg, eosinophilia, elevated immunoglobulin E, pruritic rash) prior to the development of hepatotoxicity may occur. Immediately evaluate patients with signs or symptoms of hepatitis or allergic reactions following use of maraviroc.

Indications

➤*HIV infection:* In combination with other antiretroviral agents, for treatment of adult patients infected only with chemokine receptor 5 (CCR5)–tropic HIV-1.

Administration and Dosage

➤*Adults:*

HIV infection – The recommended dose of maraviroc differs based on concomitant medications because of drug interactions.

Maraviroc Recommended Dosing Regimens

Concomitant medications	Maraviroc dosage
Potent CYP3A inhibitors (with or without a CYP3A inducer)	
Protease inhibitors (except tipranavir/ritonavir)	150 mg twice daily
Delavirdine	
Ketoconazole, itraconazole, clarithromycin	
Other potent CYP3A inhibitors (eg, nefazodone, telithromycin)	
Other concomitant medications, including tipranavir/ritonavir, nevirapine, raltegravir, all NRTIs,[a] and enfuvirtide	300 mg twice daily
Potent CYP3A inducers (without a potent CYP3A inhibitor)	
Carbamazepine, phenobarbital, phenytoin	600 mg twice daily
Efavirenz	
Etravirine	
Rifampin	

[a] NRTIs = nucleoside reverse transcriptase inhibitors.

➤*Children:*

HIV infection –

16 years of age and older: See Adults for dosing.

➤*Renal function impairment:*

Maraviroc Recommended Dosing Regimens Based on Renal Function

	Maraviroc Dosage				
	Normal	Mild	Moderate	Severe	ESRD[a]
Concomitant medications	CrCl[a] > 80 mL/min	CrCl > 50 and ≤ 80 mL/min	CrCl ≥ 30 and ≤ 50 mL/min	CrCl < 30 mL/min	On regular hemodialysis
Potent CYP3A inhibitors (with or without a CYP3A inducer)[b]	150 mg twice daily	150 mg twice daily	150 mg twice daily	Not recommended	Not recommended
Other concomitant medications[c]	300 mg twice daily	300 mg twice daily	300 mg twice daily	300 mg twice daily[d]	300 mg twice daily[d]
CYP3A inducers (without a potent CYP3A inhibitor)[e]	600 mg twice daily	600 mg twice daily	600 mg twice daily	Not recommended	Not recommended

[a] CrCl = creatinine clearance; ESRD = end-stage renal disease.
[b] Includes protease inhibitors (except tipranavir/ritonavir), clarithromycin, delavirdine, itraconazole, ketoconazole, and other potent CYP3A inhibitors (eg, nefazodone, telithromycin).
[c] Includes tipranavir/ritonavir, nevirapine, raltegravir, all NRTIs, and enfuvirtide.
[d] The maraviroc dose should be reduced to 150 mg twice daily if there are any symptoms of postural hypotension.
[e] Includes carbamazepine, efavirenz, etravirine, phenobarbital, phenytoin, and rifampin.

➤*Administration:* Maraviroc can be taken with or without food.

➤*Storage/Stability:* Store at 25°C (77°F); excursions are permitted between 15° and 30°C (59° and 86°F).

Actions

➤*Pharmacology:* Maraviroc is an antiviral drug and a member of a therapeutic class called CCR5 coreceptor antagonists. Maraviroc selectively binds to the human chemokine receptor CCR5 present on the cell membrane, preventing the interaction of HIV-1 gp120 and CCR5 necessary for CCR5-tropic HIV-1 to enter cells. Chemokine-related receptor (CXCR4)–tropic and dual-tropic HIV-1 entry is not inhibited by maraviroc.

➤*Pharmacokinetics:*

Absorption –

Mean Maraviroc Pharmacokinetic Parameters[a]

	Maraviroc dose	n	AUC_{12} (ng•h/mL)	C_{max} (ng/mL)	C_{min} (ng/mL)
Healthy volunteers (phase 1)	300 mg twice daily	64	2,908	888	43.1
Asymptomatic HIV patients (phase 2a)	300 mg twice daily	8	2,550	618	33.6
Treatment-experienced HIV patients (phase 3)[b]	300 mg twice daily	94	1,513	266	37.2
	150 mg twice daily (+ CYP3A inhibitor)	375	2,463	332	101
Treatment-naive HIV patients (phase 2b/3)[b]	300 mg twice daily	344	1,865	287	60

[a] AUC = area under the curve; C_{max} = maximal drug concentration; C_{min} = minimum plasma concentration.
[b] The estimated exposure is lower compared with other studies, possibly because of sparse sampling, food effect, compliance, and concomitant medications.

Maraviroc C_{max} is attained 0.5 to 4 hours following single oral doses of 1 to 1,200 mg administered to uninfected volunteers. The pharmacokinetics of oral maraviroc are not dose proportional over the dose range.

The absolute bioavailability of a 100 mg dose is 23% and is predicted to be 33% at 300 mg. Maraviroc is a substrate for the efflux transporter P-glycoprotein.

Effect of food: Coadministration of a 300 mg tablet with a high-fat breakfast reduced maraviroc C_{max} and AUC by 33% in healthy volunteers. There were no food restrictions in the studies that demonstrated the efficacy and safety of maraviroc. Therefore, maraviroc can be taken with or without food at the recommended dose.

MARAVIROC — ORAL

Distribution – Maraviroc is bound (approximately 76%) to human plasma proteins and shows moderate affinity for albumin and alpha-1 acid glycoprotein. The volume of distribution of maraviroc is approximately 194 L.

Metabolism – Studies in humans and in vitro studies using human liver microsomes and expressed enzymes have demonstrated that maraviroc is principally metabolized by the cytochrome P450 (CYP-450) system to metabolites that are essentially inactive against HIV-1. In vitro studies indicate that CYP3A is the major enzyme responsible for maraviroc metabolism. In vitro studies also indicate that polymorphic enzymes CYP2C9, CYP2D6, and CYP2C19 do not contribute significantly to the metabolism of maraviroc.

Maraviroc is the major circulating component (approximately 42% drug-related radioactivity) following a single oral dose of 300 mg of [^{14}C]-maraviroc. The most significant circulating metabolite in humans is a secondary amine (approximately 22% radioactivity) formed by N-dealkylation. This polar metabolite has no significant pharmacological activity. Other metabolites are products of mono-oxidation and are only minor components of plasma drug-related radioactivity.

Excretion – The terminal half-life of maraviroc following oral dosing to steady state in healthy patients was 14 to 18 hours. A mass balance/excretion study was conducted using a single 300 mg dose of ^{14}C-labeled maraviroc. Approximately 20% of the radiolabel was recovered in the urine and 76% was recovered in the feces over 168 hours. Maraviroc was the major component present in urine (mean, 8% of dose) and feces (mean, 25% of dose). The remainder was excreted as metabolites.

Special populations –

Renal function impairment: A study compared the pharmacokinetics of a single maraviroc 300 mg dose in patients with severe renal impairment (CrCl < 30 mL/min, n = 6) and ESRD (n = 6) with healthy volunteers (n = 6). Geometric mean ratios for maraviroc C_{max} and AUC_{inf} were 2.4- and 3.2-fold higher, respectively, for patients with severe renal impairment and 1.7- and 2-fold higher, respectively, for patients with ESRD as compared with patients with healthy renal function in this study. Hemodialysis had a minimal effect on maraviroc clearance and exposure in patients with ESRD. Exposures observed in patients with severe renal impairment and ESRD were within the range observed in previous maraviroc 300 mg single-dose studies in healthy volunteers with healthy renal function. However, maraviroc exposures in the patients with healthy renal function in this study were 50% lower than that observed in previous studies. Based on the results of this study, no dose adjustment is recommended for patients with renal impairment receiving maraviroc without a potent CYP3A inhibitor or inducer. However, if patients with severe renal impairment or ESRD experience any symptoms of postural hypotension while taking maraviroc 300 mg twice daily, reduce their dosage to 150 mg twice daily.

In addition, the study compared the pharmacokinetics of multiple-dose maraviroc in combination with saquinavir 1,000 mg/ritonavir 100 mg twice daily (a potent CYP3A inhibitor combination) for 7 days in patients with mild renal impairment (CrCl > 50 and ≤ 80 mL/min, n = 6) and moderate renal impairment (CrCl ≥ 30 and ≤ 50 mL/min, n = 6) with healthy volunteers with healthy renal function (n = 6). Patients received maraviroc 150 mg at different dose frequencies (healthy volunteers, every 12 hours; mild renal impairment, every 24 hours; moderate renal impairment, every 48 hours). Compared with healthy volunteers (dosed every 12 hours), geometric mean ratios for maraviroc AUC_{tau}, C_{max}, and C_{min} were 50% higher, 20% higher, and 43% lower, respectively, for patients with mild renal impairment (dosed every 24 hours). Geometric mean ratios for maraviroc AUC_{tau}, C_{max}, and C_{min} were 16% higher, 29% lower, and 85% lower, respectively, for patients with moderate renal impairment (dosed every 48 hours) compared with healthy volunteers (dosed every 12 hours). Based on the data from this study, no adjustment in dose is recommended for patients with mild or moderate renal impairment.

Hepatic function impairment: Maraviroc is primarily metabolized and eliminated by the liver. A study compared the pharmacokinetics of a single 300 mg dose of maraviroc in patients with mild (Child-Pugh class A, n = 8) and moderate (Child-Pugh class B, n = 8) hepatic impairment with pharmacokinetics in healthy patients (n = 8). The mean C_{max} and AUC were 11% and 25% higher, respectively, for patients with mild hepatic impairment and 32% and 46% higher, respectively, for patients with moderate hepatic impairment compared with patients with healthy hepatic function. These changes do not warrant a dose adjustment. Maraviroc concentrations are higher when maraviroc 150 mg is administered with a potent CYP3A inhibitor compared with following administration of 300 mg without a CYP3A inhibitor; closely monitor patients with moderate hepatic impairment who receive maraviroc 150 mg with a potent CYP3A inhibitor for maraviroc-associated adverse reactions. The pharmacokinetics of maraviroc have not been studied in patients with severe hepatic impairment.

Race: Population pharmacokinetic analysis of pooled phase 1/2a data indicated exposure was 26.5% higher in Asian patients (n = 95) compared with non-Asian patients (n = 318).

➤*Microbiology:*

Antiviral activity – Maraviroc inhibits the replication of CCR5-tropic laboratory strains and primary isolates of HIV-1 in models of acute peripheral blood leukocyte infection. The mean 50% effective concentration (EC_{50}) value for maraviroc against HIV-1 group M isolates (subtypes A to J and circulating recombinant form AE) and group O isolates ranged from 0.1 to 4.5 nM (0.05 to 2.3 ng/mL) in cell culture.

Resistance – HIV-1 variants with reduced susceptibility to maraviroc have been selected in cell culture, following serial passage of 2 CCR5-tropic viruses (CC1/85 and RU570). The maraviroc-resistant viruses remained CCR5-tropic with no evidence of a change from a CCR5-tropic virus to a CXCR4-using virus. Two amino acid residue substitutions in the V3 loop region of the HIV-1 envelope glycoprotein (gp160), A316T and I323V (HXB2 numbering), were shown to be necessary for the maraviroc-resistant phenotype in the HIV-1 isolate CC1/85. In the RU570 isolate, a 3-amino acid residue deletion in the V3 loop, ΔQAI (HXB2 positions 315-317), was associated with maraviroc resistance. The relevance of the specific gp120 mutations observed in maraviroc-resistant isolates selected in cell culture to clinical maraviroc resistance is not known. Maraviroc-resistant viruses were characterized phenotypically by concentration response curves that did not reach 100% inhibition in phenotypic drug assays, rather than increases in EC_{50} values.

Crossresistance – Maraviroc had antiviral activity against HIV-1 clinical isolates resistant to NRTIs, nonnucleoside reverse transcriptase inhibitors, protease inhibitors, and the fusion inhibitor enfuvirtide in cell culture (EC_{50} values ranged from 0.7 to 8.9 nM [0.36 to 4.57 ng/mL]). Maraviroc-resistant viruses that emerged in cell culture remained susceptible to enfuvirtide and the protease inhibitor saquinavir.

Clinical resistance – Virologic failure on maraviroc can result from genotypic and phenotypic resistance to maraviroc, through outgrowth of undetected CXCR4-using virus present before maraviroc treatment, through resistance to background therapy drugs, or because of low exposure to maraviroc.

Antiretroviral treatment–experienced patients – Week 48 data from treatment-experienced patients failing maraviroc-containing regimens with CCR5-tropic virus (n = 58) have identified 22 viruses that had decreased susceptibility to maraviroc, characterized in phenotypic drug assays by concentration response curves that did not reach 100% inhibition. Additionally, CCR5-tropic virus from 2 of these treatment-failure patients had 3-fold or greater shifts in EC_{50} values for maraviroc at the time of failure.

Fifteen of these viruses were sequenced in the gp120 encoding region, and multiple amino acid substitutions with unique patterns in the heterogeneous V3 loop region were detected. Changes at either amino acid position 308 or 323 (HXB2 numbering) were seen in the V3 loop in 7 of the patients with decreased maraviroc susceptibility. Substitutions outside the V3 loop of gp120 may also contribute to reduced susceptibility to maraviroc.

Antiretroviral treatment–naive patients – Treatment-naive patients receiving maraviroc had more virologic failures and more treatment-emergent resistance to the background regimen drugs compared with those receiving efavirenz.

Development of Resistance to Maraviroc or Efavirenz and Background Drugs in Antiretroviral Treatment–Naive Trial		
	Maraviroc	Efavirenz
Total N in dataset (as treated)	273	241
Total virologic failures (as treated)	31%	23%
Evaluable virologic failures with postbaseline genotypic and phenotypic data	73	43
Lamivudine resistance	53%	30%
Zidovudine resistance	3%	0%
Efavirenz resistance	—	53%
Phenotypic resistance to maraviroc[a]	26%	—

[a] Includes patients failing with CXCR4 or dual/mixed tropism because these viruses are not intrinsically susceptible to maraviroc.

In an as-treated analysis of treatment-naive patients at 96 weeks, 32 patients failed a maraviroc-containing regimen with CCR5-tropic virus and had a tropism result at failure; 7 of these patients had evidence of maraviroc phenotypic resistance, defined as concentration response curves that did not reach 95% inhibition. One additional subject had a 3-fold or greater shift in the EC_{50} value for maraviroc at the time of failure. A clonal analysis of the V3 loop amino acid envelope sequences was performed from 6 of the 7 patients. Changes in V3 loop amino acid sequence differed between each of these different patients, even for those infected with the same virus clade, suggesting that there are multiple diverse pathways to maraviroc resistance. The patients who failed with CCR5-tropic virus and without a detectable maraviroc shift in susceptibility were not evaluated for genotypic resistance.

Of the 32 maraviroc virologic failures failing with CCR5-tropic virus, 20 (63%) also had genotypic and/or phenotypic resistance to background drugs in the regimen (eg, lamivudine, zidovudine).

Antiretroviral treatment–naive patients – In a 96-week study of antiretroviral treatment–naive patients, 14% (12/85) who had CCR5-tropic virus at screening with an enhanced sensitivity tropism assay (*Trofile*) and who failed therapy on maraviroc had CXCR4-using virus at the time of treatment failure. A detailed clonal analysis was conducted in 2 previously antiretroviral treatment–naive patients enrolled in a phase 2a monotherapy study who had CXCR4-using virus detected after 10 days of treatment with maraviroc. Consistent with the detailed clonal analysis conducted in treatment-experienced patients, the CXCR4-using variants appear to emerge from outgrowth of a preexisting, undetected CXCR4-using virus. Screening with an enhanced sensitivity tropism assay reduced the number of maraviroc virologic failures with CXCR4- or dual/mixed-tropic virus at a failure to 12 compared with 24 when screening with the original tropism assay. All but 1 (11/12; 92%) of the maraviroc failures failing with CXCR4-or dual/mixed-tropic virus also had genotypic and phenotypic resistance to the background drug lamivudine at failure and 33% (4/12) developed zidovudine-associated resistance substitutions.

Patients who had CCR5-tropic virus at baseline and failed maraviroc therapy with CXCR4-using virus had a median increase in CD4+ cell counts from a

MARAVIROC — ORAL

baseline of +113 cells/mm^3, while those patients failing with CCR5-tropic virus has an increase of +135 cells/mm^3. The median increase in CD4+ cell count in patients failing in the efavirenz group was +95 cells/mm^3.

Contraindications

In patients with severe renal impairment or ESRD (CrCl < 30 mL/min) who are taking potent CYP3A inhibitors or inducers.

Warnings/Precautions

➤*Hepatotoxicity:* A case of possible maraviroc-induced hepatotoxicity with allergic features has been reported in a study of healthy volunteers. Consider discontinuation of maraviroc in any patient with signs or symptoms of hepatitis, or with increased liver transaminases combined with rash or other systemic symptoms.

The safety and efficacy of maraviroc have not been specifically studied in patients with significant underlying liver disorders. In studies of treatment-experienced, HIV-infected patients, approximately 6% of patients were coinfected with hepatitis B, and approximately 6% were coinfected with hepatitis C. Because of the small number of coinfected patients studied, no conclusions can be drawn regarding whether they are at an increased risk of hepatic adverse reactions with maraviroc administration. However, use caution when administering maraviroc to patients with preexisting liver impairment or who are coinfected with viral hepatitis B or C.

➤*Cardiovascular effects:*

Myocardial ischemia/infarction – Use with caution in patients at increased risk of cardiovascular events. Eleven (1.3%) patients who received maraviroc had cardiovascular events, including myocardial ischemia and/or infarction, during the phase 3, treatment-experienced studies (total exposure: 609 patient-years [300 on once-daily + 309 on twice-daily maraviroc]), while no patients who received placebo had such events (total exposure: 111 patient-years). These patients generally had cardiac disease or cardiac risk factors prior to maraviroc use, and the relative contribution of maraviroc to these events is not known.

In the phase 2b/3 study in treatment-naive patients, 0.8% of patients who received maraviroc had events related to ischemic heart disease and 1.4% of patients who received efavirenz had such events (total exposure: 506 and 508 patient-years for maraviroc and efavirenz, respectively).

Postural hypotension – When maraviroc was administered to healthy volunteers at doses higher than the recommended dose, symptomatic postural hypotension was seen at a greater frequency than in placebo. However, when maraviroc was given at the recommended dose in HIV patients in phase 3 studies, postural hypotension was seen at a rate similar to placebo (approximately 0.5%). Use caution when administering maraviroc in patients with a history of postural hypotension or on concomitant medication known to lower blood pressure.

Patients with impaired renal function may have cardiovascular comorbidities and could be at increased risk of cardiovascular adverse events triggered by postural hypotension. An increased risk of postural hypotension may occur in patients with severe renal insufficiency or in those with ESRD because of increased maraviroc exposure in some patients. Use maraviroc in patients with severe renal impairment or ESRD only if they are not receiving a concomitant potent CYP3A inhibitor or inducer. However, only consider the use of maraviroc in these patients when no alternative treatment options are available. If patients with severe renal impairment or ESRD experience any symptoms of postural hypotension while taking maraviroc 300 mg twice daily, reduce the dose to 150 mg twice daily.

➤*Immune reconstitution syndrome:* Immune reconstitution syndrome has been reported in patients treated with combination antiretroviral therapy, including maraviroc. During the initial phase of combination antiretroviral treatment, patients whose immune system responds may develop an inflammatory response to indolent or residual opportunistic infections (such as infection with *Mycobacterium avium*, cytomegalovirus, *Pneumocystis jirovecii*, or *Mycobacterium tuberculosis*, or reactivation of herpes simplex and herpes zoster), which may necessitate further evaluation and treatment.

➤*Risk of infection:* Maraviroc antagonizes the CCR5 coreceptor located on some immune cells and, therefore, could potentially increase the risk of developing infections. The overall incidence and severity of infection, as well as AIDS-defining category C infections, were comparable in the treatment groups during the phase 3 treatment-experienced studies of maraviroc. While there was a higher rate of certain upper respiratory tract infections reported in the maraviroc group compared with placebo (23% vs 13%), there was a lower rate of pneumonia (2% vs 5%) reported in patients receiving maraviroc. A higher incidence of herpes virus infections (11 per 100 patient-years) was also reported in the maraviroc group when adjusted for exposure compared with placebo (8 per 100 patient-years).

In the phase 2b/3 study in treatment-naive patients, the incidence of AIDS-defining category C events when adjusted for exposure was 1.8 for maraviroc compared with 2.4 for efavirenz per 100 patient-years of exposure.

Closely monitor patients for evidence of infections while receiving maraviroc.

➤*Risk of malignancy:* While no increase in malignancy has been observed with maraviroc, because of this drug's mechanism of action, it could affect immune surveillance and lead to an increased risk of malignancy.

The exposure-adjusted rate for malignancies per 100 patient-years of exposure in treatment-experienced patients was 4.6 for maraviroc compared with 9.3 on placebo. In treatment-naive patients, the rates were 1 and 2.4 per 100 patient-years of exposure for maraviroc and efavirenz, respectively.

Long-term follow-up is needed to more fully assess this risk.

➤*Renal function impairment:* Recommended doses of maraviroc for patients with impaired renal function (CrCl ≤ 80 mL/min) are based on the results of a pharmacokinetic study conducted in healthy patients with various degrees of renal impairment. The pharmacokinetics of maraviroc in patients with mild and moderate renal impairment was similar to that in patients with healthy renal function. A limited number of patients with mild and moderate renal impairment in the phase 3 clinical trials (n = 131 and n = 12, respectively) received the same dose of maraviroc as that administered to patients with healthy renal function. In these patients, there was no apparent difference in the adverse event profile for maraviroc compared with patients with healthy renal function.

If patients with severe renal impairment or ESRD not receiving a concomitant potent CYP3A inhibitor or inducer experience any symptoms of postural hypotension while taking maraviroc 300 mg twice daily, reduce the dose to 150 mg twice daily. No studies have been performed in patients with severe renal impairment or ESRD cotreated with potent CYP3A inhibitors or inducers. Hence, no dose of maraviroc can be recommended, and maraviroc is contraindicated for these patients.

➤*Hepatic function impairment:* Maraviroc is principally metabolized by the liver; therefore, exercise caution when administering this drug to patients with hepatic impairment because maraviroc concentrations may be increased. Maraviroc has not been studied in patients with severe hepatic impairment.

➤*Hazardous tasks:* Instruct patients who experience dizziness while taking maraviroc to avoid driving or operating machinery.

➤*Pregnancy: Category B.* There are no adequate and well-controlled studies in pregnant women. Because animal reproduction studies are not always predictive of human response, use maraviroc during pregnancy only if clearly needed.

In 2008, the updated U.S. Department of Health and Human Services guidelines for the use of antiretroviral agents in HIV-1 infected patients continued the recommendation that therapy, with the exception of efavirenz, should be continued during pregnancy. If indicated, maraviroc should not be withheld in pregnancy because the expected benefit to the HIV-positive mother outweighs the unknown risk to the fetus. Women receiving antiretroviral therapy during pregnancy should continue the therapy, but, regardless of the regimen, zidovudine administration is recommended during the intrapartum period to prevent vertical transmission of HIV to the newborn.

Antiretroviral pregnancy registry – To monitor maternal-fetal outcomes of pregnant women exposed to maraviroc and other antiretroviral agents, an antiretroviral pregnancy registry has been established. Health care providers are encouraged to register patients by calling 1-800-258-4263.

➤*Lactation:* The Centers for Disease Control and Prevention (CDC) recommend that HIV-infected mothers not breast-feed their infants to avoid risking postnatal transmission of HIV infection. Studies in lactating rats indicate that maraviroc is extensively secreted into rats milk. It is not known whether maraviroc is secreted into human milk. The molecular weight (about 514) and long elimination half-life (14 to 18 hours) suggest that the drug will be excreted into breast milk. Because of the potential for both HIV transmission and serious adverse reactions in breast-feeding infants, instruct mothers not to breast-feed if they are receiving maraviroc.

➤*Children:* The pharmacokinetics, safety, and efficacy of maraviroc in patients younger than 16 years of age have not been established. Therefore, do not use maraviroc in this patient population.

➤*Elderly:* Exercise caution when administering maraviroc in elderly patients; this reflects the greater frequency of decreased hepatic and renal function and of concomitant disease, and other drug therapy.

➤*Monitoring:* Monitor liver function tests at baseline and periodically during treatment. Monitor blood pressure in patients with a history of postural hypotension or those on antihypertensive agents. Monitor patients closely for signs of infection.

MARAVIROC — ORAL

Drug Interactions

Maraviroc Drug Interactions			
Precipitant drug	Object drug[a]		Description
Potent CYP3A inducers (eg, carbamazepine, efavirenz, etravirine, phenobarbital, phenytoin, rifampin) without a potent CYP3A inhibitor	Maraviroc	↓	Maraviroc plasma concentrations may be decreased. The recommended dosage is maraviroc 600 mg twice daily.
Potent CYP3A inhibitors (eg, clarithromycin, delavirdine, itraconazole, ketoconazole, nefazodone, protease inhibitors [except tipranavir/ ritonavir], telithromycin) with or without a CYP3 inducer	Maraviroc	↑	Maraviroc plasma concentrations may be increased. The recommended dosage is maraviroc 150 mg twice daily. Maraviroc and CYP3A inhibitors should only be administered to patients with a CrCl less than 50 mL/min if the potential benefit outweighs the risk; monitor patients for adverse reactions.
St. John's wort (*Hypericum perforatum*)	Maraviroc	↓	Maraviroc plasma concentrations may be decreased, resulting in suboptimal maraviroc concentrations and leading to loss of virologic response and possible resistance. Coadministration is not recommended.

[a] ↑ = object drug increased; ↓ = object drug decreased.

➤*Drug/Food interactions:* Coadministration of a 300 mg tablet with a high-fat breakfast reduced maraviroc C_{max} and AUC by 33% in healthy volunteers. However, maraviroc can be taken with or without food.

Adverse Reactions

➤*Treatment-experienced patients:*

Most common – The most common adverse reactions reported with maraviroc twice-daily therapy with frequency rates higher than placebo, regardless of causality, were cough, dizziness, pyrexia, rash, and upper respiratory tract infections. Additional adverse reactions that occurred with once-daily dosing at a higher rate than both placebo and twice-daily dosing were diarrhea, edema, esophageal candidiasis, influenza, parasomnias, rhinitis, sleep disorders, and urinary abnormalities. In these 2 studies, the rates of discontinuation caused by adverse reactions were 5% in patients receiving maraviroc twice daily plus optimized background therapy, as well as those who received placebo plus optimized background therapy. Most of the adverse reactions reported were judged to be mild to moderate in severity. The data described in the following sections occurred with maraviroc twice-daily dosing.

The total number of patients reporting infections were 233 (55%) and 84 (40%) in the maraviroc twice-daily and placebo groups, respectively. Correcting for the longer duration of exposure on maraviroc compared with placebo, the exposure-adjusted frequency (rate per 100 subject-years) of these reactions was 133 for both maraviroc twice daily and placebo.

Discontinuation – Dizziness or postural dizziness occurred in 8% of patients receiving maraviroc and placebo, respectively, with 2 (0.5%) patients receiving maraviroc permanently discontinuing therapy (one because of syncope, one because of orthostatic hypotension) versus 1 subject on placebo (0.5%) permanently discontinuing therapy because of dizziness.

Adverse reactions (2% or more) –

Maraviroc Adverse Reactions (≥ 2%) in Treatment-Experienced Patients				
Adverse reactions	Maraviroc twice daily[a] (n = 426)	Exposure-adjusted rate (per 100 patient-years) PYE[b] = 309	Placebo (n = 209)	Exposure-adjusted rate (per 100 patient-years) PYE = 111
CNS				
Anxiety symptoms	4%	5%	3%	7%
Depressive disorders	4%	6%	3%	5%
Disturbances in consciousness	4%	5%	3%	6%
Disturbances in initiating and maintaining sleep	8%	11%	5%	10%
Dizziness/Postural dizziness	9%	13%	8%	17%
Paresthesias and dysesthesias	5%	7%	3%	6%
Peripheral neuropathies	4%	5%	3%	6%
Sensory abnormalities	4%	6%	1%	3%
Dermatologic				
Apocrine and eccrine gland disorders	5%	7%	4%	7.5%
Erythemas	2%	3%	1%	2%
Folliculitis	4%	5%	2%	4%
Lipodystrophies	3%	5%	0.5%	1%
Pruritus	4%	5%	2%	4%
Rash	11%	16%	5%	11%
Skin neoplasms benign	3%	4%	1%	3%
GI				
Appetite disorders	8%	11%	7%	13%
Constipation	6%	9%	3%	6%
GU				
Anogenital warts	2%	3%	1%	3%
Bladder and urethral symptoms	5%	7%	1%	3%
Urinary tract signs and symptoms	3%	4%	1%	3%
Musculoskeletal				
Joint-related signs and symptoms	7%	10%	3%	5%
Muscle pains	3%	4%	0.5%	1%
Respiratory				
Breathing abnormalities	4%	5%	2%	5%
Bronchitis	7%	9%	5%	9%
Coughing and associated symptoms	14%	21%	5%	10%
Nasal congestion and inflammations	4%	6%	3%	5%
Paranasal sinus disorders	3%	4%	0.5%	1%
Pneumonia	2%	3%	5%	10%
Sinusitis	7%	10%	3%	6%
Upper respiratory tract infection	23%	37%	13%	27%
Upper respiratory tract signs and symptoms	6%	9%	3%	6%
Special senses				
Conjunctivitis	2%	3%	1%	3%
Ocular infections, inflammation, and associated manifestations	2%	3%	1%	2%
Otitis media	2%	3%	0.5%	1%
Miscellaneous				
Herpes infection	8%	11%	4%	8%
Influenza	2%	3%	0.5%	1%
Pain and discomfort	4%	5%	3%	5%
Pyrexia	13%	20%	9%	17%

MARAVIROC — ORAL

Maraviroc Adverse Reactions (≥ 2%) in Treatment-Experienced Patients				
Adverse reactions	Maraviroc twice daily[a] (n = 426)	Exposure-adjusted rate (per 100 patient-years) PYE[b] = 309	Placebo (n = 209)	Exposure-adjusted rate (per 100 patient-years) PYE = 111
Vascular hypertensive disorders	3%	4%	2%	4%

[a] 300 mg dose equivalent.
[b] PYE = patient-years of exposure.

Maraviroc Grade 3 to 4 Laboratory Abnormalities (≥ 2%) in Treatment-Experienced Patients[a,b]			
Laboratory parameter	Limit	Maraviroc twice daily + OBT (n = 421)	Placebo + OBT (n = 207)
AST	> 5 × ULN[b]	4.8%	2.9%
ALT	> 5 × ULN[b]	2.6%	3.4%
Total bilirubin	> 5 × ULN[b]	5.5%	5.3%
Amylase	> 2 × ULN[b]	5.7%	5.8%
Lipase	> 2 × ULN[b]	4.9%	6.3%
Absolute neutrophil count	< 750/mm³	4.3%	2.4%

[a] Percentages based on total patients evaluated for each laboratory parameter.
[b] OBT = optimized background therapy; ULN = upper limit of normal.

➤*Treatment-naive patients:*

Maraviroc Adverse Reactions (≥ 2%) in Treatment-Naive Patients		
Adverse reactions	Maraviroc + zidovudine/ lamivudine 300 mg twice daily (n = 360)	Efavirenz + zidovudine/ lamivudine 600 mg once daily (n = 361)
CNS		
Memory loss (excluding dementia)	3%	1%
Parasthesias and dyesthesias	4%	3%
Dermatologic		
Acne	3%	2%
Alopecias	2%	1%
Lipodystrophies	4%	3%
Nail and nail bed conditions (excluding infections and infestations)	6%	2%
GI		
Flatulence, bloating, and distention	10%	7%
GI atonic and hypomotility disorders NEC[a]	9%	5%
GI signs and symptoms NEC	3%	2%
GU		
Bladder and urethral symptoms	4%	3%
Erection and ejaculation conditions and disorders	3%	2%
Hematologic		
Anemias NEC	8%	5%
Neutropenias	4%	3%
Respiratory		
Bronchitis	13%	9%
Lower respiratory tract and lung infections	3%	2%
Upper respiratory tract infection	32%	30%
Upper respiratory tract signs and symptoms	9%	5%
Miscellaneous		
Bacterial infections NEC	6%	3%
Body temperature perception	3%	1%
Ear disorders NEC	3%	2%
Herpes infection	7%	6%
Herpes zoster/varicella	5%	4%
Joint-related signs and symptoms	6%	5%
Neisseria infections	3%	0%
Tinea infections	4%	3%
Viral infections NEC	3%	2%

[a] NEC = not elsewhere classified.

➤*Lab test abnormalities:*

Maraviroc Grade 3 to 4 Lab Test Abnormalities (≥ 2%) in Treatment-Naive Patients[a]			
Laboratory parameter	Limit	Maraviroc 300 twice daily + zidovudine/ lamivudine (n = 353)[b]	Efavirenz 600 mg once daily + zidovudine/ lamivudine (n = 350)[b]
AST	> 5× ULN	4%	4%
ALT	> 5× ULN	3.9%	4%
Creatine kinase		3.9%	4.8%
Amylase	> 2× ULN	4.3%	6%
Absolute neutrophil count	< 750/mm³	5.7%	4.9%
Hemoglobin	< 7 g/dL	2.9%	2.3%

[a] Percentages based on total patients evaluated for each laboratory parameter. If the same subject in a given treatment group has > 1 occurrence of the same abnormality, only the most severe is counted.
[b] n = total number of patients evaluable for laboratory abnormalities.

➤*Cardiovascular:* Acute cardiac failure, cerebrovascular accident, coronary artery disease, coronary artery occlusion, endocarditis, myocardial infarction, myocardial ischemia, unstable angina.

➤*CNS:* Convulsions and epilepsy, facial palsy, hemianopia, loss of consciousness, meningitis, tremor (excluding congenital), viral meningitis, visual field defect.

➤*Dermatologic:* Basal cell carcinoma, squamous cell carcinoma of skin.

➤*GI:* Abdominal neoplasm, anal cancer, *Clostridium difficile*, colitis, esophageal carcinoma, tongue neoplasm (malignant stage unspecified).

➤*Hematologic:* Hypoplastic anemia, marrow depression.

➤*Hepatic:* Bile duct neoplasms malignant, cholestatic jaundice, hepatic cirrhosis, hepatic failure, hypertransaminasemia, jaundice, metastases to liver, portal vein thrombosis.

➤*Musculoskeletal:* Blood creatine kinase increased, myositis, osteonecrosis, rhabdomyolysis.

➤*Respiratory:* Pneumonia.

➤*Miscellaneous:* Anaplastic large cell lymphomas T- and null-cell type, Bowen disease, cholangiocarcinoma, diffuse large B-cell lymphoma, endocrine neoplasms malignant and unspecified, infective myositis, lymphoma, nasopharyngeal carcinoma, septic shock, squamous cell carcinoma, treponemal infections.

➤*Postmarketing:* Stevens-Johnson syndrome.

Overdosage

➤*Symptoms:* The highest dose administered in clinical studies was 1,200 mg. The dose-limiting adverse reaction was postural hypotension, which was observed at 600 mg. While the recommended dosage for maraviroc in patients receiving a CYP3A inducer without a CYP3A inhibitor is 600 mg twice daily, this dose is appropriate because of enhanced metabolism.

Prolongation of the QT interval was seen in dogs and monkeys at plasma concentrations 6 and 12 times, respectively, those expected in humans at the intended exposure of 300 mg equivalents twice daily. However, no significant QT prolongation was seen in the studies in treatment-experienced patients with HIV using the recommended doses of maraviroc or in a specific pharmacokinetic study to evaluate the potential of maraviroc to prolong the QT interval.

➤*Treatment:* There is no specific antidote for overdose with maraviroc. Treatment of overdose should consist of general supportive measures, including keeping the patient in a supine position and careful assessment of patient vital signs, blood pressure, and electrocardiogram.

If indicated, achieve elimination of unabsorbed active maraviroc by gastric lavage. Administration of activated charcoal may also be used to aid in removal of unabsorbed drug. Because maraviroc is moderately protein bound, dialysis may be beneficial in the removal of this medicine.

Patient Information

Inform patients that if they develop signs or symptoms of hepatitis or allergic reaction (eg, abdominal pain, dark urine, rash, yellow-looking eyes or skin, vomiting) following use of maraviroc, they should discontinue maraviroc and immediately seek medical evaluation.

Cellular Chemokine Receptor (CCR5) Antagonist

MARAVIROC — ORAL

Inform patients that maraviroc is not a cure for HIV infection, and patients may still develop illnesses associated with HIV infection, including opportunistic infections. The use of maraviroc has not been shown to reduce the risk of transmission of HIV to others through sexual contact, sharing needles, or blood contamination.

Advise patients that it is important to remain under the care of a health care provider when using maraviroc and to take maraviroc every day as prescribed and in combination with other antiretroviral drugs. Advise patients to report to their health care provider the use of any other prescription or nonprescription medication or herbal products. Inform patients to tell their health care provider if they are pregnant, are planning to become pregnant, or become pregnant while taking maraviroc. Inform patients not to change the dose or dosing schedule of maraviroc or any antiretroviral medication without consulting their health care provider.

Advise patients that if they forget to take a dose, they should take the next dose of maraviroc as soon as possible and then take their next scheduled dose at its regular time. If it is less than 6 hours before their next scheduled dose, they should not take the missed dose and should instead wait and take the next dose at the regular time.

Use caution when administering maraviroc in patients with a history of postural hypotension or on concomitant medication known to lower blood pressure. Advise patients that if they experience dizziness while taking maraviroc, they should avoid driving or operating machinery.

Integrase Inhibitors

RALTEGRAVIR

Rx	**Isentress** (Merck)	**Tablets; oral:** 400 mg	Equiv. to raltegravir potassium 434.4 mg. Lactose. (227). Pink, oval. Film-coated. In 60s.

RALTEGRAVIR POTASSIUM — ORAL

Indications

➤*HIV infection:* In combination with other antiretroviral agents for the treatment of HIV-1 infection in adult patients.

Administration and Dosage

➤*General dosing considerations:* The use of other active agents with raltegravir is associated with a greater likelihood of treatment response.

➤*Adults:*

HIV infection –

Usual dosage: 400 mg twice daily.

Concomitant therapy: During coadministration with rifampin, the recommended dosage of raltegravir is 800 mg twice daily.

➤*Renal function impairment:* Because the extent to which raltegravir may be dialyzable is unknown, dosing before a dialysis session should be avoided.

➤*Administration:* Administer orally with or without food.

➤*Storage/Stability:* Store at 20° to 25°C (68° to 77°F); excursions are permitted between 15° and 30°C (59° and 86°F).

Actions

➤*Pharmacology:* Raltegravir, an HIV-1 antiviral drug, is an HIV integrase strand transfer inhibitor. Raltegravir inhibits the catalytic activity of HIV-1 integrase, an HIV-1 encoded enzyme that is required for viral replication. Inhibition of integrase prevents the covalent insertion or integration of unintegrated linear HIV-1 DNA into the host cell genome, preventing the formation of the HIV-1 provirus. The provirus is required to direct the production of progeny virus, so inhibiting integration prevents propagation of the viral infection.

➤*Pharmacokinetics:*

Absorption – Raltegravir is absorbed with a time of maximal concentration (T_{max}) of approximately 3 hours postdose in the fasted state. Raltegravir area under the curve (AUC) and maximal drug concentration (C_{max}) increase dose proportionally over the dose range of 100 to 1,600 mg. Raltegravir plasma concentration at 12 hours (C_{12h}) increases dose proportionally over the dose range of 100 to 800 mg and increases slightly less than dose proportionally over the dose range of 100 to 1,600 mg. With twice-daily dosing, pharmacokinetic steady state is achieved within approximately the first 2 days of dosing. There is little to no accumulation in AUC and C_{max}. The average accumulation ratio for C_{12h} ranged from approximately 1.2 to 1.6.

In subjects who received 400 mg twice daily alone, raltegravir drug exposures were characterized by a geometric mean AUC_{0-12h} of 14.3 mcM•h and C_{12h} of 142 nM.

Considerable variability was observed in the pharmacokinetics of raltegravir. For observed C_{12h} in protocols 018 and 019, the coefficient of variation for intersubject variability was 212% and the coefficient of variation for intrasubject variability was 122%.

Effect of food: Raltegravir C_{12h} was 66% higher and C_{max} was 5% higher following a moderate-fat meal compared with fasting. Administration of raltegravir following a high-fat meal (825 kcal, 52 g fat) increased AUC and C_{max} by approximately 2-fold and increased C_{12h} by 4.1-fold. Administration of raltegravir following a low-fat meal (300 kcal, 2.5 g fat) decreased AUC and C_{max} by 46% and 52%, respectively. C_{12h} was essentially unchanged. Food appears to increase pharmacokinetic variability relative to fasting. Raltegravir may be administered without regard to food.

Distribution – Raltegravir is approximately 83% bound to human plasma protein over the concentration range of 2 to 10 mcM.

Metabolism/Excretion – The apparent terminal half-life of raltegravir is approximately 9 hours, with a shorter alpha-phase half-life (approximately 1 hour) accounting for much of the AUC. Following administration of an oral dose of radiolabeled raltegravir, approximately 51% and 32% of the dose was excreted in feces and urine, respectively. In feces, only raltegravir was present, most of which is likely derived from hydrolysis of raltegravir-glucuronide secreted in bile, as observed in preclinical species. Two components, namely raltegravir and raltegravir-glucuronide, were detected in urine and accounted for approximately 9% and 23% of the dose, respectively. The major circulating entity was raltegravir and represented approximately 70% of the total radioactivity; the remaining radioactivity in plasma was accounted for by raltegravir-glucuronide. Studies using isoform-selective chemical inhibitors and cDNA-expressed UDP-glucuronosyltransferases (UGT) show that UGT1A1 is the main enzyme responsible for the formation of raltegravir-glucuronide. Thus, the data indicate that the major mechanism of clearance of raltegravir in humans is UGT1A1-mediated glucuronidation.

Contraindications

None well documented.

Warnings/Precautions

➤*Immune reconstitution syndrome:* During the initial phase of treatment, patients responding to antiretroviral therapy may develop an inflammatory response to indolent or residual opportunistic infections (such as *Mycobacterium avium* complex, cytomegalovirus, *Pneumocystis jiroveci* pneumonia, *Mycobacterium* tuberculosis, or reactivation of varicella zoster virus), which may necessitate further evaluation and treatment.

➤*Pregnancy: Category C.* Use raltegravir during pregnancy only if the potential benefit justifies the potential risk to the fetus. There are no adequate and well-controlled studies in pregnant women. In addition, there have been no pharmacokinetic studies conducted in pregnant patients.

Treatment-related increases over controls in the incidence of supernumerary ribs were seen in rats at 600 mg/kg/day (exposures 3-fold the exposure at the recommended human dose).

Placenta transfer of drug was demonstrated in both rats and rabbits. At a maternal dosage of 600 mg/kg/day in rats, mean drug concentrations in fetal plasma were approximately 1.5- to 2.5-fold more than in maternal plasma at 1 and 24 hours postdose, respectively. Mean drug concentrations in fetal plasma were approximately 2% of the mean maternal concentration at both 1 and 24 hours postdose at a maternal dosage of 1,000 mg/kg/day in rabbits.

Antiretroviral pregnancy registry – To monitor maternal-fetal outcomes of pregnant patients exposed to raltegravir, an antiretroviral pregnancy registry has been established. Health care providers are encouraged to register patients by calling 1-800-258-4263.

➤*Lactation:* Breast-feeding is not recommended while taking raltegravir. In addition, it is recommended that HIV-infected mothers not breast-feed their infants to avoid risking postnatal transmission of HIV.

It is not known whether raltegravir is secreted in human milk. However, raltegravir is secreted in the milk of lactating rats. Mean drug concentrations in milk were approximately 3-fold greater than those in maternal plasma at a maternal dosage of 600 mg/kg/day in rats. There were no effects in rat offspring attributable to exposure of raltegravir through the milk.

➤*Children:* Safety and effectiveness have not been established.

➤*Elderly:* In general, dose selection for an elderly patient should be cautious, reflecting the greater frequency of decreased hepatic, renal, or cardiac function, and of concomitant disease or other drug therapy.

➤*Monitoring:* Monitor CD4+ cell count and HIV RNA load.

Drug Interactions

➤*UGT1A1:* Raltegravir is eliminated mainly via UGT1A1-mediated glucuronidation pathway. Coadministration of raltegravir with drugs that inhibit UGT1A1 may increase plasma levels of raltegravir.

Raltegravir Drug Interactions

Precipitant drug	Object drug[a]		Description
Atazanavir	Raltegravir	↑	Atazanavir, a strong inhibitor of UGT1A1, increases plasma concentrations of raltegravir. No dose adjustment is recommended. Monitor the response of the patient.

RALTEGRAVIR POTASSIUM — ORAL

Raltegravir Drug Interactions			
Precipitant drug	Object drug[a]		Description
Atazanavir/ Ritonavir	Raltegravir	↑	Atazanavir/ritonavir increases plasma concentrations of raltegravir. No dose adjustment is recommended. Monitor the response of the patient.
Efavirenz	Raltegravir	↓	Efavirenz reduces plasma concentrations of raltegravir. The clinical importance is not known. Monitor the response of the patient.
Etravirine	Raltegravir	↓	Etravirine reduces plasma concentrations of raltegravir. The clinical importance is not known. Monitor the response of the patient.
Omeprazole	Raltegravir	↑	Coadministration of medications that increase gastric pH may increase raltegravir levels based on increased raltegravir solubility at higher pH. No dose adjustment is recommended. Monitor the response of the patient.
Rifampin	Raltegravir	↓	Rifampin, a strong inducer of UGT1A1, reduces plasma concentrations of raltegravir. The recommended dosage of raltegravir is 800 mg twice daily during coadministration with rifampin. Coadminister with caution.
Tipranavir/ Ritonavir	Raltegravir	↓	Tipranavir/ritonavir reduces plasma concentrations of raltegravir. No dose adjustment is recommended. Monitor the response of the patient.

[a] ↑ = object drug increased; ↓ = object drug decreased.

➤*Drug/Food interactions:* See Actions.

Adverse Reactions

➤*Treatment-naive:*

Discontinuation – In protocol 021, the rate of discontinuation of therapy because of adverse reactions was 3% in subjects receiving raltegravir + emtricitabine (+) tenofovir and 6% in subjects receiving efavirenz + emtricitabine (+) tenofovir.

Adverse reactions (at least 2%) –

Raltegravir Adverse Reactions[a,b] in Treatment-Naive Adult Patients (≥ 2%)		
	Randomized study protocol 021	
Adverse reactions	Raltegravir 400 mg twice daily + emtricitabine (+) tenofovir (n = 281)	Efavirenz 600 mg at bedtime + emtricitabine (+) tenofovir (n = 282)
CNS		
Insomnia	4%	3%

[a] Includes adverse experiences considered by investigators to be at least possibly, probably, or definitely related to the drug.
[b] Intensities are defined as follows: moderate (discomfort enough to cause, interference with usual activity); severe (incapacitating with inability to do work or do usual activity).

CNS – Abnormal dreams, fatigue (less than 2%).

➤*Treatment-experienced:*

Discontinuation – The rates of discontinuation because of adverse reactions were 2% in subjects receiving raltegravir and 3% in subjects receiving placebo.

Adverse reactions (at least 2%) –

Raltegravir Adverse Reactions in Treatment-Experienced Patients (≥ 2%)[a,b]		
	Randomized studies, protocol 018 and 019	
	Raltegravir 400 mg twice daily + optimized background therapy (n = 462)	Placebo + optimized background therapy (n = 237)
Adverse reactions	Rate per 100 patient-years	Rate per 100 patient-years
CNS		
Asthenia	2	1
Fatigue	2	1
Headache	3	1
GI		
Nausea	2	1

[a] Includes adverse reactions at least possibly, probably, or definitely related to the drug.
[b] Intensities are defined as follows: moderate (discomfort enough to cause interference with usual activity); severe (incapacitating with inability to work or do usual activity).

Other adverse reactions (less than 2%) –

GI: Abdominal pain, gastritis (less than 2%).
GU: Genital herpes, renal failure (less than 2%).
Miscellaneous: Dizziness, hepatitis, herpes zoster, hypersensitivity (less than 2%).

Cancers – Cancers were reported in treatment-experienced subjects who initiated raltegravir or placebo, both with optimized background therapy, and in treatment-naive subjects who initiated raltegravir or efavirenz, both with emtricitabine (+) tenofovir; several were recurrent. The types and rates of specific cancers were those expected in a highly immunodeficient population (many had CD4+ cell counts below 50 cells/mm^3 and most had prior AIDS diagnoses). The risk of developing cancer in these studies was similar in the group receiving raltegravir and the group receiving the comparator.

Myopathy/Rhabdomyolysis – Grades 2 to 4 creatine kinase laboratory abnormalities were observed in subjects treated with raltegravir. Myopathy and rhabdomyolysis have been reported; however, the relationship of raltegravir to these adverse reactions is not known. Use with caution in patients at increased risk of myopathy or rhabdomyolysis, such as patients receiving concomitant medications known to cause these conditions.

➤*Hepatitis B and/or hepatitis C coinfection:* In the randomized, double-blind, placebo-controlled trials, treatment-experienced subjects (16%) and treatment-naive subjects (6%) with chronic (but not acute) active HBV and/or HCV coinfection (16%) were permitted to enroll provided that baseline liver function tests did not exceed 5 times the upper limit of normal (ULN). In general, the safety profile of raltegravir in subjects with HBV and/or HCV coinfection was similar to subjects without HBV and/or HCV coinfection; although, the rates of AST and ALT abnormalities were higher in the subgroup with HBV and/or HCV coinfection for all treatment groups. In treatment-experienced subjects, grade 2 or higher laboratory abnormalities that represent a worsening grade from baseline of AST, ALT, or total bilirubin level occurred in 25%, 31%, and 12%, respectively, of raltegravir-treated coinfected subjects, compared with 8%, 7%, and 8% of all other raltegravir-treated subjects. In treatment-naive subjects, grade 2 or higher laboratory abnormalities that represent a worsening grade from baseline of AST, ALT, or total bilirubin occurred in 17%, 22%, and 11%, respectively, of coinfected subjects treated with raltegravir as compared with 4%, 4%, and 3% of all other subjects treated with raltegravir.

➤*Laboratory abnormalities:*

Treatment-naive –

Raltegravir Laboratory Abnormalities in Treatment-Naive Patients			
		Randomized study protocol 021	
Laboratory abnormality	Limit	Raltegravir 400 mg twice daily + emtricitabine (+) tenofovir (n = 281)	Efavirenz 600 mg at bedtime + emtricitabine (+) tenofovir (n = 282)
Hematology			
ANC[a] (10^3/mcL)			
Grade 2	0.75 to 0.999	3%	3%
Grade 3	0.5 to 0.749	1%	< 1%
Grade 4	< 0.5	< 1%	0%
Hemoglobin (g/dL)			
Grade 2	7.5 to 8.4	< 1%	< 1%
Grade 3	6.5 to 7.4	< 1%	< 1%
Grade 4	< 6.5	0%	0%
Platelet count (10^3/mcL)			
Grade 2	50 to 99.999	2%	0%
Grade 3	25 to 49.999	0%	< 1%
Grade 4	< 25	0%	0%

RALTEGRAVIR POTASSIUM — ORAL

Raltegravir Laboratory Abnormalities in Treatment-Naive Patients

		Randomized study protocol 021	
Laboratory abnormality	Limit	Raltegravir 400 mg twice daily + emtricitabine (+) tenofovir (n = 281)	Efavirenz 600 mg at bedtime + emtricitabine (+) tenofovir (n = 282)
Blood chemistry			
Fasting (nonrandom) serum glucose test (mg/dL)			
Grade 2	126 to 250	2%	3%
Grade 3	251 to 500	< 1%	0%
Grade 4	> 500	0%	0%
Total serum bilirubin			
Grade 2	1.6 to 2.5 × ULN	4%	0%
Grade 3	2.6 to 5 × ULN	< 1%	0%
Grade 4	> 5 × ULN	0%	0%
Serum AST			
Grade 2	2.6 to 5 × ULN	3%	4%
Grade 3	5.1 to 10 × ULN	1%	1%
Grade 4	> 10 × ULN	< 1%	< 1%
Serum ALT			
Grade 2	2.6 to 5 × ULN	4%	6%
Grade 3	5.1 to 10 × ULN	< 1%	2%
Grade 4	> 10 × ULN	< 1%	< 1%
Serum alkaline phosphatase			
Grade 2	2.6 to 5 × ULN	< 1%	2%
Grade 3	5.1 to 10 × ULN	0%	< 1%
Grade 4	> 10 × ULN	0%	0%

[a] ANC = absolute neutrophil count.

Lipids –

Raltegravir Lipid Values (Protocol 021)[a,b]

	Raltegravir 400 mg twice daily + emtricitabine (+) tenofovir (n = 281)			Efavirenz 600 mg + emtricitabine (+) tenofovir (n = 282)		
			Change from baseline at week 48			Change from baseline at week 48
Laboratory abnormality	Baseline mean (mg/dL)	Week 48 mean (mg/dL)	Mean change (mg/dL)	Baseline mean (mg/dL)	Week 48 mean (mg/dL)	Mean change (mg/dL)
LDL cholesterol[c]	97	103	6	92	108	16
HDL cholesterol[c]	38	42	4	38	48	10
Total cholesterol[c]	159	169	10	156	188	33
Triglyceride[c]	125	122	−3	136	174	37

[a] If subjects initiated or increased serum lipid-reducing agents, the last available lipid values prior to the change in therapy were used in the analysis. If the missing data was because of other reasons, subjects were censored thereafter for the analysis.At baseline, serum lipid-reducing agents were used in 5% of subjects in the group receiving raltegravir and 3% in the efavirenz group. Through week 48, serum lipid-reducing agents were used in 6% of subjects in the group receiving raltegravir and 6% in the efavirenz group.
[b] LDL = low-density lipoprotein; HDL = high-density lipoprotein.
[c] Fasting (nonrandom) laboratory tests.

Treatment-experienced –

Raltegravir Laboratory Abnormalities in Treatment-Experienced Patients

		Randomized studies, protocol 018 and 019	
Laboratory abnormality	Limit	Raltegravir 400 mg twice daily + optimized background therapy (n = 462)	Placebo + optimized background therapy (n = 237)
Hematology			
ANC (10^3/mcL)			
Grade 2	0.75 to 0.999	3%	5%
Grade 3	0.5 to 0.749	3%	3%
Grade 4	< 0.5	1%	< 1%
Hemoglobin (g/dL)			
Grade 2	7.5 to 8.4	1%	3%
Grade 3	6.5 to 7.4	1%	< 1%
Grade 4	< 6.5	< 1%	0%
Platelet count (10^3/mcL)			
Grade 2	50 to 99.999	3%	5%
Grade 3	25 to 49.999	1%	< 1%
Grade 4	< 25	1%	< 1%
Blood chemistry			
Fasting (nonrandom) serum glucose test (mg/dL)			
Grade 2	126 to 250	8%	5%
Grade 3	251 to 500	2%	1%
Grade 4	> 500	0%	0%
Total serum bilirubin			
Grade 2	1.6 to 2.5 × ULN	5%	3%
Grade 3	2.6 to 5 × ULN	2%	2%
Grade 4	> 5 × ULN	1%	0%
AST			
Grade 2	2.6 to 5 × ULN	8%	6%
Grade 3	5.1 to 10 × ULN	3%	3%
Grade 4	> 10 × ULN	< 1%	1%
ALT			
Grade 2	2.6 to 5 × ULN	7%	8%
Grade 3	5.1 to 10 × ULN	3%	2%
Grade 4	> 10 × ULN	1%	1%
Serum alkaline phosphatase			
Grade 2	2.6 to 5 × ULN	2%	< 1%
Grade 3	5.1 to 10 × ULN	< 1%	1%
Grade 4	> 10 × ULN	1%	< 1%
Serum pancreatic amylase test			
Grade 2	1.6 to 2 × ULN	2%	1%
Grade 3	2.1 to 5 × ULN	3%	3%
Grade 4	> 5 × ULN	< 1%	0%
Serum lipase test			
Grade 2	1.6 to 3 × ULN	4%	3%
Grade 3	3.1 to 5 × ULN	1%	< 1%
Grade 4	> 5 × ULN	0%	0%
Serum creatine kinase			
Grade 2	6 to 9.9 × ULN	2%	2%
Grade 3	10 to 19.9 × ULN	3%	3%
Grade 4	≥ 20 × ULN	2%	1%

➤*Postmarketing:*

CNS – Anxiety; depression (particularly in patients with a preexisting history of psychiatric illness), including suicidal ideation and behaviors; paranoia.

Dermatologic – Rash, Stevens-Johnson syndrome.

Overdosage

Patient Information

Inform patients that raltegravir is not a cure for HIV infection or AIDS. Also tell them that people taking raltegravir may still get infections or other conditions common in people with HIV (opportunistic infections). In addition, tell patients that it is very important to remain under a health care provider's care during treatment with raltegravir.

Integrase Inhibitors

RALTEGRAVIR POTASSIUM — ORAL

Inform patients that raltegravir does not reduce the chance of passing HIV to others through sexual contact, shared needles, or exposure to blood. Advise patients to continue to practice safer sex and to use latex or polyurethane condoms or other barrier methods to lower the chance of sexual contact with any body fluids, such as semen, vaginal secretions, or blood. Also advise patients to never reuse or share needles.

Instruct patients that if they miss a dose, they should take it as soon as they remember. If they do not remember until it is time for the next dose, instruct them to skip the missed dose and go back to the regular schedule. Patients should not take 2 tablets of raltegravir at the same time.

Instruct patients to read the patient package insert before starting raltegravir therapy and to reread it each time the prescription is renewed. Instruct patients to inform their health care provider or pharmacist if they develop any unusual symptom, or if any known symptom persists or worsens.

Fusion Inhibitors

ENFUVIRTIDE

Rx	Fuzeon (Hoffman-La Roche)	**Powder for injection, lyophilized:** 108 mg (≈ 90 mg/mL when reconstituted)	Preservative-free. Convenience Kit contains: Single-use vials, syringes, diluent, and alcohol wipes.

ENFUVIRTIDE — INJECTION

Indications

➤*HIV infection:* In combination with other antiretroviral agents, for the treatment of HIV-1 infection in treatment-experienced patients with evidence of HIV-1 replication despite ongoing antiretroviral therapy.

Administration and Dosage

➤*Adults:*

HIV infection – 90 mg (1 mL) twice daily injected subcutaneously into the upper arm, anterior thigh, or abdomen.

➤*Children:*

HIV infection –

16 years of age and older: See Adults for dosing.

6 to 16 years of age:

• *Usual dosage* – 2 mg/kg (up to 90 mg) twice daily injected subcutaneously into the upper arm, anterior thigh, or abdomen.

The following table contains dosing guidelines for enfuvirtide based on body weight. Weight should be monitored periodically and the enfuvirtide dose adjusted accordingly.

Enfuvirtide Pediatric Dosing Guidelines

Weight		Dose per twice daily injection (mg/dose)	Injection volume (enfuvirtide 90 mg/mL)
kg	Pounds		
≥ 42.6	> 94	90	1 mL
38.1 to 42.5	> 84 to 94	81	0.9 mL
33.6 to 38	> 74 to 84	72	0.8 mL
29.1 to 33.5	> 64 to 74	63	0.7 mL
24.6 to 29	> 54 to 64	54	0.6 mL
20.1 to 24.5	> 44 to 54	45	0.5 mL
15.6 to 20	> 34 to 44	36	0.4 mL
11 to 15.5	24 to 34	27	0.3 mL

• *Maximum dose* – 90 mg twice daily.

➤*Preparation for administration:* Enfuvirtide must be reconstituted only with 1.1 mL of sterile water for injection. After adding sterile water, the vial should be gently tapped for 10 seconds and then gently rolled between the hands to avoid foaming and to ensure all particles of the drug are in contact with the liquid and no drug remains on the vial wall. The vial should then be allowed to stand until the powder goes completely into solution, which could take up to 45 minutes. Reconstitution time can be reduced by gently rolling the vial between the hands until the product is completely dissolved. Before the solution is withdrawn for administration, the vial should be inspected visually to ensure that the contents are fully dissolved in the solution and that the solution is clear, colorless, and without bubbles or particulate matter. If there is evidence of particulate matter, the vial must not be used and should be returned to the pharmacy.

Enfuvirtide contains no preservatives. Once reconstituted, enfuvirtide should be injected immediately or kept refrigerated in the original vial until use. Reconstituted enfuvirtide must be used within 24 hours. The subsequent dose of enfuvirtide can be reconstituted in advance and must be stored in the refrigerator in the original vial and used within 24 hours. Refrigerated reconstituted solution should be brought to room temperature before injection, and the vial should be inspected visually again to ensure that the contents are fully dissolved in solution and that the solution is clear, colorless, and without bubbles or particulate matter.

➤*Administration:* The reconstituted solution should be injected subcutaneously in the upper arm, abdomen, or anterior thigh. The injection should be given at a site different from the preceding injection site and only where there is no current injection-site reaction. Also, do not inject into moles, scar tissue, bruises, or the navel. A vial is suitable for single use only; unused portions must be discarded.

➤*Storage/Stability:* Store at 25°C (77°F); excursions permitted to 15° to 30°C (59° to 86°F). Reconstituted solution should be stored under refrigeration at 2° to 8°C (36° to 46°F) and used within 24 hours.

Actions

➤*Pharmacology:* Enfuvirtide interferes with the entry of HIV-1 into cells by inhibiting fusion of viral and cellular membranes. Enfuvirtide binds to the first heptad-repeat (HR1) in the gp41 subunit of the viral envelope glycoprotein and prevents the conformational changes required for the fusion of viral and cellular membranes.

➤*Pharmacokinetics:*

Absorption – The pharmacokinetic properties of enfuvirtide were evaluated in HIV-1 infected adult and pediatric patients. Following a 90 mg single SC injection of enfuvirtide into the abdomen in 12 HIV-1 infected subjects, the mean (± SD) C_{max} was 4.59 ± 1.5 mcg/mL, the AUC was 55.8 ± 12.1 mcg•hr/mL, and the median t_{max} was 8 hours (range from 3 to 12 hours). The absolute bioavailability (using a 90 mg IV dose as a reference) was 84.3% ± 15.5%. Following 90 mg twice-daily dosing of enfuvirtide SC in combination with other antiretroviral agents in 11 HIV-1 infected subjects, the mean (±SD) steady-state C_{max} was 5 ± 1.7 mcg/mL, C_{trough} was 3.3 ± 1.6 mcg/mL, $AUC_{0\text{-}12h}$ was 48.7 ± 19.1 mcg•hr/mL, and the median t_{max} was 4 hours (ranged from 4 to 8 hours).

Absorption of the 90 mg dose was comparable when injected into the SC tissue of the abdomen, thigh or arm.

Distribution – The mean (± SD) steady-state volume of distribution after IV administration of a 90 mg dose of enfuvirtide (n = 12) was 5.5 ± 1.1 L.

Enfuvirtide is approximately 92% bound to plasma proteins in HIV-infected plasma over a concentration range of 2 to 10 mcg/mL. It is bound predominantly to albumin and to a lower extent to alpha-1-acid glycoprotein.

Metabolism/Excretion – As a peptide, enfuvirtide is expected to undergo catabolism to its constituent amino acids, with subsequent recycling of the amino acids in the body pool.

Mass-balance studies to determine elimination pathway(s) of enfuvirtide have not been performed in humans.

In vitro studies with human microsomes and hepatocytes indicate that enfuvirtide undergoes hydrolysis to form a deamidated metabolite at the C-terminal phenylalanine residue, M3. The hydrolysis reaction is not NADPH dependent. The M3 metabolite is detected in human plasma following administration of enfuvirtide, with an AUC ranging from 2.4% to 15% of the enfuvirtide AUC.

Following a 90 mg single SC dose of enfuvirtide (n = 12) the mean ± SD elimination half-life of enfuvirtide is 3.8 ± 0.6 hours and the mean ± SD apparent clearance was 24.8 ± 4.1 mL/hr/kg. Following 90 mg twice-daily dosing of enfuvirtide SC in combination with other antiretroviral agents in 11 HIV-1 infected subjects, the mean ± SD apparent clearance was 30.6 ± 10.6 mL/hr/kg.

Special populations –

Children: The pharmacokinetics of enfuvirtide have been studied in 18 pediatric subjects aged 6 through 16 years at a dose of 2 mg/kg. Enfuvirtide pharmacokinetics were determined in the presence of concomitant medications including antiretroviral agents. A dose of 2 mg/kg twice daily (maximum 90 mg twice daily) provided enfuvirtide plasma concentrations similar to those obtained in adult patients receiving 90 mg twice daily.

In the 18 pediatric subjects receiving the 2 mg/kg twice-daily dose, the mean ± SD steady-state AUC was 53.6 ± 21.4 mcg•hr/mL, C_{max} was 5.9 ± 2.2 mcg/mL, C_{trough} was 3 ± 1.5 mcg/mL, and apparent clearance was 40 ± 14 mL/hr/kg.

Gender: Analysis of plasma concentration data from subjects in clinical trials indicated that the clearance of enfuvirtide is 20% lower in females than males after adjusting for body weight.

Weight: Enfuvirtide clearance decreases with decreased body weight irrespective of gender. Relative to the clearance of a 70 kg male, a 40 kg male will have 20% lower clearance and a 110 kg male will have a 26% higher clearance. Relative to a 70 kg male, a 40 kg female will have a 36% lower clearance and a 110 kg female will have the same clearance.

No dose adjustment is recommended for weight or gender.

➤*Microbiology:*

Antiviral activity in vitro – Enfuvirtide exhibited additive to synergistic effects in cell culture assays when combined with individual members of various antiretroviral classes, including zidovudine, lamivudine, nelfinavir, indinavir, and efavirenz.

Drug resistance – In clinical trials, HIV-1 isolates with reduced susceptibility to enfuvirtide have been recovered from subjects treated with enfuvirtide in combination with other antiretroviral agents. Posttreatment HIV-1 virus from 185 subjects exhibited decreases in susceptibility to enfuvirtide ranging from 4- to 422-fold relative to their respective baseline virus and exhibited genotypic changes in gp41 amino acids 36 to 45. Substitutions

ENFUVIRTIDE — INJECTION

in this region were observed with decreasing frequency at amino acid positions 38, 43, 36, 40, 42, and 45.

Cross-resistance: HIV-1 clinical isolates resistant to nucleoside analogue reverse transcriptase inhibitors (NRTI), nonnucleoside analogue reverse transcriptase inhibitors (NNRTI), and protease inhibitors (PI) were susceptible to enfuvirtide in cell culture.

Contraindications

Hypersensitivity to enfuvirtide or any of its components.

Warnings/Precautions

➤*Local injection-site reactions:* The most common adverse reactions associated with enfuvirtide use are local injection site reactions. Manifestations may include pain and discomfort, induration, erythema, nodules and cysts, pruritus, and ecchymosis. Nine percent (9%) of patients had local reactions that required analgesics or limited usual activities. Reactions are often present at more than 1 injection site. Patients must be familiar with the enfuvirtide injection instructions in order to know how to inject enfuvirtide appropriately and how to monitor carefully for signs or symptoms of cellulitis or local infection.

➤*Pneumonia:* An increased rate of bacterial pneumonia was observed in subjects treated with enfuvirtide in the phase 3 clinical trials compared to the control arm. It is unclear if the increased incidence of pneumonia is related to enfuvirtide use. However, because of this finding, patients with HIV infection should be carefully monitored for signs and symptoms of pneumonia, especially if they have underlying conditions which may predispose them to pneumonia. Risk factors for pneumonia included low initial CD4 cell count, high initial viral load, IV drug use, smoking, and a history of lung disease.

➤*Hypersensitivity reactions:* Hypersensitivity reactions have been associated with enfuvirtide therapy and may recur on rechallenge. Hypersensitivity reactions have included the following, individually and in combination: Rash, fever, nausea and vomiting, chills, rigors, hypotension, and elevated serum liver transaminases. Other adverse reactions that may be immune mediated and have been reported in subjects receiving enfuvirtide include primary immune complex reaction, respiratory distress glomerulonephritis, and Guillain-Barre syndrome. Patients developing signs and symptoms suggestive of a systemic hypersensitivity reaction should discontinue enfuvirtide and should seek medical evaluation immediately. Therapy with enfuvirtide should not be restarted following systemic signs and symptoms consistent with a hypersensitivity reaction. Risk factors that may predict the occurrence or severity of hypersensitivity to enfuvirtide have not been identified.

➤*Hazardous tasks:* Patients should be advised that no studies have been conducted on the ability to drive or operate machinery while taking enfuvirtide. If patients experience dizziness while taking enfuvirtide, they should be advised to talk to their healthcare providers before driving or operating machinery.

➤*Pregnancy: Category B.* There are no adequate and well-controlled studies in pregnant women. Because animal reproduction studies are not always predictive of human response, this drug should be used during pregnancy only if clearly needed.

Antiretroviral pregnancy registry – To monitor maternal-fetal outcomes of pregnant women exposed to enfuvirtide and other antiretroviral drugs, an antiretroviral pregnancy registry has been established.

➤*Lactation:* The Centers for Disease Control and Prevention recommends that HIV-infected mothers not breastfeed their infants to avoid the risk of postnatal transmission of HIV. It is not known whether enfuvirtide is excreted in human milk. Because of both the potential for HIV transmission and the potential for serious adverse reactions in nursing infants, mothers should be instructed not to breastfeed if they are receiving enfuvirtide.

Studies where radiolabeled ^{3}H-enfuvirtide was administered to lactating rats indicated that radioactivity was present in the milk. It is not known whether the radioactivity in the milk was from radiolabeled enfuvirtide or from radiolabeled metabolites of enfuvirtide (ie, amino acids and peptide fragments).

➤*Children:* The safety and pharmacokinetics of enfuvirtide have not been established in pediatric subjects below 6 years of age. Limited efficacy data is available in pediatric subjects 6 years of age and older.

Thirty-five HIV-1 infected pediatric subjects ages 6 through 16 years have received enfuvirtide in 2 open-label, single-arm clinical trials. Adverse experiences were similar to those observed in adult patients.

➤*Elderly:* Clinical studies of enfuvirtide did not include sufficient numbers of subjects aged 65 years of age and over to determine whether they respond differently from younger subjects.

Drug Interactions

➤*Drug/Lab test interactions:* There is a theoretical risk that enfuvirtide use may lead to the production of antienfuvirtide antibodies which cross react with HIV gp41. This could result in a false-positive HIV test with an ELISA assay; a confirmatory western blot test would be expected to be negative. Enfuvirtide has not been studied in non-HIV-infected individuals.

Adverse Reactions

➤*Hypersensitivity:* Hypersensitivity reactions have been attributed to enfuvirtide (less than or equal to 1%) and in some cases have recurred upon rechallenge.

➤*Local:* Local injection-site reactions were the most frequent adverse events associated with the use of enfuvirtide. In phase 3 clinical studies (T20-301 and T20-302), 98% of subjects had at least 1 local injection site reaction (ISR). Three percent (3%) of subjects discontinued treatment with enfuvirtide because of ISRs. Eighty-six percent (86%) of subjects experienced their first ISR during the initial week of treatment. The majority of ISRs were associated with mild-to-moderate pain at the injection site, erythema, induration, and the presence of nodules or cysts. For most subjects the severity of signs and symptoms associated with ISRs did not change during the 24 weeks of treatment. In 17% of subjects an individual ISR lasted for longer than 7 days. Because of the frequency and duration of individual ISRs, 23% of subjects had 6 or more ongoing ISRs at any given time. Individual signs and symptoms characterizing local ISRs are summarized in the following table. Infection at the injection site (including abscess and cellulitis) was reported in 1% of subjects.

Summary of Individual Signs/Symptoms Characterizing Local Injection-Site Reactions to Enfuvirtide in Studies T20-301 and T20-302 Combined (n = 663)

Reaction category	Any severity grade	% of reactions comprising grade 3 reactions	% of reactions comprising grade 4 reactions
Pain/discomfort[a]	95%	9%	0%
Induration[b]	89%	41%	16%
Erythema[c]	89%	22%	10%
Nodules and cysts[d]	76%	26%	0%
Pruritus[e]	62%	4%	NA
Ecchymosis[f]	48%	8%	5%

[a] Grade 3 = Severe pain requiring analgesics (or narcotic analgesics for ≤ 72 hours) or limiting usual activities.Grade 4 = Severe pain requiring hospitalization or prolongation of hospitalization, resulting in death, or persistent or significant disability/incapacity, or life-threatening, or medically significant.
[b] Grade 3 = ≥ 25 mm, but < 50 mm; grade 4 = ≥ 50 mm average diameter.
[c] Grade 3 = ≥ 50 mm, but < 85 mm average diameter; grade 4 = ≥ 85 mm average diameter.
[d] Grade 3 = ≥ 3 cm; grade 4 = if draining.
[e] Grade 3 = Refractory to topical treatment or requiring oral or parenteral treatment; grade 4 = not applicable.
[f] Grade 3 = > 3 cm, but ≤ 5 cm; grade 4 = > 5 cm.

➤*Other adverse reactions:* The reactions most frequently reported in subjects receiving enfuvirtide + background regimen, excluding injection-site reactions, were diarrhea (26.8%), nausea (20.1%), and fatigue (16.1%). These events were also commonly observed in subjects that received background regimen alone: Diarrhea (33.5%), nausea (23.7%), and fatigue (17.4%).

Adults With Selected Treatment-Emergent Adverse Reactions [a] Occurring More Frequently With Enfuvirtide Treatment (Pooled Studies T20-301/T20-302 at 24 Weeks) (≥ 2%)

Adverse reaction	Enfuvirtide + background regimen (n = 663)	Background regimen (n = 334)
CNS		
Anxiety	5.7%	3%
Depression	8.6%	7.2%
Insomnia	11.3%	8.7%
Peripheral neuropathy	8.9%	6.3%
Taste disturbance	2.4%	1.5%
Dermatologic		
Pruritus not otherwise specified	5.1%	4.2%
Infections		
Herpes simplex	5%	3.9%
Influenza	3.9%	1.8%
Sinusitis	6.2%	2.1%
Skin papilloma	4.2%	1.5%
GI		
Constipation	3.9%	2.7%
Upper abdominal pain	3%	2.7%
Pancreatitis	2.4%	0.9%
Hematologic		
Lymphadenopathy	2.3%	0.3%
Musculoskeletal		
Myalgia	5%	2.4%
Ophthalmic		
Conjunctivitis	2.4%	0.9%
Respiratory		
Cough	7.4%	5.4%

ENFUVIRTIDE — INJECTION

Adults With Selected Treatment-Emergent Adverse Reactions [a] Occurring More Frequently With Enfuvirtide Treatment (Pooled Studies T20-301/T20-302 at 24 Weeks) (≥ 2%)		
Adverse reaction	Enfuvirtide + background regimen (n = 663)	Background regimen (n = 334)
Miscellaneous		
Anorexia	2.6%	1.8%
Asthenia	5.7%	4.2%
Decreased appetite	6.3%	2.4%
Decreased weight	6.5%	5.1%
Influenza-like illness	2.3%	0.9%

[a] Excludes injection-site reactions.

Respiratory – An increased rate of bacterial pneumonia was observed in subjects treated with enfuvirtide in the phase 3 clinical trials compared to the control arm (4.68 pneumonia events per 100 patient-years versus 0.61 events per 100 patient-years, respectively). Approximately half of the study subjects with pneumonia required hospitalization. One subject death in the enfuvirtide arm was attributed to pneumonia. Risk factors for pneumonia included low initial CD4 lymphocyte count, high initial viral load, IV drug use, smoking, and a history of lung disease. It is unclear if the increased incidence of pneumonia was related to enfuvirtide use. However, because of this finding patients with HIV infection should be carefully monitored for signs and symptoms of pneumonia, especially if they have underlying conditions which may predispose them to pneumonia.

➤*Less common events:* The following adverse reactions have been reported in 1 or more subjects; however, a causal relationship to enfuvirtide has not been established.

CNS – Guillain-Barre syndrome (fatal); sixth nerve palsy.

Hematologic/Lymphatic – Thrombocytopenia; neutropenia, and fever.

Hypersensitivity – Worsening abacavir hypersensitivity reaction.

Lab test abnormalities –

Treatment-Emergent Laboratory Abnormalities in Adults That Occurred More Frequently with Enfuvirtide Treatment (Pooled Studies T20-301 and T20-302 at 24 Weeks (≥ 2%)			
Laboratory parameters	Grading	Enfuvirtide + background regimen (n = 663)	Background regimen (n = 334)
Eosinophilia			
1 to 2 × ULN (0.7 × 10^9/L)	0.7-1.4 × 10^9/L	8.3%	1.5%
> 2 × ULN (0.7 × 10^9/L)	> 1.4 × 10^9/L	1.8%	0.9%
Amylase (U/L)			
Gr. 3	> 2 to 5 × ULN	6.2%	3.6%
Gr. 4	> 5 × ULN or clinical pancreatitis	0.9%	0.6%
Lipase (U/L)			
Gr. 3	> 2 to 5 × ULN	5.9%	3.6%
Gr. 4	> 5 × ULN	2.3%	1.8%
Triglycerides (mmol/L)			
Gr. 3	> 1000 mg/dL	8.9%	7.2%
ALT			
Gr. 3	> 5 to 10 × ULN	3.5%	2.1%
Gr. 4	> 10 × ULN	0.9%	0.6%
AST			
Gr. 3	> 5 to 10 × ULN	3.6%	3%
Gr. 4	> 10 × ULN	1.2%	0.6%
Creatine phosphokinase (U/L)			
Gr. 3	> 5 to 10 × ULN	5.9%	3.6%
Gr. 4	> 10 × ULN	2.3%	3.6%
GGT (U/L)			
Gr. 3	> 5 to 10 × ULN	3.5%	3.3%
Gr. 4	> 10 × ULN	2.4%	1.8%

Treatment-Emergent Laboratory Abnormalities in Adults That Occurred More Frequently with Enfuvirtide Treatment (Pooled Studies T20-301 and T20-302 at 24 Weeks (≥ 2%)			
Laboratory parameters	Grading	Enfuvirtide + background regimen (n = 663)	Background regimen (n = 334)
Hemoglobin (g/dL)			
Gr. 3	6.5 to 7.9 g/dL	1.5%	0.9%
Gr. 4	< 6.5 g/dL	0.6%	0.6%

Metabolic – Hyperglycemia.

Renal – Renal insufficiency (glomerulonephritis); renal failure.

Respiratory – Pneumonia.

Overdosage

➤*Symptoms:* There are no reports of human experience of acute overdose with enfuvirtide. The highest dose administered to 12 subjects in a clinical trial was 180 mg as a single dose SC.

➤*Treatment:* There is no specific antidote for overdose with enfuvirtide. Treatment of overdose should consist of general supportive measures.

Patient Information

To ensure safe and effective use of enfuvirtide, the following information and instructions should be given to patients:

Patients should be informed that injection-site reactions occur commonly. Patients must be familiar with the enfuvirtide injection instructions for instructions on how to appropriately inject enfuvirtide and how to carefully monitor for signs or symptoms of cellulitis or local infection. Patients should be instructed when to contact their healthcare provider about these reactions.

Patients should be made aware that an increased rate of bacterial pneumonia was observed in subjects treated with enfuvirtide in phase 3 clinical trials compared to the control arm. Patients should be advised to seek medical evaluation immediately if they develop signs or symptoms suggestive of pneumonia (cough with fever, rapid breathing, shortness of breath).

Patients should be advised of the possibility of a hypersensitivity reaction to enfuvirtide. Patients should be advised to discontinue therapy and immediately seek medical evaluation if they develop signs/symptoms of hypersensitivity. Hypersensitivity reactions have included the following, individually and in combination: Rash, fever, nausea and vomiting, chills, rigors, hypotension, and elevated serum liver transaminases.

Enfuvirtide is not a cure for HIV-1 infection and patients may continue to contract illnesses associated with HIV-1 infection. The long-term effects of enfuvirtide are unknown at this time. Enfuvirtide therapy has not been shown to reduce the risk of transmitting HIV-1 to others through sexual contact or blood contamination.

Enfuvirtide must be taken as part of a combination antiretroviral regimen. Use of enfuvirtide alone may lead to rapid development of virus resistant to enfuvirtide and possibly other agents of the same class.

Patients and caregivers must be instructed in the use of aseptic technique when administering enfuvirtide in order to avoid injection-site infections. Appropriate training for enfuvirtide reconstitution and self-injection must be given by a healthcare provider, including a careful review of the enfuvirtide patient prescribing information and enfuvirtide injection instructions. The first injection should be performed under the supervision of an appropriately qualified healthcare provider. It is recommended that the patient or caregiver's understanding and use of aseptic self-injection techniques and procedures be periodically reevaluated.

Patients should contact their healthcare providers for any questions regarding the administration of enfuvirtide. Patients should be told not to reuse needles or syringes, and be instructed in safe disposal procedures including the use of a puncture-resistant container for disposal of used needles and syringes. Patients must be instructed on the safe disposal of full containers as per local requirements. Caregivers who experience an accidental needlestick after patient injection should contact a healthcare provider immediately.

Patients should inform their healthcare providers if they are pregnant, plan to become pregnant or become pregnant while taking this medication.

Patients should inform their healthcare providers if they are breastfeeding.

Patients should not change the dose or dosing schedule of enfuvirtide or any antiretroviral medication without consulting their healthcare provider.

Patients should contact their healthcare providers immediately if they stop taking enfuvirtide or any other drug in their antiretroviral regimen.

Patients should be advised that no studies have been conducted on the ability to drive or operate machinery while taking enfuvirtide. If patients experience dizziness while taking enfuvirtide, they should be advised to talk to their healthcare provider before driving or operating machinery.

DAPSONE (DDS)

Rx	Dapsone (Jacobus)	Tablets: 25 mg	(Jacobus 25 102). White, scored. In 100s.
		100 mg	(Jacobus 100 101). White, scored. In 100s.

DAPSONE — ORAL

Indications

➤*Dermatitis herpetiformis:* Treatment of dermatitis herpetiformis (DH) and all forms of leprosy except for cases of proven dapsone resistance.

➤*Off-label uses:*

Rheumatoid arthritis – [5] = Poor documentation. Data evaluating the safety and efficacy of dapsone for the treatment of rheumatoid arthritis (RA) date back to the 1970s. The most recent American College of Rheumatology recommendations for the treatment of RA do not include dapsone. Published data are dated, show mixed results, and note safety concerns (hemolysis).

Other possible off-label uses –

Leprosy: Unlabeled uses of dapsone include treatment of relapsing polychondritis; prophylaxis of malaria; inflammatory bowel disorders; Leishmaniasis; *Pneumocystis carinii* pneumonia; rheumatic/connective tissue disorders (eg, RA, lupus erythematosus); brown recluse spider bites. Doses used generally range from 50 to 200 mg/day.

Administration and Dosage

➤*Maximum dose:*

Adults – There are no well-established maximum dosages for the approved indications according to the prescribing information.

Children – There are no well-established maximum dosages for the approved indications according to the prescribing information. However, maximum doses have been established off-label. (See Children.)

➤*Adults:*

Dermatitis herpetiformis –

Initial dosage: 50 mg daily.

Dosage titration: The dosage should be individually titrated. If full control is not achieved within the range of 50 to 300 mg daily, higher doses may be tried. Dosage should be reduced to a minimum maintenance level as soon as possible. In responsive patients, there is a prompt reduction in pruritus, followed by clearance of skin lesions. There is no effect on the GI component of the disease.

Dosage adjustment: Dapsone levels are influenced by acetylation rates. Patients with high acetylation rates or who are receiving treatment affecting acetylation may require an adjustment in dosage.

Concomitant therapy: An option for the patient to elect is a strict, gluten-free diet, permitting many patients to reduce or eliminate the need for dapsone. The average time for dosage reduction is 8 months (range, 4 months to 2.5 years), and the average time for dosage elimination is 29 months (range, 6 months to 9 years).

Leprosy – In order to reduce secondary dapsone resistance, the World Health Organization (WHO) Expert Committee on Leprosy and the United States Public Health Service (USPHS) at Carville, LA, recommended that dapsone should be commenced in combination with one or more antileprosy drugs. In the multidrug program, dapsone should be maintained at the full dosage of 100 mg daily without interruption (with corresponding smaller doses for children) and provided to all patients who have sensitive organisms with new or recrudescent disease, or who have not yet completed a 2-year course of dapsone monotherapy. For advice and other drugs, the USPHS at Carville, LA, (1-800-642-2477) should be contacted. Before using other drugs, consult appropriate product labeling.

Bacteriologically negative tuberculoid and indeterminate disease: In bacteriologically negative tuberculoid and indeterminate disease, the recommendation is the coadministration of dapsone 100 mg daily with 6 months of rifampin 600 mg daily.

Under WHO, daily rifampin may be replaced by rifampin 600 mg monthly, if supervised. The dapsone should be continued until all signs of clinical activity are controlled, usually after an additional 6 months. Then dapsone should be continued for an additional 3 years for tuberculoid and indeterminate patients and for 5 years for borderline tuberculoid patients.

Lepromatous and borderline lepromatous patients: In lepromatous and borderline lepromatous patients, the recommendation is the coadministration of dapsone 100 mg daily with 2 years of rifampin 600 mg daily. Under WHO, daily rifampin may be replaced by rifampin 600 mg monthly, if supervised. One may elect the concurrent administration of a third antileprosy drug, usually either clofazimine 50 to 100 mg daily or ethionamide 250 to 500 mg daily. Dapsone 100 mg daily is continued for 3 to 10 years until all signs of clinical activity are controlled, with negative skin scrapings and biopsies for 1 year. Dapsone should then be continued for an additional 10 years for borderline patients and for life for lepromatous patients.

Secondary dapsone resistance should be suspected whenever a lepromatous or borderline lepromatous patient receiving dapsone treatment clinically and bacteriologically relapses, solid staining bacilli being found in the smears taken from the new active lesions. If such cases show no response to regular and supervised dapsone therapy within 3 to 6 months or good compliance for the past 3 to 6 months can be ensured, dapsone resistance should be considered confirmed clinically. Determination of drug sensitivity using the mouse footpad method is recommended and, after prior arrangement, is available without charge from the USPHS, Carville, LA. Patients with proven dapsone resistance should be treated with other drugs.

Off-label dosing –

Pneumocystis pneumonia treatment: 100 mg daily with trimethoprim (see Trimethoprim for dosing).

Pneumocystis pneumonia prophylaxis:

• *Monotherapy* – 50 mg twice daily or 100 mg daily.

• *Combination therapy* – Dapsone 50 mg daily, pyrimethamine 50 mg weekly, and leucovorin 25 mg weekly; or dapsone 200 mg weekly, pyrimethamine 75 mg weekly, and leucovorin 25 mg weekly.

➤*Children:*

Dermatitis herpetiformis –

Initial dosage: The adult dosage is 50 mg daily, and the dosage for children should be correspondingly smaller.

See Adults for more information.

Leprosy – See Adults for dosing.

Off-label dosing –

Pneumocystis pneumonia:

• *Monotherapy* –

Children 1 month of age and older: 2 mg/kg daily or 4 mg/kg weekly. 100 mg daily or 200 mg weekly.

• *Combination therapy* –

Children 13 years of age or older: 100 mg once daily with trimethoprim (see Trimethoprim for dosing).

Children younger than 13 years of age: 2 mg/kg/day with trimethoprim (see Trimethoprim for dosing).

Pneumocystis pneumonia treatment:

• *Children 13 years of age or older* – 100 mg daily with trimethoprim (see Trimethoprim for dosing).

• *Children younger than 13 years of age* – 2 mg/kg/day with trimethoprim (see Trimethoprim for dosing).

Pneumocystis pneumonia prophylaxis:

• *Children 13 years of age or older* –

Monotherapy: 50 mg twice daily or 100 mg daily.

Combination therapy: Dapsone 50 mg daily, pyrimethamine 50 mg weekly, and leucovorin 25 mg weekly; or dapsone 200 mg weekly, pyrimethamine 75 mg weekly, and leucovorin 25 mg weekly.

• *Children 1 month to 13 years of age* –

Usual dosage: 2 mg/kg daily or 4 mg/kg weekly.

Maximum dose: 100 mg daily or 200 mg weekly.

➤*Storage/Stability:* Store at 20° to 25°C (68° to 77°F). Protect from light. Dispense in a well-closed, child-resistant container.

Actions

➤*Pharmacology:* The mechanism of action in dermatitis herpetiformis has not been established. By the kinetic method in mice, dapsone is bactericidal as well as bacteriostatic against *Mycobacterium leprae.*

➤*Pharmacokinetics:*

Absorption – Dapsone, when given orally, is rapidly and almost completely absorbed. Detected a few minutes after ingestion, the drug reaches peak concentration in 4 to 8 hours. Daily administration for at least 8 days is necessary to achieve a plateau level. With doses of 200 mg daily, this level averaged 2.3 mcg/mL with a range of 0.1 to 7 mcg/mL.

Excretion – The half-life in the plasma in different individuals varies from 10 to 50 hours and averages 28 hours. Repeat tests in the same individual are constant. Daily administration (50 to 100 mg) in leprosy patients will provide blood levels in excess of the usual minimum inhibitory concentration even for patients with a short dapsone half-life. Excretion of the drug is slow and a constant blood level can be maintained with the usual dosage. About 85% of the daily intake is recoverable from the urine mainly in the form of water-soluble metabolites.

Contraindications

Hypersensitivity to dapsone or its derivatives.

Warnings/Precautions

➤*Hematologic effects:* The patient should be warned to respond to the presence of clinical signs such as sore throat, fever, pallor, purpura or jaundice. Deaths associated with the administration of dapsone have been reported from agranulocytosis, aplastic anemia and other blood dyscrasias. Complete blood counts should be done frequently in patients receiving dapsone. The FDA Dermatology Advisory Committee recommended that, when feasible, counts should be done weekly for the first month, monthly for 6 months and semi-annually thereafter. If a significant reduction in leucocytes, platelets or hemopoiesis is noted, dapsone should be discontinued and the patient followed intensively. Folic acid antagonists have similar effects and may increase the incidence of hematologic reactions; if co-administered with dapsone the patient should be monitored more frequently. Patients on weekly pyrimethamine and dapsone have developed agranulocytosis during the second and third month of therapy.

Severe anemia – Severe anemia should be treated prior to initiation of therapy and hemoglobin monitored. Hemolysis and methemoglobin may be poorly tolerated by patients with severe cardiopulmonary disease.

➤*Cutaneous reactions:* Cutaneous reactions, especially bullous, include exfoliative dermatitis and are probably one of the most serious, though rare, complications of sulfone therapy. They are directly due to drug sensitization. Such reactions include toxic erythema, erythema multiforme, toxic epidermal necrolysis, morbilliform and scarlatiniform reactions, urticaria and erythema nodosum. If new or toxic dermatologic reactions occur, sulfone therapy must be promptly discontinued and appropriate therapy instituted.

DAPSONE — ORAL

➤*Leprosy reactional states:* Leprosy reactional states, including cutaneous, are not hypersensitivity reactions to dapsone and do not require discontinuation (see Administration and Dosage, Leprosy reactional states).

Abrupt changes in clinical activity occur in leprosy with any effective treatment and are known as reactional states. The majority can be classified into 2 groups.

The "reversal" reaction (Type 1) may occur in borderline or tuberculoid leprosy patients often seen after chemotherapy is started. The mechanism is presumed to result from a reduction in the antigenic load: The patient is able to mount an enhanced delayed hypersensitivity response to residual infection leading to swelling ("reversal") of existing skin and nerve lesions. If severe, or if neuritis is present, large doses of steroids should always be used. If severe, the patient should be hospitalized. In general antileprosy treatment is continued and therapy to suppress the reaction is indicated such as analgesics, steroids, or surgical decompression of swollen nerve trunks. USPHS at Carville, LA should be contacted for advice in management.

Erythema nodosum leprosum (ENL) or lepromatous reaction (Type 2 reaction) occurs mainly in lepromatous patients and small numbers of borderline patients. Approximately 50% of treated patients show this reaction in the first year. The principal clinical features are fever and tender erythematous skin nodules sometimes associated with malaise, neuritis, orchitis, albuminuria, joint swelling, iritis, epistaxis or depression. Skin lesions can become pustular or ulcerate. Histologically there is a vasculitis with an intense polymorphonuclear infiltrate. Elevated circulating immune complexes are considered to be the mechanism of reaction. If severe, patients should be hospitalized. In general, anti-leprosy treatment is continued. Analgesics, steroids, and other agents available from USPHS at Carville, LA are used to suppress the reaction.

➤*Hemolysis:* Hemolysis and Heinz body formation may be exaggerated in individuals with a glucose-6-phosphate dehydrogenase (G-6-PD) deficiency, or methemoglobin reductase deficiency, or hemoglobin M. This reaction is frequently dose-related. Dapsone should be given with caution to these patients or if the patient is exposed to other agents or conditions such as infection or diabetic ketosis capable of producing hemolysis. Drugs or chemicals which have produced significant hemolysis in G-6-PD or methemoglobin reductase-deficient patients include dapsone, sulfanilamide, nitrite, aniline, phenylhydrazine, napthalene, niridazole, nitrofurantoin and 8-aminoantimalarials such as primaquine.

➤*Hepatic effects:* Toxic hepatitis and cholestatic jaundice have been reported early in therapy. Hyperbilirubinemia may occur more often in G-6-PD-deficient patients. When feasible, baseline and subsequent monitoring of liver function is recommended: If abnormal, dapsone should be discontinued until the source of the abnormality is established.

➤*Pregnancy: Category C.* Animal reproduction studies have not been conducted with dapsone. Extensive, but uncontrolled experience and two published surveys on the use of dapsone in pregnant women have not shown that dapsone increases the risk of fetal abnormalities if administered during all trimesters of pregnancy or can affect reproduction capacity. Because of the lack of animal studies or controlled human experience, dapsone should be given to a pregnant woman only if clearly needed. In general, for leprosy, USPHS at Carville recommends maintenance of dapsone. Dapsone has been important for the management of some pregnant DH patients.

➤*Lactation:* Dapsone is excreted in breast milk in substantial amounts. Hemolytic reactions can occur in neonates (see Precautions). Because of the potential for tumorgenicity shown for dapsone in animal studies a decision should be made whether to discontinue nursing or discontinue the drug taking into account the importance of drug to the mother.

➤*Children:* Children are treated on the same schedule as adults but with correspondingly smaller doses. Dapsone is generally not considered to have an effect on the later growth, development and functional development of the child.

Drug Interactions

Dapsone Oral Drug Interactions

Precipitant drug	Object drug[a]		Description
Charcoal, activated	Dapsone	⬇	Activated charcoal may decrease dapsone's GI absorption and enterohepatic recycling.
Didanosine	Dapsone	⬇	Possible therapeutic failure of dapsone, leading to an increase in infection.
Folic acid antagonists	Dapsone	⬆	Folic acid antagonists such as pyrimethamine may increase the likelihood of hematologic reactions. Weekly concomitant use has caused agranulocytosis during the second and third months of therapy.
Para-aminobenzoic acid	Dapsone	⬇	Para-aminobenzoic acid may antagonize the effect of dapsone by interfering with the primary mechanism of action.
Probenecid	Dapsone	⬆	Probenecid reduces urinary excretion of dapsone metabolites, increasing plasma concentrations.
Rifampin	Dapsone	⬇	Rifampin lowers dapsone levels seven to tenfold by accelerating plasma clearance.
Trimethoprim	Dapsone	⬆	Increased serum levels of both drugs may occur, possibly increasing the pharmacologic and toxic effects of each drug.
Dapsone	Trimethoprim	⬆	

[a] ⬆ = object drug increased; ⬇ = object drug decreased.

Adverse Reactions

➤*Hematologic:* Dose-related hemolysis is the most common adverse effect and is seen in patients with or without G-6-PD deficiency. Almost all patients demonstrate the inter-related changes of a loss of 1 to 2 g of hemoglobin, an increase in the reticulocytes (2% to 12%), a shortened red cell life span and a rise in methemoglobin. G-6-PD deficient patients have greater responses.

➤*Miscellaneous:* In addition to the warnings and adverse effects reported above, additional adverse reactions include: Nausea, vomiting, abdominal pains, pancreatitis, vertigo, blurred vision, tinnitus, insomnia, fever, headache, psychosis, phototoxicity, pulmonary eosinophilia, tachycardia, albuminuria, the nephrotic syndrome, hypoalbuminemia without proteinuria, renal papillary necrosis, male infertility, drug-induced Lupus erythematosus and an infectious mononucleosis-like syndrome. In general, with the exception of the complications of severe anoxia from overdosage (eg, retinal and optic nerve damage) these adverse reactions have regressed following drug discontinuation.

Peripheral nervous system – Peripheral neuropathy is a definite but unusual complication of dapsone therapy in non-leprosy patients. Motor loss is predominant. If muscle weakness appears, dapsone should be withdrawn. Recovery on withdrawal is usually substantially complete. The mechanism of recovery is reported by axonal regeneration. Some recovered patients have tolerated retreatment at reduced dosage. In leprosy this complication may be difficult to distinguish from a leprosy reactional state.

Overdosage

➤*Symptoms:* Nausea, vomiting, and hyperexcitability can appear a few minutes up to 24 hours after ingestion of an overdosage. Methemoglobin induced depression, convulsions or severe cyanosis requires prompt treatment.

➤*Treatment:* In normal and methemoglobin reductase deficient patients, methylene blue, 1 to 2 mg/kg of body weight, given slowly intravenously is the treatment of choice. The effect is complete in 30 minutes, but may have to be repeated if methemoglobin reaccumulates. For non-emergencies, if treatment is needed, methylene blue may be given orally in doses of 3 to 5 mg/kg every 4 to 6 hours. Methylene blue reduction depends on G-6-PD and should not be given to fully expressed G-6-PD-deficient patients.

ANTIPROTOZOALS

NITAZOXANIDE

Rx	**Alinia** (Romark Laboratories)	**Tablets; oral:** 500 mg	Sucrose. (ALINIA 500). Yellow, round. Film-coated. In 30s and 60s.
		Suspension; oral: 100 mg per 5 mL	Sugar, sucrose. Strawberry flavor. In 60 mL.

NITAZOXANIDE — ORAL

Indications

➤*Diarrhea:* For the treatment of diarrhea caused by *Giarda lamblia* or *Cryptosporidium parvum*.

Administration and Dosage

➤*Adults:*

Diarrhea – 500 mg (1 tablet or 25 mL of oral suspension) every 12 hours for 3 days.

NITAZOXANIDE — ORAL

➤*Children:*

Diarrhea –

12 years of age and older: See Adults for dosing.
4 to 11 years of age: 200 mg (10 mL) every 12 hours for 3 days.
1 to 3 years of age: 100 mg (5 mL) every 12 hours for 3 days.
Younger than 1 year of age: Safety and effectiveness have not been studied.

➤*Preparation for administration:* Prepare a suspension at time of dispensing. The amount of water required for preparation of the suspension is 48 mL. Tap bottle until all powder flows freely. Add approximately one-half of the total amount of water required for reconstitution and shake vigorously to suspend powder. Add remainder of water and again shake vigorously. Keep container tightly closed.

➤*Administration:* Take with food. Shake the suspension well before each administration.

A single nitazoxanide tablet contains a greater amount of nitazoxanide than is recommended for children and, therefore, should not be used in children 11 years of age and younger. Oral suspension should be used for dosing nitazoxanide in children.

➤*Storage/Stability:* Store at 25°C (77°F); excursions are permitted to 15° to 30°C (59° to 86°F). The reconstituted suspension may be stored for 7 days, after which any unused portion must be discarded.

Actions

➤*Pharmacology:* The antiprotozoal activity of nitazoxanide is believed to be caused by interference with the pyruvate:ferredoxin oxidoreductase (PFOR) enzyme-dependent electron transfer reaction, which is essential to anaerobic energy metabolism. Studies have shown that the PFOR enzyme from *G. lamblia* directly reduces nitazoxanide by transfer of electrons in the absence of ferredoxin. The DNA-derived PFOR protein sequence of *C. parvum* appears to be similar to that of *G. lamblia*. Interference with the PFOR enzyme-dependent electron transfer reaction may not be the only pathway by which nitazoxanide exhibits antiprotozoal activity.

➤*Pharmacokinetics:*

Nitazoxanide Mean (±SD) Plasma Pharmacokinetic Parameters in Patients ≥ 12 Years of Age[a]

Age	Tizoxanide			Tizoxanide glucuronide		
	C_{max} (mcg/mL)	T_{max}[b] (h)	AUC_t (mcg•h/mL)	C_{max} (mcg/mL)	T_{max}[b] (h)	AUC_t (mcg•h/mL)
12 to 17 years	9.1 (6.1)	4 (1 to 4)	39.5 (24.2)	7.3 (1.9)	4 (2 to 8)	46.5 (18.2)
≥ 18 years	10.6 (2)	3 (2 to 4)	41.9 (6)	10.5 (1.4)	4.5 (4 to 6)	63 (12.3)

[a] SD = standard deviation; C_{max} = maximum plasma concentration; T_{max} = time to reach maximum plasma concentration; AUC = area under the curve.
[b] T_{max} is given as a mean (range).

Nitazoxanide Mean (± SD) Plasma Pharmacokinetic Parameters in Patients ≥ 1 Year of Age

Age	Dose	Tizoxanide			Tizoxanide glucuronide		
		C_{max} (mcg/mL)	T_{max}[a] (h)	AUC_t (mcg•h/mL)	C_{max} (mcg/mL)	T_{max}[a] (h)	AUC_t (mcg•h/mL)
1 to 3 years	100 mg	3.11 (2)	3.5 (2 to 4)	11.7 (4.46)	3.64 (1.16)	4 (3 to 4)	19 (5.03)
4 to 11 years	200 mg	3 (0.99)	2 (1 to 4)	13.5 (3.3)	2.84 (0.97)	4 (2 to 4)	16.9 (5)
≥ 18 years	500 mg	5.49 (2.06)	2.5 (1 to 5)	30.2 (12.3)	3.21 (1.05)	4 (2.5 to 6)	22.8 (6.49)

[a] T_{max} is given as mean (range).

Absorption – Following oral administration of nitazoxanide tablets or oral suspension, C_{max} of the active metabolites tizoxanide and tizoxanide glucuronide are observed within 1 to 4 hours. The parent nitazoxanide is not detected in plasma.

Nitazoxanide oral suspension is not bioequivalent to nitazoxanide tablets. The relative bioavailability of the suspension compared with the tablet was 70%.

Following oral administration of a single nitazoxanide tablet every 12 hours for 7 consecutive days, there was no significant accumulation of the nitazoxanide metabolites tizoxanide or tizoxanide glucuronide detected in plasma.

Effect of food: When nitazoxanide tablets are administered with food, the AUC_t of tizoxanide and tizoxanide glucuronide in plasma is increased almost 2-fold and the C_{max} is increased by approximately 50%.

When nitazoxanide for oral suspension was administered with food, the AUC_t of tizoxanide and tizoxanide glucuronide increased by approximately 45% to 50% and the C_{max} increased by 10% or less.

Nitazoxanide tablets and oral suspension were administered with food in clinical trials, and, therefore, they are recommended to be administered with food.

Distribution – In plasma, more than 99% of tizoxanide is bound to proteins.

Metabolism – Following oral administration in humans, nitazoxanide is rapidly hydrolyzed to an active metabolite, tizoxanide (desacetyl-nitazoxanide). Tizoxanide then undergoes conjugation, primarily by glucuronidation. In vitro metabolism studies have demonstrated that tizoxanide has no significant inhibitory effect on cytochrome P450 enzymes.

Excretion – Tizoxanide is excreted in the urine, bile, and feces, and tizoxanide glucuronide is excreted in urine and bile. Approximately two-thirds of the oral dose of nitazoxanide is excreted in the feces and one-third in the urine.

➤*Microbiology:* Nitazoxanide and its metabolite, tizoxanide, are active in vitro in inhibiting the growth of sporozoites and oocysts of *C. parvum* and trophozoites of *G. lamblia*.

Contraindications

Prior hypersensitivity to nitazoxanide or any other ingredient in the formulations.

Warnings/Precautions

➤*HIV-infected or immunodeficient patients:* Nitazoxanide has not been studied for the treatment of diarrhea caused by *G. lamblia* in HIV-infected or immunodeficient patients. Nitazoxanide has not been shown to be superior to placebo for the treatment of diarrhea caused by *C. parvum* in HIV-infected or immunodeficient patients.

➤*Renal/Hepatic function impairment:* Administer nitazoxanide with caution to patients with hepatic and biliary disease, renal disease, and combined renal and hepatic disease.

➤*Pregnancy: Category B.* There are no adequate and well-controlled studies in pregnant women. It is not known whether active metabolites of nitazoxanide cross the human placenta (nitazoxanide is not detected in the plasma). The molecular weight of one of the active metabolites, tizoxanide (approximately 265), is low enough for placental passage, but the extensive plasma protein binding will limit the amount of drug transferred to the embryo or fetus. If indicated, do not withhold nitazoxanide during pregnancy. However, until human pregnancy data are available, avoid exposure to the agent in the first trimester, if possible.

➤*Lactation:* It is not known whether nitazoxanide is excreted in human milk. The molecular weight of one of the active metabolites, tizoxanide (about 265), is low enough to pass into milk, but the extensive plasma protein binding (99.9%) will limit the amount of drug in milk. Because many drugs are excreted in human milk, exercise caution when nitazoxanide is administered to a breast-feeding woman.

➤*Children:* A single nitazoxanide tablet contains a greater amount of nitazoxanide than is recommended for children and, therefore, should not be used in children 11 years of age and younger. Use only nitazoxanide oral suspension for dosing nitazoxanide in children. Safety and effectiveness of nitazoxanide for oral suspension in children younger than 1 year of age have not been studied.

➤*Elderly:* In general, consider the greater frequency of decreased hepatic, renal, or cardiac function, and of concomitant disease or other drug therapy in elderly patients when prescribing nitazoxanide.

Drug Interactions

➤*Highly protein bound drugs:* Tizoxanide is highly bound to plasma protein (greater than 99.9%). Therefore, use caution when administering nitazoxanide concurrently with other highly plasma protein-bound drugs with narrow therapeutic indices, as competition for binding sites may occur (eg, warfarin).

➤*Drug/Food interactions:* See Actions for more information.

Adverse Reactions

➤*Tablets:*

Common adverse reactions – In controlled and uncontrolled clinical studies of 1,657 patients 12 years of age and older not infected with HIV who received various dosage regimens of nitazoxanide tablets, the most common adverse reactions reported regardless of causality assessment were abdominal pain (6.6%), diarrhea (4.2%), headache (3.1%), and nausea (3%).

The adverse reactions seen in adults treated with nitazoxanide oral suspension were similar to those observed in adults treated with nitazoxanide tablets.

Discontinuation – In the placebo-controlled trials of patients 12 years of age and older not infected with HIV who received nitazoxanide tablets for the treatment of diarrhea caused by *G. lamblia* or *C. parvum*, less than 1% of patients discontinued therapy because of an adverse reaction.

Other adverse reactions –

Cardiovascular: Hypertension, syncope, tachycardia (less than 1%).
CNS: Dizziness, hypesthesia, insomnia, somnolence, tremor (less than 1%).
Dermatologic: Pruritus, rash (less than 1%).
GI: Anorexia, constipation, dry mouth, dyspepsia, flatulence, thirst, vomiting (less than 1%).
GU: Amenorrhea, discolored urine, dysuria, edema labia, kidney pain, metrorrhagia (less than 1%).
Hematologic/Lymphatic: Anemia, leukocytosis (less than 1%).
Musculoskeletal: Back pain, leg cramps, myalgia, spontaneous bone fracture (less than 1%).
Respiratory: Epistaxis, lung disease, pharyngitis (less than 1%).
Special senses: Ear ache, eye discoloration (less than 1%).
Miscellaneous: Allergic reaction, asthenia, chills, chills and fever, fever, flu syndrome, increased ALT, pain, pelvic pain (less than 1%).

NITAZOXANIDE — ORAL

➤*Suspension:* In controlled and uncontrolled clinical studies of 613 HIV-negative children who received nitazoxanide for oral suspension, the most frequent adverse reactions reported regardless of causality assessment were abdominal pain (7.8%), diarrhea (2.1%), vomiting (1.1%), and headache (1.1%). These were typically mild and transient in nature. In placebo-controlled clinical trials, the rates of occurrence of these reactions did not differ significantly from those of placebo.

Discontinuation – None of the 613 children discontinued therapy because of adverse reactions.

Other adverse reactions –

CNS: Dizziness, malaise (less than 1%).

Dermatologic: Pruritus, sweating (less than 1%).

GI: Anorexia, appetite increase, enlarged salivary glands, flatulence, nausea (less than 1%).

Metabolic/Nutritional: Increased ALT, increased creatinine (less than 1%).

Miscellaneous: Discolored urine, eye discoloration (pale yellow), fever, infection, rhinitis (less than 1%).

Overdosage

➤*Symptoms:* Information on nitazoxanide overdosage is not available. Single oral doses of up to 4,000 mg in a tablet formulation have been administered to healthy adult volunteers without significant adverse effects.

➤*Treatment:* In the event of overdose, gastric lavage may be appropriate soon after oral administration. Observe patients carefully and give symptomatic and supportive treatment.

Patient Information

Instruct patients to take nitazoxanide with food.

Advise patients with diabetes and caregivers that the oral suspension contains sucrose 1.48 g per 5 mL.

Instruct patients to shake the suspension well before measuring their dose and to discard any remaining suspension after 7 days.

TINIDAZOLE

Rx	**Tinidazole** (BioComp)	**Tablets; oral:** 250 mg	PEG, polydextrose. (T 250). Pink, round, scored. In 40s.
Rx	**Tindamax** (Mission Pharmacal)		(TM 250). Pink, scored. In 40s.
Rx	**Tinidazole** (BioComp)	**Tablets; oral:** 500 mg	PEG, polydextrose. (T 500). Pink, oval, scored. In 20s and 60s.
Rx	**Tindamax** (Mission Pharmacal)		(TM 500). Pink, oval, scored. In 20s and 60s.

TINIDAZOLE — ORAL

WARNING

Carcinogenicity has been seen in mice and rats treated chronically with metronidazole, another nitroimidazole agent. Although such data have not been reported for tinidazole, the 2 drugs are structurally related and have similar biologic effects. Reserve its use only for the conditions for which it is indicated.

Indications

➤*Amebiasis:* For the treatment of intestinal amebiasis and amebic liver abscess caused by *Entamoeba histolytica* in adults and children older than 3 years of age. It is not indicated for the treatment of asymptomatic cyst passage.

➤*Bacterial vaginosis:* For the treatment of bacterial vaginosis (formerly referred to as *Haemophilus* vaginitis, *Gardnerella* vaginitis, nonspecific vaginitis, or anaerobic vaginosis) in nonpregnant women.

Other pathogens commonly associated with vulvovaginitis, such as *Trichomonas vaginalis, Chlamydia trachomatis, Neisseria gonorrhoeae, Candida albicans*, and *Herpes simplex* virus should be ruled out.

➤*Giardiasis:* For the treatment of giardiasis caused by *Giardiasis duodenalis* (also termed *Giardiasis lamblia*) in adults and children older than 3 years of age.

➤*Trichomoniasis:* For the treatment of trichomoniasis caused by *T. vaginalis*. The organism should be identified by appropriate diagnostic procedures. Because trichomoniasis is a sexually transmitted disease with potentially serious sequelae, treat partners of infected patients simultaneously in order to prevent reinfection.

Administration and Dosage

➤*Adults:*

Amebiasis –

Amebic liver abscess: 2 g once daily for 3 to 5 days.

Intestinal: 2 g once daily for 3 days.

Bacterial vaginosis –

Nonpregnant women: 2 g once daily for 2 days, or 1 g once daily for 5 days.

Giardiasis – 2 g (single dose).

Trichomoniasis – 2 g (single dose). Because trichomoniasis is a sexually transmitted disease, treat sexual partners with the same dose simultaneously.

➤*Children:*

Amebiasis –

3 years of age and older:

- *Amebic liver abscess* –
  - *Usual dosage:* 50 mg/kg once daily for 3 to 5 days.
  - *Maximum dose:* 2 g/day.
- *Intestinal* –
  - *Usual dosage:* 50 mg/kg once daily for 3 days.
  - *Maximum dose:* 2 g/day.

Giardiasis –

3 years of age and older:

- *Maximum dose* – 2 g.
- *Single dose* – 50 mg/kg (single dose).

➤*Renal function impairment:*

Hemodialysis – If tinidazole is administered on the same day as and prior to hemodialysis, it is recommended that an additional dose of tinidazole equivalent to one-half of the recommended dose be administered after the end of the hemodialysis.

➤*Preparation for administration:*

Extemporaneous oral suspension – For those unable to swallow tablets, tinidazole tablets may be crushed in artificial cherry syrup to be taken with food.

Pulverize four 500 mg oral tablets with a mortar and pestle. Add approximately 10 mL of cherry syrup to the powder and mix until smooth. Transfer the suspension to a graduated amber container. Use several small rinses of cherry syrup to transfer any remaining drug in the mortar to the final suspension for a final volume of 30 mL. The suspension of crushed tablets in artificial cherry syrup is stable for 7 days at room temperature. When this suspension is used, it should be shaken well before each administration.

➤*Administration:* Take tinidazole with food to minimize the incidence of epigastric discomfort and other GI adverse reactions. Food does not affect the oral bioavailability of tinidazole.

Alcoholic beverages should be avoided when taking tinidazole and for 3 days afterwards.

➤*Storage/Stability:* Store at 20° to 25°C (68° to 77°F); excursions are permitted to 15° to 30°C (59° to 86°F). Protect contents from light.

Actions

➤*Pharmacology:* Tinidazole is an antiprotozoal, antibacterial agent. The nitro group of tinidazole is reduced by cell extracts of *Trichomonas*. The free nitro radical generated as a result of this reduction may be responsible for the antiprotozoal activity. Chemically reduced tinidazole released nitrites and caused damage to purified bacterial DNA in vitro. Additionally, the drug caused DNA base changes in bacterial cells and DNA strand breakage in mammalian cells. The mechanism by which tinidazole exhibits activity against *Giardia* and *Entamoeba* species is not known.

➤*Pharmacokinetics:*

Absorption – After oral administration, tinidazole is rapidly and completely absorbed. A bioavailability study of tinidazole was conducted in adult healthy volunteers. All subjects received a single dose of tinidazole 2 g (four 500 mg tablets) orally following an overnight fast. Oral administration of four 500 mg tablets of tinidazole under fasted conditions produced a mean peak plasma concentration (C_{max}) of 47.7 (± 7.5) mcg/mL with a mean time to peak concentration (T_{max}) of 1.6 (± 0.7) hours, and a mean area under the plasma concentration-time curve ($AUC_{0-\infty}$) of 901.6 (± 126.5) mcg•h/mL at 72 hours. The elimination half-life was 13.2 (± 1.4) hours. Mean plasma levels decreased to 14.3 mcg/mL at 24 hours, 3.8 mcg/mL at 48 hours, and 0.8 mcg/mL at 72 hours following administration. Steady-state conditions are reached in 2.5 to 3 days of multi-day dosing.

Food effects: Administration of tinidazole tablets with food resulted in a delay in T_{max} of approximately 2 hours and a decline in C_{max} of approximately 10%, compared with fasted conditions. However, administration of tinidazole with food did not affect AUC or half-life in this study.

In healthy volunteers, administration of crushed tinidazole tablets in artificial cherry syrup after an overnight fast has no effect on any pharmacokinetic parameter, compared with tablets swallowed whole under fasted conditions.

Distribution – Tinidazole is distributed into virtually all tissues and body fluids and also crosses the blood-brain barrier. The apparent volume of distribution is about 50 L. Plasma protein binding of tinidazole is 12%.

Tinidazole crosses the placental barrier and is secreted in breast milk.

Metabolism – Tinidazole is significantly metabolized in humans prior to excretion. Tinidazole is partly metabolized by oxidation, hydroxylation, and conjugation. Tinidazole is the major drug-related constituent in plasma after human treatment, along with a small amount of the 2-hydroxymethyl metabolite.

TINIDAZOLE — ORAL

Tinidazole is biotransformed mainly by CYP3A4. In an in vitro metabolic drug interaction study, tinidazole concentrations of up to 75 mcg/mL did not inhibit the enzyme activities of CYP1A2, CYP2B6, CYP2C9, CYP2D6, CYP2E1, and CYP3A4.

The potential of tinidazole to induce the metabolism of other drugs has not been evaluated.

Excretion – The plasma half-life of tinidazole is approximately 12 to 14 hours. Tinidazole is excreted by the liver and the kidneys. Tinidazole is excreted in the urine mainly as unchanged drug (approximately 20% to 25% of the administered dose). Approximately 12% of the drug is excreted in feces.

Special populations –

Renal function impairment: During hemodialysis, clearance of tinidazole is significantly increased; the half-life is reduced from 12 to 4.9 hours. Approximately 43% of the amount present in the body is eliminated during a 6-hour hemodialysis session. The pharmacokinetics of tinidazole in patients undergoing routine continuous peritoneal dialysis have not been investigated.

Hepatic function impairment: There are no data on tinidazole pharmacokinetics in patients with hepatic function impairment. Reduction of metabolic elimination of metronidazole, a chemically related nitroimidazole, in patients with hepatic function impairment has been reported in several studies.

➤*Microbiology:*

Antibacterial – Culture and sensitivity testing of bacteria are not routinely performed to establish the diagnosis of bacterial vaginosis; standard methodology for the susceptibility testing of potential bacterial pathogens, *Gardnerella vaginalis*, *Mobiluncus* spp., or *Mycoplasma hominis*, has not been defined. The following in vitro data are available, but their clinical significance is unknown. Tinidazole is active in vitro against most strains of the following organisms that have been reported to be associated with bacterial vaginosis: *Bacteroides* spp., *Gardnerella vaginalis*, *Prevotella* spp.

Tinidazole does not appear to have activity against most strains of vaginal lactobacilli.

Antiprotozoal – Tinidazole demonstrates activity in vitro and in clinical infections against the following protozoa: *T. vaginalis*, *G. duodenalis* (also termed *G. lamblia*), and *E. histolytica*.

Cross-resistance – Approximately 38% of *T. vaginalis* isolates exhibiting reduced susceptibility to metronidazole also show reduced susceptibility to tinidazole in vitro. The clinical significance of such an effect is not known.

Contraindications

A previous history of hypersensitivity to tinidazole or other nitroimidazole derivatives; use during the first trimester of pregnancy.

Warnings/Precautions

➤*CNS effects:* Convulsive seizures and peripheral neuropathy, the latter characterized mainly by numbness or paresthesia of an extremity, have been reported in patients treated with tinidazole. The appearance of abnormal neurologic signs demands the prompt discontinuation of tinidazole therapy.

➤*Vaginal candidiasis:* The use of tinidazole may result in *Candida* vaginitis. In a clinical study of 235 women who received tinidazole for bacterial vaginosis, a vaginal fungal infection developed in 11 (4.7%) of all study subjects.

➤*Drug resistance:* Prescribing tinidazole in the absence of a proven or strongly suspected bacterial infection or a prophylactic indication is unlikely to provide benefit to the patient and increases the risk of the development of drug-resistant bacteria.

➤*Hematologic effects:* Tinidazole, like metronidazole, may produce transient leukopenia and neutropenia; however, no persistent hematological abnormalities attributable to tinidazole have been observed in clinical studies. Use tinidazole with caution in patients with evidence or history of blood dyscrasia.

➤*Renal function impairment:* If tinidazole is administered on the same day as and prior to hemodialysis, it is recommended that an additional dose of tinidazole equivalent to one-half of the recommended dose be administered after the end of the hemodialysis.

➤*Hepatic function impairment:* There are no data on tinidazole pharmacokinetics in patients with hepatic function impairment. Reduced elimination of metronidazole, a chemically related nitroimidazole, has been reported in this population. Administer the usual recommended doses of tinidazole with caution in patients with hepatic function impairment.

➤*Pregnancy: Category C.*

Teratogenic – The use of tinidazole in pregnant patients has not been studied. Because tinidazole crosses the placental barrier and enters fetal circulation, do not administer to pregnant patients in the first trimester.

In a study with pregnant rats, a slightly higher incidence of fetal mortality was observed at a maternal dose of 500 mg/kg (2.5-fold the highest human therapeutic dose based upon body surface area conversions).

Although there is some evidence of mutagenic potential and animal reproduction studies are not always predictive of human response, the use of tinidazole after the first trimester of pregnancy requires that the potential benefits of the drug be weighed against the possible risks to the mother and the fetus.

➤*Lactation:* Tinidazole is excreted in breast milk in concentrations similar to those seen in serum. Tinidazole can be detected in breast milk for up to 72 hours following administration. Interruption of breast-feeding is recommended during tinidazole therapy and for 3 days following the last dose.

➤*Children:* Other than for use in the treatment of giardiasis and amebiasis in children older than 3 years of age, safety and efficacy of tinidazole in children have not been established.

➤*Elderly:* In general, use caution in making dose selections for an elderly patient, reflecting the greater frequency of decreased hepatic, renal, or cardiac function, and of concomitant disease or other drug therapy.

➤*Monitoring:* Total and differential leukocyte counts are recommended if retreatment is necessary. Closely monitor children when treatment duration exceeds 3 days.

Drug Interactions

Although not studied specifically for tinidazole, the following drug interactions were reported for metronidazole, a chemically related nitroimidazole. Therefore, these drug interactions may occur with tinidazole.

Tinidazole Drug Interactions

Precipitant drug	Object drug[a]		Description
Cholestyramine	Tinidazole	⬇	Cholestyramine decreased the oral bioavailability of metronidazole 21%. Thus, consider separating the dosing of cholestyramine and tinidazole.
CYP3A4 inducers (eg, fosphenytoin, phenobarbital, rifampin, phenytoin)	Tinidazole	⬇	CYP3A4 inducers may accelerate the elimination of tinidazole, decreasing the plasma levels of tinidazole.
CYP3A4 inhibitors (eg, cimetidine, ketoconazole)	Tinidazole	⬆	CYP3A4 inhibitors may prolong the half-life and decrease plasma clearance of tinidazole.
Oxytetracycline	Tinidazole	⬇	Oxytetracycline was reported to antagonize the therapeutic effect of metronidazole.
Tinidazole	Alcohols	⬆	Avoid alcoholic beverages and preparations containing ethanol or propylene glycol during tinidazole therapy and for 3 days after discontinuation. Symptoms such as abdominal cramps, nausea, vomiting, headaches, and flushing may occur.
Tinidazole	Anticoagulants	⬆	Tinidazole may enhance the effect of warfarin and other coumarin anticoagulants, resulting in a prolongation of prothrombin time. Adjust the anticoagulant dose as needed during coadministration and up to 8 days after tinidazole discontinuation.
Tinidazole	Cyclosporine Tacrolimus	⬆	Several case reports suggest that metronidazole has the potential to increase the levels of cyclosporine and tacrolimus. During tinidazole coadministration, monitor for toxicities.
Tinidazole	Disulfiram	⬆	Psychotic reactions have been reported in alcoholic patients using metronidazole and disulfiram concurrently. Although no similar reactions have been reported with tinidazole, do not give tinidazole to patients who have taken disulfiram within the last 2 weeks.
Tinidazole	Fluorouracil	⬆	Metronidazole decreased the clearance of fluorouracil, resulting in toxicities. If concomitant use of tinidazole and fluorouracil cannot be avoided, monitor for fluorouracil toxicities.
Tinidazole	Hydantoins (eg, fosphenytoin, phenytoin)	⬆	Coadministration of oral metronidazole with intravenous phenytoin was reported to prolong the half-life and reduce the clearance of phenytoin. Orally administered phenytoin was not affected by metronidazole.

TINIDAZOLE — ORAL

Tinidazole Drug Interactions			
Precipitant drug	Object drug[a]		Description
Tinidazole	Lithium	↑	Metronidazole increased serum lithium levels. Although it is not known if tinidazole will interact with lithium, consider monitoring lithium and creatinine levels.

[a] ↑ = object drug increased; ↓ = object drug decreased.

➤*Drug/Lab test interactions:* Tinidazole, like metronidazole, may interfere with certain types of determinations of serum chemistry values, such as AST, ALT, lactate dehydrogenase, triglycerides, and hexokinase glucose. Values of zero may be observed. All of the assays in which interference has been reported involve enzymatic coupling of the assay to oxidation-reduction of nicotinamide adenine dinucleotide (NAD^+↔NADH). Potential interference is due to the similarity of absorbance peaks of NADH and tinidazole.

Adverse Reactions

Among 3,669 patients treated with a single dose of tinidazole 2 g, in controlled and uncontrolled trichomoniasis and giardiasis clinical studies, adverse reactions were reported by 11% of patients. For multi-day dosing in controlled and uncontrolled amebiasis studies, adverse reactions were reported by 13.8% of 1,765 patients.

➤*Common adverse reactions (at least 1%):*

Tinidazole Adverse Reactions		
Adverse reaction	2 g single dose	Multi-day dose
Total patients with adverse reactions	11% (403/3,669)	13.8% (244/1,765)
CNS		
Dizziness	1.1%	0.5%
Headache	1.3%	0.7%
Weakness/Fatigue/Malaise	2.1%	1.1%
GI		
Anorexia	1.5%	2.5%
Constipation	0.4%	1.4%
Dyspepsia/Cramps/Epigastric discomfort	1.8%	1.4%
Metallic/Bitter taste	3.7%	6.3%
Nausea	3.2%	4.5%
Vomiting	1.5%	0.9%

Other adverse reactions reported with tinidazole include the following:

Cardiovascular – Palpitations.

CNS – Two serious adverse reactions reported are convulsions and transient peripheral neuropathy, including numbness and paresthesia. Other CNS reports include ataxia, drowsiness, giddiness, insomnia, and vertigo.

GI – Diarrhea, stomatitis, tongue discoloration.

Hematologic – Transient leukopenia, transient neutropenia.

Hypersensitivity – Angioedema, burning sensation, dryness of mouth, fever, flushing, pruritus, rash, salivation, sweating, thirst, urticaria.

Renal – Darkened urine.

Miscellaneous – Arthralgia, arthritis, *Candida* overgrowth, hepatic abnormalities, myalgia, oral candidiasis, transaminase level raised, vaginal discharge increased.

➤*Rare adverse reactions:* Rare reported adverse reactions include bronchospasm, coma, confusion, depression, dyspnea, furry tongue, pharyngitis, and reversible thrombocytopenia.

➤*Children:* In pooled pediatric studies, adverse reactions reported in children taking tinidazole were similar in nature and frequency to adult findings, including abdominal pain, anorexia, diarrhea, nausea, taste change, and vomiting.

➤*Bacterial vaginosis:* The most common adverse reactions in treated patients (more than 2%), which were not identified in the trichomoniasis, giardiasis, and amebiasis studies, are as follows:

GI – Appetite decreased and flatulence.

GU – Menorrhagia, painful urination, pelvic pain, renal urinary tract infection, urine abnormality, vaginal odor, vulvovaginal discomfort.

Miscellaneous – Upper respiratory tract infection.

➤*Postmarketing:* The following adverse reactions have been identified and reported during post-approval use of tinidazole. Because the reports of these reactions are voluntary and the population is of uncertain size, it is not always possible to reliably estimate the frequency of the reaction or establish a causal relationship to drug exposure.

Overdosage

➤*Symptoms:* There are no reported overdoses with tinidazole in humans.

➤*Treatment:* There is no specific antidote for the treatment of overdosage with tinidazole; therefore, treatment should be symptomatic and supportive. Gastric lavage may be helpful. Hemodialysis can be considered because approximately 43% of the amount present in the body is eliminated during a 6-hour hemodialysis session.

Patient Information

Tell patients to take tinidazole with food to minimize the incidence of epigastric discomfort and other GI adverse reactions. Food does not affect the oral bioavailability of tinidazole.

Tell patients to avoid alcoholic beverages and preparations containing ethanol or propylene glycol during tinidazole therapy and for 3 days afterward because abdominal cramps, nausea, vomiting, headaches, and flushing may occur.

Counsel patients that antibacterial drugs, including tinidazole, should only be used to treat bacterial infections. They do not treat viral infections (eg, the common cold). When tinidazole is prescribed to treat a bacterial infection, tell patients that although it is common to feel better early in the course of therapy, to take the medication exactly as directed. Skipping doses or not completing the full course of therapy may decrease the efficacy of the immediate treatment and increase the likelihood that bacteria will develop resistance and will not be treatable by tinidazole or other antibacterial drugs in the future.

ATOVAQUONE

Rx	**Mepron** (GlaxoWellcome)	**Suspension**: 750 mg/5 mL	Benzyl alcohol, saccharin. Bright yellow. Citrus flavor. In 210 mL.

ATOVAQUONE — ORAL

Indications

➤*Pneumocystis carinii pneumonia:*

Prophylaxis – For the prevention of *P. carinii* pneumonia (PCP) in patients who are intolerant to trimethoprim-sulfamethoxazole (TMP-SMZ).

Treatment – For the acute oral treatment of mild-to-moderate PCP in patients who are intolerant to TMP-SMZ.

Administration and Dosage

➤*General dosing considerations:* Absorption of orally administered atovaquone is limited but can be significantly increased when the drug is taken with food. Plasma atovaquone concentrations have been shown to correlate with the likelihood of successful treatment and survival. Therefore, parenteral therapy with other agents should be considered for patients who have difficulty taking atovaquone with food. GI disorders may limit absorption of orally administered drugs. Patients with these disorders also may not achieve plasma concentrations of atovaquone associated with response to therapy in controlled trials.

➤*Adults:*

Prevention of Pneumocystis carinii pneumonia – 1,500 mg (10 mL) once daily.

Treatment of mild to moderate Pneumocystis carinii pneumonia – 750 mg (5 mL) twice daily for 21 days (total daily dose of 1,500 mg).

➤*Children:*

13 years of age and older – See Adults for dosing for children 13 years of age and older.

➤*Administration:* Take with meals because the presence of food will significantly improve the absorption of the drug. Failure to administer atovaquone suspension with meals may result in lower plasma atovaquone concentrations and may limit response to therapy.

Foil pouch – Open pouch by removing tab at perforation and tear at notch. Take entire contents by mouth. This medication can be discharged into a dosing spoon or cup or directly into the mouth.

Bottle – Shake bottle gently before using.

➤*Storage/Stability:* Store at 15° to 25°C (59° to 77°F). Do not freeze. Dispense in tight container

Actions

➤*Pharmacology:* Atovaquone is a hydroxy-1,4-naphthoquinone, an analog of ubiquinone, with antipneumocystis activity. The mechanism of action against *Pneumocystis carinii* has not been fully elucidated. In *Plasmodium* species, the site of action appears to be the cytochrome bc_1 complex (Complex III). Several metabolic enzymes are linked to the mitochondrial electron transport chain via ubiquinone. Inhibition of electron transport by atovaquone will result in indirect inhibition of these enzymes. The ultimate metabolic effects of such blockade may include inhibition of nucleic acid and ATP synthesis.

➤*Pharmacokinetics:*

Absorption – Atovaquone is a highly lipophilic compound with low aqueous solubility. The bioavailability of atovaquone is highly dependent on formulation and diet. The absolute bioavailability of a 750 mg dose of atovaquone suspension administered under fed conditions in 9 HIV-infected (CD4 greater than 100 cells/mm^3) volunteers was 47% ± 15%.

ATOVAQUONE — ORAL

Administering atovaquone with food enhances its absorption by approximately 2-fold. In 1 study, 16 healthy volunteers received a single dose of 750 mg atovaquone suspension after an overnight fast and following a standard breakfast (23 g fat, 610 kcal). The mean (± SD) area under the concentration-time curve (AUC) values were 324 ± 115 and 801 ± 320 mcg•hr/mL under fasting and fed conditions, respectively, representing a 2.6 ± 1-fold increase. The effect of food (23 g fat, 400 kcal) on plasma atovaquone concentrations was also evaluated in a multiple-dose, randomized, crossover study in 19 HIV-infected volunteers (CD4 less than 200 cells/mm^3) receiving daily doses of 500 mg atovaquone suspension. AUC was 280 ± 114 mcg•hr/mL when atovaquone was administered with food as compared to 169 ± 77 mcg•hr/mL under fasting conditions. Maximum plasma atovaquone concentration (C_{max}) was 15.1 ± 6.1 and 8.8 ± 3.7 mcg/mL when atovaquone was administered with food and under fasting conditions, respectively.

Dose proportionality: Plasma atovaquone concentrations do not increase proportionally with dose. When atovaquone suspension was administered with food at dosage regimens of 500 mg once daily, 750 mg once daily, and 1000 mg once daily, average steady-state plasma atovaquone concentrations were 11.7 ± 4.8, 12.5 ± 5.8, and 13.5 ± 5.1 mcg/mL, respectively. The corresponding C_{max} concentrations were 15.1 ± 6.1, 15.3 ± 7.6, and 16.8 ± 6.4 mcg/mL. When atovaquone suspension was administered to 5 HIV-infected volunteers at a dose of 750 mg twice daily, the average steady-state plasma atovaquone concentration was 21.0 ± 4.9 mcg/mL, and C_{max} was 24 ± 5.7 mcg/mL. The minimum plasma atovaquone concentration (C_{min}) associated with the 750 mg twice-daily regimen was 16.7 ± 4.6 mcg/mL.

Distribution – Following the IV administration of atovaquone, the volume of distribution at steady state (Vd_{ss}) was 0.6 ± 0.17 L/kg (n = 9). Atovaquone is extensively bound to plasma proteins (99.9%) over the concentration range of 1 to 90 mcg/mL. In 3 HIV-infected children who received 750 mg atovaquone as the tablet formulation 4 times daily for 2 weeks, the cerebrospinal fluid concentrations of atovaquone were 0.04, 0.14, and 0.26 mcg/mL, representing less than 1% of the plasma concentration.

Excretion – The plasma clearance of atovaquone following IV administration in 9 HIV-infected volunteers was 10.4 ± 5.5 mL/min (0.15 ± 0.09 mL/min per kg). The half-life of atovaquone was 62.5 ± 35.3 hours after IV administration and ranged from 67 ± 33.4 to 77.6 ± 23.1 hours across studies following administration of atovaquone suspension. The half-life of atovaquone is long due to presumed enterohepatic cycling and eventual fecal elimination. In a study where ^{14}C-labeled atovaquone was administered to healthy volunteers, greater than 94% of the dose was recovered as unchanged atovaquone in the feces over 21 days. There was little or no excretion of atovaquone in the urine (less than 0.6%). There is indirect evidence that atovaquone may undergo limited metabolism; however, a specific metabolite has not been identified.

Special populations –

Children: In a study of atovaquone suspension in 27 HIV-infected, asymptomatic infants and children between 1 month and 13 years of age, the pharmacokinetics of atovaquone were age-dependent. These patients were dosed once daily with food for 12 days. The average steady-state plasma atovaquone concentrations (C_{ss}, mcg/mL) in the 24 patients with available concentration data are shown in the following information. Values are mean ± SD.

- *Average steady-state plasma atovaquone concentrations in pediatric patients* – In patients aged 1 to 3 months, atovaquone 10 mg/kg resulted in an average C_{ss} = 5.9 mcg/mL (n = 1), and atovaquone 30 mg/kg resulted in an average C_{ss} = 27.8 ± 5.8 mcg/mL (n = 4).

In patients older than 3 to 24 months of age, atovaquone 10 mg/kg resulted in an average C_{ss} = 5.7 ± 5.1 mcg/mL (n = 4), atovaquone 30 mg/kg resulted in an average C_{ss} = 9.8 ± 3.2 mcg/mL (n = 4), and atovaquone 45 mg/kg resulted in an average C_{ss} = 15.4 ± 6.6 mcg/mL (n = 4).

In patients older than 2 to 13 years of age, atovaquone 10 mg/kg resulted in an average C_{ss} = 16.8 ± 6.4 mcg/mL (n = 4), and atovaquone 30 mg/kg resulted in an average C_{ss} = 37.1 ± 10.9 mcg/mL (n = 3).

➤*Microbiology:*

Drug resistance – Phenotypic resistance to atovaquone in vitro has not been demonstrated for *P. carinii*. However, in 2 patients who developed *P. carinii* pneumonia (PCP) after prophylaxis with atovaquone, DNA sequence analysis identified mutations in the predicted amino acid sequence of *P. carinii* cytochrome b (a likely target site for atovaquone). The clinical significance of this is unknown.

Contraindications

Patients who develop or have a history of potentially life-threatening allergic reactions to any of the components of the formulation.

Warnings/Precautions

➤*Severe PCP:* Clinical experience with atovaquone for the treatment of PCP has been limited to patients with mild-to-moderate PCP [(A-a)DO_2 less than or equal to 45 mmHg]. Treatment of more severe episodes of PCP has not been systematically studied with this agent. Also, the efficacy of atovaquone in patients who are failing therapy with TMP-SMZ has not been systematically studied.

➤*Concurrent pulmonary infections:* Based upon the spectrum of in vitro antimicrobial activity, atovaquone is not effective therapy for concurrent pulmonary conditions such as bacterial, viral, or fungal pneumonia or mycobacterial diseases. Clinical deterioration in patients may be due to infections with other pathogens, as well as progressive PCP. All patients with acute PCP should be carefully evaluated for other possible causes of pulmonary disease and treated with additional agents as appropriate.

➤*Hepatic function impairment:* If it is necessary to treat patients with severe hepatic impairment, caution is advised, and administration should be monitored closely.

➤*Pregnancy: Category C.* Atovaquone caused maternal toxicity in rabbits at plasma concentrations that were approximately one-half the estimated human exposure. Mean fetal body lengths and weights were decreased, and there were higher numbers of early resorption and postimplantation loss per dam. It is not clear whether these effects were caused by atovaquone directly or were secondary to maternal toxicity. Concentrations of atovaquone in rabbit fetuses averaged 30% of the concurrent maternal plasma concentrations. In a separate study in rats given a single ^{14}C-radiolabeled dose, concentrations of radiocarbon in rat fetuses were 18% (middle gestation) and 60% (late gestation) of concurrent maternal plasma concentrations. There are no adequate and well-controlled studies in pregnant women. Atovaquone should be used during pregnancy only if the potential benefit justifies the potential risk to the fetus.

➤*Lactation:* It is not known whether atovaquone is excreted into human milk. Because many drugs are excreted into human milk, caution should be exercised when atovaquone is administered to a nursing woman. In a rat study, atovaquone concentrations in the milk were 30% of the concurrent atovaquone concentrations in the maternal plasma.

➤*Children:* Evidence of safety and efficacy in pediatric patients has not been established. A relationship between plasma atovaquone concentrations and successful treatment of PCP has been established in adults (see the information below). In a study of atovaquone suspension in 27 HIV-infected, asymptomatic infants and children between 1 month and 13 years of age, the pharmacokinetics of atovaquone were age-dependent.

Average steady-state plasma atovaquone concentrations in pediatric patients – No drug-related, treatment-limiting adverse reactions were observed in the pharmacokinetic study.

See Actions for more information.

➤*Elderly:* In general, dose selection for an elderly patient should be cautious, reflecting the greater frequency of decreased hepatic, renal, or cardiac function, and of concomitant disease or other drug therapy.

Drug Interactions

➤*Plasma protein-bound drugs:* Atovaquone is highly bound to plasma protein (greater than 99.9%). Therefore, caution should be used when administering atovaquone concurrently with other highly plasma protein-bound drugs with narrow therapeutic indices, as competition for binding sites may occur. The extent of plasma protein binding of atovaquone in human plasma is not affected by the presence of therapeutic concentrations of phenytoin (15 mcg/mL), nor is the binding of phenytoin affected by the presence of atovaquone.

➤*Trimethoprim/sulfamethoxazole (TMP-SMZ):* The possible interaction between atovaquone and TMP-SMZ was evaluated in 6 HIV-infected adult volunteers as part of a larger multiple-dose, dose-escalation, and chronic-dosing study of atovaquone suspension. In this crossover study, atovaquone suspension 500 mg once daily, or TMP-SMZ tablets (160 mg trimethoprim and 800 mg sulfamethoxazole) twice daily, or the combination were administered with food to achieve steady state. No difference was observed in the average steady-state plasma atovaquone concentration after coadministration with TMP-SMZ. Coadministration of atovaquone with TMP-SMZ resulted in a 17% and 8% decrease in average steady-state concentrations of trimethoprim and sulfamethoxazole in plasma, respectively. This effect is minor and would not be expected to produce clinically significant events.

Atovaquone Drug Interactions

Precipitant drug	Object drug[a]		Description
Metoclopramide	Atovaquone	⬇	Concomitant treatment with metoclopramide has been associated with decreased bioavailability of atovaquone. Use only if other antiemetics are not available.
Rifampin Rifabutin	Atovaquone	⬇	Concomitant administration of rifampin or rifabutin is known to reduce atovaquone levels by approximately 50% and 34% respectively. The concomitant administration of these agents is not recommended. The mechanism of this interaction is unknown.
Tetracycline	Atovaquone	⬇	Concomitant treatment with tetracycline has been associated with ≈ 40% reduction in plasma concentrations of atovaquone. Closely monitor parasitemia in patients receiving tetracycline.
Atovaquone	Zidovudine	⬆	Zidovudine concentrations may be elevated, increasing the risk of zidovudine toxicity.

[a] ⬇ = object drug decreased; ⬆ = object drug increased.

➤*Drug/Lab test interactions:* It is not known if atovaquone interferes with clinical laboratory test or assay results.

Adverse Reactions

Because many patients who participated in clinical trials with atovaquone had complications of advanced HIV disease, it was often difficult to distinguish adverse events caused by atovaquone from those caused by underlying

ATOVAQUONE — ORAL

medical conditions. There were no life-threatening or fatal adverse experiences caused by atovaquone.

➤*PCP prevention studies:*

Atovaquone Treatment-Limiting Adverse Reactions in the Dapsone Comparative PCP Prevention Study

Treatment-limiting adverse reaction	All patients		Patients not taking either drug at enrollment	
	Atovaquone 1,500 mg/day (n = 536)	Dapsone 100 mg/day (n = 521)	Atovaquone 1500 mg/day (n = 238)	Dapsone 100 mg/day (n = 249)
Any event	24.4%	25.9%	20.2%	43.4%
Rash	6.3%	8.8%	7.6%	16.1%
Nausea	4.1%	0.6%	2.5%	0.8%
Diarrhea	3.2%	0.2%	2.1%	0.4%
Vomiting	2.2%	0.6%	1.3%	0.8%
Allergic reaction	1.1%	2.9%	0.8%	4.8%
Fever	0.6%	2.9%	0%	5.6%
Anemia	0%	1.5%	0%	2%

Treatment-emergent adverse reactions –

Atovaquone Treatment-Emergent Adverse Reactions in the Aerosolized Pentamidine Comparative PCP Prevention Study

Treatment-emergent adverse reaction	Atovaquone 1500 mg/day (n = 175)	Atovaquone 750 mg/day (n = 188)	Aerosolized pentamidine (n = 186)
Diarrhea	42%	42%	35%
Rash	39%	46%	28%
Headache	28%	31%	22%
Nausea	26%	32%	23%
Increased cough	25%	25%	31%
Fever	25%	31%	18%
Rhinitis	24%	18%	17%
Asthenia	22%	31%	31%
Infection	22%	18%	19%
Abdominal pain	20%	21%	20%
Dyspnea	15%	21%	16%
Vomiting	15%	22%	11%
Patients discontinuing therapy due to an adverse reaction	25%	16%	7%
Patients reporting at least 1 adverse reaction	98%	96%	89%

Other events – Other events occurring in 10% or more of the patients receiving the recommended dose of atovaquone included sweating, flu syndrome, pain, sinusitis, pruritus, insomnia, depression, and myalgia. Bronchospasm occurred more frequently in patients receiving aerosolized pentamidine (11%) than in patients receiving atovaquone 1500 mg/day (4%) and atovaquone 750 mg/day (2%).

➤*PCP treatment studies:*

Clinical adverse reactions reported by 5% or more –

Atovaquone Treatment-Emergent Adverse Reactions in the TMP-SMZ Comparative PCP Treatment Study

Treatment-emergent adverse reaction	Atovaquone (n = 203)	TMP-SMZ (n = 205)
Rash (including maculopapular)	23%	34%
Nausea	21%	44%
Diarrhea	19%	7%
Headache	16%	22%
Vomiting	14%	35%
Fever	14%	25%
Insomnia	10%	9%
Asthenia	8%	8%
Pruritus	5%	9%
Oral monilia	5%	10%
Abdominal pain	4%	7%
Constipation	3%	17%
Dizziness	3%	8%
Patients discontinuing therapy due to an adverse reaction	9%	24%

Atovaquone Treatment-Emergent Adverse Reactions in the TMP-SMZ Comparative PCP Treatment Study

Treatment-emergent adverse reaction	Atovaquone (n = 203)	TMP-SMZ (n = 205)
Patients reporting at least 1 adverse reaction	63%	65%

Discontinuation of therapy – Although an equal percentage of patients receiving atovaquone and TMP-SMZ reported at least 1 adverse reaction, more patients receiving TMP-SMZ required discontinuation of therapy due to an adverse reaction. Twenty-four percent (24%) of patients receiving TMP-SMZ were prematurely discontinued from therapy due to an adverse experience vs 9% of patients receiving atovaquone. Four percent (4%) of patients receiving atovaquone had therapy discontinued due to development of rash. The majority of cases of rash among patients receiving atovaquone were mild and did not require the discontinuation of dosing. The only other clinical adverse experience that led to premature discontinuation of dosing of atovaquone by more than 1 patient was vomiting (less than 1%). The most common adverse reaction requiring discontinuation of dosing in the TMP-SMZ group was rash (8%).

Lab test abnormalities – Laboratory test abnormalities reported for 5% or more of the study population during the treatment period are summarized in the table below. Two percent (2%) of patients treated with atovaquone and 7% of patients treated with TMP-SMZ had therapy prematurely discontinued due to elevations in ALT/AST. In general, patients treated with atovaquone developed fewer abnormalities in measures of hepatocellular function (ALT, AST, alkaline phosphatase) or amylase values than patients treated with TMP-SMZ.

Atovaquone Treatment-Emergent Laboratory Test Abnormalities in the TMP-SMZ Comparative PCP Treatment Study

Laboratory test abnormality	Atovaquone	TMP-SMZ
Anemia (Hgb < 8 g/dL)	6%	7%
Neutropenia (ANC < 750 cells/mm^3)	3%	9%
Elevated ALT (> 5 × ULN[a])	6%	16%
Elevated AST (> 5 × ULN)	4%	14%
Elevated alkaline phosphatase (> 2.5 × ULN)	8%	6%
Elevated amylase (> 1.5 × ULN)	7%	12%
Hyponatremia (< 0.96 × LLN[b])	7%	26%

[a] ULN = upper limit of normal range.
[b] LLN = lower limit of normal range.

Atovaquone Treatment-Emergent Adverse Reactions in the Pentamidine Comparative PCP Treatment Study (Primary Therapy Group)

Treatment-emergent adverse reaction	Atovaquone (n = 73)	Pentamidine (n = 71)
Fever	40%	25%
Nausea	22%	37%
Rash	22%	13%
Diarrhea	21%	31%
Insomnia	19%	14%
Headache	18%	28%
Vomiting	14%	17%
Cough	14%	1%
Abdominal pain	10%	11%
Pain	10%	10%
Sweat	10%	3%
Oral monilia	10%	3%
Asthenia	8%	14%
Dizziness	8%	14%
Anxiety	7%	10%
Anorexia	7%	10%
Sinusitis	7%	6%
Dyspepsia	5%	10%
Rhinitis	5%	7%
Taste perversion	3%	13%
Hypoglycemia	1%	15%
Hypotension	1%	10%
Patients discontinuing therapy due to an adverse reaction	7%	41%
Patients reporting at least 1 adverse reaction	63%	72%

ATOVAQUONE — ORAL

Lab test abnormalities – Laboratory test abnormalities reported in at least 5% of patients in the pentamidine comparative study are presented in the table below. Laboratory abnormality was reported as the reason for discontinuation of treatment in 2 of 73 patients who received atovaquone. One patient (1%) had elevated creatinine and BUN levels and 1 patient (1%) had elevated amylase levels. Laboratory abnormalities were the sole or contributing factor in 14 patients who prematurely discontinued pentamidine therapy. In the 71 patients who received pentamidine, laboratory parameters most frequently reported as reasons for discontinuation were hypoglycemia (11%), elevated creatinine levels (6%), and leukopenia (4%).

Atovaquone Treatment-Emergent Laboratory Test Abnormalities in the Pentamidine Comparative PCP Treatment Study

Laboratory test abnormality	Atovaquone	Pentamidine
Anemia (Hgb < 8 g/dL)	4%	9%
Neutropenia (ANC < 750 cells/mm^3)	5%	9%
Hyponatremia (< 0.96 × LLN [a])	10%	10%
Hyperkalemia (> 1.18 × ULN [b])	0%	5%
Alkaline phosphatase (> 2.5 × ULN)	5%	2%
Hyperglycemia (> 1.8 × ULN)	9%	13%
Elevated AST (> 5 × ULN)	0%	5%
Elevated amylase (> 1.5 × ULN)	8%	4%
Elevated creatinine (> 1.5 × ULN)	0%	7%

[a] LLN = lower limit of normal range.
[b] ULN = upper limit of normal range.

➤*Postmarketing:*

Dermatologic – Allergic reactions including erythema multiforme.

GU – Acute renal impairment.

Hematologic/Lymphatic – Methemoglobinemia, thrombocytopenia.

Hepatic – Pancreatitis.

Ophthalmic – Vortex keratopathy.

Overdosage

➤*Symptoms:* The median lethal dose is higher than the maximum oral dose tested in mice and rats (1825 mg/kg/day). Overdoses up to 31,500 mg of atovaquone have been reported. In 1 such patient who also took an unspecified dose of dapsone, methemoglobinemia occurred. Rash has also been reported after overdose.

➤*Treatment:* There is no known antidote for atovaquone, and it is currently unknown if atovaquone is dialyzable.

Patient Information

The importance of taking the prescribed dose of atovaquone should be stressed. Patients should be instructed to take their daily doses of atovaquone with meals, as the presence of food will significantly improve the absorption of the drug.

PENTAMIDINE ISETHIONATE

Rx	**Pentam 300** (American Pharmaceutical Partners)	**Injection**: 300 mg	In single-dose vials.
Rx	**Pentamidine Isethionate** (Abbott)	**Powder for Injection, lyophilized**: 300 mg	In single-dose flip-top vials.
Rx	**NebuPent** (American Pharmaceutical Partners)	**Aerosol**: 300 mg	In single dose vials.

PENTAMIDINE ISETHIONATE — INJECTION

Indications

➤*Pneumocystis carinii:* For the treatment of pneumonia due to *Pneumocystis carinii*.

➤*Off-label uses:* Pentamidine has been used in the treatment of trypanosomiasis and visceral leishmaniasis.

Administration and Dosage

➤*Adults:*

Pneumocystis jiroveci (formerly carinii) –

Usual dosage: 4 mg/kg once a day for 14 to 21 days.

Duration of therapy: Therapy for longer than 21 days has been used but may be associated with increased toxicity.

Off-label dosing –

Parasitic infections (Leishmaniasis): 2 to 4 mg/kg IM once daily or every other day for up to 15 to 30 doses.

Pneumocystis jiroveci:

- *Prophylactic dosage* – 4 mg/kg IM or IV once every 2 or 4 weeks.

Trypanosomiasis: 4 mg/kg once a day IM for 10 days.

➤*Children:*

Pneumocystis jiroveci (formerly carinii) –

4 months of age and older: See Adults for more information.

Off-label dosing – See Adults for more information.

➤*Renal function impairment:*

Off-label dosing –

CrCl 10 to 50 mL/min: Administer recommended dose every 24 to 36 hours.

CrCl less than 10 mL/min: Administer recommended dose every 48 hours.

➤*Preparation for administration:*

IM injection – The contents of one vial should be dissolved in 3 mL of sterile water for injection at 22° to 30°C (72° to 86°F).

IV injection – The contents of one vial should first be dissolved in 3 to 5 mL of sterile water for injection or 5% dextrose injection at 22° to 30°C (72° to 86°F).

➤*Administration:*

IM injection – The calculated daily dose should be withdrawn and administered by deep IM injection.

IV injection – The calculated dose of pentamidine should be withdrawn and diluted further in 50 to 250 mL of 5% dextrose injection. The diluted IV solutions containing pentamidine should be infused over a period of 60 to 120 minutes.

➤*Admixture compatibility:* Do not use sodium chloride injection for initial reconstitution because precipitation will occur. IV solutions of pentamidine have been shown to be incompatible with fluconazole and foscarnet sodium. IV solutions of pentamidine have been shown to be compatible with IV solutions of zidovudine and diltiazem.

➤*Storage/Stability:* Store the dry product at controlled room temperature 15° to 30°C (59° to 86°F) and protect from light. Discard unused portion. After reconstitution with sterile water, the solution is stable for 48 hours in the original vial at room temperature if protected from light. To avoid crystallization, store at 22° to 30°C (72° to 86°F). IV infusion solutions prepared in 5% dextrose injection are stable at room temperature for up to 24 hours.

Actions

➤*Pharmacology:* Pentamidine isethionate, an aromatic diamidine, is known to have activity against *Pneumocystis carinii*. The mode of action of pentamidine is not fully understood. In vitro studies indicate that the drug interferes with protozoal nuclear metabolism by inhibition of DNA, RNA, phospholipid and protein synthesis.

➤*Pharmacokinetics:*

Absorption/Distribution – Pharmacokinetic parameters following the administration of 4 mg/kg pentamidine isethionate as a single 2-hour IV infusion or after a single IM injection to 12 patients with AIDS are presented in the following table:

Pentamidine Injection Pharmacokinetic Parameters

Mean ± SD	C_{max} (ng/mL)	Clearance (L/hr)	Half-life (hours)	Vdss (L)	Concentration (ng/mL) 8 hour	24 hour
2-hour IV infusion 4 mg/kg (n = 6)	612 ± 371	248 ± 91	6.4 ± 1.3	821 ± 535	19.3 ± 16.9	2.9 ± 1.4
IM 4 mg/kg (n = 6)	209 ± 48	305 ± 81	9.4 ± 2	2724 ± 1066	22.9 ± 8	6.6 ± 3.5

In 7 patients treated with daily IM doses of pentamidine at 4 mg/kg for 10 to 12 days, plasma concentrations were between 300 to 500 ng/mL. The concentrations did not appreciably change with time after injection or from day to day. Higher plasma concentrations were encountered in patients with an elevated blood urea nitrogen.

Following multiple IV administration: Following multiple IV administration of pentamidine isethionate (3.7 to 4 mg/kg/day infused over 4 hours) to 6 patients with AIDS being treated for PCP, the pharmacokinetic parameters obtained on days 1, 4 and 7 are summarized in the following table:

Pentamidine Pharmacokinetics Following Multiple IV Administration

Mean ± SD	C_{max} [a](ng/mL)	C_{min} [a] (ng/mL)	Clearance (mL/min)	Renal clearance (mL/min/ 1.73 m^2)	Creatinine clearance (mL/min/ 1.73 m^2)
Day 1	175.3 ± 54	-	5737 ± 1878	269 ± 149	97 ± 12
Day 4	210.9 ± 80	17.6 ± 9.5	3350 ± 1944	214 ± 145	93 ± 17
Day 7	256.7 ± 89	40.8 ± 16.1	1989 ± 566	134 ± 60	69 ± 17

[a] Derived from Lidman.

PENTAMIDINE ISETHIONATE — INJECTION

Compared to the mean AUC on day 1, AUC on day 4 and day 7 were about 2- and 3-fold higher, respectively, suggesting that steady state was not achieved by day 7 of dosing.

Metabolism – In other published reports of pharmacokinetics of pentamidine following daily IV doses of 2 to 4 mg/kg/day, clearance ranged from 30 to 40 mL/min/kg, and the volume of distribution at steady state ranged from 200 to 400 L/kg. Reported values for terminal half-lives of 2.8 to 12 days is suggestive of a deep peripheral compartment. In the urine, up to 12% of the administered dose has been recovered during a dosing interval as unchanged pentamidine.

Excretion – The patients continued to excrete decreasing amounts of pentamidine in urine up to 6 to 8 weeks after cessation of the treatment.

Contraindications

History of hypersensitivity to pentamidine isethionate.

Warnings/Precautions

➤*Ulceration, tissue necrosis or sloughing at the injection site:* Extravasations have been reported which, in some instances, proceeded to ulceration, tissue necrosis or sloughing at the injection site. While not common, surgical debridement and skin grafting has been necessary in some of these cases; long-term sequelae have been reported. Prevention is the most effective means of limiting the severity of extravasation. The IV needle or catheter must be properly positioned and closely observed throughout the period of pentamidine isethionate administration. If extravasation occurs, the injection should be discontinued immediately and restarted in another vein. Because there are no known local treatment measures which have proven to be useful, management of the extravasation should be symptomatic.

➤*Hypotension:* Patients may develop sudden, severe hypotension after a single dose of pentamidine isethionate, whether given IV or IM. Therefore, patients receiving the drug should be lying down and the blood pressure should be monitored closely during administration of the drug and several times thereafter until the blood pressure is stable. Equipment for emergency resuscitation should be readily available. If pentamidine isethionate is administered IV, it should be infused over a period of 60 to 120 minutes.

➤*Hypoglycemia:* Pentamidine isethionate-induced hypoglycemia has been associated with pancreatic islet cell necrosis and inappropriately high plasma insulin concentrations. Hyperglycemia and diabetes mellitus, with or without preceding hypoglycemia, have also occurred, sometimes several months after therapy with pentamidine isethionate. Therefore, blood glucose levels should be monitored daily during therapy with pentamidine isethionate, and several times thereafter.

➤*Hypersensitivity reactions:* Fatalities due to severe hypotension, hypoglycemia, acute pancreatitis, and cardiac arrhythmias have been reported in patients treated with pentamidine isethionate, both by the IM and IV routes. Severe hypotension may result after a single IM or IV dose and is more likely with rapid IV administration (see Precautions). The administration of the drug should, therefore, be limited to the patients in whom *Pneumocystis carinii* has been demonstrated. Patients should be closely monitored for the development of serious adverse reactions (see Precautions and Adverse Reactions).

➤*Special risk:* Pentamidine isethionate should be used with caution in patients with hypertension, hypotension, ventricular tachycardia, hypoglycemia, hyperglycemia, hypocalcemia, pancreatitis, leukopenia, thrombocytopenia, anemia, hepatic or renal dysfunction and Stevens-Johnson syndrome.

➤*Pregnancy: Category C.* Animal reproduction studies have not been conducted with pentamidine isethionate. It is also not known whether pentamidine isethionate can cause fetal harm when administered to a pregnant woman or can affect reproduction capacity. Pentamidine isethionate should not be given to a pregnant woman unless the potential benefits are judged to outweigh the unknown risks.

➤*Lactation:* It is not known whether pentamidine isethionate is excreted in human milk. Because of the potential for serious adverse reactions in nursing infants from pentamidine isethionate, a decision should be made whether to discontinue nursing or to discontinue the drug, taking into account the importance of the drug to the mother. Because many drugs are excreted in human milk, pentamidine isethionate should not be given to a nursing mother unless the potential benefits are judged to outweigh the unknown risks.

➤*Children:* IV and IM pentamidine has been described as an effective treatment for *Pneumocystis carinii* pneumonia (PCP) in immunocompromised pediatric patients beyond 4 months of age. The efficacy and safety profiles in these pediatric patients were similar to those observed in adult patients (see Administration and Dosage and Overdosage).

➤*Monitoring:* The following tests should be carried out before, during and after therapy:

1.) Daily blood urea nitrogen and serum creatinine determinations.
2.) Daily blood glucose determinations.
3.) Complete blood count and platelet count.
4.) Liver function test, including serum bilirubin, alkaline phosphatase, AST, and ALT.
5.) Serum calcium determinations.
6.) ECGs.

Drug Interactions

➤*QT prolongation:* An additive effect of pentamidine with other drugs that prolong the QT interval cannot be excluded. The following drugs may prolong the QT interval and increase the risk of life-threatening cardiac arrhythmias, including torsades de pointes: Antiarrhythmic agents (eg, amiodarone, bretylium, disopyramide, dofetilide, procainamide, quinidine, and sotalol), arsenic trioxide, chlorpromazine, cisapride, dolasetron, droperidol, mefloquine, mesoridazine, moxifloxacin, pimozide, tacrolimus, thioridazine, and ziprasidone. For a more complete list of drugs that may prolong the QT interval, see the appendix, Drug-Induced Prolongation of the QT Interval and Torsades de Pointes.

➤*Other nephrotoxic drugs:* Because the nephrotoxic effects may be additive, the concomitant or sequential use of pentamidine isethionate and other nephrotoxic drugs such as aminoglycosides, amphotericin B, cisplatin, foscarnet, or vancomycin should be closely monitored and avoided, if possible.

Adverse Reactions

Fatalities due to severe hypotension, hypoglycemia, acute pancreatitis and cardiac arrhythmias have been reported in patients treated with pentamidine isethionate, both by the IM and IV routes. Nephrotoxic events (increased creatinine, impaired renal function, azotemia, and renal failure) are common with the parenteral administration of pentamidine isethionate. The administration of the drug should, therefore, be limited to the patients in whom *Pneumocystis carinii* has been demonstrated.

The most frequently reported spontaneous adverse events (1% to 30%) reported in clinical trials, regardless of their relation to pentamidine isethionate therapy were as follows (n = 424):

➤*Cardiovascular:* Hypotension, 5%.

➤*CNS:* Confusion/hallucinations, 1.7%.

➤*Dermatologic:* Rash, 3.3%.

➤*GI:* Anorexia/nausea, 5.9%.

➤*GU:* Azotemia, 8.5%; elevated serum creatinine, 23.6%; elevated blood urea nitrogen, 6.6%; impaired renal function, 28.8%.

➤*Hematologic:* Anemia, 1.2%; leukopenia, 10.4%; thrombocytopenia, 2.6%.

➤*Hepatic:* Elevated liver function tests, 8.7%.

➤*Local:* Sterile abscess or necrosis, pain, or induration at the site of IM injection, 11.1%.

➤*Metabolic:* Hypoglycemia, 5.9%.

➤*Special senses:* Bad taste, 1.7%.

➤*Adverse events (< 1%):* Adverse events with a frequency of less than 1% incidence were as follows (no causal relationship to treatment has been established for these adverse events):

Allergic – Allergic reaction (ie, urticaria, itching, rash), anaphylaxis.

Cardiovascular – Abnormal ST segment of ECG, cardiac arrhythmias, cerebrovascular accident, hypertension, palpitations, phlebitis, syncope, tachycardia, vasodilatation, vasculitis and ventricular tachycardia.

CNS – Anxiety, confusion, depression, dizziness, drowsiness, emotional lability, hypesthesia, insomnia, memory loss, neuropathy, nervousness, neuralgia, paranoia, paresthesia, peripheral neuropathy, seizure, tremors, unsteady gait, and vertigo.

Dermatologic – Desquamation, dry and breaking hair, dry skin, erythema, dermatitis, pruritus, rash, and urticaria.

GI – Abdominal pain, diarrhea, dry mouth, dyspepsia, hematochezia, hypersalivation, melena, pancreatitis, splenomegaly, and vomiting.

GU – Flank pain, hematuria, and incontinence.

Hematologic – Defibrination, eosinophilia, neutropenia, pancytopenia, and prolonged clotting time.

Hepatic – Hepatic dysfunction, hepatitis and hepatomegaly.

Metabolic – Hyperglycemia, hyperkalemia, hypocalcemia, and hypomagnesemia.

Ophthalmic – Blepharitis, blurred vision, conjunctivitis, contact lens discomfort, eye pain or discomfort.

Renal – Nephritis, renal dysfunction, and renal failure.

Respiratory – Asthma, bronchitis, bronchospasm, chest congestion, chest tightness, coryza, cyanosis, eosinophilic or interstitial pneumonitis, gagging, hemoptysis, hyperventilation, laryngitis, laryngospasm, non-specific lung disorder, nasal congestion, pleuritis, pneumothorax, rales, rhinitis, shortness of breath, and tachypnea.

Special senses – Loss of hearing, loss of taste, and loss of smell.

Miscellaneous – Arthralgia, chills, extrapulmonary pneumocystosis, headache, night sweats, and Stevens-Johnson syndrome.

➤*Postmarketing:* From postmarketing clinical experience with pentamidine isethionate, the following adverse events have been reported:

Miscellaneous – Cough, diabetes mellitus/ketoacidosis, dyspnea, infiltration (extravasation-see Warnings), and torsades de pointes.

Overdosage

➤*Symptoms:* A 17-month-old infant inadvertently received 1600 mg of IV pentamidine isethionate which was followed by renal and hepatic function impairment, hypotension and cardiopulmonary arrest.

➤*Treatment:* Treatment included cardiopulmonary resuscitation, epinephrine, atropine and intubation. In addition, a 4-hour course of charcoal hemoperfusion was accompanied by reduction of pentamidine serum concentration and stabilization of the patient's condition. The patient recovered from these adverse events, but later died due to an unknown cause.

PENTAMIDINE ISETHIONATE — INHALATIONAL

Indications

➤*Pneumocystis carinii pneumonia prophylaxis:* For the prevention of *Pneumocystis carinii* pneumonia (PCP) in high-risk, HIV-infected patients defined by 1 or both of the following criteria:

A history of 1 or more episodes of PCP.

A peripheral CD4+ (T4 helper/inducer) lymphocyte count less than or equal to 200/mm^3.

➤*Off-label uses:* Pentamidine has been used in the treatment of trypanosomiasis and visceral leishmaniasis.

Administration and Dosage

➤*Adults:*

Pneumocystis jiroveci (formerly carinii) prophylaxis – 300 mg once every 4 weeks.

➤*Children:*

Off-label dosing –

5 years of age and older:

• *Pneumocystis jiroveci (formerly carinii) prophylaxis* – 300 mg every month.

➤*Preparation for administration:* Pentamidine is considered a biohazardous agent. Follow safe handling procedures when preparing, administering, or dispensing pentamidine.

The contents of 1 vial (300 mg) must be dissolved in 6 mL sterile water for injection.

➤*Administration:* Freshly prepared solutions for aerosol use are recommended. Place the entire reconstituted contents of the vial into the *Respirgard II* nebulizer reservoir for administration. The dose should be delivered until the nebulizer chamber is empty (approximately 30 to 45 minutes). The flow rate should be 5 to 7 L per minute from a 40 to 50 pounds per square inch (PSI) air or oxygen source. Alternatively, a 40 to 50 PSI air compressor can be used with flow limited by setting the flowmeter at 5 to 7 L per minute or by setting the pressure at 22 to 25 PSI. Low pressure (less than 20 PSI) compressors should not be used.

➤*Admixture compatibility:* Do not use saline solution for reconstitution because the drug will precipitate. Do not mix the pentamidine solution with any other drugs. Do not use the *Respirgard II* nebulizer to administer a bronchodilator.

➤*Storage/Stability:* Store the dry product at controlled room temperature 15° to 30°C (59° to 86°F). Protect from light.

After reconstitution with sterile water, the pentamidine isethionate solution is stable for 48 hours in the original vial at room temperature if protected from light.

Actions

➤*Pharmacology:* Pentamidine isethionate, an aromatic diamidine, is known to have activity against *Pneumocystis carinii*. The mode of action is not fully understood. In vitro studies indicate that the drug interferes with protozoal nuclear metabolism by inhibition of DNA, RNA, phospholipid, and protein synthesis.

➤*Pharmacokinetics:*

Absorption – In 5 AIDS patients with suspected *Pneumocystis carinii* pneumonia (PCP), the mean concentrations of pentamidine determined 18 to 24 hours after inhalation therapy were 23.2 ng/mL (range 5.1 to 43 ng/mL) in bronchoalveolar lavage fluid and 705 ng/mL (range 140 to 1336 ng/mL) in sediment after administration of a 300 mg single dose via the *Respirgard II* nebulizer. In 3 AIDS patients with suspected PCP, the mean concentrations of pentamidine determined 18 to 24 hours after a 4 mg/kg intravenous dose were 2.6 ng/mL (range 1.5 to 4 ng/mL) in bronchoalveolar lavage fluid and 9.3 ng/mL (range 6.9 to 12.8 ng/mL) in sediment. In the patients who received aerosolized pentamidine, the peak plasma levels of pentamidine were at or below the lower limit of detection of the assay (2.3 ng/mL).

Following a single 2-hour intravenous infusion of 4 mg/kg of pentamidine isethionate to 6 AIDS patients, the mean plasma C_{max}, $t_{½}$ and clearance were 612 ± 371 ng/mL, 6.4 ± 1.3 hr and 248 ± 91 L/hr, respectively. In another study of aerosolized pentamidine in 13 AIDS patients with acute PCP who received 4 mg/kg/day administered via the *Ultra Vent* jet nebulizer, peak plasma levels of pentamidine averaged 18.8 ± 11.9 ng/mL after the first dose. During the next 14 days of repeated dosing, the highest observed C_{max} averaged 20.5 ± 21.2 ng/mL. In a third study, following daily administration of 600 mg of inhaled pentamidine isethionate with the *Respirgard II* nebulizer for 21 days in 11 patients with acute PCP, mean plasma levels measured shortly after the 21st dose averaged 11.8 ± 10 ng/mL.

Metabolism/Excretion – Plasma concentrations after aerosol administration are substantially lower than those observed after a comparable intravenous dose. The extent of pentamidine accumulation and distribution following chronic inhalation therapy are not known.

Contraindications

History of an anaphylactic reaction to inhaled or parenteral pentamidine isethionate.

Warnings/Precautions

➤*Development of acute PCP:* The potential for development of acute PCP still exists in patients receiving pentamidine isethionate prophylaxis. Therefore, any patient with symptoms suggestive of the presence of a pulmonary infection, including but not limited to dyspnea, fever, or cough, should receive a thorough medical evaluation and appropriate diagnostic tests for possible acute PCP as well as for other opportunistic and nonopportunistic pathogens. The use of pentamidine isethionate may alter the clinical and radiographic features of PCP and could result in an atypical presentation, including but not limited to mild disease or focal infection.

Prior to initiating pentamidine isethionate prophylaxis, symptomatic patients should be evaluated appropriately to exclude the presence of PCP. The recommended dose of pentamidine isethionate for the prevention of PCP is insufficient to treat acute PCP.

➤*Pulmonary:* Inhalation of pentamidine isethionate may induce bronchospasm or cough. This has been noted particularly in some patients who have a history of smoking or asthma. In clinical trials, cough and bronchospasm were the most frequently reported adverse experiences associated with pentamidine isethionate administration (38% and 15%, respectively, of patients receiving the 300 mg dose); however, less than 1% of the doses were interrupted or terminated due to these effects. For the majority of patients, cough and bronchospasm were controlled by administration of an aerosolized bronchodilator (only 1% of patients withdrew from the study due to treatment-associated cough or bronchospasm). In patients who experience bronchospasm or cough, administration of an inhaled bronchodilator prior to giving each pentamidine isethionate dose may minimize recurrence of the symptoms.

Extrapulmonary infection with *P. carinii* has been reported infrequently. Most, but not all, of the cases have been reported in patients who have a history of PCP. The presence of extrapulmonary pneumocystosis should be considered when evaluating patients with unexplained signs and symptoms.

➤*Pancreatitis:* Cases of acute pancreatitis have been reported in patients receiving aerosolized pentamidine. Pentamidine isethionate should be discontinued if signs or symptoms of acute pancreatitis develop.

➤*Pregnancy: Category C.* Animal reproduction studies have not been conducted with pentamidine isethionate. It is also not known whether pentamidine isethionate inhalation can cause fetal harm when administered to a pregnant woman or can affect reproduction capacity. Pentamidine isethionate inhalation should be given to a pregnant woman only if clearly needed. Pentamidine isethionate inhalation should not be given to a pregnant woman unless the potential benefits are judged to outweigh the risks.

➤*Lactation:* It is not known whether pentamidine isethionate inhalation is excreted in human milk. Because of the potential for serious adverse reactions in nursing infants from pentamidine isethionate inhalation, a decision should be made whether to discontinue nursing or to discontinue the drug, taking into account the importance of the drug to the mother. Because many drugs are excreted in human milk, pentamidine isethionate inhalation should not be given to a nursing mother unless the potential benefits are judged to outweigh the unknown risks.

➤*Children:* The safety and efficacy of pentamidine isethionate inhalation in pediatric patients (birth to 16 years of age) have not been established.

➤*Monitoring:* The extent and consequence of pentamidine accumulation following chronic inhalation therapy are not known. As a result, patients receiving pentamidine isethionate inhalation should be closely monitored for the development of serious adverse reactions that have occurred in patients receiving parenteral pentamidine, including hypotension, hypoglycemia, hyperglycemia, hypocalcemia, anemia, thrombocytopenia, leukopenia, hepatic or renal dysfunction, ventricular tachycardia, pancreatitis, Stevens-Johnson syndrome, hyperkalemia, and abnormal ST segment of ECG.

Drug Interactions

➤*QT prolongation:* An additive effect of pentamidine with other drugs that prolong the QT interval cannot be excluded. The following drugs may prolong the QT interval and increase the risk of life-threatening cardiac arrhythmias, including torsades de pointes: Antiarrhythmic agents (eg, amiodarone, bretylium, disopyramide, dofetilide, procainamide, quinidine, and sotalol), arsenic trioxide, chlorpromazine, cisapride, dolasetron, droperidol, mefloquine, mesoridazine, moxifloxacin, pimozide, tacrolimus, thioridazine, and ziprasidone. For a more complete list of drugs that may prolong the QT interval, see the appendix, Drug-Induced Prolongation of the QT Interval and Torsades de Pointes.

➤*Other nephrotoxic drugs:* Because the nephrotoxic effects may be additive, the concomitant or sequential use of pentamidine isethionate and other nephrotoxic drugs such as aminoglycosides, amphotericin B, cisplatin, foscarnet, or vancomycin should be closely monitored and avoided, if possible.

Adverse Reactions

➤*Most frequently reported adverse reactions (1% to 5%):* The most frequently reported unsolicited adverse events (1% to 5%) in clinical trials, regardless of their relation to pentamidine isethionate therapy were as follows (n = 931):

CNS – Headache.

GI – Diarrhea and nausea.

Hematologic – Anemia.

Respiratory – Chest pain, cough, and wheezing.

Special senses – Bad taste.

Miscellaneous – Night sweats.

Infection: Bronchitis, non-specific herpes, herpes zoster, non-specific influenza, oral *Candida*, pharyngitis, sinusitis, and upper respiratory tract infection.

➤*Adverse reactions with less than 1% incidence:* Adverse events of less than 1% incidence were as follows (no causal relationship to treatment has been established for these adverse events):

PENTAMIDINE ISETHIONATE — INHALATIONAL

Cardiovascular – Cerebrovascular accident, hypotension, hypertension, palpitations, poor circulation, syncope, tachycardia, vasodilatation and vasculitis.

CNS – Anxiety, confusion, depression, drowsiness, emotional lability, hallucination, hypesthesia, insomnia, memory loss, neuralgia, neuropathy, nonspecific neuropathy, nervousness, paranoia, paresthesia, peripheral neuropathy, seizure, tremors, unsteady gait, and vertigo.

Dermatologic – Desquamation, dry and breaking hair, dry skin, erythema, non-specific dermatitis, pruritus, rash, and urticaria.

GI – Abdominal cramps, abdominal pain, constipation, dry mouth, dyspepsia, gastritis, gastric ulcer, gingivitis, hiatal hernia, hypersalivation, oral ulcer/abscess, splenomegaly, and vomiting.

GU – Flank pain, incontinence, nephritis, renal failure, and renal pain.

Hematologic – Eosinophilia, neutropenia, nonspecific cytopenia, pancytopenia, and thrombocytopenia.

Hepatic – Hepatitis, hepatomegaly, and hepatic dysfunction.

Metabolic – Hyperglycemia, hypoglycemia, and hypocalcemia.

Musculoskeletal – Arthralgia, gout, and myalgia.

Respiratory – Asthma, bronchitis, bronchospasm, chest congestion, chest tightness, coryza, cyanosis, eosinophilic or interstitial pneumonitis, gagging, hemoptysis, hyperventilation, laryngitis, laryngospasm, nonspecific lung disorder, nasal congestion, pleuritis, pneumothorax, rales, rhinitis, shortness of breath, nonspecific sputum, and tachypnea.

Special senses – Blepharitis, blurred vision, conjunctivitis, contact lens discomfort, eye pain or discomfort, hemianopsia, loss of taste, nonspecific odor, and smell.

Miscellaneous – Miscarriage.

Allergic reaction, non-specific allergy, body odor, facial edema, fever, leg edema, lethargy, low body temperature, and temperature abnormality.

Infection: Bacterial pneumonia, central venous line related sepsis, cryptococcal meningitis, cytomegalovirus (CMV) colitis, CMV retinitis, esophageal *Candida*, histoplasmosis, Kaposi's sarcoma, nonspecific mycoplasma, oral herpes, nonspecific otitis, nonspecific pharyngitis, pharyngeal herpes, nonspecific serious infection, tonsillitis, tuberculosis, and viral encephalitis.

➤*Postmarketing:* From postmarketing clinical experience with pentamidine isethionate the following spontaneous adverse events have been reported: Anaphylaxis, colitis, diabetes, dyspnea, esophagitis, hematochezia, increased blood urea nitrogen (BUN) and serum creatinine levels, melena, pancreatitis, syndrome of inappropriate antidiuretic hormone (SIADH), and torsade de pointes.

Overdosage

Overdosage has not been reported with pentamidine isethionate. The symptoms and signs of overdosage are not known.

A serious overdosage, to the point of producing systemic drug levels similar to those following parenteral administration, would have the potential of producing similar types of serious systemic toxicity. Patients receiving pentamidine isethionate inhalation should be closely monitored for the development of serious adverse reactions that have occurred in patients receiving parenteral pentamidine, including hypotension, hypoglycemia, hyperglycemia, hypocalcemia, anemia, thrombocytopenia, leukopenia, hepatic or renal dysfunction, ventricular tachycardia, pancreatitis, Stevens-Johnson syndrome, hyperkalemia, and abnormal ST segment of ECG.

Available clinical pharmacology data suggest that a dose up to 40 times the recommended pentamidine isethionate dosage would be required to produce systemic levels similar to a single 4 mg/kg intravenous dose.

ANTHELMINTICS

The following table lists the major parasitic infections, causative organisms and drugs of choice for treatment. For investigational antiparasitic agents available from the Centers for Disease Control, refer to the CDC Anti-Infective Agents monograph.

	Major Parasite Infections		
	Infection (common name)	Organism	Drug(s) of Choice
Intestinal Nematodes	Ascariasis[a] (Roundworm)	*Ascaris lumbricoides*	Mebendazole or Pyrantel pamoate
	Uncinariasis (Hookworm)	*Ancylostoma duodenale* *Necator americanus*	Mebendazole or Pyrantel pamoate[b]
	Strongyloidiasis (Threadworm)	*Strongyloides stercoralis*	Thiabendazole
	Trichuriasis (Whipworm)	*Trichuris trichiura*	Mebendazole
	Enterobiasis[c] (Pinworm)	*Enterobius vermicularis*	Mebendazole, Pyrantel pamoate or Albendazole
	Capillariasis	*Capillaria philippinensis*	Mebendazole, Thiabendazole or Albendazole
Tissue Nematodes	Trichinosis	*Trichinella spiralis*	Steroids for severe symptoms plus Thiabendazole, Albendazole, Flubendazole[f] or Mebendazole[b]
	Cutaneous larva migrans (Creeping eruption)	*Ancylostoma braziliense* and others	Thiabendazole, Albendazole or Ivermectin[d]
	Onchocerciasis (River blindness)	*Onchocerca volvulus*	Suramin[e] or Ivermectin[d]
	Dracontiasis (Guinea worm)	*Dracunculus medinensis*	Thiabendazole or Mebendazole
	Angiostrongyliasis (Rat lungworm)	*Angiostrongylus cantonensis*	Thiabendazole or Mebendazole
	Loiasis	*Loa loa*	Ivermectin[b]
Cestodes	Taeniasis (Beef tapeworm)	*Taenia saginata*	Praziquantel[b] or Niclosamide[f]
	(Pork tapeworm)	*Taenia solium*	Praziquantel[b], Niclosamide[f] or Albendazole
	Diphyllobothriasis (Fish tapeworm)	*Diphyllobothrium latum*	Praziquantel[b] or Niclosamide[f]
	Dog tapeworm	*Dipylidium caninum*	Praziquantel[b]
	Hymenolepiasis (Dwarf tapeworm)	*Hymenolepis nana*	Praziquantel[b] or Niclosamide[f]
	Hydatid cysts	*Echinococcus granulosus*	Albendazole or Praziquantel
Trematodes	Schistosomiasis	*Schistosoma mansoni*	Praziquantel or Oxamniquine
		Schistosoma japonicum	Praziquantel
		Schistosoma haematobium	Praziquantel
		Schistosoma mekongi	Praziquantel
	Hermaphroditic Flukes		
	Fasciolopsiasis (Intestinal fluke)	*Fasciolopsis buski*	Praziquantel
		Heterophyes heterophyes *Metagonimus yokogawai*	Praziquantel
	Clonorchiasis (Chinese liver fluke)	*Clonorchis sinensis*	Praziquantel
	Fascioliasis (Sheep liver fluke)	*Fasciola hepatica*	Praziquantel or Bithionol[d]
	Opisthorchiasis (Liver fluke)	*Opisthorchis viverrini*	Praziquantel
	Paragonimiasis (Lung fluke)	*Paragonimus westermani*	Praziquantel or Bithionol[d] (alternate)

[a] Thiabendazole is also indicated in Ascariasis.
[b] Unlabeled use.
[c] Thiabendazole is also indicated in Enterobiasis.
[d] Available from the CDC.
[e] Available from the CDC, although generally not recommended.
[f] Not available in the US.

MEBENDAZOLE

Rx	Vermox (Janssen)	Tablets, chewable: 100 mg	(VERMOX JANSSEN). In 12s.
Rx	Mebendazole (Copley)		In 12s.

MEBENDAZOLE — ORAL

Refer to the general discussion of these products in the Anthelmintics introduction.

Indications

➤*Helminths:* For the treatment of *Enterobius vermicularis* (pinworm), *Trichuris trichiura* (whipworm), *Ascaris lumbricoides* (common roundworm), *Ancylostoma duodenale* (common hookworm), and *Necator americanus* (American hookworm) in single or mixed infections.

Administration and Dosage

➤*General dosing considerations:* If the patient is not cured 3 weeks after treatment, a second course of treatment is advised. No special procedures, such as fasting or purging, are required.

➤*Adults:*

Common roundworm (ascariasis) – 100 mg twice daily (morning and evening) for 3 consecutive days.

Hookworm – 100 mg twice daily (morning and evening) for 3 consecutive days.

Pinworm (enterobiasis) – 100 mg given as a single dose.

Whipworm (trichuriasis) – 100 mg twice daily (morning and evening) for 3 consecutive days.

➤*Children:*

2 years of age and older – See Adults for dosing.

Off-label dosing –

2 years of age and older:

- *Capillariasis* – 200 mg twice daily for 20 days.
- *Common roundworm (ascariasis)* – 500 mg as a single dose.
- *Filariasis (Mansonella perstans)* – 100 mg twice daily for 30 days.
- *Hookworm* – 500 mg as a single dose.
- *Trichinellosis* –
  Initial dosage: 200 to 400 mg 3 times daily for 3 days with steroids for severe symptoms.
  Maintenance dosage: 400 to 500 mg 3 times daily for 10 days with steroids for severe symptoms.
- *Trichostrongylus* – 100 mg twice daily for 3 days.
- *Visceral larva migrans (toxocariasis)* – 100 to 200 mg twice daily for 5 days.
- *Whipworm (trichuriasis)* – 500 mg as a single dose.

➤*Administration:* The tablet may be chewed, swallowed, or crushed and mixed with food.

➤*Storage/Stability:* Store at 15° to 25°C (59° to 77°F).

Actions

➤*Pharmacology:* Mebendazole inhibits the formation of the worms' microtubules and causes the worms' glucose depletion.

➤*Pharmacokinetics:*

Absorption – Following administration of 100 mg twice daily for 3 consecutive days, plasma levels of mebendazole and its primary metabolite, the 2-amine, do not exceed 0.03 mcg/mL and 0.09 mcg/mL respectively. All metabolites are devoid of anthelmintic activity.

Excretion – In man, ≈ 2% of administered mebendazole is excreted in urine and the remainder in the feces as unchanged drug or a primary metabolite.

Contraindications

Hypersensitivity to the drug.

Warnings/Precautions

➤*Hydatid disease:* There is no evidence that mebendazole, even at high doses, is effective for hydatid disease. There have been rare reports of neutropenia and agranulocytosis when mebendazole was taken for prolonged periods and at dosages substantially above those recommended.

➤*Pregnancy: Category C.*

Teratogenic – Mebendazole has shown embryotoxic and teratogenic activity in pregnant rats at single oral doses as low as 10 mg/kg (approximately equal to the human dose, based on mg/m^2). In view of these findings the use of mebendazole is not recommended in pregnant women. Although there are no adequate and well-controlled studies in pregnant women, a postmarketing survey has been done of a limited number of women who inadvertently had consumed mebendazole during the first trimester of pregnancy. The incidence of spontaneous abortion and malformation did not exceed that in the general population. In 170 deliveries on term, no teratogenic risk of mebendazole was identified.

➤*Lactation:* It is not known whether mebendazole is excreted in human milk. Because many drugs are excreted in human milk, caution should be exercised when mebendazole is administered to a nursing woman.

➤*Children:* The drug has not been extensively studied in children under 2 years; therefore, in the treatment of children under 2 years the relative benefit/risk should be considered.

➤*Monitoring:* Periodic assessment of organ system functions, including hematopoietic and hepatic, is advisable during prolonged therapy.

Drug Interactions

Preliminary evidence suggests that cimetidine inhibits mebendazole metabolism and may result in an increase in plasma concentrations of mebendazole.

Adverse Reactions

➤*CNS:* Very rare cases of convulsions have been reported.

➤*GI:* Transient symptoms of abdominal pain and diarrhea in cases of massive infection and expulsion of worms.

➤*Hematologic:* Neutropenia and agranulocytosis (see Warnings).

➤*Hepatic:* There have been liver function test elevations (AST [SGOT], ALT [SGPT], and GGT) and rare reports of hepatitis when mebendazole was taken for prolonged periods and at dosages substantially above those recommended.

➤*Hypersensitivity:* Rash, urticaria and angioedema have been observed on rare occasions.

Overdosage

➤*Symptoms:* In the event of accidental overdosage, GI complaints lasting up to a few hours may occur.

➤*Treatment:* Vomiting and purging should be induced.

Patient Information

Patients should be informed of the potential risk to the fetus in women taking mebendazole during pregnancy, especially during the first trimester (see Warnings, Pregnancy).

Patients should also be informed that cleanliness is important to prevent reinfection and transmission of the infection.

ALBENDAZOLE

Rx	Albenza (GlaxoSmithKline)	Tablets; oral: 200 mg	Lactose, saccharin. White to off-white, circular. Film-coated. In 112s.

ALBENDAZOLE — ORAL

Refer to the general discussion of these products in the Anthelmintics introduction.

Indications

➤*Hydatid disease:* For the treatment of cystic hydatid disease of the liver, lung, and peritoneum caused by the larval form of the dog tapeworm, *Echinococcus granulosus*.

➤*Neurocysticercosis:* For the treatment of parenchymal neurocysticercosis due to active lesions caused by larval forms of the pork tapeworm, *Taenia solium*.

➤*Off-label uses:* For the treatment of single and mixed intestinal nematode infections, including *Ancylostoma caninum*, ascariasis, enterobiasis (pinworm), hookworm, strongyloidiasis, trichuriasis, capillariasis, gnathostomiasis, gongylonemiasis, trichostrongyliasis, tissue nematode infections, cutaneous larva migrans, toxocariasis, and trichinosis; for the treatment of liver flukes; in combination with other anthelmintics in the management of the filarial nematode infection lymphatic filariasis; for microsporidial intestinal infections in patients with AIDS.

ALBENDAZOLE — ORAL

Administration and Dosage

➤*Adults:*

Hydatid disease / Neurocysticercosis –

Albendazole Dosing

Indication	Patient weight	Dosage	Duration
Hydatid disease[a]	≥ 60 kg	400 mg twice daily, with meals	28-day cycle followed by a 14-day albendazole-free interval, for a total of 3 cycles
	< 60 kg	15 mg/kg/day given in divided doses twice daily with meals (maximum total daily dose, 800 mg)	
Neurocysticercosis	≥ 60 kg	400 mg twice daily, with meals	8 to 30 days
	< 60 kg	15 mg/kg/day given in divided doses twice daily with meals (maximum total daily dose, 800 mg)	

[a] When administering albendazole in the presurgical or postsurgical setting, optimal killing of cyst contents is achieved when 3 courses of therapy have been given.

Off-label dosing –

A. caninum (eosinophilic enterocolitis), ascariasis (roundworm), hookworm (Ancylostoma duodenale, Necator americanus), Trichostrongylus: 400 mg orally once.

Cutaneous larva migrans, trichuriasis (whipworm or Trichuris trichiura), gongylonemiasis: 400 mg orally once daily for 3 days.

Enterobius vermicularis (pinworm): 400 mg orally once; repeat dose in 2 weeks.

Filariasis (Mansonella perstans), capillariasis: 400 mg orally once daily for 10 days.

Fluke (Clonorchis sinensis, Chinese liver fluke): 10 mg/kg orally once daily for 7 days.

Gnathostomiasis (Gnathostoma spinigerum): 400 mg orally once or twice daily for 21 days.

Microsporidiosis (excludes ocular infection and infection due to Enterocytozoon bieneusi or Vittaforma corneae): 400 mg orally twice daily continued until CD4+ count is more than 200 cells/mcL for more than 6 months after initiating antiretroviral therapy.

Trichinosis (Trichinella spiralis): 400 mg orally twice daily for 5 to 14 days.

Visceral larva migrans (toxocariasis): 400 mg orally twice daily for 5 days.

➤*Children:*

Hydatid disease / Neurocysticercosis – See Adults for dosing.

Off-label dosing –

A. caninum (eosinophilic enterocolitis), ascariasis (roundworm), capillariasis, cutaneous larva migrans, E. vermicularis (pinworm), filariasis (M. perstans), fluke (C. sinensis, Chinese liver fluke), hookworm (A. duodenale, N. americanus), trichinosis (T. spiralis), Trichostrongylus, trichuriasis (whipworm or T. trichiura): See Adults for dosing.

Gnathostomiasis (G. spinigerum): 400 mg orally once daily for 21 days.

Microsporidiosis (excludes ocular infection and infection due to E. bieneusi: 7.5 mg/kg (max, 400 mg) orally twice daily until immune reconstitution occurs after initiating highly active antiretroviral therapy.

Visceral larva migrans (toxocariasis): 400 mg orally once daily for 5 days.

➤*Concomitant therapy:* Patients being treated for neurocysticercosis should receive appropriate steroid and anticonvulsant therapy as required. Oral or intravenous (IV) corticosteroids should be considered to prevent cerebral hypertensive episodes during the first week of treatment.

➤*Administration:* Administer with food. In young children, the tablets should be crushed or chewed and swallowed with water.

➤*Storage / Stability:* Store between 20° and 25°C (68° and 77°F).

Actions

➤*Pharmacology:* Albendazole is a broad-spectrum anthelmintic. The principal mode of action for albendazole is by its inhibitory effect on tubulin polymerization that results in the loss of cytoplasmic microtubules.

➤*Pharmacokinetics:*

Absorption – Albendazole is poorly absorbed from the GI tract due to its low aqueous solubility.

Albendazole concentrations are negligible or undetectable in plasma because it is rapidly converted to the sulfoxide metabolite prior to reaching the systemic circulation. The systemic anthelmintic activity has been attributed to the primary metabolite, albendazole sulfoxide.

Food effects: Oral bioavailability appears to be enhanced when albendazole is coadministered with a fatty meal (estimated fat content, 40 g) as evidenced by higher plasma concentrations (up to 5-fold on average) of albendazole sulfoxide compared with the fasted state. Maximal plasma concentrations of albendazole sulfoxide are typically achieved 2 to 5 hours after dosing and are, on average, 1.31 mcg/mL (range, 0.46 to 1.58 mcg/mL) following oral doses of albendazole 400 mg in 6 patients with hydatid disease when administered with a fatty meal. Plasma concentrations of albendazole sulfoxide increase in a dose-proportional manner over the therapeutic dose range following ingestion of a fatty meal (fat content, 43.1 g).

Distribution – Albendazole sulfoxide is 70% bound to plasma protein and widely distributed throughout the body; it has been detected in urine, bile, liver, cyst wall, cyst fluid, and cerebrospinal fluid. Concentrations in plasma were 3- to 10-fold and 2- to 4-fold higher than those simultaneously determined in cyst fluid and cerebrospinal fluid, respectively. Limited in vitro and clinical data suggest that albendazole sulfoxide may be eliminated from cysts at a slower rate than observed in plasma.

Metabolism / Excretion – Albendazole is rapidly converted in the liver to its primary metabolite, albendazole sulfoxide, which is further metabolized to albendazole sulfone and other primary oxidative metabolites that have been identified in human urine. Following oral administration, albendazole has not been detected in human urine. Urinary excretion of albendazole sulfoxide is a minor elimination pathway, with less than 1% of the dose recovered in urine. Biliary elimination presumably accounts for a portion of the elimination as evidenced by biliary concentrations of albendazole sulfoxide similar to those achieved in plasma.

The mean apparent terminal elimination half-life of albendazole sulfoxide typically ranged from 8 to 12 hours in 25 healthy subjects, as well as in 14 patients with hydatid disease and 8 patients with neurocysticercosis.

Following 4 weeks of treatment with albendazole 200 mg 3 times daily, 12 patients' plasma concentrations of albendazole sulfoxide were approximately 20% lower than those observed during the first half of the treatment period, suggesting that albendazole may induce its own metabolism.

Special populations –

Hepatic function impairment: In patients with evidence of extrahepatic obstruction (n = 5), the systemic availability of albendazole sulfoxide was increased, as indicated by a 2-fold increase in maximum serum concentration and a 7-fold increase in area under the curve (AUC). The rate of absorption/conversion and elimination of albendazole sulfoxide appeared to be prolonged, with mean time to maximum plasma concentration and serum elimination half-life values of 10 and 31.7 hours, respectively.

➤*Microbiology:* In specified treatment indications, albendazole appears to be active against the larval forms of *E. granulosus* and *T. solium*.

Contraindications

Hypersensitivity to the benzimidazole class of compounds or any components of albendazole.

Warnings/Precautions

➤*Hematologic effects:* Albendazole has been shown to cause occasional (less than 1% of treated patients) reversible reductions in total white blood cell count. Rarely, more significant reductions may be encountered, including granulocytopenia, agranulocytosis, or pancytopenia. Rare fatalities associated with the use of albendazole due to granulocytopenia or pancytopenia have been reported. In all patients, perform blood cell counts at the start of each 28-day treatment cycle and every 2 weeks during each 28-day cycle.

Albendazole has been shown to cause bone marrow suppression, aplastic anemia, and agranulocytosis in patients with or without underlying hepatic dysfunction. Patients with liver disease, including hepatic echinococcosis, appear to be more at risk of bone marrow suppression leading to pancytopenia, aplastic anemia, agranulocytosis, and leukopenia attributable to albendazole and warrant closer monitoring of blood cell counts.

Discontinue albendazole in all patients if clinically significant decreases in blood cell counts occur.

➤*Concomitant therapy:* See Administration and Dosage for more information.

➤*Neurologic / Ophthalmic effects:* Preexisting neurocysticercosis may also be uncovered in patients treated with albendazole for other conditions. Patients may experience neurological symptoms (eg, seizures, increased intracranial pressure and focal signs) as a result of an inflammatory reaction caused by death of the parasite within the brain. Symptoms may occur soon after treatment; immediately start appropriate steroid and anticonvulsant therapy.

Cysticercosis may, in rare cases, involve the retina. Before initiating therapy for neurocysticercosis, examine the patient for the presence of retinal lesions. If such lesions are visualized, weigh the need for anticysticeral therapy against the possibility of retinal damage caused by albendazole-induced changes to the retinal lesion.

➤*Hepatic effects:* In clinical trials, treatment with albendazole was associated with mild to moderate elevations of hepatic enzymes in approximately 16% of patients. These elevations generally returned to normal upon discontinuation of therapy. There have been case reports of acute liver failure of uncertain causality and hepatitis.

Perform liver function tests (transaminases) before the start of each treatment cycle and at least every 2 weeks during treatment. If hepatic enzymes exceed twice the upper limit of normal (ULN), consider discontinuing albendazole therapy based on individual patient circumstances. Restarting albendazole treatment in patients whose hepatic enzymes have normalized off treatment is an individual decision that should take into account the risk and/or benefit of further albendazole usage. Frequently perform laboratory tests if albendazole treatment is restarted.

➤*Hepatic function impairment:* Patients with abnormal liver function test results are at increased risk for hepatotoxicity and bone marrow suppression. Discontinue therapy if liver enzymes are significantly increased or if clinically significant decreases in blood cell counts occur.

ALBENDAZOLE — ORAL

➤*Pregnancy: Category C.* There are no adequate and well-controlled studies of albendazole administration in pregnant women. Use albendazole during pregnancy only if the potential benefit justifies the potential risk to the fetus. It is not known if albendazole or its active metabolite, albendazole sulfoxide, crosses the placenta. The molecular weight of the parent compound (approximately 265) is low enough for transfer, but the poor oral bioavailability suggests that little, if any, of this agent reaches the plasma. There is a potential for much higher plasma concentrations of the metabolite if the drug is consumed with a fatty meal.

Do not use albendazole in pregnant women except in clinical circumstances in which no alternative management is appropriate. If albendazole is required during pregnancy, consider avoiding use during the first trimester. Patients should not become pregnant for at least 1 month following cessation of albendazole therapy. If a patient becomes pregnant while taking this drug, discontinue albendazole administration immediately. If pregnancy occurs while taking this drug, apprise the patient of the potential hazard to the fetus.

Teratogenic – Albendazole has been shown to be teratogenic (to cause embryotoxicity and skeletal malformations) in pregnant rats and rabbits. The teratogenic response in rats was shown at oral dosages of 10 and 30 mg/kg/day (0.1 times and 0.32 times the recommended human dose based on body surface area [BSA] in mg/m^2, respectively) during gestation days 6 to 15 and in pregnant rabbits at oral dosages of 30 mg/kg/day (0.6 times the recommended human dose based on BSA in mg/m^2) administered during gestation days 7 to 19. In the rabbit study, maternal toxicity (33% mortality) was noted at 30 mg/kg/day.

➤*Lactation:* Albendazole is excreted in animal milk. It is not known whether it is excreted in human milk. Although the molecular weight (approximately 265) is low enough for excretion into breast milk, the negligible bioavailability of the parent drug suggests that excretion of clinically significant amounts of this compound do not occur. However, excretion of the active metabolite (albendazole sulfoxide) into breast milk may occur. Moreover, administration of albendazole with a fatty meal will markedly increase the plasma concentration of the metabolite and, thus, may increase the amounts in milk. Because many drugs are excreted in human milk, exercise caution when albendazole is administered to a breast-feeding woman.

➤*Monitoring:* In all patients, perform blood cell counts at the start of each 28-day treatment cycle and every 2 weeks during each 28-day cycle. Patients with liver disease, including hepatic echinococcosis, appear to be more at risk of bone marrow suppression leading to pancytopenia, aplastic anemia, agranulocytosis, and leukopenia attributable to albendazole and warrant closer monitoring of blood cell counts.

Perform liver function tests (transaminases) before the start of each treatment cycle and at least every 2 weeks during treatment. If hepatic enzymes exceed twice the ULN, consider discontinuing albendazole therapy based on individual patient circumstances. Restarting albendazole treatment in patients whose hepatic enzymes have normalized off treatment is an individual decision that should take into account the risk and/or benefit of further albendazole usage. Frequently perform laboratory tests if albendazole treatment is restarted.

Drug Interactions

Albendazole Drug Interactions

Precipitant drug	Object drug[a]		Description
Cimetidine	Albendazole	↑	Albendazole sulfoxide concentrations in bile and cystic fluid were increased ≈ 2-fold in patients with hydatid cysts treated with cimetidine; however, plasma concentrations are unchanged 4 hours after dosing.
Dexamethasone	Albendazole	↑	Steady-state trough concentrations of albendazole sulfoxide were ≈ 56% higher when dexamethasone 8 mg was coadministered with each dose of albendazole (15 mg/kg/day) in 8 patients with neurocysticercosis. Monitor the patient for albendazole adverse reactions. If an interaction is suspected, adjust the albendazole dose as needed.
Praziquantel	Albendazole	↑	Praziquantel 40 mg/kg increased the mean maximum plasma concentration and AUC of albendazole sulfoxide ≈ 50% in healthy subjects. Monitor the patient for albendazole adverse reactions. If an interaction is suspected, adjust the albendazole dose as needed.
Albendazole	Theophylline	↓	Albendazole induces cytochrome P450 1A in human hepatoma cells. Monitor theophylline plasma concentrations and adjust the theophylline dose as needed.

[a] ↑ = object drug increased; ↓ = object drug decreased.

➤*Drug/Food interactions:* See Actions for more information.

Grapefruit juice – Albendazole plasma concentrations may be elevated, increasing the risk of adverse reactions. Patients should avoid grapefruit products while taking albendazole.

Adverse Reactions

➤*Adverse reactions (1% or more):*

Albendazole Adverse Reactions (≥ 1%)

Adverse reactions	Hydatid disease	Neurocysticercosis
CNS		
Dizziness/Vertigo	1.2%	< 1%
Headache	1.3%	11%
Meningeal signs	0%	1%
GI		
Abdominal pain	6%	0%
Nausea/Vomiting	3.7%	6.2%
Miscellaneous		
Abnormal liver function tests	15.6%	< 1%
Fever	1%	0%
Raised intracranial pressure	0%	1.5%
Reversible alopecia	1.6%	< 1%

Discontinuation – Treatment discontinuations were predominantly due to leukopenia (0.7%) or hepatic abnormalities (3.8% in hydatid disease).

➤*Other adverse reactions (less than 1%):*

Hematologic – Leukopenia. There have been rare reports of agranulocytosis, granulocytopenia, pancytopenia, or thrombocytopenia. Patients with liver disease, including hepatic echinococcosis, appear to be more at risk of bone marrow suppression.

Hypersensitivity – Rash, urticaria.

➤*Postmarketing:*

Dermatologic – Erythema multiforme, Stevens-Johnson syndrome.

Hematologic/Lymphatic – Aplastic anemia, bone marrow suppression, neutropenia.

Hepatic – Acute liver failure, elevations of hepatic enzymes, hepatitis.

Renal – Acute renal failure.

Overdosage

➤*Treatment:* Symptomatic therapy and general supportive measures are recommended.

Patient Information

Inform patients that albendazole may cause fetal harm; therefore, women of childbearing age should begin treatment after a negative pregnancy test.

Caution women of childbearing age against becoming pregnant while on albendazole or within 1 month of completing treatment.

Advise patients that during albendazole therapy, because of the possibility of harm to the liver or bone marrow, routine (every 2 weeks) monitoring of blood cell counts and liver function tests will take place.

Advise patients to take albendazole with food.

Advise patients that some people (particularly young children) may experience difficulties swallowing the tablets whole. In young children, the tablets should be crushed or chewed and swallowed with a drink of water.

PYRANTEL PAMOATE

otc	**Reese's Pinworm** (Reese)	**Tablets; oral:** 180 mg	Equiv. to 62.5 mg pyrantel base. Capsule shape. In 24s.
otc	**Pin-X** (Penn)	**Tablets, chewable; oral:** 720.5 mg	Equiv. to 250 mg pyrantel base. Dextrose, maltodextrin, sorbitol. (Pin-X). Orange flavor. Orange, scored. In 12s.
otc	**Pin-Rid** (Apothecary)	**Capsules, soft gel; oral:** 180 mg	Equiv. to 62.5 mg pyrantel base. In 24s.
otc	**Reese's Pinworm** (Reese)		Equiv. to 62.5 mg pyrantel base. (RC P). In 24s.
otc	**Pin-X** (Effcon)	**Suspension; oral:** 50 mg per mL	Sorbitol, parabens. Caramel flavor. In 30 mL.
otc	**Reese's Pinworm** (Reese)		In 30 mL.
otc	**Reese's Pinworm** (Reese)	**Suspension; oral:** 144 mg per mL	Equiv. to 50 mg/mL pyrantel base. Glycerin, saccharin, 4 mg/5 mL sodium, sorbitol. Banana flavor. In 30 mL with measuring cup.

PYRANTEL PAMOATE — ORAL

Refer to the general discussion of these products in the Anthelmintics introduction.

Indications

➤*Helminths:* For the treatment of ascariasis (roundworm infection) and enterobiasis (pinworm infection).

➤*Off-label uses:* Hairworm.

Administration and Dosage

➤*General dosing considerations:* Do not repeat the treatment unless directed by a doctor. When one individual in a household has pinworms, the entire household should be treated unless otherwise advised. If any worms other than pinworms are present before or after treatment, consult a doctor.

➤*Adults:*

Helminths –

Maximum dose: 1 g (16 tablets/capsules or 20 mL of suspension).

Single dose: Pyrantel base 11 mg/kg (5 mg/lb) given as a single dose. Dosages are individualized according to weight. The following single dosage should be followed according to weight. For patients weighing less than 40 kg (88 lbs), see the Children section.

Pyrantel Dosing (Give as a Single Dose) in Adults

Weight range in kg (lb)	Number of capsules/tablets	Number of chewable tablets	Amount of suspension (mL)
40 to 50 kg (88 to 112 lb)	8	2	10
51 to 62 kg (113 to 137 lb)	10	2½	12.5
63 to 73 kg (138 to 162 lb)	12	3	15
74 to 84 kg (163 to 187 lb)	14	3½	17.5
85 kg or more (188 lb or more)	16	4	20

➤*Children:*

Helminths –

2 years of age and older:

- *Maximum dose* – 1 g (16 tablets/capsules or 20 mL of suspension).
- *Single dose* – Pyrantel base 11 mg/kg (5 mg/lb) of given as a single dose.

Dosages are individualized according to weight. The following single dosage should be followed according to weight.

Pyrantel Dosing (Give as a Single Dose) in Children

Weight range in kg (lb)	Number of capsules/tablets	Number of chewable tablets	Amount of suspension (mL)
11 to 16 kg (25 to 37 lb)	2	½	2.5
17 to 28 kg (38 to 62 lb)	4	1	5
29 to 39 kg (63 to 87 lb)	6	1½	7.5
40 to 50 kg (88 to 112 lb)	8	2	10
51 to 62 kg (113 to 137 lb)	10	2½	12.5
63 to 73 kg (138 to 162 lb)	12	3	15
74 to 84 kg (163 to 187 lb)	14	3½	17.5
85 kg and more (188 lb and more)	16	4	20

➤*Hepatic function impairment:* Patients who have hepatic disease should not take pyrantel pamoate unless directed by a health care provider.

➤*Administration:* Pyrantel can be taken any time of day with or without meals. It may be taken alone or with milk or fruit juice. Use of a laxative is not necessary prior to, during, or after medication.

Shake suspension well.

Medication should only be taken 1 time as a single dose.

➤*Storage/Stability:* Store at 15° to 30° C (59° to 86° F).

Actions

➤*Pharmacology:* Pyrantel is a depolarizing neuromuscular blocking agent, resulting in spastic paralysis of the worm. It also inhibits cholinesterases. It is active against *Enterobius vermicularis* (pinworm) and *Ascaris lumbricoides* (roundworm); it is also effective against *Ancylostoma duodenale* (hookworm).

➤*Pharmacokinetics:* Pyrantel is poorly absorbed from the GI tract. Plasma levels of unchanged drug are low. Greater than 50% is excreted in feces as unchanged drug, 7% or less of the dose is found in the urine as parent drug and metabolites. Peak levels (0.05 to 0.13 mcg/mL) are reached in 1 to 3 hours.

Contraindications

Hypersensitivity to pyrantel.

Warnings/Precautions

➤*Hepatic function impairment:* Patients who have hepatic disease should not take pyrantel pamoate unless directed by a physician.

➤*Pregnancy: Category C.* Patients who are pregnant should not take pyrantel pamoate unless directed by a physician.

➤*Lactation:* No data on the transfer of pyrantel in human milk are available, but because of minimal oral absorption and low plasma levels, it is unlikely that breast milk levels would be clinically relevant.

➤*Children:* Safety and efficacy for use in children younger than 2 years of age have not been established.

Drug Interactions

➤*Piperazine:* In ascariasis (roundworm), pyrantel and piperazine are mutually antagonistic; therefore, concomitant use is unwise.

➤*Theophylline:* Serum levels increased in a pediatric patient following pyrantel pamoate administration. Further study is needed.

Adverse Reactions

Abdominal cramps, nausea, vomiting, diarrhea, headaches, or dizziness, sometimes occur after taking this drug. If any of these conditions persist consult a doctor.

Patient Information

A single dose is required. The dose is based on body weight.

May be taken with food, milk, juice, or on an empty stomach any time during the day. Be sure to take the entire dose.

Using a laxative after taking the drug to facilitate removal of the parasite is not necessary.

As with any drug, if you are pregnant or nursing a baby, seek the advise of a health professional before using this product.

Wear tight underpants both day and night. For several days after treatment clean the bedroom floor by vacuuming or damp mopping. After treatment, wash bed linens and night clothes (don't shake them). Keep toilet seats clean.

➤*Pinworms:* Many patients who have pinworms do not have symptoms, however, many will have itching in and around the rectal opening. The itching may be very annoying and continued scratching can cause an irritation in this area. The itching may be prominent at night when sleeping. That is why restless sleep is sometimes a sign of pinworms, especially in children. Other symptoms include insomnia, GI distress, irritability, enuresis (bedwetting) and secondary infection due to localized scratching. Treat with pyrantel pamoate only after pinworms have been observed and identified.

Pinworms look like tiny white threads. The female pinworm is ≈ ½ inch long (the male pinworm is shorter); they live in the bowel. Usually, at night, the female pinworm travels to the rectal opening and lays eggs within the skin folds around the opening. This usually takes place within 1 to 2 hours after the child has been put to sleep for the night. The sticky gelatin like substance in which the eggs (they are too small to see) are deposited and the movement of the female pinworm may cause annoying itching and possibly restless sleep. By checking the rectal opening at this time, you can attempt to see the pinworm as described.

Scratching will cause pinworm eggs to stick to the fingers. Reinfection will result if the fingers are placed in the mouth. The eggs, which are too small to see, contaminate whatever they come in contact with, including bed clothes, underwear, toys, hands, and food touched by contaminated hands. Even eggs floating in the air can be swallowed and cause infection. Eggs deposited can survive for as long as 3 weeks. Pinworms are highly contagious; therefore, after treatment with pyrantel pamoate you should wash hands and fingernails with soap often during the day in order to prevent spreading to others and reinfection.

PRAZIQUANTEL

Rx	**Biltricide** (Schering)	**Tablets; oral:** 600 mg	PEG. (Bayer LG). White to orange-tinged, oblong, tri-scored. Film-coated. In 6s.

PRAZIQUANTEL — ORAL

Refer to the general discussion of this product in the Anthelmintics introduction.

Indications

➤*Helminths:* For treatment of infections caused by the following: all species of schistosoma (eg, *Schistosoma mekongi, S. japonicum, S. mansoni, S. hematobium*) and the liver flukes *Clonorchis sinensis/Opisthorchis viverrini* (approval of this indication was based on studies in which the 2 species were not differentiated).

➤*Off-label uses:* Praziquantel has been used in the treatment of neurocysticercosis. It may also be beneficial in the treatment of other tissue flukes (eg, *Nanophyetus salmincola, O. felineus, Paragonimus westermani* and other species, toxemic schisto, Katayama fever), intestinal flukes (eg, *Heterophyes heterophyes, Fasciolopsis buski, Metagonimus yokogawai, P. westermani*), intestinal cestodes (eg, *Diphyllobothrium latum, Taenia saginata, T. solium, Dipylidium caninum, Hymenolepis nana, H. diminuta*), and liver flukes (eg, *Metrochis conjunctus*).

Administration and Dosage

➤*Adults:*

Clonorchiasis – 25 mg/kg given 3 times/day for 1 day. Doses should be given 4 to 6 hours apart.

Opisthorchiasis – See Clonorchiasis for dosing.

Schistosomiasis – 20 mg/kg given 3 times/day for 1 day. Doses should be given 4 to 6 hours apart.

➤*Children:*

4 years of age and older – See Adults for dosing.

➤*Administration:* Take with water during meals. Do not chew tablets. Keeping the tablets, or the segments thereof, in the mouth may reveal a bitter taste that can produce gagging or vomiting.

Tablet segments are broken off by pressing the score (notch) with thumbnails. If ¼ of a tablet is required, this is best achieved by breaking the segment from the outer end.

➤*Storage/Stability:* Store below 30°C (86°F).

Actions

➤*Pharmacology:* Praziquantel induces a rapid contraction of schistosomes by a specific effect on the permeability of the cell membrane. The drug further causes vacuolization and disintegration of the schistosome tegument.

➤*Pharmacokinetics:*

Absorption – After oral administration praziquantel is rapidly absorbed (80%). Maximal serum concentration is achieved 1 to 3 hours after dosing.

Metabolism/Excretion – Praziquantel is subjected to a first pass effect, metabolized and eliminated by the kidneys. Approximately 80% of a dose of praziquantel is excreted in the kidneys, almost exclusively (more than 99%) in the form of metabolites. The half-life of praziquantel in serum is 0.8 to 1.5 hours.

Special populations –

Renal function impairment: Excretion might be delayed in patients with impaired renal function, but accumulation of unchanged drug would not be expected. Therefore, dose adjustment for renal impairment is not considered necessary.

Hepatic function impairment: In patients with moderate to severe hepatic dysfunction (Child-Pugh class B and C), praziquantel half-life, maximum plasma concentration (C_{max}), and area under the curve (AUC) increased progressively with the degree of hepatic impairment.

Contraindications

Previous hypersensitivity to praziquantel or any of the product ingredients; ocular cysticercosis; concomitant administration with strong cytochrome P450 (CYP-450) inducers, such as rifampin (see Drug Interactions).

Warnings/Precautions

➤*Renal effects:* Nephrotoxic effects of praziquantel or its metabolites are not known.

➤*Hepatic effects:* Minimal increases in liver enzymes have occurred in some patients.

➤*Cerebral cysticercosis:* When schistosomiasis or fluke infection is found to be associated with cerebral cysticercosis, hospitalize the patient for the duration of treatment.

➤*Ocular cysticercosis:* Because parasite destruction within the eyes may cause irreparable lesions, do not treat ocular cysticercosis with praziquantel.

➤*Hepatic function impairment:* Exercise caution in the administration of the usual recommended dose of praziquantel to patients with hepatosplenic schistosomiasis with moderate to severe liver impairment (Child-Pugh class B and C). Reduced metabolism of praziquantel by the liver in these patients may lead to considerably higher and longer lasting plasma concentrations of unmetabolized praziquantel.

➤*Special risk:* Because praziquantel can exacerbate CNS pathology because of schistosomiasis, as a general rule, do not administer this drug to individuals reporting a history of epilepsy and/or other signs of potential CNS involvement, such as subcutaneous nodules suggestive of cysticercosis.

➤*Hazardous tasks:* May produce dizziness or drowsiness; observe caution while driving or performing other tasks requiring alertness on the day of and the day after treatment.

➤*Pregnancy: Category B.* There are no adequate and well-controlled studies in pregnant women. An increase of the abortion rate was found in rats at 3 times the single human therapeutic dose. While animal reproduction studies are not always predictive of human response, use this drug during pregnancy only if clearly needed.

➤*Lactation:* Praziquantel appeared in the milk of breast-feeding women at a concentration of about 25% that of maternal serum; although, it is not known whether a pharmacological effect is likely to occur in children. Women should not breast-feed on the day of praziquantel treatment and during the subsequent 72 hours.

➤*Children:* Safety in children younger than 4 years of age has not been established.

➤*Elderly:* This drug is known to be substantially excreted by the kidney. Because elderly patients are more likely to have decreased renal function, the risk of toxic reactions to this drug may be greater in these patients.

➤*Monitoring:* Monitor patients suffering from cardiac irregularities during treatment.

Drug Interactions

Praziquantel Drug Interactions

Precipitant drug	Object drug[a]		Description
Chloroquine	Praziquantel	⬇	Praziquantel blood concentrations may be reduced, decreasing the antiparasitic effect. Monitor praziquantel concentrations and adjust the dose as needed.
CYP-450 inducers (eg, carbamazepine, dexamethasone, phenobarbital, phenytoin, rifampin)	Praziquantel	⬇	Praziquantel blood concentrations may be reduced, decreasing the antiparasitic effect. Monitor praziquantel concentrations and adjust the dose as needed. Coadministration of praziquantel and strong CYP-450 inducers (eg, rifampin) is contraindicated. In patients receiving rifampin who need immediate schistosomiasis treatment, an alternative agent for praziquantel should be considered. If praziquantel treatment is necessary, rifampin should be discontinued 4 weeks before praziquantel administration. Rifampin treatment can be resumed one day after completion of praziquantel treatment.
CYP-450 inhibitors (eg, cimetidine, erythromycin, itraconazole, ketoconazole)	Praziquantel	⬆	Praziquantel plasma concentrations may be elevated, increasing the risk of adverse reactions. Monitor the patient for an increase in adverse reactions. If an interaction is suspected, it may be necessary to decrease the praziquantel dose.

[a] ⬆ = object drug increased; ⬇ = object drug decreased.

➤*Drug/Food interactions:* Grapefruit juice ingestion may increase praziquantel plasma concentrations, increasing the effectiveness and risk of adverse reactions. Advise patients taking praziquantel to avoid grapefruit products and to take praziquantel with a liquid other than grapefruit juice.

Adverse Reactions

In general, praziquantel is very well tolerated. Adverse effects are usually mild and transient and do not need treatment but may be more frequent or serious in patients with a heavy worm burden.

The following adverse reactions were observed generally, in order of severity: malaise; headache; dizziness; abdominal discomfort (with or without nausea); rising temperature; urticaria (rare). Such symptoms can, however, also result from the infection itself.

➤*Postmarketing:* Abdominal pain, allergic reaction (generalized hypersensitivity) including polyserositis, anorexia, arrhythmia (including bradycardia, ectopic rhythms, ventricular fibrillation, atrioventricular blocks), asthenia, bloody diarrhea, convulsion, eosinophilia, myalgia, pruritus, somnolence, vertigo, and vomiting.

PRAZIQUANTEL — ORAL

Overdosage

➤*Symptoms:* No data are available in humans.

➤*Treatment:* In the event of overdose, give a fast-acting laxative.

Patient Information

Instruct patients to take with water during meals. Advise patients not to chew tablets.

Warn patients not to drive a car and not to operate machinery on the day of praziquantel treatment and the following day.

IVERMECTIN

Rx	Stromectol (Merck)	Tablets: 3 mg	(MSD 32) White. In UD 20s.

IVERMECTIN — ORAL

Indications

➤*Strongyloidiasis of the intestinal tract:* For the treatment of intestinal (ie, nondisseminated) strongyloidiasis due to the nematode parasite *Strongyloides stercoralis*.

➤*Onchocerciasis:* For the treatment of onchocerciasis due to the nematode parasite *Onchocerca volvulus*.

Ivermectin has no activity against adult *Onchocerca volvulus* parasites. The adult parasites reside in SC nodules which are infrequently palpable. Surgical excision of these nodules (nodulectomy) may be considered in the management of patients with onchocerciasis, since this procedure will eliminate the microfilariae-producing adult parasites.

➤*Off-label uses:*

Head lice (Pediculosis capitis) – [3] = Safety concerns. Ivermectin appears to be effective in the treatment of head lice and the only oral alternative available. Optimal dosing regimens, particularly timing of a second dose if necessary, need to established.

Prevention of scabies – [2] = Fair documentation. Ivermectin has been used to prevent scabies infestations in nursing homes and prisons for residents and staff members in close contact with patients infested with scabies. Additional studies are needed to identify the optimal number of doses needed for prophylaxis.

Other possible off-label uses – Treatment and prophylaxis of infections with *Loa loa* and *Wucheria bancrofti* and human cutaneous larva migrans; treatment of scabies.

Administration and Dosage

➤*Adults:*

Onchocerciasis –

Single dose: Approximately 150 mcg/kg. See the table below for dosage guidelines.

Ivermectin Dosing for Onchocerciasis	
Body weight	Single oral dose
15 to 24 kg	3 mg
26 to 44 kg	6 mg
45 to 64 kg	9 mg
65 to 84 kg	12 mg
≥ 85 kg	150 mcg/kg

Retreatment: In mass-distribution campaigns in international treatment programs, the most commonly used dose interval is 12 months. For the treatment of individual patients, retreatment may be considered at intervals as short as 3 months.

Strongyloidiasis of the intestinal tract –

Single dose: Approximately 200 mcg/kg.

Ivermectin Dosing for Strongyloidiasis	
Body weight	Single oral dose
15 to 24 kg	3 mg
25 to 35 kg	6 mg
36 to 50 kg	9 mg
51 to 65 kg	12 mg
66 to 79 kg	15 mg
≥ 80 kg	200 mcg/kg

Retreatment: In general, additional doses are not necessary. However, follow-up stool examinations should be performed to verify eradication of infection.

Off-label dosing –

Head lice (Pediculosis capitis): [3] = Safety concerns. 200 mcg/kg single dose. Some studies suggested redosing after 10 days, and patients were encouraged to remove nits with a lice comb.

Prevention of scabies: [2] = Fair documentation.

- *More than 60 kg* – 18 mg.
- *60 kg or less* – 12 mg. Give as a single oral dose; dose may be repeated in 7 or 14 days.

➤*Children:*

Children weighing 15 kg or more – See Adults for dosing for children weighing 15 kg or more

➤*Administration:* Ivermectin should be taken with water.

➤*Storage/Stability:* Store at temperatures less than 30°C (86°F).

Actions

➤*Pharmacology:* Ivermectin is a member of the avermectin class of broad-spectrum antiparasitic agents which have a unique mode of action. Compounds of the class bind selectively and with high affinity to glutamate-gated chloride ion channels which occur in invertebrate nerve and muscle cells. This leads to an increase in the permeability of the cell membrane to chloride ions with hyperpolarization of the nerve or muscle cell, resulting in paralysis and death of the parasite. Compounds of this class may also interact with other ligand-gated chloride channels, such as those gated by the neurotransmitter gamma-aminobutyric acid (GABA).

The selective activity of compounds of this class is attributable to the facts that some mammals do not have glutamate-gated chloride channels and that the avermectins have a low affinity for mammalian ligand-gated chloride channels. In addition, ivermectin does not readily cross the blood-brain barrier in humans.

Ivermectin is active against various life-cycle stages of many but not all nematodes. It is active against the tissue microfilariae of *Onchocerca volvulus* but not against the adult form. Its activity against *Strongyloides stercoralis* is limited to the intestinal stages.

➤*Pharmacokinetics:*

Absorption/Distribution – Following oral administration of ivermectin, plasma concentrations are approximately proportional to the dose. In 2 studies, after single 12 mg doses of ivermectin (2 times 6 mg) in fasting healthy volunteers (representing a mean dose of 165 mcg/kg), the mean peak plasma concentrations of the major component (H_2B_{1a}) were 46.6 (± 21.9 [range 16.4 to 101.1]) and 30.6 (± 15.6 [range 13.9 to 68.4]) ng/mL respectively at ≈ 4 hours after dosing.

Metabolism/Excretion – Ivermectin is metabolized in the liver, and ivermectin or its metabolites are excreted almost exclusively in the feces over an estimated 12 days, with < 1% of the administered dose excreted in the urine. The apparent plasma half-life of ivermectin is approximately at least 16 hours following oral administration.

Contraindications

Hypersensitivity to any component of this product.

Warnings/Precautions

➤*Mazzotti reaction:* Historical data have shown that microfilaricidal drugs might cause cutaneous or systemic reactions of varying severity (the Mazzotti reaction) and ophthalmological reactions in patients with onchocerciasis. These reactions are probably due to allergic and inflammatory responses to the death of microfilariae. Patients treated with ivermectin for onchocerciasis may experience these reactions in addition to clinical adverse reactions possibly, probably, or definitely related to the drug itself (see Adverse Reactions).

The treatment of severe Mazzotti reactions has not been subjected to controlled clinical trials. Oral hydration, recumbency, IV normal saline, or parenteral corticosteroids have been used to treat postural hypotension. Antihistamines or aspirin have been used for most mild-to-moderate cases.

➤*Hyperreactive onchodermatitis:* After treatment with microfilaricidal drugs, patients with hyperreactive onchodermatitis (sowda) may be more likely than others to experience severe adverse reactions, especially edema and aggravation of onchodermatitis.

➤*Strongyloidiasis in immunocompromised hosts:* In immunocompromised (including HIV-infected) patients being treated for intestinal strongyloidiasis, repeated courses of therapy may be required. Adequate and well-controlled clinical studies have not been conducted in such patients to determine the optimal dosing regimen. Several treatments (ie, at 2-week intervals) may be required, and cure may not be achievable. Control of extraintestinal strongyloidiasis in these patients is difficult, and suppressive therapy (ie, once per month) may be helpful.

➤*Pregnancy: Category C.* Ivermectin has been shown to be teratogenic in mice, rats, and rabbits when given in repeated doses of 0.2, 8.1, and 4.5 times the maximum recommended human dose, respectively (on a mg/m²/day basis). Teratogenicity was characterized in the 3 species tested by cleft palate; clubbed forepaws were additionally observed in rabbits. These development effects were found only at or near doses that were maternotoxic to the pregnant female. Therefore, ivermectin does not appear to be selectively fetotoxic to the developing fetus. There are, however, no adequate and well-controlled studies in pregnant women. Ivermectin should not be used during pregnancy since safety in pregnancy has not been established.

➤*Lactation:* Ivermectin is excreted in human milk in low concentrations. Treatment of mothers who intend to breastfeed should only be undertaken when the risk of delayed treatment to the mother outweighs the possible risk to the newborn.

➤*Children:* Safety and effectiveness in pediatric patients weighing

IVERMECTIN — ORAL

Adverse Reactions

➤*Strongyloidiasis:*

CNS – Dizziness (2.8%); somnolence (0.9%); vertigo (0.9%); tremor (0.9%).

Dermatologic – Pruritus (2.8%); rash (0.9%); urticaria (0.9%).

GI – Anorexia (0.9%); constipation (0.9%); diarrhea (1.8%); nausea (1.8%); vomiting (0.9%).

Lab test abnormalities – In clinical trials involving 109 patients given either 1 or 2 doses of 170 to 200 mcg/kg ivermectin, the following laboratory abnormalities were seen irrespective of drug relationship: Elevation in ALT or AST (2%), and decrease in leukocyte count (3%). Leukopenia and anemia were seen in 1 patient.

Miscellaneous – Asthenia/fatigue (0.9%) and abdominal pain (0.9%).

➤*Onchocerciasis:* In clinical trials involving 963 adult patients treated with 100 to 200 mcg/kg ivermectin, worsening of the following Mazzotti reactions during the first 4 days posttreatment were reported: Arthralgia/synovitis (9.3%); axillary lymph node enlargement and tenderness (11% and 4.4%, respectively); cervical lymph node enlargement and tenderness (5.3% and 1.2%, respectively); inguinal lymph node enlargement and tenderness (12.6% and 13.9%, respectively); other lymph node enlargement and tenderness (3% and 1.9%, respectively); pruritus (27.5%); skin involvement including edema, papular and pustular or frank urticarial rash (22.7%), and fever (22.6%) (see Warnings).

Ophthalmic – In clinical trials, ophthalmological conditions were examined in 963 adult patients before treatment, at day 3, and months 3 and 6 after treatment with 100 to 200 mcg/kg ivermectin. Changes observed were primarily deterioration from baseline 3 days posttreatment. Most changes either returned to baseline condition or improved over baseline severity at the month 3 and 6 visits. The percentages of patients with worsening of the following conditions at day 3, month 3, and 6, respectively, were as follows: Limbitis, 5.5%, 4.8%, and 3.5%, and punctate opacity, 1.8%, 1.8%, and 1.4%. The corresponding percentages for patients treated with placebo were as follows: Limbitis, 6.2%, 9.9%, and 9.4%, and punctate opacity, 2%, 6.4%, and 7.2% (see Warnings).

The following ophthalmological side effects do occur due to the disease itself but have also been reported after treatment with ivermectin: Abnormal sensation in the eyes, eyelid edema, anterior uveitis, conjunctivitis, limbitis, keratitis, and chorioretinitis or choroiditis. These have rarely been severe or associated with loss of vision and have generally resolved without corticosteroid treatment.

In clinical trials involving 963 adult patients who received 100 to 200 mcg/kg ivermectin, the following clinical adverse reactions were reported as possibly, probably, or definitely related to the drug in ≥ 1% of the patients: Facial edema (1.2%), peripheral edema (3.2%), orthostatic hypotension (1.1%), and tachycardia (3.5%).

Drug-related headache and myalgia occurred in < 1% of patients (0.2% and 0.4%, respectively). However, these were the most common adverse experiences reported overall during these trials regardless of causality (22.3% and 19.7%, respectively).

A similar safety profile was observed in an open study in pediatric patients ages 6 to 13.

Additionally, hypotension (mainly orthostatic hypotension) and worsening of bronchial asthma have been reported since the drug was registered overseas.

Lab test abnormalities – In controlled clinical trials, the following laboratory adverse experiences were reported as possibly, probably, or definitely related to the drug in ≥ 1% of the patients: Eosinophilia (3%) and hemoglobin increase (1%).

Overdosage

➤*Symptoms:* In accidental intoxication with or significant exposure to unknown quantities of veterinary formulations of ivermectin in humans, either by ingestion, inhalation, injection, or exposure to body surfaces, the following adverse effects have been reported most frequently: Rash, edema, headache, dizziness, asthenia, nausea, vomiting, and diarrhea. Other adverse effects that have been reported include seizure, ataxia, dyspnea, abdominal pain, paresthesia, and urticaria.

➤*Treatment:* In case of accidental poisoning, supportive therapy, if indicated, should include parenteral fluids and electrolytes, respiratory support (oxygen and mechanical ventilation if necessary) and pressor agents if clinically significant hypotension is present. Induction of emesis or gastric lavage as soon as possible, followed by purgatives and other routine antipoison measures, may be indicated if needed to prevent absorption of ingested material.

Patient Information

Ivermectin should be taken with water.

➤*Strongyloidiasis:* The patient should be reminded of the need for repeated stool examinations to document clearance of infection with *Strongyloides stercoralis*.

➤*Onchocerciasis:* The patient should be reminded that treatment with ivermectin does not kill the adult *Onchocerca* parasites, and therefore repeated follow-up and retreatment is usually required.

The following general information applies to all immune sera. For specific information on individual agents, refer to specific monographs:

- Cytomegalovirus Immune Globulin, IV (CMV-IGIV)
- Hepatitis B Immune Globulin (HBIG)
- Immune Globulin, IM (IGIM)
- Immune Globulin, IV (IGIV)
- Immune Globulin, Subcutaneous
- Lymphocyte Immune Globulin, Antithymocyte Globulin (Equine) (ATG equine)
- Antithymocyte Globulin (Rabbit) (ATG rabbit)
- Rabies Immune Globulin (RIG)
- Rh$_o$(D) Immune Globulin, IM (Rh$_o$[D] IGIM)
- Rh$_o$(D) Immune Globulin, IV (Rh$_o$[D] IGIV)
- Rh$_o$(D) Immune Globulin Microdose (Rh$_o$[D] IG Microdose)
- Botulism Immune Globulin IV (Human) (BIG-IV)
- Vaccinia Immune Globulin Intravenous (VIGIV) (Human)

WARNING

Immune globulin IV (human) – **IGIV** (human) products have been associated with renal dysfunction, acute renal failure, osmotic nephrosis, and death. Patients predisposed to acute renal failure include patients with any degree of preexisting renal insufficiency, diabetes mellitus, volume depletion, sepsis, or paraproteinemia, patients older than 65 years of age, or patients receiving known nephrotoxic drugs. Especially in such patients, administer IGIV products at the minimum concentration available and the minimum rate of infusion practicable. While these reports of renal dysfunction and acute renal failure have been associated with the use of many of the licensed IGIV products, those containing sucrose as a stabilizer accounted for a disproportionate share of the total number. See Warnings/Precautions for important information intended to reduce the risk of acute renal failure. (*Gammagard S/D, Gamimune N, Gammaplex, Gamunex, Gamunex-C, Venoglobulin-S*, and *Iveegam* do not contain sucrose).

Rh$_o$(D) immune globulin (human) –

Intravascular hemolysis: Intravascular hemolysis leading to death has been reported in patients treated for idiopathic thrombocytopenic purpura (ITP) with *WinRho SDF*.

Intravascular hemolysis can lead to clinically compromising anemia and multisystem organ failure, including acute respiratory distress syndrome (ARDS).

Serious complications, including severe anemia, acute renal insufficiency, renal failure, and disseminated intravascular coagulation (DIC) have also been reported.

Closely monitor patients treated with *WinRho SDF* for ITP in a health care setting for at least 8 hours after administration. Perform a dipstick urinalysis at baseline, 2 and 4 hours after administration, and prior to the end of the monitoring period. Alert patients of and monitor the signs and symptoms of intravascular hemolysis, including back pain, shaking, chills, fever, and discolored urine or hematuria. Absence of these signs and/or symptoms of intravascular hemolysis within 8 hours does not indicate that intravascular hemolysis cannot occur subsequently. If signs and/or symptoms of intravascular hemolysis are present or suspected after *WinRho SDF* administration, perform posttreatment laboratory tests, including plasma hemoglobin, haptoglobin, lactate dehydrogenase (LDH), and plasma bilirubin (direct and indirect).

Antithymocyte globulin (equine) – Only health care providers experienced in immunosuppressive therapy in the treatment of renal transplant or aplastic anemia patients should use **antithymocyte globulin (equine)**.

Treat patients receiving antithymocyte globulin (equine) in facilities equipped and staffed with adequate laboratory and supportive medical resources.

Antithymocyte globulin (rabbit) – **Antithymocyte globulin (rabbit)** should only be used by health care providers experienced in immunosuppressive therapy for the management of renal transplant patients.

Indications

➤*Chronic inflammatory demyelinating polyneuropathy (Gamunex, Gamunex-C)*: For the treatment of chronic inflammatory demyelinating polyneuropathy (CIDP) to improve neuromuscular disability and impairment and for maintenance therapy to prevent relapse.

➤*Idiopathic thrombocytopenic purpura:* Treatment of nonsplenectomized, rhesus (Rh)$_o$(D)-positive children with chronic or acute ITP (*WinRho SDF* only), adults with chronic ITP (*Rhophylac* and *WinRho SDF*), or children and adults with ITP secondary to HIV infection (*WinRho SDF* only) in clinical situations requiring an increase in platelet counts to prevent excessive hemorrhage. Treatment of patients with ITP to raise platelet counts to prevent bleeding or to allow a patient with ITP to undergo surgery (*Gammagard S/D, Gamunex, Gamunex-C, Privigen*).

➤*Kawasaki syndrome (Gammagard S/D only)*: For the prevention of coronary artery aneurysms associated with Kawasaki syndrome.

➤*Passive immunization:* To provide passive immunization to greater than or equal to 1 infectious diseases. Protection derived will be of rapid onset, but of short duration (1 to 3 months). See individual monographs for specific indications.

➤*Primary humoral immunodeficiency (Carimune, Flebogamma, Gammagard, Gammagard S/D, Gammaplex, Gamunex, Gamunex-C, Hizentra 20%, Octagam, Privigen, Vivaglobin)*: For the replacement therapy of primary humoral immunodeficiency. This includes, but is not limited to, the humoral immune defect in common variable immunodeficiency, X-linked agammaglobulinemia, congenital agammaglobulinemia, Wiskott-Aldrich syndrome, and severe combined immunodeficiencies.

➤*Suppression of Rh isoimmunization:*

Pregnancy and obstetric conditions –

Rhophylac: For the suppression of Rh isoimmunization in nonsensitized Rh$_o$(D)-negative women with an Rh-incompatible pregnancy, including routine antepartum and postpartum Rh prophylaxis; and Rh prophylaxis in cases of obstetric complications (eg, miscarriage, abortion, threatened abortion, ectopic pregnancy or hydatidiform mole, transplacental hemorrhage resulting from antepartum hemorrhage), invasive procedures during pregnancy (eg, amniocentesis, chorionic biopsy), or obstetric manipulative procedures (eg, external version, abdominal trauma).

WinRho SDF: For the suppression of Rh isoimmunization in nonsensitized Rh$_o$(D)-negative women within 72 hours after spontaneous or induced abortions, amniocentesis, chorionic villus sampling, ruptured tubal pregnancy, abdominal trauma or transplacental hemorrhage, or in the normal course of pregnancy, unless the blood type of the fetus or father is known to be Rh$_o$(D)-negative. In the case of maternal bleeding because of threatened abortion, administer as soon as possible. Suppression of Rh isoimmunization reduces the likelihood of hemolytic disease in an Rh$_o$(D)-positive fetus in present and future pregnancies. Do not administer to infants born to Rh-incompatible mothers.

Transfusion (Rhophylac and WinRho SDF) – For the suppression of Rh isoimmunization in Rh$_o$(D)-negative female children and female adults in their childbearing years transfused with Rh$_o$(D)-positive red blood cells (RBCs) or blood components containing Rh$_o$(D)-positive RBCs. Initiate treatment within 72 hours of exposure.

➤*Off-label uses:*

Juvenile idiopathic arthritis –

Carimune: 5 = Poor documentation.

Gammagard: 5 = Poor documentation.

Gammagard S/D: 5 = Poor documentation.

Gammaplex: 5 = Poor documentation.

Gamunex: 5 = Poor documentation.

Octagam: 5 = Poor documentation.

Privigen: 5 = Poor documentation.

Actions

➤*Pharmacology:*

CMV-IGIV – This product contains immunoglobulin G (IgG) antibodies representative of the large number of healthy people who contributed to the plasma pools from which the product was derived. The globulin contains a relatively high concentration of antibodies directed against CMV. In people who may be exposed to CMV, this product can raise the relevant antibodies to levels sufficient to attenuate or reduce the incidence of serious CMV disease.

HBIG – HBIG provides passive immunization for individuals exposed to the hepatitis B virus (HBV). The administration of the usual recommended dose of this immune globulin generally results in a detectable level of circulating anti-HBs, which persists for approximately 2 months or longer.

IGIM – IGIM is a transient source of IgG that specifically and nonspecifically inactivates various bacteria, viruses, and fungi. IgG antibodies activate the complement system, promote opsonization, neutralize microorganisms and their toxins, and participate in antibody-dependent cytolytic reactions.

Hepatitis A: IGIM is 80% to 95% effective in preventing hepatitis A, depending on the temporal relation between administration and exposure and on the severity of exposure.

Measles: IGIM reduces the risk of clinical evidence of measles by an estimated 50%. A lower incidence of measles encephalitis also has been associated with the use of IGIM.

Varicella: IGIM reduces severity of disease, as measured by temperature and the number of pox.

IGIV – IGIV passively supplies a broad spectrum of IgG antibodies against bacterial, viral, parasitic, and mycoplasmic antigens. IGIV antibodies act through a variety of mechanisms, including antimicrobial or antitoxin neutralization. IGIV appears to work by contributing anti-idiotypic antibodies that bind and neutralize pathogenic autoantibodies. There may also be negative feedback and down-regulation of antibody production. Other mechanisms may involve binding to CD5 receptors, interleukin (IL)-1a, IL-6, tumor necrosis factor-alpha, and T-cell receptors, suppressing pathogenic cytokines and phagocytes. IGIV also interferes with pathogenic effects of products of complement activation.

Immune globulin subcutaneous – Immune globulin subcutaneous supplies a broad spectrum of opsonizing and neutralizing IgG antibodies against a wide variety of bacterial and viral agents.

ATG equine – ATG equine is a lymphocyte-selective immunosuppressant. It reduces the number of circulating, thymus-dependent lymphocytes that form rosettes with sheep erythrocytes. This antilymphocytic effect is believed to reflect an alteration of the function of the T-lymphocytes, which are responsible, in part, for cell-mediated immunity and are involved in humoral immunity. It also contains low concentrations of antibodies against other formed elements of the blood. In rhesus and cynomolgus monkeys, this drug reduces lymphocytes in the thymus-dependent areas of the spleen and lymph nodes. It also decreases the circulating sheep-erythrocyte-rosetting lymphocytes that can be detected, but ordinarily does not cause severe lymphopenia.

In general, when administered with other immunosuppressive therapy, such as antimetabolites and corticosteroids, the patient's own antibody response to horse gamma globulin is minimal.

Precise methods of determining potency have not been established; thus activity may potentially vary from lot to lot.

In general, ATG equine enables a 1 year graft survival rate of greater than or equal to 80%. Graft and patient survival are dependent on whether the transplanted organ is harvested from a living or deceased host, the degree of antigenic matching, the combination of immunosuppressive drugs delivered, and other factors.

ATG rabbit – The mechanism of action by which polyclonal antilymphocyte preparations suppress immune responses is not fully understood. Possible mechanisms by which ATG rabbit may induce immunosuppression in vivo include: T-cell clearance from the circulation and modulation of T-cell activation, homing, and cytotoxic activities. ATG rabbit includes antibodies against T-cell markers such as CD2, CD3, CD4, CD8, CD11a, CD18, CD25, CD44, CD45, HLA-DR, HLA Class 1 heavy chains, and β2 microglobulin. In vitro, ATG rabbit (concentrations greater than 0.1 mg/mL) mediates T-cell suppressive effects via inhibition of proliferative responses to several mitogens. In patients, T-cell depletion is usually observed within a day from initiating ATG rabbit therapy. ATG rabbit has not been shown to be effective for treating antibody (humoral) mediated rejections.

RIG – Rabies antibody provides passive protection when given immediately to individuals exposed to rabies virus. RIG of adequate potency was used in conjunction with rabies vaccine of duck embryo origin. When a globulin dose of 20 units/kg of rabies antibody was given simultaneously with the first dose of vaccine, levels of passive rabies antibody were detected 24 hours after injection in all individuals. There was minimal or no interference with the immune response to the initial and subsequent doses of vaccine, including booster doses. Studies of RIG given with the first of 5 doses of human diploid cell rabies vaccine (HDCV) confirmed that passive immunization with 20 units/kg of RIG provides maximum circulating antibody with minimum interference of active immunization by HDCV.

Rh_o(D) IGIM – Rh_o(D) IGIM acts by suppressing the immune response of Rh_o(D)-negative individuals to Rh_o(D)-positive RBCs. The mechanism of action of the full dose is not fully understood.

Passive immunization with Rh_o(D) prevents the formation of anti-Rh_o(D) antibodies in nonsensitized Rh_o(D) antigen-negative individuals who receive Rh_o(D) antigen-positive RBCs. Rh_o(D) antibody binds circulating antigen, thus preventing stimulation of antigen-sensitive lymphocytes and the resulting production of anti-Rh_o(D). Prevention of Rh_o(D) sensitization in turn prevents hemolytic disease of the fetus and newborn in subsequent Rh_o(D) antigen-positive children.

Rh_o(D) IGIV –

Suppression of Rh isoimmunization: Rh_o(D) IGIV is used to suppress the immune response of nonsensitized Rh_o(D)-negative individuals following Rh_o(D)-positive red blood cell exposure by fetomaternal hemorrhage during delivery of an Rh_o(D)-positive infant, abortion (spontaneous or induced), amniocentesis, abdominal trauma, or mismatched transfusion. The mechanism of action is not completely understood.

Idiopathic thrombocytopenic purpura: The mechanism of action is not completely understood, but is thought to be due to the formation of anti-Rh_o(D) (anti-D)-coated RBC complexes resulting in Fc receptor blockade, thus sparing antibody-coated platelets.

Rh_o(D) IG microdose – Rh_o(D) IG microdose is used to prevent the formation of anti-Rh_o(D) antibody in Rh_o(D)-negative women who are exposed to the Rh_o(D) antigen at the time of spontaneous or induced abortion (up to 12 weeks gestation). Rh_o(D) IG microdose suppresses the stimulation of active immunity by Rh_o(D)-positive fetal erythrocytes that may enter the maternal circulation at the time of termination of the pregnancy.

The amount of anti-Rh_o(D) in Rh_o(D) IG microdose has been shown to effectively prevent material isosensitization to the Rh_o(D) antigens following spontaneous or induced abortion occurring up to the 12th week of gestation. After the 12th week of gestation, a standard dose of Rh_o(D) IGIM full dose is indicated.

Rh_o(D) IG microdose acts by suppressing the immune response of Rh-negative individuals to Rh-positive RBCs. The risk of immunization is related to the number of D-positive RBCs received. The risk was found to be 3% when 0.1 mL of fetal RBCs is present in the mother and 65% when 5 mL is present. In the first 12 weeks of gestation, the total volume of RBCs in the fetus is estimated at less than 2.5 mL.

RSV-IGIV – RSV-IGIV is a sterile liquid IgG containing neutralizing antibody to respiratory syncytial virus (RSV). The immunoglobulin is purified from pooled adult human plasma selected for high titers of neutralizing antibody against RSV. A widely utilized solvent-detergent viral inactivation process is used to decrease the possibility of transmission of bloodborne pathogens. Each milliliter contains 50 ± 10 mg immunoglobulin, primarily IgG, and trace amounts of IgA and IgM.

➤*Pharmacokinetics:* Immunoglobulins are primarily eliminated by catabolism.

CMV-IGIV – The onset of action is rapid. The mean half-life is 21 days, shorter in transplant recipients, where half-lives have been measured as 8 days immediately after transplant, or 13 to 15 days if given greater than or equal to 60 days after transplant. The protective level is unknown.

HBIG – Antibodies appear within 1 to 6 days after IM administration and peak in 3 to 11 days. The mean half-life is 17 to 25 days (range, 6 to 35) and clinical protection typically persists for approximately 2 months. The protective level of anti-HBs titer is greater than or equal to 10 milliunit/mL. The clearance rate was 0.433 ± 0.144 L/day, with a volume of distribution of 15.3 ± 6.2 L.

IGIM – IgG titers peak 2 to 5 days after IM injection. Mean IgG half-life in circulation of people with normal IgG levels is 23 days. Protective levels are 200 mg per 100 mL of plasma as a target in immunoglobulin replacement therapy.

IGIV – The onset is rapid. In general, the mean half-life in healthy people is 18 to 35 days, although there is tremendous intersubject variability. Fever or infection may decrease antibody half-life because of increased catabolism or consumption, respectively. In ITP, the increase in platelets usually lasts from several days to several weeks, although it may rarely persist for greater than or equal to 1 year. In a group of burn patients, the half-life ranged from 47 to 154 days.

IV administration makes essentially 100% of the dose immediately available in the recipient's circulation. After approximately 6 days, approximately 50% of the body pool partitions into the extravascular space, with the balance remaining in the serum.

Expect a rapid fall in serum IgG in the first week after infusion, mainly because of equilibration of IgG between plasma and the extravascular space. The decrease averages 40% of peak level after infusion; within 24 hours, 30% of a single dose is removed from circulation to extravascular fluid, tissue, cells, and catabolism.

Immune globulin subcutaneous – Bioavailability of immune globulin subcutaneous is approximately 73% compared with IGIV. Peak serum IgG levels are lower with subcutaneous compared with IV administration. Mean peak and trough IgG levels following immune globulin subcutaneous administration are 1,163 to 1,616 mg/dL and 1,064 to 1,448 mg/dL, respectively. Steady-state serum IgG levels are relatively stable with weekly subcutaneous administration.

ATG equine – Onset is rapid. Peak plasma level of equine IgG occurs after 5 days of infusion at 10 mg/kg/day. Peak values vary depending on recipient's ability to catabolize equine IgG. In a small study, mean peak plasma value was 727 ± 310 mcg/mL. Rosette-forming cells decrease immediately after beginning therapy. Recovery to normal values after therapy cessation is dependent on recipient's catabolic rate and, in some cases, upon length of therapy. Mean half-life is approximately 5.7 days (range, 2.7 to 8.7 days).

ATG rabbit – After an IV dosage of 1.25 to 1.5 mg/kg/day (over 4 hours for 7 to 11 days) 4 to 8 hours postinfusion, ATG rabbit levels were on average 21.5 mcg/mL (10 to 40 mcg/mL) with a half-life of 2 to 3 days after the first dose, and 87 mcg/mL (23 to 170 mcg/mL) after the last dose.

RIG – Adequate levels of antibody appear in serum within 24 hours and peak within 2 to 13 days. Because rabies vaccine takes approximately 1 week to induce active immunity, the importance of RIG cannot be overemphasized. The mean serum half-life of rabies antibody is 24 days, consistent with the 21-day half-life expected of IgG.

Rh_o(D) IGIM (human) – The onset of action is prompt. The mean half-life is 23 to 26 days, with antibody titers greater than or equal to 1:5 by RFFIT indicative of adequate protection.

Rh_o(D) immune globulin, when administered within 72 hours of a full-term delivery of an Rh_o(D)-positive infant by an Rh_o(D)-negative mother, will reduce the incidence of Rh isoimmunization from between 12% and 13% to between 1% and 2%. The 1% to 2% range is due, for the most part, to isoimmunization during the last trimester of pregnancy. When treatment is given both antenatally at 28 weeks gestation and postpartum, the Rh immunization rate drops to approximately 0.1%.

When 600 units (120 mcg) of Rh_o(D) IGIV is given to pregnant women, passive anti-Rh_o(D) antibodies are not detectable in the circulation for greater than 6 weeks; therefore, give a dose of 1500 units (300 mcg) for antenatal administration.

IM vs IV administration: The absolute bioavailability of *Rhophylac* was 69%. In a clinical study involving Rh_o(D)-negative volunteers, 2 subjects were given 600 units (120 mcg) IM and 2 subjects were given this dose IV. Peak levels (36 to 48 ng/mL) were reached within 2 hours of IV administration; for IM, peak levels (18 to 19 ng/mL) were reached at 5 to 10 days. The calculated areas under the curve (AUCs) were the same for both routes of administration. The half-life was approximately 24 and 30 days following IV and IM administration, respectively. Mean systemic clearance of *Rhophylac* was 0.2 ± 0.03 mL/min, and half-life was 16 ± 4 days; mean apparent clearance was 0.29 ± 0.12 mL/min, and half-life was 18 ± 5 days.

Rh_o(D) IG microdose – Administration of Rh_o(D) IG microdose within 3 hours following abortion was 100% effective in preventing Rh immunization. Studies showed Rh_o(D) IG microdose to be effective when given as long as 72 hours after the infusion of Rh-positive red cells. A lesser degree of protection is afforded if the antibody is administered beyond this time period.

RSV-IGIV – The onset of action is rapid with the mean half-life of serum RSV neutralizing antibodies after RSV-IG infusion as 22 to 28 days. The protective level is not established. In one study, monthly doses of 750 mg/kg of RSV-IG attained trough geometric mean serum RSV neutralization antibody titers of 1:297 ± 38 (SE) 1 month after the first infusion, 1:477 ± 85 1 month after the second infusion, 1:490 ± 61 1 month after the third infusion, and 1:429 ± 23 1 month after the fourth infusion.

Contraindications

History of systemic allergic reactions following administration of human immunoglobulin preparations.

Allergic response to gamma globulin or anti-IgA antibodies.

Allergic response to thimerosal.

People with isolated IgA deficiency. Such people have the potential for developing antibodies to IgA and could have anaphylactic reactions to subsequent administration of blood products that contain IgA.

➤*IGIM:* Patients who have severe thrombocytopenia or any coagulation disorder that would contraindicate IM use.

➤*Immune globulin subcutaneous (Hizentra only):* History of anaphylactic or severe systemic response to polysorbate 80; hyperprolinemia.

➤*ATG equine:* Severe prior systemic reaction with the administration of antithymocyte globulin (equine) or other equine immunoglobulin preparations.

➤*ATG rabbit:* In patients with a history of allergy or anaphylaxis to rabbit proteins, or who have an acute viral illness.

➤*RIG (Imogam):* Rabies immune globulin should not be administered in repeated doses once vaccine treatment has been initiated. Repeating the dose may interfere with maximum active immunity expected from the vaccine.

➤*Rh_o(D) IGIV:* Known anaphylactic or severe systemic reaction to the administration of human immune globulin products.

➤*WinRho SDF:* Patients with autoimmune hemolytic anemia or preexisting hemolysis or in patients at high risk for hemolysis; in infants for the suppression of isoimmunization, Rh_o(D).

➤*Rh_o(D) IG microdose (MICRhoGAM):* Must not be used for any indication with continuation of pregnancy; not recommended for any indication beyond 12 weeks gestation.

Warnings/Precautions

➤*Renal risks:* IGIV (human) products have been reported to be associated with renal dysfunction, acute renal failure, osmotic nephrosis, and death. Patients predisposed to acute renal failure include patients with any degree of preexisting renal insufficiency, diabetes mellitus, volume depletion, sepsis, or paraproteinemia, patients who are older than 65 years of age, or patients receiving known nephrotoxic drugs. Especially in such patients, administer IGIV products at the minimum concentrations available and at the minimum rate of infusion practical. While these reports of renal dysfunction and acute renal failure have been associated with the use of many IGIV products, those containing sucrose as a stabilizer (and given at daily doses of greater than or equal to 400 mg/kg) account for a disproportionate share of the total number. See Warnings/Precautions and Administration and Dosage sections for important information intended to reduce the risk of acute renal failure.

➤*Bloodborne viral transmission:* Most of these products are made from human plasma and like other plasma products, they carry the possibility for transmission of bloodborne pathogenic agents. The risk of transmission of recognized bloodborne viruses is considered to be low because of the screening of plasma donors, and the collection and testing of plasma, through the application of viral elimination/reduction step such as alcohol fractionation, PEG/Bentonite precipitation and solvent-detergent treatment. Despite these measures, such products can still potentially transmit disease; therefore, the risk of infectious agents cannot be totally eliminated. Report all infections thought by the physician to have been possibly transmitted by these products to the manufacturer. Weigh the risks and benefits of the use of this product and discuss these with the patient.

➤*Intravascular hemolysis:* Intravascular hemolysis leading to death has been reported in patients treated for ITP.

Intravascular hemolysis can lead to clinically compromising anemia and multisystem organ failure, including ARDS.

Serious complications, including severe anemia, acute renal insufficiency, renal failure, and DIC have also been reported.

➤*Route of administration:* Administer these agents only as indicated (eg, IM or IV, subcutaneous). Inappropriate IV injections may cause a precipitous fall in blood pressure and a picture similar to anaphylaxis (ie, RIG). Administer IM.

➤*Rate of administration:* Except for hypersensitivity reactions, adverse reactions to IGIVs may be related to the rate of administration. Careful adherence to the infusion rate outlined under Administration and Dosage is therefore important. Have loop diuretics available for the management of patients who are at risk for fluid overload. Although systemic allergic reactions are rare (see Adverse Reactions), have epinephrine and diphenhydramine available for treatment of acute allergic symptoms.

➤*Immunoglobulin A deficiency:* People with isolated IgA deficiency have the potential for developing antibodies to IgA and could have anaphylactic reactions to subsequent administration of blood products that contain IgA.

➤*Aseptic meningitis syndrome:* Rare occurrences of aseptic meningitis syndrome (AMS) have been reported in association with IGIV treatment. AMS usually begins within several hours to 2 days following IGIV treatment and is characterized by symptoms including severe headache, drowsiness, fever, photophobia, painful eye movements, muscle rigidity, nausea, and vomiting. Cerebrospinal fluid studies generally demonstrate pleocytosis, predominately granulocytic, and elevated protein levels. Thoroughly evaluate patients exhibiting such signs and symptoms to rule out other causes of meningitis. AMS may occur more frequently in association with high-dose (2 g/kg) IGIV treatment and/or rapid infusion. Discontinuation of IGIV treatment has resulted in remission of AMS within several days without sequelae.

➤*Hyperproteinemia/increased serum viscosity/hyponatremia:* Hyperproteinemia, increased serum viscosity, and hyponatremia may occur in patients receiving IGIV therapy. It is critical to clinically distinguish true hyponatremia from a pseudohyponatremia that is associated with or causally related to hyperproteinemia with concomitant decreased calculated serum osmolality or elevated osmolar gap, because treatment aimed at decreasing serum free water in patients with pseudohyponatremia may lead to volume depletion, a further increase in serum viscosity, and a possible predisposition to thrombotic events.

➤*Bleeding complications:* As will all preparations administered by the IM route, bleeding complications may be encountered in patients with thrombocytopenia or other bleeding disorders.

➤*ATG equine:* Only health care providers experienced in immunosuppressive therapy in the treatment of renal transplant or aplastic anemia patients should use lymphocyte immune globulin. Treat patients receiving lymphocyte immune globulin in facilities equipped and staffed with adequate laboratory and supportive medical resources.

Discontinuation – Discontinue treatment if any of the following occurs: Anaphylaxis; severe and unremitting thrombocytopenia and severe and unremitting leukopenia in renal transplant patients.

Hemolysis: Clinically significant hemolysis is rare. Treatment may include transfusion of erythrocytes; if necessary, administer IV mannitol, furosemide, sodium bicarbonate, and fluids. Severe and unremitting hemolysis may require discontinuation of therapy.

Thrombocytopenia: Thrombocytopenia is usually transient; platelet counts generally return to adequate levels without discontinuing therapy; platelet transfusions may be necessary in patients with aplastic anemia.

➤*ATG rabbit:* ATG rabbit should only be used by health care providers experienced in immunosuppressive therapy for the treatment of renal transplant patients. Medical surveillance is required during ATG rabbit infusion.

Hematologic effects – Thrombocytopenia or neutropenia may result from cross-reactive antibodies and is reversible following dose adjustments.

➤*Criteria for Rh_o(D) IGIV administration:* The criteria for an Rh-incompatible pregnancy requiring administration of Rh_o(D) immune globulin at 28 weeks gestation and within 72 hours after delivery are the following: The mother must be Rh_o(D) antigen-negative; the mother is carrying a child whose father is either Rh_o(D) antigen-positive or Rh_o(D) unknown; the infant is either Rh_o(D) antigen-positive or Rh_o(D) unknown; and the mother must not be previously sensitized to the Rh_o(D) antigen.

Rh_oD-negative or splenectomized patients – Do not administer Rh_o(D) immune globulin IV to Rh_o(D)-negative or splenectomized individuals as its efficacy in these patients has not been demonstrated.

➤*RSV-IGIV:*

Fluid overload – Infants with underlying pulmonary disease may be sensitive to the extra fluid volume. Infusion of RSV-IGIV, particularly in children with bronchopulmonary dysplasia (BPD), may precipitate symptoms of fluid overload. Overall, 8.4% of participants (1% premature and 13% BPD) received new or extra diuretics during the period 24 hours before through 48 hours after at least one of their infusions in the PREVENT trial. RSV-IGIV-related fluid overload was reported in 3 patients (1.2%) and RSV-IGIV-related respiratory distress was reported in 4 patients (1.6%); all had underlying BPD. These children were managed with diuretics or modification of the infusion rate and went on to receive subsequent infusions.

Complications related to fluid volume were recorded as a reason for incomplete or prolonged infusion in 2% of children receiving RSV-IGIV (2.5% BPD and 1.1% premature) and in 1.5% of children receiving placebo. Children with clinically apparent fluid overload should not be infused with RSV-IGIV.

➤*Anaphylactic reactions:* Anaphylactic reactions (rare) may occur following injection of human immune globulin preparations. Anaphylaxis is more likely if immune globulin is given IV; therefore, except for IGIV, these products must only be given IM. In highly allergic individuals, repeated injections may lead to anaphylactic shock.

➤*Skin testing:* Skin testing should not be performed. Intradermal injection of concentrated gamma globulin causes a localized area of inflammation that can be misinterpreted as a positive allergic reaction. It is actually localized chemical tissue irritation. Misinterpretation can cause necessary medication to be withheld from a patient not actually allergic to this material. True allergic responses to human gamma globulin given in the prescribed IM manner are extremely rare.

➤*Mercury:* Some of these products contain mercury in the form of ethyl mercury from thimerosal. While there are no definitive data on the toxicity of ethyl mercury, literature suggests that information related to methyl mercury toxicities may be applicable.

➤*Latex sensitivity:* Certain components of some of the packaging of these products contain natural rubber latex, which may cause an allergic reaction in sensitive individuals.

➤*Maltose:* Some of these products contain maltose and have been shown to give falsely high blood glucose levels in certain types of blood glucose testing systems.

➤*Admixture incompatibilities:* Do not admix with other medications.

➤*Rh_o(D) IGIM:*

Hemorrhage – A large fetomaternal hemorrhage late in pregnancy or following delivery may cause a weak mixed field positive D^u test result. If there is any doubt about the mother's Rh type, she should be given Rh_o(D) immune globulin. A screening test to detect fetal RBCs may be helpful in such cases.

If greater than 15 mL of D-positive fetal RBCs are present in the mother's circulation, more than a single dose of Rh_o(D) immune globulin full dose is required. Failure to recognize this may result in the administration of an inadequate dose.

➤*Rh_oD IGIV:* Do not administer Rh_o(D) IGIV as immunoglobulin replacement therapy for immune globulin deficiency syndromes.

Intravascular hemolysis – Following administration of Rh_o(D) IGIV, monitor Rh_o(D)-positive patients for signs and symptoms of intravascular hemolysis (IVH), clinically compromising anemia, and renal insufficiency in patients treated for ITP. If patients are to be transfused, use Rh_o(D)-

negative packed RBCs so as not to exacerbate ongoing IVH. Platelet products may contain up to 5 mL of RBCs; thus, exercise caution if platelets from Rh_o(D)-positive donors are transfused.

Suppression of Rh isoimmunization – Do not administer Rh_o(D) IGIV to Rh_o(D)-negative individuals who are Rh immunized, as evidenced by an indirect antiglobulin (Coombs) test revealing the presence of anti-Rh_o(D) (anti-D) antibody.

Fetomaternal hemorrhage: A large fetomaternal hemorrhage late in pregnancy or following delivery may cause a weak mixed field positive D^u test result. Assess such an individual for a large fetomaternal hemorrhage and adjust the dose of Rh_o(D) immune globulin accordingly. Administer Rh_o(D) immune globulin if there is any doubt about the mother's blood type.

Hemoglobin – If a patient has a lower than normal hemoglobin level (less than 10 g/dL), give a reduced dose of 125 to 200 units/kg to minimize the risk of increasing the severity of anemia in the patient. Rh_o(D) IGIV must be used with extreme caution in patients with a hemoglobin level that is less than 8 g/dL because of the risk of increasing the severity of the anemia (see Administration and Dosage).

➤*ATG equine:*

Infection – Because this agent is ordinarily given with corticosteroids and antimetabolites, monitor patients carefully for leukopenia, thrombocytopenia, or for concurrent infection. If infection occurs, institute adjunctive therapy promptly. On the basis of the clinical circumstances, decide whether therapy will continue.

Concomitant immunosuppressive therapy – Safety and efficacy have been demonstrated in renal transplant patients who received concomitant immunosuppressive therapy and in patients with aplastic anemia.

When the dose of corticosteroids and other immunosuppressants is being reduced, some previously masked reactions to the drug may appear; observe patients carefully during therapy.

Chills and fever – Chills and fever occur frequently. ATG equine may release endogenous leukocyte pyrogens. Prophylactic or therapeutic administration of antihistamines, antipyretics, or corticosteroids generally controls this reaction.

Chemical phlebitis – Chemical phlebitis can be caused by infusion through peripheral veins. Avoid by administering the solution into a high-flow vein. An subcutaneously arterialized vein produced by a Brescia fistula is also a useful administration site.

Itching and erythema – Itching and erythema probably result from the drug's effect on blood elements. Antihistamines control the symptoms.

Serum sickness-like symptoms – Serum sickness-like symptoms in aplastic anemia patients have been treated with oral or IV corticosteroids. Resolution of symptoms has generally been prompt and long-term sequelae have not been observed. Prophylactic administration of corticosteroids may decrease the frequency of this reaction.

➤*ATG rabbit:*

Chills and fever – ATG rabbit infusion may produce fever and chills. To minimize these, infuse the first dose over a minimum of 6 hours into a high-flow vein. Also premedication with corticosteroids, acetaminophen, or an antihistamine or slowing the infusion rate may reduce reaction incidence and intensity (see Administration and Dosage).

Prolonged use or overdosage – Prolonged use or overdosage of ATG rabbit in association with other immunosuppressive agents may cause over-immunosuppression resulting in severe infections and may increase the incidence of lymphoma or posttransplant lymphoproliferative disease (PTLD) or other malignancies. Appropriate antiviral, antibacterial, antiprotozoal, or antifungal prophylaxis is recommended.

➤*RSV-IGIV:*

Rate of administration – Except for hypersensitivity reactions, adverse reactions to IGIVs may be related to the rate of administration. Careful adherence to the infusion rate outlined under Administration and Dosage is therefore important. Have loop diuretics available for the management of patients who are at risk for fluid overload. Although systemic allergic reactions are rare (see Adverse Reactions), have epinephrine and diphenhydramine available for treatment of acute allergic symptoms.

Discard after use – RSV-IGIV does not contain a preservative. Enter the single-use vial only once for administration purposes and begin the infusion within 6 hours. Closely adhere to the infusion schedule (see Administration and Dosage). Do not use if the solution is turbid.

➤*Thrombotic events:* There is clinical evidence of a possible association between IGIV administration and the potential for the development of thrombotic events. The exact cause of this is unknown; therefore, exercise caution in the prescribing and infusion of IGIV in patients with a history of and predisposing factors toward cardiovascular disease or thrombotic episodes. Patients at high risk include those with a history of atherosclerosis, multiple cardiovascular risk factors, advanced age, impaired cardiac output, coagulation disorders, prolonged periods of immobilization, and/or unknown suspected hyperviscosity. Analysis of adverse event reports has indicated that a rapid rate of infusion may be a risk factor for vascular occlusive events.

➤*Transfusion-related acute lung injury:* Noncardiogenic pulmonary edema may occur following treatment with IGIV. Symptoms usually appear within 1 to 6 hours following treatment and are characterized by fever, hypoxemia, normal left ventricular function, pulmonary edema, and severe respiratory distress. Monitor patients for pulmonary adverse reactions and manage with oxygen therapy and adequate ventilatory support.

➤*Hypersensitivity reactions:* Give with caution to patients with prior systemic allergic reactions following use of human immunoglobulin preparations. Hypersensitivity reactions are rare; the incidence may be increased by use of large IM doses or repeated injections of immune globulin. Have epinephrine available for treatment of acute allergic symptoms. Refer to Management of Acute Hypersensitivity Reactions.

Severe reactions – Severe reactions, such as anaphylaxis or angioneurotic edema, have been reported in association with IV immunoglobulins, even in patients not known to be sensitive to human immunoglobulins or blood products. If hypotension, anaphylaxis, or severe allergic reaction occurs, discontinue infusion and administer epinephrine (1:1,000) as required. Administer steroids, assist respiration, and provide other resuscitative measures. If hypotension occurs, stop infusion and stabilize blood pressure with pressors if necessary. Respiratory distress may also indicate anaphylaxis. Pain in the chest, flank, or back may indicate anaphylaxis or hemolysis. Treat appropriately with an antihistamine, epinephrine, corticosteroids, or some combination of the three. Refer to Management of Acute Hypersensitivity Reactions.

Although systemic reactions to immunoglobulin preparations are rare, epinephrine should be available for treatment of acute anaphylactic symptoms.

➤*Pregnancy: Category C.* No studies have been conducted in pregnant patients. Clinical experience suggests no adverse effects on the fetus per se; however, it is not known whether these agents can cause fetal harm.

It should be noted again that *BayRho-D Mini-Dose* is not indicated for use during pregnancy and it should be administered only postabortion or post-miscarriage.

The available evidence suggests that *Rhophylac* does not harm the fetus or affect future pregnancies or reproduction capacity when given to pregnant Rh_o(D)-negative women for suppression of Rh isoimmunization.

Intact IgG crosses the placenta significantly after 32 weeks' gestation.

➤*Lactation:* Safety for use in the nursing mother has not been established. It is not known whether immune globulin is excreted in breast milk. The World Health Organization classifies IGIV and IGIM as compatible with breast-feeding.

➤*Children:* Safety and efficacy have not been established in pediatric patients. Do not inject infants with **Rh_o(D) IGIV, Rh_o(D) IGIM**, or **Rh_o(D) IG microdose**.

ATG equine has been administered safely to a small number of pediatric renal allograft recipients and pediatric aplastic anemia patients at dosage levels comparable to those used in adults on a mg/kg basis.

RSV-IGIV is indicated for use in children less than 24 months of age. However, the safety and efficacy of RSV-IGIV in children with congenital heart disease have not been established. Although equivalent proportions of children in the RSV-IGIV and control groups in one trial had adverse events, a larger number of RSV-IGIV recipients had severe or life-threatening adverse events. These events were most frequently observed in infants with coronary heart disease (CHD) with right to left shunts who underwent cardiac surgery.

IGIV – Six pediatric patients with primary humoral immunodeficiency (2 between the ages of 9 and 10, and 4 between the ages of 12 and 16) were included within the clinical evaluation of *Gammaplex*. This number of pediatric patients was too small for separate evaluation from the adult patients for safety or efficacy.

The safety and efficacy of *Gammar-P I.V.* has not been established in neonates and infants with primary defective antibody syntheses.

High-dose administration of *Panglobulin* in pediatric patients with acute or chronic ITP did not reveal any pediatric-specific hazard.

Immune globulin subcutaneous – No specific dosage adjustments are necessary to achieve the desired serum IgG levels in children. *Hizentra* has not been evaluated in neonates or infants; *Vivaglobin* has not been evaluated in children younger than 2 years of age.

Immune globulin intravenous/subcutaneous – No pediatric-specific dose requirements are necessary when administering *Gamunex-C* to children with idiopathic thrombocytopenic purpura or primary humoral immunodeficiency. Safety and efficacy of treatment of CIDP and administration using the subcutaneous route has not been established in children.

Venoglobulin-S –

Immunodeficiency: The safety and effectiveness of *Venoglobulin-S* in the treatment of primary immunodeficiency was established in adults and a limited number of children. No infants or neonates were studied. No differences in dosing were found necessary for pediatric patients, nor were any special precautions required.

Idiopathic thrombocytopenic purpura: The safety and effectiveness of *Venoglobulin-S* was established in both pediatric and adult populations and included all pediatric age groups except neonates. No differences in dosing were found necessary for children, nor were any special precautions required.

Kawasaki disease: The safety and efficacy of *Venoglobulin* was established in pediatric populations containing all age groups except neonates.

Sandoglobulin – High-dose administration of *Sandoglobulin* in pediatric patients with acute or chronic ITP did not reveal any pediatric-specific hazard.

➤*Monitoring:* Ensure that patients are not volume depleted prior to the initiation of therapy.

Periodic monitoring of renal function tests and urine output is particularly important in patients judged to have a potential increased risk for developing acute renal failure. Renal function, including the measurement of serum urea nitrogen (BUN) or serum creatinine should be assessed prior to the initial infusion, and again at appropriate intervals thereafter. If renal function deteriorates, discontinuation of the product should be considered.

For patients judged to be at risk for developing renal dysfunction, it may be prudent to reduce the amount of product infused per unit time (see specific product inserts for measurements).

Administer **RSV-IGIV** cautiously. During administration, monitor the patient's vital signs frequently for increases in heart rate, respiratory rate, retractions, and rales. A loop diuretic such as furosemide or bumetanide should be available for management of fluid overload.

During **ATG rabbit** therapy, monitoring the lymphocyte count (eg, total lymphocyte or T-cell subset) may help assess the degree of T-cell depletion. For safety, monitor the white blood cell and platelet counts.

Following administration of Rh_o(D) immune globulin, monitor the patient for at least 8 hours post administration and perform a dipstick urinalysis at baseline, 2 and 4 hours after administration, and prior to the end of the monitoring period.

Following administration of Rh_o(D) immune globulin, monitor patients for signs or symptoms of intravascular hemolysis, clinically compromising anemia, acute renal function impairment, and DIC. Patients with ITP presenting with signs and/or symptoms of intravascular hemolysis and its complications after anti-D administration should have confirmatory laboratory testing that may include, but is not limited to, complete blood cell count (eg, Hb, platelet counts), haptoglobin, plasma Hb, urine dipstick, assessment of renal function (eg, BUN, serum creatinine), liver function (eg, LDH, direct and indirect bilirubin), and DIC-specific tests, such as D-dimer or fibrin/fibrinogen degradation products or fibrin split products.

Because of the potentially increased risk of thrombosis, consider baseline assessment of blood viscosity in patients at risk for hyperviscosity, including those with cryoglobulins, fasting chylomicronemia/markedly high triacylglycerols (triglycerides), or monoclonal gammopathies.

Drug Interactions

Immune Globulin Drug Interactions

Precipitant drug	Object drug[a]		Description
IGIV, IGIM, immune globulin subcutaneous	Hydantoins (eg, phenytoin)	⬆	The risk of hydantoin-induced hypersensitivity myocarditis may be increased. Use with caution. Monitor hematologic findings and cardiac function if these agents are coadministered.
RIG, RSV-IGIV, IGIV, immune globulin subcutaneous Rh_o(D)	Virus vaccines, live (measles/mumps/rubella vaccine)	⬇	Antibodies present in immune globulin preparations may interfere with the immune response to live virus vaccines, such as mumps, rubella and particularly, measles. As a general rule, administer live virus vaccines 14 to 30 days before or 6 to 12 weeks after immune globulin administration. Administer live virus vaccines during this interval if corresponding antibody titers are measured 3 months after **RIG** administration. For varicella vaccine, wait 5 months. For a vaccine containing the measles virus, wait 4 months. If live vaccines are given during or within 10 months after **RSV-IGIV** infusion, reimmunization is recommended, if appropriate. Do not administer within 3 months of immune globulin administration (Rh_o[D], HBIG, CMV-IGIV, IG, RIG) because antibodies in the globulin preparation may interfere with the immune response to the live virus vaccinations (eg, measles, mumps, polio, or rubella). It may be necessary to revaccinate people who received immune globulin shortly after live virus vaccination. Use of live vaccines should be deferred for ≈ 6 months after (IGIV) administration.
Rh_o(D), HBIG, CMV-IGIV, IG	Inactivated vaccines (DPT, Hib, OPV)	⬇	Responses to non-live childhood vaccines (eg, DPT) do not appear to be substantially influenced by administration of IGIVs. Limited information available from infants who receive **RSV-IGIV** concurrently with one or more doses of their primary immunization series indicates that antibody responses to diphtheria, tetanus, pertussis and *Haemophilus influenzae* b may be lower in RSV-IGIV recipients than in controls. It is not known whether antibody responses to trivalent oral polio vaccine might be affected. Consider giving a booster dose of these vaccines 3 to 4 months after the last dose of RSV-IGIV in order to ensure immunity to DPT, DTaP, Hib and OPV (oral polio virus).
RIG	Rabies vaccine	⬇	Simultaneous administration may slightly delay the antibody response to rabies vaccine; follow Centers for Disease Control and Prevention recommendations exactly and give no more than the recommended dose of **RIG**.
ATG rabbit	Immunosuppressants	⬆	Because **antithymocyte globulin (rabbit)** is administered to patients receiving a standard immunosuppressive regimen, this may predispose patients to over-immunosuppression. Many transplant centers decrease maintenance immunosuppression therapy during the period of antibody therapy. **Antithymocyte globulin (rabbit)** can stimulate the production of antibodies that cross-react with rabbit immune globulins.
ATG equine	Immunosuppressants	⬇	When dose of corticosteroids and other immunosuppressants is being reduced, some previously masked reactions to antithymocyte globulin (equine) may appear. Observe patient carefully.

[a] ⬇ = object drug decreased; ⬆ = object drug increased.

➤*Drug/Lab test interactions:* After injection of immune globulins, the transitory rise of the various passively transferred antibodies in the patient's blood may yield positive serological testing results, with the potential for misleading interpretation. Passive transmission of antibodies to erythrocyte antigens (eg, A, B, D) may cause a positive direct or indirect antiglobulin (Coombs) test.

Rh_o(D) IGIM – Babies born of women given Rh_o(D) IGIM antepartum may have a weakly positive direct antiglobulin test at birth.

Passively acquired anti-Rh_o(D) may be detected in maternal serum if antibody screening tests are performed subsequent to antepartum or postpartum administration of Rh_o(D) IGIM. This does not preclude further antepartum or postpartum prophylaxis.

Late in pregnancy or following delivery, there may be sufficient fetal RBCs in the maternal circulation to cause a positive antiglobulin test for weak $D(D^u)$. When there is any doubt as to the patient's Rh type, administer Rh_o(D) IGIM.

Elevated bilirubin levels have been reported in some individuals receiving multiple doses of Rh_o(D) IGIM following mismatched transfusions. This is believed to be caused by a relatively rapid rate of foreign red cell destruction. About 25% of a group of 22 individuals who were given multiple doses of Rh_o(D) IGIM to treat mismatched transfusions noted fever, myalgia, and lethargy, and 1 had splenomegaly.

Rh_o(D) IGIV – The presence of passively administered anti-Rh_o(D) antibodies in maternal or fetal blood can lead to a positive direct antiglobulin (Coombs) test. If there is an uncertainty about the mother's Rh group or immune status, administer Rh_o(D) immune globulin to the mother.

In addition to anti-D, Rh_o(D) IGIV contains trace amounts of anti-A, anti-B, anti-C, and anti-E antibodies. Passively acquired anti-A, anti-B, anti-C, and anti-E blood group antibodies may be detectable in direct and indirect antiglobulin (Coombs) tests obtained following Rh_o(D) IGIV administration. Interpretation of direct and indirect antiglobulin tests must be made in the context of the patients' underlying clinical condition and supporting laboratory data.

ATG rabbit – ATG rabbit has not been shown to interfere with any routine clinical laboratory tests that do not use immunoglobulins. ATG rabbit may interfere with rabbit antibody-based immunoassays and with cross-match or panel-reactive antibody cytotoxicity assays.

Adverse Reactions

There is a remote chance of an idiosyncratic or anaphylactic reaction in individuals with hypersensitivity to blood products.

➤*Local:* Tenderness, pain, muscle stiffness at injection site, urticaria, angioedema, ache, erythema, burning; may persist for several hours.

➤*Systemic:* Urticaria; angioedema; malaise, nausea, diarrhea. The most common adverse events were headache, chills, and fever. Less frequently reported reactions include the following: emesis; chills; fever; fatigue; lightheadedness; abdominal cramping; retching; myalgia; lethargy; chest tightness; nausea. Isolated cases of angioneurotic edema and nephrotic syndrome have occurred.

Systemic reactions associated with administration are extremely rare. Discomfort at the site of injection has been reported and a small number of women have noted a slight elevation in temperature. While sensitization to repeated injections is extremely rare, it has occurred.

Potential reactions for all immune globulin IV products are often related to infusion rate and may include the following: nausea, vomiting, abdominal cramps, chills, pyrexia, chest tightness, palpitations, tachycardia, blood pressure changes, edema, flushing, diaphoresis, rash, erythema, pruritus, cyanosis, dizziness, headache, backache, or other body aches, anxiety, wheezing (and other respiratory events), myalgia, shaking, fatigue, malaise, and arthralgia, usually beginning within 1 hour of the start of the infusion. Other reactions include feeling of faintness; chest tightness; shortness of breath; dyspnea; chills; headache; mild hemolysis; hypertension; pallor; irritability; pain (chest, hip, back, neck, legs); urticaria (hives); rash (rare).

➤*CMV-IGIV:* Minor reactions such as flushing, chills, muscle cramps, back pain, fever, nausea, vomiting, arthralgia, and wheezing were the most frequent adverse reactions observed during the clinical trials of CMV-IGIV. The incidence of these reactions during the clinical trials was less than 6% of all infusions and such reactions were most often related to infusion rates. A decrease in blood pressure was observed in 1 of 1039 infusions in clinical trials. If a patient develops a minor side effect, slow the rate immediately or temporarily interrupt the infusion.

Increases in serum creatinine and BUN have been observed as soon as 1 to 2 days following IGIV infusion. Progression to oliguria or anuria requiring dialysis has been observed. Types of severe renal adverse events that have been seen following IGIV therapy include acute renal failure, acute tubular necrosis, proximal tubular nephropathy, and osmotic nephrosis.

Severe reactions such as angioneurotic edema and anaphylactic shock, although not observed during clinical trials, are a possibility. Clinical anaphylaxis may occur even when the patient is not known to be sensitized to immune globulin products. A reaction may be related to the rate of infusion; therefore, carefully adhere to the infusion rates as outlined under Administration and Dosage. If anaphylaxis or drop in blood pressure occurs, discontinue infusion and use antidote such as diphenhydramine and epinephrine. Refer to the Management of Acute Hypersensitivity Reactions.

➤*IGIV:* Increases in creatinine and BUN have been observed as soon as 1 to 2 days following infusion. Progression to oliguria and anuria requiring dialysis has been observed, although some patients have improved spontaneously following cessation of treatment. Types of severe renal adverse reactions that have been seen following IGIV therapy include the following: acute renal failure, acute tubular necrosis, osmotic nephrosis, and proximal tubular nephropathy.

Gammaplex Adverse Reactions (> 5%)

Adverse reactions	Patients (n = 50)	Infusions (n = 703)
CNS		
Chills	6%	0.7%
Fatigue	6%	1.3%
Headache	36%	7.5%
Insomnia	6%	0.4%
GI		
Nausea	12%	1%
Vomiting	6%	0.4%
Respiratory		
Nasal congestion	6%	0.4%
Sinusitis	16%	1.3%
Upper respiratory tract infection	6%	0.7%
Miscellaneous		
Hypertension	6%	0.6%
Pain	10%	0.7%
Pyrexia	14%	1.4%

➤*Immune globulin subcutaneous:*

Immune Globulin Subcutaneous Adverse Reactions[a]

Adverse reactions	*Hizentra* (n = 49)	*Vivaglobin* (n = 65)
CNS		
Asthenia	–	5%
Fatigue	12.2%	–
Headache	26.5%	48%
Migraine	8.2%	–
Dermatologic		
Contusion	4.1%	–
Rash	10.2%	17%
Skin disorder	–	3%
GI		
Diarrhea	14.3%	10%
GI disorder	–	37%
Nausea	10.2%	18%
Upper abdominal pain	10.2%	–
Vomiting	6.1%	–
Musculoskeletal		
Arthralgia	8.2%	–
Back pain	10.2%	–
Pain in extremity	8.2%	–
Respiratory		
Cough	16.3%	10%
Epistaxis	8.2%	–
Pharyngolaryngeal pain	8.2%	–
Sore throat	–	17%
Miscellaneous		
Allergic reaction	–	11%
Fever	–	25%
Pain	8.2%	10%
Tachycardia	–	3%
Urine abnormality	–	3%

[a] Excluding infections.

Local – Local reactions at the injection site were the most frequent adverse reactions. For *Hizentra*, injection-site reactions, including swelling, redness, heat, pain, and itching at the injection site, comprised 98% of local reactions. Most of the local reactions were mild (93.4%) or moderate (6.3%) in intensity. For *Vivaglobin*, these consisted of mostly mild or moderate swelling, redness, and itching; no serious local site reactions were reported.

➤*Immune globulin intravenous/subcutaneous:*

***Gamunex-C* Adverse Reactions**

Adverse reactions	IV administration	Subcutaneous administration
CNS		
Asthenia	10%	–
Dizziness	6%	–
Fatigue		6.3%
Headache	58%	13%
Dermatologic		
Pruritus	8%	–
Rash	10%	–
Urticaria	5%	–
GI		
Abdominal pain	6%	–
Diarrhea	28%	–
Dyspepsia	6%	–
Nausea	21%	–
Vomiting	21%	–
Hematologic		
Anemia	6%	–
Ecchymosis, purpura	40%	–
Hemorrhage	29%	–
Petechiae	21%	–
Thrombocytopenia	15%	–

Gamunex-C Adverse Reactions		
Adverse reactions	IV administration	Subcutaneous administration
Lab test abnormalities		
Elevated ALT	18%	–
Elevated alkaline phosphatase	13%	–
Elevated AST	9%	–
Musculoskeletal		
Arthralgia	7%	6.3%
Back pain	8%	–
Neck pain	6%	–
Respiratory		
Asthma	29%	–
Cough increased	54%	–
Epistaxis	23%	–
Pharyngitis	41%	–
Rhinitis	51%	–
Miscellaneous		
Accidental injury	13%	–
Chills	8%	–
Ear pain	18%	–
Fever	28%	6.3%
Flu syndrome	6%	–
Hypertension	9%	–
Injection site reaction	5%	75%

➤*ATG equine:*

Renal transplantation – Fever (33%); chills, leukopenia (14%); dermatological reactions (eg, rash, pruritus, urticaria, wheal, flare) (13%); thrombocytopenia (11%); arthralgia, chest/back pain, clotted atrioventricular fistula, diarrhea, dyspnea, headache, hypotension, nausea, vomiting, night sweats, pain at the infusion site, peripheral thrombophlebitis, stomatitis (1% to 5%); anaphylaxis, dizziness, weakness, faintness, edema, herpes simplex reactivation, hiccoughs, epigastric pain, hyperglycemia, hypertension, iliac vein obstruction, laryngospasm, localized infection, lymphadenopathy, malaise, myalgia, paresthesia, possible serum sickness, pulmonary edema, renal artery thrombosis, seizures, systemic infection, tachycardia, toxic epidermal necrosis, wound dehiscence (less than 1%).

Aplastic anemia – Chills, arthralgia (50%); headache (17%); myalgia (10%); nausea, chest pain (7%); phlebitis (5%); diaphoresis, joint stiffness, periorbital edema, aches, edema, muscle ache, vomiting, agitation/lethargy, listlessness, lightheadedness, seizures, diarrhea, bradycardia, myocarditis, cardiac irregularity, hepatosplenomegaly, encephalitis or postviral encephalopathy, hypotension, congestive heart failure (CHF), hypertension, burning soles/palms, foot sole pain, lymphadenopathy, postcervical lymphadenopathy, tender lymph nodes, bilateral pleural effusion, respiratory distress, anaphylaxis, proteinuria (less than 5%); abnormal tests of liver function (eg, AST, ALT, alkaline phosphatase) and renal function (eg, serum creatinine). In some trials, clinical and laboratory findings of serum sickness were seen in a majority of patients.

Postmarketing experience – Fever (51%); thrombocytopenia (30%); rashes (27%); chills (16%); leukopenia (14%); systemic infection (13%); abnormal renal function tests, serum sickness-like symptoms, dyspnea or apnea, arthralgia, chest/back/flank pain, diarrhea, nausea, vomiting (5% to 10%); hypertension, herpes simplex infection, pain, swelling or redness at the infusion site, eosinophilia, headache, myalgia, leg pains, hypotension, anaphylaxis, tachycardia, edema, localized infection, malaise, seizures, GI bleeding/perforation, deep vein thrombosis, sore mouth/throat, hyperglycemia, acute renal failure, abnormal liver function tests, confusion, disorientation, cough, neutropenia, granulocytopenia, anemia, thrombophlebitis, dizziness, epigastric/stomach pain, lymphadenopathy, pulmonary edema, CHF, abdominal pain, nosebleed, vasculitis, aplasia, pancytopenia, abnormal involuntary movement, tremor, rigidity, sweating, laryngospasm, edema, hemolysis/hemolytic anemia, viral hepatitis, faintness, enlarged/ruptured kidney, paresthesias, renal artery thrombosis (less than 5%).

➤*ATG rabbit:* ATG rabbit adverse events are generally manageable or reversible. In the US phase 3 controlled clinical trial (n = 163) comparing the efficacy and safety of ATG rabbit and ATG equine, there were no significant differences in clinically significant adverse events between the 2 treatment groups. Malignancies were reported in 3 patients who received ATG rabbit and in 3 patients who received ATG equine during the 1-year follow-up period. These included 2 PTLDs in the ATG rabbit group and 2 PTLDs in the ATG equine group. Infections occurring in both treatment groups during the 3-month follow-up are summarized in the following table. No significant differences were seen between the ATG rabbit and ATG equine groups for all types of infections, and the incidence of CMV infection was equivalent in both groups. (Viral prophylaxis was by the centers discretion during antibody treatment, but all centers used ganciclovir infusion during treatment.)

Antithymocyte Globulin Adverse Reactions		
Adverse reactions	ATG rabbit (n = 82)	ATG equine (n = 81)
Cardiovascular		
Hypertension	36.6%	28.4%
Tachycardia	26.8%	23.5%
GI		
Abdominal pain	37.8%	27.2%
Diarrhea	36.6%	32.1%
Gastritis	1.2%	0%
GI moniliasis	4.9%	1.2%
Nausea	36.6%	28.4%
Oral moniliasis	3.7%	2.5%
GU		
Urinary tract infection	18.3%	25.9%
Vaginitis	0%	1.2%
Hematologic		
Leukopenia	57.3%	29.6%
Thrombocytopenia	36.6%	44.4%
Respiratory		
Dyspnea	28%	19.8%
Pneumonia	0%	1.2%
Miscellaneous		
Asthenia	26.8%	32.1%
Chills	57.3%	43.2%
Dizziness	8.5%	24.7%
Fever	63.4%	63%
Headache	40.2%	34.6%
Herpes simplex	4.9%	0%
Hyperkalemia	26.8%	18.5%
Infection	30.5%	23.5%
Infection (CMV)	13.4%	11.1%
Infection (not specified)	0%	2.5%
Infection (other)	17.1%	13.6%
Malaise	13.4%	3.7%
Moniliasis	0%	1.2%
Pain	46.3%	43.2%
Peripheral edema	34.1%	34.6%
Sepsis	12.2%	9.6%

➤*Rh_o(D) IGIV:* The most serious adverse reactions in patients receiving Rh_o(D) immune globulin have been observed in the treatment of ITP. These include intravascular hemolysis (manifested by an increase in bilirubin and a decrease in Hb), clinically compromising anemia, acute renal function impairment, DIC, and death.

The most common adverse reactions observed for all indications are abdominal or back pain, arthralgia, asthenia, chills, diarrhea, dizziness, fever, headache, hyperkinesia, hypertension, hypotension, increased LDH, injection-site pain, malaise, myalgia, nausea, pallor, pruritus, rash, somnolence, sweating, vasodilation, and vomiting.

Rh_o(D) IGIV is administered to Rh_o(D) positive patients with ITP. Adverse reactions related to the destruction of Rh_o(D)-positive red cells, such as decreased hemoglobin, can be expected. At the recommended initial IV dose of 250 units/kg, the mean maximum decrease in hemoglobin was 1.7 g/dL (range, +0.4 to -6.1 g/dL). At a reduced dose, ranging from 125 to 200 units/kg, the mean maximum decrease in hemoglobin was 0.81 g/dL (range, +0.65 to -1.9 g/dL). Only 5 of the 137 (3.7%) patients had a maximum decrease in hemoglobin of greater than 4 g/dL (range, 4.2 to 6.1 g/dL).

In most cases, the RBC destruction is believed to occur in the spleen. However, signs and symptoms consistent with IVH, including back pain, shaking chills, or hemoglobinuria have been reported, occurring within 4 hours of Rh_o(D) IGIV administration.

IVH-related complications that have been reported include death (4 cases reported between May 1996 and April 1999), acute onset or exacerbation of anemia, and acute onset or exacerbation of renal insufficiency. One patient died from complications secondary to IVH-induced exacerbation of anemia after administration of Rh_o(D) IGIV for treatment of ITP. Although the primary cause of death in the other 3 ITP patients treated with Rh_o(D) IGIV was related to underlying disease, the extent to which IVH-related clinical complications exacerbated their conditions and contributed to their deaths is unknown.

The following table shows the most common treatment-emergent adverse reactions observed in the clinical study with *Rhophylac*.

Rhophylac Adverse Reactions in Patients With Immune Thrombocytopenic Purpura		
Adverse reactions	Subjects with a treatment-emergent adverse reaction (n = 98)	Subjects with a drug-related, treatment-emergent adverse reaction[a] (n = 98)
CNS		
Headache	14.3%	11.2%
Miscellaneous		
Chills	34.7%	34.7%
Increased blood bilirubin	21.4%	21.4%
Pyrexia/Increased body temperature	32.6%	30.6%

[a] Defined as treatment-emergent adverse reactions with a possible, probable, definite, or unknown relationship to the study drug.

In addition to the adverse reactions described previously, the following have been reported infrequently in clinical trials or postmarketing experience in patients treated for ITP or Rh isoimmunization suppression and are thought to be temporally associated with Rh_o(D) IGIV use: abdominal or back pain, ARDS, arthralgia, asthenia, cardiac arrest, cardiac failure, diarrhea, dizziness, hyperkinesia, hypotension, increased LDH, jaundice, myocardial infarction, myalgia, pallor, pruritus, rash, somnolence, sweating, tachycardia, and vasodilation.

➤*RSV-IGIV:* RSV-IGIV is generally well tolerated. In the PREVENT trial of RSV-IGIV in children with BPD or prematurity, there was no difference in the proportion of children in the RSV-IGIV and placebo groups who reported adverse reactions.

RSV-IGIV Adverse Reactions		
Adverse reactions	RSV-IGIV (n = 250)	Placebo (n = 260)
Diarrhea	1%	< 1%
Fever/Pyrexia	6%	2%
Fluid overload	1%	0%
Gastroenteritis	1%	< 1%
Hypertension	1%	0%
Hypoxia/Hypoxemia	1%	1%
Injection-site inflammation	1%	1%
Overdose effect	1%	< 1%
Rales	1%	0%
Rash	1%	2%
Respiratory distress	2%	< 1%
Tachycardia/Increased pulse rate	1%	0%
Tachypnea	1%	< 1%
Vomiting/Emesis	2%	1%
Wheezing	2%	2%

Infrequent adverse reactions included: Edema, pallor, hypotension, heart murmur, gagging, cyanosis, sleepiness, cough, rhinorrhea, eczema, cold and clammy skin, conjunctival hemorrhage (less than 1%).

Reactions similar to those reported with other IGIVs may occur with RSV-IGIV. These include: Dizziness; flushing; blood pressure changes; anxiety; palpitations; chest tightness; dyspnea; abdominal cramps; pruritus; myalgia; arthralgia. Such reactions are often related to the rate of infusion. Immediate allergic, anaphylactic, or hypersensitivity reactions may be observed (see Warnings). Rarely, AMS has been reported in association with IGIV treatment, particularly at high dosage (2 g/kg; see Warnings/Precautions).

In the PREVENT trial, 3 children developed aseptic meningitis of unknown etiology. In the single-blind, controlled NIAID trial in children with BPD, CHD or prematurity, adverse reactions were reported in 3% of all RSV-IGIV infusions. Five of 160 children were considered to have had mild fluid overload associated with infusion. The remaining adverse reactions consisted of mild decreases in oxygen saturation (n = 8) and fever (n = 5). In the open-label study in children with BPD or prematurity (n = 6), infusion-associated adverse reactions were noted in 14 of 294 (4.8%) infusions. Six adverse events were considered related to infusion, including 4 mild and 2 moderate events. In the CARDIAC study, children with CHD with right to left shunts appeared to have an increased frequency of cardiac surgery and had a greater frequency of severe and life-threatening adverse events associated with cardiac surgery (see Warnings).

Overdosage

Although few data are available, clinical experience with other immune globulin preparations suggests that the major manifestations would be those related to fluid volume overload. Other reactions would include pain and tenderness at the injection site.

➤*ATG equine:* Because of its mode of action and because it is a biologic substance, the maximal tolerated dose of ATG equine solution would be expected to vary from patient to patient. To date, the largest single daily dose administered to a patient, a renal transplant recipient, was 7000 mg administered at a concentration of approximately 10 mg/mL sodium chloride injection, USP, approximately 7 times the recommended total dose and infusion concentration. In this patient, administration of ATG equine was not associated with any signs of acute intoxication.

The greatest number of doses (10 to 20 mg/kg/dose) that can be administered to a single patient has not yet been determined. Some renal transplant patients have received up to 50 doses in 4 months, and others have received 28-day courses of 21 doses followed by as many as 3 more courses for the treatment of acute rejection. The incidence of toxicologic manifestations did not increase with any of these regimens.

➤*ATG rabbit:* ATG rabbit overdosage may result in leukopenia or thrombocytopenia, which can be managed with dose reduction (see Administration and Dosage).

➤*Rh_o(D) IGIV:* There are no reports of known overdoses in patients being treated for Rh isoimmunization or ITP. In clinical studies with nonpregnant Rh_o(D) positive patients with ITP (n = 141) treated with 600 to 32,500 units (120 to 6500 mcg) of Rh_o(D) IGIV, there were no signs or symptoms that warranted medical intervention. However, these same doses were associated with a mild, transient hemolytic anemia.

Patient Information

Instruct patients to report symptoms of decreased urine output, sudden weight gain, fluid retention/edema, and/or shortness of breath (which may suggest kidney damage) immediately to their health care provider.

Instruct patients, parents, or guardians to report any serious adverse reaction to their health care provider.

Patients, parents, or guardians should be fully informed by their health care provider of the benefits and risks of these products.

Inform patients that administration of immunoglobulin may temporarily impair the efficacy of live virus vaccines (eg, measles, mumps, rubella, varicella) and instruct them to notify their immunizing health care provider of recent therapy with Rh_o(D) immune globulin.

Instruct patients being treated for ITP to immediately report symptoms of intravascular hemolysis, including back pain, decreased urine output, discolored urine, edema, fever, shaking, chills, shortness of breath, and/or sudden weight gain.

CYTOMEGALOVIRUS IMMUNE GLOBULIN INTRAVENOUS, HUMAN (CMV-IGIV)

Rx	**CytoGam** (CSL Behring)	**Solution for injection:**[a] 50 ± 10 mg/mL	In 20 and 50 mL vials.

[a] Preservative free. 5% sucrose, 1% Albumin (human). Solvent/Detergent treated.

CYTOMEGALOVIRUS IMMUNE GLOBULIN INTRAVENOUS (HUMAN) — INJECTION

For complete and comparative prescribing information, refer to the Immune Globulins group monograph.

Indications

➤*Cytomegalovirus prophylaxis:* For the prophylaxis of cytomegalovirus disease associated with transplantation of kidney, lung, liver, pancreas, and heart. In transplants of these organs other than kidney from CMV seropositive donors into seronegative recipients, prophylactic CMV-IGIV should be considered in combination with ganciclovir.

➤*Off-label uses:* For prevention or attenuation of primary CMV disease in immunosuppressed recipients of organ transplants (eg, bone marrow, liver). Also used in immunocompromised patients with CMV pneumonia or to prevent CMV disease.

Administration and Dosage

➤*Adults:*

Cytomegalovirus prophylaxis –

Usual dosage:

Cytomegalovirus Infusion Schedule		
	Type of transplant	
Administer within:	Kidney	Liver, pancreas, lung, heart
72 hours of transplant	150 mg/kg	150 mg/kg
2 weeks posttransplant	100 mg/kg	150 mg/kg
4 weeks posttransplant	100 mg/kg	150 mg/kg
6 weeks posttransplant	100 mg/kg	150 mg/kg

CYTOMEGALOVIRUS IMMUNE GLOBULIN INTRAVENOUS (HUMAN) — INJECTION

Cytomegalovirus Infusion Schedule		
Administer within:	Type of transplant	
	Kidney	Liver, pancreas, lung, heart
8 weeks posttransplant	100 mg/kg	150 mg/kg
12 weeks posttransplant	50 mg/kg	100 mg/kg
16 weeks posttransplant	50 mg/kg	100 mg/kg

Maximum dose: The maximum recommended total dosage per infusion is 150 mg/kg.

➤*Renal function impairment:* Use with caution in patients with preexisting renal insufficiency and those judged to be at increased risk of developing renal insufficiency (including, but not limited to, those with diabetes mellitus, older than 65 years of age, volume depletion, paraproteinemia, sepsis, and patients receiving known nephrotoxic drugs). In these cases especially, it is important to assure that patients are not volume depleted prior to cytomegalovirus immune globulin IV (CMV-IgIV) (human) infusion.

In the absence of prospective data, recommended doses should not be exceeded and the concentration and infusion rate selected should be the minimum practicable.

➤*Preparation for administration:* Do not shake vial; avoid foaming. Predilution of CMV-IgIV (human) before infusion is not recommended.

➤*Administration:* Administer through an IV line using an administration set that contains an in-line filter (pore size 15 microns) and a constant infusion pump (ie, IVAC pump or equivalent). A smaller in-line filter (0.2 microns) is also acceptable.

CMV-IgIV (human) should be administered through a separate IV line. If this is not possible, CMV-IgIV (human) may be piggybacked into a preexisting line if that line contains sodium chloride injection USP, or 1 of the following dextrose solutions (with or without sodium chloride added): 2.5% dextrose in water, 5% dextrose in water, 10% dextrose in water, or 20% dextrose in water. If a preexisting line must be used, the CMV-IgIV (human) should not be diluted by a ratio of more than 1:2 with any of the previously named solutions.

Infusion should begin within 6 hours after entering the vial and should be complete within 12 hours.

Vital signs should be taken preinfusion, midway, and postinfusion, as well as before any rate increase.

Initial dose – Administer IV at 15 mg/kg/h. If no adverse reactions occur after 30 minutes, the rate may be increased to 30 mg/kg/h; if no adverse reactions occur after a subsequent 30 minutes, then the infusion may be increased to 60 mg/kg/h (volume not to exceed 75 mL/h). Do not exceed this rate of administration. The patient should be monitored closely during and after each rate change.

Subsequent doses – Administer at 15 mg/kg/h for 15 minutes. If no adverse reactions occur, increase to 30 mg/kg/h for 15 minutes and then increase to a maximum rate of 60 mg/kg/h (volume not to exceed 75 mL/h). Do not exceed this rate of administration. The patient should be monitored closely during each rate change.

Infusion reactions – Potential adverse reactions are flushing, chills, muscle cramps, back pain, fever, nausea, vomiting, wheezing, and drop in blood pressure. Minor adverse reactions have been infusion rate–related; if the patient develops a minor side effect (ie, nausea, back pain, flushing), slow the rate or temporarily interrupt the infusion. If anaphylaxis or a drop in blood pressure occurs, discontinue the infusion and use an antidote, such as diphenhydramine and adrenalin.

➤*Admixture compatibility:* CMV-IgIV (human) may be piggybacked into a preexisting line if that line contains sodium chloride injection USP, or 1 of the following dextrose solutions (with or without sodium chloride added): 2.5% dextrose in water, 5% dextrose in water, 10% dextrose in water, or 20% dextrose in water. Admixtures of CMV-IgIV (human) with any other solutions have not been evaluated.

➤*Storage/Stability:* Store between 2°C and 8°C (35.6°F and 46.4°F), and used within 6 hours after entering the vial.

HEPATITIS B IMMUNE GLOBULIN (HUMAN) (HBIG)

Rx	**HyperHEP B S/D** (Talecris Biotherapeutics)	**Injection, solution**[a]: 15% to 18% protein	In 1 and 5 mL single-dose vials, 1 mL single-dose syringe, and 0.5 mL neonatal single-dose syringe.
Rx	**Nabi-HB** (Nabi Biopharmaceuticals)	**Injection, solution**[b]: 5% ± 1% protein	In 1 and 5 mL single-dose vials.
Rx	**HepaGam B** (Cangene Biopharma)	**Injection, solution**[c]: 5% (50 mg/mL) protein	In 1 and 5 mL single-dose vials.

[a] Preservative free. With 0.21 to 0.32 M glycine. Solvent/Detergent treated.
[b] Preservative free. With 0.15 M glycine, 0.01% polysorbate 80. Solvent/Detergent treated.
[c] Preservative free. With 10% maltose, 0.03% polysorbate 80. Solvent/Detergent treated.

HEPATITIS B IMMUNE GLOBULIN (HUMAN) — INJECTION

For complete and comparative prescribing information, refer to the Immune Globulins group monograph.

Indications

➤*Postexposure hepatitis B prophylaxis:*

Acute exposure to blood containing hepatitis B surface antigen (HBsAg) – After parenteral exposure (eg, needlestick, bite, sharps), direct mucous membrane contact (accidental splash), or oral ingestion (pipetting accident) involving HBsAg-positive materials such as blood, plasma, or serum.

HyperHEP B: For inadvertent percutaneous exposure, a regimen of 2 doses of hepatitis B immune globulin (HBIG) (human), 1 given after exposure and 1 a month later, is about 75% effective in preventing hepatitis B in this setting.

Household exposure to persons with acute HBV infection – For infants younger than 12 months of age whose mother or primary caregiver is positive for HBsAg and for other household contacts with an identifiable blood exposure to the index patient.

HyperHEP B: Because infants have close contact with primary caregivers and they have a higher risk of becoming HBV carriers after acute HBV infection, prophylaxis of an infant younger than 12 months of age with HBIG (human) and hepatitis B vaccine is indicated if the mother or primary caregiver has acute HBV infection.

Perinatal exposure of infants born to HBsAg-positive mothers – For infants born to mothers positive for HBsAg with or without hepatitis B e antigen (HBeAg).

Infant risk: Infants born to HBsAg-positive mothers are at risk of being infected with hepatitis B virus (HBV) and becoming chronic carriers. This risk is especially great if the mother is HBeAg-positive. Studies conducted with HBIGs similar to HBIG (human) indicated that for an infant with perinatal exposure to an HBsAg-positive or an HBeAg-positive mother, a regimen combining 1 dose of HBIG (human) at birth, with the hepatitis B vaccine series started soon after birth, is 85% to 95% effective in preventing development of the HBV carrier state. Regimens involving either multiple doses of HBIG (human) alone or the vaccine series alone have 70% to 90% efficacy, while a single dose of HBIG (human) alone has only 50% efficacy.

Sexual exposure to an HBsAg-positive person – Sex partners of HBsAg-positive persons are at increased risk of acquiring HBV infection. For sexual exposure to a person with acute hepatitis B, a single dose of HBIG (human) is 75% effective if administered within 2 weeks of last sexual exposure.

➤*Prevention of hepatitis B recurrence following liver transplantation (HepaGam B only):* For the prevention of hepatitis B recurrence following liver transplantation in HBsAg-positive liver transplant patients. *HepaGam B* should be administered intravenously (IV) for this indication.

Administration and Dosage

➤*General dosing considerations:* For greatest efficacy, passive prophylaxis with hepatitis B immune globulin (human) should be given as soon as possible after exposure and within 24 hours, if possible (its value beyond 7 days of exposure is unclear).

➤*Adults:*

Acute exposure to blood containing HBsAg –

Usual dosage:

Recommendations for Hepatitis B Prophylaxis Following Percutaneous or Permucosal Exposure		
Source	Exposed person	
	Unvaccinated	Vaccinated
HBsAg-positive	1. Hepatitis B immune globulin (human) × 1 immediately[a]	1. Test exposed person for anti-HBsAg[b]
	2. Initiate hepatitis B vaccine series[c]	2. If inadequate antibody,[d] give HBIG (human) × 1 immediately plus × 1 hepatitis B vaccine booster dose, or a second dose of HBIG (human)[a] 1 month later[e]

HEPATITIS B IMMUNE GLOBULIN (HUMAN) — INJECTION

Recommendations for Hepatitis B Prophylaxis Following Percutaneous or Permucosal Exposure		
	Exposed person	
Source	Unvaccinated	Vaccinated
Known-source – high risk for HBsAg-positive	1. Initiate hepatitis B vaccine series	1. Test source for HBsAg only if exposed person is vaccine nonresponder. If source is HBsAg-positive, give HBIG (human) × 1 immediately plus × 1 hepatitis B vaccine booster dose, or a second dose of HBIG (human)[a] 1 month later[e]
		2. Test source for HBsAg. If positive, hepatitis B immune globulin (human) × 1[a]
Known-source – low risk for HBsAg-positive	Initiate hepatitis B vaccine series	Nothing required
Unknown source	Initiate hepatitis B vaccine series	Nothing required

[a] HBIG (human) dose of 0.06 mL/kg intramuscularly (IM).
[b] Anti-HBsAg = antibody to hepatitis B surface antigen.
[c] See manufacturer's recommendation for appropriate dose (*HepaGam B, Nabi-HB*). Hepatitis B vaccine dose is 20 mcg IM for adults; 10 mcg IM for infants or children younger than 10 years of age. Give the first dose within 1 week; give the second and third doses, 1 and 6 months later (*HyperHep B*).
[d] Less than 10 milliunits/mL of anti-HBsAg by radioimmunoassay, negative by enzyme immunoassay.
[e] Two doses of hepatitis immune globulin IV (human) is preferred if no response is noted after at least 4 doses of vaccine.

Repeat dose: For persons who refuse hepatitis B vaccine or are known nonresponders to vaccine, a second dose of hepatitis B immune globulin (human) should be given 1 month after the first dose.

Household exposure to persons with acute HBV infection –

Single dose: 0.06 mL/kg IM within 14 days if they have had identifiable blood exposure to the index patient, such as by sharing toothbrushes or razors. If the index patient becomes an HBV carrier, all household contacts should receive hepatitis B vaccine.

Concomitant therapy: Administer with hepatitis B vaccine. Hepatitis B immune globulin (human) may be administered at the same time (but at a different site), or up to 1 month preceding hepatitis B vaccination without impairing the active immune response from hepatitis B vaccination.

Sexual exposure to an HBsAg-positive person –

Recommendations for Postexposure Prophylaxis for Sexual Exposure to Hepatitis B			
HBIG (human)		Vaccine	
Dose	Recommended timing	Dose	Recommended timing
0.06 mL/kg IM	Single dose within 14 days of last sexual contact	1 mL IM	First dose at time of HBIG (human) treatment[a]

[a] The first dose can be administered at the same time as the HBIG (human) dose but at a different site; subsequent doses should be administered as recommended for specific vaccine.

HBsAg-positive liver transplant patients (HepaGam B only) –

Usual dosage: 20,000 units/dose IV.

HepaGam B Dosing Regimen[a]			
Anhepatic phase	Week 1 postoperative	Weeks 2 through 12 postoperative	Month 4 onward
First dose	Daily from day 1 through 7	Every 2 weeks from day 14	Monthly

[a] Each dose should contain 20,000 units calculated from the measured potency as stamped on the vial label.

Dosage adjustment: May be required in patients who fail to reach anti-HBsAg levels of 500 units/L within the first week after liver transplantation. Patients who have surgical bleeding or abdominal fluid drainage (greater than 500 mL) or patients who undergo plasmapheresis are particularly susceptible to extensive loss of circulated anti-HBsAg. In these cases, the dosing regimen should be increased to a half-dose (10,000 units calculated from the measured potency as stamped on the vial label) IV every 6 hours until the target anti-HBsAg is reached.

➤*Children:*

Household exposure to persons with acute HBV infection –

12 months and older:

• *Single dose* – 0.06 mL/kg IM within 14 days if they have had identifiable blood exposure to the index patient, such as by sharing toothbrushes or razors. If the index patient becomes an HBV carrier, all household contacts should receive hepatitis B vaccine.

• *Concomitant therapy* – Administer with hepatitis B vaccine. Hepatitis B immune globulin (human) may be administered at the same time (but at a different site), or up to 1 month preceding hepatitis B vaccination without impairing the active immune response from hepatitis B vaccination.

11 months and younger:

• *Usual dosage* – 0.5 mL IM.

• *Concomitant therapy* – Administer with hepatitis B vaccine. Hepatitis B immune globulin (human) may be administered at the same time (but at a different site), or up to 1 month preceding hepatitis B vaccination without impairing the active immune response from hepatitis B vaccination.

Prophylaxis of infants born to HBsAg-positive mothers –

HyperHep B:

• *Usual dosage* – 0.5 mL IM after physiologic stabilization of the infant and preferably within 12 hours of birth. Hepatitis B immune globulin (human) efficacy decreases markedly if treatment is delayed beyond 48 hours.

• *Concomitant therapy* – Hepatitis B vaccine should be administered IM in 3 doses of 0.5 mL of vaccine (10 mcg) each. The first dose should be given within 7 days of birth and may be given concurrently with hepatitis B immune globulin (human) but at a separate site. The second and third doses of vaccine should be given 1 and 6 months, respectively, after the first. If administration of the first dose of hepatitis B vaccine is delayed for as long as 3 months, then a 0.5 mL dose of hepatitis B immune globulin (human) should be repeated at 3 months. If hepatitis B vaccine is refused, the 0.5 mL dose of hepatitis B immune globulin (human) should be repeated at 3 and 6 months.

HepaGam B, *Nabi-HB*:

• *Usual dosage* – 0.5 mL after physiologic stabilization of the infant and preferably within 12 hours of birth.

• *Concomitant therapy* – The hepatitis B vaccine series should be initiated simultaneously, if it is not contraindicated, with the first dose of the vaccine given concurrently with the hepatitis B immune globulin (human), but at a different site.

➤*Preparation for administration:*

HepaGam B –

HepaGam B should be administered through a separate IV line using an IV administration set via infusion pump. During preparation, do not shake vials; avoid foaming.

HyperHEP B

Remove the prefilled syringe from the package. Lift syringe by barrel, not by plunger. Twist the plunger rod clockwise until the threads are seated. With the rubber needle shield secured on the syringe tip, push the plunger rod forward a few millimeters to break any friction seal between the rubber stopper and the glass syringe barrel. Remove the needle shield and expel air bubbles. Do not remove the rubber needle shield to prepare the product for administration until immediately prior to the anticipated injection time. Proceed with hypodermic needle puncture. Aspirate prior to injection to confirm that the needle is not in a vein or artery.

➤*Administration:*

HepaGam B – Administer IM for postexposure prophylactic indications, but use IV for prevention of hepatitis B recurrence following liver transplantation. The rate of administration should be set at 2 mL/min. The rate of infusion should be decreased to 1 mL/min or slower if the patient develops discomfort or infusion-related adverse events, or if there is concern about the speed of infusion.

HyperHEP B – Inject the medication IM only. Keeping your hands behind the needle, grasp the guard with free hand and slide forward toward needle until it is completely covered and guard clicks into place. If an audible click is not heard, the guard may not be completely activated. Place entire prefilled glass syringe with guard activated into an approved sharps container for proper disposal.

Nabi-HB – For IM use only.

➤*Storage/Stability:* Store between 2° and 8°C (36° and 46°F). Do not freeze. Use *HepaGam B* and *Nabi-HB* within 6 hours after the vial has been entered. Partially used vials should be discarded immediately.

IMMUNE GLOBULIN (HUMAN) INTRAMUSCULAR (IG; IGIM; IMIG; Gamma Globulin; IgG)

Rx	**GamaSTAN S/D** (Talecris Biotherapeutics)	**Injection, solution**[a]: 15% to 18% protein	In 2 and 10 mL single-dose vials and 2 mL single-dose syringes with attached needles.

[a] Preservative and latex free. With glycine 0.21 to 0.32 M. Solvent/detergent treated.

IMMUNE GLOBULIN (HUMAN) — INTRAMUSCULAR

For complete and comparative prescribing information, refer to the Immune Globulins group monograph.

Indications

➤*Hepatitis A:* The prophylactic value of immune globulin intramuscular (IM) is greatest when given before or soon after exposure to hepatitis A. Immune globulin IM is not indicated in individuals with clinical manifestations of hepatitis A or in those who were exposed more than 2 weeks previously.

➤*Immunoglobulin deficiency:* In patients with immunoglobulin deficiencies, immune globulin IM may prevent serious infection. However, it may not prevent chronic infections of the external secretory tissues, such as the respiratory and GI tracts.

Prophylactic therapy, especially against infections caused by encapsulated bacteria, is effective in Bruton-type, sex-linked, congenital agammaglobulinemia, agammaglobulinemia associated with thymoma, and acquired agammaglobulinemia.

➤*Measles (Rubeola):* Prevention or modification of measles in a susceptible person (one who has not been vaccinated and has not had measles previously) exposed fewer than 6 days previously. Immune globulin IM may be especially indicated for susceptible household contacts of measles patients, particularly those contacts younger than 1 year of age, for whom the risk of complications is highest. Do not give immune globulin IM with measles vaccine. If a child older than 12 months of age has received immune globulin IM, give measles vaccine about 3 months later, when the measles antibody titer will have disappeared.

If a susceptible child exposed to measles is immunocompromised, administer immune globulin IM immediately. Do not give children who are immunocompromised the measles vaccine or any other live viral vaccine.

➤*Rubella:* The routine use of immune globulin IM for prophylaxis of rubella in early pregnancy is of dubious value and cannot be justified. Some studies suggest that the use of immune globulin IM in exposed, susceptible women can lessen the likelihood of infection and fetal damage; therefore, immune globulin IM may benefit those women who will not consider a therapeutic abortion.

➤*Varicella:* Passive immunization against varicella in immunosuppressed patients is best accomplished by use of varicella-zoster immune globulin (VZIG). If VZIG is unavailable, immune globulin IM, promptly given, may also modify varicella.

Administration and Dosage

➤*General dosing considerations:* Immune globulin intramuscular (IM) may prevent serious infection in patients with immunoglobulin deficiencies if circulating immunoglobulin G (IgG) levels of approximately 200 mg per 100 mL plasma are maintained.

➤*Adults:*

Hepatitis A prophylaxis – 0.02 mL/kg (0.01 mL/lb) IM for household and institutional hepatitis A case contacts. The following doses are recommended for persons who plan to travel in areas where hepatitis A is common.

Immune Globulin IM Dose for Common Hepatitis A Areas	
Length of stay	Dose
< 3 months	0.02 mL/kg IM
Prolonged (> 3 months)	0.06 mL/kg IM (repeat every 4 to 6 months)

Immunoglobulin deficiency – 0.66 mL/kg (at least 100 mg/kg) IM given every 3 to 4 weeks. A double dose is given at the onset of therapy; some patients may require more frequent injections.

Measles (rubeola) prophylaxis – 0.25 mL/kg (0.11 mL/lb) to prevent or modify measles in a susceptible person exposed fewer than 6 days previously.

Rubella prophylaxis – 0.55 mL/kg IM may benefit those women who will not consider a therapeutic abortion.

Varicella – If VZIG is unavailable, immune globulin IM at a dose of 0.6 to 1.2 mL/kg, promptly given, may also modify varicella.

➤*Children:*

Measles (rubeola) prophylaxis –

Usual dosage: A susceptible child who is exposed to measles and who is immunocompromised should receive an immune globulin IM dose of 0.5 mL/kg (maximum dose, 15 mL) immediately.

Maximum dose: 15 mL dose.

➤*Administration:* Immune globulin IM is administered IM, preferably in the anterolateral aspects of the upper thigh and the deltoid muscle of the upper arm. The gluteal region should not be used routinely as an injection site because of the risk of injury to the sciatic nerve.

Doses greater than 10 mL should be divided and injected into several muscle sites to reduce local pain and discomfort. An individual decision as to which muscle is injected must be made for each patient based on the volume of material to be administered. If the gluteal region is used when very large volumes are to be injected or multiple doses are necessary, the central region must be avoided; only the upper, outer quadrant should be used.

➤*Storage/Stability:* Store between 2° and 8°C (36° and 46°F). Do not freeze.

A number of factors could reduce the efficacy of this product or result in an ill effect following its use. These include improper storage and handling of the product after it leaves the manufacturer, diagnosis, dosage, method of administration, and biological differences in individual patients. Because of these factors, it is important that this product be stored properly and that the directions be followed carefully during use.

IMMUNE GLOBULIN INTRAVENOUS (IGIV; IVIG)

Rx	**Flebogamma 5%** (Grifols)	**Injection**: immune globulin (human) 5% (50 mg/mL)[a]	Preservative free. In 10, 50, 100, and 200 mL vials.
Rx	**Octagam** (Octapharma)	**Injection**: immune globulin (human) 5% (50 mg/mL)[b]	In 1, 2.5, 5, and 10 g single-use bottles.
Rx	**Gammagard S/D** (Baxter Healthcare)	**Injection, freeze-dried powder for solution**: immune globulin (human) 0.5 g[c]	In single-use bottles.
Rx	**Gammagard Liquid** (Baxter)	**Injection**: immune globulin (human) 10%	Preservative free. In 1, 2.5, 5, 10, and 20 g single-use bottles.
Rx	**Gamunex** (Talecris Biotherapeutics)	**Injection, solution**: immune globulin (human) 10% (100 mg/mL)[d]	Preservative free. In 10, 25, 50, 100, and 200 mL single-use vials.
Rx	**Carimune NF** (ZLB Bioplasma)	**Injection, lyophilized powder for solution**: immune globulin (human) 3, 6, 12 g[e]	Preservative free. In 3, 6, and 12 g vials.
Rx	**Privigen** (Aventis Behring)	**Injection, solution**: immune globulin (human) 10% (100 mg/mL)	Preservative free. In 5, 10, and 20 g single-use vials.
Rx	**Gammaplex** (FFF Enterprises Inc)[g]	**Injection, solution**: 5% immune globulin (human)[h]	Sorbitol, glycine, polysorbate 80. Preservative free. In 50, 100, and 200 mL single-use vials.

[a] Sorbitol 50 mg and polyethylene glycol ≤ 6 mg/mL.
[b] Maltose 100 mg.
[c] Contains glycine 22.5 mg/mL, glucose 20 mg/mL, polyethylene glycol (PEG) 2 mg/mL, and polysorbate 80 100 mcg/mL in a 5% solution.
[d] With glycine 0.16 to 0.24 M, and trace fragments of immunoglobulin (Ig) A (approximately 0.046 mg/mL) and immunoglobulin M. Caprylate/chromatography purified.
[e] With 1.67 g of sucrose per gram of protein.
[f] Glucose 50 mg and sodium chloride 3 mg.
[g] FFF Enterprises, Inc., 41093 County Center Drive, Temecula, CA 92591, phone: (800) 843-7477, fax: (800) 418-4333.
[h] Contains approximately 5 g of D-sorbitol, 0.6 g of glycine, 0.2 g of sodium acetate, 0.3 g of sodium chloride, and 5 mg of polysorbate 80 per 100 mL.

IMMUNE GLOBULIN (HUMAN) — SUBCUTANEOUS (IGSC, SCIG)

Rx	**Vivaglobin** (CSL Behring LLC)	**Injection, solution:** 16% protein (160 mg/mL)[a]	Preservative free. In 3, 10, and 20 mL single-use vials.
Rx	**Hizentra** (CSL Behring LLC)	**Injection, solution:** 20% protein (200 mg/mL)[b]	Preservative free. In 5, 10, and 20 mL single-use vials.

[a] With glycine 2.25%, sodium chloride 0.3%.

[b] Contains 210 to 290 mmol/L of L-proline and 10 to 30 mg/L of polysorbate 80.

IMMUNE GLOBULIN (HUMAN) — SUBCUTANEOUS INJECTION

For complete and comparative prescribing information, refer to the Immune Globulins class monograph.

Indications

➤*Primary immune deficiency:* For the treatment of patients with primary immune deficiency.

Administration and Dosage

➤*General dosing considerations:* The dose should be individualized based on the patient's clinical response to therapy and serum immunoglobulin G (IgG) trough levels. As there can be differences in the half-life of IgG among patients with primary immune deficiencies, the dose and dosing interval of immunoglobulin therapy may vary.

Begin treatment with immune globulin subcutaneous 1 week after the patient's last immunoglobulin intravenous (IGIV) infusion. Prior to switching treatment from IGIV to immune globulin subcutaneous, obtain the patient's serum IgG trough level to guide subsequent dose adjustments.

➤*Adults:*

Primary immune deficiency –

Initial dosage: Establish the initial weekly dose of immune globulin subcutaneous by converting the monthly IGIV dose into a weekly equivalent and increasing it using a dose adjustment factor. The goal is to achieve a systemic serum IgG exposure (area under the curve [AUC]) not inferior to that of the previous IGIV treatment.

• *Hizentra* – To calculate the initial weekly dose of *Hizentra*, multiply the previous IGIV dose in grams by the dose adjustment factor of 1.53; then divide this by the number of weeks between doses during the patients IGIV treatment (ie, 3 or 4).

Initial *Hizentra* dose = (1.53 × previous IGIV dose [in grams])/number of weeks between IGIV doses

To convert the *Hizentra* dose (in grams) to milliliters, multiply the calculated dose (in grams) by 5.

• *Vivaglobin* – The initial weekly *Vivaglobin* dose can be calculated by multiplying the previous IGIV dose by 1.37, then dividing this dose into weekly doses based on the patient's previous IGIV treatment interval; for example, if IGIV was administered every 3 weeks, divide by 3.

The recommended weekly dose of *Vivaglobin* is 100 to 200 mg/kg body weight.

Dosage adjustment: Over time, the dose may need to be adjusted to achieve the desired clinical response and serum IgG trough level. To determine if a dose adjustment may be considered, measure the patient's serum IgG trough level 2 to 3 months after switching from IGIV to immune globulin subcutaneous. However, the patient's clinical response should be the primary consideration in dose adjustment.

• *Hizentra* – The target serum IgG trough level on weekly *Hizentra* treatment is projected to be 1.3 ± 0.2 times (ie, between 1.1 and 1.5 times) the last IGIV trough level.

To adjust the dose based on trough levels, calculate the difference (in mg/dL) of the patient's serum IgG trough level from the target IgG trough level (1.3 times the last IGIV trough level). Then find this difference in the following table and the corresponding amount (in mL) by which to increase or decrease the weekly dose based on the patient's body weight.

Adjustment (± mL) of the Weekly *Hizentra* Dose Based on the Difference (± mg/dL) From the Target Serum IgG Trough Level

Difference from the target serum IgG trough level	Body weight												
	10 kg	15 kg	20 kg	30 kg	40 kg	50 kg	60 kg	70 kg	80 kg	90 kg	100 kg	110 kg	120 kg
	Dose adjustment (mL/wk)[a]												
50 mg/dL	0	1	1	1	2	2	3	3	4	4	5	5	6
100 mg/dL	1	1	2	3	4	5	6	7	8	8	9	10	11
150 mg/dL	1	2	3	4	6	7	8	10	11	13	14	15	17
200 mg/dL	2	3	4	6	8	9	11	13	15	17	19	21	23
250 mg/dL	2	4	5	7	9	12	14	16	19	21	23	26	28
300 mg/dL	3	4	6	8	11	14	17	20	23	25	28	31	34
350 mg/dL	3	5	7	10	13	16	20	23	26	30	33	36	39
400 mg/dL	4	6	8	11	15	19	23	26	30	34	38	41	45
450 mg/dL	4	6	8	13	17	21	25	30	34	38	42	46	51
500 mg/dL	5	7	9	14	19	23	28	33	38	42	47	52	56

[a] Dose adjustment in mL is based on the slope of the serum IgG trough level response to *Hizentra* dose increments (5.3 mg/dL per increment of 1 mg/kg per week).

Monitor the patient's clinical response, and repeat the dose adjustment as needed.

• *Vivaglobin* – The minimum serum concentration of IgG necessary for protection against infections has not been established in randomized and controlled clinical trials. However, based on clinical experience, a target serum IgG trough level (ie, prior to the next infusion) of at least 500 mg/dL has been proposed in the literature for IGIV therapy.

Serum IgG levels can be sampled at any time during routine weekly treatment. Subjects on *Vivaglobin* therapy maintained relatively constant IgG levels, rather than the peak and trough pattern observed with monthly IGIV therapy.

Measles exposure – If a patient is at risk of measles exposure (ie, because of an outbreak in the United States or travel to endemic areas outside of the United States), the weekly *Hizentra* dose should be a minimum of 200 mg/kg body weight for 2 consecutive weeks. If a patient has been exposed to measles, ensure this minimum dose is administered as soon as possible after exposure.

Switching from other immune globulin subcutaneous products – Dosage requirements for patients switching to *Hizentra* from another immune globulin subcutaneous product have not been studied. If a patient on *Hizentra* does not maintain an adequate clinical response or a serum IgG trough level equivalent to that of the previous immune globulin subcutaneous treatment, the health care provider may want to adjust the dose. For such patients, the previous table also provides guidance for dose adjustment if their desired immune globulin subcutaneous trough level is known.

➤*Children:*

Hizentra –

12 months of age and older: See Adults for dosing.

Vivaglobin –

2 years of age and older: See Adults for dosing.

• *Dosage adjustment* – Over time, the dose may need to be adjusted to achieve the desired clinical response and serum IgG trough level. To determine if a dose adjustment may be considered, measure the patient's serum IgG trough level 2 to 3 months after switching from IGIV to immune globulin subcutaneous. However, the patient's clinical response should be the primary consideration in dose adjustment.

The minimum serum concentration of IgG necessary for protection against infections has not been established in randomized and controlled clinical trials. However, based on clinical experience, a target serum IgG trough level (ie, prior to the next infusion) of at least 500 mg/dL has been proposed in the literature for IGIV therapy.

Serum IgG levels can be sampled at any time during routine weekly treatment. Subjects on *Vivaglobin* therapy maintained relatively constant IgG levels, rather than the peak and trough pattern observed with monthly IGIV therapy.

➤*Renal function impairment:* For patients judged to be at risk of developing renal dysfunction because of preexisting renal impairment, administer immune globulin subcutaneous at the minimum rate practicable.

➤*Administration:*

Hizentra – *Hizentra* is for subcutaneous infusion only. Do not inject into a blood vessel.

Hizentra is intended for weekly subcutaneous administration using an infusion pump. Infuse *Hizentra* in the abdomen, thigh, upper arm, and/or lateral hip. A dose may be infused into multiple injection sites. However, do not use more than 4 sites simultaneously. Injection sites should be at least 2 inches apart. Change the actual site of injection with each weekly administration. For the first infusion of *Hizentra*, do not exceed a volume of 15 mL per injection site. The volume may be increased to 20 mL per site after the fourth infusion and to a maximum of 25 mL per site as tolerated. For the first infusion of *Hizentra*, the maximum recommended flow rate is 15 mL per hour per site. For subsequent infusions, the flow rate may be increased to a maximum of 25 mL per hour per site as tolerated. However, the maximum flow rate is not to exceed a total of 50 mL per hour for all sites combined at any time.

The number and location of injection sites depends on the volume of the total dose. Infuse immune globulin subcutaneous into a maximum of 4 sites simultaneously; each injection site should be at least 2 inches apart.

Vivaglobin – Administer subcutaneously; do not inject intravenously (IV). Do not inject into a blood vessel.

In the clinical study with *Vivaglobin*, a volume of 15 mL per injection site at a rate of 20 mL per hour per site was not exceeded. Doses over 15 mL were divided and infused into several sites using an infusion pump. Multiple simultaneous injections were enabled by administration tubing and Y-site connection tubing (*CADD-Legacy* pumps were used in the study conducted in the United States and Canada). Injection sites were at least 2 inches apart.

The following areas were used for subcutaneous injection of *Vivaglobin*: abdomen, thighs, upper arms, and/or lateral hip. The actual point of injection was changed with each weekly administration.

Vivaglobin contains no preservative; discard unused product immediately after use.

Home treatment – If home administration is appropriate, provide the patient with instructions on subcutaneous infusion for home treatment. This should include the type of equipment to be used along with its maintenance, proper infusion techniques, selection of appropriate infusion sites (eg,

IMMUNE GLOBULIN (HUMAN) — SUBCUTANEOUS INJECTION

abdomen, thighs, upper arms, lateral hip), maintenance of a treatment diary, and measures to be taken in case of adverse reactions.

➤*Admixture compatibility:* Immune globulin subcutaneous must not be mixed with other products.

➤*Storage/Stability:* Store *Hizentra* at room temperature (up to 25°C [77°F]). Do not freeze. Do not use product that has been frozen. Do not shake. Keep *Hizentra* in its original carton to protect it from light.

Store *Vivaglobin* in the refrigerator at 2° to 8°C (36° to 46°F). Do not freeze. Keep vials in storage box until use.

IMMUNE GLOBULIN (HUMAN) — INTRAVENOUS/— SUBCUTANEOUS (*GAMUNEX-C*)

Rx	**Gamunex-C** (Talecris Biotherapeutics)	**Injection, solution**: immune globulin (human) 10% (100 mg/mL)[a]	Preservative free. In 10, 25, 50, 100, and 200 mL single-use vials.

[a] Each vial consists of 9% to 11% protein in 0.16 to 0.24 M of glycine.

IMMUNE GLOBULIN (HUMAN) — INTRAVENOUS/— SUBCUTANEOUS (*GAMUNEX-C*)

For complete and comparative prescribing information, refer to the Immune Globulins class monograph.

WARNING

Renal dysfunction and failure – Renal dysfunction, acute renal failure, osmotic nephrosis, and death may occur with immune globulin intravenous (IV) products in predisposed patients. Patients predisposed to renal dysfunction include those with any degree of preexisting renal insufficiency, diabetes mellitus, age older than 65 years, volume depletion, sepsis, paraproteinemia, or patients receiving known nephrotoxic drugs.

Renal dysfunction and acute renal failure occur more commonly in patients receiving immune globulin IV products containing sucrose. *Gamunex-C* does not contain sucrose.

For patients at risk of renal dysfunction or failure, administer *Gamunex-C* at the minimum concentration available and the minimum infusion rate practicable.

Indications

➤*Chronic inflammatory demyelinating polyneuropathy:* For the treatment of chronic inflammatory demyelinating polyneuropathy (CIDP) to improve neuromuscular disability and impairment and for maintenance therapy to prevent relapse.

➤*Idiopathic thrombocytopenic purpura:* For the treatment of patients with idiopathic thrombocytopenic purpura (ITP) to raise platelet counts to prevent bleeding or to allow a patient with ITP to undergo surgery.

➤*Primary humoral immunodeficiency:* As replacement therapy of primary humoral immunodeficiency. This includes, but is not limited to, congenital agammaglobulinemia, common variable immunodeficiency, X-linked agammaglobulinemia, Wiskott-Aldrich syndrome, and severe combined immunodeficiencies.

Administration and Dosage

➤*Adults:*

Chronic inflammatory demyelinating polyneuropathy –

Loading dose: 2 g/kg (20 mL/kg) IV given in divided doses over 2 to 4 consecutive days.

Maintenance dosage: 1 g/kg (10 mL/kg) administered over 1 day or divided into 2 doses of 0.5 g/kg (5 mL/kg) given on 2 consecutive days, every 3 weeks.

Idiopathic thrombocytopenic purpura –

Usual dosage: 2 g/kg IV total dose divided in 2 doses of 1 g/kg (10 mL/kg) IV given on 2 consecutive days. This regimen is not recommended for individuals with expanded fluid volumes or for patients in whom fluid volume may be a concern. (See Alternative Dosage.)

If, after administration of the first of 2 daily 1 g/kg (10 mL/kg) doses, an adequate increase in the platelet count is observed at 24 hours, the second dose of 1 g/kg (10 mL/kg) body weight may be withheld.

Forty-eight ITP subjects were treated with *Gamunex-C* 2 g/kg divided in two 1 g/kg doses (10 mL/kg) given on 2 successive days. With this dose regimen, 90% of subjects responded with a platelet count from 20×10^9/L or less to 50×10^9/L or more within 7 days after treatment.

Alternative dosage: 2 g/kg IV divided into 5 doses of 0.4 g/kg (4 mL/kg), given on 5 consecutive days.

Primary humoral immunodeficiency – Because there are significant differences in the half-life of immunoglobulin G (IgG) among patients with primary humoral immunodeficiencies, the frequency and amount of immunoglobulin therapy may vary from patient to patient. The proper amount can be determined by monitoring clinical response.

IV:

• *Usual dosage* – 300 to 600 mg/kg body weight (3 to 6 mL/kg) IV administered every 3 to 4 weeks.

• *Dosage adjustment* – The dosage may be adjusted over time to achieve the desired trough levels and clinical responses.

• *Measles exposure* – If a patient routinely receives a dose of less than 400 mg/kg of *Gamunex-C* every 3 to 4 weeks (less than 4 mL/kg) and is at risk of measles exposure (ie, traveling to a measles endemic area), administer a dose of at least 400 mg/kg (4 mL/kg) just prior to the expected measles exposure. If a patient has been exposed to measles, a dose of 400 mg/kg (4 mL/kg) should be administered as soon as possible after exposure.

Subcutaneous:

• *Initial dosage –*

Conversion from Gamunex-C IV: Establish the weekly dose of *Gamunex-C* by converting the monthly IV dose into a weekly equivalent.

Conversion from other immunoglobulin IV products: To calculate the initial weekly dose of subcutaneous administration of *Gamunex-C*, multiply the previous immune globulin IV dose in grams by the dose adjustment factor of 1.37; then divide this by the number of weeks between doses during the patient's immune globulin IV treatment (ie, 3 or 4).

Conversion from other immunoglobulin subcutaneous products: Dosage requirements for patients switching to *Gamunex-C* from another immune globulin subcutaneous product have not been studied. If a patient on *Gamunex-C* does not maintain an adequate clinical response or a serum IgG trough level equivalent to that of the previous immune globulin subcutaneous treatment, the health care provider may want to adjust the dose. For such patients, the *Gamunex-C* Weekly Subcutaneous Dosage Adjustment table also provides guidance for dose adjustment to achieve a desired immune globulin subcutaneous trough level.

• *Dosage adjustment* – Over time, the dose may need to be adjusted to achieve the desired clinical response and serum IgG trough level.

To determine if a dose adjustment may be considered, measure the patient's serum IgG trough level on immune globulin IV and as early as 5 weeks after switching from immune globulin IV to subcutaneous. The target serum IgG trough level on weekly subcutaneous treatment is projected to be the last immune globulin IV trough level plus 340 mg/dL.

To determine if further dose adjustments are necessary, monitor the patient's IgG trough level every 2 to 3 months.

To adjust the dose based on trough levels, calculate the difference (in mg/dL) of the patient's serum IgG trough level from the target IgG trough level (the last immune globulin IV trough level + 340 mg/dL). Then find this difference in the following table and the corresponding amount (in milliliters) by which to increase or decrease the weekly dose based on the patient's body weight. However, the patient's clinical response should be the primary consideration in dose adjustment. Monitor the patient's clinical response and repeat the dose adjustment as needed.

***Gamunex-C* Weekly Subcutaneous Dosage Adjustment**

Difference from target IgG trough level (mg/dL)	Body weight (kg)												
	10	15	20	30	40	50	60	70	80	90	100	110	120
	Dosage adjustment (mL/wk)[a]												
50	1	1	2	3	3	4	5	6	7	8	8	9	10
100	2	3	3	5	7	8	10	12	13	15	17	18	20
150	3	4	5	8	10	13	15	18	20	23	25	28	30
200	3	5	7	10	13	17	20	23	27	30	33	37	40
250	4	6	8	13	17	21	25	29	33	38	42	46	50
300	5	8	10	15	20	25	30	35	40	45	50	55	60
350	6	9	12	18	23	29	35	41	47	53	58	64	70
400	7	10	13	20	27	33	40	47	53	60	67	73	80
450	8	11	15	23	30	38	45	53	60	68	75	83	90
500	8	13	17	25	33	42	50	58	67	75	83	92	100

[a] Dose adjustment in mL is based on the slope of the serum IgG trough level response to subcutaneous administration of *Gamunex-C* dose increments (approximately 6 mg/dL per increment of 1 mg/kg/wk).

For example, if a patient with a body weight of 70 kg has an actual IgG trough level of 900 mg/dL and the target level is 1,000 mg/dL, this results in a difference of 100 mg/dL. Therefore, increase the weekly subcutaneous dose by 12 mL.

➤*Children:*

Idiopathic thrombocytopenic purpura – See Adults for dosing.

Primary humoral immunodeficiency –

IV: See Adults for dosing.

➤*Elderly:* Use with caution in patients 65 years of age and older who are judged to be at increased risk for developing thromboembolic events or renal insufficiency. Do not exceed recommended doses and administer at the minimum infusion rate practicable.

➤*Renal function impairment:* Ensure that patients with preexisting renal insufficiency are not volume depleted. For patients at risk of renal dysfunction or thromboembolic events, administer *Gamunex-C* at the minimum infusion rate practicable and discontinue *Gamunex-C* if renal function deteriorates.

➤*Preparation for administration:* Do not freeze. Solutions that have been frozen should not be used. The vial is for single use only and contains no preservative. Any vial that has been entered should be used promptly. Partially used vials should be discarded.

IMMUNE GLOBULIN (HUMAN) — INTRAVENOUS/— SUBCUTANEOUS (*GAMUNEX-C*)

If dilution is required, *Gamunex-C* may be diluted with dextrose 5% in water. Do not dilute with saline. Content of vials may be pooled under aseptic conditions into sterile infusion bags and infused within 8 hours after pooling.

IV – Only 18-gauge needles should be used to penetrate the stopper for dispensing product from the 10 mL vial; 16 gauge needles or dispensing pins should only be used with 25 mL vial sizes and larger. Needles or dispensing pins should only be inserted once and be within the stopper area delineated by the raised ring. The stopper should be penetrated perpendicular to the plane of the stopper within the ring.

Subcutaneous – Prior to use, allow the solution to reach ambient room temperature. Do not shake.

Follow the manufacturer's instructions for filling the pump reservoir and preparing the pump, administration tubing, and Y-site connection tubing, if needed. Be sure to prime the administration tubing to ensure that no air is left in the tubing or needle by filling the tubing/needle with *Gamunex-C*.

➤*Administration:* Administer IV for treatment of primary humoral immunodeficiency, ITP, and CIDP; may also be administered subcutaneously for the treatment of primary humoral immunodeficiency.

Gamunex-C should be infused using a separate line by itself, without mixing with other IV fluids or medications the patient might be receiving.

Gamunex-C should be at room temperature during administration.

IV – Following initial infusion, the infusion rate may be gradually increased to a maximum of 0.08 mL/kg/min (8 mg/kg/min), as tolerated.

Gamunex-C Infusion Rate Based on Indication

Indication	Initial infusion rate (first 30 minutes)	Maximum infusion rate (if tolerated)
Primary humoral immunodeficiency	1 mg/kg/min	8 mg/kg/min
Idiopathic thrombocytopenic purpura	1 mg/kg/min	8 mg/kg/min
Chronic inflammatory demyelinating polyneuropathy	2 mg/kg/min	8 mg/kg/min

Infusion reaction: Monitor patient's vital signs throughout the infusion. Slow or stop infusion if adverse reactions occur. If symptoms subside promptly, the infusion may be resumed at a lower rate that is comfortable for the patient.

Certain severe adverse drug reactions may be related to the rate of infusion. Slowing or stopping the infusion usually allows the symptoms to disappear promptly.

Subcutaneous – Select the number and location of injection sites. Cleanse the injection site(s) with antiseptic solution using a circular motion working from the center of the site and moving to the outside. Sites should be clean, dry, and at least 2 inches apart. The maximum number of infusion sites is 8. Grasp the skin between 2 fingers and insert the needle into the subcutaneous tissue. Repeat priming and needle insertion steps using a new needle, administration tubing, and a new infusion site. Secure the needle in place by applying sterile gauze or transparent dressing over the site. If using multiple, simultaneous injection sites, use Y-site connection tubing and secure to the administration tubing. Infuse *Gamunex-C* following the manufacturer's instructions for the pump.

For primary humoral immunodeficiency, it is recommended that *Gamunex-C* is infused at a rate of 20 mL/h per infusion site.

➤*Admixture compatibility:* *Gamunex-C* is not compatible with saline. If dilution is required, *Gamunex-C* may be diluted with dextrose 5% in water. Do not mix with immune globulin IV products from other manufacturers. No other drug interactions or compatibilities have been evaluated.

➤*Storage/Stability:* Vials may be stored for 36 months at 2° to 8°C (36° to 46°F) from the date of manufacture at temperatures not to exceed 25°C (77°F) for up to 6 months any time during the 36-month shelf life, after which the product must be immediately used or discarded. Do not freeze.

Actions

➤*Pharmacology:*

Chronic inflammatory demyelinating polyneuropathy – The precise mechanism of action in CIDP has not been fully elucidated.

Idiopathic thrombocytopenic purpura – The mechanism of action of high doses of immunoglobulins in the treatment of ITP has not been fully elucidated.

Primary humoral immunodeficiency – *Gamunex-C* supplies a broad spectrum of opsonic and neutralizing IgG antibodies against bacteria, viral, parasitic, mycoplasma agents, and their toxins. The mechanism of action in primary humoral immunodeficiency has not been fully elucidated.

➤*Pharmacokinetics:*

IV administration – Two randomized, pharmacokinetic, crossover trials were carried out with *Gamunex-C* in 38 subjects with primary humoral immunodeficiencies given 3 infusions 3 or 4 weeks apart of test product at a dose of 100 to 600 mg/kg body weight per infusion. One trial compared the pharmacokinetic characteristics of *Gamunex-C* with *Gamimune N, 10%*, and the other trial compared the pharmacokinetics of *Gamunex-C* (10% strength) with a 5% concentration of this product. The ratio of the geometric least square means for dose-normalized IgG peak levels of *Gamunex-C* and *Gamimune N, 10%* was 0.996. The corresponding value for the dose-normalized area under the curve (AUC) of IgG levels was 0.99. The results of both pharmacokinetic parameters were within the pre-established limits of 0.08 and 1.25. Similar results were obtained in the comparison of *Gamunex-C* 10% to a 5% concentration of *Gamunex-C*.

Pharmacokinetic Parameters of *Gamunex-C* and *Gamimune N, 10%*[a]

	Gamunex-C				Gamimune N, 10%			
	n	Mean	SD	Median	n	Mean	SD	Median
C_{max} (mg/mL)	17	19.04	3.06	19.71	17	19.31	4.17	19.3
C_{max}-norm (kg/mL)	17	0.047	0.007	0.046	17	0.047	0.008	0.047
$AUC_{(0\text{-}tn)}$[b] (mg•h/mL)	17	6,746.48	1,348.13	6,949.47	17	6,854.17	1,425.08	7,119.86
$AUC_{(0\text{-}tn)norm}$[b] (kg•h/mL)	17	16.51	1.83	16.95	17	16.69	2.04	16.99
Half-life[c] (days)	16	35.74	8.69	33.09	16	34.27	9.28	31.88

[a] SD = standard deviation; C_{max} = maximum plasma concentration.
[b] Partial AUC = predose concentration to the last concentration common across both treatment periods in the same patient.
[c] Only 15 subjects were valid for the analysis of half-life.

The 2 pharmacokinetic trials with *Gamunex-C* show the IgG concentration/time curve follows a biphasic slope, with a distribution phase of approximately 5 days characterized by a fall in serum IgG levels to approximately 65% to 75% of the peak levels achieved immediately post infusion. This phase is followed by the elimination phase, with a half-life of approximately 35 days. IgG trough levels were measured over 9 months in the therapeutic equivalence trial. Mean trough levels were 7.8 ± 1.9 mg/mL for the *Gamunex-C* treatment group and 8.2 ± 2 mg/mL for the *Gamimune N, 10%* control group.

Subcutaneous administration –

Primary humoral immunodeficiency: In a single sequence, open-label, crossover trial, the pharmacokinetics, safety, and tolerability of subcutaneously administered *Gamunex-C* in subjects with primary humoral immunodeficiency were evaluated. A total of 32 and 26 subjects received *Gamunex-C* as IV or subcutaneous for the pharmacokinetic study, respectively. Subjects received *Gamunex-C* 200 to 600 mg/kg IV every 3 to 4 weeks for at least 3 months, at which time they entered the IV phase of the study. Subjects were crossed over to weekly subcutaneous infusions. The weekly subcutaneous dose was determined by multiplying the total IV dose by 1.37 and dividing the resultant new total dose by 3 or 4, depending on the previous IV interval. The lower bound of the 90% confidence interval (CI) for the geometric mean ratio of AUC (subcutaneous vs IV) was 0.861, therefore, meeting the prespecified noninferiority margin between the 2 modes of administration.

Summary of *Gamunex-C* Pharmacokinetic End Point of AUC[a]

Route of administration	Statistics	$AUC_{0\text{-}tau,\ IV}$ (mg•h/mL)	$AUC_{0\text{-}tau,\ SC}$ (mg•h/mL)	Adjusted $AUC_{0\text{-}tau,\ SC}$[b] (mg•h/mL)
IV (n = 32)	Mean	7,640	NA[c]	NA
	%CV	15.9		
	Range	5,616 to 10,400		
Subcutaneous (n = 26)	Mean	NA	1,947	6,858
	%CV		20.4	18.1
	Range		1,300 to 2,758	5,169 to 10,364

[a] CV = coefficient of variation.
[b] Adjusted $AUC_{0\text{-}tau,\ SC}$ = adjusted steady-state area under the concentration vs time curve following subcutaneous administration based on IV dosing schedule, calculated as $AUC_{0\text{-}tau,\ SC}$ multiplied by 3 or 4 for subjects on every-3-week or every-4-week IV dosing schedule, respectively.
[c] NA = not applicable.

Gamunex-C Mean Plasma Trough Concentrations of Total IgG (mg/mL) in Plasma

	IV mean C_{trough}	Subcutaneous mean C_{trough}
n	32	28
Mean (mg/mL)	9.58	11.4
%CV	22.3	20.4
Range	6.66 to 14	8.1 to 16.2

In contrast to plasma total IgG levels observed with monthly IV *Gamunex-C* treatment (rapid peaks followed by a slow decline), the plasma IgG levels in subjects receiving weekly subcutaneous *Gamunex-C* therapy were relatively stable.

Contraindications

Anaphylactic or severe systemic reaction to the administration of human immune globulin; IgA-deficient patients with antibodies against IgA and history of hypersensitivity.

IMMUNE GLOBULIN (HUMAN) — INTRAVENOUS/—SUBCUTANEOUS (*GAMUNEX-C*)

Warnings/Precautions

➤*Renal effects:* Ensure that patients are not volume depleted prior to the initiation of the infusion of *Gamunex-C*. Periodic monitoring of renal function and urine output is particularly important in patients judged to have a potential increased risk for developing acute renal failure. Assess renal function, including measurement of serum urea nitrogen (BUN)/serum creatinine, prior to the initial infusion of *Gamunex-C* and again at appropriate intervals thereafter. If renal function deteriorates, consider discontinuation of *Gamunex-C*. For patients judged to be at risk for developing renal dysfunction, including patients with any degree of preexisting renal insufficiency, diabetes mellitus, age older than 65 years, volume depletion, sepsis, paraproteinemia, or patients receiving known nephrotoxic drugs, administer *Gamunex-C* at the minimum infusion rate practicable (less than IG 8 mg/kg/min [0.08 mL/kg/min]).

➤*Hematoma formation:* Do not administer *Gamunex-C* subcutaneously in patients with ITP because of the risk of hematoma formation.

➤*Hyperproteinemia/Increased serum viscosity/Hyponatremia:* Hyperproteinemia, increased serum viscosity, and hyponatremia may occur in patients receiving immune globulin IV treatment, including *Gamunex-C*. It is clinically critical to distinguish true hyponatremia from a pseudohyponatremia that is associated with concomitant decreased calculated serum osmolality or elevated osmolar gap, because treatment aimed at decreasing serum-free water in patients with pseudohyponatremia may lead to volume depletion, a further increase in serum viscosity, and a possible predisposition to thromboembolic events.

➤*Thrombotic events:* Thrombotic events have been reported following immune globulin IV treatment and may occur in patients receiving immune globulin IV treatment, including *Gamunex-C*. Patients at risk may include those with a history of atherosclerosis, multiple cardiovascular risk factors, advanced age, impaired cardiac output, coagulation disorders, prolonged periods of immobilization, and/or known or suspected hyperviscosity. Consider baseline assessment of blood viscosity in patients at risk for hyperviscosity, including those with cryoglobulins, fasting chylomicronemia/markedly high triacylglycerols (triglycerides), or monoclonal gammopathies. For patients judged to be at risk of developing thrombotic events, administer *Gamunex-C* at the minimum rate of infusion practicable.

➤*Aseptic meningitis syndrome:* Aseptic meningitis syndrome may occur infrequently with immune globulin IV treatment, including *Gamunex-C*. Discontinuation of immune globulin IV treatment has resulted in remission of aseptic meningitis syndrome within several days without sequelae. The syndrome usually begins within several hours to 2 days following immune globulin IV treatment. Aseptic meningitis syndrome is characterized by the following symptoms and signs: severe headache, nuchal rigidity, drowsiness, fever, photophobia, painful eye movements, nausea, and vomiting. Cerebrospinal fluid (CSF) studies are frequently positive, with pleocytosis up to several thousand cells/mm^3, predominantly from the granulocytic series, and with elevated protein levels up to several hundred mg/dL, but negative culture results. Conduct a thorough neurological examination on patients exhibiting such symptoms and signs, including CSF studies, to rule out other causes of meningitis. Aseptic meningitis syndrome may occur more frequently in association with high doses (2 g/kg) and/or rapid infusion of immune globulin IV.

➤*Hemolysis:* Immune globulin IV products, including *Gamunex-C*, may contain blood group antibodies that may act as hemolysins and induce in vivo coating of red blood cells (RBCs) with immunoglobulin, causing a positive direct antiglobulin reaction and, rarely, hemolysis. Delayed hemolytic anemia can develop subsequent to immune globulin IV therapy because of enhanced RBC sequestration, and acute hemolysis consistent with intravascular hemolysis has been reported. Monitor patients for clinical signs and symptoms of hemolysis. If signs and/or symptoms of hemolysis are present after *Gamunex-C* infusion, perform appropriate confirmatory laboratory testing.

➤*Transfusion-related acute lung injury:* Noncardiogenic pulmonary edema may occur in patients following treatment with immune globulin IV products, including *Gamunex-C*. Transfusion-related acute lung injury is characterized by severe respiratory distress, pulmonary edema, hypoxemia, normal left ventricular function, and fever. Symptoms typically occur within 1 to 6 hours after treatment.

Monitor patients for pulmonary adverse reactions. If transfusion-related acute lung injury is suspected, perform appropriate tests for the presence of antineutrophil and anti–human leukocyte antigen (HLA) antibodies in the product and patient serum. Transfusion-related acute lung injury may be managed using oxygen therapy with adequate ventilatory support.

➤*Volume overload:* The high-dose regimen (1 g/kg × 1 to 2 days) is not recommended for patients with expanded fluid volumes or where fluid volume may be a concern.

➤*Transmissible infectious agents:* Because *Gamunex-C* is made from human blood, it may carry a risk of transmitting infectious agents (eg, viruses, and theoretically, the Creutzfeldt-Jakob disease agent). No cases of transmission of viral diseases or Creutzfeldt-Jakob disease have ever been identified for *Gamunex-C*. Report all infections suspected by a health care provider possibly to have been transmitted by this product to the manufacturer at 1-800-520-2807.

➤*Vaccines:* Passive transfer of antibodies may transiently interfere with the immune response to live virus vaccines, such as measles, mumps, rubella and varicella. Inform the immunizing health care provider of recent therapy with *Gamunex-C* so that appropriate measures may be taken.

➤*Hypersensitivity reactions:* Severe hypersensitivity reactions may occur with immune globulin IV products, including *Gamunex-C*. In case of hypersensitivity, discontinue *Gamunex-C* infusion immediately and institute appropriate treatment. Medications, such as epinephrine, should be available for immediate treatment of acute hypersensitivity reaction.

Gamunex-C contains trace amounts of IgA (average, 46 micrograms/mL). Patients with known antibodies to IgA may have a greater risk of developing potentially severe hypersensitivity and anaphylactic reactions. It is contraindicated in IgA-deficient patients with antibodies against IgA and history of hypersensitivity reaction.

➤*Pregnancy: Category C.* Animal reproduction studies have not been conducted with *Gamunex-C*. It is not known whether *Gamunex-C* can cause fetal harm when administered to a pregnant woman or can affect reproduction capacity. Give *Gamunex-C* to a pregnant woman only if clearly needed. Immunoglobulins cross the placenta from maternal circulation increasingly after 30 weeks of gestation.

➤*Lactation:* Use of *Gamunex-C* has not been evaluated in breast-feeding women. The World Health Organization classifies immune globulin IV and immune globulin intramuscular as compatible with breast-feeding.

➤*Children:*

Primary humoral immunodeficiency –

IV: Pharmacokinetics, safety, and efficacy were similar to those in adults, with the exception of vomiting, which was more frequently reported in children (3/18 subjects). No pediatric-specific dose requirements were necessary to achieve serum IgG levels.

Subcutaneous: Efficacy and safety in children using the subcutaneous route of administration have not been established.

Idiopathic thrombocytopenic purpura –

Pharmacokinetics, safety, and efficacy were similar to those in adults, with the exception that fever was more frequently reported in children (6/12 subjects). No pediatric-specific dose requirements were necessary to achieve serum IgG levels. One subject, a boy 10 years of age, died suddenly from myocarditis 50 days after his second infusion of *Gamunex-C*. The death was judged to be unrelated to *Gamunex-C*.

Chronic inflammatory demyelinating polyneuropathy – The safety and effectiveness of *Gamunex-C* have not been established in children with CIDP.

➤*Elderly:* Use caution when administering *Gamunex-C* to patients 65 years of age and older who are judged to be at increased risk for developing thromboembolic events or renal insufficiency. Do not exceed recommended doses, and administer *Gamunex-C* at the minimum infusion rate practicable.

➤*Monitoring:* Assess renal function, including measurement of BUN/serum creatinine, prior to the initial infusion of *Gamunex-C* and again at appropriate intervals thereafter. Periodic monitoring of renal function and urine output is particularly important in patients judged to have a potential increased risk for developing acute renal failure.

If signs and/or symptoms of hemolysis are present after *Gamunex-C* infusion, perform appropriate confirmatory laboratory testing.

Consider baseline assessment of blood viscosity in patients at risk for hyperviscosity, including those with cryoglobulins, fasting chylomicronemia/markedly high triacylglycerols (triglycerides), or monoclonal gammopathies.

Conduct a thorough neurological examination, including CSF studies, in patients exhibiting signs and symptoms suggestive of aseptic meningitis syndrome, to rule out other causes of meningitis.

Monitor patients for pulmonary adverse reactions. If transfusion-related acute lung injury is suspected, perform appropriate tests for the presence of antineutrophil and anti-HLA antibodies in the product and patient serum. Clinically assess patients with known renal dysfunction or renal failure, including patients with preexisting renal insufficiency, diabetes mellitus, age older than 65 years, volume depletion, sepsis, paraproteinemia, or those receiving nephrotoxic agents. Monitor (BUN, creatinine), as appropriate, during therapy with *Gamunex-C*.

Drug Interactions

➤*Hydantoins (eg, phenytoin):* The risk of hydantoin-induced hypersensitivity myocarditis may be increased. Use with caution. Monitor hematologic findings and cardiac function if these agents are coadministered.

➤*Viral vaccines, live:* See Warnings/Precautions for more information.

➤*Drug/Lab test interactions:* Various passively transferred antibodies in immunoglobulin preparations can confound the results of serological testing.

Passive transmission of antibodies to erythrocyte antigens (eg, A, B, and D) may cause a positive direct or indirect antiglobulin (Coombs) test.

Adverse Reactions

➤*Primary humoral immunodeficiency:*

IV –

Most common adverse reactions: The most common adverse reactions observed at a rate of 5% or more in subjects treated with *Gamunex-C* IV for primary humoral immunodeficiency were headache, cough, injection-site reaction, nausea, pharyngitis, and urticaria.

Serious adverse reactions: The most serious adverse reaction observed in clinical study subjects receiving *Gamunex-C* IV for primary humoral immunodeficiency was an exacerbation of autoimmune pure red cell aplasia in 1 subject.

Discontinuation of therapy: In 4 different clinical trials to study primary humoral immunodeficiency, out of 157 subjects treated with *Gamunex-C*, 4 subjects discontinued because of the following adverse reactions: Coombs

IMMUNE GLOBULIN (HUMAN) — INTRAVENOUS/—SUBCUTANEOUS (*GAMUNEX-C*)

negative hypochromic anemia, autoimmune pure red cell aplasia, arthralgia/hyperhidrosis/fatigue/myalgia/nausea, and migraine.

Pretreatment medications: In a study of 87 subjects, 9 subjects in each treatment group were pretreated with nonsteroidal medication prior to infusion, such as diphenhydramine and acetaminophen.

Adverse reactions:

Gamunex-C IV Adverse Reactions in Primary Humoral Immunodeficiency (> 10%)[a]		
Adverse reactions	*Gamunex-C* (n = 87)	*Gamimune N, 10%* (n = 85)
CNS		
Asthenia	10%	15%
Headache	25%	33%
GI		
Diarrhea	28%	32%
Nausea	20%	26%
Respiratory		
Asthma	29%	20%
Cough increased	54%	54%
Pharyngitis	41%	46%
Rhinitis	51%	53%
Miscellaneous		
Ear pain	18%	14%
Fever	28%	32%

[a] Irrespective of causality.

Gamunex-C IV Adverse Reactions in Primary Humoral Immunodeficiency During 9 Months of Treatment (≥ 5%)		
Adverse reactions	*Gamunex-C* (n = 87)	*Gamimune N, 10%* (n = 85)
Respiratory		
Cough increased	7%	5%
Pharyngitis	5%	4%
Miscellaneous		
Headache	8%	9%
Injection-site reaction	5%	8%
Nausea	5%	5%
Urticaria	5%	1%

The following table lists the frequency of adverse reactions, which were reported by at least 5% of subjects, and their relationship to infusions administered.

Gamunex-C IV Adverse Reactions (≥ 5%) and Relationship to the Infusion		
Adverse reactions	*Gamunex-C* (n = 825 infusions)	*Gamimune N, 10%* (n = 865 infusions)
Respiratory		
Cough increased		
All	18.7%	17.1%
Drug related	1.7%	1.3%
Pharyngitis		
All	11.6%	11.4%
Drug related	0.8%	1%
Miscellaneous		
Headache		
All	6.9%	8%
Drug related	0.8%	1.3%
Fever		
All	5%	7.5%
Drug related	0.1%	1%
Nausea		
All	3.8%	5%
Drug related	0.5%	0.5%
Urticaria		
All	0.6%	0.9%
Drug related	0.5%	0.6%

Infusion reactions: The mean number of adverse reactions per infusion that occurred during or on the same day as an infusion was 0.21 in both the *Gamunex-C* and *Gamimune N, 10%* treatment groups.

In all 3 trials in primary humoral immunodeficiencies, the maximum infusion rate was 0.08 mL/kg/min (8 mg/kg/min). The infusion rate was reduced for 11 of 222 exposed subjects (7 *Gamunex-C*, 4 *Gamimune N, 10%*) at 17 occasions. In most instances, mild to moderate hives/urticaria, itching, pain or reaction at infusion site, anxiety, or headache was the main reason. There was 1 case of severe chills. There were no anaphylactic or anaphylactoid reactions to *Gamunex-C* or *Gamimune N, 10%* in clinical trials.

Subcutaneous –

Most common adverse reactions: The most common adverse reactions observed at a rate 5% or more of subjects treated with subcutaneous *Gamunex-C* for primary humoral immunodeficiency were arthralgia, fatigue, headache, infusion-site reactions, and pyrexia.

Adverse reactions:

Gamunex-C Subcutaneous Adverse Reactions in Primary Humoral Immunodeficiency (≥ 2% of Infusions)[a]	
Adverse reaction (n = 725 infusions)	Rate[b]
Local	
Infusion-site reactions	0.59
Mild	0.54
Moderate	0.04
Severe	0.01
Miscellaneous	
Headache	0.05
Sinusitis	0.02

[a] Irrespective of causality.
[b] Rate is calculated by the total number of reactions divided by the number of infusions received (725).

The following table lists the adverse reactions occurring in 5% or more of subjects and the frequency of adverse reactions per infusion.

Gamunex-C Subcutaneous Adverse Reactions (≥ 5% of Subjects) by Subject and Infusion[a]		
Adverse reactions	Subjects (n = 32)	Rate[b]
CNS		
Fatigue	6.3%	≤ 0.01
Headache	13%	0.03
Miscellaneous		
Arthralgia	6.3%	0.01
Local infusion-site reactions	75%	0.59
Pyrexia	6.3%	≤ 0.01

[a] All local infusion-site reactions were a priori considered drug-related.
[b] Rate is calculated by the total number of reactions divided by the number of infusions received (725).

Local: Local infusion-site reactions with subcutaneous *Gamunex-C* consisted of erythema, pain, and swelling. The majority of local infusion-site reactions resolved within 3 days. The number of subjects experiencing an infusion-site reaction and the number of infusion-site reactions decreased over time as subjects received continued weekly subcutaneous infusions. At the beginning of the subcutaneous phase (week 1), a rate of approximately 1 infusion-site reaction per infusion was reported, whereas at the end of the study (week 24), this rate was reduced to 0.5 infusion-site reactions per infusion, a reduction of 50%.

➤*Idiopathic thrombocytopenic purpura:*

Most common adverse reactions – The most common adverse reactions observed at a rate 5% or more in subjects treated with *Gamunex-C* for ITP were back pain, fever, headache, nausea, rash, and vomiting. More than 90% of the observed drug-related adverse reactions were of mild to moderate severity and of transient nature.

Discontinuation of therapy – In 2 different clinical trials to study ITP, out of 76 subjects treated with *Gamunex-C*, 2 subjects discontinued because of the following adverse events: hives and headache/fever/vomiting.

Mortality – One subject, a boy 10 years of age, died suddenly from myocarditis 50 days after his second infusion of *Gamunex-C*. The death was judged to be unrelated to *Gamunex-C*.

Pretreatment medications – No premedication with corticosteroids was permitted by the protocol. Twelve ITP subjects treated in each treatment group were pretreated with medication prior to infusion. Generally, diphenhydramine and/or acetaminophen were used.

Infusion reactions – The infusion rate was reduced for 4 of the 97 exposed subjects (1 *Gamunex-C*, 3 *Gamimune N, 10%*) on 4 occasions. Mild to moderate headache, fever, and nausea were the reported reasons.

Adverse reactions – The following table lists any adverse reactions, irrespective of the causality, reported by at least 5% of subjects during the 3-month efficacy and safety study.

Gamunex-C Adverse Reactions in Idiopathic Thrombocytopenic Purpura During a 3-Month Study (≥ 5%)[a]		
Adverse reactions	*Gamunex-C* (n = 48)	*Gamimune N, 10%* (n = 49)
CNS		
Asthenia	6%	10%
Dizziness	6%	6%
Headache	58%	61%

IMMUNE GLOBULIN (HUMAN) — INTRAVENOUS/SUBCUTANEOUS (*GAMUNEX-C*)

Gamunex-C Adverse Reactions in Idiopathic Thrombocytopenic Purpura During a 3-Month Study (≥ 5%)[a]

Adverse reactions	*Gamunex-C* (n = 48)	*Gamimune N, 10%* (n = 49)
Dermatologic		
Pruritus	8%	2%
Rash	10%	12%
GI		
Abdominal pain	6%	8%
Dyspepsia	6%	0%
Nausea	21%	14%
Vomiting	21%	20%
Hematologic		
Anemia	6%	0%
Ecchymosis, purpura	40%	51%
Hemorrhage (all systems)	29%	33%
Petechiae	21%	31%
Thrombocytopenia	15%	16%
Musculoskeletal		
Arthralgia	6%	12%
Back pain	6%	6%
Neck pain	6%	2%
Respiratory		
Epistaxis	23%	24%
Pharyngitis	10%	10%
Rhinitis	13%	12%
Miscellaneous		
Accidental injury	13%	16%
Fever	21%	14%
Flu syndrome	6%	6%

[a] Irrespective of causality.

The following table lists the adverse reactions reported by at least 5% of subjects during the 3-month efficacy and safety study.

Gamunex-C Adverse Reactions in Idiopathic Thrombocytopenic Purpura During a 3-Month Study (≥ 5%)

Adverse reactions	*Gamunex-C* (n = 48)	*Gamimune N, 10%* (n = 49)
GI		
Nausea	10%	8%
Vomiting	13%	16%
Miscellaneous		
Back pain	6%	4%
Fever	10%	10%
Headache	50%	49%
Rash	6%	0%

➤*Chronic inflammatory demyelinating polyneuropathy:*

Serious adverse reactions – The most serious adverse reaction observed in clinical study subjects receiving *Gamunex-C* for CIDP was pulmonary embolism (PE) in 1 subject with a history of PE.

Most common adverse reactions – The most common adverse reactions observed at a rate 5% or more in subjects with *Gamunex-C* for CIDP were asthenia, chills, fever, headache, hypertension, nausea, and rash.

Discontinuation of therapy –

Gamunex-C Reasons for Discontinuation Due to Adverse Reactions in CIDP

Number of subjects	Percent of subjects discontinued due to adverse reactions	Adverse event
Gamunex-C (n = 113)	2.7%	Urticaria, dyspnea, bronchopneumonia
Placebo (n = 95)	2.1%	Cerebrovascular accident, deep vein thrombosis

Adverse reactions (5% or more) –

Gamunex-C Adverse Reactions in CIDP (≥ 5%)

Adverse reactions[a]	*Gamunex-C* (n = 113)			Placebo (n = 95)		
	%	No. of adverse reactions	Incidence density[b]	%	No. of adverse reactions	Incidence density[b]
Adverse reactions	75%	377	0.344	47%	120	0.209
CNS						
Asthenia	8%	10	0.009	3%	4	0.007
Dizziness	6%	3	0.006	1%	1	0.002
Headache	32%	57	0.052	8%	15	0.026
Musculoskeletal						
Arthralgia	7%	11	0.01	1%	1	0.002
Back pain	8%	10	0.009	3%	3	0.005
Miscellaneous						
Chills	8%	10	0.009	0%	0	0
Hypertension	9%	20	0.018	4%	6	0.01
Influenza	5%	6	0.005	2%	2	0.003
Nausea	6%	9	0.008	3%	3	0.005
Pyrexia (fever)	13%	27	0.025	0%	0	0
Rash	7%	13	0.012	1%	1	0.002

[a] Reported in ≥ 5% of subjects in any treatment group irrespective of causality.
[b] Calculated by the total number of adverse reactions divided by the number of infusions received (1,096 for *Gamunex-C* and 575 for placebo).

Gamunex-C Adverse Reactions in CIDP (≥ 5%)

Adverse reactions[a]	*Gamunex-C* (n = 113)			Placebo (n = 95)		
	%	No. of adverse reactions	Incidence density[b]	%	No. of adverse reactions	Incidence density[b]
Adverse reactions	55%	194	0.177	17%	25	0.043
CNS						
Asthenia	5%	6	0.005	0%	0	0
Headache	27%	44	0.04	6%	7	0.012
Miscellaneous						
Chills	7%	9	0.008	0%	0	0
Hypertension	6%	16	0.015	3%	3	0.005
Nausea	5%	7	0.006	3%	3	0.005
Pyrexia (fever)	13%	26	0.024	0%	0	0
Rash	5%	8	0.007	1%	1	0.002

[a] Reported in ≥ 5% of subjects in any treatment group.
[b] Calculated by the total number of adverse reactions divided by the number of infusions received (1,096 for *Gamunex-C* and 575 for placebo).

➤*Lab test abnormalities:*

Hepatic – During the course of the clinical program, ALT and AST elevations were identified in some subjects. Elevations of ALT and AST were generally mild (less than 3 times the upper limit of normal [ULN]), and transient, and were not associated with obvious symptoms of liver dysfunction.

Primary humoral immunodeficiency: For ALT, in the IV primary humoral immunodeficiency study, treatment-emergent elevations above the ULN were transient and observed among 18% of subjects in the *Gamunex-C* group versus 6% of subjects in the *Gamimune N, 10%* group ($P = 0.026$).

In the subcutaneous primary humoral immunodeficiency study, treatment-emergent laboratory abnormalities during the subcutaneous phase occurred in several subjects. Thirteen percent had elevated alkaline phosphatase and 3% had a low alkaline phosphatase. Three percent had an elevated ALT, and 9% had an elevated AST. No elevations were more than 1.6 times the ULN.

Idiopathic thrombocytopenic purpura: In the ITP study, which employed a higher dose per infusion but a maximum of only 2 infusions, the reverse finding was observed among 7% subjects in the *Gamunex-C* group versus 19% of subjects in the *Gamimune N, 10%* group ($P = 0.118$).

Chronic inflammatory demyelinating polyneuropathy: In the CIDP study, 13% subjects in the *Gamunex-C* group and 7% in the placebo group ($P = 0.168$) had a treatment-emergent transient elevation of ALT.

Hematologic – *Gamunex-C* may contain low levels of anti–blood group A and B antibodies primarily of the IgG_4 class. Direct antiglobulin tests (DAT) (or direct Coombs tests), which are carried out in some centers as a safety check prior to RBC transfusions, may become positive temporarily. Hemolytic events not associated with positive DAT findings were observed in clinical trials.

➤*Postmarketing:*

Gamunex-C – Aseptic meningitis, hemolytic anemia.

IMMUNE GLOBULIN (HUMAN) — INTRAVENOUS/—SUBCUTANEOUS (*GAMUNEX-C*)

All immune globulin IV products –

Cardiovascular: Cardiac arrest, hypotension, thromboembolism, and vascular collapse.

CNS: Loss of consciousness, seizures/convulsions, tremor.

Dermatologic: Bullous dermatitis, epidermolysis, erythema multiforme, Stevens-Johnson syndrome.

Hematologic: Hemolysis, leukopenia, pancytopenia, positive direct antiglobulin (Coombs test).

Musculoskeletal: Back pain, rigors.

Respiratory: Acute respiratory distress syndrome, apnea, bronchospasm, cyanosis, dyspnea, hypoxemia, pulmonary edema, transfusion-related acute lung injury.

Miscellaneous: Abdominal pain, coma, hepatic dysfunction, pyrexia.

Overdosage

No data available.

Patient Information

Inform patients to immediately report the following signs and symptoms to their health care provider: decreased urine output, sudden weight gain, fluid retention/edema, and/or shortness of breath; acute chest pain, shortness of breath, leg pain, and swelling of the legs/feet; severe headache, neck stiffness, drowsiness, fever, sensitivity to light, painful eye movements, nausea, and vomiting; increased heart rate, fatigue, yellowing of the skin or eyes, and dark-colored urine; trouble breathing, chest pain, blue lips or extremities, and fever.

Inform patients that *Gamunex-C* is made from human plasma and may contain infectious agents that can cause disease. While the risk that *Gamunex-C* can transmit an infectious agent has been reduced by screening plasma donors for prior exposure, testing donated plasma, and inactivating or removing certain viruses during manufacturing, instruct patients to report any symptoms that concern them.

Inform patients that *Gamunex-C* can interfere with their immune response to live viral vaccines, such as measles, mumps, and rubella. Inform patients to notify their health care provider of this potential interaction when they are receiving vaccinations.

Provide the patient with instructions on subcutaneous infusion for home treatment, if the health care provider believes that home administration is appropriate for the patient. Include the type of equipment to be used along with its maintenance, proper infusion techniques, selection of appropriate infusion sites (eg, abdomen, thighs, upper arms, lateral hip), maintenance of a treatment diary, and measures to be taken in case of adverse reactions in the patient instructions.

LYMPHOCYTE IMMUNE GLOBULIN, ANTITHYMOCYTE GLOBULIN (EQUINE) (LIG, ATG, ATG equine)

Rx	**Atgam** (Pharmacia)	**Injection:**[a] 50 mg horse gamma globulin/ mL	In 5 mL amps.

[a] With 0.3 M glycine.

LYMPHOCYTE IMMUNE GLOBULIN — INJECTION

For complete and comparative prescribing information, refer to the Immune Globulins group monograph.

WARNING

Only physicians experienced in immunosuppressive therapy in the treatment of renal transplant or aplastic anemia patients should use lymphocyte immune globulin.

Patients receiving lymphocyte immune globulin should be treated in facilities equipped and staffed with adequate laboratory and supportive medical resources.

Indications

➤*Renal transplantation:* For the management of allograft rejection in renal transplant patients. When administered with conventional therapy at the time of rejection, it increases the frequency of resolution of the acute rejection episode. The drug has also been administered as an adjunct to other immunosuppressive therapy to delay the onset of the first rejection episode. Data accumulated to date have not consistently demonstrated improvement in functional graft survival associated with therapy to delay the onset of the first rejection episode.

➤*Aplastic anemia:* For the treatment of moderate-to-severe aplastic anemia in patients who are unsuitable for bone marrow transplantation.

When administered with a regimen of supportive care, lymphocyte immune globulin may induce partial or complete hematologic remission. In a controlled trial, patients receiving lymphocyte immune globulin showed a statistically significantly higher improvement rate compared with standard supportive care at 3 months. Improvement was defined in terms of sustained increase in peripheral blood counts and reduced transfusion needs.

➤*Off-label uses:*

Multiple sclerosis – [5] = Poor documentation. Data evaluating the efficacy of lymphocyte immune globulin for the treatment of multiple sclerosis (MS) are dated. No new research in the area has been published in almost 30 years, and lymphocyte immune globulin is not included as a treatment option in American Academy of Neurology practice guidelines for MS. Its use in patients with MS is not recommended.

Other possible off-label uses – As an immunosuppressant in the course of liver, bone-marrow, heart, and other organ transplants; myasthenia gravis, pure red cell aplasia, and scleroderma, although efficacy is not definitively established.

Administration and Dosage

➤*General dosing considerations:* Exercise caution during repeat courses of lymphocyte immune globulin; carefully observe patients for signs of allergic reactions.

➤*Adults:*

Aplastic anemia –

Usual dosage: 10 to 20 mg/kg/day IV.

Duration of therapy: 8 to 14 days. Additional alternate-day therapy up to a total of 21 doses can be administered.

Concomitant therapy: Because thrombocytopenia can be associated with the administration of lymphocyte immune globulin, patients receiving it for the treatment of aplastic anemia may need prophylactic platelet transfusions to maintain platelets at clinically acceptable levels.

Renal transplantation – Adult renal allograft patients have received lymphocyte immune globulin at the dosage of 10 to 30 mg/kg IV daily.

Delaying the onset of allograft rejection: 15 mg/kg/day IV for 14 days, then every other day for 14 days for a total of 21 doses in 28 days. Administer the first dose within 24 hours before or after the transplant.

Treatment of rejection: 10 to 15 mg/kg/day IV for 14 days. Additional alternate-day therapy up to a total of 21 doses can be given. The first dose of lymphocyte immune globulin can be delayed until the diagnosis of the first rejection episode.

Concomitant therapy: Usually, lymphocyte immune globulin is used concomitantly with azathioprine and corticosteroids, which are commonly used to suppress the immune response.

➤*Children:*

Aplastic anemia – See Adults for dosing.

Renal transplantation – The few children studied received 5 to 25 mg/kg daily.

See Adults for dosing.

➤*Skin testing:* Before the first infusion of lymphocyte immune globulin, the manufacturer strongly recommends that patients be tested with an intradermal injection of 0.1 mL of a 1:1000 dilution (5 mcg horse IgG) of lymphocyte immune globulin in sodium chloride injection and a contralateral sodium chloride injection control. Use only freshly diluted lymphocyte immune globulin for skin testing. The patient, and specifically the skin test, should be observed every 15 to 20 minutes over the first hour after intradermal injection. A local reaction of greater than or equal to 10 mm with a wheal or erythema, or both, with or without pseudopod formation and itching or a marked local swelling should be considered a positive test.

A systemic reaction such as a generalized rash, tachycardia, dyspnea, hypotension, or anaphylaxis precludes any additional administration of lymphocyte immune globulin.

The predictive value of this test has not been proved clinically. Allergic reactions, such as anaphylaxis, have occurred in patients whose skin test is negative. In the presence of a locally positive skin test to lymphocyte immune globulin, serious consideration to alternative forms of therapy should be given. The risk-to-benefit ratio must be carefully weighed. If therapy with lymphocyte immune globulin is deemed appropriate following a locally positive skin test, treatment should be administered in a setting where intensive life support facilities are immediately available and with a physician familiar with the treatment of potentially life-threatening allergic reactions in attendance.

➤*Discontinuation of therapy:* Discontinue treatment with lymphocyte immune globulin if symptoms of anaphylaxis or severe and unremitting thrombocytopenia and/or leukopenia in renal transplant patients occur.

➤*Preparation for administration:* Lymphocyte immune globulin is a gamma globulin product and it can be transparent to slightly opalescent, colorless to faintly pink or brown, and may develop a slight granular or flaky deposit during storage. Lymphocyte immune globulin (diluted or undiluted) should not be shaken because excessive foaming or denaturation of the protein may occur.

Dilute lymphocyte immune globulin for intravenous (IV) infusion in an inverted bottle of sterile vehicle so the undiluted lymphocyte immune globulin does not contact the air inside. Add the total daily dose of lymphocyte immune globulin to the sterile vehicle (see Admixture Compatibility). The concentration should not exceed 4 mg of lymphocyte immune globulin per mL. The diluted solution should be gently rotated or swirled to effect thorough mixing.

➤*Administration:* The diluted lymphocyte immune globulin should be allowed to reach room temperature before infusion.

Lymphocyte immune globulin is appropriately administered IV into a vascular shunt, arterial venous fistula, or a high-flow central vein through an in-line filter with a pore size of 0.2 to 1 micron. The in-line filter should be used with all infusions of lymphocyte immune globulin to prevent the administration of any insoluble material that may develop in the product during storage. The use of high-flow veins will minimize the occurrence of phlebitis and thrombosis.

Do not infuse a dose of lymphocyte immune globulin in less than 4 hours.

LYMPHOCYTE IMMUNE GLOBULIN — INJECTION

Infusion reactions – Any severe systemic reaction to the skin test, such as generalized rash, tachycardia, dyspnea, hypotension, or anaphylaxis, should preclude further therapy.

Always keep appropriate resuscitation equipment at the patient's bedside while lymphocyte immune globulin is being administered. Observe the patient continuously for possible allergic reactions throughout the infusions.

➤*Admixture compatibility:*

Compatibility – Lymphocyte immune globulin, once diluted, has been shown to be physically and chemically stable for up to 24 hours at concentrations of up to 4 mg/mL in the following diluents: sodium chloride 0.9% injection, dextrose 5% and sodium chloride 0.225% injection, and dextrose 5% and sodium chloride 0.45% injection.

Incompatibility – Adding lymphocyte immune globulin to dextrose injection is not recommended because low salt concentrations can cause precipitation. Highly acidic infusion solutions can also contribute to physical instability over time.

➤*Storage/Stability:* Store in a refrigerator at 2° to 8°C (36° to 46°F). Do not freeze.

Diluted lymphocyte immune globulin should be stored in a refrigerator if it is prepared prior to the time of infusion. Even if it is stored in a refrigerator, the total time in dilution should not exceed 24 hours (including infusion time).

ANTITHYMOCYTE GLOBULIN (RABBIT) (ATG Rabbit)

Rx	Thymoglobulin (SangStat)	Powder for Injection, lyophilized[a]: 25 mg	In 7 mL vials with 5 mL vial of diluent.

[a] 50 mg glycine, 50 mg mannitol, 10 mg NaCl.

ANTITHYMOCYTE GLOBULIN (RABBIT) — INJECTION

For complete and comparative prescribing information, refer to the Immune Globulins group monograph.

WARNING

Anti-thymocyte globulin should only be used by physicians experienced in immunosuppressive therapy for the management of renal transplant patients.

Indications

➤*Acute renal transplant rejection:* For the treatment of renal transplant acute rejection in conjunction with concomitant immunosuppression.

➤*Off-label uses:* Treatment of refractory aplastic anemia; prophylaxis and treatment of acute allograft rejection in renal-pancreatic, liver, cardiac, renal, and lung transplantation; treatment of refractory graft-vs-host disease (GVHD) in allogeneic bone marrow transplantation; prophylaxis of GVHD in allogeneic bone marrow transplantation; allogeneic bone marrow transplantation.

Administration and Dosage

➤*General dosing considerations:* Premedication may reduce the incidence and intensity of side effects during the infusion. (See Premedication.)

Overdosage of anti-thymocyte globulin may result in leukopenia or thrombocytopenia. (See Dosage Adjustment.)

➤*Adults:*

Acute renal transplant rejection –

Usual dosage: 1.5 mg/kg intravenously (IV) daily for 7 to 14 days.

Dosage adjustment: The anti-thymocyte globulin dose should be reduced by one-half if the white blood cell (WBC) count is between 2,000 and 3,000 cells/mm^3 or if the platelet count is between 50,000 and 75,000 cells/mm^3. Stopping anti-thymocyte globulin treatment should be considered if the WBC count falls below 2,000 cells/mm^3 or platelets below 50,000 cells/mm^3.

Concomitant therapy: Administration of antiviral prophylactic therapy is recommended.

➤*Premedication:* Premedication with corticosteroids, acetaminophen, or an antihistamine 1 hour prior to the infusion is recommended. Medical personnel should monitor patients for adverse events during and after infusion.

➤*Monitoring:* Monitoring T-cell counts (absolute or subsets) to assess the level of T-cell depletion is recommended. Total WBC and platelet counts should be monitored.

➤*Preparation for administration:*

Reconstitution –

Allow anti-thymocyte globulin and supplied diluent (sterile water for injection) vials to reach room temperature before reconstituting the lyophilized product. Aseptically remove caps and tabs of the aluminum seals to expose rubber stoppers. Clean stoppers with germicidal or alcohol swab. Aseptically remove 5 mL of diluent (sterile water for injection) using a sterile, single-use syringe and inject it slowly into the vial containing anti-thymocyte globulin lyophilized powder. Reconstitute each vial of anti-thymocyte globulin lyophilized powder with 5 mL of sterile diluent. Rotate vial gently until powder is completely dissolved. Each reconstituted vial contains 25 mg or 5 mg/mL of anti-thymocyte globulin. Anti-thymocyte globulin should be used within 4 hours after reconstitution if kept at room temperature.

Inspect solution for particulate matter after reconstitution. Should some particulate matter remain, continue to gently rotate the vial until no particulate matter is visible. If particulate matter persists, discard this vial.

Dilution – Transfer the contents of the calculated number of anti-thymocyte globulin vials into the bag of infusion solution (saline or dextrose). Use 50 mL of infusion solution Per 1 vial of anti-thymocyte globulin (total volume usually between 50 to 500 mL). Mix the solution by inverting the bag gently only once or twice.

➤*Administration:* The recommended route of administration is IV infusion using a high-flow vein. Anti-thymocyte globulin should be infused over a minimum of 6 hours for the first infusion and over at least 4 hours on subsequent days of therapy. Anti-thymocyte globulin should be administered through an in-line 0.22 mcm filter.

➤*Storage/Stability:* Store in refrigerator between 2° to 8°C (36° to 46°F). Protect from light. Do not freeze. Reconstituted vials of anti-thymocyte globulin should be used within 4 hours. Infusion solutions of anti-thymocyte globulin must be used immediately. Any unused drug remaining after infusion must be discarded.

RABIES IMMUNE GLOBULIN HUMAN (RIGH)

Rx	HyperRab S/D[a] (Talecris Biotherapeutics)	Injection: 150 units/mL	In 2 and 10 mL single-dose vials.
Rx	Imogam Rabies–HT[b] (Sanofi Pasteur)		In 2 and 10 mL vials.

[a] Preservative free. With 0.21 to 0.32 M glycine. Solvent/Detergent treated.

[b] Preservative free. With 0.3 M glycine. Heat treated.

RABIES IMMUNE GLOBULIN HUMAN — INJECTION

For complete and comparative prescribing information, refer to the general discussion for Rabies Prophylaxis in the Treatment Guidelines section of the Appendix.

Indications

➤*Rabies exposure:* For persons suspected of exposure to rabies, particularly severe exposure, with one exception: persons who have been previously immunized with rabies vaccine prepared from human diploid cells (HDCV) in a preexposure or postexposure treatment series should receive only vaccine. Persons who have been previously immunized with rabies vaccine other than HDCV, rabies vaccine adsorbed (RVA), or purified chick embryo cell vaccine (PCEC) vaccines should have confirmed adequate rabies antibody titers if they are to receive only vaccine.

Inject rabies immunoglobulin as promptly as possible after exposure, along with the first dose of vaccine. If initiation of treatment is delayed for any reason, rabies immune globulin, human (RIGH) and the first dose of vaccine should still be given, regardless of the interval between exposure and treatment. RIGH may be given up to 8 days after the first dose of vaccine was given.

Rabies virus is usually transmitted by the bite of a rabid animal (eg, dog, bat) but can occasionally penetrate abraded skin contaminated with the saliva of infected animals. Progress of the virus after exposure is believed to follow a neural pathway, and the time between exposure and clinical rabies is a function of the proximity of the bite (or abrasion) to the CNS and the dose of virus injected. The incubation is usually 2 to 6 weeks but can be longer. After severe bites about the face and neck and arms, it may be as short as 10 days. After initiation of the vaccine series (human diploid cell origin), it takes approximately 1 week for development of immunity to rabies; therefore, the value of immediate passive immunization with rabies antibodies in the form of RIGH cannot be overemphasized.

Recommendations for use of passive and active immunization after exposure to an animal suspected of having rabies have been detailed by the US Public Health Service Advisory Committee on Immunization Practices (ACIP).

Each exposure to possible rabies infection must be individually evaluated. Local or state public health officials should be consulted if questions arise about the need for rabies prophylaxis.

➤*Rationale of treatment:* In the United States and Canada, the following factors should be considered before specific antirabies treatment is indicated:

Species of biting animal – Carnivorous animals (especially skunks, foxes, coyotes, raccoons, dogs, bobcats, and cats) and bats are the animals most commonly infected with rabies and have caused most of the indigenous cases of human rabies in the United States since 1960. Unless the animal is tested and shown not to be rabid, postexposure prophylaxis should be initiated upon bite or nonbite exposure to these animals. If treatment has been initiated and subsequent testing in a competent laboratory shows the exposing animal is not rabid, treatment can be discontinued.

RABIES IMMUNE GLOBULIN HUMAN — INJECTION

Rats, mice, squirrels, hamsters, guinea pigs, gerbils, chipmunks, and other rodents, or rabbits and hares are rarely infected with rabies and have not been known to cause human rabies in the United States. Their bites almost never call for antirabies prophylaxis; therefore, before initiating antirabies prophylaxis, the local or state health department should be consulted.

However, from 1971 through 1988, woodchucks accounted for 70% of the 179 cases of rabies among rodents reported to Centers for Disease Control and Prevention. In these cases, the state or local health department should be consulted before a decision is made to initiate postexposure antirabies prophylaxis.

Because some bat bites may be less severe, and, therefore, more difficult to recognize, rabies postexposure treatment should be considered for any physical contact with bats when bite or mucous membrane contact cannot be excluded.

In the United States, the likelihood that a domestic dog or cat is infected with rabies varies from region to region; hence, the need for postexposure prophylaxis also varies. However, in most of Asia and all of Africa and Latin American, the dog remains the major source of human exposure; exposures to dogs in such countries represent a special threat. Travelers to those countries should be aware that more than 50% of the rabies cases among humans in the United States result from exposure to dogs outside the United States.

Circumstances of biting incident – An unprovoked attack is more likely than a provoked attack to mean that the animal is rabid. Bites during attempts to feed or handle an apparently healthy animal may generally be regarded as provoked.

Type of exposure – Rabies is commonly transmitted by inoculation with infectious saliva. Rabies is transmitted only when the virus is introduced into open cuts or wounds in skin or mucous membranes. If there has been no exposure (as described in this section), postexposure treatment is not necessary. Thus, the likelihood that rabies infection will result from exposure to a rabid animal varies with the nature and extent of the exposure. Two categories and exposure should be considered:

Bite: Any penetration of the skin by teeth. Bites to the face and hands carry the highest risk, but the site of the bite should not influence the decision to begin treatment.

Bat-associated strains of rabies can be transmitted to humans either directly through a bat's bite or indirectly through the bite of an animal previously infected by a bat. Because some bat bites may be less severe and can go completely undetected, unlike bites inflicted by larger animals, especially mammalian carnivores, rabies postexposure treatment should be considered for any physical contact with bats when bite or mucous membrane contact cannot be excluded.

Nonbite: Scratches, abrasions, open wounds, or mucous membranes contaminated with saliva or any potentially infectious material, such as brain tissue, from a rabid animal constitute nonbite exposures. If the material containing the virus is dry, the virus can be considered noninfectious.

In addition, 2 cases of rabies have been attributed to airborne exposures in laboratories and 2 cases of rabies have been attributed to probable exposures to a bat-infested cave (Frio Cave, Texas). Casual contact, such as petting a rabid animal (without a bite or nonbite exposure as previously described) and contact with blood, urine, or feces (eg, guano) of a rabid animal, does not constitute an exposure and is not an indication for prophylaxis. Instances of airborne rabies have been reported rarely. Adherence to respiratory precautions will minimize the risk of airborne exposure.

The only documented cases of rabies caused by human-to-human transmission have occurred in patients who received corneas transplanted from persons who died of rabies undiagnosed at the time of death. Stringent guidelines for acceptance of donor corneas have reduced this risk.

Bite and nonbite exposures from humans with rabies theoretically could transmit rabies, although no cases of rabies acquired this way have been documented.

➤*Vaccination status of biting animal:* A properly immunized animal has only a minimal chance of developing rabies and transmitting the virus.

➤*Presence of rabies in region:* If adequate laboratory and field records indicate that there is no rabies infection in a domestic species within a given region, local health officials are justified in considering this in making recommendations on antirabies treatment following a bite by that particular species. Such officials should be consulted for current interpretations.

➤*Local treatment of wounds:* Immediate and thorough local treatment of all bite wounds and scratches is perhaps the most effective preventive measure. The wound should be thoroughly cleansed with soap and water immediately. In experimental animals, simple local wound cleansing has been shown to reduce markedly the likelihood of rabies. Give tetanus prophylaxisand measures to control bacterial infection as indicated.

Active immunization – Active immunization should be initiated as soon as possible after exposure (within 24 hours). Many dosage schedules have been evaluated for the currently available rabies vaccines, and their respective manufacturers' literature should be consulted.

Passive immunization – A combination of active and passive immunization (vaccine and immune globulin) is considered the acceptable postexposure prophylaxis except for those persons who have been previously immunized with rabies vaccine and who have documented adequate rabies antibody titer. These persons should receive vaccine only. For passive immunization, RIGH is preferred over antirabies serum, equine. It is recommended both for treatment of all bites by animals suspected of having rabies and for nonbite exposure inflicted by animals suspected of being rabid. RIGH should be used in conjunction with rabies vaccine and can be administered through the seventh day after the first dose of vaccine is given. Beyond the seventh day, RIGH is not indicated because an antibody response to cell culture vaccine is presumed to have occurred.

➤*Specific treatment:* Postexposure antirabies vaccination with rabies vaccine should be accompanied by administration of rabies immune globulin. However, persons who have previously received complete vaccination regimens (preexposure or postexposure) with a cell culture vaccine or persons who have been vaccinated with other types of vaccines and have had documented rabies antibody titers should receive vaccine alone. The combination of rabies immune globulin and vaccine is recommended for both bite exposures and nonbite exposures, regardless of the interval between exposure and initiation of treatment.

➤*Postexposure treatment guide:* The following recommendations are only a guide. They should be applied in conjunction with knowledge of the animal species involved, circumstances of the bite or other exposure, vaccination status of the animal, and presence of rabies in the region. Consult local and state public health officials if questions arise about the need for rabies prophylaxis.

Rabies Postexposure ProphylaxisGuide, United States, 1999

Animal type	Evaluation and disposition of animal	Postexposure prophylaxis recommendations
Dogs, cats, and ferrets	Healthy and available for 10 days of observation	Persons should not begin prophylaxis unless animal develops clinical signs of rabies.[a]
	Rabid or suspected rabid	Immediately vaccinate.
	Unknown (eg, escaped)	Consult public health officials.
Skunks, raccoons, foxes, and most other carnivores; bats	Regarded as rabid unless animal proven negative by laboratory tests[b]	Consider immediate vaccination.
Livestock, small rodents, lagomorphs (rabbits and hares), large rodents (woodchucks and beavers), and other mammals	Consider individually.	Consult public health officials. Bites of squirrels, hamsters, guinea pigs, gerbils, chipmunks, rats, mice, other small rodents, rabbits, and hares almost never require antirabies postexposure prophylaxis.

[a] During the 10-day observation period, begin postexposure prophylaxis at the first sign of rabies in a dog, cat, or ferret that has bitten someone. If the animal exhibits clinical signs of rabies, it should be euthanized immediately and tested.

[b] The animal should be euthanized and tested as soon as possible. Holding for observation is not recommended. Discontinue vaccine if immunofluorescence test results of the animal are negative.

Administration and Dosage

➤*General dosing considerations:* All postexposure treatment should begin with immediate, thorough cleansing of all wounds with soap and water. If available, a virucidal agent, such as a povidone-iodine solution, should be used to irrigate the wounds.

➤*Adults:*

Rabies prophylaxis (postexposure) –

Usual dosage:

Rabies Postexposure Prophylaxis Schedule, United States 1999

Vaccination status	Treatment	Regimen[a]
Not previously vaccinated	Wound cleansing	All postexposure treatment should begin with immediate thorough cleansing of all wounds with soap and water. If available, a virucidal agent such as a povidone-iodine solution should be used to irrigate the wounds.
	RIGH	Administer 20 units/kg body weight. If anatomically feasible, the full dose should be infiltrated around the wound(s) and any remaining volume should be administered IM[b] at an anatomical site distant from vaccine administration. Also, RIGH should not be administered in the same syringe as vaccine. Because RIGH might partially suppress active production of antibody, no more than the recommended dose should be given.
	Vaccine	HDCV, RVA, or PCEC 1 mL, IM (deltoid area[c]), 1 each on days 0,[d] 3, 7, 14, and 28
Previously vaccinated[e]	Wound cleansing	All postexposure treatment should begin with immediate thorough cleansing of all wounds with soap and water. If available, a virucidal agent such as a povidone-iodine solution should be used to irrigate the wounds.
	RIGH	RIGH should not be administered.
	Vaccine	HDCV, RVA, or PCEC 1 mL, IM (deltoid area[c]), 1 each on days 0[d] and 3

[a] These regimens are applicable for all age groups, including children.

[b] IM = intramuscular.

[c] The deltoid area is the only acceptable site of vaccination for adults and older children. For younger children, the outer aspect of the thigh may be used. Vaccine should never be administered in the gluteal area.

[d] Day 0 is the day the first dose of vaccine is administered.

[e] Any person with a history of preexposure vaccination with HDCV, RVA, or PCEC; prior postexposure prophylaxis with HDCV, RVA, or PCEC; or previous vaccination with any other type of rabies vaccine and a documented history of antibody response to the prior vaccination.

RABIES IMMUNE GLOBULIN HUMAN — INJECTION

Maximum dose: 20 units/kg (0.133 mL/kg) according to the prescribing information.

➤*Children:*

Rabies prophylaxis (postexposure) –

HyperRab S/D: Safety and efficacy of *HyperRab S/D* in children have not been established.

Imogam Rabies-HT: See Adults for dosing for *Imogam Rabies-HT*.

➤*Administration:* RIGH should never be administered in the same syringe or into the same anatomical site as vaccine.

If anatomically feasible, up to the full dose of RIGH should be thoroughly infiltrated in the area around the wound, and the rest should be administered IM in the gluteal area or lateral thigh muscle. Because of risk of injury to the sciatic nerve, the central region of the gluteal area must be avoided; only the upper, outer quadrant should be used.

Do not administer RIGH intravenously because of the potential for serious reactions. Inject IM, and take care to draw back on the plunger of the syringe before injection in order to be certain that the needle is not in a blood vessel.

➤*Storage/Stability:* Store between 2° and 8°C (35° and 46°F). Do not freeze. Solution that has been frozen should not be used.

RIGH contains no preservative, and unused portion must be discarded immediately.

Rh_o(D) IMMUNE GLOBULIN

Rx	**HyperRHO S/D Full Dose** (Talecris Biotherapeutics)	**Injection (intramuscular), solution**: 15% to 18% protein (≥ 1,500 units)	Preservative free. In prefilled single-dose syringes with attached needles. In 1s.[a]
Rx	**RhoGAM Ultra Filtered Plus** (Ortho-Clinical Diagnostics)	**Injection (intramuscular), solution**: 300 mcg (1,500 units)	Preservative free. In packages with prefilled single-dose syringes, control form, and patient ID card. In 1s, 5s, and 25s.[b]
Rx	**Rhophylac** (CSL Behring)	**Injection (intravenous), solution**: 1,500 units (300 mcg)	Glycine, sodium chloride. Preservative free. In 2 mL prefilled syringes.
Rx	**WinRho SDF** (Cangene Biopharma)	**Injection (intravenous), solution**: 1,500 units (300 mcg)	Polysorbate 80. Preservative free. In single-dose vials.[c]
		2,500 units (500 mcg)	Polysorbate 80. Preservative free. In single-dose vials.[c]
		5,000 units (1,000 mcg)	Polysorbate 80. Preservative free. In single-dose vials.[c]
		15,000 units (3,000 mcg)	Polysorbate 80. Preservative free. In single-dose vials.[c]
Rx	**HyperRHO** S/D Mini-Dose (Talecris Biotherapeutics)	**Injection, solution**: 15% to 18% protein (≥ 250 units)	Preservative free. In prefilled single-dose syringes with attached needles. In 10s.[d]
Rx	**MICRhoGAM** Ultra-Filtered Plus (Ortho-Clinical Diagnostics)	**Injection, solution**: 50 mcg (250 units/dose)	Preservative free. In packages with prefilled single-dose syringes, control form, and patient ID card. In 1s, 5s, and 25s.[e]

[a] With glycine 0.21 to 0.32 M. Solvent/detergent treated.
[b] With sodium chloride 2.9 mg/mL, 0.01% polysorbate 80, glycine 15 mg/mL. 1 mcg of Rh_o(D) immune globulin = 5 units.
[c] Contains maltose 10% and 0.03% polysorbate 80.
[d] With glycine 0.21 to 0.32 M. Solvent/detergent treated.
[e] With sodium chloride 2.9 mg/mL, polysorbate 80 0.01%, glycine 15 mg/mL. Rh_o(D) immune globulin 1 mcg = 5 units.

RH_o(D) IMMUNE GLOBULIN (HUMAN) — INTRAMUSCULAR (Rh_o[D] IGIM)

For complete and comparative prescribing information, refer to the Immune Globulins group monograph.

Indications

➤*Pregnancy/Obstetric conditions:*

HyperRHO S/D Full Dose – For the prevention of Rh hemolytic disease of the newborn by its administration to the Rh_o(D)–negative mother within 72 hours of the birth of an Rh_o(D)–positive infant, provided the following criteria are met: the mother is Rh_o(D) negative and not already sensitized to the Rh_o(D) factor, and her child is Rh_o(D) positive and has a negative direct antiglobulin test.

If administered antepartum, the mother must receive another dose after delivery of an Rh_o(D)–positive infant.

If the father can be determined to be Rh_o(D) negative, Rh_o(D) immune globulin does not need to be given.

Administer Rh_o(D) immune globulin within 72 hours to all nonimmunized Rh_o(D)–negative women who have undergone spontaneous or induced abortion following ruptured tubal pregnancy, amniocentesis, or abdominal trauma, unless the blood group of the fetus or the father is known to be Rh_o(D) negative. If the fetal blood group cannot be determined, assume that it is Rh_o(D) positive and administer Rh_o(D) immune globulin to the mother.

RhoGAM Ultra Filtered Plus – For administration to Rh-negative women not previously sensitized to the Rh_o(D) factor, unless the father or baby are conclusively Rh negative, in the following situations: delivery of an Rh-positive baby irrespective of the ABO groups of the mother and baby; antepartum prophylaxis at 26 to 28 weeks of gestation; antepartum fetomaternal hemorrhage (suspected or proven) as a result of placenta previa, amniocentesis, chorionic villus sampling (CVS), percutaneous umbilical blood sampling, other obstetrical manipulative procedure (eg, version), or abdominal trauma; actual or threatened pregnancy loss at any stage of gestation; ectopic pregnancy.

➤*Transfusion:* To prevent Rh immunization in any Rh_o(D)–negative individual after incompatible transfusion of Rh-positive blood or blood products (eg, red blood cells [RBCs], platelet or granulocyte concentrates).

➤*Off-label uses:* Although controversial, some health care providers advocate administration prior to external version attempts for breech presentations (because of induced fetomaternal hemorrhage) and following tubal ligation after delivery of an Rh_o(D)–positive infant (to prevent problems should the sterilization fail or subsequent tubal reanastomoses occur).

Administration and Dosage

➤*General dosing considerations:*

Fetomaternal hemorrhage – Multiple doses are required if a fetomaternal hemorrhage exceeds 15 mL, an event that is possible, but unlikely, prior to the third trimester of pregnancy and is most likely at delivery.

To maintain an adequate level of anti-D, Rho(D) immune globulin should be administered every 12 weeks. (See Administration.)

➤*Adults:*

Pregnancy/Obstetric conditions –

Abdominal trauma (in second or third trimester):

• *Usual dosage* – Following amniocentesis at either 13 to 18 weeks of gestation or during the third trimester, abdominal trauma in the second or third trimester, obstetrical manipulation, CVS, or percutaneous umbilical blood sampling, administer 1 syringe (1,500 units) within 72 hours of suspected or proven exposure to Rh-positive RBCs.

• *Maintenance dosage* – If abdominal trauma, amniocentesis, or another adverse reaction requires the administration of Rho(D) immune globulin at 13 to 18 weeks of gestation, another dose should be given at 26 to 28 weeks of gestation.

To maintain protection throughout pregnancy, the level of passively acquired anti-Rho(D) should not be allowed to fall below the level required to prevent an immune response to Rh-positive RBCs.

• *Dosage adjustment* – If more than 15 mL of RBCs is suspected because of fetomaternal hemorrhage, the same dose modification as in postpartum prophylaxis applies.

• *Postpartum dose* – A dose of Rho(D) immune globulin should be given within 72 hours of delivery if the baby is Rh-positive. If delivery occurs within 3 weeks of the last dose, the postpartum dose may be withheld, unless there is a fetomaternal hemorrhage in excess of 15 mL of RBCs.

Amniocentesis, CVS, and percutaneous umbilical blood sampling: See Abdominal Trauma for dosing.

Antenatal prophylaxis: One syringe (1,500 units) is administered at approximately 26 to 28 weeks of gestation. This must be followed by another full dose, preferably within 72 hours of delivery, if the infant is Rh-positive.

Miscarriage, abortion, or termination of ectopic pregnancy:

• *Usual dosage* – Following miscarriage, abortion, or termination of ectopic pregnancy at or beyond 13 weeks of gestation, it is recommended that 1 syringe be given.

• *Dosage adjustment* – If more than 15 mL of RBCs is suspected because of fetomaternal hemorrhage, the same dose modification as in postpartum prophylaxis applies.

• *Alternative dosage* – If pregnancy is terminated prior to 13 weeks of gestation, where licensed, a single dose of Rho(D) immune globulin microdose may be used instead of Rho(D) immune globulin full dose.

Obstetrical manipulation: See Abdominal Trauma for dosing.

Postpartum prophylaxis:

• *Usual dosage* – Administer 1 syringe (1,500 units), preferably within 72 hours of delivery. Although a lesser degree of protection is afforded if Rh antibody is administered beyond the 72-hour period, Rho(D) immune globulin may still be given.

• *Dosage adjustment* – Full-term deliveries can vary in their dosage requirements depending on the magnitude of the fetomaternal hemorrhage. One full-dose syringe provides sufficient antibody to prevent Rh sensitization if the volume of RBCs that has entered the circulation is 15 mL or less.

In instances in which a large (more than 30 mL of whole blood or 15 mL of RBCs) fetomaternal hemorrhage is suspected, a fetal RBC count by an approved laboratory technique (eg, modified Kleihauer-Betke acid elution stain technique) should be performed to determine the dosage of immune globulin required.

Rh$_o$(D) IMMUNE GLOBULIN (HUMAN) — INTRAMUSCULAR (Rh$_o$[D] IGIM)

The RBC volume of the calculated fetomaternal hemorrhage is divided by 15 mL to obtain the number of syringes needed for administration. If more than 15 mL of RBCs is suspected or if the dose calculation results in a fraction, administer the next higher whole number of syringes (eg, if 1.4, give 2 syringes).

Multiple doses are required if a fetomaternal hemorrhage exceeds 15 mL, an event that is possible, but unlikely, prior to the third trimester of pregnancy and is most likely at delivery. Patients known or suspected to be at increased risk of fetomaternal hemorrhage should be tested for it by qualitative or quantitative methods.

In efficacy studies, Rho(D) immune globulin was shown to suppress Rh immunization in all subjects when given at a dose of at least 20 mcg/mL of Rh-positive RBCs. Thus, a single dose of Rho(D) immune globulin will suppress the immune response after exposure to 15 mL or less of Rh-positive RBCs. However, in clinical practice, laboratory methods used to determine the amount of exposure (volume of transfusion or fetomaternal hemorrhage) to Rh-positive RBCs are imprecise. Therefore, administration of more than 20 mcg of Rho(D) immune globulin per milliliter of Rh-positive RBCs should be considered whenever a large fetomaternal hemorrhage or RBC exposure is suspected or documented.

Threatened abortion:

• *Usual dosage* – Following threatened abortion at any stage of gestation with continuation of pregnancy, it is recommended that 1 syringe (1,500 units) be given.

• *Dosage adjustment* – If more than 15 mL of RBCs is suspected because of fetomaternal hemorrhage, the same dose modification as in postpartum prophylaxis applies.

Other FDA-approved uses –

Transfusions:

• *Usual dosage* – The volume of Rh-positive whole blood administered is multiplied by the hematocrit of the donor unit giving the volume of RBCs transfused. The volume of RBCs is divided by 15 mL, which provides the number of syringes of Rho(D) immune globulin to be administered. If the dose calculated results in a fraction, the next higher whole number of syringes should be administered (eg, if 1.4, give 2 syringes). Administer Rho(D) immune globulin within 72 hours of an incompatible transfusion, but preferably as soon as possible.

➤*Administration:* To maintain an adequate level of anti-D, Rho(D) immune globulin should be administered every 12 weeks. The exact timing for the injection is based on 12-week intervals starting from the administration of the first injection. If delivery of the baby does not occur 12 weeks after the administration of the standard antepartum dose (at 26 to 28 weeks), a second dose is recommended to maximize protection antepartum. If delivery occurs within 3 weeks of the last antepartum dose, the postpartum dose may be withheld, but a test for fetomaternal hemorrhage should be performed to determine if exposure to more than 15 mL of RBCs has occurred.

Never administer to the neonate. In the case of postpartum use, the product is intended for maternal administration.

Never administer Rho(D) immune globulin intravenously (IV).

Inject entire contents of the syringe intramuscularly (IM), preferably in the anterolateral aspects of the upper thigh and the deltoid muscle of the upper arm. The gluteal region should not be used routinely as an injection site because of the risk of injury to the sciatic nerve. If the gluteal region is used, the central region must be avoided; only the upper, outer quadrant should be used.

Syringe use –

Multilple-syringe dose: Multiple doses may be administered at the same time or at spaced intervals, as long as the total dose is administered within 3 days of exposure.

➤*Storage / Stability:* Store at 2° to 8°C (36° to 46°F). Do not freeze.

Rh$_o$(D) IMMUNE GLOBULIN — INTRAVENOUS (Rh$_o$[D] IGIV)

For complete and comparative prescribing information, refer to the Immune Globulins class monograph.

WARNING

Intravascular hemolysis – Intravascular hemolysis leading to death has been reported in patients treated for immune thrombocytopenic purpura (ITP) with Rh$_o$(D) immune globulin.

Intravascular hemolysis can lead to clinically compromising anemia and multisystem organ failure, including acute respiratory distress syndrome (ARDS).

Serious complications, including severe anemia, acute renal insufficiency, renal failure, and disseminated intravascular coagulation (DIC), have also been reported.

Closely monitor patients with ITP in a health care setting for at least 8 hours after administration. Perform a dipstick urinalysis at baseline, 2 and 4 hours after administration, and prior to the end of the monitoring period. Alert patients and monitor for signs and symptoms of intravascular hemolysis, including back pain, shaking chills, fever, and discolored urine or hematuria. Absence of these signs and/or symptoms of intravascular hemolysis within 8 hours do not indicate intravascular hemolysis cannot occur subsequently. If signs and/or symptoms of intravascular hemolysis are present or suspected after administration, perform posttreatment laboratory tests, including plasma hemoglobin (Hb), haptoglobin, lactate dehydrogenase (LDH), and plasma bilirubin (direct and indirect).

Indications

➤*Immune thrombocytopenic purpura:*

Rhophylac – In the treatment of Rh$_o$(D)-positive, nonsplenectomized adults with chronic ITP to raise platelet counts.

WinRho SDF – In the treatment of nonsplenectomized, Rh$_o$(D)-positive children with long-term or acute ITP, adults with long-term ITP, or children and adults with ITP secondary to HIV infection.

➤*Suppression of Rh isoimmunization:*

Pregnancy and obstetric conditions –

Rhophylac: For suppression of Rh isoimmunization in nonsensitized Rh$_o$(D)-negative women with an Rh-incompatible pregnancy, including routine antepartum and postpartum Rh prophylaxis, and Rh prophylaxis in cases of obstetric complications (eg, miscarriage, abortion, threatened abortion, ectopic pregnancy or hydatidiform mole, transplacental hemorrhage resulting from antepartum hemorrhage), invasive procedures during pregnancy (eg, amniocentesis, chorionic biopsy), or obstetric manipulative procedures (eg, external version, abdominal trauma).

WinRho SDF: For the suppression of Rh isoimmunization in nonsensitized Rh$_o$(D)-negative women within 72 hours after spontaneous or induced abortions, amniocentesis, chorionic villus sampling, ruptured tubal pregnancy, abdominal trauma or transplacental hemorrhage, or in the normal course of pregnancy, unless the blood type of the fetus or father is known to be Rh$_o$(D)-negative.

Transfusion –

Rhophylac: For the suppression of Rh isoimmunization in Rh$_o$(D)-negative individuals transfused with Rh$_o$(D)-positive red blood cells (RBCs) or blood components containing Rh$_o$(D)-positive RBCs.

WinRho SDF: For the suppression of Rh isoimmunization in Rh$_o$(D)-negative female children and women in their childbearing years transfused with Rh$_o$(D)-positive RBCs or blood components containing Rh$_o$(D)-positive RBCs.

Administration and Dosage

➤*Adults:*

Immune thrombocytopenic purpura –

Rhophylac: 250 units (50 mcg) per kg as a single intravenous (IV) injection at a rate of 2 mL per 15 to 60 seconds.

WinRho SDF:

• *Initial dosage* – 250 units (50 mcg) per kg body weight given as a single IV injection after confirming that the patient is Rh$_o$(D)-positive. The initial dose may be administered in 2 divided doses given on separate days, if desired.

• *Maintenance dosage –*

Response to initial dose: If the patient responded to initial dose with a satisfactory increase in platelets, maintenance therapy is 125 to 300 units/kg (25 to 60 mcg/kg), individualized based on platelet and Hb levels.

No response to initial dose: If no response to initial dose, administer a subsequent dose based on Hb. If Hb is between 8 and 10 g/dL, redose between 125 and 200 units/kg (25 to 40 mcg/kg). If Hb is more than 10 g/dL, redose between 250 and 300 units/kg (50 to 60 mcg/kg). If Hb is less than 8 g/dL, alternative treatments should be used. Safety and efficacy of doses exceeding 300 units/kg (60 mcg/kg) have not been established.

• *Dosage adjustment* – If Hb level is less than 10 g/dL, a reduced dose of 125 to 200 units/kg (25 to 40 mcg/kg) should be given to minimize the risk of increasing the severity of anemia in the patient.

• *Subsequent dosage* – If subsequent therapy is required to elevate platelet counts, an IV dose of 125 to 300 units per kg (25 to 60 mcg/kg) body weight is recommended.

Suppression of Rh isoimmunization –

Rhophylac:

***Rhophylac* Dosing Guidelines for Obstetric Conditions**

Indication	Timing of administration	Dose[a] (administer by IM[b] or IV injection)
Routine antepartum prophylaxis	At weeks 28 to 30 of gestation	1,500 units (300 mcg)
Postpartum prophylaxis (required only if the newborn is Rh$_o$[D]-positive)	Within 72 hours of birth	1,500 units (300 mcg)[c]
Obstetric complications (eg, miscarriage, abortion, threatened abortion, ectopic pregnancy or hydatidiform mole, transplacental hemorrhage resulting from antepartum hemorrhage)	Within 72 hours of complication	1,500 units (300 mcg)[c]

Rh_o(D) IMMUNE GLOBULIN — INTRAVENOUS (Rh_o[D] IGIV)

Rhophylac Dosing Guidelines for Obstetric Conditions		
Indication	Timing of administration	Dose[a] (administer by IM[b] or IV injection)
Invasive procedures during pregnancy (eg, amniocentesis, chorionic biopsy) or obstetric manipulative procedures (eg, external version, abdominal trauma)	Within 72 hours of procedure	1,500 units (300 mcg)[c]
Excessive fetomaternal hemorrhage (> 15 mL)	Within 72 hours of complication	1,500 units (300 mcg) plus: 100 units (20 mcg) per mL fetal RBCs in excess of 15 mL if excess transplacental bleeding is quantified, or an additional 1,500 unit (300 mcg) dose if excess transplacental bleeding cannot be quantified

[a] A 1,500 unit (300 mcg) dose of *Rhophylac* will suppress the immunizing potential of ≥ 15 mL of Rh_o(D)-positive RBCs.
[b] IM = intramuscular.
[c] The dose of *Rhophylac* must be increased if the patient is exposed to > 15 mL of Rh_o(D)-positive RBCs; in this case, follow the dosing guidelines for excessive fetomaternal hemorrhage.

WinRho SDF:

WinRho SDF Dosing Guidelines for Obstetric Conditions		
Indication	Timing of administration	Dose (administer IM or IV)
Routine antepartum prophylaxis	28 weeks' gestation[a]	1,500 units (300 mcg)
Postpartum (if newborn Rh_o[D]-positive)	Within 72 hours of birth[b]	600 units (120 mcg)
Threatened abortion at any time	Immediately	1,500 units (300 mcg)
Amniocentesis and chorionic villus sampling before 34 weeks' gestation	Immediately after procedure[c]	1,500 units (300 mcg)
Abortion, amniocentesis, or any other manipulation after 34 weeks' gestation	Within 72 hours	600 units (120 mcg)

[a] If *WinRho SDF* is administered early in the pregnancy, it is recommended that *WinRho SDF* be administered at 12-week intervals in order to maintain adequate levels of passively acquired anti-Rh.
[b] In the event the Rh status of the baby is not known at 72 hours, *WinRho SDF* should be administered to the mother 72 hours after delivery. If > 72 hours have elapsed, *WinRho SDF* should not be withheld; administer as soon as possible up to 28 days after delivery.
[c] Repeat every 12 weeks during pregnancy.

Transfusion –

Rhophylac: 100 units (200 mcg) IV or IM per 2 mL transfused blood or per 1 mL erythrocyte concentrate. Administer within 72 hours of exposure.

WinRho SDF: Administer within 72 hours after exposure for treatment of incompatible blood transfusions or massive fetal hemorrhage.

Recommended Dose of *WinRho SDF* for Transfusions		
	WinRho SDF dose	
Route of administration	If exposed to Rh_o(D)-positive whole blood	If exposed to Rh_o(D)-positive RBCs
IV[a]	45 units (9 mcg)/mL blood	90 units (18 mcg)/mL cells
IM[b]	60 units (12 mcg)/mL blood	120 units (24 mcg)/mL cells

[a] Administer 3,000 units (600 mcg) every 8 hours via the IV route until the total dose, calculated from the previous table, is administered.
[b] Administer 6,000 units (1,200 mcg) every 12 hours via the IM route until the total dose, calculated from the previous table, is administered.

➤*Children:*

Immune thrombocytopenic purpura –

WinRho SDF: See Adults for dosing.

Transfusion –

WinRho SDF: See Adults for dosing.

➤*Renal function impairment:* Use with caution. May require infusion rate reduction or discontinuation.

➤*Preparation for administration:*

Rhophylac – Bring to room temperature before use.

WinRho SDF –

The entire contents of the vial should be removed to obtain the labeled dosage. If partial vials are required for dosage calculation, the entire contents of the vial should be withdrawn to ensure accurate calculation of the dosage requirement.

➤*Administration:* As with all blood products, patients should be observed for at least 20 minutes following administration.

Rhophylac –

ITP: Administer by the IV route only at a rate of 2 mL per 15 to 60 seconds.

Suppression of Rh isoimmunization: May be administered by IM or IV injection.

If large doses (more than 5 mL) are required and IM injection is chosen, it is advisable to administer in divided doses at different sites.

WinRho SDF –

IV administration: The entire dose may be injected into a suitable vein as rapidly as over 3 to 5 minutes.

IM administration: Administer into the deltoid muscle of the upper arm or the anterolateral aspects of the upper thigh. Because of the risk of sciatic nerve injury, the gluteal region should not be used as a routine injection site. If the gluteal region is used, use only the upper, outer quadrant.

➤*Admixture compatibility:* Administer *WinRho SDF* separately from other drugs.

➤*Storage / Stability:* Store at 2° to 8°C (36° to 46°F). Discard any unused portion. Do not freeze. Keep *Rhophylac* in original carton to protect from light.

Rh_o(D) IMMUNE GLOBULIN MICRODOSE — INJECTION

For complete and comparative prescribing information, refer to the Immune Globulins group monograph.

Indications

➤*Pregnancy / Obstetric conditions:* For the prevention of isoimmunization of Rh_o(D)–negative women at the time of spontaneous or induced abortion of up to 12 weeks of gestation, provided the following criteria are met: the mother is Rh_o(D) negative and not already sensitized to the Rh_o(D) antigen; the father is not known to be Rh_o(D) negative; and/or gestation is not more than 12 weeks at termination.

Rh_o(D) immune globulin prophylaxis is not indicated if the fetus or father can be determined to be Rh negative. If the Rh status of the fetus is unknown, the fetus must be assumed to be Rh_o(D) positive, and the dose should be administered to the mother.

For abortions or miscarriages occurring after 12 weeks of gestation, a standard dose of Rh_o(D) immune globulin is indicated.

➤*Transfusion (MICRhoGAM Ultra-Filtered Plus* only): To prevent Rh immunization in any Rh_o(D)–negative individual after incompatible transfusion of Rh-positive blood or blood products (eg, red blood cells [RBCs], platelet or granulocyte concentrates).

Administration and Dosage

➤*Adults:*

Pregnancy / Obstetric conditions –

Usual dosage: See the following table.

Administer within 3 hours of or as soon as possible after spontaneous passage or surgical removal at conception, up to and including 12 weeks of gestation. If prompt administration is not possible, give the dose within 72 hours of pregnancy termination or transfusion of Rh-incompatible blood or blood products. This dose will suppress the immune response to up to 2.5 mL of Rh-positive RBCs or the equivalent (5 mL) of whole blood.

Rh_o(D) Immune Globulin Microdose Recommended Dosages in Adults		
Indication	Dosage	Notes
Actual or threatened termination of pregnancy (spontaneous or induced) ≤ 12 weeks of gestation	50 mcg (250 units) within 72 h	Full-dose Rh_o(D) immune globulin may be administered if microdose is not available.
Transfusion of Rh-incompatible blood or blood products (< 2.5 mL of Rh-positive RBCs)	50 mcg (250 units) within 72 h	

Rh_o(D) IMMUNE GLOBULIN MICRODOSE — INJECTION

Transfusion –

MICRhoGAM Ultra-Filtered Plus only: See Pregnancy/Obstetric conditions for dosing.

➤*Preparation for administration:* Parenteral drug products should be visually inspected for particulate matter, discoloration, and syringe damage prior to administration whenever solution and container permit. Do not use if particulate matter and/or discoloration are observed. The solution should appear clear or slightly opalescent.

➤*Administration:* Administer only to women postabortion or postmiscarriage of up to 12 weeks' duration.

Never administer intravenously (IV). Inject entire contents of the syringe intramuscularly (IM), preferably in the anterolateral aspects of the upper thigh and the deltoid muscle of the upper arm. The gluteal region should not be used routinely as an injection site because of the risk of injury to the sciatic nerve. If the gluteal region is used, the central region must be avoided; only the upper, outer quadrant should be used.

Syringe use –

HyperRHO S/D Mini-Dose: Remove the prefilled syringe from the package. Lift the syringe by the barrel, not by the plunger. Twist the plunger rod clockwise until the threads are seated. With the rubber needle shield secured on the syringe tip, push the plunger rod forward a few millimeters to break any friction seal between the rubber stopper and the glass syringe barrel. Remove the needle shield and expel air bubbles. Do not remove the rubber needle shield to prepare the product for administration until immediately prior to the anticipated injection time. Proceed with hypodermic needle puncture. Aspirate prior to injection to confirm that the needle is not in a vein or artery. Inject the medication. Keeping your hands behind the needle, grasp the guard with your free hand and slide it forward toward the needle until it is completely covered and the guard clicks into place. If an audible click is not heard, the guard may not be completely activated. Place the entire refilled glass syringe with the guard activated into an approved sharps container for proper disposal.

MICRhoGAM Ultra-Filtered Plus: Administer injection per the standard protocol. When administering an IM injection, place fingers in contact with the syringe barrel through windows in the shield to prevent possible premature activation of the guard. Slide the safety guard over the needle. After the injection, use your free hand to slide the safety guard over the needle. An audible click indicates proper activation. Keep your hands behind the needle at all times. Dispose of the syringe in accordance with local regulations.

➤*Storage/Stability:*

Safety and handling – A number of factors could reduce the efficacy of the product or even result in an ill effect following its use. These include improper storage and handling of the product after it leaves the manufacturer's hands, diagnosis, dosage, method of administration, and biological differences in individual patients. Because of these factors, it is important that the product be stored properly and the directions be followed carefully during use. Store at 2° to 8°C (36° to 46°F). Do not freeze.

BOTULISM IMMUNE GLOBULIN IV (HUMAN) (BIG-IV)

Rx	**BabyBIG** (California Dept. of Health Services)	**Powder for injection, lyophilized**[a]: 100 ± 20 mg (50 mg/mL when reconstituted)	Preservative-free. In single-dose vial with 2 mL vial of diluent.

[a] Contains 5% sucrose, 1% albumin (human). Solvent/detergent treated.

BOTULISM IMMUNE GLOBULIN IV (HUMAN) (BIG-IV) — INJECTION

For complete and comparative prescribing information, refer to the Immune Globulins group monograph.

Indications

➤*Botulism:* For the treatment of patients below 1 year of age with infant botulism caused by toxin type A or B.

Administration and Dosage

➤*Children:*

Botulism –

Younger than 1 year of age: 1 mL/kg (50 mg/kg), given as a single intravenous (IV) infusion as soon as the clinical diagnosis of infant botulism is made.

➤*Renal function impairment:* Use with caution in patients with preexisting renal insufficiency and in patients judged to be at increased risk of developing renal insufficiency (including, but not limited to, those with diabetes mellitus, volume depletion, paraproteinemia, sepsis, or who are receiving known nephrotoxic drugs). In the absence of prospective data allowing identification of the maximum safe dose, concentration, and rate of infusion in these patients, do not exceed the recommended dose, concentration, or rate of infusion. Especially in such patients, administer at the minimum concentration available and at the minimum rate of infusion practicable.

➤*Preparation for administration:* Remove the tab portion of the vial cap and clean the rubber stopper with 70% alcohol or equivalent. Reconstitute the lyophilized powder with 2 mL of sterile water for injection to obtain a *BabyBIG* solution of 50 mg/mL.

Rotate the container gently to wet all the powder. An approximately 30-minute interval should be allowed for dissolving the powder. Do not shake the vial, because this will cause foaming.

➤*Administration:* Administer only as an IV infusion.

The infusion should begin slowly. Administer IV at 0.5 mL/kg/h (25 mg/kg/h. If no untoward reactions occur after 15 minutes, the rate may be increased to 1 mL/kg/h (50 mg/kg/h). Do not exceed this rate of administration. The patient should be monitored closely during and after each rate change. At the recommended rates, infusion of the indicated dose should take 67.5 minutes total elapsed time.

Infusion should begin within 2 hours after reconstitution is complete and should be concluded within 4 hours of reconstitution. Vital signs should be monitored continuously during infusion. *BabyBIG* should be administered IV using low volume tubing and a constant infusion pump (ie, an IVAC pump or equivalent). Pre-dilution of *BabyBIG* before infusion is not recommended. The product should be administered through a separate IV line. If this is not possible, it may be "piggybacked" into a preexisting line if that line contains sodium chloride injection or 1 of the following dextrose solutions (with or without sodium chloride added): dextrose 2.5% in water, dextrose 5% in water, dextrose 10% in water, or dextrose 20% in water. If a preexisting line must be used, *BabyBIG* should not be diluted more than 1:2 with any of the previously named solutions. Use of an in-line or syringe-tip sterile, disposable filter (18 mcm) is recommended for the administration of *BabyBIG*.

Infusion reactions – Minor adverse reactions experienced by patients treated with IGIV products have been related to the infusion rate. If the patient develops a minor side effect (ie, flushing), slow the rate of infusion or temporarily interrupt the infusion. If anaphylaxis or a significant drop in blood pressure occurs, discontinue the infusion and administer epinephrine.

➤*Admixture compatibility: BabyBIG* may be "piggybacked" into a preexisting line if that line contains sodium chloride injection or 1 of the following dextrose solutions (with or without sodium chloride added): dextrose 2.5% in water, dextrose 5% in water, dextrose 10% in water, or dextrose 20% in water. Admixtures of *BabyBIG* with any other solutions have not been evaluated.

➤*Storage/Stability:* The product should be stored between 2° and 8°C (35.6° to 46.4°F). Reconstituted solution should be used within 2 hours. Do not store in the reconstituted state.

VACCINIA IMMUNE GLOBULIN INTRAVENOUS (VIGIV) (HUMAN)

Rx	**Vaccinia Immune Globulin Intravenous (Human)** (Dynport Vaccine Company LLC)	**Solution for injection**: 50 mg/mL (immunoglobulin 2,500 mg/vial).	With 5% sucrose and 1% albumin (human). In vials.

VACCINIA IMMUNE GLOBULIN INTRAVENOUS (VIGIV) (HUMAN) — INJECTION

WARNING

Immune globulin intravenous (human) (IGIV) products have been reported to be associated with renal dysfunction, acute renal failure, osmotic nephrosis, proximal tubular nephropathy, and death. Although the reports of renal dysfunction and acute renal failure have been associated with the use of many licensed IGIV products, those that contained sucrose as a stabilizer and were administered at daily doses of 400 mg/kg or greater have accounted for a disproportionate share of the total number. Vaccinia immune globulin intravenous (VIGIV) contains sucrose 5% as a stabilizer, and the recommended dose is 100 mg/kg. Patients predisposed to acute renal failure include the following: patients with any degree of preexisting renal insufficiency, diabetes mellitus, volume depletion, sepsis, or paraproteinemia, patients who are 65 years of age or older, or patients who are receiving known nephrotoxic drugs. In such patients, administer VIGIV at the minimum concentration available and at the minimum rate of infusion practical.

Indications

➤*Vaccinia conditions:* For the treatment and/or modification of the following conditions:

- Aberrant infections induced by vaccinia virus that include its accidental implantation in eyes (except in cases of isolated keratitis), mouth, or other areas where vaccinia infection would constitute a special hazard.
- Eczema vaccinatum
- Progressive vaccinia
- Severe generalized vaccinia, and
- Vaccinia infections in individuals who have skin conditions such as burns, impetigo, varicella-zoster, or poison ivy; or in individuals who have eczematous skin lesions because of either the activity or extensiveness of such lesions.

Perform treatment of complications that include vaccinia keratitis with VIGIV with caution because a single study in rabbits has demonstrated increased corneal scarring with intramuscular VIG administration. VIGIV is not considered to be effective in the treatment of postvaccinial encephalitis.

VACCINIA IMMUNE GLOBULIN INTRAVENOUS (VIGIV) (HUMAN) — INJECTION

Administration and Dosage

➤*Adults:*

Vaccinia conditions –

Usual dosage: When the clinical diagnosis of a severe vaccinia-related complication is established, infuse 2 mL/kg (100 mg/kg), at a rate of 1 mL/kg/h for the first 30 minutes, increased to 2 mL/kg/h for the next 30 minutes and then to 3 mL/kg/h for the remainder of the infusion, as tolerated. Do not exceed these rates of administration.

Monitor the patient closely during and after each infusion rate change. At the recommended rates, infusion at the indicated dose (100 mg/kg [2 mL/kg]) should take approximately 70 minutes.

This dose may be repeated, depending on the severity of the symptoms and response to treatment.

Dosage adjustment: The administration of higher doses (200 or 500 mg/kg) may be considered in the event that the patient does not respond to the initial 100 mg/kg dose.

➤*Renal function impairment:* For patients with renal impairment who do not respond to the 100 mg/kg dose, the concentration and infusion selected should be the minimum practicable. Most cases of renal insufficiency have occurred in patients receiving total doses of immune globulin IV containing sucrose 400 mg/kg or greater. Doses of vaccinia immune globulin IV higher than 400 mg/kg will exceed this level of sucrose and are thus not recommended in patients with potential renal problems.

➤*Preparation for administration:* Remove the tab portion of the vial cap and clean the rubber stopper with 70% alcohol or equivalent. Do not shake the vial; avoid foaming.

Predilution of vaccinia immune globulin IV before infusion is not recommended.

➤*Administration:* To prevent the transmission of hepatitis viruses or other infectious agents, use sterile, disposable syringes and needles. Never reuse the syringes and needles.

Infusion – Begin IV infusion within 6 hours after entering the vial and complete within 12 hours of entering the vial. Monitor vital signs continuously.

Administer vaccinia immune globulin IV through an IV catheter with an administration set that contains an in-line filter (pore size: 0.22 mcm) and a constant infusion pump (ie, an IVAC pump or equivalent).

Administer vaccinia immune globulin IV through a dedicated IV catheter. Otherwise, vaccinia immune globulin IV may be piggybacked into a preexisting catheter if the catheter contains either sodium chloride 0.9% for injection or 1 of the following dextrose solutions (with or without sodium chloride added): dextrose 2.5% in water, dextrose 5% in water, dextrose 10% in water, and dextrose 20% in water. If a preexisting access must be used, flush the line before use and do not dilute the vaccinia immune globulin IV more than 1:2 (v/v) with any of these solutions.

Infusion rate – Adverse reactions related to the infusion rate have been experienced by patients treated with immune globulin IV products; most infusion rate-related adverse reactions reported for other immune globulin IV products have been minor (including flushing, chills, muscle cramps, back pain, fever, nausea, vomiting, arthralgia, and wheezing). However, major adverse events are possible. Observe patients for increase in heart rate, respiratory rate, retractions, and rales. If the patient develops a minor adverse reaction (eg, flushing), slow the rate of infusion or temporarily interrupt the infusion. For serious adverse reactions, such as anaphylaxis or a significant drop in blood pressure, discontinue the infusion and administer epinephrine with or without diphenhydramine. A loop diuretic should be available for management of fluid overload during administration.

➤*Admixture compatibility:* Admixtures of vaccinia immune globulin IV with any other solutions have not been evaluated. It is recommended that vaccinia immune globulin IV be administrated separately from other drugs or medications that the patient may be receiving.

➤*Storage/Stability:* Store vaccinia immune globulin IV between 2° and 8°C (35.6° to 46.4°F). Start IV infusion within 6 hours after entering the vial.

MONOCLONAL ANTIBODY

PALIVIZUMAB

Rx	**Synagis** (MedImmune)	**Injection; solution:** 100 mg/mL	Preservative free. In 0.5[a] and 1[b] mL single-use vials.

[a] With 1.9 mg histidine and 0.06 mg glycine/mL.

[b] With 3.9 mg histidine and 0.1 mg glycine/mL.

PALIVIZUMAB — INJECTION

Indications

➤*Respiratory syncytial virus (RSV):* For the prevention of serious lower respiratory tract disease caused by RSV in pediatric patients at high risk of RSV disease. Safety and efficacy were established in infants with bronchopulmonary dysplasia (BPD), infants with a history of premature birth (≤ 35 weeks gestational age), and children with hemodynamically significant congenital heart disease (CHD).

Administration and Dosage

➤*Children:*

Respiratory syncytial virus prophylaxis –

24 months of age and younger:

- *Usual dosage* – 15 mg/kg IM monthly throughout the RSV season. Administer the first dose prior to commencement of the RSV season.
- *Cardiopulmonary bypass patients* – Administer dose as soon as possible after the procedure (even if sooner than 1 month from the previous dose). Thereafter, administer doses monthly.

➤*Preparation for administration:* Both the 50 and 100 mg vials contain an overfill to allow the withdrawal of 50 or 100 mg. Administer immediately after withdrawal from vial.

➤*Administration:* For IM use only. Administer in the anterolateral aspect of the thigh. Do not use the gluteal muscle routinely because of the risk of damage to the sciatic nerve. Give injection volumes larger than 1 mL as a divided dose.

➤*Storage/Stability:* Store between 2° and 8°C (35.6° and 46.4°F) in its original container. Do not freeze. Discard any unused portion.

Actions

➤*Pharmacology:* Palivizumab exhibits neutralizing and fusion-inhibitory activity against RSV. These activities inhibit RSV replication in laboratory experiments. Although resistant RSV strains may be isolated in laboratory studies, a panel of 57 clinical RSV isolates were all neutralized by palivizumab. Palivizumab serum concentrations equal to 40 mcg/mL have been shown to reduce pulmonary RSV replication in the cotton rat model of RSV infection by 100-fold. The in vivo neutralizing activity of the active ingredient in palivizumab was assessed in a randomized, placebo-controlled study of 35 pediatric patients tracheally intubated because of RSV disease. In these patients, palivizumab significantly reduced the quantity of RSV in the lower respiratory tract compared with control patients.

➤*Pharmacokinetics:* In pediatric patients younger than 24 months of age without CHD, the mean half-life of palivizumab was 20 days, and monthly IM doses of 15 mg/kg achieved mean ± SD 30-day trough serum drug concentrations of 37 ± 21 mcg/mL after the first injection, 57 ± 41 mcg/mL after the second injection, 68 ± 51 mcg/mL after the third injection, and 72 ± 50 mcg/mL after the fourth injection. Trough concentrations following the first and fourth palivizumab dose were similar in children with CHD and in noncardiac patients. In pediatric patients given palivizumab for a second season, the mean ± SD serum concentrations following the first and fourth injections were 61 ± 17 mcg/mL and 86 ± 31 mcg/mL, respectively.

Cardiopulmonary bypass procedure – In 139 pediatric patients 24 months of age or younger with hemodynamically significant CHD who received palivizumab and underwent cardiopulmonary bypass for open-heart surgery, the mean ± SD serum palivizumab concentration was 98 ± 52 mcg/mL before bypass and declined to 41 ± 33 mcg/mL after bypass, a reduction of 58%. The clinical significance of this reduction is unknown.

Contraindications

Pediatric patients with a history of a severe reaction to palivizumab or other components of this product.

Warnings/Precautions

➤*Established RSV disease:* The safety and efficacy of palivizumab have not been demonstrated for treatment of established RSV disease.

➤*For IM use only:* Palivizumab is for IM use only. As with any IM injection, give palivizumab with caution to patients with thrombocytopenia or any coagulation disorder.

➤*Immunogenicity:* In trial 1, the incidence of antipalivizumab antibody following the fourth injection was 1.1% in the placebo group and 0.7% in the palivizumab group. In pediatric patients receiving palivizumab for a second season, 1 of 56 patients had transient, low-titer reactivity. This reactivity was not associated with adverse reactions or alteration in palivizumab serum concentrations. Immunogenicity was not assessed in trial 2.

These data reflect the percentage of patients whose test results were considered positive for antibodies to palivizumab in an ELISA assay, and are highly dependent on the sensitivity and specificity of the assay. Additionally, the observed incidence of antibody positivity in an assay may be influenced by several factors, including, sample handling, concomitant medications, and underlying disease. For these reasons, comparison of the incidence of antibodies to palivizumab with the incidence of antibodies to other products may be misleading.

➤*Hypersensitivity reactions:* Very rare cases of anaphylaxis (less than 1 case per 100,000 patients) have been reported following reexposure to palivizumab. Rare severe acute hypersensitivity reactions also have been reported on initial exposure or reexposure to palivizumab. None of the reported hypersensitivity reactions were fatal. Hypersensitivity reactions may include dyspnea, cyanosis, respiratory failure, urticaria, pruritus, angioedema, hypotonia, and unresponsiveness. The relationship between these reactions and the development of antibodies to palivizumab is unknown. If a severe hypersensitivity reaction occurs, permanently discontinue therapy with palivizumab. If milder hypersensitivity reactions occur, use caution on readministration of palivizumab. If anaphylaxis or severe allergic reactions occur, administer appropriate medications (eg, epinephrine) and provide supportive care as required.

PALIVIZUMAB — INJECTION

➤*Pregnancy: Category C.* Palivizumab is not indicated for adult usage and animal reproduction studies have not been conducted. It also is not known whether palivizumab could affect reproductive capacity or cause fetal harm when administered to a pregnant woman.

➤*Lactation:* Palivizumab is not indicated for adult usage.

➤*Children:* Palivizumab is indicated for use in pediatric patients.

Adverse Reactions

The most serious adverse reactions occurring with palivizumab treatment are anaphylaxis and other acute hypersensitivity reactions. The adverse reactions most commonly observed in palivizumab-treated patients were the following: cough, diarrhea, fever, gastroenteritis, otitis media, rash, rhinitis, upper respiratory tract infection, vomiting, and wheezing. Upper respiratory tract infection, otitis media, fever, and rhinitis occurred at a rate of 1% or greater in the palivizumab group compared with placebo (see the following table).

The data described reflect palivizumab exposure for 1,641 pediatric patients 3 days to 24.1 months of age in trials 1 and 2. Among these patients, 496 had bronchopulmonary dysplasia, 506 were premature birth infants younger than 6 months of age, and 639 had CHD. Adverse reactions observed in the 153 patient crossover study comparing the liquid and lyophilized formulations were similar between the 2 formulations, and similar to the adverse reactions observed with palivizumab in trials 1 and 2.

Palivizumab Adverse Reactions (≥ 1%)[a]

Adverse reaction	Palivizumab (n = 1,641)	Placebo (n = 1,148)
Fever	446 (27.1%)	289 (25.2%)
Hernia	68 (4.1%)	30 (2.6%)
Otitis media	597 (36.4%)	397 (34.6%)
Rhinitis	439 (26.8%)	282 (24.6%)
AST increased	49 (3%)	20 (1.7%)
Upper respiratory tract infection	830 (50.6%)	544 (47.4%)

[a] Cyanosis (palivizumab [9.1%]/placebo [6.9%] and arrythmia (palivizumab [3.1%]/placebo [1.7%]) were reported during trial 2 in CHD patients.

➤*Postmarketing:* The following adverse reactions have been identified and reported during postapproval use of palivizumab. Because the reports of these reactions are voluntary and the population is of uncertain size, it is not always possible to reliably estimate the frequency of the reaction or establish a causal relationship to drug exposure.

Hypersensitivity – Based on experience in over 400,000 patients who have received palivizumab (greater than 2 million doses), rare severe acute hypersensitivity reactions have been reported on initial or subsequent exposure. Very rare cases of anaphylaxis (less than 1 case per 100,000 patients) also have been reported, following reexposure. None of the reported hypersensitivity reactions were fatal. Hypersensitivity reactions may include the following: angioedema, cyanosis, dyspnea, hypotonia, pruritus, respiratory failure, unresponsiveness, and urticaria. The relationship between these reactions and the development of antibodies to palivizumab is unknown.

Limited information from postmarketing reports suggests that, within a single RSV season, adverse reactions after a sixth or greater dose of palivizumab are similar in character and frequency to those after the initial 5 doses.

Overdosage

➤*Symptoms:* No data from clinical studies are available on overdosage. No toxicity was observed in rabbits administered a single IM or subcutaneous injection of palivizumab at a dose of 50 mg/kg. No data are available from human subjects who have received more than 5 monthly palivizumab doses during a single RSV season.

DENOSUMAB

Rx	**Prolia** (Amgen)	**Injection, solution:** 60 mg/mL	Preservative free. In single-use prefilled syringes and vials.
Rx	**Xgeva** (Amgen)	**Injection, solution:** 70 mg/mL	Preservative free. In single-use vials.

DENOSUMAB — INJECTION

Indications

➤*Bone metastasis from solid tumors (Xgeva only):* For the prevention of skeletal-related events in patients with bone metastases from solid tumors.

➤*Osteoporosis (Prolia only):* For the treatment of postmenopausal women with osteoporosis at high risk of fracture, defined as a history of osteoporotic fracture, or multiple risk factors for fracture; or patients who have failed or are intolerant to other available osteoporosis therapies.

Administration and Dosage

➤*General dosing considerations:* Individuals sensitive to latex should not handle the gray needle cap on the single-use prefilled syringe, which contains dry natural rubber (a derivative of latex).

➤*Adults:*

Bone metastases from solid tumors (Xgeva only) –

Usual dosage: 120 mg subcutaneously every 4 weeks.

Concomitant therapy: Administer with calcium and vitamin D as necessary to treat or prevent hypocalcemia.

Osteoporosis (Prolia only) –

Usual dosage: 60 mg subcutaneously once every 6 months.

Concomitant therapy: All patients should receive 1,000 mg of calcium daily and at least 400 units of vitamin D daily.

Missed dose: If a dose of denosumab is missed, administer the injection as soon as the patient is available. Thereafter, schedule injections every 6 months from the date of the last injection.

➤*Renal function impairment:* Consider the benefit-risk profile when administering to patients with severe renal impairment or dialysis; these patients may be at a greater risk of developing hypocalcemia.

➤*Preparation for administration:* Prior to administration, denosumab may be removed from the refrigerator and brought to room temperature (up to 25°C [77°F]) by standing in the original container. This generally takes 15 to 30 minutes. Do not warm denosumab in any other way. Avoid vigorous shaking of denosumab.

➤*Administration:* Administer denosumab via subcutaneous injection in the upper arm, upper thigh, or abdomen.

Single-use vial – Use a 27-gauge needle to withdraw and inject the dose.

➤*Storage/Stability:* Refrigerate at 2° to 8°C (36° to 46°F) in the original carton. Do not freeze. Prior to administration, denosumab may be allowed to reach up to 25°C (77°F) in the original container. Once removed from the refrigerator, denosumab must not be exposed to temperatures above 25°C (77°F) and must be used within 14 days. If not used within 14 days, discard denosumab. Protect denosumab from direct light and heat.

Actions

➤*Pharmacology:* Denosumab binds to receptor activator of nuclear factor kappa B ligand (RANKL), a transmembrane or soluble protein essential for the formation, function, and survival of osteoclasts, the cells responsible for bone resorption. Denosumab prevents RANKL from activating its receptor, RANK, on the surface of osteoclasts and their precursors. Prevention of the RANKL/RANK interaction inhibits osteoclast formation, function, and survival, thereby decreasing bone resorption and increasing bone mass and strength in both cortical and trabecular bone.

Increased osteoclast activity, stimulated by RANKL, is a mediator of bone pathology in solid tumors with osseous metastases.

➤*Pharmacokinetics:*

Absorption –

Prolia: In a study conducted in healthy men and women volunteers (n = 73; age range, 18 to 64 years) following a single subcutaneous dose of denosumab 60 mg after fasting (for at least 12 hours), the mean maximum denosumab concentration (C_{max}) was 6.75 mcg/mL (standard deviation [SD], 1.89 mcg/mL). The median time to denosumab C_{max} was 10 days (range, 3 to 21 days). After C_{max}, serum denosumab concentrations declined over a period of 4 to 5 months. The mean denosumab area under the curve (AUC) up to 16 weeks ($AUC_{0\text{-}16\ wk}$) was 316 mcg•day/mL (SD, 101 mcg•day/mL).

Xgeva: Following subcutaneous administration, bioavailability was 62%. Denosumab displayed nonlinear pharmacokinetics at doses below 60 mg, but approximately dose-proportional increases in exposure at higher doses. With multiple subcutaneous doses of 120 mg every 4 weeks in patients with cancer metastatic to the bone, up to 2.8-fold accumulation in serum denosumab concentrations was observed and steady state was achieved by 6 months. At steady state, the mean ± SD serum trough concentration was 20.5 ± 13.5 mcg/mL at the recommended denosumab dose.

Excretion – Denosumab has a mean half-life of 25.4 days (*Prolia*) (SD, 8.5 days; n = 46) to 28 days (*Xgeva*).

Contraindications

Hypocalcemia (*Prolia* only).

Warnings/Precautions

➤*Hypocalcemia and mineral metabolism:* Denosumab may exacerbate or cause severe hypocalcemia. Correct preexisting hypocalcemia prior to denosumab treatment. Monitor calcium levels and administer calcium, magnesium, and vitamin D as necessary. Monitor levels more frequently when denosumab is administered with other drugs that can also lower calcium levels. In patients predisposed to hypocalcemia and disturbances of mineral metabolism (eg, history of hypoparathyroidism, thyroid surgery, parathyroid surgery, malabsorption syndromes, excision of small intestine, severe renal impairment [creatinine clearance less than 30 mL/min] or receiving dialysis), clinical monitoring of calcium and mineral levels (phosphorus and magnesium) is highly recommended. Inform all patients with severe renal impairment, including those receiving

DENOSUMAB — INJECTION

dialysis, about the symptoms of hypocalcemia and the importance of maintaining calcium levels with adequate calcium and vitamin D supplementation. Advise patients to contact a health care provider for symptoms of hypocalcemia.

Based on clinical trials using a lower dose of denosumab, patients with a CrCl less than 30 mL/min or receiving dialysis are at a greater risk of severe hypocalcemia compared with patients with normal renal function. In a trial of 55 patients, without cancer and with varying degrees of renal impairment, who received a single dose of denosumab 60 mg, 8 of 17 patients with a CrCl less than 30 mL/min or receiving dialysis experienced corrected serum calcium levels less than 8 mg/dL when compared with 0 of 12 patients with normal renal function. The risk of hypocalcemia at the recommended dosing schedule of *Xgeva* 120 mg every 4 weeks has not been evaluated in patients with a CrCl less than 30 mL/min or receiving dialysis.

➤*Osteonecrosis of the jaw:* Osteonecrosis of the jaw, which can occur spontaneously, is generally associated with tooth extraction and/or local infection with delayed healing. Osteonecrosis of the jaw can occur in patients receiving denosumab, manifesting as jaw pain, osteomyelitis, osteitis, bone erosion, tooth or periodontal infection, toothache, gingival ulceration, or gingival erosion. Persistent pain or slow healing of the mouth or jaw after dental surgery may also be manifestations of osteonecrosis of the jaw. In clinical trials, 2.2% of patients receiving denosumab developed osteonecrosis of the jaw; of these patients, 79% had a history of tooth extraction, poor oral hygiene, or use of a dental appliance.

Prolia – Perform a routine oral exam prior to initiation. Consider a dental examination with appropriate preventive dentistry prior to treatment with initiation in patients with risk factors for osteonecrosis of the jaw, such as invasive dental procedures (eg, tooth extraction, dental implants, oral surgery), diagnosis of cancer, concomitant therapies (eg, chemotherapy, corticosteroids), poor oral hygiene, and comorbid disorders (eg, periodontal and/or other preexisting dental disease, anemia, coagulopathy, infection, ill-fitting dentures). Advise patients to maintain good oral hygiene practices during treatment with denosumab. For patients requiring invasive dental procedures, use clinical judgment to guide the management plan of each patient based on individual benefit-risk assessment. Ensure that patients who are suspected of having or who develop osteonecrosis of the jaw while taking denosumab receive care by a dentist or an oral surgeon. In these patients, extensive dental surgery to treat osteonecrosis of the jaw may exacerbate the condition. Consider discontinuation of denosumab therapy based on individual benefit-risk assessment.

Xgeva – Perform an oral examination and appropriate preventative dentistry prior to the initiation and periodically during therapy. Advise patients regarding oral hygiene practices. Avoid invasive dental procedures during treatment with denosumab. Patients who are suspected of having or who develop osteonecrosis of the jaw while taking denosumab should receive care by a dentist or an oral surgeon. In these patients, extensive dental surgery to treat osteonecrosis of the jaw may exacerbate the condition.

➤*Serious infections:*

Prolia – In a clinical trial of more than 7,800 women with postmenopausal osteoporosis, serious infections leading to hospitalization were reported more frequently in the denosumab group than in the placebo group. Serious skin infections, as well as infections of the abdomen, urinary tract, and ear, were more frequent in patients treated with denosumab. Endocarditis was also reported more frequently in denosumab-treated patients. The incidence of opportunistic infections was balanced between placebo and denosumab groups, and the overall incidence of infections was similar between the treatment groups. Advise patients to seek prompt medical attention if they develop signs or symptoms of severe infection, including cellulitis.

Patients on concomitant immunosuppressant agents or with impaired immune systems may be at increased risk for serious infections. Consider the benefit-risk profile in these patients before treating with denosumab. In patients who develop serious infections while taking denosumab, assess the need for continued denosumab therapy.

➤*Dermatologic effects:*

Prolia – In a large clinical trial of more than 7,800 women with postmenopausal osteoporosis, epidermal and dermal adverse reactions, such as dermatitis, eczema, and rashes, occurred at a significantly higher rate in the denosumab group compared with the placebo group. Most of these reactions were not specific to the injection site. Consider discontinuing denosumab if severe symptoms develop.

➤*Long-term use:*

Prolia – In clinical trials in women with postmenopausal osteoporosis, treatment with denosumab resulted in significant suppression of bone remodeling as evidenced by markers of bone turnover and bone histomorphometry. The significance of these findings and the effect of long-term treatment with denosumab are unknown. The long-term consequences of the degree of suppression of bone remodeling observed with denosumab may contribute to adverse outcomes, such as osteonecrosis of the jaw, atypical fractures, and delayed fracture healing. Monitor patients for these consequences.

➤*Immunogenicity:* Denosumab is a human monoclonal antibody. As with all therapeutic proteins, there is potential for immunogenicity. Using an electrochemiluminescent bridging immunoassay, less than 1% of patients treated with *Prolia* for up to 5 years tested positive for binding antibodies, including preexisting, transient, and developing antibodies. Similarly, less than 1% of patients with osseous metastases treated with denosumab doses ranging from 30 to 180 mg every 4 weeks or every 12 weeks for up to 3 years tested positive for binding antibodies. None of the patients tested positive for neutralizing antibodies, as was assessed using a chemiluminescent cell-based in vitro biological assay. No evidence of altered pharmacokinetic profile, toxicity profile, or clinical response was associated with binding antibody development.

The incidence of antibody formation is highly dependent on the sensitivity and specificity of the assay. Additionally, the observed incidence of a positive antibody (including neutralizing antibody) test result may be influenced by several factors, including assay methodology, sample handling, timing of sample collection, concomitant medications, and underlying disease. For these reasons, comparison of antibodies to denosumab with the incidence of antibodies to other products may be misleading.

➤*Renal function impairment:* In a trial of 55 patients without cancer and with varying degrees of renal function who received a single dose of denosumab 60 mg, patients with a CrCl of less than 30 mL/min or receiving dialysis were at greater risk of severe hypocalcemia with denosumab compared with patients with normal renal function. Consider the benefit-risk profile when administering denosumab to patients with severe renal impairment or receiving dialysis. Clinical monitoring of calcium and mineral levels (phosphorus and magnesium) is highly recommended. Adequate intake of calcium and vitamin D is important in patients with severe renal impairment or receiving dialysis.

Xgeva – The risk of hypocalcemia at the recommended dosing schedule of 120 mg every 4 weeks has not been evaluated in patients with a CrCl of less than 30 mL/min or receiving dialysis.

➤*Pregnancy:* Category C. There are no adequate and well-controlled studies of denosumab in pregnant women. Administer denosumab during pregnancy only if the potential benefit justifies the potential risk to the fetus.

In genetically-engineered mice in which RANKL was turned off by gene removal (a "knockout" mouse), absence of RANKL (the target of denosumab) caused fetal lymph node agenesis and led to postnatal impairment of dentition and bone growth. Pregnant RANKL knockout mice also showed altered maturation of the maternal mammary gland, leading to impaired lactation postpartum.

In an embryofetal developmental study, cynomolgus monkeys received subcutaneous denosumab weekly during organogenesis at doses of up to 13-fold (*Prolia*) and 6.5-fold (*Xgeva*) higher than the recommended human dose of 60 mg administered once every 6 months (*Prolia*) and 120 mg every 4 weeks (*Xgeva*) based on body weight (mg/kg). No evidence of maternal toxicity or fetal harm was observed. However, this study only assessed fetal toxicity during a period equivalent to the first trimester and fetal lymph nodes were not examined. Monoclonal antibodies are transported across the placenta in a linear fashion as pregnancy progresses, with the largest amount transferred during the third trimester. Potential adverse developmental effects resulting from exposures during the second and third trimesters have not been assessed in animals.

Pregnancy registry – Women who become pregnant during denosumab treatment are encouraged to enroll in the manufacturer's Pregnancy Surveillance Program. Patients or their health care provider should call 1-800-772-6436 to enroll.

➤*Lactation:* It is not known whether denosumab is excreted into human breast milk. Because many drugs are excreted in human milk and because of the potential for serious adverse reactions in breast-feeding infants from denosumab, decide whether to discontinue breast-feeding or the drug, taking into account the importance of the drug to the mother.

Maternal exposure to denosumab during pregnancy may impair mammary gland development and lactation based on animal studies in pregnant mice lacking the RANK/RANKL signaling pathway that have shown altered maturation of the maternal mammary gland, leading to impaired lactation postpartum.

➤*Children:* Denosumab is not recommended in children. The safety and effectiveness of denosumab in children have not been established. Treatment with denosumab may impair bone growth in children with open growth plates and may inhibit eruption of dentition.

➤*Monitoring:* Monitor patients for the development of infections. Monitor patients in long-term therapy for the development of osteonecrosis of the jaw, atypical fractures, and delayed fracture healing.

Monitor calcium levels. In patients predisposed to hypocalcemia and disturbances of mineral metabolism (eg, history of hypoparathyroidism, thyroid surgery, parathyroid surgery, malabsorption syndromes, excision of small intestine, severe renal impairment [CrCl less than 30 mL/min] or receiving dialysis), clinical monitoring of mineral levels (phosphorus and magnesium) is highly recommended.

Perform a routine oral exam prior to initiation of denosumab treatment. Consider a dental examination with appropriate preventive dentistry prior to treatment with denosumab in patients with risk factors for osteonecrosis of the jaw, such as invasive dental procedures (eg, tooth extraction, dental implants, oral surgery), diagnosis of cancer, concomitant therapies (eg, chemotherapy, corticosteroids), poor oral hygiene, and comorbid disorders (eg, periodontal and/or other preexisting dental disease, anemia, coagulopathy, infection, ill-fitting dentures).

Drug Interactions

None well documented.

Adverse Reactions

➤*Prolia*:

Most common adverse reactions – The most common adverse reactions reported with denosumab are back pain, pain in extremity, musculoskeletal pain, hypercholesterolemia, and cystitis.

DENOSUMAB — INJECTION

Discontinuation of therapy – The percentage of patients who withdrew from the study because of adverse reactions was 2.1% and 2.4% for the placebo and denosumab groups, respectively. The most common adverse reactions leading to discontinuation of denosumab are breast cancer, back pain, and constipation.

Serious adverse reactions – The incidence of all-cause mortality was 2.3% in the placebo group and 1.8% in the denosumab group. The incidence of nonfatal serious adverse reactions was 24.2% in the placebo group and 25% in the denosumab group.

Adverse reactions (2% or more) –

Denosumab (*Prolia*) Adverse Reactions (≥ 2%) in Postmenopausal Women With Osteoporosis		
Adverse reactions	Denosumab (n = 3,886)	Placebo (n = 3,876)
Cardiovascular		
Angina pectoris	2.6%	2.2%
Atrial fibrillation	2%	2%
CNS		
Asthenia	2.3%	1.9%
Insomnia	3.2%	3.1%
Sciatica	4.6%	3.8%
Vertigo	5%	4.8%
Dermatologic		
Pruritus	2.2%	2.1%
Rash	2.5%	2%
GI		
Abdominal pain, upper	3.3%	2.9%
Flatulence	2.2%	1.4%
Gastroesophageal reflux disease	2.1%	1.7%
Musculoskeletal		
Back pain	34.7%	34.6%
Bone pain	3.7%	3%
Musculoskeletal pain	7.6%	7.5%
Myalgia	2.9%	2.4%
Pain in extremity	11.7%	11.1%
Spinal osteoarthritis	2.1%	1.7%
Respiratory		
Pneumonia	3.9%	3.9%
Upper respiratory tract infection	4.9%	4.3%
Miscellaneous		
Anemia	3.3%	2.8%
Cystitis	5.9%	5.8%
Edema, peripheral	4.9%	4%
Herpes zoster	2%	1.9%
Hypercholesterolemia	7.2%	6.1%
Pharyngitis	2.3%	2%

Hypocalcemia – Decreases in serum calcium levels to less than 8.5 mg/dL were reported in 0.4% of women in the placebo group and 1.7% of women in the denosumab group at the month-1 visit. The nadir in serum calcium level occurs at approximately day 10 after denosumab dosing in patients with healthy renal function.

In clinical studies, patients with impaired renal function were more likely to have greater reductions in serum calcium levels compared with patients with healthy renal function. In a study of 55 patients with varying degrees of renal function, serum calcium levels less than 7.5 mg/dL or symptomatic hypocalcemia were observed in 5 patients. These included no patients in the healthy-renal-function group, 10% of patients in the group with CrCl 50 to 80 mL/min, 29% of patients in the group with CrCl less than 30 mL/min, and 29% of patients in the hemodialysis group. These patients did not receive calcium and vitamin D supplementation. In a study of 4,550 postmenopausal women with osteoporosis, the mean change from baseline in serum calcium level 10 days after denosumab dosing was −5.5% in patients with CrCl less than 30 mL/min versus −3.1% in patients with CrCl at least 30 mL/min.

Serious infections – RANKL is expressed on activated T and B lymphocytes and in lymph nodes. Therefore, a RANKL inhibitor, such as denosumab, may increase the risk of infection.

In the clinical study of 7,808 postmenopausal women with osteoporosis, the incidence of infections resulting in death was 0.2% in both placebo and denosumab treatment groups. However, the incidence of nonfatal serious infections was 3.3% in the placebo group and 4% in the denosumab group. Hospitalizations because of serious infections in the abdomen (0.7% placebo vs 0.9% denosumab), urinary tract (0.5% placebo vs 0.7% denosumab), and ear (0% placebo vs 0.1% denosumab) were reported. Endocarditis was reported in no placebo patients and 3 patients receiving denosumab.

Skin infections, including erysipelas and cellulitis, leading to hospitalization were reported more frequently in patients treated with denosumab (less than 0.1% placebo vs 0.4% denosumab).

Dermatologic reactions – A significantly higher number of patients treated with denosumab developed epidermal and dermal adverse reactions, such as dermatitis, eczema, and rashes; these reactions were reported in 8.2% of the placebo group and 10.8% of the denosumab group ($P < 0.0001$). Most of these reactions were not specific to the injection site.

Osteonecrosis of the jaw – See Warnings/Precautions for more information.

Pancreatitis – Pancreatitis was reported in 0.1% of patients in the placebo group and 0.2% of patients in the denosumab group. Of these reports, 1 subject in the placebo group and all 8 patients in the denosumab group had serious reactions, including 1 death in the denosumab group. Several patients had a history of pancreatitis. The time from product administration to event occurrence was variable.

New malignancies – The overall incidence of new malignancies was 4.3% in the placebo group and 4.8% in the denosumab group. New malignancies related to breast (0.7% placebo vs 0.9% denosumab), reproductive (0.2% placebo vs 0.5% denosumab), and GI systems (0.6% placebo vs 0.9% denosumab) were reported. A causal relationship to drug exposure has not been established.

➤*Xgeva*:

Most common adverse reactions – The most common adverse reactions in patients receiving denosumab (per-patient incidence of 25% or more) were fatigue/asthenia, hypophosphatemia, and nausea.

Serious adverse reactions – The most common serious adverse reaction in patients receiving denosumab was dyspnea.

Discontinuation of therapy – The most common adverse reactions resulting in discontinuation of denosumab were osteonecrosis and hypocalcemia.

Adverse reactions (10% or more) –

Denosumab (*Xgeva*)[a] Adverse Reactions (≥ 10%) (Trials 1, 2, and 3)		
Adverse reactions	Denosumab (n = 2,841)	Zoledronic acid (n = 2,836)
CNS		
Fatigue/asthenia	45%	46%
Headache	13%	14%
GI		
Diarrhea	20%	19%
Nausea	31%	32%
Metabolic		
Hypocalcemia[b]	18%	9%
Hypophosphatemia[b]	32%	20%
Respiratory		
Cough	15%	15%
Dyspnea	21%	18%

[a] Adverse reactions reported in ≥ 10% of patients receiving denosumab in trials 1, 2, and 3, and meeting 1 of the following criteria: ≥ 1% incidence in denosumab-treated patients, or between-group difference (either direction) of < 1% and > 5% incidence in patients treated with zoledronic acid compared with placebo.

[b] Laboratory-derived and below the central laboratory lower limit of normal (8.3 to 8.5 mg/dL [2.075 to 2.125 mmol/L] for calcium and 2.2 to 2.8 mg/dL [0.71 to 0.9 mmol/L] for phosphorus).

Severe mineral/electrolyte abnormalities – Severe hypocalcemia (corrected serum calcium less than 7 mg/dL or less than 1.75 mmol/L) occurred in 3.1% of patients treated with denosumab and 1.3% of patients treated with zoledronic acid. Of patients who experienced severe hypocalcemia, 33% experienced 2 or more episodes of severe hypocalcemia and 16% experienced 3 or more episodes.

Severe hypophosphatemia (serum phosphorus less than 2 mg/dL or less than 0.6 mmol/L) occurred in 15.4% of patients treated with denosumab and 7.4% of patients treated with zoledronic acid.

Osteonecrosis of the jaw – In the primary treatment phases of trials 1, 2, and 3, osteonecrosis of the jaw was confirmed in 1.8% of patients in the denosumab group and 1.3% of patients in the zoledronic acid group. When events occurring during an extended treatment phase of approximately 4 months in each trial are included, the incidence of confirmed osteonecrosis of the jaw was 2.2% in patients who received denosumab. The median time to osteonecrosis of the jaw was 14 months (range, 4 to 25).

Patient Information

Adequately supplement patients with calcium and vitamin D and instruct them on the importance of maintaining serum calcium levels while receiving denosumab. Advise patients to seek prompt medical attention if they develop signs or symptoms of hypocalcemia, including paresthesias or muscle stiffness, twitching, spasms, or cramps.

Advise patients to seek prompt medical attention if they develop signs or symptoms of infections, including cellulitis, or if they develop signs or symptoms of dermatological reactions (dermatitis, rashes, and eczema).

Advise patients to maintain good oral hygiene during treatment with denosumab and to inform their dentist prior to dental procedures that they are

DENOSUMAB — INJECTION

receiving denosumab. Advise patients to inform their health care provider or dentist if they experience persistent pain and/or slow healing of the mouth or jaw after dental surgery or if symptoms of osteonecrosis of the jaw, including pain, numbness, swelling of or drainage from the jaw, mouth, or teeth occur. Advise patients to avoid invasive dental procedures during treatment with denosumab.

Advise patients to contact their health care provider if they become pregnant or are breast-feeding.

ECULIZUMAB

Rx	**Soliris** (Alexion)	**Injection, solution, concentrate:** 10 mg/mL	Preservative free. 6.6 mg of polysorbate 80. In single-use 30 mL vials.

ECULIZUMAB — INJECTION

WARNING

Serious meningococcal infection – Eculizumab increases the risk of meningococcal infections. Meningococcal infection may become rapidly life-threatening or fatal if not recognized and treated early.

Vaccinate patients with a meningococcal vaccine at least 2 weeks prior to receiving the first dose of eculizumab; revaccinate according to current medical guidelines for vaccine use.

Monitor patients for early signs of meningococcal infections; evaluate immediately if infection is suspected and treat with antibiotics if necessary.

Indications

➤*Paroxysmal nocturnal hemoglobinuria:* For the treatment of patients with paroxysmal nocturnal hemoglobinuria (PNH) to reduce hemolysis.

Administration and Dosage

➤*General dosing considerations:* Patients must be administered a meningococcal vaccine at least 2 weeks prior to initiation of eculizumab and revaccinated according to current medical guidelines for vaccine use.

Monitor the patient for at least 1 hour following completion of the infusion for signs or symptoms of an infusion reaction.

➤*Adults:*

Paroxysmal nocturnal hemoglobinuria – 600 mg by intravenous (IV) infusion every 7 days for the first 4 weeks, followed by 900 mg for the fifth dose 7 days later, then 900 mg every 14 days thereafter. Eculizumab should be administered at the recommended dosage regimen time points or within 2 days of these time points.

➤*Preparation for administration:* Eculizumab must be diluted to a final admixture concentration of 5 mg/mL.

Withdraw the required amount of eculizumab from the vial into a sterile syringe. Transfer the recommended dose to an infusion bag. Dilute eculizumab to a final concentration of 5 mg/mL by adding the appropriate amount (equal volume of diluent to drug volume) of sodium chloride 0.9% injection, sodium chloride 0.45% injection, dextrose 5% in water, or Ringer's lactate to the infusion bag.

The final admixed eculizumab 5 mg/mL infusion volume is 120 mL for 600 mg doses or 180 mL for 900 mg doses. Gently invert the infusion bag containing the diluted eculizumab solution to ensure thorough mixing of the product and diluent. Do not shake.

Prior to administration, the admixture should be allowed to adjust to room temperature (18° to 25°C [64° to 77°F]). The admixture must not be heated in a microwave or with any heat source other than ambient air temperature.

➤*Administration:* Eculizumab should be administered by IV infusion over 35 minutes via gravity feed, a syringe-type pump, or an infusion pump. Do not administer as an IV push or bolus injection.

If an adverse reaction occurs during the administration of eculizumab, the infusion may be slowed or stopped at the discretion of the health care provider. If the infusion is slowed, the total infusion time should not exceed 2 hours.

➤*Storage / Stability:* Eculizumab vials must be stored in the original carton until time of use under refrigerated conditions at 2° to 8°C (36° to 46°F) and protected from light. Admixed solutions of eculizumab are stable for 24 hours at 2° to 8°C (36° to 46°F) and at room temperature. Do not freeze. Discard any unused portion left in a vial because the product contains no preservatives.

Actions

➤*Pharmacology:* Eculizumab is a monoclonal antibody that specifically binds to the complement protein C5 with high affinity, thereby inhibiting its cleavage to C5a and C5b and preventing the generation of the terminal complement complex C5b-9. Eculizumab inhibits terminal complement mediated intravascular hemolysis in patients with PNH.

➤*Pharmacokinetics:*

Absorption / Distribution – The mean observed peak and trough serum concentrations of eculizumab by week 26 were 194 ± 76 mcg/mL and 97 ± 60 mcg/mL, respectively. The volume of distribution was 7.7 L.

Excretion – The clearance of eculizumab for a typical PNH patient weighing 70 kg was 22 mL/h. The half-life was 272 ± 82 hours (mean ± standard deviation [SD]).

Contraindications

Unresolved serious *Neisseria meningitidis* infection; patients who are not currently vaccinated against *N. meningitidis*.

Warnings/Precautions

➤*Serious meningococcal infections:* The use of eculizumab increases a patient's susceptibility to serious meningococcal infections (septicemia and/or meningitis). All patients without a history of prior meningococcal vaccination must receive the meningococcal vaccine at least 2 weeks prior to receiving the first dose of eculizumab and be revaccinated according to current medical guidelines for vaccine use. Quadravalent, conjugated meningococcal vaccines are strongly recommended. Vaccination may not prevent meningococcal infections.

See the Warning box for more information.

In clinical studies, 2 of 196 patients with PNH developed serious meningococcal infections while receiving treatment with eculizumab; both had been vaccinated. In clinical studies among non-PNH patients, meningococcal meningitis occurred in 1 patient who was unvaccinated.

➤*Other infections:* Eculizumab blocks terminal complement; therefore, patients may have increased susceptibility to infections, especially with encapsulated bacteria. Use caution when administering eculizumab to patients with any systemic infection.

➤*Discontinuation of therapy:* Because eculizumab therapy increases the number of PNH cells (in study 1, the proportion of PNH red blood cells (RBCs) increased among eculizumab-treated patients by a median of 28% from baseline [range, −25% to 69%]), patients who discontinue treatment with eculizumab may be at increased risk for serious hemolysis. Serious hemolysis is identified by serum lactate dehydrogenase (LDH) levels greater than the pretreatment level, along with any of the following: more than 25% absolute decrease in PNH clone size (in the absence of dilution due to transfusion) in 1 week or less, a hemoglobin level of less than 5 g/dL or a decrease of more than 4 g/dL in 1 week or less, angina, change in mental status, a 50% increase in serum creatinine level, or thrombosis.

If serious hemolysis occurs after eculizumab discontinuation, consider the following procedures/treatments: blood transfusion (packed RBCs) or exchange transfusion if the PNH RBCs are greater than 50% of the total RBCs by flow cytometry, anticoagulation, corticosteroids, or reinstitution of eculizumab.

In clinical studies, 16 of 196 patients with PNH discontinued treatment with eculizumab. Patients were followed for evidence of worsening hemolysis, and no serious hemolysis was observed.

➤*Infusion reactions:* As with all protein products, administration of eculizumab may result in infusion reactions, including anaphylaxis or other hypersensitivity reactions.

In clinical trials, no patients with PNH experienced an infusion reaction that required discontinuation of eculizumab. Interrupt eculizumab administration in all patients experiencing severe infusion reactions and administer appropriate medical therapy.

➤*Immunogenicity:* As with all proteins, there is a potential for immunogenicity. Low titers of antibodies to eculizumab were detected in 2% of all patients with PNH treated with eculizumab. No apparent correlation of antibody development to clinical response was observed.

➤*Pregnancy: Category C.* PNH is a serious illness. Pregnant women with PNH and their fetuses have high rates of morbidity and mortality during pregnancy and the postpartum period. There are no adequate and well-controlled studies of eculizumab in pregnant women. Eculizumab, a recombinant immunoglobulin G (IgG) molecule (humanized anti-C5 antibody), is expected to cross the placenta. Animal studies using a mouse analogue of the eculizumab molecule (murine anti-C5 antibody) showed increased rates of developmental abnormalities and an increased rate of dead and moribund offspring at doses 2 to 8 times the human dose. Administer eculizumab during pregnancy only if the potential benefit justifies the potential risk to the fetus.

When maternal exposure to the antibody occurred during organogenesis, 2 cases of retinal dysplasia and 1 case of umbilical hernia were observed among 230 offspring born to mothers exposed to the higher antibody dose; however, the exposure did not increase fetal loss or neonatal death. When maternal exposure to the antibody occurred in the time period from implantation through weaning, a higher number of male offspring became moribund or died (controls, 1/25; low-dose group, 2/25; high-dose group, 5/25). Surviving offspring had normal development and reproductive performance.

➤*Lactation:* It is not known whether eculizumab is secreted into human milk. IgG is excreted in human milk; therefore, it is expected that eculizumab will be present in human milk. However, published data suggest that breast milk antibodies do not enter the neonatal and infant circulation in substantial amounts. Exercise caution when administering eculizumab to a breast-feeding woman. Weigh the unknown risks to the infant from GI or limited systemic exposure to eculizumab against the known benefits of breast-feeding.

➤*Children:* The safety and efficacy of eculizumab therapy in children younger than 18 years of age have not been established.

ECULIZUMAB — INJECTION

➤*Monitoring:* Monitor all patients for early signs and symptoms of meningococcal infections and evaluate immediately if an infection is suspected. Monitor the patient for at least 1 hour following completion of the infusion for signs or symptoms of an infusion reaction. Monitor any patient who discontinues eculizumab for at least 8 weeks to detect serious hemolysis and other reactions.

Serum LDH levels increase during hemolysis and may assist in monitoring eculizumab effects, including the response to discontinuation of therapy. In clinical studies, 6 patients achieved a reduction in serum LDH levels only after a decrease in the eculizumab dosing interval from 14 to 12 days. All other patients achieved a reduction in serum LDH levels with the 14-day dosing interval.

Drug Interactions

None well documented.

Adverse Reactions

➤*Adverse reactions (5% or more):*

Eculizumab Adverse Reactions (≥ 5%)		
Adverse reactions	Eculizumab (n = 43)	Placebo (n = 44)
CNS		
Fatigue	12%	2%
Headache	44%	27%
GI		
Constipation	7%	5%
Nausea	16%	11%
Musculoskeletal		
Back pain	19%	9%
Myalgia	7%	2%
Respiratory		
Cough	12%	9%
Nasopharyngitis	23%	18%
Respiratory tract infection	7%	2%
Sinusitis	7%	0%
Miscellaneous		
Herpes simplex infections	7%	0%
Influenza-like illness	5%	2%
Pain in extremity	7%	2%

➤*Serious adverse reactions:* In the placebo-controlled clinical study, serious adverse reactions occurred among 9% patients receiving eculizumab and 21% patients receiving placebo. The serious reactions included infections and progression of PNH. No deaths occurred in the study and no patients receiving eculizumab experienced a thrombotic event; 1 thrombotic event occurred in a patient receiving placebo.

Among 193 patients with PNH treated with eculizumab in the single-arm clinical study or the follow-up study, the adverse reactions were similar to those reported in the placebo-controlled clinical study. Serious adverse reactions occurred in 16% of the patients in these studies. The most common serious adverse reactions were anemia, headache, pyrexia, and viral infection (2%).

Meningococcal infections – See Warnings/Precautions for more information.

➤*Postmarketing:* Cases of serious or fatal meningococcal infections have been reported.

Patient Information

Prior to treatment, ensure that patients fully understand the risks and benefits of eculizumab, particularly the risk of meningococcal infection.

Ensure that patients receive the Medication Guide.

Inform patients that they are required to receive a meningococcal vaccination at least 2 weeks prior to receiving the first dose of eculizumab if they have not previously been vaccinated. They are required to be revaccinated according to current medical guidelines for meningococcal vaccine use while on eculizumab therapy. Inform patients that vaccination may not prevent meningococcal infection.

Educate patients about any of the signs and symptoms of meningococcal infection, and strongly advise them to seek immediate medical attention if the following signs or symptoms occur: moderate to severe headache with nausea or vomiting, moderate to severe headache and a fever, moderate to severe headache with a stiff neck or stiff back, fever of 103°F (39.4°C) or higher, fever and a rash, confusion, severe muscle aches with flu-like symptoms, and eyes sensitive to light.

Inform patients that they should be provided with the Patient Safety Card that they should carry with them at all times. This card describes symptoms that, if experienced, should prompt the patient to immediately seek medical evaluation.

Inform patients that there is a potential for serious hemolysis when eculizumab is discontinued and that they will be monitored by their health care provider for at least 8 weeks following eculizumab discontinuation.

BELIMUMAB

Rx	**Benlysta** (Human Genome Sciences[a])	**Injection, lyophilized powder for solution:** 120 mg	Latex free, preservative free. Polysorbate 80, sucrose 80 mg/mL. In single-use 5 mL vials.
		400 mg	Latex free, preservative free. Polysorbate 80, sucrose 80 mg/mL. In single-use 20 mL vials.

[a] Human Genome Sciences, 14200 Shady Grove Road, Rockville, MD 20850; 301-309-8504, fax 301-309-8512; http://www.hgsi.com.

BELIMUMAB — INJECTION

Indications

➤*Systemic lupus erythematosus:* For the treatment of adult patients with active, autoantibody-positive, systemic lupus erythematosus who are receiving standard therapy.

Administration and Dosage

➤*Adults:*

Systemic lupus erythematosus –

Usual dosage: 10 mg/kg at 2-week intervals for the first 3 doses, and at 4-week intervals thereafter.

Concomitant therapy: Consider administering premedication for prophylaxis against infusion reactions and hypersensitivity reactions.

➤*Preparation for administration:*

Reconstitution – Remove belimumab from the refrigerator and allow to stand 10 to 15 minutes for the vial to reach room temperature. Reconstitute the 120 mg vial with 1.5 mL sterile water for injection. Reconstitute the 400 mg vial with 4.8 mL sterile water for injection. The stream of sterile water should be directed toward the side of the vial to minimize foaming. Gently swirl the vial for 60 seconds. Allow the vial to sit at room temperature during reconstitution, gently swirling the vial for 60 seconds every 5 minutes until the powder is dissolved. Do not shake. Reconstitution is typically complete within 10 to 15 minutes after the sterile water has been added, but it may take up to 30 minutes. The reconstituted solution will contain a concentration of belimumab 80 mg/mL.

If a mechanical reconstitution device (swirler) is used to reconstitute belimumab, it should not exceed 500 rpm, and the vial should be swirled for no longer than 30 minutes. Once reconstitution is complete, the solution should be opalescent, colorless to pale yellow, and without particles. However, small air bubbles, are expected and acceptable.

Dilution – Belimumab should only be diluted in sodium chloride 0.9% injection. Dilute the reconstituted product to 250 mL in sodium chloride 0.9% injection for intravenous (IV) infusion. From a 250-mL infusion bag or bottle of normal saline, withdraw and discard a volume equal to the volume of the reconstituted solution of belimumab required for the patient's dose. Then add the required volume of the reconstituted solution of belimumab into the infusion bag or bottle. Gently invert the bag or bottle to mix the solution.

➤*Administration:* For IV infusion only. Do not administer as an IV push or bolus. Administer over a period of 1 hour. The infusion rate may be slowed or interrupted if the patient develops an infusion reaction. The infusion must be discontinued immediately if the patient experiences a serious hypersensitivity reaction.

➤*Admixture compatibility:* Belimumab should not be infused concomitantly in the same IV line with other agents. No physical or biochemical compatibility studies have been conducted to evaluate the coadministration of belimumab with other agents. Dextrose IV solutions are incompatible with belimumab.

➤*Storage/Stability:* Store vials between 2° and 8°C (36° and 46°F). Vials should be protected from light and stored in the original carton until use. Do not freeze. Avoid exposure to heat. The reconstituted solution, if not used immediately, should be stored, protected from direct sunlight, between 2° and 8°C (36° and 46°F). Any unused solution in the vials must be discarded. Solutions diluted in normal saline may be stored between 2° and 8°C (36° to 46°F) or room temperature. The total time from reconstitution to completion of infusion should not exceed 8 hours.

Actions

➤*Pharmacology:* Belimumab, a human immune globulin G1 lambda monoclonal antibody, is a BLyS-specific inhibitor that blocks the binding of soluble BLyS, a B-cell survival factor, to its receptors on B cells. Belimumab does not bind B cells directly, but by binding BLyS, belimumab inhibits the survival of B cells, including auto reactive B cells, and reduces the differentiation of B cells into immunoglobulin-producing plasma cells.

BELIMUMAB — INJECTION

➤*Pharmacokinetics:*

Belimumab Pharmacokinetic Parameters in Systemic Lupus Erythematosus Patients[a,b]	
Pharmacokinetic parameter	Population estimates (n = 563)
C_{max}	313 mcg/mL
$AUC_{0-\infty}$	3,083 day•mcg/mL
Distribution t½	1.75 days
Terminal t½	19.4 days
Systemic CL	215 mL/day
Vd_{ss}	5.29 L

[a] IV infusions of 10 mg/kg were administered at 2-week intervals for the first 3 doses and at 4-week intervals thereafter.
[b] C_{max} = peak plasma concentrations; AUC = area under the curve; t½ = half-life; CL = clearance; Vd_{ss} = volume of distribution at steady state.

Special populations –

Renal function impairment: Although increases in CrCl and proteinuria (more than 2 g/day) increased belimumab clearance, these effects were within the expected range of variability. Therefore, dosage adjustment in patients with renal impairment is not recommended.

Race: In trials 2 and 3, response rates for the primary end point were lower for black subjects in the belimumab group relative to black subjects in the placebo group. Use with caution in black patients.

Contraindications

Patients who have had anaphylaxis with belimumab.

Warnings/Precautions

➤*Mortality:* There were more deaths reported with belimumab than with placebo during the controlled period of the clinical trials. Out of 2,133 patients in 3 clinical trials, a total of 14 deaths occurred during the placebo-controlled, double-blind treatment periods: 0.4%, 0.7%, 0%, and 0.9% deaths in the placebo and belimumab 1, 4, and 10 mg/kg groups, respectively. No single cause of death predominated. Causes included infection, cardiovascular disease, and suicide.

➤*Serious infections:* Serious and sometimes fatal infections have been reported in patients receiving immunosuppressive agents, including belimumab. Exercise caution when considering the use of belimumab in patients with chronic infections. Patients receiving any therapy for chronic infection should not begin therapy with belimumab. Consider interrupting belimumab therapy in patients who develop a new infection while undergoing treatment with belimumab and monitor these patients closely.

In the controlled clinical trials, the overall incidence of infections was 71% in patients treated with belimumab compared with 67% in patients who received placebo. The most frequent infections (more than 5% of patients receiving belimumab) were upper respiratory tract infection, urinary tract infection, nasopharyngitis, sinusitis, bronchitis, and influenza. Serious infections occurred in 6% of patients treated with belimumab and in 5.2% of patients who received placebo. The most frequent serious infections included pneumonia, urinary tract infection, cellulitis, and bronchitis. Infections leading to discontinuation of treatment occurred in 0.7% of patients receiving belimumab and 1% of patients receiving placebo. Infections resulting in death occurred in 0.3% of patients treated with belimumab and in 0.1 % of patients receiving placebo.

➤*Malignancy:* The impact of treatment with belimumab on the development of malignancies is not known. In the controlled clinical trials, malignancies (including nonmelanoma skin cancers) were reported in 0.4% of patients receiving belimumab and 0.4% of patients receiving placebo. In the controlled clinical trials, malignancies, excluding nonmelanoma skin cancers, were observed in 0.2% and 0.3% of patients receiving belimumab and placebo, respectively. As with other immunomodulating agents, the mechanism of action of belimumab could increase the risk of the development of malignancies.

➤*Infusion reactions:* In the controlled clinical trials, adverse events associated with the infusion (occurring on the same day of the infusion) were reported in 17% of patients receiving belimumab and 15% of patients receiving placebo. Serious infusion reactions (excluding hypersensitivity reactions) were reported in 0.5% of patients receiving belimumab and 0.4% of patients receiving placebo and included bradycardia, myalgia, headache, rash, urticaria, and hypotension. The most common infusion reactions (3% or more of patients receiving belimumab) were headache, nausea, and skin reactions. Due to overlap in signs and symptoms, it was not possible to distinguish between hypersensitivity reactions and infusion reactions in all cases. Some patients (13%) received premedication, which may have mitigated or masked an infusion reaction; however, there is insufficient evidence to determine whether premedication diminishes the frequency or severity of infusion reactions.

Belimumab should be administered by health care providers prepared to manage infusion reactions. The infusion rate may be slowed or interrupted if the patient develops an infusion reaction. Be aware of the risk of hypersensitivity reactions, which may present as infusion reactions, and monitor patients closely.

➤*Psychiatric effects:* In the controlled clinical trials, psychiatric events were reported more frequently with belimumab (16%) than with placebo (12%), related primarily to depression-related events (6.3% belimumab and 4.7% placebo), insomnia (6% belimumab and 5.3% placebo), and anxiety (3.9% belimumab and 2.8% placebo). Serious psychiatric events were reported in 0.8% of patients receiving belimumab (0.6% and 1.2% with 1 and 10 mg/kg, respectively) and 0.4% of patients receiving placebo. Serious depression was reported in 0.4% of patients receiving belimumab and 0.1% of patients receiving placebo. Two suicides (0.1%) were reported in patients receiving belimumab. The majority of patients who reported serious depression or suicidal behavior had a history of depression or other serious psychiatric disorders, and most were receiving psychoactive medications. It is unknown if belimumab treatment is associated with increased risk of these events.

➤*Immunization:* Do not give live vaccines for 30 days before or concurrently with belimumab because clinical safety has not been established. No data are available on the secondary transmission of infection from persons receiving live vaccines to patients receiving belimumab or the effect of belimumab on new immunizations. Because of its mechanism of action, belimumab may interfere with the response to immunizations.

➤*Immunogenicity:* In trials 2 and 3, antibelimumab antibodies were detected in 0.7% of patients receiving belimumab 10 mg/kg and in 4.8% of patients receiving belimumab 1 mg/kg. The reported frequency for the group receiving 10 mg/kg may underestimate the actual frequency due to lower assay sensitivity in the presence of high drug concentrations. Neutralizing antibodies were detected in 3 patients receiving belimumab 1 mg/kg. Three patients with antibelimumab antibodies experienced mild infusion reactions of nausea, erythematous rash, pruritus, eyelid edema, headache, and dyspnea; none of the reactions was life-threatening. The clinical relevance of the presence of antibelimumab antibodies is not known.

The data reflect the percentage of patients whose test results were positive for antibodies to belimumab in specific assays. The observed incidence of antibody positivity in an assay is highly dependent on several factors, including assay sensitivity and specificity, assay methodology, sample handling, timing of sample collection, concomitant medications, and underlying disease. For these reasons, comparison of the incidence of antibodies to belimumab with the incidence of antibodies to other products may be misleading.

➤*Hypersensitivity reactions:* In the controlled clinical trials, hypersensitivity reactions (occurring on the same day of infusion) were reported in 13% of patients receiving belimumab and 11% of patients receiving placebo. Anaphylaxis was observed in 0.6% of patients receiving belimumab and 0.4% of patients receiving placebo. Manifestations included hypotension, angioedema, urticaria or other rash, pruritus, and dyspnea. Due to overlap in signs and symptoms, it was not possible to distinguish between hypersensitivity reactions and infusion reactions in all cases. Some patients (13%) received premedication, which may have mitigated or masked a hypersensitivity response; however, there is insufficient evidence to determine whether premedication diminishes the frequency or severity of hypersensitivity reactions.

Belimumab should be administered by health care providers prepared to manage anaphylaxis. In the event of a serious reaction, administration of belimumab must be discontinued immediately and appropriate medical therapy administered. Monitor patients during and for an appropriate period of time after administration of belimumab.

➤*Pregnancy: Category C.* There are no adequate and well-controlled clinical studies using belimumab in pregnant women. Immunoglobulin G antibodies, including belimumab, can cross the placenta. Because animal reproduction studies are not always predictive of human response, use belimumab during pregnancy only if the potential benefit to the mother justifies the potential risk to the fetus. Instruct women of childbearing potential to use adequate contraception during treatment with belimumab and for at least 4 months after the final treatment.

Nonclinical reproductive studies have been performed in pregnant cynomolgus monkeys receiving belimumab at doses of 0, 5, and 150 mg/kg by IV infusion (the high dose was approximately 9 times the anticipated maximum human exposure) every 2 weeks from gestation day 20 to 150. Belimumab was shown to cross the placenta. Belimumab was not associated with direct or indirect teratogenicity under the conditions tested. Fetal deaths were observed in 14%, 24%, and 15% of pregnant females in the 0, 5, and 150 mg/kg groups, respectively. Infant deaths occurred with an incidence of 0%, 8%, and 5%. The cause of fetal and infant deaths is not known. The relevance of these findings to humans is not known. Other treatment-related findings were limited to the expected reversible reduction of B cells in both dams and infants and reversible reduction of IgM in infant monkeys. B-cell numbers recovered after the cessation of belimumab treatment by approximately 1 year postpartum in adult monkeys and by 3 months of age in infant monkeys. Immunoglobulin M levels in infants exposed to belimumab in utero recovered by 6 months of age.

Pregnancy registry – To monitor maternal-fetal outcomes of pregnant women exposed to belimumab, a pregnancy registry has been established. Health care professionals are encouraged to register patients, and pregnant women are encouraged to enroll themselves by calling 1-877-681-6296.

➤*Lactation:* It is not known whether belimumab is excreted in human milk or absorbed systemically after ingestion. However, belimumab was excreted into the milk of cynomolgus monkeys. Because maternal antibodies are excreted in human breast milk, decide whether to discontinue breast-feeding or the drug, taking into account the importance of breast-feeding to the infant and the importance of the drug to the mother.

➤*Children:* Safety and effectiveness of belimumab have not been established in children.

➤*Monitoring:* Monitor patients closely for the development of infusion and/or hypersensitivity reactions. Monitor patients who develop a new infection while undergoing treatment carefully.

Drug Interactions

None well documented.

BELIMUMAB — INJECTION

Adverse Reactions

➤*Common adverse reactions:* In clinical trials, 93% of patients treated with belimumab reported an adverse reaction, compared with 92% treated with placebo. The most common serious adverse reactions were serious infections (6% and 5.2% in the groups receiving belimumab and placebo, respectively). The most commonly-reported adverse reactions, occurring in 5% or more of patients in clinical trials, were nausea, diarrhea, pyrexia, nasopharyngitis, bronchitis, insomnia, pain in extremity, depression, migraine, and pharyngitis.

➤*Discontinuation:* The proportion of patients who discontinued treatment due to any adverse reaction during the controlled clinical trials was 6.2% for patients receiving belimumab and 7.1% for patients receiving placebo. The most common adverse reactions resulting in discontinuation of treatment (1% or more of patients receiving belimumab or placebo) were infusion reactions (1.6% belimumab and 0.9% placebo), lupus nephritis (0.7% belimumab and 1.2% placebo), and infections (0.7% belimumab and 1% placebo).

➤*Adverse reactions (3% or more):*

Belimumab Adverse Reactions (≥ 3%)		
Adverse reactions	Belimumab 10 mg/kg + standard of care (n = 674)	Placebo + standard of care (n = 675)
CNS		
Depression	5%	4%
Insomnia	7%	5%
Migraine	5%	4%
GI		
Diarrhea	12%	9%
Gastroenteritis viral	3%	1%
Nausea	15%	12%
Respiratory		
Bronchitis	9%	5%
Nasopharyngitis	9%	7%
Pharyngitis	5%	3%
Miscellaneous		
Cystitis	4%	3%
Leukopenia	4%	2%
Pain in extremity	6%	4%
Pyrexia	10%	8%

Patient Information

Advise patients that more patients receiving belimumab in the main clinical trials died than did patients receiving placebo treatment.

Advise patients that belimumab may decrease their ability to fight infections. Ask patients if they have a history of chronic infections and if they are currently on any therapy for an infection. Instruct patients to tell their health care provider if they develop signs or symptoms of an infection.

Educate patients on the signs and symptoms of anaphylaxis, including wheezing, difficulty breathing, peri-oral or lingual edema, and rash. Instruct patients to immediately tell their health care provider if they experience symptoms of an allergic reaction during or after the administration of belimumab.

Instruct patients to contact their health care provider if they experience new or worsening depression, suicidal thoughts, or other mood changes.

Inform patients that they should not receive live vaccines while taking belimumab. Response to vaccinations could be impaired by belimumab.

Inform patients that belimumab has not been studied in pregnant women or breast-feeding mothers so the effects of belimumab on pregnant women or breast-feeding infants are not known. Instruct patients to tell their health care provider if they are pregnant, become pregnant, or are thinking about becoming pregnant. Instruct patients to tell their health care provider if they plan to breast-feed their infant.

Advise women of childbearing potential to use adequate contraception during treatment with belimumab and for at least 4 months after final treatment.

ANTITOXINS/ANTIVENINS

ANTIVENIN (*LATRODECTUS MACTANS*) (Black Widow Spider Antivenin) (Equine Origin)

Rx	**Antivenin** (*Latrodectus mactans*) (Merck)	**Powder for Injection:** ≥ 6000 antivenin units/vial[a]	In single-use vials with 1 vial diluent (2.5 mL vial of sterile water for injection) and 1 mL vial of normal horse serum[a] (1:10 dilution) for sensitivity testing.

[a] With 1:10,000 thimerosal.

ANTIVENIN (*LATRODECTUS MACTANS*) (Black Widow Spider Antivenin) (Equine Origin) — INJECTION

Indications

➤*Envenomations:* For passive, transient protection from toxic effects of bites by the black widow (*Latrodectus mactans*) and similar spiders. Emphasize early use of this antivenin for prompt relief. The best effect occurs with antivenin administration within 4 hours after envenomation.

Administration and Dosage

➤*General dosing considerations:* Prior to treatment with any product prepared from horse serum, carefully review the patient's history emphasizing prior exposure to horse serum or any allergies. Serious sickness and even death could result from the use of horse serum in a sensitive patient. Perform a skin or conjunctival test prior to administration. (See Test dose.)

If the history is positive or the results of the sensitivity tests are mildly or questionably positive, desensitization may be required. (See Desensitization.)

➤*Adults:*

Envenomations –

Usual dosage: Inject 1 vial (2.5 mL) of antivenin intramuscularly (IM), preferably in the region of the anterolateral thigh. Symptoms usually subside in 1 to 3 hours. Although 1 dose is usually adequate, a second dose may be necessary.

May also be given intravenously (IV) in 10 to 50 mL of saline over 15 minutes. This is the preferred route in severe cases, when the patient is younger than 12 years of age, or in shock. One vial is usually adequate.

Test dose –

Skin test: Inject into (not under) the skin no more than 0.02 mL of the test material (1:10 dilution of normal horse serum in physiologic saline). Evaluate result in 10 minutes. A positive reaction is an urticarial wheal surrounded by a zone of erythema. A control test using sodium chloride injection facilitates interpretation of the results.

Conjunctival test: Instill 1 drop of a 1:10 dilution of horse serum into the conjunctival sac. Itching of the eye and reddening of the conjunctiva indicate a positive reaction, usually within 10 minutes.

➤*Children:*

Envenomations –

Usual dosage: See Adults for dosing.

Test dose:

- *Skin test –* See Adults for dosing.
- *Conjunctival test –* Instill 1 drop of 1:100 dilution of horse serum into the conjunctival sac. Itching of the eye and reddening of the conjunctiva indicate a positive reaction, usually within 10 minutes.

Desensitization – Attempt desensitization only when the administration of antivenin is considered necessary to save a life. Epinephrine must be available in case of untoward reaction.

If the history is positive or the results of the sensitivity tests are mildly or questionably positive, administer antivenin as follows to reduce the risk of an immediate severe allergic reaction:

1.) In separate sterile vials or syringes, prepare 1:10 or 1:100 dilutions of antivenin in sodium chloride for injection.
2.) Allow at least 15 but preferably 30 minutes between injections and only proceed with the next dose if no reactions occurred following the previous dose.
3.) Using a tuberculin syringe, inject subcutaneously 0.1, 0.2, and 0.5 mL of the 1:100 dilution at 15- or 30-minute intervals; repeat with the 1:10 dilution, and finally the undiluted antivenin.
4.) If there is a reaction after any of the injections, place a tourniquet proximal to the sites of injection and administer epinephrine 1:1000 (0.3 to 1 mL subcutaneously, 0.05 to 0.1 mL IV), proximal to the tourniquet or into another extremity. Wait at least 30 minutes before giving another injection of antivenin, the amount of which should be the same as the last one not evoking a reaction.
5.) If no reaction has occurred after 0.5 mL of undiluted antivenin has been given, it is probably safe to continue the dose at 15-minute intervals until the entire dose has been injected.

➤*Administration:* Administer IM in the region of the anterolateral thigh so that a tourniquet may be applied in the event of a systemic reaction. May be given IV in 10 to 50 mL of saline over 15 minutes. This is the preferred route in severe cases, when the patient is younger than 12 years of age, or in shock.

➤*Storage/Stability:* Refrigerate at 2° to 8°C (36° to 46°F). Do not freeze. Discard if frozen. Do not expose to excessive heat. When reconstituted, the color of the antivenin ranges from light (straw) to very dark (iced tea), but the color has no effect on potency.

Actions

➤*Pharmacology:* Prepared from blood serum of horses immunized against black widow spider venom. Moderately effective in pain relief and can be life-saving. IV effect is rapid; concentration peaks 2 to 3 days after IM injection. Mean half-life is less than 15 days. Symptoms begin to subside within 1 to 3 hours following administration.

ANTIVENIN (*LATRODECTUS MACTANS*) (Black Widow Spider Antivenin) (Equine Origin) — INJECTION

Warnings/Precautions

➤*Serum sickness:* Observe patients for serum sickness for an average of 8 to 12 days following administration of antivenin.

➤*Pregnancy: Category C.* It is not known whether the antivenin can cause fetal harm when administered to a pregnant woman or can affect reproduction capacity. Give to a pregnant woman only if clearly needed and when potential benefits outweigh potential hazards to the fetus.

Envenomation has produced spontaneous abortion.

➤*Lactation:* It is not known whether this drug is excreted in breast milk. Use caution when administering to a nursing woman.

➤*Children:* Controlled studies have not been conducted. However, there have been virtually no adverse effects in children receiving this product.

Adverse Reactions

➤*Hypersensitivity:* Anaphylaxis and serum sickness have been reported following use of antivenin.

Patient Information

Advise patients to contact their physician immediately if they experience any signs and symptoms of delayed allergic reactions or serum sickness (eg, rash, pruritus, urticaria, muscle aches, fever) after hospital discharge.

CROTALIDAE POLYVALENT IMMUNE FAB (Ovine Origin)

Rx	**CroFab** (BTG International)	**Powder for Injection, lyophilized**	1 g total protein and thimerosal (0.11 mg mercury)/vial. Diluent not included. In single-use vials.

CROTALIDAE POLYVALENT IMMUNE FAB (Ovine Origin) — INJECTION

Indications

➤*Envenomation:* Crotalidae polyvalent immune fab (ovine) injection is indicated for the management of patients with minimal or moderate North American rattlesnake envenomation. Crotalidae polyvalent immune fab (ovine) injection was effective in neutralizing the venoms of 10 clinically important North American Crotalid snakes in a murine lethality model. Early use of Crotalidae polyvalent immune fab (ovine) injection (within 6 hours of snakebite) is advised to prevent clinical deterioration and the occurrence of systemic coagulation abnormalities.

Administration and Dosage

➤*General dosing considerations:* Reconstitute and dilute Crotalidae Polyvalent Immune Fab prior to administration (See Preparation for Administration).

Administration of antivenin should be initiated as soon as possible after crotalid snakebite in patients who develop signs of progressive envenomation (eg, worsening local injury, coagulation abnormality, systemic signs of envenomation). Crotalidae polyvalent immune fab (ovine) injection was shown in the clinical studies to be effective when given within 6 hours of snakebite.

Supportive measures are often utilized to treat certain manifestations of crotalid snake envenomation, such as pain, swelling, hypotension, and wound infection. Poison control centers are a helpful resource for individual treatment advice.

➤*Adults:*

Envenomation –

Initial dosage: Antivenin dosage requirements are contingent upon an individual patient's response; however, based on clinical experience with Crotalidae polyvalent immune fab (ovine) injection, the recommended initial dose is 4 to 6 vials. The patient should be observed for up to 1 hour following the completion of this first dose to determine if initial control of the envenomation has been achieved (as defined by complete arrest of local manifestations and return of coagulation tests and systemic signs to normal).

If initial control is not achieved by the first dose, an additional dose of 4 to 6 vials should be repeated until initial control of the envenomation syndrome has been achieved.

Maintenance dosage: After initial control has been established, additional 2-vial doses of Crotalidae polyvalent immune fab (ovine) injection every 6 hours for up to 18 hours (3 doses) is recommended. Optimal dosing following the 18-hour scheduled dose of Crotalidae polyvalent immune fab (ovine) injection has not been determined. Additional 2-vial doses may be administered as deemed necessary by the treating health care provider, based on the patient's clinical course.

➤*Children:* See Warnings/Precautions for more information.

Envenomation – See Adults for dosing.

➤*Preparation for administration:*

Reconstitution – Each vial of Crotalidae polyvalent immune fab (ovine) injection should be reconstituted with 10 mL of sterile water for injection (diluent not included) and mixed by continuous gentle swirling.

Dilution – The contents of the reconstituted vials should be further diluted in 250 mL of 0.9% sodium chloride and mixed by gently swirling. The reconstituted and diluted product should be used within 4 hours.

➤*Administration:* The initial dose of Crotalidae polyvalent immune fab (ovine) injection diluted in 250 mL of saline should be infused IV over 60 minutes. However, the infusion should proceed slowly over the first 10 minutes at a 25 to 50 mL/h rate with careful observation for any allergic reaction. If no such reaction occurs, the infusion rate may be increased to the full 250 mL/h rate until completion. Close patient monitoring is necessary.

➤*Storage/Stability:* Store at 2° to 8°C (36° to 46°F). Do not freeze. Use within 4 hours after reconstitution

Actions

➤*Pharmacology:* Crotalidae polyvalent immune fab (ovine) injection is a venom-specific fab fragment of immunoglobulin G (IgG) that works by binding and neutralizing venom toxins, facilitating their redistribution away from target tissues and their elimination from the body.

➤*Pharmacokinetics:*

Excretion – The planned pharmacokinetic study of Crotalidae polyvalent immune fab (ovine) injection was not adequately performed. A limited number of samples were collected from 3 patients. Based on these data, estimates of elimination half-life were made. The elimination half-life for total fab ranged from approximately 12 to 23 hours. These limited pharmacokinetic estimates of half-life are augmented by data obtained with an analogous ovine fab product that was produced using a similar production process. In that study, 8 healthy subjects were given 1 mg of IV digoxin followed by an approximately equimolar neutralizing dose of 76 mg of digoxin immune fab (ovine). Total fab was shown to have a volume of distribution of 0.3 L/kg, a systemic clearance of 32 mL/min (approximately 0.4 mL/min/kg) and an elimination half-life of approximately 15 hours.

Contraindications

Crotalidae polyvalent immune fab (ovine) injection should not be administered to patients with a known history of hypersensitivity to papaya or papain, unless the benefits outweigh the risks and appropriate management for anaphylactic reactions is readily available.

Warnings/Precautions

➤*Coagulopathy:* Coagulopathy is a complication noted in many victims of viper envenomation that arises due to the ability of the snake venom to interfere with the blood coagulation cascade. In clinical trials with Crotalidae polyvalent immune fab (ovine) injection, recurrent coagulopathy (the return of a coagulation abnormality after it has been successfully treated with antivenin), characterized by decreased fibrinogen, decreased platelets, and elevated prothrombin time, occurred in approximately half of patients studied. The clinical significance of these recurrent abnormalities is not known. Recurrent coagulation abnormalities were observed only in patients who experienced coagulation abnormalities during their initial hospitalizations. Optimal dosing to completely prevent recurrent coagulopathy has not been determined. Because Crotalidae polyvalent immune fab (ovine) injection has a shorter persistence in the blood than crotalid venoms that can leak from depot sites over a prolonged period of time, repeat dosing to prevent or treat such recurrence may be necessary. Additional 2-vial doses may be administered as deemed necessary by the treating physician, based on the patient's clinical course.

Recurrent coagulopathy may persist for 1 to 2 weeks or more. Patients who experience coagulopathy due to snakebite during hospitalization for initial treatment should be monitored for signs and symptoms of recurrent coagulopathy for up to 1 week or longer at the physician's discretion. During this period, the physician should carefully assess the need for retreatment with Crotalidae polyvalent immune fab (ovine) injection and use of any type of anticoagulant or antiplatelet drug.

➤*Mercury:* Crotalidae polyvalent immune fab (ovine) injection contains mercury in the form of ethyl mercury from thimerosal. The final product contains up to 104.5 mcg or approximately 0.11 mg of mercury per vial, which amounts to no more than 1.9 mg of mercury per dose (based on the maximum dose of 18 vials studied in clinical trials of Crotalidae polyvalent immune fab [ovine]injection). While there are no definitive data on the toxicity of ethyl mercury, literature suggests that information related to methyl mercury toxicities may be applicable.

➤*Hypersensitivity reactions:* Papain is used to cleave the whole antibody into fab and Fc fragments, and trace amounts of papain or inactivated papain residues may be present in Crotalidae polyvalent immune fab (ovine) injection. Patients with allergies to papain, chymopapain, other papaya extracts, or the pineapple enzyme bromelain may also be at risk for allergic reactions to Crotalidae polyvalent immune fab (ovine) injection. In addition, it has been noted in the literature that some dust mite allergens and some latex allergens share antigenic structures with papain, and patients with these allergies may be allergic to papain.

Crotalidae polyvalent immune fab (ovine) injection should not be administered to patients with known histories of hypersensitivity to papaya or papain, unless the benefits outweigh the risks and appropriate management for anaphylactic reactions is readily available.

CROTALIDAE POLYVALENT IMMUNE FAB (Ovine Origin) — INJECTION

Anaphylaxis, anaphylactoid reactions and allergic reactions – The possible risks and side effects that attend the administration of heterologous animal proteins in humans include anaphylactic and anaphylactoid reactions, delayed allergic reactions (late serum reaction or serum sickness) and possible febrile responses to immune complexes formed by animal antibodies and neutralized venom components. Although no patient in the clinical studies of Crotalidae polyvalent immune fab (ovine) injection has experienced a severe anaphylactic reaction, the possibility of an anaphylactic reaction should be considered. The patient should be informed of the possibility of an anaphylactic reaction, and close patient monitoring and readiness with IV therapy using epinephrine and diphenhydramine hydrochloride is recommended during the infusion of Crotalidae polyvalent immune fab (ovine) injection. If an anaphylactic reaction occurs during the infusion, Crotalidae polyvalent immune fab (ovine) injection administration should be terminated at once and appropriate treatment administered. Patients with known allergies to sheep protein would be particularly at risk for an anaphylactic reaction.

See Warnings/Precautions for more information.

Infusion reactions: It has been noted in the literature with the use of other antibody therapies that reactions during the infusion, such as fever, low back pain, wheezing and nausea are often related to the rate of infusion and can be controlled by decreasing the rate of administration of the solution.

Sensitivity: Patients who receive courses of treatment with foreign proteins such as Crotalidae polyvalent immune fab (ovine) injection may become sensitized to them. Therefore, caution should be used when administering a repeat course of treatment with Crotalidae polyvalent immune fab (ovine) injection for a subsequent envenomation episode.

➤*Special risk:* Because snake envenomation can cause coagulation abnormalities, the following conditions, which are also associated with coagulation defects, should be considered: Cancer, collagen disease, congestive heart failure, diarrhea, elevated temperature, hepatic disorders, hyperthyroidism, poor nutritional state, steatorrhea, vitamin K deficiency.

➤*Pregnancy: Category C.* Animal reproduction studies have not been conducted with Crotalidae polyvalent immune fab (ovine) injection. It is also not known whether Crotalidae polyvalent immune fab (ovine) injection can cause fetal harm when administered to a pregnant woman or can affect reproduction capacity. Crotalidae polyvalent immune fab (ovine) injection should be given to a pregnant woman only if clearly needed.

Crotalidae polyvalent immune fab (ovine) injection contains mercury in the form of ethyl mercury from thimerosal. The final product contains up to 104.5 mcg or approximately 0.11 mg of mercury per vial, which amounts to no more than 1.9 mg of mercury per dose (based on the maximum dose of 18 vials studied in clinical trials of Crotalidae polyvalent immune fab [ovine]injection). While there are no definitive data on the toxicity of ethyl mercury, literature suggests that information related to methyl mercury toxicities may be applicable. Developing fetuses and very young children are most susceptible and, therefore, at greater risk.

➤*Lactation:* It is not known whether Crotalidae polyvalent immune fab (ovine) injection is excreted in human breast milk. Because many drugs are excreted in human milk, caution should be exercised when Crotalidae polyvalent immune fab (ovine) injection is administered to a nursing woman.

➤*Children:* Specific studies in pediatric patients have not been conducted. The absolute venom dose following snakebite is expected to be the same in children and adults, therefore, no dosage adjustment for age should be made.

Crotalidae polyvalent immune fab (ovine) injection contains mercury in the form of ethyl mercury from thimerosal. Although there are limited toxicology data on ethyl mercury, high dose and acute exposures to methyl mercury have been associated with neurological and renal toxicities. Developing fetuses and very young children are most susceptible and, therefore, at greater risk.

➤*Monitoring:* All patients treated with antivenin should be carefully monitored for signs and symptoms of an acute allergic reaction (eg, urticaria, pruritus, erythema, angioedema, bronchospasm with wheezing or cough, stridor, laryngeal edema, hypotension, tachycardia) and treated with appropriate emergency medical care (eg, epinephrine, IV antihistamines, albuterol). All patients should be followed up for signs and symptoms of delayed allergic reactions or serum sickness (eg, rash, fever, myalgia, arthralgia) and treated appropriately, if necessary.

Adverse Reactions

The most common adverse reactions reported in the clinical studies were urticaria and rash. Adverse reactions involving the skin and appendages (primarily rash, urticaria, and pruritus) were reported in 14 of the 42 patients (see the following table).

Of the 25 patients who experienced adverse reactions, 3 patients experienced severe or serious adverse reactions. The 1 patient who experienced a serious adverse event had a recurrent coagulopathy due to envenomation, which required rehospitalization and additional antivenin administration. This patient eventually made a complete recovery. The other 2 patients that had severe adverse reactions consisted of 1 patient who developed severe hives following treatment and 1 patient who developed a severe rash and pruritus several days following treatment. Both patients recovered following treatment with antihistamines and prednisone.

One patient discontinued Crotalidae polyvalent immune fab (ovine) injection therapy due to an allergic reaction.

Incidence of Clinical Adverse Reactions in Studies of Crotalidae Polyvalent Immune Fab (Ovine) Injection by Body System

Adverse reactions	Number of reactions (n = 42[a])
Cardiovascular	
Hypotension	1
CNS	
Circumoral paresthesia	1
General paresthesia	1
Nervousness	1
Dermatologic	
Urticaria	7
Rash	5
Pruritus	3
Subcutaneous nodule	1
GI	
Nausea	3
Anorexia	1
Hematologic/Lymphatic	
Coagulation disorder	3
Ecchymosis	1
Musculoskeletal	
Myalgia	1
Respiratory	
Asthma	1
Cough	1
Increased sputum	1
Miscellaneous	
Back pain	2
Chest pain	1
Cellulitis	1
Wound infection	1
Chills	1
Allergic reaction[b]	1
Serum sickness	1

[a] Of the 42 patients receiving Crotalidae polyvalent immune fab (ovine) injection in the clinical studies, 25 experienced an adverse reaction. A total of 40 adverse reactions was experienced by these 25 patients.
[b] Allergic reactions consisted of urticaria, dyspnea, and wheezing in 1 patient.

In the 42 patients treated with Crotalidae polyvalent immune fab (ovine) injection for minimal or moderate crotalid envenomations, there were 7 reactions classified as early serum reactions and 5 reactions classified as late serum reactions, and none was serious. In the clinical studies, serum reactions consisted mainly of urticaria and rash, and all patients recovered without sequelae.

Incidence of Early and Late Serum Reactions (Reactions Associated with Crotalidae Polyvalent Immune Fab (Ovine) Injection

Serum reactions	Number of reactions (n = 42[a])
Early serum reactions	
Urticaria	5
Cough	1
Allergic reaction[b]	1
Late serum reactions	
Rash	2
Pruritus	1
Urticaria	1
Serum sickness[c]	1

[a] Six of the 42 patients experienced an adverse reaction associated with an early serum reaction, and 4 experienced an adverse reaction associated with a late serum reaction. Two additional patients were considered to have a late serum reaction by the investigator, although no associated adverse reaction was reported.
[b] Allergic reaction consisted of urticaria, dyspnea and wheezing in 1 patient.
[c] Serum sickness consisted of severe rash and pruritus in 1 patient.

Overdosage

The maximum amount of Crotalidae polyvalent immune fab (ovine) injection that can safely be administered in single or multiple doses has not been determined. Doses of up to 18 vials (approximately 13.5 g of protein) have been administered without any observed direct toxic effect.

CROTALIDAE POLYVALENT IMMUNE FAB (Ovine Origin) — INJECTION

Patient Information

Patients should be advised to contact their physicians immediately if they experience any signs and symptoms of delayed allergic reactions or serum sickness (eg, rash, pruritus, urticaria) after hospital discharge.

Patients should be advised to contact their physicians immediately if they experience unusual bruising or bleeding (eg, nosebleeds, excessive bleeding after brushing teeth, the appearance of blood in stools or urine, excessive menstrual bleeding, petechiae, excessive bruising or persistent oozing from superficial injuries) after hospital discharge, as they may need additional antivenin treatment. Such bruising or bleeding may occur for up to 1 week or longer following initial treatment, and patients should be advised to follow up with their physicians for monitoring.

ANTIVENIN (*MICRURUS FULVIUS*) (North American Coral Snake Antivenin) (Equine Origin)

Rx	**Antivenin** (*Micrurus fulvius*)[a] (Wyeth-Ayerst)	**Powder for Injection, lyophilized**[b]	In single-use vials with 1 vial diluent (10 mL Water for Injection).[c]

[a] The manufacturer is in the process of discontinuing this product; however, it will be producing enough antivenin to satisfy demand for several years.

[b] Prior to lyophilization, product contains 0.25% phenol and 0.005% thimerosal.

[c] With 1:100,000 phenylmercuric nitrate.

ANTIVENIN (*MICRURUS FULVIUS*) (North American Coral Snake Antivenin) (Equine Origin) INJECTION

Indications

➤*Envenomations:* For passive, transient protection from toxic effects of venoms of *Micrurus fulvius fulvius* (Eastern coral snake). Also neutralizes venom of *M. fulvius tenere* (Texas coral snake). If indicated, the best effect results if antivenin administration begins within 4 hours of envenomation.

This antivenin partially neutralizes the venom of *M. dumerilii carinicauda* and minimally neutralizes the venom of *M. spixii*. It may also provide some protection against the venom of *M. nigrocinctus*.

Administration and Dosage

➤*General dosing considerations:* Whenever a product containing horse serum is administered, there is a possibility of a severe immediate reaction. Have appropriate therapeutic agents available (not corticosteroids). See also Management of Acute Hypersensitivity Reactions.

Before administration of any product prepared from horse serum, take appropriate measures in an effort to detect the presence of dangerous sensitivity. A careful review of the patient's history should be noted, including any report of the following: asthma, hay fever, urticaria, or other allergic manifestations; allergic reactions upon exposure to horses; prior injections of horse serum.

Perform a skin test in every patient prior to administration, regardless of clinical history. (See Test dose.)

If the patients history is negative, and the skin test is mildly or questionably positive, desensitization may be needed to reduce the risk of a severe immediate systemic reaction. (See Desensitization.)

If symptoms or signs of envenomation occur or are already present at the time the patient is first seen, give IV antivenin promptly.

➤*Adults:*

Envenomation –

Test dose: Intracutaneously inject 0.02 to 0.03 mL of a 1:10 dilution of Normal Horse Serum or Antivenin. A control test on the opposite extremity, using Sodium Chloride Injection facilitates interpretation. Use of larger amounts for the skin-test dose increases the likelihood of false-positive reactions, and in the exquisitely sensitive patient, increases the risk of a systemic reaction from the skin-test dose. At least a 1:100 dilution should be used for preliminary skin testing if the history suggests sensitivity. A positive reaction to a skin test occurs within 5 to 30 minutes and is manifested by a wheal with or without pseudopodia and surrounding erythema. In general, the shorter the interval between injection and the beginning of the skin reaction, the greater the sensitivity.

If the history is negative for allergy and the result of a skin test is negative, proceed with administration of antivenin as outlined. If the history is positive and a skin test is strongly positive, administration may be dangerous, especially if the positive sensitivity test is accompanied by systemic allergic manifestations. In such instances, the risk of administering antivenin must be weighed against the risk of withholding it, keeping in mind that severe envenomation can be fatal.

A negative allergic history and absence of reaction to a properly applied skin test do not rule out the possibility of an immediate reaction. Also, a negative skin test has no bearing on whether or not delayed serum reactions (serum sickness) will occur after administration of the full dose.

Initial dose: If the results of appropriate tests have indicated the patient is not dangerously hypersensitive to horse serum and depending on the nature and severity of the signs and symptoms of envenomation, administer 3 to 5 vials slowly intravenously (IV), giving the first 1 to 2 mL of the antivenin dilution over 3 to 5 minutes. Watch the patient carefully for evidence of an allergic reaction. If no signs or symptoms of anaphylaxis appear, continue the injection or infusion.

Repeat dosage: Administer additional antivenin as required. Some envenomed patients may need the contents of more than 10 vials.

➤*Children:*

Envenomation – See Adults for dosing.

➤*Desensitization:* If the history is negative, and the skin test is mildly or questionably positive, administer as follows to reduce the risk of a severe immediate systemic reaction:

1.) Prepare, in separate sterile vials or syringes, 1:100 and 1:10 dilutions of antivenin.
2.) Allow at least 15 minutes between injections and proceed with the next dose if no reaction follows the previous dose.
3.) Inject subcutaneously using a tuberculin-type syringe, 0.1, 0.2, and 0.5 mL of the 1:100 dilution at 15-minute intervals; repeat with the 1:10 dilution, and finally undiluted antivenin.
4.) If a systemic reaction occurs after any injection, place a tourniquet proximal to the site of injections and administer an appropriate dose of epinephrine, 1:1000, proximal to the tourniquet or into another extremity. Wait at least 30 minutes before injecting another dose. The amount of the next dose should be the same as the last that did not evoke a reaction.
5.) If no reaction occurs after 0.5 mL of undiluted antivenin has been administered, switch to the IM route and continue doubling the dose at 15-minute intervals until the entire dose has been injected IM or proceed to the IV route.

➤*Preparation for administration:* Withdraw diluent and inject into the vial of antivenin. Gentle agitation will hasten complete dissolution of lyophilized drug. Do not shake. To avoid foaming and protein degradation, mix by gently swirling rather than shaking.

➤*Administration:* Start an IV drip of 250 to 500 mL of sodium chloride injection. If the results of appropriate tests have indicated the patient is not dangerously hypersensitive to horse serum and depending on the nature and severity of the signs and symptoms of envenomation, administer the contents of 3 to 5 vials as the initial dose IV by slow injection directly into the IV tubing or by slow IV infusion by adding to the reservoir bottle of the IV drip. In either case, give the first 1 to 2 mL of the antivenin dilution over 3 to 5 minutes and watch the patient carefully for evidence of an allergic reaction. If no signs or symptoms of anaphylaxis appear, continue the injection or infusion.

Adjust the rate of delivery by the severity of signs and symptoms of envenomation and tolerance of antivenin. Nonetheless, until the contents of 3 to 5 vials of antivenin have been given, administer at the maximum safe rate for IV fluids, based on body weight and general condition of the patient. For example, 250 to 500 mL over 30 minutes may be appropriate in a healthy adult, while small children may receive the first 100 mL rapidly, followed by a rate not to exceed 4 mL/min. Response to treatment may be rapid and dramatic.

➤*Storage/Stability:* Store at 2° to 8°C (36° to 46°F). Do not expose to temperatures greater than 40°C (104°F). Do not freeze diluent. Product can tolerate 10 days in solution at room temperature. Use reconstituted solutions within 48 hours and dilutions within 12 hours. Product shelf life expires within 60 months.

Actions

➤*Pharmacology:* Refined, concentrated, lyophilized preparation of serum globulins obtained by fractionating blood from healthy horses immunized with eastern coral snake (*Micrurus fulvius fulvius*) venom.

Two genera of coral snakes inhabit the US: *Micrurus* (including the eastern and Texas varieties), and *Micruroides* (the Arizonan or Sonoran variety). *Micrurus fulvius fulvius* inhabits an area from North Carolina south to Florida and west to the Mississippi River. *Micrurus fulvius tenere* inhabits an area west of the Mississippi River including Louisiana, Arkansas, and Texas. Several other species of coral snake inhabit much of Central and South America, including 3 genera, *Leptomicrurus*, *Micrurus*, and *Micruroides*.

Warnings/Precautions

➤*Not effective:* Not effective against the venom of *Euryxanthus* (Arizonan or Sonoran coral snake), found only in southeastern Arizona, southwestern New Mexico, and portions of Mexico. Not effective in other snakes not described above.

➤*Supportive therapy:* Appropriate tetanus prophylaxis is indicated. Morphine or other narcotics that depress respiration are contraindicated. Use sedatives with extreme caution.

If practical, immobilize victim immediately and completely. If complete immobilization is not practical, splint bitten extremity to limit spread of venom.

Hemoglobinuria has occurred in animals. Therefore, continuous bladder drainage with careful attention to urinary output and blood electrolyte balance is recommended.

➤*Hypersensitivity reactions:* The immediate reaction (eg, shock, anaphylaxis) usually occurs within 30 minutes. Symptoms and signs may include apprehension; flushing; itching; urticaria; edema of the face, tongue, and throat; cough; dyspnea; cyanosis; vomiting; and collapse.

Serum sickness – See Adverse Reactions for more information.

ANTIVENIN (*MICRURUS FULVIUS*) (North American Coral Snake Antivenin) (Equine Origin) INJECTION

➤*Pregnancy: Category C.* Use only if clearly needed, with appropriate consideration of the risk-benefit ratio. It is not known if antivenom antibodies cross the placenta. Intact IgG crosses the placenta from the maternal circulation increasingly after 30 weeks' gestation.

➤*Lactation:* It is not known if antivenom antibodies are excreted into breast milk. Problems in humans have not been documented.

➤*Children:* The pediatric dose is equivalent to the adult dose. Pediatric doses are not adjusted by the weight of the patient.

Adverse Reactions

➤*Hypersensitivity:* The immediate reaction (eg, shock, anaphylaxis) usually occurs within 30 minutes. Symptoms and signs may include apprehension; flushing; itching; urticaria; edema of the face, tongue, and throat; cough; dyspnea; cyanosis; vomiting; and collapse.

Serum sickness – Serum sickness usually occurs 5 to 24 days after administration. The incubation period may be

Patient Information

Advise patients to contact their physician immediately if they experience any signs and symptoms of delayed allergic reactions or serum sickness (eg, rash, pruritus, urticaria) after hospital discharge.

In contrast to the immune serums and antitoxins, which contain exogenous antibodies to provide passive immunity, the agents for active immunization include specific antigens that induce the endogenous production of antibodies. Agents that induce active immunity include vaccines and the subset of vaccines called toxoids.

Vaccines contain whole (killed or attenuated live) or partial microorganisms capable of inducing antibody formation, but which are not pathogenic. Toxoids are detoxified by-products derived from organisms that induce disease primarily through the elaboration of exotoxins. Although toxoids are not toxic, they are antigenic and, therefore, stimulate specific antibody production. Active immunization induced through administration of vaccines and toxoids provides prolonged immunity, whereas passive immunization with immune sera or antitoxins is of short duration.

Vaccination with any vaccine may not result in a protective antibody response in all individuals given the vaccine.

➤*Immunization schedules for children:* The following tables reflect the recommended immunization schedules for children 0 to 18 years of age and the catch-up immunization schedule for 2011 approved by the Advisory Committee on Immunization Practices (ACIP), the American Academy of Pediatrics, and the American Academy of Family Physicians (AAFP). This table is revised annually.

Recommended Immunization Schedule for Children 0 to 6 Years of Age — United States, 2011[a]

Vaccine	Birth	1 mo	2 mo	4 mo	6 mo	12 mo	15 mo	18 mo	19 to 23 mo	2 to 3 y	4 to 6 y
Hep B[b]	Hep B	Hep B			Hep B						
Rotavirus[c]			Rotavirus	Rotavirus	Rotavirus[c]						
DTaP[d]			DTaP	DTaP	DTaP	d	DTaP				DTaP
Hib[e]			Hib	Hib	Hib[e]	Hib					
Pneumococcal[f]			PCV	PCV	PCV	PCV				PPSV	
IPV[g]			IPV	IPV	IPV						IPV
Influenza[h]					Influenza (yearly)						
MMR[i]						MMR			i		MMR
Varicella[j]						Varicella			j		Varicella
Hep A[k]						Hep A (2 doses)				Hep A series	
Meningococcal[l]										MCV4	

Range of recommended ages for all children. Range of recommended ages for certain high-risk groups.

NOTE: The recommendations in the table must be read along with the following footnotes.

[a] This schedule includes recommendations in effect as of December 21, 2010. Any dose not administered at the recommended age should be administered at a subsequent visit, when indicated and feasible. The use of a combination vaccine generally is preferred over separate injections of its equivalent component vaccines. Considerations should include provider assessment, patient preference, and the potential for adverse events. Providers should consult the relevant ACIP statement for detailed recommendations: http://www.cdc.gov/vaccines/pubs/acip-list.htm. Clinically significant adverse events that follow immunization should be reported to the Vaccine Adverse Event Reporting System (VAERS) at http://www.vaers.hhs.gov or by telephone (1-800-822-7967).

[b] **Hepatitis B (Hep B) vaccine** *(minimum age, birth)*

At birth:
- Administer monovalent Hep B to all newborns before hospital discharge.
- If mother is hepatitis B surface antigen (HBsAg)-positive, administer Hep B and 0.5 mL of hepatitis B immune globulin (HBIG) within 12 hours of birth.
- If mother's HBsAg status is unknown, administer Hep B within 12 hours of birth. Determine mother's HBsAg status as soon as possible and, if HBsAg-positive, administer HBIG (no later than 1 week of age).

Doses following the birth dose:
- The second dose should be administered at 1 or 2 months of age. Monovalent Hep B should be used for doses administered before 6 weeks of age.
- Infants born to HBsAg-positive mothers should be tested for HBsAg and antibody to HBsAg 1 to 2 months after completion of at least 3 doses of the HepB series, at 9 through 18 months of age (generally at the next well-child visit).
- Administration of 4 doses of Hep B to infants is permissible when a combination vaccine containing Hep B is administered after the birth dose.
- Infants who did not receive a birth dose should receive 3 doses of Hep B on a schedule of 0, 1, and 6 months.
- The final (third or fourth) dose in the HepB series should be administered no earlier than 24 weeks of age.

[c] **Rotavirus vaccine** *(minimum age, 6 weeks)*
- Administer the first dose at 6 through 14 weeks of age (maximum age, 14 weeks 6 days). Vaccination should not be initiated for infants 15 weeks 0 days of age or older.
- The maximum age for the final dose in the series is 8 months 0 days.
- If *Rotarix* is administered at 2 and 4 months of age, a dose at 6 months is not indicated.

[d] **Diphtheria and tetanus toxoids and acellular pertussis (DTaP) vaccine** *(minimum age, 6 weeks)*
- The fourth dose may be administered as early as 12 months of age, provided at least 6 months have elapsed since the third dose.

[e] ***Haemophilus influenzae* type b (Hib) conjugate vaccine** *(minimum age, 6 weeks)*
- If PRP-OMP (*PedvaxHIB* or *Comvax* [Hep B-Hib]) is administered at 2 and 4 months of age, a dose at 6 months of age is not indicated.
- *Hiberix* should not be used for doses at 2, 4, or 6 months of age for the primary series but can be used as the final dose in children 12 months through 4 years of age.

[f] **Pneumococcal vaccine (PCV)** *(minimum age, 6 weeks for PCV; 2 years for pneumococcal polysaccharide vaccine [PPSV])*
- PCV is recommended for all children younger than 5 years. Administer 1 dose of PCV to all healthy children 24 through 59 months of age who are not completely vaccinated for their age.
- A PCV series begun with 7-valent pneumococcal vaccine (PCV7) should be completed with 13-valent pneumococcal vaccine (PCV13).
- A single supplemental dose of PCV13 is recommended for all children 14 through 59 months of age who have received an age-appropriate series of PCV7.
- A single supplemental dose of PCV13 is recommended for all children 60 through 71 months of age with underlying medical conditions who have received an age-appropriate series of PCV7.
- The supplemental dose of PCV13 should be administered at least 8 weeks after the previous dose of PCV7. See *MMWR.* 2010;59(No. RR-11).
- Administer PPSV at least 8 weeks after the last dose of PCV to children 2 years or older with certain underlying medical conditions, including a cochlear implant.

[g] **Inactivated poliovirus vaccine (IPV)** *(minimum age, 6 weeks)*
- If 4 or more doses are administered prior to 4 years of age, an additional dose should be administered at 4 through 6 years of age.
- The final dose in the series should be administered on or after the fourth birthday and at least 6 months following the previous dose.

[h] **Influenza vaccine (seasonal)** *(minimum age, 6 months for trivalent inactivated influenza vaccine [TIV]; 2 years for live attenuated influenza vaccine [LAIV])*
- For healthy children 2 years and older (ie, those who do not have underlying medical conditions that predispose them to influenza complications), either LAIV or TIV may be used, except LAIV should not be given to children 2 through 4 years of age who have had wheezing in the past 12 months.
- Administer 2 doses (separated by at least 4 weeks) to children 6 months through 8 years of age who are receiving seasonal influenza vaccine for the first time or who were vaccinated for the first time during the previous influenza season but only received 1 dose.
- Children 6 months through 8 years of age who received no doses of monovalent 2009 H1N1 vaccine should receive 2 doses of 2010–2011 seasonal influenza vaccine. See *MMWR.* 2010;59(No. RR-8):33-34.

[i] **Measles, mumps, rubella (MMR) vaccine** *(minimum age, 12 months)*
- The second dose may be administered before 4 years of age, provided at least 4 weeks have elapsed since the first dose.

[j] **Varicella vaccine** *(minimum age, 12 months)*
- The second dose may be administered before 4 years of age, provided at least 3 months have elapsed since the first dose.
- For children 12 months through 12 years of age the recommended minimum interval between doses is 3 months. However, if the second dose was administered at least 4 weeks after the first dose, it can be accepted as valid.

[k] **Hepatitis A (Hep A) vaccine** *(minimum age, 12 months)*
- Administer 2 doses at least 6 months apart.
- Hep A is recommended for children older than 23 months who live in areas where vaccination programs target older children, who are at increased risk for infection, or for whom immunity against hepatitis A is desired.

[l] **Meningococcal cojugate vaccine, quadrivalent (MCV4)** *(minimum age, 2 years)*
- Administer 2 doses of MCV4 at least 8 weeks apart to children 2 through 10 years of age with persistent complement component deficiency and anatomic or functional asplenia, and 1 dose every 5 years thereafter.
- Individuals with HIV infection who are vaccinated with MCV4 should receive 2 doses at least 8 weeks apart.
- Administer 1 dose of MCV4 to children 2 through 10 years of age who travel to countries with highly endemic or epidemic disease and during outbreaks caused by a vaccine serogroup.
- Administer MCV4 to children at continued risk for meningococcal disease who were previously vaccinated with MCV4 or meningococcal polysaccharide vaccine after 3 years if the first dose was administered at 2 through 6 years of age.

Recommended Immunization Schedule for Children 7 to 18 Years of Age — United States, 2011[a]

Vaccine	7 to 10 y	11 to 12 y	13 to 18 y
Tdap[b]	[b]	Tdap	Tdap
HPV[c]	[c]	HPV (3 doses) (females)	HPV series
MCV4[d]	MCV4	MCV4	MCV4
Influenza[e]	Influenza (yearly)		
Pneumococcal[f]	Pneumococcal		
Hep A[g]	Hep A series		
Hep B[h]	Hep B series		
IPV[i]	IPV series		
MMR[j]	MMR series		
Varicella[k]	Varicella series		

Range of recommended ages for children — Range of recommended ages for catch-up immunization — Range of recommended ages for certain high-risk groups

NOTE: The recommendations in the table must be read along with the following footnotes.

[a] **This schedule includes recommendations in effect as of December 21, 2010.** Any dose not administered at the recommended age should be administered at a subsequent visit, when indicated and feasible. The use of a combination vaccine generally is preferred over separate injections of its equivalent component vaccines. Considerations should include provider assessment, patient preference, and the potential for adverse events. Providers should consult the relevant ACIP statement for detailed recommendations: http://www.cdc.gov/vaccines/pubs/acip-list.htm. Clinically significant adverse events that follow immunization should be reported to the VAERS at http://www.vaers.hhs.gov or by telephone (1-800-822-7967).

[b] **Tetanus and diphtheria toxoids and acellular pertussis (Tdap) vaccine** *(minimum age, 10 years for Boostrix and 11 years for Adacel)*
- Individuals 11 through 18 years of age who have not received Tdap should receive a dose followed by Td booster doses every 10 years thereafter.
- Individuals 7 through 10 years of age who are not fully immunized against pertussis (including those never vaccinated or with unknown pertussis vaccination status) should receive a single dose of Tdap. Refer to the catch-up schedule if additional doses of tetanus and diphtheria toxoid–containing vaccine are needed.
- Tdap can be administered regardless of the interval since the last tetanus and diphtheria toxoid–containing vaccine.

[c] **Human papillomavirus (HPV) vaccine** *(minimum age, 9 years)*
- Quadrivalent HPV vaccine (HPV4) or bivalent HPV vaccine (HPV2) is recommended for the prevention of cervical precancers and cancers in females.
- HPV4 is recommended for prevention of cervical precancers, cancers, and genital warts in females.
- HPV4 may be administered in a 3-dose series to males 9 through 18 years of age to reduce their likelihood of genital warts.
- Administer the second dose 1 to 2 months after the first dose and the third dose 6 months after the first dose (at least 24 weeks after the first dose).

[d] **MCV4** *(minimum age, 2 years)*
- Administer MCV4 at 11 through 12 years of age with a booster dose at 16 years of age.
- Administer 1 dose at 13 through 18 years of age if not previously vaccinated.
- Individuals who received their first dose at 13 through 15 years of age should receive a booster dose at 16 through 18 years of age.
- Administer 1 dose to previously unvaccinated college freshmen living in a dormitory.
- Administer 2 doses at least 8 weeks apart to children 2 through 10 years of age with persistent complement component deficiency and anatomic or functional asplenia, and 1 dose every 5 years thereafter.
- Individuals with HIV infection who are vaccinated with MCV4 should receive 2 doses at least 8 weeks apart.
- Administer 1 dose of MCV4 to children 2 through 10 years of age who travel to countries with highly endemic or epidemic disease and during outbreaks caused by a vaccine serogroup.
- Administer MCV4 to children at continued risk for meningococcal disease who were previously vaccinated with MCV4 or meningococcal polysaccharide vaccine after 3 years (if first dose administered at 2 through 6 years of age) or after 5 years (if first dose administered at 7 years or older).

[e] **Influenza vaccine (seasonal)**
- For healthy nonpregnant individuals 7 through 18 years of age (ie, those who do not have underlying medical conditions that predispose them to influenza complications), either LAIV or TIV may be used.
- Administer 2 doses (separated by at least 4 weeks) to children 6 months through 8 years of age who are receiving seasonal influenza vaccine for the first time or who were vaccinated for the first time during the previous influenza season but only received 1 dose.
- Children 6 months through 8 years of age who received no doses of monovalent 2009 H1N1 vaccine should receive 2 doses of 2010-2011 seasonal influenza vaccine. See *MMWR*. 2010;59(No. RR-8):33-34.

[f] **Pneumococcal vaccines**
- A single dose of PCV13 may be administered to children 6 through 18 years of age who have functional or anatomic asplenia, HIV infection, or other immunocompromising condition, cochlear implant, or cerebrospinal fluid (CSF) leak. See *MMWR*. 2010;59(No. RR-11).
- The dose of PCV13 should be administered at least 8 weeks after the previous dose of PCV7.
- Administer pneumococcal polysaccharide vaccine at least 8 weeks after the last dose of PCV to children 2 years or older with certain underlying medical conditions, including a cochlear implant. A single revaccination should be administered after 5 years to children with functional or anatomic asplenia or an immunocompromising condition.

[g] **Hep A vaccine**
- Administer 2 doses at least 6 months apart.
- Hep A is recommended for children older than 23 months who live in areas where vaccination programs target older children, or who are at increased risk for infection, or for whom immunity against hepatitis A is desired.

[h] **Hep B vaccine**
- Administer the 3-dose series to those not previously vaccinated. For those with incomplete vaccination, follow the catch-up schedule.
- A 2-dose series (separated by at least 4 months) of adult formulation *Recombivax HB* is licensed for children 11 through 15 years of age.

[i] **IPV**
- The final dose in the series should be administered on or after the fourth birthday and at least 6 months following the previous dose.
- If both oral polio vaccine (OPV) and IPV were administered as part of a series, a total of 4 doses should be administered, regardless of the child's current age.

[j] **MMR vaccine**
- The minimum interval between the 2 doses of MMR is 4 weeks.

[k] **Varicella vaccine**
- For individuals 7 through 18 years of age without evidence of immunity (see *MMWR*. 2007;56[No. RR-4]), administer 2 doses if not previously vaccinated or the second dose if only 1 dose has been administered.
- For individuals 7 through 12 years of age, the recommended minimum interval between doses is 3 months. However, if the second dose was administered at least 4 weeks after the first dose, it can be accepted as valid.
- For individuals 13 years and older, the minimum interval between doses is 4 weeks.

Catch-up immunization schedule for children 4 months to 18 years of age who start late or who are more than 1 month behind — United States, 2011 – The following table provides catch-up schedules and minimum intervals between doses for children whose vaccinations have been delayed. A vaccine series does not need to be restarted, regardless of the time that has elapsed between doses. Use the section appropriate for the child's age.

Vaccine Catch-up Schedule for Children 4 Months to 6 Years of Age — United States, 2011

Vaccine	Minimum age for dose 1	Minimum interval between doses: Dose 1 to dose 2	Dose 2 to dose 3	Dose 3 to dose 4	Dose 4 to dose 5
Hep B[a]	birth	4 wk	**8 wk** (and ≥ 16 wk after first dose)		
Rotavirus[b]	6 wk	4 wk	4 wk[b]		
DTaP[c]	6 wk	4 wk	4 wk	6 mo	6 mo[c]
Hib[d]	6 wk	**4 wk:** if first dose administered at < 12 mo of age **8 wk (as final dose):** if first dose administered at 12 to 14 mo of age **No further doses needed:** if first dose administered at ≥ 15 mo of age	**4 wk[d]:** if currently < 12 mo of age **8 wk (as final dose)[d]:** if currently ≥ 12 mo of age and first dose administered at < 12 mo of age and second dose administered at < 15 mo of age **No further doses needed:** if previous dose administered at ≥ 15 mo of age	**8 wk (as final dose):** only necessary for children 12 to 59 mo of age who received 3 doses before 12 mo of age	
Pneumococcal[e]	6 wk	**4 wk:** if first dose administered at < 12 mo of age **8 wk (as final dose for healthy children):** if first dose administered at ≥ 12 mo of age or currently 24 to 59 mo of age **No further doses needed:** for healthy children if first dose administered at ≥ 24 mo of age	**4 wk:** if currently < 12 mo of age **8 wk (as final dose for healthy children):** if currently ≥ 12 mo of age **No further doses needed:** for healthy children if previous dose administered at ≥ 24 mo of age	**8 wk (as final dose):** only necessary for children 12 to 59 mo of age who received 3 doses before 12 mo of age or for high-risk children who received 3 doses at any age	
IPV[f]	6 wk	4 wk	4 wk	6 mo[f]	
MMR[g]	12 mo	4 wk			
Varicella[h]	12 mo	3 mo			
Hep A[i]	12 mo	6 mo			
Vaccine Catch-up Schedule for Children 7 to 18 Years of Age — United States, 2011					
Td/Tdap[j]	7 y[j]	4 wk	**4 wk:** if first dose administered at < 12 mo of age **6 mo:** if first dose administered at ≥ 12 mo of age	**6 mo:** if first dose administered at < 12 mo of age	
HPV[k]	9 y	Routine dosing intervals are recommended (females)[k]			
Hep A[i]	12 mo	6 mo			
Hep B[a]	birth	4 wk	**8 wk** (and 16 wk after first dose)		
IPV[f]	6 wk	4 wk	4 wk[f]	6 mo[f]	
MMR[g]	12 mo	4 wk			
Varicella[h]	12 mo	**3 mo:** if the person is < 13 y of age **4 wk:** if the person is ≥ 13 y of age			

NOTE: The recommendations in the table must be read along with the following footnotes.

[a] **Hep B vaccine**
- Administer the 3-dose series to those not previously vaccinated.
- The minimum age for the third dose of Hep B is 24 weeks.
- A 2-dose series (separated by at least 4 months) of adult formulation *Recombivax HB* is licensed for children 11 to 15 years of age.

[b] **Rotavirus vaccine**
- The maximum age for the first dose is 14 weeks 6 days. Vaccination should not be initiated for infants 15 weeks 0 days and older.
- The maximum age for the final dose in the series is 8 months 0 days.
- If *Rotarix* was administered for the first and second doses, a third dose is not indicated.

[c] **DTaP vaccine**
- The fifth dose is not necessary if the fourth dose was administered at 4 years and older.

[d] **Hib vaccine**
- 1 dose of Hib vaccine should be considered for unvaccinated individuals 5 years or older who have sickle cell disease, leukemia, or HIV infection, or who have had a splenectomy.
- If the first 2 doses were PRP-OMP (*PedvaxHIB* or *Comvax*), and administered at 11 months or younger, the third (and final) dose should be administered at 12 to 15 months of age and at least 8 weeks after the second dose.
- If the first dose was administered at 7 to 11 months of age, administer the second dose at least 4 weeks later and a final dose at 12 to 15 months of age.

[e] **Pneumococcal vaccine**
- Administer 1 dose of PCV13 to all healthy children 24 to 59 months of age with any incomplete PCV schedule (PCV7 or PCV13).
- For children 24 to 71 months of age with underlying medical conditions, administer 1 dose of PCV13 if 3 doses pf PCV were previously received or administer 2 doses of PCV13 at least 8 weeks apart if fewer than 3 doses of PCV were previously received.
- A single dose of PCV13 is recommended for certain children with underlying medical conditions through 18 years of age. See age-specific schedules for details.
- Administer PPSV to children 2 years and older with certain underlying medical conditions, including cochlear implant, at least 8 weeks after the last dose of PCV. A single revaccination should be administered after 5 years to children with functional or anatomic asplenia or an immunocompromising condition. See *MMWR*. 2010;59(No. RR-11).

[f] **IPV vaccine**
- The final dose in the series should be administered on or after the fourth birthday and at least 6 months following the previous dose.
- A fourth dose is not necessary if the third dose was administered at 4 years or older and at least 6 months following the previous dose.
- In the first 6 months of life, minimum age and minimum intervals are only recommended if the person is at risk for imminent exposure to circulating poliovirus (ie, travel to a polio endemic region or during an outbreak).

[g] **MMR vaccine**
- Administer the second dose routinely at 4 to 6 years of age. The minimum interval between the 2 doses of MMR is 4 weeks.

[h] **Varicella vaccine**
- Administer the second dose routinely at 4 to 6 years of age.
- If the second dose was administered at least 4 weeks after the first dose, it can be accepted as valid.

[i] **Hep A vaccine**
- Hep A is recommended for children older than 23 months who live in areas where vaccination programs target older children, who are at increased risk for infection, or for whom immunity against hepatitis A is desired.

[j] **Td/Tdap vaccine**
- Doses of DTaP are counted as part of the Td/Tdap series.
- Tdap should be substituted for a single dose of Td in the catch-up series for children 7 through 10 years of age or as a booster for children 11 through 18 years of age; use Td for other doses.

[k] **HPV vaccine**
- Administer the HPV vaccine series to girls 13 to 18 years of age if not previously vaccinated or have not completed the vaccine series.
- HPV4 may be administered in a 3-dose series to males 9 through 18 years of age to reduce their likelihood of genital warts.
- Use recommended routine dosing intervals for series catch-up (ie, the second and third doses should be administered at 1 to 2 and 6 months after the first dose). The minimum interval between the first and second doses is 4 weeks. The minimum interval between the second and third doses is 12 weeks, and the third dose should be given at least 24 weeks after the first dose.

Reference – Centers for Disease Control and Prevention. *Recommended Immunization Schedules for Persons Aged 0 to 18 years — United States, 2011*. http://www.cdc.gov/mmwr/preview/mmwrhtml/mm6005a6.htm?s_cid=mm6005a6_w. Published February 11, 2011. Accessed March 21, 2011.

➤*Immunization schedules for adults:* The Recommended Adult Immunization Schedule for 2011 has been approved by the ACIP, the American College of Obstetricians and Gynecologists, and the AAFP. This table is revised annually.

Recommended Adult Immunization Schedule by Vaccine and Age Group — United States, 2011

Vaccine	Age group: 19 to 26 y	27 to 49 y	50 to 59 y	60 to 64 y	≥ 65 y
Td/Tdap[a,b]	Substitute 1-time dose of Tdap for Td booster; then boost with Td every 10 y				**Td booster every 10 y**
HPV[a,c]	3 doses (females)				
Varicella[a,d]	2 doses				
Herpes zoster[e]				1 dose	
MMR[a,f]	1 or 2 doses		1 dose		
Influenza[a,g]	1 dose annually				
Pneumoccal (polysaccharide)[h,i]	1 to 2 doses				1 dose
Hep A[a,j]	2 doses				
Hep B[a,k]	3 doses				
Meningococcal[a,l]	1 or more doses				

Vaccines That Might Be Indicated for Adults Based on Medical and Other Indications — United States, 2011

Vaccine	Indication: Pregnancy	Immunocompromising conditions (excluding HIV)[n]	HIV infection[d-f,m,n] CD4+T lymphocyte count: < 200 cells/mcL	≥ 200 cells/mcL	Diabetes, heart disease, chronic lung disease, chronic alcoholism	Asplenia[n] (including elective splenectomy and persistent complement component deficiencies)	Chronic liver disease	Kidney failure, end-stage renal disease, receiving hemodialysis	Health care workers
Td/Tdap[a,b]	Td	Substitute 1-time dose of Tdap for Td booster; then boost with Td every 10 y							
HPV[a,c]		3 doses through age 26 y							
Varicella[a,d]	contraindicated			2 doses					
Herpes zoster[e]	contraindicated			1 dose					
MMR[a,f]	contraindicated			1 or 2 doses					
Influenza[a,g]	1 dose TIV annually								1 dose TIV or LAIV annually
Pneumococcal (polysaccharide)[h,i]		1 or 2 doses							
Hep A[a,j]	2 doses								
Hep B[a,k]					3 doses				
Meningococcal[a,l]	1 or more doses								

Light shading: For all individuals in this category who meet the age requirements and lack evidence of immunity (eg, lack documentation of vaccination or have no evidence of prior infection).

Dark shading: Recommended if some other risk factor is present (eg, based on medical, occupational, lifestyle, or other indications).

No shading: No recommendation.

NOTE: The recommendations in the tables must be read along with the following footnotes.

[a] Covered by the VICP.

[b] **Tetanus, diphtheria and acellular pertussis (Td/Tdap) vaccine**

- Administer a 1-time dose of Tdap to adults younger than 65 years who have not previously received Tdap or for whom vaccine status is unknown to replace 1 of the 10-year Td boosters, and as soon as feasible to all 1) postpartum women, 2) close contacts of infants younger than 12 months of age (eg, grandparents, child-care providers), and 3) health care personnel with direct patient contact. Adults 65 years and older who have not previously received Tdap and who have close contact with an infant younger than 12 months also should be vaccinated. Other adults 65 years and older may receive Tdap. Tdap can be administered regardless of interval since the most recent tetanus- or diphtheria-containing vaccine.
- Adults with uncertain or incomplete history of completing a 3-dose primary vaccination series with Td-containing vaccines should begin or complete a primary vaccination series. For unvaccinated adults, administer the first 2 doses at least 4 weeks apart and the third dose 6 to 12 months after the second. If incompletely vaccinated (ie, less than 3 doses), administer remaining doses. Substitute a 1-time dose of Tdap for 1 of the doses of Td, either in the primary series or for the routine booster, whichever comes first.
- If a woman is pregnant and received the most recent Td vaccination 10 or more years previously, administer Td during the second or third trimester. If the woman received the most recent Td vaccination less than 10 years previously, administer Tdap during the immediate postpartum period. At the clinician's discretion, Td may be deferred during pregnancy and Tdap substituted in the immediate postpartum period, or Tdap may be administered instead of Td to a pregnant woman after an informed discussion with the woman.
- The ACIP statement for recommendations for administering Td as prophylaxis in wound management is available at http://www.cdc.gov/vaccines/pubs/acip-list.htm.

[c] **HPV vaccine**

- HPV vaccination with either HPV4 vaccine or HPV2 vaccine is recommended for females at 11 or 12 years of age and catch-up vaccination for females 13 through 26 years of age.
- Ideally, vaccine should be administered before potential exposure to HPV through sexual activity; however, females who are sexually active should still be vaccinated consistent with age-based recommendations. Sexually active females who have not been infected with any of the 4 HPV vaccine types (types 6, 11, 16, and 18, all of which HPV4 prevents) or any of the 2 HPV vaccine types (types 16 and 18, both of which HPV2 prevents) receive the full benefit of the vaccination. Vaccination is less beneficial for females who have already been infected with 1 or more of the HPV vaccine types. HPV4 or HPV2 can be administered to individuals with a history of genital warts, abnormal Papanicolaou test, or positive HPV DNA test, because these conditions are not evidence of previous infection with all vaccine HPV types.
- HPV4 may be administered to males 9 through 26 years of age to reduce their likelihood of genital warts. HPV4 would be most effective when administered before exposure to HPV through sexual contact.
- A complete series for either HPV4 or HPV2 consists of 3 doses. The second dose should be administered 1 to 2 months after the first dose; the third dose should be administered 6 months after the first dose.
- Although HPV vaccination is not specifically recommended for individuals with the medical indications described in the table "Vaccines that might be indicated for adults based on medical and other indications," it may be administered to these individuals because the HPV vaccine is not a live-virus vaccine. However, the immune response and vaccine efficacy might be less for individuals with the medical indications described in this table than in individuals who do not have the medical indications described or who are immunocompetent.

[d] **Varicella vaccine**

- All adults without evidence of immunity to varicella should receive 2 doses of single-antigen varicella vaccine if not previously vaccinated or a second dose if they have received only 1 dose, unless they have a medical contraindication. Special consideration should be given to those who 1) have close contact with individuals at high risk for severe disease (eg, health care personnel, family contacts of individuals with immunocompromising conditions) or 2) are at high risk for exposure or transmission (eg, teachers; child care employees; residents and staff members of institutional settings, including correctional institutions; college students; military personnel; adolescents and adults living in households with children; nonpregnant women of childbearing age; international travelers).
- Evidence of immunity to varicella in adults includes any of the following: 1) documentation of 2 doses of varicella vaccine at least 4 weeks apart; 2) US-born before 1980 (although for health care personnel and pregnant women, birth before 1980 should not be considered evidence of immunity); 3) history of varicella based on diagnosis or verification of varicella by a health care provider (for a patient reporting a history of or having an atypical case, a mild case, or both, health care providers should seek either an epidemiologic link with a typical varicella case or to a laboratory-confirmed case or evidence of laboratory confirmation, if it was performed at the time of acute disease); 4) history of herpes zoster based on diagnosis or verification of herpes zoster by a health care provider; or 5) laboratory evidence of immunity or laboratory confirmation of disease.
- Pregnant women should be assessed for evidence of varicella immunity. Women who do not have evidence of immunity should receive the first dose of varicella vaccine upon completion or termination of pregnancy and before discharge from the health care facility. The second dose should be administered 4 to 8 weeks after the first dose.

[e] **Herpes zoster vaccine**

- A single dose of zoster vaccine is recommended for adults 60 years and older regardless of whether they report a previous episode of herpes zoster. Individuals with chronic medical conditions may be vaccinated unless their condition constitutes a contraindication.

[f] **MMR vaccine**

- Adults born before 1957 generally are considered immune to measles and mumps. All adults born in 1957 or later should have documentation of 1 or more doses of MMR vaccine unless they have a medical contraindication to the vaccine, laboratory evidence of immunity to each of the three diseases, or documentation of provider-diagnosed measles or mumps disease. For rubella, documentation of provider-diagnosed disease is not considered acceptable evidence of immunity.
- *Measles component*: A second dose of MMR vaccine, administered a minimum of 28 days after the first dose, is recommended for adults who 1) have been recently exposed to measles or are in an outbreak setting; 2) are students in postsecondary educational institutions; 3) work in a health care facility; or 4) plan to travel internationally. Individuals who received inactivated (killed) measles vaccine or measles vaccine of unknown type during 1963 to 1967 should be revaccinated with 2 doses of MMR vaccine.
- *Mumps component*: A second dose of MMR vaccine, administered a minimum of 28 days after the first dose, is recommended for adults who 1) live in a community experiencing a mumps outbreak and are in an affected age group; 2) are students in postsecondary educational institutions; 3) work in a health care facility; or 4) plan to travel internationally. Individuals vaccinated before 1979 with either killed mumps vaccine or mumps vaccine of unknown type who are at high risk for mumps infection (eg, individuals who are working in a health care facility) should be revaccinated with 2 doses of MMR vaccine.
- *Rubella component*: For women of childbearing age, regardless of birth year, rubella immunity should be determined. If there is no evidence of immunity, women who are not pregnant should be vaccinated. Pregnant women who do not have evidence of immunity should receive the MMR vaccine upon completion or termination of pregnancy and before discharge from the health care facility.
- *Health care personnel born before 1957*: For unvaccinated health care personnel born before 1957 who lack laboratory evidence of measles, mumps, and/or rubella immunity or laboratory confirmation of disease, health care facilities should 1) consider routinely vaccinating personnel with 2 doses of MMR vaccine at the appropriate interval (for measles and mumps) and 1 dose of MMR vaccine (for rubella), and 2) recommend 2 doses of MMR vaccine at the appropriate interval during an outbreak of measles or mumps, and 1 dose during an outbreak of rubella. Complete information about evidence of immunity is available at http://www.cdc.gov/vaccines/recs/provisional/default.htm.

[g] **Influenza vaccine**

- Annual vaccination against influenza is recommended for all individuals 6 months and older, including all adults. Healthy, nonpregnant adults younger than 50 years without high-risk medical conditions can receive either intranasally administered LAIV (*FluMist*) or inactivated vaccine. Other individuals should receive the inactivated vaccine. Adults 65 years and older can receive the standard influenza vaccine or the high-dose (*Fluzone*) influenza vaccine. Additional information about influenza vaccination is available at http://www.cdc.gov/vaccines/vpd-vac/flu/default.htm.

[h] **PPSV**

Vaccinate all individuals with the following indications:

- *Medical*: Chronic lung disease (including asthma); chronic cardiovascular diseases; diabetes mellitus; chronic liver diseases; cirrhosis; chronic alcoholism; functional or anatomic asplenia (eg, sickle cell disease, splenectomy [if elective splenectomy is planned, vaccinate at least 2 weeks before surgery]); immunocompromising conditions (including chronic renal failure or nephrotic syndrome); and cochlear implants and CSF leaks. Vaccinate as close to HIV diagnosis as possible.
- *Other*: Residents of nursing homes or long-term care facilities and individuals who smoke cigarettes. Routine use of PPSV is not recommended for American Indians/Alaska Natives or individuals younger than 65 years unless they have underlying medical conditions that are PPSV indications. However, public health authorities may consider recommending PPSV for American Indians/Alaska Natives and individuals 50 through 64 years of age who are living in areas where the risk for invasive pneumococcal disease is increased.

[i] **Revaccination with PPSV**

- One-time revaccination after 5 years is recommended for individuals 19 through 64 years of age with chronic renal failure or nephrotic syndrome; functional or anatomic asplenia (eg, sickle cell disease or splenectomy); and immunocompromising conditions. For individuals 65 years and older, one-time revaccination is recommended if they were vaccinated 5 or more years previously and were younger than 65 years at the time of primary vaccination.

[j] **Hep A vaccine**

- Vaccinate individuals with any of the following indications and any person seeking protection from hepatitis A virus (HAV) infection:
- *Behavioral*: Men who have sex with men and individuals who use injection drugs.
- *Occupational*: Individuals working with HAV-infected primates or with HAV in a research laboratory setting.
- *Medical*: Individuals with chronic liver disease and individuals who receive clotting factor concentrates.
- *Other*: Individuals traveling to or working in countries that have high or intermediate endemicity of hepatitis A (a list of countries is available at http://www.cdc.gov/travel/contentdiseases.aspx).
- Unvaccinated individuals who anticipate close personal contact (eg, household or regular babysitting) with an international adoptee during the first 60 days after arrival in the United States from a country with high or intermediate endemicity should be vaccinated. The first dose of the 2-dose Hep A vaccine series should be administered as soon as adoption is planned, ideally 2 or more weeks before the arrival of the adoptee.
- Single-antigen vaccine formulations should be administered in a 2-dose schedule at either 0 and 6 to 12 months (*Havrix*), or 0 and 6 to 18 months (*Vaqta*). If the combined hepatitis A and hepatitis B vaccine (*Twinrix*) is used, administer 3 doses at 0, 1, and 6 months; alternatively, a 4-dose schedule may be used, administered on days 0, 7, and 21 to 30, followed by a booster dose at month 12.

[k] **Hep B vaccine**

- Vaccinate individuals with any of the following indications and any person seeking protection from HBV infection:
- *Behavioral*: Sexually active individuals who are not in a long-term, mutually monogamous relationship (eg, individuals with more than 1 sex partner during the previous 6 months); individuals seeking evaluation or treatment for a sexually transmitted disease (STD); current or recent injection-drug users; and men who have sex with men.
- *Occupational*: Health care personnel and public-safety workers who are exposed to blood or other potentially infectious body fluids.
- *Medical*: Individuals with end-stage renal disease, including patients receiving hemodialysis; HIV infection; and chronic liver disease.
- *Other*: Household contacts and sex partners of individuals with chronic HBV infection; clients and staff members of institutions for individuals with developmental disabilities; and international travelers to countries with high or intermediate prevalence of chronic HBV infection (a list of countries is available at http://wwwn.cdc.gov/travel/contentdiseases.aspx).
- Hep B vaccination is recommended for all adults in the following settings: STD treatment facilities; HIV testing and treatment facilities; facilities providing drug-abuse treatment and prevention services; health care settings targeting services to injection-drug users or men who have sex with men; correctional facilities; end-stage renal disease programs and facilities for chronic hemodialysis patients; and institutions and nonresidential day-care facilities for individuals with developmental disabilities.
- Administer missing doses to complete a 3-dose series of Hep B vaccine to those individuals not vaccinated or not completely vaccinated. The second dose should be administered 1 month after the first dose; the third dose should be given at least 2 months after the second dose (and at least 4 months after the first dose). If the combined hepatitis A and hepatitis B vaccine (*Twinrix*) is used, administer 3 doses at 0, 1, and 6 months; alternatively, a 4-dose *Twinrix* schedule, administered on days 0, 7, and 21 to 30, followed by a booster dose at month 12 may be used.
- Adult patients receiving hemodialysis or with other immunocompromising conditions should receive 1 dose of 40 *mcg*/mL (*Recombivax HB*) administered on a 3-dose schedule or 2 doses of 20 *mcg*/mL (*Engerix-B*) administered simultaneously on a 4-dose schedule at 0, 1, 2, and 6 months.

[l] **Meningococcal vaccine**

- Meningococcal vaccine should be administered to individuals with the following indications:
- *Medical*: A 2-dose series of meningococcal conjugate vaccine is recommended for adults with anatomic or functional asplenia, or persistent complement component deficiencies. Adults with HIV infection who are vaccinated should also receive a routine 2-dose series. The 2 doses should be administered at 0 and 2 months.
- *Other*: A single dose of meningococcal vaccine is recommended for unvaccinated first-year college students living in dormitories; microbiologists routinely exposed to isolates of *Neisseria meningitidis*; military recruits; and individuals who travel to or live in countries in which meningococcal disease is hyperendemic or epidemic (eg, the "meningitis belt" of sub-Saharan Africa during the dry season [December through June]), particularly if their contact with local populations will be prolonged. Vaccination is required by the government of Saudi Arabia for all travelers to Mecca during the annual Hajj.
- MCV4 is preferred for adults with any of the preceding indications who are 55 years and younger; meningococcal polysaccharide vaccine (MPSV4) is preferred for adults 56 years and older. Revaccination with MCV4 every 5 years is recommended for adults previously vaccinated with MCV4 or MPSV4 who remain at increased risk for infection (eg, adults with anatomic or functional asplenia, persistent complement component deficiencies).

[m] **Immunocompromising conditions**

- Inactivated vaccines generally are acceptable (eg, pneumococcal, meningococcal, influenza [inactivated influenza vaccine]) and live vaccines generally are avoided in individuals with immune deficiencies or immunocompromising conditions. Information on specific conditions is available at http://www.cdc.gov/vaccines/pubs/acip-list.htm.

[n] **Selected conditions for which Hib vaccine may be used**

- 1 dose of Hib vaccine should be considered for individuals who have sickle-cell disease, leukemia, or HIV infection, or who have had a splenectomy, if they have not previously received Hib vaccine.

Reference – Centers for Disease Control and Prevention. *Recommended Adult Immunization Schedule — United States, 2011.* http://www.cdc.gov/mmwr/preview/mmwrhtml/mm6004a10.htm. Published February 4, 2011. Accessed February 7, 2011.

➤*Immunization for other diseases:* Immunization for other diseases is recommended for people with a risk of exposure. Specific immunization requirements and recommendations for international travel may be obtained from the Centers for Disease Control and Prevention (CDC) Web site (http://www.cdc.gov), including their online publication *Health Information for International Travel*. These also may be found in the following publication: Grabenstein JD. *ImmunoFacts: Vaccines & Immunologic Drugs*. St. Louis, MO: Wolters Kluwer Health Inc; 2011.

➤*Hypersensitivity to vaccine components:* Vaccine antigens produced in systems containing allergenic substances (eg, embryonated chicken eggs) may cause hypersensitivity reactions, including anaphylaxis. Do not give such vaccines to individuals with known hypersensitivity to these components. Influenza vaccine antigens (whole or split), although prepared in embryonated eggs, are highly purified and rarely associated with hypersensitivity reactions.

Live virus vaccines prepared by growing viruses in cell cultures are essentially devoid of allergenic substances. On very rare occasions, hypersensitivity reactions to measles vaccine have been reported in individuals with anaphylactic hypersensitivity to gelatin. However, measles vaccine may be given safely to egg-allergic individuals, provided the allergies are not manifested by anaphylactic symptoms. The same precautions apply to mumps and varicella vaccines.

Some vaccines contain preservatives (eg, thimerosal) or trace amounts of antibiotics (eg, neomycin) to which patients may be hypersensitive. Such allergies are relevant only if they reflect immediate hypersensitivity (eg, the airway).

Before the injection of any biological, take all precautions known for prevention of allergic or other adverse reactions, including a review of the patient's history regarding possible sensitivity, occurrence of any adverse reaction–related symptoms or signs to determine any contraindication to immunization, and a knowledge of the recent literature pertaining to the use of the biological concerned. Have epinephrine 1:1,000 available for immediate use when this product is injected. Refer to Management of Acute Hypersensitivity Reactions.

➤*Altered immunocompetence:* Microbial replication after administration of live, attenuated vaccines may be enhanced in people with immune deficiency diseases and in those with suppressed capability for immune response (eg, leukemia, lymphoma, generalized malignancy or therapy with corticosteroids, alkylating agents, antimetabolites, radiation). Do not give live, attenuated vaccines to such patients or to a member of a household in which there is a family history of congenital or hereditary immunodeficiency until the immune competence of the recipient is known.

➤*Disease transmission:* Use a separate, sterilized syringe and needle for each patient to prevent transmission of hepatitis B virus (HBV) and other infectious agents from one patient to another.

➤*Vaccine reconstitution:* When preparing injections for reconstitution, cleanse the rubber stoppers of both vials with a suitable germicide prior to reconstitution.

➤*Aspirate:* Before delivering the intramuscular or subcutaneous dose, aspirate to help avoid inadvertent injection into a blood vessel.

➤*HIV infection:* Special immunization recommendations are appropriate for patients infected with HIV.

Live bacterial or viral vaccines – Patients infected with HIV and those who have developed AIDS are theoretically at risk of disseminated infection following immunization with a live, albeit attenuated, bacterial or viral vaccine.

Inactivated vaccines or toxoids – In general, immunization with an inactivated vaccine or toxoid poses no additional risk to patients infected with HIV and those who have developed AIDS, but these patients may be less likely to develop an adequate immune response to vaccination and may remain susceptible to the disease at issue. While HIV-infected patients and AIDS patients may develop less than optimal immunity compared with uninfected people, immunization is often still recommended to confer at least partial protection. Optimally, complete the immunization of HIV-infected patients before they meet the criteria for AIDS.

Immunization of HIV-infected patients – In vitro studies demonstrate that proliferating CD4 cells are more susceptible to infection with HIV than nonproliferating cells, raising the possibility that immunization may be a cofactor in exacerbating the progression of HIV infection to AIDS. The CDC and World Health Organization continue to recommend immunization of HIV-infected patients when the benefits of immunization outweigh the risks of infection.

Summary Recommendations for Routine Immunization of HIV-infected Patients in the United States

Drug	Known asymptomatic	Symptomatic
BCG	no	no
DTP/Td/Tdap	yes	yes
e-IPV[a]	yes	yes
Hep A	yes	yes
Hep B	yes	yes
Hib[b]	yes	yes
HPV	yes	yes
Influenza, inactivated	yes[c]	yes
Japanese encephalitis	yes	yes
Meningococcal	yes	yes
MMR	yes	yes[c]
Pneumococcal	yes	yes
Poliovirus	yes (IPV only)	yes (IPV only)
Rabies	yes	yes
Rotavirus	no	no
Typhoid	yes (injection only)	yes (injection only)
Vaccinia[d]	no	no
Varicella[e]	yes	no
Yellow fever	yes, if high risk	no
Zoster	no	no

[a] For adults ≥ 18 years of age; use only if indicated.
[b] Also consider for HIV-infected adults.
[c] Consider risk and benefit.
[d] Except in an outbreak setting.
[e] Consult detailed references.

➤*Severe febrile illnesses:* Generally defer immunization of individuals with severe febrile illnesses until they have recovered.

➤*Vaccination during pregnancy:* On the grounds of a theoretical risk to the developing fetus, live, attenuated virus vaccines are not generally given to pregnant women or to those likely to become pregnant within 3 months after receiving the vaccine. With some of these vaccines, particularly rubella, measles, and mumps, pregnancy is contraindicated. When the vaccine is to be given during pregnancy, waiting until the second or third trimester to minimize any concern over teratogenicity is a reasonable precaution. However, there has been no evidence of congenital rubella syndrome in infants born to susceptible mothers who received rubella vaccine during pregnancy.

MMR or OPV may be safely administered to children of pregnant women. Experience to date has not revealed any risks of polio vaccine virus to the fetus.

There is no convincing evidence of risk to the fetus from immunization of pregnant women using inactivated virus vaccines, bacterial vaccines, or toxoids. Give tetanus and Td to inadequately immunized pregnant women because it affords protection against neonatal tetanus. Similarly, Hep B, influenza, and meningococcal vaccines may be indicated during pregnancy.

➤*Adverse reactions following immunization:* Modern vaccines are extremely safe and effective; however, adverse reactions following immunization have been reported with all vaccines. These range from frequent, minor local reactions to extremely rare, severe systemic illness, such as paralysis associated with OPV.

Provide required vaccine information with each vaccine to the patient, parent, or guardian, and inform them of the benefits and risks associated with the vaccine.

Reporting of adverse reactions – The National Vaccine Injury Compensation Program (VICP), established by the National Childhood Vaccine Injury Act of 1986, requires health care providers who administer vaccines to maintain permanent vaccination records and report occurrences of certain adverse reactions to the US Department of Health and Human Services. Reportable reactions include those listed in the Act for each vaccine and reactions specified in the package insert as contraindications to further doses of that vaccine.

Encourage patients, parents, and guardians to report all adverse reactions occurring after vaccine administration. Adverse reactions following immunization with vaccine should be reported by the health care provider to VAERS. Reporting forms and information about reporting requirements or completion of the form can be obtained from VAERS at http://www.vaers.hhs.gov or 1-800-822-7967. Also report these reactions to the manufacturer.

Record the date, lot number, and manufacturer of the vaccine as part of the patient's immunization record.

Vaccines, Bacterial

BCG VACCINE

Rx	**BCG Vaccine** (Organon)	**Powder for injection, lyophilized:** TICE strain[a] (1 to 8 × 10^8 CFU equivalent to ≈ 50 mg)	In vials.[b]

[a] Developed at the University of Illinois.
[b] Preservative free.

BCG VACCINE — INJECTION

For complete and comparative prescribing information, refer to the Agents for Active Immunization introduction. TICE BCG vaccine is also indicated for carcinoma in situ of the bladder. See individual monograph in the Antineoplastics section.

Indications

➤*Tuberculosis (TB) prevention:* For the prevention of tuberculosis (TB) in people not previously infected with *Mycobacterium tuberculosis* who are at high risk for exposure. As with any vaccine, immunization with BCG vaccine may not protect 100% of susceptible individuals.

The Advisory Committee on Immunization Practices (ACIP) and the Advisory Committee for the Elimination of Tuberculosis has recommended that BCG vaccination be considered in the following circumstances.

➤*TB exposed tuberculin skin test-negative infants and children:* BCG vaccination is recommended for infants and children with negative tuberculin skin test who are at high risk of intimate and prolonged exposure to persistently untreated or ineffectively treated patients with infectious pulmonary tuberculosis and who cannot be removed from the source of exposure and cannot be placed on long-term preventive therapy, or who are continuously exposed to people with infectious pulmonary tuberculosis who have bacilli resistant to isoniazid and rifampin.

➤*TB exposed health care workers (HCW) in high risk settings:* Consider BCG vaccination of HCWs on an individual basis in settings where a high percentage of TB patients are infected with *M. tuberculosis* strains resistant to both isoniazid and rifampin, transmission of such drug resistant *M. tuberculosis* strains to HCWs and subsequent infection are likely, and comprehensive TB infection control precautions have been implemented and have not been successful. Vaccination should not be required for employment or for assignment of HCWs in specific work areas. Counsel HCWs considered for BCG vaccination regarding the risks and benefits associated with BCG vaccinations and TB preventive therapy.

➤*Exposed HCWs in low risk settings:* BCG vaccination is not recommended for HCWs in settings in which the risk for *M. tuberculosis* transmission is low.

➤*Off-label uses:*

Prevention of leprosy – [2] = Fair documentation. The protective effect of the BCG vaccine in leprosy has been controversial since its introduction in 1939, which has been fueled by many studies providing conflicting data. The evidence provided shows little safety concern and suggests that the BCG vaccine may be effective in preventing leprosy in most patients at risk. There is a potential role for the BCG vaccine and a vaccine using killed *Mycobacterium w* bacilli as adjunct immunotherapy treatment with multidrug therapy. These vaccines are suggested to improve biological clearance of the bacteria and reduce the risk of reactions and relapses in patients with confirmed multibacillary leprosy. (See Administration and Dosage.)

Administration and Dosage

➤*General dosing considerations:* Vaccination is recommended only for those who are tuberculin negative to a recent skin test with 5 tuberculin units (5TU).

➤*Adults:*

Tuberculosis prevention – 0.2 to 0.3 mL dropped on the cleansed surface of the skin and spread over a 1 × 2 inch area using the edge of the multiple puncture device. An additional 1 to 2 drops of BCG vaccine may be added to ensure a very wet vaccination site. Repeat vaccination for those who remain tuberculin-negative to 5TU of tuberculin after 2 to 3 months.

Off-label dosing –

Prevention of leprosy: [2] = Fair documentation. Place 0.2 to 0.3 mL onto the cleansed surface of the skin and use a sterile multiple-puncture disc to percutaneously penetrate the tensed skin. Spread the vaccine as evenly as possible over the puncture area with the edge of the device. An additional 1 to 2 drops of the vaccine may be added to ensure a very wet vaccination site. No dressing is required, but the site should be kept dry for 24 hours. Although the vaccine will not survive in a dry state for long, it is a live vaccine and infection of others is possible.

➤*Children:*

Tuberculosis prevention –

1 month of age and older: See Adults for dosing.

Younger than 1 month of age: Reduce the dosage of vaccine by 50% by using 2 mL sterile water when reconstituting. If a vaccinated infant remains tuberculin negative to 5TU on skin testing, and if indications for vaccination persist, the infant should receive a full dose after 1 year of age.

Off-label dosing –

Prevention of leprosy: [2] = Fair documentation.

- *1 month of age or older* – See Adults for dosing.
- *Younger than 1 month of age* – Administer half of the adult dose by diluting the vaccine with 2 mL of the diluent rather than 1 mL.

➤*Preparation for administration:* Add 1 mL of sterile water for injection at 4° to 25°C (39° to 77°F) to 1 vial of vaccine. Gently swirl the vial until a homogeneous suspension is obtained. Avoid forceful agitation, which may cause clumping of the mycobacteria.

➤*Administration:* The vaccine is administered percutaneously utilizing a sterile multiple-puncture device. While holding the skin taut, press downward on the device, allowing the points to be well buried in the skin for 5 seconds. Do not "rock" the device. After successful puncture, spread vaccine as evenly as possible over the puncture area with the edge of the device. No dressing is required; however, it is recommended that the site be kept dry for 24 hours.

Advise the patient that the vaccine contains live organisms. Although the vaccine will not survive in a dry state for long, infection of others is possible.

➤*Storage/Stability:* Refrigerate the intact vial at 2° to 8°C (36° to 46°F). Protect from light.

Keep reconstituted vaccine refrigerated; protect from light; use within 2 hours. Freezing of the reconstituted product is not recommended.

Actions

➤*Pharmacology:* BCG vaccine for percutaneous use is an attenuated, live culture preparation of the Bacillus of Calmette and Guerin (BCG) strain of *M. bovis*. The TICE strain was developed at the University of Illinois from a strain originated at the Pasteur Institute.

Contraindications

Impaired immunologic responses because of HIV infections, congenital immunodeficiency such as chronic granulomatous disease or interferon gamma receptor deficiency, leukemia, lymphoma, or generalized malignancy; immunologic responses that have been suppressed by steroids, alkylating agents, antimetabolites, or radiation; HIV- infected or immunocompromised infants, children, or adults; hypersensitivity or history of hypersensitivity to the product; active tuberculosis. Do not use in infants, children, or adults with severe immune deficiency syndromes.

Warnings/Precautions

➤*Route of administration:* Do not inject IV, SC, or intradermally. Use percutaneous administration with the multiple puncture device (see Administration and Dosage).

➤*Immune deficiency syndromes:* Administer with caution to people in groups at high risk for HIV infection. Do not vaccinate children with a family history of immune deficiency disease. If they are, consult an infectious disease specialist and administer antituberculous therapy if clinically indicated.

➤*BCG infection:* Symptoms such as fever of 103°F or greater, or acute localized inflammation persisting longer than 2 to 3 days suggest active infections, and evaluation for serious infectious complication should be considered. If a BCG infection is suspected, the physician should consult with an infectious disease expert before therapy is initiated. Treatment should be started without delay. In patients who develop persistent fever or experience an acute febrile illness consistent with BCG infection, 2 or more antimycobacterial agents should be administered while diagnostic evaluation, including cultures, is conducted. Negative cultures do not necessarily rule out infection. The most serious complication of BCG vaccination is disseminated BCG infection. BCG osteitis affecting the epiphyses of the long bones, particularly the epiphyses of the leg can occur from 4 months to 2 years after vaccination. Fatal disseminated BCG disease has occurred at a rate of 0.06 to 1.56 cases per million doses of vaccine administered; these deaths occurred primarily among immunocompromised people.

➤*Biohazardous:* BCG contains live bacteria; use with aseptic technique. Handle and dispose of all equipment, supplies, and receptacles in contact with BCG vaccine as biohazardous.

➤*Normal reaction:* The intensity and duration of the local reaction depends on the depth of penetration of the multiple-puncture device and individual variations in patients' tissue reactions. The initial skin lesions usually appear within 10 to 14 days and consist of small red papules at the site. The papules reach maximum diameter (about 3 mm) after 4 to 6 weeks, after which they may scale and then slowly subside.

After vaccination, it is usually not possible to clearly distinguish between a tuberculin reaction caused by persistent postvaccination sensitivity and one caused by a virulent suprainfection. Caution is advised in attributing a positive skin test to BCG vaccination. Further investigate a sharp rise in the tuberculin reaction since the latest test (except in the immediate postvaccination period).

➤*Hypersensitivity reactions:* Assess the possibility of allergic reactions. Epinephrine injection (1:1000) for the control of immediate allergic reactions must be available should an acute anaphylactic reaction occur.

➤*Pregnancy: Category C.* It is not known whether BCG vaccine can cause fetal harm when administered to a pregnant woman or can affect reproduction capacity. Although no harmful effects to the fetus have been associated with BCG vaccine, its use is not recommended during pregnancy.

➤*Lactation:* It is not known whether BCG vaccine is excreted in breast milk. Because many drugs are excreted in human milk and because of the potential for serious adverse reactions in nursing infants from BCG vaccine, decide whether to discontinue nursing or not to vaccinate, taking into account the importance of tuberculosis vaccination to the mother.

➤*Children:* Take precautions with respect to infants vaccinated with BCG and exposed to individuals with active tuberculosis (see Administration and Dosage).

Drug Interactions

➤*Antimicrobial or immunosuppressive agents:* These may interfere with the development of the immune response; use only under medical supervision.

➤*Live vaccines:* Because BCG is a live vaccine, the immune response to the vaccine might be impaired if administered within 30 days of another live

BCG VACCINE — INJECTION

vaccine. However, no evidence exists for currently available vaccines to support this concern. Whenever possible, live vaccines administered on different days should be administered at least 30 days apart.

➤*Drug/Lab test interactions:* BCG vaccination results in tuberculin skin test reactivity. Tuberculin skin test reactivity as a result of BCG vaccination cannot be readily differentiated from reactivity following exposure to tuberculosis. BCG vaccination should not be administered to individuals with a positive tuberculin skin test.

Adverse Reactions

All suspected adverse reactions to BCG vaccination should be reported to Organon at (800) 842-3220 and to the Vaccine Adverse Effect Reporting System (VAERS) at (800) 822-7967. These reactions occasionally could occur more than 1 year after vaccination.

➤*Local:* Although BCG vaccination often results in local adverse effects, serious or long-term complications are rare. Reactions that can be expected after vaccination include moderate axillary or cervical lymphadenopathy and induration and subsequent pustule formation at the injection site; these reactions can persist for as long as 3 months after vaccination. More severe local reactions include ulceration at the vaccination site, regional suppurative lymphadenitis with draining sinuses, and caseous lesions or purulent drainage at the puncture site; these manifestations might occur within the 5 months after vaccination and could persist for several weeks.

➤*Systemic:* Acute, localized irritative toxicities of BCG may be accompanied by systemic manifestations, consistent with a flu-like syndrome. Systemic adverse effects of 1 to 2 days' duration such as fever, anorexia, myalgia, and neuralgia, often reflect hypersensitivity reactions.

Overdosage

➤*Symptoms:* Accidental overdosages, if treated immediately with antituberculous drugs, have not led to complications. If vaccination response is allowed to progress, it can still be treated successfully with antituberculous drugs but complications may occur (eg, regional adenitis, lupus vulgaris, SC cold abscesses, ocular lesions).

Patient Information

Keep the vaccination site clean until the local reaction has disappeared.

Following BCG vaccination, no dressing is required; however, it is recommended that the site be loosely covered and kept dry for 24 hours.

The patients should be advised that the vaccine contains live organisms. Although the vaccine will not survive in a dry state for long, infection of others is possible. Following vaccination with BCG, initial skin lesions usually appear within 10 to 14 days and consist of small red papules at the vaccination site. The papules reach a maximum diameter (about 3 mm) after 4 to 6 weeks, after which they may scale and slowly subside.

Patients may experience flu-like symptoms for 24 to 48 hours following BCG vaccination. However, the patients should consult with their physician immediately if they experience fever of 103°F or greater, or acute local reactions persisting longer than 2 to 3 days.

ANTHRAX VACCINE

Rx	**BioThrax** (Emergent BioDefense Operations Lansing Inc)	**Injection, suspension:** 83 kDa of *Bacillus anthracis*	Aluminum 1.2 mg/mL, benzethonium chloride 25 mcg/mL, formaldehyde 100 mcg/mL. In 5 mL multidose vials.

ANTHRAX VACCINE — INJECTION

Indications

➤*Anthrax immunization:* For active immunization for the prevention of the disease caused by *Bacillus anthracis* in persons between 18 and 65 years of age whose occupations or other activities place them at high risk of exposure.

Administration and Dosage

➤*General dosing considerations:* The vial stopper contains dry natural rubber. Individuals should not be considered protected until they have received the full series of vaccinations.

➤*Adults:*

Anthrax immunization – 0.5 mL intramuscularly (IM) as 5 injections at day 0, week 4, and then 6, 12, and 18 months. Yearly booster injections of 0.5 mL IM are recommended for those who remain at risk.

➤*Preparation for administration:* Shake the bottle thoroughly to ensure that the suspension is homogenous during withdrawal. Use a separate 1 or 1½ inch 23- or 25-gauge sterile needle and syringe for each patient.

➤*Administration:* Administer IM; do not inject intravenously or intradermally. Select a different injection site for each sequential injection of the vaccine.

When medically indicated, such as in persons with coagulation disorders or receiving medications that affect coagulation (eg, warfarin), anthrax vaccine may be administered by the subcutaneous route.

➤*Admixture compatibility:* Do not mix with any other product in the same syringe or vial.

➤*Storage/Stability:* Store at 2° to 8°C (36° to 46°F). Do not freeze.

Actions

➤*Pharmacology:* Anthrax is a zoonotic disease caused by the gram-positive, spore-forming bacterium *B. anthracis*. Virulence components of *B. anthracis* include an antiphagocytic polypeptide capsule and 3 proteins known as protective antigen (PA), lethal factor (LF), and edema factor (EF). Individually, these proteins are not cytotoxic, but the combination of PA with LF or EF results in the formation of the cytotoxic lethal toxin and edema toxin, respectively. Although an immune correlate of protection is unknown, antibodies raised against PA may contribute to protection by neutralizing the activities of these toxins. *B. anthracis* proteins other than PA may be present in anthrax vaccine, but their contribution to protection has not been determined.

Contraindications

History of anaphylactic or anaphylactic-like reaction following a previous dose of anthrax vaccine.

Warnings/Precautions

➤*Latex sensitivity:* Administer with caution to patients with a possible history of latex sensitivity because the vial stopper contains dry natural rubber and may cause allergic reactions.

➤*History of anthrax disease:* History of anthrax disease may increase the potential for severe local adverse reactions.

➤*Immunosuppression:* If anthrax vaccine is administered to immunocompromised persons, including those receiving immunosuppressive therapy, the immune response may be diminished.

➤*Protection:* Vaccination with anthrax vaccine may not protect all individuals. The extent to which one is protected prior to completion of the full immunization schedule is unknown.

➤*Hypersensitivity reactions:* Before administration, review the patient's medical immunization history for possible vaccine sensitivities and/or previous vaccination-related adverse reactions in order to determine the existence of any contraindications to immunization. Appropriate medical treatment and supervision must be available to manage possible anaphylactic reactions following administration of the vaccine.

➤*Pregnancy: Category D.* Do not vaccinate pregnant women against anthrax unless the potential benefits of vaccination have been determined to outweigh the potential risk to the fetus. Results of a large observational study that examined the rate of birth defects among 37,140 infants born to US military service women who received anthrax vaccine during pregnancy between 1998 and 2004 showed that birth defects were slightly more common in first trimester–exposed infants (odds ratio, 1.18; 95% confidence interval, 0.997 to 1.41) when compared with infants of women vaccinated outside of the first trimester and compared with unvaccinated women. Increased birth defect rates were not statistically significant when compared with infants born to women vaccinated outside of pregnancy.

Anthrax vaccine can cause fetal harm when administered to a pregnant woman. If this vaccine is used during pregnancy, or if the patient becomes pregnant during the immunization series, apprise the patient of the potential hazard to a fetus.

Out of a total of 44 pregnancies reported in this study, no distinct patterns of infant outcome were seen, with the majority of pregnancies uncomplicated and healthy term infants delivered. Of women who received vaccine approximately within the first trimester (n = 15), 2 reports of spontaneous abortion were reported, along with 1 report of a healthy term infant with mild right clubbed foot abnormality.

➤*Lactation:* It is not known whether anthrax vaccine is excreted in human milk. The anthrax vaccine consists mostly of protein fragments of anthrax bacteria; therefore, it is highly unlikely any vaccine would transfer into breast-milk. The Centers for Disease Control and Prevention (CDC) states that no data are available to suggest any increased risks for adverse reactions in breast-fed children. Because many drugs are excreted in human milk, exercise caution when anthrax vaccine is administered to a breast-feeding woman.

➤*Children:* Safety and effectiveness in children younger than 18 years of age have not been established.

➤*Elderly:* Subgroup analysis of study subjects younger than 30 years of age, 30 to younger than 40 years of age, 40 to younger than 50 years of age, and older than 50 years of age, indicated that subjects older than 50 years of age had statistically insignificant but numerically lower immune responses than younger subjects.

ANTHRAX VACCINE — INJECTION

Drug Interactions

Anthrax Vaccine Drug Interactions			
Precipitant drug	Object drug[a]		Description
Concomitant vaccines	Anthrax vaccine	↔	No studies to assess the concomitant use of anthrax vaccine with other vaccines have been conducted. If anthrax vaccine is to be administered at the same time as another injectable vaccine, give the vaccines at different injection sites.
Anthrax vaccine	Concomitant vaccines		
Immunosuppressive therapies (eg, chemotherapy, corticosteroids [high doses for longer than 2 weeks], radiation therapy)	Anthrax vaccine	⬇	Immune response to anthrax vaccine may be reduced.

[a] ⬇ = object drug decreased; ↔ = undetermined clinical effect.

Adverse Reactions

➤*Most common adverse reactions:* The most common (10% or more) local (injection-site) adverse reactions observed in clinical studies were tenderness, pain, erythema, and arm motion limitation. The most common (5% or more) systemic adverse reactions were muscle aches, headache, and fatigue.

Anthrax Vaccine Local Adverse Reactions[a]																
	Treatment arm															
Local adverse reactions	Group B anthrax vaccine IM weeks 0, 2, 4, 26				Group C anthrax vaccine IM weeks 0, 4, 26[b]				Group A anthrax vaccine subcutaneous weeks 0, 2, 4, 26				Placebo subcutaneous/IM weeks 0, 2, 4, 26[c]			
	n = 170				n = 501				n = 165				n = 169			
	Dose				Dose				Dose				Dose			
Number of subjects[d]	1	2	3	4	1	2[b]	3	4	1	2	3	4	1	2	3	4
Adverse reactions																
Arm motion limitation	11%	14%	5%	10%	16%	1%	16%	13%	9%	14%	6%	12%	1%	0%	2%	0%
Bruise	6%	4%	3%	3%	4%	3%	5%	4%	5%	5%	5%	3%	4%	6%	2%	4%
Edema	4%	12%	13%	16%	3%	1%	13%	11%	14%	28%	27%	29%	1%	4%	3%	2%
Erythema	13%	22%	21%	31%	10%	8%	20%	25%	52%	60%	57%	63%	12%	10%	8%	13%
Induration	5%	9%	8%	11%	4%	3%	9%	14%	26%	32%	30%	43%	1%	2%	4%	3%
Itching	1%	3%	4%	9%	0%	1%	3%	6%	4%	15%	21%	19%	0%	0%	0%	0%
Nodule	4%	2%	5%	6%	2%	1%	3%	6%	38%	45%	36%	27%	0%	1%	0%	1%
Pain	23%	23%	11%	17%	18%	4%	23%	15%	18%	24%	8%	16%	2%	2%	3%	3%
Presence of any large local adverse reaction[f]	0%	1%	3%	1%	0%	0%	1%	2%	1%	1%	5%	3%	0%	0%	0%	0%
Presence of any local adverse reaction	62%	69%	52%	62%	58%	25%	67%	68%	81%	86%	79%	81%	20%	19%	17%	23%
Presence of any moderate/severe local adverse reaction[e]	6%	9%	5%	8%	5%	1%	9%	5%	6%	16%	8%	10%	1%	0%	0%	0%
Tenderness	51%	61%	37%	42%	47%	10%	52%	51%	67%	72%	45%	60%	5%	6%	6%	9%
Warmth	4%	8%	6%	11%	3%	1%	10%	9%	28%	37%	29%	36%	2%	0%	0%	0%

[a] Per-dose statistical assessment performed on intent-to-treat population (ITT) data. Evaluations performed at 15 to 60 minutes and 1 to 3 days following each injection and prior to the next scheduled injection.
[b] Subjects received saline (instead of anthrax vaccine) for the week 2 dose.
[c] The 2 saline groups (subcutaneous and IM) were combined.
[d] The highest number per treatment arm; denominator (N) varied with dose number because of attrition over time.
[e] Moderate = causes discomfort and interferes with normal daily activities; severe = incapacitating and completely prevents performing normal daily activities.
[f] Large = an occurrence of induration, erythema, edema, nodule, and bruise with a largest diameter more than 120 mm.

Serious adverse reactions – Serious adverse reactions were infrequently reported during this study but 2 important serious adverse reactions that were noted to be possibly related to anthrax vaccine administration included a case of anaphylaxis and a case of an antinuclear antibody positive autoimmune disorder manifesting as a moderate bilateral arthralgia of the metacarpophalangeal joints. The majority of serious adverse reactions reported were unrelated to vaccination.

➤*Serious adverse reactions:* Serious allergic reactions, including anaphylactic shock, have been observed during postmarketing surveillance in individuals receiving anthrax vaccine.

➤*Open-label study:*

Local reactions – Over the course of the 5-year study, the following local reactions were reported: 24 (0.15% of doses administered) severe local reactions (defined as edema or induration measuring more than 120 mm in diameter or accompanied by marked limitation of arm motion or marked axillary node tenderness), 150 (0.94% of doses administered) moderate local reactions (edema or induration more than 30 mm but less than 120 mm in diameter), and 1,373 (8.63% of doses administered) mild local reactions (erythema only or induration measuring less than 30 mm in diameter).

Systemic reactions – During the 5-year reporting period, 4 (less than 0.06% of doses administered) cases of systemic reactions were reported. These reactions, which were reported to have been transient, included fever, chills, nausea, and general body aches.

➤*CDC study:*

Local reactions – The analysis of injection-site (local) reactions demonstrated that administration of the vaccine by the IM route, as compared with the subcutaneous route, resulted in a statistically significant reduction in reactogenicity (ie, cutaneous adverse reactions). Local adverse reactions, including warmth, tenderness, itching, erythema, induration, edema, and nodule, consistently occurred at lower frequencies and for shorter durations in participants given anthrax vaccine by the IM route. Route of administration did not statistically significantly influence the occurrence or duration of systemic adverse reactions, with the exception of muscle ache (increased occurrence only). Most local and systemic adverse reactions were mild or moderate in severity; the proportion of participants with severe adverse reactions reported was very low (less than 1%).

ANTHRAX VACCINE — INJECTION

Systemic adverse reactions –

Anthrax Vaccine Adverse Reactions[a]																
	Treatment arm															
Adverse reactions	Group B anthrax vaccine IM weeks 0, 2, 4, 26				Group C anthrax vaccine IM weeks 0, 4, 26[b]				Group A anthrax vaccine subcutaneous weeks 0, 2, 4, 26				Placebo subcutaneous/IM weeks 0, 2, 4, 26[c]			
Number of subjects[d]	n = 170				n = 501				n = 165				n = 169			
	Dose				Dose				Dose				Dose			
	1	2	3	4	1	2[b]	3	4	1	2	3	4	1	2	3	4
CNS																
Fatigue	7%	10%	12%	8%	8%	5%	12%	8%	8%	9%	7%	8%	5%	5%	6%	5%
Headache	4%	7%	9%	5%	5%	5%	7%	4%	7%	6%	8%	9%	2%	6%	3%	1%
Miscellaneous																
Fever > 100.4 °F	0%	0%	0%	0%	0%	0%	0%	0%	0%	0%	0%	0%	0%	0%	0%	0%
Muscle ache	11%	10%	6%	6%	9%	2%	14%	7%	6%	8%	3%	5%	1%	2%	3%	3%
Presence of any moderate/severe systemic adverse reactions[e]	1%	3%	3%	4%	2%	1%	6%	4%	1%	4%	3%	3%	1%	1%	3%	2%
Presence of any systemic adverse reaction	20%	22%	21%	15%	18%	10%	26%	15%	17%	17%	17%	17%	8%	10%	12%	8%
Tender/painful axillary adenopathy	0%	1%	0%	1%	0%	0%	1%	0%	1%	1%	4%	1%	0%	0%	0%	0%

[a] Per-dose statistical assessment performed on ITT population data. Evaluations performed at 15 to 60 minutes and 1 to 3 days following each injection and prior to the next scheduled injection.
[b] Subjects received saline (instead of anthrax vaccine) for the week 2 dose.
[c] The 2 saline groups (subcutaneous and IM) were combined.
[d] The highest number per treatment arm; denominator (N) varied with dose number because of attrition over time.
[e] Moderate = causes discomfort and interferes with normal daily activities; severe = incapacitating and completely prevents performing normal daily activities.

Gender – It was observed in this study that women receiving anthrax vaccine reported significantly more injection-site adverse reactions than men. This gender-related difference was seen regardless of the route of administration, but was more pronounced in those receiving the vaccine by the subcutaneous route. Women also reported more systemic adverse reactions than men (in particular, fatigue, muscle ache, and headache), but these gender differences were not influenced by route of administration. A brief pain or burning sensation, felt immediately after vaccine injection, was reported by most study participants. The pain was rated on a visual analog scale as 0 to 10. It was described as significant (more than 3) more often following subcutaneous administration (41%) than IM administration (26%). Women generally experienced a higher pain scale rating than men.

Adverse reactions (at least 2%) –

Anthrax Vaccine Adverse Reactions (> 2%)[a]				
Adverse reactions	Group B anthrax vaccine IM weeks 0, 2, 4, 26 (n = 170)	Group C anthrax vaccine IM weeks 0, 4, 26 (n = 501)	Group A anthrax vaccine subcutaneous weeks 0, 2, 4, 26 (n = 165)	Placebo subcutaneous/IM weeks 0, 2, 4, 26[b] (n = 169)
CNS				
Headache	63.5%	62.3%	67.3%	48.5%
Fatigue	61.2%	62.1%	61.2%	48.5%
GI				
Diarrhea	7.7%	6.2%	4.2%	3.6%
Nausea	5.9%	5.8%	9.1%	4.7%
Musculoskeletal				
Back pain	8.8%	7.2%	6.7%	3.6%
Joint sprain	0%	2%	0.6%	1.8%
Myalgia	61.8%	71.9%	61.2%	37.3%
Neck pain	2.9%	3.2%	0.6%	1.8%
Rigors	2.3%	1.4%	0%	1.2%
Respiratory				
Nasopharyngitis	15.3%	12.2%	10.9%	7.7%
Pharyngolaryngeal pain	12.4%	11.6%	12.1%	10.7%
Sinus headache	2.9%	1.4%	1.8%	0%
Sinusitis	7.1%	4.8%	4.2%	4.7%
Upper respiratory tract infection	1.8%	3.2%	4.2%	1.2%
Miscellaneous				
Dysmenorrhoea	7.1%	7.2%	4.2%	6.5%
Hypersensitivity	3.5%	2.4%	3.6%	0%
Influenza-like illness	1.8%	2.4%	0.6%	1.2%
Lymphadenopathy	2.9%	1.8%	3%	1.2%
Pruritus	0%	2%	1.8%	0.6%
Rash	0%	2.4%	1.8%	0.6%

[a] The adverse reactions listed are limited to those for which the adverse reaction rate for anthrax vaccine (weeks 0, 2, 4, 26 or weeks 0, 4, 26) exceeds the adverse reactions rate for placebo (weeks 0, 2, 4, 26) through month 7 irrespective of causality and severity; an adverse reaction is only listed once per subject, even if the adverse reaction occurs more than once during the 7-month observation period; reactions already listed in the second table are not listed here. The denominator includes any subject who was randomized and received at least 1 dose of vaccine.
[b] The 2 saline groups (subcutaneous and IM) were combined.

➤*Postmarketing:*

CNS – Headache, fatigue, paresthesia, tremor, ulnar nerve neuropathy.

Hypersensitivity – Allergic reactions (including anaphylaxis, angioedema, rash, urticaria, pruritus, erythema multiforme, anaphylactoid reaction, and Stevens-Johnson syndrome).

Local – Injection-site reactions (including pain, nodule, edema, induration, erythema, warmth, pruritus, and cellulitis).

Musculoskeletal – Arthralgia, arthropathy, myalgia, rhabdomyolysis.

Miscellaneous – Alopecia, flu-like symptoms, lymphadenopathy, pyrexia, syncope.

Other reactions – Infrequent reports were also received of multisystem disorders defined as chronic symptoms involving at least 2 of the following 3 categories: fatigue, mood-cognition, and musculoskeletal system.

Patient Information

Inform patients of the benefits and risks of immunization with anthrax vaccine and inform patients that the booster dose needs to be administered as scheduled in order for the vaccine to provide long-term protection.

Advise patients to report any serious adverse reaction to their health care provider.

HAEMOPHILUS B CONJUGATE VACCINE

Rx	**ActHIB** (Sanofi Pasteur)	**Injection, lyophilized powder for solution or suspension**: 10 mcg of purified *Haemophilus* b capsular polysaccharide PRP,[a] 24 mcg of inactivated tetanus toxoid per 0.5 mL	Sucrose 8.5%. Preservative free. In single-dose vials with sodium chloride 0.4% 0.6 mL as diluent and in single-dose vials with **Tripedia** vaccine 0.6 mL (DTaP[b]) as diluent.
Rx	**Hiberix** (GlaxoSmithKline)	**Injection, lyophilized powder for solution**: 10 mcg of purified *Haemophilus* b capsular polysaccharide PRP, 25 mcg of tetanus toxoid per 0.5 mL	Preservative free. Lactose. In single-dose vials with prefilled *Tip-Lok* syringe containing 0.7 mL of saline diluent.
Rx	**Liquid PedvaxHIB** (Merck)	**Injection, suspension**: 7.5 mcg of *Haemophilus* b PRP,[a] 125 mcg of *Neisseria meningitidis* OMPC[a] per 0.5 mL	Aluminum 225 mcg (as aluminum hydroxide). In single-dose vials.

[a] PRP = polyribosylribitol phosphate; OMPC = outer-membrane protein complex.
[b] DTaP = diphtheria and tetanus toxoids and acellular pertussis vaccine adsorbed.

HAEMOPHILUS B CONJUGATE VACCINE — INJECTION

For complete and comparative prescribing information, refer to the Agents for Active Immunization introduction.

Indications

➤*ActHIB*: For the active immunization of infants and children 2 to 18 months of age for the prevention of invasive disease caused by *Haemophilus influenzae* type b (Hib); for the active immunization of children 15 to 18 months of age for prevention of invasive disease caused by Hib and diphtheria, tetanus, and pertussis when reconstituted with *Tripedia* (DTaP) vaccine.

➤*Hiberix*: For active immunization as a booster dose for the prevention of invasive disease caused by Hibin children 15 months to 4 years of age (prior to fifth birthday).

➤*Liquid PedvaxHIB*: For routine vaccination against invasive disease caused by Hibin infants and children 2 to 71 months of age.

Administration and Dosage

➤*Children:*

Active immunity against Haemophilus influenzae type b –

ActHIB: The number of doses depends on the age at which immunization is begun. A child 7 to 11 months of age should receive 2 doses of *ActHIB* at 8-week intervals and a booster dose at 15 to 18 months of age. A child 12 to 14 months of age should receive 1 dose of *ActHIB*, followed by a booster 2 months later. Preterm infants should be vaccinated according to their chronological age from birth.

ActHIB and Tripedia Vaccination Recommendations for Previously Unvaccinated Infants and Children

Dose	Age	Immunization
First, second, and third	At 2, 4, and 6 months	*ActHIB* reconstituted with sodium chloride 0.4%
Fourth	At 15 to 18 months	*ActHIB* reconstituted with *Tripedia* or with sodium chloride 0.4%
Fifth	At 4 to 6 years	*Tripedia*

• *Reconstituted with Tripedia* –

15 to 18 months of age: 0.5 mL intramuscularly (IM).

• *Reconstituted with sodium chloride 0.4%* –

2 to 18 months of age: 0.5 mL IM.

Hiberix:

• *15 months to 4 years of age* –

Booster dose: 0.5 mL by IM injection.

Liquid PedvaxHIB:

Liquid PedvaxHIB Vaccination Recommendations

Age at first dose	Primary	Age at booster dose
2 to 10 months	2 doses, 2 months apart	12 to 15 months
11 to 14 months	2 doses, 2 months apart	—
15 to 71 months	1 dose	—

• *15 months to 5 years of age previously unvaccinated* – A single 0.5 mL IM injection.

• *2 to 14 months of age* – 0.5 mL, ideally beginning at 2 months of age, followed by a 0.5 mL dose 2 months later (or as soon as possible thereafter). When the primary 2-dose regimen is completed before 12 months of age, a booster dose is required. Infants born prematurely, regardless of birth weight, should be vaccinated at the same chronological age and according to the same schedule and precautions as full-term infants and children.

Booster dose: In infants completing the primary 2-dose regimen before 12 months of age, a booster dose (0.5 mL) should be administered at 12 to 15 months of age, but no earlier than 2 months after the second dose.

➤*Interchangeability: PedvaxHIB* may be interchanged with other licensed *Haemophilus* b conjugate vaccines for the primary and booster doses.

➤*Concomitant therapy:* Results from clinical studies indicate that *Liquid PedvaxHIB* can be coadministered with diphtheria and tetanus toxoids and whole-cell pertussis vaccine (DTP); oral polio vaccine (OPV); enhanced inactivated poliovirus vaccine (eIPV); varicella virus vaccine live; measles, mumps, and rubella virus vaccine live (*M-M-R II*); or hepatitis B vaccine (recombinant). No impairment of immune response to these individually tested vaccine antigens was demonstrated.

In addition, a PRP-OMPC–containing product, *Haemophilus* b conjugate (meningococcal protein conjugate) and hepatitis B (recombinant) vaccine, was given concomitantly with a booster dose of DTaP at approximately 15 months of age, using separate sites and syringes for injectable vaccines. No impairment of immune response to these individually tested vaccine antigens was demonstrated. *Haemophilus* b conjugate (meningococcal protein conjugate) and hepatitis B (recombinant) vaccine has also been coadministered with the primary series of DTaP to a limited number of infants. PRP antibody responses are satisfactory for *Haemophilus* b conjugate (meningococcal protein conjugate) and hepatitis B (recombinant) vaccine, but immune responses are currently unavailable for DTaP (see labeling for *Haemophilus* b conjugate [meningococcal protein conjugate] and hepatitis B [recombinant] vaccine). No serious vaccine-related adverse reactions were reported.

➤*Missed dose:* If there is an interruption or delay between doses in the primary series, there is no need to repeat the series, but dosing should be continued at the next clinic visit. Interruption of the recommended schedule with a delay between doses should not interfere with the final immunity.

➤*Preparation for administration:*

ActHIB –

Reconstitution with Tripedia: Cleanse both the *Tripedia* and *ActHIB* vial rubber stoppers with a suitable germicide prior to reconstitution. Thoroughly agitate the vial of *Tripedia*; then withdraw a 0.6 mL dose and inject into the vial of *ActHIB*. After reconstitution and thorough agitation, combined vaccines will appear whitish in color. Withdraw a 0.5 mL dose of the combined vaccines. Vaccine should be used immediately (within 30 minutes) after reconstitution.

Reconstitution with sodium chloride 0.4%: Using sodium chloride 0.4% diluent, cleanse the vaccine vial rubber stopper with a suitable germicide and inject the entire volume of diluent (0.6 mL) into the vial of vaccine. Thorough agitation is advised to ensure complete reconstitution. The entire volume of reconstituted vaccine is then drawn back into the syringe before injecting one 0.5 mL dose IM. The vaccine will appear clear and colorless. Vaccine should be used within 24 hours after reconstitution.

Hiberix –

Cleanse the vial stopper. Attach appropriate needle to accompanying prefilled syringe of diluent and insert into vial. Transfer entire contents of prefilled syringe into vial. With needle still inserted, vigorously shake the vial. After reconstitution, withdraw entire contents of vial (approximately 0.5 mL) and administer by IM injection. If the vaccine is not administered promptly, shake the solution vigorously again before injection.

Liquid PedvaxHIB – The vaccine should be used as supplied; no reconstitution is necessary. Shake well before withdrawal and use. Thorough agitation is necessary to maintain suspension of the vaccine.

➤*Administration:* Before injection, the skin over the site to be injected should be cleansed with a suitable germicide. The vaccines should be injected IM, preferably into the midlateral muscles of the thigh or deltoid, with care to avoid major peripheral nerve trunks. Do not inject into the gluteal area. Do not inject intravenously (IV), intradermally, or subcutaneously. After insertion of the needle, aspirate to help avoid inadvertent injection into a blood vessel. During the course of primary immunizations, injections should not be made more than once at the same site.

➤*Storage/Stability:*

ActHIB – Store between 2° and 8°C (36° and 46°F). Do not freeze. For *ActHIB* reconstituted with sodium chloride 0.4%, administer within 24 hours after reconstitution. For *ActHIB* reconstituted with *Tripedia*, administer immediately (within 30 minutes) after reconstitution.

Hiberix – Store between 2° and 8°C (36° and 46°F). Protect from light. Store diluent between 2° and 8°C (36° and 46°F) or between 20° and 25°C (68° and 77°F). Do not freeze. Discard if the diluent has been frozen. After reconstitution, administer promptly or refrigerate between 2° and 8°C (36° and 46°F) and administer within 24 hours. Discard the reconstituted vaccine if not used within 24 hours. Do not freeze; discard if the vaccine has been frozen.

Liquid PedvaxHIB – Store vaccine between 2° and 8°C (36° and 46°F). Do not freeze.

Actions

➤*Pharmacology: H. influenzae* is a gram-negative coccobacillus. Most strains of *H. influenzae* that cause invasive disease, including sepsis and meningitis, are Hib.

ActHIB – The response to *ActHIB* is typical of a T-dependent immune response to antigen. The prominent isotype of anticapsular PRP antibody induced by *ActHIB* is immunoglobulin G (IgG). A substantial booster response has been demonstrated in children 12 months of age and older who

HAEMOPHILUS B CONJUGATE VACCINE — INJECTION

previously received 2 or 3 doses. Bactericidal activity against Hib is demonstrated in serum after immunization and statistically correlates with the anti-PRP antibody response induced by *ActHIB*.

Antibody to *H. influenzae* capsular polysaccharide (anti-PRP) titers of more than 1 mcg/mL following vaccination with unconjugated PRP vaccine correlated with long-term protection against invasive Hib disease in children older than 24 months of age. Although the relevance of this threshold to clinical protection after immunization with conjugate vaccines is not known, particularly in light of the induced, immunologic memory, this level continues to be considered indicative of long-term protection. The immunogenicity and safety of *ActHIB* have been demonstrated in the United States and worldwide. *ActHIB* induced, on average, anti-PRP levels of 1 mcg/mL or more in 90% of infants after the primary series and in more than 98% of infants after a booster dose.

Hiberix – Specific levels of antibodies to anti-PRP have been shown to correlate with protection against invasive disease caused by Hib. Based on data from passive antibody studies and a clinical efficacy study with unconjugated *Haemophilus* b polysaccharide vaccine, an anti-PRP concentration of 0.15 mcg/mL has been accepted as a minimal protective level. Data from an efficacy study with unconjugated *Haemophilus* b polysaccharide vaccine indicate that an anti-PRP concentration of 1 mcg/mL or more predicts protection through at least a 1-year period. These antibody levels have been used to evaluate the effectiveness of *Hiberix*.

Liquid PedvaxHIB – An important virulence factor of the Hib bacterium is its polysaccharide capsule (PRP). Antibody to PRP (anti-PRP) has been shown to correlate with protection against Hib disease. While the anti-PRP level associated with protection using conjugated vaccines has not yet been determined, the level of anti-PRP associated with protection in studies using bacterial polysaccharide immune globulin or nonconjugated PRP vaccines ranged from more than 0.15 to more than 1 mcg/mL.

Nonconjugated PRP vaccines are capable of stimulating B lymphocytes to produce antibody without the help of T lymphocytes (T independent). The responses to many other antigens are augmented by helper T lymphocytes (T dependent). *PedvaxHIB* is a PRP-conjugate vaccine in which the PRP is covalently bound to the OMPC carrier, producing an antigen that is postulated to convert the T-independent antigen (PRP alone) into a T-dependent antigen resulting in both an enhanced antibody response and immunologic memory.

Contraindications

Hypersensitivity to any component of the vaccine or to the provided diluent.

Warnings/Precautions

➤*Latex allergy:* The stopper to the *ActHIB* diluent vial contains dry natural latex rubber. The lyophilized vaccine vial contains no rubber of any kind.

The tip caps of the *Hiberix* prefilled diluent syringes may contain natural rubber latex. The rubber plungers of the prefilled syringes and the vial stoppers do not contain latex.

➤*Antibodies: Haemophilus* b conjugate vaccine may not induce protective antibody levels immediately following vaccination.

➤*Immunosuppression:* Safety and effectiveness in immunosuppressed children have not been evaluated. If these vaccines are used in persons with malignancies or those receiving immunosuppressive therapy or who are otherwise immunocompromised, the expected immune response may not be obtained. Children with impaired immune responsiveness, whether due to the use of immunosuppressive therapy (including radiation, corticosteroids, antimetabolites, alkylating agents, and cytotoxic agents), asymptomatic or symptomatic HIV infection, severe combined immunodeficiency, hypogammaglobulinemia, agammaglobulinemia, or altered immune states caused by disease such as leukemia, lymphoma, or generalized malignancy, may have reduced antibody response to active immunization procedures. Consider deferring administration of vaccine may be considered in individuals receiving immunosuppressive therapy. Other groups should receive this vaccine according to the usual recommended schedule.

➤*HIV infection: Haemophilus* b conjugate vaccine is not contraindicated based on the presence of HIV infection.

➤*Infection:* The decision to administer or delay vaccination because of current or recent febrile illness depends on the severity of symptoms and on the etiology of the disease. The Advisory Committee on Immunization Practices (ACIP) has recommended delaying vaccination during the course of an acute febrile illness. All vaccines can be administered to persons with minor illnesses, such as diarrhea, mild upper respiratory tract infection with or without low-grade fever, or other low-grade febrile illness. Vaccinate persons with moderate or severe febrile illness as soon as they have recovered from the acute phase of the illness.

➤*Active disease:* As reported with *Haemophilus* b polysaccharide vaccines, cases of Hib disease may occur subsequent to vaccination and prior to the onset of protective effects of the vaccine. There is insufficient evidence that this vaccine given immediately after exposure to natural Hib will prevent illness.

➤*Disease transmission:* The evidence favors rejection of a causal relation between immunization with *Haemophilus* b conjugate vaccines and early-onset *Haemophilus* b disease.

➤*Guillain-Barré syndrome:* If Guillain-Barré syndrome has occurred within 6 weeks of receipt of a prior vaccine containing tetanus toxoid, base the decision to give any tetanus toxoid–containing vaccine on careful consideration of the potential benefits and possible risks.

➤*Tetanus immunization:* Immunization with *ActHIB* or *Hiberix* does not substitute for routine tetanus immunization.

➤*Hypersensitivity reactions:* Epinephrine injection (1:1000) and other appropriate agents used for the control of immediate allergic reactions must be immediately available should an acute anaphylactic or other allergic reaction occur because of any component of the vaccine.

➤*Pregnancy: Category C.* Animal reproduction studies have not been conducted. It is also not known whether these vaccines can cause fetal harm when administered to a pregnant woman or can affect reproduction capacity. These vaccines are not recommended for use in a pregnant woman and are not indicated for use in adults.

➤*Lactation:* These vaccines are not recommended for use in breast-feeding women and are not indicated for use in adults. Women who were vaccinated with *Haemophilus* b conjugate vaccine at 34 to 36 weeks' gestation had significantly higher antibody titers (more than 20-fold) in their colostrum than nonimmunized women or women who were vaccinated before pregnancy. Breast milk antibody titer were also significantly higher (more than 20-fold) than the comparison groups at 3 and 6 months after delivery. The Centers for Disease Control and Prevention and several health professional organizations state that vaccines given to a breast-feeding mother do not affect the safety of breast-feeding for mothers or infants and that breast-feeding is not a contraindication to the *Haemophilus* vaccine. Vaccinate breast-fed infants according to the recommended schedules.

➤*Children:*

ActHIB – Safety and effectiveness of *ActHIB* reconstituted with *Tripedia* in children younger than 15 months of age have not been established. Do not administer *ActHIB* combined with *Tripedia* to children younger than 15 months of age.

Safety and effectiveness of *ActHIB* reconstituted with sodium chloride 0.4% in infants younger than 6 weeks of age have not been established.

Hiberix – Safety and effectiveness of *Hiberix* in children younger than 15 months of age and in children 5 to 16 years of age have not been established.

Liquid PedvaxHIB – Safety and effectiveness in infants younger than 2 months of age and in children 6 years of age and older have not been established. In addition, do not use *Liquid PedvaxHIB* in infants younger than 6 weeks of age because this will lead to a reduced anti-PRP response and may lead to immune tolerance (impaired ability to respond to subsequent exposure to the PRP antigen). *Liquid PedvaxHIB* is not recommended for use in persons 6 years of age and older because they are generally not at risk of Hib disease.

➤*Elderly:* These vaccines are not indicated for use in adult populations.

Drug Interactions

➤*Anticoagulants:* As with other IM injections, use with caution in patients on anticoagulant therapy.

➤*Immunosuppressives:* Immunosuppressive therapies, including irradiation, antimetabolites, alkylating agents, cytotoxic drugs, and corticosteroids (used in greater than physiologic doses) may reduce the immune response to vaccines. Short-term (less than 2 weeks) corticosteroid therapy or intra-articular, bursal, or tendon injections with corticosteroids should not be immunosuppressive. Although no specific studies with pertussis vaccine are available, if immunosuppressive therapy will be discontinued shortly, it is reasonable to defer vaccination until the patient has been off therapy for 1 month; otherwise, the patient should be vaccinated while still on therapy.

If *ActHIB* reconstituted with *Tripedia* has been administered to persons receiving immunosuppressive therapy or a recent injection of immunoglobulin, or those who have an immunodeficiency disorder, an adequate immunologic response may not be obtained.

➤*Drug/Lab test interactions:* Urine antigen detection may not have a diagnostic value in suspected disease caused by Hib within 1 to 2 weeks (30 days for *PedvaxHIB*) after receipt of a Hib-containing vaccine.

Adverse Reactions

➤*ActHIB*:

Common adverse reactions – Adverse reactions commonly associated with a first *ActHIB* immunization of children 12 to 15 months of age who were not previously immunized with a *Haemophilus* b conjugate vaccine, include local pain, redness, and swelling at the injection site. Systemic reactions include fever, irritability and lethargy.

ActHIB and DTP adverse reactions –

***ActHIB* and DTP Adverse Reactions After Simultaneous Administration at Separate Sites**									
	Age at immunization								
	2 months (n = 365)			4 months (n = 364)			6 months (n = 365)		
Adverse reaction	6 h	24 h	48 h	6 h	24 h	48 h	6 h	24 h	48 h
CNS[a]									
Drowsiness	57.5%	29.9%	10.4%	44.2%	18.1%	7.4%	32.6%	13.4%	2.5%
Irritability	72.6%	21.9%	12.6%	48.4%	25%	13.2%	44.1%	25.2%	10.1%
Persistent crying	Percentage of infants within 72 h after immunization was 1.6% after dose 1, 0.6% after dose 2, and 0.3% after dose 3.								
GI[a]									
Diarrhea	4.4%	6.6%	5.2%	5%	4.7%	4.7%	4.7%	6.3%	3.6%
Vomiting	2.7%	4.1%	2.7%	2.5%	3.3%	2.8%	2.2%	2.7%	1.9%

HAEMOPHILUS B CONJUGATE VACCINE — INJECTION

ActHIB and DTP Adverse Reactions After Simultaneous Administration at Separate Sites

	Age at immunization								
	2 months (n = 365)			4 months (n = 364)			6 months (n = 365)		
Adverse reaction	6 h	24 h	48 h	6 h	24 h	48 h	6 h	24 h	48 h
Local[b]									
Erythema	14.3%	4.1%	0.3%	8.8%	5.8%	0.6%	11.5%	6.9%	1.6%
Induration	22.5%	6.3%	1.9%	12.4%	4.7%	0.8%	9.6%	3.8%	1.1%
Tenderness	46.3%	11.5%	2.2%	23.4%	7.4%	1.1%	19.2%	6%	1.1%
Miscellaneous[a]									
Anorexia	15.3%	5.8%	4.9%	8%	5%	3%	5.5%	4.9%	2.2%
Fever > 100.8°F[c]	20.1%	1.3%	0.6%	14.6%	6.6%	1.4%	15.7%	8.8%	0.8%

[a] The adverse reaction profile is defined by the concomitant use of DTP vaccine.
[b] Local reactions were evaluated at the *ActHIB* injection site.
[c] The number of individuals observed at each time point for fever varied from 357 to 363.

ActHIB Combined With DTP by Reconstitution Adverse Reactions

	Age at immunization								
	2 months (n = 204)			4 months (n = 199)			6 months (n = 200)		
Adverse reaction	6 h	24 h	48 h	6 h	24 h	48 h	6 h	24 h	48 h
CNS									
Drowsiness	60.3%	23.5%	11.3%	42.2%	20.6%	9.6%	30.3%	12.3%	5.6%
Irritability	70.6%	22.1%	12.8%	56.8%	31.2%	19.1%	40.5%	28.2%	15.9%
Persistent crying	Percentage of infants within 72 h after immunization was 0% after dose 1, 0% after dose 2, and 0.005% after dose 3.								
GI									
Diarrhea	2.5%	5.4%	1.5%	3.5%	3.5%	2.5%	2.6%	4.1%	5.6%
Vomiting	2.9%	5.4%	2.9%	3%	5%	3%	3.6%	3.6%	1.5%
Local									
Erythema > 1″	11.8%	2.5%	0%	11.6%	9.1%	2.5%	10.5%	13.5%	3.5%
Induration	31.4%	17.2%	3.9%	26.1%	20.1%	7.5%	28.5%	22.5%	10%
Tenderness	47.1%	18.6%	3.4%	33.2%	17.6%	4%	25%	17%	3.5%
Miscellaneous									
Anorexia	17.7%	6.4%	2.9%	10.1%	7.5%	5.5%	5.1%	4.6%	4.1%
Fever > 100.4°F	24.6%	2%	0.5%	15.8%	6.1%	3.6%	13%	10.3%	3.1%

Other adverse reactions: In a third US trial when *ActHIB* was combined with DTP by reconstitution, approximately 1,450 doses were administered to infants starting at 2 months of age. Adverse reactions observed at 6 and 24 hours, respectively, after the first immunization (n = 498) were tenderness, 66.9% and 30.7%; erythema (more than 1 inch), 8.6% and 2.2%; induration, 38.2% and 21.7%; irritability, 77.9% and 35.7%; drowsiness, 63.7% and 34.1%; anorexia, 26.1% and 12.9%; diarrhea, 6.8% and 9%; and vomiting, 3.4% and 3.8%. One hypotonic-hyporesponsive episode was seen in an infant following the second dose in this trial. This is consistent with the hypotonic-hyporesponsive episode incidence rate observed with DTP vaccination alone.

ActHIB and *Tripedia* adverse reactions –

ActHIB Reconstituted With Tripedia Vs. ActHIB and Tripedia Coadministered at Separate Sites

	6 hours postdose		24 hours postdose		48 hours postdose	
Adverse reaction	Separate injections[a] (n = 103 to 110)	*ActHIB* with *Tripedia* (n = 102 to 110)	Separate injections[a] (n = 105 to 110)	*ActHIB* with *Tripedia* (n = 103 to 110)	Separate injections[a] (n = 104 to 110)	*ActHIB* with *Tripedia* (n = 103 to 109)
CNS						
Drowsiness	36.4%	30.3%	17.3%	13.9%	12.7%	11%
Irritability	27.3%	22.9%	20.9%	17.6%	12.7%	10.1%
Persistent cry	0%	0%	0%	0%	0%	0%
Unusual cry	0%	0%	0%	0%	0%	0.9%
Local						
Erythema > 1 in	0.9%/ 0%	3.6%	2.7%/ 0.9%	3.6%	0.9%/ 0%	1.8%
Induration[b]	3.6%/ 5.5%	2.7%	2.7%/ 3.6%	8.2%	4.5%/ 0.9%	3.6%
Swelling	3.6%/ 3.6%	3.6%	2.7%/ 1.8%	5.5%	0.9%/ 0%	4.5%
Tenderness	17.3%/ 20%	19.1%	8.2%/ 8.2%	10%	1.8%/ 0.9%	1.8%
Miscellaneous						
Anorexia	12.7%	9.2%	10%	6.5%	6.4%	2.8%
Fever > 102.2°F	0%	2%	1%	1.9%	1.9%	0%
Vomiting	0.9%	1.8%	0.9%	1.9%	0.9%	2.8%

[a] *Tripedia*/*ActHIB* injection site.
[b] Induration is defined as hardness with or without swelling.

ActHIB combined with *Tripedia* was administered to approximately 850 children, aged 15 to 20 months. All children received 3 doses of a *Haemophilus* b conjugate vaccine and 3 doses of whole-cell DTP at approximately 2, 4, and 6 months of age. Local reactions were typically mild and usually resolved within the 24- to 48-hour period after immunization. The most common local reactions were pain and tenderness at the injection site. Systemic reactions occurring were usually mild and resolved within 72 hours of immunization. The reaction rates were similar to those observed above when *ActHIB* reconstituted with *Tripedia* was administered and when *Tripedia* was administered alone as a booster.

ActHIB and DTP versus hepatitis B vaccine with DTP: In a randomized, double-blind US clinical trial, *ActHIB* was given concomitantly with DTP to more than 5,000 infants and hepatitis B vaccine was given with DTP to a similar number. In this large study, deaths due to sudden infant death syndrome (SIDS) and other causes were observed but were not different in the 2 groups. In the first 48 hours following immunization, 2 definite and 3 possible seizures were observed after *ActHIB* and DTP in comparison with none after hepatitis B vaccine and DTP. This rate of seizures following*ActHIB* and DTP was not greater than previously reported in infants receiving DTP alone. Other adverse reactions reported with administration of other *Haemophilus* b conjugate vaccines include urticaria, seizures, hives, renal failure, and Guillain-Barré syndrome. A cause-and-effect relationship among any of these reactions and the vaccination has not been established.

➤*Hiberix:*

Adverse reactions –

Hiberix[a,b] Coadministered With DTaP-HBV-IPV[c] Adverse Reactions (N = 371)

Adverse reaction	Any	Grade 3
CNS		
Fussiness	25.9%	0.8%[d]
Restlessness	21.8%	0.5%[e]
Sleepiness	19.9%	1.1%[e]
GI		
Diarrhea	14.6%	0.8%[e]
Vomiting	4.9%	0.5%[e]
Local[f]		
Pain	20.5%	1.1%[g]
Redness	24.5%	2.4%[h]
Swelling	14.8%	2.2%[h]
Miscellaneous		
Fever[i]	34.8%	3.8%
Loss of appetite	22.9%	0.8%[e]

[a] N = all subjects for whom safety data were available. Reactions reported within 4 days of vaccination (defined as day of vaccination and the next 3 days).
[b] In this study, 92 subjects previously received 3 doses of *Hiberix* (not approved for primary immunization in the US), 96 subjects previously received 3 doses of US-licensed *Haemophilus* b conjugate vaccine (manufactured by Sanofi Pasteur SA , and 183 subjects previously received 3 doses of a *Haemophilus* b conjugate vaccine that is no longer licensed in the US.
[c] In this study, DTaP-HBV-IPV was given to subjects who previously received 3 doses of DTaP-HBV-IPV. In the US, *Pediarix* is approved for use as a 3-dose primary series; use as a fourth consecutive dose is not approved in the US.
[d] Grade 3 fussiness defined as persistent crying and could not be comforted.
[e] Grade 3 for these symptoms defined as preventing normal daily activity.
[f] Local reactions at the injection site for *Hiberix*.
[g] Grade 3 pain defined as causing crying when limb moved.
[h] Grade 3 redness or swelling defined as more than 20 mm.
[i] Fever defined as at least 38°C (100.4°F) rectally or at least 37.5°C (99.5°F) axillary, oral, or tympanic; Grade 3 fever defined as higher than 39.5°C (103.1°F) rectally or higher than 39°C (102.2°F) axillary, oral, or tympanic.

Serious adverse reactions – Two of 1,008 subjects reported a serious adverse reaction that occurred in the 31-day period following booster immunization with *Hiberix*. One subject developed bilateral pneumonia 9 days postvaccination, and 1 subject experienced asthenia following accidental drug ingestion 18 days postvaccination.

➤*PedvaxHIB:*

Liquid PedvaxHIB – During a 3-day period following primary vaccination with *Liquid PedvaxHIB*, the most frequently reported (more than 1%) adverse reactions, without regard to causality, excluding those shown in the following table, in decreasing order of frequency, were as follows: Irritability, sleepiness, injection-site pain/soreness, injection-site erythema (less than or equal to 2.5 cm diameter), injection-site swelling/induration (less than or equal to 2.5 cm diameter), unusual high-pitched crying, prolonged crying (more than 4 hours), diarrhea, vomiting, crying, pain, otitis media, rash, and upper respiratory tract infection.

HAEMOPHILUS B CONJUGATE VACCINE — INJECTION

Liquid *PedvaxHIB* Adverse Reactions in Subjects First Vaccinated at 2 to 6 Months of Age[a]								
Adverse reaction	Number of subjects evaluated	Postdose 1			Number of subjects evaluated	Postdose 2		
		6 h	24 h	48 h		6 h	24 h	48 h
Erythema > 2.5 cm diameter	674	2.2%	1%	0.5%	562	1.6%	1.1%	0.4%
Fever[b] > 38.3°C (≥ 101°F) rectal	222	18.1%	4.4%	0.5%	206	14.1%	9.4%	2.8%
Swelling > 2.5 cm diameter	674	2.5%	1.9%	0.9%	562	0.9%	0.9%	1.3%

[a] DTP and OPV were coadministered to most subjects.

[b] Fever was also measured by another method or reported as normal for an additional 345 infants after dose 1 and for an additional 249 infants after dose 2; however, these data are not included in the this table.

Lyophilized PedvaxHIB –

Only one serious reaction (tracheitis) was reported as possibly related to lyophilized *PedvaxHIB* and only one (diarrhea) as possibly related to placebo. Seizures occurred infrequently in both groups (9 occurred in vaccine recipients, 8 of whom also received DTP; 8 occurred in placebo recipients, 7 of whom also received DTP) and were not reported to be related to lyophilized *PedvaxHIB*.

In early clinical studies involving the administration of 8,086 doses of lyophilized *PedvaxHIB* alone to 5,027 healthy infants and children 2 months to 71 months of age, lyophilized *PedvaxHIB* was generally well tolerated. No serious adverse reactions were reported. In a subset of these infants, urticaria was reported in 2 children, and thrombocytopenia was seen in 1 child. A cause-and-effect relationship between these adverse effects and the vaccination has not been established.

Other adverse reactions – The use of *Haemophilus* b polysaccharide vaccines and another *Haemophilus* b conjugate vaccine has been associated with the following additional adverse reactions: early-onset Hib disease and Guillain-Barré syndrome. A cause-and-effect relationship between these adverse effects and the vaccination was not established.

➤*Postmarketing:*

CNS – Convulsions (with or without fever), febrile seizures, hypotonic-hyporesponsive episode, somnolence, syncope or vasovagal responses to injection.

Dermatologic – Rash, urticaria.

Hypersensitivity – Allergic reactions including anaphylactic and anaphylactoid reactions, angioedema.

Local – Extensive swelling of the vaccinated limb, injection-site induration, sterile injection-site abscess.

Miscellaneous – Apnea, lymphadenopathy.

Overdosage

None well documented.

Patient Information

Inform the parent, guardian, or other responsible adult of the recommended immunization schedule for protection against *Haemophilus* b disease and of the benefits and risks of the vaccine.

Prior to administration ask the parent or guardian about the recent health status of the infant or child to be immunized, previous vaccination history, and reactions to previous *Haemophilus* vaccines, if any.

Inform the parent or guardian about the significant adverse reactions that have been temporally associated with the administration of *Haemophilus* b conjugate vaccine.

Instruct the parent or guardian to report any serious adverse reactions to their health care provider.

Inform the parent or guardian that the US Department of Health and Human Services has established a new Vaccine Adverse Event Reporting System (VAERS) to accept all reports of suspected adverse reactions after the administration of any vaccine, including but not limited to the reporting of reactions required by the National Childhood Vaccine Injury Act of 1986. The toll-free number for VAERS forms and information is 1-800-822-7967.

Inform the parent or guardian of the importance of completing the immunization series.

Provide the parent or guardian with the Vaccine Information Materials (VIMs) which are required to be given with each immunization.

HAEMOPHILUS B CONJUGATE VACCINE/HEPATITIS B VACCINE

Rx	Comvax (Merck)	Injection: 7.5 mcg *Haemophilus* b PRP, 5 mcg hepatitis B surface antigen/0.5 mL[a]	In 0.5 mL single-dose vials.

[a] With 125 mcg *Neisseria meningitidis* OMPC, approximately 225 mcg aluminum (as aluminum hydroxide), and 35 mcg sodium borate (decahydrate) in 0.9% sodium chloride.

HAEMOPHILUS B CONJUGATE/HEPATITIS B — INJECTION

For complete and comparative prescribing information, refer to the Agents for Active Immunization introduction. For complete and comparative prescribing information, refer to the Haemophilus b conjugate vaccine monograph.

Indications

➤*Haemophilus b/Hepatitis B vaccination:* For vaccination against invasive disease caused by *Haemophilus influenzae* type b and against infection caused by all known subtypes of hepatitis B virus in infants 6 weeks to 15 months of age born of HBsAg negative mothers.

See Administration and Dosage for more information.

Vaccination with haemophilus b conjugate and hepatitis B should ideally begin at approximately 2 months of age or as soon thereafter as possible. In order to complete the 3-dose regimen of haemophilus b conjugate and hepatitis B, vaccination should be initiated no later than 10 months of age. Infants in whom vaccination with a PRP-OMPC-containing product (ie, *PedvaxHIB*, haemophilus b conjugate and hepatitis B) is not initiated until 11 months of age do not require 3 doses of PRP-OMPC; however, 3 doses of an HBsAg-containing product are required for complete vaccination against hepatitis B, regardless of age. For infants and children not vaccinated according to the recommended schedule see Administration and Dosage.

Haemophilus b conjugate and hepatitis B will not protect against invasive disease caused by *Haemophilus influenzae* other than type b or against invasive disease (such as meningitis or sepsis) caused by other microorganisms. Haemophilus b conjugate and hepatitis B will not prevent hepatitis caused by other viruses known to infect the liver. Because of the long incubation period for hepatitis B, it is possible for unrecognized infection to be present at the time the vaccine is given. The vaccine may not prevent hepatitis B in such patients.

➤*Use with other vaccines:* Immunogenicity results from open-labeled studies indicate that haemophilus b conjugate and hepatitis B can be administered concomitantly with DTP (diphtheria, tetanus and whole cell pertussis vaccine), DTaP (diphtheria, tetanus and acellular pertussis vaccine), OPV (oral poliomyelitis vaccine), IPV (inactivated poliomyelitis vaccine), M-M-R II (measles, mumps, and rubella virus vaccine live), and *VARIVAX* (varicella virus vaccine live) using separate sites and syringes for injectable vaccines (see Pharmacology).

Administration and Dosage

➤*Children:*

Haemophilus b/hepatitis B vaccination –

6 weeks to 15 months of age:

• *Usual dosage* – Three 0.5 mL doses of haemophilus b conjugate/hepatitis B vaccine intramuscularly (IM), ideally at 2, 4, and 12 to 15 months of age, in infants born to HBsAg-negative mothers.

If the recommended schedule cannot be followed, the interval between the first 2 doses should be at least 6 weeks and the interval between the second and third doses should be as close as possible to 8 to 11 months.

• *Modified schedule –*

Children previously vaccinated with 1 or more doses of either hepatitis B vaccine or Haemophilus b conjugate vaccine: Children who receive 1 dose of hepatitis B vaccine at or shortly after birth may be administered haemophilus b conjugate/hepatitis B vaccine on the schedule of 2, 4, and 12 to 15 months of age.

There are no data to support the use of a 3-dose series of haemophilus b conjugate/hepatitis B vaccine in infants who have previously received more than 1 dose of hepatitis B vaccine. However, haemophilus b conjugate/hepatitis B vaccine may be administered to children otherwise scheduled to receive concurrent *RECOMBIVAX HB* and *PedvaxHIB*.

Children not vaccinated according to recommended schedule for haemophilus b conjugate and hepatitis B: Vaccination schedules for children not vaccinated according to the recommended schedule should be considered on an individual basis. The number of doses of a PRP-OMPC-containing product (ie, haemophilus b conjugate/hepatitis B vaccine, *PedvaxHIB*) depends on the age that vaccination is begun. An infant 2 to 10 months of age should receive 3 doses of a product containing PRP-OMPC. An infant 11 to 14 months of age should receive 2 doses of a product containing PRP-OMPC. A child 15 to 71 months of age should receive 1 dose of a product containing PRP-OMPC. Infants and children, regardless of age, should receive 3 doses of an HBsAg-containing product.

➤*Preparation for administration:* The vaccine should be used as supplied; no reconstitution is necessary.

Shake well before withdrawal and use. Thorough agitation is necessary to maintain suspension of the vaccine.

HAEMOPHILUS B CONJUGATE/HEPATITIS B — INJECTION

➤*Administration:* For IM administration. Do not inject intravenously, intradermally, or subcutaneously.

The anterolateral thigh is the recommended site for IM injection in infants.

Injection must be accomplished with a needle long enough to ensure IM deposition of the vaccine. The Advisory Committee on Immunization Practices (ACIP) has recommended that for IM injections, the needle should be of sufficient length to reach the muscle mass itself. In a clinical trial with haemophilus b conjugate/hepatitis B vaccine, vaccination was accomplished with a needle length of ⅝ inches in accordance with ACIP recommendations in effect at that time. ACIP currently recommends that needles of longer length (⅞ to 1 inch) be used.

➤*Storage/Stability:* Store vaccine at 2° to 8°C (36° to 46°F). Storage above or below the recommended temperature may reduce potency.

Do not freeze; freezing destroys potency.

MENINGOCOCCAL VACCINE

Rx	**Menomune A/C/Y/W-135** (Sanofi Pasteur)	**Injection, lyophilized powder for solution**: When reconstituted, each 0.5 mL contains 50 mcg "isolated product" from each of groups A, C, Y, and W-135	Lactose. In single- and 10-dose vials[a,b] with diluent.
Rx	**Menactra** (Sanofi Pasteur)	**Injection, solution**: each 0.5 mL contains 4 mcg each of groups A, C, Y, and W-135[c]	Preservative free. In single-dose vials.[b]
Rx	**Menveo** (Novartis)	**Injection, lyophilized powder and solution**: each 0.5 mL contains serogroup A 10 mcg and 5 mcg each of groups C, Y, and W-135.	Preservative free. In single-dose vials.[d]

[a] Formulated to contain lactose 2.5 to 5 mg per dose. Single-dose vial supplied with 0.78 mL of preservative-free distilled water diluent; 10-dose vial supplied with 6 mL of diluent with thimerosal 1:10,000.
[b] Stopper to the vial contains dry, natural latex rubber.
[c] Conjugated to approximately 48 mcg of diphtheria toxoid protein carrier.
[d] Supplied as a vial containing group A meningococcal (MenA) lyophilized conjugate component and a vial containing MenCYW-135 liquid.

MENINGOCOCCAL POLYSACCHARIDE VACCINE — INJECTION

For complete and comparative prescribing information, refer to the Agents for Active Immunization introduction.

Indications

➤*Meningococcal disease prevention:*

Menactra – Active immunization of persons 9 months to 55 years for the prevention of invasive meningococcal disease caused by *Neisseria meningitidis* serogroups A, C, Y, and W-135.

Menactra vaccine is not indicated for the prevention of *N. meningitidis* serogroup B.

Menomune – Active immunization against invasive meningococcal disease caused by serogroups A, C, Y, and W-135 may be used to prevent and control outbreaks of serogroup C meningococcal disease.

Menomune is not indicated for infants and children younger than 2 years of age, except as short-term protection of infants at least 3 months of age against group A. For persons remaining at high risk, especially children who were first vaccinated at younger than 4 years of age, revaccination may be indicated.

As with any vaccine, vaccination with *Menomune* may not protect 100% of persons.

Menveo – Active immunization to prevent invasive meningococcal disease caused by *N. meningitidis* serogroups A, C, Y, and W-135. *Menveo* is approved for use in persons 2 to 55 years of age.

Menveo does not prevent *N. meningitidis* serogroup B infections.

Administration and Dosage

➤*Dosage:*

Menactra – 0.5 mL as a single injection intramuscularly (IM). In children 9 through 23 months of age, *Menactra* is given as a 2-dose series 3 months apart. Persons 2 through 55 years of age receive a single dose. The need for a booster dose of *Menactra* has not been determined.

Menomune – For both adults and children, the vaccine is administered subcutaneously as a single 0.5 mL dose. Protective antibody levels may be achieved within 7 to 10 days after vaccination.

Menveo – Administer as a single 0.5 mL IM injection, preferably into the deltoid muscle (upper arm). For children 2 to 5 years of age at continued high risk of meningococcal disease, a second dose may be administered 2 months after the first dose.

The duration of protection following immunization is not known.

➤*Revaccination:*

Menomune – Revaccination of a single 0.5 mL dose administered subcutaneously may be indicated for persons at high risk of infection, particularly children who were first vaccinated when they were younger than 4 years of age; such children should be considered for revaccination after 2 to 3 years if they remain at high risk. Although the need for revaccination in older children and adults has not been determined, antibody levels decline rapidly over 2 to 3 years, and, if indications still exist for immunization, revaccination may be considered within 3 to 5 years.

➤*Preparation for administration:*

Menomune – Reconstitute the vaccine using only the diluent supplied for this purpose. Draw the volume of diluent shown on the diluent label into a suitable size syringe and inject into the vial containing the vaccine. Shake vial until the vaccine is dissolved.

Menveo – *Menveo* must be prepared for administration by reconstituting the MenA lyophilized conjugate vaccine component with the MenCYW-135 liquid conjugate vaccine component. Using a graduated syringe, withdraw the entire contents of the vial of MenCYW-135 liquid conjugate component and inject into the MenA lyophilized conjugate component vial. Invert the vial and shake well until the vaccine is dissolved and then withdraw 0.5 mL of reconstituted product. Note that it is normal for a small amount of liquid to remain in the vial following withdrawal of the dose.

Following reconstitution, the vaccine is a clear, colorless solution, free from visible foreign particles.

Menactra – *Menactra* vaccine is a clear to slightly turbid solution.

➤*Administration:*

Menactra/Menveo – For IM use. Do not administer this product intravenously (IV), subcutaneously, or intradermally.

Menomune – Special care should be taken to avoid injecting the vaccine intradermally, IM, or IV because clinical studies have not been done to establish safety and efficacy of the vaccine using these different routes of administration.

➤*Coadministration with other vaccines:*

Menomune – Because of the combined endotoxin content, *Menomune* should not be administered at the same time as whole-cell pertussis or whole-cell typhoid vaccines.

➤*Incompatibilities:* Meningococcal vaccine must not be mixed with any vaccine in the same syringe. Therefore, separate injection sites and different syringes should be used in case of coadministration.

➤*Storage/Stability:*

Menactra – Store at 2° to 8°C (35° to 46°F). Do not freeze. Product that has been exposed to freezing should not be used.

Menomune – Store freeze-dried vaccine and reconstituted vaccine, when not in use, between 2° and 8°C (35° and 46°F). Discard remainder of multidose vials of vaccine within 35 days after reconstitution. Use the single-dose vial within 30 minutes after reconstitution.

Menveo – Do not freeze. Frozen/previously frozen product should not be used. Store refrigerated, away from the freezer compartment, at 2° to 8°C (36° to 46°F). Protect from light. Vaccine must be maintained at 2° to 8°C (36° to 46°F) during transport. Use the reconstituted vaccine immediately; may be held at or below 25°C (77°F) for up to 8 hours.

Actions

➤*Pharmacology:* The presence of bactericidal anticapsular meningococcal antibodies has been associated with protection from invasive meningococcal disease. Meningococcal polysaccharide diphtheria toxoid conjugate vaccine induces the production of bactericidal antibodies specific to the capsular polysaccharides of serogroups A, C, Y, and W-135.

Contraindications

➤*Menactra*: Known hypersensitivity to any component of *Menactra*, including diphtheria toxoid, or a life-threatening reaction after previous administration of a vaccine containing similar components; known history of Guillain-Barré syndrome; known hypersensitivity to dry, natural rubber latex.

➤*Menomune*: Defer use during the course of any acute illness. Do not administer to persons who are sensitive to thimerosal, which is found in the 10-dose vial, or any other component of the vaccine.

➤*Menveo*: Severe allergic reaction (eg, anaphylaxis) after a previous dose of *Menveo*, any component of this vaccine, or any other CRM_{197}, diphtheria toxoid, or meningococcal-containing vaccine.

Warnings/Precautions

➤*Guillain-Barré syndrome:* Guillain-Barré syndrome has been reported in temporal relationship following administration of *Menactra* vaccine. An evaluation of postmarketing adverse reactions suggests a potential for an increased risk of Guillain-Barré syndrome following *Menactra* vaccination. Persons previously diagnosed with Guillain-Barré syndrome should not receive *Menactra* vaccine.

MENINGOCOCCAL POLYSACCHARIDE VACCINE — INJECTION

➤*Latex sensitivity:* The stopper of the vial contains dry natural rubber latex, which may cause allergic reactions in latex-sensitive persons. There is no latex in any component of the syringe.

➤*Immunosuppressed patients:* If the vaccine is used in persons receiving immunosuppressive therapy, the expected immune response may not be obtained.

The immune response to *Menactra* administered to immunosuppressed patients has not been studied.

➤*Recent or acute illness:* The Advisory Committee on Immunization Practices has published guidelines for vaccination of persons with recent or acute illness (refer to http://www.cdc.gov).

➤*Other vaccines: Menomune* vaccine should not be give at the same time as whole-cell pertussis or whole-cell typhoid vaccines because of combined endotoxin content.

➤*Infection transmission:* Use a separate, sterile syringe and needle or a sterile disposable unit for each patient to prevent transmission of hepatitis and other infectious agents from person to person. Do not recap needles, and dispose of them according to biohazard waste guidelines.

➤*Administration:*

Menomune – Take special care to avoid injecting *Menomune* intradermally, IM, or IV because clinical studies have not been done to establish safety and efficacy of the vaccine using these routes of administration.

Menactra – Take special care to avoid injecting *Menactra* subcutaneously because clinical studies have not been conducted to establish safety and efficacy of the vaccine using this route of administration.

➤*Hypersensitivity reactions:* As a precautionary measure, epinephrine injection (1:1,000) and other appropriate agents and equipment must be immediately available in case of anaphylactic or serious allergic reactions.

➤*Pregnancy: Category C.* Animal reproduction studies have not been conducted with meningococcal vaccine. It is not known whether meningococcal vaccine can cause fetal harm when given to a pregnant woman or can affect reproduction capacity. There are no adequate and well-controlled studies in pregnant women. Give meningococcal vaccine to a pregnant woman only if clearly needed.

The effect of *Menactra* vaccine on embryo-fetal and preweaning development was evaluated in one developmental toxicity study in mice. Animals were administered *Menactra* vaccine on day 14 prior to gestation and during the period of organogenesis (gestation day 6). The total dose given per time point was 0.1 mL/mouse via IM injection (900 times the human dose, adjusted by body weight). There were no adverse effects on pregnancy, parturition, lactation, or preweaning development noted in this study. Skeletal examinations revealed 1 fetus (1 of 234 examined) in the vaccine group with a cleft palate. None were observed in the concurrent control group (0 of 174 examined). There are no data that suggest that this isolated finding is vaccine-related, and there were no vaccine-related fetal malformations or other evidence of teratogenesis observed in this study.

Pregnancy registry – Health care providers are encouraged to register pregnant women who receive *Menactra* in the manufacturer's pregnancy registry by calling 1-800-822-2463.

➤*Lactation:* It is not known whether this drug is excreted in human milk. Because many drugs are excreted in human milk, exercise caution when meningococcal vaccine is given to a breast-feeding woman.

➤*Children:* Safety and effectiveness of meningococcal vaccine in children younger than 2 years of age have not been established.

➤*Elderly:* Safety and efficacy of *Menactra* vaccine in adults older than 55 years of age have not been established.

➤*Monitoring:* Take care to ensure the safe and effective use of meningococcal vaccine.

Obtain the previous immunization history of the vaccinee, and inquire about the current health status of the vaccinee.

Before administration, take all appropriate precautions to prevent adverse reactions. This includes a review of the patient's previous immunization history, the presence of any contraindications to immunization, the patient's current health status, and history concerning possible sensitivity to the vaccine, similar vaccine, or latex.

Drug Interactions

➤*Immunosuppressive therapy:* If meningococcal vaccine is used in persons receiving immunosuppressive therapy (including irradiation, antimetabolites, alkylating agents, cytotoxic drugs, and corticosteroids [used in greater than physiologic doses]), the expected immune response may not be obtained.

➤*Other vaccines:* Do not give *Menomune* vaccine at the same time as whole-cell pertussis or whole-cell typhoid vaccines because of combined endotoxin content.

The safety and immunogenicity of coadministration of *Menactra* with vaccines other than typhoid Vi polysaccharide or tetanus and diphtheria toxoids, adsorbed (for adult use) vaccines have not been determined.

Adverse Reactions

➤*Menactra* and *Menomune*:

Serious adverse reactions – Serious adverse reactions reported within a 6-month time period following vaccination in children 2 to 10 years of age occurred at a rate of 0.6% following *Menactra* and at a rate of 0.7% following *Menomune*. Serious adverse reactions reported within a 6-month time period following vaccination in adolescents and adults occurred at a rate of 1% following *Menactra* and at a rate of 1.3% following *Menomune*.

Most common – The most frequently reported solicited local and systemic adverse reactions in US children 2 to 10 years of age were injection-site pain and irritability. Anorexia, diarrhea, and drowsiness were also common.

The most commonly reported solicited adverse reactions in adolescents 11 to 18 years of age (see the following table) and adults 18 to 55 years of age (see the second table that follows) were injection-site pain, headache, and fatigue. Except for redness in adults, local reactions were more frequently reported after *Menactra* vaccination than after *Menomune* vaccination. The majority of local and systemic reactions following *Menactra* or *Menomune* were reported as mild in intensity. No important differences in rates of anorexia, diarrhea, malaise, rash (including urticaria), or vomiting were observed between the vaccine groups.

Meningococcal Vaccine Adverse Reactions (2 to 10 Years of Age)

	Menactra (n[a] = 1,157)			*Menomune* (n[a] = 1,027)		
Reaction	Any	Moderate	Severe	Any	Moderate	Severe
CNS						
Drowsiness[b]	10.8%	2.7%	0.3%	11.2%	2.5%	0.5%
Irritability[c]	12.4%	3%	0.3%	12.2%	2.6%	0.6%
Seizure[d]	0%	—	—	0%	—	—
GI						
Anorexia[e]	8.2%	1.7%	0.4%	8.7%	1.3%	0.8%
Diarrhea[f]	11.1%	2.1%	0.2%	11.8%	2.5%	0.3%
Vomiting[g]	3%	0.7%	0.3%	2.7%	0.7%	0.6%
Local						
Induration[h]	18.9%	3.4%	1.4%	4.2%	0.6%	0%
Pain[i]	45%	4.9%	0.3%	26.1%	2.5%	0%
Rash[d]	3.4%	—	—	3%	—	—
Redness[h]	21.8%	4.6%	3.9%	7.9%	0.5%	0%
Swelling[h]	17.4%	3.9%	1.9%	2.8%	0.3%	0%
Miscellaneous						
Arthralgia[j]	6.8%	0.5%	0.2%	5.3%	0.7%	0%
Fever[k]	5.2%	1.7%	0.3%	5.2%	1.7%	0.2%

[a] n = the total number of subjects reporting at least 1 solicited reaction. The median age of participants was 6 years in both vaccine groups.
[b] Moderate: interferes with normal activities; severe: disabling, unwilling to engage in play or interact with others.
[c] Moderate: 1 to 3 hours' duration; severe: > 3 hours' duration.
[d] These solicited adverse reactions were reported as present or absent only.
[e] Moderate: skipped 2 meals; severe: skipped ≥ 3 meals.
[f] Moderate: 3 to 4 episodes; severe: ≥ 5 episodes.
[g] Moderate: 2 episodes; severe: ≥ 3 episodes.
[h] Moderate: 1 to 2 inches; severe: > 2 inches.
[i] Moderate: interferes with normal activities; severe: disabling, unwilling to move arm.
[j] Moderate: decreased range of motion due to pain or discomfort; severe: unable to move major joints due to pain.
[k] Oral equivalent temperature; moderate: 38.4° to 39.4°C; severe: ≥ 39.5°C.

Meningococcal Vaccine Adverse Reactions (11 to 18 Years of Age)

	Menactra vaccine (n[a] = 2,264)			*Menomune* vaccine (n[a] = 970)		
Adverse reaction	Any	Moderate	Severe	Any	Moderate	Severe
CNS						
Headache[b]	35.6%[c]	9.6%[c]	1.1%	29.3%	6.5%	0.4%
Seizure[d]	0%	—	—	0%	—	—
GI						
Anorexia[e]	10.7%[c]	2%	0.3%	7.7%	1.1%	0.2%
Diarrhea[f]	12%	1.6%	0.3%	10.2%	1.3%	0%
Vomiting[g]	1.9%	0.4%	0.3%	1.4%	0.5%	0.3%
Local						
Induration[h]	15.7%[c]	2.5%[c]	0.3%	5.2%	0.5%	0%
Pain[i]	59.2%[c]	12.8%[c]	0.3%	28.7%	2.6%	0%
Rash[d]	1.6%	—	—	1.4%	—	—
Redness[h]	10.9%[c]	1.6%[c]	0.6%[c]	5.7%	0.4%	0%
Swelling[h]	10.8%[c]	1.9%[c]	0.5%[c]	3.6%	0.3%	0%

MENINGOCOCCAL POLYSACCHARIDE VACCINE — INJECTION

Meningococcal Vaccine Adverse Reactions (11 to 18 Years of Age)						
	Menactra vaccine (n[a] = 2,264)			*Menomune* vaccine (n[a] = 970)		
Adverse reaction	Any	Moderate	Severe	Any	Moderate	Severe
Miscellaneous						
Arthralgia[b]	17.4%[c]	3.6%[c]	0.4%	10.2%	2.1%	0.1%
Chills[b]	7%[c]	1.7%[c]	0.2%	3.5%	0.4%	0.1%
Fatigue[b]	30%[c]	7.5%	1.1%[c]	25.1%	6.2%	0.2%
Fever[j]	5.1%[c]	0.6%	0%	3%	0.3%	0.1%
Malaise[b]	21.9%[c]	5.8%[c]	1.1%	16.8%	3.4%	0.4%

[a] n = the number of subjects with available data.
[b] Moderate: interferes with normal activities; severe: requiring bed rest.
[c] Denotes $P < 0.05$ level of significance. The P values were calculated for each category and severity using chi-square test.
[d] These solicited adverse reactions were reported as present or absent only.
[e] Moderate: skipped 2 meals; severe: skipped ≥ 3 meals.
[f] Moderate: 3 to 4 episodes; severe: ≥ 5 episodes.
[g] Moderate: 2 episodes; severe: ≥ 3 episodes.
[h] Moderate: 1 to 2 inches; severe: > 2 inches.
[i] Moderate: interferes with or limits usual arm movement; severe: disabling, unable to move arm.
[j] Oral equivalent temperature; moderate: 38.5° to 39.4°C; severe: ≥ 39.5°C.

Meningococcal Vaccine Adverse Reactions (18 to 55 Years of Age)						
	Menactra (n[a] = 1,371)			*Menomune* (n[a] = 1,159)		
Adverse reaction	Any	Moderate	Severe	Any	Moderate	Severe
CNS						
Headache[b]	41.4%	10.1%	1.2%	41.8%	8.9%	0.9%
Seizure[c]	0%	—	—	0%	—	—
GI						
Anorexia[d]	11.8%	2.3%	0.4%	9.9%	1.6%	0.4%
Diarrhea[e]	16%	2.6%	0.4%	14%	2.9%	0.3%
Vomiting[f]	2.3%	0.4%	0.2%	1.5%	0.2%	0.4%
Local						
Induration[g]	17.1%[h]	3.4%[h]	0.7%[h]	11%	1%	0%
Pain[i]	53.9%[h]	11.3%[h]	0.2%	48.1%	3.3%	0.1%
Rash[c]	1.4%	—	—	0.8%	—	—
Redness[g]	14.4%	2.9%	1.1%[h]	16%	1.9%	0.1%
Swelling[g]	12.6%[h]	2.3%[h]	0.9%[h]	7.6%	0.7%	0%
Miscellaneous						
Arthralgia[b]	19.8%[h]	4.7%[h]	0.3%	16%	2.6%	0.1%
Chills[b]	9.7%[h]	2.1%[h]	0.6%[h]	5.6%	1%	0%
Fatigue[b]	34.7%	8.3%	0.9%	32.3%	6.6%	0.4%
Fever[j]	1.5%[h]	0.3%	0%	0.5%	0.1%	0%
Malaise[b]	23.6%	6.6%[h]	1.1%	22.3%	4.7%	0.9%

[a] n = number of subjects with available data.
[b] Moderate: interferes with normal activities; severe: requiring bed rest.
[c] These solicited adverse reactions were reported as present or absent only.
[d] Moderate: skipped 2 meals; severe: skipped ≥ 3 meals.
[e] Moderate: 3 to 4 episodes; severe: ≥ 5 episodes.
[f] Moderate: 2 episodes; severe: ≥ 3 episodes.
[g] Moderate: 1 to 2 inches; severe: > 2 inches.
[h] Denotes $P < 0.05$ level of significance. The P values were calculated for each category and severity using chi-square test.
[i] Moderate: interferes with or limits usual arm movement; severe: disabling, unable to move arm.
[j] Oral equivalent temperature; moderate: 39° to 39.9°C; severe: ≥ 40°C.

➤*Concomitant vaccine adverse reactions:*

Adverse reactions when given with Td vaccine or Typhim Vi vaccine –

Local: The 2 vaccine groups reported similar frequencies of pain, induration, redness, and swelling at the *Menactra* injection site, as well as at the Td injection site and the *Typhim Vi* injection site. Pain was the most frequent local reaction reported at the *Menactra*, Td, and *Typhim Vi* injection sites. More participants experienced pain after Td vaccination and *Typhim Vi* than after *Menactra* vaccination (71% vs 53% and 76% vs 47%, respectively). The majority (66% to 77%) of local solicited reactions for both groups (Td and *Menactra*) at either injection site were reported as mild and resolved within 3 days after vaccination. The majority (70% to 77%) of local solicited reactions for both groups (*Typhim Vi* and *Menactra*) at either injection site were reported as mild and resolved within 3 days after vaccination.

Systemic: In both groups, the most common systemic reactions were headache (*Menactra* + *Typhim Vi* vaccine, 41%; *Typhim Vi* vaccine + placebo, 42%; *Menactra* vaccine alone, 33%) and fatigue (*Menactra* + *Typhim Vi* vaccine, 38%; *Typhim Vi* vaccine + placebo, 35%; *Menactra* vaccine alone, 27%). Between the groups, differences in rates of malaise, diarrhea, anorexia, or vomiting were not statistically significant. Fever 40°C or higher and seizures were not reported in either group.

➤*Menomune*: Adverse reactions to *Menomune* are mild and consist principally of pain and redness at the injection site for 1 to 2 days. Pain at the injection site is the most commonly reported adverse reaction, and a transient fever might develop in 2% or less of young children.

The following adverse reactions were reported by 150 adults following vaccination with *Menomune*. The subjects were observed for 3 weeks following vaccination. Local reactions resolved within 48 hours, and no significant systemic reactions were reported.

Menomune Adverse Reactions		
Adverse reaction	Mild	Moderate
Local		
Injection-site reactions	Diameter: < 2 inches	Diameter: ≥ 2 inches
Erythema	3.8%	1.2%
Induration	4.4%	1.2%
Pain	2.6%	2%
Tenderness	36%	9%
Systemic		
Chills	2.5%	0%
Fever	2.6% (100° to 101°F)	0.6% (> 101°F)
Headache	5.2%	1.8%
Malaise	2.5%	0%

In a clinical study involving 73 children 2 to 12 years of age who received *Menomune*, local reactions consisting of erythema or tenderness were seen in approximately 40% of the children. In another clinical study involving 53 children 4 to 6 years of age who received *Menomune*, erythema was seen in 89% of the children, swelling in 92%, and tenderness in 64%. None of these reactions was considered serious or necessitated medical intervention.

On rare occasions, immunoglobulin A nephropathy has occurred following vaccinations with *Menomune*; however, a cause-and-effect relationship has not been established.

Do not give *Menomune* vaccine at the same time as whole-cell pertussis or whole-cell typhoid vaccines because of combined endotoxin content.

Hypersensitivity – As with the administration of any vaccine, vaccine components can cause hypersensitivity reactions in some recipients.

➤*Reporting adverse reactions:* The National Vaccine Injury Compensation Program, established by the National Childhood Vaccine Injury Act of 1986, requires health care providers who administer vaccines to maintain permanent vaccination records and to report occurrences of certain adverse reactions to the US Department of Health and Human Services (DHHS). Reportable reactions include those listed in the act for each vaccine and reactions specified in the package insert as contraindications to further doses of that vaccine.

Encourage reporting by patients, parents, or guardians of all adverse reactions occurring after vaccine administration. Report adverse reactions following immunization with vaccine to the US DHHS Vaccine Adverse Event Reporting Systems (VAERS). VAERS was established by the US DHHS to accept all reports of suspected adverse reactions after administration of any vaccine. Reporting forms and information about reporting requirements or completion of the form can be obtained from VAERS through a toll-free number 1-800-822-7967 or through the Web site http://vaers.hhs.gov. Also report these reactions to the manufacturer.

➤*Postmarketing:* The following adverse reactions have been reported during postapproval use of *Menactra* vaccine. Because these reactions were reported voluntarily from a population of uncertain size, it is not always possible to reliably calculate their frequency or to establish a causal relationship to *Menactra* vaccine exposure.

CNS – Acute disseminated encephalomyelitis, facial palsy, Guillain-Barré syndrome, transverse myelitis, vasovagal syncope.

Dermatologic – Urticaria.

Musculoskeletal – Myalgia.

Patient Information

Prior to administration of meningococcal vaccine, inform the patient, parent, guardian, or other responsible adult of the potential benefits and risks to the patient and give the patient, parent, or guardian the Vaccine Information Statement, which is required by the National Childhood Vaccine Injury Act of 1986 to be given prior to immunization. These materials are available free of charge at the CDC Web site (http://www.cdc.gov/vaccines). Instruct patients, parents, or guardians to report any suspected adverse reactions to their health care provider.

Inform patients, parents, or guardians that the US DHHS has established a VAERS to accept all reports of suspected adverse reactions after the administration of any vaccine and be given the contact information for VAERS.

Inform women of childbearing potential that the manufacturer maintains a pregnancy registry to monitor fetal outcomes of pregnant women exposed to meningococcal vaccine. If they are pregnant or become aware they were pregnant at the time of meningococcal vaccine immunization, instruct them to contact their health care provider or the manufacturer.

PNEUMOCOCCAL VACCINE POLYVALENT

Rx	**Pneumovax 23** (Merck)	**Injection:** 25 mcg each of 23 polysaccharide isolates per 0.5 mL dose	In 1- and 5-dose vials.[a]

[a] With 0.25% phenol.

PNEUMOCOCCAL VACCINE POLYVALENT — INJECTION

For complete and comparative information, refer to the Agents for Active Immunization introduction.

Indications

➤*Pneumococcal disease prevention:* For vaccination against pneumococcal disease caused by those pneumococcal types included in the vaccine.

If it is known that a person has not received any pneumococcal vaccine or if earlier pneumococcal vaccination status is unknown, then persons in the categories listed should be administered pneumococcal vaccine; however, if a person has received a primary dose of pneumococcal vaccine, before administering an additional dose of vaccine, please refer to the Revaccination section.

Vaccination with pneumococcal vaccine is recommended for selected individuals as follows:

➤*Immunocompetent persons:*

- Routine vaccination for people 50 years of age and older (the Advisory Committee on Immunization Practices [ACIP] recommends routine vaccination for immunocompetent people 65 years of age and older).
- Persons 2 years of age and older with long-term cardiovascular disease (including congestive heart failure and cardiomyopathies), chronic pulmonary disease (including chronic obstructive pulmonary disease and emphysema), or diabetes mellitus.
- Persons 2 years of age and older with alcoholism, chronic liver disease (including cirrhosis), or cerebrospinal fluid leaks.
- Persons 2 years of age and older with functional or anatomic asplenia (including sickle cell disease and splenectomy).
- Persons 2 years of age and older living in special environments or social settings (including Alaskan Natives and certain American Indian populations).

➤*Immunocompromised persons:* Persons 2 years of age and older, including those with HIV infection, leukemia, lymphoma, Hodgkin disease, multiple myeloma, generalized malignancy, chronic renal failure, or nephrotic syndrome; those receiving immunosuppressive chemotherapy (including corticosteroids); and those who have received an organ or bone marrow transplant.

➤*Timing of vaccination:* Pneumococcal vaccine should be given at least 2 weeks before elective splenectomy, if possible.

For patients planning cancer chemotherapy or other immunosuppressive therapy (eg, for patients with Hodgkin disease or those who undergo organ or bone marrow transplantation), the interval between vaccination and initiation of immunosuppressive therapy should be at least 2 weeks. Vaccination during chemotherapy or radiation therapy should be avoided. Pneumococcal vaccine may be given several months following completion of chemotherapy or radiation therapy for neoplastic disease. In Hodgkin disease, immune response to vaccination may be suboptimal for 2 years or longer after intensive chemotherapy (with or without radiation). During the 2 years following the completion of chemotherapy or other immunosuppressive therapy, antibody responses improve in some patients as the interval between the end of treatment and pneumococcal vaccination increases.

Persons with asymptomatic or symptomatic HIV infection should be vaccinated as soon as possible after their diagnosis is confirmed.

➤*Use with other vaccines:* See Administration and Dosage for more information.

➤*Revaccination:* The ACIP has recommendations for revaccination against pneumococcal disease in persons at high risk who are previously vaccinated with pneumococcal vaccine or the pneumococcal conjugate vaccine.

Early studies have indicated that local reactions (ie, arthus-type reactions) among adults receiving the second dose of 14-valent vaccine within 2 years after the first dose are more severe than those occurring after initial vaccination. However, subsequent studies have suggested that revaccination after intervals of 4 years or more is not associated with an increased incidence of adverse reactions.

Routine revaccination of immunocompetent persons previously vaccinated with 23-valent polysaccharide vaccine is not recommended. However, revaccination once is recommended for persons 2 years of age and older who are at highest risk of serious pneumococcal infection and those likely to have a rapid decline in pneumococcal antibody levels, provided that at least 5 years have passed since receipt of a first dose of pneumococcal vaccine.

The highest risk group includes persons with functional or anatomic asplenia (eg, sickle cell disease or splenectomy), HIV infection, leukemia, lymphoma, Hodgkin disease, multiple myeloma, generalized malignancy, chronic renal failure, nephrotic syndrome, or other conditions associated with immunosuppression (eg, organ or bone marrow transplantation), and those receiving immunosuppressive chemotherapy (including long-term systemic corticosteroids).

For children 10 years of age and younger at time of revaccination and at highest risk of severe pneumococcal infection (eg, children with functional or anatomic asplenia, including sickle cell disease, splenectomy, or conditions associated with rapid antibody decline after initial vaccination including nephrotic syndrome, renal failure, or renal transplantation), the ACIP recommends that revaccination may be considered 3 years after the previous dose.

If prior vaccination status is unknown for patients in the high risk group, patients should be given pneumococcal vaccine.

All persons 65 years of age and older who have not received vaccine within 5 years (and were younger than 65 years of age at the time of vaccination) should receive another dose of vaccine.

Because data are insufficient concerning the safety of pneumococcal vaccine when administered 3 or more times, revaccination following a second dose is not routinely recommended.

Administration and Dosage

➤*Adults:*

Pneumococcal disease prevention – 0.5 mL subcutaneously or intramuscularly (IM).

➤*Children:*

2 years of age and older –

Pneumococcal disease prevention: See Adults for dosing.

➤*Coadministration with other vaccines:* The ACIP states that pneumococcal vaccine may be administered concurrently with other vaccines and at the same time as influenza vaccine (by separate injection in the other arm) without an increase in adverse reactions or decreased antibody response to either vaccine. In contrast to pneumococcal vaccine, influenza vaccine is recommended annually, for appropriate populations.

➤*Administration:* The vaccine is used directly as supplied. No dilution or reconstitution is necessary.

Do not inject intravenously or intradermally. Intradermally may cause severe local reactions. Use appropriate precautions to avoid intravascular administration.

Administer by IM or subcutaneously, preferably in the deltoid muscle or lateral mid-thigh.

➤*Storage/Stability:* Store unopened and opened vials at 2° to 8°C (36° to 46°F).

Actions

➤*Pharmacology:*

Immunogenicity – It has been established that the purified pneumococcal capsular polysaccharides induce antibody production and that such antibody is effective in preventing pneumococcal disease. Clinical studies have demonstrated the immunogenicity of each of the 23 capsular types when tested in polyvalent vaccines.

Studies with 12-, 14-, and 23-valent pneumococcal vaccines in children 2 years of age and older and in adults of all ages showed immunogenic responses. Protective capsular type-specific antibody levels generally develop by the third week following vaccination.

Bacterial capsular polysaccharides induce antibodies primarily by T-cell–independent mechanisms. Therefore, antibody response to most pneumococcal capsular types is generally poor or inconsistent in children younger than 2 years of age whose immune systems are immature.

Efficacy – The protective efficacy of pneumococcal vaccines containing 6 or 12 capsular polysaccharides was investigated in 2 controlled studies of young, healthy gold miners in South Africa, in whom there was a high attack rate for pneumococcal pneumonia and bacteremia. Capsular type-specific attack rates for pneumococcal pneumonia were observed for the period from 2 weeks through about 1 year after vaccination. Protective efficacy was 76% and 92%, respectively, in the 2 studies for the capsular types represented.

In similar studies using similar pneumococcal vaccines prepared for the National Institute of Allergy and Infectious Diseases, the reduction in pneumonia caused by the capsular types contained in the vaccines was 79%. Reduction in type-specific pneumococcal bacteremia was 82%.

A prospective study in France found pneumococcal vaccine to be 77% effective in reducing the incidence of pneumonia among nursing home residents.

Duration of immunity – Following pneumococcal vaccination, serotype-specific antibody levels decline after 5 to 10 years. A more rapid decline in antibody levels may occur in some groups (eg, children). Limited published data suggest that antibody levels may decline in patients older than 60 years of age.

ACIP states that these findings indicate that revaccination may be needed to provide continued protection.

The results from 1 epidemiologic study suggest that vaccination may provide protection for at least 9 years after receipt of the initial dose. Decreasing estimates of effectiveness with increasing interval since vaccination, particularly among very elderly patients (persons 85 years of age and older) have been reported.

Contraindications

Hypersensitivity to any component of the vaccine.

PNEUMOCOCCAL VACCINE POLYVALENT — INJECTION

Warnings/Precautions

➤*Timing of vaccination:* See Indications for more information.

If the vaccine is used in persons receiving immunosuppressive therapy, the expected serum antibody response may not be obtained and potential impairment of future immune responses to pneumococcal antigens may occur (see Indications, Timing of Vaccination).

➤*Antibiotic prophylaxis:* In patients who require penicillin (or other antibiotic) prophylaxis against pneumococcal infection, such prophylaxis should not be discontinued after vaccination with pneumococcal vaccine.

➤*Pneumococcal meningitis:* Pneumococcal vaccine may not be effective in preventing pneumococcal meningitis in patients who have chronic cerebrospinal fluid leakage resulting from congenital lesions, skull fractures, or neurosurgical procedures.

➤*Revaccination:* Routine revaccination of immunocompetent persons previously vaccinated with a 23-valent vaccine is not recommended. However, revaccination once is recommended for persons 2 years of age and older who are at highest risk for serious pneumococcal infections and those likely to have a rapid decline in pneumococcal antibody levels.

➤*Hypersensitivity reactions:* Epinephrine injection (1:1,000) must be immediately available should a short-term anaphylactoid reaction occur due to any component of the vaccine.

➤*Special risk:* Exercise caution and appropriate care in administering pneumococcal vaccine to individuals with severely compromised cardiovascular and/or pulmonary function in whom a systemic reaction would pose a significant risk.

Febrile illness – Any febrile respiratory illness or other active infection is reason for delaying use of pneumococcal vaccine, except when, in the opinion of the health care provider, withholding the agent entails even greater risk.

➤*Pregnancy: Category C.* It is also not known whether pneumococcal vaccine can cause fetal harm when administered to a pregnant woman or can affect reproduction capacity. Pneumococcal vaccine should be given to a pregnant woman only if clearly needed.

➤*Lactation:* It is not known whether this drug is excreted in human milk. Because many drugs are excreted in human milk, caution should be exercised when pneumococcal vaccine is administered to a breast-feeding woman.

➤*Children:* In general, children younger than 2 years of age respond poorly to the capsular types of pneumococcal vaccine that are most often the cause of pneumococcal disease in this age group. Safety and effectiveness in children younger than 2 years of age have not been established. Accordingly, pneumococcal vaccine polyvalent is not recommended in this age group.

➤*Elderly:* Because elderly individuals may not tolerate medical interventions as well as younger individuals, a higher frequency and/or a greater severity of reactions in some older individuals cannot be ruled out.

Drug Interactions

For patients planning cancer chemotherapy or other immunosuppressive therapy (eg, for patients with Hodgkin disease or those who undergo organ or bone marrow transplantation), the interval between vaccination and initiation of immunosuppressive therapy should be at least 2 weeks. Vaccination during chemotherapy or radiation therapy should be avoided. Pneumococcal vaccine may be given several months following completion of chemotherapy or radiation therapy for neoplastic disease. See Administration and Dosage for more information.

Adverse Reactions

➤*Most common adverse reactions:*

Local – Local reactions at injection site including erythema, soreness, swelling and induration, warmth; fever of 102°F or less.

➤*Other adverse reactions:*

CNS – Asthenia, decreased limb mobility, febrile convulsion, Guillain-Barré syndrome, headache, malaise, paresthesia, radiculoneuropathy.

Dermatologic – Rash, urticaria.

GI – Nausea, vomiting.

Hematologic/Lymphatic – Hemolytic anemia in patients who have had other hematologic disorders, leukocytosis, lymphadenitis, lymphadenopathy, thrombocytopenia in patients with stabilized idiopathic thrombocytopenic purpura.

Hypersensitivity – Anaphylactoid reactions, angioneurotic edema, serum sickness.

Musculoskeletal – Arthralgia, arthritis, myalgia.

Miscellaneous – Cellulitis, chills, fever (more than 102°F), increased serum C-reactive protein, pain, peripheral edema in the injected extremity.

➤*Postmarketing:*

Local – In postmarketing experience, injection-site cellulitis-like reactions were reported rarely; between 1989 and 2002, when approximately 43 million doses were distributed, the annual reporting rate was less than 2 per 100,000 doses. The cellulitis-like reactions occurred with initial and repeat vaccination at a median onset time of 2 days after vaccine administration.

In a clinical trial, an increased rate of local reactions has been observed with revaccination at 3 to 5 years following primary vaccination.

For subjects 65 years of age and older, it was reported that the overall injection-site adverse reactions rate was higher following revaccination (79.3%) than following primary vaccination (52.9%). For subjects 50 to 64 years of age, the reported overall injection-site adverse reactions rate for re-vaccinees and primary vaccinees were similar (79.6% and 72.8%, respectively).

In both age groups, re-vaccinees reported a higher rate of a composite end point (any of the following: moderate pain, severe pain, and/or large induration at the injection site) than primary vaccinees. Among subjects 65 years of age and older, the composite end point was reported by 30.6% and 10.4% of revaccination and primary vaccination subjects, respectively, while among subjects 50 to 64 years of age, the end point was reported by 35.5% and 18.9%, respectively. The injection-site reactions occurred within the 3-day monitoring period and typically resolved by day 5.

Systemic – Systemic signs and symptoms including fever, leukocytosis and an increase in the laboratory value for serum C-reactive protein may be associated with local reactions.

The rate of overall systemic adverse reactions was similar among primary vaccinees and re-vaccinees within each age group. The rate of vaccine-related systemic adverse reactions was higher following revaccination (33.1%) than following primary vaccination (21.7%) in subjects 65 years of age and older, and was similar following revaccination (37.5%) and primary vaccination (35.5%) in subjects 50 to 64 years of age. The most common systemic adverse reactions reported after pneumococcal vaccine polyvalent were as follows: asthenia/fatigue, headache, and myalgia.

Regardless of age, the observed increase in post vaccination use of analgesics (13% or less in the re-vaccinees and 4% or less in the primary vaccinees) returned to baseline by day 5.

Patient Information

Inform the patient, parent, or guardian of the benefits and risks associated with vaccination.

Tell patients, parents, and guardians that vaccination with pneumococcal vaccine may not offer 100% protection from pneumococcal infection.

Instruct the patients, parents, and guardians to report any serious adverse reactions to their health care provider who in turn should report such events to the vaccine manufacturer or the United States Department of Health and Human Services through the Vaccine Adverse Event Reporting System (VAERS), 1-800-822-7967.

PNEUMOCOCCAL CONJUGATE VACCINE

Rx	**Prevnar** (Wyeth)	**Injection, suspension:** 16 mcg of total saccharides[a] per 0.5 mL dose	(7–valent.) In 0.5 mL syringes.[b]
Rx	**Prevnar 13** (Wyeth)	**Injection, suspension:** 30.8 mcg of total saccharides[c] per 0.5 mL dose	(13–valent.) Latex free. In 0.5 mL single-dose, prefilled syringes.[d]

[a] 2 mcg each of 6 polysaccharide isolates (4, 9V, 14, 18C, 19F, and 23F); 4 mcg of serotype 6B per 0.5 mL dose.

[b] Also contains approximately 20 mcg of CRM_{197} carrier protein and 0.125 mg of aluminum per 0.5 mL dose as aluminum phosphate adjuvant.

[c] Each 0.5 mL dose contains ≈ 2.2 mcg of each of *Streptococcus pneumoniae* serotypes 1, 3, 4, 5, 6A, 7F, 9V, 14, 18C, 19A, 19F, and 23F saccharides; and 4.4 mcg of serotype 6B saccharides.

[d] Each dose also contains 34 mcg of CRM_{197} carrier protein, 100 mcg of polysorbate 80, 295 mcg of succinate buffer, and 125 mcg of aluminum as aluminum phosphate adjuvant.

PNEUMOCOCCAL CONJUGATE VACCINE, 7-VALENT (PCV7) — INJECTION

For complete and comparative prescribing information, refer to the Agents for Active Immunization introduction.

Indications

➤*Prevention of otitis media:* Active immunization of infants and toddlers against otitis media caused by serotypes included in the vaccine.

➤*Prevention of S. pneumoniae invasive disease:* Active immunization of infants and toddlers against invasive disease caused by *S. pneumoniae* due to the capsular serotypes included in the vaccine (4, 6B, 9V, 14, 18C, 19F, and 23F).

PNEUMOCOCCAL CONJUGATE VACCINE, 7-VALENT (PCV7) — INJECTION

Administration and Dosage

➤*General dosing considerations:* Safety and immunogenicity data are limited or not available for children in specific high-risk groups for invasive pneumococcal disease (eg, individuals with sickle cell disease, asplenia, HIV infection).

➤*Children:*

Prevention of otitis media or S. pneumoniae invasive disease –

Routine vaccination schedule for children 15 months of age and younger: 3 doses of 0.5 mL each at approximately 2-month intervals, followed by a fourth dose of 0.5 mL at 12 to 15 months of age.

PCV7 Vaccination Schedule for Children (≤ 15 Months of Age)[a]				
Dose	Dose 1[b,c]	Dose 2[c]	Dose 3[c]	Dose 4[d]
Age at dose	2 months	4 months	6 months	12 to 15 months

[a] PCV7 = pneumococcal conjugate vaccine 7-valent.
[b] Dose 1 may be given as early as 6 weeks of age.
[c] The recommended dosing interval is 4 to 8 weeks.
[d] The fourth dose should be administered at ≈ 12 to 15 months of age and ≥ 2 months after the third dose.

Previously unvaccinated children (at least 7 months of age): For previously unvaccinated older infants and children who are older than the age of the routine infant schedule, the following schedule applies.

PCV7 Vaccination Schedule for Previously Unvaccinated Children (≥ 7 Months of Age)	
Age at first dose	Total number of 0.5 mL doses
7 to 11 months of age	3[a]
12 to 23 months of age	2[b]
≥ 24 months through 9 years of age	1

[a] Two doses ≥ 4 weeks apart; third dose after the 1-year birthday, separated from the second dose by ≥ 2 months.
[b] Two doses ≥ 2 months apart.

Catch-up immunization schedule: The following information is based on the Advisory Committee on Immunization Practices (ACIP) recommended immunization schedule.

• *Healthy children* – For all healthy children 24 to 59 months of age who have not received at least 1 dose of PCV7 at 12 months of age or older, administer 1 dose of PCV7.

• *Children with underlying medical conditions* – For all children 24 to 59 months of age with underlying medical conditions who have received 3 doses, administer 1 dose of PCV7.

For all children 24 to 59 months of age with underlying medical conditions who have received less than 3 doses, administer 2 doses of PCV7 at least 8 weeks apart.

➤*Preparation for administration:* Because this product is a suspension containing an adjuvant, shake vigorously immediately prior to use to obtain a uniform suspension in the vaccine container. Do not use the vaccine if it cannot be resuspended. After shaking, the vaccine appears as a homogeneous, white suspension.

➤*Administration:* Administer as one 0.5 mL intramuscular (IM) injection. Do not inject intravenously (IV).

The preferred sites of IM injection are the anterolateral aspect of the thigh in infants or the deltoid muscle of the upper arm in toddlers and young children. Do not inject the vaccine in the gluteal area or areas where there may be a major nerve trunk and/or blood vessel.

➤*Admixture compatibility:* The vaccine is not to be mixed with other vaccines/products in the same syringe.

➤*Storage/Stability:* Do not freeze. Store refrigerated, away from the freezer compartment, at 2° to 8°C (36° to 46°F).

Actions

➤*Pharmacology:* PCV7 is a sterile solution of saccharides of the capsular antigens of *S. pneumoniae* serotypes 4, 6B, 9V, 14, 18C, 19F, and 23F individually conjugated to diphtheria CRM_{197} protein.

Serotypes 4, 6B, 9V, 14, 18C, 19F, and 23F have been responsible for approximately 80% of invasive pneumococcal disease in children younger than 6 years of age in the United States. These 7 serotypes also accounted for 74% of penicillin-nonsusceptible *S. pneumoniae* and 100% of pneumococci with high-level penicillin resistance isolated from children younger than 6 years of age with invasive disease during a 1993 to 1994 surveillance by the Centers for Disease Control and Prevention.

Contraindications

Hypersensitivity to any component of the vaccine, including diphtheria toxoid.

Warnings/Precautions

➤*Protection:* This vaccine will not protect against *S. pneumoniae* disease caused by serotypes unrelated to those in the vaccine, nor will it protect against other microorganisms that cause invasive infections, such as bacteremia and meningitis, or noninvasive infections, such as otitis media. This vaccine is not intended to be used for the treatment of active infection.

Immunization with PCV7 does not substitute for routine diphtheria immunization.

➤*Bleeding disorders:* Do not give this vaccine to infants or children with thrombocytopenia or any coagulation disorder that would contraindicate IM injection unless the potential benefit clearly outweighs the risk of administration. If the decision is made to administer this vaccine to children with coagulation disorders, administer it with caution.

➤*Administration:* PCV7 is for IM use only. Do not administer IV under any circumstances. The safety and immunogenicity for other routes of administration (eg, subcutaneously) have not been evaluated.

➤*Postvaccination fever and febrile seizures:* Fever and, rarely, febrile seizures have been reported in children receiving PCV7. For children at higher risk of seizures than the general population, appropriate antipyretics (dosed according to respective prescribing information) may be administered around the time of vaccination to reduce the possibility of postvaccination fever.

➤*Febrile illness:* The decision to administer or delay vaccination because of current or recent febrile illness depends largely on the severity of the symptoms and their etiology. Postpone the administration of PCV7 in subjects suffering from acute severe febrile illness. Minor illnesses, such as mild respiratory infection with or without low-grade fever, are generally not contraindications to vaccination.

➤*Patient history:* Prior to administration of any dose of this vaccine, ask the parent or guardian about the personal history, family history, and recent health status of the vaccine recipient. Ascertain previous immunization history, current health status, and occurrence of any symptoms and/or signs of an adverse reaction after previous immunizations in the child to be immunized in order to determine the existence of any contraindication to immunization with this vaccine and to allow an assessment of the risk and benefits.

➤*Immunodeficiency:* Children with impaired immune responsiveness, whether caused by the use of immunosuppressive therapy (including irradiation, corticosteroids, antimetabolites, alkylating agents, and cytotoxic agents), a genetic defect, HIV infection, or other causes, may have reduced-antibody response to active immunization.

➤*Immunogenicity:* The immunogenicity of PCV7 has been investigated in an open-label, multicenter study in 49 infants with sickle cell disease. Children in France were vaccinated according to a primary immunization schedule with PCV7 (2, 3, and 4 months of age), and 46 of these children also received a 23-valent pneumococcal polysaccharide vaccine at the age of 15 to 18 months. After the third dose, the proportion of subjects in the per-protocol population (n = 26) with an antibody response at the 0.35 mcg/mL threshold ranged from 92.3% (95% confidence interval [CI], 74.9% to 99.1%) for serotype 6B to 100% (95% CI, 86.8% to 100%) for serotypes 4, 9V, and 14. At the 1 mcg/mL threshold after the third dose, the response ranged from 92.3% (95% CI, 74.9% to 99.1%) for serotypes 6B and 18C to 100% (95% CI, 86.8% to 100%) for serotype 4. After polysaccharide vaccination, the immunoglobulin G GMC to the 7 common serotypes ranged from 6.3 mcg/mL (95% CI, 4.94% to 8.03%) for serotype 18C to 29.71 mcg/mL (95% CI, 22.67% to 38.92%) for serotype 19F. According to the study protocol, no GMC data were obtained for the remaining 16 pneumococcal serotypes.

In a randomized study, 23 children 2 years of age and older with sickle cell disease were administered either 2 doses of PCV7 followed by a dose of polysaccharide vaccine or a single dose of polysaccharide vaccine alone. In this small study, safety and immune responses with the combined schedule were similar to polysaccharide vaccine alone. However, this study was too small to achieve statistically significant results.

➤*Hypersensitivity reactions:* Before the administration of any biological, take all precautions known for the prevention of allergic or any other adverse reaction. This includes a review of the patient's history regarding possible sensitivity, the ready availability of epinephrine 1:1,000 and other appropriate agents used for the control of immediate allergic reactions, and a knowledge of the recent literature pertaining to the use of the biological concerned, including the nature and possibility of adverse reactions that may follow its use.

➤*Special risk:* The use of PCV7 does not replace the use of 23-valent pneumococcal polysaccharide vaccination in children 24 months of age and older with sickle cell disease, asplenia, HIV infection, or chronic illness, or in those who are immunocompromised. Data on sequential vaccination with PCV7 followed by 23-valent pneumococcal polysaccharide vaccine are limited.

➤*Pregnancy:* *Category C.* Animal reproductive studies have not been conducted with this product. It is not known whether PCV7 can cause fetal harm when administered to a pregnant woman or whether it can affect reproductive capacity. PCV7 is not recommended for use in pregnant women.

➤*Lactation:* It is not known whether vaccine antigens or antibodies are excreted in breast milk. This vaccine is not recommended for use in breast-feeding mothers.

➤*Children:* PCV7 has been shown to be usually well-tolerated and immunogenic in infants. The safety and efficacy of PCV7 in children younger than 6 weeks of age or on or after the 10th birthday have not been established. Immune responses elicited by PCV7 among infants born prematurely have not been adequately studied.

PNEUMOCOCCAL CONJUGATE VACCINE, 7-VALENT (PCV7) — INJECTION

➤*Elderly:* This vaccine is not recommended for use in adult populations. Do not use as a substitute for the pneumococcal polysaccharide vaccine in elderly populations.

Drug Interactions

PCV7 Drug Interactions

Precipitant drug	Object drug[a]		Description
Immunosuppressants (eg, alkylating agents, antimetabolites, large doses of corticosteroids, cytotoxic agents)	PCV7	⬇	Response to PCV7 may not be optimal.
PCV7	Anticoagulants (eg, warfarin)	⬆	Risk of bleeding may be increased. Use with caution.
PCV7	Haemophilus b conjugate vaccine (HbOC)	⬆⬇	After 3 doses of HbOC, antibody levels to *H. influenza* type b were higher when PCV7 was administered than when HbOC was given alone. After 4 doses, antibody levels were lower when HbOC was given with PCV7. However, more than 97% of children receiving HbOC with PCV7 achieved serum antibody levels of 1 mcg/mL or more.
PCV7	Pertussis	⟷	Some inconsistent differences in response to pertussis antigen were observed; however, the clinical relevance is unknown.

[a] ⬆ = object drug increased; ⬇ = object drug decreased; ⬆⬇ = object drug both increased and decreased; ⟷ = undetermined clinical effect.

Adverse Reactions

Overall, the safety of PCV7 was evaluated in a total of 5 clinical studies in the United States in which 18,168 infants and children received 58,699 doses of vaccine at 2, 4, 6, and 12 to 15 months of age. In addition, the safety of PCV7 was evaluated in 831 Finnish infants using the same schedule, and the overall safety profile was similar to that of infants in the United States. The safety of PCV7 was also evaluated in 560 children from 4 ancillary studies in the United States who started immunization at 7 months to 9 years of age.

➤*Systemic:*

PCV7 Adverse Reactions Within 2 or 3 Days of Administration to Infants as a Primary Series at 2, 4, and 6 Months of Age (US Studies)

Adverse reactions	PCV7 concurrently with DTaP[a] and HbOC (3,848 doses)[b]	DTaP and HbOC control (538 doses)[c]
CNS		
Drowsiness	32.9%	27.7%
Irritability	52.5%	45.2%
Restless sleep	20.6%	22.3%
GI		
Decreased appetite	18.1%	13.6%
Diarrhea	9.8%	4.4%
Vomiting	13.4%	9.8%
Miscellaneous		
Fever ≥ 38°C (100.4°F)	21.1%	14.2%
Fever > 39°C (102.2°F)	1.8%	0.4%
Urticaria-like rash	0.6%	0.3%

[a] DTaP = diphtheria, tetanus toxoids, and acellular pertussis.
[b] Total from which reaction data are available varies between reactions from 3,121 to 3,848 doses. Data from studies 118-8, 118-12, and 118-16.
[c] Total from which reaction data are available varies between reactions from 295 to 538 doses. Data from studies 118-12 and 118-16.

PCV7 Systemic Adverse Reactions Within 2 or 3 Days of Administration to Toddlers as a Fourth Dose at 12 to 15 Months of Age (US Studies)

Adverse reactions	PCV7 concurrently with DTaP and HbOC (270 doses)[a]	PCV7 only (727 doses)[b]
CNS		
Drowsiness	17.5%	15.9%
Irritability	45.9%	45.8%
Restless sleep	21.2%	21.2%
GI		
Decreased appetite	21.1%	18.3%
Diarrhea	13.7%	12.8%
Vomiting	5.6%	6.3%
Miscellaneous		
Fever ≥ 38°C (100.4°F)	19.6%	13.4%
Fever > 39°C (102.2°F)	1.5%	1.2%
Urticaria-like rash	0.7%	1.2%

[a] Total from which reaction data are available varies between reactions from 269 to 270 doses. Data from studies 118-7 and 118-8.
[b] Total from which reaction data are available varies between reactions from 725 to 727 doses. Data from studies 118-7 and 118-8.

PCV7 Systemic Adverse Reactions Within 2 Days of Coadministration with DTaP at 2, 4, 6, and 12 to 15 Months of Age[a,b]

Adverse reactions	Dose 1 PCV7 (n = 710)	Dose 1 Control[b] (n = 711)	Dose 2 PCV7 (n = 559)	Dose 2 Control[b] (n = 508)	Dose 3 PCV7 (n = 461)	Dose 3 Control[b] (n = 414)	Dose 4[c] PCV7 (n = 224)	Dose 4[c] Control[b] (n = 230)
CNS								
Drowsiness	40.7%	42%	25.6%	22.8%	19.5%	21.9%	17%	16.5%
Irritability	48%	48.2%	58.7%	45.3%[d]	51.2%	44.8%	44.2%	42.6%
Restless sleep	15.3%	15.1%	20.2%	19.3%	25.2%	19%[d]	20.2%	19.1%
GI								
Decreased appetite	17%	13.5%	17.4%	13.4%	20.7%	13.8%[d]	20.5%	23.1%
Diarrhea	11.9%	8.4%[d]	10.2%	9.3%	8.3%	9.4%	11.6%	9.2%
Vomiting	14.6%	14.5%	16.8%	14.4%	10.4%	11.6%	4.9%	4.8%
Miscellaneous								
Fever ≥ 38°C (100.4°F)	15.1%	9.4%[d]	23.9%	10.8%[d]	19.1%	11.8%[d]	21%	17%
Fever > 39°C (102.2°F)	0.9%	0.3%	2.5%	0.8%[d]	1.7%	0.7%	1.3%	1.7%
Urticaria-like rash	1.4%	0.3%[d]	1.3%	1.4%	0.4%	0.5%	0.5%	1.7%

[a] Approximately 75% of subjects received prophylactic or therapeutic antipyretics within 48 hours of each dose.
[b] Investigational MnCC vaccine.
[c] Most of these children had received DTP for the primary series; therefore, this is a fourth dose of a pertussis vaccine, but not of DTaP.
[d] $P < 0.05$ when PCV7 compared with control group using a chi-square test.

PNEUMOCOCCAL CONJUGATE VACCINE, 7-VALENT (PCV7) — INJECTION

PCV7 Systemic Adverse Reactions Within 3 Days of Immunization to Previously Unvaccinated Children (7 months through 9 Years of Age)

Age at first vaccination	7 to 11 months of age						12 to 23 months of age			24 to 35 months of age	36 to 59 months of age	5 to 9 years of age
Study number	118-12			118-16			118-9[a]	118-18		118-18	118-18	118-18
Dose number	1	2	3[b]	1	2	3[b]	1	1	2	1	1	1
Number of subjects	54	51	24	85	80	50	60	120	117	47	52	100
Adverse reactions												
CNS												
Drowsiness	11.1%	17.6%	16.7%	24.7%	16.3%	14%	13.3%	18.3%	11.1%	12.8%	17.3%	11%
Fussiness	29.6%	39.2%	16.7%	54.1%	41.3%	38%	40%	37.5%	36.8%	46.8%	34.6%	29.3%
GI												
Decreased appetite	9.3%	15.7%	0%	15.3%	15%	30%	25%	20.8%	16.2%	23.4%	11.5%	9%
Miscellaneous												
Fever ≥ 38°C (100.4°F)	20.8%	21.6%	25%	17.6%	18.8%	22%	36.7%	11.7%	6.8%	14.9%	11.5%	7%
Fever > 39°C (102.2°F)	1.9%	5.9%	0%	1.6%	3.9%	2.6%	0%	4.4%	0%	4.2%	2.3%	1.2%

[a] For study 118-9, 2 of 60 subjects were ≥ 24 months of age.

[b] For study 118-12, dose 3 was administered at 15 to 18 months of age. For study 118-16, dose 3 was administered at 12 to 15 months of age.

Fever – Fever (38°C [100.4°F] or higher) within 48 hours of a vaccine dose was reported by a greater proportion of subjects who received PCV7 compared with control (investigational MnCC vaccine) after each dose when coadministered with DTP-HbOC or DTaP in the efficacy study. In the Manufacturing Bridging Study, fever within 48 to 72 hours was also more commonly reported after each dose compared with infants in the control group who received only the recommended vaccines. When coadministered with DTaP in either study, fever rates among PCV7 recipients ranged from 15% to 34% and were greatest after the second dose.

➤*Local:* With vaccines in general, including PCV7, it is not uncommon for patients to note within 48 to 72 hours the following minor reactions at or around the injection site: edema; pain or tenderness; inflammation, redness, or skin discoloration; mass; local hypersensitivity reaction. Such local reactions are usually self-limited and require no therapy.

As with other aluminum-containing vaccines, a nodule may occasionally be palpable at the injection site for several weeks.

PCV7 Local Adverse Reactions Within 2 Days of Immunization at 2, 4, 6, and 12 to 15 Months of Age

Adverse reactions	Dose 1: PCV7 site[a] (n = 693)	Dose 1: DTaP[b] site (n = 693	Dose 2: PCV7[a] site (n = 526)	Dose 2: DTaP[b] site (n = 526)	Dose 3: PCV7[a] site (n = 422)	Dose 3: DTaP[b] site (n = 422)	Dose 4: PCV7[a] site (n = 165)	Dose 4: DTaP[b] site[c] (n = 165)
Erythema								
Any	10%	6.7%[d]	11.6%	10.5%	13.8%	11.4%	10.9%	3.6%[d]
2.4 cm	1.3%	0.4%[d]	0.6%	0.6%	1.4%	1%	3.6%	0.6%
Induration								
Any	9.8%	6.6%[d]	12%	10.5%	10.4%	10.4%	12.1%	5.5%[d]
2.4 cm	1.6%	0.9%	1.3%	1.7%	2.4%	1.9%	5.5%	1.8%
Tenderness								
Any	17.9%	16%	19.4%	17.3%	14.7%	13.1%	23.3%	18.4%
Interfered with limb movement	3.1%	1.8%[d]	4.1%	3.3%	2.9%	1.9%	9.2%	8%

[a] HbOC was administered in the same limb as PCV7. If reactions occurred at either or both sites on that limb, the more severe reaction was recorded.

[b] If hep B vaccine was administered simultaneously, it was administered into the same limb as DTaP. If reactions occurred at either or both sites on that limb, the more severe reaction was recorded.

[c] Subjects may have received DTP or a mixed DTP/DTaP regimen for the primary series; thus, this is the fourth dose of a pertussis vaccine, but not a fourth dose of DTaP.

[d] $P < 0.05$ when PCV7 was compared with DTaP site using the sign test.

PCV7 Local Adverse Reactions Within 3 Days of Immunization of Previously Unvaccinated Children (7 Months through 9 Years of Age)

Age at first vaccination	7 to 11 months of age						12 to 23 months of age			24 to 35 months of age	36 to 59 months of age	5 to 9 years of age
Study number	118-12			118-16			118-9[a]	118-18		118-18	118-18	118-18
Dose number	1	2	3[b]	1	2	3[b]	1	1	2	1	1	1
Number of subjects	54	51	24	81	76	50	60	114	117	46	48	49
Adverse reactions												
Erythema												
Any	16.7%	11.8%	20.8%	7.4%	7.9%	14%	48.3%	10.5%	9.4%	6.5%	29.2%	24.2%
> 2.4 cm[c]	1.9%	0%	0%	0%	0%	0%	6.7%	1.8%	1.7%	0%	8.3%	7.1%
Induration												
Any	16.7%	11.8%	8.3%	7.4%	3.9%	10%	48.3%	8.8%	6%	10.9%	22.9%	25.5%
> 2.4 cm[c]	3.7%	0%	0%	0%	0%	0%	3.3%	0.9%	0.9%	2.2%	6.3%	9.3%
Tenderness												
Any	13%	11.8%	12.5%	8.6%	10.5%	12%	46.7%	25.7%	26.5%	41.3%	58.3%	82.8%
Interfered with limb movement	1.9%	2%	4.2%	1.2%	1.3%	0%	3.3%	6.2%	8.5%	13%	20.8%	39.4%

[a] For study 118-9, 2 of 60 subjects were ≥ 24 months.

[b] For study 118-12, dose 3 was administered at 15 to 18 months of age. For study 118-16, dose 3 was administered at 12 to 15 months of age.

[c] For study 118-16 and 118-18, ≥ 2 cm.

PNEUMOCOCCAL CONJUGATE VACCINE, 7-VALENT (PCV7) — INJECTION

➤*CNS:* In the Kaiser efficacy study in which 17,066 children received a total of 55,352 doses of PCV7 and 17,080 children received a total of 55,387 doses of the control vaccine (investigational MnCC), seizures were reported in 8 PCV7 recipients and 4 control vaccine recipients within 3 days of immunization from October 1995 through April 1998. Of the 8 PCV7 recipients, 7 received concomitant DTP-containing vaccines and 1 received DTaP. Of the 4 control vaccine recipients, 3 received concomitant DTP-containing vaccines and 1 received DTaP. In the other 4 studies combined in which 1,102 children were immunized with 3,347 doses of PCV7 and 408 children were immunized with 1,310 doses of control vaccine (either investigational MnCC or concurrent vaccines), there was 1 seizure reported within 3 days of immunization. This subject received PCV7 concurrently with DTaP vaccine.

➤*Dermatologic:* In the large-scale efficacy study, urticaria-like rash was reported in 0.4% to 1.4% of children within 48 hours of immunization with PCV7 coadministered with other routine childhood vaccines. Urticaria-like rash was reported in 1.3% to 6% of children within 3 to 14 days of immunization and was most often reported following the fourth dose when it was coadministered with measles, mumps, and rubella (MMR) vaccine. Based on limited data, it appears that children with urticaria-like rash after a dose of PCV7 may be more likely to report urticaria-like rash following a subsequent dose of PCV7.

➤*Miscellaneous:* Of the 17,066 subjects who received at least 1 dose of PCV7 in the efficacy trial, there were 24 hospitalizations (for 29 diagnoses) within 3 days of a dose from October 1995 through April 1998. Diagnoses were as follows: bronchiolitis (5); congenital anomaly (4); elective procedure, urinary tract infection (3 each); acute gastroenteritis, asthma, pneumonia (2 each); aspiration, breath-holding, febrile seizure, influenza, inguinal hernia repair, otitis media, viral syndrome, well child/reassurance (1 each). There were 162 visits to the emergency room (for 182 diagnoses) within 3 days of a dose from October 1995 through April 1998. Diagnoses were as follows: febrile illness (20); acute gastroenteritis (19); trauma, upper respiratory tract infection (16 each); otitis media (15); well child (13); irritable child, viral syndrome (10 each); rash (8); croup, pneumonia (6 each); poisoning/ingestion (5); asthma, bronchiolitis (4 each); febrile seizure, urinary tract infection (3 each); breath-holding, choking, conjunctivitis, inguinal hernia repair, pharyngitis, thrush, wheezing (2 each); colic, colitis, congestive heart failure, elective procedure, hives, influenza, ingrown toenail, local swelling, roseola, sepsis (1 each).

In a review of all hospitalizations that occurred between October 1995 and August 1999 in the efficacy study for the specific diagnoses of aplastic anemia, autoimmune disease, autoimmune hemolytic anemia, diabetes mellitus, neutropenia, and thrombocytopenia, the numbers of cases were equal to or less than the expected numbers based on the 1995 Kaiser Vaccine Safety Datalink (VSD) data set.

Hypotonic-hyporesponsive episode – One case of a hypotonic-hyporesponsive episode was reported in the efficacy study following PCV7 and concurrent DTP vaccines in the study period from October 1995 through April 1998. Two additional cases of hypotonic-hyporesponsive episode were reported in 4 other studies, and these also occurred in children who received PCV7 concurrently with DTP vaccine.

Sudden infant death syndrome – Twelve deaths (5 from sudden infant death syndrome [SIDS] and 7 with clear alternative cause) occurred among subjects receiving PCV7, of which 11 (4 SIDS and 7 with clear alternative cause) occurred in the Kaiser efficacy study from October 1995 until April 20, 1999. In comparison, 21 deaths (8 SIDS, 12 with clear alternative cause, and 1 SIDS-like death in an older child) occurred in the control vaccine group during the same time period. The number of SIDS deaths in the efficacy study from October 1995 until April 20, 1999, was similar to or lower than the age and season-adjusted expected rate from the California state data from 1995 to 1997 and are presented in the following table.

Age and Season-Adjusted Comparison of SIDS Rates in PCV7 Study (NCKP Efficacy Trial) With the Expected Rate From the California State Data for 1995 to 1997[a]

Vaccine	< 1 week after immunization		≤ 2 weeks after immunization		≤ 1 month after immunization		≤ 1 year after immunization	
	Exp	Obs	Exp	Obs	Exp	Obs	Exp	Obs
PCV7	1.06	1	2.09	2	4.28	2	8.08	4
Control[b]	1.06	2	2.09	3[c]	4.28	3[c]	8.08	8[c]

[a] Exp = expected; Obs = observed.
[b] Investigational MnCC vaccine.
[c] Does not include 1 additional case of SIDS-like death in a child older than the usual SIDS age (448 days).

➤*Postmarketing:*

Hypersensitivity – Anaphylactic/anaphylactoid reaction including shock; hypersensitivity reaction including bronchospasm, dyspnea, face edema.

Local – Injection-site dermatitis, injection-site pruritus, injection-site urticaria.

Miscellaneous – Angioneurotic edema, apnea, crying, erythema multiforme, lymphadenopathy localized to the region of the injection site.

The primary safety outcomes analyses did not demonstrate a consistently elevated risk of health care utilization for allergic reactions, breath-holding, croup, gastroenteritis, seizures, or wheezing diagnoses across doses, health care settings, or multiple time windows. As in prelicensure trials, fever was associated with PCV7 administration. In analyses of secondary safety outcomes, the adjusted relative risk of hospitalization for reactive airways disease was 1.23 (95% CI, 1.11 to 1.35). Potential confounders (eg, differences in coadministered vaccines, yearly variation in respiratory infections, secular trends in reactive airways disease incidence) could not be controlled. Extended follow-up of subjects originally enrolled in the NCKP efficacy trial revealed no increased risk of reactive airways disease among PCV7 recipients. In general, the study results support the previously described safety profile of PCV7.

Overdosage

➤*Symptoms:* There have been reports of overdose with PCV7, including cases of the administration of a higher than recommended dose and cases of subsequent doses administered closer than recommended to the previous dose. Most individuals were asymptomatic. In general, adverse reactions reported with overdose have also been reported with recommended single doses of PCV7.

Patient Information

Prior to the administration of this vaccine, inform the parent, guardian, or other responsible adult of the potential benefits and risks to the patient and the importance of completing the immunization series, unless contraindicated. Instruct parents or guardians to report any suspected adverse reactions to their health care provider. Provide vaccine information prior to each vaccination.

PNEUMOCOCCAL CONJUGATE VACCINE, 13-VALENT (PCV13) — INJECTION

For complete and comparative prescribing information, refer to the Agents for Active Immunization introduction.

Indications

➤*Prevention of otitis media:* For active immunization of children 6 weeks through 5 years of age (prior to the 6th birthday) against otitis media caused by *Streptococcus pneumoniae* serotypes included in the vaccine (4, 6B, 9V, 14, 18C, 19F, and 23F).

➤*Prevention of S. pneumoniae invasive disease:* For active immunization in children 6 weeks through 5 years of age (prior to the 6th birthday) for the prevention of invasive disease caused by *S. pneumoniae* serotypes included in the vaccine (1, 3, 4, 5, 6A, 6B, 7F, 9V, 14, 18C, 19A, 19F, and 23F).

Administration and Dosage

➤*Children:*

Prevention of otitis media or S. pneumoniae invasive disease –

Routine vaccination schedule for children 15 months of age and younger: Administer as 0.5 mL/dose for a total of 4 doses at 2, 4, 6, and 12 to 15 months of age.

PCV13 Schedule for Infants and Toddlers[a]

Dose	Dose 1[b,c]	Dose 2[c]	Dose 3[c]	Dose 4[d]
Age at dose	2 months	4 months	6 months	12 to 15 months

[a] PCV13 = pneumococcal conjugate vaccine 13-valent (*Prevnar 13*).
[b] Dose 1 may be given as early as 6 weeks of age.
[c] The recommended dosing interval is 4 to 8 weeks.
[d] Dose 4 should be administered at ≈ 12 to 15 months of age and ≥ 2 months after dose 3.

Previously unvaccinated children (at least 7 months of age): For children who are beyond the age of the routine infant schedule and have not received *Prevnar* (PCV7) or *Prevnar 13* (PCV13), the following catch-up schedule applies:

PCV13 Schedule for Unvaccinated Children ≥ 7 Months of Age

Age at first dose	Total number of 0.5 mL doses
7 to 11 months	3[a]
12 to 23 months	2[b]
24 months through 5 years (prior to the 6th birthday)	1

[a] The first 2 doses ≥ 4 weeks apart; third dose after the 1-year birthday, separated from the second dose by ≥ 2 months.
[b] Two doses ≥ 2 months apart.

PCV13 schedule for children previously vaccinated with PCV7:

- *Children who previously received 1 or more doses* – Children who have received 1 or more doses of PCV7 may complete the 4-dose immunization series with PCV13.
- *Children 15 months through 5 years of age who have previously received 4 doses* – Children 15 months through 5 years of age who have received 4 doses of PCV7 may receive 1 dose of PCV13 to elicit immune responses to the 6 additional serotypes. The immune responses induced by this PCV13 transition schedule may result in lower antibody concentrations for the 6 additional serotypes (types 1, 3, 5, 6A, 7F, and 19A), compared with antibody concentrations following 4 doses of PCV13 (given at 2, 4, 6, and 12 to 15 months of age). The clinical relevance of these lower antibody responses is not known.

PNEUMOCOCCAL CONJUGATE VACCINE, 13-VALENT (PCV13) — INJECTION

➤*Preparation for administration:* Because this product is a suspension containing an adjuvant, shake vigorously immediately prior to use to obtain a homogenous, white suspension in the vaccine container. Do not use the vaccine if it cannot be resuspended.

➤*Administration:* For intramuscular (IM) injection only. Do not inject intravenously, intradermally, or subcutaneously.

Each 0.5 mL dose is to be injected IM. The preferred sites for injection are the anterolateral aspect of the thigh in infants or the deltoid muscle of the upper arm in toddlers and young children. The vaccine should not be injected in the gluteal area or areas where there may be a major nerve trunk and/or blood vessel.

➤*Admixture compatibility:* Do not mix with other vaccines/products in the same syringe.

➤*Storage/Stability:* Store refrigerated at 2° to 8°C (36° to 46°F). Do not freeze. Discard if the vaccine has been frozen.

The vial stopper and the tip cap and rubber plunger of the prefilled syringe do not contain latex.

Actions

➤*Pharmacology:* B cells produce antibodies in response to antigenic stimulation via T-dependent and T-independent mechanisms. PCV13, comprised of polysaccharides conjugated to a carrier protein, elicits a T-cell dependent immune response. Protein carrier-specific T cells provide the signals needed for maturation of the B-cell response and generation of B-cell memory. This type of response induces immune memory and elicits booster responses on re-exposure in infants and young children to pneumococcal polysaccharides.

Contraindications

Severe allergic reaction (eg, anaphylaxis) to any component of PVC13, PCV7, or any diphtheria toxoid-containing vaccine.

Warnings/Precautions

➤*Protection:* PCV13 may not protect all individuals receiving the vaccine. PCV13 will not protect against *S. pneumoniae* serotypes that are not in the vaccine or serotypes unrelated to those in the vaccine. It will also not protect against other microorganisms. This vaccine does not treat active infection.

Protection against otitis media is expected to be substantially lower than protection against invasive disease. In addition, because otitis media is caused by many organisms other than the 7 serotypes of *S. pneumoniae* included in the indication, protection against all causes of otitis media is expected to be lower than for pneumococcal otitis media caused by these 7 vaccine serotypes.

The duration of protection from immunization is not known.

➤*Immunodeficiency:* Data on the safety and effectiveness of PCV13 when administered to children in specific groups at higher risk for invasive pneumococcal disease (eg, children with congenital or acquired splenic dysfunction, HIV infection, malignancy, nephrotic syndrome) are not available.

Children in these groups may have reduced antibody response to active immunization due to impaired immune responsiveness. Consider vaccination in high-risk groups on an individual basis.

The use of pneumococcal conjugate vaccine does not replace the use of 23-valent pneumococcal polysaccharide vaccine (PPV23) in children at least 24 months of age with sickle cell disease, asplenia, HIV infection, or chronic illness, or who are otherwise immunocompromised.

➤*Premature infants:* Apnea following IM vaccination has been observed in some infants born prematurely. Base decisions about when to administer an IM vaccine, including PCV13, to infants born prematurely on consideration of the individual infant's medical status and the potential benefits and possible risks of vaccination.

➤*Hypersensitivity reactions:* Before administration of any dose, take all precautions to prevent allergic or any other adverse reactions. This includes a review of the patient immunization history for possible sensitivity to the vaccine or similar vaccines and for previous vaccination-related adverse reactions in order to determine the existence of any contraindication to immunization with PCV13 and to allow an assessment of risks and benefits. Epinephrine and other appropriate agents used for the control of immediate allergic reactions must be immediately available if an acute anaphylactic reaction occurs following the administration of the vaccine.

➤*Pregnancy: Category C.* Animal reproduction studies have not been conducted with PCV13. It is also not known whether PCV13 can cause fetal harm when administered to a pregnant woman or whether it can affect reproductive capacity.

➤*Lactation:* It is not known whether vaccine antigens or antibodies are excreted in breast milk. This vaccine is not recommended for use in breastfeeding mothers.

➤*Children:* Safety and effectiveness of PCV13 in children younger than 6 weeks of age or on or after the 6th birthday have not been established. PCV13 is not approved for use in children in these age groups.

Immune responses elicited by PCV13 among infants born prematurely have not been specifically studied.

➤*Elderly:* The safety and effectiveness of PCV13 in elderly populations have not been established. PCV13 is not to be used as a substitute for PPV23 in elderly populations.

Drug Interactions

When administering PCV13 at the same time as another injectable vaccine(s), always administer the vaccines with different syringes and at different injection sites. Do not mix PCV13 with other vaccines/products in the same syringe.

➤*Concomitant immunizations:* In children receiving PCV13, immune responses to concomitant vaccine antigens were comparable with those responses in children receiving PCV7. Responses to diphtheria toxoid, haemophilus B conjugate, hepatitis B, measles, mumps, pertussis, polio types 1, 2, and 3, rubella, tetanus toxoid, and varicella antigens in PCV13 recipients were similar to PCV7 recipients.

➤*Immunosuppressants (eg, alkylating agents, antimetabolites, large doses of corticosteroids, cytotoxic agents):* Children with impaired immune responsiveness due to the use of immunosuppressive agents may not respond optimally to PCV13.

Adverse Reactions

The safety of PCV13 was evaluated in 13 clinical trials in which 4,729 infants and toddlers received at least 1 dose of PCV13 and 2,760 infants and toddlers received at least 1 dose of PCV7 active control. Safety data for the first 3 doses are available for all 13 infant studies; dose 4 data are available for 10 studies; and data for the 6-month follow-up are available for 7 studies. The vaccination schedule and concomitant vaccinations used in these infant trials were consistent with country-specific recommendations and local clinical practice. There were no substantive differences in demographic characteristics between the vaccine groups. By race, 84% of subjects were white, 6% were black, 5.8% were Asian, and 3.8% were of other race (most of these being biracial). Overall, 52.3% of subjects were male infants.

Three studies in the United States evaluated the safety of PCV13 when coadministered with routine US pediatric vaccinations at 2, 4, 6, and 12 to 15 months of age. Solicited local and systemic adverse reactions were recorded daily by parents/guardians using an electronic diary for 7 consecutive days following each vaccination. For unsolicited adverse reactions, study subjects were monitored from administration of the first dose until 1 month after the infant series and for 1 month after the administration of the toddler dose. Information regarding unsolicited and serious adverse reactions, newly diagnosed chronic medical conditions, and hospitalizations since the last visit were collected during the clinic visit for the fourth-study dose and during a scripted telephone interview 6 months after the fourth-study dose. Serious adverse reactions were also collected throughout the study period. Overall, the safety data show a similar proportion of PCV13 and PCV7 subjects reporting serious adverse reactions. Among US study subjects, a similar proportion of PCV13 and PCV7 recipients reported solicited local and systemic adverse reactions as well as unsolicited adverse reactions.

➤*Serious adverse reactions:* Serious adverse reactions were collected throughout the study period for all 13 clinical trials. This reporting period is longer than the 30-day postvaccination period used in some vaccine trials. The longer reporting may have resulted in serious adverse reactions being reported in a higher percentage of subjects than for other vaccines. Serious adverse reactions reported following vaccination in infants and toddlers occurred in 8.2% among PCV13 recipients and 7.2% among PCV7 recipients. Serious adverse reactions observed during different study periods for PCV13 and PCV7, respectively, were as follows: 3.7% and 3.5% from dose 1 to the bleed after the infant series; 3.6% and 2.7% from the bleed after the infant series to the toddler dose; 0.9% and 0.8% from the toddler dose to the bleed after the toddler dose; and 2.5% and 2.8% during the 6-month follow-up period after the last dose.

The most commonly reported serious adverse reactions were in the infections and infestations system organ class, including bronchiolitis (0.9%, 1.1%), gastroenteritis, (0.9%, 0.9%), and pneumonia (0.9%, 0.5%) for PCV13 and PCV7, respectively.

There were 3 (0.063%) deaths among PCV13 recipients and 1 (0.036%) death in PCV7 recipients, all as a result of sudden infant death syndrome (SIDS). These SIDS rates are consistent with published age-specific background rates of SIDS from the year 2000.

PNEUMOCOCCAL CONJUGATE VACCINE, 13-VALENT (PCV13) — INJECTION

➤*Solicited adverse reactions in the 3 US infant and toddler studies:*

Local –

PCV13 and PCV7 Local Reactions at the Injection Sites Within 7 Days After Each Vaccination[a]

Adverse reactions	Dose 1		Dose 2		Dose 3		Dose 4	
	PCV13 (n[b] = 1,375 to 1,612)	PCV7 (n[b] = 516 to 606)	PCV13 (n[b] = 1,069 to 1,331)	PCV7 (n[b] = 405 to 510)	PCV13 (n[b] = 998 to 1,206)	PCV7 (n[b] = 348 to 446)	PCV13 (n[b] = 874 to 1,060)	PCV7 (n[b] = 283 to 379)
Redness[c]								
Any	24.3%	26%	33.3%	29.7%	37.1%	36.6%	42.3%	45.5%
Mild	23.1%	25.2%	31.9%	28.7%	35.3%	35.3%	39.5%	42.7%
Moderate	2.2%	1.5%	2.7%	2.2%	4.6%	5.1%	9.6%	13.4%[d]
Severe	0%	0%	0%	0%	0%	0%	0%	0%
Swelling[c]								
Any	20.1%	20.7%	25.2%	22.5%	26.8%	28.4%	31.6%	36%[d]
Mild	17.2%	18.7%	23.8%	20.5%	25.2%	27.5%	29.4%	33.8%
Moderate	4.9%	3.9%	3.7%	4.9%	3.8%	5.8%	8.3%	11.2%[d]
Severe	0%	0%	0.1%	0%	0%	0%	0%	0%
Tenderness								
Any	62.5%	64.5%	64.7%	62.9%	59.2%	60.8%	57.8%	62.5%
Interferes with limb movement	10.4%	9.6%	9%	10.5%	8.4%	9%	6.9%	5.7%

[a] Data are from 3 primary US safety studies (the US phase 2 infant study, the pivotal US noninferiority study, and the US consistency study). All infants received concomitant routine infant immunizations. Concomitant vaccines and pneumococcal conjugate vaccines were administered in different limbs.

[b] Number of patients reporting "Yes" for at least 1 day or "No" for all days.

[c] Diameters were measured in caliper units of whole numbers from 1 to 14 or 14+. One caliper unit = 0.5 cm. Measurements were rounded up to the nearest whole number. Intensity of induration and erythema were then characterized as mild (0.5 to 2 cm), moderate (2.5 to 7 cm), or severe (> 7 cm).

[d] Statistically significant difference $P < 0.05$.

Systemic –

PCV13 and PCV7 Systemic Adverse Reactions Within 7 Days After Each Vaccination[a,b]

Adverse reactions	Dose 1		Dose 2		Dose 3		Dose 4	
	PCV13 (n[a] = 1,360 to 1,707)	PCV7 (n[a] = 497 to 640)	PCV13 (n[a] = 1,084 to 1,469)	PCV7 (n[a] = 409 to 555)	PCV13 (n[a] = 997 to 1,361)	PCV7 (n[a] = 354 to 521)	PCV13 (n[a] = 850 to 1,227)	PCV7 (n[a] = 278 to 436)
Fever[c]								
Any	24.3%	22.1%	36.5%	32.8%	30.3%	31.6%	31.9%	30.6%
Mild	23.6%	21.7%	34.9%	31.6%	29.1%	30.2%	30.3%	30%
Moderate	1.1%	0.6%	3.4%	2.8%	4.2%	3.3%	4.4%	4.6%
Severe	0.1%	0.2%	0.1%	0.3%	0.1%	0.7%	1%	0%
Decreased appetite	48.3%	43.6%	47.8%	43.6%	47.6%	47.6%	51%	49.4%
Irritability	85.6%	83.6%	84.8%	80.4%	79.8%	80.8%	80.4%	77.8%
Increased sleep	71.5%	71.5%	66.6%	63.4%	57.7%	55.2%	48.7%	55.1%
Decreased sleep	42.5%	40.6%	45.6%	43.7%	46.5%	47.7%	45.3%	40.3%

[a] Number of patients reporting "Yes" for at least 1 day or "No" for all days.

[b] Data are from 3 primary US safety studies (the US phase 2 infant study, the pivotal US noninferiority study, and the US consistency study). All infants received concomitant routine infant immunizations. Concomitant vaccines and pneumococcal conjugate vaccines were administered in different limbs.

[c] Fever gradings: mild (≥ 38°C but ≤ 39°C), moderate (> 39°C but ≤ 40°C), and severe (> 40°C). No other systemic reaction other than fever was graded. Parents reported the use of antipyretic medication to treat or prevent symptoms in 62% to 75% of subjects after any of the 4 doses. There were no statistical differences between the PCV13 and PCV7 groups.

➤*Unsolicited adverse reactions in the 3 US infant and toddler safety studies:* The following were determined to be adverse drug reactions based on experience with PCV13 in clinical trials:

Reactions occurring in greater than 1% of infants and toddlers: diarrhea, vomiting, and rash.

Reactions occurring in less than 1% of infants and toddlers: crying, hypersensitivity reaction (including face edema, dyspnea, and bronchospasm), seizures (including febrile seizures), and urticaria or urticaria-like rash.

➤*Safety assessments in the catch-up studies:*

Local –

Local Adverse Reactions Within 4 Days After Each Catch-Up PCV13 Vaccination[a]

Adverse reactions	7 through 11 months			12 through 23 months		24 months through 5 years
	Dose 1 (n[b] = 86)	Dose 2 (n[b] = 86 to 87)	Dose 3 (n[b] = 78 to 82)	Dose 1 (n[b] = 108 to 110)	Dose 2 (n[b] = 98 to 106)	Dose 1 (n[b] = 147 to 149)
Redness[c]						
Any	48.8%	46%	37.8%	70%	54.7%	50%
Mild	41.9%	40.2%	31.3%	55.5%	44.7%	37.4%
Moderate	16.3%	9.3%	12.5%	38.2%	25.5%	25.7%
Severe	0%	0%	0%	0%	0%	0%

Local Adverse Reactions Within 4 Days After Each Catch-Up PCV13 Vaccination[a]

Adverse reactions	7 through 11 months			12 through 23 months		24 months through 5 years
	Dose 1 (n[b] = 86)	Dose 2 (n[b] = 86 to 87)	Dose 3 (n[b] = 78 to 82)	Dose 1 (n[b] = 108 to 110)	Dose 2 (n[b] = 98 to 106)	Dose 1 (n[b] = 147 to 149)
Swelling[c]						
Any	36%	32.2%	25%	44.5%	41%	36.9%
Mild	32.6%	28.7%	20.5%	36.7%	36.2%	28.2%
Moderate	11.6%	14%	11.3%	24.8%	12.1%	20.3%
Severe	0%	0%	0%	0%	0%	0%
Tenderness						
Any	15.1%	15.1%	15.2%	33.3%	43.7%	42.3%
Interferes with limb movement	1.2%	3.5%	6.4%	0%	4.1%	4.1%

[a] Study conducted in Poland.

[b] Number of patients reporting "Yes" for at least 1 day or "No" for all days.

[c] Diameters were measured in caliper units of whole numbers from 1 to 14 or 14+. One caliper unit = 0.5 cm. Measurements were rounded up to the nearest whole number. Intensity of redness and swelling were then characterized as mild (0.5 to 2 cm), moderate (2.5 to 7 cm), or severe (> 7 cm).

PNEUMOCOCCAL CONJUGATE VACCINE, 13-VALENT (PCV13) — INJECTION

Systemic –

Systemic Adverse Reactions Within 4 Days After Each Catch-Up PCV13 Vaccination[a]						
	7 through 11 months			12 through 23 months		24 months through 5 years
Adverse reactions	Dose 1 (n[b] = 86 to 87)	Dose 2 (n[b] = 86 to 87)	Dose 3 (n[b] = 78 to 81)	Dose 1 (n[b] = 108)	Dose 2 (n[b] = 98 to 100)	Dose 1 (n[b] = 147 to 148)
Fever[c]						
Mild	3.4%	8.1%	5.1%	3.7%	5.1%	0.7%
Moderate	1.2%	2.3%	1.3%	0.9%	0%	0.7%
Severe	0%	0%	0%	0%	0%	0%
Decreased appetite	19.5%	17.2%	17.5%	22.2%	25.5%	16.3%
Irritability	24.1%	34.5%	24.7%	30.6%	34%	14.3%
Increased sleep	9.2%	9.3%	2.6%	13%	10.1%	11.6%
Decreased sleep	24.1%	18.4%	15%	19.4%	20.4%	6.8%

[a] Study conducted in Poland.
[b] Number of subjects reporting "Yes" for at least 1 day or "No" for all days.
[c] Fever gradings: mild (≥ 38°C but 39°C or lower), moderate (> 39°C but ≤ 40°C), and severe (> 40°C). No other systemic reaction other than fever was graded.

➤*Safety assessments in the supplemental dose studies:*

Local –

Previously Vaccinated With 3 or 4 Prior Infant Doses of PCV7, Reporting Local Adverse Reactions Within 7 Days After 1 Supplemental PCV13 Vaccination			
	15 months through 23 months[a]		24 months through 59 months[b]
Adverse reactions	1 dose PCV13 3 prior PCV7 doses (n[c] = 28 to 32)	1 dose PCV13 4 prior PCV7 doses (n[c] = 62 to 76)	1 dose PCV13 3 or 4 prior PCV7 doses (n[c] = 138 to 155)
Redness[d]			
Any	46.9%	36.6%	34.9%
Mild	31%	31.4%	31.5%
Moderate	22.6%	7.9%	9.9%
Severe	0%	0%	0%
Swelling[d]			
Any	35.5%	21.2%	22.2%
Mild	26.7%	18.8%	20.3%
Moderate	13.8%	7.7%	5.7%
Severe	0%	0%	0%
Tenderness			
Any	53.1%	50%	61.9%
Interferes with limb movement	10.3%	6.3%	10.6%

[a] Dose 2 data not shown.
[b] The data for this age group are only represented as a single result because 95% of children received 4 doses of PCV7 prior to enrollment.
[c] Number of patients reporting "Yes" for ≥ 1 day or "No" for all days.
[d] Diameters were measured in caliper units of whole numbers from 1 to 14 or 14+. One caliper unit = 0.5 cm. Measurements were rounded up to the nearest whole number. Intensity of redness and swelling were then characterized as mild (0.5 to 2 cm), moderate (2.5 to 7 cm), or severe (> 7 cm).

Systemic –

Previously Vaccinated with 3 or 4 Prior Infant PCV7 Doses, Reporting Systemic Adverse Reactions Within 7 Days After 1 Supplemental PCV13 Vaccination			
	15 through 23 months[a]		24 months through 59 months[b]
Adverse reactions	1 dose PCV13 3 prior PCV7 doses (n[c] = 28 to 33)	1 dose PCV13 4 prior PCV7 doses (n[c] = 62 to 75)	1 dose PCV13 3 or 4 prior PCV7 doses (n[c] = 138 to 151)
Fever[d]			
Mild	10.7%	18.8%	5.1%
Moderate	7.1%	3.2%	0.7%
Severe	0%	0%	0.7%
Decreased appetite	56.7%	36.2%	24.8%
Irritability	66.7%	57.3%	39.7%
Increased sleep	30%	33.8%	15.9%
Decreased sleep	22.6%	22.7%	14%

[a] Dose 2 data not shown.
[b] The data for this age group are only represented as a single result because 95% of children received 4 doses of PCV7 prior to enrollment.
[c] Number of patients reporting "Yes" for ≥ 1 day or "No" for all days.
[d] Fever gradings: mild (≥ 38°C but ≤ 39°C), moderate (> 39°C but ≤ 40°C), and severe (> 40°C). No other systemic reaction other than fever was graded.

➤*PCV7 adverse reactions:* Generally, the adverse reactions reported in clinical trials with PCV13 were also reported in clinical trials with PCV7. Additionally, hypotonic-hyporesponsive episode was reported in the clinical trials with PCV7 and, therefore, is considered an adverse reaction for PCV13 as well.

Adverse reactions reported in clinical trials with PCV7 include the following:

GI – Acute gastroenteritis, colic, colitis.

GU – Inguinal hernia repair, urinary tract infection.

Respiratory – Aspiration, asthma, breath-holding, bronchiolitis, croup, upper respiratory tract infection, wheezing.

Miscellaneous – Choking, congestive heart failure, conjunctivitis, influenza, pharyngitis, roseola, sepsis, thrush, viral syndrome.

➤*Postmarketing (with PCV7):*

Dermatologic – Angioneurotic edema, erythema multiforme.

Hematologic/Lymphatic – Lymphadenopathy localized to the region of the injection site.

Hypersensitivity – Anaphylactic/anaphylactoid reaction, including shock.

Local – Injection-site dermatitis, injection-site pruritus, injection-site urticaria.

Respiratory – Apnea.

Overdosage

➤*Symptoms:* Overdose with PCV13 is unlikely because of its presentation as a prefilled syringe. However, there have been reports of overdose with PCV13 defined as subsequent doses administered closer than recommended to the previous dose. In general, adverse reactions reported with overdose are consistent with those that have been reported with doses given in the recommended schedules of PCV13.

Patient Information

Prior to administration of this vaccine, inform the parent, guardian, or other responsible adult of the potential benefits and risks to the patient and the importance of completing the immunization series unless contraindicated.

Instruct parents, guardians, or other responsible adults to report any suspected adverse reactions to their health care provider.

TYPHOID VACCINE

Rx	**Vivotif Berna** (Berna)	**Capsules, enteric-coated:** 2 to 6 × 10[9] colony-forming units of viable *Salmonella typhi* Ty21a and 5 to 50 × 10[9] bacterial cells of nonviable *S. typhi* Ty21a[a]	Salmon/White. In blister pack 4s.
Rx	**Typhim Vi** (Sanofi Pasteur)	**Injection:** 25 mcg purified Vi capsular polysaccharide/0.5 mL[b]	In 0.5 mL syringes and 20 and 50 dose vials.

[a] With 26 to 130 mg sucrose, 1 to 5 mg ascorbic acid, 1.4 to 7 mg amino acid mixture, 100 to 180 mg lactose, and 3.6 to 4.4 mg magnesium stearate.

[b] With 4.15 mg NaCl, 0.065 mg disodium phosphate, 0.023 mg monosodium phosphate, 0.5 mL sterile water for injection.

TYPHOID VACCINE

For complete and comparative prescribing information, refer to the Agents for Active Immunization introduction.

Indications

➤*Oral:* For immunization of adults and children over 6 years of age against disease caused by *Salmonella typhi*. Complete the vaccine regimen at least 1 week before potential exposure to typhoid bacteria.

➤*Parenteral:* For active immunity against typhoid fever for people 2 years of age. Complete the vaccine regimen at least 2 weeks before potential exposure to typhoid bacteria.

➤*General information:* Routine immunization against typhoid fever is not recommended in the United States. Selective immunization against typhoid fever is recommended under the following circumstances: 1) Expected intimate exposure to a household contact with typhoid fever or a known carrier; 2) travelers to typhoid-endemic areas (especially Africa, Asia, and South and Central America), especially if prolonged exposure to potentially contaminated food and water is likely, and travelers to areas of the world with a risk of exposure to typhoid fever; and 3) workers in microbiology laboratories with expected frequent contact with *S. typhi*.

➤*Off-label uses:* Parenteral typhoid vaccine may offer some cross-protection against *Salmonella paratyphi* A. These bacteria share a common O antigen factor 12 with *S. typhi*.

Administration and Dosage

➤*General dosing considerations:* Not all recipients will be fully protected against typhoid fever. Travelers should take all necessary precautions to avoid contact or ingestion of potentially contaminated food or water.

➤*Adults:*

Typhoid fever immunization –

Oral:

• *Usual dosage* – One capsule on alternate days (eg, days 1, 3, 5, and 7).

A complete immunization schedule is the ingestion of 4 vaccine capsules as described previously. Immunization (ingestion of all 4 doses should be completed at least 1 week prior to potential exposure to *S. typhi*).

Unless a complete immunization schedule is followed, an optimum immune response may not be achieved.

• *Booster dose* – The optimum booster schedule has not been determined. Efficacy persists for at least 5 years. Further, there is no experience with oral typhoid vaccine as a booster in people previously immunized with parenteral typhoid vaccine.

It is recommended that a booster dose consisting of 4 vaccine capsules taken on alternate days be given every 5 years under conditions of repeated or continued exposure to typhoid fever.

Parenteral:

• *Usual dosage* – A single 0.5 mL (25 mcg) intramuscularly (IM) dose.

• *Booster doses* – Give a single 0.5 mL (25 mcg) dose every 2 years under conditions of repeated or continued exposure. Booster doses do not elicit higher antibody levels than primary immunization with the polysaccharide antigen.

➤*Children:*

Typhoid fever immunization –

Oral:

• *6 years of age and older* – See Adults for dosing for children 6 years of age and older.

• *Younger than 6 years of age* – Safety and efficacy have not been established for the oral vaccine in children younger than 6 years of age and is, therefore, not recommended for use in this age group.

Parenteral:

• *2 years of age and older* – See Adults for dosing for children 2 years of age and older.

• *Younger than 2 years of age* – Vaccine is not recommended for children younger than 2 years of age because no safety or efficacy data are available for that age group.

➤*Administration:*

Oral – Swallow capsule whole about 1 hour before a meal with cold or lukewarm drink, not to exceed body temperature (37°C; 98.6°F). The vaccine capsule should not be chewed; swallow as soon as possible after placing in the mouth.

Parenteral – For IM use only. Do not inject IV. Inject adults in the deltoid muscle. Inject children in the deltoid or vastus lateralis. Do not inject in the gluteal area or where there may be a nerve trunk. There are no published data on safety and efficacy with administration by jet injector.

➤*Storage/Stability:*

Oral – The oral vaccine is not stable when exposed to ambient temperatures. Ship and store between 2° and 8°C (36° to 46°F). If frozen, thaw capsules before use. Product can tolerate 8 hours at 25°C (77°F). Each package of vaccine has an expiration date. This expiration date is valid only if the product has been maintained at these temperatures.

Parenteral – Store at 2° to 8°C (36° to 46°F). Discard frozen vaccine.

Actions

➤*Pharmacology:* Upon ingestion, virulent strains of *S. typhi* are able to pass through the stomach acid barrier, colonize the intestinal tract, penetrate the lumen, and enter the lymphatic system and blood stream, thereby causing disease.

The ability of *S. typhi* to cause disease and to induce a protective immune response is dependent upon the bacteria possessing a complete lipopolysaccharide. The *S. typhi* Ty21a vaccine strain is restricted in its ability to produce a complete lipopolysaccharide. However, a sufficient quantity of complete lipopolysaccharide is synthesized to evoke a protective immune response.

➤*Pharmacokinetics:*

Onset –

Oral: Finish the fourth capsule at least 1 week before travel.

Parenteral: Protective antibody titers develop within 2 weeks after a single dose.

Duration –

Oral: Approximately 5 years.

Parenteral: Approximately 2 years.

Contraindications

Typhoid fever or a chronic typhoid carrier.

➤*Oral:* Hypersensitivity to any component of the vaccine or the capsule. Do not administer the capsules during acute febrile illness or during an acute GI illness (eg, persistent diarrhea or vomiting).

Safety of the vaccine has not been demonstrated in people deficient in their ability to mount a humoral or cell-mediated immune response because of a congenital or acquired immunodeficient state, including treatment with immunosuppressive or antimitotic drugs. Do not administer the vaccine to these people regardless of benefit.

➤*Parenteral:* Hypersensitivity to any component of the vaccine. Defer administration in the presence of acute respiratory or other active infection, or intensive physical activity (particularly when environmental temperatures are high).

Warnings/Precautions

➤*Immunodeficiency:* If administered to immunosuppressed people or those receiving immunosuppressive therapy, the expected immune response may not be obtained. This includes patients with asymptomatic or symptomatic HIV infection, severe combined immunodeficiency, hypogammaglobulinemia, or agammaglobulinemia, altered immune states because of diseases such as leukemia, lymphoma, or generalized malignancy; or an immune system compromised by treatment with corticosteroids, alkylating drugs, antimetabolites, or radiation.

➤*Protection:* Not all recipients of typhoid vaccine will be fully protected against typhoid fever. Travelers should take all necessary precautions to avoid contact with or ingestion of potentially contaminated food or water sources.

➤*Latex sensitivity:* The parenteral form of this product contains dry natural latex rubber as follows: The stopper to the vial contains no rubber of any kind. In the case of the syringe, the needle cover contains dry natural latex rubber, but the plunger for the syringe contains no rubber of any kind.

➤*Infection:* Acute infection or febrile illness may be reason for delaying use of typhoid vaccine except when in the opinion of the physician, withholding the vaccine entails a greater risk.

➤*Hypersensitivity reactions:* Allergic reactions have been reported rarely in postmarketing experience. Epinephrine injection (1:1000) must be immediately available following immunization should anaphylactic or other allergic reactions occur because of any component of the vaccine.

➤*Pregnancy: Category C.* It is not known whether typhoid vaccine can cause fetal harm when administered to pregnant women or can affect reproduction capacity. Give to a pregnant woman only if clearly needed.

➤*Lactation:* There are no data to warrant the use of the product in nursing mothers. It is not known if the vaccine is excreted in breast milk.

➤*Children:*

Oral – Safety and efficacy have not been established for the oral vaccine in children under 6 years of age and is, therefore, not recommended for use in this age group.

Parenteral – Vaccine is not recommended for children under 2 years of age because no safety or efficacy data are available for that age group.

Drug Interactions

Typhoid Vaccine Drug Interactions

Precipitant drug	Object drug[a]		Description
Immunosuppressants	Typhoid vaccine	⬇	Administration of typhoid vaccine to people receiving immunosuppressant drugs, including high-dose corticosteroids or radiation therapy may result in an insufficient response to immunization. They may remain susceptible despite immunization.
Proguanil	Typhoid vaccine (oral)	⬇	Coadministration may decrease the immune response rate. Administer proguanil only if at least 10 days have elapsed since the final dose of the oral typhoid vaccine.

TYPHOID VACCINE

Typhoid Vaccine Drug Interactions

Precipitant drug	Object drug[a]		Description
Sulfonamides Antibiotics	Typhoid vaccine (oral)	⬇	Do not administer the vaccine to individuals receiving sulfonamides and antibiotics because these agents may be active against the vaccine strain and prevent a sufficient degree of multiplication to occur in order to induce a protective immune response.

[a] ⬇ = object drug decreased.

Adverse Reactions

➤*Oral:* Reported adverse reactions include the following: Nausea (5.8%), abdominal pain (6.4%), headache (4.8%), fever (3.3%), diarrhea (2.9%), vomiting (1.5%), skin rash (1%), abdominal cramps, or urticaria on the trunk or extremities. One case of nonfatal anaphylactic shock, considered to be an allergic reaction, has been reported. Only the incidence of nausea occurred at a statistically higher frequency in the vaccinated group compared with placebo.

➤*Parenteral:*

Typhoid Vaccine Adverse Reactions Occurring within 48 Hours in Adults (%)

Adverse reaction	Trial 1 Placebo (N = 54)	Trial 1 Typhoid vaccine (parenteral) (1 lot) (N = 54)	Trial 2 Typhoid vaccine (parenteral) (2 lots combined) (N = 98)
Local			
Tenderness	13	98	96.9
Pain	7.4	40.7	26.5
Induration	0	14.8	5.1

Typhoid Vaccine Adverse Reactions Occurring within 48 Hours in Adults (%)

Adverse reaction	Trial 1 Placebo (N = 54)	Trial 1 Typhoid vaccine (parenteral) (1 lot) (N = 54)	Trial 2 Typhoid vaccine (parenteral) (2 lots combined) (N = 98)
Erythema	0	3.7	5.1
Systemic			
Malaise	14.8	24	4.1
Headache	13	20.4	16.3
Diarrhea	3.7	0	3.1
Nausea	3.7	1.9	8.2
Fever ≥ 100°F	0	1.9	0
Feverish (subjective)	0	11.1	3.1
Myalgia	0	7.4	3.1
Vomiting	0	1.9	0

Patient Information

Advise vaccine recipients to take standard food and water precautions to avoid typhoid fever. Vaccine protection can be overwhelmed by swallowing a large dose of typhoid bacteria.

➤*Oral:* It is essential that all 4 doses of vaccine be taken at the prescribed alternate day interval to obtain a maximal protective immune response.

Vaccine potency is dependent upon storage under refrigeration (2° to 8°C; 36° to 46°F). Store the vaccine under refrigeration at all times. It is essential to replace unused vaccine in the refrigerator between doses.

Swallow the vaccine capsule about 1 hour before a meal with a cold or lukewarm drink, not to exceed body temperature (37°C; 98.6°F). Do not chew the vaccine capsule; swallow as soon as possible.

Vaccines, Viral

MEASLES VIRUS VACCINE LIVE ATTENUATED

Rx	**Attenuvax** (Merck)	**Powder for injection, lyophilized:** ≥ 1000 $TCID_{50}$ (tissue culture infectious doses) per 0.5 ml dose.	Preservative free. With ≈ 25 mcg neomycin, 14.5 mg sorbitol, 1.9 mg sucrose, 14.5 mg hydrolyzed gelatin, 0.3 mg human albumin, < 1 ppm fetal bovine serum per dose. In single-dose vials with diluent and 50-dose vials with 30 ml diluent.

MEASLES VIRUS VACCINE LIVE — INJECTION

For information on recommended immunization schedules, refer to the Agents for Active Immunization introduction.

Indications

➤*Measles vaccination:* For vaccination against measles in persons 12 months of age or older.

Individuals first vaccinated with the measles virus vaccine at 12 months of age or older should be revaccinated with measles, mumps, and rubella virus vaccine live prior to elementary school entry. Revaccination may seroconvert primary failures or boost antibody titers of those individuals whose titers have declined. The Advisory Committee on Immunization Practices (ACIP) recommends administration of the first dose of measles, mumps, and rubella virus vaccine live at 12 to 15 months of age and administration of the second dose of measles, mumps, and rubella virus vaccine live at 4 to 6 years of age. In addition, some public health jurisdictions mandate the age for revaccination. Consult the complete text of applicable guidelines regarding routine revaccination including that of high-risk adult populations.

➤*Measles outbreak schedule:*

Infants between 6 to 12 months of age – Local health authorities may recommend measles vaccination of infants between 6 to 12 months of age in outbreak situations. This population may fail to respond to the measles component of the vaccine. The younger the infant, the lower the likelihood of seroconversion. Such infants should receive a second dose of measles, mumps, and rubella virus vaccine live between 12 to 15 months of age followed by revaccination prior to elementary school entry.

➤*Other vaccination considerations:*

Other populations – Individuals planning travel outside the United States, if not immune, can acquire measles, mumps or rubella and import these diseases into the US. Therefore, prior to international travel, individuals known to be susceptible to one or more of these diseases can receive either a monovalent vaccine (measles, mumps or rubella), or a combination vaccine as appropriate. However, measles, mumps, and rubella virus vaccine live is preferred for persons likely to be susceptible to mumps and rubella; and if monovalent measles vaccine is not readily available, travelers should receive measles, mumps, and rubella virus vaccine live regardless of their immune status to mumps or rubella.

Vaccination is recommended for susceptible individuals in high-risk groups such as college students, healthcare workers, and military personnel.

According to ACIP recommendations, most persons born in 1956 or earlier are likely to have been infected with measles naturally and generally need not be considered susceptible. All children, adolescents, and adults born after 1956 are considered susceptible and should be vaccinated, if there are no contraindications. This includes persons who may be immune to measles but who lack adequate documentation of immunity such as:

1.) Physician-diagnosed measles.
2.) Laboratory evidence of measles immunity.
3.) Adequate immunization with live measles vaccine on or after the first birthday.

The ACIP recommends that "Persons vaccinated with inactivated vaccine followed within 3 months by live vaccine should be revaccinated with 2 doses of live vaccine. Revaccination is particularly important when the risk of exposure to natural measles virus is increased, as may occur during international travel."

Postexposure vaccination – The measles virus vaccine given immediately after exposure to natural measles may provide some protection if the vaccine can be administered within 72 hours of exposure. If, however, the vaccine is given a few days before exposure, substantial protection may be provided.

Use with other vaccines – See Administration and Dosage for more information.

Administration and Dosage

➤*Recommended dosage:* Do not inject by IV. The dose for any age is 0.5 mL administered SC, preferably into the outer aspect of the upper arm. See Indications for more information.

➤*Immune globulin:* Immune Globulin (IG) is not to be given concurrently with the measles virus vaccine.

➤*Syringe selection:* A sterile syringe free of preservatives, antiseptics, and detergents should be used for each injection or reconstitution of the vaccine because these substances may inactivate the live virus vaccine. A 25 gauge, ⅝ inch needle is recommended.

➤*Reconstitution:* To reconstitute, use only the diluent supplied, since it is free of preservatives or other antiviral substances which might inactivate the vaccine.

➤*Single-dose vial:* First withdraw the entire volume of diluent into the syringe to be used for reconstitution. Inject all the diluent in the syringe into the vial of lyophilized vaccine, and agitate to mix thoroughly. If the lyophilized vaccine cannot be dissolved, discard. Withdraw the entire contents into a syringe and inject the total volume of restored vaccine SC.

MEASLES VIRUS VACCINE LIVE — INJECTION

➤*50-dose vial (available only to government agencies/institutions):* Withdraw the entire contents (30 mL) of diluent vial into the sterile syringe to be used for reconstitution and introduce into the 50-dose vial of lyophilized vaccine. Agitate to ensure thorough mixing. If the lyophilized vaccine cannot be dissolved, discard. With full aseptic precautions, attach the vial to the sterilized multidose jet injector apparatus. Use 0.5 mL of the reconstituted vaccine for SC injection.

➤*Use with other vaccines:* The measles virus vaccine should not be given less than 1 month before or after administration of other live viral vaccines.

Routine administration of DTP (diphtheria, tetanus, pertussis) or OPV (oral poliovirus vaccine) concurrently with measles, mumps and rubella vaccines is not recommended because there are limited data relating to the simultaneous administration of these antigens.

However, other schedules have been used. The ACIP has stated, "Although data are limited concerning the simultaneous administration of the entire recommended vaccine series (ie, DTP, OPV, MMR, and Hib vaccines, with or without hepatitis B vaccine), data from numerous studies have indicated no interference between routinely recommended childhood vaccines (either live, attenuated, or killed). These findings support the simultaneous use of all vaccines as recommended."

➤*Storage/Stability:* During shipment, to ensure that there is no loss of potency, the vaccine must be maintained at a temperature of 10°C (50°F) or colder. Freezing during shipment will not affect potency.

Protect the vaccine from light at all times, since such exposure may inactivate the virus.

Before reconstitution, store the vial of lyophilized vaccine at 2° to 8°C (36° to 46°F) or colder. The diluent may be stored in the refrigerator with the lyophilized vaccine or separately at room temperature.

It is recommended that the vaccine be used as soon as possible after reconstitution. Store reconstituted vaccine in the vaccine vial in a dark place at 2° to 8°C (36° to 46°F) and discard if not used within 8 hours.

Actions

➤*Pharmacology:* Measles is a common childhood disease, caused by measles virus (paramyxovirus), that may be associated with serious complications or death. For example, pneumonia and encephalitis are caused by measles.

Contraindications

➤*Hypersensitivity:* Hypersensitivity to any component of the vaccine, including gelatin.

Anaphylactic or anaphylactoid reactions to neomycin (each dose of reconstituted vaccine contains approximately 25 mcg of neomycin).

➤*Pregnancy:* Do not give measles vaccine to pregnant females; the possible effects of the vaccine on fetal development are unknown at this time. If vaccination of postpubertal females is undertaken, pregnancy should be avoided for 3 months following vaccination (see Warnings, Pregnancy).

➤*Febrile respiratory illness or other active febrile infection:* Febrile respiratory illness or other active febrile infection. However, the ACIP has recommended that all vaccines can be administered to persons with minor illnesses such as diarrhea, mild upper respiratory infection with or without low-grade fever, or other low-grade febrile illness.

➤*Hematology issues:* Individuals with blood dyscrasias, leukemia, lymphomas of any type, or other malignant neoplasms affecting the bone marrow or lymphatic systems.

➤*Immunosuppressive or immunodeficiency states:* Patients receiving immunosuppressive therapy. This contraindication does not apply to patients who are receiving corticosteroids as replacement therapy, eg, for Addison's disease.

Primary and acquired immunodeficiency states, including patients who are immunosuppressed in association with AIDS or other clinical manifestations of infection with human immunodeficiency viruses; cellular immune deficiencies; and hypogammaglobulinemic and dysgammaglobulinemic states. Measles inclusion body encephalitis (MIBE), pneumonitis and death as a direct consequence of disseminated measles vaccine virus infection has been reported in immunocompromised individuals inadvertently vaccinated with measles-containing vaccine.

Individuals with a family history of congenital or hereditary immunodeficiency, until the immune competence of the potential vaccine recipient is demonstrated.

Warnings/Precautions

➤*Thrombocytopenia:* Individuals with current thrombocytopenia may develop more severe thrombocytopenia following vaccination. In addition, individuals who experienced thrombocytopenia with the first dose of measles, mumps, and rubella virus vaccine live (or its component vaccines) may develop thrombocytopenia with repeat doses. Serologic status may be evaluated to determine whether or not additional doses of vaccine are needed. The potential risk to benefit ratio should be carefully evaluated before considering vaccination in such cases (see Adverse Reactions).

➤*Hypersensitivity reactions:* Adequate treatment provisions including epinephrine injection (1:1000), should be available for immediate use should an anaphylactic or anaphylactoid reaction occur.

Special care should be taken to ensure that the injection does not enter a blood vessel.

Eggs – The live measles vaccine is produced in chick embryo cell culture. Persons with a history of anaphylactic, anaphylactoid or other immediate reactions (eg, hives, swelling of the mouth and throat, difficulty breathing, hypotension and shock) subsequent to egg ingestion may be at an enhanced risk of immediate-type hypersensitivity reactions after receiving vaccines containing traces of chick embryo antigen. The potential risk to benefit ratio should be carefully evaluated before considering vaccination in such cases. Such individuals may be vaccinated with extreme caution, having adequate treatment on hand should a reaction occur (see Warnings).

However, the AAP has stated, "Most children with a history of anaphylactic reactions to eggs have no untoward reactions to measles or MMR vaccine. Persons are not at increased risk if they have egg allergies that are not anaphylactic, and they should be vaccinated in the usual manner. In addition, skin testing of egg-allergic children with vaccine has not been predictive of which children will have an immediate hypersensitivity reaction...Persons with allergies to chickens or chicken feathers are not at increased risk of reaction to the vaccine."

Neomycin – The AAP states, "Persons who have experienced anaphylactic reactions to topically or systemically administered neomycin should not receive measles vaccine. Most often, however, neomycin allergy manifests as a contact dermatitis, which is a delayed-type (cell-mediated) immune response rather than anaphylaxis. In such persons, an adverse reaction to neomycin in the vaccine would be an erythematous, pruritic nodule or papule, 48 to 96 hours after vaccination. A history of contact dermatitis to neomycin is not a contraindication to receiving measles vaccine."

➤*Special risk:*

Cerebral injury/convulsions – Due caution should be employed in administration of the measles virus vaccine to persons with a history of cerebral injury, individual or family histories of convulsions, or any other condition in which stress due to fever should be avoided. The physician should be alert to the temperature elevation which may occur following vaccination (see Adverse Reactions).

➤*Pregnancy: Category C.*

Animal reproduction studies have not been conducted with the measles virus vaccine. It is also not known whether the measles virus vaccine can cause fetal harm when administered to a pregnant woman or can affect reproduction capacity. Therefore, the vaccine should not be administered to pregnant females; furthermore, pregnancy should be avoided for 3 months following vaccination (see Contraindications).

In counseling women who are inadvertently vaccinated when pregnant or who become pregnant within 3 months of vaccination, the physician should be aware that reports have indicated that contracting natural measles during pregnancy enhances fetal risk. Increased rates of spontaneous abortion, stillbirth, congenital defects and prematurity have been observed subsequent to natural measles during pregnancy. There are no adequate studies of the attenuated (vaccine) strain of measles virus in pregnancy. However, it would be prudent to assume that the vaccine strain of virus is also capable of inducing adverse fetal effects.

➤*Lactation:* It is not known whether the measles vaccine virus is secreted in human milk. Therefore, because many drugs are excreted in human milk, caution should be exercised when the measles virus vaccine is administered to a nursing woman.

➤*Children:* Safety and effectiveness in infants younger than 6 months of age have not been established.

Children with HIV – Children and young adults who are known to be infected with HIV and are not immunosuppressed may be vaccinated. However, vaccinees who are infected with HIV should be monitored closely for vaccine-preventable diseases because immunization may be less effective than for uninfected persons (see Contraindications).

Vaccination should be deferred for 3 months or longer following blood or plasma transfusions, or administration of immune globulin (human).

Children under treatment for tuberculosis – Children under treatment for tuberculosis (TB) have not experienced exacerbation of the disease when immunized with live measles virus vaccine; no studies have been reported to date of the effect of measles virus vaccines on untreated TB children. However, individuals with active untreated TB should not be vaccinated.

Drug Interactions

Measles Virus Vaccine Drug Interactions

Precipitant drug	Object drug[a]		Description
Immunosuppressants	Measles vaccine	⬇	Administration of measles vaccine to patients receiving immunosuppressants, including corticosteroids or radiation therapy, may result in insufficient response to immunization. They may remain susceptible despite immunization.

MEASLES VIRUS VACCINE LIVE — INJECTION

Measles Virus Vaccine Drug Interactions

Precipitant drug	Object drug[a]		Description
Immune globulins	Measles vaccine	↓	To avoid inactivation of the attenuated virus, administer the vaccine at least 14 to 30 days before or 6 to 8 weeks after the immune globulin. Alternately, check antibody titers or repeat the vaccine dose 3 months after immune globulin administration. Base the interval on the dose of IgG administered: 3 months for 3 to 10 mg/kg, 4 months for 20 mg/kg, 5 months for 40 mg/kg, 6 months for 60 to 100 mg/kg, 7 months for 160 mg/kg, 8 months for 300 to 400 mg/kg, 10 months for 1 g/kg, 11 months for 2 g/kg.
Interferon	Measles vaccine	↓	Concurrent use may inhibit antibody response to the vaccine.
Vitamin A	Measles vaccine	↓	Simultaneous administration of large doses of vitamin A impaired the response to Schwarz-strain measles vaccine in a group of Indonesian infants at 6 months of age.
Measles vaccine	Meningococcal vaccine	↓	Reduced seroconversion rate to meningococci may occur with concurrent immunization. If possible, separate these 2 vaccinations by ≥ 1 month.
Measles vaccine	Tuberculin skin test	↓	Measles vaccine may temporarily depress tuberculin skin sensitivity. Administer the test before or simultaneously with the vaccine.
Measles vaccine	Virus vaccines, other	↓	To avoid the hypothetical concern over antigenic competition, give measles vaccine≥ 1 month before or after other virus vaccines. However, several vaccines may be given simultaneously at separate injection sites (eg, DTP, OPV or e-IPV, MMR, Hib, hepatitis B, varicella, influenza).

[a] ↓ = Object drug decreased.

➤*Drug/Lab test interactions:* It has been reported that attenuated measles virus vaccine live may result in a temporary depression of TB skin sensitivity. Therefore, if a tuberculin test is to be done, it should be administered either before or simultaneously with the measles virus vaccine.

Adverse Reactions

The following adverse reactions are listed in decreasing order of severity, without regard to causality, within each body system category and have been reported during clinical trials, with use of the marketed vaccine, or with use of polyvalent vaccine containing measles:

➤*Cardiovascular:* Vasculitis.

➤*CNS:* Encephalitis; encephalopathy; measles inclusion body encephalitis (MIBE) (see Contraindications); subacute sclerosing panencephalitis (SSPE); Guillain-Barré syndrome (GBS); febrile convulsions; afebrile convulsions or seizures; ataxia; ocular palsies.

There have been reports of subacute sclerosing panencephalitis (SSPE) in children who did not have a history of natural measles but did receive measles vaccine. Some of these cases may have resulted from unrecognized measles in the first year of life or possibly from the measles vaccination. Based on estimated nationwide measles vaccine distribution, the association of SSPE cases to measles vaccination is about one case per million vaccine doses distributed. This is far less than the association with natural measles, 6 to 22 cases of SSPE per million cases of measles. The results of a retrospective case-controlled study conducted by the Centers for Disease Control and Prevention suggest that the overall effect of measles vaccine has been to protect against SSPE by preventing measles with its inherent higher risk of SSPE.

➤*Dermatologic:* Stevens-Johnson syndrome; erythema multiforme; urticaria; rash.

➤*GI:* Diarrhea.

➤*Hematologic/Lymphatic:* Thrombocytopenia (see Warnings, Thrombocytopenia); purpura; lymphadenopathy; leukocytosis.

➤*Hypersensitivity:* Anaphylaxis and anaphylactoid reactions have been reported as well as related phenomena such as angioneurotic edema (including peripheral or facial edema) and bronchial spasm.

➤*Local:* Burning/stinging at injection site; wheal and flare; redness (erythema); swelling; vesiculation at injection site.

➤*Ophthalmic:* Retinitis; optic neuritis; papillitis; retrobulbar neuritis; conjunctivitis.

➤*Respiratory:* Pneumonitis (see Contraindications); cough; rhinitis.

➤*Special senses:*

Ear – Nerve deafness; otitis media.

➤*Miscellaneous:* Panniculitis; atypical measles; fever; syncope; headache; dizziness; malaise; irritability.

Patient Information

The health care provider should provide the vaccine information required to be given with each vaccination to the patient, parent or guardian.

The health care provider should inform the patient, parent or guardian of the benefits and risks associated with vaccination. For risks associated with vaccination, see Warnings, Precautions, and Adverse Reactions.

➤*Adverse reactions:* Patients, parents or guardians should be instructed to report any serious adverse reactions to their health care provider who in turn should report such events to the US Department of Health and Human Services through the Vaccine Adverse Event Reporting System (VAERS), 1-800-822-7967.

Pregnancy – See Contraindications for more information.

Immunosuppressive therapy – The immune status of patients about to undergo immunosuppressive therapy should be evaluated so that the physician can consider whether vaccination prior to the initiation of treatment is indicated (see Contraindications and Precautions).

The ACIP has stated that "Patients with leukemia in remission who have not received chemotherapy for at least 3 months may receive live-virus vaccines. Short-term (less than 2 weeks), low- to moderate-dose systemic corticosteroid therapy, topical steroid therapy (eg, nasal, skin), long-term alternate-day treatment with low to moderate doses of short-acting systemic steroid, and intra-articular, bursal, or tendon injection of corticosteroids are not immunosuppressive in their usual doses and do not contraindicate the administration of measles vaccine."

Immune globulin – Administration of immune globulins concurrently with the measles virus vaccine may interfere with the expected immune response.

MEASLES, MUMPS AND RUBELLA VIRUS VACCINE, LIVE

Rx	M-M-R II (Merck)	**Powder for injection**: Mixture of 3 viruses: ≥ 1000 measles $TCID_{50}$ (tissue culture infectious doses), ≥ 20,000 mumps $TCID_{50}$ and ≥ 1000 rubella $TCID_{50}$ per 0.5 ml dose.	With 25 mcg neomycin. In single dose vials with diluent.

MEASLES, MUMPS AND RUBELLA VIRUS VACCINE, LIVE — INJECTION

For information on recommended immunization schedules, refer to the Agents for Active Immunization introduction. Consider the prescribing information for measles (rubeola) virus vaccine, mumps virus vaccine and rubella virus vaccine when using this product (see individual monographs).

Indications

➤*Measles, mumps, and rubella vaccination:* For simultaneous vaccination against measles, mumps, and rubella in individuals at least 12 months of age.

Revaccinate individuals first vaccinated at at least 12 months of age prior to elementary school entry. Revaccination may seroconvert primary failures or boost antibody titers of previously vaccinated individuals whose titers have declined. The Advisory Committee on Immunization Practices (ACIP) recommends administration of the first dose of measles, mumps and rubella virus vaccine live at 12 to 15 months of age and administration of the second dose of measles, mumps and rubella virus vaccine live at 4 to 6 years of age. In addition, some public health jurisdictions mandate the age for revaccination. Consult the complete text of applicable guidelines regarding routine revaccination including that of high-risk adult populations.

➤*Measles outbreak schedule:*

Infants between 6 and 12 months of age – Local health authorities may recommend measles vaccination of infants between 6 and 12 months of age in outbreak situations. This population may fail to respond to the components of the vaccine. Safety and efficacy of mumps and rubella vaccine in infants younger than 12 months of age have not been established. The younger the infant, the lower the likelihood of seroconversion. Such infants should receive a second dose of measles, mumps and rubella virus vaccine live between 12 and 15 months of age, followed by revaccination at elementary school entry.

➤*Other vaccination considerations:*

Nonpregnant adolescent and adult women – Immunization of susceptible nonpregnant adolescent and adult women of childbearing age with live, attenuated rubella virus vaccine is indicated if certain precautions are

MEASLES, MUMPS AND RUBELLA VIRUS VACCINE, LIVE — INJECTION

observed. Vaccinating susceptible postpubertal women confers individual protection against subsequently acquiring rubella infection during pregnancy, which in turn prevents infection of the fetus and consequent congenital rubella injury.

Advise women of childbearing age not to become pregnant for 3 months after vaccination and inform them of the reasons for this precaution. Note: The ACIP has recommended "In view of the importance of protecting this age group against rubella, reasonable practices in a rubella immunization program include asking women if they are pregnant, excluding those who say they are, explaining the concern about risk for the fetus to the others, and explaining the importance of not becoming pregnant during the 3 months following vaccination."

Postpartum women – It has been found convenient in many instances to vaccinate rubella-susceptible women in the immediate postpartum period.

Other populations – Previously unvaccinated children older than 12 months who are in contact with susceptible pregnant women should receive live, attenuated rubella vaccine (such as that contained in monovalent rubella vaccine or in measles, mumps and rubella virus vaccine live) to reduce the risk of exposure of the pregnant woman.

Individuals planning travel outside the United States, if not immune, can acquire measles, mumps or rubella and import these diseases into the United States. Therefore, prior to international travel, individuals known to be susceptible to 1 or more of these diseases can receive either a monovalent vaccine (measles, mumps or rubella), or a combination vaccine as appropriate. However, measles, mumps and rubella virus vaccine live is preferred for persons likely to be susceptible to mumps and rubella; and if monovalent measles vaccine is not readily available, travelers should receive measles, mumps and rubella virus vaccine live regardless of their immune status to mumps or rubella.

Vaccination is recommended for susceptible individuals in high-risk groups such as college students, health care workers, and military personnel.

According to ACIP recommendations, most persons born in 1956 or earlier are likely to have been infected with measles naturally and generally need not be considered susceptible. All children, adolescents, and adults born after 1956 are considered susceptible and should be vaccinated if there are no contraindications. This includes persons who may be immune to measles but who lack adequate documentation of immunity such as physician-diagnosed measles, laboratory evidence of measles immunity, or adequate immunization with live measles vaccine on or after the first birthday.

The ACIP recommends that "Persons vaccinated with inactivated vaccine followed within 3 months by live vaccine should be revaccinated with 2 doses of live vaccine. Revaccination is particularly important when the risk of exposure to natural measles virus is increased, as may occur during international travel."

➤*Postexposure vaccination:* Vaccination of individuals exposed to natural measles may provide some protection if the vaccine can be administered within 72 hours of exposure. If, however, vaccine is given a few days before exposure, substantial protection may be afforded. There is no conclusive evidence that vaccination of individuals recently exposed to natural mumps or natural rubella will provide protection.

Administration and Dosage

➤*Adults:*

Measles, mumps, and rubella vaccination – 0.5 mL administered subcutaneously.

➤*Children:*

12 months of age and older – See Adults for dosing.

Measles, mumps, and rubella vaccination:

The recommended age for primary vaccination is 12 to 15 months. Revaccination with measles, mumps, and rubella virus vaccine live is recommended prior to elementary school entry.

Children first vaccinated when younger than 12 months of age should receive another dose between 12 to 15 months of age, followed by revaccination prior to elementary school entry.

➤*Concomitant therapy:*

Use with other vaccines – Measles, mumps, and rubella virus vaccine live should be given 1 month before or after administration of other live viral vaccines.

Measles, mumps, and rubella virus vaccine live has been administered concurrently with varicella virus vaccine live and *Haemophilus B* conjugate vaccine (meningococcal protein conjugate), using separate sites and syringes. No impairment of immune response to individual tested vaccine antigens was demonstrated. The type, frequency, and severity of adverse experiences observed with measles, mumps, and rubella virus vaccine live were similar to those seen when each vaccine was given alone.

Routine administration of diphtheria, tetanus, pertussis (DTP) or oral poliovirus vaccine (OPV) concurrently with measles, mumps, and rubella vaccines is not recommended because there are limited data relating to the simultaneous administration of these antigens.

However, other schedules have been used. The ACIP has stated, "Although data are limited concerning the simultaneous administration of the entire recommended vaccine series (ie, DTP, OPV, MMR, and Hib vaccines, with or without hepatitis B vaccine), data from numerous studies have indicated no interference between routinely recommended childhood vaccines (either live, attenuated, or killed). These findings support the simultaneous use of all vaccines as recommended."

Immune globulin – Immune globulin is not to be given concurrently with measles, mumps, and rubella virus vaccine live. See Warnings/ Precautions for more information.

➤*Preparation for administration:* Measles, mumps, and rubella virus vaccine live, when reconstituted, is clear yellow.

Use a sterile syringe free of preservatives, antiseptics, and detergents for each injection or reconstitution of the vaccine because these substances may inactivate the live virus vaccine. A 25-gauge, ⅝ inch needle is recommended.

To reconstitute, use only the diluent supplied because it is free of preservatives or other antiviral substances that might inactivate the vaccine.

Single-dose vial – First, withdraw the entire volume of diluent into the syringe to be used for reconstitution. Inject all the diluent in the syringe into the vial of lyophilized vaccine, and agitate to mix thoroughly. If the lyophilized vaccine cannot be dissolved, discard. Withdraw the entire contents into a syringe and inject the total volume of restored vaccine subcutaneously.

➤*Administration:* Administer subcutaneously, preferably into the outer aspect of the upper arm. Do not administer intravenously.

➤*Storage/Stability:* During shipment, to ensure that there is no loss of potency, the vaccine must be maintained at a temperature of 10°C (50°F). Freezing during shipment will not affect potency.

Protect the vaccine from light at all times because such exposure may inactivate the virus.

Before reconstitution, store the vial of lyophilized vaccine between 2° and 8°C (36° and 46°F), or colder. The diluent may be stored in the refrigerator with the lyophilized vaccine, or separately at room temperature.

Use as soon as possible after reconstitution. Store reconstituted vaccine in the vaccine vial in a dark place between 2° and 8°C (36° and 46°F) and discard if not used within 8 hours.

MEASLES, MUMPS, RUBELLA, AND VARICELLA VIRUS VACCINE, LIVE, ATTENUATED

Rx	**ProQuad** (Merck & Co.)	**Powder for injection, lyophilized**: Mixture of 4 viruses: ≥ 3.00 $\log_{10}$ measles $TCID_{50}$ (50% tissue culture infectious doses), 4.30 $\log_{10}$ mumps $TCID_{50}$, 3.00 $\log_{10}$ rubella $TCID_{50}$, and ≥ 3.99 $\log_{10}$ varicella PFU (plaque-forming units) per 0.5 mL dose.	Preservative free.[a] In single dose vials with diluent.

[a] Sucrose, hydrolyzed gelatin, sodium chloride, sorbitol, monosodium L-glutamate, sodium phosphate dibasic, human albumin, sodium bicarbonate, potassium phosphate monobasic, potassium chloride, potassium phosphate dibasic, residual components of MRC-5 cells including DNA and protein, neomycin, bovine calf serum.

MEASLES, MUMPS, RUBELLA, AND VARICELLA VIRUS VACCINE, LIVE, ATTENUATED — INJECTION

Indications

➤*Measles, mumps, rubella, and varicella vaccination:* Measles, mumps, rubella, and varicella virus (MMRV) vaccine live is indicated for simultaneous vaccination against measles, mumps, rubella, and varicella in children 12 months to 12 years of age. It may be used in children 12 months to 12 years of age if a second dose of measles, mumps, and rubella vaccine is to be administered.

Administration and Dosage

➤*General dosing considerations:* Vaccination should be deferred for at least 3 months following blood or plasma transfusions or administration of immunoglobulin.

➤*Children:*

Measles, mumps, rubella and varicella vaccination –

12 months to 12 years of age:

• *Usual dosage* – 0.5 mL administered subcutaneously. The first dose is usually administered at 12 to 15 months of age but may be given anytime through 12 years of age. At least 1 month should elapse between a dose of a measles-containing vaccine (ie, measles, mumps, and rubella virus vaccine, live [*M-M-R II*]) and a dose of measles, mumps, rubella, and varicella vaccine. At least 3 months should elapse between a dose of varicella-containing vaccine and measles, mumps, rubella, and varicella vaccine.

• *Booster dosage* – If a second dose of measles, mumps, rubella, and varicella vaccine is needed, it is usually administered at 4 to 6 years of age.

➤*Preparation for administration:* Withdraw the entire volume of the supplied diluent into a syringe. Use only the diluent supplied with the vaccine because it is free of preservatives or other antiviral substances.

Preservatives, antiseptics, detergents, and other antiviral substances may inactivate the vaccine. Use only sterile syringes that are free of preservatives, antiseptics, detergents and other antiviral substances for reconstitution and injection of measles, mumps, rubella, and varicella vaccine.

Inject the entire content of the syringe into the vial containing the powder. Gently agitate to dissolve completely. Visually inspect the vaccine before and after reconstitution for particulate matter and discoloration prior to administration. Before reconstitution, the lyophilized vaccine is a white to pale yellow compact crystalline plug. measles, mumps, rubella, and varicella vaccine, when reconstituted, is a clear pale yellow to light pink liquid.

MEASLES, MUMPS, RUBELLA, AND VARICELLA VIRUS VACCINE, LIVE, ATTENUATED — INJECTION

Withdraw the entire amount of the reconstituted vaccine from the vial into the same syringe and inject the entire volume. When reconstituted, each vial of measles, mumps, rubella, and varicella vaccine contains a single 0.5 mL dose.

To minimize loss of potency, the vaccine should be administered immediately after reconstitution. Discard reconstituted vaccine if it is not used within 30 minutes.

➤*Administration:* For subcutaneous administration; do not inject intravascularly. The vaccine is to be injected subcutaneously in the outer aspect of the deltoid region of the upper arm or in the higher anterolateral area of the thigh.

To minimize loss of potency, administer immediately after reconstitution. Discard reconstituted vaccine if it is not used within 30 minutes.

➤*Storage/Stability:* Store between −50° and −15°C (−58° and 5°F). Use of dry ice may subject the vaccine to temperatures colder than −50°C (−58°F).

Before reconstitution, store the lyophilized vaccine continuously in a reliably maintained freezer (eg, chest, frostfree) for up to 18 months. May store at 2° to 8°C (36° to 46° F) or up to 72 hours prior to reconstitution. Discard any vaccine stored at 2° to 8°C (36° to 46°F) that is not used within 72 hours of removal from −15°C (5°F) storage.

Protect the vaccine from light at all times because such exposure may inactivate the vaccine viruses.

Discard reconstituted vaccine if it is not used within 30 minutes. Do not freeze reconstituted vaccine.

Store diluent separately at room temperature (20° to 25°C [68° to 77° F]), or in a refrigerator (2° to 8°C [36° to 46° F]).

POLIOVIRUS VACCINE, INACTIVATED (IPV)

Rx	**IPOL** (Connaught)	**Injection:** Suspension of 3 types of poliovirus (Types 1, 2 and 3) grown in monkey kidney cell cultures	In 0.5 ml single-dose syringe with integrated needle.[a]

[a] Each dose contains 0.5% 2-phenoxyethanol, a maximum of 0.02% formaldehyde and not more than 200 ng streptomycin, 25 ng polymyxin B and 5 ng neomycin.

POLIOVIRUS VACCINE, INACTIVATED (IPV) — INJECTION

For complete and comparative prescribing information, refer to the Agents for Active Immunization introduction.

Indications

➤*Poliovirus prevention:* Poliovirus vaccine, inactivated (IPV) is indicated for active immunization of infants (as young as 6 weeks of age), children and adults for the prevention of poliomyelitis caused by poliovirus types 1, 2, and 3.

➤*Infants, children, and adolescents:* It is recommended that all infants (as young as 6 weeks of age), unimmunized children, and adolescents not previously immunized be vaccinated routinely against paralytic poliomyelitis. Following the eradication of poliomyelitis caused by wild poliovirus from the Western Hemisphere (including North and South America) vaccine-associated paralytic poliomyelitis (VAPP) is the only cause of paralytic poliomyelitis in the US. The use of IPV has been suggested as a way to reduce VAPP incidence.

All children should receive 4 doses of IPV at ages 2, 4, 6 to 18 months, and 4 to 6 years. Oral poliovirus vaccine (OPV) is no longer recommended for routine immunization. In the special circumstances that OPV is acceptable, please refer to the monograph for the appropriate administration schedule and all other issues related to the use of OPV.

Children incompletely immunized – Children of all ages should have their immunization status reviewed and be considered for supplemental immunization as follows for adults. Time intervals between doses longer than those recommended for routine primary immunization do not necessitate additional doses as long as a final total of 4 doses is reached.

➤*Adults:* Routine primary poliovirus vaccination of adults (generally those 18 years of age and older) residing in the United States is not recommended. Unimmunized adults residing in a household when a child is receiving OPV or adults who have increased risk of exposure to either oral vaccine or wild poliovirus and have not been adequately immunized should receive polio vaccination in accordance with the schedule given in Administration and Dosage.

Persons with previous wild poliovirus disease, who are incompletely immunized or unimmunized, should be given additional doses of IPV if they fall into one or more categories listed previously.

The following categories of adults are at an increased risk of exposure to wild polioviruses:

- Travelers to regions or countries where poliomyelitis is endemic or epidemic.
- Healthcare workers in close contact with patients who may be excreting polioviruses.
- Laboratory workers handling specimens that may contain polioviruses.
- Members of communities or specific population groups with disease caused by wild polioviruses.
- Incompletely vaccinated or unvaccinated adults in a household (or other close contacts) with children given OPV. The adult should be informed of the risk of VAPP associated with contact of those receiving OPV.

➤*Immunodeficiency and altered immune status:* Patients with recognized immunodeficiency are at greater risk of developing paralysis when exposed to live poliovirus than persons with a healthy immune system. Under no circumstances should oral poliovirus vaccine be used in such patients or introduced into a household where such a patient resides.

IPV should be used in all patients with immunodeficiency diseases and members of such patients' households when vaccination of such persons is indicated. This includes patients with asymptomatic HIV infection, AIDS or AIDS-related complex, severe combined immunodeficiency, hypogammaglobulinemia, or agammaglobulinemia; altered immune states due to diseases such as leukemia, lymphoma, or generalized malignancy; or an immune system compromised by treatment with corticosteroids, alkylating drugs, antimetabolites, or radiation. Immunogenicity of IPV in individuals receiving immunoglobulin could be impaired and patients with an altered immune state may or may not develop a protective response against paralytic poliomyelitis after administration of IPV.

Administration and Dosage

➤*General dosing considerations:* Precaution is recommended in patients with sensitivity to natural latex rubber (see Preparation for Administration).

Health care providers should question the patient, parent, or guardian about reactions to a previous dose of this product, or similar product.

Health care providers should obtain the immunization history of the vaccinee, and inquire about the current health status of the vaccinee.

➤*Adults:*

Poliovirus prevention –

Unvaccinated adults: A primary series of IPV is recommended for unvaccinated adults at increased risk of exposure to poliovirus.

• *Usual dosage* – While the responses of adults to primary series have not been studied, the recommended schedule for adults is 2 doses given at a 1- to 2-month interval and a third dose given 6 to 12 months later. If less than 3 months but greater than 2 months are available before protection is needed, 3 doses of IPV should be given at least 1 month apart. Likewise, if only 1 or 2 months are available, 2 doses of IPV should be given at least 1 month apart. If less than 1 month is available, a single dose of IPV is recommended.

Incompletely vaccinated adults:

• *Usual dosage* – Adults who are at an increased risk of exposure to poliovirus and who have had at least 1 dose of OPV, fewer than 3 doses of conventional IPV (inactivated poliovirus vaccine available in the United States prior to 1988) or a combination of conventional IPV or OPV totaling fewer than 3 doses should receive at least 1 dose of IPV. Additional doses needed to complete a primary series should be given if time permits.

Completely vaccinated adults: Adults who are at an increased risk of exposure to poliovirus and who have previously completed a primary series with 1 or a combination of polio vaccines can be given a dose of IPV.

➤*Children:*

Poliovirus prevention –

Unvaccinated children:

• *Usual dosage* – The primary series of poliovirus vaccine, inactivated consists of three 0.5 mL doses administered intramuscularly (IM) or subcutaneously, preferably 8 or more weeks apart and usually at 2, 4, and 6 to 18 months of age. Under no circumstances should the vaccine be given more frequently than 4 weeks apart. The first immunization may be administered as early as 6 weeks of age. For this series, a booster dose of IPV is administered at 4 to 6 years of age.

• *Concomitant use with other vaccines* – From historical data on the antibody responses to diphtheria, tetanus, whole-cell or acellular pertussis, Hib, or hepatitis B vaccines used concomitantly with IPV, no interferences have been observed on the immunological end points accepted for clinical protection. If the third dose of poliovirus vaccine, inactivated is given between 12 to 18 months of age, it may be desirable to administer this dose with measles, mumps, and rubella (MMR) or other vaccines using separate syringes at separate sites, but no data on the immunological interference between IPV and these vaccines exist.

Previously vaccinated children: Children and adolescents with a previously incomplete series of IPV/OPV or IPV only should receive sufficient additional doses of poliovirus vaccine, inactivated to complete the series. OPV is no longer recommended for routine immunization and is recommended only in special circumstances.

Interruption of the recommended schedule with a delay between doses does not interfere with the final immunity. There is no need to start either series over again, regardless of the time elapsed between doses.

The need to routinely administer additional doses is unknown at this time.

➤*Administration:* A separate, sterile syringe and needle or a sterile disposable unit must be used for each patient to prevent transmission of hepatitis or other infectious agents from person to person. Needles should not be recapped and should be disposed of according to biohazard waste guidelines.

POLIOVIRUS VACCINE, INACTIVATED (IPV) — INJECTION

After preparation of the injection site, immediately administer poliovirus vaccine, inactivated IM or subcutaneously. In infants and small children, the mid-lateral aspect of the thigh is the preferred site. In older children and adults, IPV should be administered IM or subcutaneously in the deltoid area.

The preferred injection site of IPV for adults is in the tissue of the deltoid area.

Do not administer vaccine intravenously.

Care should be taken to avoid administering the injection into or near blood vessels and nerves. After aspiration, if blood or any suspicious discoloration appears in the syringe, do not inject, but discard contents and repeat procedures using a new dose of vaccine administered at a different site.

Latex allergy – Prior to an injection of any vaccine, all known precautions should be taken to prevent adverse reactions. This includes a review of the patient's history with respect to possible sensitivity to the vaccine or similar vaccines and to possible sensitivity to dry, natural latex rubber.

➤*Storage/Stability:* The vaccine is stable if stored in the refrigerator between 2° and 8°C (35° and 46°F). The vaccine must not be frozen.

Actions

➤*Pharmacology:* Poliomyelitis is caused by poliovirus Types 1, 2, or 3. It is primarily spread by the fecal-oral route of transmission but may also be spread by the pharyngeal route.

Poliovirus vaccine, inactivated induces the production of neutralizing antibodies against each type of virus which are related to protective efficacy and induces antibody responses in most children after administering fewer doses than the vaccine available in the United States prior to 1988.

IPV is able to induce secretory antibody (IgA) produced in the pharynx and gut and reduces pharyngeal excretion of poliovirus Type 1 from 75% in children with neutralizing antibodies at levels less than 1:8 to 25% in children with neutralizing antibodies at levels more than 1:64. There is also evidence of induction of herd immunity with IPV, and that this herd immunity is sufficiently maintained in a population vaccinated only with IPV.

Paralytic polio and VAPP have not been reported in association with administration of poliovirus vaccine, inactivated. It is expected that an IPV only schedule will eliminate the risk of VAPP in both recipients and contacts compared to a schedule that included OPV.

Contraindications

Poliovirus vaccine, inactivated is contraindicated in persons with a history of hypersensitivity to any component of the vaccine, including 2-phenoxyethanol, formaldehyde, neomycin, streptomycin and polymyxin B.

No further doses should be given if anaphylaxis or anaphylactic shock occurs within 24 hours of administration of 1 dose of vaccine.

Vaccination of persons with an acute, febrile illness should be deferred until after recovery; however, minor illness, such as mild upper respiratory tract infection, with or without low grade fever, are not reasons for postponing vaccine administration.

Warnings/Precautions

➤*Latex allergy:* This product contains dry, natural latex rubber as follows: The stopper to the vial contains no rubber of any kind. In the case of the syringe, the needle cover contains dry, natural latex rubber but the plunger for the syringe contains no rubber of any kind.

➤*Immunodeficiency:* Immunodeficient patients or patients under immunosuppressive therapy may not develop a protective immune response against paralytic poliomyelitis after administration of IPV.

Administration of IPV is not contraindicated in individuals infected with HIV.

➤*Hypersensitivity reactions:* Neomycin, streptomycin, polymyxin B, 2-phenoxyethanol, and formaldehyde are used in the production of this vaccine. Although purification procedures eliminate measurable amounts of these substances, traces may be present (see Ingredients) and allergic reactions may occur in persons sensitive to these substances (see Contraindications).

Although no causal relationship between IPV and Guillain-Barré syndrome (GBS) has been established, GBS has been temporally related to administration of another inactivated poliovirus vaccine. Deaths have been reported in temporal association with the administration of inactivated poliovirus vaccine (see Adverse Reactions).

Epinephrine injection (1:1000) and other appropriate agents should be available to control immediate allergic reactions.

➤*Pregnancy: Category C.*

Animal reproduction studies have not been conducted with poliovirus vaccine, inactivated. It is also not known whether IPV can cause fetal harm when administered to a pregnant woman or can affect reproduction capacity. Poliovirus vaccine, inactivated should be given to a pregnant woman only if clearly needed.

➤*Lactation:* It is not known whether IPV is excreted in human milk. Because many drugs are excreted in human milk, exercise caution when IPV is administered to a breast-feeding woman.

➤*Children:* See Indications for more information.

Drug Interactions

➤*Immunosuppressive agents:* If poliovirus vaccine, inactivated has been administered to persons receiving immunosuppressive therapy, an adequate immunologic response may not be obtained.

Adverse Reactions

In earlier studies with the vaccine grown in primary monkey kidney cells, transient local reactions at the site of injection were observed. Erythema, induration and pain occurred in 3.2%, 1%, and 13%, respectively, of vaccinees within 48 hours postvaccination. Temperatures of greater than or equal to 39°C (greater than or equal to 102°F) were reported in 38% of vaccinees. Other symptoms included irritability, sleepiness, fussiness, and crying. Because IPV was given in a different site but concurrently with diphtheria and tetanus toxoids and pertussis vaccine adsorbed (DTP), these systemic reactions could not be attributed to a specific vaccine. However, these systemic reactions were comparable in frequency and severity to that reported for DTP given alone without IPV. Although no causal relationship has been established, deaths have occurred in temporal association after vaccination of infants with IPV.

➤*IPV adverse reactions:*

IPV Adverse Reactions (Administered Intramuscularly, Concomitantly at Separate Sites with AvP[a] Whole-Cell DTP Vaccine at 2 and 4 Months of Age and with AvP Acellular Pertussis Vaccine at 18 months of age)

	Age at immunization								
	2 months (n = 211)			4 months (n = 206)			18 months[b] (n = 74)		
Reaction	6 hours	24 hours	48 hours	6 hours	24 hours	48 hours	6 hours	24 hours	48 hours
Local, IPV alone[c]									
Erythema greater than 1 inch	0.5%	0.5%	0.5%	1%	0%	0%	1.4%	0%	0%
Swelling	11.4%	5.7%	0.9%	11.2%	4.9%	1.9%	2.7%	0%	0%
Tenderness	29.4%	8.5%	2.8%	22.8%	4.4%	1%	13.5%	4.1%	0%
Systemic[d]									
Fever greater than 39°C (102.2°F)	1%	0.5%	0.5%	2%	0.5%	0%	0%	0%	4.2%
Irritability	64.5%	24.6%	17.5%	49.5%	25.7%	11.7%	14.7%	6.7%	8%
Tiredness	60.7%	31.8%	7.1%	38.8%	18.4%	6.3%	9.3%	5.3%	4%
Anorexia	16.6%	8.1%	4.3%	6.3%	4.4%	2.4%	2.7%	1.3%	2.7%
Vomiting	1.9%	2.8%	2.8%	1.9%	1.5%	1%	1.3%	1.3%	0%
Persistent crying	Percentage of infants within 72 hours after immunization was 0% after dose 1, 1.4% after dose 2, and 0% after dose 3.								

[a] AvP (Aventis Pasteur Inc) formerly known as Connaught Laboratories, Inc.
[b] Children vaccinated with DTaP vaccine.
[c] Data are from the IPV administration site, given intramuscularly.
[d] The adverse reaction profile includes the concomitant use of AvP whole-cell DTP vaccine or DTaP (diphtheria and tetanus toxoids and acellular pertussis vaccine, adsorbed) with IPV. Rates are comparable in frequency and severity to that reported for whole-cell DTP given alone.

POLIOVIRUS VACCINE, INACTIVATED (IPV) — INJECTION

➤*CNS:* See Warnings/Precautions for more information.

➤*GI:* Anorexia and vomiting occurred with frequencies not significantly different as reported when DTP was given alone without IPV or OPV.

Patient Information

Instruct patients, parents, or guardians to report any serious adverse reactions to their health care provider.

Inform the patient, parent, or guardian of the benefits and risks of the vaccine.

Inform the patient, parent, or guardian of the importance of completing the immunization series.

Provide the Vaccine Information Materials (VIMs) which are required to be given with each immunization.

INFLUENZA TYPES A AND B VACCINE

Rx	**Afluria** (CSL Biotherapies)	**Injection, suspension (purified split-virus):** 15 mcg HA[a] each of A/California/7/2009 NYMC X-181 (H1N1), A/Victoria/210/2009 NYMC X-187 (H3N2) (an A/Perth/16/2009-like strain), and B/Brisbane/60/2008 per 0.5 mL	In preservative-free, 0.5 mL prefilled, single-dose syringes and 5 mL multidose vials with preservative (thimerosal).[b,c]
Rx	**Agriflu** (Novartis Vaccines)	**Injection, suspension (purified split-virus):** 15 mcg HA each of A/California/7/2009 NYMC X-181 (H1N1), A/Victoria/210/2009 NYMC X-187 (H3N2) (an A/Perth/16/2009-like virus), and B/Brisbane/60/2008 per 0.5 mL	Preservative free. In 0.5 mL prefilled, single-dose syringes.[d]
Rx	**Fluarix** (GlaxoSmithKline)	**Injection, suspension (purified split-virus):** 15 mcg HA each of A/California/7/2009 NYMC X-181 (H1N1), A/Victoria/210/2009 NYMC X-187 (H3N2) (an A/Perth/16/2009-like virus), and B/Brisbane/60/2008 per 0.5 mL	Preservative free. In 0.5 mL prefilled, single-dose syringes.[e,f]
Rx	**FluLaval** (GlaxoSmithKline)	**Injection, suspension (purified split-virus):** 15 mcg HA each of A/California/7/2009 NYMC X-181 (H1N1), A/Victoria/210/2009 NYMC X-187 (H3N2) (an A/Perth/16/2009-like virus), and B/Brisbane/60/2008 per 0.5 mL	Thimerosal. In 5 mL multidose vials.[g,h]
Rx	**Fluvirin** (Novartis Vaccines)	**Injection, suspension (purified split-virus):** 15 mcg HA each of A/Christchurch/16/2010, NIB-74 (H1N1) (an A/California/7/2009-like virus), A/Victoria/210/2009 NYMC X-187 (H3N2) (an A/Perth/16/2009-like strain), and B/Brisbane/60/2008 per 0.5 mL	In preservative-free, 0.5 mL prefilled, single-dose syringes[i] and 5 mL multidose vials[g,j] with preservative (thimerosal).
Rx	**Fluzone** (Sanofi Pasteur)	**Injection, suspension (purified split-virus):** 15 mcg HA each of A/California/7/2009 X-179A (H1N1), A/Victoria/210/2009 X-187 (H3N2) (an A/Perth/16/2009-like virus), and B/Brisbane/60/2008 per 0.5 mL	In preservative-free, 0.25 and 0.5 mL prefilled syringes; preservative-free, 0.5 mL single-dose vials; and 5 mL multi-dose vials with preservative (thimerosal).[g,k]
Rx	**Fluzone Intradermal** (Sanofi Pasteur)	**Injection, suspension (purified split-virus):** 9 mcg HA each of A/California/7/2009 X-179A (H1N1), A/Victoria/210/2009 X-187 (H3N2) (an A/Perth/16/2009-like virus), and B/Brisbane/60/2008 per 0.1 mL	Preservative free. In 0.1 mL single-dose, prefilled microinjection systems[l]
Rx	**Fluzone High-Dose** (Sanofi Pasteur)	**Injection, suspension (purified split-virus):** 60 mcg HA each of A/California/7/2009 X-179A (H1N1), A/Victoria/210/2009 X-187 (H3N2) (an A/Perth/16/2009-like virus), and B/Brisbane/60/2008 per 0.5 mL	Preservative free. In 0.5 mL prefilled, single-dose syringes.[m]
Rx	**FluMist** (MedImmune Vaccines)	**Spray, solution; intranasal:** FFU[a] $10^{6.5-7.5}$ of A/California/7/2009 (H1N1), A/Perth/16/2009 (H3N2), and B/Brisbane/60/2008 per 0.2 mL actuation	Preservative free and latex free. In 0.2 mL prefilled, single-use sprayers.[n]

[a] HA = hemagglutinin; FFU = fluorescent focus units.
[b] Each dose may contain residual amounts of sodium taurodeoxycholate (≤ 10 ppm), ovalbumin (≤ 1 mcg), neomycin sulfate (≤ 3 nanograms), polymyxin B (≤ 0.5 nanograms), and beta-propiolactone (< 2 nanograms).
[c] With mercury 24.5 mcg/dose.
[d] Each 0.5 mL dose may contain residual amounts of egg proteins (< 0.4 mg), formaldehyde (≤ 10 mcg), kanamycin (≤ 0.03 mcg), neomycin (≤ 0.02 mcg), polysorbate 80 (≤ 50 mcg), and CTAB (≤ 12 mcg).
[e] Each 0.5 mL dose also contains octoxynol-10 ≤ 0.085 mg, alpha-tocopheryl hydrogen succinate ≤ 0.1 mg, and ≤ 0.415 mg of polysorbate 80. Each dose also may contain residual amounts of hydrocortisone ≤ 0.0016 mcg, gentamicin sulfate ≤ 0.15 mcg, ovalbumin ≤ 0.05 mcg, formaldehyde ≤ 5 mcg, and sodium deoxycholate ≤ 50 mcg.
[f] The tip caps of the prefilled syringes may contain natural latex rubber. The rubber plungers do not contain latex.
[g] With mercury 25 mcg/dose.
[h] Each dose may also contain residual amounts of egg protein (ovalbumin ≤ 1 mcg), formaldehyde ≤ 25 mcg, and sodium deoxycholate ≤ 50 mcg.
[i] The 0.5 mL prefilled syringes are formulated without preservative; however, thimerosal is used during manufacturing and is removed by subsequent purification steps to a trace amount (mercury ≤ 1 mcg per 0.5 mL dose).
[j] Each dose from the multidose vial or prefilled syringe may also contain residual amounts of ovalbumin (≤ 1 mcg), polymyxin (≤ 3.75 mcg), neomycin (≤ 2.5 mcg), betapropiolactone (≤ 0.5 mcg), and nonylphenol ethoxylate (≤ 0.015%).
[k] Each 0.5 mL dose may contain residual amounts of formaldehyde (≤ 100 mcg), octylphenol ethoxylate (≤ 100 mcg), and gelatin (0.05%).
[l] Each 0.1 mL dose contains formaldehyde (≤ 20 mcg) and octylphenol ethoxylate (≤ 50 mcg).
[m] Each 0.5 mL dose contains formaldehyde (≤ 100 mcg) and octylphenol ethoxylate (≤ 250 mcg).
[n] Each 0.2 mL dose also contains monosodium glutamate 0.188 mg, hydrolyzed porcine gelatin 2 mg, arginine 2.42 mg, sucrose 13.68 mg, dibasic potassium phosphate 2.26 mg, monobasic potassium phosphate 0.96 mg, and gentamicin sulfate < 0.015 mcg/mL.

INFLUENZA TYPES A AND B VACCINE — INJECTION

For additional information, refer to the Agents for Active Immunization introduction.

Indications

➤*Influenza vaccination:* For active immunization against influenza disease caused by influenza virus subtypes A and type B contained in the vaccine in the following persons:
- 6 months and older (*Afluria* and *Fluzone*),
- 3 years and older (*Fluarix*),
- 4 years and older (*Fluvirin*),
- 18 years and older (*Agriflu* and *FluLaval*),
- 18 through 64 years of age (*Fluzone Intradermal*),
- 65 years and older (*Fluzone High-Dose*).
- The 2011-2012 seasonal flu vaccine includes the H1N1 strain derived from the pandemic strain that circulated in 2009 to 2010.

Administration and Dosage

➤*General dosing considerations:* Annual vaccination with the current vaccine is necessary because immunity declines during the year after vaccination. Vaccine prepared for a previous season should not be administered to provide protection for the current season.

The Advisory Committee on Immunization Practices (ACIP) has issued recommendations regarding the use of the inactivated influenza virus vaccine.

Children who were given 2 doses of influenza vaccine last season or at least 1 dose 2 or more years ago should only receive 1 dose of influenza vaccine.

Children 6 months to 8 years of age who did not receive at least 1 dose of 2009 H1N1 vaccine should receive 2 doses of 2010 seasonal flu vaccine.

➤*Adults:*

Influenza – 0.5 mL intramuscularly (IM) as a single dose of *Afluria, Agriflu, Fluarix, FluLaval, Fluvirin, Fluzone,* or *Fluzone High-Dose*.

0.1 mL intradermally as a single dose of *Fluzone Intradermal*.

INFLUENZA TYPES A AND B VACCINE — INJECTION

➤*Children:*

Influenza –

Afluria:

• *9 years and older* – See Adults for dosing.

• *3 to 8 years of age* – 0.5 mL IM as a single dose. Repeat the dose approximately 4 weeks later for those who are receiving the influenza vaccine for the first time or were vaccinated for the first time last season with only 1 dose.

• *6 to 35 months of age* – 0.25 mL IM as a single dose. Repeat the dose approximately 4 weeks later for those who are receiving the influenza vaccine for the first time or were vaccinated for the first time last season with only 1 dose.

Fluarix:

• *9 years and older* – See Adults for dosing.

• *3 to younger than 9 years* – 0.5 mL IM as a single dose. Repeat the dose at least 4 weeks later for those who are receiving the influenza vaccine for the first time or were vaccinated for the first time last season with only 1 dose.

Fluvirin:

• *9 years and older* – See Adults for dosing.

• *4 to 8 years of age* – 0.5 mL IM as a single dose. Repeat the dose at least 4 weeks later for those who are receiving the influenza vaccine for the first time or were vaccinated for the first time last season with only 1 dose.

Fluzone:

• *9 years and older* – See Adults for dosing.

• *3 to 8 years of age* – 0.5 mL IM as a single dose. Repeat the dose at least 1 month later for those who are receiving the influenza vaccine for the first time or were vaccinated for the first time last season with only 1 dose.

• *6 to 35 months of age* – 0.25 mL IM as a single dose. Repeat the dose at least 1 month later for those who are receiving the influenza vaccine for the first time or were vaccinated for the first time last season with only 1 dose.

➤*Elderly:*

Fluzone High-Dose – 0.5 mL IM as a single dose.

➤*Coadministration with other vaccines:* If the influenza vaccine is to be given at the same time as another injectable vaccine(s), the vaccine(s) should always be administered at separate injection sites.

➤*Administration:* Shake the prefilled syringes, microinjection systems, and single-dose vials well before administration and the multidose vials before withdrawing each dose. Before injection, the skin over the site to be injected should be cleansed with a suitable germicide. For IM administration, after insertion of the needle, aspirate to ensure that the needle has not entered a blood vessel. It is recommended that small syringes (0.5 or 1 mL) should be used to minimize any product loss.

Adult and elderly patients – Administer as a single IM dose preferably in the deltoid muscle. A needle of 1 inch or more is preferred because needles less than 1 inch might be of insufficient length to penetrate muscle tissue in certain adults and older children.

Children – The preferred sites for IM injections are the anterolateral aspect of the thigh in infants (6 to 12 months of age) or the deltoid muscle of the upper arm in toddlers and young children (12 months to 17 years of age).

The needle size may range from ⅞ to 1¼ inches, depending on the size of the child's deltoid muscle, and should be of sufficient length to penetrate the muscle tissue. The anterolateral thigh can be used, but the needle should be longer, usually 1 inch. ACIP recommends a needle length of ⅞ to 1 inch for children younger than 12 months for IM vaccination into the anterolateral thigh.

➤*Admixture compatibility:* Influenza virus vaccine should not be mixed with any other vaccine in the same syringe or vial.

➤*Storage/Stability:* Store refrigerated between 2° and 8°C (35° and 46°F). Do not freeze. Discard if the vaccine is or has previously been frozen. Store *Afluria, Fluarix, Fluvirin,* and *FluLaval* in the original package to protect from light. Once entered, multidose vials should be discarded after 28 days. Between uses, return the multidose vial to the refrigerator at 2° and 8°C (36° to 46°F).

Contraindications

History of hypersensitivity to egg proteins (eg, eggs or egg products); hypersensitivity to any component of the vaccine, including thimerosal (a mercury derivative), or a life-threatening reaction to previous administration of the vaccine; known hypersensitivity to neomycin or polymyxin (*Afluria* only); known hypersensitivity to kanamycin or neomycin (*Agriflu* only).

Warnings/Precautions

➤*Guillain-Barré syndrome:* If Guillain-Barré syndrome has occurred within 6 weeks of receipt of a prior influenza vaccine, base the decision to give influenza vaccine on careful consideration of the potential benefits and possible risks.

➤*Immunocompromised:* If influenza vaccine is administered to immunocompromised persons, including persons receiving immunosuppressive therapy, the expected immune response may not be obtained.

➤*Bleeding disorders:* As with other IM injections, give influenza vaccine with caution to persons with bleeding disorders, such as hemophilia, or to persons on anticoagulant therapy to avoid the risk of hematoma following injection.

➤*Efficacy:* As with any vaccine, vaccination with influenza vaccine may not protect 100% of susceptible persons.

➤*Concomitant vaccines:* There are no data to assess the coadministration of influenza vaccine with other vaccines. If influenza vaccine is to be given at the same time as another injectable vaccine, always administer the vaccines at different injection sites.

➤*Hypersensitivity reactions:* Have appropriate medical treatment and supervision readily available for immediate use in case of a rare anaphylactic reaction following the administration of the vaccine.

Latex sensitivity – The tip caps of the *Fluarix, Fluvirin, Fluzone,* and *Fluzone High-Dose* prefilled syringes may contain natural latex rubber that may cause allergic reactions in latex-sensitive persons.

➤*Pregnancy: Category B (Agriflu, Fluarix, FluLaval, Fluzone Intradermal); Category C (Afluria, Fluvirin, Fluzone, Fluzone High-Dose).*

Animal reproduction studies have not been conducted with influenza vaccine. There are no adequate and well-controlled studies in pregnant women. It is not known whether influenza vaccine can cause fetal harm when administered to a pregnant woman or can affect reproduction capacity. Administer influenza vaccine to a pregnant woman only if clearly needed. According to the ACIP, vaccination is recommended in women who will be pregnant during the influenza season. The clinical judgment of the attending health care provider should prevail at all times in determining whether to administer influenza vaccine to a pregnant woman.

➤*Lactation:* Excretion in human breast milk is not known. Because many drugs are excreted in human milk, exercise caution when administering to a breast-feeding woman. The ACIP recommends vaccination in breast-feeding women who are in contact with infants or children younger than 5 years because they are more likely to require medical attention or hospitalization if infected. Breast-feeding does not affect the immune response adversely and is not a contraindication for vaccination.

➤*Children:* The ACIP recommends that all children 6 months and older receive routine influenza vaccination.

Afluria – Safety and effectiveness of *Afluria* in children younger than 6 months have not been established.

Administration of CSL's 2010 Southern Hemisphere influenza vaccine has been associated with increased postmarketing reports of fever febrile seizures in children in predominantly younger than 5 years, as compared with previous years.

Agriflu, Fluzone High-Dose, FluLaval, and *Fluzone Intradermal* – Safety and effectiveness in children have not been established.

Fluarix –

Safety and efficacy of *Fluarix* in children younger than 3 years have not been established.

Fluvirin – The safety and immunogenicity of *Fluvirin* have not been established in children younger than 4 years. *Fluvirin* is not indicated in children younger than 4 years because there is evidence of diminished immune response in this group.

Fluzone – Safety and effectiveness of *Fluzone* vaccine in infants younger than 6 months have not been established.

➤*Elderly:* HI antibody response in elderly patients was lower after administration in comparison with younger adults.

Fluzone High-Dose – *Fluzone High-Dose* is indicated for adults 65 years and older.

Fluzone Intradermal – Safety and effectiveness in persons 65 years and older have not been established.

Drug Interactions

➤*Concomitant vaccines:* See Warnings/Precautions for more information.

Influenza Vaccine Drug Interactions

Precipitant drug	Object drug[a]		Description
Immunosuppressants (eg, alkylating drugs, antimetabolites, cytotoxic drugs, corticosteroids, radiation)	Influenza vaccine	⬇	Coadministration may reduce the expected antibody response to influenza vaccine.
Influenza vaccine	Phenytoin	⬆	Data are conflicting. Influenza vaccine may inhibit the clearance of phenytoin; however, no adverse clinical effects have been shown in studies. Use with caution.
Influenza vaccine	Theophylline	⬆	Data are conflicting. Influenza vaccine may inhibit the clearance of theophylline; however, no adverse clinical effects have been shown in studies. Use with caution.
Influenza vaccine	Warfarin	⬆	Data are conflicting. Influenza vaccine may inhibit the clearance of warfarin; however, no adverse clinical effects have been shown in studies. Use with caution.

[a] ⬇ = object drug decreased; ⬆ = object drug increased.

INFLUENZA TYPES A AND B VACCINE — INJECTION

Adverse Reactions

➤*Reporting adverse reactions:* Encourage reporting by patients, parents, or guardians of all adverse reactions after vaccine administration. Report adverse reactions following immunization with vaccine to the US Department of Health and Human Services' Vaccine Adverse Event Reporting System (VAERS). Reporting forms and information about reporting requirements or completion of the form can be obtained from VAERS at 1-800-822-7967. Reporting forms may also be obtained at the VAERS Web site at http://www.vaers.hhs.gov.

➤*Afluria:*

Most common adverse reactions – In adults, the most common local (injection-site) adverse reactions observed were pain, redness (erythema), swelling, and tenderness. The most common systemic adverse reactions observed were headache, malaise, and muscle aches.

In children, the most common local (injection-site) adverse reactions observed were pain, redness, and swelling. The most common systemic adverse reactions observed were cough, fever, headache, irritability, loss of appetite, muscle aches, rhinitis, sore throat, and vomiting/diarrhea.

Hypersensitivity – Serious allergic reactions, including anaphylactic shock, have been observed during postmarketing surveillance. Administration has been associated with increased postmarketing reports of fever and febrile seizures in children predominantly younger than 5 years, as compared with previous years.

Adults –

Adverse reactions in adults within 5 days of vaccination (1% or more):

Afluria Adverse Reactions[a,b]			
	Patients 18 to < 65 years of age		Patients ≥ 65 years of age
Adverse reactions	*Afluria*[c] (n = 1,089)	Placebo[d] (n = 268)	*Afluria* (n = 206)
CNS			
Headache	26%	26%	15%
Malaise	20%	19%	10%
GI			
Nausea	6%	9%	3%
Vomiting	1%	1%	0%
Local			
Bruising	5%	1%	4%
Pain[e]	40%	9%	9%
Redness	16%	8%	23%
Swelling	9%	1%	11%
Tenderness[f]	60%	18%	34%
Miscellaneous			
Chills/Shivering	3%	2%	7%
Fever ≥ 37.7°C (99.86°F)	1%	1%	1%
Muscle aches	13%	9%	14%

[a] In study 1, 87% of solicited local and systemic adverse reactions were mild, 12% were moderate, and 1% were severe. In study 2, 76.5% were mild, 20.5% were moderate, and 3% were severe. In both studies, most solicited local and systemic adverse reactions lasted no longer than 2 days.
[b] Adverse reactions reported within 5 days after administration.
[c] Includes subjects who received either the single-dose (preservative-free) or multidose formulation of *Afluria*.
[d] Thimerosal-containing placebo.
[e] Pain defined as spontaneously painful without touch.
[f] Tenderness defined as pain on touching.

Adverse reactions in adults within 21 days of vaccination (1% or more):

Afluria Adverse Reactions (≥ 1%)[a,b]			
	Patients 18 to < 65 years of age		Patients ≥ 65 years of age
Adverse reactions	*Afluria*[c] (n = 1,089)	Placebo[d] (n = 268)	*Afluria* (n = 206)
Musculoskeletal			
Back pain	2%	0.4%	2%
Muscle spasms	0.4%	1%	0%
Myalgia	1%	1%	1%
Respiratory			
Cough	1%	0.4%	5%
Lower respiratory tract infection	0%	0%	1%
Nasal congestion	1%	1%	7%
Pharyngolaryngeal pain	3%	1%	5%
Rhinorrhea	1%	1%	5%
Upper respiratory tract infection	2%	1%	0.5%
Miscellaneous			
Diarrhea	2%	3%	1%
Headache	8%	6%	8%
Reactogenicity event	3%	3%	0%
Viral infection	0.4%	1%	0%

[a] In study 1, 63% of unsolicited adverse reactions were mild, 35% were moderate, and 2% were severe. In study 2, 47% were mild, 51% were moderate, and 3% were severe. In both studies, most unsolicited adverse reactions lasted no longer than 5 days.
[b] Adverse reactions reported within 21 days of administration.
[c] Includes subjects who received either the single-dose (preservative-free) or multidose formulation of *Afluria*.
[d] Thimerosal-containing placebo.

Children –

Adverse reactions in children within 7 days of vaccination (1% or more):

Afluria Adverse Reactions[a] in Children Within 7 Days after Vaccination (1% or more)				
	Children ≥ 6 months to < 3 years (n = 151)[b]		Children ≥ 3 to < 9 years (n = 147)[c]	
Adverse reactions	Dose 1	Dose 2	Dose 1	Dose 2
CNS				
Headache	2%[d]	3%[e]	14%	11%
Irritability	48%	41%	20%	17%
GI				
Loss of appetite	19%	24%	8%	5%
Vomiting/Diarrhea	15%	14%	8%	7%
Local				
Erythema	36%	38%	37%	46%
Pain	36%	37%	59%	62%
Swelling	16%	21%	25%	27%
Respiratory				
Cough	21%	32%	19%	19%
Wheezing/Shortness of breath	3%	9%	3%	2%
Special senses				
Earache	3%[e]	3%[f]	4%	1%
Rhinitis	37%	48%	21%	29%
Sore throat	2%[d]	5%[e]	8%	11%
Miscellaneous				
Fever[g]	23%	23%	16%	8%
Myalgia	1%[f]	3%[e]	14%	8%

[a] In study 4, 78% of all local and systemic solicited reactions experienced by children 6 months to < 3 years of age were mild, 19% were moderate, and 3% were severe; 76% of all events experienced by children 3 years to < 9 years of age were mild, 20% were moderate, and 4% severe. Severe pain was reported by < 1% of children 6 months to < 3 years of age and 3% in children 3 years to < 9 years of age. Severe fever (more than 103.1°F axillary or more than 104°F oral) was reported by less than 1% of subjects in children 6 months to < 3 years of age and 1% of subjects in children 3 years to < 9 years of age.
[b] Dosage in children 6 months to < 3 years of age was 0.25 mL.
[c] Dosage in children 3 years to < 9 years of age was 0.5 mL.
[d] Data obtained from a total of 148 subjects.
[e] Data obtained from a total of 150 subjects.
[f] Data obtained from a total of 149 subjects.
[g] Axillary temperature at least 37.5°C (99.5°F) or oral temperature at least 38°C (100.4°F).

Adverse reactions in children within 30 days of vaccination (5% or more):

Afluria Adverse Reactions[a] in Children				
	Children ≥ 6 months to < 3 years (n = 151)[b]		Children ≥ 3 to < 9 years (n = 147)[c]	
Adverse reactions	Dose 1	Dose 2	Dose 1	Dose 2
CNS				
Headache	1.3%	0.7%	6.1%	4.1%
Irritability	3.3%	5.3%	0.7%	0.7%
Respiratory				
Cough	10.6%	13.2%	10.9%	13.6%
Nasopharyngitis	5.3%	7.9%	5.4%	5.4%

INFLUENZA TYPES A AND B VACCINE — INJECTION

Afluria Adverse Reactions[a] in Children				
	Children ≥ 6 months to < 3 years (n = 151)[b]		Children ≥ 3 to < 9 years (n = 147)[c]	
Adverse reactions	Dose 1	Dose 2	Dose 1	Dose 2
Upper respiratory tract infection	9.9%	7.3%	6.1%	6.1%
Special senses				
Rhinitis	13.2%	9.9%	6.8%	10.9%
Rhinorrhea	7.3%	6%	6.8%	4.8%
Miscellaneous				
Influenza-like illness	13.9%	10.6%	6.8%	3.4%
Pyrexia	2.65	9.3%	2.7%	4.1%
Teething	14.6%	9.9%	0%	0%
Vomiting	5.3%	2.6%	2%	2.7%

[a] In study 4, for both doses and both groups combined, 47% of unsolicited adverse reactions were mild, 42% were moderate, and 12% were severe.
[b] Dosage in children 6 months to < 3 years of age was 0.25 mL.
[c] Dosage in children 3 to < 9 years of age was 0.5 mL.

Fever:

Fever[a] in Children Within 7 Days of Vaccination With *Afluria*							
	Children 6 months to < 3 years[b]		Children 3 to < 5 years[c]		Children 5 to < 9 years[d]		Children 9 to < 18 years[e]
Product	Dose 1	Dose 2	Dose 1	Dose 2	Dose 1	Dose 2	Dose 1
Afluria[f]	37%	15%	32%	14%	16%	0%	6%
Comparator[f]	14%	14%	11%	16%	9%	2%	4%

[a] Defined as ≥ 99.5°F axillary or ≥ 100.4°F orally after first or second vaccination.
[b] Dosage in subjects 6 months to < 3 years of age was one or two 0.25 mL doses (depending on vaccination history) 1 month apart. Group sizes were n = 229 for *Afluria* dose 1, n = 228 for comparator dose 1, n = 96 for *Afluria* dose 2, and n = 110 for comparator dose 2.
[c] Dosage in subjects 3 to < 5 years of age was one or two 0.5 mL doses (depending on vaccination history) 1 month apart. Group sizes were n = 91 for *Afluria* dose 1, n = 90 for comparator dose 1, n = 29 for *Afluria* dose 2, and n = 25 for comparator dose 2.
[d] Dosage in subjects 5 to < 9 years of age was one or two 0.5 mL doses (depending on vaccination history) 1 month apart. Group sizes were n = 161 for *Afluria* dose 1, n = 165 for comparator dose 1, n = 39 for *Afluria* dose 2, and n = 53 for comparator dose 2.
[e] Dosage in subjects 9 to < 18 years of age was one 0.5 mL dose. Group sizes were n = 254 for *Afluria* dose 1 and n = 250 for comparator dose 1.
[f] 2009 to 2010 formulation (A/Brisbane/59/2007, IVR-148 [H1N1], A/Uruguay/716/2007, NYMC X-175C [H3N2] [an A/Brisbane/10/2007-like strain], and B/Brisbane/60/2008).

➤*Agriflu*:

Most common adverse reactions – The most common local (injection-site) adverse reactions observed in clinical studies were pain, induration, swelling, and erythema. The most common systemic adverse reactions observed were headache, myalgia, and malaise. These reactions are typically mild. Serious allergic reactions, including anaphylactic shock, have been observed during postmarketing surveillance.

Adverse reactions days 1 to 4 after vaccination –

Agriflu Adverse Reactions Days 1 to 4 After Vaccination				
	Study 1 2007 NCT00464672 (18 to 64 years of age)		Study 2 2007 to 2008 NCT00617851 (18 to 49 years of age)	
	Agriflu (n = 460)	Comparator[a] (n = 233)	*Agriflu* (n = 1,209)	Comparator[a] (n = 202)
CNS				
Fatigue	9%	9%	8%	7%
Headache	20%	16%	22%	22%
Malaise	10%	11%	10%	12%
Dermatologic				
Sweating	4%	4%	4%	4%
Local				
Ecchymosis	< 1%	0%	0%	< 1%
Erythema	< 1%	1%	< 1%	< 1%
Injection-site pain	25%	30%	22%	20%
Severe injection-site pain[b]	< 1%	0%	< 1%	< 1%
Induration	2%	1%	1%	1%
Swelling	< 1%	1%	1%	< 1%
Musculoskeletal				
Arthralgia	5%	6%	5%	6%
Myalgia	13%	15%	16%	19%
Miscellaneous				
Chills	3%	7%	6%	8%
Fever (≥ 38°C)	1%	2%	3%	3%

[a] Comparator is US-licensed trivalent, inactivated influenza virus vaccine (*Fluvirin*).
[b] Severe injection-site pain = local reaction leading to the inability to perform normal daily activities.

Other adverse reactions (more than 1%) – Unsolicited adverse reactions were reported by subjects over a 3-week period after vaccination. Unsolicited adverse reactions that occurred in more than 1% of subjects included influenza-like illness (4% of *Agriflu* subjects and 3% of active comparator subjects) and headache (2% of *Agriflu* and comparator subjects). A total of 17% of subjects in the *Agriflu* and the comparator groups reported unsolicited adverse reactions: 15% and 16% of subjects in the *Agriflu* and in the comparator groups, respectively, had mild unsolicited adverse reactions, 2% and 1% of subjects had moderate adverse reactions, and less than 1% of subjects in both groups had severe adverse reactions.

➤*Fluarix*:

Adults – In adults, the most common local adverse reactions and general adverse reactions observed were pain and redness at the injection site, muscle aches, fatigue, and headache.

Adverse reactions within 4 days of vaccination:

Fluarix Adverse Reactions in Adults Reported Within 4 Days of Vaccination[a,b]		
Adverse reactions	*Fluarix* (n = 760)	Placebo (n = 192)
CNS		
Fatigue	20%	18%
Headache	19%	21%
Local		
Pain	55%	12%
Redness	18%	10%
Swelling	9%	6%
Musculoskeletal		
Arthralgia	6%	6%
Muscle aches	23%	12%
Miscellaneous		
Fever (≥ 100.4°F)	2%	2%
Shivering	3%	3%

[a] The 4 days included the day of vaccination and the subsequent 3 days.
[b] Total vaccinated cohort for safety included all vaccinated subjects for whom safety data were available.

- *Other adverse reactions (1% or more)* –
  GI: Diarrhea (1.6% vs 0%); vomiting (1.4% vs 0%).
  Respiratory: Nasopharyngitis (2.5% vs 1.6%); upper respiratory tract infection (3.9% vs 2.6%).
  Special senses: Nasal congestion (2.2% vs 2.1%).
  Miscellaneous: Dysmenorrhea (1.3% vs 1%); influenza-like illness (1.6% vs 0.5%).

Fluarix versus *Fluzone* adverse reactions:

Fluarix vs *Fluzone* Adverse Reactions Within 4 Days[a] of Vaccination[b]				
	18 to 64 years of age		≥ 65 years of age	
Adverse reactions	*Fluarix* (n = 315)	*Fluzone* (n = 314)	*Fluarix* (n = 601 to 602)	*Fluzone* (n = 596)
CNS				
Fatigue	21%	18%	9%	10%
Headache	20%	21%	8%	8%
Local				
Pain	48%	53%	19%	18%
Redness	13%	16%	11%	13%
Swelling	9%	11%	6%	9%
Musculoskeletal				
Arthralgia	9%	9%	6%	5%
Muscle aches	16%	13%	7%	7%

INFLUENZA TYPES A AND B VACCINE — INJECTION

Fluarix vs *Fluzone* Adverse Reactions Within 4 Days[a] of Vaccination[b]				
	18 to 64 years of age		≥ 65 years of age	
Adverse reactions	*Fluarix* (n = 315)	*Fluzone* (n = 314)	*Fluarix* (n = 601 to 602)	*Fluzone* (n = 596)
Miscellaneous				
Fever (≥ 99.5°F)	3%	1%	2%	1%
Shivering	3%	5%	2%	2%

[a] Four days included day of vaccination and the subsequent 3 days.
[b] Total vaccinated cohort for safety included all vaccinated subjects for whom safety data were available.

• *Other Fluarix versus Fluzone adverse reactions (at least 1%)* – Unsolicited adverse reactions that occurred in at least 1% of all recipients of *Fluarix* or *Fluzone* in the 21-day postvaccination period included headache (2.8% vs 2.3%), back pain (1.5% vs 0.4%), pain in extremity (1.2% vs 0.7%), pharyngolaryngeal pain (1.2% vs 0.9%), cough (1.1% vs 0.9%), fatigue (1.1% vs 0.7%), nasopharyngitis (1% vs 1.3%), nausea (0.4% vs 1%), arthralgia (0.3% vs 1%), and injection-site pruritus (0.2% vs 1%).

Adverse reactions within 21 days of vaccination: The percentage of subjects reporting at least 1 unsolicited reactions was similar among the groups (24.3% for *Fluarix* and 22.6% for placebo). Unsolicited adverse reactions that occurred in at least 1% of recipients of *Fluarix* and at a rate greater than placebo included injection-site pain (5.2% vs 1.3%), dysmenorrhea (1.3% vs 0.6%), and migraine (1% vs 0%).

• *Adverse reactions (1% or more)* –
Musculoskeletal: Musculoskeletal pain, neck pain.
Miscellaneous: Injection-site ecchymosis, injection-site induration, malaise, rhinitis, sweating.

Serious adverse reactions: In the 4 clinical trials in adults (N = 10,923), there was a single case of anaphylaxis reported with *Fluarix* (less than 0.01%).

Children –

Most common adverse reactions: In children 5 to younger than 18 years, the most common (at least 10%) local and general adverse reactions were similar to those in adults but also included swelling at the injection site. In children 3 years to younger than 5 years of age, the most common (at least 10%) local and general adverse reactions included pain, redness, and swelling at the injection site; irritability; loss of appetite; and drowsiness.

Adverse reactions within 4 days of vaccination:

Fluarix Adverse Reactions in Children Within 4 Days[a] of First Vaccination				
	Children 3 to		Children 5 to	
Adverse reactions	*Fluarix* (n = 350)	Comparator influenza vaccine (n = 341)	*Fluarix* (n = 1,348)	Comparator influenza vaccine (n = 451)
Local				
Pain	35%	38%	56%	56%
Redness	23%	20%	18%	16%
Swelling	14%	13%	14%	13%
CNS				
Drowsiness	13%	20%	—	—
Fatigue	—	—	20%	19%
Headache	—	—	15%	16%
Irritability	21%	22%	—	—
Musculoskeletal				
Arthralgia	—	—	6%	6%
Muscle aches	—	—	29%	29%
Miscellaneous				
Fever	7%	8%	4%	3%
Loss of appetite	13%	15%	—	—
Shivering	—	—	3%	4%

[a] Four days included day of vaccination and the subsequent 3 days.

Other adverse reactions (1% or more):
• *GI* – Diarrhea (2.5%); upper abdominal pain (1.4%); vomiting (3.2%).
• *Respiratory* – Cough (4.7%); nasopharyngitis (2.3%); pharyngolaryngeal pain (2.4%); upper respiratory tract congestion (1%); upper respiratory tract infection (5.5%).
• *Special senses* – Nasal congestion (1.8%); otitis media (2%); rhinorrhea (2.7%).
• *Miscellaneous* – Headache (2.8%); pyrexia (4.8%).

➤*FluLaval*:

Most common adverse reactions: In clinical trials, the most common (at least 10%) local and systemic adverse reactions were pain, redness, and/or swelling at the injection site; fatigue, headache, low-grade fever, malaise, and myalgia.

Adverse reactions within 4 days of vaccination:

FluLaval Adverse Reactions in Adults Within 4 Days of Vaccination[a]			
	US trial of adults 18 to 64 years of age (80% < 50 years)		Canadian trial of adults ≥ 50 years of age
Adverse reactions	*FluLaval* (n = 721)	*Fluzone* (n = 279)	*FluLaval*[b] (n = 328)
CNS			
Fatigue	17%	15%	10%
Headache	18%	17%	10%
Malaise	10%	10%	4%
Local			
Pain	24%	31%	21%
Redness	11%	10%	14%
Swelling	10%	10%	6%
Respiratory			
Cough	6%	7%	3%
Sore throat	9%	9%	5%
Miscellaneous			
Chest tightness	3%	1%	2%
Chills	5%	2%	3%
Facial swelling	1%	1%	1%
Fever[c]	11%	10%	1%
Myalgia	13%	16%	11%
Reddened eyes	6%	5%	3%

[a] Results > 1% reported to nearest whole percent; results > 0% but ≤ 1% reported as 1%.
[b] Includes subjects who received *FluLaval* and a similar investigational formulation of *FluLaval* with reduced thimerosal.
[c] Fever defined as 37.5°C or higher in the US study, and 38°C or higher in the Canadian study.

FluLaval versus *Fluzone* adverse reactions (5% or more):

FluLaval vs *Fluzone*Adverse Reactions[a] (≥ 5%)[b]			
	US trial of (safety follow-up 42 days) adults 18 to 64 years of age (80% < 50 years)		Canadian trial of (safety follow-up 6 months) adults ≥ 50 years of age
Adverse reactions	*FluLaval* (n = 721)	*Fluzone* (n = 279)	*FluLaval*[c] (n = 328)
CNS			
Fatigue	1%	1%	5%
Headache	7%	7%	19%
Dermatologic			
Injection-site erythema	1%	1%	5%
GI			
Diarrhea	1%	0%	5%
Nausea	1%	1%	5%
Musculoskeletal			
Arthralgia	1%	1%	8%
Back pain	1%	1%	6%
Myalgia	1%	1%	7%
Respiratory			
Cough	2%	2%	15%
Nasal congestion	1%	1%	5%
Nasopharyngitis	1%	1%	7%
Pharyngolaryngeal pain	2%	3%	12%
Upper respiratory tract infection	1%	1%	9%

[a] Adverse reactions in this table were reported spontaneously or in response to queries about changes in health status.
[b] Results > 1% reported to nearest whole percent; results > 0%, but ≤ 1% reported as 1%.
[c] Includes subjects who received *FluLaval* and a similar investigational formulation of *FluLaval* with reduced thimerosal.

➤*Fluvirin*:

Adults –

Serious adverse reactions: Serious allergic reactions, including anaphylactic shock, have been observed in individuals receiving *Fluvirin* during postmarketing surveillance.

Only 11 serious adverse reactions in patients 18 years and older have been reported to date from all the trials performed. These serious adverse reactions were a minor stroke experienced by a 67-year-old subject 14 days after vaccination (1990), death of an 82-year-old patient 35 days after vaccination (1990) in very early studies; death of a 72-year-old subject 19 days after vaccination (1998 to 1999), a hospitalization for hemorrhoidectomy of a 38-year-old man (1999 to 2000), a severe respiratory tract infection experienced by a 74-year-old patient 12 days after vaccination (2002 to 2003), a planned

INFLUENZA TYPES A AND B VACCINE — INJECTION

transurethral resection of the prostate in a patient with prior history of prostatism (2004 to 2005), 2 cases of influenza (2005 to 2006), a drug overdose (2005 to 2006), cholelithiasis (2005 to 2006), and a nasal septal operation (2005 to 2006). None of these reactions were considered causally related to vaccination.

• *Most common adverse reactions* – In adults, solicited local adverse reactions occurred with similar frequency in all trials. The most common solicited adverse reactions occurring in the first 96 hours after administration were associated with the injection site (eg, erythema, induration, mass, pain, and swelling), but were generally mild/moderate and transient. The most common solicited systemic adverse reactions were headache and myalgia.

The most common overall reactions in adults 18 to 64 years of age were fatigue, headache, injection-site reactions (erythema, induration, mass, and pain), and malaise.

Fluvirin Adverse Reactions in Adults From 1998 to 2001 (≥ 5%)[a]

Adverse reactions	1998 to 1999[b] 18 to 64 years (n = 66)	1998 to 1999[b] ≥ 65 years (n = 44)	1999 to 2000[b] 18 to 64 years (n = 76)	1999 to 2000[b] ≥ 65 years (n = 34)	2000 to 2001[b] 18 to 64 years (n = 75)	2000 to 2001[b] ≥ 65 years (n = 35)
CNS						
Fatigue	5%	5%	5%	3%	4%	—[c]
Headache	11%	2%	22%	9%	5%	—
Malaise	3%	2%	3%	3%	1%	—
Local						
Ecchymosis	6%	2%	4%	3%	5%	—
Edema	3%	2%	1%	6%	4%	3%
Hemorrhage	—	—	1%	—	—	—
Inflammation	8%	5%	8%	—	9%	3%
Mass	11%	2%	5%	—	11%	3%
Pain	24%	9%	21%	—	12%	—
Reaction	3%	—	3%	—	5%	3%
Musculoskeletal						
Arthralgia	—	2%	—	3%	—	—
Myalgia	2%	—	3%	—	—	—
Miscellaneous						
Fever (> 38°C)	2%	—	1%	—	—	—
Sweating	—	—	4%	—	1%	3%

[a] Results reported to the nearest whole percent.
[b] Solicited adverse reactions in the first 72 hours after administration.
[c] — = not reported.

Fluvirin Adverse Reactions in Adults From 2001 to 2005 (≥ 5%)[a]

Adverse reactions	2001 to 2002[b] 18 to 64 years (n = 75)	2001 to 2002[b] ≥ 65 years (n = 35)	2002 to 2003[b] 18 to 64 years (n = 107)	2002 to 2003[b] ≥ 65 years (n = 88)	2004 to 2005[b] 18 to 64 years (n = 74)	2004 to 2005[b] ≥ 65 years (n = 61)
CNS						
Fatigue	1%	3%	—[c]	—	7%	3%
Headache	11%	3%	11%	10%	19%	5%
Malaise	4%	—	3%	5%	1%	2%
Local						
Ecchymosis	3%	—	3%	3%	3%	2%
Edema	3%	3%	6%	2%	—	—
Erythema	7%	—	10%	6%	22%	8%
Induration	—	—	13%	3%	15%	2%
Mass	5%	3%	—	—	—	—
Pain	16%	3%	13%	8%	20%	15%
Pruritus	—	—	1%	—	—	—
Reaction	—	—	2%	—	—	—
Swelling	—	—	—	—	15%	7%
Musculoskeletal						
Arthralgia	—	—	2%	—	1%	—
Myalgia	4%	—	5%	3%	11%	2%
Miscellaneous						
Fever (> 38°C)	—	—	—	1%	—	—
Shivering	—	—	—	1%	—	—
Sweating	4%	3%	—	2%	—	—

[a] Results reported to the nearest whole percent.
[b] Solicited adverse reactions in the first 72 hours after administration.
[c] — = not reported.

Fluvirin Adverse Reactions in Adults from 2005 to 2006 (≥ 1%)[a]

Adverse reactions	*Fluvirin* (N = 304)
CNS	
Fatigue	18%
Headache	30%
Malaise	19%
Local	
Ecchymosis	7%
Erythema	16%
Induration	6%
Pain	55%
Swelling	5%
Musculoskeletal	
Arthralgia	7%
Myalgia	21%
Respiratory	
Chest tightness	1%
Cough	6%
Other difficulties breathing	1%
Sore throat	8%
Wheezing	1%
Miscellaneous	
Facial edema	—
Chills	7%
Nausea	7%
Sweating	6%

[a] Results reported to the nearest whole percent.

Fluvirin Adverse Reactions in Adults 1998 to 2001 (≥ 5%)[a]

Adverse reactions	1998 to 1999 18 to 64 years (n = 66)	1998 to 1999 ≥ 65 years (n = 44)	1999 to 2000 18 to 64 years (n = 76)	1999 to 2000 ≥ 65 years (n = 34)	2000 to 2001 18 to 64 years (n = 75)	2000 to 2001 ≥ 65 years (n = 35)
CNS						
Fatigue	12%	5%	11%	6%	7%	—[b]
Headache	18%	11%	29%	15%	19%	6%
Malaise	6%	9%	5%	3%	—	—
Migraine	6%	2%	—	—	—	—
Local						
Ecchymosis	6%	2%	—	—	5%	—
Edema	—	—	1%	6%	—	—
Inflammation	8%	5%	8%	—	9%	3%
Mass	11%	2%	5%	—	11%	3%
Pain	24%	9%	21%	—	12%	—
Reaction	—	—	—	—	5%	3%
Musculoskeletal						
Arthralgia	—	—	—	6%	—	—
Back pain	6%	7%	—	–	—	—
Myalgia	6%	2%	—	—	—	—
Respiratory						
Cough, increased	3%	5%	—	—	—	—
Pharyngitis	9%	2%	13%	—	8%	—
Rhinitis	5%	2%	—	—	7%	6%
Miscellaneous						
Ecchymosis	6%	2%	5%	3%	7%	—
Fever (> 38°C)	5%	—	—	—	—	—
Infection	5%	5%	—	—	—	—
Sweating	8%	2%	—	—	—	—

[a] Results reported to the nearest whole percent.
[b] Not reaching the cutoff of 5%.

INFLUENZA TYPES A AND B VACCINE — INJECTION

Fluvirin Adverse Reactions in Adults 2001 to 2005 (≥ 5%)[a]						
	2001 to 2002		2002 to 2003		2004 to 2005	
Adverse reactions	18 to 64 years (n = 75)	≥ 65 years (n = 35)	18 to 64 years (n = 107)	≥ 65 years (n = 88)	18 to 64 years (n = 74)	≥ 65 years (n = 61)
CNS						
Fatigue	7%	11%	10%	9%	5%	3%
Headache	27%	6%	33%	20%	16%	2%
Malaise	8%	3%	12%	9%	—[b]	—
Local						
Ecchymosis	5%	3%	4%	5%	—	—
Edema	—	—	6%	2%	5%	2%
Erythema	7%	6%	10%	6%	5%	—
Induration	—	—	13%	3%	9%	—
Mass	5%	3%	—	—	—	—
Pain	17%	9%	13%	8%	8%	3%
Musculoskeletal						
Arthralgia	—	—	5%	5%	—	—
Myalgia	5%	3%	9%	5%	—	—
Respiratory						
Pharyngitis	—	—	—	—	8%	—
Rhinitis	5%	—	—	—	—	—
Rhinorrhea	—	—	2%	6%	—	—
Sore throat	5%	3%	5%	5%	—	—
Miscellaneous						
Hypertension	—	—	1%	5%	—	—
Sweating	4%	9%	2%	6%	—	—

[a] Results reported to the nearest whole percent.
[b] Not reaching the cutoff of 5%.

Elderly patients: In elderly patients, solicited local and systemic adverse reactions occurred less frequently than in adults. The most common solicited local and systemic adverse reactions were injection-site pain and headache. All were considered mild/moderate and were transient.

The most common overall reactions in elderly patients 65 years and older were fatigue and headache.

Children – In 1987, a clinical study was carried out in 38 "at risk" children between 4 and 12 years of age (17 girls and 21 boys). To record the safety of *Fluvirin*, participants recorded their symptoms on a diary card during the 3 days after vaccination and noted any further symptoms they thought were attributable to the vaccine. The only reactions recorded were tenderness at the site of vaccination in 21% of the participants on day 1, which was still present in 16% on day 2 and 5% on day 3. In 1 child, the tenderness also was accompanied by redness at the site of injection for 2 days. The reactions were not age-dependent, and there was no bias toward the younger children.

➤*Fluzone:*

Adults –

Most common adverse reactions: The most common (occurring in more than 10% of the study participants in either of the 2 studies) solicited reactions were arm stiffness, headache, injection-site pain, myalgia, swelling, and tenderness. Most of the solicited injection-site and systemic adverse reactions were reported as mild and resolved within 3 days.

Serious adverse reactions: The rates of serious adverse reactions were comparable between the 2 groups; 6.1% of *Fluzone High-Dose* recipients and 7.4% of *Fluzone* recipients experienced serious adverse reactions.

No deaths were reported within 28 days postvaccination. A total of 23 deaths were reported during the follow-up period of the study; 0.6% among *Fluzone High-Dose* recipients and 0.6% among *Fluzone* recipients. The majority of these participants had medical history of cardiac, hepatic, neoplastic, renal, and/or respiratory diseases.

Adverse reactions within 7 days of vaccination:

Fluzone and *Fluzone High-Dose*[a] Adverse Reactions Within 7 Days Postvaccination		
Adverse reactions	*Fluzone High-Dose* (n = 2,573)	*Fluzone* (n = 1,260)
CNS		
Headache	16.8%	14.4%
Malaise	18%	14%
Local		
Erythema	14.9%	10.8%
Pain	35.6%	24.3%
Swelling	8.9%	5.8%
Miscellaneous		
Fever	3.6%	2.3%
Myalgia	21.4%	18.3%

[a] Solicited injection-site reactions and systemic adverse reactions were more frequent after vaccination with *Fluzone High-Dose* compared with standard *Fluzone* in adults 65 years and older.

Fluzone and *Fluzone High-Dose* Frequency and Severity of Adverse Reactions Within 7 Days Postvaccination		
Adverse reactions	*Fluzone High-Dose* (n = 2,573)	*Fluzone* (n = 1,260)
CNS		
Headache		
Mild	12.6%	11.7%
Moderate	3.1%	2.5%
Severe	1.1%	0.3%
Malaise		
Mild	11.7%	9.8%
Moderate	4.7%	3.7%
Severe	1.6%	0.6%
Local		
Injection-site erythema		
Mild	11.3%	9.4%
Moderate	1.9%	0.8%
Severe	1.8%	0.6%
Injection-site pain		
Mild	31.5%	22.5%
Moderate	3.7%	1.7%
Severe	0.3%	0.2%
Injection-site swelling		
Mild	5.8%	3.9%
Moderate	1.6%	1.3%
Severe	1.5%	0.6%
Miscellaneous		
Fever		
Mild	2.5%	2%
Moderate	1.1%	0.2%
Severe	0%	0.1%
Myalgia		
Mild	15.6%	14.8%
Moderate	4.2%	3.2%
Severe	1.6%	0.2%

➤*Fluzone Intradermal:*

Adults –

Fluzone Intradermal and *Fluzone* Adverse Reactions Within 7 Days Post-vaccination						
	Fluzone Intradermal (N[a] = 2,798 to 2,802)			*Fluzone* (N[a] = 1,392 to 1,394)		
Adverse reactions	Any	Grade 2[b]	Grade 3[c]	Any	Grade 2[b]	Grade 3[c]
CNS						
Headache	31.2%	6.4%	1.5%	30.3%	6.5%	1.6%
Malaise	23.3%	5.5%	2.2%	22.2%	5.5%	1.8%
Local						
Injection-site ecchymosis	9.3%	1.4%	0.4%	6.2%	1.1%	0.4%
Injection-site erythema	76.4%	28.8%	13%	13.2%	2.1%	0.9%
Injection-site induration	58.4%	13%	3.4%	10%	2.3%	0.5%
Injection-site pain	51%	4.4%	0.6%	53.7%	5.8%	0.8%
Injection-site pruritus	46.9%	4.1%	1.1%	9.3%	0.4%	0%

INFLUENZA TYPES A AND B VACCINE — INJECTION

Fluzone Intradermal and Fluzone Adverse Reactions Within 7 Days Post-vaccination

	Fluzone Intradermal (N[a] = 2,798 to 2,802)			Fluzone (N[a] = 1,392 to 1,394)		
Adverse reactions	Any	Grade 2[b]	Grade 3[c]	Any	Grade 2[b]	Grade 3[c]
Injection-site swelling	56.8%	13.4%	5.4%	8.4%	2.1%	0.9%
Miscellaneous						
Fever[d]	3.9%	0.6%	0.1%	2.6%	0.4%	0.2%
Myalgia	26.5%	4.6%	1.5%	30.8%	5.5%	1.8%
Shivering	7.3%	1.5%	0.7%	6.2%	1.1%	0.6%

[a] N is the number of vaccinated subjects with available data for the events listed.
[b] Grade 2 - Injection-site erythema, Injection-site induration, Injection-site swelling, and Injection-site ecchymosis: ≥ 2.5 cm to < 5 cm; Injection-site pain and Injection-site pruritus: sufficiently discomforting to interfere with normal behavior or activities; Fever: > 100.4°F to ≤ 102.2°F; Headache, Myalgia, Malaise, and Shivering: interferes with daily activities.
[c] Grade 3 - Injection-site erythema, Injection-site induration, Injection-site swelling, and Injection-site ecchymosis: ≥ 5 cm; Injection-site pain: incapacitating, unable to perform usual activities; Injection-site pruritus: incapacitating, unable to perform usual activities, may have/or required medical care or absenteeism; Fever: > 102.2°F; Headache, Myalgia, Malaise, and Shivering: prevents daily activities.
[d] Fever - Any Fever indications ≥ 99.5°F. The percentage of temperature measurements that were taken by oral or axillary routes, or not recorded were 99.9%, < 0.1%, and 0.1%, respectively for *Fluzone Intradermal*; and 99.6%, 0%, and 0.4%, respectively for *Fluzone*.

Serious adverse reactions: Within 28 days post-vaccination, a serious adverse reaction was reported by 0.4% of *Fluzone Intradermal* recipients and 0.4% of *Fluzone* recipients. Within 6 months post-vaccination, a serious adverse reaction was reported by 1.6% of *Fluzone Intradermal* recipients and 1.4% of *Fluzone* recipients. No deaths were reported during the 6 months post-vaccination. Throughout the study, one reported serious adverse reaction was considered to be caused by vaccination: a pruritic rash on the extremities and torso that began 48 hours after receipt of *Fluzone Intradermal* and resulted in hospitalization and treatment with an antihistamine and steroids.

➤*Other adverse reactions:*

Cardiovascular – Microscopic polyangiitis (vasculitis) has been reported temporally associated with influenza vaccination.

CNS –

Guillain-Barré syndrome: The 1976 swine influenza vaccine was associated with an increased frequency of Guillain-Barré syndrome. Evidence for a causal relation of Guillain-Barré syndrome with subsequent vaccines prepared from other influenza vaccine is unclear. If influenza vaccine does pose a risk, it is probably slightly more than 1 additional case per 1 million persons vaccinated.

Other CNS disorders: Neurological disorders temporally associated with influenza vaccination, such as brachial plexus neuropathy, encephalopathy, optic neuritis/neuropathy, and partial facial paralysis, have been reported.

Hypersensitivity – Immediate, presumably allergic, reactions (eg, allergic asthma, angioedema, hives, systemic anaphylaxis) rarely occur after influenza vaccination. Two patients experienced urticaria in clinical trials of *Fluarix*. These reactions probably resulted from hypersensitivity to certain vaccine components, such as residual egg protein. Although influenza vaccines contain only a limited quantity of egg protein, this protein can induce immediate hypersensitivity reactions among persons who have severe egg allergy.

➤*Postmarketing:*

Cardiovascular – Henoch-Schönlein purpura, tachycardia, vasculitis with transient renal involvement.

CNS – Abnormal gait, asthenia, confusion, convulsions (including febrile seizures), dizziness, encephalopathy, fatigue, headache, hypesthesia, hypokinesia, Guillian-Barré syndrome, insomnia, malaise, neuralgia, neuritis or neuropathy (including brachial plexus neuropathy), paralysis (including Bell palsy and other cranial or facial nerve paralyses), paresthesia, myelitis (including encephalomyelitis and transverse myelitis), somnolence, syncope shortly after vaccination, tremor, vertigo.

Dermatologic – Angioedema, erythema, erythema multiforme, facial swelling, pallor, pruritus, rash (including nonspecific, maculopapular, and vesiculobullous), Stevens-Johnson syndrome, sweating, urticaria.

GI – Abdominal pain or discomfort, diarrhea, dysphagia, loss of appetite, nausea, vomiting.

Hematologic / Lymphatic – Lymphadenopathy, thrombocytopenia.

Hypersensitivity – Allergic reactions, including anaphylaxis, anaphylactic shock, throat, tongue, and/or mouth edema, and serum sickness. In rare cases, hypersensitivity reactions have led to death.

Local – Local injection-site reactions, including pain, pain-limiting limb movement, redness, swelling, warmth, ecchymosis, induration, local lymphadenopathy, abscess, bruising, cellulitis, inflammation, mass, rash, or warmth.

Musculoskeletal – Arthralgia, arthritis, back pain, limb paralysis, muscle weakness, myalgia, myasthenia, pain in extremity, rigors.

Respiratory – Asthma, bronchospasm, cough, dysphonia, dyspnea, laryngitis, pharyngitis, respiratory distress, rhinitis, stridor, throat tightness.

Special senses – Conjunctivitis, eye irritation, eye pain, eye redness, eye swelling, eyelid swelling, periorbital edema, photophobia, tonsillitis.

Miscellaneous – Body aches, cellulitis, chest pain, chills, facial edema, feeling hot, fever, hot flush, influenza-type symptoms, shivering.

Patient Information

Fully inform patients, parents, or guardians of the benefits and risks of immunization with influenza vaccine. When educating vaccine recipients and guardians regarding potential adverse reactions, emphasize that influenza vaccine contains noninfectious killed viruses and cannot cause influenza and that coincidental respiratory disease unrelated to influenza vaccine can occur after vaccination. The influenza vaccine is intended to provide protection and illness caused by influenza virus only and cannot provide protection against all respiratory illness.

Inform vaccine recipients and guardians that the full effect of the vaccine is generally achieved approximately 3 weeks after vaccination. Annual revaccination is recommended.

Instruct patients, parents, or guardians to report any serious adverse reactions to their health care provider.

Provide the vaccine recipients or guardian with the vaccine information statements, which are required by the National Childhood Vaccine Injury Act of 1986 to be given prior to immunization. These materials are available free of charge at the Centers for Disease Control and Prevention Web site at http://www.cdc.gov/vaccines.

INFLUENZA TYPES A AND B VACCINE LIVE — INTRANASAL

For additional information, refer to the Agents for Active Immunization introduction.

Indications

➤*Influenza vaccination:* For the active immunization of individuals 2 to 49 years of age against influenza disease caused by influenza virus subtypes A and type B contained in the vaccine.

The 2010 to 2011 intranasal seasonal flu vaccine includes the 2009 pandemic A/H1N1 (ie, "swine flu") influenza vaccine strain that was released as a monovalent vaccine in 2009.

Administration and Dosage

➤*General dosing considerations:* Intranasal influenza vaccine should be administered prior to exposure to influenza. Annual revaccination with influenza vaccine is recommended.

For intranasal administration by a health care provider. Active inhalation (sniffing) is not required by the patient during intranasal influenza vaccine administration.

➤*Adults:*

Influenza –

49 years and younger: 0.2 mL dose (0.1 mL per nostril) intranasally.

➤*Children:*

Influenza –

9 years and older: See Adults for dosing.

2 to 8 years of age:

• *Previously vaccinated with influenza vaccine* – 0.2 mL dose (0.1 mL per nostril) intranasally.

• *Not previously vaccinated with influenza vaccine* – 0.2 mL dose (0.1 mL per nostril) intranasally followed by a second 0.2 mL dose (0.1 mL per nostril) given at least 1 month later.

➤*Administration:* Each sprayer contains a single dose of intranasal influenza vaccine; approximately one-half of the contents should be administered into each nostril. Administer 0.1 mL (ie, half of the dose from a single intranasal influenza vaccine sprayer) into each nostril while the recipient is in an upright position. Insert the tip of the sprayer just inside the nose and rapidly depress the plunger until the dose-divider clip stops the plunger. The dose-divider clip is removed from the sprayer to administer the second half of the dose (0.1 mL) into the other nostril.

➤*Storage / Stability:* Store in a refrigerator between 2° and 8°C (35° and 46°F) upon receipt and until use. Do not freeze. The cold chain (2° to 8°C) should be maintained when transporting intranasal influenza vaccine.

Once intranasal influenza vaccine has been administered, the sprayer should be disposed of according to the standard procedures for medical waste (eg, sharps or biohazard container).

Actions

➤*Pharmacology:* Immune mechanisms conferring protection against influenza following receipt of intranasal influenza vaccine are not fully understood. Likewise, naturally acquired immunity to wild-type influenza has not been completely elucidated. Serum antibodies, mucosal antibodies, and influenza-specific T cells may play a role in prevention and recovery from infection.

Influenza illness and its complications follow infection with influenza viruses. Global surveillance of influenza identifies yearly antigenic variants. For example, since 1977, antigenic variants of influenza A (H1N1 and H3N2) viruses and influenza B viruses have been in global circulation. Antibody against 1 influenza virus type or subtype confers limited or no protection against another. Furthermore, antibody to 1 antigenic variant of influenza virus might not protect against a new antigenic variant of the same type or subtype. Frequent development of antigenic variants through antigenic drift is the virologic basis for seasonal epidemics and the reason for the usual

INFLUENZA TYPES A AND B VACCINE LIVE — INTRANASAL

change of 1 or more new strains in each year's influenza vaccine. Therefore, influenza vaccines are standardized to contain the strains (ie, typically 2 type A and 1 type B) representing the influenza viruses likely to be circulating in the United States in the upcoming winter.

Annual revaccination with the current vaccine is recommended because immunity declines during the year after vaccination, and because circulating strains of influenza virus change from year to year.

Contraindications

History of hypersensitivity, especially anaphylactic reactions, to eggs, egg proteins, gentamicin, gelatin, or arginine; or with life-threatening reactions to previous influenza vaccination; children and adolescents (2 to 17 years of age) receiving aspirin therapy or aspirin-containing therapy because of the association of Reye syndrome with aspirin and wild-type influenza infection.

Warnings/Precautions

➤*Asthma/Recurrent wheezing:* Do not administer intranasal influenza vaccine to any individuals with asthma or to children younger than 5 years with recurrent wheezing, because of the potential for increased risk of wheezing postvaccination, unless the potential benefit outweighs the potential risk.

Do not administer intranasal influenza vaccine to individuals with severe asthma or active wheezing because these individuals have not been studied in clinical trials.

➤*Guillain-Barré syndrome:* If Guillain-Barré syndrome has occurred within 6 weeks of any prior influenza vaccination, base the decision to give intranasal influenza vaccine on careful consideration of the potential benefits and risks.

➤*Immunocompromised individuals:* Base administration of intranasal influenza vaccine, a live virus vaccine, to immunocompromised individuals on careful consideration of potential benefits and risks. Although intranasal influenza vaccine was studied in 57 asymptomatic or mildly symptomatic adults with HIV infection, data supporting the safety and effectiveness of intranasal influenza vaccine administration in immunocompromised individuals are limited.

➤*Protection:* Intranasal influenza vaccine may not protect all individuals receiving the vaccine.

➤*Concomitant vaccines:*

Inactivated vaccines – The safety and immunogenicity of intranasal influenza vaccine when coadministered with inactivated vaccines have not been determined. Studies of intranasal influenza vaccine excluded subjects who received any inactivated or subunit vaccine within 2 weeks of enrollment. Therefore, consider the risks and benefits of coadministration of intranasal influenza vaccine with inactivated vaccines.

Live vaccines – Coadministration of intranasal influenza vaccine with the measles, mumps, and rubella vaccine and the varicella vaccine was studied in 1,245 children 12 to 15 months of age. Adverse reactions were similar to those seen in other clinical trials with intranasal influenza vaccine. No evidence of interference with immune responses to measles, mumps, rubella, varicella, and intranasal influenza vaccines was observed. Coadministration of intranasal influenza vaccine with the measles, mumps, and rubella vaccine and the varicella vaccine in children older than 15 months have not been studied.

➤*Hypersensitivity reactions:* Prior to vaccination, review the individual's medical history for possible sensitivity to influenza vaccine or vaccine components. Treatment must be readily available in the event of an acute anaphylactic reaction following vaccination.

➤*Special risk:* The safety of intranasal influenza vaccine in individuals with underlying medical conditions that may predispose them to complications following wild-type influenza infection has not been established. Do not administer intranasal influenza vaccine unless the potential benefit outweighs the potential risk.

➤*Pregnancy: Category C.* Animal reproduction studies have not been conducted with intranasal influenza vaccine. It is not known whether intranasal influenza vaccine can cause fetal harm when administered to a pregnant woman or can affect reproductive capacity. Administer intranasal influenza vaccine to a pregnant woman only if clearly needed.

➤*Lactation:* It is not known whether intranasal influenza vaccine is excreted in human breast milk. Therefore, because some viruses are excreted in human breast milk, exercise caution if intranasal influenza vaccine is administered to breast-feeding women.

➤*Children:* Do not administer intranasal influenza vaccine to children younger than 24 months. In clinical trials, an increased risk of hospitalizations and wheezing postvaccination was observed in intranasal influenza vaccine recipients younger than 24 months.

Safety and effectiveness of the vaccine have been demonstrated for children 2 years and older with reduction in culture-confirmed influenza rates compared with active control and placebo.

➤*Elderly:* Intranasal influenza vaccine is not indicated for use in individuals 65 years and older. Subjects with underlying high-risk medical conditions (n = 200) were studied for safety. Compared with controls, intranasal influenza vaccine recipients had a higher rate of sore throat.

Adults 50 to 64 years of age – Intranasal influenza vaccine is not indicated for use in individuals 50 to 64 years of age. In study AV009, effectiveness was not demonstrated in individuals 50 to 64 years of age (n = 641). Solicited adverse reactions were similar in type and frequency to those reported in younger adults.

Drug Interactions

➤*Concomitant vaccines:*

Inactivated vaccines – See Warnings/Precautions for more information.

Live vaccines – See Warnings/Precautions for more information.

Intranasal Influenza Vaccine Drug Interactions

Precipitant drug	Object drug[a]		Description
Antiviral agents (eg, amantadine, oseltamivir, rimantadine)	Intranasal influenza vaccine	⬇	Based on the potential for interference between intranasal influenza vaccine and antiviral agents active against influenza A and B, do not administer intranasal influenza vaccine until 48 hours after the cessation of antiviral therapy, and do not administer antiviral agents until 2 weeks after administration of intranasal influenza vaccine unless medically indicated.
Aspirin	Intranasal influenza vaccine	⬆	Intranasal influenza vaccine is contraindicated in children and adolescents receiving aspirin therapy because of the association of Reye syndrome with aspirin and wild-type influenza infection.
Immunosuppressants (eg, alkylating drugs, antimetabolites, radiation, systemic corticosteroids)	Intranasal influenza vaccine	⬆	Because intranasal influenza vaccine is a live vaccine, the risk of dissemination may be increased in patients receiving immunosuppressant agents or in patients who are immunocompromised. Avoid coadministration.

[a] ⬇ = object drug decreased; ⬆ = object drug increased.

Adverse Reactions

➤*Children and adolescents:* Intranasal influenza vaccine is not indicated in children younger than 24 months. In a clinical trial among children 6 to 23 months of age, wheezing requiring bronchodilator therapy or with significant respiratory symptoms occurred in 5.9% of intranasal influenza vaccine recipients compared with 3.8% of active control recipients (relative risk, 1.5; 95% confidence interval [CI], 1.2 to 2.1). Wheezing was not increased in children 24 months and older.

In a placebo-controlled safety study (AV019) conducted in a large health maintenance organization in children 1 to 17 years of age (n = 9,689), an increase in asthma events, captured by review of diagnostic codes, was observed in children younger than 5 years (relative risk, 3.53; 90% CI, 1.1 to 15.7). This observation was prospectively evaluated in study MI-CP111.

In MI-CP111, an active-controlled study, increases in wheezing and hospitalization (for any cause) were observed in children younger than 24 months.

Children With Hospitalizations and Wheezing After Influenza Vaccine Administration

Adverse reactions	Age group	Intranasal influenza vaccine	Active control[a]
Hospitalizations[b]	6 to 23 months (n = 3,967)	4.2%	3.2%
	24 to 59 months (n = 4,385)	2.1%	2.5%
Wheezing[c]	6 to 23 months (n = 3,967)	5.9%	3.8%
	24 to 59 months (n = 4,385)	2.1%	2.5%

[a] Injectable influenza vaccine.
[b] From randomization through 180 days after last vaccination.
[c] Wheezing requiring bronchodilator therapy or with significant respiratory symptoms evaluated from randomization through 42 days after last vaccination.

INFLUENZA TYPES A AND B VACCINE LIVE — INTRANASAL

Most hospitalizations observed were because of GI and respiratory tract infections and occurred more than 6 weeks postvaccination. In posthoc analysis, rates of hospitalization in children 6 to 11 months of age (n = 1,376) were 6.1% in intranasal influenza vaccine recipients and 2.6% in active control recipients.

Influenza Intranasal Vaccine[a] Adverse Reactions Observed Within 10 Days After Dose 1 in Children 2 to 6 Years of Age

Adverse reactions	D153-P501 & AV006		MI-CP111	
	Intranasal influenza vaccine (n = 876 to 1,759)[b]	Placebo (n = 424 to 1,034)[b]	Intranasal influenza vaccine (n = 2,170)[b]	Active control[c] (n = 2,165)[b]
CNS				
Decreased activity (lethargy)	14%	11%	7%	6%
Headache	9%	7%	3%	3%
Irritability	21%	19%	12%	11%
Respiratory				
Runny nose/ nasal congestion	58%	50%	51%	42%
Sore throat	11%	9%	5%	6%
Miscellaneous				
Chills	4%	3%	2%	2%
Decreased appetite	21%	17%	13%	12%
Fever				
100° to 101°F oral	9%	6%	6%	4%
101° to 102°F oral	4%	3%	4%	3%
Muscle aches	6%	3%	2%	2%

[a] Frozen formulation used in AV006; refrigerated formulation used in D153-P501 and MI-CP111.
[b] Number of evaluable subjects (those who returned diary cards) for each event. Range reflects differences in data collection between the 2 pooled studies.
[c] Injectable influenza vaccine.

Other adverse reactions – In clinical studies D153-P501 and AV006, other adverse reactions in children occurring in at least 1% of intranasal influenza vaccine recipients and at a higher rate compared with placebo were abdominal pain (2% intranasal influenza vaccine vs 0% placebo) and otitis media (3% intranasal influenza vaccine vs 1% placebo).

An additional adverse reaction identified in the MI-CP111 active-controlled trial, occurring in at least 1% of intranasal influenza vaccine recipients and at a higher rate compared with active control was sneezing (2% intranasal influenza vaccine vs 1% active control).

In a separate trial (MI-CP112) that compared the refrigerated and frozen formulations of intranasal influenza vaccine in children and adults 5 to 49 years of age, the solicited reactions and other adverse reactions were consistent with observations from previous trials. Fever of higher than 103°F was observed in 1% to 2% of children 5 to 8 years of age.

➤*Adults:* In adults 18 to 49 years of age in study AV009, the summary of solicited adverse reactions occurring in at least 1% of intranasal influenza vaccine recipients and at a higher rate compared with placebo included runny nose (44% intranasal influenza vaccine vs 27% placebo), headache (40% intranasal influenza vaccine vs 38% placebo), sore throat (28% intranasal influenza vaccine vs 17% placebo), tiredness/weakness (26% intranasal influenza vaccine vs 22% placebo), muscle aches (17% intranasal influenza vaccine vs 15% placebo), cough (14% intranasal influenza vaccine vs 11% placebo), and chills (9% intranasal influenza vaccine vs 6% placebo).

In addition to the solicited reactions, other adverse reactions from study AV009 occurring in at least 1% of intranasal influenza vaccine recipients and at a higher rate compared with placebo were nasal congestion (9% intranasal influenza vaccine vs 2% placebo) and sinusitis (4% intranasal influenza vaccine vs 2% placebo).

➤*Postmarketing:*

CNS – Bell palsy, Guillain-Barré syndrome, meningitis, eosinophilic meningitis, vaccine-associated encephalitis.

GI – Diarrhea, nausea, vomiting.

Hypersensitivity – Hypersensitivity reactions, including anaphylactic reaction, facial edema, and urticaria.

Miscellaneous – Epistaxis, exacerbation of symptoms of mitochondrial encephalomyopathy (Leigh syndrome), pericarditis, rash.

Patient Information

Inform vaccine recipients or their parents/guardians of the potential benefits and risks of intranasal influenza vaccine and the need for 2 doses at least 1 month apart in children 2 to 8 years of age who have not previously received influenza vaccine.

Ask vaccine recipients or their parents/guardians if the vaccine recipient has asthma. For children younger than 5 years, also ask if the vaccine recipient has recurrent wheezing because this may be an asthma equivalent in this age group.

Inform vaccine recipients or their parents/guardians that intranasal influenza vaccine is an attenuated live virus vaccine and has the potential for transmission to immunocompromised household contacts.

Inform vaccine recipients or their parents/guardians accompanying the vaccine recipient to report any suspected adverse reaction to the health care provider or clinic where the vaccine was administered.

H5N1 INFLUENZA VACCINE

Rx	**H5N1 Influenza Vaccine** (Sanofi Pasteur)	**Injection, suspension (purified split-virus):** 90 mcg HA of strain A/Vietnam/1203/2004 (H5N1, clade 1) per mL.	Thimerosal.[a] In 5 mL multidose vials.[b]

[a] Each 1 mL dose is formulated to contain not more than 98.2 mcg thimerosal (approximately 50 mcg mercury per dose).

[b] Each dose may also contain residual amounts of formaldehyde (not more than 200 mcg), polyethylene glycol p-isooctylphenyl ether (not more than 0.05%), and sucrose (not more than 2%).

H5N1 INFLUENZA VACCINE — INJECTION

Indications

➤*Avian influenza:* For active immunization of persons 18 to 64 years of age at increased risk of exposure to the H5N1 influenza virus subtype contained in the inactivated monovalent vaccine.

This indication is based on immune response and not on demonstration of decreased influenza disease after vaccination with H5N1 influenza vaccine.

Administration and Dosage

➤*Adults:*

Avian influenza –

18 to 64 years of age: 1 mL injected IM. A second 1 mL dose of vaccine should be administered approximately 28 days later (window, 21 to 35 days).

➤*Preparation for administration:* Shake the multidose vial vigorously each time before withdrawing a dose of vaccine. Between uses, return the multidose vial to the recommended storage conditions.

➤*Administration:* Administer the vaccine by IM injection, preferably in the lateral aspect of the deltoid muscle of the upper arm. The vaccine should not be injected in the gluteal region or areas where there may be a major nerve trunk. A needle of at least 1 inch is preferred because needles less than 1 inch might be of insufficient length to penetrate the muscle tissue in certain adults.

➤*Storage/Stability:* Store in a refrigerator at 2° to 8°C (35° to 46°F). Do not freeze. Discard if the vaccine has been frozen. Protect from light.

Actions

➤*Pharmacology:* The mechanism of action of type A (H5N1) influenza virus vaccines is not well understood. Influenza vaccines induce antibodies against the viral HA in the vaccine, thereby blocking viral attachment to human respiratory epithelial cells. Specific levels of hemagglutinin inhibition (HI) antibody titer post-vaccination with inactive influenza virus vaccines, including H5N1 influenza virus vaccines, have not been correlated with protection from influenza illness but the antibody titers have been used as a measure of vaccine activity. In some human challenge studies of other influenza viruses, antibody titers of at least 1:40 have been associated with protection from influenza illness in up to 50% of subjects.

Antibody against one influenza virus type or subtype confers little or no protection against viruses from other types or subtypes. Furthermore, antibody to one antigenic variant of influenza virus might not protect against a new antigenic variant of the same type or subtype. Frequent development of antigenic variants through antigenic drift is the virological basis for seasonal epidemics and the reason for the usual change of one or more new strains in each year's influenza vaccine.

Global surveillance of influenza identifies yearly antigenic variants. An influenza pandemic occurs when humans have little or no immunity to an influenza virus strain and this virus strain is rapidly transmitted from human to human. Antigenic variants of H5N1 viruses have been in circulation in the avian species globally, with rare transmission to humans. However, these avian H5N1 viruses may acquire mutations that facilitate transmission among humans.

Contraindications

None known.

Warnings/Precautions

➤*Guillain-Barré syndrome:* If Guillain-Barré syndrome has occurred within 6 weeks of receipt of prior influenza vaccine, base the decision to give H5N1 influenza vaccine on careful consideration of the potential benefits and risks.

➤*Altered immunocompetence:* If H5N1 influenza vaccine is administered to immunocompromised persons, including persons receiving immunosuppressive therapy, the expected immune response may not be obtained.

➤*Hypersensitivity reactions:* H5N1 influenza vaccine, contains chicken and egg proteins. Base the decision to give H5N1 influenza vaccine to persons with known systemic hypersensitivity reactions to egg proteins or life-threatening reactions to previous influenza vaccinations on careful considerations of risks and benefits.

Prior to administration of H5N1 influenza vaccine, the healthcare provider should review the patient's prior immunization history for possible adverse reactions, to allow an assessment of benefits and risks. Epinephrine injection (1:1,000) and other appropriate agents used for the control of immediate allergic reactions must be immediately available should an acute anaphylactic reaction occur.

➤*Pregnancy: Category C.* Animal reproductive studies have not been conducted with H5N1 influenza vaccine. It is not known whether H5N1 influenza vaccine can cause fetal harm when administered to a pregnant woman or can affect reproduction capacity. Give H5N1 influenza vaccine to a pregnant woman only if clearly needed.

➤*Lactation:* It is not known whether H5N1 influenza vaccine is excreted in human milk. Because many drugs are excreted in human milk, exercise caution the H5N1 influenza vaccine is administered to a breast-feeding mother.

➤*Children:* No data are available for children (younger than 18 years of age). Safety and efficacy of H5N1 influenza vaccine in children have not been established.

➤*Elderly:* Clinical studies of H5N1 influenza vaccine did not include subjects 65 years of age and older to determine whether they respond differently from younger subjects. Other reported clinical experience has identified differences in immune response between elderly and younger patients to inactivated influenza vaccines.

Drug Interactions

➤*Other vaccines:* There are no data to assess the coadministration of H5N1 influenza vaccine with other vaccines. If H5N1 influenza vaccine is to be given at the same time as another injectable vaccine(s), the vaccines should always be administered at different injection sites. Do not mix H5N1 influenza vaccine with any other vaccine in the same syringe or vial.

➤*Immunosuppressive therapies:* Immunosuppressive therapies, including irradiation, antimetabolites, alkylating agents, cytotoxic drugs, and corticosteroids (used in greater than physiologic doses), may reduce the immune response to H5N1 influenza vaccine.

Adverse Reactions

Four serious adverse reactions, all considered unrelated to vaccine, occurred after vaccination including 1 death and 3 other serious adverse reactions (1 each: menorrhagia, cerebrovascular event, and breast cancer).

The following table summarizes the frequencies of the solicited adverse reactions that were recorded following any vaccination.

Frequencies of Solicited Adverse Events for H5N1 Influenza Vaccine[a,b]

Adverse reaction	Placebo (n = 48)	H5N1 influenza vaccine 7.5 mcg (n = 101)	15 mcg (n = 101)	45 mcg (n = 98)	90 mcg (n = 103)
Local					
Erythema/Redness	14.6%	14.9%	10.9%	18.4%	20.4%
Induration/Swelling	8.3%	7.9%	7.9%	10.2%	14.6%
Pain	18.8%	27.7%	44.6%	61.2%	73.8%
Tenderness	27.1%	30.7%	43.6%	57.1%	69.9%
Systemic					
Fever	8.3%	8.9%	10.9%	2%	6.8%
Headache	37.5%	27.7%	34.7%	22.4%	35.9%
Malaise	29.2%	23.8%	25.7%	13.3%	22.3%
Myalgia	29.2%	12.9%	19.8%	15.3%	15.5%
Nausea	6.3%	10.9%	14.9%	5.1%	9.7%

[a] All solicited events are considered to be reactions.

[b] Note: Immediate reactions are included, except for immediate redness and swelling, as no severity grade was assigned.

Most of the solicited injection site reactions were of mild to moderate severity and resolved within 3 days of vaccination. Most of the solicited systemic reactions were also of mild to moderate severity.

The following table summarizes the frequencies of the unsolicited adverse reactions that were recorded throughout the study.

Unsolicited Adverse Reactions of H5N1 Influenza Vaccine (≥ 5%)[a]

Adverse reaction	Placebo (n = 48)	H5N1 Influenza Vaccine 7.5 mcg (n = 101)	15 mcg (n = 101)	45 mcg (n = 98)	90 mcg (n = 103)
CNS					
Headache	2.1%	1%	5%	3.1%	2.9%
GI					
Diarrhea	2.1%	4%	4%	2%	5.8%
Respiratory					
Nasal congestion	0%	5%	2%	1%	1%
Nasopharyngitis	8.3%	4%	4%	1%	1.9%
Pharyngolaryngeal pain	2.1%	2%	5%	1%	4.9%
Upper respiratory tract infection	4.2%	5%	2%	2%	1.9%

H5N1 INFLUENZA VACCINE — INJECTION

Unsolicited Adverse Reactions of H5N1 Influenza Vaccine (≥ 5%)[a]					
		H5N1 Influenza Vaccine			
Adverse reaction	Placebo (n = 48)	7.5 mcg (n = 101)	15 mcg (n = 101)	45 mcg (n = 98)	90 mcg (n = 103)
Miscellaneous					
Pyrexia	6.3%	0%	0%	0%	0%

[a] For unsolicited events, the denominator for percentages is the number of vaccinated subjects for whom safety data are available (safety analysis set).

➤*Adverse reactions associated with influenza vaccines:*

CNS – Neurological disorders temporally associated with influenza vaccination such as encephalopathy, optic neuritis/neuropathy, partial facial paralysis, and brachial plexus neuropathy have been reported.

Cardiovascular – Microscopic polyangitis (vasculitis) has been reported temporally associated with influenza vaccination.

Hypersensitivity – Anaphylaxis has been reported after administration of influenza vaccines. Although H5N1 influenza vaccine contains only a limited quantity of egg protein, this protein can induce immediate hypersensitivity reactions among persons who have severe egg allergy. Allergic reactions include hives, angioedema, allergic asthma, and systemic anaphylaxis.

Miscellaneous – The 1976 swine influenza vaccine was associated with an increased frequency of Guillain-Barré syndrome. Evidence for a causal relation of Guillain-Barré syndrome with subsequent vaccines prepared from other influenza viruses is unclear.

Patient Information

Inform patients, parents, or guardians of the benefits and risks of immunization with H5N1 influenza vaccine. When educating vaccine recipients and guardians regarding the potential side effects, emphasize that H5N1 influenza vaccine contains noninfectious particles.

Instruct patients, parents, or guardians to report any serious adverse reaction to their health care provider.

Inform patient, parents, or guardian that product contains chicken and egg proteins. Persons with known hypersensitivity reactions to egg proteins should use vaccine with caution.

JAPANESE ENCEPHALITIS VIRUS VACCINE

Rx	**JE-Vax** (Sanofi Pasteur)	**Injection, lyophilized powder for suspension**[a,b]	In single-dose vial with 1.3 mL diluent (sterile water for injection).
	Ixiaro (Novartis)	**Injection, suspension:** 6 mcg per 0.5 mL[c,d]	Preservative free. In 0.5 mL single-dose prefilled syringes.

[a] Potency is determined by immunizing mice with either the test vaccine or the Japanese encephalitis reference vaccine. Neutralizing antibodies are measured in a plaque-neutralization assay performed on sera from the immunized mice. The potency of the test vaccine must be no less than that of the reference vaccine.

[b] With thimerosal 0.007%. Each 1 mL dose contains gelatin ≈ 500 mcg, formaldehyde < 100 mcg, polysorbate 80 < 0.0007%, and mouse serum protein

[c] Contains ≈ 6 mcg of purified inactivated Japanese encephalitis virus proteins and 250 mcg aluminum hydroxide.

[d] Each 0.5 mL dose contains formaldehyde ≤ 200 ppm, bovine serum albumin ≤ 100 ng/mL, host cell DNA ≤ 200 pg/mL, sodium metabisulfite ≤ 200 ppm, host cell proteins ≤ 300 ng/mL, and protamine sulfate ≤ 1 mcg/mL.

JAPANESE ENCEPHALITIS VIRUS VACCINE

For complete and comparative prescribing information, refer to the Agents for Active Immunization introduction.

Indications

➤*Japanese encephalitis vaccination:* For active immunization against Japanese encephalitis for persons 1 year of age and older (*JE-Vax*) and for persons 17 years of age and older (*Ixiaro*).

➤*Research laboratory workers:* Laboratory-acquired Japanese encephalitis has been reported in 22 cases. JEV may be transmitted in a laboratory setting through needle sticks and other accidental exposures. Vaccine-derived immunity presumably protects against exposure through these percutaneous routes. Exposure to aerosolized JEV, and particularly to high concentrations of virus, such as may occur during viral purification, potentially could lead to infection through mucous membranes and possibly directly into the CNS through the olfactory mucosa. It is unknown whether vaccine-derived immunity protects against such exposures, but immunization is recommended for all laboratory workers with a potential for exposure to infectious JEV.

➤*Protection:* As with any vaccine, vaccination with Japanese encephalitis vaccine may not result in protection in all individuals. Long-term protection, as demonstrated by persistence of neutralizing antibody for more than 2 years, has not yet been shown.

Administration and Dosage

➤*Maximum dose:*

JE-Vax –

Adults and children 3 years of age and older: 1 mL per subcutaneous dose according to the prescribing information.

Children 1 to 3 years of age: 0.5 mL per subcutaneous dose according to the prescribing information.

Ixiaro –

Adults: 1 mL per IM dose according to the prescribing information.

➤*General dosing considerations:* For persons 3 years of age and older, a single dose is 1 mL of vaccine. For children 1 to 3 years of age, a single dose is 0.5 mL of vaccine (*JE-Vax* only).

The last dose of *JE-Vax* should be given at least 10 days before the commencement of international travel to ensure an adequate immune response and access to medical care in the event of delayed adverse reactions.

Immunization series with *Ixiaro* should be completed at least 1 week prior to potential exposure to JEV.

➤*Adults:*

Japanese encephalitis vaccination –

JE-Vax:

• *Primary immunization schedule* – 3 doses of 1 mL each given subcutaneously on days 0, 7, and 30. The last dose should be given at least 10 days before travel.

An abbreviated schedule of days 0, 7, and 14 can be used when the longer schedule is impractical because of time constraints.

Booster dose: A booster dose of 1 mL may be given after 2 years.

Ixiaro: 2 doses of 0.5 mL administered intramuscularly (IM) 28 days apart. Complete immunization at least 1 week before exposure to JEV.

➤*Children:*

Japanese encephalitis vaccination –

JE-Vax:

• *3 years of age and older* – See Adults for dosing.

• *1 to 3 years of age* –

Primary immunization schedule: 3 doses of 0.5 mL each given subcutaneously on days 0, 7, and 30. The last dose should be given at least 10 days before travel.

An abbreviated schedule of days 0, 7, and 14 can be used when the longer schedule is impractical because of time constraints.

Booster dose: A booster dose of 0.5 mL may be given after 2 years.

➤*Preparation for administration:*

JE-Vax –

Remove plastic tab of flip-off cap. Do not remove rubber stopper. Cleanse stopper with a suitable disinfectant. Reconstitute only with the supplied 1.3 mL of diluent (sterile water for injection). Shake vial thoroughly.

Ixiaro – Before administration, shake the syringe well to obtain a white, opaque, homogeneous suspension. Do not administer if particulate matter remains following shaking or if discoloration is observed.

➤*Administration:* When Japanese encephalitis vaccine and any other vaccines are given concurrently, separate syringes and separate sites should be used.

JE-Vax – The vaccine should be given by subcutaneous administration only. Shake vial well.

Ixiaro – Each 0.5 mL dose is administered IM into the deltoid muscle. Do not administer intravenously, intradermally, or subcutaneously.

➤*Admixture compatibility:* Do not mix with any other vaccine in the same syringe or vial.

➤*Storage/Stability:*

JE-Vax – Store the vaccine between 2° and 8°C (35° and 46°F). Do not freeze. After reconstitution, store the vaccine between 2° and 8°C (35° and 46°F) and use it within 8 hours. Do not freeze reconstituted vaccine.

Ixiaro – Store the vaccine between 2° and 8°C (35° and 46°F). Do not freeze. Store in the original package in order to protect from light. During storage, a clear liquid with a white precipitate can be observed.

Actions

➤*Pharmacology:* Japanese encephalitis is a disease caused by the mosquito-borne arboviral *Flavivirus* infection. The JEV vaccine acts by inducing antibodies that neutralize live JE.

Contraindications

➤*JE-Vax*: Adverse reactions to a prior dose of *JE-Vax* manifesting as generalized urticaria and angioedema; proven or suspected hypersensitivity to proteins of rodent or neural origin; hypersensitivity to thimerosal.

➤*Ixiaro*: Severe allergic reaction (eg, anaphylaxis) after a previous dose of *Ixiaro*.

JAPANESE ENCEPHALITIS VIRUS VACCINE

Warnings/Precautions

➤*Vaccine efficacy:*

JE-Vax – Although substantial neutralizing antibody titers are elicited by *JE-Vax* in more than 90% of US travelers without history of Japanese encephalitis immunization or of exposure to JE, the precise relationship between antibody level and efficacy has not been established even though these titers persisted for at least 2 years after immunization.

Ixiaro – Vaccinees who receive only 1 dose of *Ixiaro* may have a suboptimal response and may therefore incur higher risk if exposed to JE, compared with vaccinees who receive both doses. Vaccination with *Ixiaro* may not result in protection in all cases. *Ixiaro* will not protect against encephalitis caused by viruses/pathogens other than JE.

➤*Immunocompromised persons:* There are no safety or efficacy data regarding the use of *Ixiaro* in immunocompromised persons. Immunocompromised persons may have a diminished immune response to *Ixiaro*.

➤*Hypersensitivity reactions:*

JE-Vax –

Persons with a history of urticaria after hymenoptera envenomation, drug administration, physical or other provocations, or of idiopathic cause appear to have a greater risk of developing reactions to *JE-Vax* (relative risk, 9.1; 95% CI, 1.8 to 50.9). Consider this history when weighing risks and benefits of the vaccine for an individual patient. When patients with such a history are offered *JE-Vax*, they should be alerted to their increased risk for reaction and monitored appropriately. There are no data supporting the efficacy of prophylactic antihistamines or steroids in preventing *JE-Vax*–related allergic reactions.

Another case control study consisting of 5 cases and 15 controls identified an increased risk of hypersensitivity reactions to *JE-Vax* in persons who had unusual alcohol consumption during the 2 days following vaccination ($P = 0.005$). Advise recipients should be advised to avoid more than the usual alcohol intake during the 48 hours following Japanese encephalitis vaccination.

In the same study an increased risk for hypersensitivity reactions was seen in persons who received other vaccines within the 7-day period prior to receipt of *JE-Vax*. When possible, coadminister *JE-Vax* with other vaccines.

Epinephrine injection (1:1,000) must be immediately available should an acute anaphylactic reaction occur due to any component of the vaccine.

Ixiaro – *Ixiaro* contains protamine sulfate, a compound known to cause hypersensitivity reactions in some persons . Appropriate medical care should be readily available in case of anaphylactic reaction.

➤*Pregnancy:* Category C (*JE-Vax*), Category B (*Ixiaro*).

JE-Vax – Animal reproduction studies have not been conducted with *JE-Vax*. It is not known whether *JE-Vax* can cause fetal harm when administered to a pregnant woman or can affect reproductive capacity. Japanese encephalitis acquired during the first or second trimesters of pregnancy may cause intrauterine infection and miscarriage. Infections that occur during the third trimester of pregnancy have not been associated with adverse outcomes in newborns. Immunize pregnant women who must travel to an area where risk of Japanese encephalitis is high when the theoretical risks of immunization are outweighed by the risk of infection to the mother and developing fetus. Give *JE-Vax* to a pregnant woman only if clearly needed.

Ixiaro – There are no adequate and well-controlled studies in pregnant women. Because animal reproduction studies are not always predictive of human response, use *Ixiaro* during pregnancy only if clearly needed.

➤*Lactation:* It is not known whether Japanese encephalitis vaccine is excreted in human milk. Because many drugs are excreted in human milk, use caution when Japanese encephalitis vaccine is administered to a breastfeeding woman.

➤*Children:* Safety and effectiveness of *JE-Vax* in infants younger than 1 year of age have not been established. Safety and effectiveness of *Ixiaro* in children younger than 17 years of age have not been established.

➤*Elderly:* Five serious adverse events were reported. Four (3.4%) subjects who received *Ixiaro*, no subjects who received *JE-Vax*, and 1 (5.9%) subject who received the control 0.5 mL of phosphate buffered saline with aluminum hydroxide 0.1% experienced an adverse event. The serious adverse events occurring in the *Ixiaro* group were as follows: 1 case each of rectal hemorrhage, pancreatic adenocarcinoma, and breast cancer; death occurred in a subject with metastatic lung adenocarcinoma, which occurred 4 months after the subject completed the 2-dose regimen.

➤*Monitoring:* Observe vaccinees for 30 minutes after vaccination with *JE-Vax* and warn about the possibility of delayed generalized urticaria, often in a generalized distribution or angioedema of the extremities, face, and oropharynx, especially of the lips.

Drug Interactions

None known.

Adverse Reactions

➤*JE-Vax*: Japanese encephalitis vaccine is associated with a moderate frequency of local and mild systemic adverse reactions. Tenderness, redness, swelling, and other local effects have been reported in about 20% of vaccinees (less than 1% to 31%). Systemic side effects, principally fever, headache, malaise, rash, and other reactions, (eg, chills, dizziness, myalgia, nausea, vomiting, abdominal pain) have been reported in approximately 10% of vaccinees.

In a study conducted by the CDC, less than 5% of the 1,756 US travelers immunized with a 3-dose regimen of the vaccine reported headache, flu-like symptoms, fever, and other systemic complaints. Hives and facial swelling were reported in 0.2% and 0.1% of vaccinees, respectively. Local soreness occurred in 5.9% and local redness in 2.9%. There was no increase in the number or severity of reactions with increasing numbers of doses.

The US Army studied 4,034 personnel from 1987 to 1989. Using a 2- or 3-dose regimen of *JE-Vax* arm soreness was described in 22.7%, local redness in 4.8%, headache in 15.2%, and a febrile episode in 5.5%. In another trial evaluating the safety and immunogenicity of a 3-dose immunizing series (day 0, 7, and 30 or day 0, 7, and 14), in 538 adult volunteers in 1990, the Army determined that local soreness and redness occurred in 21% of vaccinees after the first dose, then decreased with subsequent injections ($P < 0.0001$, chi-square for downward trend). Systemic symptoms including feverishness, headache, and rash occurred in 5% of vaccinees after the first dose, then decreased with subsequent injections ($P < 0.001$, chi-square for downward trend). Participants who received the third dose on day 14 reported more side effects than those who received the injection on day 30. Among these volunteers, 252 received a booster injection of vaccine 1 year after receiving the first dose of the primary series. Side effects reported after the booster injection included local symptoms of soreness (24.5%) and redness (6.1%) at the injection site and systemic complaints of headache (4.9%), fever (1.6%), and rash (0.8%). Less than 1% of all reported symptoms were graded as severe. No generalized urticaria or anaphylaxis was reported.

Hypersensitivity reactions – Since 1989, an apparently new pattern of adverse reactions has been reported among vaccinees in Europe, North America, and Australia. The reactions have been characterized by urticaria, often in a generalized distribution, or angioedema of the extremities and face, especially of the lips and oropharynx. Three vaccine recipients developed respiratory distress. Distress or collapse caused by hypotension or other causes led to hospitalization in several cases. Most reactions were treated successfully with antihistamines or oral steroids; however, some patients were hospitalized for parenteral steroid therapy. Three patients developed an erythema multiforme or erythema nodosum and some patients have had joint swelling. Some vaccinees complained of generalized itching without objective evidence of a rash.

An important feature of the reactions has been the interval between vaccination and onset of symptoms. Reactions after a first vaccine dose occurred after a median of 12 hours after immunization (88% of reactions occurred within 3 days). The interval between administration of a second dose and onset of symptoms generally was longer (median 3 days and possibly as long as 2 weeks). Reactions have occurred after a second or third dose, when preceding doses were received uneventfully.

A case-control study conducted as part of the Japanese encephalitis immunization campaign in Okinawa found that people developing these reactions after Japanese encephalitis vaccination were more likely to have had a history of urticaria after hymenoptera envenomation, drugs, physical or other provocations, or of idiopathic origins (relative risk, 9.1; 95% CI, 1.8 to 50.9). The vaccine constituents responsible for these adverse reactions have not been identified.

Other serious adverse reactions – Other serious adverse events reported following vaccination include 1 case of Guillain-Barré syndrome after Japanese encephalitis vaccination reported in the United States since 1984 (this patient was diagnosed as having mononucleosis 3 weeks before the onset of weakness); 1 case of urticaria, hepatitis, and respiratory failure 1 week after dose 2 (this person showed effusion and infiltrate on chest x-ray and eosinophilia); 1 case of respiratory and renal failure 1 week after a dose (this 26-month-old male had infiltrate on chest x-ray and acid fast bacilli in sputum); and 1 case of newly diagnosed hypertension in a young men presenting with a headache several hours after receiving dose 1. The relationship of *JE-Vax* to the etiology of these adverse events is unknown.

Optic neuritis has been reported for 1 patient. In addition to *JE-Vax*, this patient concurrently received a number of other vaccines.

Fatal myocarditis has been reported in a patient who had recently been given meningococcal vaccine and at least 1 dose of Japanese encephalitis vaccine. Any causal role for the vaccines is unclear.

Sudden death occurred approximately 60 hours after receiving the first dose of *JE-Vax* in a 21-year-old US military person with a history of recurrent hypersensitivity and an episode of possible anaphylaxis. This person also received the third dose of plague vaccine approximately 12 to 15 hours prior to the death. There was no evidence of urticaria or angioedema. Cause of death was not established at autopsy.

Surveillance of *JE-Vax*–related complications in Japan from 1965 to 1973 disclosed neurologic events (primarily encephalitis, encephalopathy, seizures, and peripheral neuropathy) in 1 to 2.3 per million vaccinees. Very rarely, deaths occurred with vaccine-associated encephalitis. Between 1987 and 1989, 2 cases of neurologic dysfunction were reported from Japan; 1 of these was a transverse myelitis, while the second included seizures, cranial nerve paresis, cerebellar ataxia, and behavior disorder. In 1992, 2 cases of acute disseminated encephalomyelitis were reported from Japan; 1 occurred 14 days after the second dose and the second occurred 17 days after a booster dose of Japanese encephalitis vaccine. Both cases recovered. One case of Bell palsy was reported from Thailand.

➤*Ixiaro*:

Most common adverse reactions – The most common (more than 10%) systemic adverse events observed in clinical trials with *Ixiaro* were headache and myalgia. The most common (more than 10%) local reactions after *Ixiaro* administration were pain and tenderness.

Serious adverse reactions – In 5 clinical studies conducted in North America, Europe, Australia, and New Zealand, a total of 3,558 adults 18 to 86 years of age received at least 1 dose of *Ixiaro* (92% completed the 2-dose

JAPANESE ENCEPHALITIS VIRUS VACCINE

series) and were followed up for safety for at least 6 months after the first dose. In this pooled dataset of subjects who received *Ixiaro*, 1 death occurred in a subject with metastatic lung adenocarcinoma 4 months after completing the 2-dose regimen. Approximately 1% of subjects who received *Ixiaro* experienced a serious adverse event, including 1 case of multiple sclerosis. Approximately 1% of subjects who received *Ixiaro* discontinued because of adverse events.

Comparison with control – The safety of *Ixiaro* was evaluated in a randomized, controlled, double-blind clinical trial in healthy men and women. *Ixiaro* was compared with a control: phosphate buffered saline containing aluminum hydroxide 0.1% 0.5 mL of phosphate buffered saline with aluminum hydroxide 0.1%.

Systemic adverse reactions:

Ixiaro Adverse Reactions (≥ 1%)[a,b]						
	First vaccination period (day 0 to day 28)		Second vaccination period (day 28 to day 56)		Total vaccination period (day 0 to day 56)	
Adverse reaction	*Ixiaro* (n = 1,993)	PBS + $Al(OH)_3$[a] (n = 657)	*Ixiaro* (n = 1,968)	PBS + $Al(OH)_3$ (n = 645)	*Ixiaro* (n = 1993)	PBS + $Al(OH)_3$ (n = 657)
CNS						
Fatigue[c]	8.6%	8.7%	5.2%	5.9%	11.3%	11.7%
Headache[c]	21.6%	20.2%	13.4%	13%	27.9%	26.2%
GI						
Diarrhea	0.8%	0.8%	0.7%	0.3%	1.5%	1.1%
Nausea[c]	4.7%	5.3%	2.6%	3.7%	6.6%	7.5%
Vomiting[c]	0.6%	0.8%	0.8%	0.9%	1.4%	1.7%
Respiratory						
Cough	0.8%	0.8%	0.6%	0.6%	1.2%	1.2%
Nasopharyngitis	2.3%	1.8%	2.6%	2.3%	4.7%	4%
Pharyngolaryngeal pain	0.8%	0.9%	1%	0.5%	1.6%	1.4%
Rhinitis	1%	0.8%	0.5%	0.6%	1.4%	1.4%
Upper respiratory tract infection	0.9%	0.9%	0.8%	0.9%	1.7%	2%
Miscellaneous						
Back pain	0.8%	0.9%	0.6%	0.2%	1.3%	1.1%
Influenza-like illness[c]	8.2%	8.5%	5.8%	4.3%	12.3%	11.7%
Myalgia[c]	13.3%	12.9%	5.6%	5.3%	15.6%	15.5%
Pyrexia[c]	1.9%	2.1%	1.5%	1.7%	3.2%	3%
Rash[c]	0.8%	0.9%	0.7%	0.8%	1.3%	1.5%

[a] The adverse events in this table are those observed at an incidence of ≥ 1% in the *Ixiaro* or phosphate buffered saline with aluminum hydroxide 0.1% groups.
[b] N = number of subjects in the safety population (subjects treated with at least 1 dose) who received the respective dose.
[c] These symptoms were solicited in a subject diary card. Percentages include unsolicited events that occurred after the 7-day period covered by the diary card.

Injection-site reactions:

Ixiaro Injection-Site Adverse Reactions[a,b,c]						
	Postdose 1		Postdose 2		Postdose 1 or dose 2	
Adverse reaction	*Ixiaro* (n = 1,963)	PBS + $Al(OH)_3$ (n = 645)	*Ixiaro* (n = 1,951)	PBS + $Al(OH)_3$ (n = 638)	*Ixiaro* (n = 1,963)	PBS + $Al(OH)_3$ (n = 645)
Any reaction	48.5%	47.7%	32.6%	32.2%	55.4%	56.2%

Ixiaro Injection-Site Adverse Reactions[a,b,c]						
	Postdose 1		Postdose 2		Postdose 1 or dose 2	
Adverse reaction	*Ixiaro* (n = 1,963)	PBS + $Al(OH)_3$ (n = 645)	*Ixiaro* (n = 1,951)	PBS + $Al(OH)_3$ (n = 638)	*Ixiaro* (n = 1,963)	PBS + $Al(OH)_3$ (n = 645)
Edema	2.4%	3.3%	2.3%	1.6%	4.2%	4.6%
Erythema	6.8%	5.4%	4.6%	4.1%	9.6%	7.4%
Induration	4.8%	5.3%	4%	3%	7.5%	7.4%
Pain	27.7%	28.2%	17.7%	18.2%	33%	35.8%
Pruritus	2.6%	3.3%	1.6%	1.9%	3.8%	4.5%
Tenderness	28.8%	26.9%	22.5%	18.1%	35.9%	32.6%

[a] Injection-site reactions were assessed for 7 days after each dose.
[b] Denominators used to calculate percentages were based on the number of evaluable diary card entries (defined as documented presence on any day (ie, entry of yes) or absence on all days (ie, entry of no) for each individual symptom and observation period.
[c] N = number of subjects who returned diary cards after each dose

Serious adverse events: The serious adverse events occurring in the *Ixiaro* group were as follows: dermatomyositis, appendicitis, rectal hemorrhage, limb abscess (contralateral to the injected arm), chest pain, ovarian torsion, ruptured corpus luteal cyst, and 3 orthopedic injuries.

Comparison with JE-Vax: No deaths occurred during this trial. One serious adverse event occurred in this trial in a subject with a history of myocardial infarction who experienced an myocardial infarction 3 weeks after receiving the second dose of *Ixiaro*. The most common adverse events after immunization occurring in less than 1% of subjects were headache, myalgia, fatigue, influenza-like illness, nausea, nasopharyngitis, pyrexia, pharyngolaryngeal pain, cough, rash, diarrhea, sinusitis, upper respiratory tract infection, back pain, migraine, vomiting and influenza, which occurred with similar frequency in both treatment groups. Local injection-site reactions solicited in diary cards were observed at a rate of 54% in the *Ixiaro* group (n = 428) compared with a rate of 69.1% in the *JE-Vax* group (n = 435).

Overdosage

None reported.

Patient Information

Instruct patients that a 3-dose immunizing series should be completed, except in unusual circumstances.

Advise patients that Japanese encephalitis vaccine should be given to a pregnant woman only if, in the opinion of a health care provider, withholding the vaccine entails even greater risk.

Advise patients to report any adverse events following Japanese encephalitis vaccine through the VAERS at 1-800-822-7967 after contacting the health care provider immediately.

Advise patients with a history of urticaria (hives) following hymenoptera envenomation, drug administration, physical or other provocation, or of idiopathic origin that adverse effects are more likely.

Educate patients that adverse events consisting of arm soreness and local redness can occur shortly after vaccination.

Educate patients that adverse events consisting of headache, rash, edema, and generalized urticaria or angioedema may occur shortly after vaccination or up to 17 days (usually within 10 days) following vaccination.

Inform patients that international travel should not be initiated within 10 days of vaccination with *JE-Vax* vaccine because of the possibility of delayed adverse reactions. Instruct patients to seek medical attention immediately upon onset of any adverse reaction.

Inform patients that Japanese encephalitis vaccines may not fully protect everyone who receives the vaccine. Personal precautions should be taken to avoid exposure to mosquito bites by the use of insect repellents, mosquito nets, and protective clothing. Avoiding outdoor activity, especially during twilight periods and in the evening, will reduce risk even further.

ROTAVIRUS VACCINE, LIVE

Rx	**Rotarix** (GlaxoSmithKline)	**Lyophilized powder for suspension; oral:** rotavirus human 89-12 strain (G1P[8] type); ≥ 10^6 cell culture infective dose per 1 mL (after reconstitution)[a]	Preservative free. Dextran, D-glucose, sorbitol, sucrose. In vials with 1 mL of prefilled liquid diluent and transfer adapter for reconstitution.
Rx	**RotaTeq** (Merck)	**Suspension; oral:** rotavirus outer capsid protein (2.2×10^6 infectious units of G1, 2.8×10^6 infectious units of G2, 2.2×10^6 infectious units of G3, and 2×10^6 infectious units of G4) and 2.3×10^6 infectious units of rotavirus attachment protein P1A[8] per 2 mL[b]	Preservative free. Sucrose. In 2 mL single-dose tubes.

[a] Attenuated. The tip cap and rubber plunger of the oral applicator contain dry natural latex rubber. The vial stopper and transfer adaptor are latex free.

[b] Pentavalent. Contains 5 live reassortant rotaviruses.

ROTAVIRUS VACCINE, LIVE — ORAL

Indications

➤*Rotavirus gastroenteritis:*

Rotarix – For the prevention of rotavirus gastroenteritis in infants 6 to 24 weeks of age caused by G1 and non-G1 (G3, G4, and G9) types when administered as a 2-dose series.

RotaTeq – For the prevention of rotavirus gastroenteritis in infants and children caused by the serotypes G1, G2, G3, and G4 when administered as a 3-dose series to infants between 6 and 32 weeks of age. Administer the first dose of rotavirus vaccine when the patient is between 6 and 12 weeks of age.

Administration and Dosage

➤*Children:*

Rotavirus gastroenteritis prevention –

Rotarix:

• *6 to 24 weeks of age* – The vaccination series consists of two 1 mL oral doses. The first dose should be administered to infants beginning at 6 weeks of age. There should be an interval of at least 4 weeks between the first and second doses. The 2-dose series should be completed by 24 weeks of age.

RotaTeq:

• *6 to 32 weeks of age* – The vaccination series consists of 3 oral doses starting when the patient is 6 to 12 weeks of age, with the subsequent doses administered at 4- to 10-week intervals. The third dose should not be given after the patient reaches 32 weeks of age.

➤*Preparation for administration:*

Rotarix – Reconstitute only with the accompanying diluent. Remove the vial cap and push the transfer adapter onto the vial (lyophilized vaccine). Shake the diluent in the oral applicator (white, turbid suspension). Connect the oral applicator to the transfer adapter. Push the plunger of the oral applicator to transfer the diluent into the vial. The suspension will appear white and turbid. Withdraw vaccine into the oral applicator. Twist and remove the oral applicator. Administer within 24 hours of reconstitution.

RotaTeq –

Tear open the pouch and remove the dosing tube. Clear the fluid from the dispensing tip by holding the tube vertically and tapping the cap. Open the dosing tube in 2 easy motions (puncture the dispensing tip by screwing the cap clockwise until it becomes tight and then remove the cap by turning it counterclockwise).

➤*Administration:* For oral use only. Not for injection.

Rotarix – In the event that the infant spits out or regurgitates most of the vaccine dose, a single replacement dose may be considered at the same vaccination visit.

RotaTeq – Administer the dose by gently squeezing the liquid into the infant's mouth toward the inner cheek until the dosing tube is empty. A residual drop may remain in the tip of the tube. If for any reason an incomplete dose is administered (eg, infant spits or regurgitates the vaccine), a replacement dose is not recommended because such dosing was not studied in the clinical trials. The infant should continue to receive any remaining doses in the recommended series.

➤*Admixture compatibility:* Do not mix rotavirus vaccine with any other vaccines or solutions.

➤*Storage/Stability:*

Rotarix – Store the unreconstituted vials at 2° to 8°C (36° to 46°F). The diluent may be stored at 20° to 25°C (68° to 77°F). Do not freeze. Discard the vaccine if it has been frozen. Protect vials from light. *Rotarix* should be administered within 24 hours of reconstitution. It may be stored at 2° to 8°C (36° to 46°F) or at room temperature up to 25°C (77°F) after reconstitution. If not used within 24 hours, discard. Do not freeze. Discard if the vaccine has been frozen.

RotaTeq – Store at 2° to 8°C (36° to 46°F). Administer *RotaTeq* as soon as possible after being removed from refrigeration. Protect from light. For information regarding stability under conditions other than those recommended, call 1-800-637-2590.

Actions

➤*Pharmacology:* The exact immunologic mechanism by which rotavirus vaccine protects against rotavirus gastroenteritis is unknown. Rotavirus vaccine is a live, viral vaccine that replicates in the small intestine and induces immunity.

Contraindications

A demonstrated history of hypersensitivity to any component of the vaccine; history of uncorrected congenital malformation of the GI tract (such as Meckel diverticulum) that would predispose the infant for intussusception (*Rotarix* only); history of intussusception (*Rotarix* only); severe combined immunodeficiency disease.

Warnings/Precautions

➤*Immunodeficiency:*

Rotarix – Safety and effectiveness in infants with known primary or secondary immunodeficiencies, including infants with HIV, infants on immunosuppressive therapy, or infants with malignant neoplasms affecting the bone marrow or lymphatic system, have not been evaluated.

RotaTeq – No safety or efficacy data are available from clinical trials regarding administration to infants who are potentially immunocompromised, including infants with blood dyscrasias, leukemia, lymphomas of any type, or other malignant neoplasms affecting the bone marrow or lymphatic system; and infants on immunosuppressive therapy (including high-dose systemic corticosteroids). *RotaTeq* may be administered to infants who are being treated with topical corticosteroids or inhaled steroids; and to infants with primary and acquired immunodeficiency states, including HIV/AIDS or other clinical manifestations of infection with human immunodeficiency viruses, cellular immune deficiencies, and hypogammaglobulinemic and dysgammaglobulinemic states. There are insufficient data from the clinical trials to support administration of rotavirus vaccine to infants with indeterminate HIV status who are born to mothers with HIV/AIDS; infants who have received a blood transfusion or blood products, including immunoglobulins, within 42 days.

➤*GI disorders:*

Rotarix – Delay administration in infants suffering from acute diarrhea or vomiting.

Safety and effectiveness in infants with chronic GI disorders have not been evaluated.

RotaTeq – No safety or efficacy data are available for administration to infants with a history of GI disorders, including infants with active acute GI illness, infants with chronic diarrhea and failure to thrive, and infants with a history of congenital abdominal disorders, abdominal surgery, and intussusception. Therefore, use caution when considering administration of rotavirus vaccine to these infants.

➤*Intussusception:* Following administration of a previously licensed oral live rhesus rotavirus-based vaccine, an increased risk of intussusception was observed. In postmarketing experience, cases of intussusception have been reported.

➤*Shedding and transmission:* Caution is advised when considering whether to administer to individuals with immunodeficient close contacts, such as individuals with malignancies or who are otherwise immunocompromised, or those who are receiving immunosuppressive therapy.

Rotavirus vaccine is a solution of live reassortant rotaviruses and can potentially be transmitted to persons who have contact with the vaccine. Weigh the potential risk of transmission of vaccine virus against the risk of acquiring and transmitting natural rotavirus.

➤*Febrile illness:* Febrile illness may be reason for delaying use of rotavirus vaccine except when, in the opinion of the health care provider, withholding the vaccine entails a greater risk. Low-grade fever (less than 38.1°C [100.5°F]) itself and mild upper respiratory infection do not preclude vaccination.

➤*Level of protection:* The clinical studies were not designed to assess the level of protection provided by only 1 or 2 doses of *RotaTeq*. *RotaTeq* may not protect all vaccine recipients against rotavirus.

➤*Postexposure prophylaxis:* Safety and effectiveness of *Rotarix* when administered after exposure to rotavirus have not been evaluated. No clinical data are available for *RotaTeq* when administered after exposure to rotavirus.

➤*Hypersensitivity reactions:* Do not give further doses to infants who develop symptoms suggestive of hypersensitivity after receiving a dose of rotavirus vaccine.

➤*Pregnancy: Category C.* Animal reproduction studies have not been conducted with rotavirus vaccine. It is also not known whether rotavirus vaccine can cause fetal harm when administered to a pregnant woman or can affect reproduction capacity. Rotavirus vaccine is not indicated in women of childbearing age; do not administer to pregnant women.

ROTAVIRUS VACCINE, LIVE — ORAL

➤*Lactation:* Rotavirus vaccine is not indicated in women of childbearing age; do not administer to breast-feeding women.

➤*Children:* Safety and effectiveness of *Rotarix* in infants younger than 6 weeks of age or older than 24 weeks of age have not been evaluated. Safety and efficacy of *RotaTeq* have not been established in infants younger than 6 weeks of age or older than 32 weeks of age.

➤*Monitoring:* Prior to administration of rotavirus vaccine, determine the current health status and previous vaccination history of the infant, including whether there has been a reaction to a previous dose of this rotavirus vaccine or other types of rotavirus vaccines (eg, rhesus rotavirus-based product).

Drug Interactions

➤*Immunosuppressive therapies:* Immunosuppressive therapies, including irradiation, antimetabolites, alkylating agents, cytotoxic drugs, and corticosteroids (used in more than physiologic doses), may reduce the immune response to either formulation of rotavirus vaccine. Use with caution.

➤*Severe adverse reactions:* The risk of live rotavirus vaccine-induced severe adverse reactions may be increased by coadministration of live rotavirus vaccine with antineoplastic agents, busulfan, docetaxel, epothilones (eg, ixabepilone), melphalan, nitrosoureas (eg, carmustine), paclitaxel, thiopurines (eg, azathioprine), or thiotepa. Concurrent use of live rotavirus live vaccine with one of these agents is not recommended under most circumstances. Defer administration of live rotavirus vaccine.

Adverse Reactions

➤*Rotarix:*

Solicited adverse reactions –

Rotarix Solicited Adverse Reactions[a]

	Dose 1		Dose 2	
Adverse reactions	*Rotarix* (n = 3,284)	Placebo (n = 2,013)	*Rotarix* (n = 3,201)	Placebo (n = 1,973)
GI				
Diarrhea	4%	3%	3%	3%
Loss of appetite[b]	25%	25%	21%	21%
Vomiting	13%	11%	8%	8%
Miscellaneous				
Cough/Runny nose[c]	28%	30%	31%	33%
Fever[d]	25%	33%	28%	34%
Fussiness/Irritability[e]	52%	52%	42%	42%

[a] n = number of infants for whom at least 1 symptom sheet was completed.
[b] Defined as eating less than usual.
[c] Data not collected in 1 of 7 studies; dose 1: *Rotarix*, n = 2,583 and placebo, n = 1,897; dose 2: *Rotarix*, n = 2,522 and placebo, n = 11,863.
[d] Defined as a rectal temperature of 100.4°F (38°C) or more or an oral temperature of 99.5°F (37.5°C) or more.
[e] Defined as crying more than usual.

Unsolicited adverse reactions – Infants were monitored for unsolicited serious and nonserious adverse reactions that occurred in the 31-day period following vaccination in 7 clinical studies. The following adverse reactions occurred at a statistically higher incidence (95% CI of relative risk [RR] excluding 1) among recipients of *Rotarix* (n = 5,082) compared with placebo recipients (n = 2,902): irritability (*Rotarix*, 11.4%; placebo, 8.7%) and flatulence (*Rotarix*, 2.2%; placebo, 1.3%).

Serious adverse reactions – Infants were monitored for serious adverse reactions that occurred in the 31-day period following vaccination in 8 clinical studies. Serious adverse reactions occurred in 1.7% of recipients of *Rotarix* (n = 36,755) compared with 1.9% of placebo recipients (n = 34,454). Among placebo recipients, diarrhea (placebo, 0.07%; *Rotarix*, 0.02%), dehydration (placebo, 0.06%; *Rotarix*, 0.02%), and gastroenteritis (placebo,0.3; *Rotarix*, 0.2%) occurred at a statistically higher incidence (95% CI of RR excluding 1) compared with recipients of *Rotarix*.

Deaths – During the entire course of 8 clinical studies, there were 68 (0.19%) deaths following administration of *Rotarix* (n = 36,755) and 50 (0.15%) deaths following placebo administration (n = 34,454). The most commonly reported cause of death following vaccination was pneumonia, which was observed in 0.05% of recipients of *Rotarix* and 0.03% of placebo recipients (RR, 1.74; 95% CI, 0.76 to 4.23).

Intussusception –

No increased risk of intussusception following administration of *Rotarix* was observed within a 31-day period following any dose, and rates were comparable with the placebo group after a median of 100 days. In the subset of 20,169 infants followed up to 1 year after dose 1, there were 4 cases of intussusception with *Rotarix* compared with 14 cases of intussusception with placebo (RR, 0.28; 95% CI, 0.1 to 0.81). All of the infants who developed intussusception recovered without sequelae.

Intussusception and Relative Risk With Rotarix

Confirmed cases of intussusception	*Rotarix* (n = 31,673)	Placebo (n = 31,552)
Within 31 days of diagnosis after any dose	6	7
RR (95% CI)	0.85 (0.3 to 2.42)	
Within 100 days of dose 1[a]	9	16
RR (95% CI)	0.56 (0.25 to 1.24)	

[a] Median duration after dose 1 (follow-up visit at 30 to 90 days after dose 2).

Kawasaki disease – Kawasaki disease has been reported in 0.035% of recipients of *Rotarix* and 0.021% of placebo recipients from 16 completed or ongoing clinical trials. Of the 27 cases, 5 occurred following *Rotarix* in clinical trials that were either not placebo controlled or 1:1 randomized. In placebo-controlled trials, Kawasaki disease was reported in 17 recipients of *Rotarix* and 9 placebo recipients (RR, 1.71; 95% CI, 0.71 to 4.38). 11.1% of cases were reported within 30 days postvaccination: 2 cases (*Rotarix* = 1, placebo = 1) were from placebo-controlled trials (RR, 1; 95% CI, 0.01 to 78.35), and 1 case following *Rotarix* was from a nonplacebo-controlled trial. Among recipients of *Rotarix*, the time of onset after study dose ranged 3 days to 19 months.

➤*RotaTeq:*

Serious adverse reactions – Serious adverse reactions occurred in 2.4% of recipients of *RotaTeq* compared with 2.6% of placebo recipients within the 42-day period of a dose in the phase 3 clinical studies of *RotaTeq*. The most frequently reported serious adverse reactions for *RotaTeq* compared with placebo were bronchiolitis (0.6% *RotaTeq* vs 0.7% placebo), gastroenteritis (0.2% *RotaTeq* vs 0.3% placebo), pneumonia (0.2% *RotaTeq* vs 0.2% placebo), fever (0.1% *RotaTeq* vs 0.1% placebo), and urinary tract infection (0.1% *RotaTeq* vs 0.1% placebo).

Deaths – Across the clinical studies, 52 deaths were reported. There were 25 deaths in the *RotaTeq* recipients compared with 27 deaths in the placebo recipients. The most commonly reported cause of death was sudden infant death syndrome (SIDS), which was observed in 8 recipients of *RotaTeq* and 9 recipients of placebo.

Intussusception –

Intussusception With RotaTeq

	RotaTeq (n = 34,837)	Placebo (n = 34,788)
Confirmed intussusception cases within 42 days of any dose	6	5
RR (95% CI)[a]	1.6 (0.4 to 6.4)	
Confirmed intussusception cases within 365 days of dose 1	13	15
RR (95% CI)	0.9 (0.4 to 1.9)	

[a] RR and 95% CI based on group-sequential design-stopping criteria employed in the Rotavirus Efficacy and Safety Trial (REST).

All of the children who developed intussusception recovered without sequelae with the exception of a male infant 9 months of age who developed intussusception 98 days after dose 3 and died of postoperative sepsis. There was a single case of intussusception among the 2,470 recipients of *RotaTeq* in a male infant 7 months of age in the phase 1 and 2 studies (716 placebo recipients).

Hematochezia – Hematochezia reported as an adverse reaction occurred in 0.6% of vaccine and 0.6% of placebo recipients within 42 days of any dose. Hematochezia reported as a serious adverse reaction occurred in less than 0.1% of vaccine and less than 0.1% of placebo recipients within 42 days of any dose.

Seizures –

Reported Seizures With RotaTeq

Day range	1 to 7	1 to 14	1 to 42
RotaTeq	10	15	33
Placebo	5	8	24

Seizures reported as serious adverse reactions occurred in less than 0.1% of vaccine and less than 0.1% of placebo recipients (not significant). Ten febrile seizures were reported as serious adverse reactions, 5 were observed in vaccine recipients and 5 in placebo recipients.

Kawasaki disease – In the phase 3 clinical trials, infants were followed for up to 42 days of vaccine dose. Kawasaki disease was reported in 5 of vaccine recipients and in 1 of placebo recipients with unadjusted relative risk of 4.9 (95% CI, 0.6 to 239.1).

ROTAVIRUS VACCINE, LIVE — ORAL

Most common adverse reactions –

RotaTeq Adverse Reactions Occurring in the First Week						
Adverse reactions	Dose 1		Dose 2		Dose 3	
	RotaTeq	Placebo	*RotaTeq*	Placebo	*RotaTeq*	Placebo
	(n = 5,616)	(n = 5,077)	(n = 5,215)	(n = 4,725)	(n = 4,865)	(n = 4,382)
Elevated temperature[a]	17.1%	16.2%	20%	19.4%	18.2%	17.6%
	(n = 6,130)	(n = 5,560)	(n = 5,703)	(n = 5,173)	(n = 5,496)	(n = 4,989)
Diarrhea	10.4%	9.1%	8.6%	6.4%	6.1%	5.4%
Irritability	7.1%	7.1%	6%	6.5%	4.3%	4.5%
Vomiting	6.7%	5.4%	5%	4.4%	3.6%	3.2%

[a] Temperature of at least 100.5°F (38.1°C) rectal equivalent obtained by adding 1°F to otic and oral temperatures and 2°F to axillary temperatures.

Other adverse reactions –

Fever was observed at similar rates in vaccine (n = 6,138) and placebo (n = 5,573) recipients (42.6% vs 42.8%). Adverse reactions that occurred at a statistically higher incidence (ie, 2-sided P value < 0.05) within the 42 days of any dose among recipients of *RotaTeq* compared with placebo recipients are provided.

RotaTeq Adverse Reactions Occurring Within 42 Days of Any Dose		
Adverse reactions	*RotaTeq* (n = 6,138)	Placebo (n = 5,573)
GI		
Diarrhea	24.1%	21.3%
Vomiting	15.2%	13.6%
Respiratory		
Bronchospasm	1.1%	0.7%
Nasopharyngitis	6.9%	5.8%
Special senses		
Otitis media	14.5%	13%

Preterm infants – *RotaTeq* or placebo was administered to 2,070 preterm infants (25 to 36 weeks' gestational age; median, 34 weeks) according to their age in weeks since birth in REST. All preterm infants were followed for serious adverse reactions; a subset of 308 infants was monitored for all adverse reactions. There were 4 deaths throughout the study, 2 among vaccine recipients (1 sudden infant death syndrome [SIDS] and 1 motor vehicle accident) and 2 among placebo recipients (1 SIDS and 1 unknown cause). No cases of intussusception were reported. Serious adverse reactions occurred in 5.5% of vaccine and 5.8% of placebo recipients. The most common serious adverse reaction was bronchiolitis, which occurred in 1.4% of vaccine and 2% of placebo recipients. Parents/guardians were asked to record the child's temperature and any episodes of vomiting and diarrhea daily for the first week following vaccination. The frequencies of these adverse reactions and irritability within the week after dose 1 are provided.

RotaTeq Adverse Reactions in Preterm Infants						
Adverse reactions	Dose 1		Dose 2		Dose 3	
	RotaTeq	Placebo	*RotaTeq*	Placebo	*RotaTeq*	Placebo
	(n = 127)	(n = 133)	(n = 124)	(n = 121)	(n = 115)	(n = 108)
Elevated temperature[a]	18.1%	17.3%	25%	28.1%	14.8%	20.4%
	(n = 154)	(n = 154)	(n = 137)	(n = 137)	(n = 135)	(n = 129)
Diarrhea	6.5%	5.8%	7.3%	7.3%	3.7%	3.9%
Irritability	3.9%	5.2%	2.9%	4.4%	8.1%	5.4%
Vomiting	5.8%	7.8%	2.9%	2.2%	4.4%	4.7%

[a] Temperature of 100.5°F (38.1°C) or more, rectal equivalent obtained by adding 1°F to otic and oral temperatures and 2°F to axillary temperatures.

➤*Postmarketing:*

Dermatologic – Urticaria.

GI – Gastroenteritis with vaccine shedding in infants with severe combined immunodeficiency disease, hematochezia, intussusception (including death).

Miscellaneous – Idiopathic thrombocytopenia purpura, Kawasaki disease, maladministration.

Patient Information

Inform parents or guardians of the potential benefits and risks of immunization with rotavirus vaccine, and of the importance of completing the immunization series.

Inform parents or guardians about the potential for adverse reactions that have been temporally associated with administration of rotavirus vaccine or other vaccines containing similar components.

Give the parent or guardian the Vaccine Information Statements, which are required by the National Childhood Vaccine Injury Act of 1986 to be given prior to immunization. These materials are available free of charge at the Centers for Disease Control and Prevention (CDC) Web site (http://www.cdc.gov/vaccines). Encourage parents and/or guardians to read the patient information that describes the benefits and risks associated with the vaccine and to ask any questions they may have during the visit.

Instruct parents or guardians to report any adverse reactions to their health care provider. Report all adverse reactions to the US Department of Health and Human Services' VAERS. VAERS accepts all reports of suspected adverse reactions after the administration of any vaccine, including, but not limited to, the reporting of reactions required by the National Childhood Vaccine Injury Act of 1986. For information or a copy of the vaccine reporting form, call VAERS toll-free number at 1-800-822-7967 or report online to http://www.vaers.hhs.gov.

YELLOW FEVER VACCINE

Rx	**YF-Vax**[a] (Sanofi Pasteur)	**Lyophilized Powder for Injection:** Not less than 4.74 $\log_{10}$ plaque-forming units (PFU) per 0.5 mL dose when reconstituted[b]	In single-dose vials with 0.6 mL diluent, and 5-dose vials with 3 mL of diluent.

[a] Supplied only to designated Yellow Fever Vaccination Centers authorized to issue certificates of Yellow Fever Vaccination.

[b] With gelatin and sorbitol.

YELLOW FEVER VACCINE — INJECTION

Indications

➤*General information:* As with any vaccine, vaccination with yellow fever vaccine may not protect 100% of susceptible individuals.

➤*Yellow fever vaccination:* For active immunization of persons 9 months of age and older in the following categories:

Persons living in or traveling to endemic areas – While the actual risk for contracting yellow fever during travel is probably low, variability of itineraries and behaviors and the seasonal incidence of disease make it difficult to predict the actual risk for a given individual traveling to a known endemic or epidemic area. Vaccinate persons 9 months of age and older traveling to or living in areas of South America and Africa where yellow fever infection is officially reported at the time of travel. Vaccination is also recommended for travel outside the urban areas of countries that do not officially report the disease but lie in a yellow fever endemic zone.

Persons traveling internationally – Yellow fever vaccination may be required for international travel. Some countries in Africa require evidence of vaccination from all entering travelers and some countries may waive the requirements for travelers staying less than 2 weeks that are coming from areas where there is no current evidence of significant risk for contracting yellow fever. Some countries require an individual, even if only in transit, to have a valid International Certificate of Vaccination if the individual has been in countries either known or thought to harbor yellow fever virus. The certificate becomes valid 10 days after vaccination with yellow fever vaccine.

Laboratory personnel – Vaccinate those laboratory personnel who might be exposed to virulent yellow fever virus or concentrated preparations of the yellow fever vaccine strain by direct or indirect contact or by aerosols.

Administration and Dosage

➤*General dosing considerations:* If immunization is imperative and the individual has a history of severe egg sensitivity and has a positive skin test to the vaccine, a desensitization procedure may be used to administer the vaccine (See Administration: Desensitization).

➤*Adults:*

Yellow fever vaccination –

Usual dosage:

• *Primary vaccination* – For all eligible persons, a single subcutaneous injection of 0.5 mL of reconstituted vaccine (formulated to contain not less than 4.74 $\log_{10}$ plaque-forming units [PFU]) should be administered. Immunity develops by the 10th day after primary vaccination.

• *Booster doses* – Re-immunization is recommended every 10 years for those at continuing risk of exposure and is required by International Health Regulations. Revaccination boosts antibody titer, although evidence from several studies suggests that yellow fever vaccine immunity persists for at least 30 to 35 years and probably for life, and epidemiologic data suggest that a single infection with wild-type yellow fever virus provides lifelong immunity against illness due to subsequent exposure.

• *Concomitant therapy with other vaccines* – Determination of whether to administer yellow fever vaccine and other immunobiologics simultaneously should be made on the basis of convenience to the traveler in completing the desired vaccinations before travel and on information regarding possible interference. Limited data are available related to administration of yellow fever vaccine with other vaccines. In those specific instances in which vaccines may be given concurrently, injections should be administered at separate sites. When there are no data to support administration of yellow fever vaccine concurrently with other vaccines, 4 weeks should elapse between sequential vaccinations.

YELLOW FEVER VACCINE — INJECTION

➤*Children:*

Yellow fever vaccination –

9 months of age and older: See Adults for dosing for patients 9 months of age and older.

Younger than 9 months of age: Vaccination of infants younger than 9 months of age is contraindicated because of the risk of encephalitis.

➤*Elderly:* Limit vaccination of subjects older than 65 years of age to individuals who are traveling to or reside in known yellow fever endemic or epidemic areas because of the increased risk for systemic adverse reactions in this age group.

➤*Preparation for administration:* A separate, sterile syringe and needle should be used for each patient to prevent transmission of hepatitis or other infectious agents from person to person. Needles should not be recapped and should be properly disposed (eg, sterilized, disposed in red hazardous waste containers).

Reconstitution – Reconstitute the vaccine using only the diluent supplied (0.6 mL vial of sodium chloride injection for single dose vial of vaccine and 3 mL vial of sodium chloride injection for 5-dose vial of vaccine). Draw the volume of the diluent, shown on the diluent label, into a suitable size syringe and slowly inject into the vial containing the vaccine. Allow the reconstituted vaccine to sit for 1 to 2 minutes and then carefully swirl mixture until a uniform suspension is achieved. Avoid vigorous shaking as this tends to cause foaming of the suspension. Do not dilute reconstituted vaccine. Swirl vaccine well before withdrawing each dose.

➤*Administration:* Administer the single immunizing dose of 0.5 mL subcutaneously using a 5/8- to 3/4-inch long needle within 60 minutes of reconstituting the vial. Properly dispose of all reconstituted vaccine and containers that remain unused after 1 hour (eg, sterilized, disposed in red hazardous waste containers).

Desensitization – If immunization is imperative and the individual has a history of severe egg sensitivity and has a positive skin test to the vaccine, this desensitization procedure may be used to administer the vaccine.

Desensitization should only be performed under the direct supervision of a health care provider experienced in the management of anaphylaxis with necessary emergency equipment immediately available.

The following successive doses should be administered subcutaneously at 15- to 20-minute intervals:

- 0.05 mL of 1:10 dilution
- 0.05 mL of full strength
- 0.1 mL of full strength
- 0.15 mL of full strength
- 0.2 mL of full strength

➤*Storage/Stability:* Yellow fever vaccine is shipped frozen in a container with solid carbon dioxide; do not use unless the shipping case contains some dry ice upon arrival.

Upon receipt, lyophilized vaccine must be maintained continuously at 0° to 5°C (32° to 41°F). Do not refreeze.

Yellow fever vaccine does not contain a preservative; therefore, all reconstituted vaccine and containers that remain unused after 1 hour must be properly disposed (eg, sterilized, disposed in red hazardous waste containers).

The following stability information for yellow fever vaccine is provided for those countries or areas of the world where an adequate cold chain is a problem and inadvertent exposure to abnormal temperatures has occurred.

Actions

➤*Pharmacology:* Vaccination with 17D strain viruses is predicted to elicit an immune response identical in quality to that induced by wild-type infection. This response is presumed to result from initial infection of cells in the dermis or other subcutaneous tissues near the injection site, with subsequent replication and limited spread of virus leading to the processing and presentation of viral antigens to the immune system, as would occur during infection with wild-type yellow fever virus. The humoral immune response to the viral structural proteins, as opposed to a cell-mediated response, is most important in the protective effect induced by 17D vaccines. Yellow fever antibodies with specificities that prevent or abort infection of cells are detected as neutralizing antibodies in assays that measure the ability of serum to reduce plaque formation in tissue culture cells. The titer of virus-neutralizing antibodies in sera of vaccinees is a surrogate for efficacy. A $\log_{10}$ neutralization index (LNI; measured by a plaque reduction assay) of 0.7 or greater was shown to protect 90% of monkeys from lethal intracerebral challenge. This is the definition of seroconversion adopted for clinical trials of yellow fever vaccine. The standard has also been adopted by WHO for efficacy of yellow fever vaccines in humans.

Contraindications

➤*Hypersensitivity reactions:* Because the yellow fever virus used in the production of this vaccine is propagated in chicken embryos, do not administer yellow fever vaccine to anyone with a history of acute hypersensitivity to eggs or egg products; anaphylaxis may occur. Less severe or localized manifestations of allergy to eggs or feathers are not contraindications to vaccine administration and do not usually warrant vaccine skin testing. Generally, persons who are able to eat eggs or egg products may receive the vaccine.

➤*Children:* Vaccination of infants younger than 9 months of age is contraindicated because of the risk of encephalitis, and travel of such persons to rural areas in yellow fever endemic zones or to countries experiencing an epidemic should be postponed or avoided whenever possible.

➤*Immunodeficiency:* Exposure to yellow fever vaccine, which is a live virus vaccine, poses a risk of encephalitis or other serious adverse reactions to patients with illnesses that commonly result in immunosuppression (eg, AIDS or other manifestations of HIV infection, leukemia, lymphoma, thymoma, generalized malignancy) or patients whose immunologic responses are suppressed by drug therapy (eg, corticosteroids, alkylating drugs, antimetabolites) or radiation. Therefore, do not immunize immunosuppressed subjects, and such persons' travel to yellow fever endemic areas should be postponed or avoided. If travel to a yellow fever-infected zone is unavoidable, advise immunosuppressed patients of the risk, instruct them in methods for avoiding vector mosquitoes, and supply them with vaccination waiver letters by their health care providers.

Family members of immunosuppressed persons, who themselves have no contraindications, may receive yellow fever vaccine.

Warnings/Precautions

➤*Viscerotropic disease:* Yellow fever vaccines must be considered as a possible, but rare, cause of vaccine-associated viscerotropic disease (previously described as multiple organ system failure), which is similar to fulminant yellow fever caused by wild-type yellow fever virus. Available evidence suggests that the occurrence of this syndrome may depend upon the presence of undefined host factors, rather than intrinsic virulence of the yellow fever strain 17D vaccine viruses isolated from subjects with vaccine-associated viscerotropic disease.

➤*Neurotropic disease:* Vaccine-associated neurotropic disease (previously described as postvaccinal encephalitis) is a known rare adverse reaction associated with yellow fever vaccination. Age younger than 9 months and immunosuppression are known risk factors for this adverse reaction.

➤*Immunodeficiency:* Exposure to yellow fever vaccine, which is a live virus vaccine, poses a risk of encephalitis or other serious adverse reactions to patients with illnesses that commonly result in immunosuppression (eg, AIDS or other manifestations of HIV infection, leukemia, lymphoma, thymoma, generalized malignancy) or patients whose immunologic responses are suppressed by drug therapy (eg, corticosteroids, alkylating drugs, antimetabolites) or radiation. Therefore, do not immunize immunosuppressed subjects, and such persons' travel to yellow fever endemic areas should be postponed or avoided. If travel to a yellow fever-infected zone is unavoidable, advise immunosuppressed patients of the risk, instruct them in methods for avoiding vector mosquitoes, and supply them with vaccination waiver letters by their health care providers.

Family members of immunosuppressed persons, who themselves have no contraindications, may receive yellow fever vaccine.

➤*Latex sensitivity:* The stopper of the vial contains dry natural latex rubber, which may cause allergic reactions. In some instances in which symptoms appear soon after a vaccine is administered, differentiation between allergic reaction to the vaccine and reaction to an environmental allergen may not be possible.

➤*Revaccination:* Existing data suggest that the small percentage of immunologically healthy subjects who fail to develop an immune response to an initial vaccination may do so upon revaccination.

➤*HIV infection:* Subjects with asymptomatic HIV infection who have had recent laboratory verification of adequate immune system function and who cannot avoid potential exposure to yellow fever virus should be offered the choice of vaccination. Monitor vaccinees for possible adverse reactions. The seroconversion rate to 17D vaccines is likely to be reduced in these patients. Therefore, documentation of a protective antibody response is recommended before travel.

➤*Hypersensitivity reactions:* Anaphylaxis may occur following the use of yellow fever vaccine, even in individuals with no prior history of hypersensitivity to the vaccine components.

Epinephrine injection (1:1,000) should always be immediately available in case of an unexpected anaphylactic or other serious allergic reaction.

Do not administer yellow fever vaccine to an individual with a history of hypersensitivity to egg or chicken protein. Less severe or localized manifestations of allergy to eggs or feathers are not contraindications to vaccine administration and do not usually warrant vaccine skin testing. Generally, persons who are able to eat eggs or egg products may receive the vaccine. However, if a subject is suspect as being an egg-sensitive individual, the following test can be performed before the vaccine is administered:

1.) Scratch, prick, or puncture test: Place a drop of a 1:10 dilution of the vaccine in physiologic saline on a superficial scratch, prick, or puncture on the volar surface of the forearm. Also use positive (histamine) and negative (physiologic saline) controls. The test is read after 15 to 20 minutes. A positive test is a wheal 3 mm larger than that of the saline control, usually with surrounding erythema. The histamine control must be positive for valid interpretation. If the result of this test is negative, perform an intradermal (ID) test.
2.) Intradermal test: Inject a dose of 0.02 mL of a 1:100 dilution of the vaccine in physiologic saline. Perform positive and negative control skin tests concurrently. A wheal 5 mm or larger than the negative control with surrounding erythema is considered a positive reaction.

If vaccination is considered essential, despite a positive skin test, then desensitization can be considered.

➤*Pregnancy: Category C.* Safety of yellow fever vaccine was evaluated in a study involving 101 Nigerian women, the majority of whom (88%) were in the third trimester of pregnancy. In this study, it appeared that vaccinating pregnant women with the 17D-204 strain of yellow fever vaccine was not associated with adverse reactions affecting the mother or fetus. There were no adverse reactions among 40 infants who were carefully followed up for

YELLOW FEVER VACCINE — INJECTION

1 year after birth, and none of these infants tested positive for immunoglobulin M (IgM) antibodies as a criterion for transplacental infection. However, the percentage of pregnant women who seroconverted was significantly reduced compared with a nonpregnant control group (38.6% vs 81.5%).

Following a mass immunization campaign in Trinidad, during which 100 to 200 pregnant women were immunized, no adverse reactions related to pregnancy were reported. In addition, 41 cord blood samples were obtained from infants born to mothers immunized during the first trimester. One of these infants tested positive for IgM antibodies in cord blood. The infant appeared normal at delivery and no subsequent adverse sequelae of infection were reported. However, this result suggests that transplacental infection with 17D vaccine viruses can occur.

A recent case-control study of spontaneous abortion following vaccination of Brazilian women found no significant difference in the odds ratio among vaccinated women compared with a similar unvaccinated group.

Animal reproduction studies have not been conducted with yellow fever vaccine. It is also not known whether yellow fever vaccine can cause fetal harm when administered to a pregnant woman or can affect reproductive capacity. Because of the lack of large-scale controlled studies to verify its safety in pregnancy, give yellow fever vaccine to a pregnant woman only if clearly needed. The seroconversion rate to 17D vaccines is markedly reduced in pregnant women.

➤*Lactation:* It is not known whether this vaccine is excreted in human milk. There have been no reports of adverse reactions or transmission of 17D vaccine virus from breast-feeding mother to infant. However, avoid vaccination of breast-feeding mothers when possible because of the theoretical risk of the transmission of 17D virus to the breast-fed infant. When travel of breast-feeding mothers to high-risk yellow fever endemic areas cannot be avoided or postponed, such individuals may be immunized.

➤*Children:* See Contraindications for more information.

➤*Elderly:* Limit vaccination of subjects older than 65 years of age to individuals who are traveling to or reside in known yellow fever endemic or epidemic areas because of the increased risk for systemic adverse reactions in this age group. When vaccination is deemed necessary, evaluate the health status of such individuals prior to vaccination. Additionally, if vaccinated, carefully monitor elderly subjects for adverse reactions for 10 days postvaccination.

➤*Monitoring:* Prior to an injection of any vaccine, all known precautions should be taken to prevent adverse reactions. Review the patient's previous immunization history, current health status, and medical history for previous hypersensitivity reactions and other adverse reactions related to this vaccine or similar vaccines. Monitor all vaccinees for possible adverse reactions.

Adverse Reactions

➤*Reporting of adverse reactions:* The US Department of Health and Human Services (DHHS) has established a Vaccine Adverse Event Reporting System (VAERS) to accept all reports of suspected adverse reactions after the administration of any vaccine, including but not limited to the reporting of events required by the National Childhood Vaccine Injury Act of 1986. Reporting by patients, parents, or guardians of all adverse reactions occurring after vaccine administration is encouraged. Adverse reactions following immunization with vaccine should be reported by the health care provider to the US DHHS VAERS. The VAERS toll-free number for forms and information is 1-800-822-7967. Forms may also be available for downloading at the DHHS Web site http://www.hhs.gov.

Also report adverse reactions to the Pharmacovigilance Department, Aventis Pasteur Inc., Discovery Drive, Swiftwater, PA 18370, or call 1-800-822-2463.

➤*Adverse reactions:* Adverse reactions to 17D yellow fever vaccine include mild headaches, myalgia, low-grade fevers, or other minor symptoms for 5 to 10 days. Local reactions, including edema, hypersensitivity, or pain or mass at the injection site, have also been reported following yellow fever vaccine administration. Immediate hypersensitivity reactions, characterized by rash, urticaria, and/or asthma, are uncommon and occur principally among persons with histories of egg allergy.

No placebo-controlled trials to assess the safety of yellow fever 17D vaccines have been performed. However, between 1953 and 1994, reactogenicity of 17D-204 vaccine was monitored in 10 uncontrolled clinical trials. The trials included a total of 3,933 adults and 264 infants older than 4 months of age residing in Europe or yellow fever endemic areas. Self-limited and mild local reactions consisting of erythema and pain at the injection site and systemic reactions consisting of headache and/or fever occurred in a minority of subjects (typically less than 5%) 5 to 7 days after immunization. In one study involving 115 infants 4 to 24 months of age, the incidence of fever was as high as 21%. Also in this study, reactogenicity of the vaccine was markedly reduced among a subset of subjects who had serological evidence of previous exposure to yellow fever virus. Only 2 of the 10 studies provided diary cards for daily reporting; this method resulted in a slightly higher incidence of local and systemic complaints.

In 2001, yellow fever vaccine was used as a control in a double-blind, randomized, comparative trial with another 17D-204 vaccine, conducted at 9 centers in the United States. Yellow fever vaccine was administered to 725 adults at least 18 years of age (mean age, 38 years). Safety data were collected by diary card for days 1 through 10 after vaccination and by interview on days 5, 11, and 31. Among subjects who received yellow fever vaccine, there were no serious adverse reactions, and 71.9% experienced nonserious adverse reactions judged to have been related to vaccination. Most of these were injection site reactions of mild to moderate severity. Four such local reactions were considered severe. Rash occurred in 3.2% and urticaria in 2 subjects. Systemic reactions (headache, myalgia, malaise, and asthenia) were usually mild and occurred in 10% to 30% of subjects during the first few days after vaccination. The incidence of nonserious adverse reactions, including headache, malaise, injection site edema, and pain, was significantly lower in subjects older than 60 years of age compared with younger subjects. Adverse reactions were less frequent in the 1.7% of vaccinated subjects who had preexisting immunity to yellow fever virus, compared with those who had not been previously exposed.

➤*Elderly:* A Centers for Disease Control (CDC) analysis of data submitted to the VAERS between 1990 and 1998 suggests that patients 65 years of age or older are at increased risk for systemic adverse reactions temporally associated with vaccination, compared with the group 25 to 44 years of age. The rate of systemic adverse reactions occurring postvaccination in patients 65 to 74 years of age was 2.5 times higher than the rate occurring in patients 25 to 44 years of age, based on incidence rates of 6.21 and 2.49 per 100,000 doses of vaccine in the 2 groups, respectively.

➤*Neurotropic disease:* Vaccine-associated neurotropic disease (previously described as postvaccinal encephalitis) is a known rare serious adverse reaction associated with 17D vaccination. Age younger than 9 months and immunosuppression are known risk factors. Twenty-one cases of vaccine-associated neurotropic disease associated with all licensed 17D vaccines have been reported between 1952 and the present, 18 in children or adolescents. Fifteen of these cases occurred prior to 1960, 13 of which occurred in infants 4 months of age or younger, and 2 of which occurred in infants 6 and 7 months of age. Six cases were reported between 1960 and 1996 worldwide. Three occurred in children, including an infant 1 month of age, a 3-year-old, and a 13-year-old. The 3-year-old died of encephalitis, and a genetic variant of the vaccine virus was isolated from the brain in this case. This is the only verified fatality due to yellow fever vaccine-associated neurotropic disease. The 3 remaining cases of vaccine-associated neurotropic disease since 1960 occurred in adults.

The incidence of vaccine-associated neurotropic disease in infants younger than 4 months of age is estimated to be between 0.5 and 4 per 1,000, based on 2 historical reports where denominators are available. No data are available for calculation of an age-specific incidence rate in the group 4 to 9 months of age. A study in Senegal described 2 fatal cases of encephalitis possibly associated with 17D-204 vaccination among 67,325 children between the ages of 6 months and 2 years, for an incidence rate of 3 per 100,000. One study conducted in Kenya in 1993 detected 4 cases of encephalitis temporally associated with vaccination, 1 in a child 2 years of age and 3 in adults, for an incidence of 5.3 cases per million vaccinees of all ages.

➤*Viscerotropic disease:* Between 1996 and 1998, four patients, 63, 67, 76, and 79 years of age, became severely ill 2 to 5 days after vaccination with yellow fever vaccine. Three of these 4 subjects died. The clinical presentations were characterized by a nonspecific febrile syndrome with fatigue, myalgia, and headache, rapidly progressing to a severe illness including respiratory failure, elevated hepatocellular enzymes, lymphocytopenia and thrombocytopenia, hyperbilirubinemia, and renal failure requiring hemodialysis. None of these subjects had vaccine-associated neurotropic disease. This severe adverse reaction is known as "vaccine-associated viscerotropic disease" (previously described as multiple organ system failure). No cause-and-effect relationship has been established between vaccination and these subsequent illnesses. In 2 cases in which vaccine virus was recovered from serum, limited nucleotide sequence analysis of the viral genome suggested that the isolates had not undergone a mutation associated with an increase in virulence. The incidence rate for these serious adverse reactions was estimated at 1 per 400,000 doses of yellow fever vaccine, based on the total number of doses administered in the US civilian population during the surveillance period.

Vaccine-associated viscerotropic disease temporally associated with yellow fever vaccination has also been reported in Australia and Brazil. One Australian citizen became ill after receiving an immunization with the 17D-204 strain of yellow fever vaccine in his home country, and 2 Brazilian citizens (5 and 22 years of age) became ill 3 to 4 days after receiving 17DD vaccine in Brazil. In the Brazilian and Australian cases, histopathologic changes in the liver included midzonal necrosis, microvesicular fatty change, and Councilman bodies, which are characteristic of wild-type yellow fever. Vaccine-type yellow fever virus was isolated from blood and autopsy material (ie, brain, liver, kidney, spleen, lung, skeletal muscle, skin) of each of these 3 persons, all of whom died 8 to 11 days after vaccination. In Brazil, an estimated 23 million vaccine doses were administered during the 15-month period during which the 2 cases of multiple organ system failure were reported.

In view of the data cited, both the 17D-204 and 17DD yellow fever vaccines may be considered as a possible, but rare, cause of vaccine-associated viscerotropic disease that is similar to fulminant yellow fever caused by wild-type yellow fever virus. All available evidence from complete nucleotide sequence analysis and testing in experimental animals of vaccine-type yellow fever viruses isolated from the Brazilian subjects suggests that the occurrences are due to undefined host factors, rather than to intrinsic virulence of the 17DD vaccine viruses.

Patient Information

Prior to administration of yellow fever vaccine, ask potential vaccinees or their parents or guardians about their recent health status. Fully inform all potential vaccinees or their parents or guardians of the benefits and risks of immunization and potential for adverse reactions that have been temporally associated with yellow fever vaccine administration. Instruct vaccinees or their parents or guardians to report all serious adverse reactions that occur up to 30 days postvaccination to their health care providers.

All travelers should seek information regarding vaccination requirements by consulting local health departments, the CDC, and WHO. Travel agencies, international airlines, and/or shipping lines may also have up-to-date

YELLOW FEVER VACCINE — INJECTION

information. Such requirements may be strictly enforced, particularly for persons traveling from Africa or South America to Asia. Consult the latest published version of Health Information for International Travel to determine requirements and regulations for vaccination.

An International Certificate of Vaccination must be completed, signed, and validated with the center's stamp where the vaccine is administered and provided to all vaccinees. The immunization record contains the date, lot number, and manufacturer of the vaccine administered. Inform subjects that US vaccination certificates are valid for a period of 10 years commencing 10 days after initial vaccination or revaccination.

HEPATITIS B VACCINE RECOMBINANT

Rx	**Recombivax HB** (Merck)	**Injection (adult formulation):** 10 mcg hepatitis B surface antigen/mL	Preservative free. In 1 mL single-dose vials, 3 mL multi-dose vials, and 1 mL prefilled single-dose syringes.
		Injection (pediatric/adolescent formulation): 5 mcg hepatitis B surface antigen/0.5 mL	Preservative free. In 0.5 mL single-dose vials.
		Injection (dialysis formulation): 40 mcg hepatitis B surface antigen/mL	Preservative free. In 1 mL single-dose vials.
Rx	**Engerix-B** (GlaxoSmithKline)	**Injection (adult formulation):** 20 mcg hepatitis B surface antigen/mL	Preservative free. In single-dose vials.

HEPATITIS B VACCINE RECOMBINANT — INJECTION

For complete and comparative prescribing information, refer to the Agents for Active Immunization introduction.

Indications

➤*Hepatitis B vaccination:* For immunization against infection caused by all known subtypes of hepatitis B virus. As hepatitis D (caused by the delta virus) does not occur in the absence of hepatitis B infection, it can be expected that hepatitis D will also be prevented by hepatitis B vaccination.

Hepatitis B vaccination will not prevent hepatitis caused by other agents, such as hepatitis A, C and E viruses, or other pathogens known to infect the liver.

Immunization is recommended for persons of all ages, especially those who are, or will be, at increased risk of exposure to hepatitis B virus.

➤*Patient selection:* Vaccination with hepatitis B vaccine (recombinant) is recommended for: infants, including those born of HBsAg-positive mothers, whether HBsAg-positive or -negative; children born after November 21, 1991; adolescents.

Other persons of all ages in areas of high prevalence or those who are or may be at increased risk of infection with hepatitis B virus, such as:

➤*Healthcare personnel:* Dentists and oral surgeons; physicians and surgeons; nurses; paramedical personnel and custodial staff who may be exposed to the virus via blood or other patient specimens; dental hygienists and dental nurses; laboratory personnel handling blood, blood products, and other patient populations; dental, medical and nursing students.

➤*Selected patients and patient contacts:* Staff in hemodialysis units and hematology/oncology units; hemodialysis patients and patients with early renal failure before they require hemodialysis; patients requiring frequent or large volume blood transfusions or clotting factor concentrates (eg, persons with hemophilia, thalassemia, sickle-cell anemia, cirrhosis); individuals with hepatitis C virus infection; clients (residents) and staff of institutions for the mentally handicapped; classroom contacts of deinstitutionalized mentally handicapped persons who have persistent hepatitis B surface antigenemia and who show aggressive behavior; household and other intimate contacts of persons with persistent hepatitis B surface antigenemia.

➤*Subpopulations with a known high incidence of the disease:* Persons who may be exposed to the hepatitis B virus by travel to high-risk areas. HBV infection is highly endemic in China and Southeast Asia, most of Africa, most Pacific Islands, parts of the Middle East, and in the Amazon Basin. In these areas, most persons acquire infection at birth or during childhood, and 8% to 15% of the population are chronically infected with HBV. Police and fire department personnel who render first aid or medical assistance, and any others who, through their work or personal lifestyles, may be exposed to the hepatitis B virus; Alaskan Natives, Pacific Islanders, Indochinese immigrants, and Haitian immigrants; refugees from areas where HBV is endemic; all infants of women born in areas where the infection is highly endemic; adoptees from countries where hepatitis B virus infection is endemic; international travelers; military personnel identified as being at increased risk; morticians and embalmers; blood bank and plasma fractionation workers

➤*Persons at increased risk of the disease due to their sexual practices:* Persons who have heterosexual activity with multiple partners (greater than 1 sexual partner in a 6-month period); persons who repeatedly contract sexually transmitted diseases; homosexual and bisexual adolescent and adult men; female prostitutes; prisoners; injection drug users.

➤*Individuals with chronic hepatitis C:* Risk factors for hepatitis C are similar to those for hepatitis B. Consequently, immunization with hepatitis B vaccine is recommended for individuals with chronic hepatitis C.

➤*Indications for Recombivax HB* dialysis formulation (40 mcg/mL): Vaccination of adult predialysis (eg, patients with early renal failure before they require hemodialysis) and dialysis patients.

➤*Use with other vaccines:* The Advisory Committee on Immunization Practices (ACIP) states that, in general, simultaneous administration of certain live and inactivated pediatric vaccines has not resulted in impaired antibody responses or increased rates of adverse reactions. Separate sites and syringes should be used for simultaneous administration of injectable vaccines.

➤*Off-label uses:* Hepatitis B vaccination is appropriate for people expected to receive human alpha-1 proteinase inhibitor that is produced from heat-treated, pooled human plasma that may contain the causative agents of hepatitis and other viral diseases.

Administration and Dosage

➤*General dosing considerations: Recombivax HB* hepatitis B vaccine (recombinant) dialysis formulation (40 mcg/mL) is intended only for adult predialysis/dialysis patients.

Recombivax HB hepatitis B vaccine (recombinant) pediatric/adolescent and adult formulations are not intended for use in predialysis/dialysis patients.

➤*Adults:*

Hepatitis B vaccination –

Engerix-B:

• *Usual dosage –*

***Engerix-B* Dosage and Administration Schedule for Adults and Hemodialysis Patients**		
Group	Dose	Schedules
Adults (> 19 years)	20 mcg/mL	0, 1, 6 months
Adult hemodialysis	40 mcg/2 mL[a] IM	0, 1, 2, 6 months

[a] Two × 20 mcg in 1 or 2 injections.

• *Alternate schedule* – 20 mcg/mL per dose administered IM on a 0, 1, 2, 12 month schedule. This alternate schedule may be used for specific populations (eg, persons who have or might been recently exposed to the virus, travelers to high risk areas). An additional dose at 12 months is recommended for prolonged maintenance of protective titers.

• *Booster dosage* – Whenever administration of a booster dose is appropriate, the dose of *Engerix-B* is 20 mcg for adults.

For hemodialysis patients, in whom vaccine-induced protection is less complete and may persist only as long as antibody levels remain above 10 mIU/mL, the need for booster doses should be assessed by annual antibody testing. Forty (40) mcg (2 × 20 mcg) booster doses with *Engerix-B* should be given when antibody levels decline below 10 mIU/mL.

Recombivax HB:

• *Usual dosage* – Vaccination regimen consists of 3 doses of vaccine given on the elected date, followed by the second dose 1 month later, and the third dose 6 months after the first dose.

***Recombivax HB* Dose and Formulation for Adults and Predialysis/Dialysis Patients Regardless of the Risk of Infection With Hepatitis B Virus**			
Group	Dose/regimen	Formulation	Color code
Adults ≥ 20 years of age	10 mcg[a] (1 mL) 3 × 10 mcg	Adult	Green
Predialysis and dialysis patients[b]	40 mcg (1 mL) 3 × 40 mcg	Dialysis	Blue

[a] If the suggested formulation is not available, the appropriate dosage can be achieved from another formulation provided that the total volume of vaccine administered does not exceed 1 mL. However, the dialysis formulation may be used only for adult predialysis/dialysis patients.

[b] See also recommendations for revaccination of predialysis and dialysis patients.

• *Booster dose* – A booster dose or revaccination with *Recombivax HB Dialysis Formulation* (blue color code) may be considered in predialysis/dialysis patients if the anti-HBs level is less than 10 mIU/mL 1 to 2 months after the third dose. The ACIP recommends that the need for booster doses of vaccine should be assessed by annual antibody testing and a booster dose given when antibody levels decline to less than 10 mIU/mL.

HEPATITIS B VACCINE RECOMBINANT — INJECTION

➤*Children:*

Hepatitis B vaccination –

Engerix-B:

• *Usual dosage* – 0.5 mL administered IM on a 0, 1, and 6 month schedule.

• *Alternate schedule –*

Engerix-B Alternate Dosage and Administration Schedules[a]		
Group	Dose	Schedules
Infants born of:		
HBsAg-positive mothers	0.5 mL IM	0, 1, 2, and 12 months[a]
Children:		
Birth through 10 years of age	0.5 mL IM	0, 1, 2, and 12 months[a]
5 though 10 years of age	0.5 mL IM	0, 12, and 24 months[b]
Adolescents:		
11 through 16 years of age	0.5 mL IM	0, 12, and 24 months[b]
11 through 19 years of age	1 mL IM	0, 1, 6 months
11 through 19 years of age	1 mL IM	0, 1, 2, and 12 months[b]

[a] This alternate schedule may be used for certain populations (eg, neonates born of hepatitis B–infected mothers, persons who have or might been recently exposed to the virus, travelers to high-risk areas). On this alternate schedule, an additional dose at 12 months is recommended for prolonged maintenance of protective titers.

[b] For children and adolescents for whom an extended administration schedule is acceptable based on risk of exposure.

• *Booster dose* – Whenever administration of a booster dose is appropriate, the dose of *Engerix-B* is 10 mcg for children 10 years or younger; 20 mcg for adolescents 11 through 19 years of age.

Recombivax HB:

Recombivax HB for Infants, Children, and Adolescents, Regardless of the Risk of Infection with Hepatitis B Virus			
Group	Dose/regimen	Formulation	Color code
Infants, children, and adolescents 0 to 19 years of age	5 mcg (0.5 mL) IM 3 × 5 mcg	Pediatric/ adolescent	Yellow
Adolescents 11 through 15 years of age[a]	10 mcg[b] (1 mL) IM 2 × 10 mcg	Adult	Green

[a] Adolescents (11 through 15 years of age) may receive either regimen: The 3 × 5 mcg (pediatric/adolescent formulation) or the 2 × 10 mcg (adult formulation).

[b] If the suggested formulation is not available, the appropriate dosage can be achieved from another formulation provided that the total volume of vaccine administered does not exceed 1 mL. However, the dialysis formulation may be used only for adult predialysis/dialysis patients.

• *3-Dose regimen* – Vaccination regimen consists of 3 doses of vaccine given on the elected date, followed by the second dose 1 month later, and the third dose 6 months after the first dose.

• *2-Dose regimen* – An alternate 2-dose regimen is available for routine vaccination of adolescents (11 to 15 years of age). The regimen consists of 2 doses of vaccine (10 mcg) given according to the following schedule: First injection, at elected date; second injection, 4 to 6 months later.

• *Infants born of HBsAg-positive mothers or mothers of unknown HBsAg status* – Each infant should receive 3 *Recombivax HB* 5 mcg doses irrespective of the mother's HBsAg status (see previous table). The ACIP recommends that if the mother is determined to be HBsAg-positive within 7 days of delivery, the infant also should be given a dose of HBIG (0.5 mL) immediately. The first dose of *Recombivax HB* may be given at the same time as HBIG, but it should be administered in the opposite anterolateral thigh.

• *Booster dose* – The ACIP recommends that the need for booster doses of vaccine should be assessed by annual antibody testing and a booster dose given when antibody levels decline to less than 10 mIU/mL.

➤*Known or presumed exposure to hepatitis B virus:*

Engerix-B – Unprotected individuals with known or presumed exposure to the hepatitis B virus (eg, neonates born of infected mothers, others experiencing percutaneous or permucosal exposure) should be given hepatitis B immune globulin (HBIG) in addition to *Engerix-B* in accordance with ACIP recommendations and with the monograph for HBIG. *Engerix-B* can be given on either dosing schedule.

Recombivax HB – There are no prospective studies directly testing the efficacy of a combination of HBIG and *Recombivax HB* in preventing clinical hepatitis B following percutaneous, ocular, or mucous membrane exposure to hepatitis B virus. However, since most persons with such exposures (eg, healthcare workers) are candidates for *Recombivax HB*, and since combined HBIG plus vaccine is more efficacious than HBIG alone in perinatal exposures, the following guidelines are recommended for persons who have been exposed to hepatitis B virus such as through percutaneous (needlestick), ocular, mucous membrane exposure to blood known or presumed to contain HBsAg, human bites by known or presumed HBsAg carriers, that penetrate the skin, or following intimate sexual contact with known or presumed HBsAg carriers.

HBIG (0.06 mL/kg) should be given IM as soon as possible after exposure and within 24 hours if possible. *Recombivax HB* (see dosage recommendation) should be given IM at a separate site within 7 days of exposure and second and third doses given 1 and 6 months, respectively, after the first dose.

➤*Preparation for administration:* Shake well before withdrawal and use. With thorough agitation, *Engerix-B* is a slightly turbid white suspension and *Recombivax HB* is a slightly opaque, white suspension. Discard if it appears otherwise. The vaccine should be used as supplied; no dilution is necessary. Any vaccine remaining in a single-dose vial should be discarded.

Withdraw the recommended dose from the vial using a sterile needle and a syringe free of preservatives, antiseptics, and detergents. It is important to use a separate sterile syringe and needle for each individual patient to prevent transmission of hepatitis and other infectious agents from one person to another. Needles should be disposed of properly and should not be recapped.

➤*Administration:* Hepatitis B vaccine (recombinant) should be administered by IM injection. Do not inject IV or intradermally. In adults, the injection should be given in the deltoid region, but it may be preferable to inject in the anterolateral thigh in neonates and infants, who have smaller deltoid muscles. Hepatitis B vaccine (recombinant) should not be administered in the gluteal region; such injections may result in suboptimal response and a lower seroconversion rate than expected.

Hepatitis B vaccine (recombinant) may be administered subcutaneously to persons at risk of hemorrhage (eg, hemophiliacs). However, hepatitis B vaccines administered subcutaneously are known to result in lower geometric mean antibody titers (GMTs). Additionally, when other aluminum-adsorbed vaccines have been administered subcutaneously, an increased incidence of local reactions including subcutaneous nodules has been observed. Therefore, subcutaneous administration should be used only in persons who are at risk of hemorrhage with IM injections.

➤*Storage / Stability:* Store between 2° and 8°C (36° and 46°F). Storage above or below the recommended temperature may reduce potency. Do not freeze; discard if product has been frozen because freezing destroys potency.

Actions

➤*Pharmacology:* Hepatitis B virus is 1 of several hepatitis viruses that cause a systemic infection, with a major pathology in the liver. These include hepatitis A virus, hepatitis D virus, and hepatitis C and E viruses, previously referred to as non-A, non-B hepatitis viruses.

Reduced risk of hepatocellular carcinoma – Hepatocellular carcinoma is another serious complication of hepatitis B virus infection. Studies have demonstrated the link between chronic hepatitis B infection and hepatocellular carcinoma; 80% of primary liver cancers are caused by hepatitis B virus infection. The CDC has recognized hepatitis B vaccine as the first anticancer vaccine because it can prevent primary liver cancer.

Contraindications

Hypersensitivity to yeast or any other component of the vaccine; hypersensitivity to any hepatitis B-containing vaccine. Patients experiencing hypersensitivity after a hepatitis B vaccine (recombinant) injection should not receive further injections of hepatitis B vaccine (recombinant).

Warnings/Precautions

➤*Engerix-B*: The vial stopper is latex-free. The tip cap and the rubber plunger of the needleless prefilled syringes contain dry natural latex rubber that may cause allergic reactions in latex-sensitive individuals.

➤*Active infection:* Because of the long incubation period for hepatitis B, it is possible for unrecognized infection to be present at the time the vaccine is given. The vaccine may not prevent hepatitis B in such patients.

➤*Postponing vaccination:* As with other vaccines, although a moderate or severe febrile illness is sufficient reason to postpone vaccination, minor illnesses such as mild upper respiratory tract infections, with or without low-grade fever, are not contraindications.

Any serious active infection (including febrile illness) is reason for delaying use of the vaccine, except when, in the opinion of the physician, withholding the vaccine entails a greater risk.

➤*Administration precautions:* Special care should be taken to prevent injection into a blood vessel.

➤*Immunosuppressed patients:* As with any vaccine administered to immunosuppressed persons or persons receiving immunosuppressive therapy, the expected immune response may not be obtained. For individuals receiving immunosuppressive therapy, deferral of vaccination for at least 3 months after therapy may be considered.

➤*Multiple sclerosis:* Although no causal relationship has been established, rare instances of exacerbation of multiple sclerosis have been reported following administration of hepatitis B vaccines and other vaccines. In persons with multiple sclerosis, the benefit of immunization for prevention of hepatitis B infection and sequelae must be weighed against the risk of exacerbation of the disease.

➤*Hypersensitivity reactions:* Patients who develop symptoms suggestive of hypersensitivity after an injection should not receive further injections of the vaccine.

HEPATITIS B VACCINE RECOMBINANT — INJECTION

As with any percutaneous vaccine, epinephrine (1:1000) should be available for immediate use in case of anaphylaxis or an anaphylactoid reaction.

➤*Special risk:* Caution and appropriate care should be exercised in administering the vaccine to individuals with severely compromised cardiopulmonary status or to others in whom a febrile or systemic reaction could pose a significant risk.

➤*Pregnancy: Category C.* Animal reproduction studies have not been conducted with hepatitis B vaccine (recombinant). It is also not known whether this vaccine can cause fetal harm when administered to a pregnant woman or can affect reproduction capacity. Hepatitis B vaccine (recombinant) should be given to a pregnant woman only if clearly needed.

➤*Lactation:* It is not known whether hepatitis B vaccine (recombinant) is excreted in human milk. Because many drugs are excreted in human milk, caution should be exercised when hepatitis B vaccine (recombinant) is administered to a nursing woman.

➤*Children:* Hepatitis B vaccine (recombinant) has been shown to be well tolerated and highly immunogenic in infants and children of all ages. Newborns also respond well; maternally transferred antibodies do not interfere with the active immune response to the vaccine. The safety and efficacy of *Recombivax HB Dialysis Formulation* in children have not been established.

➤*Elderly:* Clinical trials of *Recombivax HB* did not include sufficient numbers of subjects aged 65 years and over to determine whether they respond differently from younger subjects. Other reports from the clinical literature indicate that hepatitis B vaccines are less immunogenic in adults aged 65 years or older than in younger individuals. No overall differences in safety were observed between these subjects and younger subjects.

Drug Interactions

Hepatitis B Vaccine (HBV) Drug Interactions

Precipitant drug	Object drug[a]		Description
Immunosuppressants	HBV	⬇	Administration of HBV to people receiving immunosuppressant drugs, including high-dose corticosteroids or radiation therapy, may result in an inadequate response to immunization.
HBV	Yellow fever vaccine	⬇	In 1 study, concurrent vaccination against hepatitis B and yellow fever viruses reduced the antibody titer otherwise expected from yellow fever vaccine. Separate these vaccines by a month, if possible.
Interleukin-2	HBV	⬌	Natural interleukin 2 may boost systemic immune response to HBsAg in immunodeficient nonresponders to hepatitis B vaccination, but recombinant interleukin 2 did not augment response to hepatitis B vaccine in healthy adults in 1 study.

[a] ⬇ = object drug decreased; ⬌ = undetermined clinical effect.

Adverse Reactions

Using a symptom checklist, the most frequently reported adverse reactions were injection site soreness (22%) and fatigue (14%). Parents or guardians completed forms for children and neonates. The neonatal checklist did not include headache, fatigue or dizziness. Other reactions are listed below.

➤*Cardiovascular:*
Less than 1% – Hypotension.

➤*CNS:*
1% to 10% – Headache; dizziness.
Less than 1% – Somnolence, insomnia, irritability, agitation.

➤*Dermatologic:*
Less than 1% – Rash, urticaria, petechiae, pruritus, erythema.

➤*GI:*
Less than 1% – Nausea, anorexia, abdominal pain/cramps, vomiting, constipation, diarrhea.

➤*Local:*
1% to 10% – Induration, erythema, swelling.
Less than 1% – Pain, pruritus, ecchymosis at injection site.

➤*Lymphatic:*
Less than 1% – Lymphadenopathy.

➤*Musculoskeletal:*
Less than 1% – Pain/stiffness in arm, shoulder or neck, arthralgia, myalgia, back pain.

➤*Respiratory:*
Less than 1% – Influenza-like symptoms, upper respiratory tract illnesses.

➤*Systemic:*
1% to 10% – Fever (greater than 37.5°C [99.5°F]).
Less than 1% – Sweating, malaise, chills, weakness, flushing, tingling.

➤*Postmarketing experience with Engerix-B:* Additional adverse reactions have been reported with the commercial use of *Engerix-B*. Those listed below are to serve as alerting information to physicians.

Cardiovascular – Tachycardia/palpitations.

CNS – Migraine; syncope; paresis; neuropathy including hypoesthesia, paresthesia, Guillain-Barré syndrome and Bell's palsy, transverse myelitis; optic neuritis; multiple sclerosis; seizures.

Dermatologic – Eczema; purpura; herpes zoster; erythema nodosum; alopecia.

GI – Abnormal liver function tests; dyspepsia.

Hematologic – Thrombocytopenia.

Hypersensitivity – Anaphylaxis; erythema multiforme including Stevens-Johnson syndrome; angioedema; arthritis. An apparent hypersensitivity syndrome (serum-sickness-like) of delayed onset has been reported days to weeks after vaccination, including arthralgia/arthritis (usually transient), fever, and dermatologic reactions such as urticaria, erythema multiforme, ecchymoses and erythema nodosum.

Patients who have experienced a hypersensitivity reaction after a hepatitis B (recombinant) vaccine injection should not receive further injections of hepatitis B (recombinant) vaccine.

Respiratory – Bronchospasm including asthma-like symptoms.

Special senses – Conjunctivitis; keratitis; visual disturbances; vertigo; tinnitus; earache.

➤*Recombivax HB*: *Recombivax HB* and *Recombivax HB Dialysis Formulation* are generally well tolerated. No serious adverse reactions attributable to the vaccine have been reported during the course of clinical trials. No adverse experiences were reported during clinical trials which could be related to changes in the titers of antibodies to yeast. As with any vaccine, there is the possibility that broad use of the vaccine could reveal adverse reactions not observed in clinical trials.

In 3 clinical studies, 434 doses of *Recombivax HB*, 5 mcg, were administered to 147 healthy infants and children (up to 10 years of age) who were monitored for 5 days after each dose. Injection site reactions and systemic complaints were reported following 0.2% and 10.4% of the injections, respectively. The most frequently reported systemic adverse reactions (greater than 1% of injections), in decreasing order of frequency, were irritability, fever (greater than or equal to 38.3°C [101°F] oral equivalent), diarrhea, fatigue/weakness, diminished appetite, and rhinitis.

In a study that compared the 3-dose regimen (5 mcg) with the 2-dose regimen (10 mcg) of *Recombivax HB* in adolescents, the overall frequency of adverse reactions was generally similar.

In a group of studies, 3258 doses of *Recombivax HB*, 10 mcg, were administered to 1252 healthy adults who were monitored for 5 days after each dose. Injection site reactions and systemic complaints were reported following 17% and 15% of the injections, respectively. The following adverse reactions were reported:

Cardiovascular –
Less than 1%: Hypotension.

CNS –
Less than 1%: Vertigo/dizziness, and paresthesia.

Dermatologic –
Less than 1%: Pruritus, rash (nonspecified), angioedema, and urticaria.

GI –
Greater than or equal to 1%: Nausea and diarrhea.
Less than 1%: Vomiting, abdominal pains/cramps, dyspepsia, and diminished appetite.

GU –
Less than 1%: Dysuria.

Hematologic/Lymphatic –
Less than 1%: Lymphadenopathy.

Local –
Greater than or equal to 1%: Injection site reactions consisting principally of soreness, and including pain, tenderness, pruritus, erythema, ecchymosis, swelling, warmth, and nodule formation.

Musculoskeletal –
Less than 1%: Arthralgia including monoarticular, myalgia, back pain, neck pain, shoulder pain, and neck stiffness.

Psychiatric –
Less than 1%: Insomnia/disturbed sleep.

Respiratory –
Greater than or equal to 1%: Pharyngitis and upper respiratory tract infection.
Less than 1%: Rhinitis, influenza, and cough.

Special senses –
Less than 1%: Earache.

Miscellaneous –
Greater than or equal to 1%: The most frequent systemic complaints include fatigue/weakness, headache, fever (greater than or equal to 37.7°C [100°F]), and malaise.

HEPATITIS B VACCINE RECOMBINANT — INJECTION

Less than 1%: Sweating, achiness, sensation of warmth, lightheadedness, chills, and flushing.

➤*Postmarketing experience with Recombivax HB*: The following additional adverse reactions have been reported with use of the marketed vaccine. In many instances, the relationship to the vaccine was unclear.

Cardiovascular – Syncope; tachycardia.

CNS – Guillain-Barré syndrome; multiple sclerosis; exacerbation of multiple sclerosis; myelitis, including transverse myelitis; seizure; febrile seizure; peripheral neuropathy including Bell's palsy; radiculopathy; herpes zoster; migraine; muscle weakness; hypesthesia; encephalitis.

Dermatologic – Stevens-Johnson syndrome; alopecia; petechiae.

Hematologic – Increased erythrocyte sedimentation rate; thrombocytopenia.

Hypersensitivity – Anaphylaxis and symptoms of immediate hypersensitivity reactions including rash, pruritus, urticaria, edema, angioedema, dyspnea, chest discomfort, bronchial spasm, palpitation, or symptoms consistent with a hypotensive episode have been reported within the first few hours after vaccination. An apparent hypersensitivity syndrome (serum-sickness-like) of delayed onset has been reported days to weeks after vaccination, including arthralgia/arthritis (usually transient), fever, and dermatologic reactions such as urticaria, erythema multiforme, ecchymoses, and erythema nodosum.

Patients who experience a hypersensitivity reaction to hepatitis B vaccine (recombinant) should not receive further doses of hepatitis B vaccine (recombinant).

GI – Elevation of liver enzymes; constipation.

Musculoskeletal – Arthritis.

Psychiatric – Irritability; agitation; somnolence.

Special senses – Optic neuritis; tinnitus; conjunctivitis; visual disturbances.

Systemic – Systemic lupus erythematosus (SLE); lupus-like syndrome; vasculitis.

Miscellaneous – The following adverse reaction has been reported with another hepatitis B vaccine (recombinant) but not with *Recombivax HB*: Keratitis. Patients, parents and guardians should be instructed to report any serious adverse reactions to their healthcare provider.

Patient Information

The healthcare provider should provide the vaccine information required to be given with each vaccination to the patient, parent or guardian.

The healthcare provider should inform the patient, parent or guardian of the benefits and risks associated with vaccination, as well as the importance of completing the immunization series.

Patients, parents and guardians should be instructed to report any serious adverse reactions to their healthcare providers.

HEPATITIS A VACCINE, INACTIVATED

Rx	**Havrix** (GlaxoSmithKline)	**Injection, suspension:** 720 ELU hepatitis A viral antigen per 0.5 mL[a]	Pediatric formulation.[b] Preservative free. In 0.5 mL single-dose vials and prefilled syringes.[c]
		Injection, suspension: 1,440 ELU hepatitis A viral antigen per 1 mL[a]	Adult formulation.[d] Preservative free. In 1 mL single-dose vials and prefilled syringes.[c]
Rx	**Vaqta** (Merck)	**Injection, suspension:** ≈ 25 units hepatitis A virus antigen per 0.5 mL	Pediatric/adolescent formulation.[e] In 0.5 mL single-dose vials and prefilled syringes.[f]
		Injection, suspension: ≈ 50 units hepatitis A virus antigen per 1 mL	Adult formulation.[g] Preservative free. In 1 mL single-dose vials and prefilled syringes.[f]

[a] ELU = enzyme-linked immunosorbent assay (ELISA) units.
[b] Antigen is adsorbed onto aluminum 0.25 mg (as aluminum hydroxide). Also contains residual neomycin.
[c] Tip cap and rubber plunger of the needleless prefilled syringes contain dry natural latex rubber.
[d] Antigen is adsorbed onto ≈ 0.5 mg of aluminum (as aluminum hydroxide). Also contains residual neomycin.
[e] Antigen is adsorbed onto ≈ 0.225 mg of aluminum (as amorphous aluminum hydroxyphosphate sulfate).
[f] Vial stopper and the syringe plunger stopper contain dry natural latex rubber.
[g] Antigen is adsorbed onto ≈ 0.45 mg of aluminum (as amorphous aluminum hydroxyphosphate sulfate).

HEPATITIS A VACCINE, INACTIVATED — INJECTION

For complete and comparative prescribing information, refer to the Agents for Active Immunization introduction.

Indications

➤*Hepatitis A virus (HAV):* For active immunization of persons 12 months of age and older against disease caused by HAV. Primary immunization should be administered at least 2 weeks prior to expected exposure to HAV.

Administration and Dosage

➤*General dosing considerations:*

Known or presumed exposure to HAV/travel to endemic areas – For individuals requiring either postexposure prophylaxis or combined immediate and longer-term protection (eg, travelers departing on short notice to endemic areas), hepatitis A vaccine may be coadministered with immune globulin using separate sites and syringes.

According to the Centers for Disease Control and Prevention (CDC), the first dose of hepatitis A vaccine should be administered as soon as travel is considered for all susceptible persons traveling to countries that have high or intermediate hepatitis A endemicity. For most healthy persons 40 years of age and younger, one dose of hepatitis A vaccine administered at any time before departure can provide adequate protection. Completion of the vaccine series is necessary for long-term protection.

➤*Adults:*

Hepatitis A Virus –

Havrix: A single 1 mL dose injected IM at elected date and a 1 mL booster dose administered anytime between 6 and 12 months later.

Vaqta: A single 1 mL dose injected IM at elected date and a 1 mL booster dose anytime between 6 to 18 months later.

➤*Children:*

Hepatitis A Virus –

Havrix:

• *12 months to 18 years of age* – A single 0.5 mL dose injected IM at elected date, and a 0.5 mL booster dose administered anytime 6 and 12 months later.

Vaqta:

• *12 months to 18 years of age* – A single 0.5 mL dose (approximately 25 units) injected IM at elected date and a booster dose of 0.5 mL (approximately 25 units) 6 to 18 months later.

➤*Concomitant Therapy:*

Havrix –

Children 12 months to 18 years of age: Havrix may be given concurrently with *Haemophilus influenzae* type b (Hib) conjugate vaccine (tetanus toxoid conjugate) (PRP-T) (Sanofi Pasteur SA) in children 15 to 18 months of age. *Havrix* may also be given concurrently with the fourth dose of pneumococcal 7-valent conjugate vaccine (Wyeth) in children 15 months of age (age range, 14 to 16 months).

The safety of *Havrix* given concomitantly with diphtheria and tetanus toxoids and acellular pertussis vaccine, adsorbed (DTaP) (*Infanrix*) has been evaluated. Insufficient data are available to assess the immune response of a fourth dose of DTaP when administered with *Havrix*.

Vaqta –

Adults and Children 12 months to 18 years of age: Vaqta may be given concomitantly with typhoid and yellow fever vaccines and measles, mumps, and rubella virus vaccine (*M-M-R II*).

The geometric mean titers (GMTs) for hepatitis A when *Vaqta*, typhoid, and yellow fever vaccines were coadministered were reduced when compared with *Vaqta* alone. Following receipt of the booster dose of *Vaqta*, the GMTs for hepatitis A in these 2 groups were observed to be comparable.

Use with immune globulin – Hepatitis A vaccine may be coadministered with immune globulin. When coadministration of immune globulin is required, the vaccines should be given with different syringes and at different injection sites.

The vaccination regimen should be followed as previously stated. Consult the manufacturer for the appropriate dosage of immune globulin. A booster dose should be administered at the appropriate time as previously outlined.

CDC recommendations – According to the CDC, hepatitis A vaccine may be administered simultaneously with the following vaccines when indicated: DTaP; Hib; hepatitis B; measles, mumps, and rubella (MMR); diphtheria; poliovirus (oral and inactivated); tetanus; typhoic (oral and IM); cholera; Japanese encephalitis; rabies; or yellow fever vaccines.

➤*Interchangeability:* According to the manufacturer, a booster dose of *Vaqta* may be given 6 to 12 months following the initial dose of other inactivated hepatitis A vaccines (eg, *Havrix*).

According to the CDC, using the vaccines according to the licensed schedule is preferable; however, data indicate that the 2 brands of hepatitis A vaccine can be considered to be interchangeable.

➤*Preparation for administration:* Use vaccine as supplied; no dilution or reconstitution is necessary. The full recommended dose of the vaccine should be used. After removal of the appropriate volume from a single-dose vial, discard any vaccine remaining in the vial.

Shake well before withdrawal and use. Agitate thoroughly to maintain suspension of the vaccine. After thorough agitation, *Havrix* is a homogeneous, turbid, white suspension and *Vaqta* is a slightly opaque, white suspension. Discard if it appears otherwise.

HEPATITIS A VACCINE, INACTIVATED — INJECTION

➤*Administration:* The following are the Advisory Committee on Immunization Practices (ACIP) and American Academy of Family Physicians recommendations for all IM injections: For administration of hepatitis A vaccine for children and adolescents (persons 12 months to 18 years of age), the deltoid muscle can be used if the muscle mass is adequate. The needle size can range form 22- to 25-gauge and from ⅞ to 1¼ inches, on the basis of the size of the muscle. For toddlers, the anterolateral thigh can be used, but the needle should be longer, usually 1 inch.

For adults (persons older than 18 years of age), the deltoid muscle is recommended for routine IM vaccinations, but the anterolateral thigh can be used. The suggested needle size is 1 to 1.5 inches and 22- to 25-gauge.

Havrix –

Adults: Inject IM, preferably into the deltoid muscle. Do not administer in the gluteal region; such injections may result in suboptimal response.

Children:

- *12 months to 18 years of age* – Inject IM into the anterolateral aspect of the thigh in infants and young children or the deltoid muscle in older children.

Vaqta – For adults and children older than 2 years of age, the deltoid muscle is the preferred site for IM injections. For children 12 through 23 months of age, the anterolateral area of the thigh is the preferred site for IM injections.

➤*Storage/Stability:* Store refrigerated between 2° and 8°C (36° and 46°F). Do not freeze because freezing destroys potency; discard if product has been frozen. Do not dilute to administer.

Actions

➤*Pharmacology:* The presence of antibodies to HAV (anti-HAV) confers protection against hepatitis A infection. However, the lowest titer needed to confer protection has not been determined.

Protection after vaccination with *Vaqta* has been associated with the onset of seroconversion (10 milliunits or more per mL of hepatitis A antibody, measured by a modification of the *HAVAB* radioimmunoassay) and with an anamnestic antibody response following booster vaccination with *Vaqta*.

Contraindications

Hypersensitivity to any component of the vaccine, including neomycin; history of a severe reaction to a prior dose of hepatitis A vaccine or to a vaccine component.

Warnings/Precautions

➤*Latex sensitivity:* Certain components of the *Havrix* packaging (the tip cap and the rubber plunger of the needleless prefilled syringes) and the *Vaqta* packaging (the vial stopper and the syringe plunger stopper) contain dry natural latex rubber that may cause allergic reactions in latex-sensitive individuals. The *Havrix* vial stopper is latex free.

➤*Immunocompromised patients:* As with any vaccine, if administered to immunocompromised persons, including individuals receiving immunosuppressive therapy, the expected immune response may not be obtained.

➤*Protection:* Hepatitis A has a relatively long incubation period (15 to 50 days). Hepatitis A vaccine may not prevent hepatitis A infection in individuals who have an unrecognized hepatitis A infection at the time of vaccination. Additionally, it may not prevent infection in individuals who do not achieve protective antibody titers (although the lowest titer needed to confer protection has not been determined).

As with any vaccine, vaccination with hepatitis A vaccine may not result in a protective response in all susceptible vaccinees.

➤*Patient history:* Prior to immunization with hepatitis A vaccine, inactivated, review the patient's current health status and medical history. Review the patient's immunization history for possible vaccine sensitivity, previous vaccination-related adverse reactions, and occurrence of any adverse reaction-related symptoms and/or signs in order to determine the existence of any contraindication to immunization with hepatitis A vaccine, inactivated and to allow an assessment of benefits and risks.

➤*Administration:* Use a separate, sterile syringe and needle or a sterile disposable unit for each patient to prevent the transmission of other infectious agents from person to person. Dispose of needles properly and do not recap them.

➤*Bleeding disorders:* As with other IM injections, do not administer hepatitis A vaccine to individuals with bleeding disorders such as hemophilia or thrombocytopenia or to persons on anticoagulant therapy unless the potential benefits clearly outweigh the risk of administration. If the decision is made to administer the vaccine to such persons, give it with caution and take steps to avoid the risk of hematoma following the injection.

➤*Acute infection/febrile illness:* An acute infection or febrile illness may be reason for delaying use of hepatitis A vaccine, inactivated except when, in the opinion of the health care provider, withholding the vaccine entails a greater risk.

➤*Hypersensitivity reactions:* Do not give further injections of hepatitis A vaccine to individuals who develop symptoms suggestive of hypersensitivity after an injection of hepatitis A vaccine.

There have been postmarketing reports of anaphylaxis/anaphylactoid reactions following commercial use of the vaccine. Appropriate medical treatment and supervision must be readily available to manage possible anaphylactic reactions following the administration of the vaccine. Epinephrine injection (1:1,000) and other appropriate agents used for the control of immediate allergic reactions must be immediately available.

➤*Hepatic function impairment:* Subjects with chronic liver disease had a lower antibody response to *Havrix* than healthy subjects.

➤*Pregnancy: Category C.* Animal reproduction studies have not been conducted with hepatitis A vaccine, inactivated. It is also not known whether hepatitis A vaccine, inactivated can cause fetal harm when administered to a pregnant woman or can affect reproduction capacity. Give hepatitis A vaccine, inactivated to a pregnant woman only if clearly needed.

According to the CDC, the theoretical risk to the developing fetus is expected to be low because hepatitis A vaccine is produced from inactivated HAV. The risk associated with vaccination should be weighed against the risk for hepatitis A in pregnant women who might be at high risk for exposure to HAV.

➤*Lactation:* It is not known whether hepatitis A vaccine, inactivated is excreted in human milk. However, hepatitis A vaccine does not appear to be contraindicated in breast-feeding women based on other inactivated viral vaccines. Because many drugs are excreted in human milk, exercise caution when hepatitis A vaccine, inactivated is administered to a woman who is breast-feeding.

➤*Children:* The safety and efficacy of hepatitis A vaccine, inactivated have not been established in subjects younger than 12 months of age.

➤*Elderly:*

Havrix – Clinical studies of *Havrix* did not include sufficient numbers of subjects 65 years of age and older to determine whether they respond differently from younger subjects. Other reported clinical experience has not identified differences in overall safety between these subjects and younger adult subjects.

Vaqta – Of the total number of adults in clinical studies of *Vaqta*, conducted pre- and postlicensure, 68 were 65 years of age or older, 10 of whom were 75 years of age or older. No overall differences in safety and immunogenicity were observed between these subjects and younger subjects; however, greater sensitivity of some older individuals cannot be ruled out. In a large, postmarketing safety study in 42,110 individuals 2 years of age and older, 4,769 were 65 years of age or older, 1,073 of whom were 75 years of age or older. There were no adverse reactions judged by the investigator to be vaccine related in the geriatric study population. Other reported clinical experience has not identified differences in responses between the elderly and younger subjects.

Drug Interactions

➤*Use with other vaccines:* See Administration and Dosage for more information.

Havrix – See Administration and Dosage for more information.

Vaqta – See Administration and Dosage for more information.

Adverse Reactions

➤*Reporting of adverse reactions:* The US Department of Health and Human Services has established the Vaccine Adverse Events Reporting System (VAERS) to accept all reports of suspected adverse reactions after the administration of any vaccine including, but not limited to, the reporting of events required by the National Childhood Vaccine Injury Act of 1986. The toll-free number for VAERS is 1-800-822-7967. Reporting forms may also be obtained at the VAERS Web site at http://www.vaers.org.

➤*Havrix*: The frequency of solicited adverse reactions tended to decrease with successive doses of *Havrix*.

The following are solicited and unsolicited reactions occurring during clinical trials:

CNS – Headache was reported by 14% of adults and less than 9% of children. Malaise (1% to 10%); hypertonia, insomnia, vertigo (less than 1%).

Dermatologic – Pruritus, rash, urticaria (less than 1%).

GI – Anorexia, nausea (1% to 10%); abdominal pain, diarrhea, dysgeusia, vomiting (less than 1%).

Hematologic/Lymphatic – Lymphadenopathy (less than 1%).

Local – Injection-site soreness occurred (56% of adults and 21% of children); however, less than 0.5% of soreness was reported as severe. Induration, redness, swelling (1% to 10%); hematoma (less than 1%) also were reported.

Musculoskeletal – Arthralgia, myalgia (less than 1%).

Respiratory – Pharyngitis, upper respiratory tract infections (less than 1%).

Miscellaneous – Fatigue, fever (greater than 37.5°C [99.5°F]) (1% to 10%); elevation of creatine phosphokinase, photophobia (less than 1%).

➤*Additional safety data (Havrix)*: Safety data were obtained from 2 additional sources in which large populations were vaccinated. In an outbreak setting in which 4,930 individuals were immunized with a single dose of either 720 or 1,440 ELU of *Havrix*, no serious adverse reactions due to vaccination were reported. Overall, less than 10% of vaccinees reported solicited general adverse reactions following the vaccine. The most common solicited local adverse reaction was pain at the injection site, reported in 22.3% of subjects at 24 hours and decreasing to 2.4% by 72 hours.

In a field efficacy trial, 19,037 children received the 360 ELU dose of *Havrix*. The most commonly reported adverse reactions following administration of *Havrix* were injection site pain (9.5%) and tenderness (8.1%), which were reported following first doses of *Havrix*. Other adverse reactions were infrequent and comparable with the control vaccine hepatitis B vaccine, recombinant. Additionally, no serious adverse reactions due to the vaccine were

HEPATITIS A VACCINE, INACTIVATED — INJECTION

reported. The large trial further allowed for analysis of rare adverse reactions, including hospitalization and death. No significant differences were found between the cohorts.

In subjects with chronic liver disease, local injection-site reactions were similar among all 4 groups, and no serious adverse reactions attributed to the vaccine were reported in subjects with chronic liver disease.

Safety data for Havrix 720 ELU per 0.5 mL beginning at 11 months of age – In the multicenter study, parents/guardians recorded local and general symptoms on diary cards for 4 days (days 0 to 3) after vaccination. In the 3 groups of children who received *Havrix* alone, safety data were available for 723 children who received 1,396 documented doses of *Havrix*. Additional safety data were available for 181 children who received *Havrix* coadministered with DTaP and Hib conjugate vaccine (PRP-T). The frequencies of solicited local and systemic reactions following receipt of *Havrix* were monitored during the 4-day observation period.

The following ranges of solicited adverse reaction rates were observed among 3 groups of children who received their first dose of *Havrix* alone between 11 and 25 months of age: injection-site pain in 15% to 21% of subjects, redness in 16% to 21% of subjects, and swelling in 8% of subjects, irritability in 24% to 36% of subjects, loss of appetite in 16% to 19% of subjects, drowsiness in 15% to 17% of subjects, and fever greater than 39.5°C (103.1°F) in 2% or less of subjects. Following the booster dose of *Havrix*, among local reactions, pain was reported in 16% to 21% of subjects, redness in 17% to 22%, and swelling in 8% to 10% of subjects. Following the booster dose of *Havrix*, among general reactions, irritability was reported in 19% to 29% of subjects, loss of appetite in 14% to 18% of subjects, drowsiness in 13% to 16% of subjects, and fever greater than 39.5°C (103.1°F) in 1% or less of subjects.

Drowsiness and loss of appetite occurred at statistically significantly higher rates in subjects 15 to 18 months of age who received Hib conjugate vaccine (PRP-T) and DTaP concomitantly with *Havrix* as compared with subjects 15 to 18 months of age who received Hib conjugate vaccine (PRP-T) and DTaP (drowsiness 34% and 22% and loss of appetite 29% and 19%, respectively). With the exception of fever (greater than 39.5°C [103.1°F]), the solicited general symptoms occurred at statistically significantly higher rates in subjects 15 to 18 months of age who received Hib conjugate vaccine (PRP-T) and DTaP concomitantly with *Havrix* as compared with subjects 15 to 18 months of age who received *Havrix* alone (irritability 46% and 30%, drowsiness 34% and 17%, and loss of appetite 29% and 17%, respectively).

A febrile seizure was reported in a subject 18 months of age 2 days after receiving the first dose of *Havrix*. Other serious adverse reactions reported during the course of this study included a single case each of hepatitis approximately 5 months after dose 1, insulin-dependent diabetes approximately 4 months after dose 1, and Kawasaki disease approximately 3.5 months after dose 1. The association of these events with vaccination is unknown.

In a US multicenter study, children 15 months of age (range, 14 to 16 months) received either *Havrix* coadministered with a US-licensed pneumococcal 7-valent conjugate vaccine followed by a second dose of *Havrix* 6 to 9 months later; *Havrix* administered alone followed by a second dose of *Havrix* 6 to 9 months later; or pneumococcal 7-valent conjugate vaccine administered alone followed by a first dose of *Havrix* 1 month later and a second dose of *Havrix* 6 to 9 months after the first. Parents/guardians recorded local and general symptoms on diary cards for 4 days (days 0 to 3) after vaccination.

Solicited local adverse events were reported as follows among children who received the first dose *Havrix* coadministered with pneumococcal 7-valent conjugate vaccine: Pain was reported in 36% of subjects, redness in 41% of subjects, and swelling in 29% of subjects. The reported rates of these local adverse reactions were similar to those reported in children who received the first dose of pneumococcal 7-valent conjugate vaccine alone (44%, 46%, and 27%, respectively). Among children who received the first dose of *Havrix* alone, pain was reported in 28% of subjects, redness in 22% of subjects, and swelling in 7% of subjects.

Solicited general adverse reactions were reported as follows among children who received the first dose *Havrix* coadministered with pneumococcal 7-valent conjugate vaccine: Irritability was reported in 35% of subjects, drowsiness in 26% of subjects, loss of appetite in 25% of subjects, and fever in 14% of subjects. The reported rates of these general adverse reactions were similar to those reported in children who received the first dose of pneumococcal 7-valent conjugate vaccine alone (41%, 32%, 25%, and 16% respectively). Among children who received the first dose of *Havrix* alone, irritability was reported in 35% of subjects, drowsiness in 29% of subjects, loss of appetite in 26% of subjects, and fever in 9% of subjects.

➤*Postmarketing (Havrix)*:

CNS – Convulsions, dizziness, encephalopathy, Guillain-Barré syndrome, multiple sclerosis, myelitis, neuropathy, paresthesia, somnolence, syncope.

Dermatologic – Erythema multiforme, hyperhydrosis.

Hepatic – Hepatitis, jaundice.

Hypersensitivity – Anaphylaxis/anaphylactoid reactions, angioedema.

Miscellaneous – Congenital anomaly, dyspnea, local swelling, thrombocytopenia.

➤*Vaqta*: The safety of *Vaqta* has been evaluated in more than 10,000 subjects 1 to 85 years of age. Subjects were given 1 or 2 doses of the vaccine. The second (booster dose) was given 6 months or more after the first dose. As with any vaccine, there is the possibility that use of *Vaqta* in very large populations might reveal adverse reactions not observed in clinical trials.

➤*Children (12 through 23 months of age) (Vaqta)*: In combined clinical trials involving 706 healthy children 12 through 23 months of age who received 1 or more doses of approximately 25 units, subjects were monitored for local adverse reactions and fever for 5 days after each vaccination and systemic adverse reactions for 14 days after each vaccination by diary cards. Some of these children received *Vaqta* in combination with other routinely recommended pediatric vaccines. The following information lists the complaints (with 95% CI) for all solicited reactions and for unsolicited reactions reported at 1% or more without regard to causality.

Vaqta Adverse Reactions in Children 12 through 23 Months of Age		
	Vaqta	
	Dose 1	Booster
Adverse reactions	Adverse reaction rate (95% CI)	
Local		
Erythema	1.3% (0.6% to 2.6%)	1.6% (0.8% to 3%)
Pain/Tenderness/ Soreness	3.5% (2.3% to 5.2%)	3.1% (1.9% to 4.9%)
Swelling	1.6% (0.8% to 2.9%)	1.3% (0.6% to 2.6%)
Warmth	0.9% (0.4% to 2%)	0.8% (0.3% to 2%)
Miscellaneous		
Fever ≥ 38°C (100.4°F), oral	9.1% (7.1% to 11.6%)	11.3% (9% to 14.1%)
Fever ≥ 38.9°C (102°F), oral	3.8% (2.5% to 5.6%)	3.1% (1.9% to 4.9%)
Rash, measles-like/rubella-like	1% (0.4% to 2%)	
Rash, varicella-like	0.9% (0.3% to 2%)	—

➤*Unsolicited adverse reactions of 1% or more in children 12 to 23 months of age (95% CI) (Vaqta)*:

CNS – Crying 1.8% (1% to 3.2%); irritability 10.8% (8.6% to 13.4%).

Dermatologic – Rash 4.5% (3.1% to 6.4%); viral exanthema 1% (0.4% to 2.2%).

GI – Anorexia 1.2% (0.6% to 2.4%); diarrhea 5.9% (4.3% to 8%); vomiting 4% (2.7% to 5.8%).

Local – Ecchymosis 1% (0.4% to 2.2%).

Respiratory – Cough 5.1% (3.6% to 7.1%); laryngotracheobronchitis 1.2% (0.6% to 2.4%); nasal congestion 1.2% (0.6% to 2.4%); respiratory congestion 1.6% (0.8% to 2.9%); rhinorrhea 5.7% (4.1% to 7.8%); upper respiratory tract infection 10.1% (8% to 12.7%).

Special senses – Conjunctivitis 1.3% (0.6% to 2.6%); otitis 1.8% (1% to 3.2%); otitis media 7.6% (5.8% to 9.9%).

Serious adverse reactions (Vaqta) – There were 7 children who experienced 9 seizures during the entire study period. Seizures were reported between 9 and 81 days following the administration of *Vaqta*. Some subjects had received concomitant or nonconcomitant immunization with measles, mumps, and rubella virus vaccine and varicella virus vaccine live. None of the events were considered to be related to *Vaqta* by the investigator. Other serious reactions that occurred during the study included bronchiolitis, dehydration, right lower lobe pneumonia, asthma, and asthma exacerbation, which were also considered by the investigator to be unrelated to *Vaqta*. These events occurred 9 to 46 days following the administration of *Vaqta*. Some subjects received concomitant or nonconcomitant immunization with MMR virus vaccine and varicella virus vaccine live or DTaP, and/or inactivated polio vaccine (IPV).

➤*Children/Adolescents 2 through 18 years of age (safety data gathered from The Monroe Efficacy Study) (Vaqta)*: In The Monroe Efficacy study, 1,037 healthy children and adolescents 2 through 16 years of age received a primary dose of approximately 25 units of *Vaqta* and a booster 6, 12, or 18 months later, or placebo. Subjects were followed during a 5-day period for fever and local complaints and during a 14-day period for systemic complaints. Injection-site complaints, generally mild and transient, were the most frequently reported complaints. The following table summarizes the local and systemic complaints (1% or greater) reported in this study, without regard to causality. There were no significant differences in the rates of any complaints between vaccine and placebo recipients after dose 1.

HEPATITIS A VACCINE, INACTIVATED — INJECTION

Vaqta Adverse Reactions in Children and Adolescents From the Monroe Efficacy Study (≥ 1%)

Adverse reactions	Vaqta		
	Dose 1[a]	Booster	Placebo [a,b]
Local			
Erythema	1.9%	0.8%	1.8%
Pain	6.4%	3.4%	6.3%
Swelling	1.7%	1.5%	1.6%
Tenderness	4.9%	1.7%	6.1%
Warmth	1.7%	0.6%	1.6%
Miscellaneous			
Abdominal pain	1.2%	1.1%	1%
Headache	0.4%	0.8%	1%
Pharyngitis	1.2%	0%	0.8%

[a] No statistically significant differences between the groups.
[b] Second injection of placebo not administered because the code for the trial was broken.

➤*Children / Adolescents (2 through 18 years of age) (combined clinical trials) (Vaqta)*: In combined clinical trials (including The Monroe Efficacy Study participants) involving 2,615 healthy children (2 years of age and older) who received 1 or more doses of approximately 25 units of *Vaqta*, subjects were followed for fever and local complaints during a 5-day period postvaccination and systemic complaints during a 14-day period postvaccination. Injection-site complaints, generally mild and transient, were the most frequently reported complaints. The following adverse reactions are the complaints reported by 1% or more of subjects, without regard to causality.

GI – Abdominal pain (1.6%); diarrhea (1%); vomiting (1%).

Lab test abnormalities – Very few laboratory abnormalities were reported and included isolated reports of elevated liver function tests, eosinophilia, and increased urine protein.

Local – Ecchymosis (1.3%); erythema (7.5%); pain (18.7%); swelling (7.3%); tenderness (16.9%); warmth (8.6%).

Respiratory – Cough (1%); pharyngitis (1.5%); upper respiratory tract infection (1.1%).

Miscellaneous – Headache (2.3%); fever (38.8°C [102°F] or higher, oral) (3.1%).

➤*Adults (19 years of age or older) (Vaqta)*: In combined clinical trials involving 1,512 healthy adults who received 1 or more doses of approximately 50 units of *Vaqta*, subjects were followed for fever and local complaints during a 5-day period postvaccination and systemic complaints during a 14–day period postvaccination. Injection-site complaints, generally mild and transient, were the most frequently reported complaints. Listed below are the complaints reported by 1% or more of subjects, without regard to causality.

CNS – Asthenia/fatigue (3.9%); headache (16%).

GI – Abdominal pain (1.3%); diarrhea (2.5%); nausea (2.3%).

Local – Ecchymosis (1.5%); erythema (13.1%); pain (51.1%); pain/soreness (1.2%); swelling (13.8%); tenderness (52.7%); warmth (17.4%).

Musculoskeletal – Arm pain (1.3%); back pain (1.1%); myalgia (1.9%); stiffness (1%).

Respiratory – Nasal congestion (1.1%); pharyngitis (2.7%); upper respiratory tract infection (2.7%).

Miscellaneous – Fever (2.7%); menstruation disorder (1.1%).

➤*Hypersensitivity (Vaqta)*: Local and/or systemic allergic reactions that occurred in less than 1% of children/adolescents or adults in clinical trials regardless of causality included the following:

Local – Injection-site pruritus and/or rash (less than 1%).

Systemic – Asthma, bronchial constriction, dermatitis, edema/swelling, eye irritation/itching, generalized erythema, pruritus, rash, urticaria, wheezing (less than 1%).

➤*Postmarketing (Vaqta)*:

CNS – Very rarely, Guillain-Barré syndrome, cerebellar ataxia, and encephalitis.

Hematologic – Very rarely, thrombocytopenia.

Miscellaneous – In a postmarketing short-term safety surveillance study conducted at a large health maintenance organization in the United States, a total of 42,110 individuals 2 years of age and older received 1 or 2 doses of *Vaqta* (13,735 children/adolescents and 28,375 adult subjects). Safety was passively monitored by electronic search of the automated medical records database for emergency room and outpatient visits, hospitalizations, and deaths. Medical charts were reviewed when indicated. There was no serious, vaccine-related adverse reaction identified among the 42,110 vaccine recipients in this study. Diarrhea/gastroenteritis, resulting in outpatient visits, was determined by the investigator to be the only vaccine-related, nonserious adverse reaction in the study. There was no vaccine-related adverse reaction identified that had not been reported in earlier clinical trials with *Vaqta*.

Patient Information

Inform vaccine recipients, parents, or guardians of the potential benefits and risks of immunization with hepatitis A vaccine. When educating vaccine recipients, parents or guardians regarding potential adverse reactions, emphasize that hepatitis A vaccine contains noninfectious killed viruses and cannot cause hepatitis A infection. It is important to question the vaccine recipient, parent, or guardian concerning the occurrence of any symptoms and/or signs of an adverse reaction after a previous dose of hepatitis A vaccine. Inform the patients, parents, or guardians about the potential for adverse reactions that have been temporally associated with administration of hepatitis A vaccine. Instruct the patient, parent, or guardian accompanying the recipient to report severe or unusual adverse reactions to the health care provider or clinic where the vaccine was administered.

Give vaccine recipients, parents, or guardians the vaccine information statements, which are required by the National Childhood Vaccine Injury Act of 1986 to be given prior to immunization. These materials are available free of charge at the CDC Web site (http://www.cdc.gov/nip). The US Department of Health and Human Services has established a VAERS to accept all reports of suspected adverse reactions after the administration of any vaccine including, but not limited to, the reporting of events required by the National Childhood Vaccine Injury Act of 1986. The VAERS toll-free number is 1–800–822–7967. Reporting forms also may be obtained at the VAERS Web site at http://www.vaers.org.

HEPATITIS A (INACTIVATED)/HEPATITIS B (RECOMBINANT) VACCINE

Rx	**Twinrix** (GlaxoSmithKline)	**Injection, suspension**: 720 EL.U.[a] inactivated hepatitis A virus, 20 mcg recombinant HBsAg[b] protein/mL	Preservative free. In single-dose vials and prefilled, disposable *TIP-LOK* syringes without needles.

[a] EL.U. = enzyme-linked immunosorbent assay (ELISA) units.
[b] HBsAg = hepatitis B surface antigen.

HEPATITIS A (INACTIVATED)/HEPATITIS B (RECOMBINANT) VACCINE — INJECTION

For complete and comparative prescribing information, refer to the Agents for Active Immunization introduction and the individual Hepatitis A, Inactivated and Hepatitis B, Recombinant monographs.

Indications

➤*Hepatitis A and B vaccination:* For active immunization of persons 18 years of age and older against disease caused by hepatitis A virus (HAV) and infection by all known subtypes of hepatitis B virus (HBV). As with any vaccine, vaccination with this product may not protect 100% of recipients. Because hepatitis D (caused by the delta virus) does not occur in the absence of HBV infection, it can be expected that hepatitis D also will be prevented by vaccination with this product.

Administration and Dosage

➤*Adults:*

Hepatitis A and hepatitis B vaccination –
Usual dosage: 1 mL injected intramuscularly (IM), given on a 0-, 1-, and 6-month schedule.

Alternative dosage: Inject 1 mL IM, on days 0, 7, and 21 to 30, followed by a booster dose at month 12.

➤*Preparation for administration:* Shake the vial or syringe well before withdrawal and use. With thorough agitation, the vaccine is a slightly turbid white suspension. Discard if it appears otherwise.

Use the vaccine as supplied; no dilution or reconstitution is necessary. Use the full recommended dose. After removal of the appropriate volume from a single-dose vial, discard any vaccine remaining in the vial.

➤*Administration:* Administer by IM injection into the deltoid region. Do not inject into the gluteal region; such injections may result in a suboptimal response. Do not inject intravenously or intradermally.

➤*Storage / Stability:* Store refrigerated between 2° and 8°C (36° and 46°F). Do not freeze; discard if product has been frozen.

HUMAN PAPILLOMAVIRUS (TYPES 16, 18) BIVALENT VACCINE, RECOMBINANT

Rx	Cervarix (GlaxoSmithKline)	**Injection, suspension:** ≈ 20 mcg of HPV[a] 16 L1 protein, 20 mcg of HPV 18 L1 protein per 0.5 mL[b]	Preservative free. 0.5 mL single-dose vials and prefilled *TIP-LOK* syringes.[c]

[a] HPV = human papillomavirus.
[b] Each 0.5 mL dose contains approximately 50 mcg of 3–O-desacyl-4′-monophosphoryl lipid A (MPL), 0.5 mg of aluminum hydroxide, 4.4 mg of sodium chloride, and 0.624 mg of sodium dihydrogen phosphate dihydrate.
[c] The tip cap and the rubber plunger of the needleless prefilled syringes contain dry natural latex rubber.

HUMAN PAPILLOMAVIRUS (TYPES 16, 18) BIVALENT VACCINE, RECOMBINANT — INJECTION

Indications

➤*Prevention of human papillomavirus:* Prevention in girls and women 10 to 25 years of age of the following diseases caused by oncogenic HPV types 16 and 18: cervical cancer, cervical intraepithelial neoplasia (CIN) grade 2 or worse and adenocarcinoma in situ, and CIN grade 1.

Administration and Dosage

➤*Adults:*

Prevention of human papillomavirus – 0.5 mL intramuscularly (IM) given as 3 doses according to the following schedule: 0, 1, and 6 months.

➤*Children:*

10 years of age and older – See Adults for dosing.

➤*Administration:* Administer IM in the deltoid region of the upper arm. Do not administer intravenously, intradermally, or subcutaneously.

➤*Admixture compatibility:* Do not mix HPV vaccine with any other vaccine in the same syringe or vial.

➤*Storage/Stability:* Store refrigerated between 2° and 8°C (36° and 46°F). Do not freeze. Discard if the vaccine has been frozen. Upon storage, a fine, white deposit with a clear, colorless supernatant may be observed. This does not constitute a sign of deterioration.

Actions

➤*Pharmacology:* Animal studies suggest that the efficacy of L1 VLP vaccines may be mediated by the development of immunoglobulin G neutralizing antibodies directed against HPV-L1 capsid proteins generated as a result of vaccination.

Contraindications

Severe allergic reactions (eg, anaphylaxis) to any component of HPV vaccine.

Warnings/Precautions

➤*Syncope:* Because vaccinees may develop syncope, sometimes resulting in falling with injury, observation for 15 minutes after administration is recommended. Syncope, sometimes associated with tonic-clonic movements and other seizure-like activity, has been reported following vaccination with HPV vaccine. When syncope is associated with tonic-clonic movements, the activity is usually transient and typically responds to restoring cerebral perfusion by maintaining a supine or Trendelenburg position.

➤*Limitations of use and effectiveness:* HPV vaccine does not provide protection against disease caused by all HPV types.

HPV vaccine has not been demonstrated to provide protection against disease from vaccine and nonvaccine HPV types to which a woman has previously been exposed through sexual activity.

Women should continue to adhere to recommended cervical cancer screening procedures.

Vaccination with HPV vaccine may not result in protection in all vaccine recipients.

➤*Immunocompromised patients:* The immune response to HPV vaccine may be diminished in immunocompromised persons.

➤*Latex sensitivity:* The tip cap and the rubber plunger of the needleless, prefilled syringes contain dry natural latex rubber that may cause allergic reactions in latex-sensitive persons. The vial stopper does not contain latex.

➤*Hypersensitivity reactions:* Prior to administration, the health care provider should review the immunization history for possible vaccine hypersensitivity and previous vaccination-related adverse reactions to allow an assessment of benefits and risks. Appropriate medical treatment and supervision should be readily available in case of anaphylactic reactions following administration of HPV vaccine.

➤*Pregnancy: Category B.* There are no adequate and well-controlled studies in pregnant women. Because animal reproduction studies are not always predictive of human response, this drug should be used during pregnancy only if clearly needed. Reproduction studies have been performed in rats at a dose approximately 47 times the human dose (on a mg/kg basis) and revealed no evidence of impaired fertility or harm to the fetus caused by HPV vaccine.

In clinical studies, pregnancy testing was performed prior to each vaccine administration and vaccination was discontinued if a subject had a positive pregnancy test. In all clinical trials, subjects were instructed to take precautions to avoid pregnancy until 2 months after the last vaccination. During prelicensure clinical development, 7,276 pregnancies were reported among 3,696 women receiving HPV vaccine and 3,580 women receiving a control (hepatitis A vaccine 360 EL.U, hepatitis A vaccine 720 EL.U, or 500 mcg of $Al(OH)_3$). The overall proportions of pregnancy outcomes were similar between treatment groups. The majority of women gave birth to healthy infants (62.2% and 62.6% of recipients of HPV vaccine and control, respectively). Other outcomes included spontaneous abortion (11% and 10.8% of recipients of HPV vaccine and control, respectively), elective termination (5.8% and 6.1% of recipients of HPV vaccine and control, respectively), abnormal infant other than congenital anomaly (2.8% and 3.2% of recipients of HPV vaccine and control, respectively), and premature birth (2% and 1.7% of recipients of HPV vaccine and control, respectively). Other outcomes (congenital anomaly, stillbirth, ectopic pregnancy, and therapeutic abortion) were reported less frequently in 0.1% to 0.8% of pregnancies in both groups.

It is not known whether the observed numerical imbalance in spontaneous abortions in pregnancies which occurred around the time of vaccination is because of a vaccine-related effect.

Pregnancy registry – Health care providers are encouraged to register pregnant women who inadvertently receive HPV vaccine in the manufacturer's vaccination pregnancy registry by calling 1-888-452-9622.

➤*Lactation:* In nonclinical studies in rats, serological data suggest a transfer of anti–HPV-16 and anti–HPV-18 antibodies via milk during lactation in rats. Excretion of vaccine-induced antibodies in human milk has not been studied for HPV vaccine. Because many drugs are excreted in human milk, exercise caution when HPV vaccine is administered to a breast-feeding woman.

➤*Children:* Safety and effectiveness in children younger than 10 years of age have not been established.

➤*Elderly:* HPV vaccine is not approved for use in subjects 65 years of age and older.

➤*Monitoring:* Observe patients for 15 minutes after administration for signs of syncope.

Drug Interactions

➤*Immunosuppressive drugs:* Immunosuppressive therapies, including irradiation, antimetabolites, alkylating agents, cytotoxic drugs, and corticosteroids (used in greater than physiologic doses), may reduce the immune response to HPV vaccine.

Adverse Reactions

➤*Most common adverse reactions:* The most common local adverse reactions (at least 20% of subjects) were pain, redness, and swelling at the injection site.

The most common general adverse events (at least 20% of subjects) were arthralgia, fatigue, GI symptoms, headache, and myalgia.

➤*Clinical studies experience:*

Local and systemic adverse reactions – The reported frequencies of solicited local injection site reactions (pain, redness, and swelling) and general adverse events (fatigue, fever, GI symptoms, headache, arthralgia, myalgia, and urticaria) within 7 days after vaccination in women 10 to 25 years of age are presented in the following table. Local reactions were reported more frequently with HPV vaccine when compared with the control groups; in at least 84% of recipients of HPV vaccine, these local reactions were mild to moderate in intensity. Compared with dose 1, pain was reported less frequently after doses 2 and 3 of HPV vaccine, in contrast to redness and swelling where there was a small increased incidence. There was no increase in the frequency of general adverse events with successive doses.

HPV Vaccine Local and Systemic Adverse Reactions in Women (10 to 25 Years of Age) Within 7 Days of Vaccination[a]

Adverse reaction	HPV vaccine (10 to 25 years)	HAV 720[b] (15 to 25 years)	HAV 360[c] (10 to 14 years)	$Al(OH)_3$ control[d] (15 to 25 years)
Local adverse reaction	n = 6,431	n = 3,079	n = 1,027	n = 549
Pain	91.8%	78%	64.2%	87.2%
Redness	48%	27.6%	25.2%	24.4%
Swelling	44.1%	19.8%	17.3%	21.3%
Systemic adverse reaction	n = 6,432	n = 3,079	n = 1,027	n = 549
Fatigue	55%	53.7%	42.3%	53.6%
Headache	53.4%	51.3%	45.2%	61.4%
GI[e]	27.8%	27.3%	24.6%	32.8%
Fever (≥ 99.5°F)	12.8%	10.9%	16%	13.5%

HUMAN PAPILLOMAVIRUS (TYPES 16, 18) BIVALENT VACCINE, RECOMBINANT — INJECTION

HPV Vaccine Local and Systemic Adverse Reactions in Women (10 to 25 Years of Age) Within 7 Days of Vaccination[a]

Adverse reaction	HPV vaccine (10 to 25 years)	HAV 720[b] (15 to 25 years)	HAV 360[c] (10 to 14 years)	$Al(OH)_3$ control[d] (15 to 25 years)
Rash	9.6%	8.4%	6.7%	10%
	n = 5,881	n = 3,079	n = 1,027	—
Myalgia[f]	49.1%	44.9%	33.1%	—
Arthralgia[f]	20.8%	17.9%	19.9%	—

HPV Vaccine Local and Systemic Adverse Reactions in Women (10 to 25 Years of Age) Within 7 Days of Vaccination[a]

Adverse reaction	HPV vaccine (10 to 25 years)	HAV 720[b] (15 to 25 years)	HAV 360[c] (10 to 14 years)	$Al(OH)_3$ control[d] (15 to 25 years)
Urticaria[f]	7.4%	7.9%	5.4%	—

[a] Total vaccinated cohort included subjects with at least 1 documented dose (n).
[b] HAV 720 = hepatitis A vaccine control group (720 EL.U of antigen and 500 mcg of $Al(OH)_3$).
[c] HAV 360 = hepatitis A vaccine control group (360 EL.U of antigen and 250 mcg of $Al(OH)_3$).
[d] $Al(OH)_3$ control = control containing 500 mcg of $Al(OH)_3$.
[e] GI symptoms include nausea, vomiting, diarrhea, and/or abdominal pain.
[f] Adverse reactions solicited in a subset of subjects.

HPV Vaccine Local Adverse Reactions in Women (10 to 25 Years of Age) by Dose Within 7 Days of Vaccination[a]

	HPV vaccine (10 to 25 years)			HAV 720[b] (15 to 25 years)			HAV 360[c] (10 to 14 years)			$Al(OH)_3$ control[d] (15 to 25 years)		
	Postdose			Postdose			Postdose			Postdose		
Adverse reaction	1	2	3	1	2	3	1	2	3	1	2	3
n	6,415	6,197	5,936	3,070	2,919	2,758	1,027	1,021	1,011	546	521	500
Pain	86.9%	76.2%	78.7%	65.6%	54.4%	56.1%	48.5%	38.5%	36.9%	79.1%	66.8%	72.4%
Pain, grade 3[e]	7.5%	5.7%	7.7%	2%	1.4%	2%	0.8%	0.2%	1.6%	9%	6%	8.6%
Redness	27.8%	29.6%	35.6%	16.6%	15.2%	16.1%	15.6%	13.3%	12.1%	11.5%	11.5%	15.6%
Redness, > 50 mm	0.2%	0.5%	1%	0.1%	0.1%	0%	0.1%	0.2%	0.1%	0.2%	0%	0%
Swelling	22.7%	25.2%	32.7%	10.5%	9.4%	10.5%	9.4%	8.6%	7.6%	10.3%	10.4%	12%
Swelling, > 50 mm	1.2%	1%	1.3%	0.2%	0.2%	0.2%	0.4%	0.3%	0%	0%	0%	0%

[a] Total vaccinated cohort included subjects with at least 1 documented dose (n).
[b] HAV 720 = hepatitis A vaccine control group (720 EL.U of antigen and 500 mcg of $Al(OH)_3$).
[c] HAV 360 = hepatitis A vaccine control group (360 EL.U of antigen and 250 mcg of $Al(OH)_3$).
[d] $Al(OH)_3$ control = control containing 500 mcg of $Al(OH)_3$.
[e] Defined as spontaneously painful or pain that prevented normal daily activities.

The pattern of solicited local adverse reactions and general adverse events following administration of HPV vaccine was similar between the age cohorts (10 to 14 years of age and 15 to 25 years of age).

Other adverse reactions –

HPV Vaccine Adverse Reactions in Women (10 to 25 Years of Age) Within 30 Days of Vaccination (≥ 1%)[a]

Adverse reaction	HPV vaccine (n = 6,654)	HAV 720[b] (n = 3,186)	HAV 360[c] (n = 1,032)	$Al(OH)_3$ control[d] (n = 581)
CNS				
Dizziness	2.2%	2.6%	1.5%	3.1%
Headache	5.3%	7.6%	3.3%	9.3%
GU				
Dysmenorrhea	2%	2.3%	1.9%	4%
Urinary tract infection	1%	1.4%	0.3%	1.2%
Vaginal infection	1.4%	2.2%	0.1%	0.9%
Respiratory				
Influenza	3.2%	5.6%	1.3%	1.9%
Nasopharyngitis	3.6%	3.4%	5.9%	3.3%
Pharyngitis	1.5%	1.8%	2.2%	0.5%
Upper respiratory infection	2%	1.3%	6.7%	1.5%
Local				
Injection-site bruising	1.4%	1.8%	0.7%	1.5%
Injection-site pruritus	1.3%	0.5%	0.6%	0.2%
Miscellaneous				
Back pain	1.1%	1.3%	0.7%	3.1%
Chlamydia infection	2%	4.4%	0%	0%
Pharyngolaryngeal pain	2.9%	2.7%	2.2%	2.2%

[a] Total vaccinated cohort included subjects with at least 1 dose administered (n).
[b] HAV 720 = hepatitis A vaccine control group (720 EL.U of antigen and 500 mcg of $Al(OH)_3$).
[c] HAV 360 = hepatitis A vaccine control group (360 EL.U of antigen and 250 mcg of $Al(OH)_3$).
[d] $Al(OH)_3$ Control = control containing 500 mcg $Al(OH)_3$.

Systemic autoimmune diseases –

HPV Vaccine Systemic Autoimmune Disease Adverse Reactions in Women 10 to 25 Years of Age[a]

	HPV vaccine (n = 12,533)[c]	Pooled control group[b] (n = 10,730)[c]
Total number of subjects with at least 1 medical condition	0.8%	0.8%
Arthritis[d]	0%	0%
Celiac disease	0%	0%
Dermatomyositis	0%	0%
Diabetes mellitus insulin-dependent (type 1 or unspecified)	0%	0%
Erythema nodosum	0%	0%
Hyperthyroidism[e]	0.1%	0.1%
Hypothyroidism[f]	0.2%	0.3%
Inflammatory bowel disease[g]	0.1%	0%
Multiple sclerosis	0%	0%
Myelitis transverse	0%	0%
Optic neuritis/Optic neuritis retrobulbar	0%	0%
Psoriasis[h]	0.1%	0.1%
Raynaud phenomenon	0%	0%
Rheumatoid arthritis	0%	0%
Systemic lupus erythematosus[i]	0%	0%
Thrombocytopenia[j]	0%	0%
Vasculitis[k]	0%	0%
Vitiligo	0%	0%

[a] Total vaccinated cohort included subjects with at least 1 documented dose (n).
[b] Pooled control group = hepatitis A vaccine control group (720 EL.U of antigen and 500 mcg of $Al(OH)_3$), hepatitis A vaccine control group (360 EL.U of antigen and 250 mcg of $Al(OH)_3$), and a control containing 500 mcg of $Al(OH)_3$.
[c] n (%): number and percentage of subjects with medical condition.
[d] Term includes reactive arthritis and arthritis.
[e] Term includes Basedow disease, goiter, and hyperthyroidism.
[f] Term includes thyroiditis, autoimmune thyroiditis, and hypothyroidism.
[g] Term includes colitis ulcerative, Crohn disease, proctitis ulcerative, and inflammatory bowel disease.
[h] Term includes psoriatic arthropathy, nail psoriasis, guttate psoriasis, and psoriasis.
[i] Term includes systemic lupus erythematosus and cutaneous lupus erythematosus.
[j] Term includes idiopathic thrombocytopenic purpura and thrombocytopenia.
[k] Term includes leukocytoclastic vasculitis and vasculitis.

HUMAN PAPILLOMAVIRUS (TYPES 16, 18) BIVALENT VACCINE, RECOMBINANT — INJECTION

➤*Serious adverse reactions:* In the pooled safety database, inclusive of controlled and uncontrolled studies, which enrolled women 10 to 72 years of age, 5.3% (862/16,142) of subjects who received HPV vaccine and 5.9% (814/13,811) of subjects who received control reported at least 1 serious adverse event, without regard to causality, during the entire follow-up period (up to 7.4 years). Among women 10 to 25 years of age enrolled in these clinical studies, 6.4% of subjects who received HPV vaccine and 7.2% of subjects who received the control reported at least 1 serious adverse event during the entire follow-up period (up to 7.4 years).

➤*Deaths:* The most common causes of death were motor vehicle accident (5 subjects who received HPV vaccine; 5 subjects who received control) and suicide (2 subjects who received HPV vaccine; 5 subjects who received control), followed by neoplasm (3 subjects who received HPV vaccine; 2 subjects who received control), autoimmune disease (3 subjects who received HPV vaccine; 1 subject who received control), infectious disease (3 subjects who received HPV vaccine; 1 subject who received control), homicide (2 subjects who received HPV vaccine; 1 subject who received control), cardiovascular disorders (2 subjects who received HPV vaccine), and death of unknown cause (2 subjects who received control). Among women 10 to 25 years of age, 31 deaths were reported (0.05%; 16/29,467 of subjects who received HPV vaccine, and 0.07%; 15/20,192 of subjects who received control.

➤*Postmarketing:*

CNS – Syncope or vasovagal responses to injection (sometimes accompanied by tonic-clonic movements).

Hypersensitivity – Allergic reactions (including anaphylactic and anaphylactoid reactions), angioedema, erythema multiforme.

Overdosage

None well documented.

Patient Information

Provide the Vaccine Information Statements prior to immunization. This is required by the National Childhood Vaccine Injury Act of 1986 and are available free of charge at the Centers for Disease Control and Prevention (CDC) Web site (http://www.cdc.gov/vaccines).

Inform the patient, parent, or guardian that vaccination does not substitute for routine cervical cancer screening. Women who receive HPV vaccine should continue to undergo cervical cancer screening per standard of care. HPV vaccine does not protect against disease from HPV types to which a woman has previously been exposed through sexual activity.

Inform patients that syncope has been reported following vaccination in young women, sometimes resulting in falling with injury; observation for 15 minutes after administration is recommended.

Inform patient, parent, or guardian of the potential benefits and risks associated with vaccination.

Advise patients to report any adverse events to their health care provider.

Safety has not been established in pregnant women. Inform patients that the HPV vaccine is not recommended for use in pregnant women or women planning to become pregnant during the vaccination course. Register women who receive HPV vaccine while pregnant in the pregnancy registry by calling 1-888-452-9622.

HUMAN PAPILLOMAVIRUS QUADRIVALENT VACCINE, RECOMBINANT

Rx	**Gardasil** (Merck)	**Injection, suspension:** ≈ 20 mcg of HPV[a] 6 L1 protein, 40 mcg of HPV 11 L1 protein, 40 mcg of HPV 16 L1 protein, and 20 mcg of HPV 18 L1 protein per 0.5 mL[b]	Preservative free. In single-dose vials and prefilled syringes.

[a] HPV = human papillomavirus.

[b] Each 0.5 mL dose contains 225 mcg of aluminum, 9.56 mg of sodium chloride, 0.78 mg of L-histidine, 50 mcg of polysorbate eighty, 35 mcg of sodium borate, and less than 7 mcg/dose of yeast protein.

HUMAN PAPILLOMAVIRUS QUADRIVALENT VACCINE, RECOMBINANT — INJECTION

For additional information, refer to the Agents for Active Immunization introduction.

Indications

➤*Prevention of human papillomavirus:*

Females – For the prevention of the following diseases caused by HPV in females 9 to 26 years of age: cervical, vulvar, vaginal, and anal cancer caused by HPV types 16 and 18; and genital warts (condyloma acuminatum) caused by HPV types 6 and 11; for the prevention of the following precancerous or dysplastic lesions caused by HPV types 6, 11, 16, and 18 in females 9 to 26 years of age: cervical intraepithelial neoplasia (CIN) grade 2/3 and cervical adenocarcinoma in situ; CIN grade 1; vulvar intraepithelial neoplasia grade 2 and 3; vaginal intraepithelial neoplasia grade 2 and 3; and anal intraepithelial neoplasia grades 1, 2, and 3.

Males – For the prevention of the following diseases caused by HPV in males 9 through 26 years of age: anal cancer caused by HPV types 16 and 18; genital warts (condyloma acuminata) caused by HPV types 6 and 11; for the prevention of the following precancerous or dysplastic lesions caused by HPV types 6, 11, 16, and 18: anal intraepithelial neoplasia grades 1, 2, and 3.

Administration and Dosage

➤*Adults:*

Human papillomavirus prevention –

26 years of age and younger: 0.5 mL intramuscularly (IM). Administer a second dose 2 months after the first dose and a third dose 6 months after the first dose.

➤*Children:*

Human papillomavirus prevention –

9 years of age and older: See Adults for dosing.

➤*Preparation for administration:* Shake well before use. Thorough agitation immediately before administration is necessary to maintain suspension of the vaccine. After thorough agitation, the HPV vaccine is a white, cloudy liquid. Use promptly.

➤*Administration:* Administer the entire dose IM in the deltoid region of the upper arm or in the higher anterolateral area of the thigh. Do not administer intravenously, intradermally, or subcutaneously.

➤*Admixture compatibility:* May be coadministered (at a separate injection site) with *Recombivax HB*, *Menactra*, and *Adacel*. The HPV vaccine should not be diluted or mixed with other vaccines.

➤*Storage / Stability:* Store refrigerated at 2° to 8°C (36° to 46°F). Do not freeze. Protect from light. Administer as soon as possible after removing it from refrigeration; can be out of refrigeration (at temperatures at or below 25°C [77°F]) for a total time of not more than 72 hours.

Actions

➤*Pharmacology:* The HPV vaccine is a quadrivalent (types 6, 11, 16, and 18) recombinant vaccine for the prevention of HPV. HPV only infects humans, but animal studies with analogous animal papillomaviruses suggest that the efficacy of L1 virus-like particle vaccines may involve the development of humoral immune responses. Humans develop a humoral immune response to the vaccine, although the exact mechanism of protection is unknown.

Contraindications

Hypersensitivity, including severe allergic reactions to yeast (a vaccine component), or after a previous dose of HPV vaccine.

Warnings/Precautions

➤*Syncope:* Because vaccinees may experience syncope, sometimes resulting in falling with injury, observation for 15 minutes after administration is recommended. Syncope, sometimes associated with tonic-clonic movements and other seizure-like activity, has been reported following vaccination with HPV vaccine. When syncope is associated with tonic-clonic movements, the activity is usually transient and typically responds to restoring cerebral perfusion by maintaining a supine or Trendelenburg position.

➤*Immunocompromised patients:* The immunologic response to HPV vaccine may be diminished in immunocompromised individuals.

➤*Hypersensitivity reactions:* Appropriate medical treatment and supervision must be readily available in case of anaphylactic reactions following the administration of HPV vaccine.

➤*Pregnancy: Category B.* There are no adequate and well-controlled studies in pregnant women. Because animal reproduction studies are not always predictive of human responses, use HPV vaccine during pregnancy only if clearly needed.

Further subanalyses were conducted to evaluate pregnancies with estimated onset within 30 days or more than 30 days from administration of a dose of the HPV vaccine or amorphous aluminum hydroxyphosphate sulfate control or saline placebo. For pregnancies with estimated onset within 30 days of vaccination, 5 cases of congenital anomaly were observed in the group that received the HPV vaccine compared with 1 case of congenital anomaly in the group that received amorphous aluminum hydroxyphosphate sulfate control or saline placebo. The congenital anomalies seen in pregnancies with estimated onset within 30 days of vaccination included pyloric stenosis, congenital megacolon, congenital hydronephrosis, hip dysplasia, and club foot.

Conversely, in pregnancies with onset more than 30 days following vaccination, 35 cases of congenital anomaly were observed in the group that received the HPV vaccine compared with 29 cases of congenital anomaly in the group that received amorphous aluminum hydroxyphosphate sulfate control or saline placebo.

Pregnancy registry – There is a pregnancy registry to monitor fetal outcomes of pregnant women exposed to the HPV vaccine. Patients and health care providers are encouraged to report any exposure to the HPV vaccine during pregnancy by calling 1-800-986-8999.

➤*Lactation:* It is not known whether the HPV vaccine is excreted in human milk. Because many drugs are excreted in human milk, exercise caution when the HPV vaccine is administered to a breast-feeding woman.

HUMAN PAPILLOMAVIRUS QUADRIVALENT VACCINE, RECOMBINANT — INJECTION

In a post-hoc analysis of clinical studies, a higher number of breast-feeding infants (n = 6) whose mothers received the HPV vaccine had acute respiratory illnesses within 30 days postvaccination of the mother compared with infants (n = 2) whose mothers received amorphous aluminum hydroxyphosphate sulfate control.

➤*Children:* The safety and effectiveness of the HPV vaccine have not been established in children younger than 9 years of age.

➤*Monitoring:* Observe patient for 15 minutes after administration for signs of syncope.

Drug Interactions

➤*Immunosuppressive drugs:* Immunosuppressive therapies, including irradiation, antimetabolites, alkylating agents, cytotoxic drugs, and corticosteroids (used in greater than physiologic doses), may reduce the immune responses to vaccines.

Adverse Reactions

➤*Common injection-site adverse reactions:*

Females –

HPV Vaccine Injection-Site Adverse Reactions (≥ 1%)[a] in Females 9 Through 26 Years of Age

Adverse reactions (1 to 5 days postvaccination)	HPV vaccine (n = 5,088)	Amorphous aluminum hydroxyphosphate sulfate control (n = 3,470)	Saline placebo (n = 320)
Bruising	2.8%	3.2%	1.6%
Erythema	24.7%	18.4%	12.1%
Pain	83.9%	75.4%	48.6%
Pruritus	3.2%	2.8%	0.6%
Swelling	25.4%	15.8%	7.3%

[a] The injection-site adverse reactions that were observed among recipients of the HPV vaccine were at a frequency of ≥ 1% and also at a greater frequency than that observed among amorphous aluminum hydroxyphosphate sulfate control or saline placebo recipients.

Males –

HPV Vaccine Injection-Site Adverse Reactions (≥ 1%)[a] in Males 9 Through 26 Years of Age

Adverse reactions (1 to 5 days postvaccination)	HPV vaccine (n = 3,093)	Amorphous aluminum hydroxyphosphate sulfate control (n = 2,029)	Saline placebo (n = 274)
Erythema	16.7%	14.1%	14.5%
Hematoma	1%	0.3%	3.3%
Pain	61.4 %	50.8%	41.6%
Swelling	13.9%	9.6%	8.2%

[a] The injection site adverse reactions that were observed among recipients of the HPV vaccine were at a frequency of at least 1% and also at a greater frequency than that observed among amorphous aluminum hydroxyphosphate sulfate control or saline placebo recipients.

➤*Common systemic adverse reactions:*

Females –

HPV Vaccine Systemic Adverse Reactions (≥ 1%)[a] in Females 9 Through 26 Years of Age

Adverse reactions (1 to 15 days postvaccination)	HPV vaccine (n = 5,088)	Amorphous aluminum hydroxyphosphate sulfate control or saline placebo (n = 3,790)
CNS		
Headache	28.2%	28.4%
Insomnia	1.2%	0.9%
Malaise	1.4%	1.2%
GI		
Diarrhea	3.6%	3.5%
Nausea	6.7%	6.5%
Toothache	1.5%	1.4%
Vomiting	2.4%	1.9%
Respiratory		
Cough	2%	1.5%
Nasal congestion	1.1%	0.9%
Upper respiratory tract infection	1.5%	1.5%
Miscellaneous		
Arthralgia	1.2%	0.9%
Pyrexia	13%	11.2%

[a] The adverse reactions are those observed among recipients of the HPV vaccine at a frequency of at least 1% and greater than or equal to those observed among amorphous aluminum hydroxyphosphate sulfate control or saline placebo recipients.

Males –

HPV Vaccine Systemic Adverse Reactions (≥ 1%)[a] in Males 9 Through 26 Years of Age

Adverse reactions (1 to 15 days postvaccination)	HPV vaccine (n = 3,093)	Amorphous aluminum hydroxyphosphate sulfate control or saline placebo (n = 2,303)
CNS		
Dizziness	1.2%	0.9%
Headache	12.3%	11.2%
GI		
Abdominal pain, upper	1.4%	1.4%
Diarrhea	2.7%	2.2%
Nausea	2%	1%
Vomiting	1%	0.8%
Respiratory		
Nasopharyngitis	2.6%	2.6%
Oropharyngeal pain	2.8%	2.1%
Upper respiratory tract infection	1.5%	1%
Miscellaneous		
Myalgia	1.3%	0.7%
Pyrexia	8.3%	6.5%

[a] The adverse reactions are those observed among recipients of HPV vaccine at a frequency of at least 1% and greater than or equal to those observed among amorphous aluminum hydroxyphosphate sulfate control or saline placebo recipients.

➤*Serious adverse reactions:* Across the clinical studies, 0.8% (HPV vaccine) and 1% (control or placebo) reported a serious systemic adverse reaction. Of the entire study population, 0.04% of the reported serious systemic adverse reactions were judged to be vaccine related by the study investigator. The most frequently reported serious systemic adverse reactions (frequency of 4 cases or greater with either HPV vaccine, amorphous aluminum hydroxyphosphate sulfate control, saline placebo, or the total of all 3) and regardless of causality were as follows:

CNS – Headache (0.02% vs 0.02% control).

GI – Appendicitis (0.03% vs 0.01% control); gastroenteritis (0.02 vs 0.02% control).

GU – Pelvic inflammatory disease (0.02% vs 0.03% control); pyelonephritis, urinary tract infection (0.01% vs 0.02% control).

Local – One subject in the clinical trials in the group that received HPV vaccine reported 2 injection-site serious adverse reactions (injection-site pain and injection-site joint movement impairment).

Respiratory – Asthma (0.01% vs 0% control), pneumonia, pulmonary embolism (0.01% vs 0.02% control); bronchospasm (0.006% vs 0% control).

➤*Deaths:* The most common cause of death was motor vehicle accident (5 subjects who received the HPV vaccine and 4 amorphous aluminum hydroxyphosphate sulfate control subjects), followed by drug overdose/suicide (2 subjects who received HPV vaccine and 6 subjects who received amorphous aluminum hydroxyphosphate sulfate control), gun shot wound (1 subject who received HPV vaccine and 3 who received amorphous aluminum hydroxyphosphate sulfate control), and pulmonary embolism/deep vein thrombosis (1 subject who received the HPV vaccine and 1 amorphous aluminum hydroxyphosphate sulfate subject). In addition, there were 2 cases of sepsis, 1 case of pancreatic cancer, 1 case of arrhythmia, 1 case of pulmonary tuberculosis, 1 case of hyperthyroidism, 1 case of postoperative pulmonary embolism and acute renal failure, 1 case of traumatic brain injury/cardiac arrest, and 1 case of systemic lupus erythematosus, cerebrovascular accident, breast cancer, and nasopharyngeal cancer in the group that received HPV vaccine; 1 case of asphyxia, 1 case of acute lymphocytic leukemia, 1 case of chemical poisoning, and 1 case of myocardial ischemia in the amorphous aluminum hydroxyphosphate sulfate control; and 1 case of medulloblastoma in the saline placebo group.

HUMAN PAPILLOMAVIRUS QUADRIVALENT VACCINE, RECOMBINANT — INJECTION

➤*Systemic autoimmune disorders:*

Females –

HPV Vaccine Systemic Autoimmune Disorder Adverse Reactions[a] in Females 9 Through 26 Years of Age

Adverse reactions	HPV vaccine (n = 10,706)	Amorphous aluminum hydroxyphosphate sulfate control or saline placebo (n = 9,412)
GI		
Celiac disease	0.1%	0.1%
Inflammatory bowel disease[b]	0.1%	0.1%
Endocrine		
Hyperthyroidism[c]	0.3%	0.2%
Hypothyroidism[d]	0.3%	0.4%
Musculoskeletal		
Arthralgia/Arthritis/Arthropathy[e]	1.1%	1%
Rheumatoid arthritis[f]	0.1%	0%
Miscellaneous		
Nephritis[g]	0%	0.1%
Psoriasis[h]	0.1%	0.2%
All conditions	2.3%	2.3%

[a] Percent represents subjects with specific new medical conditions. Although a subject may have had ≥ 2 new medical conditions, the subject is counted only once within a category. The same subject may appear in different categories. This population includes all females who received at least 1 dose of HPV vaccine or amorphous aluminum hydroxyphosphate sulfate control or saline placebo and had safety data available.
[b] Inflammatory bowel disease includes the following terms: colitis ulcerative, Crohn disease, and inflammatory bowel disease.
[c] Hyperthyroidism includes the following terms: Basedow disease, goiter, toxic nodular goiter, and hyperthyroidism.
[d] Hypothyroidism includes the following terms: hypothyroidism and thyroiditis.
[e] Arthralgia/Arthritis/Arthropathy includes the following terms: arthralgia, arthritis, arthropathy, and reactive arthritis.
[f] Rheumatoid arthritis includes juvenile rheumatoid arthritis. One subject counted in the rheumatoid arthritis group reported rheumatoid arthritis as an adverse reaction at day 130.
[g] Nephritis includes the following terms: nephritis, glomerulonephritis minimal lesion, and glomerulonephritis proliferative.
[h] Psoriasis includes the following terms: psoriasis, pustular psoriasis, and psoriatic arthropathy.

Males –

HPV Vaccine Systemic Autoimmune Disorder Adverse Reactions[a] in Males 9 Through 26 Years of Age

Adverse reactions	HPV vaccine (n = 3,093)	Amorphous aluminum hydroxyphosphate sulfate control or saline placebo (n = 2,303)
Dermatological		
Alopecia areata	0.1%	0%
Psoriasis	0%	0.2%
Vitiligo	0.1%	0.2%
Endocrine		
Diabetes mellitus type 1	0.1%	0.1%
Hypothyroidism[b]	0.1%	0%
Musculoskeletal		
Ankylosing spondylitis	0%	0.1%
Arthralgia/Arthritis/Reactive arthritis	1%	0.7%
Miscellaneous		
Inflammatory bowel disease[c]	0%	0.1%
All conditions	1.5%	1.5%

[a] Percent represents subjects with specific new medical conditions who received 1 dose or more of either vaccine or placebo. Although a subject may have had 2 or more new medical conditions, the subject is counted only once within a category. The same subject may appear in different categories. This population includes all males who received at least 1 dose of HPV vaccine or amorphous aluminum hydroxyphosphate sulfate control or saline placebo and had safety data available.
[b] Hypothyroidism includes the following terms: autoimmune thyroiditis and hypothyroidism.
[c] Inflammatory bowel disease includes the following terms: colitis ulcerative and Crohn disease.

➤*Postmarketing:*

Cardiovascular – Deep venous thrombosis, pulmonary embolus.

CNS – Acute disseminated encephalomyelitis, asthenia, chills, dizziness, fatigue, Guillain-Barré syndrome, headache, malaise, motor neuron disease, paralysis, seizures, syncope (including syncope associated with tonic-clonic movements and other seizure-like activity) sometimes resulting in falling with injury, transverse myelitis.

GI – Nausea, pancreatitis, vomiting.

Hematologic/Lymphatic – Autoimmune hemolytic anemia, idiopathic thrombocytopenic purpura, lymphadenopathy.

Hypersensitivity – Hypersensitivity reactions including anaphylactic/anaphylactoid reaction, bronchospasm, urticaria.

Musculoskeletal – Arthralgia, myalgia.

Miscellaneous – Autoimmune disease, cellulitis, death.

Patient Information

Inform the patient, parent, or guardian that vaccination does not substitute for routine cervical cancer screening. Women who receive the HPV vaccine should continue to undergo cervical cancer screening per standard of care.

Advise recipients of HPV vaccine not to discontinue anal cancer screening if it has been recommended by their health care provider.

HPV vaccine has not been demonstrated to provide protection against disease from vaccine and nonvaccine HPV types to which a person has previously been exposed through sexual activity.

Advise patients that syncope has been reported following vaccination, sometimes resulting in falling with injury; observation for 15 minutes after administration is recommended.

Provide the vaccine information required with each vaccination to the patient, parent, or guardian.

Inform the patient, parent, or guardian of the benefits and risks associated with vaccination.

The HPV vaccine is not recommended for use in pregnant women.

Inform the patient, parent, or guardian of the importance of completing the immunization series, unless contraindicated.

Instruct patients, parents, and guardians to report any adverse reactions to their health care provider.

There is a pregnancy registry to monitor fetal outcomes of pregnant women exposed to the HPV vaccine. Patients and health care providers are encouraged to report any exposure to the HPV vaccine during pregnancy by calling 1-800-986-8999.

ZOSTER VACCINE, LIVE, ATTENUATED (OKA/MERCK)

Rx	**Zostavax** (Merck)	**Injection, lyophilized powder for suspension:** ≥ 19,400 PFU[a] of Oka/Merck varicella-zoster virus per 0.65 mL	Sucrose. Preservative free. In single-dose vials of 1s and 10s.

[a] PFU = plaque-forming units.

ZOSTER VACCINE, LIVE, ATTENUATED (OKA/MERCK) — INJECTION

Indications

➤*Herpes zoster prevention:* For prevention of herpes zoster (shingles) in persons 50 years and older.

Administration and Dosage

➤*Adults:*

Herpes zoster prevention –

50 years and older: 0.65 mL as a single dose subcutaneously.

➤*Children:* Do not administer zoster vaccine in children.

➤*Elderly:*

Herpes zoster prevention – 0.65 mL as a single dose subcutaneously.

➤*Preparation for administration:* Use only sterile syringes free of preservatives, antiseptics, and detergents for each injection and/or reconstitution of zoster vaccine. Preservatives, antiseptics, and detergents may inactivate the vaccine virus.

Zoster vaccine, when reconstituted, is a semi-hazy to translucent, off-white to pale yellow liquid.

ZOSTER VACCINE, LIVE, ATTENUATED (OKA/MERCK) — INJECTION

Reconstitution – Zoster vaccine is stored frozen and should be reconstituted immediately upon removal from the freezer. Reconstitute the vaccine using only the diluent supplied. Withdraw the entire contents of the diluent vial into a syringe. To avoid excessive foaming, slowly inject all of the diluent in the syringe into the vial of lyophilized vaccine and gently agitate to mix thoroughly. Withdraw the entire contents of reconstituted vaccine into a syringe and inject the total volume subcutaneously. The vaccine should be administered immediately after reconstitution to minimize loss of potency. Discard reconstituted vaccine if it is not used within 30 minutes. Do not freeze reconstituted vaccine.

➤*Administration:* Administer as a single dose subcutaneously in the deltoid region of the upper arm.

➤*Storage/Stability:* To maintain potency, the vaccine must be stored frozen between −50° and −15°C (−58° and +5°F). Use of dry ice may subject the vaccine to temperatures colder than −50°C (−58°F).

Before reconstitution, the vaccine should be stored frozen at a temperature between −50° and −15°C (−58° and +5°F) until it is reconstituted for injection. Any freezer, including frost-free, that has a separate sealed freezer door and reliably maintains a temperature between −50° and −15°C (−58° and +5°F) is acceptable for storing the vaccine.

Zoster vaccine may be stored and/or transported at refrigerator temperature between 2° and 8°C (36° and 46°F) for up to 72 continuous hours prior to reconstitution. Vaccine stored between 2° and 8°C (36° and 46°F) that is not used within 72 hours of removal from −15°C (+5°F) storage should be discarded. Zoster vaccine should be reconstituted immediately upon removal from the freezer. The diluent should be stored separately at room temperature (20° to 25°C [68° to 77°F]), or in the refrigerator (2° to 8°C [36° to 46°F]).

Before reconstitution, protect from light. Do not freeze reconstituted vaccine.

Actions

➤*Pharmacology:* The risk of developing zoster appears to be related to a decline in varicella-zoster virus–specific immunity. Zoster vaccine was shown to boost varicella-zoster virus–specific immunity, which is thought to be the mechanism by which it protects against zoster and its complications.

Contraindications

History of anaphylactic/anaphylactoid reaction to gelatin, neomycin, or any other component of the vaccine; immunosuppression or immunodeficiency, including a history of primary or acquired immunodeficiency states, leukemia, lymphoma, or other malignant neoplasms affecting the bone marrow or lymphatic system, AIDS or other clinical manifestations of infection with HIV; persons on immunosuppressive therapy; pregnancy during or within 3 months of treatment.

Warnings/Precautions

➤*Immunosuppression:* Vaccination with a live attenuated vaccine, such as zoster vaccine, may result in a more extensive vaccine-associated rash or disseminated disease in patients who are immunosuppressed. Safety and efficacy of zoster vaccine have not been evaluated in patients on immunosuppressive therapy, nor in patients receiving daily topical or inhaled corticosteroids or low-dose oral corticosteroids.

➤*Neomycin allergy:* Neomycin allergy commonly manifests as a contact dermatitis, which is not a contraindication to receiving this vaccine. Do not give zoster vaccine to persons with a history of anaphylactic reaction to topically or systemically administered neomycin.

➤*Anaphylactoid reactions:* As with any vaccine, make adequate treatment provisions, including epinephrine injection (1:1,000), available for immediate use should an anaphylactic/anaphylactoid reaction occur.

➤*Varicella virus:* Zoster vaccine is not a substitute for varicella virus vaccine.

➤*Acute illness:* Consider deferral of vaccination in acute illness, for example, in the presence of fever higher than 38.5°C (higher than 101.3°F).

➤*Duration:* The duration of protection after vaccination with zoster vaccine is unknown. In the Shingles Prevention Study (SPS), protection from zoster was demonstrated through 4 years of follow-up. The need for revaccination has not been defined.

➤*Protection:* As with any vaccine, vaccination with zoster vaccine may not result in protection of all vaccine recipients.

➤*Transmission:* In clinical trials with zoster vaccine, transmission of the vaccine virus has not been reported. However, postmarketing experience with varicella vaccines suggests that transmission of the vaccine virus may occur rarely between vaccinees who develop a varicella-like rash and susceptible contacts. Transmission of the vaccine virus from varicella vaccine recipients without a varicella-zoster virus–like rash has been reported but has not been confirmed. Weigh the risk of transmitting the attenuated vaccine virus to a susceptible person against the risk of developing natural zoster that could be transmitted to a susceptible person.

➤*Pregnancy: Category C.* Animal reproduction studies have not been conducted with zoster vaccine. It is also not known whether zoster vaccine can cause fetal harm when administered to a pregnant woman or can affect reproduction capacity. However, naturally occurring varicella-zoster virus infection is known to sometimes cause fetal harm. Therefore, do not administer zoster vaccine to a pregnant woman; furthermore, pregnancy should be avoided for 3 months following vaccination.

Pregnancy registry – Vaccinees and health care providers are encouraged to report any exposure to zoster vaccine during pregnancy by calling 1-800-986-8999.

➤*Lactation:* Some viruses are excreted in human milk; however, it is not known whether varicella-zoster virus is secreted in human milk. Therefore, because some viruses are secreted in human milk, exercise caution if zoster vaccine is administered to a breast-feeding woman.

➤*Children:* Do not administer zoster vaccine in children.

Adverse Reactions

The remainder of subjects in the SPS (n = 15,925 received zoster vaccine and n = 16,005 received placebo) were actively followed for safety outcomes through day 42 postvaccination and passively followed for safety after day 42.

Because clinical trials are conducted under conditions that may not be typical of those observed in clinical practice, the adverse reaction rates presented below may not be reflective of those observed in clinical practice.

➤*Serious adverse reactions:* The following table displays selected cardiovascular serious adverse reactions (SARs) occurring in the SPS within 42 days postvaccination.

Zoster Vaccine Cardiovascular Adverse Reactions

	Adverse Event Monitoring Substudy		Entire study cohort	
	Zoster vaccine 3,326[a] n[b]	Placebo 3,249[a] n[b]	Zoster vaccine 18,671[a] n[b]	Placebo 18,717[a] n[b]
Overall cardiovascular reactions by body system	20 (0.6%)	12 (0.4%)	81 (0.4%)	72 (0.4%)
Coronary artery disease–related conditions[c]	10 (0.3%)	5 (0.2%)	45 (0.2%)	35 (0.2%)

[a] Number of subjects with safety follow-up.
[b] n = number of subjects reporting SARs within the category.
[c] Angina pectoris, coronary artery disease, coronary occlusion, cardiovascular disorder, myocardial ischemia, and myocardial infarction

Investigator-determined, vaccine-related serious adverse reactions were reported for 2 subjects vaccinated with zoster vaccine (asthma exacerbation and polymyalgia rheumatica) and 3 subjects who received placebo (Goodpasture syndrome, anaphylactic reaction, and polymyalgia rheumatica).

➤*Deaths:* The overall incidence of death occurring days 0 to 42 postvaccination was similar between vaccination groups during the days 0 to 42 postvaccination period; 14 deaths occurred in the group of subjects who received zoster vaccine, and 16 deaths occurred in the group of subjects who received placebo. The most common reported cause of death was cardiovascular disease (10 in the group of subjects who received zoster vaccine, 8 in the group of subjects who received placebo). The overall incidence of death occurring at any time during the study was similar between vaccination groups: 793 deaths (4.1%) occurred in subjects who received zoster vaccine and 795 deaths (4.1%) in subjects who received placebo.

➤*Most common adverse reactions:*

Zoster Vaccine Adverse Reactions (≥ 1%)

Adverse reaction	Zoster vaccine (3,345)	Placebo (3,271)
CNS		
Headache	1.4%	0.8%
Local		
Erythema[a]	33.7%	6.4%
Hematoma	1.4%	1.4%
Pain/tenderness[a]	33.4%	8.3%
Pruritus	6.6%	1%
Swelling[a]	24.9%	4.3%
Warmth	1.5%	0.3%

[a] Designates a solicited adverse reaction. Injection-site adverse reactions were solicited only from days 0 to 4 postvaccination.

The following adverse reactions in the Adverse Event Monitoring Substudy of the SPS (days 0 to 42 postvaccination) were reported at an incidence of 1% or greater in subjects who received zoster vaccine than in subjects who received placebo, respectively.

➤*CNS:* Asthenia (32 [1%] vs 14 [0.4%]).

➤*Dermatologic:* Skin disorder (35 [1.1%] vs 31 [1%])

➤*GI:* Diarrhea (51 [1.5%] vs 41 [1.3%])

➤*Respiratory:* Respiratory disorder (35 [1.1%] vs 27 [0.8%]), respiratory infection (65 [1.9%] vs 55 [1.7%]), rhinitis (46 [1.4%] vs 36 [1.1%])

➤*Miscellaneous:* Fever (59 [1.8%] vs 53 [1.6%]), flu syndrome (57 [1.7%] vs 52 [1.6%])

➤*Adverse reactions occurring after day 42 postvaccination:* Over the course of the study (4.9 years), 51 subjects (1.5%) receiving zoster vaccine

ZOSTER VACCINE, LIVE, ATTENUATED (OKA/MERCK) — INJECTION

were reported to have congestive heart failure (CHF) or pulmonary edema compared with 39 subjects (1.2%) receiving placebo in the Adverse Event Monitoring Substudy; 58 subjects (0.3%) receiving zoster vaccine were reported to have CHF or pulmonary edema compared with 45 (0.2%) subjects receiving placebo in the overall study.

➤*Varicella-zoster virus rashes following vaccination:* Within the 42-day postvaccination reporting period in the SPS, noninjection-site, zoster-like rashes were reported by 53 subjects (17 for zoster vaccine and 36 for placebo). Of 41 specimens that were adequate for polymerase chain reaction (PCR) testing, wild-type varicella-zoster virus was detected in 25 (5 for zoster vaccine, 20 for placebo) of these specimens. The Oka/Merck strain of varicella-zoster virus was not detected from any of these specimens.

Of reported varicella-like rashes (n = 59), 10 had specimens that were available and adequate for PCR testing. Varicella-zoster virus was not detected in any of these specimens.

In all other clinical trials in support of zoster vaccine, the reported rates of noninjection-site, zoster-like and varicella-like rashes within 42 days postvaccination were also low in both zoster vaccine recipients and placebo recipients. Of the 17 reported varicella-like rashes and noninjection-site, zoster-like rashes, 10 specimens were available and adequate for PCR testing. The Oka/Merck strain was identified by PCR analysis from the lesion specimens of 2 subjects who reported varicella-like rashes (onset on day 8 and 17).

➤*Reporting adverse reactions:* The US Department of Health and Human Services has established a Vaccine Adverse Event Reporting System (VAERS) to accept all reports of suspected adverse reactions after the administration of any vaccine. For information or a copy of the vaccine reporting form, call the VAERS toll-free number at 1-800-822-7967 or report online to http://www.vaers.hhs.gov.

Patient Information

Question the vaccine recipient about reactions to previous vaccines. Inform the vaccine recipient of the benefits and risks of zoster vaccine. Provide a copy of the patient information sheet and an opportunity to discuss any questions or concerns.

Inform vaccinees of the theoretical risk of transmitting the vaccine virus to varicella-susceptible persons, including pregnant women who have not had chickenpox. Advise patients that pregnancy should be avoided for 3 months following vaccination.

Advise patients to report any adverse reactions to their health care provider.

VARICELLA VIRUS VACCINE

Rx	**Varivax** (Merck)	**Powder for Injection:** 1350 PFU of Oka/Merck varicella virus (live)	Sucrose. In single-dose vials of 1s and 10s.

VARICELLA VIRUS VACCINE LIVE — INJECTION

For complete and comparative prescribing information, refer to the Agents for Active Immunization introduction.

Indications

➤*Varicella vaccination:* Varicella virus vaccine live is indicated for vaccination against varicella in individuals 12 months of age and older.

➤*Revaccination:* The duration of protection of varicella virus vaccine live is unknown at present and the need for booster doses is not defined. However, a boost in antibody levels has been observed in vaccinees following exposure to natural varicella as well as following a booster dose of varicella virus vaccine live administered 4 to 6 years postvaccination.

In a highly vaccinated population, immunity for some individuals may wane due to lack of exposure to natural varicella as a result of shifting epidemiology. Postmarketing surveillance studies are ongoing to evaluate the need and timing for booster vaccination.

➤*Protection:* Vaccination with varicella virus vaccine live may not result in protection of all healthy, susceptible children, adolescents, and adults.

➤*Off-label uses:*

Immunization (infants) – [2] = Fair documentation. The seronegativity rate at baseline in reviewed studies suggests that most 9-month-old infants have lost any maternally derived immunity and are susceptible to varicella. Although the decision to vaccinate after exposure should be made on a case-by-case basis after considering individual risk, studies to date have found that vaccination was associated with an adequate immune response and an acceptable safety profile in infants as young as 9 months of age.

Administration and Dosage

➤*General dosing considerations:* Varicella virus vaccine live should be stored frozen at an average temperature of −15°C (5°F) or colder until it is reconstituted for injection. (See Storage and Stability).

Do not give immune globulin including varicella-zoster immune globulin concurrently with varicella virus vaccine live (See Administration: Use with other vaccines).

➤*Adults:*

Varicella vaccination – A 0.5 mL dose administered subcutaneously at elected date and a second 0.5 mL dose 4 to 8 weeks later.

➤*Children:*

Varicella vaccination –

Usual dosage:

• *13 years of age and older* – A 0.5 mL dose administered subcutaneously at elected date and a second 0.5 mL dose 4 to 8 weeks later.

• *12 months to 12 years of age* – A single 0.5 mL dose administered subcutaneously.

• *Younger than 12 months of age* – Administration to infants under 12 months of age is not recommended.

Off-label dosing –

Immunization (infants): [2] = Fair documentation.

• *Children 9 to 12 months of age* – One subcutaneous dose of live, attenuated varicella virus vaccine within 3 days of exposure to chickenpox.

➤*Preparation for administration:* It is important to use a separate sterile syringe and needle for each patient to prevent transmission of infectious agents from one individual to another.

To reconstitute the vaccine, use only the sterile diluent supplied with varicella virus vaccine live, measles, mumps, and rubella virus vaccine live, or the component vaccines of measles, mumps, and rubella virus vaccine live, because it is free of preservatives or other antiviral substances that might inactivate the vaccine virus.

To reconstitute the vaccine, first withdraw 0.7 mL of diluent into the syringe to be used for reconstitution. Inject all the diluent in the syringe into the vial of lyophilized vaccine and gently agitate to mix thoroughly. Withdraw the entire contents into a syringe and inject the total volume (about 0.5 mL) of reconstituted vaccine subcutaneously, preferably into the outer aspect of the upper arm (deltoid) or the anterolateral thigh. It is recommended that the vaccine be administered immediately after reconstitution, to minimize loss of potency. Discard if reconstituted vaccine is not used within 30 minutes.

Do not freeze reconstituted vaccine.

➤*Administration:* Varicella virus vaccine live is for subcutaneous administration.

Do not inject intravenously.

The outer aspect of the upper arm (deltoid) is the preferred site of injection.

➤*Admixture compatibility:* Do not give immune globulin including varicella-zoster immune globulin concurrently with varicella virus vaccine live. Vaccination should be deferred for at least 5 months following blood or plasma transfusions, or administration of immune globulin or varicella-zoster immune globulin. Following administration of varicella virus vaccine live, any immune globulin including varicella-zoster immune globulin should not be given for 2 months thereafter unless its use outweighs the benefits of vaccination.

Caution – A sterile syringe free of preservatives, antiseptics, and detergents should be used for each injection or reconstitution of varicella virus vaccine live because these substances may inactivate the vaccine virus.

➤*Storage/Stability:* Varicella virus vaccine live retains a potency level of 1,500 plaque-forming units (PFU) or higher per dose for at least 24 months in a frost-free freezer with an average temperature of −15°C (5°F) or colder.

Varicella virus vaccine live has a minimum potency level of approximately 1,350 PFU 30 minutes after reconstitution at room temperature (20° to 25°C; 68° to 77°F).

Prior to reconstitution, varicella virus vaccine live retains potency when stored for up to 72 continuous hours at refrigerator temperature (2° to 8°C; 36° to 46°F).

For information regarding stability under conditions other than those recommended, call 1-800-9-VARIVAX.

During shipment, to ensure that there is no loss of potency, the vaccine must be maintained at a temperature of −20°C (−4°F) or colder.

Before reconstitution, store the lyophilized vaccine in a freezer at an average temperature of −15°C (5°F) or colder. Any freezer (eg, chest, frost-free) that reliably maintains an average temperature of −15°C (5°F) and has a separate sealed freezer door is acceptable for storing varicella virus vaccine live.

Varicella virus vaccine live may be stored at refrigerator temperature (2° to 8°C; 36° to 46°F) for up to 72 continuous hours prior to reconstitution. Vaccine stored at 2° to 8°C that is not used within 72 hours of removal from −15°C storage should be discarded.

Before reconstitution, protect from light.

The diluent should be stored separately at room temperature (20° to 25°C; 68° to 77°F), or in the refrigerator.

Contraindications

Hypersensitivity to any component of the vaccine, including gelatin; anaphylactoid reaction to neomycin (each dose of reconstituted vaccine contains trace quantities of neomycin); blood dyscrasias, leukemia, lymphomas of any type, or other malignant neoplasms affecting the bone marrow or lymphatic systems; active untreated tuberculosis; any febrile respiratory illness or other active febrile infection.

Individuals receiving immunosuppressive therapy. Individuals who are on immunosuppressant drugs are more susceptible to infections than healthy

VARICELLA VIRUS VACCINE LIVE — INJECTION

individuals. Vaccination with live attenuated varicella vaccine can result in a more extensive vaccine-associated rash or disseminated disease in individuals on immunosuppressant doses of corticosteroids.

Individuals with primary and acquired immunodeficiency states, including those who are immunosuppressed in association with AIDS or other clinical manifestations of infection with human immunodeficiency virus; cellular immune deficiencies; and hypogammaglobulinemic and dysgammaglobulinemic states.

A family history of congenital or hereditary immunodeficiency, unless the immune competence of the potential vaccine recipient is demonstrated.

➤*Pregnancy:* The possible effects of the vaccine on fetal development are unknown at this time. However, natural varicella is known to sometimes cause fetal harm. If vaccination of postpubertal females is undertaken, pregnancy should be avoided for 3 months following vaccination.

Warnings/Precautions

➤*Acute lymphoblastic leukemia:* Children and adolescents with acute lymphoblastic leukemia (ALL) in remission can receive the vaccine under an investigational protocol. More information is available by contacting the varicella virus vaccine live coordinating center, Omnicare Clinical Research, Inc., 630 Allendale Road, King of Prussia, PA 19406, (484) 679-2856.

➤*Anaphylactoid reactions:* See Warnings/Precautions for more information.

➤*Protection:* The duration of protection from varicella infection after vaccination with varicella virus vaccine live is unknown.

➤*Live virus:* It is not known whether varicella virus vaccine live given immediately after exposure to natural varicella virus will prevent illness.

➤*Use with other vaccines:* See Drug Interactions for more information.

➤*Immunosuppression:* The safety and efficacy of varicella virus vaccine live have not been established in children and young adults who are known to be infected with human immunodeficiency viruses with and without evidence of immunosuppression. These patients should not receive varicella virus vaccine live.

➤*Patient history:* The healthcare provider should question the patient, parent, or guardian about reactions to a previous dose of varicella virus vaccine live or a similar product.

➤*Administration precautions:* Varicella virus vaccine live should not be injected into a blood vessel.

➤*Congenital immunodeficiency:* Vaccination should be deferred in patients with a family history of congenital or hereditary immunodeficiency until the patient's own immune system has been evaluated.

➤*Transmission:* Postmarketing experience suggests that transmission of vaccine virus may occur rarely between healthy vaccinees who develop a varicella-like rash and healthy susceptible contacts. Transmission of vaccine virus from vaccinees without a varicella-like rash has been reported but has not been confirmed.

Therefore, vaccine recipients should attempt to avoid, whenever possible, close association with susceptible high-risk individuals for up to 6 weeks. In circumstances where contact with high-risk individuals is unavoidable, the potential risk of transmission of vaccine virus should be weighed against the risk of acquiring and transmitting natural varicella virus. Susceptible high risk individuals include:

- Immunocompromised individuals.
- Pregnant women without documented history of chickenpox or laboratory evidence of prior infection.
- Newborn infants of mothers without documented history of chickenpox or laboratory evidence of prior infection.

➤*Hypersensitivity reactions:* Adequate treatment provisions, including epinephrine injection (1:1000), should be available for immediate use should an anaphylactoid reaction occur.

➤*Pregnancy:* Category C. Animal reproduction studies have not been conducted with varicella virus vaccine live. It is also not known whether varicella virus vaccine live can cause fetal harm when administered to a pregnant woman or can affect reproduction capacity. Therefore, varicella virus vaccine live should not be administered to pregnant females; furthermore, pregnancy should be avoided for 3 months following vaccination. Merck & Co, Inc. maintains a Pregnancy Registry to monitor fetal outcomes of pregnant women exposed to varicella virus vaccine live. Patients and health care providers are encouraged to report any exposure to varicella virus vaccine live during pregnancy by calling (800) 986-8999.

➤*Lactation:* It is not known whether varicella vaccine virus is secreted in human milk. Therefore, because some viruses are secreted in human milk, caution should be exercised if varicella virus vaccine live is administered to a nursing woman.

➤*Children:* No clinical data are available on safety or efficacy of varicella virus vaccine live in children less than 1 year of age and administration to infants under 12 months of age is not recommended.

Drug Interactions

➤*Use with other vaccines:* Vaccination should be deferred for at least 5 months following blood or plasma transfusions, or administration of immune globulin or varicella-zoster immune globulin (VZIG).

Varicella Vaccine Drug Interactions

Precipitant drug	Object drug[a]		Description
Immune globulins	Varicella vaccine	↔	Defer vaccination for at least 5 months following blood or plasma transfusions, or administration of immune globulin or varicella-zoster immune globulin (VZIG). Following administration of varicella vaccine, do not give any immune globulin, including VZIG, for 2 months thereafter unless its use outweighs the benefits of vaccination.
Immunosuppressants	Varicella vaccine	⬇	Individuals who are on immunosuppressant drugs are more susceptible to infections than healthy individuals. Vaccination with live attenuated varicella vaccine can result in a more extensive vaccine-associated rash or disseminated disease in individuals on immunosuppressant doses of corticosteroids.
Salicylates	Varicella vaccine	⬆	Avoid use of salicylates for 6 weeks after varicella vaccine; Reye syndrome has been reported following salicylate use during natural varicella infections.

[a] ⬆ = object drug increased; ⬇ = object drug decreased; ↔ = undetermined clinical effect.

Adverse Reactions

➤*Children 1 to 12 years of age:* In clinical trials involving healthy children monitored for up to 42 days after a single dose of varicella virus vaccine live, the frequency of fever, injection-site complaints, or rashes were reported as follows:

Fever, Local Reactions, or Rashes (%) in Children 0 To 42 Days Postvaccination With Varicella Virus Vaccine Live

Reaction	N	Post dose 1	Peak occurrence in postvaccination days
Fever ≥ 39°C (102°F) oral	8827	14.7%	0 to 42
Injection-site complaints (pain/soreness, swelling or erythema, rash, pruritus, hematoma, induration, stiffness)	8916	19.3%	0 to 2
Varicella-like rash (injection site)	8916	3.4%	8 to 19
Varicella-like rash (injection site) (median number of lesions)		2	
Varicella-like rash (generalized)	8916	3.8%	5 to 26
Varicella-like rash (generalized) (median number of lesions)		5	

In addition, the most frequently (greater than or equal to 1%) reported adverse experiences, without regard to causality, are listed in decreasing order of frequency: Upper respiratory tract illness, cough, irritability/nervousness, fatigue, disturbed sleep, diarrhea, loss of appetite, vomiting, otitis, diaper rash/contact rash, headache, teething, malaise, abdominal pain, other rash, nausea, eye complaints, chills, lymphadenopathy, myalgia, lower respiratory tract illness, allergic reactions (including allergic rash, hives), stiff neck, heat rash/prickly heat, arthralgia, eczema/dry skin/dermatitis, constipation, itching.

Pneumonitis has been reported rarely (less than 1%) in children vaccinated with varicella virus vaccine live; a causal relationship has not been established.

Febrile seizures have occurred rarely (less than 0.1%) in children vaccinated with varicella virus vaccine live; a causal relationship has not been established.

➤*Adolescents and adults 13 years of age and older:* In clinical trials involving healthy adolescents and adults, the majority of whom received 2 doses of varicella virus vaccine live and were monitored for up to 42 days

VARICELLA VIRUS VACCINE LIVE — INJECTION

after any dose, the frequency of fever, injection-site complaints, or rashes were reported as follows:

Fever, Local Reactions, or Rashes (%) in Adolescents and Adults 0 To 42 Days Postvaccination With Varicella Virus Vaccine Live

Reaction	N	Post dose 1	Peak occurrence in post-vaccination days	N	Post dose 2	Peak occurrence in post-vaccination days
Fever ≥ 37.7°C (100°F) oral	1584	10.2%	14 to 27	956	9.5%	0 to 42
Injection-site complaints (soreness, erythema, swelling, rash, pruritus, pyrexia, hematoma, induration, numbness)	1606	24.4%	0 to 2	955	32.5%	0 to 2
Varicella-like rash (injection site)	1606	3%	6 to 20	955	1%	0 to 6
Varicella-like rash (injection site) (median number of lesions)		2			2	
Varicella-like rash (generalized)	1606	5.5%	7 to 21	955	0.9%	0 to 23
Varicella-like rash (generalized) (median number of lesions)		5			5.5	

In addition, the most frequently (greater than or equal to 1%) reported adverse experiences, without regard to causality, are listed in decreasing order of frequency: Upper respiratory tract illness, headache, fatigue, cough, myalgia, disturbed sleep, nausea, malaise, diarrhea, stiff neck, irritability/nervousness, lymphadenopathy, chills, eye complaints, abdominal pain, loss of appetite, arthralgia, otitis, itching, vomiting, other rashes, constipation, lower respiratory tract illness, allergic reactions (including allergic rash, hives), contact rash, cold/canker sore. As with any vaccine, there is the possibility that broad use of the vaccine could reveal adverse reactions not observed in clinical trials.

➤*Postmarketing reports:* The following additional adverse reactions have been reported since the vaccine has been marketed:

CNS – Encephalitis; cerebrovascular accident; non-febrile seizures; Guillain-Barré syndrome; transverse myelitis; Bell's palsy; ataxia; dizziness; paresthesia.

Dermatologic – Stevens-Johnson syndrome; erythema multiforme; Henoch-Schönlein purpura; secondary bacterial infections of skin and soft tissue, including impetigo and cellulitis; herpes zoster.

Hematologic / Lymphatic – Thrombocytopenia.

Hypersensitivity – Anaphylaxis in individuals with or without an allergic history.

Respiratory – Pharyngitis.

Patient Information

The healthcare provider should inform the patient, parent or guardian of the benefits and risks of varicella virus vaccine live.

Patients, parents, or guardians should be instructed to report any adverse reactions to their healthcare provider.

The US Department of Health and Human Services has established a Vaccine Adverse Event Reporting System (VAERS) to accept all reports of suspected adverse events after the administration of any vaccine, including but not limited to the reporting of events required by the National Childhood Vaccine Injury Act of 1986. The VAERS toll-free number for VAERS forms and information is 1-800-822-7967.Pregnancy should be avoided for 3 months following vaccination.

RABIES VACCINE

Rx	**Imovax Rabies Vaccine (Human Diploid Cell)** (Aventis Pasteur)	**Injection, lyophilized powder for reconstitution**[a]:	Contains ≥ 2.5 international units rabies antigen per mL	Preservative free. In single-dose vial[b] with disposable needle and syringe containing diluent and disposable needle for administration.
Rx	**RabAvert** (Chiron Corporation)	**Injection, lyophilized powder for reconstitution**[c]:	Contains ≥ 2.5 international units rabies antigen per mL	Preservative free. In single-dose vial[d] with 1 vial diluent, 1 disposable syringe, 1 longer needle for reconstitution, and 1 smaller needle for injection.

[a] Freeze-dried suspension of Wistar rabies virus strain PM-1503-3M grown in human diploid cell cultures (inactivated whole virus).
[b] With < 100 mg human albumin, < 150 mcg neomycin sulfate, and 20 mcg phenol red indicator.
[c] Freeze-dried, fixed-virus strain Flury LEP grown in cultures of chicken fibroblasts.
[d] With < 0.3 mg human albumin, < 3 ng ovalbumin, < 12 mg processed bovine gelatin, 1 mg potassium glutamate, 0.3 mg sodium EDTA, < 1 mcg neomycin, < 20 ng chlortetracycline, and

RABIES VACCINE — INJECTION

Refer to the general discussion in the Rabies Prophylaxis Products appendix.

Indications

➤*Rabies vaccination:* For preexposure vaccination, in both primary series and booster dose, and for postexposure prophylaxis against rabies in all age groups. Usually an immunization series is initiated and completed with 1 vaccine product.

➤*Rationale of treatment:* Health care providers must evaluate each possible rabies exposure. Consult local or state public health officials if questions arise about the need for prophylaxis.

Administration and Dosage

➤*General dosing considerations:* Booster immunization is given to people who have received previous rabies immunization and remain at increased risk of rabies exposure for reasons of occupation or avocation.

Because the antibody response following the recommended vaccination regimen with *Imovax* and *RabAvert* has been so satisfactory, routine postvaccination serologic testing is not recommended. Serologic testing is indicated in unusual circumstances, such as when the patient is immunosuppressed. Contact the state health department or Centers for Disease Control and Prevention (CDC) for recommendations.

➤*Adults:*

Imovax –

Preexposure rabies vaccination:

• *Primary immunization* – In the United States, the Advisory Committee on Immunization Practices (ACIP) recommends 3 injections of 1 mL each: 1 injection on day 0, 1 on day 7, and 1 on either day 21 or 28.

• *Booster immunization* – People who work with live rabies virus in research laboratories or vaccine production facilities should have a serum sample tested for rabies antibodies every 6 months and boosters given as needed to maintain an adequate titer. Only laboratory workers, such as those doing rabies diagnostic tests, spelunkers, veterinarians, and animal control and wildlife officers in areas where rabies is epizootic, should have boosters every 2 years or have their serum tested for antibodies every 2 years, and, if the titer is inadequate, have a booster dose. Veterinarians and animal control and wildlife officers, if working in areas of low rabies endemicity, do not require routine booster doses of *Imovax* after completion of primary preexposure immunization.

People who have experienced "immune complex–like" hypersensitivity reactions should receive no further doses of *Imovax* unless they are exposed to rabies or they are likely to be inapparently and/or unavoidably exposed to the rabies virus and have unsatisfactory antibody titers.

Postexposure prophylaxis:

• *Unimmunized patients –*

Usual dosage:

Based on these data, the ACIP recommends a 5-dose regimen for postexposure situations. Five 1 mL doses are given intramuscularly (IM) on days 0, 3, 7, 14, and 28 in conjunction with rabies immune globulin (RIG) on day 0.

Alternative dosage: The World Health Organization (WHO) established a recommendation for 6 IM doses of *Imovax* based on studies in Germany and Iran. Used in this way, a total of 6 injections of a 1 mL dose of vaccine are given according to the following schedule: on days 0, 3, 7, 14, 30, and 90. The first dose should be accompanied by RIG or antirabies serum (ARS). If possible, up to half the dose of RIG or ARS should be used to infiltrate the wound, and the rest should be administered IM in a different site from the rabies vaccine, preferably in the gluteal region.

• *Immunized patients* – 1 mL IM of *Imovax*, on day 0 and day 3 when rabies exposure occurs in a previously vaccinated person.

RabAvert –

Preexposure rabies vaccination:

• *Primary immunization* – See *Imovax*.

• *Booster immunization* – The individual booster is 1 mL given IM.

People who work with live rabies virus in research laboratories or vaccine production facilities should have a serum sample tested for rabies antibodies every 6 months. The minimum acceptable antibody level is complete virus neutralization at a 1:5 serum dilution by the rapid fluorescent focus inhibition test (RFFIT). A booster dose should be administered if the titer falls below this level.

The frequent-risk category includes other laboratory workers, such as those doing rabies diagnostic testing, spelunkers, veterinarians and their staff, and animal control and wildlife officers in areas where rabies is epizootic. People in the frequent-risk category should have a serum sample test for rabies antibodies every 2 years and, if the titer is less than complete neutralization at a 1:5 serum dilution by RFFIT, should have a booster dose of vaccine. Alternatively, a booster can be administered in the absence of a titer determination.

People in the infrequent-risk category, including veterinarians, animal control and wildlife officers working in areas of low rabies enzooticity (infrequent-exposure group), and international travelers to rabies enzootic areas, do not require preexposure booster doses of *RabAvert* after completion of a full primary preexposure vaccination scheme.

Postexposure prophylaxis:

• *Unimmunized patients* – Begin immunization as soon as possible after exposure. A complete course of immunization consists of a total of 5 injec-

RABIES VACCINE — INJECTION

tions of 1 mL each: 1 injection on days 0, 3, 7, 14, and 28 in conjunction with the administration of human rabies immune globulin on day 0.

• *Immunized patients* – 1 mL IM of *RabAvert* on day 0 and day 3 when rabies exposure occurs in a previously vaccinated person.

➤*Children:* See Adults for dosing.

➤*Preparation for administration:* A separate sterile syringe and needle or a sterile disposable unit should be used for each patient to prevent transmission of hepatitis and other infectious agents from person to person. Needles should not be recapped and should be disposed of properly.

The reconstituted vaccine should be used immediately.

Reconstitution –

Imovax: The package contains a vial of freeze-dried vaccine, a syringe containing 1 mL of diluent, a plunger for the syringe, and a needle for reconstitution.

Attach the plunger and reconstitution needle to the syringe and reconstitute the freeze-dried vaccine by injecting the diluent into the vaccine vial. Gently swirl the contents until completely dissolved and withdraw the total contents of the vial into the syringe. Remove the reconstitution needle and discard. For administration, use a needle of choice that is suitable for IM injection.

The freeze-dried vaccine is creamy white to orange. After reconstitution, it is pink to red.

RabAvert: Using the longest of the 2 needles supplied, withdraw the entire contents of the sterile diluent for *RabAvert* into the syringe. Insert the needle at a 45° angle and slowly inject the entire contents of the diluent vial into the vaccine vial. Mix gently to avoid foaming. The white, freeze-dried vaccine dissolves to give a clear or slightly opaque suspension. Withdraw the total amount of dissolved vaccine into the syringe and replace the long needle with the smaller needle for IM injection.

The lyophilization of the vaccine is performed under reduced pressure, and the subsequent closure of the vials needs to be done under vacuum. Additionally, if there is no negative pressure in the vial, injection of sterile diluent for *RabAvert* would lead to an excess of positive pressure in the vial. After reconstitution of the vaccine, it is recommended to unscrew the syringe from the needle to eliminate the negative pressure. After that, the vaccine can be easily withdrawn from the vial. It is not recommended to induce excess pressure, because over-pressurization will create problems in withdrawing the proper amount of the vaccine.

➤*Administration:* The individual dose for adults, children, and infants is 1 mL given IM.

In adults, administer the vaccine by IM injection into the deltoid muscle. In small children and infants, administer the vaccine into the anterolateral zone of the thigh. The gluteal area should be avoided for vaccine injection because administration in this area may result in lower neutralizing antibody titers. Care should be taken to avoid injection into or near blood vessels and nerves. After aspiration, if blood or any suspicious discoloration appears in the syringe, do not inject, but discard the contents and repeat the procedure using a new dose of vaccine at a different site.

➤*Storage/Stability:*

Imovax – The freeze-dried vaccine is stable if stored in the refrigerator between 2° and 8°C (35° and 46°F). Do not freeze.

RabAvert – Store between 2° and 8°C (36° and 46°F). Protect from light. After reconstitution, use the vaccine immediately. The vaccine may not be used after the expiration date given on the package and container.

Actions

➤*Pharmacology:*

Rabies in the United States – Over the last 100 years, the epidemiology of rabies in animals in the United States has changed dramatically. More than 90% of all animal rabies cases reported annually to the CDC occur in wildlife, whereas before 1960, the majority were in domestic animals. The principal rabies hosts today are wild terrestrial carnivores and bats. Annual human deaths have fallen from more than 100 at the turn of the century to 1 to 2 per year, despite major epizootics of animal rabies in several geographic areas. Within the United States, only Hawaii has remained rabies-free. Although rabies among humans is rare in the United States, tens of thousands of people receive rabies vaccine for postexposure prophylaxis every year.

Rabies is a viral infection transmitted via the saliva of infected mammals. The virus enters the CNS of the host, causing an encephalomyelitis that is almost invariably fatal. The incubation period varies between 5 days and several years, but is usually between 20 and 60 days. Clinical rabies presents in a furious or paralytic form. Clinical illness most often starts with prodromal complaints of malaise, anorexia, fatigue, headache, and fever, followed by pain or paresthesia at the site of exposure. Anxiety, agitation, and irritability may be prominent during this period, followed by hyperactivity, disorientation, seizures, aero- and hydrophobia, hypersalivation, and eventually paralysis, coma, and death.

Modern-day prophylaxis has proven nearly 100% successful; most human fatalities now occur in people who fail to seek medical treatment, usually because they do not recognize a risk in the animal contact leading to the infection. Inappropriate postexposure prophylaxis may also result in clinical rabies. Survival after clinical rabies is extremely rare and is associated with severe brain damage and permanent disability.

RabAvert (in combination with passive immunization with HRIG and local wound treatment) in postexposure treatment against rabies protected patients of all age groups from rabies when the vaccine was administered according to the CDC's ACIP or WHO guidelines as soon as possible after rabid animal contact. Antirabies antibody titers after immunization have been shown to reach levels well above the minimum antibody titer accepted as seroconversion (protective titer) within 14 days after initiating the postexposure treatment series. The minimum antibody titer accepted as seroconversion is a 1:5 titer (complete inhibition in the RFFIT at 1:5 dilution), as specified by the CDC, or 0.5 international units/mL or more, as specified by the WHO.

Contraindications

➤*Imovax*: For postexposure treatment, there are no known specific contraindications. In cases of preexposure immunization, there are no known specific contraindications other than situations, such as developing febrile illness.

➤*RabAvert*: In view of the almost invariable fatal outcome of rabies, there is no contraindication to postexposure prophylaxis, including pregnancy.

Hypersensitivity – History of anaphylaxis to the vaccine or any of the vaccine components constitutes a contraindication to preexposure vaccination with this vaccine.

In case of postexposure prophylaxis, if an alternative product is not available, vaccinate the patient with caution with the necessary medical equipment and emergency supplies available, and observe the patient carefully after vaccination. A patient's risk of acquiring rabies must be carefully considered before deciding to discontinue vaccination. Advice and assistance on the management of serious adverse reactions for people receiving rabies vaccines may be sought from the state health department or CDC.

Warnings/Precautions

➤*Imovax*:

Injection site – Rabies vaccine in this package is a unit dose to be delivered IM in the deltoid area.

This vaccine must not be used intradermally or as a multiple-dose dispensing unit. For pre- and postexposure immunization, give the full 1 mL dose IM.

In adults and children, inject the vaccine into the deltoid muscle. In infants and small children, the midlateral aspect of the thigh may be preferable.

Immune complex–like reactions – In the case of preexposure immunization, recently a significant increase has been noted in "immune complex–like" reactions in people receiving booster doses of *Imovax*. The illness, characterized by onset 2 to 21 days postbooster, presents with a generalized urticaria and may also include angioedema, arthralgia, arthritis, fever, malaise, nausea, and vomiting. In no cases were the illnesses life-threatening. Preliminary data suggest this "immune complex–like" illness may occur in up to 6% of people receiving booster vaccines and much less frequently in people receiving primary immunization. Additional experience with this vaccine is needed to define more clearly the risk of these adverse reactions.

CNS disorder: Two cases of neurologic illness resembling Guillain-Barré syndrome, a transient neuroparalytic illness, that resolved without sequelae in 12 weeks and a focal subacute CNS disorder temporally associated with *Imovax* have been reported.

Immediately report all serious systemic, neuroparalytic, or anaphylactic reactions to a rabies vaccine to the state health department or Aventis Pasteur at 1-800-822-2463.

➤*RabAvert*:

Serious adverse reactions – Anaphylaxis; encephalitis, including death; meningitis; neuroparalytic reactions, such as encephalitis, transient paralysis, Guillain-Barré Syndrome, myelitis, and retrobulbar neuritis; and multiple sclerosis have been reported to be temporally associated with the use of rabies vaccine. However, carefully consider a patient's risk of developing rabies before deciding to discontinue immunization.

Injection route – *RabAvert* must not be used subcutaneously or intradermally. *RabAvert* must be injected IM. For adults, the deltoid area is the preferred site of immunization; for small children and infants, administration into the anterolateral zone of the thigh is preferred. Avoid the use of the gluteal region, because administration in this area may result in lower neutralizing antibody titers.

Do not inject intravascularly. Unintentional intravascular injection may result in systemic reactions, including shock. Immediate measures include catecholamines, volume replacement, high doses of corticosteroids, and oxygen. Development of active immunity after vaccination may be impaired in immune-compromised individuals.

Transmission of viral diseases – This product contains albumin, a derivative of human blood. It is present in *RabAvert* at concentrations of less than 0.3 mg/dose. Based on effective donor screening and product manufacturing processes, it carries an extremely remote risk of transmission of viral diseases. A theoretical risk for transmission of Creutzfeld-Jakob disease (CJD) also is considered extremely remote. No cases of transmission of viral diseases or CJD have ever been identified for albumin.

General – Take care for the safe and effective use of the product. Question the patient, parent, or guardian about the following: the current health status of the vaccinee and reactions to a previous dose of rabies vaccine or a similar product. Postpone preexposure vaccination in the case of sick and convalescent persons and in those considered to be in the incubation stage of an infectious disease. Use a separate sterile syringe and needle or a sterile disposable unit for each patient to prevent transmission of hepatitis and other infectious agents from person to person. Do not recap needles; dispose of them properly. As with any rabies vaccine, vaccination with rabies vaccine may not protect 100% of susceptible individuals.

➤*Hypersensitivity reactions:* When a person with a history of hypersensitivity must be given rabies vaccine, antihistamines may be given. Epi-

RABIES VACCINE — INJECTION

nephrine (1:1,000) should be readily available to counteract anaphylactic reactions; observe the person carefully after immunization.

Imovax – While the concentration of antibiotics in each dose of vaccine is extremely small, people with known hypersensitivity to any of these agents could manifest an allergic reaction. While the risk is small, it should be weighed in light of the potential risk of contracting rabies.

RabAvert – At present, there is no evidence that people are at increased risk if they have egg hypersensitivities that are not anaphylactic or anaphylactoid in nature. Although there is no safety data regarding the use of *RabAvert* in patients with egg allergies, experience with other vaccines derived from primary cultures of chick embryo fibroblasts demonstrates that documented egg hypersensitivity does not necessarily predict an increased likelihood of adverse reactions. There is no evidence to indicate that people with allergies to chickens or feathers are at increased risk of reaction to vaccines produced in primary cultures of chick embryo fibroblasts.

Reconstituted *RabAvert* contains processed bovine gelatin and trace amounts of chicken protein, neomycin, chlortetracycline, and amphotericin B; when administering the vaccine, consider the possibility of allergic reactions in individuals hypersensitive to these substances.

➤*Pregnancy: Category C.* Animal reproduction studies have not been conducted with *Imovax* or *RabAvert*. It is also not known whether either product can cause fetal harm when administered to a pregnant woman or can affect reproductive capacity. Give the rabies vaccine to a pregnant woman only if clearly needed. The ACIP has issued recommendations for use of rabies vaccine in pregnant women.

Because of the potential consequences of inadequately treated rabies exposure and limited data that indicate that fetal abnormalities have not been associated with rabies vaccination, pregnancy is not considered a contraindication to postexposure prophylaxis. If there is substantial risk of exposure to rabies, preexposure prophylaxis may also be indicated during pregnancy.

➤*Lactation:* It is not known whether rabies vaccines are excreted in animal or human milk, but many drugs are excreted in human milk. Although there are no data, because of the potential consequences of inadequately treated rabies exposure, breast-feeding is not considered a contraindication to postexposure prophylaxis. If the risk of exposure to rabies is substantial, preexposure vaccination might also be indicated during breast-feeding.

➤*Children:* Safety and efficacy of *Imovax* and *RabAvert* in children have been established. Children and infants receive the same dose as adults, 1 mL given IM. Only limited data on the safety and efficacy of rabies vaccine in the pediatric age group are available. However, in 3 studies, some preexposure and postexposure experience has been gained.

Drug Interactions

Rabies Vaccine Drug Interactions

Precipitant drug	Object drug[a]		Description
Immunosuppressants	Rabies vaccine	⬇	Like all inactivated vaccines, administration of rabies vaccine to people receiving immunosuppressants, including high-dose corticosteroids, or radiation therapy, may result in an insufficient response to immunization. They may remain susceptible despite immunization. Do not give immunosuppressives during postexposure therapy unless essential. It may be helpful to test steroid-treated patients for development of antirabies antibodies.
RIG	Rabies vaccine	⬇	Simultaneous administration may slightly delay the antibody response to rabies vaccine. Because of this possibility, follow CDC recommendations exactly and give no more than the recommended dose of RIG.

[a] ⬇ = object drug decreased.

Adverse Reactions

➤*Imovax:* Once initiated, do not interrupt or discontinue rabies prophylaxis because of local or mild systemic adverse reactions to rabies vaccine. Usually such reactions can be managed successfully with anti-inflammatory and antipyretic agents (eg, aspirin).

Reactions after vaccination with *Imovax* are less common than with previously available vaccines. In a study using 5 doses of *Imovax*, local reactions, such as pain, erythema, and swelling or itching at the injection site, were reported in approximately 25% of recipients of *Imovax*, and mild systemic reactions, such as headache, nausea, abdominal pain, muscle aches, and dizziness, were reported in approximately 20% of recipients.

Serious systemic, anaphylactic, or neuroparalytic reactions occurring during the administration of *Imovax* pose a dilemma for the attending health care provider. Carefully consider a patient's risk of developing rabies before deciding to discontinue vaccination. Moreover, the use of corticosteroids to treat life-threatening neuroparalytic reactions carries the risk of inhibiting the development of active immunity to rabies. It is especially important in these cases that the serum of the patient be tested for rabies antibodies. Advice and assistance on the management of serious adverse reactions in people receiving rabies vaccines may be sought from the state health department.

➤*RabAvert*: In very rare cases, neurological and neuroparalytical reactions have been reported in temporal association with administration of *RabAvert*. These include cases of hypersensitivity.

The most commonly occurring adverse reactions are injection site reactions, such as injection site erythema, induration, and pain; flu-like symptoms, such as asthenia, fatigue, fever, headache, myalgia, and malaise; arthralgia; dizziness; lymphadenopathy; nausea; and rash. Carefully consider a patient's risk of acquiring rabies before deciding to discontinue vaccination. Advice and assistance on the management of serious adverse reactions for people receiving rabies vaccines may be sought from the state health department or CDC.

Local reactions, such as induration, swelling, and reddening, have been reported more often than systemic reactions. In a comparative trial in normal volunteers, study 1 described an experience with *RabAvert* compared with *Imovax*.

Rabies Vaccine Adverse Reactions

	Study 1		US study	
Adverse reaction	*Imovax* (n = 20)	*RabAvert* (n = 19)	*Imovax* (n = 82)	*RabAvert* (n = 83)
CNS				
Dizziness	10%	15%	—	—
Headache	20%	10%	45%	52%
Malaise	25%	15%	17%	20%
Local				
Injection site pain	45%	34%	80%	84%
Localized lymphadenopathy	15%	15%	—	—
Miscellaneous				
Myalgia	—	—	38%	53%

None of the adverse reactions were serious; almost all adverse reactions were of mild or moderate intensity. Statistically significant differences between vaccination groups were not found. Both vaccines were generally well tolerated.

Uncommonly observed adverse reactions include temperatures higher than 38°C (100°F), swollen lymph nodes, pain in limbs, and GI complaints. In rare cases, patients have experienced severe headache, fatigue, circulatory reactions, sweating, chills, monoarthritis, and allergic reactions; transient paresthesias and 1 case of suspected urticaria pigmentosa have also been reported.

Postmarketing – The following adverse reactions have been identified during postapproval use of *RabAvert*. Because these reactions are reported voluntarily from a population of uncertain size, estimates of frequency cannot be made. These reactions have been chosen for inclusion because of their seriousness, frequency of reporting, causal connection to rabies vaccine, or a combination of these factors.

Cardiovascular: Hot flush, palpitations.

CNS: Encephalitis, Guillain-Barré syndrome, meningitis, multiple sclerosis, myelitis, neuroparalysis, retrobulbar neuritis, transient paralysis, vertigo, visual disturbance.

Hypersensitivity: Anaphylaxis, bronchospasm, edema, pruritus, type III hypersensitivity-like reactions, urticaria.

Local: Extensive limb swelling. The use of corticosteroids to treat life-threatening neuroparalytic reactions may inhibit the development of immunity to rabies. Once initiated, do not interrupt or discontinue rabies prophylaxis because of local or mild systemic adverse reactions to rabies vaccine. Usually, such reactions can be managed successfully with anti-inflammatory and antipyretic agents.

Reporting adverse reactions – The patient or health care provider should report adverse reactions to the US Department of Health and Human Services Vaccine Adverse Event Reporting System (VAERS). Report forms and information about reporting requirements or completion of the form can be obtained from VAERS by calling the toll-free number 1-800-822-7967.

DIPHTHERIA TOXOID/TETANUS TOXOID/ACELLULAR PERTUSSIS, ADSORBED/INACTIVATED POLIOVIRUS COMBINATION VACCINE (DTaP/IPV)

Rx	**Kinrix** (GlaxoSmithKline)	**Injection, suspension**: diphtheria toxoid 25 Lf, tetanus toxoid 10 Lf, inactivated pertussis toxin (PT) 25 mcg, filamentous hemaglutinin (FHA) 25 mcg, pertactin 8 mcg, type 1 poliovirus (Mahoney) 40 D-antigen units (DU), type 2 poliovirus (MEF-1) 8 DU, type 3 poliovirus (Saukett) 32 DU per 0.5 mL[a]	Preservative free. In 0.5 mL single-dose vials and prefilled *Tip-Lok* syringes.[b]

[a] Each 0.5 mL dose contains sodium chloride 4.5 mg, alumin adjuvant (≤ 0.6 mg aluminum by assay), residual formaldehyde ≤ 100 mcg, polysorbate 80 (*Tween 80*) ≤ 100 mcg, neomycin ≤ 0.05 ng, and polymyxin B ≤ 0.01 ng per dose.

[b] The tip cap and the rubber plunger of the needleless, prefilled syringes contain dry natural latex rubber that may cause allergic reactions in latex sensitive individuals. The vial stopper is latex free.

DIPHTHERIA TOXOID/TETANUS TOXOID/ACELLULAR PERTUSSIS, ADSORBED/INACTIVATED POLIOVIRUS COMBINATION VACCINE — INJECTION

Indications

➤*Immunization:* For active immunization against diphtheria, tetanus, pertussis, and poliomyelitis as the fifth dose in the diphtheria, tetanus, and acellular pertussis (DTaP) vaccine series and the fourth dose in the inactivated poliovirus vaccine (IPV) series in children 4 through 6 years of age whose previous DTaP vaccine doses have been with *Infanrix* (diphtheria and tetanus toxoids and acellular pertussis vaccine adsorbed) and/or *Pediarix* (diphtheria and tetanus toxoids and acellular pertussis adsorbed, hepatitis B, recombinant, and inactivated poliovirus vaccine combined) for the first 3 doses and *Infanrix* for the fourth dose.

Administration and Dosage

➤*Children:*

Immunization –

4 through 6 years of age (prior to the seventh birthday): 0.5 mL IM as the fifth dose in the DTaP immunization series and the fourth dose in the IPV immunization series in children whose previous DTaP vaccine doses have been with *Infanrix* and/or *Pediarix* for the first 3 doses and *Infanrix* for the fourth dose.

➤*Concomitant therapy:* When DTaP/IPV is coadministered with other injectable vaccines, they should be given with separate syringes.

➤*Preparation for administration:* Shake vigorously to obtain a homogenous, turbid, white suspension. Do not use if resuspension does not occur with vigorous shaking. After removal of the dose, any vaccine remaining in the vial should be discarded.

➤*Administration:* Administer by IM injection. Do not administer this product intravenously, intradermally, or subcutaneously.

The preferred site of administration is the deltoid muscle of the upper arm.

➤*Admixture compatibility:* DTaP/IPV should not be mixed with any other vaccine in the same syringe or vial.

➤*Storage/Stability:* Store refrigerated between 2° and 8°C (36° and 46°F). Do not freeze. Discard if the vaccine has been frozen.

Actions

➤*Pharmacology:*

Diphtheria – Diphtheria is an acute toxin-mediated infectious disease caused by toxigenic strains of *Corynebacterium diphtheriae*. Protection against disease is because of the development of neutralizing antibodies to the diphtheria toxin. A serum diphtheria antitoxin level of 0.01 units/mL is the lowest level giving some degree of protection; a level of 0.1 units/mL is regarded as protective.

Tetanus – Tetanus is an acute toxin-mediated disease caused by a potent exotoxin released by *C. tetani*. Protection against disease is because of the development of neutralizing antibodies to the tetanus toxin. A serum tetanus antitoxin level of at least 0.01 units/mL, measured by neutralization assays, is considered the minimum protective level. A level of at least 0.1 units/mL is considered protective.

Pertussis – Pertussis (whooping cough) is a disease of the respiratory tract caused by *B. pertussis*. The role of the different components produced by *B. pertussis* in either the pathogenesis of, or the immunity to, pertussis is not well understood. There is no well-established serological correlate of protection for pertussis. The efficacy of the pertussis component of DTaP/IPV was determined in clinical trials of *Infanrix* administered as a 3-dose series in infants (see the *Infanrix* monograph).

Poliomyelitis – Poliovirus is an enterovirus that belongs to the Picornavirus family. Three serotypes of poliovirus have been identified (types 1, 2, and 3). Neutralizing antibodies against the 3 poliovirus serotypes are recognized as conferring protection against poliomyelitis disease.

Contraindications

Severe allergic reaction (eg, anaphylaxis) after a previous dose of any diphtheria toxoid, tetanus toxoid, pertussis- or poliovirus-containing vaccine, or to any component of DTaP/IPV, including neomycin and polymyxin B; encephalopathy (eg, coma, decreased level of consciousness, prolonged seizures) within 7 days of administration of a previous dose of a pertussis-containing vaccine that is not attributable to another identifiable cause; progressive neurologic disorder, including infantile spasms, uncontrolled epilepsy, or progressive encephalopathy.

Warnings/Precautions

➤*Guillain-Barré syndrome:* If Guillain-Barré syndrome occurs within 6 weeks of receipt of a prior vaccine containing tetanus toxoid, base the decision to give any tetanus toxoid-containing vaccine, including DTaP/IPV, on careful consideration of the potential benefits and possible risks. When a decision is made to withhold tetanus toxoid, give other available vaccines as indicated.

➤*Latex sensitivity:* The tip cap and the rubber plunger of the needleless, prefilled syringes contain dry natural latex rubber that may cause allergic reactions in latex-sensitive individuals. The vial stopper is latex-free.

➤*Postvaccination effects:* If any of the following reactions occur in temporal relation to receipt of a pertussis-containing vaccine, base the decision to give any pertussis-containing vaccine, including DTaP/IPV, on careful consideration of the potential benefits and possible risks:

1.) temperature of 40.5°C (105°F) or higher within 48 hours not due to another identifiable cause;
2.) collapse or shock-like state (hypotonic-hyporesponsive episode) within 48 hours;
3.) persistent, inconsolable crying lasting at least 3 hours, occurring within 48 hours;
4.) seizures with or without fever occurring within 3 days.

When a decision is made to withhold pertussis vaccination, give other available vaccines as indicated.

➤*Seizure:* For children at higher risk for seizures than the general population, an appropriate antipyretic may be administered at the time of vaccination with a pertussis-containing vaccine, including DTaP/IPV, and for the ensuing 24 hours to reduce the possibility of postvaccination fever.

➤*Patient history:* Prior to administration, review the patient's immunization history for possible vaccine sensitivity and previous vaccination-related adverse reactions to allow an assessment of benefits and risks. Epinephrine and other appropriate agents used for the control of immediate allergic reactions must be immediately available should an acute anaphylactic reaction occur.

➤*Pregnancy: Category C.* Animal reproduction studies have not been conducted with DTaP/IPV. It also is not known whether DTaP/IPV can cause fetal harm when administered to a pregnant woman or can affect reproduction capacity.

➤*Children:* Safety and effectiveness of DTaP/IPV in children younger than 4 years of age and children 7 to 16 years of age have not been evaluated. DTaP/IPV is not approved for use in persons in these age groups.

Drug Interactions

➤*Vaccine coadministration:* In clinical trials, DTaP/IPV was coadministered with the second dose of measles, mumps, and rubella (MMR) vaccine.

Data are not available on concomitant use of DTaP/IPV and varicella vaccine.

➤*Immunosuppressive therapies:* Immunosuppressive therapies, including irradiation, antimetabolites, alkylating agents, cytotoxic drugs, and corticosteroids (used in greater than physiologic doses), may reduce the immune response to DTaP/IPV.

Adverse Reactions

DTaP/IPV Adverse Reactions (Children 4 to 6 Years of Age) Within 4 Days of Vaccination or Separate Coadministration of *Infanrix* and IPV When Coadministered With MMR Vaccine[a,b]

	DTaP/IPV	*Infanrix* + IPV
Local[c]	*(N = 3,121 to 3,128)*	*(N = 1,039 to 1,043)*
Pain, any	57%[d]	53.3%
Pain, grade 2 or 3[e]	13.7%	12%
Pain, grade 3[e]	1.6%[d]	0.6%
Redness, any	36.6%	36.6%
Redness, ≥ 50 mm	17.6%	20%
Redness, ≥ 110 mm	2.9%	4.1%
Arm circumference increase, any	36%	37.8%
Arm circumference increase, > 20 mm	6.9%	7.4%
Arm circumference increase, > 30 mm	2.4%	3.2%
Swelling, any	26%	27%
Swelling, ≥ 50 mm	10.2%	11.5%
Swelling, ≥ 110 mm	1.4%	1.8%

DIPHTHERIA TOXOID/TETANUS TOXOID/ ACELLULAR PERTUSSIS, ADSORBED/INACTIVATED POLIOVIRUS COMBINATION VACCINE — INJECTION

DTaP/IPV Adverse Reactions (Children 4 to 6 Years of Age) Within 4 Days of Vaccination or Separate Coadministration of *Infanrix* and IPV When Coadministered With MMR Vaccine[a,b]

	DTaP/IPV	*Infanrix* + IPV
Miscellaneous	*(N = 3,037 to 3,120)*	*(N = 993 to 1,036)*
Drowsiness, any	19.1%	17.5%
Drowsiness, grade 3[f]	0.8%	0.8%
Fever, ≥ 99.5°F	16%	14.8%
Fever, > 100.4°F	6.5%[d]	4.4%
Fever, > 102.2°F	1.1%	1.1%
Fever, > 104°F	0.1%	0%
Loss of appetite, any	15.5%	16%
Loss of appetite, grade 3[g]	0.8%	0.6%

[a] Total vaccinated cohort = all vaccinated subjects for whom safety data were available; N = number of children with evaluable data for the reactions listed.
[b] Within 4 days of vaccination defined as day of vaccination and the next 3 days.
[c] Local reactions at the injection site for DTaP/IPV or *Infanrix*.
[d] Statistically higher than comparator group ($P < 0.05$).
[e] Grade 2 defined as painful when the limb was moved; grade 3 defined as preventing normal daily activities.
[f] Grade 3 defined as preventing normal daily activities.
[g] Grade 3 defined as not eating at all.

In study 048, DTaP/IPV was noninferior to *Infanrix* with regard to swelling that involved more than 50% of the injected upper arm length and that was associated with a more than 30 mm increase in mid-upper arm circumference within 4 days following vaccination (upper limit of 2-sided 95% CI for difference in percentage of DTaP/IPV [0.6%, n = 20] minus *Infanrix* [1%, n = 11] 2% or less).

➤*Serious adverse reactions:* Within the 31-day period following study vaccination in 3 studies (study 046, 047, and 048), in which all subjects received concomitant MMR vaccine (US-licensed MMR vaccine [Merck] in study 047 and 048; non-US licensed MMR vaccine in study 046), 3 subjects (0.1% [3/3,537]) who received DTaP/IPV reported serious adverse reactions (dehydration and hypernatremia, cerebrovascular accident, dehydration, gastroenteritis) and 4 subjects (0.3% [4/1,434]) who received *Infanrix* and IPV (Sanofi Pasteur SA) reported serious adverse reactions (cellulitis, constipation, foreign body trauma, fever without identified etiology).

➤*Postmarketing:*

Dermatologic – Injection site vesicles; pruritus.

Additional adverse reactions reported following postmarketing use of *Infanrix*, for which a causal relationship to vaccination is plausible, are allergic reactions (including anaphylactoid reactions, anaphylaxis, angioedema, and urticaria), apnea, collapse or shock-like state (hypotonic-hyporesponsive episode), convulsions (with or without fever), lymphadenopathy, and thrombocytopenia.

Patient Information

Inform parents or guardians of the potential benefits and risks of immunization with DTaP/IPV.

Inform parents or guardians about the potential for adverse reactions that have been temporally associated with administration of DTaP/IPV or other vaccines containing similar components.

Instruct the parent or guardian accompanying the recipient to report any adverse reactions to their health care provider where the vaccine was administered.

Give the parent or guardian the Vaccine Information Statements, which are required by the National Childhood Vaccine Injury Act of 1986 to be given prior to immunization. These materials are available free of charge at the Centers for Disease Control and Prevention (CDC) website (http://www.cdc.gov/nip).

The US Department of Health and Human Services has established a Vaccine Adverse Event Reporting System (VAERS) to accept all reports of suspected adverse reactions after the administration of any vaccine, including, but not limited to, the reporting of reactions required by the National Childhood Vaccine Injury Act of 1986. The VAERS toll-free number is 1-800-822-7967. Reporting forms may be obtained at the VAERS Web site at http://www.vaers.org.

DIPHTHERIA AND TETANUS TOXOIDS/ACELLULAR PERTUSSIS ADSORBED/INACTIVATED POLIOVIRUS/ HAEMOPHILUS INFLUENZAE TYPE B CONJUGATE VACCINE COMBINED

Rx	**Pentacel** (Sanofi Pasteur)	**Injection, suspension:** diphtheria toxoid 15 Lf, tetanus toxoid 5 Lf, pertussis toxin detoxified 20 mcg, filamentous hemagglutinin 20 mcg, pertactin 3 mcg, fimbriae types 2 and 3 five mcg, 40 D-antigen units type 1 inactivated poliovirus (Mahoney), 8 D-antigen units type 2 inactivated poliovirus (MEF-1), 32 D-antigen units type 3 inactivated poliovirus (Saukett), and lyophilized polyribosyl-ribilol-phosphate of *Haemophilus influenzae* type B 10 mcg bound to tetanus toxoid 24 mcg per 0.5 mL[a]	Formaldehyde, phenoxyethanol. In single-dose vials for reconstitution. Preservative free.

[a] Each 0.5 mL dose also contains 1.5 mg aluminum phosphate (0.33 mg aluminum), 5 mcg or less residual formaldehyde, less than 50 ng residual glutaraldehyde, 50 ng or less residual bovine serum albumin, 3.3 mg (0.6% v/v) 2-phenoxyethanol, less than 4 pg neomycin, less than 4 pg polymyxin B sulfate.

DIPHTHERIA AND TETANUS TOXOIDS/ACELLULAR PERTUSSIS ADSORBED/INACTIVATED POLIOVIRUS/ HAEMOPHILUS INFLUENZAE TYPE B CONJUGATE VACCINE COMBINED — INJECTION

For complete prescribing information, refer to the Haemophilus b Conjugate Vaccine; Diphtheria and Tetanus Toxoids and Acellular Pertussis Vaccine, Adsorbed; and Poliovirus Vaccine, Inactivated monographs. For additional information, refer to the Agents for Active Immunization introduction.

Indications

➤*Immunization:* For active immunization against diphtheria, tetanus, pertussis, poliomyelitis, and invasive disease caused by *Haemophilus influenzae* type b (Hib) in children between 6 weeks and 4 years of age (prior to fifth birthday).

Administration and Dosage

➤*General dosing considerations:* Four doses of *Pentacel* constitute a primary immunization against pertussis. Three doses constitute a primary immunization course against diphtheria, tetanus, *H. influenzae* type b invasive disease, and poliomyelitis; the fourth dose is a booster for diphtheria, tetanus, *H. influenzae* type b invasive disease, and poliomyelitis immunizations.

Pentacel may be used to complete the first 4 doses of the 5-dose diphtheria and tetanus toxoids and acellular pertussis adsorbed (DTaP) series in infants and children who have received 1 or more doses of *Daptacel* and are also scheduled to receive the other antigens of *Pentacel*.

Pentacel may be used to complete the vaccination series in infants and children previously vaccinated with 1 or more doses of *Haemophilus* b conjugate vaccine (separately administered or as part of another combination vaccine), who are also scheduled to receive the other antigens of *Pentacel*. If different brands of *Haemophilus* b conjugate vaccine are administered to complete the series, 3 primary immunizing doses are needed, followed by a booster dose.

Pentacel may be used in infants and children who have received 1 or more doses of another licensed inactivated poliovirus (IPV) vaccine and are scheduled to receive the antigens of *Pentacel*.

➤*Children:*

Immunization –

6 weeks through 4 years of age (prior to fifth birthday):

• *Usual dosage* – 0.5 mL IM at 2, 4, 6, and 15 to 18 months of age. The first dose may be given as early as 6 weeks of age.

• *Booster dose* – Children who have completed a 4-dose series with *Pentacel* should receive a fifth dose of DTaP vaccine using *Daptacel* at 4 to 6 years of age.

When *Pentacel* is administered at ages 2, 4, 6, and 15 to 18 months, an additional booster dose of IPV vaccine should be administered at 4 to 6 years of age.

➤*Concomitant therapy:* In clinical trials, *Pentacel* was routinely coadministered, at separate sites, with 1 or more of the following vaccines: hepatitis B, 7-valent pneumococcal conjugate, measles/mumps/rubella, and varicella. When *Pentacel* is given at the same time as another injectable vaccine, the vaccines should be given with different syringes.

➤*Preparation for administration:* Thoroughly but gently shake the vial of DTaP-IPV component, withdraw the entire liquid content, and inject into the vial of the lyophilized *Haemophilus* b conjugate vaccine (tetanus toxoid conjugate) component. Shake the vial now containing *Pentacel* thoroughly until a cloudy, uniform, white to off-white (yellow tinge) suspension results. *Pentacel* should be used immediately after reconstitution.

➤*Administration:* Administer IM. Do not administer this product intravenously or subcutaneously. In infants younger than 1 year of age, the anterolateral aspect of the thigh provides the largest muscle and is the preferred site of injection. In older children, the deltoid muscle is usually large enough for injection. The vaccine should not be injected into the gluteal area or into areas where there may be a major nerve trunk.

➤*Admixture compatibility: Pentacel* should not be mixed in the same syringe with other parenteral products.

➤*Storage/Stability:* Store between 2° and 8°C (35° and 46°F). Do not freeze. Discard the product if exposed to freezing.

Actions

➤*Pharmacology: Pentacel* for IM use is a vaccine for protection against diphtheria, tetanus, pertussis, poliovirus, and invasive disease caused by Hib.

Diphtheria – Diphtheria is an acute toxin-mediated disease caused by toxigenic strains of *Corynebacterium diphtheriae*. Protection against disease is due to the development of neutralizing antibodies to diphtheria toxin. A serum diphtheria antitoxin level of 0.01 unit/mL is the lowest level giving

DIPHTHERIA AND TETANUS TOXOIDS/ACELLULAR PERTUSSIS ADSORBED/INACTIVATED POLIOVIRUS/HAEMOPHILUS INFLUENZAE TYPE B CONJUGATE VACCINE COMBINED — INJECTION

some degree of protection. Antitoxin levels of at least 0.1 unit/mL are generally regarded as protective. Levels of 1 unit/mL have been associated with long-term protection.

Tetanus – Tetanus is an acute disease caused by an extremely potent neurotoxin produced by *Clostridium tetani*. Protection against disease is due to the development of neutralizing antibodies to tetanus toxin. A serum tetanus antitoxin level of at least 0.01 unit/mL, measured by neutralization assay, is considered the minimum protective level. A tetanus antitoxoid level of 0.1 unit/mL or greater as measured by the enzyme-linked immunosorbent assay (ELISA) used in clinical studies of *Pentacel* is considered protective.

Pertussis – Pertussis (whooping cough) is a respiratory disease caused by *Bordetella pertussis*. This gram-negative coccobacillus produces a variety of biologically active components, although their role in either the pathogenesis of or immunity to pertussis has not been clearly defined.

Poliomyelitis – Polioviruses, of which there are 3 serotypes (1, 2, and 3) are enteroviruses. The presence of poliovirus type–specific neutralizing antibodies has been correlated with protection against poliomyelitis.

Invasive disease caused by Hib – Hib can cause invasive disease, such as meningitis and sepsis. Anti–polyribosyl-ribitol-phosphate (PRP) antibody has been shown to correlate with protection against invasive disease caused by Hib. Based on data from passive antibody studies and an efficacy study with Hib polysaccharide vaccine in Finland, a postvaccination anti-PRP level of 0.15 mcg/mL has been accepted as a minimal protective level. Data from an efficacy study with Hib polysaccharide vaccine in Finland indicate that a level of more than 1 mcg/mL 3 weeks after vaccination predicts protection through a subsequent 1-year period. These levels have been used to evaluate the effectiveness of *Haemophilus* b conjugate vaccines, including the *ActHIB* vaccine component of *Pentacel*.

Contraindications

A severe allergic reaction (eg, anaphylaxis) after a previous dose of *Pentacel*, any ingredient of this vaccine, or any other tetanus toxoid, diphtheria toxoid, pertussis-containing vaccine, inactivated poliovirus vaccine, or Hib vaccine; encephalopathy (eg, coma, decreased level of consciousness, prolonged seizures) within 7 days of a previous dose of a pertussis containing vaccine that is not attributable to another identifiable cause; progressive neurologic disorder, including infantile spasms, uncontrolled epilepsy, progressive encephalopathy. Do not administer pertussis vaccine to individuals with such conditions until the neurologic status is clarified and stabilized.

Warnings/Precautions

➤*Postvaccination effects:* If any of the following reactions occur within the specified period after administration of a whole-cell pertussis or acellular pertussis-containing vaccine, base the decision to administer *Pentacel* or any pertussis-containing vaccine on careful consideration of potential benefits and possible risks.

- Temperature of 40.5°C (105°F) or higher within 48 hours, not attributable to another identifiable cause.
- Collapse or shock-like state (hypotonic-hyporesponsive episode) within 48 hours.
- Persistent, inconsolable crying lasting 3 hours or more within 48 hours.
- Seizure with or without fever within 3 days.

➤*Guillain-Barré syndrome:* A review by the Institute of Medicine found evidence for a causal relation between tetanus toxoid and brachial neuritis, Guillain-Barré syndrome, and anaphylaxis. If Guillain-Barré syndrome occurred within 6 weeks of receipt of a prior vaccine containing tetanus toxoid, base the decision to give *Pentacel* or any vaccine containing tetanus toxoid on careful consideration of the potential benefits and possible risks.

➤*Protection:* Vaccination with *Pentacel* may not protect all individuals.

➤*Patient history:* Before administration of *Pentacel*, review the patient's current health status and medical history in order to determine whether any contraindications exist and to assess the benefits and risks of vaccination.

➤*Seizure:* For infants or children at higher risk for seizures than the general population, an appropriate antipyretic may be administered (in the dosage recommended in its prescribing information) at the time of vaccination with an acellular pertussis-containing vaccine (including *Pentacel*) and for the following 24 hours to reduce the possibility of postvaccination fever.

➤*Immunodeficiency:* If *Pentacel* is administered to immunocompromised persons, including persons receiving immunosuppressive therapy, the expected immune response may not be obtained.

➤*Hypersensitivity reactions:* Ensure that epinephrine solution (1:1,000) and other appropriate agents and equipment are available for immediate use in case an anaphylactic or acute hypersensitivity reaction occurs.

➤*Pregnancy: Category C.* Animal reproduction studies have not been conducted with *Pentacel*. It is not known whether *Pentacel* can cause fetal harm when administered to a pregnant woman or affect reproduction capacity. *Pentacel* is not approved for use in women of childbearing age.

➤*Lactation: Pentacel* is not approved for use in women of childbearing age.

➤*Children:* The safety and effectiveness of *Pentacel* was established in children between 6 weeks and 18 months of age on the basis of clinical studies. The safety and effectiveness of *Pentacel* in the children between 19 months and 4 years of age is supported by evidence in children 6 weeks through 18 months of age. The safety and effectiveness of *Pentacel* in infants younger than 6 weeks of age and in children 5 to 16 years of age have not been established. *Pentacel* is not approved for use in persons 5 years of age and older.

Drug Interactions

➤*Immunosuppressants:* Immunosuppressive therapies, including irradiation, antimetabolites, alkylating agents, cytotoxic drugs, and corticosteroids (used in greater than physiologic doses), may reduce the immune response to *Pentacel*.

➤*Other vaccines:* See Dosage and Administration for more information.

➤*Drug/Lab test interactions:* Antigenuria has been detected in some instances following receipt of *ActHIB*. Urine antigen detection may not have definite diagnostic value in suspected Hib disease within 1 week following receipt of *Pentacel*.

Adverse Reactions

➤*Solicited adverse reactions:*

Pentacel Adverse Reactions								
	Pentacel				*Daptacel*			
	Dose 1	Dose 2	Dose 3	Dose 4	Dose 1	Dose 2	Dose 3	Dose 4
Injection-site reactions								
Redness								
> 5 mm	7.1%	8.4%	8.7%	17.3%	6.2%	7.1%	9.6%	16.4%
> 25 mm	2.8%	1.8%	1.8%	9.2%	1%	0.6%	1.9%	7.9%
> 50 mm	0.6%	0.2%	0%	2.3%	0.4%	0.1%	0%	2.4%
Swelling								
> 5 mm	7.5%	7.3%	5%	9.7%	4%	4%	6.5%	10.3%
> 25 mm	3%	2%	1.6%	3.8%	1.6%	0.7%	1.1%	4%
> 50 mm	0.9%	0%	0%	0.8%	0.4%	0.1%	0.1%	1.3%
Tenderness[a]								
Any	47.5%	39.2%	42.7%	56.1%	48.8%	38.2%	40.9%	51.1%
Moderate or severe	19.6%	10.6%	11.6%	16.7%	20.7%	12.2%	12.3%	15.8%
Severe	5.4%	1.6%	1.4%	3.3%	4.1%	2.3%	1.7%	2.4%
Increase in arm circumference								
> 5 mm				36.6%				30.6%
> 20 mm				4.7%				6.9%
> 40 mm				0.5%				0.8%
	Pentacel				*Daptacel*			*Daptacel + ActHIB*
	Dose 1	Dose 2	Dose 3	Dose 4	Dose 1	Dose 2	Dose 3	Dose 4
Systemic reactions								
Fever[b,c]								
≥ 38°C	5.8%	10.9%	16.3%	13.4%	9.3%	16.1%	15.8%	8.7%
> 38.5°C	1.3%	2.4%	4.4%	5.1%	1.6%	4.3%	5.1%	3.2%
> 39.5°C	0.4%	0%	0.7%	0.3%	0.1%	0.4%	0.3%	0.8%
Decreased activity/lethargy[d]								
Any	45.8%	32.7%	32.5%	24.1%	51.1%	37.4%	33.2%	24.1%
Moderate or severe	22.9%	12.4%	12.7%	9.8%	24.3%	15.8%	12.7%	9.2%
Severe	2.1%	0.7%	0.2%	2.5%	1.2%	1.4%	0.6%	0.3%
Inconsolable crying								
Any	59.3%	49.8%	47.3%	35.9%	58.5%	51.4%	47.9%	36.2%
≥ 1 hour	19.7%	10.6%	13.6%	11.8%	16.4%	16%	12.2%	10.5%
> 3 hours	1.9%	0.9%	1.1%	2.3%	2.2%	3.4%	1.4%	1.8%
Fussiness/Irritability								
Any	76.9%	71.2%	68%	53.5%	75.8%	70.7%	67.1%	53.8%
≥ 1 hour	34.5%	27%	26.4%	23.6%	33.3%	30.5%	26.2%	19.4%
> 3 hours	4.3%	4%	5%	5.3%	5.6%	5.5%	4.3%	4.5%

[a] Any: mild, moderate, or severe; mild: subject whimpers when site is touched; moderate: subject cries when site is touched; severe: subject cries when leg or arm is moved.

[b] Fever is based upon actual temperatures recorded with no adjustments to the measurement route.

[c] Following doses 1 to 3 combined, the proportion of temperature measurements that were taken by axillary, rectal, or other routes, or not recorded were 46%, 53%, 1%, and 0%, respectively, for *Pentacel* and 44.8%, 54%, 1%, and 0.1%, respectively, for *Daptacel + IPOL + ActHIB*. Following dose 4, the proportion of temperature measurements that were taken by axillary, rectal, or other routes, or not recorded were 62.7%, 34.4%, 2.4% and 0.5%, respectively, for *Pentacel*, and 61.1%, 36.6%, 1.7% and 0.5%, respectively, for *Daptacel + ActHIB*.

[d] Moderate: interferes with or limits usual daily activity; severe: disabling, not interested in usual daily activity.

DIPHTHERIA AND TETANUS TOXOIDS/ACELLULAR PERTUSSIS ADSORBED/INACTIVATED POLIOVIRUS/ HAEMOPHILUS INFLUENZAE TYPE B CONJUGATE VACCINE COMBINED — INJECTION

➤*Hypotonic hyporesponsive episodes:* In study P3T06, the diary cards included questions pertaining to hypotonic hyporesponsive episodes. In studies 494-01, 494-03, and 5A9908, a question about the occurrence of fainting or change in mental status was asked during postvaccination phone calls. Across these 4 studies, no hypotonic hyporesponsive episodes, as defined in a report of a US Public Health Service workshop, were reported among participants who received *Pentacel* (n = 5,979), separately administered HCPDT + *POLIOVAX* + *ActHIB* (n = 1,032), or separately administered *Daptacel* + *IPOL* + *ActHIB* (n = 1,455). Hypotonia not fulfilling hypotonic hyporesponsive episode criteria within 7 days following vaccination was reported in 4 participants after the administration of *Pentacel* (1 on the same day as the first dose; 3 on the same day as the third dose) and in 1 participant after the administration of *Daptacel* + *IPOL* + *ActHIB* (4 days following the first dose).

➤*Seizures:* Across studies 494-01, 494-03, 5A9908, and P3T06, a total of 8 participants experienced a seizure within 7 days following either *Pentacel* (4 participants; n = 4,197 for at least 1 of doses 1 to 3; n = 5,033 for dose 4), separately administered HCPDT + *POLIOVAX* + *ActHIB* (3 participants; n = 1,032 for at least 1 of doses 1 to 3, n = 739 for dose 4), separately administered *Daptacel* + *IPOL* + *ActHIB* (1 participant; n = 1,455 for at least 1 of doses 1 to 3), or separately administered *Daptacel* + *ActHIB* (0 participants; n = 418 for dose 4). Among the 4 participants who experienced a seizure within 7 days following *Pentacel*, 1 participant in study 494-01 had an afebrile seizure 6 days after the first dose, 1 participant in study 494-01 had a possible seizure the same day as the third dose, and 2 participants in study 5A9908 had a febrile seizure 2 and 4 days, respectively, after the fourth dose. Among the 4 participants who experienced a seizure within 7 days following control vaccines, 1 participant had an afebrile seizure the same day as the first dose of *Daptacel* + *IPOL* + *ActHIB*, 1 participant had an afebrile seizure the same day as the second dose of HCPDT + *POLIOVAX* + *ActHIB*, and 2 participants had a febrile seizure 6 and 7 days, respectively, after the fourth dose of HCPDT + *POLIOVAX* + *ActHIB*.

➤*Serious adverse reactions:* In study P3T06, within 30 days following any of doses 1 to 3 of *Pentacel* or control vaccines, 19 of 484 (3.9%) participants who received *Pentacel* and 50 of 1,455 (3.4%) participants who received *Daptacel* + *IPOL* + *ActHIB* experienced a serious adverse reaction. Within 30 days following dose 4 of *Pentacel* or control vaccines, 5 of 431 (1.2%) participants who received *Pentacel* and 4 of 418 (1%) participants who received *Daptacel* + *ActHIB* experienced a serious adverse reaction. In study 494-01, within 30 days following any of doses 1 to 3 of *Pentacel* or control vaccines, 23 of 2,506 (0.9%) participants who received *Pentacel* and 11 of 1,032 (1.1%) participants who received HCPDT + *POLIOVAX* + *ActHIB* experienced a serious adverse reaction. Within 30 days following dose 4 of *Pentacel* or control vaccines, 6 of 1,862 (0.3%) participants who received *Pentacel* and 2 of 739 (0.3%) participants who received HCPDT + *POLIOVAX* + *ActHIB* experienced a serious adverse reaction.

Across studies 494-01, 494-03, and P3T06, within 30 days following any of doses 1 to 3 of *Pentacel* or control vaccines, overall, the most frequently reported serious adverse reactions were bronchiolitis, dehydration, pneumonia, and gastroenteritis. Across studies 494-01, 494-03, 5A9908, and P3T06, within 30 days following dose 4 of *Pentacel* or control vaccines, overall, the most frequently reported serious adverse reactions were dehydration, gastroenteritis, asthma, and pneumonia.

Across studies 494-01, 494-03, 5A9908, and P3T06, 2 cases of encephalopathy were reported, both in participants who had received *Pentacel* (n = 5,979). One case occurred 30 days postvaccination and was secondary to cardiac arrest following cardiac surgery. One infant who had onset of neurologic symptoms 8 days postvaccination was subsequently found to have structural cerebral abnormalities and was diagnosed with congenital encephalopathy.

A total of 5 deaths occurred during studies 494-01, 494-03, 5A9908, and P3T06: 4 in children who had received *Pentacel* (n = 5,979) and 1 in a participant who had received *Daptacel* + *IPOL* + *ActHIB* (n = 1,455). There were no deaths reported in children who received HCPDT + *POLIOVAX* + *ActHIB* (n = 1,032). Causes of death among children who received *Pentacel* were asphyxia caused by suffocation, head trauma, Sudden Infant Death syndrome, and neuroblastoma (8, 23, 52, and 256 days postvaccination, respectively). One participant with ependymoma died secondary to aspiration 222 days following *Daptacel* + *IPOL* + *ActHIB*.

➤*Postmarketing:*

CNS – Depressed level of consciousness, hemiconvulsion-hemiplegia-epilepsy syndrome, screaming, somnolence.

Dermatologic – Erythema, skin discoloration.

GI – Diarrhea, vomiting.

Hypersensitivity – Rash, urticaria.

Respiratory – Apnea, cough.

Miscellaneous – Cyanosis, decreased appetite, extensive swelling of the injected limb (including swelling that involved adjacent joints), injection-site reactions (including abscess and sterile abscess, inflammation, and mass), meningitis, pallor, rhinitis, vaccination failure/therapeutic response decreased (invasive Hib disease), viral infection.

➤*Reporting of adverse reactions:* The National Childhood Vaccine Injury Act of 1986 requires health care providers who administer vaccines to maintain in the recipient's permanent medical record the manufacturer, lot number, date of administration, and the name, address, and title of the person administering the vaccine. The Act further requires the health care provider to report to the US Department of Health and Human Services the occurrence of certain adverse reactions following immunization. For *Pentacel*, reactions required to be reported are anaphylaxis or anaphylactic shock within 7 days, brachial neuritis within 2 to 28 days, encephalopathy or encephalitis within 7 days following vaccination, or any acute complication or sequela (including death) of these reactions, or any contraindicating reaction listed in the contraindications section. Report these reactions and other suspected adverse reactions to Vaccine Adverse Events Reporting System at 1-800-822-7967 or http://www.vaers.hhs.gov, and to Sanofi Pasteur at 1-800-822-2463.

Patient Information

Before administration of *Pentacel*, inform the parent or guardian of the benefits and risks of the vaccine and the importance of completing the immunization series unless a contraindication to further immunization exists.

Inform the parent or guardian about the potential for adverse reactions that have been temporally associated with *Pentacel* or other vaccines containing similar ingredients. Provide the Vaccine Information Statements, which are required by the National Childhood Vaccine Injury Act of 1986 to be given with each immunization. Instruct the parent or guardian to report adverse reactions to their health care provider.

DIPHTHERIA AND TETANUS TOXOIDS ADSORBED

Rx	**Decavac** (Sanofi Pasteur)	**Injection:** 2 Lf units diphtheria and 5 Lf units tetanus per 0.5 mL dose	Preservative free. In 0.5 mL *Luer-Lok* syringe.[b]
Rx	**Diphtheria & Tetanus Toxoids, Adult** (Merck)	**Injection:** 2 Lf units diphtheria and 2 Lf units tetanus per 0.5 mL dose	In 0.5 mL single-dose vials.[c]
Rx	**Diphtheria & Tetanus Toxoids, Pediatric** (Sanofi Pasteur)	**Injection:** 6.7 Lf units diphtheria and 5 Lf units tetanus per 0.5 mL dose	In 5 mL multidose vials.[a]

[a] With aluminum potassium sulfate, thimerosal.
[b] With ≤ 0.28 mg of aluminum and trace thimerosal (≤ 0.3 mcg mercury/dose).
[c] With ≤ 0.53 mg aluminum, < 100 mcg (0.02%) formaldehyde, and trace thimerosal (≤ 0.3 mcg mercury/dose).

DIPHTHERIA AND TETANUS TOXOIDS ADSORBED — INJECTION

Indications

➤*Diphtheria and tetanus toxoids adsorbed for pediatric use (DT):* Diphtheria and tetanus toxoids adsorbed for pediatric use (DT) is indicated for active immunization against diphtheria and tetanus diseases in infants and children from 2 months of age up to 7 years of age (prior to their seventh birthday) for whom the use of a combined vaccine containing pertussis antigen is contraindicated (see Administration and Dosage).

Protection against diphtheria and tetanus is based on a full course of immunization.

DT is intended only for active immunization against diphtheria and tetanus and is not to be used for treatment of actual infection or in people 7 years of age or older.

Persons recovering from tetanus or diphtheria – Diphtheria or tetanus infection may not confer immunity; therefore, initiation or completion of active immunization is indicated at the time of recovery from these infections.

If a contraindication to using tetanus toxoid-containing preparations exists in a person who has not completed a primary immunizing course of tetanus toxoid, and other than a clean minor wound is sustained, only passive immunization should be given using human tetanus immune globulin (TIG).

If passive immunization for diphtheria is needed, equine diphtheria antitoxin is recommended (see Administration and Dosage).

As with any vaccine, DT may not protect 100% of individuals receiving the vaccine.

➤*Tetanus and diphtheria toxoids adsorbed for adult use (Td):* Tetanus and diphtheria toxoids adsorbed for adult use (Td) is indicated for active immunization of children 7 years of age or older and adults against tetanus and diphtheria. Td is the preparation of choice for vaccination of all persons 7 years of age or older because side effects from higher doses of diphtheria toxoid are more common in this group than they are among younger children.

➤*Pregnancy:* See Warnings/Precautions for more information.

➤*Active infection:* This vaccine is not to be used for the treatment of tetanus or diphtheria infection.

➤*Children:* See Warnings/Precautions for more information.

➤*Protection:* As with any vaccine, vaccination with Td may not protect 100% of susceptible individuals.

➤*Passive immunization:* See Administration and Dosage for more information.

DIPHTHERIA AND TETANUS TOXOIDS ADSORBED — INJECTION

Administration and Dosage

➤*General dosing considerations:* Td vaccine is approved for administration in persons 7 years of age and older who have not been immunized previously against tetanus and diphtheria, as a primary immunization series, and as booster immunization in those who have completed primary immunization against tetanus and diphtheria.

DT vaccine is recommended for children 6 weeks through 6 years of age (up to the seventh birthday), ideally beginning when the child is 6 weeks to 2 months of age. Persons 7 years of age and older should not be immunized with DT vaccine.

Interruption of the recommended schedule with a delay between doses does not interfere with the final immunity achieved with DT vaccine. There is no need to restart the series, regardless of the length of time between doses.

➤*Adults:*

Immunization (Td vaccine only) –

Primary immunization: Three 0.5 mL IM doses. The interval between doses recommended by the ACIP is 4 to 8 weeks between the first and second dose and 6 to 12 months between the second and third dose.

Booster immunization: 0.5 mL IM administered every 10 years.

If a dose of tetanus and diphtheria toxoid-containing vaccine is given sooner than 10 years, as part of wound management or on exposure to diphtheria, the next booster is not needed for 10 years thereafter.

Tetanus prophylaxis in wound management:

• *Primary immunization complete* –

Minor, uncontaminated wounds: Administer a booster dose of a tetanus toxoid–containing preparation only if the individual has not received tetanus toxoid within the preceding 10 years.

Tetanus-prone wounds: For tetanus-prone wounds (eg, wounds contaminated with dirt, feces, soil, and saliva; puncture wounds; avulsions; wounds resulting from missiles, crushing, burns, and frostbite), a booster is appropriate if the patient has not received a tetanus toxoid–containing preparation within the preceding 5 years.

• *Primary immunization incomplete or unknown* – Immunize with a tetanus toxoid–containing product and ensure completion of primary immunization thereafter.

In addition, if these individuals have sustained a tetanus-prone wound, the use of TIG is recommended. If a contraindication to using tetanus toxoid–containing preparations exists in a person who has not completed a primary immunizing course of tetanus toxoid, only passive immunization with TIG should be given.

➤*Children:*

Immunization –

7 years of age and older (Td vaccine only):

• *Primary immunization* – See Adults for dosing.

• *Booster immunization* – 0.5 mL IM in patients 11 to 12 years of age, if at least 5 years have elapsed since the last dose of tetanus and diphtheria toxoid-containing vaccine. Subsequent routine booster immunization is recommended every 10 years.

If a dose of tetanus and diphtheria toxoid-containing vaccine is given sooner than 10 years, as part of wound management or on exposure to diphtheria, the next booster is not needed for 10 years thereafter.

• *Tetanus prophylaxis in wound management* – See Adults for dosing

1 year up to 7 years of age (DT vaccine only):

• *Primary immunization* – Two 0.5 mL IM doses, 4 to 8 weeks apart, followed by a third 0.5 mL dose 6 to 12 months after the second injection.

In the event that the final immunizing dose would be given after the seventh birthday, Td vaccine should be used.

• *Booster immunization* – 0.5 mL IM in patients 4 to 6 years of age (preferably at the time of kindergarten or elementary school entrance).

Those who received all 4 primary immunizing doses before their fourth birthday should receive a single dose of DT vaccine just before entering kindergarten or elementary school.

The booster dose is not necessary if the fourth dose of the primary immunizing series was given after the fourth birthday.

Subsequent booster doses are recommended at intervals of 10 years.

6 weeks up to 1 year of age (DT vaccine only):

• *Primary immunization* – Three 0.5 mL IM doses, 4 to 8 weeks apart, followed by a fourth 0.5 mL dose 6 to 12 months after the third injection.

➤*Concomitant therapy:*

DT – The simultaneous administration of DT vaccine, oral polio virus vaccine (OPV), and measles-mumps-rubella vaccine (MMR) has resulted in seroconversion rates and rates of side effects similar to those observed when the vaccines are administered separately. Simultaneous vaccination (at separate sites and separate syringes) with DT, MMR, OPV, or inactivated poliovirus vaccine (IPV), and *Haemophilus* b conjugate vaccine (HbCV) is also acceptable. The ACIP recommends the simultaneous administration, at separate sites and separate syringes, of all vaccines appropriate to the age and previous vaccination status of the recipients including the special circumstance of simultaneous administration of DT, OPV, HbCV, and MMR at 15 months of age or older.

➤*Preparation for administration:* Shake vial or syringe well before withdrawing or administering a dose. Discard vial or syringe if vaccine cannot be resuspended.

➤*Administration:* For IM administration only. Do not administer intravenously or subcutaneously.

DT – The preferred IM injection sites are the anterolateral aspect of the thigh and the deltoid muscle of the upper arm. The vaccine should not be injected into the gluteal area or areas where there may be a major nerve trunk. During the course of primary immunizations, injections should not be made more than once at the same site.

Td – Inject IM in the area of the vastus lateralis (mid-thigh laterally) or deltoid. Do not inject into the gluteal area or areas where there may be a major nerve trunk.

The needle length should be sufficient to deliver the vaccine IM, but not so long as to involve the underlying nerves and blood vessels or bone. The health care professional should determine the appropriate size and length of the needle for individual patients.

➤*Storage / Stability:* Store at 2° to 8°C (35° to 46°F). Do not freeze.

Actions

➤*Pharmacology:* The potency of tetanus and diphtheria toxoids was determined on the basis of immunogenicity studies, with a comparison to a serological correlate of protection (0.01 antitoxin units/mL) established by the Panel on Review of Bacterial Vaccines and Toxoids.

A clinical study to evaluate the serological responses and adverse reactions was performed in 58 individuals 6 years of age or older. The results indicated protective levels of antibody were achieved in more than 90% of the study population after primary immunization with both components. Booster effects were achieved in 100% of the individuals with preexisting antibody responses.

Contraindications

Hypersensitivity to any component of the vaccine, including thimerosal, a mercury derivative, is a contraindication.

A history of systemic allergic or neurologic reactions following a previous dose of Td is an absolute contraindication for further use.

The decision to administer or delay vaccination because of a current or recent febrile illness depends largely on the severity of symptoms and their etiology. Although a moderate or severe febrile illness is sufficient reason to postpone vaccination, minor illnesses such as a mild upper respiratory tract infection with or without low-grade fever are not contraindications.

Routine immunization should be deferred during an outbreak of poliomyelitis, provided the patient has not sustained an injury that increases the risk of tetanus and provided an outbreak of diphtheria disease does not occur simultaneously.

If a contraindication to using tetanus toxoid-containing preparations exists in a person who has not completed a primary immunizing course of tetanus toxoid and other than a clean, minor wound is sustained, only passive immunization should be given using human TIG.

Warnings/Precautions

➤*DT for pediatric use:* This product is not recommended for immunizing persons on or after their seventh birthday.

For individuals 7 years of age or older, tetanus and diphtheria toxoids adsorbed, for adult use (Td), should be used instead of DT. The concentration of diphtheria toxoid in preparations intended for use in persons 7 years of age or older is approximately 80% lower than that of the pediatric formulation. The lower dosage of diphtheria toxoid is recommended for persons 7 years of age or older because adverse reactions to the diphtheria component are thought to be related to both dose and age.

➤*Td for adult use:* A routine booster should not be given more frequently than every 10 years. This guideline should not preclude wound management considerations.

➤*Both DT and Td:* DT or Td should not be given to infants, children, or adults with thrombocytopenia or any coagulation disorder that would contraindicate IM injection unless the potential benefits clearly outweigh the risk of administration. If the decision is made to administer DT or Td, it should be given with caution (see Drug Interactions).

Deaths have been reported in temporal association with the administration of preparations containing diphtheria or tetanus antigens; however, no causal relationship was proven (see Adverse Reactions).

➤*Before administration:* Before the injection of any biological, the healthcare professional should take all precautions known for prevention of allergic or any other adverse reactions. These should include the following: A review of the patient's history regarding possible sensitivity and any previous adverse reactions to the vaccine or similar vaccine or to dry natural latex rubber; the ready availability of epinephrine 1:1000 (should an acute anaphylactic reaction occur due to any component of the vaccine) and other appropriate agents used for control of immediate allergic reactions; a current knowledge of the literature concerning the use of the vaccine under consideration.

➤*HIV infection:* These products (DT and Td) are not contraindicated for use in individuals with HIV infection.

➤*Administration precautions:* Special care should be taken to prevent injection into or near a blood vessel or nerve.

➤*DT for pediatric use:*

Immunodeficiency – See Drug Interactions for more information.

➤*Td for adult use:*

Immunodeficiency – Immunosuppressive therapies including radiation, corticosteroids, antimetabolites, alkylating agents, and cytotoxic drugs may reduce the immune response to vaccines. Therefore, routine vaccination

DIPHTHERIA AND TETANUS TOXOIDS ADSORBED — INJECTION

should be deferred, if possible, while patients are receiving such therapy. If Td has been administered to persons receiving immunosuppressive therapy, or having an immunodeficiency disorder, an adequate antibody response may not be obtained. When possible, immunosuppressive treatment should be interrupted when immunization is required due to a tetanus-prone wound.

Wound prophylaxis – It is advisable to use Td (for adult use in those 7 years of age or older) in wound prophylaxis instead of tetanus toxoid alone in order to maintain adequate levels of diphtheria immunity.

➤*Latex allergy:* Healthcare professionals should prescribe or administer this product with caution to patients with a possible history of latex sensitivity since this packaging contains dry natural rubber.

➤*Guillain-Barre syndrome:* Healthcare professionals should administer these products with caution to patients with a history of Guillain-Barre syndrome (see Adverse Reactions).

➤*Hypersensitivity reactions:*

Both DT and Td – Persons who experience Arthus-type hypersensitivity reactions or temperatures higher than 39.4°C (103°F) after a previous dose of tetanus toxoid usually have very high serum tetanus antibody levels and should not be given even emergency doses of a tetanus toxoid-containing preparation more frequently than every 10 years, even if they have a wound that is neither clean nor minor.

➤*Pregnancy:*

DT for pediatric use – *Category C.* Animal reproduction studies have not been conducted with DT vaccine. It is not known whether DT vaccine can cause fetal harm when administered to a pregnant woman or can affect reproductive capacity. DT is not recommended for use in a pregnant woman. This product is not recommended for use in individuals 7 years of age or older.

Td for adult use – Animal reproduction studies have not been conducted with Td vaccine. It is also not known whether Td vaccine can cause fetal harm when administered to a pregnant woman or can affect reproduction capacity. Td vaccine should be given to a pregnant woman only if clearly needed.

Adequate immunization by routine boosters in nonpregnant women of childbearing age can obviate the need to vaccinate women during pregnancy (see Administration and Dosage).

However, the ACIP recommends the following: A previously unvaccinated pregnant woman whose child might be born under unhygienic circumstances (without sterile technique) should receive 2 doses of Td 4 to 8 weeks apart before delivery, preferably during the last 2 trimesters. Pregnant women in similar circumstances who have not had a complete vaccination series should complete the 3-dose series. Those vaccinated more than 10 years previously should have a booster dose. No evidence exists to indicate that tetanus and diphtheria toxoids administered during pregnancy are teratogenic.

It has been reported that tetanus toxoid administered to pregnant women prevents neonatal tetanus in newborns. However, the data reported on the safety of tetanus toxoid when so used is inconclusive because the incidence of neonatal deaths in New Guinea was significantly higher than in the United States. A prospective study in the US has not been done to confirm these reports.

➤*Lactation:*

DT for pediatric use – This product is not recommended for use in individuals 7 years of age or older.

➤*Children:*

DT for pediatric use – The safety and efficacy of DT for pediatric use, in children younger than 6 weeks of age have not been established (see Administration and Dosage).

Td for adult use – Safety and efficacy of Td for adult use in children younger than 7 years of age have not been established.

In children younger than 7 years of age, either diphtheria and tetanus toxoids and acellular pertussis vaccine adsorbed (DTaP) or diphtheria and tetanus toxoids and pertussis vaccine adsorbed USP (for pediatric use) (DTP) is recommended. If a contraindication to pertussis immunization exists, the recommended vaccine is DT.

➤*Elderly:*

DT for pediatric use – This vaccine is not recommended for use in adult populations.

Drug Interactions

➤*Anticoagulants:* As with other IM injections, DT or Td should be given with caution to patients on anticoagulant therapy.

➤*Human TIG/equine diphtheria antitoxin:* Human TIG or equine diphtheria antitoxin, if used, should be given in a separate site with a separate needle and syringe.

➤*DT for pediatric use:*

Immunosuppressive therapy – Infants or children receiving immunosuppressive therapy (including irradiation, systemic corticosteroids, antimetabolites, alkylating agents, and cytotoxic agents) may have a reduced response to active immunization procedures. Although no specific studies are available, if immunosuppressive therapy will be discontinued shortly, it would be reasonable to defer immunization until the patient has been off therapy for 1 month; otherwise the patient should be vaccinated while still on therapy.

➤*Passive immunization:* See Administration and Dosage for more information.

Immunosuppressants – See Warnings/Precautions for more information.

Adverse Reactions

➤*DT for pediatric use:* In a prospective study that compared the reaction rates of a similar diphtheria and tetanus toxoid-containing vaccine to diphtheria and tetanus toxoids and pertussis vaccine (DTP), 784 children 0 to 6 years of age who were scheduled to receive routine DTP immunization instead received a dose of DT vaccine. Of these children, 684 and 110 were enrolled in the open-label and double-blind portions of the study, respectively. Most (98.8%) of the children received DT vaccine as a first, second, or third dose of the primary immunization series; the remainder of the immunizations were administered as a booster (fourth or fifth) dose. Local and systemic reactions that occurred within 48 hours of immunization were reported by parents through home visit, telephone call or mail-in questionnaire.

Local – Local reactions occurring within 48 hours following immunization for both the blinded and unblinded groups included redness (7.6%), swelling (7.6%), and pain (9.9%).

Systemic – Systemic symptoms included drowsiness (14.9%), fretfulness (22.6%), vomiting (2.6%), anorexia (7%), and persistent crying (0.7%). The incidence rates of fever 38° C (100.4°F) or higher and 39°C (102.2°F) or higher, reported in a subset of children (n = 292) three to 6 hours postimmunization, were 9.3% and 0.7%, respectively.

➤*Td for adult use:* In a clinical study involving 58 individuals 6 years of age or older, 19% of the individuals noted local reactions consisting of erythema, tenderness and induration at the injection site and 2% systemic reactions consisting of headache, malaise and temperature elevations.

Cardiovascular – Acute anaphylactic reactions may occur rarely following administration of tetanus and diphtheria antigens which may cause acute hives and cardiovascular collapse.

Adverse reactions to diphtheria toxoid in adults are minimized by the small amount of the antigen (not more than 2 Lf units per dose) contained in Td.

Epinephrine injection (1:1000) must be immediately available should an acute anaphylactic reaction occur due to any component of the vaccine.

➤*CNS:*

DT for pediatric use – Neurological complications, such as convulsions, encephalopathy, and various mono- and polyneuropathies, including Guillain-Barre syndrome (GBS), have been reported following administration of preparations containing diphtheria or tetanus antigens. A review by the Institute Of Medicine (IOM) found evidence of a causal relation between tetanus toxoid and brachial neuritis and GBS, but did not find evidence of a causal relation between DT and sudden infant death syndrome (SIDS).

Td for adult use – The following neurologic illnesses have been reported as temporally associated with vaccines containing tetanus toxoid: Neurological complications, including cochlear lesions, brachial plexus neuropathies, paralysis of the radial nerve, paralysis of the recurrent nerve, accommodation paresis, Guillain-Barre syndrome (GBS), and EEG disturbances with encephalopathy. The IOM following review of the reports of neurologic events following vaccination with tetanus toxoid, Td or DT, concluded the evidence favored acceptance of a causal relationship between tetanus toxoid and brachial neuritis and GBS.

➤*Hypersensitivity:* Allergic and hypersensitivity reactions, urticaria, erythema multiforme or other rash, arthralgias and, more rarely, a severe anaphylactic reaction (ie, urticaria with swelling of the mouth, difficulty breathing, hypotension, shock, or death) have been reported following administration of preparations containing diphtheria or tetanus antigens.

Deaths have been reported in temporal association to receipt of preparations containing tetanus and diphtheria toxoids. The IOM found inadequate evidence to accept or reject a causal relationship between tetanus toxoid-containing products and death from causes other than anaphylaxis or GBS.

See Warnings/Precautions for more information.

➤*Local:* Local reactions, manifested by varying degree of erythema, warmth, edema, induration with or without tenderness, as well as urticaria and rash may occur after administration of DT or Td. With vaccines in general, it is not uncommon for patients to note within 48 to 72 hours at or around the injection site the following minor reactions: Edema; pain or tenderness; redness, inflammation or skin discoloration; mass or induration; local hypersensitivity. Such local reactions are usually self-limited and require no therapy. As with other aluminum-containing vaccines, a nodule may occasionally be palpable at the injection site for several weeks. Sterile abscess formation or subcutaneous atrophy at the injection site may also occur.

➤*Miscellaneous:* Other adverse events which have been reported in temporal association with various tetanus toxoid-containing products include the following: Warmth, swelling, cellulitis, malaise, weakness or fatigue, dizziness, irritability, aches and pains, arthralgia, flushing, tachycardia, syncope, nausea, vomiting, lymphadenopathy, phlebitis, pruritis/itching, hives, sweating, acute midbrain syndrome, EEG disturbances, accommodation pareses, paresthesia, radiculopathy, brachial plexus neuropathy, cranial nerve pareses, myelopathy, myelitis, and cochlear lesions.

Pallor, coldness, and hyporesponsiveness have been reported in a child receiving a DT vaccine.

DIPHTHERIA AND TETANUS TOXOIDS ADSORBED — INJECTION

Patient Information

Prior to the administration of these vaccines, healthcare professionals should inform the parent or guardian or adult patient of the recommended immunization schedule for protection against tetanus and diphtheria diseases and the benefits and risks of vaccination against tetanus and diphtheria diseases, and also inquire about the recent health status of the patient to be injected.

As part of the child's or adult's permanent immunization record, the date, lot number and manufacturer of the vaccine administered must be recorded.

The healthcare provider should inform the parent, guardian or adult patient about the potential for adverse reactions that have been temporally associated with the administration of these vaccines.

It is extremely important that when the parent, guardian or adult patient returns for the next dose in the series, the parent, guardian or adult patient should be questioned concerning occurrence of any symptoms or signs of an adverse reaction after the previous dose.

Guidance should be provided on measures to be taken by the parent or guardian should suspected adverse events occur, such as antipyretic measures for elevated temperatures and the need to report any suspected adverse occurrences to the healthcare professional. Parents or guardians should be provided with vaccine information statements prior to the time of vaccination, as required by the National Childhood Vaccine Injury Act (see previous information). The healthcare provider should provide the Vaccine Information Materials (VIMs) which are required to be given with each immunization.

The healthcare professional should inform the parent or guardian of the importance of completing the immunization series unless contraindicated.

DIPHTHERIA TOXOID/TETANUS TOXOID/ACELLULAR PERTUSSIS VACCINE, ADSORBED (DTaP/Tdap)

Rx	**Adacel**[a] (Sanofi Pasteur)	**Injection, suspension**: diphtheria toxoid 2 limits of flocculation (Lf) units, tetanus toxoid 5 Lf units, acellular pertussis antigens (pertactin 3 mcg, FHA[b] 5 mcg, detoxified pertussis toxins 2.5 mcg, fimbriae types two and three 5 mcg) per 0.5 mL	Aluminum phosphate 1.5 mg (aluminum 0.33 mg), residual formaldehyde, residual glutaraldehyde, phenoxyethanol. In single-dose vials.
Rx	**Boostrix**[a] (GlaxoSmithKline)	**Injection, suspension**: diphtheria toxoid 2.5 Lf units, tetanus toxoid 5 Lf units, acellular pertussis antigens (pertactin 2.5 mcg, FHA 8 mcg, inactivated pertussis toxins 8 mcg) per 0.5 mL	Aluminum adjuvant (aluminum ≤ 0.39 mg), residual formaldehyde, sodium chloride. In single-dose vials and disposable prefilled *Tip-Lok* syringes.[c]
Rx	**Daptacel**[d] (Sanofi Pasteur)	**Injection, suspension**: diphtheria toxoid 15 Lf units, tetanus toxoid 5 Lf units, acellular pertussis antigens (pertussis toxoid 10 mcg, FHA 5 mcg, pertactin 3 mcg, fimbriae types two and three 5 mcg) per 0.5 mL	Aluminum phosphate 1.5 mg (aluminum 0.33 mg), phenoxyethanol, residual formaldehyde, residual glutaraldehyde. In single-dose vials.[c]
Rx	**Infanrix**[d] (GlaxoSmithKline)	**Injection, suspension**: diphtheria toxoid 25 Lf units, tetanus toxoid 10 Lf units, acellular pertussis antigens (inactivated pertussis toxin 25 mcg, FHA 25 mcg, pertactin 8 mcg) per 0.5 mL	Preservative free. Aluminum adjuvant (aluminum ≤ 0.625 mg), residual formaldehyde, sodium chloride. In single-dose vials and disposable, prefilled *Tip-Lok* syringes.[c]
Rx	**Tripedia**[d] (Sanofi Pasteur)	**Injection, suspension**: diphtheria toxoid 6.7 Lf units, tetanus toxoid 5 Lf units, pertussis antigens 46.8 mcg (≈ 23.4 mcg each of inactivated pertussis toxin and FHA) per 0.5 mL	Aluminum ≤ 0.17 mg, residual formaldehyde. In preservative-free[e] single-dose vials.[c]

[a] Tdap - per Centers for Disease Control and Prevention (CDC), for use in older children and adults (10 to 64 years of age for *Boostrix* and 11 to 64 years of age for *Adacel*).
[b] FHA = filamentous hemagglutinin.
[c] Contains dry natural latex rubber.
[d] DTaP - per CDC, for use in infants and young children (younger than 7 years of age).
[e] With thimerosal (not more than mercury 0.3 mcg/dose).

TETANUS TOXOID/REDUCED DIPHTHERIA TOXOID/ACELLULAR PERTUSSIS VACCINE, ADSORBED (Tdap) — INJECTION

For additional information, refer to the Agents for Active Immunization introduction.

Indications

➤*Immunization:* For active booster immunization for the prevention of tetanus, diphtheria, and pertussis (whooping cough) as a single dose in persons 10 to 64 years of age (*Boostrix*) or persons 11 to 64 years of age (*Adacel*).

Administration and Dosage

➤*General dosing considerations:* Tdap (*Adacel*, *Boostrix*) is indicated for use in adults and adolescents only. For children, see the DTaP monograph.

Five years should have elapsed since the recipient's last dose of tetanus toxoid–, diphtheria toxoid–, and/or pertussis-containing vaccine.

➤*Adults:*

Immunization – Administer a single dose of *Adacel* or *Boostrix* (0.5 mL) intramuscularly (IM), preferably into the deltoid muscle.

➤*Children:*

Immunization – See Adults for dosing for children 10 years of age and older (*Boostrix*) or 11 years of age and older (*Adacel*).

➤*Vaccine coadministration:* When coadministration of other vaccines is required, they should be given with separate syringes and at different injection sites.

Several routine vaccines may safely be administered simultaneously at separate injection sites (eg, meningococcal, influenza, hepatitis B). Minor interferences with tetanus antitoxin levels and responses to pertactin were noted when *Adacel* and influenza vaccine were coadministered, but these effects are not expected to affect protective efficacy. National authorities recommend simultaneous immunization at separate sites as indicated.

➤*Diphtheria prophylaxis for case contacts:* The Advisory Committee on Immunization Practices (ACIP) has published recommendations on vaccination for diphtheria prophylaxis in persons who have had contact with a person with confirmed or suspected diphtheria. These recommendations are available at http://www.cdc.gov/vaccines/pubs/acip-list.htm.

➤*Tetanus prophylaxis in wound management:* Clinicians should refer to guidelines for tetanus prophylaxis in routine wound management.

A thorough attempt must be made to determine whether a patient has completed primary immunization. Persons who have completed primary immunization against tetanus and who sustain wounds that are minor and uncontaminated should receive a booster dose of a tetanus toxoid–containing preparation if they have not received tetanus toxoid within the preceding 10 years. For tetanus-prone wounds (eg, wounds contaminated with dirt, feces, soil, or saliva; puncture wounds; avulsions; wounds resulting from missiles, crushing, burns, or frostbite), a booster is appropriate if the patient has not received a tetanus toxoid–containing preparation within the preceding 5 years.

Tdap can be used as a one-time alternative to tetanus and diphtheria toxoids for adult use (Td) vaccine in patients for whom the pertussis component is also indicated.

If passive protection against tetanus is required, tetanus immune globulin (human) may be administered at a separate site with a separate needle and syringe.

➤*Preparation for administration:* Just before use, shake well until a uniform, white, cloudy suspension results. Do not use if resuspension does not occur with vigorous shaking. Visually inspect for particulate matter, discoloration, or cracks in the vial or syringe prior to administration whenever solution and container permit. If any of these conditions exist, the vaccine should not be administered.

After removal of the dose, any vaccine remaining in the vial should be discarded.

When administering a dose of *Adacel* from a stoppered vial, do not remove the stopper or the metal seal holding it in place.

➤*Administration:* Administer IM, preferably into the deltoid muscle. Do not inject into the gluteal area or other areas where there may be a major nerve trunk. Do not administer intravenously (IV), intradermally, or subcutaneously.

➤*Admixture compatibility:* Tdap should not be combined through reconstitution or mixed with any other vaccines.

➤*Storage/Stability:* Store between 2° and 8°C (35° and 46°F). Do not freeze. Discard if vaccine has been frozen.

Actions

➤*Pharmacology:*

Tetanus –

Protection against disease is caused by the development of neutralizing antibodies to the tetanus toxin. A serum tetanus antitoxin level of at least 0.01 unit/mL, measured by neutralization assays, is considered the minimum protective level. A level of 0.1 unit/mL or more has been considered as protective.

Diphtheria –

Protection against disease is due to the development of neutralizing antibody to diphtheria toxin. Following adequate immunization with diphtheria toxoid, protection persists for at least 10 years. A serum diphtheria antitoxin level of 0.01 units/mL is the lowest level providing some degree of protection; a level of 0.1 units/mL is regarded as protective. Levels of 1 unit/mL are associated with long-term protection. Immunization with diphtheria toxoid does not, however, eliminate carriage of *Corynebacterium diphtheriae* in the pharynx or nose or on the skin.

TETANUS TOXOID/REDUCED DIPHTHERIA TOXOID/ ACELLULAR PERTUSSIS VACCINE, ADSORBED (Tdap) — INJECTION

Pertussis –

The mechanism of protection from *Bordetella pertussis* disease is not well understood. However, the pertussis components in *Adacel* have been shown to prevent pertussis in infants in a clinical trial with *Daptacel* vaccine.

Contraindications

Severe allergic reaction(eg, anaphylaxis) after a previous dose of any tetanus toxoid–, diphtheria toxoid–, or pertussis antigen–containing vaccine or any component of the vaccine . Because of the uncertainty about which component of the vaccine might be responsible, do not administer vaccine with any of these components. Alternatively, refer such persons to an allergist for evaluation if immunizations are to be considered.

Encephalopathy (eg, coma, decreased level of consciousness, prolonged seizures) within 7 days of administration of a previous dose of a pertussis antigen–containing vaccine that is not attributable to another identifiable cause.

Warnings/Precautions

➤*Guillain-Barré syndrome and brachial neuritis:* If Guillain-Barré syndrome has occurred within 6 weeks of receipt of a prior vaccine containing tetanus toxoid, base the decision to give Tdap or any vaccine containing tetanus toxoid on careful consideration of the potential benefits and possible risks. A review by the Institute of Medicine found evidence for a causal relationship between receipt of tetanus toxoid and brachial neuritis and Guillain-Barré syndrome.

➤*Progressive or unstable neurologic disorders:* Progressive neurologic disorder, uncontrolled epilepsy, progressive encephalopathy, or unstable neurological conditions (eg, cerebrovascular events and acute encephalopathic conditions) are considered reasons to defer Tdap vaccination. In these situations, base administration of any pertussis antigen–containing vaccine on careful consideration of the potential benefits and possible risks.

➤*Acute illness:* Defer vaccination during the course of a moderate or severe illness with or without fever until the acute illness resolves.

➤*Immunodeficiency:* If Tdap vaccine is administered to persons receiving immunosuppressive therapy, including irradiation, antimetabolites, alkylating agents, cytotoxic drugs, and corticosteroids (used in greater than physiologic doses), or who have an immunodeficiency disorder, the expected immune response may not be obtained.

➤*Latex sensitivity:* The tip cap and rubber plunger of the *Boostrix* needleless prefilled syringes contain dry natural latex rubber, which may cause allergic reactions in latex-sensitive persons. The vial stopper is latex free.

➤*Patient history:* Prior to immunization, review the patient's current health status and medical history. Review the patient's immunization history for possible vaccine sensitivity and previous vaccination-related adverse reactions to determine the existence of any contraindication to immunization with Tdap and to allow an assessment of benefits and risks.

➤*Hypersensitivity reactions:* See Adverse Reactions for more information.

Epinephrine injection (1:1,000) and other appropriate agents and equipment used for the control of the immediate allergic reactions must be immediately available if an acute anaphylactic or acute hypersensitivity reaction occurs.

Persons who experienced Arthus-type hypersensitivity reactions (eg, severe local reactions associated with systemic symptoms) following a prior dose of tetanus toxoid usually have high serum tetanus antitoxin levels and should not be given emergency doses of tetanus toxoid–containing vaccines more frequently than every 10 years, even if the wound is neither clean nor minor.

➤*Pregnancy: Category C.* According to the CDC, pregnancy is not a contraindication for use of Tdap. Data on safety, immunogenicity, and the outcomes of pregnancy are not available for pregnant women who receive Tdap. When Tdap is administered during pregnancy, transplacental maternal antibodies might protect the infant against pertussis in early life. They also could interfere with the infant's immune response to infant doses of DTaP, and leave the infant less well-protected against pertussis. ACIP recommends Td when tetanus and diphtheria protection is required during pregnancy. In some situations, health care providers can choose to administer Tdap instead of Td to add protection against pertussis. When Td or Tdap is administered during pregnancy, the second or third trimester is preferred.

According to the manufacturers, animal reproduction studies have not been conducted with *Adacel* or *Boostrix*. It is not known whether these vaccines can cause fetal harm when administered to a pregnant woman or can affect reproduction capacity. Give Tdap to a pregnant woman only if clearly needed.

Adacel – The effect of *Adacel* on embryofetal and preweaning development was evaluated in 2 developmental toxicity studies using pregnant rabbits. Animals were administered *Adacel* twice prior to gestation, during the period of organogenesis (gestation day 6), and later during pregnancy on the twenty-ninth day of gestation, 0.5 mL per rabbit per occasion (a 17-fold increase compared with the human dose of *Adacel* on a body weight basis) by IM injection. No adverse effects on pregnancy, parturition, lactation, or embryofetal or preweaning development were observed. There were no vaccine-related fetal malformations or other evidence of teratogenesis noted in this study.

Boostrix – In a developmental toxicity study, the effect of *Boostrix* on embryofetal and preweaning development was evaluated in pregnant rats. Animals were administered *Infanrix* prior to gestation and *Boostrix* during the period of organogenesis (gestation days 6, 8, and 11) and later in pregnancy (gestation day 15), 0.1 mL/rat/occasion (a 45-fold increase compared with the human dose of *Boostrix* on a body weight basis), by IM injection. No adverse effect on pregnancy and lactation parameters or embryofetal or preweaning development was observed. There were no fetal malformations or other evidence of teratogenesis noted in this study.

Pregnancy registry – Health care providers are encouraged to register pregnant women who receive this vaccination.
Adacel: 1-800-822-2463.
Boostrix: 1-888-452-9622.

➤*Lactation:* It is not known if Tdap is excreted in human milk. However, according to the CDC, neither inactivated nor live vaccines administered to a lactating woman affect the safety of breast-feeding for mothers or infants. Breast-feeding does not adversely affect immunization and is not a contraindication for any vaccine, with the exception of smallpox vaccine. Exercise caution when Tdap is administered to a breast-feeding woman.

➤*Children:* For immunization of persons 6 weeks to 6 years of age against diphtheria, tetanus, and pertussis, refer to the manufacturers' package inserts for DTaP vaccines. *Boostrix* is not indicated for use in persons younger than 10 years of age. *Adacel* vaccine is not indicated for persons younger than 11 years of age.

➤*Elderly:* Tdap vaccine is not indicated for persons 65 years of age and older. Clinical studies did not include sufficient numbers of subjects older than 65 years of age to determine whether they respond differently from younger subjects.

Drug Interactions

➤*Immunosuppressants:* Immunosuppressive therapies, including irradiation, antimetabolites, alkylating agents, cytotoxic drugs, and corticosteroids (used in greater than physiologic doses), may reduce the immune response to vaccines.

➤*Concomitant vaccines:* See also Administration and Dosage.

Adverse Reactions

Arthus-type hypersensitivity reactions, characterized by severe local reactions (generally starting 2 to 8 hours after an injection), may follow receipt of tetanus toxoid. Such reactions may be associated with high levels of circulating antitoxin in persons who have had overly frequent injections of tetanus toxoid. (See also Warnings/Precautions.)

Persistent nodules at the site of injection have been reported following the use of adsorbed products.

Certain neurological conditions have been reported in temporal association with some tetanus toxoid–containing vaccines or tetanus- and diphtheria toxoid–containing vaccines. A review by the IOM found evidence for a causal relationship between receipt of tetanus toxoid and brachial neuritis and Guillain-Barré syndrome. Other neurological conditions that have been reported include demyelinating diseases of the CNS, peripheral mononeuropathies, and cranial mononeuropathies. The IOM concluded that the evidence was inadequate to accept or reject a causal relationship.

TETANUS TOXOID/REDUCED DIPHTHERIA TOXOID/ACELLULAR PERTUSSIS VACCINE, ADSORBED (Tdap) — INJECTION

➤*Adacel:*

Solicited adverse reactions in the principal safety study –

Adacel Injection-Site Reactions and Fever Following a Single Dose					
		Adolescents 11 to 17 years of age		Adults 18 to 64 years of age	
Adverse reactions[a]		*Adacel* (n = 1,170 to 1,175)	Td (n = 783 to 787)	*Adacel* (n = 1,688 to 1,698)	Td (n = 551 to 561)
Injection-site pain	Any	77.8%[b]	71%	65.7%	62.9%
	Moderate[c]	18%	15.6%	15.1%	10.2%
	Severe[d]	1.5%	0.6%	1.1%	0.9%
Injection-site swelling	Any	20.9%	18.3%	21%	17.3%
	Moderate[c]				
	1 to 3.4 cm	6.5%	5.7%	7.6%	5.4%
	Severe[d]				
	≥ 3.5 cm	6.4%	5.5%	5.8%	5.5%
	≥ 5 cm (2 in)	2.8%	3.6%	3.2%	2.7%
Injection-site erythema	Any	20.8%	19.7%	24.7%	21.6%
	Moderate[c]				
	1 to 3.4 cm	5.9%	4.6%	8%	8.4%
	Severe[d]				
	≥ 3.5 cm	6%	5.3%	6.2%	4.8%
	≥ 5 cm (2 in)	2.7%	2.9%	4%	3%
Fever	≥ 38°C (≥ 100.4°F)	5%[b]	2.7%	1.4%	1.1%
	≥ 38.8° to ≤ 39.4°C (≥ 102° to ≤103°F)	0.9%	0.6%	0.4%	0.2%
	≥ 39.5°C (103.1°F)	0.2%	0.1%	0%	0.2%

[a] Sample size was designed to detect > 10% differences between *Adacel* and Td vaccines for events of any intensity.

[b] *Adacel* did not meet the noninferiority criterion for rates of any pain in adolescents compared with Td vaccine rates (upper limit of the 95% CI on the difference for *Adacel* minus Td vaccine was 10.7%, whereas the criterion was < 10%). For any fever, the noninferiority criteria was met; however, any fever was statistically higher in adolescents receiving *Adacel*.

[c] Interfered with activities, but did not necessitate medical care or absenteeism.

[d] Incapacitating, prevented the performance of usual activities, may have or did necessitate medical care or absenteeism.

Other *Adacel* Adverse Reactions Following a Single Dose					
		Adolescents 11 to 17 years of age		Adults 18 to 64 years of age	
Adverse reactions		*Adacel* (n = 1,174 to 1,175)	Td (n = 787)	*Adacel* (n = 1,697 to 1,698)	Td (n = 560 to 561)
GI					
Diarrhea	Any	10.3%	10.2%	10.3%	11.3%
	Moderate[a]	1.9%	2%	2.2%	2.7%
	Severe[b]	0.3%	0%	0.5%	0.5%
Nausea	Any	13.3%	12.3%	9.2%	7.9%
	Moderate[a]	3.2%	3.2%	2.5%	1.8%
	Severe[b]	1%	0.6%	0.8%	0.5%
Vomiting	Any	4.6%	2.8%	3%	1.8%
	Moderate[a]	1.2%	1.1%	1%	0.9%
	Severe[b]	0.5%	0.3%	0.5%	0.2%
Musculoskeletal					
Body ache or muscle weakness	Any	30.4%	29.9%	21.9%	18.8%
	Moderate[a]	8.5%	6.9%	6.1%	5.7%
	Severe[b]	1.3%	0.9%	1.2%	0.9%
Sore and swollen joints	Any	11.3%	11.7%	9.1%	7%
	Moderate[a]	2.6%	2.5%	2.5%	2.1%
	Severe[b]	0.3%	0.1%	0.5%	0.5%
Miscellaneous					
Chills	Any	15.1%	12.6%	8.1%	6.6%
	Moderate[a]	3.2%	2.5%	1.3%	1.6%
	Severe[b]	0.5%	0.1%	0.7%	0.5%
Headache	Any	43.7%	40.4%	33.9%	34.1%
	Moderate[a]	14.2%	11.1%	11.4%	10.5%
	Severe[b]	2%	1.5%	2.8%	2.1%
Lymph node swelling	Any	6.6%	5.3%	6.5%	4.1%
	Moderate[a]	1%	0.5%	1.2%	0.5%
	Severe[b]	0.1%	0%	0.1%	0%
Rash	Any	2.7%	2%	2%	2.3%

TETANUS TOXOID/REDUCED DIPHTHERIA TOXOID/ACELLULAR PERTUSSIS VACCINE, ADSORBED (Tdap) — INJECTION

Other *Adacel* Adverse Reactions Following a Single Dose					
		Adolescents 11 to 17 years of age		Adults 18 to 64 years of age	
Adverse reactions		*Adacel* (n = 1,174 to 1,175)	Td (n = 787)	*Adacel* (n = 1,697 to 1,698)	Td (n = 560 to 561)
Tiredness	Any	30.2%	27.3%	24.3%	20.7%
	Moderate[a]	9.8%	7.5%	6.9%	6.1%
	Severe[b]	1.2%	1%	1.3%	0.5%

[a] Interfered with activities, but did not necessitate medical care or absenteeism.
[b] Incapacitating, prevented the performance of usual activities, may have or did necessitate medical care or absenteeism.

Local and systemic solicited reactions occurred at similar rates in *Adacel* and Td vaccine recipients in the 3-day postvaccination period. Most local reactions occurred within the first 3 days after vaccination (with a mean duration of less than 3 days).

Adverse reactions in the concomitant vaccine studies –

Hepatitis B vaccine: The rates reported for fever and injection-site pain at the *Adacel* administration site were similar when *Adacel* and hepatitis B vaccines were given concurrently or separately. However, the rates of injection-site erythema (23.4% for concomitant vaccination and 21.4% for separate administration) and swelling (23.9% for concomitant vaccination and 17.9% for separate administration) at the *Adacel* administration site were increased when coadministered. Swollen and/or sore joints were reported by 22.5% for concomitant vaccination and 17.9% for separate administration. The rates of generalized body aches in the persons who reported swollen and/or sore joints were 86.7% for concomitant vaccination and 72.2% for separate administration. Most joint complaints were mild in intensity with a mean duration of 1.8 days. The incidence of other solicited and unsolicited adverse reactions were not different between the 2 study groups.

Trivalent inactivated influenza vaccine: The rates of fever and injection-site erythema and swelling were similar for recipients of concurrent and separate administration of *Adacel* and trivalent inactivated influenza vaccine. However, pain at the *Adacel* injection site occurred at statistically higher rates following coadministration (66.6%) versus separate administration (60.8%). The rates of sore and/or swollen joints were 13% for coadministration and 9% for separate administration. Most joint complaints were mild in intensity with a mean duration of 2 days. The incidence of other solicited and unsolicited adverse reactions were similar between the 2 study groups.

Additional studies – An additional 1,806 adolescents received *Adacel* as part of the lot consistency study used to support *Adacel* licensure. This study was a randomized, double-blind, multicenter trial designed to assess lot consistency as measured by the safety and immunogenicity of 3 lots of *Adacel* when given as a booster dose to adolescents 11 to 17 years of age inclusive. Local and systemic adverse reactions were monitored for 14 days postvaccination using a diary card. Unsolicited adverse reactions and serious adverse reactions were collected for 28 days postvaccination. Pain was the most frequently reported local adverse reaction occurring in approximately 80% of all subjects. Headache was the most frequently reported systemic reaction occurring in approximately 44% of all subjects. Sore and/or swollen joints were reported by approximately 14% of participants. Most joint complaints were mild in intensity with a mean duration of 2 days.

An additional 962 adolescents and adults received *Adacel* in 3 supportive Canadian studies used as the basis for licensure in other countries. Within these clinical trials, the rates of local and systemic reactions following *Adacel* were similar to those reported in the 4 principal trials in the United States, with the exception of a higher rate (86%) of adults experiencing any local injection-site pain. The rate of severe pain (0.8%), however, was comparable with the rates reported in the 4 principal trials conducted in the United States. There was 1 spontaneous report of whole-arm swelling of the injected limb among the 277 Td vaccine recipients and 2 spontaneous reports among the 962 *Adacel* recipients in the supportive Canadian studies.

Postmarketing (Adacel) –

Cardiovascular: Myocarditis.

CNS: Convulsion, facial palsy, Guillain-Barré syndrome, hypesthesia, myelitis, paresthesia, syncope.

Dermatologic: Pruritus, urticaria.

Hypersensitivity: Anaphylactic reaction, hypersensitivity reaction (angioedema, edema, hypotension, rash).

Local: Extensive limb swelling from the injection site beyond 1 or both joints, injection-site bruising, large injection-site reactions (more than 50 mm), sterile abscess.

Musculoskeletal: Muscle spasm, myositis.

➤*Boostrix:*

Adverse reactions in the US adolescent safety study –

Boostrix Solicited Local Adverse Reactions or General Adverse Reactions (Within 15 Days Postvaccination) in Children 10 to 18 Years of Age[a]		
Adverse reactions	*Boostrix* (n = 3,032)	Td (n = 1,013)
CNS		
Headache, any	43.1%	41.5%
Headache,[b] grade 2[c] or 3[d]	15.7%	12.7%
Headache, grade 3	3.7%	2.7%
GI		
GI symptoms,[e] any	26%	25.8%
GI symptoms,[e] grade 2 or 3	9.8%	9.7%
GI symptoms,[e] grade 3	3%	3.2%
Local		
Arm circumference increase,[f] > 5 mm	28.3%	29.5%
Arm circumference increase,[f] > 20 mm	2%	2.2%
Arm circumference increase,[f] > 40 mm	0.5%	0.3%
Pain,[b] any	75.3%	71.7%
Pain,[b] grade 2 or 3	51.2%	42.5%
Pain,[g] grade 3	4.6%	4%
Redness, any	22.5%	19.8%
Redness, > 20 mm	4.1%	3.9%
Redness, ≥ 50 mm	1.7%	1.6%
Swelling, any	21.1%	20.1%
Swelling, >20 mm	5.3%	4.9%
Swelling, ≥ 50 mm	2.5%	3.2%
Miscellaneous		
Fatigue, any	37%	36.7%
Fatigue, grade 2 or 3	14.4%	12.9%
Fatigue, grade 3	3.7%	3.2%
Fever,[h] ≥ 37.5°C (99.5°F)	13.5%	13.1%
Fever,[h] > 38°C (100.4°F)	5%	4.7%
Fever,[h] > 39°C (102.2°F)	1.4%	1%

[a] Day of vaccination and the next 14 days.
[b] Statistically significantly higher ($P < 0.05$) following *Boostrix* as compared with Td vaccine.
[c] Grade 2 = local: painful when the limb was moved; general: interfered with normal activity.
[d] Grade 3 = local: spontaneously painful and/or prevented normal activity; general: prevented normal activity.
[e] GI symptoms included abdominal pain, diarrhea, nausea, and/or vomiting.
[f] Mid-upper region of the vaccinated arm.
[g] Grade 3 injection-site pain following *Boostrix* was not inferior to Td (upper limit of 2-sided 95% CI for the difference in the percentage of subjects ≤ 4%).
[h] Oral temperatures or axillary temperatures.

Adverse reactions in the German adolescent safety study –

No cases of whole-arm swelling were reported. Two individuals (2 of 193) reported large injection-site swelling (range, 110 to 200 mm diameter) in 1 case associated with grade 3 pain. Neither individual sought medical attention. These episodes were reported to resolve without sequelae within 5 days.

Boostrix Solicited Adverse Reactions (Within 15 Days Postvaccination) in Children 10 to 12 Years of Age	
Adverse reactions	*Boostrix* (n = 193)
Local	
Pain, any	62.2%
Pain, grade 2 or 3	33.2%
Pain, grade 3	5.7%
Redness, any	47.7%
Redness, > 20 mm	15%
Redness, ≥ 50 mm	10.9%

TETANUS TOXOID/REDUCED DIPHTHERIA TOXOID/ ACELLULAR PERTUSSIS VACCINE, ADSORBED (Tdap) — INJECTION

Boostrix Solicited Adverse Reactions (Within 15 Days Postvaccination) in Children 10 to 12 Years of Age

Adverse reactions	*Boostrix* (n = 193)
Swelling, any	38.9%
Swelling, > 20 mm	17.6%
Swelling, ≥ 50 mm	14%
Miscellaneous	
Fever, ≥ 37.5°C (99.5°F)[a]	8.8%
Fever > 38°C (100.4°F)[a]	4.1%
Fever, > 39°C (102.2°F)[a]	1%

[a] Oral temperatures or axillary temperatures.

Adverse reactions in the US adult safety study –

Boostrix Local or General Adverse Reactions (Within 15 Days Postvaccination) in Adults

Adverse reactions	*Boostrix* (n = 1,480)	Tdap (n = 741)
CNS		
Headache, any	30.1%	31%
Headache, grade 2 or 3	11.1%	10.5%
Headache, grade 3	2.2%	1.5%
GI		
GI symptoms, any[a]	15.9%	17.5%
GI symptoms, grade 2 or 3[a]	4.3%	5.7%
GI symptoms, grade 3[a]	1.2%	1.3%
Local		
Pain, any	61%	69.2%
Pain, grade 2 or 3	35.1%	44.4%
Pain, grade 3	1.6%	2.3%
Redness, any	21.1%	27.1%
Redness, > 20 mm	4%	6.2%
Redness, ≥ 50 mm	1.6%	2.3%
Swelling, any	17.6%	25.6%
Swelling, > 20 mm	3.9%	6.3%
Swelling, ≥ 50 mm	1.4%	2.8%
Miscellaneous		
Fatigue, any	28.1%	28.9%
Fatigue, grade 2 or 3	9.1%	9.4%
Fatigue, grade 3	2.5%	1.2%
Fever, ≥ 37.5°C (99.5°F)[b]	5.5%	8%
Fever, > 38°C (100.4°F)[b]	1%	1.5%
Fever, > 39°C (102.2°F)[b]	0.1%	0.4%

[a] GI symptoms included abdominal pain, diarrhea, nausea, and/or vomiting.
[b] Oral temperatures.

Serious adverse reactions – In the US and German adolescent safety studies, no serious adverse reactions were reported to occur within 31 days of vaccination. During the 6-month extended safety evaluation period, no serious adverse reactions that were of potential autoimmune origin or new-onset and chronic in nature were reported to occur. In non-US adolescent studies in which serious adverse reactions were monitored for up to 37 days, 1 subject was diagnosed with insulin-dependent diabetes 20 days following administration of *Boostrix*. No other serious adverse reactions of potential autoimmune origin or that were new-onset and chronic in nature were reported to occur in these studies. In the US adult safety study, serious adverse reactions were reported to occur during the entire study period (0 to 6 months) by 1.4% and 1.7% of subjects who received *Boostrix* and the comparator Tdap vaccine, respectively. During the 6-month extended safety evaluation period, no serious adverse reactions of a neuroinflammatory nature or with information suggesting an autoimmune etiology were reported in subjects who received *Boostrix*.

Postmarketing (Boostrix) –
Cardiovascular: Myocarditis.
CNS: Convulsion, encephalitis, facial palsy, paresthesia.
Dermatologic: Exanthem, Henoch-Schönlein purpura, rash, urticaria.
Hematologic/Lymphatic: Lymphadenitis, lymphadenopathy.
Local: Extensive swelling of the injected limb, induration, inflammation, injection-site pruritus, local reaction, mass, nodule, warmth.
Musculoskeletal: Arthralgia, back pain, myalgia.

Patient Information

Inform women of childbearing potential that the manufacturers maintain a pregnancy surveillance system to collect data on pregnancy outcomes and newborn health status outcomes following administration with Tdap vaccine during pregnancy. Inform women that if they are pregnant or become aware that they are pregnant at the time of Tdap vaccine immunization to contact their health care provider.

Inform patients, parents, or guardians of the potential benefits and risks of the vaccine. It is important to question the vaccine recipient, parent, or guardian concerning occurrence of any symptoms and/or signs of an adverse reaction after a previous dose of a diphtheria, tetanus, and pertussis vaccine. Inform the patients, parents, or guardians about the potential for adverse reactions that have been temporally associated with administration of Tdap or other vaccines containing similar components.

Give the patient, parent, or guardian the Vaccine Information statements that are required by the National Childhood Vaccine Injury Act of 1986 to be given prior to immunization. These materials are available free of charge at the CDC Web site (http://www.cdc.gov/vaccines/).

DIPHTHERIA TOXOID/TETANUS TOXOID/ACELLULAR PERTUSSIS VACCINE, ADSORBED (DTaP) — INJECTION

For additional information, refer to the Agents for Active Immunization introduction.

Indications

➤*Immunization:* For active immunization against diphtheria, tetanus, and pertussis as a 5-dose series in infants and children 6 weeks to 7 years of age (prior to seventh birthday). Because of the substantial risks of complications from pertussis disease in infants, completion of a primary series of vaccine early in life is strongly recommended.

When Haemophilus b conjugate vaccine (tetanus toxoid conjugate) (*ActHIB*) is reconstituted with *Tripedia* vaccine (*TriHIBit* vaccine), the combined vaccines are indicated for the active immunization of children 15 to 18 months of age who have been immunized previously against diphtheria, tetanus, and pertussis with 3 doses consisting of either whole-cell pertussis (DTP) vaccine or *Tripedia* vaccine and 3 or fewer doses of *ActHIB* vaccine within the first year of life for the prevention of diphtheria, tetanus, pertussis, and invasive diseases caused by *Haemophilus influenzae* type b (Hib).

Children who have had well-documented pertussis (ie, positive culture for *Bordetella pertussis* or epidemiologic linkage to a culture-positive case) should complete the vaccination series with diphtheria-tetanus (DT). Some experts recommend including the pertussis component as well (ie, administration of diphtheria, tetanus, and acellular pertussis [DTaP] vaccine). Although well-documented pertussis disease is likely to confer immunity against pertussis, the duration of such immunity is unknown.

If passive immunization is needed for tetanus prophylaxis or for treatment of diphtheria, tetanus immune globulin (TIG) or diphtheria antitoxin, respectively, should be administered as required.

Administration and Dosage

➤*General dosing considerations:* DTaP (*Daptacel, Infanrix, Tripedia*) is indicated for use in children only. For adults and adolescents, see the Tdap monograph.

DTaP is administered as a 5-dose series. Four doses constitute a primary immunization course for pertussis. The fifth dose is a booster for pertussis. Three doses of DTaP constitute a primary immunization course for diphtheria and tetanus. The fourth and fifth doses are boosters for diphtheria and tetanus.

If any recommended dose of pertussis vaccine cannot be given, DT (for pediatric use) vaccine should be given as needed to complete the series.

Preterm infants should be vaccinated according to their chronological age from birth.

Interruption of the recommended schedule with a delay between doses should not interfere with the final immunity achieved with the vaccine and does not require restarting the series.

➤*Children:*

Immunization –

6 weeks up to 7 years of age: Administer a single dose (0.5 mL) intramuscularly (IM) according to the schedule in the following table.

The customary age for the first dose is 2 months of age, but it may be given as early as 6 weeks of age and up to the seventh birthday. Preterm infants should be vaccinated according to their chronological age from birth.

DIPHTHERIA TOXOID/TETANUS TOXOID/ ACELLULAR PERTUSSIS VACCINE, ADSORBED (DTaP) — INJECTION

DTaP Vaccination Schedule				
Dose	CDC recommendations	*Daptacel*	*Infanrix*	*Tripedia*
1 to 3	2, 4, and 6 months of age	2, 4, and 6 months of age[a]	2, 4, and 6 months of age[b]	2, 4, and 6 months of age[b]
4	15 to 18 months of age[c]	15 to 20 months of age	15 to 20 months of age	15 to 18 months of age[d]
5	4 to 6 years of age	4 to 6 years of age	4 to 6 years of age	4 to 6 years of age[e]

[a] 6- to 8-week intervals.
[b] 4- to 8-week intervals.
[c] May be administered as early as 12 months of age, provided 6 months have elapsed since the third dose.
[d] Administered 6 to 12 months after third dose.
[e] Recommended before entry into kindergarten or elementary school, and is not needed if the fourth dose was given after the fourth birthday.

➤*Interchanging vaccines:* According to the CDC, the same brand of DTaP vaccine should be used for all doses of the vaccination series, when feasible. If the type of DTaP vaccine previously administered is not known, then any DTaP vaccine should be used to continue or complete the series.

According to the manufacturers of *Infanrix* and *Tripedia*, interchanging DTaP vaccines from different manufacturers for successive doses of the vaccination series is not recommended because data are limited regarding the safety and efficacy of such regimens.

Infanrix may be used to complete a DTaP vaccination series initiated with *Pediarix*.

Tripedia used to reconstitute *ActHIB* vaccine (*TriHIBit* vaccine) may be administered at 15 to 18 months of age for the fourth dose.

Daptacel or *Tripedia* may be used to complete the immunization series in infants and children who have received one or more doses or whole-cell pertussis DTP vaccine. However, the safety and efficacy have not been evaluated.

➤*Concomitant vaccine administration:* When concomitant administration of other vaccines or TIG is required, they should be given with separate syringes and at different injection sites.

The CDC recommends routinely administering all age-appropriate doses of vaccines simultaneously for children for whom no specific contraindications exist at the time of the visit. Children 12 to 15 months of age may receive up to 9 injections during a single visit (DTaP, measles-mumps-rubella, varicella, Hib, pneumococcal conjugate, inactivated poliovirus vaccine [IPV], hepatitis A, hepatitis B, and seasonal influenza).

See also Drug Interactions.

➤*Preparation for administration:* Just before use, shake well until a uniform, white, cloudy suspension results. Do not use if resuspension does not occur with vigorous shaking. Visually inspect for particulate matter, discoloration, or cracks in the vial or syringe prior to administration whenever solution and container permit. If any of these conditions exist, the vaccine should not be administered.

After removal of the dose, any vaccine remaining in the vial should be discarded.

When administering a dose of *Daptacel* from a stoppered vial, do not remove the stopper or the metal seal holding it in place.

➤*Administration:* Administer IM only; do not administer intravenously (IV), intradermally, or subcutaneously. The anterolateral aspect of the thigh (for most children younger than 1 year of age [ie, infants]) or the deltoid muscle of the upper arm (for most older children) is preferred.

Do not inject in the gluteal area or other areas where there may be a major nerve trunk.

➤*Admixture compatibility: Daptacel* and *Infanrix* should not be combined through reconstitution or mixed with any other vaccine in the same syringe or vial.

Tripedia should not be combined through reconstitution with any other vaccine for administration to infants younger than 15 months of age. Available serologic data do not support the use of *Tripedia* to reconstitute *ActHIB* (*TriHIBit*) for primary immunization.

➤*Storage/Stability:* Store between 2° and 8°C (35° and 46°F). Do not freeze. Discard if vaccine has been frozen.

Actions

➤*Pharmacology:* Simultaneous immunization of infants and children against diphtheria, tetanus, and pertussis has been a routine practice in the United States since the late 1940s. This has played a major role in markedly reducing disease and deaths from these infections.

Diphtheria –

Protection against disease is due to the development of neutralizing antibody to diphtheria toxin. Following adequate immunization with diphtheria toxoid, protection persists for at least 10 years. A serum diphtheria antitoxin level of 0.01 units/mL is the lowest level giving some degree of protection. Antitoxin levels of at least 0.1 units/mL are regarded as protective. Levels of 1 unit/mL are associated with long-term protection. Immunization with diphtheria toxoid does not, however, eliminate carriage of *C. diphtheriae* in the pharynx or nares or on the skin.

Tetanus –

Protection against disease is caused by the development of neutralizing antibodies to the tetanus toxin. Following adequate immunization with tetanus toxoid, it is thought that protection persists for at least 10 years. A serum tetanus antitoxin level of at least 0.01 units/mL, measured by neutralization assays, is considered the minimum protective level. More recently, a level of at least 0.1 to 0.2 units/mL has been considered as protective.

Pertussis –

There is no well-established serological correlate of protection for pertussis.

Contraindications

Serious allergic reaction (eg, anaphylaxis) temporally associated with a previous dose of DTaP or with any components of this vaccine (including thimerosal and gelatin in *Tripedia*). Because of the uncertainty as to which component of the vaccine might be responsible, do not administer the vaccine with any of these components. Alternatively, refer such persons to an allergist for evaluation if immunizations are to be considered.

In addition, the following events are contraindications to administration of any pertussis-containing vaccine: encephalopathy (eg, coma, decreased level of consciousness, prolonged seizures) within 7 days of administration of a previous dose of a pertussis-containing vaccine that is not attributable to another identifiable cause; and progressive neurologic disorders, including infantile spasms, uncontrolled epilepsy, or progressive encephalopathy. Do not administer pertussis vaccine to persons with such conditions until a treatment regimen has been established, the condition has stabilized, and the benefit clearly outweighs the risk.

If a contraindication to the pertussis vaccine component occurs, substitute DT for each of the remaining doses.

Warnings/Precautions

➤*Guillain-Barré syndrome and brachial neuritis:* A review by the Institute of Medicine (IOM) found evidence for a causal relation between tetanus toxoid and both brachial neuritis and Guillain-Barré syndrome. If Guillain-Barré syndrome has occurred within 6 weeks of receipt of prior vaccine containing tetanus toxoid, base the decision to give subsequent doses of DTaP or any vaccine containing tetanus toxoid on careful consideration of the potential benefits and possible risks.

➤*Acute illness:* Do not delay vaccination because of the presence of mild respiratory tract illness or other acute illness (eg, diarrhea) with or without fever. Vaccinate persons with moderate or severe acute illness as soon as the acute illness has improved.

➤*Latex sensitivity:* The stopper of the *Tripedia* and *Daptacel* vials and the tip cap and rubber plunger of the *Infanrix* needleless prefilled syringes contain dry natural latex rubber, which may cause allergic reactions in latex-sensitive persons. The vial stopper of *Infanrix* does not contain latex.

➤*Postvaccination effects:* If any of the following events occurs in temporal relation with the receipt of a pertussis-containing vaccine, carefully consider the decision to administer subsequent doses of vaccine containing the pertussis component on careful consideration of potential benefits and possible risks:

1.) temperature of at least 40.5°C (105°F) within 48 hours, not caused by another identifiable cause
2.) collapse or shock-like state (hypotonic-hyporesponsive episode) within 48 hours
3.) persistent, inconsolable crying lasting at least 3 hours, occurring within 48 hours
4.) seizure or convulsions, with or without fever, occurring within 3 days.

When the decision is made to withhold the pertussis component, consider giving immunization with DT vaccine.

➤*Convulsions and other CNS disorders:* The decision to administer a pertussis-containing vaccine to persons with stable CNS disorders must be made by the health care provider on an individual basis, with consideration of all relevant factors and assessment of potential risk and benefits for that individual. The ACIP and the Committee on Infectious Diseases of the American Academy of Pediatrics (AAP) have issued guidelines for such persons.

For infants or children at higher risk of seizures than the general population or who have a history of seizures, an appropriate antipyretic may be administered at the time of vaccination with a vaccine containing an acellular pertussis component (including DTaP) and for the ensuing 24 hours to reduce the possibility of postvaccination fever.

➤*Immunodeficiency:* Persons receiving immunosuppressive therapy, including irradiation, antimetabolites, alkylating agents, cytotoxic drugs, and corticosteroids (used in greater than physiologic doses), or with other immunodeficiencies may have diminished antibody response to active immunization. If DTaP vaccine has been administered to persons who are receiving immunosuppressive therapy, have had a recent injection of immune globulin, or have an immunodeficiency disorder, an adequate immunological response may not be obtained.

➤*Bleeding disorders:* Because of the risk of hemorrhage, do not give DTaP to infants or children with any coagulation disorder (such as thrombocytopenia) that would contraindicate IM injection or to persons on anticoagulant therapy, unless the potential benefit clearly outweighs the risk of administration. If the decision is made to administer DTaP to such persons, administer the vaccine with caution and take steps to avoid the risk of bleeding and hematoma following the injection.

DIPHTHERIA TOXOID/TETANUS TOXOID/ ACELLULAR PERTUSSIS VACCINE, ADSORBED (DTaP) — INJECTION

➤*Patient history:* Before the injection of any vaccine, take all known precautions to prevent allergic or other adverse reactions. Be sure to have a current knowledge of the literature concerning the use of the vaccine under consideration, including the nature of the adverse reactions that may follow its use.

Prior to immunization, review the patient's current health status and medical history. Review the patient's immunization history for possible vaccine sensitivity, previous vaccination-related adverse reactions, and occurrence of any adverse reaction–related symptoms and/or signs in order to determine the existence of any contraindication to immunization with DTaP and to allow an assessment of benefits and risks.

➤*Hypersensitivity reactions:* See Adverse Reactions for more information.

Epinephrine injection (1:1,000) and other appropriate agents used for the control of the immediate allergic reactions must be immediately available if an acute anaphylactic or acute hypersensitivity reaction occurs.

➤*Pregnancy: Category C.* Animal reproduction studies have not been conducted with *Daptacel*, *Infanrix*, and/or *Tripedia*. It is not known if any of these vaccines can cause fetal harm when administered to a pregnant woman or if they can affect reproductive capacity; they are not indicated for women of childbearing age. See the Tdap monograph for more information.

➤*Children:* DTaP is not indicated for infants younger than 6 weeks of age or children 7 years of age or older. Safety and effectiveness in these age groups have not been established.

➤*Elderly:* DTaP is not indicated for use in adults.

Drug Interactions

➤*Immunosuppressants:* Immunosuppressive therapies, including irradiation, antimetabolites, alkylating agents, cytotoxic drugs, and corticosteroids (used in greater than physiologic doses), may reduce the immune response to vaccines.

➤*Concomitant vaccines:* See also Administration and Dosage.

Tripedia – Except for reconstitution of *Tripedia* vaccine with *ActHIB* (*TriHIBit*), do not combine *Tripedia* vaccine through reconstitution with any vaccine. Because recent clinical trials in infants younger than 15 months of age have indicated that *TriHIBit* vaccine may induce a lower immune response to the Hib vaccine component than *ActHIB* given separately, this combination should not be used in infants for the first 3 doses. Only use *TriHIBit* vaccine for the booster dose at 15 to 18 months of age.

If *Tripedia* and TIG are coadministered, use separate syringes and separate sites.

Adverse Reactions

➤*Daptacel:*

Sweden I Efficacy Trial –

***Daptacel* Adverse Reactions (Within 24 Hours Postdose) From Sweden I Efficacy Trial**

Adverse reaction	Dose 1 (2 months of age)			Dose 2 (4 months of age)			Dose 3 (6 months of age)		
	Daptacel (n[a] = 2,587)	DT (n = 2,574)	DTP (n = 2,102)	*Daptacel* (n = 2,563)	DT (n = 2,555)	DTP (n = 2,040)	*Daptacel* (n = 2,549)	DT (n = 2,538)	DTP (n = 2,001)
CNS									
Crying (≥ 1 hour)	1.7%[b]	1.6%	11.8%	2.5%[b]	2.7%	9.3%	1.2%[b]	1%	3.3%
Drowsiness	32.7%[b]	32%	56.9%	25.9%[b]	25.6%	50.6%	18.9%[b]	20.6%	37.6%
Fretfulness[c]	32.3%	33%	82.1%	39.6%	39.8%	85.4%	35.9%	37.7%	73%
GI									
Anorexia	11.2%[b]	10.3%	39.2%	9.1%[b]	8.1%	25.6%	8.4%[b]	7.7%	17.5%
Vomiting	6.9%[b]	6.3%	9.5%	5.2%[d]	5.8%	7.4%	4.3%	5.2%	5.5%
Local									
Redness (≥ 2 cm)	0.3%[b]	0.3%	6%	1%[b]	0.8%	5.1%	3.7%[b]	2.4%	6.4%
Swelling (≥ 2 cm)	0.9%[b]	0.7%	10.6%	1.6%[b]	2%	10%	6.3%[b,e]	3.9%	10.5%
Tenderness (any)	8%[b]	8.4%	59.5%	10.1%[b]	10.3%	60.2%	10.8%[b]	10%	50%
Miscellaneous									
Fever (≥ 38°C [100.4°F])[f]	7.8%[b]	7.6%	72.3%	19.1%[b]	18.4%	74.3%	23.6%[b]	22.1%	65.1%

[a] n = number of evaluable subjects.
[b] $P < 0.001$: *Daptacel* vs whole-cell DTP.
[c] Statistical comparisons were not made for this variable.
[d] $P < 0.003$: *Daptacel* vs whole-cell DTP.
[e] $P < 0.0001$: *Daptacel* vs DT.
[f] Rectal temperature.

***Daptacel* Select Systemic Reactions in Sweden I Efficacy Trial (Rates Per 1,000 Doses)**

Adverse reaction	Dose 1 (2 months of age)			Dose 2 (4 months of age)			Dose 3 (6 months of age)		
	Daptacel (n[a] = 2,587)	DT (n = 2,574)	DTP (n = (2,102)	*Daptacel* (n = 2,565)	DT (n = 2,556)	DTP (n = 2,040)	*Daptacel* (n = 2,551)	DT (n = 2,539)	DTP (n = 2,002)
CNS									
Hypotonic-hyporesponsive episode within 24 hours of vaccination	0%	0%	1.9%	0%	0%	0.49%	0.39%	0%	0%
Persistent crying ≥ 3 hours within 24 hours of vaccination	1.16%	0%	8.09%	0.39%	0.39%	1.96%	0%	0%	1%
Seizures within 72 hours of vaccination	0%	0.39%	0%	0%	0.39%	0.49%	0%	0.39%	0%
Miscellaneous									
Rectal temperature ≥ 40°C (104°F) within 48 hours of vaccination	0.39%	0.78%	3.33%	0%	0.78%	3.43%	0.39%	1.18%	6.99%

[a] n = number of evaluable subjects.

In the Sweden I Efficacy trial, 1 case of whole limb swelling and generalized symptoms, with resolution within 24 hours, was observed following dose 2 of *Daptacel*. No episodes of anaphylaxis or encephalopathy were observed. No seizures were reported within 3 days of vaccination with *Daptacel*. Throughout the entire study period, 6 seizures were reported in the *Daptacel* group, 9 in the DT group, and 3 in the whole-cell pertussis DTP group, for overall rates of 2.3, 3.5, and 1.4 per 1,000 vaccinees, respectively. One case of infantile spasms was reported in the *Daptacel* group. There were no instances of invasive bacterial infection or death.

US studies –

The incidence of redness, tenderness, and swelling at the *Daptacel* injection site increased with the fourth and fifth doses, with the highest rates reported after the fifth dose.

DIPHTHERIA TOXOID/TETANUS TOXOID/ACELLULAR PERTUSSIS VACCINE, ADSORBED (DTaP) — INJECTION

Daptacel Local and Systemic Adverse Reactions in US Studies (0 to 3 Days Postdose) in Children

Adverse reaction	Dose 1[a] (n = 1,390 to 1,406)	Dose 2[a] (n = 1,346 to 1,360)	Dose 3[a] (n = 1,301 to 1,312)	Dose 4[a] (n = 1,118 to 1,144)	Dose 5[a] (n = 473 to 481)
CNS					
Decreased activity/lethargy[b] (any)	51.1%	37.4%	33.2%	25.3%	21%
Decreased activity/lethargy[b] (moderate)	23%	14.4%	12.1%	8.2%	5.8%
Decreased activity/lethargy[b] (severe)	1.2%	1.4%	0.6%	1%	0.8%
Fussiness/Irritability[c] (any)	75.8%	70.7%	67.1%	54.4%	34.9%
Fussiness/Irritability[c] (moderate)	27.7%	25%	22%	16.3%	7.5%
Fussiness/Irritability[c] (severe)	5.6%	5.5%	4.3%	3.9%	0.4%
Inconsolable crying[d] (any)	58.5%	51.4%	47.9%	37.1%	14.1%
Inconsolable crying[d] (moderate)	14.2%	12.6%	10.8%	7.7%	3.5%
Inconsolable crying[d] (severe)	2.2%	3.4%	1.4%	1.5%	0.4%
Local					
Increase in arm circumference[e] > 5 mm	–	–	–	30.1%	38.3%
Increase in arm circumference[e] 20 to 40 mm	–	–	–	7%	14%
Increase in arm circumference[e] > 40 mm	–	–	–	0.4%	1.5%
Interference with normal activity of the arm[f] (any)	–	–	–	–	20.4%
Interference with normal activity of the arm[f] (moderate)	–	–	–	–	5.6%
Interference with normal activity of the arm[f] (severe)	–	–	–	–	0.4%
Redness > 5 mm	6.2%	7.1%	9.6%	17.3%	35.8%
Redness 25 to 50 mm	0.6%	0.5%	1.9%	6.3%	10.4%
Redness > 50 mm	0.4%	0.1%	0%	3.1%	15.8%
Swelling > 5 mm	4%	4%	6.5%	11.7%	23.9%
Swelling 25 to 50 mm	1.2%	0.6%	1%	3.2%	5.8%
Swelling > 50 mm	0.4%	0.1%	0.1%	1.6%	7.7%
Tenderness[g] (any)	48.8%	38.2%	40.9%	49.5%	61.5%
Tenderness[g] (moderate)	16.5%	9.9%	10.6%	12.3%	11.2%
Tenderness[g] (severe)	4.1%	2.3%	1.7%	2.2%	1.7%

Daptacel Local and Systemic Adverse Reactions in US Studies (0 to 3 Days Postdose) in Children

Adverse reaction	Dose 1[a] (n = 1,390 to 1,406)	Dose 2[a] (n = 1,346 to 1,360)	Dose 3[a] (n = 1,301 to 1,312)	Dose 4[a] (n = 1,118 to 1,144)	Dose 5[a] (n = 473 to 481)
Miscellaneous					
Fever[h] ≥ 38°C (100.4°F)	9.3%	16.1%	15.8%	10.5%	6.1%
Fever[h] > 38.5° to 39.5°C (101.3° to 103.1°F)	1.5%	3.9%	4.8%	2.7%	2.1%
Fever[h] > 39.5°C (103.1°F)	0.1%	0.4%	0.3%	0.7%	0.2%

[a] In 1 US study, children received 4 doses of *Daptacel*. A nonrandom subset of these children received a fifth dose of *Daptacel* in a subsequent study.

[b] Dose 1 to 4: moderate = interferes with and limits daily activity, less interactive; severe = disabling (not interested in usual daily activity, subject cannot be coaxed to interact with caregiver). Dose 5: moderate = interfered with activities, but did not require medical care or absenteeism; severe = incapacitating, unable to perform usual activities, may have/or required medical care or absenteeism.

[c] Doses 1 to 4: moderate = irritability for 1 to 3 hours; severe = irritability for more than 3 hours. Dose 5: moderate = interfered with activities, but did not require medical care or absenteeism; severe = incapacitating, unable to perform usual activities, may have/or required medical care or absenteeism.

[d] Doses 1 to 4: moderate = 1 to 3 hours inconsolable crying; severe = more than 3 hours inconsolable crying. Dose 5: moderate = interfered with activities, but did not require medical care or absenteeism; severe = incapacitating, unable to perform usual activities, may have/or required medical care or absenteeism.

[e] The circumference of the *Daptacel*-injected arm at the level of the axilla was monitored following the fourth and fifth doses only. Increase in arm circumference was calculated by subtracting the baseline circumference prevaccination (day 0) from the circumference postvaccination.

[f] Moderate = decreased use of arm, but did not require medical care or absenteeism; severe = incapacitating, refusal to move arm, may have/or required medical care or absenteeism.

[g] Doses 1 to 4: moderate = subject cries when site is touched; severe = subject cries when leg or arm is moved. Dose 5: moderate = interfered with activities, but did not require medical care or absenteeism; severe = incapacitating, unable to perform usual activities, may have/or required medical care or absenteeism.

[h] For doses 1 to 3, 53.7% of temperatures were measured rectally, 45.1% were measured axillary, 1% were measured orally, and 0.1% were measured by an unspecified route. For dose 4, 35.7% were measured rectally, 62.3% were measured axillary, 1.5% were measured orally, and 0.5% were measured by an unspecified route. For dose 5, 0.2% of temperatures were measured rectally, 11.3% were measured axillary, and 88.4% were measured orally. Fever is based upon actual temperatures recorded with no adjustments to the measurement for route.

In the US study in which children received 4 doses of *Daptacel*, 1,454 subjects received *Daptacel*, of which, 5 (0.3%) subjects experienced a seizure within 60 days following any dose of *Daptacel*. One seizure occurred within 7 days postvaccination: an infant who experienced an afebrile seizure with apnea on the day of the first vaccination. Three other cases of seizures occurred between 8 and 30 days postvaccination. Of the seizures that occurred within 60 days postvaccination, 3 were associated with fever. In this study, there were no reported cases of hypotensive-hyporesponsive episodes following *Daptacel*. There was 1 death caused by aspiration 222 days postvaccination in a subject with ependymoma. Within 30 days following any dose of *Daptacel*, 57 (3.9%) subjects reported at least 1 serious adverse reaction. During this period, the most frequently reported serious adverse reaction was bronchiolitis, reported in 28 (1.9%) subjects. Other serious adverse reactions that occurred within 30 days following *Daptacel* include 3 cases of pneumonia, 2 cases of meningitis, and 1 case each of sepsis, pertussis (postdose 1), irritability, and unresponsiveness.

In the fifth dose study of *Daptacel* vaccine in the United States, within 30 days following the fifth dose consecutive dose of *Daptacel*, 1 (0.2%) subject reported 2 serious adverse reactions (bronchospasm and hypoxia).

Postmarketing (Daptacel) –

CNS: Febrile convulsion, grand mal convulsion, hypotonic-hyporesponsive episodes, hypotonia, partial seizures, screaming, somnolence.

GI: Diarrhea, nausea.

Hypersensitivity: Allergic reaction, anaphylactic reaction (edema, face edema, face swelling, generalized rash, pruritus), hypersensitivity, rash (erythematous, macular, maculopapular).

Local: Extensive swelling of injected limb (including swelling that involves adjacent joints), injection-site abscess, injection-site cellulitis, injection-site mass, injection-site nodule, injection-site pain, injection-site rash.

Miscellaneous: Cellulitis, cyanosis.

DIPHTHERIA TOXOID/TETANUS TOXOID/ ACELLULAR PERTUSSIS VACCINE, ADSORBED (DTaP) — INJECTION

➤*Infanrix*:

***Infanrix* Adverse Reactions (Within 4 Days of Vaccination) When Given Concomitantly With Other Vaccines[a] (Modified Intent-to-Treat Cohort)[b]**

Adverse reaction	*Infanrix*, hepatitis B (recombinant), IPV, Hib, and PCV7		
	Dose 1	Dose 2	Dose 3
CNS	(n = 335)[c]	(n = 323)[c]	(n = 315)[c]
Drowsiness, any	54%	48.3%	38.4%
Drowsiness, grade 2[d] or 3[e]	17.6%	12.4%	11.1%
Drowsiness, grade 3[e]	3.6%	0.6%	1.9%
Irritability/Fussiness, any	61.5%	61.6%	56.5%
Irritability/Fussiness, grade 2[d] or 3[e]	19.4%	21.1%	19.4%
Irritability/Fussiness, grade 3[e]	3.9%	3.4%	3.2%
GI	(n = 335)[c]	(n = 323)[c]	(n = 315)[c]
Loss of appetite, any	27.8%	26.6%	23.8%
Loss of appetite, grade 2[d] or 3[e]	5.1%	3.4%	5.4%
Loss of appetite, grade 3[e]	0.6%	0.3%	0%
Local[f]	(n = 335)[c]	(n = 323)[c]	(n = 315)[c]
Pain, any	31.9%	30%	29.8%
Pain, grade 2[d] or 3[e]	9%	8.7%	8.9%
Pain, grade 3[e]	2.7%	1.5%	1.3%
Redness, any	18.2%	32.8%	39%
Redness, > 20 mm	0.3%	0%	1.9%
Swelling, any	9.6%	20.4%	24.8%
Swelling, > 20 mm	0.6%	0%	1.3%
Miscellaneous	(n = 333)[g]	(n = 321)[g]	(n = 311)[g]
Fever ≥ 38°C (100.4°F)[h]	19.8%	30.2%	23.8%
Fever > 38.5°C (101.3°F)[h]	4.5%	9.7%	5.8%
Fever > 39°C (102.2°F)[h]	0.3%	3.1%	2.3%
Fever > 39.5°C (103.1°F)[h]	0%	0.3%	0.3%

[a] Within 4 days of vaccination, defined as day of vaccination and the next 3 days.
[b] Modified intent-to-treat (ITT) cohort = all vaccinated subjects for whom safety data were obtained.
[c] Number of infants for whom at least 1 symptom sheet was completed.
[d] Grade 2: pain, defined as cried/protested on touch; drowsiness, defined as interfered with normal daily activities; irritability/fussiness, defined as crying more than usual/interfered with normal daily activities; loss of appetite, defined as eating less than usual/interfered with normal daily activities.
[e] Grade 3: pain, defined as cried when limb was moved/spontaneously painful; drowsiness, defined as prevented normal daily activities; irritability/fussiness, defined as crying that could not be comforted/prevented normal daily activities; loss of appetite, defined as not eating at all.
[f] Local reactions at the injection site for *Infanrix*.
[g] Number of infants for whom at least 1 symptom sheet was completed; for fever, numbers exclude missing temperature recordings or tympanic measurements.
[h] Rectal temperatures or axillary temperatures increased by 1°C to derive equivalent rectal temperature.

***Infanrix* Adverse Reactions Within 4 Days of Vaccination With a Fourth Consecutive Dose [a] (Total Vaccinated Cohort)**

Adverse reaction	Group primed with *Infanrix*[b] (n = 247)	Group primed with *Pediarix*[c] (n = 553)
CNS		
Drowsiness, any	35.6%	31.3%
Drowsiness, grade 2[d] or 3[e]	9.3%	6.7%
Drowsiness, grade 3[e]	2.4%	1.3%
Irritability, any	52.2%	53.9%
Irritability, grade 2[d] or 3[e]	18.2%	19.7%
Irritability, grade 3[e]	3.2%	1.4%
GI		
Loss of appetite, any	24.7%	23.3%
Loss of appetite, grade 2[d] or 3[e]	5.3%	4.9%
Loss of appetite, grade 3[e]	2.4%	0.5%
Local[f]		
Increase in mid-thigh circumference, any	33.2%	26.2%
Increase in mid-thigh circumference, > 40 mm	0%	1.3%
Pain, any	44.5%	48.3%
Pain, grade 2[d] or 3[e]	19%	18.6%
Pain, grade 3[e]	3.6%	3.4%
Redness, any	48.2%	49.9%
Redness, > 20 mm	6.1%	6%
Swelling, any	32.8%	32.7%
Swelling, > 20 mm	3.6%	5.2%
Miscellaneous		
Fever >37.5°C (99.5°F)[g]	8.9%	15.4%
Fever > 38°C (100.4°F)[g]	4.5%	6.7%
Fever > 38.5°C (101.3°F)[g]	2%	2%

[a] Within 4 days of vaccination, defined as day of vaccination and the next 3 days.
[b] Received *Infanrix*, hepatitis B vaccine, IPV, PCV7 vaccine, and Hib conjugate vaccine at 2, 4, and 6 months of age.
[c] Received *Pediarix*, PCV7 vaccine, and Hib conjugate vaccine at 2, 4, and 6 months of age or PCV7 vaccine within 2 weeks later.
[d] Grade 2: pain, defined as cried/protested on touch; drowsiness, defined as interfered with normal daily activities; irritability, defined as crying more than usual/interfered with normal daily activities; loss of appetite, defined as eating less than usual/no effect on normal daily activities.
[e] Grade 3: pain, defined as cried when limb was moved/spontaneously painful; drowsiness, defined as prevented normal daily activities; irritability, defined as crying that could not be comforted/prevented normal daily activities; loss of appetite, defined as eating less than usual/interfered with normal daily activities.
[f] Local reactions at the injection site for *Infanrix*.
[g] Axillary temperatures.

***Infanrix* Adverse Reactions (Within 4 Days of Vaccination) With a Fifth Consecutive Dose When Given Concomitantly With Other Vaccines[a,b] (Total Vaccinated Cohort)**

Adverse reaction	Children with evaluable data
CNS	n = 993 to 1,036
Drowsiness, any	17.5%
Drowsiness, grade 3[c]	0.8%
GI	n = 993 to 1,036
Loss of appetite, any	16%
Loss of appetite, grade 3[d]	0.6%
Local[e]	n = 1,039 to 1,043
Arm circumference increase, any	38.1%
Arm circumference increase, > 20 mm	7.4%
Arm circumference increase, > 30 mm	3.2%
Pain, any	53.3%
Pain, grade 2 or 3[f]	12%
Pain, grade 3[f]	0.6%
Redness, any	36.6%
Redness, ≥ 50 mm	20%
Redness, ≥ 110 mm	4.1%
Swelling, any	27%
Swelling, ≥ 50 mm	11.5%
Swelling, ≥ 110 mm	1.8%
Miscellaneous	n = 993 to 1,036
Fever ≥ 37.5°C (99.5°F)	14.8%
Fever > 38°C (100.4°F)	4.4%
Fever > 39°C (102.2°F)	1.1%
Fever > 40°C (104°F)	0%

[a] Within 4 days of vaccination, defined as day of vaccination and the next 3 days.
[b] Coadministered with a fourth dose of IPV and a second dose of MMR vaccine.
[c] Grade 3, defined as preventing normal daily activities.
[d] Grade 3, defined as not eating at all.
[e] Local reactions at the injection site for *Infanrix*.
[f] Grade 2, defined as painful when limb was moved; grade 3, defined as preventing normal daily activities.

In the US booster immunization studies in which *Infanrix* was administered as the fourth or fifth dose in the DTaP series following previous doses with *Infanrix* or *Pediarix*, large swelling reactions of the limb injected with *Infanrix* were assessed.

In the fourth dose study, a large swelling reaction was defined as injection-site swelling with a diameter more than 50 mm, a more than 50 mm increase in the mid-thigh circumference compared with the prevaccination measurement, and/or any diffuse swelling that interfered with or prevented daily activities. The overall incidence of large swelling reactions occurring within 4 days (day 0 to 3) following *Infanrix* was 2.3%.

DIPHTHERIA TOXOID/TETANUS TOXOID/ ACELLULAR PERTUSSIS VACCINE, ADSORBED (DTaP) — INJECTION

In the fifth dose study, a large swelling reaction was defined as swelling that involved more than 50% of the injected upper arm length and that was associated with a more than 30 mm increase in mid-upper arm circumference within 4 days following vaccination. The incidence of large swelling reactions following the fifth consecutive dose of *Infanrix* was 1%.

***Infanrix* Adverse Reactions Compared With Whole-Cell DTP Vaccine**

Adverse reaction	*Infanrix* (n = 13,761 doses)		Whole-cell DTP vaccine (n = 13,520 doses)	
	Number	Rate per 1,000 doses	Number	Rate per 1,000 doses
Fever ≥ 40°C (104°F)[a,b]	5	0.36	32	2.4
Hypotonic-hyporesponsive episode[c]	0	0	9	0.67
Persistent crying ≥ 3 hours[a]	6	0.44	54	4
Seizures[d]	1[e]	0.07	3[f]	0.22

[a] $P < 0.001$.
[b] Rectal temperatures.
[c] $P = 0.002$.
[d] Not statistically significant at $P < 0.05$.
[e] Maximum rectal temperature within 72 hours of vaccination = 39.5°C (103.1°F).
[f] Maximum rectal temperature within 72 hours of vaccination = 37.5°C (99.5°F), 38.5°C (101.3°F), and 39°C (102.2°F).

Postmarketing (Infanrix) –

CNS: Encephalopathy, hypotonia.
Dermatologic: Erythema, pruritus, rash, urticaria.
Hematologic/Lymphatic: Lymphadenopathy, thrombocytopenia.
Hypersensitivity: Anaphylactic reaction, hypersensitivity.
Miscellaneous: Cellulitis, cyanosis, ear pain, injection-site reactions, respiratory tract infection, sudden infant death syndrome.

➤*Tripedia*:

***Tripedia* Adverse Reactions (Within 72 Hours Postvaccination) in Infants 2 to 6 Months of Age**

Adverse reaction[a]	*Tripedia* vaccine reaction Dose 1 (n = 505)	Dose 2 (n = 499)	Dose 3 (n = 490)	Whole-cell pertussis DTP vaccine reaction Dose 1 (n = 167)	Dose 2 (n = 159)	Dose 3 (n = 152)
CNS						
Drowsiness[b]	39.4%	17.6%	15.9%	59.6%	45.2%	25.5%
High-pitched cry	2.4%	1%	1.4%	10.8%	5.8%	3.4%
Irritability[b]	35.3%	30.1%	27.1%	72.9%	71.8%	57.7%
Persistent cry	0.2%	0.2%	0.8%	3%	1.3%	2%
GI						
Anorexia[b]	6%	5.3%	5.7%	26.5%	20%	18.8%
Vomiting	6%[c]	5.5%	3.7%	10.8%	7.1%	2.7%
Local						
Erythema[b]	9%	9.8%	16.9%	28.3%	32.9%	32.9%
Erythema > 1 in[b]	1.2%	1.8%	2.2%	7.8%	8.4%	7.4%
Swelling[b]	6.4%	4.5%	6.5%	28.3%	23.9%	27.5%
Swelling > 1 in[b]	1.4%	0.6%	1%	12.7%	11%	11.4%
Tenderness[b]	11.8%	6.7%	7.1%	50.6%	44.2%	42.6%
Miscellaneous						
Fever (> 38.3°C [101°F]) (rectal)[b]	0.4%	1.6%	3.5%	3.6%	7.5%	11.2%

[a] For certain adverse reactions, information was not available for a small number of infants.
[b] $P < 0.01$ when compared with whole-cell DTP vaccine for all doses.
[c] $P < 0.05$ when compared with whole-cell DTP vaccine.

***Tripedia* Adverse Reactions in Infants Following Any of the First 3 Doses**

Adverse reaction	*Tripedia* (n = 135)	Whole-cell pertussis DTP vaccine (n = 371)
CNS		
Drowsiness	41.5%[a]	62%
Fussiness[b]	19.3%[a]	41.5%
GI		
Anorexia	22.2%[a]	35%
Vomiting	7.4%	13.7%
Local		
Erythema	32.6%[a]	72.7%
Pain[c]	9.6%[a]	40.2%
Swelling	20%[a]	60.9%
Miscellaneous		
Fever > 38.3°C (101°F)[d]	5.2%[a]	15.9%

[a] $P < 0.01$ when compared with whole-cell DTP vaccine.
[b] Moderate or severe = prolonged or persistent crying that could not be comforted and refusal to play.
[c] Moderate or severe = cried or protested to touch or when leg moved.
[d] Rectal temperatures.

***Tripedia* Adverse Reactions[a] When Administered for All Doses**

Adverse reaction	Primary (n = 135 infants) Dose 1 (2 months of age)	Dose 2 (4 months of age)	Dose 3 (6 months of age)	Booster Dose 4 (15 to 20 months of age (n = 82)	Dose 5 (4 to 6 years of age (n = 18)
CNS					
Drowsiness	28.9%	17.9%	4.6%	6.1%	5.6%
Irritability[b]	8.1%	7.4%	7.6%	3.7%	0%
GI					
Anorexia	8.1%	9.7%	9.9%	8.5%	0%
Vomiting	5.2%	1.5%	2.3%	2.4%	0%
Local					
Pain[c]	8.1%	3.7%	2.3%	7.3%	11.1%
Redness					
Any	12.6%	12.7%	19.1%	17.1%	33.3%
> 20 mm	2.2%	0%	3.8%	NA[de]	22.2%[e]
Swelling					
Any	8.8%	8.2%	10.7%	15.9%	27.8%
> 20 mm	0.7%	0.7%	3.1%	NA[e]	16.7%[e]
Miscellaneous					
Fever (> 38.3°C [101°F][f])	0.7%	1.4%	3.1%	2.4%	5.6%

[a] Occurring within 72 hours postvaccination.
[b] Moderate or severe = prolonged or persistent crying that could not be comforted and refusal to play.
[c] Moderate or severe = cried or protested to touch or when limb moved.
[d] NA = not applicable.
[e] Following dose 4, percent redness or swelling more than 20 mm was not available; following dose 4, 1.2% of subjects had redness more than 50 mm and 3.8% had swelling more than 50 mm. Following dose 5, 5.6% of children had redness more than 50 mm, and none had swelling that exceeded 50 mm.
[f] Rectal temperatures for primary series, oral temperatures for doses 4 and 5. Dose 5 reported as at least 38.3°C (100.1°F).

***Tripedia* Adverse Reactions (Within 3 Days Postvaccination) in Children 15 to 18 Months of Age**

Adverse reaction	*Tripedia*[a] fourth dose (n = 1,010)
CNS	
Irritability	250/1,005 (24.9%)
Persistent crying > 3 hours	8/1,005 (0.8%)
Local	
Any reaction	481/1,008 (47.7%)
Pain	214/1,002 (21.4%)
Redness	
Any size	390/1,007 (38.7%)
< 2.5 cm	257/1,007 (25.5%)
> 2.5 cm	133/1,002 (13.3%)
Swelling, any size	218/1,004 (21.7%)
Miscellaneous	
Loss of appetite	146/1,003 (14.6%)
Temperature (> 38°C [100.4°F])[b]	242/968 (25%)

[a] Subset of 12,514 subjects who received 3 doses of *Tripedia* in a German case-control study of vaccine efficacy.
[b] Temperatures measured orally.

DIPHTHERIA TOXOID/TETANUS TOXOID/ ACELLULAR PERTUSSIS VACCINE, ADSORBED (DTaP) — INJECTION

Tripedia Adverse Reactions (Within 72 Hours Postvaccination) in Children 15 to 20 Months of Age[a]

Adverse reaction	Tripedia primed (n = 109)	Whole-cell pertussis DTP vaccine primed (n = 30)
Local		
Erythema ≥ 1 inch	30.3%	23.3%
Pain	19.3%	10.3%
Swelling ≥ 1 inch	29.4%	20%
Miscellaneous		
Irritability	19.3%	13.3%
Temperature (≥ 38.3°C [101°F])[b]	5.5%	3.3%

[a] Children had received 3 previous doses of *Tripedia* or 3 doses of whole-cell pertussis DTP vaccine.
[b] Temperatures measured rectally.

The frequency of adverse reactions following a fifth consecutive dose of *Tripedia* administered to German children 4 to 6 years of age is shown in the following table. This fifth dose study was an open-label study that enrolled 580 subjects from 24 sites. These subjects were recruited from subjects who had participated in the case-control study of the efficacy of *Tripedia* in which more than 12,000 infants received 3 doses of *Tripedia*. In the fifth dose study, information on systemic and local reactions was collected on diary forms for 3 days following vaccination for all subjects and for 14 days following vaccination for a subset of 241 subjects. For 490 subjects, the actual sizes of local reactions more than 5 cm, as measured by the parents, were also documented on the diary forms. Local reactions, including those measured as at least 11 cm, typically had an onset within the first 3 days after vaccination and generally resolved within 5 days. Three subjects had a local reaction that lasted more than 21 days, 1 subject had swelling for 25 days, 1 subject had redness for 26 days, and 1 subject had redness for 28 days. Twenty-eight of 580 (4.8%) subjects had redness or swelling that led to a medical visit. There were no reported permanent sequelae associated with any local reactions. Thirty-two of 490 (6.5%) subjects had swelling reported as at least 11 cm, including 14 (2.9%) subjects who reported swelling of the entire upper arm. Swelling of the entire upper arm was not specifically solicited. Of 32 subjects with swelling reported as at least 11 cm, 19 also reported pain, 30 had redness, and 2 had fever more than 38°C (100.4°F). All cases of swelling 11 cm or more resolved spontaneously without treatment, except for a few subjects who were treated with cool packs. The subjects in the fifth dose study are not necessarily a subset of the 1,010 German children for whom safety data following the fourth dose of *Tripedia* are available. However, children in both the fourth and fifth dose studies were recruited from subjects who had participated in the German case-control study. Available data from these studies suggest an increased frequency and severity of local reactions following the fifth successive dose of *Tripedia* compared with the fourth dose. Additional safety data in 96 US children who received a fifth dose of *Tripedia* following 4 previous doses of *Tripedia* or *TriHIBit* also demonstrated an increase in the frequency and severity of local reactions following the fifth dose, compared with the first 3 doses.

Tripedia Adverse Reactions (Within 72 Hours Postvaccination) Following a Fifth Dose in Children 4 to 6 Years of Age[a,b]

Adverse reaction	Tripedia[c] (n = 490 to 580)
CNS	
Drowsiness	15.5%
Fussiness[d]	5.9%
GI	
Loss of appetite	7.3%
Vomiting	2.2%
Local	
Pain/Tenderness[e]	20.5%
Redness (any)	59.8%
Redness > 5 cm	31%
Redness ≥ 11 cm	6.1%
Swelling (any)	61.4%
Swelling > 5 cm	25%
Swelling ≥ 11 cm	6.5%
Miscellaneous	
Fever (> 38°C [100.4°F])[f]	3.8%

[a] Note: 1 child was a protocol violation because he had received 4 doses of whole-cell DTP vaccine previously.
[b] These subjects are a subset of 12,514 subjects who had received the first 3 doses of *Tripedia* in the German case-control study of vaccine efficacy.
[c] Redness ≥ 11 cm and swelling ≥ 11 cm available for 490 subjects; information on other reactions was available for 580 subjects.
[d] Moderate or severe = prolonged irritability, occasional crying, and refusal to play or prolonged irritability, frequent crying, and bed rest.
[e] Moderate or severe = crying or protesting to touch or crying when arm moved.
[f] Temperatures measured orally.

Tripedia Adverse Reactions (Within 72 Hours Postvaccination) When Given at 15 to 20 Months of Age and 4 to 6 Years of Age[a]

Adverse reaction	3 previous whole-cell pertussis DTP vaccine doses at 15 to 20 months of age (n = 372)	4 previous whole-cell pertussis DTP vaccine doses at 4 to 6 years of age (n = 240)
CNS		
Drowsiness	12.4%	15%
High-pitched, unusual cry	1.1%	NA[b]
Irritability	21.2%	15.8%
GI		
Anorexia	7.8%	5.4%
Diarrhea	6.3%	0.8%
Vomiting	2.2%	1.7%
Local		
Erythema[c]	18.3%	31.3%
Swelling[d]	10.8%	27.9%
Tenderness	14.2%	46.2%
Miscellaneous		
Fever (> 38.3°C [101°F])[e]	4.7%	4.8%

[a] Children had received 3 or 4 doses of whole-cell pertussis DTP vaccine.
[b] NA = data not collected in this age group.
[c] Includes all occurrences of erythema.
[d] Includes all occurrences of swelling.
[e] Temperatures measured rectally for children 15 to 20 months of age and measured orally for children 4 to 6 years of age.

Tripedia Moderately Severe Adverse Reactions (Within 48 Hours Postvaccination) When Given at 2, 4, or 6 Months of Age (N = 7,102 Doses)

Adverse reactions	Number	Rate per 1,000 doses
CNS		
Convulsions[a]	0	0
Hypotonic-hyporesponsive episode	1	0.14
Persistent cry ≥ 3 hours	4	0.56
Miscellaneous		
Fever (≥ 40.5°C [105°F])	2	0.28

[a] One seizure episode was noted between 48 and 72 hours.

In the German case-control efficacy study that enrolled 16,780 infants (12,514 of whom received 41,615 doses of *Tripedia*), hospitalization rates and death rates were similar between *Tripedia* and DT vaccine recipients. Adverse reactions were monitored by spontaneous reporting by parents and a medical history obtained at each subsequent vaccination. Adverse reactions (rates per 1,000 doses) occurring within 7 days following vaccination with *Tripedia* included the following: unusual cry (0.96), persistent cry more than 3 hours (0.12), febrile seizure (0.05), afebrile seizure (0.02), and hypotonic-hyporesponsive episodes (0.05).

In the German case-control study and US open-label safety study in which 14,971 infants received *Tripedia*, 13 deaths in *Tripedia* recipients were reported. Causes of death included 7 cases of sudden infant death syndrome (SIDS), and 1 of each of the following: accidental drowning, adrenogenital syndrome, cardiac arrest, enteritis, Leigh syndrome, and motor vehicle accident. All of these events occurred more than 2 weeks past immunization. The rate of SIDS observed in the German case-control study was 0.4 per

DIPHTHERIA TOXOID/TETANUS TOXOID/ ACELLULAR PERTUSSIS VACCINE, ADSORBED (DTaP) — INJECTION

1,000 vaccinated infants. The rate of SIDS observed in the US open-label safety study was 0.8 per 1,000 vaccinated infants, and the reported rate of SIDS in the US from 1985 to 1991 was 1.5 per 1,000 live births. By chance alone, some cases of SIDS can be expected to follow receipt of whole-cell DTP or DTaP vaccines.

Postmarketing (Tripedia) – Anaphylactic reaction, apnea, autism, cellulitis, convulsion/tonic-clonic convulsion, encephalopathy, hypotonia, idiopathic thrombocytopenic purpura, neuropathy, SIDS, and somnolence.

➤*Additional adverse reactions:* As with other aluminum-containing vaccines, a nodule may be palpable at the injection sites for several weeks. Sterile abscess formation at the site of injection has been reported.

Rarely, an anaphylactic reaction (eg, hives, swelling of the mouth, difficulty breathing, hypotension, shock) has been reported after receiving preparations containing diphtheria, tetanus, and/or pertussis antigens.

Arthus-type hypersensitivity reactions, characterized by severe local reactions (generally starting 2 to 8 hours after an injection), may follow receipt of tetanus toxoid.

A few cases of peripheral mononeuropathy and of cranial mononeuropathy have been reported following tetanus toxoid administration, although available evidence is inadequate to accept or reject a causal relation.

A review by the IOM found evidence for a causal relationship between tetanus toxoid and both brachial neuritis and Guillain-Barré syndrome.

Patient Information

DTaP is used to immunize children 6 weeks to 7 years of age (before the seventh birthday) against diphtheria, tetanus, and pertussis (whooping cough). Do not use to treat diphtheria or tetanus or to vaccinate persons older than 7 years of age.

Inform the parent or guardian of the importance of completing the pertussis immunization series, unless a contraindication to further immunization exists.

Inform patients, parents, or guardians of the potential benefits and risks of the vaccine. It is important to question the vaccine recipient, parent, or guardian concerning occurrence of any symptoms and/or signs of an adverse reaction after a previous dose of a DTaP vaccine. Inform the patients, parents, or guardians about the potential for adverse reactions that have been temporally associated with administration of DTaP, Tdap, or other vaccines containing similar components. Tell the patient or parent or guardian accompanying the recipient to report severe or unusual adverse reactions to the health care provider or clinic where the vaccine was administered.

Give the patient, parent, or guardian the vaccine information statements, which are required by the National Childhood Vaccine Injury Act of 1986 to be given prior to immunization. These materials are available free of charge at the CDC Web site (http://www.cdc.gov/vaccines/).

Advise the parent or guardian to contact a health care provider at once if the vaccine recipient develops the following signs of encephalopathy within 7 days of receiving a vaccination: changes in alertness, unresponsiveness, seizure activity.

Advise the parent or guardian to contact a health care provider at once if the vaccine recipient develops a fever of 40.5°C (105°F) or more, faints, persistently cries for more than 3 hours within 48 hours of receiving this vaccine, or has a seizure with or without fever within 3 days of receiving this vaccine.

Controlling fever is especially important for children who have had seizures for any reason. Reduce fever by giving the child an aspirin-free pain reliever when the vaccine is given and for the next 24 hours, following the package instructions.

DIPHTHERIA AND TETANUS TOXOIDS AND ACELLULAR PERTUSSIS ADSORBED, HEPATITIS B (RECOMBINANT) AND INACTIVATED POLIOVIRUS VACCINE COMBINED

Rx	**Pediarix** (GlaxoSmithKline)	**Injection, suspension:** diphtheria toxoid 25 Lf, tetanus toxoid 10 Lf, inactivated pertussis toxin (PT) 25 mcg, filamentous hemagglutinin (FHA) 25 mcg, pertactin 8 mcg, hepatitis B surface antigen (HBsAg) 10 mcg, type 1 poliovirus 40 D-antigen units, type 2 poliovirus 8 D-antigen units, and type 3 poliovirus 32 D-antigen units per 0.5 mL.[a]	Preservative free. ≤ 5% yeast protein. In single-dose 0.5 mL vials and prefilled *Tip-Lok* syringes (without needles).

[a] Each 0.5 mL dose also contains sodium chloride 4.5 mg and aluminum adjuvant (≤ 0.85 mg aluminum by assay). Each dose also contains residual formaldehyde 100 mcg or less and polysorbate 80 (*Tween 80*) 100 mcg or less. In addition, neomycin 0.05 ng or less and polymyxin B 0.01 ng or less may be present.

DIPHTHERIA AND TETANUS TOXOIDS AND ACELLULAR PERTUSSIS ADSORBED, HEPATITIS B (RECOMBINANT) AND INACTIVATED POLIOVIRUS VACCINE COMBINED — INJECTION

For complete and comparative prescribing information, refer to the Diphtheria and Tetanus Toxoids and Acellular Pertussis Vaccine, Hepatitis B Recombinant Vaccine, and Poliovirus Inactivated Vaccine monographs. For additional information, also refer to the Agents for Active Immunization introduction.

Indications

➤*Immunization:* For active immunization against diphtheria, tetanus, pertussis(whooping cough), all known subtypes of hepatitis B virus, and poliomyelitis caused by poliovirus types 1, 2, and 3 as a 3-dose primary series in infants born of HBsAg-negative mothers, beginning as early as 6 weeks of age.

Administration and Dosage

➤*General dosing considerations:* It is recommended that *Pediarix* be given for all 3 doses because data are limited regarding the safety and efficacy of using diphtheria, tetanus toxoids, and acellular pertussis (DTaP) vaccines from different manufacturers for successive doses of the pertussis vaccination series. *Pediarix* is not recommended for completion of the first 3 doses of the DTaP vaccination series initiated with a DTaP vaccine from a different manufacturer because no data are available regarding the safety or efficacy of using such a regimen.

Pediarix may be used to complete a hepatitis B vaccination series initiated with a licensed hepatitis B vaccine (recombinant) from a different manufacturer.

Pediarix may be used to complete the first 3 doses of the inactivated poliovirus vaccine (IPV) vaccination series initiated with IPV from a different manufacturer.

➤*Children:*

Immunization –

6 weeks of age to 6 years of age:

• *Usual dosage* – 3 doses of 0.5 mL intramuscularly (IM) at 6- to 8-week intervals (preferably 8 weeks).

➤*HBsAg maternal status:* Infants born of HBsAg-positive mothers should receive hepatitis B immune globulin and hepatitis B vaccine (recombinant) within 12 hours of birth at separate sites and should complete the hepatitis B vaccination series according to a particular schedule. Infants born of mothers of unknown HBsAg status should receive hepatitis B vaccine (recombinant) within 12 hours of birth and should complete the hepatitis B vaccination series according to a particular schedule.

➤*Previously vaccinated children:*

Hepatitis B vaccine – Infants born of HBsAg-negative mothers and who received a dose of hepatitis B vaccine at or shortly after birth may be administered 3 doses of *Pediarix* according to the recommended schedule. However, data are limited regarding the safety of *Pediarix* in these infants. There are no data to support the use of a 3-dose series of *Pediarix* in infants who have previously received more than 1 dose of hepatitis B vaccine. *Pediarix* may be used to complete a hepatitis B vaccination series in infants who have received 1 or more doses of hepatitis B vaccine (recombinant) and who are also scheduled to receive the other vaccine components of *Pediarix*. However, the safety and efficacy of *Pediarix* in these infants have not been studied.

Infanrix – *Pediarix* may be used to complete the first 3 doses of the DTaP series in infants who have received 1 or 2 doses of *Infanrix* and also are scheduled to receive the other vaccine components of *Pediarix*. However, the safety and efficacy of *Pediarix* in these infants have not been studied.

Inactivated poliovirus vaccine – *Pediarix* may be used to complete the first 3 doses of the IPV series in infants who have received 1 or 2 doses of IPV and also are scheduled to receive the other vaccine components of *Pediarix*. However, the safety and efficacy of *Pediarix* in these infants have not been studied.

➤*Preparation for administration:* *Pediarix* contains an adjuvant; therefore, shake vigorously to obtain a homogeneous, turbid, white suspension. Do not use if resuspension does not occur with vigorous shaking.

➤*Administration:* Administer by IM injection. Do not administer this product subcutaneously, intravenously, or intradermally. Take special care to prevent injection into a blood vessel. The preferred administration site is the anterolateral aspects of the thigh for children younger than 1 year of age. In older children, the deltoid muscle is usually large enough for an IM injection. The vaccine should not be injected into the gluteal area or areas where there may be a major nerve trunk. Gluteal injections may result in suboptimal hepatitis B immune response.

When coadministration of other vaccines is required, they should be given with separate syringes and at different injection sites.

➤*Admixture compatibility:* Do not mix with any other vaccine in the same syringe or vial.

➤*Storage/Stability:* Refrigerate between 2° and 8°C (36° and 46°F). Do not freeze. Discard if the vaccine has been frozen. Discard any vaccine remaining in the vial after administration.

Actions

➤*Pharmacology:*

Diphtheria – Diphtheria is an acute toxin-mediated infectious disease caused by toxigenic strains of *Corynebacterium diphtheriae*. Diphtheria in the US has been controlled through the use of diphtheria toxoid–containing vaccines. Protection against disease is due to the development of 2 neutralizing antibodies to the diphtheria toxin. Following adequate immunization with diphtheria toxoid, protection lasts for at least 10 years. A serum diphtheria antitoxin level of 0.01 units/mL is the lowest level giving some degree of protection; a level of 0.1 units/mL is regarded as protective. Levels of 1 unit/mL are associated with long-term protection. Immunization with diph-

DIPHTHERIA AND TETANUS TOXOIDS AND ACELLULAR PERTUSSIS ADSORBED, HEPATITIS B (RECOMBINANT) AND INACTIVATED POLIOVIRUS VACCINE COMBINED — INJECTION

theria toxoid does not, however, eliminate carriage of *C. diphtheriae* in the pharynx or nares or on the skin.

Tetanus – Tetanus is a condition manifested primarily by neuromuscular dysfunction caused by a potent exotoxin released by *Clostridium tetani*. Spores of *C. tetani* are ubiquitous. Naturally acquired immunity to tetanus toxin does not occur. Thus, universal primary immunization and timed booster doses to maintain adequate tetanus antitoxin levels are necessary to protect all age groups. Protection against disease is due to the development of neutralizing antibodies to the tetanus toxin. A serum tetanus antitoxin level of at least 0.01 unit/mL measured by neutralization assays is considered the minimum protective level. A level of at least 0.1 to 0.2 units/mL has been considered protective. Following immunization, protection lasts for at least 10 years.

Pertussis – Pertussis (whooping cough) is a disease of the respiratory tract caused by *Bordetella pertussis*. The role of the different components produced by *B. pertussis* in either the pathogenesis of, or the immunity to, pertussis is not well understood.

Hepatitis B – Infection with hepatitis B virus can have serious consequences, including acute massive hepatic necrosis and chronic active hepatitis. Chronically infected people are at increased risk for cirrhosis and hepatocellular carcinoma. According to the Centers for Disease Control and Prevention (CDC), the hepatitis B vaccine is recognized as an anticancer vaccine because it can prevent primary liver cancer. In a Taiwanese study, the institution of universal childhood immunization against hepatitis B virus has been shown to decrease the incidence of hepatocellular carcinoma among children. In a Korean study in adult men, vaccination against the hepatitis B virus has been shown to decrease the incidence and risk of developing hepatocellular carcinoma in adults. Antibody concentrations of 10 milliunits/mL or more against HBsAg are recognized as conferring protection against hepatitis B.

Poliomyelitis – Poliovirus is an enterovirus that belongs to the picornavirus family. Three serotypes of poliovirus have been identified (types 1, 2, and 3). Whereas poliovirus infections are usually asymptomatic or cause nonspecific symptoms, up to 2% of infected people have CNS involvement and develop paralytic disease. IPV induces the production of neutralizing antibodies against each poliovirus serotype; these neutralizing antibodies are recognized as conferring protection against poliomyelitis disease.

Contraindications

Hypersensitivity to any component of the vaccine, including yeast, neomycin, and polymyxin B; serious allergic reactions (eg, anaphylaxis) temporally associated with a previous dose of this vaccine or with any components of this vaccine; encephalopathy (eg, coma, decreased level of consciousness, prolonged seizures) within 7 days of administration of a previous dose of a pertussis-containing vaccine that is not attributable to another identifiable cause; progressive neurologic disorder, including infantile spasms, uncontrolled epilepsy, or progressive encephalopathy.

Warnings/Precautions

➤*Fever:* Administration of *Pediarix* is associated with higher rates of fever relative to separately administered vaccines. In a safety study that evaluated medically attended fever after *Pediarix* or separately administered vaccines when coadministered with pneumococcal 7-valent conjugate vaccine (PCV7) and *Haemophilus influenzae* type b (Hib) conjugate vaccine, infants who received *Pediarix* had a higher rate of medical encounters for fever within the first 4 days following the first vaccination. In some infants, these encounters included the use of diagnostic studies to evaluate other causes of fever.

➤*Latex sensitivity:* The tip cap and rubber plunger of the needleless prefilled syringes contain dry natural latex rubber that may cause allergic reactions in latex-sensitive individuals. The vial stopper is latex free.

➤*Postvaccination effects:* If any of the following reactions occur in temporal relation to the receipt of DTaP or a vaccine containing an acellular pertussis component, base the decision to give any pertussis vaccine, including *Pediarix*, on careful consideration of the potential benefits and possible risks: temperature of 40.5°C (105°F) or more within 48 hours not due to another identifiable cause; collapse or shock-like state (hypotonic-hyporesponsive episode) within 48 hours; persistent, inconsolable crying lasting 3 hours or more occurring within 48 hours; and seizures with or without fever occurring within 3 days. When a decision is made to withhold pertussis vaccination, give diphtheria and tetanus toxoid (DT) vaccine, hepatitis B vaccine, and IPV as indicated.

➤*Guillain-Barré syndrome:* If Guillain-Barré syndrome occurs within 6 weeks of the receipt of a prior vaccine containing tetanus toxoid, base the decision to give any tetanus toxoid–containing vaccine, including *Pediarix*, on careful consideration of the potential benefits and possible risks. If tetanus toxoid is withheld, give other available vaccines as indicated.

➤*CNS disorders:* The decision to administer a pertussis-containing vaccine to individuals with stable CNS disorders must be made by the health care provider on an individual basis with consideration of all relevant factors and assessment of potential risks and benefits for that individual. The Advisory Committee on Immunization Practices (ACIP) has issued guidelines for these individuals. Advise the parent or guardian of the potential increased risk involved.

➤*Seizure:* For children at higher risk of seizures than the general population, an appropriate antipyretic may be administered at the time of vaccination with a vaccine containing an acellular pertussis component (including *Pediarix*) and for the ensuing 24 hours according to the respective prescribing information recommended dosage to reduce the possibility of postvaccination fever.

➤*Recent/Acute illness:* The ACIP has published guidelines for vaccination of people with recent or acute illness (www.cdc.gov/vaccines).

➤*Bleeding disorders:* Give *Pediarix* with caution to children with bleeding disorders, such as hemophilia or thrombocytopenia, and in children taking anticoagulant therapy, with steps taken to avoid the risk of hematoma following the injection.

➤*Patient history:* Before the injection of any biological, take all reasonable precautions to prevent allergic or other adverse reactions, including understanding the use of the biological concerned and the nature of the adverse reactions that may follow its use.

Prior to immunization, review the patient's current health status and medical history. Review the patient's immunization history for possible vaccine sensitivity, previous vaccination-related adverse reactions, and occurrence of any adverse reaction–related symptoms and/or signs to determine the existence of any contraindication to immunization with *Pediarix* and to allow an assessment of benefits and risks.

➤*Immunosuppression:* As with any vaccine, if administered to immunosuppressed people, including individuals receiving immunosuppressive therapy, the expected immune response may not be obtained.

➤*Hypersensitivity reactions:* Epinephrine injection (1:1,000) and other appropriate agents used for the control of immediate allergic reactions must be immediately available in case an acute anaphylactic reaction occurs.

➤*Pregnancy: Category C.* This vaccine is not indicated for women of childbearing age. Animal reproduction studies have not been conducted. It is not known whether this vaccine can cause fetal harm when administered to a pregnant woman or if it can affect reproductive capacity.

➤*Lactation:* This vaccine is not indicated for women of childbearing age.

➤*Children:* Safety and effectiveness in infants younger than 6 weeks of age have not been evaluated and the vaccination is not recommended for children 7 years of age or older.

Consider the potential risk of apnea and the need for respiratory monitoring for 48 to 72 hours when administering the primary immunization series to very premature infants (born 28 weeks or less of gestation) who remain hospitalized at the time of vaccination, and particularly for those with a previous history of respiratory immaturity. It is generally understood that the benefit of vaccination is high in very premature infants. Base the decision to vaccinate on careful consideration of the potential benefits and possible risks.

➤*Elderly:* This vaccine is not indicated for use in adult populations.

Drug Interactions

DTaP Adsorbed, Hepatitis B (Recombinant), and Inactivated Polio Vaccine Combined Drug Interactions

Precipitant drug	Object drug[a]		Description
Concomitant vaccines	DTaP adsorbed, hepatitis B (recombinant), and IPV combined	⟷	If DTaP adsorbed, hepatitis B (recombinant), and IPV combined is to be coadministered with another injectable vaccine, do not mix any other vaccine in the same syringe or vial.
Immunosuppressive therapies (eg, alkylating agents, antimetabolites, corticosteroids [at greater than physiologic doses], cytotoxic drugs, radiation therapy)	DTaP, hepatitis B (recombinant), and IPV combined	⬇	Immune response to DTaP adsorbed, hepatitis B (recombinant), and IPV combined may be reduced.

[a] ⬇ = object drug decreased; ⟷ = undetermined clinical effect.

Adverse Reactions

➤*Common adverse reactions:* The most common adverse reactions observed in clinical trials were local injection-site reactions (pain, redness, or swelling), fever, and fussiness. In comparative studies, *Pediarix* was associated with higher rates of fever relative to separately administered vaccines. The prevalence of fever was highest on the day of vaccination and the day following vaccination. More than 96% of fever episodes resolved within the 4-day period following vaccination (ie, the period including the day of vaccination and the next 3 days).

Deaths – In 14 clinical trials, 0.06% of deaths were reported among recipients of *Pediarix* and 0.04% of deaths were reported among recipients of comparator vaccines. Causes of death in the group that received *Pediarix* included 2 cases of sudden infant death syndrome (SIDS) and 1 case of each of the following: convulsive disorder, congenital immunodeficiency with sepsis, and neuroblastoma. One case of SIDS was reported in the comparator group. The rate of SIDS among all recipients of *Pediarix* across the 14 trials was 0.025%. The rate of SIDS observed for recipients of *Pediarix* in the German safety study was 0.02% of infants (reported rate of SIDS in Germany in

DIPHTHERIA AND TETANUS TOXOIDS AND ACELLULAR PERTUSSIS ADSORBED, HEPATITIS B (RECOMBINANT) AND INACTIVATED POLIOVIRUS VACCINE COMBINED — INJECTION

the latter part of the 1990s was 0.07% of newborns). The reported rate of SIDS in the US from 1990 to 1994 was 0.12% of live births. By chance alone, some cases of SIDS can be expected to follow receipt of pertussis-containing vaccines.

➤*Serious adverse reactions:* Within 30 days following any dose of vaccine in the US safety study in which all subjects received concomitant pneumococcal and Hib conjugate vaccines, serious adverse reactions were reported in 1% of patients who received *Pediarix* (1 case each of pyrexia, gastroenteritis, and culture-negative clinical sepsis, and 4 cases of bronchiolitis) and in 1% of patients who received *Infanrix, Engerix-B*, and IPV (uteropelvic junction obstruction and testicular atrophy in 1 subject and 3 cases of bronchiolitis).

Onset of chronic illnesses – In the US safety study in which all subjects received concomitant pneumococcal and Hib conjugate vaccines, 3% of patients who received *Pediarix* and 4% of patients who received *Infanrix, Engerix-B*, and IPV reported new onset of a chronic illness during the period from 1 to 6 months following the last dose of study vaccines. Among the chronic illnesses reported in the subjects who received *Pediarix*, there were 4 cases of asthma and 1 case each of diabetes mellitus and chronic neutropenia. There were 4 cases of asthma in subjects who received *Infanrix, Engerix-B*, and IPV.

Seizures – In the German safety study over the entire study period, 6 subjects in the group who received *Pediarix* reported seizures. Two of these subjects had a febrile seizure, 1 of whom also developed afebrile seizures. The remaining 4 subjects had afebrile seizures, including 2 with infantile spasms. Two subjects reported seizures within 7 days following vaccination (1 subject had febrile and afebrile seizures, and 1 subject had afebrile seizures), corresponding to a rate of 0.022% (febrile seizures, 0.007%; afebrile seizures, 0.014%). No subject who received concomitant *Infanrix*, Hib vaccine, and oral polio vaccine reported seizures. In a separate German study that evaluated the safety of *Infanrix* in 22,505 infants who received 66,867 doses of *Infanrix* administered as a 3-dose primary series, the rate of seizures within 7 days of vaccination with *Infanrix* was 0.013% (febrile seizures, 0%; afebrile seizures, 0.013%).

Over the entire study period in the US safety study in which all subjects received concomitant pneumococcal and Hib conjugate vaccines, 4 subjects in the group that received *Pediarix* reported seizures. Three of these subjects had a febrile seizure and 1 had an afebrile seizure. Over the entire study period, 2 subjects in the group that received *Infanrix, Engerix-B*, and IPV reported febrile seizures. There were no afebrile seizures in this group. No subject in either study group had seizures within 7 days following vaccination.

➤*Local and systemic adverse reactions:*

Pediarix With Hib Conjugate Vaccine and PCV7 Adverse Reactions[a,b]

	Pediarix, Hib vaccine, and PCV7			*Infanrix, Engerix-B*, IPV, Hib vaccine, and PCV7		
	Dose 1	Dose 2	Dose 3	Dose 1	Dose 2	Dose 3
Local[c]						
	(n = 671)	(n = 653)	(n = 648)	(n = 335)	(n = 323)	(n = 315)
Pain, any	36.1%	36.1%	31.2%	31.9%	30%	29.8%
Pain, grade 2 or 3	11.5%	10.9%	10.6%	9%	8.7%	8.9%
Pain, grade 3	2.4%	2.5%	1.7%	2.7%	1.5%	1.3%
Redness, any	24.9%[d]	37.2%	40.1%	18.2%	32.8%	39%
Redness, > 5 mm	6%[d]	9.6%[d]	12.7%[d]	1.8%	5.9%	7.3%
Redness, > 20 mm	0.9%	1.2%[d]	2.8%	0.3%	0%	1.9%
Swelling, any	17.3%[d]	26.5%[d]	28.7%	9.6%	20.4%	24.8%
Swelling, > 5 mm	5.8%[d]	9.6%[d]	9.3%[d]	1.8%	5%	4.1%
Swelling, > 20 mm	1.9%	2.5%[d]	3.1%	0.6%	0%	1.3%
Systemic						
	(n = 667)	(n = 644)	(n = 645)	(n = 333)	(n = 321)	(n = 311)
Fever,[e] ≥ 100.4°F	27.9%[d]	38.8%[d]	33.5%[d]	19.8%	30.2%	23.8%
Fever,[e] > 101.3°F	7%	14.1%[d]	8.8%	4.5%	9.7%	5.8%
Fever,[e] > 102.2°F	2.2%[d]	3.6%	3.4%	0.3%	3.1%	2.3%
Fever,[e] > 103.1°F	0.4%	1.4%	1.1%	0%	0.3%	0.3%
Fever,[e] MA	1.2%[d]	0.2%	0.8%	0%	0.6%	0%
	(n = 671)	(n = 653)	(n = 648)	(n = 335)	(n = 323)	(n = 315)
Drowsiness, any	57.2%	51.6%	40.9%	54%	48.3%	38.4%
Drowsiness, grade 2 or 3	15.8%	13.8%	11.4%	17.6%	12.4%	11.1%
Drowsiness, grade 3	2.5%	1.2%	0.9%	3.6%	0.6%	1.9%
Irritability/ Fussiness, any	60.5%	64.9%	61.1%	61.5%	61.6%	56.5%
Irritability/ Fussiness, grade 2 or 3	19.8%	27.9%[d]	25.2%[d]	19.4%	21.1%	19.4%
Irritability/ Fussiness, grade 3	3.4%	4.4%	3.5%	3.9%	3.4%	3.2%
Loss of appetite, any	30.4%	30.6%	26.2%	27.8%	26.6%	23.8%
Loss of appetite, grade 2 or 3	6.6%	7.8%[d]	5.9%	5.1%	3.4%	5.4%
Loss of appetite, grade 3	0.7%	0.3%	0.2%	0.6%	0.3%	0%

[a] Modified intent-to-treat cohort = all vaccinated subjects for whom safety data were available; n = number of infants for whom at least 1 symptom sheet was completed (for fever, numbers exclude missing temperature recordings or tympanic measurements); MA = medically attended (a visit to or from medical personnel); grade 2 = sufficiently discomforting to interfere with daily activities; grade 3 = preventing normal daily activities.
[b] Within 4 days of vaccination defined as day of vaccination and the next 3 days.
[c] Local reactions at the injection site for *Pediarix* or *Infanrix*.
[d] Rate significantly higher in the group that received *Pediarix* compared with separately administered vaccines ($P < 0.05$ [2-sided Fisher Exact test] or the 95% confidence interval on the difference between groups [separate minus *Pediarix*] does not include 0).
[e] Axillary temperatures increased by 1°C (34°F) and oral temperatures increased by 0.5°C (33°F) to derive equivalent rectal temperature.

➤*CNS:* A review by the Institute of Medicine (IOM) found evidence for a causal relationship between the receipt of tetanus toxoid and both brachial neuritis and Guillain-Barré syndrome. A few cases of demyelinating diseases of the CNS have been reported following some tetanus toxoid–containing vaccines or DT-containing vaccines, although the IOM concluded that the evidence was inadequate to accept or reject a causal relationship. A few cases of peripheral mononeuropathy and cranial mononeuropathy have been reported following tetanus toxoid administration, although the IOM concluded that the evidence was inadequate to accept or reject a causal relationship.

➤*Hypersensitivity:* Rarely, an anaphylactic reaction (eg, hives, swelling of the mouth, difficulty breathing, hypotension, shock) has been reported after receiving preparations containing diphtheria, tetanus, and/or pertussis antigens. Arthus-type hypersensitivity reactions, characterized by severe local reactions, may follow receipt of tetanus toxoid.

➤*Postmarketing:*

CNS – Bulging fontanelle, convulsions, crying, depressed level of consciousness, fatigue, febrile convulsion, hypotonia, hypotonic-hyporesponsive episode, insomnia, irritability, lethargy, nervousness, restlessness, screaming, somnolence, unusual crying.

Dermatologic – Cyanosis, erythema, pallor, petechiae, rash, urticaria.

Hypersensitivity – Anaphylactic reaction, anaphylactoid reaction, angioedema, hypersensitivity.

GI – Anorexia, diarrhea, vomiting.

Local – Injection-site cellulitis, induration, itching, nodule/lump, pain, reaction, redness, swelling, vesicles, and warmth.

Musculoskeletal – Limb pain, limb swelling.

Respiratory – Apnea, cough, dyspnea, upper respiratory tract infection.

Miscellaneous – Abnormal liver function tests, pyrexia, SIDS.

➤*Reporting adverse reactions:* The National Childhood Vaccine Injury Act requires that the manufacturer and lot number of the vaccine administered be recorded by the health care provider in the vaccine recipient's per-

DIPHTHERIA AND TETANUS TOXOIDS AND ACELLULAR PERTUSSIS ADSORBED, HEPATITIS B (RECOMBINANT) AND INACTIVATED POLIOVIRUS VACCINE COMBINED — INJECTION

manent medical record, along with the date of administration of the vaccine and the name, address, and title of the person administering the vaccine. The Act further requires the health care provider to report to the US Department of Health and Human Services the occurrence following immunization of any reaction set forth in the Vaccine Injury Table, including anaphylaxis or anaphylactic shock within 7 days; encephalopathy or encephalitis within 7 days; brachial neuritis within 28 days; an acute complication or sequelae (including death) of an illness, disability, injury, or condition referred to previously; or any reactions that would contraindicate further doses of vaccine, according to this prescribing information. These reactions should be reported to the Vaccine Adverse Event Reporting System (VAERS). The VAERS toll-free number is 1-800-822-7967. Reporting forms may also be obtained at the VAERS Web site at www.vaers.hhs.gov.

Patient Information

Inform caregivers that children with a minor illness, such as a cold, may be vaccinated. Wait to vaccinate children who are moderately or severely ill until they recover.

Advise caregivers to contact their child's heath care provider at once if the child develops a fever of 40.5°C (105°F) or more, faints, persistently cries for more than 3 hours within 48 hours of receiving this vaccine, has a seizure with or without fever within 3 days of receiving this vaccine, or changes in mental alertness or responsiveness occur within 7 days of receiving this vaccine.

Advise caregivers to use nonaspirin-containing over-the-counter analgesics (eg, acetaminophen) for fever, pain, or discomfort at the injection site.

Inform parents or guardians of the potential benefits and risks of the vaccine and of the importance of completing the immunization series. Inform the parents or guardians about the potential for adverse reactions that have been temporally associated with administration of *Pediarix* or other vaccines containing similar components. Tell the parent or guardian accompanying the recipient to report severe or unusual adverse reactions to the health care provider or clinic where the vaccine was administered.

Give the parent or guardian the Vaccine Information Statements, which are required by the National Childhood Vaccine Injury Act of 1986 to be given prior to immunization. These materials are available free of charge at the CDC Web site (www.cdc.gov/vaccines).

ALLERGENIC EXTRACTS

Indications

➤*Diagnosis of specific allergies:* Diagnosis of specific allergies, when properly diluted.

➤*Relief of allergic symptoms:* Relief of allergic symptoms (eg, hay fever, rhinitis, allergic asthma, insect-sting anaphylaxis) due to specifically identified materials by means of a graduated schedule of doses.

Administration and Dosage

Begin immunotherapy with very small doses; increase progressively until maintenance levels are reached. Dosages vary depending on the type of standardization used. Individualize dosage.

Do not inject IV. SC injection is preferable because it is less painful, allows better delineation of reaction size and slows the absorption rate, thus lowering the likelihood of an anaphylactic reaction. Although IM administration is acceptable, it is more painful and more difficult to assess the local reaction.

➤*Combining allergens:* Do not combine allergens to which the patient is extremely sensitive with allergens for which only a nominal sensitivity is shown. Distinct treatment schedules for each formula are frequently employed. (See Precautions.)

➤*Children:* Dosage is the same as for adults; divide large volume doses among several injection sites.

➤*Diagnostic testing:* Perform puncture (prick) or intradermal testing with appropriate dilutions, employing positive and negative controls. Consult manufacturer's literature for each allergen. Do not conduct test with alum-precipitated allergen extracts.

➤*Therapeutic dosing:* Typical doses are given SC every 3 to 14 days (or 7 to 14 days with alum-precipitated allergen extracts). Progress to the maximum tolerated dose or a weekly maintenance dose. Consult manufacturer's literature for each allergen.

➤*Admixtures:* Limit combinations of allergens so that each allergen will be present at a therapeutic concentration. Do not combine allergens of different standardization types. Stability varies with diluent, storage condition and concentration. Stability will be shortest in the low concentration ranges.

➤*Storage/Stability:* Store between 2° and 8°C (36° to 46°F).

Actions

➤*Pharmacology:* Allergenic extracts are derived individually from various biological sources containing antigens that possess immunologic activity. They are categorized based standardization and doseform. Standardization systems include the following: 1) Standardized by biological activity (in allergenic units, AU), 2) weight-to-volume (w/v) standardized, and 3) protein nitrogen unit (PNU) standardized. Doseforms include: 1) aqueous, 2) glycerinated and 3) alum-precipitated.

The mechanism of action is not completely defined. Specific immunoglobulin G (IgG) appears in the serum following injection of allergenic extracts. IgG competes with specific IgE for a specific antigen. Bound to receptors on mast cell membranes, IgE produces an allergenic reaction by releasing histamine and other agents upon coupling with an antigen. Serum IgE levels decrease over time. Decreased leukocyte sensitivity to allergens and increased numbers of T-suppressor cells for IgE-producing plasma cells are also noted. The histamine release response of circulating basophils to a specific allergen may be reduced in some patients by hyposensitization.

Onset/Duration – Relief of symptoms is dose-related. It is rarely achieved before maintenance dosage levels are reached, which often takes 4 to 6 months, sometimes 12 months. Serum IgG levels remain elevated for weeks to months following injection and vary markedly between individuals.

Contraindications

As initial therapy when an allergen can be environmentally avoided.

Frequent large local reactions or systemic reactions are relative contraindications for continued immunotherapy.

Foodstuff allergen extracts are diagnostic tools; efficacy for hyposensitization immunotherapy has not been demonstrated.

Warnings/Precautions

➤*Cross-sensitivity:* Cross-immunoreactivity has been documented within botanical genus groups, especially among grasses. Exercise caution in prescribing since the additive effects could precipitate an allergic reaction. Markedly increased exposure to allergens in the environment may have an additive effect when coupled with an allergen extract injection. Dosage reduction may be necessary.

➤*Mixed allergens:* Mixed allergens are not to be used for skin testing. In the case of a negative reaction, a mixture fails to indicate whether one of the individual components at the full labeled concentration is capable of evoking a positive reaction. If the patient responds positively, there is no indication which component of the mixture produced the antigenic response. Treatment with nonreactive allergens can lead to sensitization and induction of IgE production.

➤*Combining allergens:* Do not combine allergens to which the patient is extremely sensitive with allergens for which only a nominal sensitivity is shown. Administer separately to individualize and better control dosage.

➤*Seasonal exposure:* Delay the start of immunotherapy until after any period of symptoms from seasonal environmental exposure. Typical allergic symptoms may follow shortly after an injection, particularly when the sum of the antigen load from the environment and from the injection exceeds the patient's antigen tolerance.

➤*Routine immunizations:* While routine immunizations may theoretically exacerbate autoimmune diseases, studies have failed to demonstrate this. Give hyposensitization cautiously to patients with autoimmune diseases and only if the risk from exposure exceeds the risk of exacerbating the underlying condition.

➤*Hypersensitivity reactions:* Anaphylactic reactions may occur with an overdose or in extremely sensitive individuals. Administer allergen extracts only where emergency facilities are immediately available. Refer to Management of Acute Hypersensitivity Reactions.

➤*Pregnancy: Category C.* Controlled studies of hyposensitization with allergen extracts throughout pregnancy failed to demonstrate any fetal or maternal risk. Because histamine can produce uterine contraction, avoid any reaction that releases significant amounts of histamine, whether from natural allergen exposure or from hyposensitization overdose. IgG crosses the placenta, especially in the third trimester. Administer during pregnancy only if clearly needed and with caution. Although pregnancy is not an indication to stop allergen extract therapy in women receiving maintenance doses without side effects, some allergists empirically decrease the maintenance dose by 50% throughout gestation.

➤*Lactation:* Minimal amounts of IgG are excreted in breast milk. No problems in humans have been documented. Various nutritional, immunologic and other advantages of breastfeeding have been described, especially in children of atopic mothers.

➤*Children:* Dosage for children is generally the same as for adults. The larger dosage volumes may produce relatively greater discomfort. To achieve the total dose required, the volume of the dose may be distributed among several injection sites.

Drug Interactions

➤*Drug/Lab test interactions:* **Histamine H_1 antagonists** and **tricyclic antidepressants** may produce a false-negative reaction to cutaneous diagnostic testing with allergen extracts, unless a 72-hour period of antihistamine abstinence is observed. Long-acting antihistamines may interfere for weeks. **H_2 antagonists** do not decrease skin-test responsiveness alone, but may enhance suppression synergistically with H_1 antihistamines. **Topical corticosteroids** suppress dermal reactivity to allergen extracts locally.

Adverse Reactions

Most serious reactions begin within 30 minutes of an injection. Observe patients for at least 30 minutes after every injection, even once they have achieved maintenance therapy.

➤*Local:* Erythema and swelling at the injection site are common, but not significant unless they persist > 24 hours or exceed the diameter of a nickel (about 2 cm).

➤*Systemic:* Anaphylaxis, including fainting, pallor, bradycardia, hypotension, angioedema, wheezing, cough, conjunctivitis, rhinitis, generalized urticaria (see Warnings).

Patient Information

Comply with full course of therapy. To achieve efficacy, take regularly and in the proper dosage. Medication will not cure allergies, but will help control them.

Notify physician of increased environmental exposure to natural allergens; a dosage reduction may be required.

➤*Missed dose:* Depending on the amount of time elapsed, dosage reduction may be required. Do *not* double the dose to make up for the missed dose. More frequent injections may be necessary to return to maintenance doses.

Notify physician if erythema, swelling or generalized urticaria persists.

Notify physician immediately if fainting, wheezing, hypotension or bradycardia occurs.

AQUEOUS AND GLYCERINATED ALLERGENIC EXTRACTS

Rx	**Allergenic Extracts, Aqueous and Glycerinated** (Various, eg, ALK, Allergy Laboratories, Allermed, ALO, Center, Greer, Meridian, Miles, Nelco)	**Injection:** Over 900 distinct allergens available in these categories: Animal products, foods, grass pollens, insect products, molds, tree pollens, weed pollens and other inhalants	Extracts supplied in various aqueous diluents or with varying concentrations of glycerin. In multidose vials of 2, 5, 10, 20, 30 and 50 ml.

For complete and comparative prescribing information, refer to the Allergenic Extracts group monograph.

ALUM-PRECIPITATED ALLERGENIC EXTRACTS

Rx	**Allpyral** (Miles)	**Injection:** Alum-precipitated extracts, prepared by pyridine extraction	In multidose vials of 10 and 30 ml at 5000, 10,000 and 20,000 PNU/ml.
Rx	**Center-Al** (Center)	**Injection:** Alum-precipitated extracts	In multidose vials of 10 and 30 ml at 10,000 and 20,000 PNU/ml.

For complete and comparative prescribing information, refer to the Allergenic Extracts group monograph.

HYMENOPTERA VENOM/VENOM PROTEIN

Rx	**Pharmalgen** (ALK)	**Injection:** Purified venoms of honey bee, wasp, white faced hornet, yellow hornet, yellow jacket and mixed vespids (both hornets and yellow jackets)	In vials of 120 and 1100 mcg.

For complete and comparative prescribing information, refer to the Allergenic Extracts group monograph.

IMMUNOLOGIC AGENTS

Immunostimulants

PEGADEMASE BOVINE

Rx	**Adagen** (Enzon)	**Injection:** 250 units[a]/mL	In 1.5 mL vials.[b]

[a] One unit of activity is defined as the amount of ADA that converts 1 mcM of adenosine to inosine per minute at 25°C and pH 7.3.

[b] With 1.2 mg monobasic sodium phosphate, 5.58 mg dibasic sodium phosphate, 8.5 mg sodium chloride and water for injection.

PEGADEMASE BOVINE — INJECTION

Indications

➤*Adenosine deaminase deficiency:* For enzyme replacement therapy for adenosine deaminase (ADA) deficiency in patients with severe combined immunodeficiency disease who are not suitable candidates for or who have failed bone marrow transplantation. Pegademase bovine is recommended for use in infants from birth or in children of any age at the time of diagnosis. It is not intended as a replacement for HLA identical bone marrow transplant therapy, and it is also not intended to replace continued close medical supervision and the initiation of appropriate diagnostic tests and therapy (eg, antibiotics, nutrition, oxygen, gammaglobulin) as indicated for intercurrent illnesses.

Administration and Dosage

➤*Dose:* Administer every 7 days as an IM injection. Individualize the dosage.

First dose – 10 U/kg.

Second dose – 15 U/kg.

Third dose – 20 U/kg.

Usual maintenance dose – 20 U/kg/week. Further increases of 5 U/kg/week may be necessary, but a maximum single dose of 30 U/kg should not be exceeded.

➤*Plasma levels:* Plasma levels of ADA more than twice the upper limit of 35 mcmol/hr/mL have occurred on occasion in several patients, and have been maintained for several weeks in one patient who received twice weekly injections (20 U/kg per dose). No adverse effects have been observed at these higher levels; there is no evidence that maintaining preinjection plasma ADA > 35 mcmol/hr/mL produces any additional clinical benefits.

➤*Administration precautions:* Dose proportionality has not been established; closely monitor patients when the dosage is increased. Pegademase bovine is not recommended for IV administration.

Establish the optimal dosage and schedule of administration for each patient based on monitoring of plasma ADA activity levels (trough levels before maintenance injection), biochemical markers of ADA deficiency (primarily red cell deoxyadenosine triphosphate [dATP] content). Since improvement in immune function follows correction of metabolic abnormalities, maintenance dosage in individual patients should be aimed at achieving the following biochemical goals: 1) Maintain plasma ADA activity (trough levels before maintenance injection) in the range of 15 to 35 mcmol/hr/mL (assayed at 37°C [98.6°F]); and 2) decline in erythrocyte dATP to ≤ 0.005 to 0.015 mcmol/mL packed erythrocytes, or ≤ 1% of the total erythrocyte adenine nucleotide (ATP = dATP) content, with a normal ATP level, as measured in a preinjection sample. In addition, continued monitoring of immune function and clinical status is essential in any patient with a primary immunodeficiency disease and should be continued in patients being treated with pegademase bovine.

➤*Admixture incompatibility:* Pegademase bovine should not be diluted nor mixed with any other drug prior to administration.

➤*Storage / Stability:* Refrigerate. Store between 2°C and 8°C (36°F and 46°F). Do not freeze. Pegademase bovine should not be stored at room temperature. This product should not be used if there are any indications that it may have been frozen.

Actions

➤*Pharmacology:* Pegademase bovine is a modified enzyme used for enzyme replacement therapy for the treatment of severe combined immunodeficiency disease (SCID) associated with a deficiency of adenosine deaminase. The drug will not benefit patients with immunodeficiency due to other causes. It is a conjugate of numerous strands of monomethoxypolyethylene glycol (PEG), covalently attached to the enzyme ADA. ADA, used in the manufacture of pegademase bovine, is derived from bovine intestine.

Pegademase bovine provides specific replacement of the deficient enzyme. In the absence of the enzyme ADA, the purine substrates adenosine, 2′-deoxyadenosine and their metabolites are toxic to lymphocytes. The direct action of pegademase bovine is the correction of these metabolic abnormalities. Improvement in immune function and diminished frequency of opportunistic infections only occurs after metabolic abnormalities are corrected. There is a lag between the correction of the metabolic abnormalities and improved immune function. This period of time is variable, from a few weeks to as long as 6 months. In contrast to the natural history of combined immunodeficiency disease due to ADA deficiency, a trend toward diminished frequency of opportunistic infections and fewer complications of infections has occurred in patients receiving pegademase bovine.

SCID associated with ADA deficiency is a rare, inherited and often fatal disease. In the absence of ADA enzyme, purine substrates adenosine and 2′-deoxyadenosine accumulate, causing metabolic abnormalities that are directly toxic to lymphocytes.

The immune deficiency can be cured by bone marrow transplantation. When a suitable bone marrow donor is unavailable or when bone marrow transplantation fails, non-selective replacement of the ADA enzyme has been provided by periodic irradiated red blood cell transfusions. However, transmission of viral infections and iron overload are serious risks, and relatively few ADA-deficient patients have benefited from chronic transfusion therapy.

➤*Pharmacokinetics:* Pharmacokinetics and biochemical effects have been studied in six children ranging in age from 6 weeks to 12 years with SCID associated with ADA deficiency. After IM injection, peak plasma ADA activ-

PEGADEMASE BOVINE — INJECTION

ity levels were reached in 2 to 3 days. ADA plasma elimination half-life of was variable, even for the same child. Range was 3 to > 6 days. Following weekly injections of 15 U/kg, average trough level of ADA activity in plasma was between 20 and 25 mcmol/hr/mL.

The changes in red blood cell deoxyadenosine nucleotide (ie, dATP) and S-adenosylhomocysteine hydrolase (SAHase) have been evaluated. In patients with ADA deficiency, inadequate elimination of 2′-deoxyadenosine caused a marked elevation in dATP and a decrease in SAHase level in red blood cells. Prior to treatment with pegademase bovine, the levels of dATP in the red blood cells ranged from 0.056 to 0.899 mcmol/mL of erythrocytes. After 2 months of maintenance treatment, the levels decreased to 0.007 to 0.015 mcmol/mL. The normal value of dATP is below 0.001 mcmol/mL. In the same period of time, SAHase increased from pretreatment range of 0.09 to 0.22 nmol/hr/mg protein to 2.37 to 5.16 nmol/hr/mg protein. Normal value for SAHase is 4.18 ± 1.9 nmol/hr/mg protein.

Contraindications

There is no evidence to support the safety and efficacy of pegademase bovine as preparatory or support therapy for bone marrow transplantation. Since the drug is administered by IM injection, use with caution in patients with thrombocytopenia and do not use if thrombocytopenia is severe.

Warnings/Precautions

➤*Product potency:* Product potency testing prior to distribution may not assure the initial and continuing potency of each new lot of pegademase bovine. Report any laboratory or clinical indication of a decrease in potency immediately by telephone to Enzon (732-980-4500).

➤*Immunodeficiency:* Maintain appropriate care to protect immune-deficient patients until improvement in immune function has been documented. The degree of immune function improvement may vary from patient to patient and, therefore, each patient will require appropriate care consistent with immunologic status.

➤*Immune function:* Immune function, including the ability to produce antibodies, generally improves after 2 to 6 months of therapy, and matures over a longer period. Compared with the natural history of combined immunodeficiency disease due to ADA deficiency, a trend toward diminished frequency of opportunistic infections and fewer complications of infections has occurred in patients receiving pegademase bovine. However, the lag between the correction of the metabolic abnormalities and improved immune function with a trend toward diminished frequency of infections and complications of infection is variable, and has ranged from a few weeks to approximately 6 months. Improvement in the general clinical status of the patient may be gradual (as evidenced by improvement in various clinical parameters) but should be apparent by the end of the first year of therapy.

A decline in immune function, with increased risk of opportunistic infections and complications of infection, will result from failure to maintain adequate levels of plasma ADA activity (whether due to the development of antibody, improper calculation of dosage, interruption of treatment or to improper storage with subsequent loss of activity). If a persistent decline in plasma ADA activity occurs, monitor immune function and clinical status closely and take precautions to minimize the risk of infection. If antibody to ADA or pegademase bovine is found to be the cause of a persistent fall in plasma ADA activity, then adjustment in the dosage and other measures may be taken to induce tolerance and restore adequate ADA activity.

➤*Antibody:* Antibody to pegademase bovine may develop in patients and may result in more rapid clearance of the drug. Suspect antibody to pegademase bovine if a persistent fall in preinjection level of plasma ADA to < 10 mcmol/hr/mL occurs. If other causes for a decline in plasma ADA levels can be ruled out (eg, improper storage of vials [freezing or prolonged storage at temperatures > 4°C], or improper handling of plasma samples [eg, repeated freezing and thawing during transport to laboratory]), then perform a specific assay for antibody to ADA and pegademase bovine (ELISA, enzyme inhibition).

One of 12 patients showed an enhanced rate of clearance of plasma ADA activity after 5 months of therapy at 15 U/kg/week. Enhanced clearance was correlated with the appearance of an antibody that directly inhibited both unmodified ADA and pegademase bovine. Subsequently, the patient was treated with twice weekly IM injections at an increased dose of 20 U/kg, or a total weekly dose of 40 U/kg. No adverse effects were observed at the higher dose and effective levels of plasma ADA were restored. After 4 months, the patient returned to a weekly dosage schedule of 20 U/kg and effective plasma levels have been maintained.

➤*Pregnancy: Category C.* It is not known whether pegademase bovine can cause fetal harm when administered to a pregnant woman or can affect reproduction capacity. Give to a pregnant woman only if clearly needed.

➤*Lactation:* It is not known whether pegademase bovine is excreted in breast milk. Exercise caution when administering to a nursing woman.

➤*Monitoring:* Monitor the treatment of SCID associated with ADA deficiency with pegademase bovine by measuring plasma ADA activity and red blood cell dATP levels.

Determine plasma ADA activity and red cell dATP prior to treatment. Once treatment has been initiated, a desirable range of plasma ADA activity (trough level before maintenance injection) should be 15 to 35 mcmol/hr/mL. This minimum trough level will ensure that plasma ADA activity from injection to injection is maintained above the level of total erythrocyte ADA activity in the blood of normal individuals.

Determine plasma ADA activity (preinjection) every 1 to 2 weeks during the first 8 to 12 weeks of treatment in order to establish an effective dose. After 2 months of maintenance treatment, red cell dATP levels should decrease to a range of ≤ 0.005 to 0.015 mcmol/mL. The normal value of dATP is below 0.001 mcmol/mL. Once the level of dATP has fallen adequately, measure 2 to 4 times during the remainder of the first year and 2 to 3 times a year thereafter, assuming no interruption in therapy.

Between 3 and 9 months, determine plasma ADA twice a month, then monthly until after 18 to 24 months of treatment. In patients who have successfully been maintained on therapy for 2 years, continue to have plasma ADA measured every 2 to 4 months and red cell dATP measured twice yearly. More frequent monitoring would be necessary if therapy were interrupted or if an enhanced rate of clearance of plasma ADA activity develops.

Once effective ADA plasma levels have been established, should a patient's plasma ADA activity level fall below 10 mcmol/hr/mL (which cannot be attributed to improper dosing, sample handling or antibody development) then all patients receiving this lot of pegademase bovine will be required to have a blood sample for plasma ADA determination taken prior to their next injection. The index patient will require retesting for determination of plasma ADA activity prior to their next injection. If this value, as well as the value from one of the other patients from a different site, is < 10 mcmol/hr/mL, then the lot in use will be recalled and replaced with a new clinical lot by Enzon.

Drug Interactions

➤*Vidarabine:* Vidarabine is a substrate for ADA and **2′-deoxycoformycin** is a potent inhibitor of ADA. Thus, the activities of these drugs and pegademase bovine could be substantially altered if they are used in combination with one another.

Adverse Reactions

Clinical experience is limited. The following adverse reactions have occurred: Headache (1 patient) and pain at the injection site (2 patients).

Overdosage

An intraperitoneal dose of 50,000 U/kg of pegademase bovine in mice resulted in weight loss up to 9%.

ALEFACEPT

Rx	**Amevive** (Biogen Idec)	**Powder for injection, lyophilized:** 15 mg	12.5 mg sucrose. Preservative-free. In dose pack 1s and 4s.[a]

[a] In single-use vials with 10 mL single-use diluent (sterile water for injection).

ALEFACEPT — INJECTION

Indications

➤*Plaque psoriasis:* Treatment of adult patients with moderate to severe chronic plaque psoriasis who are candidates for systemic therapy or phototherapy.

Administration and Dosage

➤*Adults:*

Plaque psoriasis –

Usual dosage: 15 mg given once weekly as an intramuscular (IM) injection.

Duration of therapy: The recommended regimen is a course of 12 weekly injections. Re-treatment with an additional 12-week course may be initiated provided that CD4+ T lymphocyte counts are within the normal range, and a minimum of 12-weeks have passed since the previous course of treatment.

Discontinuation of therapy: Alefacept should be discontinued if the CD4+ T lymphocyte counts remain below 250 cells/mcL for 1 month.

➤*Monitoring:* The CD4+ T lymphocyte counts of patients receiving alefacept should be monitored before initiating dosing and every 2 weeks throughout the course of the 12-week dosing regimen. If CD4+ T lymphocyte counts are below 250 cells/mcL, alefacept dosing should be withheld and weekly monitoring instituted. Alefacept should be discontinued if the counts remain below 250 cells/mcL for 1 month.

➤*Preparation for administration:* Each vial is intended for single patient use only.

Using the supplied syringe and 1 of the supplied needles, withdraw only 0.6 mL of the supplied diluent (sterile water for injection). Keeping the needle pointed at the sidewall of the vial, slowly inject the diluent into the vial of alefacept. Some foaming will occur, which is normal. To avoid excessive foaming, do not shake or vigorously agitate. The contents should be swirled gently during dissolution. Generally, dissolution of alefacept takes less than 2 minutes. The reconstituted solution should be clear and colorless to slightly yellow. The solution should be used as soon as possible after

ALEFACEPT — INJECTION

reconstitution. The reconstituted solution contains alefacept 15 mg per 0.5 mL. Do not filter reconstituted solution during preparation or administration.

Remove the needle used for reconstitution and attach the other supplied needle. Withdraw 0.5 mL of the alefacept solution into the syringe. Some foam or bubbles may remain in the vial.

➤*Administration:* For IM use. Inject the full 0.5 mL of solution. Rotate injection sites so that a different site is used for each new injection. New injections should be given at least 1 inch from an old site and never into areas where the skin is tender, bruised, red, or hard.

➤*Admixture compatibility:* Do not add other medications to solutions containing alefacept. Do not reconstitute alefacept with diluents other than the supplied diluent.

➤*Storage/Stability:* Store the drug/diluent pack containing alefacept (lyophilized powder) in a refrigerator between 2° and 8°C (36° and 46°F). Protect from light. Retain in drug/diluent pack until time of use. Following reconstitution, the product should be used immediately or within 4 hours if stored in the vial at 2° to 8°C (36° to 46°F). Alefacept not used within 4 hours of reconstitution should be discarded.

Actions

➤*Pharmacology:* Alefacept interferes with lymphocyte activation by specifically binding to the lymphocyte antigen, CD2, and inhibiting leukocyte function antigen-3 (LFA-3)/CD2 interaction. Activation of T lymphocytes involving the interaction between LFA-3 on antigen-presenting cells and CD2 on T lymphocytes plays a role in the pathophysiology of chronic plaque psoriasis. The majority of T lymphocytes in psoriatic lesions are of the memory effector phenotype characterized by the presence of the CD45RO marker, express activation markers (eg, CD25, CD69) and release inflammatory cytokines, such as interferon γ.

Alefacept also causes a reduction in subsets of CD2+ T lymphocytes (primarily CD45RO+), presumably by bridging between CD2 on target lymphocytes and immunoglobulin Fc receptors on cytotoxic cells, such as natural killer cells. Treatment with alefacept results in a reduction in circulating total CD4+ and CD8+ T lymphocyte counts. CD2 is also expressed at low levels on the surface of natural killer cells and certain bone marrow B lymphocytes. Therefore, the potential exists for alefacept to affect the activation and numbers of cells other than T lymphocytes. In clinical studies of alefacept, minor changes in the numbers of circulating cells other than T lymphocytes have been observed.

➤*Pharmacokinetics:*

Absorption – Following an IM injection, bioavailability was 63%.

Distribution – In patients with moderate to severe plaque psoriasis, following a 7.5 mg intravenous (IV) administration, the mean volume of distribution of alefacept was 94 mL/kg.

Excretion – The mean clearance was 0.25 mL/h/kg and the mean elimination half-life was approximately 270 hours.

Contraindications

Do not administer alefacept to patients infected with HIV. Alefacept reduces CD4+ T lymphocyte counts, which might accelerate disease progression or increase complications of disease in these patients. Do not administer alefacept to patients with known hypersensitivity to alefacept or any of its components.

Warnings/Precautions

➤*Lymphopenia:* Alefacept induces dose-dependent reductions in circulating CD4+ and CD8+ T lymphocyte counts.

Do not initiate a course of alefacept therapy in patients with a CD4+ T lymphocyte count below normal.

See Warnings/Precautions for more information.

➤*Malignancies:* Alefacept may increase the risk of malignancies. In the 24-week period constituting the first course of placebo-controlled studies, 13 malignancies were diagnosed in 11 alefacept-treated patients. The incidence of malignancies was 1.3% (11/876) for alefacept-treated patients, compared with 0.5% (2/413) in the placebo group. In preclinical studies, animals developed B cell hyperplasia, and 1 animal developed a lymphoma. Do not administer alefacept to patients with a history of systemic malignancy. Exercise caution when considering the use of alefacept in patients at high risk for malignancy. If a patient develops a malignancy, discontinue alefacept.

➤*Serious infections:* Alefacept is an immunosuppressive agent and, therefore, has the potential to increase the risk of infection and reactivate latent, chronic infections. Do not administer alefacept to patients with a clinically important infection. Exercise caution when considering the use of alefacept in patients with chronic infections or a history of recurrent infection. Monitor patients for signs and symptoms of infection during or after a course of alefacept. Closely monitor new infections. If a patient develops a serious infection, discontinue alefacept. In the 24-week period constituting the first course of placebo-controlled studies, serious infections (infections requiring hospitalization) were observed at a rate of 0.9% (8/876) in alefacept-treated patients and 0.2% (1/413) in the placebo group.

➤*Phototherapy:* Patients receiving phototherapy should not receive concurrent therapy with alefacept because of the possibility of excessive immunosuppression.

➤*Hepatic injury:* In postmarketing experience, there have been reports of liver injury, including asymptomatic transaminase elevation, fatty infiltration of the liver, hepatitis, decompensation of cirrhosis with liver failure, and acute liver failure. Two cases of liver failure were reported with concomitant alcohol use. In the 24-week period constituting the first course of placebo-controlled studies, 1.7% (15/876) of alefacept-treated patients and 1.2% (5/413) of the placebo group experienced ALT and/or AST elevations of at least 3 times the upper limit of normal. While the exact relationship of these occurrences with the use of alefacept has not been established, fully evaluate patients with signs or symptoms of liver injury. Discontinue alefacept in patients who develop significant clinical signs of liver injury.

➤*Immunogenicity:* Approximately 3% (40/1,357) of patients receiving alefacept developed low-titer antibodies to alefacept. No apparent correlation of antibody development and clinical response or adverse reactions was observed. The long-term immunogenicity of alefacept is unknown.

The data reflect the percentage of patients whose test results were considered positive for antibodies to alefacept in an enzyme-linked immunosorbent assay (ELISA), and are highly dependent on the sensitivity and specificity of the assay. Additionally, the observed incidence of antibody positivity in an assay may be influenced by several factors, including sample handling, timing of sample collection, concomitant medications, and underlying disease. For these reasons, comparison of the incidence of antibodies to alefacept with the incidence of antibodies to other products may be misleading.

➤*Hypersensitivity reactions:* Hypersensitivity reactions (urticaria, angioedema) were associated with the administration of alefacept. If an anaphylactic reaction or other serious allergic reaction occurs, discontinue administration of alefacept immediately and initiate appropriate therapy.

➤*Pregnancy: Category B.* Women of childbearing potential make up a considerable segment of the patient population affected by psoriasis. Because the effect of alefacept on pregnancy and fetal development, including immune system development, is not known, health care providers are encouraged to enroll patients taking alefacept who become pregnant into the manufacturer's pregnancy registry by calling 1-866-263-8483.

Animal reproduction studies, however, are not always predictive of human response and there are no adequate and well-controlled studies in pregnant women. Because the risk to the development of the fetal immune system and postnatal immune function in humans is unknown, use alefacept during pregnancy only if clearly needed. If pregnancy occurs while taking alefacept, assess continued use of the drug.

➤*Lactation:* It is not known whether alefacept is excreted in human milk. Because many drugs are excreted in human milk, and because there exists the potential for serious adverse reactions in breast-feeding infants from alefacept, decide whether to discontinue breast-feeding during drug therapy or to discontinue the use of the drug, taking into account the importance of the drug to the mother.

➤*Children:* The safety and efficacy of alefacept in children have not been studied. Alefacept is not indicated for children.

➤*Elderly:* Because the incidence of infections and certain malignancies is higher in the elderly population, in general, use caution in treating the elderly.

➤*Monitoring:* Monitor CD4+ T lymphocyte counts weekly before initiating dosing and every 2 weeks throughout the 12-week dosing period and use them to guide dosing. Patients should have normal CD4+ T lymphocyte counts prior to an initial or a subsequent course of treatment with alefacept. If CD4+ T lymphocyte counts are below 250 cells/mcL, withhold alefacept dosing and institute weekly monitoring. Discontinue alefacept if CD4+ T lymphocyte counts remain below 250 cells/mcL for 1 month.

Monitor patients for signs and symptoms of infection during or after a course of alefacept. Closely monitor new infections.

Drug Interactions

No formal interaction studies have been performed.

➤*Immunosuppressants:* Patients receiving other immunosuppressive agents should not receive concurrent therapy with alefacept because of the possibility of excessive immunosuppression.

➤*Vaccines:* The safety and efficacy of vaccines, specifically live or live-attenuated vaccines, administered to patients being treated with alefacept have not been studied. In a study of 46 patients with chronic plaque psoriasis, the ability to mount immunity to tetanus toxoid (recall antigen) and an experimental neo-antigen was preserved in those patients undergoing alefacept therapy.

Adverse Reactions

Commonly observed adverse reactions seen in the first course of placebo-controlled clinical trials with at least a 2% higher incidence in the alefacept-treated patients compared with placebo-treated patients were pharyngitis, dizziness, increased cough, nausea, pruritus, myalgia, chills, injection site pain, injection site inflammation, and accidental injury. The only adverse reaction that occurred at a 5% or higher incidence among alefacept-treated patients compared with placebo-treated patients was chills (1% placebo vs 6% alefacept), which occurred predominantly with IV administration.

The adverse reactions that most commonly resulted in clinical intervention were cardiovascular events, including coronary artery disorder in less than 1% of patients and myocardial infarct in less than 1% of patients. These reactions were not observed in any of the 413 placebo-treated patients. The total number of patients hospitalized for cardiovascular events in the alefacept-treated group was 1.2% (11/876).

The most common reactions resulting in discontinuation of treatment with alefacept were CD4+ T lymphocyte levels below 250 cells/mcgL, headache (0.2%), and nausea (0.2%).

ALEFACEPT — INJECTION

The most serious adverse reactions were lymphopenia, malignancies, serious infections requiring hospitalization, and hypersensitivity reactions.

➤*Lymphopenia:* In the IM study (study 2), 4% of patients temporarily discontinued treatment and no patients permanently discontinued treatment due to CD4+ T lymphocyte counts below the specified threshold of 250 cells/mcL. In study 2, 10%, 28%, and 42% of patients had total lymphocyte, CD4+, and CD8+ T lymphocyte counts below normal, respectively. Twelve weeks after a course of therapy (12 weekly doses), 2%, 8%, and 21% of patients had total lymphocyte, CD4+, and CD8+ T cell counts below normal.

In the first course of the IV study (study 1), 10% of patients temporarily discontinued treatment and 2% permanently discontinued treatment due to CD4+ T lymphocyte counts below the specified threshold of 250 cells/mcL. During the first course of study 1, 22% of patients had total lymphocyte counts below normal, 48% had CD4+ T lymphocyte counts below normal and 59% had CD8+ T lymphocyte counts below normal. The maximal effect on lymphocytes was observed within 6 to 8 weeks of initiation of treatment. Twelve weeks after a course of therapy (12 weekly doses), 4% of patients had total lymphocyte counts below normal, 19% had CD4+ T lymphocyte counts below normal, and 36% had CD8+ T lymphocyte counts below normal.

For patients receiving a second course of alefacept in study 1, 17% of patients had total lymphocyte counts below normal, 44% had CD4+ T lymphocyte counts below normal, and 56% had CD8+ T lymphocyte counts below normal. Twelve weeks after completing dosing, 3% of patients had total lymphocyte counts below normal, 17% had CD4+ T lymphocyte counts below normal, and 35% had CD8+ T lymphocyte counts below normal.

➤*Malignancies:* See Warnings/Precautions for more information.

Among 1,869 patients who received alefacept at any dose in clinical trials, 43 patients were diagnosed with 63 treatment-emergent malignancies. The majority of the malignancies were nonmelanoma skin cancers: 46 cases (20 basal cell, 26 squamous cell carcinomas) in 27 patients. Other malignancies observed in alefacept-treated patients included melanoma (n = 3), solid organ malignancies (n = 12 in 11 patients), and lymphomas (n = 5); the latter consisted of 2 Hodgkin and 2 non-Hodgkin lymphomas, and 1 cutaneous T cell lymphoma (mycosis fungoides).

➤*Hypersensitivity:* In clinical studies, 4 of 1,869 (0.2%) patients were reported to experience angioedema: 2 of these patients were hospitalized. In the 24-week period constituting the first course of placebo-controlled studies, urticaria was reported in 6 (less than 1%) alefacept-treated patients versus 1 patient in the control group. Urticaria resulted in discontinuation of therapy in 1 of the alefacept-treated patients.

➤*Hepatic:* See Precautions for more information.

➤*Infections:* In the 24-week period constituting the first course of placebo-controlled studies, serious infections (infections requiring hospitalization) were seen at a rate of 0.9% (8/876) in alefacept-treated patients and 0.2% (1/413) in the placebo group. In patients receiving repeated courses of alefacept therapy, the rates of serious infections remained similar across courses of therapy. Serious infections among 1,869 alefacept-treated patients included cellulitis, abscesses, wound infections, toxic shock, pneumonia, appendicitis, cholecystitis, gastroenteritis, and herpes infections.

➤*Local:* In the IM study (study 2), 16% of alefacept-treated patients and 8% of placebo-treated patients reported injection site reactions. In patients receiving repeated courses of alefacept IM therapy, the incidence of injection site reactions remained similar across courses of therapy. Reactions at the site of injection were generally mild, typically occurred on single occasions, and included either pain (7%), inflammation (4%), bleeding (4%), edema (2%), nonspecific reaction (2%), mass (1%), or skin hypersensitivity (less than 1%). In the clinical trials, a single case of injection site reaction led to the discontinuation of alefacept.

➤*Postmarketing:* In postmarketing experience there have been reports of asymptomatic transaminase elevation, fatty infiltration of the liver, hepatitis, and severe liver failure.

Overdosage

➤*Symptoms:* The highest dose tested in humans (0.75 mg/kg IV) was associated with chills, headache, arthralgia, and sinusitis within 1 day of dosing.

➤*Treatment:* Closely monitor patients who have been inadvertently administered an excess of the recommended dose for effects on total lymphocyte count and CD4+ T lymphocyte count.

Patient Information

Inform patients of the need for regular monitoring of white blood cell (lymphocyte) counts during therapy and that alefacept must be administered under the supervision of a health care provider. Also inform patients that alefacept reduces lymphocyte counts, which could increase their chances of developing an infection or a malignancy. Advise patients to inform their health care provider promptly if they develop any signs of an infection or malignancy while undergoing a course of treatment with alefacept.

Also advise female patients to notify their health care provider if they become pregnant while taking alefacept (or within 8 weeks of discontinuing alefacept). Advise them of the existence of and encourage them to enroll in the manufacturer's pregnancy registry. Call 1-866-263-8483 to enroll into the registry.

Advise patients that serious liver injury has been reported in patients receiving alefacept. Advise patients to report to their health care provider persistent nausea, anorexia, fatigue, vomiting, abdominal pain, jaundice, easy bruising, dark urine, or pale stools.

AZATHIOPRINE

Rx	Azathioprine (aaiPharma)	Tablets: 50 mg	In 100s.
Rx	Imuran (Prometheus)		(Imuran 50). Yellow to off-white, scored. In 100s and UD 100s.
Rx	Azasan (aaiPharma)	Tablets: 75 mg	Lactose. Yellow, triangular, scored. In 100s.
Rx	Azasan (aaiPharma)	Tablets: 100 mg	Lactose. Yellow, diamond shape, scored. In 100s.
Rx	Azathioprine Sodium (Various, eg, Bedford)	Injection: 100 mg (as sodium) per vial	In 20 ml vials.

AZATHIOPRINE — ORAL

WARNING

Chronic immunosuppression with this purine antimetabolite increases risk of neoplasia in humans. Physicians using this drug should be very familiar with this risk as well as with the mutagenic potential to both men and women and with possible hematologic toxicities (see Warnings/Precautions).

Indications

➤*Renal homotransplantation:* Adjunct for the prevention of rejection in renal homotransplantation. Experience with more than 16,000 transplants shows a 5 year patient survival of 35% to 55%, but this is dependent on donor, match for HLA antigens, anti-donor or anti-B-cell alicantigen antibody, and other variables. The effect of azathioprine on these variables has not been tested in controlled trials.

➤*Rheumatoid arthritis:* Azathioprine is indicated only in adult patients meeting criteria for classic or definite rheumatoid arthritis as specified by the American Rheumatism Association. Azathioprine should be restricted to patients with severe, active and erosive disease not responsive to conventional management including rest, aspirin, or other nonsteroidal drugs, or to agents in the class of which gold is an example. Rest, physiotherapy, and salicylates should be continued while azathioprine is given, but it may be possible to reduce the dose of corticosteroids in patients on azathioprine. The combined use of azathioprine with gold, antimalarials, or penicillamine has not been studied for either added benefit or unexpected adverse effects. The use of azathioprine with these agents cannot be recommended.

➤*Off-label uses:*

Juvenile idiopathic arthritis – [3] = Safety concerns. Data evaluating the safety and efficacy of azathioprine for the treatment of juvenile idiopathic arthritis (JIA) are limited and show conflicting results. In addition, there are significant safety concerns with azathioprine use, including risk for neoplasia and pancytopenia. For these reasons, it is recommended that azathioprine not be routinely used for the treatment of JIA.

Multiple sclerosis – [2] = Fair documentation. Azathioprine has been used for the treatment of multiple sclerosis (MS) for more than 30 years and, while it is not approved for this indication in the United States, it is approved for this use in Europe. Currently available data and consensus guidelines state that azathioprine therapy appears to reduce the relapse rate in patients with MS. However, evidence supporting an effect on slowing disease progression is currently lacking. Avoid long-term use because of the potential for increased risk of carcinoma.

Psoriasis – [2] = Fair documentation. According to the American Academy of Dermatology guidelines, methotrexate, cyclosporine, and acitretin are considered first-line systemic agents for the treatment of psoriasis, but azathioprine may be an appropriate alternative for certain patients.

Other possible off-label uses –

Immunosuppression (children): Azathioprine has been used in children for immunosuppression.

Administration and Dosage

➤*Adults:*

Renal homotransplantation –

Initial dosage: 3 to 5 mg/kg daily given as a single daily dose on the day of, and in a minority of cases 1 to 3 days before, transplantation.

Maintenance dosage: 1 to 3 mg/kg daily. The dose should not be increased to toxic levels because of threatened rejection.

Conversion: Often initiated with the intravenous (IV) administration of the sodium salt, with subsequent use of tablets (at the same dose level) after the postoperative period. IV use of sodium salt is indicated only in patients unable to tolerate oral medications.

Discontinuation of therapy: Discontinuation may be necessary for severe hematologic or other toxicity, even if rejection of the homograft may be a consequence of drug withdrawal.

AZATHIOPRINE — ORAL

Rheumatoid arthritis –

Maximum dose: 2.5 mg/kg per day.

Initial dosage: 1 mg/kg (50 to 100 mg) given once or twice a day.

Maintenance dosage: Maintenance therapy should be at the lowest effective dose, and the dose given can be lowered decrementally with changes of 0.5 mg/kg or approximately 25 mg daily every 4 weeks while other therapy is kept constant.

Dosage adjustment: The dose may be increased by 0.5 mg/kg/day at 6 to 8 weeks and thereafter by 4-week intervals, up to a maximum dose of 2.5 mg/kg per day, if there are no serious toxicities and if initial response is unsatisfactory.

Duration of therapy: The optimum duration of maintenance has not been determined. Therapy may be continued long-term in patients with clinical response, but patients should be monitored carefully, and gradual dosage reduction should be attempted to reduce risk of toxicities.

Discontinuation of therapy: Can be discontinued abruptly, but delayed effects are possible.

Off-label dosing –

Multiple sclerosis: [2] = Fair documentation. 2 to 3 mg/kg daily, alone or in combination with other immunosuppressive or immunomodulating agents.

Psoriasis: [2] = Fair documentation. The recommended initial dose is 0.5 mg/kg, after which patients should be monitored for cytopenia. If cytopenia is not observed, the dosage may be increased by 0.5 mg/kg/day after 6 to 8 weeks, if needed, and then increased further by 0.5 mg/kg/day every 4 weeks thereafter. The usual dosage is 75 to 150 mg/day; however, dosages up to 300 mg/day have been used in a limited number of patients. Alternatively, dosing may be guided by thiopurine methyltransferase levels.

➤*Children:*

Off-label dosing –

Immunosuppression:

- *Initial dosage* – 3 to 5 mg/kg daily.
- *Maintenance dosage* – 1 to 3 mg/kg daily.

Juvenile idiopathic arthritis: [3] = Safety concerns.

- *Patients 1 to 20 years of age* – For patients 1 to 20 years of age with refractory JIA, the most common dosages studied were 1 to 3 mg/kg orally once daily, to a maximum dosage of 5 mg/kg daily. Therapy continued for several years in 1 report.

➤*Renal function impairment:* Give lower doses.

➤*Preparation for administration:* Azathioprine is an immunosuppressant agent and is also considered a potential teratogen and mutagen. Follow safe handling procedures when preparing, administering, or dispensing azathioprine.

➤*Administration:* Administer with food to decrease GI discomfort.

➤*Storage/Stability:* Store at 15° to 25°C (59° to 77°F) in a dry place and protect from light.

Actions

➤*Pharmacology:*

Homograft survival – Summary information from transplant centers and registries indicates relatively universal use of azathioprine with or without other immunosuppressive agents. Although the use of azathioprine for inhibition of renal homograft rejection is well established, the mechanism(s) for this action are somewhat obscure. The drug suppresses hypersensitivities of the cell-mediated type and causes variable alterations in antibody production. Suppression of T-cell effects, including ablation of T-cell suppression, is dependent on the temporal relationship to antigenic stimulus or engraftment. This agent has little effect on established graft rejections or secondary responses.

Alterations in specific immune responses or immunologic functions in transplant recipients are difficult to relate specifically to immunosuppression by azathioprine. These patients have subnormal responses to vaccines, low numbers of T-cells, and abnormal phagocytosis by peripheral blood cells, but their mitogenic responses, serum immunoglobulins, and secondary antibody responses are usually normal.

Immunoinflammatory response – Azathioprine suppresses disease manifestations as well as underlying pathology in animal models of autoimmune disease. For example, the severity of adjuvant arthritis is reduced by azathioprine.

The mechanisms whereby azathioprine affects autoimmune diseases are not known. Azathioprine is immunosuppressive, delayed hypersensitivity and cellular cytotoxicity tests being suppressed to a greater degree than are antibody responses. In the rat model of adjuvant arthritis, azathioprine has been shown to inhibit the lymph node hyperplasia, which precedes the onset of the signs of the disease. Both the immunosuppressive and therapeutic effects in animal models are dose-related. Azathioprine is considered a slow-acting drug and effects may persist after the drug has been discontinued.

➤*Pharmacokinetics:* Azathioprine is well absorbed following oral administration. Maximum serum radioactivity occurs at 1 to 2 hours after oral ^{35}S-azathioprine and decays with a half-life of 5 hours. This is not an estimate of the half-life of azathioprine itself, but is the decay rate for all ^{35}S-containing metabolites of the drug. Because of extensive metabolism, only a fraction of the radioactivity is present as azathioprine. Usual doses produce blood levels of azathioprine, and of mercaptopurine derived from it, which are low (less than 1 mcg/mL). Blood levels are of little predictive value for therapy since the magnitude and duration of clinical effects correlate with thiopurine nucleotide levels in tissues rather than with plasma drug levels. Azathioprine and mercaptopurine are moderately bound to serum proteins (30%) and are partially dialyzable.

Azathioprine is cleaved in vivo to mercaptopurine. Both compounds are rapidly eliminated from blood and are oxidized or methylated in erythrocytes and liver; no azathioprine or mercaptopurine is detectable in urine after 8 hours. Conversion to inactive 6-thiouric acid by xanthine oxidase is an important degradative pathway, and the inhibition of this pathway in patients receiving allopurinol is the basis for the azathioprine dosage reduction required in these patients. Patients receiving azathioprine and allopurinol concomitantly should have a dose reduction of azathioprine, to approximately ⅓ to ¼ the usual dose. Proportions of metabolites are different in individual patients, and this presumably accounts for variable magnitude and duration of drug effects. Renal clearance is probably not important in predicting biological effectiveness or toxicities, although dose reduction is practiced in patients with poor renal function.

Contraindications

Hypersensitivity to the drug.

Treating rheumatoid arthritis in pregnant women.

Patients with rheumatoid arthritis previously treated with alkylating agents (cycloposphamide, chlorambucil, melphalan, or others) may have a prohibitive risk of neoplasia if treated with azathioprine.

Warnings/Precautions

➤*Mercaptopurine/Azathioprine:* Mercaptopurine is a metabolite of azathioprine; therefore, avoid coadministration due to the risk of severe myelosuppression.

➤*Hematologic effects:* Severe leukopenia or thrombocytopenia may occur in patients on azathioprine. Macrocytic anemia and severe bone marrow depression may also occur. Hematologic toxicities are dose-related and may be more severe in renal transplant patients whose homograft is undergoing rejection. It is suggested that patients on azathioprine have complete blood counts, including platelet counts, weekly during the first month, twice monthly for the second and third months of treatment, then monthly or more frequently if dosage alterations or other therapy changes are necessary. Delayed hematologic suppression may occur. Prompt reduction in dosage or temporary withdrawal of the drug may be necessary if there is a rapid fall in or persistently low leukocyte count, or other evidence of bone marrow depression. Leukopenia does not correlate with therapeutic effect; therefore the dose should not be increased intentionally to lower the white blood cell count.

➤*Serious infections:* Serious infections are a constant hazard for patients receiving chronic immunosuppression, especially for homograft recipients. Fungal, viral, bacterial, and protozoal infections may be fatal and should be treated vigorously. Reduction of azathioprine dosage or use of other drugs should be considered.

➤*GI effects:* A GI hypersensitivity reaction characterized by severe nausea and vomiting has been reported. These symptoms may also be accompanied by diarrhea, rash, fever, malaise, myalgias, elevations in liver enzymes, and occasionally, hypotension. Symptoms of gastrointestinal toxicity most often develop within the first several weeks of therapy with azathioprine and are reversible upon discontinuation of the drug. The reaction can recur within hours after rechallenge with a single dose of azathioprine.

➤*Pregnancy: Category D.* Azathioprine can cause fetal harm when administered to a pregnant woman. Azathioprine should not be given during pregnancy without careful weighing of risk versus benefit. Whenever possible, use of azathioprine in pregnant patients should be avoided. This drug should not be used for treating rheumatoid arthritis in pregnant women.

Azathioprine is teratogenic in rabbits and mice when given in doses equivalent to the human dose (5 mg/kg daily). Abnormalities included skeletal malformations and visceral anomalies.

Limited immunologic and other abnormalities have occurred in a few infants born of renal allograft recipients on azathioprine, in a detailed case report, documented lymphopenia, diminished IgG and IgM levels, CMV infection, and a decreased thymic shadow were noted in an infant born to a mother receiving 150 mg azathioprine and 30 mg prednisone daily throughout pregnancy. At 10 weeks most features were normalized. DeWitte et al reported pancytopenia and severe immune deficiency in a preterm infant whose mother received 125 mg azathioprine and 12.5 mg prednisone daily. There have been 2 published reports of abnormal physical findings. Williamson and Karp described an infant born with preaxial polydactyly whose mother received azathioprine 200 mg daily and prednisone 20 mg every other day during pregnancy. Tallent et al described an infant with a large myelomeningocele in the upper lumbar region, bilateral dislocated hips, and bilateral talipes equinovarus. The father was on long-term azathioprine therapy.

Benefit versus risk must be weighed carefully before use of azathioprine in patients of reproductive potential. There are no adequate and well-controlled studies in pregnant women. If this drug is used during pregnancy or if the patient becomes pregnant while taking this drug, the patient should be apprised of the potential hazard to the fetus. Women of childbearing age should be advised to avoid becoming pregnant.

➤*Lactation:* The use of azathioprine in nursing mothers is not recommended. Azathioprine or its metabolites are transferred at low levels, both transplacentally and in breast milk. Because of the potential for tumorigenicity shown for azathioprine, a decision should be made whether to discontinue nursing or discontinue the drug, taking into account the importance of the drug to the mother.

➤*Children:* Safety and efficacy of azathioprine in children have not been established.

AZATHIOPRINE — ORAL

Drug Interactions

➤*Other agents affecting myeloposis:* Drugs that may affect leukocyte production, including cotrimoxazole, may lead to exaggerated leukopenia, especially in renal transplant recipients.

Azathioprine Drug Interactions			
Precipitant drug	Object drug[a]		Description
ACE inhibitors	Azathioprine	↑	Concurrent use may induce severe leukopenia.
Allopurinol	Azathioprine	↑	Allopurinol may increase the pharmacologic and toxic effects of azathioprine. Patients receiving azathioprine and allopurinol concomitantly should have a dose reduction of azathioprine, to approximately ⅓ to ¼ the usual dose.
Methotrexate	Azathioprine	↑	Plasma levels of the 6-MP metabolite may be increased.
Azathioprine	Anticoagulants	↓	Azathioprine may decrease the action of the anticoagulants.
Azathioprine	Cyclosporine	↓	Cyclosporine plasma levels may be decreased.
Azathioprine	Nondepolarizing neuromuscular blockers	↓	Pharmacologic actions of the neuromuscular blockers may be decreased or reversed.

[a] ↑ = object drug increased; ↓ = object drug decreased.

Adverse Reactions

The principal and potentially serious toxic effects of azathioprine are hematologic and gastrointestinal. The risks of secondary infection and neoplasia are also significant (see Warnings/Precautions). The frequency and severity of adverse reactions depend on the dose and duration of azathioprine as well as on the patient's underlying disease or concomitant therapies. The incidence of hematologic toxicities and neoplasia encountered in groups of renal homograft recipients is significantly higher than that in studies employing azathioprine for rheumatoid arthritis. The relative incidences in clinical studies are summarized below:

Azathioprine Toxicities		
Toxicity	Renal homograft	Rheumatoid arthritis
Leukopenia (any degree)	> 50%	28%
< 2500 cells/mm^3	18%	5.3%
Infections	20%	< 1%
Neoplasia		[a]
Lymphoma	0.5%	
Others	2.8%	

[a] Data on the rate and risk of neoplasia among persons with rheumatoid arthritis are limited. The incidence of lymphoproliferative disease in patients with rheumatoid arthritis appears to be significantly higher than that in the general population. In 1 completed study, the rate of lymphoproliferative disease in RA patients receiving higher than recommended doses of azathioprine (5 mg/kg per day) was 1.8 cases per 1000 patient-years of follow-up, compared with 0.8 cases per 1000 patient-years of follow-up in those not receiving azathioprine. However, the proportion of the increased risk attributable to the azathioprine dosage or to other therapies (ie, alkylating agents) received by patients treated with azathioprine cannot be determined.

➤*GI:* Nausea and vomiting may occur within the first few months of therapy with azathioprine, and occurred in approximately 12% of 676 rheumatoid arthritis patients. The frequency of gastric disturbance often can be reduced by administration of the drug in divided doses or after meals. However, in some patients, nausea and vomiting may be severe and may be accompanied by symptoms such as diarrhea, fever, malaise, and myalgias (see Precautions). Vomiting with abdominal pain may occur rarely with a hypersensitivity pancreatitis. Hepatotoxicity manifest by elevation of serum alkaline phosphatase, bilirubin, or serum transaminases is known to occur following azathioprine use, primarily in allograft recipients. Hepatotoxicity has been uncommon (< 1%) in rheumatoid arthritis patients. Hepatotoxicity following transplantation most often occurs within 5 months of transplantation and is generally reversible after interruption of azathioprine. A rare, but life-threatening hepatic veno-occlusive disease associated with chronic administration of azathioprine has been described in transplant patients and in 1 patient receiving azathioprine for panuveitis. Periodic measurement of serum transaminases, alkaline phosphatase, and bilirubin is indicated for early detection of hepatotoxicity. If hepatic veno-occlusive disease is clinically suspected, azathioprine should be permanently withdrawn.

➤*Hematologic:* Leukopenia or thrombocytopenia are dose-dependent and may occur late in the course of therapy with azathioprine. Dose reduction or temporary withdrawal allows reversal of these toxicities. Infection may occur as a secondary manifestation of bone marrow suppression or leukopenia, but the incidence of infection in renal homotransplantation is 30 to 60 times that in rheumatoid arthritis. Macrocytic anemia or bleeding have been reported.

There are rare individuals with an inherited deficiency of the enzyme thiopurine methyltransferase (TPMT) who may be unusually sensitive to the myelosuppressive effect of azathioprine and prone to developing rapid bone marrow suppression following the initiation of treatment with azathioprine.

➤*Miscellaneous:* Additional side effects of low frequency have been reported. Those include skin rashes, alopecia, fever, arthralgias, diarrhea, steatorrhea, negative nitrogen balance, and reversible interstitial pneumonitis.

Overdosage

➤*Symptoms:* The oral LD_{50}s for single doses of azathioprine in mice and rats are 2500 mg/kg and 400 mg/kg, respectively. Very large doses of this antimetabolite may lead to marrow hypoplasia, bleeding, infection, and death. About 30% of azathioprine is bound to serum proteins, but approximately 45% is removed during an 8 hour hemodialysis. A single case has been reported of a renal transplant patient who ingested a single dose of 7500 mg azathioprine. The immediate toxic reactions were nausea, vomiting, and diarrhea, followed by mild leukopenia and mild abnormalities in liver function. The white blood cell count, AST, and bilirubin returned to normal 6 days after the overdose.

Patient Information

Patients being started on azathioprine should be informed of the necessity of periodic blood counts while they are receiving the drug and should be encouraged to report any unusual bleeding or bruising to their physician. They should be informed of the danger of infection while receiving azathioprine and asked to report signs and symptoms of infection to their physician. Careful dosage instructions should be given to the patient, especially when azathioprine is being administered in the presence of impaired renal function or concomitantly with allopurinol (see Administration and Dosage and Drug Interactions). Patients should be advised of the potential risks of the use of azathioprine during pregnancy and during the nursing period. The increased risk of neoplasia following therapy with azathioprine should be explained to the patient.

AZATHIOPRINE — INJECTION

WARNING

Chronic immunosuppression with this purine antimetabolite increases risk of neoplasia in humans. Physicians using this drug should be very familiar with this risk as well as with the mutagenic potential to both men and women and with possible hematologic toxicities (See Warnings/Precautions).

Indications

➤*Renal homotransplantation:* Adjunct for the prevention of rejection in renal homotransplantation. Experience with over 16,000 transplants shows a 5 year patient survival of 35% to 55%, but this is dependent on donor, match for HLA antigens, anti-donor or anti-B-cell alicantigen antibody, and other variables. The effect of azathioprine on these variables has not been tested in controlled trials.

➤*Rheumatoid arthritis:* Azathioprine is indicated only in adult patients meeting criteria for classic or definite rheumatoid arthritis as specified by the American Rheumatism Association. Azathioprine should be restricted to patients with severe, active and erosive disease not responsive to conventional management including rest, aspirin, or other nonsteroidal drugs, or to agents in the class of which gold is an example. Rest, physiotherapy, and salicylates should be continued while azathioprine is given, but it may be possible to reduce the dose of corticosteroids in patients on azathioprine. The combined use of azathioprine with gold, antimalarials, or penicillamine has not been studied for either added benefit or unexpected adverse effects. The use of azathioprine with these agents cannot be recommended.

➤*Off-label uses:*

Other possible off-label uses – For immunosuppression in children. (See Administration and Dosage.)

Administration and Dosage

➤*Adults:*

Renal homotransplantation –

Initial dosage: 3 to 5 mg/kg daily given as a single daily dose on the day of, and in a minority of cases 1 to 3 days before, transplantation.

Maintenance dosage: 1 to 3 mg/kg daily. The dose should not be increased to toxic levels because of threatened rejection.

Conversion: Often initiated with the intravenous (IV) administration of the sodium salt, with subsequent use of tablets (at the same dose level) after the postoperative period. IV use of sodium salt is indicated only in patients unable to tolerate oral medications.

Discontinuation of therapy: Discontinuation may be necessary for severe hematologic or other toxicity, even if rejection of the homograft may be a consequence of drug withdrawal.

Rheumatoid arthritis –

Maximum dose: 2.5 mg/kg per day.

Initial dosage: 1 mg/kg (50 to 100 mg) once or twice a day.

AZATHIOPRINE — INJECTION

Maintenance dosage: Maintenance therapy should be at the lowest effective dose, and the dose given can be lowered decrementally with changes of 0.5 mg/kg or approximately 25 mg daily every 4 weeks while other therapy is kept constant.

Dosage adjustment: The dosage may be increased by 0.5 mg/kg daily at 6 to 8 weeks and thereafter by 4 week intervals, up to a maximum dosage of 2.5 mg/kg per day, if there are no serious toxicities and if initial response is unsatisfactory.

Duration of therapy: The optimum duration of maintenance has not been determined. May be continued long-term in patients with clinical response, but patients should be monitored carefully and gradual dosage reduction should be attempted to reduce risk of toxicities.

Discontinuation of therapy: Can be discontinued abruptly, but delayed effects are possible.

➤*Children:*

Off-label dosing –

Immunosuppression:

- *Initial dosage* – 3 to 5 mg/kg IV daily.
- *Maintenance dosage* – 1 to 3 mg/kg IV daily.

➤*Renal function impairment:* Give lower doses.

➤*Preparation for administration:* Add 10 mL of sterile water for injection and swirl until a clear solution results. This solution (equivalent to azathioprine 100 mg) has a pH of approximately 9.6 and it should be used within 24 hours. Further dilution into sterile saline or dextrose is usually made for infusion; the final volume depends on time for the infusion, usually 30 to 60 minutes, but as short as 5 minutes and as long as 8 hours for the daily dose.

Azathioprine is an immunosuppressant agent and is also considered a potential teratogen and mutagen. Follow safe handling procedures when preparing, administering, or dispensing azathioprine.

➤*Administration:* For IV use only. Time for infusion is usually 30 to 60 minutes, but as short as 5 minutes and as long as 8 hours for the daily dose.

➤*Storage/Stability:* Store at 15°C to 25°C (59°F to 77°F) in a dry place and protect from light. Diluted solution should be used within 24 hours.

Actions

➤*Pharmacology:*

Homograft survival – Summary information from transplant centers and registries indicates relatively universal use of azathioprine with or without other immunosuppressive agents. Although the use of azathioprine for inhibition of renal homograft rejection is well established, the mechanism(s) for this action are somewhat obscure. The drug suppresses hypersensitivities of the cell-mediated type and causes variable alterations in antibody production. Suppression of T-cell effects, including ablation of T-cell suppression, is dependent on the temporal relationship to antigenic stimulus or engraftment. This agent has little effect on established graft rejections or secondary responses.

Alterations in specific immune responses or immunologic functions in transplant recipients are difficult to relate specifically to immunosuppression by azathioprine. These patients have subnormal responses to vaccines, low numbers of T-cells, and abnormal phagocytosis by peripheral blood cells, but their mitogenic responses, serum immunoglobulins, and secondary antibody responses are usually normal.

Immunoinflammatory response – Azathioprine suppresses disease manifestations as well as underlying pathology in animal models of autoimmune disease. For example, the severity of adjuvant arthritis is reduced by azathioprine.

The mechanisms whereby azathioprine affects autoimmune diseases are not known. Azathioprine is immunosuppressive, delayed hypersensitivity and cellular cytotoxicity tests being suppressed to a greater degree than are antibody responses. In the rat model of adjuvant arthritis, azathioprine has been shown to inhibit the lymph node hyperplasia which precedes the onset of the signs of the disease. Both the immunosuppressive and therapeutic effects in animal models are dose-related. Azathioprine is considered a slow-acting drug and effects may persist after the drug has been discontinued.

➤*Pharmacokinetics:*

Metabolism – Usual doses produce blood levels of azathioprine, and of mercaptopurine derived from it, which are low (< 1 mcg/mL). Blood levels are of little predictive value for therapy since the magnitude and duration of clinical effects correlate with thiopurine nucleotide levels in tissues rather than with plasma drug levels. Azathioprine and mercaptopurine are moderately bound to serum proteins (30%) and are partially dialyzable.

Azathioprine is cleaved in vivo to mercaptopurine. Both compounds are rapidly eliminated from blood and are oxidized or methylated in erythrocytes and liver; no azathioprine or mercaptopurine is detectable in urine after 8 hours. Conversion to inactive 6-thiouric acid by xanthine oxidase is an important degradative pathway, and the inhibition of this pathway in patients receiving allopurinol is the basis for the azathioprine dosage reduction required in these patients (see Drug Interactions). Proportions of metabolites are different in individual patients, and this presumably accounts for variable magnitude and duration of drug effects. Renal clearance is probably not important in predicting biological effectiveness or toxicities, although dose reduction is practiced in patients with poor renal function.

Contraindications

Hypersensitivity to the drug.

Treating rheumatoid arthritis in pregnant women.

Patients with rheumatoid arthritis previously treated with alkylating agents (cyclophosphamide, chlorambucil, melphalan, or others) may have a prohibitive risk of neoplasia if treated with azathioprine.

Warnings/Precautions

➤*Mercaptopurine/Azathioprine:* Mercaptopurine is a metabolite of azathioprine; therefore, avoid coadministration due to the risk of severe myelosuppression.

➤*Hematologic effects:* Severe leukopenia or thrombocytopenia may occur in patients on azathioprine. Macrocytic anemia and severe bone marrow depression may also occur. Hematologic toxicities are dose-related and may be more severe in renal transplant patients whose homograft is undergoing rejection. It is suggested that patients on azathioprine have complete blood counts, including platelet counts, weekly during the first month, twice monthly for the second and third months of treatment, then monthly or more frequently if dosage alterations or other therapy changes are necessary. Delayed hematologic suppression may occur. Prompt reduction in dosage or temporary withdrawal of the drug may be necessary if there is a rapid fall in or persistently low leukocyte count, or other evidence of bone marrow depression. Leukopenia does not correlate with therapeutic effect; therefore the dose should not be increased intentionally to lower the white blood cell count.

➤*Serious infections:* Serious infections are a constant hazard for patients receiving chronic immunosuppression, especially for homograft recipients. Fungal viral, bacterial, and protozoal infections may be fatal and should be treated vigorously. Reduction of azathioprine dosage or use of other drugs should be considered.

➤*GI toxicity:* A gastrointestinal hypersensitivity reaction characterized by severe nausea and vomiting has been reported. These symptoms may also be accompanied by diarrhea, rash, fever, malaise, myalgias, elevations in liver enzymes, and occasionally, hypotension. Symptoms of GI toxicity most often develop within the first several weeks of therapy with azathioprine and are reversible upon discontinuation of the drug. The reaction can recur within hours after rechallenge with a single dose of azathioprine.

➤*Pregnancy:* *Category D.* Azathioprine can cause fetal harm when administered to a pregnant woman. Azathioprine should not be given during pregnancy without careful weighing of risk versus benefit. Whenever possible, use of azathioprine in pregnant patients should be avoided. This drug should not be used for treating rheumatoid arthritis in pregnant women.

Azathioprine is teratogenic in rabbits and mice when given in doses equivalent to the human dose (5 mg/kg daily). Abnormalities included skeletal malformations and visceral anomalies.

Limited immunologic and other abnormalities have occurred in a few infants born of renal allograft recipients on azathioprine, in a detailed case report, documented lymphopenia, diminished IgG and IgM levels, CMV infection, and a decreased thymic shadow were noted in an infant born to a mother receiving 150 mg azathioprine and 30 mg prednisone daily throughout pregnancy. At 10 weeks most features were normalized. DeWitte et al reported pancytopenia and severe immune deficiency in a preterm infant whose mother received 125 mg azathioprine and 12.5 mg prednisone daily. There have been 2 published reports of abnormal physical findings. Williamson and Karp described an infant born with preaxial polydactyly whose mother received azathioprine 200 mg daily and prednisone 20 mg every other day during pregnancy. Tallent et al described an infant with a large myelomeningocele in the upper lumbar region, bilateral dislocated hips, and bilateral talipes equinovarus. The father was on long-term azathioprine therapy.

Benefit vs risk must be weighed carefully before use of azathioprine in patients of reproductive potential. There are no adequate and well-controlled studies in pregnant women. If this drug is used during pregnancy or if the patient becomes pregnant while taking this drug, the patient should be apprised of the potential hazard to the fetus. Women of childbearing age should be advised to avoid becoming pregnant.

➤*Lactation:* The use of azathioprine in nursing mothers is not recommended. Azathioprine or its metabolites are transferred at low levels, both transplacentally and in breast milk. Because of the potential for tumorigenicity shown for azathioprine, a decision should be made whether to discontinue nursing or discontinue the drug, taking into account the importance of the drug to the mother.

➤*Children:* Safety and efficacy of azathioprine in children have not been established.

Drug Interactions

➤*Other agents affecting myeloposis:* Drugs that may affect leukocyte production, including cotrimoxazole, may lead to exaggerated leukopenia, especially in renal transplant recipients.

AZATHIOPRINE — INJECTION

Azathioprine Drug Interactions

Precipitant drug	Object drug[a]		Description
ACE inhibitors	Azathioprine	↑	Concurrent use may induce severe leukopenia.
Allopurinol	Azathioprine	↑	Allopurinol may increase the pharmacologic and toxic effects of azathioprine. Patients receiving azathioprine and allopurinol concomitantly should have a dose reduction of azathioprine, to approximately ¼ to ⅓ the usual dose.
Methotrexate	Azathioprine	↑	Plasma levels of the 6-MP metabolite may be increased.
Azathioprine	Anticoagulants	↓	Azathioprine may decrease the action of the anticoagulants.
Azathioprine	Cyclosporine	↓	Cyclosporine plasma levels may be decreased.
Azathioprine	Nondepolarizing neuromuscular blockers	↓	Pharmacologic actions of the neuromuscular blockers may be decreased or reversed.

[a] ↑ = object drug increased; ↓ = object drug decreased.

Adverse Reactions

The principal and potentially serious toxic effects of azathioprine are hematologic and GI. The risks of secondary infection and neoplasia are also significant (see Warnings/Precautions). The frequency and severity of adverse reactions depend on the dose and duration of azathioprine and on the patient's underlying disease or concomitant therapies. The incidence of hematologic toxicities and neoplasia encountered in groups of renal homograft recipients is significantly higher than that in studies employing azathioprine for rheumatoid arthritis. The relative incidences in clinical studies are summarized below.

Azathioprine Toxicities

Toxicity	Renal homograft	Rheumatoid arthritis
Leukopenia (any degree)	> 50%	28%
< 2500/mm³	16%	5.3%
Infections	20%	< 1%
Neoplasia		[a]
Lymphoma	0.5%	
Others	2.8%	

[a] Data on the rate and risk of neoplasm among persons with rheumatoid arthritis treated with azathioprine are limited. The incidence of lymphoproliferative disease in patients with RA appears to be significantly higher than that in the general population. In one completed study, the rate of lymphoproliferative disease in RA patients receiving higher than recommended doses of azathioprine (5 mg/kg/day) was 1.8 cases per 1000 patient-years of follow-up, compared to 0.8 cases per 1000 patient-years of follow-up in those not receiving azathioprine. However, the proportion of the increased risk attributable to the azathioprine dosage or to other therapies (ie, alkylating agents) received by patients treated with azathioprine cannot be determined.

➤*GI:* Nausea and vomiting may occur within the first few months of therapy with azathioprine, and occurred in approximately 12% of 676 rheumatoid arthritis patients. The frequency of gastric disturbance often can be reduced by administration of the drug in divided doses or after meals. However, in some patients, nausea and vomiting may be severe and may be accompanied by symptoms such as diarrhea, fever, malaise, and myalgias (see Precautions). Vomiting with abdominal pain may occur rarely with a hypersensitivity pancreatitis. Hepatotoxicity manifest by elevation of serum alkaline phosphatase, bilirubin, or serum transaminases is known to occur following azathioprine use, primarily in allograft recipients. Hepatotoxicity has been uncommon (< 1%) in rheumatoid arthritis patients. Hepatotoxicity following transplantation most often occurs within 5 months of transplantation and is generally reversible after interruption of azathioprine. A rare, but life-threatening hepatic veno-occlusive disease associated with chronic administration of azathioprine has been described in transplant patients and in one patient receiving azathioprine for panuveitis. Periodic measurement of serum transaminases, alkaline phosphatase, and bilirubin is indicated for early detection of hepatotoxicity. If hepatic veno-occlusive disease is clinically suspected, azathioprine should be permanently withdrawn.

➤*Hematologic:* Leukopenia or thrombocytopenia are dose-dependent and may occur late in the course of therapy with azathioprine. Dose reduction or temporary withdrawal allows reversal of these toxicities. Infection may occur as a secondary manifestation of bone marrow suppression or leukopenia, but the incidence of infection in renal homotransplantation is 30 to 60 times that in rheumatoid arthritis. Macrocytic anemia or bleeding have been reported.

There are rare individuals with an inherited deficiency of the enzyme thiopurine methyltransferase (TPMT) who may be unusually sensitive to the myelosuppressive effect of azathioprine and prone to developing rapid bone marrow suppression following the initiation of treatment with azathioprine.

➤*Miscellaneous:* Additional side effects of low frequency have been reported. Those include skin rashes, alopecia, fever, arthralgias, diarrhea, steatorrhea, negative nitrogen balance, and reversible interstitial pneumonitis.

Overdosage

➤*Symptoms:* The oral LD_{50}s for single doses of azathioprine in mice and rats are 2500 mg/kg and 400 mg/kg, respectively. Very large doses of this antimetabolite may lead to marrow hypoplasia, bleeding, infection, and death. About 30% of azathioprine is bound to serum proteins, but approximately 45% is removed during an 8 hour hemodialysis. A single case has been reported of a renal transplant patient who ingested a single dose of 7500 mg azathioprine. The immediate toxic reactions were nausea, vomiting, and diarrhea, followed by mild leukopenia and mild abnormalities in liver function. The white blood cell count, AST, and bilirubin returned to normal 6 days after the overdose.

Patient Information

Patients being started on azathioprine should be informed of the necessity of periodic blood counts while they are receiving the drug and should be encouraged to report any unusual bleeding or bruising to their physician. They should be informed of the danger of infection while receiving azathioprine and asked to report signs and symptoms of infection to their physician. Careful dosage instructions should be given to the patient, especially when azathioprine is being administered in the presence of impaired renal function or concomitantly with allopurinol (see Administration and Dosage and Drug Interactions). Patients should be advised of the potential risks of the use of azathioprine during pregnancy and during the nursing period. The increased risk of neoplasia following therapy with azathioprine should be explained to the patient.

BASILIXIMAB

Rx	**Simulect** (Novartis)	**Powder for injection, lyophilized:** 20 mg	Preservative free. Sucrose, mannitol, potassium phosphate, sodium chloride. In single-use vials.

BASILIXIMAB — INJECTION

WARNING

Only physicians experienced in immunosuppression therapy and management of organ transplantation patients should prescribe basiliximab. The physician responsible for basiliximab administration should have complete information requisite for the follow-up of the patient. Patients receiving the drug should be managed in facilities equipped with adequate laboratory and supportive medical resources.

Indications

➤*Organ rejection:* For the prophylaxis of acute organ rejection in patients receiving renal transplantation when used as part of an immunosuppressive regimen that includes cyclosporine and corticosteroids.

The efficacy of basiliximab for the prophylaxis of acute rejection in recipients of other solid organ allografts has not been demonstrated.

Administration and Dosage

➤*General dosing considerations:* Patients previously administered basiliximab should only be re-exposed to a subsequent course of therapy with extreme caution.

➤*Adults:*

Organ rejection – 20 mg IV administered within 2 hours prior to transplantation surgery. A second 20 mg IV dose should be administered 4 days after transplantation. Withhold the second dose if complications such as severe hypersensitivity reactions to basiliximab or graft loss occur.

➤*Children:*

Organ rejection –

Patients weighing 35 kg or more: See Adults for dosing.

Patients weighing less than 35 kg: 10 mg IV administered within 2 hours prior to transplantation surgery. A second 10 mg IV dose should be administered 4 days after transplantation. Withhold the second dose if complications such as severe hypersensitivity reactions to basiliximab or graft loss occur.

➤*Concomitant therapy:* Basiliximab is used as part of an immunosuppressive regimen that includes cyclosporine (modified) and corticosteroids.

➤*Preparation for administration:* To prepare the reconstituted solution, add 2.5 mL (10 mg vial) or 5 mL (20 mg vial) of sterile water for injection, using aseptic technique, to the vial containing the basiliximab powder. Shake the vial gently to dissolve the powder.

The reconstituted solution is isotonic and may be given either as a bolus injection or diluted to a volume of 25 mL (10 mg vial) or 50 mL (20 mg vial) with normal saline or dextrose 5% for infusion. When mixing the solution, gently invert the bag in order to avoid foaming; do not shake.

➤*Administration:* Basiliximab is for central or peripheral IV administration only.

BASILIXIMAB — INJECTION

Reconstituted basiliximab should be given either as a bolus injection or diluted as previously described and administered as an IV infusion over 20 to 30 minutes.

Bolus administration may be associated with nausea, vomiting, and local reactions, including pain.

➤*Admixture compatibility:* No incompatibility between basiliximab and polyvinyl chloride bags or infusion sets has been observed. No data are available on the compatibility of basiliximab with other IV substances. Other drug substances should not be added or infused simultaneously through the same IV line.

➤*Storage / Stability:* Store lyophilized basiliximab under refrigerated conditions (2° to 8°C; 36° to 46°F). It is recommended that after reconstitution, the solution should be used immediately. If not used immediately, it can be stored between 2° and 8°C (35.6° and 46.4°F) for 24 hours or at room temperature for 4 hours. Discard the reconstituted solution if not used within 24 hours.

Actions

➤*Pharmacology:* Basiliximab functions as an IL-2 receptor antagonist by binding with high affinity ($K_a = 1 \bullet 10^{10}\ M^{-1}$) to the alpha chain of the high affinity IL-2 receptor complex and inhibiting IL-2 binding. Basiliximab is specifically targeted against IL-2Rα, which is selectively expressed on the surface of activated T-lymphocytes. This specific high affinity binding of basiliximab to IL-2Rα competitively inhibits IL-2-mediated activation of lymphocytes, a critical pathway in the cellular immune response involved in allograft rejection. While in the circulation, basiliximab impairs the response of the immune system to antigenic challenges. Whether the ability to respond to repeated or ongoing challenges with those antigens returns to normal after basiliximab is cleared is unknown.

Pharmacodynamics – Complete and consistent binding to IL-2Rα in adults is maintained as long as serum basiliximab levels exceed 0.2 mcg/mL. As concentrations fall below this threshold, the IL-2Rα sites are no longer fully bound and the number of T-cells expressing unbound IL-2Rα returns to pretherapy values within 1 to 2 weeks. The relationship between serum concentration and receptor saturation was assessed in 13 pediatric patients and was similar to that characterized in adult renal transplantation patients. In vitro studies using human tissues indicate that basiliximab binds only to lymphocytes.

The duration of clinically relevant IL-2 receptor blockade after the recommended course of basiliximab is not known. When basiliximab was added to a regimen of cyclosporine (modified) and corticosteroids in adult patients, the duration of IL-2Rα saturation was 36 ± 14 days (mean ± SD), similar to that observed in pediatric patients (36 ± 14 days). When basiliximab was added to a triple therapy regimen consisting of cyclosporine (modified), corticosteroids, and azathioprine in adults, the duration was 50 ± 20 days and when added to cyclosporine (modified), corticosteroids, and mycophenolate mofetil in adults, the duration was 59 ± 17 days. No significant changes to circulating lymphocyte numbers or cell phenotypes were observed by flow cytometry.

➤*Pharmacokinetics:*

Adults – Single-dose and multiple-dose pharmacokinetic studies have been conducted in patients undergoing first kidney transplantation. Cumulative doses ranged from 15 mg up to 150 mg. Peak mean ± SD serum concentration following intravenous infusion of 20 mg over 30 minutes is 7.1 ± 5.1 mg/L. There is a dose-proportional increase in C_{max} and AUC up to the highest tested single dose of 60 mg. The volume of distribution at steady state is 8.6 ± 4.1 L. The extent and degree of distribution to various body compartments have not been fully studied. The terminal half-life is 7.2 ± 3.2 days. Total body clearance is 41 ± 19 mL/hr. No clinically relevant influence of body weight or gender on distribution volume or clearance has been observed in adult patients. Elimination half-life was not influenced by age (20 to 69 years), gender, or race.

Children – The pharmacokinetics of basiliximab have been assessed in 39 pediatric patients undergoing renal transplantation. In infants and children (1 to 11 years of age, n = 25), the distribution volume and clearance were reduced by about 50% compared to adult renal transplantation patients. The volume of distribution at steady state was 4.8 ± 2.1 L, half-life was 9.5 ± 4.5 days and clearance was 17 ± 6 mL/hr. Disposition parameters were not influenced to a clinically relevant extent by age (1 to 11 years of age), body weight (9 to 37 kg) or body surface area (0.44 to 1.2 m^2) in this age group. In adolescents (12 to 16 years of age, n = 14), disposition was similar to that in adult renal transplantation patients. The volume of distribution at steady state was 7.8 ± 5.1 L, half-life was 9.1 ± 3.9 days and clearance was 31 ± 19 mL/hr.

Contraindications

Basiliximab is contraindicated in patients with known hypersensitivity to basiliximab or any other component of the formulation.

Warnings/Precautions

➤*Administration and usage:* See the Warning box for more information.

➤*Opportunistic infections / lymphoproliferative disorders:* While neither the incidence of lymphoproliferative disorders nor of opportunistic infections was higher in basiliximab-treated patients than in placebo-treated patients, patients on immunosuppressive therapy are at increased risk for developing these complications and should be monitored accordingly.

➤*Infectious episodes:* See Adverse Reactions for more information.

➤*Immunogenicity:* Of renal transplantation patients treated with basiliximab and tested for anti-idiotype antibodies, 4 out of 339 developed an anti-idiotype antibody response, with no deleterious clinical effect upon the patient. In none of these cases was there evidence that the presence of anti-idiotype antibody accelerated basiliximab clearance or decreased the period of receptor saturation. In study 2, the incidence of human anti-murine antibody (HAMA) in renal transplantation patients treated with basiliximab was 2 out of 138 in patients not exposed to muromonab-CD3 and 4 out of 34 in patients who subsequently received muromonab-CD3. The available clinical data on the use of muromonab-CD3 in patients previously treated with basiliximab suggest that subsequent use of muromonab-CD3 or other murine anti-lymphocytic antibody preparations is not precluded.

These data reflect the percentage of patients whose test results were considered positive for antibodies to basiliximab in an ELISA assay, and are highly dependent on the sensitivity and specificity of the assay. Additionally the observed incidence of antibody positivity in an assay may be influenced by several factors including sample handling, concomitant medications, and underlying disease. For these reasons, comparison of the incidence of antibodies to basiliximab with the incidence of antibodies to other products may be misleading.

➤*Immunogenicity:* See Warnings/Precautions for more information.

➤*Hypersensitivity reactions:* Severe acute (onset within 24 hours) hypersensitivity reactions including anaphylaxis have been observed both on initial exposure to basiliximab or following re-exposure after several months. These reactions may include hypotension, tachycardia, cardiac failure, dyspnea, wheezing, bronchospasm, pulmonary edema, respiratory failure, urticaria, rash, pruritus, or sneezing. If a severe hypersensitivity reaction occurs, therapy with basiliximab should be permanently discontinued. Medications for the treatment of severe hypersensitivity reactions including anaphylaxis should be available for immediate use. Patients previously administered basiliximab should only be re-exposed to a subsequent course of therapy with extreme caution. The potential risks of such re-administration, specifically those associated with immunosuppression, are not known.

Anaphylactoid reactions following the administration of basiliximab have not been observed but can occur following the administration of proteins.

➤*Pregnancy: Category B.* There are no adequate and well-controlled studies in pregnant women.

Because IgG molecules are known to cross the placental barrier, because IL-2 receptor may play an important role in development of the immune system, and because animal reproduction studies are not always predictive of human response, basiliximab should only be used in pregnant women when the potential benefit justifies the potential risk to the fetus. Women of childbearing potential should use effective contraception before beginning basiliximab therapy, during therapy, and for 4 months after completion of basiliximab therapy.

➤*Lactation:* It is not known whether basiliximab is excreted in human milk. Because many drugs including human antibodies are excreted in human milk, and because of the potential for adverse reactions, a decision should be made to discontinue nursing or to discontinue the drug, taking into account the importance of the drug to the mother.

Adverse Reactions

The most frequently reported adverse reactions were gastrointestinal disorders, reported in 69% of basiliximab-treated patients and 67% of placebo-treated patients.

➤*The following adverse reactions occurred in greater than or equal to 10% of basiliximab-treated patients:* The incidence and types of adverse reactions were similar in basiliximab-treated and placebo-treated patients.

Cardiovascular – Hypertension.

CNS – Headache, tremor.

Dermatologic – Acne.

GI – Constipation, nausea, abdominal pain, vomiting, diarrhea, dyspepsia.

GU – Urinary tract infection.

Hematologic – Anemia.

Metabolic / Nutritional – Hyperkalemia, hypokalemia, hyperglycemia, hypercholesterolemia, hypophosphatemia, hyperuricemia.

Psychiatric – Insomnia.

Respiratory – Dyspnea, upper respiratory tract infection.

Miscellaneous – Surgical wound complications, pain, peripheral edema, fever, viral infection.

➤*Adverse reactions, not mentioned above, reported with an incidence of greater than or equal to 3% and less than 10% in patients:* The following adverse reactions, not mentioned above, were reported with an incidence of greater than or equal to 3% and less than 10% in pooled analysis of patients treated with basiliximab in the 4 controlled clinical trials, or in an analysis of the 2 dual-therapy trials:

Cardiovascular – Arrhythmia, atrial fibrillation, tachycardia, vascular disorder, abnormal heart sounds, aggravated hypertension, angina pectoris, cardiac failure, chest pain, hypotension.

CNS – Dizziness, neuropathy, paraesthesia, hypoesthesia.

Dermatologic – Cyst, herpes simplex, herpes zoster, hypertrichosis, pruritus, rash, skin disorder, skin ulceration.

Endocrine – Increased glucocorticoids.

BASILIXIMAB — INJECTION

GI – Enlarged abdomen, esophagitis, flatulence, gastrointestinal disorder, gastroenteritis, GI hemorrhage, gum hyperplasia, melena, moniliasis, ulcerative stomatitis.

GU – Albuminuria, bladder disorder, dysuria, frequent micturition, hematuria, increased non-protein nitrogen, oliguria, abnormal renal function, renal tubular necrosis, surgery, ureteral disorder, urinary retention.
Male: Genital edema, impotence.

Hematologic – Hematoma, hemorrhage, purpura, thrombocytopenia, thrombosis. White blood cell: Leucopenia. Red blood cell: Polycythemia

Among these reactions, leukopenia and hypertriglyceridemia occurred more frequently in the 2 triple-therapy studies using azathioprine and mycophenolate mofetil than in the dual-therapy studies.

Metabolic/Nutritional – Acidosis, dehydration, diabetes mellitus, fluid overload, hypercalcemia, hyperlipemia, hypertriglyceridemia, hypocalcemia, hypoglycemia, hypomagnesemia, hypoproteinemia, weight increase.

Musculoskeletal – Arthralgia, arthropathy, back pain, bone fracture, cramps, hernia, myalgia, leg pain.

Psychiatric – Agitation, anxiety, depression.

Respiratory – Bronchitis, bronchospasm, abnormal chest sounds, coughing, pharyngitis, pneumonia, pulmonary disorder, pulmonary edema, rhinitis, sinusitis.

Special senses – Cataract, conjunctivitis, abnormal vision.

Miscellaneous – Accidental trauma, asthenia, chest pain, increased drug level, infection, face edema, fatigue, dependent edema, generalized edema, leg edema, malaise, rigors, sepsis.

➤*Malignancies:* The overall incidence of malignancies among all patients in the controlled studies was not significantly different between the basiliximab- and placebo-treatment groups. Overall, lymphoma/lymphoproliferative disease occurred in 1 out of 590 patients in the basiliximab group compared with 3 out of 594 patients in the placebo group. Other malignancies were reported among 8 out of 590 patients in the basiliximab group compared with 9 out of 594 patients in the placebo group.

➤*Infections:* The overall incidence of cytomegalovirus infection was similar in basiliximab- and placebo-treated patients (15% vs 17%) receiving a dual- or triple-immunosuppression regimen. However, in patients receiving a triple-immunosuppression regimen, the incidence of serious cytomegalovirus infection was higher in basiliximab-treated patients compared to placebo-treated patients (11% vs 5%). The rates of infections, serious infections, and infectious organisms were similar in the basiliximab- and placebo-treatment groups among dual- and triple-therapy treated patients.

➤*Postmarketing experience:* Severe acute hypersensitivity reactions including anaphylaxis characterized by hypotension, tachycardia, cardiac failure, dyspnea, wheezing, bronchospasm, pulmonary edema, respiratory failure, urticaria, rash, pruritus, or sneezing, as well as capillary leak syndrome and cytokine release syndrome, have been reported during postmarketing experience with basiliximab.

Overdosage

A maximum tolerated dose of basiliximab has not been determined in patients. During the course of clinical studies, basiliximab has been administered to adult renal transplantation patients in single doses of up to 60 mg, or in divided doses over 3 to 5 days of up to 120 mg, without any associated serious adverse reactions. There has been 1 spontaneous report of a pediatric renal transplantation patient who received a single 20 mg dose (2.3 mg/kg) without adverse reactions.

CYCLOSPORINE (Cyclosporin A)

Rx	**Cyclosporine** (Apotex)	**Capsules; oral:** 25 mg	May contain methanol. In 30s, 500s, 1,000s.
Rx	**Gengraf** (Abbott)	**Capsules; oral:** 25 mg (as cyclosporine modified)	Alcohol 12.8%, castor oil, PEG, sorbitan. (25 mg OR). White, oval. In UD 30s.
Rx	**Cyclosporine** (Apotex)	**Capsules; oral:** 100 mg	May contain methanol. In 30s, 500s, 1,000s.
Rx	**Gengraf** (Abbott)	**Capsules; oral:** 100 mg (as cyclosporine modified)	Alcohol 12.8%, castor oil, PEG, sorbitan. (100 mg OT). White, oval. In UD 30s.
Rx	**Cyclosporine Modified** (eg, Watson, Sandoz, Teva)	**Capsules, soft-gelatin; oral:** 25 mg (as cyclosporine modified)	May contain alcohol, castor oil, sorbitol. In UD 30s.
Rx	**Neoral** (Novartis)		Castor oil, corn oil, dehydrated alcohol 11.9%. (Neoral 25 mg). Blue-gray, oval. In UD 30s.
Rx	**Sandimmune** (Novartis)	**Capsules, soft-gelatin; oral:** 25 mg	Corn oil, dehydrated alcohol ≤ 12.7%, sorbitol. (78/240). Pink, oblong. In UD 30s.
Rx	**Cyclosporine Modified** (Teva)	**Capsules, soft-gelatin; oral:** 50 mg (as cyclosporine modified)	May contain alcohol, sorbitol. In UD 30s.
Rx	**Cyclosporine Modified** (eg, Watson, Sandoz, Teva)	**Capsules, soft-gelatin; oral:** 100 mg (as cyclosporine modified)	May contain alcohol, castor oil, sorbitol. In UD 30s.
Rx	**Neoral** (Novartis)		Castor oil, corn oil, dehydrated alcohol 11.9%. (Neoral 100 mg). Blue-gray, oblong. In UD 30s.
Rx	**Sandimmune** (Novartis)	**Capsules, soft-gelatin; oral:** 100 mg	Corn oil, dehydrated alcohol ≤ 12.7%, sorbitol. (78/241). Rose, oblong. In UD 30s.
Rx	**Cyclosporine Modified** (eg, Apotex, Watson)	**Solution; oral:** 100 mg/mL (as cyclosporine modified)	May contain castor oil. In 50 mL.
Rx	**Gengraf** (Abbott)		Castor oil, propylene glycol, sorbitan. In 50 mL with syringe.
Rx	**Neoral** (Novartis)		Castor oil, corn oil, dehydrated alcohol 11.9%, propylene glycol. In 50 mL.
Rx	**Cyclosporine** (Wockhardt)	**Solution; oral:** 100 mg/mL	May contain alcohol. In 50 mL.
Rx	**Sandimmune** (Novartis)		Alcohol 12.5%, olive oil. In 50 mL with syringe.
Rx	**Cyclosporine** (Paddock)	**Injection, solution, concentrate:** 50 mg/mL	May contain alcohol, polyoxyethylated castor oil. In 5 mL ampules.
Rx	**Sandimmune** (Novartis)		Alcohol 32.9%, olive oil, polyoxyethylated castor oil. In 5 mL amps.

[a] Product tables do not imply bioequivalence. Also refer to Bioequivalency (in Administration and Dosage).

CYCLOSPORINE — ORAL

WARNING

Only health care providers experienced in immunosuppressive therapy and management of organ transplant patients should prescribe cyclosporine. Manage patients receiving the drug in facilities equipped and staffed with adequate laboratory and supportive medical resources. The health care provider responsible for maintenance therapy should have complete information requisite for the follow-up of the patient.

Administer *Sandimmune* with adrenal corticosteroids but not with other immunosuppressive agents. Increased susceptibility to infection and possible development of lymphoma may result from immunosuppression.

Neoral and *Gengraf* may increase the susceptibility to infection and the development of neoplasia. In kidney, liver, and heart transplant patients, *Gengraf* and *Neoral* may be administered with other immunosuppressive agents. Increased susceptibility to infection and the possible development of lymphoma and other neoplasms may result from the increase in the degree of immunosuppression in transplant patients.

The absorption of *Sandimmune* during long-term administration was found to be erratic. It is recommended that patients taking *Sandimmune* over a period of time be monitored at repeated intervals for cyclosporine blood levels and that subsequent dose adjustments be made to avoid toxicity from high levels and possible organ rejection from low absorption of cyclosporine. This is of special importance in liver transplants. Numerous assays are being developed to measure blood levels of cyclosporine.

Sandimmune capsules and oral solution have decreased bioavailability in comparison with *Neoral* capsules, *Neoral* oral solution, *Gengraf* capsules, and *Gengraf* oral solution. *Gengraf* and *Neoral* are not bioequivalent to *Sandimmune*; advise patients not to use them interchangeably without the supervision of a health care provider. For given trough concentrations, cyclosporine exposure will be greater with *Neoral* and *Gengraf* than with *Sandimmune*. If a patient receiving exceptionally high doses of *Sandimmune* is converted to *Neoral* or *Gengraf*, exercise particular caution. Monitor cyclosporine blood concentrations in transplant and rheumatoid arthritis (RA) patients taking *Gengraf* and *Neoral* to avoid toxicity due to high concentrations. Make dose adjustments in transplant patients to minimize possible organ rejection due to low concentrations. Comparison of blood concentrations in the published literature with blood concentrations obtained using current assays must be done with detailed knowledge of the assay methods employed.

Psoriasis – Psoriasis patients previously treated with psoralens plus ultraviolet A (PUVA) and, to a lesser extent, methotrexate or other immunosuppressive agents, ultraviolet B (UVB), coal tar, or radiation therapy, are at an increased risk of developing skin malignancies when taking *Neoral* or *Gengraf*.

Cyclosporine, in recommended doses, can cause systemic hypertension and nephrotoxicity. The risk increases with increasing dose and duration of cyclosporine therapy. Renal dysfunction, including structural kidney damage, is a potential consequence of cyclosporine and, therefore, renal function must be monitored during therapy.

Indications

➤*Allogeneic transplants:* For prophylaxis of organ rejection in kidney, liver, and heart allogeneic transplants. *Gengraf* and *Neoral* have been used in combination with azathioprine and corticosteroids. *Sandimmune* is always to be used with adrenal corticosteroids. *Sandimmune* also may be used in the treatment of chronic rejection in patients previously treated with other immunosuppressive agents.

➤*Psoriasis (Neoral* and *Gengraf* only*)*: For the treatment of adult, nonimmunocompromised patients with severe (ie, extensive and/or disabling), recalcitrant plaque psoriasis who have failed to respond to at least 1 systemic therapy (eg, PUVA, retinoids, methotrexate) or in patients for whom other systemic therapies are contraindicated or cannot be tolerated. While rebound rarely occurs, most patients will experience relapse with *Neoral* or *Gengraf*, as with other therapies, upon cessation of treatment.

➤*Rheumatoid arthritis (Neoral* and *Gengraf* only*)*: For the treatment of patients with severe, active RA in which the disease has not adequately responded to methotrexate. *Neoral* and *Gengraf* can be used in combination with methotrexate in RA patients who do not respond adequately to methotrexate alone.

➤*Off-label uses:*

Juvenile idiopathic arthritis – [3] = Safety concerns. Data evaluating the safety and efficacy of cyclosporine for the treatment of juvenile idiopathic arthritis are limited and show conflicting results. In most cases, cyclosporine was add-on therapy for patients with refractory disease. Although some reports show promise, there are concerns about potential significant toxicity.

Multiple sclerosis – [3] = Safety concerns. Studies evaluating the efficacy of cyclosporine in patients with multiple sclerosis (MS) have shown modest clinical benefit. However, there are significant safety concerns with its use, most notably nephrotoxicity, decreased serum magnesium levels, and hypertension. Because of the significant safety concerns, cyclosporine is not recommended as a treatment option for MS.

Psoriasis (children) – [3] = Safety concerns. American Academy of Dermatology guidelines state that the evidence for use in pediatric psoriasis is limited. A review of its use in children with several different rheumatologic and dermatologic conditions suggested that the adverse effect profile was similar in adults and children. It was concluded that cyclosporine may be considered for children with severe psoriasis.

Other possible off-label uses – Prevention and treatment of acute graft-versus-host disease (GVHD) following bone marrow transplantation; aplastic anemia; resistant leukemias.

Administration and Dosage

➤*General dosing considerations:*

Bioequivalency – Cyclosporine (*Sandimmune*) capsules and oral solution have decreased bioavailability in comparison with cyclosporine modified (*Neoral* or *Gengraf*) capsules and oral solutions. *Gengraf* and *Neoral* are not bioequivalent to *Sandimmune* and cannot be used interchangeably without the supervision of a health care provider.

Because *Sandimmune* is not bioequivalent to *Neoral* or *Gengraf*, conversion from *Neoral* or *Gengraf* to *Sandimmune* using a 1:1 ratio (mg/kg/day) may result in lower cyclosporine blood concentration. Conversion from *Neoral* or *Gengraf* to *Sandimmune* should be made with increased blood concentration monitoring to avoid the potential of underdosing.

➤*Adults:*

Allogeneic transplants – See also Off-Label Dosing for additional renal transplantation recommendations.

Cyclosporine (Sandimmune):

• *Initial dosage* – A single dose of 15 mg/kg given 4 to 12 hours prior to transplantation. Although a single daily dose of 14 to 18 mg/kg was used in most clinical trials, few centers continue to use the highest dose, and most favor the lower end of the scale. There is a trend towards use of even lower initial doses for renal transplantation in the range of 10 to 14 mg/kg/day.

• *Maintenance dosage* – The initial single daily dose is continued postoperatively for 1 to 2 weeks and then tapered by 5% per week to a maintenance dosage of 5 to 10 mg/kg/day. Some centers have successfully tapered the maintenance dosage to as low as 3 mg/kg/day in selected renal transplant patients without an apparent rise in rejection rate.

• *Adjunct therapy* – Adjunct therapy with adrenal corticosteroids is recommended. Different tapering dosage schedules of prednisone appear to achieve similar results. A dosage schedule based on the patient's weight started with 2 mg/kg/day for the first 4 days tapered to 1 mg/kg/day by 1 week, 0.6 mg/kg/day by 2 weeks, 0.3 mg/kg/day by 1 month, and 0.15 mg/kg/day by 2 months and continued thereafter as a maintenance dosage. Another center started with an initial dose of 200 mg tapered by 40 mg/day until reaching 20 mg/day. After 2 months at this dose, a further reduction to 10 mg/day was made. Adjustments in dosage of prednisone must be made according to the clinical situation.

Cyclosporine modified (Gengraf or *Neoral)*:

• *Initial dosage* – In newly transplanted patients, the initial oral dose of *Neoral* and *Gengraf* are the same as the initial dose of *Sandimmune*. The initial dose varies depending on the transplanted organ and the other immunosuppressive agents included in the immunosuppressive protocol. Give the initial dose 4 to 12 hours prior to transplantation, or postoperatively.

Suggested initial doses are available from the results of a 1994 survey of the use of *Sandimmune* in US transplant centers. The mean ± standard deviation (SD) initial dosages were 9 ± 3 mg/kg/day for renal transplant patients (75 centers), 8 ± 4 mg/kg/day for liver transplant patients (30 centers), and 7 ± 3 mg/kg/day for heart transplant patients (24 centers). Total daily doses were divided into 2 equal daily doses.

• *Dosage adjustment* – The dosage is subsequently adjusted to achieve a predefined cyclosporine blood concentration. Using the same trough concentration target as for *Sandimmune* results in greater cyclosporine exposure when *Neoral* and *Gengraf* are administered. Titrate dosing based on clinical assessments of rejection and tolerability. Lower *Neoral* and *Gengraf* doses may be sufficient as maintenance therapy.

• *Adjunct therapy* – Adjunct therapy with adrenal corticosteroids is recommended initially. Different tapering dosage schedules of prednisone appear to achieve similar results. A representative dosage schedule based on the patient's weight started with 2 mg/kg/day for the first 4 days tapered to 1 mg/kg/day by 1 week, 0.6 mg/kg/day by 2 weeks, 0.3 mg/kg/day by 1 month, and 0.15 mg/kg/day by 2 months and continued thereafter as a maintenance dosage. Steroid doses may be further tapered on an individualized basis depending on status of patient and function of graft. Adjustments in dosage of prednisone must be made according to the clinical situation.

• *Conversion from Sandimmune* – In transplanted patients who are considered for conversion to *Neoral* or *Gengraf* from *Sandimmune*, start with the same daily dose as was previously used with *Sandimmune* (1:1 dose conversion). Subsequently, adjust the *Neoral* or *Gengraf* dose to attain the preconversion cyclosporine blood trough concentration. Using the same trough concentration target range as for *Sandimmune* results in greater cyclosporine exposure when *Neoral* and *Gengraf* are administered. Patients with suspected poor absorption of *Sandimmune* require different dosing strategies. In some patients, the increase in blood trough concentration is more pronounced and may be of clinical significance.

Until the blood trough concentration attains the preconversion value, it is strongly recommended that the cyclosporine blood-trough concentration be monitored every 4 to 7 days after conversion to *Neoral* or *Gengraf*. In addition, monitor clinical safety parameters, such as serum creatinine and blood pressure, every 2 weeks during the first 2 months after conversion. If the blood trough concentrations are outside the desired range and/or if the clinical safety parameters worsen, adjust the dosage accordingly.

• *Poor Sandimmune absorption* – Patients with lower than expected cyclosporine blood trough concentrations in relation to the oral dose of *Sandimmune* may have poor or inconsistent absorption of cyclosporine from *Sandimmune*. After conversion to *Neoral* or *Gengraf*, patients tend to have higher cyclosporine concentrations. Due to the increase in bioavailability of cyclosporine following conversion to *Neoral* or *Gengraf*, exercise caution because the cyclosporine blood trough concentration may exceed the target

CYCLOSPORINE — ORAL

range. Exercise particular caution when converting patients to *Neoral* or *Gengraf* at dosages greater than 10 mg/kg/day. Individually titrate the dose based on cyclosporine trough concentrations, tolerability, and clinical response. In this population, measure the cyclosporine trough concentrations more frequently, at least twice per week (daily, if initial dosage exceeds 10 mg/kg/day), until the concentration stabilizes within the desired range.

Psoriasis (Gengraf and *Neoral* only) –

Maximum dose: 4 mg/kg/day.

Initial dosage: 2.5 mg/kg/day, as a divided (1.25 mg/kg twice daily) oral dose. Keep patients at the initial dose for at least 4 weeks, barring adverse reactions.

Dosage titration: Increase dosage at 2-week intervals if significant clinical improvement has not occurred by that time. Based on patient response, make dosage increases of approximately 0.5 mg/kg/day to a maximum of 4 mg/kg/day.

Maintenance dosage: Once a patient is adequately controlled and appears stable, the dosage should be lowered and the patient treated with the lowest dosage that maintains an adequate response (this should not necessarily be total clearing of the patient).

Dosage adjustment: Make dosage decreases by 25% to 50% at any time to control adverse reactions, such as hypertension, serum creatinine elevations (25% or more above the patient's pretreatment level), or clinically significant laboratory abnormalities. If dose reduction is not effective in controlling abnormalities, or if the adverse reaction or abnormality is severe, discontinue therapy.

Duration of therapy: Long-term experience in psoriasis patients is limited, and continuous treatment for extended periods (longer than 1 year) is not recommended. Consider alternating with other forms of treatment in the long-term management of patients with lifelong disease.

Discontinuation of therapy: Discontinue treatment if satisfactory response cannot be achieved after 6 weeks at 4 mg/kg/day or the patient's maximum tolerated dosage.

Upon stopping treatment with cyclosporine, relapse will occur in approximately 6 weeks (50% of patients) to 16 weeks (75% of patients). In the majority of patients, rebound does not occur after cessation of treatment with cyclosporine. Thirteen cases of transformation of chronic plaque psoriasis to more severe forms of psoriasis have been reported. There were 9 cases of pustular and 4 cases of erythrodermic psoriasis.

Rheumatoid arthritis (Gengraf and *Neoral* only) –

Maximum dose: 4 mg/kg/day.

Initial dosage: 2.5 mg/kg/day, taken twice daily as a divided dose. Onset of action generally occurs between 4 and 8 weeks.

Dosage titration: If sufficient clinical benefit is seen and tolerability is good (including serum creatinine less than 30% above baseline), the dosage may be increased by 0.5 to 0.75 mg/kg/day after 8 weeks and again after 12 weeks to a maximum of 4 mg/kg/day.

Dosage adjustment: Make dosage decreases by 25% to 50% at any time to control adverse reactions, such as hypertension, serum creatinine elevations (30% above the patient's pretreatment level), or clinically significant laboratory abnormalities. If dosage reduction is not effective in controlling abnormalities, or if the adverse reaction or abnormality is severe, discontinue therapy.

Duration of therapy: There is limited long-term treatment data. Recurrence of RA disease activity is generally apparent within 4 weeks after stopping cyclosporine.

Concomitant therapy: Salicylates, nonsteroidal anti-inflammatory drugs (NSAIDs), and oral corticosteroids may be continued.

• *Use with methotrexate* – Use the same initial dose and dose range if combined with the recommended dose of methotrexate. Most patients can be treated with *Gengraf* or *Neoral* dosages of 3 mg/kg/day or less when combined with methotrexate dosages of up to 15 mg/wk.

Discontinuation of therapy: If no benefit is seen by 16 weeks of therapy, discontinue therapy.

Off-label dosing –

Multiple sclerosis: [3] = Safety concerns. Administer at a starting dosage of 6 mg/kg/day, with dosage adjustments to maintain a trough level between 300 and 500 ng/mL to minimize renal toxicity.

Prevention of acute graft-versus-host disease: 1.5 mg/kg intravenous (IV) given every 12 hours in combination with methotrexate, beginning 1 day prior to hematopoietic stem cell transplantation. Dosages are adjusted based on clinical status. When oral therapy is tolerated, 12.5 mg/kg/day is given in 2 divided doses.

Renal transplantation: One reference suggests 8 to 12 mg/kg/day in 1 or 2 divided doses starting immediately prior to transplantation, decreased to a maintenance dosage of 3 to 5 mg/kg/day by 3 months posttransplant.

Resistant leukemias: Initiate therapy with cyclosporine 5 to 6 mg/kg/day (mean dosage, 300 mg/day). Titrate dose to achieve a whole blood trough level between 400 and 600 mg/mL.

➤*Children:*

Allogeneic transplants – See Adults for dosing.

In children, the same dose and dosing regimen may be used as in adults; although, in several studies, children have required and tolerated higher doses than those used in adults.

Off-label dosing –

Juvenile idiopathic arthritis: [3] = Safety concerns. For patients 2 to 18 years of age with refractory juvenile idiopathic arthritis, oral dosages ranged from 1.2 to 6.7 mg/kg daily. Therapy continued for more than 7 years in 1 report. In most cases, cyclosporine was added to an existing drug regimen.

Psoriasis: [3] = Safety concerns. Per psoriasis guidelines, the adult dosage is 2.5 to 5 mg/kg/day in 2 divided doses. The dose may be adjusted downward by 0.5 to 1 mg/kg when clearance is achieved or when adverse effects are observed. The manufacturer's prescribing information states that when used for transplants, the same dose and dosing regimen may be used in children as in adults; although in several studies, children have required and tolerated higher doses than those used in adults.

In the treatment of psoriasis, cyclosporine was recommended for intermittent interventional therapy, with repeat courses allowed after a rest period. Long-term continuous use was not advised because of the potential for toxicity.

➤*Renal function impairment:* Impaired renal function at any time requires close monitoring, and frequent dosage adjustment may be indicated.

➤*Therapeutic drug monitoring:* Transplant centers have found blood concentration monitoring of cyclosporine to be an essential component of patient management. Of importance to blood concentration analysis are the type of assay used, the transplanted organ, and other immunosuppressant agents being administered. While no fixed relationship has been established, blood concentration monitoring may assist in the clinical evaluation of rejection and toxicity, dose adjustments, and the assessment of compliance. In one series of 375 consecutive cadaveric renal transplant recipients, dosage was adjusted to achieve specific whole blood 24-hour trough levels of 100 to 200 ng/mL, as determined by high-pressure liquid chromatography (HPLC). These levels are specific to the parent cyclosporine molecule and correlate directly to the monoclonal specific radioimmunoassays (mRIA-sp).

Various assays have been used to measure blood concentrations of cyclosporine. Older studies using a nonspecific assay often cited concentrations that were roughly twice those of specific assays. Therefore, comparison between concentrations in the published literature and an individual patient concentration using current assays must be made with detailed knowledge of the assay methods employed. Current assay results are also not interchangeable and their use should be guided by their approved labeling. If plasma specimens are employed, levels will vary with the temperature at the time of separation from whole blood. Plasma levels may range from one-half to one-fifth of whole blood levels. A discussion of the different assay methods is contained in *Annals of Clinical Biochemistry* 1994;31:420-446. While several assays and assay matrices are available, there is a consensus that parent compound–specific assays correlate best with clinical events. Of these, HPLC is the standard reference, but the monoclonal antibody RIAs and the monoclonal antibody fluorescent polarization immunoassay (FPIA) offer sensitivity, reproducibility, and convenience. Most clinicians base their monitoring on trough cyclosporine concentrations. *Transplantation Proceedings* (June 1990) contains position papers and a broad consensus generated at the Cyclosporine Therapeutic Drug Monitoring conference that year. *Applied Pharmacokinetics: Principles of Therapeutic Drug Monitoring* (1992) contains a broad discussion of cyclosporine pharmacokinetics and drug monitoring techniques. Blood level monitoring is not a replacement for renal function monitoring or tissue biopsies.

Approximate therapeutic ranges in renal transplantation – One reference suggests the following therapeutic ranges for cyclosporine in renal transplant patients.

Trough levels:

• *0 to 2 months posttransplant* – 150 to 350 ng/mL by HPLC and enzyme-multiplied immunoassay technique (EMIT) or 250 to 450 ng/mL by FPIA.

• *2 to 6 months posttransplant* – 100 to 250 ng/mL by HPLC and EMIT or 175 to 350 ng/mL by FPIA.

• *More than 6 months posttransplant* – Approximately 100 ng/mL by HPLC and EMIT or approximately 150 ng/mL by FPIA.

• *C2 levels* – Monitoring with 2-hour peak levels (C2 levels) may be more useful than traditional trough level monitoring. Levels are drawn within 15 minutes to 2 hours after the cyclosporine dose.

0 to 2 months posttransplant: 1.5 to 2 ng/mL.

2 to 6 months posttransplant: 1.1 to 1.5 ng/mL.

More than 6 months posttransplant: 0.8 to 1 ng/mL.

➤*Preparation for administration:* Cyclosporine is an immunosuppressant and is also considered a potential teratogen and a potential mutagen. Follow safe handling procedures when preparing, administering, or dispensing cyclosporine.

Oral solution preparation –

Sandimmune: To make *Sandimmune* oral solution more palatable, it may be diluted with milk, chocolate milk, or orange juice, preferably at room temperature. Instruct patients to stir well and drink at once, not allowing the solution to stand before drinking. It is best to use a glass container and to rinse it with more diluent to ensure that the total dose is taken. After use, instruct patients to replace the dosage syringe in the protective cover. Instruct patients to not rinse the dosage syringe with water or other cleaning agents either before or after use. If the dosage syringe requires cleaning, it must be completely dry before resuming use. Introduction of water into the product by any means will cause variation in dose. Patients should avoid switching diluents frequently.

Gengraf or *Neoral*: To make *Neoral* or *Gengraf* more palatable, it should be diluted with orange or apple juice that is at room temperature. Instruct patients not to switch diluents frequently. Grapefruit and grapefruit juice affect metabolism, increasing blood concentration of cyclosporine, and should be avoided. The combination of *Neoral* or *Gengraf* solution with milk can be unpalatable.

Instruct patients to remove the protective cover from the dosing syringe supplied, and transfer the solution to a glass of orange or apple juice. Advise patients to stir well and drink at once, not allowing the diluted solution to stand before drinking. A glass container, not plastic, should be used. Tell patients to rinse the glass with more diluent to ensure that the total dose is consumed. After use, the outside of the dosing syringe should be dried with

CYCLOSPORINE — ORAL

a clean towel and the protective cover should be replaced. The dosing syringe should not be rinsed with water or other cleaning agents. If the syringe requires cleaning, it must be completely dry before resuming use.

➤*Administration:*

Sandimmune – Administer capsules and oral solution on a consistent schedule with regard to time of day and relation to meals.

Gengraf and *Neoral* – Always give the daily dosage in 2 divided doses on a consistent schedule with regard to time of day and relation to meals.

➤*Storage / Stability:*

Gengraf and *Neoral* –

Capsules: Store in the original unit-dose container at 20° to 25°C (68° to 77°F).

Oral solution: Store in the original container at 20° to 25°C (68° to 77°F). Do not store in the refrigerator. Once opened, the contents must be used within 2 months. At temperatures below 20°C (68°F), the solution may gel; light flocculation or the formation of a light sediment also may occur. There is no impact on product performance or dosing using the syringe provided. Allow to warm to room temperature (25°C [77°F]) to reverse these changes.

Sandimmune –

Capsules: Store at 25°C (77°F); excursions are permitted between 15° and 30°C (59° and 86°F). An odor may be detected upon opening the unit-dose container, which will dissipate shortly thereafter. This odor does not affect the quality of the product.

Oral solution: Store in the original container at temperatures below 30°C (86°F). Do not store in the refrigerator. Protect from freezing. Once opened, the contents must be used within 2 months.

Actions

➤*Pharmacology:* Cyclosporine is a potent immunosuppressive agent that in animals prolongs survival of allogeneic transplants involving the skin, kidney, liver, heart, pancreas, bone marrow, small intestine, and lung. Cyclosporine has been demonstrated to suppress some humoral immunity and, to a greater extent, cell-mediated immune reactions, such as allograft rejection, delayed hypersensitivity, experimental allergic encephalomyelitis, Freund adjuvant arthritis, and GVHD, in many animal species for a variety of organs.

Successful kidney, liver, and heart allogeneic transplants have been performed in humans using *Sandimmune*.

Experimental evidence suggests that the effectiveness of cyclosporine results from specific and reversible inhibition of immunocompetent lymphocytes in the G_0 and G_1 phase of the cell cycle. T-lymphocytes are preferentially inhibited. The T-helper cell is the main target, although the T-suppressor cell also may be suppressed. Cyclosporine also inhibits lymphokine production and release, including interleukin-2 or T-cell growth factor.

➤*Pharmacokinetics:*

Pharmacokinetic Parameters of *Gengraf* and *Neoral* (Mean ± SD)[a]

Patient population	Dose/day[b] (mg/day)	Dose/weight (mg/kg/day)	AUC[c] (ng•h/mL)	C_{max} (ng/mL)	Trough[d] (ng/mL)	CL/F (mL/min)	CL/F (mL/min/kg)
De novo renal transplant[e] week 4 (n = 37)	597 ± 174	7.95 ± 2.81	8,772 ± 2,089	1,802 ± 428	361 ± 129	593 ± 204	7.8 ± 2.9
Stable renal transplant[e] (n = 55)	344 ± 122	4.1 ± 1.58	6,035 ± 2,194	1,333 ± 469	251 ± 116	492 ± 140	5.9 ± 2.1
De novo liver transplant[f] week 4 (n = 18)	458 ± 190	6.89 ± 3.68	7,187 ± 2,816	1,555 ± 740	268 ± 101	577 ± 309	8.6 ± 5.7
De novo RA[g] (n = 23)	182 ± 55.6	2.37 ± 0.36	2,641 ± 877	728 ± 263	96.4 ± 37.7	613 ± 196	8.3 ± 2.8
De novo psoriasis[g] Week 4 (n = 18)	189 ± 69.8	2.48 ± 0.65	2,324 ± 1,048	655 ± 186	74.9 ± 46.7	723 ± 186	10.2 ± 3.9

[a] AUC = area under the curve; C_{max} = maximum drug concentration; CL/F = apparent total clearance of the drug from plasma after oral administration.
[b] Total daily dose was divided into 2 doses administered every 12 hours.
[c] AUC was measured over 1 dosing interval.
[d] Trough concentration was measured just prior to the morning *Gengraf* or *Neoral* dose, approximately 12 hours after the previous dose.
[e] Assay: *TDx* specific monoclonal fluorescence polarization immunoassay.
[f] Assay: *Cyclo-Trac* specific monoclonal radioimmunoassay.
[g] Assay: *Incstar* specific monoclonal radioimmunoassay.

Absorption – The absorption of cyclosporine from the GI tract is incomplete and variable. The extent of absorption of cyclosporine is dependent on the individual patient, the patient population, and the formulation.

Gengraf and *Neoral*: *Gengraf* and *Neoral* have increased bioavailability compared with *Sandimmune*. The absolute bioavailability of cyclosporine administered as*Gengraf* or *Neoral* has not been determined in adults. In studies of renal transplant, RA, and psoriasis patients, the mean cyclosporine AUC was approximately 20% to 50% greater, and the cyclosporine blood C_{max} was approximately 40% to 106% greater following administration of *Gengraf* or *Neoral* compared with following administration of *Sandimmune*. The dose-normalized AUC in de novo liver transplant patients administered *Gengraf* or*Neoral* 28 days after transplantation was 50% greater, and C_{max} was 90% greater than in those patients administered *Sandimmune*. AUC and C_{max} are also increased (*Gengraf* and *Neoral* relative to *Sandimmune*) in heart transplant patients, but data are very limited. Although the AUC and C_{max} values are higher when taking *Gengraf* or *Neoral* relative to *Sandimmune*, the predose trough concentrations (dose normalized) are similar for the 2 formulations.

Following oral administration of *Gengraf* and *Neoral*, the time to peak blood cyclosporine concentrations (T_{max}) ranged from 1.5 to 2 hours. *Gengraf* and *Neoral* capsules and oral solutions are bioequivalent. *Gengraf* and *Neoral* oral solution diluted with orange or apple juice is bioequivalent to *Gengraf* and *Neoral* oral solution diluted with water. The effect of milk on the bioavailability of cyclosporine when administered as *Gengraf* and *Neoral* oral solution has not been evaluated.

The relationship between administered dose and exposure (AUC) is linear within the therapeutic dose range. The intersubject variability (total, percent coefficient of variation [CV]) of cyclosporine exposure (AUC) when cyclosporine is administered ranges from approximately 20% to 50% in renal transplant patients. This intersubject variability contributes to the need for individualization of the dosing regimen for optimal therapy. Intrasubject variability of AUC in renal transplant recipients (percentage CV) was 9% to 21% for *Gengraf* and *Neoral*, and 19% to 26% for *Sandimmune*. In the same studies, intrasubject variability of trough concentrations (percentage CV) was 17% to 30% for *Gengraf* and *Neoral* and 16% to 38% for *Sandimmune*.

The effect of T-tube diversion of bile on the absorption of cyclosporine from *Gengraf* or *Neoral* was investigated in 11 de novo liver transplant patients. When the patients were administered *Gengraf* or *Neoral* with and without T-tube diversion of bile, very little difference in absorption was observed, as measured by the change in cyclosporine blood C_{max} from predose values with the T-tube closed relative to when it was open (6.9% ± 41%; range, −55% to 68%).

Sandimmune: The absolute bioavailability of cyclosporine administered as *Sandimmune* is dependent on the patient population, estimated to be less than 10% in liver transplant patients and as great as 89% in some renal transplant patients.

C_{max} in blood and plasma is achieved at approximately 3.5 hours. C_{max} and AUC increase with the administered dose; for blood, the relationship is curvilinear (parabolic) between 0 and 1,400 mg. As determined by a specific assay, C_{max} is approximately 1 ng/mL/mg for plasma and 2.7 to 1.4 ng/mL/mg for blood (for low to high doses). Compared with an IV infusion, the absolute bioavailability of the oral solution is approximately 30% based on results in 2 patients. The bioavailability of *Sandimmune* capsules is equivalent to the oral solution.

Effect of food: The administration of food with *Gengraf* or *Neoral* decreases the cyclosporine AUC and C_{max}. A high-fat meal (669 kcal, 45 g fat) consumed within one-half hour before *Gengraf* or *Neoral* administration decreased the AUC by 13% and C_{max} by 33%. The effects of a low-fat meal (667 kcal, 15 g fat) were similar.

Distribution – Cyclosporine is distributed largely outside the blood volume; approximately 33% to 47% is in plasma, 4% to 9% in lymphocytes, 5% to 12% in granulocytes, and 41% to 58% in erythrocytes. At high concentrations, the binding capacity of leukocytes and erythrocytes becomes saturated. In plasma, approximately 90% is bound to proteins, primarily lipoproteins. The steady-state volume of distribution during IV dosing has been reported as 3 to 5 L/kg in solid organ transplant recipients. In blood, the distribution is concentration-dependent.

Metabolism – Cyclosporine is extensively metabolized by the CYP3A4 enzyme system in the liver and, to a lesser degree, in the GI tract and the kidney. The immunosuppressive activity of cyclosporine is primarily due to parent drug. At least 25 metabolites have been identified from human bile, feces, blood, and urine. The biological activity of the metabolites and their contributions to toxicity are considerably less than those of the parent compound. The major metabolites (M1, M9, and M4N) result from oxidation at the 1-beta, 9-gamma, and 4-N–demethylated positions, respectively. At steady state following the oral administration of *Sandimmune*, the mean AUCs for blood concentrations of the major metabolites M1, M9, and M4N are approximately 70%, 21%, and 7.5% of the AUC for blood cyclosporine concentrations, respectively. Based on blood concentration data from stable renal transplant patients (13 patients administered *Neoral* and *Sandimmune* in a crossover study) and bile concentration data from de novo liver transplant patients (4 administered *Neoral*, 3 administered *Sandimmune*), the percentage of dose present as M1, M9, and M4N metabolites is similar when *Neoral* or *Sandimmune* is administered.

Of 15 metabolites characterized in human urine, 9 have been assigned structures. The major pathways consist of hydroxylation of the C-gamma-carbon of 2 of the leucine residues, C-eta-carbon hydroxylation, and cyclic

CYCLOSPORINE — ORAL

ether formation (with oxidation of the double bond) in the side chain of the amino acid 3-hydroxyl-N,4-dimethyl-L-2-amino-6-octenoic acid and N-demethylation of N-methyl leucine residues. Hydrolysis of the cyclic peptide chain or conjugation of the aforementioned metabolites do not appear to be important biotransformation pathways.

Excretion – Only 0.1% of a dose is excreted unchanged in the urine. Excretion is primarily biliary, with only 6% of the dose (parent drug and metabolites) excreted in urine. Neither dialysis nor renal failure alter cyclosporine clearance significantly.

The disposition of cyclosporine from blood is generally biphasic, with a terminal half-life of approximately 8.4 hours (19 hours for *Sandimmune*) (range, 5 to 18 hours [10 to 27 hours for *Sandimmune*]). Following IV administration, the blood clearance of cyclosporine (assay: HPLC) is approximately 5 to 7 mL/min/kg in adult recipients of renal or liver allografts. Blood cyclosporine clearance appears to be slightly slower in cardiac transplant patients.

Contraindications

Hypersensitivity to cyclosporine, or any component of the products; *Gengraf* and *Neoral* in psoriasis or RA patients with abnormal renal function, uncontrolled hypertension, or malignancies; *Gengraf* and *Neoral* concomitantly with PUVA or UVB, methotrexate or other immunosuppressive agents, or coal tar or radiation therapy in psoriasis patients.

Warnings/Precautions

➤*Renal effects:* Cyclosporine can cause nephrotoxicity when used in high doses. The risk increases with increasing doses of cyclosporine. Renal dysfunction, including structural kidney damage, is a potential consequence of cyclosporine and, therefore, renal function must be monitored during therapy.

An increase in serum creatinine and serum urea nitrogen (BUN) may occur during cyclosporine therapy and reflects a reduction in the glomerular filtration rate. These elevations in renal transplant patients do not necessarily indicate rejection, and each patient must be fully evaluated before dosage adjustment is initiated. Impaired renal function at any time requires close monitoring, and frequent dosage adjustments may be indicated. The frequency and severity of serum creatinine elevations increase with dose and duration of cyclosporine therapy. These elevations are likely to become more pronounced without dose reduction or discontinuation.

Allogeneic transplants – Based on the historical *Sandimmune* experience with oral solution, nephrotoxicity associated with cyclosporine has been noted in 25% of cases of renal transplantation, 38% of cases of cardiac transplantation, and 37% of cases of liver transplantation. Mild nephrotoxicity was generally noted 2 to 3 months after transplant and consisted of an arrest in the fall of the preoperative elevations of BUN and creatinine at a range of 35 to 45 mg/dL and 2 to 2.5 mg/dL, respectively. These elevations are often responsive to dosage reductions.

More overt nephrotoxicity was seen early after transplantation and was characterized by a rapidly rising BUN and creatinine. Because these events are similar to rejection episodes, care must be taken to differentiate between them. This form of toxicity is usually responsive to cyclosporine dosage reduction.

Although specific diagnostic criteria that reliably differentiate renal graft rejection from drug toxicity have not been found, a number of parameters have been significantly associated to one or the other. However, up to 20% of patients may have simultaneous nephrotoxicity and rejection.

A form of chronic progressive cyclosporine-associated nephrotoxicity is characterized by serial deterioration in renal function and morphologic changes in the kidneys. From 5% to 15% of transplant patients who have received cyclosporine will fail to show a reduction in rising serum creatinine despite a decrease or discontinuation of cyclosporine therapy. Renal biopsies from these patients will demonstrate one or several of the following alterations: interstitial fibrosis with tubular atrophy, toxic tubulopathy, tubular vacuolization, tubular microcalcifications, peritubular capillary congestion, arteriolopathy, and a striped form of interstitial fibrosis with tubular atrophy. Although none of these morphologic changes are entirely specific, a histologic diagnosis of chronic progressive cyclosporine-associated structural nephrotoxicity requires evidence of these findings.

When considering the development of chronic nephrotoxicity, it is noteworthy that several authors have reported an association between the appearance of interstitial fibrosis and higher cumulative doses or persistently high circulating trough levels of cyclosporine. This is particularly true during the first 6 posttransplant months when the dosage tends to be highest and when, in kidney recipients, the organ appears to be most vulnerable to the toxic effects of cyclosporine. Among other contributing factors to the development of interstitial fibrosis in these patients are prolonged perfusion time, warm ischemia time, as well as episodes of acute toxicity, and acute and chronic rejection. The reversibility of interstitial fibrosis and its correlation to renal function have not yet been determined. Reversibility of arteriolopathy has been reported after stopping cyclosporine and lowering the dosage.

In patients with persistent high elevations of BUN and creatinine unresponsive to dosage adjustments, consider switching to other immunosuppressive therapy. In the event of severe and unremitting rejection, when rescue therapy with pulse steroids and monoclonal antibodies fails to reverse the rejection episode, it is preferable to switch to alternative immunosuppressive therapy or allow the kidney transplant to be rejected and removed rather than increase the dosage to a very high level in an attempt to reverse the rejection.

Psoriasis – The risk of cyclosporine nephropathy in psoriasis patients is reduced when the starting dosage is low (2.5 mg/kg/day), the maximum dosage does not exceed 4 mg/kg/day, serum creatinine is monitored regularly while cyclosporine is administered, and the dose of cyclosporine is decreased when the rise in creatinine is 25% or more above the patient's pretreatment level. The increase in creatinine is generally reversible upon timely decrease of the dose of cyclosporine or its discontinuation. Kidney biopsies from 86 psoriasis patients treated for a mean duration of 23 months with cyclosporine 1.2 to 7.6 mg/kg/day showed evidence of cyclosporine nephropathy in 21% of patients. The pathology consisted of renal tubular atrophy and interstitial fibrosis. Upon repeat biopsy of 13 of these patients maintained on various dosages of cyclosporine for a mean of 2 additional years, the number with cyclosporine-induced nephropathy rose to 30%. The majority of patients (19/26) were receiving a dosage of 5 mg/kg/day or more (the highest recommended dosage is 4 mg/kg/day). The patients were also receiving cyclosporine for longer than 15 months (18/26) and/or had a clinically significant increase for longer than 1 month (21/26). Creatinine levels returned to normal in 7 of 11 patients in whom cyclosporine therapy was discontinued.

Rheumatoid arthritis – Cyclosporine nephropathy was detected in renal biopsies in 10% of RA patients after an average treatment duration of 19 months. Only 1 of these 6 patients was treated with a dosage of 4 mg/kg/day or less. Serum creatinine improved in all but 1 patient after discontinuation of cyclosporine. The maximal creatinine increase appeared to be a factor in predicting cyclosporine nephropathy.

➤*Hematologic effects:* Occasionally, patients have developed a syndrome of thrombocytopenia and microangiopathic hemolytic anemia that may result in graft failure. The vasculopathy can occur in the absence of rejection and is accompanied by avid platelet consumption within the graft, as demonstrated by indium 111–labeled platelet studies. Neither the pathogenesis nor the management of this syndrome is clear. Although resolution has occurred after reduction or discontinuation of cyclosporine and administration of streptokinase and heparin, or plasmapheresis, this appears to depend upon early detection with indium 111 platelet scans.

➤*Metabolic effects:* Significant hyperkalemia (sometimes associated with hyperchloremic metabolic acidosis) and hyperuricemia have been seen occasionally in individual patients.

➤*Hepatotoxicity:* Cyclosporine can cause hepatotoxicity when used in high doses. The risk increases with increased dosing of cyclosporine. Hepatotoxicity has been noted in 4% of cases of renal transplantation, 7% of cases of cardiac transplantation, and 4% of cases of liver transplantation. This was usually noted during the first month of therapy, when high doses of cyclosporine were used, and consisted of elevations of hepatic enzymes and bilirubin. The chemistry elevations usually decreased with a reduction in dosage.

➤*Malignancies:* As in patients receiving other immunosuppressants, those receiving cyclosporine are at increased risk of development of lymphomas and other malignancies, particularly those of the skin. Warn patients taking cyclosporine to avoid excess UV light exposure. The increased risk appears to be related to the intensity and duration of immunosuppression rather than to the use of specific agents. Because of the danger of oversuppression of the immune system, resulting in increased risk of infection or malignancy, use a treatment regimen containing multiple immunosuppressants with caution; do not administer *Sandimmune* with other immunosuppressive agents, except adrenal corticoids. The efficacy and safety of cyclosporine in combination with other immunosuppressive agents have not been determined. Some malignancies may be fatal. Transplant patients receiving cyclosporine are at increased risk for serious infection with fatal outcome. Reduction or discontinuation of immunosuppression may cause the lesions to regress.

Psoriasis – There is an increased risk for the development of skin and lymphoproliferative malignancies in cyclosporine-treated psoriasis patients. The relative risk of malignancies is comparable with that observed in psoriasis patients treated with other immunosuppressive agents.

Do not treat patients for psoriasis concurrently with cyclosporine and PUVA or UVB, other radiation therapy, or other immunosuppressive agents because of the possibility of excessive immunosuppression and the subsequent risk of malignancies. Also warn patients to protect themselves appropriately when in the sun and to avoid excessive sun exposure. Thoroughly evaluate patients before and during treatment for the presence of malignancies, remembering that malignant lesions may be hidden by psoriatic plaques. Biopsy skin lesions not typical of psoriasis before starting treatment. Treat patients with cyclosporine only after complete resolution of suspicious lesions, and only if there are no other treatment options.

Rheumatoid arthritis –
Thoroughly evaluate patients before and during cyclosporine treatment for the development of malignancies. Use of cyclosporine therapy with other immunosuppressive agents may induce an excessive immunosuppression that is known to increase the risk of malignancy.

➤*Latent viral infections:* Immunosuppressed patients are at increased risk for opportunistic infections, including activation of latent viral infections. These include BK virus–associated nephropathy, which has been observed in patients receiving immunosuppressants, including cyclosporine. This infection is associated with serious outcomes, including deteriorating renal function and renal graft loss. Patient monitoring may help detect patients at risk of BK virus–associated nephropathy. Consider reduction in immunosuppression for patients who develop evidence of BK virus–associated nephropathy.

➤*Convulsions:* There have been reports of convulsions in adults and children receiving cyclosporine, particularly in combination with high-dose methylprednisolone.

CYCLOSPORINE — ORAL

➤*Encephalopathy:* Encephalopathy has been described in postmarketing reports and in the literature. Manifestations include impaired consciousness, convulsions, visual disturbances (including blindness), loss of motor function, movement disorders, and psychiatric disturbances. In many cases, changes in the white matter have been detected using imaging techniques and pathologic specimens. Predisposing factors, such as hypertension, hypomagnesemia, hypocholesterolemia, high-dose corticosteroids, high cyclosporine blood concentrations, and GVHD, have been noted in many, but not all, reported cases. The changes in most cases have been reversible upon discontinuation of cyclosporine and, in some cases, improvement was noted after reduction of dose. It appears that patients receiving liver transplants are more susceptible to encephalopathy than those receiving kidney transplants. Another rare manifestation of cyclosporine-induced neurotoxicity, occurring in transplant patients more frequently than in other indications, is optic disc edema, including papilloedema with possible visual impairment secondary to benign intracranial hypertension.

➤*Psoriasis patients:* See the Warning box for more information.

➤*Bioequivalency:* See Administration and Dosage for more information.

➤*Malabsorption:* Patients with malabsorption may have difficulty achieving therapeutic levels with *Sandimmune* capsules or oral solution.

➤*Hypertension:* Hypertension is a common adverse effect of cyclosporine therapy that may persist. Mild or moderate hypertension is encountered more frequently than severe hypertension, and the incidence decreases over time. In recipients of kidney, liver, and heart allografts treated with cyclosporine, antihypertensive therapy may be required. Control of blood pressure can be accomplished with any of the common antihypertensive agents. However, because cyclosporine may cause hyperkalemia, do not use potassium-sparing diuretics. While calcium antagonists can be effective agents in treating cyclosporine-associated hypertension, care should be taken because interference with cyclosporine metabolism may require dosage adjustment.

Rheumatoid arthritis – In placebo-controlled trials of RA patients, systolic hypertension (defined as an occurrence of 2 systolic blood pressure readings of more than 140 mm Hg) and diastolic hypertension (defined as 2 diastolic blood pressure readings of more than 90 mm Hg) occurred in 33% and 19% of patients treated with cyclosporine, respectively. The corresponding placebo rates were 22% and 8%.

➤*Vaccination:* During treatment with cyclosporine, vaccination may be less effective; avoid the use of live attenuated vaccines.

➤*Glomerular capillary thrombosis:* See Adverse Reactions for more information.

➤*Hypomagnesemia:* See Adverse Reactions for more information.

➤*Hypersensitivity reactions:* Anaphylactic reactions have not been reported with *Sandimmune* capsules or oral solution, which lack *Cremophor EL* (polyoxyethylated castor oil). Patients experiencing anaphylactic reactions have been treated subsequently with the soft-gelatin capsules or oral solution without incident.

➤*Renal function impairment:* Renal function impairment requires close monitoring and possible frequent dosage adjustment.

➤*Pregnancy: Category C.* There are no adequate and well-controlled studies in pregnant women. Use during pregnancy only if the potential benefit justifies the risk to the fetus.

In pregnant transplant recipients who are being treated with immunosuppressants, the risk of premature birth is increased. The following data represent the reported outcomes of 116 pregnancies in women receiving cyclosporine during pregnancy, 90% of whom were transplant patients and most of whom received cyclosporine throughout the entire gestational period. Because most of the patients were not prospectively identified, the results are likely to be biased toward negative outcomes. The only consistent patterns of abnormality were premature birth (gestational period of 28 to 36 weeks) and low birth weight for gestational age. It is not possible to separate the effects of the other immunosuppressants, the underlying maternal disorders, or other aspects of the transplantation milieu. Sixteen fetal losses occurred. Most of the pregnancies (85/100) were complicated by disorders, including preeclampsia, eclampsia, premature labor, abruptio placentae, oligohydramnios, Rh incompatibility, and fetoplacental dysfunction. Preterm delivery occurred in 47%. Seven malformations were reported in 5 viable infants and in 2 cases of fetal loss. Twenty-eight percent of the infants were small for gestational age. Neonatal complications occurred in 27%. In a report of 23 children followed for up to 4 years, postnatal development was said to be normal. More information on cyclosporine use during pregnancy is available from the manufacturer. Weigh the risks and benefits of using cyclosporine during pregnancy.

A limited number of observations in children exposed to cyclosporine in utero are available, up to an age of approximately 7 years. Renal function and blood pressure in these children were healthy.

Because of the possible disruption of maternal-fetal interaction, carefully weigh the risk-to-benefit ratio of using cyclosporine in psoriasis patients during pregnancy, with serious consideration for discontinuation of cyclosporine.

➤*Lactation:* Cyclosporine is excreted in breast milk; advise mothers receiving cyclosporine treatment not to breast-feed.

The American Academy of Pediatrics classifies cyclosporine as a drug that may interfere with cellular metabolism in the breast-feeding infant.

➤*Children:* Although no adequate and well-controlled studies have been completed in children, patients as young as 6 months of age have received *Sandimmune* with no unusual adverse effects. Transplant recipients as young as 1 year of age have received *Gengraf* or *Neoral* with no unusual adverse effects.

The safety and efficacy of *Gengraf* or *Neoral* treatment in children younger than 18 years of age with juvenile RA or psoriasis have not been established.

➤*Elderly:* In RA clinical trials with cyclosporine, 17.5% of patients were 65 years of age and older. These patients were more likely to develop systolic hypertension on therapy and more likely to show serum creatinine rises of 50% or more above the baseline after 3 to 4 months of therapy. Monitor elderly patients with particular care because decreases in renal function also occur with age. If patients are not properly monitored and dosages are not properly adjusted, cyclosporine therapy can cause structural kidney damage and persistent renal dysfunction.

Clinical studies of cyclosporine in transplant and psoriasis patients did not include sufficient numbers of subjects 65 years of age and older to determine whether they respond differently from younger patients. Other reported clinical experience has not identified differences in responses between elderly and younger patients. In general, use caution in dose selection for an elderly patient, usually starting at the low end of the dosing range, reflecting the greater frequency of decreased hepatic, renal, or cardiac function, and of concomitant disease or other drug therapy.

➤*Monitoring:* Assess renal and liver functions repeatedly by measurement of BUN, serum creatinine, serum bilirubin, and liver enzymes. Also monitor serum lipids, magnesium, and potassium. Routinely monitor cyclosporine blood concentrations in transplant patients and periodically in RA patients.

Blood levels – See Administration and Dosage for more information.

Rheumatoid arthritis (Gengraf and *Neoral)* – Before initiating treatment, perform a careful physical exam, including blood pressure measurements (on at least 2 occasions) and 2 creatinine levels to estimate baseline. Evaluate blood pressure and serum creatinine every 2 weeks during the initial 3 months, and then monthly if the patient is stable. It is advisable to monitor serum creatinine and blood pressure after an increase of the dose of NSAIDs and after initiation of new NSAID therapy during cyclosporine treatment. If coadministered with methotrexate, it is recommended that complete blood cell count (CBC) and liver function tests be monitored monthly.

Psoriasis (Gengraf and *Neoral)* – Before initiating treatment, perform a careful dermatological and physical examination, including blood pressure measurements (on at least 2 occasions). Evaluate patients for the presence of occult infection on the first physical examination, and for the presence of tumors initially and throughout treatment with cyclosporine. Biopsy skin lesions not typical for psoriasis before starting cyclosporine. Treat patients with malignant or premalignant changes of the skin with cyclosporine only after appropriate treatment of such lesions and if no other treatment option exists. Baseline laboratories include serum creatinine (on 2 occasions), BUN, CBC, serum magnesium, potassium, uric acid, and lipids.

Evaluate serum creatinine and BUN every 2 weeks during the initial 3 months of therapy and then monthly if the patient is stable. If the serum creatinine is 25% or more above the patient's pretreatment level, repeat serum creatinine within 2 weeks. If the change in serum creatinine remains at 25% or more above baseline, reduce cyclosporine by 25% to 50%. If at any time the serum creatinine increases by 50% or more above the pretreatment level, reduce cyclosporine by 25% to 50%. Discontinue cyclosporine if reversibility (within 25% of baseline) of serum creatinine is not achievable after 2 dosage modifications. It is advisable to monitor serum creatinine after an increase of the dose of NSAID and after initiation of new NSAID therapy during cyclosporine treatment.

Evaluate blood pressure every 2 weeks during the initial 3 months of therapy and then monthly if the patient is stable or more frequently when dosage adjustments are made. Reduce the drug by 25% to 50% in patients without a history of hypertension before initiation of treatment with cyclosporine if they are found to have sustained hypertension. If the patient continues to be hypertensive despite multiple reductions of cyclosporine, discontinue cyclosporine. For patients with treated hypertension, before the initiation of cyclosporine therapy, adjust medication to control hypertension while taking cyclosporine. Discontinue cyclosporine if a change in hypertension management is not effective or tolerable.

Also monitor CBC, uric acid, potassium, lipids, and magnesium every 2 weeks for the first 3 months of therapy, and then monthly if the patient is stable or more frequently when dosage adjustments are made. Reduce the cyclosporine dosage by 25% to 50% for any abnormality of clinical concern.

Drug Interactions

➤*Cytochrome P450 system:* Because cyclosporine is metabolized mainly by the CYP3A enzyme systems, substances known to inhibit these enzymes may decrease metabolism or increase bioavailability of cyclosporine, as indicated by increased whole blood or plasma concentrations. Drugs known to induce these enzyme systems may result in an increased metabolism of cyclosporine or decreased bioavailability, as indicated by decreased whole blood or plasma concentrations. Monitoring of blood concentrations and appropriate dosage adjustments are essential when such drugs are used concomitantly.

➤*Vaccinations:* See Warnings/Precautions for more information.

CYCLOSPORINE — ORAL

Cyclosporine Drug Interactions

Precipitant drug	Object drug[a]		Description
Allopurinol	Cyclosporine	↑	Coadministration may increase cyclosporine concentrations, possibly increasing the risk of nephrotoxicity. Closely monitor cyclosporine concentrations when allopurinol is started or stopped. If an interaction is suspected, adjust the cyclosporine dose as needed.
Aluminum salts	Cyclosporine	↓	Aluminum salts may decrease plasma concentrations and pharmacologic effects of oral cyclosporine. Do not coadminister.
Aminoglycosides (eg, gentamicin, tobramycin, vancomycin)	Cyclosporine	↑	The risk of renal dysfunction may be increased. Monitor cyclosporine concentrations and renal function. Adjust the cyclosporine dose as needed.
Amiodarone	Cyclosporine	↑	Amiodarone may increase cyclosporine blood levels, possibly increasing the risk of nephrotoxicity. Closely monitor cyclosporine concentrations and the patient for signs of toxicity. Adjust the cyclosporine dose as needed.
Amphotericin B	Cyclosporine	↑	Concomitant use of cyclosporine and amphotericin B may increase the risk of nephrotoxicity and neurotoxicity. Closely monitor the patient and renal function. If renal function declines or neurotoxicity occurs, decrease the cyclosporine dose or stop one or both drugs.
Androgens (eg, danazol, methyltestosterone)	Cyclosporine	↑	Increased cyclosporine blood concentrations and possible nephrotoxicity may occur. Closely monitor cyclosporine concentrations and the patient for signs of toxicity. Adjust the cyclosporine dose as needed.
Anticonvulsants (eg, barbiturates [eg, phenobarbital], carbamazepine, hydantoins [eg, phenytoin], oxcarbazepine)	Cyclosporine	↓	Cyclosporine levels may be decreased, resulting in a reduction in the pharmacologic effects (eg, graft loss, transplanted organ rejection). Monitor cyclosporine concentrations and observe the patient for signs of rejection or toxicity when the anticonvulsant is started or stopped, respectively. Adjust the cyclosporine dose as needed.
Azole antifungals (eg, fluconazole, itraconazole, ketoconazole, posaconazole, voriconazole)	Cyclosporine	↑	Cyclosporine levels and toxicity may increase 1 to 3 days after starting therapy and persist more than 1 week after stopping antifungal therapy. Monitor cyclosporine concentrations and serum creatinine. Adjust the cyclosporine dose as needed. When administering posaconazole, reduce the cyclosporine dose 25% and frequently monitor cyclosporine whole blood trough concentrations during posaconazole administration and after discontinuation.
Berberine	Cyclosporine	↑	Elevated cyclosporine concentrations with a risk of toxicity (eg, nephrotoxicity) may occur. Advise patients receiving cyclosporine to avoid berberine and caution them not to use herbal products without consulting their health care provider.
Beta-blockers (eg, carvedilol)	Cyclosporine	↑	Elevated cyclosporine concentrations with a risk of nephrotoxicity and neurotoxicity may occur. Closely monitor cyclosporine concentrations and the patient for signs of toxicity. Adjust the cyclosporine dose as needed.
Bortezomib	Cyclosporine	↑	Neurotoxicity of both drugs may be increased. Closely monitor the patient and adjust treatment as needed.
Cyclosporine	Bortezomib		
Bosentan	Cyclosporine	↓	Trough concentrations of bosentan may be elevated, increasing the risk of adverse effects, while cyclosporine plasma levels may be decreased. Coadministration is contraindicated.
Cyclosporine	Bosentan	↑	
Bromocriptine	Cyclosporine	↑	Coadministration may increase cyclosporine concentrations. Closely monitor cyclosporine concentrations and the patient for signs of toxicity. Adjust the cyclosporine dose as needed.
Calcium channel blockers (eg, diltiazem, nicardipine, verapamil)	Cyclosporine	↑	Increased cyclosporine levels with possible nephrotoxicity may occur. However, administration of verapamil before cyclosporine may be nephroprotective. The interaction is typically observed within 7 days of starting verapamil and may abate within 1 week after discontinuation. Use with caution. Monitor cyclosporine concentrations when the calcium channel blocker is started, stopped, or the dose is changed. Adjust the cyclosporine dose as needed.
Cyclosporine	Calcium channel blockers (ie, nifedipine)		Frequent gingival hyperplasia has been reported with coadministration of cyclosporine and nifedipine.
Chamomile	Cyclosporine	↑	Elevated cyclosporine concentrations with a risk of toxicity (eg, nephrotoxicity) may occur. Advise patients receiving cyclosporine to avoid chamomile and caution them not to use herbal products without consulting their health care provider.
Chloramphenicol	Cyclosporine	↑	Cyclosporine concentrations may be elevated, increasing the risk of toxicity (eg, nephrotoxicity). Closely monitor cyclosporine concentrations and the patient for signs of toxicity. Adjust the cyclosporine dose as needed.
Chloroquine	Cyclosporine	↑	Cyclosporine concentrations may be elevated, increasing the risk of toxicity (eg, nephrotoxicity). Closely monitor cyclosporine concentrations and the patient for signs of toxicity. Adjust the cyclosporine dose as needed.
Clindamycin	Cyclosporine	↓	Cyclosporine concentrations may be decreased, resulting in a reduction in the pharmacologic effects (eg, graft loss, transplanted organ rejection). Monitor cyclosporine concentrations and observe the patient for signs of rejection or toxicity when clindamycin is started or stopped, respectively. Adjust the cyclosporine dose as needed.
Clonidine	Cyclosporine	↑	Cyclosporine concentrations may be elevated, increasing the risk of toxicity (eg, nephrotoxicity). Closely monitor cyclosporine concentrations and the patient for signs of toxicity. Adjust the cyclosporine dose as needed.

CYCLOSPORINE — ORAL

Cyclosporine Drug Interactions

Precipitant drug	Object drug[a]		Description
Colchicine	Cyclosporine	↑	Severe adverse clinical symptoms, including GI, hepatic, renal, and neuromuscular toxicity, may occur during coadministration. Coadministration of cyclosporine and colchicine is contraindicated in patients with hepatic or renal impairment. In patients with healthy hepatic or renal function, use with caution at a maximum dosage of colchicine 0.3 mg twice daily. Cyclosporine may increase the risk of colchicine toxicity (eg, myopathy, neuropathy), especially in patients with renal dysfunction. Closely monitor the clinical response of the patient and for adverse reactions. Adjust therapy as needed.
Cyclosporine	Colchicine		
Contraceptives, hormonal	Cyclosporine	↑	Hormonal contraceptives may increase cyclosporine blood levels, possibly increasing the risk of nephrotoxicity. Closely monitor cyclosporine concentrations and the patient for signs of toxicity. Adjust the cyclosporine dose as needed.
Corticosteroids (eg, methylprednisolone)	Cyclosporine	↑	Although this combination is therapeutically beneficial for organ transplants, toxicity of both agents may be enhanced. If an interaction is suspected (eg, convulsions, increased serum creatinine, cushingoid symptoms), consider decreasing the dose of one or both drugs.
Cyclosporine	Corticosteroids (eg, methylprednisolone)		
Efavirenz	Cyclosporine	↓	Cyclosporine levels may be decreased, resulting in a reduction in the pharmacologic effects (eg, graft loss, transplanted organ rejection). Larger doses of cyclosporine may be needed after starting efavirenz. Monitor cyclosporine concentrations and observe the patient for signs of rejection or toxicity when efavirenz is started or stopped, respectively. Adjust the cyclosporine dose as needed.
Ezetimibe	Cyclosporine	↑	Cyclosporine and ezetimibe concentrations may be elevated, increasing the pharmacologic effects and risk of adverse reactions. Monitor cyclosporine concentrations when ezetimibe is coadministered. Adjust the cyclosporine dose as needed. In addition, monitor patients for cyclosporine or ezetimibe adverse reactions.
Cyclosporine	Ezetimibe		
Fenofibrate	Cyclosporine	↑	The risk of renal dysfunction may be increased. Monitor cyclosporine concentrations and renal function. Adjust the cyclosporine dose as needed.
Fluoroquinolones (eg, ciprofloxacin)	Cyclosporine	↑	Cyclosporine blood concentrations may be elevated, increasing the risk of toxicity (eg, renal dysfunction). Monitor cyclosporine concentrations and renal function. If an interaction is suspected, adjust the cyclosporine dose or consider administering an alternative antibiotic.
Foscarnet	Cyclosporine	↑	The risk of renal failure may be increased due to additive or synergistic nephrotoxicity. Closely monitor renal function. If nephrotoxicity occurs, it may be necessary to discontinue foscarnet.
Cyclosporine	Foscarnet		
Gemfibrozil	Cyclosporine	↓	Cyclosporine concentrations may be decreased, resulting in a reduction in the pharmacologic effects (eg, graft loss, transplanted organ rejection). Monitor cyclosporine concentrations and observe the patient for signs of rejection or toxicity when gemfibrozil is started or stopped, respectively. Adjust the cyclosporine dose as needed.
Griseofulvin	Cyclosporine	↓	Cyclosporine concentrations may be decreased, resulting in a reduction in the pharmacologic effects (eg, graft loss, transplanted organ rejection). Monitor cyclosporine concentrations and observe the patient for signs of rejection or toxicity when griseofulvin is started or stopped, respectively. Adjust the cyclosporine dose as needed.
Histamine H_2 antagonists (eg, cimetidine, ranitidine)	Cyclosporine	↑	The risk of renal dysfunction may be increased. Monitor cyclosporine concentrations and renal function. Adjust the cyclosporine dose as needed.
Imatinib	Cyclosporine	↑	Imatinib may increase cyclosporine blood levels, possibly increasing the risk of nephrotoxicity. Closely monitor cyclosporine concentrations and the patient for signs of toxicity. Adjust the cyclosporine dose as needed.
Imipenem/Cilastatin	Cyclosporine	↑	The neurotoxicity of both agents may be increased. Close clinical and plasma concentration monitoring are indicated. If an interaction is suspected, decrease the cyclosporine dosage and consider an alternative antimicrobial agent.
Cyclosporine	Imipenem/Cilastatin		
Immunosuppressive agents, radiation therapy (eg, PUVA, UV light treatment)	Cyclosporine	↑	Avoid concurrent treatment because of the possibility of excessive immunosuppression.
Cyclosporine	Immunosuppressive agents, radiation therapy (eg, PUVA, UV light treatment)		
Macrolide antibiotics (eg, azithromycin, clarithromycin, erythromycin, telithromycin)	Cyclosporine	↑	Elevated cyclosporine levels may occur, increasing the risk of nephrotoxicity and neurotoxicity. Closely monitor cyclosporine concentrations and serum creatinine, and monitor for toxicity. Adjust the cyclosporine dose as needed.
Melphalan	Cyclosporine	↑	The risk of renal dysfunction may be increased. Monitor cyclosporine concentrations and renal function. Adjust the cyclosporine dose as needed.
Methoxsalen	Cyclosporine	↑	Methoxsalen may increase cyclosporine blood levels, increasing the risk of nephrotoxicity. Closely monitor cyclosporine concentrations and the response of the patient when methoxsalen is started or stopped. Adjust the cyclosporine dose as needed.

CYCLOSPORINE — ORAL

Cyclosporine Drug Interactions			
Precipitant drug	Object drug[a]		Description
Metoclopramide	Cyclosporine	↑	An increase in the immunosuppressive and toxic effects of cyclosporine may result with metoclopramide coadministration. Monitor cyclosporine concentrations and the response of the patient when starting or stopping metoclopramide. Adjust the cyclosporine dose as needed.
Metronidazole	Cyclosporine	↑	Cyclosporine concentrations may be elevated, increasing the risk of toxicity (eg, nephrotoxicity). Closely monitor cyclosporine concentrations and the patient for signs of toxicity. Adjust the cyclosporine dose as needed.
Mibefradil	Cyclosporine	↑	Mibefradil may increase cyclosporine blood levels, possibly increasing the risk of nephrotoxicity. Closely monitor cyclosporine concentrations and the response of the patient when mibefradil is started or stopped. Adjust the cyclosporine dose as needed.
Micafungin	Cyclosporine	↑	Micafungin may increase cyclosporine blood levels, possibly increasing the risk of nephrotoxicity. Closely monitor cyclosporine concentrations when micafungin is started or stopped. Adjust the cyclosporine dose as needed.
Nafcillin	Cyclosporine	↓	Coadministration may decrease cyclosporine concentrations. If an alternative antibiotic is not available, monitor cyclosporine concentrations and adjust the cyclosporine dose as needed.
Nefazodone	Cyclosporine	↑	Cyclosporine concentrations and toxicity may be increased. Closely monitor cyclosporine concentrations and the patient for signs of toxicity (eg, nephrotoxicity). Adjust the cyclosporine dose as needed.
NSAIDs (eg, diclofenac, naproxen, sulindac)	Cyclosporine	↑	The risk of renal dysfunction may be increased, especially in patients with dehydration. Closely monitor cyclosporine concentrations and renal function. Adjust the cyclosporine dose as needed.
Octreotide	Cyclosporine	↓	Cyclosporine levels may be decreased, resulting in a reduction in the pharmacologic effects (eg, graft loss, transplanted organ rejection). Monitor cyclosporine concentrations and observe the clinical response of the patient when starting or stopping octreotide. Adjust the cyclosporine dose as needed.
Omeprazole	Cyclosporine	↑↓	Cyclosporine levels may be increased, decreased, or unchanged. Monitor cyclosporine concentrations and observe the clinical response of the patient when starting or stopping omeprazole. Adjust the cyclosporine dose as needed.
Orlistat	Cyclosporine	↓	Whole blood cyclosporine concentrations may be decreased, possibly resulting in a decrease in the immunosuppressive action of cyclosporine. If coadministration cannot be avoided, give cyclosporine at least 2 hours before or after orlistat.

Cyclosporine Drug Interactions			
Precipitant drug	Object drug[a]		Description
Propafenone	Cyclosporine	↑	Cyclosporine blood concentrations may be elevated, increasing the risk of toxicity (eg, renal dysfunction). Monitor cyclosporine concentrations and renal function. If an interaction is suspected, adjust the cyclosporine dose as needed.
Protease inhibitors (eg, indinavir, nelfinavir, ritonavir, saquinavir)	Cyclosporine	↑	Plasma concentrations and pharmacologic effects of both drugs may increase when cyclosporine and protease inhibitors are coadministered. Toxicity may occur. Closely monitor cyclosporine concentrations and the clinical response of the patient to both agents. Adjust the dose of cyclosporine and the protease inhibitor as needed.
Cyclosporine	Protease inhibitors (eg, indinavir, nelfinavir, ritonavir, saquinavir)		
Quercetin	Cyclosporine	↑	Elevated cyclosporine concentrations with a risk of toxicity (eg, nephrotoxicity) may occur. Advise patients receiving cyclosporine to avoid quercetin and caution them not to use herbal products without consulting their health care provider.
Quinupristin/ Dalfopristin	Cyclosporine	↑	Cyclosporine blood concentrations may be elevated, increasing the risk of toxicity (eg, renal dysfunction). Closely monitor cyclosporine concentrations and for toxicity. Adjust the cyclosporine dose as needed.
Rifamycins (ie, rifabutin, rifampin)	Cyclosporine	↓	The immunosuppressive effect of cyclosporine may be reduced. This appears to occur as early as 2 days following the initiation of rifamycins and may persist for 1 to 3 weeks after their discontinuation. If coadministration cannot be avoided, closely monitor cyclosporine concentrations and serum creatinine. Adjust the cyclosporine dose as needed.
SSRIs[b] (eg, fluoxetine, fluvoxamine, sertraline)	Cyclosporine	↑	SSRIs may increase cyclosporine concentrations and toxicity (eg, nephrotoxicity). Monitor cyclosporine concentrations and renal function. Adjust the cyclosporine dose as needed.
St. John's wort	Cyclosporine	↓	Decreased cyclosporine levels and efficacy (eg, graft loss, transplanted organ rejection) may occur with coadministration. If coadministration cannot be avoided, closely monitor cyclosporine concentrations and the clinical response of the patient when St. John's wort is started or stopped. Adjust the cyclosporine dose as needed.
Sulfonamides (eg, sulfadiazine, sulfasalazine, sulfamethoxazole/trimethoprim)	Cyclosporine	↓↑	The action of cyclosporine may be reduced. Oral sulfonamides may increase the risk of nephrotoxicity. If coadministration cannot be avoided, closely monitor cyclosporine concentrations and serum creatinine. Adjust the cyclosporine dose as needed.
Sulfonylureas (eg, glipizide, glyburide)	Cyclosporine	↑	Sulfonylureas may increase cyclosporine blood levels, possibly increasing the risk of nephrotoxicity. Closely monitor cyclosporine concentrations when the sulfonylurea is started or stopped. If an interaction is suspected, adjust the cyclosporine dose as needed.

CYCLOSPORINE — ORAL

Cyclosporine Drug Interactions

Precipitant drug	Object drug[a]		Description
Tacrolimus	Cyclosporine	⬆	Additive or synergistic toxicity may occur, increasing the risk of renal toxicity. Avoid coadministration of cyclosporine and tacrolimus. Discontinue cyclosporine or tacrolimus at least 24 hours prior to initiating treatment with the other agent.
Cyclosporine	Tacrolimus		
Terbinafine	Cyclosporine	⬇	Terbinafine may decrease cyclosporine concentrations, producing a decrease in efficacy (eg, resulting in graft rejection or transplanted organ rejection). Monitor cyclosporine concentrations and the clinical response of the patient. Adjust the cyclosporine dose as needed.
Ticlopidine	Cyclosporine	⬇	Cyclosporine whole blood concentrations may decrease, producing a decrease in pharmacologic effects (eg, resulting in graft rejection or transplanted organ rejection). Monitor cyclosporine concentrations and the clinical response of the patient. Adjust the cyclosporine dose as needed.
Tigecycline	Cyclosporine	⬆	Tigecycline may increase cyclosporine blood levels, possibly increasing the risk of toxicity (eg, nephrotoxicity). Closely monitor cyclosporine concentrations when tigecycline is started or stopped. Adjust the cyclosporine dose as needed.
Trimethoprim	Cyclosporine	⬇⬆	Both a decrease in the immunosuppressive action of cyclosporine and an increase in the risk of nephrotoxicity have been reported during coadministration of trimethoprim. Close clinical and laboratory monitoring of cyclosporine is indicated. If an interaction is suspected, consider substituting another antimicrobial agent for trimethoprim.
Troglitazone	Cyclosporine	⬇	Cyclosporine whole blood concentrations may decrease, producing a decrease in pharmacologic effects (eg, resulting in graft rejection or transplanted organ rejection). Monitor cyclosporine concentrations and the clinical response of the patient. Adjust the cyclosporine dose as needed.
Vitamin E	Cyclosporine	⬆	Vitamin E may increase cyclosporine blood levels. Closely monitor cyclosporine concentrations when vitamin E is started or stopped. Adjust the cyclosporine dose as needed.
Cyclosporine	ACE[b] inhibitors (eg, captopril)	⬆	The risk of hyperkalemia may be increased. Use with caution. Closely monitor potassium concentrations. In addition, acute renal failure has been reported with coadministration of ACE inhibitors and cyclosporine. If an interaction is suspected, discontinue the ACE inhibitor. Dose reduction or discontinuation of cyclosporine may also be necessary.
Cyclosporine	Aliskiren	⬆	Pharmacologic effects and plasma concentrations of aliskiren may be increased by cyclosporine. Coadministration is not recommended.
Cyclosporine	Caspofungin	⬆	Pharmacologic effects and plasma concentrations of caspofungin may be increased by cyclosporine. Coadministration is not recommended.
Cyclosporine	Digoxin	⬆	Elevated digoxin levels with toxicity may occur. In patients receiving digoxin, severe digitalis toxicity has been seen within days of starting cyclosporine. Closely monitor the clinical response of the patient and discontinue digoxin or adjust the dose as needed.
Cyclosporine	Doxorubicin	⬆	Doxorubicin serum concentration may be elevated, resulting in increased toxicity. Monitor the clinical response of the patient, including CBC, and adjust the doxorubicin dose as needed.
Cyclosporine	Etoposide	⬆	Serum etoposide concentration may be elevated, resulting in increased toxicity. Monitor the clinical response of the patient, including CBC, and adjust the etoposide dose as needed.
Cyclosporine	Everolimus	⬆	Serum everolimus concentrations may be elevated, increasing the pharmacologic effects and risk of adverse reactions. Monitor the clinical response of the patient (including renal function and hematologic parameters) when the cyclosporine dose is started, stopped, or changed. Adjust the everolimus dose as needed.
Cyclosporine	HMG-CoA reductase inhibitors (eg, lovastatin, simvastatin)	⬆	Severe myopathy or rhabdomyolysis may occur with coadministration. When cyclosporine is coadministered, reduce the dose of the HMG-CoA reductase inhibitor according to the label recommendations. In patients with signs and symptoms of myopathy or those at risk of severe renal injury secondary to rhabdomyolysis, temporarily withhold or discontinue the HMG-CoA reductase inhibitor.
Cyclosporine	Meglitinides (eg, nateglinide, repaglinide)	⬆	Meglitinide plasma concentrations may be elevated, increasing the pharmacologic effect and risk of hypoglycemia. Coadministration of cyclosporine and repaglinide to healthy men increased the repaglinide mean C_{max} and AUC 1.8- and 2.4-fold, respectively. Closely monitor blood glucose and adjust the meglitinide dose as needed.
Cyclosporine	Methotrexate	⬆	Coadministration resulted in an increase of methotrexate AUC by ≈ 30% and the AUC of its metabolite was decreased ≈ 80%. Monitor the clinical response of the patient when cyclosporine is started or stopped. Adjust the methotrexate dose as needed.
Cyclosporine	Mycophenolate	⬇	Plasma concentrations and pharmacologic effects of mycophenolate may be decreased by cyclosporine. Larger mycophenolate doses may be needed after starting cyclosporine. Monitor mycophenolic acid concentrations and the clinical response of the patient when starting or stopping cyclosporine. Adjust the mycophenolate dose as needed.

CYCLOSPORINE — ORAL

Cyclosporine Drug Interactions

Precipitant drug	Object drug[a]		Description
Cyclosporine	Nondepolarizing muscle relaxants (eg, vecuronium)	⬆	Cyclosporine may prolong the neuromuscular blocking effects of nondepolarizing muscle relaxants. Closely monitor the extent and duration of neuromuscular blockade. Be prepared to decrease the dosage of nondepolarizing agent and provide mechanical respiratory support as needed.
Cyclosporine	Potassium-containing drugs (eg, potassium penicillin)	⬆	The risk of hyperkalemia may be increased. Use with caution. Closely monitor potassium concentrations.
Cyclosporine	Potassium-sparing diuretics (eg, spironolactone)	⬆	Coadministration may lead to hyperkalemia. Avoid concomitant use.
Cyclosporine	Red yeast rice	⬆	Red yeast rice contains HMG-CoA reductase inhibitor–like components. The risk of HMG-CoA reductase inhibitor–like adverse reactions (eg, rhabdomyolysis) may be increased with coadministration of cyclosporine. Advise patients receiving cyclosporine to avoid red yeast rice and caution them not to use herbal products without consulting their health care provider.
Cyclosporine	Sirolimus	⬆	Sirolimus plasma concentrations may be increased, resulting in increased toxicity. Administer sirolimus 4 hours after cyclosporine to prevent variations in sirolimus concentrations.
Cyclosporine	Vinca alkaloids (eg, vinblastine, vincristine)	⬆	The pharmacologic and toxic effects of vinca alkaloids may be increased by cyclosporine. Use with caution. Monitor the clinical response of the patient and adjust the vinca alkaloid dose as needed.

[a] ⬆ = object drug increased; ⬇ = object drug decreased; ⬆⬇ = object drug both increased and decreased.

[b] ACE = angiotensin-converting enzyme; SSRIs = selective serotonin reuptake inhibitors.

➤*Drug/Food interactions:* See Actions for more information.

Grapefruit may increase cyclosporine concentrations. Unless patients have been instructed by a health care provider to take cyclosporine with grapefruit juice, caution them to avoid grapefruit juice while taking cyclosporine. Potassium-rich diets may increase the risk of hypokalemia. Closely monitor potassium concentrations. Pomelo juice may elevate cyclosporine concentrations, increasing the risk of toxicity (eg, nephrotoxicity). Advise patients to avoid pomelo juice while taking cyclosporine. Red wine may decrease cyclosporine concentrations, decreasing pharmacologic effects. Advise patients to avoid red wine while taking cyclosporine.

Adverse Reactions

➤*Allogeneic transplant:*

Most common adverse reactions – The principal adverse reactions of cyclosporine therapy are gum hyperplasia, hirsutism, hypertension, renal dysfunction, and tremor.

Hypertension – Hypertension, which is usually mild to moderate, may occur in approximately 50% of patients following renal transplantation and in most cardiac transplant patients.

Glomerular capillary thrombosis – Glomerular capillary thrombosis has been found in patients treated with cyclosporine and may progress to graft failure. The pathologic changes resemble those seen in the hemolytic-uremic syndrome, and include thrombosis of the renal microvasculature, with platelet-fibrin thrombi occluding glomerular capillaries and afferent arterioles, microangiopathic hemolytic anemia, thrombocytopenia, and decreased renal function. Similar findings have been observed when other immunosuppressives have been employed posttransplantation.

Hypomagnesemia – Hypomagnesemia has been reported in some, but not all, patients exhibiting convulsions while on cyclosporine therapy. Although magnesium depletion studies in healthy subjects suggest that hypomagnesemia is associated with neurologic disorders, multiple factors, including high-dose methylprednisolone, hypertension, hypocholesterolemia, and nephrotoxicity associated with high plasma concentrations of cyclosporine, appear to be related to the neurological manifestations of cyclosporine toxicity.

Adverse reactions (3% or more) –

***Sandimmune* Adverse Reactions (≥ 3%)**

Adverse reaction	Randomized kidney transplant patients		All *Sandimmune* patients		
	Sandimmune (n = 227)	Azathioprine (n = 228)	Kidney (n =705)	Heart (n = 112)	Liver (n = 75)
Cardiovascular					
Flushing	< 1%	0%	4%	0%	4%
Hypertension	26%	18%	13%	53%	27%
CNS					
Convulsions	3%	1%	1%	4%	5%
Headache	2%	< 1%	2%	15%	4%
Paresthesia	3%	0%	1%	2%	1%
Tremor	12%	0%	21%	31%	55%
Dermatologic					
Acne	6%	8%	2%	2%	1%
Hirsutism	21%	< 1%	21%	28%	45%
GI					
Abdominal discomfort	< 1%	0%	< 1%	7%	0%
Diarrhea	3%	< 1%	3%	4%	8%
Gum hyperplasia	4%	0%	9%	5%	16%
Hepatotoxicity	< 1%	< 1%	4%	7%	4%
Nausea/Vomiting	2%	< 1%	4%	10%	4%
GU					
Gynecomastia	< 1%	0%	< 1%	4%	3%
Renal dysfunction	32%	6%	25%	38%	37%
Hematologic					
Leukopenia	2%	19%	< 1%	6%	0%
Lymphoma	< 1%	0%	1%	6%	1%

CYCLOSPORINE — ORAL

Sandimmune Adverse Reactions (≥ 3%)					
Adverse reaction	Randomized kidney transplant patients: *Sandimmune* (n = 227)	Randomized kidney transplant patients: Azathioprine (n = 228)	All *Sandimmune* patients: Kidney (n =705)	All *Sandimmune* patients: Heart (n = 112)	All *Sandimmune* patients: Liver (n = 75)
Miscellaneous					
Cramps	4%	< 1%	2%	< 1%	0%
Sinusitis	< 1%	0%	4%	3%	7%

Other adverse reactions (2% or less) – The following adverse reactions occurred in 2% or fewer patients: allergic reactions, anemia, anorexia, brittle fingernails, confusion, conjunctivitis, edema, fever, gastritis, hearing loss, hiccups, hyperglycemia, muscle pain, peptic ulcer, thrombocytopenia, tinnitus.

Rare adverse reactions – The following reactions occurred rarely: anxiety, chest pain, constipation, depression, hair breaking, hematuria, joint pain, lethargy, mouth sores, myocardial infarction (MI), night sweats, pancreatitis, pruritus, swallowing difficulty, tingling, upper GI bleeding, visual disturbance, weakness, weight loss.

Discontinuation of therapy –

Adverse Reactions Associated With Discontinuation of *Sandimmune* in Renal Transplant Patients[a]			
Reason for discontinuation	Randomized patients: *Sandimmune* (n = 227)	Randomized patients: Azathioprine (n = 228)	All *Sandimmune* patients (n = 705)
GU			
Acute tubular necrosis	2.6%	0%	1%
Renal toxicity	5.7%	0%	5.4%
Hematologic			
Hematological abnormalities	0%	0.4%	0%
Lymphoma/ Lymphoproliferative disease	0.4%	0%	0.3%
Miscellaneous	0%	0%	0.7%
Hypertension	0%	0%	0.3%
Infection	0%	0.4%	0.9%
Lack of efficacy	2.6%	0.9%	1.4%

[a] *Sandimmune* was discontinued on a temporary basis and then restarted in 18 additional patients.

Infection – Patients receiving immunosuppressive therapies, including cyclosporine and cyclosporine-containing regimens, are at increased risk of infections (viral, bacterial, fungal, parasitic). Both generalized and localized infections can occur. Preexisting infections may also be aggravated. Fatal outcomes have been reported.

Infectious Complications in Renal Transplant Patients		
Complication	*Sandimmune* (n = 227)	Azathioprine with steroids[a] (n = 228)
Abscess	4.4%	5.3%
Cytomegalovirus	4.8%	12.3%
Local fungal infections	7.5%	9.6%
Pneumonia	6.2%	9.2%
Septicemia	5.3%	4.8%
Systemic fungal infections	2.2%	3.9%
Urinary tract infections	21.1%	20.2%
Other viral infections	15.9%	18.4%
Wound and skin infections	7%	10.1%

[a] Some patients also received antilymphocytic globulin.

➤*Psoriasis:*

Most common adverse reactions – The principal adverse reactions associated with the use of cyclosporine in patients with psoriasis are abdominal discomfort, diarrhea, headache, hirsutism/hypertrichosis, hypertension, hypertriglyceridemia, influenza-like symptoms, lethargy, musculoskeletal or joint pain, nausea/vomiting, paresthesia or hyperesthesia, and renal dysfunction.

Discontinuation of therapy – In psoriasis patients treated in US controlled trials within the recommended dose range, cyclosporine therapy was discontinued in 1% of patients because of hypertension and in 5.4% of patients because of increased creatinine. In the majority of cases, these changes were reversible after dosage reduction or discontinuation of cyclosporine. The frequency and severity of serum creatinine elevations increases with dose and duration of cyclosporine therapy. These elevations are likely to become more pronounced and may result in irreversible renal damage without dose reduction or discontinuation.

Mortality – There has been 1 reported death associated with the use of cyclosporine in psoriasis. A 27-year-old man developed renal deterioration and was continued on cyclosporine. He had progressive renal failure leading to death.

Adverse reactions (3% or more) –

Neoral/*Sandimmune* Adverse Reactions in Psoriasis Patients (≥ 3%)		
Adverse reaction[a]	*Neoral* (n = 182)	*Sandimmune* (n = 185)
Cardiovascular	28%	25.4%
Hypertension[b]	27.5%	25.4%
CNS	26.4%	20.5%
Headache	15.9%	14%
Paresthesia	7.1%	4.8%
Psychiatric adverse reactions	5%	3.8%
Dermatologic	17.6%	15.1%
Hypertrichosis	6.6%	5.4%
GI	19.8%	28.7%
Abdominal pain	2.7%	6%
Diarrhea	5%	5.9%
Dyspepsia	2.2%	3.2%
Gum hyperplasia	3.8%	6%
Nausea	5.5%	5.9%
GU	24.2%	16.2%
Increased creatinine	19.8%	15.7%
Reproductive (women)	8.5%	11.5%
Musculoskeletal	13.2%	8.7%
Arthralgia	6%	1.1%
Respiratory	5%	6.5%
Bronchospasm, coughing, dyspnea, rhinitis	5%	4.9%
Upper respiratory tract infection	7.7%	11.3%
Miscellaneous	29.1%	22.2%
Infection or potential infection	24.7%	24.3%
Influenza-like symptoms	9.9%	8.1%
Metabolic/Nutritional adverse reactions	9.3%	9.7%
Pain	4.4%	3.2%
Resistance mechanism	18.7%	21.1%
White cell and reticuloendothelial system adverse reactions	4.4%	2.7%

[a] Total percentages of reactions within the system shown.
[b] Newly occurring hypertension = systolic blood pressure ≥ 160 mm Hg and/or diastolic blood pressure ≥ 90 mm Hg.

Adverse reactions (1% to less than 3%) –

CNS: Appetite increased, dizziness, insomnia, nervousness, vertigo.
Dermatologic: Acne, dry skin, folliculitis, keratosis, pruritus, rash.
GI: Abdominal distention, constipation, gingival bleeding.
Hematologic: Platelet, bleeding, and clotting disorders; red blood cell disorder.
Respiratory: Infection (viral and other infection).
Miscellaneous: Abnormal vision, chest pain, fever, flushes, hot flushes, hyperbilirubinemia, micturition frequency, skin malignancies (squamous cell [0.9%] and basal cell [0.4%] carcinomas).

Lab test abnormalities – Mild hypomagnesemia and hyperkalemia may occur but are asymptomatic. Increases in uric acid may occur and attacks of gout have been reported rarely. A minor dose-related hyperbilirubinemia has been observed in the absence of hepatocellular damage. Cyclosporine therapy may be associated with a modest increase of serum triglycerides and cholesterol. Elevations of triglycerides (more than 750 mg/dL) occur in approximately 15% of psoriasis patients; elevations of cholesterol (more than 300 mg/dL) are observed in less than 3% of psoriasis patients. Generally, these laboratory abnormalities are reversible upon dose reduction or discontinuation of cyclosporine.

CYCLOSPORINE — ORAL

➤*Rheumatoid arthritis:*

Most common adverse reactions – The principal adverse reactions associated with the use of cyclosporine in RA are renal dysfunction, hypertension, headache, GI disturbances, and hirsutism/hypertrichosis.

Discontinuation of therapy – In RA patients treated in clinical trials within the recommended dose range, cyclosporine was discontinued in 5.3% of patients because of hypertension and in 7% of patients because of increased creatinine. These changes are usually reversible with timely dose decreases or discontinuation. The frequency and severity of serum creatinine elevations increase with dose and duration of cyclosporine therapy. These elevations are likely to become more pronounced without dose reduction or discontinuation.

Adverse reactions (3% or more) –

Neoral/Sandimmune Rheumatoid Arthritis Adverse Reactions (≥ 3%)						
	Studies 651, 652, and 2008	Study 302	Study 654	Study 654	Study 302	Studies 651, 652, and 2008.
Adverse reaction	*Sandimmune*[a] (n = 269)	*Sandimmune* (n = 155)	Methotrexate + *Sandimmune* (n = 74)	Methotrexate + placebo (n = 73)	*Neoral* (n = 143)	Placebo (n = 201)
Cardiovascular						
Arrhythmia	2%	5%	5%	6%	2%	1%
Chest pain	4%	5%	1%	1%	6%	1%
Flushing	2%	2%	3%	0%	5%	2%
Hypertension	8%	26%	16%	12%	25%	2%
CNS						
Depression	3%	6%	3%	1%	1%	2%
Dizziness	8%	6%	7%	3%	8%	3%
Fatigue	6%	3%	8%	12%	3%	7%
Headache	17%	23%	22%	11%	25%	9%
Insomnia	4%	1%	1%	0%	3%	2%
Migraine	2%	3%	0%	0%	3%	1%
Paresthesia	8%	7%	8%	4%	11%	1%
Tremor	8%	7%	7%	3%	13%	4%
Dermatologic						
Alopecia	3%	0%	1%	1%	4%	4%
Bullous eruptions	1%	0%	4%	1%	1%	1%
Hypertrichosis	19%	17%	12%	0%	15%	3%
Purpura	3%	4%	1%	1%	2%	0%
Rash	7%	12%	10%	7%	8%	10%
Skin ulceration	1%	1%	3%	4%	0%	2%
GI						
Abdominal pain	15%	15%	15%	7%	15%	10%
Anorexia	3%	3%	1%	0%	3%	3%
Diarrhea	12%	12%	18%	15%	13%	8%
Dyspepsia	12%	12%	10%	8%	8%	4%
Flatulence	5%	5%	5%	4%	4%	1%
GI disorder NOS[b]	0%	2%	1%	4%	4%	0%
Gingivitis	4%	3%	0%	0%	0%	1%
Gum hyperplasia	2%	4%	1%	3%	4%	1%
Nausea	23%	14%	24%	15%	18%	14%
Rectal hemorrhage	0%	3%	0%	0%	1%	1%
Stomatitis	7%	5%	16%	12%	6%	8%
Vomiting	9%	8%	14%	7%	6%	5%
GU						
Dysuria	0%	0%	11%	3%	1%	2%
Leukorrhea	1%	0%	4%	0%	1%	0%
Menstrual disorder	3%	2%	1%	0%	1%	1%
Micturition frequency	2%	4%	3%	1%	2%	2%
Nonprotein nitrogen increased	0%	19%	12%	0%	18%	0%
UTI[b]	0%	3%	5%	4%	3%	0%
Lab test abnormalities						
Creatinine elevations ≥ 30%	43%	39%	55%	19%	48%	13%
Creatinine elevations ≥ 50%	24%	18%	26%	8%	18%	3%
Hypomagnesemia	0%	4%	0%	0%	6%	0%
Musculoskeletal						
Arthropathy	0%	5%	0%	1%	4%	0%
Leg cramps/involuntary muscle contractions	2%	11%	11%	3%	12%	1%
Rigors	1%	1%	4%	0%	3%	1%

CYCLOSPORINE — ORAL

Neoral/*Sandimmune* Rheumatoid Arthritis Adverse Reactions (≥ 3%)						
Adverse reaction	Studies 651, 652, and 2008 *Sandimmune*[a] (n = 269)	Study 302 *Sandimmune* (n = 155)	Study 654 Methotrexate + *Sandimmune* (n = 74)	Study 654 Methotrexate + placebo (n = 73)	Study 302 *Neoral* (n = 143)	Studies 651, 652, and 2008. Placebo (n = 201)
Respiratory						
Bronchitis	1%	3%	1%	0%	1%	3%
Coughing	5%	3%	5%	7%	4%	4%
Dyspnea	5%	1%	3%	3%	1%	2%
Infection NOS	9%	5%	0%	7%	3%	10%
Pharyngitis	3%	5%	5%	6%	4%	4%
Pneumonia	1%	0%	4%	0%	1%	1%
Rhinitis	0%	3%	11%	10%	1%	0%
Sinusitis	4%	4%	8%	4%	3%	3%
Upper respiratory tract infection	0%%	14%	23%	15%	13%	0%
Miscellaneous						
Accidental trauma	0%	1%	10%	4%	4%	0%
Ear disorder NOS	0%	5%	0%	0%	1%	0%
Edema NOS	5%	14%	12%	4%	10%	< 1%
Fever	2%	3%	0%	0%	2%	4%
Influenza-like symptoms	< 1%	6%	1%	0%	3%	2%
Pain	6%	9%	10%	15%	13%	4%

[a] Includes patients in 2.5 mg/kg/day dosage group only.
[b] NOS = not otherwise specified; UTI = urinary tract infection.

Other adverse reactions (1% to less than 3%) –

Cardiovascular: Abnormal heart sounds, cardiac failure, MI, peripheral ischemia.

CNS: Anxiety, asthenia, confusion, decreased libido, emotional lability, hypoesthesia, impaired concentration, increased libido, malaise, nervousness, neuropathy, paranoia, somnolence, vertigo.

Dermatologic: Abnormal pigmentation, angioedema, dermatitis, dry skin, eczema, increased sweating, nail disorder, pruritus, skin disorder, urticaria.

GI: Constipation, dry mouth, dysphagia, enanthema, eructation, esophagitis, gastric ulcer, gastritis, gastroenteritis, gingival bleeding, glossitis, peptic ulcer, salivary gland enlargement, tongue disorder, tooth disorder.

GU: Abnormal urine, breast fibroadenosis, breast pain, hematuria, increased BUN, micturition urgency, nocturia, polyuria, pyelonephritis, renal abscess, urinary incontinence, uterine hemorrhage.

Hematologic: Anemia, epistaxis, leukopenia, lymphadenopathy.

Metabolic/Nutritional: Diabetes mellitus, hyperkalemia, hyperuricemia, hypoglycemia, weight decrease, weight increase.

Musculoskeletal: Arthralgia, bone fracture, bursitis, joint dislocation, myalgia, stiffness, synovial cyst, tendon disorder.

Respiratory: Abnormal chest sounds, bronchospasm, tonsillitis.

Special senses: Abnormal vision, cataract, conjunctivitis, deafness, eye pain, taste perversion, tinnitus, vestibular disorder.

Miscellaneous: Abscess, allergy, bacterial infection, bilirubinemia, carcinoma, cellulitis, folliculitis, fungal infection, goiter, herpes simplex, herpes zoster, hot flushes, moniliasis, overdose, procedure NOS, tumor NOS, viral infection.

➤*Postmarketing:* BK virus–associated nephropathy has been observed in patients receiving immunosuppressants, including cyclosporine. This infection is associated with serious outcomes, including deteriorating renal function and renal graft loss.

Overdosage

➤*Symptoms:* There is minimal experience with cyclosporine overdosage. Transient hepatotoxicity and nephrotoxicity may occur, which should resolve following drug withdrawal. Oral doses of cyclosporine up to 10 g (approximately 150 mg/kg) have been tolerated with relatively minor clinical consequences, such as vomiting, drowsiness, headache, tachycardia, and, in a few patients, moderately severe, reversible impairment of renal function. However, serious symptoms of intoxication have been reported following accidental parenteral overdosage with cyclosporine in premature neonates.

➤*Treatment:* Gastric lavage can be of value up to 2 hours after administration of cyclosporine. Follow general supportive measures and symptomatic treatment in all cases of overdosage. Cyclosporine is not dialyzable to any great extent, nor is it cleared well by charcoal hemoperfusion.

Patient Information

Advise patients to make any change of cyclosporine formulation cautiously and only under their health care provider's supervision because a change in the formulation may result in the need for a change in dosage.

Inform patients of the necessity of repeated laboratory tests while they are receiving cyclosporine. Give patients careful dosage instructions, and inform them of the potential risks during pregnancy and of the risk of neoplasia. Also inform patients of the risk of hypertension and renal dysfunction.

Caution patients using cyclosporine oral solution with its accompanying syringe for dosage measurement not to rinse the syringe before or after use. Introduction of water into the product by any means will cause variation in dose.

Advise patients that during treatment with cyclosporine, vaccination may be less effective, and advise them to avoid use of live attenuated vaccines.

Give patients careful dosing instructions. Instruct patients to dilute *Gengraf* or *Neoral* oral solution with orange or apple juice that is at room temperature; inform them that *Sandimmune* oral solution may be diluted with milk, chocolate milk, or orange juice, preferably at room temperature.

Advise patients to take cyclosporine on a consistent schedule with regard to time of day and in relation to meals. Advise patients to avoid grapefruit and grapefruit juice because they affect metabolism, increasing blood concentration of cyclosporine.

Instruct patients to contact their health care provider if fever, sore throat, tiredness, unusual bleeding or bruising, decreased urination, or yellow skin/eyes occurs.

An odor may be present upon opening the *Sandimmune* package. The odor will disappear shortly after opening and does not mean that there is anything wrong with the medicine.

Cyclosporine may increase skin cancer risk. Advise patients to avoid prolonged exposure to the sun and other UV light and to use sunscreens and wear protective clothing while taking this medicine. Patients who are being treated for psoriasis will need to have at least 2 careful skin and physical examinations, including blood pressure measurements, before starting cyclosporine.

Inform patients that cyclosporine may increase risk of high blood pressure and abnormal kidney function.

Inform patients that cyclosporine may affect blood sugar level in diabetic patients.

CYCLOSPORINE — INJECTION

WARNING

Only health care providers experienced in immunosuppressive therapy and management of organ transplant patients should prescribe cyclosporine. Patients receiving the drug should be managed in facilities equipped and staffed with adequate laboratory and supportive medical resources. The health care provider responsible for maintenance therapy should have complete information requisite for the follow-up of the patient.

Administer cyclosporine with adrenal corticosteroids but not with other immunosuppressive agents. Increased susceptibility to infection and other possible development of lymphoma may result from immunosuppression.

Indications

➤*Allogeneic transplants:* For prophylaxis of organ rejection in kidney, liver, and heart allogeneic transplants. Cyclosporine always is to be used with adrenal corticosteroids. Cyclosporine also may be used in the treatment of chronic rejection in patients previously treated with other immunosuppressive agents. Because of the risk of anaphylaxis, reserve cyclosporine injection for patients who are unable to take the soft-gelatin capsule or oral solution.

➤*Off-label uses:* Prevention and treatment of acute graft-versus-host disease (GVHD) following bone marrow transplantation; aplastic anemia; resistant leukemias.

Administration and Dosage

➤*General dosing considerations:* Anaphylactic reactions have occurred with cyclosporine injection.

➤*Adults:*

Allogeneic transplant – See also Off-Label Dosing for additional renal transplantation recommendations.

Usual dosage: Cyclosporine injection is administered at one-third the oral dose.

Initial dosage: A single intravenous (IV) dose of 5 to 6 mg/kg/day given 4 to 12 hours prior to transplantation. This single dose is continued postoperatively until the patient can tolerate oral therapy. Switch patients to oral therapy as soon as possible after surgery.

Adjunct therapy: Adjunct therapy with adrenal corticosteroids is recommended. Different tapering dosage schedules of prednisone appear to achieve similar results. A dosage schedule based on the patient's weight started with 2 mg/kg/day for the first 4 days and tapered to 1 mg/kg/day by 1 week, 0.6 mg/kg/day by 2 weeks, 0.3 mg/kg/day by 1 month, and 0.15 mg/kg/day by 2 months and thereafter as a maintenance dose. Another center started with an initial dose of 200 mg and tapered by 40 mg/day until reaching 20 mg/day. After 2 months at this dose, a further reduction to 10 mg/day was made. Adjustments in dosage of prednisone must be made according to the clinical situation.

Off-label dosing –

Prevention of acute graft-versus host disease: 1.5 mg/kg IV given every 12 hours in combination with methotrexate, beginning 1 day prior to hematopoietic stem cell transplantation (HSCT). Doses are adjusted based on clinical status. When oral therapy is tolerated, 12.5 mg/kg/day is given in 2 divided doses.

Renal transplantation: One reference suggests 3 to 4 mg/kg/day in 1 or 2 divided doses starting immediately prior to transplantation, as an IV infusion over at least 4 hours or as a continuous infusion over 24 hours.

➤*Children:*

Allogeneic transplant – See Adults for dosing.

In children, the same dose and dosing regimen as adults may be used, although higher doses may be required.

➤*Renal function impairment:* Impaired renal function at any time requires close monitoring, and frequent dosage adjustment may be indicated.

➤*Therapeutic drug monitoring:* Several study centers have found blood concentration monitoring of cyclosporine useful in patient management. While no fixed relationship has been established, in 1 series of 375 consecutive cadaveric renal transplant recipients, dosage was adjusted to achieve specific whole blood 24-hour trough levels of 100 to 200 ng/mL as determined by high-pressure liquid chromatography (HPLC).

Of major importance to blood level analysis is the type of assay used. The above levels are specific to the parent cyclosporine molecule and correlate directly to the new monoclonal specific radioimmunoassays (mRIA-sp). Nonspecific assays that detect the parent compound molecule and various of its metabolites are also available. Older studies often cited levels using a nonspecific assay that were roughly twice those of specific assays. Assay results are not interchangeable and their use should be guided by their approved labeling. If plasma specimens are employed, levels will vary with the temperature at the time of separation from whole blood. Plasma levels may range from one-half to one-fifth of whole blood levels. Refer to individual assay labeling for complete instructions. In addition, *Transplantation Proceedings* (June 1990) contains position papers and a broad consensus generated at the Cyclosporine Therapeutic Drug Monitoring conference that year. Blood level monitoring is not a replacement for renal function monitoring or tissue biopsies.

Approximate therapeutic ranges in renal transplantation – One reference suggests the following therapeutic ranges for cyclosporine in renal transplant patients.

Trough levels:

- *0 to 2 months posttransplant* – 150 to 350 ng/mL by HPLC and enzyme-multiplied immunoassay technique (EMIT) or 250 to 450 ng/mL by fluorescent polarization immunoassay (FPIA).
- *2 to 6 months posttransplant* – 100 to 250 ng/mL by HPLC and EMIT or 175 to 350 ng/mL by FPIA.
- *More than 6 months posttransplant* – Approximately 100 ng/mL by HPLC and EMIT or approximately 150 ng/mL by FPIA.

C2 levels: Monitoring with 2-hour peak levels (C2 levels) may be more useful than traditional trough level monitoring. Levels are drawn within 15 minutes to 2 hours after cyclosporine dose.

- *0 to 2 months posttransplant* – 1.5 to 2 ng/mL.
- *2 to 6 months posttransplant* – 1.1 to 1.5 ng/mL.
- *More than 6 months posttransplant* – 0.8 to 1 ng/mL.

➤*Preparation for administration:* Cyclosporine is an immunosuppressant agent and is also considered a potential teratogen and a potential mutagen. Follow safe handling procedures when preparing, administering, or dispensing cyclosporine.

Immediately before use, dilute 1 mL of cyclosporine IV concentrate in 20 to 100 mL of sodium chloride 0.9% injection or dextrose 5% injection.

The *Cremophor EL* (polyoxyethylated castor oil) contained in the concentrate for IV infusion can cause phthalate stripping from polyvinyl chloride (PVC).

➤*Administration:* For IV infusion only. Administer as a slow IV infusion over approximately 2 to 6 hours.

➤*Storage/Stability:* Store at temperatures below 30°C (86°F) and protect from light. Discard diluted infusion solutions after 24 hours.

Actions

➤*Pharmacology:* Cyclosporine is a potent immunosuppressive agent that in animals prolongs survival of allogeneic transplants involving skin, kidney, heart, pancreas, bone marrow, small intestine, and lung. Cyclosporine has been demonstrated to suppress some humoral immunity and to a greater extent, cell-mediated reactions, such as allograft rejection, delayed hypersensitivity, experimental allergic encephalomyelitis, Freund adjuvant arthritis, and GVHD, in many animal species for a variety of organs.

Successful kidney, liver, and heart allogeneic transplants have been performed in humans using cyclosporine.

The exact mechanism of action of cyclosporine is not known. Experimental evidence suggests that the effectiveness of cyclosporine is due to specific and reversible inhibition of immunocompetent lymphocytes in the G_0 or G_1 phase of the cell cycle. T-lymphocytes are preferentially inhibited. The T-helper cell is the main target, although the T-suppressor cell may also be suppressed. Cyclosporine also inhibits lymphokine production and release, including interleukin-2 or T-cell growth factor.

➤*Pharmacokinetics:*

Distribution – Cyclosporine is distributed largely outside the blood volume; approximately 33% to 47% is in plasma, 4% to 9% in lymphocytes, 5% to 12% in granulocytes, and 41% to 58% in erythrocytes. At high concentrations, the uptake by leukocytes and erythrocytes becomes saturated. In plasma, approximately 90% is bound to proteins, primarily lipoproteins. In blood, the distribution is concentration dependent.

Metabolism – Cyclosporine is extensively metabolized, but there is no major metabolic pathway.

Of 15 metabolites characterized in human urine, 9 have been assigned structures. The major pathways consist of hydroxylation of the C-gamma-carbon of 2 of the leucine residues, C-eta-carbon hydroxylation, and cyclic ether formation (with oxidation of the double bond) in the side chain of the amino acid 3-hydroxyl-N,4-dimethyl-L-2-amino-6-octenoic acid and N-demethylation of N-methyl leucine residues. Hydrolysis of the cyclic peptide chain or conjugation of the aforementioned metabolites do not appear to be important biotransformation pathways.

Excretion – The disposition of cyclosporine from blood is biphasic, with a terminal half-life of approximately 19 hours (range, 10 to 27 hours.) Elimination is primarily biliary, with only 6% of the dose excreted in the urine.

Only 0.1% of the dose is excreted in the urine as unchanged drug.

Contraindications

Hypersensitivity to *Cremophor EL* (polyoxyethylated castor oil) or cyclosporine.

Warnings/Precautions

➤*Renal effects:*

Elevated serum urea nitrogen and serum creatinine – It is not unusual for serum creatinine and serum urea nitrogen (BUN) levels to be elevated during cyclosporine therapy. These elevations in renal transplant patients do not necessarily indicate rejection, and each patient must be fully evaluated before dosage adjustment is initiated.

Impaired renal function at any time requires close monitoring, and frequent dosage adjustments may be indicated.

Nephrotoxicity – Cyclosporine, when used in high doses, can cause nephrotoxicity. Nephrotoxicity has been noted in 25% of cases of renal transplantation, 38% of cases of cardiac transplantation, and 37% of cases of liver

CYCLOSPORINE — INJECTION

transplantation. Mild nephrotoxicity was generally noted 2 to 3 months posttransplant and consisted of an arrest in the fall of the preoperative elevations of BUN and creatinine at a range of 35 to 45 mg/dL and 2 to 2.5 mg/dL, respectively. These elevations are often responsive to dosage reductions. More overt nephrotoxicity was seen early after transplantation and was characterized by a rapidly rising BUN and creatinine. Because these events are similar to rejection episodes, care must be taken to differentiate between them. This form of nephrotoxicity is usually responsive to cyclosporine dosage reduction.

Although specific diagnostic criteria that reliably differentiate renal graft rejection from drug toxicity have not been found, a number of parameters have been significantly associated to one or the other. However, up to 20% of patients may have simultaneous nephrotoxicity and rejection.

A form of chronic progressive cyclosporine-associated nephrotoxicity is characterized by serial deterioration in renal function and morphologic changes in the kidneys. From 5% to 15% of transplant patients who have received cyclosporine will fail to show a reduction in rising serum creatinine despite a decrease or discontinuation of cyclosporine therapy. Renal biopsies from these patients will demonstrate an interstitial fibrosis with tubular atrophy. In addition, toxic tubulopathy, peritubular capillary congestion, arteriolopathy, and a striped form of interstitial fibrosis with tubular atrophy may be present. Although none of these morphologic changes are entirely specific, a histologic diagnosis of chronic progressive cyclosporine-associated nephrotoxicity requires evidence of these findings.

When considering the development of chronic nephrotoxicity, it is noteworthy that several authors have reported an association between the appearance of interstitial fibrosis and higher cumulative doses or persistently high circulating trough levels of cyclosporine. This is particularly true during the first 6 posttransplant months when the dosage tends to be highest and when, in kidney recipients, the organ appears to be most vulnerable to the toxic effects of cyclosporine. Among other contributing factors to the development of interstitial fibrosis in these patients are prolonged perfusion time, warm ischemia time, as well as episodes of acute toxicity, and acute and chronic rejection. The reversibility of interstitial fibrosis and its correlation to renal function have not yet been determined.

In patients with persistent high elevations of BUN and creatinine who are unresponsive to dosage adjustments, consider switching to other immunosuppressive therapy. In the event of severe and unremitting rejection, it is preferable to allow the kidney transplant to be rejected and removed rather than increase the cyclosporine dosage to a very high level in an attempt to reverse the rejection.

Diagnostic Criteria Differentiating Nephrotoxicity From Rejection[a]

Parameter	Nephrotoxicity	Rejection
History	• Donor > 50 years of age or hypotensive, • Prolonged kidney preservation, • Prolonged anastomosis time, • Concomitant nephrotoxic drugs	• Antidonor immune response, • Retransplant patient
Clinical	• Often > 6 weeks after surgery,[b] • Prolonged initial nonfunction (acute tubular necrosis)	• Often [b] • Fever > 37.5°C, • Weight gain > 0.5 kg, • Graft swelling and tenderness, • Decrease in daily urine volume > 500 mL (or 50%)
Laboratory	• Cyclosporine A serum trough level > 200 ng/mL, • Gradual rise in creatinine (< 0.15 mg/dL/day),[c] • Creatinine plateau < 25% above baseline, • BUN/creatinine ≥ 20	• Cyclosporine A serum trough level < 150 ng/mL, • Rapid rise in creatinine (> 0.3 mg/dL/day),[c] • Creatinine > 25% above baseline, • BUN/creatinine < 20
Biopsy	• Arteriolopathy (medial hypertrophy,[c] hyalinosis, nodular deposits, intimal thickening, endothelial vacuolization, progressive scarring), • Tubular atrophy, isometric vacuolization, isolated calcifications, • Minimal edema, • Mild focal infiltrates,[d] • Diffuse interstitial fibrosis, often striped form	• Endovasculitis[d] (proliferation,[c] intimal arteritis,[b] necrosis, sclerosis), • Tubulitis with RBC[b] and WBC[b] casts, some irregular vacuolization, • Interstitial edema[d] and hemorrhage,[b] • Diffuse moderate to severe mononuclear infiltrates,[e] • Glomerulitis (mononuclear cells)[d]
Aspiration cytology	• Cyclosporine A deposits in tubular and endothelial cells, • Fine isometric vacuolization of tubular cells	• Inflammatory infiltrate with mononuclear phagocytes, macrophages, lymphoblastoid cells, and activated T cells, • These strongly express HLA-DR antigens
Urine cytology	• Tubular cells with vacuolization and granularization	• Degenerative tubular cells, plasma cells and lymphocyturia > 20% of sediment
Manometry	• Intracapsular pressure < 40 mm Hg[b]	• Intracapsular pressure > 40 mm Hg[b]
Ultrasonography	• Unchanged graft cross sectional area	• Increase in graft cross sectional area, • Anteroposterior diameter ≥ transverse diameter
MRI	• Normal appearance	• Loss of distinct corticomedullary junction, swelling image intensity of parachyma approaching that of psoas, loss of hilar fat
Radionuclide scan	• Normal or generally decreased perfusion, • Decrease in tubular function, • (^{131}I-hippuran) > decrease in perfusion (^{99m}Tc DTPA)	• Patchy arterial flow, • Decrease in perfusion > decrease in tubular function, • Increased uptake of indium 111 labeled platelets or Tc-99m in colloid
Therapy	• Responds to decreased cyclosporine	• Responds to increased steroids or antilymphocyte globulin

[a] RBC = red blood cell count; WBC = white blood cell count; HLA-DR = varieties of human leukocyte antigen; MRI = magnetic resonance imaging; DTPA = diethylenetriamine pentaacetic acid.
[b] $P < 0.01$.
[c] $P < 0.05$.
[d] $P < 0.001$.
[e] $P < 0.0001$.

➤*Hematologic effects:* Occasionally, patients have developed a syndrome of thrombocytopenia and microangiopathic hemolytic anemia that may result in graft failure. The vasculopathy can occur in the absence of rejection and is accompanied by avid platelet consumption within the graft, as demonstrated by indium 111–labeled platelet studies. Neither the pathogenesis nor the management of this syndrome is clear. Although resolution has occurred after reduction or discontinuation of cyclosporine and administration of streptokinase and heparin, or plasmapheresis, this appears to depend upon early detection with indium 111 platelet scans.

➤*Metabolic effects:* Significant hyperkalemia (sometimes associated with hyperchloremic metabolic acidosis) and hyperuricemia have been seen occasionally in individual patients.

➤*Hepatotoxicity:* Cyclosporine, when used in high doses, can cause hepatotoxicity. Hepatotoxicity has been noted in 4% of cases of renal transplantation, 7% of cases of cardiac transplantation, and 4% of cases of liver transplantation. This was usually noted during the first month of therapy, when high doses of cyclosporine were used, and consisted of elevations of hepatic enzymes and bilirubin. The chemistry elevations usually decreased with a reduction in dosage.

➤*Malignancies:* As in patients receiving other immunosuppressants, those receiving cyclosporine are at increased risk of development of lymphomas and other malignancies, particularly those of the skin. The increased risk appears to be related to the intensity and duration of immunosuppression rather than to the use of specific agents. Because of the danger of oversuppression of the immune system, which can also increase susceptibility to infection, do not administer cyclosporine with other immunosuppressive agents, except adrenal corticosteroids. The efficacy and safety of cyclosporine in combination with other immunosuppressive agents have not been determined. Some malignancies may be fatal. Transplant patients receiving cyclosporine are at increased risk for serious infection with fatal outcome. Reduction or discontinuation of immunosuppression may cause the lesions to regress.

CYCLOSPORINE — INJECTION

➤*Latent viral infections:* Immunosuppressed patients are at increased risk for opportunistic infections, including activation of latent viral infections. These include BK virus–associated nephropathy, which has been observed in patients receiving immunosuppressants, including cyclosporine. This infection is associated with serious outcomes, including deteriorating renal function and renal graft loss. Patient monitoring may help detect patients at risk of BK virus–associated nephropathy. Consider reduction in immunosuppression for patients who develop evidence of BK virus–associated nephropathy.

➤*Convulsions:* Convulsions have occurred in adults and children receiving cyclosporine, particularly in combination with high-dose methylprednisolone.

➤*Encephalopathy:* Encephalopathy has been described in postmarketing reports and in the literature. Manifestations include impaired consciousness, convulsions, visual disturbances (including blindness), loss of motor function, movement disorders, and psychiatric disturbances. In many cases, changes in the white matter have been detected using imaging techniques and pathologic specimens. Predisposing factors, such as hypertension, hypomagnesemia, hypocholesterolemia, high-dose corticosteroids, high cyclosporine blood concentrations, and GVHD have been noted in many, but not all, of the reported cases. The changes in most cases have been reversible upon discontinuation of cyclosporine and, in some cases, improvement was noted after reduction of dose. It appears that patients receiving liver transplants are more susceptible to encephalopathy than those receiving kidney transplants. Another rare manifestation of cyclosporine-induced neurotoxicity is optic disc edema, including papilloedema, with possible visual impairment, secondary to benign intracranial hypertension.

➤*Vaccination:* During treatment with cyclosporine, vaccination may be less effective; avoid the use of live attenuated vaccines.

➤*Glomerular capillary thrombosis:* See Adverse Reactions for more information.

➤*Hypomagnesemia:* See Adverse Reactions for more information.

➤*Hypertension:* Hypertension is a common adverse effect of cyclosporine therapy. Mild or moderate hypertension is encountered more frequently than severe hypertension, and the incidence decreases over time. Antihypertensive therapy may be required. Control of blood pressure can be accomplished with any of the common antihypertensive agents. However, because cyclosporine may cause hyperkalemia, do not use potassium-sparing diuretics. While calcium antagonists can be effective agents in treating cyclosporine-associated hypertension, care should be taken because interference with cyclosporine metabolism may require a dosage adjustment.

➤*Hypersensitivity reactions:* Rarely (approximately 1 in 1,000), patients receiving cyclosporine injection have experienced anaphylactic reactions. Although the exact cause of these reactions is unknown, it is believed to be due to the *Cremophor EL* (polyoxyethylated castor oil) used as the vehicle for the IV formulation. These reactions have consisted of flushing of the face and upper thorax, acute respiratory distress, dyspnea, wheezing, blood pressure changes, and tachycardia. One patient died after respiratory arrest and aspiration pneumonia. In some cases, the reaction subsided after the infusion stopped. Continually observe patients receiving cyclosporine injection for at least the first 30 minutes following the start of the infusion and at frequent intervals thereafter. If anaphylaxis occurs, stop the infusion. Ensure that an aqueous solution of epinephrine 1:1,000, as well as a source of oxygen, is available at the bedside.

Anaphylactic reactions have not been reported with the capsules or oral solution, which lack *Cremophor EL* (polyoxyethylated castor oil). Patients experiencing anaphylactic reactions have been treated subsequently with the capsules or oral solution without incident.

➤*Renal function impairment:* Renal function impairment requires close monitoring and possibly frequent dosage adjustment.

➤*Pregnancy: Category C.* There are no adequate and well-controlled studies in pregnant women. Use during pregnancy only if the potential benefit justifies the risk to the fetus.

In pregnant transplant recipients who are being treated with immunosuppressants, the risk of premature birth is increased. The following data represent the reported outcomes of 116 pregnancies in women receiving cyclosporine during pregnancy, 90% of whom were transplant patients and most of whom received cyclosporine throughout the entire gestational period. Because most of the patients were not prospectively identified, the results are likely to be biased toward negative outcomes. The only consistent patterns of abnormality were premature birth (gestational period of 28 to 36 weeks) and low birth weight for gestational age. It is not possible to separate the effects of cyclosporine on these pregnancies from the effects of the other immunosuppressants, the underlying maternal disorders, or other aspects of the transplantation milieu. Sixteen fetal losses occurred. Most of the pregnancies (85/100) were complicated by disorders, including preeclampsia, eclampsia, premature labor, abruptio placentae, oligohydramnios, Rh incompatibility, and fetoplacental dysfunction. Preterm delivery occurred in 47%. Seven malformations were reported in 5 viable infants and in 2 cases of fetal loss. Twenty-eight percent of the infants were small for gestational age. Neonatal complications occurred in 27%. In a report of 23 children, followed for up to 4 years, postnatal development was said to be normal. More information on cyclosporine use in pregnancy is available from the manufacturer.

A limited number of observations in children exposed to cyclosporine in utero are available, up to an age of approximately 7 years. Renal function and blood pressure in these children were healthy.

➤*Lactation:* Cyclosporine passes into breast milk. Advise mothers receiving treatment with cyclosporine not to breast-feed.

The American Academy of Pediatrics classifies cyclosporine as a drug that may interfere with cellular metabolism in the breast-feeding infant.

➤*Children:* Although no adequate and well-controlled studies have been completed in children, patients as young as 6 months of age have received cyclosporine with no unusual adverse effects.

➤*Elderly:* In general, use caution in dose selection for an elderly patient, usually starting at the low end of the dosing range, reflecting the greater frequency of decreased hepatic, renal, or cardiac function, and of concomitant disease or other drug therapy.

➤*Monitoring:* Continually observe patients receiving cyclosporine injection for at least the first 30 minutes following the start of the infusion and at frequent intervals thereafter.

Assess renal and liver functions repeatedly by measurement of BUN, serum creatinine, serum bilirubin, and liver enzymes. Also monitor blood pressure and serum lipids, magnesium, and potassium.

Blood levels – See Administration and Dosage for more information.

Drug Interactions

➤*Cytochrome P450 system:* Because cyclosporine is metabolized mainly by the CYP3A enzyme systems, substances known to inhibit these enzymes may decrease metabolism or increase bioavailability of cyclosporine, as indicated by increased whole blood or plasma concentrations. Drugs known to induce these enzyme systems may result in an increased metabolism of cyclosporine or decreased bioavailability, as indicated by decreased whole blood or plasma concentrations. Monitoring of blood concentrations and appropriate dosage adjustments are essential when such drugs are used concomitantly.

➤*Vaccinations:* See Warnings/Precautions for more information.

Cyclosporine Drug Interactions

Precipitant drug	Object drug[a]		Description
Allopurinol	Cyclosporine	⬆	Coadministration may increase cyclosporine concentrations, possibly increasing the risk of nephrotoxicity. Closely monitor cyclosporine concentrations when allopurinol is started or stopped. If an interaction is suspected, adjust the cyclosporine dose as needed.
Aminoglycosides (eg, gentamicin, tobramycin, vancomycin)	Cyclosporine	⬆	The risk of renal dysfunction may be increased. Monitor cyclosporine concentrations and renal function. Adjust the cyclosporine dose as needed.
Amiodarone	Cyclosporine	⬆	Amiodarone may increase cyclosporine blood levels, possibly increasing the risk of nephrotoxicity. Closely monitor cyclosporine concentrations and the patient for signs of toxicity. Adjust the cyclosporine dose as needed.
Amphotericin B	Cyclosporine	⬆	Concomitant use of cyclosporine and amphotericin B may increase the risk of nephrotoxicity and neurotoxicity. Closely monitor the patient and renal function. If renal function declines or neurotoxicity occurs, decrease the cyclosporine dose or stop one or both drugs.
Androgens (eg, danazol, methyltestosterone)	Cyclosporine	⬆	Increased cyclosporine blood concentrations and possible nephrotoxicity may occur. Closely monitor cyclosporine concentrations and the patient for signs of toxicity. Adjust the cyclosporine dose as needed.
Anticonvulsants (eg, barbiturates [eg, phenobarbital], carbamazepine, hydantoins [eg, phenytoin], oxcarbazepine)	Cyclosporine	⬇	Cyclosporine levels may be decreased, resulting in a reduction in the pharmacologic effects (eg, graft loss, transplanted organ rejection). Monitor cyclosporine concentrations and observe the patient for signs of rejection or toxicity when the anticonvulsant is started or stopped, respectively. Adjust the cyclosporine dose as needed.

CYCLOSPORINE — INJECTION

Cyclosporine Drug Interactions			
Precipitant drug	Object drug[a]		Description
Azole antifungals (eg, fluconazole, itraconazole, ketoconazole, posaconazole, voriconazole)	Cyclosporine	↑	Cyclosporine levels and toxicity may increase 1 to 3 days after starting therapy and persist more than 1 week after stopping antifungal therapy. Monitor cyclosporine concentrations and serum creatinine. Adjust the cyclosporine dose as needed. When administering posaconazole, reduce the cyclosporine dose 25% and frequently monitor cyclosporine whole blood trough concentrations during posaconazole administration and after discontinuation.
Berberine	Cyclosporine	↑	Elevated cyclosporine concentrations with a risk of toxicity (eg, nephrotoxicity) may occur. Advise patients receiving cyclosporine to avoid berberine, and caution them not to use herbal products without consulting their health care provider.
Beta-blockers (eg, carvedilol)	Cyclosporine	↑	Elevated cyclosporine concentrations with a risk of nephrotoxicity and neurotoxicity may occur. Closely monitor cyclosporine concentrations and the patient for signs of toxicity. Adjust the cyclosporine dose as needed.
Bortezomib	Cyclosporine	↑	Neurotoxicity of both drugs may be increased. Closely monitor the patient and adjust treatment as needed.
Cyclosporine	Bortezomib		
Bosentan	Cyclosporine	↓	Trough concentrations of bosentan may be elevated, increasing the risk of adverse effects, while cyclosporine plasma levels may be decreased. Coadministration is contraindicated.
Cyclosporine	Bosentan	↑	
Bromocriptine	Cyclosporine	↑	Coadministration may increase cyclosporine concentrations. Closely monitor cyclosporine concentrations and the patient for signs of toxicity. Adjust the cyclosporine dose as needed.
Calcium channel blockers (eg, diltiazem, nicardipine, verapamil)	Cyclosporine	↑	Increased cyclosporine levels with possible nephrotoxicity may occur. However, administration of verapamil before cyclosporine may be nephroprotective. The interaction is typically observed within 7 days of starting verapamil and may abate within 1 week after discontinuation. Use with caution. Monitor cyclosporine concentrations when the calcium channel blocker is started, stopped, or the dose is changed. Adjust the cyclosporine dose as needed. Frequent gingival hyperplasia has been reported with coadministration of cyclosporine and nifedipine.
Cyclosporine	Calcium channel blockers (ie, nifedipine)		
Chamomile	Cyclosporine	↑	Elevated cyclosporine concentrations with a risk of toxicity (eg, nephrotoxicity) may occur. Advise patients receiving cyclosporine to avoid chamomile and caution them not to use herbal products without consulting their health care provider.
Chloramphenicol	Cyclosporine	↑	Cyclosporine concentrations may be elevated, increasing the risk of toxicity (eg, nephrotoxicity). Closely monitor cyclosporine concentrations and the patient for signs of toxicity. Adjust the cyclosporine dose as needed.

Cyclosporine Drug Interactions			
Precipitant drug	Object drug[a]		Description
Chloroquine	Cyclosporine	↑	Cyclosporine concentrations may be elevated, increasing the risk of toxicity (eg, nephrotoxicity). Closely monitor cyclosporine concentrations and the patient for signs of toxicity. Adjust the cyclosporine dose as needed.
Clindamycin	Cyclosporine	↓	Cyclosporine concentrations may be decreased, resulting in a reduction in the pharmacologic effects (eg, graft loss, transplanted organ rejection). Monitor cyclosporine concentrations and observe the patient for signs of rejection or toxicity when clindamycin is started or stopped, respectively. Adjust the cyclosporine dose as needed.
Clonidine	Cyclosporine	↑	Cyclosporine concentrations may be elevated, increasing the risk of toxicity (eg, nephrotoxicity). Closely monitor cyclosporine concentrations and the patient for signs of toxicity. Adjust the cyclosporine dose as needed.
Colchicine	Cyclosporine	↑	Severe adverse clinical symptoms, including GI, hepatic, renal, and neuromuscular toxicity, may occur during coadministration. Coadministration of cyclosporine and colchicine is contraindicated in patients with hepatic or renal impairment. In patients with healthy hepatic or renal function, use with caution at a maximum dosage of colchicine 0.3 mg twice daily. Cyclosporine may increase the risk of colchicine toxicity (eg, myopathy, neuropathy), especially in patients with renal dysfunction. Closely monitor the clinical response of the patient and for adverse reactions. Adjust therapy as needed.
Cyclosporine	Colchicine		
Contraceptives, hormonal	Cyclosporine	↑	Hormonal contraceptives may increase cyclosporine blood levels, possibly increasing the risk of nephrotoxicity. Closely monitor cyclosporine concentrations and the patient for signs of toxicity. Adjust the cyclosporine dose as needed.
Corticosteroids (eg, methylprednisolone)	Cyclosporine	↑	Although this combination is therapeutically beneficial for organ transplants, toxicity of both agents may be enhanced. If an interaction is suspected (eg, convulsions, increased serum creatinine, cushingoid symptoms) consider decreasing the dose of one or both drugs.
Cyclosporine	Corticosteroids (eg, methylprednisolone)		
Efavirenz	Cyclosporine	↓	Cyclosporine levels may be decreased, resulting in a reduction in the pharmacologic effects (eg, graft loss, transplanted organ rejection). Larger doses of cyclosporine may be needed after starting efavirenz. Monitor cyclosporine concentrations and observe the patient for signs of rejection or toxicity when efavirenz is started or stopped, respectively. Adjust the cyclosporine dose as needed.

CYCLOSPORINE — INJECTION

Cyclosporine Drug Interactions

Precipitant drug	Object drug[a]		Description
Ezetimibe	Cyclosporine	↑	Cyclosporine and ezetimibe concentrations may be elevated, increasing the pharmacologic effects and risk of adverse reactions. Monitor cyclosporine concentrations when ezetimibe is coadministered. Adjust the cyclosporine dose as needed. In addition, monitor patients for cyclosporine or ezetimibe adverse reactions.
Cyclosporine	Ezetimibe		
Fenofibrate	Cyclosporine	↑	The risk of renal dysfunction may be increased. Monitor cyclosporine concentrations and renal function. Adjust the cyclosporine dose as needed.
Fluoroquinolones (eg, ciprofloxacin)	Cyclosporine	↑	Cyclosporine blood concentrations may be elevated, increasing the risk of toxicity (eg, renal dysfunction). Monitor cyclosporine concentrations and renal function. If an interaction is suspected, adjust the cyclosporine dose or consider administering an alternative antibiotic.
Foscarnet	Cyclosporine	↑	The risk of renal failure may be increased due to additive or synergistic nephrotoxicity. Closely monitor renal function. If nephrotoxicity occurs, it may be necessary to discontinue foscarnet.
Cyclosporine	Foscarnet		
Gemfibrozil	Cyclosporine	↓	Cyclosporine concentrations may be decreased, resulting in a reduction in the pharmacologic effects (eg, graft loss, transplanted organ rejection). Monitor cyclosporine concentrations and observe the patient for signs of rejection or toxicity when gemfibrozil is started or stopped, respectively. Adjust the cyclosporine dose as needed.
Griseofulvin	Cyclosporine	↓	Cyclosporine concentrations may be decreased, resulting in a reduction in the pharmacologic effects (eg, graft loss, transplanted organ rejection). Monitor cyclosporine concentrations and observe the patient for signs of rejection or toxicity when griseofulvin is started or stopped, respectively. Adjust the cyclosporine dose as needed.
Histamine H_2 antagonists (eg, cimetidine, ranitidine)	Cyclosporine	↑	The risk of renal dysfunction may be increased. Monitor cyclosporine concentrations and renal function. Adjust the cyclosporine dose as needed.
Imatinib	Cyclosporine	↑	Imatinib may increase cyclosporine blood levels, possibly increasing the risk of nephrotoxicity. Closely monitor cyclosporine concentrations and the patient for signs of toxicity. Adjust the cyclosporine dose as needed.
Imipenem/Cilastatin	Cyclosporine	↑	The neurotoxicity of both agents may be increased. Close clinical and plasma concentration monitoring are indicated. If an interaction is suspected, decrease the cyclosporine dosage and consider an alternative antimicrobial agent.
Cyclosporine	Imipenem/Cilastatin		
Immunosuppressive agents, radiation therapy (eg, psoralens + ultraviolet A, ultraviolet light treatment)	Cyclosporine	↑	Avoid concurrent treatment because of the possibility of excessive immunosuppression.
Cyclosporine	Immunosuppressive agents, radiation therapy (eg, psoralens + ultraviolet A, ultraviolet light treatment)		
Macrolide antibiotics (eg, azithromycin, clarithromycin, erythromycin, telithromycin)	Cyclosporine	↑	Elevated cyclosporine levels may occur, increasing the risk of nephrotoxicity and neurotoxicity. Closely monitor cyclosporine concentrations and serum creatinine, and monitor for toxicity. Adjust the cyclosporine dose as needed.
Melphalan	Cyclosporine	↑	The risk of renal dysfunction may be increased. Monitor cyclosporine concentrations and renal function. Adjust the cyclosporine dose as needed.
Metoclopramide	Cyclosporine	↑	An increase in the immunosuppressive and toxic effects of cyclosporine may result with metoclopramide coadministration. Monitor cyclosporine concentrations and the response of the patient when starting or stopping metoclopramide. Adjust the cyclosporine dose as needed.
Metronidazole	Cyclosporine	↑	Cyclosporine concentrations may be elevated, increasing the risk of toxicity (eg, nephrotoxicity). Closely monitor cyclosporine concentrations and the patient for signs of toxicity. Adjust the cyclosporine dose as needed.
Mibefradil	Cyclosporine	↑	Mibefradil may increase cyclosporine blood levels, possibly increasing the risk of nephrotoxicity. Closely monitor cyclosporine concentrations and the response of the patient when mibefradil is started or stopped. Adjust the cyclosporine dose as needed.
Micafungin	Cyclosporine	↑	Micafungin may increase cyclosporine blood levels, possibly increasing the risk of nephrotoxicity. Closely monitor cyclosporine concentrations when micafungin is started or stopped. Adjust the cyclosporine dose as needed.
Nafcillin	Cyclosporine	↓	Coadministration may decrease cyclosporine concentrations. If an alternative antibiotic is not available, monitor cyclosporine concentrations and adjust the cyclosporine dose as needed.
Nefazodone	Cyclosporine	↑	Cyclosporine concentrations and toxicity may be increased. Closely monitor cyclosporine concentrations and the patient for signs of toxicity (eg, nephrotoxicity). Adjust the cyclosporine dose as needed.
NSAIDs (eg, diclofenac, naproxen, sulindac)	Cyclosporine	↑	The risk of renal dysfunction may be increased, especially in patients with dehydration. Closely monitor cyclosporine concentrations and renal function. Adjust the cyclosporine dose as needed.

CYCLOSPORINE — INJECTION

Cyclosporine Drug Interactions			
Precipitant drug	Object drug[a]		Description
Octreotide	Cyclosporine	↓	Cyclosporine levels may be decreased, resulting in a reduction in the pharmacologic effects (eg, graft loss, transplanted organ rejection). Monitor cyclosporine concentrations and observe the clinical response of the patient when starting or stopping octreotide. Adjust the cyclosporine dose as needed.
Omeprazole	Cyclosporine	↑↓	Cyclosporine levels may be increased, decreased, or unchanged. Monitor cyclosporine concentrations and observe the clinical response of the patient when starting or stopping omeprazole. Adjust the cyclosporine dose as needed.
Propafenone	Cyclosporine	↑	Cyclosporine blood concentrations may be elevated, increasing the risk of toxicity (eg, renal dysfunction). Monitor cyclosporine concentrations and renal function. If an interaction is suspected, adjust the cyclosporine dose as needed.
Protease inhibitors (eg, indinavir, nelfinavir, ritonavir, saquinavir)	Cyclosporine	↑	Plasma concentrations and pharmacologic effects of both drugs may increase when cyclosporine and protease inhibitors are coadministered. Toxicity may occur. Closely monitor cyclosporine concentrations and the clinical response of the patient to both agents. Adjust the dose of cyclosporine and the protease inhibitor as needed.
Cyclosporine	Protease inhibitors (eg, indinavir, nelfinavir, ritonavir, saquinavir)		
Quercetin	Cyclosporine	↑	Elevated cyclosporine concentrations with a risk of toxicity (eg, nephrotoxicity) may occur. Advise patients receiving cyclosporine to avoid quercetin and caution them not to use herbal products without consulting their health care provider.
Quinupristin/ Dalfopristin	Cyclosporine	↑	Cyclosporine blood concentrations may be elevated, increasing the risk of toxicity (eg, renal dysfunction). Closely monitor cyclosporine concentrations and for toxicity. Adjust the cyclosporine dose as needed.
Rifamycins (ie, rifabutin, rifampin)	Cyclosporine	↓	The immunosuppressive effect of cyclosporine may be reduced. This appears to occur as early as 2 days following the initiation of rifamycins and may persist for 1 to 3 weeks after their discontinuation. If coadministration cannot be avoided, closely monitor cyclosporine concentrations and serum creatinine. Adjust the cyclosporine dose as needed.
SSRIs[b] (eg, fluoxetine, fluvoxamine, sertraline)	Cyclosporine	↑	SSRIs may increase cyclosporine concentrations and toxicity (eg, nephrotoxicity). Monitor cyclosporine concentrations and renal function. Adjust the cyclosporine dose as needed.
St. John's wort	Cyclosporine	↓	Decreased cyclosporine levels and efficacy (eg, graft loss, transplanted organ rejection) may occur with coadministration. If coadministration cannot be avoided, closely monitor cyclosporine concentrations and the clinical response of the patient when St. John's wort is started or stopped. Adjust the cyclosporine dose as needed.
Sulfonamides (eg, sulfadiazine, sulfamethoxazole/trimethoprim, sulfasalazine)	Cyclosporine	↓↑	The action of cyclosporine may be reduced. Oral sulfonamides may increase the risk of nephrotoxicity. If coadministration cannot be avoided, closely monitor cyclosporine concentrations and serum creatinine. Adjust the cyclosporine dose as needed.
Sulfonylureas (eg, glipizide, glyburide)	Cyclosporine	↑	Sulfonylureas may increase cyclosporine blood levels, possibly increasing the risk of nephrotoxicity. Closely monitor cyclosporine concentrations when the sulfonylurea is started or stopped. If an interaction is suspected, adjust the cyclosporine dose as needed.
Tacrolimus	Cyclosporine	↑	Additive or synergistic toxicity may occur, increasing the risk of renal toxicity. Avoid coadministration of cyclosporine and tacrolimus. Discontinue cyclosporine or tacrolimus at least 24 hours prior to initiating treatment with the other agent.
Cyclosporine	Tacrolimus		
Terbinafine	Cyclosporine	↓	Terbinafine may decrease cyclosporine concentrations, producing a decrease in efficacy (eg, resulting in graft rejection or transplanted organ rejection). Monitor cyclosporine concentrations and the clinical response of the patient. Adjust the cyclosporine dose as needed.
Ticlopidine	Cyclosporine	↓	Cyclosporine whole blood concentrations may decrease, producing a decrease in pharmacologic effects (eg, resulting in graft rejection or transplanted organ rejection). Monitor cyclosporine concentrations and the clinical response of the patient. Adjust the cyclosporine dose as needed.
Tigecycline	Cyclosporine	↑	Tigecycline may increase cyclosporine blood levels, possibly increasing the risk of toxicity (eg, nephrotoxicity). Closely monitor cyclosporine concentrations when tigecycline is started or stopped. Adjust the cyclosporine dose as needed.
Trimethoprim	Cyclosporine	↓↑	Both a decrease in the immunosuppressive action of cyclosporine and an increase in the risk of nephrotoxicity have been reported during coadministration of trimethoprim. Close clinical and laboratory monitoring of cyclosporine is indicated. If an interaction is suspected, consider substituting another antimicrobial agent for trimethoprim.

CYCLOSPORINE — INJECTION

Cyclosporine Drug Interactions			
Precipitant drug	Object drug[a]		Description
Troglitazone	Cyclosporine	⬇	Cyclosporine whole blood concentrations may decrease, producing a decrease in pharmacologic effects (eg, resulting in graft rejection or transplanted organ rejection). Monitor cyclosporine concentrations and the clinical response of the patient. Adjust the cyclosporine dose as needed.
Cyclosporine	ACE[b] inhibitors (eg, captopril)	⬆	The risk of hyperkalemia may be increased. Use with caution. Closely monitor potassium concentrations. In addition, acute renal failure has been reported with coadministration of ACE inhibitors and cyclosporine. If an interaction is suspected, discontinue the ACE inhibitor. Dose reduction or discontinuation of cyclosporine may also be necessary.
Cyclosporine	Aliskiren	⬆	Pharmacologic effects and plasma concentrations of aliskiren may be increased by cyclosporine. Coadministration is not recommended.
Cyclosporine	Caspofungin	⬆	Pharmacologic effects and plasma concentrations of caspofungin may be increased by cyclosporine. Coadministration is not recommended.
Cyclosporine	Digoxin	⬆	Elevated digoxin levels with toxicity may occur. In patients receiving digoxin, severe digitalis toxicity has been seen within days of starting cyclosporine. Closely monitor the clinical response of the patient and discontinue digoxin or adjust the dose as needed.
Cyclosporine	Doxorubicin	⬆	Doxorubicin serum concentration may be elevated, resulting in increased toxicity. Monitor the clinical response of the patient, including CBC[b], and adjust the doxorubicin dose as needed.
Cyclosporine	Etoposide	⬆	Serum etoposide concentration may be elevated, resulting in increased toxicity. Monitor the clinical response of the patient, including CBC, and adjust the etoposide dose as needed.
Cyclosporine	Everolimus	⬆	Serum everolimus concentrations may be elevated, increasing the pharmacologic effects and risk of adverse reactions. Monitor the clinical response of the patient (including renal function and hematologic parameters) when the cyclosporine dose is started, stopped, or changed. Adjust the everolimus dose as needed.
Cyclosporine	HMG-CoA reductase inhibitors (eg, lovastatin, simvastatin)	⬆	Severe myopathy or rhabdomyolysis may occur with coadministration. When cyclosporine is coadministered, reduce the dose of the HMG-CoA reductase inhibitor according to the label recommendations. In patients with signs and symptoms of myopathy or those at risk of severe renal injury secondary to rhabdomyolysis, temporarily withhold or discontinue the HMG-CoA reductase inhibitor.
Cyclosporine	Meglitinides (eg, nateglinide, repaglinide)	⬆	Meglitinide plasma concentrations may be elevated, increasing the pharmacologic effect and risk of hypoglycemia. Coadministration of cyclosporine and repaglinide to healthy men increased the repaglinide mean C_{max} and AUC 1.8- and 2.4-fold, respectively. Closely monitor blood glucose and adjust the meglitinide dose as needed.
Cyclosporine	Methotrexate	⬆	Coadministration resulted in an increase of methotrexate AUC by ≈ 30% and the AUC of its metabolite was decreased ≈ 80%. Monitor the clinical response of the patient when cyclosporine is started or stopped. Adjust the methotrexate dose as needed.
Cyclosporine	Mycophenolate	⬇	Plasma concentrations and pharmacologic effects of mycophenolate may be decreased by cyclosporine. Larger mycophenolate doses may be needed after starting cyclosporine. Monitor mycophenolic acid concentrations and the clinical response of the patient when starting or stopping cyclosporine. Adjust the mycophenolate dose as needed.
Cyclosporine	Nondepolarizing muscle relaxants (eg, vecuronium)	⬆	Cyclosporine may prolong the neuromuscular blocking effects of nondepolarizing muscle relaxants. Closely monitor the extent and duration of neuromuscular blockade. Be prepared to decrease the dosage of nondepolarizing agent and provide mechanical respiratory support as needed.
Cyclosporine	Potassium-containing drugs (eg, potassium penicillin)	⬆	The risk of hyperkalemia may be increased. Use with caution. Closely monitor potassium concentrations.
Cyclosporine	Potassium-sparing diuretics (eg, spironolactone)	⬆	Coadministration may lead to hyperkalemia. Avoid concomitant use.
Cyclosporine	Red yeast rice	⬆	Red yeast rice contains HMG-CoA reductase inhibitor–like components. The risk of HMG-CoA reductase inhibitor–like adverse reactions (eg, rhabdomyolysis) may be increased with coadministration of cyclosporine. Advise patients receiving cyclosporine to avoid red yeast rice and caution them not to use herbal products without consulting their health care provider.
Cyclosporine	Sirolimus	⬆	Sirolimus plasma concentrations may be increased, resulting in increased toxicity. Administer sirolimus 4 hours after cyclosporine to prevent variations in sirolimus concentrations.
Cyclosporine	Vinca alkaloids (eg, vinblastine, vincristine)	⬆	The pharmacologic and toxic effects of vinca alkaloids may be increased by cyclosporine. Use with caution. Monitor the clinical response of the patient and adjust the vinca alkaloid dose as needed.

[a] ⬆ = object drug increased; ⬇ = object drug decreased; ⬆⬇ = object drug both increased and decreased.
[b] ACE = angiotensin-converting enzyme; SSRIs = selective serotonin reuptake inhibitors; CBC = complete blood cell count.

➤*Drug/Food interactions:* Potassium-rich diets may increase the risk of hypokalemia. Closely monitor potassium concentrations.

CYCLOSPORINE — INJECTION

Adverse Reactions

➤*Most common:* The principal adverse reactions of cyclosporine therapy are renal dysfunction, tremor, hirsutism, hypertension, and gum hyperplasia.

➤*Hypertension:* Hypertension, which is usually mild to moderate, may occur in approximately 50% of patients following renal transplantation and in most cardiac transplant patients.

➤*Glomerular capillary thrombosis:* Glomerular capillary thrombosis has been found in patients treated with cyclosporine and may progress to graft failure. The pathologic changes resemble those seen in the hemolytic-uremic syndrome and include thrombosis of the renal microvasculature, with platelet-fibrin thrombi occluding glomerular capillaries and afferent arterioles, microangiopathic hemolytic anemia, thrombocytopenia, and decreased renal function. Similar findings have been observed when other immunosuppressives have been employed posttransplantation.

➤*Hypomagnesemia:* Hypomagnesemia has been reported in some, but not all, patients exhibiting convulsions while receiving cyclosporine therapy. Although magnesium-depletion studies in healthy subjects suggest that hypomagnesemia is associated with neurologic disorders, multiple factors, including hypertension, high-dose methylprednisolone, hypocholesterolemia, and nephrotoxicity associated with high plasma concentrations of cyclosporine appear to be related to the neurological manifestations of cyclosporine toxicity.

➤*Adverse reactions (3% or more):*

Cyclosporine Adverse Reactions (≥ 3%)

Adverse reaction	Randomized kidney transplant patients: Cyclosporine (n = 227)	Randomized kidney transplant patients: Azathioprine (n = 228)	All cyclosporine patients: Kidney transplant (n =705)	All cyclosporine patients: Heart transplant (n = 112)	All cyclosporine patients: Liver transplant (n = 75)
Cardiovascular					
Flushing	< 1%	0%	4%	0%	4%
Hypertension	26%	18%	13%	53%	27%
CNS					
Convulsions	3%	1%	1%	4%	5%
Headache	2%	< 1%	2%	15%	4%
Paresthesia	3%	0%	1%	2%	1%
Tremor	12%	0%	21%	31%	55%
Dermatologic					
Acne	6%	8%	2%	2%	1%
Hirsutism	21%	< 1%	21%	28%	45%
GI					
Abdominal discomfort	< 1%	0%	< 1%	7%	0%
Diarrhea	3%	< 1%	3%	4%	8%
Gum hyperplasia	4%	0%	9%	5%	16%
Hepatotoxicity	< 1%	< 1%	4%	7%	4%
Nausea/Vomiting	2%	< 1%	4%	10%	4%
GU					
Gynecomastia	< 1%	0%	< 1%	4%	3%
Renal dysfunction	32%	6%	25%	38%	37%
Hematologic					
Leukopenia	2%	19%	< 1%	6%	0%
Lymphoma	< 1%	0%	1%	6%	1%
Miscellaneous					
Cramps	4%	< 1%	2%	< 1%	0%
Sinusitis	< 1%	0%	4%	3%	7%

➤*Other adverse reactions (2% or less):* The following reactions occurred in 2% or fewer patients: allergic reactions, anemia, anorexia, confusion, conjunctivitis, edema, fever, brittle fingernails, gastritis, hearing loss, hiccups, hyperglycemia, muscle pain, peptic ulcer, thrombocytopenia, tinnitus.

➤*Rare adverse reactions:* The following reactions occurred rarely: anxiety, chest pain, constipation, depression, hair breaking, hematuria, joint pain, lethargy, mouth sores, myocardial infarction, night sweats, pancreatitis, pruritus, swallowing difficulty, tingling, upper GI bleeding, visual disturbance, weakness, weight loss.

➤*Discontinuation of therapy:*

Adverse Reactions Associated With Discontinuation of Cyclosporine in Renal Transplant Patients[a]

Reason for discontinuation	Randomized patients: Cyclosporine (n = 227)	Randomized patients: Azathioprine (n = 228)	All cyclosporine patients (n = 705)
GU			
Acute tubular necrosis	2.6%	0%	1%
Renal toxicity	5.7%	0%	5.4%
Hematologic			
Hematological abnormalities	0%	0.4%	0%
Lymphoma/ lymphoproliferative disease	0.4%	0%	0.3%
Miscellaneous			
Other	0%	0%	0.7%

Adverse Reactions Associated With Discontinuation of Cyclosporine in Renal Transplant Patients[a]

Reason for discontinuation	Randomized patients: Cyclosporine (n = 227)	Randomized patients: Azathioprine (n = 228)	All cyclosporine patients (n = 705)
Hypertension	0%	0%	0.3%
Infection	0%	0.4%	0.9%
Lack of efficacy	2.6%	0.9%	1.4%

[a] Cyclosporine was discontinued on a temporary basis and then restarted in 18 additional patients.

➤*Infection:* Patients receiving immunosuppressive therapies, including cyclosporine and cyclosporine-containing regimens, are at increased risk of infections (viral, bacterial, fungal, parasitic). Both generalized and localized infections can occur. Preexisting infections may also be aggravated. Fatal outcomes have been reported.

Infectious Complications in Randomized Renal Transplant Patients

Complication	Cyclosporine (n = 227)	Standard treatment[a] (n = 228)
Abscess	4.4%	5.3%
Cytomegalovirus	4.8%	12.3%
Local fungal infections	7.5%	9.6%
Pneumonia	6.2%	9.2%
Septicemia	5.3%	4.8%
Systemic fungal infections	2.2%	3.9%

CYCLOSPORINE — INJECTION

Infectious Complications in Randomized Renal Transplant Patients		
Complication	Cyclosporine (n = 227)	Standard treatment[a] (n = 228)
Urinary tract infections	21.1%	20.2%
Other viral infections	15.9%	18.4%
Wound and skin infections	7%	10.1%

[a] Some patients also received antilymphocytic globulin.

➤*Polyoxyethylated castor oil: Cremophor EL* (polyoxyethylated castor oil) is known to cause hyperlipidemia and electrophoretic abnormalities of lipoproteins. These effects are reversible upon discontinuation of treatment but are usually not a reason to stop treatment.

➤*Postmarketing:* BK virus–associated nephropathy has been observed in patients receiving immunosuppressants, including cyclosporine. This infection is associated with serious outcomes, including deteriorating renal function and renal graft loss.

Overdosage

➤*Symptoms:* There is minimal experience with cyclosporine overdosage. Transient hepatotoxicity and nephrotoxicity may occur, which should resolve following drug withdrawal. Oral doses of cyclosporine up to 10 g (approximately 150 mg/kg) have been tolerated with relatively minor clinical consequences, such as vomiting, drowsiness, headache, tachycardia, and, in a few patients, moderately severe, reversible impairment of renal function. However, serious symptoms of intoxication have been reported following accidental parenteral overdosage with cyclosporine in premature neonates.

➤*Treatment:* Follow general supportive measures and symptomatic treatment in all cases of overdosage. Cyclosporine is not dialyzable to any great extent, nor is it cleared well by charcoal hemoperfusion.

Patient Information

Advise patients to make any change of cyclosporine formulation cautiously and only under the supervision of their health care provider because it may result in the need for a change in dosage.

Inform patients of the necessity of repeated laboratory tests while they are receiving the drug. Give patients careful dosage instructions, and inform them of the potential risks during pregnancy and of the risk of neoplasia.

Instruct patients to contact their health care provider if fever, sore throat, tiredness, unusual bleeding or bruising, decreased urination, or yellow skin/eyes occurs.

Cyclosporine may increase skin cancer risk. Advise patients to avoid prolonged exposure to the sun and other ultraviolet light and to use sunscreens and wear protective clothing while taking this medicine. Patients who are being treated for psoriasis will need to have at least 2 careful skin and physical examinations, including blood pressure measurements, before starting cyclosporine.

Advise patients to avoid live vaccines (eg, measles, mumps, oral polio) while taking cyclosporine. The vaccination may be less effective.

Inform patients that cyclosporine may increase risk of high blood pressure and abnormal kidney function.

Inform patients that cyclosporine may affect blood sugar level in diabetic patients.

GLATIRAMER ACETATE

Rx	**Copaxone** (Teva)	**Injection, solution:** 20 mg/mL	Mannitol 40 mg. Preservative free. In single-use prefilled syringes.

GLATIRAMER ACETATE — INJECTION

Indications

➤*Multiple sclerosis:* For the reduction of the frequency of relapses in patients with relapsing remitting multiple sclerosis (MS), including patients who have experienced a first clinical episode and have magnetic resonance imaging (MRI) features consistent with MS.

Administration and Dosage

➤*Adults:*

Multiple sclerosis – 20 mg/day subcutaneously.

➤*Administration:* Administer subcutaneously only. Glatiramer should not be administered intravenously.

Sites for self-injection include arms, abdomen, hips, and thighs. One blister that contains the syringe from the glatiramer prefilled syringes package should be removed. Because this product should be refrigerated, the prefilled syringe should stand at room temperature for 20 minutes to allow the solution to warm to room temperature. The prefilled syringe is for single use only; any unused portion should be discarded.

➤*Storage/Stability:* The recommended storage condition is refrigeration (2° to 8°C; 36° to 46°F). Excursions to 15° to 30°C (59° to 86°F) for up to 1 month had no adverse impact on the product. Avoid exposure to higher temperatures or intense light. Glatiramer should not be frozen. If a glatiramer syringe freezes, it should be discarded.

Actions

➤*Pharmacology:* The mechanism(s) by which glatiramer exerts its effects in patients with MS are not fully understood. However, it is thought to act by modifying immune processes that are currently believed to be responsible for the pathogenesis of MS. This hypothesis is supported by findings of studies that have been carried out to explore the pathogenesis of experimental autoimmune encephalomyelitis, a condition induced in animals through immunization against CNS-derived material containing myelin and often used as an experimental animal model of MS. Studies in animals and in vitro systems suggest that upon its administration, glatiramer-specific suppressor T cells are induced and activated in the periphery.

Because glatiramer can modify immune functions, concerns exist about its potential to alter naturally occurring immune responses. There is no evidence that glatiramer does this, but this has not been systematically evaluated.

➤*Pharmacokinetics:* Results obtained in pharmacokinetic studies performed in humans (healthy volunteers) and animals support that a substantial fraction of the therapeutic dose delivered to patients subcutaneously is hydrolyzed locally. Larger fragments of glatiramer can be recognized by glatiramer-reactive antibodies. Some fraction of the injected material, either intact or partially hydrolyzed, is presumed to enter the lymphatic circulation, enabling it to reach regional lymph nodes, and some may enter the systemic circulation intact.

Contraindications

Hypersensitivity to glatiramer or mannitol.

Warnings/Precautions

➤*Immediate postinjection reaction:* Approximately 16% of patients exposed to glatiramer in the 5 placebo-controlled trials compared with 4% of those on placebo experienced a constellation of symptoms immediately after injection that included at least 2 of the following: anxiety, chest pain, constriction of the throat, dyspnea, flushing, palpitations, and urticaria. In clinical trials, the symptoms were generally transient and self-limited and did not require specific treatment. In general, these symptoms have their onset several months after the initiation of treatment, although they may occur earlier, and a given patient may experience 1 or several episodes of these symptoms. Whether or not any of these symptoms actually represent a specific syndrome is uncertain. During the postmarketing period, there have been reports of patients with similar symptoms who received emergency medical care.

➤*Chest pain:* Approximately 13% of glatiramer patients in the 5 placebo-controlled studies compared with 6% of placebo patients experienced at least 1 episode of what was described as transient chest pain. While some of these episodes occurred in the context of the immediate postinjection reaction previously described, many did not. The temporal relationship of this chest pain to an injection of glatiramer was not always known. The pain was transient (usually lasting only a few minutes), often unassociated with other symptoms, and appeared to have no important clinical sequelae. Some patients experienced more than 1 such episode, and episodes usually began at least 1 month after the initiation of treatment. The pathogenesis of this symptom is unknown.

➤*Lipoatrophy and skin necrosis:* Localized lipoatrophy and, rarely, injection site skin necrosis at injection sites have been reported during the postmarketing experience. Lipoatrophy may occur at various times after treatment onset (sometimes after several months) and is thought to be permanent. There is no known therapy for lipoatrophy. To assist in possibly minimizing these events, advise the patient to follow proper injection technique and to rotate injection sites daily.

➤*Immunosuppression:* Because glatiramer can modify immune response, it may interfere with immune functions. For example, treatment with glatiramer may interfere with the recognition of foreign antigens in a way that would undermine the body's tumor surveillance and its defenses against infection. There is no evidence that glatiramer does this, but there has not been a systematic evaluation of this risk. Because glatiramer is an antigenic material, it is possible that its use may lead to the induction of host responses that are untoward, but systematic surveillance for these effects has not been undertaken.

Although glatiramer is intended to minimize the autoimmune response to myelin, there is the possibility that continued alteration of cellular immunity caused by chronic treatment with glatiramer may result in untoward effects.

Glatiramer-reactive antibodies are formed in most patients exposed to daily treatment with the recommended dose. Studies in the rat and monkey have suggested that immune complexes are deposited in the renal glomeruli. Furthermore, in a controlled trial of 125 relapsing remitting MS patients given glatiramer 20 mg subcutaneously every day for 2 years, serum immunoglobulin G (IgG) levels reached at least 3 times baseline values in 80% of patients by 3 months of initiation of treatment. However, by 12 months of treatment, 30% of patients still had IgG levels at least 3 times baseline values, and 90% had levels above baseline by 12 months. The antibodies are exclusively of the IgG subtype and predominantly of the IgG-1 subtype. No IgE-type antibodies could be detected in any of the 94 sera tested; nevertheless, anaphylaxis can be associated with the administration of most any foreign substance, and therefore, this risk cannot be excluded.

GLATIRAMER ACETATE — INJECTION

➤*Pregnancy: Category B.*

➤*Lactation:* It is not known whether glatiramer is excreted in human milk. No reports describing the use of glatiramer during lactation have been located. Because of the high molecular weight (4,700 to 11,000), it is doubtful that the unmetabolized agent is excreted into breast milk. Because many drugs are excreted in human milk, exercise caution when administering glatiramer to a breast-feeding woman.

➤*Children:* The safety and efficacy of glatiramer have not been established in patients younger than 18 years of age.

Drug Interactions

None known.

Adverse Reactions

➤*Discontinuation of treatment:* Among 563 patients treated with glatiramer in blind placebo-controlled trials, approximately 5% of the subjects discontinued treatment because of an adverse reaction. The adverse reactions most commonly associated with discontinuation were: dyspnea, hypersensitivity, injection site reactions, urticaria, and vasodilation.

➤*Common adverse reactions:* The most common adverse reactions were chest pain, dyspnea, injection site reactions, rash, and vasodilation.

Glatiramer Adverse Reactions (≥ 2%)[a]

Adverse reactions	Glatiramer 20 mg (n = 563)	Placebo (n = 564)
Cardiovascular		
Palpitations	9%	4%
Syncope	3%	2%
Tachycardia	5%	2%
Vasodilation	20%	5%
CNS		
Anxiety	13%	10%
Asthenia	22%	21%
Chills	3%	1%
Migraine	4%	2%
Nervousness	2%	1%
Speech disorder	2%	1%
Tremor	4%	2%
Dermatologic		
Benign neoplasm of skin	2%	1%
Hyperhidrosis	7%	5%
Pruritus	5%	4%
Rash	19%	11%
Skin disorder	3%	1%
Urticaria	3%	1%
GI		
Dysphagia	2%	1%
Gastroenteritis	6%	4%
Nausea	15%	11%
Vomiting	7%	4%
GU		
Micturition urgency	5%	4%
Vaginal candidiasis	4%	2%
Local reactions		
Injection site atrophy[b]	2%	0%
Injection site edema	19%	4%
Injection site erythema	43%	10%
Injection site fibrosis	2%	1%
Injection site hypersensitivity	4%	0%
Injection site inflammation	9%	1%
Injection site mass	26%	6%
Injection site pain	40%	20%
Injection site pruritus	27%	4%
Injection site reaction	8%	1%
Local reaction	3%	1%
Metabolic/Nutritional		
Edema	8%	2%
Face edema	3%	1%
Peripheral edema	3%	2%
Weight gain	3%	1%
Respiratory		
Bronchitis	6%	5%
Cough	6%	5%
Dyspnea	14%	4%
Laryngospasm	2%	1%
Rhinitis	7%	5%
Special senses		
Diplopia	3%	2%
Eye disorder	3%	1%
Miscellaneous		
Back pain	12%	10%
Chest pain	13%	6%
Hypersensitivity	3%	2%
Infection	30%	28%
Influenza	14%	13%
Lymphadenopathy	7%	3%
Pain	20%	17%
Pyrexia	6%	5%

[a] Adverse reactions were usually mild in intensity.
[b] Injection site atrophy comprises terms relating to localized lipoatrophy at injection site.

Miscellaneous – Adverse reactions that occurred only in 4 to 5 more subjects in the glatiramer group than in the placebo group (less than 1% difference), but for which a relationship to glatiramer could not be excluded, were arthralgia and herpes simplex.

➤*Other adverse reactions:*

Cardiovascular – Hypertension (1% or more); atrial fibrillation, bradycardia, fourth heart sound, hypotension, midsystolic click, postural hypotension, systolic murmur, varicose veins (0.1% to 1%).

CNS – Abnormal dreams, emotional lability, stupor (1% or more); aphasia, ataxia, circumoral paresthesia, coma, concentration disorder, convulsion, decreased libido, depersonalization, facial paralysis, hallucinations, hostility, hypokinesia, manic reaction, memory impairment, myoclonus, neuralgia, paranoid reaction, paraplegia, psychotic depression, suicide attempt, transient stupor (0.1% to 1%).

Dermatologic – Eczema, herpes zoster, pustular rash, skin atrophy, warts (1% or more); angioedema, benign skin neoplasm, contact dermatitis, dermatitis, dry skin, erythema nodosum, fungal dermatitis, furunculosis, maculopapular rash, pigmentation, psoriasis, skin carcinoma, skin hypertrophy, skin striae, vesiculobullous rash (0.1% to 1%).

Endocrine – Goiter, hyperthyroidism, hypothyroidism (0.1% to 1%).

GI – Bowel urgency, oral moniliasis, salivary gland enlargement, tooth caries, ulcerative stomatitis (1% or more); burning sensation on tongue, cholecystitis, colitis, dry mouth, duodenal ulcer, esophageal ulcer, esophagitis, GI carcinoma, gum hemorrhage, hepatomegaly, increased appetite, melena, mouth ulceration, pancreas disorder, pancreatitis, rectal hemorrhage, stomatitis, tenesmus, tongue discoloration (0.1% to 1%).

GU – Amenorrhea, hematuria, impotence, menorrhagia, suspicious papanicolaou smear, urinary frequency, vaginal hemorrhage (1% or more); abnormal sexual function, abortion, breast engorgement, breast enlargement, carcinoma in situ cervix, fibrocystic breast, flank pain (kidney), kidney calculus, nocturia, ovarian cyst, priapism, pyelonephritis, urethritis, vaginitis (0.1% to 1%).

Hematologic/Lymphatic – Anemia, cyanosis, eosinophilia, hematemesis, leukopenia, lymphedema, pancytopenia, splenomegaly (0.1% to 1%).

Local – Abscess, injection site atrophy, injection site edema, injection site hypersensitivity (1% or more); injection site abscess, injection site fibrosis, injection site hematoma, injection site hypertrophy, injection site melanosis (0.1% to 1%).

Metabolic/Nutritional – Abnormal healing, alcohol intolerance, Cushing syndrome, gout, weight loss, xanthoma (0.1% to 1%).

Musculoskeletal – Arthritis, bone pain, bursitis, kidney pain, muscle atrophy, muscle disorder, myopathy, osteomyelitis, tendon pain, tenosynovitis (0.1% to 1%).

Respiratory – Hay fever, hyperventilation (1% or more); asthma, epistaxis, hypoventilation, pneumonia, voice alteration (0.1% to 1%).

Special senses – Visual field defect (1% or more); cataract, corneal ulcer, dry eyes, mydriasis, optic neuritis, otitis externa, photophobia, ptosis, taste loss (0.1% to 1%).

Miscellaneous – Cellulitis, generalized edema, hernia, lipoma, moon face, photosensitivity reaction, serum sickness (0.1% to 1%).

➤*Postmarketing:*

Cardiovascular – Angina pectoris, arrhythmia, cardiomegaly, cardiomyopathy, cerebrovascular accident, congestive heart failure, coronary occlu-

GLATIRAMER ACETATE — INJECTION

sion, deep thrombophlebitis, myocardial infarct, pericardial effusion, peripheral vascular disease, thrombosis.

CNS – Abnormal dreams, aphasia, brain edema, CNS neoplasm, convulsion, meningitis, myelitis, neuralgia.

GI – Cholelithiasis, cirrhosis of the liver, enlarged abdomen, eructation, hemorrhage, hepatitis, liver damage, liver function abnormality, stomach ulcer, tongue edema.

GU – Bladder carcinoma, breast carcinoma, kidney failure, nephrosis, ovarian carcinoma, urinary frequency, urine abnormality, urogenital neoplasm.

Hematologic/Lymphatic – Acute leukemia, lymphoma-like reaction, thrombocytopenia.

Musculoskeletal – Generalized spasm, rheumatoid arthritis.

Ophthalmic – Blindness, glaucoma, visual field defect.

Respiratory – Carcinoma of lung, hay fever, pleural effusion, pulmonary embolus.

Miscellaneous – Allergic reaction, anaphylactoid reaction, hydrocephalus, hypercholesterolemia, injection site hypersensitivity, sepsis, systemic lupus erythematosus.

Patient Information

Instruct patients to inform their health care provider if they are pregnant or plan to become pregnant while taking glatiramer.

Advise patients that glatiramer may cause various symptoms after injection, including flushing, chest pain, palpitations, anxiety, dyspnea, constriction of the throat, and urticaria. These symptoms are generally transient and self-limited and do not require specific treatment. Inform patients that these symptoms may occur early or may have their onset several months after the initiation of treatment. A patient may experience one or several episodes of these symptoms.

Advise patients that they may experience transient chest pain either as part of the immediate postinjection reaction or in isolation. Inform patients that the pain should be transient (usually only lasting a few minutes). Some patients may experience more than 1 such episode, usually beginning at least 1 month after the initiation of treatment. Advise patients to seek medical attention if they experience chest pain of unusual duration or intensity.

Advise patients that localized lipoatrophy, and rarely, injection site necrosis may occur at injection sites. Instruct patients to follow proper injection technique and to rotate injection areas and sites on a daily basis.

Instruct patients to read the glatiramer patient information leaflet carefully. Caution patients to use aseptic technique. The first injection should be performed under the supervision of a health care professional. Instruct patients to rotate injection areas and sites on a daily basis. Caution patients against the reuse of needles or syringes. Instruct patients in safe disposal procedures.

Advise patients that the recommended storage condition for glatiramer is refrigeration (2° to 8°C; 36° to 46°F), although glatiramer can be stored at room temperature (15° to 30°C; 59° to 86°F) for up to 1 month. Glatiramer should not be exposed to higher temperatures or intense light.

MUROMONAB-CD3

Rx	**Orthoclone OKT3** (Ortho Biotech)	**Injection:** 5 mg per 5 ml	With 1 mg polysorbate 80. In 5 ml amps.

MUROMONAB-CD3 — INJECTION

WARNING

Only physicians experienced in immunosuppressive therapy and management of solid organ transplant patients should use muromonab-CD3.

Anaphylactic or anaphylactoid reactions may occur following administration of any dose or course of muromonab-CD3. Serious and occasionally life-threatening systemic, cardiovascular and CNS reactions have been reported. These have included: Pulmonary edema, especially in patients with volume overload; shock; cardiovascular collapse; cardiac or respiratory arrest; seizures; coma. Hence, a patient being treated with muromonab-CD3 must be managed in a facility equipped and staffed for cardiopulmonary resuscitation.

Indications

➤*Renal allograft rejection:* Treatment of acute allograft rejection in renal transplant patients.

➤*Cardiac/Hepatic allograft rejection:* Treatment of steroid-resistant acute allograft rejection in cardiac and hepatic transplant patients.

➤*Off-label uses:* Prophylaxis and treatment of acute graft-versus-host disease (GVHD) in allogenic bone marrow transplantation.

Administration and Dosage

➤*General dosing considerations:* Premedication prior to muromonab-CD3 administration is strongly recommended. (See Premedication.)

Reduce the dose of concomitant immunosuppressive drugs during muromonab-CD3 administration. (See Concomitant Therapy.)

➤*Adults:*

Cardiac allograft rejection, steroid resistant –
Usual dosage: 5 mg/day for 10 to 14 days. Begin treatment when it is determined that a rejection has not been reversed by an adequate course of corticosteroid therapy.

Hepatic allograft rejection, steroid resistant – See Cardiac allograft rejection for dosing.

Renal allograft rejection, acute –
Usual dosage: 5 mg/day for 10 to 14 days. Begin treatment once acute renal rejection is diagnosed.

➤*Premedication:* Monitor patients closely for the first few doses. Methylprednisolone sodium succinate 8 mg/kg IV given 1 to 4 hours prior to muromonab-CD3 administration is strongly recommended to decrease the incidence of reactions to the first dose. Acetaminophen and antihistamines, given concomitantly, may reduce early reactions. Patient temperature should not exceed 37.8°C (100°F) prior to first administration.

➤*Concomitant therapy:* Reduce the dose of concomitant immunosuppressive drugs during muromonab-CD3 administration to the lowest level compatible with an effective therapeutic response. Resume maintenance immunosuppression for approximately 3 days prior to cessation of muromonab-CD3.

➤*Preparation for administration:* Draw solution into a syringe through a low protein-binding 0.2 or 0.22 micrometer filter.

➤*Administration:* Administer as an IV bolus in less than 1 minute. Do not give by IV infusion or in conjunction with other drug solutions.

➤*Admixture compatibility:* Do not add or infuse other drugs simultaneously through the same IV line. If the same IV line is used for sequential infusion of several different drugs, flush with saline before and after infusion of muromonab-CD3.

➤*Storage/Stability:* Refrigerate at 2° to 8°C (36° to 46°F). Do not freeze or shake. Because this drug is a protein solution, it may develop a few fine translucent particles, which do not affect its potency. Because no bacteriostatic agent is present in this product, use the amp immediately once opened and discard the unused portion.

Actions

➤*Pharmacology:* Muromonab-CD3 is a murine monoclonal antibody to the T3 (CD3) antigen of human T-cells that functions as an immunosuppressant. Muromonab-CD3 is for IV use only. The antibody is a biochemically purified IgG_{2a} immunoglobulin. It reverses graft rejection, probably by blocking the T-cell function, which plays a major role in acute allograft rejection. The drug reacts with, and blocks the function of, a molecule (CD3) in the membrane of human T-cells that is associated with the antigen recognition structure of T-cells and is essential for signal transduction. Muromonab-CD3 blocks all known T-cell functions and reacts with most peripheral T-cells in blood and in body tissues. Following termination of therapy, T-cell function usually returns to normal within 1 week.

A rapid concomitant decrease in the number of circulating CD2, CD3, CD4 and CD8 positive T-cells was observed within minutes after administration. This decrease in the number of CD3 positive T-cells results from the specific interaction between muromonab-CD3 and the CD3 antigen on the surface of all T-lymphocytes. T-cell activation results in the release of numerous cytokines/lymphokines, which are thought to be responsible for many of the acute clinical manifestations seen following muromonab-CD3 therapy (see Warnings).

Between days 2 and 7, increasing numbers of circulating CD4 and CD8 positive cells have been observed, although CD3 positive cells are not detectable. CD3 positive cells reappear rapidly and reach pretreatment levels within a week after therapy termination. Increasing numbers of CD3 positive cells have been observed in patients prior to termination of therapy, possibly caused by the development of neutralizing antibodies.

Antibodies have occurred (incidence of 21% for IgM, 86% for IgG and 29% for IgE). Mean time of appearance of IgG antibodies was 20 days. Early IgG antibodies occur towards the end of the second week of treatment in 3% of patients.

➤*Pharmacokinetics:* Serum levels are measured with an enzyme-linked immunosorbent assay (ELISA). During treatment with 5 mg/day for 14 days, mean serum trough levels rose over the first 3 days and then averaged 0.9 mcg/mL on days 3 to 14. Circulating serum levels ≥ 0.8 mcg/mL block the function of cytotoxic T-cells in vitro and in vivo.

Contraindications

Hypersensitivity to this or any product of murine origin; anti-mouse antibody titers ≥ 1:1000; patients in fluid overload or uncompensated heart failure, as evidenced by chest x-ray or > 3% weight gain within the week prior to treatment; history of seizures or predisposition to seizures; pregnancy, breastfeeding (see Warnings).

Warnings/Precautions

➤*Cytokine release syndrome (CRS):* Temporally associated with the administration of the first few doses of muromonab-CD3 (particularly, the first two to three doses), most patients have developed an acute clinical syndrome (CRS) that has been attributed to the release of cytokines by activated lymphocytes or monocytes. This clinical syndrome has ranged from a

MUROMONAB-CD3 — INJECTION

more frequently reported mild, self-limited, "flu-like" illness to a less frequently reported severe, life-threatening shock-like reaction, which may include serious cardiovascular and CNS manifestations. The syndrome typically begins approximately 30 to 60 minutes after administration of a dose (but may occur later) and may persist for several hours. The frequency and severity of this symptom complex is usually greatest with the first dose. With each successive dose, both the frequency and severity of the CRS tend to diminish. Increasing the amount of a dose or resuming treatment after a hiatus may result in a reappearance of the CRS.

Common clinical manifestations – High fever (often spiking, up to 107°F); chills/rigors; headache; tremor; nausea/vomiting; diarrhea; abdominal pain; malaise; muscle/joint aches and pains; generalized weakness. Less frequently reported adverse experiences include minor dermatologic reactions (eg, rash, pruritus) and a spectrum of often serious, occasionally fatal, cardiorespiratory and neuro-psychiatric adverse experiences.

Cardiorespiratory – Cardiorespiratory findings may include the following: Dyspnea; shortness of breath; bronchospasm/wheezing; tachypnea; respiratory arrest/failure/distress; cardiovascular collapse; cardiac arrest; angina/MI; chest pain/tightness; tachycardia (including ventricular); hypertension; hemodynamic instability; hypotension, including profound shock; heart failure; pulmonary edema (cardiogenic and non-cardiogenic); adult respiratory distress syndrome; hypoxemia; apnea; arrhythmias.

Pulmonary edema – In the initial renal rejection studies, potentially fatal, severe pulmonary edema, the most serious postdose reaction, occurred in 4.7% of the initial 107 patients. Fluid overload was present before treatment in all of these cases. However, it occurred in none of the subsequent 311 patients treated with first-dose volume/weight restrictions. In subsequent trials and in postmarketing experience, severe pulmonary edema has occurred in patients who appeared to be euvolemic. The pathogenesis of pulmonary edema may involve all or some of the following: Volume overload; increased pulmonary vascular permeability; reduced left ventricular compliance/contractility.

Serum creatinine – During the first 1 to 3 days of therapy, some patients have experienced an acute and transient decline in the glomerular filtration rate and diminished urine output with a resulting increase in the level of serum creatinine. Massive release of cytokines appears to lead to reversible renal function impairment or delayed renal allograft function. Similarly, transient elevations in hepatic transaminases have been reported following administration of the first few doses.

Fluid status – Prior to administration, assess the patient's volume (fluid) status carefully. It is imperative, especially prior to the first few doses, that there be no clinical evidence of volume overload or uncompensated heart failure, including a clear chest X-ray and weight restriction of ≤ 3% above the patient's minimum weight during the week prior to injection.

Prevention/Minimization of CRS – Manifestations of the CRS may be prevented or minimized by pretreatment with 8 mg/kg methylprednisolone (ie, high-dose steroids), given 1 to 4 hours prior to administration of the first dose of muromonab-CD3 and by closely following recommendations for dosage and treatment duration. If any of the more serious presentations of the CRS occur, intensive treatment including oxygen, IV fluids, corticosteroids, pressor amines, antihistamines, and intubation may be required.

➤*Neuropsychiatric events:* Seizures, encephalopathy, cerebral edema, aseptic meningitis, and headaches have occurred during therapy with muromonab-CD3, even following the first dose, resulting in part from T-cell activation and subsequent systemic release of cytokines.

Seizures – Seizures, some accompanied by loss of consciousness or cardiorespiratory arrest, or death, have occurred independently or in conjunction with any of the neurologic syndromes described below. Patients predisposed to seizures may include those with the following conditions: Acute tubular necrosis/uremia; fever; infection; a precipitous fall in serum calcium; fluid overload; hypertension; hypoglycemia, history of seizures and electrolyte imbalances; those who are taking a medication concomitantly that may, by itself, cause seizures. The number and regularity of seizure reports indicate that this hazard appears not to be rare. Anticipate convulsions clinically with appropriate patient monitoring.

Encephalopathy – Manifestations may include the following: Impaired cognition; confusion; obtundation; altered mental status; auditory/visual hallucinations; psychosis (delirium, paranoia); mood changes (eg, mania, agitation, combativeness); diffuse hypotonus; hyperreflexia; myoclonus; tremor; asterixis; involuntary movements; major motor seizures; lethargy/stupor/coma; diffuse weakness. Approximately one-third of patients with a diagnosis of encephalopathy may have had coexisting aseptic meningitis syndrome.

Cerebral edema – Cerebral edema and other signs of increased vascular permeability (eg, otitis media, nasal and ear stuffiness) have been seen in patients treated with muromonab-CD3 and may accompany some of the other neurologic manifestations.

Aseptic meningitis syndrome – The incidence of this syndrome was 6%. Fever (89%), headache (44%), meningismus (ie, neck stiffness; 14%) and photophobia (10%) were the most commonly reported symptoms; a combination of these 4 symptoms occurred in 5% of patients. Diagnosis is confirmed by CSF analysis demonstrating leukocytosis with pleocytosis, elevated protein and normal or decreased glucose, with negative viral, bacterial, and fungal cultures. In any immunosuppressed transplant patient with clinical findings suggesting meningitis, evaluate the possibility of infection. Approximately one-third of the patients with a diagnosis of aseptic meningitis had coexisting signs and symptoms of encephalopathy. Most patients with the aseptic meningitis syndrome had a benign course and recovered without any permanent sequelae during therapy or subsequent to its completion or discontinuation.

Headache – Headache is frequently seen after any of the first few doses and may occur in any of the aforementioned neurologic syndromes or by itself.

The following additional neurologic events have been reported occasionally: Irreversible blindness; impaired vision; quadri- or paraparesis/plegia; cerebrovascular accident (hemiparesis/-plegia); aphasia; transient ischemic attack; subarachnoid hemorrhage; palsy of the VI cranial nerve; hearing loss.

Signs or symptoms of encephalopathy, meningitis, seizures, and cerebral edema, with or without headache, have typically been reversible. Headache, aseptic meningitis, seizures, and less severe forms of encephalopathy resolved in most patients despite continued treatment. However, some events have been irreversible.

CNS adverse experiences – Patients who may be at greater risk for CNS adverse experiences include the following: Known or suspected CNS disorders (eg, history of seizure disorder); cerebrovascular disease (small or large vessel); conditions having associated neurologic problems (eg, head trauma, uremia); underlying vascular diseases; concomitant medication that may, by itself, affect the CNS.

➤*Infections:* Muromonab-CD3 is usually added to immunosuppressive therapeutic regimens, thereby augmenting the degree of immunosuppression. This increase in the total burden of immunosuppression may alter the spectrum of infections observed and increase the risk, the severity and the potential gravity (morbidity) of infectious complications. Approximately 1 to 6 months posttransplant, patients are at risk for viral infections (eg, cytomegalovirus, Epstein-Barr virus, herpes simplex virus), which produce serious systemic disease and also increase the overall state of immunosuppression. Multiple or intensive courses of any anti-T cell antibody preparation, including muromonab-CD3, which produce profound impairment of cell-mediated immunity, further increase the risk of (opportunistic) infection, especially with the herpes viruses and fungi. Anti-infective prophylaxis may reduce the morbidity associated with certain potential pathogens and should be considered for high-risk patients.

➤*Intravascular thrombosis:* As with other immunosuppressive therapies, arterial, or venous thrombosis of allografts and other vascular beds (eg, heart, lungs, brain, bowel) have been reported. Consider these findings when deciding to use muromonab-CD3 in patients with a history of thrombotic events or underlying vascular disease. Consider concomitant use of prophylactic anti-thrombotic interventions (eg, minidose heparin).

➤*Hypersensitivity reactions:* Serious and occasionally fatal, immediate (usually within 10 minutes) hypersensitivity (anaphylactic) reactions have occurred. Manifestations of anaphylaxis may appear similar to manifestations of the CRS. It may be impossible to determine the mechanism responsible for any systemic reaction(s). Reactions attributed to hypersensitivity have been reported less frequently than those attributed to cytokine release. Acute hypersensitivity reactions may be characterized by the following: Cardiovascular collapse; cardiorespiratory arrest; loss of consciousness; hypotension/shock; tachycardia; tingling; angioedema (including laryngeal, pharyngeal or facial edema); airway obstruction; bronchospasm; dyspnea; urticaria; pruritus.

Serious allergic events, including anaphylactic or anaphylactoid reactions, have been reported in patients re-exposed to muromonab-CD3 subsequent to their initial course of therapy. Pretreatment with antihistamines or steroids may not reliably prevent anaphylaxis in this setting. Weigh the possible allergic hazards of retreatment against expected therapeutic benefits and alternatives. If retreatment is employed, have epinephrine and other emergency life-support equipment available, and monitor the patient closely.

If hypersensitivity is suspected, discontinue the drug immediately and do not resume therapy or re-expose the patient to muromonab-CD3. Serious acute hypersensitivity reactions may require emergency treatment with 0.3 to 0.5 mL aqueous epinephrine (1:1000 dilution) SC and other resuscitative measures. Refer to Management of Acute Hypersensitivity Reactions.

➤*Special risk:* Patients at risk for more serious complications of the CRS may include those with the following conditions: Unstable angina; recent MI or symptomatic ischemic heart disease; heart failure of any etiology; pulmonary edema of any etiology; any form of chronic obstructive pulmonary disease; intravascular volume overload or depletion of any etiology (eg, excessive dialysis, recent intensive diuresis, blood loss); cerebrovascular disease; patients with advanced symptomatic vascular disease or neuropathy; history of seizures; septic shock. Make efforts to correct or stabilize background conditions prior to the initiation of therapy.

➤*Pregnancy: Category C.* It is not known whether muromonab-CD3 can cause fetal harm when administered to a pregnant woman or can affect reproduction capacity. However, it is an IgG antibody and may cross the placenta. If this drug is used during pregnancy, or the patient becomes pregnant while taking this drug, apprise the patient of the potential hazard to the fetus.

➤*Lactation:* It is not known whether muromonab-CD3 is excreted in breast milk. Because of the potential for serious adverse reactions/oncogenesis, decide whether to discontinue nursing or to discontinue the drug, taking into account the importance of the drug to the mother.

➤*Children:* Safety and efficacy in children have not been established. Muromonab-CD3 has been used in infants/children, beginning with a dose of 5 mg or less. Based on immunologic monitoring, the dosage has been adjusted accordingly. Pediatric recipients may be significantly immunosuppressed for a prolonged period of time and therefore require close monitoring

MUROMONAB-CD3 — INJECTION

posttherapy for opportunistic infection, particularly varicella (VZV), which poses an infectious complication unique to this population. GI fluid loss secondary to diarrhea or vomiting resulting from the CRS may be significant when treating small children and may require parenteral hydration. It is unknown whether there may be significant long-term sequelae (eg, neurodevelopmental language difficulties in infants younger than 1 year of age) related to the occurrence of seizures, high fever, CNS infections, or aseptic meningitis following muromonab-CD3 treatment. In cases where administration would be deemed medically appropriate, more vigilant and frequent monitoring is required for children than in adults.

➤*Monitoring:* Monitor the following tests prior to and during therapy:

Renal – BUN, serum creatinine.

Hepatic – Transaminases, alkaline phosphatase, bilirubin.

Hematopoietic – WBCs and differential, platelet count.

Chest X-ray – Within 24 hours before initiating treatment, which should be free of any evidence of heart failure or fluid overload.

Monitor one of the following immunologic tests during therapy:

Plasma levels determined by an ELISA (target levels should be ≥ 800 ng/mL); or

Quantitative T-lymphocyte surface phenotyping (CD3, CD4, CD8); target CD3 positive T-cells < 25 cells/mm^3.

Testing for human-mouse antibody titers is strongly recommended; a titer ≥1:1000 is a contraindication for use.

Drug Interactions

➤*Indomethacin:* Encephalopathy and other CNS effects have occurred with concurrent use.

Adverse Reactions

➤*Cytokine release syndrome:* See Warnings. In trials, the majority of patients experienced pyrexia (90%), of which 19% were ≥ 40°C (104°F), and chills (59%). Other adverse experiences occurring in ≥ 8% during the first 2 days included the following: Dyspnea (21%); nausea, vomiting (19%); chest pain, diarrhea (14%); tremor, wheezing (13%); headache (11%); tachycardia (10%); rigor, hypertension (8%).

➤*Infections:* See Warnings.

Renal rejection trial – The most common infections during the first 45 days of therapy were due to herpes simplex (27%) and cytomegalovirus (CMV; 19%). Other severe and life-threatening infections were *Staphylococcus epidermidis* (4.8%), *Pneumocystis carinii* (3.1%), *Legionella*, *Cryptococcus*, *Serratia*, and gram-negative bacteria (1.6%).

Hepatic rejection trial – The most common infections during the first 45 days of treatment were CMV (15.7%), fungal infections (14.9%) and herpes simplex (7.5%). Other severe and life-threatening infections were gram-positive (9%), gram-negative (7.5%), viral (1.5%), *Legionella* (0.7%). In another hepatic rejection trial, incidence of fungal infections was 34% and of herpes simplex virus infections was 31%.

Cardiac rejection trial – The most common infections reported during the first 45 days of treatment were herpes simplex (5%), fungal (4%), and CMV (3%).

➤*Neoplasia:* See Warnings.

➤*Neuropsychiatric:* See Warnings.

➤*Hypersensitivity:* See Warnings.

➤*Other:*

Cardiovascular – Cardiac arrest; hypotension/shock; heart failure; cardiovascular collapse; angina/MI; tachycardia; bradycardia; hemodynamic instability; hypertension; left ventricular dysfunction; arrhythmias; chest pain/tightness.

Dermatologic – Rash; Stevens-Johnson syndrome; urticaria; pruritus; erythema; flushing; diaphoresis.

GI – Diarrhea; nausea/vomiting; abdominal pain; bowel infarction; GI hemorrhage.

Hepatic – Increases in transaminases (eg, AST, ALT); hepato/splenomegaly or hepatitis, usually secondary to viral infection or lymphoma.

Musculoskeletal – Arthralgia; arthritis; myalgia; stiffness/aches/pains.

Renal – Anuria/oliguria; delayed graft function; transient and reversible increases in BUN and serum creatinine; abnormal urinary cytology, including exfoliation of damaged lymphocytes, collecting duct cells and cellular casts.

Respiratory – Respiratory arrest; adult respiratory distress syndrome (ARDS); respiratory failure; pulmonary edema (cardiogenic or noncardiogenic); apnea; dyspnea; bronchospasm; wheezing; shortness of breath; hypoxemia; tachypnea/hyperventilation; abnormal chest sounds; pneumonia/pneumonitis.

Special senses – Blindness; blurred vision; diplopia; hearing loss; otitis media; tinnitus; vertigo; VI cranial nerve palsy; photophobia; conjunctivitis; nasal/ear stuffiness.

Miscellaneous – Pancytopenia; aplastic anemia; neutropenia; leukopenia; thrombocytopenia; lymphopenia; leukocytosis; lymphadenopathy; arterial and venous thrombosis of allografts and other vascular beds (eg, heart, lung, brain, bowel); disturbances of coagulation; fever (including spiking temperatures as high as 107°F); chills/rigors; flu-like syndrome; fatigue/malaise; generalized weakness; anorexia.

Overdosage

Symptoms of overdose may include hyperthermia, severe chills, myalgia, vomiting, diarrhea, edema, oliguria, pulmonary edema, and acute renal failure. A high incidence (5%) of microangiopathic hemolytic anemia/HUS syndrome in patients receiving 10 mg/day was also reported. In the event of acute overdosage, carefully observe the patient and give symptomatic and supportive treatment.

Patient Information

Advise patients of the signs and symptoms associated with the cytokine release syndrome, including the potentially serious nature of this symptom complex (eg, systemic, cardiovascular, neuro-psychiatric events).

Advise patients to seek medical attention at the first sign of skin rash, urticaria, rapid heartbeat, difficulty in swallowing and breathing, or any swelling that may suggest angioedema or other allergic reaction.

Patients should know how they might react before operating an automobile or machinery, or engaging in activities requiring mental alertness, coordination, or physical dexterity.

MYCOPHENOLATE

Rx	**Mycophenolate** (Various, eg, Accord)	**Capsules; oral:** 250 mg	As mycophenolate mofetil. In 100s, 120s, 500s, 1,000s, and UD 100s.
Rx	**CellCept** (Roche)		As mycophenolate mofetil. (CellCept 250 Roche). Blue/Brown. In 100s, 120s, and 500s.
Rx	**Mycophenolate** (Various, eg, Accord)	**Tablets; oral:** 500 mg	As mycophenolate mofetil. In 100s, 500s, 1,000s, and UD 100s.
Rx	**CellCept** (Roche)		As mycophenolate mofetil. PEG. (CellCept 500 Roche). Lavender, capsule shape. Film-coated. In 100s and 500s.
Rx	**Myfortic** (Novartis)	**Tablets, delayed-release; oral:** 180 mg	As mycophenolate sodium. Lactose. (C). Lime green, round. Film-coated. In 120s.
		360 mg	As mycophenolate sodium. Lactose. (CT). Pale orange-red, oval. Film-coated. In 120s.
Rx	**CellCept** (Roche)	**Suspension, powder for reconstitution; oral:** 200 mg/mL	As mycophenolate mofetil. Aspartame, methylparaben, phenylalanine 0.56 mg/mL, sorbitol. Mixed fruit flavor. In 225 mL.
Rx	**CellCept** (Roche)	**Injection, lyophilized powder for solution, concentrate:** 500 mg	As mycophenolate mofetil hydrochloride. Preservative free. Polysorbate 80. In 20 mL vials.

MYCOPHENOLATE MOFETIL — ORAL

WARNING

Immunosuppression may lead to increased susceptibility to infection and the possible development of lymphoma. Only health care providers experienced in immunosuppressive therapy and management of renal, cardiac, or hepatic transplant patients should use mycophenolate. Manage patients receiving the drug in facilities equipped and staffed with adequate laboratory and supportive medical resources. The health care provider responsible for maintenance therapy should have complete information requisite for the follow-up of the patient.

Women of childbearing potential must use contraception. Use of mycophenolate during pregnancy is associated with and increased risk of miscarriage and congenital malformations.

Indications

➤*Renal, cardiac, and hepatic transplantation:* For the prophylaxis of organ rejection in patients receiving allogeneic renal, cardiac, or hepatic transplants. Use mycophenolate concomitantly with cyclosporine and corticosteroids.

➤*Off-label uses:*

Lupus nephritis – [3] = Safety concerns. Guidelines, meta-analyses, and systematic reviews of the studies to date with mycophenolate have characterized the results as encouraging or promising. Mycophenolate appeared to be associated with higher rates of complete and partial response than the standard of care (cyclophosphamide). The incidence of adverse effects and death was also lower with mycophenolate than with cyclophosphamide. Some authors have concluded that mycophenolate would be an appropriate first-line agent in patients with less severe lupus nephritis. However, because long-term efficacy has been demonstrated only with cyclophosphamide-based regimens, other authors, including the authors of the European League Against Rheumatism guidelines, recommend mycophenolate only as an alternative agent, unless or until long-term outcome data become available.

Other possible off-label uses – Refractory uveitis (2 g/day or in combination with previous corticosteroid, cyclosporine, or tacrolimus therapy); second-line therapy for Churg-Strauss syndrome; in combination with prednisolone for the treatment of diffuse proliferative lupus nephritis.

Administration and Dosage

➤*Adults:*

Cardiac transplantation – 1.5 g twice a day.

Hepatic transplantation – 1.5 g twice a day.

Renal transplantation – 1 g twice a day.

Off-label dosing –

Lupus nephritis: [3] = Safety concerns. 1 to 3 g/day, divided for twice-daily administration. Maintenance treatment continues indefinitely; however, if an adequate response to therapy is not observed within the first 6 months, a more intense treatment approach should be considered.

➤*Children:*

Renal transplantation –

3 months to 18 years of age:

- *Usual dosage* –
  Suspension: 600 mg/m^2 twice a day.
  Capsules/Tablets: Patients with a body surface area (BSA) of 1.25 to 1.5 m^2 may be dosed with capsules at a dosage of 750 mg twice a day. Patients with a BSA greater than 1.5 m^2 may be dosed with capsules or tablets at a dosage of 1 g twice a day.
- *Maximum dose* –
  Suspension: 2 g per 10 mL day.

➤*Renal function impairment:* In renal transplant patients with severe chronic renal impairment (glomerular filtration rate [GFR] less than 25 mL/min/1.73 m^2) outside the immediate posttransplant period, avoid doses of mycophenolate greater than 1 g administered twice a day. Carefully observe these patients.

➤*Neutropenia:* If neutropenia develops (absolute neutrophil counts [ANC] less than 1.3 × 10^3/mcL), interrupt dosing or reduce the dosage of mycophenolate, perform appropriate diagnostic tests, and manage the patient appropriately.

➤*Preparation for administration:*

Suspension – Tap the closed bottle several times to loosen the powder. Measure 94 mL of water in a graduated cylinder. Add approximately half the total amount of water for reconstitution to the bottle and shake the closed bottle well for about 1 minute. Remove the child-resistant cap and push bottle adapter into neck of bottle. Close bottle with child-resistant cap tightly. This will ensure the proper seating of the bottle adapter in the bottle and child-resistant status of the cap.

➤*Administration:* Give the initial dose as soon as possible following renal, cardiac, or hepatic transplantation. Food has been shown to decrease mycophenolic acid maximum plasma concentration by 40%. Therefore, it is recommended that mycophenolate be administered on an empty stomach. However, in stable renal transplant patients, mycophenolate may be administered with food if necessary.

Capsules/Tablets – Do not crush mycophenolate tablets; do not open or crush mycophenolate capsules.

Suspension – Can be administered via a nasogastric tube with a minimum size of 8 French (minimum of 1.7 mm interior diameter).

➤*Admixture compatibility:* Do not mix the oral suspension with any other medication.

➤*Storage/Stability:* Store at 25°C (77°F); excursions are permitted between 15° and 30°C (59° and 86°F). Protect from light. Store reconstituted suspension at 25°C (77°F); excursions are permitted between 15° and 30°C (59° and 86°F). Storage in a refrigerator at 2° to 8°C (36° to 46°F) is acceptable. Do not freeze. Discard any unused portion 60 days after reconstitution.

Handling and disposal – Exercise caution in the handling and preparation of mycophenolate. Avoid inhalation or direct contact of the powder contained in the capsules and oral suspension (before and after reconstitution) with skin or mucous membranes. If such contact occurs, wash thoroughly with soap and water; rinse eyes with plain water. If a spill occurs, wipe up using paper towels wetted with water to remove spilled powder or suspension.

Actions

➤*Pharmacology:* Mycophenolic acid, the hydrolyzed form of mycophenolate, is a potent, selective, uncompetitive, and reversible inhibitor of inosine monophosphate dehydrogenase (IMPDH), and, therefore, inhibits the de novo pathway of guanosine nucleotide synthesis without incorporation into DNA. Because T- and B-lymphocytes are critically dependent for their proliferation on de novo synthesis of purines, whereas other cell types can utilize salvage pathways, mycophenolic acid has potent cytostatic effects on lymphocytes. Mycophenolic acid inhibits proliferative responses of T- and B-lymphocytes to both mitogenic and allospecific stimulation. Addition of guanosine or deoxyguanosine reverses the cytostatic effects of mycophenolic acid on lymphocytes. Mycophenolic acid also suppresses antibody formation by B-lymphocytes. Mycophenolic acid prevents the glycosylation of lymphocyte and monocyte glycoproteins that are involved in intercellular adhesion to endothelial cells and may inhibit recruitment of leukocytes into sites of inflammation and graft rejection. Mycophenolate mofetil did not inhibit early events in the activation of human peripheral blood mononuclear cells (eg, the production of interleukin-1 and interleukin-2), but did block the coupling of these events to DNA synthesis and proliferation.

➤*Pharmacokinetics:*

Renal, cardiac, and hepatic transplant patients –

Mycophenolic Acid Pharmacokinetic Parameters (Mean ± SD)[a]

Parameter	Dose/Route	T_{max} (h)	C_{max} (mcg/mL)	AUC (mcg•h/mL)
Healthy volunteers (single dose)	1 g/oral	0.8 (± 0.36) (n = 129)	24.5 (± 9.5) (n = 129)	63.9 (± 16.2) (n = 117)
Renal transplant patients (twice-daily dosing) Time after transplantation				
5 days (n = 31)	1 g/IV	1.58 (± 0.46)	12 (± 3.82)	40.8 (± 11.4)[b]
6 days (n = 31)	1 g/oral	1.33 (± 1.05)	10.7 (± 4.83)	32.9 (± 15)[b]
Early (< 40 days) (n = 25)	1 g/oral	1.31 (± 0.76)	8.16 (± 4.5)	27.3 (± 10.9)[b]
Early (< 40 days) (n = 27)	1.5 g/oral	1.21 (± 0.81)	13.5 (± 8.18)	38.4 (± 15.4)[b]
Late (> 3 months) (n = 23)	1.5 g/oral	0.9 (± 0.24)	24.1 (± 12.1)	65.3 (± 35.4)[b]
Cardiac transplant patients (twice-daily dosing) Time after transplantation				
Early (day before discharge)	1.5 g/oral	1.8 (± 1.3) (n = 11)	11.5 (± 6.8) (n = 11)	43.3 (± 20.8)[b] (n = 9)
Late (> 6 months)	1.5 g/oral	1.1 (± 0.7) (n = 52)	20 (± 9.4) (n = 52)	54.1 (± 20.4)[c] (n = 49)
Hepatic transplant patients (twice-daily dosing) Time after transplantation				
4 to 9 days (n = 22)	1 g/IV	1.5 (± 0.517)	17 (± 12.7)	34 (± 17.4)[b]
Early (5 to 8 days) (n = 20)	1.5 g/oral	1.15 (± 0.432)	13.1 (± 6.76)	29.2 (± 11.9)[b]
Late (> 6 months) (n = 6)	1.5 g/oral	1.54 (± 0.51)	19.3 (± 11.7)	49.3 (± 14.8)[b]

[a] SD = standard deviation; T_{max} = time of maximal concentration; C_{max} = maximal drug concentration; AUC = area under the curve; IV = intravenous.
[b] Interdosing interval $AUC_{0\text{-}12h}$.
[c] $AUC_{0\text{-}12h}$ values quoted are extrapolated from data from samples collected over 4 hours.

Bioequivalence – Two 500 mg tablets have been shown to be bioequivalent to four 250 mg capsules. Five mL of the 200 mg/mL reconstituted oral suspension have been shown to be bioequivalent to four 250 mg capsules.

Absorption – Oral absorption of the drug is rapid and essentially complete. Mycophenolate can be measured systemically during the IV infusion; however, shortly (approximately 5 minutes) after the infusion is stopped or after oral administration, mycophenolate concentration is below the limit of

MYCOPHENOLATE MOFETIL — ORAL

quantitation (0.4 mcg/mL). Following oral administration, mycophenolate mofetil undergoes rapid and complete metabolism to mycophenolic acid, the active metabolite.

In 12 healthy volunteers, the mean absolute bioavailability of oral mycophenolate relative to IV mycophenolate (based on mycophenolic AUC) was 94%. The AUC for mycophenolic acid appears to increase in a dose-proportional fashion in renal transplant patients receiving multiple doses of mycophenolate up to a daily dosage of 3 g.

Secondary peaks in the plasma mycophenolic acid concentration-time profile are usually observed 6 to 12 hours postdose. The coadministration of cholestyramine (4 g 3 times daily) resulted in an approximately 40% decrease in the mycophenolic acid AUC (largely as a consequence of lower concentrations in the terminal portion of the profile). These observations suggest that enterohepatic recirculation contributes to mycophenolic acid plasma concentrations.

Effect of food: Food (27 g fat, 650 calories) had no effect on the extent of absorption (mycophenolic acid AUC) of mycophenolate when administered at dosages of 1.5 g twice daily to renal transplant patients. However, mycophenolic acid C_{max} was decreased by 40% in the presence of food.

Distribution – The mean (± SD) apparent volume of distribution of mycophenolic acid in 12 healthy volunteers is approximately 4 (± 1.2) L/kg following oral administration. Mycophenolic acid, at clinically relevant concentrations, is 97% bound to plasma albumin. Mycophenolic acid glucuronate is 82% bound to plasma albumin at mycophenolic acid glucuronate concentration ranges that are normally seen in stable renal transplant patients; however, at higher mycophenolic acid glucuronate concentrations (observed in patients with renal impairment or delayed renal graft function), the binding of mycophenolic acid may be reduced as a result of competition between mycophenolic acid glucuronate and mycophenolic acid for protein binding. Mean blood-to-plasma ratio of radioactivity concentrations was approximately 0.6, indicating that mycophenolic acid and mycophenolic acid glucuronate do not distribute extensively into the cellular fractions of blood.

Metabolism – Following oral dosing, mycophenolate mofetil undergoes complete metabolism to mycophenolic acid, the active metabolite. Metabolism to mycophenolic acid occurs presystemically after oral dosing. Mycophenolic acid is metabolized principally by glucuronyl transferase to form the phenolic glucuronide of mycophenolic acid (mycophenolic acid glucuronate), which is not pharmacologically active. In vivo, mycophenolic acid glucuronate is converted to mycophenolic acid via enterohepatic recirculation. The following metabolites of the 2-hydroxyethyl-morpholino moiety are also recovered in the urine following oral administration of mycophenolate to healthy subjects: N-(2-carboxymethyl)-morpholine, N-(2-hydroxyethyl)-morpholine, and the N-oxide of N-(2-hydroxyethyl)-morpholine.

Excretion – A negligible amount of the drug is excreted as mycophenolic acid (less than 1% of the dose) in the urine. Orally administered radiolabeled mycophenolate mofetil resulted in complete recovery of the administered dose, with 93% of the administered dose recovered in the urine and 6% recovered in feces. Most (approximately 87%) of the administered dose is excreted in the urine as mycophenolic acid glucuronate. At clinically encountered concentrations, mycophenolic acid and mycophenolic acid glucuronate are usually not removed by hemodialysis. However, at high mycophenolic acid glucuronate plasma concentrations (more than 100 mcg/mL), small amounts of mycophenolic acid glucuronate are removed. Bile acid sequestrants, such as cholestyramine, reduce mycophenolic acid AUC by interfering with enterohepatic circulation of the drug.

Mean (± SD) apparent half-life and plasma clearance of mycophenolic acid are 17.9 (± 6.5) hours and 193 (± 48) mL/min following oral administration.

Special populations –

Children:

Pharmacokinetic Parameters for Mycophenolic Acid in Children Mean (± SD)

Age (years)	n	Time	T_{max} (h)	Dosage adjusted[a] C_{max} (mcg/mL)	Dosage adjusted[a] $AUC_{0\text{-}12h}$ (mcg•h/mL)
1 to < 2	6[b]	Early (day 7)	3.03 (4.7)	10.3 (5.8)	22.5 (6.66)
1 to < 6	17		1.63 (2.85)	13.2 (7.16)	27.4 (9.54)
6 to < 12	16		0.94 (0.546)	13.1 (6.3)	33.2 (12.1)
12 to 18	21		1.16 (0.83)	11.7 (10.7)	26.3 (9.14)[c]
1 to < 2	4[b]	Late (month 3)	0.725 (0.276)	23.8 (13.4)	47.4 (14.7)
1 to < 6	15		0.989 (0.511)	22.7 (10.1)	49.7 (18.2)
6 to < 12	14		1.21 (0.532)	27.8 (14.3)	61.9 (19.6)
12 to 18	17		0.978 (0.484)	17.9 (9.57)	53.6 (20.3)[d]
1 to < 2	4[b]	Late (month 9)	0.604 (0.208)	25.6 (4.25)	55.8 (11.6)
1 to < 6	12		0.869 (0.479)	30.4 (9.16)	61 (10.7)
6 to < 12	11		1.12 (0.462)	29.2 (12.6)	66.8 (21.2)
12 to 18	14		1.09 (0.518)	18.1 (7.29)	56.7 (14)

[a] Adjusted to a dosage of 600 mg/m^2.
[b] A subset of 1 to < 6 years.
[c] n = 20.
[d] n = 16.

Renal/Hepatic function impairment: Increased plasma concentrations of mycophenolate metabolites (mycophenolic acid increased 50% and mycophenolic acid glucuronate increased about 3- to 6-fold) are observed in patients with renal insufficiency.

Mycophenolate Oral Pharmacokinetic Parameters (Mean ± SD) in Chronic Renal and Hepatic Impairment

Parameter	Dosage	T_{max} (h)	C_{max} (mcg/mL)	AUC (mcg•h/mL)
Renal impairment				
Healthy volunteers GFR > 80 mL/min/1.73 m^2 (n = 6)	1 g	0.75 (± 0.27)	25.3 (± 7.99)	45 (± 22.6)[a]
Mild renal impairment GFR 50 to 80 mL/min/1.73 m^2 (n = 6)	1 g	0.75 (± 0.27)	26 (± 3.82)	59.9 (± 12.9)[a]
Moderate renal impairment GFR 25 to 49 mL/min/1.73 m^2 (n = 6)	1 g	0.75 (± 0.27)	19 (± 13.2)	52.9 (± 25.5)[a]
Severe renal impairment GFR[2] (n = 7)	1 g	1 (± 0.41)	16.3 (± 10.8)	78.6 (± 46.4)[a]
Hepatic impairment				
Healthy volunteers (n = 6)	1 g	0.63 (± 0.14)	24.3 (± 5.73)	29 (± 5.78)[b]
Alcoholic cirrhosis (n = 18)	1 g	0.85 (± 0.58)	22.4 (± 10.1)	29.8 (± 10.7)[b]

[a] Interdosing interval $AUC_{0\text{-}96h}$.
[b] Interdosing interval $AUC_{0\text{-}48h}$.

In 8 patients with primary nonfunction of the organ following renal transplantation, plasma concentrations of mycophenolic acid glucuronate accumulated about 6- to 8-fold after multiple dosing for 28 days. Accumulation of mycophenolic acid was about 1- to 2-fold.

Contraindications

Hypersensitivity to mycophenolate, mycophenolic acid, or any component of the drug product.

Warnings/Precautions

➤*Lymphomas/Malignancies:* Patients receiving immunosuppressive regimens involving combinations of drugs, including mycophenolate, as part of an immunosuppressive regimen are at an increased risk of developing lymphomas and other malignancies, particularly of the skin. The risk appears to be related to the intensity and duration of immunosuppression rather than to the use of any specific agent.

As usual for patients with increased risk for skin cancer, limit exposure to sunlight and ultraviolet light by wearing protective clothing and using a sunscreen with a high protection factor.

Lymphoproliferative disease or lymphoma developed in 0.4% to 1% of patients receiving mycophenolate (2 or 3 g) with other immunosuppressive agents in controlled clinical trials of renal, cardiac, and hepatic transplant patients.

In children, no other malignancies besides lymphoproliferative disorder (2/148 patients) have been observed.

➤*Other immunosuppressive agents:* Mycophenolate has been administered in combination with the following agents in clinical trials: antithymocyte globulin, muromonab-CD3, cyclosporine, and corticosteroids. The efficacy and safety of the use of mycophenolate in combination with other immunosuppressive agents have not been determined.

➤*Infection:* Oversuppression of the immune system can also increase susceptibility to infection, including opportunistic infections, fatal infections, and sepsis. In patients receiving mycophenolate (2 or 3 g) in controlled studies for prevention of renal, cardiac, or hepatic rejection, fatal infection/sepsis occurred in approximately 2% of renal and cardiac patients and in 5% of hepatic patients.

In cardiac transplant patients, the overall incidence of opportunistic infections was approximately 10% higher in patients treated with mycophenolate than in those receiving azathioprine therapy, but this difference was not associated with excess mortality due to infection/sepsis among patients treated with mycophenolate.

There were more herpes virus (herpes simplex, herpes zoster, and cytomegalovirus) infections in cardiac transplant patients treated with mycophenolate compared with those treated with azathioprine.

Latent viral infections – Immunosuppressed patients are at increased risk for opportunistic infections, including activation of latent viral infections. These include cases of progressive multifocal leukoencephalopathy (PML) and BK virus–associated nephropathy (BKVAN), which have been observed in patients receiving immunosuppressants, including mycophenolate.

Cases of PML, sometimes fatal, have been reported in patients treated with mycophenolate. Apathy, ataxia, cognitive deficiencies, confusion, and hemiparesis were the most frequent clinical features observed. The reported cases generally had risk factors for PML, including treatment with immunosuppressant therapies and impairment of immune function. In immunosuppressed patients, consider PML in the differential diagnosis in patients reporting neurological symptoms and consider consultation with a neurologist as clinically indicated. Give consideration to reducing the amount of immunosuppression in patients who develop PML. In transplant patients, consider the risk that reduced immunosuppression represents to the graft.

BKVAN is associated with serious outcomes, including deteriorating renal function and renal graft loss. Patient monitoring may help detect patients at risk for BKVAN. Consider reduction in immunosuppression for patients who develop evidence of BKVAN.

MYCOPHENOLATE MOFETIL — ORAL

➤*Neutropenia:* Severe neutropenia (ANC less than 0.5 × 10^3/mcL) developed in up to 2% of renal, up to 2.8% of cardiac, and up to 3.6% of hepatic transplant patients receiving mycophenolate 3 g daily. Monitor patients receiving mycophenolate for neutropenia. The development of neutropenia may be related to mycophenolate itself, concomitant medications, viral infections, or some combination of these causes. If neutropenia develops (ANC less than 1.3 × 10^3/mcL), interrupt dosing with mycophenolate or reduce the dosage, perform appropriate diagnostic tests, and manage the patient appropriately. Neutropenia has been observed most frequently 31 to 180 days posttransplant in patients treated for prevention of renal, cardiac, and hepatic rejection.

➤*Pure red cell aplasia:* Cases of pure red cell aplasia (PRCA) have been reported in patients treated with mycophenolate in combination with other immunosuppressive agents. The mechanism for mycophenolate-induced PRCA is unknown; the relative contribution of other immunosuppressants and their combinations in an immunosuppression regimen are also unknown. In some cases, PRCA was found to be reversible with dose reduction or cessation of mycophenolate therapy. In transplant patients, however, reduced immunosuppression may place the graft at risk.

➤*GI effects:* GI bleeding (requiring hospitalization) has been observed in approximately 3% of renal, 1.7% of cardiac, and 5.4% of hepatic transplant patients treated with mycophenolate 3 g daily. In pediatric renal transplant patients, 5 of 148 cases of GI bleeding (requiring hospitalization) were observed.

GI perforations have been observed rarely. Most patients receiving mycophenolate were also receiving other drugs known to be associated with these complications. Patients with active peptic ulcer disease were excluded from enrollment in studies with mycophenolate. Because mycophenolate has been associated with an increased incidence of digestive system adverse reactions, including infrequent cases of GI tract ulceration, hemorrhage, and perforation, administer mycophenolate with caution in patients with active serious digestive system disease.

➤*Rare hereditary deficiency:* On theoretical grounds, because mycophenolate is an IMPDH inhibitor, avoid its use in patients with rare hereditary hypoxanthine-guanine phosphoribosyltransferase (HGPRT) deficiency, such as Lesch-Nyhan and Kelley-Seegmiller syndrome.

➤*Vaccines:* During treatment with mycophenolate, avoid the use of live, attenuated vaccines and advise patients that vaccinations may be less effective.

➤*Phenylketonurics:* Mycophenolate oral suspension contains aspartame, a source of phenylalanine (phenylalanine 0.56 mg/mL of suspension). Therefore, take care if mycophenolate oral suspension is administered to patients with phenylketonuria.

➤*Renal function impairment:* Patients with severe chronic renal impairment (GFR less than 25 mL/min/1.73 m^2) who have received single doses of mycophenolate showed higher plasma mycophenolic acid and mycophenolic acid glucuronate AUCs relative to subjects with lesser degrees of renal impairment or healthy volunteers. No data are available on the safety of long-term exposure to these levels of mycophenolic acid glucuronate. Avoid doses of more than 1 g of mycophenolate twice daily in renal transplant patients and carefully observe these patients.

No data are available for cardiac or hepatic transplant patients with severe chronic renal impairment. Mycophenolate may be used for cardiac or hepatic transplant patients with severe chronic renal impairment if the potential benefits outweigh the potential risks.

In the 3 controlled studies of prevention of renal rejection, 20% of patients had delayed graft function. Although patients with delayed graft function have a higher incidence of certain adverse reactions (eg, anemia, hyperkalemia, thrombocytopenia) than patients without delayed graft function, these events were not more frequent in patients receiving mycophenolate than azathioprine or placebo. No dosage adjustment is recommended for these patients; however, carefully observe them.

➤*Pregnancy: Category D.* It is not known if mycophenolate mofetil or mycophenolic acid cross the human placenta to the fetus. The molecular weight of mycophenolate (about 434) is low enough that exposure of the embryo and fetus probably occurs. Mycophenolate can cause fetal harm when administered to a pregnant woman. Use of mycophenolate during pregnancy is associated with an increased risk of first trimester pregnancy loss and an increased risk of congenital malformations, especially external ear and other facial abnormalities, including cleft lip and palate, and anomalies of the distal limbs, heart, esophagus, and kidney. In the National Transplantation Pregnancy Registry, there were data on 33 mycophenolate mofetil–exposed pregnancies in 24 transplant patients; there were 15 spontaneous abortions (45%) and 18 live-born infants; 22% of the live-born infants had structural malformations. In postmarketing data (collected from 1995 to 2007) on 77 women exposed to systemic mycophenolate during pregnancy, 25 had spontaneous abortions and 14 had a malformed infant or fetus. Six of 14 malformed offspring had ear abnormalities. Because these postmarketing data are reported voluntarily, it is not always possible to reliably estimate the frequency of particular adverse outcomes. The malformations seen in these offspring were similar to findings in animal reproductive toxicology studies. For comparison, the background rate for congenital abnormalities in the United States is about 3% and National Transplantation Pregnancy Registry data show a rate of 4% to 5% among babies born to organ transplant patients using other immunosuppressive drugs.

In animal reproductive toxicology studies, there were increased rates of fetal resorptions and malformations in the absence of maternal toxicity. Female rats and rabbits received mycophenolate doses equivalent to 0.02 and 0.9 times the recommended human dose for renal and cardiac transplant patients, based on BSA conversions. In rat offspring, malformations included agnathia, anophthalmia, and hydrocephaly. In rabbit offspring, malformations included ectopia cordis, ectopic kidneys, diaphragmatic hernia, and umbilical hernia.

If this drug is used during pregnancy or if the patient becomes pregnant while taking this drug, apprise the patient of the potential hazard to the fetus. In certain situations, the patient and her health care provider may decide that the maternal benefits outweigh the risks to the fetus. Encourage women using mycophenolate at any time during pregnancy to enroll in the National Transplantation Pregnancy Registry.

Advise women of childbearing potential to have a negative serum or urine pregnancy test with a sensitivity of at least 25 milliunits/mL within 1 week prior to beginning therapy. Do not initiate mycophenolate until a negative pregnancy test report is obtained.

Women of childbearing potential (including pubertal girls and perimenopausal women) taking mycophenolate must receive contraceptive counseling and use effective contraception. Advise the patient to begin using her 2 chosen methods of contraception 4 weeks prior to starting mycophenolate therapy, unless abstinence is the chosen method. She should continue contraceptive use during therapy and for 6 weeks after stopping mycophenolate. Patients should be aware that mycophenolate reduces blood levels of the hormones in the oral contraceptive pill and could theoretically reduce its effectiveness.

➤*Lactation:* Studies in rats treated with mycophenolate have shown mycophenolic acid to be excreted in milk. It is not known whether this drug is excreted in human milk. The molecular weight of the prodrug mycophenolate (about 434) is low enough that passage of mycophenolate and/or mycophenolic acid into breast milk should be expected. Because many drugs are excreted in human milk, and because of the potential for serious adverse reactions in breast-feeding infants from mycophenolate, decide whether to discontinue breast-feeding or the drug, taking into account the importance of the drug to the mother.

➤*Children:* Safety and efficacy in children receiving allogeneic cardiac or hepatic transplants or in renal transplantation children younger than 3 months of age have not been established.

➤*Elderly:* In general, use cautious dosage selection for an elderly patient, reflecting the greater frequency of decreased hepatic, renal, or cardiac function and of concomitant or other drug therapy. Elderly patients may be at an increased risk of adverse reactions compared with younger individuals.

Elderly patients (65 years of age and older), particularly those who are receiving mycophenolate as part of a combination immunosuppressive regimen, may be at increased risk of certain infections (including cytomegalovirus tissue-invasive disease) and possibly GI hemorrhage and pulmonary edema, compared with younger individuals.

➤*Monitoring:* Perform complete blood cell counts weekly during the first month, twice monthly for the second and third months of treatment, then monthly through the first year. Monitor patients for signs and symptoms of bacterial, viral, or fungal infections, and for signs and symptoms of organ rejection. Monitor neurological status as needed. Carefully follow patients with severe chronic renal impairment (GFR less than 25 mL/min/1.73 m^2 BSA) for potential adverse reactions.

Drug Interactions

➤*Drugs that alter the GI flora:* Drugs that alter the GI flora may interact with mycophenolate by disrupting enterohepatic recirculation. Interference of mycophenolic acid glucuronide hydrolysis may lead to less mycophenolic acid available for absorption.

➤*Vaccines:* See Warnings/Precautions for more information. Influenza vaccination may be of value. Refer to national guidelines for influenza vaccination.

Mycophenolate Mofetil Oral Drug Interactions

Precipitant drug	Object drug[a]		Description
Acyclovir, ganciclovir, valacyclovir	Mycophenolate	⬆	Mycophenolic acid glucuronide and acyclovir plasma AUCs were increased 10.6% and 21.9%, respectively. Because mycophenolic acid glucuronide plasma concentrations are increased in the presence of renal impairment, as are acyclovir, ganciclovir, and valacyclovir concentrations, the potential exists for these drugs to compete for tubular secretion, further increasing the concentrations of these drugs. Carefully monitor patients with renal impairment when these agents are coadministered.
Mycophenolate	Acyclovir, ganciclovir, valacyclovir		
Antacids	Mycophenolate	⬇	Absorption of a single mycophenolate dose was decreased when coadministered with an aluminum/magnesium hydroxide antacid. The C_{max} and AUC for mycophenolic acid were 33% and 17% lower, respectively, than when mycophenolate was given alone. Avoid coadministration.

MYCOPHENOLATE MOFETIL — ORAL

Mycophenolate Mofetil Oral Drug Interactions			
Precipitant drug	Object drug[a]		Description
Amoxicillin plus clavulanic acid	Mycophenolate	↓	Mycophenolic acid concentrations were reduced approximately 50% 3 days after the start of amoxicillin plus clavulanic acid. The decrease tended to diminish within 14 days of starting the antibiotic and ceased within 3 days of stopping the antibiotic. The suspected mechanism is decreased mycophenolic acid enterohepatic recirculation. The clinical importance of this change is not known. Monitor the response of the patient. If an interaction is suspected, adjust the mycophenolate dose as needed.
Azathioprine	Mycophenolate	↔	Avoid concomitant use because of a potentially increased risk of bone marrow suppression.
Cholestyramine	Mycophenolate	↓	Following coadministration, mycophenolic acid AUC decreased ≈ 40%. Do not give with cholestyramine or agents that may interfere with enterohepatic recirculation.
Ciprofloxacin	Mycophenolate	↓	Mycophenolic acid concentrations were reduced ≈ 50% 3 days after the start of ciprofloxacin. The decrease tended to diminish within 14 days of starting ciprofloxacin and ceased within 3 days of stopping the antibiotic. The suspected mechanism is decreased mycophenolic acid enterohepatic recirculation. The clinical importance of this change is not known. Monitor the response of the patient. If an interaction is suspected, adjust the mycophenolate dose as needed.
Cyclosporine	Mycophenolate	↓	Coadministration may reduce enterohepatic recirculation of mycophenolate. Monitor mycophenolic acid concentrations and response to therapy. Adjust the mycophenolate dose as needed.
Immunosuppressive agents (eg, sirolimus, tacrolimus)	Mycophenolate	↑	Mycophenolic acid trough plasma concentrations may be elevated, increasing the risk of adverse reactions. Monitor plasma mycophenolate levels and adjust dose as needed.
Iron	Mycophenolate	↓	Following coadministration, mycophenolate absorption and mycophenolic acid AUC were significantly decreased. Avoid coadministration.
Metronidazole, Norfloxacin	Mycophenolate	↓	Coadministration may reduce plasma concentrations of mycophenolic acid, if metronidazole and norfloxacin are coadministered. Avoid coadministration.
Probenecid	Mycophenolate	↑	In animals, coadministration resulted in a 3-fold increase in plasma mycophenolic acid glucuronide AUC and a 2-fold increase in plasma mycophenolic acid AUC.
Rifamycins (eg, rifabutin, rifampin)	Mycophenolate	↓	Rifamycins may reduce mycophenolic acid plasma concentrations. Closely monitor mycophenolic acid concentrations and adjust the dose as needed. Coadministration of rifampin and mycophenolate is not recommended.
Salicylates	Mycophenolate	↑	Coadministration increased the free fraction of mycophenolic acid.
Sevelamer	Mycophenolate	↓	Sevelamer may decrease the plasma concentrations of mycophenolic acid. Administer sevelamer 2 hours after mycophenolate.
Mycophenolate	Contraceptives, hormonal	↓	Coadministration of mycophenolate and hormonal contraceptives containing levonorgestrel produced a significant decrease in the levonorgestrel AUC by ≈ 15%. Mean serum levels of luteinizing hormone, follicle-stimulating hormone, and progesterone were not significantly affected. Administer with caution and consider additional birth control methods.
Mycophenolate	Phenytoin	↑	Mycophenolic acid decreased protein binding of phenytoin and may, therefore, increase free phenytoin levels.
Mycophenolate	Theophylline	↑	Mycophenolic acid decreased protein binding of theophylline and may, therefore, increase free theophylline levels.

[a] ↑ = object drug increased; ↓ = object drug decreased; ↔ = undetermined clinical effect.

➤*Drug/Food interactions:* Mycophenolic acid C_{max} was decreased by 40% in the presence of food.

Adverse Reactions

Mycophenolate Mofetil Oral Adverse Reactions (≥ 20%)							
	Renal studies			Cardiac study		Hepatic study	
Adverse reactions	Mycophenolate 2 g/day (n = 336)	Mycophenolate 3 g/day (n = 330)	Azathioprine 1 to 2 mg/kg/day or 100 to 150 mg/day (n = 326)	Mycophenolate 3 g/day (n = 289)	Azathioprine 1.5 to 3 mg/kg/day (n = 289)	Mycophenolate 3 g/day (n = 277)	Azathioprine 1 to 2 mg/kg/day (n = 287)
Cardiovascular							
Cardiovascular disorder	—	—	—	25.6%	24.2%	—	—
Hypertension	32.4%	28.2%	32.2%	77.5%	72.3%	62.1%	59.6%
Hypotension	—	—	—	32.5%	36%	—	—
Tachycardia	—	—	—	20.1%	18%	22%	15.7%
CNS							
Anxiety	—	—	—	28.4%	23.9%	—	—
Asthenia	—	—	—	43.3%	36.3%	35.4%	33.8%
Dizziness	—	—	—	28.7%	27.7%	—	—
Headache	21.1%	16.1%	21.2%	54.3%	51.9%	53.8%	49.1%
Insomnia	—	—	—	40.8%	37.7%	52.3%	47%

MYCOPHENOLATE MOFETIL — ORAL

Mycophenolate Mofetil Oral Adverse Reactions (≥ 20%)							
	Renal studies			Cardiac study		Hepatic study	
Adverse reactions	Mycophenolate 2 g/day (n = 336)	Mycophenolate 3 g/day (n = 330)	Azathioprine 1 to 2 mg/kg/day or 100 to 150 mg/day (n = 326)	Mycophenolate 3 g/day (n = 289)	Azathioprine 1.5 to 3 mg/kg/day (n = 289)	Mycophenolate 3 g/day (n = 277)	Azathioprine 1 to 2 mg/kg/day (n = 287)
Paresthesia	—	—	—	20.8%	18%	—	—
Tremor	—	—	—	24.2%	23.9%	33.9%	35.5%
GI							
Abdominal pain	24.7%	27.6%	23%	33.9%	33.2%	62.5%	51.2%
Anorexia	—	—	—	—	—	25.3%	17.1%
Ascites	—	—	—	—	—	24.2%	22.6%
Constipation	22.9%	18.5%	22.4%	41.2%	37.7%	37.9%	38.3%
Diarrhea	31%	36.1%	20.9%	45.3%	34.3%	51.3%	49.8%
Dyspepsia	—	—	—	—	—	22.4%	20.9%
Liver function tests abnormal	—	—	—	—	—	24.9%	19.2%
Nausea	19.9%	23.6%	24.5%	54%	54.3%	54.5%	51.2%
Vomiting	—	—	—	33.9%	28.4%	32.9%	33.4%
GU							
Kidney function abnormal	—	—	—	21.8%	26.3%	25.6%	28.9%
Urinary tract infection	37.2%	37%	33.7%	—	—	—	—
Hematologic/Lymphatic							
Anemia	25.6%	25.8%	23.6%	42.9%	43.9%	43%	53%
Hypochromic anemia	—	—	—	24.6%	23.5%	—	—
Leukocytosis	—	—	—	40.5%	35.6%	22.4%	21.3%
Leukopenia	23.2%	34.5%	24.8%	30.4%	39.1%	45.8%	39%
Thrombocytopenia	—	—	—	23.5%	27%	38.3%	42.2%
Metabolic/Nutritional							
Creatinine increased	—	—	—	39.4%	36%	—	—
Edema	—	—	—	26.6%	25.6%	28.2%	28.2%
Hypercholesterolemia	—	—	—	41.2%	38.4%	—	—
Hyperglycemia	—	—	—	46.7%	52.6%	43.7%	48.8%
Hyperkalemia	—	—	—	—	—	22%	23.7%
Hypocalcemia	—	—	—	—	—	30%	30%
Hypokalemia	—	—	—	31.8%	25.6%	37.2%	41.1%
Hypomagnesemia	—	—	—	—	—	39%	37.6%
Lactic dehydrogenase increased	—	—	—	23.2%	17%	—	—
Peripheral edema	28.6%	27%	28.2%	64%	53.3%	48.4%	47.7%
Serum urea nitrogen (BUN) increased	—	—	—	34.6%	32.5%	—	—
Respiratory							
Cough increased	—	—	—	31.1%	25.6%	—	—
Dyspnea	—	—	—	36.7%	36.3%	31%	30.3%
Infection	22%	23.9%	19.6%	37%	35.3%	—	—
Lung disorder	—	—	—	30.1%	29.1%	22%	18.8%
Pleural effusion	—	—	—	—	—	34.3%	35.9%
Sinusitis	—	—	—	26%	19%	—	—
Miscellaneous							
Back pain	—	—	—	34.6%	28.4%	46.6%	47.4%
Chest pain	—	—	—	26.3%	26%	—	—
Fever	21.4%	23.3%	23.3%	47.4%	46.4%	52.3%	56.1%
Infection	18.2%	20.9%	19.9%	25.6%	19.4%	27.1%	25.1%
Pain	33%	31.2%	32.2%	75.8%	74.7%	74%	77.7%
Rash	—	—	—	22.1%	18%	—	—
Sepsis	—	—	—	—	—	27.4%	26.5%

➤*Lymphomas/Malignancies:* Patients receiving mycophenolate alone or as part of an immunosuppressive regimen are at increased risk of developing lymphomas and other malignancies, particularly of the skin. The incidence of malignancies among the 1,483 patients treated in controlled trials for the prevention of renal allograft rejection who were followed for 1 year or more was similar to the incidence reported in the literature for renal allograft recipients.

Lymphoproliferative disease or lymphoma developed in 0.4% to 1% of patients receiving mycophenolate (2 or 3 g daily) with other immunosuppressive agents in controlled clinical trials of renal, cardiac, and hepatic transplant patients followed for at least 1 year. Nonmelanoma skin carcinomas occurred in 1.6% to 4.2% of patients; other types of malignancy occurred in 0.7% to 2.1% of patients. Three-year safety data in renal and cardiac transplant patients did not reveal any unexpected changes in the incidence of malignancy compared with the 1-year data.

➤*Neutropenia:* See Warnings/Precautions for more information.

➤*Infections:* All transplant patients are at increased risk of opportunistic infections. The risk increases with total immunosuppressive load.

MYCOPHENOLATE MOFETIL — ORAL

Mycophenolate Mofetil Oral Viral and Fungal Infections							
	Renal studies			Cardiac study		Hepatic study	
Infections	Mycophenolate 2 g/day (n = 336)	Mycophenolate 3 g/day (n = 330)	Azathioprine 1 to 2 mg/kg/day or 100 to 150 mg/day (n = 326)	Mycophenolate 3 g/day (n = 289)	Azathioprine 1.5 to 3 mg/kg/day (n = 289)	Mycophenolate 3 g/day (n = 277)	Azathioprine 1 to 2 mg/kg/day (n = 287)
Candida	17%	17.3%	18.1%	18.7%	17.6%	22.4%	24.4%
Mucocutaneous	15.5%	16.4%	15.3%	18%	17.3%	18.4%	17.4%
Cytomegalovirus							
Viremia/Syndrome	13.4%	12.4%	13.8%	12.1%	10%	14.1%	12.2%
Tissue-invasive disease	8.3%	11.5%	6.1%	11.4%	8.7%	5.8%	8%
Herpes simplex	16.7%	20%	19%	20.8%	14.5%	10.1%	5.9%
Herpes zoster	6%	7.6%	5.8%	10.7%	5.9%	4.3%	4.9%
Cutaneous disease	6%	7.3%	5.5%	10%	5.5%	4.3%	4.9%

The following other opportunistic infections occurred with an incidence of less than 4% in mycophenolate patients in the previously described azathioprine-controlled studies: herpes zoster, visceral disease; *Candida*, urinary tract infection, fungemia/disseminated disease, tissue-invasive disease; cryptococcosis; *Aspergillus/Mucor*; *Pneumocystis carinii*.

In patients receiving mycophenolate (2 or 3 g) in controlled studies for prevention of renal, cardiac, or hepatic rejection, fatal infection/sepsis occurred in approximately 2% of renal and cardiac patients and in 5% of hepatic patients.

In cardiac transplant patients, the overall incidence of opportunistic infections was approximately 10% higher in patients treated with mycophenolate than in those receiving azathioprine, but this difference was not associated with excess mortality due to infection/sepsis among patients treated with mycophenolate.

➤*Other adverse reactions (3% to less than 20%):*

Mycophenolate Mofetil Oral Adverse Reactions (3% to < 20%) in Combination With Cyclosporine and Corticosteroids	
Body system	Adverse reaction
Cardiovascular	Angina pectoris, arrhythmia, arterial thrombosis, atrial fibrillation, atrial flutter, bradycardia, cardiovascular disorder, congestive heart failure, extrasystole, heart arrest, heart failure, hypotension, pallor, palpitation, pericardial effusion, peripheral vascular disorder, postural hypotension, pulmonary hypertension, supraventricular extrasystoles, supraventricular tachycardia, syncope, tachycardia, thrombosis, vasodilation, vasospasm, ventricular extrasystole, ventricular tachycardia, venous pressure increased
CNS	Agitation, anxiety, confusion, convulsion, delirium, depression, emotional lability, hallucinations, hypertonia, hypesthesia, nervousness, neuropathy, paresthesia, psychosis, somnolence, thinking abnormal, vertigo
Dermatologic	Acne, alopecia, cellulitis, fungal dermatitis, hemorrhage, hirsutism, pruritus, rash, skin carcinoma, skin disorder, skin hypertrophy, skin neoplasm benign, skin ulcer, sweating, vesiculobullous rash
Endocrine	Cushing syndrome, diabetes mellitus, hypothyroidism, parathyroid disorder
GI	Anorexia, cholangitis, cholestatic jaundice, dry mouth, dysphagia, esophagitis, flatulence, gastritis, gastroenteritis, GI disorder, GI hemorrhage, GI moniliasis, gingivitis, gum hyperplasia, hepatitis, hernia, ileus, infection, jaundice, liver damage, liver function tests abnormal, melena, mouth ulceration, nausea and vomiting, oral moniliasis, peritonitis, rectal disorder, stomach ulcer, stomatitis
GU	Acute kidney failure, albuminuria, dysuria, hematuria, hydronephrosis, impotence, kidney failure, kidney tubular necrosis, nocturia, oliguria, pain, pelvic pain, prostatic disorder, pyelonephritis, scrotal edema, urinary frequency, urinary incontinence, urinary retention, urinary tract disorder, urine abnormality
Hematologic/Lymphatic	Coagulation disorder, ecchymosis, pancytopenia, petechia, polycythemia, prothrombin time increased, thromboplastin time increased

Mycophenolate Mofetil Oral Adverse Reactions (3% to < 20%) in Combination With Cyclosporine and Corticosteroids	
Body system	Adverse reaction
Metabolic/Nutritional	Abnormal healing, acidosis, alkaline phosphatase increased, alkalosis, ALT increased, AST increased, bilirubinemia, creatinine increased, dehydration, gamma-glutamyl transpeptidase increased, generalized edema, gout, hypercalcemia, hypercholesteremia, hyperlipemia, hyperphosphatemia, hyperuricemia, hypervolemia, hypocalcemia, hypochloremia, hypoglycemia, hyponatremia, hypophosphatemia, hypoproteinemia, hypovolemia, hypoxia, lactic dehydrogenase increased, respiratory acidosis, thirst, weight gain, weight loss
Musculoskeletal	Arthralgia, joint disorder, leg cramps, myalgia, myasthenia, neck pain, osteoporosis
Respiratory	Apnea, asthma, atelectasis, bronchitis, epistaxis, hemoptysis, hiccup, hyperventilation, lung disorder, lung edema, neoplasm, pain, pharyngitis, pleural effusion, pneumonia, pneumothorax, respiratory disorder, respiratory moniliasis, rhinitis, sinusitis, sputum increased, voice alteration
Special senses	Abnormal vision, amblyopia, cataract (not specified), conjunctivitis, deafness, ear disorder, ear pain, eye hemorrhage, lacrimation disorder, tinnitus
Miscellaneous	Abdomen enlarged, abscess, accidental injury, chills occurring with fever, cyst, face edema, flu syndrome, hemorrhage, lab test abnormal, malaise

➤*Children:* The type and frequency of adverse reactions in a clinical study of 100 children 3 months to 18 years of age dosed with mycophenolate oral suspension 600 mg/m^2 twice daily (up to 1 g twice daily) were generally similar to those observed in adult patients dosed with mycophenolate capsules at a dose of 1 g twice daily, with the exception of abdominal pain, anemia, diarrhea, fever, hypertension, infection, leukopenia, pain, pharyngitis, respiratory tract infection, sepsis, and vomiting, which were observed in a higher proportion in children.

➤*Postmarketing:*

GI – Colitis (sometimes caused by cytomegalovirus), isolated cases of intestinal villous atrophy, pancreatitis.

Hematologic/Lymphatic – Cases of PRCA have been reported in patients treated with mycophenolate in combination with other immunosuppressive agents.

Respiratory – Interstitial lung disorders, including fatal pulmonary fibrosis, have been reported rarely and should be considered in the differential diagnosis of pulmonary symptoms, ranging from dyspnea to respiratory failure in posttransplant patients receiving mycophenolate.

Miscellaneous – Serious life-threatening infections, such as meningitis and infectious endocarditis, have been reported occasionally. There is evidence of a higher frequency of certain types of serious infections, such as tuberculosis and atypical mycobacterial infection. Cases of PML, sometimes fatal, have been reported in patients treated with mycophenolate. The reported cases generally had risk factors for PML, including treatment with immunosuppressant therapies and impairment of immune function. BK virus–associated nephropathy has been observed in patients receiving immunosuppressants, including mycophenolate. This infection is associated with serious outcomes, including deteriorating renal function and renal graft loss.

Congenital malformations, including ear malformations, have been reported in offspring of patients exposed to mycophenolate during pregnancy.

MYCOPHENOLATE MOFETIL — ORAL

Overdosage

➤*Symptoms:* The experience with overdose of mycophenolate in humans is very limited. The events received from reports of overdose fall within the known safety profile of the drug. The highest dosage administered to renal transplant patients in clinical trials has been 4 g/day. In limited experience with cardiac and hepatic transplant patients in clinical trials, the highest dosages used were 4 or 5 g/day. At dosages of 4 or 5 g/day, there appears to be a higher rate (compared with the use of 3 g/day or less) of GI intolerance (eg, diarrhea, nausea, vomiting), and occasional hematologic abnormalities, principally neutropenia, leading to a need to reduce or discontinue dosing.

➤*Treatment:* Mycophenolic acid and mycophenolic acid glucuronate are usually not removed by hemodialysis. However, at high mycophenolic acid glucuronate plasma concentrations (more than 100 mcg/mL), small amounts of mycophenolic acid glucuronate are removed. By increasing excretion of the drug, mycophenolic acid can be removed by bile acid sequestrants (eg, cholestyramine).

Patient Information

Instruct patients or their caregivers to read the Medication Guide before stating therapy and to reread it with each refill.

Inform patients of the need for repeated appropriate laboratory tests while they are receiving mycophenolate.

Give patients complete dosage instructions and inform them of the increased risk of lymphoproliferative disease and certain other malignancies.

Inform women of childbearing potential that use of mycophenolate in pregnancy is associated with an increased risk of first trimester pregnancy loss and an increased risk of birth defects, and that they must use effective contraception. Discuss pregnancy plans with women of childbearing potential.

Any woman of childbearing potential must use highly effective (2 methods) contraception 4 weeks prior to starting mycophenolate therapy and continue contraception until 6 weeks after stopping mycophenolate treatment, unless abstinence is the chosen method. A patient who is planning a pregnancy should not use mycophenolate unless she cannot be successfully treated with other immunosuppressant drugs.

Instruct patients receiving mycophenolate to report immediately any evidence of infection, unexpected bruising, bleeding, or any other manifestation of bone marrow depression.

Advise patients with increased risk for skin cancer to limit exposure to sunlight and ultraviolet light by wearing protective clothing and using sunscreen with a high protection factor.

Advise phenylketonuric patients that the oral suspension contains aspartame, a source of phenylalanine (phenylalanine 0.56 mg/mL of suspension).

MYCOPHENOLATE MOFETIL HYDROCHLORIDE — INJECTION

WARNING

Immunosuppression may lead to increased susceptibility to infection and the possible development of lymphoma. Only health care providers experienced in immunosuppressive therapy and management of renal, cardiac, or hepatic transplant patients should use mycophenolate. Manage patients receiving the drug in facilities equipped and staffed with adequate laboratory and supportive medical resources. The health care provider responsible for maintenance therapy should have complete information requisite for the follow-up of the patient.

Female users of childbearing potential must use contraception. Use of mycophenolate during pregnancy is associated with increased risk of miscarriage and congenital malformations.

Indications

➤*Renal, cardiac, and hepatic transplantation:* For the prophylaxis of organ rejection in patients receiving allogeneic renal, cardiac, or hepatic transplants. Use mycophenolate concomitantly with cyclosporine and corticosteroids.

➤*Off-label uses:* Refractory uveitis (2 g/day alone or in combination with previous corticosteroid, cyclosporine, or tacrolimus therapy); second-line therapy for Churg-Strauss syndrome; in combination with prednisolone for the treatment of diffuse proliferative lupus nephritis.

Administration and Dosage

➤*General dosing considerations:* Mycophenolate intravenous (IV) is an alternative dosage form to mycophenolate oral recommended for patients unable to take oral mycophenolate.

Mycophenolate IV can be administered for up to 14 days; patients should be switched to oral mycophenolate as soon as they can tolerate oral medication.

➤*Adults:*

Cardiac transplantation – 1.5 g twice a day IV (over no less than 2 hours).

Hepatic transplantation – 1 g twice a day IV (over no less than 2 hours).

Renal transplantation – 1 g twice a day IV (over no less than 2 hours).

➤*Renal function impairment:* In renal transplant patients with severe chronic renal impairment (glomerular filtration rate [GFR] less than 25 mL/min/1.73 m^2) outside the immediate posttransplant period, avoid doses of mycophenolate greater than 1 g administered twice a day. Carefully observe these patients.

➤*Neutropenia:* If neutropenia develops (absolute neutrophil count [ANC] less than 1.3×10^3/mcL), interrupt dosing or reduce the dosage of mycophenolate, perform appropriate diagnostic tests, and manage the patient appropriately.

➤*Preparation for administration:* Reconstitute and dilute mycophenolate to a concentration of 6 mg/mL using dextrose 5% injection.

Reconstitution – Two vials of mycophenolate are used for preparing each 1 g dose, whereas 3 vials are needed for each 1.5 g dose. Reconstitute the contents of each vial by injecting 14 mL of dextrose 5% injection. Gently shake the vial to dissolve the drug.

Dilution – To prepare a 1 g dose, further dilute the contents of the 2 reconstituted vials (approximately 2 × 15 mL) into 140 mL of dextrose 5% injection. To prepare a 1.5 g dose, further dilute the contents of the 3 reconstituted vials (approximately 3 × 15 mL) into 210 mL of dextrose 5% injection. The final concentration of both solutions is mycophenolate 6 mg/mL.

➤*Administration:* Following reconstitution, administer by slow IV infusion over a period of no less than 2 hours by either peripheral or central vein. Never administer by rapid or bolus IV injection. Administer within 24 hours of transplantation.

➤*Admixture compatibility:* Mycophenolate is incompatible with other IV infusion solutions. Do not administer mycophenolate or coadminister via the same infusion catheter with other IV drugs or infusion admixtures.

➤*Storage/Stability:* Store powder and reconstituted/infusion solutions at 25°C (77°F); excursions are permitted between 15° and 30°C (59° and 86°F). If the infusion solution is not prepared immediately prior to administration, commence administration of the infusion solution within 4 hours from reconstitution and dilution of the drug product.

Handling/Disposal – Exercise caution in the handling and preparation of solutions of mycophenolate. Avoid direct contact of the prepared solution of mycophenolate with skin or mucous membranes. If such contact occurs, wash thoroughly with soap and water; rinse eyes with plain water.

Actions

➤*Pharmacology:* Mycophenolic acid, the hydrolyzed form of mycophenolate, is a potent, selective, uncompetitive, and reversible inhibitor of inosine monophosphate dehydrogenase (IMPDH), and, therefore, inhibits the de novo pathway of guanosine nucleotide synthesis without incorporation into DNA. Because T- and B-lymphocytes are critically dependent for their proliferation on de novo synthesis of purines, whereas other cell types can utilize salvage pathways, mycophenolic acid has potent cytostatic effects on lymphocytes. Mycophenolic acid inhibits proliferative responses of T- and B-lymphocytes to both mitogenic and allospecific stimulation. Addition of guanosine or deoxyguanosine reverses the cytostatic effects of mycophenolic acid on lymphocytes. Mycophenolic acid also suppresses antibody formation by B-lymphocytes. Mycophenolic acid prevents the glycosylation of lymphocyte and monocyte glycoproteins that are involved in intercellular adhesion to endothelial cells and may inhibit recruitment of leukocytes into sites of inflammation and graft rejection. Mycophenolate did not inhibit early events in the activation of human peripheral blood mononuclear cells, such as the production of interleukin-1 (IL-1) and interleukin-2 (IL-2), but did block the coupling of these events to DNA synthesis and proliferation.

➤*Pharmacokinetics:*

Renal, cardiac, and hepatic transplant patients –

Mycophenolic Acid Pharmacokinetic Parameters (Mean ± SD)[a]

Parameter	Dose/Route	T_{max} (h)	C_{max} (mcg/mL)	AUC (mcg•h/mL)
Healthy volunteers (single dose)	1 g/oral	0.8 (± 0.36) (n = 129)	24.5 (± 9.5) (n = 129)	63.9 (± 16.2) (n = 117)
Renal transplant patients (twice-daily dosing) Time after transplantation				
5 days (n = 31)	1 g/IV	1.58 (± 0.46)	12 (± 3.82)	40.8 (± 11.4)[b]
6 days (n = 31)	1 g/oral	1.33 (± 1.05)	10.7 (± 4.83)	32.9 (± 15)[b]
Early (< 40 days) (n = 25)	1 g/oral	1.31 (± 0.76)	8.16 (± 4.5)	27.3 (± 10.9)[b]
Early (< 40 days) (n = 27)	1.5 g/oral	1.21 (± 0.81)	13.5 (± 8.18)	38.4 (± 15.4)[b]
Late (> 3 months) (n = 23)	1.5 g/oral	0.9 (± 0.24)	24.1 (± 12.1)	65.3 (± 35.4)[b]
Cardiac transplant patients (twice-daily dosing) Time after transplantation				
Early (day before discharge)	1.5 g/oral	1.8 (± 1.3) (n = 11)	11.5 (± 6.8) (n = 11)	43.3 (± 20.8)[b] (n = 9)
Late (> 6 months)	1.5 g/oral	1.1 (± 0.7) (n = 52)	20 (± 9.4) (n = 52)	54.1 (± 20.4)[c] (n = 49)
Hepatic transplant patients (twice-daily dosing) Time after transplantation				
4 to 9 days (n = 22)	1 g/IV	1.5 (± 0.517)	17 (± 12.7)	34 (± 17.4)[b]

MYCOPHENOLATE MOFETIL HYDROCHLORIDE — INJECTION

Mycophenolic Acid Pharmacokinetic Parameters (Mean ± SD)[a]				
Parameter	Dose/Route	T_{max} (h)	C_{max} (mcg/mL)	AUC (mcg•h/mL)
Early (5 to 8 days) (n = 20)	1.5 g/oral	1.15 (± 0.432)	13.1 (± 6.76)	29.2 (± 11.9)[b]
Late (> 6 months) (n = 6)	1.5 g/oral	1.54 (± 0.51)	19.3 (± 11.7)	49.3 (± 14.8)[b]

[a] SD = standard deviation; T_{max} = time of maximal concentration; C_{max} = maximal drug concentration; AUC = area under the curve.
[b] Interdosing interval AUC_{0-12h}.
[c] AUC_{0-12h} values quoted are extrapolated from data from samples collected over 4 hours.

Absorption – Following IV administration, mycophenolate undergoes rapid and complete metabolism to mycophenolic acid, the active metabolite. The parent drug, mycophenolate mofetil, can be measured systemically during IV infusion; however, shortly (approximately 5 minutes) after the infusion is stopped, mycophenolate mofetil concentration is below the limit of quantitation (0.4 mcg/mL).

In 12 healthy volunteers, the mean absolute bioavailability of oral mycophenolate relative to IV mycophenolate mofetil (based on mycophenolic acid AUC) was 94%. The AUC for mycophenolic acid appears to increase in a dose-proportional fashion in renal transplant patients receiving multiple doses of mycophenolate mofetil up to a daily dosage of 3 g.

Secondary peaks in the plasma mycophenolic acid concentration-time profile are usually observed 6 to 12 hours postdose. The coadministration of cholestyramine (4 g 3 times daily) resulted in approximately a 40% decrease in the mycophenolic acid AUC (largely as a consequence of lower concentrations in the terminal portion of the profile). These observations suggest that enterohepatic recirculation contributes to mycophenolic acid plasma concentrations.

Distribution – The mean (± SD) apparent volume of distribution of mycophenolic acid in 12 healthy volunteers is approximately 3.6 (± 1.5) L/kg following IV administration. Mycophenolic acid, at clinically relevant concentrations, is 97% bound to plasma albumin. Mycophenolic acid glucuronide is 82% bound to plasma albumin at mycophenolic acid glucuronide concentration ranges that are normally seen in stable renal transplant patients; however, at higher mycophenolic acid glucuronide concentrations (observed in patients with renal impairment or delayed graft function), the binding of mycophenolic acid may be reduced as a result of competition between mycophenolic acid glucuronide and mycophenolic acid for protein binding. Mean blood-to-plasma ratio of radioactivity concentrations was approximately 0.6, indicating that mycophenolic acid and mycophenolic acid glucuronide do not distribute extensively into the cellular fractions of blood.

Metabolism – Following IV administration, mycophenolate undergoes complete metabolism to mycophenolic acid, the active metabolite. Mycophenolic acid is metabolized principally by glucuronyl transferase to form the phenolic glucuronide of mycophenolic acid (mycophenolic acid glucuronide) which is not pharmacologically active. In vivo, mycophenolic acid glucuronide is converted to mycophenolic acid via enterohepatic recirculation.

Excretion – A negligible amount of the drug is excreted as mycophenolic acid (less than 1% of dose) in the urine. Oral radiolabeled mycophenolate resulted in complete recovery of the administered dose, with 93% of the administered dose recovered in the urine and 6% recovered in feces. Most (approximately 87%) of the administered dose is excreted in the urine as mycophenolic acid glucuronide. At clinically encountered concentrations, mycophenolic acid and mycophenolic acid glucuronide are usually not removed by hemodialysis. However, at high mycophenolic acid glucuronide plasma concentrations (more than 100 mcg/mL), small amounts of mycophenolic acid glucuronide are removed. Bile acid sequestrants, such as cholestyramine, reduce mycophenolic acid AUC by interfering with enterohepatic circulation of the drug.

Mean (± SD) apparent half-life and plasma clearance of mycophenolic acid are 16.6 (± 5.8) hours and 177 (± 31) mL/min following IV administration, respectively.

Special populations –

Renal function impairment: Increased plasma concentrations of mycophenolate mofetil metabolites (mycophenolic acid 50% increase and mycophenolic acid glucuronide approximately a 3- to 6-fold increase) are observed in patients with renal insufficiency.

In a single-dose study, mycophenolate was administered as an IV infusion over 40 minutes. Plasma mycophenolic acid AUC observed after single-dose (1 g) IV dosing to volunteers (n = 4) with severe chronic renal impairment (GFR less than 25 mL/min/1.73 m^2) was 62.4 mcg•h/mL (± 19.3). Multiple dosing of mycophenolate in patients with severe chronic renal impairment has not been studied.

In 8 patients with primary nonfunction of the organ following renal transplantation, plasma concentrations of mycophenolic acid glucuronide accumulated about 6- to 8-fold after multiple dosing for 28 days. Accumulation of mycophenolic acid was about 1- to 2-fold.

Hepatic function impairment: In a single-dose (1 g) IV study of 6 volunteers with severe hepatic impairment (aminopyrine breath test less than 0.2% of dose) due to alcoholic cirrhosis, mycophenolate was rapidly converted to mycophenolic acid. Mycophenolic acid AUC was 44.1 mcg•h/mL (± 15.5).

Contraindications

Hypersensitivity to mycophenolate, mycophenolic acid, any component of the drug product, or polysorbate 80 (*Tween* 80).

Warnings/Precautions

➤*Lymphomas/Malignancies:* Patients receiving immunosuppressive regimens involving combinations of drugs, including mycophenolate, as part of an immunosuppressive regimen are at increased risk of developing lymphomas and other malignancies, particularly of the skin. The risk appears to be related to the intensity and duration of immunosuppression rather than to the use of any specific agent.

As usual for patients with increased risk for skin cancer, they should limit exposure to sunlight and ultraviolet light by wearing protective clothing and using a sunscreen with a high protection factor.

Lymphoproliferative disease or lymphoma developed in 0.4% to 1% of patients receiving mycophenolate (2 or 3 g) with other immunosuppressive agents in controlled clinical trials of renal, cardiac, and hepatic transplant patients.

➤*Other immunosuppressive agents:* Mycophenolate has been administered in combination with the following agents in clinical trials: antithymocyte globulin, muromonab-CD3, cyclosporine, and corticosteroids. The efficacy and safety of the use of mycophenolate in combination with other immunosuppressive agents have not been determined.

➤*Infection:* Oversuppression of the immune system can also increase susceptibility to infection, including opportunistic infections, fatal infections, and sepsis. In patients receiving mycophenolate (2 or 3 g) in controlled studies for prevention of renal, cardiac, or hepatic rejection, fatal infection/sepsis occurred in approximately 2% of renal and cardiac patients and in 5% of hepatic patients.

In cardiac transplant patients, the overall incidence of opportunistic infections was approximately 10% higher in patients treated with mycophenolate than in those receiving azathioprine therapy, but this difference was not associated with excess mortality due to infection/sepsis among patients treated with mycophenolate.

There were more herpes virus (eg, herpes simplex, herpes zoster, and cytomegalovirus) infections in cardiac transplant patients treated with mycophenolate compared with those treated with azathioprine.

Latent viral infections – Immunosuppressed patients are at increased risk for opportunistic infections, including activation of latent viral infections. These include cases of progressive multifocal leukoencephalopathy (PML) and BK virus–associated nephropathy (BKVAN), which have been observed in patients receiving immunosuppressants, including mycophenolate.

Cases of PML, sometimes fatal, have been reported in patients treated with mycophenolate. Apathy, ataxia, cognitive deficiencies, confusion, and hemiparesis were the most frequent clinical features observed. The reported cases generally had risk factors for PML, including treatment with immunosuppressant therapies and impairment of immune function. In immunosuppressed patients, consider PML in the differential diagnosis in patients reporting neurological symptoms and consider consultation with a neurologist as clinically indicated. Give consideration to reducing the amount of immunosuppression in patients who develop PML. In transplant patients, consider the risk that reduced immunosuppression represents to the graft.

BKVAN is associated with serious outcomes, including deteriorating renal function and renal graft loss. Patient monitoring may help detect patients at risk for BKVAN. Consider reduction in immunosuppression for patients who develop evidence of BKVAN.

➤*Neutropenia:* Severe neutropenia (ANC less than 0.5 × 10^3/mcL) developed in up to 2% of renal, up to 2.8% of cardiac, and up to 3.6% of hepatic transplant patients receiving mycophenolate 3 g daily. Monitor patients receiving mycophenolate for neutropenia. The development of neutropenia may be related to mycophenolate itself, concomitant medications, viral infections, or some combination of these causes. If neutropenia develops (ANC less than 1.3 × 10^3/mcL), interrupt dosing or reduce the dosage of mycophenolate, perform appropriate diagnostic tests, and manage the patient appropriately. Neutropenia has been observed most frequently in the period from 31 to 180 days posttransplant in patients treated for prevention of renal, cardiac, and hepatic rejection.

➤*Pure red cell aplasia:* Cases of pure red cell aplasia (PRCA) have been reported in patients treated with mycophenolate in combination with other immunosuppressive agents. The mechanism for mycophenolate-induced PRCA is unknown; the relative contribution of other immunosuppressants and their combinations in an immunosuppression regimen are also unknown. In some cases, PRCA was found to be reversible with dose reduction or cessation of mycophenolate therapy. In transplant patients, however, reduced immunosuppression may place the graft at risk.

➤*Administration:* Never administer mycophenolate by rapid or bolus IV injection.

➤*GI effects:* GI bleeding (requiring hospitalization) has been observed in approximately 3% of renal, 1.7% of cardiac, and 5.4% of hepatic transplant patients treated with mycophenolate 3 g daily.

GI perforations have been observed rarely. Most patients receiving mycophenolate were also receiving other drugs known to be associated with these complications. Patients with active peptic ulcer disease were excluded from enrollment in studies with mycophenolate. Because mycophenolate has been associated with an increased incidence of digestive system adverse reactions, including infrequent cases of GI tract ulceration, hemorrhage, and

MYCOPHENOLATE MOFETIL HYDROCHLORIDE — INJECTION

perforation, administer mycophenolate with caution in patients with active serious digestive system disease.

➤*Rare hereditary deficiency:* On theoretical grounds, because mycophenolate is an IMPDH inhibitor, avoid use in patients with rare hereditary hypoxanthine-guanine phosphoribosyl-transferase (HGPRT) deficiency , such as Lesch-Nyhan and Kelley-Seegmiller syndrome.

➤*Vaccines:* During treatment with mycophenolate, avoid the use of live, attenuated vaccines and advise patients that vaccinations may be less effective.

➤*Renal function impairment:* Patients with severe chronic renal impairment (GFR less than 25 mL/min/1.73 m^2) who have received single doses of mycophenolate showed higher plasma mycophenolic acid and mycophenolic acid glucuronide AUCs relative to patients with lesser degrees of renal impairment or healthy volunteers. No data are available on the safety of long-term exposure to these levels of mycophenolic acid glucuronide. Avoid doses of mycophenolate more than 1 g twice daily to renal transplant patients, and carefully observe these patients.

No data are available for cardiac or hepatic transplant patients with severe chronic renal impairment. Mycophenolate may be used for cardiac or hepatic transplant patients with severe chronic renal impairment if the potential benefits outweigh the potential risks.

In the 3 controlled studies of prevention of renal rejection, 20% of patients had delayed graft function. Although patients with delayed graft function have a higher incidence of certain adverse reactions (eg, anemia, hyperkalemia, thrombocytopenia) than patients without delayed graft function, these reactions were not more frequent in patients receiving mycophenolate than azathioprine or placebo. No dosage adjustment is recommended; however, carefully observe these patients.

➤*Pregnancy: Category D.* It is not known if mycophenolate mofetil or mycophenolic acid crosses the human placenta to the fetus. The molecular weight of mycophenolate (about 434) is low enough that exposure to the embryo and fetus probably occurs. Mycophenolate can cause fetal harm when administered to a pregnant woman. Use of mycophenolate during pregnancy is associated with an increased risk of first trimester miscarriage and an increased risk of congenital malformations, especially external ear and other facial abnormalities, including cleft lip and palate, and anomalies of the distal limbs, heart, esophagus, and kidney. In the National Transplantation Pregnancy Registry, there were data on 33 mycophenolate-exposed pregnancies in 24 transplant patients; there were 15 spontaneous abortions (45%) and 18 live-born infants. 22% of the live-born infants had structural malformations. In postmarketing data (collected from 1995 to 2007) on 77 women exposed to systemic mycophenolate during pregnancy, 25 had spontaneous abortions and 14 had a malformed infant or fetus. Six of 14 malformed offspring had ear abnormalities. Because these postmarketing data are reported voluntarily, it is not always possible to reliably estimate the frequency of particular adverse outcomes. The malformations seen in these offspring were similar to findings in animal reproductive toxicology studies. For comparison, the background rate for congenital abnormalities in the United States is about 3%, and National Transplantation Pregnancy Registry data show a rate of 4% to 5% among babies born to organ transplant patients using other immunosuppressive drugs.

In animal reproductive toxicology studies, there were increased rates of fetal resorptions and malformations in the absence of maternal toxicity. Female rats and rabbits received mycophenolate doses equivalent to 0.02 and 0.9 times the recommended human dose for renal and cardiac transplant patients, based on BSA conversions. In rat offspring, malformations included agnathia, anophthalmia, and hydrocephaly. In rabbit offspring, malformations included ectopia cordis, ectopic kidneys, diaphragmatic hernia, and umbilical hernia.

If this drug is used during pregnancy or if the patient becomes pregnant while taking this drug, apprise the patient of the potential hazard to the fetus. In certain situations, the patient and her health care provider may decide that the maternal benefits outweigh the risks to the fetus. Encourage women using mycophenolate at any time during pregnancy to enroll in the National Transplantation Pregnancy Registry.

Advise women of childbearing potential to have a negative serum or urine pregnancy test with a sensitivity of at least 25 milliunits/mL within 1 week prior to beginning therapy. Do not initiate mycophenolate mofetil therapy until a negative pregnancy test report is obtained.

Women of childbearing potential (including pubertal girls and perimenopausal women) taking mycophenolate must receive contraceptive counseling and use effective contraception. Advise the patient to begin using her 2 chosen methods of contraception 4 weeks prior to starting mycophenolate therapy, unless abstinence is the chosen method. She should continue contraceptive use during therapy and for 6 weeks after stopping mycophenolate. Make patients aware that mycophenolate reduces blood levels of the hormones in the oral contraceptive pill and could theoretically reduce its effectiveness.

➤*Lactation:* Studies in rats treated with mycophenolate have shown mycophenolic acid to be excreted in milk. It is not known whether this drug is excreted in human milk. The molecular weight of the prodrug mycophenolate (about 434) is low enough that passage of mycophenolate and/or mycophenolic acid into breast milk should be expected. Because many drugs are excreted in human milk, and because of the potential for serious adverse reactions in breast-feeding infants from mycophenolate, decide whether to discontinue breast-feeding or the drug, taking into account the importance of the drug to the mother.

➤*Children:* Safety and efficacy of mycophenolic IV in children have not been established.

➤*Elderly:* In general, use cautious dosage selection for an elderly patient, reflecting the greater frequency of decreased hepatic, renal, or cardiac function and of concomitant or other drug therapy. Elderly patients may be at an increased risk of adverse reactions compared with younger individuals.

Elderly patients (65 years of age and older), particularly those who are receiving mycophenolate as part of a combination immunosuppressive regimen, may be at increased risk of certain infections (including cytomegalovirus tissue-invasive disease) and possibly GI hemorrhage and pulmonary edema, compared with younger individuals.

➤*Monitoring:* Perform complete blood cell counts weekly during the first month, twice monthly for the second and third months of treatment, then monthly through the first year. Monitor patients for signs and symptoms of bacterial, viral, or fungal infections and for signs and symptoms of organ rejection. Monitor neurological status as needed. Carefully follow patients with severe chronic renal impairment (GFR less than 25 mL/min/1.73 m^2 BSA) for potential adverse reactions.

Drug Interactions

➤*Drugs that alter the GI flora:* Drugs that alter the GI flora may interact with mycophenolate by disrupting enterohepatic recirculation. Interference of mycophenolic acid glucuronide hydrolysis may lead to less mycophenolic acid available for absorption.

➤*Vaccines:* See Warnings/Precautions for more information. Influenza vaccination may be of value. Refer to national guidelines for influenza vaccination.

Mycophenolate Mofetil Hydrochloride Injection Drug Interactions

Precipitant drug	Object drug[a]		Description
Acyclovir, ganciclovir, valacyclovir	Mycophenolate	⬆	Mycophenolic acid glucuronide and acyclovir plasma AUCs were increased 10.6% and 21.9%, respectively. Because mycophenolic acid glucuronide plasma concentrations are increased in the presence of renal impairment, as are acyclovir, ganciclovir, and valacyclovir concentrations, the potential exists for these drugs to compete for tubular secretion, further increasing the concentrations of these drugs. Carefully monitor patients with renal impairment when these agents are coadministered.
Mycophenolate	Acyclovir, ganciclovir, valacyclovir		
Amoxicillin plus clavulanic acid	Mycophenolate	⬇	Mycophenolate acid concentrations were reduced ≈ 50% 3 days after the start of amoxicillin plus clavulanic acid. The decrease tended to diminish within 14 days of starting the antibiotic and ceased within 3 days of stopping the antibiotic. The suspected mechanism is decreased mycophenolic acid enterohepatic recirculation. The clinical importance of this change is not known. Monitor the response of the patient. If an interaction is suspected, adjust the mycophenolate dose as needed.
Azathioprine	Mycophenolate	⟷	Avoid concomitant use because of a potentially increased risk of bone marrow suppression.
Cholestyramine	Mycophenolate	⬇	Following coadministration, mycophenolic acid AUC decreased ≈ 40%. Do not give with cholestyramine or agents that may interfere with enterohepatic recirculation.
Ciprofloxacin	Mycophenolate	⬇	Mycophenolate acid concentrations were reduced ≈ 50% 3 days after the start of ciprofloxacin. The decrease tended to diminish within 14 days of starting the antibiotic and ceased within 3 days of stopping the antibiotic. The suspected mechanism is decreased mycophenolic acid enterohepatic recirculation. The clinical importance of this change is not known. Monitor the response of the patient. If an interaction is suspected, adjust the mycophenolate dose as needed.

MYCOPHENOLATE MOFETIL HYDROCHLORIDE — INJECTION

Mycophenolate Mofetil Hydrochloride Injection Drug Interactions			
Precipitant drug	Object drug[a]		Description
Cyclosporine	Mycophenolate	⬇	Coadministration may reduce enterohepatic recirculation of mycophenolate. Monitor mycophenolic acid concentrations and response to therapy.
Immunosuppressives (eg, sirolimus, tacrolimus)	Mycophenolate	⬆	Mycophenolic acid trough plasma concentrations may be elevated, increasing the risk of adverse reactions. Monitor plasma mycophenolate levels and adjust dose as needed.
Probenecid	Mycophenolate	⬆	In animals, coadministration resulted in a 3-fold increase in plasma mycophenolic acid glucuronide AUC and a 2-fold increase in plasma mycophenolic acid AUC.
Rifamycins (eg, rifabutin, rifampin)	Mycophenolate	⬇	Rifamycins may reduce mycophenolic acid plasma concentrations. Closely monitor mycophenolic acid concentrations and adjust dose as needed. Coadministration of rifampin and mycophenolate is not recommended.
Salicylates	Mycophenolate	⬆	Coadministration increased the free fraction of mycophenolic acid.
Mycophenolate	Contraceptives, hormonal	⬇	Coadministration of mycophenolate and hormonal contraceptives containing levonorgestrel produced a significant decrease in the levonorgestrel AUC by ≈ 15%. Mean serum levels of luteinizing hormone, follicle-stimulating hormone, and progesterone were not significantly affected. Administer with caution and consider additional birth control methods.
Mycophenolate	Phenytoin	⬆	Mycophenolic acid decreased protein binding of phenytoin and may, therefore, increase free phenytoin levels.
Mycophenolate	Theophylline	⬆	Mycophenolic acid decreased protein binding of theophylline and may, therefore, increase free theophylline levels.

[a] ⬆ = object drug increased; ⬇ = object drug decreased; ⬌ = undetermined clinical effect.

Adverse Reactions

The principal adverse reactions associated with the administration of mycophenolate include diarrhea, leukopenia, sepsis, and vomiting, and there is evidence of a higher frequency of certain types of infections (eg, opportunistic infection). The adverse reaction profile associated with the administration of mycophenolate IV has been shown to be similar to that observed after administration of oral dosage forms of mycophenolate.

For more adverse reaction information, refer to the mycophenolate mofetil oral monograph.

The adverse reaction profile of mycophenolate IV was determined from a single, double-blind, controlled comparative study of the safety of mycophenolate 2 g/day IV and oral in renal transplant patients in the immediate posttransplant period (administered for the first 5 days). The potential venous irritation of mycophenolate IV was evaluated by comparing the adverse reactions attributable to peripheral venous infusion of mycophenolate IV with those observed in the IV placebo group; patients in this group received active medication by the oral route.

➤*Local:* Adverse reactions attributable to peripheral venous infusion were phlebitis and thrombosis, both observed in 4% of patients treated with mycophenolate IV.

➤*Postmarketing:*

GI – Colitis (sometimes caused by cytomegalovirus), isolated cases of intestinal villous atrophy, pancreatitis.

Hematologic/Lymphatic – Cases of PRCA have been reported in patients treated with mycophenolate in combination with other immunosuppressive agents.

Respiratory – Interstitial lung disorders, including fatal pulmonary fibrosis, have been reported rarely; consider these in the differential diagnosis of pulmonary symptoms ranging from dyspnea to respiratory failure in posttransplant patients receiving mycophenolate.

Miscellaneous – Serious life-threatening infections, such as meningitis and infectious endocarditis, have been reported occasionally, and there is evidence of a higher frequency of certain types of serious infections, such as tuberculosis and atypical mycobacterial infection. Cases of PML, sometimes fatal, have been reported. The reported cases generally had risk factors for PML, including treatment with immunosuppressant therapies and impairment of immune function. BK virus–associated nephropathy has been observed in patients receiving immunosuppressants, including mycophenolate. This infection is associated with serious outcomes, including deteriorating renal function and renal graft loss.

Congenital malformations, including ear malformations, have been reported in the offspring of patients exposed to mycophenolate during pregnancy.

Overdosage

➤*Symptoms:* The experience with overdose of mycophenolate in humans is very limited. The events received from reports of overdose fall within the known safety profile of the drug. The highest dosage administered to renal transplant patients in clinical trials has been 4 g/day. In limited experience with cardiac and hepatic transplant patients in clinical trials, the highest dosages used were 4 or 5 g/day. At dosages of 4 or 5 g/day, there appears to be a higher rate (compared with the use of 3 g/day or less) of GI intolerance (eg, diarrhea, nausea, and/or vomiting), and occasional hematologic abnormalities, principally neutropenia, leading to a need to reduce or discontinue dosing.

➤*Treatment:* Mycophenolic acid and mycophenolic acid glucuronide are usually not removed by hemodialysis. However, at high mycophenolic acid glucuronide plasma concentrations (more than 100 mcg/mL), small amounts of mycophenolic acid glucuronide are removed. By increasing excretion of the drug, mycophenolic acid can be removed by bile acid sequestrants, such as cholestyramine.

Patient Information

Instruct patients to read the Medication Guide before starting therapy.

Inform patients of the need for repeated appropriate laboratory tests while they are receiving mycophenolate.

Give patients complete dosage instructions and inform them of the increased risk of lymphoproliferative disease and certain other malignancies.

Instruct patients receiving mycophenolate to immediately report any evidence of infection, unexpected bruising, bleeding, or any other manifestation of bone marrow depression.

Inform women of childbearing potential that use of mycophenolate in pregnancy is associated with an increased risk of first trimester pregnancy loss and an increased risk of birth defects, and that they must use effective contraception. Discuss pregnancy plans with women of childbearing potential.

Any woman of childbearing potential must use highly effective (2 methods) contraception 4 weeks prior to starting mycophenolate therapy and continue contraception until 6 weeks after stopping mycophenolate treatment, unless abstinence is the chosen method. A patient who is planning a pregnancy should not use mycophenolate unless she cannot be successfully treated with other immunosuppressant drugs.

MYCOPHENOLATE SODIUM — ORAL

WARNING

Immunosuppression may lead to increased susceptibility to infection and the possible development of lymphoma and other neoplasms. Only health care providers experienced in immunosuppressive therapy and management of organ transplant recipients should use mycophenolate. Manage patients receiving mycophenolate in facilities equipped and staffed with adequate laboratory and supportive medical resources. The health care provider responsible for maintenance therapy should have complete information requisite for the follow-up of the patient.

Women of childbearing potential must use contraception. Use of mycophenolate during pregnancy is associated with increased risks of pregnancy loss and congenital malformations.

Indications

➤*Renal transplantation:* For the prophylaxis of organ rejection in patients receiving allogeneic renal transplants, administered in combination with cyclosporine and corticosteroids.

➤*Off-label uses:*

Lupus nephritis – [3] = Safety concerns. Guidelines, meta-analyses, and systematic reviews of the studies to date with mycophenolate have characterized the results as encouraging or promising. Mycophenolate appeared to be associated with higher rates of complete and partial response than the standard of care (cyclophosphamide). The incidence of adverse effects and death was also lower with mycophenolate than with cyclophosphamide. Some authors have concluded that mycophenolate would be an appropriate first-line agent in patients with less severe lupus nephritis. However, because long-term efficacy has been demonstrated only with cyclophosphamide-based regimens, other authors, including the authors of

MYCOPHENOLATE SODIUM — ORAL

the European League Against Rheumatism guidelines, recommend mycophenolate only as an alternative agent, unless or until long-term outcome data become available.

Administration and Dosage

➤*General dosing considerations:* Renal transplant rejection does not lead to changes in mycophenolic acid pharmacokinetics; dosage reduction or interruption of mycophenolate is not required.

Mycophenolate sodium and mycophenolate mofetil should not be used interchangeably without health care provider supervision because the rate of absorption following the administration of these 2 products is not equivalent.

➤*Adults:*

Renal transplantation – 720 mg twice daily.

Off-label dosing –

Lupus nephritis: [3] = Safety concerns. 1 to 3 g/day, divided for twice-daily administration. Maintenance treatment continues indefinitely; however, if an adequate response to therapy is not observed within the first 6 months, a more intense treatment approach should be considered.

➤*Children:*

Renal transplantation –

5 to 16 years of age:

- *Usual dosage* – 400 mg/m² body surface area (BSA) twice daily.
- *Maximum dose* – 720 mg twice daily.

➤*Elderly:* The maximum recommended dosage is 720 mg twice daily. In general, be cautious in dose selection for an elderly patient, reflecting the greater frequency of decreased hepatic, renal, or cardiac function, and of concomitant disease or other drug therapy.

➤*Administration:* Administer on an empty stomach 1 hour before or 2 hours after food intake. Do not crush, chew, or cut tablets prior to ingesting. Swallow the tablets whole in order to maintain the integrity of the enteric coating.

Children – Children with a BSA of 1.19 to 1.58 m² may be dosed with 3 mycophenolate 180 mg tablets or 1 mycophenolate 180 mg tablet plus 1 mycophenolate 360 mg tablet twice daily. Patients with a BSA of more than 1.58 m² may be dosed with 4 mycophenolate 180 mg tablets or 2 mycophenolate 360 mg tablets twice daily. Doses for children with a BSA of less than 1.19 m² cannot be accurately administered using currently available formulations of mycophenolate.

➤*Storage/Stability:* Store at 25°C (77°F); excursions are permitted between 15° and 30°C (59° and 86°F). Protect from moisture.

Actions

➤*Pharmacology:* Mycophenolic acid is an uncompetitive and reversible inhibitor of inosine monophosphate dehydrogenase and, therefore, inhibits the de novo pathway of guanosine nucleotide synthesis without incorporation to DNA. Because T- and B-lymphocytes are critically dependent for their proliferation on de novo synthesis of purines, whereas other cell types can utilize salvage pathways, mycophenolic acid has a potent cytostatic effect on lymphocytes.

➤*Pharmacokinetics:*

Renal transplant patients –

Mycophenolic Acid Pharmacokinetic Parameters in Renal Transplant Patients[a,b]

Population	Mycophenolate dosing	Dose (mg)	T_{max}[c] (h)	C_{max} (mcg/mL)	AUC_{0-12h} (mcg•h/mL)
Adults (n = 24)	Single	720	2 (0.8 to 8)	26.1 ± 12	66.5 ± 22.6[d]
Children[e] (n = 10)	Single	450/m²	2.5 (1.5 to 24)	36.3 ± 20.9	74.3 ± 22.5[d]
Adults (n = 10)	Multiple × 6 days, twice daily	720	2 (1.5 to 3)	37 ± 13.3	67.9 ± 20.3
Adults (n = 36)	Multiple × 28 days, twice daily	720	2.5 (1.5 to 8)	31.2 ± 18.1	71.2 ± 26.3
Adults (n = 12)	*Chronic, multiple dose, twice daily*				
	2 weeks posttransplant	720	1.8 (1 to 5.3)	15 ± 10.7	28.6 ± 11.5
	3 months posttransplant	720	2 (0.5 to 2.5)	26.2 ± 12.7	52.3 ± 17.4
	6 months posttransplant	720	2 (0 to 3)	24.1 ± 9.6	57.2 ± 15.3
Adults (n = 18)	Chronic, multiple dose, twice daily	720	1.5 (0 to 6)	18.9 ± 7.9	57.4 ± 15

[a] Renal transplant patients on modified cyclosporine-based immunosuppression.
[b] T_{max} = time of maximal concentration; C_{max} = maximal drug concentration; AUC = area under the curve.
[c] Median (range).
[d] $AUC_{0-\infty}$.
[e] Range, 5 to 16 years of age.

Absorption – In vitro studies demonstrated that enteric-coated mycophenolate tablets do not release mycophenolic acid under acidic conditions (pH less than 5), as in the stomach, but are highly soluble in neutral pH conditions, as in the intestine. Following mycophenolate oral administration without food in several pharmacokinetic studies conducted in renal transplant patients, consistent with its enteric-coated formulation, the median delay in the rise of mycophenolic acid concentration ranged between 0.25 and 1.25 hours and the median T_{max} of mycophenolic acid ranged between 1.5 and 2.75 hours. In comparison, following the administration of mycophenolate mofetil, the median T_{max} ranged between 0.5 and 1 hour. In stable renal transplant patients on modified cyclosporine–based immunosuppression, GI absorption and absolute bioavailability of mycophenolic acid following the administration of mycophenolate were 93% and 72%, respectively. Mycophenolate pharmacokinetics are dose proportional over the dose range of 360 to 2,160 mg.

Effect of food: Compared with the fasting state, administration of mycophenolate 720 mg with a high-fat meal (55 g fat, 1,000 calories) had no effect on the systemic exposure (AUC) of mycophenolic acid. However, there was a 33% decrease in the C_{max}, a 3.5-hour delay in the median delay (range, −6 to 18 hours), and a 5-hour delay in the T_{max} (range, −9 to 20 hours) of mycophenolic acid. To avoid the variability in mycophenolic acid absorption between doses, advise patients to take mycophenolate on an empty stomach.

Distribution – The mean (± standard deviation [SD]) volume of distribution at steady state and elimination phase for mycophenolic acid is 54 ± 25 L and 112 ± 48 L, respectively. Mycophenolic acid is highly protein bound to albumin (more than 98%). The protein binding of mycophenolic acid glucuronide is 82%. The free mycophenolic acid concentration may increase under conditions of decreased protein binding (eg, hepatic failure, hypoalbuminemia, uremia).

Metabolism – Mycophenolic acid is metabolized principally by glucuronyl transferase to glucuronidated metabolites. The phenolic glucuronide of mycophenolic acid, mycophenolic acid glucuronide, is the predominant metabolite of mycophenolic acid and does not manifest pharmacological activity. The acyl glucuronide is a minor metabolite and has comparable pharmacological activity with mycophenolic acid. In stable renal transplant patients on modified cyclosporine-based immunosuppression, approximately 28% of the oral mycophenolate dose was converted to mycophenolic acid glucuronate by presystemic metabolism. The AUC ratio of mycophenolic acid:mycophenolic acid glucuronide:acyl glucuronide is approximately 1:24:0.28 at steady state. The mean clearance of mycophenolic acid was 140 ± 30 mL/min.

Excretion – The majority of mycophenolic acid dose administered is eliminated in the urine primarily as mycophenolic acid glucuronide (more than 60%) and approximately 3% as unchanged mycophenolic acid following mycophenolate administration to stable renal transplant patients. The mean renal clearance of mycophenolic acid glucuronide was 15.5 ± 5.9 mL/min. Mycophenolic acid glucuronide also is secreted in the bile and available for deconjugation by gut flora. Mycophenolic acid resulting from the deconjugation may then be reabsorbed and produce a second peak of mycophenolic acid approximately 6 to 8 hours after mycophenolate dosing. The mean elimination half-life of mycophenolic acid and mycophenolic acid glucuronide ranged between 8 and 16 hours and 13 and 17 hours, respectively.

Special populations –

Renal function impairment: Mycophenolic acid glucuronide exposure would be increased markedly with decreased renal function, mycophenolic acid glucuronide exposure being approximately 8-fold higher in the setting of anuria. Although dialysis may be used to remove the inactive metabolite mycophenolic acid glucuronide, it would not be expected to remove clinically significant amounts of the active moiety mycophenolic acid. This is in large part because of the high plasma protein binding of mycophenolic acid.

Children: Limited data are available for stable pediatric renal transplant patients 5 to 16 years of age on the use of mycophenolate at a dose of 450 mg/m² BSA. At the same dose administered based on BSA, the respective mean C_{max} and AUC of mycophenolic acid determined in children were higher by 33% and 18% than those determined for adults. The clinical impact of the increase in mycophenolic acid exposure is not known.

Contraindications

Hypersensitivity to mycophenolate sodium, mycophenolic acid, mycophenolate mofetil, or any of its excipients.

Warnings/Precautions

➤*Lymphomas/Malignancies:* Patients receiving immunosuppressive regimens involving combinations of drugs, including mycophenolate, as part of an immunosuppressive regimen are at increased risk of developing lymphomas and other malignancies, particularly of the skin. The risk appears to be related to the intensity and duration of immunosuppression rather than to the use of any specific agent.

As usual, for patients with increased risk for skin cancer, limit exposure to sunlight and ultraviolet light by wearing protective clothing and using sunscreen with a high protection factor.

➤*Infections:* Oversuppression of the immune system can also increase susceptibility to infection, including opportunistic infections, fatal infections, and sepsis. Fatal infections can occur in patients receiving immunosuppressive therapy.

Latent viral infections – Immunosuppressed patients are increased risk for opportunistic infections, including activation of latent viral infections. These include cases of progressive multifocal leukoencephalopathy (PML) and BK virus–associated nephropathy (BKVAN), which have been observed in patients receiving immunosuppressants, including mycophenolate.

Cases of PML, sometimes fatal, have been reported in patients treated with mycophenolate mofetil. Apathy, ataxia, cognitive deficiencies, confusion, and hemiparesis were the most frequent clinical features observed. Mycophenolate mofetil is metabolized to mycophenolic acid, the active ingredient in mycophenolate sodium and the active form of the drug. The reported cases

MYCOPHENOLATE SODIUM — ORAL

generally had risk factors for PML, including treatment with immunosuppressant therapies and impairment of immune functions. In immunosuppressed patients, consider PML in the differential diagnosis in patients reporting neurological symptoms and consider consultation with a neurologist as clinically indicated. Consider reducing the amount of immunosuppression in patients who develop PML. In transplant patients, consider the risk that reduced immunosuppression represents to the graft.

BKVAN is associated with serious outcomes, including deteriorating renal function and renal graft loss. Patient monitoring may help detect patients at risk for BKVAN. Consider reduction in immunosuppression for patients who develop evidence of BKVAN.

➤*Pure red cell aplasia:* Cases of pure red cell aplasia (PRCA) have been reported in patients treated with mycophenolate mofetil in combination with other immunosuppressive agents. The mechanism for mycophenolate mofetil-induced PRCA is unknown; the relative contribution of other immunosuppressants and their combinations in an immunosuppressive regimen are also unknown. In some cases, PRCA was found to be reversible with dose reduction or cessation of mycophenolate mofetil therapy. In transplant patients, however, reduced immunosuppression may place the graft at risk. Undertake changes to mycophenolate acid therapy under appropriate supervision in transplant recipients in order to minimize the risk of graft rejection.

➤*Other immunosuppressive agents:* Mycophenolate has been administered in combination with the following agents in clinical trials: antithymocyte/lymphocyte immunoglobulin, muromonab-CD3, basiliximab, daclizumab, cyclosporine, and corticosteroids. The efficacy and safety of mycophenolate acid in combination with other immunosuppression agents have not been determined.

➤*Neutropenia:* Monitor patients receiving mycophenolate for neutropenia. The development of neutropenia may be related to mycophenolate itself, concomitant medications, viral infections, or some combination of these reactions. If neutropenia develops (absolute neutrophil count [ANC] less than 1.3×10^3/mcL), interrupt or reduce the dose of mycophenolate acid, perform appropriate diagnostic tests, and mange the patient appropriately.

➤*GI effects:* GI bleeding (requiring hospitalization) has been reported in de novo renal transplant patients (1%) and maintenance patients (1.3%) treated with mycophenolate (for up to 12 months). Duodenal ulcers, gastric ulcers, GI hemorrhage, and intestinal perforations have rarely been observed. Most patients receiving mycophenolate also were receiving other drugs known to be associated with these complications. Patients with active peptic ulcer disease were excluded from enrollment in studies with mycophenolate. Because mycophenolic acid derivatives have been associated with an increased incidence of digestive system adverse reactions, including infrequent cases of GI tract ulceration, hemorrhage, and perforation, administer mycophenolate with caution in patients with active serious digestive system disease.

➤*Delayed graft function:* In the de novo study, 18.3% of mycophenolate sodium–treated patients versus 16.7% in the mycophenolate mofetil group experienced delayed graft function. Although patients with delayed graft function experienced a higher incidence of certain adverse reactions (eg, anemia, hyperkalemia, leukopenia) than patients without delayed graft function, these reactions in delayed graft function patients were not more frequent in patients receiving mycophenolate sodium compared with mycophenolate mofetil. No dose adjustment is recommended for these patients; however, carefully observe such patients.

➤*Hereditary deficiency:* On theoretical grounds, because mycophenolate is an inosine monophosphate dehydrogenase inhibitor, avoid use in patients with rare hereditary deficiency of hypoxanthine-guanine phosphoribosyltransferase, such as Lesch-Nyhan and Kelley-Seegmiller syndrome.

➤*Vaccines:* During treatment with mycophenolate, avoid the use of live attenuated vaccines and advise patients that vaccinations may be less effective.

➤*Renal function impairment:* Subjects with severe chronic renal impairment (GFR less than 25 mL/min/1.73 m^2) may present higher plasma mycophenolic acid and mycophenolic acid glucuronide AUCs relative to subjects with lesser degrees of renal impairment or healthy volunteers. No data are available on the safety of long-term exposure to these levels of mycophenolic acid glucuronide.

➤*Pregnancy: Category D.* It is not known if mycophenolate crosses the human placenta to the fetus. The molecular weight of mycophenolate (about 434) is low enough that exposure of the embryo and fetus probably occurs. Mycophenolate mofetil can cause fetal harm when administered to a pregnant woman. Following oral or IV administration, mycophenolate mofetil is metabolized to mycophenolic acid, the active ingredient in mycophenolate sodium and the active form of the drug. Use of mycophenolate during pregnancy is associated with an increased risk of first-trimester pregnancy loss and an increased risk of congenital malformations, especially external ear and other facial abnormalities, including cleft lip and palate, and anomalies of the distal limbs, heart, esophagus, and kidney. In the National Transplantation Pregnancy Registry, there were data on 33 mycophenolate mofetil–exposed pregnancies in 24 transplant patients; there were 15 spontaneous abortions (45%) and 18 live-born infants; 22% of the live-born infants had structural malformations. In postmarketing data (collected from 1995 to 2007) on 77 women exposed to systemic mycophenolate mofetil during pregnancy, 25 had spontaneous abortions and 14 had a malformed infant or fetus. Six of 14 malformed offspring had ear abnormalities. Because these postmarketing data are reported voluntarily, it is not always possible to reliably estimate the frequency of particular adverse reactions. These malformations are similar to findings in animal reproductive toxicology studies. For comparison, the background rate for congenital anomalies in the United States is about 3%, and National Transplantation Pregnancy Registry data show a rate of 4% to 5% among babies born to organ transplant patients using other immunosuppressive drugs.

If this drug is used during pregnancy or if the patient becomes pregnant while taking this drug, apprise the patient of the potential hazard to the fetus. In certain situations, the patient and her health care provider may decide that the maternal benefits outweigh the risks to the fetus. Encourage women using mycophenolate at any time during pregnancy to enroll in the National Transplantation Pregnancy Registry.

Advise women of childbearing potential to have a negative serum or urine pregnancy test with a sensitivity of at least 25 milliunits/mL within 1 week prior to beginning therapy. Do not initiate mycophenolate therapy until a report of a negative pregnancy test has been obtained.

Women of childbearing potential (including pubertal girls and perimenopausal women) taking mycophenolate must receive contraceptive counseling and use effective contraception. Instruct the patient to begin using her 2 chosen methods of contraception 4 weeks prior to starting mycophenolate therapy, unless abstinence is the chosen method. Instruct her to continue contraceptive use during therapy and for 6 weeks after stopping mycophenolate. Make patients aware that mycophenolate reduces blood levels of hormones in the oral contraceptive pill and could theoretically reduce its effectiveness.

Teratogenic – In a teratology study performed with mycophenolate sodium in rats at a dose as low as 1 mg/kg, malformations in offspring were observed, including anophthalmia, exencephaly, and umbilical hernia. The systemic exposure at this dose represents 0.05 times the clinical exposure at the dosage of mycophenolate 1.44 g/day. In teratology studies in rabbits, fetal resorptions and malformations occurred from 80 mg/kg/day in the absence of maternal toxicity (dose levels are equivalent to approximately 0.8 times the recommended clinical dose, corrected for BSA). There are no relevant qualitative or quantitative differences in the teratogenic potential of mycophenolate sodium and mycophenolate mofetil.

➤*Lactation:* It is not known whether mycophenolic acid is excreted in human milk. However, mycophenolate is expected to pass into breast milk because the drug's molecular weight (about 434) is considered to be low enough. Because of the potential for serious adverse reactions in breast-feeding infants from mycophenolic acid, decide whether to discontinue the drug or breast-feeding while on treatment or within 6 weeks after stopping therapy, taking into account the importance of the drug to the mother.

➤*Children:* The safety and effectiveness of mycophenolate in de novo pediatric renal transplant patients or in stable renal transplant patients younger than 5 years of age have not been established.

➤*Elderly:* Patients 65 years of age and older generally may be at increased risk of adverse drug reactions caused by immunosuppression. In general, be cautious in dose selection for an elderly patient, reflecting the greater frequency of decreased hepatic, renal, or cardiac function, and of concomitant disease or other drug therapy.

➤*Monitoring:* Perform a complete blood cell count weekly during the first month of treatment, twice monthly for the second and the third months, then monthly through the first year. Carefully follow patients with severe chronic renal impairment (GFR less than 25 mL/min/1.73 m^2 BSA) for potential adverse reactions caused by an increase in free mycophenolic acid and total mycophenolic acid glucuronide concentrations. Monitor for signs and symptoms of bacterial, viral, or fungal infections and for signs and symptoms of organ rejection. Monitor neurological status as needed.

Drug Interactions

➤*Drugs that alter the GI flora:* Drugs that alter the GI flora may interact with mycophenolate by disrupting enterohepatic recirculation. Interference of mycophenolic acid glucuronide hydrolysis may lead to less mycophenolic acid available for absorption.

➤*Vaccines:* See Warnings/Precautions for more information. Influenza vaccination may be of value. Refer to national guidelines for influenza vaccination.

Mycophenolate Sodium Drug Interactions

Precipitant drug	Object drug[a]		Description
Acyclovir Ganciclovir	Mycophenolate	⬆	Both acyclovir/ganciclovir and mycophenolic acid glucuronide concentrations are increased in the presence of renal impairment; their coexistence may compete for tubular secretion and further increase their concentrations. Monitor blood cell counts during concomitant therapy.
Mycophenolate	Acyclovir Ganciclovir		
Antacids	Mycophenolate	⬇	Absorption of mycophenolic acid may be decreased. The C_{max} and AUC values for mycophenolic acid were 25% and 37% lower, respectively, when coadministered with aluminum/magnesium antacids than when administered alone under fasting conditions. Avoid coadministration.

MYCOPHENOLATE SODIUM — ORAL

Mycophenolate Sodium Drug Interactions

Precipitant drug	Object drug[a]		Description
Azathioprine	Mycophenolate	↔	Given that azathioprine and mycophenolate mofetil inhibit purine metabolism, do not coadminister mycophenolate sodium with azathioprine and/or mycophenolate mofetil.
Bile acid sequestrants (eg, cholestyramine)	Mycophenolate	↓	Bile acid sequestrants interrupt enterohepatic recirculation and reduce mycophenolic acid exposure. Do not coadminister because of the potential to reduce mycophenolate efficacy.
Charcoal, activated	Mycophenolate	↓	Coadministration may interrupt enterohepatic recirculation and reduce mycophenolic acid exposure. Do not coadminister because of the potential to reduce mycophenolate efficacy.
Cyclosporine	Mycophenolate	↓	Coadministration may interrupt enterohepatic recirculation and reduce mycophenolic acid exposure. Monitor the patient. Larger dosages of mycophenolate sodium may be needed upon the addition of cyclosporine.
Immunosuppressive agents (eg, sirolimus, tacrolimus)	Mycophenolate	↑	Mycophenolic acid trough plasma concentrations may be elevated, increasing the risk of adverse reactions. Monitor levels and adjust the dose as needed.
Iron salts (eg, ferrous fumarate, ferrous sulfate, iron polysaccharide)	Mycophenolate	↓	Data are conflicting. Absorption of mycophenolate may be decreased, possibly by the formation of a drug-iron complex. Avoid coadministration. Separate administration by as much time as possible.
Metronidazole, Norfloxacin	Mycophenolate	↓	Coadministration may reduce plasma concentrations of mycophenolic acid if metronidazole and norfloxacin are given concurrently. Avoid coadministration.
Rifamycins (eg, rifabutin, rifampin)	Mycophenolate	↓	Rifamycins may reduce mycophenolic acid plasma concentrations. Monitor and adjust the dose as needed. Coadministration of rifampin and mycophenolate sodium is not recommended.
Sevelamer	Mycophenolate	↓	Sevelamer may reduce mycophenolic acid plasma concentrations. Administer sevelamer 2 hours after mycophenolate sodium.
Mycophenolate	Contraceptives, hormonal	↓	Coadministration of mycophenolate mofetil and hormonal contraceptives containing levonorgestrel produced a decrease in the levonorgestrel AUC by ≈ 15%. Administer hormonal contraceptives with caution. Patients must use 2 methods of highly effective contraception because of the risk of mycophenolate-induced fetal harm.

[a] ↑ = object drug increased; ↓ = object drug decreased; ↔ = undetermined clinical effect.

➤*Drug/Food interactions:* See Actions for more information.

Adverse Reactions

Mycophenolate Sodium Adverse Reactions (≥ 20%)

Adverse reactions	De novo renal study: Mycophenolate sodium[a] 1.44 g/day (n = 213)	De novo renal study: Mycophenolate mofetil[a] 2 g/day (n = 210)	Maintenance renal study: Mycophenolate sodium[a] 1.44 g/day (n = 159)	Maintenance renal study: Mycophenolate mofetil[a] 2 g/day (n = 163)
GI				
Constipation	38%	39.5%	—	—
Diarrhea	23.5%	24.8%	21.4%	24.5%
Dyspepsia	22.5%	19%	—	—
Nausea	29.1%	27.1%	24.5%	19%
Vomiting	23%	20%	—	—
Hematologic				
Anemia	21.6%	21.9%	—	—
Leukopenia	19.2%	20.5%	—	—
Miscellaneous				
Any cytomegalovirus[b] infection[c]	21.6%	20.5%	1.9%	1.8%
Any fungal infection[b]	10.8%	11.9%	2.5%	1.8%
Candida NOS[b,c]	5.6%	6.2%	0%	1.8%
Candida albicans infection[b]	2.3%	3.8%	0.6%	0%
Cytomegalovirus disease[b]	4.7%	4.3%	0%	0.6%
Cytomegalovirus infection	20.2%	18.1%	—	—
Herpes simplex[b]	8%	6.2%	1.3%	2.5%
Herpes zoster[b]	4.7%	3.8%	1.9%	3.1%
Insomnia	23.5%	23.8%	—	—
Postoperative pain	23.9%	18.6%	—	—
Urinary tract infection	29.1%	33.3%		

[a] In combination with modified cyclosporine and corticosteroids.
[b] Reported over 0 to 12 months.
[c] NOS = not otherwise specified.

The following opportunistic infections occurred rarely in the previous controlled trials: *Aspergillus* and *Cryptococcus*.

➤*Lymphomas/Malignancies:* The incidence of malignancies and lymphomas is consistent with that reported in the literature for this patient population. Lymphoma developed in 0.9% of de novo patients (1 diagnosed 9 days after treatment initiation) and 1.3% of maintenance patients (1 was AIDS-related) receiving mycophenolate with other immunosuppressive agents in the 12-month controlled clinical trials. Nonmelanoma skin carcinoma occurred in 0.9% of de novo patients and 1.8% of maintenance patients. Other types of malignancy occurred in 0.5% of de novo patients and 0.6% of maintenance patients.

➤*Adverse reactions (3% to less than 20%):*

Mycophenolate Sodium in Combination With Cyclosporine[a] and Corticosteroids Adverse Reactions (3% to < 20%)

Body system	De novo renal study	Maintenance renal study
Cardiovascular	Blood pressure increased, hypertension, hypertension aggravated, hypotension, tachycardia	Hypertension
CNS	Anxiety, dizziness (excluding vertigo), fatigue, headache, tremor	Depression, dizziness, fatigue, headache, insomnia
Dermatologic	Acne, pruritus	Contusion, rash
Endocrine	Cushingoid, hirsutism	—
GI	Abdominal distension, abdominal pain, abdominal pain lower, abdominal pain upper, flatulence, gingival hyperplasia, loose stool, oral candidiasis, sore throat	Abdominal pain, abdominal pain upper, constipation, dyspepsia, flatulence, gastroesophageal reflux disease, loose stool, vomiting
GU	Bladder spasm, dysuria, hematuria, hydronephrosis, renal impairment, renal tubular necrosis, urinary retention	Urinary tract infection
Hematologic/Lymphatic	Hemoglobin decrease, lymphocele, thrombocytopenia	Anemia, leukopenia
Metabolic/Nutritional	Blood creatinine increased, diabetes mellitus, edema (eg, lower limb, peripheral), dehydration, fluid overload, hypercalcemia hypercholesterolemia, hyperglycemia, hyperkalemia, hyperlipidemia, hyperphosphatemia, hyperuricemia, hypocalcemia, hypokalemia, hypomagnesemia, hypophosphatemia	Blood creatinine increase, dehydration, edema, hypercholesterolemia, hypokalemia, peripheral edema, weight increase

MYCOPHENOLATE SODIUM — ORAL

Mycophenolate Sodium in Combination With Cyclosporine[a] and Corticosteroids Adverse Reactions (3% to < 20%)		
Body system	De novo renal study	Maintenance renal study
Musculoskeletal	Arthralgia, back pain, muscle cramps, myalgia, pain in limb	Arthralgia, back pain, muscle cramps, myalgia, pain in limb, peripheral swelling
Respiratory	Cough, dyspnea, dyspnea exertional, nasopharyngitis, pneumonia, sinusitis, upper respiratory tract infection	Cough, dyspnea, nasopharyngitis, pharyngolaryngeal pain, sinus congestion, sinusitis, upper respiratory tract infection
Miscellaneous	Chest pain, complications of transplant surgery, drug toxicity, herpes simplex, herpes zoster, implant infection, liver function tests abnormal, pain, postoperative complications, postoperative wound complication, pyrexia, vision blurred, wound infection	Chest pain, influenza, postprocedural pain, pyrexia

[a] Modified.

➤*Other adverse reactions:*

GI – Colitis (sometimes caused by cytomegalovirus), duodenal ulcers, esophagitis, gastric ulcers, GI hemorrhage, ileus, intestinal perforation, pancreatitis.

Respiratory – Interstitial lung disorders, including fatal pulmonary fibrosis, have been reported rarely with mycophenolic acid administration and should be considered in the differential diagnosis of pulmonary symptoms ranging from dyspnea to respiratory failure in posttransplant patients receiving mycophenolic acid derivatives.

Miscellaneous – Serious, life-threatening infections, such as infectious endocarditis and meningitis, have been reported occasionally. There is evidence of a higher frequency of certain types of serious infections, such as atypical mycobacterial infection and tuberculosis.

➤*Postmarketing:* Cases of PML, sometimes fatal, have been reported in patients treated with mycophenolate mofetil.

BKVAN has been observed in patients receiving immunosuppressants, including mycophenolate acid.

Congenital malformations have been reported in the offspring of patients exposed to mycophenolate mofetil during pregnancy.

Cases of PRCA have been reported in patients treated with mycophenolate mofetil in combination with other immunosuppressive agents.

Overdosage

➤*Symptoms:* Possible signs and symptoms of acute overdose could include the following: hematological abnormalities, such as leukopenia and neutropenia, and GI symptoms, such as abdominal pain, diarrhea, dyspepsia, and nausea and vomiting.

➤*Treatment:* Follow general supportive measures and symptomatic treatment in all cases of overdosage. Although dialysis may be used to remove the inactive metabolite mycophenolic acid glucuronide, it would not be expected to remove clinically significant amounts of the active moiety mycophenolic acid because of the 98% plasma protein binding of mycophenolic acid. By interfering with enterohepatic circulation of mycophenolic acid, activated charcoal or bile acid sequestrants, such as cholestyramine, may reduce the systemic mycophenolic acid exposure.

Patient Information

Instruct patients or their caregivers to read the Medication Guide before starting therapy and to reread it with each refill.

Administer mycophenolate on an empty stomach 1 hour before or 2 hours after food intake.

In order to maintain the integrity of the enteric coating of the tablet, instruct patients not to crush, chew, or cut tablets and to swallow the tablets whole.

Inform patients of the need for repeated appropriate laboratory tests while they are receiving mycophenolate.

Give patients complete dosage instructions and inform them of the increased risk of lymphoproliferative disease and certain other malignancies.

Inform women of childbearing potential that use of mycophenolate in pregnancy is associated with an increased risk of first-trimester pregnancy loss and birth defects and that they must use effective contraception. Discuss pregnancy plans with female patients of childbearing potential.

All women of childbearing potential must begin use of 2 methods of highly effective contraception 4 weeks prior to starting mycophenolate therapy and continue contraception until 6 weeks after stopping treatment, unless abstinence is the chosen method. A negative pregnancy test report must be obtained within 1 week prior to beginning therapy.

Discuss the risks and benefits of mycophenolate and alternative immunosuppressants with patients planning a pregnancy. Instruct women who are planning a pregnancy not to use mycophenolate, unless they cannot be successfully treated with other immunosuppressive drugs.

Instruct patients receiving mycophenolate to immediately report any evidence of infection, unexpected bruising, bleeding, or any other manifestation of bone marrow suppression.

Advise patients with increased risk for skin cancer to limit exposure to sunlight and ultraviolet light by wearing protective clothing and using sunscreen with a high protection factor.

TACROLIMUS

Rx	**Tacrolimus** (Various, eg, Sandoz)	**Capsules; oral:** 0.5 mg	May contain lactose. In 100s.
Rx	**Prograf** (Astellas)		Lactose. (f 607). Light yellow, oblong. In 100s and UD 100s.
Rx	**Tacrolimus** (Various, eg, Sandoz)	**Capsules; oral:** 1 mg	May contain lactose. In 100s.
Rx	**Prograf** (Astellas)		Lactose. (f 617). White, oblong. In 100s and UD 100s.
Rx	**Tacrolimus** (Astellas)	**Capsules; oral:** 5 mg	May contain lactose. In 100s.
Rx	**Prograf** (Astellas)		Lactose. (f 657). Grayish/red, oblong. In 100s and UD 100s.
Rx	**Prograf** (Astellas)	**Injection, solution, concentrate:** 5 mg/mL	In 1 mL amps.[a]

[a] Contains 200 mg/mL of polyoxyl 60 hydrogenated castor oil (HCO-60) and dehydrated alcohol 80%.

TACROLIMUS — ORAL

Tacrolimus also is available as an ointment for use in mild to moderate atopic dermatitis. For complete and comparative prescribing information for the ointment, refer to the Dermatological Agents chapter.

WARNING

Increased susceptibility to infection and the possible development of lymphoma may result from immunosuppression. Only health care providers experienced in immunosuppressive therapy and management of organ transplant patients should prescribe tacrolimus. Manage patients receiving the drug in facilities equipped and staffed with adequate laboratory and supportive medical resources. The health care provider responsible for maintenance therapy should have complete information requisite for the follow-up of the patient.

Indications

➤*Organ rejection prophylaxis:* For the prophylaxis of organ rejection in patients receiving allogeneic liver, kidney, or heart transplants. It is recommended that tacrolimus be used concomitantly with adrenal corticosteroids. In heart and kidney transplant recipients, it is recommended that tacrolimus be used in conjunction with azathioprine or mycophenolate mofetil.

➤*Off-label uses:*

Crohn disease – [3] = Safety concerns. According to an American Gastroenterological Association position statement, the potential toxicities of tacrolimus make it appropriate for use in the treatment of Crohn disease only in patients with complex perianal fistulas who have failed multiple other treatments. Although some studies have enrolled children, the majority of reported experience is in patients 12 years of age and older.

Psoriasis – [3] = Safety concerns. Guidelines from the American Academy of Dermatology identified methotrexate, cyclosporine, and acitretin as first-tier, traditional systemic therapies for the treatment of psoriasis. Tacrolimus was among the Academy's second-tier therapies, agents for which the level of evidence supporting their use was of lesser quality than for methotrexate, cyclosporine, and acitretin.

Pyoderma gangrenosum – [4] = Insufficient documentation. Initial positive results from a limited number of individual case reports suggest oral tacrolimus may be an effective treatment for pyoderma gangrenosum.

Rheumatoid arthritis – [3] = Safety concerns. Results from controlled trials suggest tacrolimus may be effective for the treatment of rheumatoid arthritis (RA). However, there are safety concerns with its use. The American College of Rheumatology (ACR) treatment recommendations do not include recommendations or a review of the data for tacrolimus because of the high incidence of adverse events associated with its use.

TACROLIMUS — ORAL

Other possible off-label uses – Prevention and treatment of acute graft-versus-host disease (GVHD) following hematopoietic stem cell transplantation.

Administration and Dosage

➤*Adults:*

Heart transplant –

Initial dosage: 0.075 mg/kg/day administered every 12 hours in 2 divided doses. The initial dose of tacrolimus should be administered no sooner than 6 hours after transplantation. In a patient receiving an intravenous (IV) infusion, the first dose of oral therapy should be given 8 to 12 hours after discontinuing the IV infusion.

Dosage titration: Dosing should be titrated based on clinical assessments of rejection and tolerability.

Maintenance dosage: Lower tacrolimus dosages may be sufficient as maintenance therapy.

Concomitant therapy: Adjunct therapy with adrenal corticosteroids is recommended early posttransplant. It is recommended that tacrolimus be used in conjunction with azathioprine or mycophenolate mofetil.

Conversion: If possible, initiating oral therapy with tacrolimus capsules is recommended. If IV therapy is necessary, conversion from IV to oral tacrolimus is recommended as soon as oral therapy can be tolerated. This usually occurs within 2 to 3 days.

Kidney transplant –

Initial dosage: 0.2 mg/kg/day in combination with azathioprine or 0.1 mg/kg/day when used in combination with mycophenolate mofetil and interleukin-2 receptor antagonist. Administer in 2 divided doses, given every 12 hours.

Initial dose may be administered within 24 hours of transplantation but should be delayed until renal function has recovered (eg, serum creatinine less than or equal to 4 mg/dL).

Black patients may require higher doses to achieve comparable blood concentrations. See also Therapeutic Drug Monitoring.

Concomitant therapy: It is recommended that tacrolimus be used in conjunction with azathioprine or mycophenolate mofetil and interleukin-2 receptor antagonist.

Liver transplant –

Initial dosage: 0.1 to 0.15 mg/kg/day administered in 2 divided daily doses every 12 hours. The initial dose should be administered no sooner than 6 hours after transplantation. In a patient receiving an IV infusion, the first dose of oral therapy should be given 8 to 12 hours after discontinuing the IV infusion.

Dosage titration: Dosing should be titrated based on clinical assessments of rejection and tolerability.

Maintenance dosage: Lower tacrolimus dosages may be sufficient as maintenance therapy.

Concomitant therapy: Adjunct therapy with adrenal corticosteroids is recommended early posttransplant.

Coadministered grapefruit juice has been reported to increase tacrolimus blood trough concentrations in liver transplant patients. Grapefruit juice affects CYP3A-mediated metabolism and should be avoided.

Conversion: If IV therapy is necessary, conversion from IV to oral tacrolimus is recommended as soon as oral therapy can be tolerated. This usually occurs within 2 to 3 days.

Off-label dosing –

Crohn disease: [3] = Safety concerns. Tacrolimus 0.1 mg/kg orally twice daily, adjusted to maintain serum concentrations of 10 to 20 ng/mL, or 1 g topically twice daily. Therapy can continue until maximal benefit is achieved and then be discontinued, or it may be continued long term for maintenance therapy.

Psoriasis: [3] = Safety concerns. 0.05 to 0.15 mg/kg/day; the appropriate duration of therapy is unknown.

Pyoderma gangrenosum: [4] = Insufficient documentation. 0.1 mg/kg/day for 3 months as adjunctive therapy or monotherapy (range, 0.1 to 0.3 mg/kg/day in divided doses for 1 month to 2 years).

Rheumatoid arthritis: [3] = Safety concerns. 1 to 3 mg orally daily for up to 18 months.

➤*Children:*

Liver transplant –

Initial dosage: 0.15 to 0.2 mg/kg/day in 2 divided doses every 12 hours.

Pediatric liver transplantation patients without preexisting renal or hepatic dysfunction have required and tolerated higher doses than adults to achieve similar blood concentrations.

Dosage adjustment: Dosage adjustment may be required.

➤*Renal function impairment:* Because of the potential for nephrotoxicity, patients with renal impairment should receive doses at the lowest value of the recommended oral dosing ranges. Further reductions in dose below these ranges may be required.

➤*Hepatic function impairment:* Because of the reduced clearance and prolonged half-life, patients with severe hepatic impairment (Child-Pugh score of 10 or more) may require lower doses of tacrolimus. Close monitoring of blood concentrations is warranted.

Because of the potential for nephrotoxicity, patients with hepatic impairment should receive doses at the lowest value of the recommended oral dosing ranges. Further reductions in dose below these ranges may be required. Tacrolimus therapy usually should be delayed up to 48 hours or longer in patients with postoperative oliguria.

➤*Conversion from another immunosuppressive therapy:* Tacrolimus should not be used simultaneously with cyclosporine. Tacrolimus or cyclosporine should be discontinued at least 24 hours before initiating the other. In the presence of elevated tacrolimus or cyclosporine concentrations, dosing with the other drug usually should be further delayed.

➤*Therapeutic drug monitoring:*

Kidney/Liver/Heart Transplant Tacrolimus Observed Whole Blood Trough Concentrations

Patient population	Typical whole blood trough concentrations
Adult kidney transplant patients in combination with azathioprine	Months 1 to 3: 7 to 20 ng/mL Months 4 to 12: 5 to 15 ng/mL
Adult kidney transplant patients in combination with mycophenolate mofetil and interleukin-2 receptor antagonist[a]	Months 1 to 12: 4 to 11 ng/mL
Adult liver transplant patients	Months 1 to 12: 5 to 20 ng/mL
Pediatric liver transplant patients	Months 1 to 12: 5 to 20 ng/mL
Adult heart transplant patients	Months 1 to 3: 10 to 20 ng/mL Months ≥ 4: 5 to 15 ng/mL

[a] In a second smaller study, the initial dosage of tacrolimus was 0.15 to 0.2 mg/kg/day and observed tacrolimus concentrations were 6 to 16 ng/mL during month 1 to 3 and 5 to 12 ng/mL during months 4 to 12.

Tacrolimus Dosing and Trough Concentrations by Race

	White (n = 114)		Black (n = 56)	
Time after transplant	Dose (mg/kg)	Trough concentrations (ng/mL)	Dose (mg/kg)	Trough concentrations (ng/mL)
Day 7	0.18	12	0.23	10.9
Month 1	0.17	12.8	0.26	12.9
Month 6	0.14	11.8	0.24	11.5
Month 12	0.13	10.1	0.19	11

➤*Preparation for administration:*

Extemporaneous compounding – For tacrolimus 0.5 mg/mL oral suspension, open 6 of the 5 mg oral capsules and pour out capsule contents. Combine into a paste with equal amounts of *Ora-Plus* and simple syrup, then further dilute with equal amounts of *Ora-Plus* and simple syrup for a final total volume of 60 mL. Extemporaneous oral suspension is stable for 56 days at room temperature in amber glass or plastic bottles.

➤*Administration:* Avoid coadministration of tacrolimus with grapefruit juice. Grapefruit juice has been reported to increase tacrolimus blood trough concentrations in liver transplant patients.

If dosed twice daily, doses should be administered 12 hours apart.

➤*Storage/Stability:* Store at 25°C (77°F); excursions are permitted between 15° and 30°C (59° and 86°F).

Extemporaneous oral suspension (0.5 mg/mL) is stable for 56 days at room temperature in amber glass or plastic bottles.

Actions

➤*Pharmacology:* Tacrolimus, previously known as FK506, is a macrolide immunosuppressant produced by *Streptomyces tsukubaensis*. Tacrolimus prolongs the survival of the host and transplanted graft in animal transplant models of liver, kidney, heart, bone marrow, small bowel and pancreas, lung and trachea, skin, cornea, and limb.

In animals, tacrolimus has been demonstrated to suppress some humoral immunity and, to a greater extent, cell-mediated reactions such as allograft rejection, delayed-type hypersensitivity, collagen-induced arthritis, experimental allergic encephalomyelitis, and GVHD.

Tacrolimus inhibits T-lymphocyte activation, although the exact mechanism of action is not known. Experimental evidence suggests that tacrolimus binds to an intracellular protein, FKBP-12. A complex of tacrolimus-FKBP-12, calcium, calmodulin, and calcineurin is then formed and the phosphatase activity of calcineurin inhibited. This effect may prevent the dephosphorylation and translocation of nuclear factor of activated T cells, a nuclear component thought to initiate gene transcription for the formation of lymphokines (such as interleukin-2, gamma interferon). The net result is the inhibition of T-lymphocyte activation (ie, immunosuppression).

TACROLIMUS — ORAL

➤*Pharmacokinetics:*

Pharmacokinetic Parameters of Tacrolimus Oral[a]								
Population	N	Route (dose)	C_{max} (ng/mL)	T_{max} (h)	AUC (ng•h/mL)	Half-life (h)	Clearance (L/h/kg)	Volume (L/kg)
Healthy volunteers	16	Orally (5 mg)	≈ 29.7 ± 7.2	≈ 1.6 ± 0.7	≈ 243[b] ± 73	≈ 34.8 ± 11.4	≈ 0.041[c] ± 0.008	≈ 1.94[c] ± 0.53
Kidney transplant patients	26	Orally (0.2 mg/kg/day)	≈ 19.2 ± 10.3	3	≈ 203[d] ± 42	NA[e]	NA	NA
		Orally (0.3 mg/kg/day)	≈ 24.2 ± 15.8	1.5	≈ 288[d] ± 93	NA	NA	NA
Liver transplant patients	17	Orally (0.3 mg/kg/day)	≈ 68.5 ± 30	≈ 2.3 ± 1.5	≈ 519[d] ± 179	NA	NA	NA
Heart transplant patients	11	Orally (0.075 mg/kg/day)[f]	14.7 ± 7.79	2.1 [0.5 to 6][g]	82.7[h] ± 63.2	—	NA	NA
	14	Orally (0.15 mg/kg/day)[f]	24.5 ± 13.7	1.5 [0.4 to 4][g]	142[h] ± 116	—	NA	NA

[a] C_{max} = maximum plasma concentration; T_{max} = time to reach maximum plasma concentration; AUC = area under the curve.
[b] AUC_{0-72}.
[c] Corrected for individual bioavailability.
[d] $AUC_{0-\infty}$.
[e] — = Not available
[f] Determined after the first dose.
[g] Median [range].
[h] AUC_{0-12}.

Because of intersubject variability in tacrolimus pharmacokinetics, individualization of dosing regimen is necessary for optimal therapy. Pharmacokinetic data indicate that whole blood concentrations, rather than plasma concentrations, serve as the more appropriate sampling compartment to describe tacrolimus pharmacokinetics.

Absorption – Absorption of tacrolimus from the GI tract after oral administration is incomplete and variable. The absolute bioavailability of tacrolimus was 17% ± 10% in adult kidney transplant patients (n = 26), 22% ± 6% in adult liver transplant patients (n = 17), 23% ± 9% in adult heart transplant patients (n = 11), and 18% ± 5% in healthy volunteers (n = 16).

A single-dose study conducted in 32 healthy volunteers established the bioequivalence of the 1 and 5 mg capsules. Another single-dose study in 32 healthy volunteers established the bioequivalence of the 0.5 and 1 mg capsules. Tacrolimus C_{max} and AUC appeared to increase in a dose-proportional fashion in 18 fasted, healthy volunteers receiving a single oral dose of 3, 7, and 10 mg.

In 18 kidney transplant patients, tacrolimus trough concentrations from 3 to 30 ng/mL measured at 10 to 12 hours postdose (minimum plasma concentration [C_{min}] correlated well with the AUC (correlation coefficient, 0.93). In 24 liver transplant patients over a concentration range of 10 to 60 ng/mL, the correlation coefficient was 0.94. In 25 heart transplant patients over a concentration range of 2 to 24 ng/mL, the correlation coefficient was 0.89 after an oral dosage of 0.075 or 0.15 mg/kg/day at steady state.

Food effects: The effect was most pronounced with a high-fat meal (848 kcal, 46% fat): mean AUC and C_{max} were decreased 37% and 77%, respectively; time to C_{max} was lengthened 5-fold. A high-carbohydrate meal (668 kcal, 85% carbohydrate) decreased mean AUC and mean C_{max} by 28% and 65%, respectively.

In 11 liver transplant patients, tacrolimus administered 15 minutes after a high-fat breakfast (400 kcal, 34% fat) resulted in decreased AUC (27 ± 18%) and C_{max} (50 ± 19%), as compared with a fasted state.

Distribution – The plasma protein binding of tacrolimus is approximately 99% and is independent of concentration over a range of 5 to 50 ng/mL. Tacrolimus is bound mainly to albumin and alpha-1 acid glycoprotein and has a high level of association with erythrocytes. The distribution of tacrolimus between whole blood and plasma depends on several factors such as hematocrit, temperature at the time of plasma separation, drug concentration, and plasma protein concentration. In a US study, the ratio of whole blood concentration to plasma concentration averaged 35 (range, 12 to 67).

Metabolism – Tacrolimus is extensively metabolized by the mixed-function oxidase system, primarily the cytochrome P450 (CYP-450) system (CYP3A). A metabolic pathway leading to the formation of 8 possible metabolites has been proposed. Demethylation and hydroxylation were identified as the primary mechanisms of biotransformation in vitro. The major metabolite identified in incubations with human liver microsomes is 13-demethyl tacrolimus. In in vitro studies, a 31-demethyl metabolite has been reported to have the same activity as tacrolimus.

Excretion – When administered orally, the mean recovery of radiolabeled tacrolimus was 94.9% ± 30.7%. Fecal elimination accounted for 92.6% ± 30.7%, urinary elimination accounted for 2.3% ± 1.1%, and the elimination half-life based on radioactivity was 31.9 ± 10.5 hours, whereas it was 48.4 ± 12.3 hours based on tacrolimus concentrations. The mean clearance of radiolabel was 0.226 ± 0.116 L/h/kg, and clearance of tacrolimus was 0.172 ± 0.088 L/h/kg.

Special populations –

Renal function impairment: Tacrolimus pharmacokinetics following a single IV administration were determined in 12 patients (7 not on dialysis and 5 on dialysis, serum creatinine of 3.9 ± 1.6 and 12 ± 2.4 mg/dL, respectively) prior to their kidney transplants. The pharmacokinetic parameters obtained were similar for both groups.

Tacrolimus Injection Pharmacokinetics in Patients With Hepatic Impairment					
Population (Number of patients)	Dose	$AUC_{(0-t)}$ (ng•h/mL)	Half-life (h)	Volume of distribution (L/kg)	Clearance (L/h/kg)
Renal impairment (n = 12)	0.02 mg/kg per 4 h IV	393 ± 123 (t = 60 h)	26.3 ± 9.2	1.07 ± 0.2	0.038 ± 0.014

Hepatic function impairment: Tacrolimus pharmacokinetics have been determined in 6 patients with mild hepatic dysfunction (mean Child-Pugh score of 6.2) following single IV and oral administrations. The mean clearance of tacrolimus in patients with mild hepatic dysfunction was not substantially different from that in healthy volunteers.

Tacrolimus pharmacokinetics were studied in 6 patients with severe hepatic dysfunction (mean Child-Pugh score greater than 10). The mean clearance was substantially lower in patients with severe hepatic dysfunction, irrespective of the route of administration.

Tacrolimus Pharmacokinetics in Patients With Hepatic Impairment					
Population (Number of patients)	Dose	$AUC_{(0 \text{ to } t)}$ (ng•h/mL)	Half-life (h)	Volume of distribution (L/kg)	Clearance (L/h/kg)
Renal impairment (n = 12)	0.02 mg/kg per 4 h IV	393 ± 123 (t = 60 h)	26.3 ± 9.2	1.07 ± 0.2	0.038 ± 0.014
Mild hepatic impairment IV (n = 6)	0.02 mg/kg per 4 h IV	367 ± 107 (t = 72 h)	60.6 ± 43.8 Range, 27.8 to 141	3.1 ± 1.6	0.042 ± 0.02
	7.7 mg orally	488 ± 320 (t = 72 h)	66.1 ± 44.8 Range, 29.5 to 138	3.7 ± 4.7[a]	0.034 ± 0.019[b]
Severe hepatic impairment (n = 6)	0.02 mg/kg per 4 h IV (n = 2)	762 ± 204 (t = 120 h)	198 ± 158 Range, 81 to 436	3.9 ± 1	0.017 ± 0.013
	0.01 mg/kg per 8 h IV (n = 4)	289±117 (t = 144 h)			
Orally (n = 5)[b]	8 mg orally (n = 1)	658 (t = 120 h)	119±35 Range, 85 to 178	3.1 ± 3.4[a]	0.016 ± 0.011[b]
	5 mg orally (n = 4)	533 ± 156 (t = 144 h)			
	4 mg orally (n = 1)				

[a] Corrected for bioavailability.
[b] One patient did not receive the oral dose.

Children: Pharmacokinetics of tacrolimus have been studied in liver transplantation patients 0.7 to 13.2 years of age. Following oral administration to 9 patients, mean AUC and C_{max} were 337 ± 167 ng•h/mL and 48.4 ± 27.9 ng/mL, respectively. The absolute bioavailability was 31% ± 24%.

Whole blood C_{min} from 31 patients younger than 12 years of age showed that children needed higher doses than adults to achieve similar tacrolimus C_{min}.

Race: A formal study to evaluate the pharmacokinetic disposition of tacrolimus in black transplant patients has not been conducted. However, a retrospective comparison of black and white kidney transplant patients indicated that black patients required higher tacrolimus doses to attain similar trough concentrations. (See Administration and Dosage.)

Contraindications

Hypersensitivity to tacrolimus.

Warnings/Precautions

➤*Posttransplant diabetes mellitus:* Insulin-dependent posttransplant diabetes mellitus was reported in 20% of tacrolimus-treated kidney transplant patients without pretransplant history of diabetes mellitus in the phase 3 study. The median time to onset of posttransplant diabetes mellitus was 68 days. Insulin dependence was reversible in 15% of these patients at 1 year and in 50% at 2 years posttransplant. Black and Hispanic kidney transplant patients were at an increased risk of development of posttransplant diabetes mellitus.

Tacrolimus Post Kidney Transplant Diabetes Mellitus		
Status of posttransplant diabetes mellitus[a]	Tacrolimus	Cyclosporine-based immunosuppressive regimen
Patients without pretransplant history of diabetes mellitus	151	151
New onset of posttransplant diabetes mellitus[a], first year	20%	4%
Still insulin-dependent at 1 year in those without history of diabetes	17%	3%
New onset of posttransplant diabetes mellitus[a] after 1 year	1	0
Patients with posttransplant diabetes mellitus[a] at 2 years	11%	3%

[a] Use of insulin for 30 or more consecutive days, with less than a 5-day gap, without a history of insulin-dependent diabetes mellitus or non–insulin-dependent diabetes mellitus.

TACROLIMUS — ORAL

Tacrolimus Post Kidney Transplant Diabetes Mellitus By Race				
	Tacrolimus		Cyclosporine-based immunosuppressive regimen	
Patient race	Number of patients at risk	Patients who developed posttransplant diabetes mellitus[a]	Number of patients at risk	Patients who developed posttransplant diabetes mellitus[a]
Black	41	37%	36	8%
Hispanic	17	29%	18	6%
White	82	12%	87	1%
Other	11	0%	10	10%
Total	151	20%	151	4%

[a] Use of insulin for 30 or more consecutive days, with less than a 5-day gap, without a history of insulin-dependent diabetes mellitus or non–insulin-dependent diabetes mellitus.

Insulin-dependent posttransplant diabetes mellitus was reported in 18% and 11% of tacrolimus-treated liver transplant patients and was reversible in 45% and 31% of these patients at 1 year posttransplant in the US and European randomized studies, respectively. Hyperglycemia was associated with the use of tacrolimus in 47% and 33% of liver transplant recipients in the US and European randomized studies, respectively, and may require treatment.

Tacrolimus Post Liver Transplant Diabetes Mellitus				
	United States study		European study	
Status of Posttransplant Diabetes Mellitus[a]	Tacrolimus	Cyclosporine-based immunosuppressive regimen	Tacrolimus	Cyclosporine-based immunosuppressive regimen
Patients at risk[b]	239	236	239	249
New-onset Posttransplant Diabetes Mellitus[a]	18%	13%	11%	5%
Patients still on insulin at 1 yr	10%	8%	8%	2%

[a] Use of insulin for 30 or more consecutive days, with less than a 5-day gap, without a history of insulin-dependent diabetes mellitus or non–insulin-dependent diabetes mellitus.
[b] Patients without a pretransplant history of diabetes mellitus.

Insulin-dependent posttransplant diabetes mellitus was reported in 13% and 22% of tacrolimus-treated heart transplant patients receiving mycophenolate mofetil or azathioprine and was reversible in 30% and 17% of these patients at 1 year posttransplant in the US and European randomized studies, respectively. Hyperglycemia, defined as two fasting plasma glucose levels of 126 mg/dL or greater, was reported with the use of tacrolimus plus mycophenolate mofetil or azathioprine in 32% and 35% of heart transplant recipients in the US and European randomized studies, respectively, and may require treatment.

Tacrolimus Post Heart Transplant Diabetes Mellitus					
	United States study			European study	
Status of Posttransplant Diabetes Mellitus[a]	Tacrolimus/ Sirolimus	Tacrolimus/ Mycophenolate mofetil	Cyclosporine/ Mycophenolate mofetil	Tacrolimus/ Azathioprine	Cyclosporine/ Azathioprine
Patients at risk[b]	85	75	83	132	138
New-onset Posttransplant Diabetes Mellitus[a]	25%	13%	7%	22%	4%
Patients still on insulin at 1 year[c]	12%	9%	1%	18%	3%

[a] Use of insulin for 30 or more consecutive days without a history of insulin-dependent diabetes mellitus or non–insulin-dependent diabetes mellitus.
[b] Patients without pretransplant history of diabetes mellitus.
[c] Seven to 12 months for the US study.

➤*Nephrotoxicity:* Tacrolimus can cause nephrotoxicity, particularly when used in high doses. Nephrotoxicity was reported in approximately 52% of kidney transplantation patients and in 40% and 36% of liver transplantation patients receiving tacrolimus in the US and European randomized trials, respectively, and in 59% of heart transplant patients in a European randomized trial. Use of tacrolimus with sirolimus in heart transplantation patients in a US study was associated with an increased risk of renal impairment and is not recommended. More overt nephrotoxicity is seen early after transplantation, characterized by increasing serum creatinine and a decrease in urine output. Closely monitor patients with impaired renal function, as the dosage of tacrolimus may need to be reduced. In patients with persistent elevations of serum creatinine who are unresponsive to dosage adjustments, consider changing to another immunosuppressive therapy. Take care in using tacrolimus with other nephrotoxic drugs. In particular, to avoid excess nephrotoxicity, do not use tacrolimus simultaneously with cyclosporine. Discontinue tacrolimus at least 24 hours prior to initiating the other. In the presence of elevated tacrolimus or cyclosporine concentrations, dosing with the other drug usually should be further delayed.

➤*Hyperkalemia:* Mild to severe hyperkalemia was reported in 31% of kidney transplant recipients and in 45% and 13% of liver transplant recipients treated with tacrolimus in the US and European randomized trials, respectively, and in 8% of heart transplant recipients in a European randomized trial, and may require treatment. Monitor serum potassium levels, and potassium-sparing diuretics should not be used during tacrolimus therapy.

➤*Neurotoxicity:* Tacrolimus can cause neurotoxicity, particularly when used in high doses. Neurotoxicity, including tremor, headache, and other changes in motor function, mental status, and sensory function, was reported in approximately 55% of liver transplant recipients in the 2 randomized studies. Tremor occurred more often in tacrolimus-treated kidney transplant patients (54%) and heart transplant patients (15%), compared with cyclosporine-treated patients. The incidence of other neurological events in kidney and heart transplant patients was similar in the 2 treatment groups. Tremor and headache have been associated with high whole-blood concentrations of tacrolimus and may respond to dosage adjustment. Seizures have occurred in adults and children receiving tacrolimus. Coma and delirium also have been associated with high plasma concentrations of tacrolimus.

Patients treated with tacrolimus have been reported to develop posterior reversible encephalopathy syndrome. Symptoms indicating posterior reversible encephalopathy syndrome include altered mental status, headache, hypertension, seizures, and visual disturbances. Diagnosis may be confirmed by radiological procedure. If posterior reversible encephalopathy syndrome is suspected or diagnosed, blood pressure control should be maintained and immediate reduction of immunosuppression is advised. This syndrome is characterized by reversal of symptoms upon reduction or discontinuation of immunosuppression.

➤*Lymphomas and other malignancies:* As in patients receiving other immunosuppressants, patients receiving tacrolimus are at increased risk of developing lymphomas and other malignancies, particularly of the skin. The risk appears to be related to the intensity and duration of immunosuppression rather than to the use of any specific agent.

➤*Infections:*

Epstein-Barr virus – A lymphoproliferative disorder related to Epstein-Barr virus infection has been reported in immunosuppressed organ transplant recipients. The risk of lymphoproliferative disorder appears greatest in young children who are at risk for primary Epstein-Barr virus infection while immunosuppressed or who are switched to tacrolimus following long-term immunosuppression therapy. Because of the danger of oversuppression of the immune system, which can increase susceptibility to infection, use combination immunosuppressant therapy with caution.

Latent viral infections – Immunosuppressed patients are at increased risk for opportunistic infections, including activation of latent viral infections. These include BK virus–associated neuropathy and JC virus–associated progressive multifocal leukoencephalopathy (PML), which have been observed in patients receiving tacrolimus. These infections may lead to serious, including fatal, outcomes.

➤*Tacrolimus in combination with sirolimus:* The use of full-dose tacrolimus with sirolimus (2 mg per day) in heart transplant recipients was associated with an increased risk of wound healing complications, renal impairment, and insulin-dependent posttransplant diabetes mellitus, and is not recommended.

➤*Hypertension:* Hypertension is a common adverse reaction of tacrolimus therapy. Mild or moderate hypertension is more frequently reported than severe hypertension. Antihypertensive therapy may be required; the control of blood pressure can be accomplished with any of the common antihypertensive agents. Since tacrolimus may cause hyperkalemia, avoid potassium-sparing diuretics. While calcium-channel blocking agents can be effective in treating tacrolimus-associated hypertension, interference with tacrolimus metabolism may require a dosage reduction.

➤*Myocardial hypertrophy:* Myocardial hypertrophy has been reported in association with the administration of tacrolimus and is generally manifested by echocardiographically demonstrated concentric increases in left ventricular posterior wall and interventricular septum thickness. Hypertrophy has been observed in infants, children, and adults. This condition appears reversible in most cases following dose reduction or discontinuance of therapy. In a group of 20 patients with pre- and posttreatment echocardiograms who showed evidence of myocardial hypertrophy, mean tacrolimus whole blood concentrations during the period prior to diagnosis of myocardial hypertrophy ranged from 11 to 53 ng/mL in infants (n = 10; range, 0.4 to 2 years of age), 4 to 46 ng/mL in children (n = 7; range, 2 to 15 years of age), and 11 to 24 ng/mL in adults (n = 3; range, 37 to 53 years of age).

In patients who develop renal failure or clinical manifestations of ventricular dysfunction while receiving tacrolimus therapy, consider echocardiographic evaluation.

If myocardial hypertrophy is diagnosed, consider dosage reduction or discontinuation of tacrolimus.

➤*Renal/Hepatic function impairment:* For patients with renal insufficiency, some evidence suggests that lower doses should be used.

See Administration and Dosage for more information.

The use of tacrolimus in liver transplant recipients experiencing posttransplant hepatic impairment may be associated with an increased risk of developing renal insufficiency related to high whole blood levels of tacrolimus. Closely monitor these patients, and consider dosage adjustments. Some evidence suggests that lower doses should be used in these patients.

➤*Photosensitivity:* As with other immunosuppressive agents, owing to the potential risk of malignant skin changes, patients should limit their exposure to sunlight and ultraviolet light by wearing protective clothing and using a sunscreen with a high sun protection factor.

TACROLIMUS — ORAL

➤*Pregnancy: Category C.* There are no adequate and well-controlled studies in pregnant women. Tacrolimus is transferred across the placenta. The use of tacrolimus during pregnancy has been associated with neonatal hyperkalemia and renal dysfunction. Administer tacrolimus during pregnancy only if the potential benefit to the mother justifies potential risk to the fetus.

In reproduction studies in rats and rabbits, adverse reactions on the fetus were observed mainly at dose levels that were toxic to dams. Tacrolimus at oral doses of 0.32 and 1 mg/kg during organogenesis in rabbits was associated with maternal toxicity as well as an increase in incidence of abortions; these doses are equivalent to 0.5 to 1 times and 1.6 to 3.3 times the recommended clinical dosage range (0.1 to 0.2 mg/kg) based on body surface area corrections. At the higher dose only, an increased incidence of malformations and developmental variations was also seen. Tacrolimus, at oral doses of 3.2 mg/kg during organogenesis in rats, was associated with maternal toxicity and caused an increase in late resorptions, decreased numbers of live births, and decreased pup weight and viability. Tacrolimus, given orally at 1 and 3.2 mg/kg (equivalent to 0.7 to 1.4 times and 2.3 to 4.6 times the recommended clinical dose range based on body surface area corrections) to pregnant rats after organogenesis and during lactation, was associated with reduced pup weights.

➤*Lactation:* Because tacrolimus is excreted in human milk, advise patients to avoid breast-feeding.

➤*Children:* Experience with tacrolimus in pediatric kidney and heart transplant patients is limited. Successful liver transplants have been performed in children (up to 16 years of age) using tacrolimus. Children generally required higher doses of tacrolimus to maintain blood trough concentrations of tacrolimus similar to those of adult patients.

The 2 randomized, active-controlled trials of tacrolimus in primary liver transplantation included 56 children. Thirty-one patients were randomized to tacrolimus-based and 25 to cyclosporine-based therapies. Additionally, a minimum of 122 children were studied in an uncontrolled trial of tacrolimus in living related-donor liver transplantation.

➤*Monitoring:* The relative risk of toxicity is increased with higher trough concentrations. Therefore, monitoring of whole blood trough concentrations is recommended to assist in the clinical evaluation of toxicity.

Assess serum creatinine, potassium, and fasting glucose regularly. Perform routine monitoring of metabolic and hematologic systems as clinically warranted.

Drug Interactions

➤*Cytochrome P450 system:* Since tacrolimus is metabolized mainly by the CYP3A enzyme systems, substances known to inhibit these enzymes may decrease metabolism or increase bioavailability of tacrolimus, as indicated by increased whole blood or plasma concentrations. Drugs known to induce these enzyme systems may result in an increased metabolism of tacrolimus or decreased bioavailability, as indicated by decreased whole blood or plasma concentrations. Monitoring of blood concentrations and appropriate dosage adjustments are essential when such drugs are used concomitantly.

➤*Drugs that prolong the QT interval:* An additive effect of tacrolimus with other drugs that prolong the QT interval cannot be excluded. The following drugs may prolong the QT interval and increase the risk of life-threatening cardiac arrhythmias, including torsades de pointes: antiarrhythmic agents (eg, amiodarone, bretylium, disopyramide, dofetilide, flecainide, procainamide, quinidine, sotalol), arsenic trioxide, chlorpromazine, cisapride, dolasetron, droperidol, lapatinib, mefloquine, mesoridazine, methadone, moxifloxacin, nilotinib, paliperidone, pentamidine, perflutren, pimozide, propafenone, quinupristin/dalfopristin, tetrabenazine, thioridazine, and ziprasidone. For a more complete list of drugs that may prolong the QT interval, see the appendix "Drug-Induced Prolongation of the QT Interval and Torsades de Pointes".

➤*Vaccinations:* Immunosuppressants may affect vaccination. Therefore, during treatment with tacrolimus, vaccination may be less effective. Avoid the use of live vaccines (eg, measles, mumps, rubella, oral polio, BCG, yellow fever, and TY 21a typhoid).

Tacrolimus Drug Interactions

Precipitant drug	Object drug[a]		Description
Amiodarone	Tacrolimus	⬆	Tacrolimus plasma concentration may be increased, increasing the risk of toxicity. Consider lower doses of tacrolimus and monitoring of plasma concentrations.
Anticonvulsants (ie, carbamazepine, fosphenytoin, phenobarbital, phenytoin)	Tacrolimus	⬇⬆	These anticonvulsants may decrease tacrolimus blood levels, increasing the risk of organ transplant rejection. Phenytoin serum concentrations may be increased by tacrolimus.
Tacrolimus	Phenytoin		
Antifungal agents (eg, clotrimazole, fluconazole, itraconazole, ketoconazole, voriconazole)	Tacrolimus	⬆	Tacrolimus blood levels may be increased, increasing the risk of toxicity.
Bromocriptine	Tacrolimus	⬆	Tacrolimus blood levels may be increased, increasing the risk of toxicity.
Calcium channel blockers (eg, diltiazem, nicardipine, nifedipine, verapamil)	Tacrolimus	⬆	Tacrolimus blood levels may be increased, increasing the risk of toxicity.
Caspofungin	Tacrolimus	⬇	Tacrolimus blood levels may be decreased, increasing the risk of organ transplant rejection.
Chloramphenicol	Tacrolimus	⬆	Tacrolimus blood levels may be increased, increasing the risk of toxicity.
Cimetidine	Tacrolimus	⬆	Tacrolimus blood levels may be increased, increasing the risk of toxicity.
Cisapride[b]	Tacrolimus	⬆	Tacrolimus blood levels may be increased, increasing the risk of toxicity.
Danazol	Tacrolimus	⬆	Tacrolimus blood levels may be increased, increasing the risk of toxicity.
Ethinyl estradiol	Tacrolimus	⬆	Tacrolimus blood levels may be increased, increasing the risk of toxicity.
Macrolide antibiotics (eg, clarithromycin, erythromycin, troleandomycin[c])	Tacrolimus	⬆	Tacrolimus blood levels may be increased, increasing the risk of toxicity.
Magnesium-aluminum hydroxide antacid	Tacrolimus	⬆⬇	Coadministration of tacrolimus and magnesium-aluminum hydroxide resulted in a 21% increase in the mean tacrolimus AUC and a 10% decrease in the mean tacrolimus C_{max} relative to tacrolimus administration alone.
Methylprednisolone	Tacrolimus	⬆	Tacrolimus blood levels may be increased, increasing the risk of toxicity.
Metoclopramide	Tacrolimus	⬆	Tacrolimus blood levels may be increased, increasing the risk of toxicity.
Nefazodone	Tacrolimus	⬆	Tacrolimus blood levels may be increased, increasing the risk of toxicity.
Nephrotoxic agents (eg, aminoglycosides, amphotericin B, cisplatin, cyclosporine)	Tacrolimus	⬆	Because of the potential for additive or synergistic impairment of renal function, take care when administering tacrolimus with drugs that may be associated with renal dysfunction. Coadministration with cyclosporine resulted in additive/synergistic nephrotoxicity; tacrolimus blood levels also may be increased. Give the first tacrolimus dose no sooner than 24 hours after the last cyclosporine dose.
Tacrolimus	Nephrotoxic agents (eg, aminoglycosides, amphotericin B, cisplatin, cyclosporine)		
Protease inhibitors (eg, nelfinavir, ritonavir)	Tacrolimus	⬆	Tacrolimus blood levels may be increased, increasing the risk of toxicity.

TACROLIMUS — ORAL

Tacrolimus Drug Interactions			
Precipitant drug	Object drug[a]		Description
Proton pump inhibitors (eg, lansoprazole, omeprazole)	Tacrolimus	↑	Tacrolimus blood levels may be increased, increasing the risk of toxicity.
Rifabutin, Rifampin	Tacrolimus	↓	Tacrolimus bioavailability may be decreased and clearance increased with coadministration.
Sirolimus	Tacrolimus	↑↓	Trough concentrations of tacrolimus may be decreased by sirolimus, resulting in a reduced pharmacologic effect of tacrolimus. In addition, coadministration of tacrolimus and sirolimus in combination with corticosteroids has been associated with fatal cases of bronchial anastomotic dehiscence in lung transplant patients. The safety and efficacy of tacrolimus used in combination with sirolimus have not been established and the combination is not recommended.
St. John's wort	Tacrolimus	↓	St. John's wort induces CYP3A4 and P-glycoprotein. Because tacrolimus is a substrate for CYP3A4, tacrolimus blood levels may decrease.
Tacrolimus	Mycophenolate mofetil	↑	Mycophenolate trough plasma concentrations may be elevated, increasing the risk of adverse reactions.
Tacrolimus	Phenytoin	↑↓	Phenytoin serum concentrations may be increased by tacrolimus. Phenytoin may also reduce tacrolimus plasma concentrations and pharmacologic effects.
Phenytoin	Tacrolimus		
Tacrolimus	Potassium-sparing diuretics	↑	Because tacrolimus can cause hyperkalemia, avoid using potassium-sparing diuretics.
Potassium-sparing diuretics	Tacrolimus		
Tacrolimus	Statins (eg, lovastatin, simvastatin)	↑	Coadministration may increase both plasma concentrations of tacrolimus and certain statins. Fluvastatin or pravastatin may be less likely to interact and may be safer alternatives.
Statins (eg, lovastatin, simvastatin)	Tacrolimus		
Tacrolimus	Ziprasidone	↑	The risk of life-threatening cardiac arrhythmias, including torsades de pointes, may be increased. Coadministration is contraindicated.

[a] ↑ = object drug increased; ↓ = object drug decreased; ↑↓ = object drug both increased and decreased.
[b] Available from the manufacturer on a limited-access protocol.
[c] No longer marketed in the United States.

➤*Drug/Food interactions:* The rate and extent of tacrolimus absorption were greatest under fasted conditions. The presence and composition of food decreased both the rate and extent of tacrolimus absorption. The effect was most pronounced with a high-fat meal (848 kcal, 46% fat): mean AUC and C_{max} were decreased 37% and 77%, respectively; T_{max} was lengthened 5-fold. A high-carbohydrate meal (668 kcal, 85% carbohydrate) decreased mean AUC and mean C_{max} by 28% and 65%, respectively.

Coadministered grapefruit juice has been reported to increase tacrolimus blood trough concentrations in liver transplant patients. Grapefruit juice affects CYP3A-mediated metabolism and should be avoided.

Adverse Reactions

➤*Kidney/Liver/Heart transplant adverse reactions:*

Tacrolimus Adverse Reactions in Kidney/Liver/Heart Transplant Patients (≥ 15%)						
	Liver transplant patients[a]		Kidney transplant patients		Heart transplant patients	
Adverse reaction	Tacrolimus + steroids (n = 514)	Cyclosporine based regimen (n = 515)	Tacrolimus + azathioprine (n = 205)	Cyclosporine based regimen (n = 207)	Tacrolimus + azathioprine (n = 157)	Cyclosporine + azathioprine (n = 157)
Cardiovascular						
Chest pain	—	—	19%	13%	—	—
Hypertension[b]	38% to 47%	43% to 56%	50%	52%	62%	69%
Pericardial effusion	—	—	—	—	15%	14%
CNS						
Asthenia	11% to 52%	7% to 48%	34%	30%	—	—
Dizziness	—	—	19%	16%	—	—
Headache[b]	37% to 64%	26% to 60%	44%	38%	—	—
Insomnia	32% to 64%	23% to 68%	32%	30%	—	—
Paresthesia	17% to 40%	17% to 30%	23%	16%	—	—
Tremor[b]	48% to 56%	32% to 46%	54%	34%	15%	6%
Dermatologic						
Pruritus	15% to 36%	7% to 20%	15%	7%	—	—
Rash	10% to 24%	4% to 19%	17%	12%	—	—
GI						
Abdominal pain	29% to 59%	22% to 54%	33%	31%	—	—
Anorexia	7% to 34%	5% to 24%	—	—	—	—
Constipation	23% to 24%	21% to 27%	35%	43%	—	—
Diarrhea	37% to 72%	27% to 47%	44%	41%	—	—
Dyspepsia	—	—	28%	20%	—	—
Liver function tests abnormal	6% to 36%	5% to 30%	—	—	—	—
Nausea	32% to 46%	27% to 37%	38%	36%	—	—
Vomiting	14% to 27%	11% to 15%	29%	23%	—	—
GU						
Creatinine increased[b]	24% to 39%	19% to 25%	45%	42%	—	—
Kidney function abnormal[b]	36% to 40%	23% to 27%	—	—	56%	57%
Oliguria	18% to 19%	12% to 15%	—	—	—	—
Serum urea nitrogen increased[b]	12% to 30%	9% to 22%	—	—	—	—
Urinary tract infection	16% to 21%	18% to 19%	34%	35%	16%	12%

TACROLIMUS — ORAL

Tacrolimus Adverse Reactions in Kidney/Liver/Heart Transplant Patients (≥ 15%)						
	Liver transplant patients[a]		Kidney transplant patients		Heart transplant patients	
Adverse reaction	Tacrolimus + steroids (n = 514)	Cyclosporine based regimen (n = 515)	Tacrolimus + azathioprine (n = 205)	Cyclosporine based regimen (n = 207)	Tacrolimus + azathioprine (n = 157)	Cyclosporine + azathioprine (n = 157)
Hematologic/Lymphatic						
Anemia	5% to 47%	1% to 38%	30%	24%	50%	36%
Leukocytosis	8% to 32%	8% to 26%	—	—	—	—
Leukopenia	—	—	15%	17%	48%	39%
Thrombocytopenia	14% to 24%	19% to 20%	—	—	—	—
Metabolic/Nutritional						
Diabetes mellitus[b]	—	—	24%	9%	26%	16%
Edema	—	—	18%	19%	—	—
Hyperglycemia[b]	33% to 47%	22% to 38%	22%	16%	23%	17%
Hyperkalemia[b]	13% to 45%	9% to 26%	31%	32%	—	—
Hyperlipemia	—	—	31%	38%	18%	27%
Hypokalemia	13% to 29%	16% to 34%	22%	25%	—	—
Hypomagnesemia	16% to 48%	9% to 45%	34%	17%	—	—
Hypophosphatemia	—	—	49%	53%	—	—
Peripheral edema	12% to 26%	14% to 26%	36%	48%	—	—
Respiratory						
Atelectasis	5% to 28%	4% to 30%	—	—	—	—
Bronchitis	—	—	—	—	17%	18%
Cough increased	—	—	18%	15%	—	—
Dyspnea	5% to 29%	4 to 23%	22%	18%	—	—
Pleural effusion	30% to 36%	32% to 35%	—	—	—	—
Miscellaneous						
Arthralgia	—	—	25%	24%	—	—
Ascites	7% to 27%	8% to 22%	—	—	—	—
Back pain	17% to 30%	17% to 29%	24%	20%	—	—
Cytomegalovirus infection	—	—	—	—	32%	30%
Fever	19% to 48%	22% to 56%	29%	29%	—	—
Infection	—	—	45%	49%	24%	21%
Pain	24% to 63%	22% to 57%	32%	30%	—	—

[a] Data are pooled from separate US and European studies and are not necessarily comparable.
[b] See Warnings/Precautions.

➤*Kidney transplant:* The most common adverse reactions reported in kidney transplant patients were infection, tremor, hypertension, abnormal renal function, constipation, diarrhea, headache, abdominal pain, and insomnia.

Adverse reactions that occurred in 10% or more of kidney transplant patients treated with tacrolimus in conjunction with mycophenolate mofetil in study 1 are presented in the following table. Study 1 was conducted entirely outside the United States and such studies often report a lower incidence of adverse reactions in comparison with United States studies.

Kidney Transplantation: Adverse Reactions Occurring in of Tacrolimus-Treated Patients (≥ 10%)			
Adverse reaction	Tacrolimus (group C) (n = 403)	Cyclosporine (group A) (n = 384)	Cyclosporine (group B) (n = 408)
Hematological			
Anemia	17%	19%	17%
Leukopenia	13%	10%	10%
Metabolic/Nutritional			
Edema peripheral	11%	12%	13%
Hyperlipidemia	10%	15%	13%
Miscellaneous			
Diarrhea	25%	16%	13%
Hypertension	13%	14%	12%
Urinary tract infection	24%	28%	24%

Kidney Transplantation: Adverse Reactions Occurring in Tacrolimus-Treated Patients (≥ 15%)		
Adverse reaction	Tacrolimus + mycophenolate mofetil (n = 212)	Cyclosporine (n = 212)
CNS		
Headache	24%	25%
Insomnia	30%	21%
Tremor	34%	20%
GI		
Constipation	36%	41%
Diarrhea	44%	26%
Dyspepsia	18%	15%
Nausea	39%	47%
Vomiting	26%	25%
Hematologic/Lymphatic		
Anemia	30%	28%
Leukopenia	16%	12%
Metabolic/Nutrition		
Edema peripheral	35%	46%
Hyperglycemia	21%	15%
Hyperkalemia	26%	19%
Hyperlipidemia	18%	25%
Hypokalemia	16%	18%
Hypomagnesemia	28%	22%
Hypophosphatemia	28%	21%
Miscellaneous		
Blood creatinine increased	23%	23%
Graft dysfunction	24%	18%
Hypertension	32%	35%
Incision-site complication	28%	23%
Postprocedural pain	29%	27%
Urinary tract infection	26%	22%

Less frequently observed adverse reactions in both liver transplantation and kidney transplantation patients are described in the following sections.

➤*Liver transplant:* The principal adverse reactions of tacrolimus are tremor, headache, diarrhea, hypertension, nausea, and renal dysfunction. These adverse reactions may respond to a reduction in dosing. Diarrhea was sometimes associated with other GI complaints such as nausea and vomiting.

Hyperkalemia and hypomagnesemia have occurred. Hyperglycemia has been noted in many patients; some may require insulin therapy.

The incidence of adverse reactions was determined in 2 randomized, comparative liver transplant trials among 514 patients receiving tacrolimus and steroids and 515 patients receiving a cyclosporine-based regimen. The proportion of patients reporting more than 1 adverse reaction was 99.8% in the tacrolimus group and 99.6% in the cyclosporine-based regimen group. Precautions must be taken when comparing the incidence of adverse reactions in the US study to that in the European study. The 12-month posttransplant information from the US study and from the European study is presented in the first table in Adverse Reactions. The 2 studies also included different patient populations and patients were treated with immunosuppressive regimens of differing intensities.

➤*Heart transplant:* The more common adverse reactions in tacrolimus-treated heart transplant recipients were abnormal renal function, hyperten-

TACROLIMUS — ORAL

sion, diabetes mellitus, cytomegalovirus infection, tremor, hyperglycemia, leukopenia, infection, and hyperlipemia.

In the European study, the cyclosporine trough concentrations were above the predefined target range (ie, 100 to 200 ng/mL) at day 122 and beyond in 32% to 68% of the patients in the cyclosporine treatment arm, whereas the tacrolimus trough concentrations were within the predefined target range (ie, 5 to 15 ng/mL) in 74% to 86% of the patients in the tacrolimus treatment arm.

Only selected targeted treatment-emergent adverse reactions were collected in the US heart transplantation study. Those reactions that were reported at a rate of 15% or greater in patients treated with tacrolimus and mycophenolate mofetil include the following: any target adverse reactions (99.1%), hypertension (88.8%), hyperglycemia requiring antihyperglycemic therapy (70.1%), hypertriglyceridemia (65.4%), anemia (hemoglobin less than 10 g/dL) (65.4%), fasting blood glucose greater than 140 mg/dL (on 2 separate occasions) (60.7%), hypercholesterolemia (57%), hyperlipidemia (33.6%), white blood cell count less than 3,000 cells/mcL (33.6%), serious bacterial infections (29.9%), magnesium less than 1.2 mEq/L (24.3%), platelet count less than 75,000 cells/mcL (18.7%), and other opportunistic infections (15%).

Other targeted treatment-emergent adverse reactions in tacrolimus-treated patients occurred at a rate of less than 15% and include the following: cushingoid features, impaired wound healing, hyperkalemia, *Candida* infection, and cytomegalovirus infection/syndrome.

➤*Other liver/kidney/heart transplant adverse reactions:*

Cardiovascular – Abnormal electrocardiogram (ECG), angina pectoris, arrhythmia, atrial fibrillation, atrial flutter, bradycardia, cardiac fibrillation, cardiopulmonary failure, cardiovascular disorder, chest pain, congestive heart failure, deep thrombophlebitis, ECG QRS complex abnormal, ECG ST segment abnormal, echocardiogram abnormal, heart failure, heart rate decreased, hemorrhage, hypotension, peripheral vascular disorder, phlebitis, postural hypotension, syncope, tachycardia, thrombosis, vasodilation.

CNS – Abnormal dreams, agitation, amnesia, anxiety, asthenia, chills, confusion, convulsion, crying, depression, dizziness, elevated mood, emotional lability, encephalopathy, feeling abnormal, hallucinations, headache, hemorrhagic stroke, hypertonia, incoordination, insomnia, monoparesis, myoclonus, nerve compression, nervousness, neuralgia, neuropathy, paralysis flaccid, paresthesia, psychomotor skills impaired, psychosis, quadriparesis, somnolence, thinking abnormal, vertigo, writing impaired.

Dermatologic – Acne, alopecia, exfoliative dermatitis, fungal dermatitis, herpes simplex, herpes zoster, hirsutism, neoplasm (skin, benign), photosensitivity reaction, skin discoloration, skin disorder, skin ulcer, sweating.

Endocrine – Cushing syndrome, diabetes mellitus.

GI – Abdomen enlarged, abdominal pain, anorexia, cholangitis, cholestatic jaundice, diarrhea, duodenitis, dyspepsia, dysphagia, esophagitis, esophagitis ulcerative, flatulence, gastritis, gastroesophagitis, GI disorder, GI hemorrhage, GI perforation, hepatitis, hepatitis granulomatous, ileus, increased appetite, jaundice, liver damage, liver function test abnormal, nausea, nausea and vomiting, oral moniliasis, pancreatic pseudocyst, rectal disorder, stomatitis, vomiting.

GU – Acute kidney failure, albuminuria, BK neuropathy, bladder spasm, cystitis, dysuria, hematuria, hydronephrosis, kidney failure, kidney tubular necrosis, nocturia, oliguria, pyuria, toxic nephropathy, urge incontinence, urinary frequency, urinary incontinence, urinary retention, vaginitis.

Hematologic/Lymphatic – Coagulation disorder, ecchymosis, hematocrit increased, hemoglobin abnormal, hypochromic anemia, leukocytosis, leukopenia, polycythemia, prothrombin decreased, serum iron decreased, thrombocytopenia.

Hepatic – Cholestatic jaundice, hepatitis, hepatitis granulomatous, liver damage, liver function test abnormal.

Metabolic/Nutritional – Acidosis, alkaline phosphatase increased, alkalosis, ALT increased, AST increased, bicarbonate decreased, bilirubinemia, dehydration, edema, gamma-glutamyl transpeptidase increased, gout, hypercalcemia, hypercholesterolemia, hyperkalemia, hyperlipidemia, hyperphosphatemia, hyperuricemia, hypervolemia, hypocalcemia, hypoglycemia, hypokalemia, hypomagnesemia hyponatremia, hypophosphatemia, hypoproteinemia, lactic dehydrogenase increased, peripheral edema, serum urea nitrogen increased, weight gain.

Musculoskeletal – Arthralgia, back pain, cramps, generalized spasm, joint disorder, leg cramps, myalgia, myasthenia, osteoporosis.

Respiratory – Asthma, bronchitis, cough increased, dyspnea, emphysema, hiccups, lung disorder, lung function decreased, pharyngitis, pleural effusion, pneumonia, pneumothorax, pulmonary edema, respiratory disorder, rhinitis, sinusitis, voice alteration.

Special senses – Abnormal vision, amblyopia, ear pain, otitis media, tinnitus.

Miscellaneous – Abscess, accidental injury, allergic reaction, cellulitis, fall, fever, flu syndrome, generalized edema, healing abnormal, hernia, mobility decreased, pain, peritonitis, sepsis, temperature intolerance, ulcer.

➤*Postmarketing:*

Cardiovascular – Atrial fibrillation, atrial flutter, cardiac arrhythmia, cardiac arrest, ECG T wave abnormal, flushing, myocardial infarction, myocardial ischemia, pericardial effusion, QT prolongation, syncope, torsades de pointes, venous thrombosis deep limb, ventricular extrasystoles, ventricular fibrillation.

There have been rare, spontaneous reports of myocardial hypertrophy associated with clinically manifested ventricular dysfunction in patients receiving tacrolimus therapy.

CNS – Carpal tunnel syndrome, cerebral infection, feeling jittery, hemiparesis, leukoencephalopathy, mental disorder, mutism, PML, posterior reversible encephalopathy syndrome, quadriplegia, speech disorder.

Dermatologic – Stevens-Johnson syndrome, toxic epidermal necrolysis.

GI – Bile duct stenosis, colitis, enterocolitis, gastroenteritis, gastroesophageal reflux disease, impaired gastric emptying, mouth ulceration, pancreatitis hemorrhagic, pancreatitis necrotizing, stomach ulcer.

GU – Acute renal failure, cystitis hemorrhagic, hemolytic-uremic syndrome, micturition disorder.

Hematologic/Lymphatic – Disseminated intravascular coagulation, neutropenia, pancytopenia, thrombocytopenic purpura, thrombotic thrombocytopenic purpura.

Hepatic – Hepatic cytolysis, hepatic necrosis, hepatotoxicity, liver fatty, venoocclusive liver disease.

Metabolic/Nutritional – Glycosuria, increased amylase including pancreatitis, weight decreased.

Respiratory – Acute respiratory distress syndrome, interstitial lung disease, lung infiltration, respiratory distress, respiratory failure.

Special senses – Blindness, blindness cortical, hearing loss including deafness, photophobia.

Miscellaneous – Feeling hot and cold, hot flushes, multiorgan failure, primary graft dysfunction.

Overdosage

➤*Symptoms:* Limited overdosage experience is available. Acute overdosages of up to 30 times the intended dose have been reported. Almost all cases have been asymptomatic, and all patients recovered with no sequelae. Occasionally, acute overdosage has been followed by tacrolimus adverse reactions, except in 1 case where transient urticaria and lethargy were observed.

➤*Treatment:* Based on the poor aqueous solubility and extensive erythrocyte and plasma protein binding, it is anticipated that tacrolimus is not dialyzable to any significant extent; there is no experience with charcoal hemoperfusion. The oral use of activated charcoal has been reported in treating acute overdoses, but experience has not been sufficient to warrant recommending its use. Follow general supportive measures and treatment of specific symptoms in all cases of overdosage.

Patient Information

Inform patients of the need for repeated appropriate laboratory tests while they are receiving tacrolimus. Give patients complete dosage instructions, advise them of the potential risks during pregnancy, and inform them of the increased risk of neoplasia.

Inform patients not to undertake changes in dosage without first consulting their health care provider.

Inform patients that tacrolimus can cause diabetes mellitus and advise them of the need to see their health care provider if they develop frequent urination or increased thirst or hunger.

Advise patients to limit exposure to sunlight and ultraviolet light by wearing protective clothing and using a sunscreen with a high protection factor because of the increased risk for skin cancer.

TACROLIMUS — INJECTION

Tacrolimus also is available as an ointment for use in mild to moderate atopic dermatitis. For complete and comparative prescribing information for the ointment, refer to the Dermatological Agents chapter.

WARNING

Increased susceptibility to infection and the possible development of lymphoma may result from immunosuppression. Only health care providers experienced in immunosuppressive therapy and management of organ transplant patients should prescribe tacrolimus. Manage patients receiving the drug in facilities equipped and staffed with adequate laboratory and supportive medical resources. The health care provider responsible for maintenance therapy should have complete information necessary for the follow-up of the patient.

Indications

➤*Organ rejection prophylaxis:* For the prophylaxis of organ rejection in patients receiving allogeneic liver, kidney, or heart transplants. It is recommended that tacrolimus be used concomitantly with adrenal corticosteroids. Because of the risk of anaphylaxis, reserve tacrolimus injection for patients unable to take tacrolimus capsules orally. In heart and kidney transplant recipients, it is recommended that tacrolimus be used in conjunction with azathioprine or mycophenolate mofetil.

➤*Off-label uses:* Tacrolimus may be beneficial for the treatment of autoimmune disease (ie, rheumatoid arthritis); for the prevention and treatment of acute graft-versus-host disease (GVHD) following hematopoietic stem cell transplantation.

TACROLIMUS — INJECTION

Administration and Dosage

➤*General dosing considerations:* In patients unable to take the capsules, therapy may be initiated with the injection.

Anaphylactic reactions have occurred with injectables containing castor oil derivatives.

Give adult patients doses at the lower end of the dosing range.

➤*Adults:*

Heart transplant –

Initial dosage: 0.01 mg/kg/day as a continuous intravenous (IV) infusion. Administer the initial dose no sooner than 6 hours after transplantation.

• *Duration of therapy* – Continue continuous IV infusion only until the patient can tolerate oral administration.

Concomitant therapy: Concomitant adrenal corticosteroid therapy is recommended early posttransplantation.

Kidney transplant –

Initial dosage: 0.03 to 0.05 mg/kg/day as a continuous IV infusion. Administer the initial dose no sooner than 6 hours after transplantation.

• *Duration of therapy* – Continue continuous IV infusion only until the patient can tolerate oral administration.

Concomitant therapy: Concomitant adrenal corticosteroid therapy is recommended early posttransplantation.

Liver transplant –

Initial dosage: 0.03 to 0.05 mg/kg/day as a continuous IV infusion. Administer the initial dose no sooner than 6 hours after transplantation.

Continue continuous IV infusion only until the patient can tolerate oral administration.

Concomitant therapy: Concomitant adrenal corticosteroid therapy is recommended early posttransplantation.

➤*Children:*

Liver transplant –

Initial dosage: 0.03 to 0.05 mg/kg/day as a continuous IV infusion. Tacrolimus has been given at 0.03 to 0.15 mg/kg/day as a continuous infusion.

Pediatric liver transplantation patients without preexisting renal or hepatic dysfunction have required and tolerated higher doses than adults to achieve similar blood concentrations.

Dosage adjustment: Dose adjustments may be required.

Off-label dosing –

Cardiac transplant: 0.05 to 0.15 mg/kg/day IV starting no sooner than 6 hours after transplantation. Urine output should be more than 1 mL/kg/h and monitor blood concentrations initially at 12 h.

Graft-versus-host disease after bone marrow transplant: 0.03 mg/kg IV of tacrolimus administered with mycophenolate mofetil or methotrexate. Initiate treatment as a 24-hour continuous infusion starting on the day before the transplant for GVHD prophylaxis.

Renal transplant: 0.03 to 0.15 mg/kg/day as a continuous IV infusion given over at least 12 hours. Administer the first dose within 24 hours of the kidney transplant as long as renal function has recovered (serum creatinine less than 4 mg/dL).

Postpone therapy more than 48 hours in patients with postoperative oliguria.

➤*Renal function impairment:* Because of the potential for nephrotoxicity, give patients with renal impairment doses at the lowest value of the recommended IV dosing ranges. Further reductions in dose below these ranges may be required. Therapy may need to be delayed by up to 48 hours or longer in patients with postoperative oliguria.

➤*Hepatic function impairment:* Because of the reduced clearance and prolonged half-life, patients with severe hepatic impairment (Child-Pugh score of 10 or more) may require lower doses of tacrolimus. Close monitoring of blood concentrations is warranted.

Because of the potential for nephrotoxicity, give patients with hepatic impairment doses at the lowest value of the recommended IV dosing ranges. Further reductions in dose below these ranges may be required.

➤*Conversion from another immunosuppressive therapy:* Do not use tacrolimus simultaneously with cyclosporine. Discontinue either agent at least 24 hours before initiating the other. In the presence of elevated tacrolimus or cyclosporine concentrations, dosing with the other drug usually should be further delayed.

➤*Preparation for administration:* Tacrolimus must be diluted with sodium chloride 0.9% injection or dextrose 5% injection to a concentration between 0.004 and 0.02 mg/mL prior to use. In situations in which more dilute solutions are utilized (eg, pediatric dosing), polyvinyl chloride (PVC-)–free tubing should likewise be used to minimize the potential for significant drug adsorption onto the tubing.

➤*Administration:* For IV infusion only.

Continuously observe patients receiving the injection for at least the first 30 minutes following the start of the infusion and at frequent intervals thereafter. If signs or symptoms of anaphylaxis occur, stop the infusion. Have an aqueous solution of epinephrine available at the bedside as well as a source of oxygen.

➤*Admixture compatibility:* Because of the chemical instability of tacrolimus in alkaline media, tacrolimus injection should not be mixed or coinfused with solutions of pH 9 or greater (eg, acyclovir, ganciclovir).

➤*Storage/Stability:* Store between 5° and 25°C (41° and 77°F). Store diluted infusion solution in glass or polyethylene containers and discard after 24 hours. Do not store the diluted infusion solution in a PVC container because of decreased stability and the potential for extraction of phthalates.

Actions

➤*Pharmacokinetics:*

Pharmacokinetic Parameters of Tacrolimus Injection[a]

Population	N	Route (dose)	C_{max} (ng/mL)	T_{max} (h)	AUC (ng•h/mL)	Half-life (h)	Clearance (L/h/kg)	Volume of distribution (L/kg)
Healthy volunteers	8	IV (0.025 mg/kg per 4 h)	—[b]	—	≈ 598[c] ± 125	≈ 34.2 ± 7.7	≈ 0.04 ± 0.009	≈ 1.91 ± 0.31
Kidney transplant patients	26	IV (0.02 mg/kg per 12 h)	—	—	≈ 294[d] ± 262	≈ 18.8 ± 16.7	≈ 0.083 ± 0.05	1.41 ± 0.66
Liver transplant patients	17	IV (0.05 mg/kg per 12 h)	—	—	≈ 3,300[d] ± 2,130	≈ 11.7 ± 3.9	≈ 0.053 ± 0.017	≈ 0.85 ± 0.3
Heart transplant patients	11	IV (0.01 mg/kg/day) as a continuous infusion	—	—	954[e] ± 334	23.6 ± 9.22	0.051 ± 0.015	NA

[a] C_{max} = maximum plasma concentration; T_{max} = time to reach maximum plasma concentration; AUC = area under the curve.
[b] — = Not applicable.
[c] AUC_{0-120}.
[d] $AUC_{0-\infty}$.
[e] AUC_{0-t}.

Because of intersubject variability in tacrolimus pharmacokinetics, individualization of dosing regimen is necessary for optimal therapy. Pharmacokinetic data indicate that whole blood concentrations rather than plasma concentrations serve as the more appropriate sampling compartment to describe tacrolimus pharmacokinetics.

Absorption – Absorption of tacrolimus from the GI tract after oral administration is incomplete and variable. The absolute bioavailability of tacrolimus was approximately 17% ± 10% in adult kidney transplant patients (n = 26), approximately 22% ± 6% in adult liver transplant patients (n = 17), 23 ± 9% in adult heart transplant patients (n = 11), and approximately 18% ± 5% in healthy volunteers (n = 16). Tacrolimus C_{max} and AUC appeared to increase in a dose-proportional fashion in 18 fasted healthy volunteers receiving a single oral dose of 3, 7, and 10 mg.

In 18 kidney transplant patients, tacrolimus trough concentrations from 3 to 30 ng/mL measured at 10 to 12 hours postdose (C_{min}) correlated well with the AUC (correlation coefficient, 0.93). In 24 liver transplant patients over a concentration range of 10 to 60 ng/mL, the correlation coefficient was 0.94. In 25 heart transplant patients over a concentration range of 2 to 24 ng/mL, the correlation coefficient was 0.89 after an oral dose of 0.075 or 0.15 mg/kg/day at steady state.

Distribution – The plasma protein binding of tacrolimus is approximately 99% and is independent of concentration over a range of 5 to 50 ng/mL. Tacrolimus is bound mainly to albumin and alpha-1 acid glycoprotein and has a high level of association with erythrocytes. The distribution of tacrolimus between whole blood and plasma depends on several factors, such as hematocrit, temperature at the time of plasma separation, drug concentration, and plasma protein concentration. In a United States study, the ratio of whole blood concentration to plasma concentration averaged 35 (range, 12 to 67).

Metabolism – Tacrolimus is extensively metabolized by the mixed-function oxidase system, primarily the cytochrome P450 (CYP-450) system (CYP3A). A metabolic pathway leading to the formation of 8 possible metabolites has been proposed. Demethylation and hydroxylation were identified as the primary mechanisms of biotransformation in vitro. The major metabolite identified is 13-demethyl tacrolimus. In in vitro studies, a 31-demethyl metabolite has been reported to have the same activity as tacrolimus.

Excretion – The mean clearance following IV administration of tacrolimus is 0.04, 0.083, 0.053, and 0.051 L/h/kg in healthy volunteers, adult kidney transplant patients, adult liver transplant patients, and adult heart transplant patients, respectively. Less than 1% of the dose administered is excreted unchanged in urine.

In a mass balance study of IV-administered radiolabeled tacrolimus to 6 healthy volunteers, the mean recovery of radiolabel was 77.8% ± 12.7%. Fecal elimination accounted for approximately 92.4% ± 1%, and the elimination half-life was approximately 48.1 ± 15.9 hours, whereas it was approximately 43.5 ± 11.6 hours based on tacrolimus concentrations. The mean clearance of radiolabel was 0.029 ± 0.015 L/h/kg, and clearance of tacrolimus was 0.029 ± 0.009 L/h/kg.

Special populations –

Renal function impairment: Tacrolimus pharmacokinetics following a single IV administration were determined in 12 patients (7 not on dialysis and 5 on dialysis, serum creatinine of 3.9±1.6 and 12±2.4 mg/dL, respectively) prior to their kidney transplants. The pharmacokinetic parameters obtained were similar for both groups.

The mean clearance of tacrolimus in patients with renal dysfunction was similar to that in healthy volunteers.

TACROLIMUS — INJECTION

Hepatic function impairment:

Tacrolimus Injection Pharmacokinetics in Patients With Hepatic Impairment					
Population (Number of patients)	Dose	$AUC_{(0-t)}$ (ng•h/mL)	Half-life (h)	Volume of distribution (L/kg)	Clearance (L/h/kg)
Renal impairment (n = 12)	0.02 mg/kg/4 h IV	393 ± 123 (t = 60 h)	26.3 ± 9.2	1.07 ± 0.2	0.038 ± 0.014

Tacrolimus pharmacokinetics have been determined in 6 patients with mild hepatic dysfunction (mean Child-Pugh score of 6.2) following single IV and oral administrations. The mean clearance of tacrolimus in patients with mild hepatic dysfunction was not substantially different from that in healthy volunteers. Tacrolimus pharmacokinetics were studied in 6 patients with severe hepatic dysfunction (mean Child-Pugh score greater than 10). The mean clearance was substantially lower in patients with severe hepatic dysfunction, irrespective of the route of administration.

Tacrolimus Pharmacokinetics in Patients With Hepatic Impairment					
Population (Number of patients)	Dose	$AUC_{(0-t)}$ (ng•h/mL)	Half-life (h)	Volume of distribution (L/kg)	Clearance (L/h/kg)
Renal impairment (n = 12)	0.02 mg/kg/4 h IV	393 ± 123 (t = 60 h)	26.3 ± 9.2	1.07 ± 0.2	0.038 ± 0.014
Mild hepatic impairment (n = 6)	0.02 mg/kg/4 h IV	367 ± 107 (t = 72 h)	60.6 ± 43.8 Range, 27.8 to 141	3.1 ± 1.6	0.042 ± 0.02
	7.7 mg orally	488 ± 320 (t = 72 h)	66.1 ± 44.8 Range, 29.5 to 138	3.7 ± 4.7[a]	0.034 ± 0.019[a]
Severe hepatic impairment IV (n = 6)	0.02 mg/kg/4 h IV (n = 2)	762 ± 204 (t = 120 h)	198 ± 158 Range, 81 to 436	3.9 ± 1	0.017 ± 0.013
	0.01 mg/kg/8 h IV (n = 4)	289±117 (t = 144 h)			
Orally (n = 5)[b]	8 mg orally (n = 1)	658 (t = 120 h)	119±35 Range, 85 to 178	3.1 ± 3.4[a]	0.016 ± 0.011[a]
	5 mg orally (n = 4)	533 ± 156 (t = 144 h)			
	4 mg orally (n = 1)				

[a] Corrected for bioavailability.
[b] One patient did not receive the oral dose.

Children: Pharmacokinetics of tacrolimus have been studied in liver transplantation patients 0.7 to 13.2 years of age. Following IV administration of a 0.037 mg/kg/day dose to 12 pediatric patients, mean terminal half-life, volume of distribution, and clearance were 11.5 ± 3.8 hours, 2.6 ± 2.1 L/kg, and 0.138 ± 0.071 L/h/kg, respectively.

Whole blood C_{min} obtained from 31 children younger than 12 years of age showed that children need higher doses than adults to achieve similar trough concentrations.

Race: A formal study to evaluate the pharmacokinetic disposition of tacrolimus in black transplant patients has not been conducted. However, a retrospective comparison of black and white kidney transplant patients indicated that black patients required higher tacrolimus doses to attain similar trough concentrations.

Contraindications

Hypersensitivity to tacrolimus; hypersensitivity to polyoxyl 60 hydrogenated castor oil (HCO-60) (used in vehicle for injection).

Warnings/Precautions

➤*Posttransplant diabetes mellitus:* Insulin-dependent posttransplant diabetes mellitus was reported in 20% of tacrolimus-treated kidney patients without pretransplant history of diabetes mellitus in the phase 3 study. The median time to onset of posttransplant diabetes mellitus was 68 days. Insulin dependence was reversible in 15% of these posttransplant diabetes mellitus patients at 1 year and in 50% at 2 years posttransplant. Black and Hispanic kidney transplant patients were at an increased risk of development of posttransplant diabetes mellitus.

Tacrolimus Post Kidney Transplant Diabetes Mellitus		
Status of posttransplant diabetes mellitus[a]	Tacrolimus	Cyclosporine-based immunosuppressive regimen
Patients without pretransplant history of diabetes mellitus	151	151
New-onset posttransplant diabetes mellitus[a], 1st year	20%	4%
Still insulin-dependent at 1 year in those without history of diabetes	17%	3%
New onset of posttransplant diabetes mellitus[a] after 1 year	1	0

Tacrolimus Post Kidney Transplant Diabetes Mellitus		
Status of posttransplant diabetes mellitus[a]	Tacrolimus	Cyclosporine-based immunosuppressive regimen
Patients with posttransplant diabetes mellitus [a] at 2 years	11%	3%

[a] Use of insulin for 30 or more consecutive days, with less than a 5-day gap, without a prior history of insulin-dependent diabetes mellitus or non-insulin–dependent diabetes mellitus.

Tacrolimus Post Kidney Transplant Diabetes Mellitus By Race				
	Tacrolimus		Cyclosporine-based immunosuppressive regimen	
Patient race	No. of patients at risk	Patients who developed Posttransplant Diabetes Mellitus[a]	No. of patients at risk	Patients who developed Posttransplant Diabetes Mellitus[a]
Black	41	37%	36	8%
Hispanic	17	29%	18	6%
White	82	12%	87	1%
Other	11	0%	10	10%
Total	151	20%	151	4%

[a] Use of insulin for 30 or more consecutive days, with less than a 5-day gap, without a history of insulin-dependent diabetes mellitus or non–insulin-dependent diabetes mellitus.

Insulin-dependent Posttransplant Diabetes Mellitus was reported in 18% and 11% of tacrolimus-treated liver transplant patients and was reversible in 45% and 31% of these patients at 1 year posttransplant in the United States and European randomized studies, respectively. Hyperglycemia was associated with the use of tacrolimus in 47% and 33% of liver transplant recipients in the United States and European randomized studies, respectively, and may require treatment.

Tacrolimus Post Liver Transplant Diabetes Mellitus				
	United States study		European study	
Status of Posttransplant Diabetes Mellitus[a]	Tacrolimus	Cyclosporine-based immunosuppressive regimen	Tacrolimus	Cyclosporine-based immunosuppressive regimen
Patients at risk[b]	239	236	239	249
New-onset Posttransplant Diabetes Mellitus[a]	18%	13%	11%	5%
Patients still on insulin at 1 year	10%	8%	8%	2%

[a] Use of insulin for 30 or more consecutive days, with less than a 5-day gap, without a prior history of insulin-dependent diabetes mellitus or non-insulin–dependent diabetes mellitus.
[b] Patients without pretransplant history of diabetes mellitus.

Insulin-dependent posttransplant diabetes mellitus was reported in 13% and 22% of tacrolimus-treated heart transplant patients receiving mycophenolate mofetil or azathioprine and was reversible in 30% and 17% of these patients at 1 year posttransplant in the United States and European randomized studies, respectively. Hyperglycemia defined as 2 fasting plasma glucose levels of 26 mg/dL or more was reported with the use of tacrolimus plus mycophenolate mofetil or azathioprine in 32% and 35% of heart transplant recipients in the United States and European randomized studies, respectively, and may require treatment.

Tacrolimus Post Heart Transplant Diabetes Mellitus					
	United States Study			European Study	
Status of Posttransplant Diabetes Mellitus[a]	Tacrolimus/ Sirolimus	Tacrolimus/ Mycophenolate mofetil	Cyclosporine/ Mycophenolate mofetil	Tacrolimus/ Azathioprine	Cyclosporine/ Azathioprine
Patients at risk[b]	85	75	83	132	138
New-onset Posttransplant Diabetes Mellitus[a]	25%	13%	7%	22%	4%
Patients still on insulin at 1 year[c]	12%	9%	1%	18%	3%

[a] Use of insulin for 30 or more consecutive days without a history of insulin-dependent diabetes mellitus or non–insulin-dependent diabetes mellitus.
[b] Patients without pretransplant history of diabetes mellitus.
[c] Seven to 12 months for the United States study.

➤*Nephrotoxicity:* Tacrolimus can cause nephrotoxicity, particularly when used in high doses. Nephrotoxicity has been noted in approximately 52% of kidney transplantation patients and in 36% to 40% of liver transplantation patients receiving the drug, and in 59% of heart transplantation patients in a European randomized trial. Use of tacrolimus with sirolimus in heart transplant patients in a United States study was associated with an increased risk of renal impairment and is not recommended. More overt nephrotoxicity is seen early after transplantation, characterized by increasing serum creatinine and a decrease in urine output. Closely monitor patients with impaired renal function; the dosage may need to be reduced. In patients with persistent elevations of serum creatinine who are unre-

TACROLIMUS — INJECTION

sponsive to dosage adjustments, consider changing to another immunosuppressive therapy. Take care in using tacrolimus with other nephrotoxic drugs; in particular, to avoid excess nephrotoxicity, do not use simultaneously with cyclosporine. Discontinue tacrolimus or cyclosporine at least 24 hours prior to initiating the other. In the presence of elevated tacrolimus or cyclosporine concentrations, usually delay dosing with the other drug.

➤*Hyperkalemia:* Mild to severe hyperkalemia that may require treatment has been noted in 31% of kidney transplant recipients and in 13% to 45% of liver transplant recipients treated with tacrolimus, and in 8% of heart transplant recipients in a European randomized trial. Monitor serum potassium levels, and potassium-sparing diuretics should not be used during tacrolimus therapy.

➤*Neurotoxicity:* Tacrolimus can cause neurotoxicity, particularly when used in high doses. Neurotoxicity, including tremor, headache, and other changes in motor function, mental status, and sensory function, occurred in approximately 55% of liver transplant recipients. Tremor occurred more often in tacrolimus-treated kidney transplant patients (54%) and heart transplant patients (15%) compared with cyclosporine-treated patients. The incidence of other neurological events in kidney transplant and heart transplant patients was similar in the 2 treatment groups. Tremor and headache have been associated with high whole blood concentrations of tacrolimus and may respond to dosage adjustment. Seizures have occurred in adult and pediatric patients. Coma and delirium also have been associated with high plasma concentrations of tacrolimus.

Patients treated with tacrolimus have been reported to develop posterior reversible encephalopathy syndrome. Symptoms indicating posterior reversible encephalopathy syndrome include altered mental status, headache, hypertension, seizures, and visual disturbances. Diagnosis may be confirmed by radiological procedure. If posterior reversible encephalopathy syndrome is suspected or diagnosed, blood pressure control should be maintained and immediate reduction of immunosuppression is advised. This syndrome is characterized by reversal of symptoms upon reduction or discontinuation of immunosuppression.

➤*Lymphomas and other malignancies:* As with other immunosuppressants, patients receiving tacrolimus are at increased risk of developing lymphomas and other malignancies, particularly of the skin. The risk appears to be related to the intensity and duration of immunosuppression rather than to the use of any specific agent.

➤*Infections:*

Epstein-Barr virus – A lymphoproliferative disorder related to Epstein-Barr virus infection has been reported in immunosuppressed organ transplant recipients. The risk of lymphoproliferative disorder appears greatest in young children who are at risk for primary Epstein-Barr virus infection while immunosuppressed or who are switched to tacrolimus following long-term immunosuppressive therapy. Because of the danger of oversuppression of the immune system, which can increase susceptibility to infection, use combination immunosuppressant therapy with caution.

Latent viral infections – Immunosuppressed patients are at increased risk for opportunistic infections, including activation of latent viral infections. These include BK virus–associated neuropathy and JC virus–associated progressive multifocal leukoencephalopathy (PML), which have been observed in patients receiving tacrolimus. These infections may lead to serious, including fatal, outcomes.

➤*Tacrolimus in combination with sirolimus:* The use of full-dose tacrolimus with sirolimus (2 mg per day) in heart transplant recipients was associated with an increased risk of wound healing complications, renal impairment, and insulin-dependent posttransplant diabetes mellitus, and is not recommended.

➤*Hypertension:* Hypertension is a common adverse reaction of tacrolimus therapy. Mild or moderate hypertension is more frequently reported than severe hypertension. Antihypertensive therapy may be required; the control of blood pressure can be accomplished with any of the common antihypertensive agents. Because tacrolimus may cause hyperkalemia, avoid potassium-sparing diuretics. While calcium-channel blocking agents can be effective in treating tacrolimus-associated hypertension, interference with tacrolimus metabolism may require a dosage reduction.

➤*Myocardial hypertrophy:* Myocardial hypertrophy has been reported in association with the administration of tacrolimus and is generally manifested by echocardiographically demonstrated concentric increases in left ventricular posterior wall and interventricular septum thickness. Hypertrophy has been observed in infants, children, and adults. This condition appears reversible in most cases following dose reduction or discontinuance of therapy. In a group of 20 patients with pretreatment and posttreatment echocardiograms who showed evidence of myocardial hypertrophy, mean tacrolimus whole blood concentrations during the period prior to diagnosis of myocardial hypertrophy ranged from 11 to 53 ng/mL in infants (n = 10; range, 0.4 to 2 years of age), 4 to 46 ng/mL in children (n = 7; range, 2 to 15 years of age), and 11 to 24 ng/mL in adults (n = 3; range, 37 to 53 years of age).

In patients who develop renal failure or clinical manifestations of ventricular dysfunction while receiving tacrolimus therapy, consider echocardiographic evaluation. If myocardial hypertrophy is diagnosed, consider dosage reduction or discontinuation of tacrolimus.

➤*Hypersensitivity reactions:* A few patients receiving tacrolimus injection have experienced anaphylactic reactions. Although the exact cause of these reactions is not known, other drugs with castor oil derivatives in the formulation have been associated with anaphylaxis in a small percentage of patients. Because of this potential risk of anaphylaxis, reserve the injection for patients who are unable to take capsules.

Continuously observe patients receiving the injection for at least the first 30 minutes following the start of the infusion and at frequent intervals thereafter. If signs or symptoms of anaphylaxis occur, stop the infusion. Have an aqueous solution of epinephrine available at the bedside as well as a source of oxygen.

➤*Renal/Hepatic function impairment:* For patients with renal insufficiency, some evidence suggests that lower doses should be used.

The use of tacrolimus in liver transplant recipients experiencing posttransplant hepatic impairment may be associated with an increased risk of developing renal insufficiency related to high whole-blood levels of tacrolimus. Monitor these patients closely and consider dosage adjustments. Some evidence suggests that lower doses should be used in these patients.

➤*Photosensitivity:* As with other immunosuppressive agents, owing to the potential risk of malignant skin changes, patients should limit their exposure to sunlight and ultraviolet light by wearing protective clothing and using a sunscreen with a high sun protection factor.

➤*Pregnancy:* *Category C.* There are no adequate and well-controlled studies in pregnant women. Tacrolimus is transferred across the placenta. The use of tacrolimus during pregnancy has been associated with neonatal hyperkalemia and renal dysfunction. Administer during pregnancy only if the potential benefit to the mother justifies potential risk to the fetus.

In reproduction studies in rats and rabbits, adverse reactions on the fetus were observed, mainly at dose levels that were toxic to dams. Tacrolimus at oral doses of 0.32 and 1 mg/kg during organogenesis in rabbits was associated with maternal toxicity as well as an increase in incidence of abortions; these doses are equivalent to 0.5 to 1 times and 1.6 to 3.3 times the recommended clinical dose range (0.1 to 0.2 mg/kg) based on body surface area corrections. At the higher dose only, an increased incidence of malformations and developmental variations was also seen. Tacrolimus at oral doses of 3.2 mg/kg during organogenesis in rats was associated with maternal toxicity and caused an increase in late resorptions, decreased numbers of live births, and decreased pup weight and viability. Oral tacrolimus 1 and 3.2 mg/kg (equivalent to 0.7 to 1.4 times and 2.3 to 4.6 times the recommended clinical dose range based on body surface area corrections) given to pregnant rats after organogenesis and during lactation was associated with reduced pup weights. No reduction in male or female fertility was evident.

➤*Lactation:* Tacrolimus is excreted in breast milk; patients should avoid breast-feeding.

➤*Children:* Experience with tacrolimus in pediatric kidney and heart transplant patients is limited. Successful liver transplants have been performed in children (up to 16 years of age) using tacrolimus. Children generally require higher doses to maintain blood trough levels of tacrolimus similar to adult patients.

Two randomized, active-controlled trials of tacrolimus in primary liver transplantation included 56 children. Thirty-one patients were randomized to tacrolimus-based therapy and 25 to cyclosporine-based. Additionally, a minimum of 122 children were studied in an uncontrolled trial of tacrolimus in living related-donor liver transplantation.

➤*Monitoring:* Regularly assess serum creatinine, potassium, and fasting glucose. Perform routine monitoring of metabolic and hematologic systems as clinically warranted.

Continuously observe patients receiving tacrolimus injection for at least the first 30 minutes following the start of the infusion and at frequent intervals thereafter.

The relative risk of toxicity is increased with higher trough concentrations; therefore, monitoring of whole blood trough concentrations is recommended to assist in the clinical evaluation of toxicity.

Drug Interactions

➤*Cytochrome P450 system:* Since tacrolimus is metabolized mainly by the CYP3A enzyme systems, substances known to inhibit these enzymes may decrease metabolism or increase bioavailability of tacrolimus, as indicated by increased whole blood or plasma concentrations. Drugs known to induce these enzyme systems may result in an increased metabolism of tacrolimus or decreased bioavailability, as indicated by decreased whole blood or plasma concentrations. Monitoring of blood concentrations and appropriate dosage adjustments are essential when such drugs are used concomitantly.

➤*Drugs that prolong the QT interval:* An additive effect of tacrolimus with other drugs that prolong the QT interval cannot be excluded. The following drugs may prolong the QT interval and increase the risk of life-threatening cardiac arrhythmias, including torsades de pointes: antiarrhythmic agents (eg, amiodarone, bretylium, disopyramide, dofetilide, flecainide, procainamide, quinidine, sotalol), arsenic trioxide, chlorpromazine, cisapride, dolasetron, droperidol, lapatinib, mefloquine, mesoridazine, methadone, moxifloxacin, nilotinib, paliperidone, pentamidine, perflutren, pimozide, propafenone, quinupristin-dalfopristin, tetrabenazine, thioridazine, and ziprasidone. For a more complete list of drugs that may prolong the QT interval, see the appendix "Drug-Induced Prolongation of the QT Interval and Torsades de Pointes."

➤*Vaccinations:* Immunosuppressants may affect vaccination. Therefore, during treatment with tacrolimus, vaccination may be less effective. Avoid the use of live vaccines (ie, measles, mumps, rubella, oral polio, BCG, yellow fever, and TY 21a typhoid).

TACROLIMUS — INJECTION

Tacrolimus Drug Interactions

Precipitant drug	Object drug[a]		Description
Amiodarone	Tacrolimus	↑	Tacrolimus plasma concentration may be increased, increasing the risk of toxicity. Consider lower doses of tacrolimus and monitoring of plasma concentrations.
Anticonvulsants (ie, carbamazepine, fosphenytoin, phenobarbital, phenytoin)	Tacrolimus	↓↑	These anticonvulsants may decrease tacrolimus blood levels, increasing the risk of organ transplant rejection. Phenytoin serum concentrations may be increased by tacrolimus.
Tacrolimus	Phenytoin		
Antifungal agents (eg, clotrimazole, fluconazole, itraconazole, ketoconazole, voriconazole)	Tacrolimus	↑	Tacrolimus blood levels may be increased, increasing the risk of toxicity.
Bromocriptine	Tacrolimus	↑	Tacrolimus blood levels may be increased, increasing the risk of toxicity.
Calcium channel blockers (eg, diltiazem, nicardipine, nifedipine, verapamil)	Tacrolimus	↑	Tacrolimus blood levels may be increased, increasing the risk of toxicity.
Caspofungin	Tacrolimus	↓	Tacrolimus blood levels may be decreased, increasing the risk of organ transplant rejection.
Chloramphenicol	Tacrolimus	↑	Tacrolimus blood levels may be increased, increasing the risk of toxicity.
Cimetidine	Tacrolimus	↑	Tacrolimus blood levels may be increased, increasing the risk of toxicity.
Cisapride[b]	Tacrolimus	↑	Tacrolimus blood levels may be increased, increasing the risk of toxicity.
Danazol	Tacrolimus	↑	Tacrolimus blood levels may be increased, increasing the risk of toxicity.
Ethinyl estradiol	Tacrolimus	↑	Tacrolimus blood levels may be increased, increasing the risk of toxicity.
Macrolide antibiotics (eg, clarithromycin, erythromycin, troleandomycin[c])	Tacrolimus	↑	Tacrolimus blood levels may be increased, increasing the risk of toxicity.
Magnesium-aluminum-hydroxide antacid	Tacrolimus	↑↓	Coadministration of tacrolimus and magnesium-aluminum-hydroxide resulted in a 21% increase in the mean tacrolimus AUC and a 10% decrease in the mean tacrolimus C_{max} relative to tacrolimus administration alone.
Methylprednisolone	Tacrolimus	↑	Tacrolimus blood levels may be increased, increasing the risk of toxicity.
Metoclopramide	Tacrolimus	↑	Tacrolimus blood levels may be increased, increasing the risk of toxicity.
Nefazodone	Tacrolimus	↑	Tacrolimus blood levels may be increased, increasing the risk of toxicity.
Nephrotoxic agents (eg, aminoglycosides, amphotericin B, cisplatin, cyclosporine)	Tacrolimus	↑	Because of the potential for additive or synergistic impairment of renal function, take care when administering tacrolimus with drugs that may be associated with renal dysfunction. Coadministration with cyclosporine resulted in additive/synergistic nephrotoxicity; tacrolimus blood levels also may be increased. Give the first tacrolimus dose no sooner than 24 hours after the last cyclosporine dose.
Tacrolimus	Nephrotoxic agents (eg, aminoglycosides, amphotericin B, cisplatin, cyclosporine)		
Protease inhibitors (eg, nelfinavir, ritonavir)	Tacrolimus	↑	Tacrolimus blood levels may be increased, increasing the risk of toxicity.
Proton pump inhibitors (eg, lansoprazole, omeprazole)	Tacrolimus	↑	Tacrolimus blood levels may be increased, increasing the risk of toxicity.
Rifabutin, rifampin	Tacrolimus	↓	Tacrolimus bioavailability may be decreased and clearance increased with coadministration.
Sirolimus	Tacrolimus	↑↓	Trough concentrations of tacrolimus may be decreased by sirolimus resulting in a reduced pharmacologic effect of tacrolimus. In addition, coadministration of tacrolimus and sirolimus in combination with corticosteroids has been associated with fatal cases of bronchial anastomotic dehiscence in lung transplant patients. The safety and efficacy of tacrolimus used in combination with sirolimus have not been established and the combination is not recommended.
St. John's wort	Tacrolimus	↓	St. John's wort induces CYP3A4 and P-glycoprotein. Because tacrolimus is a substrate for CYP3A4, tacrolimus blood levels may decrease.
Tacrolimus	Mycophenolate mofetil	↑	Mycophenolate trough plasma concentrations may be elevated, increasing the risk of adverse reactions.
Tacrolimus	Phenytoin	↑↓	Phenytoin serum concentrations may be increased by tacrolimus. Phenytoin may also reduce tacrolimus plasma concentrations and pharmacologic effects.
Phenytoin	Tacrolimus		
Tacrolimus	Potassium-sparing diuretics	↑	Because tacrolimus can cause hyperkalemia, avoid using potassium-sparing diuretics.
Potassium-sparing diuretics	Tacrolimus		
Tacrolimus	Statins (eg, lovastatin, simvastatin)	↑	Coadministration may increase both plasma concentrations of tacrolimus and certain statins. Fluvastatin or pravastatin may be less likely to interact and may be safer alternatives.
Statins (eg, lovastatin, simvastatin)	Tacrolimus		
Tacrolimus	Ziprasidone	↑	The risk of life-threatening cardiac arrhythmias, including torsades de pointes, may be increased. Coadministration is contraindicated.

[a] ↑ = object drug increased; ↓ = object drug decreased; ↑↓ = object drug both increased and decreased.

[b] Available from the manufacturer on a limited-access protocol.

[c] No longer marketed in the United States.

➤*Drug/Food interactions:* Coadministered grapefruit juice has been reported to increase tacrolimus blood trough concentrations in liver transplant patients. Grapefruit juice affects CYP3A-mediated metabolism and should be avoided.

TACROLIMUS – INJECTION

Adverse Reactions

➤*Kidney / Liver / Heart transplant adverse reactions:*

Tacrolimus Adverse Reactions in Kidney/Liver/Heart Transplant Patients (≥ 15%)[a]

Adverse reaction	Liver transplant patients[a]		Kidney transplant patients		Heart transplant patients	
	Tacrolimus + steroids (n = 514)	Cyclosporine based regimen (n = 515)	Tacrolimus + azathioprine (n = 205)	Cyclosporine based regimen (n = 207)	Tacrolimus + azathioprine (n = 157)	Cyclosporine + azathioprine (n = 157)
Cardiovascular						
Chest pain	—	—	19%	13%	—	—
Hypertension[b]	38% to 47%	43% to 56%	50%	52%	62%	69%
Pericardial effusion	—	—	—	—	15%	14%
CNS						
Asthenia	11% to 52%	7% 48%	34%	30%	—	—
Dizziness	—	—	19%	16%	—	—
Headache[b]	37% to 64%	26% to 60%	44%	38%	—	—
Insomnia	32% to 64%	23% to 68%	32%	30%	—	—
Paresthesia	17% to 40%	17% to 30%	23%	16%	—	—
Tremor[b]	48% to 56%	32% to 46%	54%	34%	15%	6%
Dermatologic						
Pruritus	15% to 36%	7% to 20%	15%	7%	—	—
Rash	10% to 24%	4% to 19%	17%	12%	—	—
GI						
Abdominal pain	29% to 59%	22% to 54%	33%	31%	—	—
Anorexia	7% to 34%	5% to 24%	—	—	—	—
Constipation	23% to 24%	21% to 27%	35%	43%	—	—
Diarrhea	37% to 72%	27% to 47%	44%	41%	—	—
Dyspepsia	—	—	28%	20%	—	—
Liver function tests abnormal	6% to 36%	5% to 30%				
Nausea	32% to 46%	27% to 37%	38%	36%	—	—
Vomiting	14% to 27%	11% to 15%	29%	23%	—	—
GU						
Creatinine increased[b]	24% to 39%	19% to 25%	45%	42%	—	—
Kidney function abnormal[b]	36% to 40%	23% to 27%	—	—	56%	57%
Oliguria	18% to 19%	12% to 15%	—	—	—	—
Serum urea nitrogen increased[b]	12% to 30%	9% to 22%	—	—	—	—
Urinary tract infection	16% to 21%	18% to 19%	34%	35%	16%	12%
Hematologic/Lymphatic						
Anemia	5% to 47%	1% to 38%	30%	24%	50%	36%
Leukocytosis	8% to 32%	8% to 26%	—	—	—	—
Leukopenia	—	—	15%	17%	48%	39%
Thrombocytopenia	14% to 24%	19% to 20%	—	—	—	—
Metabolic/Nutritional						
Diabetes mellitus[b]	—	—	24%	9%	26%	16%
Edema	—	—	18%	19%	—	—
Hyperglycemia[b]	33% to 47%	22% to 38%	22%	16%	23%	17%
Hyperkalemia[b]	13% to 45%	9% to 26%	31%	32%	—	—
Hyperlipemia	—	—	31%	38%	18%	27%
Hypokalemia	13% to 29%	16% to 34%	22%	25%	—	—
Hypomagnesemia	16% to 48%	9% to 45%	34%	17%	—	—
Hypophosphatemia	—	—	49%	53%	—	—
Peripheral edema	12% to 26%	14% to 26%	36%	48%	—	—
Respiratory						
Atelectasis	5% to 28%	4% to 30%	—	—	—	—
Bronchitis	—	—	—	—	17%	18%
Cough increased	—	—	18%	15%	—	—
Dyspnea	5% to 29%	4% to 23%	22%	18%	—	—
Pleural effusion	30% to 36%	32% to 35%	—	—	—	—
Miscellaneous						
Arthralgia	—	—	25%	24%	—	—
Ascites	7% to 27%	8% to 22%	—	—	—	—
Back pain	17% to 30%	17% to 29%	24%	20%	—	—
Cytomegalovirus infection	—	—	—	—	32%	30%
Fever	19% to 48%	22% to 56%	29%	29%	—	—
Infection	—	—	45%	49%	24%	21%
Pain	24% to 63%	22% to 57%	32%	30%	—	—

[a] Data are pooled from separate United States and European studies and are not necessarily comparable.
[b] See Warnings/Precautions.

➤*Kidney Transplant:* The most common adverse reactions reported in kidney transplant patients were abdominal pain, abnormal renal function, constipation, diarrhea, headache, hypertension, infection, insomnia, and tremor.

Adverse reactions that occurred in 10% or more of kidney transplant patients treated with tacrolimus in conjunction with mycophenolate mofetil in study 1 are presented in the following table. Study 1 was conducted entirely outside the United States and such studies often report a lower incidence of adverse reactions in comparison to United States studies.

Kidney Transplantation: Adverse Reactions Occurring in Tacrolimus-Treated Patients (≥ 10%)

Adverse reaction	Tacrolimus (Group C) (n = 403)	Cyclosporine (Group A) (n = 384)	Cyclosporine (Group B) (n = 408)
Hematologic			
Anemia	17%	19%	17%
Leukopenia	13%	10%	10%
Metabolic/Nutritional			
Edema peripheral	11%	12%	13%
Hyperlipidemia	10%	15%	13%

TACROLIMUS — INJECTION

Kidney Transplantation: Adverse Reactions Occurring in Tacrolimus-Treated Patients (≥ 10%)			
Adverse reaction	Tacrolimus (Group C) (n = 403)	Cyclosporine (Group A) (n = 384)	Cyclosporine (Group B) (n = 408)
Miscellaneous			
Diarrhea	25%	16%	13%
Hypertension	13%	14%	12%
Urinary tract infection	24%	28%	24%

Kidney Transplantation: Adverse Reactions Occurring in Tacrolimus-Treated Patients (≥ 15%)		
Adverse reaction	Tacrolimus and mycophenolate mofetil (n = 212)	Cyclosporine (n = 212)
CNS		
Headache	24%	25%
Insomnia	30%	21%
Tremor	34%	20%
GI		
Constipation	36%	41%
Diarrhea	44%	26%
Dyspepsia	18%	15%
Nausea	39%	47%
Vomiting	26%	25%
Hematologic/Lymphatic		
Anemia	30%	28%
Leukopenia	16%	12%
Metabolic/Nutritional		
Edema peripheral	35%	46%
Hyperglycemia	21%	15%
Hyperkalemia	26%	19%
Hyperlipidemia	18%	25%
Hypokalemia	16%	18%
Hypomagnesemia	28%	22%
Hypophosphatemia	28%	21%
Miscellaneous		
Blood creatinine increased	23%	23%
Graft dysfunction	24%	18%
Hypertension	32%	35%
Incision-site complication	28%	23%
Postprocedural pain	29%	27%
Urinary tract infection	26%	22%

Liver transplant – The principal adverse reactions of tacrolimus are abnormal renal function, diarrhea, headache, hypertension, nausea, and tremor. These adverse reactions may respond to a reduction in dosing. Diarrhea was sometimes associated with other GI complaints, such as nausea and vomiting.

Hyperkalemia and hypomagnesemia have occurred. Hyperglycemia has been noted in many patients; some may require insulin therapy.

The incidence of adverse reactions was determined in 2 randomized, comparative liver transplant trials among 514 patients receiving tacrolimus and steroids and 515 patients receiving a cyclosporine-based regimen. The proportion of patients reporting more than 1 adverse reaction was 99.8% in the tacrolimus group and 99.6% in the cyclosporine-based regimen group. Precautions must be taken when comparing the incidence of adverse reactions in the United States study with that in the European study. The 12-month posttransplant information from the United States study and from the European study are presented in the first table in the Adverse Reactions sections. The 2 studies also included different patient populations and patients were treated with immunosuppressive regimens of differing intensities.

Heart transplant – The more common adverse reactions in tacrolimus-treated heart transplant recipients were abnormal renal function, cytomegalovirus infection, diabetes mellitus, hyperglycemia, hyperlipemia, hypertension, infection, leukopenia, and tremor.

In the European study, the cyclosporine trough concentrations were above the predefined target range (ie, 100 to 200 ng/mL) at day 122 and beyond in 32% to 68% of the patients in the cyclosporine treatment arm, whereas the tacrolimus trough concentrations were within the predefined target range (ie, 5 to 15 ng/mL) in 74% to 86% of the patients in the tacrolimus treatment arm.

Only selected targeted treatment-emergent adverse reactions were collected in the United States heart transplantation study. Those reactions that were reported at a rate of 15% or greater in patients treated with tacrolimus and mycophenolate mofetil include the following: any target adverse reactions (99.1%), hypertension (88.8%), hyperglycemia requiring antihyperglycemic therapy (70.1%), hypertriglyceridemia (65.4%), anemia (hemoglobin less than 10 g/dL) (65.4%), fasting blood glucose greater than 140 mg/dL (on 2 separate occasions) (60.7%), hypercholesterolemia (57%), hyperlipidemia (33.6%), white blood cell count less than 3,000 cells/mcL (33.6%), serious bacterial infections (29.9%), magnesium less than 1.2 mEq/L (24.3%), platelet count less than 75,000 cells/mcL (18.7%), and other opportunistic infections (15%).

Other targeted treatment-emergent adverse reactions in tacrolimus-treated patients occurred at a rate of less than 15%, and include the following: *Candida* infection, cytomegalovirus infection/syndrome, cushingoid features, hyperkalemia, and impaired wound healing.

➤*Other liver/kidney/heart transplant adverse reactions:*

Cardiovascular – Angina pectoris, arrhythmia, atrial fibrillation, atrial flutter, abnormal electrocardiogram (ECG), bradycardia, cardiac fibrillation, cardiopulmonary failure, cardiovascular disorder, chest pain, congestive heart failure, deep thrombophlebitis, ECG QRS complex abnormal, ECG ST segment abnormal, echocardiogram abnormal, heart failure, heart rate decreased, hemorrhage, hypotension, peripheral vascular disorder, phlebitis, postural hypotension, syncope, tachycardia, thrombosis, vasodilation.

CNS – Abnormal dreams, agitation, amnesia, anxiety, asthenia, chills, confusion, convulsion, crying, depression, dizziness, elevated mood, emotional lability, encephalopathy, feeling abnormal, hallucinations, headache, hemorrhagic stroke, hypertonia, incoordination, insomnia, monoparesis, myoclonus, nerve compression, nervousness, neuralgia, neuropathy, paralysis flaccid, paresthesia, psychomotor skills impaired, psychosis, quadriparesis, somnolence, thinking abnormal, vertigo, writing impaired.

Dermatologic – Acne, alopecia, exfoliative dermatitis, fungal dermatitis, herpes simplex, herpes zoster, hirsutism, neoplasm (skin, benign), photosensitivity reaction, skin discoloration, skin disorder, skin ulcer, sweating.

Endocrine – Cushing syndrome, diabetes mellitus.

GI – Abdomen enlarged, anorexia, cholangitis, diarrhea, duodenitis, dyspepsia, dysphagia, esophagitis, esophagitis ulcerative, flatulence, gastritis, gastroesophagitis, GI disorder, GI hemorrhage, GI perforation, ileus, increased appetite, jaundice, nausea, nausea and vomiting, oral moniliasis, pancreatic pseudocyst, rectal disorder, stomatitis, vomiting.

GU – Acute kidney failure, albuminuria, BK neuropathy, bladder spasm, cystitis, dysuria, hematuria, hydronephrosis, kidney failure, kidney tubular necrosis, nocturia, oliguria, pyuria, toxic nephropathy, urge incontinence, urinary frequency, urinary incontinence, urinary retention, vaginitis.

Hematologic/Lymphatic – Coagulation disorder, ecchymosis, hematocrit increased, hemoglobin abnormal, hypochromic anemia, leukocytosis, leukopenia, polycythemia, prothrombin decreased, serum iron decreased, thrombocytopenia.

Hepatic – Cholestatic jaundice, hepatitis, hepatitis granulomatous, liver damage, liver function tests abnormal.

Metabolic/Nutritional – Acidosis, alkaline phosphatase increased, alkalosis, ALT increased, AST increased, bicarbonate decreased, bilirubinemia, dehydration, edema, gamma glutamyl transpeptidase increased, gout, hypercalcemia, hypercholesterolemia, hyperkalemia, hyperlipidemia, hyperphosphatemia, hyperuricemia, hypervolemia, hypocalcemia, hypoglycemia, hypokalemia, hypomagnesemia, hyponatremia, hypophosphatemia, hypoproteinemia, lactic dehydrogenase increase, peripheral edema, serum urea nitrogen increased, weight gain.

Musculoskeletal – Arthralgia, back pain, cramps, generalized spasm, joint disorder, leg cramps, myalgia, myasthenia, osteoporosis.

Respiratory – Asthma, bronchitis, cough increased, dyspnea, emphysema, hiccups, lung disorder, lung function decreased, pharyngitis, pleural effusion, pneumonia, pneumothorax, pulmonary edema, respiratory disorder, rhinitis, sinusitis, voice alteration.

Special senses – Abnormal vision, amblyopia, ear pain, otitis media, tinnitus.

Miscellaneous – Abdominal pain, abscess, accidental injury, allergic reaction, cellulitis, fall, fever, flu syndrome, generalized edema, healing abnormal, hernia, mobility decreased, pain, peritonitis, sepsis, temperature intolerance, ulcer.

➤*Postmarketing:*

Cardiovascular – Atrial fibrillation, atrial flutter, cardiac arrhythmia, cardiac arrest, ECG T-wave abnormal, flushing, myocardial infarction, myocardial ischemia, pericardial effusion, QT prolongation, syncope, torsades de pointes, venous thrombosis deep limb, ventricular extrasystoles, ventricular fibrillation.

There have been rare, spontaneous reports of myocardial hypertrophy associated with clinically manifested ventricular dysfunction in patients receiving tacrolimus therapy.

CNS – Carpal tunnel syndrome, cerebral infection, feeling jittery, hemiparesis, leukoencephalopathy, mental disorder, mutism, posterior reversible encephalopathy syndrome, PML, quadriplegia, speech disorder.

Dermatologic – Stevens-Johnson syndrome, toxic epidermal necrolysis.

GI – Bile duct stenosis, colitis, enterocolitis, gastroenteritis, gastroesophageal reflux disease, hepatotoxicity, impaired gastric emptying, mouth ulceration, pancreatitis hemorrhagic, pancreatitis necrotizing, stomach ulcer.

TACROLIMUS — INJECTION

GU – Acute renal failure, cystitis hemorrhagic, hemolytic-uremic syndrome, micturition disorder.

Hematologic/Lymphatic – Disseminated intravascular coagulation, neutropenia, pancytopenia, thrombocytopenic purpura, thrombotic thrombocytopenic purpura.

Hepatic – Hepatic cytolysis, hepatic necrosis, liver fatty, venoocclusive liver disease.

Metabolic/Nutritional – Glycosuria, increased amylase including pancreatitis, weight decreased.

Respiratory – Acute respiratory distress syndrome, interstitial lung disease, lung infiltration, respiratory distress, respiratory failure.

Special senses – Blindness; blindness cortical; hearing loss, including deafness; photophobia.

Miscellaneous – Feeling hot and cold, hot flushes, multiorgan failure, primary graft dysfunction.

Overdosage

➤*Symptoms:* There is limited experience with overdosage. Acute overdosages of up to 30 times the intended dose have been reported. Almost all cases have been asymptomatic and all patients recovered with no sequelae. Occasionally, acute overdosage has been followed by adverse reactions consistent with tacrolimus, except in one case where transient urticaria and lethargy were observed.

➤*Treatment:* Based on the poor aqueous solubility and extensive erythrocyte and plasma protein binding, it is anticipated that tacrolimus is not dialyzable to any significant extent; there is no experience with charcoal hemoperfusion. The oral use of activated charcoal has been reported in treating acute overdoses, but experience has not been sufficient to warrant recommending its use. Follow general supportive measures in all cases of overdosage.

Patient Information

Inform patients of the need for repeated appropriate lab tests while they are receiving tacrolimus. Give patients complete dosage instructions, advise them of potential risks during pregnancy, and inform them of the increased risk of neoplasia.

Inform patients to not undertake changes in dosage without first consulting their health care provider.

Inform patients that tacrolimus can cause diabetes mellitus and advise them of the need to see their health care provider if they develop frequent urination or increased thirst or hunger.

Advise patients to limit exposure to sunlight and ultraviolet light by wearing protective clothing and using a sunscreen with a high protection factor because of the increased risk for skin cancer.

SIROLIMUS

Rx	**Rapamune** (Wyeth)	**Tablets; oral:** 0.5 mg	Lactose, PEG, sucrose. (RAPAMUNE 0.5 mg). Tan, triangular. In 100s and *Redipak* UD 100s.
		1 mg	Lactose, PEG, sucrose. (RAPAMUNE 1 mg). White, triangular. In 100s and *Redipak* UD 100s.
		2 mg	Lactose, PEG, sucrose. (RAPAMUNE 2 mg). Yellow to beige, triangular. In 100s.
Rx	**Rapamune** (Wyeth)	**Solution; oral:** 1 mg/mL	Ethanol 1.5% to 2.5%, polysorbate 80, propylene glycol. In 60 mL glass bottle with oral syringe adapter and disposable oral syringes.

SIROLIMUS — ORAL

WARNING

Immunosuppression – Increased susceptibility to infection and development of lymphoma may result from immunosuppression. Only health care providers experienced in immunosuppressive therapy and management of renal transplant patients should use sirolimus. Manage patients receiving the drug in facilities equipped and staffed with adequate laboratory and supportive medical resources. The health care provider responsible for maintenance therapy should have complete information requisite for the follow-up of the patient.

Liver transplantation –

Excess mortality, graft loss, and hepatic artery thrombosis: The use of sirolimus in combination with tacrolimus was associated with excess mortality and graft loss in a study in de novo liver transplant recipients. Many of these patients had evidence of infection at or near the time of death.

In this and another study in de novo liver transplant recipients, the use of sirolimus in combination with cyclosporine or tacrolimus was associated with an increase in hepatic artery thrombosis; most cases of hepatic artery thrombosis occurred within 30 days posttransplantation, and most led to graft loss or death. The safety and efficacy of sirolimus as immunosuppressive therapy have not been established in liver transplant patients; therefore, use in these patients is not recommended.

Lung transplantation –

Bronchial anastomotic dehiscence: Cases of bronchial anastomotic dehiscence, most fatal, have been reported in de novo lung transplant patients when sirolimus has been used as part of an immunosuppressive regimen. The safety and efficacy of sirolimus as immunosuppressive therapy have not been established in lung transplant patients; therefore, use in these patients is not recommended.

Indications

➤*Renal transplantation:* For the prophylaxis of organ rejection in patients 13 years of age and older who are receiving renal transplants. Therapeutic drug monitoring is recommended for all patients receiving sirolimus.

➤*Off-label uses:*

Psoriasis – [2] = Fair documentation. Sirolimus as monotherapy for psoriasis has not proven to be as effective as cyclosporine monotherapy for the treatment of severe psoriasis; however, its use in combination with subtherapeutic levels of cyclosporine has been effective. The 2 drugs, when given together, can lead to a beneficial drug interaction, leading to a synergistic effect on sirolimus and, ultimately, to decreased toxicities of both drugs. The combination may be considered in patients at increased risk for cyclosporine nephrotoxicity.

Administration and Dosage

➤*General dosing considerations:* Therapeutic drug monitoring should be used to maintain sirolimus drug concentrations within the target range. (See Therapeutic drug monitoring.)

The initial dose should be administered as soon as possible after transplantation.

2 mg of the oral solution has been demonstrated to be clinically equivalent to 2 mg tablets; therefore, they are interchangeable on a milligram-to-milligram basis. However, it is not known whether higher doses of solution are clinically equivalent to higher doses of tablets on a milligram-to-milligram basis.

It is recommended that sirolimus be used in combination with cyclosporine and corticosteroids.

➤*Adults:*

Renal transplantation –

High immunologic risk:

- *Maximum dose* – 40 mg/day.
- *Loading dose* – Up to 15 mg on day 1 posttransplantation.
- *Maintenance dosage* – 5 mg/day beginning on day 2. A trough level should be obtained between days 5 and 7, and the daily dose of sirolimus should be adjusted thereafter.
- *Dosage adjustment* –

Once the maintenance dosage is adjusted, patients should continue on the new maintenance dosage for at least 7 to 14 days before further dosage adjustment with concentration monitoring. In most patients, dosage adjustments can be based on a simple proportion: new dose = current dose × (target concentration/current concentration). A loading dose should be considered in addition to a new maintenance dosage when it is necessary to increase sirolimus trough concentrations: sirolimus loading dose = 3 × (new maintenance dose – current maintenance dose). If an estimated daily dose exceeds 40 mg because of the addition of a loading dose, the loading dose should be administered over 2 days.

- *Concomitant therapy* – Use in combination with cyclosporine and corticosteroids for the first 12 months following transplantation. The starting dosage of cyclosporine should be up to 7 mg/kg/day in divided doses and the dosage should subsequently be adjusted to achieve target whole blood trough concentrations. Prednisone should be administered at a minimum of 5 mg/day. Antibody induction therapy may be used.

Low to moderate immunologic risk:

- *Maximum dose* – 40 mg/day.
- *Loading dose* – 6 mg.
- *Maintenance dosage* – 2 mg/day.
- *Dosage adjustment* – See High Immunologic Risk for dosage adjustment.
- *Concomitant therapy* – It is recommended that sirolimus be used initially in a regimen with cyclosporine and corticosteroids. At 2 to 4 months following transplantation, cyclosporine should be progressively discontinued over 4 to 8 weeks, and the sirolimus dose should be adjusted to obtain whole blood trough concentrations within the target range. Because cyclosporine inhibits the metabolism and transport of sirolimus, sirolimus concentrations may decrease when cyclosporine is discontinued unless the sirolimus dose is increased.

Off-label dosing –

Psoriasis: [2] = Fair documentation. Used in combination therapy at a dosage of 3 mg/m^2 daily orally, along with subtherapeutic doses of cyclosporine.

➤*Children:*

Renal transplantation –

Low to moderate immunologic risk:

- *13 years of age and older* –

Maximum dose: 40 mg daily.

SIROLIMUS — ORAL

Loading dose: 6 mg for patients weighing 40 kg or more; 3 mg/m² for patients weighing less than 40 kg.

Maintenance dosage: 2 mg for patients weighing 40 kg or more; 1 mg/m² for patients weighing less than 40 kg.

Dosage adjustment: See Adults Low to Moderate Immunologic Risk for dosage adjustment.

Concomitant therapy: See Adults Low to Moderate Immunologic Risk for concomitant therapy.

➤*Hepatic function impairment:* It is recommended that the maintenance dose of sirolimus be reduced by approximately one-third in patients with mild or moderate hepatic impairment and by approximately one-half in patients with severe hepatic impairment. It is not necessary to modify the loading dose.

➤*Therapeutic drug monitoring:* Monitoring of sirolimus trough concentrations is recommended for all patients, especially in those patients likely to have altered drug metabolism, in patients 13 years of age and older who weigh less than 40 kg, in patients with hepatic impairment, when a change in the sirolimus dosage form is made, and during coadministration of strong CYP3A4 inducers and inhibitors. Therapeutic drug monitoring should not be the sole basis for adjusting therapy. Careful attention should be paid to clinical signs/symptoms, tissue biopsy findings, and laboratory parameters. Sirolimus trough concentrations should be monitored at least 3 to 4 days after a loading dose(s).

When used in combination with cyclosporine, sirolimus trough concentrations should be maintained within the target range. Following cyclosporine withdrawal in transplant patients at low to moderate immunologic risk, the target sirolimus trough concentrations should be 16 to 24 ng/mL for the first year following transplantation. Thereafter, the target sirolimus concentrations should be 12 to 20 ng/mL.

The above recommended 24-hour trough concentration ranges for sirolimus are based on chromatographic methods. On average, chromatographic methods (high-performance liquid chromatography with ultraviolet light or liquid chromatography/tandem mass spectrometry) yield results that are approximately 20% lower than the immunoassay for whole blood concentration determinants. Currently in clinical practice, sirolimus whole blood concentrations are being measured by both chromatographic and immunoassay methodologies. Because the measured whole blood concentrations depend on the type of assay used, the concentrations obtained by these different methodologies are not interchangeable. Adjustments to the targeted range should be made according to the assay used to determine sirolimus trough concentrations. Because results are assay and laboratory dependent and the results may change over time, adjustments to the targeted therapeutic range must be made with a detailed knowledge of the site-specific assay used.

➤*Preparation for administration:* Sirolimus is an immunosuppressant agent. Follow safe handling procedures when preparing, administering, or dispensing sirolimus.

Sirolimus is not absorbed through the skin; however, if direct contact with the skin or mucous membranes occurs, wash thoroughly with soap and water. Rinse eyes with plain water.

➤*Administration:* Administer orally once daily consistently with or without food. It is recommended that sirolimus be taken 4 hours after administration of cyclosporine (modified).

Solution – The amber oral dose syringe should be used to withdraw the prescribed amount of solution from the bottle. Empty the correct amount of sirolimus from the syringe into a glass or plastic container holding at least 60 mL of water or orange juice. No other liquids, especially grapefruit juice, should be used for dilution. Stir vigorously and drink at once. Refill the container with an additional volume (minimum of 120 mL) of water or orange juice, stir vigorously, and drink at once.

The solution contains polysorbate 80, which is known to increase the rate of di-(2-ethylhexyl)phthalate extraction from polyvinyl chloride. This should be considered during the preparation and administration of the solution. It is important that the recommendations for administration be followed closely.

Tablets – Tablets should not be crushed, chewed, or split. Patients unable to take the tablets should be prescribed the solution.

➤*Storage/Stability:*

Solution – Store at 2° to 8°C (36° to 46°F). Protect from light. Once the bottle is opened, use the contents within 1 month. If necessary, the patient may store the bottles at up to 25°C (77°F) for a short period of time (not more than 15 days). An amber syringe and cap are provided for dosing, and the product may be kept in the syringe for a maximum of 24 hours at up to 25°C (77°F) or refrigerated at 2° to 8°C (36° to 46°F). Discard the syringe after 1 use. After dilution, use the preparation immediately. Sirolimus oral solution provided in bottles may develop a slight haze when refrigerated. If such a haze occurs, allow the product to stand at room temperature and shake gently until the haze disappears. The presence of this haze does not affect the quality of the product.

Tablets – Store at 20° to 25°C (68° to 77°F). Use cartons to protect blister cards and strips from light.

Actions

➤*Pharmacology:* Sirolimus is an immunosuppressive agent. It inhibits T-lymphocyte activation and proliferation that occurs in response to antigenic and cytokine (interleukin [IL]–2, IL-4, and IL-15) stimulation by a mechanism that is distinct from that of other immunosuppressants. Sirolimus also inhibits antibody production. In cells, sirolimus binds to the immunophilin FK-binding protein-12 (FKBP-12) to generate an immunosuppressive complex. The sirolimus:FKBP-12 complex has no effect on calcineurin activity. This complex binds to and inhibits the activation of the mammalian target of rapamycin (mTOR), a key regulatory kinase. This inhibition suppresses cytokine-driven T-cell proliferation, inhibiting the progression from the G_1 to the S-phase of the cell cycle.

Orally administered sirolimus, at dosages of 2 and 5 mg/day, significantly reduced the incidence of organ rejection in renal transplant patients at low to moderate immunologic risk at 6 months following transplantation compared with azathioprine or placebo. There was no demonstrable efficacy advantage of a daily maintenance dose of 5 mg with a loading dose of 15 mg compared with a daily maintenance dose of 2 mg with a loading dose of 6 mg. Use therapeutic drug monitoring to maintain sirolimus drug levels within the target range.

➤*Pharmacokinetics:*

Sirolimus Pharmacokinetics in Renal Transplant Adults at Low to Moderate Immunologic Risk[a,b,c]

Pharmacokinetic parameter	Multiple-dose (2 mg daily) oral solution	Multiple-dose (2 mg daily) tablets
C_{max} (ng/mL)	14.4 ± 5.3	15 ± 4.9
T_{max} (h)	2.1 ± 0.8	3.5 ± 2.4
AUC (ng•h/mL)	194 ± 78	230 ± 67
C_{min} (ng/mL)[d]	7.1 ± 3.5	7.6 ± 3.1
CL/F (mL/h/kg)	173 ± 50	139 ± 63

[a] C_{max} = maximum plasma concentration; T_{max} = time to maximal drug concentration; AUC = area under the curve; C_{min} = minimal drug concentration; CL/F = apparent clearance.
[b] In presence of cyclosporine administered 4 h before sirolimus dosing.
[c] Based on data collected at months 1 and 3 posttransplantation.
[d] Average C_{min} over 6 months.

Absorption – Following administration of sirolimus oral solution, the mean T_{max} of sirolimus is approximately 1 and 2 hours in healthy subjects and renal transplant patients, respectively. The systemic availability of sirolimus is low and was estimated to be approximately 14% after the administration of sirolimus oral solution. In healthy subjects, the mean bioavailability of sirolimus after administration of the tablet is approximately 27% higher relative to the solution. Sirolimus tablets are not bioequivalent to the solution; however, clinical equivalence has been demonstrated at the 2 mg dose level. Sirolimus concentrations following the administration of sirolimus oral solution to stable renal transplant patients are dose proportional between 3 and 12 mg/m².

Effect of food: To minimize variability in sirolimus concentrations, instruct patients to take both sirolimus oral solution and tablets consistently with or without food. In healthy subjects, a high-fat meal (861.8 kcal, 54.9% kcal from fat) increased the mean total exposure (AUC) of sirolimus by 23% to 35% compared with fasting. The effect of food on the mean sirolimus C_{max} was inconsistent depending on the sirolimus dosage form evaluated.

Whole blood trough sirolimus concentrations, as measured by liquid chromatography/tandem mass spectrometry in transplant patients, were significantly correlated with $AUC_{\tau\text{ to steady state}}$). Upon repeated, twice-daily administration without an initial loading dose in a multiple-dose study, the average trough concentration of sirolimus increases approximately 2- to 3-fold over the initial 6 days of therapy, at which time steady state is reached. A loading dose of 3 times the maintenance dose will provide near steady-state concentrations within 1 day in most patients.

Sirolimus concentrations: The withdrawal of cyclosporine and concurrent increases in sirolimus trough concentrations to steady state required approximately 6 weeks. Following cyclosporine withdrawal, larger sirolimus doses were required because of the absence of the inhibition of sirolimus metabolism and transport by cyclosporine, and to achieve higher target sirolimus trough concentrations during concentration-controlled administration.

Sirolimus Whole Blood Trough Concentrations in Renal Transplant Patients Enrolled in Phase 3 Studies

		Year 1		Year 3	
Patient population (study number)	Treatment	Mean (ng/mL)	10th to 90th percentiles (ng/mL)	Mean (ng/mL)	10th to 90th percentiles (ng/mL)
Low to moderate risk (studies 1/2)	Sirolimus 2 mg/day plus cyclosporine A	7.2	3.6 to 11	—	—
	Sirolimus 5 mg/day plus cyclosporine A	14	8 to 22	—	—
Low to moderate risk (study 3)	Sirolimus plus cyclosporine A	8.6	5 to 13[a]	9.1	5.4 to 14
	Sirolimus alone	19	14 to 22[a]	16	11 to 22
High risk (study 4)	Sirolimus plus cyclosporine A	15.7	5.4 to 27.3[b]	—	—
		11.8	6.2 to 16.9[c]	—	—
		11.5	6.3 to 17.3[d]	—	—

[a] Months 4 through 12.
[b] Up to wk 2; observed cyclosporine A C_{min} was 217 ng/mL (range, 56 to 432 ng/mL).
[c] Wk 2 to 26; observed cyclosporine A C_{min} was 174 ng/mL (range, 71 to 288 ng/mL).
[d] Wk 26 to 52; observed cyclosporine A C_{min} was 136 ng/mL (range, 54.5 to 218 ng/mL).

Distribution – The mean (± standard deviation [SD]) blood-to-plasma ratio of sirolimus was 36 (± 18) in stable renal allograft patients, indicating

SIROLIMUS — ORAL

that sirolimus is extensively partitioned into formed blood elements. The mean volume of distribution of sirolimus is 12 ± 8 L/kg. Sirolimus is extensively bound (approximately 92%) to human plasma proteins, mainly serum albumin (97%), alpha-1 acid glycoprotein, and lipoproteins.

Metabolism – Sirolimus is a substrate for CYP3A4 and P-glycoprotein (P-gp). Sirolimus is extensively metabolized in the intestinal wall and liver and undergoes countertransport from enterocytes of the small intestine into the gut lumen. Inhibitors of CYP3A4 and P-gp increase sirolimus concentrations. Inducers of CYP3A4 and P-gp decrease sirolimus concentrations. Sirolimus is extensively metabolized by O-demethylation and/or hydroxylation. Seven major metabolites, including hydroxy, demethyl, and hydroxydemethyl, are identifiable in whole blood. Some of these metabolites are also detectable in plasma, fecal, and urine samples. Sirolimus is the major component in human whole blood and contributes to more than 90% of the immunosuppressive activity.

Excretion – After a single dose of [^{14}C] sirolimus oral solution in healthy volunteers, the majority (91%) of radioactivity was recovered from the feces, and only a minor amount (2.2%) was excreted in urine. The mean ± SD half-life of sirolimus after multiple dosing in stable renal transplant patients was estimated to be approximately 62 ± 16 hours.

Special populations –

Hepatic function impairment: Sirolimus was administered as a single oral dose to subjects with healthy hepatic function and to patients with Child-Pugh class A (mild), B (moderate), or C (severe) hepatic impairment. Compared with the values in the healthy hepatic function group, the patients with mild, moderate, and severe hepatic impairment had 43%, 94%, and 189% higher mean values for sirolimus AUC, respectively, with no statistically significant differences in mean C_{max}. As the severity of hepatic impairment increased, there were steady increases in mean sirolimus half-life and decreases in the mean sirolimus clearance normalized for body weight.

See Administration and Dosage for more information.

Children:

Sirolimus[a] Pharmacokinetic Parameters (Mean ± SD) in Pediatric Renal Transplant Patients[b] (Multiple-Dose Concentration Control)[c]

Age (y)	Body weight (kg)	$C_{max\ to\ ss}$ (ng/mL)	$T_{max\ to\ ss}$ (h)	$C_{min\ to\ ss}$ (ng/mL)	$AUC_{\tau\ to\ ss}$ (ng•h/mL)	CL/F[d] (mL/h/kg)	CL/F[d] (L/h/m²)
6 to 11 (n = 8)	27 ± 10	22.1 ± 8.9	5.88 ± 4.05	10.6 ± 4.3	356 ± 127	214 ± 129	5.4 ± 2.8
12 to 18 (n = 14)	52 ± 15	34.5 ± 12.2	2.7 ± 1.5	14.7 ± 8.6	466 ± 236	136 ± 57	4.7 ± 1.9

[a] Coadministered with cyclosporine oral solution (modified) and/or cyclosporine capsules (modified).
[b] As measured by liquid chromatography/tandem mass spectrometry.
[c] ss = steady state.
[d] Oral dose clearance adjusted either by body weight (kg) or by body surface area (BSA) (m^2).

Sirolimus Pharmacokinetic Parameters (Mean ± SD) in Children With End-Stage Kidney Disease Maintained on Hemodialysis or Peritoneal Dialysis (1, 3, 9, 15 mg/m² Single Dose)[a]

Age group (years)	T_{max} (h)	Half-life (h)	CL/F/WT (mL/h/kg)
5 to 11 (n = 9)	1.1 ± 0.5	71 ± 40	580 ± 450
12 to 18 (n = 11)	0.79 ± 0.17	55 ± 18	450 ± 232

[a] All subjects received sirolimus oral solution.

Gender: Sirolimus clearance in men was 12% lower than in women; men had a significantly longer half-life than women (72.3 vs 61.3 h). Dosage adjustments based on gender are not recommended.

Contraindications

Hypersensitivity to sirolimus.

Warnings/Precautions

➤*Infection/Lymphoma/Other malignancies:* Increased susceptibility to infection and the possible development of lymphoma and other malignancies, particularly of the skin, may result from immunosuppression. The rates of lymphoma/lymphoproliferative disease observed in studies 1 and 2 were 0.7% to 3.2% (for sirolimus-treated patients) versus 0.6% to 0.8% (azathioprine and placebo control). Oversuppression of the immune system can also increase susceptibility to infections, including opportunistic infections such as tuberculosis, fatal infections, and sepsis. Only health care providers experienced in immunosuppressive therapy and management of organ transplant patients should use sirolimus. Manage patients receiving the drug in facilities equipped and staffed with adequate laboratory and supportive medical resources. The health care provider responsible for maintenance therapy should have complete information requisite for the follow-up of the patient.

➤*Liver transplantation:* The safety and efficacy of sirolimus as immunosuppressive therapy have not been established in liver transplant patients; therefore, such use is not recommended. The use of sirolimus has been associated with adverse outcomes in patients following liver transplantation, including excess mortality, graft loss, and hepatic artery thrombosis.

The use of sirolimus in combination with tacrolimus was associated with excess mortality and graft loss in a study in de novo liver transplant patients (22% in combination vs 9% on tacrolimus alone). Many of these patients had evidence of infection at or near the time of death. In this and another study in de novo liver transplant patients, the use of sirolimus in combination with cyclosporine or tacrolimus was associated with an increase in hepatic artery thrombosis (7% in combination vs 2% in the control arm); most cases of hepatic artery thrombosis occurred within 30 days posttransplantation and most led to graft loss or death.

➤*Lung transplantation:* Cases of bronchial anastomotic dehiscence, most fatal, have been reported in de novo lung transplant patients when sirolimus has been used as part of an immunosuppressive regimen.

The safety and efficacy of sirolimus as immunosuppressive therapy have not been established in lung transplant patients; therefore, such use is not recommended.

➤*Angioedema:* Sirolimus has been associated with the development of angioedema. The concomitant use of sirolimus with other drugs known to cause angioedema, such as angiotensin-converting enzyme (ACE) inhibitors, may increase the risk of developing angioedema.

➤*Wound healing:* There have been reports of impaired or delayed wound healing in patients receiving sirolimus, including lymphocele and wound dehiscence. mTOR inhibitors, such as sirolimus, have been shown in vitro to inhibit production of certain growth factors that may affect angiogenesis, fibroblast proliferation, and vascular permeability. Lymphocele, a known surgical complication of renal transplantation, occurred significantly more often in a dose-related manner in patients treated with sirolimus. Consider appropriate measures to minimize such complications. Patients with a body mass index greater than 30 kg/m² may be at increased risk of abnormal wound healing based on data from the medical literature.

➤*Fluid accumulation:* There have been reports of fluid accumulation, including peripheral edema, lymphedema, pleural effusion, and pericardial effusions (including hemodynamically significant effusions and tamponade requiring intervention in children and adults) in patients receiving sirolimus.

➤*Hyperlipidemia:* Increased serum cholesterol and triglycerides requiring treatment occurred more frequently in patients treated with sirolimus compared with azathioprine or placebo controls in studies 1 and 2. There were increased incidences of hypercholesterolemia (43% to 46%) and/or hypertriglyceridemia (45% to 57%) in patients receiving sirolimus compared with placebo controls (each 23%). Carefully consider the risk-benefit ratio in patients with established hyperlipidemia before initiating an immunosuppressive regimen that includes sirolimus.

Monitor any patient who is administered sirolimus for hyperlipidemia. If detected, initiate interventions such as diet, exercise, and lipid-lowering agents as outlined by the National Cholesterol Education Program guidelines.

During sirolimus therapy with cyclosporine, monitor patients administered an HMG-CoA reductase inhibitor and/or fibrate for the possible development of rhabdomyolysis and other adverse reactions as described in the respective monographs for these agents.

➤*Renal effects:* Closely monitor renal function during the coadministration of sirolimus with cyclosporine because long-term administration can be associated with deterioration of renal function. Patients treated with cyclosporine and sirolimus were noted to have higher serum creatinine levels and lower GFRs compared with patients treated with cyclosporine and placebo or azathioprine controls (studies 1 and 2). The rate of decline in renal function in these studies was greater in patients receiving sirolimus and cyclosporine compared with control therapies.

Consider appropriate adjustment of the immunosuppression regimen, including discontinuation of sirolimus and/or cyclosporine, in patients with elevated or increasing serum creatinine levels. In patients at low to moderate immunologic risk, only consider continuation of combination therapy with cyclosporine beyond 4 months following transplantation when the benefits outweigh the risks of this combination for the individual patient. Exercise caution when using agents (eg, aminoglycosides, amphotericin B) that are known to have a deleterious effect on renal function.

In patients with delayed graft function, sirolimus may delay recovery of renal function.

➤*Proteinuria:* Periodic quantitative monitoring of urinary protein excretion is recommended. In a study evaluating conversion from calcineurin inhibitors to sirolimus in maintenance renal transplant patients 6 to 120 months after transplant, increased urinary protein excretion was commonly observed from 6 through 24 months after conversion to sirolimus compared with calcineurin inhibitor continuation. Patients with the greatest amount of urinary protein excretion prior to sirolimus conversion were those whose protein excretion increased the most after conversion. New-onset nephrosis (nephrotic syndrome) was also reported as a treatment-emergent adverse reaction in 2.2% of the sirolimus conversion group patients in comparison with 0.4% in the calcineurin inhibitor continuation group of patients. Nephrotic-range proteinuria (defined as urinary protein-to-creatinine ratio greater than 3.5) was also reported in 9.2% in the sirolimus conversion group of patients in comparison with 3.7% in the calcineurin inhibitor continuation group of patients. In some patients, reduction in the degree of urinary protein excretion was observed for individual patients following discontinuation of sirolimus. The safety and efficacy of conversion from calcineurin inhibitors to sirolimus in maintenance renal transplant patients have not been established.

➤*Latent viral infections:* Immunosuppressed patients are at increased risk for opportunistic infections, including activation of latent viral infections. These include BK virus–associated nephropathy, which has been observed in patients receiving immunosuppressants, including sirolimus. This infection may be associated with serious outcomes, including deteriorating renal function and renal graft loss. Patient monitoring may help detect patients at risk for BK virus–associated nephropathy. Consider reduction in immunosuppression for patients who develop evidence of BK virus–associated nephropathy.

SIROLIMUS — ORAL

➤*Interstitial lung disease:* Cases of interstitial lung disease (eg, pneumonitis, bronchiolitis obliterans-organizing pneumonia, pulmonary fibrosis), some fatal, with no identified infectious etiology, have occurred in patients receiving immunosuppressive regimens, including sirolimus. In some cases, the interstitial lung disease has resolved upon discontinuation or dose reduction of sirolimus. The risk may be increased as the trough sirolimus concentration increases.

➤*Use without cyclosporine:* The safety and efficacy of de novo use of sirolimus without cyclosporine have not been established in renal transplant patients. In a multicenter clinical study, de novo renal transplant patients treated with sirolimus, mycophenolate mofetil, steroids, and an IL-2 receptor antagonist had significantly higher acute rejection rates and numerically higher death rates compared with patients treated with cyclosporine, mycophenolate mofetil, steroids, and IL-2 receptor antagonist. A benefit, in terms of better renal function, was not apparent in the treatment arm with de novo use of sirolimus without cyclosporine. These findings were also observed in a similar treatment group of another clinical trial.

➤*Calcineurin inhibitor–induced reactions:* The concomitant use of sirolimus with a calcineurin inhibitor (eg, cyclosporine, tacrolimus) may increase the risk of calcineurin inhibitor–induced hemolytic uremic syndrome/thrombotic thrombocytopenic purpura/thrombotic microangiopathy.

➤*Antimicrobial prophylaxis:* Cases of *Pneumocystis carinii* pneumonia have been reported in patients not receiving antimicrobial prophylaxis. Therefore, administer antimicrobial prophylaxis for *P. carinii* pneumonia for 1 year following transplantation. Cytomegalovirus (CMV) prophylaxis is recommended for 3 months after transplantation, particularly for patients at increased risk for CMV disease.

➤*Skin cancer:* Patients on immunosuppressive therapy are at increased risk for skin cancer and should limit exposure to sunlight and ultraviolet (UV) light by wearing protective clothing and using a sunscreen with a high protective factor.

➤*Vaccines:* Immunosuppressants may affect response to vaccination. Therefore, during treatment with sirolimus, vaccination may be less effective. The use of live vaccines should be avoided. Live vaccines may include, but are not limited to, measles, mumps, rubella, oral polio, Bacillus Calmette-Guérin, yellow fever, varicella, and TY21a typhoid.

➤*Hypersensitivity reactions:* Hypersensitivity reactions, including anaphylactic/anaphylactoid reactions, angioedema, exfoliative dermatitis, and hypersensitivity vasculitis, have been associated with the administration of sirolimus.

➤*Hepatic function impairment:* See Administration and Dosage for more information.

➤*Pregnancy: Category C.* Sirolimus was embryo/fetotoxic in rats when given in doses approximately 0.2 to 0.5 the human doses (adjusted for body surface area [BSA]). Embryo/fetotoxicity was manifested as mortality and reduced fetal weights (with associated delays in skeletal ossification). However, no teratogenesis was evident. In combination with cyclosporine, rats had increased embryo/fetal mortality compared with sirolimus alone. There were no effects on rabbit development at a maternally toxic dosage approximately 0.3 to 0.8 times the human dose (adjusted for BSA). There are no adequate and well-controlled studies in pregnant women. It is not known if sirolimus crosses the human placenta. The molecular weight (approximately 914) is within the range for passive diffusion, and the elimination half-life will allow the drug to be present at the maternal-fetal interface for a long interval. However, the high protein binding should limit the amount of drug available to cross the placenta. Effective contraception must be initiated before sirolimus therapy, during sirolimus therapy, and for 12 weeks after sirolimus therapy has been stopped. Only use sirolimus during pregnancy if the potential benefit outweighs the potential risk to the embryo/fetus.

➤*Lactation:* Sirolimus is excreted in trace amounts in milk of lactating rats. It is not known whether sirolimus is excreted in human milk. The molecular weight (approximately 914) and prolonged half-life suggest that the drug will be excreted into breast milk. The pharmacokinetic and safety profiles of sirolimus in infants are not known. Because many drugs are excreted in human milk and because of the potential for adverse reactions in breast-feeding infants from sirolimus, make a decision whether to discontinue breast-feeding or the drug, taking into account the importance of the drug to the mother.

➤*Children:* The safety and efficacy of sirolimus in children younger than 13 years of age or in pediatric renal transplant patients younger than 18 years considered at high immunologic risk have not been established.

➤*Elderly:* Ensure that dose selection for an elderly patient is cautious, usually starting at the low end of the dosing range, reflecting the greater frequency of decreased hepatic or cardiac function, and of concomitant disease or other drug therapy.

➤*Monitoring:* Monitoring of sirolimus trough concentrations is recommended for all patients, especially in those patients likely to have altered drug metabolism, in patients 13 years of age or older who weigh less than 40 kg, in patients with hepatic impairment, and during coadministration of strong CYP3A4 inducers and inhibitors.

Therapeutic drug monitoring should not be the sole basis for adjusting sirolimus therapy. Pay particular attention to clinical signs/symptoms, tissue biopsy findings, and laboratory parameters.

When used in combination with cyclosporine, maintain sirolimus trough concentrations within the target range. Following cyclosporine withdrawal in transplant patients at low to moderate immunologic risk, ensure the target sirolimus trough concentrations are 16 to 24 ng/mL for the first year following transplantation. Thereafter, ensure the target sirolimus concentrations are 12 to 20 ng/mL.

The previously recommended 24-hour trough concentration ranges for sirolimus are based on chromatographic methods. On average, chromatographic methods (high-performance liquid chromatography with UV light or liquid chromatography/tandem mass spectrometry) yield results that are approximately 20% lower than the immunoassay for whole blood concentration determinants. Currently in clinical practice, sirolimus whole blood concentrations are being measured by both chromatographic and immunoassay methodologies. Because the measured sirolimus whole blood concentrations depend on the type of assay used, the concentrations obtained by these different methodologies are not interchangeable. Make adjustments to the targeted range according to the assay used to determine sirolimus trough concentrations.

Closely monitor renal function during the administration of sirolimus in combination with cyclosporine.

Monitor all patients for hyperlipidemia and infections.

Periodic quantitative monitoring of urinary protein excretion is recommended.

During sirolimus therapy with cyclosporine, monitor patients administered an HMG-CoA reductase inhibitor and/or fibrate for the possible development of rhabdomyolysis and other adverse reactions.

Drug Interactions

➤*Cytochrome P450 system:* Because sirolimus is metabolized mainly by the CYP3A4 and P-gp enzyme systems, substances known to inhibit these enzymes may decrease metabolism or increase bioavailability of sirolimus, as indicated by increased whole blood or plasma concentrations. Drugs known to induce these enzyme systems may result in an increased metabolism of sirolimus or decreased bioavailability, as indicated by decreased whole blood or plasma concentrations. Monitoring of blood concentrations and appropriate dosage adjustments are essential when such drugs are used concomitantly.

➤*Vaccines:* See Warnings/Precautions for more information.

Sirolimus Drug Interactions

Precipitant drug	Object drug[a]		Description
Amiodarone	Sirolimus	↑	Sirolimus blood concentrations may be elevated, increasing the risk of toxicity. Consider prospectively lowering the sirolimus dose and frequently monitoring blood concentrations in order to minimize prolonged periods of increased concentrations and related toxicities.
Cyclosporine	Sirolimus	↑	Sirolimus plasma concentrations may be increased, resulting in increased toxicity. Administer sirolimus 4 h after cyclosporine (modified) to prevent variations in sirolimus concentrations. Monitor sirolimus levels and adjust dosage as needed.
CYP3A4 and/or P-gp strong inducers (eg, rifabutin, rifampin)	Sirolimus	↓	Concomitant use may increase the metabolism of sirolimus, decreasing sirolimus concentration levels and efficacy. Avoid coadministration.
CYP3A4 and/or P-gp strong inhibitors (eg, clarithromycin, erythromycin, itraconazole, ketoconazole, telithromycin, voriconazole)	Sirolimus	↑	Concomitant use may decrease the metabolism of sirolimus, increasing sirolimus concentrations and the risk of toxicity. Avoid coadministration.
CYP3A4 inducers (eg, carbamazepine, phenobarbital, phenytoin, rifapentine)	Sirolimus	↓	Concomitant use may increase metabolism of sirolimus and decrease sirolimus levels and efficacy. Use with caution. Monitor sirolimus concentrations and adjust the dose as needed.

SIROLIMUS — ORAL

Sirolimus Drug Interactions

Precipitant drug	Object drug[a]		Description
CYP3A4 inhibitors (eg, bromocriptine, cimetidine, cisapride[b], clotrimazole, danazol, metoclopramide, nicardipine, protease inhibitors [eg, indinavir, ritonavir], troleandomycin)	Sirolimus	↑	Concomitant use may decrease the metabolism of sirolimus and increase sirolimus levels and the risk of adverse reactions. Use with caution. Monitor sirolimus concentrations and adjust the dose as needed.
Diltiazem	Sirolimus	↑	Sirolimus C_{max}, T_{max}, and AUC were increased 1.4-, 1.3-, and 1.6-fold, respectively, following coadministration of sirolimus and diltiazem. Monitor sirolimus concentrations; a dosage adjustment may be necessary.
Erythromycin	Sirolimus	↑	Sirolimus C_{max} and AUC were increased 4.4- and 4.2-fold, respectively, and T_{max} was increased by 0.4 h. Erythromycin C_{max} and AUC were increased 1.6- and 1.7-fold, respectively, and T_{max} was increased by 0.3 h. Coadministration is not recommended.
Sirolimus	Erythromycin		
St. John's wort	Sirolimus	↓	Sirolimus concentrations may be reduced, resulting in organ transplant rejection. Use with caution. Monitor sirolimus concentrations and adjust the dose as needed.
Streptogramins (eg, dalfopristin/quinupristin)	Sirolimus	↑	Sirolimus concentrations may be elevated, increasing the pharmacologic effects and risk of adverse reactions. Monitor sirolimus concentrations and observe the patient for adverse reactions. Adjust the sirolimus dose as needed.
Verapamil	Sirolimus	↑	Sirolimus C_{max} and AUC were increased 2.3- and 2.2-fold, respectively. C_{max} and AUC of the S (-) enantiomer of verapamil increased by 1.5-fold, and T_{max} was decreased by 1.2 h. Monitor sirolimus concentrations and adjust dosage as needed.
Sirolimus	Verapamil		
Sirolimus	ACE inhibitors (eg, enalapril)	↔	Coadministration may increase the risk for developing angioedema. Monitor the response of the patient. If an interaction is suspected, provide treatment as indicated.
Sirolimus	Calcineurin inhibitors (eg, cyclosporine, pimecrolimus, tacrolimus)	↑	Risk of calcineurin-induced hemolytic uremic syndrome, thrombotic thrombocytopenic purpura, and thrombotic microangiopathy may be increased. Closely monitor the response of the patient. If an interaction is suspected, provide treatment as indicated.
Sirolimus	Disulfiram, furazolidone, metronidazole	↑	Because sirolimus oral solution contains alcohol, coadministration with disulfiram, furazolidone, or metronidazole may produce acute and severe alcohol intolerance. Avoid coadministration.
Sirolimus	Mycophenolate mofetil	↑	Mycophenolic acid trough concentrations may be elevated, increasing the risk of adverse reactions. Monitor mycophenolic acid concentrations and adjust the dose as needed.
Sirolimus	Tacrolimus	↑↓	Tacrolimus trough concentrations may be reduced, increasing the risk for organ transplant rejection. In addition, coadministration of tacrolimus and sirolimus in combination with corticosteroids has been associated with fatal cases of bronchial anastomotic dehiscence in lung transplant patients. Use with caution.

[a] ↑ = object drug increased; ↓ = object drug decreased; ↑↓ = object drug both increased and decreased; ↔ = undetermined clinical effect.
[b] Available from the manufacturer on a limited-access protocol.

➤*Drug/Food interactions:* Grapefruit juice reduces CYP3A4-mediated metabolism of sirolimus and must not be taken with or used for dilution of drug.

See Actions for more information.

Adverse Reactions

➤*Discontinuation of treatment:* The following adverse reactions resulted in a rate of discontinuation of more than 5% in clinical trials: creatinine increased, hypertriglyceridemia, and thrombotic thrombocytopenic purpura.

➤*Most common adverse reaction:* The most common (30% or more) adverse reactions observed with sirolimus in clinical trials are abdominal pain, anemia, arthralgia, constipation, creatinine increased, diarrhea, fever, headache, hypercholesterolemia, hypertension, hypertriglyceridemia, nausea, pain, peripheral edema, thrombocytopenia, and urinary tract infection.

➤*Prophylaxis of organ rejection following renal transplantation:* In general, adverse reactions related to the administration of sirolimus were dependent on dose/concentration. Although a daily maintenance dose of 5 mg, with a loading dose of 15 mg, was shown to be safe and effective, no efficacy advantage over the 2 mg dose could be established for renal transplant patients. Patients receiving sirolimus 2 mg/day oral solution demonstrated an overall better safety profile than did patients receiving sirolimus 5 mg/day oral solution.

Adverse reactions (20% or more) –

Sirolimus Adverse Reactions (≥ 20%) in Prophylaxis of Organ Rejection Following Renal Transplantation[a]

Adverse reactions	Sirolimus 2 mg/day oral solution (n = 218)	Sirolimus 5 mg/day oral solution (n = 208)	Placebo (n = 124)
Dermatologic			
Acne	22%	22%	19%
Rash	10%	20%	6%
GI			
Abdominal pain	29%	36%	30%
Constipation	36%	38%	31%
Diarrhea	25%	35%	27%
Nausea	25%	31%	29%
Hematologic/Lymphatic			
Anemia	23%	33%	21%
Thrombocytopenia	14%	30%	9%
Metabolic/Nutritional			
Creatinine increased	39%	40%	38%
Edema	20%	18%	15%
Hypercholesterolemia	43%	46%	23%
Hypertriglyceridemia	45%	57%	23%
Peripheral edema	54%	58%	48%
Miscellaneous			
Arthralgia	25%	31%	18%
Fever	23%	34%	35%
Headache	34%	34%	31%
Hypertension	45%	49%	48%
Pain	33%	29%	25%
Urinary tract infection	26%	33%	26%

[a] Patients received cyclosporine and corticosteroids.

Adverse reactions (at least 3% and less than 20%) –

Cardiovascular: Tachycardia, venous thromboembolism (including pulmonary embolism and deep venous thrombosis).

Dermatologic: Basal cell carcinoma, melanoma, squamous cell carcinoma.

SIROLIMUS — ORAL

GU: Decline in renal function (creatinine increased) in long-term combination of cyclosporine with sirolimus, pyelonephritis.

Hematologic/Lymphatic: Leukopenia, thrombotic thrombocytopenic purpura/hemolytic uremic syndrome.

Metabolic/Nutritional: Hypokalemia, increased lactate dehydrogenase.

Respiratory: Epistaxis, pneumonia.

Miscellaneous: Abnormal healing, bone necrosis, herpes simplex, herpes zoster, lymphocele, sepsis, stomatitis.

Adverse reactions (less than 3%): CMV infections, Epstein-Barr virus infections, lymphoma/posttransplant lymphoproliferative disorder, mycobacterial infections (including *Mycobacterium tuberculosis*), and pancreatitis.

Hyperlipidemia – The use of sirolimus in renal transplant patients was associated with increased serum cholesterol and triglycerides, which may require treatment.

In studies 1 and 2, in de novo renal transplant patients who began the study with fasting total serum cholesterol less than 200 mg/dL, or fasting total serum triglycerides less than 200 mg/dL, there was an increased incidence of hypercholesterolemia (fasting serum cholesterol more than 240 mg/dL) or hypertriglyceridemia (fasting serum triglycerides more than 500 mg/dL), respectively, in patients receiving both sirolimus 2 and 5 mg compared with azathioprine and placebo controls.

Treatment of new-onset hypercholesterolemia with lipid-lowering agents was required in 42% to 52% of patients enrolled in the sirolimus arms of studies 1 and 2 compared with 16% of patients in the placebo arm and 22% of patients in the azathioprine arm.

Abnormal healing – Abnormal healing events following transplant surgery include anastomosis disruption (eg, airway, biliary, ureteral, vascular, wound), fascial dehiscence, and incisional hernia.

Malignancies –

Incidence of Malignancies With Sirolimus Use For the Prevention of Acute Rejection[a,b]

Malignancy	Sirolimus 2 mg/day oral solution Study 1 (n = 284)	Sirolimus 2 mg/day oral solution Study 2 (n = 227)	Sirolimus 5 mg/day oral solution Study 1 (n = 274)	Sirolimus 5 mg/day oral solution Study 2 (n = 219)	Azathioprine 2 to 3 mg/kg/day Study 1 (n = 161)	Placebo Study 2 (n = 130)
Lymphoma/Lymphoproliferative disease	0.7%	1.8%	1.1%	3.2%	0.6%	0.8%
Skin carcinoma						
Any squamous cell[c]	0.4%	2.7%	2.2%	0.9%	3.8%	3%
Any basal cell[c]	0.7%	2.2%	1.5%	1.8%	2.5%	5.3%
Melanoma	0%	0.4%	0%	1.4%	0%	0%
Miscellaneous/Not specified	0%	0%	0%	0%	0%	0.8%
Total	1.1%	4.4%	3.3%	4.1%	4.3%	7.7%
Other malignancy	1.1%	2.2%	1.5%	1.4%	0.6%	2.3%

[a] Patients received cyclosporine and corticosteroids.
[b] Includes patients who discontinued treatment prematurely.
[c] Patients may be counted in more than 1 category.

➤*Sirolimus following cyclosporine withdrawal:* Following randomization (at 3 months), patients who had cyclosporine eliminated from their therapy experienced significantly higher incidences of abnormal healing, abnormal liver function tests (including increased AST and increased ALT), hypokalemia, and thrombocytopenia. Conversely, the incidence of abnormal kidney function, cyclosporine toxicity, edema, gum hyperplasia, hyperkalemia, hypertension, hyperuricemia, increased creatinine, and toxic nephropathy was higher in patients who remained on cyclosporine than those who had cyclosporine withdrawn from therapy. Mean systolic and diastolic blood pressure improved significantly following cyclosporine withdrawal.

Malignancies –

Incidence of Malignancies with Sirolimus Following Cyclosporine Withdrawal[a,b]

Malignancy	Nonrandomized (n = 95)	Sirolimus with cyclosporine therapy (n = 215)	Sirolimus following cyclosporine withdrawal (n = 215)
Lymphoma/Lymphoproliferative disease	1.1%	1.4%	0.5%
Skin carcinoma			
Any squamous cell[c]	3.2%	3.3%	2.3%
Any basal cell[c]	3.2%	6.5%	2.3%
Melanoma	0%	0.5%	0%
Miscellaneous/Not specified	1.1%	0.9%	0%
Total	4.2%	7.9%	3.7%
Other malignancy	3.2%	3.3%	1.9%

[a] Patients received cyclosporine and corticosteroids.
[b] Includes patients who discontinued treatment prematurely.
[c] Patients may be counted in more than 1 category.

➤*High immunologic risk patients:* Safety was assessed in 224 patients who received at least 1 dose of sirolimus with cyclosporine. Overall, the incidence and nature of adverse reactions were similar to those seen in previous combination studies with sirolimus. The incidence of malignancy was 1.3% at 12 months.

➤*Conversion from calcineurin inhibitors to sirolimus:* The safety and efficacy of conversion from calcineurin inhibitors to sirolimus in maintenance renal transplant population have not been established. In an ongoing study evaluating the safety and efficacy of conversion from calcineurin inhibitors to sirolimus (initial target sirolimus concentrations of 12 to 20 ng/mL, and then 8 to 20 ng/mL, by chromatographic assay) in maintenance renal transplant patients, enrollment was stopped in the subset of patients (n = 87) with a baseline GFR of less than 40 mL/min. There was a higher rate of serious adverse reactions, including acute rejection, graft loss, pneumonia, and death, in this stratum of the sirolimus treatment arm.

Overall in this study, a 5-fold increase in the reports of tuberculosis among sirolimus (11/551) and comparator (1/273) treatment groups was observed with a 2:1 randomization scheme.

➤*Children:* Safety was assessed in a controlled clinical trial in pediatric (younger than 18 years of age) renal transplant patients considered at high immunologic risk, defined as a history of 1 or more acute allograft rejection episodes and/or the presence of chronic allograft nephropathy on a renal biopsy. The use of sirolimus in combination with calcineurin inhibitors and corticosteroids was associated with a higher incidence of deterioration of renal function (creatinine increased) compared with calcineurin inhibitor–based therapy, serum lipid abnormalities (including, but not limited to, increased serum triglycerides and cholesterol), and urinary tract infections.

➤*Postmarketing:*

Cardiovascular – Pericardial effusion (including hemodynamically significant effusions and tamponade requiring intervention in children and adults).

GU – Focal segmental glomerulosclerosis, nephrotic syndrome, proteinuria. Azoospermia has been reported with the use of sirolimus and has been reversible upon discontinuation of sirolimus in most cases.

Hematologic/Lymphatic – The concomitant use of sirolimus with a calcineurin inhibitor may increase the risk of calcineurin inhibitor–induced hemolytic uremic syndrome/thrombotic thrombocytopenic purpura/thrombotic microangiopathy; neutropenia, pancytopenia.

Hepatic – Hepatotoxicity, including fatal hepatic necrosis with elevated sirolimus trough concentrations.

Hypersensitivity – Hypersensitivity reactions, including anaphylactic/anaphylactoid reactions, angioedema, and hypersensitivity vasculitis.

Metabolic/Nutritional – Abnormal liver function tests, hyperglycemia, hypophosphatemia, increased ALT/AST.

Respiratory – Alveolar proteinosis, pleural effusion, pulmonary hemorrhage, tuberculosis. Cases of interstitial lung disease (including bronchiolitis obliterans–organizing pneumonia, pneumonitis, and pulmonary fibrosis), some fatal with no identified infectious etiology, have occurred in patients receiving immunosuppressive regimens including sirolimus. In some cases, the interstitial lung disease has resolved upon discontinuation or dose reduction of sirolimus. The risk may be increased as the sirolimus trough concentration increases.

Miscellaneous – BK virus–associated nephropathy has been observed in patients receiving immunosuppressants, including sirolimus. This infection may be associated with serious outcomes, including deteriorating renal function and renal graft loss. Exfoliative dermatitis, lymphedema, and tuberculosis have also been reported.

Overdosage

➤*Treatment:* Follow general supportive measures in all cases of overdosage. Based on the low aqueous solubility and high erythrocyte and plasma protein binding of sirolimus, it is anticipated that sirolimus is not dialyzable to any significant extent.

Patient Information

Give patients complete dosage instructions.

Instruct patients to take each dose consistently with or without food.

Advise patients taking cyclosporine (modified) to take sirolimus 4 hours after taking cyclosporine.

Inform women of childbearing potential of the potential risks during pregnancy and instruct them to use effective contraception prior to initiation of sirolimus therapy, during sirolimus therapy, and for 12 weeks after sirolimus therapy has been stopped.

Instruct patients to limit exposure to sunlight and UV light by wearing protective clothing and using a sunscreen with a high protection factor because of the increased risk for skin cancer.

Advise patients to avoid grapefruit juice while taking sirolimus.

PEGINTERFERON ALFA-2a

Rx	**Pegasys** (Roche)	**Injection:** 180 mcg	In 1 mL single-use vials[a] and 0.5 mL prefilled syringes.[b] Available in vial[c] and prefilled syringe[d] monthly convenience packs.

[a] With sodium chloride 8 mg, polysorbate 80 0.05 mg, and benzyl alcohol 10 mg.
[b] With sodium chloride 4 mg, polysorbate 80 0.025 mg, and benzyl alcohol 5 mg.
[c] Contains 4 single-use vials, four 1 mL syringes with needles, and 8 alcohol swabs.
[d] Contains 4 single-use prefilled syringes, 4 needles, and 4 alcohol swabs.

PEGINTERFERON ALFA-2a — INJECTION

For complete and comparative prescribing information, refer to the Ribavirin monograph.

WARNING

Alpha interferons, including peginterferon alfa-2a, may cause or aggravate fatal or life-threatening neuropsychiatric, autoimmune, ischemic, and infectious disorders. Monitor patients closely with periodic clinical and laboratory evaluations. Withdraw therapy in patients with persistently severe or worsening signs or symptoms of these conditions. In many, but not all, cases these disorders resolve after stopping peginterferon alfa-2a therapy.

Combination therapy with ribavirin – Ribavirin may cause birth defects and/or death of the fetus. Extreme care must be taken to avoid pregnancy in women taking peginterferon alfa-2a and in female partners of men taking peginterferon alfa-2a. Ribavirin causes hemolytic anemia. The anemia associated with ribavirin therapy may result in a worsening of cardiac disease. Because ribavirin is genotoxic and mutagenic, consider it a potential carcinogen.

Indications

➤*Chronic hepatitis B:* For the treatment of adult patients with HBeAg-positive and HBeAG-negativechronic hepatitis B virus (HBV) infection who have compensated liver disease and evidence of viral replication and liver inflammation.

➤*Chronic hepatitis C:* For the treatment of adults with chronic hepatitis C virus (HCV) infection who have compensated liver disease and have not been previously treated with interferon alpha. Patients in whom efficacy was demonstrated included patients with compensated liver disease and histological evidence of cirrhosis (Child-Pugh class A), and patients with HIV disease that is clinically stable (ie, antiretroviral therapy not required, receiving stable antiretroviral therapy).

➤*Off-label uses:* Renal cell carcinoma, chronic myelogenous leukemia.

Administration and Dosage

➤*Adults:*

Chronic hepatitis B virus infection –

Usual dosage:

• *Monotherapy* – 180 mcg (1 mL vial or 0.5 mL prefilled syringe) once weekly for 48 weeks.

Chronic hepatitis C virus infection –

Usual dosage:

• *Monotherapy* – 180 mcg (1 mL vial or 0.5 mL prefilled syringe) once weekly for 48 weeks.

• *Combination therapy with ribavirin* – 180 mcg (1 mL vial or 0.5 mL prefilled syringe) subcutaneously once weekly.

The daily dose of ribavirin is 800 to 1,200 mg administered orally in 2 divided doses. Individualize the dose to the patient depending on baseline disease characteristics (eg, genotype), response to therapy, and tolerability of the regimen.

The recommended dose of ribavirin and duration for peginterferon alfa-2a/ribavirin therapy is based on viral genotype (see the following table).

Peginterferon Alfa-2a and Ribavirin Dosing Recommendations

Genotype	Peginterferon alfa-2a dose	Ribavirin dose	Duration
Genotypes 1, 4	180 mcg	< 75 kg = 1,000 mg	48 weeks
		≥ 75 kg = 1,200 mg	48 weeks
Genotypes 2, 3	180 mcg	800 mg	24 weeks

Genotypes 2 and 3 showed no increased response to treatment beyond 24 weeks. Data on genotypes 5 and 6 are insufficient for dosing recommendations.

Discontinuation of therapy: If severe adverse reactions or laboratory abnormalities develop during combination ribavirin/peginterferon alfa-2a therapy, modify, or discontinue if appropriate, the dose until the adverse reactions abate. If intolerance persists after dose adjustment, discontinue ribavirin/peginterferon alfa-2a therapy.

Chronic hepatitis C virus with HIV coinfection –

Usual dosage:

• *Monotherapy* – 180 mcg (1 mL vial or 0.5 mL prefilled syringe) once weekly for 48 weeks.

• *Combination therapy with ribavirin* – 180 mcg subcutaneously once weekly and ribavirin 800 mg daily given orally in 2 divided doses for a total of 48 weeks, regardless of genotype.

Discontinuation of therapy: If severe adverse reactions or laboratory abnormalities develop during combination ribavirin/peginterferon alfa-2a therapy, modify, or discontinue if appropriate, the dose until the adverse reactions abate. If intolerance persists after dose adjustment, discontinue ribavirin/peginterferon alfa-2a therapy.

➤*Renal function impairment:*

Peginterferon alfa-2a – Use peginterferon alfa-2a with caution in patients with creatinine clearance (CrCl) less than 50 mL/min.

In patients with impaired renal function, closely monitor for signs and symptoms of interferon toxicity. Adjust doses of peginterferon alfa-2a accordingly.

In patients with end-stage renal disease requiring hemodialysis, dose reduction to peginterferon alfa-2a 135 mcg is recommended. Monitor signs and symptoms of interferon toxicity closely.

Ribavirin – It is recommended that renal function be evaluated in all patients started on ribavirin. Do not administer ribavirin to patients with CrCl less than 50 mL/min.

➤*Hepatic function impairment:* In patients with persistent, severe (ALT greater than 10 times above the upper limit of normal [ULN]) hepatitis B flares, give consideration to discontinuation of treatment.

If ALT increases are progressive despite dose reduction or accompanied by increased bilirubin or evidence of hepatic decompensation, discontinue therapy immediately.

Chronic hepatitis B virus – In chronic HBV patients with elevations in ALT (greater than 5 times the ULN), perform more frequent monitoring of liver function and consider either reducing the dose of peginterferon alfa-2a to 135 mcg or temporarily discontinuing treatment. After peginterferon alfa-2a dose reduction or withholding, therapy can be resumed after ALT flares subside.

Chronic hepatitis C virus – In chronic HCV patients with progressive ALT increases above baseline values, reduce the dose of peginterferon alfa-2a to 135 mcg and perform more frequent monitoring of liver function. After peginterferon alfa-2a dose reduction or withholding, therapy can be resumed after ALT flares subside.

➤*Dose adjustment:* When dose modification is required for moderate to severe adverse reactions (clinical and/or laboratory), initial dose reduction to 135 mcg (0.75 mL for the vials or adjustment to the corresponding graduation mark for the syringes) is generally adequate. However, in some cases, dose reduction to 90 mcg (0.5 mL for the vials or adjustment to the corresponding graduation mark for the syringes) may be needed. Following improvement of the adverse reaction, re-escalation of the dose may be considered. (See the following tables.)

Peginterferon Alfa-2a Hematological Dose Modification Guidelines

Laboratory values	Peginterferon alfa-2a dose	Discontinue peginterferon alfa-2a
ANC[a] ≥ 750/mm³	Maintain 180 mcg	ANC < 500/mm³, suspend treatment until ANC values return to more than 1,000/mm³; reinstitute at 90 mcg and monitor ANC.
ANC < 750/mm³	Reduce to 135 mcg	
Platelet ≥ 50,000/mm³	Maintain 180 mcg	Platelet count < 25,000/mm³
Platelet < 50,000/mm³	Reduce to 90 mcg	

[a] ANC = absolute neutrophil count.

PEGINTERFERON ALFA-2a — INJECTION

Guidelines for Modification or Discontinuation of Peginterferon Alfa-2a and for Scheduling Visits for Patients With Depression

Depression severity	Initial management (4 to 8 weeks)		Depression		
	Dose modification	Visit schedule	Remains stable	Improves	Worsens
Mild	No change.	Evaluate once weekly by visit and/or phone.	Continue weekly visit schedule.	Resume normal visit schedule.	(See moderate or severe depression)
Moderate	Decrease peginterferon alfa-2a dose to 135 mcg (in some cases, dose reduction to 90 mcg may be needed).	Evaluate once weekly (office visit at least every other week).	Consider psychiatric consultation. Continue reduced dosing.	If symptoms improve and are stable for 4 weeks, may resume normal visit schedule. Continue reduced dosing or return to normal dose.	(See severe depression)
Severe	Discontinue peginterferon alfa-2a permanently.	Obtain immediate psychiatric consultation.	Psychiatric therapy necessary.		

Ribavirin Dosage Modification Guidelines

Laboratory values	Reduce only ribavirin dosage to 600 mg/day[a]	Discontinue ribavirin
Hgb[b] in patients with no cardiac disease	< 10 g/dL	< 8.5 g/dL
Hgb in patients with history of stable cardiac disease	≥ 2 g/dL decrease in Hgb during any 4-week period treatment	< 12 g/dL despite 4 weeks at reduced dose

[a] One 200 mg tablet in the morning and two 200 mg tablets in the evening.
[b] Hgb = hemoglobin.

Once ribavirin has been withheld because of a laboratory abnormality or clinical manifestation, an attempt may be made to restart ribavirin at 600 mg daily and further increase the dosage to 800 mg daily depending upon the health care provider's judgment. However, it is not recommended that ribavirin be increased to the original dose (1,000 or 1,200 mg).

➤*Duration of therapy:* There are no safety and efficacy data on treatment of chronic HCV or HBV for longer than 48 weeks. For patients with HCV, consider discontinuing therapy after 12 to 24 weeks of therapy if the patient has failed to demonstrate an early virologic response, defined as undetectable HCV ribonucleic acid (RNA) or at least a 2 $\log_{10}$ reduction from baseline in HCV RNA titer by 12 weeks of therapy.

➤*Administration:*

Self-injection – A patient should only self-inject peginterferon alfa-2a if the health care provider determines that it is appropriate, the patient agrees to medical follow-up as necessary, and training in proper injection technique has been provided to the patient.

Administer by subcutaneous injection in the abdomen or thigh.

Because ribavirin absorption increases when administered with a meal, patients are advised to take ribavirin with food.

➤*Storage/Stability:* Refrigerate at 2° to 8°C (36° to 46°F). Do not freeze or shake. Protect from light. Vials and prefilled syringes are for single use only. Discard any unused portion.

Actions

➤*Pharmacology:* Interferons bind to specific receptors on the cell surface initiating intracellular signaling via a complex cascade of protein-protein interactions leading to rapid activation of gene transcription. Interferon-stimulated genes modulate many biological effects, including the inhibition of viral replication in infected cells, inhibition of cell proliferation, and immunomodulation. The clinical relevance of these in vitro activities is not known.

Peginterferon alfa-2a stimulates the production of effector proteins, such as serum neopterin and 2′,5′-oligoadenylate synthetase.

➤*Pharmacokinetics:*

Absorption/Distribution – Maximum serum concentrations (C_{max}) and area under the plasma concentration-time curve (AUC) increased in a nonlinear dose-related manner following administration of 90 to 270 mcg of peginterferon alfa-2a. C_{max} occurs between 72 and 96 hours postdose. Week 48 mean trough concentrations (16 ng/mL; range, 4 to 28) at 168 hours postdose are approximately 2-fold higher than week 1 mean trough concentrations (9 ng/mL; range, 0 to 15). Steady-state serum levels are reached within 5 to 8 weeks of once-weekly dosing. The peak-to-trough ratio at week 48 is approximately 2.

Effect of food on absorption of ribavirin: Bioavailability of a single oral dose of ribavirin was increased by coadministration with a high-fat meal. The absorption was slowed (time to maximum concentration was doubled), and the $AUC_{0\text{-}192\ h}$ and C_{max} increased by 42% and 66%, respectively, when ribavirin was taken with a high-fat meal compared with fasting conditions. Because ribavirin absorption increases when administered with a meal, advise patients to take ribavirin with food.

Metabolism/Excretion – The mean systemic clearance in healthy subjects given peginterferon alfa-2a was 94 mL/h, which is approximately 100-fold lower than that for interferon alfa-2a. The mean terminal half-life after subcutaneous dosing in patients with chronic HCV was 80 hours (range, 50 to 140 hours) compared with 5.1 hours (range, 3.7 to 8.5 hours) for interferon alfa-2a.

Special populations –

Renal function impairment: In patients with end-stage renal disease undergoing hemodialysis, there is a 25% to 45% reduction in peginterferon alfa-2a clearance.

The pharmacokinetics of ribavirin following administration of ribavirin have not been studied in patients with renal impairment and there are limited data from clinical trials on administration of ribavirin in patients with Ccr less than 50 mL/min. Therefore, do not treat patients with Ccr less than 50 mL/min with ribavirin.

Elderly: The AUC was increased from 1,295 to 1,663 ng•h/mL in subjects older than 62 years of age taking peginterferon alfa-2a 180 mcg, but peak concentrations were similar (9 vs 10 ng/mL) in those older and younger than 62 years of age.

Children: In a population pharmacokinetics study, 14 children 2 to 8 years of age with chronic HCV received peginterferon alfa-2a based on their body surface area (BSA) of the child × 180 mcg/1.73 m^2. The clearance of peginterferon alfa-2a in children was nearly 4-fold lower compared with the clearance reported in adults.

Steady-state trough levels in children with the BSA-adjusted dosing were similar to trough levels observed in adults with 180 mcg fixed dosing. Time to reach the steady state in children is approximately 12 weeks, whereas in adults, steady state is reached within 5 to 8 weeks. In these children receiving the BSA-adjusted dose, the mean exposure AUC during the dosing interval is predicted to be 25% to 70% higher than that observed in adults receiving 180 mcg fixed dosing. The safety and efficacy of peginterferon alfa-2a in patients younger than 18 years of age have not been established.

Contraindications

Hypersensitivity to peginterferon alfa-2a or any of its components; autoimmune hepatitis; hepatic decompensation (Child-Pugh score greater than 6 [class B and C]) in cirrhotic patients before or during treatment; hepatic decompensation with Child-Pugh score greater than or equal to 6 in cirrhotic chronic HCV patients coinfected with HIV before or during treatment; in neonates and infants because it contains benzyl alcohol. Benzyl alcohol is associated with an increased incidence of neurologic and other complications that are sometimes fatal in neonates and infants.

➤*Combination therapy with ribavirin:* Hypersensitivity to ribavirin or any component of the tablet; women who are pregnant; men whose female partners are pregnant; patients with hemoglobinopathies (eg, thalassemia major, sickle cell anemia).

Warnings/Precautions

➤*Neuropsychiatric reactions:* Life-threatening or fatal neuropsychiatric reactions may manifest in patients receiving peginterferon alfa-2a therapy and include suicide, suicidal ideation, homicidal ideation, depression, relapse of drug addiction, and drug overdose. These reactions may occur in patients with and without previous psychiatric illness.

Use peginterferon alfa-2a with extreme caution in patients who report history of depression. Neuropsychiatric adverse reactions observed with alpha interferon treatment include aggressive behavior, psychoses, hallucinations, bipolar disorders, and mania. Monitor all patients for evidence of depression and other psychiatric symptoms. Advise patients to report any sign or symptom of depression or suicidal ideation to their health care provider. In severe cases, stop therapy immediately and institute psychiatric intervention.

➤*Infections:* Serious and severe bacterial infections, some fatal, have been observed in patients treated with alpha interferons, including peginterferon alfa-2a. Some of the infections have been associated with neutropenia. Discontinue peginterferon alfa-2a in patients who develop severe infections and institute appropriate antibiotic therapy.

➤*Bone marrow toxicity:* Peginterferon alfa-2a suppresses bone marrow function and may result in severe cytopenias. Ribavirin may potentiate the neutropenia and lymphopenia induced by alpha interferons including peginterferon alfa-2a. Very rarely, alpha interferons may be associated with aplastic anemia. Obtain complete blood cell counts (CBCs) pretreatment and monitor routinely during therapy.

Use peginterferon alfa-2a and ribavirin with caution in patients with baseline neutrophil counts less than 1,500 cells/mm^3, baseline platelet counts less than 90,000 cells/mm^3, or baseline hemoglobin (Hgb) less than 10 g/dL. Discontinue peginterferon alfa-2a therapy, at least temporarily, in patients who develop severe decreases in neutrophil and/or platelet counts.

Severe neutropenia and thrombocytopenia occur with a greater incidence in HIV-coinfected patients than monoinfected patients and may result in serious infections or bleeding.

PEGINTERFERON ALFA-2a — INJECTION

➤*Cardiovascular effects:* Hypertension, supraventricular arrhythmias, chest pain, and myocardial infarction have been observed in patients treated with peginterferon alfa-2a.

Administer peginterferon alfa-2a with caution to patients with preexisting cardiac disease. Because cardiac disease may be worsened by ribavirin-induced anemia, do not use ribavirin in patients with a history of significant or unstable cardiac disease.

Fatal and nonfatal myocardial infarctions have been reported in patients with anemia caused by ribavirin. Assess patients for underlying cardiac disease before initiation of ribavirin therapy. Before treatment, administer electrocardiograms to patients with preexisting cardiac disease and monitor these patients during therapy. If there is any deterioration of cardiovascular status, suspend or discontinue therapy. Because cardiac disease may be worsened by drug-induced anemia, do not use ribavirin in patients with a history of significant or unstable cardiac disease.

➤*Hepatitis exacerbations:* Exacerbations of hepatitis during hepatitis B therapy are not uncommon and are characterized by transient and potentially severe increases in serum ALT. Chronic HBV patients experienced transient acute exacerbations (flares) of hepatitis B (ALT elevation greater than 10-fold higher than the ULN) during peginterferon alfa-2a treatment (12% and 18%) and posttreatment (7% and 12%) in HBeAg-negative and HBeAg-positive patients, respectively. Marked transaminase flares while on peginterferon alfa-2a therapy have been accompanied by other liver test abnormalities. Monitor liver function more frequently in patients experiencing ALT flares. Consider peginterferon alfa-2a dose reduction in patients experiencing transaminase flares. If ALT increases are progressive despite reduction of peginterferon alfa-2a dose or are accompanied by increased bilirubin or evidence of hepatic decompensation, discontinue peginterferon alfa-2a immediately.

➤*Endocrine disorders:* Peginterferon alfa-2a causes or aggravates hypothyroidism and hyperthyroidism. Hyperglycemia, hypoglycemia, and diabetes mellitus have been observed to develop in patients treated with peginterferon alfa-2a. Do not begin peginterferon alfa-2a therapy in patients with these conditions at baseline who cannot be effectively treated by medication. Patients who develop these conditions during treatment and cannot be controlled with medication may require discontinuation of peginterferon alfa-2a therapy.

➤*Autoimmune disorders:* Development or exacerbation of autoimmune disorders, including hepatitis, idiopathic thrombocytopenia purpura, interstitial nephritis, myositis, psoriasis, rheumatoid arthritis, systemic lupus erythematosus, thrombotic thrombocytopenic purpura, and thyroiditis, have been reported in patients receiving alpha interferons. Use peginterferon alfa-2a therapy with caution in patients with autoimmune disorders.

➤*Pulmonary disorders:* Bronchiolitis obliterans, dyspnea, interstitial pneumonitis, pneumonia, pulmonary infiltrates, and sarcoidosis, some resulting in respiratory failure and/or death, may be induced or aggravated by peginterferon alfa-2a or alpha interferon therapy. Discontinue peginterferon alfa-2a treatment in patients who develop persistent or unexplained pulmonary infiltrates or pulmonary function impairment.

➤*Colitis:* Ulcerative and hemorrhagic/ischemic colitis, sometimes fatal, has been observed within 12 weeks of starting alpha interferon treatment. Abdominal pain, bloody diarrhea, and fever are the typical manifestations of colitis. Immediately discontinue peginterferon alfa-2a if these symptoms develop. The colitis usually resolves within 1 to 3 weeks of discontinuation of alpha interferon.

➤*Pancreatitis:* Pancreatitis, sometimes fatal, has occurred during alpha interferon and ribavirin treatment. Suspend peginterferon alfa-2a and ribavirin if symptoms or signs suggestive of pancreatitis are observed. Discontinue peginterferon alfa-2a and ribavirin in patients diagnosed with pancreatitis.

➤*Ophthalmologic disorders:* Decrease or loss of vision; retinopathy, including macular edema; retinal artery or vein thrombosis; retinal hemorrhages and cotton wool spots; optic neuritis; and papilledema are induced or aggravated by treatment with peginterferon alfa-2a or other alpha interferons. Give all patients an eye examination at baseline. Give patients with preexisting ophthalmologic disorders (eg, diabetic, hypertensive retinopathy) periodic ophthalmologic exams during interferon alfa treatment. Give any patient who develops ocular symptoms a prompt and complete eye examination. Discontinue peginterferon alfa-2a treatment in patients who develop new or worsening ophthalmologic disorders.

➤*Hemolytic anemia:* The primary toxicity of ribavirin is hemolytic anemia. Hgb less than 10 g/dL was observed in approximately 13% of ribavirin and peginterferon alfa-2a–treated patients in chronic HCV clinical trials. The anemia associated with ribavirin occurs within 1 to 2 weeks of initiation of therapy with maximum drop in Hgb observed during the first 8 weeks. Because the initial drop in Hgb may be significant, it is advised that Hgb or hematocrit be obtained pretreatment and at week 2 and week 4 of therapy or more frequently if clinically indicated. Follow patients as clinically appropriate.

➤*Fever:* While fever is commonly caused by peginterferon alfa-2a therapy, other causes of persistent fever must be ruled out, particularly in patients with neutropenia.

➤*Clinical study criteria:* The following entrance criteria used for the clinical studies of peginterferon alfa-2a may be considered as a guideline to acceptable baseline values for initiation of treatment:

- platelet count greater than or equal to 90,000 cells/mm^3 (as low as 75,000 cells/mm^3 in HCV patients with cirrhosis or 70,000 cells/mm^3 in patients with chronic HCV and HIV)
- ANC greater than or equal to 1,500 cells/mm^3
- serum creatinine concentration less than 1.5 times the ULN
- TSH and thyroxine (T_4) within normal limits or adequately controlled thyroid function
- CD4+ cell count at least 200 cells/mcL or CD4+ cell count at least 100 cells/mcL but less than 200 cells/mcL and HIV-1 RNA less than 5,000 copies/mL in patients coinfected with HIV
- Hgb at least 12 g/dL for women and at least 13 g/dL for men in chronic HCV monoinfected patients
- Hgb at least 11 g/dL for women and at least 12 g/dL for men in patients with chronic HCV and HIV

➤*Hypersensitivity reactions:* Severe acute hypersensitivity reactions (eg, anaphylaxis, angioedema, bronchoconstriction, urticaria) have been rarely observed during alpha interferon and ribavirin therapy. If such reactions occur, discontinue therapy with peginterferon alfa-2a and ribavirin and immediately institute appropriate medical therapy.

➤*Renal function impairment:* A 25% to 45% higher exposure to peginterferon alfa-2a is seen in subjects undergoing hemodialysis. In patients with impaired renal function, closely monitor for signs and symptoms of interferon toxicity. Adjust doses of peginterferon alfa-2a accordingly. Use peginterferon alfa-2a with caution in patients with Ccr less than 50 mL/min.

It is recommended that renal function be evaluated in all patients started on ribavirin. Do not administer ribavirin to patients with Ccr less than 50 mL/min.

➤*Hepatic function impairment:* Chronic HCV patients with cirrhosis may be at risk of hepatic decompensation and death when treated with alpha interferons, including peginterferon alfa-2a. Cirrhotic chronic HCV patients coinfected with HIV receiving highly active antiretroviral therapy (HAART) and interferon alfa-2a with or without ribavirin appear to be at increased risk for the development of hepatic decompensation, compared with patients not receiving HAART. In study 6, among 129 chronic HCV/HIV cirrhotic patients receiving HAART, 14 (11%) of these patients across all treatment arms developed hepatic decompensation, resulting in 6 deaths. All 14 patients were on nucleoside reverse transcriptase inhibitors (NRTIs), including abacavir, didanosine, lamivudine, stavudine, and zidovudine. These small numbers of patients do not permit discrimination between specific NRTIs for the associated risk. During treatment, closely monitor patients' clinical status and hepatic function, and discontinue peginterferon alfa-2a treatment if decompensation (Child-Pugh score at least 6) is observed.

➤*Special risk:* The safety and efficacy of peginterferon alfa-2a alone or in combination with ribavirin have not been established for the treatment of chronic HCV in the following instances:

- those who have failed alpha interferon- or alpha interferon and ribavirin treatment
- liver or other organ transplant recipients
- hepatitis B patients coinfected with HCV or HIV
- hepatitis C patients coinfected with HBV or HIV with a CD4+ cell count less than 100 cells/mcL

Exercise caution when initiating treatment in any patient with baseline risk of severe anemia (eg, spherocytosis, history of GI bleeding).

➤*Hazardous tasks:* Caution patients who develop dizziness, confusion, somnolence, and fatigue to avoid driving or operating machinery.

➤*Pregnancy: Category C.* Peginterferon alfa-2a has not been studied for its teratogenic effects. Nonpegylated interferon alfa-2a treatment of pregnant Rhesus monkeys at approximately 20 to 500 times the human weekly dose resulted in a statistically significant increase in abortions. No teratogenic effects were seen in the offspring delivered at term. Assume peginterferon alfa-2a to have abortifacient potential. There are no adequate and well-controlled studies of peginterferon alfa-2a in pregnant women. Use peginterferon alfa-2a during pregnancy only if the potential benefit justifies the potential risk to the fetus. Peginterferon alfa-2a is recommended for use in women of childbearing potential only when they are using effective contraception during therapy.

Fertility impairment – Peginterferon alfa-2a may impair fertility in women. The effects of peginterferon alfa-2a on male fertility have not been studied. However, no adverse reactions on fertility were observed in male rhesus monkeys treated with nonpegylated interferon alfa-2a for 5 months at dosages up to 25 × 106 units/kg/day.

Combination therapy with ribavirin – *Category X.* Significant teratogenic and/or embryocidal effects have been demonstrated in all animal species exposed to ribavirin. Ribavirin therapy is contraindicated in women who are pregnant and in the male partners of women who are pregnant.

Ribavirin may cause birth defects and/or death in the exposed fetus. Take extreme care to avoid pregnancy in women and in female partners of men taking peginterferon alfa-2a and ribavirin combination therapy. Do not start

PEGINTERFERON ALFA-2a — INJECTION

ribavirin therapy unless a report of a negative pregnancy test has been obtained immediately prior to initiation of therapy. Women of childbearing potential and men must use 2 forms of effective contraception during treatment and for at least 6 months after conclusion of treatment. Routine monthly pregnancy tests must be performed during this time.

Ribavirin pregnancy registry – A ribavirin pregnancy registry has been established to monitor maternal and fetal outcomes of pregnancies of women and female partners of men exposed to ribavirin during treatment and for 6 months following cessation of treatment. Health care providers and patients are strongly encouraged to report such cases by calling 1-800-593-2214.

➤*Lactation:* It is not known whether peginterferon alfa-2a or ribavirin or its components are excreted in human milk. The effect of orally ingested peginterferon alfa-2a or ribavirin from breast milk on the breast-feeding infant has not been evaluated. Because of the potential for adverse reactions from the drug in breast-feeding infants, decide whether to discontinue breast-feeding or peginterferon alfa-2a and ribavirin treatment.

➤*Children:* The safety and efficacy of peginterferon alfa-2a alone or in combination with ribavirin in patients younger than 18 years of age have not been established.

Benzyl alcohol – Peginterferon alfa-2a contains benzyl alcohol. Benzyl alcohol has been reported to be associated with an increased incidence of neurological and other complications that can be fatal in neonates and infants.

➤*Elderly:* Younger patients have higher virologic response rates than older patients. Clinical studies of peginterferon alfa-2a alone or in combination with ribavirin did not include sufficient numbers of subjects 65 years of age and older to determine whether they respond differently from younger subjects. Adverse reactions related to alpha interferons, such as CNS, cardiac, and systemic (eg, flu-like) effects, may be more severe in the elderly; exercise caution when using peginterferon alfa-2a in this population. Peginterferon alfa-2a and ribavirin are known to be excreted by the kidney, and the risk of toxic reactions to this therapy may be greater in patients with impaired renal function. Because elderly patients are more likely to have decreased renal function, take care in dose selection; it may be useful to monitor renal function. Use peginterferon alfa-2a with caution in patients with Ccr less than 50 mL/min. Do not administer ribavirin to patients with Ccr less than 50 mL/min.

➤*Lab test abnormalities:*

Hematologic abnormalities – Peginterferon alfa-2a treatment was associated with decreases in WBC, ANC, lymphocytes, and platelet counts often starting within the first 2 weeks of treatment. Dose reduction is recommended in patients with hematologic abnormalities.

Hepatic effects – In chronic HCV, transient elevations in ALT (2- to 5-fold above baseline) were observed in some patients receiving peginterferon alfa-2a, and were not associated with deterioration of other liver function tests. When the increase in ALT levels is progressive despite dose reduction or is accompanied by increased bilirubin, discontinue peginterferon alfa-2a therapy.

Unlike hepatitis C, during hepatitis B therapy follow-up, transient elevations in ALT of 5 to 10 times the ULN were observed in 25% and 27% and of greater than 10 times the ULN were observed in 12% and 18%, of HBeAg-negative and HBeAg-positive patients, respectively. These ALT elevations have been accompanied by other liver test abnormalities.

Immunogenicity –

Chronic HBV: Twenty-nine percent (42/143) of hepatitis B patients treated with peginterferon alfa-2a for 24 weeks developed binding antibodies to interferon alfa-, as assessed by an enzyme-linked immunosorbent assay (ELISA). Thirteen percent of patients (19/143) receiving peginterferon alfa-2a developed low-titer neutralizing antibodies (using an assay with a sensitivity of 100 interferon neutralizing units/mL).

Chronic HCV: Nine percent (71/834) of patients treated with peginterferon alfa-2a with or without ribavirin developed binding antibodies to interferon alfa-2a, as assessed by an ELISA. Three percent of patients (25/835) receiving peginterferon alfa-2a with or without ribavirin developed low-titer neutralizing antibodies (using an assay of a sensitivity of 100 interferon neutralizing units/mL).

➤*Monitoring:* Before beginning peginterferon alfa-2a or peginterferon alfa-2a and ribavirin combination therapy, standard hematological and biochemical laboratory tests are recommended for all patients. Pregnancy screening for women of childbearing potential must be performed. Monitor all patients for evidence of depression and other psychiatric symptoms. In patients with impaired renal function, closely monitor for signs and symptoms of interferon toxicity. Patients with preexisting ophthalmologic disorders (eg, diabetic or hypertensive retinopathy) should receive periodic ophthalmologic exams during interferon-alfa treatment. Before treatment, administer electrocardiograms to patients with preexisting cardiac disease, and monitor during therapy.

After initiation of therapy, perform hematological tests at 2 and 4 weeks, and perform biochemical tests at 4 weeks. Perform additional testing periodically during therapy. In the clinical studies, the CBC (including Hgb level, white blood cell count [WBC], and platelet count) and chemistries (including liver function tests and uric acid) were measured at 1, 2, 4, 6, and 8, and then every 4 to 6 weeks, or more frequently if abnormalities were found. Thyrotropin (TSH) was measured every 12 weeks. Perform monthly pregnancy testing during combination therapy and for 6 months after discontinuing therapy.

Drug Interactions

Peginterferon Alfa-2a Drug Interactions

Precipitant drug	Object drug[a]		Description
Peginterferon alfa-2a	Methadone	↑	Concomitant treatment with peginterferon alfa-2a once weekly for 4 weeks was associated with methadone levels that were 10% to 15% higher than at baseline.
Peginterferon alfa-2a	NRTIs (eg, didanosine, zidovudine, stavudine)	↑	Coadministration may increase toxicities, such as hematologic toxicities. Cases of hepatic decomposition (some fatal) were observed.
Peginterferon alfa-2a	Theophylline	↑	Coadministration with peginterferon alfa-2a was associated with an inhibition of CYP1A2 and a 25% increase in theophylline AUC. Monitor theophylline levels and adjust dose as needed.

[a] ↑ = object drug increased.

Adverse Reactions

Peginterferon alfa-2a alone or in combination with ribavirin causes a broad variety of serious adverse reactions. The most common life-threatening or fatal reactions induced or aggravated by peginterferon alfa-2a and ribavirin were depression, suicide, relapse of drug abuse/overdose, and bacterial infections, each occurring at a frequency of less than 1%. Hepatic decompensation occurred in 2% (10/574) of chronic HCV/HIV patients.

➤*Hepatitis C studies:* In all hepatitis C studies, 1 or more serious adverse reaction occurred in 10% of chronic HCV monoinfected patients and in 19% of chronic HCV/HIV patients receiving peginterferon alfa-2a alone or in combination with ribavirin. The most common serious adverse reaction (3% in chronic HCV and 5% in chronic HCV/HIV) was bacterial infection (eg, endocarditis, osteomyelitis, pneumonia, pyelonephritis, sepsis). Other serious adverse reactions occurred at a frequency of less than 1% and included aggression, angina, anxiety, aplastic anemia, arrhythmia, autoimmune phenomena (eg, hyperthyroidism, hypothyroidism, sarcoidosis, systemic lupus erythematosus, rheumatoid arthritis), cerebral hemorrhage, cholangitis, colitis, coma, corneal ulcer, diabetes mellitus, drug abuse and drug overdose, fatty liver, GI bleeding, hepatic dysfunction, myositis, pancreatitis, peptic ulcer, peripheral neuropathy, psychosis, pulmonary embolism, suicidal ideation, suicide, and thrombotic thrombocytopenic purpura.

Nearly all hepatitis C patients in clinical trials experienced 1 or more adverse reaction. The most commonly reported adverse reactions were psychiatric reactions, including anxiety, depression, insomnia, and irritability, and flu-like symptoms (eg, fatigue, headache, myalgia, pyrexia, rigors). Other common reactions were alopecia, anorexia, arthralgia, diarrhea, injection site reactions, nausea and vomiting, and pruritus.

Overall, 11% of chronic HCV monoinfected patients receiving 48 weeks of therapy with peginterferon alfa-2a either alone or in combination with ribavirin discontinued therapy; 16% of chronic HCV/HIV coinfected patients discontinued therapy. The most common reasons for discontinuation of therapy were psychiatric, flu-like syndrome (eg, lethargy, fatigue, headache), dermatologic, and GI disorders and laboratory abnormalities (thrombocytopenia, neutropenia, and anemia).

Overall, 39% of patients with chronic HCV or chronic HCV/HIV required modification of peginterferon alfa-2a and/or ribavirin therapy. The most common reason for dose modification of peginterferon alfa-2a in chronic HCV and chronic HCV/HIV patients was for laboratory abnormalities: neutropenia (20% and 27%, respectively) and thrombocytopenia (4% and 6%, respectively). The most common reason for dose modification of ribavirin in chronic HCV and chronic HCV/HIV patients was anemia (22% and 16%, respectively).

Peginterferon alfa-2a dose was reduced in 12% of patients receiving ribavirin 1,000 to 1,200 mg for 48 weeks and in 7% of patients receiving ribavirin 800 mg for 24 weeks. Ribavirin dose was reduced in 21% of patients receiving ribavirin 1,000 to 1,200 mg for 48 weeks and 12% in patients receiving ribavirin 800 mg for 24 weeks.

Chronic HCV monoinfected patients treated for 24 weeks with peginterferon alfa-2a and ribavirin 800 mg were observed to have lower incidence of serious adverse reactions (3% vs 10%), Hgb less than 10 g/dL (3% vs 15%), dose modification of peginterferon alfa-2a (30% vs 36%) and ribavirin (19% vs 38%), and of withdrawal from treatment (5% vs 15%), compared with patients treated for 48 weeks with peginterferon alfa-2a and ribavirin 1,000 or 1,200 mg. On the other hand, the overall incidence of adverse reactions appeared to be similar in the 2 treatment groups.

Because clinical trials are conducted under widely varying and controlled conditions, adverse reaction rates observed in clinical trials of a drug cannot be directly compared with rates in the clinical trials of another drug. Also, the adverse reaction rates listed here may not predict the rates observed in a broader patient population in clinical practice.

PEGINTERFERON ALFA-2a — INJECTION

Peginterferon Alfa-2a Adverse Reactions in Chronic HCV Patients (≥ 5%)				
	Chronic hepatitis C monotherapy (pooled studies 1 to 3)		Chronic hepatitis C combination therapy (study 4)	
Adverse reaction	Peginterferon alfa-2a 180 mcg (48 weeks)[a] (n = 559)	Interferon alfa-2a recombinant[a,b] (n = 554)	Peginterferon alfa-2a 180 mcg + ribavirin 1,000 or 1,200 mg (48 weeks) (n = 451)	Interferon alfa-2b, recombinant + ribavirin 1,000 or 1,200 mg (48 weeks) (n = 443)
CNS				
Concentration impairment	8%	10%	10%	13%
Depression	18%	19%	20%	28%
Dizziness (excluding vertigo)	16%	12%	14%	14%
Fatigue/ Asthenia	56%	57%	65%	68%
Headache	54%	58%	43%	49%
Insomnia	19%	23%	30%	37%
Irritability/ Anxiety/ Nervousness	19%	22%	33%	38%
Memory impairment	5%	4%	6%	5%
Mood alteration	3%	2%	5%	6%
Dermatologic				
Alopecia	23%	30%	28%	33%
Dermatitis	8%	3%	16%	13%
Dry skin	4%	3%	10%	13%
Eczema	1%	1%	5%	4%
Increased sweating	6%	7%	6%	5%
Pruritus	12%	8%	19%	18%
Rash	5%	4%	8%	5%
Endocrine				
Hypothyroidism	3%	2%	4%	5%
GI				
Abdominal pain	15%	15%	8%	9%
Diarrhea	16%	16%	11%	10%
Dry mouth	6%	3%	4%	7%
Dyspepsia	< 1%	1%	6%	5%
Nausea/ Vomiting	24%	33%	25%	29%
Hematologic[c]				
Anemia	2%	1%	11%	11%
Lymphopenia	3%	5%	14%	12%
Neutropenia	21%	8%	27%	8%
Thrombocytopenia	5%	2%	5%	< 1%
Metabolic/Nutritional				
Anorexia	17%	17%	24%	26%
Weight decrease	4%	3%	10%	10%
Musculoskeletal				
Arthralgia	28%	29%	22%	23%
Back pain	9%	10%	5%	5%
Myalgia	37%	38%	40%	49%
Resistance mechanism disorders				
Overall	10%	6%	12%	10%
Respiratory				
Cough	4%	3%	10%	7%
Dyspnea	4%	2%	13%	14%
Dyspnea, exertional	< 1%	< 1%	4%	7%
Miscellaneous				
Blurred vision	4%	2%	5%	2%
Injection site reaction	22%	18%	23%	16%
Pain	11%	12%	10%	9%
Pyrexia	37%	41%	41%	55%
Rigors	35%	44%	25%	37%

[a] Pooled studies 1, 2, and 3.
[b] Either 3 million units or 6 million units 3 times a week for 12 weeks, followed by 3 million units 3 times a week for 36 weeks of interferon alfa-2a, recombinant.
[c] Severe hematologic abnormalities (lymphocytes $< 0.5 \times 10^9$/L; Hgb < 10 g/dL; neutrophils $< 0.75 \times 10^9$/L; platelets $< 50 \times 10^9$/L).

➤***Chronic HCV with HIV coinfection:*** The adverse reaction profile of coinfected patients treated with peginterferon alfa-2a and ribavirin in study 6 was generally similar to that shown for monoinfected patients in study 4. Events occurring more frequently in coinfected patients were neutropenia (40%), anemia (14%), thrombocytopenia (8%), weight decrease (16%), and mood alteration (9%).

➤***Chronic HBV:*** In clinical trials of 48-week treatment duration, the adverse reaction profile of peginterferon alfa-2a in chronic HBV was similar to that seen in chronic HCV peginterferon alfa-2a monotherapy use, except for exacerbations of hepatitis. Six percent of peginterferon alfa-2a-treated patients in the hepatitis B studies experienced 1 or more serious adverse reactions.

The most common or important serious adverse reactions in the hepatitis B studies were infections (appendicitis, influenza, sepsis, tuberculosis), hepatitis B flares, anaphylactic shock, thrombotic thrombocytopenic purpura.

The most commonly observed adverse reactions were pyrexia (54% vs 4%), headache (27% vs 9%), fatigue (24% vs 10%), myalgia (26% vs 4%), alopecia (18% vs 2%), and anorexia (16% vs 3%) in the peginterferon alfa-2a and lamivudine groups respectively.

Overall 5% of hepatitis B patients discontinued peginterferon alfa-2a therapy and 40% of patients required modification of peginterferon alfa-2a dose. The most common reason for dose modification in patients receiving peginterferon alfa-2a therapy was for laboratory abnormalities including neutropenia (20%), thrombocytopenia (13%), and ALT disorders (11%).

➤***Lab test abnormalities:*** The laboratory test values observed in the hepatitis B trials (except where noted below) were similar to those seen in the peginterferon alfa-2a monotherapy hepatitis C trials.

ALT elevations –

Chronic HBV: Transient ALT elevations are common during hepatitis B therapy with peginterferon alfa-2a. Twenty-five percent and 27% of patients experienced elevations of 5 to 10 times the ULN and 12% and 18% had elevations of greater than 10 times the ULN during treatment of HBeAg-negative and HBeAg-positive disease, respectively. Flares have been accompanied by elevations of total bilirubin and alkaline phosphatase and less commonly with prolongation of prothrombin time and reduced albumin levels. Eleven percent of patients had dose modifications due to ALT flares and less than 1% of patients were withdrawn from treatment.

ALT flares of 5 to 10 times the ULN occurred in 13% and 16% of patients, while ALT flares of greater than 10 times the ULN occurred in 7% and 12% of patients in HBeAg-negative and HBeAg-positive disease, respectively, after discontinuation of peginterferon alfa-2a therapy.

Chronic HCV: One percent of patients in the hepatitis C trials experienced marked elevations (5- to 10-fold above the ULN) in ALT levels during treatment and follow-up. On occasion, these transaminase elevations were associated with hyperbilirubinemia and were managed by dose reduction or discontinuation of study treatment. Liver function test abnormalities were generally transient. One case was attributed to autoimmune hepatitis, which persisted beyond study medication discontinuation.

Hemoglobin – In hepatitis C studies, the Hgb concentration decreased below 12 g/dL in 17% (median Hgb reduction of 2.2 g/dL) of monotherapy and 52% (median Hgb reduction of 3.7 g/dL) of combination therapy patients. Severe anemia (Hgb less than 10 g/dL) was encountered in 13% of all patients receiving combination therapy and in 2% of chronic HCV patients and 8% of chronic HCV/HIV patients receiving peginterferon alfa-2a monotherapy. Dose modification for anemia in ribavirin recipients treated for 48 weeks occurred in 22% of chronic HCV patients and 16% of chronic HCV/HIV patients.

PEGINTERFERON ALFA-2a — INJECTION

Immunogenicity –

Chronic HBV: See Warnings/Precautions for more information.
Chronic HCV: See Warnings/Precautions for more information.

Lymphocytes – Decreases in lymphocyte count are induced by interferon alpha therapy. Peginterferon alfa-2a plus ribavirin combination therapy induced decreases in median total lymphocyte counts (56% in chronic HCV and 40% in chronic HCV/HIV, with median decrease of 1,170 cells/mm^3 in chronic HCV and 800 cells/mm^3 in chronic HCV/HIV). In hepatitis C studies, lymphopenia was observed during monotherapy (81%) and combination therapy with peginterferon alfa-2a and ribavirin (91%). Severe lymphopenia (less than 0.5 × 10^9/L) occurred in approximately 5% of all monotherapy patients and 14% of all combination peginterferon alfa-2a and ribavirin therapy recipients. Dose adjustments were not required by protocol. The clinical significance of the lymphopenia is not known.

In chronic HCV with HIV coinfection, CD4 counts decreased 29% from baseline (median decreases of 137 cells/mm^3), and CD8 counts decreased 44% from baseline (median decrease of 389 cells/mm^3) in the peginterferon alfa-2a plus ribavirin combination therapy arm. Median lymphocyte CD4 and CD8 counts returned to pretreatment levels after 4 to 12 weeks of the cessation of therapy. CD4 percent did not decrease during treatment.

Neutrophils – In the hepatitis C studies, decreases in neutrophil count below normal were observed in 95% of all patients treated with peginterferon alfa-2a either alone or in combination with ribavirin. Severe, potentially life-threatening neutropenia (ANC less than 0.5 × 10^9/L) occurred in 5% of chronic HCV patients and 12% of chronic HCV/HIV patients receiving peginterferon alfa-2a either alone or in combination with ribavirin. Modification of peginterferon alfa-2a dose for neutropenia occurred in 17% of patients receiving peginterferon alfa-2a monotherapy and 22% of patients receiving peginterferon alfa-2a/ribavirin combination therapy. In the chronic HCV/HIV patients, 27% required modification of interferon dosage for neutropenia. Two percent of patients with chronic HCV and 10% of patients with chronic HCV/HIV required permanent reductions of peginterferon alfa-2a dosage, and less than 1% required permanent discontinuation. Median neutrophil counts returned to pretreatment levels 4 weeks after cessation of therapy.

Platelets – In hepatitis C studies, platelet counts decreased in 52% of chronic HCV patients and 51% of chronic HCV/HIV patients treated with peginterferon alfa-2a alone (median decrease of 41% and 35% from baseline, respectively), and in 33% of chronic HCV patients and 47% of chronic HCV/HIV patients receiving combination therapy with ribavirin (median decrease of 30% from baseline). Moderate to severe thrombocytopenia (less than 50,000/mm^3) was observed in 4% of chronic HCV and 8% of chronic HCV/HIV patients. Median platelet counts returned to pretreatment levels 4 weeks after the cessation of therapy.

Postmarketing – The following adverse reactions have been identified and reported during postapproval use of peginterferon alfa-2a therapy: hearing impairment, hearing loss.

Triglycerides: Triglyceride levels are elevated in patients receiving alpha interferon therapy and were elevated in the majority of patients participating in clinical studies receiving either peginterferon alfa-2a alone or in combination with ribavirin. Random levels greater than or equal to 400 mg/dL were observed in about 20% of chronic HCV patients. Severe elevations of triglycerides (more than 1,000 mg/dL) occurred in 2% of monoinfected patients.

In HCV/HIV coinfected patients, fasting levels at least 400 mg/dL were observed in up to 36% of patients receiving either peginterferon alfa-2a alone or in combination with ribavirin. Severe elevations of triglycerides (more than 1,000 mg/dL) occurred in 7% of coinfected patients.

Thyroid function: Peginterferon alfa-2a alone or in combination with ribavirin was associated with the development of abnormalities in thyroid laboratory values, some with associated clinical manifestations. In hepatitis C studies, hypothyroidism or hyperthyroidism requiring treatment, dose modification, or discontinuation occurred in 4% and 1% of peginterferon alfa-2a treated patients and 4% and 2% of peginterferon alfa-2a- and ribavirin-treated patients, respectively. Among the patients who developed thyroid abnormalities during peginterferon alfa-2a treatment, approximately half still had abnormalities during the follow-up period.

Overdosage

➤*Symptoms:* There is limited experience with overdosage. The maximum dosage received by any patient was 7 times the intended dosage of peginterferon alfa-2a (180 mcg/day for 7 days). There were no serious reactions attributed to overdosages. Weekly doses of up to 630 mcg have been administered to patients with cancer. Dose-limiting toxicities were fatigue, elevated liver enzymes, neutropenia, and thrombocytopenia.

➤*Treatment:* There is no specific antidote for peginterferon alfa-2a. Hemodialysis and peritoneal dialysis are not effective.

Patient Information

Direct patients receiving peginterferon alfa-2a alone or in combination with ribavirin in its appropriate use, inform them of the benefits and risks associated with treatment, and refer them to the peginterferon alfa-2a and, if applicable, ribavirin medication guides.

Peginterferon alfa-2a and ribavirin combination therapy must not be used by women who are pregnant or by men whose female partners are pregnant. Do not initiate ribavirin therapy until a report of a negative pregnancy test has been obtained immediately before starting therapy. Advise women of childbearing potential and men with female partners of childbearing potential of the teratogenic/embryocidal risks, and instruct them to practice effective contraception during ribavirin therapy and for 6 months posttherapy. Advise patients to notify their health care provider immediately in the event of a pregnancy.

Women of childbearing potential and men must use 2 forms of effective contraception during treatment and during the 6 months after treatment has been stopped; routine monthly pregnancy tests must be performed during this time.

To monitor maternal and fetal outcomes of pregnant women exposed to ribavirin, a ribavirin pregnancy registry has been established. Strongly encourage patients to register by calling 1-800-593-2214.

Advise patients that laboratory evaluations are required before starting therapy and periodically thereafter. Instruct patients to remain well hydrated, especially during the initial stages of treatment. Advise patients to take ribavirin with food.

Inform patients that it is not known if therapy with peginterferon alfa-2a alone or in combination with ribavirin will prevent transmission of HCV or HBV infection to others or prevent cirrhosis, liver failure, or liver cancer that might result from HCV or HBV infection.

Caution patients who develop dizziness, confusion, somnolence, and fatigue to avoid driving or operating machinery.

If home use is prescribed, supply a puncture-resistant container for the disposal of used needles and syringes to the patients. Thoroughly instruct patients in the importance of proper disposal; caution against any reuse of needles and syringes. Advise patients to dispose of the full container according to the directions provided by their health care provider.

Advise patients to report any signs or symptoms of depression or suicidal ideation to their health care provider.

INTERFERON ALFA-2B, RECOMBINANT (IFN-alpha 2; rIFN-α2; α-2-interferon)

Rx	**Intron A**[a] (Schering)	**Injection, powder for solution:**[b] 10 million units/vial	In vials with 1 mL diluent vial.[c]
		18 million units/vial	In vials with 1 mL diluent vial.[c]
		50 million units/vial	In vials with 1 mL diluent vial.[c]
		Injection, solution:[d] 3 million units/dose	In multidose pens (6 doses; 22.5 million units per 1.5 mL/pen) with needles.
		5 million units/dose	In multidose pens (6 doses; 37.5 million units per 1.5 mL/pen) with needles.
		10 million units/dose	In multidose pens (6 doses; 75 million units per 1.5 mL/pen) with needles. In vials, Pak-10 (6 vials, 6 BD Safety-Lok syringes).
		18 million units/vial	In multidose vials (22.8 million units per 3.8 mL/vial).
		25 million units/vial	In multidose vials (32 million units per 3.2 mL/vial).

[a] Not all dosage forms and strengths are appropriate for some indications.
[b] Each milliliter includes 1 mg human albumin, 20 mg glycine, 2.3 mg sodium phosphate dibasic, 0.55 mg sodium phosphate monobasic.
[c] Diluent is sterile water for injection.
[d] Each milliliter contains 7.5 mg sodium chloride, 1.8 mg sodium phosphate dibasic, 1.3 mg sodium phosphate monobasic, 0.1 mg EDTA, 0.1 mg polysorbate 80, and 1.5 mg m-cresol as a preservative.

INTERFERON ALFA-2B, RECOMBINANT — INJECTION

WARNING

Alpha interferons, including interferon alfa-2b, cause or aggravate fatal or life-threatening neuropsychiatric, autoimmune, ischemic, and infectious disorders. Monitor patients closely with periodic clinical and laboratory evaluations. Withdraw therapy from patients with persistently severe or worsening signs or symptoms of these conditions. In many but not all cases these disorders resolve after stopping interferon alfa-2b therapy.

Indications

➤*AIDS-related Kaposi sarcoma (KS):* For the treatment of selected patients 18 years of age and older with AIDS-related KS. The likelihood of response to interferon alfa-2b therapy is greater in patients who are without systemic symptoms, who have limited lymphadenopathy, and who have a relatively intact immune system as indicated by total CD4 count.

➤*Chronic hepatitis B:* For the treatment of chronic hepatitis B in patients 1 year of age and older with compensated liver disease. Patients who have been serum hepatitis B surface antigen (HBsAg) positive for at

INTERFERON ALFA-2B, RECOMBINANT — INJECTION

least 6 months and have evidence of hepatitis B virus (HBV) replication (serum hepatitis B e antigen [HBeAg] positive) with elevated serum ALT are candidates for treatment.

Patients with causes of chronic hepatitis other than chronic hepatitis B or chronic hepatitis C should not be treated with interferon alfa-2b therapy.

ALT flares – A transient increase in ALT 2 or more times baseline value (flare) can occur during interferon alfa-2b therapy for chronic hepatitis B. In clinical trials in adults and children, this flare generally occurred 8 to 12 weeks after initiation of therapy and was more frequent in interferon alfa-2b responders (adults 63%, 24 of 38; children 59%, 10 of 17) than in nonresponders (adults 27%, 13 of 48; children 35%, 19 of 55). However, in adults and children, elevations in bilirubin of 3 mg/dL or more (at least 2 times the upper limit of normal [ULN]) occurred infrequently (adults 2%, 2 of 86; children 3%, 2 of 72) during therapy. When ALT flare occurs, in general, continue interferon alfa-2b therapy unless signs and symptoms of liver failure are observed. During ALT flare, monitor clinical symptomatology and liver function tests, including ALT, prothrombin time, alkaline phosphatase, albumin, and bilirubin, at approximately 2-week intervals.

➤*Chronic hepatitis C:* For the treatment of chronic hepatitis C in patients 18 years of age and older with compensated liver disease who have a history of blood or blood-product exposure and/or are hepatitis C virus (HCV) antibody–positive.

Interferon alfa-2b in combination with ribavirin capsules is indicated for the treatment of chronic hepatitis C in patients with compensated liver disease previously untreated with alpha interferon therapy or who have relapsed following alpha interferon therapy.

➤*Condylomata acuminata:* For intralesional treatment of selected patients 18 years of age and older with condylomata acuminata involving external surfaces of the genital and perianal areas.

➤*Follicular lymphoma:* For the initial treatment of clinically aggressive follicular non-Hodgkin lymphoma in conjunction with anthracycline-containing combination chemotherapy in patients 18 years of age and older.

➤*Hairy cell leukemia:* For the treatment of patients 18 years of age and older with hairy cell leukemia.

➤*Malignant melanoma:* Adjuvant to surgical treatment in patients 18 years of age and older with malignant melanoma who are free of disease but at high risk for systemic recurrence, within 56 days of surgery.

➤*Off-label uses:* Treatment of angiomatous disorders; mycosis fungoides; ovarian and cervical carcinoma; renal cell carcinoma; basal and squamous cell skin cancer; bladder tumors (local use for superficial tumors); chronic myelogenous leukemia; cutaneous T-cell lymphoma; non-Hodgkin lymphoma; multiple myeloma; carcinoid tumor; papillomaviruses; West Nile virus infection.

Administration and Dosage

➤*General dosing considerations:*

Pretreatment – To reduce the incidence of certain adverse reactions, acetaminophen may be administered at the time of injection.

➤*Adults:*

AIDS-related Kaposi sarcoma –

Usual dosage: 30 million units/m^2 per dose 3 times a week administered subcutaneously or intramuscularly (IM) until disease progression or maximal response has been achieved after 16 weeks of treatment.

Dosage adjustment: Dose reduction is frequently required. Reduce dosage by 50% or withhold for severe adverse reactions. Resume at a reduced dose if severe adverse reactions abate with interruption of dosing.

Discontinuation of therapy: Permanently discontinue if severe adverse reactions persist or if they recur in patients receiving a reduced dose.

Recommended dosage forms:

Appropriate Interferon Alfa-2b Dosage Forms for AIDS-Related Kaposi Sarcoma

Dosage form	Route
Powder 50 million units	IM, subcutaneously

Chronic hepatitis B –

Usual dosage: 5 million units daily or 10 million units 3 times a week (for a total of 30 to 35 million units per week), administered subcutaneously or IM.

Dosage adjustment: Reduce dose by 50% if severe adverse reactions or laboratory abnormalities develop or discontinue if appropriate, until the adverse reactions abate.

For patients with decreases in white blood cell count (WBC), granulocyte count, or platelet count, the following guidelines for dose modification should be followed:

Interferon Alfa-2b Dose Modification Guidelines

Interferon alfa-2b dose	WBC	Granulocyte count	Platelet count
Reduce 50%	$< 1.5 \times 10^9$/L	$< 0.75 \times 10^9$/L	$< 50 \times 10^9$/L

Duration of therapy: 16 weeks.

Discontinuation of therapy: Discontinue if intolerance persists after dose adjustment.

For patients with decreases in WBC, granulocyte count, or platelet count, the following guidelines for therapy discontinuation should be followed:

Interferon Alfa-2b Discontinuation Guidelines

Interferon alfa-2b dose	WBC	Granulocyte count	Platelet count
Permanently discontinue	$< 1 \times 10^9$/L	$< 0.5 \times 10^9$/L	$< 25 \times 10^9$/L

Resumption of therapy: Resume at up to 100% of the initial dose when WBC, granulocyte, and/or platelet counts returned to normal or baseline values.

Recommended dosage forms:

Appropriate Interferon Alfa-2b Dosage Forms for Chronic Hepatitis B

Dosage form	Route
Powder 10 million units (single dose)	IM, subcutaneously
Solution 25 million units multidose	IM, subcutaneously
Pen 5 million units/dose multidose	Subcutaneously
Pen 10 million units/dose multidose	Subcutaneously

Chronic hepatitis C –

Usual dosage: 3 million units 3 times a week administered IM or subcutaneously.

Dosage adjustment: Reduce dose by 50% if severe adverse reactions develop or temporarily discontinue until the adverse reactions abate.

Duration of therapy: In patients tolerating therapy with normalization of ALT at 16 weeks of treatment, extend treatment to 18 to 24 months (72 to 96 weeks) at 3 million units 3 times a week to improve the sustained response rate.

Discontinuation of therapy: Consider discontinuing therapy in patients who can not normalize their ALT and have persistently high levels of HCV RNA after 16 weeks of therapy, because they rarely achieve a sustained response with extension of treatment.

Discontinue treatment if intolerance persists after dose adjustment.

Combination therapy: See the interferon alfa-2b/ribavirin combination therapy monograph for dosing when used in combination with ribavirin capsules.

Recommended dosage forms:

Appropriate Interferon Alfa-2b Dosage Forms for Chronic Hepatitis C

Dosage form	Route
Solution 18 million units multidose	IM, subcutaneously
Pen 3 million units/dose multidose	Subcutaneously

Condylomata acuminata –

Usual dosage: 1 million units per lesion in a maximum of 5 lesions in a single course 3 times weekly on alternate days.

Duration of therapy: 3 weeks. An additional course may be administered at 12 to 16 weeks.

Recommended dosage forms:

Appropriate Interferon Alfa-2b Dosage Forms for Condylomata Acuminata

Dosage form	Route
Powder 10 million units (single dose)	Intralesionally
Solution 25 million units multidose	Intralesionally

Follicular lymphoma –

Usual dosage: 5 million units subcutaneously 3 times per week.

Dosage adjustment: Reduce interferon alfa-2b by 50% (2.5 million units 3 times a week) for a neutrophil count more than 1,000/mm^3 but less than 1,500/mm^3. May re-escalate interferon alfa-2b dose to the starting dose (5 million units 3 times a week) after resolution of hematologic toxicity (absolute neutrophil count more than 1,500/mm^3).

Withhold interferon alfa-2b if neutrophil count is less than 1,000/mm^3, or platelet count less than 50,000/mm^3.

Duration of therapy: Up to 18 months.

Concomitant therapy: Administer in conjunction with an anthracycline-containing chemotherapy regimen and following completion of the chemotherapy regimen.

The doses of myelosuppressive drugs were reduced by 25% from those utilized in a full-dose cyclophosphamide, doxorubicin, vincristine, and prednisone (CHOP) regimen, and cycle length increased by 33% (eg, from 21 to 28 days) when alpha interferon was added to the regimen.

The chemotherapy regimen was delayed if either the neutrophil count was less than 1,500/mm^3 or the platelet count was less than 75,000/mm^3.

Discontinuation of therapy: Discontinue if AST exceeds more than 5 times the ULN or serum creatinine more than 2 mg/dL.

Recommended dosage forms:

Appropriate Interferon Alfa-2b Dosage Forms for Follicular Lymphoma

Dosage form	Route
Powder 10 million units (single dose)	Subcutaneously
Solution 18 million units multidose	Subcutaneously
Solution 25 million units multidose	Subcutaneously
Pen 5 million units/dose multidose	Subcutaneously
Pen 10 million units/dose multidose	Subcutaneously

INTERFERON ALFA-2B, RECOMBINANT — INJECTION

Hairy cell leukemia –

Usual dosage:

• *Platelet counts 50,000/mm³ or more* – 2 million units/m² administered IM or subcutaneously 3 times a week.

• *Platelet counts less than 50,000/mm³* – 2 million units/m² administered subcutaneously 3 times a week. Do not administer intramuscularly.

Dosage adjustment: Reduce dose by 50% if severe adverse reactions develop or temporarily discontinue until the adverse reactions abate, and then resume at 50% (1 million units/m² 3 times a week).

Duration of therapy: Up to 6 months. Responding patients may benefit from continued treatment.

Discontinuation of therapy: Permanently discontinue if severe adverse reactions persist or recur following dosage adjustment. Discontinue if progressive disease or failure to respond after 6 months of treatment.

Recommended dosage forms:

Appropriate Interferon Alfa-2b Dosage Forms for Hairy Cell Leukemia	
Dosage form	Route
Powder 10 million units (single dose)	IM, subcutaneously
Solution 18 million units multidose	IM, subcutaneously
Solution 25 million units multidose	IM, subcutaneously
Pen 3 million units/dose multidose	Subcutaneously
Pen 5 million units/dose multidose	Subcutaneously

Malignant melanoma –

Initial dosage: For induction phase, 20 million units/m² as an intravenous (IV) infusion, over 20 minutes, 5 consecutive days per week.

Maintenance dosage: For maintenance phase, 10 million units/m² as a subcutaneous injection 3 times a week.

Dosage adjustment: Withhold if severe adverse reactions develop, including granulocyte counts more than 250/mm³ but less than 500/mm³ or ALT/AST of more than 5 to 10 times the ULN, until adverse reactions abate. Restart at 50% of the previous dose.

Regular laboratory testing should be performed to monitor laboratory abnormalities for the purposes of dose modification.

Duration of therapy:

• *Induction Phase* – 4 weeks.

• *Maintenance Phase* – 48 weeks

Discontinuation of therapy: Permanently discontinue for toxicity that does not abate after withholding therapy, severe adverse reactions that recur in patients receiving reduced dose, and granulocyte count less than 250/mm³ or ALT/AST of more than 10 times the ULN.

• *Recommended dosage forms –*

Appropriate Interferon Alfa-2b Dosage Forms for Malignant Melanoma	
Dosage form	Route
Induction dose	
Powder 10 million units	IV
Powder 18 million units	IV
Powder 50 million units	IV
Maintenance dose	
Powder 10 million units (single dose)[a]	Subcutaneously
Powder 18 million units (single dose)[b]	Subcutaneously
Solution 18 million units multidose	Subcutaneously
Solution 25 million units multidose	Subcutaneously
Pen 3 million units/dose multidose[a]	Subcutaneously
Pen 5 million units/dose multidose	Subcutaneously
Pen 10 million units/dose multidose	Subcutaneously

[a] Patients receiving 50% dose reduction only.
[b] Patients receiving full dose only.

➤*Children:*

Chronic hepatitis B –

One to 17 years of age:

• *Usual dosage* – 3 million units/m_2 3 times a week for the first week of therapy followed by dose escalation to 6 million units/m² 3 times a week administered subcutaneously.

• *Maximum dose* – 10 million units 3 times a week.

• *Dosage adjustment* – See Adults for dosage adjustment.

• *Duration of therapy* – 16 to 24 weeks.

• *Discontinuation of therapy* – See Adults for discontinuation of therapy.

• *Resumption of therapy* – Resume at up to 100% of the initial dose when WBC, granulocyte, and/or platelet counts returned to normal or baseline values.

• *Recommended dosage forms –*

Appropriate Interferon Alfa-2b Dosage Forms for Chronic Hepatitis B	
Dosage form	Route
Powder 10 million units (single dose)	Subcutaneously
Solution 10 million units (single dose)	Subcutaneously
Pen 3 million units/dose multidose	Subcutaneously
Pen 5 million units/dose multidose	Subcutaneously
Pen 10 million units/dose multidose	Subcutaneously

➤*Renal function impairment:* Interferon/alfa-2b/ribavirin combination therapy is not recommended in patients with severe renal function impairment. Use with caution in patients with moderate renal function impairment.

➤*Hepatic function impairment:* Do not treat patients with decompensated liver disease, autoimmune hepatitis, or a history of autoimmune disease, or patients who are immunosuppressed transplant recipients, with interferon alfa-2b. Discontinue therapy for any patient developing signs and symptoms of liver failure.

➤*Preparation for administration:*

Powder for injection –

Intramuscular, subcutaneous or intralesional administration: Inject 1 mL of diluent (sterile water for injection) into the interferon alfa-2b vial. Swirl gently to hasten complete dissolution of the powder. Withdraw the appropriate dose and inject IM, subcutaneously, or intralesionally as indicated.

The interferon alfa-2b powder reconstituted with sterile water for injection is a single-use vial and does not contain a preservative. The reconstituted solution is clear and colorless to light yellow. Do not reenter vial after withdrawing the dose. Discard unused portion. Once the dose from the single-dose vial has been withdrawn, the sterility of any remaining product can no longer be guaranteed. Pooling of unused portions of some medications has been linked to bacterial contamination and morbidity.

IV infusion: Prepare the infusion solution immediately prior to use. Based on the desired dose, the appropriate vial strength(s) of interferon alfa-2b powder for injection should be reconstituted with the diluent provided. Inject 1 mL of diluent (sterile water for injection) into the interferon alfa-2b vial. Swirl gently to hasten complete dissolution of the powder. Withdraw the appropriate dose and inject into a 100 mL bag of sodium chloride 0.9% injection. The final concentration of interferon alfa-2b for injection should be not less than 10 million units per 100 mL.

Solution for injection in vials – Interferon alfa-2b solution for injection is supplied in 2 different strengths of multidose vials. The solutions for injection does not require reconstitution prior to administration; the solution is clear and colorless. Withdraw the appropriate dose and inject IM, subcutaneously, or intralessionally. Interferon alfa-2b solution for injection is not recommended for IV administration.

Multidose injection pens – The interferon alfa-2b solution for injection multidose pens are designed to deliver 3 to 12 doses, depending on the individual dose, using a simple dial mechanism and are for subcutaneous injections only. Interferon alfa-2b multidose pens are not recommended for intravenous administration. Only the needles provided in the packaging should be used with the multidose pen. A new needle is to be used each time a dose is delivered using the pen. To avoid the possible transmission of disease, each multidose pen is for single patient use only.

➤*Administration:* To enhance the tolerability of interferon alfa-2b, administer injections in the evening when possible.

AIDS-related Kaposi sarcoma – Administer IM or subcutaneously.

Chronic hepatitis B – In adults, administer IM (powder for injection or solution for injection only) or subcutaneously. In children, administer subcutaneously.

Chronic hepatitis C – Administer IM (solution for injection only) or subcutaneously.

Condylomata Acuminata – Administer intralesionally using a tuberculin or similar syringe and a 25- to 30-gauge needle. Direct the needle at the center of the base of the wart and at an angle almost parallel to the plane of the skin (approximately that in the commonly used purified protein derivative [PDD] test). This will deliver the interferon to the dermal core of the lesion, infiltrating the lesion and causing a small wheal. Do not go beneath the lesion too deeply; avoid subcutaneous injection, because this area is below the base of the lesion. Do not inject too superficially since this will result in possible leakage, infiltrating only the keratinized layer and not the dermal core.

Follicular lymphoma – Administer subcutaneously.

Hairy cell leukemia –

Platelet counts 50,000/mm³ or more: Administer IM or subcutaneously.

Platelet counts less than 50,000/mm³: Administer subcutaneously. Do not administer IM.

Malignant melanoma –

Induction phase: Administer by intravenous infusion.

Maintenance phase: Administer subcutaneously.

INTERFERON ALFA-2B, RECOMBINANT — INJECTION

➤*Storage/Stability:* Store interferon alfa-2b (powder for injection and solution for injection in vials and multidose pens) between 2° and 8°C (36° and 46°F). After reconstitution of the powder for injection, the solution should be used immediately but may be stored up to 24 hours at 2° and 8°C (36° and 46°F).

Actions

➤*Pharmacology:* The interferons are a family of naturally occurring small proteins and glycoproteins with molecular weights of approximately 15,000 to 27,600 daltons produced and secreted by cells in response to viral infections and to synthetic or biological inducers.

Interferons exert their cellular activities by binding to specific membrane receptors on the cell surface. Once bound to the cell membrane, interferons initiate a complex sequence of intracellular reactions. In vitro studies demonstrated that these include the induction of certain enzymes, suppression of cell proliferation, immunomodulating activities such as enhancement of the phagocytic activity of macrophages and augmentation of the specific cytotoxicity of lymphocytes for target cells, and inhibition of virus replication in virus-infected cells.

In a study using human hepatoblastoma cell line, HB 611, the in vitro antiviral activity of alpha interferon was demonstrated by its inhibition of HBV replication.

➤*Pharmacokinetics:*

Absorption/Distribution – The mean serum interferon alfa-2b concentrations following IM and subcutaneous injections were comparable. The maximum serum concentrations obtained via these routes were approximately 18 to 116 units/mL and occurred 3 to 12 hours after administration.

After IV administration, serum interferon alfa-2b concentrations peaked (135 to 273 units/mL) by the end of the 30-minute infusion, then declined at a slightly more rapid rate than after IM or subcutaneous drug administration, becoming undetectable 4 hours after the infusion. Serum concentrations were undetectable by 16 hours after the injections.

Metabolism/Excretion – Urine interferon alfa-2b concentrations following a single dose (5 million units/m^2) were not detectable after any of the parenteral routes of administration. This result was expected since preliminary studies with isolated and perfused rabbit kidneys have shown that the kidney may be the main site of interferon catabolism.

The elimination half-life of interferon alfa-2b following both IM and subcutaneous injections was approximately 2 to 3 hours. The elimination half-life was approximately 2 hours.

Contraindications

Hypersensitivity to interferon alfa or any component of the injection.

The combination therapy containing interferon alfa-2b and ribavirin capsules must not be used by women who are pregnant or by men whose female partners are pregnant. Extreme care must be taken to avoid pregnancy in women and in female partners of patients taking combination interferon alfa-2b and ribavirin therapy. Patients with autoimmune hepatitis must not be treated with combination interferon alfa-2b and ribavirin therapy.

Warnings/Precautions

➤*Fever/Flu-like symptoms:* Moderate to severe adverse reactions may require modification of the patient's dosage regimen or, in some cases, termination of interferon alfa-2b therapy. Because of the fever and other "flu-like" symptoms associated with interferon alfa-2b administration, use interferon alfa-2b cautiously in patients with debilitating medical conditions, such as those with a history of pulmonary disease (eg, chronic obstructive pulmonary disease), or diabetes mellitus prone to ketoacidosis. Also observe caution in patients with coagulation disorders (eg, pulmonary embolism, thrombophlebitis) or severe myelosuppression.

While fever may be related to the flu-like syndrome reported commonly in patients treated with interferon, rule out other causes of persistent fever.

➤*Cardiovascular effects:* Use interferon alfa-2b therapy cautiously in patients with a history of cardiovascular disease. Closely monitor those patients with a history of myocardial infarction (MI) and/or previous or current arrhythmic disorder who require interferon alfa-2b therapy. Cardiovascular adverse reactions, which include hypotension, arrhythmia, or tachycardia of 150 beats/minute or more, and, rarely, cardiomyopathy and MI, have been observed in some interferon alfa-2b–treated patients. Some patients with these adverse reactions had no history of cardiovascular disease. Transient cardiomyopathy was reported in approximately 2% of the AIDS-related KS patients treated with interferon alfa-2b. Hypotension may occur during interferon alfa-2b administration, or up to 2 days posttherapy, and may require supportive therapy, including fluid replacement, to maintain intravascular volume.

Supraventricular arrhythmias occurred rarely and appeared to be correlated with preexisting conditions and prior therapy with cardiotoxic agents. These adverse reactions were controlled by modifying the dose or discontinuing treatment, but may require specific additional therapy.

➤*Neuropsychiatric reactions:* Depression and suicidal behavior, including suicidal ideation, suicidal attempts, and completed suicides, have been reported in association with treatment with alpha interferons, including interferon alfa-2b therapy. Do not treat patients with a preexisting psychiatric condition, especially depression, or a history of severe psychiatric disorder with interferon alfa-2b. Discontinue interferon alfa-2b therapy for any patient developing severe depression or other psychiatric disorder during treatment. Obtundation and coma have also been observed in some patients, usually elderly patients, treated at higher doses. While these reactions are usually rapidly reversible upon discontinuation of therapy, full resolution of symptoms has taken up to 3 weeks in a few severe episodes. Narcotics, hypnotics, or sedatives may be used concurrently with caution; closely monitor patients until the adverse reactions have resolved.

➤*Hematological effects:* Interferon alfa-2b therapy suppresses bone marrow function and may result in severe cytopenias, including very rare events of aplastic anemia. It is advised that complete blood cell counts (CBCs) be obtained pretreatment and monitored routinely during therapy. Discontinue interferon alfa-2b therapy in patients who develop severe decreases in neutrophil (less than 0.5×10^9/L) or platelet counts (less than 25×10^9 /L).

Combination therapy containing interferon alfa-2b and ribavirin capsules was associated with hemolytic anemia. Hemoglobin less than 10 g/dL was observed in approximately 10% of patients in clinical trials. Anemia occurred within 1 to 2 weeks of initiation of ribavirin therapy.

➤*Ophthalmic effects:* Decrease or loss of vision, retinopathy, including macular edema, retinal artery or vein thrombosis, retinal hemorrhages, and cotton wool spots; optic neuritis and papilledema may be induced or aggravated by treatment with interferon alfa-2b or other alpha interferons. All patients should receive an eye examination at baseline. Patients with preexisting ophthalmic disorders (eg, diabetic or hypertensive retinopathy) should receive periodic ophthalmologic exams during interferon alpha treatment. Any patient who develops ocular symptoms should receive a prompt and complete eye examination. Discontinue interferon alfa-2b treatment in patients who develop new or worsening ophthalmologic disorders.

➤*Thyroid abnormalities:* Infrequently, patients receiving interferon alfa-2b therapy developed thyroid abnormalities, either hypothyroid or hyperthyroid. The mechanism by which interferon alfa-2b may alter thyroid status is unknown. Patients with preexisting thyroid abnormalities may be treated if thyroid-stimulating hormone (TSH) levels can be maintained in the normal range by medication. Do not treat patients with preexisting thyroid abnormalities whose thyroid function cannot be maintained in the normal range by medication with interferon alfa-2b. Prior to initiation of interferon alfa-2b therapy, evaluate serum TSH. TSH levels must be within normal limits upon initiation of interferon alfa-2b treatment; repeat TSH testing at 3 and 6 months. Evaluate thyroid function and institute appropriate treatment in patients developing symptoms consistent with possible thyroid dysfunction during the course of interferon alfa-2b therapy. Discontinue therapy for patients developing thyroid abnormalities during treatment whose thyroid function cannot be normalized by medication. Discontinuation of interferon alfa-2b therapy has not always reversed thyroid dysfunction occurring during treatment.

➤*Hepatoxicity:* Hepatotoxicity, including fatality, has been observed in interferon alpha–treated patients, including those treated with interferon alfa-2b for injection. Closely monitor and, if appropriate, discontinue treatment in any patient developing liver function abnormalities during treatment.

➤*Pulmonary effects:* Pulmonary infiltrates, pneumonitis, and pneumonia, including fatality, have been observed in interferon alpha–treated patients, including those treated with interferon alfa-2b. The etiologic explanation for these pulmonary findings has yet to be established. Any patient developing fever, cough, dyspnea, or other respiratory symptoms should have a chest X-ray taken. If the chest X-ray shows pulmonary infiltrates or there is evidence of pulmonary function impairment, monitor the patient closely and, if appropriate, discontinue interferon alpha treatment. While this has been reported more often in patients with chronic hepatitis C treated with interferon alpha, it has also been reported in patients with oncologic diseases treated with interferon alpha.

➤*Autoimmune disorders:* Rare cases of autoimmune diseases, including thrombocytopenia, vasculitis, Raynaud phenomenon, rheumatoid arthritis, lupus erythematosus, and rhabdomyolysis, have been observed in patients treated with alpha interferons, including patients treated with interferon alfa-2b. In very rare cases, the reaction resulted in fatality. The mechanism by which these reactions develop and their relationship to interferon alpha therapy is not clear. Closely monitor any patient developing an autoimmune disorder during treatment and, if appropriate, discontinue treatment.

➤*Hyperglycemia:* Diabetes mellitus and hyperglycemia have been observed rarely in patients treated with interferon alfa-2b. Measure blood glucose in symptomatic patients and follow up accordingly. Patients with diabetes mellitus may require adjustment of their antidiabetic regimen.

➤*Albumin risks:* The powder formulations of this product contain albumin, a derivative of human blood. Based on effective donor screening and product manufacturing processes, it carries an extremely remote risk for transmission of viral diseases. A theoretical risk for transmission of Creutzfeldt-Jakob disease (CJD) is also considered extremely remote. No cases of transmission of viral diseases or CJD have ever been identified for albumin.

➤*AIDS-related KS:* Do not use interferon alfa-2b therapy for patients with rapidly progressive visceral disease. Also of note, there may be synergistic adverse reactions between interferon alfa-2b and zidovudine. Patients receiving concomitant zidovudine have had a higher incidence of neutropenia than that expected with zidovudine alone. Careful monitoring of the WBC count is indicated in all patients who are myelosuppressed and in all patients receiving other myelosuppressive medications. The effects of interferon alfa-2b when combined with other drugs used in the treatment of AIDS-related disease are unknown.

➤*Psoriasis/Sarcoidosis:* There have been reports of interferon, including interferon alfa-2b, exacerbating preexisting psoriasis and sarcoidosis, as well as development of new sarcoidosis. Therefore, use interferon alfa-2b therapy in these patients only if the potential benefit justifies the risk.

INTERFERON ALFA-2B, RECOMBINANT — INJECTION

➤*Product interchangeability:* Variations in dosage, routes of administration, and adverse reactions exist among different brands of interferon. Therefore, do not use different brands of interferon in any single-treatment regimen.

➤*Triglycerides:* Elevated triglyceride levels have been observed in patients treated with interferons, including interferon alfa-2b therapy. Manage elevated triglyceride levels as clinically appropriate. Hypertriglyceridemia may result in pancreatitis. Consider discontinuation of interferon alfa-2b therapy for patients with persistently elevated triglycerides (eg, triglycerides more than 1,000 mg/dL) associated with symptoms of potential pancreatitis, such as abdominal pain, nausea, or vomiting.

➤*Hypersensitivity reactions:* Acute serious hypersensitivity reactions (eg, anaphylaxis, angioedema, bronchoconstriction, urticaria) have been observed rarely in interferon alfa-2b–treated patients; if such an acute reaction develops, discontinue the drug immediately and institute appropriate medical therapy. Transient rashes have occurred in some patients following injection, but have not necessitated treatment interruption.

➤*Renal function impairment:* Interferon alfa-2b/ribavirin combination therapy is not recommended in patients with severe renal function impairment. Use with caution in patients with moderate renal function impairment.

➤*Hepatic function impairment:* Do not treat patients with decompensated liver disease, autoimmune hepatitis, or a history of autoimmune disease, or patients who are immunosuppressed transplant recipients, with interferon alfa-2b. There are reports of worsening liver disease, including jaundice, hepatic encephalopathy, hepatic failure, and death, following interferon alfa-2b therapy in such patients. Discontinue therapy for any patient developing signs and symptoms of liver failure.

Chronic hepatitis B patients with evidence of decreasing hepatic synthetic functions, such as decreasing albumin levels or prolongation of prothrombin time, who nevertheless meet the entry criteria to start therapy, may be at increased risk of clinical decompensation if a flare of aminotransferases occurs during interferon alfa-2b treatment. In such patients, carefully follow them if increases in ALT occur during interferon alfa-2b therapy for chronic hepatitis B, including close monitoring of clinical symptomatology and liver function tests, including ALT, prothrombin time, alkaline phosphatase, albumin, and bilirubin. In considering these patients for interferon alfa-2b therapy, the potential risks must be evaluated against the potential benefits of treatment.

➤*Pregnancy: Category C.* Interferon alfa-2b has been shown to have abortifacient effects in *Macaca mulatta* (rhesus monkeys) at 15 and 30 million units/kg (estimated human equivalent of 5 and 10 million units/kg, based on body surface area adjustment for a 60 kg adult). There are no adequate and well-controlled studies in pregnant women. Use interferon alfa-2b therapy during pregnancy only if the potential benefit justifies the potential risk to the fetus.

Fertility impairment – Interferon may impair fertility. Decreases in serum estradiol and progesterone concentrations have been reported in women treated with human leukocyte interferon. Therefore, fertile women should not receive interferon alfa-2b therapy unless they are using effective contraception during the therapy period. Use interferon alfa-2b therapy with caution in fertile men.

Combination therapy – Category X. This pregnancy category applies to the combination therapy containing interferon alfa-2b and ribavirin capsules. See the interferon alfa-2b/ribavirin combination therapy monograph for additional information.

➤*Lactation:* It is not known whether this drug is excreted in human milk. However, studies in mice have shown that mouse interferons are excreted into the milk. Because of the potential for serious adverse reactions from the drug in breast-feeding infants, decide whether to discontinue breast-feeding or interferon alfa-2b therapy, taking into account the importance of the drug to the mother.

➤*Children:* Safety and effectiveness in children younger than 18 years of age have not been established for indications other than chronic hepatitis B.

Chronic hepatitis B – Safety and effectiveness in children ranging from 1 to 17 years of age have been established based upon one controlled clinical trial. Safety and effectiveness in children younger than 1 year of age have not been established.

➤*Elderly:* In all clinical studies of interferon alfa-2b, including studies as monotherapy and in combination with ribavirin capsules, only a small percentage of the subjects were 65 years of age and older. These numbers were too few to determine if they respond differently from younger subjects except for the clinical trials of interferon alfa-2b in combination with ribavirin, where elderly subjects had a higher frequency of anemia (67%) compared with younger patients (28%).

In a database consisting of clinical study and postmarketing reports for various indications, cardiovascular adverse reactions and confusion were reported more frequently in elderly patients receiving interferon alfa-2b therapy compared with younger patients.

In general, administer interferon alfa-2b therapy to elderly patients cautiously, reflecting the greater frequency of decreased hepatic, renal, bone marrow, and/or cardiac function, and concomitant disease or other drug therapy. Interferon alfa-2b is known to be substantially excreted by the kidney, and the risk of adverse reactions to interferon alfa-2b may be greater in patients with renal function impairment. Because elderly patients often have decreased renal function, carefully monitor patients during treatment and make dose adjustments based on symptoms and/or laboratory abnormalities.

➤*Monitoring:* Mild to moderate leukopenia and elevated serum liver enzyme levels (AST) have been reported with intralesional administration of interferon alfa-2b; therefore, consider monitoring these laboratory parameters.

In addition to those tests normally required for monitoring patients, the following laboratory tests are recommended for all patients on interferon alfa-2b therapy, prior to beginning treatment and then periodically thereafter: standard hematologic tests, including hemoglobin, complete and differential WBC counts, and platelet count; and blood chemistries, including electrolytes, liver function tests, and thyroid-stimulating hormone.

Those patients who have preexisting cardiac abnormalities and/or are in advanced stages of cancer should have electrocardiograms taken prior to and during the course of treatment.

Baseline chest x-rays are suggested; repeat if clinically indicated.

For malignant melanoma patients, monitor differential WBC count and liver function tests weekly during the induction phase of therapy and monthly during the maintenance phase of therapy.

Prior to initiation of interferon alfa-2b therapy in chronic hepatitis C patients, evaluate CBC and platelet counts in order to establish baselines for monitoring potential toxicity. Repeat these tests at weeks 1 and 2 following initiation of interferon alfa-2b therapy, and monthly thereafter. Evaluate serum ALT at approximately 3-month intervals to assess response to treatment.

In chronic hepatitis B patients, evaluate CBC and platelet counts prior to initiation of interferon alfa-2b therapy in order to establish baselines for monitoring potential toxicity. Repeat these tests at treatment weeks 1, 2, 4, 8, 12, and 16. Evaluate liver function tests, including serum ALT, albumin, and bilirubin, at treatment weeks 1, 2, 4, 8, 12, and 16. Evaluate HBeAg, HBsAg, and ALT at the end of therapy, as well as 3- and 6-months posttherapy, since patients may become virologic responders during the 6-month period following the end of treatment. In clinical studies in adults, 39% (15/38) of responding patients lost HBeAg 1 to 6 months following the end of interferon alfa-2b therapy. Of responding patients who lost HBsAg, 58% (7/12) did so 1 to 6 months posttreatment.

Drug Interactions

Interferon Alfa-2b Drug Interactions

Precipitant drug	Object drug[a]		Description
Interferon alfa-2b	Myelosuppressive agents (eg, zidovudine)	↑	There may be synergistic adverse reactions between interferon alfa-2b and zidovudine. Patients have had a higher incidence of neutropenia than that expected with zidovudine alone. Carefully monitor WBC count in myelosuppressed patients or those receiving myelosuppressive agents.
Interferon alfa-2b	Theophyllines	↑	Concomitant use significantly reduces theophylline clearance, resulting in a 100% increase in serum theophylline levels.

[a] ↑ = object drug increased.

Adverse Reactions

The most frequently reported adverse reactions were "flu-like" symptoms, particularly fever, headache, chills, myalgia, and fatigue. More severe toxicities are observed generally at higher doses and may be difficult for patients to tolerate.

In addition, the following spontaneous adverse reactions have been reported during the marketing surveillance of interferon alfa-2b: nephrotic syndrome, pancreatitis, psychosis (including hallucinations), renal failure, and renal function impairment. Very rarely, interferon alfa-2b used alone or in combination with ribavirin capsules may be associated with aplastic anemia. Rarely, sarcoidosis or exacerbation of sarcoidosis has been reported.

INTERFERON ALFA-2B, RECOMBINANT — INJECTION

Interferon Alfa-2b Adverse Reactions[a,b]

Adverse reaction	Malignant melanoma: 20 million units/m^2 induction (IV) 10 million units/m^2 maintenance (subcutaneously) (n = 143)	Follicular lymphoma: 5 million units 3 times a week/ subcutaneously (n = 135)	Hairy cell leukemia: 2 million units/m^2 3 times a week/ subcutaneously (n = 145)	Condylomata acuminata: 1 million units/lesion (n = 352)	AIDS-related KS: 30 million units/m^2 3 times a week/ subcutaneously (n = 74)	AIDS-related KS: 3 million units once daily/ subcutaneously (n = 29)	Chronic hepatitis C[c]: 3 million units 3 times a week (n = 183)	Chronic hepatitis B, Adults: 5 million units once daily (n = 101)	Chronic hepatitis B, Adults: 10 million units 3 times a week (n = 78)	Chronic hepatitis B, Children: 6 million units/m^2 3 times a week (n = 116)
Cardiovascular										
< 5%	Angina, arrhythmia, atrial fibrillation, bradycardia, cardiac failure, cardiomegaly, cardiomyopathy, coronary artery disorder, extrasystoles, heart valve disorder, hematoma, hypertension (9% in chronic hepatitis C), hypotension, palpitations, peripheral ischemia, phlebitis, poor peripheral circulation, postural hypotension, pulmonary embolism, Raynaud disease, tachycardia, thrombosis, varicose vein									
CNS										
Amnesia	[d]	1%	< 5%	—	—	14%	—	—	—	—
Anxiety	1%	9%	5%	< 1%	1%	3%	5%	2%		3%
Asthenia	—	63%	7%	—	11%	—	40%	5%	15%	5%
Confusion	8%	2%	< 5%	4%	12%	10%	1%	—	—	2%
Decreased libido	1%	1%	< 5%	—	—	—	1%	5%	1%	—
Depression	40%	9%	6%	3%	9%	28%	19%	17%	6%	4%
Dizziness	23%	—	12%	9%	7%	24%	9%	13%	10%	8%
Headache	62%	21%	39%	47%	36%	21%	43%	61%	44%	57%
Hypesthesia	—	1%	< 5%	1%	—	10%	—	—	—	—
Impaired concentration	—	1%	—	< 1%	3%	14%	3%	8%	5%	3%
Insomnia	5%	4%	—	< 1%	3%	3%	12%	11%	6%	8%
Irritability	1%	1%	—	—	—	—	13%	16%	12%	22%
Nervousness	1%	1%	—	1%	—	3%	2%	3%	—	3%
Paresthesia	13%	13%	6%	1%	3%	21%	5%	6%	3%	< 1%
Somnolence	1%	2%	< 5%	3%	3%	—	33%[e]	14%	9%	5%
Other (< 5%)	Abnormal coordination, abnormal dreaming, abnormal gait, abnormal thinking, aggravated depression, aggressive reaction, agitation (7% in chronic hepatitis B children), alcohol intolerance, apathy, aphasia, ataxia, Bell palsy, CNS dysfunction, coma, convulsions, delirium, dysphonia, emotional lability, extrapyramidal disorder, feeling of ebriety, flushing, hearing disorder, hearing impairment, hot flashes, hyperesthesia, hyperkinesia, hypertonia, hypokinesia, impaired consciousness, labyrinthine disorder, loss of consciousness, manic depression, manic reaction, migraine, neuralgia, neuritis, neuropathy, neurosis, paresis, paroniria, parosmia, personality disorder, polyneuropathy, psychosis, speech disorder, stroke, suicidal ideation, suicide attempt, syncope, tinnitus, tremor, twitching, vertigo (8% in follicular lymphoma)									
Dermatological										
Alopecia	29%	23%	8%	—	12%	31%	28%	26%	38%	17%
Dermatitis	1%	—	8%	—	—	—	2%	1%	—	
Dry skin	1%	3%	9%	—	9%	10%	4%	3%	—	< 1%
Increased sweating	6%	13%	8%	2%	4%	21%	4%	1%	1%	3%
Pruritus	—	10%	11%	1%	7%	—	9%	6%	4%	3%
Rash	19%	13%	25%	—	9%	10%	5%	8%	1%	5%
Other (< 5%)	Abnormal hair texture, acne, cellulitis, cold and clammy skin, cyanosis of the hand, dermatitis lichenoides, eczema, epidermal necrolysis, erythema, erythema nodosum, folliculitis, furunculosis, genital pruritus, increased hair growth, lacrimal gland disorder, lacrimation, lipoma, maculopapular rash, melanosis, nail disorders, nonherpetic cold sores, pallor, photosensitivity, psoriasis, psoriasis aggravated, purpura (5% in chronic hepatitis C), rash erythematous, sebaceous cyst, skin depigmentation, skin discoloration, skin nodule, urticaria, vitiligo									
Endocrine										
< 5%	Aggravation of diabetes mellitus, goiter, gynecomastia, hyperglycemia, hyperthyroidism, hypertriglyceridemia, hypothyroidism, virilism									
GI										
Abdominal pain	2%	20%	< 5%	1%	5%	21%	16%	5%	4%	23%
Anorexia	69%	21%	19%	1%	38%	41%	14%	43%	53%	43%
Constipation	1%	14%	< 1%	—	1%	10%	4%	5%	—	2%
Diarrhea	35%	19%	18%	2%	18%	45%	13%	19%	8%	12%
Dry mouth	1%	2%	19%	—	22%	28%	5%	6%	5%	—
Dyspepsia	—	2%	—	2%	4%	—	7%	3%	8%	3%
Gingivitis	2%[f]	7%[f]	—	—	—	14%	—	1%	—	—
Loose stools	—	1%	—	< 1%	—	10%	2%	2%		2%
Nausea	66%	24%	21%	17%	28%	21%	19%	50%	33%	18%
Taste alteration	24%	2%	13%	< 1%	5%	7%	2%	10%	—	—

INTERFERON ALFA-2B, RECOMBINANT — INJECTION

Interferon Alfa-2b Adverse Reactions[a,b]

Adverse reaction	Malignant melanoma 20 million units/m² induction (IV) 10 million units/m² maintenance (subcutaneously) (n = 143)	Follicular lymphoma 5 million units 3 times a week/ subcutaneously (n = 135)	Hairy cell leukemia 2 million units/m² 3 times a week/ subcutaneously (n = 145)	Condylomata acuminata 1 million units/lesion (n = 352)	AIDS-related KS 30 million units/m² 3 times a week/ subcutaneously (n = 74)	AIDS-related KS 3 million units once daily/ subcutaneously (n = 29)	Chronic hepatitis C[c] 3 million units 3 times a week (n = 183)	Chronic hepatitis B Adults 5 million units once daily (n = 101)	Chronic hepatitis B Adults 10 million units 3 times a week (n = 78)	Chronic hepatitis B Children 6 million units/m² 3 times a week (n = 116)
Vomiting	[g]	32%	6%	2%	11%	14%	8%	7%	10%	27%
Other (< 5%)	Abdominal ascites, abdominal distension, colitis, dysphagia, eructation, esophagitis, flatulence, gallstones, gastric ulcer, gastritis, gastroenteritis, GI disorder (7% in follicular lymphoma), GI hemorrhage, GI mucosal discoloration, gingival bleeding, gum hyperplasia, halitosis, hemorrhoids, increased appetite, increased saliva, intestinal disorder, melena, mouth ulceration, mucositis, oral hemorrhage, oral leukoplakia, rectal bleeding after stool, rectal hemorrhage, stomatitis, stomatitis ulcerative, taste loss, tongue disorder, tooth disorder									
GU										
< 5%	Albumin/protein in urine, amenorrhea (12% in follicular lymphoma), cystitis, dysmenorrhea, dysuria, hematuria, impotence, incontinence, increased BUN, leukorrhea, menorrhagia, menstrual irregularity, micturition disorder, micturition frequency, nocturia, pelvic pain, penis disorder, polyuria (10% in follicular lymphoma), renal function impairment, sexual dysfunction, urinary tract infection (5% in chronic hepatitis C), uterine bleeding, vaginal dryness									
Hematologic										
ALT	2%	—	13%	—	10%	15%	—	—	—	—
AST	63%	24%	4%	12%	11%	41%	—	—	—	—
Alkaline phosphatase	13%	—	4%	—	—	—	—	8%	4%	0%
Hemoglobin	22%	8%	NA	—	1%	15%	26%[h]	32%[i]	23%[i]	17%[j]
Granulocyte count										
Total	92%	36%	NA	—	31%	39%	45%[k]	75%[k]	61%[k]	70%[k]
1,000 to 1,500/mm³	66%	—	—	—	—	—	32%	30%	32%	43%
750 to < 1,000/mm³	—	21%	—	—	—	—	10%	24%	18%	18%
500 to 750/mm³	25%	—	—	—	—	—	1%	17%	9%	7%
< 500/mm³	1%	13%	—				2%	4%	2%	2%
Lactate dehydrogenase	1%	—	0%	—	—	—				
Platelet count	15%	13%	NA	—	0%	8%	15%[l]	12%[l]	5%[l]	1%[l]
Serum creatinine	3%	2%	0%	—	—	—	6%	3%	0%	3%
Serum urea nitrogen	12%	4%	0%	—	—	—	—	2%	0%	2%
WBC	[m]	—	NA	17%	10%	22%	26%[n]	68%[n]	34%[n]	9%[n]
< 5%	Anemia, anemia hypochromic, granulocytopenia, hemolytic anemia, leukopenia, lymphocytosis, neutropenia (9% in chronic hepatitis C, 14% in chronic hepatitis B children), thrombocytopenia (10% in chronic hepatitis C) (bleeding 8% in malignant melanoma), thrombocytopenic purpura									
Hepatic										
< 5%	Abnormal hepatic function tests, biliary pain, bilirubinemia, hepatitis, increased lactate dehydrogenase, increased transaminases (AST/ALT) (elevated AST 63% in malignant melanoma and 24% in follicular lymphoma), jaundice, right upper quadrant pain (15% in chronic hepatitis C), and, very rarely, hepatic encephalopathy, hepatic failure, and death									
Local										
Application site disorder	—	—	20%	—	—	—	—	—	—	
Injection-site inflammation	—	1%	—	—	—	—	5%	3%	—	—
Other (≤ 5%)	Burning, injection-site bleeding, injection-site pain, injection-site reaction (5% in chronic hepatitis B children), itching									
Musculoskeletal										
Arthralgia	6%	8%	8%	9%	—	3%	16%	19%	8%	15%
Back pain	—	15%	19%	6%	1%	3%	—	—	—	—
Musculoskeletal pain	—	18%	—	—	—	—	21%	9%	1%	10%
Myalgia	75%	16%	39%	44%	34%	28%	43%	59%	40%	27%
Other (< 5%)	Arteritis, arthritis, arthritis aggravated, arthrosis, bone disorder, bone pain, carpal tunnel syndrome, hyporeflexia, leg cramps, muscle atrophy, muscle weakness, polyarteritis nodosa, rheumatoid arthritis, spondylitis, tendonitis									
Ophthalmic										
< 5%	Abnormal vision, blurred vision, diplopia, dry eyes, eye pain, nystagmus, photophobia									
Respiratory										
Coughing	6%	13%	< 1%	—	—	31%	1%	4%	—	5%

INTERFERON ALFA-2B, RECOMBINANT — INJECTION

Interferon Alfa-2b Adverse Reactions[a,b]

Adverse reaction	Malignant melanoma	Follicular lymphoma	Hairy cell leukemia	Condylomata acuminata	AIDS-related KS		Chronic hepatitis C[c]	Chronic hepatitis B		
								Adults		Children
	20 million units/m² induction (IV) 10 million units/m² maintenance (subcutaneously) (n = 143)	5 million units 3 times a week/ subcutaneously (n = 135)	2 million units/m² 3 times a week/ subcutaneously (n = 145)	1 million units/lesion (n = 352)	30 million units/m² 3 times a week/ subcutaneously (n = 74)	3 million units once daily/ subcutaneously (n = 29)	3 million units 3 times a week (n = 183)	5 million units once daily (n = 101)	10 million units 3 times a week (n = 78)	6 million units/m² 3 times a week (n = 116)
Dyspnea	15%	14%	< 1%	—	1%	34%	3%	5%	—	—
Nasal congestion	1%	7%	—	1%	—	10%	< 1%	4%	—	—
Nonproductive coughing	2%	7%	—	—	—	14%	0%	1%	—	—
Pharyngitis	2%	8%	< 5%	1%	1%	31%	3%	7%	1%	7%
Sinusitis	1%	4%	—	—	—	21%	2%	—	—	—
Other (≤ 5%)	Asthma, bronchitis (10% in follicular lymphoma), bronchospasm, cyanosis, epistaxis (7% in chronic hepatitis B children), hemoptysis, hypoventilation, laryngitis, lung fibrosis, orthopnea, pleural effusion, pleural pain, pneumonia, pneumonitis, pneumothorax, rales, respiratory disorder, respiratory function impairment, rhinitis, rhinorrhea, sneezing, tonsillitis, tracheitis, upper respiratory tract infection, wheezing									
Miscellaneous										
Chest pain	2%	8%	< 1%	< 1%	1%	28%	4%	4%	—	—
Chills	54%	—	46%	45%	—	—	—	—	—	—
Facial edema	—	1%	—	< 1%	—	10%	< 1%	3%	1%	< 1%
Fatigue	96%	8%	61%	18%	84%	48%	23%	75%	69%	71%
Fever	81%	56%	68%	56%	47%	55%	34%	66%	86%	94%
Herpes simplex	1%	2%	—	1%	—	3%	1%	5%	—	—
Influenza-like symptoms	10%	18%	37%	—	45%	79%	26%	5%	—	< 1%
Malaise	6%	—	—	14%	5%	—	13%	9%	6%	3%
Moniliasis	—	1%	—	< 1%	—	17%	—	—	—	—
Pain (unspecified)	15%	9%	18%	3%	3%	3%	—	—	—	—
Rigors	2%	7%	—	—	30%	14%	16%	38%	42%	30%
Weight decrease	3%	13%	< 1%	< 1%	5%	3%	10%	2%	5%	3%
Other (≤ 5%)	Abscess, allergic reaction, bacterial infection, cachexia, chest pain, substernal, conjunctivitis, dehydration, earache, edema, fungal infection, hemophilus, hernia, herpes zoster, hypercalcemia, hyperthermia, hypothermia, infection, lymphadenitis, lymphadenopathy, mastitis, nonspecific infection (7% in follicular lymphoma), nonspecific inflammation, otitis media, parasitic infection, periorbital edema, peripheral edema (6% in follicular lymphoma), scrotal/penile edema, sepsis, stye, superficial phlebitis, thirst, trichomonas, viral infection (7% in chronic hepatitis C), weakness, weight increase									

[a] Dash (—) indicates not reported.
[b] NA = not applicable. Patients' initial hematologic laboratory test values were abnormal because of their condition.
[c] Percentages based upon a summary of all adverse reactions during 18 to 24 months of treatment.
[d] Amnesia was reported with confusion as a single term.
[e] Predominantly lethargy.
[f] Includes stomatitis/mucositis.
[g] Vomiting was reported with nausea as a single term.
[h] Decrease of at least 2 g/dL; 20% two to less than three g/dL; 6% at least 3 g/dL.
[i] Decrease of at least 2 g/dL
[j] Decrease of at least 2 g/dL; 14% two to less than three g/dL; 3% at least 3 g/dL.
[k] Neutrophils plus bands.
[l] Decrease to less than 70,000/mm³.
[m] WBC was reported as neutropenia.
[n] Decrease to less than 3,000/mm³.

➤*Hairy cell leukemia:* The adverse reactions most frequently reported during clinical trials in 145 patients with hairy cell leukemia were the "flu-like" symptoms of fatigue (61%), fever (68%), and chills (46%).

➤*Malignant melanoma:* The interferon alfa-2b dose was modified because of adverse reactions in 65% (n = 93) of patients. Interferon alfa-2b therapy was discontinued because of adverse reactions in 8% of patients during induction and 18% of patients during maintenance. The most frequently reported adverse reaction was fatigue, which was observed in 96% of patients. Other adverse reactions that were recorded in more than 20% of interferon alfa-2b–treated patients included alopecia (29%), altered taste sensation (24%), anemia (22%), anorexia (69%), chills (54%), depression (40%), diarrhea (35%), dizziness/vertigo (23%), fever (81%), headache (62%), increased AST (63%), myalgia (75%), neutropenia (92%), and vomiting/nausea (66%).

Adverse reactions classified as severe or life-threatening (Eastern Cooperative Oncology Group toxicity criteria grade 3 or 4) were recorded in 66% and 14% of interferon alfa-2b treated patients, respectively. Severe adverse reactions recorded in more than 10% of interferon alfa-2b treated patients included chills (16%), fatigue (23%), fever (18%), headache (17%), increased AST (14%), myalgia (17%), and neutropenia/leukopenia (26%). Grade 4 fatigue was recorded in 4% and grade 4 depression was recorded in 2% of interferon alfa-2b treated patients. No other grade 4 adverse reaction was reported in more than 2 interferon alfa-2b–treated patients. Lethal hepatotoxicity occurred in 2 interferon alfa-2b–treated patients early in the clinical trial. No subsequent lethal hepatotoxicities were observed with adequate monitoring of liver function tests.

➤*Follicular lymphoma:* Ninety-six percent of patients treated with cyclophosphamide, doxorubicin, teniposide, prednisone plus interferon alfa-2b therapy and 91% of patients treated with cyclophosphamide, doxorubicin, teniposide, prednisone alone reported an adverse reaction of any severity. Alopecia, anorexia, asthenia, dyspnea, fever, "flu-like" symptoms, headache, increased hepatic enzymes, myalgia, neutropenia, paresthesia, polyuria, and thrombocytopenia occurred more frequently in the cyclophosphamide, doxorubicin, teniposide, prednisone plus interferon alfa-2b treated patients than in patients treated with cyclophosphamide, doxorubicin, teniposide, prednisone alone. Adverse reactions classified as severe or life threatening (World Health Organization [WHO] grade 3 or 4) recorded in more than 5% of cyclophosphamide, doxorubicin, teniposide, prednisone plus interferon alfa-2b treated patients included asthenia (10%), neutropenia (34%), and vomiting (10%). The incidence of neutropenic infection was 6% in cyclophosphamide, doxorubicin, teniposide, prednisone plus interferon alfa-2b versus 2% in cyclophosphamide, doxorubicin, teniposide, prednisone alone. One patient in each treatment group required hospitalization.

Twenty-eight percent of cyclophosphamide, doxorubicin, teniposide, prednisone plus interferon alfa-2b–treated patients had a temporary modification/interruption of their interferon alfa-2b therapy, but only 13 (10%) patients permanently stopped interferon alfa-2b therapy because of toxicity. There were 4 deaths on study; 2 patients committed suicide in the cyclophosphamide, doxorubicin, teniposide, prednisone plus interferon alfa-2b arm and 2 patients in the cyclophosphamide, doxorubicin, teniposide, prednisone arm had unwitnessed sudden death. Three patients with hepatitis B (one of whom also had alcoholic cirrhosis) developed hepatotoxicity leading to discontinuation of interferon alfa-2b. Other reasons for discontinuation

INTERFERON ALFA-2B, RECOMBINANT — INJECTION

included intolerable asthenia (5/135), severe flu symptoms (2/135), and 1 patient each with exacerbation of ankylosing spondylitis, psychosis, and decreased ejection fraction.

➤*Condylomata acuminata:* Eighty-eight percent (311/352) of patients treated with interferon alfa-2b for condylomata acuminata who were evaluable for safety reported an adverse reaction during treatment. The incidence of the adverse reactions reported increased when the number of treated lesions increased from 1 to 5. All 40 patients who had 5 warts treated reported some type of adverse reaction during treatment.

Adverse reactions and abnormal laboratory test values reported by patients who were re-treated were qualitatively and quantitatively similar to those reported during the initial interferon alfa-2b treatment period.

➤*AIDS-related KS:* In patients with AIDS-related KS, some type of adverse reaction occurred in 100% of the 74 patients treated with 30 million units/m^2 three times a week and in 97% of the 29 patients treated with 35 million units/day.

Of these adverse reactions, those classified as severe (WHO grade 3 or 4) were reported in 27% to 55% of patients. Severe adverse reactions in the 30 million units/m^2 3 times a week study included the following: anorexia (12%), confusion (3%), dry mouth (4%), fatigue (20%), fever (3%), headache (4%), influenza-like symptoms (15%), myalgia (3%), and nausea and vomiting (1% each). Severe adverse reactions for patients who received the 35 million units every day included the following: dyspnea (14%), fatigue (17%), fever (24%), headache (10%), influenza-like symptoms (14%), pharyngitis (7%), and abnormal hepatic function, ataxia, cardiomyopathy, chest pain, confusion, coughing, depression, dysphagia, emotional lability, face edema, GI hemorrhage, increased AST, myalgia, and suicide attempt (1 patient each). Overall, the incidence of severe toxicity was higher among patients who received the 35 million units per day dose.

➤*Chronic hepatitis C:* Two studies of extended treatment (18 to 24 months) with interferon alfa-2b showed that approximately 95% of all patients treated experienced some type of adverse reaction and that patients treated for extended duration continued to experience adverse reactions throughout treatment. Most adverse reactions reported were mild to moderate in severity. However, 29 of 152 (19%) of patients treated for 18 to 24 months experienced a serious adverse reaction compared with 11 of 163 (7%) of those treated for 6 months. Adverse reactions that occur or persist during extended treatment are similar in type and severity to those occurring during short-course therapy.

Of the patients achieving a complete response after 6 months of therapy, 12 of 79 (15%) subsequently discontinued interferon alfa-2b treatment during extended therapy because of adverse reactions, and 23 of 79 (29%) experienced severe adverse reactions (WHO grade 3 or 4) during extended therapy.

In patients using the combination therapy containing interferon alfa-2b and ribavirin, the primary toxicity observed was hemolytic anemia. Reductions in hemoglobin levels occurred within the first 1 to 2 weeks of therapy. Cardiac and pulmonary reactions associated with anemia occurred in approximately 10% of patients treated with interferon alfa-2b/ribavirin therapy.

➤*Chronic hepatitis B:*

Adults – In patients with chronic hepatitis B, some type of adverse reaction occurred in 98% of the 101 patients treated at 5 million units every day and 90% of the 78 patients treated at 10 million units 3 times weekly. Most of these adverse reactions were mild to moderate in severity, were manageable, and were reversible following the end of therapy.

Adverse reactions classified as severe (causing a significant interference with normal daily activities or clinical state) were reported in 21% to 44% of patients. The severe adverse reactions reported most frequently were fatigue (15%), "flu-like" symptoms of fever (28%), fatigue (15%), headache (5%), myalgia (4%), rigors (4%), and other severe "flu-like" symptoms, which occurred in 1% to 3% of patients. Other severe adverse reactions occurring in more than 1 patient were alopecia (8%), anorexia (6%), depression (3%), nausea (3%), and vomiting (2%).

To manage adverse reactions, the dose was reduced, or interferon alfa-2b therapy was interrupted in 25% to 38% of patients. Five percent of patients discontinued treatment because of adverse reactions.

Children – In children, the most frequently reported adverse reactions were those commonly associated with interferon treatment: flu-like symptoms (100%), GI system disorders (46%), and nausea and vomiting (40%). Neutropenia (13%) and thrombocytopenia (3%) were also reported. None of the adverse reactions were life-threatening. The majority were moderate to severe and resolved upon dose reduction or drug discontinuation.

Overdosage

➤*Symptoms:* There is limited experience with overdosage. Postmarketing surveillance includes reports of patients receiving a single dose as great as 10 times the recommended dose. In general, the primary effects of an overdose are consistent with the effects seen with therapeutic doses of interferon alfa-2b. Hepatic enzyme abnormalities, renal failure, hemorrhage, and MI have been reported with single administration overdoses and/or with longer durations of treatment than prescribed. Toxic effects after ingestion of interferon alfa-2b are not expected because interferons are poorly absorbed orally.

➤*Treatment:* Consultation with a poison control center is recommended. There is no specific antidote for interferon alfa-2b. Hemodialysis and peritoneal dialysis are not considered effective for treatment of overdose.

Patient Information

Inform patients receiving interferon alfa-2b treatment alone or in combination with ribavirin capsules of the benefits and risks associated with treatment, and instruct patients on proper use of the product. To supplement your discussion with a patient, provide patients with a Medication Guide.

Inform patients of symptoms and advise them to seek medical attention for symptoms indicative of serious adverse reactions associated with this product. Such adverse reactions may include depression (suicidal ideation), cardiovascular (chest pain), ophthalmologic toxicity (decrease in/loss of vision), pancreatitis or colitis (severe abdominal pain), and cytopenias (high persistent fevers, bruising, dyspnea). Advise patients that some side effects such as fatigue and decreased concentration might interfere with the ability to perform certain tasks. Inform patients who are not taking interferon alfa-2b in combination with ribavirin capsules of the risks to a fetus. Tell women and female partners of men to use 2 forms of birth control during treatment and for 6 months after therapy is discontinued.

Advise patients to remain well hydrated during the initial stages of treatment and that use of an antipyretic may ameliorate some of the flu-like symptoms.

If a decision is made to allow a patient to self-administer interferon alfa-2b, supply a puncture-resistant container for the disposal of needles and syringes. Instruct patients self-administering interferon alfa-2b on the proper disposal of needles and syringes and caution against reuse.

PEGINTERFERON ALFA-2b

Rx	**PEG-Intron** (Schering)	**Injection, lyophilized powder for solution:** 50 mcg per 0.5 mL (when reconstituted)	In preservative-free 2 mL single-use vials[a] with 1.25 mL diluent vial, 2 syringes, and 2 alcohol swabs, and *Redipen*[b] with 1 BD needle and 2 alcohol swabs.
		80 mcg per 0.5 mL (when reconstituted)	In preservative-free 2 mL single-use vials[a] with 1.25 mL diluent vial, 2 syringes, and 2 alcohol swabs, and *Redipen*[b] with 1 BD needle and 2 alcohol swabs.
		120 mcg per 0.5 mL (when reconstituted)	In preservative-free 2 mL single-use vials[a] with 1.25 mL diluent vial, 2 syringes, and 2 alcohol swabs, and *Redipen*[b] with 1 BD needle and 2 alcohol swabs.
		150 mcg per 0.5 mL (when reconstituted)	In preservative-free 2 mL single-use vials[a] with 1.25 mL diluent vial, 2 syringes, and 2 alcohol swabs, and *Redipen*[b] with 1 BD needle and 2 alcohol swabs.
Rx	**Sylatron** (Schering)	**Injection, lyophilized powder for solution:** 40 mcg per 0.1 mL (when reconstituted)	In single-use vials[a] with 1.25 mL diluent vial, 2 BD *Safety Lok* syringes, and 2 alcohol swabs; and boxes of 4 single-use vials[a] with four 1.25 mL diluent vials, 8 BD *Safety Lok* syringes, and 8 alcohol swabs.
		60 mcg per 0.1 mL (when reconstituted)	In single-use vials[a] with 1.25 mL diluent vial, 2 BD *Safety Lok* syringes, and 2 alcohol swabs; and boxes of 4 single-use vials[a] with four 1.25 mL diluent vials, 8 BD *Safety Lok* syringes, and 8 alcohol swabs.
		120 mcg per 0.1 mL (when reconstituted)	In single-use vials[a] with 1.25 mL diluent vial, 2 BD *Safety Lok* syringes, and 2 alcohol swabs; and boxes of 4 single-use vials[a] with four 1.25 mL diluent vials, 8 BD *Safety Lok* syringes, and 8 alcohol swabs.

[a] Contains dibasic sodium phosphate anhydrous 1.11 mg, monobasic sodium phosphate dihydrate 1.11 mg, 0.074 mg of polysorbate 80, and sucrose 59.2 mg.

[b] Contains dibasic sodium phosphate anhydrous 1.013 mg, monobasic sodium phosphate dihydrate 1.013 mg, 0.0675 mg of polysorbate 80, and sucrose 54 mg.

PEGINTERFERON ALFA-2b — INJECTION

WARNING

PEG-Intron – Alpha interferons, including *PEG-Intron*, may cause or aggravate fatal or life-threatening neuropsychiatric, autoimmune, ischemic, and infectious disorders. Closely monitor patients with periodic clinical and laboratory evaluations. Withdraw patients with persistently severe or worsening signs or symptoms of these conditions from therapy. In many, but not all cases, these disorders resolve after stopping *PEG-Intron* therapy (see Warnings/Precautions, Adverse Reactions).

Ribavirin use: Ribavirin may cause birth defects and/or death of the fetus. Take extreme care to avoid pregnancy in women and in female partners of men. Ribavirin causes hemolytic anemia. The anemia associated with ribavirin therapy may result in a worsening of cardiac disease. Ribavirin is genotoxic and mutagenic; consider it a potential carcinogen.

Sylatron –

Depression and other neuropsychiatric disorders: The risk of serious depression with suicidal ideation and completed suicides and other serious neuropsychiatric disorders are increased with alpha interferons, including *Sylatron*. Permanently discontinue *Sylatron* in patients with persistently severe or worsening signs or symptoms of depression, psychosis, or encephalopathy. These disorders may not resolve after stopping *Sylatron*.

Indications

➤*PEG-Intron*:

Chronic hepatitis C –

Monotherapy (for patients who are intolerant to ribavirin): For use alone for the treatment of chronic hepatitis C in patients with compensated liver disease who have not been previously treated with interferon alfa and who are 18 years and older.

Combination therapy: For use in combination with ribavirin capsules for the treatment of chronic hepatitis C in patients with compensated liver disease who are 3 years and older. When initiating therapy with peginterferon alfa-2b, consider that these indications are based on achieving undetectable hepatitis C virus (HCV) RNA after treatment for 24 or 48 weeks and maintaining a sustained virologic response 24 weeks after that last dose. Patients with the following characteristics are less likely to benefit from re-treatment after failing a course of therapy: previous nonresponse, previous pegylated interferon treatment, significant bridging fibrosis or cirrhosis, and genotype 1 infection. No safety and efficacy data are available for treatment longer than 1 year.

➤*Sylatron*:

Melanoma – For the adjuvant treatment of melanoma with microscopic or gross nodal involvement within 84 days of definitive surgical resection including complete lymphadenectomy.

➤*Off-label uses:* Treatment of renal cell carcinoma, chronic myelogenous leukemia, metastatic melanoma.

Administration and Dosage

➤*Adults:*

Chronic hepatitis C (PEG-Intron only) –

Monotherapy:

• *Usual dosage* – 1 mcg/kg/wk subcutaneously for 1 year. Administer the dose on the same day of the week. The volume of peginterferon alfa-2b to be injected depends on the patient's weight.

Recommended Dosing of Peginterferon Alfa-2b Monotherapy

Body weight	*Redipen* or vial strength to use	Amount of peginterferon alfa-2b to administer	Volume[a] of peginterferon alfa-2b to administer
≤ 45 kg (≤ 100 lbs)	50 mcg per 0.5 mL	40 mcg	0.4 mL
46 to 56 kg (101 to 124 lbs)		50 mcg	0.5 mL
57 to 72 kg (125 to 159 lbs)	80 mcg per 0.5 mL	64 mcg	0.4 mL
73 to 88 kg (160 to 195 lbs)		80 mcg	0.5 mL
89 to 106 kg (196 to 234 lbs)	120 mcg per 0.5 mL	96 mcg	0.4 mL
107 to 136 kg (235 to 300 lbs)		120 mcg	0.5 mL
137 to 160 kg (301 to 353 lbs)	150 mcg per 0.5 mL	150 mcg	0.5 mL

[a] When reconstituted as directed

• *Discontinuation of therapy* – Discontinuation of therapy should be considered in patients who do not achieve at least a 2 $\log_{10}$ drop or loss of HCV RNA at 12 weeks of therapy, or whose HCV RNA levels remain detectable after 24 weeks of therapy.

Combination therapy with ribavirin capsules:

• *Usual dosage* – 1.5 mcg/kg/wk of peginterferon alfa-2b subcutaneously when administered in combination with ribavirin 800 to 1,400 mg capsules.

Recommended Peginterferon Alfa-2b Combination Therapy Dosing

Body weight	*Redipen* or vial strength to use	Amount of peginterferon alfa-2b to administer	Volume[a] of peginterferon alfa-2b to administer	Ribavirin daily dosage	Number of ribavirin 200 mg capsules
< 40 kg (< 88 lbs)	50 mcg per 0.5 mL	50 mcg	0.5 mL	800 mg/day	2 in the AM 2 in the PM
40 to 50 kg (88 to 111 lbs)	80 mcg per 0.5 mL	64 mcg	0.4 mL	800 mg/day	2 in the AM 2 in the PM
51 to 60 kg (112 to 133 lbs)		80 mcg	0.5 mL	800 mg/day	2 in the AM 2 in the PM
61 to 65 kg (134 to 144 lbs)	120 mcg per 0.5 mL	96 mcg	0.4 mL	800 mg/day	2 in the AM 2 in the PM
66 to 75 kg (145 to 166 lbs)		96 mcg	0.4 mL	1,000 mg/day	2 in the AM 3 in the PM
76 to 80 kg (167 to 177 lbs)		120 mcg	0.5 mL	1,000 mg/day	2 in the AM 3 in the PM
81 to 85 kg (178 to 187 lbs)		120 mcg	0.5 mL	1,200 mg/day	3 in the AM 3 in the PM
86 to 105 kg (188 to 231 lbs)	150 mcg per 0.5 mL	150 mcg	0.5 mL	1,200 mg/day	3 in the AM 3 in the PM
> 105 kg (> 231 lbs)		[b]	[b]	1,400 mg/day	3 in the AM 4 in the PM

[a] When reconstituted as directed.

[b] For patients weighing more than 105 kg (> 231 lbs), the peginterferon alfa-2b dosage of 1.5 mcg/kg/wk should be calculated based on the individual patient's weight. Two vials of peginterferon alfa-2b may be necessary to provide the dose.

• *Duration of therapy* –

Interferon alfa–naive patients: The treatment duration for patients with genotype 1 is 48 weeks. Patients with genotype 2 and 3 should be treated for 24 weeks.

Re-treatment with peginterferon alfa-2b/ribavirin of prior treatment failures: The duration of treatment for patients who previously failed therapy is 48 weeks, regardless of HCV genotype.

• *Discontinuation of therapy* –

Interferon alfa–naive patients (HCV genotype 1): Discontinuation of therapy should be considered in patients who do not achieve at least a 2 $\log_{10}$ drop or loss of HCV RNA at 12 weeks, or if HCV RNA remains detectable after 24 weeks of therapy.

Re-treatment with peginterferon alfa-2b/ribavirin of prior treatment failures: Re-treated patients who fail to achieve undetectable HCV RNA at week 12, or whose HCV RNA remains detectable after 24 weeks of therapy, are highly unlikely to achieve sustained virologic response and discontinuation of therapy should be considered.

Melanoma (Sylatron only) –

Usual dosage: 6 mcg/kg/wk subcutaneously for 8 doses, followed by 3 mcg/kg/wk subcutaneously for up to 5 years.

• *Premedication* – Premedicate with acetaminophen 500 to 1,000 mg orally 30 minutes prior to the first dose of peginterferon alfa-2b and as needed for subsequent doses.

➤*Children:*

Chronic hepatitis C (PEG-Intron only) –

Combination therapy:

• *3 to 17 years of age* –

Usual dosage: 60 mcg/m^2/wk subcutaneously in combination with ribavirin 15 mg/kg/day orally in 2 divided doses. Dosing for children is determined by body surface area (BSA) for peginterferon alfa-2b and by body weight for ribavirin. Patients who reach 18 years of age while receiving combination therapy should remain on the pediatric dosing regimen.

PEGINTERFERON ALFA-2b — INJECTION

Recommended Ribavirin[a] Dosing in Combination Therapy for Children		
Body weight	Ribavirin daily dosage	Number of ribavirin 200 mg capsules
< 47 kg (< 103 lbs)	15 mg/kg/day	Use oral solution[b]
47 to 59 kg (103 to 131 lbs)	800 mg/day	2 in the AM 2 in the PM
60 to 73 kg (132 to 162 lbs)	1,000 mg/day	2 in the AM 3 in the PM
> 73 kg (> 162 lbs)	1,200 mg/day	3 in the AM 3 in the PM

[a] To be used in combination with peginterferon alfa-2b 60 mcg/m²/wk.
[b] Ribavirin oral solution may be used for any patient, regardless of body weight.

Duration of therapy: The treatment duration for patients with genotype 1 is 48 weeks. Patients with genotypes 2 and 3 should be treated for 24 weeks.

Discontinuation of therapy: It is recommended that patients receiving peginterferon alfa-2b in combination with ribavirin (excluding those with HCV genotype 2 and 3) be discontinued from therapy at 12 weeks if their treatment week 12 HCV RNA dropped below 2 $\log_{10}$ compared with pretreatment, or at 24 weeks if they have detectable HCV RNA at treatment week 24.

➤*Renal function impairment:*

PEG-Intron – If renal function decreases during treatment, peginterferon alfa-2b therapy should be discontinued. When peginterferon alfa-2b is administered in combination with ribavirin, patients with renal impairment or those older than 50 years should be more carefully monitored with respect to the development of anemia.

Moderate renal impairment (creatinine clearance [CrCl] 30 to 50 mL/min): Reduce dose by 25%.

Severe renal impairment (CrCl 10 to 29 mL/min) and hemodialysis: Reduce dose by 50%.

• *CrCl less than 50 mL/min* – Peginterferon alfa-2b/ribavirin should not be used.

Children: If creatinine is more than 2 mg/dL, permanently discontinue peginterferon alfa-2b and ribavirin capsules.

➤*Dosage adjustment:*

Chronic hepatitis C (PEG-Intron only) –

Adults on monotherapy: Dosage reduction in patients on peginterferon alfa-2b monotherapy is accomplished by reducing the original starting dosage of 1 mcg/kg/wk to 0.5 mcg/kg/wk.

Reduced Peginterferon Alfa-2b Dose (0.5 mcg/kg) for (1 mcg/kg) Monotherapy in Adults			
Redipen or vial strength to use	Body weight	Amount of peginterferon alfa-2b to administer	Volume[a] of peginterferon alfa-2b to administer
50 mcg per 0.5 mL[b]	< 45 kg	20 mcg	0.2 mL
50 mcg per 0.5 mL	46 to 56 kg	25 mcg	0.25 mL
	57 to 72 kg	30 mcg	0.3 mL
	73 to 88 kg	40 mcg	0.4 mL

Reduced Peginterferon Alfa-2b Dose (0.5 mcg/kg) for (1 mcg/kg) Monotherapy in Adults			
Redipen or vial strength to use	Body weight	Amount of peginterferon alfa-2b to administer	Volume[a] of peginterferon alfa-2b to administer
50 mcg per 0.5 mL	89 to 106 kg	50 mcg	0.5 mL
80 mcg per 0.5 mL	107 to 136 kg	64 mcg	0.4 mL
	≥ 137 kg	80 mcg	0.5 mL

[a] When reconstituted as directed.
[b] Must use vial. Minimum delivery for *Redipen* is 0.3 mL.

Adults on combination therapy: Dosage reduction of peginterferon alfa-2b in adults on combination therapy with ribavirin is accomplished in a 2-step process from the original starting dosage of 1.5 mcg/kg/wk to 1 mcg/kg/wk and then to 0.5 mcg/kg/wk, if needed.

Two-Step Dose Reduction of Peginterferon Alfa-2b Combination Therapy in Adults							
First dose reduction to 1 mcg/kg				Second dose reduction to 0.5 mcg/kg			
Redipen or vial strength to use	Body weight	Amount of peginterferon alfa-2b to administer	Volume[a] of peginterferon alfa-2b to administer	*Redipen* or vial strength to use	Body weight	Amount of peginterferon alfa-2b to administer	Volume[a] of peginterferon alfa-2b to administer
50 mcg per 0.5 mL	< 40 kg	35 mcg	0.35 mL	50 mcg per 0.5 mL[b]	< 40 kg	20 mcg	0.2 mL
	40 to 50 kg	45 mcg	0.45 mL		40 to 50 kg	25 mcg	0.25 mL
	51 to 60 kg	50 mcg	0.5 mL	50 mcg per 0.5 mL	51 to 60 kg	30 mcg	0.3 mL
80 mcg per 0.5 mL	61 to 75 kg	64 mcg	0.4 mL		61 to 75 kg	35 mcg	0.35 mL
	76 to 85 kg	80 mcg	0.5 mL		76 to 85 kg	45 mcg	0.45 mL
120 mcg per 0.5 mL	86 to 104 kg	96 mcg	0.4 mL		86 to 104 kg	50 mcg	0.5 mL
	105 to 125 kg	108 mcg	0.45 mL	80 mcg per 0.5 mL	105 to 125 kg	64 mcg	0.4 mL
150 mcg per 0.5 mL	> 125 kg	135 mcg	0.45 mL		> 125 kg	72 mcg	0.45 mL

[a] When reconstituted as directed.
[b] Must use vial. Minimum delivery for *Redipen* is 0.3 mL.

Children on combination therapy: Dosage reduction of peginterferon alfa-2b in children is accomplished by modifying the recommended dosage in a 2-step process from the original starting dosage of 60 mcg/m²/wk to 40 mcg/m²/wk, then to 20 mcg/m²/wk, if needed.

Serious adverse reactions: If a serious adverse reaction develops during the course of treatment (see Warnings/Precautions), discontinue or modify the dosage of peginterferon alfa-2b and/or ribavirin capsules until the adverse reaction abates or decreases in severity. If persistent or recurrent serious adverse reactions develop despite adequate dosage adjustment, discontinue treatment. Decreases in hemoglobin, neutrophils, and platelets may require dose reduction or permanent discontinuation from therapy.

Patients with depression:

Guidelines for Modification or Discontinuation of Peginterferon Alfa-2b or Peginterferon Alfa-2b/Ribavirin Capsules and for Scheduling Visits for Patients With Depression					
	Initial management (4 to 8 weeks)		Depression		
Depression severity[a,b]	Dose modification	Visit schedule	Remains stable	Improves	Worsens
Mild	No change.	Evaluate once weekly by visit or phone.	Continue weekly visit schedule.	Resume normal visit schedule.	See moderate or severe depression.
Moderate	Adults: Adjust dose. Children: Decrease IFN[c] dosage to 40 mcg/m²/wk, then to 20 mcg/m²/wk if needed.	Evaluate once weekly (office visit at least every other week).	Consider psychiatric consultation. Continue reduced dosing.	If symptoms improve and are stable for 4 weeks, may resume normal visit schedule. Continue reduced dosing or return to normal dose.	See severe depression.
Severe	Discontinue IFN/R[c] permanently.	Obtain immediate psychiatric consultation.	Psychiatric therapy as necessary.		

[a] For patients on peginterferon alfa-2b/ribavirin combination therapy, the first dosage reduction of peginterferon alfa-2b is to 1 mcg/kg/wk and the second dosage reduction (if needed) of peginterferon alfa-2b is to 0.5 mcg/kg/wk. For patients on peginterferon alfa-2b monotherapy, decrease peginterferon alfa-2b dosage to 0.5 mcg/kg/wk.
[b] See *Diagnostic and Statistical Manual of Mental Disorders* (Fourth Edition) for definitions.
[c] IFN = interferon; R = ribavirin.

PEGINTERFERON ALFA-2b — INJECTION

Hematologic:

Guidelines for Dose Modification and Discontinuation of Peginterferon Alfa-2b or Peginterferon Alfa-2b/Ribavirin Capsules Based on Laboratory Parameters

Laboratory values		Peginterferon alfa-2b		Ribavirin capsules	
		Adults	Children	Adults	Children
Hemoglobin	< 10 g/dL	For patients with cardiac disease, reduce by 50%.[a]	—[a]	Adjust dose.[b]	First reduction to 12 mg/kg /day, second reduction to 8 mg/kg /day
	< 8.5 g/dL	Permanently discontinue.	Permanently discontinue.	Permanently discontinue.	Permanently discontinue.
WBC[c]	< 1.5 × 10^9/L	Adjust dose.[d]	First reduction to 40 mcg/m^2/wk, second reduction to 20 mcg/m^2/wk	No change	No change
	< 1 × 10^9/L	Permanently discontinue.	Permanently discontinue.	Permanently discontinue.	Permanently discontinue.
Neutrophils	< 0.75 × 10^9/L	Adjust dose.[d]	First reduction to 40 mcg/m^2/wk, second reduction to 20 mcg/m^2/wk	No change	No change
	< 0.5 × 10^9/L	Permanently discontinue.	Permanently discontinue.	Permanently discontinue.	Permanently discontinue.
Platelets	< 70 × 10^9/L (children)		First reduction to 40 mcg/ m^2/wk, second reduction to 20 mcg/ m^2/wk		No change
	< 50 × 10^9/L	Adjust dose.[d]	Permanently discontinue.	No change	Permanently discontinue.
	< 25 × 10^9/L (adults)	Permanently discontinue.	—	Permanently discontinue.	

[a] For patients with a history of stable cardiac disease receiving peginterferon alfa-2b in combination with ribavirin capsules, reduce the peginterferon alfa-2b dose by half and the ribavirin capsule dosage by 200 mg/day if more than a 2 g/dL decrease in hemoglobin is observed during any 4-week period. Permanently discontinue peginterferon alfa-2b and ribavirin capsules if patient has hemoglobin levels of less than 12 g/dL after this ribavirin dose reduction. Children who have preexisting cardiac conditions and experience a hemoglobin decrease of 2 g/dL or more during any 4-week period during treatment should have weekly evaluations and hematology testing.

[b] First dosage reduction of ribavirin is by 200 mg/day, except in patients receiving the 1,400 mg dose it is by 400 mg/day; second dosage reduction of ribavirin (if needed) is by an additional 200 mg/day.

[c] WBC = white blood cells.

[d] For patients on peginterferon alfa-2b/ribavirin combination therapy, first dosage reduction of peginterferon alfa-2b is to 1 mcg/kg/wk; second dosage reduction (if needed) of peginterferon alfa-2b is to 0.5 mcg/kg/wk. For patients on peginterferon alfa-2b monotherapy, decrease the peginterferon dosage to 0.5 mcg/kg/wk.

Melanoma (Sylatron only) – The following guidelines for dose modification are based on the National Cancer Institute Common Terminology Criteria for Adverse Events (NCI-CTCAE Version 2.0):

Permanently discontinue peginterferon alfa-2b for persistent or worsening severe neuropsychiatric disorders; grade 4 nonhematologic toxicity; inability to tolerate a dose of 1 mcg/kg/week; new or worsening retinopathy.

Withhold peginterferon alfa-2b dose for any of the following: absolute neutrophil count (ANC) less than 0.5 × 10^9/L; platelet count less than 50 × 10^9/L; ECOG performance status of 2 or more; nonhematologic toxicity of grade 3 or more.

Resume dosing at a reduced dose (see the following table) when all of the following are present: ANC of at least 0.5 × 10^9/L; platelet count of at least 50 × 10^9/L; ECOG performance status of 0 to 1; nonhematologic toxicity has completely resolved or improved to grade 1.

Peginterferon Alfa-2b Dose Modifications in Patients With Melanoma

Starting dose	Dose modification
Doses 1 to 8	
6 mcg/kg/wk	First dose modification: 3 mcg/kg/wk
	Second dose modification: 2 mcg/kg/wk
	Third dose modification: 1 mcg/kg/wk
	Permanently discontinue is unable to tolerate 1 mcg/kg/wk
Doses 9 to 260	
3 mcg/kg/wk	First dose modification: 2 mcg/kg/wk
	Second dose modification: 1 mcg/kg/wk
	Permanently discontinue if unable to tolerate 1 mcg/kg/wk

➤*Preparation for administration:*

PEG-Intron –

Redipen: Peginterferon alfa-2b *Redipen* consists of a dual-chamber glass cartridge with sterile, lyophilized peginterferon alfa-2b in the active chamber and sterile water for injection in the diluent chamber. The peginterferon alfa-2b in the glass cartridge should appear as a white to off-white, tablet-shaped solid that is whole or in pieces or powder.

To reconstitute the lyophilized peginterferon alfa-2b in the *Redipen*, hold the *Redipen* upright (dose button down) and press the 2 halves of the pen together until there is an audible click. Gently invert the pen to mix the solution. Do not shake. The reconstituted solution has a concentration of 50, 80, 120, or 150 mcg per 0.5 mL for a single subcutaneous injection. Keeping the pen upright, attach the supplied needle and select the appropriate peginterferon alfa-2b dose by pulling back on the dosing button until the dark bands are visible and turning the button until the dark band is aligned with the correct dose. The *Redipen* is a single pen and does not contain preservatives. Do not reuse the *Redipen*. Discard the unused portion. The sterility of any remaining product can no longer be guaranteed.

Vials: Two *BD Safety-Lok* syringes are provided in the package; one syringe is for the reconstitution steps and one is for the patient injection. There is a plastic safety sleeve to be pulled over the needle after use. The syringe locks with an audible click when the green stripe on the safety sleeve covers the red stripe on the needle.

Reconstitute the peginterferon alfa-2b lyophilized product with only 0.7 mL of supplied diluent (sterile water for injection). The diluent vial is for single use only and does not contain a preservative. Discard the remaining diluent. Do not add any other medication to solutions containing peginterferon alfa-2b, and do not reconstitute peginterferon alfa-2b with other diluents. Swirl gently to hasten complete dissolution of the powder. Do not reuse the vial. Discard the unused portion. The sterility of any remaining product can no longer be guaranteed.

Sylatron – Reconstitute with 0.7 mL of sterile water for injection. Upon reconstitution, the final concentration of peginterferon alfa-2b will be 40 mcg per each 0.1 mL, 60 mcg per each 0.1 mL, or 120 mcg per each 0.1 mL.

Swirl gently to dissolve the lyophilized powder. Do not shake.

Do not withdraw more than 0.5 mL of reconstituted solution from each vial. For single-use only. Discard any unused portion.

➤*Administration:* The prepared peginterferon alfa-2b solution is to be injected subcutaneously. Rotate injection sites.

PEG-Intron – When taken as combination therapy, ribavirin should be taken with food.

➤*Storage/Stability:*

PEG-Interon –

Redipen: Store at 2° to 8°C (36° to 46°F). After reconstitution, use the solution immediately, or it may be stored for up to 24 hours at 2° to 8°C (36° to 46°F). The reconstituted solution contains no preservative and is clear and colorless. Do not freeze.

Vials: Store at 25°C (77°F); excursions are permitted to 15° to 30°C (59° to 86°F). After reconstitution with supplied diluent, use the solution immediately, or it may be stored for up to 24 hours at 2° to 8°C (36° to 46°F). The reconstituted solution contains no preservative and is clear and colorless. Do not freeze.

Sylatron – Store at 25°C (77°F); excursions are permitted between 15° and 30°C (59° and 86°F). If reconstituted solution is not used immediately, store at 2° to 8°C (36° to 46°F) for no more than 24 hours. Discard reconstituted solution after 24 hours. Do not freeze.

Actions

➤*Pharmacology:* Pegylated recombinant human interferon alfa-2b is an inducer of the innate antiviral immune response. The biological activity of peginterferon alfa-2b is derived from its interferon alfa-2b moiety. Peginterferon alfa-2b binds to and activates the human type 1 interferon receptor. Upon binding, the receptor subunits dimerize and activate multiple intracellular signal transduction pathways. Signal transduction is initially mediated by the JAK/STAT activation, which may occur in a wide variety of cells. Interferon receptor activation also activates nuclear factor kappa B in many cell types. Given the diversity of cell types that respond to interferon alfa-2b and the multiplicity of potential intracellular responses to interferon receptor activation, peginterferon alfa-2b is expected to have pleiotropic biological effects in the body.

The mechanism by which ribavirin contributes to its antiviral efficacy in the clinic is not fully understood. Ribavirin has direct antiviral activity in tissue culture against many RNA viruses. Ribavirin increases the mutation frequency in the genomes of several viruses, and ribavirin triphosphate inhibits HCV polymerase in a biochemical reaction.

➤*Pharmacokinetics:*

Absorption/Distribution – Following a single subcutaneous dose of peginterferon alfa-2b, the mean absorption half-life was 4.6 hours. Maximal serum concentrations (C_{max}) occur between 15 and 44 hours postdose and are sustained for up to 48 to 72 hours. The C_{max} and area under the curve (AUC) measurements of peginterferon alfa-2b increase in a dose-related manner. After multiple dosing, there is an increase in bioavailability of

PEGINTERFERON ALFA-2b — INJECTION

peginterferon alfa-2b. Week 48 mean trough concentrations (320 pg/mL; range, 0 to 2,960) are approximately 3-fold higher than week 4 mean trough concentrations (94 pg/mL; range, 0 to 416).

At effective therapeutic doses, peginterferon alfa-2b has approximately 10-fold greater C_{max} and 50-fold greater AUC than interferon alfa-2b.

Effects of food on ribavirin: Both AUC_{tf} and C_{max} increased by 70% when ribavirin capsules were administered with a high-fat meal (841 kcal, 53.8 g of fat, 31.6 g of protein, 57.4 g of carbohydrate) in a single-dose pharmacokinetic study.

Metabolism/Excretion – The mean peginterferon alfa-2b elimination half-life is approximately 40 hours (range, 22 to 60 hours) in patients with HCV infection. The apparent clearance of peginterferon alfa-2b is estimated to be approximately 22 mL/h•kg. Renal elimination accounts for 30% of the clearance.

Pegylation of interferon alfa-2b produces a product (peginterferon alfa-2b) with a clearance lower than that of nonpegylated interferon alfa-2b. When compared with interferon alfa-2b, peginterferon alfa-2b (1 mcg/kg) has an approximately 7-fold lower mean apparent clearance and a 5-fold greater mean half-life, permitting a reduced dosing frequency.

Special populations –

Renal function impairment: Following multiple dosing of peginterferon alfa-2b (1 mcg/kg subcutaneously given every week for 4 weeks), the clearance of peginterferon alfa-2b is reduced by a mean of 17% in subjects with moderate renal impairment (CrCl 30 to 49 mL/min) and by a mean of 44% in subjects with severe renal impairment (CrCl 10 to 29 mL/min), compared with subjects with healthy renal function. Clearance was similar in subjects with severe renal impairment not on dialysis and subjects who are receiving hemodialysis. The dose of peginterferon alfa-2b for monotherapy should be reduced in patients with moderate or severe renal impairment. Ribavirin should not be used in patients with CrCl less than 50 mL/min.

Children: Population pharmacokinetics for peginterferon alfa-2b and ribavirin (capsules and oral solution) were evaluated in children between 3 and 17 years of age with chronic hepatitis C. In children receiving peginterferon alfa-2b 60 mcg/m^2/wk subcutaneously, exposure may be approximately 50% higher than that observed in adults receiving 1.5 mcg/kg/wk subcutaneously.

Contraindications

➤*PEG-Intron:*

Peginterferon alfa-2b – Hypersensitivity to interferon alfa or any component of the product; autoimmune hepatitis; decompensated liver disease (Child-Pugh score more than 6 [class B and C]) in cirrhotic chronic hepatitis C patients before or during treatment.

Peginterferon alfa-2b/ribavirin capsules combination (additionally) – Hypersensitivity to ribavirin capsules or any other component of the product; men whose female partners are pregnant; patients with hemoglobinopathies (eg, thalassemia major, sickle-cell anemia); CrCl less than 50 mL/min.

➤*Sylatron:* History of anaphylaxis to peginterferon alfa-2b or interferon alfa-2b; autoimmune hepatitis; hepatic decompensation (Child-Pugh score greater than 6 [class B and C]).

Warnings/Precautions

➤*Anemia:* Ribavirin caused hemolytic anemia in 10% of peginterferon alfa-2b/ribavirin capsule–treated patients within 1 to 4 weeks of initiation of therapy. Obtain complete blood cell counts (CBCs) before treatment and at weeks 2 and 4 of therapy or more frequently if clinically indicated. Anemia associated with ribavirin capsule therapy may result in a worsening of cardiac disease. Decrease in dosage or discontinuation of ribavirin capsules may be necessary.

➤*Neuropsychiatric effects:* Life-threatening or fatal neuropsychiatric events, including suicide, suicidal and homicidal ideation, depression, relapse of drug addiction/overdose, and aggressive behavior, have occurred in patients with and without a previous psychiatric disorder during peginterferon alfa-2b treatment and follow-up. Psychoses, hallucinations, bipolar disorders, and mania have been observed in patients treated with alpha interferons. Use peginterferon alfa-2b with extreme caution in patients with a history of psychiatric disorders. Advise patients to report immediately any symptoms of depression and/or suicidal ideation to their prescribing health care providers. Monitor all patients for evidence of depression and other psychiatric symptoms. If patients develop psychiatric problems, including clinical depression, carefully monitor patients during treatment and in the 6-month follow-up period. If psychiatric symptoms persist or worsen, or if suicidal ideation or aggressive behavior towards others is identified, discontinue treatment with peginterferon alfa-2b and follow the patient, with psychiatric intervention as appropriate. In severe cases, stop peginterferon alfa-2b immediately and institute psychiatric intervention. Cases of encephalopathy have been observed in some patients, usually elderly patients, treated at higher doses of peginterferon alfa-2b.

➤*Cardiovascular effects:* Cardiovascular events, including hypotension, arrhythmia, tachycardia, cardiomyopathy, angina pectoris, and myocardial infarction (MI) have been observed in patients treated with peginterferon alfa-2b. Use peginterferon alfa-2b cautiously in patients with cardiovascular disease. Closely monitor patients with a history of MI and arrhythmic disorder who require peginterferon alfa-2b therapy. Do not treat patients with a history of significant or unstable cardiac disease with peginterferon/ribavirin capsules combination therapy.

➤*Endocrine disorders:* Peginterferon alfa-2b causes or aggravates hypothyroidism and hyperthyroidism. Hyperglycemia has been observed in patients treated with peginterferon alfa-2b. Diabetes mellitus has been observed in patients treated with alpha interferons. Do not begin peginterferon alfa-2b therapy in patients with these conditions who cannot be effectively treated by medication. Do not continue peginterferon alfa-2b therapy in patients who develop these conditions during treatment and cannot be controlled with medication.

➤*Ophthalmic effects:* Decreased or loss of vision, retinopathy (including macular edema), retinal artery or vein thrombosis, retinal hemorrhages and cotton wool spots, optic neuritis, papilledema, and serous retinal detachment may be induced or aggravated by treatment with peginterferon alfa-2b or other alpha interferons. Ensure that all patients receive an eye examination at baseline, and that patients with preexisting ophthalmologic disorders (eg, diabetic or hypertensive retinopathy) receive periodic ophthalmologic exams during interferon alpha treatment. Give any patient who develops ocular symptoms a prompt and complete eye examination. Discontinue peginterferon alfa-2b treatment in patients who develop new or worsening ophthalmologic disorders.

➤*Cerebrovascular disorders:* Ischemic and hemorrhagic cerebrovascular events have been observed in patients treated with interferon alfa–based therapies, including peginterferon alfa-2b. Events occurred in patients with few or no reported risk factors for stroke, including patients younger than 45 years of age. Because these are spontaneous reports, estimates of frequency cannot be made and a causal relationship between interferon alfa–based therapies and these events is difficult to establish.

➤*Bone marrow toxicity:* Peginterferon alfa-2b suppresses bone marrow function, sometimes resulting in severe cytopenias. Discontinue peginterferon alfa-2b in patients who develop severe decreases in neutrophil or platelet counts. Ribavirin may potentiate the neutropenia induced by interferon alpha. Very rarely, alpha interferons may be associated with aplastic anemia.

➤*Autoimmune disorders:* Development or exacerbation of autoimmune disorders (eg, thyroiditis, thrombotic thrombocytopenic purpura, idiopathic thrombocytopenic purpura, rheumatoid arthritis, interstitial nephritis, systemic lupus erythematosus, psoriasis) has been observed in patients receiving peginterferon alfa-2b. Use peginterferon alfa-2b with caution in patients with autoimmune disorders.

➤*Pancreatitis:* Fatal and nonfatal pancreatitis has been observed in patients treated with alpha interferons. Suspend peginterferon alfa-2b therapy in patients with signs and symptoms suggestive of pancreatitis, and discontinue in patients diagnosed with pancreatitis.

➤*Colitis:* Fatal and nonfatal ulcerative or hemorrhagic/ischemic colitis has been observed within 12 weeks of the start of alpha interferon treatment. Abdominal pain, bloody diarrhea, and fever are the typical manifestations. Immediately discontinue peginterferon alfa-2b in patients who develop these symptoms and signs. Colitis usually resolves within 1 to 3 weeks of discontinuation of alpha interferons.

➤*Pulmonary disorders:* Dyspnea, pulmonary infiltrates, pneumonia, bronchiolitis obliterans, interstitial pneumonitis, pulmonary hypertension, and sarcoidosis, some resulting in respiratory failure and/or patient deaths, may be induced or aggravated by peginterferon alfa-2b or alpha interferon therapy. Recurrence of respiratory failure has been observed with interferon rechallenge. Suspend peginterferon alfa-2b combination treatment in patients who develop pulmonary infiltrates or pulmonary function impairment. Closely monitor patients who resume interferon treatment.

➤*Hepatic effects:* Chronic hepatitis C patients with cirrhosis may be at risk of hepatic decompensation and death when treated with alpha interferons, including peginterferon alfa-2b. Cirrhotic chronic hepatitis C patients coinfected with HIV receiving highly active antiretroviral therapy (HAART) and alpha interferons with or without ribavirin appear to be at increased risk for the development of hepatic decompensation compared with patients not receiving HAART. During treatment, closely monitor patients' clinical status and hepatic function, and immediately discontinue peginterferon alfa-2b treatment if decompensation (Child-Pugh score more than 6) is observed.

➤*Dental and periodontal disorders:* Dental and periodontal disorders have been reported in patients receiving peginterferon alfa-2b/ribavirin combination therapy. In addition, dry mouth could have a damaging effect on teeth and mucous membranes of the mouth during long-term treatment with the combination of ribavirin and peginterferon alfa-2b. Advise patients to brush their teeth thoroughly twice daily and have regular dental examinations. If vomiting occurs, advise patients to rinse out their mouth thoroughly afterwards.

➤*Triglycerides:* Elevated triglyceride levels have been observed in patients treated with interferons, including peginterferon alfa-2b therapy. Manage elevated triglyceride levels as clinically appropriate. Hypertriglyceridemia may result in pancreatitis. Consider discontinuation of peginterferon alfa-2b therapy for patients with persistently elevated triglycerides (ie, triglycerides greater than 1,000 mg/dL) associated with symptoms of potential pancreatitis, such as abdominal pain, nausea, or vomiting.

➤*Peripheral neuropathy:* Peripheral neuropathy has been reported when alpha interferons were given in combination with telbivudine. In one clinical trial, an increased risk and severity of peripheral neuropathy was observed with the combination use of telbivudine and pegylated interferon alfa-2a as compared to telbivudine alone. The safety and efficacy of telbivudine in combination with interferons for the treatment of chronic hepatitis B has not been demonstrated

➤*Immunogenicity:* As with all therapeutic proteins, there is potential for immunogenicity. Approximately 2% of patients receiving peginterferon alfa-2b or interferon alfa-2b with or without ribavirin capsules developed low-titer (160 or less) neutralizing antibodies to peginterferon alfa-2b or

PEGINTERFERON ALFA-2b — INJECTION

interferon alfa-2b. The clinical and pathological significance of the appearance of serum neutralizing antibodies is unknown. The incidence of antibody formation is highly dependent on the sensitivity and specificity of the assay. Additionally, the observed incidence of antibody (including neutralizing antibody) positivity in an assay may be influenced by several factors, including assay methodology, sample handling, timing of sample collection, concomitant medications, and underlying disease. For these reasons, comparison of the incidence of antibodies to peginterferon alfa-2b with the incidence of antibodies to other products may be misleading.

➤*Organ transplants:* The safety and efficacy of peginterferon alfa-2b alone or in combination with ribavirin capsules for the treatment of hepatitis C in patients who have received liver or other organ transplants have not been studied. In a small (n = 16) single-center, uncontrolled case experience, renal failure in renal allograft recipients receiving interferon alpha and ribavirin combination therapy was more frequent than expected from the center's previous experience with renal allograft recipients not receiving combination therapy. The relationship of renal failure to renal allograft rejection is not clear.

➤*Hypersensitivity reactions:* Serious, acute hypersensitivity reactions (eg, urticaria, angioedema, bronchoconstriction, anaphylaxis) and cutaneous eruptions (Stevens-Johnson syndrome and toxic epidermal necrolysis) rarely have been observed during alpha interferon therapy. If such a reaction develops during treatment with peginterferon alfa-2b, discontinue treatment and immediately institute appropriate medical therapy. Transient rashes do not necessitate interruption of treatment.

➤*Renal function impairment:* Increases in serum creatinine levels have been observed in patients treated with interferons, including peginterferon alfa-2b therapy. Closely monitor patients with impairment of renal function for signs and symptoms of interferon toxicity, including increases in serum creatinine, and adjust doses of peginterferon alfa-2b accordingly. Use peginterferon alfa-2b with caution in patients with CrCl less than 50 mL/min; weigh the potential risks against the potential benefits in these patients. Do not use ribavirin in patients with CrCl less than 50 mL/min.

➤*Pregnancy: Category C.* Assume that peginterferon alfa-2b has abortifacient potential. There are no adequate and well-controlled studies in pregnant women. Use during pregnancy only if the potential benefit justifies the potential risk to the fetus. Peginterferon alfa-2b is recommended for use in fertile women only when they are using effective contraception during the treatment period.

Nonpegylated interferon alfa-2b has been shown to have abortifacient effects in *Macaca mulatta* (rhesus monkeys) at 15 and 30 million units/kg (estimated human equivalent of 5 and 10 million units/kg based on BSA adjustment for a 60 kg adult).

Use with ribavirin – Category X.

Ribavirin capsules may cause birth defects and/or death of the fetus. Do not start ribavirin therapy until a report of a negative pregnancy test has been obtained immediately prior to planned initiation of therapy. Instruct patients to use at least 2 forms of contraception and have monthly pregnancy tests (see Warning Box, Contraindications).

Significant teratogenic and/or embryocidal effects have been demonstrated in all animal species exposed to ribavirin. Ribavirin therapy is contraindicated in women who are pregnant and in the male partners of women who are pregnant.

➤*Lactation:* Interferon alfa is excreted in breast milk. The American Academy of Pediatrics classifies interferon alfa as compatible with breastfeeding.

It is not known whether the components of peginterferon alfa-2b and/or ribavirin are excreted in human milk. Studies in mice have shown that mouse interferons are excreted in breast milk. Because of the potential for adverse reactions from the drug in breast-feeding infants, decide whether to discontinue breast-feeding or the peginterferon alfa-2b and ribavirin treatment, taking into account the importance of the drug to the mother.

➤*Children:* Safety and efficacy in children younger than 3 years of age have not been established. Clinical trials in children younger than 3 years of age are not considered feasible because of the small proportion of patients in this age group that require treatment for chronic hepatitis C.

Impact on growth – Data on the effects of peginterferon alfa-2b plus ribavirin on growth come from an open-label study in subjects 3 to 17 years of age, and weight and height changes are compared with US normative population data. In general, the weight and height gain of children treated with peginterferon alfa-2b plus ribavirin lags behind that predicted by normative population data for the entire length of treatment. Approximately 6 months posttreatment (follow-up week 24), subjects had weight gain rebounds and regained their weight to the 53rd percentile, above the average of the normative population and similar to that predicted by their average baseline weight (57th percentile). Approximately 6 months posttreatment, height gain stabilized and subjects treated with peginterferon alfa-2b plus ribavirin had an average height percentile of the 44th percentile, which was less than the average of the normative population and less than their average baseline height (51st percentile). Severely inhibited growth velocity (less than 3rd percentile) was observed in 70% of subjects while on treatment. Of the subjects experiencing severely inhibited growth, 20% had continued inhibited growth velocity (less than 3rd percentile) after 6 months of follow-up.

Among the boys studied, the age groups of 3 to 11 years and 12 to 17 years had similar height percentile decreases of approximately 5 percentiles after 6 months posttreatment; weight gain continued to be similar to their average baseline percentile. Girls who were 3 to 11 years of age and treated for 48 weeks had the largest average drop in height and weight percentiles (13 and 7 percentiles, respectively), whereas girls 12 to 17 years of age continued along their average baseline height and weight percentiles after 6 months posttreatment.

➤*Elderly:* Treatment with alpha interferons, including peginterferon alfa-2b, is associated with neuropsychiatric, cardiac, pulmonary, GI, and systemic (flu-like) adverse effects. Because these adverse reactions may be more severe in elderly patients, exercise caution when using peginterferon alfa-2b in this population. This drug is known to be substantially excreted by the kidney. Because elderly patients are more likely to have decreased renal function, the risk of toxic reactions to this drug may be greater in patients with impaired renal function.

➤*Lab test abnormalities:* Peginterferon alfa-2b alone or in combination with ribavirin capsules may cause severe decreases in neutrophil and platelet counts and hematologic, endocrine (eg, thyroid-stimulating hormone [TSH]), and hepatic abnormalities. In 10% of patients treated with peginterferon alfa-2b, ALT levels rose 2- to 5-fold above baseline. The elevations were transient and were not associated with deterioration of other liver functions. Triglyceride levels are frequently elevated in patients receiving alpha interferon therapy, including peginterferon alfa-2b, and should be periodically monitored.

In the adult clinical trial, CBC (including hemoglobin, neutrophil, and platelet counts) and chemistries (including AST, ALT, bilirubin, and uric acid) were measured during the treatment period at weeks 2, 4, 8, 12, and then at 6-week intervals or more frequently if abnormalities developed. In children, the same laboratory parameters were evaluated with additional assessment of hemoglobin at treatment week 6. TSH levels were measured every 12 weeks during the treatment period. Measure HCV RNA periodically during treatment.

➤*Monitoring:* Monitor patients for worsening depression, suicidal thoughts or ideation, aggressive behavior, or other psychiatric symptoms. Withdraw patients with persistently severe or worsening signs or symptoms from therapy.

Monitor patients with a history of MI or arrhythmic disorder. Monitor blood glucose more frequently in patients with diabetes.

Patients on peginterferon alfa-2b or peginterferon alfa-2b/ribavirin capsules combination therapy should have hematology and blood chemistry testing, including creatine, liver function, and lipids, before the start of treatment and then periodically thereafter. Obtain CBC pretreatment and at weeks 2 and 4 of therapy, or more frequently if clinically indicated, in patients on peginterferon alfa-2b and ribavirin capsules. Administer an electrocardiogram to patients who have preexisting cardiac abnormalities before treatment with peginterferon alfa-2b/ribavirin capsules.

Ensure that all patients receive an eye exam prior to start of therapy and periodically thereafter in patients with diabetic or hypertensive retinopathy.

Monitor clinical status and hepatic function closely in patients with chronic hepatitis C with cirrhosis.

Drug Interactions

Peginterferon Alfa-2b Drug Interactions			
Precipitant drug	Object drug[a]		Description
Peginterferon alfa-2b	CYP2C8/9 substrates (eg, phenytoin, warfarin)	⬇	Plasma concentrations of these substrates may be reduced, decreasing the pharmacologic effects. Evaluate the response of the patient and adjust the dose of the substrate as needed.
Peginterferon alfa-2b	CYP2D6 substrates (eg, flecainide)	⬇	Plasma concentrations of these substrates may be reduced, decreasing the pharmacologic effects. Evaluate the response of the patient and adjust the dose of the substrate as needed.
Peginterferon alfa-2b	Methadone	⬆	Methadone plasma concentrations may be elevated, increasing the pharmacologic effects and adverse reactions. Monitor patients for signs and symptoms of increased narcotic effect and adjust the methadone dose as needed.
Peginterferon alfa-2b with or without ribavirin	NRTIs[b]	⬆	Closely monitor for treatment-associated toxicities (eg, hepatic decompensation, anemia) especially in cirrhotic HIV/HCV coinfected patients. Discontinue the NRTI as medically appropriate. Reduce the dose or discontinue interferon, ribavirin, or both if toxicities develop.

PEGINTERFERON ALFA-2b — INJECTION

Peginterferon Alfa-2b Drug Interactions

Precipitant drug	Object drug[a]		Description
Peginterferon alfa-2b with ribavirin	Didanosine	↑	Coadministration of ribavirin and didanosine is not recommended. Reports of fatal hepatic failure, as well as peripheral neuropathy, pancreatitis, and symptomatic hyperlactatemia/lactic acidosis have been reported.
Peginterferon alfa-2b with ribavirin	Pyrimidine nucleoside analogs (eg, lamivudine, stavudine, zidovudine)	↑	Severe neutropenia and severe anemia may develop in HIV/HCV coinfected patients. Closely monitor the patient.

[a] ↑ = object drug increased; ↓ = object drug decreased.
[b] NRTIs = nucleoside reverse transcriptase inhibitors.

Adverse Reactions

➤*Discontinuation:* In the monotherapy study and the combination study comparing peginterferon alfa-2b/ribavirin with interferon alfa-2b/ribavirin, 10% to 14% of patients receiving peginterferon alfa-2b, alone or in combination with ribavirin capsules, discontinued therapy, compared with 6% treated with interferon alfa-2b alone and 13% treated with interferon alfa-2b in combination with ribavirin capsules. In the weight-based/flat-dose trial, 15% of subjects receiving peginterferon alfa-2b in combination with weight-based ribavirin and 14% of subjects receiving peginterferon alfa-2b and flat-dose ribavirin discontinued therapy because of an adverse reaction. The most common reasons for discontinuation of therapy were related to psychiatric, systemic (eg, fatigue, headache), or GI adverse reactions. In the combination therapy trial using interferon alfa-2b as the comparator, 13% of subjects in the peginterferon alfa-2b 1.5 mcg/ribavirin arm, 10% in the peginterferon alfa-2b 1 mcg/ribavirin arm, and 13% in the peginterferon alfa-2a 180 mcg/ribavirin tablets arm discontinued because of adverse events.

➤*Combination therapy:* In the combination therapy trial using interferon alfa-2b as the comparator, dose reductions caused by adverse reactions occurred in 42% of patients receiving peginterferon alfa-2b (1.5 mcg/kg)/ribavirin capsules and in 34% of those receiving interferon alfa-2b/ribavirin capsules. The majority of patients (57%) weighing 60 kg or less receiving peginterferon alfa-2b (1.5 mcg/kg)/ribavirin capsules required dose reduction. Reduction of interferon was dose-related (peginterferon alfa-2b 1.5 mcg/kg greater than peginterferon alfa-2b 0.5 mcg/kg or interferon alfa-2b; 40%, 27%, 28%, respectively). Dose reduction for ribavirin capsules was similar across all 3 groups: 33% to 35%. The most common reasons for dose modifications were neutropenia (18%) or anemia (9%). Other common reasons included depression, fatigue, nausea, and thrombocytopenia. In the combination study using peginterferon alfa-2a/ribavirin as the comparator, 16% of subjects had a dose reduction of peginterferon alfa-2b to 1 mcg/kg in combination with ribavirin, with an additional 4% requiring the second dose reduction of peginterferon alfa-2b to 0.5 mcg/kg due to adverse events, compared to 15% of subjects in the peginterferon alfa-2a/ribavirin tablets arm, who required a dose reduction to 135 mcg/week with peginterferon alfa-2a, with an additional 7% in the peginterferon alfa-2a/ribavirin tablets arm requiring a second dose reduction to 90 mcg/week with peginterferon alfa-2a.

CNS – In the peginterferon alfa-2b/ribavirin capsules combination trial, the most common adverse events were psychiatric, occurring among 77% of patients, and included most commonly depression, irritability, and insomnia, each reported by approximately 30% to 40% of subjects in all treatment groups. Suicidal behavior (eg, ideation, attempts, suicides) occurred in 2% of all patients during treatment or during follow-up after treatment cessation. In the combination study using peginterferon alfa-2a/ribavirin as the comparator, psychiatric adverse reactions occurred in 58% of subjects in the peginterferon alfa-2b 1.5 mcg/ribavirin arm, 55% of subjects in the peginterferon alfa-2b 1 mcg/ribavirin arm, and 57% of subjects in the peginterferon alfa-2a 180 mcg/ribavirin tablets arm.

Peginterferon alfa-2b induced fatigue or headache in approximately two-thirds of patients and induced fever or rigors in approximately 50% of patients. The severity of some of these systemic symptoms (eg, fever, headache) tended to decrease as treatment continued.

Local – Application-site inflammation and reaction (eg, bruising, itchiness, irritation) occurred at approximately twice the incidence with peginterferon alfa-2b therapies (in up to 75% of patients) compared with interferon alfa-2b. However, injection-site pain was infrequent (2% to 3%) in all groups. Many patients continued to experience adverse reactions several months after discontinuation of therapy. By the end of the 6-month follow-up period, the incidence of ongoing adverse reactions by body class in the peginterferon alfa-2b 1.5/ribavirin capsules group was 33% (psychiatric), 20% (musculoskeletal), and 10% (for endocrine and for GI). In approximately 10% to 15% of patients, weight loss, fatigue, and headache had not resolved.

➤*Weight-based versus flat-dose trials:* In the peginterferon alfa-2b/ribavirin combination trials, the most common adverse reactions were psychiatric, which occurred among 77% of subjects and 68% to 69% of subjects in the weight-based/flat-dose trial. These psychiatric adverse reactions included most commonly depression, irritability, and insomnia, each reported by approximately 30% to 40% of subjects in all treatment groups. Suicidal behavior (ideation, attempts, and suicides) occurred in 2% of all subjects during treatment or during follow-up after treatment cessation.

The adverse reaction profile in a study that compared peginterferon alfa-2b/weight-based ribavirin combination with peginterferon alfa-2b/flat-dose ribavirin regimen revealed an increased rate of anemia with weight-based dosing (29% vs 19% for weight-based vs flat-dose regimens, respectively). However, the majority of cases of anemia were mild and responded to dose reductions. There was a similar incidence of serious adverse reactions reported for the weight-based group (12%) and with the flat-dose regimen. Dose modifications because of adverse reactions occurred more frequently in the weight-based group compared with the flat-dose group (29% and 23%, respectively). There was a 23% to 24% incidence overall for injection-site reactions or inflammation in the weight-based/flat-dose trial.

➤*Mortality:* There have been 31 subject deaths that occurred during treatment or during follow-up in these clinical trials. In the monotherapy trial, there was 1 suicide in a subject receiving peginterferon alfa-2b and 2 deaths among subjects receiving interferon alfa-2b (1 murder/suicide and 1 sudden death). In a combination therapy study, there was 1 suicide in a subject receiving peginterferon alfa-2b/ribavirin, and 1 subject death in the interferon alfa-2b/ribavirin group (motor vehicle accident). In the weight-based/flat-dose trial, there were 14 deaths, 2 of which were probable suicides and 1 being an unexplained death in a person with a relevant medical history of depression. In the combination therapy trial using interferon alfa-2b as the comparator, there were 12 deaths, 6 of which occurred in subjects who received peginterferon alfa-2b/ribavirin combination therapy, 5 in the peginterferon alfa-2b 1.5 mcg/ribavirin arm (n = 1,019) and 1 in the peginterferon alfa-2b 1 mcg/ribavirin arm (n = 1,016), and 6 of which occurred in subjects receiving peginterferon alfa-2a/ribavirin tablets (n = 1,035). There were 3 suicides that occurred during the off-treatment follow-up period in subjects who received peginterferon alfa-2b (1.5 mcg/kg)/ribavirin combination therapy.

➤*Common adverse reactions:* More than 96% of all subjects in clinical trials experienced 1 or more adverse reaction. The most commonly reported adverse reactions in adult subjects receiving either peginterferon alfa-2b or peginterferon alfa-2b/ribavirin were injection-site inflammation/reaction, fatigue/asthenia, headache, rigors, fevers, nausea, myalgia, and emotional liability/irritability.

Peginterferon Alfa-2b Adverse Reactions (> 5%)[a]

	Study 1		Study 2	
Adverse reaction	Peginterferon alfa-2b 1 mcg/kg (n = 297)	Interferon alfa-2b 3 million units (n = 303)	Peginterferon alfa-2b (1.5 mcg/kg)/ribavirin capsules (n = 511)	Interferon alfa-2b/ribavirin capsules (n = 505)
CNS				
Agitation	2%	2%	8%	5%
Anxiety/Emotional lability/Irritability	28%	34%	47%	47%
Concentration impaired	10%	8%	17%	21%
Depression	29%	25%	31%	34%
Dizziness	12%	10%	21%	17%
Fatigue/Asthenia	52%	54%	66%	63%
Headache	56%	52%	62%	58%
Insomnia	23%	23%	40%	41%
Malaise	7%	6%	4%	6%
Nervousness	4%	3%	6%	6%
Rigors	23%	19%	48%	41%
Dermatologic				
Alopecia	22%	22%	36%	32%
Dry skin	11%	9%	24%	23%
Flushing	6%	3%	4%	3%
Pruritus	12%	8%	29%	28%
Rash	6%	7%	24%	23%
Sweating increased	6%	7%	11%	7%
GI				
Abdominal pain	15%	11%	13%	13%
Anorexia	20%	17%	32%	27%
Constipation	1%	3%	5%	5%
Diarrhea	18%	16%	22%	17%
Dry mouth	6%	7%	12%	8%
Dyspepsia	6%	7%	9%	8%
Nausea	26%	20%	43%	33%
Vomiting	7%	6%	14%	12%
Hematologic				
Anemia	0%	0%	12%	17%
Leukopenia	< 1%	0%	6%	5%
Neutropenia	6%	2%	26%	14%

PEGINTERFERON ALFA-2b — INJECTION

Peginterferon Alfa-2b Adverse Reactions (> 5%)[a]				
	Study 1		Study 2	
Adverse reaction	Peginterferon alfa-2b 1 mcg/kg (n = 297)	Interferon alfa-2b 3 million units (n = 303)	Peginterferon alfa-2b (1.5 mcg/kg)/ ribavirin capsules (n = 511)	Interferon alfa-2b/ ribavirin capsules (n = 505)
Thrombocytopenia	7%	< 1%	5%	2%
Musculoskeletal				
Arthralgia	23%	27%	34%	28%
Musculoskeletal pain	28%	22%	21%	19%
Myalgia	54%	53%	56%	50%
Respiratory				
Coughing	8%	5%	23%	16%
Dyspnea	4%	2%	26%	24%
Pharyngitis	10%	7%	12%	13%
Rhinitis	2%	2%	8%	6%
Sinusitis	7%	7%	6%	5%
Special senses				
Conjunctivitis	4%	2%	4%	5%
Taste perversion	< 1%	2%	9%	4%
Vision blurred	2%	3%	5%	6%
Miscellaneous				
Chest pain	6%	4%	8%	7%
Fever	22%	12%	46%	33%
Hepatomegaly	6%	5%	4%	4%
Hypothyroidism	5%	3%	5%	4%
Infection, fungal	< 1%	3%	6%	1%
Infection, viral	11%	10%	12%	12%
Injection-site inflammation/ reaction	47%	20%	75%	49%
Menstrual disorder	4%	3%	7%	6%
Right upper quadrant pain	8%	8%	12%	6%
Weight loss	11%	13%	29%	20%

[a] Patients reporting 1 or more adverse reaction. A patient may have reported more than 1 adverse reaction within a body system/organ class category.

Peginterferon Alfa-2b Adverse Reactions (≥ 10%)			
Adverse reaction	Peginterferon alfa-2b 1.5 mcg/kg with ribavirin (n = 1,019)	Peginterferon alfa-2b 1 mcg/kg with ribavirin (n = 1,016)	Peginterferon alfa-2a 180 mcg with ribavirin tablets (n = 1,035)
CNS			
Anxiety	11%	11%	10%
Depression	25%	19%	20%
Dizziness	16%	14%	13%
Fatigue	67%	68%	64%
Headache	50%	47%	41%
Insomnia	38%	37%	41%
Irritability	25%	25%	25%
Dermatologic			
Alopecia	23%	20%	17%
Dry skin	11%	11%	12%
Rash	29%	25%	34%
GI			
Abdominal pain	10%	10%	10%
Anorexia	29%	25%	21%
Diarrhea	15%	16%	14%
Nausea	40%	35%	34%
Vomiting	12%	10%	9%
Hematologic			
Anemia	35%	30%	34%
Leukopenia	9%	7%	10%
Neutropenia	26%	19%	31%
Musculoskeletal			
Arthralgia	21%	22%	22%
Myalgia	27%	26%	22%
Respiratory			
Cough	15%	16%	17%
Dyspnea	21%	20%	22%
Miscellaneous			
Chills	39%	36%	23%
Injection-site reactions	34%	35%	23%
Pyrexia	35%	32%	21%
Pruritus	18%	15%	19%
Influenza-like illness	16%	15%	15%
Weight decreased	13%	10%	10%
Unspecified pain	12%	13%	9%

➤*Serious adverse reactions:* Serious adverse reactions have occurred in approximately 12% of subjects in clinical trials with peginterferon alfa-2b with or without ribavirin. The most common serious events occurring in subjects treated with peginterferon alfa-2b and ribavirin were depression and suicidal ideation, each occurring at a frequency of less than 1%. The most common fatal events occurring in subjects treated with peginterferon alfa-2b and ribavirin were cardiac arrest, suicidal ideation, and suicide attempt, all occurring in less than 1% of subjects. Individual serious adverse reactions occurred at a frequency of 1% or less.

In the peginterferon alfa-2b monotherapy trial, the incidence of serious adverse reactions was similar (approximately 12%) in all treatment groups. In the peginterferon alfa-2b/ribavirin capsules trial, the incidence of serious adverse reactions was 17% in the peginterferon alfa-2b/ribavirin capsules groups, compared with 14% in the interferon alfa-2b/ribavirin capsules group.

In many but not all cases, adverse reactions resolved after dose reduction or discontinuation of therapy. Some patients experienced ongoing or new serious adverse reactions during the 6-month follow-up period.

Individual serious adverse reactions in clinical trials comparing peginterferon alfa-2b and ribavirin with interferon alfa-2b and ribavirin occurred at a frequency of 1% or less and included the following.

Cardiovascular – Angina, cardiomyopathy, MI, pericardial effusion, supraventricular arrhythmias, transient ischemic attack, vasculitis (1% or less).

CNS – Aggressive reaction, loss of consciousness, nerve palsy (eg, facial, oculomotor), psychosis, relapse of drug addiction/overdose, severe depression, suicidal ideation, suicide attempt (1% or less).

Dermatologic – Aggravated psoriasis, injection-site necrosis, phototoxicity, urticaria (1% or less).

Hematologic – Autoimmune thrombocytopenia with or without purpura, neutropenia (1% or less).

Metabolic – Gout, hyperglycemia, hyperthyroidism, hypothyroidism (1% or less).

Respiratory – Bronchiolitis obliterans, emphysema, pleural effusion (1% or less).

Special senses – Blindness, decreased visual acuity, optic neuritis, retinal artery or vein thrombosis, retinal ischemia (1% or less).

Miscellaneous – Gastroenteritis, infection (eg, abscess, cellulitis, pneumonia, sepsis), interstitial nephritis, lupus-like syndrome, pancreatitis, rheumatoid arthritis, sarcoidosis (1% or less).

➤*Children:* In general, the adverse reaction profile in children was similar to that observed in adults.

The majority of adverse reactions reported in the study were mild or moderate in severity. Severe adverse reactions were reported in 7% of all subjects and included pyrexia (4%), injection-site pain (1%), pain in extremity (1%), headache (1%), and neutropenia (1%). Important adverse reactions that occurred in this subject population were nervousness (7%), aggression (3%), anger (2%), and depression (1%). Five subjects received levothyroxine treatment, 3 with clinical hyperthyroidism and 2 with asymptomatic TSH elevations.

Dose modifications were required in 25% of subjects, most commonly for anemia, neutropenia, and weight loss. Two (2% [2/107]) subjects discontinued therapy as the result of an adverse reaction.

PEGINTERFERON ALFA-2b — INJECTION

Peginterferon Alfa-2b Adverse Reactions in Children (≥ 10%)	
Adverse reaction	Peginterferon alfa-2b in children (n = 107)
CNS	
Asthenia	15%
Dizziness	14%
Fatigue	30%
Headache	62%
Irritability	14%
Dermatologic	
Alopecia	17%
GI	
Abdominal pain	21%
Abdominal pain, upper	12%
Nausea	18%
Vomiting	27%
Hematologic	
Anemia	11%
Leukopenia	10%
Neutropenia	33%
Metabolic/Nutritional	
Anorexia	29%
Decreased appetite	22%
Weight decreased	19%
Musculoskeletal	
Arthralgia	17%
Myalgia	17%
Miscellaneous	
Chills	21%
Injection-site erythema	29%
Pyrexia	80%

➤*Lab test abnormalities:* Changes in selected laboratory values during treatment with peginterferon alone or in combination with ribavirin treatment are described. Decreases in hemoglobin, neutrophils, and platelets may require dose reduction or permanent discontinuation from therapy.

Hemoglobin – Hemoglobin levels decreased to less than 11 g/dL in approximately 30% of patients in the combination study using interferon alfa 2b/ribavirin as the comparator. Dose modification was required in 9% and 13% of patients in the peginterferon alfa-2b/ribavirin capsule and interferon alfa-2b/ribavirin capsule groups, respectively. In the weight-based/flat-dose study, 47% of subjects receiving weight-based ribavirin and 33% on flat-dose ribavirin had decreases in hemoglobin levels of less than 11 g/dL. Reductions in hemoglobin to less than 9 g/dL occurred more frequently in subjects receiving weight-based compared with flat dosing (4% and 2%, respectively). In the combination study using peginterferon alfa-2a/ribavirin as the comparator, patients receiving peginterferon alfa-2b 1.5 mcg/kg/ribavirin had decreases in hemoglobin levels to between 8.5 to less than 10 mg/dL (28%) and less than 8.5 mg/dL (3%), whereas in patients receiving peginterferon alfa-2a 180 mcg/ribavirin, these decreases occurred in 26% and 4% of patients, respectively. Hemoglobin levels become stable by treatment weeks 4 to 6 on average. The typical pattern observed was a decrease in hemoglobin levels by treatment week 4, followed by stabilization and a plateau, which was maintained to the end of treatment. In the peginterferon monotherapy trial, hemoglobin decreases were generally mild and dose modifications were rarely necessary.

Neutrophils – Decreases in neutrophil counts were observed in a majority of patients treated with peginterferon alfa-2b alone (70%) or as combination therapy with ribavirin capsules (85%) and interferon alfa-2b/ribavarin capsules (60%) in combination study. Severe and potentially life-threatening neutropenia (less than 0.5×10^9/L) occurred in 1% of patients treated with peginterferon alfa-2b monotherapy, 2% of patients treated with interferon alfa-2b/ribavirin capsules, and in 4% of patients treated with peginterferon alfa-2b/ribavirin capsules. Two percent of patients receiving peginterferon alfa-2b monotherapy and 18% of patients receiving peginterferon alfa-2b/ribavirin capsules required modification of interferon dosage. Few patients (1% or less) required permanent discontinuation of treatment. Neutrophil counts generally return to pretreatment levels within 4 weeks of cessation of therapy.

Platelets – Platelet counts decrease to less than 100,000/mm^3 in approximately 20% of patients treated with peginterferon alfa-2b alone or with ribavirin capsules and in 6% of patients treated with interferon alfa-2b/ribavirin capsules. Severe decreases in platelet counts (less than 50,000/mm^3) occur in less than 4% of patients. Patients may require discontinuation or dose modification as a result of platelet decreases. In the peginterferon alfa-2b/ribavirin capsules combination therapy trial, 1% or 3% of patients required dose modification of interferon alfa-2b or peginterferon alfa-2b, respectively. Platelet counts generally returned to pretreatment levels within 4 weeks of the cessation of therapy.

Triglycerides – Elevated triglyceride levels have been observed in patients treated with interferon alphas, including peginterferon alfa-2b.

Thyroid function – Development of TSH abnormalities, with and without clinical manifestations, is associated with interferon therapies. Clinically apparent thyroid disorders occur among patients treated with either interferon alfa-2b or peginterferon alfa-2b (with or without ribavirin capsules) at a similar incidence (5% for hypothyroidism and 3% for hyperthyroidism). Subjects developed new-onset TSH abnormalities while on treatment and during the follow-up period. At the end of the follow-up period, 7% of subjects still had abnormal TSH values.

Bilirubin and uric acid – In the peginterferon alfa-2b/ribavirin capsules trial using interferon alfa-2a as the comparator, 10% to 14% of patients developed hyperbilirubinemia and 33% to 38% developed hyperuricemia in association with hemolysis. Six patients developed mild to moderate gout.

Children – Decreases in hemoglobin, white blood cells, platelets, and neutrophils may require dose reduction or permanent discontinuation from therapy. Changes in selected laboratory values during treatment of 107 children with peginterferon alfa-2b are described. Most of the changes in laboratory values in this study were mild or moderate.

Selected Hematological Abnormalities During Treatment Phase With Peginterferon Alfa-2b Plus Ribavirin in Previously Untreated Children	
Laboratory parameter[a]	Peginterferon alfa-2b + ribavirin (N = 107)
Hemoglobin (g/dL)	
9.5 to < 11	30%
8 to < 9.5	2%
WBC (× 10⁹/L)	
2 to 2.9	39%
1.5 to < 2	3%
Platelets (× 10⁹/L)	
70 to 100	1%
50 to < 70	—
25 to < 50	1%
Neutrophils	
1 to 1.5	35%
0.75 to < 1	26%
0.5 to < 0.75	13%
< 0.5	3%
Total bilirubin	
1.26 to 2.59 × ULN[b]	7%
Evidence of hepatic failure	—

[a] The table summarizes the worst category observed within the period per subject per laboratory test. Only subjects with at least one treatment value for a given laboratory test are included.
[b] ULN = upper limit of normal.

➤*Postmarketing:*

Cardiovascular – Palpitations, hypertension, hypotension.

CNS – Asthenic conditions (including asthenia, malaise, fatigue), homicidal ideation, memory loss, migraine headache, paresthesia, peripheral neuropathy, seizures, vertigo.

Dermatologic – Erythema multiforme, psoriasis, Stevens-Johnson syndrome, toxic epidermal necrolysis.

Endocrine – Diabetic ketoacidosis, diabetes.

GU – Renal failure, renal insufficiency.

Hematologic/Lymphatic – Pure red cell aplasia, thrombotic thrombocytopenic purpura.

Hypersensitivity – Cases of acute hypersensitivity reactions (including anaphylaxis, angioedema, urticaria).

Metabolic – Dehydration, hypertriglyceridemia.

Musculoskeletal – Myositis, rhabdomyolysis.

Special senses – Hearing impairment, hearing loss, serous retinal detachment, Vogt-Koyanagi-Harada syndrome.

Miscellaneous – Aphthous stomatitis, pulmonary hypertension, systemic lupus erythematosus, bacterial infection including sepsis.

Overdosage

➤*Symptoms:* There is limited experience with overdosage. In clinical studies, a few patients accidentally received a dose greater than that prescribed. There were no instances in which a participant in the monotherapy or combination therapy trials received more than 10.5 times the intended dose of peginterferon alfa-2b. The maximum dose received by any patient was 3.45 mcg/kg weekly over a period of approximately 12 weeks. The maximum known overdosage of ribavirin capsules was an intentional ingestion of 10 g (fifty 200 mg capsules). There were no serious reactions attributed to these overdosages.

PEGINTERFERON ALFA-2b — INJECTION

➤*Treatment:* In cases of overdosing, symptomatic treatment and close observation of the patient are recommended.

Patient Information

Instruct the patient to self-inject only if it has been determined that it is appropriate and the patient agrees to medical follow-up as necessary and training in proper injection technique has been given.

Direct patients receiving peginterferon alfa-2b alone or in combination with ribavirin capsules in its appropriate use, inform them of the benefits and risks associated with treatment, and refer them to the Medication Guide.

Advise patients to use a puncture-resistant container for the disposal of used syringes, needles, and the *Redipen*. Thoroughly instruct patients in the importance of proper disposal, and caution them against any reuse of needles, syringes, or the *Redipen*. Instruct patients to dispose of the full container in accordance with state and local laws.

Inform patients that there are no data evaluating whether peginterferon alfa-2b therapy will prevent transmission of HCV infection to others. Also, it is not known if treatment with peginterferon alfa-2b will cure hepatitis C, or prevent cirrhosis, liver failure, or liver cancer that may result from infection with HCV.

Advise patients that laboratory evaluations are required before starting therapy and periodically thereafter. It is advised that patients be well-hydrated, especially during the initial stages of treatment. Flu-like symptoms associated with administration of peginterferon alfa-2b may be minimized by bedtime administration or by use of antipyretics.

Inform patients that ribavirin may cause birth defects and/or death of the fetus. Extreme care must be taken to avoid pregnancy in women and in female partners of men during treatment with combination peginterferon alfa-2b/ribavirin capsules therapy and for 6 months posttherapy. Do not initiate combination peginterferon alfa-2b/ribavirin capsule therapy until a report of a negative pregnancy test has been obtained immediately prior to initiation of therapy. It is recommended that patients undergo monthly pregnancy tests during therapy and for 6 months posttherapy.

Advise patients to brush their teeth thoroughly twice daily and to have regular dental examinations. If vomiting occurs, advise patients to rinse our their mouth thoroughly afterwards.

INTERFERON ALFACON-1

Rx	**Infergen** (Three Rivers Pharmaceuticals)	**Injection, solution:** 9 mcg per 0.3 mL	Preservative free. In 0.3 mL single-dose vials.[a]
		15 mcg per 0.5 mL	Preservative free. In 0.5 mL single-dose vials.[a]

[a] With sodium chloride 5.9 mg/mL and sodium phosphate 3.8 mg/mL.

INTERFERON ALFACON-1 — INJECTION

WARNING

Fatal or life-threatening disorders – Alpha interferons, including interferon alfacon-1, may cause or aggravate fatal or life-threatening neuropsychiatric, autoimmune, ischemic, and infectious disorders.

Monitor patients closely with periodic clinical and laboratory evaluations. Patients with persistently severe or worsening symptoms of these conditions should be withdrawn from therapy. In many but not all cases, these disorders resolve after stopping interferon alfacon-1 therapy.

Use with ribavirin – Ribavirin may cause birth defects and/or death of the fetus. Extreme care must be taken to avoid pregnancy in female patients and in female partners of male patients. Ribavirin causes hemolytic anemia. The anemia associated with ribavirin therapy may result in a worsening of cardiac disease. Ribavirin is genotoxic and mutagenic and should be considered a potential carcinogen.

Indications

➤*Chronic hepatitis C:* For the treatment of chronic hepatitis C virus (HCV) infection in patients 18 years of age and older with compensated liver disease.

Administration and Dosage

➤*Adults:*

Chronic hepatitis C –

Usual dosage:

• *Monotherapy* – 9 mcg 3 times per week subcutaneously as a single injection for 24 weeks.

• *Depression* –

Interferon Alfacon-1/Ribavirin Dosage Modifications in Patients With Depression

Depression severity[a]	Initial management (4 to 8 weeks)		
	Dose modification		Visit schedule
Mild	No change to interferon alfacon-1 dose or ribavirin dose.		Evaluate once weekly by visit and/or phone.
Moderate	Decrease interferon alfacon-1 dose from 15 to 9 mcg or from 9 to 6 mcg; no change to ribavirin dose.		Evaluate once weekly (office visit at least every other week).
Severe	Discontinue interferon alfacon-1 and ribavirin permanently.		Not applicable.
Depression severity[a]	Depression		
	Remains stable	Improves	Improves
Mild	Continue weekly visit schedule.	Resume normal visit schedule.	(See moderate or severe depression.)
Moderate	Consider psychiatric consultation. Continue reduced dosing.	If symptoms improve and are stable for 4 weeks, may resume normal visit schedule. Continue reduced interferon alfacon-1 dosing or return to normal interferon alfacon-1 dose.	(See severe depression.)
Severe	Psychiatric therapy necessary.	Not applicable.	Not applicable.

[a] See *Diagnostic and Statistical Manual of Mental Disorders* (Fourth Edition) (*DSM-IV*) for definitions.

Nonresponders/Relapse: 15 mcg 3 times per week subcutaneously as a single injection for up to 48 weeks.

Combination therapy with ribavirin: 15 mcg daily subcutaneously in combination with weight-based ribavirin at 1,000 to 1,200 mg (less than 75 kg and at least 75 kg) orally in 2 divided doses for up to 48 weeks.

➤*Renal function impairment:* Interferon alfacon-1/ribavirin should not be used in patients with creatinine clearance (CrCl) less than 50 mL/min.

➤*Hepatic function impairment:* Contraindicated in patients with hepatic decompensation (Child Pugh score more than 5) and/or autoimmune hepatitis.

➤*Dosage adjustment:* If a serious adverse reaction develops during the course of treatment, discontinue or modify the dosage of interferon alfacon-1 and/or ribavirin until the adverse reaction abates or decreases in severity. If persistent or recurrent serious adverse reactions develop despite adequate dosage adjustment, discontinue treatment. Upon resolution or improvement of the adverse reaction, resuming interferon alfacon-1 and/or ribavirin may be considered.

Monotherapy – Dosage reduction to 7.5 mcg may be necessary following a serious adverse reaction. If serious adverse reactions continue to occur, dosing should be interrupted or discontinued, because the efficacy of lower doses has not been established.

Combination therapy with ribavirin:

• *Serious adverse reactions* – Stepwise dose reduction from 15 to 9 mcg and from 9 to 6 mcg may be necessary for serious adverse reactions.

INTERFERON ALFACON-1 — INJECTION

• *Hematologic toxicities –*

Interferon Alfacon-1/ Ribavirin Dosage Modification for Patients with Hematologic Toxicities	
Laboratory value	Action
ANC[a] < 0.75 × 10^9/L	Reduce interferon alfacon-1 dose from 15 to 9 mcg, or from 9 to 6 mcg; maintain ribavirin dose at 1,200 or 1,000 mg.
ANC < 50 × 10^9/L	Interferon alfacon-1 and ribavirin treatment should be suspended until ANC values return to more than 1,000/mm³.
Platelet count < 50 × 10^9/L	Reduce interferon alfacon-1 dose from 15 to 9 mcg or from 9 to 6 mcg; maintain ribavirin dose at 1,200 or 1,000 mg.
Platelet count < 25 × 10^9/L	Interferon alfacon-1 and ribavirin treatment should be discontinued.

[a] ANC = absolute neutrophil count.

• *Anemia –*

Interferon Alfacon-1/Ribavirin Dosage Modification for Patients With Anemia[a]		
Condition	Interferon alfacon-1	Ribavirin
Hgb[b] < 10 g/dL	History of cardiac or cerebrovascular disease, reduce dose of interferon alfacon-1.	Adjust dose.[c]
Hgb < 8.5 g/dL	Permanently discontinue.	Permanently discontinue.

[a] For adult patients with a history of stable cardiac disease receiving interferon alfacon-1 in combination with ribavirin, the interferon alfacon-1 dose should be reduced from 15 to 9 mcg or 9 to 6 mcg and the ribavirin dose by 200 mg/day if a decrease more than 2 g/dL in hemoglobin is observed during any 4-week period. Both interferon alfacon-1 and ribavirin should be permanently discontinued if patients have hemoglobin levels less than 12 g/dL after this ribavirin dose reduction.
[b] Hgb = hemoglobin.
[c] The first dose reduction of ribavirin is by 200 mg/day. The second dose reduction of ribavirin (if needed) is by an additional 200 mg/day.

➤*Discontinuation of therapy:* Patients who fail to achieve at least a 2 $\log_{10}$ drop for at least 12 weeks or undetectable HCV RNA at week 24 are highly unlikely to achieve sustained viral response and discontinuation of therapy should be considered.

➤*Preparation for administration:* Just prior to injection, interferon alfacon-1 may be allowed to reach room temperature. Use only 1 vial per dose; do not re-enter the vial. Discard unused portions. Do not save unused drug for later administration.

➤*Administration:* Administer undiluted by subcutaneous injection. Avoid vigorous shaking.

When interferon alfacon-1 is administered in combination therapy, ribavirin should be taken with food.

➤*Storage/Stability:* Store vials in the refrigerator at 2° to 8°C (36° to 46°F). Do not freeze. Avoid exposure to direct sunlight.

Actions

➤*Pharmacology:* Interferon alfacon-1, a recombinant hybrid protein based on the consensus amino acid sequence of naturally occurring human type-1 interferon alphas, is an inducer of the innate antiviral immune response. Type-1 interferons are a family of small protein molecules with molecular weights of 15,000 to 21,000 Da that are produced and secreted by cells in response to viral infections or to various synthetic and biological inducers. Interferons do not act directly on the virus but bind to the interferon cell-surface receptor leading to the production of several interferon-stimulated gene products. Interferons induce pleiotropic biological responses, which include antiviral, antiproliferative, and immunomodulatory effects, regulation of cell surface major histocompatibility antigen (HLA [human leukocyte antigen] class I and class II) expression and regulation of cytokine expression.

➤*Pharmacokinetics:*

Absorption – Analysis of interferon alfacon-1–induced cellular products (induction of 2′5′-oligoadenylate synthetase (OAS) and beta-2 microglobulin) after treatment in these subjects revealed a statistically significant, dose-related increase in the area under the curve for the levels of 2′5′-OAS or beta-2 microglobulin induced over time. Concentrations of 2′5′-OAS were maximal at 24 hours after dosing, while serum levels of beta-2 microglobulin appeared to reach a maximum 24 to 36 hours after dosing. The dose-response relationships observed for 2′5′-OAS and beta-2 microglobulin were indicative of biological activity after subcutaneous administration of 1 to 9 mcg of interferon alfacon-1.

Special populations –

Renal function impairment: Patients with CrCl less than 50 mL/min should not be treated with ribavirin.

Contraindications

Hepatic decompensation (Child-Pugh score of more than 5 [class B and C]); autoimmune hepatitis; known hypersensitivity to interferon alphas or to any component of the product.

Warnings/Precautions

➤*CNS effects:* Severe psychiatric adverse reactions may manifest in patients receiving therapy with alpha interferons, including interferon alfacon-1. Depression, suicidal ideation, suicide attempt, suicide, and homicidal ideation may occur. Use interferon alfacon-1 with caution in patients who report a history of depression; monitor all patients for evidence of depression and other psychiatric symptoms. Inform patients of the possible development of depression prior to initiation of interferon alfacon-1 therapy, and instruct patients to report any sign or symptom of depression and/or suicidal ideation immediately. Other prominent psychiatric adverse reactions may also occur, including abnormal thinking, aggressive behavior, agitation, anxiety, apathy, emotional lability, nervousness, psychosis, and relapse of drug addiction. If patients develop psychiatric problems, including clinical depression, carefully monitor patients during treatment and in the 6-month follow-up period. If psychiatric symptoms persist or worsen or suicidal ideation or aggressive behavior toward others are identified, discontinue treatment with interferon alfacon-1, and follow the patient with psychiatric intervention as appropriate. In severe cases, stop interferon alfacon-1 immediately and institute psychiatric intervention.

➤*Cardiovascular effects:* Cardiovascular events, including angina pectoris, arrhythmia, cardiomyopathy, hypotension, myocardial infarction (MI), and tachycardia, have been observed. Administer with caution to patients with cardiovascular disease. Closely monitor patients with a history of MI and arrhythmic disorder. Do not treat patients with a history of significant or unstable cardiac disease with interferon alfacon-1/ribavirin combination therapy.

➤*Pulmonary effects:* Bronchiolitis obliterans, dyspnea, interstitial pneumonitis, pneumonia, pulmonary hypertension, pulmonary infiltrates, and sarcoidosis, some resulting in respiratory failure and/or death, may be induced or aggravated by interferon alpha therapy, including interferon alfacon-1. Discontinue interferon alfacon-1 treatment in patients who develop persistent or unexplained pulmonary infiltrates or pulmonary impairment. Recurrence of respiratory failure has been observed with interferon rechallenge. Suspend interferon alfacon-1 treatment in patients who develop pulmonary infiltrates or pulmonary impairment. Closely monitor patients who resume interferon treatment.

➤*Hepatic failure:* Chronic hepatitis C patients with cirrhosis may be at risk of hepatic decompensation when treated with interferon alphas, including interferon alfacon-1. During treatment, closely monitor patient clinical status and hepatic function, and immediately discontinue interferon alfacon-1 treatment if symptoms of hepatic decompensation, such as jaundice, ascites, coagulopathy, or decreased serum albumin, are observed.

➤*Renal effects:* Increases in serum creatinine levels, including renal failure, have been observed. Interferon alfacon-1 has not been studied in patients with renal insufficiency. It is recommended that renal function be evaluated in all patients starting interferon alfacon-1 alone or with ribavirin therapy. Closely monitor patients with impaired renal function for signs and symptoms of interferon toxicity, including increases in serum creatinine. Do not use combination treatment with interferon alfacon-1/ribavirin in patients with CrCl less than 50 mL/min.

➤*Cerebrovascular disorders:* Ischemic and hemorrhagic cerebrovascular events have been observed in patients treated with interferon alpha–based therapies, including interferon alfacon-1. Events occurred in patients with few or no reported risk factors for stroke, including patients younger than 45 years of age. Because these are spontaneous reports, estimates of frequency cannot be made and a causal relationship between interferon alpha–based therapies and these events is difficult to establish.

➤*Bone marrow toxicity:* Alpha interferons suppress bone marrow function and may result in severe cytopenias including aplastic anemia. It is advised that CBCs be obtained pretreatment and monitored routinely during therapy. Discontinue interferon alfacon-1 therapy in patients who develop severe decreases in neutrophil (less than 0.5 × 10^9/L) or platelet counts (less than 25 × 10^9/L).

Cautiously use interferon alfacon-1 in patients with abnormally low peripheral blood cell counts or who are receiving agents that are known to cause myelosuppression. Use caution when treating transplantation patients or other chronically immunosuppressed patients with interferon alpha therapy.

➤*Colitis:* Hemorrhagic/ischemic colitis, sometimes fatal, has been observed within 12 weeks of interferon alpha therapies and has been reported in patients treated with interferon alfacon-1. Immediately discontinue interferon alfacon-1 treatment in patients who develop signs and symptoms of colitis.

➤*Pancreatitis:* Pancreatitis, sometimes fatal, has been observed in patients treated with interferon alphas, including interferon alfacon-1. Suspend interferon alfacon-1 in patients with signs and symptoms suggestive of pancreatitis and discontinue in patients diagnosed with pancreatitis.

➤*Autoimmune disease:* Development or exacerbation of autoimmune disorders (eg, autoimmune thrombocytopenia, idiopathic thrombocytopenic purpura, psoriasis, rheumatoid arthritis, thyroiditis, interstitial nephritis, systemic lupus erythematosus) has been reported in patients receiving interferon alpha therapies, including interferon alfacon-1. Do not use interferon alfacon-1 in patients with autoimmune hepatitis and use with caution in patients with other autoimmune disorders.

➤*Ophthalmologic disorders:* Decrease or loss of vision, retinopathy including macular edema, retinal artery or vein thrombosis, retinal hemorrhages and cotton wool spots, optic neuritis, papilledema, and serious retinal detachment are induced or aggravated by treatment with interferon alfacon-1 or other alpha interferons. All patients should receive an eye

INTERFERON ALFACON-1 — INJECTION

examination at baseline. Patients with preexisting ophthalmologic disorders (eg, diabetic or hypertensive retinopathy) should receive periodic ophthalmologic exams during interferon alpha treatment. Any patient who develops ocular symptoms should receive a prompt and complete eye examination. Discontinue interferon alfacon-1 therapy in patients who develop new or worsening ophthalmologic disorders.

➤*Peripheral neuropathy:* Peripheral neuropathy has been reported when interferon alphas were given in combination with telbivudine. In 1 clinical trial, an increased risk and severity of peripheral neuropathy was observed with the combination use of telbivudine and pegylated interferon alfa-2a as compared with telbivudine alone. The safety and efficacy of telbivudine in combination with interferons for the treatment of chronic hepatitis B has not been demonstrated.

➤*Endocrine disorders:* Administer interferon alfacon-1 with caution to patients with a history of endocrine disorders. Occurrence or aggravation of hyperthyroidism or hypothyroidism have been reported with interferon alfacon-1. Hyperglycemia and diabetes mellitus have also been observed in patients treated with interferon alfacon-1. Patients who develop these conditions during treatment that cannot be controlled with medication should not continue interferon alfacon-1 therapy.

➤*Immunogenicity:* The number of subjects developing positive binding antibody responses was similar in the 9 mcg of interferon alfacon-1 (11%) and interferon alfa-2b 3 million units (15%) groups in monotherapy studies. The titer of neutralizing antibodies to interferon was not measured. Following cessation of interferon therapy, the number of subjects with a positive antibody response declined.

➤*Hypersensitivity reactions:* Serious acute hypersensitivity reactions have been reported following treatment with alpha interferons. If hypersensitivity reactions occur (eg, anaphylaxis, angioedema, bronchoconstriction, urticaria), immediately discontinue the drug and institute appropriate medical treatment.

➤*Renal function impairment:* In patients with impaired renal function, closely monitor signs and symptoms of interferon toxicity and adjust the interferon alfacon-1 dose. Do not administer interferon alfacon-1/ribavirin to patients with CrCl less than 50 mL/min.

➤*Hepatic function impairment:* See Contraindications for more information.

➤*Special risk:* The safety and efficacy of interferon alfacon-1, alone or in combination with ribavirin, for the treatment of chronic HCV infection in liver or other organ transplant recipients or in patients coinfected with HIV or HBV have not been evaluated.

➤*Pregnancy: Category C.* Interferon alfacon-1 has been shown to have embryolethal or abortifacient effects in golden Syrian hamsters when given at doses of more than 150 mcg/kg/day (135 times the human dose) and in cynomolgus and rhesus monkeys when given at doses of 3 mcg/kg/day and 10 mcg/kg/day (9 to 81 times the human dose), respectively (based on body surface area), the human dose. There are no adequate and well-controlled studies in pregnant women. Interferon alfacon-1 should not be used during pregnancy. If a woman becomes pregnant or plans to become pregnant while taking interferon alfacon-1, she should be informed of the potential hazards to the fetus. Advise men and women treated with interferon alfacon-1 to use effective contraception.

➤*Lactation:* It is not known whether interferon alfacon-1 is excreted in human milk. Because many drugs are excreted in human milk, exercise caution if interferon alfacon-1 is administered to a breast-feeding woman. The effect of oral interferon alfacon-1 in breast milk on the breast-feeding neonate has not been evaluated. Interferon alfa, a closely related drug, is excreted in breast-milk in low amounts and is considered to be compatible with breast-feeding according to the American Academy of Pediatrics. Any interferon in breast-milk is most likely destroyed in the infant's (except neonates) GI tract and not absorbed.

➤*Children:* The safety and effectiveness of interferon alfacon-1 has not been established in patients younger than 18 years of age and is not recommended in children.

➤*Elderly:* Treatment with interferons, including interferon alfacon-1, is associated with psychiatric, cardiac, and systemic (flu-like) adverse reactions. Because decreased hepatic, renal, or cardiac function; concomitant disease; and the use of other drug therapies in elderly patients may produce adverse reactions of greater severity, exercise caution in the use of interferon alfacon-1 and interferon alfacon-1/ribavirin in this population.

➤*Monitoring:* Monitor patient's clinical status closely. Laboratory tests (eg, hepatic function tests, renal function tests, CBCs, lipid panel, thyroid function tests) are recommended for all patients, prior to beginning treatment, 2 weeks after initiation of therapy, and periodically thereafter during the 24 or 48 weeks of therapy. Following completion of therapy, periodically monitor any abnormal test values.

The entrance criteria that were used for the clinical study may be considered as a guideline to acceptable baseline values for initiation of treatment: Platelet count of at least 75×10^9/L; hemoglobin concentration at least 100 g/L; ANC of at least 1,500 $\times 10^6$/L; serum creatinine concentration less than 180 mcmol/L (less than 2 mg/dL) or CrCl greater than 0.83 mL/second (greater than 50 mL/min); serum albumin concentration at least 25 g/L; bilirubin within normal limits; thyroid stimulating hormone and T_4 within normal limits.

Patients who have preexisting cardiac abnormalities (eg, arrhythmic disorders, MI) should have an electrocardiogram before treatment and periodically during treatment. Monitor all patients for evidence of depression and other psychiatric symptoms. If patients develop psychiatric problems, monitor carefully during treatment and during the 6 month follow-up period. Monitor all patients for signs and symptoms of colitis, pancreatitis, and/or hypersensitivity reactions. All patients should have an eye exam at baseline. Patients with preexisting ophthalmologic disorders (eg, diabetic or hypertensive retinopathy) should receive periodic ophthalmologic exams.

Drug Interactions

No formal drug interaction studies have been conducted with interferon alfacon-1. Use caution when administering with other agents known to cause myelosuppression.

Adverse Reactions

➤*Monotherapy:*

Most frequent adverse reactions – Flu-like symptoms (eg, headache, fatigue, fever, rigors, myalgia, increased sweating, arthralgia) were the most frequently reported treatment-related adverse reactions. Most were short-lived and could be treated symptomatically.

Depression – Depression of any severity was reported in 26% of patients who received 9 mcg of interferon alfacon-1 monotherapy and was the most common adverse reaction resulting in study drug discontinuation.

Hematologic – Monotherapy of 15 mcg 3 times a week of interferon alfacon-1 as subsequent treatment was associated with a greater incidence of leukopenia and granulocytopenia. One or more dose reductions for any cause were required in up to 36% of subjects.

Adverse reactions (10% or more) –

Interferon Alfacon-1 Adverse Reactions (≥ 10%)

Adverse reactions	Initial treatment		Subsequent treatment	
	Interferon alfacon-1 9 mcg (n = 231)	Interferon alfa-2b (n = 236)	Interferon alfacon-1 15 mcg, 24 weeks (n = 165)	Interferon alfacon-1 15 mcg, 48 weeks (n = 168)
CNS				
Amnesia	10%	6%	2%	5%
Anxiety	19%	18%	9%	14%
Asthenia	9%	11%	10%	7%
Dizziness	22%	25%	18%	25%
Depression	26%	25%	18%	19%
Emotional lability	12%	11%	6%	3%
Fatigue	69%	67%	65%	71%
Headache	82%	83%	78%	80%
Hypoesthesia	10%	8%	8%	10%
Insomnia	39%	30%	24%	28%
Malaise	11%	10%	2%	5%
Nervousness	31%	29%	16%	22%
Paresthesia	13%	10%	9%	9%
Thinking abnormal	8%	12%	10%	20%
Dermatologic				
Alopecia	14%	25%	10%	13%
Pruritus	14%	14%	11%	10%
Rash	13%	15%	13%	10%
Sweating increased	12%	11%	13%	11%
GI				
Abdominal pain	41%	40%	24%	32%
Anorexia	24%	17%	21%	14%
Diarrhea	29%	24%	24%	22%
Dyspepsia	21%	18%	12%	10%
Nausea	40%	36%	30%	36%
Vomiting	12%	11%	13%	11%
Musculoskeletal				
Arthralgia	51%	44%	43%	46%
Back pain	42%	37%	29%	23%
Limb pain	26%	25%	13%	23%
Myalgia	58%	56%	51%	55%
Neck pain	14%	13%	8%	5%
Rigors	57%	45%	62%	66%
Skeletal pain	14%	14%	10%	12%
Respiratory				
Cough	22%	17%	12%	11%
Dyspnea	7%	12%	8%	7%
Pharyngitis	34%	31%	17%	21%
Sinusitis	17%	22%	12%	16%

INTERFERON ALFACON-1 — INJECTION

Interferon Alfacon-1 Adverse Reactions (≥ 10%)				
	Initial treatment		Subsequent treatment	
Adverse reactions	Interferon alfacon-1 9 mcg (n = 231)	Interferon alfa-2b (n = 236)	Interferon alfacon-1 15 mcg, 24 weeks (n = 165)	Interferon alfacon-1 15 mcg, 48 weeks (n = 168)
Miscellaneous				
Body pain	54%	45%	39%	51%
Chest pain	13%	14%	5%	9%
Fever	61%	45%	58%	55%
Hot flushes	13%	7%	7%	4%
Influenza-like symptoms	15%	11%	8%	8%
Injection-site erythema	23%	15%	17%	22%

➤*Lab test abnormalities:*

Hemoglobin and hematocrit – Treatment with interferon alfacon-1 alone or in combination with ribavirin was associated with decreases in mean values for hemoglobin and hematocrit. In the interferon alfacon-1 monotherapy trials, 4% and 5% of subjects had decreases in hemoglobin and hematocrit levels. Decreases from baseline of 20% or more in hemoglobin or hematocrit were seen in 1% or less of subjects.

White blood cells – Interferon alfacon-1 treatment was associated with decreases in mean values for both total white blood cell (WBC) count and ANC. By the end of initial monotherapy treatment, mean decreases from baseline of 19% for WBCs and 23% for ANC were observed. These effects reversed during the posttreatment observation period. In 2 interferon alfacon-1 monotherapy-treated patients, decreases in ANC to levels of less than 500 × 10^3 cells/mcL were seen. In both cases, the ANC returned to clinically acceptable levels with reduction of the dose of interferon alfacon-1, and were not associated with infections.

Mean decreases from baseline up to 23% for WBCs and up to 27% for ANC were observed for subjects subsequently re-treated with interferon alfacon-1 monotherapy. Two subjects experienced reversible reductions in ANC to less than 500 × 10^6 cells/L.

Platelets – Interferon alfacon-1 treatment was associated with alterations in platelet count. Decreases in mean platelet count of 16% compared with baseline were seen by the end of interferon alfacon-1 monotherapy treatment. These decreases were reversed during the posttreatment observation period. Three percent of patients had platelets decrease to less than 50 × 10^9 cells/L, which necessitated dose reduction.

Triglycerides – Mean values for serum triglycerides increased shortly after the start of administration of interferon alfacon-1 monotherapy, with increases of 41%, compared with baseline, at the end of the treatment period. Seven percent (7%) of patients developed values which were at least 3 times above pretreatment levels during treatment. This effect was reversed after discontinuation of treatment.

Thyroid function – Interferon alfacon-1 monotherapy treatment was associated with biochemical changes consistent with hypothyroidism including increases in thyroid stimulating hormone and decreases in T_4 mean values. Increases in thyroid stimulating hormone to greater than 7 million units/L were seen in 10% of interferon alfacon-1 9 mcg-treated patients either during the treatment period or the 24-week posttreatment observation period. Thyroid supplements were instituted in approximately one-third of these patients.

➤*Postmarketing:*

CNS – Ataxia, convulsions, delusions, gait abnormal, hallucinations, loss of consciousness, memory impairment, speech disorder, tremors, visual field defect.

Dermatologic – Bruising, pyoderma gangrenosum, toxic epidermal necrolysis.

GI – Abdominal distention, GI bleeding, gastritis.

Hepatic – Abnormal hepatic function; ascites; hepatic encephalopathy; hepatic enzyme elevations, including ALT and AST elevation; hyperbilirubinemia; jaundice.

Local – Injection-site reaction, including injection-site necrosis ulcer and bruising.

Musculoskeletal – Arthritis, bone pain, rhabdomyolysis.

Special senses – Hearing impairment, hearing loss.

Miscellaneous – Dehydration, hemorrhage, sepsis.

Overdosage

➤*Symptoms:* In interferon alfacon-1 trials, the maximum overdose reported was a dose of 150 mcg of interferon alfacon-1 administered subcutaneously in a patient enrolled in a phase 1 advanced malignancy trial. The patient received 10 times the prescribed dosage for 3 days. The patient experienced a mild increase in anorexia, chills, fever, and myalgia. Increases in ALT (15 to 127 units/L), AST (15 to 164 units/L), and lactic dehydrogenase (183 to 281 units/L) were reported. These laboratory values returned to normal or to the patient's baseline values within 30 days.

Patient Information

Instruct patients about appropriate use by a health care professional. Patients receiving interferon alfacon-1 alone or in combination with ribavirin must be instructed as to the proper dosage and administration, and informed of the benefits and risks associated with treatment. Information included in the Medication Guide should be reviewed fully with the patient; it is not a disclosure of all or possible adverse reactions.

Inform patients that there are no data regarding whether interferon alfacon-1 therapy will prevent transmission of HCV infection to others. Also, it is not known if treatment with interferon alfacon-1 will cure hepatitis C or prevent cirrhosis, liver failure, or liver cancer that may be the result of infection with the hepatitis C virus.

Advise patients that the most common adverse reactions are flu-like symptoms including fatigue, fever, nausea, headache, arthralgia, myalgia, rigors, and increased sweating. Nonnarcotic analgesics and bedtime administration of interferon alfacon-1 may be used to prevent or lessen some of these symptoms. Other common adverse reactions are neutropenia, insomnia, leukopenia, and depression.

Inform patients that while fever may be related to the flu-like symptoms reported in patients treated with interferon alfacon-1, when fever occurs, other possible causes of persistent fever should be ruled out.

Patients must be thoroughly instructed in the importance of proper disposal procedures and cautioned against the reuse of needles, syringes, or re-entry of the vial. A puncture-resistant container for the disposal of used syringes and needles should be used by the patient and should be disposed of according to the directions provided by the health care provider.

Advise patients that laboratory evaluations are required before starting therapy and periodically thereafter.

Inform patients it is advised that they be well hydrated, especially during the initial stages of treatment.

INTERFERON ALFA-N3 (HUMAN LEUKOCYTE DERIVED)

Rx	**Alferon N** (Hemispherx Biopharma)	**Injection:** 5 million IU/ml	8 mg NaCl, 1.74 mg Na phosphate dibasic, 0.2 mg K phosphate monobasic, 0.2 mg KCl. In 1 ml vials.

INTERFERON ALFA-N3 — INJECTION

Indications

➤*Condylomata acuminata:* For the intralesional treatment of refractory or recurring external condylomata acuminata in patients 18 years of age or older (see Administration and Dosage).

The physician should select patients for treatment with interferon alfa-n3 (human leukocyte derived) after consideration of a number of factors: The locations and sizes of the lesions, past treatment and response thereto, and the patient's ability to comply with the treatment regimen. Interferon alfa-n3 (human leukocyte derived) is particularly useful for patients who have not responded satisfactorily to other treatment modalities (eg, podophyllin resin, surgery, laser or cryotherapy).

Administration and Dosage

➤*Adults:*

Condylomata acuminata –

Usual dosage: 0.05 mL (250,000 units) per wart twice weekly.

Dosage adjustment: Moderate to severe adverse experiences may require modification of the dosage regimen, or, in some cases, termination of therapy with interferon alfa-n3 (human leukocyte derived).

Duration of therapy: Up to 8 weeks. Genital warts usually begin to disappear after several weeks of treatment with interferon alfa-n3 (human leukocyte derived).

It is recommended that no further therapy (interferon alfa-n3 [human leukocyte derived] or conventional therapy) be administered for 3 months after the initial 8-week course of treatment unless the warts enlarge or new warts appear.

➤*Administration:* Inject into the base of each wart, preferably using a 30-gauge needle. For large warts, interferon alfa-n3 (human leukocyte derived) may be injected at several points around the periphery of the wart, using a total dose of 0.05 mL per wart.

➤*Storage/Stability:* Store between 2° and 8°C (36° and 46°F). Do not freeze. Do not shake.

Actions

➤*Pharmacology:* Interferons are naturally occurring proteins with antiviral, antiproliferative and immunoregulatory properties. They are produced and secreted in response to viral infections and to a variety of other synthetic and biological inducers. Four major families of interferons have been identified: Alpha, beta, gamma and omega. The interferon alpha family contains 13 different nonallelic molecular species. Their molecular weights range from 16,000 to 27,000 daltons.

INTERFERON ALFA-N3 — INJECTION

Interferons bind to specific membrane receptors on cell surfaces. Interferon alfa-n3 has been shown to bind to the same receptors as Interferon alfa-2b. The receptors have a high degree of selectivity for the binding of human but not mouse interferon. This correlates with the high species specificity found in laboratory studies.

Binding of interferon to membrane receptors initiates a series of events including induction of protein synthesis. These actions are followed by a variety of cellular responses, including inhibition of virus replication and suppression of cell proliferation. Immunomodulation, including enhancement of phagocytosis by macrophages, augmentation of the cytotoxicity of lymphocytes and enhancement of human leukocyte antigen expression occurs in response to exposure to interferons. One or more of these activities may contribute to the therapeutic effect of interferon.

➤*Pharmacokinetics:* In a study of intralesional use of interferon alfa-n3 (human leukocyte derived) for the treatment of condylomata acuminata, plasma concentrations of interferon were below the detection limit of the assay, ie, less than 3 IU/mL. Minor systemic effects (eg, myalgias, fever, and headaches) were noted, indicating that some of the injected interferon entered the systemic circulation (see Adverse Reactions).

Contraindications

Hypersensitivity to human interferon alpha proteins or any component of the product. The product is also contraindicated in patients who have anaphylactic sensitivity to mouse immunoglobulin (IgG), egg protein or neomycin.

Warnings/Precautions

➤*Interchangeability:* Patients being treated with interferon alfa-n3 (human leukocyte derived) should be informed of the benefits and risks associated with the treatment. Because the manufacturing process, strength, and type of interferon (eg, natural, human leukocyte interferon versus single-species recombinant interferon) may vary for different interferon formulations, changing brands may require a change in dosage. Therefore, physicians are cautioned not to change from one interferon product to another without considering these factors.

➤*Special risk:* Because of the fever and other "flu-like" symptoms associated with interferon alfa-n3 (human leukocyte derived) (see Adverse Reactions), it should be used cautiously in patients with debilitating medical conditions such as cardiovascular disease (eg, unstable angina and uncontrolled congestive heart failure), severe pulmonary disease (eg, chronic obstructive pulmonary disease), or diabetes mellitus with ketoacidosis.

Interferon alfa-n3 (human leukocyte derived) should be used cautiously in patients with coagulation disorders (eg, thrombophlebitis, pulmonary embolism and hemophilia), severe myelosuppression, or seizure disorders. Acute, serious hypersensitivity reactions (eg, urticaria, angioedema, bronchoconstriction, and anaphylaxis) have not been observed in patients receiving interferon alfa-n3 (human leukocyte derived). However, if such reactions develop, drug administration should be discontinued immediately and appropriate medical therapy should be instituted.

Because this product is made from human blood, it may carry a risk of transmitting infectious agents (eg, viruses) and theoretically, the Creutzfeldt-Jakob disease (CJD) agent.

➤*Pregnancy: Category C.*

Animal reproduction studies have not been conducted with interferon alfa-n3 (human leukocyte derived). It is also not known whether interferon alfa-n3 (human leukocyte derived) can cause fetal harm when administered to a pregnant woman or can affect reproductive capacity. Interferon alfa-n3 (human leukocyte derived) should be given to a pregnant woman only if clearly needed.

Changes in the menstrual cycle and abortions have been reported to occur in non-human primates given extremely high doses of recombinant interferon alpha. In these studies, Macaca mulatta (rhesus monkeys) were given interferon daily by intramuscular injection. Abortifacient effects were noted when the recombinant interferon alpha was given daily during early to mid-gestation at intramuscular doses of 978 times the average intralesional dose of interferon alfa-n3 (human leukocyte derived) (360 times the maximum recommended dose).

Fertility impairment – In studies with adult females, interferon alpha has been shown to affect the menstrual cycle and decrease serum estradiol and progesterone levels. Interferon alfa-n3 should be used with caution in fertile men. Fertile women should be cautioned to use effective contraception while being treated with interferon alfa-n3.

➤*Lactation:* It is not known whether interferon alfa-n3 (human leukocyte derived) is excreted in human milk. Studies in mice have shown that mouse interferons are excreted in milk. Because many drugs are excreted in human milk and because of the potential for serious adverse reactions in nursing infants, a decision should be made whether to discontinue nursing or to not initiate drug treatment, taking into account the importance of the drug to the mother and the potential risks to the infant.

➤*Children:* Safety and effectiveness have not been established in patients less than 18 years of age.

Adverse Reactions

➤*Adverse reactions in patients with condylomata acuminata:* The "flu-like" adverse reactions, consisting of fever, myalgias, or headache, occurred primarily after the first treatment session and were reported by 30% of the patients. The frequency of "flu-like" adverse reactions abated with repeated dosing of interferon alfa-n3 (human leukocyte derived) so that the incidences due to interferon alfa-n3 (human leukocyte derived) and placebo were similar after 3 to 4 weeks of treatment (after 6 to 8 treatment sessions). "Flu-like" symptoms were relieved by administration of acetaminophen.

Adverse reactions were reported at least once during the course of treatment in the following percentages of patients in each treatment group:

Interferon Alfa-n3 Adverse Reactions		
Adverse reactions	Interferon alfa-n3 (n = 104)	Placebo (n = 85)
Autonomic nervous system		
Sweating	2%	1%
Vasovagal reaction	2%	0%
CNS		
Depression	2%	1%
Dizziness	9%	4%
Insomnia	2%	1%
Dermatologic		
Generalized pruritus	2%	0%
GI		
Diarrhea	2%	2%
Dyspepsia/heartburn	3%	1%
Nausea	4%	7%
Vomiting	3%	0%
Musculoskeletal		
Arthralgia	5%	1%
Back pain	4%	1%
Headache	31%	15%
Myalgias	45%	15%
Nasopharyngeal		
Drainage	2%	2%
Miscellaneous		
Chills	14%	2%
Fatigue	14%	6%
Fever	40%	19%
Malaise	9%	9%

Most of the systemic adverse reactions were mild or moderate. Severe systemic adverse reactions were reported by 18% of interferon alfa-n3 (human leukocyte derived)-treated patients and 13% of placebo-treated patients (not a statistically significant difference). Most of the severe systemic adverse reactions reported were "flu-like". Other severe systemic adverse reactions included back pain, insomnia, and sensitivity to allergens. Those adverse reactions which were reported by 1% of patients treated with interferon alfa-n3 (human leukocyte derived) in the double-blind trial include: Left groin lymph node swelling, tongue hyperaesthesia, thirst, tingling of legs/feet, hot sensation on bottom of feet, strange taste in mouth, increased salivation, heat intolerance, visual disturbances, pharyngitis, sensitivity to allergens, muscle cramps, nosebleed, throat tightness, and papular rash on neck. Additional adverse reactions which were reported by 1% of patients treated with placebo include: Pharyngitis, oral pain, penile discharge, cold, knuckle stiffness, herpes outbreak, cough, disorientation, and weight/appetite loss.

Additional adverse reactions which occurred only in open clinical trials of intralesional use of interferon alfa-n3 (human leukocyte derived) for treatment of condylomata acuminata were herpes labialis, hot flashes, nervousness, decrease in concentration, dysuria, photosensitivity, and swollen lymph nodes. These reactions occurred in 1% of the patients. One patient with a history of epilepsy, who was not taking anticonvulsant medication, had a grand mal seizure while being treated with interferon alfa-n3 (human leukocyte derived); this seizure was judged to be unrelated to interferon alfa-n3 (human leukocyte derived) administration.

➤*Local:* The frequency of application site disorders (such as itching and pain) for patients treated with interferon alfa-n3 (human leukocyte derived) was significantly less than that reported with placebo (12% versus 26%). No severe application site disorders were reported by patients treated with interferon alfa-n3 (human leukocyte derived), while 7% of placebo-treated patients reported severe disorders.

➤*Lab test abnormalities:* Abnormalities were seen with statistically equivalent frequencies in both the interferon alfa-n3 (human leukocyte derived) and placebo groups. None of the laboratory abnormalities were considered clinically significant. The abnormalities in the interferon alfa-n3 (human leukocyte derived)-treated patients consisted primarily of decreased WBC (11%). Decreases also occurred in 4% of the placebo patients (not a statistically significant difference). The abnormalities in interferon alfa-n3 (human leukocyte derived)-treated patients involved increases of only one WHO grade.

➤*Adverse reactions in patients with cancer:* The following adverse reactions were reported at least once (the percentage of patients experiencing the reaction is indicated in parenthesis): Chills (87%), fever (81%), anorexia (68%), malaise (65%), nausea (48%), vomiting (29%), myalgias (16%), arthralgia (10%), chest pains (10%), soreness at injection site (10%),

INTERFERON ALFA-N3 — INJECTION

sleepiness (10%), headache (10%), diarrhea (6%), fatigue (6%), low blood pressure (6%), sore mouth/stomatitis (6%), and blurred vision (6%). Those adverse reactions which were each reported by only one patient treated with interferon alfa-n3 (human leukocyte derived) include the following: Stiff shoulders, flushed face, edema, dry mouth, mucositis, coughing, numbness, numbness in hands, numbness in fingers, pain on ocular rotation, shakes/shivers, ringing in ears, cramps, constipation, muscle soreness, confusion, lightheadedness, depression, upset stomach, and sweating. The following adverse reactions were reported as severe by at least 1 patient (the percentage of patients experiencing the reaction is indicated in parentheses): Fever (55%), malaise (54%), anorexia (45%), chills (45%), nausea (16%), myalgias (13%), vomiting (10%), fatigue (6%), low blood pressure (6%), chest pains (6%), sore mouth/stomatitis (6%), headache (3%), diarrhea (3%), sleepiness (3%), arthralgia (3%), blurred vision (3%), stiff shoulders (3%), numbness (3%), pain on ocular rotation (3%), muscle soreness (3%), confusion (3%), lightheadedness (3%), depression (3%), and sweating (3%).

The number and percentage of patients with cancer who experienced a significant abnormal laboratory test value (values that changed from WHO Grades 0, 1, or 2 at baseline to WHO Grades 3 or 4 during or after treatment) at least once during the trials are shown in the following table:

Abnormal Laboratory Test Values with Interferon Alfa-n3 Administration

Laboratory test	Cancer (n = 31)
Hemoglobin level	2 (7%)
White blood cell count	1 (3%)
Platelet count	1 (3%)
GGT	1 (6%)
AST	1 (3%)
Alkaline phosphatase	2 (8%)
Total bilirubin	1 (4%)

Patient Information

Patients should be informed of the early signs of hypersensitivity reactions including hives, generalized urticaria, tightness of the chest, wheezing, hypotension and anaphylaxis, and should be advised to contact their physician if these symptoms occur.

Patients being treated with interferon alfa-n3 (human leukocyte derived) should be informed of benefits and risks associated with treatment. Patients should be cautioned not to change brands of interferon without medical consultation, as a change in dosage may occur.

INTERFERON GAMMA-1B

Rx	**Actimmune** (InterMune)	**Injection, solution:** 100 mcg (2 million units) per 0.5 mL	Preservative free. In single-dose vials.[a]

[a] With 20 mg mannitol, 0.36 mg sodium succinate, and 0.05 mg polysorbate 20.

INTERFERON GAMMA-1B — INJECTION

Indications

➤*Chronic granulomatous disease:* For reducing the frequency and severity of serious infections associated with chronic granulomatous disease.

➤*Malignant osteopetrosis:* For delaying time to disease progression in patients with severe, malignant osteopetrosis.

Administration and Dosage

➤*Maximum dose:*

BSA greater than 0.5 m² – 50 mcg/m²/dose.

BSA 0.5 m² or less – 1.5 mcg/kg/dose.

➤*Adults:*

Chronic granulomatous disease –

Usual dosage:

• *BSA greater than 0.5 m²* – 50 mcg/m² (1 million units/m²) subcutaneously 3 times a week (ie, Monday, Wednesday, Friday).

• *BSA 0.5 m² or less* – 1.5 mcg/kg/dose subcutaneously 3 times a week (ie, Monday, Wednesday, Friday).

Maximum dose:

• *BSA greater than 0.5 m²* – 50 mcg/m²/dose.

• *BSA 0.5 m² or less* – 1.5 mcg/kg/dose.

Malignant osteopetrosis – See Chronic granulomatous disease for dosing.

➤*Children:* See Adults for dosing.

➤*Dosage adjustment:* If a severe reaction occurs, the dosage should be reduced by 50% or therapy should be discontinued until the adverse reaction abates.

➤*Administration:* Administer by subcutaneous injection. Avoid excessive or vigorous agitation. Interferon gamma-1b may be administered using either sterilized glass or plastic disposable syringes. The optimal sites of injection are the right and left deltoid and anterior thigh.

➤*Admixture compatibility:* Interferon gamma-1b should not be mixed with other drugs in the same syringe.

➤*Storage/Stability:* Vials of interferon gamma-1b must be placed in a 2° to 8°C (36° to 46°F) refrigerator immediately upon receipt to ensure optimal retention of physical and biochemical integrity. Do not freeze. Do not shake. Do not leave an unentered vial of interferon gamma-1b at room temperature for a total time exceeding 12 hours prior to use. Do not return vials exceeding this time period to the refrigerator; discard such vials.

The formulation does not contain a preservative. A vial of interferon gamma-1b is suitable for a single dose only. The unused portion of any vial should be discarded.

Actions

➤*Pharmacology:* Interferons bind to specific cell surface receptors and initiate a sequence of intracellular events that lead to the transcription of interferon-stimulated genes. The 3 major groups of interferons (ie, alpha, beta, gamma) have partially overlapping biological activities that include immunoregulation, such as increased resistance to microbial pathogens and inhibition of cell proliferation. Type 1 interferons (alpha and beta) bind to the alpha/beta receptor. Interferon-gamma binds to a different cell surface receptor and is classified as a type 2 interferon. Specific effects of interferon-gamma include the enhancement of the oxidative metabolism of macrophages, antibody-dependent cellular cytotoxicity, activation of natural killer cells, and the expression of Fc receptors and major histocompatibility antigens.

Chronic granulomatous disease is an inherited disorder of leukocyte function caused by defects in the enzyme complex responsible for phagocyte superoxide generation. Interferon gamma-1b does not increase phagocyte superoxide production even in treatment responders.

In severe, malignant osteopetrosis (an inherited disorder characterized by an osteoclast defect leading to bone overgrowth and by deficient phagocyte oxidative metabolism), a treatment-related enhancement of superoxide production by phagocytes was observed. Interferon gamma-1b was found to enhance osteoclast function in vivo.

In both disorders, the exact mechanism(s) by which interferon gamma-1b has a treatment effect has not been established. Changes in superoxide levels during interferon gamma-1b therapy do not predict efficacy; do not use these levels to assess patient response to therapy.

➤*Pharmacokinetics:*

Absorption – The intravenous (IV), intramuscular (IM), and subcutaneous pharmacokinetics of interferon gamma-1b have been investigated in 24 healthy men following single-dose administration of 100 mcg/m².

Interferon gamma-1b is rapidly cleared after IV administration (1.4 L/min) and slowly absorbed after IM or subcutaneous injection. After IM or subcutaneous injection, the apparent fraction of dose absorbed was more than 89%.

Peak plasma concentrations, determined by enzyme-linked immunosorbent assay, occurred approximately 4 hours (1.5 ng/mL) after IM dosing and 7 hours (0.6 ng/mL) after subcutaneous dosing.

Multiple-dose subcutaneous pharmacokinetic studies were conducted in 38 healthy men. There was no accumulation of interferon gamma-1b after 12 consecutive daily injections of 100 mcg/m².

Pharmacokinetic studies in patients with chronic granulomatous disease have not been performed.

Excretion – The mean elimination half-life after IV administration of 100 mcg/m² in healthy male subjects was 38 minutes. The mean elimination half-lives for IM and subcutaneous dosing with 100 mcg/m² were 2.9 and 5.9 hours, respectively.

Interferon-gamma was not detected in the urine of healthy human volunteers following administration of 100 mcg/m² of interferon gamma-1b by the IV, IM, and subcutaneous routes.

Contraindications

Hypersensitivity to interferon-gamma, *Escherichia coli*-derived products, or any component of the product.

Warnings/Precautions

➤*Cardiac effects:* Acute and transient "flu-like" symptoms, such as fever and chills induced by interferon gamma-1b at doses of 250 mcg/m²/day (more than 10 times the weekly recommended dose) or higher may exacerbate preexisting cardiac conditions. Use interferon gamma-1b with caution in patients with preexisting cardiac conditions, including ischemia, congestive heart failure, or arrhythmia.

➤*CNS effects:* Exercise caution when treating patients with seizure disorders or compromised CNS function. Decreased mental status, gait disturbance, and dizziness have been observed, particularly in patients receiving doses more than 250 mcg/m²/day (more than 10 times the weekly recommended dose). Most of these abnormalities were mild and reversible within a few days upon dose reduction or discontinuation of therapy.

➤*Hematologic effects:* Exercise caution when administering interferon gamma-1b to patients with myelosuppression. Reversible neutropenia and

INTERFERON GAMMA-1B — INJECTION

thrombocytopenia that can be severe and possibly dose related have been observed during interferon gamma-1b therapy.

➤*Antibody formation:* No neutralizing antibodies to interferon gamma-1b have been detected in any patients with chronic granulomatous disease receiving interferon gamma-1b.

➤*Hepatic effects:* Elevations of AST and/or ALT (25-fold or less) have been observed during interferon gamma-1b therapy. The incidence appeared to be higher in patients younger than 1 year of age than in older children. The transaminase elevations were reversible with reduction in dosage or interruption of interferon gamma-1b treatment. Patients begun on interferon gamma-1b younger than 1 year of age should receive monthly assessments of liver function. If severe hepatic enzyme elevations develop, modify interferon gamma-1b dosage.

➤*Hypersensitivity reactions:* Isolated cases of acute serious hypersensitivity reactions have been observed in patients receiving interferon gamma-1b. If such an acute reaction develops, discontinue the drug immediately and institute appropriate medical therapy. Transient cutaneous rashes have occurred in some patients following injection but have rarely necessitated treatment interruption.

➤*Pregnancy: Category C.*

Teratogenic – Interferon gamma-1b has shown an increased incidence of abortions in primates when given in doses approximately 100 times the human dose.

Female mice treated subcutaneously with rmuIFN-gamma at 280 times the maximum recommended clinical dose of interferon gamma-1b from shortly after birth through puberty, but not during pregnancy, had offspring that exhibited decreased body weight during the lactation period. The clinical significance of this finding observed following treatment of mice with rmuIFN-gamma is uncertain.

There are no adequate and well-controlled studies in pregnant women. Use interferon gamma-1b during pregnancy only if the potential benefit justifies the potential risk to the fetus.

➤*Lactation:* It is not known whether interferon gamma-1b is excreted in human milk. Because many drugs are excreted in human milk and because of the potential for serious adverse reactions in breast-feeding infants from interferon gamma-1b, decide whether to discontinue breast-feeding or the drug, depending upon the importance of the drug to the mother.

➤*Monitoring:* The following laboratory tests are recommended for all patients on interferon gamma-1b therapy prior to the beginning of, and at 3-month intervals during, treatment: hematologic tests, including complete blood counts, differential and platelet counts; blood chemistries, including renal and liver function tests; and urinalysis. In patients younger than 1 year of age, measure liver function tests monthly.

Drug Interactions

➤*Myelosuppressive agents:* Exercise caution when administering interferon gamma-1b in combination with other potentially myelosuppressive agents.

➤*CYP-450 system:* Preclinical studies in rodents using species-specific interferon-gamma have demonstrated a decrease in hepatic microsomal CYP-450 concentrations. This could potentially lead to a depression of the hepatic metabolism of certain drugs that use this degradative pathway.

Adverse Reactions

➤*Chronic granulomatous disease:* The most common adverse reactions observed in patients with chronic granulomatous disease are shown in the following table.

Interferon Gamma-1b Adverse Reactions in Patients With Chronic Granulomatous Disease

Adverse reaction	Interferon gamma-1b (n = 63)	Placebo (n = 65)
CNS		
Fatigue	14%	11%
Headache	33%	9%
GI		
Diarrhea	14%	12%
Nausea	10%	2%
Vomiting	13%	5%
Local		
Injection-site erythema or tenderness	14%	2%
Injection-site pain	0%	2%
Musculoskeletal		
Arthralgia	2%	0%
Myalgia	6%	0%
Miscellaneous		
Chills	14%	0%
Fever	52%	28%
Rash	17%	6%

Miscellaneous adverse reactions that occurred infrequently in patients with chronic granulomatous disease and may have been related to underlying disease included abdominal pain (8% vs 3%), back pain (2% vs 0%), and depression (3% vs 0%) for interferon gamma-1b- and placebo-treated patients, respectively.

➤*Malignant osteopetrosis:* Similar safety data were observed in 34 patients with severe, malignant osteopetrosis.

➤*Other adverse reactions:* Interferon gamma-1b also has been evaluated in additional disease states in studies in which patients have generally received higher doses (more than 100 mcg/m^2 3 times weekly) administered by IM or subcutaneous injection or IV infusion. All of the previously described adverse reactions that occurred in patients with chronic granulomatous disease also have been observed in patients receiving higher doses. Adverse reactions not observed in patients with chronic granulomatous disease but reported in patients receiving interferon gamma-1b in other studies included the following:

Cardiovascular – Heart block, heart failure, hypotension, myocardial infarction, syncope, tachyarrhythmia.

CNS – Confusion, disorientation, gait disturbance, hallucinations, parkinsonian symptoms, seizure, transient ischemic attacks.

GI – GI bleeding; hepatic function impairment; pancreatitis, including pancreatitis with fatal outcome.

Hematologic – Deep venous thrombosis, pulmonary embolism.

Lab test abnormalities – Elevations of ALT and AST, neutropenia, proteinuria, thrombocytopenia.

Metabolic – Hyperglycemia, hypertriglyceridemia, hyponatremia,

Pulmonary – Bronchospasm, interstitial pneumonitis, tachypnea.

Miscellaneous – Chest discomfort, exacerbation of dermatomyositis, increased autoantibodies, lupus-like syndrome, reversible renal function impairment.

➤*Postmarketing:* Data on the safety and activity of interferon gamma-1b in 37 patients younger than 3 years of age was pooled from 4 uncontrolled postmarketing studies. The rate of serious infections per patient year in this uncontrolled group was similar to the rate observed in the interferon gamma-1b treatment groups in controlled trials. Developmental parameters (height, weight, and endocrine maturation) for this uncontrolled group conformed to national normative scales before and during interferon gamma-1b therapy.

In 6 of the 10 patients younger than 1 year of age receiving interferon gamma-1b therapy, 2- to 25-fold elevations from baseline of AST and/or ALT were observed. These elevations occurred as early as 7 days after starting treatment. Treatment with interferon gamma-1b was interrupted in all 6 of these patients and was restarted at a reduced dosage in 4 patients. Liver transaminase values returned to baseline in all patients and transaminase elevation recurred in one patient upon interferon gamma-1b rechallenge. An 11-fold alkaline phosphatase elevation and hypokalemia in one patient and neutropenia (absolute neutrophil count = 525 cells/mm^3) in another patient resolved with interruption of interferon gamma-1b treatment and did not recur with rechallenge.

In the postmarketing safety database, clinically significant adverse reactions observed during interferon gamma-1b therapy in children younger than 3 years of age (n = 14) included the following: 2 cases of hepatomegaly, and 1 case each of atopic dermatitis, granulomatous colitis, Stevens-Johnson syndrome, and urticaria.

Overdosage

➤*Symptoms:* CNS adverse reactions, including decreased mental status, dizziness, and gait disturbance, have been observed, particularly in cancer patients receiving doses of more than 100 mcg/m^2/day by IV or IM administration. These abnormalities were reversible within a few days upon dose reduction or discontinuation of therapy. Elevation of hepatic enzymes and of triglycerides, reversible neutropenia, and thrombocytopenia have also been observed.

Patient Information

Inform patients being treated with interferon gamma-1b and/or their parents about the potential benefits and risks associated with treatment. If home use is determined to be desirable by the health care provider, give instructions on appropriate use, including review of the contents of the patient information insert. This information is intended to aid in the safe and effective use of the medication. It is not a disclosure of all possible adverse or intended reactions.

If home use is prescribed, supply the patient with a puncture-resistant container for the disposal of used syringes and needles. Thoroughly instruct patients in the importance of proper disposal and caution against any reuse of needles and syringes. Dispose of the full container according to the directions provided by the health care provider.

The most common adverse reactions occurring with interferon gamma-1b therapy are "flu-like" or constitutional symptoms, such as fever, headache, chills, myalgia, or fatigue, which may decrease in severity as treatment continues. Some of the "flu-like" symptoms may be minimized by bedtime administration (ie, acetaminophen may also be used to prevent or partially alleviate the fever and headache).

The long-term effects of interferon gamma-1b therapy on growth, development, or other parameters are not known.

INTERFERON BETA

Indications

➤*Multiple sclerosis (MS):* Treatment of MS. See individual monographs for specific indications.

Actions

➤*Pharmacology:* **Interferon beta-1a** is a 166 amino acid glycoprotein. It is produced by mammalian cells (Chinese hamster ovary cells) into which the human interferon beta gene has been introduced. The amino acid sequence of interferon beta-1a is identical to that of natural human interferon beta. **Interferon beta-1b** is manufactured by bacterial fermentation of a strain of *Escherichia coli* that bears a genetically engineered plasmid containing the gene for human interferon $beta_{ser17}$. Interferon beta-1b is a purified protein that has 165 amino acids. It does not include the carbohydrate side chains found in the natural material.

Interferons are a family of naturally occurring proteins and glycoproteins that are produced by eukaryotic cells in response to viral infection and other biological inducers. Interferon beta is produced by various cell types including fibroblasts and macrophages. Three major classes of interferons have been identified: Alpha, beta, and gamma; they each have overlapping yet distinct biologic activities.

Interferon beta has antiviral, antiproliferative, and immunoregulatory activities. The mechanisms by which it exerts its actions in MS are not clearly understood. However, it is known that the binding of interferon beta to its receptors initiates a complex cascade of intracellular events that leads to the expression of numerous interferon-induced gene products and markers, including 2′,5′-oligoadenylate synthetase, beta 2-microglobulin, and neopterin, which may mediate some of the biological activities.

➤*Pharmacokinetics:*

Interferon beta-1a – Biological response markers (eg, neopterin and β_2-microglobulin) are induced by interferon beta-1a following parenteral doses of 15 to 75 mcg in healthy subjects and treated patients. Biological response marker levels increase within 12 hours of dosing and remain elevated for at least 4 days. Peak biological response marker levels are typically observed 48 hours after dosing.

Interferon Beta-1a Pharmacokinetic Parameters[a]

Route	Mean C_{max} (IU/mL)	T_{max} (h)	Mean AUC (IU•h/mL)	t½ (h)
IM	4.9	3 to 15	65	10
SC[b]	5.1	16 (median)	294	69

[a] Data are pooled from different studies and are not necessarily comparable.
[b] Based on a single dose of 60 mcg.

Interferon beta-1b – Because serum concentrations of interferon beta-1b are low or not detectable following SC administration of up to 0.25 mg, pharmacokinetic information in patients with MS receiving the recommended dose is not available. Following single and multiple daily SC administrations of 0.5 mg (16 mIU) to healthy volunteers (n = 12), serum concentrations were generally less than 100 IU/mL. Peak serum concentrations occurred between 1 to 8 hours, with a mean peak serum concentration of 40 IU/mL. Bioavailability, based on a total dose of 0.5 mg given as 2 SC injections at different sites, was approximately 50%.

After IV administration (0.006 to 2 mg), similar pharmacokinetic profiles were obtained from healthy volunteers (n = 12) and from patients with diseases other than MS (n = 142). In patients receiving single IV doses up to 2 mg, increases in serum concentrations were dose-proportional. Mean serum clearance values ranged from 9.4 to 28.9 mL/min/kg and were independent of dose. Mean terminal elimination half-life values ranged from 8 minutes to 4.3 hours and mean steady-state volume of distribution values ranged from 0.25 to 2.88 L/kg. IV dosing 3 times/week for 2 weeks resulted in no accumulation of interferon beta-1b in the serum of patients. Pharmacokinetic parameters after single and multiple IV doses were comparable.

Following SC administration every other day, biologic response marker levels increased significantly above baseline 6 to 12 hours after the first dose. Peak biologic response marker levels usually occur between 40 and 124 hours after dosing and remain elevated for at least 7 days.

Contraindications

Hypersensitivity to natural or recombinant interferon beta, human albumin, or any other component of the formulations.

Warnings/Precautions

➤*Chronic progressive MS:* The safety and efficacy of interferon beta in chronic progressive MS have not been evaluated.

➤*Depression:* Use interferon beta with caution in patients with depression or other mood disorders, conditions that are common with MS. Depression and suicide have been reported in patients receiving interferon compounds. Depression, suicidal ideation, and suicidal attempts are known to occur at an increased frequency in patients receiving interferon compounds. Additionally, there have been postmarketing reports of depression, suicidal ideation, and/or development of new or worsening pre-existing psychiatric disorders, including psychosis. Some of these patients improved upon cessation of dosing.

Advise patients treated with interferon beta to immediately report any symptoms of depression or suicidal ideation. If a patient develops depression or other severe psychiatric symptoms, consider cessation of therapy.

➤*Injection-site necrosis (ISN):* ISN has been reported. Typically, ISN occurs within the first 4 months of therapy, although postmarketing reports have been received of ISN occurring over 1 year after initiation of therapy. Necrosis may occur at a single or multiple injection sites. The necrotic lesions are typically 3 cm or less in diameter, but larger areas have been reported. Generally, the necrosis has extended only to subcutaneous fat. However, there also are reports of necrosis extending to and including fascia overlaying muscle. In some lesions where biopsy results are available, vasculitis has been reported. For some lesions, debridement and, infrequently, skin grafting have been required.

As with any open lesion, it is important to avoid infection and, if it occurs, to treat the infection. Time to healing varied depending on the severity of the necrosis at the time of treatment. In most cases, healing was associated with scarring.

Some patients have experienced healing of necrotic skin lesions while **interferon beta-1b** therapy continued; others have not. Whether to discontinue therapy following a single site of necrosis is dependent on the extent of necrosis. For patients who continue therapy with interferon beta-1b after ISN has occurred, do not administer interferon beta -1b into the affected area until it is fully healed. If multiple lesions occur, discontinue therapy until healing occurs.

Periodically re-evaluate patient understanding and use of aseptic self-injection techniques, particularly if ISN has occurred.

➤*Anaphylaxis:* Anaphylaxis has been reported as a rare complication of interferon beta use. Other allergic reactions have included dyspnea, bronchospasm, tongue edema, orolingual edema, skin rash, and urticaria, and have ranged from mild to severe without a clear relationship to dose or duration of exposure. Several allergic reactions, some severe, have occurred after prolonged use.

➤*Decreased peripheral blood counts:* Decreased peripheral blood counts in all cell lines, including rare pancytopenia and thrombocytopenia, have been reported from postmarketing experience. Some cases of thrombocytopenia have had nadirs below 10,000/mcL. Some cases reoccur with rechallenge. Monitor patients for signs of these disorders.

➤*Albumin (human):* Some of these products contain albumin, a derivative of human blood. Based on effective donor screening and product manufacturing processes, it carries an extremely remote risk for transmission of viral diseases. A theoretical risk for transmission of Creutzfeldt-Jakob disease (CJD) also is considered extremely remote. No cases of transmission of viral diseases or CJD have been identified for albumin.

➤*Special risk patients:* Exercise caution when administering **interferon beta-1a** to patients with pre-existing seizure disorders. Seizures have been associated with the use of beta interferons. A relationship between occurrence of seizures and the use of interferon beta has not been established. Leukopenia and new or worsening thyroid abnormalities have developed in some patients treated with interferon beta. Regular monitoring for these conditions is recommended.

➤*Cardiac disease:* Closely monitor patients with cardiac disease, such as angina, CHF, or arrhythmia, for worsening of their clinical condition during initiation and continued treatment. While interferon beta does not have any known direct-acting cardiac toxicity, during the postmarketing period infrequent cases of CHF, cardiomyopathy, and cardiomyopathy with CHF have been reported in patients without known predisposition to these events and without other known etiologies being established. In rare cases, these events have been temporally related to the administration of interferon beta. In some of these instances, recurrence upon rechallenge was observed.

➤*Self-administration:* Instruct patients in injection techniques to ensure the safe self-administration of interferon beta. A patient information sheet is provided with the product.

➤*Flu-like symptoms complex:* Flu-like symptoms, including headache, fever, fatigue, rigors, chest pain, back pain, and myalgia, have been commonly reported with interferon beta therapy. Symptoms usually occur 4 hours after injection and subside within 24 hours. Acetaminophen or NSAIDs prior to and/or following injection may help to prevent or treat these symptoms.

➤*Autoimmune disorders:* Autoimmune disorders of multiple target organs have been reported postmarketing, including idiopathic thrombocytopenia, hyper- and hypothyroidism, and rare cases of autoimmune hepatitis. Monitor patients for signs of these disorders and implement appropriate treatment when observed.

➤*Hepatic injury:* Hepatic injury, including elevated serum hepatic enzyme levels and hepatitis, some of which have been severe, has been reported postmarketing. In some patients, a recurrence of elevated serum levels of hepatic enzymes has occurred upon rechallenge. In some cases, these events have occurred in the presence of other drugs associated with hepatic injury. The potential of additive effects from multiple drugs or other hepatotoxic agents (eg, alcohol) has not been determined. Monitor patients for signs of hepatic injury and exercise caution when interferons are used concomitantly with other drugs associated with hepatic injury.

➤*Immunogenicity:* As with all therapeutic proteins, there is a potential for immunogenicity. Antibodies to interferon beta have developed during therapy. The relationship between antibody formation and clinical safety or efficacy is unknown.

➤*Latex sensitivity:* Administer with caution to patients with a possible history of latex sensitivity; packaging may contain dry natural rubber.

➤*Hepatic function impairment:* Severe liver dysfunction, leading to hepatic failure requiring liver transplantation, has been reported very rarely in patients taking interferon beta. Symptomatic hepatic dysfunction (including hepatitis), primarily presenting as jaundice, has been reported as

INTERFERON BETA

a rare complication of use. Asymptomatic elevation of hepatic transaminases (particularly ALT) is common with interferon therapy. Initiate therapy with caution in patients with active liver disease, alcohol abuse, increased serum ALT (greater than 2.5 times the upper limit of normal [ULN]), or a history of significant liver disease. Consider dose reduction if ALT rises above 5 times the ULN. The dose may be re-escalated gradually once the enzyme levels have normalized. Stop treatment if jaundice or other clinical symptoms of liver dysfunction appear.

➤*Photosensitivity:* Photosensitization (photoallergy or phototoxicity) may occur; therefore, caution patients to take protective measures (ie, sunscreens, protective clothing) against exposure to sunlight or ultraviolet light (eg, tanning beds) until tolerance is determined.

➤*Pregnancy: Category C.* There are no adequate and well-controlled studies in pregnant women. Abortifacient activity has been shown in animals and 6 spontaneous abortions were reported in patients on interferon beta therapy during the clinical trials. If the patient becomes pregnant or plans to become pregnant while taking interferon beta, apprise the patient of the potential hazards to the fetus and recommend that the patient discontinue therapy.

➤*Lactation:* It is not known whether interferon beta is excreted in breast milk. Decide whether to discontinue nursing or discontinue the drug, taking into account the importance of the drug to the mother.

➤*Children:* Safety and efficacy in children younger than 18 years of age have not been established.

➤*Monitoring:* In addition to the laboratory tests normally required for monitoring patients with MS, blood cell counts and liver function tests are recommended at baseline and regular intervals (1, 3, and 6 months) following introduction of interferon beta therapy and then periodically thereafter in the absence of clinical symptoms. Thyroid function tests are recommended every 6 months in patients with a history of thyroid dysfunction or as clinically indicated. Patients with myelosuppression may require more intensive monitoring of complete blood cell counts, with differential and platelet counts.

Drug Interactions

➤*Myelosuppressive agents:* Because of the potential of **interferon beta-1a** to cause neutropenia and lymphopenia, proper monitoring is required if administered concomitantly with myelosuppressive agents.

Adverse Reactions

The most serious adverse reactions associated with interferon beta therapy were depression, suicidal ideation, and ISN (see Warnings). The most commonly reported adverse reactions were asthenia, flu-like symptoms complex (see Precautions), headache, injection site reaction, lymphopenia (lymphocytes less than 1500/mm^3), and pain. The most frequently reported adverse reactions resulting in clinical intervention (ie, discontinuation of therapy, adjustment in dosage, or the need for concomitant medication to treat an adverse reaction symptom) were asthenia, depression, flu-like symptoms complex, hypertonia, injection site reactions, increased liver enzymes, leukopenia, and myasthenia.

Interferon Beta Adverse Reactions (%)[a]

Adverse reactions	*Avonex* (n = 351)	*Rebif* 22 mcg 3 times/week (n = 189)	*Rebif* 44 mcg 3 times/week (n = 184)	Interferon beta-1b (n = 1115)
Cardiovascular				
Hypertension	–	–	–	7
Migraine	5	–	–	–
Palpitations	–	–	–	4
Peripheral edema	–	–	–	15
Peripheral vascular disorder	–	–	–	6
Tachycardia	–	–	–	4
Vasodilation	2	–	–	8
CNS				
Anxiety	–	–	–	10
Asthenia	24	–	–	61
Convulsions	–	5	4	–
Depression	18	–	–	–
Dizziness	14	–	–	24
Fatigue	–	33	41	–
Headache	58	65	70	57
Incoordination	–	5	4	21
Nervousness	–	–	–	7
Hypertonia	–	7	6	50
Sleep difficulty	–	–	–	24
Somnolence	–	4	5	–
Dermatologic				
Alopecia	4	–	–	4
Rash (erythematous, maculopapular)	–	5-7	4-5	24
Skin disorder	–	–	–	12
Sweating	–	–	–	8
GI				
Abdominal pain	8	22	20	19
Constipation	–	–	–	20
Diarrhea	–	–	–	19
Dry mouth	–	1	5	–
Dyspepsia	–	–	–	14
Nausea	23	–	–	27
GU				
Dysmenorrhea[b]	–	–	–	7
Impotence[c]	–	–	–	9
Menorrhagia[b]	–	–	–	8
Metrorrhagia[b]	–	–	–	11
Prostatic disorder[c]	–	–	–	3
Urinary frequency	–	2	7	7
Urinary incontinence	–	4	2	–
Urinary urgency	–	–	–	13
Urine constituents, abnormal	3	–	–	–
UTI	17	–	–	–
Hemic/Lymphatic				
ANC < 1500/mm^3	–	–	–	14
Anemia	4	3	5	–
Leukopenia	–	28	36	–
Lymphadenopathy	–	11	12	8
Lymphocytes < 1500/mm^3	–	–	–	88
Thrombocytopenia	–	2	8	–
WBC < 3000/mm^3	–	–	–	14
Hepatic				
ALT > 5 × baseline	–	20	27	10
AST > 5 × baseline	–	10	17	3
Bilirubinemia	–	3	2	–
Hepatic function abnormal	–	4	9	–
Musculoskeletal				
Arthralgia	9	–	–	31
Back pain	–	23	25	–
Myalgia	29	25	25	27
Myasthenia	–	–	–	46
Skeletal pain	–	15	10	–
Respiratory				
Bronchitis	8	–	–	–
Dyspnea	–	–	–	7
Sinusitis	14	–	–	–
Upper respiratory tract infection	14	–	–	–
Special senses				
Eye disorder	4	–	–	–
Vision abnormal	–	7	13	–
Xerophthalmia	–	3	1	–
Miscellaneous				
Chest pain	5	6	8	11
Chills	19	–	–	25
Fever	20	25	28	36
Flu-like symptoms	49	56	59	60
Infection	7	–	–	–
ISN/inflammation/ecchymosis	6	1	3	5
Injection site reaction/pain	3-8	89	92	85

INTERFERON BETA

Interferon Beta Adverse Reactions (%)[a]

Adverse reactions	*Avonex* (n = 351)	*Rebif* 22 mcg 3 times/week (n = 189)	*Rebif* 44 mcg 3 times/week (n = 184)	Interferon beta-1b (n = 1115)
Leg cramps	–	–	–	4
Malaise	–	4	5	8
Pain	23	–	–	51
Rigors	–	6	13	–
Thyroid disorder	–	4	6	–
Toothache	3	–	–	–
Weight gain		–	–	7

[a] Data are pooled from separate studies and are not necessarily comparable.
[b] Premenopausal patients.Male patients
– = Not reported.

➤*Postmarketing:*

Interferon beta-1a –

Cardiovascular: CHF, cardiomyopathy, cardiomyopathy with CHF.
CNS: New or worsening psychiatric disorders, seizures in patients without history.
GU: Menorrhagia, metrorrhagia.
Hematologic: Decreased peripheral blood counts, including pancytopenia (rare); thrombocytopenia (some cases with nadirs below 10,000/mcL and have reoccurred upon rechallenge); idiopathic thrombocytopenia.
Hepatic: Autoimmune hepatitis; hepatic injury, including elevated serum hepatic enzyme levels; hepatitis.
Miscellaneous: Anaphylaxis, hyper- and hypothyroidism.

Interferon beta-1b –

Cardiovascular: Cardiomyopathy, deep vein thrombosis, pulmonary embolism.
CNS: Ataxia, confusion, convulsion, depersonalization, emotional lability, paresthesia.
Dermatologic: Pruritus, skin discoloration, urticaria.
Endocrine: Hypothyroidism, hyperthyroidism, thyroid dysfunction.
GU: UTI, urosepsis.
Hemic/Lymphatic: Anemia, thrombocytopenia.
Metabolic/Nutritional: Gamma GT increase, hypocalcemia, hyperuricemia, triglyceride increase.
Respiratory: Bronchospasm, pneumonia.
Miscellaneous: Fatal capillary leak syndrome (may appear in patients with a pre-existing monoclonal gammopathy); hepatitis; pancreatitis; vomiting.

Patient Information

➤*Instruction on self-injection technique and procedures:* Instruct patients in the use of aseptic technique when administering interferon beta. Give appropriate instruction for reconstitution of the product and self-injection, including careful review of the patient information sheet that is provided. If possible, perform the first injection under the supervision of an appropriately qualified health care professional.

➤*Dosage schedule:* Caution patients not to change the dosage or the schedule of administration without medical consultation.

➤*Disposal:* Caution patients against the re-use of needles or syringes and instruct them in safe disposal procedures. Supply the patient with a puncture-resistant container for disposal of used needles/syringes along with instructions for safe disposal of containers.

➤*Injection site reactions:* Injection site reactions may occur at least one time during therapy. In general, these are transient and do not require discontinuation of therapy, but carefully assess the nature and severity of all reported reactions. Periodically re-evaluate patient understanding and use of aseptic self-injection technique and procedures.

Advise patients to promptly report any break in the skin, which may be associated with blue-black discoloration, swelling, or drainage of fluid from the injection site, prior to continuing interferon beta therapy.

➤*Flu-like symptoms:* Flu-like symptoms are common following initiation of therapy. Symptoms of flu syndrome are most prominent at the initiation of therapy and decrease in frequency with continued treatment. Concurrent use of analgesics and/or antipyretics may help ameliorate flu-like symptoms on treatment days.

➤*Depression/Suicide:* Caution patients to report depression or suicidal ideation.

➤*Abortifacient potential:* Advise patients about the abortifacient potential.

➤*Photosensitivity:* Advise patients to avoid prolonged exposure to sunlight or sunlamps; interferon beta may cause photosensitivity.

➤*Latex sensitivity:* Some of the packaging may contain latex; caution patients with a possible history of latex allergy.

INTERFERON BETA-1a

Rx	**Rebif** (Serono)	**Injection:** 8.8 mcg per 0.2 mL (2.4 million units)	Preservative free. In prefilled single-use syringes. In *Titration Pack* 6s.[a]
		22 mcg per 0.5 mL (6 million units)	Preservative free. In prefilled single-use syringes. In 1s and 12s.[b]
		44 mcg per 0.5 mL (12 million units)	Preservative free. In prefilled single-use syringes. In 1s and 12s.[c]
Rx	**Avonex** (Biogen Idec)	**Powder for injection, lyophilized:** 33 mcg (6.6 million units [30 mcg/vial when reconstituted])	Preservative free. In administration dose packs (single-use vial with diluent [sterile water for injection], alcohol wipes, gauze pad, syringe, *Micro Pin* vial access pin, needle, and bandage).[d]
		Prefilled syringe: 30 mcg per 0.5 mL	Albumin free. In administration dose packs (single-use syringe, needle, reclose-able accessory pouch, alcohol wipes, gauze pads, and bandages).[e]

[a] With 0.8 mg human albumin, 10.9 mg mannitol, and 0.16 mg sodium acetate in water for injection.
[b] With 2 mg human albumin, 27.3 mg mannitol, and 0.4 mg sodium acetate in water for injection.
[c] With 4 mg human albumin, 27.3 mg mannitol, and 0.4 mg sodium acetate in water for injection.
[d] With 16.5 mg human albumin, 6.4 mg sodium chloride, 6.3 mg dibasic sodium phosphate, and 1.3 mg monobasic sodium phosphate/vial.
[e] With 0.79 mg sodium acetate trihydrate, 0.25 mg glacial acetic acid, 15.8 mg arginine HCl, and 0.025 mg polysorbate 20 in water for injection.

INTERFERON BETA-1a — INJECTION

Indications

➤*Multiple sclerosis (MS):* For the treatment of patients with relapsing forms of MS to slow the accumulation of physical disability and decrease the frequency of clinical exacerbations.

Administration and Dosage

➤*Adults:*

Multiple sclerosis –

Avonex: 30 mcg injected intramuscularly (IM) once a week.
Rebif:

- *Usual dosage* – 22 or 44 mcg injected subcutaneously 3 times per week.
- *Initial dosage* – 20% of the prescribed dose subcutaneously 3 times per week.
- *Dosage titration* – Increase over a 4-week period to the targeted dose, either 22 or 44 mcg 3 times per week.

***Rebif* Schedule for Patient Titration**

	Recommended titration (% of final dose)	Titration dose for *Rebif* 22 mcg	Titration dose for *Rebif* 44 mcg	Injection volume
Weeks 1 to 2	20%	4.4 mcg	8.8 mcg	0.1 mL
Weeks 3 to 4	50%	11 mcg	22 mcg	0.25 mL
Weeks 5+	100%	22 mcg	44 mcg	0.5 mL

- *Dosage adjustment* – Leukopenia or elevated liver function tests may necessitate dose reduction or discontinuation of *Rebif* administration until toxicity is resolved.
- *Concomitant therapy* – Concurrent use of analgesics and/or antipyretics may help ameliorate flu-like symptoms on treatment days.

➤*Hepatic function impairment:*

Rebif – Initiate *Rebif* with caution in patients with active liver disease, alcohol abuse, increased serum ALT (greater than 2.5 times the upper limit of normal [ULN]), or histories of significant liver disease. Consider dose reduction if ALT rises above 5 times the ULN. The dose may be gradually reescalated when enzyme levels have normalized. Stop treatment if jaundice or other clinical symptoms of liver dysfunction appear.

➤*Preparation for administration:*

Avonex –

Powder for injection:
To reconstitute lyophilized *Avonex*, use a sterile syringe and *Micro Pin* to inject 1.1 mL of the supplied diluent, sterile water for injection, into the vial. Gently swirl the vial of *Avonex* to dissolve the drug completely. Do not shake. Withdraw 1 mL of reconstituted solution from the vial into a sterile syringe. The reconstituted solution should be clear to slightly yellow without particles. Each vial of reconstituted solution contains interferon beta-1a 30 mcg/mL. Replace the cover on the *Micro Pin* and attach the sterile 23-gauge, 1.25-inch needle and inject the solution IM.

INTERFERON BETA-1a — INJECTION

Prefilled syringes: Hold the *Avonex* prefilled syringe upright (rubber cap facing up). Remove the protective cover by turning and gently pulling the rubber cap in a clockwise motion. Attach the 23-gauge, 1.25-inch needle and inject the solution IM.

➤*Administration:*

Avonex – Administer IM into the thigh or upper arm.

Do not substitute subcutaneous administration of *Avonex* for IM administration. Subcutaneous and IM administration have been observed to have nonequivalent pharmacokinetic and pharmacodynamic parameters following administration to healthy volunteers.

Rebif – Administer by subcutaneous injection. If possible, at the same time (preferably in the late afternoon or evening) on the same 3 days (eg, Monday, Wednesday, Friday) at least 48 hours apart each week. Advise patients to rotate injection sites.

➤*Storage/Stability:* Store in refrigerator at 2° to 8°C (36° to 46°F). Do not expose to high temperatures. Do not freeze. Protect from light.

Avonex –

Powder for reconstitution: Should refrigeration be unavailable, store vials of *Avonex* at 25°C (77°F) for a period of up to 30 days. Following reconstitution, it is recommended the product be used as soon as possible within 6 hours of being stored at 2° to 8°C (36° to 46°F). Do not freeze reconstituted *Avonex*. The *Avonex* and diluent vials are for single-use only; discard unused portions.

Prefilled syringes: Once removed from the refrigerator, allow *Avonex* in a prefilled syringe to warm to room temperature (about 30 minutes) and use within 12 hours. Do not use external heat sources such as hot water to warm *Avonex* in a prefilled syringe. The prefilled syringe is for single use only.

Rebif – If a refrigerator is not available, store *Rebif* at or below 25°C (77°F) for up to 30 days and away from heat and light. *Rebif* contains no preservatives. Each syringe is intended for single use. Unused portions should be discarded.

INTERFERON BETA-1b

Rx	**Betaseron** (Bayer)	**Injection, lyophilized powder for solution:** 0.3 mg	Preservative free. In single-use 3 mL capacity vials with 1.2 mL prefilled syringe of diluent (sodium chloride 0.54%),[a] alcohol prep pads, and vial adaptor with attached needle for each drug vial. In blister unit 14s.
Rx	**Extavia** (Novartis)		Preservative free. In single-use 3 mL capacity vials with 1.2 mL prefilled syringe of diluent (sodium chloride 0.54%),[a] alcohol prep pads, and vial adaptor with attached needle for each drug vial. In blister unit 15s.

[a] With 15 mg human albumin, 15 mg mannitol per vial.

INTERFERON BETA-1b — INJECTION

Indications

➤*Multiple sclerosis (MS):* For the treatment of relapsing forms of MS to reduce the frequency of clinical exacerbations. Patients with MS in whom efficacy has been demonstrated include patients who have experienced a first clinical episode and have magnetic resonance imaging (MRI) features consistent with MS.

Administration and Dosage

➤*Adults:*

Multiple sclerosis –

Usual dosage: 0.25 mg injected subcutaneously every other day.

Dosage titration: Start at 0.0625 mg subcutaneously every other day and increased over a 6-week period to 0.25 mg every other day.

Interferon Beta-1b Dose Titration Schedule

	Recommended titration	Interferon beta-1b dose	Volume
Weeks 1 to 2	25%	0.0625 mg	0.25 mL
Weeks 3 to 4	50%	0.125 mg	0.5 mL
Weeks 5 to 6	75%	0.1875 mg	0.75 mL
Week 7+	100%	0.25 mg	1 mL

Concomitant therapy: Concurrent use of analgesics and/or antipyretics may help ameliorate flu-like symptoms on treatment days.

➤*Preparation for administration:* To reconstitute interferon beta-1b, attach the prefilled syringe containing the diluent (sodium chloride 0.54% solution) to the interferon beta-1b vial using the vial adapter. Slowly inject 1.2 mL of diluent into the interferon beta-1b vial. Gently swirl the vial to dissolve the drug completely; do not shake. Foaming may occur during reconstitution or if the vial is swirled or shaken too vigorously. If foaming occurs, allow the vial to sit undisturbed until the foam settles. Keeping the syringe and vial adapter in place, turn the assembly over so the vial is on top. Withdraw the appropriate dose of interferon beta-1b solution. Remove the vial from the vial adapter before injecting interferon beta-1b. Reconstituted interferon beta-1b solution contains interferon beta-1b 0.25 mg/mL.

➤*Administration:* Administer subcutaneously. Patients should be advised to rotate sites for subcutaneous injections.

➤*Storage/Stability:* Before reconstitution with diluent, store interferon beta-1b at room temperature, 25°C (77°F). Excursions of 15° to 30°C (59° to 86°F) are permitted. After reconstitution, if not used immediately, the product should be refrigerated and used within 3 hours. The reconstituted product contains no preservative. Do not freeze. Unused portions should be discarded.

ETANERCEPT

Rx	**Enbrel** (Amgen)	**Injection, solution:** 25 mg per 0.5 mL	Preservative free. Sodium chloride, sodium phosphate. In single-use prefilled syringes.
		50 mg/mL	Preservative free. Sodium chloride, sodium phosphate. In single-use prefilled syringes and single-use prefilled *SureClick* autoinjectors.
		Injection, lyophilized powder for solution: 25 mg	Preservative free. In multiple-use vials. Diluent contains benzyl alcohol.

ETANERCEPT — INJECTION

WARNING

Risk of serious infections – Patients treated with etanercept are at increased risk for developing serious infections that may lead to hospitalization or death (see Warnings/Precautions and Adverse Reactions).

Most patients who developed these infections were taking concomitant immunosuppressants such as methotrexate or corticosteroids.

Discontinue etanercept if a patient develops a serious infection or sepsis.

Reported infections include the following:

- Active tuberculosis (TB), including reactivation of latent TB. Patients with TB have frequently presented with disseminated or extrapulmonary disease. Patients should be tested for latent TB before etanercept use and during therapy. Treatment for latent infection should be initiated prior to etanercept use.

WARNING (cont.)

- Invasive fungal infections, including histoplasmosis, coccidioidomycosis, candidiasis, aspergillosis, blastomycosis, and pneumocystosis. Patients with histoplasmosis or other invasive fungal infections may present with disseminated, rather than localized, disease. Antigen and antibody testing for histoplasmosis may be negative in some patients with active infection. Consider empiric antifungal therapy in patients at risk for invasive fungal infections who develop severe systemic illness.
- Bacterial, viral, and other infections caused by opportunistic pathogens.

Carefully consider the risks and benefits of treatment with etanercept prior to initiating therapy in patients with chronic or recurrent infections.

Closely monitor patients for the development of signs and symptoms of infection during and after treatment with etanercept, including the possible development of TB in patients who tested negative for latent TB infection prior to initiating therapy.

ETANERCEPT — INJECTION

Indications

➤*Ankylosing spondylitis:* For reducing signs and symptoms in patients with active ankylosing spondylitis.

➤*Plaque psoriasis:* For treatment of adults 18 years of age and older with chronic moderate to severe plaque psoriasis who are candidates for systemic therapy or phototherapy.

➤*Polyarticular juvenile idiopathic arthritis:* For reducing signs and symptoms of moderately to severely active polyarticular juvenile idiopathic arthritis in patients 2 years of age and older.

➤*Psoriatic arthritis:* For reducing signs and symptoms, inhibiting the progression of structural damage of active arthritis, and improving physical function in patients with psoriatic arthritis. Etanercept can be used in combination with methotrexate in patients who do not respond adequately to methotrexate alone.

➤*Rheumatoid arthritis:* For reducing signs and symptoms, inducing major clinical response, inhibiting the progression of structural damage, and improving physical function in patients with moderately to severely active rheumatoid arthritis (RA). Etanercept can be initiated in combination with methotrexate or used alone.

➤*Off-label uses:*

Congestive heart failure – [5] = Poor documentation. Although animal models and in vitro studies have suggested that tumornecrosis factor (TNF) may contribute to heart failure progression, it currently is unclear if TNF antagonists are clinically beneficial in heart patients. A small multidose study demonstrated that twice-weekly subcutaneous injections are well tolerated and suggested that some improvements in clinical end points may be observed. However, a full profile of safety data associated with long-term dosing and optimal dosing regimens has yet to be determined. In early 2001, Immunex notified health care providers about the discontinuation of two phase 2/3 trials in New York Heart Association (NYHA) congestive heart failure (CHF) patients because of a lack of efficacy. This preliminary analysis of data suggests that the drug may be ineffective in the treatment of CHF. Full publication of the results is pending.

Crohn disease – [4] = Insufficient documentation. To date there is limited published information regarding the use of etanercept for the treatment of Crohn disease. The 2 studies published have demonstrated conflicting results in benefit. Both studies used dosing recommendations for arthritis. These data may suggest that optimal dosing, dosing frequency, or best candidates have not been established.

Graft versus host disease – Initial results suggest that etanercept may be a beneficial adjunctive therapy in the management of graft versus host disease (GVHD). A consistent increase in response rates compared with conventional immunosuppresive therapy has been observed in controlled and noncontrolled studies, but these trials are limited by small patient samples, patient heterogeneity, and variations in conditioning, prophylaxis, and treatment protocols between study sites. Larger, controlled trials are needed to investigate both efficacy and safety, especially with regard to the risk of infection. In addition, etanercept is associated with significant safety risks, as evidenced by a black box warning.

Graft versus host disease (adults): [3] = Safety concerns.

Graft versus host disease (children/adolescents): [3] = Safety concerns.

Hidradenitis suppurativa – [4] = Insufficient documentation. Initial data suggest that etanercept may have benefit as monotherapy in the management of severe, refractory hidradenitis suppurativa. A consistent decrease in the extent of hidradenitis suppurativa and improvements in patient quality of life have been observed in published, noncontrolled studies, but these trials are limited by small patient samples, limited follow-up periods, and nonstandardized scoring of disease activity. In addition to these limitations, preliminary data suggest that long-term treatment would be required to maintain patients in remission; thus, larger, controlled trials are needed to investigate both efficacy and long-term safety.

Nephrotic syndrome – [4] = Insufficient documentation. Although etanercept appears to be a promising therapeutic option in the limited number of cases reported, routine use cannot be recommended because of the small population that has been treated. In addition, the mechanism of action of etanercept in the management of nephrotic syndrome has not been fully elucidated, and nephrotic syndrome can spontaneously regress despite persistent evidence of renal amyloidosis.

Pyoderma gangrenosum – [4] = Insufficient documentation. Initial data suggest that etanercept may have some benefit in patients with pyoderma gangrenosum. However, some case reports have shown no benefit of using etanercept in pyoderma gangrenosum treatment.

Uveitis – Although a meta-analysis of controlled and uncontrolled trials suggested that etanercept may have a role in the management of uveitis resulting from inflammatory disease, carefully controlled studies have not consistently observed a benefit with therapy. Of note, etanercept has also been implicated as a possible cause of new-onset or worsening uveitis or optic neuritis in case reports and case series. Based on these conflicting data, which suggest that etanercept treatment of uveitis may possibly be ineffective or unsafe, use cannot be recommended.

Uveitis (adults): [5] = Poor documentation.

Uveitis (children/adolescents): [5] = Poor documentation.

Wegener granulomatosis – [5] = Poor documentation. Based on the lack of efficacy in a large, well-controlled, long-term prospective clinical trial, etanercept is not indicated for the treatment of Wegener granulomatosis. The addition of etanercept to standard therapy may increase the risk of developing solid tumors. Adverse effects, including life-threatening and fatal events, have been reported during treatment of Wegener granulomatosis with etanercept.

Administration and Dosage

➤*General dosing considerations:* In adults, methotrexate, glucocorticoids, salicylates, nonsteroidal anti-inflammatory drugs (NSAIDs), or analgesics may be continued during treatment with etanercept.

In children 2 to 17 years of age, glucocorticoids, NSAIDs, or analgesics may be continued during treatment with etanercept. Concurrent use with methotrexate and higher doses of etanercept have not been studied in children.

➤*Adults:*

Ankylosing spondylitis – 50 mg/week by subcutaneous injection.

Plaque psoriasis –

Usual dosage: 50 mg twice weekly (administered 3 or 4 days apart) by subcutaneous injection for 3 months, followed by a reduction to a maintenance dosage of 50 mg/week by subcutaneous injection.

Alternative dosage: Starting dosages of etanercept 25 or 50 mg/week by subcutaneous injection were also shown to be efficacious. The proportion of responders were related to etanercept dosage.

Psoriatic arthritis – 50 mg/week by subcutaneous injection.

Rheumatoid arthritis –

Usual dosage: 50 mg/week by subcutaneous injection.

Maximum dose: Dosages higher than 50 mg weekly are not recommended.

Off-label dosing –

Crohn disease: [4] = Insufficient documentation. 25 mg subcutaneous injections twice per week for 8 to 12 weeks.

Graft versus host disease (adults): [3] = Safety concerns. 0.4 mg/kg as a subcutaneous injection twice weekly for 4 weeks, followed by once weekly for 4 weeks or 0.4 mg/kg twice weekly for 8 weeks. The maximum reported duration of therapy was more than 5 months. Some authors limited the maximum dose to 25 mg or used a flat dose of 25 mg. In one study, 16 mg/m^2 per injection was administered on days 1, 5, 9, 13, and 17.

Hidradenitis suppurativa: [4] = Insufficient documentation. 25 mg subcutaneously twice weekly or 50 mg subcutaneously once weekly. The range is 25 to 50 mg subcutaneously twice weekly. Patients have been treated with 50 mg subcutaneously twice weekly for more than 40 weeks.

Nephrotic syndrome: [4] = Insufficient documentation. 25 mg subcutaneously twice a week. Treatment has been continued for more than 4 years in case reports. Lifelong therapy may be needed to prevent progression to end-stage renal disease.

Pyoderma gangrenosum: [4] = Insufficient documentation. 25 to 50 mg subcutaneously twice weekly. Some dosages were given as 50 mg subcutaneously once per week. Although some patients respond and can discontinue therapy upon remission, long-term therapy may be needed to maintain remission.

➤*Children:*

Juvenile idiopathic arthritis –

2 to 17 years of age:

- *Usual dosage* – 0.8 mg/kg weekly by subcutaneous injection.
- *Maximum dose* – 50 mg weekly by subcutaneous injection.

Off-label dosing –

Graft versus host disease (children/adolescents): [3] = Safety concerns. 0.4 mg/kg as a subcutaneous injection twice weekly for 4 weeks, followed by once weekly for 4 weeks or 0.4 mg/kg twice weekly for 8 weeks. Some authors limited the maximum dose to 25 mg or used a flat dose of 25 mg.

Juvenile idiopathic arthritis:

- *4 to 17 years of age* –

  Usual dosage: 0.4 mg/kg subcutaneously twice weekly given 72 to 96 hours apart. Alternate with once weekly dose of 0.8 mg/kg.

  Maximum dose: 25 mg/single dose; 50 mg/week.

➤*Preparation for administration:*

Single-use prefilled syringe – Before injection, etanercept may be allowed to reach room temperature (approximately 15 to 30 minutes). Do not remove the needle cover while allowing the prefilled syringe to reach room temperature.

Prior to administration, visually inspect the solution for particulate matter and discoloration. There may be small white particles of protein in the solution. This is not unusual for proteinaceous solutions. The solution should not be used if it is discolored or cloudy, or if foreign particulate matter is present. Check to see if the amount of liquid in the prefilled syringe falls between the 2 purple fill level indicator lines on the syringe. If the syringe does not have the right amount of liquid, do not use that syringe.

Single-use prefilled SureClick autoinjector – Before injection, etanercept may be allowed to reach room temperature (approximately 15 to 30 minutes). Do not remove the needle shield while allowing the *SureClick* autoinjector to reach room temperature.

Prior to administration, visually inspect the solution for particulate matter and discoloration. There may be small white particles of protein in the solution. This is not unusual for proteinaceous solutions. The solution should not be used if it is discolored or cloudy, or if foreign particulate matter is present.

Multiple-use vial – Reconstitute etanercept aseptically with 1 mL of the supplied sterile bacteriostatic water for injection (benzyl alcohol 0.9%), giving a solution of 1 mL containing etanercept 25 mg.

A vial adapter is supplied for use when reconstituting the lyophilized powder. However, do not use the vial adapter if multiple doses are going to be

ETANERCEPT — INJECTION

withdrawn from the vial. If the vial will be used for multiple doses, a 25-gauge needle should be used for reconstituting and withdrawing etanercept; the supplied "Mixing Date" sticker should also be attached to the vial, and the date of reconstitution should be entered. Reconstitution with the supplied bacteriostatic water for injection, using a 25-gauge needle, yields a preserved, multiple-use solution that must be used within 14 days.

If using the vial adapter, twist the vial adapter onto the diluent syringe. Then, place the vial adapter over the etanercept vial, and insert the vial adapter into the vial stopper. Push down on the plunger to inject the diluent into the etanercept vial. It is normal for some foaming to occur. Keeping the diluent syringe in place, gently swirl the contents of the etanercept vial during dissolution. To avoid excessive foaming, do not shake or agitate vigorously.

If using a 25-gauge needle to reconstitute and withdraw etanercept, the diluent should be injected very slowly into the etanercept vial. It is normal for some foaming to occur. Swirl the contents gently during dissolution. To avoid excessive foaming, do not shake or agitate vigorously.

Generally, dissolution of etanercept takes less than 10 minutes. The solution should not be used if it is discolored or cloudy, or if particulate matter remains.

Withdraw the correct dose of reconstituted solution into the syringe. Some foam or bubbles may remain in the vial. Remove the syringe from the vial adapter or remove the 25-gauge needle from the syringe. Attach a 27-gauge needle to inject etanercept.

Do not mix the contents of 1 vial of etanercept solution with, or transfer into, the contents of another vial of etanercept.

Do not filter reconstituted solution during preparation or administration.

Reconstitution with the supplied sterile bacteriostatic water for injection using a 25-gauge needle yields a preserved, multiple-use solution that must be used within 14 days. Discard reconstituted solution after 14 days. Product stability and sterility cannot be ensured after 14 days.

➤*Administration:* The 25 mg prefilled syringe is not recommended for children weighing less than 31 kg (68 pounds). The 50 mg prefilled syringe or *SureClick* autoinjector may be used for children weighing 63 kg (138 pounds) or more.

A 50 mg dose should be given as 1 subcutaneous injection using a 50 mg single-use prefilled syringe or a 50 mg single-use prefilled *SureClick* autoinjector.

A 50 mg dose can also be given as two 25 mg subcutaneous injections using 25 mg single-use prefilled syringes or multiple-use vials. The two 25 mg injections should be given either on the same day or 3 or 4 days apart.

Sites for injection (thigh, abdomen, or upper arm) should be rotated. Never inject into areas where the skin is tender, bruised, red, or hard.

➤*Admixture compatibility:* Do not add other medications to solutions containing etanercept, and do not reconstitute etanercept with other diluents.

➤*Storage/Stability:*

Single-use prefilled syringe and single-use prefilled SureClick autoinjector – Do not use etanercept beyond the expiration date stamped on the carton or syringe barrel label. Etanercept must be refrigerated at 2° to 8°C (36° to 46°F). Do not freeze. Keep the etanercept prefilled syringes in the original carton to protect from light until the time of use. Do not shake.

Multiple-use vial – Do not use a dose tray beyond the date stamped on the carton, dose tray label, vial label, or diluent syringe label. The dose tray containing etanercept (sterile powder) must be refrigerated at 2° to 8°C (36° to 46°F). Do not freeze.

Reconstituted solutions of etanercept prepared with the supplied bacteriostatic water for injection (benzyl alcohol 0.9%), using a 25-gauge needle, may be stored for up to 14 days if refrigerated at 2° to 8°C (36° to 46°F). Discard reconstituted solution after 14 days. Product stability and sterility cannot be ensured after 14 days.

Actions

➤*Pharmacology:* Etanercept binds specifically to TNF and blocks its interaction with cell surface TNF receptors (TNFRs). TNF is a naturally occurring cytokine that is involved in normal inflammatory and immune responses. It plays an important role in the inflammatory processes of RA, polyarticular course juvenile idiopathic arthritis, and ankylosing spondylitis and the resulting joint pathology. In addition, TNF plays a role in the inflammatory process of plaque psoriasis. Elevated levels of TNF are found in involved tissues and fluids of patients with RA, psoriatic arthritis, ankylosing spondylitis, and plaque psoriasis.

Two distinct TNFRs, a 55 kDa protein (p55) and a 75 kDa protein (p75), exist naturally as monomeric molecules on cell surfaces and in soluble forms. Biological activity of TNF is dependent upon binding to either cell surface TNFR.

Etanercept is a dimeric soluble form of the p75 TNFR that can bind to 2 TNF molecules. It inhibits the activity of TNF in vitro and has been shown to affect several animal models of inflammation, including murine collagen-induced arthritis. Etanercept inhibits binding of both TNF-alpha and TNF-beta (lymphotoxin alpha) to cell surface TNFRs, rendering TNF biologically inactive. Cells expressing transmembrane TNF that bind etanercept are not lysed in vitro in the presence or absence of complement.

Etanercept can also modulate biological responses that are induced or regulated by TNF, including expression of adhesion molecules responsible for leukocyte migration (ie, E-selectin and, to a lesser extent, intercellular adhesion molecule-1), serum levels of cytokines (eg, interleukin-6), and serum levels of matrix metalloproteinase-3 (stromelysin).

➤*Pharmacokinetics:*

Absorption/Distribution – After administration of etanercept 25 mg by a single subcutaneous injection to 25 patients with RA, a maximum serum concentration (C_{max}) of 1.1 ± 0.6 mcg/mL and time to C_{max} of 69 ± 34 hours were observed in these patients following a single 25 mg dose. After 6 months of twice-weekly 25 mg doses in these same RA patients, the mean C_{max} was 2.4 ± 1 mcg/mL (n = 23). Patients exhibited a 2- to 7-fold increase in peak serum concentrations and approximately 4-fold increase in area under the curve (AUC_{0-72h}) (range, 1- to 17-fold) with repeated dosing. Serum concentrations in patients with RA have not been measured for periods of dosing that exceed 6 months. The pharmacokinetic parameters in patients with plaque psoriasis were similar to those seen in patients with RA.

In another study, serum concentration profiles at steady-state were comparable among patients with RA treated with etanercept 50 mg once weekly and those treated with etanercept 25 mg twice weekly. The mean (± standard deviation [SD]) C_{max}, minimum serum concentration (C_{min}), and partial AUC were 2.4 ± 1.5 mg/L, 1.2 ± 0.7 mg/L, and 297 ± 166 mg•h/L, respectively, for patients treated with etanercept 50 mg once weekly (n = 21); and 2.6 ± 1.2 mg/L, 1.4 ± 0.7 mg/L, and 316 ± 135 mg•h/L, respectively, for patients treated with etanercept 25 mg twice weekly (n = 16).

Metabolism/Excretion – After administration of etanercept 25 mg by a single subcutaneous injection to 25 patients with RA, a mean ± SD half-life of 102 ± 30 hours was observed, with a clearance of 160 ± 80 mL/h.

Special populations –

Children: Patients 4 to 17 years of age with juvenile idiopathic arthritis were administered 0.4 mg/kg twice weekly for up to 18 weeks. The mean serum concentration after repeated subcutaneous dosing was 2.1 mcg/mL, with a range of 0.7 to 4.3 mcg/mL. Limited data suggest that the clearance of etanercept is reduced slightly in children 4 to 8 years of age. Population pharmacokinetic analyses predict that administration of etanercept 0.8 mg/kg once weekly will result in C_{max} 11% higher, and C_{min} 20% lower at steady state compared with administration of etanercept 0.4 mg/kg twice weekly. The predicted pharmacokinetic differences between the regimens in juvenile idiopathic arthritis patients are of the same magnitude as the differences observed between twice-weekly and weekly regimens in adult RA patients.

Contraindications

Sepsis; known hypersensitivity to etanercept or any of its components.

Warnings/Precautions

➤*Serious infections:* Serious and sometimes fatal infections caused by bacterial, mycobacterial, invasive fungal, viral, or other opportunistic pathogens have been reported in patients receiving TNF-blocking agents. Among opportunistic infections, TB, histoplasmosis, aspergillosis, candidiasis, coccidioidomycosis, listeriosis, and pneumocystosis were the most commonly reported. Patients have frequently presented with disseminated rather than localized disease, and are often taking concomitant immunosuppressants, such as methotrexate or corticosteroids, with etanercept.

Do not initiate treatment with etanercept in patients with an active infection, including clinically important localized infections. Consider the risks and benefits of treatment prior to initiating therapy in patients with chronic or recurrent infection; who have been exposed to TB; who have resided or traveled in areas of endemic TB or endemic mycoses, such as histoplasmosis, coccidioidomycosis, or blastomycosis; or with an underlying conditions that may predispose them to infection, such as advanced or poorly controlled diabetes.

Cases of reactivation of TB or new TB infections have been observed in patients receiving etanercept, including patients who have previously received treatment for latent or active TB. Data from clinical trials and preclinical studies suggest that the risk of reactivation of latent TB infection is lower with etanercept than with TNF-blocking monoclonal antibodies. Nonetheless, postmarketing cases of TB reactivation have been reported for TNF blockers, including etanercept. Evaluate patients for TB risk factors and test for latent infection prior to initiating etanercept and periodically during therapy.

Treatment of latent TB infection prior to therapy with TNF-blocking agents has been shown to reduce the risk of TB reactivation during therapy. Induration of 5 mm or more with tuberculin skin testing should be considered a positive test result when assessing if treatment for latent TB is needed prior to initiating etanercept, even for patients previously vaccinated with Bacille Calmette-Guérin.

Consider anti-TB therapy prior to initiation of etanercept in patients with a history of latent or active TB in whom an adequate course of treatment cannot be confirmed, and for patients with a negative test for latent TB but having risk factors for TB infection. Consultation with a health care provider with expertise in the treatment of TB is recommended to aid in the decision whether initiating anti-TB therapy is appropriate for an individual patient.

Strongly consider TB in patients who develop a new infection during etanercept treatment, especially in patients who have previously or recently traveled to countries with a higher prevalence of TB, or who have had close contact with a person with active TB.

Closely monitor patients for the development of signs and symptoms of infection during and after treatment with etanercept, including the development of TB in patients who tested negative for latent TB infection prior to initiating therapy. Tests for latent TB infection may be falsely negative while on therapy with etanercept.

ETANERCEPT — INJECTION

Discontinue etanercept if a patient develops a serious infection or sepsis. Closely monitor a patient who develops a new infection during treatment with etanercept and have the patient undergo a prompt and complete diagnostic workup appropriate for an immunocompromised patient, and initiate appropriate antimicrobial therapy.

Nonetheless, postmarketing cases of serious and sometimes fatal fungal infections, including histoplasmosis, have been reported with TNF blockers, including etanercept. For patients who reside or travel in regions where mycoses are endemic, suspect invasive fungal infection if they develop a serious systemic illness. Consider appropriate empiric antifungal therapy while a diagnostic workup is being performed. Antigen and antibody testing for histoplasmosis may be negative in some patients with active infection. When feasible, make a decision to administer empiric antifungal therapy in these patients in consultation with a health care provider with expertise in the diagnosis and treatment of invasive fungal infections, and take into account both the risk for severe fungal infection and the risks of antifungal therapy.

➤*Neurologic effects:* Treatment with etanercept and other agents that inhibit TNF has been associated with rare cases of new-onset or exacerbation of CNS-demyelinating disorders, some presenting with mental status changes and some associated with permanent disability. Cases of transverse myelitis, optic neuritis, multiple sclerosis, and new-onset or exacerbation of seizure disorders have been observed in association with etanercept therapy. The causal relationship to etanercept therapy remains unclear. While no clinical trials have been performed evaluating etanercept therapy in patients with multiple sclerosis, other TNF antagonists administered to patients with multiple sclerosis have been associated with increases in disease activity. Exercise caution in considering the use of etanercept in patients with preexisting or recent-onset CNS-demyelinating disorders.

➤*Hematologic effects:* Rare reports of pancytopenia, including aplastic anemia, some with a fatal outcome, have been reported in patients treated with etanercept. The causal relationship to etanercept therapy remains unclear. Although no high-risk group has been identified, exercise caution in patients being treated with etanercept who have a history of significant hematologic abnormalities. Advise all patients to seek immediate medical attention if they develop signs and symptoms suggestive of blood dyscrasias or infection (eg, bleeding, bruising, pallor, persistent fever) while on etanercept. Consider discontinuation of etanercept therapy in patients with confirmed significant hematologic abnormalities.

➤*Malignancies:* In the controlled portions of clinical trials of all the TNF-blocking agents, more cases of lymphoma have been observed among patients receiving the TNF blocker compared with control patients. During the controlled portions of etanercept trials, 3 lymphomas were observed among 4,509 etanercept-treated patients versus 0 among 2,040 control patients (mean duration of controlled treatment ranged from 3 to 24 months). In the controlled and open-label portions of clinical trials of etanercept, 9 lymphomas were observed in 5,723 patients over approximately 11,201 patient-years of therapy. This is 3-fold higher than that expected in the general population. While patients with RA or psoriasis, particularly those with highly active disease, may be at a higher risk (up to several-fold) for the development of lymphoma, the potential role of TNF-blocking therapy in the development of malignancies is not known.

In a randomized, placebo-controlled study of 180 patients with Wegener granulomatosis in which etanercept was added to standard treatment (including cyclophosphamide, methotrexate, and corticosteroids), the patients receiving etanercept experienced more noncutaneous solid malignancies than patients receiving placebo. The addition of etanercept to standard treatment was not associated with improved clinical outcomes when compared with standard therapy alone. The use of etanercept in patients with Wegener granulomatosis receiving immunosuppressive agents is not recommended. The use of etanercept in patients receiving concurrent cyclophosphamide therapy is not recommended.

➤*Hepatitis B virus reactivation:* Use of TNF blockers, including etanercept, has been associated with reactivation of hepatitis B virus (HBV) in patients who are chronic carriers of this virus. In some instances, HBV reactivation occurring in conjunction with TNF-blocker therapy has been fatal. The majority of these reports have occurred in patients concomitantly receiving other medications that suppress the immune system, which may also contribute to HBV reactivation. Prior to initiating TNF-blocker therapy, evaluate patients at risk for HBV infection for prior evidence of HBV infection. Exercise caution in prescribing TNF blockers for patients identified as carriers of HBV. Adequate data are not available on the safety or efficacy of treating patients who are carriers of HBV with antiviral therapy in conjunction with TNF-blocker therapy to prevent HBV reactivation. Closely monitor patients who are carriers of HBV and require treatment with etanercept for clinical and laboratory signs of active HBV infection throughout therapy and for several months following termination of therapy. In patients who develop HBV reactivation, consider stopping etanercept and initiating antiviral therapy with appropriate supportive treatment. The safety of resuming etanercept therapy after HBV reactivation is controlled is not known. Therefore, weigh the risks and benefits when considering resumption of therapy in this situation.

➤*Heart failure:* Two large clinical trials evaluating the use of etanercept in the treatment of heart failure were terminated early because of lack of efficacy. Results of one study suggested higher mortality in patients treated with etanercept compared with placebo. Results of the second study did not corroborate these observations. Analyses did not identify specific factors associated with increased risk of adverse outcomes in patients with heart failure treated with etanercept. There have been postmarketing reports of worsening of CHF, with and without identifiable precipitating factors, in patients taking etanercept. There have also been rare reports of new-onset CHF, including CHF in patients without known preexisting cardiovascular disease. Some of these patients have been younger than 50 years of age. Exercise caution when using etanercept in patients who also have heart failure, and monitor patients carefully.

➤*Immunosuppression:* Anti-TNF therapies, including etanercept, affect host defenses against infections and malignancies because TNF mediates inflammation and modulates cellular immune responses. In a study of 49 patients with RA treated with etanercept, there was no evidence of depression of delayed-type hypersensitivity, depression of immunoglobulin levels, or change in enumeration of effector cell populations. The impact of treatment with etanercept on the development and course of malignancies, as well as active or chronic infections, is not fully understood. The safety and efficacy of etanercept in patients with immunosuppression or chronic infections have not been evaluated.

➤*Immunizations:* Patients receiving etanercept may receive concurrent vaccinations, except for live vaccines. No data are available on the secondary transmission of infection by live vaccines in patients receiving etanercept.

It is recommended that patients with juvenile idiopathic arthritis, if possible, be brought up to date with all immunizations in agreement with current immunization guidelines prior to initiating etanercept therapy. Temporarily discontinue etanercept therapy in patients with a significant exposure to varicella virus and consider prophylactic treatment with varicella-zoster immune globulin.

➤*Autoimmunity:* Treatment with etanercept may result in the formation of autoantibodies and, rarely, in the development of a lupus-like syndrome or autoimmune hepatitis that may resolve following withdrawal of etanercept. If a patient develops symptoms and findings suggestive of a lupus-like syndrome or autoimmune hepatitis following treatment with etanercept, discontinue treatment and carefully evaluate the patient.

➤*Immunogenicity:* Patients with RA, psoriatic arthritis, ankylosing spondylitis, or plaque psoriasis were tested at multiple time points for antibodies to etanercept. Antibodies to the TNFR portion or other protein components of the etanercept drug product, all nonneutralizing, were detected at least once in sera of approximately 6% of adult patients with RA, psoriatic arthritis, ankylosing spondylitis, or plaque psoriasis. These antibodies were all nonneutralizing. No apparent correlation of antibody development to clinical response or adverse reactions was observed. Results from patients with juvenile idiopathic arthritis were similar to those seen in adult patients with RA treated with etanercept. The long-term immunogenicity of etanercept is unknown.

➤*Benzyl alcohol:* The diluent for etanercept multiple-use vials containing lyophilized powder contains benzyl alcohol. Benzyl alcohol has been associated with a fatal "gasping syndrome" in premature infants.

➤*Latex allergy:* The needle cover of the prefilled syringe and the *SureClick* autoinjector contain dry natural rubber (a derivative of latex), which may cause allergic reactions in individuals sensitive to latex.

➤*Hypersensitivity reactions:* Allergic reactions associated with administration of etanercept during clinical trials have been reported in less than 2% of patients. If an anaphylactic reaction or other serious allergic reaction occurs, discontinue administration of etanercept immediately and initiate appropriate therapy.

➤*Pregnancy: Category B.* There are no studies in pregnant women. Although the human pregnancy experience is very limited, there is no evidence of embryofetal harm. However, the human data are too limited for an assessment of the risk. Use this drug during pregnancy only if clearly needed

Pregnancy registry – To monitor outcomes of pregnant women exposed to etanercept, a pregnancy registry has been established. Register patients by calling 1-877-311-8972.

➤*Lactation:* It is not known whether etanercept is excreted in human milk or absorbed systemically after ingestion. Because etanercept is a protein, it most likely would be digested in the infant's stomach and not absorbed systemically. Because many drugs and immunoglobulins are excreted in human milk, and because of the potential for serious adverse reactions from etanercept in breast-feeding infants, decide whether to discontinue breast-feeding or the drug.

➤*Children:* Etanercept is indicated for treatment of polyarticular-course juvenile idiopathic arthritis in patients 2 years of age and older. Etanercept has not been studied in children younger than 2 years of age.

➤*Elderly:* Because there is a higher incidence of infections in the elderly population in general, use caution in treating elderly patients.

➤*Monitoring:* Closely monitor patients for the development of signs and symptoms of infection during and after treatment with etanercept, including the development of TB in patients who tested negative for latent TB infection prior to initiating therapy. Closely monitor a patient who develops a new infection during treatment with etanercept and have the patient undergo a prompt and complete diagnostic workup appropriate for an immunocompromised patient, and initiate appropriate antimicrobial therapy. Closely monitor patients who develop a new infection while undergoing treatment with etanercept. Discontinue administration of etanercept if a patient develops a serious infection or sepsis. Do not initiate treatment with etanercept in patients with active infections, including chronic or localized infections. Exercise caution when considering the use of etanercept in patients with a history of recurring infections or with underlying conditions that may predispose patients to infections, such as advanced or poorly controlled diabetes. Evaluate patients for TB risk factors and test for latent infection prior to initiating etanercept and periodically during therapy. Closely monitor patients who are carriers of HBV and require treatment

ETANERCEPT — INJECTION

with etanercept for clinical and laboratory signs of active HBV infection throughout therapy and for several months following termination of therapy.

Drug Interactions

➤*Immunizations:* See Warnings/Precautions.

Etanercept Drug Interactions			
Precipitant drug	Object drug[a]		Description
Anakinra	Etanercept	⬆	Concurrent etanercept and anakinra therapy produced a 7% rate of serious infection, which was higher than that observed with etanercept alone (0%). Concurrent therapy is not recommended.
Sulfasalazine	Etanercept	⬆	Concomitant use may cause a mild decrease in mean neutrophil counts. The clinical significance of this observation is unknown.
Etanercept	Sulfasalazine		
Etanercept	Cyclophosphamide	⬆	In a study of patients with Wegener granulomatosis, the addition of etanercept to standard treatment (including cyclophosphamide, methotrexate, and corticosteroids) was associated with a higher incidence of noncutaneous solid malignancies. Concurrent use of cyclophosphamide is not recommended.
Etanercept	Immunosuppressive agents	⬆	The use of etanercept in patients with Wegener granulomatosis receiving immunosuppressive agents is not recommended.

[a] ⬆ = object drug increased.

Adverse Reactions

➤*Rheumatoid arthritis, psoriatic arthritis, ankylosing spondylitis, or plaque psoriasis:*

Injection-site reactions – In controlled trials in rheumatologic indications, approximately 37% of patients treated with etanercept developed injection-site reactions. In controlled trials in patients with plaque psoriasis, 14% of patients treated with etanercept developed injection-site reactions during the first 3 months of treatment. All injection-site reactions were described as mild to moderate (eg, erythema or itching, pain, swelling) and generally did not necessitate drug discontinuation. Injection-site reactions generally occurred in the first month and subsequently decreased in frequency. The mean duration of injection-site reactions was 3 to 5 days. Seven percent of patients experienced redness at a previous injection site when subsequent injections were given. In postmarketing experience, injection-site bleeding and bruising have also been observed in conjunction with etanercept therapy.

Infections – In controlled trials, there were no differences in rates of infection among patients with RA, psoriatic arthritis, ankylosing spondylitis, and plaque psoriasis treated with etanercept and those treated with placebo (or methotrexate for patients with RA and psoriatic arthritis). The most common type of infection was upper respiratory tract infection, which occurred at a rate of approximately 20% among both etanercept- and placebo-treated patients in RA, psoriatic arthritis, and ankylosing spondylitis trials, and at a rate of approximately 12% among both etanercept- and placebo-treated patients in plaque psoriasis trials in the first 3 months of treatment.

In placebo-controlled trials in RA, psoriatic arthritis, ankylosing spondylitis, and plaque psoriasis, no increase in the incidence of serious infections was observed (approximately 1% in both placebo- and etanercept-treated groups). In all clinical trials in RA, serious infections experienced by patients included pyelonephritis, bronchitis, septic arthritis, abdominal abscess, cellulitis, osteomyelitis, wound infection, pneumonia, foot abscess, leg ulcer, diarrhea, sinusitis, and sepsis. The rate of serious infections has not increased in open-label extension trials, and is similar to that observed in etanercept- and placebo-treated patients from controlled trials. Serious infections, including sepsis and death, have also been reported during postmarketing use of etanercept. Some have occurred within a few weeks after initiating treatment with etanercept. Many of the patients had underlying conditions (eg, diabetes, CHF, history of active or chronic infections) in addition to RA. Data from a sepsis clinical trial not specifically in patients with RA suggest that etanercept treatment may increase mortality in patients with established sepsis.

In patients who received both etanercept and anakinra for up to 24 weeks, the incidence of serious infections was 7%. The most common infections consisted of bacterial pneumonia (4 cases) and cellulitis (4 cases). One patient with pulmonary fibrosis and pneumonia died because of respiratory failure.

In postmarketing experience in rheumatologic indications, infections have been observed with various pathogens, including viral, bacterial, fungal, and protozoal organisms. Infections have been noted in all organ systems and have been reported in patients receiving etanercept alone or in combination with immunosuppressive agents.

In clinical trials in plaque psoriasis, serious infections experienced by etanercept-treated patients have included cellulitis, gastroenteritis, pneumonia, abscess, and osteomyelitis.

In global clinical studies of 20,070 patients (23,308 patient-years of therapy), TB was observed in approximately 0.01% of patients. In 15,438 patients (23,524 patient-years of therapy) from clinical studies in the US and Canada, TB was observed in approximately 0.007% of patients. These studies include reports of pulmonary and extrapulmonary TB.

Malignancies – Patients have been observed in clinical trials with etanercept for more than 5 years. Among 4,462 patients with RA treated with etanercept in clinical trials for a mean of 27 months (approximately 10,000 patient-years of therapy), 9 lymphomas were observed for a rate of 0.09 cases per 100 patient-years. This is 3-fold higher than the rate of lymphomas expected in the general population based on the Surveillance, Epidemiology, and End Results Database. An increased rate of lymphoma up to several-fold has been reported in the RA patient population, and may be further increased in patients with more severe disease activity. Sixty-seven malignancies other than lymphoma were observed. Of these, the most common malignancies were colon, breast, lung, and prostate, which were similar in type and number to what would be expected in the general population. Analysis of the cancer rates at 6-month intervals suggest constant rates throughout 5 years of observation.

In the placebo-controlled portions of the psoriasis studies, 8 of 933 patients who received etanercept at any dose were diagnosed with a malignancy compared with 1 of 414 patients who received placebo. Among the 1,261 patients with psoriasis who received etanercept at any dose in the controlled and uncontrolled portions of the psoriasis studies (1,062 patient-years), a total of 22 patients were diagnosed with 23 malignancies: 9 patients with noncutaneous solid tumors, 12 patients with 13 nonmelanoma skin cancers (8 basal, 5 squamous), and 1 patient with non-Hodgkin lymphoma. Among the placebo-treated patients (90 patient-years of observation), 1 patient was diagnosed with 2 squamous cell cancers. The size of the placebo group and limited duration of the controlled portions of studies precludes the ability to draw firm conclusions.

See Warnings/Precautions for more information.

Autoantibodies – Patients with RA had serum samples tested for autoantibodies at multiple time points. In RA studies 1 and 2, the percentage of patients evaluated for antinuclear antibodies (ANA) who developed new positive ANA (titer of 1:40 or more) was higher in patients treated with etanercept (11%) than in placebo-treated patients (5%). The percentage of patients who developed new positive anti–double-stranded DNA antibodies was also higher by radioimmunoassay (15% of patients treated with etanercept compared with 4% of placebo-treated patients) and by crithidia lucilae assay (3% of patients treated with etanercept compared with none of the placebo-treated patients). The proportion of patients treated with etanercept who developed anticardiolipin antibodies was similarly increased compared with placebo-treated patients. In study 3, no pattern of increased autoantibody development was seen in etanercept patients compared with methotrexate patients.

Other adverse reactions – In placebo-controlled plaque psoriasis trials, the percentages of patients reporting injection-site reactions were lower in the placebo dose group (6.4%) than in the etanercept dose groups (15.5%) in studies 1 and 2. Otherwise, the percentages of patients reporting adverse reactions in the 50 mg twice-weekly dose group were similar to those observed in the 25 mg twice-weekly dose group or placebo group. In psoriasis study 1, there were no serious adverse reactions of worsening psoriasis following withdrawal of study drug. However, adverse reactions of worsening psoriasis, including 3 serious adverse reactions, were observed during the course of the clinical trials. Urticaria and noninfectious hepatitis were observed in a small number of patients, and angioedema was observed in 1 patient in clinical studies. Urticaria and angioedema have also been reported in spontaneous postmarketing reports. Adverse reactions in psoriatic arthritis, ankylosing spondylitis, and plaque psoriasis trials were similar to those reported in RA clinical trials.

Etanercept Adverse Reactions in Patients With RA (≥ 3%)[a]				
	Placebo-controlled		Active-controlled (study 3)	
Adverse reactions	Etanercept (n = 349)	Placebo[b] (n = 152)	Etanercept (n = 415)	Methotrexate (n = 217)
CNS				
Asthenia	5%	3%	11%	12%
Dizziness	7%	5%	8%	11%
Headache	17%	13%	24%	27%
Dermatologic				
Alopecia	1%	1%	6%	12%
Rash	5%	3%	14%	23%
GI				
Abdominal pain	5%	3%	10%	10%
Dyspepsia	4%	1%	11%	10%
Mouth ulcer	2%	1%	6%	14%
Nausea	9%	10%	15%	29%
Vomiting	3%		5%	8%

ETANERCEPT — INJECTION

Etanercept Adverse Reactions in Patients With RA (≥ 3%)[a]				
	Placebo-controlled		Active-controlled (study 3)	
Adverse reactions	Etanercept (n = 349)	Placebo[b] (n = 152)	Etanercept (n = 415)	Methotrexate (n = 217)
Respiratory				
Cough	6%	3%	5%	6%
Pharyngitis	7%	5%	6%	9%
Pneumonitis ("methotrexate lung")			0%	2%
Respiratory disorder	5%	1%	NA[c]	NA
Rhinitis	12%	8%	16%	14%
Sinusitis	3%	2%	5%	3%
Upper respiratory tract infection[d]	29%	16%	31%	39%
Miscellaneous				
Infection (total)[d]	35%	32%	64%	72%
Injection-site reaction	37%	10%	34%	7%
Non-upper respiratory tract infection[d]	38%	32%	51%	60%
Peripheral edema	2%	3%	8%	4%

[a] Includes data from the 6-month study in which patients received concurrent methotrexate therapy.
[b] The duration of exposure for patients receiving placebo was less than the etanercept-treated patients.
[c] NA = not applicable.
[d] Infection (total) includes data from all 3 placebo-controlled trials. Non-upper respiratory tract infection and upper respiratory tract infection include data only from the 2 placebo-controlled trials in which infections were collected separately from adverse reactions (placebo, n = 110; etanercept, n = 213).

Serious adverse infections: In controlled trials of RA and psoriatic arthritis, rates of serious adverse reactions were seen at a frequency of approximately 5% among etanercept- and control-treated patients. In controlled trials of plaque psoriasis, rates of serious adverse reactions were seen at a frequency of less than 1.5% among etanercept- and placebo-treated patients in the first 3 months of treatment. Among patients with RA in placebo-controlled, active-controlled, and open-label trials of etanercept, malignancies and infections were the most common serious adverse reactions observed. The following other infrequent serious adverse reactions observed in RA, psoriatic arthritis, ankylosing spondylitis, and plaque psoriasis clinical trials are listed by body system in the following sections.

• *Cardiovascular* – Deep vein thrombosis, heart failure, hypertension, hypotension, myocardial infarction, myocardial ischemia, thrombophlebitis.
• *CNS* – Cerebral ischemia, depression, multiple sclerosis.
• *GI* – Appendicitis, cholecystitis, GI hemorrhage, pancreatitis.
• *GU* – Kidney calculus, membranous glomerulonephropathy.
• *Musculoskeletal* – Bursitis, polymyositis.
• *Respiratory* – Dyspnea, pulmonary embolism, sarcoidosis.
• *Miscellaneous* – Lymphadenopathy, worsening psoriasis. In a randomized, controlled trial in which 51 patients with RA received etanercept 50 mg twice weekly and 25 patients received etanercept 25 mg twice weekly, the following serious adverse reactions were observed in the 50 mg twice-weekly arm: GI bleeding, normal pressure hydrocephalous, seizure, and stroke. No serious adverse reactions were observed in the 25 mg arm.

➤*Juvenile idiopathic arthritis:*

Severe adverse reactions – Severe adverse reactions reported in 69 patients 4 to 17 years of age with juvenile idiopathic arthritis included varicella, gastroenteritis, depression/personality disorder, cutaneous ulcer, esophagitis/gastritis, group A streptococcal septic shock, type 1 diabetes mellitus, and soft tissue and postoperative wound infection.

Infection – Of 69 children with juvenile idiopathic arthritis, 43 (62%) experienced an infection while receiving etanercept during 3 months of the study (part 1 open-label), and the frequency and severity of infections were similar in 58 patients completing 12 months of open-label extension therapy. The types of infections reported in juvenile idiopathic arthritis patients were generally mild and consistent with those commonly seen in outpatient pediatric populations. Two juvenile idiopathic arthritis patients developed varicella infection and signs and symptoms of aseptic meningitis that resolved without sequelae.

Common adverse reactions – The following adverse reactions were reported more commonly in 69 patients with juvenile idiopathic arthritis receiving 3 months of etanercept compared with the 349 adult patients with RA in placebo-controlled trials: headache (19% of patients; 1.7 events per patient-year), nausea (9%; 1 event per patient-year), abdominal pain (19%; 0.74 events per patient-year), and vomiting (13%; 0.74 events per patient-year).

➤*Postmarketing:*

Adults –

Cardiovascular: Chest pain, new-onset CHF, stroke, vasodilation (flushing).

CNS: Fatigue, paresthesias, seizures and CNS events suggestive of multiple sclerosis or isolated demyelinating conditions such as transverse myelitis or optic neuritis.

Dermatologic: Cutaneous vasculitis, erythema multiforme, pruritus, Stevens-Johnson syndrome, subcutaneous nodules, toxic epidermal necrolysis, urticaria.

GI: Altered sense of taste, anorexia, diarrhea, dry mouth, intestinal perforation.

Hematologic: Adenopathy, anemia, aplastic anemia, leukopenia, neutropenia, pancytopenia, thrombocytopenia.

Musculoskeletal: Joint pain, lupus-like syndrome with manifestations including rash consistent with subacute or discoid lupus.

Ophthalmic: Dry eyes, ocular inflammation.

Respiratory: Dyspnea, interstitial lung disease, pulmonary disease, worsening of prior lung disorder.

Miscellaneous: Angioedema, autoimmune hepatitis, fever, flu syndrome, generalized pain, weight gain.

Children – In postmarketing experience, the following additional serious adverse reactions have been reported in children: abscess with bacteremia, coagulopathy, cutaneous vasculitis, optic neuritis, pancytopenia, seizures, transaminase elevations, tuberculous arthritis, and urinary tract infection. The frequency of these reactions and their causal relationship to etanercept therapy are unknown.

Patient Information

Instruct patients to seek medical evaluation immediately if they develop signs and symptoms of infection.

Instruct patients or caregivers that the needle cover on the single-use prefilled syringe and on the *SureClick* autoinjector contains dry natural rubber (a derivative of latex), which should not be handled by persons sensitive to this substance.

If a patient or caregiver is to administer etanercept, instruct the patient or caregiver in injection techniques and how to measure and administer the correct dose. Have the patient or caregiver perform the first injection under the supervision of a qualified health care provider. Assess the patient's or caregiver's ability to inject subcutaneously. Instruct patients and caregivers in the technique, as well as proper syringe and needle disposal, and caution them against reuse of needles and syringes.

Advise patients to use a puncture-resistant container for disposal of needles and syringes. If the product is intended for multiple use, additional syringes, needles, and alcohol swabs will be required.

Instruct patients to rotate the site for each injection. Instruct patients not to inject into areas where the skin is tender, bruised, red, or hard, and to avoid areas with scars or stretch marks.

For patients with psoriasis, instruct the patient not to inject directly into any raised, thick, red, or scaly skin patches ("psoriasis skin lesions").

ANAKINRA

Rx	**Kineret** (Biovitrum AB)	**Injection:** 100 mg per 0.67 mL	Preservative free. Disodium EDTA, polysorbate 80, sodium chloride. In 1 mL single-use prefilled syringe with 27-gauge needle.

ANAKINRA — INJECTION

Indications

➤*Rheumatoid arthritis:* For the reduction in signs and symptoms and slowing the progression of structural damage of moderately to severely active rheumatoid arthritis (RA) in patients 18 years of age and older who have failed 1 or more disease-modifying antirheumatic drugs (DMARDs). Anakinra can be used alone or in combination with DMARDs other than tumor necrosis factor (TNF)-blocking agents.

➤*Off-label uses:*

Juvenile idiopathic arthritis – [4] = Insufficient documentation. The data evaluating the safety and efficacy of anakinra for the treatment of systemic-onset juvenile idiopathic arthritis (JIA) are limited to case reports and retrospective evaluations. The most recent consensus statement considers anakinra to be effective in some children with systemic-onset JIA. Until additional data are available, the use of anakinra for JIA is not routinely recommended but can be considered in children who are refractory to other treatment options.

Administration and Dosage

➤*Adults:*

Rheumatoid arthritis – 100 mg daily by subcutaneous injection.

➤*Children:*

Off-label dosing –

Juvenile idiopathic arthritis: [4] = Insufficient documentation.

• *Children 4 to 17 years of age* – 1 to 2 mg/kg daily by subcutaneous injection, with a maximum dosage of 100 mg daily. Dosages of up to 100 mg

ANAKINRA — INJECTION

twice daily were used in select children. Therapy continued for more than 12 months in some reports.

➤*Renal function impairment:* Consider a dose of anakinra 100 mg administered every other day for patients with RA who have severe renal insufficiency or end-stage renal disease (defined as creatinine clearance less than 30 mL/min, as estimated from serum creatinine levels).

➤*Administration:* Administer the dose at approximately the same time every day. Administer only 1 dose (the entire contents of 1 prefilled glass syringe) per day.

Instructions on appropriate use should be given by the health care provider to the patients or caregiver. Patients or caregivers should not be allowed to administer anakinra until they have demonstrated a thorough understanding of procedures and an ability to inject the product.

There may be trace amounts of small, translucent-to-white amorphous particles of protein in the solution. The prefilled syringe should not be used if the solution is discolored or cloudy, or if foreign particulate matter is present. If the number of translucent-to-white amorphous particles in a given syringe appears excessive, do not use this syringe.

➤*Storage/Stability:* Store anakinra in the refrigerator at 2° to 8°C (36° to 46°F). Do not freeze or shake. Protect from light.

Actions

➤*Pharmacology:* Anakinra is a recombinant, nonglycosylated form of the human interleukin-1 receptor antagonist (IL-1Ra). Anakinra differs from native human IL-1Ra in that it has the addition of a single methionine residue at its amino terminus. Anakinra consists of 153 amino acids and has a molecular weight of 17.3 kilodaltons. It is produced by recombinant DNA technology using an *Escherichia coli* bacterial expression system.

Anakinra blocks the biologic activity of IL-1 by competitively inhibiting IL-1 binding to the interleukin-1 type I receptor (IL-1RI), which is expressed in a wide variety of tissues and organs.

IL-1 production is induced in response to inflammatory stimuli and mediates various physiologic responses including inflammatory and immunological responses. IL-1 has a broad range of activities, including cartilage degradation by its induction of the rapid loss of proteoglycans and stimulation of bone resorption. The levels of the naturally occurring IL-1Ra in synovium and synovial fluid from RA patients are not sufficient to compete with the elevated amount of locally produced IL-1.

➤*Pharmacokinetics:* The absolute bioavailability of anakinra after a 70 mg SC bolus injection in healthy subjects (n = 11) is 95%. In subjects with RA, maximum plasma concentrations of anakinra occurred 3 to 7 hours after SC administration of anakinra at clinically relevant doses (1 to 2 mg/kg; n = 18); the terminal half-life ranged from 4 to 6 hours. In RA patients, no unexpected accumulation of anakinra was observed after daily SC doses for up to 24 weeks. The estimated anakinra clearance increased with increasing Ccr and body weight.

Special populations –

Renal function impairment: The mean plasma clearance of anakinra decreased 70% to 75% in normal subjects with severe or end-stage renal disease (defined as Ccr less than 30 mL/min, as estimated from serum creatinine levels). No formal studies have been conducted examining the pharmacokinetics of anakinra administered SC in RA patients with renal impairment.

Contraindications

Known hypersensitivity to *E. coli*-derived proteins, anakinra, or any component of the product.

Warnings/Precautions

➤*Infections:* Anakinra has been associated with an increased incidence of serious infections (2%) vs placebo (less than 1%). Discontinue administration of anakinra if a patient develops a serious infection. Do not initiate treatment with anakinra in patients with active infections. The safety and efficacy of anakinra in immunocompromised patients or in patients with chronic infections have not been evaluated. In a 24-week study of concurrent etanercept and anakinra therapy, the rate of serious infections in the combination arm (7%) was higher than with etanercept alone (0%). The combination of anakinra and etanercept did not result in higher ACR response rates compared to etanercept alone. Coadministration of anakinra and etanercept has not demonstrated increased clinical benefit. Carefully monitor patients when considering initiation of anakinra therapy concurrently with etanercept therapy.

➤*Immunosuppression:* The impact of treatment with anakinra on active and/or chronic infections and the development of malignancies is unknown.

➤*Vaccinations:* No data are available on the effects of vaccination in patients receiving anakinra. Do not give live vaccines concurrently with anakinra. No data are available on the secondary transmission of infections by live vaccines in patients receiving anakinra. Because anakinra interferes with normal immune response mechanisms to new antigens such as vaccines, vaccination may not be effective in patients receiving anakinra.

➤*Hematologic events:* See Adverse Reactions for more information.

➤*Immunogenicity:* In 2 studies, 26% of patients tested positive for anti-anakinra antibodies at month 12 in a highly sensitive, anakinra-binding biosensor assay. Of the 1318 subjects with available data at week 12 or later, 1% were seropositive in a cell-based bioassay for antibodies capable of neutralizing the biologic effects of anakinra. Two of the 15 of these subjects were positive for neutralizing antibodies at more than 1 time point up to the week 52 visit and 4 were positive at week 52. No correlation between antibody development, clinical response, or adverse events was observed. The long-term immunogenicity of anakinra is unknown.

➤*Hypersensitivity reactions:* Hypersensitivity reactions associated with anakinra administration are rare. If a severe hypersensitivity reaction occurs, discontinue anakinra administration and initiate appropriate therapy.

➤*Renal function impairment:* This drug is known to be substantially excreted by the kidney; the risk of toxic reactions to this drug may be greater in patients with impaired renal function.

➤*Pregnancy: Category B.* Reproductive studies have been conducted with anakinra on rats and rabbits at doses up to 100 times the human dose and have revealed no evidence of impaired fertility or harm to the fetus. However, there are no adequate and well-controlled studies in pregnant women. Because animal reproduction studies are not always predictive of human response, use anakinra during pregnancy only if clearly needed.

➤*Lactation:* It is not known whether anakinra is secreted in human milk. Because many drugs are secreted in human milk, exercise caution if anakinra is administered to nursing women.

➤*Children:* The safety and efficacy of anakinra in patients with juvenile RA have not been established.

➤*Elderly:* Greater sensitivity of some older individuals cannot be ruled out. Because there is a higher incidence of infections in the elderly population in general, use caution in treating the elderly.

➤*Monitoring:* Assess neutrophil counts prior to initiating anakinra treatment, while receiving anakinra monthly for 3 months, and quarterly for a period up to 1 year thereafter.

Adverse Reactions

Anakinra Adverse Reactions Occurring in ≥ 5% of RA Patients (%)		
Adverse reaction	Anakinra 100 mg/day (n = 1565)	Placebo (n = 733)
Injection-site reaction	71	29
Worsening of RA	19	29
Upper respiratory tract infection	14	17
Headache	12	9
Nausea	8	7
Diarrhea	7	5
Sinusitis	7	7
Arthralgia	6	6
Influenza-like symptoms	6	6
Pain, abdominal	5	5

The most serious adverse reactions were serious infection and neutropenia, particularly when used in combination with TNF-blocking agents. The most common adverse reaction with anakinra is injection-site reactions (ISRs). These reactions were the most common reason for withdrawing from studies.

➤*Infections:* In 2 combined studies, the incidence of infection was 39% in the anakinra-treated patients and 37% in placebo-treated patients. The incidence of serious infections was 2% in anakinra-treated patients and 1% in placebo-treated patients over 6 months. The incidence of serious infection over 1 year was 3% in anakinra-treated patients and 2% in patients receiving placebo. These infections consisted primarily of bacterial events such as cellulitis, pneumonia, and bone and joint infections, rather than unusual, opportunistic, fungal, or viral infections. Patients with asthma appeared to be at higher risk of developing serious infections; anakinra 4% vs placebo 0%. Most patients continued on study drug after the infection resolved. There were no on-study deaths caused by serious infectious episodes in either study.

In 2 studies in which patients were receiving etanercept and anakinra for up to 24 weeks, the incidence of serious infections was 7%. The common infections consisted of bacterial pneumonia (4 cases) and cellulitis (4 cases). One patient with pulmonary fibrosis and pneumonia died because of respiratory failure.

➤*Hematologic:* In placebo-controlled studies with anakinra, treatment was associated with small reductions in the mean values for total white blood count, platelets, and ANC, and a small increase in the mean eosinophil differential percentage.

In all placebo-controlled studies, 8% of patients receiving anakinra had decreases in ANC of at least 1 WHO toxicity grade, compared with 2% of placebo patients. Nine anakinra-treated patients (0.4%) developed neutropenia (ANC less than 1×10^9/L). Additional patients treated with anakinra plus etanercept (2%) developed ANC less than 1×10^9/L. One neutropenic patient developed cellulitis and recovered with antibiotic therapy.

➤*Malignancies:* Twenty-three malignancies of various types were observed in 2730 RA patients treated in clinical trials with anakinra for up to 60 months. The observed rates and incidences were similar to those expected for the population studied.

ANAKINRA — INJECTION

➤*Injection-site reaction:* The most common and consistently reported treatment-related adverse event associated with anakinra is an ISR. The majority of ISRs were reported as mild. These typically lasted for 14 to 28 days and were characterized by: Erythema, ecchymosis, inflammation, and/or pain. In 2 studies, 71% of patients developed an ISR, which was typically reported within the first 4 weeks of therapy. The development of ISRs in patients who had not previously experienced ISRs was uncommon after the first month of therapy.

Patient Information

Instruct patients and their caregivers on the proper dosage and administration of anakinra. Provide all patients with the "Information for Patients and Caregivers' insert.

Inform patients of the signs and symptoms of allergic and other adverse drug reactions, and advise patients on appropriate actions. Thoroughly instruct patients and their caregivers on the importance of proper disposal and caution against the reuse of needles, syringes, and drug product. Have a puncture-resistance container available for the patient for the disposal of used syringes.

ADALIMUMAB

Rx	**Humira** (Abbott)	**Injection, solution:** 20 mg per 0.4 mL	Mannitol, polysorbate 80. Preservative free. In single-use prefilled syringes.[a]
		40 mg per 0.8 mL	Mannitol, polysorbate 80. Preservative free. In single-use prefilled syringes or single-use prefilled pens.[a]

[a] Each dose tray consists of a single-use syringe or pen with a fixed 27-gauge, ½-inch needle.

ADALIMUMAB — INJECTION

WARNING

Risk of serious infections – Patients treated with adalimumab are at increased risk of developing serious infections that may lead to hospitalization or death. Most patients who developed these infections were taking concomitant immunosuppressants, such as methotrexate or corticosteroids.

Discontinue adalimumab if a patient develops a serious infection or sepsis. Reported infections include the following:

- Active tuberculosis (TB), including reactivation of latent TB. Patients with TB frequently have presented with disseminated or extrapulmonary disease. Test patients for latent TB before adalimumab use and during therapy. Initiate treatment for latent infection prior to adalimumab use.
- Invasive fungal infections, including histoplasmosis, coccidioidomycosis, candidiasis, aspergillosis, blastomycosis, and pneumocystosis. Patients with histoplasmosis or other invasive fungal infections may present with disseminated, rather than localized, disease. Antigen and antibody testing for histoplasmosis may be negative in some patients with active infection. Consider empiric antifungal therapy in patients at risk of invasive fungal infections who develop severe systemic illness.
- Bacterial, viral, and other infections caused by opportunistic pathogens.

Carefully consider the risks and benefits of treatment with adalimumab prior to initiating therapy in patients with chronic or recurrent infection.

Closely monitor patients for the development of signs and symptoms of infection during and after treatment with adalimumab, including the possible development of TB in patients who tested negative for latent TB infection prior to initiating therapy.

Malignancy – Lymphoma and other malignancies, some fatal, have been reported in children and adolescents treated with tumor necrosis factor (TNF) blockers, of which adalimumab is a member. Postmarketing cases of hepatosplenic T-cell lymphoma (HSTCL), a rare type of T-cell lymphoma, have been reported in patients treated with TNF blockers, including adalimumab. These cases have had a very aggressive disease course and have been fatal. The majority of reported TNF blocker cases has occurred in patients with Crohn disease or ulcerative colitis and the majority were in adolescent and young adult males. Almost all these patients had received treatment with azathioprine or 6-mercaptopurine concomitantly with a TNF blocker at or prior to diagnosis. It is uncertain whether the occurrence of HSTCL is related to use of a TNF blocker or a TNF blocker in combination with these other immunosuppressants.

Indications

➤*Ankylosing spondylitis:* For reducing signs and symptoms in adults with active ankylosing spondylitis.

➤*Crohn disease:* For reducing signs and symptoms, as well as inducing and maintaining clinical remission, in adults with moderately to severely active Crohn disease who have had an inadequate response to conventional therapy; for reducing signs and symptoms, as well as inducing clinical remission, in these patients if they have also lost response to or are intolerant to infliximab.

➤*Juvenile idiopathic arthritis:* For reducing signs and symptoms of moderately to severely active polyarticular juvenile idiopathic arthritis in patients 4 years and older, alone or in combination with methotrexate.

➤*Plaque psoriasis:* For the treatment of adults with moderate to severe chronic plaque psoriasis who are candidates for systemic therapy or phototherapy, and when other systemic therapies are medically less appropriate.

➤*Psoriatic arthritis:* For reducing signs and symptoms, inhibiting the progression of structural damage, and improving physical function in adults with active psoriatic arthritis, alone or in combination with nonbiologic disease-modifying antirheumatic drugs (DMARDs).

➤*Rheumatoid arthritis:* For reducing signs and symptoms, inducing major clinical response, inhibiting the progression of structural damage, and improving physical function in adults with moderately to severely active rheumatoid arthritis (RA), alone or in combination with methotrexate or other nonbiologic DMARDs.

➤*Off-label uses:*

Pyoderma gangrenosum – [4] = Insufficient documentation. Preliminary data suggest that adalimumab could be successful as an adjunct therapy or monotherapy for the treatment of severe pyoderma gangrenosum. Adalimumab has been shown to be beneficial in refractory pyoderma gangrenosum in cases in which infliximab and etanercept have failed.

Administration and Dosage

➤*General dosing considerations:* Aminosalicylates, corticosteroids, methotrexate, salicylates, nonsteroidal anti-inflammatory drugs, analgesics, immunomodulatory agents (eg, 6-mercaptopurine, azathioprine), and/or other nonbiologic DMARDs may be continued during treatment with adalimumab.

Prior to initiating adalimumab and periodically during therapy, patients should be evaluated for active tuberculosis and tested for latent infection.

➤*Adults:*

Ankylosing spondylitis – 40 mg subcutaneously every other week.

Crohn disease –

Initial dosage: 160 mg subcutaneously on day 1 (four 40 mg injections in 1 day or two 40 mg injections per day for 2 consecutive days), followed by 80 mg subcutaneously 2 weeks later (day 15).

Maintenance dosage: Two weeks later (day 29), begin a maintenance dosage of 40 mg subcutaneously every other week.

Plaque psoriasis –

Initial dosage: 80 mg subcutaneously.

Maintenance dosage: 40 mg subcutaneously every other week starting 1 week after the initial dose.

Duration of therapy: Use beyond 1 year has not been evaluated in controlled clinical studies.

Psoriatic arthritis – 40 mg subcutaneously every other week.

Rheumatoid arthritis –

Usual dosage: 40 mg subcutaneously every other week.

Alternative dosage: Some patients not taking concomitant methotrexate may benefit from increasing the dosing frequency to 40 mg every week.

Off-label dosing –

Pyoderma gangrenosum: [4] = Insufficient documentation. 40 to 80 mg subcutaneously every week or every other week.

➤*Children:*

Juvenile idiopathic arthritis –

4 to 17 years of age:

- *Usual dosage* – See also Off-Label Uses.

Adalimumab Dosage in Children 4 to 17 Years of Age	
Weight	Dosage
≥ 30 kg	40 mg subcutaneously every other wk
15[a] to < 30 kg	20 mg subcutaneously every other wk

[a] Limited data are available for treatment in children who weigh

Off-label dosing –

Juvenile idiopathic arthritis (older than 4 years):

- *Maximum dose* – 40 mg subcutaneously every other week.
- *Alternative dosage* – 24 mg/m^2 subcutaneously every other week.

Pyoderma gangrenosum: [4] = Insufficient documentation. 25 to 70 mg/m^2 subcutaneously every 2 weeks.

➤*Preparation for administration:* The needle cover of the syringe contains dry rubber (latex), which should not be handled by persons sensitive to this substance.

➤*Administration:* Administer by subcutaneous injection. Injection sites should be rotated, and injections should never be given into areas where the skin is tender, bruised, red, or hard.

➤*Storage/Stability:* Refrigerate at 2° to 8°C (36° to 46°F). Do not freeze. Do not use if frozen even if it has been thawed. When traveling, adalimumab should be stored in a cool carrier with an ice pack. Protect the prefilled syringe from exposure to light. Store in the original carton until time of administration. Discard unused portions of the drug remaining from the syringe.

ADALIMUMAB — INJECTION

Actions

➤*Pharmacology:* Adalimumab, a recombinant human immunoglobulin G1 (IgG1), binds specifically to TNF-alpha and blocks its interaction with the p55 and p75 cell surface TNF receptors. Adalimumab also lyses surface TNF-expressing cells in vitro in the presence of a complement. Adalimumab does not bind or inactivate lymphotoxin (TNF-beta). TNF is a naturally occurring cytokine that is involved in healthy inflammatory and immune responses. Elevated levels of TNF are found in the synovial fluid of RA, including juvenile idiopathic arthritis, psoriatic arthritis, and ankylosing spondylitis patients; they play an important role in the pathologic inflammation and joint destruction that are hallmarks of these diseases. Increased levels of TNF are also found in psoriasis plaques. In plaque psoriasis, treatment with adalimumab may reduce the epidermal thickness and infiltration of inflammatory cells. The relationship between these pharmacodynamic activities and the mechanism(s) by which adalimumab exerts its clinical effects is unknown.

Adalimumab also modulates biological responses that are induced or regulated by TNF, including changes in the levels of adhesion molecules responsible for leukocyte migration (ELAM-1, VCAM-1, and ICAM-1 with a 50% inhibitory concentration of 1 to 2 × 10^{-10}M).

➤*Pharmacokinetics:*

Absorption – The maximum serum concentration (C_{max}) and the time to reach the C_{max} were 4.7 ± 1.6 mcg/mL and 131 ± 56 hours, respectively, following a single subcutaneous administration of adalimumab 40 mg to healthy adults. The average absolute bioavailability of adalimumab estimated from 3 studies following a single 40 mg subcutaneous dose was 64%.

Distribution – The distribution volume ranged from 4.7 to 6 L. Adalimumab concentrations in the synovial fluid from 5 patients with RA ranged from 31% to 96% of those in serum.

Excretion – The systemic clearance of adalimumab is approximately 12 mL/h. The mean terminal half-life was approximately 2 weeks, ranging from 10 to 20 days across studies.

Special populations –

Elderly: Population pharmacokinetic analyses in patients with RA revealed a trend toward higher apparent clearance of adalimumab in the presence of anti-adalimumab antibodies and lower clearance with increasing age in patients 40 to 75 years of age and older.

Children: In subjects with juvenile idiopathic arthritis (4 to 17 years of age), the mean steady-state trough serum adalimumab concentrations for subjects weighing less than 30 kg receiving adalimumab 20 mg subcutaneously every other week as monotherapy or with concomitant methotrexate were 6.8 and 10.9 mcg/mL, respectively. The mean steady-state trough serum adalimumab concentrations for subjects weighing 30 kg or more receiving adalimumab 40 mg subcutaneously every other week as monotherapy or with concomitant methotrexate were 6.6 and 8.1 mcg/mL, respectively.

Contraindications

None well documented.

Warnings/Precautions

➤*Serious infections:* Serious and sometimes fatal infections caused by bacterial, mycobacterial, invasive fungal, viral, or other opportunistic pathogens have been reported in patients receiving TNF-blocking agents. Among opportunistic infections, TB, histoplasmosis, aspergillosis, candidiasis, coccidioidomycosis, listeriosis, and pneumocystosis were the most commonly reported. Patients have frequently presented with disseminated rather than localized disease and are often taking concomitant immunosuppressants, such as methotrexate or corticosteroids with adalimumab.

Do not initiate treatment with adalimumab in patients with an active infection, including localized infections. Consider the risks and benefits of treatment prior to initiating therapy in patients with chronic or recurrent infection; who have been exposed to TB; who have resided or traveled in areas of endemic TB or endemic mycoses, such as histoplasmosis, coccidioidomycosis, or blastomycosis; or with underlying conditions that may predispose them to infection.

Closely monitor patients for the development of signs and symptoms of infection during and after treatment with adalimumab.

Discontinue adalimumab if a patient develops a serious infection or sepsis. Closely monitor a patient who develops a new infection during treatment with adalimumab, perform a prompt and complete diagnostic workup appropriate for an immunocompromised patient, and initiate appropriate antimicrobial therapy.

For patients who reside or travel in regions where mycoses are endemic, suspect invasive fungal infection if they develop a serious systemic illness. Consider appropriate empiric antifungal therapy while a diagnostic workup is being performed. Antigen and antibody testing for histoplasmosis may be negative in some patients with active infection. When feasible, make the decision to administer empiric antifungal therapy in these patients in consultation with a health care provider with expertise in the diagnosis and treatment of invasive fungal infections and take into account both the risk of severe fungal infection and the risk of antifungal therapy.

➤*Tuberculosis:* Cases of reactivation of TB or new TB infections have been observed in patients receiving adalimumab, including patients who have previously received treatment for latent or active TB. Evaluate patients for TB risk factors and test for latent infection prior to initiating adalimumab and periodically during therapy.

Treatment of latent TB infection prior to therapy with TNF-blocking agents reduced the risk of TB reactivation during therapy. Consider induration of 5 mm or more with tuberculin skin testing a positive test result when assessing if treatment for latent TB is needed prior to initiating adalimumab, even for patients previously vaccinated with Bacille Calmette-Guerin (BCG).

Also consider antituberculosis therapy prior to initiation of adalimumab in patients with a history of latent or active TB in whom an adequate course of treatment cannot be confirmed and for patients with a negative test for latent TB but having risk factors of TB infection. Consultation with a health care provider with expertise in the treatment of TB is recommended to aid in the decision to initiate antituberculosis therapy.

Strongly consider TB in patients who develop a new infection during adalimumab treatment, especially in patients who have previously or recently traveled to countries with a high prevalence of TB or who have had close contact with a person with active TB.

Closely monitor patients for the development of signs and symptoms of infection during and after treatment with adalimumab, including the development of TB in patients who tested negative for latent TB infection prior to initiating therapy. Tests for latent TB infection may also be falsely negative while on therapy with adalimumab.

➤*Malignancies:* In the controlled portions of clinical trials of some TNF-blocking agents, including adalimumab, more cases of malignancies have been observed among patients receiving those TNF blockers compared with control patients.

During the controlled portions of adalimumab trials in patients with RA, psoriatic arthritis, ankylosing spondylitis, Crohn disease, and plaque psoriasis, malignancies other than lymphoma and nonmelanoma (basal cell and squamous cell) skin cancer were observed at a rate (95% confidence interval [CI]) of 0.6 (0.3 to 1) per 100 patient-years among 3,853 adalimumab-treated patients versus a rate of 0.4 (0.2 to 1) per 100 patient-years among 2,183 control patients (median duration of treatment of 5.5 months for adalimumab-treated patients and 3.9 months for control-treated patients). The size of the control group and limited duration of the controlled portions of studies precludes the ability to draw firm conclusions.

Malignancies, some fatal, have been reported among children, adolescents, and young adults who received treatment with TNF-blocking agents (initiation of therapy 18 years and younger), of which adalimumab is a member. Approximately 50% of the cases were lymphomas, including Hodgkin and non-Hodgkin lymphoma. The other cases represented a variety of different malignancies and included rare malignancies usually associated with immunosuppression and malignancies that are not usually observed in children and adolescents. The malignancies occurred after a median of 30 months of therapy (range, 1 to 84 months). Most of the patients were receiving concomitant immunosuppressants. These cases were reported postmarketing and are derived from a variety of sources including registries and spontaneous postmarketing results.

Patients with RA, particularly those with highly active disease, are at a higher risk of the development of lymphoma. Cases of acute and chronic leukemia have been reported in association with postmarketing TNF blocker use in RA and other indications. Even in the absence of TNF blocker therapy, patients with RA may be at a higher risk (approximately 2-fold) than the general population for the development of leukemia.

➤*Hepatitis B virus reactivation:* Use of TNF blockers, including adalimumab, may increase the risk of reactivation of hepatitis B virus (HBV) in patients who are chronic carriers of this virus. In some instances, HBV reactivation occurring in conjunction with TNF blocker therapy has been fatal. The majority of these reports have occurred in patients concomitantly receiving other medications that suppress the immune system, which also may contribute to HBV reactivation. Evaluate patients at risk of HBV infection for prior evidence of HBV infection before initiating TNF blocker therapy. Exercise caution in prescribing TNF blockers for patients identified as carriers of HBV. Adequate data are not available on the safety or efficacy of treating patients who are carriers of HBV with antiviral therapy in conjunction with TNF blocker therapy to prevent HBV reactivation. Closely monitor patients who are carriers of HBV and require treatment with TNF blockers for clinical and laboratory signs of active HBV infections throughout therapy and for several months following termination of therapy. In patients who develop HBV reactivation, stop adalimumab and initiate effective antiviral therapy with appropriate supportive treatment. The safety of resuming TNF blocker therapy after HBV reactivation is controlled is not known. Therefore, exercise caution when considering resumption of adalimumab therapy in this situation and monitor patients closely.

➤*Neurologic effects:* Use of TNF-blocking agents, including adalimumab, has been associated with rare cases of new onset or exacerbation of clinical symptoms and/or radiographic evidence of CNS demyelinating disease, including multiple sclerosis, and peripheral demyelinating disease, including Guillain-Barré syndrome. Exercise caution in considering the use of adalimumab in patients with preexisting or recent-onset CNS demyelinating disorders.

➤*Hematologic effects:* Rare reports of pancytopenia, including aplastic anemia, have been reported with TNF-blocking agents. Adverse reactions of the hematologic system, including medically significant cytopenia (eg, leukopenia, thrombocytopenia), have been reported infrequently with adalimumab. The causal relationship of these reports to adalimumab remains unclear. Advise patients to seek immediate medical attention if they develop signs and symptoms suggestive of blood dyscrasias or infection (eg, bleeding, bruising, pallor, persistent fever) while taking adalimumab. Consider discontinuation of adalimumab therapy in patients with confirmed significant hematologic abnormalities.

ADALIMUMAB — INJECTION

➤*Congestive heart failure:* Cases of worsening congestive heart failure (CHF) and new-onset CHF have been reported with TNF blockers. Cases of worsening CHF have also been observed with adalimumab. Adalimumab has not been formally studied in patients with CHF; however, in clinical trials of another TNF blocker, a higher rate of serious CHF-related adverse reactions was observed. Exercise caution when using adalimumab in patients who have heart failure and monitor them carefully.

➤*Autoimmunity:* See Adverse Reactions for more information.

➤*Immunizations:* Patients on adalimumab may receive concurrent vaccinations, except for live vaccines. No data are available on the secondary transmission of infection by live vaccines in patients receiving adalimumab. It is recommended that juvenile idiopathic arthritis patients, if possible, be brought up to date with all immunizations in agreement with current immunization guidelines prior to initiating adalimumab therapy.

➤*Immunosuppression:* The possibility exists for TNF-blocking agents, including adalimumab, to affect host defenses against infections and malignancies because TNF mediates inflammation and modulates cellular immune responses.

➤*Immunogenicity:* Patients in studies RA-I, RA-II, and RA-III were tested at multiple time points for antibodies to adalimumab during the 6- to 12-month period. Approximately 5% of adult RA patients receiving adalimumab developed low-titer antibodies to adalimumab at least once during treatment, which were neutralizing in vitro. Patients treated with concomitant methotrexate had a lower rate of antibody development than patients on adalimumab monotherapy (1% vs 12%). No apparent correlation of antibody development to adverse reactions was observed. With monotherapy, patients receiving every-other-week dosing may develop antibodies more frequently than those receiving weekly dosing. In patients receiving the recommended dosage of 40 mg every other week as monotherapy, the American College of Rheumatology (ACR) 20 response was lower among antibody-positive patients than among antibody-negative patients. The long-term immunogenicity of adalimumab is unknown.

In patients with juvenile idiopathic arthritis, adalimumab antibodies were identified in 16% of adalimumab-treated patients. In patients receiving concomitant methotrexate, the incidence was 6% compared with 26% receiving adalimumab monotherapy.

In patients with ankylosing spondylitis, the rate of development of antibodies to adalimumab in adalimumab-treated patients was comparable with patients with RA. In patients with psoriatic arthritis, the rate of antibody development in patients receiving adalimumab monotherapy was comparable with patients with RA; however, in patients receiving concomitant methotrexate, the rate was 7% compared with 1% in RA. In patients with Crohn disease, the rate of antibody development was 2.6%. The immunogenicity rate was 8% for plaque psoriasis patients who were treated with adalimumab monotherapy.

➤*Hypersensitivity reactions:* In postmarketing experience, anaphylaxis and angioneurotic edema have been reported rarely following adalimumab administration. If an anaphylactic or other serious allergic reaction occurs, discontinue administration of adalimumab immediately and institute appropriate therapy. In adults in clinical trials of adalimumab, allergic reactions (eg, allergic rash, anaphylactoid reaction, fixed drug reaction, nonspecified drug reaction, urticaria) have been observed in approximately 1% of patients.

➤*Pregnancy:* *Category B.* There are no adequate and well-controlled studies in pregnant women. It is not known if adalimumab crosses the human placenta. The molecular weight is very high (about 148,000), but immunoglobulin G has been shown to cross the placenta late in pregnancy. Because animal reproduction and developmental studies are not always predictive of human response, use adalimumab during pregnancy only if clearly needed.

Pregnancy registry – To monitor outcomes of pregnant women exposed to adalimumab, a pregnancy registry has been established. Health care providers are encouraged to register patients by calling 1-877-311-8972.

➤*Lactation:* It is not known whether adalimumab is excreted in human breast milk or absorbed systemically after ingestion. The molecular weight is very high (approximately 148,000), but immunoglobulins are excreted into breast milk. Thus, adalimumab might be excreted also, but the amount and the systemic bioavailability are unknown. Because many drugs and immunoglobulins are excreted in human breast milk and because of the potential for serious adverse reactions in breast-feeding infants from adalimumab, decide whether to discontinue breast-feeding or the drug, taking into account the importance of the drug to the mother.

➤*Children:* Safety and effectiveness of adalimumab in children for uses other than juvenile idiopathic arthritis have not been established. Adalimumab has not been studied in children younger than 4 years of age, and there are limited data on adalimumab treatment in children weighing less than 15 kg.

➤*Elderly:* The frequency of serious infection and malignancy among adalimumab-treated subjects older than 65 years was higher than for those younger than 65 years. Because there is a higher incidence of infections and malignancies in the elderly population in general, use caution when treating elderly patients.

➤*Monitoring:* Closely monitor patients for the development of signs and symptoms of infection during and after treatment with adalimumab. Monitor patients for signs and symptoms of active TB, including patients who had a negative tuberculin skin test prior to initiating therapy and periodically thereafter. Closely monitor a patient who develops a new infection during treatment and perform a prompt and complete diagnostic workup appropriate for an immunocompromised patient, and initiate appropriate antimicrobial therapy. Monitor heart failure patients carefully. Closely monitor patients who are carriers of HBV and require treatment with TNF blockers for clinical and laboratory signs of active HBV infections throughout therapy and for several months following termination of therapy.

Drug Interactions

➤*Live vaccines:* See Warnings/Precautions for more information.

Adalimumab Drug Interactions

Precipitant drug	Object drug[a]		Description
Abatacept	Adalimumab	⬆	An increased rate of infection may occur. Concurrent therapy is not recommended. If coadministration occurs, closely monitor for signs of infection.
Adalimumab	Abatacept		
Anakinra	Adalimumab	⬆	Coadministration of anakinra with another TNF-blocking agent has been associated with an increased risk of serious infections and an increased risk of neutropenia. Concurrent use is not recommended.
Adalimumab	Anakinra		
Methotrexate	Adalimumab	⬆	Methotrexate reduced adalimumab apparent clearance after single and multiple dosing by 29% and 44%, respectively. Dosage adjustment is not needed.
Tocilizumab	Adalimumab	⬆	An increased rate of infection may occur. Concurrent use is not recommended.
Adalimumab	Tocilizumab		

[a] ⬆ = object drug increased.

Adverse Reactions

➤*Serious adverse reactions:* The most serious adverse reactions were serious infections, neurologic reactions, and malignancies.

➤*Common adverse reactions:* The most common adverse reaction was injection-site reactions. In placebo-controlled trials, 20% of patients treated with adalimumab developed injection-site reactions (eg, erythema and/or itching, hemorrhage, pain, swelling) compared with 14% of patients receiving placebo. Most injection-site reactions were described as mild and generally did not necessitate drug discontinuation.

➤*Discontinuation of treatment:* The proportion of patients who discontinued treatment because of adverse reactions during the double-blind, placebo-controlled portion of studies RA-I, RA-II, RA-III, and RA-IV was 7% for patients taking adalimumab and 4% for placebo-treated patients. The most common adverse reactions leading to discontinuation of adalimumab were clinical flare reaction (0.7%), rash (0.3%), and pneumonia (0.3%).

➤*Infections:* In placebo-controlled RA trials, the rate of infection was 1 per patient-year in the adalimumab-treated patients and 0.9 per patient-year in the placebo-treated patients. The infections consisted primarily of bronchitis, upper respiratory tract infections, and urinary tract infections. Most patients continued on adalimumab after the infection resolved. The incidence of serious infections was 0.04 per patient-year in adalimumab-treated patients and 0.02 per patient-year in placebo-treated patients. Serious infections observed included cellulitis, diverticulitis, erysipelas, pneumonia, prosthetic and postsurgical infections, pyelonephritis, and septic arthritis.

➤*Tuberculosis and opportunistic infections:* In completed and ongoing global clinical studies that include more than 13,000 patients, the overall rate of TB is approximately 0.26 per 100 patient-years. In more than 4,500 patients in the United States and Canada, the rate is approximately 0.07 per 100 patient-years. These studies include reports of miliary, lymphatic, and peritoneal, as well as pulmonary. Most of the cases of TB occurred within the first 8 months after initiation of therapy and may reflect recrudescence of latent disease. Cases of opportunistic infections have also been reported in these clinical trials at an overall rate of approximately 0.075 per 100 patient-years. Some cases of opportunistic infections and TB have been fatal.

➤*Malignancies:* See Warnings/Precautions for more information.

➤*Autoantibodies:* In the RA controlled trials, 12% of patients treated with adalimumab and 7% of placebo-treated patients that had negative baseline antinuclear antibody titers developed positive titers at week 24. Two patients out of 3,046 treated with adalimumab developed clinical signs suggestive of new-onset lupus-like syndrome. The patients improved following discontinuation of therapy.

ADALIMUMAB — INJECTION

➤*Rheumatoid arthritis:*

Adverse reactions (5% or more) –

Adalimumab Adverse Reactions in Rheumatoid Arthritis (≥ 5%)		
Adverse reactions	Adalimumab 40 mg subcutaneous every other week (n = 705)	Placebo (n = 690)
GI		
Abdominal pain	7%	4%
Nausea	9%	8%
GU		
Hematuria	5%	4%
Urinary tract infection	8%	5%
Lab test abnormalities[a]		
Alkaline phosphatase increased	5%	3%
Hypercholesterolemia	6%	4%
Hyperlipidemia	7%	5%
Laboratory test abnormal	8%	7%
Local		
Injection-site pain	12%	12%
Injection-site reaction[b]	8%	1%
Respiratory		
Sinusitis	11%	9%
Upper respiratory tract infection	17%	13%
Miscellaneous		
Accidental injury	10%	8%
Back pain	6%	4%
Flu syndrome	7%	6%
Headache	12%	8%
Hypertension	5%	3%
Rash	12%	6%

[a] Laboratory test abnormalities were reported as adverse reactions in European trials.
[b] Does not include erythema and/or itching, hemorrhage, pain, or swelling.

Other adverse reactions (less than 5%) –

Cardiovascular: Arrhythmia, atrial fibrillation, cardiovascular disorder, chest pain, CHF, coronary artery disorder, heart arrest, hypertensive encephalopathy, myocardial infarction, palpitation, pericardial effusion, pericarditis, syncope, tachycardia, thrombosis leg, vascular disorder (less than 5%).

CNS: Confusion, multiple sclerosis, paresthesia, subdural hematoma, tremor (less than 5%).

Dermatologic: Cellulitis, erysipelas, herpes zoster (less than 5%).

GI: Cholecystitis, cholelithiasis, esophagitis, gastroenteritis, GI disorder, GI hemorrhage, hepatic necrosis, vomiting (less than 5%).

GU: Cystitis, kidney calculus, menstrual disorder, pyelonephritis (less than 5%).

Hematologic/Lymphatic: Agranulocytosis, granulocytopenia, leukopenia, lymphoma-like reaction, pancytopenia, polycythemia (less than 5%).

Metabolic/Nutritional: Dehydration, healing abnormal, ketosis, paraproteinemia, peripheral edema (less than 5%).

Musculoskeletal: Arthritis, bone disorder, bone fracture (not spontaneous), bone necrosis, joint disorder, muscle cramps, myasthenia, pyogenic arthritis, synovitis, tendon disorder (less than 5%).

Respiratory: Asthma, bronchospasm, dyspnea, lung disorder, lung function decreased, pleural effusion, pneumonia (less than 5%).

Miscellaneous: Adenoma, carcinomas (eg, breast, GI, skin, urogenital), cataract, fever, infection, lupus erythematous syndrome, lymphoma and melanoma, pain in extremity, parathyroid disorder, pelvic pain, sepsis, surgery, TB reactivated, thorax pain (less than 5%).

➤*Juvenile idiopathic arthritis:*

Severe adverse reactions – Severe adverse reactions reported in the study included appendicitis, herpes zoster, increased aminotransferases, metrorrhagia, myositis, neutropenia, and streptococcal pharyngitis.

Serious infection – Serious infections were observed in 4% of patients within approximately 2 years of initiation of treatment with adalimumab and included cases of herpes simplex, herpes zoster, pharyngitis, pneumonia, and urinary tract infection. A total of 45% of children experienced an infection while receiving adalimumab with or without concomitant methotrexate in the first 16 weeks of treatment. The types of infections reported in juvenile idiopathic arthritis patients were generally similar to those commonly seen in outpatient juvenile idiopathic arthritis populations.

Common adverse reactions – Upon initiation of treatment, the most common adverse reactions occurring in children treated with adalimumab were injection-site pain and injection-site reaction (19% and 16%, respectively).

Granuloma annulare – A less commonly reported adverse reaction in children receiving adalimumab was granuloma annulare, which did not lead to discontinuation of adalimumab treatment.

Hypersensitivity reactions – In the first 48 weeks of treatment, nonserious hypersensitivity reactions were seen in approximately 6% of children and included primarily localized allergic hypersensitivity reactions and allergic rash.

Hepatic – Isolated mild to moderate elevations of liver aminotransferases (ALT more common than AST) were observed in children with juvenile idiopathic arthritis exposed to adalimumab alone; liver function test elevations were more frequent among those treated with the combination of adalimumab and methotrexate. In general, these elevations did not lead to discontinuation of adalimumab treatment.

Autoantibodies – In the juvenile idiopathic arthritis trial, 10% of patients treated with adalimumab who had negative baseline anti-dsDNA (double-stranded) antibodies developed positive titers after 48 weeks of treatment. No patient developed clinical signs of autoimmunity during the clinical trial.

Creatine phosphokinase – Approximately 15% of children treated with adalimumab developed mild to moderate elevations of creatine phosphokinase (CPK). Elevations exceeding 5 times the upper limit of normal (ULN) were observed in several patients. CPK levels decreased or returned to normal in all patients. Most patients were able to continue adalimumab without interruption.

➤*Psoriatic arthritis/ankylosing spondylitis:*

Laboratory abnormalities – In the clinical trials of patients with psoriatic arthritis and ankylosing spondylitis, elevations of aminotransferase were observed (ALT more common than AST) in a greater proportion of patients receiving adalimumab than in controls, both when adalimumab was given as monotherapy and when it was used in combination with other immunosuppressive agents. Most elevations of ALT and AST observed were in the range of 1.5 to 3 times the ULN. In general, patients who develop ALT and AST elevations were asymptomatic, and the abnormalities decreased or resolved with either continuation or discontinuation of adalimumab, or modification of concomitant medications.

➤*Plaque psoriasis:*

Musculoskeletal – In the placebo-controlled portions of the clinical trials in plaque psoriasis patients, adalimumab-treated patients had a higher incidence of arthralgia when compared with controls (3% vs 1%).

Laboratory abnormalities – Elevations of aminotransferases were observed (ALT more common than AST) in a greater proportion of patients receiving adalimumab than in controls. Most elevations of ALT and AST observed were in the range of 1.5 to 3 times the ULN. In general, patients who developed ALT and AST elevations were asymptomatic, and most of the abnormalities decreased or resolved with continuation or discontinuation of adalimumab.

➤*Postmarketing:*

Dermatologic – Cutaneous vasculitis, erythema multiforme, new or worsening psoriasis (all sub-types including pustular and palmoplantar).

Hematologic – Thrombocytopenia.

Hypersensitivity – Anaphylaxis, angioneurotic edema.

Respiratory – Interstitial lung disease, including pulmonary fibrosis.

Overdosage

➤*Treatment:* In a case of overdosage, monitor the patient for any signs or symptoms of adverse reactions or effects and immediately institute appropriate symptomatic treatment.

Patient Information

Advise patients of the potential benefits and risks of adalimumab.

Inform patients that adalimumab may lower the ability of their immune system to fight infections. Instruct patients of the importance of contacting their health care provider if they develop any symptoms of infection, including TB and reactivation of HBV infections.

Advise patients to report any signs of new or worsening medical conditions such as heart disease, neurological disease, or autoimmune disorders. Advise patients to report any symptoms suggestive of a cytopenia such as bruising, bleeding, or persistent fever.

Counsel patients about the risk of lymphoma and other malignancies while receiving adalimumab.

Advise patients to seek immediate medical attention if they experience any symptoms of severe allergic reactions. Advise latex-sensitive patients that the needle cap of the prefilled syringe contains latex.

Perform the first injection under the supervision of a qualified health care provider. If a patient or caregiver is to administer adalimumab, instruct them in injection techniques and assess their ability to inject subcutaneously to ensure the proper administration of adalimumab.

Use a puncture-resistant container for disposal of needles and syringes. Instruct patients or caregivers in the technique, as well as proper syringe and needle disposal, and caution them against reuse of these items.

NATALIZUMAB

Rx	Tysabri[a] (Elan)	Injection, solution, concentrate: 20 mg/mL	Preservative free. Polysorbate 80, sodium chloride. In single-use 15 mL vials.

[a] Only available through a special restricted distribution program (the TOUCH prescribing program). See Warnings/Precautions for more information.

NATALIZUMAB — INJECTION

WARNING

Progressive multifocal leukoencephalopathy – Natalizumab increases the risk of progressive multifocal leukoencephalopathy (PML), an opportunistic viral infection of the brain that usually leads to death or severe disability. Cases of PML have been reported in patients taking natalizumab who were recently or concomitantly treated with immunomodulators or immunosuppressants, as well as in patients receiving natalizumab as monotherapy.

Because of the risk of PML, natalizumab is available only through a special restricted distribution program called the TOUCH prescribing program. Under the TOUCH prescribing program, only prescribers, infusion centers, and pharmacies associated with infusion centers registered with the program are able to prescribe, distribute, or infuse the product. In addition, natalizumab must be administered only to patients who are enrolled in and meet all the conditions of the TOUCH prescribing program.

Monitor patients on natalizumab for any new sign or symptom that may be suggestive of PML. Withhold natalizumab dosing immediately at the first sign or symptom suggestive of PML. For diagnosis, an evaluation that includes a gadolinium-enhanced magnetic resonance imaging (MRI) scan of the brain and, when indicated, cerebrospinal fluid analysis for John Cunningham viral DNA are recommended.

Indications

➤*Crohn disease:* For inducing and maintaining clinical response and remission in adult patients with moderately to severely active Crohn disease with evidence of inflammation who have had an inadequate response to, or are unable to tolerate, conventional Crohn disease therapies and inhibitors of tumor necrosis factor–alpha (TNF-alpha).

➤*Multiple sclerosis (adults):* As monotherapy for the treatment of patients with relapsing forms of multiple sclerosis to delay the accumulation of physical disability and reduce the frequency of clinical exacerbations.

Administration and Dosage

➤*General dosing considerations:* Only prescribers registered in the TOUCH prescribing program may prescribe natalizumab.

➤*Adults:*

Crohn disease –

Usual dosage: 300 mg intravenous (IV) infusion over 1 hour every 4 weeks.

Concomitant therapy: Do not use with concomitant immunosuppressants (eg, azathioprine, cyclosporine, methotrexate, 6-mercaptopurine) or concomitant inhibitors of TNF-alpha. Aminosalicylates may be continued during treatment with natalizumab.

Discontinuation of therapy: If the patient has not experienced therapeutic benefit by 12 weeks of induction therapy, discontinue natalizumab. For patients who start natalizumab while on chronic oral corticosteroids, commence steroid tapering as soon as a therapeutic benefit of natalizumab has occurred; if the patient cannot be tapered off oral corticosteroids within 6 months of starting natalizumab, discontinue natalizumab. Other than the initial 6-month taper, consider discontinuing natalizumab for patients who require additional steroid use that exceeds 3 months in a calendar year to control their Crohn disease.

Multiple sclerosis – 300 mg IV infusion over 1 hour every 4 weeks.

➤*Preparation for administration:* To prepare the solution, withdraw 15 mL of natalizumab concentrate from the vial using a sterile needle and syringe. Inject the concentrate into 100 mL of sodium chloride 0.9% injection. No other IV diluents may be used to prepare the natalizumab solution.

Gently invert the natalizumab solution to mix completely. Do not shake.

The final dosage solution has a concentration of 2.6 mg/mL.

➤*Administration:* Infuse natalizumab 300 mg in 100 mL of sodium chloride 0.9% injection over approximately 1 hour (infusion rate, approximately 5 mg/min). Do not administer natalizumab as an IV push or bolus injection. After the infusion is complete, flush with sodium chloride 0.9% injection.

Observe patients during the infusion and for 1 hour after the infusion is complete. Promptly discontinue the infusion upon the first observation of any signs or symptoms consistent with a hypersensitivity-type reaction.

➤*Admixture compatibility:* Do not inject other medications into infusion set side ports or mix them with natalizumab.

➤*Storage/Stability:* Refrigerate undiluted vials between 2° and 8°C (36° and 46°F). Do not shake or freeze. Protect from light.

Following dilution, infuse natalizumab solution immediately, or refrigerate solution at 2° to 8°C (36° to 46°F) and use within 8 hours. If stored at 2° to 8°C (36° to 46°F), allow the solution to warm to room temperature prior to infusion. Do not freeze.

Actions

➤*Pharmacology:* Natalizumab is a recombinant humanized immunoglobulin G4-kappa monoclonal antibody produced in murine myeloma cells. Natalizumab binds to the alpha-4 subunit of alpha-4 beta-1 and alpha-4 beta-7 integrins expressed on the surface of all leukocytes except neutrophils and inhibits the alpha-4–mediated adhesion of leukocytes to their counter-receptor(s). The receptors for the alpha-4 family of integrins include vascular cell adhesion molecule 1 (VCAM-1), which is expressed on activated vascular endothelium, and mucosal addressin cell adhesion molecule 1 (MAdCAM-1) present on vascular endothelial cells of the GI tract. Disruption of these molecular interactions prevents transmigration of leukocytes across the endothelium into inflamed parenchymal tissue. In vitro, anti–alpha-4 integrin antibodies also block alpha-4–mediated cell binding to ligands, such as osteopontin and an alternatively spliced domain of fibronectin, connecting segment 1. In vivo, natalizumab may further act to inhibit the interaction of alpha-4–expressing leukocytes with their ligand(s) in the extracellular matrix and on parenchymal cells, thereby inhibiting further recruitment and inflammatory activity of activated immune cells.

Multiple sclerosis – In multiple sclerosis, lesions are believed to occur when activated inflammatory cells, including T-lymphocytes, cross the blood-brain barrier. Leukocyte migration across the blood-brain barrier involves interaction between adhesion molecules on inflammatory cells and their counter-receptors present on endothelial cells of the vessel wall. The clinical effect of natalizumab in multiple sclerosis may be secondary to blockade of the molecular interaction of alpha-4 beta-1 integrin expressed by inflammatory cells with VCAM-1 on vascular endothelial cells, and with connecting segment 1 and/or osteopontin expressed by parenchymal cells in the brain. Data from an experimental autoimmune encephalitis animal model of multiple sclerosis demonstrate reduction of leukocyte migration into brain parenchyma and reduction of plaque formation, detected by MRI following repeated administration of natalizumab. The clinical significance of these animal data is unknown.

Crohn disease – In Crohn disease, the interaction of the alpha-4 beta-7 integrin with the endothelial receptor MAdCAM-1 has been implicated as an important contributor to the chronic inflammation that is a hallmark of the disease. MAdCAM-1 is mainly expressed on gut endothelial cells and plays a critical role in the homing of T-lymphocytes to gut lymph tissue found in Peyer patches. MAdCAM-1 expression increased at active sites of inflammation in patients with Crohn disease, which suggests it may play a role in the recruitment of leukocytes to the mucosa and contribute to the inflammatory response characteristic of Crohn disease. The clinical effect of natalizumab in Crohn disease may therefore be secondary to blockade of the molecular interaction of the alpha-4 beta-7 integrin receptor with MAdCAM-1 expressed on the venular endothelium at inflammatory foci. VCAM-1 expression upregulated on colonic endothelial cells in a mouse model of inflammatory bowel disease and appears to play a role in leukocyte recruitment to sites of inflammation. However, the role of VCAM-1 in Crohn disease is not clear.

➤*Pharmacokinetics:*

Absorption/Distribution –

Multiple sclerosis: In patients with multiple sclerosis, following the repeat IV administration of a dose of natalizumab 300 mg, the mean ± standard deviation (SD) maximum observed serum concentration was 110 ± 52 mcg/mL. Mean average steady-state trough concentrations ranged from 23 to 29 mcg/mL. The observed time to steady state was approximately 24 weeks after every 4 weeks of dosing. The mean ± SD volume of distribution of natalizumab was 5.7 ± 1.9 L.

Crohn disease: In patients with Crohn disease, following the repeat IV administration of a dose of natalizumab 300 mg, the mean ± SD maximum observed serum concentration was 101 ± 34 mcg/mL. The mean ± SD average steady-state trough concentration was 10 ± 9 mcg/mL. The estimated time to steady state was approximately 16 to 24 weeks after every 4 weeks of dosing. The mean ± SD volume of distribution of natalizumab was 5.2 ± 2.8 L.

Excretion –

Multiple sclerosis: The mean ± SD half-life and clearance of natalizumab were 11 ± 4 days and 16 ± 5 mL/h, respectively.

Crohn disease: The mean ± SD half-life and clearance of natalizumab were 10 ± 7 days and 22 ± 22 mL/h, respectively.

Contraindications

Patients who have or have had PML; hypersensitivity to natalizumab.

Warnings/Precautions

➤*Progressive multifocal leukoencephalopathy:* PML, an opportunistic infection caused by the John Cunningham virus and that typically only occurs in patients who are immunocompromised, developed in 3 patients who received natalizumab in clinical trials. Two cases of PML were observed in 1,869 patients with multiple sclerosis treated for a median of 120 weeks. The third case occurred among 1,043 patients with Crohn disease after the patient received 8 doses. Both patients with multiple sclerosis were receiving concomitant immunomodulatory therapy, and the Crohn disease patient had been treated in the past with immunosuppressive therapy.

In the postmarketing setting, additional cases of PML have been reported in patients with multiple sclerosis who were not receiving concomitant immunomodulatory therapy. In patients treated with natalizumab, the risk of developing PML increases with longer treatment duration; for patients treated 24 to 36 months, it is generally similar to rates seen in clinical trials. There is limited experience beyond 3 years of treatment. There are no known interventions that can reliably prevent PML or adequately treat PML if it occurs. It is not known whether early detection of PML and discontinuation of natalizumab will mitigate the disease.

NATALIZUMAB — INJECTION

Ordinarily, do not treat patients receiving chronic immunosuppressant or immunomodulatory therapy or who have systemic medical conditions resulting in significantly compromised immune system function with natalizumab.

In patients with multiple sclerosis, obtain an MRI scan prior to initiating therapy with natalizumab. This MRI may be helpful in differentiating subsequent multiple sclerosis symptoms from PML.

See the Warning box for more information.

Immune reconstitution inflammatory syndrome has been reported in natalizumab-treated patients who developed PML and subsequently discontinued natalizumab. In almost all cases, immune reconstitution inflammatory syndrome occurred after plasma exchange was used to eliminate circulating natalizumab. It presents as an unanticipated clinical decline in the patient's condition after return of immune function (and in some cases after apparent clinical improvement) and, in the case of PML, is often followed by characteristic changes in the MRI. Natalizumab has not been associated with immune reconstitution inflammatory syndrome in patients discontinuing treatment with natalizumab for reasons unrelated to PML. In natalizumab-treated patients with PML, immune reconstitution inflammatory syndrome has been reported within days to several weeks after plasma exchange. Monitor for development of immune reconstitution inflammatory syndrome and institute appropriate treatment of the associated inflammation.

➤*Distribution program for natalizumab:* Natalizumab is available only under a special restricted distribution program called the TOUCH Prescribing Program. Under the TOUCH Prescribing Program, only prescribers, infusion centers, and pharmacies associated with infusion centers registered with the program are able to prescribe, distribute, or infuse the product. For prescribers and patients, the TOUCH prescribing program has 2 components: MS TOUCH (for patients with multiple sclerosis) and CD TOUCH (for patients with Crohn disease). Natalizumab must be administered only to patients who are enrolled in and meet all the conditions of the MS or CD TOUCH Prescribing Program. Contact the TOUCH Prescribing Program at 1-800-456-2255.

➤*Immunosuppression/Infections:* The immune system effects of natalizumab may increase the risk of infections. In study MS1, certain types of infections, including pneumonias and urinary tract infections (including serious cases), gastroenteritis, vaginal infections, tooth infections, tonsillitis, and herpes infections, occurred more often in natalizumab-treated patients than in placebo-treated patients. One opportunistic infection, a cryptosporidial gastroenteritis with a prolonged course, was observed in a patient who received natalizumab in the multiple sclerosis monotherapy study.

In studies MS1 and MS2, an increase in infections was seen in patients concurrently receiving short courses of corticosteroids. However, the increase in infections in natalizumab-treated patients who received steroids was similar to the increase in placebo-treated patients who received steroids.

In Crohn disease clinical studies, opportunistic infections (*Pneumocystis carinii* pneumonia, pulmonary *Mycobacterium avium-intracellulare*, bronchopulmonary aspergillosis, and *Burkholderia cepacia*) have been observed in less than 1% of natalizumab-treated patients; some of these patients were receiving concurrent immunosuppressants.

In studies CD1 and CD2, an increase in infections was seen in patients concurrently receiving corticosteroids. However, the increase in infections was similar in placebo- and natalizumab-treated patients who received steroids.

Concurrent use of antineoplastic, immunosuppressant, or immunomodulating agents may further increase the risk of infections, including PML and other opportunistic infections, over the risk observed with use of natalizumab alone. The safety and efficacy of natalizumab in combination with antineoplastic, immunosuppressant, or immunomodulating agents have not been established. Ordinarily, do not treat patients receiving chronic immunosuppressant or immunomodulatory therapy or who have systemic medical conditions resulting in significantly compromised immune system function with natalizumab.

For patients with Crohn disease who start natalizumab while on chronic corticosteroids, commence steroid withdrawal as soon as a therapeutic benefit has occurred. If the patient cannot discontinue systemic corticosteroids within 6 months, discontinue natalizumab.

➤*Immunogenicity:* If the presence of persistent antibodies is suspected, perform antibody testing. Antibodies may be detected and confirmed with sequential serum antibody tests. Antibodies detected early in the treatment course (eg, within the first 6 months) may be transient and disappear with continued dosing. Repeat testing at 3 months after the initial positive result is recommended in patients in whom antibodies are detected to confirm that antibodies are persistent. Consider the overall benefits and risks of natalizumab in a patient with persistent antibodies.

Experience with monoclonal antibodies, including natalizumab, suggests that patients who receive therapeutic monoclonal antibodies after an extended period without treatment may be at higher risk of hypersensitivity reactions than patients who received regularly scheduled treatment. Given that patients with persistent antibodies to natalizumab experience reduced efficacy, and that hypersensitivity reactions are more common in these patients, consider testing for the presence of antibodies in patients who wish to recommence therapy following a dose interruption. Following a period of dose interruption, patients testing negative for antibodies prior to redosing have a risk of antibody development with re-treatment that is similar to natalizumab-naive patients.

Multiple sclerosis – Patients in study MS1 were tested for antibodies to natalizumab every 12 weeks. The assays used were unable to detect low to moderate levels of antibodies to natalizumab. Approximately 9% of patients receiving natalizumab developed detectable antibodies at least once during treatment. Approximately 6% of patients had positive antibodies on more than one occasion. Approximately 82% of patients who became persistently antibody-positive developed detectable antibodies by 12 weeks. Antinatalizumab antibodies were neutralizing in vitro.

The presence of antinatalizumab antibodies was correlated with a reduction in serum natalizumab levels. In study MS1, the week 12 preinfusion mean natalizumab serum concentration in antibody-negative patients was 15 mcg/mL compared with 1.3 mcg/mL in antibody-positive patients. Persistent antibody positivity resulted in a substantial decrease in the effectiveness of natalizumab. The risk of increased disability and the annualized relapse rate were similar in persistently antibody-positive natalizumab-treated patients and patients who received placebo. A similar phenomenon was also observed in study MS2.

Crohn disease – Patients in Crohn disease studies were first tested for antibodies at week 12; in a substantial proportion of patients, this was the only test performed because of the 12-week duration of placebo-controlled studies. Approximately 10% of patients had antinatalizumab antibodies on at least 1 occasion. On more than 1 occasion, 5% of patients had positive antibodies. Persistent antibodies resulted in reduced efficacy and an increase in infusion-related reactions with symptoms that include dyspnea, flushing, nausea, pruritus, and urticaria.

➤*Hepatic effects:* Clinically significant liver injury has been reported in patients treated with natalizumab in the postmarketing setting. Signs of liver injury, including markedly elevated serum hepatic enzymes and elevated total bilirubin, occurred as early as 6 days after the first dose; signs of liver injury have also been reported for the first time after multiple doses. In some patients, liver injury recurred upon rechallenge, providing evidence that natalizumab caused the injury. The combination of transaminase elevations and elevated bilirubin without evidence of obstruction is generally recognized as an important predictor of severe liver injury that may lead to death or the need for a liver transplant in some patients. Discontinue natalizumab in patients with jaundice or other evidence of significant liver injury (eg, laboratory evidence).

➤*Immunizations:* See Drug Interactions for more information.

➤*Hypersensitivity reactions:* Hypersensitivity reactions occurring in patients receiving natalizumab included serious systemic reactions (eg, anaphylaxis) at an incidence of less than 1%. These reactions usually occur within 2 hours of the start of the infusion. Symptoms associated with these reactions can include chest pain, dizziness, dyspnea, fever, flushing, hypotension, nausea, pruritus, rash, rigors, and urticaria. Generally, these reactions are associated with antibodies to natalizumab.

If a hypersensitivity reaction occurs, discontinue administration of natalizumab and initiate appropriate therapy. Do not re-treat patients who experience a hypersensitivity reaction with natalizumab. Hypersensitivity reactions were more frequent in patients with antibodies to natalizumab compared with patients who did not develop antibodies to natalizumab in both multiple sclerosis and Crohn disease studies. Therefore, consider the possibility of antibodies to natalizumab in patients who have hypersensitivity reactions.

➤*Pregnancy: Category C.* There are no adequate and well-controlled studies in pregnant women. Natalizumab reduced pup survival in guinea pigs when given in doses 7 times the human dose and had hematologic effects on the fetus in monkeys when given in doses 2.3 times the human dose. Use natalizumab during pregnancy only if the potential benefit justifies the potential risk to the fetus.

In one study in which female guinea pigs were exposed to natalizumab during the second half of pregnancy, a small reduction in pup survival was noted at postnatal day 14 with respect to control (3 pups/litter for the group treated with natalizumab 30 mg/kg and 4.3 pups/litter for the control group). In 1 of 5 studies that exposed monkeys or guinea pigs during pregnancy, the number of abortions in natalizumab-treated (30 mg/kg) monkeys was 33% versus 17% in controls. No effects on abortion rates were noted in any other study. Natalizumab underwent transplacental transfer and produced in utero exposure in developing guinea pigs and cynomolgus monkeys. When pregnant dams were exposed to natalizumab at approximately 7-fold the clinical dose, serum levels in fetal animals at delivery were approximately 35% of maternal serum natalizumab levels. A study in pregnant cynomolgus monkeys treated at 2.3-fold the clinical dose demonstrated natalizumab-related changes in the fetus. These changes included mild anemia, reduced platelet count, increased spleen weights, and reduced liver and thymus weights associated with increased splenic extramedullary hematopoiesis, thymic atrophy, and decreased hepatic hematopoiesis. In offspring born to mothers treated with natalizumab at 7-fold the clinical dose, platelet counts were also reduced. This effect was reversed upon clearance of natalizumab. There was no evidence of anemia in these offspring. Offspring exposed in utero and via breast milk had no natalizumab-related changes in the lymphoid organs and had normal immune response to challenge with a T cell–dependent antigen.

Pregnancy registry – If a woman becomes pregnant while taking natalizumab, consider enrolling her in the natalizumab pregnancy exposure registry by calling 1-800-456-2255.

➤*Lactation:* It is not known whether this drug is excreted in human breast milk. The molecular weight of natalizumab is very high (approximately 149,000), but immunoglobulins are excreted into breast milk. The long elimination half-life (10 to 11 days) will assure that the drug is available for excretion throughout the dosing period. The effects of this potential exposure on a beast-feeding infant are unknown. Because many drugs are excreted in human milk and because of the potential for serious adverse

NATALIZUMAB — INJECTION

reactions in breast-feeding infants from natalizumab, decide whether to discontinue breast-feeding or the drug, taking into account the importance of the drug to the mother.

➤*Children:* Safety and effectiveness of natalizumab in children younger than 18 years of age with multiple sclerosis or Crohn disease have not been established. Natalizumab is not indicated for use in children.

➤*Lab test abnormalities:* Natalizumab induces increases in circulating lymphocytes, monocytes, eosinophils, basophils, and nucleated red blood cells. Observed changes persist during natalizumab exposure but are reversible, returning to baseline levels usually within 16 weeks after the last dose. Elevations of neutrophils are not observed. Natalizumab induces mild decreases in hemoglobin levels that are frequently transient.

➤*Monitoring:* Observe patients during the infusion and for 1 hour after the infusion is complete. Evaluate the patient 3 months after the first infusion, 6 months after the first infusion, and every 6 months thereafter.

Monitor patients on natalizumab for any new sign or symptom that may be suggestive of PML. In patients with multiple sclerosis, obtain an MRI scan prior to initiating therapy with natalizumab. This MRI may be helpful in differentiating subsequent multiple sclerosis symptoms from PML. In patients with Crohn disease, a baseline brain MRI may also be helpful to distinguish preexistent lesions from newly developed lesions; however, brain lesions at baseline that could cause diagnostic difficulty while on natalizumab therapy are uncommon.

Monitor patients for development of infections.

Drug Interactions

➤*Live vaccines:* The use of live vaccines during administration of drugs that may reduce immunocompetence (eg, natalizumab) may cause reduced effectiveness of the vaccine. Additionally, patients with altered immunocompetence may be at increased risk of vaccine-induced infection. Live vaccines should generally be deferred until immune function has improved. Immune globulin or inactivated vaccines, if available, may be effective immunization alternatives.

Natalizumab Drug Interactions

Precipitant drug	Object drug[a]		Description
Antineoplastic agents	Natalizumab	↔	The risk of infection may be increased.
Natalizumab	Antineoplastic agents		
Corticosteroids	Natalizumab	↑	The risk of infection may be increased. patients with Crohn disease who start natalizumab while receiving corticosteroids, begin steroid withdrawal as soon as therapeutic benefit occurs. If systemic corticosteroid cannot be discontinued within 6 months, discontinue natalizumab.
Natalizumab	Corticosteroids		
Immunomodulating agents (eg, peginterferon alfa-2a)	Natalizumab	↔	Because of the potential for increased risk of PML and other infections, do not treat patients with Crohn disease receiving natalizumab with concomitant immunosuppressants. Ordinarily, do not administer natalizumab to patients with multiple sclerosis receiving chronic immunomodulating therapy.
Natalizumab	Immunomodulating agents (eg, peginterferon alfa-2a)		
Immunosuppressants (eg, azathioprine, cyclosporine, 6-mercaptopurine, methotrexate)	Natalizumab	↔	Because of the potential for increased risk of PML and other infections, do not treat patients with Crohn disease receiving natalizumab with concomitant immunosuppressants. Ordinarily, do not administer natalizumab to patients with multiple sclerosis receiving chronic immunosuppressant therapy.
Natalizumab	Immunosuppressants (eg, azathioprine, cyclosporine, 6-mercaptopurine, methotrexate)		
TNF-alpha inhibitors (eg, golimumab, infliximab)	Natalizumab	↑	Because of the potential for increased risk of PML and other infections, do not treat patients receiving natalizumab with concomitant TNF-alpha inhibitors.
Natalizumab	TNF-alpha inhibitors (eg, golimumab, infliximab)		

[a] ↑ = object drug increased; ↔ = undetermined clinical effect.

Adverse Reactions

➤*Most common:* The most common adverse reactions (incidence of at least 10%) were headache and fatigue in both the multiple sclerosis and Crohn disease studies. Other common adverse reactions (incidence of at least 10%) in the multiple sclerosis population were abdominal discomfort, arthralgia, depression, diarrhea not otherwise specified (NOS), gastroenteritis, lower respiratory tract infection, pain in extremity, rash, urinary tract infection, and vaginitis. Other common adverse reactions (incidence of at least 10%) in the Crohn disease population were upper respiratory tract infections and nausea.

➤*Discontinuation:* The most frequently reported adverse reactions resulting in clinical intervention (ie, discontinuation of natalizumab) in the multiple sclerosis studies were urticaria (1%) and other hypersensitivity reactions (1%), and in the 2 Crohn disease studies were the exacerbation of Crohn disease (4.2%) and acute hypersensitivity reactions (1.5%).

➤*Multiple sclerosis:* The most frequently reported serious adverse reactions in study MS1 were infections (3.2% vs 2.6% in placebo, including urinary tract infection [0.8% vs 0.3%] and pneumonia [0.6% vs 0%]), acute hypersensitivity reactions (1.1% vs 0.3%, including anaphylaxis/anaphylactoid reaction [0.8% vs 0%]), depression (1% vs 1%, including suicidal ideation or attempt [0.6% vs 0.3%]), and cholelithiasis (1% vs 0.3%). In study MS2, serious adverse reactions of appendicitis were also more common in patients who received natalizumab (0.8% vs 0.2% in placebo).

Study MS1 –

Natalizumab Adverse Reactions in Patients With Multiple Sclerosis

Adverse reactions	Natalizumab (n = 627)	Placebo (n = 312)
CNS		
Depression	19%	16%
Fatigue	27%	21%
Headache	38%	33%
Somnolence	2%	< 1%
Vertigo	6%	5%
Dermatologic		
Dermatitis	7%	4%
Night sweats	1%	0%
Pruritus	4%	2%
Rash	12%	9%
Skin laceration	2%	< 1%
Thermal burn	1%	< 1%
GI		
Abdominal discomfort	11%	10%
Abnormal liver function test	5%	4%
Diarrhea NOS	10%	9%
Gastroenteritis	11%	9%
GU		
Amenorrhea[a]	2%	1%
Dysmenorrhea[a]	3%	< 1%
Irregular menstruation[a]	5%	4%
Ovarian cyst[a]	2%	< 1%
Urinary incontinence	4%	3%
Urinary tract infection	21%	17%
Urinary urgency/frequency	9%	7%
Vaginitis[a]	10%	6%
Hypersensitivity		
Acute hypersensitivity reactions[b]	4%	< 1%
Other hypersensitivity reactions[b]	5%	2%
Metabolic		
Weight decreased	2%	< 1%
Weight increased	2%	< 1%
Musculoskeletal		
Arthralgia	19%	14%
Joint swelling	2%	1%
Limb injury NOS	3%	2%
Muscle cramp	5%	3%
Pain in extremity	16%	14%

NATALIZUMAB — INJECTION

Natalizumab Adverse Reactions in Patients With Multiple Sclerosis		
Adverse reactions	Natalizumab (n = 627)	Placebo (n = 312)
Miscellaneous		
Chest discomfort	5%	3%
Herpes	8%	7%
Lower respiratory tract infection	17%	16%
Rigors	3%	< 1%
Seasonal allergy	3%	2%
Tonsillitis	7%	5%
Tooth infections	9%	7%

[a] Percentage based on female patients only.
[b] Acute other hypersensitivity reactions are defined as occurring within 2 hours postinfusion vs > 2 hours.

Study MS2 – In study MS2, peripheral edema was more common in patients who received natalizumab (5% vs 1% in placebo).

➤*Crohn disease:* The following serious adverse reactions in the induction studies CD1 and CD2 were reported more commonly with natalizumab than placebo and occurred at an incidence of at least 0.3%: intestinal obstruction or stenosis (2% vs 1% in placebo), acute hypersensitivity reactions (0.5% vs 0%), abdominal adhesions (0.3% vs 0%), and cholelithiasis (0.3% vs 0%). Similar serious adverse reactions were seen in the maintenance study CD3.

Studies CD1 and CD2 –

Natalizumab Adverse Reactions in Patients With Crohn Disease		
Adverse reactions[a]	Natalizumab (n = 983)	Placebo (n = 431)
CNS		
Fatigue	10%	8%
Headache	32%	23%
Tremor	1%	< 1%
Dermatologic		
Dry skin	1%	0%
Rash	6%	4%
GI		
Aphthous stomatitis	2%	< 1%
Constipation	4%	2%
Dyspepsia	5%	3%
Flatulence	3%	2%
Nausea	17%	15%
GU		
Dysmenorrhea[b]	2%	< 1%
Urinary tract infection	3%	1%
Vaginal infections[b]	4%	2%
Respiratory		
Cough	3%	< 1%
Pharyngolaryngeal pain	6%	4%
Upper respiratory tract infection	22%	16%
Miscellaneous		
Acute hypersensitivity reactions	2%	< 1%
Arthralgia	8%	6%
Influenza-like illness	5%	4%
Viral infection	3%	2%

[a] Occurred at an incidence of ≥ 1% higher in natalizumab-treated patients than placebo-treated patients.
[b] Percentage based on female patients only.

Study CD3 –

Natalizumab Adverse Reactions in Patients With Crohn Disease		
Adverse reactions[a]	Natalizumab (n = 214)	Placebo (n = 214)
GU		
Dysmenorrhea[b]	6%	3%
Vaginal infections[b]	8%	< 1%
Respiratory		
Cough	7%	5%
Sinusitis	8%	4%

Natalizumab Adverse Reactions in Patients With Crohn Disease		
Adverse reactions[a]	Natalizumab (n = 214)	Placebo (n = 214)
Miscellaneous		
Back pain	12%	8%
Headache	37%	31%
Influenza	12%	5%
Influenza-like illness	11%	6%
Lower abdominal pain	4%	2%
Peripheral edema	6%	3%
Toothache	4%	< 1%
Viral infection	7%	3%

[a] Occurred at an incidence of ≥ 2% higher in natalizumab-treated patients than placebo-treated patients.
[b] Percentage based on female patients only.

➤*Infections:* PML has occurred in 3 patients who received natalizumab in clinical trials. Two cases of PML were observed in the 1,869 patients with multiple sclerosis who were treated for a median of 120 weeks. These 2 patients had received natalizumab in addition to interferon beta-1a. The third case occurred after 8 doses in 1 of the 1,043 patients with Crohn disease who were evaluated for PML. In the postmarketing setting, additional cases of PML have been reported in natalizumab-treated patients with multiple sclerosis who were not receiving concomitant immunomodulatory therapy. See Warnings/Precautions for more information.

In studies MS1 and MS2, the rate of any type of infection was approximately 1.5 per patient-year in natalizumab-treated patients and placebo-treated patients. The infections were predominately influenza, upper respiratory tract infections, and urinary tract infections. In study MS1, the incidence of serious infection was approximately 3% in natalizumab-treated patients and placebo-treated patients. Most patients did not interrupt treatment with natalizumab during infections. The only opportunistic infection in the multiple sclerosis clinical trials was a case of cryptosporidial gastroenteritis with a prolonged course.

In studies CD1 and CD2, the rate of any type of infection was 1.7 per patient-year in natalizumab-treated patients and 1.4 per patient-year in placebo-treated patients. In study CD3, the incidence of any type of infection was 1.7 per patient-year in natalizumab-treated patients and was similar in placebo-treated patients. The most common infections were influenza, nasopharyngitis, and upper respiratory tract infection. The majority of patients did not interrupt natalizumab therapy during infections and recovery occurred with appropriate treatment. Concurrent use of natalizumab in Crohn disease clinical trials with chronic steroids and/or methotrexate, 6-mercaptopurine, and azathioprine did not result in an increase in overall infections compared with natalizumab alone; however, the concomitant use of these agents could lead to an increased risk of serious infections.

In studies CD1 and CD2, the incidence of serious infection was approximately 2.1% in both natalizumab-treated patients and placebo-treated patients. In study CD3, the incidence of serious infection was approximately 3.3% in natalizumab-treated patients and approximately 2.8% in placebo-treated patients.

In clinical studies for Crohn disease, opportunistic infections (*P. carinii* pneumonia, pulmonary *M. avium-intracellulare*, bronchopulmonary aspergillosis, and *B. cepacia*) have been observed in less than 1% of natalizumab-treated patients; some of these patients were receiving concurrent immunosuppressants. Two serious nonbacterial meningitides occurred in natalizumab-treated patients compared with none in placebo-treated patients.

➤*Infusion-related reactions:* An infusion-related reaction was defined in clinical trials as any adverse reaction occurring within 2 hours of the start of an infusion. In multiple sclerosis clinical trials, approximately 24% of natalizumab-treated patients with multiple sclerosis experienced an infusion-related reaction compared with 18% of placebo-treated patients. In the controlled Crohn disease clinical trials, infusion-related reactions occurred in approximately 11% of patients treated with natalizumab compared with 7% of placebo-treated patients. Reactions more common in the natalizumab-treated patients with multiple sclerosis compared with the placebo-treated patients with multiple sclerosis included dizziness, fatigue, headache, pruritus, rigors, and urticaria. Acute urticaria was observed in approximately 2% of patients. Other hypersensitivity reactions were observed in 1% of patients receiving natalizumab. Serious systemic hypersensitivity infusion reactions occurred in less than 1% of patients. All patients recovered with treatment and/or discontinuation of the infusion.

Infusion-related reactions more common in patients with Crohn disease receiving natalizumab than those receiving placebo included flushing, headache, nausea, pruritus, and urticaria. Serious infusion reactions occurred in studies CD1, CD2, and CD3 at an incidence of less than 1% in natalizumab-treated patients.

Multiple sclerosis patients and Crohn disease patients who became persistently positive for antibodies to natalizumab were more likely to have an infusion-related reaction than those who were antibody-negative.

➤*Postmarketing:* One multiple sclerosis patient who received natalizumab developed herpes encephalitis and died; a second multiple sclerosis patient developed herpes meningitis and recovered with appropriate treatment. PML has been reported with natalizumab monotherapy.

NATALIZUMAB — INJECTION

Patient Information

Instruct patients to promptly report any new or continuously worsening symptoms that persist over several days to their health care provider.

Inform patients that PML has occurred in patients who received natalizumab. Inform patients of the importance of contacting their health care provider if they develop any symptoms suggestive of PML. Instruct patients that typical symptoms associated with PML are diverse, progress over days to weeks, and include progressive weakness on one side of the body or clumsiness of limbs, disturbance of vision, and changes in thinking, memory, and orientation leading to confusion and personality changes. Instruct patients that the progression of deficits usually leads to death or severe disability over weeks or months.

Inform patients that they will need to see their health care provider 3 months after the first infusion, 6 months after the first infusion, and at least as frequently as every 6 months thereafter.

Instruct patients to immediately report any symptoms they experience that are consistent with a hypersensitivity reaction (eg, urticaria with or without associated symptoms) during or following an infusion of natalizumab.

Inform patients that natalizumab may lower the ability of their immune system to fight infections. Instruct patients of the importance of contacting their health care provider if they develop any symptoms of infection.

Inform patients that natalizumab may cause liver injury. Instruct patients to contact their health care provider if they develop symptoms of hepatotoxicity.

GOLIMUMAB

Rx	Simponi (Centocor Ortho Biotech)	**Injection, solution:** 50 mg per 0.5 mL	Preservative free. In single-dose prefilled syringes[a] and prefilled *SmartJect* autoinjectors.

[a] The needle shield is made of dry natural rubber, containing latex.

GOLIMUMAB — INJECTION

WARNING

Serious infection – Patients treated with golimumab are at increased risk for developing serious infections that may lead to hospitalization or death. Most patients who developed these infections were taking concomitant immunosuppressants such as methotrexate or corticosteroids.

Discontinue golimumab if a patient develops a serious infection.

Reported infections include the following:

- Active tuberculosis (TB), including reactivation of latent TB. Patients with TB have frequently presented with disseminated or extrapulmonary disease. Patients should be tested for latent TB before golimumab use and during therapy. Initiate treatment for latent infection prior to golimumab use.
- Invasive fungal infections, including histoplasmosis, coccidioidomycosis, and pneumocystosis. Patients with histoplasmosis or other invasive fungal infections may present with disseminated, rather than localized, disease. Antigen and antibody testing for histoplasmosis may be negative in some patients with active infection. Consider empiric antifungal therapy in patients at risk for invasive fungal infections who develop severe systemic illness.
- Bacterial, viral, and other infections due to opportunistic pathogens.

Carefully consider the risks and benefits of treatment with golimumab prior to initiating therapy in patients with chronic or recurrent infection.

Monitor patients closely for the development of signs and symptoms of infection during and after treatment with golimumab, including the possible development of TB in patients who tested negative for latent TB infection prior to initiating therapy.

Malignancy – Lymphoma and other malignancies, some fatal, have been reported in children and adolescents treated with tumor necrosis factor (TNF) blockers, including golimumab.

Indications

➤*Ankylosing spondylitis:* For the treatment of adults with active ankylosing spondylitis.

➤*Psoriatic arthritis:* For the treatment of adults with active psoriatic arthritis, used alone or in combination with methotrexate.

➤*Rheumatoid arthritis:* For the treatment of adults with moderately to severely active rheumatoid arthritis (RA), in combination with methotrexate.

Administration and Dosage

➤*Adults:*

Ankylosing spondylitis –

Usual dosage: 50 mg subcutaneously once a month.

Concomitant therapy: May be given with or without methotrexate or other nonbiologic disease-modifying antirheumatic drugs (DMARDs). Corticosteroids, nonbiologic DMARDs, and/or nonsteroidal anti-inflammatory drugs (NSAIDs) may be continued during treatment with golimumab.

Psoriatic arthritis – See Ankylosing Spondylitis for dosing.

Rheumatoid arthritis –

Usual dosage: 50 mg subcutaneously once a month.

Concomitant therapy: Should be given in combination with methotrexate. Corticosteroids, nonbiologic DMARDs, and/or NSAIDs may be continued during treatment with golimumab.

➤*Preparation for administration:* Allow the prefilled syringe or autoinjector to sit at room temperature outside the carton for 30 minutes prior to subcutaneous injection. Do not warm golimumab in any other way. Do not shake.

Any leftover product remaining in the prefilled syringe or prefilled autoinjector should not be used.

The needle cover on the prefilled syringe, as well as the prefilled syringe in the autoinjector, contains dry natural rubber (a derivative of latex), which should not be handled by persons sensitive to latex.

➤*Administration:* Administer by subcutaneous injection. Injection sites should be rotated and injections should never be given into areas where the skin is tender, bruised, red, or hard.

➤*Storage/Stability:* Refrigerate at 2° to 8°C (36° to 46°F) and protect from light. Do not freeze. Keep the product in the original carton to protect from light until the time of use.

Actions

➤*Pharmacology:* Golimumab is a human monoclonal antibody that binds to both the soluble and transmembrane bioactive forms of human TNF-alpha. This interaction prevents the binding of TNF-alpha to its receptors, thereby inhibiting the biological activity of TNF-alpha (a cytokine protein). There was no evidence of the golimumab antibody binding to other TNF superfamily ligands; in particular, the golimumab antibody did not bind or neutralize human lymphotoxin. Golimumab did not lyse human monocytes expressing transmembrane TNF in the presence of complement or effector cells.

Elevated TNF-alpha levels in the blood, synovium, and joints have been implicated in the pathophysiology of several chronic inflammatory diseases, such as RA, psoriatic arthritis, and ankylosing spondylitis. TNF-alpha is an important mediator of the articular inflammation that is characteristic of these diseases. Golimumab modulated the in vitro biological effects mediated by TNF in several bioassays, including the expression of adhesion proteins responsible for leukocyte infiltration (E-selectin, intercellular adhesion molecule 1 [ICAM-1] and vascular cell adhesion molecule 1 [VCAM-1]) and the secretion of proinflammatory cytokines (interleukin [IL]–6, IL-8, granulocyte colony-stimulating factor [G-CSF], and granulocyte-macrophage colony-stimulating factor [6M-CSF]).

Pharmacodynamics – In clinical studies, decreases in C-reactive protein (CRP), IL-6, matrix metalloproteinase (MMP-3), ICAM-1, and vascular endothelial growth factor (VEGF) were observed following golimumab administration in patients with RA, psoriatic arthritis, and ankylosing spondylitis.

➤*Pharmacokinetics:* Golimumab exhibited dose-proportional pharmacokinetics in patients with active RA over the dose range of 0.1 to 10 mg/kg following a single intravenous (IV) dose.

Absorption – Following subcutaneous administration of golimumab to healthy subjects and patients with active RA, the median time to reach maximum serum concentrations (T_{max}) ranged from 2 to 6 days. A subcutaneous injection of golimumab 50 mg to healthy subjects produced a mean maximum serum concentration (C_{max}) of approximately 2.5 mcg/mL. By cross-study comparisons of mean area under curve (AUC_{inf}) values following an IV or subcutaneous administration of golimumab, the absolute bioavailability of subcutaneous golimumab was estimated to be approximately 53%.

When golimumab 50 mg was administered subcutaneously to patients with RA, psoriatic arthritis, or ankylosing spondylitis every 4 weeks, serum concentrations appeared to reach steady state by week 12. With concomitant use of methotrexate, treatment with golimumab 50 mg subcutaneously every 4 weeks resulted in a mean steady-state trough serum concentration of approximately 0.4 to 0.6 mcg/mL in patients with active RA, approximately 0.5 mcg/mL in patients with active psoriatic arthritis, and approximately 0.8 mcg/mL in patients with active ankylosing spondylitis. Patients with RA, psoriatic arthritis, and ankylosing spondylitis treated with golimumab 50 mg and methotrexate had approximately 52%, 36%, and 21% higher mean steady-state trough concentrations of golimumab, respectively, compared with those treated with golimumab 50 mg without methotrexate. The presence of methotrexate also decreased anti-golimumab antibody incidence from 7% to 2%. For RA, use golimumab with methotrexate. In the psoriatic arthritis and ankylosing spondylitis trials, the presence or absence of concomitant methotrexate did not appear to influence clinical efficacy and safety parameters.

Patients who developed anti-golimumab antibodies generally had lower steady-state serum trough concentrations of golimumab.

Distribution – Following a single IV administration over the same dose range in patients with active RA, mean volume of distribution ranged from 58 to 126 mL/kg. The volume of distribution for golimumab indicates that golimumab is distributed primarily in the circulatory system, with limited extravascular distribution.

GOLIMUMAB — INJECTION

Excretion – Mean systemic clearance of golimumab was estimated to be 4.9 to 6.7 mL/day/kg. Median terminal half-life values were estimated to be approximately 2 weeks in healthy subjects and patients with active RA, psoriatic arthritis, or ankylosing spondylitis.

Contraindications

None well documented.

Warnings/Precautions

➤*Serious infections:* Serious and sometimes fatal infections caused by bacterial, mycobacterial, invasive fungal, viral, protozoal, or other opportunistic pathogens have been reported in patients receiving TNF-blockers, including golimumab. Among opportunistic infections, TB, histoplasmosis, aspergillosis, candidiasis, coccidioidomycosis, listeriosis, and pneumocystosis were the most commonly reported with TNF-blockers. Patients have frequently presented with disseminated, rather than localized, disease and were often taking concomitant immunosuppressants such as methotrexate or corticosteroids. The concomitant use of a TNF-blocker and abatacept or anakinra was associated with a higher risk of serious infections; therefore, the concomitant use of golimumab and these biologic products is not recommended.

Do not initiate treatment with golimumab in patients with an active infection, including clinically important localized infections. Consider the risks and benefits of treatment prior to initiating golimumab in patients with chronic or recurrent infection; patients who have been exposed to TB; patients with a history of an opportunistic infection; patients who have resided or traveled in areas of endemic TB or endemic mycoses, such as histoplasmosis, coccidioidomycosis, or blastomycosis; or patients with underlying conditions that may predispose them to infection. See Monitoring for more information.

➤*Tuberculosis:* Cases of reactivation of TB or new TB infections have been observed in patients receiving TNF-blockers, including patients who have previously received treatment for latent or active TB. Evaluate patients for TB risk factors and test for latent infection prior to initiating golimumab and periodically during therapy.

Treatment of latent TB infection prior to therapy with TNF-blockers has been shown to reduce the risk of TB reactivation during therapy. Consider induration of 5 mm or more with tuberculin skin testing a positive test result when assessing if treatment for latent TB is needed prior to initiating golimumab, even for patients previously vaccinated with Bacille Calmette-Guérin (BCG).

Also consider anti-TB therapy prior to initiation of golimumab in patients with a history of latent or active TB in whom an adequate course of treatment cannot be confirmed, and for patients with a negative test for latent TB but having risk factors for TB infection. Consultation with a health care provider with expertise in the treatment of TB is recommended to aid in the decision of whether initiating anti-TB therapy is appropriate for an individual patient.

Closely monitor patients for the development of signs and symptoms of TB, including patients who tested negative for latent TB infection prior to initiating therapy.

TB should be strongly considered in patients who develop a new infection during golimumab treatment, especially in patients who have previously or recently traveled to countries with a high prevalence of TB or who have had close contact with a person with active TB.

➤*Invasive fungal infections:* For golimumab-treated patients who reside or travel in regions where mycoses are endemic, suspect invasive fungal infection if they develop a serious systemic illness. Consider appropriate empiric antifungal therapy while a diagnostic workup is being performed. Antigen and antibody testing for histoplasmosis may be negative in some patients with active infection. When feasible, make the decision to administer empiric antifungal therapy in these patients in consultation with a health care provider with expertise in the diagnosis and treatment of invasive fungal infections, and take into account both the risk for severe fungal infection and the risks of antifungal therapy.

➤*Hepatitis B virus reactivation:* The use of TNF-blockers, including golimumab, has been associated with reactivation of hepatitis B virus (HBV) in patients who are chronic hepatitis B carriers (ie, surface-antigen positive). In some instances, HBV reactivation occurring in conjunction with TNF-blocker therapy has been fatal. The majority of these reports have occurred in patients who received concomitant immunosuppressants.

Evaluate patients at risk for HBV infection for prior evidence of HBV infection before initiating TNF-blocker therapy. Consider the risks and benefits of treatment prior to prescribing TNF-blockers, including golimumab, to patients who are carriers of HBV. Adequate data are not available on whether antiviral therapy can reduce the risk of HBV reactivation in HBV carriers who are treated with TNF-blockers. Closely monitor patients who are carriers of HBV and require treatment with TNF-blockers for clinical and laboratory signs of active HBV infection throughout therapy and for several months following termination of therapy.

In patients who develop HBV reactivation, stop TNF-blockers and antiviral therapy and initiate appropriate supportive treatment. The safety of resuming TNF-blockers after HBV reactivation has been controlled is not known. Therefore, exercise caution when considering resumption of TNF-blockers in this situation, and monitor patients closely.

➤*Malignancies:* Malignancies, some fatal, have been reported among children, adolescents, and young adults who received treatment with TNF-blocking agents (initiation of therapy 18 years of age and younger), of which golimumab is a member. Approximately half the cases were lymphomas, including Hodgkin and non-Hodgkin lymphoma. The other cases represented a variety of malignancies, including rare malignancies that are usually associated with immunosuppression and malignancies that are not usually observed in children and adolescents. The malignancies occurred after a median of 30 months (range, 1 to 84 months) after the first dose of TNF-blocker therapy. Most of the patients were receiving concomitant immunosuppressants. These cases were reported postmarketing and are derived from a variety of sources, including registries and spontaneous postmarketing reports.

Consider the risks and benefits of TNF-blocker treatment, including golimumab, prior to initiating therapy in patients with a known malignancy other than a successfully treated nonmelanoma skin cancer or when considering continuing a TNF-blocker in patients who develop a malignancy.

➤*Congestive heart failure:* Cases of worsening congestive heart failure (CHF) and new-onset CHF have been reported with TNF-blockers. In several exploratory trials of other TNF-blockers in the treatment of CHF, there were greater proportions of TNF-blocker–treated patients who had CHF exacerbations requiring hospitalization or increased mortality. Golimumab has not been studied in patients with a history of CHF; use with caution in patients with CHF. If a decision is made to administer golimumab to patients with CHF, closely monitor these patients during therapy, and discontinue golimumab if new or worsening symptoms of CHF appear.

➤*Demyelinating disorders:* Use of TNF-blockers has been associated with cases of new onset or exacerbation of CNS demyelinating disorders, including multiple sclerosis (MS). While no trials have been performed evaluating golimumab in the treatment of patients with MS, another TNF-blocker was associated with increased disease activity in patients with MS. Therefore, exercise caution in considering the use of TNF-blockers, including golimumab, in patients with CNS demyelinating disorders, including MS.

➤*Immunogenicity:* Antibodies to golimumab were detected in 4% of golimumab-treated patients across the phase 3 RA, psoriatic arthritis, and ankylosing spondylitis trials through week 24. Similar rates were observed in each of the 3 indications. Patients who received golimumab with concomitant methotrexate had a lower proportion of antibodies to golimumab than patients who received golimumab without methotrexate (approximately 2% vs 7%, respectively). Of the patients with a positive antibody response to golimumab in the phase 2 and 3 trials, most were determined to have neutralizing antibodies to golimumab as measured by a cell-based functional assay. The small number of patients positive for antibodies to golimumab limits the ability to draw definitive conclusions regarding the relationship between antibodies to golimumab and clinical efficacy or safety measures.

➤*Hematologic effects:* There have been postmarketing reports of pancytopenia, leukopenia, neutropenia, aplastic anemia, and thrombocytopenia in patients receiving TNF-blockers. Although there were no cases of severe cytopenias seen in the golimumab clinical trials, exercise caution when using TNF-blockers, including golimumab, in patients who have significant cytopenias.

➤*Latex sensitivity:* The needle cover on the prefilled syringe as well as the prefilled syringe in the autoinjector contains dry natural rubber (a derivative of latex), which should not be handled by people sensitive to latex.

➤*Vaccinations:* Patients treated with golimumab may receive vaccinations, except for live vaccines. No data are available on the response to live vaccination, the risk of infection, or the transmission of infection after the administration of live vaccines to patients receiving golimumab. In the phase 3 psoriatic arthritis study, after pneumococcal vaccination, a similar proportion of golimumab- and placebo-treated patients were able to mount an adequate immune response of at least a 2-fold increase in antibody titers to pneumococcal polysaccharide vaccine. In both golimumab- and placebo-treated patients, the proportions of patients with response to pneumococcal vaccine were lower among patients receiving methotrexate compared with patients not receiving methotrexate. The data suggest that golimumab does not suppress the humoral immune response to the pneumococcal vaccine.

➤*Pregnancy: Category B.* There are no adequate and well-controlled studies of golimumab in pregnant women. Because animal reproduction and developmental studies are not always predictive of human response, it is not known whether golimumab can cause fetal harm when administered to a pregnant woman or can affect reproduction capacity. Only use golimumab during pregnancy if clearly needed.

➤*Lactation:* It is not known whether golimumab is excreted in human milk or absorbed systemically after ingestion. Because many drugs and immunoglobulins are excreted in human milk, and because of the potential for adverse reactions in breast-feeding infants from golimumab, decide whether to discontinue breast-feeding or the drug, taking into account the importance of the drug to the mother.

In the prenatal and postnatal development study in cynomolgus monkeys in which golimumab was administered subcutaneously during pregnancy and lactation, golimumab was detected in the breast milk at concentrations that were approximately 400-fold lower than the maternal serum concentrations.

➤*Children:* Safety and effectiveness of golimumab in children younger than 18 years of age have not been established.

➤*Elderly:* Because there is a higher incidence of infections in the elderly population in general, use caution in treating elderly patients with golimumab.

➤*Monitoring:* Closely monitor patients for the development of signs and symptoms of infection during and after treatment with golimumab. Discontinue golimumab if a patient develops a serious infection, an opportunistic infection, or sepsis. A patient who develops a new infection during treatment with golimumab should undergo a prompt and complete diagnostic workup

GOLIMUMAB — INJECTION

appropriate for an immunocompromised patient, appropriate antimicrobial therapy should be initiated, and the patient should be closely monitored.

Closely monitor patients for the development of signs and symptoms of TB, including patients who tested negative for latent TB infection prior to initiating therapy. Closely monitor patients with CHF and discontinue treatment if new or worsening symptoms of CHF appear.

Closely monitor patients who are carriers of HBV and require treatment with TNF-blockers for clinical and laboratory signs of active HBV infection throughout therapy and for several months following termination of therapy.

Drug Interactions

➤*Live vaccines:* See Warnings/Precautions for more information.

Golimumab Drug Interactions

Precipitant drug	Object drug[a]		Description
Abatacept	Golimumab	↑	The risk of serious infection may be increased. Use of TNF-blockers and abatacept is not recommended.
Golimumab	Abatacept		
Anakinra	Golimumab	↑	The risk of serious infection and neutropenia may be increased. Use of TNF-blockers and anakinra is not recommended.
Golimumab	Anakinra		
Rituximab	Golimumab	↑	The risk of serious infection may be increased. Consider avoiding concurrent use of golimumab and rituximab.
Golimumab	Rituximab		
TNF-blocker (eg, adalimumab, certolizumab, etanercept, infliximab)	Golimumab	↑	Risk of serious infection may be increased. Avoid coadministration of golimumab and another TNF-blocker.
Golimumab	TNF-blockers (eg, adalimumab, certolizumab, etanercept, infliximab)		
Golimumab	Cytochrome P450 substrates (eg, cyclosporine, theophylline, warfarin)	↑↓	Monitor the effects and plasma concentrations of drugs with a narrow therapeutic index when golimumab is started or stopped. Dose adjustments may be needed.
Golimumab	Live vaccines (eg, intranasal flu vaccine)	↔	There are no data on the response to live vaccination, the risk of infection, or transmission of infection after administration of live vaccines to patients receiving golimumab. Avoid administration of live vaccines.

[a] ↑ = object drug increased; ↑↓ = object drug both increased and decreased; ↔ = undetermined clinical effect.

Adverse Reactions

➤*Serious adverse reactions:* The most serious adverse reactions were serious infections and malignancies.

➤*Common adverse reactions:* Upper respiratory tract infection and nasopharyngitis were the most common adverse reactions reported in the combined phase 3 RA, psoriatic arthritis, and ankylosing spondylitis trials through week 16, occurring in 7% and 6% of golimumab-treated patients compared with 6% and 5% of control-treated patients, respectively.

➤*Discontinuation of treatment:* The proportion of patients who discontinued treatment because of adverse reactions in the controlled phase 3 trials through week 16 in RA, psoriatic arthritis, and ankylosing spondylitis was 2% for golimumab-treated patients and 3% for placebo-treated patients. The most common adverse reactions leading to discontinuation of golimumab in the controlled phase 3 trials through week 16 were sepsis (0.2%), ALT increased (0.2%), and AST increased (0.2%).

➤*Clinical studies experience:*

Golimumab Adverse Reactions (≥ 1%)[a]

Adverse reactions	Golimumab ± DMARDs (n = 1,659)	Placebo ± DMARDs (n = 639)
CNS		
Dizziness	2%	1%
Paresthesia	1%	< 1%
Hepatic		
ALT increased	4%	3%
AST increased	3%	2%
Respiratory		
Bronchitis	2%	1%
Nasopharyngitis	6%	5%
Pharyngitis	1%	1%
Rhinitis	1%	< 1%
Sinusitis	2%	1%
Upper respiratory tract infection	7%	6%
Miscellaneous		
Hypertension	3%	1%
Influenza	2%	1%
Injection-site erythema	3%	1%
Oral herpes	1%	< 1%
Pyrexia	1%	< 1%

[a] Patients may have taken concomitant methotrexate, sulfasalazine, hydroxychloroquine, low-dose corticosteroids (10 mg or less of prednisone/day or equivalent), and/or NSAIDs during the trials.

➤*Infections:* In controlled phase 3 trials through week 16 in RA, psoriatic arthritis, and ankylosing spondylitis, infections were observed in 28% of golimumab-treated patients compared with 25% of control-treated patients.

➤*Liver enzyme elevations:* There have been reports of severe hepatic reactions, including acute liver failure, in patients receiving TNF-blockers. In controlled phase 3 trials of golimumab in patients with RA, psoriatic arthritis, and ankylosing spondylitis through week 16, ALT elevations at least 5 times upper limits of normal (ULN) occurred in 0.2% of control-treated patients and 0.7% of golimumab-treated patients, and ALT elevations 3 times ULN or more occurred in 2% of control-treated patients and 2% of golimumab-treated patients. Because many of the patients in the phase 3 trials were also taking medications that cause liver enzyme elevations (eg, NSAIDs, methotrexate), the relationship between golimumab and liver elevation is not clear.

➤*Autoimmune disorders and autoantibodies:* The use of TNF-blockers has been associated with the formation of autoantibodies and, rarely, with the development of a lupus-like syndrome. In the controlled phase 3 trials in patients with RA, psoriatic arthritis, and ankylosing spondylitis through week 14, there was no association of golimumab treatment and the development of newly positive anti–double-stranded DNA antibodies.

➤*Injection-site reactions:* In controlled phase 3 trials through week 16 in RA, psoriatic arthritis, and ankylosing spondylitis, 6% of golimumab-treated patients had injection-site reactions compared with 2% of control-treated patients. The majority of the injection-site reactions were mild and the most frequent manifestation was injection-site erythema. In controlled phase 2 and 3 trials in RA, psoriatic arthritis, and ankylosing spondylitis, no patients treated with golimumab developed anaphylactic reactions.

➤*Dermatologic effects:* Cases of new-onset psoriasis, including pustular psoriasis and palmoplantar psoriasis, have been reported with the use of TNF-blockers, including golimumab. Cases of exacerbation of preexisting psoriasis have also been reported with the use of TNF-blockers. Many of these patients were taking concomitant immunosuppressants (eg, methotrexate, corticosteroids). Some of these patients required hospitalization. Most patients had improvement of their psoriasis following discontinuation of their TNF-blocker. Some patients have had recurrences of the psoriasis when they were rechallenged with a different TNF-blocker. Consider discontinuation of golimumab for severe cases and those that do not improve or that worsen despite topical treatments.

Patient Information

Advise patients of the potential benefits and risks of golimumab. Instruct patients to read the Medication Guide before starting golimumab therapy and to read it each time the prescription is renewed.

Inform patients that golimumab may lower the ability of their immune system to fight infections. Instruct the patient of the importance of contacting their health care provider if they develop any symptoms of infection, including TB, invasive fungal infections, and hepatitis B reactivation.

Counsel patients about the risk of lymphoma and other malignancies while receiving golimumab.

Advise latex-sensitive patients that the needle cover on the prefilled syringe as well as the prefilled syringe in the prefilled *SmartJect* autoinjector contains dry natural rubber (a derivative of latex).

Advise patients to report any signs or worsening medical conditions, such as CHF, demyelinating disorders, autoimmune disease, liver disease, cytopenias, or psoriasis.

Patients should perform the first self-injection under the supervision of a qualified health care provider. If a patient or caregiver is to administer golimumab, instruct him/her in injection techniques and assess his/her ability to inject subcutaneously to ensure the proper administration of golimumab. Prior to use, remove the prefilled syringe or the prefilled *SmartJect* autoinjector from the refrigerator and allow golimumab to sit at room temperature outside of the carton for 30 minutes and out of the reach of children. Do not warm golimumab in any other way. For example, do not warm golimumab in a microwave or in hot water. Do not remove the prefilled syringe needle cover or *SmartJect* autoinjector cap while allowing golimumab to reach room temperature. Remove these immediately before injection. Do not pull the autoinjector away from the skin until you hear a first click sound and then a second click sound (the injection is finished and the needle is pulled back). It usually takes about 3 to 6 seconds, but may take up to 15 seconds to hear the second click after the first click. If the autoinjector is pulled away from the skin before the injection is completed, a full dose of golimumab may not be administered. Use a puncture-resistant container for disposal of needles and syringes. Instruct patients or caregivers in the technique of proper syringe and needle disposal, and advise them not to reuse these items.

INFLIXIMAB

Rx	**Remicade** (Centocor)	**Injection, lyophilized powder for solution:** 100 mg	Preservative free. Sucrose 500 mg. In 20 mL single-use vials.

INFLIXIMAB — INJECTION

WARNING

Risk of serious infections – Patients treated with infliximab are at an increased risk for developing serious infections that may lead to hospitalization or death. Most patients who developed these infections were taking concomitant immunosuppressants such as methotrexate or corticosteroids.

Discontinue infliximab if a patient develops a serious infection or sepsis.

Reported infections include:

- Active tuberculosis (TB), including reactivation of latent TB. Patients with TB have frequently presented with disseminated or extrapulmonary disease. Test patients for latent TB before infliximab use and during therapy. Initiate treatment for latent infection prior to infliximab use.
- Invasive fungal infections, including histoplasmosis, coccidioidomycosis, candidiasis, aspergillosis, blastomycosis, and pneumocystosis. Patients with histoplasmosis or other invasive fungal infections may present with disseminated, rather than localized, disease. Antigen and antibody testing for histoplasmosis may be negative in some patients with active infection. Empiric antifungal therapy should be considered in patients who develop severe systemic illness.
- Bacterial, viral, and other infections caused by opportunistic pathogens.

Carefully consider the risks and benefits of treatment with infliximab prior to initiating therapy in patients with long-term or recurrent infection.

Closely monitor patients for the development of signs and symptoms of infection during and after treatment with infliximab, including the possible development of TB in patients who tested negative for latent TB infection prior to initiating therapy.

Malignancy – Lymphoma and other malignancies, some fatal, have been reported in children and adolescent patients treated with tumor necrosis factor (TNF) blockers, including infliximab.

Postmarketing cases of hepatosplenic T-cell lymphoma, a rare type of T-cell lymphoma, have been reported in patients treated with TNF blockers, including infliximab. These cases had a very aggressive disease course and have been fatal. All reported infliximab cases have occurred in patients with Crohn disease or ulcerative colitis, and the majority were in adolescent and young adult males. All of these patients received treatment with azathioprine or 6-mercaptopurine concomitantly with infliximab at or prior to diagnosis.

Indications

➤*Ankylosing spondylitis:* Reducing signs and symptoms in patients with active ankylosing spondylitis.

➤*Crohn disease:* Reducing the signs and symptoms and inducing and maintaining clinical remission in adults and children with moderately to severely active Crohn disease who have had inadequate responses to conventional therapy.

Fistulizing Crohn disease – Reducing the number of draining enterocutaneous and rectovaginal fistulas and maintaining fistula closure in adult patients with fistulizing Crohn disease.

➤*Plaque psoriasis:* Treatment of adult patients with chronic, severe (ie, extensive and/or disabling) plaque psoriasis who are candidates for systemic therapy and when other systemic therapies are medically less appropriate.

➤*Psoriatic arthritis:* Reducing signs and symptoms of active arthritis, inhibiting the progression of structural damage, and improving physical function in patients with psoriatic arthritis.

➤*Rheumatoid arthritis:* In combination with methotrexate for reducing signs and symptoms, inhibiting the progression of structural damage, and improving physical function in patients with moderately to severely active rheumatoid arthritis (RA).

➤*Ulcerative colitis:* Reducing signs and symptoms, inducing and maintaining clinical remission and mucosal healing, and eliminating corticosteroid use in patients with moderately to severely active ulcerative colitis who have had an inadequate response to conventional therapy.

➤*Off-label uses:*

Behçet syndrome uveitis – [2] = Fair documentation. Initial data from 3 case series suggest that intravenous (IV) infliximab may play a beneficial role in the management of uveitis associated with Behçet syndrome. Additional controlled trials are needed to verify these results.

Celiac sprue – [3] = Safety concerns. In published cases, infliximab was used to treat cases of refractory sprue in patients unresponsive to a gluten-free diet and immunotherapy. Significant improvement in refractory sprue was noted in a handful of patients following a single infusion of infliximab. Infliximab has a black box warning for increased risk of infections and hepatosplenic T-cell lymphomas and may have contributed to the development of cytomegalovirus infection and enteropathy-associated T-cell lymphoma in 2 cases. Controlled clinical trials are needed to verify the long-term safety and efficacy of infliximab in treating patients with refractory sprue.

Erythrodermic psoriasis – [4] = Insufficient documentation. IV infliximab for the treatment of erythrodermic psoriasis has been evaluated in 19 patients in case reports or case series. Although all patients showed short-term symptomatic improvement, infliximab cannot be recommended based on these limited data and short-term follow-up. Larger, controlled trials are needed to establish the efficacy, long-term benefits, and safety profile.

Giant cell arteritis – [5] = Poor documentation. Benefits of infliximab therapy in the management of giant cell arteritis have been observed only in noncontrolled trials and case reports. The 1 large, well-controlled study of infliximab for giant cell arteritis was halted early because of a lack of efficacy. Lack of efficacy was also observed in a controlled study of infliximab treatment for polymyalgia rheumatica, a disorder with many similarities to giant cell arteritis. In addition, new-onset giant cell arteritis has been reported as a possible adverse effect with other TNF blockers. Finally, infliximab has a black box warning regarding the risk of potentially serious infections or lymphomas that may occur during use. Because of its potential lack of efficacy and serious safety concerns, infliximab use cannot be recommended for the treatment of giant cell arteritis.

Graft-versus-host disease (adults) – [3] = Safety concerns. Infliximab does not appear to provide added benefit when used as graft-versus-host disease (GVHD) prophylaxis, although it is active for the acute control of steroid-resistant GVHD as an adjunctive treatment. The high incidence of bacterial and invasive fungal infections is of concern. Currently available studies are limited by small patient samples, patient heterogeneity, and variations in treatment protocols between study sites. Larger, controlled trials evaluating infliximab treatment of steroid-resistant GVHD are needed to provide better estimations of treatment benefit versus risk, particularly with respect to infectious complications.

Graft-versus-host disease (children/adolescents) – [3] = Safety concerns. Infliximab may be beneficial in the acute control of steroid-resistant GVHD as an adjunctive treatment. The high incidence of bacterial and invasive fungal infections is of concern. Currently available studies are limited by small patient samples and patient heterogeneity. Larger, controlled trials evaluating infliximab treatment of steroid-resistant GVHD are needed to provide better estimations of treatment benefit versus risks, particularly with respect to infectious complications.

Hidradenitis suppurativa (adults) – [3] = Safety concerns. Although the limited research indicates a possible role for infliximab in the management of hidradenitis suppurativa, controlled trial data are lacking. In addition, some authors have reported only short-term, transient improvements in disease severity after infliximab, necessitating ongoing treatment. Carefully consider the expense of this agent and its significant safety risks before routine use.

Juvenile idiopathic arthritis – [2] = Fair documentation. Results of studies involving infliximab for the treatment of juvenile idiopathic arthritis (JIA) have been mixed. In the only randomized trial to date, infliximab plus methotrexate was no more effective than placebo plus methotrexate at week 14, the a priori end point. In 1 open-label study, infliximab combined with disease-modifying antirheumatic drugs (DMARDs) or corticosteroids was found to be effective, but this regimen was no more effective than etanercept combined with DMARDs or corticosteroids. In other open-label studies in small numbers of patients, the combination of infliximab plus methotrexate appeared to be effective. Two TNF-alpha inhibitors, etanercept and adalimumab, have received Food and Drug Administration (FDA) approval for treatment of JIA. The 2009 consensus statement on the use of biological agents for the treatment of rheumatic disease considers TNF-alpha inhibitors to be beneficial at improving clinical symptoms, restoring growth velocity, and improving bone mineral density in patients with polyarticular JIA. However, they state there is no evidence to suggest one TNF blocker is more effective than any other. TNF-alpha inhibitors have a black box warning about the increased risk of hepatosplenic T-cell lymphoma and/or the risk of infections. Further data are required to establish the efficacy, safety, and optimal dosage of infliximab in patients with JIA.

Pustular psoriasis – [4] = Insufficient documentation. IV infliximab for the treatment of pustular psoriasis has been evaluated in 11 patients. All patients showed short-term symptomatic improvement; however, larger, controlled trials are needed to establish the efficacy, long-term benefits, and safety profile.

Pyoderma gangrenosum – [3] = Safety concerns. Initial data suggest that infliximab may be beneficial in the treatment of refractory pyoderma gangrenosum.

Sarcoidosis – [4] = Insufficient documentation. Contrary to the beneficial effect in small numbers of patients in the case reports, data from the 2 small trials did not support the use of infliximab in the treatment of sarcoidosis. In the presence of equivocal data and a black box warning for increased risk of infections and lymphomas, more studies are needed to determine the usefulness of infliximab in the treatment of sarcoidosis, a disease with diverse presentation and frequent periods of potential remission or stabilization without drug therapy.

Uveitis (adults) – [3] = Safety concerns. Large-scale, controlled clinical trials are lacking, but existing studies consistently found improvements in uveitis with infliximab compared with placebo or etanercept. Infliximab has a black box warning regarding the potential risk of infection and lymphomas. When used for the prevention or management of uveitis, infliximab has been associated with serious infectious and allergic adverse effects requiring treatment discontinuation.

Uveitis (children/adolescents) – [3] = Safety concerns. Several retrospective case series have concluded that infliximab is effective in treating childhood uveitis. However, no prospective studies or controlled clinical tri-

INFLIXIMAB — INJECTION

als have been performed. Infliximab has several safety concerns, including a black box warning regarding serious infections and hepatosplenic T-cell lymphomas. Further data are needed to establish the efficacy, safety, and optimal dosage of infliximab in children with uveitis.

Wegener granulomatosis – [3] = Safety concerns. Based on guidelines and results from limited noncontrolled studies and case series, infliximab may be considered as an adjunctive therapy for patients with active Wegener granulomatosis (Wegener granulomatosis) who are refractory to standard steroids and immunosuppressive regimens. The interpretation of many of the studies conducted to date was confounded by the inclusion of different subcategories of systemic necrotizing vasculitis, not just Wegener granulomatosis. The possible increased risk of serious infection, especially with prolonged treatment, is of concern and requires careful monitoring. Larger, controlled trials are needed before widespread use of infliximab for Wegener granulomatosis can be recommended.

Administration and Dosage

➤*Adults:*

Ankylosing spondylitis – 5 mg/kg given as an IV infusion followed by additional similar doses 2 and 6 weeks after the first infusion, and every 6 weeks thereafter.

Crohn disease or fistulizing Crohn disease –

Initial dosage: 5 mg/kg given as an IV induction regimen at 0, 2, and 6 weeks.

Maintenance dosage: After initial dosage, follow with a maintenance regimen of 5 mg/kg every 8 weeks thereafter.

Dosage adjustment: For adult patients who respond and then lose their response, consider treatment with 10 mg/kg.

Discontinuation of therapy: Patients who do not respond by week 14 are unlikely to respond with continued dosing; consider discontinuing infliximab in these patients.

Plaque psoriasis – 5 mg/kg given as an IV infusion followed by additional doses at 2 and 6 weeks after the first infusion, then every 8 weeks thereafter.

Psoriatic arthritis –

Usual dosage: 5 mg/kg given as an IV infusion followed by additional similar doses at 2 and 6 weeks after the first infusion, then every 8 weeks thereafter.

Concomitant therapy: Infliximab can be used with or without methotrexate.

Rheumatoid arthritis –

Usual dosage: 3 mg/kg given as an IV infusion followed by additional similar doses at 2 and 6 weeks after the first infusion, then every 8 weeks thereafter.

Dosage adjustment: For patients who have incomplete responses, consider adjusting the dose up to 10 mg/kg or treating as often as every 4 weeks, bearing in mind that risk of serious infections is increased at higher doses.

Concomitant therapy: Give infliximab in combination with methotrexate.

Ulcerative colitis –

Initial dosage: 5 mg/kg given as an induction regimen at 0, 2, and 6 weeks.

Maintenance dosage: After initial dosage, follow with a maintenance regimen of 5 mg/kg every 8 weeks thereafter.

Off-label dosing –

Behçet syndrome uveitis: [2] = Fair documentation. 3 to 5 mg/kg IV infusion over 2 hours, given at weeks 0, 2, and 6, and continued every 6 to 8 weeks.

Celiac sprue: [3] = Safety concerns. One infusion of infliximab 5 mg/kg IV over 2 hours followed by maintenance therapy with azathioprine. Therapy was continued every 8 weeks for 1 year in 1 case report.

Erythrodermic psoriasis: [4] = Insufficient documentation. 2.7 to 10 mg/kg administered by IV infusion over 3 to 4 hours. Case series duration ranged from 4 weeks to 7 months.

Graft-versus-host disease (adults): [3] = Safety concerns. 10 mg/kg/dose (maximum, 15 mg/kg/dose) infused IV over 1 to 2 hours. Repeat doses were given weekly or according to clinical judgment.

Hidradenitis suppurativa (adults): [3] = Safety concerns. 5 mg/kg IV at weeks 0, 2, and 6. Some authors reported using maintenance doses of 5 mg/kg every 4 to 8 weeks. Maintenance doses have been administered for as long as 2 years.

Pustular psoriasis: [4] = Insufficient documentation. 3 to 5 mg/kg administered by IV infusion over 3 to 4 hours. Case series treatment duration ranged from 4 weeks to 6 years.

Pyoderma gangrenosum: [3] = Safety concerns. Induction therapy of 5 mg/kg IV over 2 hours at weeks 0, 2, and 6 (variable), and then maintenance therapy of 5 mg/kg IV over 2 hours every 4 to 12 weeks. Although some patients respond and can discontinue therapy upon remission, long-term therapy may be needed to maintain remission for others.

Sarcoidosis: [4] = Insufficient documentation. Infliximab 3 or 5 mg/kg by IV infusion over a 2-hour interval. Study duration has ranged from 6 to 52 weeks.

Uveitis (adults): [3] = Safety concerns. 3 to 5 mg/kg IV at weeks 0, 2, and 6. Additional maintenance doses have been administered at 4- to 8-week intervals for up to 72 weeks.

Wegener granulomatosis: [3] = Safety concerns. 3 to 5 mg/kg by IV infusion at weeks 0, 2, and 6 and then every 4 to 8 weeks until remission. Infliximab is typically used as adjunctive therapy.

➤*Children:*

Crohn disease –

6 years of age and older:

• *Initial dosage* – 5 mg/kg given as an IV induction regimen at 0, 2, and 6 weeks.

• *Maintenance dosage* – After initial dosage, follow with a maintenance regimen of 5 mg/kg every 8 weeks.

Off-label dosing –

Graft-versus-host disease (children/adolescents): [3] = Safety concerns. Infliximab administered as 10 mg/kg/dose infused IV over 1 to 2 hours or 10 to 15 mg/kg up to 3 times per week.

Juvenile idiopathic arthritis: [2] = Fair documentation. 3 to 10 mg/kg IV at weeks 0, 2, and 6, and every 4 to 10 weeks thereafter, given in combination with corticosteroids and/or DMARDs. Therapy continued for up to 4 years in 1 long-term extension trial. Consensus guidelines consider infliximab to be effective for polyarticular JIA at a dose of 6 mg/kg (category A, evidence from at least 1 randomized, controlled trial).

Juvenile idiopathic arthritis uveitis:

• *Usual dose* – 5 to 10 mg/kg at weeks 0, 2, and 4 followed by infusions every 6 to 8 weeks with a more rapid infusion rate based on tolerance.

• *Alternative dosage* – All patients responded to 5 to 10 mg/kg at 2- to 8-week intervals in a case series of pediatric patients with uveitis with or without associated JIA.

Refractory juvenile idiopathic arthritis:

• *Initial dosage* – 3 to 4 mg/kg initially or at weeks 0, 2, and 6.

• *Maintenance dosage* – After initial dosage, follow with a maintenance regimen of up to 10 mg/kg every 4 to 8 weeks.

Refractory Kawasaki syndrome: Single infusion of 5 to 10 mg/kg. This may be beneficial in patients who have not responded to 2 doses of immune globulin IV and daily high-dose aspirin therapy.

Ulcerative colitis:

• *Initial dosage* – 5 mg/kg initially followed by 5 to 10 mg/kg in 2 weeks or 5 mg/kg as induction therapy at 0, 2, and 6 weeks.

• *Maintenance dosage* – After initial dosage, follow with a maintenance regimen every 6 to 8 weeks.

Uveitis (children/adolescents): [3] = Safety concerns. 3 to 20 mg/kg IV at varying intervals (every 2 to 6 weeks) in conjunction with other immunomodulatory agents.

➤*Elderly:* Because there is a higher incidence of infections in the elderly population in general, use caution in treating elderly patients.

➤*Preparation for administration:* Use aseptic technique.

Infliximab vials do not contain antibacterial preservatives; therefore, after reconstitution the vials should be used immediately, not reentered or stored. The diluent to be used for reconstitution is 10 mL of sterile water for injection. The total dose of the reconstituted product must be further diluted to 250 mL with sodium chloride 0.9% injection. The infusion concentration should range between 0.4 and 4 mg/mL. The infliximab infusion should begin within 3 hours of preparation.

1.) Calculate the dose and the number of infliximab vials needed. Each infliximab vial contains infliximab 100 mg. Calculate the total volume of reconstituted infliximab solution required.
2.) Reconstitute each infliximab vial with 10 mL of sterile water for injection, using a syringe equipped with a 21-gauge or smaller needle. Remove the flip-top from the vial and wipe the top with an alcohol swab. Insert the syringe needle into the vial through the center of the rubber stopper and direct the stream of sterile water for injection to the glass wall of the vial. Do not use the vial if the vacuum is not present. Gently swirl the solution by rotating the vial to dissolve the lyophilized powder. Avoid prolonged or vigorous agitation. Do not shake. Foaming of the solution on reconstitution is not unusual. Allow the reconstituted solution to stand for 5 minutes. The solution should be colorless to light yellow and opalescent and may develop a few translucent particles because infliximab is a protein. Do not use if opaque particles, discoloration, or other foreign particles are present.
3.) Dilute the total volume of the reconstituted infliximab solution dose to 250 mL with sodium chloride 0.9% injection by withdrawing a volume of sodium chloride 0.9% injection equal to the volume of reconstituted infliximab from the sodium chloride 0.9% injection 250 mL bottle or bag. Slowly add the total volume of reconstituted infliximab solution to the 250 mL infusion bottle or bag. Gently mix.

➤*Administration:* The infusion solution must be administered over a period of at least 2 hours and must use an infusion set with an in-line, sterile, nonpyrogenic, low protein-binding filter (pore size of 1.2 mcm or less). Any unused portion of the infusion solution should not be stored for reuse.

Premedication – Prior to infusion with infliximab, premedication may be administered at the health care provider's discretion. Premedication could include antihistamines (anti-H_1 ± anti-H_2), acetaminophen, and/or corticosteroids.

Infusion reaction – Adverse reactions during administration of infliximab included flu-like symptoms, headache, dyspnea, hypotension, transient fever, chills, GI symptoms, and skin rashes. Anaphylaxis might occur at any time during infliximab infusion. Approximately 20% of infliximab-treated patients in all clinical trials experienced an infusion reaction, compared with 10% of placebo-treated patients.

Mild to moderate infusion reaction: During infusion, mild to moderate infusion reactions may improve following slowing or suspension of the infusion, and, upon resolution of the reaction, reinitiation at a lower infusion rate and/or therapeutic administration of antihistamines, acetaminophen, and/or corticosteroids. For patients who do not tolerate the infusion following these interventions, infliximab should be discontinued.

INFLIXIMAB — INJECTION

Severe infusion reaction: During or following infusion, patients that have severe infusion-related hypersensitivity reactions should discontinue further infliximab treatment. The management of severe infusion reactions should be dictated by the signs and symptoms of the reaction. Appropriate personnel and medication should be available to treat anaphylaxis if it occurs.

➤*Admixture compatibility:* No physical biochemical compatibility studies have been conducted to evaluate the coadministration of infliximab with other agents. Infliximab should not be infused concomitantly in the same IV line with other agents.

➤*Storage / Stability:* Store the lyophilized product under refrigeration at 2° to 8°C (36° to 46°F). This product contains no preservatives.

Actions

➤*Pharmacology:* Infliximab neutralizes the biological activity of TNF-alpha by binding with high affinity to the soluble and transmembrane forms of TNF-alpha and inhibits binding of TNF-alpha with its receptors. Infliximab does not neutralize TNF-beta (lymphotoxin-alpha), a related cytokine that utilizes the same receptors as TNF-alpha. Biological activities attributed to TNF-alpha include the following: induction of proinflammatory cytokines such as interleukins 1 and 6; enhancement of leukocyte migration by increasing endothelial layer permeability and expression of adhesion molecules by endothelial cells and leukocytes; activation of neutrophil and eosinophil functional activity; and induction of acute phase reactants and other liver proteins, as well as tissue-degrading enzymes produced by synoviocytes and/or chondrocytes. Cells expressing transmembrane TNF-alpha bound by infliximab can be lysed in vitro or in vivo. Infliximab inhibits the functional activity of TNF-alpha in a wide variety of in vitro bioassays utilizing human fibroblasts, endothelial cells, neutrophils, B and T lymphocytes, and epithelial cells. The relationship of these biological response markers to the mechanism(s) by which infliximab exerts its clinical effects is unknown. Anti–TNF-alpha antibodies reduce disease activity in the cotton-top tamarin colitis model and decrease synovitis and joint erosions in a murine model of collagen-induced arthritis. Infliximab prevents disease in transgenic mice that develop polyarthritis as a result of constitutive expression of human TNF-alpha and, when administered after disease onset, allows eroded joints to heal.

Pharmacodynamics – Elevated concentrations of TNF-alpha have been found in involved tissues and fluids of patients with RA, Crohn disease, ulcerative colitis, ankylosing spondylitis, psoriatic arthritis, and plaque psoriasis. In RA, treatment with infliximab reduced infiltration of inflammatory cells in inflamed areas of the joint, as well as expression of molecules mediating cellular adhesion (E-selectin, intercellular adhesion molecule-1, and vascular cell adhesion molecule-1), chemoattraction (interleukin-8 and monocyte chemotactic protein), and tissue degradation (matrix metalloproteinase 1 and 3). In Crohn disease, treatment with infliximab reduced infiltration of inflammatory cells and TNF-alpha production in inflamed areas of the intestine and reduced the proportion of mononuclear cells from the lamina propria able to express TNF-alpha and interferon.

After treatment with infliximab, patients with RA or Crohn disease exhibited decreased levels of serum interleukin-6 and C-reactive protein compared with baseline. Peripheral blood lymphocytes from infliximab-treated patients showed no significant decrease in number or in proliferative responses to in vitro mitogenic stimulation, compared with cells from untreated patients. In psoriatic arthritis, treatment with infliximab resulted in a reduction of the number of T cells and blood vessels in the synovium and psoriatic skin lesions, as well as a reduction of macrophages in the synovium. In plaque psoriasis, infliximab treatment may reduce the epidermal thickness and infiltration of inflammatory cells. The relationship between these pharmacodynamic activities and the mechanism(s) by which infliximab exerts its clinical effects is not known.

➤*Pharmacokinetics:*

Absorption / Distribution – In adults, single IV infusions of 3 to 20 mg/kg showed a linear relationship between the dose administered and the maximum serum concentration. The volume of distribution at steady state was independent of dose and indicated that infliximab was distributed primarily within the vascular compartment.

Following an initial dose of infliximab, repeated infusions at 2 and 6 weeks resulted in predictable concentration-time profiles following each treatment. No systemic accumulation of infliximab occurred upon continued repeated treatment with 3 or 10 mg/kg at 4- or 8-week intervals. At 8 weeks after a maintenance dose of 3 to 10 mg/kg of infliximab, median infliximab serum concentrations ranged from approximately 0.5 to 6 mcg/mL; however, infliximab concentrations were not detectable (less than 0.1 mcg/mL) in patients who became positive for antibodies to infliximab.

Excretion – Pharmacokinetic results for single doses of 3 to 10 mg/kg in RA, 5 mg/kg in Crohn disease, and 3 to 5 mg/kg in plaque psoriasis indicate that the median terminal half-life of infliximab is 7.7 to 9.5 days.

Development of antibodies to infliximab increased infliximab clearance.

Contraindications

Administration of doses greater than 5 mg/kg to patients with moderate to severe heart failure; readministration to patients who have experienced a severe hypersensitivity reaction to infliximab; known hypersensitivity to inactive components of the product or to any murine proteins.

Warnings/Precautions

➤*Risk of serious infections:* Serious and sometimes fatal infections caused by bacterial, mycobacterial, invasive fungal, viral, or other opportunistic pathogens have been reported in patients receiving TNF-blocking agents. Among opportunistic infections, TB, histoplasmosis, aspergillosis, candidiasis, coccidioidomycosis, listeriosis, and pneumocystosis were the most commonly reported. Patients have frequently presented with disseminated rather than localized disease, and are often taking concomitant immunosuppressants, such as methotrexate or corticosteroids, with infliximab.

Treatment with infliximab should not be initiated in patients with an active infection, including clinically important localized infections. Consider the risks and benefits of treatment prior to initiating therapy in patients with long-term or recurrent infection; who have been exposed to TB; who have resided or traveled in areas of endemic TB or endemic mycoses, such as histoplasmosis, coccidioidomycosis, or blastomycosis; or with underlying conditions that may predispose them to infection.

Cases of reactivation of TB or new TB infections have been observed in patients receiving infliximab, including patients who have previously received treatment for latent or active TB. Evaluate patients for TB risk factors and test for latent infection prior to initiating infliximab and periodically during therapy.

Treatment of latent TB infection prior to therapy with TNF-blocking agents has been shown to reduce the risk of TB reactivation during therapy. Induration of 5 mm or greater with tuberculin skin testing should be considered a positive test result when assessing if treatment for latent TB is needed prior to initiating infliximab, even for patients previously vaccinated with Bacille Calmette-Guerin.

Also consider anti-TB therapy prior to initiation of infliximab in patients with a history of latent or active TB in whom an adequate course of treatment cannot be confirmed, and for patients with a negative test for latent TB but having risk factors for TB infection. Consultation with a health care provider with expertise in the treatment of TB is recommended to aid in the decision of whether initiating anti-TB therapy is appropriate for an individual patient.

Strongly consider TB in patients who develop a new infection during infliximab treatment, especially in patients who have previously or recently traveled to countries with a high prevalence of TB, or who have had close contact with a person with active TB.

Closely monitor patients for the development of signs and symptoms of infection during and after treatment with infliximab, including the development of TB in patients who tested negative for latent TB infection prior to initiating therapy. Tests for latent TB infection may also be falsely negative while on therapy with infliximab.

Discontinue infliximab if a patient develops a serious infection or sepsis. Closely monitor a patient who develops a new infection during treatment with infliximab, and undergoes a prompt and complete diagnostic workup appropriate for an immunocompromised patient, and initiate appropriate antimicrobial therapy.

For patients who reside or travel in regions where mycoses are endemic, invasive fungal infection should be suspected if they develop a serious systemic illness. Consider appropriate empiric antifungal therapy while a diagnostic workup is being performed. Antigen and antibody testing for histoplasmosis may be negative in some patients with active infection. When feasible, the decision to administer empiric antifungal therapy in these patients should be made in consultation with a health care provider with expertise in the diagnosis and treatment of invasive fungal infections and should take into account both the risk for severe fungal infection and the risks of antifungal therapy.

Serious infections were seen in clinical studies with concurrent use of anakinra and another TNF-alpha–blocking agent, etanercept, with no added clinical benefit compared with etanercept alone. Because of the nature of the adverse reactions seen with combination of etanercept and anakinra therapy, similar toxicities may also result from the combination of anakinra and other TNF-alpha–blocking agents. Therefore, the combination of infliximab and anakinra is not recommended.

➤*Malignancies:* Malignancies, some fatal, have been reported among children, adolescents and young adults who received treatment with TNF-blocking agents (initiation of therapy, 18 years of age or younger), including infliximab. Approximately half of these cases were lymphomas, including Hodgkin and non-Hodgkin lymphomas. The other cases represented a variety of malignancies, including rare malignancies that are usually associated with immunosuppression and malignancies that are not usually observed in children and adolescents. The malignancies occurred after a median of 30 months (range, 1 to 84 months) after the first dose of TNF blocker therapy. Most of the patients were receiving concomitant immunosuppressants. These cases were reported postmarketing and were derived from a variety of sources, including registries and spontaneous postmarketing reports.

Postmarketing cases of hepatosplenic T-cell lymphomas, a rare type of T-cell lymphoma, have been reported in patients treated with TNF blockers, including infliximab. These cases have had a very aggressive disease course and have been fatal. All reported infliximab cases have occurred in patients with Crohn disease or ulcerative colitis, and the majority were in adolescent and young adult males. All of these patients had received treatment with the immunosuppressants azathioprine or 6-mercaptopurine concomitantly with infliximab at or prior to diagnosis. It is uncertain whether the occurrence of hepatosplenic T-cell lymphomas is related to infliximab or infliximab in combination with these other immunosuppressants.

In the controlled portions of clinical trials of some TNF-blocking agents, including infliximab, more malignancies (excluding lymphoma and non-melanoma skin cancer) have been observed in patients receiving TNF blockers, compared with control patients. During the controlled portions of infliximab trials in patients with moderately to severely active RA, Crohn disease, psoriatic arthritis, ankylosing spondylitis, ulcerative colitis, and plaque psoriasis, 14 patients were diagnosed with malignancies (excluding

INFLIXIMAB — INJECTION

lymphoma and nonmelanoma skin cancer) among 4,019 infliximab-treated patients versus 1 among 1,597 control patients (at a rate of 0.52 per 100 patient-years among infliximab-treated patients vs a rate of 0.11 per 100 patient-years among control patients), with median duration of follow-up 0.5 years for infliximab-treated patients and 0.4 years for control patients. Of these, the most common malignancies were breast, colorectal, and melanoma. The rate of malignancies among infliximab-treated patients was similar to that expected in the general population, whereas the rate in control patients was lower than expected.

In the controlled portions of clinical trials of all the TNF-blocking agents, more cases of lymphoma have been observed among patients receiving a TNF blocker, compared with control patients. In the controlled and open-label portions of infliximab clinical trials, 5 patients developed lymphomas among 5,707 patients treated with infliximab (median duration of follow-up, 1 year) versus 0 lymphomas in 1,600 control patients (median duration of follow-up, 0.4 years). In patients with RA, 2 lymphomas were observed for a rate of 0.08 cases per 100 patient-years of follow-up, which is approximately 3-fold higher than expected in the general population. In the combined clinical trial population for RA, Crohn disease, psoriatic arthritis, ankylosing spondylitis, ulcerative colitis, and plaque psoriasis, 5 lymphomas were observed for a rate of 0.1 cases per 100 patient-years of follow-up, which is approximately 4-fold higher than expected in the general population. Patients with Crohn disease, RA, or plaque psoriasis, particularly patients with highly active disease and/or chronic exposure to immunosuppressant therapies, may be at a higher risk (up to several-fold) than the general population for the development of lymphoma, even in the absence of TNF-blocking therapy. Cases of acute and chronic leukemia have been reported with postmarketing TNF blocker use in RA and other indications. Even in the absence of TNF blocker therapy, patients with RA may be at higher risk (approximately 2–fold) than the general population for the development of leukemia.

In a clinical trial exploring the use of infliximab in patients with moderate to severe chronic obstructive pulmonary disease (COPD), more malignancies, the majority of lung or head and neck origin, were reported in infliximab-treated patients, compared with control patients. All patients had a history of heavy smoking. Exercise caution when considering the use of infliximab in patients with moderate to severe COPD.

Monitor psoriasis patients for nonmelanoma skin cancers, particularly patients who have had prior prolonged phototherapy treatment. In the maintenance portion of clinical trials for infliximab, nonmelanoma skin cancers were more common in patients with previous phototherapy.

The potential role of TNF-blocking therapy in the development of malignancies is not known. Rates in clinical trials for infliximab cannot be compared with rates in clinical trials of other TNF blockers and may not predict rates observed in a broader patient population. Exercise caution in considering infliximab treatment in patients with a history of malignancy or in continuing treatment in patients who develop malignancy while receiving infliximab.

➤*Hepatitis B virus reactivation:* Use of TNF blockers, including infliximab, has been associated with reactivation of hepatitis B virus (HBV) in patients who are chronic carriers of this virus. In some instances, HBV reactivation occurring in conjunction with TNF blocker therapy has been fatal. The majority of these reports have occurred in patients concomitantly receiving other medications that suppress the immune system, which also may contribute to HBV reactivation. Evaluate patients at risk for HBV infection for prior evidence of HBV infection before initiating TNF blocker therapy. Exercise caution in prescribing TNF blockers, including infliximab, for patients identified as carriers of HBV. Adequate data are not available on the safety or efficacy of treating patients who are carriers of HBV with antiviral therapy in conjunction with TNF blocker therapy to prevent HBV reactivation. Closely monitor patients who are carriers of HBV and require treatment with TNF blockers for clinical and laboratory signs of active HBV infection throughout therapy and for several months following termination of therapy. In patients who develop HBV reactivation, stop TNF blockers and initiate antiviral therapy with appropriate supportive treatment. The safety of resuming TNF blocker therapy after HBV reactivation is controlled is not known. Therefore, exercise caution when considering resumption of TNF blocker therapy in this situation, and monitor patients closely.

➤*Hepatotoxicity:* Severe hepatic reactions, including acute liver failure, jaundice, hepatitis, and cholestasis, have been reported rarely in postmarketing data in patients receiving infliximab. Autoimmune hepatitis has been diagnosed in some of these cases. Severe hepatic reactions occurred between 2 weeks and more than a year after initiation of infliximab; elevations in hepatic aminotransferase levels were not noted prior to discovery of the liver injury in many of these cases. Some of these cases were fatal or necessitated liver transplantation. Evaluate patients with symptoms or signs of liver function impairment for evidence of liver injury. If jaundice and/or marked liver enzyme elevations (eg, 5 times the upper limit of normal [ULN] or more) develop, discontinue infliximab and investigate the abnormality thoroughly. In clinical trials, mild or moderate elevations of ALT and AST have been observed in patients receiving infliximab without progression to severe hepatic injury.

➤*Heart failure:* Infliximab has been associated with adverse outcomes in patients with heart failure and use in patients with heart failure only after consideration of other treatment options. The results of a randomized study evaluating the use of infliximab in patients with heart failure (New York Heart Association [NYHA] functional class III/IV) suggested higher mortality in patients who received infliximab 10 mg/kg and higher rates of cardiovascular adverse reactions at doses of 5 and 10 mg/kg. There have been postmarketing reports of worsening heart failure, with and without identifiable precipitating factors, in patients taking infliximab. There have also been rare postmarketing reports of new-onset heart failure, including heart failure in patients without known preexisting cardiovascular disease. Some of these patients were younger than 50 years of age. If a decision is made to administer infliximab to patients with heart failure, closely monitor them during therapy and discontinue infliximab if new or worsening symptoms of heart failure appear.

➤*Hematologic effects:* Cases of leukopenia, neutropenia, thrombocytopenia, and pancytopenia, some with a fatal outcome, have been reported in patients receiving infliximab. The causal relationship to infliximab therapy remains unclear. Although no high-risk group has been identified, exercise caution in patients being treated with infliximab who have ongoing or histories of significant hematologic abnormalities. Advise all patients to seek immediate medical attention if they develop signs and symptoms suggestive of blood dyscrasias or infection (eg, persistent fever) while on infliximab. Consider discontinuation of infliximab therapy in patients who develop significant hematologic abnormalities.

➤*CNS effects:* Infliximab and other agents that inhibit TNF have been associated in rare cases with optic neuritis, seizure, and new onset or exacerbation of clinical symptoms and/or radiographic evidence of CNS-demyelinating disorders, including multiple sclerosis and CNS manifestations of systemic vasculitis and peripheral demyelinating disorders, including Guillain-Barré syndrome. Exercise caution when considering the use of infliximab in patients with preexisting or recent onset of CNS-demyelinating or seizure disorders. Consider discontinuation of infliximab in patients who develop significant CNS adverse reactions.

➤*Autoimmunity:* Treatment with infliximab may result in the formation of autoantibodies and, rarely, in the development of a lupus-like syndrome. If a patient develops symptoms suggestive of a lupus-like syndrome following treatment with infliximab, discontinue treatment.

➤*Vaccinations:* No data are available on the response to vaccination with live vaccines or on the secondary transmission of infection by live vaccines in patients receiving anti-TNF therapy. It is recommended that live vaccines not be given concurrently.

It is recommended that all children with Crohn disease be brought up to date with all vaccinations prior to initiating infliximab therapy. The interval between vaccination and initiation of infliximab therapy should be in accordance with current vaccination guidelines.

➤*Immunogenicity:* Treatment with infliximab can be associated with the development of antibodies to infliximab. The incidence of antibodies to infliximab in patients given a 3-dose induction regimen followed by maintenance dosing was approximately 10%, as assessed through 1 to 2 years of infliximab treatment. A higher incidence of antibodies to infliximab was observed in patients with Crohn disease receiving infliximab after drug-free intervals greater than 16 weeks. In a study of psoriatic arthritis, in which 191 patients received 5 mg/kg with or without methotrexate, antibodies to infliximab occurred in 15% of patients. The majority of antibody-positive patients had low titers. Patients who were antibody positive were more likely to have higher rates of clearance, and reduced efficacy, and to experience an infusion reaction than were patients who were antibody negative. Antibody development was lower among patients with RA and Crohn disease receiving immunosuppressive therapies, such as 6-mercaptopurine/azathioprine or methotrexate.

In the psoriasis study II, which included both the 5 and 3 mg/kg doses, antibodies were observed in 36% of patients treated with 5 mg/kg every 8 weeks for 1 year and in 51% of patients treated with 3 mg/kg every 8 weeks for 1 year. In the psoriasis study III, which also included both the 5 and 3 mg/kg doses, antibodies were observed in 20% of patients treated with 5 mg/kg induction (weeks 0, 2, and 6), and in 27% of patients treated with 3 mg/kg induction. Despite the increase in antibody formation, the infusion reaction rates in studies I and II (in patients treated with 5 mg/kg induction followed by every 8 week maintenance for 1 year) and in study III (in patients treated with 5 mg/kg induction [14.1% to 23%]) and serious infusion reaction rates (less than 1%) were similar to those observed in other study populations. The clinical significance of apparent increased immunogenicity on efficacy and infusion reactions in psoriasis patients compared with patients with other diseases treated with infliximab long-term is not known.

➤*Hypersensitivity reactions:* Infliximab has been associated with hypersensitivity reactions that varied in times of onset and required hospitalization in some cases. Most hypersensitivity reactions, which include urticaria, dyspnea, and/or hypotension, occurred during or within 2 hours of infliximab infusion.

However, in some cases, serum sickness–like reactions have been observed in patients after initial infliximab therapy (as early as after the second dose) and when infliximab therapy was reinstituted following an extended period without infliximab treatment. Symptoms associated with these reactions include fever, rash, headache, sore throat, myalgias, polyarthralgias, hand and facial edema, and/or dysphagia. These reactions were associated with marked increase in antibodies to infliximab, loss of detectable serum concentrations of infliximab, and possible loss of drug efficacy.

For severe hypersensitivity reactions, discontinue infliximab. Have medications for the treatment of hypersensitivity reactions (eg, acetaminophen, antihistamines, corticosteroids, epinephrine) available for immediate use in the event of a reaction.

➤*Pregnancy: Category B.* Because infliximab does not crossreact with TNF-alpha in species other than humans and chimpanzees, animal reproduction studies have not been conducted with infliximab.

It is not known if infliximab crosses the human placenta to the fetus. Limited human pregnancy data are inadequate to assess the embryo/fetal risk. It is not known if infliximab can cause fetal harm when administered to a

INFLIXIMAB — INJECTION

pregnant woman or can affect reproduction capacity. Give infliximab to a pregnant woman only if clearly needed.

➤*Lactation:* It is not known if infliximab is excreted in human milk or absorbed systemically after ingestion. Infliximab would not be expected to be excreted in breast-milk because of its high molecular weight (149,100). Even if it were excreted into breast milk, the antibody would probably be digested in the GI tract. Therefore, the risk of toxicity in a breast-feeding infant from exposure via milk would most likely be next to nothing. The manufacturer recommends that, because many drugs and immunoglobulins are excreted in human milk, and the potential for adverse reactions in breast-feeding infants from infliximab, women should not breast-feed their infants while taking infliximab. Decide whether to discontinue breast-feeding or the drug, taking into account the importance of the drug to the mother.

➤*Children:* Infliximab is indicated for reducing signs and symptoms and inducing and maintaining clinical remission in children with moderately to severely active Crohn disease who have had an inadequate response to conventional therapy. Infliximab has been studied only in combinations with conventional immunosuppressive therapy in children with Crohn disease.

Infliximab has not been studied in children with Crohn disease younger than 6 years of age. The long-term (more than 1 year) safety and effectiveness of infliximab in children with Crohn disease have not been established in clinical trials.

Safety and efficacy of infliximab in children with ulcerative colitis and plaque psoriasis have not been established.

The safety and efficacy of infliximab in patients with juvenile RA were evaluated in a multicenter, randomized, placebo-controlled, double-blind study for 14 weeks, followed by a double-blind, all-active treatment extension for a maximum of 44 weeks.

The study failed to establish the efficacy of infliximab in the treatment of juvenile RA. Key observations in the study included a high placebo response rate and a higher rate of immunogenicity than what has been observed in adults. Additionally, a higher rate of clearance of infliximab was observed than had been observed in adults.

A total of 60 patients with juvenile RA were treated with doses of 3 mg/kg and 57 patients were treated with doses of 6 mg/kg. The proportion of patients with infusion reactions who received infliximab 3 mg/kg was 35% over 52 weeks, compared with 18% in patients who received 6 mg/kg over 38 weeks. The most common infusion reactions reported were vomiting, fever, headache, and hypotension. In the infliximab 3 mg/kg group, 4 patients had a serious infusion reaction, and 3 patients reported a possible anaphylactic reaction (2 of which were among the serious infusion reactions). In the infliximab 6 mg/kg group, 2 patients had a serious infusion reaction, 1 of whom had a possible anaphylactic reaction. Two of the 6 patients who experienced serious infusion reactions received infliximab by rapid infusion (duration, less than 2 hours). Antibodies to infliximab developed in 38% (20/53) of patients who received infliximab 3 mg/kg, compared with 12% (6/49) of patients who received 6 mg/kg.

A total of 68% of patients who received infliximab 3 mg/kg in combination with methotrexate experienced an infection over 52 weeks, compared with 65% of patients who received infliximab 6 mg/kg in combination with methotrexate over 38 weeks. The most commonly reported infections were upper respiratory tract infection and pharyngitis and the most commonly reported serious infection was pneumonia. Other notable infections included primary varicella infection in 1 patient and herpes zoster in 1 patient.

➤*Elderly:* In RA and plaque psoriasis clinical trials, no overall differences were observed in efficacy or safety in 181 patients with RA and 75 patients with plaque psoriasis 65 years of age and older who received infliximab, compared with younger patients, although the incidence of serious adverse reactions in patients 65 years of age and older was higher in both infliximab and control groups, compared with younger patients. In Crohn disease, ulcerative colitis, ankylosing spondylitis, and psoriatic arthritis studies, there were insufficient numbers of patients 65 years of age and older to determine whether they respond differently from patients 18 to 65 years of age. Because there is a higher incidence of infections in the elderly population in general, use caution in treating elderly patients.

➤*Monitoring:* Monitor patients for signs and symptoms of infection, including TB, during or after treatment with infliximab. Perform tuberculin skin tests before and during treatment with infliximab.

Closely monitor new infections. If a patient develops a serious infection, discontinue infliximab therapy. Appropriately evaluate and monitor chronic carriers of hepatitis B prior to the initiation of and during treatment with infliximab.

Closely monitor patients with heart failure during therapy, and discontinue infliximab if new or worsening symptoms of heart failure appear.

Evaluate patients with symptoms or signs of liver dysfunction for evidence of liver injury.

Monitor psoriasis patients for nonmelanoma skin cancers, particularly patients who have had prior prolonged phototherapy treatment.

Drug Interactions

➤*Vaccinations:* See Warnings/Precautions for more information.

Infliximab Drug Interactions

Precipitant drug	Object drug[a]		Description
Abatacept	Infliximab	↑	An increased rate of infection may occur with coadministration of infliximab and costimulation modulators (eg, abatacept). Concurrent use is not recommended. May result in similar toxicities.
Infliximab	Abatacept		
Anakinra	Infliximab	↑	Coadministration of etanercept (another TNF-blocking agent) and anakinra (an interleukin-1 antagonist) has been associated with an increased risk of serious infections and neutropenia; the combination has no additional benefit compared with these medicinal products alone. Other TNF-blocking agents (including infliximab) used in combination with anakinra also may result in similar toxicities.
Infliximab	Anakinra		
Azathioprine and 6-mercaptopurine	Infliximab	↑	Rare postmarketing cases of hepatosplenic T-cell lymphoma have been reported in adolescent and young adult patients with Crohn disease treated with infliximab. This rare type of T-cell lymphoma has a very aggressive disease course and is usually fatal. All of these hepatosplenic T-cell lymphomas with infliximab have occurred in patients on concomitant treatment with azathioprine or 6-mercaptopurine.
TNF blockers (eg, adalimumab, certolizumab, etanercept, golimumab)	Infliximab	↑	Risk of serious infection may be increased. Avoid coadministration of infliximab and another TNF blocker.
Infliximab	TNF blockers (eg, adalimumab, certolizumab, etanercept, golimumab)		
Tocilizumab	Infliximab	↑	Coadministration of tocilizumab with biologic DMARDs, such as infliximab, may increase the risk of serious infection, avoid coadministration.
Infliximab	Tocilizumab		

[a] ↑ = object drug increased.

Adverse Reactions

➤*Discontinuation of therapy:* One of the most common reasons for discontinuation of treatment was infusion-related reactions (eg, dyspnea, flushing, headache, rash).

➤*Dose-related adverse reactions:* Adverse reactions have been reported in a higher proportion of patients with RA receiving the 10 mg/kg dose than the 3 mg/kg dose; however, no differences were observed in a frequency of adverse reactions between the 5 mg/kg dose and the 10 mg/kg dose in patients with Crohn disease.

➤*Infusion-related reactions:*

Acute infusion reactions – An infusion reaction was defined in clinical trials as any adverse reaction occurring during the infusion or within 1 to 2 hours of an infusion. Approximately 20% of infliximab-treated patients in all clinical trials experienced infusion reactions, compared with approximately 10% of placebo-treated patients. Among all infliximab infusions, 3% were accompanied by nonspecific symptoms such as fever or chills, 1% were accompanied by cardiopulmonary reactions (primarily chest pain, hypotension, hypertension, or dyspnea), and less than 1% were accompanied by pruritus, urticaria, or the combined symptoms of pruritus/urticaria and cardiopulmonary reactions. Serious infusion reactions occurred in less than 1% of patients and included anaphylaxis, convulsions, erythematous rash, and hypotension. Approximately 3% of patients discontinued infliximab because of infusion reactions, and all patients recovered with treatment

INFLIXIMAB — INJECTION

and/or discontinuation of infusion. Infliximab infusions beyond the initial infusion were not associated with a higher incidence of reactions. The infusion reaction rates remained stable in psoriasis through 1 year in psoriasis study I. In psoriasis study II, the rates were variable over time and somewhat higher following the final infusion than after the initial infusion. Across the 3 psoriasis studies, the percent of total infusions resulting in infusion reactions was 7% in the 3 mg/kg group, 4% in the 5 mg/kg group, and 1% in the placebo group.

Patients who became positive for antibodies to infliximab were more likely (approximately 2- to 3-fold) to have an infusion reaction than were those who were negative. Use of concomitant immunosuppressive agents appeared to reduce the frequency of both antibodies to infliximab and infusion reactions.

Delayed reactions / reactions following readministration –

Plaque psoriasis: In psoriasis studies, approximately 1% of infliximab-treated patients experienced a possible delayed hypersensitivity reaction, generally reported as serum sickness or a combination of arthralgia and/or myalgia with fever and/or rash. These reactions generally occurred within 2 weeks after repeat infusion.

Crohn disease: In a study in which 37 of 41 patients with Crohn disease were re-treated with infliximab following a 2- to 4-year period without infliximab treatment, 10 patients experienced adverse reactions manifesting 3 to 12 days following infusion, of which 6 were considered serious. Signs and symptoms included the following: myalgia and/or arthralgia with fever and/or rash, with some patients also experiencing pruritus; facial, hand, or lip edema; dysphagia; urticaria; sore throat; and headache. Patients experiencing these adverse reactions had not experienced infusion-related adverse reactions associated with initial infliximab therapy. These adverse reactions occurred in 39% (9/23) who had received liquid formulation, which is no longer in use, and 7% (1/14) of patients who received lyophilized formulation. The clinical data are not adequate to determine if occurrence of these reactions is due to differences in formulation. Patients' signs and symptoms improved substantially or resolved with treatment in all cases. There are insufficient data on the incidence of these reactions after drug-free intervals of 1 to 2 years; however, these reactions have been observed only infrequently in clinical trials and postmarketing surveillance with re-treatment intervals for up to 1 year.

➤*Infections:* In infliximab clinical studies, treated infections were reported in 36% of infliximab-treated patients (average, 51 weeks of follow-up) and in 25% of placebo-treated patients (average, 37 weeks of follow-up). The infections most frequently reported were respiratory tract infections (including sinusitis, pharyngitis, and bronchitis) and urinary tract infections. Among infliximab-treated patients, serious infections included pneumonia, cellulitis, abscess, skin ulceration, sepsis, and bacterial infection. In clinical trials, 7 opportunistic infections were reported; 2 cases each of coccidioidomycosis (1 case was fatal) and histoplasmosis (1 case was fatal), and 1 case each of pneumocystosis, nocardiosis, and cytomegalovirus. TB was reported in 14 patients, 4 of whom died because of miliary TB. Other cases of TB, including disseminated TB, also have been reported postmarketing. Most of the cases of TB occurred within the first 2 months after initiation of therapy with infliximab and may reflect recrudescence of latent disease. In the 1-year, placebo-controlled studies RA I and RA II, 5.3% of patients receiving infliximab every 8 weeks with methotrexate developed serious infections, compared with 3.4% of placebo patients receiving methotrexate. Of 924 patients receiving infliximab, 1.7% developed pneumonia and 0.4% developed TB, when compared with 0.3% and 0% in the placebo arm, respectively. In a shorter (22-week) placebo-controlled study of 1,082 patients with RA randomized to receive placebo, infliximab 3 or 10 mg/kg infusions at 0, 2, and 6 weeks, followed by every 8 weeks with methotrexate, serious infections were more frequent in the infliximab 10 mg/kg group (5.3%) than the 3 mg/kg or placebo groups (1.7% in both). During the 54-week Crohn II study, 15% of patients with fistulizing Crohn disease developed a new fistula-related abscess.

In infliximab clinical studies in patients with ulcerative colitis, infections treated with antimicrobials were reported in 27% of infliximab-treated patients (average, 41 weeks of follow-up) and in 18% of placebo-treated patients (average, 32 weeks of follow-up). The types of infections, including serious infections, reported in patients with ulcerative colitis were similar to those reported in other clinical studies.

The onset of serious infections may be preceded by constitutional symptoms, such as fever, chills, weight loss, and fatigue. However, the majority of serious infections may also be preceded by signs or symptoms localized to the site of the infection.

➤*Autoantibodies / Lupus-like syndrome:* Approximately half of infliximab-treated patients in clinical trials who were antinuclear antibody negative at baseline developed a positive antinuclear antibody during the trial, compared with approximately one-fifth of placebo-treated patients. Anti–double-stranded DNA antibodies were newly detected in approximately one-fifth of infliximab-treated patients, compared with 0% of placebo-treated patients. However, reports of lupus and lupus-like syndromes remain uncommon.

➤*Malignancies:* In controlled trials, more infliximab-treated patients developed malignancies than placebo-treated patients.

In a randomized, controlled, clinical trial exploring the use of infliximab in patients with moderate to severe COPD who were either current smokers or ex-smokers, 157 patients were treated with infliximab at doses similar to those used in RA and Crohn disease. Nine of these infliximab-treated patients developed a malignancy, including 1 lymphoma, for a rate of 7.67 cases per 100 patient-years of follow-up (median duration of follow-up, 0.8 years; 95% confidence interval [CI], 3.51 to 14.56). There was 1 reported malignancy among 77 control patients for a rate of 1.63 cases per 100 patient-years of follow-up (median duration of follow-up, 0.8 years; 95% CI, 0.04 to 9.1). The majority of the malignancies developed in the lung or head and neck.

Malignancies, including non-Hodgkin lymphoma and Hodgkin disease, have also been reported in patients receiving infliximab during postapproval use.

➤*Heart failure:* In a randomized study evaluating infliximab in moderate to severe heart failure (NYHA class III/IV; left ventricular ejection fraction of 35% or less), 150 patients were randomized to receive treatment with 3 infusions of infliximab 10 mg/kg, 5 mg/kg, or placebo, at 0, 2, and 6 weeks. Higher incidences of mortality and hospitalization because of worsening heart failure were observed in patients receiving the infliximab 10 mg/kg dose. At 1 year, 8 patients in the infliximab 10 mg/kg group had died, compared with 4 deaths each in the infliximab 5 mg/kg and the placebo groups. There were trends toward increased dyspnea, hypotension, angina, and dizziness in both the infliximab 5 and 10 mg/kg treatment groups versus placebo. Infliximab has not been studied in patients with mild heart failure (NYHA class I/II).

➤*Hepatotoxicity:* Severe liver injury, including acute liver failure and autoimmune hepatitis, has been reported rarely in patients receiving infliximab. Reactivation of HBV has occurred in patients receiving TNF-blocking agents, including infliximab, who are chronic carriers of this virus.

In clinical trials in RA, Crohn disease, ulcerative colitis, ankylosing spondylitis, plaque psoriasis, and psoriatic arthritis, elevations of aminotransferases were observed (ALT more common than AST) in a greater proportion of patients receiving infliximab than in controls, both when infliximab was given as monotherapy and when it was used in combination with other immunosuppressive agents. In general, patients who developed ALT and AST elevations were asymptomatic, and the abnormalities decreased or resolved with either continuation or discontinuation of infliximab or modification of concomitant medications.

Infliximab ALT Elevations

	Proportion of patients with elevated ALT					
	> 1 to		≥ 3 × ULN		≥ 5 × ULN	
	Infliximab	Placebo	Infliximab	Placebo	Infliximab	Placebo
Ankylosing spondylitis[a]	51%	15%	10%	0%	4%	0%
Crohn disease[b]	39%	34%	5%	4%	2%	0%
Plaque psoriasis[c]	49%	24%	8%	< 1%	3%	0%
Psoriatic arthritis[d]	50%	16%	7%	0%	2%	0%
RA[e]	34%	24%	4%	3%	< 1%	< 1%
Ulcerative colitis[f]	17%	12%	2%	1%	< 1%	< 1%

[a] Median follow-up was 24 weeks for placebo group and 102 weeks for infliximab group.
[b] Placebo patients in the 2 phase 3 trials in Crohn disease received an initial dose of infliximab 5 mg/kg at study start and were on placebo in the maintenance phase. Patients who were randomized to the placebo maintenance group and then later crossed over to infliximab are included in the infliximab group in ALT analysis. Median follow-up was 54 weeks.
[c] ALT values are obtained in two phase 3 psoriasis studies, with median follow-up of 50 weeks for infliximab and 16 weeks for placebo.
[d] Median follow-up was 39 weeks for infliximab group and 18 weeks for placebo group.
[e] Placebo patients received methotrexate, while infliximab patients received both infliximab and methotrexate. Median follow-up was 58 weeks.
[f] Median follow-up was 30 weeks. Specifically, the median duration of follow-up was 30 weeks for placebo and 31 weeks for infliximab.

➤*Crohn disease in children:*

Most common adverse reactions – The following adverse reactions were reported more commonly in 103 randomized children with Crohn disease administered infliximab 5 mg/kg through 54 weeks than in 385 adult Crohn disease patients receiving a similar treatment regimen: anemia (11%); blood the in stool (10%); flushing, leukopenia (9%); viral infection (8%); bone fracture, neutropenia (7%); bacterial infection, respiratory tract allergic reactions (6%).

Infections – Infections were reported in 56% of randomized children in Study Peds Crohn and in 50% of adult patients in Study Crohn I. In Study Peds Crohn, infections were reported more frequently for patients who received every 8 week infusions, as opposed to every 12 week infusions (74% and 38%, respectively), while serious infections were reported for 3 patients in the every 8 week maintenance treatment group and 4 patients in the every 12 week maintenance treatment group. The most commonly reported infections were upper respiratory tract infections and pharyngitis, and the most commonly reported serious infection was abscess. Pneumonia was reported for 3 patients (2 in the every 8 week maintenance treatment group and 1 in the every 12 week maintenance treatment group). Herpes zoster was reported for 2 patients in the every 8 week maintenance treatment group.

Infusion reactions – In Study Peds Crohn, 18% of randomized patients experienced 1 or more infusion reactions, with no notable difference between treatment groups. Of the 112 patients in Study Peds Crohn, there were no serious infusion reactions, and 2 patients had nonserious anaphylactoid reactions.

Immunogenicity – Antibodies to infliximab developed in 3% of children in Study Peds Crohn.

INFLIXIMAB — INJECTION

Hepatic – Elevations of ALT up to 3 times the ULN were seen in 18% of children in Crohn disease clinical trials; 4% had ALT elevations greater than or equal to 3 times ULN, and 1% had elevations of greater than or equal to 5 times ULN. Median follow-up was 53 weeks.

➤*Plaque psoriasis:*

Serious adverse reactions – During the placebo-controlled portion across the 3 clinical trials up to week 16, the proportion of patients who experienced at least 1 serious adverse reaction (defined as resulting in death, life-threatening, requiring hospitalization, or resulting in persistent or significant disability/incapacity) was 1.7% in the infliximab 3 mg/kg group, 3.2% in the placebo group, and 3.9% in the infliximab 5 mg/kg group.

Among patients in the two phase 3 studies, 12.4% of patients receiving infliximab 5 mg/kg every 8 weeks through 1 year of maintenance treatment experienced at least 1 serious adverse reaction in study I. In study II, 4.1% and 4.7% of patients receiving infliximab 3 and 5 mg/kg every 8 weeks, respectively, through 1 year of maintenance treatment experienced at least 1 serious adverse reaction.

Infections – One death caused by bacterial sepsis occurred 25 days after the second infusion of infliximab 5 mg/kg. Serious infections included sepsis and abscesses. In study I, 2.7% of patients receiving infliximab 5 mg/kg every 8 weeks through 1 year of maintenance treatment experienced at least 1 serious infection. In Study II, 1% and 1.3% of patients receiving infliximab 3 and 5 mg/kg, respectively, through 1 year of treatment experienced at least 1 serious infection. The most common serious infections (requiring hospitalization) were abscesses (skin, throat, and perirectal) reported by 5 (0.7%) patients in the infliximab 5 mg/kg group. Two active cases of TB were reported at 6 weeks and 34 weeks after starting infliximab.

Malignancies – In the placebo-controlled portion of the psoriasis studies, 7 of 1,123 patients who received infliximab at any dose were diagnosed with at least 1 nonmelanoma skin cancer, compared with 0 of 334 patients who received placebo.

Serum sickness – In the psoriasis studies, 1% (15/1,373) of patients experienced serum sickness or a combination of arthralgia and/or myalgia with fever, and/or rash, usually early in the treatment course. Of these patients, 6 required hospitalization because of fever, severe myalgia, arthralgia, swollen joints, and immobility.

➤*Other adverse reactions:* Adverse reactions reported in 5% or more of all patients with RA receiving 4 or more infusions are in the following table. The types and frequencies of adverse reactions observed were similar in infliximab-treated RA, ankylosing spondylitis, psoriatic arthritis, plaque psoriasis, and Crohn disease patients, except for abdominal pain, which occurred in 26% of infliximab-treated patients with Crohn disease. In the Crohn disease studies, there were insufficient numbers and duration of follow-up for patients who never received infliximab to provide meaningful comparisons.

Infliximab Adverse Reactions in Rheumatoid Arthritis Patients (≥ 5%)

Adverse reactions	Infliximab (n = 1,129)	Placebo (n = 350)
Average weeks of follow-up	66	59
CNS		
Fatigue	9%	7%
Headache	18%	14%
Dermatologic		
Pruritus	7%	2%
Rash	10%	5%
GI		
Abdominal pain	12%	8%
Diarrhea	12%	12%
Dyspepsia	10%	7%
Nausea	21%	20%
Musculoskeletal		
Arthralgia	8%	7%
Back pain	8%	5%
Respiratory		
Bronchitis	10%	9%
Coughing	12%	8%
Pharyngitis	12%	8%
Rhinitis	8%	5%
Sinusitis	14%	8%
Upper respiratory tract infection	32%	25%
Miscellaneous		
Fever	7%	4%
Hypertension	7%	5%
Moniliasis	5%	3%
Pain	8%	7%
Urinary tract infection	8%	6%

The most common serious adverse reactions observed in clinical trials were infections. Other serious, medically relevant adverse reactions of at least 0.2% or clinically significant adverse reactions by body system were as follows:

Cardiovascular – Arrhythmia, bradycardia, brain infarction, cardiac arrest, circulatory failure, hypotension, myocardial infarction, syncope, tachycardia, thrombophlebitis.

CNS – Confusion, dizziness, meningitis, neuritis, peripheral neuropathy, suicide attempt.

Dermatologic – Increased sweating, ulceration.

GI – Constipation, GI hemorrhage, ileus, intestinal obstruction, intestinal perforation, intestinal stenosis, pancreatitis, peritonitis, proctalgia.

GU – Menstrual irregularity, renal calculus, renal failure.

Hematologic/Lymphatic – Anemia, hemolytic anemia, leukopenia, lymphadenopathy, pancytopenia, thrombocytopenia.

Hepatic – Biliary pain, cholecystitis, cholelithiasis, hepatitis.

Musculoskeletal – Intervertebral disk herniation, tendon disorder.

Respiratory – Adult respiratory distress syndrome, lower respiratory tract infection (including pneumonia), pleural effusion, pleurisy, pulmonary edema, pulmonary embolism, respiratory insufficiency.

Miscellaneous – Allergic reaction; basal cell, breast, or lymphoma neoplasms; cellulitis; dehydration; diaphragmatic hernia; edema; sepsis; serum sickness; surgical/procedural sequela.

➤*Postmarketing:* The following adverse reactions (some with fatal outcomes) have been reported during postapproval use of infliximab: acute liver failure, cholestasis, erythema multiforme, hepatitis, idiopathic thrombocytopenic purpura, interstitial lung disease (including pulmonary fibrosis/interstitial pneumonitis and very rare rapidly progressive disease), jaundice, neuropathies (additional neurologic events also have been observed), neutropenia, pericardial effusion, Stevens-Johnson syndrome, systemic and cutaneous vasculitis, thrombocytopenic purpura, thrombotic thrombocytopenic purpura, toxic epidermal necrolysis, peripheral demyelinating disorders (such as Guillain-Barré syndrome, chronic inflammatory demyelinating polyneuropathy, and multifocal motor neuropathy), new-onset and worsening psoriasis (including pustular, primarily palmar/plantar), and transverse myelitis. Because these reactions are reported voluntarily from a population of uncertain size, it is not always possible to reliably estimate their frequency or establish a causal relationship to infliximab exposure.

In postmarketing experience, cases of anaphylactic-like reactions, including laryngeal/pharyngeal edema, severe bronchospasm, and seizure have been associated with infliximab administration.

In postmarketing experience in the various indications, infections have been observed with various pathogens, including viral, bacterial, fungal, and protozoal organisms. Infections have been noted in all organ systems and have been reported in patients receiving infliximab alone or in combination with immunosuppressive agents.

The following serious adverse reactions reported in the postmarketing experience in children were infections (some fatal), including opportunistic infections and TB, infusion reactions, and hypersensitivity reactions.

Serious adverse reactions in the postmarketing experience with infliximab in children have also included malignancies, including hepatosplenic T-cell lymphomas, transient hepatic enzyme abnormalities, lupus-like syndromes, and the development of autoantibodies.

Overdosage

➤*Symptoms:* Single doses of up to 20 mg/kg have been administered without any direct toxic effect.

➤*Treatment:* In case of overdosage, monitor the patient for any signs or symptoms of adverse reactions, and institute appropriate symptomatic treatment immediately.

Patient Information

Advise patients developing signs and symptoms of infection to seek medical evaluation immediately.

Provide patients or their caregivers with the infliximab Medication Guide and an opportunity to read it and ask questions prior to each treatment infusion session. Exercise caution in administering infliximab to patients with clinically important active infections; it is important that the patient's overall health be assessed at each treatment visit and any questions resulting from the patient's or caregiver's reading of the Medication Guide be discussed.

Advise patients to notify their health care provider immediately if they experience bleeding or unusual bruising, dark urine, difficulty breathing or unexplained shortness of breath, paleness, right upper stomach pain, or yellowing of the skin or eyes.

Advise patients with heart failure to notify their health care provider immediately if new or worsening symptoms of heart failure develop.

Advise patients not to receive live vaccines during infliximab therapy. Children with Crohn disease should be brought up to date with all vaccinations prior to initiating infliximab therapy.

CERTOLIZUMAB PEGOL

Rx	Cimzia (UCB)	Injection, lyophilized powder for solution: 200 mg	Preservative free. In single-use vials.[a]
		Injection, solution: 200 mg	Preservative free. In 1 mL single-use, prefilled syringe.

[a] Also contains sucrose 100 mg, lactic acid 0.9 mg, and polysorbate 0.1 mg.

CERTOLIZUMAB PEGOL — INJECTION

WARNING

Serious infections – Patients treated with certolizumab are at an increased risk for developing serious infections that may lead to hospitalization or death. Most patients who developed these infections were taking concomitant immunosuppressants, such as methotrexate or corticosteroids.

Discontinue certolizumab if a patient develops a serious infection or sepsis.

Reported infections include the following:

- Active tuberculosis (TB), including reactivation of latent TB. Patients with TB have frequently presented with disseminated or extrapulmonary disease. Test patients for latent TB before certolizumab use and during therapy. Initiate treatment for latent infections prior to certolizumab use.
- Invasive fungal infections, including histoplasmosis, coccidioidomycosis, candidiasis, aspergillosis, blastomycosis, and pneumocystosis. Patients with histoplasmosis or other invasive fungal infections may present with disseminated rather than localized disease. Antigen and antibody testing for histoplasmosis may be negative in some patients with active infection. Consider empiric antifungal therapy in patients at risk for invasive fungal infections who develop severe systemic illness.
- Bacterial, viral, and other infections caused by opportunistic pathogens.

Carefully consider the risks and benefits of treatment with certolizumab prior to initiating therapy in patients with chronic or recurrent infection.

Closely monitor patients for the development of signs and symptoms of infection during and after treatment with certolizumab, including the possible development of TB in patients who tested negative for latent TB infection prior to initiating therapy.

Malignancy – Lymphoma and other malignancies, some fatal, have been reported in children and adolescent patients treated with tumor necrosis factor (TNF) blockers, of which certolizumab is a member. Certolizumab is not indicated for use in children.

Indications

➤*Crohn disease:* For reducing signs and symptoms of Crohn disease and maintaining clinical response in adult patients with moderately to severely active disease who have had an inadequate response to conventional therapy.

➤*Rheumatoid arthritis:* For the treatment of adults with moderately to severely active rheumatoid arthritis (RA).

Administration and Dosage

➤*General dosing considerations:* Before initiation of therapy, evaluate all patients for active and inactive (latent) TB infection. Consider the possibility of undetected latent TB in patients who have immigrated from or traveled to countries with a high prevalence of TB or had close contact with a person with active TB. Perform appropriate screening tests (eg, tuberculin skin test, chest x-ray) in all patients.

➤*Adults:*

Crohn disease –

Initial dosage: 400 mg (given as 2 subcutaneous injections of 200 mg) initially and at weeks 2 and 4.

Maintenance dosage: 400 mg every 4 weeks in patients who obtain a clinical response.

Rheumatoid arthritis –

Initial dosage: 400 mg (given as 2 subcutaneous injections of 200 mg) initially and at weeks 2 and 4, followed by 200 mg every other week.

Maintenance dosage: 400 mg every 4 weeks can be considered.

➤*Concomitant medications:* Certolizumab may be used as monotherapy or concomitantly with nonbiological disease-modifying antirheumatic drugs (DMARDs). In RA clinical studies, patients on certolizumab therapy also took concomitant methotrexate with the recommended certolizumab dose of 200 mg every other week. Certolizumab should not be used in combination with biological DMARDs or other TNF-blocker therapy.

➤*Preparation for administration:*

Powder for solution –

Bring certolizumab to room temperature before reconstituting to facilitate dissolution. Reconstitute each vial using appropriate aseptic technique, with 1 mL of sterile water for injection and a syringe with a 20-gauge needle. Gently swirl each vial without shaking so that all of the powder comes into contact with the sterile water. Leave the vials undisturbed to fully reconstitute (this may take up to 30 minutes). Reconstituted certolizumab has a concentration of approximately 200 mg/mL. Once reconstituted, certolizumab is a clear to opalescent, colorless to pale yellow liquid essentially free from particulates.

Prior to injecting, reconstituted certolizumab should be at room temperature. Do not leave reconstituted certolizumab at room temperature for more than 2 hours prior to administration. Using a new 20-gauge (reconstitution) needle for each vial, withdraw the reconstituted solution into a separate syringe for each vial, so that each syringe contains certolizumab 1 mL (200 mg). Switch each 20-gauge needle to a 23-gauge (dosing) needle and inject the full contents of each syringe subcutaneously into the thigh or abdomen. Where a 400 mg dose is required, separate sites should be used for each 200 mg injection.

Prefilled syringe –

Instruct patients using certolizumab to inject the full amount in the syringe (1 mL).

➤*Administration:* Certolizumab is administered by subcutaneous injection. Rotate injection sites and do not give injections into areas where the skin is tender, bruised, red, or hard. When a 400 mg dose is needed (given as 2 subcutaneous injections of 200 mg), injections should occur at separate sites in the thigh or abdomen.

➤*Storage/Stability:* Refrigerate intact carton at 2° to 8°C (36° to 46°F). Do not freeze. Do not separate contents of carton prior to use. Protect solution from light.

Once reconstituted, certolizumab can be stored in the vials for up to 24 hours at 2° to 8°C (36° to 46°F) prior to injection. Do not freeze. Certolizumab does not contain preservatives; therefore, unused portions of the drug remaining in the syringe or vial should be discarded.

Actions

➤*Pharmacology:* Certolizumab binds to human TNF-alpha with a dissociation constant (KD) of 90 pM. TNF-alpha is a key proinflammatory cytokine with a central role in inflammatory processes. Certolizumab selectively neutralizes TNF-alpha (inhibitory concentration [IC_{90}] of 4 ng/mL for inhibition of human TNF-alpha in the in vitro L929 murine fibrosarcoma cytotoxicity assay) but does not neutralize lymphotoxin alpha (TNF-beta). Certolizumab cross-reacts poorly with TNF from rodents and rabbits; therefore, in vivo efficacy was evaluated using animal models in which human TNF-alpha was the physiologically active molecule.

Certolizumab was shown to neutralize membrane-associated and soluble human TNF-alpha in a dose-dependent manner. Incubation of monocytes with certolizumab resulted in a dose-dependent inhibition of lipopolysaccharide-induced TNF-alpha and interleukin-1 beta production in human monocytes.

➤*Pharmacokinetics:*

Absorption – A mean C_{max} of approximately 43 to 49 mcg/mL occurred at week 5 during the initial loading dose period using the recommended dose regimen for the treatment of patients with RA (400 mg subcutaneously at weeks 0, 2, and 4 followed by 200 mg every other week).

Following subcutaneous administration, peak plasma concentrations of certolizumab were attained between 54 and 171 hours postinjection. Certolizumab has a bioavailability of approximately 80% (range, 76% to 88%) following subcutaneous administration compared with intravenous (IV) administration.

Distribution – The steady-state volume of distribution was estimated as 6 to 8 L in the population pharmacokinetic analysis for patients with Crohn disease and patients with RA.

Metabolism – The metabolism of certolizumab has not been studied in human subjects. Data from animals indicate that once cleaved from the Fab' fragment the polyethylene glycol moiety is mainly excreted in urine without further metabolism.

Excretion – Pegylation, the covalent attachment of polyethylene glycol polymers to peptides, delays the metabolism and elimination of these entities from the circulation by a variety of mechanisms, including decreased renal clearance, proteolysis, and immunogenicity. Accordingly, certolizumab is an antibody Fab fragment conjugated with polyethylene glycol in order to extend the terminal plasma elimination half-life of the Fab. The terminal elimination phase half-life was approximately 14 days for all doses tested. The clearance following IV administration to healthy subjects ranged from 9.21 to 14.38 mL/h. The clearance following subcutaneous dosing was estimated as 17 mL/h in the Crohn disease population pharmacokinetic analysis, with an intersubject variability of 38% (coefficient of variation [CV]) and an interoccasion variability of 16%.

Similarly, the clearance following subcutaneous dosing was estimated as 21 mL/h in the RA population pharmacokinetic analysis, with an intersubject variability of 30.8% (%CV) and interoccasion variability of 22%. The route of elimination of certolizumab has not been studied in human subjects. Studies in animals indicate that the major route of elimination of the polyethylene glycol component is via urinary excretion.

Special populations –

Antibodies: The presence of anti-certolizumab antibodies was associated with a 3.6-fold increase in clearance.

Body weight: Body weight significantly affected certolizumab pharmacokinetics. Pharmacokinetic exposure was inversely related to body weight, but pharmacodynamic exposure-response analysis showed that no additional therapeutic benefit would be expected from a weight-adjusted dose regimen.

Contraindications

None well documented.

CERTOLIZUMAB PEGOL — INJECTION

Warnings/Precautions

➤*Serious infections:* Serious and sometimes fatal infection caused by bacterial, mycobacterial, invasive fungal, viral, or other opportunistic pathogens has been reported in patients receiving TNF-blocking agents. Among opportunistic infections, TB, histoplasmosis, aspergillosis, candidiasis, coccidioidomycosis, listeriosis, and pneumocystosis were the most common. Patients have frequently presented with disseminated rather than localized disease and are often taking concomitant immunosuppressants, such as methotrexate or corticosteroids, with certolizumab.

Do not initiate treatment with certolizumab in patients with an active infection, including clinically important localized infections. Consider the risks and benefits of treatment prior to initiating therapy in patients with chronic or recurrent infection; patients who have been exposed to TB; patients who have resided or traveled in areas of endemic TB or endemic mycoses, such as histoplasmosis, coccidioidomycosis, or blastomycosis; and patients with underlying conditions that may predispose them to infection.

Cases of reactivation of TB or new TB infections have been observed in patients receiving certolizumab, including patients who have previously received treatment for latent or active TB. Evaluate patients for TB risk factors and test for latent infection prior to initiating certolizumab and periodically during therapy.

Treatment of latent TB infection prior to therapy with TNF-blocking agents has been shown to reduce the risk of TB reactivation during therapy. Induration of 5 mm or greater with tuberculin skin testing should be considered a positive test result when assessing if treatment for latent TB is needed prior to initiating certolizumab, even for patients previously vaccinated with Bacille Calmette-Guérin (BCG).

Consider anti-TB therapy prior to initiation of certolizumab in patients with a history of latent or active TB in whom an adequate course of treatment cannot be confirmed, and for patients with a negative test for latent TB but who have risk factors for TB infection. Consultation with a health care provider with expertise in the treatment of TB is recommended to aid in the decision of whether initiating anti-TB therapy is appropriate for an individual patient.

Strongly consider the presence of TB in patients who develop a new infection during certolizumab treatment, especially in patients who have previously or recently traveled to countries with a high prevalence of TB or have had close contact with a person with active TB.

Closely monitor patients for the development of signs and symptoms of infection during and after treatment with certolizumab, including the development of TB in patients who tested negative for latent TB infection prior to initiating therapy. Tests for latent TB infection also may be falsely negative while patients are taking certolizumab.

Discontinue certolizumab if a patient develops a serious infection or sepsis. A patient who develops a new infection during treatment with certolizumab should be closely monitored, undergo a prompt and complete diagnostic workup appropriate for an immunocompromised patient, and appropriate antimicrobial therapy should be initiated.

For patients who reside or travel in regions where mycoses are endemic, suspect the presence of invasive fungal infection if a serious systemic illness develops. Consider appropriate empiric antifungal therapy while a diagnostic workup is being performed. Antigen and antibody testing for histoplasmosis may be negative in some patients with active infection. When feasible, make the decision to administer empiric antifungal therapy in these patients in consultation with a health care provider with expertise in the diagnosis and treatment of invasive fungal infections and take into account both the risk for severe fungal infection and risks of antifungal therapy.

➤*Malignancies:* In the controlled portions of clinical studies of some TNF blockers, more cases of malignancies have been observed among patients receiving TNF blockers compared with control patients.

Malignancies, some fatal, have been reported among children, adolescents, and young adults who received treatment with TNF-blocking agents (initiation of therapy at 18 years of age or younger), of which certolizumab is a member. Approximately half the cases were lymphomas, including Hodgkin and non-Hodgkin lymphoma. The other cases represented a variety of different malignancies and included rare malignancies usually associated with immunosuppression and malignancies that are not usually observed in children and adolescents. The malignancies occurred after a median of 30 months of therapy (range, 1 to 84 months). Most of the patients were receiving concomitant immunosuppressants. These cases were reported postmarketing and are derived from a variety of sources, including registries and spontaneous postmarketing reports.

In the controlled portions of clinical trials of all TNF blockers, more cases of lymphoma have been observed among patients receiving TNF blockers compared with control patients. In controlled studies of certolizumab for Crohn disease and other investigational uses, there was 1 case of lymphoma among 2,657 certolizumab-treated patients and 1 case of Hodgkin lymphoma among 1,319 placebo-treated patients.

In the certolizumab RA clinical trials (placebo-controlled and open-label), 3 cases of lymphoma were observed among 2,367 patients. This is approximately 2-fold higher than expected in the general population. Patients with RA, particularly those with highly active disease, are at a higher risk for the development of lymphoma.

Rates in clinical studies for certolizumab cannot be compared with the rates of clinical trials of other TNF blockers and may not predict the rates observed when certolizumab is used in a broader patient population. Patients with Crohn disease or other diseases that require long-term exposure to immunosuppressant therapies may be at higher risk than the general population for the development of lymphoma, even in the absence of TNF-blocker therapy. The potential role of TNF-blocker therapy in the development of malignancies in adults is not known.

Cases of acute and chronic leukemia have been reported in association with postmarketing TNF-blocker use in RA and other indications. Even in the absence of TNF-blocker therapy, patients with RA may be at a higher risk (approximately 2-fold) than the general population for the development of leukemia.

➤*Heart failure:* Cases of worsening congestive heart failure (CHF) and new-onset CHF have been reported with TNF blockers, including certolizumab. Certolizumab has not been formally studied in patients with CHF; however, in clinical studies in patients with CHF with another TNF blocker, worsening CHF and increased mortality caused by CHF were observed. Exercise caution when using certolizumab in patients who have heart failure and monitor them carefully.

➤*Hepatitis B virus reactivation:* Use of TNF blockers, including certolizumab, may increase the risk of reactivation of hepatitis B virus (HBV) in patients who are chronic carriers of this virus. In some instances, HBV reactivation occurring in conjunction with TNF-blocker therapy has been fatal. The majority of reports have occurred in patients concomitantly receiving other medications that suppress the immune system, which may also contribute to HBV reactivation.

Evaluate patients at risk for HBV infection for prior evidence of HBV infection before initiating certolizumab therapy. Exercise caution in prescribing certolizumab for patients identified as carriers of HBV. Adequate data are not available on the safety or efficacy of treating patients who are carriers of HBV with antiviral therapy in conjunction with TNF-blocker therapy to prevent HBV reactivation. Closely monitor patients who are carriers of HBV and require treatment with certolizumab for clinical and laboratory signs of active HBV infection throughout therapy and for several months following termination of therapy.

In patients who develop HBV reactivation, discontinue certolizumab and initiate effective antiviral therapy with appropriate supportive treatment. The safety of resuming TNF-blocker therapy after HBV reactivation is controlled is not known; therefore, exercise caution when considering resumption of certolizumab therapy in this situation and monitor patients closely.

➤*CNS effects:* Use of TNF blockers, including certolizumab, has been associated with rare cases of new onset or exacerbation of clinical symptoms and/or radiographic evidence of demyelinating disease. Exercise caution in considering the use of certolizumab in patients with preexisting or recent-onset CNS demyelinating disorders. Rare cases of neurological disorders, including seizure disorder, optic neuritis, and peripheral neuropathy, have been reported in patients treated with certolizumab; the causal relationship to certolizumab remains unclear.

➤*Hematologic effects:* Rare reports of pancytopenia, including aplastic anemia, have been reported with TNF blockers. Adverse reactions of the hematologic system, including medically significant cytopenia (eg, leukopenia, pancytopenia, thrombocytopenia), have been infrequently reported with certolizumab. The causal relationship of these events to certolizumab remains unclear.

Although no high-risk group has been identified, exercise caution in patients being treated with certolizumab who have ongoing, or a history of, significant hematologic abnormalities. Advise all patients to seek immediate medical attention if they develop signs and symptoms suggestive of blood dyscrasias or infection (eg, bleeding, bruising, pallor, persistent fever) while on certolizumab. Consider discontinuation of certolizumab therapy in patients with confirmed significant hematologic abnormalities.

➤*Autoimmunity:* Treatment with certolizumab may result in the formation of autoantibodies and, rarely, in the development of a lupus-like syndrome. If a patient develops symptoms suggestive of a lupus-like syndrome following treatment with certolizumab, discontinue treatment.

➤*Vaccinations:* No data are available on the response to vaccinations or the secondary transmission of infection by live vaccines in patients receiving certolizumab. Do not coadminister live vaccines or attenuated vaccines with certolizumab.

➤*Immunosuppression:* Because TNF mediates inflammation and modulates cellular immune responses, the possibility exists for TNF blockers, including certolizumab, to affect host defenses against infections and malignancies. The impact of treatment with certolizumab on the development and course of malignancies, as well as active and/or chronic infections, is not fully understood. The safety and efficacy of certolizumab in patients with immunosuppression have not been formally evaluated.

➤*Immunogenicity:* Patients were tested at multiple time points for antibodies to certolizumab during studies CD1 and CD2. The overall percentage of antibody-positive patients was 8% in patients continuously exposed to certolizumab, of which approximately 6% were neutralizing in vitro. No apparent correlation of antibody development to adverse reactions or efficacy was observed. Patients treated with concomitant immunosuppressants had a lower rate of antibody development than patients not taking immunosuppressants at baseline (3% and 11%, respectively).

The following adverse reactions were reported in Crohn disease patients who were antibody-positive patients (n = 100) at an incidence at least 3% compared with antibody-negative patients (n = 1,242): abdominal pain, arthralgia, erythema nodosum, injection-site erythema, injection-site pain, pain in extremity, peripheral edema, and upper respiratory tract infection.

The overall percentage of patients with antibodies to certolizumab detectable on at least 1 occasion was 7% (105/1,509) in the RA placebo-controlled trials. Approximately one-third (3%, 39/1,509) of these patients had antibodies with neutralizing activity in vitro. Patients treated with concomitant

CERTOLIZUMAB PEGOL — INJECTION

immunosuppressants (methotrexate) had a lower rate of antibody development than patients not taking immunosuppressants at baseline. Patients treated with concomitant immunosuppressant therapy (methotrexate) in RA-1, RA-2, and RA-3 had a lower rate of neutralizing antibody formation overall than patients treated with certolizumab monotherapy in RA-4 (2% vs 8%). Both the loading dose of 400 mg every other week at weeks 0, 2, and 4 and concomitant use of methotrexate were associated with reduced immunogenicity.

Antibody formation was associated with lowered drug plasma concentration and reduced efficacy. In patients receiving the recommended certolizumab dosage of 200 mg every other week with concomitant methotrexate, the ACR 20 response was lower among antibody-positive patients than among antibody-negative patients (study RA-1, 48% vs 60%; study RA-2, 35% vs 59%, respectively). In study RA-3, too few patients developed antibodies to allow for meaningful analysis of ACR 20 response by antibody status. In study RA-4 (monotherapy), the ACR 20 response was 33% versus 56%, antibody-positive versus antibody-negative status, respectively. No association was seen between antibody development and the development of adverse reactions.

➤*Hypersensitivity reactions:* The following symptoms that could be compatible with hypersensitivity reactions have been reported rarely following certolizumab administration to patients: angioedema, dyspnea, hypotension, rash, serum sickness, and urticaria. If such reactions occur, discontinue further administration of certolizumab and institute appropriate therapy. There are no data on the risks of using certolizumab in patients who have experienced a severe hypersensitivity reaction towards another TNF blocker; in these patients, caution is needed.

➤*Pregnancy:* Category B.

There are no adequate and well-controlled studies of certolizumab in pregnant women. Because animal reproduction studies are not always predictive of human response, use this drug during pregnancy only if clearly needed.

There is some similarity between the action of immunomodulators with anti-TNF-alpha activity and the human teratogen thalidomide, a drug that also decreases the activity of TNF-alpha. However, decreased production of TNF-alpha may not be a primary cause of the teratogenicity of thalidomide. Theoretically, TNF-alpha antagonists could interfere with implantation and ovulation, but this has not been shown clinically. Until adequate human data is available, the safest course is to avoid the drug during organogenesis (20 to 55 days after conception or 34 to 69 days from the first day of the last menstrual period).

➤*Lactation:* It is not known whether this drug is excreted in human milk. The molecular weight is high (about 91,000), but the terminal half-life is long (14 days). If certolizumab is excreted, the effects, if any, on a nursing infant are unknown, but serious infections and other adverse effects have been observed in adults treated with SC doses of the antibody. Because many drugs are excreted in human milk and because of the potential for serious adverse reactions in breast-feeding infants from certolizumab, decide whether to discontinue breast-feeding or the drug, taking into account the importance of the drug to the mother.

➤*Children:* Safety and effectiveness in children have not been established.

➤*Elderly:* Because there is a higher incidence of infections in the elderly population in general, use caution when treating elderly patients.

➤*Monitoring:* Monitor patients for signs and symptoms of infection during and after treatment with certolizumab. Closely monitor patients who develop a new infection while undergoing treatment with certolizumab. Monitor patients receiving certolizumab for signs and symptoms of active TB, particularly because tests for latent TB infection may be falsely negative.

Closely monitor patients who are carriers of HBV and require treatment with certolizumab for clinical and laboratory signs of active HBV infection throughout therapy and for several months following termination of therapy.

Exercise caution when using certolizumab in patients who have heart failure and monitor carefully.

Drug Interactions

➤*Abatacept, anakinra, natalizumab, rituximab:* An increased risk of serious infections has been seen in clinical studies of other TNF-blocking agents used in combination with anakinra or abatacept, with no added benefit. Formal drug interaction studies have not been performed with rituximab or natalizumab. Because of the nature of the adverse events seen with these combinations with TNF-blocker therapy, similar toxicities also may result from the use of certolizumab in these combinations. There is not enough information to assess the safety and efficacy of such combination therapy; therefore, the use of certolizumab in combination with abatacept, anakinra, natalizumab, or rituximab is not recommended.

➤*Live vaccines:* See Warnings/Precautions for more information.

➤*Drug/Lab test interactions:* Interference with certain coagulation assays has been detected in patients treated with certolizumab. Certolizumab may cause erroneously elevated activated partial thromboplastin time (aPTT) assay results in patients without coagulation abnormalities. This effect has been observed with the PTT-LA test from Diagnostica Stago and the *HemosIL* APTT-SP liquid and *HemosIL* lyophilized silica tests from Instrumentation Laboratories. Other aPTT assays may be affected as well. Interference with thrombin time and prothrombin time assays has not been observed. There is no evidence that certolizumab therapy has an effect on in vivo coagulation.

Adverse Reactions

➤*Common adverse reactions:* In premarketing controlled trials of all patient populations combined, the most common adverse reactions (at least 8%) were upper respiratory infections (18%), rash (9%), and urinary tract infections (8%).

➤*Discontinuation of therapy:* The proportion of patients with Crohn disease who discontinued treatment because of adverse reactions in the controlled clinical studies was 8% for certolizumab and 7% for placebo. The most common adverse reactions leading to the discontinuation of certolizumab (for at least 2 patients and with a higher incidence than placebo) were abdominal pain (0.4% certolizumab, 0.2% placebo), diarrhea (0.4% certolizumab, 0% placebo), and intestinal obstruction (0.4% certolizumab, 0% placebo).

The proportion of patients with RA who discontinued treatment because of adverse reactions in the controlled clinical studies was 5% for certolizumab and 2.5% for placebo. The most common adverse reactions leading to discontinuation of certolizumab were TB infections (0.5%); and pneumonia, pyrexia, rash, and urticaria (0.3%).

➤*Crohn disease:* During controlled clinical studies, the proportion of patients with serious adverse reactions was 10% for certolizumab and 9% for placebo. The most common adverse reactions (occurring in 5% or more of certolizumab-treated patients and with a higher incidence compared with placebo) in controlled clinical studies with certolizumab were upper respiratory infection (eg, laryngitis, nasopharyngitis, viral infection) (20% certolizumab, 13% placebo), urinary tract infection (eg, bacteriuria, bladder infection, cystitis) (7% certolizumab, 6% placebo), and arthralgia (6% certolizumab, 4% placebo).

Cardiovascular – Angina pectoris, arrhythmias, atrial fibrillation, cardiac failure, hypertensive heart disease, myocardial infarction, myocardial ischemia, pericardial effusion, pericarditis, stroke, thrombophlebitis, transient ischemic attack, vasculitis.

CNS – Anxiety, bipolar disorder, suicide attempt.

Dermatologic – Dermatitis, erythema nodosum, urticaria.

GU – Menstrual disorder, nephrotic syndrome, renal failure.

Hematologic/Lymphatic – Anemia, leukopenia, lymphadenopathy, pancytopenia, thrombophilia.

Hepatic – Elevated liver enzymes, hepatitis.

Ophthalmic – Optic neuritis, retinal hemorrhage, uveitis.

Miscellaneous – Alopecia totalis, bleeding, injection-site reactions.

➤*Rheumatoid arthritis:*

Certolizumab With Concomitant Methotrexate Adverse Reactions in Patients With Rheumatoid Arthritis (≥ 3%)

Adverse reactions	Certolizumab 200 mg every other week + methotrexate (n = 640)	Placebo + methotrexate (n = 324)
CNS		
Fatigue	3%	2%
Headache	5%	4%
Respiratory		
Acute bronchitis	3%	1%
Nasopharyngitis	5%	1%
Pharyngitis	3%	1%
Upper respiratory tract infection	6%	2%
Miscellaneous		
Back pain	4%	1%
Hypertension	5%	2%
Pyrexia	3%	2%
Rash	3%	1%

Hypertensive adverse reactions were observed more frequently in patients receiving certolizumab than in controls. These adverse reactions occurred more frequently among patients with a baseline history of hypertension and among patients receiving concomitant corticosteroids and nonsteroidal anti-inflammatory drugs.

➤*Infections:*

Crohn disease – The incidence of infections in controlled studies in Crohn disease was 38% for certolizumab-treated patients and 30% for placebo-treated patients. The infections consisted primarily of upper respiratory infection (20% certolizumab, 13% placebo). The incidence of serious infections during the controlled clinical studies was 3% per patient-year for certolizumab-treated patients and 1% for placebo-treated patients. Serious infections observed included bacterial and viral infections, pneumonia, and pyelonephritis.

Rheumatoid arthritis – The incidence of new cases of infections in controlled clinical studies in RA was 0.91 per patient-year for all certolizumab-treated patients and 0.72 per patient-year for placebo-treated patients. The infections consisted primarily of upper respiratory tract infections, herpes

CERTOLIZUMAB PEGOL — INJECTION

infections, urinary tract infections, and lower respiratory tract infections. In the controlled RA studies, there were more new cases of serious infection adverse reactions in the certolizumab treatment groups compared with the placebo groups (0.06 per patient-year for all certolizumab doses vs 0.02 per patient-year for placebo). Rates of serious infections in the 200 mg every-other-week dose group were 0.06 per patient-year and in the 400 mg every-4-weeks dose group were 0.04 per patient-year. Serious infections included cellulitis, pneumonia, pyelonephritis, and TB. In the placebo group, no serious infection occurred in more than 1 subject. There is no evidence of increased risk of infections with continued exposure over time.

TB and opportunistic infections – In completed and ongoing global clinical studies in all indications, including 5,118 certolizumab-treated patients, the overall rate of TB is approximately 0.61 per 100 patient-years across all indications.

The majority of cases occurred in countries with high endemic rates of TB. No cases of TB (0/980) have been reported in the United States or Canada across all indications. Reports include cases of miliary, lymphatic, peritoneal, as well as pulmonary TB. The median time to onset of TB for all patients exposed to certolizumab across all indications was 345 days. In the studies with certolizumab in RA, there were 36 cases of TB among 2,367 exposed patients, including some fatal cases. Rare cases of opportunistic infections also have been reported in these clinical trials.

➤*Malignancies:* In clinical studies of certolizumab, the overall incidence rate of malignancies was similar for certolizumab-treated and control patients. For some TNF blockers, more cases of malignancies have been observed among patients receiving those TNF blockers compared with control patients.

➤*Heart failure:* In placebo-controlled and open-label RA studies, cases of new or worsening heart failure have been reported for certolizumab-treated patients. The majority of these cases were mild to moderate and occurred during the first year of exposure.

➤*Autoantibodies:* In clinical studies in Crohn disease, 4% of patients treated with certolizumab and 2% of patients treated with placebo who had negative baseline antinuclear autoantibody titers developed positive titers during the studies. One of the 1,564 Crohn disease patients treated with certolizumab developed symptoms of a lupus-like syndrome.

In clinical trials of TNF blockers, including certolizumab, in patients with RA, some patients developed antinuclear antibodies. Four patients out of 2,367 treated with certolizumab in RA clinical studies developed clinical signs suggestive of a lupus-like syndrome. The impact of long-term treatment with certolizumab on the development of autoimmune diseases is unknown.

➤*Hypersensitivity:* The following symptoms that could be compatible with hypersensitivity reactions have been reported rarely following certolizumab administration: angioedema, dermatitis allergic, dizziness (postural), dyspnea, hot flush, hypotension, injection-site reactions, malaise, pyrexia, rash, serum sickness, and (vasovagal) syncope.

➤*Postmarketing:* Cases of severe skin reactions, including erythema multiforme, Stevens-Johnson syndrome, toxic epidermal necrolysis, and new or worsening psoriasis (all subtypes including pustular and palmoplantar), have been identified during postapproval use of other TNF blockers.

Overdosage

➤*Symptoms:* The maximum tolerated dose of certolizumab has not been established. Doses of up to 800 mg subcutaneous and 20 mg/kg IV have been administered without evidence of dose-limiting toxicities.

➤*Treatment:* In cases of overdosage, monitor patients closely for any adverse reactions and immediately institute appropriate symptomatic treatment.

Patient Information

Exercise caution in administering certolizumab to patients with clinically important active infections, and advise patients of the importance of informing their health care providers about all aspects of their health.

Inform patients that certolizumab may lower the ability of the immune system to fight infections. Instruct patients of the importance of contacting their health care provider if they develop any symptoms of infection, including TB and reactivation of HBV infections.

Counsel patients about the possible risk of lymphoma and other malignancies while receiving certolizumab.

Advise patients to seek immediate medical attention if they experience any symptoms of severe allergic reactions. The prefilled syringe components do not contain any latex or dry natural rubber.

Advise patients to report any signs of new or worsening medical conditions, such as autoimmune disorders, heart disease, or neurological disease. Advise patients to report promptly any symptoms suggestive of a cytopenia such as bleeding, bruising, or persistent fever.

In the event that the patient or caregiver is giving the certolizumab injection, they need to be instructed by a qualified health care provider in proper injection technique, and their ability to administer certolizumab subcutaneous injections should be checked to ensure correct administration. Suitable sites for injection include the thigh or abdomen. Certolizumab should be injected when the liquid is at room temperature.

To avoid needle-stick injury, patients and health care providers should not attempt to place the needle cover back on the syringe or otherwise recap the needle. Be sure to properly dispose of needles and syringes in a puncture-proof container, and instruct patients and caregivers in proper syringe and needle disposal technique. Actively discourage any reuse of the injection materials.

USTEKINUMAB

Rx	**Stelara** (Centocor Ortho Biotech)	**Injection, solution:** 90 mg per 1 mL	Preservative free. In single-use vial.[b]

[a] Contains sucrose 38 mg, L-histidine 0.5 mg, and 0.02 mg of polysorbate 80 to fill to a final volume of 0.5 mL.

[b] Contains sucrose 76 mg, L-histidine 1 mg, and 0.04 mg of polysorbate 80 to fill to a final volume of 1 mL.

USTEKINUMAB — INJECTION

Indications

➤*Plaque psoriasis:* For the treatment of adults (18 years of age and older) with moderate to severe plaque psoriasis who are candidates for phototherapy or systemic therapy.

Administration and Dosage

➤*Adults:*

Plaque psoriasis –

Patient weight of 100 kg or less: 45 mg subcutaneously initially and 4 weeks later, followed by 45 mg every 12 weeks.

Patient weight of more than 100 kg: 90 mg subcutaneously initially and 4 weeks later, followed by 90 mg every 12 weeks. The 45 mg dose was also shown to be efficacious; however, 90 mg resulted in greater efficacy.

➤*Administration:* Administered by subcutaneous injection. Do not shake. It is recommended each injection be administered using a 27-gauge, ½-inch needle at a different anatomic location (such as upper arms, gluteal regions, thighs, or any quadrant of abdomen) than the previous injection, and not into areas where the skin is tender, bruised, erythematous, or indurated.

➤*Storage/Stability:* Store upright at 2° to 8°C (36° to 46°F). Keep the product in the original carton to protect from light until the time of use. Do not freeze. Discard any unused portion.

Actions

➤*Pharmacology:* Ustekinumab is a human immunoglobulin G1 (IgG1) kappa monoclonal antibody that binds with high affinity and specificity to the p40 protein subunit used by both the interleukin (IL)-12 and IL-23 cytokines. IL-12 and IL-23 are naturally occurring cytokines that are involved in inflammatory and immune responses, such as natural killer cell activation and CD4+ T-cell differentiation and activation. In in vitro models, ustekinumab was shown to disrupt IL-12 and IL-23 mediated signaling and cytokine cascades by disrupting the interaction of these cytokines with a shared cell-surface receptor chain, IL-12 beta 1.

➤*Pharmacokinetics:*

Absorption – In psoriasis subjects, the median time to reach the maximum serum concentration (T_{max}) was 13.5 days and 7 days, respectively, after a single subcutaneous administration of ustekinumab 45 mg (n = 22) and 90 mg (n = 24). In healthy subjects (n = 30), the median T_{max} value (8.5 days) following a single subcutaneous administration of ustekinumab 90 mg was comparable with that observed in psoriasis subjects. Following multiple subcutaneous doses of ustekinumab, the steady-state serum concentrations of ustekinumab were achieved by week 28. The mean (± standard deviation [SD]) steady-state trough serum concentration ranged from 0.31 ± 0.33 mcg/mL (45 mg) to 0.64 ± 0.64 mcg/mL (90 mg). There was no apparent accumulation in serum ustekinumab concentration over time when given subcutaneously every 12 weeks.

Distribution – Following subcutaneous administration of ustekinumab 45 mg (n = 18) and 90 mg (n = 21) to psoriasis subjects, the mean (± SD) apparent volume of distribution during the terminal phase (Vz/F) was 161 ± 65 mL/kg and 179 ± 85 mL/kg, respectively. The mean (± SD) volume of distribution during the terminal phase (Vz) following a single intravenous (IV) administration to subjects with psoriasis ranged from 56.1 ± 6.5 to 82.1 ± 23.6 mL/kg.

Metabolism – The metabolic pathway of ustekinumab has not been characterized. As a human IgG1 kappa monoclonal antibody ustekinumab is expected to be degraded into small peptides and amino acids via catabolic pathways in the same manner as endogenous IgG.

Excretion – The mean (± SD) systemic clearance (CL) following a single IV administration of ustekinumab to psoriasis subjects ranged from 1.9 ± 0.28 to 2.22 ± 0.63 mL/day/kg. The mean (± SD) half-life ranged from 14.9 ± 4.6 to 45.6 ± 80.2 days across all psoriasis subjects following IV and subcutaneous administration.

Special populations –

Weight: When given the same dose, subjects weighing more than 100 kg had lower median serum ustekinumab concentrations compared with those subjects weighing 100 kg or less.

USTEKINUMAB — INJECTION

Contraindications

None known.

Warnings/Precautions

➤*Infections:* Ustekinumab may increase the risk of infections and reactivation of latent infections. Serious bacterial, fungal, and viral infections were observed in subjects receiving ustekinumab.

Do not give ustekinumab to patients with any clinically important active infection. Do not administer ustekinumab until the infection resolves or is adequately treated. Instruct patients to seek medical advice if signs or symptoms suggestive of an infection occur. Exercise caution when considering the use of ustekinumab in patients with a chronic infection or a history of recurrent infection.

Serious infections requiring hospitalization occurred in the psoriasis development program. These serious infections included cellulitis, diverticulitis, osteomyelitis, viral infections, gastroenteritis, pneumonia, and urinary tract infections.

Individuals genetically deficient in IL-12/IL-23 are particularly vulnerable to disseminated infections from mycobacteria (including nontuberculous, environmental mycobacteria), salmonella (including nontyphi strains), and Bacillus Calmette-Guerin (BCG) vaccinations. Serious infections and fatal outcomes have been reported in such patients.

It is not known whether patients with pharmacologic blockade of IL-12/IL-23 from treatment with ustekinumab will be susceptible to these types of infections. Appropriate diagnostic testing should be considered (eg, tissue culture, stool culture) as dictated by clinical circumstances.

➤*Tuberculosis:* Evaluate patients for tuberculosis infection prior to initiating treatment with ustekinumab. Do not administer ustekinumab to patients with active tuberculosis. Initiate treatment of latent tuberculosis prior to administering ustekinumab. Consider antituberculosis therapy prior to initiation of ustekinumab in patients with a history of latent or active tuberculosis in whom an adequate course of treatment cannot be confirmed. Closely monitor patients receiving ustekinumab for signs and symptoms of active tuberculosis during and after treatment.

➤*Malignancies:* Ustekinumab is an immunosuppressant and may increase the risk of malignancy. Malignancies were reported among subjects who received ustekinumab in clinical studies. In rodent models, inhibition of IL-12/IL-23 p40 increased the risk of malignancy.

➤*Reversible posterior leukoencephalopathy syndrome:* One case of reversible posterior leukoencephalopathy syndrome (RPLS) was observed during the clinical development program, which included 3,523 ustekinumab-treated subjects. The subject, who had received 12 doses of ustekinumab over approximately 2 years, presented with headache, seizures, and confusion. No additional ustekinumab injections were administered and the subject fully recovered with appropriate treatment.

If RPLS is suspected, discontinue ustekinumab and administer appropriate treatment.

➤*Immunizations:* Prior to initiating therapy with ustekinumab, patients should receive all immunizations appropriate for age as recommended by current immunization guidelines. Patients being treated with ustekinumab should not receive live vaccines. Do not give BCG vaccines during treatment with ustekinumab or for 1 year prior to initiating treatment or 1 year following discontinuation of treatment. Caution is advised when administering live vaccines to household contacts of patients receiving ustekinumab because of the potential risk for shedding from the household contact and transmission to patient.

Nonlive vaccinations received during a course of ustekinumab may not elicit an immune response sufficient to prevent disease.

➤*Immunogenicity:* The presence of ustekinumab in the serum can interfere with the detection of anti-ustekinumab antibodies resulting in inconclusive results due to assay interference. In studies 1 and 2, antibody testing was done at time points when ustekinumab may have been present in the serum. In study 1 the last ustekinumab injection was between weeks 28 and 48 and the last test for anti-ustekinumab antibodies was at week 52. In study 2 the last ustekinumab injection was at week 16 and the last test for anti-ustekinumab antibodies was at week 24.

Ustekinumab Antibody Results

Antibody results	Study 1 (N = 743)	Study 2 (N = 1,198)
Positive	5%	3%
Negative	47%	8%
Inconclusive	48%	90%

➤*Pregnancy: Category B.* There are no studies of ustekinumab in pregnant women. Use ustekinumab during pregnancy only if the potential benefit justifies the potential risk to the fetus.

Fetal losses occurred in 6 control monkeys, 6 ustekinumab 22.5 mg/kg-treated monkeys, and 5 ustekinumab 45 mg/kg-treated monkeys. Neonatal deaths occurred in 1 ustekinumab 22.5 mg/kg-treated monkey and in 1 ustekinumab 45 mg/kg-treated monkey.

➤*Lactation:* Exercise caution when ustekinumab is administered to a breast-feeding woman. Weigh the unknown risks to the infant from GI or systemic exposure to ustekinumab against the known benefits of breast-feeding. Ustekinumab is excreted in the milk of lactating monkeys administered ustekinumab. IgG is excreted in human milk, so it is expected that ustekinumab will be present in human milk. It is not known if ustekinumab is absorbed systemically after ingestion; however, published data suggest that antibodies in breast milk do not enter the neonatal and infant circulation in substantial amounts.

➤*Children:* Safety and effectiveness in children have not been evaluated.

➤*Monitoring:* Monitor patients closely for signs and symptoms of active tuberculosis and infection during and after treatment.

Drug Interactions

➤*Immunosuppressive agents/phototherapy:* The safety of ustekinumab in combination with other immunosuppressive agents or phototherapy has not been evaluated. Ultraviolet-induced skin cancers developed earlier and more frequently in mice genetically manipulated to be deficient in both IL-12 and IL-23 or IL-12 alone.

➤*Cytochrome P450 substrates:* The formation of cytochrome P450 (CYP-450) enzymes can be altered by increased levels of certain cytokines (eg, IL-1, IL-6, IL-10, tumor necrosis factor-alpha, IFN) during chronic inflammation. Thus, ustekinumab could normalize the formation of CYP-450 enzymes. A role for IL-12 or IL-23 in the regulation of CYP-450 enzymes has not been reported. However, upon initiation of ustekinumab in patients who are receiving concomitant CYP-450 substrates, particularly those with a narrow therapeutic index, consider monitoring for therapeutic effect (eg, for warfarin) or drug concentration (eg, for cyclosporine) and adjust the individual dose of the drug as needed.

➤*Vaccines:* See Warnings/Precautions for more information.

Adverse Reactions

➤*Adverse reactions (at least 1%):*

Ustekinumab Adverse Reactions (≥ 1%)

Adverse reactions	Ustekinumab 45 mg (n = 664)	Ustekinumab 90 mg (n = 666)	Placebo (n = 665)
CNS			
Depression	1%	1%	< 1%
Dizziness	1%	2%	1%
Fatigue	3%	3%	2%
Headache	5%	5%	3%
Dermatologic			
Injection-site erythema	1%	2%	< 1%
Pruritus	2%	1%	1%
Musculoskeletal			
Back pain	1%	2%	1%
Myalgia	1%	1%	1%
Respiratory			
Nasopharyngitis	8%	7%	8%
Upper respiratory tract infection	5%	4%	5%
Miscellaneous			
Diarrhea	2%	2%	2%
Pharyngolaryngeal pain	1%	2%	1%

➤*Adverse reactions (less than 1%):* Adverse drug reactions that occurred at rates less than 1% included: cellulitis and certain injection-site reactions (bruising, hemorrhage, induration, irritation, pain, pruritus, and swelling). One case of RPLS occurred during clinical trials.

➤*Infections:* In the placebo-controlled period of clinical studies of psoriasis subjects (average follow-up of 12.6 weeks for placebo-treated subjects and 13.4 weeks for ustekinumab-treated subjects), 27% of ustekinumab-treated subjects reported infections (1.39 per subject-year of follow-up) compared with 24% of placebo-treated subjects (1.21 per subject-year of follow-up). Serious infections occurred in 0.3% of ustekinumab-treated subjects (0.01 per subject-year of follow-up) and in 0.4% of placebo-treated subjects (0.02 per subject-year of follow-up).

In the controlled and noncontrolled portions of psoriasis clinical trials, 61% of ustekinumab-treated subjects reported infections (1.24 per subject-year of follow-up). Serious infections were reported in 0.9% of subjects (0.01 per subject-year of follow-up).

➤*Malignancies:* In the controlled and noncontrolled portions of psoriasis clinical trials, 0.4% of ustekinumab-treated subjects reported malignancies excluding nonmelanoma skin cancers (0.36 per 100 subject-years of follow-up). Nonmelanoma skin cancer was reported in 0.8% of ustekinumab-treated subjects (0.8 per 100 subject-years of follow-up).

Serious malignancies included breast, colon, head and neck, kidney, prostate, and thyroid cancers.

Overdosage

Single doses of up to 4.5 mg/kg IV have been administered in clinical studies without dose-limiting toxicity.

USTEKINUMAB — INJECTION

➤*Treatment:* In case of overdosage, it is recommended that the patient be monitored for any signs or symptoms of adverse reactions or effects and appropriate symptomatic treatment be instituted immediately.

Patient Information

Instruct patients to read the Medication Guide before starting ustekinumab therapy and to reread the Medication Guide each time the prescription is renewed.

Inform patients that ustekinumab may lower the ability of their immune system to fight infections. Instruct patients of the importance of communicating any history of infections to their health care provider, and of contacting their health care provider if they develop any symptoms of infection.

Counsel patients about the risk of malignancies while receiving ustekinumab.

TOCILIZUMAB

Rx	Actemra (Genentech)	Injection, solution, concentrate: 20 mg/mL	Preservative free. Polysorbate 80, sucrose 50 mg/mL. In 4, 10, and 20 mL single-use vials.

TOCILIZUMAB — INJECTION

WARNING

Risk of serious infections – Patients treated with tocilizumab are at increased risk for developing serious infections that may lead to hospitalization or death. Most patients who developed these infections were taking concomitant immunosuppressants, such as methotrexate or corticosteroids.

If a serious infection develops, interrupt tocilizumab until the infection is controlled.

Reported infections include the following: 1) Active tuberculosis, which may present with pulmonary or extrapulmonary disease. Test patients for latent tuberculosis before tocilizumab use and during therapy. Initiate treatment for latent infection prior to tocilizumab use. 2) Invasive fungal infections, including candidiasis, aspergillosis, and pneumocystis. Patients with invasive fungal infections may present with disseminated, rather than localized, disease. 3) Bacterial, viral, and other infections caused by opportunistic pathogens. Carefully consider the risks and benefits of treatment with tocilizumab prior to initiating therapy in patients with chronic or recurrent infection. Closely monitor patients for the development of signs and symptoms of infection during and after treatment with tocilizumab, including the possible development of tuberculosis in patients who tested negative for latent tuberculosis infection prior to initiating therapy.

Indications

➤*Rheumatoid arthritis:* For the treatment of adults with moderately to severely active rheumatoid arthritis (RA) who have had an inadequate response to one or more tumor necrosis factor (TNF) antagonist therapies.

➤*Systemic juvenile idiopathic arthritis:* For the treatment of active systemic juvenile idiopathic arthritis in patients 2 years and older.

Administration and Dosage

➤*General dosing considerations:* Tocilizumab may be used as monotherapy or concomitantly with methotrexate or other disease-modifying antirheumatic drugs (DMARDs). Tocilizumab has not been studied and its use should be avoided in combination with biological DMARDs such as TNF antagonists, interleukin 1 receptor (IL-1R) antagonists, anti-CD20 monoclonal antibodies, and selective costimulation modulators because of the possibility of increased immunosuppression and increased risk of infection.

It is recommended that tocilizumab not be initiated in patients with an absolute neutrophil count (ANC) below 2,000/mm³, platelet count below 100,000 mm³, or ALT or AST approximately 1.5 times the upper limit of normal (ULN).

Tocilizumab treatment should be interrupted if a patient develops a serious infection until the infection is controlled.

Reduction of dose is recommended for management of certain dose-related laboratory changes, including elevated liver enzymes, neutropenia, and thrombocytopenia (see Dosage Adjustment). Tocilizumab requires further dilution (see Preparation for Administration).

➤*Adults:*

Rheumatoid arthritis –

Usual dosage: 4 mg/kg once every 4 weeks as a 60-minute single intravenous (IV) drip infusion.

Maximum dose: 800 mg per infusion.

Dosage titration: Increase to 8 mg/kg based on clinical response.

Dosage adjustment: Reduction of dose from 8 to 4 mg/kg is recommended for management of certain dose-related laboratory changes, including elevated liver enzymes, neutropenia, and thrombocytopenia.

Tocilizumab Dosage Modifications

Laboratory value	Recommendation
Liver enzymes abnormalities	
> 1 to 3 × ULN	Dose modify concomitant DMARDs if appropriate. For persistent increases in this range, reduce tocilizumab dose to 4 mg/kg or interrupt tocilizumab until ALT/AST have normalized.
> 3 to 5 × ULN (confirmed by repeat testing)	Interrupt tocilizumab dosing until < 3 × ULN and follow previous recommendations for > 1 to 3 × ULN. For persistent increases > 3 × ULN, discontinue tocilizumab.
> 5 × ULN	Discontinue tocilizumab.
Neutropenia	
ANC > 1,000 cells/mm³	Maintain dose.
ANC 500 to 1,000 cells/mm³	Interrupt tocilizumab dosing. When ANC is > 1,000 cells/mm³, resume tocilizumab at 4 mg/kg and increase to 8 mg/kg as clinically appropriate.
ANC < 500 cells/mm³	Discontinue tocilizumab.
Thrombocytopenia	
Platelets 50,000 to 100,000 cells/mm³	Interrupt tocilizumab dosing. When platelet count is > 100,000 cells/mm³, resume tocilizumab at 4 mg/kg and increase to 8 mg/kg as clinically appropriate.
Platelets < 50,000 cells/mm³	Discontinue tocilizumab.

➤*Children:*

Systemic juvenile idiopathic arthritis – The recommended dose of tocilizumab for systemic juvenile idiopathic arthritis patients given once every 2 weeks as a 60-minute single IV drip infusion is 12 mg/kg in patients weighing less than 30 kg and 8 mg/kg in patients weighing 30 kg or more. A change in dose should not be made based solely on a single visit body weight measurement, as weight may fluctuate. Interruption of dosing may be needed for management of dose-related laboratory abnormalities, including elevated liver enzymes, neutropenia, and thrombocytopenia. (Refer to Rheumatoid Arthritis Dosage Adjustment.)

➤*Hepatic function impairment:* Not recommended in patients with active hepatic disease or hepatic impairment.

➤*Preparation for administration:* Tocilizumab should be diluted to 50 or 100 mL using aseptic technique. From a 100 mL infusion bag or bottle, withdraw a volume of sodium chloride 0.9% injection equal to the volume of the tocilizumab solution required for the patient's dose. Slowly add tocilizumab from each vial into the infusion bag or bottle. To mix the solution, gently invert the bag to avoid foaming.

➤*Administration:* Allow the fully diluted tocilizumab solution to reach room temperature prior to infusion. The infusion should be administered over 60 minutes and must be administered with an infusion set. Do not administer as an IV push or bolus.

➤*Admixture compatibility:* Fully diluted solutions are compatible with polypropylene, polyethylene, and polyvinyl chloride infusion bags, and polypropylene, polyethylene, and glass infusion bottles. Tocilizumab should not be infused concomitantly in the same IV line with other drugs.

➤*Storage/Stability:* Refrigerate at 2° to 8°C (36° to 46°F). Do not freeze. Protect the vials from light by storage in the original package until time of use. The fully diluted tocilizumab solutions may be stored at 2° to 8° C (36° to 46°F) or room temperature for up to 24 hours and should be protected from light. Unused product remaining in the vials should not be used.

Actions

➤*Pharmacology:* Tocilizumab, a recombinant humanized antihuman IL-6 receptor monoclonal antibody, binds specifically to both soluble and membrane-bound IL-6 receptors (sIL-6R and mIL-6R) and has been shown to inhibit IL-6–mediated signaling through these receptors. IL-6 is a pleiotropic proinflammatory cytokine produced by a variety of cell types, including T- and B-cells, lymphocytes, monocytes, and fibroblasts. IL-6 has been shown to be involved in diverse physiological processes such as T-cell activation, induction of immunoglobulin secretion, initiation of hepatic acute phase protein synthesis, and stimulation of hematopoietic precursor cell proliferation and differentiation. IL-6 is also produced by synovial and endothelial cells, leading to local production of IL-6 in joints affected by inflammatory processes such as RA.

TOCILIZUMAB — INJECTION

➤*Pharmacokinetics:*

Absorption – The pharmacokinetic parameters of tocilizumab did not change with time. A more than dose-proportional increase in area under the curve (AUC) and trough concentration (C_{min}) was observed for doses of 4 and 8 mg/kg every 4 weeks. Maximum concentration (C_{max}) increased dose proportionally. At steady state, predicted AUC and C_{min} were 2.7- and 6.5-fold higher at 8 mg/kg compared with 4 mg/kg, respectively.

For doses of tocilizumab 4 mg/kg given every 4 weeks, the predicted mean (± standard deviation [SD]) steady-state AUC, C_{min}, and C_{max} of tocilizumab were 13,000 ± 5,800 mcg•h/mL, 1.49 ± 2.13 mcg/mL, and 88.3 ± 41.4 mcg/mL, respectively. The accumulation ratios for AUC and C_{max} were 1.11 and 1.02, respectively. The accumulation ratio was higher for C_{min} (1.96). Steady state was reached following the first administration for C_{max} and AUC, respectively, and after 16 weeks for C_{min}.

For doses of tocilizumab 8 mg/kg given every 4 weeks, the predicted mean (± SD) steady-state AUC, C_{min}, and C_{max} of tocilizumab were 35,000 ± 15,500 mcg•h/mL, 9.74 ± 10.5 mcg/mL, and 183 ± 85.6 mcg/mL, respectively. The accumulation ratios for AUC and C_{max} were 1.22 and 1.06, respectively. The accumulation ratio was higher for C_{min} (2.35). Steady state was reached following the first administration and after 8 and 20 weeks for C_{max}, AUC, and C_{min}, respectively.

Distribution – Following IV dosing, tocilizumab undergoes biphasic elimination from the circulation. In RA patients, the central volume of distribution was 3.5 L, and the peripheral volume of distribution was 2.9 L, resulting in a volume of distribution at steady state of 6.4 L.

Excretion – The total clearance of tocilizumab is concentration dependent and is the sum of the linear clearance and the nonlinear clearance. The clearance of tocilizumab decreased with increased dose. The linear clearance was estimated to be 12.5 mL/h in the population pharmacokinetic analysis. The concentration-dependent nonlinear clearance plays a major role at low tocilizumab concentrations. Once the nonlinear clearance pathway is saturated, at higher tocilizumab concentrations, clearance is mainly determined by the linear clearance.

The terminal half-life of tocilizumab is concentration dependent. The concentration-dependent apparent terminal half-life is up to 11 days for 4 mg/kg and up to 13 days for 8 mg/kg every 4 weeks at steady state. At the 10 mg/kg single dose in RA patients, mean clearance was 0.29 ± 0.1 mL/h/kg, and mean apparent terminal half-life was 151 ± 59 hours (6.3 days).

Special populations –

Weight: Linear clearance was found to increase with body size. The body weight–based dose (8 mg/kg) resulted in approximately 86% higher exposure in patients who weighed more than 100 kg in comparison with patients who weighed less than 60 kg. Tocilizumab AUC, C_{min}, and C_{max} increased with increase of body weight. At body weight at least 100 kg, the predicted mean (± SD) steady-state AUC, C_{min}, and C_{max} of tocilizumab were 55,500 ± 14,100 mcg•h/mL, 19 ± 12 mcg/mL, and 269 ± 57 mcg/mL, respectively, which are higher than mean exposure values for the patient population.

Contraindications

Known hypersensitivity to tocilizumab.

Warnings/Precautions

➤*Serious infections:* Serious and sometimes fatal infections caused by bacterial, mycobacterial, invasive fungal, viral, protozoal, or other opportunistic pathogens have been reported in patients receiving immunosuppressive agents, including tocilizumab for RA. The most common serious infections included pneumonia, urinary tract infection, cellulitis, herpes zoster, gastroenteritis, diverticulitis, sepsis, and bacterial arthritis. Among opportunistic infections, tuberculosis, cryptococcus, aspergillosis, candidiasis, and pneumocystosis were reported with tocilizumab. Other serious infections not reported in clinical studies may also occur (eg, histoplasmosis, coccidioidomycosis, listeriosis). Patients have presented with disseminated, rather than localized, disease and were often taking concomitant immunosuppressants such as methotrexate or corticosteroids, which, in addition to RA, may predispose them to infections.

Tocilizumab should not be administered in patients with an active infection, including localized infections. Consider the risks and benefits of treatment prior to initiating tocilizumab in patients with chronic or recurrent infection, who have been exposed to tuberculosis, with a history of serious or an opportunistic infection, who have resided or traveled in areas of endemic tuberculosis or endemic mycoses, or with underlying conditions that may predispose them to infection.

Closely monitor patients for the development of signs and symptoms of infection during and after treatment with tocilizumab, as signs and symptoms of acute inflammation may be lessened because of suppression of the acute-phase reactants.

Interrupt tocilizumab if a patient develops a serious infection, an opportunistic infection, or sepsis. A patient who develops a new infection during treatment with tocilizumab should undergo a prompt and complete diagnostic workup appropriate for an immunocompromised patient; initiate appropriate antimicrobial therapy, and closely monitor the patient.

Tuberculosis – Evaluate patients for tuberculosis risk factors and test for latent infection prior to initiating tocilizumab.

Consider antituberculosis therapy prior to initiation of tocilizumab in patients with a history of latent or active tuberculosis, in whom an adequate course of treatment cannot be confirmed, and for patients with a negative test for latent tuberculosis but having risk factors for tuberculosis infection. Consultation with a health care provider with expertise in the treatment of tuberculosis is recommended to aid in the decision of whether initiating antituberculosis therapy is appropriate for an individual patient.

Closely monitor patients for the development of signs and symptoms of tuberculosis including patients who tested negative for latent tuberculosis infection prior to initiating therapy.

It is recommended that patients be screened for latent tuberculosis infection prior to starting tocilizumab. The incidence of tuberculosis in worldwide clinical development programs is 0.1%. Treat patients with latent tuberculosis with standard antimycobacterial therapy before initiating tocilizumab.

➤*Viral reactivation:* Viral reactivation has been reported with immunosuppressive biologic therapies, and cases of herpes zoster exacerbation were observed in clinical studies with tocilizumab. No cases of hepatitis B reactivation were observed in the trials; however, patients who screened positive for hepatitis were excluded.

➤*GI perforations:* Events of GI perforation have been reported in clinical trials, primarily as complications of diverticulitis. Use tocilizumab with caution in patients who may be at increased risk for GI perforation. Promptly evaluate patients presenting with new-onset abdominal symptoms for early identification of GI perforation.

➤*Hematological effects:*

Neutropenia – Treatment with tocilizumab was associated with a higher incidence of neutropenia. Infections have been uncommonly reported in association with treatment-related neutropenia in long-term extension studies and postmarketing clinical experience. It is not recommended to initiate tocilizumab treatment in patients with a low neutrophil count (ie, ANC less than 2,000/mm^3). In patients who develop an ANC less than 500/mm^3, treatment is not recommended. Monitor neutrophils every 4 to 8 weeks.

Thrombocytopenia – Treatment with tocilizumab was associated with a reduction in platelet counts. Treatment-related reduction in platelets was not associated with serious bleeding events in clinical trials. It is not recommended to initiate tocilizumab treatment in patients with a platelet count below 100,000/mm^3. In patients who develop a platelet count less than 50,000/mm^3, treatment is not recommended. Monitor platelets every 4 to 8 weeks.

➤*Hepatic effects:* Treatment with tocilizumab was associated with a higher incidence of transaminase elevations. These elevations did not result in apparent permanent or clinically evident hepatic injury in clinical trials. Increased frequency and magnitude of these elevations were observed when potentially hepatotoxic drugs (eg, methotrexate) were used in combination with tocilizumab.

In one case, a patient who had received tocilizumab 8 mg/kg monotherapy without elevations in transaminases experienced elevation in AST to above 10 times the ULN and elevation in ALT to above 16 times the ULN when methotrexate was initiated in combination with tocilizumab. Transaminases normalized when both treatments were held, but elevations recurred when methotrexate and tocilizumab were restarted at lower doses. Elevations resolved when methotrexate and tocilizumab were discontinued.

It is not recommended to initiate tocilizumab treatment in patients with elevated transaminases ALT or AST more than 1.5 times the ULN. In patients who develop elevated ALT or AST greater than 5 times the ULN, treatment is not recommended. Monitor ALT and AST levels every 4 to 8 weeks. When clinically indicated, consider other liver function tests, such as bilirubin.

➤*Lipids:* Treatment with tocilizumab was associated with increases in lipid parameters such as total cholesterol, triglycerides, low-density lipoprotein (LDL) cholesterol, and/or high-density lipoprotein (HDL) cholesterol. Perform assessment of lipid parameters approximately 4 to 8 weeks following initiation of tocilizumab therapy, then at approximately 6-month intervals. Manage patients according to clinical guidelines (eg, National Cholesterol Educational Program [(NCEP)]) for the management of hyperlipidemia.

➤*Malignancy:* The impact of treatment with tocilizumab on the development of malignancies is not known but malignancies were observed in clinical studies. Tocilizumab is an immunosuppressant, and treatment with immunosuppressants may result in an increased risk of malignancies.

➤*Demyelinating disorders:* The impact of treatment with tocilizumab on demyelinating disorders is not known, but multiple sclerosis and chronic inflammatory demyelinating polyneuropathy were reported rarely in clinical studies. Exercise caution in considering the use of tocilizumab in patients with preexisting or recent-onset demyelinating disorders.

➤*Vaccinations:* Do not give live vaccines concurrently with tocilizumab, as clinical safety has not been established. No data are available on the secondary transmission of infection from persons receiving live vaccines to patients receiving tocilizumab. No data are available on the effectiveness of vaccination in patients receiving tocilizumab. Because IL-6 inhibition may interfere with the normal immune response to new antigens, bring patients up to date on all recommended vaccinations, except for live vaccines, prior to initiation of therapy with tocilizumab.

➤*Immunogenicity:* In the 6-month, controlled clinical studies, 2,876 patients have been tested for anti-tocilizumab antibodies. Two percent of patients developed positive anti-tocilizumab antibodies, of whom 5 had an associated, medically significant hypersensitivity reaction leading to withdrawal. One percent of patients developed neutralizing antibodies.

➤*Hypersensitivity reactions:* Serious hypersensitivity reactions, including anaphylaxis, have been reported in association with infusion of tocilizumab. Appropriate medical treatment should be available for immediate use in the event of an anaphylactic reaction during administration of tocilizumab.

TOCILIZUMAB — INJECTION

➤*Hepatic function impairment:* The safety and efficacy of tocilizumab have not been studied in patients with hepatic impairment, including patients with positive hepatitis B virus and hepatitis C virus serology. Treatment with tocilizumab is not recommended in patients with active hepatic disease or hepatic impairment.

➤*Pregnancy: Category C.* There are no adequate and well-controlled studies in pregnant women. Use tocilizumab during pregnancy only if the potential benefit justifies the potential risk to the fetus.

Tocilizumab produced an increase in the incidence of abortion/embryofetal death at 10 and 50 mg/kg doses (1.25 and 6.25 times the human dose of 8 mg/kg every 4 weeks based on a mg/kg comparison).

Pregnancy registry – To monitor the outcomes of pregnant women exposed to tocilizumab, a pregnancy registry has been established. Health care providers are encouraged to register patients and pregnant women are encouraged to register themselves by calling 1-877-311-8972.

➤*Lactation:* It is not known whether tocilizumab is excreted in human milk or absorbed systemically after ingestion. Because many drugs are excreted in human milk, and because of the potential for serious adverse reactions in breast-feeding infants from tocilizumab, decide whether to discontinue breastfeeding or the drug, taking into account the importance of the drug to the mother.

➤*Children:* Safety and effectiveness of tocilizumab in children have not been established.

➤*Elderly:* The frequency of serious infection among tocilizumab-treated subjects 65 years of age and older was higher than those under the age of 65. As there is a higher incidence of infections in the elderly population in general, use caution when treating elderly patients.

➤*Monitoring:* Monitor neutrophils, platelets, ALT, and AST every 4 to 8 weeks. Monitor lipid panel approximately 4 to 8 weeks following initiation of therapy, then at approximately 6-month intervals.

Closely monitor patients for the development of signs and symptoms of infection during and after treatment with tocilizumab.

Closely monitor patients for the development of signs and symptoms of tuberculosis, including patients who tested negative for latent tuberculosis infection prior to initiating therapy.

Closely monitor patients for signs and symptoms potentially indicative of demyelinating disorders.

Drug Interactions

➤*Cytochrome P450 system:* Cytochrome P450s (CYP-450) in the liver are down-regulated by infection and inflammation stimuli, including cytokines such as IL-6. Tocilizumab may restore CYP-450 activities to higher levels than those in the absence of tocilizumab, leading to increased metabolism of drugs that are CYP-450 substrates. The effect of tocilizumab on CYP enzymes may be clinically important for CYP-450 substrates with narrow therapeutic index, where the dose is individually adjusted. Upon initiation or discontinuation of tocilizumab in patients treated with these types of agents, perform therapeutic monitoring of effects or drug concentration and adjust the dose of the agent as needed. The effect of tocilizumab on CYP-450 enzyme activity may persist for several weeks after stopping therapy.

Live vaccines – See Warnings/Precautions for more information.

Tocilizumab Drug Interactions

Precipitant drug	Object drug[a]		Description
Anti-CD20 monoclonal antibodies (eg, rituximab)	Tocilizumab	⬆	There is a possibility of increased immunosuppression and increased risk of infection. Avoid coadministration.
Tocilizumab	Anti-CD20 monoclonal antibodies (eg, rituximab)		
IL-1 receptor antagonists (eg, anakinra)	Tocilizumab	⬆	There is a possibility of increased immunosuppression and increased risk of infection. Avoid coadministration.
Tocilizumab	IL-1 receptor antagonists (eg, anakinra)		
Immunosuppressants (eg, corticosteroids, methotrexate)	Tocilizumab	⬆	May predispose patients to infections and malignancy. Monitor patients and adjust treatment as needed.
Selective costimulation modulators (eg, abatacept)	Tocilizumab	⬆	There is a possibility of increased immunosuppression and increased risk of infection. Avoid coadministration.
Tocilizumab	Selective costimulation modulators (eg, abatacept)		
TNF antagonists (eg, infliximab)	Tocilizumab	⬆	There is a possibility of increased immunosuppression and increased risk of infection. Avoid coadministration.
Tocilizumab	TNF antagonists (eg, infliximab)		
Tocilizumab	Contraceptives, hormonal	⬇	The pharmacologic effect of the hormonal contraceptives may be decreased. Inform women of the possible increased risk of hormonal contraceptive failure. Consider an alternative nonhormonal contraceptive or an additional method of contraception.
Tocilizumab	Cyclosporine	⬇	The pharmacologic effect of cyclosporine may be decreased. Closely measure cyclosporine concentrations when starting or stopping tocilizumab. Adjust the cyclosporine dose as needed.
Tocilizumab	Dextromethorphan	⬇	The pharmacologic effect of dextromethorphan may be decreased. One week following infusion of a single dose of tocilizumab 8 mg/kg, dextromethorphan exposure was decreased approximately 5%, while that of its metabolite was decreased 29%. Monitor the response to dextromethorphan when starting or stopping tocilizumab. Adjust the dextromethorphan dose as needed.
Tocilizumab	HMG-CoA[b] reductase inhibitors (eg, lovastatin, simvastatin)	⬇	The pharmacologic effect of the HMG-CoA reductase inhibitor may be decreased. One week following infusion of a single dose of tocilizumab 10 mg/kg, exposure to simvastatin and simvastatin acid decreased 57% and 39%, respectively. Exposure increased when tocilizumab was discontinued. Monitor the response of the patient when starting or stopping tocilizumab and adjust the HMG-CoA reductase inhibitor dose as needed.
Tocilizumab	Proton pump inhibitors (eg, omeprazole)	⬇	The pharmacologic effect of proton pump inhibitors may be decreased. One week following infusion of a single dose of tocilizumab 8 mg/kg, omeprazole AUC decreased 12% for poor and intermediate metabolizers and 28% for extensive metabolizers. Monitor the response of the patient when starting or stopping tocilizumab and adjust the proton pump inhibitor dose as needed.
Tocilizumab	Theophylline	⬇	The pharmacologic effect of theophylline may be decreased. Closely measure theophylline concentrations when starting or stopping tocilizumab. Adjust the theophylline dose as needed.
Tocilizumab	Warfarin	⬇	The anticoagulant effect of warfarin may be decreased. Monitor coagulation parameters more closely when starting or stopping tocilizumab. Adjust the warfarin dose as needed.

[a] ⬆ = object drug increased; ⬇ = object drug decreased.
[b] HMG CoA = 3-hydroxy-3-methylglutaryl coenzyme A.

Adverse Reactions

➤*Common adverse reactions:* The most common serious adverse reactions were serious infections. The most commonly reported adverse reactions in controlled studies up to 6 months (occurring in at least 5% of patients treated with tocilizumab monotherapy or in combination with DMARDs) were headache, hypertension, increased ALT, nasopharyngitis, and upper respiratory tract infections.

➤*Discontinuation:* The proportion of patients who discontinued treatment because of any adverse reactions during the double-blind, placebo-

TOCILIZUMAB — INJECTION

controlled studies was 5% for patients taking tocilizumab and 3% for placebo-treated patients. The most common adverse reactions that required discontinuation of tocilizumab were increased hepatic transaminase values (per protocol requirement) and serious infections.

➤*Infections:* In the 6-month, controlled clinical studies, the rate of infections in the tocilizumab monotherapy group was 119 events per 100 patient-years and was similar in the methotrexate monotherapy group. The rate of infections in the tocilizumab 4 and 8 mg/kg plus DMARD group was 133 and 127 events per 100 patient-years, respectively, compared with 112 events per 100 patient-years in the placebo plus DMARD group. The most commonly reported infections (5 to 8% of patients) were upper respiratory tract infections and nasopharyngitis.

The overall rate of infections with tocilizumab in the all-exposure population was 108 events per 100 patient-years.

Serious infections – In the 6-month, controlled clinical studies, the rate of serious infections in the tocilizumab monotherapy group was 3.6 per 100 patient-years compared with 1.5 per 100 patient-years in the methotrexate group. The rate of serious infections in the tocilizumab 4 and 8 mg/kg plus DMARD group was 4.4 and 5.3 events per 100 patient-years, respectively, compared with 3.9 events per 100 patient-years in the placebo plus DMARD group.

In the all-exposure population, the overall rate of serious infections was 4.7 events per 100 patient-years. The most common serious infections included bacterial arthritis, cellulitis, diverticulitis, gastroenteritis, herpes zoster, pneumonia, sepsis, and urinary tract infection. The overall rate of fatal serious infections was 0.13 per 100 patient-years. Cases of opportunistic infections have been reported.

➤*GI perforations:* During the 6-month, controlled clinical trials, the overall rate of GI perforation was 0.26 events per 100 patient-years with tocilizumab therapy.

In the all-exposure population, the overall rate of GI perforation was 0.28 events per 100 patient-years. Reports of GI perforation were primarily reported as complications of diverticulitis, including generalized purulent peritonitis, lower GI perforation, fistula, and abscess. Most patients who developed GI perforations were taking concomitant nonsteroidal anti-inflammatory drugs (NSAIDs), corticosteroids, or methotrexate. The relative contribution of these concomitant medications versus tocilizumab to the development of GI perforations is not known.

➤*Infusion reactions:* In the 6-month, controlled clinical studies, adverse reactions associated with the infusion (occurring during or within 24 hours of the start of infusion) were reported in 8% and 7% of patients in the tocilizumab 4 and 8 mg/kg plus DMARD group, respectively, compared with 5% of patients in the placebo plus DMARD group. The most frequently reported reaction on the 4 and 8 mg/kg dose during the infusion was hypertension (1% for both doses), while the most frequently reported reaction occurring within 24 hours of finishing an infusion were headache (1% for both doses) and skin reactions (1% for both doses), including pruritus, rash, and urticaria. These reactions were not treatment limiting.

➤*Hypersensitivity:* Clinically significant hypersensitivity reactions (eg, anaphylactoid and anaphylactic reactions) associated with tocilizumab and requiring treatment discontinuation were reported in 0.1% in the 6-month controlled trials and in 0.2% in the all-exposure population. These reactions were generally observed during the second to fourth infusion of tocilizumab. Appropriate medical treatment should be available for immediate use in the event of a serious hypersensitivity reaction.

➤*Malignancies:* During the 6-month, controlled period of the studies, 15 malignancies were diagnosed in patients receiving tocilizumab compared with 8 malignancies in patients in the control groups. Exposure-adjusted incidence was similar in the tocilizumab groups (1.32 events per 100 patient-years) and in the placebo plus DMARD group (1.37 events per 100 patient-years).

➤*Other adverse reactions (2% or more):*

Tocilizumab Adverse Reactions (≥ 1%)					
	6-month, phase 3, controlled study population				
Adverse reactions	Tocilizumab 8 mg/kg (n = 288)	Methotrexate (n = 284)	Tocilizumab 4 mg/kg + DMARDs (n = 774)	Tocilizumab 8 mg/kg + DMARDs (n = 1,582)	Placebo + DMARDs (n = 1,170)
GI					
Headache	7%	2%	6%	5%	3%
Dizziness	3%	1%	2%	3%	2%
CNS					
Abdominal pain upper	2%	2%	3%	3%	2%
Gastritis	1%	2%	1%	2%	1%
Hepatic					
ALT increased	6%	4%	3%	3%	1%
Transaminase increased	1%	5%	2%	2%	1%
Respiratory					
Bronchitis	3%	2%	4%	3%	3%
Nasopharyngitis	7%	6%	4%	6%	4%
Upper respiratory tract infection	7%	5%	6%	8%	6%
Miscellaneous					
Hypertension	6%	2%	4%	4%	3%
Mouth ulceration	2%	2%	1%	2%	1%
Rash	2%	1%	4%	3%	1%

➤*Lab test abnormalities:*

Neutropenia – In the 6-month, controlled clinical studies, decreases in neutrophil counts below 1,000/mm³ occurred in 1.8% and 3.4% of patients in the tocilizumab 4 and 8 mg/kg plus DMARD group, respectively, compared with 0.1% of patients in the placebo plus DMARD group. Approximately half of the instances of ANC below 1,000/mm³ occurred within 8 weeks of starting therapy. Decreases in neutrophil counts below 500/mm³ occurred in 0.4% and 0.3% of patients in the tocilizumab 4 and 8 mg/kg plus a DMARD, respectively, compared with 0.1% of patients in the placebo plus DMARD group. There was no clear relationship between decreases in neutrophils below 1,000/mm³ and the occurrence of serious infections.

Platelets – In the 6-month, controlled clinical studies, decreases in platelet counts below 100,000/mm³ occurred in 1.3% and 1.7% of patients receiving tocilizumab 4 and 8 mg/kg plus a DMARD, respectively, compared with 0.5% of patients receiving placebo plus DMARD without associated bleeding reactions.

Liver function tests – In patients experiencing liver enzyme elevation, modification of treatment regimen, such as reduction in the dose of a concomitant DMARDs, interruption of tocilizumab, or reduction in tocilizumab dose resulted in decrease or normalization of liver enzymes. These elevations were not associated with clinically relevant increases in direct bilirubin, nor were they associated with clinical evidence of hepatitis or hepatic insufficiency.

Tocilizumab Liver Enzyme Abnormalities					
	Tocilizumab 8 mg/kg (n = 288)	Methotrexate (n = 284)	Tocilizumab 4 mg/kg + DMARDs (n = 774)	Tocilizumab 8 mg/kg + DMARDs (n = 1,582)	Placebo + DMARDs (n = 1,170)
AST (units/L)					
> ULN to 3 × ULN	22%	26%	34%	41%	17%
> 3 × ULN to 5× ULN	0.3%	2%	1%	2%	0.3%
> 5 × ULN	0.7%	0.4%	0.1%	0.2%	< 0.1%
ALT (U/L)					
> ULN to 3 × ULN	36%	33%	45%	48%	23%
> 3 × ULN to 5 × ULN	1%	4%	5%	5%	1%
> 5 × ULN	0.7%	1%	1.3%	1.5%	0.3%

Lipids – Elevations in lipid parameters (total cholesterol, LDL, HDL, triglycerides) were first assessed at 6 weeks following initiation of tocilizumab

TOCILIZUMAB — INJECTION

in the controlled 6-month clinical trials. Increases were observed at this time point and remained stable thereafter. Increases in triglycerides to levels above 500 mg/dL were rarely observed. Changes in other lipid parameters from baseline to week 24 are summarized: Mean LDL increased by 13 mg/dL in the tocilizumab 4 mg/kg plus DMARD arm, 20 mg/dL in the tocilizumab 8 mg/kg plus DMARD arm, and 25 mg/dL in tocilizumab 8 mg/kg monotherapy. Mean HDL increased by 3 mg/dL in the tocilizumab 4 mg/kg plus DMARD arm, 5 mg/dL in the tocilizumab 8 mg/kg plus DMARD arm, and 4 mg/dL in tocilizumab 8 mg/kg monotherapy. Mean LDL/HDL ratio increased by an average of 0.14 in the tocilizumab 4 mg/kg plus DMARD arm, 0.15 in the tocilizumab 8 mg/kg plus DMARD arm, and 0.26 in tocilizumab 8 mg/kg monotherapy. ApoB/ApoA1 ratios were essentially unchanged in tocilizumab-treated patients. Elevated lipids responded to lipid lowering agents.

Overdosage

➤*Treatment:* In case of an overdose, it is recommended that the patient be monitored for signs and symptoms of adverse reactions. Patients who develop adverse reactions should receive appropriate symptomatic treatment.

Patient Information

Inform patients that tocilizumab may lower their resistance to infections. Instruct patients of the importance of contacting their health care provider immediately when symptoms suggesting infection appear in order to ensure rapid evaluation and appropriate treatment.

Inform patients that some patients who have been treated with tocilizumab have had serious side effects in the stomach and intestines. Instruct patients of the importance of contacting their health care provider immediately when symptoms of severe, persistent abdominal pain appear to ensure rapid evaluation and appropriate treatment.

ABATACEPT

Rx	**Orencia** (Bristol-Myers Squibb)	**Injection, lyophilized powder for solution:** 250 mg	Preservative free. Maltose 500 mg, monobasic sodium phosphate 17.2 mg, sodium chloride 14.6 mg. In 15 mL single-use vials with syringe.

ABATACEPT — INJECTION

Indications

➤*Adult rheumatoid arthritis (RA):* For reducing signs and symptoms, inducing major clinical response, inhibiting the progression of structural damage, and improving physical function in adult patients with moderately to severely active RA. Abatacept may be used as monotherapy or concomitantly with disease-modifying antirheumatic drugs (DMARDs) other than tumor necrosis factor (TNF) antagonists.

➤*Juvenile idiopathic arthritis:* For reducing signs and symptoms in children 6 years of age and older with moderately to severely active polyarticular juvenile idiopathic arthritis. Abatacept may be used as monotherapy or concomitantly with methotrexate.

➤*General information:* Do not coadminister abatacept with TNF antagonists. Abatacept is not recommended for use concomitantly with other biologic RA therapy, such as anakinra.

Administration and Dosage

➤*Adults:*

Rheumatoid arthritis – Dosage is based on weight. Following the initial administration, abatacept should be given at 2 and 4 weeks after the first infusion, then every 4 weeks thereafter.

Abatacept Dosing in Adults With Rheumatoid Arthritis

Body weight	Dose	Number of vials[a]
< 60 kg	500 mg	2
60 to 100 kg	750 mg	3
> 100 kg	1,000 mg	4

[a] Each vial provides abatacept 250 mg for administration.

➤*Children:*

Juvenile idiopathic arthritis –

6 to 17 years of age:

• *Usual dosage* – For juvenile idiopathic arthritis, a dose calculated based on each patient's body weight is used. Following the initial administration, abatacept should be given at 2 and 4 weeks after the first infusion, then every 4 weeks thereafter.

Weighing less than 75 kg: 10 mg/kg calculated based on the patient's body weight at each administration.

Weighing 75 kg or more: Administer abatacept following the adult dosing regimen.

• *Maximum dose* – Do not exceed a maximum dose of 1,000 mg.

➤*Preparation for administration:* Each vial must be reconstituted with 10 mL of sterile water for injection using only the silicone-free disposable syringe provided with each vial and an 18- to 21-gauge needle. After reconstitution, the concentration of abatacept in the vial will be 25 mg/mL. If the abatacept powder is accidentally reconstituted using a siliconized syringe, the solution may develop a few translucent particles. Discard any solutions prepared using siliconized syringes.

If the silicone-free disposable syringe is dropped or becomes contaminated, use a new silicone-free disposable syringe from inventory. For information on obtaining additional silicone-free disposable syringes, contact the manufacturer at 1-800-673-6242.

During reconstitution, to minimize foam formation in solutions of abatacept, the vials should be rotated with gentle swirling until the contents are completely dissolved. Avoid prolonged or vigorous agitation. Do not shake. The solution should be clear and colorless to pale yellow. Do not use if opaque particles, discoloration, or other foreign particles are present.

The reconstituted abatacept solution must be further diluted to 100 mL.

1.) To reconstitute abatacept powder, remove the flip top from the vial and wipe the top with an alcohol swab. Insert the syringe needle into the vial through the center of the rubber stopper and direct the stream of sterile water for injection to the glass wall of the vial. Do not use the vial if the vacuum is not present. Rotate the vial with gentle swirling until the contents are completely dissolved.

2.) Upon complete dissolution of the lyophilized powder, the vial should be vented with a needle to dissipate any foam that may be present. After reconstitution, each milliliter will contain 25 mg (250 mg per 10 mL).

3.) The reconstituted abatacept solution must be further diluted to 100 mL as follows. From a 100 mL infusion bag or bottle, withdraw a volume of sodium chloride 0.9% injection equal to the volume of the reconstituted abatacept solution required for the patient's dose. Slowly add the reconstituted abatacept solution from each vial into the infusion bag or bottle using the same silicone-free disposable syringe provided with each vial. Gently mix. Do not shake the bag or bottle. The final concentration of abatacept in the bag or bottle will depend upon the amount of drug added but will be no more than 10 mg/mL. Any unused portion in the vials must be immediately discarded.

➤*Administration:* Abatacept should be administered as a 30-minute intravenous (IV) infusion utilizing the weight range-based dosing. Following the initial administration, abatacept should be given at 2 and 4 weeks after the first infusion, then every 4 weeks thereafter.

The entire fully diluted abatacept solution must be administered with an infusion set and a sterile nonpyrogenic, low-protein–binding filter (pore size of 0.2 to 1.2 mcm).

The infusion of the fully diluted abatacept solution must be completed within 24 hours of reconstitution of the abatacept vials.

➤*Admixture compatibility:* Abatacept should not be infused concomitantly in the same IV line with other agents.

➤*Storage/Stability:* Store vials in a refrigerator at 2° to 8°C (36° to 46°F). Protect the vials from light by storing them in the original package until time of use. The fully diluted solution may be stored at room temperature or refrigerated at 2° to 8°C (36° to 46°F) before use. Infusion must be completed within 24 hours of reconstitution of the vials.

Actions

➤*Pharmacology:* Abatacept, a selective costimulation modulator, inhibits T-cell (T-lymphocyte) activation by binding to CD80 and CD86, thereby blocking interaction with CD28. This interaction provides a costimulatory signal necessary for full activation of T-lymphocytes. Activated T-lymphocytes are implicated in the pathogenesis of RA and are found in the synovium of patients with RA.

In vitro, abatacept decreases T-cell proliferation and inhibits the production of the cytokines TNF-alpha, interferon-gamma, and interleukin-2. In a rat collagen-induced arthritis model, abatacept suppresses inflammation, decreases anticollagen antibody production, and reduces antigen-specific production of interferon-gamma. The relationship of these biological response markers to the mechanisms by which abatacept exerts its effects in RA is unknown.

Pharmacodynamics – In clinical trials with abatacept at doses approximating 10 mg/kg, decreases were observed in serum levels of soluble interleukin-2 receptor, interleukin-6, rheumatoid factor, C-reactive protein (CRP), matrix metalloproteinase-3, and TNF-alpha. The relationship of these biological response markers to the mechanisms by which abatacept exerts its effects in RA is unknown.

➤*Pharmacokinetics:*

Adult RA – The pharmacokinetics of abatacept were studied in healthy adult subjects after a single 10 mg/kg IV infusion and in patients with RA after multiple 10 mg/kg IV infusions (see the following table).

Abatacept Pharmacokinetic Parameters (Mean, Range) in Healthy Subjects and Patients With RA After 10 mg/kg IV Infusion(s)

Pharmacokinetic parameter	Healthy subjects (after 10 mg/kg single dose) (n = 13)	RA patients (after 10 mg/kg multiple doses[a]) (n = 14)
Peak concentration (C_{max}[b]) (mcg/mL)	292 (175 to 427)	295 (171 to 398)
Terminal half-life (days)	16.7 (12 to 23)	13.1 (8 to 25)

ABATACEPT — INJECTION

Abatacept Pharmacokinetic Parameters (Mean, Range) in Healthy Subjects and Patients With RA After 10 mg/kg IV Infusion(s)

Pharmacokinetic parameter	Healthy subjects (after 10 mg/kg single dose) (n = 13)	RA patients (after 10 mg/kg multiple doses[a]) (n = 14)
Systemic clearance (mL/h/kg)	0.23 (0.16 to 0.3)	0.22 (0.13 to 0.47)
Volume of distribution (L/kg)	0.09 (0.06 to 0.13)	0.07 (0.02 to 0.13)

[a] Multiple IV infusions were administered at days 1, 15, and 30 and monthly thereafter.
[b] C_{max} = maximal drug concentration.

Absorption/Distribution –

Adult RA: The pharmacokinetics of abatacept in patients with RA and healthy subjects appeared to be comparable. In patients with RA, after multiple IV infusions, the pharmacokinetics of abatacept showed proportional increases of C_{max} and area under the curve (AUC) over the dose range of 2 to 10 mg/kg. At 10 mg/kg, serum concentration appeared to reach steady state by day 60, with a mean (range) trough concentration of 24 mcg/mL (1 to 66 mcg/mL). No systemic accumulation of abatacept occurred upon continued repeated treatment with 10 mg/kg at monthly intervals in patients with RA.

Juvenile idiopathic arthritis: In patients 6 to 17 years of age, the mean (range) steady-state serum peak and trough concentrations of abatacept were 217 mcg/mL (57 to 700 mcg/mL) and 11.9 mcg/mL (0.15 to 44.6 mcg/mL).

Excretion –

Juvenile idiopathic arthritis: Population pharmacokinetic analyses of the serum concentration data showed that clearance of abatacept increased with baseline body weight. The estimated mean (range) clearance of abatacept in juvenile idiopathic arthritis patients was 0.4 mL/h/kg (0.2 to 1.12 mL/h/kg).

Special populations –

Body weight: Population pharmacokinetic analyses in patients with RA revealed that there was a trend toward higher clearance of abatacept with increasing body weight.

Contraindications

None known.

Warnings/Precautions

➤*Concomitant use with TNF antagonists:* In controlled clinical trials in patients with adult RA, patients receiving concomitant abatacept and TNF antagonist therapy experienced more infections (63%) and serious infections (4.4%) compared with patients treated with only TNF antagonists (43% and 0.8%, respectively). These trials failed to demonstrate an important enhancement of efficacy with coadministration of abatacept and a TNF antagonist; therefore, concurrent therapy with abatacept and a TNF antagonist is not recommended. While transitioning from TNF antagonist therapy to abatacept therapy, monitor patients for signs of infection.

➤*Infections:* Exercise caution when considering the use of abatacept in patients with a history of recurrent infections, underlying conditions that may predispose them to infections, or chronic, latent, or localized infections. Closely monitor patients who develop a new infection while undergoing treatment with abatacept. Discontinue administration of abatacept if a patient develops a serious infection. A higher rate of serious infections has been observed in patients treated with concurrent TNF antagonists and abatacept.

Prior to initiating immunomodulatory therapies, including abatacept, screen patients for latent tuberculosis (TB) infection with a tuberculin skin test. Abatacept has not been studied in patients with a positive TB screen, and the safety of abatacept in individuals with latent TB infection is unknown. Treat patients testing positive in TB screening by standard medical practice prior to therapy with abatacept.

Antirheumatic therapies have been associated with hepatitis B reactivation. Therefore, perform screening for viral hepatitis in accordance with published guidelines before starting therapy with abatacept. In clinical studies with abatacept, patients who screened positive for hepatitis were excluded from study.

➤*Immunizations:* Do not give live vaccines concurrently with abatacept or within 3 months of its discontinuation. No data are available on the secondary transmission of infection from persons receiving live vaccines to patients receiving abatacept. The efficacy of vaccination in patients receiving abatacept is not known. Based on its mechanism of action, abatacept may blunt the efficacy of some immunizations.

It is recommended that patients with juvenile idiopathic arthritis be brought up to date with all immunizations in agreement with current immunization guidelines prior to initiating abatacept therapy.

➤*Chronic obstructive pulmonary disease (COPD):* Adult patients with COPD treated with abatacept developed adverse reactions more frequently than those treated with placebo, including COPD exacerbations, cough, rhonchi, and dyspnea. Undertake use of abatacept with caution in patients with RA and COPD and monitor such patients for worsening of respiratory status.

➤*Immunosuppression:* The possibility exists for drugs inhibiting T-cell activation, including abatacept, to affect host defenses against infections and malignancies because T cells mediate cellular immune responses. The impact of treatment with abatacept on the development and course of malignancies is not fully understood. In clinical trials, a higher rate of infections was seen in abatacept-treated patients compared with placebo-treated patients.

➤*Hypersensitivity reactions:* See Adverse Reactions for more information.

➤*Pregnancy: Category C.* There are no adequate and well-controlled studies of abatacept use in pregnant women. Abatacept has been shown to cross the placenta in animals; in animal reproduction studies, alterations in immune function occurred. Use abatacept during pregnancy only if the potential benefit to the mother justifies the potential risk to the fetus.

Abatacept was not teratogenic when administered to pregnant mice at doses of up to 300 mg/kg and in pregnant rats and rabbits at doses of up to 200 mg/kg daily, representing approximately 29 times the exposure associated with the MRHD of 10 mg/kg based on AUC.

Abatacept administered to female rats every 3 days during early gestation and throughout the lactation period produced no adverse reactions in offspring at doses of up to 45 mg/kg, representing 3 times the exposure associated with the MRHD of 10 mg/kg based on AUC. However, at 200 mg/kg, 11 times the MRHD exposure, alterations in immune function were observed consisting of a 9-fold increase in T-cell-dependent antibody response in female pups and thyroid inflammation in 1 female pup. It is not known whether these findings indicate a risk for development of autoimmune diseases in humans exposed in utero to abatacept. However, exposure to abatacept in juvenile rats, which may be more representative of the fetal immune system state in humans, resulted in immune system abnormalities, including inflammation of the thyroid and pancreas.

Pregnancy registry – To monitor maternal–fetal outcomes of pregnant women exposed to abatacept, a pregnancy registry has been established. Health care providers are encouraged to register patients and pregnant women are encouraged to enroll themselves by calling 1-877-311-8972.

➤*Lactation:* It is not known whether abatacept is excreted into human milk or absorbed systemically after ingestion by a breast-feeding infant. However, abatacept was excreted in rat milk. Because many drugs are excreted in human milk, and because of the potential for serious adverse reactions in breast-feeding infants from abatacept, decide whether to discontinue breast-feeding or the drug, taking into account the importance of the drug to the mother.

➤*Children:* Abatacept is indicated for reducing signs and symptoms in children 6 years of age and older with moderately to severely active polyarticular juvenile idiopathic arthritis. Abatacept may be used as monotherapy or concomitantly with methotrexate.

Studies in juvenile rats exposed to abatacept prior to immune system maturity have shown immune system abnormalities, including an increase in the incidence of infections leading to death, as well as inflammation of the thyroid and pancreas. Studies in adult mice and monkeys have not demonstrated similar findings. As the immune system of rats is undeveloped in the first few weeks after birth, the relevance of these results to humans older than 6 years of age (when the immune system is largely developed) is unknown.

The safety and effectiveness of abatacept in children younger than 6 years of age have not been established. Therefore, abatacept is not recommended for use in patients younger than 6 years of age.

The safety and efficacy of abatacept in children for uses other than juvenile idiopathic arthritis have not been established.

➤*Elderly:* The frequency of serious infection and malignancy among abatacept-treated patients older than 65 years of age was higher than for those younger than 65 years of age. Because there is a higher incidence of infections and malignancies in the elderly population in general, exercise caution when treating elderly patients.

➤*Monitoring:* While transitioning from TNF antagonist therapy to abatacept therapy, monitor patients for signs of infection.

Prior to initiating immunomodulatory therapies, including abatacept, screen patients for latent TB infection with a tuberculin skin test. Monitor patients with COPD for worsening of respiratory status.

Antirheumatic therapies have been associated with hepatitis B reactivation. Therefore, perform screening for viral hepatitis in accordance with published guidelines before starting therapy with abatacept.

Drug Interactions

Formal drug interaction studies have not been conducted with abatacept.

➤*TNF antagonists:* Coadministration of a TNF antagonist with abatacept has been associated with an increased risk of serious infections and no significant additional efficacy over use of the TNF antagonists alone. Concurrent therapy with abatacept and TNF antagonists is not recommended.

➤*Anakinra:* There is insufficient experience to assess the safety and efficacy of abatacept coadministered with other biologic RA therapy, such as anakinra, and therefore such use is not recommended.

➤*Drug/Lab test interactions:* Parenteral drug products containing maltose can interfere with the readings of blood glucose monitors that use test strips with glucose dehydrogenase pyrroloquinolinequinone (GDH-PQQ). The GDH-PQQ–based glucose monitoring systems may react with the maltose present in abatacept, resulting in falsely elevated blood glucose readings on the day of infusion. When receiving abatacept, advise patients who require blood glucose monitoring to consider methods that do not react with maltose, such as those based on glucose dehydrogenase nicotine adenine dinucleotide (GDH-NAD), glucose oxidase, or glucose hexokinase test methods.

ABATACEPT — INJECTION

Adverse Reactions

➤*Adult RA:* The most serious adverse reactions were serious infections and malignancies. The most commonly reported adverse reactions (occurring in at least 10% of patients treated with abatacept) were headache, nasopharyngitis, nausea, and upper respiratory tract infection.

The adverse reactions most frequently resulting in clinical intervention (interruption or discontinuation of abatacept) were caused by infection. The most frequently reported infections resulting in dose interruption were upper respiratory tract infection (1%), bronchitis (0.7%), and herpes zoster (0.7%). The most frequent infections resulting in discontinuation were localized infection (0.2%), pneumonia (0.2%), and bronchitis (0.1%).

Infections – In the placebo-controlled trials, infections were reported in 54% of abatacept-treated patients and 48% of placebo-treated patients. The most commonly reported infections (5% to 13%) were bronchitis, influenza, nasopharyngitis, sinusitis, upper respiratory tract infection, and urinary tract infection. Other infections reported in less than 5% of patients at a higher frequency (more than 0.5%) with abatacept compared with placebo were herpes simplex, pneumonia, and rhinitis.

Serious infections were reported in 3% of patients treated with abatacept and 1.9% of patients treated with placebo. The most common (0.2% to 0.5%) serious infections reported with abatacept were acute pyelonephritis, bronchitis, cellulitis, diverticulitis, pneumonia, and urinary tract infection.

Malignancies – In the placebo-controlled portions of the clinical trials (1,955 patients treated with abatacept for a median of 12 months), the overall frequencies of malignancies were similar in the abatacept- and placebo-treated patients (1.3% and 1.1%, respectively). However, more cases of lung cancer were observed in abatacept-treated patients (4 [0.2%]) than placebo-treated patients (0). In the cumulative abatacept clinical trials (placebo-controlled and uncontrolled, open-label), 8 cases of lung cancer (0.21 cases per 100 patient-years) and 4 lymphomas (0.10 cases per 100 patient-years) were observed in 2,688 patients (3,827 patient-years). The rate observed for lymphoma is approximately 3.5-fold higher than expected in an age- and gender-matched general population based on the Surveillance, Epidemiology, and End Results Database. Patients with RA, particularly those with highly active disease, are at a higher risk for the development of lymphoma. Other malignancies included breast, bile duct, bladder, cervical, endometrial, lymphoma, melanoma, myelodysplastic syndrome, ovarian, prostate, renal, skin, thyroid, and uterine cancers. The potential role of abatacept in the development of malignancies in humans is unknown.

Acute infusion reactions – Acute infusion-related reactions (adverse reactions occurring within 1 hour of the start of the infusion) in studies 3, 4, and 5 were more common in the abatacept-treated patients than the placebo-treated patients (9% for abatacept, 6% for placebo). The most frequently reported reactions (1% to 2%) were dizziness, headache, and hypertension.

Acute infusion-related reactions that were reported in more than 0.1% and 1% or less of patients treated with abatacept included cardiopulmonary symptoms, such as hypotension, increased blood pressure, and dyspnea; other symptoms included cough, flushing, hypersensitivity, nausea, pruritus, rash, urticaria, and wheezing. Most of these reactions were mild to moderate. Less than 1% of abatacept-treated patients discontinued because of an acute infusion-related reaction. In controlled trials, 6 abatacept-treated patients compared with 2 placebo-treated patients discontinued study treatment because of acute infusion-related reactions.

Hypersensitivity reactions: Of 2,688 patients treated with abatacept in clinical trials, there were 2 cases of anaphylaxis or anaphylactoid reactions. Other reactions potentially associated with drug hypersensitivity, such as dyspnea, hypotension, and urticaria, occurred in less than 0.9% of abatacept-treated patients and generally occurred within 24 hours of abatacept infusion. Appropriate medical support measures for the treatment of hypersensitivity reactions should be available for immediate use in the event of a reaction.

COPD – In study 5, there were 37 patients with COPD who were treated with abatacept and 17 patients with COPD who were treated with placebo. The COPD patients treated with abatacept developed adverse reactions more frequently than those treated with placebo (97% versus 88%, respectively). Respiratory disorders occurred more frequently in abatacept-treated patients compared with placebo-treated patients (43% versus 24%, respectively), including COPD exacerbation, cough, dyspnea, and rhonchi. A higher percentage of abatacept-treated patients developed a serious adverse reaction compared with placebo-treated patients (27% vs 6%), including COPD exacerbation (3 of 37 patients [8%]) and pneumonia (1 of 37 patients [3%]).

Other adverse reactions – Adverse reactions occurring in 3% or more of patients and at least 1% more frequently in abatacept-treated patients during placebo-controlled RA studies are summarized in the following table.

Abatacept Adverse Reactions in RA Studies (≥ 3%)

Adverse reaction	Abatacept (n = 1,955)[a]	Placebo (n = 989)[b]
CNS		
Dizziness	9%	7%
Headache	18%	13%
Dermatologic		
Rash	4%	3%
GI		
Dyspepsia	6%	4%
Respiratory		
Cough	8%	7%
Nasopharyngitis	12%	9%
Miscellaneous		
Back pain	7%	6%
Hypertension	7%	4%
Pain in extremity	3%	2%
Urinary tract infection	6%	5%

[a] Includes 204 patients on concomitant biologic DMARDs (adalimumab, anakinra, etanercept, or infliximab).
[b] Includes 134 patients on concomitant biologic DMARDs (adalimumab, anakinra, etanercept, or infliximab).

Immunogenicity – Antibodies directed against the entire abatacept molecule or to the cytotoxic T-lymphocyte-associated antigen 4 (CTLA-4) portion of abatacept were assessed by enzyme-linked immunoabsorbent assays (ELISA) in patients with RA for up to 2 years following repeated treatment with abatacept. Thirty-four of 1,993 (1.7%) patients developed binding antibodies to the entire abatacept molecule or to the CTLA-4 portion of abatacept. Because trough levels of abatacept can interfere with assay results, a subset analysis was performed. In this analysis, it was observed that 9 of 154 (5.8%) patients who had discontinued treatment with abatacept for more than 56 days developed antibodies.

Samples with confirmed binding activity to CTLA-4 were assessed for the presence of neutralizing antibodies in a cell-based luciferase reporter assay. Six of 9 (67%) evaluable patients were shown to possess neutralizing antibodies. No correlation of antibody development to clinical response or adverse reactions was observed.

The data reflect the percentage of patients whose test results were positive for antibodies to abatacept in specific assays. The observed incidence of antibody (including neutralizing antibody) positivity in an assay is highly dependent on several factors, including assay sensitivity and specificity, assay methodology, sample handling, timing of sample collection, concomitant medication, and underlying disease. For these reasons, comparison of the incidence of antibodies to abatacept with the incidence of antibodies to other products may be misleading.

➤*Juvenile idiopathic arthritis:* In general, the adverse reactions in children were similar in frequency and type to those seen in adult patients.

Abatacept has been studied in 190 children 6 to 17 years of age with polyarticular juvenile idiopathic arthritis. Overall frequency of adverse reactions in the 4-month, lead-in, open-label period of the study was 70%; infections occurred at a frequency of 36%. The most common infections were nasopharyngitis and upper respiratory tract infection. The infections resolved without sequelae, and the types of infections were consistent with those commonly seen in outpatient pediatric populations. Other reactions that occurred at a prevalence of at least 5% were abdominal pain, cough, diarrhea, headache, nausea, and pyrexia.

Six serious adverse reactions (acute lymphocytic leukemia, disease flare [2], joint wear, ovarian cyst, and varicella infection) were reported during the initial 4 months of treatment with abatacept.

Of the 190 patients with juvenile idiopathic arthritis treated with abatacept in clinical trials, there was 1 case of a hypersensitivity reaction (0.5%). During periods A, B, and C, acute infusion-related reactions occurred at a frequency of 4%, 2%, and 3%, respectively, and were consistent with the types of reactions reported in adults.

Upon continued treatment in the open-label extension period, the types of adverse reactions were similar in frequency and type to those seen in adult patients, except for a single patient diagnosed with multiple sclerosis while on open-label treatment.

Immunogenicity – Antibodies directed against the entire abatacept molecule or to the CTLA-4 portion of abatacept were assessed by ELISA assays in patients with juvenile idiopathic arthritis following repeated treatment with abatacept throughout the open-label period. For patients who were withdrawn from therapy for up to 6 months during the double-blind period, the rate of antibody formation to the CTLA-4 portion of the molecule was 41% (22/54), while for those who remained on therapy, the rate was 13% (7/54).

The presence of antibodies was generally transient and titers were low. The presence of antibodies was not associated with adverse reactions, changes in efficacy, or an effect on serum concentrations of abatacept. For patients who were withdrawn from abatacept during the double-blind period for up to 6 months, no serious acute infusion-related reactions were observed upon reinitiation of abatacept therapy.

➤*Postmarketing:* Adverse reactions have been reported during postapproval use of abatacept. Because these reactions are reported voluntarily from a population of uncertain size, it is not always possible to reliably estimate their frequency or establish a causal relationship to abatacept. Based on the postmarketing experience with abatacept in adult patients with RA, the adverse reaction profile of abatacept does not differ from that previously listed/discussed.

ABATACEPT — INJECTION

Overdosage

➤*Animal toxicology:* A juvenile animal study was conducted in rats dosed with abatacept from 4 to 94 days of age in which an increase in the incidence of infections leading to death occurred at all doses compared with controls. Altered T-cell subsets, including increased T-helper cells and reduced T-regulatory cells, were observed. In addition, inhibition of T-cell-dependent antibody responses was observed. Upon following these animals into adulthood, lymphocytic inflammation of the thyroid and pancreatic islets was observed.

In studies of adult mice and monkeys, inhibition of T-cell-dependent antibody responses was apparent. However, infection and mortality, altered T-helper cells, and inflammation of the thyroid and pancreas were not observed.

➤*Symptoms:* Abatacept is administered as an IV infusion under medically controlled conditions. Doses of up to 50 mg/kg have been administered without apparent toxic effect.

➤*Treatment:* In case of overdosage, it is recommended that the patient be monitored for any signs or symptoms of adverse reactions and that appropriate symptomatic treatment be instituted.

Patient Information

Inform patients that they should not receive abatacept treatment concomitantly with a TNF antagonist, such as adalimumab, etanercept, and infliximab, because such combination therapy may increase their risk for infections. Also inform them that they should not receive abatacept concomitantly with other biologic RA therapy, such as anakinra, because there is not enough information to assess the safety and efficacy of such combination therapy.

Instruct patients to immediately tell their health care provider if they experience symptoms of an allergic reaction during or for the first day after the administration of abatacept.

Ask patients if they have a history of recurrent infections, have underlying conditions that may predispose them to infections, or have chronic, latent, or localized infections. Ask patients if they have had TB, a positive skin test for TB, or recently have been in close contact with someone who has had TB. Instruct patients that they may be tested for TB before they receive abatacept. Inform patients to tell their health care provider if they develop an infection during therapy with abatacept.

Inform patients that live vaccines should not be given concurrently with abatacept or within 3 months of its discontinuation. Inform caregivers of patients with juvenile idiopathic arthritis that the patients should be brought up to date with all immunizations in agreement with current immunization guidelines prior to initiating abatacept therapy; tell patients to discuss with their health care provider how best to handle future immunizations once abatacept therapy has been initiated.

Inform patients that abatacept has not been studied in pregnant women or breast-feeding mothers so the effects of abatacept on pregnant women or breast-feeding infants are not known. Also instruct patients to tell their health care provider if they are pregnant, become pregnant, or are thinking about becoming pregnant. Instruct patients to tell their health care provider if they plan to breast-feed their infant.

Ask patients if they have diabetes. Maltose contained in abatacept can give falsely elevated blood glucose readings with certain blood glucose monitors on the day of abatacept infusion. If a patient is using such a monitor, advise the patient to discuss with their health care provider methods that do not react with maltose.

THALIDOMIDE

Rx	**Thalomid**[a] (Celgene)	**Capsules:** 50 mg	(Celgene/50 mg). White, opaque. In blister pack 28s and 280s.
		100 mg	(Celgene/100 mg). Tan. In blister pack 28s and 140s.
		200 mg	(Celgene/200 mg). Blue. In blister pack 28s and 84s.

[a] Available only to be prescribed and dispensed under the terms of the System for Thalidomide Education and Prescribing Safety (S.T.E.P.S.) restricted distribution program.

THALIDOMIDE — ORAL

WARNING

Severe, life-threatening human birth defects – If thalidomide is taken during pregnancy, it can cause severe birth defects or death to a fetus. Thalidomide should never be used by women who are pregnant or who could become pregnant while taking the drug. Even a single dose (one 50, 100, or 200 mg capsule) taken by a pregnant woman can cause severe birth defects. Because of this toxicity and in an effort to make the chance of fetal exposure to thalidomide as negligible as possible, thalidomide is approved for marketing only under a special restricted distribution program approved by the Food and Drug Administration (FDA). This program is called the System for Thalidomide Education and Prescribing Safety (S.T.E.P.S.). Under this restricted distribution program, only prescribers and pharmacists registered with the program are allowed to prescribe and dispense the product. In addition, patients must be advised of, agree to, and comply with the requirements of the S.T.E.P.S. program in order to receive the product.

Prescribers – Thalidomide may be prescribed only by licensed prescribers who are registered in the S.T.E.P.S. program and understand the risk of teratogenicity if thalidomide is used during pregnancy. The following major human fetal abnormalities related to thalidomide administration during pregnancy have been documented: absence of bones, amelia (absence of limbs), congenital heart defects, external ear abnormalities (including anotia, micro pinna, small or absent external auditory canals), eye abnormalities (anophthalmos, microphthalmos), facial palsy, hypoplasticity of the bones, and phocomelia (short limbs). Alimentary tract, urinary tract, and genital malformations also have been documented. Mortality at or shortly after birth has been reported at about 40%. Effective contraception must be used for at least 4 weeks before beginning thalidomide therapy, during therapy, and for 4 weeks following discontinuation of therapy. Reliable contraception is indicated even where there has been a history of infertility, unless the patient has had a hysterectomy or has been postmenopausal for at least 24 months. Two reliable forms of contraception must be used simultaneously unless continuous abstinence from heterosexual sexual intercourse is the chosen method. Refer women of childbearing potential to a qualified provider of contraceptive methods, if needed. Sexually mature women who have not undergone a hysterectomy or who have not been postmenopausal for at least 24 consecutive months (ie, who have had menses at some time in the preceding 24 consecutive months) are considered to be women of childbearing potential.

WARNING (cont.)

Before starting treatment, administer a pregnancy test (sensitivity of at least 50 milliunits/mL) to women of childbearing potential. Perform the test within the 24 hours prior to beginning therapy. A prescription for thalidomide for a woman of childbearing potential must not be issued until a written report of a negative pregnancy test has been obtained by the prescriber. Once treatment has started, test for pregnancy weekly during the first 4 weeks of use, then repeat pregnancy testing at 4 weeks in women with regular menstrual cycles. If menstrual cycles are irregular, test for pregnancy every 2 weeks. Perform pregnancy testing and counseling if a patient misses her period or if there is any abnormality in menstrual bleeding.

If pregnancy occurs during thalidomide treatment, discontinue the drug immediately.

Report any suspected fetal exposure to thalidomide to the FDA immediately via MedWatch at 1-800-FDA-1088 and also to the manufacturer. Refer the patient to an obstetrician/gynecologist experienced in reproductive toxicity for further evaluation and counseling.

Men – Because thalidomide is present in the semen of patients receiving the drug, men receiving thalidomide must always use a latex condom during any sexual contact with women of childbearing potential, even if he has undergone a successful vasectomy.

Thalidomide is contraindicated in sexually mature men unless the patient meets ALL of the following conditions:

- He understands and can reliably carry out instructions.
- He is capable of complying with the mandatory contraceptive measures that are appropriate for men, patient registration, and patient survey as described in the S.T.E.P.S. program.
- He has received both oral and written warnings of the hazards of taking thalidomide and exposing a fetus to the drug.
- He has received both oral and written warnings of the risk of possible contraception failure and of the presence of thalidomide in semen. He has been instructed that he must always use a latex condom during any sexual contact with women of childbearing potential, even if he has undergone successful vasectomy.
- He acknowledges, in writing, his understanding of these warnings and of the need to use a latex condom during any sexual contact with women of childbearing potential, even if he has undergone a successful vasectomy, when having sexual intercourse with women of childbearing potential. Sexually mature women who have not undergone a hysterectomy or who have not been postmenopausal for at least 24 consecutive months (ie, who have had menses at some time in the preceding 24 consecutive months) are considered to be women of childbearing potential.

THALIDOMIDE — ORAL

WARNING (cont.)

- If the patient is between 12 and 18 years of age, his parent or legal guardian must have read this material and agreed to ensure compliance.

Women – Thalidomide is contraindicated in women of childbearing potential unless alternative therapies are considered inappropriate and the patient meets all of the following conditions (ie, she is essentially unable to become pregnant while on thalidomide therapy):

- She understands and can reliably carry out instructions.
- She is capable of complying with the mandatory contraceptive measures, pregnancy testing, patient registration, and patient survey as described in the S.T.E.P.S. program.
- She has received both oral and written warnings of the hazards of taking thalidomide during pregnancy and of exposing a fetus to the drug.
- She has received both oral and written warnings of the risk of possible contraception failure and of the need to use 2 reliable forms of contraception simultaneously, unless continuous abstinence from heterosexual sexual intercourse is the chosen method. Sexually mature women who have not undergone a hysterectomy or who have not been postmenopausal for at least 24 consecutive months (ie, who have had menses at some time in the preceding 24 consecutive months) are considered to be women of childbearing potential.
- She acknowledges, in writing, her understanding of these warnings and of the need for using 2 reliable methods of contraception for 4 weeks prior to starting thalidomide therapy, during thalidomide therapy, and for 4 weeks after stopping thalidomide therapy.
- She has had a negative pregnancy test, with a sensitivity of at least 50 milliunits/mL, within the 24 hours prior to beginning therapy.
- If the patient is between 12 and 18 years of age, her parent or legal guardian must have read this material and agreed to ensure compliance.

Venous thromboembolic events – The use of thalidomide in multiple myeloma results in an increased risk of venous thromboembolic events, such as deep venous thrombosis and pulmonary embolus. This risk increases significantly when thalidomide is used in combination with standard chemotherapeutic agents, including dexamethasone. In one controlled trial, the rate of venous thromboembolic events was 22.5% in patients receiving thalidomide in combination with dexamethasone, compared with 4.9% in patients receiving dexamethasone alone (P = 0.002). Patients and health care providers are advised to be observant for the signs and symptoms of thromboembolism. Instruct patients to seek medical care if they develop symptoms such as arm or leg swelling, chest pain, or shortness of breath. Preliminary data suggest that patients who are appropriate candidates may benefit from concurrent prophylactic anticoagulation or aspirin treatment.

Indications

➤*Multiple myeloma:* In combination with dexamethasone, for the treatment of patients with newly diagnosed multiple myeloma.

➤*Erythema nodosum leprosum:*

Acute treatment – Acute treatment of the cutaneous manifestations of moderate to severe erythema nodosum leprosum. Not indicated as monotherapy for such erythema nodosum leprosum treatment in the presence of moderate to severe neuritis.

Maintenance therapy – For prevention and suppression of the cutaneous manifestations of erythema nodosum leprosum recurrence.

➤*Off-label uses:*

Aphthous ulcers – [3] = Safety concerns. Thalidomide appears to be an effective treatment option for aphthous ulcers in healthy patients and those with HIV infections. Careful consideration is needed when deciding to use thalidomide because of its adverse event profile and black box warning regarding the high risk of birth defects when used by women or men. Larger studies are needed to study risks of longer-term therapy and optimal dosing.

Behçet syndrome – [3] = Safety concerns. Studies have confirmed a therapeutic role for thalidomide in patients with Behçet syndrome who have been unresponsive to conventional therapy or who have suffered intolerable adverse reactions. However, larger, controlled trials are needed.

Cachexia – [3] = Safety concerns. Limited data suggest that short-term treatment of cachexia with thalidomide results in significant weight gain and increases in lean body mass in patients with cancer but may not increase lean body mass in AIDS-associated wasting. Thalidomide has a black box warning for men and women regarding severe teratogenic potential and requires a restricted dispensing program that should be discussed with patients when weighing the benefits and risks of therapy. Larger studies are needed to identify appropriate candidates as well as optimal dosage and duration of thalidomide therapy in patients with cachexia caused by cancer, HIV/AIDS, and other chronic diseases.

Cholestatic pruritus (adults) – [5] = Poor documentation. Data regarding thalidomide, a recognized teratogen, in the treatment of cholestatic pruritus are limited. Despite apparent benefits observed in a small number of patients, several other treatment modalities with more benign safety profiles are available.

Crohn disease – [3] = Safety concerns. Case reports have shown thalidomide to be effective in reversing oral and colonic ulcerations. Symptomatic improvement has occurred within 2 to 4 weeks, and continued therapy has reduced recurrences. Full publication of abstract data and presentations will clarify the initial beneficial results observed in case reports.

Generalized pruritus – [3] = Safety concerns. Data regarding thalidomide, a recognized teratogen, in the treatment of pruritus are limited. Despite apparent benefits observed in a small number of patients, several other treatment modalities with more benign safety profiles are available.

GI bleeding – [3] = Safety concerns. Published information regarding the use of thalidomide in the treatment of severe GI bleeding related to angiodysplasias and other causes is limited to case report data. In all published cases, thalidomide resulted in either dramatic improvement or resolution of intestinal bleeding.

Juvenile idiopathic arthritis – [4] = Insufficient documentation. Data evaluating the safety and efficacy of thalidomide for the treatment of systemic-onset juvenile idiopathic arthritis (JIA) are limited to a handful of case reports. Although these reports show potential promise, additional studies are needed to define the optimal dose and patient population that would most benefit from therapy. Given the safety concerns associated with thalidomide therapy, routine use in patients with systemic-onset JIA should be avoided until additional data are available. Currently, there are no national guidelines for the management of JIA.

Rheumatoid arthritis – [3] = Safety concerns. Clinical trials evaluating the efficacy of thalidomide for the treatment of rheumatoid arthritis (RA) show limited to no clinical benefit and considerable toxicity. The most recent American College of Rheumatology (ACR) recommendations for the treatment of RA do not include thalidomide. Given the safety concerns and available treatment options with demonstrated efficacy, its use is not recommended.

Uremic pruritus – [3] = Safety concerns. Data regarding thalidomide, a recognized teratogen, in the treatment of pruritus are limited. Despite apparent benefits observed in a small number of patients, several other treatment modalities with more benign safety profiles are available.

Other possible off-label uses – Graft versus host disease after bone marrow transplantation; refractory multiple myeloma; primary brain tumors; prostate cancer (in combination with docetaxel).

Administration and Dosage

➤*General dosing considerations:* Thalidomide must only be administered in compliance with all of the terms outlined in the S.T.E.P.S. program. Thalidomide may only be prescribed by health care providers registered with the S.T.E.P.S. program and dispensed by pharmacists registered with the S.T.E.P.S. program.

Prescribing thalidomide to women of childbearing potential is contingent upon initial and continued confirmed negative results of pregnancy testing.

Dispensing instructions – This product is only supplied to pharmacists registered with the S.T.E.P.S. program (see the Warning Box). Pharmacist's note: Before dispensing thalidomide, activate the authorization number on every prescription by calling the manufacturer's customer center at 1-888-423-5436 and obtaining a confirmation number. Write the confirmation number on the prescription. Accept a thalidomide prescription only if it has been issued within the previous 7 days (telephone prescriptions are not permitted); dispense no more than a 4-week (28-day) supply. A new prescription is required for further dispensing. Dispense blister packs intact (capsules cannot be repackaged). Dispense subsequent prescriptions only if fewer than 7 days of therapy remain on the previous prescription, and educate all staff pharmacists about the dispensing procedure for thalidomide.

➤*Adults:*

Multiple myeloma –

Usual dosage: 200 mg orally, once daily with water, preferably at bedtime, and at least 1 hour after the evening meal.

Concomitant therapy: Administer in combination with dexamethasone in 28-day treatment cycles. The dosage of dexamethasone is 40 mg daily administered orally on days 1 to 4, 9 to 12, and 17 to 20 every 28 days.

Discontinuation of therapy: Patients who develop adverse reactions such as constipation, oversedation, or peripheral neuropathy may benefit by either temporarily discontinuing the drug or continuing at a lower dose. With the abatement of these adverse reactions, the drug may be started at a lower dose or at the previous dose, based on clinical judgement.

Erythema nodosum leprosum –

Initial dosage: 100 to 300 mg/day, once daily with water, preferably at bedtime, and at least 1 hour after the evening meal. Start patients weighing less than 50 kg (110 lb) at the low end of the dose range.

In patients with a severe cutaneous erythema nodosum leprosum reaction, or in those who have previously required higher doses to control the reaction, thalidomide dosing may be initiated at higher doses, up to 400 mg/day once daily at bedtime or in divided doses with water at least 1 hour after meals.

Maintenance dosage: Maintain patients who have a documented history of requiring prolonged maintenance treatment to prevent the recurrence of cutaneous erythema nodosum leprosum or who flare during tapering on the minimum dose necessary to control the reaction. Attempt tapering of medication every 3 to 6 months in decrements of 50 mg every 2 to 4 weeks.

Duration of therapy: Continue dosing with thalidomide until signs and symptoms of active reaction have subsided, usually at least 2 weeks. Patients then may be tapered off medication in 50 mg decrements every 2 to 4 weeks.

Concomitant therapy: In patients with moderate to severe neuritis associated with a severe erythema nodosum leprosum reaction, corticosteroids may be started concomitantly with thalidomide. Steroid usage can be tapered and discontinued when the neuritis has ameliorated.

THALIDOMIDE — ORAL

Off-label dosing –

Aphthous ulcers: [3] = Safety concerns. 100 to 400 mg/day given orally either once daily or in divided doses twice daily. Low-dose therapy of 50 mg/day has also been effective. Benefit is seen within 1 to 3 weeks of therapy, and recurrence typically occurs within a few weeks of discontinuing thalidomide.

Behçet syndrome: [3] = Safety concerns. 50 to 400 mg daily orally.

Cachexia: [3] = Safety concerns. 200 mg orally given once daily for 8 to 24 weeks.

Crohn disease: [3] = Safety concerns. 25 to 300 mg/day for up to 1 year.

Generalized pruritus: [3] = Safety concerns. 200 mg nightly for 2 nights.

GI bleeding: [3] = Safety concerns. Initial doses range from 100 to 400 mg daily. In 1 case series, patients treated with initial doses of 300 mg daily were tapered to 100 mg daily after 3 months. Treatment duration was several months in some patients.

Juvenile idiopathic arthritis: [4] = Insufficient documentation.

• *Patients 3 to 23 years of age* – 2 mg/kg daily (range, 1.5 to 5 mg/kg), with doses typically rounded to the nearest 50 mg. Duration of therapy was not reported.

Rheumatoid arthritis: [3] = Safety concerns. 100 to 600 mg daily, with higher doses titrated over several weeks. Treatment continued for up to 20 weeks in 1 study.

Uremic pruritus: [3] = Safety concerns. 100 mg nightly for 7 days.

➤*Children:*

12 years of age and older –

Erythema nodosum leprosum: See Adults for dosing.

Off-label dosing –

Juvenile idiopathic arthritis: [4] = Insufficient documentation.

• *Patients 3 to 23 years of age* – 2 mg/kg daily (range, 1.5 to 5 mg/kg), with doses typically rounded to the nearest 50 mg. Duration of therapy was not reported.

➤*Preparation for administration:* Thalidomide is considered a cytotoxic agent and a teratogen. Follow safe handling procedures when preparing, administering, or dispensing thalidomide.

➤*Storage/Stability:* Store at 25°C (77°F); excursions are permitted to 15° to 30°C (59° to 86°F). Protect from light.

Actions

➤*Pharmacology:* The mechanism of action of thalidomide is not fully understood. Thalidomide possesses immunomodulatory, anti-inflammatory, and antiangiogenic properties.

Data suggest that the immunologic effects of thalidomide can vary substantially under different conditions, but may be related to suppression of excessive tumor necrosis factor-alpha (TNF-α) production and down-modulation of selected cell surface adhesion molecules involved in leukocyte migration. For example, administration of thalidomide has been reported to decrease circulating levels of TNF-α in patients with erythema nodosum leprosum; however, it also has been shown to increase plasma TNF-α levels in HIV-seropositive patients. Other anti-inflammatory and immunomodulatory properties of thalidomide may include suppression of macrophage involvement in prostaglandin synthesis and modulation of interleukin-10 and interleukin-12 production by peripheral blood mononuclear cells. Thalidomide treatment of multiple myeloma patients is accompanied by an increase in the number of circulating natural killer cells, and an increase in plasma levels of interleukin-2 and interferon-gamma (T-cell-derived cytokines associated with cytotoxic activity). Thalidomide was found to inhibit angiogenesis in a human umbilical artery explant model in vitro. The cellular processes of angiogenesis inhibited by thalidomide may include the proliferation of endothelial cells.

➤*Pharmacokinetics:*

Absorption – The absolute bioavailability of oral thalidomide has not yet been characterized in human subjects because of its poor aqueous solubility. However, the capsules are 90% bioavailable relative to oral polyethylene glycol solution. In studies of healthy volunteers and subjects with Hansen disease, the mean time to peak plasma concentrations (T_{max}) of thalidomide ranged from 2.9 to 5.7 hours, indicating that thalidomide is slowly absorbed from the GI tract. While the extent of absorption as measured by the area under the curve (AUC) is proportional to the dose in healthy subjects, the maximum plasma concentration (C_{max}) increased in a less than proportional manner (see the following table). This lack of C_{max} dose proportionality, coupled with the observed increase in T_{max} values, suggests that the poor solubility of thalidomide in aqueous media may be hindering the rate of absorption.

Various Thalidomide Pharmacokinetic Parameters (Mean)

Population/ single dose	$AUC_{0-\infty}$ (mcg•h/mL)	C_{max} (mcg/mL)	T_{max} (h)	Half-life (h)
Healthy subjects (n = 14)				
50 mg	4.9 (16%)	0.62 (52%)	2.9 (66%)	5.52 (37%)
200 mg	18.9 (17%)	1.76 (30%)	3.5 (57%)	5.53 (25%)
400 mg	36.4 (26%)	2.82 (28%)	4.3 (37%)	7.29 (36%)
Patients with Hansen disease (n = 6)				
400 mg	46.4 (44.1%)	3.44 (52.6%)	5.7 (27%)	6.86 (17%)

Coadministration of thalidomide with a high-fat meal causes minor (less than 10%) changes in the observed AUC and C_{max} values; however, it causes an increase in T_{max} to approximately 6 hours.

Distribution – In human blood plasma, the geometric mean plasma protein binding was 55% and 66%, respectively, for (+)-(R)- and (−)-(S)-thalidomide. In a pharmacokinetic study of thalidomide in HIV-seropositive men receiving thalidomide 100 mg/day, thalidomide was detectable in the semen.

Metabolism – The exact metabolic route and fate of thalidomide is not known. Thalidomide does not appear to be hepatically metabolized to any large extent, but appears to undergo nonenzymatic hydrolysis in plasma to multiple products. In a repeat dose study in which thalidomide 200 mg was given to 10 healthy women for 18 days, thalidomide showed similar pharmacokinetic profiles on the first and last day of dosing. Thalidomide does not appear to induce or inhibit its own metabolism.

Excretion – As indicated in the previous table, the mean elimination half-life ranges from approximately 5 to 7 hours after a single dose and is not altered by multiple dosing. Thalidomide has a renal clearance of 1.15 mL/min with less than 0.7% of the dose excreted in the urine as unchanged drug. Following a single dose, urinary levels of thalidomide were undetectable 48 hours after dosing. Although thalidomide is thought to be hydrolyzed to a number of metabolites, only a very small amount (0.02% of the administered dose) of 4-OH-thalidomide was identified in the urine of subjects 12 to 24 hours after dosing.

Special populations –

Renal function impairment: The pharmacokinetics of thalidomide in patients with renal function impairment have not been determined. In a study of 6 patients with end-stage renal disease, thalidomide 200 mg/day was administered on a nondialysis day and on a dialysis day. Comparison of concentration-time profiles in a nondialysis day and during dialysis where blood samples were collected at least 10 hours following the dose, showed that the mean total clearance increased by a factor of 2.5 during hemodialysis. Because the dialysis was performed 10 hours following administration of the dose, the drug-concentration time curves were not statistically significantly different for days patients were on and off of dialysis. Thus, no dosage adjustment is needed for patients with renal function impairment on dialysis.

Children: No pharmacokinetic data are available in subjects younger than 18 years of age.

Patients with Hansen disease: Analysis of data from a small study in patients with Hansen disease suggests that these patients, relative to healthy subjects, may have an increased bioavailability of thalidomide. The increase is reflected in increased AUC and in increased peak plasma levels. The clinical significance of this reason is unknown.

Contraindications

Pregnancy (*Category X*; see Warning Box and Warnings); hypersensitivity to the drug and its components.

Warnings/Precautions

➤*Severe birth defects:* See the Warning box for more information.

➤*Drowsiness and somnolence:* Thalidomide frequently causes drowsiness and somnolence. Instruct patients to avoid situations in which drowsiness may be a problem and not to take other medications that may cause drowsiness without adequate medical advice. Advise patients about the possible impairment of mental or physical abilities required for the performance of hazardous tasks, such as driving a car or operating other complex or dangerous machinery.

➤*Peripheral neuropathy:* Thalidomide is known to cause nerve damage that may be permanent. Peripheral neuropathy is a common, potentially severe, and irreversible side effect of treatment with thalidomide. Peripheral neuropathy generally occurs following chronic use over a period of months; however, reports following relatively short-term use also exist. The correlation with cumulative dose is unclear. Symptoms may occur some time after thalidomide treatment has been stopped and may resolve slowly or not at all. Few reports of neuropathy have arisen in the treatment of erythema nodosum leprosum despite long-term thalidomide treatment. However, the clinical inability to differentiate thalidomide neuropathy from the neuropathy often seen in Hansen disease makes it difficult to accurately determine the incidence of thalidomide-related neuropathy in patients with erythema nodosum leprosum.

See Drug Interactions for more information.

➤*Dizziness/orthostatic hypotension:* Thalidomide may cause dizziness and orthostatic hypotension. Advise patients to sit upright for a few minutes prior to standing up from a recumbent position.

➤*Neutropenia:* Decreased white blood cell counts, including neutropenia, have been reported. Do not initiate treatment in patients with an absolute neutrophil count (ANC) of less than 750/mm^3. Monitor white blood cell count and differential on an ongoing basis, especially in patients who may be more prone to neutropenia, such as patients who are HIV-seropositive. If ANC decreases to less than 750/mm^3 while on treatment, reevaluate the patient's medication regimen and, if neutropenia persists, consider withholding thalidomide if clinically appropriate.

➤*Patients with HIV:* In a randomized, placebo-controlled trial of thalidomide in HIV-seropositive patients, plasma HIV RNA levels were found to increase (median change, 0.42 $\log_{10}$ copies HIV RNA/mL; $P = 0.04$) compared with placebo. A similar trend was observed in a second, unpublished study conducted in patients who were HIV-seropositive. The clinical significance of this increase is unknown. Both studies were conducted prior to availability of highly active antiretroviral therapy. Until the clinical signifi-

THALIDOMIDE — ORAL

cance of this finding in HIV-seropositive patients is further understood, measure viral load after the first and third months of treatment and every 3 months thereafter.

➤*Thrombotic events:* See the Warning box for more information.

➤*Exposure:* The only type of thalidomide exposure known to result in drug-associated birth defects are as a result of direct oral ingestion of thalidomide. Currently, no specific data are available regarding the cutaneous absorption or inhalation of thalidomide in women of childbearing potential and whether these exposures may result in any birth defects. Instruct patients not to extensively handle or open thalidomide capsules and to maintain storage of capsules in blister packs until ingestion. If there is contact with nonintact thalidomide capsules or the powder contents, wash the exposed area with soap and water.

Thalidomide has been shown to be present in the serum and semen of patients receiving thalidomide. If health care providers or other caregivers are exposed to body fluids from patients receiving thalidomide, utilize appropriate precautions, such as wearing gloves, to prevent the potential cutaneous exposure to thalidomide or wash the exposed area with soap and water.

➤*Bradycardia:* Bradycardia in association with thalidomide use has been reported. There have been reports of cases of bradycardia requiring medical intervention. The clinical significance and underlying etiology of the bradycardia in some thalidomide-treated patients are unknown.

➤*Serious dermatological reactions:* Serious dermatological reactions, including Stevens-Johnson syndrome and toxic epidermal necrolysis, which may be fatal, have been reported. Discontinue thalidomide if a skin rash occurs and only resume following appropriate clinical evaluation. If the rash is exfoliative, purpuric, or bullous, or if Stevens-Johnson syndrome or toxic epidermal necrolysis is suspected, do not resume use of thalidomide.

➤*Seizures:* Although not reported from premarketing controlled clinical trials, seizures, including generalized tonic-clonic seizures, have been reported during postapproval use of thalidomide in clinical practice. Because these reactions are reported voluntarily from a population of unknown size, estimates of frequency cannot be made. Most patients had disorders that may have predisposed them to seizure activity, and it is not currently known whether thalidomide has any epileptogenic influence. During therapy with thalidomide, closely monitor patients with a history of seizures or with other risk factors for the development of seizures for clinical changes that could precipitate acute seizure activity.

➤*Hypersensitivity reactions:* Hypersensitivity to thalidomide has been reported. Signs and symptoms have included the occurrence of erythematous macular rash, possibly associated with fever, tachycardia, and hypotension. May necessitate interruption of therapy if severe. If the reaction recurs when dosing is resumed, discontinue thalidomide. SeeManagement of Acute Hypersensitivity Reactions.

➤*Pregnancy:* Category X.

Because of the known human teratogenicity of thalidomide, thalidomide is contraindicated in women who are pregnant or may become pregnant, and who are not using the 2 required types of birth control or who are not continually abstaining from heterosexual sexual contact. If thalidomide is taken during pregnancy, it can cause severe birth defects or death to a fetus. Thalidomide should never be used by women who are pregnant or who could become pregnant while taking the drug. Even a single dose (one 50, 100, or 200 mg capsule) taken by a pregnant woman can cause birth defects. If pregnancy does occur during treatment, immediately discontinue the drug. Under these conditions, refer the patient to an obstetrician/gynecologist experienced in reproductive toxicity for further evaluation and counseling. Any suspected fetal exposure to thalidomide must be reported to the FDA via the MedWatch program at 1-800-FDA-1088 and also to the manufacturer.

Because thalidomide is present in the semen of patients receiving the drug, men receiving thalidomide must always use a latex condom during any sexual contact with women of childbearing potential. The risk to the fetus from the semen of men taking thalidomide is unknown.

A pre- and postnasal reproductive toxicity study was conducted in pregnant female rabbits. Compound-related increased abortion incidences and elevated fetotoxicity were observed at the lowest oral dose level of 30 mg/kg/day (approximately 1.5-fold the maximum human dose based upon BSA) and all higher dose levels. Neonatal mortality was elevated at oral dose levels to the lactating female rabbits at least 150 mg/kg/day (approximately 7.5-fold the maximum human dose based upon BSA). No delay in postnatal development, including learning and memory functions, was noted at the oral dose level to the lactating female rabbits of 150 mg/kg/day (average thalidomide concentrations in milk ranged from 22 to 36 mcg/mL).

➤*Lactation:* It is not known whether thalidomide is excreted in breast milk. Because of the potential for serious adverse reactions in breast-feeding infants from thalidomide, either discontinue breast-feeding or the drug, taking into account the importance of the drug to the mother.

➤*Children:* Safety and efficacy in children younger than 12 years of age have not been established.

➤*Elderly:* Of the total number of subjects in the clinical study of thalidomide and dexamethasone combination, 50% were 65 years of age and older, while 15% were 75 years of age and older. No overall differences in safety and efficacy were observed between these subjects and younger subjects. Other reported clinical experience has not identified differences in responses between the elderly and younger patients, but greater sensitivity of some older individuals cannot be ruled out.

➤*Monitoring:* Perform pregnancy testing (sensitivity of at least 50 milliunits/mL) on women of childbearing potential. Perform the test within the 24 hours prior to beginning thalidomide therapy, weekly during the first month of use, then monthly thereafter in women with regular menstrual cycles or every 2 weeks in women with irregular menstrual cycles. Also perform pregnancy testing if a patient misses her period or if there is any abnormality in menstrual bleeding.

Monitor white blood cell and differential on an ongoing basis. Monitor for signs of neuropathy (numbness, tingling, or pain in hands and feet) at monthly intervals for the first 3 months of therapy. Monitor viral load of HIV-seropositive patients after first and third months of therapy and every 3 months thereafter.

Drug Interactions

Thalidomide Drug Interactions

Precipitant drug	Object drug[a]		Description
Thalidomide	Alcohol Barbiturates Chlorpromazine Reserpine	⬆	Thalidomide may enhance sedative activity of these agents.
Thalidomide	Medication associated with peripheral neuropathy (eg, metronidazole, vincristine, isoniazid)	⬆	Symptoms of peripheral neuropathy may be enhanced when thalidomide is taken with other medications known to cause peripheral neuropathy. Use caution when coadministering.
Medication associated with peripheral neuropathy (eg, metronidazole, vincristine, isoniazid)	Thalidomide		

[a] ⬆ = object drug increased.

➤*Drugs that interfere with hormonal contraceptives:* Concomitant use of carbamazepine, griseofulvin, HIV-protease inhibitors, modafinil, penicillins, rifabutin, rifampin, phenytoin, or certain herbal supplements, such as St. John's wort, with hormonal contraceptive agents may reduce the efficacy of the contraception for up to 1 month after discontinuation of these concomitant therapies. Therefore, women requiring treatment with 1 or more of these drugs must use 2 other effective or highly effective methods of contraception or abstain from heterosexual sexual contact while taking thalidomide.

➤*Drug/Food interactions:* See Actions for more information.

Adverse Reactions

See the Warning box for more information.

Thalidomide is considered to have very low emetogenic potential (less than 10% incidence of emesis).

Thalidomide is associated with bradycardia, dizziness/orthostatic hypotension, drowsiness/somnolence, HIV viral load increase, hypersensitivity, neutropenia, and peripheral neuropathy. Dizziness, rash, and somnolence are the most commonly observed adverse reactions associated with the use of thalidomide. Thalidomide has been studied in controlled and uncontrolled clinical trials in patients with multiple myeloma and erythema nodosum leprosum, and in people who are HIV-seropositive. In addition, thalidomide has been administered investigationally for more than 20 years in numerous indications. Adverse reaction profiles from these uses are summarized in the following information.

Because of the nature of the longitudinal data that form the basis of this product's safety evaluation, no determination has been made of the causal relationship between the reported adverse reactions listed in the following information and thalidomide. These lists are of various adverse reactions noted by investigators in patients to whom they had administered thalidomide under various conditions. The use of thalidomide may not limit disease progression and/or death.

➤*Multiple myeloma controlled clinical trial:* The safety analysis was conducted in 204 patients who received study drugs in the randomized trial. The following table lists the most common treatment-emergent signs and symptoms (occurring in at least 10% of patients) that were observed. The most frequently reported adverse reactions were confusion, constipation, dyspnea, edema, hypocalcemia, sensory neuropathy, thrombosis/embolism, and rash/desquamation (occurring in at least 20% of patients and with a frequency of at least 10% in patients treated with thalidomide and dexamethasone compared with dexamethasone alone).

Twenty-three percent of patients (47/204) discontinued because of adverse reactions: 30% (31/102) from the thalidomide and dexamethasone arm and 16% (16/102) from the dexamethasone alone arm.

THALIDOMIDE — ORAL

Thalidomide Adverse Reactions in Multiple Myeloma Trial (≥ 10%)						
Adverse reactions	Thalidomide + dexamethasone (n = 102)			Dexamethasone alone (n = 102)		
	All reactions	Grade 3 reactions	Grade 4 reactions	All reactions	Grade 3 reactions	Grade 4 reactions
Cardiovascular	70 (68.6%)	24 (23.5%)	14 (13.7%)	60 (58.8%)	17 (16.7%)	5 (4.9%)
Hypertension	11 (10.8%)	1 (1%)	0 (0%)	12 (11.8%)	9 (8.8%)	0 (0%)
Hypotension	16 (15.7%)	7 (6.9%)	2 (2%)	15 (14.7%)	2 (2%)	3 (2.9%)
Thrombosis/ embolism	23 (22.5%)	13 (12.7%)	9 (8.8%)	5 (4.9%)	3 (2.9%)	2 (2%)
CNS	92 (90.2%)	27 (26.5%)	5 (4.9%)	76 (74.5%)	15 (14.7%)	4 (3.9%)
Anxiety/ agitation	26 (25.5%)	1 (1%)	0 (0%)	14 (13.7%)	3 (2.9%)	0 (0%)
Confusion	29 (28.4%)	6 (5.9%)	3 (2.9%)	12 (11.8%)	2 (2%)	3 (2.9%)
Depression	22 (21.6%)	2 (2%)	0 (0%)	24 (23.5%)	1 (1%)	0 (0%)
Dizziness/ light-headedness	20 (19.6%)	1 (1%)	0 (0%)	14 (13.7%)	0 (0%)	0 (0%)
Insomnia	23 (22.5%)	0 (0%)	0 (0%)	48 (47.1%)	5 (4.9%)	0 (0%)
Neuropathy (motor)	22 (21.6%)	7 (6.9%)	1 (1%)	16 (15.7%)	5 (4.9%)	1 (1%)
Neuropathy (sensory)	55 (53.9%)	3 (2.9%)	1 (1%)	28 (27.5%)	1 (1%)	0 (0%)
Tremor	26 (25.5%)	1 (1%)	0 (0%)	6 (5.9%)	0 (0%)	0 (0%)
Dermatologic	48 (47.1%)	5 (4.9%)	1 (1%)	35 (34.3%)	2 (2%)	0 (0%)
Dry skin	21 (20.6%)	0 (0%)	0 (0%)	11 (10.8%)	0 (0%)	0 (0%)
Rash/ desquamation	31 (30.4%)	4 (3.9%)	0 (0%)	18 (17.6%)	2 (2%)	0 (0%)
GI	83 (81.4%)	19 (18.6%)	3 (2.9%)	70 (68.6%)	8 (7.8%)	0 (0%)
Anorexia	29 (28.4%)	4 (3.9%)	0 (0%)	25 (24.5%)	2 (2%)	0 (0%)
Constipation	56 (54.9%)	8 (7.8%)	0 (0%)	29 (28.4%)	1 (1%)	0 (0%)
Diarrhea	12 (11.8%)	1 (1%)	0 (0%)	17 (16.7%)	3 (2.9%)	0 (0%)
Dyspepsia	8 (7.8%)	1 (1%)	0 (0%)	19 (18.6%)	1 (1%)	0 (0%)
Nausea	29 (28.4%)	5 (4.9%)	0 (0%)	23 (22.5%)	1 (1%)	0 (0%)
Vomiting	12 (11.8%)	2 (2%)	0 (0%)	12 (11.8%)	1 (1%)	0 (0%)
GU	43 (42.2%)	3 (2.9%)	3 (2.9%)	49 (48%)	4 (3.9%)	3 (2.9%)
Creatinine	36 (35.3%)	1 (1%)	1 (1%)	43 (42.2%)	2 (2%)	2 (2%)
Hematologic	88 (86.3%)	25 (24.5%)	9 (8.8%)	96 (94.1%)	10 (9.8%)	10 (9.8%)
Hemoglobin decreased	79 (77.5%)	13 (12.7%)	3 (2.9%)	88 (86.3%)	5 (4.9%)	1 (1%)
Leukocytes decreased	36 (35.3%)	6 (5.9%)	1 (1%)	30 (29.4%)	1 (1%)	2 (2%)
Neutrophils decreased	32 (31.4%)	8 (7.8%)	5 (4.9%)	24 (23.5%)	3 (2.9%)	8 (7.8%)
Platelets decreased	24 (23.5%)	2 (2%)	2 (2%)	34 (33.3%)	3 (2.9%)	0 (0%)
Hepatic	47 (46.1%)	5 (4.9%)	2 (2%)	45 (44.1%)	3 (2.9%)	1 (1%)
Alkaline phosphatase increased	27 (26.5%)	0 (0%)	0 (0%)	29 (28.4%)	1 (1%)	0 (0%)
AST increased	25 (24.5%)	1 (1%)	1 (1%)	24 (23.5%)	1 (1%)	1 (1%)
Bilirubin increased	14 (13.7%)	1 (1%)	1 (1%)	10 (9.8%)	1 (1%)	1 (1%)
Metabolic/ laboratory	97 (95.1%)	30 (29.4%)	15 (14.7%)	96 (94.1%)	28 (27.5%)	6 (5.9%)
Hyperglycemia	74 (72.5%)	12 (11.8%)	4 (3.9%)	81 (79.4%)	17 (16.7%)	2 (2%)

Thalidomide Adverse Reactions in Multiple Myeloma Trial (≥ 10%)						
Adverse reactions	Thalidomide + dexamethasone (n = 102)			Dexamethasone alone (n = 102)		
	All reactions	Grade 3 reactions	Grade 4 reactions	All reactions	Grade 3 reactions	Grade 4 reactions
Hyperkalemia	19 (18.6%)	1 (1%)	2 (2%)	20 (19.6%)	2 (2%)	0 (0%)
Hypocalcemia	73 (71.6%)	9 (8.8%)	6 (5.9%)	60 (58.8%)	4 (3.9%)	1 (1%)
Hypokalemia	23 (22.5%)	4 (3.9%)	1 (1%)	23 (22.5%)	0 (0%)	1 (1%)
Hyponatremia	44 (43.1%)	11 (10.8%)	2 (2%)	49 (48%)	13 (12.7%)	2 (2%)
Musculoskeletal	42 (41.2%)	8 (7.8%)	2 (2%)	41 (40.2%)	11 (10.8%)	3 (2.9%)
Muscle weakness	41 (40.2%)	6 (5.9%)	1 (1%)	38 (37.3%)	10 (9.8%)	3 (2.9%)
Pain	64 (62.7%)	8 (7.8%)	2 (2%)	66 (64.7%)	15 (14.7%)	0 (0%)
Arthralgia	13 (12.7%)	0 (0%)	0 (0%)	10 (9.8%)	2 (2%)	0 (0%)
Bone pain	31 (30.4%)	3 (2.9%)	2 (2%)	37 (36.3%)	11 (10.8%)	0 (0%)
Headache	20 (19.6%)	3 (2.9%)	0 (0%)	23 (22.5%)	0 (0%)	0 (0%)
Myalgia	17 (16.7%)	0 (0%)	0 (0%)	14 (13.7%)	1 (1%)	0 (0%)
Pain, other	25 (24.5%)	4 (3.9%)	0 (0%)	26 (25.5%)	3 (2.9%)	0 (0%)
Pulmonary	52 (51%)	15 (14.7%)	6 (5.9%)	51 (50%)	15 (14.7%)	5 (4.9%)
Cough	15 (14.7%)	0 (0%)	0 (0%)	19 (18.6%)	0 (0%)	0 (0%)
Dyspnea	43 (42.2%)	10 (9.8%)	3 (2.9%)	32 (31.4%)	12 (11.8%)	4 (3.9%)
Miscellaneous	91 (89.2%)	17 (16.7%)	3 (2.9%)	84 (82.4%)	15 (14.7%)	2 (2%)
Edema	58 (56.9%)	6 (5.9%)	0 (0%)	47 (46.1%)	4 (3.9%)	0 (0%)
Fatigue	81 (79.4%)	14 (13.7%)	3 (2.9%)	72 (70.6%)	12 (11.8%)	2 (2%)
Fever	24 (23.5%)	1 (1%)	0 (0%)	20 (19.6%)	3 (2.9%)	0 (0%)
Infection/ febrile neutropenia	23 (22.5%)	5 (4.9%)	2 (2%)	28 (27.5%)	6 (5.9%)	6 (5.9%)
Infection without neutropenia	19 (17.6%)	4 (3.9%)	1 (1%)	18 (17.6%)	4 (3.9%)	2 (2%)
Weight gain	22 (21.6%)	1 (1%)	0 (0%)	13 (12.7%)	0 (0%)	0 (0%)
Weight loss	23 (22.5%)	1 (1%)	0 (0%)	21 (20.6%)	2 (2%)	0 (0%)

➤*Erythema nodosum leprosum controlled clinical trials:* The following table lists treatment-emergent signs and symptoms that occurred in thalidomide-treated patients in controlled clinical trials in erythema nodosum leprosum. Doses ranged from 50 to 300 mg/day. All adverse reactions were mild to moderate in severity, and none resulted in discontinuation. The following table also lists treatment-emergent adverse reactions that occurred in at least 3 of the thalidomide-treated, HIV-seropositive patients who participated in an 8-week, placebo-controlled, clinical trial. Reactions that were more frequent in the placebo-treated group are not included.

Thalidomide Adverse Reactions in Erythema Nodosum Leprosum Trial				
Adverse reaction	All adverse reactions reported in erythema nodosum leprosum patients	Adverse reactions reported in ≥ 3 HIV-seropositive patients		
		Thalidomide		Placebo
	50 to 300 mg/day (n = 24)	100 mg/day (n = 36)	200 mg/day (n = 32)	(n = 35)
CNS	13 (54.2%)	19 (52.8%)	18 (56.3%)	12 (34.3%)
Agitation	0 (0%)	0 (0%)	3 (9.4%)	0 (0%)
Dizziness	1 (4.2%)	7 (19.4%)	6 (18.7%)	0 (0%)
Headache	3 (12.5%)	6 (16.7%)	6 (18.7%)	4 (11.4%)
Insomnia	0 (0%)	0 (0%)	3 (9.4%)	2 (5.7%)
Nervousness	0 (0%)	1 (2.8%)	3 (9.4%)	0 (0%)
Neuropathy	0 (0%)	3 (8.3%)	0 (0%)	0 (0%)

THALIDOMIDE — ORAL

Thalidomide Adverse Reactions in Erythema Nodosum Leprosum Trial				
	All adverse reactions reported in erythema nodosum leprosum patients	Adverse reactions reported in ≥ 3 HIV-seropositive patients		
		Thalidomide		Placebo
Adverse reaction	50 to 300 mg/day (n = 24)	100 mg/day (n = 36)	200 mg/day (n = 32)	(n = 35)
Paresthesia	0 (0%)	2 (5.6%)	5 (15.6%)	4 (11.4%)
Somnolence	9 (37.5%)	13 (36.1%)	12 (37.5%)	4 (11.4%)
Tremor	1 (4.2%)	0 (0%)	0 (0%)	0 (0%)
Vertigo	2 (8.3%)	0 (0%)	0 (0%)	0 (0%)
Dermatologic	10 (41.7%)	17 (47.2%)	18 (56.3%)	19 (54.3%)
Acne	0 (0%)	4 (11.1%)	1 (3.1%)	0 (0%)
Dermatitis, fungal	1 (4.2%)	2 (5.6%)	3 (9.4%)	0 (0%)
Nail disorder	1 (4.2%)	0 (0%)	1 (3.1%)	0 (0%)
Pruritus	2 (8.3%)	1 (2.8%)	2 (6.3%)	2 (5.7%)
Rash	5 (20.8%)	9 (25%)	8 (25%)	11 (31.4%)
Rash, maculopapular	1 (4.2%)	6 (16.7%)	6 (18.7%)	2 (5.7%)
Sweating	0 (0%)	0 (0%)	4 (12.5%)	4 (11.4%)
GI	5 (20.8%)	16 (44.4%)	16 (50%)	15 (42.9%)
Abdominal pain	1 (4.2%)	1 (2.8%)	1 (3.1%)	4 (11.4%)
Anorexia	0 (0%)	1 (2.8%)	3 (9.4%)	2 (5.7%)
Constipation	1 (4.2%)	1 (2.8%)	3 (9.4%)	0 (0%)
Diarrhea	1 (4.2%)	4 (11.1%)	6 (18.7%)	6 (17.1%)
Dry mouth	0 (0%)	3 (8.3%)	3 (9.4%)	2 (5.7%)
Flatulence	0 (0%)	3 (8.3%)	0 (0%)	2 (5.7%)
Nausea	1 (4.2%)	0 (0%)	4 (12.5%)	1 (2.9%)
Oral moniliasis	1 (4.2%)	4 (11.1%)	2 (6.3%)	0 (0%)
Tooth pain	1 (4.2%)	0 (0%)	0 (0%)	0 (0%)
GU	2 (8.3%)	6 (16.7%)	2 (6.3%)	4 (11.4%)
Albuminuria	0 (0%)	3 (8.3%)	1 (3.1%)	2 (5.7%)
Hematuria	0 (0%)	4 (11.1%)	0 (0%)	1 (2.9%)
Impotence	2 (8.3%)	1 (2.8%)	0 (0%)	0 (0%)
Hematologic/ lymphatic	0 (0%)	8 (22.2%)	13 (40.6%)	10 (28.6%)
Anemia	0 (0%)	2 (5.6%)	4 (12.5%)	3 (8.6%)
Leukopenia	0 (0%)	6 (16.7%)	8 (25%)	3 (8.6%)
Lymphadenopathy	0 (0%)	2 (5.6%)	4 (12.5%)	3 (8.6%)
Metabolic/ endocrine	1 (4.2%)	8 (22.2%)	12 (37.5%)	8 (22.9%)
AST increased	0 (0%)	1 (2.8%)	4 (12.5%)	2 (5.7%)
Edema, peripheral	1 (4.2%)	3 (8.3%)	1 (3.1%)	0 (0%)
Hyperlipemia	0 (0%)	2 (5.6%)	3 (9.4%)	1 (2.9%)
Liver function tests (multiple abnormalities)	0 (0%)	0 (0%)	3 (9.4%)	0 (0%)
Respiratory	3 (12.5%)	9 (25%)	6 (18.7%)	9 (25.7%)
Pharyngitis	1 (4.2%)	3 (8.3%)	2 (6.3%)	2 (5.7%)
Rhinitis	1 (4.2%)	0 (0%)	0 (0%)	4 (11.4%)
Sinusitis	1 (4.2%)	3 (8.3%)	1 (3.1%)	2 (5.7%)
Miscellaneous	16 (66.7%)	18 (50%)	19 (59.4%)	13 (37.1%)
Accidental injury	1 (4.2%)	2 (5.6%)	0 (0%)	1 (2.9%)
Asthenia	2 (8.3%)	2 (5.6%)	7 (21.9%)	1 (2.9%)
Back pain	1 (4.2%)	2 (5.6%)	0 (0%)	0 (0%)
Chills	1 (4.2%)	0 (0%)	3 (9.4%)	4 (11.4%)
Facial edema	1 (4.2%)	0 (0%)	0 (0%)	0 (0%)
Fever	0 (0%)	7 (19.4%)	7 (21.9%)	6 (17.1%)
Infection	0 (0%)	3 (8.3%)	2 (6.3%)	1 (2.9%)
Malaise	2 (8.3%)	0 (0%)	0 (0%)	0 (0%)
Neck pain	1 (4.2%)	0 (0%)	0 (0%)	0 (0%)
Neck rigidity	1 (4.2%)	0 (0%)	0 (0%)	0 (0%)
Pain	2 (8.3%)	0 (0%)	1 (3.1%)	2 (5.7%)

➤*Other adverse reactions observed in patients with erythema nodosum leprosum:* Thalidomide in doses up to 400 mg/day has been administered investigationally in the United States over a 19-year period in 1,465 patients with erythema nodosum leprosum. The published literature describes the treatment of an additional 1,678 patients. All reported reactions are included except those already listed in the previous table. Because these data were collected from uncontrolled studies, the incidence rate cannot be determined.

Cardiovascular – Bradycardia, hypertension, hypotension, peripheral vascular disorder, tachycardia, vasodilation.

CNS – Abnormal thinking, agitation, amnesia, anxiety, causalgia, circumoral paresthesia, confusion, depression, euphoria, hyperesthesia, insomnia, nervousness, neuralgia, neuritis, neuropathy, paresthesia, peripheral neuritis, psychosis.

Dermatologic – Acne, alopecia, dry skin, eczematous rash, exfoliative dermatitis, ichthyosis, perifollicular thickening, photosensitivity, skin necrosis, seborrhea, sweating, urticaria, vesiculobullous rash.

GI – Anorexia, appetite increase/weight gain, dry mouth, dyspepsia, enlarged liver, eructation, flatulence, intestinal obstruction, vomiting.

GU – Hematuria, orchitis, proteinuria, pyuria, urinary frequency.

Hematologic/Lymphatic – Eosinophilia, erythrocyte sedimentation rate decrease, granulocytopenia, hypochromic anemia, leukemia, leukocytosis, leukopenia, mean corpuscular volume elevated, red blood cell count abnormal, spleen palpable, thrombocytopenia.

Lab test abnormalities – ALT increased, creatinine increased, decreased creatinine clearance, electrolyte abnormalities, increased liver function tests, lactic dehydrogenase increased, phosphorus decreased, serum urea nitrogen (BUN) increased.

Metabolic – Amyloidosis, antidiuretic hormone inappropriate, bilirubinemia, cyanosis, diabetes, edema, hyperglycemia, hyperkalemia, hyperuricemia, hypocalcemia, hypoproteinemia.

Musculoskeletal – Arthritis, bone tenderness, hypertonia, joint disorder, leg cramps, myalgia, myasthenia, periosteal disorder.

Respiratory – Cough, emphysema, epistaxis, pulmonary embolus, rales, upper respiratory tract infection, voice alteration.

Special senses – Amblyopia, deafness, dry eye, eye pain, tinnitus.

Miscellaneous – Abdomen enlarged, fever, upper extremity pain.

➤*Other adverse reactions observed in HIV-seropositive patients:*

Cardiovascular – Angina pectoris, arrhythmia, atrial fibrillation, bradycardia, cerebral ischemia, cerebrovascular accident, congestive heart failure, deep thrombophlebitis, heart arrest, heart failure, hypertension, hypotension, murmur, myocardial infarction, palpitation, pericarditis, peripheral vascular disorder, postural hypotension, syncope, tachycardia, thrombophlebitis, thrombosis.

CNS – Abnormal gait, ataxia, decreased libido, decreased reflexes, dementia, dysesthesia, dyskinesia, emotional lability, hostility, hypalgesia, hyperkinesia, incoordination, meningitis, neurologic disorder, tremor, vertigo.

Dermatologic – Angioedema, benign skin neoplasm, eczema, herpes simplex, incomplete Stevens-Johnson syndrome, nail disorder, photosensitivity reaction, pruritus, psoriasis, skin discoloration, skin disorder.

GI – Cholangitis, cholestatic jaundice, colitis, dyspepsia, dysphagia, esophagitis, gastroenteritis, GI disorder, GI hemorrhage, gum disorder, hepatitis, pancreatitis, parotid gland enlargement, periodontitis, stomatitis, tongue discoloration, tooth disorder.

Hematologic/Lymphatic – Aplastic anemia, macrocytic anemia, megaloblastic anemia, microcytic anemia.

Metabolic – Avitaminosis, bilirubinemia, dehydration, hypercholesteremia, hypoglycemia, increased alkaline phosphatase, increased lipase, increased serum creatinine, peripheral edema.

Musculoskeletal – Myalgia, myasthenia.

Respiratory – Apnea, bronchitis, lung disorder, lung edema, pneumonia (including *Pneumocystis carinii* pneumonia), rhinitis.

Special senses – Conjunctivitis, eye disorder, lacrimation disorder, retinitis, taste perversion.

Miscellaneous – AIDS, allergic reaction, ascites, cellulitis, chest pain, chills and fever, cyst, decreased CD4 count, facial edema, flu syndrome, hernia, thyroid hormone level altered, moniliasis, sarcoma, sepsis, viral infection.

Other adverse reactions in the published literature or from spontaneous reports from other sources – Acute renal failure, amenorrhea, aphthous stomatitis, bile duct obstruction, carpal tunnel, chronic myelogenous leukemia, diplopia, dysesthesia, dyspnea, enuresis, erythema nodosum, erythroleukemia, foot drop, galactorrhea, gynecomastia, hangover effect, hypomagnesemia, hypothyroidism, lymphedema, lymphopenia, metrorrhagia, migraine, myxedema, nodular sclerosing Hodgkin disease, nystagmus, oliguria, pancytopenia, petechiae, purpura, Raynaud syndrome, stomach ulcer, suicide attempt.

➤*Postmarketing:*

Cardiovascular – Cardiac arrhythmias, including atrial fibrillation; bradycardia; electrocardiogram abnormalities; sick sinus syndrome; tachycardia.

Dermatologic – Erythema multiforme.

CNS – Changes in mental status or mood, including depression and suicide attempts; disturbances in consciousness, including lethargy, loss of con-

THALIDOMIDE — ORAL

sciousness, or stupor; seizures, including generalized tonic-clonic seizures; status epilepticus; syncope.

GI – Intestinal perforation.

Hematologic/Lymphatic – Decreased white blood cell counts, including neutropenia and febrile neutropenia; changes in prothrombin time.

Metabolic/endocrine – Electrolyte imbalance, including hypercalcemia and hypocalcemia; hyperkalemia; hypokalemia; hyponatremia; hypothyroidism; increased alkaline phosphatase; tumor lysis syndrome.

Respiratory – Pleural effusion.

Overdosage

There have been 3 cases of overdose reported, all attempted suicides. There have been no reported fatalities in doses of up to 14.4 g, and all patients recovered without reported sequelae.

Patient Information

Instruct patients about the potential teratogenicity of thalidomide and the precautions that must be taken to preclude fetal exposure as per the S.T.E.P.S. program. Patients should take thalidomide only as prescribed in compliance with all of the provisions of the S.T.E.P.S. Restricted Distribution Program.

Instruct patients not to extensively handle or open thalidomide capsules and to maintain storage of capsules in blister packs until ingestion.

Instruct patients not to share their medication with anyone else.

Thalidomide frequently causes drowsiness and somnolence. Instruct patients to avoid situations in which drowsiness may be a problem and not to take other medications that may cause drowsiness without adequate medical advice. Advise patients as to the possible impairment of mental or physical abilities required for the performance of hazardous tasks, such as driving a car or operating other complex machinery. Thalidomide may potentiate the somnolence caused by alcohol.

Thalidomide may cause photosensitivity (sensitivity to sunlight). Instruct patients to avoid prolonged exposure to the sun and other ultraviolet light. Instruct patients to use sunscreens and wear protective clothing until tolerance is determined.

Thalidomide can cause peripheral neuropathies that may be initially signaled by numbness, tingling, pain, or a burning sensation in the feet or hands. Instruct patients to report such occurrences to their health care provider immediately.

Thalidomide may cause dizziness and orthostatic hypotension. Instruct patients to sit upright for a few minutes prior to standing from a recumbent position.

Educate patients about the signs and symptoms of thromboembolism and instruct them to seek medical care if they develop symptoms such as arm or leg swelling, chest pain, or shortness of breath.

Patients are not permitted to donate blood while taking thalidomide. In addition, instruct male patients not to donate sperm while taking thalidomide.

LENALIDOMIDE

Rx	**Revlimid** (Celgene Corp)	**Capsules; oral:** 5 mg	Lactose. (REV 5 mg). White. In 28s and 100s.
		10 mg	Lactose. (REV 10 mg). Blue/green and pale yellow. In 28s and 100s.
		15 mg	Lactose. (REV 15 mg). Powder blue and white. In 21s and 100s.
		25 mg	Lactose. (REV 25 mg). White. In 21s and 100s.

LENALIDOMIDE — ORAL

WARNING

Potential for human birth defects – Lenalidomide is an analog of thalidomide. Thalidomide is a known human teratogen that causes severe, life-threatening human birth defects. If lenalidomide is taken during pregnancy, it may cause birth defects or death to a fetus. Advise women to avoid pregnancy while taking lenalidomide.

Special prescribing requirements: Because of this potential toxicity and to avoid fetal exposure to lenalidomide, lenalidomide is only available under a special restricted distribution program called *RevAssist*. Under this program, only health care providers and pharmacists registered with the program are able to prescribe and dispense the product. In addition, lenalidomide must only be dispensed to patients who are registered and meet all the conditions of the *RevAssist* program.

See the following information for health care providers and patients about this restricted distribution program.

RevAssist program –

Prescribers: Lenalidomide can only be prescribed by licensed health care providers who are registered in the *RevAssist* program and understand the potential risk of teratogenicity if lenalidomide is used during pregnancy.

Effective contraception must be used by patients for at least 4 weeks before beginning lenalidomide therapy, during therapy, during dose interruptions, and for 4 weeks following discontinuation of therapy. Reliable contraception is indicated even if the patient has a history of infertility, unless infertility is because of hysterectomy or because the patient has been postmenopausal naturally for at least 24 consecutive months. Two reliable forms of contraception must be used simultaneously unless continuous abstinence from heterosexual sexual contact is the chosen method. Refer women of childbearing potential to a qualified provider of contraceptive methods, if needed. Sexually mature women who have not undergone a hysterectomy, have not had a bilateral oophorectomy, or who have not been postmenopausal naturally for at least 24 consecutive months (ie, who have had menses at some time in the preceding 24 consecutive months) are considered to be women of childbearing potential.

Before prescribing lenalidomide, women of childbearing potential should have 2 negative pregnancy tests (sensitivity of at least 50 milliunits/mL). Perform the first test within 10 to 14 days and the second test within 24 hours prior to prescribing lenalidomide. A prescription for lenalidomide for a woman of childbearing potential must not be issued by the health care provider until negative pregnancy tests have been verified by the health care provider.

It is not known whether lenalidomide is present in the semen of patients receiving the drug; therefore, men receiving lenalidomide must always use a latex condom during any sexual contact with women of childbearing potential, even if they have undergone a successful vasectomy.

WARNING (cont.)

Once treatment has started and during dose interruptions, pregnancy testing for women of childbearing potential should occur weekly during the first 4 weeks of use, and should then be repeated every 4 weeks in women with regular menstrual cycles. If menstrual cycles are irregular, the pregnancy testing should occur every 2 weeks. Perform pregnancy testing and counseling if a patient misses her period or if there is any abnormality in her pregnancy test or in her menstrual bleeding. Lenalidomide treatment must be discontinued during this evaluation.

If pregnancy does occur during lenalidomide treatment, lenalidomide must be discontinued immediately.

Report any suspected fetal exposure to lenalidomide to the Food and Drug Administration (FDA) via the MedWatch number at 1-800-332-1088 and also to the manufacturer at 1-888-423-5436. Refer the patient to an obstetrician/gynecologist experienced in reproductive toxicity for further evaluation and counseling.

Female patients: Use lenalidomide in women of childbearing potential only when the patient meets all of the following conditions (ie, she is unable to become pregnant while on lenalidomide therapy):

- She understands the risks associated with the drug and can reliably carry out instructions.
- She is capable of complying with the contraceptive measures, pregnancy testing, patient registration, and patient survey as described in the *RevAssist* program.
- She has received both oral and written warnings of the potential risks of taking lenalidomide during pregnancy and of exposing a fetus to the drug.
- She has received both oral and written warnings of the risk of possible contraception failure and of the need to use 2 reliable forms of contraception simultaneously, unless continuous abstinence from heterosexual sexual contact is the chosen method. Sexually mature women who have not undergone a hysterectomy, who have not been postmenopausal for at least 24 consecutive months (ie, who have had menses at some time in the preceding 24 consecutive months), or who have not had a bilateral oophorectomy are considered to be women of childbearing potential.
- She acknowledges in writing her understanding of these warnings and of the need for using 2 reliable methods of contraception for 4 weeks prior to beginning lenalidomide therapy, during lenalidomide therapy, during dose interruptions, and for 4 weeks after discontinuation of lenalidomide therapy.
- She has had 2 negative pregnancy tests with a sensitivity of at least 50 milliunits/mL within 10 to 14 days and 24 hours prior to beginning therapy.
- If the patient is between 12 and 18 years of age, her parent or legal guardian is to read the educational materials and agree to try to ensure compliance with all conditions.

LENALIDOMIDE — ORAL

WARNING (cont.)

Male patients: Use lenalidomide in sexually active men when the patient meets all of the following conditions:
- He understands the risks associated with the drug and can reliably carry out instructions.
- He is capable of complying with the mandatory contraceptive measures that are appropriate for men, patient registration, and patient survey as described in the *RevAssist* program.
- He has received and understands both oral and written warnings of the potential risks of taking lenalidomide and exposing a fetus to the drug.
- He has received both oral and written warnings of the risk of possible contraception failure and that it is unknown whether lenalidomide is present in semen. He has been instructed that he must always use a latex condom during any sexual contact with women of childbearing potential, even if he has undergone a successful vasectomy.
- He acknowledges in writing his understanding of these warnings and of the need to use a latex condom during any sexual contact with women of childbearing potential, even if he has undergone a successful vasectomy. Women of childbearing potential are considered to be sexually mature women who have not undergone a hysterectomy, have not had a bilateral oophorectomy, or who have not been postmenopausal for at least 24 consecutive months (ie, who have had menses at any time in the preceding 24 consecutive months).
- If the patient is between 12 and 18 years of age, his parent or legal guardian is to read the educational materials and agree to try to ensure compliance with all conditions.

Hematologic toxicity (neutropenia and thrombocytopenia) – Lenalidomide is associated with significant neutropenia and thrombocytopenia. Eighty percent of patients with deletion 5q myelodysplastic syndromes (MDS) had to have a dose delay/reduction during the major study. Thirty-four percent of patients had to have a second dose delay/reduction. Grade 3 or 4 hematologic toxicity was seen in 80% of patients enrolled in the study. Patients on therapy for deletion 5q MDS should have their complete blood cell count (CBC) monitored weekly for the first 8 weeks of therapy and at least monthly thereafter. Patients may require dose interruption and/or reduction. Patients may require use of blood product support and/or growth factors.

Deep vein thrombosis and pulmonary embolism – Lenalidomide has demonstrated a significantly increased risk of deep vein thrombosis (DVT) and pulmonary embolism (PE) in patients with multiple myeloma who were treated with lenalidomide combination therapy. Patients and health care providers are advised to be observant for the signs and symptoms of thromboembolism. Instruct patients to seek medical care if they develop symptoms such as shortness of breath, chest pain, or arm or leg swelling. It is not known whether prophylactic anticoagulation or antiplatelet therapy prescribed in conjunction with lenalidomide may lessen the potential for venous thromboembolic events. The decision to take prophylactic measures should be done carefully after an assessment of an individual patient's underlying risk factors.

Information about lenalidomide and the *RevAssist* program can be obtained at http://www.revlimid.com or by calling the manufacturer's toll-free number 1-888-423-5436.

Indications

➤*Multiple myeloma:* In combination with dexamethasone for the treatment of multiple myeloma patients who have received at least 1 prior therapy.

➤*Myelodysplastic syndromes:* For the treatment of patients with transfusion-dependent anemia because of low- or intermediate-1–risk MDS associated with a deletion 5q cytogenetic abnormality with or without additional cytogenetic abnormalities.

➤*Off-label uses:*

Behçet syndrome – [3] = Safety concerns. Beneficial results from case report data indicate possible benefit of lenalidomide in the treatment of Behçet syndrome. Larger controlled trials using lenalidomide for longer periods of time are needed. (See Administration and Dosage.)

Multiple myeloma (induction therapy) – [2] = Fair documentation. Some guidelines support the combination of lenalidomide and dexamethasone as an option for induction therapy for multiple myeloma. Lenalidomide may be better tolerated than thalidomide and can be used in patients who were resistant to previous thalidomide therapy. Further studies are needed to evaluate the effectiveness of lenalidomide as a single agent for induction and maintenance therapy.

Administration and Dosage

➤*Adults:*

Multiple myeloma –

Usual dosage: 25 mg/day with water orally administered as a single 25 mg capsule on days 1 through 21 of repeated 28-day cycles.

Dosage adjustment:

- *Grade 3 or 4 thrombocytopenia* –

Lenalidomide Dosage Adjustments for Thrombocytopenia

Platelet counts	Recommended course
When platelets fall to < 30,000/mcL	Interrupt lenalidomide treatment, follow CBC weekly.
When platelets return to ≥ 30,000/mcL	Restart lenalidomide at 15 mg daily.
For each subsequent platelet count drop to < 30,000/mcL	Interrupt lenalidomide treatment.
When platelet counts return to ≥ 30,000/mcL after subsequent drops	Resume lenalidomide treatment at 5 mg less than the previous dose. Do not dose below 5 mg daily.

- *Grade 3 or 4 neutropenia* –

Lenalidomide Dosage Adjustments for Neutropenia

ANC	Recommended course
When neutrophils fall to < 1,000/mcL	Interrupt lenalidomide treatment, add G-CSF,[a] follow CBC weekly.
When neutrophils return to ≥ 1,000/mcL and neutropenia is the only toxicity	Resume lenalidomide at 25 mg daily.
When neutrophils return to ≥ 1,000/mcL and if other toxicity exists	Resume lenalidomide at 15 mg daily.
For each subsequent neutrophil count drop to < 1,000/mcL	Interrupt lenalidomide treatment.
When neutrophils return to ≥ 1,000/mcL after subsequent drops	Resume lenalidomide at 5 mg less than the previous dose. Do not dose below 5 mg daily.

[a] G-CSF = granulocyte colony-stimulating factor.

- *Other grade 3/4 toxicities* – For other grade 3/4 toxicities judged to be related to lenalidomide, hold treatment and restart at the next lower dose level when toxicity has resolved to grade 2 or less.

Concomitant therapy: The recommended dosage of dexamethasone is 40 mg/day on days 1 through 4, 9 through 12, and 17 through 20 of each 28-day cycle for the first 4 cycles of therapy and then 40 mg/day orally on days 1 through 4 every 28 days. Dosing is continued or modified based upon clinical and laboratory findings.

Myelodysplastic syndromes –

Usual dosage: 10 mg daily with water. Dosing is continued or modified based on clinical and laboratory findings.

Dosage adjustment:

- *Patients who are dosed initially at 10 mg and experience thrombocytopenia* –

Lenalidomide 10 mg Dosage Adjustments for Thrombocytopenia

Platelet counts	Recommended course
If thrombocytopenia develops within 4 weeks of starting treatment at 10 mg daily	
If baseline ≥ 100,000/mcL	
When platelets fall to < 50,000/mcL	Interrupt lenalidomide treatment.
When platelets return to ≥ 50,000/mcL	Resume lenalidomide at 5 mg daily.
If baseline < 100,000/mcL	
When platelets fall to 50% of baseline value	Interrupt lenalidomide treatment.
If baseline is ≥ 60,000/mcL and returns to ≥ 50,000/mcL	Resume lenalidomide at 5 mg daily.
If baseline is < 60,000/mcL and returns to ≥ 30,000/mcL	Resume lenalidomide at 5 mg daily.
If thrombocytopenia develops after 4 weeks of starting treatment at 10 mg daily	
When platelets are < 30,000/mcL or	Interrupt lenalidomide treatment.
When platelets return to ≥ 30,000/mcL (without hemostatic failure)	Resume lenalidomide at 5 mg daily.

- *Patients who experience thrombocytopenia at 5 mg daily* –

Lenalidomide 5 mg Dosage Adjustments for Thrombocytopenia

Platelet count	Recommended course
If thrombocytopenia develops during treatment at 5 mg daily	
When platelets are < 30,000/mcL or < 50,000/mcL and platelet transfusions	Interrupt lenalidomide treatment.
When platelets return to ≥ 30,000/mcL (without hemostatic failure)	Resume lenalidomide at 5 mg every other day.

LENALIDOMIDE — ORAL

• *Patients who are dosed initially at 10 mg and experience neutropenia –*

Lenalidomide 10 mg Dosage Adjustments for Neutropenia	
ANC[a]	Recommended course
If neutropenia develops within 4 weeks of starting treatment at 10 mg daily	
If baseline ANC ≥ 1,000/mcL	
When neutrophils fall to < 750/mcL	Interrupt lenalidomide treatment.
When neutrophils return to ≥ 1,000/mcL	Resume lenalidomide at 5 mg daily.
If baseline ANC < 1,000/mcL	
When neutrophils fall to < 500/mcL	Interrupt lenalidomide treatment.
When neutrophils return to ≥ 500/mcL	Resume lenalidomide at 5 mg daily.
If neutropenia develops after 4 weeks of starting treatment at 10 mg daily	
When neutrophils are < 500/mcL for ≥ 7 days or neutrophils are < 500/mcL associated with fever (≥ 38.5°C [101°F])	Interrupt lenalidomide treatment.
When neutrophils return to ≥ 500/mcL	Resume lenalidomide at 5 mg daily.

[a] ANC = absolute neutrophil count.

• *Patients who experience neutropenia at 5 mg daily –*

Lenalidomide 5 mg Dosage Adjustments for Neutropenia	
ANC	Recommended course
If neutropenia develops during treatment at 5 mg daily	
When neutrophils are < 500/mcL for ≥ 7 days or neutrophils are < 500/mcL associated with fever (≥ 38.5°C [101°F])	Interrupt lenalidomide treatment.
When neutrophils return to ≥ 500/mcL	Resume lenalidomide at 5 mg every other day.

Off-label dosing –

Behçet syndrome: [3] = Safety concerns. 25 mg daily for up to 15 months.

Multiple myeloma (induction therapy): [2] = Fair documentation. 25 mg orally every day for 21 days of a 28-day cycle. In patients who respond to treatment, therapy should be continued until relapse occurs.

➤*Elderly:* Because elderly patients are more likely to have decreased renal function, care should be taken in dose selection, and it would be prudent to monitor renal function. See Adults for dosing.

➤*Renal function impairment:* Because lenalidomide is primarily excreted unchanged by the kidney, adjustments to the starting dose of lenalidomide are recommended to provide appropriate drug exposure in patients with moderate or severe renal impairment or in patients on dialysis. Based on a pharmacokinetic study in patients with renal impairment because of nonmalignant conditions, lenalidomide starting dose adjustment is recommended for patients with creatinine clearance (CrCl) of less than 60 mL/min. Patients not on dialysis with CrCl less than 11 mL/min and dialysis patients with CrCl less that 7 mL/min have not been studied. The recommendations for initial starting doses for patients with multiple myeloma and MDS are as follows.

Lenalidomide Renal Function Impairment Starting Dose			
Category	Renal function (Cockcroft-Gault CrCl)	Multiple myeloma	MDS
Moderate renal impairment	CrCl > 30 to 59 mL/min	10 mg every 24 hours	5 mg every 24 hours
Severe renal impairment	CrCl < 30 mL/min (not requiring dialysis)	15 mg every 48 hours	5 mg every 48 hours
End-stage renal disease	CrCl < 30 mL/min (requiring dialysis)	5 mg once daily. On dialysis days, the dose should be administered following dialysis.	5 mg 3 times per week following each dialysis

After initiation of lenalidomide therapy, subsequent lenalidomide dose modification should be based on individual patient treatment tolerance, as described elsewhere in this section.

➤*Preparation for administration:* Lenalidomide is considered a cytotoxic agent and is also considered a teratogen. Follow safe handling procedures when preparing, administering, or dispensing lenalidomide.

➤*Administration:* Patients should take the capsules daily with water and should not break, chew, or open the capsules.

Dispense no more than a 28-day supply.

➤*Storage/Stability:* Store at 25°C (77°F); excursions are permitted between 15° and 30°C (59° and 86°F).

Actions

➤*Pharmacology:* The mechanism of action of lenalidomide remains to be fully characterized. Lenalidomide possesses antineoplastic, immunomodulatory, and antiangiogenic properties. Lenalidomide inhibited the secretion of proinflammatory cytokines and increased the secretion of anti-inflammatory cytokines from peripheral blood mononuclear cells. Lenalidomide inhibited cell proliferation with varying efficacy (50% inhibitory concentrations) in some but not all cell lines. Of cell lines tested, lenalidomide was effective in inhibiting growth of Namalwa cells (a human B cell lymphoma cell line with a deletion of one chromosome 5), but was much less effective in inhibiting growth of KG-1 cells (human myeloblastic cell line, also with a deletion of one chromosome 5) and other cell lines without chromosome 5 deletions. Lenalidomide inhibited the growth of multiple myeloma cells from patients, as well as MM.1S cells (a human multiple myeloma cell line), by inducing cell cycle arrest and apoptosis.

Lenalidomide inhibited the expression of cyclooxygenase-2 (COX-2) but not COX-1 in vitro.

➤*Pharmacokinetics:*

Absorption – Lenalidomide, in healthy volunteers, is rapidly absorbed following oral administration, with maximum plasma concentrations (C_{max}) occurring between 0.625 and 1.5 hours postdose. Coadministration with food does not alter the extent of absorption (area under the curve [AUC]) but does reduce the C_{max} by 36%. The pharmacokinetic disposition of lenalidomide is linear. C_{max} and AUC increase proportionately with increases in dose. Multiple dosing at the recommended dose regimen does not result in drug accumulation.

Pharmacokinetic sampling in MDS patients was not performed. In multiple myeloma patients, C_{max} occurred between 0.5 and 4 hours postdose on days 1 and 28. AUC and C_{max} values increase proportionally with dose following single and multiple doses. Exposure (AUC) in multiple myeloma patients is 57% higher than in healthy men.

Distribution – In vitro, (^{14}C)-lenalidomide binding to plasma proteins is approximately 30%.

Metabolism/Excretion – The metabolic profile of lenalidomide in humans has not been studied. In healthy volunteers, approximately two-thirds of lenalidomide is eliminated unchanged through urinary excretion. The process exceeds the glomerular filtration rate and, therefore, is partially or entirely active. Half-life of elimination is approximately 3 hours.

Special populations –

Renal function impairment: The pharmacokinetics of lenalidomide were studied in patients with renal impairment caused by nonmalignant conditions. In this study, 5 patients with mild renal impairment (CrCl 57 to 74 mL/min), 6 patients with moderate renal impairment (CrCl 33 to 46 mL/min), 6 patients with severe renal impairment (CrCl 17 to 29 mL/min), and 6 patients with end-stage renal disease requiring dialysis were administered a single oral dose of lenalidomide 25 mg. As a control group comparator, 7 healthy subjects of similar age with healthy renal function (CrCl 83 to 145 mL/min) were also administered a single oral dose of lenalidomide 25 mg.

As CrCl decreased from mild to severe impairment, half-life increased and drug clearance decreased linearly. Patients with moderate and severe renal impairment had a 3-fold increase in half-life and a 66% to 75% decrease in drug clearance compared with healthy subjects.

Adjustment of the starting dose of lenalidomide is recommended in patients with moderate or severe (CrCl less than 60 mL/min) renal impairment and in patients on dialysis. In multiple myeloma patients, those patients with mild renal impairment had an AUC 56% greater than those with healthy renal function.

• *Hemodialysis* – Patients on hemodialysis (n = 6) given a single dose of lenalidomide 25 mg had an approximate 4.5-fold increase in half-life and an 80% decrease in drug clearance compared with healthy subjects. Approximately 40% of the administered dose was removed from the body during a single dialysis session.

Contraindications

Demonstrated hypersensitivity to the drug or its components; pregnancy and women of childbearing potential (see Warnbox and Warnings/Precautions).

Warnings/Precautions

➤*Hematologic toxicity (neutropenia and thrombocytopenia):* This drug is associated with significant neutropenia and thrombocytopenia. Eighty percent of patients with deletion 5q MDS had to have a dose delay or reduction during the major study for the indication. Thirty-four percent of patients had to have a second dose delay/reduction. Grade 3 or 4 hematologic toxicity was seen in 80% of patients enrolled in the study. In the 48% of patients who developed grade 3 or 4 neutropenia, the median time to onset was 42 days (range, 14 to 411 days), and the median time to documented recovery was 17 days (range, 2 to 170 days). In the 54% of patients who developed grade 3 or 4 thrombocytopenia, the median time to onset was 28 days (range, 8 to 290 days), and the median time to documented recovery was 22 days (range, 5 to 224 days). Patients on therapy for deletion 5q MDS should have their CBC monitored weekly for the first 8 weeks of therapy and at least monthly thereafter. Patients may require dose interruption and/or reduction. Patients may require use of blood product support and/or growth factors.

In the pooled multiple myeloma studies, grade 3 and 4 hematologic toxicities were more frequent in patients treated with the combination of lenalidomide and dexamethasone than in patients treated with dexamethasone alone.

LENALIDOMIDE — ORAL

Monitor CBC every 2 weeks for the first 12 weeks and then monthly thereafter in patients on therapy. Patients may require dose interruption and/or dose reduction.

➤*Deep vein thrombosis and pulmonary embolism:* See the Warning box for more information.

➤*Dermatologic reactions:* Angioedema and serious dermatological reactions, including Stevens-Johnson syndrome and toxic epidermal necrolysis (TEN), have been reported. These events can be fatal. Do not prescribe lenalidomide to patients with a history of grade 4 rash associated with thalidomide treatment. Consider lenalidomide interruption or discontinuation for grade 2 to 3 skin rash. Lenalidomide must be discontinued for angioedema, grade 4 rash, exfoliative or bullous rash, or if Stevens-Johnson syndrome or TEN is suspected; do not resume following discontinuation for these reactions.

➤*Tumor lysis syndrome:* Lenalidomide has antineoplastic activity and, therefore, the complications of tumor lysis syndrome may occur. The patients at risk of tumor lysis syndrome are those with high tumor burden prior to treatment. Monitor these patients closely and take appropriate precautions.

➤*Renal function impairment:* No formal studies have been conducted in patients with renal function impairment. This drug is known to be substantially excreted by the kidney and the risk of adverse reactions to this drug may be greater in patients with impaired renal function. Take care in dose selection and monitor renal function. Because lenalidomide is primarily excreted unchanged by the kidney, adjustments to the starting dose of lenalidomide are recommended to provide appropriate drug exposure in patients with moderate or severe (CrCl less than 60 mL/min) renal impairment and in patients on dialysis.

➤*Pregnancy: Category X.* There are no adequate and well-controlled studies in pregnant women. Lenalidomide may cause fetal harm when administered to a pregnant woman. Advise women of childbearing potential to avoid pregnancy while on lenalidomide. Use 2 effective contraceptive methods for at least 4 weeks before starting lenalidomide therapy, during therapy, during therapy interruptions, and for at least 4 weeks after completing therapy.

See the Warning box for more information.

Lenalidomide is an analog of thalidomide. Thalidomide is a known human teratogen that causes life-threatening human birth defects. An embryofetal developmental study in nonhuman primates indicates that lenalidomide produced malformations in the offspring of female monkeys who received the drug during pregnancy, similar to birth defects observed in humans following exposure to thalidomide during pregnancy. The teratogenic effect of lenalidomide in humans cannot be ruled out.

Lenalidomide has been shown to have an embryocidal effect in rabbits at a dose of 50 mg/kg (approximately 120 times the human dose of 10 mg based on body surface area [BSA]).

An embryofetal development study in rats revealed no teratogenic effects at the highest dose of 500 mg/kg (approximately 600 times the human dose of 10 mg based on BSA). At 100, 300, or 500 mg/kg/day there was minimal maternal toxicity that included slight, transient reduction in mean body weight gain and food intake. However, this animal model may not adequately address the full spectrum of the potential embryofetal developmental effects of lenalidomide.

A pre- and postnatal development study in rats revealed few adverse effects on the offspring of female rats treated with lenalidomide at dosages of up to 500 mg/kg (approximately 600 times the human dose of 10 mg based on BSA). The male offspring exhibited slightly delayed sexual maturation and the female offspring had slightly lower body weight gains during gestation when bred to male offspring. Reproductive effects of lenalidomide have not been thoroughly assessed. The structural similarity of lenalidomide to thalidomide, a known human teratogen, as well as malformations seen in the offspring of female monkeys administered lenalidomide during pregnancy, suggests a potential risk to the developing fetus.

See the Warning box for more information.

➤*Lactation:* It is not known whether this drug is excreted in human milk. However, the molecular weight (approximately 259), moderate metabolism (approximately one-third) and plasma protein binding (approximately 30%), and the elimination half-life (approximately 3 hours) suggest that lenalidomide will be excreted into breast milk. Because of the uncertainty regarding the amount of drug in milk and the potential for severe toxicity, instruct women being treated with lenalidomide not to breast-feed.

➤*Children:* Safety and effectiveness in children younger than 18 years of age have not been established.

➤*Elderly:* In both MDS and multiple myeloma studies, patients older than 65 years of age were more likely than patients 65 years of age and younger to experience diarrhea, fatigue, PE, and syncope following use of lenalidomide. No differences in efficacy were observed between patients older than 65 years of age and younger patients.

This drug is known to be substantially excreted by the kidney, and the risk of toxic reactions to this drug may be greater in patients with impaired renal function. Because elderly patients are more likely to have decreased renal function, take care in dose selection and monitor renal function.

➤*Monitoring:*

Myelodysplastic syndromes – Perform a CBC, including white blood cell count with differential, platelet count, hemoglobin, and hematocrit, weekly for the first 8 weeks of lenalidomide treatment and monthly thereafter to monitor for cytopenias.

Multiple myeloma – Perform a CBC every 2 weeks for the first 3 months and at least monthly thereafter to monitor for cytopenias.

Drug Interactions

➤*Digoxin:* When digoxin was coadministered with lenalidomide, the digoxin AUC was not significantly different; however, the digoxin C_{max} was increased by 14%. Periodic monitoring of digoxin plasma levels, in accordance with clinical judgment and based on standard clinical practice in patients receiving this medication, is recommended during administration of lenalidomide.

➤*Drug/Food interactions:* Coadministration with food does not alter the extent of absorption, but does reduce the C_{max} by 36%.

Adverse Reactions

➤*Myelodysplastic syndromes:* The following table summarizes the adverse reactions that were reported in at least 5% of the lenalidomide-treated patients in the deletion 5q MDS clinical study. The subsequent table summarizes the most frequently observed grade 3 and 4 adverse reactions regardless of relationship to treatment with lenalidomide. In the single-arm studies conducted, it is often not possible to distinguish adverse reactions that are drug-related and those that reflect the patient's underlying disease.

Lenalidomide Grade 3 and 4 Adverse Reactions (≥ 5%)

Adverse reaction[a]	10 mg overall (N = 148)
Cardiovascular	
Hypertension, NOS[b]	6.1%
Palpitations	5.4%
CNS	
Asthenia	14.9%
Depression	5.4%
Dizziness	19.6%
Fatigue	31.1%
Headache	19.6%
Hypoesthesia	6.8%
Insomnia	10.1%
Peripheral neuropathy, NOS	5.4%
Rigors	6.1%
Dermatologic	
Cellulitis	5.4%
Dry skin	14.2%
Ecchymosis	5.4%
Erythema	5.4%
Night sweats	8.1%
Pruritus	41.9%
Rash, NOS	35.8%
Sweating increased	6.8%
GI	
Abdominal pain, NOS	12.2%
Abdominal pain upper	8.1%
Anorexia	10.1%
Constipation	23.6%
Diarrhea, NOS	48.6%
Dry mouth	6.8%
Dysgeusia	6.1%
Loose stools	6.1%
Nausea	23.6%
Vomiting, NOS	10.1%
GU	
Dysuria	6.8%
Urinary tract infection, NOS	10.8%
Hematologic/Lymphatic	
Anemia, NOS	11.5%
Febrile neutropenia	5.4%
Leukopenia, NOS	8.1%
Neutropenia	58.8%
Thrombocytopenia	61.5%
Metabolic/Nutritional	
Acquired hypothyroidism	6.8%
Edema, NOS	10.1%

LENALIDOMIDE — ORAL

Lenalidomide Grade 3 and 4 Adverse Reactions (≥ 5%)	
Adverse reaction[a]	10 mg overall (N = 148)
Edema peripheral	20.3%
Hypokalemia	10.8%
Hypomagnesemia	6.1%
Peripheral swelling	8.1%
Musculoskeletal	
Arthralgia	21.6%
Back pain	20.9%
Muscle cramp	18.2%
Myalgia	8.8%
Pain in limb	10.8%
Respiratory	
Bronchitis, NOS	6.1%
Cough	19.6%
Dyspnea, NOS	16.9%
Dyspnea, exertional	6.8%
Epistaxis	14.9%
Nasopharyngitis	23%
Pharyngitis	15.5%
Pneumonia, NOS	11.5%
Rhinitis, NOS	6.8%
Sinusitis, NOS	8.1%
Upper respiratory tract infection, NOS	14.9%
Miscellaneous	
ALT increased	8.1%
Chest pain	5.4%
Contusion	8.1%
Pain, NOS	6.8%
Pyrexia	20.9%

[a] System organ classes and preferred terms are coded using the *Medical Dictionary for Regulatory Activities* (*MedDRA*). A patient with multiple occurrences of an adverse reaction is counted only once in the adverse reaction category.
[b] NOS = not otherwise specified.

Lenalidomide Grade 3 and 4 Adverse Reactions[a]	
Adverse reaction[b]	10 mg (N = 148)
Patients with at least 1 grade 3 or 4 adverse reaction	88.5%
Cardiovascular	
PE	2%
Pulmonary hypertension, NOS	1.4%
Syncope	1.4%
CNS	
Asthenia	1.4%
Dizziness	2.7%
Fatigue	4.7%
Headache	1.4%
Dermatologic	
Pruritus	2%
Rash, NOS	6.8%
Sweating increased	1.4%
GI	
Diarrhea, NOS	3.4%
Nausea	4.1%
Vomiting, NOS	1.4%
Hematologic/Lymphatic	
Anemia, NOS	6.1%
Febrile neutropenia	4.1%
Granulocytopenia	2%
Leukopenia, NOS	5.4%
Neutropenia	53.4%
Pancytopenia	2%
Thrombocytopenia	50%
Musculoskeletal	
Arthralgia	1.4%
Back pain	4.7%
Muscle cramp	2%
Pain in limb	1.4%
Respiratory	
Dyspnea	4.7%
Epistaxis	1.4%
Hypoxia	1.4%
Pleural effusion	1.4%
Pneumonia, NOS	7.4%
Pneumonitis, NOS	1.4%
Respiratory distress	2%
Respiratory tract infection	1.4%
Upper respiratory tract infection	1.4%
Miscellaneous	
Chest pain	2%
Multiorgan failure	1.4%
Pyrexia	3.4%
Sepsis	2.7%

[a] Adverse reactions with a frequency of at least 1% in the 10 mg overall group. Grade 3 and 4 are based on National Cancer Institute Common Toxicity Criteria version 2.0.
[b] Preferred terms are coded using the *MedDRA* dictionary. A patient with multiple occurrences of an adverse reaction is counted only once in the adverse reaction category.

In other clinical studies of lenalidomide in MDS patients, the following serious adverse reactions (regardless of relationship to study drug treatment) not described in the previous tables were reported:

Cardiovascular – Angina pectoris, aortic disorder, atrial fibrillation, atrial fibrillation aggravated, bradycardia (NOS), cardiac arrest, cardiac failure (NOS), cardiac failure congestive, cardiogenic shock, cardiomyopathy (NOS), cardiorespiratory arrest, cerebellar infarction, cerebral infarction, cerebrovascular accident, DVT, hypotension (NOS), ischemia (NOS), myocardial infarction, myocardial ischemia, pulmonary edema (NOS), subarachnoid hemorrhage (NOS), supraventricular arrhythmia (NOS), tachyarrhythmia, thrombophlebitis superficial, thrombosis, transient ischemic attack, ventricular dysfunction.

CNS – Aphasia, confusional state, depressed level of consciousness, dysarthria, fall, gait abnormal, migraine (NOS), spinal cord compression (NOS), vertigo.

Dermatologic – Acute febrile neutrophilic dermatosis.

GI – Colitis ischemic, colonic polyp, diverticulitis (NOS), dysphagia, gastritis (NOS), gastroenteritis (NOS), gastroesophageal reflux disease, GI hemorrhage (NOS), intestinal perforation (NOS), irritable bowel syndrome, melena, obstructive inguinal hernia, oral infection, pancreatitis (NOS), pancreatitis due to biliary obstruction, perirectal abscess, rectal hemorrhage, small intestinal obstruction (NOS), upper GI hemorrhage.

GU – Hematuria, pelvic pain (NOS), prostate cancer metastatic, urosepsis.

Hematologic/Lymphatic – Acute leukemia (NOS), acute myeloid leukemia (NOS), anemia, bone marrow depression (NOS), coagulopathy, hemolysis (NOS), hemolytic anemia (NOS), lymphoma (NOS), refractory anemia, splenic infarction, warm-type hemolytic anemia.

Hepatic – Cholecystitis (NOS), cholecystitis acute (NOS), hepatic failure, hyperbilirubinemia.

Lab test abnormalities – Blood creatinine increased, culture negative (NOS), hemoglobin decreased, liver function tests abnormal (NOS), troponin I increased.

Metabolic/Nutritional – Dehydration, hypernatremia, hypoglycemia (NOS).

Musculoskeletal – Arthritis (NOS), arthritis aggravated (NOS), gouty arthritis, neck pain, rigors.

Renal – Azotemia, calculus ureteric, kidney infection (NOS), renal failure (NOS), renal failure acute, renal mass (NOS).

Respiratory – Bronchitis (NOS), bronchoalveolar carcinoma, chronic obstructive airways disease exacerbated, dyspnea exacerbated, ear infection, interstitial lung disease, lobar pneumonia (NOS), lung cancer metastatic, lung infiltration (NOS), respiratory failure, sinusitis (NOS), sinusitis acute (NOS), wheezing.

Miscellaneous – Bacteremia, Basedow disease, central line infection, cervical vertebral fracture, chondrocalcinosis pyrophosphate, clostridial infection (NOS), disease progression (NOS), ear infection (NOS), *Enterobacter* sepsis, femoral neck fracture, femur fracture, fractured pelvis (NOS), fungal infection (NOS), gout, herpes viral infection (NOS), hip fracture, hypersensitivity (NOS), infection (NOS), influenza, intermittent pyrexia, *Klebsiella* sepsis, localized infection, nodule, overdose (NOS), postprocedural hemor-

LENALIDOMIDE — ORAL

rhage, *Pseudomonas* infection (NOS), rib fracture, road traffic accident, septic shock, spinal compression fracture, *Staphylococcal* infection, sudden death, transfusion reaction.

➤*Multiple myeloma:* The following table summarizes the number and percentage of patients with grade 1 to 4 adverse reactions reported in at least 10% of patients in either treatment group in studies 1 and 2.

Lenalidomide/Dexamethasone Adverse Reactions (≥ 10%)		
Adverse reaction	Lenalidomide/ Dexamethasone (n = 346)	Placebo/ Dexamethasone (n = 345)
Subjects with ≥ 1 adverse reaction	100%	99.7%
Cardiovascular		
DVT	7.8%	3.2%
PE	3.2%	0.9%
CNS		
Asthenia	23.4%	24.9%
Dizziness	20.8%	15.4%
Fatigue	38.4%	37.4%
Headache	21.4%	21.4%
Insomnia	32.1%	37.1%
Paresthesia	11.6%	12.5%
Tremor	19.7%	7%
GI		
Anorexia	13.6%	8.7%
Constipation	38.7%	18.6%
Diarrhea, NOS	29.2%	24.6%
Dysgeusia	13.3%	9.3%
Dyspepsia	13.9%	13.3%
Nausea	22%	19.1%
Vomiting, NOS	10.1%	8.1%
Hematologic/Lymphatic		
Anemia, NOS	24.3%	17.4%
Neutropenia	27.7%	4.6%
Thrombocytopenia	17.1%	9.9%
Metabolism/Nutrition		
Edema peripheral	21.1%	18.8%
Hyperglycemia, NOS	15%	14.2%
Hypokalemia	11.3%	5.2%
Weight decreased	18.2%	13.9%
Musculoskeletal		
Arthralgia	10.4%	14.8%
Back pain	15.3%	14.2%
Muscle cramp	30.1%	20.6%
Muscle weakness, NOS	15%	15.4%
Respiratory		
Cough	14.5%	20.6%
Dyspnea, NOS	20.2%	15.4%
Pneumonia, NOS	11.3%	7.5%
Upper respiratory tract infection	13.6%	12.5%
Miscellaneous		
Pyrexia	23.1%	19.4%
Rash	15.9%	8.1%
Vision blurred	14.7%	10.4%

Lenalidomide/Dexamethasone Grade 3 and 4 Adverse Reactions (≥ 2%)				
	Lenalidomide/ Dexamethasone (n = 346)		Placebo/ Dexamethasone (n = 345)	
Adverse reaction	Grade 3 n (%)	Grade 4 n (%)	Grade 3 n (%)	Grade 4 n (%)
Patients with at least one grade 3 or 4 event	65%	7.2%	53.9%	9%
Cardiovascular				
Atrial fibrillation	2.6%	0.3%	0.6%	0.3%
DVT	6.6%	0.3%	2.6%	0.3%
PE	0.6%	2.6%	0.3%	0.6%
Syncope	2%	0%	0.9%	0%
CNS				
Asthenia	4%	0%	4.6%	0%
Confusional state	1.7%	0%	2.3%	0%
Depression	2.6%	0%	1.4%	0.3%
Fatigue	5.8%	0.3%	3.8%	0%
Neuropathy, NOS[a]	2%	0%	0.6%	0%
GI				
Constipation	2%	0%	0.3%	0%
Diarrhea, NOS	2.3%	0%	0.6%	0%
Hematologic/Lymphatic				
Anemia, NOS	7.2%	1.2%	2.9%	0.6%
Leukopenia, NOS	3.5%	0%	0.3%	0%
Lymphopenia	2.3%	0%	1.2%	0%
Neutropenia	17.3%	3.8%	2.3%	0.6%
Thrombocytopenia	9%	1.2%	4.6%	0.9%
Metabolism/Nutrition				
Hyperglycemia, NOS	6.5%	1.2%	5.5%	2%
Hypocalcemia	2.3%	1.4%	1.2%	0.3%
Hypokalemia	2.6%	0.3%	1.4%	0%
Respiratory				
Dyspnea, NOS	1.7%	0.9%	2%	0.3%
Pneumonia, NOS	5.2%	1.2%	14.3%	0.9%
Miscellaneous				
Muscle weakness, NOS	5.2%	0%	2.9%	0%
Pyrexia	1.2%	0%	2.3%	0%

[a] NOS = not otherwise specified.

In these and other clinical studies of lenalidomide in patients with multiple myeloma, the following serious adverse reactions (considered related to study drug treatment) not described in the previous table were reported.

Cardiovascular – Atrial flutter, cardiac failure congestive, cerebral infarction, cerebral ischemia, cerebrovascular accident, circulatory collapse, hypertension (NOS), hypotension (NOS), intracranial hemorrhage (NOS), intracranial venous sinus thrombosis (NOS), orthostatic hypotension, peripheral ischemia, phlebitis (NOS), pulmonary edema, subacute endocarditis, venous thrombosis limb (NOS).

In the pooled analysis, thrombotic or thromboembolic events, including DVT, PE, thrombosis, and intracranial venous sinus thrombosis, were reported more frequently in patients treated with the lenalidomide/dexamethasone combination. The number of patients experiencing a thrombotic event in the combination arm were 43 of 346 (12%), compared with 14 of 345 (4%) of those in the placebo/dexamethasone arm.

CNS – Brain edema, delirium, delusion (NOS), dizziness, encephalitis (NOS), insomnia, leukoencephalopathy, memory impairment, mental status changes, performance status decreased, psychotic disorder (NOS), somnolence, tremor.

Dermatologic – Cellulitis, rash (NOS), skin desquamation (NOS).

Endocrine – Acquired hypothyroidism, adrenal insufficiency (NOS).

GI – Abdominal pain (NOS), colitis pseudomembranous, gastritis (NOS), GI hemorrhage (NOS), GI infection (NOS), peptic ulcer hemorrhage, upper GI hemorrhage.

GU – Hematuria, urinary retention, urinary tract infection (NOS).

Hematologic / Lymphatic – Anemia (NOS) aggravated, neutropenic sepsis, pancytopenia.

LENALIDOMIDE — ORAL

Hepatic – Hepatic failure, hepatitis toxic.

Lab test abnormalities – Blood creatinine increased, body temperature increased, C-reactive protein increased, hemoglobin decreased, international normalized ratio increased, weight decreased, white blood cell count decreased.

Metabolic/Nutritional – Dehydration, diabetes mellitus (NOS), diabetes with hyperosmolarity, diabetic ketoacidosis.

Musculoskeletal – Back pain, myopathy, myopathy steroid.

Renal – Fanconi syndrome acquired, renal failure (NOS), renal failure acute, renal tubular necrosis.

Respiratory – Bronchopneumonia (NOS), bronchopneumopathy, hypoxia, lung infection (NOS), *Pneumocystis carnii* pneumonia, pneumonia bacterial (NOS), pneumonia cytomegaloviral, pneumonia pneumococcal, pneumonia primary atypical, pneumonia staphylococcal.

Special senses – Blindness, herpes zoster ophthalmic.

Miscellaneous – Bursitis infective (NOS), cellulitis, cellulitis staphylococcal, *Enterobacter* bacteremia, *Escherichia* sepsis, herpes zoster, infection (NOS), sepsis (NOS), septic shock, streptococcal sepsis.

Overdosage

No cases of overdose have been reported during the clinical studies.

Patient Information

Counsel patients on lenalidomide's potential risk of teratogenicity because of its structural similarity to thalidomide. Patients may only acquire a prescription for lenalidomide therapy through a controlled distribution program (*RevAssist*) through contracted pharmacies. Women of childbearing potential will be educated and counseled on the requirements of the *RevAssist* program and the precautions to be taken to preclude fetal exposure to lenalidomide. Familiarize patients with the lenalidomide *RevAssist* educational materials and patient Medication Guide, and advise them to direct any questions to their doctor or pharmacist prior to starting lenalidomide therapy.

➤*Warning: potential for human birth defects:* Lenalidomide is an analogue of thalidomide. Thalidomide is a known human teratogen that causes life-threatening human birth defects. If lenalidomide is taken during pregnancy, it may cause birth defects or death to a fetus. Advise women to avoid pregnancy while on lenalidomide.

RILONACEPT

Rx	**Arcalyst** (Regeneron)	**Injection, lyophilized, powder for solution:** 220 mg	Preservative free. PEG 3350, sucrose. In 20 mL single-use vials.

RILONACEPT — INJECTION

Indications

➤*Cryopyrin-associated periodic syndromes:* For the treatment of cryopyrin-associated periodic syndromes, including familial cold autoinflammatory syndrome and Muckle-Wells syndrome in adults and children 12 years of age and older.

Administration and Dosage

➤*Adults:*

Cryopyrin-associated periodic syndromes –

18 years of age and older:

• *Initial dosage* – Treatment should be initiated with a loading dose of 320 mg delivered as two, 2 mL, subcutaneous injections of 160 mg each given on the same day at 2 different sites.

• *Maintenance dosage* – Dosing should be continued with a once-weekly injection of 160 mg administered as a single, 2 mL, subcutaneous injection.

Rilonacept should not be given more often than once weekly.

➤*Children:*

Cryopyrin-associated periodic syndromes –

18 years of age and older: See Adults for dosing.

12 to 17 years of age:

• *Maximum dose* –

Initial dose: 320 mg.

Maintenance dose: 160 mg.

• *Initial dosage* – Treatment should be initiated with a loading dose of 4.4 mg/kg, up to a maximum of 320 mg, delivered as 1 or 2 subcutaneous injections, with a maximum single-injection volume of 2 mL.

If the initial dose is given as 2 injections, they should be given on the same day at 2 different sites.

• *Maintenance dosage* – Dosing should be continued with a once-weekly injection of 2.2 mg/kg, up to a maximum of 160 mg, administered as a single subcutaneous injection, up to 2 mL.

Rilonacept should not be given more often than once weekly.

➤*Preparation for administration:* Each single-use vial of rilonacept contains a sterile, white to off-white, preservative-free, lyophilized powder. Reconstitution with 2.3 mL of preservative-free sterile water for injection (supplied separately) is required prior to subcutaneous administration of the drug.

Using aseptic technique, withdraw 2.3 mL of preservative-free sterile water for injection through a 27-gauge, ½-inch needle attached to a 3 mL syringe and inject the preservative-free sterile water for injection into the drug product vial for reconstitution. The needle and syringe used for reconstitution with preservative-free sterile water for injection should then be discarded and should not be used for subcutaneous injections. After the addition of preservative-free sterile water for injection, the vial contents should be reconstituted by shaking the vial for approximately 1 minute and then allowing it to sit for 1 minute. The resulting 80 mg/mL solution is sufficient to allow a withdrawal volume of up to 2 mL for subcutaneous administration.

Using aseptic technique, withdraw the recommended dose volume, up to 2 mL (160 mg), of the solution with a new 27-gauge, ½-inch needle attached to a new 3 mL syringe for subcutaneous injection. Each vial should be used for a single dose only. Discard the vial after withdrawal of the drug.

➤*Administration:* Injection is for subcutaneous use only.

Sites for subcutaneous injection, such as the abdomen, thigh, or upper arm, should be rotated. Injections should never be made at sites that are bruised, red, tender, or hard.

➤*Storage/Stability:* Store refrigerated at 2° to 8°C (36° to 46°F) inside the original carton to protect it from light. After reconstitution, keep rilonacept at room temperature, protect from light, and use within 3 hours of reconstitution.

Rilonacept does not contain preservatives; therefore, discard unused portions of rilonacept. Each vial should be used for a single dose only; discard the vial after withdrawal of the drug.

Actions

➤*Pharmacology:* Rilonacept is a dimeric fusion protein consisting of the ligand-binding domains of the extracellular portions of the human interleukin-1 receptor component (IL-1RI) and IL-1 receptor accessory protein (IL-1RAcP) linked in-line to the Fc portion of human immunoglobin G1 (IgG1).

Cryopyrin-associated periodic syndromes refer to rare genetic syndromes generally caused by mutations in the nucleotide-binding domain, leucine rich family, pyrin domain containing 3 (NLRP-3) gene (also known as cold-induced autoinflammatory syndrome 1). Cryopyrin-associated periodic syndromes disorders are inherited in an autosomal dominant pattern with male and female offspring equally affected. Features common to all disorders include fever, urticaria-like rash, arthralgia, myalgia, fatigue, and conjunctivitis.

In most cases, inflammation in cryopyrin-associated periodic syndromes is associated with mutations in the NLRP-3 gene, which encodes the protein cryopyrin, an important component of the inflammasome. Cryopyrin regulates the protease caspase-1 and controls the activation of interleukin-1 beta (IL-1β). Mutations in NLRP-3 gene result in an overactive inflammasome, resulting in excessive release of activated IL-1β that drives inflammation.

Rilonacept blocks IL-1β signaling by acting as a soluble decoy receptor that binds IL-1β and prevents its interaction with cell surface receptors. Rilonacept also binds IL-1α and IL-1 receptor antagonist (IL-1ra) with reduced affinity. The equilibrium dissociation constants for rilonacept binding to IL-1β, IL-1α, and IL-1ra were 0.5, 1.4, and 6.1 pM, respectively.

Pharmacodynamics – C-reactive protein (CRP) and serum amyloid A are indicators of inflammatory disease activity that are elevated in patients with cryopyrin-associated periodic syndromes. Elevated serum amyloid A has been associated with the development of systemic amyloidosis in patients with cryopyrin-associated periodic syndromes. Compared with placebo, treatment with rilonacept resulted in sustained reductions from baseline in mean serum CRP and serum amyloid A to normal levels during the clinical trial. Rilonacept also normalized mean serum amyloid A from elevated levels.

➤*Pharmacokinetics:*

Absorption – The average trough levels of rilonacept were approximately 24 mcg/mL at steady state following weekly subcutaneous doses of 160 mg for up to 48 weeks in patients with cryopyrin-associated periodic syndromes. The steady state appeared to be reached by 6 weeks.

Contraindications

None.

Warnings/Precautions

➤*Infections:* IL-1 blockade may interfere with the immune response to infections. Treatment with another medication that works through inhibition of IL-1 has been associated with an increased risk of serious infections, and serious infections have been reported in patients taking rilonacept. There was a greater incidence of infections in patients on rilonacept compared with placebo. In the controlled portion of the study, 1 infection was reported as severe, which was bronchitis in a patient on rilonacept.

In an open-label extension study, 1 patient developed bacterial meningitis and died. Discontinue rilonacept if a patient develops a serious infection. Do not initiate treatment with rilonacept in patients with an active or chronic infection.

In clinical studies, rilonacept has not been coadministered with tumor necrosis factor (TNF) inhibitors. An increased incidence of serious infections has been associated with administration of an IL-1 blocker in combination

RILONACEPT — INJECTION

with TNF inhibitors. Taking rilonacept with TNF inhibitors is not recommended because this may increase the risk of serious infections.

Drugs that affect the immune system by blocking TNF have been associated with an increased risk of reactivation of latent tuberculosis (TB). It is possible that taking drugs such as rilonacept that block IL-1 increases the risk of TB or other atypical or opportunistic infections. Follow current Centers for Disease Control and Prevention (CDC) guidelines to evaluate for and to treat possible latent TB infections before initiating therapy with rilonacept.

➤*Immunosuppression:* The impact of treatment with rilonacept on active and/or chronic infections and the development of malignancies is not known. However, treatment with immunosuppressants, including rilonacept, may result in an increase in the risk of malignancies.

➤*Immunizations:* Because data are not available on either the efficacy of live vaccines or on the risks of secondary transmission of infection by live vaccines in patients receiving rilonacept, do not give live vaccines concurrently with rilonacept. In addition, because rilonacept may interfere with normal immune response to new antigens, vaccinations may not be effective in patients receiving rilonacept. No data are available on the effectiveness of vaccination with inactivated (killed) antigens in patients receiving rilonacept.

Because IL-1 blockade may interfere with immune response to infections, it is recommended that prior to initiation of therapy with rilonacept adult and children receive all recommended vaccinations, as appropriate, including pneumococcal vaccine and inactivated influenza vaccine (see current recommended immunizations schedules at the Web site of the CDC http://www.cdc.gov/vaccines/recs/schedules/).

➤*Hypersensitivity reactions:* Hypersensitivity reactions associated with rilonacept administration in the clinical studies were rare. If a hypersensitivity reaction occurs, discontinue administration of rilonacept and initiate appropriate therapy.

➤*Pregnancy: Category C.* There are no adequate and well-controlled studies of rilonacept in pregnant women. Based on animal data, rilonacept may cause fetal harm. An embryo-fetal developmental toxicity study was performed in cynomolgus monkeys treated with 0, 5, 15, or 30 mg/kg given twice a week (the highest dose is approximately 3.7-fold higher than the human doses of 160 mg based on body surface area [BSA]). The fetus of the only monkey with exposure to rilonacept during the later period of gestation showed multiple fusions and absences of the ribs and thoracic vertebral bodies and arches. Exposure to rilonacept during this time period was below that expected clinically. Likewise, in the cynomolgus monkey, all doses of rilonacept reduced serum levels of estradiol up to 64% compared with controls and increased the incidence of lumbar ribs compared with both control animals and historical control incidences. In perinatal and postnatal developmental toxicology studies in the mouse model using a murine analog of rilonacept (0, 20, 100, or 200 mg/kg), there was a 3-fold increase in the number of stillbirths in dams treated with 200 mg/kg 3 times per week (the highest dose is approximately 6-fold higher than the 160 mg maintenance dose based on BSA). Use rilonacept during pregnancy only if the benefit justifies the potential risk to the fetus.

Nonteratogenic – A perinatal and postnatal reproductive toxicology study was performed in which mice were subcutaneously administered a murine analog of rilonacept at doses of 20, 100, and 200 mg/kg 3 times per week (the highest dose is approximately 6-fold higher than the 160 mg maintenance dose based on BSA). Results indicated an increased incidence in unscheduled deaths of the F_1 offspring during maturation at all doses tested.

➤*Lactation:* It is not known whether rilonacept is excreted in human milk. Because many drugs are excreted in human milk, exercise caution when rilonacept is administered to a breast-feeding woman.

➤*Children:* Six children and adolescents with cryopyrin-associated periodic syndromes between 12 and 16 years of age were treated with rilonacept at a weekly, subcutaneous dose of 2.2 mg/kg (up to a maximum of 160 mg) for 24 weeks during the open-label extension phase. These patients showed improvement from baseline in their symptom scores and in objective markers of inflammation (eg, serum amyloid A and CRP). The adverse reactions included injection-site reactions and upper respiratory tract symptoms, as were commonly seen in the adults.

The trough drug levels for 4 children measured at the end of the weekly dose interval (mean, 20 mcg/mL; range, 3.6 to 33 mcg/mL) were similar to those observed in adults with cryopyrin-associated periodic syndromes (mean, 24 mcg/mL; range, 7 to 56 mcg/mL).

Safety and effectiveness in children younger than 12 years of age have not been established.

When administered to pregnant primates, rilonacept treatment may have contributed to alterations in bone ossification in the fetus. It is not known if rilonacept will alter bone development in children. Monitor children treated with rilonacept for growth and development.

➤*Elderly:* In the placebo-controlled clinical studies in patients with cryopyrin-associated periodic syndromes and other indications, 70 patients randomized to treatment with rilonacept were 65 years of age and older, and 6 were 75 years of age and older. In the cryopyrin-associated periodic syndromes clinical trial, efficacy, safety, and tolerability were generally similar in elderly patients as compared with younger adults; however, only 10 patients 65 years of age and older participated in the trial.

In an open-label extension study of cryopyrin-associated periodic syndromes, a woman 71 years of age developed bacterial meningitis and died. Age did not appear to have a significant effect on steady-state trough concentrations in the clinical study.

➤*Monitoring:* Monitor patients for changes in their lipid profiles and provide with medical treatment if warranted. Monitor children treated with rilonacept for growth and development.

Drug Interactions

➤*CYP-450 substrates:* The formation of CYP-450 enzymes is suppressed by increased levels of cytokines (eg, IL-1) during chronic inflammation. Thus, it is expected that for a molecule that binds to IL-1, such as rilonacept, the formation of CYP-450 enzymes could be normalized. This is clinically relevant for CYP-450 substrates with a narrow therapeutic index, where the dose is individually adjusted (eg, warfarin). Upon initiation of rilonacept in patients being treated with these types of medicinal products, perform therapeutic monitoring of the effect or drug concentration and adjust the individual dose of the medicinal product as needed.

Rilonacept Drug Interactions

Precipitant drug	Object drug[a]		Description
TNF-blocking agent (eg, adalimumab)	Rilonacept	↑	Coadministration of rilonacept with TNF-blocking agents may result in an increased risk of serious infections and neutropenia. Coadministration is not recommended.
Rilonacept	TNF-blocking agent (eg, adalimumab)		
IL-1–blocking agents (eg, anakinra)	Rilonacept	↑	Coadministration of rilonacept and other agents that block IL-1 or its receptors is not recommended.
Rilonacept	IL-1–blocking agents (eg, anakinra)		

[a] ↑ = object drug increased.

Adverse Reactions

➤*Serious adverse reactions:* Six serious adverse reactions were reported by 4 patients during the clinical program. These serious adverse reactions were bronchitis, colitis, GI bleeding, *Mycobacterium intracellulare* infection, sinusitis, and *Streptococcus pneumoniae* meningitis.

➤*Common adverse reactions:* The most commonly reported adverse reaction associated with rilonacept was injection-site reaction. The next most commonly reported adverse reaction was upper respiratory tract infection.

➤*Clinical trial experience:*

Rilonacept Most Frequent Adverse Reactions (Part A, Reported by at Least 2 Patients)

Adverse reaction	Rilonacept 160 mg (n = 23)	Placebo (n = 24)
Any adverse reaction	74%	54%
CNS		
Hypesthesia	9%	0%
GI		
Abdominal pain, upper	0%	8%
Diarrhea	4%	13%
Nausea	4%	13%
Stomach discomfort	4%	4%
GU		
Urinary tract infection	4%	4%
Local		
Injection-site reactions	48%	13%
Respiratory		
Cough	9%	0%
Sinusitis	9%	4%
Upper respiratory tract infection	26%	4%

➤*Injection-site reactions:* In patients with cryopyrin-associated periodic syndromes, the most common and consistently reported adverse reaction associated with rilonacept was injection-site reaction. The injection-site reaction included erythema, swelling, pruritus, mass, bruising, inflammation, pain, edema, dermatitis, discomfort, urticaria, vesicles, warmth, and hemorrhage. Most injection-site reactions lasted for 1 to 2 days. No injection-site reactions were assessed as severe, and no patient discontinued study participation because of an injection-site reaction.

➤*Infections:* During part A, the incidence of patients reporting infections was greater with rilonacept (48%) than with placebo (17%). In part B, randomized withdrawal, the incidence of infections were similar in the rilonacept (18%) and the placebo patients (22%). Part A of the trial was initiated in the winter months, while part B was predominantly performed in the summer months.

In placebo-controlled studies across a variety of patient populations encompassing 360 patients treated with rilonacept and 179 patients treated with placebo, the incidence of infections was 34% and 27% (2.15 and 1.81 per patient-exposure year), respectively, for rilonacept and placebo.

RILONACEPT — INJECTION

Serious infections – One subject receiving rilonacept for an unapproved indication in another study developed an infection in his olecranon bursa with *M. intracellulare*. The patient was on chronic glucocorticoid treatment. The infection occurred after an intra-articular glucocorticoid injection into the bursa with subsequent local exposure to a suspected source of mycobacteria. The patient recovered after the administration of the appropriate antimicrobial therapy. One patient treated for another unapproved indication developed bronchitis/sinusitis that resulted in hospitalization. One patient died in an open-label study of cryopyrin-associated periodic syndromes from *S. pneumoniae* meningitis.

➤*Hematologic reactions:* One patient in a study in an unapproved indication developed transient neutropenia (absolute neutrophil count [ANC] less than 1×10^9/L) after receiving a large dose (2,000 mg intravenously [IV]) of rilonacept. The patient did not experience any infection associated with the neutropenia.

➤*Immunogenicity:* Antibodies directed against the receptor domains of rilonacept were detected by an enzyme-linked immunosorbent (immunoabsorbent) assay in patients with cryopyrin-associated periodic syndromes after treatment with rilonacept. Nineteen of 55 (35%) subjects who had received rilonacept for at least 6 weeks tested positive for treatment-emergent binding antibodies on at least 1 occasion. Of the 19, seven tested positive at the last assessment (week 18 or 24 of the open-label extension period), and 5 subjects tested positive for neutralizing antibodies on at least 1 occasion. There was no correlation of antibody activity and clinical effectiveness or safety.

➤*Lipid profiles:* Cholesterol and lipid levels may be reduced in patients with chronic inflammation. Patients with cryopyrin-associated periodic syndromes treated with rilonacept experienced increases in their mean total cholesterol, high-density lipoprotein (HDL) cholesterol, low-density lipoprotein (LDL) cholesterol, and triglycerides. The mean increases from baseline for total cholesterol, HDL cholesterol, LDL cholesterol, and triglycerides were 19, 2, 10, and 57 mg/dL, respectively, after 6 weeks of open-label therapy. Monitor the lipid profiles of patients (eg, after 2 to 3 months) and consider lipid-lowering therapies as needed based upon cardiovascular risk factors and current guidelines.

Overdosage

There have been no reports of overdose with rilonacept. Maximum weekly doses of up to 320 mg have been administered subcutaneously for up to approximately 18 months in a small number of patients with cryopyrin-associated periodic syndromes and up to 6 months in patients with an unapproved indication in clinical trials without evidence of dose-limiting toxicities. In addition, rilonacept given IV at doses of up to 2,000 mg monthly in another patient population for up to 6 months were tolerated without dose-limiting toxicities. The maximum amount of rilonacept that can be safely administered has not been determined.

➤*Treatment:* In case of overdose, it is recommended that the subject be monitored for any signs or symptoms of adverse reactions or effects, and appropriate symptomatic treatment instituted immediately.

Patient Information

Perform the first injection of rilonacept under the supervision of a qualified health care provider. If a patient or caregiver is to administer rilonacept, instruct him/her on aseptic reconstitution of the lyophilized product and injection technique. Assess the ability to inject subcutaneously to ensure proper administration of rilonacept, including rotation of injection sites. Reconstitute rilonacept with preservative-free sterile water for injection to be provided by the pharmacy. Use a puncture-resistant container for disposal of vials, needles and syringes. Instruct patients or caregivers in proper vial, syringe, and needle disposal, and caution against reuse of these items.

Inform patients that almost half of the patients in the clinical trials experienced a reaction at the injection site. Injection-site reactions may include pain, erythema, swelling, pruritus, bruising, mass, inflammation, dermatitis, edema, urticaria, vesicles, warmth, and hemorrhage. Caution patients to avoid injecting into an area that is already swollen or red. Advise patients to inform their health care provider of any persistent injection-site reaction.

Caution patients that rilonacept has been associated with serious, life-threatening infections, and not to initiate treatment with rilonacept if they have a chronic or active infection. Counsel patients to contact their health care provider immediately if they develop an infection after starting rilonacept. Discontinue treatment with rilonacept if a patient develops a serious infection. Counsel patients not to take any IL-1–blocking drug, including rilonacept, if they are also taking a drug that blocks TNF, such as etanercept, infliximab, or adalimumab. Use of rilonacept with other IL-1–blocking agents, such as anakinra, is not recommended.

Inform patients that prior to initiation of therapy with rilonacept, health care providers should review with adults and children their vaccination history relative to current medical guidelines for vaccine use, including taking into account the potential of increased risk of infection during treatment with rilonacept.

CANAKINUMAB

Rx	**Ilaris** (Novartis)	**Injection, lyophilized powder for solution:** 180 mg	Preservative free. In 6 mL single-use vials.

CANAKINUMAB — INJECTION

Indications

➤*Cryopyrin-associated periodic syndromes:* For the treatment of cryopyrin-associated periodic syndromes in adults and children 4 years of age and older, including familial cold autoinflammatory syndrome and Muckle-Wells syndrome.

Administration and Dosage

➤*Adults:*

Cryopyrin-associated periodic syndromes –

Body weight greater than 40 kg: 150 mg every 8 weeks via subcutaneous injection.

Body weight between 15 and 40 kg: 2 mg/kg every 8 weeks via subcutaneous injection.

➤*Children:*

Cryopyrin-associated periodic syndromes –

4 years of age and older:

- *Body weight greater than 40 kg* – See Adults for dosing.
- *Body weight between 15 and 40 kg* –

  Usual dosage: 2 mg/kg every 8 weeks via subcutaneous injection.

  Dosage adjustment: The dose can be increased to 3 mg/kg for children with an inadequate response.

➤*Preparation for administration:* Using aseptic technique, reconstitute each vial of canakinumab by slowly injecting 1 mL of preservative-free sterile water for injection with a 1 mL syringe and an 18 G × 2 inch needle. Swirl the vial slowly at an angle of approximately 45° for approximately 1 minute and allow to stand for 5 minutes. Then gently turn the vial upside down and back again 10 times. Avoid touching the rubber stopper with your fingers. Allow to stand for approximately 15 minutes at room temperature to obtain a clear solution. Do not shake. Tap the side of the vial to remove any residual liquid from the stopper. Slight foaming of the product upon reconstitution is not unusual.

Using a sterile syringe and needle, carefully withdraw the required volume depending on the dose to be administered (0.2 to 1 mL). Each vial after reconstitution results in a 150 mg/mL solution.

➤*Administration:* Inject subcutaneously only using a 27 G × 0.5 inch needle. Injection into scar tissue should be avoided because this may result in insufficient exposure to canakinumab.

➤*Storage/Stability:* The unopened vial must be stored refrigerated at 2° to 8°C (36° to 46°F). Do not freeze. Store in the original carton to protect from light. Do not use beyond the date stamped on the label. After reconstitution, canakinumab should be kept from light and can be kept at room temperature if used within 60 minutes of reconstitution. Otherwise, it should be refrigerated at 2° to 8°C (36° to 46°F) and used within 4 hours of reconstitution. Unused portions of canakinumab should be discarded.

Actions

➤*Pharmacology:* Cryopyrin-associated periodic syndromes refer to rare genetic syndromes generally caused by mutations in the nucleotide-binding domain, leucine rich family (NLR), pyrin domain containing 3 (NLRP-3) gene (also known as cold-induced autoinflammatory syndrome-1). Cryopyrin-associated periodic syndrome disorders are inherited in an autosomal dominant pattern with male and female offspring equally affected. Features common to all disorders include fever, urticaria-like rash, arthralgia, myalgia, fatigue, and conjunctivitis.

The NLRP-3 gene encodes the protein cryopyrin, an important component of the inflammasome. Cryopyrin regulates the protease caspase-1 and controls the activation of interleukin-1 beta (IL-1 beta). Mutations in NLRP-3 result in an overactive inflammasome, resulting in excessive release of activated IL-1 beta that drives inflammation.

Canakinumab is a human monoclonal anti-IL-1 beta antibody of the IgG1/κ isotype. Canakinumab binds to human IL-1β and neutralizes its activity by blocking its interaction with IL-1 receptors, but it does not bind IL-1 alpha or IL-1 receptor antagonist.

➤*Pharmacokinetics:*

Absorption – The peak serum canakinumab concentration (C_{max}) of 16 ± 3.5 mcg/mL occurred approximately 7 days after subcutaneous administration of a single 150 mg subcutaneous dose to adults with cryopyrin-associated periodic syndromes. The absolute bioavailability of subcutaneous canakinumab was estimated to be 70%. Exposure parameters (such as area under the curve [AUC] and C_{max}) increased in proportion to dose over the dose range of 0.3 to 10 mg/kg given as an intravenous (IV) infusion or from 150 to 300 mg as a subcutaneous injection.

Distribution – Canakinumab binds to serum IL-1 beta. Canakinumab volume of distribution at steady state varied according to body weight and was estimated to be 6.01 L in a typical patient with cryopyrin-associated periodic syndromes weighing 70 kg. The expected accumulation ratio was 1.3-fold following 6 months of subcutaneous dosing of canakinumab 150 mg every 8 weeks.

Excretion – Clearance of canakinumab varied according to body weight and was estimated to be 0.174 L/day in a typical patient with cryopyrin-associated periodic syndromes weighing 70 kg. There was no indication of accelerated clearance or time-dependent change in the pharmacokinetic

CANAKINUMAB — INJECTION

properties of canakinumab following repeated administration. The mean terminal half-life was 26 days.

Contraindications

None known.

Warnings/Precautions

➤*Serious infections:* Canakinumab may be associated with an increased risk of serious infections. Exercise caution when administering canakinumab to patients with infections, a history of recurring infections, or underlying conditions that may predispose them to infections. Do not initiate treatment with canakinumab in patients with active infection requiring medical intervention. Discontinue administration of canakinumab if a patient develops a serious infection.

Infections, predominantly of the upper respiratory tract, in some instances serious, have been reported with canakinumab. The observed infections responded to standard therapy. No unusual or opportunistic infections were reported with canakinumab. In clinical trials, canakinumab has not been coadministered with tumor necrosis factor (TNF) inhibitors. An increased incidence of serious infections has been associated with administration of another IL-1 blocker in combination with TNF inhibitors. Taking canakinumab with TNF inhibitors is not recommended because this may increase the risk of serious infections.

Tuberculosis – Drugs that affect the immune system by blocking TNF have been associated with an increased risk of reactivation of latent tuberculosis (TB). It is possible that taking drugs such as canakinumab that block IL-1 increases the risk of TB or other atypical or opportunistic infections.

Prior to initiating immunomodulatory therapies, including canakinumab, test patients for latent TB infection. Canakinumab has not been studied in patients with a positive TB screen, and the safety of canakinumab in patients with latent TB infection is unknown. Patients testing positive in TB screening should be treated by standard medical practice prior to therapy with canakinumab.

Follow current Centers for Disease Control and Prevention (CDC) guidelines both to evaluate for and to treat possible latent TB infections before initiating therapy with canakinumab.

➤*Immunosuppression:* The impact of treatment with anti–IL-1 therapy on the development of malignancies is not known. However, treatment with immunosuppressants, including canakinumab, may result in an increase in the risk of malignancies.

➤*Vaccines:* Do not give live vaccines concurrently with canakinumab. Because no data are available on either the efficacy or risks of secondary transmission of infection by live vaccines in patients receiving canakinumab, do not give live vaccines concurrently with canakinumab. In addition, because canakinumab may interfere with normal immune response to new antigens, vaccinations may not be effective in patients receiving canakinumab. No data are available on the effectiveness of vaccinations with inactivated (killed) antigens in patients receiving canakinumab.

Because IL-1 blockade may interfere with immune response to infections, it is recommended that prior to initiation of therapy with canakinumab, adult and pediatric patients receive all recommended vaccinations, as appropriate, including pneumococcal vaccine and inactivated influenza vaccine. (See current recommended immunization schedules at the CDC Web site, http://www.cdc.gov/vaccines/recs/schedules/.)

➤*Pregnancy: Category C.* Canakinumab has been shown to produce delays in fetal skeletal development when evaluated in marmoset monkeys using doses 23-fold the maximum recommended human dose (MRHD) and greater (based on a plasma AUC comparison). Doses producing exposures within the clinical exposure range at the MHRD were not evaluated. Similar delays in fetal skeletal development were observed in mice administered a murine analog of canakinumab. There are no adequate and well-controlled studies of canakinumab in pregnant women. Because animal reproduction studies are not always predictive of human response, use this drug during pregnancy only if clearly needed.

There were increases in the incidence of incomplete ossification of the terminal caudal vertebra and misaligned and/or bipartite vertebra in fetuses at all dose levels when compared with concurrent controls suggestive of delay in skeletal development in the marmoset. Because canakinumab does not cross-react with mouse or rat IL-1, pregnant mice were subcutaneously administered a murine analog of canakinumab at doses of 15, 50, or 150 mg/kg on gestation days 6, 11, and 17. The incidence of incomplete ossification of the parietal and frontal skull bones of fetuses was increased in a dose-dependent manner at all dose levels tested.

➤*Lactation:* It is not known whether canakinumab is excreted in human milk. Because many drugs are excreted in human milk, exercise caution when canakinumab is administered to a breast-feeding woman.

➤*Children:* The safety and effectiveness of canakinumab in patients younger than 4 years of age have not been established.

Drug Interactions

➤*Cytochrome P450 substrates:* The formation of cytochrome P450 (CYP-450) enzymes is suppressed by increased levels of cytokines (eg, IL-1) during chronic inflammation. Thus it is expected that for a molecule that binds to IL-1, such as canakinumab, the formation of CYP-450 enzymes could be normalized. This is clinically relevant for CYP-450 substrates with a narrow therapeutic index, where the dose is individually adjusted (eg, warfarin). Upon initiation of canakinumab in patients being treated with these types of medicinal products, perform therapeutic monitoring of the effect or drug concentration; the individual dose of the medicinal product may need to be adjusted as needed.

➤*TNF-blocker and IL-1 blocking agent:* An increased incidence of serious infections and an increased risk of neutropenia have been associated with administration of another IL-1 blocker in combination with TNF inhibitors in another patient population. Use of canakinumab with TNF inhibitors may also result in similar toxicities and is not recommended because this may increase the risk of serious infections.

The coadministration of canakinumab with other drugs that block IL-1 has not been studied. Based on the potential for pharmacological interactions between canakinumab and a recombinant IL-1ra, coadministration of canakinumab and other agents that block IL-1 or its receptors is not recommended.

➤*Vaccines:* See Warnings/Precautions for more information.

Adverse Reactions

Canakinumab Adverse Reactions (≥ 10%)	
Adverse reaction	Canakinumab (n = 35)
Any adverse reaction	100%
CNS	
Headache	14%
Vertigo	11%
GI	
Diarrhea	20%
Nausea	14%
Gastroenteritis	11%
Respiratory	
Bronchitis	11%
Nasopharyngitis	34%
Pharyngitis	11%
Rhinitis	17%
Miscellaneous	
Influenza	17%
Weight increased	11%
Musculoskeletal pain	11%

➤*Vertigo:* Vertigo has been reported in 9% to 14% of patients in cryopyrin-associated periodic syndromes studies, exclusively in patients with Muckle-Wells syndrome, and reported as a serious adverse reaction in 2 cases. All reactions resolved with continued treatment with canakinumab.

➤*Injection-site reactions:* In study 1, subcutaneous injection-site reactions were observed in 9% of patients in part 1 with mild tolerability reactions; in part 2, one patient each (7%) had a mild or a moderate tolerability reaction and, in part 3, one patient had a mild local tolerability reaction. No severe injection-site reactions were reported and none led to discontinuation of treatment.

Overdosage

➤*Treatment:* In the case of overdose, it is recommended that the subject be monitored for any signs and symptoms of adverse reactions or effects, and that appropriate symptomatic treatment be instituted immediately.

Patient Information

Caution patients that canakinumab use has been associated with serious infections. Instruct patients to contact their health care provider immediately if they develop an infection after starting canakinumab. Instruct patients to discontinue treatment with canakinumab if they develop a serious infection. Counsel patients not to take any IL-1–blocking drug, including canakinumab, if they are also taking a drug that blocks TNF, such as etanercept, infliximab, or adalimumab. Use of canakinumab with other IL-1–blocking agents, such as rilonacept and anakinra, is not recommended. Caution patients not to initiate treatment with canakinumab if they have a chronic or active infection, including HIV or hepatitis B or C.

Prior to initiation of therapy with canakinumab, review with adult and pediatric patients their vaccination history relative to current medical guidelines for vaccine use, taking into account the potential of increased risk of infection during treatment with canakinumab.

Explain to patients that a very small number of patients in the clinical trials experienced a reaction at the subcutaneous injection site. Injection-site reactions may include pain, erythema, swelling, pruritus, bruising, mass, inflammation, dermatitis, edema, urticaria, vesicles, warmth, and hemorrhage. Avoid injecting into an area that is already swollen or red. Advise patients that any persistent reaction should be brought to the attention of the prescribing health care provider.

MITOXANTRONE HYDROCHLORIDE

For complete prescribing information, see the Mitoxantrone monograph in the Antineoplastics chapter.

FINGOLIMOD

Rx	**Gilenya** (Novartis)	**Capsules; oral:** 0.5 mg	Equiv. to fingolimod hydrochloride 0.56 mg. Mannitol. (FTY 0.5 mg). Opaque white/yellow. In UD 7s and 28s.

FINGOLIMOD HYDROCHLORIDE — ORAL

Indications

➤*Multiple sclerosis:* For the treatment of patients with relapsing forms of multiple sclerosis (MS) to reduce the frequency of clinical exacerbations and to delay the accumulation of physical disability.

Administration and Dosage

➤*General dosing considerations:* Observe patients for 6 hours after the first dose to monitor for signs and symptoms of bradycardia.

➤*Adults:*

Multiple sclerosis – 0.5 mg once daily.

➤*Hepatic function impairment:* Closely monitor patients with severe hepatic impairment because adverse reactions may be greater.

➤*Administration:* Administer with or without food.

➤*Storage/Stability:* Store at 25°C (77°F); excursions are permitted between 15° and 30°C (59° and 86°F). Protect from moisture.

Actions

➤*Pharmacology:* Fingolimod is metabolized by sphingosine kinase to the active metabolite, fingolimod-phosphate. Fingolimod-phosphate is a sphingosine 1-phosphate receptor modulator, and binds with high affinity to sphingosine 1-phosphate receptors 1, 3, 4, and 5. Fingolimod-phosphate blocks the capacity of lymphocytes to egress from lymph nodes, reducing the number of lymphocytes in peripheral blood. The mechanism by which fingolimod exerts therapeutic effects in MS is unknown, but may involve reduction of lymphocyte migration into the central nervous system.

Pharmacodynamics –

Electrophysiology:

• *Heart rate and rhythm* – Fingolimod causes a transient reduction in heart rate and atrioventricular (AV) conduction at treatment initiation. The maximal decline of heart rate is seen in the first 6 hours postdose, with 70% of the negative chronotropic effect achieved on the first day. Heart rate progressively increases after the first day, returning to baseline values within 1 month of the start of long-term treatment.

• *Potential to prolong the QT interval* – In a thorough QT interval study of doses of fingolimod 1.25 or 2.5 mg at steady state, when a negative chronotropic effect of fingolimod was still present, fingolimod treatment resulted in a prolongation of QTc, with the upper bound of the 90% confidence interval (CI) of 14.0 ms. There is no consistent signal of increased incidence of QTc outliers, either absolute or change from baseline, associated with fingolimod treatment. In MS studies, there was no clinically relevant prolongation of QT interval, but patients at risk of QT prolongation were not included in clinical studies.

Immune system:

• *Immune cell numbers* – In a study in which 12 subjects received fingolimod 0.5 mg daily, the lymphocyte count decreased to approximately 60% of baseline within 4 to 6 hours after the first dose. With continued daily dosing, the lymphocyte count continued to decrease over a 2-week period, reaching a nadir count of approximately 500 cells/mcL or approximately 30% of baseline. In a placebo-controlled study in 1,272 MS patients (of whom 425 received fingolimod 0.5 mg daily and 418 received placebo), 18% of patients on fingolimod 0.5 mg reached a nadir count of fewer than 200 cells/mcL on at least 1 occasion. No patient on placebo reached a nadir count of fewer than 200 cells/mcL. Low lymphocyte counts are maintained with long-term daily dosing of fingolimod 0.5 mg daily.

Long-term fingolimod dosing leads to a mild decrease in the neutrophil count to approximately 80% of baseline. Monocytes are unaffected by fingolimod.

Peripheral lymphocyte count increases are evident within days of stopping fingolimod treatment and typically normal counts are reached within 1 to 2 months.

• *Antibody response* – The immunogenicity of keyhole-limpet hemocyanin (KLH) and pneumococcal polysaccharide vaccine (PPV-23) immunization were assessed by immunoglobulin M (IgM) and immunoglobulin G (IgG) titers in a steady-state, randomized, placebo-controlled study in healthy volunteers. Compared with placebo, antigen-specific IgM titers were decreased by 91% and 25% in response to KLH and PPV, respectively, in subjects receiving fingolimod 0.5 mg. Similarly, IgG titers were decreased by 45% and 50% in response to KLH and PPV, respectively, in subjects receiving fingolimod 0.5 mg daily compared with placebo. The responder rate for fingolimod 0.5 mg as measured by the number of subjects with a greater than 4-fold increase in KLH IgG was comparable with placebo and 25% lower for PPV-23 IgG, while the number of subjects with a more than 4-fold increase in KLH and PPV-23 IgM was 75% and 40% lower, respectively, compared with placebo. The capacity to mount a skin delayed-type hypersensitivity reaction to *Candida* and tetanus toxoid was decreased by approximately 30% in subjects receiving fingolimod 0.5 mg daily compared with placebo. Immunologic responses were further decreased with fingolimod 1.25 mg (a dose higher than recommended in MS).

Pulmonary function: Single fingolimod doses of at least 5 mg (10-fold the recommended dose) are associated with a dose-dependent increase in airway resistance. In a 14-day study of 0.5, 1.25, or 5 mg/day, fingolimod was not associated with impaired oxygenation or oxygen desaturation with exercise or an increase in airway responsiveness to methacholine. Subjects on fingolimod treatment had a normal bronchodilator response to inhaled beta-agonists.

In a 14-day placebo-controlled study of patients with moderate asthma, no effect was seen for fingolimod 0.5 mg (recommended dose in MS). A 10% reduction in mean forced expiratory volume at 1 second (FEV-1) at 6 hours after dosing was observed in patients receiving fingolimod 1.25 mg (a dose higher than recommended for use in MS) on day 10 of treatment. Fingolimod 1.25 mg was associated with a 5-fold increase in the use of rescue short-acting beta-agonists.

➤*Pharmacokinetics:*

Absorption – The time to maximum concentration (T_{max}) of fingolimod is 12 to 16 hours. The apparent absolute oral bioavailability is 93%.

Steady-state blood concentrations are reached within 1 to 2 months following once-daily administration, and steady-state levels are approximately 10-fold greater than with the initial dose.

Effect of food: Food intake does not alter maximal plasma concentration (C_{max}) or exposure (area under the curve [AUC]) of fingolimod or fingolimod-phosphate. Therefore fingolimod may be taken without regard to meals.

Distribution – Fingolimod highly (86%) distributes in red blood cells. Fingolimod-phosphate has a smaller uptake in blood cells of less than 17%. Fingolimod and fingolimod-phosphate are more than 99.7% protein bound. Fingolimod and fingolimod-phosphate protein binding is not altered by renal or hepatic impairment.

Fingolimod is extensively distributed to body tissues with a volume of distribution of about 1,200 ± 260 L.

Metabolism – The biotransformation of fingolimod in humans occurs by 3 main pathways: by reversible stereoselective phosphorylation to the pharmacologically active (S)-enantiomer of fingolimod-phosphate, by oxidative biotransformation mainly via the cytochrome P450 (CYP-450) 4F2 isoenzyme and subsequent fatty acid–like degradation to inactive metabolites, and by formation of pharmacologically inactive nonpolar ceramide analogs of fingolimod.

Fingolimod is primarily metabolized via human CYP4F2, with a minor contribution of CYP2D6, 2E1, 3A4, and 4F12. Inhibitors or inducers of these isozymes might alter the exposure of fingolimod or fingolimod-phosphate. The involvement of multiple CYP isoenzymes in the oxidation of fingolimod suggests that the metabolism of fingolimod will not be subject to substantial inhibition in the presence of an inhibitor of a single specific CYP isozyme.

Following single oral administration of [^{14}C] fingolimod, the major fingolimod-related components in blood, as judged from their contribution to the AUC up to 816 hours postdose of total radiolabeled components, are fingolimod itself (23.3%), fingolimod-phosphate (10.3%), and inactive metabolites (M3 carboxylic acid metabolite [8.3%], M29 ceramide metabolite [8.9%], and M30 ceramide metabolite [7.3%]).

Excretion – Fingolimod blood clearance is 6.3 ± 2.3 L/h, and the average apparent terminal half-life is 6 to 9 days. Blood levels of fingolimod-phosphate decline in parallel with those of fingolimod in the terminal phase, yielding similar half-lives for both. After oral administration, approximately 81% of the dose is slowly excreted in the urine as inactive metabolites. Fingolimod and fingolimod-phosphate are not excreted intact in urine but are the major components in the feces, with amounts of each representing less than 2.5% of the dose.

Special populations –

Renal function impairment: In patients with severe renal impairment, fingolimod C_{max} and AUC are increased by 32% and 43%, respectively, and fingolimod-phosphate C_{max} and AUC are increased by 25% and 14%, respectively, with no change in apparent elimination half-life. Based on these findings, the fingolimod 0.5 mg dose is appropriate for use in patients with renal impairment. The systemic exposure of 2 metabolites (M2 and M3) is increased by 3- and 13-fold, respectively. The toxicity of these metabolites has not been fully characterized.

Hepatic function impairment: In subjects with mild, moderate, or severe hepatic impairment, no change in fingolimod C_{max} was observed, but fingolimod AUC was increased, respectively, by 12%, 44%, and 103%. In patients with severe hepatic impairment, fingolimod-phosphate C_{max} was decreased by 22% and AUC was not substantially changed. The pharmacokinetics of fingolimod-phosphate were not evaluated in patients with mild or moderate hepatic impairment. The apparent elimination half-life of fingolimod is unchanged in subjects with mild hepatic impairment, but is prolonged by about 50% in patients with moderate or severe hepatic impairment.

Closely monitor patients with severe hepatic impairment because the risk of adverse reactions is greater.

Elderly: The mechanism for elimination and results from population pharmacokinetics suggest that dose adjustment would not be necessary in elderly patients. However, clinical experience in patients older than 65 years of age is limited.

Contraindications

None well documented.

FINGOLIMOD HYDROCHLORIDE — ORAL

Warnings/Precautions

➤*Cardiovascular effects:*

Bradycardia – Initiation of fingolimod treatment results in a decrease in heart rate. Observe all patients for a period of 6 hours for signs and symptoms of bradycardia. If postdose bradyarrhythmia-related symptoms occur, initiate appropriate management and continue observation until the symptoms have resolved.

To identify underlying risk factors of bradycardia and AV block, if a recent electrocardiogram (ECG) (ie, within 6 months) is not available, obtain one in patients using antiarrhythmics including beta-blockers and calcium channel blockers, those with cardiac risk factors, and those who upon examination have a slow or irregular heartbeat prior to starting fingolimod.

Experience with fingolimod in patients receiving concurrent therapy with beta-blockers or in those with a history of syncope is limited. Fingolimod has not been studied in patients with sitting heart rate less than 55 beats per minute (bpm). Fingolimod has not been studied in patients with second-degree or higher AV block, sick sinus syndrome, prolonged QT interval, ischemic cardiac disease, or congestive heart failure. Fingolimod has not been studied in patients with arrhythmias requiring treatment with class Ia (eg, quinidine, procainamide) or class III (eg, amiodarone, sotalol) antiarrhythmic drugs. Class Ia and class III antiarrhythmic drugs have been associated with cases of torsades de pointes in patients with bradycardia.

After the first dose of fingolimod, the heart rate decrease starts within an hour and the day 1 decline is maximal at approximately 6 hours. Following the second dose a further decrease in heart rate may occur when compared with the heart rate prior to the second dose, but this change is of a smaller magnitude than that observed following the first dose. With continued dosing, the heart rate returns to baseline within 1 month of long-term treatment. The mean decrease in heart rate in patients on fingolimod 0.5 mg at 6 hours after the first dose was approximately 13 bpm. Heart rates lower than 40 bpm were rarely observed. Adverse reactions of bradycardia following the first dose were reported in 0.5% of patients receiving fingolimod 0.5 mg, but in no patient on placebo. Patients who experienced bradycardia were generally asymptomatic, but some patients experienced mild to moderate dizziness, fatigue, palpitations, and chest pain that resolved within the first 24 hours of treatment.

Atrioventricular blocks – Initiation of fingolimod treatment has resulted in transient AV conduction delays. In controlled clinical trials, adverse reactions of first-degree AV block (prolonged PR interval on ECG) following the first dose were reported in 0.1% of patients receiving fingolimod 0.5 mg, but in no patient on placebo. Second-degree AV blocks following the first dose were also identified in 0.1% of patients receiving fingolimod 0.5 mg, but in no patient on placebo. In a study of 698 patients with available 24-hour Holter monitoring data after their first dose (n = 351 on fingolimod 0.5 mg and n = 347 on placebo), second-degree AV blocks, usually Mobitz type I (Wenckebach) were reported in 3.7% of patients receiving fingolimod 0.5 mg and 2% of patients on placebo. The conduction abnormalities were usually transient and asymptomatic, and resolved within the first 24 hours on treatment, but they occasionally required treatment with atropine or isoproterenol. One patient developed syncope and complete AV block following the first dose of fingolimod 1.25 mg (a dose higher than recommended) in an uncontrolled study.

Re-initiation of therapy following discontinuation – If fingolimod therapy is discontinued for more than 2 weeks, the effects on heart rate and AV conduction may recur upon reintroduction of fingolimod treatment, and the same precautions as for initial dosing should apply.

Blood pressure effects – In MS clinical trials, patients treated with fingolimod 0.5 mg had an average increase of approximately 2 mm Hg in systolic pressure and approximately 1 mmHg in diastolic pressure, first detected after approximately 2 months of treatment initiation and persisting with continued treatment. In controlled studies involving 854 MS patients receiving fingolimod 0.5 mg and 511 MS patients receiving placebo, hypertension was reported as an adverse reaction in 5% of patients receiving fingolimod 0.5 mg and in 3% of patients on placebo. Monitor blood pressure during treatment with fingolimod.

➤*Infections:* Fingolimod causes a dose-dependent reduction in peripheral lymphocyte count to 20% to 30% of baseline values because of reversible sequestration of lymphocytes in lymphoid tissues. Fingolimod may, therefore, increase the risk of infections, some serious in nature.

Risk of infections – Before initiating treatment with fingolimod, ensure that a recent complete blood cell count (CBC) (ie, within 6 months) is available. Consider suspending treatment with fingolimod if a patient develops a serious infection, and reassess the benefits and risks prior to re-initiation of therapy. Because the elimination of fingolimod after discontinuation may take up to 2 months, continue monitoring for infections throughout this period. Instruct patients receiving fingolimod to report symptoms of infections to a health care provider. Do not start patients with active acute or chronic infections on treatment until the infection(s) is resolved.

Two patients died of herpetic infections during fingolimod controlled studies in the premarketing database (1 disseminated primary herpes zoster and 1 herpes simplex encephalitis). In both cases, the patients were receiving a fingolimod dose (1.25 mg) higher than recommended for the treatment of MS (0.5 mg), and had received high-dose corticosteroid therapy for suspected MS relapse. No deaths due to viral infections occurred in patients treated with fingolimod 0.5 mg in the premarketing database.

In MS controlled studies, the overall rate of infections (72%) and serious infections (2%) with fingolimod 0.5 mg was similar to placebo. However, bronchitis and, to a lesser extent, pneumonia were more common in fingolimod-treated patients.

Varicella zoster virus antibody testing/vaccination – As for any immune modulating drug, before initiating fingolimod therapy, test patients without a history of chickenpox or without vaccination against varicella zoster virus (VZV) for antibodies to VZV. Consider VZV vaccination of antibody-negative patients prior to commencing treatment with fingolimod, following which postpone the initiation of treatment with fingolimod for 1 month to allow the full effect of vaccination to occur.

Vaccines – Vaccination may be less effective during and for up to 2 months after discontinuing fingolimod. Avoid live attenuated vaccine administration during this period.

Immune system effects following discontinuation – Fingolimod remains in the blood and has pharmacodynamic effects, including decreased lymphocyte counts, for up to 2 months following the last dose of fingolimod. Lymphocyte counts generally return to the normal range within 1 to 2 months of stopping therapy. Because of the continuing pharmacodynamic effects of fingolimod, initiating other drugs during this period warrants the same considerations needed for coadministration (eg, risk of additive immunosuppressant effects).

➤*Macular edema:* In patients receiving fingolimod 0.5 mg, macular edema occurred in 0.4% of patients. Perform an adequate ophthalmologic evaluation at baseline and 3 to 4 months after treatment initiation. If patients report visual disturbances at any time while on fingolimod therapy, undertake additional ophthalmologic evaluation.

In MS controlled studies involving 1,204 patients treated with fingolimod 0.5 mg and 861 patients treated with placebo, macular edema with or without visual symptoms was reported in 0.4% of patients treated with fingolimod 0.5 mg and 0.1% of patients treated with placebo; it occurred predominantly in the first 3 to 4 months of therapy. Some patients had blurred vision or decreased visual acuity, but others were asymptomatic and diagnosed on routine ophthalmologic examination. Macular edema generally improved or resolved with or without treatment after drug discontinuation, but some patients had residual visual acuity loss even after resolution of macular edema.

Continuation of fingolimod in patients who develop macular edema has not been evaluated. When deciding whether or not to discontinue fingolimod therapy, include an assessment of the potential benefits and risks for the individual patient. The risk of recurrence after rechallenge has not been evaluated.

Patients with a history of uveitis or diabetes mellitus – Patients with a history of uveitis and patients with diabetes mellitus are at an increased risk of macular edema during fingolimod therapy. The incidence of macular edema is also increased in MS patients with a history of uveitis. The rate was approximately 20% in patients with a history of uveitis versus 0.6% in those without a history of uveitis in the combined experience with all doses of fingolimod. Ensure that MS patients with diabetes mellitus or a history of uveitis undergo an ophthalmologic evaluation prior to initiating fingolimod therapy and have regular follow-up ophthalmologic evaluations while receiving fingolimod therapy. Fingolimod has not been tested in MS patients with diabetes mellitus.

➤*Respiratory effects:* Dose-dependent reductions in FEV-1 and diffusing lung capacity for carbon monoxide (DL_{CO}) were observed in patients treated with fingolimod as early as 1 month after treatment initiation. At month 24, the reduction from baseline in the percent of predicted values for FEV-1 was 3.1% for fingolimod 0.5 mg and 2% for placebo. For DL_{CO}, the reductions from baseline in percent of predicted values at month 24 were 3.8% for fingolimod 0.5 mg and 2.7% for placebo. The changes in FEV-1 appear to be reversible after treatment discontinuation. There is insufficient information to determine the reversibility of the decrease of DL_{CO} after drug discontinuation. In MS controlled trials, dyspnea was reported in 5% of patients receiving fingolimod 0.5 mg and 4% of patients receiving placebo. Several patients discontinued fingolimod because of unexplained dyspnea during the extension (uncontrolled) studies. Fingolimod has not been tested in MS patients with compromised respiratory function.

Perform a spirometric evaluation of respiratory function and evaluation of DL_{CO} during therapy with fingolimod if clinically indicated.

➤*Hepatic effects:* Elevations of liver enzymes may occur in patients receiving fingolimod. Ensure recent (ie, within last 6 months) transaminase and bilirubin levels are available before initiation of fingolimod therapy.

During clinical trials, 3-fold the upper limit of normal (ULN) or greater elevation in liver transaminases occurred in 8% of patients treated with fingolimod 0.5 mg compared with 2% of patients on placebo. Elevations 5-fold the ULN occurred in 2% of patients on fingolimod and 1% of patients on placebo. In clinical trials, fingolimod was discontinued if the elevation exceeded 5 times the ULN. Recurrence of liver transaminase elevations occurred with rechallenge in some patients, supporting a relationship to drug. The majority of elevations occurred within 3 to 4 months. Serum transaminase levels returned to normal within approximately 2 months after discontinuation of fingolimod.

Monitor liver enzymes in patients who develop symptoms suggestive of hepatic dysfunction, such as unexplained nausea, vomiting, abdominal pain, fatigue, anorexia, or jaundice and/or dark urine. Discontinue fingolimod if significant liver injury is confirmed. Patients with preexisting liver disease may be at increased risk of developing elevated liver enzymes when taking fingolimod.

Because fingolimod exposure is doubled in patients with severe hepatic impairment, closely monitor these patients because the risk of adverse reactions is higher.

FINGOLIMOD HYDROCHLORIDE — ORAL

➤*Renal function impairment:* The blood level of some fingolimod metabolites is increased (up to 13-fold) in patients with severe renal impairment. The toxicity of these metabolites has not been fully explored. The blood level of these metabolites has not been assessed in patients with mild or moderate renal impairment.

➤*Hepatic function impairment:* Because fingolimod, but not fingolimod-phosphate, exposure is doubled in patients with severe hepatic impairment, closely monitor patients with severe hepatic impairment because the risk of adverse reactions may be greater. Patients with preexisting liver disease may be at increased risk of developing elevated liver enzymes when taking fingolimod.

➤*Pregnancy: Category C.* There are no adequate and well-controlled studies in pregnant women. Based on animal studies, fingolimod may cause fetal harm. Because it takes approximately 2 months to eliminate fingolimod from the body, potential risks to the fetus may persist after treatment ends. Advise women of childbearing potential to use effective contraception to avoid pregnancy during and for 2 months after stopping fingolimod treatment. Use fingolimod during pregnancy only if the potential benefit justifies the potential risk to the fetus.

In oral studies conducted in rats and rabbits, fingolimod demonstrated developmental toxicity, including teratogenicity (rats) and embryolethality, when given to pregnant animals. In rats, the highest no-effect dose was less than the RHD of 0.5 mg/day on a body surface area (mg/m^2) basis. The most common fetal visceral malformations in rats included persistent truncus arteriosus and ventricular septal defect. The receptor affected by fingolimod (sphingosine 1-phosphate receptor) is known to be involved in vascular formation during embryogenesis.

When fingolimod was orally administered to pregnant rats during the period of organogenesis (0, 0.03, 0.1, and 0.3 mg/kg/day or 0, 1, 3, and 10 mg/kg/day), increased incidences of fetal malformations and embryofetal deaths were observed at all but the lowest dose tested (0.03 mg/kg/day), which is less than the RHD on a mg/m^2 basis. Oral administration to pregnant rabbits during organogenesis (0, 0.5, 1.5, and 5 mg/kg/day) resulted in increased incidences of embryofetal mortality and fetal growth retardation at the mid and high doses. The no-effect dose for these effects in rabbits (0.5 mg/kg/day) is approximately 20 times the RHD on a mg/m^2 basis.

When fingolimod was orally administered to female rats during pregnancy and lactation (0, 0.05, 0.15, and 0.5 mg/kg/day), pup survival was decreased at all doses and a neurobehavioral (learning) deficit was seen in offspring at the high dose. The low-effect dose of 0.05 mg/kg/day is similar to the RHD on a mg/m^2 basis.

Pregnancy registry – A pregnancy registry has been established to collect information about the effect of fingolimod use during pregnancy. Health care providers are encouraged to enroll pregnant patients, or pregnant women may enroll themselves in the fingolimod pregnancy registry by calling 1-877-598-7237.

➤*Lactation:* Fingolimod is excreted in the milk of treated rats. It is not known whether this drug is excreted in human milk. Because many drugs are excreted in human milk and because of the potential for serious adverse reactions in breast-feeding infants from fingolimod, decide whether to discontinue breast-feeding or the drug, taking into account the importance of the drug to the mother.

➤*Children:* The safety and effectiveness of fingolimod in children with MS younger than 18 years of age have not been established.

➤*Elderly:* Clinical MS studies of fingolimod did not include sufficient numbers of patients 65 years of age and older to determine whether they respond differently than younger patients. Use fingolimod with caution in patients 65 years of age and older, reflecting the greater frequency of decreased hepatic or renal function, and of concomitant disease or other drug therapy.

➤*Monitoring:* Before initiating fingolimod therapy, test patients without a history of chickenpox or without vaccination against VZV for antibodies to VZV.

Perform an adequate ophthalmologic evaluation at baseline and 3 to 4 months after treatment initiation. If patients report visual disturbances at any time while on fingolimod therapy, undertake additional ophthalmologic evaluation. Ensure that MS patients with diabetes mellitus or a history of uveitis undergo an ophthalmologic evaluation prior to initiating fingolimod therapy and have regular follow-up ophthalmologic evaluations while receiving fingolimod therapy.

Spirometric evaluation of respiratory function and evaluation of DL_{CO} should be performed during therapy with fingolimod if clinically indicated.

Ensure that recent (ie, within last 6 months) transaminase and bilirubin levels are available before initiation of fingolimod therapy. Monitor liver enzymes in patients who develop symptoms suggestive of hepatic dysfunction.

Observe all patients for a period of 6 hours after the first dose for signs and symptoms of bradycardia. If a recent ECG (within 6 hours) is not available, obtain one in patients using antiarrhythmics, those with cardiac risk factors, and those who have a slow or irregular heartbeat prior to starting fingolimod. Monitor blood pressure during treatment with fingolimod.

Before initiating treatment with fingolimod, ensure that a recent CBC (ie, within 6 months) is available. Monitor patients for infection during treatment and for at least 2 months after discontinuation.

Drug Interactions

➤*QT prolongation:* An additive effect of fingolimod with other drugs that prolong the QT interval cannot be excluded. The following drugs may prolong the QT interval and increase the risk of life-threatening cardiac arrhythmias, including torsades de pointes: antiarrhythmic agents (eg, amiodarone, bretylium, disopyramide, dofetilide, procainamide, quinidine, sotalol), arsenic trioxide, chlorpromazine, cisapride, dolasetron, droperidol, gatifloxacin, halofantrine, levomethadyl, mefloquine, mesoridazine, moxifloxacin, pentamidine, pimozide, probucol, sparfloxacin, thioridazine, and ziprasidone.

➤*Vaccines:* See Warnings/Precautions for more information.

Fingolimod Drug Interactions

Precipitant drug	Object drug[a]		Description
Antineoplastics, immune modulating therapies, immunosuppressives	Fingolimod	↑	Concurrent use with fingolimod may increase the risk of immunosuppression and infection. Use caution when switching patients from long-acting therapies with immune effects (eg, mitoxantrone, natalizumab).
Beta-blockers (eg, atenolol)	Fingolimod	↑	The heart rate–lowering effects may be increased. Carefully monitor patients during initiation of therapy.
Fingolimod	Beta-blockers (eg, atenolol)		
Class Ia (eg, procainamide, quinidine) and class III (eg, amiodarone, sotalol)	Fingolimod	↑	Class Ia and class III antiarrhythmic agents have been associated with torsades de pointes in patients with bradycardia. Because initiation of fingolimod treatment results in decreased heart rate, closely monitor patients receiving class Ia or class III antiarrhythmics.
Diltiazem	Fingolimod	↑	The heart rate–lowering effects may be increased. Carefully monitor patients during initiation of therapy.
Fingolimod	Diltiazem		
Ketoconazole (oral)	Fingolimod	↑	Fingolimod and fingolimod-phosphate blood concentrations are increased 1.7-fold when ketoconazole is given concomitantly. The risk of adverse reactions may be increased. Closely monitor the clinical response.
Fingolimod	Vaccines	↓	Vaccination may be less effective during and for up to 2 months after discontinuing fingolimod. Avoid live attenuated vaccine administration during this period.

[a] ↑ = object drug increased; ↓ = object drug decreased.

➤*Drug/Lab test interactions:* Because fingolimod reduces blood lymphocyte counts via redistribution in secondary lymphoid organs, peripheral blood lymphocyte counts cannot be used to evaluate the lymphocyte subset status. Ensure that a recent CBC is available before starting fingolimod treatment.

Adverse Reactions

➤*Most common adverse reactions:* The most frequent adverse reactions (incidence at least 10% and higher than placebo) for fingolimod 0.5 mg were back pain, diarrhea, headache, influenza, liver enzyme elevations, and cough. The only adverse reaction leading to treatment interruption reported at an incidence of more than 1% for fingolimod 0.5 mg was serum transaminase elevations (3.8%).

➤*Adverse reactions (1% or more):*

Fingolimod Adverse Reactions in Study 1 (≥ 1%)

Adverse reactions	Fingolimod 0.5 mg (n = 425)	Placebo (n = 418)
Cardiovascular		
Bradycardia	4%	1%
Hypertension	6%	4%
CNS		
Asthenia	3%	1%
Depression	8%	7%
Dizziness	7%	6%
Headache	25%	23%
Migraine	5%	1%
Paresthesia	5%	4%

FINGOLIMOD HYDROCHLORIDE — ORAL

Fingolimod Adverse Reactions in Study 1 (≥ 1%)		
Adverse reactions	Fingolimod 0.5 mg (n = 425)	Placebo (n = 418)
Dermatologic		
Alopecia	4%	2%
Eczema	3%	2%
Pruritus	3%	1%
GI		
Diarrhea	12%	7%
Gastroenteritis	5%	3%
Hematologic		
Leukopenia	3%	< 1%
Lymphopenia	4%	1%
Laboratory test abnormalities		
ALT/AST increased	14%	5%
Blood triglycerides increased	3%	1%
GGT[a] increased	5%	1%
Respiratory		
Bronchitis	8%	4%
Cough	10%	8%
Dyspnea	8%	5%
Sinusitis	7%	5%
Special senses		
Eye pain	3%	1%
Vision blurred	4%	1%
Miscellaneous		
Back pain	12%	7%
Herpes viral infections	9%	8%
Influenza viral infections	13%	10%
Tinea infections	4%	1%
Weight decreased	5%	3%

[a] GGT = gamma glutamyl transferase.

Adverse reactions in study 2, a 1-year active-controlled (vs interferon beta-1a, n = 431) study, including 849 patients with MS treated with fingolimod, were generally similar to those in study 1.

Vascular events – Vascular events, including ischemic and hemorrhagic strokes, peripheral arterial occlusive disease and posterior reversible encephalopathy syndrome were reported in premarketing clinical trials in patients who received fingolimod doses (1.25 to 5 mg) higher than recommended for use in MS. No vascular events were observed with fingolimod 0.5 mg in the premarketing database.

Lymphomas – Cases of lymphoma (cutaneous T-cell lymphoproliferative disorders or diffuse B-cell lymphoma) were reported in premarketing clinical trials in MS patients receiving fingolimod at, or above, the recommended dose of 0.5 mg. Based on the small number of cases and short duration of exposure, the relationship to fingolimod remains uncertain.

Overdosage

➤*Symptoms:* No cases of overdosage have been reported. However, single doses of up to 80-fold the recommended dose (0.5 mg) resulted in no clinically significant adverse reactions. At 40 mg, 5 of 6 subjects reported mild chest tightness or discomfort that was clinically consistent with small airway reactivity.

➤*Treatment:* Neither dialysis nor plasma exchange results in removal of fingolimod from the body.

Patient Information

Encourage patients to read the Medication Guide before starting therapy and with each refill.

inform patients of the benefits and potential risks of treatment with fingolimod. Advise patients to take fingolimod once daily as prescribed. Instruct patients not to discontinue fingolimod without first discussing this with the prescribing health care provider.

Advise patients that initiation of fingolimod treatment results in a transient decrease in heart rate. Inform patients that they will need to be observed in the health care provider's office or other facility for 6 hours after the first dose. Advise patients that if fingolimod is discontinued for more than 2 weeks, effects similar to those observed upon treatment initiation may be seen and observation for 6 hours will be needed upon treatment reinitiation.

Inform patients that they may be more likely to get infections when taking fingolimod, and to contact their health care provider if they develop symptoms of infection. Advise patients to avoid the use of some vaccines during treatment with fingolimod and for 2 months after discontinuation. Advise patients who have not had chickenpox or vaccination to consider VZV vaccination prior to commencing treatment with fingolimod.

Advise patients that fingolimod may cause macular edema, and to contact their health care provider if they experience any changes in their vision. Inform patients with diabetes mellitus or a history of uveitis that their risk of macular edema is increased.

Advise patients to contact their health care provider if they experience new-onset or worsening of dyspnea.

Inform patients that fingolimod may increase liver enzymes. Advise patients to contact their health care provider if they have any unexplained nausea, vomiting, abdominal pain, fatigue, anorexia, jaundice, and/or dark urine.

Inform patients that, based on animal studies, fingolimod may cause fetal harm. Women of childbearing age should discuss whether they are pregnant, might be pregnant, or are trying to become pregnant. Advise women of childbearing age of the need for effective contraception during fingolimod treatment and for 2 months after stopping fingolimod. Advise patients to immediately inform their health care provider if they become pregnant.

Advise patients that fingolimod remains in the blood and continues to have effects, including decreased blood lymphocyte counts, for up to 2 months following the last dose.

ANTIRHEUMATIC AGENTS

HYDROXYCHLOROQUINE SULFATE

Rx	**Hydroxychloroquine Sulfate** (Various, eg, Geneva, Mylan, Teva, Watson)	**Tablets**: 200 mg (equivalent to 155 mg base)	In 100s, 500s, and 1000s.
Rx	**Plaquenil** (Sanofi Synthelabo)		(PLAQUENIL). White to off-white. Film-coated. In 100s.

HYDROXYCHLOROQUINE SULFATE — ORAL

WARNING

Physicians should completely familiarize themselves with the complete contents of the package insert before prescribing hydroxychloroquine.

Indications

➤*Lupus erythematosus:* For the treatment of chronic discoid and systemic lupus erythematosus (SLE) in patients who have not responded satisfactorily to drugs with less potential for serious side effects.

➤*Malaria:* For the suppressive treatment and treatment of acute attacks of malaria caused by *Plasmodium vivax*, *P. malariae*, *P. ovale*, and susceptible strains of *P. falciparum*.

➤*Rheumatoid arthritis (RA):* For the treatment of acute or chronic RA in patients who have not responded satisfactorily to drugs with less potential for serious side effects.

Administration and Dosage

➤*Lupus erythematosus:* Initially, 400 mg once or twice daily in adults, continued for several weeks or months depending on response. For prolonged maintenance therapy, a smaller dose (200 to 400 mg daily) frequently will suffice. The incidence of retinopathy reportedly has been higher when the maintenance dose is exceeded.

➤*RA:*

Initial dosage – 400 to 600 mg daily, taken with a meal or a glass of milk. Side effects may require temporary reduction. Later (usually from 5 to 10 days), dose may be increased gradually to optimum response level, often without return of side effects.

Maintenance dosage – When a good response is obtained (usually in 4 to 12 weeks), reduce dosage by 50% and continue at a level of 200 to 400 mg daily. Incidence of retinopathy is higher when this dose is exceeded.

Duration of therapy – The compound is cumulative and requires several weeks to exert therapeutic effects; minor side effects may occur early. Maximum effects may not be obtained for several months. If objective improvement (reduced joint swelling, increased mobility) does not occur within 6 months, discontinue the drug. Safe use of hydroxychloroquine to treat juvenile rheumatoid arthritis (JRA) has not been established.

Relapse – If relapse occurs after drug withdrawal, resume therapy or continue on an intermittent schedule if there are no ocular contraindications.

Corticosteroid dose reduction – Corticosteroids and salicylates may be used with this compound; generally they can be decreased gradually or eliminated after hydroxychloroquine has been used for several weeks. When gradual reduction of steroid dosage is indicated, reduce (every 4 to 5 days) dose of cortisone by no more than 5 to 15 mg; hydrocortisone by 5 to 10 mg;

HYDROXYCHLOROQUINE SULFATE — ORAL

prednisolone and prednisone by 1 to 2.5 mg; methylprednisolone and triamcinolone by 1 to 2 mg; or dexamethasone by 0.25 to 0.5 mg.

➤*Malaria:* Hydroxychloroquine sulfate 200 mg is equivalent to 155 mg hydroxychloroquine base and 250 mg chloroquine phosphate.

Children's doses – Expressed in mg/kg, these should not exceed the recommended adult dose.

Suppression –

Adults: 310 mg base weekly on the same day each week. Begin 1 to 2 weeks prior to exposure; continue for 4 weeks after leaving endemic area. If suppressive therapy is not begun prior to exposure, double the initial loading dose (adults – 620 mg base; children – 10 mg base/kg) and give in 2 doses, 6 hours apart.

Children: Administer 5 mg base/kg weekly, up to a maximum adult dose.

Children's Hydroxychloroquine Dose Based on Age

Age (years)	Hydroxychloroquine base equivalent
< 1	37.5 mg
1 to 3	75 mg
4 to 6	100 mg
7 to 10	150 mg
11 to 16	225 mg

Acute attack –

Hydroxychloroquine Dose in Acute Malarial Attack

Dose	Time	Dosage (mg of base) Adults	Children
Initial dose	Day 1	620 mg	10 mg/kg
2nd dose	6 hours later	310 mg	5 mg/kg
3rd dose	Day 2	310 mg	5 mg/kg
4th dose	Day 3	310 mg	5 mg/kg

An alternative method, using a single dose of 620 mg base, has also been proven effective.

➤*Storage/Stability:* Store at room temperature, up to 30°C (86°F). Dispense in a tight, light-resistant container.

Actions

➤*Pharmacology:* Inhibition of heme polymerization appears crucial for antimalarial action. Hydroxychloroquine binds initially to heme and then prevents further heme polymerization by incorporating as heme-quinoline complexes into growing heme polymer chains. It is unknown whether the accumulation of heme, heme-quinoline complexes, or both suffices to kill the parasites or if other actions of the antimalarial quinolones are required.

➤*Pharmacokinetics:*

Absorption/Distribution – Pharmacokinetics of hydroxychloroquine are similar to chloroquine. Both drugs are absorbed very rapidly and almost completely after oral administration. Hydroxychloroquine is distributed widely into body tissues and concentrates in the spleen, liver, kidney, melanin-containing tissues, lungs, and, to a lesser extent, the spinal cord and brain. It has a large apparent volume of distribution (more than 100 L/kg). It is bound approximately 60% to plasma proteins.

Metabolism/Excretion – Chloroquine is extensively metabolized in the liver. The renal clearance is approximately half of its total systemic clearance. Renal excretion is increased by acidification of the urine. The terminal half-life ranges from 30 to 60 days, and traces of the drug can be found in the urine for years after a therapeutic regimen.

Contraindications

Retinal or visual field changes attributable to any 4-aminoquinoline compound; hypersensitivity to 4-aminoquinoline compounds; long-term therapy in children.

Warnings/Precautions

➤*Psoriasis:* Use in patients with psoriasis may precipitate a severe attack. Porphyria may be exacerbated. Do not use unless the benefit to the patient outweighs possible risks.

➤*Ophthalmic effects:* Irreversible retinal damage has been observed in some patients who had received long-term or high-dosage 4-aminoquinoline therapy for discoid and SLE or RA. Retinopathy has been reported to be dose-related. When prolonged therapy is contemplated, perform initial (baseline) and periodic (every 3 months) ophthalmologic examinations (including visual acuity, expert slit-lamp, funduscopic, and visual field tests). If there is any indication of abnormality in the visual acuity, visual field, or retinal macular areas (eg, pigmentary changes, loss of foveal reflex) or any visual symptoms (eg, light flashes or streaks) not fully explainable by difficulties of accommodation or corneal opacities, discontinue drug immediately and observe patient for possible progression (see Adverse Reactions).

Retinal changes – See Adverse Reactions for more information.

Chloroquine retinopathy – Methods recommended for early diagnosis of "chloroquine retinopathy" consist of (1) funduscopic examination of macula for fine pigmentary disturbances or loss of the foveal reflex and (2) examination of central visual field with a small red test object for pericentral or paracentral scotoma or determination of retinal thresholds to red. Regard unexplained visual symptoms (eg, light flashes or streaks) as possible manifestations of retinopathy.

➤*Muscular weakness:* Examine patients on long-term therapy periodically, and test knee and ankle reflexes to detect evidence of muscular weakness. If weakness occurs, discontinue drug.

➤*Hepatic disease:* Use with caution in patients with hepatic disease or in conjunction with hepatotoxic drugs.

➤*Alcoholism:* Use with caution in patients with alcoholism.

➤*Dermatologic reactions:* Dermatologic reactions may occur; exercise care when given to any patient receiving a drug with significant tendency to produce dermatitis.

➤*Toxic symptoms:* If serious toxic symptoms occur, administer ammonium chloride (8 g daily in divided doses for adults) 3 or 4 days a week for several months after therapy has been stopped; acidification of the urine increases renal excretion by 20% to 90%. Exercise caution in renal function impairment and/or metabolic acidosis.

➤*Renal/Hepatic function impairment:* Use with caution.

➤*Pregnancy:* According to *Drugs in Pregnancy and Lactation* by Briggs, the pregnancy risk factor is a *C*. The Centers for Disease Control and Prevention recommends use for prophylaxis in pregnant women who are traveling to areas with chloroquine-sensitive *P. falciparum* malaria.

Avoid use during pregnancy, except in the suppression of malaria when the benefit outweighs the possible hazard. Chloroquine administered IV to pregnant mice rapidly crossed the placenta, accumulated selectively in the melanin structures of the fetal eyes, and was retained in the ocular tissues for 5 months after the drug was eliminated from the rest of the body.

➤*Lactation:* The drug has been detected in breast milk from 2 mothers receiving 400 mg daily doses for SLE or RA.

➤*Children:* Children are especially sensitive to 4-aminoquinolines. A number of fatalities have been reported following ingestion of chloroquine in small doses (0.75 g or 1 g in one 3-year-old).

Safe use of the drug in the treatment of JRA and SLE has not been established.

➤*Monitoring:* Perform periodic blood cell counts during prolonged therapy. If a severe blood disorder appears, consider discontinuation. Use caution in glucose-6-phosphate dehydrogenase (G-6-PD) deficiency.

Drug Interactions

Hydroxychloroquine Drug Interactions

Precipitant drug	Object drug[a]		Description
Cimetidine	Aminoquinolones (eg, hydroxychloroquine)	↑	The hydroxychloroquine dose may need to be lowered during coadministration because of increased pharmacologic effects of the hydroxychloroquine.
Aminoquinolones (eg, hydroxychloroquine)	Beta-blockers (eg, metoprolol)	↑	Plasma concentrations and cardiovascular effects of certain beta-blockers may be increased. Carefully monitor patients when hydroxychloroquine is started or stopped with concomitant use of certain beta-blockers (eg, metoprolol). Consider use of an alternative beta-blocker (eg, atenolol).
Aminoquinolones (eg, hydroxychloroquine)	Cyclosporine	↑	Elevated cyclosporine concentrations may occur, increasing the risk of nephrotoxicity. Consider monitoring cyclosporine and serum creatinine levels. Adjust cyclosporine dose accordingly.
Aminoquinolones (eg, hydroxychloroquine)	Digoxin	↑	Serum levels and actions of digoxin may be increased. Monitor for signs/symptoms of digoxin toxicity; reduce dosage if necessary.
Aminoquinolones (eg, hydroxychloroquine)	Magnesium salts	↓	Oral magnesium salts may decrease the absorption and effect of hydroxychloroquine. The antacid activity of magnesium salts also may be reduced. Separate doses of each drug by 2 to 4 hours. It may be necessary to increase the hydroxychloroquine dose.
Aminoquinolones (eg, hydroxychloroquine)	Mefloquine	↑	Coadministration may lead to an increased risk of seizures.

[a] ↑ = Object drug increased. ↓ = Object drug decreased.

HYDROXYCHLOROQUINE SULFATE — ORAL

Adverse Reactions

The following have occurred with 1 or more of the 4-aminoquinoline compounds.

➤*Cardiovascular:* Cardiomyopathy has been reported rarely with high daily doses of hydroxychloroquine.

➤*CNS:* Ataxia; convulsions; dizziness; emotional changes; headache; irritability; nerve deafness; nervousness; nightmares; nystagmus; psychosis; tinnitus; vertigo.

➤*Dermatologic:* Alopecia; bleaching of hair; photosensitivity; precipitation of nonlight-sensitive psoriasis; pruritus; skin and mucosal pigmentation; skin eruptions (urticarial, morbilliform, lichenoid, maculopapular, purpuric, erythema annulare centrifugum, Stevens-Johnson syndrome, acute generalized exanthematous pustulosis, and exfoliative dermatitis).

➤*GI:* Abdominal cramps; anorexia; diarrhea; nausea; vomiting. Isolated cases of abnormal liver function and fulminant hepatic failure.

➤*Hematologic:* Agranulocytosis; aplastic anemia; hemolysis in individuals with G-6-PD deficiency; leukopenia; thrombocytopenia.

➤*Musculoskeletal:* Skeletal muscle palsies, myopathy, or neuromyopathy leading to progressive weakness and atrophy of proximal muscle groups which may be associated with mild sensory changes, depression of tendon reflexes, and abnormal nerve conduction.

➤*Ophthalmic:*

Ciliary body – See Warnings. Disturbance of accommodation with blurred vision. This reaction is dose-related and reversible with cessation of therapy.

Cornea – Decreased corneal sensitivity; punctate to lineal opacities; transient edema. The corneal changes, with or without accompanying symptoms (eg, blurred vision, halos around lights, photophobia), are fairly common but reversible. Corneal deposits may appear as early as 3 weeks following initiation of therapy. The incidence of corneal changes and visual side effects appears to be considerably lower with hydroxychloroquine than with chloroquine.

Retina – Abnormal pigmentation (mild pigment stippling to a "bull's eye" appearance); atrophy; edema; elevated retinal threshold to red light in macular, paramacular, and peripheral retinal areas; increased macular recovery time following exposure to a bright light (photo-stress test); loss of foveal reflex.

Retinopathy – The most common visual symptoms attributed to retinopathy are: Reading and seeing difficulties (ie, words, letters, or parts of objects missing); photophobia; blurred distance vision; missing or blacked out areas in the central or peripheral visual field; light flashes and streaks. Retinopathy appears to be dose-related and has occurred within several months (rarely) to several years of daily therapy; a few cases have been reported several years after the drug was discontinued.

Patients with retinal changes may have visual symptoms or may be asymptomatic (with or without visual field changes). Rarely, scotomatous vision or field defects may occur without obvious retinal change. Retinopathy may progress even after the drug is discontinued. In a number of patients, early retinopathy (macular pigmentation sometimes with central field defects) diminished or regressed completely after therapy was discontinued. Paracentral scotoma to red targets ("premaculopathy") is indicative of early retinal dysfunction, which is usually reversible with cessation of therapy.

A small number of cases of retinal changes have occurred in patients who received only hydroxychloroquine. These usually consisted of alteration in retinal pigmentation that was detected on periodic ophthalmologic examination; visual field defects also were present in some. A case of delayed retinopathy has been reported with vision loss starting 1 year after the drug was discontinued.

Other fundus changes – Attenuation of retinal arterioles; fine granular pigmentary disturbances in the peripheral retina; optic disc pallor and atrophy; prominent choroidal patterns in advanced stage.

Visual field defects – Central scotoma with decreased visual acuity; field constriction (rare); pericentral or paracentral scotoma.

➤*Miscellaneous:* Weight loss; lassitude; exacerbation or precipitation of porphyria.

Overdosage

➤*Symptoms:* Toxic symptoms may occur within 30 minutes and consist of headache, drowsiness, visual disturbances, cardiovascular collapse, and convulsions, followed by sudden and early respiratory and cardiac arrest. Electrocardiogram may reveal atrial standstill, nodal rhythm, prolonged intraventricular conduction time, and progressive bradycardia leading to ventricular fibrillation and/or arrest. Rarely, these symptoms occur with lower doses in hypersensitive patients.

➤*Treatment:* Treatment is symptomatic and must be prompt, with immediate evacuation of the stomach by emesis or gastric lavage. Treatment includes usual supportive measures. Refer to General Management of Acute Overdosage. Activated charcoal, in a dose at least 5 times the estimated dose ingested, may inhibit further intestinal absorption if introduced by stomach tube after lavage within 30 minutes after ingestion. Control convulsions before attempting gastric lavage. If caused by cerebral stimulation, attempt cautious administration of an ultrashort-acting barbiturate; if caused by anoxia, correct with oxygen, artificial respiration, or, in shock with hypotension, use vasopressor therapy. Perform tracheal intubation or tracheostomy followed by gastric lavage if necessary. Exchange transfusions have been used to reduce the level of the drug in the blood. Closely observe, for at least 6 hours, patients surviving the acute phase who are asymptomatic. Fluids may be forced. Sufficient ammonium chloride (8 g daily in divided doses for adults) administered for a few days will acidify the urine and help promote urinary excretion.

Patient Information

May cause GI upset; instruct patients to take with food or milk.

Instruct patients to notify physician if any of the following occur: Blurring or other vision changes; ringing in the ears or hearing loss; fever; sore throat; unusual bleeding or bruising; unusual pigmentation (blue-black) of the skin; muscle weakness; bleaching or loss of hair; mood or mental changes.

Advise the patient to stop taking this medicine for RA if there is no improvement (reduced joint swelling, increased mobility) within 6 months.

If RA recurs after the medicine has been stopped, this medicine may be resumed or taken on a periodic basis if there are no existing vision problems.

This medicine may cause dizziness. Instruct patients to use caution while driving or performing other tasks requiring alertness, coordination, or physical dexterity.

Lab tests, including eye exams, may be required to monitor therapy. Instruct patients to be sure to keep appointments.

Gold Compounds

WARNING

Signs of gold toxicity include the following: Fall in hemoglobin, leukopenia ^{3}, granulocytes $< 1500/mm^3$, platelets $< 100{,}000$ to $150{,}000/mm^3$, proteinuria, hematuria, pruritus, rash, stomatitis or persistent diarrhea. Review recommended laboratory work results before instituting therapy and before each injection or written prescription for oral gold. See patient before each injection to determine presence or absence of adverse reactions; some of these can be severe or even fatal. Physicians planning to use gold compounds should be experienced with chrysotherapy and thoroughly familiar with both toxicity and benefits of gold.

Explain the possibility of adverse reactions to patients before starting therapy.

Advise patients to report promptly any toxicity symptoms (see Patient Information).

Indications

➤*Rheumatoid arthritis:*

Parenteral – Active early rheumatoid arthritis, both adult and juvenile types (cases not adequately controlled by other anti-inflammatory agents or conservative measures). Use only as one part of therapy program; alone, it is not a complete treatment.

Oral – Management of adults with active classical or definite rheumatoid arthritis (ARA criteria) with insufficient therapeutic response to or intolerant of an adequate trial of full doses of one or more NSAIDs. Add **auranofin** to baseline program; include non-drug therapies.

➤*Off-label uses:* Refer to individual monographs for further information.

Juvenile idiopathic arthritis –

Auranofin: [5] = Poor documentation.

Pemphigus vulgaris –

Gold sodium thiomalate: [2] = Fair documentation.

Psoriatic arthritis –

Auranofin: [5] = Poor documentation.

Actions

➤*Pharmacology:* Gold suppresses or prevents, but does not cure, arthritis and synovitis. It is taken up by macrophages, resulting in inhibition of phagocytosis and possibly, lysosomal enzyme activity. Gold decreases concentrations of rheumatoid factor and immunoglobulins. The exact mode of action in rheumatoid arthritis is unknown; however, gold compounds may decrease synovial inflammation and retard cartilage and bone destruction. No substantial evidence exists that gold induces remission of rheumatoid arthritis.

Therapeutic effects from gold compounds occur slowly. Early improvement, often limited to reduction in morning stiffness, may begin after 6 to 8 weeks of treatment with **gold sodium thiomalate**, but beneficial effects may not be observed until after months of therapy. Therapeutic effects from **auranofin** may be seen after 3 to 4 months of treatment, but in some patients, not before 6 months.

➤*Pharmacokinetics:* Due to differences in administration routes (IM vs oral), dosage regimens (weekly vs daily), and actual quantity of gold administered to the patient, expect differences in the pharmacokinetic parameters of injectable and oral gold.

After initial injection, serum levels of gold rise sharply and decline over the next week. Peak levels of aqueous preparations are higher and decline faster than oily preparations. After a standard weekly dose, considerable individual variation in levels of gold has been found. Small amounts are found in the serum for months after discontinuation.

Although parenteral gold is widely distributed in body tissues, highest concentrations occur in the reticuloendothelial system and in adrenal and renal cortices. Binding of gold to red blood cells from injectable gold compounds is lower compared with **auranofin**-derived gold. Blood to synovial fluid ratios are similar, ≈ 1.7:1, and synovial fluid levels are ≈ 50% of the blood concentrations. No correlation between blood-gold concentrations and safety or efficacy has been established.

Major pharmacokinetic differences are summarized in the table below:

Pharmacokinetics of Auranofin and Injectable Gold Compounds								
Drug	Gold content (%)	Absorbed (%)	Time to peak (h)	Mean steady-state plasma levels (mcg/mL)	Protein binding (%)	Plasma half-life (days)	Excreted in urine (%)	Excreted in feces (%)
Auranofin	29	25 (15-33)	1-2	0.2-1	60	26 (21-31)	60[a]	85-95
Gold sodium thiomalate	50	nd	2-6	1-5	95-99	up to 168 (11th dose)	70	30

[a] 60% of the absorbed gold (15% of administered dose). nd – No data.

Contraindications

➤*Parenteral:* Hypersensitivity to any component; uncontrolled diabetes mellitus; severe debilitation; renal disease; hepatic dysfunction or history of infectious hepatitis; marked hypertension; uncontrolled CHF; systemic lupus erythematosus; agranulocytosis or hemorrhagic diathesis; blood dyscrasias; patients recently radiated; those with severe toxicity from previous exposure to gold or other heavy metals; urticaria; eczema; colitis; pregnancy (see Warnings).

➤*Oral:* A history of any of the following gold-induced disorders: Anaphylactic reactions, necrotizing enterocolitis, pulmonary fibrosis, exfoliative dermatitis, bone marrow aplasia or other severe hematologic disorders; pregnancy (see Warnings).

Warnings/Precautions

➤*Active disease:* When cartilage and bone damage has already occurred, gold cannot reverse structural damage to joints caused by previous disease. The greatest potential benefit occurs in patients with active synovitis, particularly in its early stage.

➤*Thrombocytopenia:* Thrombocytopenia has occurred in 1% to 3% of patients treated with **auranofin**, some of whom developed bleeding. It appears peripheral in origin and is usually reversible upon withdrawal. Onset is not related to duration of therapy; its course may be rapid. Monitor platelet counts at least monthly; however, if a precipitous decline in platelets or a platelet count < 100,000/mm^3 occurs or if signs and symptoms of thrombocytopenia (eg, purpura, ecchymoses or petechiae) occur, immediately withdraw auranofin and other therapies; obtain additional platelet counts. Do not reinstate auranofin unless thrombocytopenia resolves and studies show that it was not due to gold therapy.

➤*Immediate effects:* Immediate effects following injection, or at any time during therapy include the following: anaphylactic shock, syncope, bradycardia, thickening of the tongue, difficulty swallowing or breathing, and angioneurotic edema. These effects may occur immediately after injection or as late as 10 minutes after injection. If such effects occur, discontinue treatment.

➤*Proteinuria:*

Auranofin – Proteinuria has developed in 3% to 9% of auranofin patients. If clinically significant proteinuria or microscopic hematuria is found, immediately stop auranofin and other therapies with the potential to cause proteinuria or microscopic hematuria.

➤*Concomitant antirheumatic therapy:* Use of salicylates, NSAIDs and systemic corticosteroids may be continued when parenteral gold therapy is instituted. After improvement begins, slowly discontinue analgesics and NSAIDs as symptoms permit. Do not use penicillamine with gold salts.

➤*Nonvasomotor postinjection reaction:* Arthralgia may occur for a day or two after injection; it usually subsides after the first few injections. The mechanism of the transient increase in rheumatic symptoms after gold injection is unknown. These reactions are usually mild, but occasionally may be so severe that treatment is stopped prematurely.

➤*Renal/Hepatic function impairment:* Weigh the potential benefits of using **auranofin** in patients with progressive renal disease or significant hepatocellular disease against potential risks of gold toxicity on compromised organ systems and the difficulty in quickly detecting and correctly attributing the toxic effect.

➤*Special risk:* Control diabetes mellitus or CHF before gold therapy begins.

Extreme caution is indicated in patients with any of the following: History of blood dyscrasias such as agranulocytopenia or anemia caused by drug sensitivity; allergy or hypersensitivity to medications; skin rash; previous kidney or liver disease; marked hypertension; compromised cerebral or cardiovascular circulation.

Weigh the potential benefits of using auranofin in patients with inflammatory bowel disease, skin rash or history of bone marrow depression against potential risks of gold toxicity on compromised organ systems and the difficulty in quickly detecting and correctly attributing the toxic effect.

➤*Pregnancy: Category C.* Gold crosses the placenta. The placenta showed gold deposits; smaller amounts were detected in fetal liver and kidneys. Gold therapy is usually contraindicated in pregnant patients. Warn the patient about the hazards of becoming pregnant while on gold therapy. Rheumatoid arthritis frequently improves when a patient becomes pregnant. Do not superimpose the potential nephrotoxicity of gold on the increased renal burden which normally occurs in pregnancy. Discontinue therapy upon recognition of pregnancy, if possible. Consider slow excretion of gold and its persistence in body tissues after discontinuing treatment when a woman receiving gold plans to become pregnant.

Animals – **Gold sodium thiomalate** was teratogenic during the organogenic period in small animals when given in doses 140 to 175 times the usual human dose. **Auranofin** showed impaired food intake, decreased maternal and fetal weights, and increased resorptions, abortions, and congenital abnormalities, mainly abdominal defects (eg, gastroschisis, umbilical hernia).

There are no adequate, well controlled studies in pregnant women.Use only when benefits outweigh potential hazards to the fetus.

➤*Lactation:* Injectable gold is excreted in breast milk. Following **auranofin** administration, gold is excreted in the milk of rodents; human data are not available. Trace amounts appear in the serum and red blood cells of nursing offspring. This may cause rashes, nephritis, hepatitis and hematologic aberrations in nursing infants. Decide whether to discontinue nursing or to discontinue parenteral gold, taking into account the importance of the drug to the mother. Nursing during auranofin therapy is not recommended. Consider the slow excretion and persistence of gold in the mother even after therapy is discontinued.

➤*Children:* **Auranofin** is not recommended for use in children; safety and efficacy have not been established (however, see Administration and Dosage).

➤*Elderly:* Tolerance to gold usually decreases with advancing age.

➤*Monitoring:* Before instituting treatment, rule out pregnancy; perform CBC with differential, platelet, hemoglobin, WBC and erythrocyte counts, urinalysis and renal and liver function tests. Perform urinalysis for protein and sediment changes prior to each injection. Perform CBC, including platelet estimation, before every second injection (every 2 weeks) throughout treatment. Purpura or ecchymoses always require a platelet count. Inquire regarding pruritus, rash, sore mouth, metallic taste and indigestion before each injection. Observe patient at least 15 minutes after each injection. For patients on auranofin, monitor CBC with differential, platelet count and urinalysis at least monthly.

Rapid reduction of hemoglobin, granulocytes < 1500/mm^3, leukopenia < 4000 WBC/mm^3, eosinophilia > 5%, platelets < 100,000 to 150,000/mm^3, albuminuria, hematuria, rash, dermatitis, pruritus, skin eruption, stomatitis, persistent diarrhea, jaundice or petechiae are signs of possible gold toxicity. Do not give additional therapy unless further studies show these abnormalities to be caused by conditions other than gold toxicity. Monitor patients with GI symptoms for GI bleeding (**auranofin**).

Drug Interactions

➤*Phenytoin:* One report suggests coadministration with auranofin may increase phenytoin blood levels.

Adverse Reactions

Adverse reactions to gold therapy may occur during treatment or many months after discontinuation. Incidence of toxic reactions is apparently unrelated to gold plasma levels, but may relate to cumulative body content of gold. Higher than conventional dosages may increase occurrence and severity of toxicity. Adverse reactions are most frequent when cumulative dose is 400 to 800 mg (**gold sodium thiomalate**). **Auranofin** appears to cause fewer adverse reactions than injectable gold; however, therapeutic efficacy may also be less.

Adverse Reactions of Oral vs Parenteral Gold (%)		
Adverse reaction	Auranofin (oral gold) (n = 445)	Injectable gold (n = 445)
Diarrhea	42.5	13
Rash	26	39
Stomatitis	13	18
Anemia	3.1	2.7
Elevated liver function tests	1.9	1.7

Adverse Reactions of Oral vs Parenteral Gold (%)		
Adverse reaction	Auranofin (oral gold) (n = 445)	Injectable gold (n = 445)
Leukopenia	1.3	2.2
Proteinuria	0.9	5.4
Thrombocytopenia	0.9	2.2
Pulmonary	0.2	0.2

➤*Dermatologic:* Dermatitis is the most common reaction to **injectable gold** and second most common to **auranofin**. Any eruption, especially pruritic, is considered to be a reaction until proven otherwise. Rash, urticaria (auranofin, 1 to 3%) and angioedema (auranofin, < 0.1%) may occur. Pruritus (auranofin, 17%) often exists before dermatitis, and is a warning of reaction. Erythema, and occasionally more severe reactions, such as papular, vesicular and exfoliative dermatitis leading to alopecia and nail shedding, may occur. Chrysiasis (gray-to-blue pigmentation caused by gold deposits in tissues) has occurred, especially on photoexposed areas. Gold dermatitis may be aggravated by exposure to sunlight or an actinic rash may develop.

➤*Renal:* Gold may produce a nephrotic syndrome or glomerulitis with proteinuria and hematuria; these are usually relatively mild and subside completely if recognized early and treatment is discontinued. They may become severe and chronic if treatment continues after onset. Acute renal failure secondary to acute tubular necrosis, acute nephritis or degeneration of proximal tubular epithelium may occur; perform regular urinalysis and discontinue treatment immediately if proteinuria or hematuria develop. Hematuria (1% to 3%) and proteinuria (3% to 9%) occur with **auranofin**.

➤*Hematologic:*

Auranofin – Thrombocytopenia (with or without purpura), leukopenia, eosinophilia, anemia (1% to 3%); neutropenia (0.1% to 1%); agranulocytosis, pancytopenia, hypoplastic anemia, aplastic anemia, pure red cell aplasia (< 0.1%). Granulocytopenia; panmyelopathy; hemorrhagic diathesis. Constantly monitor patients throughout treatment for blood dyscrasias of the formed elements of the blood (see Warnings and Precautions). Though rare, these reactions have potentially serious consequences. These reactions may occur separately or in combination at any time during treatment.

➤*Hepatic:* Elevated liver enzymes (**auranofin** 1% to 3%), jaundice (auranofin < 0.1%) with or without cholestasis, hepatitis with jaundice, toxic hepatitis, intrahepatic cholestasis.

➤*GI:*

Auranofin – Diarrhea/loose stools (50%), generally manageable by reducing the dose (eg, from 6 to 3 mg/day), and only 6% need permanent drug discontinuation; abdominal pain (14%); nausea (10%); anorexia, flatulence, dyspepsia (3% to 9%); constipation, dysgeusia (1% to 3%); GI bleeding, melena, positive stool for occult blood (0.1% to 1%); ulcerative enterocolitis (can be severe or fatal), dysphagia (

➤*CNS:* Confusion; hallucinations; seizures.

➤*Miscellaneous:* Iritis, corneal ulcers and gold deposits in ocular tissues (**gold sodium thiomalate**; rare). These include deposits in the lens or cornea unassociated clinically with eye disorders or visual impairment (**auranofin** incidence < 0.1%). Acute yellow atrophy; encephalitis; immunological destruction of the synovia; EEG abnormalities; peripheral neuropathy (auranofin < 0.1%) with and without fasciculations or neuritis; partial or complete hair loss (auranofin 1% to 3%); fever; headache; sensorimotor effects (including Guillain-Barre syndrome) and elevated spinal fluid protein have occurred (gold sodium thiomalate rare).

Mucous membranes – Stomatitis, the second most common adverse reaction with **injectable gold,** is also seen with **auranofin** (13%). It may be manifested by shallow ulcers on buccal membranes, on borders of tongue and on palate or in pharynx and may be the only adverse reaction or occur with dermatitis. Diffuse glossitis or gingivitis may develop. Metallic taste may precede these reactions. Careful oral hygiene is important. Inflammation of upper respiratory tract, pharyngitis, gastritis, colitis, tracheitis, vaginitis and rarely, conjunctivitis (auranofin 3% to 9%) have been reported. Glossitis (auranofin 1% to 3%), gingivitis (auranofin 0.1% to 1%) and thickening of the tongue have occurred.

Pulmonary – Pulmonary injury may be shown by gold bronchitis, interstitial pneumonitis (**auranofin** < 0.1%) or fibrosis, fever and partial or complete hair loss.

Nitritoid and allergic (parenteral) – Reactions of the "nitritoid type" may resemble anaphylactoid effects. Flushing, fainting, dizziness and sweating are most frequent. Other symptoms may include nausea, vomiting, malaise, headache and weakness.

Management of adverse reactions – Discontinue immediately if toxic reactions occur. Minor complications (ie, localized dermatitis, mild stomatitis, slight proteinuria) generally require no other therapy and resolve spontaneously with therapy suspension. For mild reactions, it may be sufficient to briefly stop use and then resume with smaller doses. Moderately severe skin and mucous membrane reactions often benefit from topical corticosteroids, oral antihistamines and anesthetic lotions.

If stomatitis or dermatitis become severe or more generalized, systemic corticosteroids (generally, 10 to 40 mg prednisone daily in divided doses) may provide symptomatic relief.

For serious renal, hematologic, pulmonary and enterocolitic complications, use high doses of systemic corticosteroids (40 to 100 mg prednisone daily in divided doses). The duration of corticosteroid treatment varies. Larger doses and a longer treatment period may be required than for dermatologic reactions. Often this treatment may be required for many months because of the slow elimination of gold from the body. Therapy may also be required for months when adverse effects are unusually severe or progressive.

In high-dose gold patients whose serious adverse reactions do not improve with high-dose corticosteroids, or who develop significant steroid-related adverse reactions, a chelating agent may be given to enhance gold excretion (eg, dimercaprol, penicillamine). Monitor patients given dimercaprol carefully; untoward reactions may occur. Corticosteroids and a chelating agent may be coadministered. Adjunctive use of an anabolic steroid with other drugs (eg, dimercaprol, penicillamine, corticosteroids) may contribute to recovery of bone marrow deficiency.

Do not reinstitute after severe or idiosyncratic reactions: After resolution of mild reactions, reduced doses may be given. If test dose of 5 mg is well tolerated, give progressively larger doses (5 to 10 mg increments) at weekly to monthly intervals until 25 to 50 mg is reached.

Overdosage

➤*Symptoms:* Overdosage from too rapid increases in dosing are manifested by rapid appearance of toxic reactions, particularly renal damage (eg, hematuria, proteinuria), and hematologic effects (eg, thrombocytopenia, granulocytopenia). Other toxic effects include fever, nausea, vomiting, diarrhea and skin disorders (eg, papulovesicular lesions, urticaria and exfoliative dermatitis, all with severe pruritus).

Auranofin overdosage – Auranofin overdosage experience is limited. A 50-year-old female took 27 mg daily for 10 days and developed encephalopathy and peripheral neuropathy. Auranofin was discontinued, and she eventually recovered.

➤*Treatment:* Promptly discontinue; give dimercaprol. Use specific supportive therapy for renal/hematologic complications. Refer to General Management of Acute Overdosage. Chelating agents are used with injectable gold; consider their use also for **auranofin** overdosage. In acute overdosage, immediately induce emesis or perform gastric lavage with supportive therapy.

Patient Information

Patient package insert is available with **auranofin**.

Notify physician of the following: Itching, rash, sore mouth, indigestion, metallic taste, easy bruising or nosebleed.

Increased joint pain may continue 1 or 2 days after an injection and usually subsides after the first few injections.

Chrysiasis (gray-to-blue pigmentation) may occur, especially on photoexposed areas. Minimize exposure to sunlight or artificial ultraviolet light.

Observe careful oral hygiene in conjunction with therapy.

Warn women of childbearing potential of the risks of using gold therapy during pregnancy.

AURANOFIN (29% Gold)

Rx	**Ridaura** (SK-Beecham)	**Capsules:** 3 mg	(Ridaura SKF). Tan and brown. In 60s.

AURANOFIN (29% Gold) — ORAL

For complete and comparative prescribing information, refer to the Gold Compounds group monograph.

WARNING

Auranofin contains gold and, like other gold-containing drugs, can cause gold toxicity, signs of which include: Fall in hemoglobin, leukopenia < 4000 WBC/mm^3, granulocytes < 1500/mm^3, decrease in platelets < 150,000/mm^3, proteinuria, hematuria, pruritus, rash, stomatitis or persistent diarrhea. Therefore, the results of recommended laboratory work (see Precautions) should be reviewed before writing each auranofin prescription. Like other gold preparations, auranofin is only indicated for use in selected patients with active rheumatoid arthritis. Physicians planning to use auranofin should be experienced with chrysotherapy and should thoroughly familiarize themselves with the toxicity and benefits of auranofin. In addition, the following precautions should be routinely employed: The possibility of adverse reactions should be explained to patients before starting therapy. Patients should be advised to report promptly any symptoms suggesting toxicity (see Precautions).

Indications

➤*Rheumatoid arthritis:* Auranofin is indicated in the management of adults with active classical or definite rheumatoid arthritis (ARA criteria) who have had an insufficient therapeutic response to, or are intolerant of, an adequate trial of full doses of one or more nonsteroidal anti-inflammatory drugs. Auranofin should be added to a comprehensive baseline program, including nondrug therapies.

Unlike anti-inflammatory drugs, auranofin does not produce an immediate response. Therapeutic effects may be seen after 3 to 4 months of treatment, although improvement has not been seen in some patients before 6 months.

When cartilage and bone damage have already occurred, gold cannot reverse structural damage to joints caused by previous disease. The greatest potential benefit occurs in patients with active synovitis, particularly in its early stage.

In controlled clinical trials comparing auranofin with injectable gold, auranofin was associated with fewer dropouts due to adverse reactions, while injectable gold was associated with fewer dropouts for inadequate or poor therapeutic effect. Physicians should consider these findings when deciding on the use of auranofin in patients who are candidates for chrysotherapy.

➤*Off-label uses:*

Juvenile idiopathic arthritis – [5] = Poor documentation. Data evaluating the safety and efficacy of auranofin for the treatment of juvenile idiopathic arthritis (JIA) are limited and show conflicting results. No benefit was observed in a placebo-controlled trial. In addition, there are significant safety concerns with auranofin therapy. For these reasons, it is recommended that auranofin not be routinely used for the treatment of JIA.

Psoriatic arthritis – [5] = Poor documentation. Auranofin has not demonstrated superiority over placebo in the treatment of psoriatic arthritis and is associated with the potential for severe toxicity. Alternative treatment options demonstrating effectiveness are available.

Other possible off-label uses – Alternative or adjuvant to corticosteroids in treatment of pemphigus.

Administration and Dosage

➤*Adults:*

Rheumatoid arthritis –

Initial dosage: 6 mg daily, given either as 3 mg twice daily or 6 mg once daily. Initiation of therapy at dosages exceeding 6 mg daily is not recommended because it is associated with an increased incidence of diarrhea.

Dosage titration: If response is inadequate after 6 months, an increase to 9 mg (3 mg 3 times daily) may be tolerated.

Discontinuation of therapy: If response remains inadequate after a 3-month trial of 9 mg daily, auranofin therapy should be discontinued.

Off-label dosing –

➤*Children:*

Off-label dosing –

➤*Transferring from injectable gold:* In controlled clinical studies, patients on injectable gold have been transferred to auranofin by discontinuing the injectable agent and starting oral therapy with auranofin 6 mg daily.

➤*Storage/Stability:* Store between 15° and 30°C (59° and 86°F). Dispense in a tight, light-resistant container.

GOLD SODIUM THIOMALATE (≈ 50% Gold)

Rx	**Gold Sodium Thiomalate** (Parenta)	**Injection, solution:** 50 mg/ml[a]	In 2 ml and 1 ml fill in 2 ml single-dose vials and 10 ml multiple-dose vials.
Rx	**Aurolate** (Pasadena)		In 2 and 10 ml vials.
Rx	**Myochrysine** (Akorn)		In 2 and 10 ml vials.

[a] With 0.5% benzyl alcohol.

GOLD SODIUM THIOMALATE — INJECTION

For complete and comparative prescribing information, refer to the Gold Compounds group monograph.

WARNING

Physicians planning to use gold sodium thiomalate should thoroughly familiarize themselves with its toxicity and its benefits. The possibility of toxic reactions should always be explained to the patient before starting therapy. Patients should be warned to report promptly any symptoms suggesting toxicity. Before each injection of gold sodium thiomalate, the physician should review the results of laboratory work, and see the patient to determine the presence or absence of adverse reactions since some of these can be severe or even fatal.

Indications

➤*Rheumatoid arthritis:* Gold sodium thiomalate is indicated in the treatment of selected cases of active rheumatoid arthritis is both adult and juvenile type. The greatest benefit occurs in the early active stage. In late stages of the illness when cartilage and bone damage have occurred, gold can only check the progression of rheumatoid arthritis and prevent further structural damage to joints. It cannot repair damage caused by previously active disease.

Gold sodium thiomalate should be used only as one part of a complete program of therapy; alone it is not a complete treatment.

➤*Off-label uses:*

Pemphigus vulgaris – [2] = Fair documentation. Although gold sodium thiomalate has demonstrated efficacy in noncontrolled trials for the treatment of pemphigus vulgaris, the incidence of toxicity and consequent treatment withdrawal limits its use. Larger, controlled trials are needed to better define its role in treatment. (See Administration and Dosage.)

Administration and Dosage

➤*Adults:*

Rheumatoid arthritis –

Maximum dose: 100 mg intramuscularly (IM) (single dose).

Initial dosage: 10 mg IM on week 1; 25 mg IM on week 2; 25 to 50 mg IM on week 3 and subsequent weeks until there is toxicity or major clinical improvement, or, in the absence of either of these, the cumulative dose reaches 1 g. If significant clinical improvement occurs before a cumulative dose of 1 g has been administered, the dose may be decreased or the interval between injections increased, as with maintenance therapy.

Maintenance dosage: 25 to 50 mg every other week for 2 to 20 weeks. If the clinical course remains stable, 25 to 50 mg may be given every third and subsequently every fourth week indefinitely. Some patients may require maintenance treatment at intervals of 1 to 3 weeks. Should the arthritis exacerbate during maintenance therapy, weekly injections may be resumed temporarily until disease activity is suppressed.

Treatment failure: Should a patient fail to improve during initial therapy (cumulative dose of 1 g), several options are available: The patient may be considered to be unresponsive and gold is discontinued; the same dose (25 to 50 mg) may be continued for approximately 10 additional weeks; or the dose may be increased by increments of 10 mg every 1 to 4 weeks, not to exceed 100 mg in a single injection.

If significant clinical improvement occurs, the maintenance schedule described previously should be initiated. If there is no significant improvement or if toxicity occurs, therapy should be stopped.

Off-label dosing –

Pemphigus vulgaris: [2] = Fair documentation. 50 mg intramuscularly once weekly after toleration of a test dose.

GOLD SODIUM THIOMALATE — INJECTION

➤*Children:*

Juvenile rheumatoid arthritis –

The guidelines given above for administration to adults also apply to children.

Maximum dose: 50 mg (single injection).

Initial dosage: 10 mg.

Maintenance dosage: 1 mg/kg.

➤*Concomitant therapy:* Gold salts should not be used concomitantly with penicillamine. Other measures, such as salicylates, other nonsteroidal anti-inflammatory drugs, or systemic corticosteroids, may be continued when gold sodium thiomalate is initiated. After improvement commences, analgesic and anti-inflammatory drugs may be discontinued slowly, as symptoms permit.

➤*Administration:* Administer only by IM injection, preferably intragluteally. Give with the patient lying down. The patient should remain recumbent for approximately 10 minutes after the injection.

➤*Storage/Stability:* Store at 20° to 25°C (68° to 77°F). Protect from light. Store container in carton until contents have been used.

ANTIRHEUMATIC AGENTS

METHOTREXATE (Amethopterin; MTX)

See the Methotrexate monograph in the Antineoplastic Agents chapter.

SULFASALAZINE

See the Sulfasalazine monograph in the GI chapter.

LEFLUNOMIDE

Rx	**Leflunomide** (Various, eg, Prasco, Sandoz, Teva)	**Tablets; oral:** 10 mg	May contain lactose, PEG. In 30s.
Rx	**Arava** (Sanofi-Aventis)		Lactose, PEG. (ZBN). White, round. Film-coated. In 30s.
Rx	**Leflunomide** (Various, eg, Prasco, Sandoz, Teva)	**Tablets; oral:** 20 mg	May contain lactose, PEG. In 30s.
Rx	**Arava** (Sanofi-Aventis)		Lactose, PEG. (ZBO). Light yellow, triangular. Film-coated. In 30s.
Rx	**Arava** (Sanofi-Aventis)	**Tablets; oral:** 100 mg	Lactose, PEG. (ZBP). White, round. Film-coated. In UD 3s.

LEFLUNOMIDE — ORAL

WARNING

Pregnancy – Pregnancy must be excluded before the start of treatment with leflunomide. Leflunomide is contraindicated in pregnant women and women of childbearing potential who are not using reliable contraception. Pregnancy must be avoided during leflunomide treatment or prior to the completion of the drug elimination procedure after leflunomide treatment.

Hepatotoxicity – Severe liver injury, including fatal liver failure, has been reported in some patients treated with leflunomide. Patients with preexisting acute or chronic liver disease, or those with ALT more than twice the upper limit of normal (ULN) before initiating treatment, should not be treated with leflunomide. Use caution when leflunomide is given with other potentially hepatotoxic drugs.

Monitoring ALT levels is recommended at least monthly for 6 months after starting leflunomide, and every 6 to 8 weeks thereafter . If ALT elevation greater than 3 × the ULN occurs, interrupt leflunomide therapy while investigating the probable cause of the ALT elevation by close observation and additional tests. If the ALT elevation is likely leflunomide-induced, start cholestyramine washout and monitor liver tests weekly until normal. If leflunomide-induced liver injury is unlikely because another probable cause has been found, resumption of leflunomide therapy may be considered.

Indications

➤*Rheumatoid arthritis:* For the treatment of active rheumatoid arthritis (RA) in adults to reduce signs and symptoms, to inhibit structural damageas evidenced by x-ray erosions and joint-space narrowing, and to improve physical function.

➤*Off-label uses:*

Juvenile idiopathic arthritis – [4] = Insufficient documentation. Data evaluating the safety and efficacy of leflunomide for the treatment of juvenile idiopathic arthritis (JIA) are limited to an open-label study and a controlled trial. While these reports show promise, additional studies are needed to define the optimal dose and patient population that would most benefit from therapy. Currently, there are no national guidelines for the management of JIA.

Administration and Dosage

➤*General dosing considerations:* Due to the long half-life in patients with RA and recommended dosing interval (24 hours), a loading dose is needed to provide steady-state concentrations more rapidly. (See Loading dose.)

➤*Adults:*

Rheumatoid arthritis –

Maximum dose: 20 mg/day.

Loading dose: 100 mg once daily for 3 days.

Elimination of the loading dose regimen may decrease the risk of adverse reactions. This may be important for patients at increased risk of hematologic or hepatic toxicity, such as those receiving concomitant treatment with methotrexate or other immunosuppressive agents or who have taken such medications in the recent past.

Maintenance dosage: 20 mg once daily.

Dosage adjustment: If dosing at 20 mg/day is not well tolerated clinically, the dosage may be decreased to 10 mg daily. Carefully observe patients after dose reduction because it may take several weeks for metabolite levels to decline.

➤*Children:*

Off-label dosing –

Juvenile idiopathic arthritis: [4] = Insufficient documentation.

• *3 to 17 years of age –* 100 mg loading dose for 1 to 3 days, followed by maintenance doses of 10 mg every other day to 20 mg daily, depending on patient weight. Therapy was continued for up to 30 months in clinical trials.

➤*Hepatic function impairment:* Not recommended for patients with hepatic impairment.

➤*Preparation for administration:* Leflunomide is an immunosuppressant agent and is also considered a teratogen. Follow safe handling procedures when preparing, administering, or dispensing leflunomide.

➤*Administration:* Leflunomide should be taken orally with or without food.

➤*Storage/Stability:* Store at 25°C (77°F); excursions are permitted to 15° to 30°C (59° to 86°F). Protect from light.

Actions

➤*Pharmacology:* Leflunomide, a pyrimidine synthesis inhibitor, is an isoxazole immunomodulatory agent that inhibits dihydroorotate dehydrogenase (an enzyme involved in de novo pyrimidine synthesis) and has antiproliferative activity. Several in vivo and in vitro experimental models have demonstrated an anti-inflammatory effect.

➤*Pharmacokinetics:* Following oral administration, leflunomide is metabolized to an active metabolite A77 1726 (hereafter referred to as M1), which is responsible for essentially all of its activity in vivo. Plasma levels of leflunomide are occasionally seen at very low levels. Studies of the pharmacokinetics of leflunomide have primarily examined the plasma concentrations of this active metabolite.

M1 Pharmacokinetic Parameters After 24 Weeks (N = 54) (Mean ± SD)[a]

Pharmacokinetic parameter	Maintenance (loading) dose		
	5 mg (50 mg)	10 mg (100 mg)	25 mg (100 mg)
C_{24} (day 1) (mcg/mL)[b]	4 ± 0.6	8.4 ± 2.1	8.5 ± 2.2
C_{24} (ss) (mcg/mL)[c]	8.8 ± 2.9	18 ± 9.6	63 ± 36
$t_{½}$ (days)	15 ± 3	14 ± 5	18 ± 9

[a] SD = standard deviation; C = concentration; $t_{½}$ = half-life.
[b] Concentration at 24 hours after loading dose.
[c] Concentration at 24 hours after maintenance doses at steady state.

Absorption – Following oral administration, peak levels of M1 occurred 6 to 12 hours after dosing. Without a loading dose, it is estimated that attainment of steady-state plasma concentrations would require nearly 2 months of dosing. The resulting plasma concentrations following loading doses and continued clinical dosing indicate that M1 plasma levels are dose proportional. Relative to an oral solution, leflunomide tablets are 80% bioavailable.

Effect of food: Coadministration of leflunomide with a high-fat meal did not have a significant impact on M1 plasma levels.

Distribution – M1 has a low volume of distribution (VSS = 0.13 L/kg) and is extensively bound (more than 99.3%) to albumin in healthy subjects. Protein binding has been shown to be linear at therapeutic concentrations. The free fraction of M1 is slightly higher in patients with rheumatoid arthritis; the mechanism and significance of this increase is unknown.

Metabolism – Leflunomide is metabolized to one primary (M1) and many minor metabolites. Of these minor metabolites, only 4-trifluoromethylaniline (TFMA) is quantifiable, occurring at low levels in the plasma of some patients. The parent compound is rarely detectable in plasma. At the present time, the

LEFLUNOMIDE — ORAL

specific site of leflunomide metabolism is unknown. In vivo and in vitro studies suggest a role for the GI wall and liver in drug metabolism. No specific enzyme has been identified as the primary route of metabolism for leflunomide; however, hepatic cytosolic and microsomal cellular fractions have been identified as sites of drug metabolism.

Excretion – The active M1 metabolite is eliminated by further metabolism and subsequent renal excretion as well as by direct biliary excretion. In a 28-day study of drug elimination (n = 3) using a single dose of radiolabeled compound, approximately 43% of the total radioactivity was eliminated in the urine and 48% was eliminated in the feces. Subsequent analysis of the samples revealed the primary urinary metabolites to be leflunomide glucuronides and an oxanilic acid derivative of M1. The primary fecal metabolite was M1. Of these 2 routes of elimination, renal elimination is more significant over the first 96 hours, after which fecal elimination begins to predominate. In a study involving the intravenous administration of M1, the clearance was estimated to be 31 mL/hr.

The active metabolite of leflunomide is eliminated slowly from the plasma. In instances of serious toxicity from leflunomide, including hypersensitivity, use of a drug elimination procedure is highly recommended to reduce the drug concentration more rapidly after stopping leflunomide therapy. In small studies using activated charcoal (n = 1) or cholestyramine (n = 3) to facilitate drug elimination, the in vivo plasma half-life of M1 was reduced from more than 1 week to approximately 1 day. Similar reductions in plasma half-life were observed for a series of volunteers (N = 96) enrolled in pharmacokinetic trials who were given cholestyramine. This suggests that biliary recycling is a major contributor to the long elimination half-life (approximately 2 weeks) of M1. Studies of hemodialysis and chronic ambulatory peritoneal dialysis (CAPD) indicate that M1 is not dialyzable.

Special populations –

Renal function impairment: In single-dose studies in patients (n = 6) with chronic renal insufficiency requiring either CAPD or hemodialysis, neither had a significant impact on circulating levels of M1. The free fraction of M1 was almost doubled, but the mechanism of this increase is not known. Because the kidney plays a role in drug elimination and without adequate studies of leflunomide use in subjects with renal insufficiency, caution should be used when leflunomide is administered to these patients.

Hepatic function impairment: Given the need to metabolize leflunomide into the active species, the role of the liver in drug elimination/recycling, and the possible risk of increased hepatic toxicity, the use of leflunomide in patients with hepatic insufficiency is not recommended.

Children: The pharmacokinetics of M1 following oral administration of leflunomide have been investigated in 73 children with polyarticular course juvenile RA who ranged in age from 3 to 17 years. The results of a population pharmacokinetic analysis of these trials demonstrated that children with body weights of no more than 40 kg have a reduced clearance of M1 relative to adult RA patients.

M1 Clearance in Children (Mean ±SD [Range])

Body weight	CL[a] (mL/h)
< 20 kg (n = 10)	18 ± 9.8 (6.8 to 37)
20 to 40 kg (n = 30)	18 ± 9.5 (4.2 to 43)
> 40 kg (n = 33)	26 ± 16 (9.7 to 93.6)

[a] CL = clearance.

Contraindications

Hypersensitivity to leflunomide or any of the other components of the medication; women who are or may become pregnant.

Warnings/Precautions

➤*Hepatotoxicity:* See the Warning box for more information.

In clinical trials, leflunomide treatment as monotherapy or in combination with methotrexate was associated with elevations of liver enzymes, primarily ALT and AST, in a significant number of patients; these effects were generally reversible. Most transaminase elevations were mild (2 × the ULN or less) and usually resolved while continuing treatment. Marked elevations (more than 3 × the ULN) occurred infrequently and reversed with dose reduction or discontinuation of treatment.

Leflunomide Liver Enzyme Elevations > 3 × the ULN

	Study US301			Study MN301			Study MN302[a]	
	Leflunomide	Placebo	Methotrexate	Leflunomide	Placebo	Sulfasalazine	Leflunomide	Methotrexate
ALT								
> 3 × ULN	4.4%	2.5%	2.7%	1.5%	1.1%	1.5%	2.6%	16.7%
Reversed to ≤ 2 × ULN	n = 8	n = 3	n = 5	n = 2	n = 1	n = 2	n = 12	n = 82

Leflunomide Liver Enzyme Elevations > 3 × the ULN

	Study US301			Study MN301			Study MN302[a]	
	Leflunomide	Placebo	Methotrexate	Leflunomide	Placebo	Sulfasalazine	Leflunomide	Methotrexate
Timing of elevation								
0 to 3 months	6	1	1	2	1	2	7	27
4 to 6 months	1	1	3	–	–	–	1	34
7 to 9 months	1	1	1	–	–	–	–	16
10 to 12 months	–	–	–	–	–	–	5	6

[a] Only 10% of patients in study MN302 received folate. All patients in study US301 received folate.

It was notable that the absence of folate use in study MN302 was associated with a considerably greater incidence of liver enzyme elevation on methotrexate therapy.

In a 6-month study of 263 patients with persistent active RA despite methotrexate therapy and with normal liver function tests, leflunomide was added to a group of 130 patients starting at 10 mg/day and increased to 20 mg as needed. An increase in ALT 3 × the ULN or more was observed in 3.8% of patients compared with 0.8% in 133 patients continued on methotrexate with placebo added.

➤*Immunosuppression:* Leflunomide is not recommended for patients with severe immunodeficiency, bone marrow dysplasia, or severe, uncontrolled infections. In the event that a serious infection occurs, it may be necessary to interrupt therapy with leflunomide and administer cholestyramine or charcoal. Medications like leflunomide that have immunosuppression potential may cause patients to be more susceptible to infections, including opportunistic infections, especially *Pneumocystis jiroveci* pneumonia, tuberculosis (including extra-pulmonary tuberculosis), and aspergillosis. Severe infections including sepsis, which may be fatal, have been reported in patients receiving leflunomide, especially *Pneumocystis jiroveci* pneumonia and aspergillosis. Most of the reports were confounded by concomitant immunosuppressant therapy or comorbid illness which, in addition to rheumatoid disease, may predispose patients to infection.

There have been rare reports of pancytopenia, agranulocytosis, and thrombocytopenia in patients receiving leflunomide alone. These events have been reported most frequently in patients who received concomitant treatment with methotrexate or other immunosuppressive agents, or who had recently discontinued these therapies; in some cases, patients had a history of a significant hematologic abnormality.

Patients taking leflunomide should have platelet, white blood cell count, and hemoglobin or hematocrit monitored at baseline and monthly for 6 months following initiation of therapy and every 6 to 8 weeks thereafter. If used with concomitant methotrexate and/or other potential immunosuppressive agents, chronic monitoring should be monthly. If evidence of bone marrow suppression occurs in a patient taking leflunomide, discontinue treatment with leflunomide, and use cholestyramine or charcoal to reduce the plasma concentration of M1.

Monitor patients for hematologic toxicity if a decision is made to switch from leflunomide to another antirheumatic agent with known potential for hematologic suppression; there will be overlap of systemic exposure to both compounds. Leflunomide washout with cholestyramine or charcoal may decrease this risk, but also may induce disease worsening if the patient had been responding to leflunomide treatment.

➤*Malignancy:* The risk of malignancy, particularly lymphoproliferative disorders, is increased with the use of some immunosuppressive medications. There is a potential for immunosuppression with leflunomide. No apparent increase in the incidence of malignancies and lymphoproliferative disorders was reported in the clinical trials of leflunomide, but larger and longer-term studies would be needed to determine whether there is an increased risk of these occurrences.

➤*Need for drug elimination:* M1 is eliminated slowly from the plasma. In instances of any serious toxicity from leflunomide, including hypersensitivity, use of a drug elimination procedure is highly recommended to reduce the drug concentration more rapidly after stopping leflunomide therapy. If hypersensitivity is the suspected clinical mechanism, more prolonged cholestyramine or charcoal administration may be necessary to achieve rapid and sufficient clearance. The duration may be modified based on the clinical status of the patient. These drug elimination procedures may be repeated if clinically necessary.

➤*Drug elimination procedure:* The following drug elimination procedure is recommended to achieve nondetectable plasma levels less than 0.02 mg/L (0.02 mcg/mL) after stopping treatment with leflunomide: administer cholestyramine 8 g 3 times daily for 11 days (the 11 days do not need to be consecutive unless there is a need to lower the plasma level rapidly); verify plasma levels less than 0.02 mg/L (0.02 mcg/mL) by 2 separate tests at least 14 days apart (if plasma levels are higher than 0.02 mg/L, additional cholestyramine treatment should be considered).

LEFLUNOMIDE — ORAL

Without the drug elimination procedure, it may take up to 2 years to reach plasma M1 metabolite levels less than 0.02 mg/L due to individual variation in drug clearance.

➤*Respiratory effects:* Interstitial lung disease has been reported during treatment with leflunomide and has been associated with fatal outcomes. Interstitial lung disease is a potentially fatal disorder, which may occur acutely at any time during therapy and has a variable clinical presentation. New onset or worsening pulmonary symptoms, such as cough and dyspnea with or without associated fever, may be a reason for discontinuation of therapy and for further investigation as appropriate. If discontinuation of the drug is necessary, initiation of wash out procedures should be considered.

➤*Tuberculosis reactivation:* Prior to initiating immunomodulatory therapies, including leflunomide, screen patients for latent tuberculosis infection with a tuberculin skin test. Leflunomide has not been studied in patients with a positive tuberculosis screen, and the safety of leflunomide in individuals with latent tuberculosis infection is unknown. Patients testing positive in a tuberculosis screening should be treated by standard medical practice prior to therapy with leflunomide.

➤*Vaccinations:* No clinical data are available regarding the efficacy and safety of vaccination during leflunomide treatment. However, vaccination with live vaccines is not recommended. Consider the long half-life of leflunomide when contemplating administration of a live vaccine after discontinuing leflunomide.

➤*Renal effects:* Due to a specific effect on the brush border of the renal proximal tubule, leflunomide has a uricosuric effect. A separate effect of hypophosphaturia is seen in some patients. These effects have not been seen together nor have there been alterations in renal function.

➤*Hypersensitivity reactions:* Rare cases of Stevens-Johnson syndrome and toxic epidermal necrolysis have been reported in patients receiving leflunomide. If a patient taking leflunomide develops any of these conditions, leflunomide therapy should be stopped, and a drug elimination procedure is recommended.

➤*Renal function impairment:* See Actions for more information.

➤*Hepatic function impairment:* The use of leflunomide is not recommended in patients with hepatic impairment.

➤*Pregnancy: Category X.* Leflunomide is contraindicated in women who are or may become pregnant. If this drug is used during pregnancy or if the patient becomes pregnant while taking this drug, the patient should be apprised of the potential hazard to the fetus.

There are no adequate and well-controlled studies evaluating leflunomide in pregnant women. However, based on animal studies, leflunomide may increase the risk of fetal death or teratogenic effects when administered to a pregnant woman. Women of childbearing potential must not be started on leflunomide until pregnancy is excluded and it has been confirmed that they are using reliable contraception. Before starting treatment with leflunomide, patients must be fully counseled on the potential for serious risks to the fetus.

The patient must be advised that if there is any delay in onset of menses or any other reason to suspect pregnancy, they must notify the physician immediately for pregnancy testing, and if positive, the physician and patient must discuss the risk to the pregnancy. It is possible that rapidly lowering the blood level of the active metabolite, by instituting the drug elimination procedure at the first delay of menses, may decrease the risk to the fetus from leflunomide.

Upon discontinuing leflunomide, it is recommended that all women of childbearing potential undergo the drug elimination procedure. Women receiving leflunomide treatment who wish to become pregnant must discontinue leflunomide and undergo the drug elimination procedure, which includes verification of M1 metabolite plasma levels less than 0.02 mg/L (0.02 mcg/mL). Human plasma levels of M1 less than 0.02 mg/L (0.02 mcg/mL) are expected to have minimal risk based on available animal data.

Leflunomide, when administered orally to rats during organogenesis at a dose of 15 mg/kg, was teratogenic (most notably causing anophthalmia or microphthalmia and internal hydrocephalus). The systemic exposure of rats at this dose was approximately 1/10 the human exposure level based on the area under the curve (AUC). Under these exposure conditions, leflunomide also caused a decrease in the maternal body weight and an increase in embryolethality with a decrease in fetal body weight for surviving fetuses. In rabbits, oral treatment with leflunomide 10 mg/kg during organogenesis resulted in fused, dysplastic sternebrae. The exposure level at this dose was essentially equivalent to the maximum human exposure level based on AUC. At a 1 mg/kg dose, leflunomide was not teratogenic in rats and rabbits.

When female rats were treated with leflunomide 1.25 mg/kg beginning 14 days before mating and continuing until the end of lactation, the offspring exhibited marked (greater than 90%) decreases in postnatal survival. The systemic exposure level at 1.25 mg/kg was approximately 1/100 the human exposure level based on AUC.

Pregnancy registry – To monitor fetal outcomes, health care providers are encouraged to register pregnant women exposed to leflunomide by calling 1-877-311-8972.

Use in males – Available information does not suggest that leflunomide would be associated with an increased risk of male-mediated fetal toxicity. However, animal studies to evaluate this specific risk have not been conducted. To minimize any possible risk, men wishing to father a child should consider discontinuing use of leflunomide and taking cholestyramine 8 g 3 times daily for 11 days.

➤*Lactation:* Leflunomide should not be used by breast-feeding mothers. It is not known whether leflunomide is excreted in human breast milk. The molecular weight (about 270) is low enough that excretion into breast milk should be expected. Many drugs are excreted in human breast milk, and there is a potential for serious adverse reactions in breast-feeding infants from leflunomide. Therefore, a decision should be made whether to proceed with breast-feeding or to initiate treatment with leflunomide, taking into account the importance of the drug to the mother.

➤*Children:* The safety and efficacy of leflunomide in children with polyarticular course juvenile RA have not been fully evaluated.

➤*Monitoring:* Monitor platelet, white blood cell count, and hemoglobin or hematocrit at baseline and monthly for 6 months following initiation of therapy and every 6 to 8 weeks thereafter. If used concomitantly with immunosuppressants, such as methotrexate, chronic monitoring should be monthly.

At minimum, ALT must be performed at baseline and monitored at monthly intervals during the first 6 months, then, if stable, every 6 to 8 weeks thereafter. If methotrexate is given concomitantly, ACR guidelines for monitoring methotrexate liver toxicity must be followed with ALT, AST, and serum albumin testing every month.

Blood pressure should be checked before starting leflunomide treatment and periodically thereafter.

Drug Interactions

➤*Vaccines:* See Warnings/Precautions for more information.

Leflunomide Drug Interactions

Precipitant drug	Object drug[a]		Description
Cholestyramine Charcoal	Leflunomide	⬇	Coadministration resulted in a rapid and significant decrease in the active metabolite of leflunomide. Unless being used to treat leflunomide toxicity or hypersensitivity, avoid cholestyramine in patients receiving leflunomide.
Hepatotoxic drugs (eg, methotrexate)	Leflunomide	⬆	Increased adverse effects may occur with coadministration. This is also to be considered when leflunomide treatment is followed by such drugs without a drug elimination procedure. Concomitant use resulted in a 2- to 3-fold elevation in liver enzymes in 5 of 30 patients. A > 3-fold increase was seen in another 5 patients. All of these resolved. Close clinical and laboratory monitoring are indicated during coadministration.
Leflunomide	Hepatotoxic drugs (eg, methotrexate)		
Rifampin	Leflunomide	⬆	Following administration of a single dose of leflunomide to subjects receiving multiple doses of rifampin, M1 peak levels were increased (40%). Because of the potential for leflunomide levels to continue to increase with multiple dosing, coadminister with caution. Close clinical and laboratory monitoring are indicated during coadministration.
Leflunomide	NSAIDs[b] (eg, diclofenac, ibuprofen)	⬌	In vitro, M1 caused an increase (13% to 50%) in the free fraction of diclofenac and ibuprofen. In vitro studies indicate that M1 inhibits CYP2C9, which is responsible for the metabolism of many NSAIDs. The clinical significance of this finding is unknown. However, there was extensive concomitant use of NSAIDs in the clinical studies and no differential effect was observed. Monitor the clinical response and adjust the NSAID dose as needed.
Leflunomide	Tolbutamide	⬌	In vitro, M1 caused increases (13% to 50%) in the free fraction of tolbutamide at concentrations in the clinical range. The clinical significance of this finding is unknown.

LEFLUNOMIDE — ORAL

Leflunomide Drug Interactions			
Precipitant drug	Object drug[a]		Description
Leflunomide	Warfarin	↑	Increased INR[b] when leflunomide and warfarin were given concurrently has been reported rarely. Because warfarin has a narrow therapeutic index, closely monitor coagulation parameters when starting, stopping, or changing the dose of leflunomide. Adjust the warfarin dose as needed.

[a] ↑ = object drug increased; ↓ = object drug decreased; ↔ = undetermined clinical effect.
[b] NSAIDS = nonsteroidal anti-inflammatory drugs; INR = international normalized ratio.

Adverse Reactions

➤*Adults:* Adverse reactions associated with the use of leflunomide in rheumatoid arthritis include diarrhea, elevated liver enzymes (ALT and AST), alopecia, and rash.

Adverse reactions after 1 year of treatment –

Leflunomide Adverse Reactions (≥ 3%) After 1 Year of Treatment							
	All RA studies	Placebo-controlled trials MN301 and US301				Active-controlled trials MN302[a]	
Adverse reactions	Leflunomide (n = 1339)[b]	Leflunomide (n = 315)	Placebo (n = 210)	Sulfasalazine (n = 133)	Methotrexate (n = 182)	Leflunomide (n = 501)	Methotrexate (n = 498)
Cardiovascular							
Chest pain	2%	4%	2%	2%	4%	1%	2%
Hypertension[c]	10%	9%	4%	4%	3%	10%	4%
New onset of hypertension	—	1%	< 1%	0%	2%	2%	< 1%
CNS							
Asthenia	3%	6%	4%	5%	6%	3%	3%
Dizziness	4%	5%	3%	6%	5%	7%	6%
Headache	7%	13%	11%	12%	21%	10%	8%
Paresthesia	2%	3%	1%	1%	2%	4%	3%
Dermatologic							
Alopecia	10%	9%	1%	6%	6%	17%	10%
Dry skin	2%	3%	2%	2%	0%	3%	1%
Eczema	2%	1%	1%	1%	1%	3%	2%
Pruritus	4%	5%	2%	3%	2%	6%	2%
Rash	10%	12%	7%	11%	9%	11%	10%
GI							
Abdominal pain	6%	5%	4%	4%	8%	6%	4%
Abnormal liver enzymes	5%	10%	2%	4%	10%	6%	17%
Anorexia	3%	3%	2%	5%	2%	3%	3%
Diarrhea	17%	27%	12%	10%	20%	22%	10%
Dyspepsia	5%	10%	10%	9%	13%	6%	7%
Gastroenteritis	3%	1%	1%	0%	6%	3%	3%
GI/Abdominal pain	5%	6%	4%	7%	8%	8%	8%
Mouth ulcer	3%	5%	4%	3%	10%	3%	6%
Nausea	9%	13%	11%	19%	18%	13%	18%
Vomiting	3%	5%	4%	4%	3%	3%	3%
Metabolic/Nutritional							
Hypokalemia	1%	3%	1%	1%	1%	1%	< 1%
Weight loss[d]	4%	2%	1%	2%	0%	2%	2%
Musculoskeletal							
Arthralgia	1%	4%	3%	0%	9%	< 1%	1%
Back pain	5%	6%	3%	4%	9%	8%	7%
Joint disorder	4%	2%	2%	2%	2%	8%	6%
Leg cramps	1%	4%	2%	2%	6%	0%	0%
Synovitis	2%	< 1%	1%	0%	2%	4%	2%
Tenosynovitis	3%	2%	0%	1%	2%	5%	1%
Respiratory							
Bronchitis	7%	5%	2%	4%	7%	8%	7%
Increased cough	3%	4%	5%	3%	6%	5%	7%
Infection, upper respiratory	4%	0%	0%	0%	0%	0%	0%
Pharyngitis	3%	2%	1%	2%	1%	3%	3%
Pneumonia	2%	3%	0%	0%	1%	2%	2%
Respiratory tract infection	15%	21%	21%	20%	32%	27%	25%
Rhinitis	2%	5%	2%	4%	3%	2%	2%
Sinusitis	2%	5%	5%	0%	10%	1%	1%
Miscellaneous							
Allergic reaction	2%	5%	2%	0%	6%	1%	2%
Flu syndrome	2%	4%	2%	0%	7%	0%	0%
Injury accident	5%	7%	5%	3%	11%	6%	7%
Pain	2%	4%	2%	2%	5%	1%	< 1%
Urinary tract infection	5%	5%	7%	4%	2%	5%	6%

[a] Only 10% of patients in study MN302 received folate. All patients in study US301 received folate; none in study MN301 received folate.
[b] Includes all controlled and uncontrolled trials with leflunomide (duration up to 12 months).
[c] Hypertension as a preexisting condition was overrepresented in all leflunomide treatment groups in phase III trials.
[d] In a meta-analysis of all phase II and III studies, during the first 6 months in patients receiving leflunomide, 10% lost 10 to 19 lb (24 cases per 100 patient years) and 2% lost at least 20 lb (4 cases per 100 patient years). Of patients receiving leflunomide, 4% lost 10% of their baseline weight during the first 6 months of treatment.

Adverse reactions (1% to less than 3%) – The following adverse reactions occurred in 1% to less than 3% of patients.

Cardiovascular: Angina pectoris, palpitation, tachycardia, varicose veins, vasculitis, vasodilation.

CNS: Anxiety, depression, insomnia, malaise, migraine, neuralgia, neuritis, sleep disorder, vertigo.

Dermatologic: Acne, contact dermatitis, fungal dermatitis, hair discoloration, hematoma, herpes simplex, herpes zoster, nail disorder, skin nodule, subcutaneous nodule, maculopapular rash, skin discoloration, skin disorder, sweating increased, ulcer skin.

Endocrine: Diabetes mellitus, hyperthyroidism.

GI: Cholelithiasis, colitis, constipation, dry mouth, esophagitis, flatulence, gastritis, gingivitis, melena, oral moniliasis, salivary gland enlarged, stomatitis (or aphthous stomatitis), tooth disorder.

GU: Albuminuria, cystitis, dysuria, hematuria, menstrual disorder, pelvic pain, prostate disorder, urinary frequency, vaginal moniliasis.

Hematologic: Anemia (including iron deficiency anemia), ecchymosis.

Metabolic/Nutritional: Creatine phosphokinase increased, hyperglycemia, hyperlipidemia, peripheral edema.

Musculoskeletal: Arthrosis, bone pain, bursitis, muscle cramps, myalgia, neck pain, bone necrosis, tendon rupture.

Respiratory: Asthma, dyspnea, epistaxis, lung disorder.

Special senses: Blurred vision, cataract, conjunctivitis, eye disorder, pharyngitis, taste perversion.

Miscellaneous: Abscess, cyst, fever, hernia, pain.

Other less common adverse reactions – Other less common adverse reactions included the following.

Hypersensitivity: One case of anaphylactic reaction occurred in phase 2 trials following rechallenge of the drug after withdrawal due to rash (rare); urticaria.

Hematologic/Lymphatic: Eosinophilia; transient thrombocytopenia (rare); and leukopenia less than 2,000 white blood cells/mm^3 (rare).

➤*Postmarketing:*

Dermatologic – Erythema multiforme, Stevens-Johnson syndrome, toxic epidermal necrolysis, vasculitis including cutaneous necrotizing vasculitis.

Hematologic – Agranulocytosis, leukopenia, neutropenia, pancytopenia, thrombocytopenia.

Hepatic – Hepatitis, jaundice/cholestasis, severe liver injury such as hepatic failure and acute hepatic necrosis that may be fatal.

Respiratory – Interstitial lung disease, such as interstitial pneumonitis and pulmonary fibrosis, that may be fatal.

LEFLUNOMIDE — ORAL

Miscellaneous – Angioedema, opportunistic infections, pancreatitis, peripheral neuropathy, severe infections including sepsis that may be fatal.

Overdosage

➤*Symptoms:* There have been reports of chronic overdose in patients taking leflunomide at daily doses of up to 5 times the recommended daily dose and reports of acute overdose in adults and children. There were no adverse reactions reported in the majority of case reports of overdose. Adverse reactions were consistent with the safety profile for leflunomide. The most frequent adverse reactions observed were diarrhea, abdominal pain, leukopenia, anemia, and elevated liver function tests.

➤*Treatment:* In the event of a significant overdose or toxicity, cholestyramine or charcoal administration is recommended to accelerate elimination. The active metabolite of leflunomide is eliminated slowly from the plasma. In instances of any serious toxicity from leflunomide, including hypersensitivity, use of a drug elimination procedure is highly recommended to reduce the drug concentration more rapidly after stopping leflunomide therapy. If hypersensitivity is the suspected clinical mechanism, more prolonged cholestyramine or charcoal administration may be necessary to achieve rapid and sufficient clearance. The duration may be modified based on the clinical status of the patient (see Warnings/Precautions).

Patient Information

Discuss the potential for increased risk of birth defects with female patients of childbearing potential. Advise women that they may be at increased risk of having a child with birth defects if they are pregnant when taking leflunomide, become pregnant while taking leflunomide, or do not wait to become pregnant until they have stopped taking leflunomide and followed the drug elimination procedure.

Advise men wishing to father a child not to do so unless they have stopped the drug and have taken cholestyramine as part of the drug elimination procedure for 11 days.

Advise patients of the possibility of rare, serious skin reactions. Instruct patients to inform their health care provider promptly if they develop a skin rash or mucous membrane lesions.

Advise patients of the potential hepatotoxic effects of leflunomide and of the need for monitoring liver enzymes. Instruct patients to notify their health care provider if they develop symptoms such as unusual tiredness, abdominal pain, or jaundice.

Advise patients that they may develop a lowering of their blood counts and should have frequent hematologic monitoring. This is particularly important for patients who are receiving other immunosuppressive therapy concurrently with leflunomide, who have recently discontinued such therapy before starting treatment with leflunomide, or who have had a history of significant hematologic abnormality. Instruct patients to notify their health care provider if they notice symptoms of pancytopenia (eg, easy bruising or bleeding, recurrent infections, fever, paleness, unusual tiredness).

Inform patients about the early warning signs of interstitial lung disease and advise them to contact their health care providers as soon as possible if these symptoms appear or worsen during therapy.

KERATINOCYTE GROWTH FACTORS

PALIFERMIN

Rx	**Kepivance** (Biovitrum AB)	**Powder for injection:** 6.25 mg	Sucrose. Preservative free. Single-use vials.

PALIFERMIN — INJECTION

Indications

➤*Oral mucositis:* Palifermin is indicated to decrease the incidence and duration of severe oral mucositis in patients with hematologic malignancies who are receiving myelotoxic therapy requiring hematopoietic stem cell support.

Administration and Dosage

➤*Adults:*

Oral mucositis –

Usual dosage: The recommended dosage of palifermin is 60 mcg/kg/day, administered as an intravenous (IV) bolus injection for 3 consecutive days before and 3 consecutive days after myelotoxic therapy, for a total of 6 doses.

➤*Preparation for administration:* Reconstitute palifermin lyophilized powder only with sterile water for injection (not supplied). Aseptically reconstitute palifermin by slowly injecting sterile water for injection 1.2 mL (not supplied) to yield a final concentration of 5 mg/mL. Gently swirl the contents during dissolution. Do not shake or vigorously agitate the vial.

Generally, dissolution of palifermin takes less than 3 minutes.

Do not filter the reconstituted solution during preparation or administration.

➤*Administration:* If heparin is used to maintain an IV line, use saline to rinse the line prior to and after palifermin administration because palifermin has been shown to bind to heparin in vitro.

Following reconstitution, it is recommended that the product be used immediately.

Administer palifermin by IV bolus injection.

Premyelotoxic therapy – Administer the first 3 doses prior to myelotoxic therapy, with the third dose 24 to 48 hours before myelotoxic therapy.

Postmyelotoxic therapy – Administer the last 3 doses following myelotoxic therapy; administer the first of these doses after, but on the same day of, hematopoietic stem cell infusion and at least 4 days after the most recent administration of palifermin.

➤*Storage/Stability:* Store the dispensing pack containing palifermin lyophilized powder in its carton and refrigerate at 2° to 8°C (36° to 46°F). Protect from light. Keep vials in pack until time of use.

The reconstituted solution contains no preservatives and is intended for single use only. If not used immediately, the reconstituted solution of palifermin may be stored refrigerated in its carton at 2° to 8°C (36° to 46°F) for up to 24 hours. Prior to injection, palifermin may be allowed to reach room temperature for a maximum of 1 hour, but it should be protected from light. Discard palifermin left at room temperature for more than 1 hour. Do not freeze the reconstituted solution.

Do not use palifermin beyond the date stamped on the vial label.

Actions

➤*Pharmacology:* KGF is an endogenous protein in the fibroblast growth factor (FGF) family that binds to the KGF receptor. Binding of KGF to its receptor has been reported to result in proliferation, differentiation, and migration of epithelial cells. The KGF receptor, 1 of 4 receptors in the FGF family, has been reported to be present on epithelial cells in many tissues examined, including the tongue, buccal mucosa, esophagus, stomach, intestine, salivary gland, lung, liver, pancreas, kidney, bladder, mammary gland, skin (hair follicles and sebaceous gland), and the lens of the eye. The KGF receptor has been reported to not be present on cells of the hematopoietic lineage. Endogenous KGF is produced by mesenchymal cells and is upregulated in response to epithelial tissue injury.

Palifermin has been shown to enhance the growth of human epithelial tumor cell lines in vitro at concentrations at least 10 mcg/mL (more than 15-fold higher than average therapeutic concentrations in humans). In nude mouse xenograft models, 3 consecutive daily treatments of palifermin at doses of 1,500 and 4,000 mcg/kg (25- and 67-fold higher than the recommended human dose, respectively) repeated weekly for 4 to 6 weeks were associated with a dose-dependent increase in the growth rate of 1 of 7 KGF receptor-expressing human tumor cell lines.

Pharmacodynamics – Epithelial cell proliferation was assessed by Ki67 immunohistochemical staining in healthy subjects. A 3-fold or greater increase in Ki67 staining was observed in buccal biopsies from 3 of 6 healthy subjects given palifermin at 40 mcg/kg/day IV for 3 days, when measured 24 hours after the third dose. Dose-dependent epithelial cell proliferation was observed in healthy subjects given single IV doses of 120 to 250 mcg/kg 48 hours post-dosing.

➤*Pharmacokinetics:*

Absorption/Distribution – The pharmacokinetics of palifermin were studied in healthy subjects and patients with hematologic malignancies. After single IV doses of 20 to 250 mcg/kg (healthy subjects) and 60 mcg/kg (cancer patients), palifermin concentrations declined rapidly (over 95% decrease) in the first 30 minutes postdose. A slight increase or plateau in concentration occurred at approximately 1 to 4 hours, followed by a terminal decline phase. Palifermin exhibited linear pharmacokinetics with extravascular distribution.

Metabolism/Excretion – On average, total body clearance appeared to be 2- to 4-fold higher and volume of distribution at steady state to be 2-fold higher in cancer patients compared with healthy subjects after a 60 mcg/kg single dose of palifermin. The elimination half-life was similar between healthy subjects and cancer patients (average, 4.5 hours; range, 3.3 to 5.7 hours). No accumulation of palifermin occurred after 3 consecutive daily doses of 20 and 40 mcg/kg in healthy volunteers or 60 mcg/kg in cancer patients.

Contraindications

Hypersensitivity to *E. coli*-derived proteins, palifermin, or any other component of the product.

Warnings/Precautions

➤*Potential for stimulation of tumor growth:* The safety and efficacy of palifermin have not been established in patients with nonhematologic malignancies. The effects of palifermin on stimulation of KGF receptor-expressing, nonhematopoietic tumors in patients are not known. Palifermin has been shown to enhance the growth of human epithelial tumor cell lines in vitro and to increase the rate of tumor cell line growth in a human carcinoma xenograft model.

➤*Pregnancy: Category C.* Palifermin has been shown to be embryotoxic in rabbits and rats when given in doses that are 2.5 and 8 times the human dose, respectively.

Increased postimplantation loss and decreased fetal body weights were observed when palifermin was administered to pregnant rabbits from days 6 to 18 of gestation at IV dosages 150 mcg/kg/day or higher (2.5-fold higher than the recommended human dosage). However, treatment with these doses also was associated with maternal toxicity (clinical signs and

PALIFERMIN — INJECTION

reductions in body weight gain/food consumption). No evidence of developmental toxicity was observed in rabbits at dosages up to 60 mcg/kg/day.

Increased postimplantation loss, decreased fetal body weight, and/or increased skeletal variations were observed when palifermin was administered to pregnant rats from days 6 to 17 or 19 of gestation at IV dosages 500 mcg/kg/day or higher (more than 8-fold higher than the recommended human dose). Treatment with these doses was also frequently associated with maternal toxicity (clinical signs and body weight effects). No evidence of developmental toxicity was observed in rats at dosages up to 300 mcg/kg/day.

There are no adequate and well-controlled studies in pregnant women. Use palifermin during pregnancy only if the potential benefit justifies the potential risk to the fetus.

➤*Lactation:* It is not known whether palifermin is excreted in human milk. Because many drugs are excreted in human milk, exercise caution when palifermin is administered to a breast-feeding woman.

➤*Children:* The safety and efficacy of palifermin in pediatric patients have not been established.

Drug Interactions

➤*Heparin:* Palifermin has been shown to bind to heparin in vitro. Therefore, if heparin is used to maintain an IV line, use saline to rinse the line prior to and after palifermin administration.

➤*Chemotherapy:* Do not administer palifermin within 24 hours before, during infusion of, or within 24 hours after administration of myelotoxic chemotherapy. In a clinical trial, administration of palifermin within 24 hours of chemotherapy resulted in increased severity and duration of oral mucositis.

Adverse Reactions

Safety data are based upon 409 patients with hematologic malignancies (NHL, Hodgkin disease, AML, ALL, CML, CLL, or multiple myeloma) who received palifermin and 241 patients who received placebo in 3 randomized, placebo-controlled clinical studies and a pharmacokinetic study. Patients received palifermin either before, or before and after, regimens of myelotoxic chemotherapy, with or without TBI, followed by PBPC support. The patients were predominantly between 41 and 60 years of age (median age, 48 years), male (62%), and white (83%). NHL was the most common malignancy, followed by Hodgkin disease, multiple myeloma, and leukemia.

➤*Serious adverse reactions:* The most common serious adverse reaction attributed to palifermin was skin rash, which was reported in less than 1% (3/409) of patients treated with palifermin. Grade 3 skin rashes occurred in 14 patients, 9 of 409 (3%) receiving palifermin and 5 of 241 (2%) receiving placebo. In 7 patients (5 palifermin, 2 placebo), study drug was discontinued because of skin rash. Other serious adverse reactions occurred at a similar rate in patients who received palifermin (20%) or placebo (21%). The most frequently reported serious adverse reactions in palifermin and placebo-treated patients were fever, GI events, and respiratory events.

➤*Most common:* The most common adverse reactions attributed to palifermin were dysesthesia, oral toxicities (eg, alteration of taste, dysesthesia, tongue discoloration, tongue thickening), pain arthralgias, and skin toxicities (eg, edema, erythema, pruritus, rash). The median time-to-onset of cutaneous toxicity was 6 days following the first of 3 consecutive daily doses of palifermin, with a median duration of 5 days. In patients receiving palifermin, dysesthesia (including hyperesthesia, hypesthesia, and paresthesia) was usually localized to the perioral region, whereas in patients receiving placebo, dysesthesias were more likely to occur in extremities. Adverse reactions occurring more frequently in palifermin-treated patients as compared with placebo-treated patients (a higher incidence of at least 5%) are listed in the following table.

Palifermin Adverse Reactions (≥ 5%)

Adverse reaction	Palifermin (n = 409)	Placebo (n = 241)
CNS		
Dysesthesia (hyperesthesia/hypesthesia/paresthesia)	12%	7%
Dermatologic		
Erythema	32%	22%
Pruritus	35%	24%
Rash	62%	50%
GI		
Mouth/tongue thickness or discoloration	17%	8%
Taste altered	16%	8%
Metabolic		
Elevated serum amylase (grade 3/4)	62% (38%)	54% (31%)
Elevated serum lipase (grade 3/4)	28% (11%)	23% (5%)
Musculoskeletal		
Arthralgia	10%	5%
Miscellaneous		
Edema	28%	21%
Fever	39%	34%
Pain	16%	11%

➤*Cardiovascular:* In a phase 1, placebo-controlled study in patients undergoing hematopoietic transplantation and receiving palifermin (3 doses premyelotoxic therapy and 3 doses posttransplant), the proportion of palifermin-treated patients reporting an adverse reaction of hypertension in the palifermin 60 mcg/kg/day and 80 mcg/kg/day cohorts was greater than in the placebo group (2/15 [13%], 2/14 [14%], and 2/23 [9%] patients, respectively). These reactions were transient and did not require treatment discontinuation in any patient. In an integrated analysis of adverse reactions across palifermin studies in the hematology transplant setting, hypertensive events were reported in 30/409 palifermin (7%) patients and 13/241 placebo (5%) patients.

➤*Miscellaneous:*

Proteinuria – In a placebo-controlled study conducted in 145 patients with metastatic colorectal cancer receiving multicycle chemotherapy (5-fluorouracil/leucovorin), serial urine specimens were collected for 27 placebo-treated and 54 palifermin-treated patients. Among the 54 palifermin-treated patients, 9 patients with a baseline urinalysis negative for protein subsequently developed 2+ or greater proteinuria after treatment with palifermin. Among the 27 placebo-treated patients evaluated, none developed 2+ or greater proteinuria. Because of the study design, the number of cycles with urine analysis data collected was higher in the palifermin-treated patients. In addition, for the 9 patients with proteinuria, underlying medical conditions known to be associated with proteinuria were present at baseline. A causal relationship between palifermin and proteinuria has not been established.

➤*Lab test abnormalities:* Reversible elevations in serum lipase and amylase, which did not require treatment intervention, are shown in the preceding table. In general, peak increases were observed during the period of cytotoxic therapy and returned to baseline by the day of PBPC infusion. Fractionation of amylase revealed it to be predominantly salivary in origin.

➤*Immunogenicity:* As with all therapeutic proteins, there is a potential for immunogenicity. The clinical significance of antibodies to palifermin is unknown but may include lessened activity and/or cross-reactivity with other members of the FGF family of growth factors.

A sensitive electrochemiluminescence-based binding assay was performed on posttreatment sera from 645 patients treated with palifermin in clinical studies. Twelve (2%) of these 645 patients tested positive for antibodies to palifermin following treatment. None of the samples had evidence of neutralizing activity in a cell-based assay.

The incidence of antibody positivity is highly dependent on the specific assay and its sensitivity. Additionally, the observed incidence of antibody positivity in an assay may be influenced by several factors, including sample handling, timing of sample collection, concomitant medications, and underlying disease. For these reasons, comparison of the incidence of antibodies to palifermin with the incidence of antibodies to other products may be misleading.

Overdosage

The maximum amount of palifermin that can be safely administered in a single dose has not been determined. Single doses of 250 mcg/kg have been administered IV to 8 healthy volunteers without severe or serious adverse reactions. Five of 14 patients receiving 6 dosages of 80 mcg/kg/day administered IV over 2 weeks (3 doses preceding and 3 doses following myeloablative chemotherapy/TBI) experienced serious or severe adverse reactions. These reactions were consistent with those observed at the recommended dose but were generally more severe.

Patient Information

Inform patients of the possible side effects of palifermin, including mucocutaneous adverse effects. These include rash, erythema, edema, pruritus, oral/perioral dysesthesia, tongue discoloration, tongue thickening, and alteration of taste. Instruct patients to report these side effects, or any others, to their health care provider.

The safety and efficacy of palifermin have not been established in patients with nonhematologic malignancies. Inform patients of the evidence of tumor growth and stimulation in cell culture and in animal models of nonhematopoietic human tumors.

ANTIHISTAMINE-CONTAINING PREPARATIONS

otc	**Dermamycin** (Pfeiffer)	**Cream; topical**: 2% diphenhydramine HCl, parabens, polyethylene glycol monostearate, propylene glycol	In 28.35 g.
		Spray; topical: 2% diphenhydramine HCl, 1% menthol, alcohol, methylparaben	In 60 mL.
otc	**Maximum Strength Benadryl Itch Relief** (Pfeiffer)	**Cream; topical**: 2% diphenhydramine HCl, 0.1% zinc acetate, parabens, aloe vera	In 14.2 g.
		Stick; topical: 2% diphenhydramine HCl, 0.1% zinc acetate, 73.5% alcohol, aloe vera	In 14 mL.
otc	**Anti-Itch** (Taro)	**Cream; topical**: 2% diphenhydramine HCl, 0.1% zinc acetate, parabens	In 28.4 g.
otc	**Ziradryl** (Parke-Davis)	**Lotion; topical**: 1% diphenhydramine HCl, 2% zinc oxide, 2% alcohol, camphor, parabens	In 180 mL.
otc	**Benadryl** (Parke-Davis)	**Cream; topical**: 1% diphenhydramine HCl, parabens in a greaseless base	In 15 g.
		Spray, non-aerosol; topical: 1% diphenhydramine HCl, 85% alcohol	In 60 mL.
otc	**Di-Delamine** (Del Pharmaceuticals)	**Gel and Spray, non-aerosol; topical**: 1% diphenhydramine HCl, 0.5% tripelennamine HCl, 0.12% benzalkonium Cl, menthol, EDTA	**Gel**: In 37.5 g. **Spray**: In 120 mL.
otc	**Sting-Eze** (Wisconsin Pharm)	**Concentrate; topical**: Diphenhydramine HCl, camphor, phenol, benzocaine, eucalyptol	In 15 mL.
otc	**Derma-Pax** (Recsei Labs)	**Lotion; topical**: 0.5% diphenydramine HCl	Benzyl alcohol. In 118 mL.
otc	**Z-Xtra** (Magna)	**Lotion; topical**: 2.07 mg pyrilamine maleate, 41.35 mg zinc oxide/mL. Benzocaine, apple blossom oil, silicone oil, lanolin oil, Wysteria oil, isopropanol, camphor, menthol, parabens	In 118 mL.
otc	**Calamycin** (Pfeiffer)	**Lotion; topical**: Zinc oxide and 10% calamine, benzocaine, chloroxylenol, pyrilamine maleate, 2% isopropyl alcohol	In 120 mL.
otc	**Benadryl Itch Stopping Maximum Strength** (Warner Wellcome)	**Gel; topical**: 2% diphenhydramine HCl, 1% zinc acetate, camphor, parabens	In 118 g.
otc	**Dermarest** (Del)	**Gel; topical**: 2% diphenhydramine HCl, 2% resorcinol, aloe vera gel, benzalkonium chloride, EDTA, menthol, methylparaben, propylene glycol	In 29.25 and 56.25 g.
otc	**Dermarest Plus** (Del)	**Gel; topical**: 2% diphenhydramine HCl, 1% menthol, aloe vera gel, benzalkonium chloride, isopropyl alcohol, methylparaben, propylene glycol	In 15 and 30 g.
		Spray; topical: 2% diphenhydramine HCl, 1% menthol, aloe vera gel, benzalkonium chloride, methylparaben, propylene glycol, SD alcohol 40, EDTA	In 15 and 30 g.
otc	**Clearly Cala-gel** (Tec Labs)	**Gel; topical**: Diphenhydramine HCl, zinc acetate, menthol, EDTA	Clear. In 180 g.
otc	**Calagel Maximum Strength** (Tec Labs)	**Gel; topical**: 2% diphenhydramine HCl, 0.15% benzethonium chloride, 0.215% zinc acetate, disodium edetate, menthol	In 177.44 mL.
otc	**Benadryl Itch Relief** (GlaxoWellcome)	**Spray; topical**: 2% diphenhydramine HCl, 0.1% zinc acetate, 73.6% alcohol, aloe vera	In 59 mL.
otc	**Benadryl Itch Relief Children's** (GlaxoWellcome)	**Cream; topical**: 1% diphenhydramine HCl, 0.1% zinc acetate, aloe vera, cetyl alcohol, parabens	In 14.2 g.
		Spray; topical: 1% diphenhydramine HCl, 0.1% zinc acetate, 73.6% alcohol, aloe vera, povidone	In 59 mL.
otc	**Benadryl Itch Stopping Spray, Extra Strength** (Warner Lambert)	**Spray; topical**: 2% diphenhydramine HCl, 0.1% zinc acetate, 73.5% v/v alcohol, glycerin, tromethamine	In 59 mL.
otc	**Benadryl Itch Stopping Spray, Original Strength** (Warner Lambert)	**Spray; topical**: 1% diphenhydramine HCl, 0.1% zinc acetate, 73.6% v/v alcohol, glycerin, tromethamine	In 59 mL.
Rx	**Prudoxin** (HealthPoint Medical)	**Cream; topical**: 5% doxepin	In 45 g.

ANTIHISTAMINE-CONTAINING PREPARATIONS — TOPICAL

Indications

➤*Itching:* Temporary relief of itching due to minor skin disorders, ivy, sumac and oak poisoning, sunburn, insect bites (nonpoisonous) and stings.

Actions

➤*Pharmacology:* Topical antihistamines have some local anesthetic activity and are used to relieve itching. Some transdermal absorption may occur, but not in sufficient quantities to produce systemic side effects. They may cause local irritation and sensitization, especially with prolonged use. Refer to Antihistamine monograph in Respiratory Drugs chapter for further information on systemic antihistamines.

Warnings/Precautions

➤*Do not apply:* To blistered, raw or oozing areas of the skin, or around the eyes or other mucous membranes (eg, nose, mouth).

➤*For external use only:* Avoid contact with the eyes.

➤*Discontinue use:* If the condition persists, recurs after a few days or irritation develops.

➤*Avoid prolonged use:* For more than 7 days or use on extensive skin areas.

➤*Pregnancy: Category B.* The are no adequate and well-controlled studies in pregnant women. This drug should be used in pregnancy only if clearly needed.

➤*Lactation:* Doxepin is excreted in human milk after oral administration and significant systemic levels of doxepin are obtained after topical administration. Therefore, it is possible that doxepin could be secreted in human milk following topical administration. Because of the potential for serious adverse reactions in breast-feeding infants, a decision should be made whether to discontinue breast-feeding or to discontinue the drug, taking into account the importance of the drug to the mother.

DOXEPIN HYDROCHLORIDE

Rx	**Prudoxin** (Healthpoint)	**Cream; topical**: 5%	In 45 g.
Rx	**Zonalon** (Bioglan)		Cetyl alcohol, petrolatum, benzyl alcohol, titanium dioxide. In 30 g.

DOXEPIN HYDROCHLORIDE — TOPICAL

For information on the systemic use of doxepin, refer to the individual monographs in the CNS Drugs chapter.

Indications

➤*Pruritus:* Short-term (up to 8 days) management of moderate pruritus in adult patients with atopic dermatitis or lichen simplex chronicus.

Administration and Dosage

➤*General dosing considerations:* The risk for sedation may increase with greater body surface area application of doxepin cream. Clinical experience has shown that drowsiness is significantly more common in patients applying doxepin cream to more than 10% of the body surface area; therefore, especially caution patients with greater than 10% of body surface area affected about possible drowsiness and other systemic adverse effects of doxepin.

DOXEPIN HYDROCHLORIDE — TOPICAL

Occlusive dressing – Occlusive dressings may increase the absorption of most topical drugs; therefore, do not use occlusive dressings with doxepin cream.

➤*Adults:*

Pruritis –

Usual dosage: Apply a thin film of doxepin cream 4 times each day with at least a 3- to 4-hour interval between applications.

Duration of therapy: Long-term use longer than 8 days may result in higher systemic levels and should be avoided. Use of doxepin cream for longer than 8 days may result in an increased likelihood of contact sensitization.

Discontinuation of therapy: If excessive drowsiness occurs, it may be necessary to do 1 or more of the following: reduce the body surface area treated, reduce the number of applications per day, reduce the amount of cream applied, or discontinue the drug.

➤*Elderly:* Sedating drugs may cause confusion and oversedation in elderly patients; elderly patients generally should be observed closely for confusion and oversedation when started on doxepin cream.

➤*Administration:* For topical, dermatologic use only. Not for ophthalmic, oral, or intravaginal use.

➤*Storage/Stability:* Store at or below 27°C (80°F).

Actions

➤*Pharmacology:* Although doxepin does have H1 and H2 histamine receptor blocking actions, the exact mechanism by which doxepin exerts its antipruritic effect is unknown. Doxepin cream can produce drowsiness in significant numbers of patients, and this sedation may reduce awareness, including awareness of pruritic symptoms.

➤*Pharmacokinetics:*

Absorption – In 19 pruritic eczema patients treated with doxepin cream, plasma doxepin concentrations ranged from nondetectable to 47 ng/mL from percutaneous absorption. Plasma levels from topical application of doxepin cream can result in CNS and other systemic side effects.

Metabolism/Excretion – Once absorbed into the systemic circulation, doxepin undergoes hepatic metabolism that results in conversion to pharmacologically active desmethyldoxepin. Further glucuronidation results in urinary excretion of the parent drug and its metabolites. Desmethyldoxepin has a half-life that ranges from 28 to 52 hours and is not affected by multiple dosing. Plasma levels of both doxepin and desmethyldoxepin are highly variable and are poorly correlated with dosage. Wide distribution occurs in body tissues including lungs, heart, brain, and liver. Renal disease, genetic factors, age, and other medications affect the metabolism and subsequent elimination of doxepin.

Contraindications

Untreated narrow angle glaucoma or a tendency to urinary retention; sensitivity to any of its components.

Warnings/Precautions

➤*Drowsiness:* See Administration and Dosage for more information.

The sedating effects of alcoholic beverages, antihistamines, and other CNS depressants may be potentiated when doxepin cream is used.

If excessive drowsiness occurs, it may be necessary to reduce the frequency of applications, the amount of cream applied, and/or the percentage of body surface area treated, or discontinue the drug. However, the efficacy with reduced frequency of applications has not been established. Keep this product away from the eyes.

➤*Hypersensitivity reactions:* Use of doxepin cream can cause Type IV hypersensitivity reactions (contact sensitization) to doxepin.

➤*Hazardous tasks:*

Drowsiness – See Warnings/Precautions for more information.

➤*Pregnancy: Category B.* There are no adequate and well-controlled studies in pregnant women. Use this drug during pregnancy only if clearly needed.

➤*Lactation:* Doxepin is excreted in human milk after oral administration. It is possible that doxepin may also be excreted in human milk following topical application of doxepin cream.

One case has been reported of apnea and drowsiness in a nursing infant whose mother was taking an oral dosage form of doxepin.

Because of the potential for serious adverse reactions in nursing infants from doxepin, a decision should be made whether to discontinue nursing or to discontinue the drug, taking into account the importance of the drug to the mother.

➤*Children:* The use of doxepin cream in pediatric patients is not recommended. Safe conditions for use of doxepin cream in children have not been established. One case has been reported of a 2.5-year-old child who developed somnolence, grand mal seizure, respiratory depression, ECG abnormalities, and coma after treatment with doxepin cream. A total of 27 g had been applied over 3 days for eczema. He was treated with supportive care, activated charcoal, and systemic alkalization, and he recovered.

➤*Elderly:* Clinical studies of doxepin cream did not include sufficient numbers of subjects aged 65 years and over to determine whether they respond differently from younger subjects. Other reported clinical experience has not identified differences in responses between the elderly and younger patients. In general, dose selection for an elderly patient should be cautious, usually starting at the low end of the dosing range, reflecting the greater frequency of decreased hepatic, renal or cardiac function, and of concomitant disease or other drug therapy.

The extent of renal excretion of doxepin has not been determined. Because elderly patients are more likely to have decreased renal function, take care in dose selections.

Sedating drugs may cause confusion and oversedation in the elderly; elderly patients generally should be observed closely for confusion and oversedation when started on doxepin cream. An 80-year-old male nursing home patient developed probable systemic anticholinergic toxicity which included urinary retention and delirium after doxepin cream had been applied to his arms, legs and back 3 times daily for 2 days.

Drug Interactions

➤*Drugs metabolized by P450 2D6:* Concomitant use of tricyclic antidepressants with drugs that can inhibit cytochrome P450 2D6 may require lower doses than usually prescribed for either the tricyclic antidepressant or the other drug. It is desirable to monitor TCA plasma levels whenever a TCA is going to be coadministered with another drug known to be an inhibitor of P450 2D6.

➤*MAO inhibitors:* Serious side effects and even death have been reported following the concomitant use of certain drugs with MAO inhibitors. Therefore, discontinue MAO inhibitors at least 2 weeks prior to the cautious initiation of therapy with doxepin cream. The exact length of time may vary and is dependent upon the particular MAO inhibitor being used, the length of time it has been administered, and the dosage involved.

➤*Cimetidine:* Serious anticholinergic symptoms (ie, severe dry mouth, urinary retention and blurred vision) have been associated with elevations in the serum levels of tricyclic antidepressant when cimetidine therapy is initiated. Additionally, higher than expected tricyclic antidepressant levels have been observed when they are begun in patients already taking cimetidine.

➤*CNS depressants:* See Warnings/Precautions for more information.

➤*Tolazamide:* A case of severe hypoglycemia has been reported in a type 2 diabetes patient maintained on tolazamide (1 g/day) 11 days after the addition of oral doxepin (75 mg/day).

Adverse Reactions

➤*Controlled clinical trials:*

Systemic adverse effects – In controlled clinical trials of patients treated with doxepin cream, the most common systemic adverse event reported was drowsiness. Drowsiness occurred in 71 of 330 (22%) of patients treated with doxepin cream compared to 7 of 334 (2%) of patients treated with vehicle cream. Drowsiness resulted in the premature discontinuation of the drug in approximately 5% of patients treated with doxepin cream in controlled clinical trials.

Local site adverse effects – In controlled clinical trials of patients treated with doxepin cream, the most common local site adverse event reported was burning or stinging at the site of application. These occurred in 76 of 330 (23%) of patients treated with doxepin cream compared to 54 of 334 (16%) of patients treated with vehicle cream. Most of these reactions were categorized as "mild"; however, approximately 25% of patients who reported burning and/or stinging reported the reaction as "severe". Four patients treated with doxepin cream withdrew from the study because of the burning and/or stinging.

Doxepin Adverse Reactions (≥ 1%)

Adverse reaction	Doxepin (n = 330)	Vehicle (n = 334)
Burning/stinging	76 (23%)	54 (16.2%)
Dizziness[a]	7 (2.1%)	3 (0.9%)
Drowsiness	71 (21.5%)	7 (2.1%)
Dry mouth[b]	32 (9.7%)	4 (1.2%)
Edema	4 (1.2%)	1 (0.3%)
Exacerbated eczema	10 (3%)	8 (2.4%)
Fatigue/ tiredness	10 (3%)	5 (1.5%)
Headache	3 (0.9%)	14 (4.2%)
Mental emotional changes	6 (1.8%)	1 (0.3%)
Other application site reaction[c]	10 (3%)	16 (4.8%)
Pruritus[d]	13 (3.9%)	20 (6%)
Taste perversion[e]	5 (1.5%)	1 (0.3%)

[a] Includes reports of "lightheadedness" and "dizziness/vertigo."
[b] Includes reports of "dry lips", "dry throat", and "thirst."
[c] Includes reports of "increased irritation at application site."
[d] Includes reports of "pruritus exacerbated."
[e] Includes reports of "bitter taste" and "metallic taste in mouth."

Adverse events occurring in 0.5% to less than 1% of doxepin-cream-treated patients in the controlled clinical trials included nervousness/anxiety, tongue numbness, fever, and nausea.

DOXEPIN HYDROCHLORIDE — TOPICAL

➤*Postmarketing experience:* Twenty-six cases of allergic contact dermatitis have been reported in patients using doxepin cream, 20 of which were documented by positive patch test to doxepin 5% cream.

Overdosage

➤*Symptoms:* Should overdosage with topical application of doxepin cream occur, the signs and symptoms may include cardiac dysrhythmias, severe hypotension, convulsions, and CNS depression, including coma. Changes in the electrocardiogram, particularly in QRS axis or width, are clinically significant indicators of tricyclic antidepressant toxicity.

Other signs of overdose may include confusion, disturbed concentration, transient visual hallucinations, dilated pupils, agitation, hyperactive reflexes, stupor, drowsiness, muscle rigidity, vomiting, hypothermia, hyperpyrexia, or any other doxepin topical adverse reactions.

➤*Treatment:*

General recommendations – Obtain an ECG, and immediately initiate cardiac monitoring. Protect the patient's airway, establish an IV line, and initiate gastric decontamination. A minimum of 6 hours of observation with cardiac monitoring and observation for signs of CNS or respiratory depression, hypotension, cardiac dysrhythmias and/or conduction blocks, and seizures is strongly advised. If signs of toxicity occur at any time during this period, extended monitoring is recommended. There are case reports of patients succumbing to fatal dysrhythmias late after overdose; these patients had clinical evidence of significant poisoning prior to death and most received inadequate gastrointestinal decontamination. Monitoring of plasma drug levels should not guide management of the patient.

Cardiovascular – A maximal limb-lead QRS duration of greater than or equal to 0.1 seconds may be the best indication of the severity of the overdose. Use IV sodium bicarbonate to maintain the serum pH in the range of 7.45 to 7.55. If the pH response is inadequate, hyperventilation may also be used. Concomitant use of hyperventilation and sodium bicarbonate should be done with extreme caution, with frequent pH monitoring. A pH greater than 7.6 or a pCO_2 less than 20 mm Hg is undesirable. Dysrhythmias unresponsive to sodium bicarbonate therapy/hyperventilation may respond to lidocaine, bretylium or phenytoin.

Type 1A and 1C antiarrhythmics are generally contraindicated (eg, quinidine, disopyramide, and procainamide).

In rare instances, hemoperfusion may be beneficial in acute refractory cardiovascular instability in patients with acute toxicity. However, hemodialysis, peritoneal dialysis, exchange transfusions, and forced diuresis generally have been reported as ineffective in tricyclic antidepressant poisoning.

CNS – In patients with CNS depression, early intubation is advised because of the potential for abrupt deterioration. Control seizures with benzodiazepines, or if these are ineffective, other anticonvulsants (eg, phenobarbital, phenytoin). Physostigmine is not recommended except to treat life-threatening symptoms that have been unresponsive to other therapies, and then only in consultation with a poison control center.

Pediatric management – The principles of management of child and adult overdosages are similar. It is strongly recommended that the physician contact the local poison control center for specific pediatric treatment.

Patient Information

Since drowsiness may occur with the use of doxepin cream, warn patients of the possibility and caution them against driving a car or operating dangerous machinery while using this drug. Also caution patients that their responses to alcohol may be potentiated.

ANTI-INFECTIVES, TOPICAL

Antibiotic Agents

GENTAMICIN SULFATE

Rx	**Gentamicin** (Various, eg, Fougera)	**Ointment:** 0.1% (as base)	May contain white petrolatum, parabens. In 15 g.
		Cream: 0.1% (as base)	May contain propylene glycol, parabens. In 15 g.

GENTAMICIN SULFATE — TOPICAL

Indications

➤*Primary skin infections:* Impetigo contagiosa, superficial folliculitis, ecthyma, furunculosis, sycosis barbae, and pyoderma gangrenosum.

➤*Secondary skin infections:* Infectious eczematoid dermatitis, pustular acne, pustular psoriasis, infected seborrheic dermatitis, infected contact dermatitis (including poison ivy), infected excoriations, and bacterial superinfections of fungal or viral infections.

➤*Other infections:* Treatment of infected skin cysts and certain other skin abscesses when preceded by incision and drainage to permit adequate contact between the antibiotic and the infecting bacteria. Good results have been obtained in the treatment of infected stasis and other skin ulcers, infected superficial burns, paronychia, infected insect bites and stings, infected lacerations and abrasions, and wounds from minor surgery. Patients sensitive to neomycin can be treated with gentamicin, although regular observation of patients sensitive to topical antibiotics is advisable when such patients are treated with any topical antibiotic.

➤*Ointment:* Gentamicin sulfate ointment helps retain moisture and has been useful in infection on dry eczematous or psoriatic skin.

➤*Cream:* For wet, oozing primary infections and greasy, secondary infections, such as pustular acne or infected seborrheic dermatitis. If a water-washable preparation is desired, gentamicin sulfate cream is preferable.

Administration and Dosage

➤*General dosing considerations:* The area treated may be covered with a gauze dressing if desired.

Care should be exercised to avoid further contamination of the infected skin.

Infected stasis ulcers have responded well to gentamicin sulfate under gelatin packing.

➤*Adults:*

Skin infection – Apply a small amount of cream or ointment gently to the lesions 3 or 4 times daily. In impetigo contagiosa, the crusts should be removed before application of gentamicin sulfate to permit maximum contact between the antibiotic and the infection.

➤*Children:*

1 year of age or older – See Adults for dosing.

➤*Storage/Stability:* Store between 2° and 30°C (36° and 86°F).

Actions

➤*Pharmacology:* Gentamicin sulfate, a wide-spectrum antibiotic, provides highly effective topical treatment in primary and secondary bacterial infections of the skin. Gentamicin sulfate may clear infections that have not responded to other topical antibiotic agents. In impetigo contagiosa and other primary skin infections, treatment three or four times daily with gentamicin sulfate usually clears the lesions promptly. In secondary skin infections, gentamicin sulfate facilitates the treatment of the underlying dermatosis by controlling the infection. Bacteria susceptible to the action of gentamicin sulfate include sensitive strains of streptococci (group A beta-hemolytic, alpha-hemolytic), *Staphylococcus aureus* (coagulase-positive, coagulase-negative, and some penicillinase-producing strains), and the gram-negative bacteria, *Pseudomonas aeruginosa*, *Aerobacter aerogenes*, *Escherichia coli*, *Proteus vulgaris*, and *Klebsiella pneumoniae*.

Contraindications

History of sensitivity reactions to any of its components.

Warnings/Precautions

➤*Superinfection:* Use of topical antibiotics occasionally allows overgrowth of nonsusceptible organisms, including fungi. If this occurs, or if irritation, sensitization, or superinfection develops, treatment with gentamicin should be discontinued and appropriate therapy instituted.

➤*Pregnancy:* Category C (per Briggs' *Drugs in Pregnancy and Lactation*). Gentamicin rapidly crosses the placenta into fetal circulation and amniotic fluid.

➤*Lactation:* Small amounts of gentamicin are excreted into breast milk and absorbed by the breast-feeding infant. The American Academy of Pediatrics classifies gentamicin as compatible with breast-feeding.

Adverse Reactions

In patients with dermatoses treated with gentamicin, irritation (erythema and pruritus) that did not usually require discontinuance of treatment has been reported in a small percentage of cases. There was no evidence of irritation or sensitization, however, in any of these patients patch-tested subsequently with gentamicin on normal skin. Possible photosensitization has been reported in several patients but could not be elicited in these patients by reapplication of gentamicin followed by exposure to ultraviolet radiation.

BACITRACIN

otc	**Bacitracin** (Various, eg, Fougera, Ivax)	**Ointment:** 500 units/g	May contain mineral oil or white petrolatum. In 14, 28, 120, and 454 g and UD 144s.

BACITRACIN ZINC — TOPICAL

Indications

➤*Topical infection:* A first aid antibiotic to help prevent infection in minor cuts, scrapes, and burns.

Administration and Dosage

➤*General dosing considerations:* The affected area may be covered with a sterile bandage.

BACITRACIN ZINC — TOPICAL

➤*Adults:*

Topical infection –

Usual dosage: Clean the affected area. Apply a small amount of product (an amount equal to the surface area of the tip of a finger) on the area 1 to 3 times daily.

Duration of therapy: Do not use longer than 1 week unless directed by a health care provider.

➤*Administration:* Bacitracin is for external use only. Do not use in or near the eyes, nose, mouth, mucous membranes, or apply over large areas of the body.

➤*Storage/Stability:* Store at 15° to 25°C (59° to 77°F).

Actions

➤*Pharmacology:* Bacitracin is believed to be bactericidal or bacteriostatic in action depending on the concentration of the drip and the susceptibility of the organism. Bacitracin inhibits cell-wall synthesis by preventing amino acids and nucleotides into the cell. Absorption is reported to be negligible following topical administration.

Contraindications

Known hypersensitivity to any of the ingredients; use in the eyes.

Warnings/Precautions

➤*Systemic therapy:* Deeper cutaneous infections may require systemic antibiotic therapy in addition to local treatment. Use caution when applying over large areas of the body for deep puncture wounds, animal bites, or serious burns.

➤*External use:* Bacitracin zinc is for external use only. Do not use in or near the eyes, nose, mouth, mucous membranes, or apply over large areas of the body.

➤*Hypersensitivity reactions:* Stop use if a rash or other allergic reaction occurs.

➤*Pregnancy: Category C.* There are no adequate and well controlled studies in pregnant women. Use during pregnancy only when clearly needed.

➤*Lactation:* It is not known whether bacitracin is excreted in breast milk. Use caution when applying on a breastfeeding woman.

Adverse Reactions

Rash; hypersensitivity reaction (rare).

Patient Information

For external use only.

Do not use:

- In the eyes
- If you are allergic to any of the ingredients
- Over large areas of the body
- Longer than 1 week unless directed by a doctor

Ask a doctor before use in case of deep or puncture wounds, animal bites, or serious burns

Stop use and ask a doctor if:

- The condition persists or gets worse.
- A rash or other allergic reaction develops.

Keep out of reach of children. If swallowed, get medical help or contact a poison control center right away.

AZELAIC ACID

Rx	Azelex (Allergan)	Cream; topical: 20%	Glycerin, cetearyl alcohol, benzoic acid. In 30 and 50 g.
Rx	Finacea (Intendis)	Gel; topical: 15%	Benzoic acid, EDTA. In 30 g.

AZELAIC ACID — TOPICAL

Indications

➤*Cream:* For the topical treatment of mild-to-moderate inflammatory acne vulgaris.

➤*Gel:* For topical treatment of inflammatory papules and pustules of mild to moderate rosacea. Patients should be instructed to avoid spicy foods, thermally hot foods and drinks, alcoholic beverages, and to use only very mild soaps or soapless cleansing lotion for facial cleansing.

Administration and Dosage

➤*Adults:*

Mild to moderate inflammatory acne vulgaris –

Cream:

- *Usual dosage* – Apply a thin film to the affected areas twice daily, in the morning and evening.
- *Duration of therapy* – The duration of use of azelaic acid can vary from person to person and depends on the severity of the acne. Improvement of the condition occurs in the majority of patients with inflammatory lesions within 4 weeks.

Inflammatory papules and pustules of mild to moderate rosacea –

Gel:

- *Usual dosage* – Apply a thin layer to affected areas on the face twice daily, evening and morning.
- *Duration of therapy* – Azelaic acid gel 15% has only been studied up to 12 weeks in patients with mild to moderate rosacea.

➤*Children:*

Mild to moderate inflammatory acne vulgaris –

12 years of age or older: See Adults for dosing.

➤*Administration:*

Cream – After the skin is thoroughly washed and patted dry, a thin film of azelaic acid should be gently but thoroughly massaged into the affected areas twice daily, in the morning and evening. The hands should be washed following application.

Gel – Massage a thin layer gently into the affected areas on the face twice daily, in the morning and evening.

➤*Storage/Stability:*

Cream – Store between 15° and 30°C (59° and 86°F). Protect from freezing.

Gel – Store at 25°C (77°F); excursions are permitted between 15° and 30°C (59° and 86°F).

Actions

➤*Pharmacology:* The exact mechanism of action of azelaic acid is not known. The following in vitro data are available, but their clinical significance is unknown. Azelaic acid has been shown to possess antimicrobial activity against *Propionibacterium acnes* and *Staphylococcus epidermidis*. The antimicrobial action may be attributable to inhibition of microbial cellular protein synthesis. A normalization of keratinization leading to an anticomedonal effect of azelaic acid may also contribute to its clinical activity. Electron microscopic and immunohistochemical evaluation of skin biopsies from human subjects treated with azelaic acid demonstrated a reduction in the thickness of the stratum corneum, a reduction in number and size of keratohyalin granules, and a reduction in the amount and distribution of filaggrin (a protein component of keratohyalin) in epidermal layers. This is suggestive of the ability to decrease microcomedo formation.

➤*Pharmacokinetics:*

Cream – Following a single application of azelaic acid to human skin in vitro, azelaic acid penetrates into the stratum corneum (approximately 3% to 5% of the applied dose) and other viable skin layers (up to 10% of the dose is found in the epidermis and dermis). Negligible cutaneous metabolism occurs after topical application. Approximately 4% of the topically applied azelaic acid is systemically absorbed. Azelaic acid is mainly excreted unchanged in the urine but undergoes some oxidation to shorter chain dicarboxylic acids. The observed half-lives in healthy subjects are approximately 45 minutes after oral dosing and 12 hours after topical dosing, indicating percutaneous absorption rate-limited kinetics. Azelaic acid is a dietary constituent (whole grain cereals and animal products), and can be formed endogenously from longer-chain dicarboxylic acids, metabolism of oleic acid, and oxidation of monocarboxylic acids. Endogenous plasma concentration (20 to 80 ng/mL) and daily urinary excretion (4 to 28 mg) of azelaic acid are highly dependent on dietary intake, After topical treatment with azelaic acid in humans, plasma concentration and urinary excretion of azelaic acid are not significantly different from baseline levels.

Gel – The percutaneous absorption of azelaic acid after topical application of azelaic acid gel, 15%, could not be reliably determined. Mean plasma azelaic acid concentrations in rosacea patients treated with azelaic acid gel, 15%, twice daily for at least 8 weeks are in the range of 42 to 63.1 ng/mL. These values are within the maximum concentration range of 24 to 90.5 ng/mL observed in rosacea patients treated with vehicle only. This indicates that azelaic acid gel, 15%, does not increase plasma azelaic acid concentration beyond the range derived from nutrition and endogenous metabolism.

In vitro and human data suggest negligible cutaneous metabolism of ^{3}H-azelaic acid 20% cream after topical application. Azelaic acid is mainly excreted unchanged in the urine, but undergoes some β-oxidation to shorter chain dicarboxylic acids.

Contraindications

Hypersensitivity to any of its components.

Warnings/Precautions

➤*Hypopigmentation:* There have been isolated reports of hypopigmentation after use of azelaic acid. Since azelaic acid has not been well studied in patients with dark complexions, these patients should be monitored for early signs of hypopigmentation.

➤*Hypersensitivity:* If sensitivity or severe irritation develop with the use of azelaic acid treatment should be discontinued and appropriate therapy instituted.

➤*Pregnancy: Category B.* Embryotoxic effects were observed in Segment 1 and Segment 11 oral studies with rats receiving 2500 mg/kg/day of azelaic

AZELAIC ACID — TOPICAL

acid. Similar effects were observed in Segment 11 studies in rabbits given 150 to 500 mg/kg/day and in monkeys given 500 mg/kg/day. The doses at which these effects were noted were all within toxic dose ranges for the dams. No teratogenic effects were observed. There are, however, no adequate and well controlled studies in pregnant women. Because animal reproduction studies are not always predictive of human response, this drug should be used during pregnancy only if clearly needed.

➤*Lactation:* Equilibrium dialysis was used to assess human milk partitioning in vitro. At an azelaic acid concentration of 25 mcg/mL, the milk/plasma distribution coefficient was 0.7 and the milk/buffer distribution was 1), indicating that passage of drug into maternal milk may occur. Since less than 4% of a topically applied dose of azelaic acid is systemically absorbed, the uptake of azelaic acid into maternal milk is not expected to cause a significant change from baseline azelaic acid levels in the milk. However, caution should be exercised when azelaic acid is administered to a nursing mother.

➤*Children:*

Cream – Safety and efficacy in pediatric patients under 12 years of age have not been established.

Gel – Safety and efficacy of azelaic acid, 15%, in pediatric patients have not been established.

Drug Interactions

None known.

Adverse Reactions

➤*Cream:* During US clinical trials with azelaic acid, adverse reactions were generally mild and transient in nature. The most common adverse reactions occurring in approximately 1% to 5% of patients were pruritus, burning, stinging and tingling. Other adverse reactions such as erythema, dryness, rash, peeling, irritation, dermatitis, and contact dermatitis were reported in less than 1% of subjects. There is the potential for experiencing allergic reactions with use of azelaic acid. In patients using azelaic acid formulations, the following additional adverse experiences have been reported rarely: Worsening of asthma, vitiligo depigmentation, small depigmented spots, hypertrichosis, reddening (signs of keratosis pilaris), and exacerbation of recurrent herpes labialis.

➤*Gel:*

Azelaic Acid Cutaneous Adverse Reactions Occurring In ≥ 1% of Subjects In the Rosacea Trials by Treatment Group and Maximum Intensity[a]

	Azelaic acid gel, 15% n = 333 (100%)			Vehicle n = 331 (100%)		
Adverse reaction	Mild (n = 86) (26%)	Moderate (n = 44) (13%)	Severe (n = 20) (6%)	Mild (n = 49) (15%)	Moderate (n = 27) (8%)	Severe (n = 5) (2%)
Burning/ stinging/ tingling	66 (20%)	30 (9%)	12 (4%)	8 (2%)	6 (2%)	2 (1%)
Pruritus	24 (7%)	14 (4%)	3 (1%)	9 (3%)	6 (2%)	0 (0%)
Scaling/ dry skin/ xerosis	21 (6%)	8 (2%)	4 (1%)	33 (10%)	12 (4%)	1 (0%)
Erythema/ irritation	6 (2%)	6 (2%)	1 (0%)	8 (2%)	4 (1%)	2 (1%)
Edema	3 (1%)	2 (1%)	0 (0%)	3 (1%)	0 (0%)	0 (0%)
Contact dermatitis	2 (1%)	2 (1%)	0 (0%)	1 (0%)	0 (0%)	0 (0%)
Acne	2 (1%)	1 (0%)	0 (0%)	1 (0%)	0 (0%)	0 (0%)
Seborrhea	2 (1%)	0 (0%)	0 (0%)	0 (0%)	0 (0%)	0 (0%)
Photosensitivity	1 (0%)	0 (0%)	0 (0%)	3 (1%)	1 (0%)	1 (0%)

Azelaic Acid Cutaneous Adverse Reactions Occurring In ≥ 1% of Subjects In the Rosacea Trials by Treatment Group and Maximum Intensity[a]

	Azelaic acid gel, 15% n = 333 (100%)			Vehicle n = 331 (100%)		
Adverse reaction	Mild (n = 86) (26%)	Moderate (n = 44) (13%)	Severe (n = 20) (6%)	Mild (n = 49) (15%)	Moderate (n = 27) (8%)	Severe (n = 5) (2%)
Skin disease	1 (0%)	0 (0%)	0 (0%)	1 (0%)	2 (1%)	0 (0%)

[a] Subjects may have greater than 1 cutaneous adverse reaction; thus, the sum of the frequencies of preferred terms may exceed the number of subjects with at least 1 cutaneous adverse reaction.

Azelaic acid gel, 15%, and its vehicle caused irritant reactions at the application sitein human dermal safety studies. Azelaic acid gel, 15%, caused significantly more irritation than its vehicle in a cumulative irritation study. Some improvement in irritation was demonstrated over the course of the clinical studies, but this improvement might be attributed to subject dropouts. No phototoxicity or photoallergenicity were reported in human dermal safety studies.

In patients using azelaic acid formulations, the following additional adverse reactions have been reported rarely: Worsening of asthma, vitiligo depigmentation, small depigmented spots, hypertrichosis, reddening (signs of keratosis pilaris), and exacerbation of recurrent herpes labialis.

Overdosage

➤*Gel:* Azelaic acid gel, 15%, is intended for cutaneous use only. If pronounced local irritation occurs, patients should be directed to discontinue use and appropriate therapy should be instituted.

Patient Information

➤*Cream:* Patients should be told:

1.) To use azelaic acid for the full prescribed treatment period.
2.) To avoid the use of occlusive dressings or wrappings.
3.) To keep azelaic acid away from the mouth, eyes and other mucous membranes. If it does come in contact with the eyes, they should wash their eyes with large amounts of water and consult a physician if eye irritation persists.
4.) If they have dark complexions, to report abnormal changes in skin color to their physician.
5.) Due in part to the low pH of azelaic acid, temporary skin irritation (pruritus, burning, or stinging) may occur when azelaic acid is applied to broken or inflamed skin, usually at the start of treatment. However, this irritation commonly subsides if treatment is continued. If it continues, azelaic acid should be applied only once a day, or the treatment should be stopped until these effects have subsided. If troublesome irritation persists, use should be discontinued, and patients should consult their physician.

➤*Gel:* Azelaic acid gel, 15%, is to be used only as directed by the physician.

Azelaic acid gel, 15%, is for external use only. It is not to be used orally, intravaginally, or for the eyes.

Cleanse affected area(s) with a very mild soap or a soapless cleansing lotion and pat dry with a soft towel before applying azelaic acid gel, 15%. Avoid alcoholic cleansers, tinctures and astringents, abrasives and peeling agents.

Avoid contact of azelaic acid gel, 15%, with the mouth, eyes, and other mucous membranes. If it does come in contact with the eyes, wash the eyes with large amounts of water and consult a physician if eye irritation persists.

The hands should be washed following application of azelaic acid gel, 15%.

Cosmetics may be applied after azelaic acid gel, 15%, has dried.

Skin irritation (eg, pruritus, burning, stinging) may occur during use of azelaic acid gel, 15%, usually during the first few weeks of treatment. If irritation is excessive or persists, use of azelaic acid gel, 15%, should be discontinued, and patients should consult their physician.

Avoid any foods and beverages that might provoke erythema, flushing, and blushing (including spicy food, alcoholic beverages, and thermally hot drinks, including hot coffee and tea).

Patients should report abnormal changes in skin color to their physician.

Avoid the use of occlusive dressings or wrappings.

BENZOYL PEROXIDE

Rx	**Benzoyl Peroxide 2½% Wash** (Various, eg, Glades)	**Liquid; topical:** 2.5%	In 237 mL.
otc	**PanOxyl 2.5% Acne Spot Treatment** (GlaxoSmithKline)		Edetate disodium, glycerin. In 60 g.
Rx	**Triaz** (Medicis)	**Liquid; topical:** 3%	Glycerin, petrolatum, lavender extract, menthol. In 170.3 and 340.2 g.
Rx	**Benzac AC Wash 5** (Galderma)	**Liquid; topical:** 5%	Glycerin, water based. In 240 mL.
Rx	**Benzac W Wash 5** (Galderma)		Water based. In 120 and 240 mL.
Rx	**Benzoyl Peroxide 5% Wash** (Various, eg, Glades)		In 118, 148, and 237 mL.
Rx	**Triaz** (Medicis)	**Liquid; topical:** 6%	Glycerin, petrolatum, lavender extract, menthol. In 170.3 and 340.2 g.
Rx	**Triaz** (Medicis)	**Liquid; topical:** 9%	Glycerin, white petrolatum, zinc lactate, lavender extract, menthol. In 340.2 g.

BENZOYL PEROXIDE

Rx	**Benzac AC Wash 10** (Galderma)	**Liquid; topical:** 10%	Glycerin, water based. In 240 mL.
Rx	**Benzac W Wash 10** (Galderma)		Water based. In 240 mL.
Rx	**Benzoyl Peroxide 10% Wash** (Various, eg, Glades)		In 148 and 237 mL.
otc	**Oxy Oil-Free Maximum Strength Acne Wash** (GlaxoSmithKline)		Parabens, diazolidinyl urea. In 237 mL.
otc	**Maximum Strength PanOxyl Acne Foam Wash** (GlaxoSmithKline)		Cetearyl alcohol, glycerin, hydrogenated castor oil, lactic acid, methylparaben, mineral oil, PEG-14M. In 156 g.
otc	**PanOxyl** (GlaxoSmithKline)	**Bar; topical:** 5%	Cetearyl alcohol, glycerin, castor oil, lactic acid, mineral oil, PEG-14M. In 113 g.
Rx	**Desquam-X 10** (Westwood Squibb)	**Bar; topical:** 10%	Lactic acid, EDTA, sorbitol. In 106 g.
otc	**Maximum Strength PanOxyl Acne Cleansing** (GlaxoSmithKline)		Cetearyl alcohol, glycerin, hydrogenated castor oil, lactic acid, mineral oil, PEG-14M. In 113 g.
otc	**PanOxyl Acne Facial Wash** (GlaxoSmithKline)	**Cleanser; topical:** 2.5%	Cetearyl alcohol, glycerin, hydrogenated castor oil, lactic acid, mineral oil, PEG-14M. In 156 g.
Rx	**TL 4.25% BPO MX** (Trigen Labs)	**Cleanser; topical:** 4.25%	Aloe, cetyl alcohol, disodium EDTA, glycerin, glyceryl, green tea, PEG-100, propylene glycol. In 473 mL.
Rx	**Benzoyl Peroxide** (Fougera)	**Cleanser; topical:** 4.5%	Cetyl alcohol, disodium EDTA, glycerin, glyceryl stearate, PEG-100, urea 10%. In 400 mL.
Rx	**Zoderm** (Doak)		Urea, glycerin, cetyl alcohol, glyceryl stearate, EDTA. In 400 mL.
Rx	**Zoderm** (Doak)	**Cleanser; topical:** 5.75%	Urea, glycerin, cetyl alcohol, glyceryl stearate, PEG-100, EDTA. In 473 mL.
Rx	**Benzoyl Peroxide** (Fougera)	**Cleanser; topical:** 6.5%	Cetyl alcohol, disodium EDTA, glycerin, glyceryl stearate, PEG-100, urea 10%. In 400 mL.
Rx	**Zoderm** (Doak)		Urea, glycerin, cetyl alcohol, glyceryl stearate, EDTA. In 400 mL.
Rx	**Benzoyl Peroxide** (Fougera)	**Cleanser; topical:** 8.5%	Cetyl alcohol, disodium EDTA, glycerin, glyceryl stearate, PEG-100, urea 10%. In 400 mL.
Rx	**Zoderm** (Doak)		Urea, glycerin, cetyl alcohol, glyceryl stearate, EDTA. In 400 mL.
otc	**Neutrogena Clear Pore** (Neutrogena)	**Cleanser/Mask; topical:** 3.5%	Glycerin, titanium dioxide, EDTA, menthol. In 125 mL.
Rx	**Triaz Cleanser** (Medicis)	**Lotion; topical:** 3%	Glycerin, glycolic acid, petrolatum, zinc lactate, menthol. In 170 and 340 g.
Rx	**Delos** (Rochester Pharmaceuticals)	**Lotion; topical:** 3.5%	Alcohols, aloe, caprylic/capric triglyceride, edetate disodium, glycerin, parabens, soya sterols. In 45 g.
Rx	**Brevoxyl 4 Cleansing** (GlaxoSmithKline)	**Lotion; topical:** 4%	Cetyl alcohol. In 297 g.
Rx	**Benzoyl Peroxide** (Kylemore Pharmaceuticals)		Alcohol, propylene glycol. In 297 g.
Rx[a]	**Benzoyl Peroxide** (Various, eg, Thames)	**Lotion; topical:** 5%	In 30 mL.
Rx	**Triaz Cleanser** (Medicis)	**Lotion; topical:** 6%	Glycerin, glycolic acid, petrolatum, zinc lactate, menthol. In 170 and 340 g.
Rx	**Brevoxyl 8 Cleansing** (GlaxoSmithKline)	**Lotion; topical:** 8%	Cetyl alcohol. In 297 g.
Rx	**Benzoyl Peroxide** (Kylemore Pharmaceuticals)		Alcohol, propylene glycol. In 297 g.
Rx[a]	**Benzoyl Peroxide** (Various, eg, Thames)	**Lotion; topical:** 10%	In 30 mL.
Rx	**Triaz Cleanser** (Medicis)		Glycerin, glycolic acid, petrolatum, zinc lactate, menthol. In 85, 170, and 340 g.
Rx	**NeoBenz Micro** (SkinMedica)	**Cream; topical:** 3.5%	Cetyl alcohol, stearyl alcohol, parabens. In 45 g.
Rx	**NeoBenz Micro SD** (SkinMedica)		Cetyl alcohol, stearyl alcohol, parabens. In 0.5 g 30s.
Rx	**RE Benzoyl Peroxide** (River's Edge)		Cetyl alcohol, cetearyl alcohol, glycerin, glyceryl, PEG-3, parabens, stearyl alcohol. In 45 g.
Rx	**Brevoxyl-4 Acne Wash Kit** (GlaxoSmithKline)	**Cream; topical:** 4%	Castor oil, cetostearyl alcohol, glycerin, mineral oil, parabens. In 170 g. In kits with SFC lotion (106.6 mL).
Rx	**NeoBenz Micro** (SkinMedica)	**Cream; topical:** 5.5%	Cetyl alcohol, stearyl alcohol, parabens. In 45 g.
Rx	**NeoBenz Micro SD** (SkinMedica)		Cetyl alcohol, stearyl alcohol, parabens. In 0.5 g 30s.
Rx	**RE Benzoyl Peroxide** (River's Edge)		Cetyl alcohol, cetearyl alcohol, glycerin, glyceryl, PEG-3, parabens, stearyl alcohol. In 45 g.
Rx	**Brevoxyl-8 Acne Wash Kit** (GlaxoSmithKline)	**Cream; topical:** 8%	Castor oil, cetostearyl alcohol, glycerin, mineral oil, parabens. In 170 g. In kits with SFC lotion (106.6 mL).
Rx	**NeoBenz Micro** (SkinMedica)	**Cream; topical:** 8.5%	Cetyl alcohol, dimethicone, stearyl alcohol, parabens. In 45 g.
Rx	**NeoBenz Micro SD** (SkinMedica)		Cetyl alcohol, dimethicone, stearyl alcohol, parabens. In 0.5 g 30s.
Rx	**RE Benzoyl Peroxide** (River's Edge)		Cetyl alcohol, cetearyl alcohol, glycerin, glyceryl, PEG-3, parabens, stearyl alcohol. In 45 g.
Rx	**Zoderm** (Doak)	**Cream; topical:** 4.5%	Urea, glyceryl stearate, cetearyl alcohol, cetyl alcohol, EDTA. In 125 mL.
		6.5%	Urea, glyceryl stearate, cetearyl alcohol, cetyl alcohol, EDTA. In 125 mL.
		8.5%	Urea, glyceryl stearate, cetearyl alcohol, cetyl alcohol, EDTA. In 125 mL.
otc	**Clearasil Maximum Strength Acne Treatment** (Boots Healthcare)	**Cream; topical:** 10%	Parabens. Vanishing. In 18 g.
Rx[a]	**Benzoyl Peroxide** (Various, eg, Glades)	**Gel; topical:** 2.5%	In 60 g.
Rx	**Benziq LS** (Graceway Pharmaceuticals)	**Gel; topical:** 2.75%	Benzyl alcohol, disodium EDTA, glycerin. In 50 g.

BENZOYL PEROXIDE

Rx	**Triaz** (Medicis)	**Gel; topical:** 3%	Glycerin, zinc lactate, EDTA. In 42.5 g.
Rx	**Benzoyl Peroxide** (Glades)	**Gel; topical:** 4%	Cetyl alcohol, stearyl alcohol. In 42.5 g.
Rx	**Brevoxyl-4** (GlaxoSmithKline)		Cetyl alcohol, stearyl alcohol. In 42.5 and 90 g.
Rx	**Zoderm** (Doak)	**Gel; topical:** 4.5%	Urea, EDTA, glycerin. In 125 mL.
Rx[a]	**Benzoyl Peroxide** (Various, eg, Glades)	**Gel; topical:** 5%	In 60 and 90 g.
Rx	**Benzac AC 5** (Galderma)		Glycerin, EDTA, water based. In 60 and 90 g.
Rx	**Benzac 5** (Galderma)		12% alcohol. In 60 g.
Rx	**Soluclenz** (Obagi Medical Products)		Benzyl benzoate. In 27 mL.
Rx	**Benziq** (Graceway Pharmaceuticals)	**Gel; topical:** 5.25%	Benzyl alcohol, disodium EDTA, glycerin. In 50 g.
Rx	**Triaz** (Medicis)	**Gel; topical:** 6%	Glycerin, cetyl stearyl alcohol, zinc lactate, EDTA. In 42.5 g.
Rx	**Zoderm** (Doak)	**Gel; topical:** 6.5%	Urea, EDTA, glycerin. In 125 mL.
Rx	**Clinac BPO** (Ferndale)	**Gel; topical:** 7%	EDTA. In 45 and 90 g.
Rx	**Benzoyl Peroxide** (Glades)	**Gel; topical:** 8%	Cetyl alcohol, stearyl alcohol. In 42.5 g.
Rx	**Brevoxyl-8** (GlaxoSmithKline)		Cetyl alcohol, stearyl alcohol. In 42.5 and 90 g.
Rx	**Zoderm** (Doak)	**Gel; topical:** 8.5%	Urea, EDTA, glycerin. In 125 mL.
Rx	**Triaz** (Medicis)	**Gel; topical:** 9%	Cetyl stearyl alcohol, glycolic acid, zinc lactate, EDTA. In 42.5 g.
otc	**Acne Clear** (Altaire)	**Gel; topical:** 10%	EDTA. In 45 g.
Rx[a]	**Benzoyl Peroxide** (Various, eg, Glades)		In 60 and 90 g.
Rx	**Benzac AC 10** (Galderma)		Glycerin, EDTA, water based. In 60 and 90 g.
Rx	**Benzac 10** (Galderma)		12% alcohol. In 60 g.
Rx	**Benzagel Wash** (Dermik)		14% alcohol. In 60 g.
Rx	**Desquam-E 10** (Westwood Squibb)		EDTA, water based. In 42.5 g.
otc	**PanOxyl Maximum Strength Acne Spot Treatment** (GlaxoSmithKline)		Edetate disodium, glycerin, methylparaben. In 42.5 g.
Rx	**Triaz** (Medicis)		Glycerin, glycolic acid, cetyl stearyl alcohol, zinc lactate, EDTA. In 42.5 g.
Rx	**BenzEFoam** (Onset Therapeutics)	**Foam; topical:** 5.3%	Cetearyl alcohol, disodium EDTA, glycerin, parabens. In 60 g.
otc	**PanOxyl 10% Acne Treatment Foam** (GlaxoSmithKline)	**Foam; topical:** 10%	Edetate disodium. In 75 g.
Rx	**Benziq** (Graceway Pharmaceuticals)	**Soap; topical:** 5.25%	Benzyl alcohol, cetyl alcohol, disodium EDTA, glycerin, PEG-100. In 175 g.
Rx	**Benzoyl Peroxide** (River's Edge Pharmaceuticals)	**Soap; topical:** 5.75%	Cetyl alcohol, disodium EDTA, glycerin, urea 10%. In 473 mL.
Rx	**Benzoyl Peroxide** (River's Edge)	**Soap; topical:** 7%	Castor oil, ceteary alcohol, disodium edetate, glycerin, methylparaben, PEG-3, PEG-6, PEG-40, PEG-150. In 180 g.
Rx	**Benzoyl Peroxide Wash 7%** (Kylemore Pharmaceuticals)		Alcohol, castor oil, disodium EDTA, glycerin, methylparaben, PEG. In 180 g.
Rx	**BP 7% Wash** (River's Edge)		*Aloe barbadensis* leaf, benzyl alcohol, *Camellia oleifera* leaf, cetyl alcohol, PEG-100, glycerin. In 473 mL.
Rx	**BP 7% Wash Kit** (Various, eg Kylemore Pharmaceuticals, River's Edge Pharmaceuticals)		Alcohol, castor oil, disodium EDTA, glycerin, methylparaben, PEG. In 180 g kits with benzoyl peroxide 5.5% cream. Alcohols, parabens, PEG. In UD 7s.
Rx	**NeoBenz Micro Wash** (SkinMedica)		Castor oil, edetate disodium, methylparaben, PEG-6, PEG-15, PEG-40. In 180 g.
Rx	**SE BPO 7% Wash** (Seton Pharmaceuticals)		Castor oil, dimethicone, edetate disodium, glycerin, methylparaben, PEG-15, PEG-40. In 180 g.
Rx	**Inova Easy Pad** (JSJ Pharmaceuticals)	**Pad; topical:** 4%	Disodium EDTA, glycerin, methylparaben, 5% tocopherol. In 30s in kits with 28 topical tocopherol capsules.
Rx	**Pacnex LP Cleansing Pads** (Medimetriks Pharmaceuticals)	**Pad; topical:** 4.25%	Alcohol, aloe, edetate disodium, glycerin, glyceryl, green tea, PEG, propylene glycol. In UD 60s.
Rx	**Pacnex HP Cleansing Pads** (Medimetriks Pharmaceuticals)	**Pad; topical:** 7%	Alcohol, aloe, edetate disodium, glycerin, glyceryl, green tea, PEG, propylene glycol. In UD 60s.
Rx	**Inova Easy Pad** (JSJ Pharmaceuticals)	**Pad; topical:** 8%	Disodium EDTA, glycerin, methylparaben, 5% tocopherol. In 30s in kits with 28 topical tocopherol capsules.
Rx	**SE BPO 3%** (Seton Pharmaceuticals)	**Cloths; topical:** 3%	Cetyl alcohol, glycerin, sodium hyaluronate, zinc. In UD 60s.
Rx	**Triaz** (Medicis)		Cetyl alcohol, glycerin, glycolic acid, sodium hyaluronate, zinc. In 60s.
Rx	**SE BPO 6%** (Seton Pharmaceuticals)	**Cloths; topical:** 6%	Cetyl alcohol, glycerin, sodium hyaluronate, zinc. In UD 60s.
Rx	**Triaz** (Medicis)		Cetyl alcohol, EDTA, glycerin, glycolic acid, sodium hyaluronate, zinc. In 60s.
Rx	**SE BPO 9%** (Seton Pharmaceuticals)	**Cloths; topical:** 9%	Cetyl alcohol, glycerin, sodium hyaluronate, zinc. In UD 60s.
Rx	**Triaz** (Medicis)		Cetyl alcohol, EDTA, glycerin, glycolic acid, sodium hyaluronate, zinc. In 60s.

[a] Product available *otc* or *Rx*, depending on product labeling.

BENZOYL PEROXIDE — TOPICAL

Indications

➤*Acne:* Treatment of mild to moderate acne vulgaris.

Administration and Dosage

➤*Adults:*

Acne –

Cleansers: Wash once or twice daily. Control amount of drying or peeling by modifying dose frequency or concentration.

BENZOYL PEROXIDE — TOPICAL

Adjust frequency of use to obtain the desired clinical response. Clinically visible improvement will normally occur by the third week of therapy. Maximum lesion reduction may be expected after approximately 8 to 12 weeks of drug use. Continuing use of the drug is normally required to maintain a satisfactory clinical response.

Cloths: Use as a wash once or twice daily.

Pads: In the morning, wash the treatment area with a mild non-irritating cleanser, rinse and pat dry. Apply the vitamin E capsule to the entire treatment area.

Thirty minutes before bed wash the treatment area with a mild non-irritating cleanser, rinse and pat dry. Your doctor may recommend a mild cleanser specifically for your skin type. Apply the blue pad (benzoyl peroxide) to your face in the evening.

Other doseforms: Apply once or twice daily. After cleansing skin, smooth small amount over affected area.

➤*Children:*

Acne –

12 years of age or older: See Adults for dosing.

• *Cloths –*

Safety and efficacy in children have not been established for *Triaz* cloths.

➤*Administration:*

Cleansers – Wet skin areas to be treated prior to administration. Rinse thoroughly and pat dry.

Cloths – Wet face with water. Wet cloth with a little water and work into a full lather. Cleanse face with cloth for 10 to 20 seconds. Avoid eyes or mucous membranes. Rinse thoroughly and pat dry. Throw away cloth; do not flush.

Pads – Apply the vitamin E capsule to the entire treatment area. Twist off the small end to release the product. Use your fingertips to distribute evenly across the treatment area.

Apply the blue pad (benzoyl peroxide) to your face in the evening. Evenly distribute the medication around the treatment area avoiding scrubbing or strong pressure while applying. Avoid hair, clothing, and eyes as benzoyl peroxide may cause bleaching on contact.

Other doseforms – After cleansing skin, smooth small amount over affected area. If bothersome dryness or peeling occurs, reduce dose frequency or drug concentration. If excessive stinging or burning occurs after any single application, remove with mild soap and water; resume use the next day.

➤*Storage / Stability:* Store at 15° to 30°C (59° to 86°F).

Actions

➤*Pharmacology:* The effectiveness of benzoyl peroxide in the treatment of acne vulgaris is primarily attributable to its antibacterial activity, especially with respect to *Propionibacterium acnes*, the predominant organism in sebaceous follicles and comedones. The antibacterial activity of this compound is presumably because of the release of active or free-radical oxygen capable of oxidizing bacterial proteins. In acne patients treated topically with benzoyl peroxide, resolution of the acne usually coincides with reduction in the levels of *P. acnes* and free fatty acids (FFA). Mild desquamation is another observed action of topically applied benzoyl peroxide and may also play a role in the drug's effectiveness in acne. Studies also indicate that topical benzoyl peroxide may exert a sebostatic effect with a resultant reduction of skin surface lipids.

➤*Pharmacokinetics:* Benzoyl peroxide is absorbed by the skin, where it is metabolized to benzoic acid and then excreted as benzoate in the urine.

Contraindications

Hypersensitivity to benzoyl peroxide or any components of the products. Cross-sensitivity may occur with benzoic acid derivatives (see Precautions).

Warnings/Precautions

➤*Sun exposure:* When using this product, avoid unnecessary sun exposure and use a sunscreen.

➤*External use only:* Avoid contact with eyes, eyelids, lips, mucous membranes, and highly inflamed or damaged skin. If accidental contact occurs, rinse with water.

➤*Irritation:* If severe irritation develops, consult a doctor, discontinue use, and institute appropriate therapy. After the reaction clears, treatment may often be resumed with less frequent application.

➤*Bleaching effect:* Benzoyl peroxide is an oxidizing agent; it may bleach hair and colored fabric.

➤*Cross-sensitization:* With benzoic acid derivatives (eg, cinnamon, certain topical anesthetics), cross-sensitization may occur.

➤*Pregnancy: Category C.* It is not known whether benzoyl peroxide can cause fetal harm when administered to a pregnant woman or can affect reproductive capacity. However, there are no available data on the effect of benzoyl peroxide on the later growth, development, and functional maturation of the unborn child. Use in pregnant women only if clearly needed.

➤*Lactation:* It is not known whether this drug is excreted in breast milk. Administer with caution to nursing mothers.

➤*Children:* Safety and efficacy in children younger than 12 years of age have not been established; safety and efficacy in children have not been established for *Triaz* cloths.

Drug Interactions

➤*Tretinoin:* Concomitant use may cause significant skin irritation.

Adverse Reactions

Excessive drying, manifested by marked peeling, erythema, possible edema, and allergic contact sensitization/dermatitis.

Overdosage

➤*Symptoms:* Excessive scaling, erythema, or edema.

➤*Treatment:* Discontinue use. If reaction is caused by excessive use and not allergy, cautiously reinstate at reduced dosage after signs and symptoms subside. To hasten resolution of adverse effects, use emollients, cool compresses, and/or topical corticosteroids.

Patient Information

Keep away from eyes, mouth, inside of nose and mucous membranes. If contact occurs, rinse with water.

May cause transitory feeling of warmth or slight stinging. Expect dryness and peeling; if excessive redness or discomfort occurs, decrease or discontinue use temporarily. If excessive irritation develops, discontinue use and contact a physician.

Avoid other sources of skin irritation (eg, sunlight, sun lamps, other topical acne medications) unless directed by a physician.

Avoid contact with hair or colored fabric; bleaching may occur.

Normal use of water-based cosmetics is permissible.

RETAPAMULIN

Rx	**Altabax** (GlaxoSmithKline)	**Ointment; topical:** 1%	White petrolatum. In 15 and 30 g tubes.

RETAPAMULIN — TOPICAL

Indications

➤*Impetigo:* For the topical treatment of impetigo due to *Staphylococcus aureus* (methicillin-susceptible isolates only) or *Streptococcus pyogenes* in adults and children 9 months of age and older.

Administration and Dosage

➤*General dosing considerations:* The treated area may be covered with a sterile bandage or gauze dressing if desired.

➤*Adults:*

Impetigo –

Usual dosage: Apply a thin layer to the affected area (up to 100 cm^2 in total body surface area [BSA]) twice daily.

Maximum dose: Total treatment area should not exceed 100 cm^2 in total BSA.

Duration of therapy: 5 days.

➤*Children:*

Impetigo –

9 months of age and older:

• *Usual dosage* – Apply a thin layer to the affected area (up to 2% of total BSA) twice daily.

• *Maximum dose* – Total treatment area should not exceed 2% of total BSA.

• *Duration of therapy* – 5 days.

➤*Administration:* For external use only. Retapamulin is not intended for ingestion or for oral, intranasal, ophthalmic, or intravaginal use.

➤*Storage / Stability:* Store at 25°C (77°F); excursions are permitted between 15° and 30°C (59° and 86°F).

Actions

➤*Pharmacology:* Retapamulin is an antibacterial agent. It is a semisynthetic derivative of the compound pleuromutilin, which is isolated through fermentation from *Clitopilus passeckerianus* (formerly *Pleurotus passeckerianus*). In vitro activity of retapamulin against isolates of *S. aureus* as well as *S. pyogenes* has been demonstrated.

Retapamulin selectively inhibits bacterial protein synthesis by interacting at a site on the 50S subunit of the bacterial ribosome through an interaction that is different from that of other antibiotics. This binding site involves ribosomal protein L3 and is in the region of the ribosomal P site and peptidyl transferase center. By virtue of binding to this site, pleuromutilins inhibit peptidyl transfer, block P-site interactions, and prevent the normal formation of active 50S ribosomal subunits.

➤*Pharmacokinetics:*

Absorption – In a study of healthy adult subjects, retapamulin was applied once daily to intact skin (800 cm^2 surface area) and to abraded skin (200 cm^2 surface area) under occlusion for up to 7 days. Systemic exposure following topical application of retapamulin through intact and abraded skin was low. Three percent of blood samples obtained on day 1 after topical application to intact skin had measurable retapamulin concentrations (lower limit of quantitation, 0.5 ng/mL); thus maximal drug concentration

RETAPAMULIN — TOPICAL

(C_{max}) values on day 1 could not be determined. Eighty-two percent of blood samples obtained on day 7 after topical application to intact skin and 97% and 100% of blood samples obtained after topical application to abraded skin on days 1 and 7, respectively, had measurable retapamulin concentrations. The median C_{max} value in plasma after application to 800 cm^2 of intact skin was 3.5 ng/mL on day 7 (range, 1.2 to 7.8 ng/mL). The median C_{max} value in plasma after application to 200 cm^2 of abraded skin was 11.7 ng/mL on day 1 (range, 5.6 to 22.1 ng/mL) and 9 ng/mL on day 7 (range, 6.7 to 12.8 ng/mL).

Plasma samples were obtained from 380 adult patients and 136 children (2 to 17 years of age) who were receiving topical treatment with retapamulin twice daily. Eleven percent had measurable retapamulin concentrations (lower limit of quantitation, 0.5 ng/mL), of which the median concentration was 0.8 ng/mL. The maximum measured retapamulin concentration was 10.7 ng/mL in adults and 18.5 ng/mL in children.

Distribution – Retapamulin is approximately 94% bound to human plasma proteins, and the protein binding is independent of concentration.

Metabolism – In vitro studies with human hepatocytes showed that the main routes of metabolism were monooxygenation and dioxygenation. In vitro studies with human liver microsomes demonstrated that retapamulin is extensively metabolized to numerous metabolites, of which the predominant routes of metabolism were monooxygenation and N-demethylation. The major enzyme responsible for metabolism of retapamulin in human liver microsomes is cytochrome P450 3A4 (CYP3A4).

Excretion – Retapamulin elimination in humans has not been investigated because of low systemic exposure after topical application.

Contraindications

None well documented.

Warnings/Precautions

➤*Local effects:* In the event of sensitization or severe local irritation from retapamulin, discontinue usage, wipe off the ointment, and institute an appropriate alternative therapy for the infection.

➤*Administration:* Retapamulin has not been evaluated for use on mucosal surfaces. Epistaxis has been reported with the use of retapamulin on nasal mucosa.

➤*Superinfection:* The use of antibiotics may promote the selection of nonsusceptible organisms. If superinfection occurs during therapy, take appropriate measures.

Prescribing retapamulin in the absence of a proven or strongly suspected bacterial infection is unlikely to benefit the patient and increases the risk of developing drug-resistant bacteria.

➤*Pregnancy: Category B.* There are no adequate and well-controlled studies in pregnant women. Because animal reproduction studies are not always predictive of human response, use retapamulin during pregnancy only when the potential benefits outweigh the potential risks.

Effects on embryofetal development were assessed in pregnant rats given 50, 150, or 450 mg/kg/day by oral gavage on days 6 to 17 postcoitus. Maternal toxicity (decreased body weight gain and food consumption) and developmental toxicity (decreased fetal body weight and delayed skeletal ossification) were evident at dosages of 150 mg/kg/day or more. There were no treatment-related malformations observed in fetal rats.

Retapamulin was given as a continuous intravenous infusion to pregnant rabbits at dosages of 2.4, 7.2, or 24 mg/kg/day from day 7 to 19 of gestation. Maternal toxicity (decreased body weight gain, food consumption, and abortions) was demonstrated at dosages of 7.2 mg/kg/day or more (8-fold the estimated maximum achievable human exposure, based on area under the curve [AUC], at 7.2 mg/kg/day). There was no treatment-related effect on embryofetal development.

➤*Lactation:* It is not known whether retapamulin is excreted in human milk. Because retapamulin is minimally absorbed systemically when applied topically, this medication would probably be safe for use in breast-feeding mothers. Because many drugs are excreted in human milk, exercise caution when administering retapamulin to a breast-feeding woman. The safe use of retapamulin during breast-feeding has not been established.

➤*Children:* The safety and efficacy of retapamulin in the treatment of impetigo have been established in children 9 months to 17 years of age. The safety and efficacy of retapamulin in children younger than 9 months of age have not been established.

Drug Interactions

➤*Ketoconazole, oral:* Coadministration of oral ketoconazole 200 mg twice daily increased retapamulin geometric mean $AUC_{(0-24)}$ and C_{max} by 81% after topical application of retapamulin 1% ointment on the abraded skin of healthy adult males. Because of low systemic exposure to retapamulin following topical application, dosage adjustments for retapamulin are unnecessary when it is coadministered with CYP3A4 inhibitors such as ketoconazole.

Adverse Reactions

➤*Common adverse reactions:* Adverse reactions rated by investigators as drug-related occurred in 5.5% of patients treated with retapamulin, 6.6% of patients receiving cephalexin, and 2.8% of patients receiving placebo. The most common drug-related adverse reactions (at least 1% of patients) were diarrhea (1.7%) in the cephalexin group, application-site irritation (1.4%) in the retapamulin group, and application-site pruritus and application-site paresthesia (1.4%) in the placebo group.

➤*Adults:*

Retapamulin Adverse Reactions in Adults (≥ 1%)		
Adverse reaction	Retapamulin (n = 1,527)	Cephalexin (n = 698)
CNS		
Headache	2%	2%
GI		
Diarrhea	1.4%	2.3%
Nausea	1.2%	1.9%
Miscellaneous		
Application-site irritation	1.6%	< 1%
Creatinine phosphokinase increased	< 1%	1%
Nasopharyngitis	1.2%	< 1%

➤*Children:*

Retapamulin Adverse Reactions in Children (9 Months to 17 Years of Age) (≥ 1%)			
Adverse reaction	Retapamulin (n = 588)	Cephalexin (n = 121)	Placebo (n = 64)
Dermatologic			
Application-site pruritus	1.9%	0%	0%
Eczema	1%	0%	0%
Pruritus	1.5%	1%	1.6%
Miscellaneous			
Diarrhea	1.7%	5%	0%
Headache	1.2%	1.7%	0%
Nasopharyngitis	1.5%	1.7%	0%
Pyrexia	1.2%	< 1%	1.6%

➤*Other adverse reactions:* Application-site pain, contact dermatitis, and erythema were reported in less than 1% of patients in clinical studies.

Overdosage

➤*Symptoms:* Overdosage with retapamulin has not been reported.

➤*Treatment:* There is no known antidote for overdoses of retapamulin. Symptomatically treat any signs or symptoms of overdose, either topically or by accidental ingestion, with good clinical practice.

Patient Information

Advise patients to use retapamulin as directed by their health care provider. As with any topical medication, instruct patients and caregivers to wash their hands after application if the hands are not the area for treatment.

Inform patients that retapamulin is for external use only. Instruct patients not to swallow retapamulin, use it in the eyes, on the mouth or lips, inside the nose, or inside the female genital area.

Inform patients that the treated area may be covered by a sterile bandage or gauze dressing, if desired. This may also be helpful for infants and young children who accidentally touch or lick the lesion site. A bandage will protect the treated area and avoid accidental transfer of ointment to the eyes or other areas.

Instruct patients to use the medication for the full time recommended by their health care provider, even though symptoms may have improved.

Instruct patients to notify their health care provider if there is no improvement in symptoms within 3 to 4 days after starting use of retapamulin.

Inform patients that retapamulin may cause reactions at the site of application of the ointment. Instruct patients to inform their health care provider if the area of application worsens in irritation, redness, itching, burning, swelling, blistering, or oozing.

CLINDAMYCIN

Rx	**Clindamycin Phosphate** (Various, eg, Fougera)	**Gel; topical:** 1%	In 30 and 60 g.
Rx	**Cleocin T** (Pharmacia & Upjohn)		Methylparaben. In 30 and 60 g.
Rx	**Clindagel** (Galderma)		Methylparaben. In 7.5, 42, and 77 g.
Rx	**ClindaMax** (PharmaDerm)		Methylparaben. In 30 and 60 g.

CLINDAMYCIN

Rx	**Clindamycin Phosphate** (Various, eg, Fougera)	**Lotion; topical:** 1%	In 60 mL.
Rx	**Cleocin T** (Pharmacia & Upjohn)		2.5% cetostearyl alcohol, glycerin, 2.5% isostearyl alcohol, 0.3% methylparaben. In 60 mL.
Rx	**ClindaMax** (PharmaDerm)		2.5% cetostearyl alcohol, glycerin, 2.5% isostearyl alcohol, 0.3% methylparaben. In 60 mL.
Rx	**Clindamycin Phosphate** (Various, eg, Fougera, Morton Groves)	**Solution; topical:** 1%	In 30 and 60 mL.
Rx	**Cleocin T** (Pharmacia & Upjohn)		50% isopropyl alcohol. In 30 and 60 mL and single-use pledget applicators.
Rx	**Clindamycin Phosphate** (VersaPharm)	**Pledget; topical:** 1%	50% isopropyl alcohol, propylene glycol. In 60s.
Rx	**PledgaClin** (JSJ Pharmaceuticals)		50% isopropyl alcohol, propylene glycol. In 69s.
Rx	**Evoclin** (Stiefel)	**Aerosol, foam; topical:** 1%	Cetyl alcohol, dehydrated alcohol (ethanol 58%), stearyl alcohol. In 50 g.[a]

[a] Pressurized with a hydrocarbon (propane/butane) propellant.

CLINDAMYCIN PHOSPHATE — TOPICAL

Indications

➤*Acne:* Treatment of acne vulgaris. In view of the potential for diarrhea, bloody diarrhea, and pseudomembranous colitis, consider whether other agents are more appropriate.

➤*Off-label uses:*

Rosacea – [2] = Fair documentation. Although limited, trial data suggest that topical clindamycin may be effective in the treatment of rosacea. A head-to-head trial with topical clindamycin and standard oral tetracycline showed similar rates of efficacy. Larger, controlled studies are needed to evaluate long-term outcomes and compare topical clindamycin with other widely used antimicrobial agents.

Administration and Dosage

➤*Adults:*

Gel, lotion, pledget, solution –

Acne: Apply a thin film (except *Clindagel*) twice daily to the affected area. More than 1 pledget may be used.

Foam, Clindagel gel –

Acne: Apply a thin film of *Clindagel* gel or clindamycin topical foam once daily to the affected areas. Use enough to cover the affected area lightly.

Off-label dosing –

Rosacea: [2] = Fair documentation. Clindamycin 1% in a base or vehicle, applied topically once or twice daily for 12 weeks.

➤*Children:* See Adults for dosing in children 12 years of age and older.

➤*Administration:*

Foam – Apply once daily to affected area after the skin is washed with mild soap and allowed to fully dry. Use enough to cover the entire affected area.

To use clindamycin foam:

1.) Do not dispense clindamycin foam directly onto your hands or face, because the foam will begin to melt on contact with warm skin.
2.) Remove the clear cap. Align the black mark with the nozzle of the actuator.
3.) Hold the can at an upright angle and then press firmly to dispense. Dispense an amount directly into the cap or onto a cool surface. Dispense an amount of clindamycin that will cover the affected area. If the can is warm or the foam is runny, run the can under cold water.
4.) Pick up small amounts of clindamycin topical foam with your fingertips and gently massage into the affected area until the foam disappears.

Throw away any of the unused medicine that you dispensed out of the can. Avoid contact of clindamycin topical foam with eyes. If contact occurs, rinse eyes thoroughly with water.

Lotion – Shake well immediately before using.

Pledget – More than 1 pledget may be used. Each pledget should be used only once and then discarded. Remove pledget from foil just before use. Do not use if the seal is broken.

➤*Storage/Stability:* Store clindamycin gel, lotion, and solution at controlled room temperature, 20° to 25°C (68° to 77°F). Protect from freezing. Do not store *Clindagel* in direct sunlight. Store *Clindamax* gel, *Clindamax* lotion, and *Clindets* at controlled room temperature, 15° to 30°C (59° to 86°F). Protect from freezing.

Foam – Do not expose to heat or store at temperature above 49°C (120°F). Flammable. Avoid fire, flame, or smoking during and immediately following application. Contents under pressure. Do not puncture or incinerate. Keep out of the reach of children.

Actions

➤*Pharmacology:* Although clindamycin phosphate is inactive in vitro, rapid in vivo hydrolysis converts this compound to the antibacterially active clindamycin.

Cross resistance has been demonstrated between clindamycin and lincomycin.

Antagonism has been demonstrated between clindamycin and erythromycin.

Clindamycin activity has been demonstrated in comedones from acne patients. Clindamycin in vitro inhibits all *Propionibacterium acnes* cultures tested (minimum inhibitory concentrations [MICs], 0.4 mcg/mL). Free fatty acids on the skin surface have been decreased from approximately 14% to 2% following application of clindamycin.

➤*Pharmacokinetics:*

Absorption/Distribution – Following multiple topical applications of clindamycin phosphate at a concentration equivalent to clindamycin 10 mg/mL in an isopropyl alcohol and water solution, very low levels of clindamycin are present in the serum (0 to 3 ng/mL), and less than 0.2% of the dose is recovered in urine as clindamycin.

The mean concentration of antibiotic activity in extracted comedones after application of clindamycin topical solution for 4 weeks was 597 mcg/g of comedonal material (range, 0 to 1,490).

Clindagel: In an open-label, parallel-group study of 24 patients with acne vulgaris, once-daily topical administration of approximately 3 to 12 g/day of clindamycin gel for 5 days resulted in peak plasma clindamycin concentrations that were less than 5.5 ng/mL.

Foam: In an open-label, parallel-group study in 24 patients with acne vulgaris, 12 patients (3 men and 9 women) applied 4 g of clindamycin foam once daily for 5 days, and 12 patients (7 men and 5 women) applied 4 g of *Clindagel* (1%) once daily for 5 days. On day 5, the mean peak drug concentration (C_{max}) and area under the curve ($AUC_{0\ to\ 12}$) were 23% and 9% lower, respectively, for clindamycin foam than for clindamycin 1% topical gel.

Excretion –

Gel: Following multiple applications of clindamycin gel, less than 0.04% of the total dose was excreted in the urine.

Foam: Following multiple applications of clindamycin foam, less than 0.024% of the total dose was excreted unchanged in the urine over 12 hours on day 5.

➤*Microbiology:* Although clindamycin phosphate is inactive in vitro, rapid in vivo hydrolysis converts this compound to clindamycin, which has antibacterial activity. Clindamycin inhibits bacteria protein synthesis at the ribosomal level by binding to the 50S ribosomal subunit and affecting the process of peptide chain initiation. In vitro studies indicated that clindamycin inhibited all tested *Propionibacterium acnes* cultures at an MIC of 0.4 mcg/mL. Cross-resistance has been demonstrated between clindamycin and erythromycin.

Contraindications

Hypersensitivity to preparations containing clindamycin or lincomycin, history of regional enteritis or ulcerative colitis, or history of antibiotic-associated colitis.

Warnings/Precautions

➤*Colitis:* Orally and parenterally administered clindamycin has been associated with severe colitis, which may result in patient death. Use of the topical formulation of clindamycin results in absorption of the antibiotic from the skin surface. Diarrhea, bloody diarrhea, and colitis (including pseudomembranous colitis) have been reported with the use of topical and systemic clindamycin.

Studies indicate a toxin(s) produced by *Clostridia* is a primary cause of antibiotic-associated colitis. The colitis is usually characterized by severe persistent diarrhea and severe abdominal cramps and may be associated with the passage of blood and mucus. Endoscopic examination may reveal pseudomembranous colitis. Stool culture for *Clostridium difficile* and stool assay for *C. difficile* toxin may be helpful diagnostically.

When significant diarrhea occurs, discontinue the drug. Consider large bowel endoscopy to establish a definitive diagnosis in cases of severe diarrhea.

Antiperistaltic agents (eg, opiates, diphenoxylate with atropine) may prolong and worsen the condition. Vancomycin has been found to be effective in the treatment of antibiotic-associated pseudomembranous colitis produced by *C. difficile*. The usual adult dosage is 500 mg to 2 g of vancomycin orally per day in 3 to 4 divided doses administered for 7 to 10 days. Cholestyramine or colestipol resins bind vancomycin in vitro. If a resin and vancomycin are to be administered concurrently, it may be advisable to separate the time of administration of each drug.

CLINDAMYCIN PHOSPHATE — TOPICAL

Diarrhea, colitis, and pseudomembranous colitis have been observed to begin up to several weeks following cessation of oral and parenteral therapy with clindamycin.

Foam – Mild cases of pseudomembranous colitis usually respond to drug discontinuation alone. In moderate to severe cases, consider management with fluids and electrolytes, protein supplementation, and treatment with an antibacterial drug clinically effective against *C. difficile* colitis.

➤*For external use only:* Clindamycin topical solution (including pledgets) contains an alcohol base that will cause burning and irritation of the eye. In the event of accidental contact with sensitive surfaces (eg, abraded skin, eye, mucous membranes), bathe with copious amounts of cool tap water. The solution has an unpleasant taste; exercise caution when applying medication around the mouth.

Avoid contact of clindamycin foam with eyes. If contact occurs, rinse eyes thoroughly with water.

➤*Special risk:* Prescribe clindamycin with caution in atopic individuals.

➤*Pregnancy: Category B.* There are no adequate and well-controlled studies in pregnant women. Because animal reproduction studies are not always predictive of human response, use this drug during pregnancy only if clearly needed.

➤*Lactation:* It is not known whether clindamycin is excreted in human milk. However, orally and parenterally administered clindamycin has been reported to appear in breast milk. Because of the potential for serious adverse reactions in breast-feeding infants, decide whether to discontinue breast-feeding or the drug, taking into account the importance of the drug to the mother.

➤*Children:* Safety and efficacy in children younger than 12 years of age have not been established.

Drug Interactions

➤*Neuromuscular-blocking agents:* Clindamycin has been shown to have neuromuscular-blocking properties that may enhance the action of other neuromuscular-blocking agents; use clindamcyin with caution in patients receiving such agents.

Adverse Reactions

See Warnings/Precautions for more information.

Abdominal pain and GI disturbances, as well as gram-negative folliculitis, have been reported in association with the use of topical formulations of clindamycin.

➤*Dermatologic:*

Topical Clindamycin Adverse Reactions

Treatment-emergent adverse reaction	Number of patients reporting reactions		
	Solution (n = 553) (%)	Gel (n = 148) (%)	Lotion (n = 160) (%)
Burning	62 (11%)	15 (10%)	17 (11%)
Burning/itching	60 (11%)	NR[a]	NR
Dryness	105 (19%)	34 (23%)	29 (18%)
Erythema	86 (16%)	10 (7%)	22 (14%)
Itching	36 (7%)	15 (10%)	17 (11%)
Oiliness/Oily skin	8 (1%)	26 (18%)	12[b] (10%)
Peeling	61 (11%)	NR	11 (7%)

[a] NR = not recorded.
[b] Of 126 subjects.

➤*Clindagel:*

***Clindagel* Adverse Reactions in ≥ 1% of Patients**

Adverse reaction	Number (%) of patients	
	Clindagel (once daily) (n = 168)	Vehicle gel (once daily) (n = 84)
Contact dermatitis	0 (0%)	1 (1.2%)
Dermatitis	0 (0%)	1 (1.2%)
Dry skin	0 (0%)	0 (0%)
Erythematous rash	0 (0%)	0 (0%)
Folliculitis	0 (0%)	1 (1.2%)
Fungal dermatitis	0 (0%)	1 (1.2%)
Peeling	1 (0.6%)	0 (0%)
Photosensitivity reaction	0 (0%)	1 (1.2%)
Pruritus	1 (0.6%)	1 (1.2%)
Skin and appendage disorders	0 (0%)	1 (1.2%)

➤*Foam:*

Clindamycin Foam Adverse Reactions Occurring in ≥ 1% of Patients

Adverse reaction	Number (%) of patients	
	Clindamycin foam (n = 439)	Vehicle foam (n = 154)
Application site burning	27 (6%)	14 (9%)
Application site dryness	4 (1%)	5 (3%)
Application site pruritus	5 (1%)	5 (3%)
Application site reaction, not otherwise specified	3 (1%)	4 (3%)
Headache	12 (3%)	1 (1%)

Overdosage

➤*Symptoms:* Topically applied clindamycin may be absorbed in sufficient amounts to produce systemic effects.

Patient Information

This medicine is for external use only. Advise patients to avoid contact with the eyes because burning or irritation can occur. Advise patients to wash the area with cool tap water if contact with the eyes or sensitive surfaces (eg, mucous membranes, scraped skin) occurs.

Advise patients that this medicine is not for ophthalmic, oral, or intravaginal use.

Advise patients that this medicine has an unpleasant taste and to use caution when applying this medicine around the mouth.

Advise patients to keep clindamycin out of the reach of children.

Advise patients to contact their doctors at once if severe diarrhea, stomach cramps/pain, or bloody stools occur. This could be a symptom of a serious side effect requiring immediate medical attention. Advise patients not to treat diarrhea without consulting their doctors.

➤*Foam:* Contents under pressure. Advise patients not to puncture or incinerate container, expose to heat, or store at temperatures above 49°C (120°F).

Advise patients not to dispense clindamycin foam directly onto hands or face, because the foam will begin to melt on contact with warm skin.

ERYTHROMYCIN

Rx	**Erythromycin** (Various, eg, Morton Grove)	**Solution; topical:** 2%	Contains alcohol. In 60 mL.
Rx	**A/T/S** (Medicis)		66% alcohol. In 60 mL.
Rx	**Eryderm 2%** (Abbott)		77% alcohol. In 60 mL with applicator.
Rx	**A/T/S** (Medicis)	**Gel; topical:** 2%	92% alcohol. In 30 g.
Rx	**Emgel** (GlaxoSmithKline)		77% alcohol. In 27 and 50 g.
Rx	**Erygel** (Merz Pharmaceutical)		92% alcohol. In 30 g.
Rx	**Erythromycin** (Various, eg, Glades)		Contains alcohol. In 30 and 60 g.
Rx	**Akne-Mycin** (Coria Labs)	**Ointment; topical:** 2%	Cetostearyl alcohol, petrolatum, mineral oil. In 25 g.
Rx	**Ery Pads** (Perrigo)	**Pledgets; topical:** 2%	60.5% alcohol. In 60s.

ERYTHROMYCIN — TOPICAL

Indications

➤*Acne:* For the treatment of acne vulgaris.

Administration and Dosage

➤*Adults:*

Acne –

Gel: Apply sparingly as a thin film to affected area(s) once or twice a day after the skin is thoroughly cleansed and patted dry. If there has been no improvement after 6 to 8 weeks, or if the condition becomes worse, treatment should be discontinued and the health care provider should be reconsulted.

Topical solution: Apply to the affected area(s) each morning and evening after the skin is thoroughly washed with warm water and soap and patted dry. Use enough solution to thoroughly wet the affected area(s). The hands should be washed after application. Acne lesions on the face, neck, shoulder, chest, and back may be treated in this manner.

Pledgets: Rub over the affected area twice a day after skin is thoroughly washed with warm water and soap and patted dry. Acne lesions on the face, neck, shoulder, chest, and back may be treated in this manner. Additional pledgets may be used, if needed.

Ointment: Apply to the affected area twice daily, morning and evening.

➤*Administration:*

Gel – Spread the medication lightly rather than rubbing it in.

Topical solution – When using the *Dab-O-Matic* applicator to apply erythromycin topical solution, it should be moistened first by holding the bottle upside down and pressing once on the applicator surface with a clean finger. Then erythromycin topical solution can be applied with the applicator to the affected area(s) using a dabbing motion. The bottle should be closed tightly after each use.

Pledgets – Each pledget should be used once and discarded. Close jar tightly after each use.

➤*Storage/Stability:*

Gel – This medication is flammable; keep away from heat and flame. Store and dispense in original container. Keep tube tightly closed. Store between 15° and 25°C (59° and 77°F).

Topical solution – This medication is flammable; keep away from heat and flame. Store in a tight, light-resistant container at controlled room temperature, 15° to 30°C (59° to 86°F).

Pledgets – Keep jar tightly closed. Store at controlled room temperature, between 15° and 30°C (59° and 86°F).

Ointment – Store below 27°C (80°F).

Actions

➤*Pharmacology:* The exact mechanism by which topical erythromycin reduces lesions of acne vulgaris is not fully known; however, the effect appears to be caused by part to the antibacterial activity of the drug.

➤*Microbiology:* Erythromycin acts by inhibition of protein synthesis in susceptible organisms by reversibly binding to 50 S ribosomal subunits, thereby inhibiting translocation of aminoacyl transfer-RNA and inhibiting polypeptide synthesis. Antagonism has been demonstrated in vitro between erythromycin, and lincomycin, chloramphenicol, and clindamycin.

Contraindications

Hypersensitivity to erythromycin or to any of the other listed ingredients in the various preparations.

Warnings/Precautions

➤*Pseudomembranous colitis:* Pseudomembranous colitis has been reported with nearly all antibacterial agents, including erythromycin, and may range in severity from mild to life-threatening. Therefore, it is important to consider this diagnosis in patients who present with diarrhea subsequent to the administration of antibacterial agents.

Treatment with antibacterial agents alters the normal flora of the colon and may permit overgrowth of clostridia. Studies indicate that a toxin produced by *Clostridium difficile* is 1 primary cause of "antibiotic-associated" colitis.

After the diagnosis of pseudomembranous colitis has been established, therapeutic measures should be initiated. Mild cases of pseudomembranous colitis usually respond to drug discontinuation alone. In moderate to severe cases, consider management with fluids and electrolytes, protein supplementation, and treatment with an antibacterial drug clinically effective against *C. difficile* colitis.

➤*For external use only:* These formulations of erythromycin are for topical use only; they are not for ophthalmic use. Keep them out of the eyes, nose, and mouth and all mucous membranes. Use concomitant topical therapy with caution because a possible cumulative irritancy effect may occur, especially with the use of peeling, desquamating or abrasive agents.

Avoid contact with eyes and all mucous membranes.

➤*Superinfection:* The use of antibiotic agents may be associated with the overgrowth of antibiotic-resistant organisms. If this occurs, discontinue administration of the drug and take appropriate measures.

➤*Pregnancy: Category C* (topical solution) and *Category B* (other topical preparations).

There are no adequate and well-controlled studies in pregnant women. Because animal reproduction studies are not always predictive of human response, only use this drug in pregnancy if clearly needed. Erythromycin has been reported to cross the placental barrier in humans, but fetal plasma levels are generally low.

The safe use of topical erythromycin during pregnancy has not been established.

➤*Lactation:* It is not known whether erythromycin is excreted in human milk after topical application of gel, pledgets, or ointment. Erythromycin topical solution is excreted in breast milk, and erythromycin is excreted in human milk following oral and parenteral erythromycin administration. Therefore, caution should be exercised when erythromycin is administered to a breast-feeding woman.

The safe use of topical erythromycin during lactation has not been established.

➤*Children:* Safety and efficacy in children have not been established.

Adverse Reactions

The following local adverse reactions have been reported occasionally: peeling, dryness, burning, itching, desquamation, erythema, and oiliness. Irritation of the eyes and tenderness of the skin have also been reported with the topical use of erythromycin. A generalized urticarial reaction, possibly related to the use of erythromycin, which required systemic steroid therapy has been reported.

➤*Dermatologic:*

Gel – In controlled clinical trials, the incidence of burning associated with erythromycin topical gel was approximately 25%.

Ointment – In clinical trials, there was 1 report of a possible contact sensitization, which could not be confirmed. There were isolated reports of skin irritation, such as erythema and peeling.

Patient Information

- Patients should wash, rinse, and dry affected areas before application.
- Advise patients to wash their hands after application of medicine.
- This medication is to be used as directed by the physician. It is for external use only. Patients should avoid contact with the eyes, nose, mouth, and all mucous membranes.
- This medication should not be used for any disorder other than that for which it was prescribed.
- Patients should not use any other topical acne medication unless otherwise directed by their physicians.
- Patients should report to their physicians any signs of local adverse reactions.

METRONIDAZOLE

Rx	**Metronidazole** (Various, eg, Fougera, Glades)	**Lotion; topical:** 0.75%	May contain benzyl alcohol. In 59 mL.
Rx	**MetroLotion** (Galderma)		Benzyl alcohol, stearyl alcohol, glycerin, mineral oil. In 59 mL.
Rx	**Metronidazole** (Fougera)	**Cream; topical:** 0.75%	Glycerin, benzyl alcohol, lactic acid. In 45 g.
Rx	**MetroCream** (Galderma)		Glycerin, benzyl alcohol. In 45 g.
Rx	**Vitazol** (Rochester Pharmaceuticals)		Benzyl alcohol, emulsifying wax, glycerin, lactic acid. In 60 g.
Rx	**Noritate** (Dermik Labs)	**Cream; topical:** 1%	Parabens, glycerin. In 30 g.
Rx	**Metronidazole** (Fougera)	**Gel; topical:** 0.75%	EDTA, parabens. In 45 g.
Rx	**MetroGel** (Galderma)	**Gel; topical:** 1%	EDTA, parabens. In 45 g tube.

METRONIDAZOLE — TOPICAL

Indications

➤*Rosacea:* Treatment of inflammatory papules, pustules, and erythema of rosacea.

➤*Off-label uses:* Topical metronidazole has been used as a gel or 1% solution or suspension to treat infected decubitus ulcers; perioral dermatitis has been treated with topical metronidazole gel or cream.

Administration and Dosage

➤*General dosing considerations:* For external use only. Avoid contact with the eyes.

Cleanse areas to be treated before application of topical metronidazole.

Patients may use cosmetics after application of topical metronidazole 5 minutes after allowing medication to dry.

➤*Adults:*

Rosacea – Apply and rub in a thin film once (1% cream or gel) or twice daily, morning and evening, to entire affected areas after washing.

➤*Children:*

Off-label dosing – Apply and rub a thin film to affected areas.

0.75% cream/gel/lotion: Apply twice daily.

1% cream/gel: Apply once daily.

➤*Storage/Stability:* Store at 15° to 30°C (59° to 86°F) for 0.75% cream and gel and 20° to 25°C (68° to 77°F) for 0.75% lotion and 1% cream.

Actions

➤*Pharmacology:* Metronidazole is classified therapeutically as an antiprotozoal and antibacterial agent. The mechanisms by which topical metronidazole acts in reducing inflammatory lesions of acne rosacea are unknown, but may include an antibacterial or an anti-inflammatory effect.

➤*Pharmacokinetics:* Bioavailability studies on administration of 1 g topical metronidazole (7.5 mg metronidazole) to the faces of 10 rosacea patients showed a maximum serum concentration of 66 ng/mL. This is about 100 times less than concentrations afforded by a single 250 mg oral tablet. Three patients had no detectable serum concentrations of metronidazole. The mean dose of gel applied during clinical studies was 600 mg (4.5 mg metronidazole) per application. Therefore, under normal usage levels, the formulation affords minimal serum concentrations. The time to peak plasma concentration (T_{max}) with detectable metronidazole was 8 to 12 hours after topical application.

Contraindications

History of hypersensitivity to metronidazole, parabens, or other ingredients.

Warnings/Precautions

➤*Conjunctivitis:* Conjunctivitis associated with topical use of metronidazole on the face has been reported.

➤*For external use only:* Tearing of the eyes has occurred; avoid eye contact. If a reaction suggesting local irritation occurs, direct patients to use the medication less frequently, discontinue use temporarily, or discontinue use until further instructions.

➤*Blood dyscrasia:* Metronidazole is a nitroimidazole; use with care in patients with evidence of, or history of, blood dyscrasia.

➤*Pregnancy: Category B.* There has been no experience to date with the use of topical metronidazole in pregnant women. Metronidazole crosses the placental barrier and enters the fetal circulation rapidly. Since oral metronidazole is a carcinogen in some rodents, use during pregnancy only if clearly needed.

➤*Lactation:* After oral administration, metronidazole is excreted in breast milk in concentrations similar to those in plasma. Even though metronidazole blood levels are significantly lower than those achieved after oral metronidazole, discontinue nursing or the drug, taking into account the importance of the drug to the mother.

➤*Children:* Safety and efficacy in children have not been established.

Drug Interactions

➤*Anticoagulants:* Drug interactions are less likely with topical administration but should be kept in mind when topical metronidazole is prescribed for patients who are receiving anticoagulant treatment. Oral metronidazole may potentiate the anticoagulant effect of warfarin and coumarin resulting in a prolongation of prothrombin time.

Adverse Reactions

Topical Metronidazole Adverse Events (%)[a]

Adverse reaction	0.75% cream	1% cream (N = 200)	0.75% lotion (N = 71)	0.75% gel
Acne	–	✓	–	–
Burning/stinging	–	–	1	✓
Conjunctivitis	–	✓	–	–
Constipation	–	✓	–	–
Contact dermatitis	–	–	3	–
Dryness	✓	✓	0	✓
Erythema	< 3		6	
Eye irritation (eg, watering/tearing)	✓	✓	✓	✓
Headache	–	✓	–	–
Local allergic reaction	–	✓	3	–
Metallic taste	✓	–	✓	✓
Nausea	✓	✓	✓	✓
Paresthesia	–	✓	–	–
Pruritus	< 3	–	1	–
Rash	–	✓	–	–
Severe flare of comedonal acne	–	✓	–	–
Skin irritation	< 3	✓	✓	✓
Tingling/numbness of extremities	✓	✓	✓	✓
Transient redness	✓	–	✓	✓
Worsening of rosacea	< 3	✓	1	–

[a] All events; data are pooled from separate studies and are not necessarily comparable.
✓ = Incidence not provided.
– = not applicable.

Patient Information

For external use only. Avoid contact with the eyes.

Cleanse affected area(s) before applying the medication. Report any adverse reaction or irritation to your physician.

May apply cosmetics to face after medication is dry.

MUPIROCIN (Pseudomonic Acid A)

Rx	**Mupirocin** (Various, eg, Clay-Park, Teva)	**Ointment; topical:** 2%	Polyethylene glycol. In 15, 22, and 30 g.
Rx	**Bactroban** (GlaxoSmithKline)		Polyethylene glycol. In 22 g.
Rx	**Bactroban Nasal** (GlaxoSmithKline)		Glycerin. In 1 g.
Rx	**Centany** (Medimetriks Pharmaceuticals)		Alcohol, caprylic/capric/myristic/stearic triglyceride, castor oil, propylene glycol. In 30 g and in kits with gauze pads and latex-free cloth tape strips.
Rx	**Bactroban** (GlaxoSmithKline)	**Cream; topical:** 2%	Benzyl alcohol, cetyl alcohol, stearyl alcohol. In 15 and 30 g.

MUPIROCIN (Pseudomonic Acid A) — TOPICAL

Indications

➤*Topical infection:*

Topical ointment – Impetigo caused by *Staphylococcus aureus*, beta-hemolytic streptococcus, and *Streptococcus pyogenes*.

Topical cream – Treatment of secondarily infected traumatic skin lesions (up to 10 cm in length or 100 cm^2 in area) caused by susceptible strains of *S. aureus* and *S. pyogenes*.

Nasal – Eradication of nasal colonization with methicillin-resistant *S. aureus* in adult patients and health care workers as part of a comprehensive infection control program to reduce infection risk among patients at high risk of methicillin-resistant *S. aureus* infection during institutional outbreaks of infections with this pathogen.

➤*Off-label uses:* Topical mupirocin may be effective in treating diaper dermatitis caused by *Candida*; decolonization (neonatal intensive care use).

Administration and Dosage

➤*Adults:*

Impetigo –

Ointment:

• *Usual dosage* – Apply a small amount to the affected area 3 times daily. The area may be covered with gauze dressing. Reevaluate those not showing a response in 3 to 5 days.

MUPIROCIN (Pseudomonic Acid A) — TOPICAL

• *Duration of therapy* – 5 to 14 days.

Secondarily infected traumatic skin lesions –
Cream:
• *Usual dosage* – Apply a small amount to the affected area 3 times daily for 10 days. The area may be covered with gauze dressing. Reevaluate those not showing a response in 3 to 5 days.
• *Duration of therapy* – One source suggests treatment for 5 to 14 days.

Eradication of nasal colonization –
Nasal ointment:
• *Usual dosage* – Divide approximately one half of the ointment from the single-use tube between the nostrils and apply twice daily (morning and evening) for 5 days.
• *Duration of therapy* – One source suggests treatment for 5 to 14 days.

➤*Children:*

Impetigo –
2 months to 16 years of age:
• *Ointment* – See Adults for dosing.

Secondarily infected traumatic skin lesions –
2 months to 16 years of age and older:
• *Cream* – See Adults for dosing.

Eradication of nasal colonization –
12 years of age or older:
Nasal ointment: See Adults for dosing.

Off-label dosing –
Decolonization (neonatal intensive care use): Apply small amount to anterior nares twice daily for 5 to 7 days. Not recommended for routine use in decolonization.

➤*Renal function impairment:* Polyethylene glycol can be absorbed from open wounds and damaged skin and is excreted by the kidney. Do not use if absorption of large quantities of polyethylene glycol is possible, especially if there is evidence of moderate or severe renal impairment.

➤*Administration:* Avoid mucosal surfaces and contact with the eyes. May cover topically treated areas with gauze dressing.

Nasal ointment – After application, close nostrils by pressing together and releasing sides of the nose repeatedly for about 1 minute. The single-use tube will deliver a total of approximately 0.5 g of the ointment (approximately 0.25 g/nostril).

➤*Storage/Stability:* Store the topical ointment between 20° and 25°C (68° and 77°F); store the nasal ointment and topical cream at or below 25°C (77°F). Do not freeze the cream.

Actions

➤*Pharmacology:* Mupirocin is an antibacterial agent produced by fermentation using the organism *Pseudomonas fluorescens*. Mupirocin is considered a topical antibacterial structurally unrelated to other agents, inhibits bacterial protein synthesis by reversibly and specifically binding to bacterial isoleucyl transfer-RNA synthetase. Mupirocin demonstrates no in vitro cross-resistance with other antimicrobials. However, when resistance does occur, it appears to result from the production of a modified isoleucyl-tRNA synthetase. High level plasmid-mediated resistance (MIC greater than 1024 mcg/mL) has been reported in some strains of *S. aureus* and coagulase negative staphylococci.

➤*Pharmacokinetics:*

Absorption/Distribution –
Cream: Systemic absorption of mupirocin through human intact skin is minimal. Systemic absorption was studied following application of mupirocin cream 3 times/day for 5 days to various skin lesions (greater than 10 cm in length or 100 cm^2 in area) in 16 adults (29 to 60 years of age) and 10 children (3 to 12 years of age). Some systemic absorption was observed by detection of the metabolite, monic acid in urine. More frequent occurrence of percutaneous absorption in children (90%) was found compared with adults (44%). However, urinary concentrations in children and adults were within range. Mupirocin is highly protein bound (more than 97%), and the effect of wound secretions on the MICs of mupirocin has not been determined.
Ointment: Mupirocin ointment applied to the lower arm of healthy male subjects followed by occlusion for 24 hours showed no measurable systemic absorption (less than 1.1 ng mupirocin/mL of whole blood).
Nasal: Following single or repeated intranasal applications of 0.2 g of mupirocin nasal 3 times/day for 3 days to adults showed no evidence of systemic absorption. A study in neonates and premature infants indicated that, unlike adults, significant systemic absorption occurred following intranasal administration. Mupirocin nasal has not been adequately studied in children less than 12 years of age.

Metabolism/Excretion – Any mupirocin reaching the systemic circulation is rapidly metabolized, predominantly to inactive monic acid which is eliminated by renal excretion and demonstrates no antibacterial activity. The elimination half-life after IV administration was 20 to 40 minutes for mupirocin and 30 to 80 minutes for monic acid.

➤*Microbiology:* The aerobic isolates of *Staphylococcus aureus* (including methicillin-resistant and β-lactamase producing strains), *S. epidermidis*, *S. saprophyticus*, and *Streptococcus pyogenes* are susceptible to mupirocin in vitro. Mupirocin also has been found to be active against certain gram-negative bacteria.

Contraindications

Hypersensitivity reactions to any components of the products.

Warnings/Precautions

➤*For external use only:* Avoid mucosal surfaces and contact with the eyes.

➤*Open wounds:* Polyethylene glycol can be absorbed from open wounds and damaged skin and is excreted by the kidney. Do not use if absorption of large quantities of polyethylene glycol is possible, especially if there is evidence of moderate or severe renal impairment.

➤*Prophylaxis:* There are insufficient data at this time to recommend use of mupirocin nasal for general prophylaxis of any infection in any patient population or to establish that this product is safe and effective as part of an intervention program to prevent autoinfection of high-risk patients from their own nasal colonization.

➤*Sensitivity reaction:* If a reaction suggesting sensitivity or chemical irritation occurs, discontinue treatment and institute appropriate alternative therapy.

➤*Superinfection:* Prolonged use of antibiotics may result in overgrowth of nonsusceptible organisms, including fungi.

➤*Pregnancy: Category B.* There are no adequate and well-controlled studies in pregnant women. Use during pregnancy only if clearly needed.

➤*Lactation:* It is not known whether mupirocin is excreted in breast milk. The molecular weight of the free acid (about 501) is low enough for excretion into breast milk, but the minimal plasma concentrations and rapid metabolism and elimination suggest that clinically significant amounts of the antibiotic will not reach the milk. Exercise caution when administering to a nursing woman.

➤*Children:* Safety and efficacy of mupirocin ointment and cream have been established in children 2 months to 16 years of age.

Safety in children younger than 12 years of age has not been established for mupirocin nasal.

Drug Interactions

Do not use mupirocin nasal concurrently with any other nasal products.

Adverse Reactions

➤*Topical ointment:* Burning, stinging, or pain (1.5%); itching (1%); rash, nausea, erythema, dry skin, tenderness, swelling, contact dermatitis, and increased exudate (less than 1%); systemic reactions (rare).

➤*Topical cream:* Headache (1.7%); rash, nausea (1.1%); abdominal pain, burning at application site, cellulitis, dermatitis, dizziness, pruritus, secondary wound infection, and ulcerative stomatitis (less than 1%).

Secondarily infected eczema – Adverse events thought to be possibly or probably drug-related are as follows: Nausea (4.9%); headache and burning at application site (3.6%); pruritus (2.4%); 1 report each of abdominal pain, bleeding secondary to eczema, pain secondary to eczema, hives, dry skin, and rash.

➤*Nasal:* Headache (9%); rhinitis (6%); respiratory disorder including upper respiratory tract congestion (5%); pharyngitis (4%); taste perversion (3%); burning/stinging, cough (2%); pruritus (1%); blepharitis, diarrhea, dry mouth, ear pain, epistaxis, nausea, rash (less than 1%).

Patient Information

This medication is for external use only. Avoid eyes and mucosal membranes.

Stop the medication and contact your doctor if irritation, severe itching or rash occurs.

If no improvement is seen within 3 to 5 days, contact your doctor.

The treated area may be covered by a gauze dressing.

➤*Nasal:* Press the sides of the nose together and gently massage after application to spread the ointment throughout the inside of the nostrils.

SULFACETAMIDE SODIUM

Rx	**Ovace Plus** (Tiber)	**Cream; topical:** 10%	Cetearyl alcohol, cetyl alcohol, disodium EDTA, glycerin, glyceryl monostearate, mineral oil, parabens, PEG-3, PEG-100. In 45 g.
Rx	**Sulfacetamide Sodium** (Various, eg, River's Edge, Taro)	**Lotion; topical:** 10%	May contain disodium EDTA, PEG 400, methylparaben, urea. In 89 and 118 mL.
Rx	**Carmol Scalp Treatment** (Doak Dermatologics)		EDTA, methylparaben, urea 10%. In 85 g.
Rx	**Ovace Plus** (Tiber)	**Shampoo; topical:** 10%	PEG-150. In 227 g.

SULFACETAMIDE SODIUM

Rx	**Seb-Prev** (Perrigo)	**Gel; topical:** 10%	EDTA, methylparaben. In 30 and 60 g.
Rx	**Ovace** (Tiber)	**Aerosol, foam; topical:** 10%	Edetate disodium, glycerin, lactic acid, lauryl/myristyl alcohol, methylparaben. In 100 g.
Rx	**Sodium Sulfacetamide Medicated Pads** (A. Aarons)	**Pads; topical:** 10%	EDTA, urea 10%. In 30s.
Rx	**Sodium Sulfacetamide** (Acella Pharmaceuticals)	**Soap; topical:** 10%	Disodium EDTA, methylparaben, PEG. In 473 mL.
Rx	**Ovace Plus Wash** (Tiber)		Cetearyl alcohol, edetate disodium, glyceryl, methylparaben, PEG-3, PEG-6, PEG-150. In 340 g.
Rx	**Seb-Prev Wash** (Perrigo)		Edetate disodium, PEG-6, PEG-60, PEG-150, methylparaben. In 170 and 340 mL.

SULFACETAMIDE SODIUM — TOPICAL

Indications

➤*Bacterial infections:* For the treatment of secondary bacterial infections of the skin due to organisms susceptible to sulfonamides.

➤*Seborrheic dermatitis and seborrhea sicca:* For topical application in the following scaling dermatoses: seborrheic dermatitis and seborrhea sicca (dandruff).

Administration and Dosage

➤*Adults:*

Bacterial infections –

Foam: Dispense small amount of foam onto hand. The exact amount needed will vary according to the size of the affected area. With fingers, gently massage foam into affected areas until foam disappears. Repeat application as described for 8 to 10 days.

Lotion: Apply to the affected areas 2 to 4 times daily until the infection has cleared.

Pads: Apply to the affected areas 1 to 2 times daily or as directed by a health care provider until the infection has cleared.

Soap: Wet skin and liberally apply to areas to be cleansed, massage gently into skin working into a full lather, rinse thoroughly and pat dry. Repeat application as described for 8 to 10 days.

Seborrheic dermatitis –

Foam: Dispense small amount of foam onto hand. The exact amount needed will vary according to the size of the affected area. With fingers, gently massage foam into affected areas until foam disappears.

Use twice daily or as directed by a health care provider. Repeat application as described for 8 to 10 days.

As the condition subsides, the interval between applications may be lengthened. Applications once or twice weekly or every other week may prevent recurrence. Should the condition recur after stopping therapy, the application of the foam should be reinitiated as the beginning of treatment.

Lotion: In mild cases involving the scalp and adjacent skin areas, including non-inflammatory types with scaling (dandruff), the lotion should be applied as directed by a health care provider, with best results occurring when applied at bedtime and allowed to remain overnight. Its application should be preceded by a shampoo if the hair and scalp are oily or greasy, or if there are considerable debris.

In severe cases with crusting, heavy scaling, and inflammation involving the scalp or the scalp and other skin, the lotion should be applied twice daily. Initially, the hair and scalp should be cleansed with a nonirritating shampoo, such as *Carmol* deep cleansing antibacterial shampoo (urea 10% base). To ensure intimate contact of the medication with the affected skin, cleansing should be repeated as frequently as necessary thereafter.

The application of the lotion, as described, should be repeated 8 to 10 times.

Pads: Apply to the skin or scalp 1 to 2 times daily or as directed by a health care provider.

Soap: Wash affected areas twice daily (morning and evening), or as directed by your health care provider. Repeat application as described for 8 to 10 days.

Seborrheic sicca – See Seborrheic Dermatitis for dosing.

➤*Children:*

Bacterial infections –

12 years of age and older: See Adults for dosing.

Seborrheic dermatitis –

12 years of age and older: See Adults for dosing.

Seborrheic sicca –

12 years of age and older: See Adults for dosing.

➤*Administration:*

Foam – For proper dispensing, the can must be inverted. Shake well before use.

Hair should be towel-dried or dry before applying to scalp.

Wash hands after applying the foam.

Allow the treated area to air dry. Do not wash the treated area immediately after applying the foam. Hair styling products can be used as usual after the foam has been applied.

Lotion – The applicator tip of the plastic tube is convenient for applying sulfacetamide, especially for patients with thick hair. Part hair one section at a time and apply a small amount of lotion along the part line. Repeat until the scalp is moistened, then massage into the scalp thoroughly with fingers. Remove excess lotion or large scales by gently brushing scalp. Leave lotion on overnight or as directed by a health care provider. Shampooing following treatment is not necessary but hair should be washed at least once a week. (A thorough brushing or rinsing with plain water will remove any excess medication.)

Soap – Avoid contact with eyes or mucous membranes. Wet skin and liberally apply to areas to be cleansed, massage gently into skin working into a full lather, rinse thoroughly and pat dry. Rinsing with plain water will remove any excess medication. If skin dryness occurs it may be controlled by rinsing cleanser off sooner or using less frequently.

For seborrheic dermatitis and seborrhea sicca, regular shampooing following sulfacetamide soap is not necessary, but the hair should be shampooed at least once a week.

➤*Storage/Stability:*

Foam – Store at 20° to 25°C (68° to 77°F). Store upright.

Lotion and pads – Store at 15° to 30°C (59° to 86°F). Protect from freezing. The products may tend to darken slightly on prolonged standing. Slight discoloration does not impair the efficacy or safety of the product.

Actions

➤*Pharmacology:* Sulfacetamide exerts a bacteriostatic effect against sulfonamide-sensitive gram-positive and gram-negative microorganisms commonly isolated from secondary cutaneous pyrogenic infections. It acts by restricting the synthesis of folic acid required by bacteria for growth by its competition with para-aminobenzoic acid.

➤*Pharmacokinetics:* There are no clinical data available on the degree and rate of systemic absorption of sulfacetamide when applied to the skin of the scalp. However, significant absorption of sulfacetamide through the skin has been reported.

➤*Microbiology:* The following in vitro data are available but their clinical significance is unknown. Organisms that show susceptibility to sulfacetamide are the following: *Streptococci, Staphylococci, Escherichia coli, Klebsiella pneumoniae, Pseudomonas pyocyanea, Salmonella* species, *Proteus vulgaris, Nocardia*, and *Acitomyces*.

Contraindications

Known or suspected hypersensitivity to sulfonamides or to any of the ingredients of the preparation.

Warnings/Precautions

➤*Stevens-Johnson syndrome:* Sulfonamides are known to cause Stevens-Johnson syndrome in hypersensitive individuals. Stevens-Johnson syndrome also has been reported following topical use of sulfacetamide.

➤*Drug-induced systemic lupus erythematous (SLE):* Cases of drug-induced SLE from topical sulfacetamide have been reported. In one of these cases, there was a fatal outcome.

➤*Systemic absorption:* Systemic absorption of topical sulfonamides is greater following application to large, infected, abraded, denuded, or severely burned areas. Under these circumstances, potentially any of the adverse reactions produced by systemic administration of these agents could occur; perform appropriate observations and laboratory determinations.

➤*Hypersensitivity reactions:* Hypersensitivity reactions may recur when a sulfonamide is readministered, irrespective of the route of administration, and cross-hypersensitivity between different sulfonamides may occur. If sulfacetamide produces signs of hypersensitivity or other untoward reactions, discontinue use of the preparation.

➤*Superinfection:* Nonsusceptible organisms, including fungi, may proliferate with the use of this preparation.

➤*Pregnancy: Category C.* Animal reproduction studies have not been conducted with sulfacetamide. It is also not known whether sulfacetamide can cause fetal harm when administered to a pregnant woman or can affect reproduction capacity. Use sulfacetamide in pregnancy only if clearly needed.

➤*Lactation:* It is not known whether this drug is excreted in human milk. Because many drugs are excreted in human milk, exercise caution when administering sulfacetamide to a breast-feeding woman.

➤*Children:* Safety and efficacy in children younger than 12 years of age have not been established.

SULFACETAMIDE SODIUM — TOPICAL

Drug Interactions

Sulfacetamide is incompatible with silver preparations.

Adverse Reactions

➤*Local:* Reports of irritation and hypersensitivity to sulfacetamide are uncommon.

➤*Reactions with use of ophthalmic sulfacetamide:* The following adverse reactions, reported after administration of sterile ophthalmic sulfacetamide, are noteworthy: instances of Stevens-Johnson syndrome and local hypersensitivity, which progressed to a syndrome resembling SLE; in 1 case, a fatal outcome has been reported.

Overdosage

➤*Symptoms:* Overdosage may cause nausea and vomiting. Large doses may cause hematuria, crystalluria, and renal shutdown because of precipitation of sulfa crystals in renal tubules and urinary tract.

➤*Treatment:* In the event of overdosage, start emergency treatment immediately. Induce vomiting in the patient, even if emesis has occurred spontaneously. Pharmacologic vomiting by the administration of ipecac syrup is a preferred method. However, do not induce vomiting in patients with impaired consciousness. The action of ipecac is facilitated by physical activity and by the administration of 8 to 12 fluid ounces of water. If emesis does not occur within 15 minutes, repeat the dose of ipecac. Take precautions against aspiration, especially in infants and children. Following emesis, any drug remaining in the stomach may be absorbed by activated charcoal administered as a slurry with water. If vomiting is unsuccessful or contraindicated, perform gastric lavage. Isotonic and one-half isotonic saline are the lavage solutions of choice. Saline cathartics, such as milk of magnesia, draw water into the bowel by osmosis and, therefore, may be valuable for their action in rapid dilution of bowel content. After emergency treatment, continue to medically monitor the patient.

Observe kidney function for up to 1 week and have the patient ingest copious amounts of fluid during this period. Mannitol infusions may be helpful at the first sign of oliguria. Alkalinization of the urine by ingestion of bicarbonate is very helpful in preventing crystallization of sulfa drug in the kidney.

Patient Information

Instruct the patient to discontinue use of sulfacetamide if the condition becomes worse or if a rash develops in the area being treated or elsewhere. Instruct the patient to promptly discontinue sulfacetamide and notify their health care provider if any arthritis, fever, or sores in the mouth develop.

ANTIBIOTIC COMBINATIONS

	Product and Distributor	Polymyxin B Sulfate (units/g)	Neomycin (mg/g)[a]	Bacitracin Zinc (units/g)	Other	How Supplied
otc	**Lanabiotic Ointment** (Combe)	10,000	3.5	500	40 mg lidocaine	Aloe, lanolin, mineral oil, petrolatum. In 28 g.
otc	**ProCoMycin Ointment** (Physicians Science And Nature)					Aloe, avocado oil, cetearyl alcohol, parabens. In 15 g.
otc	**Tri-Biozene Ointment** (Reese)				10 mg pramoxine HCl/g	White petrolatum. In 15 g.
otc	**Neosporin Plus Pain Relief Ointment** (Pfizer)					White petrolatum. In 15 and 30 g.
otc	**Double Antibiotic Ointment** (Fougera)			500		In ≈ 15 and ≈ 30 g, UD 0.9 g (144s).
otc	**Polysporin Ointment** (Pfizer)					White petrolatum base. In ≈ 15 and ≈ 30 g.
otc	**Neosporin Plus Pain Relief Cream** (Pfizer)		3.5		10 mg pramoxine HCl/g	Methylparaben, mineral oil, white petrolatum. In 15 g.
otc	**Neosporin Original Ointment** (Pfizer)	5000		400		Cocoa butter, cottonseed oil, olive oil, white petrolatum. In 14 and 28 g, UD 0.9 g (10s).
otc	**Triple Antibiotic Ointment** (Various, eg, Alpharma)					In 15, 30, and 454 g.

[a] As base; equivalent to 5 mg neomycin sulfate.

ANTIBIOTIC COMBINATIONS — TOPICAL

Indications

➤*Topical infection/Pain:* Used as a first aid to help prevent skin infection and for the temporary relief of pain in minor cuts, wounds, scrapes, and burns.

Administration and Dosage

➤*General dosing considerations:* The affected area may be covered with a sterile bandage.

➤*Adults:*

Topical infection/Pain –

Usual dosage: Clean the affected area. Apply a small amount of the antibiotic on the area 1 to 3 times/day.

Duration of therapy: Do not use for longer than 1 week unless consulted by a health care provider.

➤*Children:*

2 years of age or older – See Adults for dosing for children 2 years of age or older.

➤*Renal function impairment:* If the product contains neomycin, do not apply more than once daily in burn cases where more than 20% of the body is affected, especially if the patient has impaired renal function.

➤*Administration:* For external use only. Do not use in or near the eyes, nose, mouth, or mucous membranes, or apply over large areas of the body.

Actions

➤*Pharmacology:* The topical anti-infectives may be either bactericidal or bacteriostatic. Most inhibit protein synthesis. **Bacitracin** inhibits cell-wall synthesis.

Contraindications

Known sensitivity to any of the ingredients; use in the eyes.

Warnings/Precautions

➤*Systemic therapy:* Deeper cutaneous infections may require systemic antibiotic therapy in addition to local treatment. Use caution when applying over large areas of the body for deep puncture wounds, animal bites, or serious burns.

➤*Neomycin toxicity:* Because of the potential nephrotoxicity and ototoxicity of neomycin, use with care in treating extensive burns, trophic ulceration, or other extensive conditions where absorption is possible. Do not apply more than once daily in burn cases where more than 20% of the body is affected. Especially if the patient has impaired renal function.

➤*External use:* For external use only. Do not use in or near the eyes, nose, mouth, mucous membranes, or apply over large areas of the body.

➤*Neomycin hypersensitivity:* Chronic application of neomycin sulfate to inflamed skin of individuals with allergic contact dermatitis and chronic dermatoses (eg, chronic otitis externa, stasis dermatitis) increases the possibility of sensitization. Low grade reddening with swelling, dry scaling, itching, or a failure to heal are usually manifestations of this hypersensitivity. Discontinue use if these symptoms appear and avoid neomycin-containing products thereafter.

➤*Superinfection:* Prolonged use of antibiotics may result in overgrowth of nonsusceptible organisms, particularly fungi. Such overgrowth may lead to a secondary infection. Discontinue the drug and take appropriate measures if superinfection occurs.

➤*Pregnancy: Category C* (bacitracin zinc/neomycin). There are no adequate and well-controlled studies in pregnant women. Use only when clearly needed and when the potential benefits outweigh the unknown potential hazards to the fetus. Ototoxicity is known to occur after oral, parenteral, and topical neomycin; however, it has not been reported to affect in utero exposure. Cranial nerve toxicity has been reported in the fetus following exposure to other aminoglycosides (eg, kanamycin, streptomycin) and may potentially occur with neomycin.

Category B (polymyxin B). There are no adequate and well-controlled studies in pregnant women. Use during pregnancy only if clearly needed.

➤*Lactation:* It is not known whether **bacitracin zinc**, **polymyxin B**, or **neomycin** are excreted in breast milk. Exercise caution when applying on a breastfeeding woman. Neomycin has been reported to be excreted into the milk of lactating cows and ewes after a single 10 mg/kg IM dose; also small amounts of other aminoglycosides (eg, gentamicin) are excreted into breast milk and absorbed by the nursing infant.

➤*Children:* Safety and efficacy in children younger than 2 years of age have not been established.

Antibiotic Agents

ANTIBIOTIC COMBINATIONS — TOPICAL

Adverse Reactions

Bacitracin ointment – Allergic contact dermatitis has occurred.

Neomycin – Hypersensitivity (see Warnings/Precautions); ototoxicity and nephrotoxicity have occurred (see Warnings/Precautions).

Patient Information

Discontinue use of medication if rash or other allergic reaction develops or if condition persists or worsens.

For external use only. Cleanse affected area prior to application of medicine.

Notify physician if condition worsens or if rash or irritation develops.

Not for prolonged use. Do not use for longer than 1 week unless directed by a physician.

Antifungal Agents

BUTENAFINE HYDROCHLORIDE

otc	**Lotrimin Ultra** (Schering Plough)	**Cream; topical:** 1% butenafine hydrochloride	Benzyl alcohol, cetyl alcohol, glycerin, white petrolatum. In 12 and 24 g.
Rx	**Mentax** (Mylan)		Benzyl and cetyl alcohol, glycerin, white petrolatum. In 15 and 30 g.

BUTENAFINE HYDROCHLORIDE — TOPICAL

Indications

➤*Topical infections:* For the treatment of the following dermatologic infections: Tinea (pityriasis) versicolor due to *M. furfur* (formerly *P. orbiculare*), interdigital tinea pedis (athlete's foot), tinea corporis (ringworm) and tinea cruris (jock itch) due to *E. floccosum*, *T. mentagrophytes*, *T. rubrum*, and *T. tonsurans*.

Administration and Dosage

➤*General dosing considerations:* If a patient shows no clinical improvement after the treatment period, the diagnosis and therapy should be reviewed.

➤*Adults:*

Interdigital tinea pedis – Apply twice daily for 7 days or once daily for 4 weeks.

Tinea corporis or tinea cruris – Apply once daily for 2 weeks.

Tinea (pityriasis) versicolor – Apply once daily for 2 weeks.

➤*Children:*

12 years of age and older – See Adults for dosing.

➤*Discontinuation of therapy:* If irritation or sensitivity develops with the use of butenafine hydrochloride cream 1%, treatment should be discontinued and appropriate therapy instituted.

➤*Administration:* For external use only.

Sufficient butenafine cream should be applied to cover affected areas and immediately surrounding skin of patients with tinea versicolor, interdigital tinea pedis, tinea corporis, and tinea cruris.

➤*Storage/Stability:* Store between 5° and 30°C (41° and 86°F).

Actions

➤*Pharmacokinetics:*

Absorption/Distribution – In 1 study conducted in healthy subjects for 14 days, 6 g of butenafine hydrochloride cream 1% was applied once daily to the dorsal skin (3000 cm^2) of 7 subjects, and 20 g of the cream was applied once daily to the arms, trunk and groin areas (10,000 cm^2) of another 12 subjects. After 14 days of topical applications, the 6 g dose group yielded a mean peak plasma butenafine hydrochloride concentration, C_{max}, of 1.4 ± 0.8 ng/mL, occurring at a mean time to the peak plasma concentration, t_{max}, of 15 ± 8 hours, and a mean area under the plasma concentration-time curve, $AUC_{0\text{-}24\ hrs}$ of 23.9 ± 11.3 ng•hr/mL. For the 20 g dose group, the mean C_{max} was 5 ± 2 ng/mL, occurring at a mean t_{max} of 6 ± 6 hours, and the mean $AUC_{0\text{-}24\ hrs}$ was 87.8 ± 45.3 ng•hr/mL. A biphasic decline of plasma butenafine hydrochloride concentrations was observed with the half-lives estimated to be 35 hours and greater than 150 hours, respectively.

At 72 hours after the last dose application, the mean plasma concentrations decreased to 0.3 ± 0.2 ng/mL for the 6 g dose group and 1.1 ± 0.9 ng/mL for the 20 g dose group. Low levels of butenafine hydrochloride remained in the plasma 7 days after the last dose application (mean: 0.1 ± 0.2 ng/mL for the 6 g dose group, and 0.7 ± 0.5 ng/mL for the 20 g dose group). The total amount (or % dose) of butenafine hydrochloride absorbed through the skin into the systemic circulation has not been quantitated.

In 11 patients with tinea pedis, butenafine hydrochloride cream 1% was applied by the patients to cover the affected and immediately surrounding skin area once daily for 4 weeks, and a single blood sample was collected between 10 and 20 hours following dosing at 1, 2, and 4 weeks after treatment. The plasma butenafine hydrochloride concentration ranged from undetectable to 0.3 ng/mL.

In 24 patients with tinea cruris, butenafine hydrochloride cream 1% was applied by the patients to cover the affected and immediately surrounding skin area once daily for 2 weeks (mean average daily dose: 1.3 ± 0.2 g). A single blood sample was collected between 0.5 and 65 hours after the last dose, and the plasma butenafine hydrochloride concentration ranged from undetectable to 2.52 ng/mL (mean ± SD: 0.91 ± 0.15 ng/mL). Four weeks after cessation of treatment, the plasma butenafine hydrochloride concentration ranged from undetectable to 0.28 ng/mL.

Metabolism/Excretion – It was determined that the primary metabolite in urine was formed through hydroxylation at the terminal t-butyl side-chain.

➤*Microbiology:* Butenafine hydrochloride is a benzylamine derivative with a mode of action similar to that of the allylamine class of antifungal drugs. Butenafine hydrochloride is hypothesized to act by inhibiting the epoxidation of squalene, thus blocking the biosynthesis of ergosterol, an essential component of fungal cell membranes. The benzylamine derivatives, like the allylamines, act at an earlier step in the ergosterol biosynthesis pathway than the azole class of anti-fungal drugs. Depending on the concentration of the drug and the fungal species tested, butenafine hydrochloride may be fungicidal in vitro. However, the clinical significance of these in vitro data is unknown.

Butenafine hydrochloride has been shown to be active against most strains of the following microorganisms, both in vitro and in clinical infections: *Epidermophyton floccosum*, *Malassezia furfur*, *Trichophyton mentagrophytes*, *Trichophyton rubrum*, and *trichophyton tonsurans*.

Contraindications

Known or suspected sensitivity to butenafine hydrochloride cream 1% or any of its components.

Warnings/Precautions

➤*For dermatologic use only:* Butenafine hydrochloride cream 1% is not for ophthalmic, oral, or intravaginal use.

➤*Irritation/diagnosis:* Butenafine hydrochloride cream 1% is for external use only. If irritation or sensitivity develops with the use of butenafine hydrochloride cream 1%, treatment should be discontinued and appropriate therapy instituted. Diagnosis of the disease should be confirmed either by culture or an appropriate medium, (except *M. furfur* [formerly *P. orbiculare*]) or by direct microscopic examination of infected superficial epidermal tissue in a solution of potassium hydroxide.

➤*Mucous membranes:* Use butenafine hydrochloride cream 1% as directed by the physician, and avoid contact with the eyes, nose, and mouth, and other mucous membranes.

➤*Special risk:* Patients who are known to be sensitive to allylamine antifungals should use butenafine hydrochloride cream 1% with caution, since cross-reactivity may occur.

➤*Pregnancy: Category B.*

➤*Lactation:* It is not known if butenafine hydrochloride is excreted in human milk. Because many drugs are excreted in human milk, caution should be exercised in prescribing butenafine hydrochloride cream 1% to a nursing woman. Nursing mothers should avoid application of butenafine hydrochloride cream 1% to the breast.

➤*Children:* Safety and efficacy in pediatric patients below the age of 12 years have not been studied. Use of butenafine hydrochloride cream 1% in pediatric patients 12 to 16 years of age is supported by evidence from adequate and well-controlled studies of butenafine hydrochloride cream 1% in adults.

Drug Interactions

None known.

Adverse Reactions

In controlled clinical trials, 9 (approximately 1%) of 815 patients treated with butenafine hydrochloride cream 1%, reported adverse reactions related to the skin. These included burning/stinging, itching, and worsening of the condition. No patient treated with butenafine hydrochloride cream 1% discontinued treatment due to an adverse reaction. In the vehicle-treated patients, 2 of 718 patients discontinued because of treatment site adverse reactions, 1 of which was severe burning/stinging and itching at the site of application.

In uncontrolled clinical trials, the most frequently reported adverse reactions in patients treated with butenafine hydrochloride cream 1% were contact dermatitis, erythema, irritation, and itching, each occurring in less than 2% of patients.

➤*Hypersensitivity:* In provocative testing in over 200 subjects, there was no evidence of allergic contact sensitization for either cream or vehicle base for butenafine hydrochloride cream 1%.

Patient Information

Use butenafine hydrochloride cream 1% as directed by the physician. The hands should be washed after applying the medication to the affected area(s). Avoid contact with the eyes, nose, mouth, and other mucous membranes. Butenafine hydrochloride cream 1% is for external use only.

BUTENAFINE HYDROCHLORIDE — TOPICAL

Dry the affected area(s) thoroughly before application if you wish to apply butenafine hydrochloride cream 1% after bathing.

Use the medication for the full treatment time recommended by the physician, even though symptoms may have improved. Notify the physician if there is no improvement after the end of the prescribed treatment period, or sooner, if the condition worsens (see below).

Inform the physician if the area of application shows signs of increased irritation, redness, itching, burning, blistering, swelling, or oozing.

Avoid the use of occlusive dressings unless otherwise directed by the physician.

Do not use this medication for any disorder other than that for which it was prescribed.

CICLOPIROX

Rx	**Ciclopirox** (Various, eg, Fougera, Glenmark)	**Cream; topical:** 0.77%	As ciclopirox olamine. May contain alcohol. In 15, 30, and 90 g.
Rx	**Ciclopirox** (Paddock)	**Gel; topical:** 0.77%	Isopropyl alcohol. In 30, 45, and 100 g.
Rx	**Loprox** (Medicis)		Isopropyl alcohol. In 30, 45, and 100 g.
Rx	**Ciclopirox** (Paddock)	**Shampoo; topical:** 1%	In 120 mL.
Rx	**Loprox** (Medicis)		In 120 mL.
Rx	**Ciclopirox** (Various, eg, Fougera)	**Suspension; topical:** 0.77%	As ciclopirox olamine. May contain alcohol. In 30 and 60 mL bottles.
Rx	**Ciclopirox Nail Lacquer** (Various, eg, Actavis Mid Atlantic, Apotex, Harris, Sandoz, Taro, Teva)	**Solution; topical:** 8%	May contain isopropyl alcohol. In 3.3 and 6.6 mL with brushes.
Rx	**CNL8 Nail Kit** (JSJ Pharmaceutical)		Isopropyl alcohol. In kits containing 3 5 mL bottles of nail lacquer, remover swabs, emery board, and 28 topical vitamin E 5% capsules.
Rx	**Penlac Nail Lacquer** (Dermik Labs.)		Isopropyl alcohol. In 3.3 and 6.6 mL with brushes.

CICLOPIROX — TOPICAL

Indications

➤*Nail lacquer topical solution:* As a component of a comprehensive management program for topical treatment of immunocompetent patients with mild to moderate onychomycosis of fingernails and toenails, without lunula involvement, due to *Trichophyton rubrum*. The comprehensive management program includes removal of the unattached, infected nails as frequently as monthly, by a health care provider who has special competence in the diagnosis and treatment of nail disorders, including minor nail procedures.

➤*Suspension:* For the topical treatment of the following dermal infections: tinea pedis, tinea cruris, and tinea corporis due to *Trichophyton rubrum*, *T. mentagrophytes*, *Epidermophyton floccosum*, and *Microsporum canis*; cutaneous candidiasis (moniliasis) due to *Candida albicans*; and tinea (pityriasis) versicolor due to *Malassezia furfur*.

➤*Gel:* For the topical treatment of interdigital tinea pedis and tinea corporis due to *T. rubrum*, *T. mentagrophytes*, or *E. floccosum*; and seborrheic dermatitis of the scalp.

➤*Shampoo:* For the treatment of seborrheic dermatitis of the scalp in adults.

Administration and Dosage

➤*General dosing considerations:* If a patient shows no clinical improvement after 4 weeks of treatment with the gel, shampoo, or suspension, the diagnosis should be reviewed.

Use the ciclopirox nail lacquer topical solution as a component of a comprehensive management program for onychomycosis. Integral parts of the therapy include removal of the unattached, infected nail (as frequently as monthly) by a health care provider, weekly trimming by the patient, and daily application of the medication. Give careful consideration of the appropriate nail management program to patients with diabetes.

➤*Adults:*

Dermal infections – See Indications for specific uses.

Suspension: Gently massage into the affected and surrounding skin areas twice daily, in the morning and evening. Clinical improvement with relief of pruritus and other symptoms usually occurs within the first week of treatment.

Patients with tinea versicolor usually exhibit clinical and mycological clearing after 2 weeks of treatment.

Onychomycosis of fingernails and toenails, mild to moderate –

Nail lacquer topical solution: Apply once daily (preferably at bedtime or 8 hours before washing) to all affected nails with the applicator brush provided. Apply evenly over the entire nail plate.

The nail lacquer topical solution should not be removed on a daily basis. Daily applications should be made over the previous coat and removed with alcohol every 7 days. This cycle should be repeated throughout the duration of therapy.

Seborrheic dermatitis of the scalp –

Gel: Apply to affected scalp areas twice daily, in the morning and evening, for 4 weeks. Clinical improvement usually occurs within the first week, with continuing resolution of signs and symptoms through the fourth week of treatment.

Shampoo: Wet hair and apply approximately 5 mL of ciclopirox shampoo to the scalp. Up to 10 mL may be used for long hair. Lather and leave on hair and scalp for 3 minutes. Avoid contact with eyes. Rinse off. Repeat treatment twice per week for 4 weeks, with a minimum of 3 days between applications.

Superficial dermatophyte infections (interdigital tinea pedis, tinea corporis) –

Gel: Gently massage into the affected areas and surrounding skin twice daily, in the morning and evening, immediately after cleaning or washing the areas to be treated. Interdigital tinea pedis and tinea corporis should be treated for 4 weeks.

➤*Children:*

Dermal infections –

10 years of age or older: See Adults for dosing.

Seborrheic dermatitis of the scalp –

16 years of age and older: See Adults for dosing.

Superficial dermatophyte infections (interdigital tinea pedis, tinea corporis) –

16 years of age and older: See Adults for dosing.

➤*Administration:*

Nail lacquer topical solution –

Nail care by health care providers: Removal of the unattached, infected nail (as frequently as monthly), trimming of onycholytic nail, and filing of excess horny material should be performed by professionals trained in treatment of nail disorders.

Nail care by patient: Every 7 days after ciclopirox 8% topical solution nail lacquer is removed with alcohol, or as directed by the health care provider, patients should file away (with an emery board) loose nail material and trim nails, as required.

If possible, ciclopirox 8% topical solution nail lacquer should be applied to the nail bed, hyponychium, and the under surface of the nail plate when it is free of the nail bed (eg, onycholysis).

➤*Storage/Stability:*

Nail lacquer topical solution – Store between 15° and 30°C (59° and 86°F). Protect from light (eg, store the bottle in the carton after every use). Keep away from heat and flame.

Lotion – Store between 5° and 25°C (41° and 77°F).

Cream, gel, and shampoo – Store at 15° to 30°C.

Actions

➤*Pharmacology:* Ciclopirox olamine is a broad-spectrum antifungal agent that inhibits the growth of pathogenic dermatophytes, yeasts, and *M. furfur*. Ciclopirox exhibits fungicidal activity in vitro against isolates of *T. rubrum*, *T. mentagrophytes*, *E. floccosum*, *M. canis*, and *C. albicans*.

Ciclopirox acts by chelation of polyvalent cations (Fe^{3+} or $A1^{3+}$) resulting in the inhibition of the metal-dependent enzymes that are responsible for the degradation of peroxides within the fungal cell.

In vitro studies showed that ciclopirox inhibited the formation of 5-lipoxygenase-inflammatory mediators (5-HETE and LTB_4) and also inhibited PGE_2 release in a cell culture model. In vivo ciclopirox inhibited inflammation in an arachidonic acid-induced murine ear edema model. The clinical significance of these findings is unknown.

➤*Pharmacokinetics:*

Suspension – Penetration studies in human cadaverous skin from the back, with ciclopirox 0.77% cream with tagged ciclopirox showed the presence of 0.8% to 1.6% of the dose in the stratum corneum 1.5 to 6 hours after application. The levels in the dermis were still 10 to 15 times above the minimum inhibitory concentrations.

CICLOPIROX — TOPICAL

Pharmacokinetic studies in men with radiolabeled ciclopirox solution in polythylene glycol 400 showed an average of 1.3% absorption of the dose when it was applied topically to 750 cm^2 on the back followed by occlusion for 6 hours. The biological half-life was 1.7 hours and excretion occurred via the kidney. Two days after application, only 0.01% of the dose applied could be found in the urine. Fecal excretion was negligible. Autoradiographic studies with human cadaver skin showed that ciclopirox penetrates into the hair and through the epidermis and hair follicles into the sebaceous glands and dermis, while a portion of the drug remains in the stratum corneum.

Gel – A comparative study of the pharmacokinetics of ciclopirox 0.77% gel and 0.77% cream in 18 healthy males indicated that systemic absorption of ciclopirox from ciclopirox gel was higher than that of ciclopirox cream. A 5 g dose of ciclopirox gel produced a mean (± SD) peak serum concentration of 25.02 (± 20.6) ng/mL total ciclopirox and 5 g of ciclopirox cream produced 18.62 (± 13.56) ng/mL total ciclopirox. Approximately 3% of the applied ciclopirox was excreted in the urine within 48 hours after application, with a renal elimination half-life of about 5.5 hours. In a study of ciclopirox gel, 16 men with moderate to severe tinea cruris applied approximately 15 g/day of the gel for 14.5 days. The mean (± SD) dose-normalized values of C_{max} for total ciclopirox in serum were 100 (± 42) ng/mL on day 1 and 238 (± 144) ng/mL on day 15. During the 10 hours after dosing on day 1, approximately 10% of the administered dose was excreted in the urine.

Nail lacquer topical solution – As demonstrated in pharmacokinetic studies in animals and man, ciclopirox olamine is rapidly absorbed after oral administration and completely eliminated in all species via feces and urine. Most of the compound is excreted either unchanged or as glucuronide. After oral administration of 10 mg of radiolabeled drug (14C-ciclopirox) to healthy volunteers, approximately 96% of the radioactivity was excreted renally within 12 hours of administration. Ninety-four percent (94%) of the renally excreted radioactivity was in the form of glucuronides. Thus, glucuronidation is the main metabolic pathway of this compound.

Systemic absorption of ciclopirox was determined in 5 patients with dermatophytic onychomycoses, after application of ciclopirox 8% topical solution nail lacquer to all 20 digits and adjacent 5 mm of skin once daily for 6 months. Random serum concentrations and 24 hour urinary excretion of ciclopirox olamine were determined at 2 weeks and at 1, 2, 4, and 6 months after initiation of treatment and 4 weeks posttreatment. In this study, ciclopirox serum levels ranged from 12 to 80 ng/mL. Based on urinary data, mean absorption of ciclopirox from the dosage form was less than 5% of the applied dose. One month after cessation of treatment, serum and urine levels of ciclopirox olamine were below the limit of detection.

In 2 vehicle-controlled trials, patients applied ciclopirox 8% topical solution nail lacquer to all toenails and affected fingernails. Out of a total of 66 randomly selected patients on active treatment, 24 had detectable serum ciclopirox concentrations at some point during the dosing interval (range, 10 to 24.6 ng/mL). It should be noted that 11 of these 24 patients used concomitant medication containing ciclopirox as ciclopirox 0.77% cream.

The penetration of the ciclopirox 8% topical solution nail lacquer was evaluated in an in vitro investigation. Radiolabeled ciclopirox applied once to onychomycotic toenails that were avulsed demonstrated penetration up to a depth of approximately 0.4 mm. As expected, nail plate concentrations decreased as a function of nail depth. The clinical significance of these findings in nail plates is unknown. Nail bed concentrations were not determined.

Contraindications

Hypersensitivity to any of its components.

Warnings/Precautions

➤*For external use only:* Ciclopirox is not for ophthalmic, oral, or intravaginal use.

➤*Nail lacquer topical solution:* For use on nails and immediately adjacent skin only.

➤*Diabetes:* So far there is no relevant clinical experience with patients with type 1 diabetes or who have diabetic neuropathy. Carefully consider the risk of removal of the unattached, infected nail by the health care provider and trimming by the patient, before prescribing to patients with a history of type 1 diabetes mellitus or diabetic neuropathy.

➤*Gel:* A transient burning sensation may occur, especially after application to sensitive areas. Avoid contact with eyes. Efficacy of ciclopirox gel in immunosuppressed individuals has not been studied. Seborrheic dermatitis in association with acne, atopic dermatitis, parkinsonism, psoriasis, and rosacea has not been studied with ciclopirox gel. Efficacy in the treatment of plantar and vesicular types of tinea pedis has not been established.

➤*Hypersensitivity reactions:* If a reaction suggesting sensitivity or chemical irritation should occur with the use of ciclopirox, discontinue treatment and institute appropriate therapy.

➤*Pregnancy: Category B.* There are no adequate or well-controlled studies of topically applied ciclopirox in pregnant women. Use during pregnancy only if the potential benefit justifies the potential risk to the fetus.

➤*Lactation:* It is not known whether this drug is excreted in human milk. Since many drugs are excreted in human milk, exercise caution when is administering to a nursing woman.

➤*Children:*

Nail lacquer topical solution – Safety and efficacy in pediatric patients have not been established.

Gel and shampoo – Safety and efficacy in pediatric patients younger than 16 years of age have not been established.

Suspension – Safety and efficacy in pediatric patients younger than 10 years of age have not been established.

Drug Interactions

➤*Systemic antifungals:* No studies have been conducted to determine whether ciclopirox might reduce the efficacy of systemic antifungal agents for onychomycosis. Therefore, the concomitant use of ciclopirox 8% topical solution and systemic antifungal agents for onychomycosis is not recommended.

Adverse Reactions

➤*Nail lacquer topical solution:*

Dermatologic – In the vehicle-controlled clinical trials conducted in the US, 9% (30/327) of patients treated with ciclopirox topical solution nail lacquer and 7% (23/328) of patients treated with vehicle reported treatment-emergent adverse reactions considered by the investigator to be causally related to the test material.

The incidence of these adverse reactions within each body system was similar between the treatment groups except for dermatologic; 8% (27/327) and 4% (14/328) of subjects in the ciclopirox and vehicle groups reported at least 1 adverse reaction, respectively. The most common were rash-related adverse events: periungual erythema and erythema of the proximal nail fold were reported more frequently in patients treated with ciclopirox 8% topical solution nail lacquer (5% [16/327]) than in patients treated with vehicle (1% [3/328]). Other treatment-emergent adverse reactions thought to be causally related included nail disorders such as shape change, irritation, ingrown toenail, and discoloration.

The incidence of nail disorders was similar between the treatment groups (2% [6/327] in the ciclopirox 8% topical solution nail lacquer group and 2% [7/328] in the vehicle group). Moreover, application site reactions and/or burning of the skin occurred in 1% of patients treated with ciclopirox 8% topical solution nail lacquer (3/327) and vehicle (4/328).

A 21-Day Cumulative Irritancy study was conducted under conditions of semi-occlusion. Mild reactions were seen in 46% of patients with the ciclopirox 8% topical solution nail lacquer, 32% with the vehicle and 2% with the negative control, but all were reactions of mild transient erythema. There was no evidence of allergic contact sensitization for either the ciclopirox 8% topical solution nail lacquer or the vehicle base. In the vehicle-controlled studies, 1 patient treated with ciclopirox 8% topical solution nail lacquer discontinued treatment due to a rash localized to the palm (causal relation to test material undetermined).

Use of ciclopirox 8% topical solution nail lacquer for 48 additional weeks was evaluated in an open-label extension study conducted in patients previously treated in the vehicle-controlled studies. Three percent (9/281) of subjects treated with ciclopirox 8% topical solution nail lacquer experienced at least 1 treatment-emergent adverse reaction that the investigator thought was causally related to the test material. Mild rash in the form of periungual erythema (1% [2/281]) and nail disorders (1% [4/281]) were the most frequently reported. Four patients discontinued because of treatment-emergent adverse reactions. Two of the 4 had events considered to be related to test material: 1 patient's great toenail "broke away" and another had an elevated creatine phosphokinase level on day 1 (after 48 weeks of treatment with vehicle in the previous vehicle-controlled study).

➤*Suspension:*

Dermatologic – In the controlled clinical trial with 89 patients using ciclopirox suspension and 89 patients using the vehicle, the incidence of adverse reactions was low. Those considered possibly related to treatment or occurring in more than 1 patient were pruritus, which occurred in 2 patients using ciclopirox suspension and 1 patient using the suspension vehicle, and burning, which occurred in 1 patient using ciclopirox suspension.

➤*Gel:*

Dermatologic – In clinical trials, 140 (39%) of 359 subjects treated with ciclopirox gel reported adverse reactions, irrespective of relationship to test materials, that resulted in 8 subjects discontinuing treatment. The most frequent reaction reported was skin burning sensation upon application, which occurred in approximately 34% of seborrheic dermatitis patients and 7% of tinea pedis patients. Adverse reactions occurring between 1% to 5% were contact dermatitis and pruritus. Other reactions that occurred in less than 1% included dry skin, acne, rash, alopecia, pain upon application, eye pain, and facial edema.

Patient Information

➤*Nail lacquer topical solution:* Patients should have detailed instructions regarding the use of ciclopirox 8% topical solution nail lacquer as a component of a comprehensive management program for onychomycosis in order to achieve maximum benefit with the use of this product.

Tell the patient to:

1.) Use ciclopirox 8% topical solution nail lacquer as directed by a health care provider.
2.) Avoid contact with eyes and mucous membranes.
3.) Avoid contact with skin other than skin immediately surrounding the treated nail(s).

Apply ciclopirox 8% topical solution nail lacquer evenly over the entire nail plate and 5 mm of surrounding skin. If possible, apply ciclopirox 8% topical solution nail lacquer to the nail bed, hyponychium, and the under surface of the nail plate when it is free of the nail bed (eg, onycholysis). Contact with the surrounding skin may produce mild, transient irritation (redness).

CICLOPIROX — TOPICAL

Do not use this medication for any disorder other than that for which it is prescribed.

Discuss your treatment plan with your doctor for regular removal of the unattached, infected nail.

Before using this medication, tell your doctor if you are pregnant or nursing, are a type 1 diabetic or have diabetic neuropathy, have a history of immunosuppression, are immunocompromised (eg, received an organ transplant), require medication to control epilepsy, use or require topical corticosteroids on a repeated monthly basis, or use steroid inhalers on a regular basis.

1.) Avoid contact with the eyes and mucous membranes.
2.) Removal of the unattached, infected nail, as frequently as monthly, by a doctor is needed with use of this medication. Inform a doctor if you have diabetes or problems with numbness in your toes or fingers for consideration of the appropriate nail management program (before trimming your nails or removing nail material).
3.) Inform your doctor if the area of application shows signs of increased irritation (ie, redness, itching, burning, blistering, swelling, oozing).
4.) Up to 48 weeks of daily applications with ciclopirox 8% topical solution nail lacquer and professional removal, as frequently as monthly, of the unattached, infected nail are considered the full treatment time to achieve a clear or almost clear nail (defined as 10% or less residual nail involvement). Six months of therapy with professional removal of the unattached, infected nail may be required before initial improvement of symptoms is noticed.
5.) A completely clear nail may not be achieved with use of this medication. In clinical studies, less than 12% of patients were able to achieve either a clear or almost clear toenail.
6.) Do not use nail polish or other nail cosmetic products on the treated nails.
7.) Avoid use near heat or open flame because product is flammable.

Patient Instructions – Before starting treatment, remove any loose nail or nail material using nail clippers or nail files. If you have diabetes or problems with numbness in your toes or fingers, talk to your doctor before trimming your nails or removing any nail material.

Apply once daily (preferably at bedtime) to all affected nails with the applicator brush provided. Apply the lacquer evenly over the entire nail. Where possible, apply nail lacquer to the underside of the nail and to the skin beneath it. Allow lacquer to dry (approximately 30 seconds) before putting on socks or stockings. After applying medication, wait 8 hours before taking a bath or shower.

Apply ciclopirox 8% topical solution nail lacquer daily over the previous coat.

Once a week, remove the ciclopirox 8% topical solution nail lacquer with alcohol. Remove as much as possible of the damaged nail using nail clippers or nail files.

Repeat process (steps 2 through 4).

To prevent screw cap from sticking to the bottle, do not allow solution to get into the bottle threads.

To prevent the solution from drying out, bottle should be closed tightly after every use.

To protect from light, replace bottle into carton after each use.

➤*Suspension:*

1.) Use the medication for the full treatment time even though signs/symptoms may have improved; notify your doctor if there is no improvement after 4 weeks.
2.) Inform your doctor if the area of application shows signs of increased irritation (ie, redness, itching, burning, blistering, swelling, oozing) indicative of possible sensitization.
3.) Avoid the use of occlusive wrappings or dressings.

CLOTRIMAZOLE

otc/Rx[a]	**Clotrimazole** (Various, eg Taro)	**Cream:** 1%	1% benzyl alcohol, cetostearyl alcohol. Vanishing base. In 15, 30, 45, and 2 x 45 g tubes.
otc	**Cruex** (Novartis Consumer Health)		1% benzyl alcohol, cetostearyl alcohol. In 15 g.
otc	**Lotrimin AF** (Schering-Plough)		Benzyl alcohol, cetearyl alcohol. In 12 and 24 g.
otc	**Desenex** (Novartis Consumer Health)		1% benzyl alcohol, cetostearyl alcohol. In 15 and 30 g.
otc	**Lotrimin AF** (Schering-Plough)	**Lotion:** 1%	Benzyl alcohol, cetearyl alcohol. In 20 mL.
otc/Rx[a]	**Clotrimazole** (Various, eg Taro)	**Solution, topical:** 1%	PEG 400. In 30 mL.
otc	**Lotrimin AF** (Schering-Plough)		PEG. In 10 mL.
otc	**Fungi Cure Intensive** (Alva-Amco)	**Spray, solution; topical:** 1%	Alcohol. In 60 mL pump spray.

[a] Products are available *OTC* or *Rx*, depending on product labeling.

CLOTRIMAZOLE — TOPICAL

Indications

➤*Fungal infections:*

OTC products – Clotrimazole is an antifungal that cures most jock itch (tinea cruris), athlete's foot (tinea pedis), and ringworm (tinea corporis) due to *Trichophyton rubrum*, *Trichophyton mentagrophytes*, *Epidermophyton floccosum*, and *Microsporum canis*. Relieves itching, burning, cracking, and discomfort which can accompany these conditions.

Rx products – Topical treatments of candidiasis due to *Candida albicans* and tinea versicolor due to *Malassezia furfur*.

Administration and Dosage

➤*General dosing considerations:* For athlete's foot, wear well-fitting, ventilated shoes and change shoes and socks at least once a day.

OTC products – Not effective on scalp or nails.

➤*Adults:*

OTC –

Tinea corporis (Ringworm):
• *2 years of age and older* –
Cream: Apply a thin layer over affected area morning and evening for 4 weeks or as directed by a health care provider.

Tinea cruris (Jock itch):
• *2 years of age and older* –
Cream: Apply a thin layer over affected area morning and evening for 2 weeks or as directed by a health care provider.

Tinea pedis (Athlete's foot):
• *2 years of age and older* –
Cream: Apply a thin layer over affected area morning and evening for 4 weeks or as directed by a health care provider. For athlete's foot, pay special attention to the spaces between the toes.

Rx –

Candidiasis:
• *Solution or cream* – Gently massage sufficient clotrimazole into the affected and surrounding skin areas twice a day, in the morning and evening.

Clinical improvement, with relief of pruritus, usually occurs within the first week of treatment with clotrimazole. If the patient shows no clinical improvement after 4 weeks of treatment with clotrimazole, the diagnosis should be reviewed.

Tinea versicolor:
• *Solution or cream* – See Candidiasis for dosing.

➤*Children:*

OTC –

Tinea corporis (Ringworm):
• *2 years of age and older* – See Adults for dosing.

Tinea cruris (Jock itch):
• *2 years of age and older* – See Adults for dosing.

Tinea pedis (Athlete's foot):
• *2 years of age and older* – See Adults for dosing.

Rx –

Candidiasis:
• *Solution or cream* – See Adults for dosing.

Tinea versicolor:
• *Solution or cream* – See Adults for dosing.

➤*Administration:*

Cream (OTC) – Use tip of cap to break the seal and open the tube. Wash the affected skin with soap and water and dry completely before applying.

➤*Storage/Stability:* Store between 20° and 25°C (68° and 77°F). Do not use if seal is broken or is not visible. See tube crimp for lot number and expiration date.

Actions

➤*Pharmacology:* Clotrimazole is a broad-spectrum antifungal agent that is used for the treatment of dermal infections caused by various species of pathogenic dermatophytes, yeasts, and *Malassezia furfur*. The primary action of clotrimazole is against dividing and growing organisms.

In vitro, clotrimazole exhibits fungistatic and fungicidal activity against isolates of *Trichophyton rubrum*, *Trichophyton mentagrophytes*, *Epidermophyton floccosum*, *Microsporum canis*, and *Candida* species, including *Candida albicans*. In general, the in vitro activity of clotrimazole corresponds to that of tolnaftate and griseofulvin against the mycelia of dermatophytes (*Trichophyton*, *Microsporum*, and *Epidermophyton*), and to that of the polyenes (amphotericin B and nystatin) against budding fungi (*Candida*). Using an in vivo (mouse) and an in vitro (mouse kidney homogenate) testing system, clotrimazole and miconazole were equally effective in preventing the growth of the pseudomycelia and mycelia of *Candida albicans*.

CLOTRIMAZOLE — TOPICAL

➤*Pharmacokinetics:* Clotrimazole appears to be well absorbed in humans following oral administration and is eliminated mainly as inactive metabolites. Following topical and vaginal administration, however, clotrimazole appears to be minimally absorbed.

Six hours after the application of radioactive clotrimazole 1% cream and 1% solution onto intact and acutely inflamed skin, the concentration of clotrimazole varied from 100 mcg/cm^3, in the stratum corneum to 0.5 to 1 mcg/cm^3 in the stratum reticulare, and 0.1 mcg/cm^3 in the subcutis. No measurable amount of radioactivity (less than 0.001 mcg/mL) was found in the serum within 48 hours after application under occlusive dressing of 0.5 mL of the solution or 0.8 g of the cream. Only 0.5% or less of the applied radioactivity was excreted in the urine.

Contraindications

Hypersensitivity to any of their components.

Warnings/Precautions

➤*Sensitivity:* If irritation or sensitivity develops with the use of clotrimazole, treatment should be discontinued and appropriate therapy instituted.

➤*For external use only:* For external use only. Avoid contact with the eyes.

➤*Pregnancy: Category B.* The disposition of ^{14}C-clotrimazole has been studied in humans and animals. Clotrimazole is very poorly absorbed following dermal application or intravaginal administration to humans.

In clinical trials, use of vaginally applied clotrimazole in pregnant women in their second and third trimesters has not been associated with ill effects. There are, however, no adequate and well-controlled studies in pregnant women during the first trimester of pregnancy.

High oral doses of clotrimazole in rats and mice ranging from 50 to 120 mg/kg resulted in embryotoxicity (possibly secondary to maternal toxicity), impairment of mating, decreased litter size and number of viable young and decreased pup survival to weaning. However, clotrimazole was not teratogenic in mice, rabbits and rats at oral doses up to 200, 180, and 100 mg/kg, respectively. Oral absorption in the rat amounts to approximately 90% of the administered dose.

Because animal reproduction studies are not always predictive of human response, this drug should be used only if clearly indicated during the first trimester of pregnancy.

➤*Lactation:* It is not known whether this drug is excreted in human milk. Because many drugs are excreted in human milk, caution should be exercised when clotrimazole is used by a nursing woman.

➤*Children:* Do not use in children younger than 2 years of age unless directed by a physician.

➤*Monitoring:* If there is lack of response to clotrimazole, appropriate microbiological studies should be repeated to confirm the diagnosis and rule out other pathogens before instituting another course of antimycotic therapy.

Drug Interactions

None known.

Adverse Reactions

➤*Dermatologic:* Erythema, stinging, blistering, peeling, edema, pruritus, urticaria, burning, and general skin irritation.

Overdosage

Acute overdosage with topical application of clotrimazole is unlikely and would not be expected to lead to a life-threatening situation.

Patient Information

This information is intended to aid in the safe and effective use of this medication. It is not a disclosure of all possible adverse or intended effects.

For external use only.

Keep out of reach of children. If swallowed, get medical help or contact a poison control center right away.

Use the medication for the full treatment time even though the symptoms may have improved. Notify the physician if there is no improvement after 4 weeks of treatment.

Inform the physician if the area of application shows signs of increased irritation (eg, redness, itching, burning, blistering, swelling, oozing) indicative of possible sensitization.

Avoid use of occlusive wrappings/dressings.

Avoid sources of infection or reinfection.

➤*Do not use:*
- In or near the mouth or the eyes.
- For vaginal yeast infections.
- On nails or scalp.

ECONAZOLE NITRATE

Rx	**Econazole Nitrate** (Various, eg, Fougera, Taro)	**Cream:** 1%	In 15, 30, and 85 g.
Rx	**Spectazole** (Ortho Pharm. Corp.)		Water miscible base. Mineral oil. In 15, 30, and 85 g.

ECONAZOLE NITRATE — TOPICAL

Indications

➤*Fungal infection:* For treatment of tinea pedis, tinea cruris, and tinea corporis caused by *Trichophyton rubrum, Trichophyton mentagrophytes, Trichophyton tonsurans, Microsporum canis, Microsporum audouini, Microsporum gypseum,* and *Epidermophyton floccosum* in the treatment of cutaneous candidiasis, and in the treatment of tinea versicolor.

Administration and Dosage

➤*Adults:*

Tinea infection – Apply sufficient cream to affected areas once daily.

Cutaneous candidiasis – Apply sufficient cream to affected areas twice daily (morning and evening).

➤*Children:* See Adults for dosing.

➤*Duration of therapy:* Early relief of symptoms is experienced by the majority of patients, and clinical improvement may be seen fairly soon after treatment is begun; however, candidal infections and tinea cruris and corporis should be treated for 2 weeks and tinea pedis for 1 month in order to reduce the possibility of recurrence. Patients with tinea versicolor usually exhibit clinical and mycological clearing after 2 weeks of treatment.

➤*Administration:* For topical use only. Not for ophthalmic use.

➤*Storage/Stability:* Store below 30°C (86°F).

Actions

➤*Pharmacokinetics:*

Absorption – After topical application to the skin of healthy subjects, systemic absorption of econazole nitrate is extremely low.

Distribution – Although most of the applied drug remains on the skin surface, drug concentrations were found in the stratum corneum which, by far, exceeded the minimum inhibitory concentration for dermatophytes. Inhibitory concentrations were achieved in the epidermis and as deep as the middle region of the dermis.

Excretion – Less than 1% of the applied dose was recovered in the urine and feces.

➤*Microbiology:* Econazole nitrate has been shown to be active against most strains of the following microorganisms, both in vitro and in clinical infections.

Dermatophytes – *Epidermophyton floccosum, Microsporum audouini, Microsporum canis, Microsporum gypseum, Trichophyton mentagrophytes, Trichophyton rubrum, Trichophyton tonsurans, Trichophyton verrucosum.*

Yeasts – *Candida albicans, Candida guillermondii, Candida parapsilosis, Candida tropicalis, Malassezia furfur.*

Contraindications

Hypersensitivity to econazole or any of its ingredients.

Warnings/Precautions

➤*For external use only:* Econazole nitrate is not for ophthalmic use.

➤*Sensitivity:* If a reaction suggesting sensitivity or chemical irritation should occur, use of the medication should be discontinued.

➤*Pregnancy: Category C.* Econazole nitrate should be used in the first trimester of pregnancy only when the physician considers it essential to the welfare of the patient. The drug should be used during the second and third trimesters of pregnancy only if clearly needed.

➤*Lactation:* It is not known whether econazole nitrate is excreted in human milk. Following oral administration of econazole nitrate to lactating rats, econazole and/or metabolites were excreted in milk and were found in nursing pups. Also, in lactating rats receiving large oral doses (40 or 80 times the human dermal dose), there was a reduction in postpartum viability of pups and survival to weaning; however, at these high doses, maternal toxicity was present and may have been a contributing factor. Caution should be exercised when econazole nitrate is administered to a nursing woman.

Adverse Reactions

During clinical trials, approximately 3% of patients treated with econazole nitrate 1% cream reported side effects thought possibly to be due to the drug, consisting mainly of burning, itching, stinging, and erythema. One case of pruritic rash has also been reported.

ECONAZOLE NITRATE — TOPICAL

Overdosage

Overdosage of econazole nitrate in humans has not been reported to date. In mice, rats, guinea pigs and dogs, the oral LD_{50} values were found to be 462, 668, 272, and greater than 160 mg/kg, respectively.

Patient Information

For external use only. Avoid introduction of econazole nitrate cream into the eyes.

GENTIAN VIOLET

otc	**Gentian Violet** (Various, eg, Humco)	**Solution, topical:** 1%	In 30 mL.
		2%	In 30 mL.

GENTIAN VIOLET — TOPICAL

Indications

➤*Topical infection:* An antiseptic for the external treatment of abrasions, minor cuts, surface injuries, and superficial fungus infections of the skin.

Administration and Dosage

➤*General dosing considerations:* Medication will stain skin and clothing.

➤*Adults:*

Topical infection –

Usual dosage: Clean the wound and apply gentian violet directly to the wound, or use a cotton-tipped applicator once or twice daily. Do not bandage.

Discontinuation of therapy: If redness, irritation, swelling, or pain persists or increases, or if infection occurs, the patient should discontinue use and consult a health care provider.

➤*Administration:* This medication is for external use only.

Not for application to an ulcerative lesion, as this may result in "tattooing" of the skin.

Not for use in the eyes. In case of deep or puncture wounds or serious burns, the patient should consult a health care provider.

Actions

➤*Pharmacology:* Gentian violet is an antibacterial and antifungal dye. It is active against some gram-positive bacteria, especially *Staphylococcus* species. It inhibits the growth of *Candida*, *Cryptococcus*, *Epidermophyton*, and *Trichophyton*. Because of its staining properties and the availability of effective alternatives, gentian violet has generally been replaced in practice by other agents.

Warnings/Precautions

➤*General:* This medication is for external use only. Medication will stain skin and clothing. Do not apply to an ulcerative lesion as this may result in "tattooing" of the skin. Do not use in the eyes. In case of deep or puncture wounds or serious burns, consult a physician. If redness, irritation, swelling or pain persists or increases, or if infection occurs, discontinue use and consult a physician.

➤*Pregnancy: Category C* (per Briggs' *Drugs in Pregnancy and Lactation*).

Evidence has been found to suggest a relationship to malformations based on defects in patients who had first-trimester exposure to gentian violet.

➤*Lactation:* There are not data available on gentian violet in breast-feeding patients. Per Briggs' *Drugs in Pregnancy and Lactation*, there is potential toxicity when using gentian violet in breast-feeding patients.

Overdosage

In case of accidental ingestion, seek professional assistance or contact a poison control center immediately.

Patient Information

Gentian violet topical solution is an antiseptic for the external treatment of abrasions, minor cuts, surface injuries, and superficial fungus infections of the skin.

This medication contains gentian violet 1% or 2%, ethyl alcohol 10% (preservative), and purified water.

This medication is for external use only. Medication will stain skin and clothing. Do not apply to an ulcerative lesion as this may result in "tattooing" of the skin. Do not use in the eyes. In case of deep or puncture wounds or serious burns, consult a physician. If redness, irritation, swelling or pain persists or increases, or if infection occurs, discontinue use and consult a physician.

SERTACONAZOLE NITRATE

Rx	**Ertaczo** (OrthoNeutrogena)	**Cream:** 2%	Lt. mineral oil, methylparaben. In 15 and 30 g tubes.

SERTACONAZOLE NITRATE — TOPICAL

Indications

➤*Tinea pedis:* For the topical treatment of interdigital tinea pedis in immunocompetent patients 12 years of age and older, caused by *Trichophyton rubrum*, *Trichophyton mentagrophytes*, and *Epidermophyton floccosum*.

Administration and Dosage

➤*Adults:*

Tinea pedis –

Usual dosage: Apply twice daily for 4 weeks. A sufficient amount of cream should be applied to cover the affected areas between the toes and the immediately surrounding healthy skin of patients with interdigital tinea pedis.

If a patient shows no clinical improvement 2 weeks after the treatment period, the diagnosis should be reviewed.

Duration of therapy: 4 weeks.

➤*Children:*

Tinea pedis –

12 years of age and older: See Adults for dosing.

➤*Storage/Stability:* Store at 25°C (77°F); excursions are permitted between 15° and 30°C (59° and 86°F).

Actions

➤*Pharmacokinetics:* In a multiple-dose pharmacokinetic study that included 5 male patients with interdigital tinea pedis (range of diseased area, 42 to 140 cm^2; mean, 93 cm^2), sertaconazole nitrate 2% cream was applied topically every 12 hours for a total of 13 doses to the diseased skin (0.5 g sertaconazole nitrate per 100 cm^2). Sertaconazole concentrations in plasma measured by serial blood sampling for 72 hours after the 13th dose were below the limit of quantitation (2.5 ng/mL) of the analytical method used.

➤*Microbiology:* Sertaconazole is an antifungal that belongs to the imidazole class of antifungals. While the exact mechanism of action of this class of antifungals is not known, it is believed that they act primarily by inhibiting the cytochrome P-450-dependent synthesis of ergosterol. Ergosterol is a key component of the cell membrane of fungi, and lack of this component leads to fungal cell injury primarily by leakage of key constituents in the cytoplasm from the cell.

Activity in vivo – Sertaconazole nitrate has been shown to be active against isolates of the following microorganisms in clinical infections: *Trichophyton rubrum*, *Trichophyton mentagrophytes*, and *Epidermophyton floccosum*.

Contraindications

Sensitivity to sertaconazole nitrate or any of its components or to other imidazoles.

Warnings/Precautions

➤*For external use only:* Sertaconazole nitrate 2% cream is not indicated for ophthalmic, oral, or intravaginal use.

➤*Sensitivity:* Sertaconazole nitrate 2% cream is for use on the skin only. If irritation or sensitivity develops, treatment should be discontinued and appropriate therapy instituted.

➤*Diagnosis:* Diagnosis of the disease should be confirmed either by direct microscopic examination of infected superficial epidermal tissue in a solution of potassium hydroxide or by culture on an appropriate medium.

➤*Hypersensitivity reactions:* Physicians should exercise caution when prescribing sertaconazole nitrate 2% cream to patients known to be sensitive to imidazole antifungals, since cross-reactivity may occur.

➤*Special risk:* Physicians should exercise caution when prescribing sertaconazole nitrate 2% cream to patients known to be sensitive to imidazole antifungals, since cross-reactivity may occur.

➤*Pregnancy: Category C.* In an oral peripostnatal study in rats, a reduction in live birth indices and an increase in the number of still-born pups was seen at 80 and 160 mg/kg/day.

There are no adequate and well-controlled studies that have been conducted on topically applied sertaconazole nitrate 2% cream in pregnant women. Because animal reproduction studies are not always predictive of human response, sertaconazole nitrate 2% cream should be used during pregnancy only if clearly needed.

➤*Lactation:* It is not known if sertaconazole is excreted in human milk. Because many drugs are excreted in human milk, caution should be exercised when prescribing sertaconazole nitrate 2% cream to a nursing woman.

SERTACONAZOLE NITRATE — TOPICAL

➤*Children:* The efficacy and safety have not been established in pediatric patients below the age of 12 years.

Drug Interactions

None known.

Adverse Reactions

➤*Dermatologic:* In clinical trials, cutaneous adverse events occurred in 7 of 297 (2%) patients (2 of them severe) receiving sertaconazole nitrate 2% cream and in 7 of 291 (2%) patients (2 of them severe) receiving vehicle. These reported cutaneous adverse events included contact dermatitis, dry skin, burning skin, application site reaction and skin tenderness.

In a dermal sensitization study, 8 of 202 evaluable patients tested with sertaconazole nitrate 2% cream and 4 of 202 evaluable patients tested with vehicle, exhibited a slight erythematous reaction in the challenge phase. There was no evidence of cumulative irritation or contact sensitization in a repeated insult patch test involving 202 healthy volunteers. In non-US postmarketing surveillance for sertaconazole nitrate 2% cream, the following cutaneous adverse events were reported: Contact dermatitis, erythema, pruritus, vesiculation, desquamation, and hyperpigmentation.

Overdosage

Overdosage with sertaconazole nitrate 2% cream has not been reported to date. Sertaconazole nitrate 2% cream is intended for topical dermatologic use only. It is not for oral, ophthalmic, or intravaginal use.

Patient Information

Use sertaconazole nitrate 2% cream as directed by the physician. The hands should be washed after applying the medication to the affected area(s). Avoid contact with the eyes, nose, mouth and other mucous membranes. Sertaconazole nitrate 2% cream is for external use only.

Dry the affected area(s) thoroughly before application, if you wish to use sertaconazole nitrate 2% cream after bathing.

Use the medication for the full treatment time recommended by the physician, even though symptoms may have improved. Notify the physician if there is no improvement after the end of the prescribed treatment period, or sooner, if the condition worsens.

Inform the physician if the area of application shows signs of increased irritation, redness, itching, burning, blistering, swelling or oozing.

Avoid the use of occlusive dressings unless otherwise directed by the physician.

Do not use this medication for any disorder other than that for which it was prescribed.

KETOCONAZOLE

Rx	**Ketoconazole** (Various, eg, Fougera, Taro, Teva)	**Cream; topical:** 2%	Cetyl alcohol, sodium sulfite, stearyl alcohol. In 15, 30, and 60 g.
Rx	**Extina** (GlaxoSmithKline)	**Foam; topical** : 2%	Cetyl alcohol, ethanol 58%, stearyl alcohol. In 50 and 100 g.
Rx	**Xolegel** (GlaxoSmithKline)	**Gel; topical:** 2%	Dehydrated alcohol 34%, glycerin. In 2 and 15 g tubes.
otc	**Nizoral A-D** (McNeil Consumer)	**Shampoo; topical:** 1%	Tetrasodium EDTA. In 207 mL.
Rx	**Ketoconazole** (Various, eg, Patriot, Perrigo, Sandoz)	**Shampoo; topical:** 2%	In 120 mL.
Rx	**Nizoral** (McNeil Consumer)		In 120 mL.

KETOCONAZOLE — TOPICAL

Indications

➤*Cream:* For topical treatment of tinea corporis (ringworm), tinea cruris (jock itch), and tinea pedis (athlete's foot) caused by *Trichophyton rubrum*, *Trichophyton mentagrophytes*, and *Epidermophyton floccosum*; tinea (pityriasis) versicolor caused by *Pityrosporum orbiculare* (also known as *Malassezia furfur*); cutaneous candidiasis caused by *Candida* sp.; and seborrheic dermatitis.

➤*Foam / Gel:* For the topical treatment of seborrheic dermatitis in immunocompetent adults and children 12 years of age and older.

➤*Shampoo 1%:* Controls flaking, scaling, and itching associated with dandruff.

➤*Shampoo 2%:* For the treatment of tinea versicolor caused by or presumed to be caused by *P. orbiculare* (*M. furfur* or *Malassezia orbiculare*).

Tinea versicolor may give rise to hyperpigmented or hypopigmented patches on the trunk, which may extend to the neck, arms, and upper thighs. Treatment of the infection may not immediately result in normalization of pigment to the affected sites. Normalization of pigment following successful therapy is variable and may take months, depending on individual skin type and incidental sun exposure. Although tinea versicolor is not contagious, it may recur because the organism that causes the disease is part of the normal skin flora.

Administration and Dosage

➤*Adults:*

Cutaneous candidiasis –

Cream:

• *Usual dosage* – Apply once daily to cover the affected and immediate surrounding area.

• *Duration of therapy* – Clinical improvement may be seen fairly soon after treatment is begun; however, treat candidal infections for 2 weeks in order to reduce the possibility of recurrence.

Dandruff –

Shampoo 1%: Wet hair thoroughly. Apply shampoo, generously lather, and rinse thoroughly. Repeat use every 3 to 4 days for up to 8 weeks or as directed by a doctor. Then use only as needed to control dandruff.

Seborrheic dermatitis –

Cream: Apply to the affected area twice daily for 4 weeks or until clinical clearing. If the patient shows no clinical improvement after the treatment period, redetermine the diagnosis.

Foam: Apply to the affected area twice daily for 4 weeks.

Gel: Apply once daily to the affected area for 2 weeks.

Tinea corporis, tinea cruris, and tinea pedis –

Cream:

• *Usual dosage* – Apply once daily to cover the affected and immediate surrounding area.

• *Duration of therapy* – Clinical improvement may be seen fairly soon after treatment is begun; however, treat tinea cruris and corporis for 2 weeks in order to reduce the possibility of recurrence. Patients with tinea pedis require 6 weeks of treatment.

Tinea versicolor –

Cream:

• *Usual dosage* – Apply once daily to cover the affected and immediate surrounding area.

• *Duration of therapy* – Patients with tinea versicolor usually require 2 weeks of treatment.

Shampoo 2%: Apply the shampoo to the damp skin of the affected area and a wide margin surrounding this area. Lather, leave in place for 5 minutes, and rinse off with water. One application of the shampoo should be sufficient.

➤*Children:*

Dandruff –

12 years of age or older:

• *Shampoo 1%* – See Adults for dosing.

Seborrheic dermatitis –

12 years of age or older:

• *Foam* – Apply to the affected area twice daily for 4 weeks.

• *Gel* – Apply once daily to the affected area for 2 weeks.

➤*Administration:* Avoid contact with the eyes and other mucous membranes. Not for ophthalmic, oral, or intravaginal use.

Foam – Hold the container upright and dispense ketoconazole foam into the cap of the can or other cool surface in an amount sufficient to cover the affected area(s). Dispensing directly onto hands is not recommended because the foam will begin to melt immediately upon contact with warm skin. Pick up small amounts of ketoconazole foam with the fingertips and gently massage into the affected area until the foam disappears. For hair-bearing areas, part the hair so that ketoconazole foam may be applied directly to the skin (rather than on the hair).

Shampoo – Do not use on areas of the scalp that are broken or inflamed.

➤*Storage / Stability:*

Cream – Store at 20° to 25°C (68° to 77°F). Do not store above 25°C (77°F).

Foam – Store at controlled room temperature, 20° to 25°C (68° to 77°F). Do not store under refrigerated conditions. Do not expose containers to heat and/or store at temperatures above 49°C (120°F). Do not store in direct sunlight. Contents are flammable. Contents are under pressure. Do not puncture and/or incinerate the container. Keep out of the reach of children.

Gel – Store at 25°C (77°F); excursions are permitted between 15° and 30°C (59° and 86°F). Keep out of the reach of children.

Shampoo 1% – Store between 2° and 30°C (35° and 86°F). Protect from light and freezing.

Shampoo 2% – Do not store at temperatures above 25°C (77°F). Protect from light.

KETOCONAZOLE — TOPICAL

Actions

➤*Pharmacology:* Ketoconazole is a broad spectrum synthetic antifungal agent. In vitro/in vivo studies suggest it impairs ergosterol synthesis, which is a vital component of fungal cell membranes. The therapeutic effect in seborrheic dermatitis and dandruff may be due to reduction of *Pityrosporum ovale* (*Malassezia ovale*), but this has not yet been proven.

It is postulated, but not proven, that the therapeutic effect of ketoconazole in tinea versicolor is due to the reduction of *P. orbiculare* (*M. furfur*).

Hypersensitivity/Phototoxicity –
Cream: Two dermal irritancy studies, a human sensitization test, a phototoxicity study, and a photoallergy study conducted in 38 men and 62 women showed no contact sensitization of the delayed hypersensitivity type, no irritation, no phototoxicity, and no photoallergenic potential caused by ketoconazole cream.

Shampoo 2%: An exaggerated use washing test on the sensitive antecubital skin of 10 subjects twice daily for 5 consecutive days showed that the irritancy potential of ketoconazole shampoo 2% was significantly less than that of selenium sulfide shampoo 2.5%.

A human sensitization test, a phototoxicity study, and a photoallergy study conducted in 38 men and 22 women showed no contact sensitization of the delayed hypersensitivity type, no phototoxicity, and no photoallergenic potential caused by ketoconazole shampoo 2%.

➤*Pharmacokinetics:*
Absorption –
Cream: After a single topical application of ketoconazole cream to the chest, back, and arms of healthy volunteers, systemic absorption of ketoconazole was not detected at the 5 ng/mL level in blood over a 72-hour period.

Foam: In a bioavailability study, 12 subjects with moderate to severe seborrheic dermatitis applied 3 g of ketoconazole foam twice daily for 4 weeks. Circulating plasma levels of ketoconazole were less than 6 ng/mL for a majority of subjects (75%), with a maximum level of 11 ng/mL observed in 1 subject.

Gel: In a pharmacokinetic absorption study, 18 subjects (both men and women) with severe seborrheic dermatitis (range, 1% to 14% of body surface area) applied ketoconazole gel once daily for 2 weeks. The median total amount of gel applied was 4.6 g (range, 1.65 to 46.3 g). Daily doses ranged from 0.05 to 3.47 g. Mean (± standard deviation [SD]) peak plasma levels were 1.35 ng/mL (± 3.18 ng/mL) on day 7 (range, from less than 0.1 to 13.9 ng/mL) and 0.8 ng/mL (± 1.22 ng/mL) on day 14 (range, from less than 0.1 to 5.4 ng/mL). Median time to peak concentration was 8 hours on day 7 and 7 hours on day 14. Mean (± SD) area under the curve (AUC_{0-24}) values were 20.8 ng•h/mL (± 44.7 ng/mL) and 15.6 ng•h/mL (± 26.4 ng/mL) on days 7 and 14, respectively.

The plasma levels from an oral dose of ketoconazole 200 mg taken with a meal are approximately 250 times higher than the resulting plasma levels of ketoconazole following topical application of ketoconazole gel.

Shampoo 2%: Ketoconazole was not detected in plasma in 39 patients who shampooed 4 to 10 times per week for 6 months or in 33 patients who shampooed 2 to 3 times per week for 3 to 26 months (mean, 16 months).

➤*Microbiology:* Ketoconazole inhibits the in vitro growth of the following common dermatophytes and yeasts by altering the permeability of the cell membrane. Dermatophytes: *T. rubrum*, *T. mentagrophytes*, *Trichophyton tonsurans*, *Microsporum canis*, *Microsporum audouinii*, *Microsporum gypseum*, and *Epidermophyton floccosum*. Yeasts: *Candida albicans*, *Candida tropicalis*, *P. ovale* (*M. ovale*); and *P. orbiculare* (*M. furfur*. Only those organisms listed in the indications section have been proven to be clinically affected.

Contraindications

Hypersensitivity to ketoconazole or any component of the product(s).

Warnings/Precautions

➤*For external use only:* Avoid contact with the eyes and other mucous membranes. Not for ophthalmic, oral, or intravaginal use. If irritation occurs or the disease worsens, instruct patients to discontinue the medication and contact their health care provider.

Flammable contents (foam/gel) – The contents of ketoconazole foam include alcohol and propane/butane and ketoconazole gel includes alcohol. These contents are flammable. Avoid fire, flame, and/or smoking during and immediately following applications of ketoconazole foam or gel. Do not puncture and/or incinerate the foam containers. Do not expose foam containers to heat and/or store at temperatures above 49°C (120°F).

Shampoo – If product gets into the eyes, instruct patient to rinse them thoroughly with water. Do not use on areas of the scalp that are broken or inflamed.

➤*Systemic effects:* Hepatitis has been seen with orally administered ketoconazole (1:10,000 reported incidence). Lowered testosterone and adrenocorticotropic hormone–induced corticosteroid serum levels have been seen with high doses of orally administered ketoconazole. These effects have not been seen with topical ketoconazole.

➤*Hypersensitivity reactions:* Topical ketoconazole use may result in contact sensitization, including photoallergenicity. Discontinue topical ketoconazole product if a reaction suggesting sensitivity or chemical irritation occurs.

➤*Sulfite sensitivity:* Ketoconazole cream contains sulfites that may cause allergic-type reactions, including anaphylactic symptoms and life-threatening or less severe asthmatic episodes in certain susceptible persons. The overall prevalence of sulfite sensitivity in the general population is unknown and probably low. It is seen more frequently in asthmatic than nonasthmatic persons.

➤*Pregnancy: Category C.* There are no adequate and well-controlled studies in pregnant women. Use ketoconazole during pregnancy only if the potential benefit justifies the potential risk to the fetus.

Teratogenic – In rats, ketoconazole has been shown to be teratogenic (syndactylia and oligodactylia) when given orally in the diet at 80 mg/kg/day and embryotoxic at 160 mg/kg/day. However, these effects may be related to maternal toxicity, which was seen at this and higher dose levels.

Nonteratogenic – Oral doses of 10, 20, 40, 80, and 160 mg/kg were studied in prenatal and postnatal development studies in rats. Doses of 40 mg/kg (38 times the human dose) and higher were associated with maternal toxicity, an increase in the length of gestation, and an increase in the number of stillborn fetuses. These doses of ketoconazole were also toxic to the offspring, resulting in a decrease in fetal/pup weights and viability.

➤*Lactation:* It is not known whether ketoconazole administered topically could result in sufficient systemic absorption to produce detectable quantities in breast milk. Nevertheless, decide whether to discontinue breastfeeding or the drug, taking into account the importance of the drug to the mother. Exercise caution when administering ketoconazole to a breastfeeding woman.

➤*Children:*
Cream/Shampoo 2% – Safety and efficacy in children have not been established.

Foam/Gel/Shampoo 1% – Safety and efficacy in children younger than 12 years of age have not been established.

➤*Elderly:* No overall differences in safety or efficacy were observed between elderly and younger subjects, but greater sensitivity of some older individuals cannot be ruled out.

Drug Interactions

None known.

Adverse Reactions

➤*Cream:* Pruritus, severe irritation, stinging (5%); painful allergic reaction (1 patient).

➤*Foam:*

Ketoconazole Foam Adverse Reactions (> 1%)[a]

Adverse reaction	Ketoconazole foam (n = 672)	Vehicle foam (n = 497)
Subjects with an adverse reaction	28%	25%
Application-site burning	10%	10%
Application-site reaction	6%	5%

[a] Application-site reactions that were reported in 1% or less of subjects were dryness, erythema, irritation, paresthesia, pruritus, rash, and warmth.

Hypersensitivity – In a photoallergenicity study, 9 of 53 (17%) subjects had reactions during the challenge period at both the irradiated and nonirradiated sites treated with ketoconazole foam. Ketoconazole foam may cause contact sensitization.

➤*Gel:*

Ketoconazole Gel Adverse Reactions (> 1%)[a]

Adverse reaction	Ketoconazole gel (n = 545)	Gel vehicle (n = 388)
Any adverse reaction	16.3%	17.3%
Application-site burning	4.2%	3.1%
Headache	1.1%	0.8%

[a] The same adverse reaction recorded by a subject at different visits count as 1 reaction for that subject, and the strongest intensity and relationship to treatment is used. At each level of summarization (system organ class and preferred term), subjects are only counted once.

The most common treatment-related adverse reaction was application-site burning (see the previous table). Treatment-related application-site reactions that were reported in less than 1% of subjects were dermatitis, discharge, dryness, erythema, irritation, pain, pruritus, and pustules. Other treatment-related adverse reactions that were reported in less than 1% of subjects were acne, dizziness, eye irritation, eye swelling, facial swelling, headache, impetigo, keratoconjunctivitis sicca, nail discoloration, paresthesia, and pyogenic granuloma.

Hypersensitivity – Contact sensitization, cumulative irritation, photoallergy, and phototoxicity studies were conducted with ketoconazole gel. Under the conditions of study, ketoconazole gel did not demonstrate contact sensitization, photoallergenicity, or phototoxicity but did demonstrate potential to cause irritation.

➤*Shampoo 1%:* Increased or abnormal hair loss; itching; mild irritation or stinging; oiliness and dryness of hair and scalp; reddening, blistering, peeling, itching, or burning of skin.

KETOCONAZOLE — TOPICAL

➤*Shampoo 2%:* Application-site reaction, dry skin, pruritus (less than 3%); increase in normal hair loss, irritation (less than 1%); abnormal hair texture, itching, mild dryness of the skin, oiliness/dryness of hair and scalp, scalp pustules.

➤*Postmarketing:*

Cream – Contact dermatitis has been reported rarely and associated with ketoconazole cream or one of its excipients, namely sodium sulfite or propylene glycol.

Shampoo – Hair discoloration (rare).

Overdosage

➤*Treatment:* Topical ketoconazole products are intended for external use only. In the event of accidental ingestion, instruct patients to contact a health care provider or poison control center and employ supportive measures. Avoid induced emesis and gastric lavage.

Patient Information

Ketoconazole is for external use only. It may be irritating to mucous membranes. Avoid contact with the eyes, nostrils, and mouth.

As with any topical medication, instruct patients to wash their hands before and after application.

Instruct patients not to use this medication for any disorder other than that for which it has been prescribed and to use it only as directed by their health care provider.

Instruct patients to report any signs of adverse reactions or increased irritation in the area of application to their health care provider.

➤*Foam:* Avoid fire, flame, and/or smoking during and immediately following application.

Do not apply foam directly to hands. Dispense onto a cool surface and apply to the affected areas using the fingertips.

Foam may cause irritation (application-site burning and/or reactions).

Foam may cause contact sensitization.

➤*Shampoo:* Inform patients that removal of the curl from permanently waved hair may occur.

MICONAZOLE NITRATE

otc	**Aloe Vesta** (ConvaTec)	**Ointment; topical:** 2%	Aloe, mineral oil, white petrolatum. In 56 and 141 g.
otc	**Triple Paste AF** (Summers Labs)		Beeswax, lanolin, stearyl alcohol, white petrolatum, zinc oxide. In 56.7 g.
otc	**Tetterine** (S.S.S. Company)		Petrolatum. In 28.4 g.
otc	**Miconazole Nitrate** (Taro)	**Cream; topical:** 2%	Benzoic acid, mineral oil, apricot kernal oil. In 15 and 30 g.
otc	**Micatin** (Ortho)		Mineral oil. In 15 and 30 g.
otc	**Neosporin AF** (Pfizer Consumer Healthcare)		Mineral oil. In 14 g.
otc	**Desenex** (Novartis Consumer Health)	**Powder; topical:** 2%	Talc. In 43 and 85 g.
otc	**Micatin** (Ortho)		In 90 g.
otc	**Lotrimin AF** (Schering-Plough)		Talc. In 90 g.
otc	**Zeasorb-AF** (GlaxoSmithKline)		Talc. In 71 g.
otc	**Cruex** (Novartis)	**Aerosol, powder; topical:** 2%	Aloe, 10% SD alcohol. In 85 g.
otc	**Lotrimin AF** (Schering-Plough)		10% SD alcohol 40. In 100 g.
otc	**Micatin** (Ortho)		Alcohol. Available with and without deodorant. In 90 g.
otc	**Ting** (Insight Pharmaceuticals)		10% SD alcohol 40, aloe vera gel. In 85 g.
otc	**Desenex Liquid Spray** (Novartis Consumer Health)	**Aerosol, spray; topical:** 2%	PEG 300, SD alcohol 40-B. In 133 g.
otc	**Micatin** (Ortho)		Alcohol. In 105 mL.
otc	**Lotrimin AF** (Schering-Plough)		17% SD alcohol 40. In 113 mL.
otc	**Neosporin AF** (Schering-Plough)		Alcohol. In 105 g.
otc	**Fungoid Tincture** (Pedinol)	**Solution; topical:** 2%	Alcohol. In 7.39 and 29.57 mL with brush applicator.
otc	**Zeasorb-AF** (GlaxoSmithKline)	**Gel; topical:** 2%	Alcohol. In 24 g.

MICONAZOLE NITRATE — TOPICAL

Indications

Treatment of athlete's foot (tinea pedis), jock itch (tinea cruris) and ringworm (tinea corporis). For effective relief of the itching, burning, cracking and scaling which can accompany these conditions.

Administration and Dosage

➤*General dosing considerations:* This product is not effective on the scalp or nails.

➤*Adults:*

Athlete's foot (tinea pedis) –

Usual dosage: Apply a thin layer twice a day, or as directed by a health care provider.

Duration of therapy: Use daily for 4 weeks. If condition persists longer, consult a health care provider.

Jock itch (tinea cruris) –

Usual dosage: Apply a thin layer twice a day, or as directed by a health care provider.

Duration of therapy: Use daily for 2 weeks. If condition persists longer, consult a health care provider.

Ringworm (tinea corporis) – See Athlete's Foot (Tinea Pedis) for dosing.

➤*Children:*

2 years of age and older – See Adults for dosing.

➤*Administration:* Clean the affected area and dry thoroughly. Shake spray can well, hold 4 to 6 inches from skin. Apply or spray a thin layer of the product over affected area twice daily (morning and night) or as directed by a health care provider.

For athlete's foot, pay special attention to the spaces between the toes. Wear well-fitting, ventilated shoes, and change shoes and socks at least once daily.

➤*Storage/Stability:* Store at room temperature, 15° to 30°C (59°to 86°F).

Sprays – Contents under pressure. Do not puncture or incinerate. Flammable mixture, do not use near fire or flame. Do not expose to heat or temperatures above 49°C (120°F). Use only as directed. Intentional misuse by deliberately concentrating and inhaling the contents can be harmful or fatal.

Warnings/Precautions

➤*For external use only:* Avoid contact with the eyes or other mucous membranes.

➤*Irritation:* If irritation occurs, discontinue use and consult a doctor. Use only as directed.

➤*Pregnancy: Category C.* If pregnant, ask a health professional before use. Briggs' *Drugs in Pregnancy and Lactation* lists topical miconazole as compatible with pregnancy.

➤*Lactation:* Because miconazole has poor oral bioavailability, it is unlikely to adversely affect the breast-fed infant, including topical application to the nipples. Instruct the patient to remove any excess cream or ointment from the nipples before breast-feeding.

➤*Children:* Do not use on children under 2 years of age unless directed by a doctor. Keep this and all drugs out of the reach of children. In case of accidental ingestion, seek professional assistance or contact a poison control center immediately.

NAFTIFINE HYDROCHLORIDE

Rx	**Naftin** (Merz Pharmaceutical)	**Cream:** 1%	In 15, 30 and 60 g.
		Gel: 1%	In 20, 40 and 60 g.

NAFTIFINE HYDROCHLORIDE — TOPICAL

Indications

➤*Fungal infection:* For the topical treatment of tinea pedis, tinea cruris, and tinea corporis caused by the organisms *Trichophyton rubrum, Trichophyton mentagrophytes, Trichophyton tonsurans* and *Epidermophyton floccosum.* Efficacy for these organisms in this organ system was studied in fewer than 10 infections.

Administration and Dosage

➤*Adults:*

Fungal infection – A sufficient quantity should be gently massaged into the affected and surrounding skin areas once a day in the morning and evening.

If no clinical improvement is seen after 4 weeks of treatment with naftifine hydrochloride gel or cream 1%, the patient should be re-evaluated.

➤*Administration:* Apply topically once daily in the morning and evening. The hands should be washed after application.

➤*Storage/Stability:*

Gel – Store at room temperature.

Cream – Store below 30°C (86°F).

Actions

➤*Pharmacology:* Naftifine hydrochloride is a synthetic, allylamine derivative. The following in vitro data are available, but their clinical significance is unknown. Naftifine hydrochloride has been shown to exhibit fungicidal activity in vitro against a broad spectrum of organisms including *Trichophyton rubrum, Trichophyton mentagrophytes, Trichophyton tonsurans, Epidermophyton floccosum,* and *Microsporum canis, Microsporum audouini,* and *Microsporum gypseum*; and fungistatic activity against *Candida* species including *Candida albicans.* Naftifine hydrochloride gel and cream 1% have only been shown to be clinically effective against the disease entities listed in the Indications.

Although the exact mechanism of action against fungi is not known, naftifine hydrochloride appears to interfere with sterol biosynthesis by inhibiting the enzyme squalene 2,3-epoxidase. This inhibition of enzyme activity results in decreased amounts of sterols, especially ergosterol, and a corresponding accumulation of squalene in the cells.

➤*Pharmacokinetics:* In vitro and in vivo bioavailability studies have demonstrated that naftifine penetrates the stratum corneum in sufficient concentration to inhibit the growth of dermatophytes.

Following a single topical application of 1% naftifine cream to the skin of healthy subjects, systemic absorption was approximately 6% of the applied dose.

Following single topical applications of ^{3}H-labeled naftifine gel 1% to the skin of healthy subjects, up to 4.2% of the applied dose was absorbed. Naftifine and/or its metabolites are excreted via the urine and feces with a half-life of approximately two to three days.

Contraindications

Hypersensitivity to any of its components.

Warnings/Precautions

➤*For external use only:* Naftifine hydrochloride gel and cream 1% are for topical use only and not for ophthalmic use.

➤*Irritation/diagnosis:* Naftifine hydrochloride gel and cream 1% are for external use only. If irritation or sensitivity develop with the use of naftifine hydrochloride gel or cream 1%, treatment should be discontinued and appropriate therapy instituted. Diagnosis of the disease should be confirmed either by direct microscopic examination of a mounting of infected tissue in a solution of potassium hydroxide or by culture on an appropriate medium.

➤*Pregnancy: Category B.* There are no adequate and well-controlled studies in pregnant women. This drug should be used during pregnancy only if clearly needed.

➤*Lactation:* It is not known whether this drug is excreted in human milk. Because many drugs are excreted in human milk, caution should be exercised when naftifine hydrochloride gel or cream 1% is administered to a nursing woman.

➤*Children:* Safety and effectiveness in pediatric patients have not been established.

Adverse Reactions

➤*Gel:*

Dermatologic – During clinical trials, the incidence of adverse reactions was as follows: Burning/stinging (5%), itching (1%), erythema (0.5%), rash (0.5%), skin tenderness (0.5%).

➤*Cream:*

Dermatologic – During clinical trials, the incidence of adverse reactions was as follows: Burning/stinging (6%), dryness (3%), erythema (2%), itching (2%), local irritation (2%).

Patient Information

Avoid the use of occlusive dressings or wrappings unless otherwise directed by the physician.

Keep naftifine hydrochloride gel or cream 1% away from the eyes, nose, mouth and other mucous membranes.

NYSTATIN

Rx	**Nystatin** (Various, eg, Major, NMC)	**Cream:** 100,000 units/g	In 15 and 30 g.
Rx	**Pediaderm AF** (Arbor Pharmaceuticals)		Aluminum hydroxide gel, medical antifoam AF emulsion, parabens, PEG 400, propylene glycol, titanium dioxide, white petrolatum. In 30 g with Diaper Defense Cream (beeswax, lt. mineral oil, parabens, paraffin, PEG-30, vitamin E, white petrolatum, zinc oxide).
Rx	**Mycostatin** (Westwood Squibb)		Aqueous vanishing cream base. In 15 and 30 g.
Rx	**Nystatin** (Various, eg, Goldline, Major, Moore, NMC)	**Ointment:** 100,000 units/g	In 15 and 30 g.
Rx	**Mycostatin** (Westwood Squibb)		Polyethylene and mineral oil gel base. In 15 and 30 g.
Rx	**Nystatin** (Various, eg, Par)	**Powder:** 100,000 units/g	Dispersed in talc. In 15 and 60 g.
Rx	**Mycostatin** (Westwood Squibb)		Dispersed in talc. In 15 g.
Rx	**Nystop** (Paddock)		Dispersed in talc. In 15 and 30 g.
Rx	**Pedi-Dri** (Pedinol)		Dispersed in talc. In 56.7 g.

NYSTATIN — TOPICAL

Indications

➤*Mycotic infections:* Treatment of cutaneous or mucocutaneous mycotic infections, caused by *Candida (Monilia) albicans* and other *Candida* species. Conditions such as athlete's foot (dermatophytosis), perleche, paronychia, intertrigo, diaper rash, and other cutaneous lesions can be expected to respond. The cream is usually preferred to the ointment in moniliasis involving intertriginous areas.

Administration and Dosage

➤*General dosing considerations:* Nystatin cream is usually preferred to nystatin ointment in candidiasis involving intertriginous areas; however, very moist lesions are best treated with nystatin topical powder.

➤*Adults:*

Mycotic infections –

Cream and ointment: Apply liberally to the affected areas twice daily or as indicated until healing is complete.

Powder: Apply to candidal lesions 2 or 3 times daily until lesions have healed. For fungal infection of the feet caused by *Candida* species, the powder should be dusted freely on the feet as well as in shoes and socks.

➤*Children:*

Off-label dosing –

Mucocutaneous candidal infections (neonatal):

• *Cream and ointment* – Apply to the affected areas every 6 hours. Continue treatment until 3 days after symptoms have subsided.

➤*Storage/Stability:*

Cream and topical powder – Store at controlled room temperature, 15° to 30°C (59° to 86°F). Avoid exposure to excessive heat, 40°C (104°F).

Ointment – Store at room temperature not exceeding 25°C (77°F). Avoid excessive heat.

Actions

➤*Pharmacology:* Nystatin is an antibiotic with antifungal activity against a wide variety of yeasts and yeast-like fungi. It probably acts by binding to sterols in the cell membrane of the fungus with a resultant change in membrane permeability, allowing leakage of intracellular components. Nystatin is a polyene antibiotic of undetermined structural formula that is obtained from *Streptomyces noursei* and is the first well tolerated antifungal antibiotic of dependable efficacy for the treatment of cutaneous, oral and intestinal infections caused by *Candida (Monilia) albicans* and other *Candida* species. Nystatin exhibits no appreciable activity against bacteria.

Nystatin provides specific therapy for all localized forms of candidiasis. Symptomatic relief is rapid, often occurring within 24 to 72 hours after the

NYSTATIN — TOPICAL

initiation of treatment. Cure is effected both clinically and mycologically in most cases of localized candidiasis.

Contraindications

History of hypersensitivity to any component.

Warnings/Precautions

➤*Adverse reactions:* Nystatin is virtually nontoxic and nonsensitising and is well-tolerated by all age groups including debilitated infants, even on prolonged administration. Large oral doses have occasionally produced diarrhea and gastrointestinal disturbance. If local sensitization develops, treatment should be discontinued.

➤*For external use only:* This preparation is not for ophthalmic use.

➤*Hypersensitivity reactions:* Should a reaction of hypersensitivity occur, the drug should be immediately withdrawn and appropriate measures taken.

➤*Pregnancy: Category C.*

➤*Lactation:* It is not known whether nystatin is excreted in human milk. Caution should be exercised when nystatin is prescribed for a nursing woman.

Overdosage

Treatment of overdosage should be symptomatic and supportive.

OXICONAZOLE NITRATE

Rx	**Oxistat** (Pharmaderm)	**Cream; topical:** 1%	White petrolatum, propylene glycol, stearyl alcohol NF, cetyl alcohol NF, 0.2% benzoic acid. In 15, 30 and 60 g tubes.
		Lotion; topical: 1%	White petrolatum, propylene glycol, stearyl alcohol NF, cetyl alcohol NF, 0.2% benzoic acid. In 30 mL.

OXICONAZOLE NITRATE — TOPICAL

Indications

➤*Fungal infections:* For the treatment of the following dermal infections: Tinea pedis, tinea cruris, and tinea corporis due to *Trichophyton rubrum*, *Trichophyton mentagrophytes*, or *Epidermophyton floccosum*.

Cream – For the treatment of tinea (pityriasis) versicolor due to *Malassezia furfur*.

Oxiconazole cream may be used in children for tinea corporis, tinea cruris, tinea pedis, and tinea (pityriasis) versicolor; however, these indications for which oxiconazole cream has been shown to be effective rarely occur in children younger than 12 years of age.

Administration and Dosage

➤*General dosing considerations:* Tinea (pityriasis) versicolor may give rise to hyperpigmented or hypopigmented patches on the trunk that may extend to the neck, arms, and upper thighs. Treatment of the infection may not immediately result in restoration of pigment to the affected sites. Normalization of pigment following successful therapy is variable and may take months, depending on individual skin type and incidental sun exposure. Although tinea (pityriasis) versicolor is not contagious, it may recur because the organism that causes the disease is part of the normal skin flora.

➤*Adults:*

Tinea pedis –

Cream or lotion:

• *Usual dosage* – Apply to the affected and immediately surrounding areas once to twice daily.

• *Duration of therapy* – Treat for 1 month to reduce the possibility of recurrence. If a patient shows no clinical improvement after the treatment period, the diagnosis should be reviewed.

Tinea corporis or tinea cruris –

Cream or lotion:

• *Usual dosage* – Apply to the affected and immediately surrounding areas once to twice daily.

• *Duration of therapy* – Treat for 2 weeks to reduce the possibility of recurrence. If a patient shows no clinical improvement after the treatment period, the diagnosis should be reviewed.

Tinea (pityriasis) versicolor –

Cream:

• *Usual dosage* – Apply once daily.

• *Duration of therapy* – Treat for 2 weeks to reduce the possibility of recurrence. If a patient shows no clinical improvement after the treatment period, the diagnosis should be reviewed.

➤*Children:* Oxiconazole cream may be used in pediatric patients for tinea corporis, tinea cruris, tinea pedis, and tinea (pityriasis) versicolor; however, the indications for which oxiconazole cream has been shown to be effective rarely occur in children younger than 12 years of age.

Tinea pedis – See Adults for dosing.

Tinea corporis or tinea cruris – See Adults for dosing.

Tinea (pityriasis) versicolor – See Adults for dosing.

➤*Storage/Stability:* Store between 15° and 30°C (59° and 86°F).

Actions

➤*Pharmacokinetics:* The penetration of oxiconazole nitrate into different layers of the skin was assessed using an in vitro permeation technique with human skin. Five hours after application of 2.5 mg/cm² of oxiconazole nitrate cream onto human skin, the concentration of oxiconazole nitrate was demonstrated to be 16.2 mcmol in the epidermis, 3.64 mcmol in the upper corium, and 1.29 mcmol in the deeper corium. Systemic absorption of oxiconazole nitrate is low. Using radiolabeled drug, less than 0.3% of the applied dose of oxiconazole nitrate was recovered in the urine of volunteer subjects up to 5 days after application of the cream formulation.

➤*Microbiology:* Oxiconazole nitrate is an imidazole derivative whose antifungal activity is derived primarily from the inhibition of ergosterol biosynthesis, which is critical for cellular membrane integrity. It has in vitro activity against a wide range of pathogenic fungi.

Oxiconazole has been shown to be active against most strains of the following organisms both in vitro and in clinical infections at indicated body sites (see Indications): *Epidermophyton floccosum*, *Trichophyton mentagrophytes*, *Trichophyton rubrum*, and *Malassezia furfur*.

Contraindications

Hypersensitivity to any of their components.

Warnings/Precautions

➤*For external use only:* Oxiconazole cream and lotion are not for ophthalmic or intravaginal use.

➤*Irritation:* Oxiconazole cream and lotion are for external dermal use only. Avoid introduction of oxiconazole cream or lotion into the eyes or vagina. If a reaction suggesting sensitivity or chemical irritation should occur with the use of oxiconazole cream or lotion, treatment should be discontinued and appropriate therapy instituted. If signs of epidermal irritation should occur, the drug should be discontinued.

➤*Pregnancy: Category B.* There are no adequate and well-controlled studies in pregnant women. This drug should be used during pregnancy only if clearly needed.

➤*Lactation:* Because oxiconazole is excreted in human milk, caution should be exercised when the drug is administered to a nursing woman.

➤*Children:* Oxiconazole cream may be used in pediatric patients for tinea corporis, tinea cruris, tinea pedis, and tinea (pityriasis) versicolor; however, these indications for which oxiconazole cream has been shown to be effective rarely occur in children < 12 years of age.

Drug Interactions

None known.

Adverse Reactions

➤*Cream:* During clinical trials, of 955 patients treated with oxiconazole nitrate cream, 1%, 41 (4.3%) reported adverse reactions thought to be related to drug therapy. These reactions included pruritus (1.6%); burning (1.4%); irritation and allergic contact dermatitis (0.4% each); folliculitis (0.3%); erythema (0.2%); and papules, fissure, maceration, rash, stinging, and nodules (0.1% each).

➤*Lotion:* In a controlled, multicenter clinical trial of 269 patients treated with oxiconazole nitrate lotion, 1%, 7 (2.6%) reported adverse reactions thought to be related to drug therapy. These reactions included burning and stinging (0.7% each) and pruritus, scaling, tingling, pain, and dyshidrotic eczema (0.4% each).

Overdosage

When 5% oxiconazole cream (5 times the concentration of the marketed product) was applied at a rate of 1 g/kg to ≈ 10% of body surface area of a group of 40 male and female rats for 35 days, 3 deaths and severe dermal inflammation were reported. No overdoses in humans have been reported with use of oxiconazole nitrate cream or lotion.

Patient Information

Use oxiconazole as directed by the physician. The hands should be washed after applying the medication to the affected area(s). Avoid contact with the eyes, nose, mouth, and other mucous membranes. Oxiconazole is for external use only.

Use the medication for the full treatment time recommended by the physician, even though symptoms may have improved. Notify the physician if there is no improvement after 2 to 4 weeks, or sooner if the condition worsens (see below).

Inform the physician if the area of application shows signs of increased irritation, itching, burning, blistering, swelling, or oozing.

Avoid the use of occlusive dressings unless otherwise directed by the physician.

Do not use this medication for any disorder other than that for which it was prescribed.

SULCONAZOLE NITRATE

Rx	Exelderm (Ranbaxy Labs)	Cream: 1%	In 15, 30 and 60 g tubes.
		Solution: 1%	In 30 mL.

SULCONAZOLE NITRATE — TOPICAL

Indications

➤*Fungal infections:*

Cream – For the treatment of tinea pedis (athlete's foot), tinea cruris, and tinea corporis caused by *Trichophyton rubrum*, *Trichophyton mentagrophytes*, *Epidermophyton floccosum*, and *Microsporum canis* (Efficacy for this organism in the organ system was studied in less than 10 infections), and for the treatment of tinea versicolor.

Solution – For the treatment of tinea cruris and tinea corporis caused by *Trichophyton rubrum*, *Trichophyton mentagrophytes*, *Epidermophyton floccosum*, and *Microsporum canis*; and for the treatment of tinea versicolor. Effectiveness has not been proven in tinea pedis (athlete's foot).

Administration and Dosage

➤*General dosing considerations:* If significant clinical improvement is not seen after 4 weeks of treatment, an alternate diagnosis should be considered.

➤*Adults:*

Tinea corporis –

Cream:

• *Usual dosage* – A small amount of cream should be gently massaged into the affected and surrounding skin areas once or twice daily.

• *Duration of therapy* – Early relief of symptoms is experienced by the majority of patients and clinical improvement may be seen fairly soon after treatment is begun; however treat for 3 weeks to reduce the possibility of recurrence.

Solution:

• *Usual dosage* – A small amount of the solution should be gently massaged into the affected and surrounding skin areas once or twice daily.

• *Duration of therapy* – Symptomatic relief usually occurs within a few days and clinical improvement usually occurs within 1 week. To reduce the possibility of recurrence, treat for 3 weeks.

Tinea cruris – See Tinea coroporis.

Tinea pedis –

Cream:

• *Usual dosage* – A small amount of cream should be gently massaged into the affected and surrounding skin areas twice daily.

• *Duration of therapy* – Early relief of symptoms is experienced by the majority of patients and clinical improvement may be seen fairly soon after treatment is begun; however, treat for 4 weeks to reduce the possibility of recurrence.

Tinea versicolor – See Tinea coroporis.

➤*Storage/Stability:* Avoid excessive heat, above 40°C (104°F), and protect from light.

Actions

➤*Pharmacology:* Sulconazole nitrate is an imidazole derivative that inhibits the growth of the common pathogenic dermatophytes including *Trichophyton rubrum*, *Trichophyton mentagrophytes*, *Epidermophyton floccosum*, and *Microsporum canis*. It also inhibits the organism responsible for tinea versicolor, *Malassezia furfur*, and certain gram positive bacteria.

Contraindications

Hypersensitivity to any of the ingredients.

Warnings/Precautions

➤*For external use only:* Avoid contact with the eyes. If irritation develops, the solution or cream should be discontinued and appropriate therapy instituted.

➤*Pregnancy: Category C.* Sulconazole nitrate has been shown to be embryotoxic in rats when given in doses 125 times the human dose (in mg/kg). The drug at this dose given orally to rats also resulted in prolonged gestation and dystocia. Several females died during the perinatal period, most likely due to labor complications. Sulconazole nitrate was not teratogenic in rats or rabbits at oral doses of 50 mg/kg/day.

There are no adequate and well-controlled studies in pregnant women. Sulconazole nitrate should be used during pregnancy only if the potential benefit justifies the potential risk to the fetus.

➤*Lactation:* It is not known whether this drug is excreted in human milk. The molecular weight (about 461) suggests that the drug will be excreted into breast milk. Because many drugs are excreted in human milk, caution should be exercised when sulconazole nitrate is administered to a nursing woman. Because the systemic absorption was the highest known among similar agents, other imidazole antifungals might be more appropriate if a nursing woman requires topical antifungal therapy.

➤*Children:* Safety and effectiveness have not been established.

Adverse Reactions

➤*Cream:* There were no systemic effects and only infrequent cutaneous adverse reactions in 1185 patients treated with sulconazole nitrate cream in controlled clinical trials. Approximately 3% of these patients reported itching, 3% burning or stinging, and 1% redness. These complaints did not usually interfere with treatment.

➤*Solution:* There were no systemic effects and only infrequent cutaneous adverse reactions in 370 patients treated with sulconazole nitrate solution in controlled clinical trials. Approximately 1% of these patients reported itching and 1% burning or stinging. These complaints did not usually interfere with treatment.

Patient Information

Use sulconazole nitrate as directed by the physician, only use it externally, and avoid contact with the eyes.

TERBINAFINE

otc	Terbinafine Hydrochloride (Taro)	Cream; topical: 1%	Benzyl alcohol, cetyl alcohol, stearyl alcohol. In 24 g.
otc	Lamisil AT (Novartis)		With benzyl alcohol, cetyl alcohol and stearyl alcohol. In 15 and 30 g.
otc	Lamisil AT (Novartis)	Gel; topical: 1%	Ethanol. Benzyl alcohol. In 6 and 12 g.
otc	Lamisil AT (Novartis)	Spray; topical: 1%	Ethanol, propylene glycol. In 30 mL.

TERBINAFINE — TOPICAL

For complete and comparative prescribing information, refer to the Terbinafine Oral monograph.

Indications

➤*Dermatologic infections:* For the topical treatment of the following dermatologic infections: Tinea (pityriasis) versicolor due to *Malassezia furfur* (formerly *Pityrosporum ovale*), and tinea pedis (athlete's foot), tinea cruris (jock itch), or tinea corporis (ringworm), due to *Trichophyton rubrum*, *Trichophyton mentagrophytes*, or *Epidermophyton floccosum* (see Administration and Dosage). Diagnosis of disease should be confirmed either by culture (except *Malassezia furfur* [formerly *Pityrosporum ovale*]) or direct microscopic examination of scrapings from infected tissue mounted in a solution of potassium hydroxide.

Administration and Dosage

➤*Adults:*

Dermatologic infections –

Cream, gel, or spray:

• *Athlete's foot* – For athlete's foot between the toes only, apply twice a day (morning and night) for 1 week or as directed by a health care provider. For athlete's foot on the bottom or sides of the foot, apply twice a day (morning and night) for 2 weeks or as directed by a health care provider.

• *Jock itch* – Apply once a day (morning or night) for 1 week or as directed by a health care provider.

• *Ringworm* – Apply once a day (morning or night) for 1 week or as directed by a health care provider.

➤*Children:*

Dermatologic infections –

Cream, gel, or spray:

• *12 years of age and older* – See Adults for dosing.

➤*Administration:* Use the tip of the cap to break the seal and open the tube of the cream. For the cream or spray use the following directions. Wash the affected skin with soap and water and dry completely before applying.

Wash hands after each use.

For athlete's foot, wear well-fitting, ventilated shoes. Change shoes and socks at least once daily.

➤*Storage/Stability:*

Cream/Gel – Store between 5° and 30°C (41° to 86°F). See box or tube crimp for lot number and expiration date. Do not use if seal on tube is broken or is not visible.

Spray – Store at 8° to 25°C (46° to 77°F).

TERBINAFINE — TOPICAL

Actions

➤*Pharmacokinetics:*

Absorption – In a study of 10 patients with tinea cruris, once-daily application of terbinafine hydrochloride solution for 7 days (total amount of terbinafine hydrochloride applied averaged 0.8 g) resulted in plasma concentrations of terbinafine of up to 21 ng/mL on day 7, representing ≈ 2% of plasma concentrations achieved with a 250 mg terbinafine hydrochloride tablet. Plasma concentrations of the N-demethylated metabolite of terbinafine ranged up to 14 ng/mL in these patients. In subjects with healthy skin, neither the parent nor the N-demethylated metabolite were detected in the plasma following once-daily dosing for seven days with 0.3 g of 1% terbinafine hydrochloride solution.

Distribution – The skin pharmacokinetics of terbinafine hydrochloride solution, delivered by spray was compared to the 1% cream in 36 healthy subjects following both single and multiple applications (≈ 5 mg of terbinafine hydrochloride was applied to roughly a 190 cm^2 area on the back). Maximum mean total stratum corneum drug concentrations (C_{max}) averaged 720 and 810 ng/cm^2 on days 1 and 7, respectively. No significant differences in total stratum corneum AUC (area under the curve), C_{max} and half-life were seen between the 1% spray and the 1% cream after 1 or 7 days of treatment. Similar skin levels of terbinafine are achieved by delivery of terbinafine hydrochloride solution from the spray bottle or from application of terbinafine hydrochloride cream.

Metabolism – It is unknown whether or not there is any significant skin metabolism of topically applied terbinafine. Radiolabeled studies with oral dosage forms indicate that terbinafine is highly metabolized into a number of metabolites which undergo conjugation and excretion into the urine. The primary metabolite seen in the urine (10% of the oral dose) is N-demethyl terbinafine.

Excretion – The half-life of terbinafine when absorbed through the skin, regardless of the method of topical administration, is ≈ 21 hours. Approximately 75% of cutaneously absorbed terbinafine is eliminated in the urine, predominately as metabolites.

➤*Microbiology:* Terbinafine hydrochloride is a synthetic allylamine derivative. Terbinafine hydrochloride is hypothesized to act by inhibiting the epoxidation of squalene, thus blocking the biosynthesis of ergosterol, an essential component of fungal cell membranes. The allylamine derivatives, like the benzylamines, act at an earlier step in the ergosterol biosynthesis pathway than the azole class of antifungal drugs. Depending on the concentration of the drug and the fungal species tested in vitro, terbinafine hydrochloride may be fungicidal. However, the clinical significance of in vitro data is unknown.

Terbinafine has been shown to be active against most strains of the following organisms both in vitro and in clinical infections as described in Indications: *Epidermophyton floccosum*, *Malassezia furfur* (formerly *Pityrosporum ovale*), *Trichophyton mentagrophytes*, and *Trichophyton rubrum*.

Contraindications

Known or suspected hypersensitivity to terbinafine or any other of its components.

Warnings/Precautions

➤*For external use only:* Terbinafine is not for ophthalmic, oral, or intravaginal use.

➤*Pregnancy: Category B.* There are no adequate and well-controlled studies in pregnant women. Only use terbinafine hydrochloride if clearly indicated during pregnancy.

➤*Lactation:* After a single oral dose of 500 mg of terbinafine hydrochloride to 2 volunteers, the total dose of terbinafine secreted in human milk during the 72-hour post-dosing period was 0.65 mg in 1 person and 0.15 mg in the other. The total excretion of terbinafine in human milk was 0.13% and 0.03% of the administered dose, respectively. This 500 mg dose represents about 50 times the percutaneous exposure as described in the previous paragraph. The concentrations of the N-demethylated metabolite measured in the human milk of these 2 volunteers were below the detection limit of the assay used (150 ng/mL of milk).

Because of the small amount of data on human neonatal exposure, a decision should be made whether to discontinue nursing or to discontinue the drug, taking into account the importance of the drug to the mother.

Nursing mothers should avoid application of terbinafine hydrochloride solution to the breast.

➤*Children:* Safety and efficacy have not been established in children.

Drug Interactions

None known.

Adverse Reactions

➤*Local:* Burning or irritation (1.3%); itching (1.1%); skin exfoliation (1%); rash (0.9%).

Patient Information

Use terbinafine hydrochloride as directed by the physician and avoid contact with the eyes, nose, mouth, or other mucous membranes. The spray form should not be used on the face. In case of accidental contact with the eyes, rinse eyes thoroughly with running water and consult a physician if any symptoms persist.

Use the medication for the full treatment time even though symptoms may have improved.

Inform the physician if the area of application shows signs of increased irritation or possible sensitization (redness, itching, burning, blistering, swelling, or oozing).

Avoid the use of occlusive dressings unless otherwise directed by the physician.

TOLNAFTATE

otc	**Tolnaftate** (Various, eg, Fougera, Goldline, IDE, Moore, Parmed, NMC, UDL)	**Cream; topical:** 1%	In 15 g.
otc	**Absorbine Athlete's Foot Cream** (W.F. Young)		Parabens. In 21.3 g.
otc	**Genaspor** (Goldline)		In 15 g.
otc	**Tinactin** (Schering-Plough)		In 15 and 30 g.
otc	**Tinactin for Jock Itch** (Schering-Plough)		Petrolatum, mineral oil. In 15 g.
otc	**Ting** (Insight)		In 15 g.
otc	**Tolnaftate** (Various, eg, Copley, Fougera, Goldline, Major, Moore, Parmed)	**Solution; topical:** 1%	In 10 mL.
otc	**Tinactin** (Schering-Plough)		In 10 mL.
otc	**Blis-to-Sol** (Chattem)	**Liquid; topical:** 1%	In 30 mL.
otc	**Aftate for Athlete's Foot** (Schering-Plough)	**Gel; topical:** 1%	In 15 g.
otc	**Aftate for Jock Itch** (Schering-Plough)		In 15 g.
otc	**Lamisil AF Defense** (Novartis Consumer Health)	**Powder; topical:** 1%	Talc. In 113 g.
otc	**Tolnaftate** (Various)		In 45 g.
otc	**Quinsana Plus** (Stephan)		Cornstarch, talc. In 90 g.
otc	**Tinactin** (Schering-Plough)		Talc. In 45 and 90 g.
otc	**Aftate for Athlete's Foot** (Schering-Plough)	**Spray Powder; topical:** 1%	14% alcohol, talc. In 105 g.
otc	**Aftate for Jock Itch** (Schering-Plough)		14% alcohol. In 105 g.
otc	**Tinactin** (Schering-Plough)		14% alcohol, talc. **Deodorant:** In 100 g. **Regular:** In 100, 150 g.
otc	**Tinactin for Jock Itch** (Schering-Plough)		14% alcohol, talc. In 100 g.
otc	**Aftate for Athlete's Foot** (Schering-Plough)	**Spray Liquid; topical:** 1%	36% alcohol. In 120 mL.
otc	**Tinactin** (Schering-Plough)		36% alcohol. In 120 mL.
otc	**Ting** (Insight)		41% SD alcohol, PEG-400. In 128 g.

TOLNAFTATE — TOPICAL

Indications

➤*Fungal infection:* Treatment of tinea pedis (athlete's foot), tinea cruris (jock itch) or tinea corporis (ringworm) due to infection with *Trichophyton rubrum, T. mentagrophytes, T. tonsurans, Microsporum canis, M. audouini,* and *Epidermophyton floccosum* and for tinea versicolor due to *Malassezia furfur.*

In onychomycosis, in chronic scalp infections in which fungi are numerous and widely distributed in skin and hair follicles, where kerion has formed and in fungus infections of palms and soles, use tolnaftate concurrently for adjunctive local benefit in these lesions.

Powder and powder aerosol – Also effective prophylactically against athlete's foot.

Administration and Dosage

➤*General dosing considerations:* The choice of vehicle is important for these products. Ointments, creams, and liquids are used as primary therapy. In general, powders are used as adjunctive therapy, but they may be acceptable as primary therapy in very mild conditions.

Certain products are not effective on the scalp or nails.

Do not miss any doses.

For athlete's foot, wear well-fitting, ventilated shoes; change shoes and socks at least once a day.

➤*Adults:*

Athlete's foot –

Usual dosage: Use daily for 4 weeks. Pay special attention to the spaces between the toes when applying tolnaftate.

To prevent athlete's foot, apply the powder or liquid or powder spray forms of this medicine once or twice daily (morning and/or night).

Concomitant therapy: For athlete's foot, wear well-fitting, ventilated shoes; change shoes and socks at least once a day.

Fungal infection – Apply to the affected area(s) of the skin 2 times per day (morning and night).

Jock itch – Use daily for 2 weeks.

Ringworm – Use daily for 4 weeks.

➤*Children:*

Fungal infection –

2 years of age and older: See Adults for dosing.

➤*Duration of therapy:* Only small quantities are required. Treatment twice a day for 2 or 3 weeks is usually adequate, although 4 to 6 weeks may be required if the skin has thickened. Continue treatment to maintain remission.

➤*Preparation for administration:* Before applying tolnaftate, wash the affected area with soap and water and dry thoroughly. Then apply enough medicine to cover the affected area.

➤*Administration:*

Aerosol powder – Shake well before using.

From a distance of 6 to 10 inches, spray the powder on the affected areas. If it is used on the feet, spray it between the toes, on the feet, and in socks and shoes.

Do not inhale the powder.

Do not use near heat, open flame, or while smoking.

Aerosol solution or liquid spray – Shake well before using.

From a distance of 6 to 10 inches, spray the solution on the affected area. If it is used on the feet, spray it between the toes and on the feet.

Do not inhale the vapors from the spray.

Do not use near heat, open flame, or while smoking.

Powder – If powder is used on the feet, sprinkle it between the toes, on feet, and in socks and shoes.

Premeasured unit-dose swabs – Hold the swab vertically with the color band tip upwards. Bend the tip at the color band to one side until it snaps.

Discard swab after use.

Solution – If the solution becomes a solid, it may be dissolved by warming the closed container of medicine in warm water.

➤*Storage/Stability:* Store at 15° to 30°C (59° to 86°F). Store away from excessive heat, direct light, and cold.

Do not puncture, break, or burn the aerosol powder or aerosol solution container. Do not store at temperatures above 48.9°C (120°F).

Solution – Store at 15° to 30°C (59° to 86°F). Store away from excessive heat, direct light, and cold.

The solution solidifies at low temperatures and liquifies readily when warmed, retaining its potency. Protect from freezing.

Actions

➤*Pharmacology:* Effective in the treatment of superficial fungal infections of the skin.

Warnings/Precautions

➤*Discontinuation:* If symptoms do not improve after 10 days of use as recommended by the labeling, discontinue use unless otherwise directed.

➤*Sensitization or irritation:* Persons younger than 18 years of age or those with sensitive or allergic skin should only use as directed by a doctor. Discontinue treatment if sensitization or irritation develops.

➤*Nail/Scalp infections:* Not recommended for these infections except as adjunctive therapy to systemic treatment.

➤*For external use only:* Keep out of the eyes.

➤*Prophylaxis:* To help prevent reinfection after the period of treatment with this medicine, the powder or spray powder forms of tolnaftate may be used each day after bathing and carefully drying the affected area.

➤*Reevaluate patient:* If no improvement or worsening occurs after 4 weeks, reevaluate patient.

➤*Pregnancy: Category: Undetermined.* Consult a health care provider before using in pregnant women.

➤*Lactation:* Topical tolnaftate has not been studied during breast-feeding and no data are available on the extent of its absorption after topical application. Because it is probably poorly absorbed after topical application, it is considered a low risk to the nursing infant. Avoid application to the nipple area and ensure that the infant's skin does not come into direct contact with the areas of skin that have been treated.

➤*Children:* Do not use in children younger than 2 years of age.

Adverse Reactions

➤*Sensitivity:* A few cases of sensitization have been confirmed; mild irritation has occurred.

➤*Local:* A mild temporary stinging may be expected when applying the aerosol solution form of tolnaftate.

Patient Information

For external use only. Avoid contact with the eyes.

Before applying tolnaftate, wash the affected area with soap and water and dry thoroughly. Then apply enough medicine to cover the affected area.

Do not miss any doses.

Stop use and ask a doctor:

- If irritation occurs.
- If there is no improvement within 4 weeks (for athlete's foot and ringworm) or within 2 weeks (for jock itch).

➤*Dosing:* Some products are not affected on the scalp or nails. See individual product labeling.

Persons younger than 18 years of age or those with highly sensitive or allergic skin should only use as directed by a doctor. Tell your doctor if you have ever had an allergic reaction to tolnaftate or if you are allergic to any other substances, such as preservatives or dyes.

Supervise children in the use of this product.

If you are pregnant, planning to become pregnant, or breastfeeding, ask a doctor before using this medicine.

Tell your doctor if you are using any other topical prescription or nonprescription (OTC) medicine that will be applied to the same area of skin.

Keep out of reach of children. If swallowed, get medical help or contact a poison control center right away.

UNDECYLENIC ACID AND DERIVATIVES

otc	**Caldesene** (Insight)	**Powder; topical**: 10% calcium undecylenate	In 60 and 120 g.
otc	**Cruex** (Novartis Consumer Health)		Talc. In 45 g.
otc	**Cruex Aerosol** (Novartis Consumer Health)	**Powder; topical**: 19% total undecylenate as undecylenic acid and zinc undecylenate	Menthol, talc. In 54, 105 and 165 g.
otc	**Phicon F** (T.E. Williams)	**Cream; topical**: 8% undecylenic acid, 0.05% pramoxine HCl	In 60 g.
otc	**DiabetiDerm** (Health Care Products)	**Cream; topical**: 10% undecylenic acid	Aloe, cetyl alcohol, clotrimazole, disodium EDTA, glyceryl, lavender oil, parabens, PEG-100, tea tree oil, triethanolamine, urea. In 42 g.
otc	**Blis-To-Sol** (Oakhurst)	**Powder; topical**: 12% zinc undecylenate	Bentonite, talc, zinc oxide. In 60 g.

Antifungal Agents

UNDECYLENIC ACID AND DERIVATIVES

otc	**Cruex** (Novartis Consumer Health)	**Cream; topical:** 20% total undecylenate as undecylenic acid and zinc undecylenate	Lanolin, parabens, white petrolatum. In 15 g.
otc	**Elon Dual Defense Anti-Fungal Formula** (Dartmouth)	**Solution; topical:** 25% undecylenic acid	Alcohol. In 30 mL.
otc	**Fungoid AF** (Pedinol)	**Solution; topical:** 25% undecylenic acid	In 30 mL.
otc	**Gordochom** (Gordon)	**Solution; topical:** 25% undecylenic acid and chloroxylenol in an oily base	In 30 mL.
otc	**Desenex** (Novartis Consumer Health)	**Soap; topical:** undecylenic acid	In 97.5 g.
otc	**Fungi Cure Maximum Strength** (Alva-Amco)	**Liquid; topical:** 25% undecylenic acid	Aloe vera, isopropyl alcohol 70%. In 30 mL.

UNDECYLENIC ACID — TOPICAL

Indications

➤*Fungal infections:* Undecylenic acid eliminates fungal infections of the skin by inhibiting the growth and reproduction of fungal cells.

Undecylenic acid is formulated to cure most ringworm (tinea corporis) and athlete's foot (tinea pedis) affecting the finger and toe areas, including the skin around the nails. Undecylenic acid also helps to relieve the itching, scaling, cracking, burning, redness, soreness, irritations, and other related discomforts which may accompany these conditions.

This product is not effective on scalp or nails.

Administration and Dosage

➤*General dosing considerations:* The choice of vehicle is important for these products. Ointments, creams, and liquids are used as primary therapy. In general, powders are used as adjunctive therapy, but they may be acceptable as primary therapy in very mild conditions.

For athlete's foot, pay special attention to spaces between the toes. Wear well-fitting, ventilated shoes, and change shoes and socks at least once daily.

➤*Adults:*

Fungal infections –

Usual dosage: Clean affected area with soap and warm water and dry thoroughly. Apply a thin layer of undecylenic acid solution over affected area twice daily (morning and night) or as directed by a health care provider.

Duration of therapy: For athlete's foot and ringworm, use daily for 4 weeks. If condition persists longer, consult a health care provider.

➤*Children:*

Fungal infections –

2 years of age and older: See Adults for dosing.

➤*Administration:* For external use only; avoid contact with eyes.

➤*Storage/Stability:* Protect from freezing. If freezing occurs, warm to room temperature 21° to 27°C (70° to 80°F).

Actions

➤*Pharmacology:* Eliminates fungal infections of the skin by inhibiting the growth and reproduction of fungal cells.

Warnings/Precautions

➤*For external use only:* Avoid contact with eyes.

➤*Accidental ingestion:* Stop use and contact a physician, emergency care facility or poison control center immediately for advice in case of accidental ingestion.

➤*Pregnancy: Category: Undetermined.* Consult a health care provider before administering to a pregnant woman.

➤*Lactation:* Consult a health care provider before administering to a breast-feeding woman.

➤*Children:* Keep this and all medication out of the reach of children.

Do not use on children under 2 years of age unless directed by a doctor. If irritation occurs or if there is no improvement within 4 weeks, discontinue use and consult a doctor.

Patient Information

➤*General information about undecylenic acid:* For many years, physicians and pharmacists have recommended undecylenic acid for treating infections of the nails and surrounding tissue. However, in 1994 the FDA ruled that no over-the-counter antifungal product is effective on the nails. It was the FDA's opinion that products available without a prescription could not penetrate the nails, and were therefore ineffective in treating them. A statement reading "this product not effective on scalp or nails" was subsequently required on the labels of all over the counter antifungal products.

➤*Important tips on using undecylenic acid:* Use undecylenic acid as soon as an infection is detected. This will kill fungus before it gets out of control and prevents it from spreading to other areas.

ANTIFUNGAL COMBINATIONS

Rx	**Bensal HP** (7 Oaks Pharmaceutical Co.)	**Ointment:** 6% benzoic acid and 3% salicylic acid	Extract of oak bark. In 15 and 30 g tubes and 30 and 60 g jars.
otc	**Whitfield's** (Various, eg, Dixon-Shane, Fougera, Goldline, Lannett, Lilly, Moore, NMC, URL)		In 30 g and 1 lb.
Rx	**Versiclear** (Hope Pharmaceuticals)	**Lotion:** 25% sodium thiosulfate, 1% salicylic acid, 10% isopropyl alcohol, menthol, propylene glycol, EDTA and colloidal alumina	In 120 mL.
Rx	**Castellani Paint Modified** (Pedinol)	**Liquid:** Basic fuchsin, phenol, resorcinol and acetone	In 30 and 480 mL.
		Also available as a colorless solution with alcohol and without basic fuchsin.	In 30 and 480 mL.
otc	**Fungi-Nail** (Kramer)	**Liquid:** 1% resorcinol, 2% salicylic acid, 2% chloroxylenol, 0.5% benzocaine, 50% isopropyl alcohol	In 30 mL.
otc	**Exoderm** (A.G. Marin Pharmaceuticals)	**Soap; topical:** 10% sulfur, 3% salicylic acid	In 91.67 mL.

ANTIFUNGAL COMBINATIONS — TOPICAL

Active Ingredients

The principal active components of these formulations include:

➤*Antifungal agents: UNDECYLENIC ACID* (see individual monograph), *SODIUM PROPIONATE, BENZOIC ACID, SODIUM THIOSULFATE.*

➤*Other components include:*

SALICYLIC ACID and SULFUR – For its topical keratolytic action (see individual monograph).

BORIC ACID – As an astringent and antiseptic.

CHLOROXYLENOL – As an antiseptic.

BENZOCAINE – As an anesthetic (see individual monograph).

MENTHOL and PHENOL – For their antipruritic, anesthetic and antiseptic effects.

RESORCINOL – As an antipruritic and antiseptic.

CHLOROPHYLL DERIVATIVES – To promote healing, although there is no evidence to support this effect. These agents do have a deodorant action.

BASIC FUCHSIN – For its antifungal and antibacterial activity.

➤*Note:* The choice of vehicle is important for these products. Ointments, creams and liquids are used as primary therapy. In general, powders are used as adjunctive therapy, but they may be acceptable as primary therapy in very mild conditions.

BENZALKONIUM CHLORIDE (BAC)

otc	**Pedi-Pro** (Pedinol)	**Powder:** 1%	Menthol. In 56.7 g.
otc	**Benzalkonium Chloride** (Various, eg, A-A Spectrum)	**Concentrate:** 17%	In 500 mL and 4 L.
otc	**Remedy** (Medline)	**Cleanser:** 0.12%	Aloe barbadensis, citrus oils, tetrasodium EDTA, glycerin, parabens, urea. In 236 mL.
otc	**Benza** (Century)	**Solution:** 1:750	In 60 and 120 mL.
		Disinfectant concentrate: 17%	In 120 mL and gal.
		Tincture: 1:750	In gal.
		Tissue: 1:750. With chlorothymol, isopropyl alcohol and alcohol (20%)	In individual single use packets.
otc	**Mycocide NS** (Woodward)	**Solution:** Benzalkonium chloride, propylene glycol, diazolidinyl urea, methylparaben	In 30 mL.
otc	**no more germies towelettes** (Johnson & Johnson)	**Towelettes:** Benzalkonium chloride, aloe vera gel, EDTA, methylparaben, 15% SD alcohol 40.	In 24 individually wrapped towelettes.

BENZALKONIUM CHLORIDE — TOPICAL

Indications

➤*Aqueous solutions:* For the antisepsis of skin, mucous membranes, and wounds. They are used for preoperative preparation of the skin, surgeons' hand and arm soaks, treatment of wounds, preservation of ophthalmic solutions, irrigations of the eye, body cavities, bladder, urethra, and vaginal douching.

➤*1% topical solution:* To soften and rejuvenate nails. The topical 1% solution also softens and rejuvenates feet and helps guard against bacterial contamination that potentially can cause skin infection.

➤*0.13% topical solution:* External first aid antiseptic.

➤*1% topical foot powder:* To help guard against bacterial contamination that potentially can cause skin infection. This medication is a drying, absorbing, and deodorizing topical powder.

Administration and Dosage

➤*General dosing considerations:* Benzalkonium chloride solutions must be prepared, stored, and used correctly to achieve and maintain their antiseptic action. Serious inactivation and contamination of benzalkonium chloride solutions may occur with misuse.

➤*Adults:*

Antiseptic on skin, mucous membranes, and wounds –

Aqueous solutions: Liberal use of the solution is recommended to compensate for any adsorption of benzalkonium chloride by cotton or other materials.

- *Surgery –*
  - *Preoperative preparation of skin:* Aqueous solution 1:750.
  - *Surgeons' hand and arm soaks:* Aqueous solution 1:750.
  - *Irrigation of deep infected wounds:* Aqueous solution 1:3,000 to 1:20,000
  - *Denuded skin and mucous membranes:* Aqueous solution 1:5,000 to 1:10,000.
- *Obstetrics and gynecology –*
  - *Preoperative preparation of skin:* Aqueous solution 1:750.
  - *Vaginal douche and irrigation:* Aqueous solution 1:2,000 to 1:5,000.
  - *Postepisiotomy care:* Aqueous solution 1:5,000 to 1:10,000.
  - *Breast and nipple hygiene:* Aqueous solution 1:1,000 to 1:2,000.
- *Urology –*
  - *Bladder and urethral irrigation:* Aqueous solution 1:5,000 to 1:20,000.
  - *Bladder retention lavage:* Aqueous solution 1:20,000 to 1:40,000.
- *Dermatology –*
  - *Oozing and open infections:* Aqueous solution 1:2,000 to 1:5,000.
  - *Wet dressings by irrigation or open dressing:* Use in occlusive dressings is inadvisable. Aqueous solution 1:5,000 or less.
- *Ophthalmology –*
  - *Eye irrigation:* Aqueous solution 1:5,000 to 1:10,000.
  - *Preservation of ophthalmic solutions:* Aqueous solution 1:5,000 to 1:7,500.

External first aid antiseptic –

0.13% topical solution: Apply a small amount of 0.13% topical solution to the area 1 to 3 times daily. The area may be covered with a sterile bandage. If bandaged, the patient should let it dry first.

Softening and rejuvenation of nails and feet –

1% topical solution: Clean and dry affected areas. Apply a small amount to the affected area twice a day, morning and evening, or as recommended by a podiatrist or health care provider.

To help guard against bacterial contamination that potentially can cause skin infection –

1% topical foot powder: For best results, use twice a day, morning and evening. Gently squeeze the bottle or shake the powder onto feet, between toes, and in socks, shoes, and sneakers to help guard against bacterial contamination and to aid in drying, moisture absorption, deodorizing, and cooling of the feet.

1% topical solution: Clean and dry affected areas. Apply a small amount to the affected area twice a day, morning and evening, or as recommended by a podiatrist or health care provider.

➤*Children:*

2 years of age or older –

External first aid antiseptic: See Adults for dosing

➤*Preparation for administration:*

Correct diluent – Sterile water for injection is recommended for irrigation of body cavities.

Sterile distilled water is recommended for irrigating traumatized tissue and in the eye.

Resin deionized water should not be used because the deionizing resins can carry pathogens (especially gram-negative bacteria); they also inactivate quaternary ammonium compounds.

Stored water is not recommended because it may contain many organisms.

Saline should not be used because it may decrease the antibacterial potency of benzalkonium chloride solutions.

Dilution –

Dilutions of Benzalkonium Chloride Aqueous Solution 1:750

Final dilution	Benzalkonium chloride aqueous solution 1:750 (parts)	Sterile water for injection or sterile distilled water (parts)
1:1,000	3	1
1:2,000	3	5
1:2,500	3	7
1:3,000	3	9
1:4,000	3	13
1:5,000	3	17
1:10,000	3	37
1:20,000	3	77
1:40,000	3	157

➤*Administration:*

Preoperative preparation of skin (aqueous solutions) – Benzalkonium chloride solutions 1:750 is recommended as an antiseptic for use on unbroken skin in the preoperative preparation of the surgical field. Detergents and soaps should be thoroughly rinsed from the skin before applying benzalkonium chloride solutions. The detergent action of benzalkonium chloride solutions, particularly when used alternately with alcohol, leaves the skin smooth and clean. When benzalkonium chloride solutions are applied by friction (using several changes of sponges), dirt, skin fats, desquamating epithelium, and superficial bacteria are effectively removed, thus exposing the underlying skin to the antiseptic activity of the solutions.

➤*Admixture compatibility:* Under certain circumstances the following commonly encountered substances are incompatible with benzalkonium chloride solutions: iodine, silver nitrate, fluorescein, nitrates, peroxide, lanolin, potassium permanganate, aluminum, caramel, kaolin, pine oil, zinc sulfate, zinc oxide, and yellow oxide of mercury.

Anionic detergents and soaps should be thoroughly rinsed from the skin or other areas prior to use of benzalkonium chloride solutions because they reduce its antibacterial activity.

Serum and protein material also decrease the activity of benzalkonium chloride.

Corks should not be used with stopper bottles containing benzalkonium chloride solutions.

Fibers or fabrics (eg, cotton, wool, rubber materials, gauze sponges, rayon) absorb benzalkonium chloride.

Applicators or sponges, intended for a skin prep, should be stored separately and dipped in benzalkonium chloride solutions immediately before use.

➤*Storage/Stability:*

Aqueous solutions – Store at 25°C (77°F); excursions are permitted to 15° to 30°C (59° to 86°F).

1% topical solution and foot powder – Store at 15° to 30°C (59° to 86°F).

BENZALKONIUM CHLORIDE — TOPICAL

Actions

➤*Pharmacology:* Benzalkonium chloride solutions are rapidly acting anti-infective agents with a moderately long duration of action. They are active against bacteria and some viruses, fungi, and protozoa. Bacterial spores are considered to be resistant. Solutions are bacteriostatic or bactericidal according to their concentration. The exact mechanism of bactericidal action is unknown but is thought to be due to enzyme inactivation. Activity generally increases with increasing temperature and pH. Gram-positive bacteria are more susceptible than gram-negative bacteria.

Highest Dilution of Benzalkonium Chloride Aqueous Solutions Destroying The Organism in 10 Minutes but Not in 5 Minutes

Organisms	20°C (68°F)
Streptococcus pyogenes	1:75,000
Staphylococcus aureus	1:52,500
Salmonella typhosa	1:37,500
Escherichia coli	1:10,500

Pseudomonas is the most resistant gram-negative genus. Using the AOAC Use-Dilution Confirmation Method, no growth was obtained when *Staphylococcus aureus, Salmonella choleraesuis,* and *Pseudomonas aeruginosa* (strain PRD-10) were exposed for 10 minutes at 20°C (68°F) to benzalkonium chloride aqueous solution 1:750.

Benzalkonium chloride aqueous solution 1:750 has been shown to retain its bactericidal activity following autoclaving for 30 minutes at 15 lb pressure, freezing, and then thawing.

The tubercle bacillus may be resistant to aqueous benzalkonium chloride solutions.

Benzalkonium chloride solutions also demonstrate deodorant, wetting, detergent, keratolytic, and emulsifying activity.

Contraindications

Use in occlusive dressings, casts, and anal or vaginal packs; sensitivity to any of the ingredients in the product.

Warnings/Precautions

➤*Soaps/anionic detergents:* Since benzalkonium chloride is inactivated by soaps and anionic detergents, thorough rinsing is necessary if these agents are employed prior to their use.

➤*Aqueous solutions:* Sterile water for injection should be used as diluent in preparing diluted aqueous solutions intended for use on deep wounds or for irrigation of body cavities. Otherwise, freshly distilled water should be used. Tap water, containing metallic ions and organic matter, may reduce antibacterial potency. Resin deionized water should not be used since it may contain pathogenic bacteria.

Organic, inorganic, and synthetic materials and surfaces may adsorb sufficient quantities of benzalkonium chloride to significantly reduce its antibacterial potency in solutions. This has resulted in serious contamination of benzalkonium chloride solutions with viable pathogenic bacteria. Solutions should not be stored in bottles stoppered with cork closures, but rather in those equipped with appropriate screw-caps. Cotton, wool, rayon, and other materials should not be stored in benzalkonium chloride solutions. Gauze sponges and fiber pledgets used to apply solutions of benzalkonium chloride to the skin should be sterilized and stored in separate containers. Only immediately prior to application should they be immersed in benzalkonium chloride solutions.

Antiseptics such as benzalkonium chloride solutions must not be relied upon to achieve complete sterilization, because they do not destroy bacterial spores and certain viruses, including the etiologic agent of infectious hepatitis, and may not destroy *Mycobacterium tuberculosis* and other rare bacterial strains.

If solutions stronger than 1:3000 enter the eyes, irrigate immediately and repeatedly with water. Prompt medical attention should then be obtained. Concentrations greater than 1:5000 should not be used on mucous membranes, with the exception of the vaginal mucosa.

➤*Accidental ingestion:* In case of accidental ingestion, the patient should seek professional assistance or contact a poison control center immediately.

➤*Preoperative antisepsis:* In preoperative antisepsis of the skin, benzalkonium chloride solutions should not be permitted to remain in prolonged contact with the patient's skin. Avoid pooling of the solution on the operating table.

➤*Inflamed/irritated tissues:* Benzalkonium chloride solutions that are used on inflamed or irritated tissues must be more dilute than those used on normal tissues.

➤*Preoperative preparation:* Benzalkonium chloride solutions used in skin preparation have a tendency to "run off" the skin. It may be preferable to use alternately with alcohol in preoperative preparation of the skin.

Preoperative periorbital skin or head prep should be performed only before the patient, or eye, is anesthetized.

➤*Pregnancy: Category: Undetermined.*

➤*Lactation:* Topical maternal application of benzalkonium chloride would not be expected to cause any adverse effects in breast-fed infants.

Overdosage

➤*Symptoms:* If benzalkonium chloride solution, particularly a concentrated solution, is ingested, marked local irritation of the GI tract, manifested by nausea and vomiting, may occur. Signs of systemic toxicity include restlessness, apprehension, weakness, confusion, dyspnea, cyanosis, collapse, convulsions, and coma. Death occurs as a result of paralysis of the respiratory muscles.

➤*Treatment:* Immediate administration of several glasses of a mild soap solution, milk, or egg whites beaten in water is recommended. This may be followed by gastric lavage with a mild soap solution. Alcohol should be avoided as it promotes absorption.

To support respiration, the airway should be clear and oxygen should be administered, employing artificial respiration if necessary. If convulsions occur, a short-acting barbiturate may be given parenterally with caution.

Patient Information

➤*1% topical solution, 0.13% topical solution, 1% topical foot powder:* This medication is for external use only. Keep out of the reach of children. Do not use in the eyes or apply over large areas of the body. In cases of deep or puncture wounds, animal bites, or serious burns, consult a podiatrist, physician, or pharmacist. Stop use and consult a podiatrist, physician, or pharmacist if redness, swelling or pain persists or increases or if the condition persists, gets worse or if irritation occurs. Do not use in large quantities, particularly over raw surfaces or blistered areas. The 1% topical foot powder is not for use for longer than 1 week unless directed by a podiatrist, physician, or pharmacist. Do not bandage. Do not use if known to be sensitive to any of the ingredients in this product.

In case of accidental ingestion, seek professional assistance or contact your poison control center immediately.

CHLORHEXIDINE GLUCONATE

otc	**BactoShield 2** (Amsco)	**Solution; topical:** 2% with 4% isopropyl alcohol	In 960 mL.
otc	**Dyna-Hex 2 Skin Cleanser** (Western Medical)	**Liquid; topical:** 2% with 4% isopropyl alcohol	In 120, 240, 480 and 960 mL and gal.
otc	**Betasept** (Purdue Frederick)	**Liquid; topical:** 4% with 4% isopropyl alcohol	In 946 mL.
otc	**Dyna-Hex Skin Cleanser** (Western Medical)		In 120, 240 and 480 mL and gal.
otc	**Exidine Skin Cleanser** (Baxter Health Care)		In 120 and 240 mL, qt and gal.
otc	**Hibistat Germicidal Hand Rinse** (Stuart)	**Rinse; topical:** 0.5% with 70% isopropanol and emollients	In 120 and 240 mL.
otc	**Hibistat Towelettes** (Stuart)	**Wipes; topical:** 0.5% with 70% isopropanol	In 50s.
otc	**Chlorhexidine** (Sage Products)	**Cloth; topical:** 2% with aloe vera, glycerin	Alcohol free, rinse free. In 6s.
otc	**Bactoshield** (Amsco)	**Foam; topical:** 4% with 4% isopropyl alcohol	In 180 mL aerosol.

CHLORHEXIDINE GLUCONATE — TOPICAL

Indications

➤*Cleanser:* As a surgical hand scrub, skin wound and general skin cleanser, health care personnel hand wash, and for preoperative skin preparation. Chlorhexidine gluconate significantly reduces the number of microorganisms on the hands and forearms prior to surgery or patient care.

Administration and Dosage

➤*General dosing considerations:* Chlorhexidine gluconate should not be used for repeated general skin cleansing of large body areas except in those patients whose underlying condition makes it necessary to reduce the bacterial population of the skin.

CHLORHEXIDINE GLUCONATE — TOPICAL

Wounds that involve more than the superficial layers of the skin should not be routinely treated with chlorhexidine gluconate.

➤*Adults:*

Health care personnel hand wash – Wet hands with water. Dispense approximately 5 mL of chlorhexidine gluconate into cupped hands and wash in a vigorous manner for 15 seconds. Rinse and thoroughly dry.

Preoperative skin preparation – Apply chlorhexidine gluconate liberally to surgical site and swab for at least 2 minutes. Dry with a sterile towel. Repeat procedure for an additional 2 minutes and dry with a sterile towel.

Skin wound and general skin cleansing – Thoroughly rinse the area to be cleansed with water. Apply the minimum amount of chlorhexidine gluconate necessary to cover the skin or wound area and wash gently. Rinse thoroughly again.

Surgical hand scrub (brush-sponge and nail cleaner) – Clean under nails with the nail pick provided. Nails should be maintained with a 1 millimeter free edge. Wet hands and forearms to the elbows with warm water. Wet sponge and squeeze to work up lather with about 5 mL of chlorhexidine gluconate. Discard brush-sponge. Rinse hands and forearms thoroughly and dry with a sterile towel.

➤*Storage/Stability:* Store between 20° to 25°C (68° to 77°F). Avoid freezing and excessive heat above 40°C (104°F). Keep out of the reach of children.

Warnings/Precautions

➤*For external use only:* For external use only. Keep out of eyes, ears, and mouth. Chlorhexidine gluconate should not be used as a preoperative skin preparation of the face or head. Misuse of products containing chlorhexidine gluconate has been reported to cause serious and permanent eye injury when it has been permitted to enter and remain in the eye during surgical procedures. If chlorhexidine gluconate should contact these areas, rinse out promptly and thoroughly with cold water. Avoid contact with meninges. Do not use in the genital area.

➤*Deep wounds:* Do not use chlorhexidine gluconate routinely if you have wounds that involve more than the superficial layers of the skin.

➤*Sensitivity:* Chlorhexidine gluconate should not be used by persons who have a sensitivity to it or its components.

➤*Deafness:* Chlorhexidine gluconate has been reported to cause deafness when instilled in the middle ear through perforated ear drums.

➤*Hypersensitivity reactions:* Irritation, sensitization, and generalized allergic reactions have been reported with chlorhexidine-containing products, especially in the genital areas. If adverse reactions occur and last more than 72 hours, discontinue use immediately and, if severe, contact a health care provider.

➤*Pregnancy: Category B* (per Briggs' *Drugs in Pregnancy and Lactation*). No reports of adverse effects in newborns have been reported, even though chlorhexidine is commonly used during labor and in the neonate. Moreover, only very small amounts of disinfectant reach the maternal circulation and the fetus.

➤*Lactation:* No reports describing the excretion of chlorhexidine into milk have been located.

➤*Children:* Keep out of reach of children. If swallowed, get medical help or contact a poison control center right away.

Adverse Reactions

Irritation, sensitization, and generalized allergic reactions have been reported with chlorhexidine-containing products, especially in the genital areas. If adverse reactions occur and last more than 72 hours, discontinue use immediately and, if severe, contact a physician.

Overdosage

In case of accidental ingestion, seek professional assistance or contact a poison control center immediately.

If swallowed, get medical help or contact a poison control center right away.

Patient Information

When using this product, keep out of eyes, ears and mouth. May cause serious and permanent eye injury if permitted to enter or allowed to remain. If contact occurs, rinse with cold water right away.

Do not use routinely if you have wounds which involve more than the superficial layers of the skin.

Stop use and ask a doctor if irritation, sensitization or allergic reaction occurs and lasts more than 72 hours.

Keep out of reach of children. If swallowed, get medical help or contact a poison control center right away.

HEXACHLOROPHENE

Rx	**pHisoHex** (Winthrop Pharm.)	**Liquid:** 3%	Petrolatum, lanolin, PEG. In 150 mL, pt and gal and UD 8 mL (50s).

HEXACHLOROPHENE — TOPICAL

Indications

➤*Bacteriostatic skin cleanser:* For use as a surgical scrub and a bacteriostatic skin cleanser. It may also be used to control an outbreak of gram-positive infection where other infection control procedures have been unsuccessful. Use only as long as necessary for infection control.

Administration and Dosage

➤*Adults:*

Bacteriostatic skin cleanser – Wet the hands with water. Dispense approximately 5 mL of hexachlorophene onto the palm, work up a lather with water, and apply to the area to be cleansed. Rinse thoroughly after each washing.

Surgical hand scrub –

1.) Wet hands and forearms with water. Apply approximately 5 mL of hexachlorophene over the hands and rub into a copious lather by adding small amounts of water. Spread the suds over the hands and forearms and scrub well with a wet brush for 3 minutes. Pay particular attention to the nails and interdigital spaces. A separate nail cleaner may be used. Rinse thoroughly under running water.
2.) Apply 5 mL of hexachlorophene to hands again and scrub as above for another 3 minutes. Rinse thoroughly with running water and dry.
3.) For repeat surgical scrubs during the day, scrub thoroughly with the same amount of hexachlorophene for 3 minutes only. Rinse thoroughly with water and dry.

➤*Children:* Hexachlorophene should not be used routinely for bathing infants. Use of baby skin products containing alcohol may decrease the antibacterial action of hexachlorophene.

Bacteriostatic skin cleanser – See Adults.

➤*Administration:* Hexachlorophene is intended for external use only.

Rinse thoroughly after use, especially from sensitive areas, such as the scrotum and perineum.

➤*Storage/Stability:* Store at room temperature up to 25° C (77°F).

Prolonged direct exposure of hexachlorophene to strong light may cause brownish surface discoloration, but does not affect its antibacterial or detergent properties. Shaking will disperse the color. If hexachlorophene is spilled or splashed on porous surfaces, rinse it off to avoid discoloration.

Hexachlorophene should not be dispensed from or stored in containers with ordinary metal parts. A special type of stainless steel must be used, or undesirable discoloration of the product or oxidation of metal may occur.

Directions for cleaning dispensers – Before initial installation and use, run an antiseptic, such as an aqueous solution of benzalkonium chloride, NF, 1:500 to 1:750 or alcohol, through the working parts; rinse with sterile water. At weekly intervals thereafter, remove the dispenser and pour off the remainder of the hexachlorophene emulsion. Rinse the empty dispenser with water. Run water through the working parts by operating the dispenser. Sanitize as described above. Rinse thoroughly with sterile water.

Actions

➤*Pharmacology:* Hexachlorophene is a bacteriostatic cleansing agent. It cleanses the skin thoroughly and has bacteriostatic action against staphylococci and other gram-positive bacteria. Cumulative antibacterial action develops with repeated use. Cleansing with alcohol or soaps containing alcohol removes the antibacterial residue.

Detectable blood levels of hexachlorophene following absorption through intact skin have been found in subjects who regularly scrubbed with hexachlorophene emulsion 3%. (See Warnings.)

Hexachlorophene has the same slight acidity as normal skin (pH value 5.0 to 6.0).

Contraindications

On burned or denuded skin; as an occlusive dressing, wet pack, or lotion; routinely for prophylactic total body bathing; as a vaginal pack or tampon; or on any mucous membranes; sensitivity to any of its components; primary light sensitivity to halogenated phenol derivatives because of the possibility of cross-sensitivity to hexachlorophene.

Warnings/Precautions

➤*Monitoring:* Patients should be closely monitored and use should be immediately discontinued at the first sign of any of the symptoms described below.

➤*Rapid absorption:* Rapid absorption of hexachlorophene may occur with resultant toxic blood levels when preparations containing hexachlorophene are applied to skin lesions such as ichthyosis congenita, the dermatitis of Letterer-Siwe's syndrome, or other generalized dermatological conditions. Application to burns has also produced neurotoxicity and death.

➤*Cerebral irritability:* Hexachlorophene should be discontinued promptly if signs or symptoms of cerebral irritability occur. Infants, especially those who weigh less than 1,200 g and those with a gestational age of less than 35 weeks or those with dermatoses, are particularly susceptible to hexachlorophene absorption. Systemic toxicity may be manifested by signs of stimulation (irritation) of the central nervous system, sometimes with convulsions.

HEXACHLOROPHENE — TOPICAL

➤*Infant adverse reactions:* Infants have developed dermatitis, irritability, generalized clonic muscular contractions and decerebrate rigidity following application of a 6% hexachlorophene powder. Examination of brainstems of those infants revealed vacuolization like that which can be produced in newborn experimental animals following repeated topical application of 3% hexachlorophene. Moreover, a study of histologic sections of premature infants who died of unrelated causes has shown a positive correlation between hexachlorophene baths and lesions in white matter of brains.

➤*Eye contact:* Avoid accidental contact of hexachlorophene with the eyes.

If contact occurs, promptly rinse thoroughly with water. To assist in the detection of ocular irritation, applications to the head and periorbital skin areas should be performed only in responsive patients with unanesthetized eyes.

➤*After use:* Rinse thoroughly after use, especially from sensitive areas such as the scrotum and perineum.

➤*For external use only:* Hexachlorophene is intended for external use only. If swallowed, hexachlorophene is harmful, especially to infants and children. Hexachlorophene should not be poured into measuring cups, medicine bottles, or similar containers since it may be mistaken for baby formula or other medications.

➤*Pregnancy:* Category C. There are no adequate and well-controlled studies in pregnant women. Hexachlorophene should be used during pregnancy only if the potential benefit justifies potential risk to the fetus. Hexachlorophene is not recommended as an antiseptic lubricant for vaginal exams during labor because appreciable amounts have been detected in maternal and cord serum.

Hexachlorophene has been shown to be teratogenic and embryotoxic in rats when given by mouth or instilled into the vagina in large doses.

Administration of 500 mg/kg diet or 20 to 30 mg/kg bw/day by gavage to rats caused some malformations (angulated ribs, cleft palate, micro and anophthalmia) and reduction in litter size.

Teratogenic – Placental transfer and excretion in milk of hexachlorophene has been demonstrated in rats.

Hexachlorophene is embryotoxic and produces some teratogenic effects.

➤*Lactation:* It is not known whether this drug is excreted in human milk. Because many drugs are excreted in human milk and because of the potential for serious adverse reactions in nursing infants from hexachlorophene, a decision should be made whether to discontinue nursing or to discontinue the drug taking into account the importance of the drug to the mother.

➤*Children:* Hexachlorophene should not be used routinely for bathing premature or term infants.

Adverse Reactions

Dermatitis and photosensitivity. Sensitivity to hexachlorophene is rare; however, persons who have developed photoallergy to similar compounds also may become sensitive to hexachlorophene.

In persons with highly sensitive skin, the use of hexachlorophene may at times produce a reaction characterized by redness or mild scaling or dryness, especially when it is combined with such mechanical factors as excessive rubbing or exposure to heat or cold.

Overdosage

➤*Symptoms:* The accidental ingestion of hexachlorophene in amounts from 1 oz to 4 oz has caused anorexia, vomiting, abdominal cramps, diarrhea, dehydration, convulsions, hypotension, and shock, and in several reported instances, fatalities.

➤*Treatment:* If patients are seen early, the stomach should be evacuated by emesis or gastric lavage. Olive oil or vegetable oil (60 mL or 2 fl oz) may then be given to delay absorption of hexachlorophene, followed by a saline cathartic to hasten removal. Treatment is symptomatic and supportive; intravenous fluids (5 percent dextrose in physiologic saline solution) may be given for dehydration. Any other electrolyte derangement should be corrected. If marked hypotension occurs, vasopressor therapy is indicated. Use of opiates may be considered if gastrointestinal symptoms (cramping, diarrhea) are severe. Scheduled medical or surgical procedures should be postponed until the patient's condition has been evaluated and stabilized.

IODINE COMPOUNDS

IODINE

otc	**Iodine Topical** (Various, eg, AA–Spectrum)	**Solution; topical**: 2% iodine and 2.4% sodium iodide in purified water	In 500 and 4,000 mL.
otc[a]	**Strong Iodine (Lugol's Solution)** (Various, eg, Lannett)	**Solution; topical**: 5% iodine and 10% potassium iodide in water	In pt and gal.
otc	**Iodine Tincture** (Various, eg, Century, Lannett)	**Solution; topical**: 2% iodine and 2.4% sodium iodide in 47% alcohol, purified water	In pt and gal.
otc	**Strong Iodine Tincture** (Various, eg, A-A Spectrum)	**Solution; topical**: 7% iodine and 5% potassium iodide in 83% alcohol	In 500 and 4,000 mL.

[a] Some of these products may be available *Rx*, depending on distributor discretion.

IODINE — TOPICAL

Indications

➤*Antiseptic:* Iodine preparations are used externally for their broad microbicidal spectrum against bacteria, fungi, viruses, spores, protozoa and yeasts. Iodine may be used to disinfect intact skin preoperatively. Potassium iodide is added to increase the solubility of the iodine. Sodium iodide is present to stabilize the tincture and make it miscible with water in all proportions.

Contraindications

Hypersensitivity to iodine.

Warnings/Precautions

➤*For external use only:* Avoid contact with the eyes and mucous membranes.

➤*Highly toxic if ingested:* Sodium thiosulfate is the most effective chemical antidote.

➤*Staining:* Iodine preparations stain skin and clothing.

➤*Occlusive dressings:* Do not use.

➤*Pregnancy:* Category: *Undetermined*. Consult a health care provider before using in pregnant women.

➤*Lactation:* The use of iodine in the mother near term and during breast-feeding can increase breast-milk iodine levels and cause transient hypothyroidism in breast-fed infants. The absorption of iodine can be marked after application to open wounds or mucous membranes. Exposure of mothers to iodine who are or will be breast-feeding should be avoided or minimized to the extent possible by avoiding its use on maternal mucous membranes (eg, vaginal use, wound therapy), avoiding prolonged contact time, avoiding repeated applications, and applying it to the smallest possible surface areas of the body. It is possible that maternal exposure to iodine near term could interfere with thyroid studies done as a part of newborn screening tests.

POVIDONE IODINE

otc	**Povidone-Iodine** (Various, eg, Humco, IDE, Major)	**Ointment**: 10%	In 30 g and lb.
		Solution: 10%	In pt and gal.
		Liquid: 10%	In pt.
		Spray: 10%	In 2 oz.

POVIDONE IODINE

otc	**Betadine** (Purdue Frederick)	**Aerosol**: 5%. Glycerin, dibasic sodium phosphate	In 88.7 mL.
		Ointment: 10%. Polyethylene glycols.	In 28 g tube, lb jar and 0.94 and 3.8 g packets.
		Skin cleanser, foam: 7.5%. Ammonium nonoxynol-4-sulfate, lauramide DEA	In 170 g.
		Solution: 10%. Citric acid, dibasic sodium phosphate, glycerin	In 15, 120 and 237 mL, pt, qt, gal and 30 mL packets.
		Solution, swab aid: 10%. Citric acid, dibasic sodium phosphate, glycerin	In 100s.
		Solution, swabsticks: 10%. Citric acid, dibasic sodium phosphate, glycerin	In packets of 1 (200s) or 3 (50s).
		Surgical scrub: 7.5%. Ammonium nonoxynol-4-sulfate, lauramide DEA	In pt with or without pump, qt, gal and 15 mL packets.
otc	**Betagen** (Goldline)	**Surgical scrub**: 7.5%	In pt.
otc	**Biodine Topical 1%** (Major)	**Solution**: 1% iodine	In pt and gal.
otc	**Etodine** (Fougera)	**Ointment**: 1% available iodine	In 30 g, lb and 0.94 g (144s).
otc	**Minidyne** (Pedinol)	**Solution**: 10%. Citric acid and sodium phosphate dibasic	In 15 mL.
otc	**Polydine** (Century)	**Ointment**	In 30 and 120 g & lb.
		Ointment: 10%	In 28.4 g and lb.
		Solution: 10%	In pt and gal.
		Surgical scrub: 5.5	In pt and gal.
		Scrub	In 30, 120 and 240 mL, pt and gal.
		Solution	In 30, 120 and 240 mL, pt and gal.
otc	**Curity Sponge Sticks** (Kendall)	**Sticks; topical**: 1% iodine	Latex free. In 2s.
Rx	**Curity Wet Skin Scrub Pack** (Kendall)	**Solution; topical**: 0.75% to 1%	Latex free. In kits with 2 winged grip sponges, 2 sponge sticks, wrap, gloves, applicators, and towel.

POVIDONE IODINE — TOPICAL

Indications

➤*Professional and hospital use:*

Ointment, swabs, aerosol spray – Povidone-iodine kills pathogens in primary or secondary topical infection, first-, second-, and third-degree burns, surgical incisions, decubitus or stasis ulcers, and traumatic lesions.

Use prophylactically to help prevent microbial infection in incisions, burns, and topical lesions.

Surgical scrub – Povidone-iodine surgical scrub is used for preparation of the skin prior to surgery, to help reduce bacteria that potentially can cause skin infection, for handwashing to reduce bacteria on the skin, and to reduce the number of microorganisms on the hands and forearms prior to surgery or patient care.

Swabsticks – This medication is for professional and hospital use as an bactericidal/virucidal antiseptic.

➤*Over-the-counter (OTC) products:* First aid to help prevent infection in minor cuts, scrapes, and burns.

Administration and Dosage

➤*Adults:*

Antibacterial (over-the-counter use) –

Ointment: Clean the affected area. Apply a small amount of this product to the area 1 to 3 times daily. The area may be covered with a sterile bandage. If bandaged, let dry first.

Skin cleanser solution: Wet skin and apply a sufficient amount to work up a rich, golden lather. Allow lather to remain for about 3 minutes and rinse off. Repeat 2 to 3 times a day or as directed by a health care provider.

Solution: See Ointment for dosing.

Antibacterial/antiseptic (professional and hospital use) –

Aerosol spray: Hold container about 10 inches from skin. Press valve firmly with index finger, spraying to cover desired area. Allow to dry. Replace cap after use. If actuator clogs, remove and soak in warm water.

Ointment: Apply directly to affected area as needed. The affected area may be bandaged.

Swabs: Tear notch; pull top of packette up and away, exposing pad. Use the pad to swab area thoroughly. Repeat on the other side if necessary. Use 1 time only.

Swabsticks: Tear at notch; pull top of packette across, exposing end of swabstick. Remove povidone-iodine solution swabstick and apply as needed. Use 1 time only.

Surgical scrub (professional and hospital use) –

Patient surgical pre-op: Apply scrub (1 mL is sufficient to cover an area of 20 to 30 square inches), develop lather, and scrub thoroughly for about 5 minutes.

Surgical hand scrub: Pour about 5 mL on the palm of the hand and spread over both hands. Scrub thoroughly for about 5 minutes. Repeat procedure 1 time.

➤*Children:*

Antibacterial (over-the-counter use) – See Adults for dosing.

Antibacterial/antiseptic (professional and hospital use) – See Adults for dosing.

➤*Administration:*

Surgical hand scrub –

1.) Wet hands with water.
2.) Pour about 5 mL (1 teaspoonful) of scrub on the palm of the hand and spread over both hands.
3.) Without adding more water, scrub thoroughly for about 5 minutes.
4.) Use a brush if desired. Clean thoroughly under fingernails.
5.) Add a little water and develop copious suds. Rinse thoroughly under running water.
6.) Repeat the entire procedure using another 5 mL of scrub.

Patient preoperative skin preparation –

1.) After the skin is shaved, wet it with water.
2.) Apply scrub (1 mL is sufficient to cover an area of 20 to 30 square inches), develop lather, and scrub thoroughly for about 5 minutes.
3.) Rinse off using sterile gauze saturated with water.
4.) Paint the area with povidone-iodine solution or spray with povidone-iodine aerosol spray and allow to dry.

➤*Storage/Stability:* Patients should avoid storing at excessive heat. Store in original container.

This medication does not stain skin and natural fabrics. Contents of aerosol spray are under pressure.

Aerosol spray – This product contains dry natural rubber. The contents are under pressure. The hole in the bottom is part of the aerosol system. The product contains no chlorofluorocarbons.

Warnings/Precautions

➤*External use only:* Povidone-iodine topical products are for external use only. Do not use these products in the eyes or over large areas of the body. Avoid spraying the aerosol in the eyes.

➤*Preoperative prepping:* In preoperative prepping, avoid "pooling" beneath the patient.

➤*Long term use:* Do not use these products for longer than 1 week unless directed by a doctor.

Prolonged exposure may cause irritation, or, rarely, severe skin reactions.

➤*Heating:* Do not heat prior to application.

➤*Pregnancy:* *Category D.* (per Briggs' *Drugs in Pregnancy and Lactation*). Iodide readily crosses the placenta to the fetus. When used for prolonged periods or close to term, iodide may cause hypothyroidism and goiter in the fetus and newborn. Short-term use, such as a 10-day preparation course for maternal thyroid surgery, does not carry this risk and is apparently safe.

Because many prescription and over-the-counter medications contain iodide or iodine, pregnant patients should consult with their physician before using these products.

➤*Lactation:* The use of povidone-iodine in the mother near term and during breast-feeding can increase breast milk iodine levels and cause transient hypothyroidism in breast-fed infants. The absorption of povidone-iodine is little through intact adult skin, but can be marked with vaginal use. Exposure of mothers who are or will be breast-feeding to povidone-iodine should be minimized to the extent possible by avoiding it on maternal mucous membranes (eg, douching, tampons), avoiding prolonged contact time, avoiding

POVIDONE IODINE — TOPICAL

repeated applications, using lower concentrations of povidone-iodine, and applying it to the smallest possible surface areas of the body. It is possible that maternal exposure to povidone-iodine near term could interfere with thyroid studies done as a part of newborn screening tests.

Patient Information

Povidone-iodine topical products are for external use only.

Do not use these products in the eyes or over large areas of the body.

Avoid spraying the aerosol in the eyes.

In preoperative prepping, avoid "pooling" beneath the patient.

Do not use these products for longer than 1 week unless directed by a doctor.

Prolonged exposure may cause irritation, or, rarely, severe skin reactions.

Do not heat prior to application.

OXYCHLOROSENE SODIUM

otc	**Clorpactin WCS-90** (Guardian)	**Powder for Solution:** 2 g sodium oxychlorosene	In 2 g bottles (5s).

OXYCHLOROSENE SODIUM — TOPICAL

Indications

➤*Localized infection:* Used for treating localized infections, particularly when resistant organisms are present; to remove necrotic debris in massive infections or from radiation necrosis; to counteract odorous discharges; as a preoperative and postoperative irrigant and for the cleansing and disinfection of fistulae, sinus tract, empyemas, and wounds.

Administration and Dosage

➤*Adults:*

Localized infection – Apply topically as the 0.4% solution in water or isotonic saline. Use dilutions of 0.1% to 0.2% in urology and ophthalmology.

Preoperative skin preparation and postoperative protection – See Localized Infection for dosing.

➤*Preparation for administration:* Add the powder to the required amount of cool or lukewarm water (not hot). Saline solution may be used where indicated. Stir or shake for a minute or two. Allow solution to stand for several minutes, then stir (or shake) for an additional 2 or 3 minutes. The solution may be used as such (disregarding any residue still left), or it may be allowed to settle for several minutes and the clear solution decanted for use.

This entire procedure should require no more than 10 to 15 minutes, and the resultant solution has been shown to contain more than 95% of the hypochlorous acid (based on the theoretical evaluation).

To endeavor to dissolve the product completely would require an hour or more and offer no advantages.

➤*Administration:* Apply by irrigations, instillation, spray, soaks, or wet compresses, preferably thoroughly cleansing with gravity flow irrigation or syringe to provide copious quantities of fresh solution to remove organic wastes and debris.

➤*Storage/Stability:* Oxychlorosene sodium solutions should be used as soon as possible after preparation. If, however, the solution must be stored, it should be kept refrigerated at 4° to 8°C (39.2° to 46.5°F) in a capped or sealed plastic or glass container with a non-metallic cap and used within 14 days of preparation. If stored at a room temperature of 23°C (73.4°F), solution should be used within 7 days after preparation.

Actions

➤*Pharmacology:* Oxychlorosene is a complex of the sodium salt of dodecylbenzenesulfonic acid and hypochlorous acid. Its action is markedly cidal, rapid and complete against both gram-negative and gram-positive bacteria, fungi, yeast, mold, viruses and spores.

Contraindications

Infection sites not exposed to direct contact with the solution; systemic use.

Warnings/Precautions

➤*Bladder/eye installation:* Instillation of 0.2% solution, particularly into the bladder or into the eye, may cause severe discomfort. Pretreat the eye with a topical anesthetic. In the bladder, use a 0.1% concentration for the first treatment, instilling the solution to the capacity of the bladder without over-distention.

➤*Pregnancy:* *Category: Undetermined.* Consult a health care provider before using in pregnant women.

➤*Lactation:* Consult a health care provider before using in breast-feeding.

SILVER NITRATE

Rx	**Silver Nitrate** (Gordon Labs)	**Solution:** 10%	In 30 mL.
		25%	In 30 mL.
		50%	In 30 mL.

SILVER NITRATE — TOPICAL

Indications

➤*General information:* To treat indolent wounds, destroy exuberant granulations, freshen the edges of ulcers and fissures, touch the bases of vesicular, bullous or aphthous lesions and provide styptic action.

➤*10% Ointment:*

Podiatry – To treat neurovascular helomas; to cauterize and destroy small nerve endings and blood vessels. It forms a protective covering after the removal of corns and calluses.

➤*10% Solution:* Impetigo vulgaris.

Podiatry – Helomas.

➤*25% Solution:* Pruritus.

Podiatry – Plantar warts.

➤*50% Solution:*

Podiatry – Plantar warts; granulation tissue; papillomatous growths; granuloma pyogenicum.

➤*Off-label uses:* Concentrations of 0.1% to 0.5% are used as wet dressings in burns and on lesions.

Administration and Dosage

➤*Adults:*

Helomas –

Ointment: Apply in apertured pad on affected area for approximately 5 days, as needed.

Solution 10%: Apply a cotton applicator dipped in solution on the affected area or lesion 2 or 3 times a week for 2 or 3 weeks, as needed.

Impetigo vulgaris –

Solution 10%: See Helomas for dosing.

Plantar warts –

Solution 25% and 50%: See Helomas for dosing.

Pruritis –

Solution 25%: See Helomas for dosing.

Actions

➤*Pharmacology:* Silver nitrate is a strong caustic and escharotic providing antiseptic, astringent, germicidal, local (epithelial) stimulant or caustic action externally.

The attachment of silver to a reactive group of a protein sharply decreases the protein's solubility; the protein's conformation may also be altered and denaturation may occur. Precipitation of the protein generally results. At low concentrations of silver, precipitation is confined to proteins in the interstices and an astringent action occurs. At high concentrations, membrane and intracellular structures are damaged and there is a caustic or corrosive effect.

Because silver ions attach so readily to the various groups of proteins, the ions are captured before they diffuse far into tissues. Precipitation of silver as silver chloride also limits extent of ion movement. Thus, local effects of silver are self-limiting and spread of damage occurs only when the dose overwhelms the capacity of tissues to fix the ion at the application site. Antiseptic effects of silver may derive in part from the reaction with bacterial and viral proteins.

Contraindications

Application on wounds, cuts or broken skin.

Warnings/Precautions

➤*Skin discoloration:* Prolonged or frequent use may permanently discolor skin due to deposition of reduced silver. However, topical silver nitrate for local application to suppress granulation tissue apparently does not produce argyria.

➤*Staining of clothes:* Will stain clothing and linens.

➤*Electrolyte abnormalities:* If wet dressings are used over extensive areas or prolonged periods, electrolyte abnormalities can result. Sodium and chloride leach into the dressing and hyponatremia or hypochloremia can occur. Absorbed nitrate can cause methemoglobinemia.

➤*Irritation:* Discontinue use if redness or irritation occurs.

➤*For external use only:* Avoid contact with the eyes.

SILVER NITRATE — TOPICAL

➤*Pregnancy: Category: Undetermined.* There are no information regarding silver nitrate in pregnant women.

➤*Lactation:* There are no information regarding silver nitrate in breast-feeding women.

Overdosage

➤*Symptoms:* The fatal dose of silver nitrate may be as low as 2 g. Oral intake of silver nitrate causes a local corrosive effect including pain and burning of mouth, salivation, vomiting, diarrhea progressing to anuria, shock, coma, convulsions and death. Blackening of skin and mucous membranes occurs (sometimes permanent).

➤*Treatment:* Give NaCl in water, 10 g/L, to precipitate silver Cl. Follow with catharsis, including NaCl solution. Also attend to shock and methemoglobinemia if present.

If splashed in eyes, wash with copious amounts of water and see a physician.

SODIUM HYPOCHLORITE

otc	**Dakin's** (Century Pharm.)	**Solution:** 0.25%	In pt.
		0.5%	In pt and gal.

SODIUM HYPOCHLORITE — TOPICAL

Indications

➤*Antiseptic:* Applied topically to the skin as an antiseptic.

Actions

➤*Pharmacology:* Sodium hypochlorite has germicidal, deodorizing and bleaching properties. It is effective against vegetative bacteria and viruses, and also, to some degree, against spores and fungi.

Warnings/Precautions

➤*Chemical burns:* May be produced; avoid skin or eye contact with this solution.

➤*Pregnancy: Category: Undetermined.* Consult a health care provider before using in pregnant women.

➤*Lactation:* Consult a health care provider before using in breast-feeding patients.

TRICLOSAN (Irgasan)

otc	**Ca-Rezz** (FNC Medical Corporation)	**Soap; topical:** 0.2%	Alcohol, aloe vera, parabens, polysorbate 80, propylene glycol, urea. In 237 mL.
otc	**Sarna** (GlaxoSmithKline)		Fragrance free. Benzyl alcohol, parabens, PEG-75, stearyl alcohol. In 237 mL.
otc	**Ca-Rezz** (FNC Medical Corporation)	**Soap; topical:** 0.25%	Alcohol, aloe vera, parabens, polysorbate 80, propylene glycol. In 361 mL.
otc	**Clean and Clear Foaming Facial Cleanser** (Johnson & Johnson)		Oil free. BHT, glycerin, parabens, triethanolamine. In 240 mL.
otc	**no more germies** (J & J)		EDTA, PEG. In 237 mL.
otc	**Septi-Soft** (Calgon Vestal)		Emollients, glycerin. In 240 mL, qt, gal.
otc	**Septisol** (Calgon Vestal)		Emollients, glycerin. In 240 mL, qt, gal.
otc	**ASC Lotionized** (Geritrex)	**Soap; topical:** 0.3%	Aloe vera gel, parabens, sweet almond oil, tartrazine. In 8 oz.
otc	**Ca-Rezz** (FNC Medical Corporation)		Disodium EDTA, parabens, propylene glycol, urea. In 355 mL.
otc	**Clearasil Daily Face Wash** (Procter & Gamble)		Aloe vera gel, EDTA, glycerin. In 135 mL.
otc	**Oxy ResiDon't** (SK Beecham)	**Soap; topical:** 0.6%	Diazolidinyl urea. In 240 mL.
otc	**Stridex Face Wash** (Sterling Health)	**Soap; topical:** 1%	EDTA, glycerin. Alcohol free. In 237 mL.
otc	**Ca-Rezz** (FNC Medical Corporation)	**Cream; topical:** 0.3%	Alcohol, aloe vera, glyceryl, mineral oil, parabens, PEG, propylene glycol, safflower oil, triethanolamine, urea, vitamins A, D, E. In 275 g.

TRICLOSAN (Irgasan) — TOPICAL

Indications

➤*Skin cleanser:* For use as a skin cleanser.

Ca-Rezz 0.25% soap, Ca-Rezz 0.2% soap – For ostomy or incontinent care.

Ca-Rezz 0.3% cream – To protect and soothe skin tissue irritated by diaper rash, psoriasis, minor burns, chafing, and itching.

Septi-Soft – Skin cleanser. May use as hand/body wash, shampoo, bed or towel bath.

Septisol – Healthcare personnel handwash and skin degermer.

Administration and Dosage

➤*Adults:*

Skin cleanser –

Septisol: Dispense a small amount (5 mL) on hands, rub thoroughly for 30 seconds, rinse thoroughly, dry.

Septi-Soft: Dispense a small amount (5 mL) on hands, rub thoroughly for 30 seconds, rinse thoroughly, dry. May also be used as hand or body wash, shampoo, bed or towel bath.

Actions

➤*Pharmacology:* Triclosan, a bis-phenol disinfectant, is a bacteriostatic agent with activity against a wide range of gram-positive and gram-negative bacteria.

Contraindications

Use on burned or denuded skin or mucous membranes; routine prophylactic total body bathing.

➤*Septi-Soft:* Not a surgical scrub; do not use in preparation for surgery.

Warnings/Precautions

➤*External use only:* For external use only. Avoid contact with the eyes.

➤*Pregnancy: Category: Undetermined.* Consult a health care provider before administering to a pregnant woman.

➤*Lactation:* Consult a health care provider before administering to a breast-feeding woman.

MISCELLANEOUS ANTISEPTICS

otc	**Stat•One Isopropyl Rubbing Alcohol** (Continental)	**Gel; topical:** 70% isopropyl rubbing alcohol	In 28.4 g.
otc	**Stat•One Hydrogen Peroxide** (Continental)	**Gel; topical:** 3% hydrogen peroxide	In 28.4 g.
otc	**S.T. 37** (Numark Labs)	**Solution; topical:** 0.1% hexylresorcinol	Glycerin, EDTA. In 236.5 and 473 mL.

Antiseptics and Germicides

MISCELLANEOUS ANTISEPTICS

otc	**Tincture of Green Soap** (Paddock)	**Liquid; topical:** With 28% to 32% alcohol	In gal.
otc	**Antiseptic Wound & Skin Cleanser** (MPM Medical)	**Liquid; topical:** 0.1% benzethonium chloride	EDTA, glycerin, methylparaben. In 120 mL.
otc	**B.F.I. Antiseptic** (Numark Labs)	**Powder; topical:** 16% bismuth-formic-iodide, zinc phenol sulfonate, potassium alum, bismuth subgallate, boric acid, menthol, eucalyptol, thymol	In 35.4 g.
otc	**Alco-Gel** (Tweezerman)	**Gel; topical:** 60% ethyl alcohol	In 60 and 480 g.
Rx	**Arzol Silver Nitrate Applicators** (Arzol)	**Swab; topical:** 75% silver nitrate, 25% potassium nitrate	In 100s.
Rx	**Grafco** (Graham-Field)		In 100s.
otc	**Gold Bond Antiseptic First Aid Quick Spray** (Chattem)	**Spray; topical:** 0.13% benzethonium chloride, 1% menthol	Glycerin, parabens, SD alcohol 40, urea. In 60 mL.

Antiviral Agents

ACYCLOVIR (Acycloguanosine)

Rx	**Zovirax** (Biovail)	**Ointment:** 5% (50 mg/g)	In a polyethylene glycol base. In 15 g tubes.
		Cream: 5% (50 mg/g)	Cetostearyl alcohol, mineral oil, in an aqueous cream base. In 2 g tubes.

ACYCLOVIR — TOPICAL

Indications

➤*Herpes virus:*

Ointment – Management of initial genital herpes and in limited non-life-threatening mucocutaneous herpes simplex virus infections in immunocompromised patients.

Cream – Treatment of recurrent herpes labialis (cold sores) in adults and adolescents (12 years of age and older).

Administration and Dosage

➤*General dosing considerations:* Initiate therapy as early as possible following onset of signs and symptoms.

➤*Adults:*

Cream – Apply 5 times per day for 4 days (ie, during the prodrome or when lesions appear).

Ointment – Apply sufficient quantity to adequately cover all lesions every 3 hours 6 times per day for 7 days. The dose size per application will vary depending upon the total lesion area, but should approximate a one-half inch ribbon of ointment per 4 square inches of surface area.

➤*Children:*

Cream –

Recurrent herpes labialis (cold sores):

• *12 years of age and older* – Apply 5 times per day for 4 days (ie, during the prodrome or when lesions appear).

Off-label dosing –

Ointment:

• *Usual dose* – Apply 0.5 inch ribbon for 4-inch square surface area 6 times a day.

• *Duration of therapy* – 7 days.

➤*Administration:* A finger cot or rubber glove should be used when applying acyclovir to prevent autoinoculation of other body sites and transmission of infection to other persons.

➤*Storage/Stability:*

Cream – Store at or below 25°C (77°F); excursions permitted between 15° and 30°C (59° and 86°F).

Ointment – Store at 15° to 25°C (59° to 77°F) in a dry place.

Actions

➤*Pharmacology:*

Virology –

Mechanism of antiviral action: Acyclovir is a synthetic purine nucleoside analogue with in vitro and in vivo inhibitory activity against herpes simplex virus types 1 (HSV-1), 2 (HSV-2), and varicella-zoster virus (VZV).

The inhibitory activity of acyclovir is highly selective due to its affinity for the enzyme thymidine kinase (TK) encoded by HSV and VZV. This viral enzyme converts acyclovir into acyclovir monophosphate, a nucleotide analogue. The monophosphate is further converted into diphosphate by cellular guanylate kinase and into triphosphate by a number of cellular enzymes. In vitro, acyclovir triphosphate stops replication of herpes viral DNA. This is accomplished in 3 ways:

1.) Competitive inhibition of viral DNA polymerase,
2.) Incorporation into and termination of the growing viral DNA chain, and
3.) Inactivation of the viral DNA polymerase. The greater antiviral activity of acyclovir against HSV compared to VZV is due to its more efficient phosphorylation by the viral TK.

Drug resistance: Resistance of HSV and VZV to acyclovir can result from qualitative and quantitative changes in the viral TK and/or DNA polymerase. Clinical isolates of HSV and VZV with reduced susceptibility to acyclovir have been recovered from immunocompromised patients, especially with advanced HIV infection. While most of the acyclovir-resistant mutants isolated thus far from immunocompromised patients have been found to be TK-deficient mutants, other mutants involving the viral TK gene (TK partial and TK altered) and DNA polymerase have been isolated. TK-negative mutants may cause severe disease in infants and immunocompromised adults. The possibility of viral resistance to acyclovir should be considered in patients who show poor clinical response during therapy.

➤*Pharmacokinetics:*

Absorption/Distribution –

Ointment: A study included 11 patients with localized varicella-zoster. In this uncontrolled study, acyclovir was detected in the blood of 9 patients and in the urine of all patients tested. Acyclovir levels in plasma ranged from less than 0.01 to 0.28 mcg/mL in 8 patients with normal renal function, and from less than 0.01 to 0.78 mcg/mL in 1 patient with renal function impairment.

Cream:

• *Adults* – A clinical pharmacology study was performed with acyclovir cream in adult volunteers to evaluate the percutaneous absorption of acyclovir. In this study, which included 6 male volunteers, the cream was applied to an area of 710 cm^2 on the backs of the volunteers 5 times daily at intervals of 2 hours for a total of 4 days. The weight of cream applied and urinary excretion of acyclovir were measured daily. Plasma concentration of acyclovir was assayed 1 hour after the final application. Plasma acyclovir concentrations were below the limit of detection (0.01 mcM) in 5 subjects and barely detectable (0.014 mcM) in 1 subject. Systemic absorption of acyclovir from acyclovir cream is minimal in adults.

Excretion –

Ointment: Acyclovir excreted in the urine ranged from less than 0.02% to 9.4% of the daily dose. Therefore, systemic absorption of acyclovir after topical application is minimal.

Cream: The average daily urinary excretion of acyclovir was approximately 0.04% of the daily applied dose.

Contraindications

Hypersensitivity or chemical intolerance to the components of the formulation.

Warnings/Precautions

➤*Cutaneous use only:* Acyclovir ointment or cream is intended for cutaneous use only and should not be used in the eye.

➤*Ointment:* The recommended dosage, frequency of applications, and length of treatment should not be exceeded. There exist no data which demonstrate that the use of acyclovir ointment 5% will either prevent transmission of infection to other persons or prevent recurrent infections when applied in the absence of signs and symptoms. Acyclovir ointment 5% should not be used for the prevention of recurrent HSV infections. Although clinically significant viral resistance associated with the use of acyclovir ointment 5% has not been observed, this possibility exists.

➤*Cream:* Acyclovir cream is intended for cutaneous use only and should not be used in the eye or inside the mouth or nose. Acyclovir cream should only be used on herpes labialis on the affected external aspects of the lips and face. Because no data are available, application to human mucous membranes is not recommended. Acyclovir cream has a potential for irritation and contact sensitization. The effect of acyclovir cream has not been established in immunocompromised patients.

➤*Pregnancy: Category B.* Acyclovir should be used during pregnancy only if the potential benefit justifies the potential risk to the fetus.

➤*Lactation:* It is not known whether topically applied acyclovir is excreted in breast milk. Systemic exposure following topical administration is mini-

ACYCLOVIR — TOPICAL

mal. After oral administration of acyclovir, acyclovir concentrations have been documented in breast milk in 2 women and ranged from 0.6 to 4.1 times the corresponding plasma levels. These concentrations would potentially expose the nursing infant to a dose of acyclovir up to 0.3 mg/kg per day. Nursing mothers who have active herpetic lesions near or on the breast should avoid nursing.

➤*Children:*

Ointment – Safety and effectiveness in pediatric patients have not been established.

Cream – Safety and effectiveness in pediatric patients less than 12 years of age have not been established.

Drug Interactions

None known.

Adverse Reactions

➤*Ointment:* In the controlled clinical trials, mild pain (including transient burning and stinging) was reported by about 30% of patients in both the active and placebo arms; treatment was discontinued in 2 of these patients. Local pruritus occurred in 4% of these patients. In all studies, there was no significant difference between the drug and placebo group in the rate or type of reported adverse reactions nor were there any differences in abnormal clinical laboratory findings.

➤*Observed during clinical practice:*

Dermatologic – Pruritus, rash.

Miscellaneous – Edema or pain at the application site.

➤*Cream:* In 5 double-blind, placebo-controlled trials, 1124 patients were treated with acyclovir cream and 1161 with placebo (vehicle) cream. Acyclovir cream was well tolerated; 5% of patients on acyclovir cream and 4% of patients on placebo reported local application site reactions.

The most common adverse reactions at the site of topical application were dry lips, desquamation, dryness of skin, cracked lips, burning skin, pruritus, flakiness of skin, and stinging on skin; each event occurred in less than 1% of patients receiving acyclovir cream and vehicle. Three patients on acyclovir cream and 1 patient on placebo discontinued treatment due to an adverse event.

An additional study, enrolling 22 healthy adults, was conducted to evaluate the dermal tolerance of acyclovir cream compared with vehicle using single occluded and semi-occluded patch testing methodology. Both acyclovir cream and vehicle showed a high and cumulative irritation potential. Another study, enrolling 251 healthy adults, was conducted to evaluate the contact sensitization potential of acyclovir cream using repeat insult patch testing methodology. Of 202 evaluable subjects, possible cutaneous sensitization reactions were observed in the same 4 (2%) subjects with both acyclovir cream and vehicle, and these reactions to both acyclovir cream and vehicle were confirmed in 3 subjects upon rechallenge. The sensitizing ingredient(s) has not been identified.

The safety profile in patients 12 to 17 years of age was similar to that observed in adults.

➤*Observed during clinical practice:*

Dermatologic – Contact dermatitis, eczema, application site reactions including signs and symptoms of inflammation.

Miscellaneous – Angioedema, anaphylaxis.

Overdosage

Overdosage by topical application is unlikely.

Patient Information

Use only for cold sores. For external use only.

PENCICLOVIR

Rx	**Denavir** (Novartis)	**Cream:** 1% (10 mg/g)	Cetostearyl alcohol, mineral oil, white petrolatum. In 1.5 g tubes.

PENCICLOVIR — TOPICAL

Indications

➤*Herpes labialis:* Treatment of recurrent herpes labialis (cold sores) in adults.

Administration and Dosage

➤*Adults:*

Herpes labialis – Apply every 2 hours during waking hours for a period of 4 days. Treatment should be started as early as possible (ie, during the prodrome or when lesions appear).

➤*Administration:* Apply only on herpes labialis on the lips and face.

➤*Storage/Stability:* Store at 20° to 25°C (68° to 77°F).

Actions

➤*Pharmacokinetics:*

Excretion – Measurable penciclovir concentrations were not detected in plasma or urine of healthy male volunteers (n = 12) following single or repeat application of the 1% cream at a dose of 180 mg penciclovir daily (approximately 67 times the estimated usual clinical dose).

➤*Microbiology:* The antiviral compound penciclovir has in vitro inhibitory activity against herpes simplex virus types 1 (HSV-1) and 2 (HSV-2). In cells infected with HSV-1 or HSV-2, viral thymidine kinase phosphorylates penciclovir to a monophosphate form which, in turn, is converted to penciclovir triphosphate by cellular kinases. In vitro studies demonstrate that penciclovir triphosphate inhibits HSV polymerase competitively with deoxyguanosine triphosphate. Consequently, herpes viral DNA synthesis and, therefore, replication are selectively inhibited.

Drug resistance – Penciclovir-resistant mutants of HSV can result from qualitative changes in viral thymidine kinase or DNA polymerase. The most commonly encountered acyclovir-resistant mutants that are deficient in viral thymidine kinase are also resistant to penciclovir.

Contraindications

Hypersensitivity to the product or any of its components.

Warnings/Precautions

➤*General:* Penciclovir should only be used on herpes labialis on the lips and face. Because no data are available, application to human mucous membranes is not recommended. Particular care should be taken to avoid application in or near the eyes since it may cause irritation. The effect of penciclovir has not been established in immunocompromised patients.

➤*Pregnancy: Category B.* There are no adequate and well-controlled studies in pregnant women. Use during pregnancy only if clearly needed.

➤*Lactation:* There is no information on whether penciclovir is excreted in human milk after topical administration. However, following oral administration of famciclovir (the oral prodrug of penciclovir) to lactating rats, penciclovir was excreted in breast milk at concentrations higher than those seen in the plasma. Therefore, a decision should be made whether to discontinue the drug, taking into account the importance of the drug to the mother. There are no data on the safety of penciclovir in newborns.

➤*Children:* Safety and effectiveness in pediatric patients have not been established.

Adverse Reactions

In two double-blind, placebo-controlled trials, 1516 patients were treated with penciclovir cream and 1541 with placebo. The most frequently reported adverse event was headache, which occurred in 5.3% of the patients treated with penciclovir and 5.8% of the placebo-treated patients. The rates of reported local adverse reactions are shown in the data below. One or more local adverse reactions were reported by 2.7% of the patients treated with penciclovir and 3.9% of placebo-treated patients.

Local Adverse Reactions Reported with Penciclovir in Phase III Trials

Adverse reaction	Penciclovir (n = 1516)	Placebo (n = 1541)
Application site reaction	1.3%	1.8%
Hypesthesia/local anesthesia	0.9%	1.4%
Taste perversion	0.2%	0.3%
Pruritus	0%	0.3%
Pain	0%	0.1%
Rash (erythematous)	0.1%	0.1%
Allergic reaction	0%	0.1%

Two studies, enrolling 108 healthy subjects, were conducted to evaluate the dermal tolerance of 5% penciclovir cream (a 5-fold higher concentration than the commercial formulation) compared to vehicle using repeated occluded patch testing methodology. The 5% penciclovir cream induced mild erythema in approximately one-half of the subjects exposed, an irritancy profile similar to the vehicle control in terms of severity and proportion of subjects with a response. No evidence of sensitization was observed.

ANTIVIRAL COMBINATION

Rx	**Xerese** (Meda Pharmaceuticals)	**Cream; topical:** acyclovir 5%, hydrocortisone 1%	Cetostearyl alcohol, mineral oil, propylene glycol, white petrolatum. In 2 or 5 g.

MAFENIDE

Rx	Sulfamylon (UDL)	Powder for solution; topical: 5%	As mafenide acetate. In 50 g packets.
		Cream; topical: 85 mg/g	As mafenide acetate. Cetyl alcohol, edetate disodium, parabens, sodium metabisulfite, stearyl alcohol. In 56.7, 113.4, and 453.6 g.

MAFENIDE ACETATE — TOPICAL

Indications

➤*Burn treatment:* For adjunctive therapy of patients with second- and third-degree burns (cream); for use as an adjunctive topical antimicrobial agent to control bacterial infection when used under moist dressings over meshed autografts on excised burn wounds (solution).

Administration and Dosage

➤*General dosing considerations:* When feasible, the patient should be bathed daily to aid in debridement. A whirlpool bath is particularly helpful, but the patient may be bathed in bed or in a shower.

Prompt institution of appropriate measures for controlling shock and pain is of prime importance.

➤*Adults:*

Burn treatment –

Cream:

• *Usual dosage* – Apply once or twice daily, to a thickness of approximately 1/16 inch.

• *Duration of therapy* – The duration of therapy with mafenide cream depends on each patient's requirements. Treatment is usually continued until healing is progressing well or until the burn site is ready for grafting.

• *Discontinuation of therapy* – Mafenide should not be withdrawn from the therapeutic regimen while there is the possibility of infection. However, if allergic manifestations occur during treatment with mafenide cream, discontinuation of treatment should be considered.

• *Interruption of therapy* – If acidosis occurs and becomes difficult to control, particularly in patients with pulmonary dysfunction, discontinuing therapy with mafenide cream for 24 to 48 hours while continuing fluid therapy may aid in restoring acid-base balance.

Solution:

• *Usual dosage* – Wet burn dressings with mafenide solution using an irrigation syringe and/or irrigation tubing until leaking is noticeable. The gauze dressing should be kept wet.

• *Duration of therapy* – Treatment is usually continued until autograft vascularization occurs and healing is progressing (typically occurring in about 5 days).

• *Discontinuation of therapy* – If allergic manifestations occur during treatment with mafenide solution, discontinuation of treatment should be considered.

• *Interruption of therapy* – If acidosis occurs and becomes difficult to control, particularly in patients with pulmonary dysfunction, discontinuing the soaks with the mafenide solution for 24 to 48 hours may aid in restoring acid-base balance.

➤*Children:*

Burn treatment –

3 months to 16 years of age: See Adults for dosing.

➤*Renal function impairment:* Use mafenide with caution in burn patients with acute renal failure.

➤*Preparation for administration:*

Solution – Mafenide topical solution is supplied as a sterile powder and is to be reconstituted with sterile water for irrigation or sodium chloride 0.9% irrigation. Aseptic techniques should be observed during preparation of the solution. Premeasured quantities of mafenide 50 g powder are provided in packets. The entire packet should be emptied into a suitable container that contains sterile water for irrigation 1,000 mL or sodium chloride 0.9% irrigation and mixed until completely dissolved.

➤*Administration:* Mafenide is not for injection; for topical use only.

Cream – The burn wounds are cleansed and debrided, and mafenide cream is applied with a sterile gloved hand. Satisfactory results can be achieved with application of the cream once or twice daily to a thickness of approximately 1/16 inch; thicker application is not recommended. The burned areas should be covered with mafenide cream at all times. Therefore, whenever necessary, the cream should be reapplied to any areas from which it has been removed (eg, by patient activity). The routine of administration can be accomplished in minimal time because dressings usually are not required. However, if individual patient demands make them necessary, only a thin layer of dressing should be used.

Solution – The grafted area should be covered with 1 layer of fine mesh gauze. An 8-ply burn dressing should be cut to the size of the graft and wetted with mafenide solution using an irrigation syringe and/or irrigation tubing until leaking is noticeable. If irrigation tubing is used, the tubing should be placed over the burn dressing in contact with the wound and covered with a second piece of 8-ply dressing. The irrigation dressing should be secured with a bolster dressing and wrapped as appropriate. The gauze dressing should be kept wet. In clinical studies, this has been accomplished by irrigating with a syringe or injecting the solution into the irrigation tubing every 4 hours or as necessary. If irrigation tubing is not used, the gauze dressing may be moistened every 6 to 8 hours or as necessary to keep wet.

Wound dressings may be left undisturbed, except for the irrigations, for up to 5 days. Additional soaks may be initiated until graft take is complete. Maceration of skin may result from wet dressings applied for intervals as short as 24 hours. Dressing changes and monitoring the site for bacterial growth during this interruption should be adjusted accordingly.

➤*Storage/Stability:*

Cream – Avoid exposure to excessive heat (temperatures above 40°C [104°F]).

Solution – Store packets in a dry place at room temperature 15° to 30°C (59° to 86°F). Store prepared solution at 20° to 25°C (68° to 77°F); excursions are permitted to 15° to 30°C (59° to 86°F). The solution may be held for up to 28 days if stored in unopened containers. Once a container is opened, any unused solution must be discarded within 48 hours.

Actions

➤*Pharmacology:* The mechanism of action of mafenide is not known but is different from that of sulfonamides. Mafenide is not antagonized by para-aminobenzoic acid, serum, or pus or tissue exudates, and there is no correlation between bacterial sensitivities to mafenide and to the sulfonamides. Its activity is not altered by changes in the acidity of the environment. The osmolality of the 5% topical solution is approximately 340 mOsm/kg.

Mafenide cream, applied topically, produces a marked reduction in the bacterial population present in the avascular tissues of second- and third-degree burns. Reduction in bacterial growth after application of mafenide cream has also been reported to permit spontaneous healing of deep partial-thickness burns, and thus prevent conversion of burn wounds from partial thickness to full thickness. However, it should be noted that delayed eschar separation has occurred in some cases.

➤*Pharmacokinetics:*

Absorption/Distribution –

Cream: Applied topically, mafenide cream diffuses through devascularized areas and is absorbed.

Clinical studies have shown that when applied topically to burns as a mafenide 11.2% cream, blood levels of the parent drug peaked at 2 hours following application, ranging from 26 to 197 mcg/mL for single mafenide doses of 14 to 77 g. Metabolite levels peaked at 3 hours, ranging from 10 to 340 mcg/mL. Twenty-four hours after application, combined parent and metabolite blood levels had fallen to pretreatment levels.

Mafenide is active in the presence of pus and serum, and its activity is not altered by changes in the acidity of the environment.

Solution: Applied topically, mafenide solution diffuses through devascularized areas. Approximately 80% of a mafenide dose is delivered to burned tissue over 4 hours following topical application of the 5% solution.

Cream and solution: Following application of mafenide cream and solution, peak mafenide concentrations in human burned skin tissue occur at 2 and 4 hours, respectively. Peak tissue concentrations are similar following administration of the solution or cream.

Metabolism/Excretion –

Cream and solution: Once absorbed, mafenide is rapidly converted to an inactive metabolite (p-carboxybenzenesulfonamide), which is cleared through the kidneys.

➤*Microbiology:* Mafenide exerts broad bacteriostatic action against many gram-negative and gram-positive organisms, including *Pseudomonas aeruginosa* and certain strains of anaerobes.

Contraindications

Hypersensitivity to mafenide.

Warnings/Precautions

➤*Fatal hemolytic anemia:* Fatal hemolytic anemia with disseminated intravascular coagulation, presumably related to a glucose-6-phosphate dehydrogenase deficiency, has been reported following therapy with mafenide.

➤*Metabolic acidosis:* Mafenide and its metabolite, p-carboxybenzenesulfonamide, inhibit carbonic anhydrase, which may result in metabolic acidosis, usually compensated by hyperventilation. In the presence of renal function impairment, high blood levels of mafenide and its metabolite may exaggerate the carbonic anhydrase inhibition. Therefore, close monitoring of acid-base balance is necessary, particularly in patients with extensive second-degree or partial-thickness burns and in those with pulmonary or renal dysfunction. Some burn patients treated with mafenide have also been reported to manifest an unexplained syndrome of masked hyperventilation with resulting respiratory alkalosis (slightly alkaline blood pH, low arterial partial pressure of carbon dioxide [(pCO_2)], and decreased total CO_2); change in arterial partial pressure of oxygen is variable. The etiology and significance of these findings are unknown.

➤*Administration:* For external use only. Avoid contact with eyes. The solution is not for injection.

➤*Hypersensitivity reactions:* Administer mafenide with caution to patients with history of hypersensitivity to the drug. If allergic manifestations occur during treatment with mafenide, consider discontinuation of treatment. It is not known whether there is cross-sensitivity to other sulfonamides.

MAFENIDE ACETATE — TOPICAL

➤*Sulfite sensitivity:* Mafenide cream contains sodium metabisulfite, a sulfite that may cause allergic-type reactions, including anaphylactic symptoms and life-threatening or less severe asthmatic episodes, in certain susceptible people. The overall prevalence of sulfite sensitivity in the general population is unknown and probably low. Sulfite sensitivity is seen more frequently in asthmatic than in nonasthmatic people.

➤*Renal function impairment:* Use mafenide with caution in burn patients with acute renal failure.

➤*Superinfection:* Fungal colonization in and below the eschar may occur concomitantly with reduction of bacterial growth in the burn wound. However, systemic fungal infection through the infected burn wound is rare.

➤*Pregnancy: Category C.* Animal reproduction studies have not been conducted with mafenide. It is also not known whether mafenide cream can cause fetal harm when administered to a pregnant woman or can affect reproduction capacity. Therefore, the cream preparation is not recommended for treatment in women of childbearing potential unless the burned area covers more than 20% of the total body surface or the need for the therapeutic benefit of mafenide is, in the health care provider's judgment, greater than the possible risk to the fetus.

➤*Lactation:* It is not known whether mafenide is excreted in human milk. The molecular weight of the free base (about 186) is low enough that excretion into breast milk should be expected. Because many drugs are excreted in human milk and because of the potential for serious adverse reactions in breast-feeding infants from mafenide, decide whether to discontinue breast-feeding or the drug, taking into account the importance of the drug to the mother.

➤*Children:* For mafenide cream, use the same administration and dosage as for adults. The safety and efficacy of mafenide solution have been established in children 3 months to 16 years of age.

➤*Monitoring:* Close monitoring of acid-base balance is necessary, particularly in patients with extensive second-degree or partial-thickness burns and in those with pulmonary or renal function impairment.

Monitor the site for bacterial growth during dressing changes.

Adverse Reactions

➤*Dermatologic:*

Cream – The most frequently reported reaction was pain on application or a burning sensation. Rare occurrences are excoriation of new skin and bleeding of skin.

Solution – Blisters, eosinophilia, erythema, facial edema, hives, pain or burning sensation, rash and pruritus (often localized to the area covered by the wound dressing), skin maceration from prolonged wet dressings, swelling.

➤*Hematologic:* A single case of bone marrow depression and a single case of an acute attack of porphyria have been reported following therapy with mafenide. Fatal hemolytic anemia with disseminated intravascular coagulation, presumably related to a glucose-6-phosphate dehydrogenase deficiency, has been reported following therapy with mafenide.

➤*Hypersensitivity:* Blisters, eosinophilia, erythema, facial edema, hives, itching, rash, swelling.

➤*Metabolic:* Acidosis, increase in serum chloride.

➤*Respiratory:* Decrease in arterial pCO_2, hyperventilation, tachypnea.

➤*Miscellaneous:* Accidental ingestion of mafenide cream has been reported to cause diarrhea.

➤*Children:* In a clinical study of children with acute burns requiring autografts who received mafenide solution in addition to double antibiotic solution wound therapy (neomycin sulfate 40 mg and polymyxin B 200,000 units/L), the incidence of rash (4.6%) and itching (2.8%) in the group that received mafenide solution was not different from that experienced with double antibiotic solution dressings alone (5.7% and 1.3%, respectively).

Patient Information

Advise patients to notify their health care provider if condition worsens, if irritation occurs, or if hyperventilation occurs.

➤*Cream:* Bathe the burned area daily; a whirlpool bath is particularly helpful. Continue treatment until healing occurs or until site is ready for grafting.

SILVER SULFADIAZINE

Rx	**SSD Cream** (Par)	**Cream; topical:** 10 mg per g in a water-miscible base[a]	Cetyl alcohol. In 25, 50, 85, 400 and 1,000 g.
Rx	**Silvadene** (Hoescht Marion Roussel)		In 20, 50, 85, 400 and 1,000 g.
Rx	**Thermazene** (Ascend Labs)		In 50, 400 and 1,000 g.
Rx	**SSD AF Cream** (Par)		In 50, 400 and 1,000 g.

[a] Contains white petrolatum, stearyl alcohol, 0.3% methylparaben.

SILVER SULFADIAZINE — TOPICAL

Indications

➤*Burn treatment:* As an adjunct for the prevention and treatment of wound sepsis in patients with second- and third-degree burns.

Administration and Dosage

➤*Adults:*

Burn treatment –

Usual dosage: The burn areas should be covered with silver sulfadiazine cream at all times. The cream should be applied once to twice daily to a thickness of approximately 1/16 inch. Whenever necessary, the cream should be reapplied to any areas from which it has been removed by patient activity.

Duration of therapy: Treatment should be continued until satisfactory healing has occurred, or until the burn site is ready for grafting. The drug should not be withdrawn from the therapeutic regimen while there remains the possibility of infection except if a significant adverse reaction occurs.

➤*Children:* Use of silver sulfadiazine is contraindicated in premature infants or in newborn infants during the first 2 months of life.

Off-label dosing –

Children older than 2 months of age:

• *Burn treatment* – Apply 1/16 inch of cream to the burn area once to twice daily. The burn areas should be covered completely.

➤*Renal function impairment:* If renal functions become impaired and elimination of drug decreases, accumulation may occur and discontinuation should be weighed against the therapeutic benefit being achieved.

➤*Hepatic function impairment:* If hepatic functions become impaired and elimination of drug decreases, accumulation may occur and discontinuation should be weighed against the therapeutic benefit being achieved.

➤*Administration:* For topical use only. Not for ophthalmic use. Cleanse and debride the wound bed and apply silver sulfadiazine under sterile conditions. Administration may be accomplished in minimal time because dressings are not required. However, if individual patient requirements make dressings necessary, they may be used.

Hydrotherapy – Reapply immediately after hydrotherapy.

➤*Storage/Stability:* Store at 15° to 30°C (59° to 86°F).

Actions

➤*Pharmacology:* Silver sulfadiazine has broad antimicrobial activity. It is bactericidal for many gram-negative and gram-positive bacteria as well as being effective against yeast. Results from in vitro testing are listed below.

Sufficient data have been obtained to demonstrate that silver sulfadiazine will inhibit bacteria that are resistant to other antimicrobial agents and that the compound is superior to sulfadiazine.

Studies using radioactive micronized silver sulfadiazine, electron microscopy, and biochemical techniques have revealed that the mechanism of action of silver sulfadiazine on bacteria differs from silver nitrate and sodium sulfadiazine. Silver sulfadiazine acts only on the cell membrane and cell wall to produce its bactericidal effect.

1% Silver Sulfadiazine Cream In Vitro Testing

Genus and species	# of Sensitive Strains/Total # of Strains Tested	
	50 mcg/mL	100 mcg/mL
Pseudomonas aeruginosa	130/130	130/130
Xanthomonas (Pseudomonas) maltophilia	7/7	7/7
Enterobacter species	48/50	50/50
Enterobacter cloacae	24/24	24/24
Klebsiella species	53/54	54/54
Escherichia coli	63/63	63/63
Serratia species	27/28	28/28
Proteus mirabilis	53/53	53/53
Morganella morganii	10/10	10/10
Providencia rettgeri	2/2	2/2
Providencia species	1/1	1/1
Proteus vulgaris	2/2	2/2
Citrobacter species	10/10	10/10
Acinetobacter calcoaceticus	10/11	11/11
Staphylococcus aureus	100/101	100/101
Staphylococcus epidermidis	51/51	51/51
β-hemolytic *Streptococcus*	4/4	4/4
Enterococcus species	52/53	53/53
Corynebacterium diphtheriae	2/2	2/2
Clostridium perfringens	0/2	2/2
Candida albicans	43/50	50/50

SILVER SULFADIAZINE — TOPICAL

Silver sulfadiazine is not a carbonic anhydrase inhibitor and may be useful in situations where such agents are contraindicated.

Contraindications

Hypersensitivity to silver sulfadiazine or any of the other ingredients in the preparation; pregnant women approaching or at term; on premature infants; on newborn infants during the first 2 months of life.

Warnings/Precautions

➤*Cross-sensitivity:* There is potential cross-sensitivity between silver sulfadiazine and other sulfonamides. If allergic reactions attributable to treatment with silver sulfadiazine occur, continuation of therapy must be weighed against the potential hazards of the particular allergic reaction.

➤*Hemolysis:* The use of silver sulfadiazine cream in some cases of glucose-6-phosphate dehydrogenase-deficient individuals may be hazardous, as hemolysis may occur.

➤*Topical proteolytic enzymes:* In considering the use of topical proteolytic enzymes in conjunction with silver sulfadiazine cream, the possibility should be noted that silver may inactive such enzymes.

➤*Renal/Hepatic function impairment:* If hepatic and renal functions become impaired and elimination of drug decreases, accumulation may occur and discontinuation of silver sulfadiazine cream should be weighed against the therapeutic benefit being achieved.

➤*Superinfection:* Fungal proliferation in and below the eschar may occur. However, the incidence of clinically reported fungal superinfection is low.

➤*Pregnancy: Category B.* There are no adequate and well-controlled studies in pregnant women. Use during pregnancy only if clearly justified. Use of silver sulfadiazine is contraindicated in pregnant women approaching or at term.

➤*Lactation:* It is not known whether silver sulfadiazine is excreted in human milk. However, sulfonamides are known to be excreted in human milk, and all sulfonamide derivatives are known to increase the possibility of kernicterus. Because of the possibility for serious adverse reactions in nursing infants from sulfonamides, a decision should be made whether to discontinue nursing or to discontinue the drug, taking into account the importance of the drug to the mother.

➤*Children:* Safety and effectiveness in pediatric patients have not been established. Use of silver sulfadiazine is contraindicated in premature infants or in newborn infants during the first 2 months of life.

➤*Lab test abnormalities:* In the treatment of burn wounds involving extensive areas of the body, the serum sulfa concentrations may approach adult therapeutic levels (8% to 12%). Therefore, in these patients it would be advisable to monitor serum sulfa concentrations. Renal function should be carefully monitored and the urine should be checked for sulfa crystals. Absorption of the propylene glycol vehicle has been reported to affect serum osmolality, which may affect the interpretation of laboratory tests.

Adverse Reactions

Reduction in bacterial growth after application of topical antibacterial agents has been reported to permit spontaneous healing of deep partial-thickness burns by preventing conversion of the partial thickness to full thickness by sepsis. However, reduction in bacterial colonization has caused delayed separation, in some cases necessitating escharotomy in order to prevent contracture.

Absorption of silver sulfadiazine varies depending upon the percent of body surface area and the extent of the tissue damage. Although few have been reported, it is possible that any adverse reaction associated with sulfonamides may occur.

➤*Dermatologic:* Infrequently occurring events include skin necrosis, erythema multiforme, skin discoloration, burning sensation, rashes, and interstitial nephritis.

➤*Hematologic:* Several cases of transient leukopenia have been reported in patients receiving silver sulfadiazine therapy. Leukopenia associated with silver sulfadiazine administration is primarily characterized by decreased neutrophil count. Maximal white blood cell depression occurs within 2 to 4 days of initiation of therapy. Rebound to normal leukocyte levels follows onset within 2 to 3 days. Recovery is not influenced by continuation of silver sulfadiazine therapy. The incidence of leukopenia in various reports averages about 20%. A higher incidence of leukopenia has been seen in patients treated concurrently with cimetidine.

➤*Miscellaneous:* Some of the reactions that have been associated with sulfonamides are as follows: Blood dyscrasias including agranulocytosis, aplastic anemia, thrombocytopenia, leukopenia, and hemolytic anemia; dermatologic and allergic reactions, including Stevens-Johnson syndrome and exfoliative dermatitis; GI reactions; hepatitis and hepatocellular necrosis; CNS reactions; toxic nephrosis.

DAPSONE

Rx	**Aczone** (Allergan)	**Gel; topical:** 5%	Methylparaben. In 30 g.

DAPSONE — TOPICAL

Indications

➤*Acne vulgaris:* For the topical treatment of acne vulgaris.

Administration and Dosage

➤*Adults:*

Acne vulgaris – After the skin is gently washed and patted dry, apply approximately a pea-sized amount of dapsone in a thin layer to the acne-affected areas twice daily. Rub in dapsone gently and completely.

➤*Children:*

Acne vulgaris –

12 to 17 years of age: See Adults for dosing.

➤*Duration of therapy:* If there is no improvement after 12 weeks, treatment with dapsone should be reassessed.

➤*Administration:* For topical use only. Not for oral, ophthalmic, or intravaginal use. Wash hands after application of dapsone.

➤*Storage/Stability:* Store at 20° to 25°C (68° to 76°F); excursions are permitted between 15° and 30°C (59° and 86°F). Protect from freezing.

Actions

➤*Pharmacology:* The mechanism of action of dapsone in treating acne vulgaris is not known.

➤*Pharmacokinetics:*

Absorption – An open-label study compared the pharmacokinetics of dapsone after dapsone gel (110 ± 60 mg/day) was applied twice daily (approximate body surface area, 22.5%) for 14 days (n = 18) with a single oral dapsone 100 mg dose administered to a subgroup of patients (n = 10) in a crossover design. On day 14, the mean dapsone area under the curve from 0 to 24 hours ($AUC_{0\text{-}24\ h}$) was 415 ± 224 ng•h/mL for the gel; whereas, following a single oral dapsone 100 mg dose, the $AUC_{0\text{-}infinity}$ was 52,641 ± 36,223 ng•h/mL. Exposure after oral dapsone 100 mg was approximately 100 times greater than after dapsone gel twice daily.

Contraindications

None known.

Warnings/Precautions

➤*Hematological effects:* Oral dapsone treatment has produced dose-related hemolysis and hemolytic anemia. Persons with glucose-6-phosphate dehydrogenase (G6PD) deficiency are more prone to hemolysis with the use of certain drugs. G6PD deficiency is most prevalent in populations of African, South Asian, Middle Eastern, and Mediterranean ancestry.

There was no evidence of clinically relevant hemolysis or anemia in patients treated with dapsone gel, including patients who were G6PD deficient. Some subjects with G6PD deficiency using dapsone gel developed laboratory changes suggestive of mild hemolysis.

If signs and symptoms suggestive of hemolytic anemia occur, patients should discontinue dapsone. Do not use dapsone in patients who are taking oral dapsone or antimalarial medications because of the potential for hemolytic reactions. Combination of dapsone with trimethoprim/sulfamethoxazole may increase the likelihood of hemolysis in patients with G6PD deficiency.

➤*Peripheral neuropathy:* Peripheral neuropathy (motor loss and muscle weakness) has been reported with oral dapsone. No events of peripheral neuropathy were observed in clinical trials with topical dapsone.

➤*Dermatological effects:* Skin reactions (bullous and exfoliative dermatitis, erythema multiforme, erythema nodosum, morbilliform and scarlatiniform reactions, toxic epidermal necrolysis, and urticaria) have been reported with oral dapsone. These types of skin reactions were not observed in clinical trials with topical dapsone treatment.

➤*G6PD deficiency:* Dapsone gel and vehicle were evaluated in a randomized, double-blind, crossover design clinical study of 64 patients with G6PD deficiency and acne vulgaris. Subjects were 88% black, 6% Asian, 2% Hispanic, or of other racial origin (5%). Blood samples were taken at baseline, week 2, and week 12 during both vehicle and dapsone treatment periods. There were 56 out of 64 subjects who had a week 2 blood draw and applied at least 50% of treatment applications. The following table contains results from testing of relevant hematology parameters for these 2 treatment periods. Dapsone was associated with a 0.32 g/dL drop in hemoglobin after 2 weeks of treatment, but hemoglobin levels generally returned to baseline levels at week 12.

DAPSONE — TOPICAL

Mean Hemoglobin, Bilirubin, and Reticulocyte Levels in Acne Subjects with G6PD Deficiency in Dapsone Crossover Study					
		Dapsone		Vehicle	
		n	Mean	n	Mean
Hemoglobin (g/dL)	Pretreatment	53	13.44	56	13.36
	2 weeks	53	13.12	55	13.34
	12 weeks	50	13.42	50	13.37
Bilirubin (mg/dL)	Pretreatment	54	0.58	56	0.55
	2 weeks	53	0.65	55	0.56
	12 weeks	50	0.61	50	0.62
Reticulocytes (%)	Pretreatment	53	1.3	55	1.34
	2 weeks	53	1.51	55	1.34
	12 weeks	50	1.48	50	1.41

➤*Pregnancy:* Category C. There are no adequate and well-controlled studies in pregnant women. Dapsone has been shown to have an embryocidal effect in rats and rabbits when administered orally in doses of 75 and 150 mg/kg/day (approximately 800 and 500 times the systemic exposure observed in human females as a result of use of the maximum recommended topical dose, based on AUC comparisons, respectively). These effects were probably secondary to maternal toxicity. Use dapsone during pregnancy only if the potential benefit justifies the potential risk to the fetus.

➤*Lactation:* Although systemic absorption of dapsone following topical application is minimal relative to oral dapsone administration, it is known that dapsone is excreted in human milk. Because of the potential for oral dapsone to cause adverse reactions in breast-feeding infants, decide whether to discontinue breast-feeding or dapsone, taking into account the importance of the drug to the mother.

➤*Children:* Safety and efficacy were not studied in children younger than 12 years of age; therefore, dapsone is not recommended for use in this age group.

Drug Interactions

Dapsone Topical Drug Interactions			
Precipitant drug	Object drug[a]		Description
Antimalarial agents	Dapsone	↑	Do not use concurrently because of the potential for hemolytic reactions.
Benzoyl peroxide	Dapsone	↔	Topical application of dapsone followed by benzoyl peroxide may result in a temporary yellow or orange discoloration of the skin and facial hair, with resolution in 4 to 57 days.
Dapsone, oral	Dapsone, topical	↑	Do not use oral dapsone with topical dapsone because of the potential for hemolytic reactions.
Dapsone, topical	Dapsone, oral		
Trimethoprim/ Sulfamethoxazole	Dapsone	↑	Coadministration may increase the likelihood of hemolysis in patients with G6PD deficiency. Systemic exposure of dapsone increased by about 40% during coadministration.

[a] ↑ = object drug increased; ↔ = undetermined clinical effect.

Adverse Reactions

➤*Serious adverse reactions:*

CNS – Suicide attempt, tonic clonic movements.

In the clinical trials, a total of 12 out of 4,032 patients were reported to have depression (3/1,660 treated with vehicle and 9/2,372 treated with dapsone gel). Psychosis was reported in 2 of 2,372 patients treated with dapsone and in 0 of 1,660 patients treated with vehicle.

Dermatologic – Combined contact sensitization/irritation studies with dapsone gel in 253 healthy subjects resulted in at least 3 subjects with moderate erythema. Dapsone did not induce phototoxicity or photoallergy in human dermal safety studies.

GI – Abdominal pain, pancreatitis, severe vomiting.

Miscellaneous – Severe pharyngitis.

➤*Common adverse reactions:*

Dapsone Adverse Reactions						
	Dapsone (n = 1,819)			Vehicle (n = 1,660)		
Adverse reaction	Mild	Moderate	Severe	Mild	Moderate	Severe
Dermatologic						
Dryness	14%	3%	< 1%	14%	4%	< 1%
Erythema	9%	5%	< 1%	9%	6%	< 1%
Oiliness/Peeling	13%	6%	< 1%	15%	6%	< 1%

➤*Other adverse reactions (at least 1%):*

Dapsone Adverse Reactions (≥ 1%)		
Adverse reaction	Dapsone (n = 1,819)	Vehicle (n = 1,660)
CNS		
Headache	4%	4%
Dermatologic		
Application-site burning	1%	2%
Application-site dryness	16%	17%
Application-site erythema	13%	14%
Application-site pruritus	1%	1%
Application-site reaction	18%	20%
Respiratory		
Cough	2%	2%
Nasopharyngitis	5%	6%
Pharyngitis	2%	2%
Sinusitis	2%	1%
Upper respiratory tract infection	3%	3%
Miscellaneous		
Influenza	1%	1%
Joint sprain	1%	1%
Pyrexia	1%	1%

One patient treated with dapsone gel in the clinical trials had facial swelling, which led to discontinuation of medication.

➤*Oral dapsone:* Although not observed in the clinical trials with dapsone gel, serious adverse reactions have been reported with oral use of dapsone, including agranulocytosis, hemolytic anemia, peripheral neuropathy (motor loss and muscle weakness), and skin reactions (bullous and exfoliative dermatitis, erythema multiforme, erythema nodosum, morbilliform and scarlatiniform reactions, toxic epidermal necrolysis, and urticaria).

Overdosage

➤*Treatment:* If oral ingestion occurs, patients should seek medical advice.

Patient Information

Inform patients to use dapsone as directed by their health care provider. Dapsone is for external topical use only and is not for oral, ophthalmic, or intravaginal use.

Instruct patients not to use this medication for any disorder other than that for which it was prescribed.

Advise patients to report any signs of adverse reactions to their health care provider.

Protect dapsone from freezing.

See patient labeling for additional information on safety, efficacy, general use, and storage of dapsone.

ANTI-INFLAMMATORY AGENTS

Corticosteroids, Topical

Indications

➤*Relief of inflammatory and pruritic manifestations of corticosteroid-responsive dermatoses:* Some of the conditions in which topical corticosteroids have been proven effective include: Contact dermatitis, atopic dermatitis, nummular eczema, stasis eczema, asteatotic eczema, lichen planus, lichen simplex chronicus, insect and arthropod bite reactions, first- and second-degree localized burns and sunburns.

➤*Alternative/Adjunctive treatment:* Psoriasis, seborrheic dermatitis, severe diaper rash, dysidrosis, nodular prurigo, chronic discoid lupus erythematosus, alopecia areata, lymphocytic infiltration of the skin, mycosis fungoides and familial benign pemphigus of Hailey-Hailey.

➤*Possibly effective in the following conditions:* Bullous pemphigoid, cutaneous mastocytosis, lichen sclerosus et atrophicus and vitiligo.

Topical corticosteroids relieve inflammatory symptoms associated with dermatophyte and yeast infections of the skin and may be used concomitantly with antifungal agents for initial treatment.

The use of topical corticosteroids in combination with antibiotics in secondary infected dermatoses remains controversial.

➤*Nonprescription hydrocortisone preparations:* Temporary relief of itching associated with minor skin irritations, inflammation and rashes due to eczema, insect bites, poison ivy, poison oak, poison sumac, soaps, detergents, cosmetics, jewelry, seborrheic dermatitis, psoriasis and external genital and anal itching.

Administration and Dosage

➤*Usual dose:* Apply sparingly to affected areas 2 to 4 times daily.

➤*General considerations:* Topical corticosteroids have a repository effect; with continuous use, one or two applications per day may be as effective as three or more. Many clinicians advise applying twice daily until clinical response is achieved, and then only as frequently as needed to control the condition.

Short term or intermittent therapy using high potency agents (eg, every other day, 3 to 4 consecutive days per week, or once per week) may be more effective and cause fewer adverse effects than continuous regimens using lower potency products.

Do not discontinue treatment abruptly. After long-term use or after using a potent agent, in order to prevent a rebound effect, switch to a less potent agent or alternate use of topical corticosteroids and emollient products.

Use low potency agents in children, on large areas, and on body sites especially prone to steroid damage such as the face, scrotum, axilla, flexures and skin folds. Reserve higher potency agents for areas and conditions resistant to treatment with milder agents; they may be alternated with milder agents.

Perform appropriate clinical and laboratory tests if a topical corticosteroid is used for long periods or over large areas of the body.

Treatment with very high potency topical corticosteroids should not exceed 2 consecutive weeks and the total dosage should not exceed 50 g per week because of the potential for these drugs to suppress the HPA axis.

➤*Occlusive dressing technique:*

1.) Soak the area in water or wash it well.
2.) While the skin is still moist, gently rub medication into the affected areas.
3.) Cover the area with a plastic wrap (eg, *Saran Wrap*, *Handi Wrap*). Alternatively, plastic gloves may be used for hands, plastic bags for feet, or a bathing cap for scalp.
4.) Seal edges with tape or bandage, ensuring that the wrap adheres closely to the skin.
5.) Leave in place overnight or at least 6 hours. Do not use for more than 12 hours in a 24 hour period. Do not use this technique with very high potency topical corticosteroids.

Actions

➤*Pharmacology:* Topical corticosteroids are adrenocorticosteroid derivatives incorporated into a vehicle suitable for application to skin or external mucous membranes. Modifications of the essential 4-ring steroid structure such as hydroxylation, methylation, fluorination or esterification are often made to increase lipid solubility and potency and decrease mineralocorticoid effects.

The primary therapeutic effects of the topical corticosteroids are due to their anti-inflammatory activity which is non-specific (ie, they act against most causes of inflammation including mechanical, chemical, microbiological and immunological).

Topically applied corticosteroids diffuse across cell membranes to interact with cytoplasmic receptors located in both the dermal and intradermal cells. The intracellular effects are similar to those that occur with systemically administered corticosteroids.

At the cellular level, corticosteroids appear to induce phospholipase A_2 inhibitory proteins (lipocortins), thus depressing formation, release and activity of the endogenous mediators of inflammation such as prostaglandins, kinins, histamine, liposomal enzymes and the complement system.

When corticosteroids are applied to inflamed skin, they inhibit the migration of macrophages and leukocytes into the area by reversing vascular dilation and permeability. The clinical result is a decrease in edema, erythema and pruritus.

By suppressing DNA synthesis, topically applied corticosteroids have an antimitotic effect on epidermal cells. This property is useful in proliferative disorders such as psoriasis, but also can be demonstrated in normal skin.

➤*Pharmacokinetics:* The amount of corticosteroid absorbed from the skin depends on the intrinsic properties of the drug itself, the vehicle used, the duration of exposure and the surface area and condition of the skin to which it is applied. In general, absorption will be enhanced by increased skin temperature, hydration, application to inflamed or denuded skin, intertriginous areas (eg, eyelids, groin, axilla) or skin surfaces with a thin stratum corneum layer (eg, face, scrotum). Palms, soles and crusted surfaces are less permeable. Occlusive dressings greatly enhance skin penetration and, therefore, increase drug absorption.

Infants and children have a higher total body surface to body weight ratio that decreases with age. Therefore, proportionately more topically applied medications will be absorbed systemically in this population, putting them at a greater risk for systemic effects.

Following topical absorption, corticosteroids enter the systemic circulation and are metabolized and excreted via pathways described for systemically administered corticosteroids.

Vehicles – Ointments are more occlusive and are preferred for dry scaly lesions. Use creams on oozing lesions or in intertriginous areas where the occlusive effects of ointments may cause maceration and folliculitis. Creams are often preferred by patients for aesthetic reasons even though their water content makes them more drying than ointments. Gels, aerosols, lotions and solutions are useful on hairy areas. Urea enhances the penetration of hydrocortisone and selected steroids by hydrating the skin. As a general rule, ointments and gels are more potent than creams or lotions. However, optimized vehicles that have been formulated for some products have demonstrated equal potency in cream, gel and ointment forms. Steroid impregnated tapes are useful for occlusive therapy in small areas.

Occlusive dressings – Occlusive dressings such as a plastic wrap increase skin penetration approximately tenfold by increasing the moisture content of the stratum corneum. Occlusion can be beneficial in resistant cases but it may also lead to sweat retention and increased bacterial and fungal infections. Additionally, increased absorption of the corticosteroid may produce systemic side effects. Therefore, do not use occlusive dressings for more than 12 hours per day and when using very potent topical corticosteroids.

Relative potency – The relative potency of a product depends on several factors including the characteristics and concentration of the drug and the vehicle used. Vasoconstrictor assays are used to measure the relative potency of the commercially available products. The estimated relative potency of selected topical corticosteroid preparations is given in the following table. Ranking is based on vasoconstrictor assays of brand name products. In some cases, generic "equivalents" have less vasoconstrictive activity.

Relative Potency of Selected Topical Corticosteroid Products

Drug		Dosage Form	Strength
I.	*Very high potency*		
	Augmented betamethasone dipropionate	Ointment	0.05%
	Clobetasol propionate	Cream, Ointment	0.05%
	Diflorasone diacetate	Ointment	0.05%
	Halobetasol propionate	Cream, Ointment	0.05%
II.	*High potency*		
	Amcinonide	Cream, Lotion, Ointment	0.1%
	Augmented betamethasone dipropionate	Cream	0.05%
	Betamethasone dipropionate	Cream, Ointment	0.05%
	Betamethasone valerate	Ointment	0.1%
	Desoximetasone	Cream, Ointment	0.25%
		Gel	0.05%
	Diflorasone diacetate	Cream, Ointment (emollient base)	0.05%
	Fluocinolone acetonide	Cream	0.2%
	Fluocinonide	Cream, Ointment, Gel	0.05%
	Halcinonide	Cream, Ointment	0.1%
	Triamcinolone acetonide	Cream, Ointment	0.5%
III.	*Medium potency*		
	Betamethasone benzoate	Cream, Gel, Lotion	0.025%
	Betamethasone dipropionate	Lotion	0.05%
	Betamethasone valerate	Cream	0.1%
	Clocortolone pivalate	Cream	0.1%
	Desoximetasone	Cream	0.05%
	Fluocinolone acetonide	Cream, Ointment	0.025%
	Flurandrenolide	Cream, Ointment	0.025%
		Cream, Ointment, Lotion	0.05%
		Tape	4 mcg/cm^2
	Fluticasone propionate	Cream	0.05%
		Ointment	0.005%
	Hydrocortisone butyrate	Ointment, Solution	0.1%
	Hydrocortisone valerate	Cream, Ointment	0.2%
	Mometasone furoate	Cream, Ointment, Lotion	0.1%
	Triamcinolone acetonide	Cream, Ointment, Lotion	0.025%
		Cream, Ointment, Lotion	0.1%
IV.	*Low potency*		
	Aclometasone dipropionate	Cream, Ointment	0.05%
	Desonide	Cream	0.05%
	Dexamethasone	Aerosol	0.01%
		Aerosol	0.04%
	Dexamethasone sodium phosphate	Cream	0.1%
	Fluocinolone acetonide	Cream, Solution	0.01%
	Hydrocortisone	Lotion	0.25%
		Cream, Ointment, Lotion, Aerosol	0.5%
		Cream, Ointment, Lotion, Solution	1%
		Cream, Ointment, Lotion	2.5%
	Hydrocortisone acetate	Cream, Ointment	0.5%
		Cream, Ointment	1%

Contraindications

Hypersensitivity to any component; monotherapy in primary bacterial infections such as impetigo, paronychia, erysipelas, cellulitis, angular cheilitis, erythrasma (clobetasol); treatment of rosacea, perioral dermatitis or acne; use on the face, groin or axilla (very high or high potency agents); ophthalmic use (prolonged ocular exposure may cause steroid-induced glaucoma and cataracts). When applied to the eyelids or skin near the eyes, the drug may enter the eyes.

Warnings/Precautions

➤*Systemic effects:* Systemic absorption of topical corticosteroids has produced reversible HPA axis suppression, Cushing's syndrome, hyperglycemia and glycosuria. Conditions that augment systemic absorption include the application of the more potent steroids, use over large surface areas, prolonged use and the addition of occlusive dressings.

Periodically evaluate patients for evidence of HPA axis suppression by using morning plasma cortisol, urinary free cortisol and ACTH stimulation tests. If HPA axis suppression is noted, attempt to withdraw the drug, reduce the frequency of application, substitute a less potent steroid or use a sequential approach with the occlusive technique. Also test for impairment of thermal homeostasis.

Recovery of HPA axis function and thermal homeostasis are generally prompt and complete upon discontinuation of the drug. Infrequently, signs and symptoms of steroid withdrawal may occur, requiring supplemental systemic corticosteroids.

Clobetasol suppresses the HPA axis at doses as low as 2 g per day.

Children – They may absorb proportionally larger amounts of topical corticosteroids and may be more susceptible to systemic toxicity (see Warnings).

As a general rule, little effect on the HPA axis will occur with use of a potent topical corticosteroid in amounts of less than 50 g weekly for an adult and 15 g weekly for a small child, without occlusion. To cover the adult body one time requires 12 to 26 g.

For information regarding systemic corticosteroids, refer to the Adrenal Cortical Steroids, Glucocorticoids group monograph in the Endocrine and Metabolic Agents chapter.

➤*Local irritation:* If local irritation develops, discontinue use and institute appropriate therapy. Medications containing alcohol may produce dry skin or burning sensations/irritation in open lesions. Allergic contact dermatitis is usually diagnosed by observing failure to heal rather than noting clinical exacerbation as with most topical products not containing corticosteroids. Corroborate such an observation with diagnostic patch testing.

Skin atrophy – This is common and may be clinically significant in 3 to 4 weeks with potent preparations. Atrophy occurs most readily at sites where percutaneous absorption is high.

Take care when using periorbitally or in the genital area. Avoid use of high potency topical corticosteroids on the face and in intertriginous areas because of resulting striae.

➤*Psoriasis:* Do not use topical corticosteroids as sole therapy in widespread plaque psoriasis.

In rare instances, treatment (or withdrawal of treatment) of psoriasis with corticosteroids is thought to have provoked the pustular form of the disease.

➤*Atrophic changes:* Certain areas of the body, such as the face, groin and axillae, are more prone to atrophic changes than other areas of the body following treatment with corticosteroids. Frequent observation of the patient is important if these areas are to be treated.

➤*Infections:* In the presence of an infection, institute therapy with an antifungal or antibacterial agent. If a favorable response does not occur promptly, discontinue the corticosteroid until the infection has been controlled. Treating skin infections with topical corticosteroids can extensively worsen the infection.

➤*For external use only:* Avoid inhalation of aerosols, ingestion or contact with eyes.

➤*Vehicles:* Many topical corticosteroids are in specially formulated bases designed to maximize their release and potency. Mixing with other bases or vehicles may affect potency far beyond that normally expected from the dilution. Exercise caution before mixing; if necessary, contact the manufacturer to determine if there may be an incompatibility.

➤*Occlusive therapy:* Discontinue the use of occlusive dressings if infection develops, and institute appropriate antimicrobial therapy.

Occasionally, a patient may develop a sensitivity reaction to a particular occlusive dressing material or adhesive; a substitute material may be necessary.

Do not use occlusive dressings in **augmented betamethasone dipropionate, betamethasone dipropionate, clobetasol, halobetasol propionate** and **mometasone** treatment regimens.

➤*Pregnancy:* *Category C.* Corticosteroids are teratogenic in animals when administered systemically at relatively low dosages. The more potent corticosteroids are teratogenic after dermal application in animals. There are no adequate and well controlled studies in pregnant women. Therefore, use during pregnancy only if the potential benefits outweigh the potential hazards to the fetus. In pregnant patients, do not use extensively; do not use in large amounts or for prolonged periods of time.

➤*Lactation:* It is not known whether topical corticosteroids could result in sufficient systemic absorption to produce detectable quantities in breast milk. Systemic corticosteroids are secreted into breast milk in quantities not likely to have a deleterious effect on the infant. Nevertheless, exercise caution when administering topical corticosteroids to a nursing mother.

➤*Children:* Children may be more susceptible to topical corticosteroid-induced hypothalamic-pituitary-adrenal (HPA) axis suppression and Cushing's syndrome than adults because of a larger skin surface area to body weight ratio.

HPA axis suppression, Cushing's syndrome and intracranial hypertension have occurred in children receiving topical corticosteroids. Manifestations of adrenal suppression include linear growth retardation, delayed weight gain, low plasma cortisol levels and absence of response to ACTH stimulation. Manifestations of intracranial hypertension include bulging fontanelles, headaches and bilateral papilledema.

Limit administration to the least amount compatible with effective therapy. Chronic corticosteroid therapy may interfere with the growth and development of children.

Do not use potent topical corticosteroids to treat diaper dermatoses in infants.

Safety and efficacy of augmented betamethasone dipropionate, clobetasol, fluticasone propionate, desoximetasone and halobetasol propionate are not established.

Adverse Reactions

➤*Local:* Burning; itching; irritation; erythema; dryness; folliculitis; hypertrichosis; pruritus; acneiform eruptions; hypopigmentation; perioral dermatitis; allergic contact dermatitis; numbness of fingers; stinging and cracking/tightening of skin; maceration of the skin; secondary infection; skin atrophy; striae; miliaria; telangiectasia. These may occur more frequently with occlusive dressings.

Also, there have been reports of development of pustular psoriasis from chronic plaque psoriasis following reduction or discontinuation of potent topical corticosteroids.

Sensitivity to a particular dressing material or adhesive may occur occasionally.

➤*Systemic:* Systemic absorption of topical corticosteroids has produced reversible HPA axis suppression, manifestations of Cushing's syndrome, hyperglycemia and glycosuria (see Precautions). This is more likely to occur with occlusive dressings and with the more potent steroids. Patients with liver failure or children (see Warnings) may be at at higher risk. Lightheadedness and hives have been reported rarely.

Following prolonged application around the eyes, cataracts and glaucoma may develop. In diffusely atrophied skin, blood vessels may become visible on the skin surface; telangiectasia and purpura may occur at the site of trauma.

The risk of adverse reactions may be minimized by changing to a less potent agent, reducing the dosage or using intermittent therapy.

Overdosage

Topical corticosteroids can be absorbed in sufficient amounts to produce systemic effects (see Precautions).

Patient Information

Apply ointments, creams or gels sparingly in a light film; rub in gently. Washing or soaking the area before application may increase drug penetration.

To use a lotion, solution or gel on your scalp, part your hair, apply a small amount of the medicine on the affected area and rub it in gently. Protect the area from washing, clothing, rubbing, etc until the lotion dries. You may wash your hair as usual but not right after applying the medicine.

To apply aerosols, shake well and spray on affected area holding container about 3 to 6 inches away. Spray for about 2 seconds to cover an area the size of your hand. Take care not to inhale the vapors. If you are spraying your face or near your face, cover your eyes.

Use only as directed. Do not put bandages, dressing, cosmetics or other skin products over the treated area unless directed by your physician.

Notify your physician if the condition being treated gets worse, or if burning, swelling or redness develop.

Avoid prolonged use around the eyes, in the genital and rectal areas, on the face, armpits and in skin creases unless directed by your physician. Avoid contact with the eyes.

If you forget a dose, apply it as soon as you remember and continue on your regular schedule. If it is almost time for the next application, wait and continue on your regular schedule. Do not apply double doses.

For parents of pediatric patients: Do not use tight-fitting diapers or plastic pants on a child treated in the diaper area; these garments may work like occlusive dressings and cause more of the drug to be absorbed into your child's body.

ALCLOMETASONE DIPROPIONATE

Rx	**Alclometasone Dipropionate** (Various, eg, Taro)	**Ointment**: 0.05%	In 15, 45, and 60 g.
Rx	**Aclovate** (Pharmaderm)		Hexylene glycol, white wax, propylene glycol stearate, white petrolatum. In 15 and 45 g.
Rx	**Alclometasone Dipropionate** (E. Fougera)	**Cream**: 0.05%	Hydrophilic, emollient base. White petrolatum, cetostearyl alcohol. In 15, 45, and 60 g.
Rx	**Aclovate** (Pharmaderm)		Hydrophilic, emollient base. Propylene glycol, white petrolatum, glyceryl stearate, PEG-100 stearate, chlorocresol. In 15 and 45 g.

ALCLOMETASONE DIPROPIONATE — TOPICAL

Complete prescribing information begins in the Topical Corticosteroids group monograph.

AMCINONIDE

Rx	**Amcinonide** (Taro)	**Ointment**: 0.1%	White petrolatum, benzyl alcohol 2.2%. In 15, 30, and 60 g.
Rx	**Amcinonide** (Taro)	**Cream**: 0.1%	Benzyl alcohol, glycerin. In 4, 15, 30, and 60 g.

AMCINONIDE — TOPICAL

Complete prescribing information begins in the Topical Corticosteroids group monograph.

BETAMETHASONE DIPROPIONATE

Rx	**Betamethasone Dipropionate** (Various, eg, NMC)	**Ointment; topical**: 0.05%	In 15 and 45 g.
Rx	**Betamethasone Dipropionate, Augmented** (Various, eg, Alpharma, Fougera, Warrick)		In an optimized vehicle. Propylene glycol, propylene glycol stearate, white wax, white petrolatum. In 15, 45, and 50 g.
Rx	**Diprolene** (Schering)		Augmented betamethasone. In an optimized vehicle. Propylene glycol, propylene glycol stearate, white wax, white petrolatum. In 15 and 45 g.
Rx	**Betamethasone Dipropionate** (Various, eg, NMC, Schein)	**Cream; topical**: 0.05%	In 15 and 45 g.
Rx	**Betamethasone Dipropionate, Augmented** (Various, eg, Fougera, Sandoz)		Propylene glycol, sorbitol solution, white petrolatum. In 15 and 50 g.
Rx	**Diprolene AF** (Schering)		Augmented betamethasone. Emollient base. Chlorocresol, propylene glycol, white petrolatum, white wax. In 15 and 45 g.
Rx	**Betamethasone Dipropionate** (Various, eg, Goldline, Major, Moore)	**Lotion; topical**: 0.05%	In 20 and 60 mL.
Rx	**Betamethasone Dipropionate, Augmented** (Fougera)		Hydroxypropylcellulose, 30% isopropyl alcohol, propylene glycol. In 30 and 60 mL.
Rx	**Diprolene** (Schering)		Augmented betamethasone. 30% isopropyl alcohol, hydroxypropylcellulose, propylene glycol. In 30 and 60 mL.
Rx	**Betamethasone Dipropionate, Augmented** (Various, eg, Fougera, Sandoz)	**Gel; topical**: 0.05%	Propylene glycol. In 15 and 50 g.
Rx	**Diprolene** (Schering)		Augmented betamethasone. Propylene glycol. In 15 and 45 g.

BETAMETHASONE DIPROPIONATE — TOPICAL

Complete prescribing information begins in the Topical Corticosteroids group monograph.

BETAMETHASONE DIPROPIONATE, AUGMENTED — TOPICAL

Complete prescribing information begins in the Topical Corticosteroids group monograph.

BETAMETHASONE VALERATE

Rx	**Betamethasone Valerate** (Various, eg, Genetco, Goldline, Major, Taro)	**Ointment; topical**: 0.1%	In 15 and 45 g.
Rx	**Psorion Cream** (ICN)	**Cream; topical**: 0.05%	Mineral oil, white petrolatum, propylene glycol. In 15 and 45 g.
Rx	**Betamethasone Valerate** (Various, eg, Genetco, Major, Moore, Taro)	**Cream; topical**: 0.1%	In 15 and 45 g.
Rx	**Beta-Val** (Lemmon)		Aqueous, vanishing base. Mineral oil, white petrolatum, 4-chloro-m-cresol. In 15 and 45 g.
Rx	**Betamethasone Valerate** (Various, eg, Moore)	**Lotion; topical**: 0.1%	In 60 mL.
Rx	**Beta-Val** (Lemmon)		47.5% isopropyl alcohol. In 60 mL.
Rx	**Luxiq** (GlaxoSmithKline)	**Foam; topical**: 1.2 mg/g	60.4% ethanol, cetyl alcohol, stearyl alcohol. In 100 g.
Rx	**Betamethasone Valerate** (Paddock)	**Powder for compounding; topical**	In micronized 5 and 10 g.

BETAMETHASONE VALERATE — TOPICAL

Complete prescribing information begins in the Topical Corticosteroids group monograph.

CLOBETASOL PROPIONATE

Rx	**Clobetasol Propionate** (Various, eg, Copley, NMC Labs)	**Ointment; topical:** 0.05%	In 15, 30, and 45 g.
Rx	**Temovate** (Pharmaderm)		White petrolatum, sorbitan sesquioleate. In 15, 30, and 45 g.
Rx	**Clobetasol Propionate** (Various, eg, Copley, NMC Labs)	**Cream; topical:** 0.05%	May have an emollient base. In 15, 30, and 45 g.
Rx	**Cormax** (Watson)		White petrolatum, cetyl alcohol, stearyl alcohol, lanolin oil, parabens. In 30 and 45 g.
Rx	**Temovate** (Pharmaderm)		Chlorocresol. In 15, 30, and 45 g.
Rx	**Temovate Emollient** (Pharmaderm)		Emollient base. In 15, 30, and 60 g.
Rx	**Clobex** (Galderma)	**Lotion; topical:** 0.05%	Mineral oil. In 15, 30, 59, and 118 mL.
Rx	**Temovate** (Pharmaderm)	**Scalp application; topical:** 0.05%	39.3% isopropyl alcohol. In 25 and 50 mL.
Rx	**Clobetasol Propionate** (Various, eg, Fougera, Glades)	**Gel; topical:** 0.05%	In 15, 30, and 60 g.
Rx	**Temovate** (Pharmaderm)		In 15, 30, and 60 g.
Rx	**Clobetasol Propionate** (Glades Pharmaceuticals)	**Foam; topical:** 0.05%	60% ethanol, cetyl alcohol, stearyl alcohol. In 50 and 100 g.
Rx	**Olux** (GlaxoSmithKline)		60% ethanol, cetyl alcohol, stearyl alcohol. In 100g.
Rx	**Olux-E** (GlaxoSmithKline)		Cetyl alcohol, light mineral oil, white petrolatum. In 100 g.
Rx	**Clobex** (Galderma)	**Shampoo; topical:** 0.05%	Alcohol. In 118 mL.
Rx	**Clobex** (Galderma)	**Spray; topical:** 0.05%	Alcohol. In 60 mL.
Rx	**Clobetasol Propionate** (Taro)	**Solution; topical:** 0.05%	39.3% isopropyl alcohol. In 25 and 50 mL.
Rx	**Cormax** (Watson)		40% isopropyl alcohol. In 25 and 50 mL.

CLOBETASOL PROPIONATE — TOPICAL

Complete prescribing information begins in the Topical Corticosteroids group monograph.

CLOCORTOLONE PIVALATE

Rx	**Cloderm** (Valeant)	**Cream; topical:** 0.1%	White petrolatum, mineral oil, EDTA, parabens, and stearyl alcohol. In 45 g and 90 g tubes and 30 g pump bottle.

CLOCORTOLONE PIVALATE — TOPICAL

Complete prescribing information begins in the Topical Corticosteroids group monograph.

DESONIDE

Rx	**Desonide** (Various, eg, Fougera, Taro)	**Ointment; topical:** 0.05%	In 15 g, 60 g, and 1 kg.
Rx	**DesOwen** (Galderma)		Mineral oil. In 60 g.
Rx	**Desonide** (Various, eg, Taro, Teva)	**Cream; topical:** 0.05%	May contain methylparaben. In 15 and 60 g.
Rx	**DesOwen** (Galderma)		In 60 g.
Rx	**Desonide** (Various, eg, Fougera, Glades)	**Lotion; topical:** 0.05%	May contain cetyl alcohol, EDTA, light mineral oil, parabens, and stearyl alcohol. In 59 and 118 mL.
Rx	**DesOwen** (Galderma)		Cetyl alcohol, EDTA, light mineral oil, parabens, and stearyl alcohol. In 60 and 120 mL.
Rx	**LoKara** (PharmaDerm)		Cetyl alcohol, EDTA, light mineral oil, parabens, and stearyl alcohol. In 59 and 118 mL.
Rx	**Desonate** (Intendis)	**Gel; topical:** 0.05%	Edetate disodium dihydrate, parabens. In 15, 30, and 60 g.
Rx	**Verdeso** (GlaxoSmithKline)	**Foam; topical:** 0.05%	Cetyl alcohol, light mineral oil, white petrolatum. In 100 g.

DESONIDE — TOPICAL

Complete prescribing information begins in the Topical Corticosteroids group monograph.

DESOXIMETASONE

Rx	**Desoximetasone** (Various, eg, Perrigo, Taro)	**Ointment:** 0.25%	May contain sorbitan sesquioleate, white petrolatum. In 15 and 60 g.
Rx	**Topicort** (Taro)		White petrolatum, sorbitan sesquioleate. In 15 and 60 g.
Rx	**Desoximetasone** (Various, eg, Taro)	**Cream:** 0.05%	Emollient base. White petrolatum, lanolin alcohols, mineral oil, EDTA. In 15 and 60 g.
Rx	**Topicort LP** (Taro)		Emollient. White petrolatum, mineral oil, lanolin alcohols, EDTA. In 15 and 60 g.
Rx	**Desoximetasone** (Various, eg, Taro)	**Cream:** 0.25%	Emollient base. White petrolatum, lanolin alcohols, mineral oil. In 15 and 60 g.
Rx	**Topicort** (Taro)		Emollient. White petrolatum, mineral oil, lanolin alcohols. In 15, 60, 120 g.
Rx	**Desoximetasone** (Various, eg, Perrigo, Taro)	**Gel:** 0.05%	May contain 20% SD alcohol, docusate sodium, EDTA, trolamine. In 15 and 60 g.
Rx	**Topicort** (Taro)		20% SD alcohol 40, EDTA, docusate sodium, trolamine. In 15 and 60 g.

DESOXIMETASONE — TOPICAL

Complete prescribing information begins in the Topical Corticosteroids group monograph.

DIFLORASONE DIACETATE

Rx	**ApexiCon** (PharmaDerm)	**Ointment:** 0.05%	White petrolatum. In 30 and 60 g.
Rx	**Diflorasone Diacetate** (Taro)		In 15, 30, and 60 g tubes.
Rx	**Maxiflor** (Allergan)		Emollient, occlusive base. Lanolin alcohol, white petrolatum. In 15, 30 and 60 g.
Rx	**Psorcon E** (Dermik)		Emollient, occlusive base. Lanolin alcohol, white petrolatum. In 15, 30 and 60 g.
Rx	**ApexiCon E** (PharmaDerm)	**Cream:** 0.05%	Stearyl alcohol, mineral oil, cetyl alcohol. In 30 and 60 g.
Rx	**Diflorasone Diacetate** (Taro)		In 15, 30, and 60 g tubes.
Rx	**Florone** (Dermik)		Emulsified, hydrophilic base. Propylene glycol. In 30 and 60 g.
Rx	**Florone E** (Dermik)		Emollient, hydrophilic vanishing base. Mineral oil. In 15, 30 and 60 g.
Rx	**Maxiflor** (Allergan)		Emulsified, hydrophilic base. 15% propylene glycol. In 15, 30 and 60 g.
Rx	**Psorcon E** (Dermik)		Hydrophilic base. Stearyl alcohol, cetyl alcohol, mineral oil. In 15 and 30 g.

DIFLORASONE DIACETATE — TOPICAL

Complete prescribing information begins in the Topical Corticosteroids group monograph.

FLUOCINOLONE ACETONIDE

Rx	**Fluocinolone** (Various, eg, Fougera, Goldline, Moore)	**Ointment; topical:** 0.025%	In 15 and 60 g.
Rx	**Fluocinolone** (Various, eg, Fougera, Geneva, Goldline, Major, Moore, NMC)	**Cream; topical:** 0.01%	In 15 and 60 g.
Rx	**Fluocinolone** (Various, eg, Fougera, Geneva, Goldline, Major, Moore)	**Cream; topical:** 0.025%	In 15 and 60 g.
Rx	**Fluocinolone** (Various, eg, Fougera, Goldline, Major, Moore)	**Solution; topical:** 0.01%	In 20 and 60 mL.
Rx	**Capex** (Galderma)	**Shampoo; topical:** 0.01%	In 12 mg capsule with shampoo base to be mixed by pharmacist before dispensing. Dibasic calcium phosphate dihydrate 5.48 mg. In 180 mL.
Rx	**Derma-Smoothe/FS (Body Oil)** (Hill)	**Oil; topical:** 0.01%	Isopropyl alcohol; a blend of oils, including lt. mineral oil and 48% refined peanut oil. In 120 mL.
Rx	**Derma-Smoothe/FS (Scalp Oil)** (Hill)	**Oil; topical:** 0.01%	Isopropyl alcohol; a blend of oils, including lt. mineral oil and 48% refined peanut oil. In 120 mL with 2 shower caps.

FLUOCINOLONE ACETONIDE — TOPICAL

Complete prescribing information begins in the Topical Corticosteroids group monograph.

FLUOCINONIDE

Rx	**Fluocinonide** (Various, eg, Goldline, Lemmon, Taro)	**Cream:** 0.05%	In 15, 30, 60 and 120 g.
Rx	**Fluocinonide "E" Cream** (Various, eg, Goldline, Taro, URL)		In 15, 30, 60 and 120 g.
Rx	**Fluonex** (ICN)		Greaseless, anhydrous, water-washable. In 15 and 30 g.
Rx	**Lidex** (Syntex)		Water-miscible, emollient, hydrophilic, anhydrous, greaseless. In 15, 30, 60 and 120 g.
Rx	**Lidex-E** (Syntex)		Water-washable, aqueous emollient base. Mineral oil. In 15, 30 and 60 g.
Rx	**Vanos** (Medicis)	**Cream:** 0.1%	In 30 and 60 g.
Rx	**Fluocinonide** (Various, eg, Lemmon, Taro)	**Ointment:** 0.05%	In 15, 30 and 60 g.
Rx	**Lidex** (Syntex)		Occlusive, emollient. White petrolatum. In 15, 30, 60 and 120 g.
Rx	**Fluocinonide** (Various, eg, Fougera, Goldline, Lemmon, Major, Moore)	**Solution:** 0.05%	In 60 mL.
Rx	**Lidex** (Syntex)		35% alcohol. In 20 and 60 mL.
Rx	**Fluocinonide** (Various, eg, Fougera, Lemmon, Moore)	**Gel:** 0.05%	In 60 g.
Rx	**Lidex** (Syntex)		Water-miscible, greaseless. EDTA. In 15, 30, 60, and 120 g.

FLUOCINONIDE — TOPICAL

Complete prescribing information begins in the Topical Corticosteroids group monograph.

FLURANDRENOLIDE

Rx	**Cordran** (Aqua Pharmaceutical)	**Ointment; topical:** 0.025%	White petrolatum. In 30 and 60 g.
		Ointment; topical: 0.05%	White petrolatum. In 15, 30 and 60 g.
Rx	**Cordran SP** (Aqua Pharmaceutical)	**Cream; topical:** 0.025%	Emulsified base. Cetyl alcohol, mineral oil. In 30 and 60 g.
		Cream; topical: 0.05%	Emulsified base. Cetyl alcohol, mineral oil. In 15, 30 and 60 g.
Rx	**Flurandrenolide** (Various, eg, Barre-National)	**Lotion; topical:** 0.05%	In 60 mL.
Rx	**Cordran** (Aqua Pharmaceutical)		Oil-in-water base. Mineral oil, glycerin, menthol, benzyl alcohol. In 15 and 60 mL.
Rx	**Cordran** (Watson Labs)	**Tape; topical:** 4 mcg per cm^2	In 24″ × 3″ and 80″ × 3″ rolls.

FLURANDRENOLIDE — TOPICAL

Complete prescribing information begins in the Topical Corticosteroids group monograph.

FLUTICASONE PROPIONATE

Rx	**Fluticasone Propionate** (Sandoz)	**Cream; topical:** 0.05%	Cetostearyl alcohol, mineral oil. In 15, 30, and 60 g tubes.
	Cutivate (Pharmaderm)		Mineral oil base. Imidurea. In 15, 30 and 60 g.
Rx	**Fluticasone Propionate** (Fougera)	**Ointment; topical:** 0.005%	In 15, 30, and 60 g tubes.
	Cutivate (Pharmaderm)		In 15 and 60 g.
Rx	**Cutivate** (Pharmaderm)	**Lotion; topical:** 0.05%	Cetostearyl alcohol, parabens. In 60 mL.

FLUTICASONE PROPIONATE — TOPICAL

Complete prescribing information begins in the Topical Corticosteroids group monograph.

HALCINONIDE

Rx	**Halog** (Ranbaxy)	**Ointment:** 0.1%	Polyethylene and mineral oil gel base. In 15, 30, 60, and 240 g.
		Cream: 0.1%	Titanium dioxide, cetyl alcohol. In 15, 30, 60, and 216 g.
		Solution: 0.1%	EDTA. In 20 and 60 mL.

HALCINONIDE — TOPICAL

Complete prescribing information begins in the Topical Corticosteroids group monograph.

HALOBETASOL PROPIONATE

Rx	**Halobetasol Propionate** (Various, eg, Clay Park, Fougera, Taro)	**Ointment; topical:** 0.05%	In 15 and 50 g.
Rx	**Halac Kit** (Acella)		Beeswax, petrolatum, propylene glycol. In 50 g with 225 g ammonium lactate lotion 12%.
Rx	**Halonate** (JSJ Pharmaceuticals)		Beeswax, petrolatum. In 50 g with 120 mL ammonium lactate mousse 12%.
Rx	**Ultravate** (Ranbaxy)		Petrolatum. In 15 and 45 g.
Rx	**Halobetasol Propionate** (Various, eg, Clay Park, Fougera, Glades)	**Cream; topical:** 0.05%	In 15 and 50 g.
Rx	**Ultravate** (Ranbaxy)		Glycerin, diazolidinyl urea. In 15 and 45 g.
Rx	**Ultravate PAC** (Ranbaxy)		Beeswax, petrolatum, propylene glycol. In 50 g with 225 g ammonium lactate lotion 12%.

HALOBETASOL PROPIONATE — TOPICAL

Complete prescribing information begins in the Topical Corticosteroids group monograph.

HYDROCORTISONE

Rx[a]	**Hydrocortisone** (Various, eg, Carolina Medical, Fougera, Parmed[b], URL)	**Ointment; topical:** 0.5%	In 30 g.
otc	**Cortizone-5** (Pfizer Consumer)		White petrolatum. In 28 g.
Rx[a]	**Hydrocortisone** (Various, eg, Carolina Medical[c], Fougera, Major, Parmed, URL)	**Ointment; topical:** 1%	In 20, 30, and 120 g and lb.
otc	**Hydrocortisone with Aloe** (G & W Labs)		Mineral oil, white petrolatum, parabens. In 28.4 g.
otc	**Cortizone-10** (Pfizer Consumer)		White petrolatum. In 30 g.
Rx	**Hycort** (Everett)		White petrolatum and mineral oil base. In 30 g.
otc	**Tegrin-HC** (Block)		Mineral oil, white petrolatum. In 28 g.
Rx	**1% HC** (C & M)		Washable. Petrolatum base. In 15, 20, 30, 60, 120, and 240 g and lb.
Rx	**Hydrocortisone** (Various, eg, Major, Parmed, URL)	**Ointment; topical:** 2.5%	In 20 g.
Rx	**Hytone** (Dermik)		Emollient base. Mineral oil, white petrolatum. In 30 g.
Rx[a]	**Hydrocortisone** (Various, eg, Fougera, Geneva, Major, Roberts Hauck, URL)	**Cream; topical:** 0.5%	In 15, 30, and 120 g and lb.
otc	**Cortizone for Kids** (Pfizer)		Parabens, ceteryl alcohol, glycerin, white petrolatum. In 14 g.
otc	**Dermolate** (Schering-Plough)		Greaseless, vanishing. Petrolatum, mineral oil, chlorocresol. In 15 and 30 g.
otc	**HydroTex** (Syosset)		In 30 and 60 g.

HYDROCORTISONE

Rx[a]	**Hydrocortisone** (Various, eg, Fougera, Geneva, Goldline, Major, Moore, Parmed, Roberts Hauck, URL[b])	**Cream; topical:** 1%	In 20, 30, and 120 g and lb.
otc	**HydroSkin** (Rugby)		Mineral oil, lanolin alcohol, cetyl alcohol, parabens. In 113.4 g.
Rx	**Ala-Cort** (Del-Ray)		Glycerin. In 30 and 90 g.
otc	**Maximum Strength Bactine** (Miles Inc.)		Glycerin, lt. mineral oil, methylparaben, white petrolatum. In 30 g.
Rx	**Cort-Dome** (Miles Inc.)		Glycerin, white petrolatum, lt. mineral oil, methylparaben. In 30 g.
Rx	**Hi-Cor 1.0** (C & M)		Washable. Petrolatum, glycerin. In 15, 20, 30, 60, 120, and 240 g and lb.
Rx	**Hytone** (Dermik)		Water-washable. Cholesterol. In 30 and 120 g.
otc	**Procort** (Roberts)		In 30 g.
Rx	**Synacort** (Syntex)		Mineral oil. In 15, 30, and 60 g.
otc	**Maximum Strength KeriCort-10** (Bristol-Myers Squibb)		Parabens, cetyl alcohol, stearyl alcohol. In 56.7 g.
otc	**Cortaid Intensive Therapy** (Pharmacia & Upjohn)		Alcohol, parabens. In 56 g tubes.
otc	**Cortizone-10** (Pfizer Consumer)		Aloe, cetearyl alcohol, glycerin, mineral oil, parabens, petrolatum. In 14, 28, and 57 g.
otc	**Cortizone-10 Plus** (Pfizer Consumer)		Alcohol, aloe, glycerin, mineral oil, parabens, petrolatum. In 28 and 57 g.
otc	**Cortizone-10 External Anal Itch** (Pfizer Consumer)		Cetearyl alcohol, glycerin mineral oil, parabens, petrolatum. In 28 g.
Rx	**Hydrocortisone** (Various, eg, Geneva, Goldline, King, Major, Moore, NMC, URL)	**Cream; topical:** 2.5%	In 20 and 30 g and lb.
Rx	**Anusol-HC** (Salix)		Water-washable. Benzyl and stearyl alcohols, petrolatum, EDTA. In 30 g.
Rx	**Eldecort** (ICN)		Lt. mineral oil, propylene glycol, allantoin. In 15 and 30 g.
Rx	**Hi-Cor 2.5** (C & M)		Washable. Petrolatum, glycerin. In 15, 20, 30, 60, 120, and 240 g and lb.
Rx	**Hydrocort** (Parmed)		In 20 and 30 g and lb.
Rx	**Hytone** (Dermik)		Water-washable base. Cholesterol. In 30 and 60 g.
Rx	**Synacort** (Syntex)		Mineral oil. In 30 g.
Rx	**proctoCream•HC 2.5%** (Schwarz Pharma)		Glyceryl monostearate, glycerin, stearyl alcohol, benzyl alcohol. In 30 g tubes.
Rx	**Cetacort** (Owen/Galderma)	**Lotion; topical:** 0.25%	Parabens. In 120 mL.
Rx[a]	**Hydrocortisone** (Various, eg, Goldline, Mericon, Parmed, URL)	**Lotion; topical:** 0.5%	In 30, 60, and 120 mL.
Rx	**Cetacort** (Owen/Galderma)		Parabens. In 60 mL.
otc[a]	**Hydrocortisone** (Various, eg, Geneva, Glades, Mericon)	**Lotion; topical:** 1%	In 120 mL.
otc	**HydroSkin** (Rugby)		Cetyl alcohol, parabens. In 118 mL.
Rx	**Acticort 100** (Baker Cummins)		In 60 mL.
Rx	**Ala-Cort** (Del-Ray)		Lt. mineral oil, glycerin. In 118 mL.
Rx	**Ala Scalp** (Del-Ray)	**Lotion; topical:** 2%	Isopropyl alcohol, benzalkonium chloride. In 30 mL.
Rx	**NuCort** (WraSer Pharmaceuticals)		Aloe, benzyl alcohol, camphor, cetyl alcohol, glycerin, glyceryl stearate, PEG-7. In 60 mL.
Rx	**Scalacort DK** (Avidas)		Benzalkonium chloride, isopropyl alcohol. In 29.6 mL and shampoo.
Rx	**Hydrocortisone** (Glades)	**Lotion; topical:** 2.5%	Stearyl alcohol, cetyl alcohol, lt. mineral oil. In 59 and 120 mL.
Rx	**Hytone** (Dermik)		Cholesterol, triethanolamine. In 60 mL.
otc	**Cortizone 10** (Chattem)	**Liquid; topical:** 1%	Aloe, disodium EDTA, glycerin, PEG-8, 2% SD alcohol. In 36 mL.
otc	**Scalpicin** (Combe)		Menthol, SD alcohol 40. In 45, 75, and 120 mL.
otc	**T/Scalp** (Neutrogena)		Greaseless. In 60 and 600 mL.
otc	**Extra Strength CortaGel** (Norstar)	**Gel; topical:** 1%	Greaseless. EDTA. In 15 and 30 g.
Rx	**Penecort** (Allergan)	**Solution; topical:** 1%	Alcohol, petrolatum, propylene glycol. In 30 and 60 mL.
Rx	**Texacort** (JSJ Pharm[d])	**Solution; topical:** 2.5%	Alcohol. In 30 mL.
otc	**Maximum Strength Cortaid** (Pharmacia & Upjohn)	**Pump spray; topical:** 1%	55% alcohol, glycerin, methylparaben. In 45 mL.
otc	**Procort** (Roberts)	**Spray; topical:** 1%	In 45 mL.
otc	**Cortizone-10 Quickshot** (Pfizer Consumer)		Alcohols. In 44 mL.
otc	**Itch-X** (B.F. Ascher)	**Foam; topical:** 1%	Cetyl alcohol, mineral oil, parabens, white petrolatum. In 88.7 mL.
otc	**Maximum Strength Cortaid Faststick** (Pharmacia & Upjohn)	**Stick, roll-on; topical:** 1%	55% alcohol, glycerin, methylparaben. In 14 g.

[a] Products are available *otc* or *Rx* depending on product labeling.
[b] Also available with aloe.
[c] In *Absorbase* (a water-in-oil emulsion of cholesterolized petrolatum and purified water).
[d] JSJ Pharmaceuticals, 3655 Route 202, Suite 116, Doylestown PA 18901; 1-(267) 880-2360; FAX 1-(215) 348-9186.

HYDROCORTISONE — TOPICAL

Complete prescribing information begins in the Topical Corticosteroids group monograph.

HYDROCORTISONE ACETATE

otc	**Lanacort-5** (Combe)	**Ointment; topical:** 0.5%	Acetylated lanolin alcohols, aloe, petrolatum. In 15 g.
otc	**Cortaid with Aloe** (Pharmacia & Upjohn)	**Cream; topical:** 0.5%	Aloe vera, parabens. In 15 and 30 g.
otc	**Cortef Feminine Itch** (Pharmacia & Upjohn)		Vanishing. Aloe vera, parabens. In 15 g.
otc	**Lanacort-5 Creme** (Combe)		Aloe, parabens. In 15 and 22.5 g.
otc	**Tucks** (Pfizer Consumer Health)	**Ointment; topical:** 1%	Parabens, mineral oil, white petrolatum. In 19.8 g.
otc	**Maximum Strength Cortaid** (Pharmacia & Upjohn)		Mineral oil, parabens, cholesterol, white petrolatum. In 30 g.
otc	**Maximum Strength Hydrocortisone Acetate** (Clay-Park Labs)		Aloe extract, white petrolatum. In 28 g.
Rx[a]	**Hydrocortisone Acetate** (Various, eg, Thames)	**Cream; topical:** 1%	Mineral oil, parabens. In 20, 30 and 120 g.
otc	**Gynecort Female Creme** (Combe)		Parabens, sorbitol, zinc pyrithione. In 15 g.
otc	**Lanacort 10 Creme** (Combe)		Parabens. In 15 and 30 g.
otc	**Maximum Strength Cortaid** (Pharmacia & Upjohn)		Parabens, glycerin, white petrolatum. In 15 g.
otc	**Maximum Strength Caldecort** (Insight Pharmaceuticals)		Cetostearyl alcohol, white petrolatum. In 14 g.
Rx	**U-cort** (Taro)		10% Urea, alcohol, EDTA. In 28.35 and 7 g.
Rx	**Hydrocortisone Acetate With Aloe** (River's Edge)	**Lotion; topical:** 2%	Aloe, benzyl alcohol, camphor, cetyl alcohol, dimethicone, glycerin, menthol, PEG-7, triethanolamine. In 59.14 mL.
Rx	**NuCort** (Gentex Pharma)		Aloe, benzyl alcohol, camphor, cetyl alcohol, glycerin, glyceryl, menthol, PEG-7, triethanolamine. In 59.14 mL.

[a] Products are available *otc* or *Rx* depending on product labeling.

HYDROCORTISONE ACETATE — TOPICAL

Complete prescribing information begins in the Topical Corticosteroids group monograph.

HYDROCORTISONE PROBUTATE

Rx	**Pandel** (Collagenex)	**Cream:** 0.1%	In 15, 45, and 80 g.

HYDROCORTISONE PROBUTATE — TOPICAL

Complete prescribing information begins in the Topical Corticosteroids group monograph.

HYDROCORTISONE BUTYRATE

Rx	**Hydrocortisone Butyrate** (Taro)	**Ointment; topical:** 0.1%	Mineral oil. In 5, 10, 15, 30, and 45 g.
Rx	**Locoid** (Triax)		Mineral oil. In 15 and 45 g.
Rx	**Hydrocortisone Butyrate** (Taro)	**Cream; topical:** 0.1%	In a hydrophilic base. Alcohol, lt. mineral oil, parabens, white petrolatum. In 5, 10, 15, 30, and 45 g.
Rx	**Locoid** (Triax)		Alcohol, mineral oil, parabens, white petrolatum. In 15 and 45 g.
Rx	**Locoid Lipocream** (Triax)		Alcohol, mineral oil, parabens, white petrolatum. In 15 and 45 g.
Rx	**Locoid** (Triax)	**Lotion; topical:** 0.1%	Cetostearyl alcohol, lt. mineral oil, parabens, safflower oil, white petrolatum. In 60 and 120 mL.
Rx	**Hydrocortisone Butyrate** (Taro)	**Solution; topical:** 0.1%	50% isopropyl alcohol, glycerin. In 20 and 60 mL.
Rx	**Locoid** (Triax)		50% alcohol, glycerin. In 20 and 60 mL.

HYDROCORTISONE BUTYRATE — TOPICAL

Complete prescribing information begins in the Topical Corticosteroids group monograph.

HYDROCORTISONE VALERATE

Rx	**Hydrocortisone Valerate** (Taro)	**Ointment; topical:** 0.2%	Hydrophilic base. White petrolatum, alcohol, mineral oil. In 15, 45, and 60 g.
Rx	**Westcort** (Ranbaxy)		Hydrophilic base. White petrolatum, mineral oil. In 15, 45, and 60 g.
Rx	**Hydrocortisone Valerate** (Copley)	**Cream; topical:** 0.2%	Hydrophilic base. White petrolatum, alcohol. In 15, 45, and 60 g.
Rx	**Westcort** (Westwood Squibb)		Hydrophilic base. White petrolatum. In 15, 45, 60, and 120 g.

HYDROCORTISONE VALERATE — TOPICAL

Complete prescribing information begins in the Topical Corticosteroids group monograph.

MOMETASONE FUROATE

Rx	**Mometasone Furoate** (Various, eg, Sandoz, Taro)	**Ointment; topical:** 0.1%	In 15 and 45 g.
Rx	**Elocon** (Schering)		White petrolatum. In 15 and 45 g.
Rx	**Mometasone Furoate** (Clay Park)	**Cream; topical:** 0.1%	White petrolatum, stearyl alcohol. In 15 and 45 g.
Rx	**Elocon** (Schering)		White petrolatum. In 15 and 45 g.
Rx	**Momexin** (JSJ Pharmaceuticals)		Stearyl alcohol, titanium dioxide, white petrolatum, white wax. In 45 g.
Rx	**Mometasone Furoate** (Taro)	**Lotion; topical:** 0.1%	Isopropyl alcohol. In 30 and 60 mL bottles.
Rx	**Elocon** (Schering)		40% isopropyl alcohol. In 27.5 and 55 mL.
Rx	**Mometasone Furoate** (Clay Park)	**Solution; topical:** 0.1%	40% isopropyl alcohol, glycerin. In 30 and 60 mL.

MOMETASONE FUROATE — TOPICAL

Complete prescribing information begins in the Topical Corticosteroids group monograph.

PREDNICARBATE

Rx	**Prednicarbate** (Fougera)	**Cream; topical:** 0.1% prednicarbate	Cetostearyl alcohol, EDTA, lanolin alcohols, mineral oil, white petrolatum. In 15 and 60 g.
Rx	**Dermatop E** (Dermik)		White petrolatum, mineral oil, EDTA, lanolin alcohols, cetostearyl alcohol, lactic acid. In 15 and 60 g.
Rx	**Prednicarbate** (Fougera)	**Ointment; topical:** 0.1% prednicarbate	Glyceryl, white petrolatum. In 15 and 60 g.
Rx	**Dermatop E** (Dermik)		White petrolatum, glycerin. In 15 and 60 g.

PREDNICARBATE — TOPICAL

Complete prescribing information begins in the Topical Corticosteroids group monograph.

TRIAMCINOLONE ACETONIDE

Rx	**Triamcinolone Acetonide** (Various, eg, Fougera, Goldline, Moore, URL)	**Ointment; topical:** 0.025%	In 15, 80 and 454 g.
Rx	**Triamcinolone Acetonide** (Various, eg, Fougera, Goldline, Moore, NMC, URL)	**Ointment; topical:** 0.1%	In 15 and 80 g and lb.
Rx	**Triamcinolone Acetonide** (Various, eg, URL)	**Ointment; topical:** 0.5%	In 15 g.
Rx	**Triamcinolone Acetonide** (Various, eg, Goldline, Major, Moore, Schein, URL)	**Cream; topical:** 0.025%	In 15, 80 and 454 g.
Rx	**Triamcinolone Acetonide** (Various, eg, Fougera, Goldline)	**Cream; topical:** 0.1%	In 15, 80 and 454 g.
Rx	**Kenonel** (Marnel)		In 20 g.
Rx	**Triderm** (Del-Ray)		Mineral oil. In 30 and 90 g.
Rx	**pediaderm TA** (Arbor Pharmaceuticals)		Cetyl alcohol, cetyl esters wax, glyceryl, polysorbate 80, propylene glycol. In 30 g with protective emollient (cetyl alcohol, glycerin, mineral oil, parabens, petrolatum).
Rx	**Triamcinolone Acetonide** (Various, eg, Fougera, Goldline, Moore, URL)	**Cream; topical:** 0.5%	In 15 g.
Rx	**Triamcinolone Acetonide** (Various, eg, Major, Morton Grove)	**Lotion; topical:** 0.025%	In 60 mL.
Rx	**Triamcinolone Acetonide** (Various, eg, Goldline, Morton Grove, Moore, PBI)	**Lotion; topical:** 0.1%	In 60 mL.
Rx	**Kenalog** (Ranbaxy Labs)	**Aerosol, foam; topical:** (2 sec. spray)	Alcohol 10.3%. In 23 and 63 g.

TRIAMCINOLONE ACETONIDE — TOPICAL

Complete prescribing information begins in the Topical Corticosteroids group monograph.

CORTICOSTEROID COMBINATIONS

	Product & Distributor	Hydrocortisone (%)	Clioquinol (%)	Pramoxine (%)	Other Content and How Supplied
Rx	**Hydrocortisone with Clioquinol Cream** (Various, eg, Moore)	0.5	3		In 30 g.
Rx	**Ala-Quin Cream** (Del-Ray)				Glycerin. In 30 g.
Rx	**Hydrocortisone with Clioquinol Cream** (Various, eg, Goldline, Moore, Schein, URL)	1	3		In 20, 30 and 300 g.
Rx	**Corque Cream** (Geneva)				In 20 g.
Rx	**Hysone Cream** (Roberts Med)				In 20 g tube.
Rx	**Hydrocortisone with Clioquinol Ointment** (Various, eg, Moore)				In 20 and 30 g.
Rx	**1 + 1-F Creme** (Dunhall)	1	3	1	Mineral oil, lanolin alcohol, parabens. In 30 g.
Rx	**Analpram-HC Cream** (Ferndale)	1[a]		1	0.1% potassium sorbate, 0.1% sorbic acid. In 30 g.
Rx	**Enzone Cream** (UAD)				Hydrophilic. 0.1% K sorbate, 0.1% sorbic acid. In 30 g.
Rx	**Pramosone Cream** (Ferndale)				Hydrophilic base. 0.1% potassium sorbate, 0.1% sorbic acid. In 30, 60 and 120 g.
Rx	**Pramosone Ointment** (Ferndale)				Emollient base. White petrolatum. In 30 and 120 g.
Rx	**Pramosone Lotion** (Ferndale)				Hydrophilic. Glycerin, 0.1% potassium sorbate, 0.1% sorbic acid. In 60, 120, 240 mL.
Rx	**Epifoam Aerosol Foam** (Alaven Pharmaceuticals)				Parabens, propylene glycol. In 10 g.
Rx	**ProctoFoam-HC Aerosol Foam** (Alaven Pharmaceuticals)				Hydrophilic base. Parabens. In 10 g.
Rx	**Cortane-B Lotion** (Blansett)	1		1	0.1% chloroxylenol. Benzalkonium Cl. In 60 mL.
Rx	**Carmol HC Cream** (Doak)	1[a]			Water-washable, vanishing. 10% urea, sodium metabisulfite. In 30 and 120 g.
Rx	**Keratol HC Cream** (Breckenridge)				Water-washable, vanishing. Cetyl alcohol, disodium edetate, 10% urea. In 28.3 and 95 g.

CORTICOSTEROID COMBINATIONS

	Product & Distributor	Hydrocortisone (%)	Clioquinol (%)	Pramoxine (%)	Other Content and How Supplied
Rx	**Hydrocortisone Iodoquinol 1% Cream** (Various, eg, Cypress, Glades)	1			1% iodoquinol. In 30 g.
Rx	**Vytone Cream** (Aventis)				Greaseless. 1% iodoquinol, propylene glycol, cetyl alcohol. In 30 g.
Rx	**Novacort Gel** (Primus)	2		1	Alcohols, aloe, glycerin. In 29 g tubes.
Rx	**Alcortin** (Primus)	2			1% iodoquinol. Alcohols, aloe, glycerin. In 2 g.
Rx	**Lidocaine/Hydrocortisone Acetate Cream Kit** (River's Edge)	2			2% lidocaine, cetyl alcohol, mineral oil, parabens, stearyl alcohol, white petrolatum. In 7 g tubes with applicators and cleansing wipes.
Rx	**Hydro-Iodoquinol 2-1 Gel** (Seton Pharmaceuticals)	2			Aloe polysaccharide 1%, amino methylpropanol 95%, benzyl alcohol, glycerin, glyceryl, iodoquinol 1%, propylene glycol, SD alcohol. In 2 g packettes.
Rx	**Alcortin A Gel** (Primus Pharmaceuticals)	2			Aloe polysaccharide 1%, benzyl alcohol, glycerin, iodoquinol 1%, amino methylpropanol, propylene glycol, SD alcohol. In 2 g individual packs.
Rx	**Lidocaine/Hydrocortisone Acetate Gel Kit** (River's Edge)	2.5			3% lidocaine, cetyl alcohol, mineral oil, parabens, stearyl alcohol, white petolatum. In 7 g tubes with applicators and cleansing wipes.
Rx	**Zypram Cream** (Vertical Pharmaceuticals)	2.35[a]		1	Benzyl alcohol, cetearyl alcohol, glycerin, glyceryl, methylparaben, PEG-12, white petrolatum. In 30 g with 2 wipes and 1 applicator.
Rx	**Hydrocortisone Acetate 2.5%/Pramoxine HCl 1%** (Brookstone)	2.5[a]		1	Cetostearyl alcohol, lanolin alcohol, mineral oil, parabens, PEG-40, white petrolatum. In 4 g.
Rx	**Analpram-E Cream** (Ferndale)				Cetostearyl alcohol, mineral oil, propylparaben, white petrolatum. In kits with 30 4 g single-use tubes of cream and 18 *Prax* wipes.
Rx	**Analpram-HC Cream** (Ferndale)				In 30 g.
Rx	**Pramosone Cream** (Ferndale)				Hydrophilic. 0.1% K sorbate, 0.1% sorbic acid. In 30, 120 g.
Rx	**Pramosone Ointment** (Ferndale)				Emollient base. White petrolatum. In 30 and 120 g.
Rx	**Pramosone E Cream** (Ferndale)				*Hydrolipid* base. Cetostearyl alcohol, mineral oil, propylparaben, triethanolamine, white petrolatum. In 28.4 and 57 g.
Rx	**Pramosone Lotion** (Ferndale)				Hydrophilic. Glycerin, 0.1% potassium sorbate, 0.1% sorbic acid. In 60 and 120 mL.
Rx	**Zone-A Forte Lotion** (UAD)				Hydrophilic. Glycerin, triethanolamine, 0.1% K sorbate, 0.1% sorbic acid. In 60 mL.
Rx	**Lidocaine/Hydrocortisone Cream** (River's Edge)	0.5[a]			3% lidocaine hydrochloride, aluminum sulfate, alcohols, glycerin, lt. mineral oil, parabens, petrolatum. In 28.5 and 85 g.
Rx	**AnaMantle HC Cream** (Bradley)				3% lidocaine HCl, cetyl alcohol, light mineral oil, parabens, glycerin, stearyl alcohol, petrolatum. In kits of 7 g tubes with single-use applicators (14s).
Rx	**Lidocaine/Hydrocortisone Acetate Cream Kit** (River's Edge)	0.5			3% lidocaine hydrochloride, aluminum sulfate, alcohols, glycerin, lt. mineral oil, parabens, petrolatum. In 20 single use 7 g tubes with applicators and cleansing wipes.
Rx	**Lidocaine/Hydrocortisone Acetate Cream Kit** (River's Edge)	1			3 % lidocaine hydrochloride, cetyl alcohol, mineral oil, parabens, stearyl alcohol, white petrolatum. In 20 single dose use 7 g tubes with applicators and cleansing wipes.
Rx	**Xyralid Cream** (Auriga)				3% lidocaine hydrochloride, cetyl alcohol, mineral oil, parabens, stearyl alcohol, white petrolatum. In 85 g.
Rx	**Lida-Mantle-HC Cream** (Doak)				3% lidocaine HCl, glycerin, parabens. In 30 g.
Rx	**LidaMantle HC Lotion** (Doak)				3% lidocaine HCl, cetyl alcohol, mineral oil, methylparaben, petrolatum. In 177 mL.
otc	**HC Derma-Pax Liquid** (Recsei)	0.5[a]			0.44% pyrilamine maleate, 0.06% chlorophenothane maleate, 1% benzyl alcohol, 35% isopropanol, 25% chlorobutanol. In 60 and 120 mL.
otc	**Massengill Medicated Towelettes** (SK-Beecham)				Diazolidinyl urea, parabens, propylene glycol. In 10 and 16 softcloth towelettes.
Rx	**Cortamox Lotion** (River's Edge)	1		1	50% benzalkonium chloride , 0.1% chloroxylenol, disodium EDTA, lactic acid, PEG-6. In 60 mL dropper bottles.

[a] Hydrocortisone acetate.

These products contain corticosteroids in combination with various other components. They are indicated for a variety of specific and nonspecific dermatoses. For further information see individual monographs.

CORTICOSTEROID AND ANTIBIOTIC COMBINATIONS

		Dosage form	Corticosteroid	Neomycin sulfate	Other	Base/How Supplied
Rx	**Cortisporin** (Monarch)	Cream	0.5% hydrocortisone acetate	0.5%	10,000 units polymyxin B sulfate and neomycin sulfate equiv. to 3.5 mg neomycin base per g; white, liquid petrolatum; 0.25% methylparaben	In 7.5 g.
Rx	**Myco-Biotic** II (Moore)		0.1% triamcinolone acetonide		Aqueous vanishing. 100,000 units nystatin per g, white petrolatum	In 15, 30 and 60 g and lb.
Rx	**Hydrocortisone-Neomycin** (Various)	Ointment	1% hydrocortisone	0.5%	White petrolatum, mineral oil	In 20 g.
Rx	**Cortisporin** (Monarch)				400 units bacitracin zinc, white petrolatum, and 5000 units polymyxin B and neomycin sulfate equiv. to 3.5 mg neomycin base per g	In 14 g with applicator tip.

Consider the information for Topical Corticosteroids, Antibiotics and Antifungals when using these products (see individual monographs).

CORTICOSTEROID AND ANTIFUNGAL COMBINATIONS

		Dosage form	Corticosteroid	Antifungal	Base/How Supplied
Rx	**Clotrimazole/ Betamethasone Dipropionate** (Fougera)	Cream	0.05% betamethasone (as dipropionate)	1% clotrimazole	Mineral oil, white petrolatum, cetearyl alcohol, benzyl alcohol. In 15 and 45 g.
Rx	**Nystatin/ Triamcinolone Acetonide** (Various, eg, Fougera, Taro)		0.1% triamcinolone acetonide	100,000 units nystatin per g	In 15, 30 and 60 g and UD 1.5 g.
Rx	**Mycogen** II (Goldline)				In 15, 30, 60 and 120 g.
Rx	**Mycolog-II** (B-M Squibb)				Vanishing base. White petrolatum. In 15, 30, 60 and 120 g.
Rx	**Myconel** (Marnel)				In 20 g.
Rx	**Myco-Triacet** II (Lemmon)				Aqueous, vanishing base. White petrolatum, parabens. In 15, 30 and 60 g.
Rx	**Tri-Statin** II (Rugby)				Vanishing base. White petrolatum. In 15, 30 and 60 g.
Rx	**Clotrimazole/ Betamethasone Dipropionate** (Fougera)	Lotion	0.05% betamethasone (as dipropionate)	1% clotrimazole	Hydrophilic. Mineral oil, white petrolatum, alcohols. In 30 mL.
Rx	**Lotrisone** (Schering)				Hydrophilic. Mineral oil, white petrolatum, alcohols. In 30 mL.
Rx	**Nystatin/ Triamcinolone Acetonide** (Various, eg, Fougera)	Ointment	0.1% triamcinolone acetonide	100,000 units nystatin per g	In 15, 30 and 60 g.
Rx	**Mycogen** II (Goldline)				In 15, 30 and 60 g.
Rx	**Mycolog-II** (B-M Squibb)				Mineral oil, gel base. In 15, 30, 60 and 120 g.
Rx	**Myco-Triacet** II (Lemmon)				Vanishing base. White petrolatum and mineral oil. In 15 and 30 g.

Consider the information given for Topical Corticosteroids and Topical Antifungals when using these products.

DICLOFENAC

Rx	**Pennsaid** (Mallinckrodt Brand Pharmaceuticals)	**Solution; topical:** 1.5%[a]	As diclofenac sodium. Alcohol, glycerin, propylene glycol. In 150 mL.
Rx	**Voltaren** (Novartis)	**Gel; topical:** 1%[b]	As diclofenac sodium. Isopropyl alcohol, mineral oil, propylene glycol. In 100 g tubes.
Rx	**Solaraze** (PharmaDerm)	**Gel; topical:** 3%[c]	As diclofenac sodium. Benzyl alcohol, PEG. In 100 g.
Rx	**Flector** (King Pharmaceuticals)	**Patch; topical:** 1.3%[d]	As diclofenac epolamine 13 mg/g. Disodium edetate, parabens. In 5s.

[a] 1 mL contains diclofenac sodium 16.05 mg.
[b] 1 g contains diclofenac sodium 10 mg.
[c] 1 g contains diclofenac sodium 30 mg.
[d] 180 mg per patch.

DICLOFENAC SODIUM — TRANSDERMAL

For information on CNS and ophthalmic/otic uses of diclofenac sodium, refer to individual monographs.

WARNING

Cardiovascular and GI risk (Voltaren and *Pennsaid* only) –

Cardiovascular risk: Nonsteroidal anti-inflammatory drugs (NSAIDs) may cause an increased risk of serious cardiovascular thrombotic events, myocardial infarction (MI), and stroke, which can be fatal. This risk may increase with duration of use. Patients with cardiovascular disease or risk factors for cardiovascular disease may be at greater risk.

Diclofenac is contraindicated for the treatment of perioperative pain in the setting of coronary artery bypass graft (CABG) surgery.

GI risk: NSAIDs cause an increased risk of serious GI adverse reactions, including bleeding, ulceration, and perforation of the stomach or intestines, which can be fatal. These reactions can occur at any time during use and without warning symptoms. Elderly patients are at greater risk of serious GI reactions.

Indications

➤*Actinic keratoses (Solaraze* only): For the topical treatment of actinic keratoses. Sun avoidance is indicated during therapy.

➤*Osteoarthritis (Voltaren* and *Pennsaid* only): For the relief of the pain of osteoarthritis of joints amenable to topical treatment, such as the knees and joints of the hands. *Pennsaid* is indicated for the treatment of signs and symptoms of osteoarthritis of the knee(s) only. *Voltaren* gel has not been evaluated for use on the spine, hip, or shoulder.

➤*Off-label uses:*

Postherpetic neuralgia (topical) – [5] = Poor documentation. Topical diclofenac (extemporaneously compounded) has been studied in 1 controlled trial. While the degree of pain relief was not significantly different from that seen with placebo, the duration of pain relief was significantly longer. American Academy of Neurology clinical practice guidelines do not have a statement on the use of topical diclofenac.

Administration and Dosage

➤*Adults:*

Actinic keratoses –

Solaraze:

• *Usual dosage* – Apply to lesion areas twice daily. The amount needed depends on the size of the lesion site. Normally, 0.5 g of gel is used on each 5 cm × 5 cm lesion site.

• *Duration of therapy* – 60 to 90 days. Complete healing of the lesion(s) or optimal therapeutic effect may not be evident for up to 30 days following cessation of therapy. Lesions that do not respond to therapy must be carefully reevaluated and management reconsidered.

• *Concomitant therapy* – The safety of the concomitant use of sunscreens, cosmetics, or other topical medications is unknown.

Osteoarthritis –

Pennsaid:

• *Usual dosage* – 40 drops per knee 4 times a day.

Voltaren:

• *Maximum dose* – 32 g/day over all affected joints.

• *Concomitant therapy* – Concomitant use of diclofenac gel with oral NSAIDs has not been evaluated and may increase adverse NSAID effects.

Diclofenac gel should not be used concomitantly with sunscreens, cosmetics, lotions, moisturizers, insect repellants, or other topical medications on the same skin sites, as this has not been evaluated.

• *Lower extremities, including the knees, ankles, and feet* –

Usual dosage: Apply 4 g to the affected foot, knee, or ankle 4 times daily.

Maximum dose: 16 g/day to any single joint of the lower extremities.

• *Upper extremities, including the elbows, wrists, and hands* –

Usual dosage: Apply 2 g to the affected hand, elbow, or wrist 4 times daily.

Maximum dose: 8 g/day to any single joint of the upper extremities.

➤*Administration:*

Pennsaid – Apply to clean, dry skin. To avoid spillage, dispense 10 drops at a time either directly onto the knee or first into the hand and then onto the knee. Spread evenly around front, back, and sides of the knee. Repeat this procedure until 40 drops have been applied and the knee is completely covered with solution. To treat the other knee, if symptomatic, repeat the procedure. Do not apply more or less than the recommended dose.

Avoid showering/bathing for at least 30 minutes after the application. Wash and dry hands after use.

Do not apply to open wounds. Avoid contact with eyes and mucous membranes. Do not apply external heat and/or occlusive dressings to treated knees. Avoid wearing clothing over the treated knee(s) until the treated knee is dry. Protect the treated knee(s) from sunlight. Wait until the treated area is dry before applying sunscreen, insect repellant, lotion, moisturizer, cosmetics, or other topical medication.

Solaraze – Smooth onto the affected area gently. Ensure that enough gel is applied to adequately cover each lesion. Do not apply to open skin wounds, infections, or exfoliative dermatitis. Avoid contact with the eyes.

Voltaren – Gently massage into the skin, ensuring the application covers the entire affected area. The entire foot includes the sole, top of the foot, and the toes. The entire hand includes the palm, back of the hands, and the fingers. The proper amount should be measured using the dosing cards supplied in the drug product carton. One dosing card should be used for each application of drug product. The gel should be applied within the oblong area of the dosing card up to the 2 or 4 g line (2 g for each elbow, wrist, or hand, and 4 g for each knee, ankle, or foot). The dosing card containing diclofenac can be used to apply the gel.

Showering/bathing should be avoided for at least 1 hour after the application. Patients should wash their hands after use, unless the hands are the treated joint. If diclofenac is applied to the hand(s) for treatment, patients should not wash the treated hand(s) for at least 1 hour after the application.

Do not apply to open wounds. Contact with eyes and mucous membranes should be avoided. External heat and/or occlusive dressings should not be applied to treated joints. Exposure of the treated joint(s) to sunlight should be avoided. Wearing of clothing or gloves should be avoided for at least 10 minutes after application.

➤*Storage / Stability:*

Pennsaid – Store at 25°C (77°F); excursions are permitted between 15° and 30°C (59° and 86°F).

Solaraze – Store at 20° to 25°C (68° to 77°F); excursions are permitted between 15° and 30°C (59° and 86°F). Protect from heat. Avoid freezing.

Voltaren – Store at 25°C (77°F); excursions are permitted between 15° and 30°C (59° and 86°F). Keep from freezing.

Actions

➤*Pharmacology:*

Solaraze – The mechanism of action of diclofenac in the treatment of actinic keratoses is unknown. The contribution to efficacy of individual components of the vehicle has not been established.

Voltaren and *Pennsaid* – The mechanism of action of diclofenac is similar to that of other NSAIDs. Diclofenac inhibits the enzyme cyclooxygenase (COX), an early component of the arachidonic acid cascade, resulting in the reduced formation of prostaglandins, thromboxanes, and prostacyclin. It is not completely understood how reduced synthesis of these compounds results in therapeutic efficacy.

➤*Pharmacokinetics:*

Pennsaid – After topical administration to healthy human volunteers of single and multiple maximum doses of diclofenac, 40 drops (approximately 1.2 mL) to each knee (80 drops total dose), the following diclofenac pharmacokinetic parameters were obtained.

Diclofenac Topical Solution Pharmacokinetic Parameters[a]

Pharmacokinetic parameter	Healthy adults 18 to 55 years of age (n = 18) Diclofenac single dose	Healthy adults 18 to 55 years of age (n = 19) Diclofenac multiple dose (4 times daily for 7 days)
AUC_{0-t}	177.5 ± 72.6 ng•h/mL	695.4 ± 348.9 ng•h/mL
$AUC_{0-\infty}$	196.3 ± 68.5 ng•h/mL	745.2 ± 374.7 ng•h/mL
Plasma C_{max}	8.1 ± 5.9 ng/mL	19.4 ± 9.3 ng/mL
Plasma T_{max} (h)	11 ± 6.4	4 ± 6.5
Plasma t½ (h)	36.7 ± 20.8	79 ± 38.1
Kel (h^{-1})	0.024 ± 0.01	0.011 ± 0.004
CL/F (L/h)	244.7 ± 84.7	—

[a] AUC = area under the curve; C_{max} = maximal drug concentration; T_{max} = time to maximal drug concentration; t½ = half-life; kel = elimination rate constant; CL/F = apparent total body clearance.

Voltaren – The pharmacokinetics of diclofenac were assessed in healthy volunteers following repeated applications during 7 days of diclofenac to 1 knee (4 × 4 g/day) or to 2 knees and 2 hands (4 × 12 g/day) versus the recommended oral dose of diclofenac sodium for the treatment of osteoarthritis (3 × 50 mg/day).

Pharmacokinetic Parameters and Comparison of Topical Diclofenac Gel With Oral Diclofenac After Repeated Administration[a]

Treatment	C_{max} (ng/mL) Mean ± SD Percentage of oral (CI)	T_{max} (h) Median (range)	AUC_{0-24} (ng•h/mL) Mean ± SD Percentage of oral (CI)
Diclofenac gel 4 × 4 g/day (diclofenac 160 mg/day)	15 ± 7.3 0.6% (0.5% to 0.7%)	14 (0 to 24)	233 ± 128 5.8% (5% to 6.7%)
Diclofenac gel 4 × 12 g/day (diclofenac 480 mg/day)	53.8 ± 32 2.2% (1.9% to 2.6%)	10 (0 to 24)	807 ± 478 19.7% (17% to 22.8%)
Diclofenac tablets, orally 3 × 50 mg/day (diclofenac 150 mg/day)	2,270 ± 778 100%	6.5 (1 to 14)	3,890 ±1,710 100%

[a] SD = standard deviation; CI = confidence interval.

DICLOFENAC SODIUM — TRANSDERMAL

Absorption –

Pennsaid: Diclofenac systemic exposure from diclofenac topical solution application (4 times daily for 1 week) was approximately one-third of the diclofenac systemic exposure from the *Solaraze* application (twice daily for 4 weeks).

Solaraze: When diclofenac gel is applied topically, it is absorbed into the epidermis. In a study in patients with compromised skin (mainly atopic dermatitis and other dermatitic conditions) of the hands, arms, or face, approximately 10% of the applied dose (2 g of 3% gel over 100 cm^2) of diclofenac was absorbed systemically in normal and compromised epidermis after 7 days, with 4-times-daily applications.

After topical application of diclofenac 2 g gel 3 times daily for 6 days to the calf of the leg in healthy subjects, diclofenac could be detected in plasma. Mean bioavailability parameters were $AUC_{0\text{-}t}$ 9 ± 19 ng•h/mL (mean ± SD), with a C_{max} of 4 ± 5 ng/mL and a T_{max} of 4.5 ± 8 hours. In comparison, a single oral dose of diclofenac sodium 75 mg delayed-release tablets produced an AUC of 1,600 ng•h/mL. Therefore, the systemic bioavailability after topical application of diclofenac gel is lower than after oral dosing.

Blood drawn at the end of treatment from 60 patients with actinic keratoses lesions treated with diclofenac gel in 3 adequate and well-controlled clinical trials was assayed for diclofenac levels. Each patient was administered diclofenac 0.5 g gel twice a day for up to 105 days. There were up to three 5 cm × 5 cm treatment sites per patient on the face, forehead, hands, forearm, and scalp. Serum concentrations of diclofenac were on average at or below 20 ng/mL. These data indicate that systemic absorption of diclofenac in patients treated topically with diclofenac gel is much lower than that occurring after oral daily dosing of diclofenac sodium.

Voltaren: Systemic exposure (AUC) and C_{max} of diclofenac are significantly lower with diclofenac gel than with comparable oral treatment of diclofenac sodium.

Systemic exposure with recommended use of diclofenac (4 × 4 g/day applied to 1 knee) is on average 17 times lower than with oral treatment. The amount of diclofenac that is systemically absorbed from diclofenac gel is on average 6% of the systemic exposure from an oral form of diclofenac.

The average C_{max} with recommended use of diclofenac gel (4 × 4 g/day applied to 1 knee) is 158 times lower than with the oral treatment.

The pharmacokinetics of diclofenac gel have been tested under conditions of moderate heat (application of a heat patch for 15 minutes prior to gel application) and of moderate exercise (first gel application followed by a 20-minute treadmill exercise). No clinically relevant differences of systemic absorption and of tolerability were found between applications of diclofenac gel (4 × 4 g/day on 1 knee) with and under the conditions tested. However, the pharmacokinetics of diclofenac gel were not tested under the condition of heat application following gel application. Therefore, concurrent use of diclofenac gel and heat is not recommended.

Distribution – Diclofenac is more than 99% bound to human serum proteins, primarily to albumin. Diclofenac's volume of distribution following oral administration is approximately 550 mL/kg.

Pennsaid: Diclofenac diffuses into and out of the synovial fluid. Diffusion into the joint occurs when plasma levels are higher than those in the synovial fluid, after which the process reverses and synovial fluid levels are higher than plasma levels. It is not known whether diffusion into the joint plays a role in the effectiveness of diclofenac.

Metabolism – Biotransformation of diclofenac following oral administration involves conjugation at the carboxyl group of the side chain or single or multiple hydroxylations resulting in several phenolic metabolites, most of which are converted to glucuronide conjugates. Five diclofenac metabolites have been identified in human plasma and urine. The metabolites include 4'-hydroxy-, 5-hydroxy-, 3'-hydroxy-, 4',5-dihydroxy- and 3'-hydroxy-4'-methoxydiclofenac. The major diclofenac metabolite, 4'-hydroxydiclofenac, has very weak pharmacologic activity. The formation of 4'-hydroxydiclofenac is primarily mediated by CYP2C9. Both diclofenac and its oxidative metabolites undergo glucuronidation or sulfation followed by biliary excretion. Acylglucuronidation mediated by UGT2B7 and oxidation mediated by CYP2C8 may also play a role in diclofenac metabolism. CYP3A4 is responsible for the formation of minor metabolites, 5-hydroxy and 3'-hydroxydiclofenac.

Metabolism following topical administration is thought to be similar to that after oral administration. The small amounts of diclofenac and its metabolites appearing in the plasma following topical administration makes the quantification of specific metabolites imprecise.

Excretion – Diclofenac is eliminated through metabolism and subsequent urinary and biliary excretion of the glucuronide and the sulfate conjugates of the metabolites. Diclofenac and its metabolites are excreted mainly in the urine after oral dosing.

Little or no free unchanged diclofenac is excreted in the urine.

Systemic clearance of diclofenac from plasma is 263 ± 56 mL/min (mean ± SD). The terminal plasma half-life is 1 to 2 hours. Four of the metabolites also have short terminal half-lives of 1 to 3 hours.

Contraindications

Known hypersensitivity to diclofenac sodium or any other component of diclofenac; patients who have experienced asthma, urticaria, or allergic-type reactions after taking aspirin or other NSAIDs; in the setting of CABG surgery.

Warnings/Precautions

➤*Cardiovascular effects:*

Cardiovascular thrombotic events – Clinical trials of several COX-2–selective and nonselective NSAIDs of up to 3 years' duration have shown an increased risk of serious cardiovascular thrombotic events, MI, and stroke, which can be fatal. All NSAIDs, both COX-2 selective and nonselective, may have a similar risk. Patients with known cardiovascular disease or risk factors of cardiovascular disease may be at greater risk. To minimize the potential risk of an adverse cardiovascular event in patients treated with NSAIDs, the lowest effective dose should be used for the shortest duration possible. Health care providers and patients should remain alert for the development of such events, even in the absence of previous cardiovascular symptoms. Inform patients about the signs and/or symptoms of serious cardiovascular toxicity and the steps to take if they occur.

There is no consistent evidence that concurrent use of aspirin mitigates the increased risk of serious cardiovascular thrombotic events associated with NSAIDs use. The concurrent use of aspirin and NSAIDs such as diclofenac does increase the risk of serious GI events.

Two large, controlled clinical trials of a COX-2–selective NSAID for the treatment of pain in the first 10 to 14 days following CABG surgery found an increased incidence of MI and stroke.

Hypertension – NSAIDs, including diclofenac, can lead to the onset of new hypertension or worsening of preexisting hypertension, either of which may contribute to the increased incidence of cardiovascular events. Patients taking thiazides or loop diuretics may have impaired response to these therapies when taking NSAIDs. Use NSAIDs, including diclofenac, with caution in patients with hypertension. Monitor blood pressure closely during the initiation of therapy with diclofenac and throughout the course of therapy.

Congestive heart failure and edema – Fluid retention and edema have been observed in some patients treated with NSAIDs, including diclofenac. Use diclofenac with caution in patients with fluid retention or heart failure.

➤*GI effects:* NSAIDs, including diclofenac, can cause serious GI events, including bleeding, ulceration, and perforation of the stomach, small intestine, or large intestine, which can be fatal. These serious adverse events can occur at any time, with or without warning symptoms, in patients treated with NSAIDs. Only 1 in 5 patients who develop a serious upper GI adverse event on NSAID therapy is symptomatic. Upper GI ulcers, gross bleeding, or perforation caused by NSAIDs occur in approximately 1% of patients treated for 3 to 6 months, and in approximately 2% to 4% of patients treated for 1 year. These trends continue with longer duration of use, increasing the likelihood of developing a serious GI event at some time during the course of therapy. However, even short-term therapy is not without risk.

Prescribe NSAIDs with extreme caution in patients with a history of ulcer disease or GI bleeding. Patients with a history of peptic ulcer disease and/or GI bleeding who use NSAIDs have a greater than 10-fold increased risk for developing a GI bleed compared with patients with neither of these risk factors. Other factors that increase the risk of GI bleeding in patients treated with NSAIDs include concomitant use of oral corticosteroids or anticoagulants, longer duration of NSAID therapy, smoking, use of alcohol, older age, and poor general health status. Most spontaneous reports of fatal GI events are in elderly or debilitated patients; therefore, take special care in treating this population.

To minimize the potential risk of an adverse GI event, use the lowest effective dose for the shortest possible duration. Health care providers and patients should remain alert for signs and symptoms of GI ulceration and bleeding during diclofenac therapy; promptly initiate additional evaluation and treatment if a serious GI adverse event is suspected. For high-risk patients, consider alternative therapies that do not involve NSAIDs.

➤*Hepatic effects:* Elevations of one or more liver tests may occur during therapy with diclofenac. These laboratory abnormalities may progress, may remain unchanged, or may be transient with continued therapy. Borderline elevations (ie, less than 3 times the upper limit of normal [ULN] range) or greater elevations of transaminases occurred in approximately 15% of diclofenac-treated patients. Of the markers of hepatic function, ALT is recommended for the monitoring of liver injury.

Almost all meaningful elevations in transaminases were detected before patients became symptomatic. In all trials, abnormal tests occurred during the first 2 months of therapy with diclofenac in 42 of the 51 patients who developed marked transaminase elevations.

In postmarketing reports, cases of drug-induced hepatotoxicity have been reported in the first month and, in some cases, the first 2 months of therapy, but can occur at any time during treatment with diclofenac. Postmarketing surveillance has reported cases of severe hepatic reactions, including liver necrosis, jaundice, fulminant hepatitis with and without jaundice, and liver failure. Some of these reported cases resulted in fatalities or liver transplantation.

Measure transaminases periodically in patients receiving long-term therapy with diclofenac because severe hepatotoxicity may develop without a prodrome of distinguishing symptoms. The optimum times for making the first and subsequent transaminase measurements are not known. Based on clinical trial data and postmarketing experiences, monitor transaminases within 4 to 8 weeks after initiating treatment with diclofenac. However, severe hepatic reactions can occur at any time during treatment with diclofenac.

If abnormal liver tests persist or worsen, if clinical signs and/or symptoms consistent with liver disease develop, or if systemic manifestations occur (eg, eosinophilia, rash, abdominal pain, diarrhea, dark urine), discontinue diclofenac immediately. To minimize the possibility that hepatic injury will become severe between transaminase measurements, inform patients of the warning signs and symptoms of hepatotoxicity (eg, nausea, fatigue, lethargy, diarrhea, pruritus, jaundice, right upper quadrant tenderness, flu-like symptoms), and advise patients of the appropriate action to take if these signs and symptoms appear.

DICLOFENAC SODIUM — TRANSDERMAL

To minimize the potential risk for an adverse liver-related event in patients treated with diclofenac, use the lowest effective dose for the shortest duration possible. Exercise caution in prescribing diclofenac with concomitant drugs that are known to be potentially hepatotoxic (eg, antibiotics, antiepileptics). Caution patients to avoid taking unprescribed acetaminophen while using diclofenac.

➤*Renal effects:* Use caution when initiating treatment with diclofenac in patients with considerable dehydration.

Long-term administration of NSAIDs has resulted in renal papillary necrosis and other renal injury. Renal toxicity has also been seen in patients in whom renal prostaglandins have a compensatory role in the maintenance of renal perfusion. In these patients, administration of an NSAID may cause a dose-dependent reduction in prostaglandin formation and, secondarily, in renal blood flow, which may precipitate overt renal decompensation. Patients at greatest risk of this reaction are those with impaired renal function, heart failure, liver dysfunction, those taking diuretics and angiotensin-converting enzyme (ACE) inhibitors, and elderly patients. Discontinuation of NSAID therapy is usually followed by recovery to the pretreatment state.

➤*Corticosteroid use:* Diclofenac cannot be expected to substitute for corticosteroids or to treat corticosteroid insufficiency. Abrupt discontinuation of corticosteroids may lead to exacerbation of corticosteroid-responsive illness. For patients on prolonged corticosteroid therapy, taper slowly if a decision is made to discontinue corticosteroids.

➤*Inflammation and fever:* The pharmacological activity of diclofenac in reducing inflammation, and possibly fever, may diminish the utility of these diagnostic signs in detecting infectious complications of presumed noninfectious, painful conditions.

➤*Hematological effects:* Anemia is sometimes seen in patients receiving NSAIDs. This may be due to fluid retention, occult or gross GI blood loss, or an incompletely described effect on erythropoiesis. Check hemoglobin or hematocrit of patients on long-term treatment with NSAIDS, including diclofenac, if they exhibit any signs or symptoms of anemia or blood loss.

NSAIDs inhibit platelet aggregation and have been shown to prolong bleeding time in some patients. Unlike aspirin, their effect on platelet function is quantitatively less, of shorter duration, and reversible. Carefully monitor patients receiving diclofenac who may be adversely affected by alterations in platelet function, such as those with coagulation disorders or patients receiving anticoagulants.

➤*Preexisting asthma:* Patients with asthma may have aspirin-sensitive asthma. The use of aspirin in patients with aspirin-sensitive asthma has been associated with severe bronchospasm, which can be fatal. Because cross-reactivity, including bronchospasm, between aspirin and other NSAIDs has been reported in such aspirin-sensitive patients, do not administer diclofenac to patients with this form of aspirin sensitivity, and use caution in patients with preexisting asthma.

➤*Eye exposure:* Avoid contact of diclofenac with eyes and mucosa. Advise patients that if eye contact occurs, they should immediately wash out the eye with water or saline and consult their health care provider if irritation persists for more than an hour.

➤*Hypersensitivity reactions:*

Anaphylactoid reactions – As with other NSAIDs, anaphylactoid reactions may occur in patients without prior exposure to diclofenac. Do not give diclofenac to patients with the aspirin triad. The triad typically occurs in asthmatic patients who experience rhinitis with or without nasal polyps, or who exhibit severe, potentially fatal bronchospasm after taking aspirin or other NSAIDs. Severe, rarely fatal anaphylactic-like reactions to NSAIDs have been reported in such patients. Advise patients to seek emergency help in cases in which an anaphylactoid reaction occurs.

Dermatologic reactions – NSAIDs, including diclofenac, can cause serious skin adverse events such as exfoliative dermatitis, Stevens-Johnson syndrome, and toxic epidermal necrolysis, which can be fatal. These serious events may occur without warning. Inform patients about the signs and symptoms of serious skin manifestations; discontinue diclofenac at the first appearance of skin rash or any other signs of hypersensitivity.

➤*Renal function impairment:* No information is available from controlled clinical studies regarding the use of diclofenac in patients with advanced renal disease. Therefore, treatment with diclofenac is not recommended in patients with advanced renal disease. If diclofenac therapy is initiated, close monitoring of the patient's renal function is advisable.

➤*Hepatic function impairment:* Use diclofenac with caution in patients with severe hepatic impairment.

➤*Photosensitivity:* Advise patients to minimize or avoid exposure to natural or artificial sunlight on treated areas because studies in animals indicated topical diclofenac treatment resulted in an earlier onset of ultraviolet light-induced skin tumors. The potential effects of diclofenac on skin response to ultraviolet damage in humans are not known.

➤*Pregnancy:* There are no adequate and well-controlled studies in pregnant women. Diclofenac has been shown to cross the placental barrier in mice and rats. Because animal reproduction studies are not always predictive of human response, do not use during pregnancy unless the benefits to the mother justify the potential risk to the fetus. Because of the risk to the fetus, resulting in premature closure of the ductus arteriosus, avoid diclofenac in late pregnancy (ie, starting at 30 weeks' gestation).

In rats, maternally toxic doses of diclofenac were associated with dystocia, prolonged gestation, reduced fetal weights and growth, and reduced fetal survival.

Pennsaid – *Category C* prior to 30 weeks' gestation. *Category D* starting at 30 weeks' gestation.

Solaraze – *Category B.*

Voltaren – *Category C.*

Labor and delivery – The effects of diclofenac on labor and delivery in pregnant women are unknown. Because of the known effects of prostaglandin-inhibiting drugs on the fetal cardiovascular system (closure of ductus arteriosus), avoid use of diclofenac during late pregnancy. As with other NSAIDs, it is possible that diclofenac may inhibit uterine contractions and delay parturition.

In rat studies with oral NSAIDs, including diclofenac, as with other drugs known to inhibit prostaglandin synthesis, there is an increased incidence of dystocia and delayed parturition corresponding to a human equivalent dose approximately similar to the maximum recommended clinical dose (based on bioavailability and BSA comparison). In rat studies, maternal exposure to diclofenac, as with other NSAID drugs known to inhibit prostaglandin synthesis, increased the incidence of decreased offspring survival.

➤*Lactation:* It is not known whether diclofenac is excreted in human milk; however, there is a case report in the literature indicating that diclofenac can be detected at low levels in breast milk. Studies in animals detected diclofenac in the milk after oral administration. Because of the potential for serious adverse reactions in breast-feeding infants from diclofenac, decide whether to discontinue breast-feeding or the drug, taking into account the importance of the drug to the mother. Due to its short adult serum half-life (1.1 hours), diclofenac has been classified as a low-risk alternative if an NSAID is required during breast-feeding.

➤*Children:* Safety and effectiveness of *Pennsaid* and *Voltaren* in children have not been established. Actinic keratoses is not a condition seen within the pediatric population; do not use *Solaraze* in children.

➤*Elderly:* No overall differences in safety or effectiveness were observed between elderly and younger subjects, and other reported clinical experience has not identified differences in responses between elderly and younger patients, but greater sensitivity of some older individuals cannot be ruled out.

Diclofenac, as with any NSAID, is known to be substantially excreted by the kidney, and the risk of toxic reactions to diclofenac may be greater in patients with impaired renal function. Because elderly patients are more likely to have decreased renal function, take care when using diclofenac in elderly patients, and it may be useful to monitor renal function.

➤*Monitoring:* Monitor for signs or symptoms of GI bleeding. Patients on long-term treatment with NSAIDs should have a complete blood cell count and a chemistry profile checked periodically. If abnormal liver tests or renal tests persist or worsen, discontinue diclofenac.

Monitor blood pressure closely during the initiation of therapy with diclofenac and throughout the course of therapy.

Carefully monitor patients receiving diclofenac who may be adversely affected by alterations in platelet function, such as those with coagulation disorders or patients receiving anticoagulants.

Drug Interactions

➤*NSAIDs:* Although the systemic absorption of diclofenac is low, minimize concomitant oral administration of other NSAIDs such as aspirin at anti-inflammatory/analgesic doses. Concomitant use of oral NSAIDs with diclofenac topical solution has been evaluated. Combined use of oral NSAIDs and diclofenac topical solution resulted in a higher rate of rectal hemorrhage and more frequent abnormal creatinine, urea, and hemoglobin compared with oral diclofenac alone. Therefore, do not coadminister oral NSAIDs and topical diclofenac unless the benefit outweighs the risk and perform periodic laboratory evaluations.

Drug interactions with the use of topical diclofenac have not been studied. The following drug interactions are noted with oral diclofenac sodium and potassium.

Diclofenac Drug Interactions

Precipitant drug	Object drug[a]		Description
ACE[b] inhibitors (eg, enalapril)	Diclofenac	⬇⬆	NSAIDs may decrease the antihypertensive effect of ACE inhibitors. In addition, the risk of nephrotoxicity associated with ACE inhibitors or diclofenac may be increased. If blood pressure control decreases, it may be necessary to discontinue diclofenac. Periodic measurement of renal function may be necessary.
Diclofenac	ACE inhibitors (eg, enalapril)		
Alcohol	Diclofenac	⬆	The risk of GI bleeding may be increased. Use with caution.

DICLOFENAC SODIUM — TRANSDERMAL

Precipitant drug	Object drug[a]		Description
Anticoagulants (eg, heparin, warfarin)	Diclofenac	↑	The effects of heparin or warfarin and NSAIDs on GI bleeding are synergistic. The risk of serious GI bleeding is higher than with either drug alone. Closely monitor coagulation status and adjust the dosage of anticoagulants accordingly. Monitor for signs of GI bleeding. Advise patients about the signs and symptoms of GI bleeding.
Diclofenac	Anticoagulants (eg, heparin, warfarin)		
Antiplatelet agents (eg, clopidogrel)	Diclofenac	↑	The risk of bleeding may be increased. Coadminister with caution. Closely monitor for signs of bleeding.
Diclofenac	Antiplatelet agents (eg, clopidogrel)		
Azole antifungal agents (eg, voriconazole)	Diclofenac	↑	Diclofenac concentrations may be elevated, increasing the pharmacologic effects and risk of adverse reactions. Observe the clinical response of the patient and adjust the diclofenac dose as needed.
Corticosteroids (eg, prednisone)	Diclofenac	↑	The risk of GI bleeding may be increased. Use with caution. Advise patients about the signs and symptoms of GI bleeding.
Cyclosporine	Diclofenac	↑	The nephrotoxicity of both agents may be increased. Use with caution and closely monitor for nephrotoxicity.
Diclofenac	Cyclosporine		
Hepatotoxic agents (eg, acetaminophen, certain antibiotics and antiepileptic agents)	Diclofenac	↑	The risk of hepatotoxicity may be increased. Use with caution. Closely monitor for signs and symptoms of hepatotoxicity.
Diclofenac	Hepatotoxic agents (eg, acetaminophen, certain antibiotics and antiepileptic agents)		
Hibiscus sabdariffa	Diclofenac	↑	Diclofenac urinary excretion may be reduced, increasing diclofenac concentrations and risk of adverse reactions. Patients taking diclofenac should avoid beverages made from *Hibiscus sabdariffa* flowers.
Salicylates (eg, aspirin)	Diclofenac	↔	Salicylates may decrease the protein binding of diclofenac. The clinical importance of this interaction is not known; however, as with other NSAIDs, coadministration is not generally recommended because of the potential for increased adverse effects.
Serotonin-norepinephrine reuptake inhibitors (eg, venlafaxine), SSRIs[b] (eg, citalopram, fluoxetine)	Diclofenac	↑	The risk of upper GI bleeding may be increased. Use with caution. Closely monitor for signs of GI bleeding. Advise patients about the signs and symptoms of GI bleeding.
Diclofenac	Serotonin-norepinephrine reuptake inhibitors (eg, venlafaxine), SSRIs (eg, citalopram, fluoxetine)		
Smoking	Diclofenac	↑	The risk of GI bleeding may be increased. Use with caution.
Diclofenac	Aminoglycosides (eg, amikacin, gentamicin)	↑	Aminoglycoside concentrations may be elevated, increasing the risk of acute renal insufficiency. If coadministration cannot be avoided, reduce the aminoglycoside dose before starting diclofenac. Monitor renal function and aminoglycoside serum concentrations and adjust the dose as needed.
Diclofenac	Diuretics (eg, loop diuretics [eg, furosemide], thiazide diuretics [eg, hydrochlorothiazide])	↓	Diclofenac may reduce the natriuretic effect of furosemide and thiazide diuretics in some patients. This response has been attributed to inhibition of renal prostaglandin synthesis. During concomitant therapy with NSAIDs, closely observe the patient for signs of renal failure, as well as to ensure diuretic efficacy.
Diclofenac	Lithium	↑	NSAIDs have produced an elevation of plasma lithium levels and a reduction in renal lithium clearance. These effects have been attributed to inhibition of renal prostaglandin synthesis by the NSAID. Closely monitor for signs of lithium toxicity.
Diclofenac	Methotrexate	↑	Methotrexate toxicity may be increased. Coadminister with caution.
Diclofenac	Quinolones (eg, levofloxacin)	↑	Risk of CNS stimulation and seizures from quinolones may be increased. In addition, quinolone plasma concentrations may be increased. Use with caution.
Diclofenac	Tenofovir	↑	Pharmacologic and toxic effects (eg, nephrotoxicity) of tenofovir may be increased. Use with caution. Consider use of an analgesic other than an NSAID.
Diclofenac	Triamterene	↑	Coadministration of diclofenac and triamterene may cause a sudden onset of nephrotoxicity. If renal function deteriorates during coadministration of these agents, consider stopping one or both drugs.

[a] ↑ = object drug increased; ↓ = object drug decreased; ↔ = undetermined clinical effect.
[b] ACE = angiotensin-converting enzyme; SSRIs = selective serotonin reuptake inhibitors.

Adverse Reactions

➤*Pennsaid:*

Most common – The most common adverse events with diclofenac topical solution were application-site skin reactions. These events were the most common reason for withdrawing from the studies.

Local: Application-site reactions were characterized by one or more of the following: acne, dryness, erythema, induration, paresthesia, pruritus, urticaria, vasodilation, and vesicles. The most frequent of these reactions were dry skin (32%), contact dermatitis characterized by skin erythema and induration (9%), pruritus (4%), and contact dermatitis with vesicles (2%). In one controlled trial, a higher rate of contact dermatitis with vesicles (4%) was observed after treatment of 152 subjects with the combination of diclofenac topical solution and oral diclofenac. In the open-label, uncontrolled long-term safety study, contact dermatitis occurred in 13% and contact dermatitis with vesicles in 10% of patients, generally within the first 6 months of exposure, leading to a withdrawal rate for an application-site reaction of 14%.

Adverse reactions common to the NSAID class: In controlled trials, subjects treated with diclofenac topical solution experienced some adverse reactions associated with the NSAID class more frequently than subjects using placebo (abdominal pain, constipation, diarrhea, dyspepsia, edema, flatulence, nausea). The combination of diclofenac topical solution and oral diclofenac compared with oral diclofenac alone resulted in a higher rate of rectal hemorrhage (3% vs less than 1%), and more frequent abnormal creatinine (12% vs 7%), urea (20% vs 12%), and hemoglobin (13% vs 9%), but no difference in elevation of liver transaminases.

DICLOFENAC SODIUM — TRANSDERMAL

Adverse reactions (1% or more) –

Diclofenac Topical Solution Adverse Reactions (≥ 1%)		
Adverse reactions	Diclofenac topical solution (n = 911)	Placebo (n = 332)
Dermatologic		
Dry skin	2%	< 1%
Ecchymosis	2%	< 1%
Pruritus	2%	< 1%
Rash	3%	2%
GI		
Abdominal pain	6%	3%
Constipation	3%	< 1%
Diarrhea	4%	2%
Dyspepsia	8%	4%
Flatulence	4%	< 1%
Nausea	4%	1%
Local		
Application-site reaction (NOS[a])	1%	< 1%
Contact dermatitis	9%	2%
Contact dermatitis, vesicles	2%	0%
Dry skin	32%	5%
Pruritus	4%	2%
Respiratory		
Pharyngitis	4%	4%
Sinusitis	1%	< 1%
Miscellaneous		
Accidental injury	2%	2%
Edema	3%	0%
Halitosis	1%	< 1%
Infection	3%	2%
Paresthesia	2%	< 1%

[a] NOS = not otherwise specified.

➤*Solaraze*:

Discontinuation – Eighteen percent of diclofenac gel–treated patients and 4% of vehicle-treated patients discontinued from the clinical trials because of adverse reactions (whether considered related to treatment or not). These discontinuations were mainly caused by skin irritation or related cutaneous adverse reactions.

Most common – Of the 211 patients treated with diclofenac gel, 82% experienced adverse reactions involving skin and the application site compared with 75% of the vehicle-treated patients. Application-site reactions were the most frequent adverse reactions in both groups. Contact dermatitis, dry skin, exfoliation (scaling), and rash were significantly more prevalent in the diclofenac gel group than in the vehicle-treated patients.

Adverse reactions (greater than 1%) –

Diclofenac Gel Adverse Reactions (> 1%)				
	60-day treatment		90-day treatment	
Adverse reactions	Diclofenac gel (n = 48)	Gel vehicle (n = 49)	Diclofenac gel (n = 114)	Gel vehicle (n = 114)
Cardiovascular, NOS	2%	4%	3%	1%
Hypertension	2%	0%	1%	0%
Phlebitis	0%	2%	0%	0%
CNS, NOS	2%	2%	2%	5%
Anxiety	0%	2%	0%	1%
Asthenia	0%	0%	2%	0%
Dizziness	0%	0%	0%	4%
Headache	0%	6%	7%	6%
Hypokinesia	2%	0%	0%	0%
Migraine	0%	2%	1%	0%
Dermatologic, NOS	75%	86%	86%	71%
Acne	0%	2%	0%	1%
Contact dermatitis	2%	0%	0%	0%
Dry skin	0%	4%	3%	0%
Herpes simplex	0%	2%	0%	0%
Maculopapular rash	0%	2%	0%	0%
Pain	2%	2%	1%	0%

Diclofenac Gel Adverse Reactions (> 1%)				
	60-day treatment		90-day treatment	
Adverse reactions	Diclofenac gel (n = 48)	Gel vehicle (n = 49)	Diclofenac gel (n = 114)	Gel vehicle (n = 114)
Pruritus	4%	6%	4%	1%
Rash	2%	10%	4%	0%
Skin carcinoma	0%	6%	2%	2%
Skin nodule	0%	2%	0%	0%
Skin ulcer	2%	0%	1%	0%
GI, NOS	4%	0%	6%	8%
Abdominal pain	2%	0%	1%	0%
Constipation	0%	0%	0%	2%
Diarrhea	2%	0%	2%	3%
Dyspepsia	2%	0%	3%	4%
GU, NOS	0%	0%	4%	5%
Hematuria	0%	0%	2%	1%
Local, NOS	75%	71%	84%	70%
Acne	0%	4%	1%	0%
Alopecia	2%	0%	1%	1%
Contact dermatitis	19%	4%	33%	4%
Dry skin	27%	12%	25%	17%
Edema	4%	0%	3%	0%
Exfoliation	6%	4%	24%	13%
Hyperesthesia	0%	0%	3%	1%
Pain	15%	22%	26%	30%
Paresthesia	8%	4%	20%	20%
Photosensitivity reaction	0%	2%	3%	0%
Pruritus	31%	59%	52%	45%
Rash	35%	20%	46%	17%
Vesiculobullous rash	0%	0%	4%	1%
Metabolic/ Nutritional, NOS	2%	8%	7%	2%
ALT increased	0%	0%	2%	0%
AST increased	0%	0%	3%	0%
Edema	0%	2%	0%	0%
Increased creatinine	2%	2%	0%	1%
Increased creatine phosphokinase	0%	0%	4%	1%
Hypercholesteremia	0%	2%	1%	0%
Hyperglycemia	0%	2%	1%	0%
Musculoskeletal, NOS	4%	0%	3%	4%
Arthralgia	2%	0%	0%	2%
Arthrosis	2%	0%	0%	0%
Back pain	4%	0%	2%	2%
Myalgia	2%	0%	3%	1%
Neck pain	0%	0%	2%	0%
Respiratory, NOS	8%	8%	7%	6%
Asthma	2%	0%	0%	0%
Dyspnea	2%	0%	2%	0%
Pharyngitis	2%	8%	2%	4%
Pneumonia	2%	0%	0%	1%
Rhinitis	2%	2%	2%	2%
Sinusitis	0%	0%	2%	0%
Special senses, NOS	2%	0%	4%	2%
Conjunctivitis	2%	0%	4%	1%
Eye pain	0%	2%	2%	0%
Miscellaneous, NOS	21%	20%	20%	18%
Accidental injury	0%	0%	4%	2%
Allergic reaction	0%	0%	1%	3%
Chest pain	2%	0%	1%	0%
Chills	0%	2%	0%	0%
Flu syndrome	10%	6%	1%	4%
Infection	4%	6%	4%	5%

DICLOFENAC SODIUM — TRANSDERMAL

Diclofenac Gel Adverse Reactions (> 1%)				
	60-day treatment		90-day treatment	
Adverse reactions	Diclofenac gel (n = 48)	Gel vehicle (n = 49)	Diclofenac gel (n = 114)	Gel vehicle (n = 114)
Pain	2%	0%	2%	2%
Procedure	0%	0%	0%	3%

Dermatologic – Application-site reactions (hypertonia, maculopapular rash, purpuric rash, skin carcinoma, skin hypertrophy lacrimation disorder, vasodilation), paresthesia, seborrhea, skin hypertrophy, urticaria (less than 1%).

➤*Voltaren*:

Adverse reactions (1% or more) – Nonserious adverse reactions that were reported during the short-term, placebo-controlled studies comparing diclofenac gel and placebo (vehicle gel) over study periods of 8 to 12 weeks (16 g/day) were application-site reactions. These were the only adverse reactions that occurred in more than 1% of treated patients with a greater frequency in the diclofenac gel group (7%) than the placebo group (2%).

Diclofenac Gel Application-Site Adverse Reactions (≥ 1%)		
Adverse reactions	Diclofenac gel (n = 913)	Placebo (n = 876)
Any application-site reaction	7%	2%
Application-site dermatitis	4%	< 1%
Application-site dryness	< 1%	< 1%
Application-site erythema	< 1%	< 1%
Application-site irritation	< 1%	0%
Application-site papules	< 1%	0%
Application-site paresthesia	< 1%	< 1%
Application-site pruritus	< 1%	< 1%
Application-site vesicles	< 1%	0%

Discontinuation – In the placebo-controlled trials, the discontinuation rate due to adverse reactions was 5% for patients treated with diclofenac, and 3% for patients in the placebo group. Application-site reactions, including application-site dermatitis, were the most frequent reason for treatment discontinuation.

Long-term use – In the open-label, long-term safety study, distribution of adverse reactions was similar to that in the placebo-controlled studies. In this study, in which patients were treated for up to 1 year with diclofenac gel of up to 32 g/day, application-site dermatitis was observed in 11% of patients. Twelve percent of patients experienced adverse reactions that led to discontinuation of the study drug. The most common adverse reaction that led to discontinuation of the study was application-site dermatitis, which was experienced by 6% of patients.

➤*Postmarketing:*

Pennsaid –

Cardiovascular: Cardiovascular disorder, palpitation.

CNS: Asthenia, depression, dizziness, drowsiness, headache, lethargy, paresthesia, paresthesia at application site.

Dermatologic: Eczema, pruritus, rash, skin discoloration, urticaria.

GI: Abdominal pain, decreased appetite, diarrhea, dry mouth, dyspepsia, gastroenteritis, mouth ulceration, nausea, rectal hemorrhage, ulcerative stomatitis.

Local: Contact dermatitis, contact dermatitis with vesicles, dry skin, pruritus, rash.

Metabolic/Nutritional: Creatinine increased, edema.

Musculoskeletal: Back pain, leg cramps, myalgia, neck rigidity.

Respiratory: Asthma, dyspnea, laryngismus, laryngitis, pharyngitis.

Special senses: Abnormal vision, blurred vision, cataract, ear pain, eye disorder, eye pain, taste perversion.

Miscellaneous: Accidental injury, allergic reaction, body odor, chest pain, face edema, halitosis, lack of drug effect, pain.

Overdosage

➤*Symptoms:* Because of the low systemic absorption of topically applied diclofenac, overdosage is unlikely. There have been no known experiences of overdose with *Pennsaid* or *Voltaren* gel. There have been no reports of ingestion of *Solaraze* or *Voltaren* gel. Effects similar to those observed after an overdose of diclofenac tablets can be expected if substantial amounts of topical diclofenac are ingested. Symptoms following acute oral NSAID overdoses are usually limited to lethargy, drowsiness, nausea, vomiting, and epigastric pain, which are generally reversible with supportive care. GI bleeding can occur. Hypertension, acute renal failure, respiratory depression, and coma may occur but are rare. Anaphylactoid reactions have been reported with therapeutic ingestion of NSAIDs and may occur after an overdose.

➤*Treatment:* Manage patients using symptomatic and supportive care following an NSAID overdose. There are no specific antidotes for diclofenac. In the event of oral ingestion of topical diclofenac, resulting in significant systemic adverse effects, it is recommended that the stomach be emptied by lavage. Emesis is not recommended due to a possibility of aspiration and subsequent respiratory irritation due to dimethylsulfoxide found in some of the products. Forced diuresis may theoretically be beneficial because the drug is excreted in the urine. The effect of dialysis or hemoperfusion in the elimination of diclofenac (99% protein bound) remains unproven. In addition to supportive measures, activated charcoal (60 to 100 g in adults, 1 to 2 g/kg in children) and/or osmotic cathartic may be indicated in patients seen within 4 hours of ingestion with symptoms or following a large overdose (5 to 10 times the usual dose). Give supportive and symptomatic treatment for complications such as renal failure, convulsions, GI irritation, and respiratory depression. Forced diuresis or alkalinization of urine may not be useful due to high protein binding.

Patient Information

Inform patients that localized dermal adverse effects such as contact dermatitis, exfoliation, dry skin, and rash were found in patients treated with diclofenac at a higher incidence than in those treated with placebo.

Inform patients of and make sure they understand the importance of monitoring and follow-up evaluation, the signs and symptoms of dermal adverse reactions, and the possibility of irritant or allergic contact dermatitis. If severe dermal reactions occur, treatment with diclofenac may be interrupted until the condition subsides.

Advise patients to avoid exposure to sunlight and the use of sunlamps.

Inform patients that the safety and efficacy of the use of *Solaraze* or *Voltaren* gel together with other dermal products, including cosmetics, sunscreens, and other topical medications, on the area being treated have not been studied; use should be avoided. Instruct patients to wait until the area treated with *Pennsaid* is completely dry before applying sunscreen, insect repellant, lotion, moisturizer, cosmetics, or other topical medication.

Advise patients that diclofenac, like other NSAIDs, may cause serious cardiovascular adverse effects, such as MI or stroke, which may result in hospitalization and even death. Although serious cardiovascular events can occur without warning symptoms, advise patients to be alert for the signs and symptoms of chest pain, shortness of breath, weakness, and slurring of speech, and instruct them to seek medical advice when observing any indicative sign or symptoms. Apprise patients of the importance of this follow-up.

Advise patients that diclofenac, like other NSAIDs, can cause GI discomfort and, rarely, more serious GI adverse effects, such as ulcers and bleeding, which may result in hospitalization and even death. Although serious GI tract ulcerations and bleeding can occur without warning symptoms, advise patients to be alert for the signs and symptoms of ulcerations and bleeding, and instruct them to seek medical advice when observing any indicative sign or symptoms, including epigastric pain, dyspepsia, melena, and hematemesis. Apprise patients of the importance of this follow-up.

Inform patients of the warning signs and symptoms of hepatotoxicity (eg, nausea, fatigue, lethargy, diarrhea, pruritus, jaundice, right upper quadrant tenderness, flu-like symptoms). If these occur, instruct patients to stop therapy with diclofenac and seek immediate medical therapy.

Advise patients that diclofenac, like other NSAIDs, can cause serious skin adverse effects, such as exfoliative dermatitis, Stevens-Johnson syndrome, and toxic epidermal necrolysis, which may result in hospitalizations and even death. Although serious skin reactions may occur without warning, advise patients to be alert for the signs and symptoms of skin rash and blisters, fever, or other signs of hypersensitivity, such as itching, and advise them to seek medical advice when observing any indicative signs or symptoms.

Advise patients to stop diclofenac immediately if they develop any type of rash and advise them to contact their health care provider as soon as possible.

Instruct patients not to apply diclofenac to open skin wounds, infections, inflammations, or exfoliative dermatitis, as it may affect absorption and tolerability of the drug. Avoid the use of diclofenac under occlusive dressings.

Advise patients to promptly report to their health care provider signs or symptoms of unexplained weight gain or edema following treatment with diclofenac.

Inform patients of the signs of an anaphylactoid reaction (eg, difficulty breathing, swelling of the face or throat). If these occur, instruct patients to seek immediate emergency help.

In late pregnancy, as with other NSAIDs, avoid diclofenac because it will cause premature closure of the ductus arteriosus.

Although not studied, instruct patients to avoid contact of diclofenac with the eyes and mucosa. Advise patients that if eye contact occurs, they should immediately wash out the eye with water or saline and consult their health care provider if irritation persists for more than an hour.

Advise patients to minimize concomitant oral administration of NSAIDs, such as aspirin at anti-inflammatory/analgesic doses during treatment with topical diclofenac.

DICLOFENAC EPOLAMINE — TRANSDERMAL

WARNING

Cardiovascular risk – Nonsteroidal anti-inflammatory drugs (NSAIDs) may cause an increased risk of serious cardiovascular thrombotic events, myocardial infarction (MI), and stroke, which can be fatal. This risk may increase with duration of use. Patients with cardiovascular disease or risk factors for cardiovascular disease may be at greater risk.

Diclofenac is contraindicated for the treatment of perioperative pain in the setting of coronary artery bypass graft (CABG) surgery.

GI risk – NSAIDs cause an increased risk of serious GI adverse events, including bleeding, ulceration, and perforation of the stomach or intestines, which can be fatal. These reactions can occur at any time during use and without warning symptoms. Elderly patients are at greater risk for serious GI events.

Indications

➤*Acute pain:* For the topical treatment of acute pain due to minor strains, sprains, and contusions.

➤*Off-label uses:*

Postherpetic neuralgia (topical) – [5] = Poor documentation. Topical diclofenac (extemporaneously compounded) has been studied in 1 controlled trial. While the degree of pain relief was not significantly different from that seen with placebo, the duration of pain relief was significantly longer. American Academy of Neurology clinical practice guidelines do not have a statement on the use of topical diclofenac.

Administration and Dosage

➤*General dosing considerations:* Use the lowest effective dose for the shortest duration consistent with individual patient treatment goals.

➤*Adults:*

Acute pain – Apply 1 patch to the most painful area twice a day.

Off-label dosing –

➤*Renal function impairment:* Not recommended in patients with advanced renal disease.

➤*Administration:* The diclofenac patch should not be applied to damaged or nonintact skin, or worn when bathing or showering. Patients and caregivers should wash their hands after applying, handling, or removing the patch. Eye contact should be avoided. The product is intended for topical use only.

➤*Storage/Stability:* Store at 25°C (77°F); excursions are permitted between 15° and 30°C (59° and 86°F). The envelopes should be sealed at all times when not in use.

Actions

➤*Pharmacology:* Diclofenac patch, when applied to intact skin, provides local analgesia by releasing diclofenac from the patch into the skin. Diclofenac is an NSAID. In pharmacologic studies, diclofenac has shown anti-inflammatory, analgesic, and antipyretic activity. As with other NSAIDs, its mode of action is not known; however, its ability to inhibit prostaglandin synthesis may involve its anti-inflammatory activity, as well as contribute to its efficacy in relieving pain associated with inflammation.

➤*Pharmacokinetics:*

Absorption – Following a single application of diclofenac patch on the upper inner arm, peak plasma concentrations of diclofenac (range, 0.7 to 6 ng/mL) were noted between 10 and 20 hours of application. Plasma concentrations of diclofenac in the range of 1.3 to 8.8 ng/mL were noted after 5 days with twice-daily diclofenac patch application.

Systemic exposure (AUC) and maximum plasma concentrations of diclofenac after repeated dosing for 4 days with the diclofenac patch were lower (less than 1%) than after a single oral 50 mg diclofenac sodium tablet.

The pharmacokinetics of diclofenac patch have been tested in healthy volunteers at rest or undergoing moderate exercise (cycling 20 min/h for 12 hours at a mean heart rate of 100.3 beats per minute). No clinically relevant differences in systemic absorption were observed, with peak plasma concentrations in the range of 2.2 to 8.1 ng/mL while resting and 2.7 to 7.2 ng/mL during exercise.

Distribution – Diclofenac has a very high affinity (greater than 99%) for human serum albumin.

Metabolism/Excretion – The plasma elimination half-life of diclofenac after application of the diclofenac patch is approximately 12 hours. Diclofenac is eliminated through metabolism and subsequent urinary and biliary excretion of the glucuronide and sulfate conjugates of the metabolites.

Contraindications

Hypersensitivity to diclofenac; treatment of perioperative pain in the setting of CABG surgery; patients who have experienced asthma, urticaria, or allergic-type reactions after taking aspirin or other NSAIDs; application to nonintact or damaged skin resulting from any etiology (eg, exudative dermatitis, eczema, infected lesion, burns, wounds).

Warnings/Precautions

➤*Cardiovascular effects:*

Cardiovascular thrombotic events – Clinical trials of several cyclooxygenase-2 (COX-2) selective and nonselective NSAIDs of up to 3 years' duration have shown an increased risk of serious cardiovascular thrombotic events, MI, and stroke, which can be fatal. All NSAIDs, both COX-2 selective and nonselective, may have a similar risk. Patients with known cardiovascular disease or risk factors for cardiovascular disease may be at greater risk. To minimize the potential risk for a cardiovascular adverse event in patients treated with an NSAID, use the lowest effective dose for the shortest duration possible. Remain alert for the development of such events, even in the absence of previous cardiovascular symptoms. Inform patients about the signs and/or symptoms of serious cardiovascular events and the steps to take if they occur.

There is no consistent evidence that concurrent use of aspirin mitigates the increased risk of serious cardiovascular thrombotic reactions associated with NSAID use. The concurrent use of aspirin and an NSAID does increase the risk of serious GI reactions.

Two large, controlled clinical trials of a COX-2–selective NSAID for the treatment of pain in the first 10 to 14 days following CABG surgery found an increased incidence of MI and stroke.

Hypertension – NSAIDs, including diclofenac, can lead to onset of new hypertension or worsening of preexisting hypertension, either of which may contribute to the increased incidence of cardiovascular reactions. Patients taking thiazides or loop diuretics may have impaired response to these therapies when taking NSAIDs. Use all NSAIDs, including diclofenac, with caution in patients with hypertension. Monitor blood pressure closely during the initiation of NSAID treatment and throughout the course of therapy.

Congestive heart failure and edema – Fluid retention and edema have been observed in some patients taking NSAIDs. Use diclofenac with caution in patients with fluid retention or heart failure.

➤*GI effects:* NSAIDs, including diclofenac, can cause serious GI adverse events, including inflammation, bleeding, ulceration, and perforation of the stomach, small intestine, or large intestine, which can be fatal. These serious adverse events can occur at any time with or without warning symptoms in patients treated with NSAIDs. Only 1 in 5 patients who develop a serious upper GI adverse reaction when receiving NSAID therapy is symptomatic. Upper GI ulcers, gross bleeding, or perforation caused by NSAIDs occur in approximately 1% of patients treated for 3 to 6 months, and in approximately 2% to 4% of patients treated for 1 year. These trends continue with longer duration of use, increasing the likelihood of developing a serious GI reaction at some time during the course of therapy. However, even short-term therapy is not without risk.

Prescribe NSAIDs with extreme caution in patients with a history of ulcer disease or GI bleeding. Patients with a history of peptic ulcer disease and/or GI bleeding who use NSAIDs have a greater than 10-fold increased risk for developing a GI bleed compared with patients with neither of these risk factors. Other factors that increase the risk for GI bleeding in patients treated with NSAIDs include concomitant use of oral corticosteroids or anticoagulants, longer duration of NSAID therapy, smoking, use of alcohol, older age, and poor general health status. Most spontaneous reports of fatal GI reactions are in elderly or debilitated patients; therefore, take special care in treating these populations.

To minimize the potential risk for an adverse GI reaction in patients treated with an NSAID, use the lowest effective dose for the shortest possible duration. Remain alert for signs and symptoms of GI ulceration and bleeding during NSAID therapy, and promptly initiate additional evaluation and treatment if a serious GI adverse reaction is suspected. This includes discontinuation of the NSAID until a serious GI adverse reaction is ruled out. For high-risk patients, consider alternate therapies that do not involve NSAIDs.

➤*Renal effects:* Long-term administration of NSAIDs has resulted in renal papillary necrosis and other renal injury. Renal toxicity has also been seen in patients in whom renal prostaglandins have a compensatory role in the maintenance of renal perfusion. In these patients, administration of an NSAID may cause a dose-dependent reduction in prostaglandin formation and, secondarily, in renal blood flow, which may precipitate overt renal decompensation. Patients at greatest risk of this reaction are those with impaired renal function, heart failure, liver dysfunction, those taking diuretics and angiotensin-converting enzyme (ACE) inhibitors, and elderly patients. Discontinuation of NSAID therapy is usually followed by recovery to the pretreatment state.

➤*Hepatic effects:* Elevations of 1 or more liver tests may occur during therapy with the diclofenac patch. These laboratory abnormalities may progress, remain unchanged, or be transient with continued therapy. Borderline elevations (ie, less than 3 times the upper limit of normal [ULN]) or greater elevations of transaminases occurred in approximately 15% of diclofenac-treated patients. Of the markers of hepatic function, ALT is recommended for the monitoring of liver injury.

Almost all meaningful elevations in transaminases were detected before patients became symptomatic. In all trials, abnormal tests occurred during the first 2 months of therapy with diclofenac in 42 of the 51 patients who developed marked transaminase elevations.

In postmarketing reports, cases of drug-induced hepatotoxicity have been reported in the first month and, in some cases, the first 2 months of therapy, but can occur at any time during treatment with diclofenac. Postmarketing surveillance has reported cases of severe hepatic reactions, including liver necrosis, jaundice, fulminant hepatitis with and without jaundice, and liver failure. Some of these reported cases resulted in fatalities or liver transplantation.

Measure transaminases periodically in patients receiving long-term therapy with diclofenac because severe hepatotoxicity may develop without a prodrome of distinguishing symptoms. The optimum times for making the first and subsequent transaminase measurements are not known. Based on clini-

DICLOFENAC EPOLAMINE — TRANSDERMAL

cal trial data and postmarketing experiences, monitor transaminases within 4 to 8 weeks after initiating treatment with diclofenac. However, severe hepatic reactions can occur at any time during treatment with diclofenac.

If abnormal liver tests persist or worsen, if clinical signs and/or symptoms consistent with liver disease develop, or if systemic manifestations occur (eg, eosinophilia, rash, abdominal pain, diarrhea, dark urine), discontinue the diclofenac patch immediately. To minimize the possibility that hepatic injury will become severe between transaminase measurements, inform patients of the warning signs and symptoms of hepatotoxicity (eg, nausea, fatigue, lethargy, diarrhea, pruritus, jaundice, right upper quadrant tenderness, flu-like symptoms), and inform them of the appropriate action to take if these signs and symptoms appear.

To minimize the potential risk for an adverse liver-related event in patients treated with the diclofenac patch, use the lowest effective dose for the shortest duration possible. Exercise caution in prescribing the diclofenac patch with concomitant drugs that are known to be potentially hepatotoxic (eg, antibiotics, antiepileptics).

➤*Corticosteroid use:* Diclofenac cannot be expected to substitute for corticosteroids or to treat corticosteroid insufficiency. Abrupt discontinuation of corticosteroids may lead to disease exacerbation. Slowly taper therapy for patients on prolonged corticosteroid therapy if a decision is made to discontinue corticosteroids.

➤*Inflammation:* The pharmacological activity of diclofenac in reducing inflammation may diminish the utility of these diagnostic signs in detecting complications of presumed noninfectious, painful conditions.

➤*Hematological effects:* Anemia is sometimes seen in patients receiving NSAIDs. This may be due to fluid retention, occult or gross GI blood loss, or an incompletely described effect upon erythropoiesis. If patients receiving long-term treatment with NSAIDs, including the diclofenac patch, exhibit any signs or symptoms of anemia, check their hemoglobin or hematocrit.

NSAIDs inhibit platelet aggregation and have been shown to prolong bleeding time in some patients. Unlike aspirin, the effect of NSAIDs on platelet function is quantitatively less, of shorter duration, and reversible. Carefully monitor patients receiving diclofenac who may be adversely affected by alterations in platelet function, such as those with coagulation disorders or patients receiving anticoagulants.

➤*Preexisting asthma:* Patients with asthma may have aspirin-sensitive asthma. The use of aspirin in patients with aspirin-sensitive asthma has been associated with severe bronchospasm, which can be fatal. Since cross-reactivity, including bronchospasm, between aspirin and other NSAIDs has been reported in such aspirin-sensitive patients, do not administer diclofenac to patients with this form of aspirin sensitivity, and use diclofenac with caution in patients with preexisting asthma.

➤*Eye exposure:* Although not studied, avoid contact of diclofenac patch with eyes and mucosa. If eye contact occurs, immediately wash out the eye with water or saline. Instruct patients to consult a health care provider if irritation persists for more than an hour.

➤*Accidental exposure:* Even a used diclofenac patch contains a large amount of diclofenac (as much as 170 mg). Therefore, the potential exists for a small child or pet to suffer serious adverse reactions from chewing or ingesting a new or used diclofenac patch. It is important for patients to store and dispose of diclofenac patches out of the reach of children and away from pets.

➤*Hypersensitivity reactions:*

Dermatologic reactions – NSAIDs, including diclofenac, can cause serious skin adverse reactions such as exfoliative dermatitis, Stevens-Johnson syndrome, and toxic epidermal necrolysis, which can be fatal. These serious reactions may occur without warning. Inform patients about the signs and symptoms of serious skin manifestations, and discontinue use of the drug at the first appearance of skin rash or any other sign of hypersensitivity.

Anaphylactoid reactions – As with other NSAIDs, anaphylactoid reactions may occur in patients without known prior exposure to diclofenac. Do not give diclofenac to patients with the aspirin triad. This symptom complex typically occurs in asthmatic patients who experience rhinitis with or without nasal polyps, or who exhibit severe, potentially fatal bronchospasm after taking aspirin or other NSAIDs. Severe, rarely fatal anaphylactic-like reactions to NSAIDs have been reported in such patients. Seek emergency help in cases in which an anaphylactoid reaction occurs.

➤*Renal function impairment:* No information is available from controlled clinical studies regarding the use of diclofenac in patients with advanced renal disease. Therefore, treatment with diclofenac is not recommended in patients with advanced renal disease. If diclofenac therapy is initiated, close monitoring of the patient's renal function is advisable.

➤*Pregnancy:* Category C. Category B (Category D if used in the third trimester or near delivery) (per Briggs' *Drugs in Pregnancy and Lactation*). There are no adequate and well-controlled studies in pregnant women. Use diclofenac during pregnancy only if the potential benefit justifies the potential risk to the fetus. In late pregnancy, as with other NSAIDs, avoid using diclofenac because it may cause premature closure of the ductus arteriosus.

Teratogenic – Pregnant Sprague Dawley rats were administered diclofenac epolamine 1, 3, or 6 mg/kg via oral gavage daily from gestation days 6 to 15. Maternal toxicity, embryotoxicity, and increased incidence of skeletal anomalies were noted with diclofenac epolamine 6 mg/kg/day, which corresponds to 3 times the maximum recommended daily exposure in humans based on a body surface area comparison. Pregnant New Zealand white rabbits were administered diclofenac epolamine 1, 3, or 6 mg/kg via oral gavage daily from gestation days 6 to 18. No maternal toxicity was noted; however, embryotoxicity was evident in the 6 mg/kg/day group, which corresponds to 6.5 times the maximum recommended daily exposure in humans based on a body surface area comparison.

Nonteratogenic – Male rats were orally administered diclofenac epolamine (1, 3, 6 mg/kg) for 60 days prior to mating and throughout the mating period, and females were given the same doses 14 days prior to mating and through mating, gestation, and lactation. Embryotoxicity was observed with diclofenac epolamine 6 mg/kg (3 times the maximum recommended daily exposure in humans based on a body surface area comparison) and was manifested as an increase in early resorption, postimplantation losses, and a decrease in live fetuses. The number of live born and total born were also reduced, as was F1 postnatal survival, but the physical and behavioral development of surviving F1 pups in all groups was the same as the deionized water control, and reproductive performance was not adversely affected despite a slight treatment-related reduction in body weight.

Labor and delivery – In rat studies with NSAIDs, as with other drugs known to inhibit prostaglandin synthesis, an increased incidence of dystocia, delayed parturition, and decreased pup survival occurred. The effects of diclofenac on labor and delivery in pregnant women are unknown.

➤*Lactation:* It is not known whether this drug is excreted in human milk. Because many drugs are excreted in human milk and because of the potential for serious adverse reactions in breast-feeding infants from diclofenac, decide whether to discontinue breast-feeding or the drug, taking into account the importance of the drug to the mother. Because of its short adult serum half-life (1.1 hours), diclofenac has been classified as a low-risk alternative if an NSAID is required during breast-feeding.

➤*Children:* Safety and efficacy in children have not been established.

➤*Elderly:* Diclofenac, as with any NSAID, is known to be substantially excreted by the kidney and the risk of toxic reactions to diclofenac may be greater in patients with renal impairment. Because elderly patients are more likely to have decreased renal function, use caution when administering the diclofenac patch to elderly patients, and it may be useful to monitor renal function.

➤*Monitoring:* Because serious GI tract ulcerations and bleeding can occur without warning symptoms, monitor for signs or symptoms of GI bleeding. Periodically check complete blood cell counts and chemistry profiles of patients on long-term treatment with NSAIDs. If clinical signs and symptoms consistent with liver or renal disease develop, systemic manifestations occur (eg, eosinophilia, rash), or if abnormal liver tests persist or worsen, discontinue the diclofenac patch. Monitor blood pressure closely during the initiation of NSAID treatment and throughout the course of therapy.

Evaluate patients with symptoms and/or signs suggesting hepatic impairment, or in whom an abnormal liver test has occurred, for evidence of the development of a more severe hepatic reaction while on therapy with diclofenac.

Carefully monitor patients receiving diclofenac who may be adversely affected by alterations in platelet function, such as those with coagulation disorders or patients receiving anticoagulants.

Drug Interactions

Diclofenac Drug Interactions

Precipitant drug	Object drug[a]		Description
ACE inhibitors (eg, enalapril)	Diclofenac	↓↑	NSAIDs may diminish the antihypertensive effect of ACE inhibitors. In addition, the risk of nephrotoxicity associated with ACE inhibitors or diclofenac may be increased. If blood pressure control decreases, it may be necessary to discontinue diclofenac. Periodic measurement of renal function may be necessary.
Diclofenac	ACE inhibitors (eg, enalapril)		
Alcohol	Diclofenac	↑	The risk of GI bleeding may be increased. Use with caution.
Anticoagulants (eg, heparin, warfarin)	Diclofenac	↑	The effects of heparin or warfarin and NSAIDs on GI bleeding are synergistic. The risk of serious GI bleeding is higher than with either drug alone. Closely monitor coagulation status and adjust the dosage of anticoagulants accordingly. Monitor for signs of GI bleeding. Advise patients about the signs and symptoms of GI bleeding.
Diclofenac	Anticoagulants (eg, heparin, warfarin)		
Antiplatelet agents (eg, clopidogrel)	Diclofenac	↑	The risk of bleeding may be increased. Coadminister with caution. Closely monitor for signs of bleeding.
Diclofenac	Antiplatelet agents (eg, clopidogrel)		

DICLOFENAC EPOLAMINE — TRANSDERMAL

Diclofenac Drug Interactions			
Precipitant drug	Object drug[a]		Description
Azole antifungal agents (eg, voriconazole)	Diclofenac	↑	Diclofenac concentrations may be elevated, increasing the pharmacologic effects and risk of adverse reactions. Observe the clinical response of the patient and adjust the diclofenac dose as needed.
Corticosteroids (eg, prednisone)	Diclofenac	↑	The risk of GI bleeding may be increased. Use with caution. Advise patients about the signs and symptoms of GI bleeding.
Cyclosporine	Diclofenac	↑	Coadministration may increase the nephrotoxicity of both agents. Use with caution and monitor renal function closely.
Diclofenac	Cyclosporine		
Hepatotoxic agents (eg, acetaminophen, certain antibiotics and antiepileptic agents)	Diclofenac	↑	The risk of hepatotoxicity may be increased. Use with caution. Closely monitor for signs and symptoms of hepatotoxicity.
Diclofenac	Hepatotoxic agents (eg, acetaminophen, certain antibiotics and antiepileptic agents)		
Hibiscus sabdariffa	Diclofenac	↑	Diclofenac urinary excretion may be reduced, increasing diclofenac concentrations and risk of adverse reactions. Patients taking diclofenac should avoid beverages made from *Hibiscus sabdariffa* flowers.
Salicylates (eg, aspirin)	Diclofenac	↔	Coadministration may cause reduced protein binding of diclofenac, although the clearance of free diclofenac is not altered; clinical importance is unknown. However, coadministration is generally not recommended because of the potential of increased adverse reactions.
Serotonin norepinephrine reuptake inhibitors (eg, venlafaxine), SSRIs[b] (eg, citalopram, fluoxetine)	Diclofenac	↑	Coadministration may increase the risk of upper GI bleeding. Use with caution. Closely monitor for signs of GI bleeding. Advise patients about the signs and symptoms of GI bleeding.
Diclofenac	Serotonin norepinephrine reuptake inhibitors (eg, venlafaxine), SSRIs (eg, citalopram, fluoxetine)		
Smoking	Diclofenac	↑	The risk of GI bleeding may be increased. Use with caution.
Diclofenac	Aminoglycosides (eg, amikacin, gentamicin)	↑	Aminoglycoside concentrations may be elevated, increasing the risk of acute renal insufficiency. If concomitant use cannot be avoided, reduce the aminoglycoside dose prior to starting diclofenac. Monitor renal function and aminoglycoside serum levels and adjust the dose as needed.
Diclofenac	Diuretics (eg, loop diuretics [eg, furosemide], thiazide diuretics [eg, hydrochlorothiazide])	↓	Diclofenac may reduce the natriuretic effect of furosemide and thiazide diuretics in some patients. This response has been attributed to inhibition of renal prostaglandin synthesis. Observe patients closely for signs of renal failure and to ensure diuretic efficacy.
Diclofenac	Lithium	↑	NSAIDs have produced an elevation of plasma lithium levels and a reduction in renal lithium clearance. These effects have been attributed to inhibition of renal prostaglandin synthesis by the NSAID. Monitor for signs of lithium toxicity.
Diclofenac	Methotrexate	↑	Methotrexate toxicity may be increased. Coadminister with caution.
Diclofenac	Quinolones (eg, levofloxacin)	↑	Risk of CNS stimulation and seizures from quinolones may be increased. In addition, quinolone plasma concentrations may be increased. Use with caution.
Diclofenac	Tenofovir	↑	Pharmacologic and toxic effects (eg, nephrotoxicity) of tenofovir may be increased. Use with caution. Consider use of an analgesic other than an NSAID.
Diclofenac	Triamterene	↑	Coadministration of diclofenac and triamterene may cause a sudden onset of nephrotoxicity. If renal function deteriorates during coadministration of these agents, consider stopping one or both drugs.

[a] ↑ = object drug increased; ↓ = object drug decreased; ↔ = undetermined clinical effect.
[b] SSRIs = selective serotonin reuptake inhibitors.

Adverse Reactions

➤*Discontinuation of treatment:* In the controlled trials, 3% of patients in both the diclofenac and placebo patch groups discontinued treatment because of an adverse reaction. The most common adverse reactions leading to discontinuation were application-site reactions, occurring in 2% of both the diclofenac and placebo patch groups. Application-site reactions leading to dropout included burning, dermatitis, and pruritus.

➤*Common adverse reactions:* Overall, the most common adverse reactions associated with diclofenac patch treatment were skin reactions at the site of treatment.

➤*Adverse reactions (1% or more):*

Diclofenac Patch Common Adverse Reactions (≥ 1%)[a]		
Adverse reactions	Diclofenac patch (n = 572)	Placebo (n = 564)
CNS	2%	3%
Headache	1%	2%
Paresthesia	1%	1%
Somnolence	1%	1%
Other[b]	1%	< 1%
Local	11%	12%
Burning	< 1%	1%
Dermatitis	2%	< 1%
Pruritus	5%	8%
Other[c]	4%	3%
GI	9%	6%
Dysgeusia	2%	< 1%
Dyspepsia	1%	1%
Nausea	3%	2%
Other[d]	3%	2%

[a] The table lists adverse reactions occurring in placebo-treated patients because the placebo patch was comprised of the same ingredients as the diclofenac patch except for diclofenac. Adverse reactions in the placebo group may therefore reflect effects of the nonactive ingredients.
[b] Includes dizziness, hyperkinesia, and hypoesthesia.
[c] Includes application-site dryness, atrophy, discoloration, erythema, hyperhidrosis, irritation, and vesicles.
[d] Includes constipation, diarrhea, dry mouth, gastritis, upper abdominal pain, and vomiting.

➤*Other adverse reactions:* Foreign labeling describes that dermal allergic reactions may occur with diclofenac patch treatment. Additionally, the treated area may become irritated or develop itching, erythema, edema, vesicles, or abnormal sensation.

DICLOFENAC EPOLAMINE — TRANSDERMAL

Overdosage

➤*Symptoms:* There is limited experience with overdose of diclofenac patch. In clinical studies, the maximum single dose administered was 1 diclofenac patch containing diclofenac epolamine 180 mg. There were no serious adverse reactions.

➤*Treatment:* If systemic adverse reactions occur because of incorrect use or accidental overdose of this product, take the general measures recommended for intoxication with NSAIDs.

Patient Information

Inform patients that diclofenac, like other NSAIDs, may cause serious cardiovascular adverse reactions, such as MI or stroke, which may result in hospitalization and even death. Although serious cardiovascular reactions can occur without warning symptoms, advise patients to be alert for the signs and symptoms of chest pain, shortness of breath, weakness, or slurring of speech, and instruct patients to ask for medical advice if any indicative signs or symptoms are observed. Inform patients of the importance of this follow-up.

Inform patients that diclofenac, like other NSAIDs, may cause GI discomfort and, rarely, serious GI adverse reactions, such as ulcers and bleeding, which may result in hospitalization and even death. Although serious GI tract ulcerations and bleeding can occur without warning symptoms, advise patients to be alert for the signs and symptoms of ulcerations and bleeding, and instruct patients to ask for medical advice when observing any indicative sign or symptoms, including epigastric pain, dyspepsia, melena, and hematemesis. Inform patients of the importance of this follow-up.

Inform patients that diclofenac, like other NSAIDs, may cause serious skin adverse reactions such as exfoliative dermatitis, Stevens-Johnson syndrome, and toxic epidermal necrolysis, which may result in hospitalizations and even death. Although serious skin reactions may occur without warning, advise patients to be alert for the signs and symptoms of skin rash and blisters, fever, or other signs of hypersensitivity such as itching, and instruct patients to ask for medical advice if any indicative signs or symptoms are observed. Advise patients to stop the drug immediately if they develop any type of rash and to contact their health care provider as soon as possible.

Instruct patients to promptly report signs or symptoms of unexplained weight gain or edema to their health care provider.

Inform patients of the warning signs and symptoms of hepatotoxicity (eg, nausea, fatigue, lethargy, pruritus, jaundice, right upper quadrant tenderness, flu-like symptoms). If these occur, instruct patients to stop therapy and seek immediate medical attention.

Inform patients of the signs of an anaphylactoid reaction (eg, difficulty breathing, swelling of the face or throat). If these occur, instruct patients to seek immediate emergency help.

In late pregnancy, as with other NSAIDs, avoid using diclofenac because it may cause premature closure of the ductus arteriosus.

Advise patients not to use diclofenac if they have aspirin-sensitive asthma. Diclofenac, like other NSAIDs, could cause severe and even fatal bronchospasm in these patients. Instruct patients to discontinue use of diclofenac and immediately seek emergency help if they experience wheezing or shortness of breath.

Instruct patients to only apply diclofenac patch on intact skin.

Advise patients to avoid contact of diclofenac patch with eyes and mucosa. Instruct patients that if eye contact occurs, to immediately wash out the eye with water or saline and to consult a health care provider if irritation persists for more than an hour.

Instruct patients and caregivers to wash their hands after applying, handling, or removing the patch.

Inform patients that if the diclofenac patch begins to peel off, the edges of the patch may be taped down.

Instruct patients not to wear the diclofenac patch while bathing or showering. Advise patients to bathe in between scheduled patch removal and application.

Advise patients to store new patches and discard used patches out of the reach of children and away from pets. If a child or pet accidentally ingests diclofenac patch, instruct the patient to immediately seek medical help.

ANTI-PSORIATIC AGENTS

In addition to the products described here, other products for treatment of psoriasis include: Coal tar; corticosteroids; salicylic acid. Refer to individual monographs.

ANTHRALIN (Dithranol)

Rx	**Dritho-Scalp** (Summers Labs)	**Cream; topical:** 0.5%	White petrolatum, cetostearyl alcohol. In 50 g.
Rx	**Anthralin** (Rising Pharmaceuticals)	**Cream; topical:** 1%	In 50 g.
Rx	**Zithranol-RR** (Elorac)	**Cream; topical:** 1.2%	Preservative free. Rapid release. In 15 and 45 g.

ANTHRALIN — TOPICAL

Indications

➤*Psoriasis:* Treatment of quiescent or chronic psoriasis of the scalp. Continue treatment until the skin is entirely clear (ie, when there is nothing to feel with the fingers and the texture is normal).

Administration and Dosage

➤*Adults:*

Psoriasis –

1% and 1.2% cream:

• *For the skin –* Apply sparingly only to the psoriatic lesions and rub gently and carefully into the skin. Avoid applying an excessive quantity, which may cause unnecessary soiling and staining of the clothing or bed linen. At the end of each period of treatment, rinse the skin thoroughly with cool to lukewarm water before washing with soap. The margins of the lesions may gradually become stained purple/brown as treatment progresses, but this will disappear after cessation of treatment.

• *For the scalp –* Wash the hair with shampoo, rinse with water, and apply anthralin cream while the hair is still damp. Rub the cream well into the psoriatic lesions. Keep anthralin cream away from the eyes. Take care to avoid application of the cream to uninvolved scalp margins. Rinse hair and scalp thoroughly with cool to lukewarm water and then shampoo the hair and scalp to remove any surplus cream (which may have changed in color). This treatment may be repeated on alternate days if necessary.

0.5% scalp cream: Apply as directed and remove by washing or showering. The optimal period of contact will vary according to the strength used and the patient's response to treatment.

Comb the hair to remove scalar debris and, after suitably parting, apply anthralin only to the lesions and rub in well, taking care to prevent the cream spreading onto the forehead.

Avoid application of the cream to uninvolved scalp margins. Remove any unintended residue that may be deposited behind the ears. At the end of each period of contact, wash the hair and scalp to remove any surplus cream (which may have become red/brown in color).

➤*Administration:* Generally, it is recommended that anthralin be applied once a day or as directed by a health care provider. Anthralin is known to be a potential skin irritant. The irritant potential of anthralin is directly related to the strength being used, the time of contact, and each patient's individual tolerance. Therefore, where the response to anthralin treatment has not previously been established, always commence treatment using a short contact time of 5 to 10 minutes for at least 1 week. When a short contact time is used initially, it can be increased stepwise to 20 to 30 minutes before removing the cream by thoroughly washing or showering.

Avoid contact with the eyes or mucous membranes. Exercise caution when applying anthralin cream to the face or intertriginous skin areas. Anthralin should not normally be applied to intertriginous skin areas and high strengths should not be used on these sites. Remove any unintended residue that may be deposited behind the ears. Avoid applying to the folds and creases of the skin.

Keep anthralin well away from the eyes. Always wash hands thoroughly after use.

➤*Storage / Stability:* Store at 15° to 30°C (59° to 86°F).

Actions

➤*Pharmacology:* Although the precise mechanism of anthralin's antipsoriatic action is not fully understood, in vitro evidence suggests that its antimitotic effect results from inhibition of DNA synthesis. Additionally, the chemically reducing properties of anthralin may upset oxidative metabolic processes, providing a further slowing down of epidermal mitosis.

Absorption has not been finally determined, but in a limited clinical study of anthralin cream, no traces of anthraquinone metabolites were detected in the urine of subjects treated; however, caution is advised in patients with renal disease.

Contraindications

Acute or actively inflamed psoriatic eruptions; hypersensitivity to any of the ingredients.

Warnings/Precautions

➤*For external use only:* Avoid contact with the eyes or mucous membranes. Exercise caution when applying anthralin cream to the face or intertriginous skin areas. Anthralin should not normally be applied to intertriginous skin areas and high strengths should not be used on these sites. Remove any unintended residue that may be deposited behind the ears. Avoid applying to the folds and creases of the skin.

➤*Sensitivity reaction:* Discontinue use if a sensitivity reaction occurs or if excessive irritation develops on uninvolved skin areas.

➤*Staining:* Anthralin may stain the hair; apply sparingly and carefully to psoriatic lesions only. Contact with fabrics, plastics, and other materials may cause staining and should be avoided. To prevent the possibility of discoloration, always rinse the bath/shower with hot water immediately after

ANTHRALIN — TOPICAL

washing/showering and then use a suitable cleanser to remove any deposit on the surface of the bath or shower. To prevent the possibility of staining clothing or bed linen while gaining experience in using anthralin, it may be advisable to use protective dressings. Always wash hands thoroughly after use.

➤*Long-term use of topical corticosteroids:* Because long-term use of topical corticosteroids may destabilize psoriasis, and withdrawal may also give rise to a "rebound" phenomenon, allow an interval of at least 1 week between the discontinuance of such steroids and the commencement of anthralin therapy. Application of petrolatum or a suitably bland emollient may be useful during the intervening period.

➤*Pregnancy: Category C.* Animal reproduction studies have not been conducted with anthralin. It is also not known whether anthralin can cause fetal harm when administered to a pregnant woman or can affect reproduction capacity. Anthralin should be given to a pregnant woman only if clearly needed.

➤*Lactation:* It is not known whether this drug is excreted in human milk. Because many drugs are excreted in milk and because of the potential for tumorigenicity shown for anthralin in animal studies, decide whether to discontinue breastfeeding or the drug, taking into account the importance of the drug to the mother.

➤*Children:* Safety and efficacy in pediatric patients have not been established.

Drug Interactions

➤*Topical corticosteroids:* Because long-term use of topical corticosteroids may destabilize psoriasis, and withdrawal may also give rise to a "rebound" phenomenon, allow an interval of at least 1 week between the discontinuance of such steroids and the commencement of anthralin therapy.

Adverse Reactions

Very few instances of contact allergic reactions to anthralin have been reported. However, transient primary irritation of the healthy or uninvolved skin surrounding the treated lesions is more frequently seen and may occasionally be severe. Application of anthralin must be restricted to the psoriatic lesions. If the initial treatment produces excessive soreness or if the lesions spread, reduce frequency of application and, in extreme cases, discontinue use and consult health care provider. Some temporary discoloration of hair and fingernails may arise during the period of treatment but should be minimized by careful application. Anthralin may stain skin, hair, or fabrics. Staining of fabrics may be permanent, so contact should be avoided.

Patient Information

Anthralin cream is for external use only. It is not for ophthalmic use. Avoid contact with the eyes or mucous membranes. Use care when applying anthralin cream to any facial area, uninvolved scalp margins, behind the ears, or in other sensitive areas such as skin folds. As with any other prescription drug, discontinue use if you experience any unexpected reaction or discomfort and immediately consult your doctor.

➤*Staining:* Anthralin cream may stain skin, hair, or fabrics. Some temporary discoloration of hair and nails may arise during the period of treatment but should be minimized by careful application. Staining of fabrics may be permanent, so contact should be avoided.

➤*Avoiding staining to clothes, bath or shower:* As anthralin cream may stain, follow directions carefully to avoid exposure to clothes, bath, or shower.

Clothing – Thoroughly rinse exposed clothing with cool or lukewarm water only. Wash with detergent and water as usual. The suggested water temperature should be warm (not above 86°F) or cold.

Bath and shower – To reduce the possibility of discoloration to the bath or shower, always rinse well with cool or lukewarm water only. Use a suitable cleaner to remove any deposit left on the surface.

➤*Application to skin:*

1.) While avoiding normal skin, apply small amount to the psoriatic lesions. Thoroughly and carefully rub the cream into the skin until it no longer smears.
2.) Immediately following application, wash your hands with cool or lukewarm water only.
3.) Leave anthralin cream on for the prescribed amount of time. Your doctor may recommend a short contact period at first, and then gradually increase the contact time
4.) After prescribed amount of time, rinse anthralin cream off the skin thoroughly using cool or lukewarm water only. Avoid hot water and soaps as they could cause product to stain or irritate.
5.) After anthralin cream has been thoroughly washed off, shower using soap and water.

➤*Application to scalp:*

1.) Wash the hair with shampoo and rinse with water.
2.) Part the hair away from the psoriatic scalp lesion. Apply anthralin cream and rub thoroughly into the psoriatic scalp lesions while the hair is still damp. Remove any unintended residue that may be deposited behind the ears.
3.) Immediately following application, wash your hands with cool or lukewarm water only.
4.) Leave anthralin cream on the prescribed amount of time. Your doctor may recommend a short contact period at first, and then gradually increase the contact time.
5.) After prescribed amount of time, rinse hair and scalp with cool or lukewarm water only. Avoid hot water and shampoo as they could cause product to stain or irritate.
6.) Following thorough removal of anthralin cream, shampoo and water may be used on the hair and scalp.

CALCIPOTRIENE

Rx	**Calcipotriene** (Taro Pharmaceuticals)	**Ointment; topical:** 0.005%	Alpha-tocopherol, edetate disodium, mineral oil, petrolatum, propylene glycol. In 60 g.
Rx	**Dovonex** (Westwood Squibb)		In 30, 60 and 100 g.
Rx	**Dovonex** (Leo Pharma)	**Cream; topical:** 0.005%	In 30, 60 and 100 g.
Rx	**Calcipotriene** (Various, eg, Fougera, Hi-Tech)	**Solution; topical:** 0.005%	May contain menthol. In 60 mL.
Rx	**Dovonex** (Leo Pharma)		Menthol. In 60 mL.

CALCIPOTRIENE — TOPICAL

Indications

➤*Plaque Psoriasis:* Calcipotriene cream and ointment are indicated for the treatment of plaque psoriasis in adults. The safety and effectiveness of topical calcipotriene in dermatoses other than psoriasis have not been established.

➤*Psoriasis of the scalp:* Calcipotriene scalp solution is indicated for the topical treatment of chronic, moderately severe psoriasis of the scalp. The safety and effectiveness of topical calcipotriene in dermatoses other than psoriasis have not been established.

Administration and Dosage

➤*Adults:*

Plaque psoriasis –

Cream and ointment: Apply a thin layer of calcipotriene cream or ointment to the affected skin once or twice daily and rub in gently and completely.

Psoriasis of the scalp –

Scalp solution: Comb the hair to remove scaly debris and after suitably parting, apply calcipotriene scalp solution twice daily, only to the lesions, and rub in gently and completely, taking care to prevent the solution from spreading onto the forehead.

➤*Administration:* For topical dermatologic use only.

Keep calcipotriene scalp solution well away from the eyes. Avoid application of the solution to uninvolved scalp margins. Always wash hands thoroughly after use.

➤*Storage/Stability:* Store at 15° to 25°C (59° to 77°F). Do not freeze. Avoid exposing the scalp solution to sunlight.

Scalp solution – Drug product is flammable. Keep away from open flame.

Actions

➤*Pharmacology:* In humans, the natural supply of vitamin D depends mainly on exposure to the ultraviolet rays of the sun for conversion of 7-dehydrocholesterol to vitamin D_3 (cholecalciferol) in the skin. Calcipotriene is a synthetic analog of vitamin D_3.

Vitamin D3 receptors, proteins that bind chemically to calcitriol, occur in many parts of the body, including the skin cells known as keratinocytes. The scaly red patches of psoriasis are caused by the abnormal growth and production of the keratinocytes. Calcipotriene regulates skin cell production and development.

Although the precise mechanism of calcipotriene's antipsoriatic action is not fully understood, in vitro evidence suggests that calcipotriene is roughly equipotent to the natural vitamin in its effects on proliferation and differentiation of a variety of cell types. Calcipotriene has also been shown, in animal studies, to be 100-200 times less potent in its effects on calcium utilization than the natural hormone.

➤*Pharmacokinetics:*

Absorption/Distribution – There is evidence that maternal 1,25-dihydroxy vitamin D_3 (calcitriol) may enter the fetal circulation, but it is not known whether it is excreted in human milk. The systemic disposition of calcipotriene is expected to be similar to that of the naturally occurring vitamin.

Cream and Ointment: Clinical studies with radiolabelled ointment indicate that approximately 6% (±3%, SD) of the applied dose of calcipotriene is absorbed systemically when the ointment is applied topically to psoriasis plaques or 5% (±2.6%, SD) when applied to normal skin, and much of the absorbed active is converted to inactive metabolites within 24 hours of application.

Scalp Solution: Clinical studies with radiolabelled calcipotriene solution indicate that less than 1% of the applied dose of calcipotriene is absorbed through the scalp when the solution (2.0 mL) is applied topically to normal

CALCIPOTRIENE — TOPICAL

skin or psoriasis plaques (160 cm^2) for 12 hours, and that much of the absorbed calcipotriene is converted to inactive metabolites within 24 hours of application.

Metabolism / Excretion – Vitamin D and its metabolites are transported in the blood, bound to specific plasma proteins. After entering the bloodstream, it is metabolized in the liver and kidneys to its active form, the hormone calcitriol. The active form of the vitamin, 1,25-dihydroxy vitamin D_3 (calcitriol), is known to be recycled via the liver and excreted in the bile. Calcipotriene metabolism following systemic uptake is rapid, and occurs via a similar pathway to the natural hormone.

The primary metabolites are much less potent than the parent compound.

Contraindications

➤*Cream and ointment:* Hypersensitivity to any of the components of the preparation; hypercalcemia or evidence of vitamin D toxicity. Do not use calcipotriene cream and ointment on the face.

➤*Scalp solution:* Acute psoriatic eruptions; hypersensitivity to any of the components of the preparations; hypercalcemia or evidence of vitamin D toxicity.

Warnings/Precautions

➤*Scalp Solution:* Avoid contact with the eyes or mucous membranes. Discontinue use if a sensitivity reaction occurs or if excessive irritation develops on uninvolved skin areas.

Drug product is flammable. Keep away from open flame.

➤*Irritation:* Use of calcipotriene may cause irritation of lesions and surrounding uninvolved skin. If irritation develops, calcipotriene should be discontinued.

➤*Hypercalcemia:* Reversible elevation of serum calcium has occurred with use of topical calcipotriene. If elevation in serum calcium outside the normal range should occur, discontinue treatment until normal calcium levels are restored.

➤*Pregnancy: Category C.* Studies of teratogenicity were done by the oral route where bioavailability is expected to be approximately 40–60% of the administered dose. In rabbits, increased maternal and fetal toxicity were noted at a dosage of 12 mcg/kg/day (132 mcg/m^2/day); a dosage of 36 mcg/kg/day (396 mcg/m^2/day) resulted in a significant increase in the incidence of incomplete ossification of the pubic bones and forelimb phalanges of fetuses. In a rat study, a dosage of 54 mcg/kg/day (318 mcg/m^2/day) resulted in a significantly increased incidence of skeletal abnormalities (enlarged fontanelles and extra ribs). The enlarged fontanelles are most likely due to calcipotriene's effect upon calcium metabolism. The estimated maternal and fetal no-effect exposure levels in the rat (43.2 mcg/m^2/day) and rabbit (17.6 mcg/m^2/day) studies are approximately equal to the expected human systemic exposure level (18.5 mcg/m^2/day) from dermal application. There are no adequate and well-controlled studies in pregnant women. Therefore, calcipotriene should be used during pregnancy only if the potential benefit justifies the potential risk to the fetus.

➤*Lactation:* There is evidence that maternal 1,25-dihydroxy vitamin D3 (calcitriol) may enter the fetal circulation, but it is not known whether it is excreted in human milk. The systemic disposition of calcipotriene is expected to be similar to that of the naturally occurring vitamin. Because many drugs are excreted in human milk, caution should be exercised when calcipotriene cream, ointment, or scalp solution is administered to a nursing woman.

➤*Children:* Safety and effectiveness of calcipotriene in pediatric patients have not been established. Because of a higher ratio of skin surface area to body mass, pediatric patients are at greater risk than adults of systemic adverse effects when they are treated with topical medication.

➤*Elderly:*

Ointment only – Of the total number of patients in clinical studies of calcipotriene ointment, approximately 12% were 65 or older, while approximately 4% were 75 or older. The results of an analysis of severity of skin-related adverse events showed a statistically significant difference for subjects over 65 years (more severe) compared to those under 65 years (less severe).

Adverse Reactions

➤*Cream and ointment:* In controlled clinical trials, the most frequent adverse reactions reported for calcipotriene cream and ointment were burning, itching, and skin irritation, which occurred in approximately 10%-15% of patients. Erythema, dry skin, peeling, rash, dermatitis, worsening of psoriasis including development of facial/scalp psoriasis were reported in 1% to 10% of patients. Other experiences reported in less than 1% of patients included skin atrophy, hyperpigmentation, hypercalcemia, and folliculitis. Once daily dosing has not been shown to be superior in safety to twice daily dosing.

➤*Scalp solution:* In controlled clinical trials, the most frequent adverse reactions reported to be related to calcipotriene scalp solution use were transient burning, stinging and tingling, which occurred in approximately 23% of patients. Rash was reported in about 11% of patients. Dry skin, irritation and worsening of psoriasis was reported in 1%-5% of patients. Skin atrophy, hyperpigmentation, hypercalcemia, and folliculitis were not observed in these studies, but cannot be excluded.

Overdosage

Topically applied calcipotriene can be absorbed in sufficient amounts to produce systemic effects. Elevated serum calcium has been observed with excessive use of topical calcipotriene. If elevation in serum calcium should occur, discontinue treatment until normal calcium levels are restored.

Patient Information

This medication is to be used as directed by the physician and should not be used for any disorder other than that for which it was prescribed. It is for external use only. Avoid contact with the face or eyes. As with any topical medication, patients should wash hands after application. Patients should report to their physician any signs of local adverse reactions.

CALCIPOTRIENE/BETAMETHASONE DIPROPIONATE

Rx	**Taclonex** (Leo Pharma)	**Ointment; topical:** calcipotriene 0.005%/ betamethasone dipropionate 0.064%	Equiv. to calcipotriene hydrate 52.18 mcg and betamethasone 0.5 mg. Mineral oil, white petrolatum. In 60 and 100 g.
Rx	**Taclonex Scalp** (Leo Pharma)	**Suspension; topical:** calcipotriene 0.005%/ betamethasone dipropionate 0.64%	Equiv to calcipotriene hydrate 52.18 mcg and betamethasone 0.5 mg. Castor oil, mineral oil. In 15, 30, and 60 g.

CALCIPOTRIENE/BETAMETHASONE DIPROPIONATE — TOPICAL

Indications

➤*Psoriasis vulgaris:* For the topical treatment of psoriasis vulgaris in adults 18 years of age and older.

Administration and Dosage

➤*Adults:*

Psoriasis vulgaris –

Ointment:

• *Usual dosage* – Apply an adequate layer of ointment to the affected area(s) once daily for up to 4 weeks. The ointment should be rubbed in gently and completely.

Treatment of more than 30% body surface area is not recommended.

• *Maximum dose* – The maximum weekly dose should not exceed 100 g.

Suspension:

• *Usual dosage* – Apply to affected areas on the scalp once daily for 2 weeks or until cleared. Treatment may be continued for up to 8 weeks.

• *Maximum dose* – The maximum weekly dose should not exceed 100 g.

➤*Administration:*

Ointment – Do not apply to the face, axillae, or groin.

Suspension – Patients should shake the bottle prior to using the product and wash their hands after applying topical suspension.

➤*Storage / Stability:* Store between 20° and 25°C (68° and 77°F); excursions are permitted between 15° and 30°C (59° and 86°F). Do not refrigerate. Use suspension within 3 months after it has been opened.

CALCITRIOL

Rx	**Vectical** (Galderma Laboratories, Inc)	**Ointment; topical:** 0.0003%	Mineral oil, white petrolatum. In 5 and 100 g tubes.

CALCITRIOL — TOPICAL

Indications

➤*Plaque psoriasis:* For the topical treatment of mild to moderate plaque psoriasis in adults 18 years of age and older.

➤*Off-label uses:*

Psoriasis (children / adolescents) – [1] = Good documentation. Among topical therapies for plaque-type psoriasis, the American Academy of Dermatology assigned a level A recommendation, defined as a recommendation based on consistent and good-quality patient-oriented evidence, to vitamin D analogues (eg, calcitriol); tazarotene; or corticosteroids alone or in combination with vitamin D analogues or tazarotene.

Administration and Dosage

➤*Adults:*

Plaque psoriasis –

Usual dosage: Apply to affected areas twice daily, morning and evening.

Maximum dose: 200 g weekly.

CALCITRIOL — TOPICAL

➤*Children:*

Off-label dosing –

Psoriasis (children/adolescents): [1] = Good documentation. A sufficient quantity to cover the affected area, applied twice daily. When used as needed for 52 weeks, no serious drug-related adverse effects were observed.

➤*Administration:* Ointment is not for oral, ophthalmic, or intravaginal use. Calcitriol should not be applied to the eyes, lips, or facial skin.

➤*Storage/Stability:* Store at 25°C (77°F); excursions are permitted to 15° to 30°C (59° to 86°F). Do not freeze or refrigerate.

Actions

➤*Pharmacology:* The mechanism of action of calcitriol in the treatment of psoriasis has not been established.

➤*Pharmacokinetics:*

Absorption – At day 21, the geometric mean plasma concentration values of the maximal drug concentration (C_{max}) increased by approximately 36% over baseline, and the geometric mean value of the area under the curve ($AUC_{(0\text{-}12h)}$) increased by 44%.

Contraindications

None known.

Warnings/Precautions

➤*Hypercalcemia:* In controlled clinical trials with calcitriol among subjects receiving laboratory monitoring, hypercalcemia was observed in 24% (18/74) of subjects exposed to active drug and 16% (13/79) of subjects exposed to vehicle. However, the increases in calcium and albumin-adjusted calcium levels were less than 10% above the upper limit of normal (ULN).

If aberrations in parameters of calcium metabolism occur, discontinue treatment until these parameters have normalized. The effects of calcitriol on calcium metabolism following treatment durations of more than 52 weeks have not been evaluated. Increased absorption may occur with occlusive use.

➤*Special risk:* The safety and effectiveness of calcitriol in patients with known or suspected disorders of calcium metabolism have not been evaluated. The safety and effectiveness of calcitriol in patients with erythrodermic, exfoliative, or pustular psoriasis have not been evaluated.

➤*Photosensitivity:* Animal data suggest that the vehicle of calcitriol may enhance the ability of ultraviolet radiation (UVR) to induce skin tumors.

Subjects who apply calcitriol to exposed skin should avoid excessive exposure of the treated areas to natural or artificial sunlight, including tanning booths and sun lamps. Health care providers may wish to limit or avoid use of phototherapy in patients who use calcitriol.

➤*Pregnancy: Category C.* Calcitriol has been shown to be fetotoxic. There are no adequate and well-controlled studies for calcitriol in pregnant women. Use calcitriol ointment during pregnancy only if the potential benefit to the patient justifies the potential risk to the fetus.

Teratogenic – In rabbits, topically applied calcitriol induced a significantly elevated mean postimplantation loss and an increased incidence of minor skeletal abnormalities due to retarded ossification of the pubic bones. A slightly increased incidence of skeletal variation (extra thirteenth rib, reduced ossification of epiphyses) was also observed. These effects may have been secondary to maternal toxicity. Based on the recommended human dose and instructions for use, it is not possible to calculate human dose equivalents for animal exposures in these studies.

➤*Lactation:* It is not known whether calcitriol is excreted in human milk. Because many drugs are excreted in human milk, exercise caution when calcitriol is administered to a breast-feeding woman.

➤*Children:* Safety and effectiveness in children have not been established.

Drug Interactions

Calcitriol Topical Drug Interactions

Precipitant drug	Object drug[a]		Description
Calcium supplements	Calcitriol	↑	The biological actions of vitamin D may be enhanced. Hypercalcemia could manifest. Use with caution and consider monitoring serum calcium levels.
Thiazide diuretics (eg, chlorothiazide)	Calcitriol		
Vitamin D	Calcitriol		

[a] ↑ = object drug increased.

Adverse Reactions

Calcitriol Topical Adverse Reactions (≥ 1%)

Adverse reaction	Calcitriol (n = 419)	Vehicle (n = 420)
Discomfort skin	3%	2%
Pruritus	1%	1%

➤*Hypercalcemia:* See Warnings/Precautions for more information.

➤*Adverse reactions (3% or more):*

Dermatologic – Psoriasis (4%), pruritus (3%).

GU – Urine abnormality (4%). Kidney stones were reported in 3 subjects and confirmed in 2 subjects.

Miscellaneous – Lab test abnormality (8%), hypercalciuria (3%).

➤*Postmarketing:*

Dermatologic – Acute blistering dermatitis, erythema, pruritus, skin burning sensation, and skin discomfort.

Overdosage

➤*Symptoms:* Topically applied calcitriol can be absorbed in sufficient amounts to produce systemic effects.

Patient Information

This medication is to be used as directed by a health care provider. It is for external use only. This medication is to be applied only to areas of the skin affected by psoriasis, as directed. Advise patients to gently rub it into the skin so that no medication remains visible.

Advise patients to report any signs of adverse reactions to their health care provider.

Advise patients to avoid excess exposure of the treated areas to natural or artificial sunlight, including tanning booths and sunlamps.

METHOTREXATE (Amethopterin; MTX)

See the Methotrexate monograph in the Antineoplastic Agents chapter.

SELENIUM SULFIDE

otc	**Selenium Sulfide** (Various)	**Lotion/Shampoo; topical:** 1%	In 210 mL.
otc	**Head & Shoulders Intensive Treatment** (Procter & Gamble)		In 400 mL.
otc	**Selsun Blue Medicated Treatment** (Chattem)		Menthol. In 325 mL.
Rx	**Selenos** (Breckenridge Pharmaceutical)	**Shampoo, suspension; topical:** 2.25%	Caprylic/capric triglyceride, edetate disodium, parabens, propylene glycol, urea, zinc. In 180 mL.
Rx	**Selenium Sulfide** (Various, eg, Clay-Park)	**Lotion; topical:** 2.5%	In 120 mL.
Rx	**Selsun** (Abbott)		In 120 mL.

SELENIUM SULFIDE — TOPICAL

Indications

➤*Dandruff, seborrheic dermatitis of the scalp, tinea versicolor:* For the treatment of dandruff, seborrheic dermatitis of the scalp, and tinea versicolor.

➤*Off-label uses:* Adjunctive therapy for tinea capitis.

Administration and Dosage

➤*Adults:*

Dandruff and seborrheic dermatitis –

Usual dosage: 2 applications each week for 2 weeks will afford control. After this, the lotion or shampoo may be used at less frequent intervals.

Maintenance dosage: Weekly, every 2 weeks, or even every 3 or 4 weeks in some cases. The preparation should not be applied more frequently than required to maintain control.

OTC 1%: Use at least twice per week or as directed by a doctor. For maximum dandruff control, use every time hair is shampooed.

Tinea versicolor – Apply to affected areas and lather with a small amount of water. Allow product to remain on skin for 10 minutes, then rinse the body thoroughly. Repeat this procedure once a day for 7 days.

➤*Children:*

Off-label dosing –

Seborrhea/dandruff:

• *Usual dose –* Massage 5 to 10 mL of 1% or 2.5% into wet scalp and leave on scalp for 2 to 3 minutes. Rinse thoroughly and repeat.

• *Maintenance dosage –* Shampoo twice weekly for 2 weeks then once every 1 to 4 weeks.

Tinea versicolor:

• *Usual dose –* Apply 2.5% lotion to affected areas of skin. Allow to remain on skin for 30 minutes. Rinse thoroughly. Repeat daily for 7 days.

• *Maintenance dosage –* Follow with monthly applications for 3 months to prevent recurrences.

➤*Administration:* Keep tightly capped. Shake well before using. Product may damage jewelry; remove jewelry before use.

SELENIUM SULFIDE — TOPICAL

Dandruff and seborrheic dermatitis of the scalp –

1.) Massage about 5 or 10 mL (1 or 2 teaspoonfuls) of shampoo into wet scalp.
2.) Allow to remain on scalp for 2 to 3 minutes.
3.) Rinse scalp thoroughly.
4.) Repeat application and rinse thoroughly.
5.) After treatment, wash hands well.
6.) Repeat treatments as directed by health care provider.

Lotion/Shampoo 1% – Shake well before use. Use only enough shampoo to lather and rinse. Repeat application and rinse thoroughly. If used on bleached, tinted, grey, or permed hair, rinse for 5 minutes in cool running water.

Tinea versicolor –

1.) Apply to affected areas and lather with a small amount of water.
2.) Allow to remain on skin for 10 minutes.
3.) Rinse body thoroughly.
4.) Repeat this procedure once a day for 7 days.

➤*Storage/Stability:* Store at controlled room temperature 15° to 30°C (59° to 86°F).

Protect from heat. Keep tightly closed. Keep this and all medications out of the reach of children.

Actions

➤*Pharmacology:* Selenium sulfide appears to have a cytostatic effect on cells of the epidermis and follicular epithelium, thus reducing corneocyte production.

Contraindications

Allergies to any of its components.

Warnings/Precautions

➤*Acute inflammation/exudation:* Do not use when acute inflammation or exudation is present as increased absorption may occur.

➤*For external use only:* Avoid contact with the eyes.

➤*Irritation:* Selenium sulfide may irritate the skin, especially in the genital area and in skin folds. Rinse these areas thoroughly after application.

➤*Hypersensitivity reactions:* If sensitivity reactions occur, discontinue use.

➤*Pregnancy: Category C* (tinea versicolor). When used on body surfaces for the treatment of tinea versicolor, selenium sulfide is classified as pregnancy *Category C*. Under ordinary circumstances, selenium sulfide lotion should not be used for the treatment of tinea versicolor in pregnant women.

Animal reproduction studies have not been conducted with selenium sulfide. It is also not known whether selenium sulfide can cause fetal harm when applied to body surfaces of a pregnant woman or can affect reproduction capacity.

➤*Lactation:* There is no data on the transfer of selenium sulfide into human milk. Do not apply directly to the nipple as enhanced absorption by the infant could occur.

➤*Children:* Safety and effectiveness in infants have not been established.

Adverse Reactions

➤*In decreasing order of severity:* Skin irritation; occasional reports of increase in amount of normal hair loss; discoloration of hair (can be avoided or minimized by thorough rinsing of hair after treatment).

As with other shampoos, oiliness or dryness of hair and scalp may occur.

Overdosage

➤*Symptoms:* Selenium sulfide shampoos have generally low toxicity if ingested. Nausea, vomiting, and diarrhea usually occur after oral ingestion. There may also be a burning sensation in the mouth and a garlic-like taste/smell to the breath. The detergents found in selenium sulfide shampoos may act as emetics, thereby preventing significant GI absorption of selenium.

➤*Treatment:* There have been no documented reports of serious toxicity in humans resulting from acute ingestion of selenium sulfide; however, acute toxicity studies in animals suggest that ingestion of large amounts could result in potential human toxicity. For this reason, evacuation of the stomach contents should be considered in cases of acute oral ingestion.

Patient Information

Application to skin or scalp may produce skin irritation or sensitization. If sensitivity reactions occur, use should be discontinued. May be irritating to mucous membranes of the eyes and contact with this area should be avoided. Thoroughly rinse after application.

For external use only. Do not use on broken skin or inflamed areas. If allergic reactions occur, discontinue use. Avoid getting shampoo or lotion in eyes or in contact with genital area as it may cause irritation and burning.

May damage jewelry; remove before using.

If using before or after bleaching, tinting, or permanent waving, rinse hair for at least 5 minutes in cool running water.

When applied to the body for treatment of tinea versicolor, selenium sulfide may produce skin irritation, especially in the genital area and where skin folds occur. These areas should be thoroughly rinsed after application.

Keep out of the reach of children. If swallowed, get medical help or contact a poison control center right away.

➤*Shampoo:* Ask a doctor before use if you have seborrheic dermatitis in areas other than the scalp.

For color-treated or permed hair, rinse thoroughly.

Stop use and ask a doctor if condition worsens or does not improve after regular use of this product as directed.

ANTISEBORRHEIC PRODUCTS

Antiseborrheic Combinations

Active Ingredients

➤*SALICYLIC ACID and SULFUR (see individual monographs):* These are used for antiseborrheic and keratolytic/keratoplastic actions.

➤*TAR PREPARATIONS, PYRITHIONE ZINC (see individual monographs) and MYRISTYLTRIMETHYLAMMONIUM BROMIDE:* These are used for their antipruritic, antibacterial or antiseborrheic actions.

➤*MENTHOL:* This is used as an antipruritic.

➤*BENZALKONIUM CHLORIDE, ISOPROPYL ALCOHOL, PHENOL and MENTHOL:* These are used as antiseptics.

➤*IODOQUINOL and BENZYL ALCOHOL:* These are antimicrobial agents.

Warnings/Precautions

➤*For external use only:* Avoid contact with eyes; in case of contact, flush with water.

➤*Irritation/Staining/Discoloration:* If undue skin irritation develops or increases, discontinue use and consult physician. Preparations containing tar may temporarily discolor blond, bleached or tinted hair. Slight staining of clothing may also occur.

ANTISEBORRHEIC SHAMPOOS

otc	**Maximum Strength Meted** (Sirius Labs)	**Shampoo; topical:** 5% sulfur and 3% salicylic acid	In 118 mL.
otc	**MG217 Medicated Tar-Free Shampoo** (Triton)		In 4 and 8 oz.
otc	**MG400** (Triton)	**Shampoo; topical:** 3% salicylic acid, 5% colloidal sulfur in Guy-Base II.	In 240 mL and pt.
otc	**Scalpicin** (Combe)	**Shampoo; topical:** 3% salicylic acid, menthol	SD alcohol 40. In 45 and 75 mL.
otc	**Sebex** (Rugby)	**Shampoo; topical:** 2% sulfur and 2% salicylic acid	In 118 mL.
otc	**Ala seb t** (Del-Ray Labs)	**Shampoo; topical:** 2% sulfur, 2% salicylic acid, 1% coal tar, PEG-20	In 118 mL.
otc	**Sulfoam** (Doak)	**Shampoo; topical:** 2% sulfur	In 237 mL.
otc	**P & S** (Baker Cummins)	**Shampoo; topical:** 2% salicylic acid	In 120 mL.
otc	**Neutrogena T/Sal** (Triton)	**Shampoo; topical:** 2% salicylic acid, 2% solubilized coal tar extract	In 135 mL.
otc	**Ionil** (Owen/Galderma)	**Shampoo; topical:** Salicylic acid, benzalkonium chloride, EDTA	In 120 and 240 mL, pt and qt.
otc	**X•Seb** (Baker Cummins)	**Shampoo; topical:** 4% salicylic acid	In 120 mL.
otc	**Tarsum** (Summers)	**Shampoo/Gel; topical:** 10% crude coal tar and 5% salicylic acid	In 120 and 240 mL.
otc	**X•Seb T** (Baker Cummins)	**Shampoo; topical:** 10% coal tar solution, 4% salicylic acid	In 120 mL.

Antiseborrheic Combinations

ANTISEBORRHEIC SHAMPOOS

otc	**X•Seb T Plus** (Ivax)	**Shampoo; topical:** 10% coal tar solution, 0.4% salicylic acid, EDTA	In 118 and 236 mL.
otc	**Ionil T** (Owen/Galderma)	**Shampoo; topical:** Coal tar solution, salicylic acid, benzalkonium chloride	In 120 and 240 mL, pt and qt.
otc	**Sebaquin** (Summers)	**Shampoo; topical:** 3% iodoquinol, lanolin	In 120 mL.
otc	**X•Seb Plus** (Baker Cummins)	**Shampoo; topical:** 1% pyrithione zinc and 2% salicylic acid	In 120 mL.
Rx	**Xolegel Duo** (Barrier)	**Shampoo; topical:** 1% pyrithione zinc and **Gel; topical:** 2% ketoconazole	**Shampoo:** Cetyl alcohol, benzyl alcohol. In 120 mL. **Gel:** 34% dehydrated alcohol. In 15 g.

Complete prescribing information begins in the Antiseborrheic Combinations introduction.

ANTISEBORRHEIC COMBINATION PRODUCTS

Rx	**Xolegel CorePak** (Barrier Therapeutics)	**Gel; topical: Xolegel:** Ketoconazole 2%, alcohol 34%, glycerin **Xebcort:** Hydrocortisone 1%, castor oil, menthol, SD alcohol 40-B 20%	**Xolegel** in 45 g. **Xebcort** in 22.7 g.

Complete prescribing information begins in the Antiseborrheic Combinations introduction.

MEDICATED HAIR DRESSINGS

Rx	**Sal-Oil-T** (Syosset)	**Solution:** 10% crude coal tar, 6% salicylic acid, vegetable oil	In 59.14 mL
otc	**P & S** (Baker Cummins)	**Liquid:** Phenol, mineral oil and glycerin	In 120 and 240 mL

Complete prescribing information begins in the Antiseborrheic Combinations introduction.

TAR-CONTAINING PREPARATIONS

TAR-CONTAINING PRODUCTS

otc	**Medotar** (Medco)	**Ointment; topical:** 1% coal tar	Octoxynol-5, zinc oxide, white petrolatum. In 454 g.
otc	**Taraphilic** (Medco)	**Ointment; topical:** 1% coal tar distillate	Stearyl alcohol, petrolatum, parabens. In 454 g.
otc	**MG217 Medicated Tar** (Triton)	**Ointment; topical:** 10% coal tar solution USP (equivalent to 2% coal tar)	Petrolatum, cetyl alcohol. In 107 g.
otc	**Fototar** (ICN Pharm)	**Cream; topical:** coal tar extract (equivalent to 2% coal tar)	Emollient moisturizing base. In 85 and 454 g.
otc	**MG217 Medicated Tar Lotion** (Triton)	**Lotion; topical:** 5% coal tar solution (equivalent to 1% coal tar)	Moisturizing base. Cetyl alcohol, mineral oil. In 120 mL.
otc	**Oxipor VHC** (Medtech)	**Lotion; topical:** 25% coal tar solution (equivalent to 5% coal tar)	79% alcohol. In 56 mL.
otc	**Psorent** (NeoStrata)	**Solution; topical:** 15% coal tar solution (equivalent to 2.3% coal tar)	In 100 mL.
otc	**Balnetar** (Westwood Squibb)	**Liquid; topical:** 2.5% coal tar	Bath preparation. Lanolin oil, mineral oil. In 221 mL.
otc	**Cutar Emulsion** (Summers)	**Liquid; topical:** 7.5% LCD (1.5% coal tar)	Bath preparation. Lanolin alcohols extract, mineral oil, parabens. In 177 mL and 1 gal.
otc	**Grandpa's Wonder Pine Tar Conditioner** (Grandpa Brands)	**Liquid; topical:** Pine tar oil	Cetearyl alcohol, glyceryl, sunflower seed oil. In 237 mL.
otc	**DHS Tar** (Person & Covey)	**Shampoo; topical:** 0.5% coal tar	**Liquid:** In 120, 240 & 480 mL. **Gel:** In 240 g.
otc	**Tera-Gel** (Geritrex)		EDTA, parabens. In 114 mL.
otc	**PC-Tar** (Geritrex)	**Shampoo; topical:** 1% coal tar	EDTA. In 180 mL.
otc	**Zetar** (Dermik)		In 177 mL.
otc	**Doak Tar** (Doak)	**Shampoo; topical:** 1.2% coal tar	Isopropyl alcohol. In 237 mL.
otc	**Ionil T Plus** (Healthpoint)	**Shampoo; topical:** 2% coal tar	In 120 and 240 mL.
otc	**Neutrogena T/Gel Original** (Neutrogena Corp.)	**Shampoo; topical:** 2% coal tar extract	In 132, 255, 480 mL.
otc	**Pentrax** (Medicis)	**Shampoo; topical:** 5% coal tar	In 236 mL.
otc	**MG 217 Medicated Tar** (Triton)	**Shampoo; topical:** 15% coal tar solution (3% coal tar)	In 120 and 240 mL.
otc	**Polytar** (GlaxoSmithKline)	**Shampoo; topical:** 4.5% polytar (coal tar solution, solubilized crude coal tar equivalent to 0.5% coal tar)	Lanolin. In 177 and 355 mL.
otc	**Polytar** (GlaxoSmithKline)	**Soap; topical:** 2.5% coal tar solution (equivalent to 0.5% coal tar)	Glycerin, ethyl alcohol, peanut oil. In 113 g.
otc	**Doak Tar Oil** (Doak)	**Oil; topical:** 2% doak tar distillate (equivalent to 0.8% coal tar)	Bath preparation. Mineral oil. In 237 mL.

TAR DERIVATIVES, SHAMPOOS — TOPICAL

Indications

➤*Itchy conditions of the body and scalp:* For treatment of scalp psoriasis, seborrheic dermatitis, dandruff, cradle cap, and other oily, itchy conditions of the body and scalp.

Administration and Dosage

➤*Adults:*

Itchy conditions of the body and scalp – Refer to specific product labeling. Rub shampoo liberally into wet hair and scalp. Leave on for several minutes. Rinse thoroughly. Repeat and rinse. Depending on product, use from once daily to at least twice a week or as directed by a health care provider. For severe scalp problems, use daily.

➤*Children:*

2 years of age and older – See Adults for dosing.

Actions

➤*Pharmacology:* Tar derivatives have antiseptic, antibacterial, and antiseborrheic properties and loosen and soften scales and crusts.

Contraindications

Acute inflammation; open or infected lesions.

TAR DERIVATIVES, SHAMPOOS — TOPICAL

Warnings/Precautions

➤*For external use only:* Avoid contact with eyes. If contact occurs, rinse eyes thoroughly with water. Do not use in or around the rectum or in the genital or groin area.

➤*Irritation:* Discontinue if irritation develops and contact a physician. In rare instances, temporary discoloration of blond, bleached, or tinted hair may occur.

➤*If condition worsens or does not improve:* After regular use as directed, if excessive dryness or any undesirable effect occurs, discontinue use and contact physician.

➤*Other treatment:* Do not use this product with other forms of psoriasis therapy, such as ultraviolet radiation or prescription drugs, unless directed to do so by a physician.

➤*Photosensitivity:* Use caution in exposing skin to sunlight after application. It may increase sunburn for up to 24 hours after application.

➤*Pregnancy: Category: Undetermined.* Consult a health care provider before using in pregnant women.

➤*Lactation:* Consult a health care provider before using in breast-feeding women.

➤*Children:* Use on children less than 2 years of age only as directed by a physician.

Adverse Reactions

Minor dermatologic side effects include rash or burning sensation. Photosensitivity may occur. May discolor skin.

Patient Information

For external use only. Avoid contact with the eyes.

Use caution in the sunlight after applying; it may increase the tendency to sunburn up to 24 hours after application.

Do not use for prolonged periods without consulting physician.

If condition covers a large part of the body, consult a physician before using.

TAR-CONTAINING BATH PREPARATIONS — TOPICAL

Indications

➤*Pruritic dermatoses:* These products contain tar derivatives, which have keratoplastic, antieczematous, and antipruritic effects. They are used as adjuncts in a wide range of pruritic dermatoses including psoriasis and seborrheic dermatitis.

Administration and Dosage

➤*Adults:*

Pruritic dermatoses – Add to bath water. Soak 10 to 20 minutes and then pat dry.

Contraindications

Hypersensitivity to any ingredient of the product.

Warnings/Precautions

➤*For external use only:* Avoid contact with the eyes. If contact occurs, rinse with water and contact physician.

➤*Use caution:* To avoid slipping in the bathtub.

➤*Staining:* May occur on plastic or fiberglass tubs.

➤*Irritation:* If irritation persists, discontinue use. Coal tar may cause allergic irritation.

➤*Application considerations:* Do not apply to acutely inflamed or broken skin or to the genital or rectal areas.

➤*Photosensitivity:* Coal tar is photosensitizing; for 24 hours after use, avoid exposure to direct sunlight or sunlamps.

➤*Pregnancy: Category: Undetermined.* Consult a health care provider before using in pregnant women.

➤*Lactation:* Consult a health care provider before using in breast-feeding women.

Adverse Reactions

Dermatitis; allergic sensitization; folliculitis; photosensitization (see Precautions).

Patient Information

Discontinue use and consult with physician if condition worsens or does not improve after regular use, covers a large area of the body, or causes irritation or allergic reaction.

Discontinue use and consult with physician if used for a prolonged period of time.

TAR-CONTAINING PRODUCTS, MISCELLANEOUS — TOPICAL

Indications

➤*Psoriasis / Seborrheic dermatitis:* For the relief and control of itching, irritation, and skin flaking associated with psoriasis and seborrheic dermatitis.

Administration and Dosage

➤*Adults:*

Psoriasis – Refer to specific product labeling. Depending on product, use from 1 to 4 times/day.

Seborrheic dermatitis – Refer to specific product labeling. Depending on product, use from 1 to 4 times/day.

Contraindications

Hypersensitivity to any ingredient in the product.

Warnings/Precautions

➤*For external use only:* Avoid contact with the eyes. If contact occurs, rinse eyes thoroughly with water and contact physician.

➤*Application considerations:* Do not apply preparations to acutely inflamed or broken skin or to the genital or rectal areas except on the advice of a physician.

➤*Discoloration / Staining:* Staining of clothing may occur which is normally removed by standard laundry methods. Use on the scalp may cause temporary staining of light colored hair.

➤*Other treatment:* Do not use with other forms of psoriasis therapy (eg, ultraviolet radiation, drug therapy) unless directed to do so by a physician.

➤*Flammable:* Some coal tar products are extremely flammable. Keep away from fire and flame.

➤*Photosensitivity:* Avoid exposure to sunlight for up to 24 hours as it may increase tendency to sunburn. Do not use on patients who have a disease characterized by photosensitivity (eg, lupus erythematosus, sunlight allergy).

➤*Pregnancy: Category: Undetermined.* Consult a health care provider before using in pregnant women.

➤*Lactation:* Consult a health care provider before using in breast-feeding women.

Patient Information

Do not use for prolonged periods without consulting physician.

If condition worsens or does not improve after regular use, consult physician.

If condition covers a large part of the body, consult physician before using.

ARNICA

ARNICA

otc	**Arnica** (Various, eg, Humco)	**Tincture:** 20%	In 30, 60, 120 mL, pt, gal.

ARNICA — TOPICAL

Indications

➤*Pain:* Relief of pain from sprains and bruises; of doubtful value.

Administration and Dosage

➤*Adults:*

Pain – Apply locally with massage 2 or 3 times daily.

➤*Administration:* For external use only. Avoid getting into eyes or mucous membranes.

Do not apply to irritated skin or if excessive irritation develops.

Warnings/Precautions

➤*For external use only:* Avoid getting into eyes or mucous membranes.

➤*Irritation:* Do not apply to irritated skin or if excessive irritation develops.

➤*Pregnancy: Category: Undetermined.* Uterine stimulant action has been documented. Avoid use.

➤*Lactation:* No data are available for the use of arnica in breast-feeding women.

Adverse Reactions

Arnica is an irritant to mucous membranes; when ingested, it has produced severe gastroenteritis, nervous disturbances, tachycardia, bradycardia and collapse.

Arnica may cause dermatitis in sensitive persons.

ALUMINUM ACETATE SOLUTION (Burow's or Modified Burow's Solution)

otc	**Buro-Sol** (Doak)	**Powder**: 0.23% aluminum acetate	In 12 packets.
otc	**Burow's Solution** (Various, eg, Paddock)	Aluminum acetate solution	In 480 mL.
otc	**Domeboro Powder and Tablets** (Miles)	Aluminum sulfate and calcium acetate. One packet or tablet in a pint of water produces a modified 1:40 Burow's solution. Apply every 15 to 30 minutes for 4 to 8 hours.	**Effervescent tablets**: In 12s and 100s. **Powder packets**: In 12s and 100s.
otc	**Bite Rx** (International Lab. Tech. Corp.)[a]	**Solution**: 0.5% w/w aluminum acetate	Benzalkonium chloride. In 120 mL.

[a] (954) 893-1118

ALUMINUM ACETATE SOLUTION (Burow's or Modified Burow's Solution) — TOPICAL

Indications

➤*Inflammatory conditions of the skin:* An astringent wet dressing for relief of inflammatory conditions of the skin, such as insect bites, poison ivy, swelling, allergy, bruises and athlete's foot.

Administration and Dosage

➤*Adults:*

Inflammatory skin conditions –

Compress/wet dressing: Saturate the cloth in the solution every 15 to 30 minutes and apply to affected area. Repeat as often as necessary.

Soak: Soak affected area in the solution for 15 to 30 minutes. Repeat 3 times a day as needed.

➤*Preparation for administration:* Dissolve 1 to 3 packets in 473 mL (16 oz) of water or 1 or 2 tablets in 355 mL (12 oz) of water and stir until fully dissolved. One *Domeboro* tablet dissolved in 355 mL of water produces a modified 1:40 Burow's solution.

For use as a compress or wet dressing, saturate a clean, soft cloth in the solution; gently squeeze.

➤*Administration:* For use as a compress or wet dressing, apply saturated cloth loosely to the affected area. Saturate the cloth in the solution every 15 to 30 minutes and reapply. Do not cover compress or wet dressing with plastic to prevent evaporation.

For use as a soak, soak the affected area in the solution for 15 to 30 minutes. Repeat 3 times a day as needed.

Discard solution after each use.

➤*Storage/Stability:* The unused portion of the solution may be stored at room temperature in a clean, capped container for up to 7 days.

Warnings/Precautions

➤*Discontinue use:* If intolerance, irritation or extension of inflammatory condition being treated occurs. If symptoms persist more than 7 days, discontinue use and consult physician.

➤*Do not use plastic:* Do not use plastic nor any other impervious material to prevent evaporation.

➤*For external use only:* Avoid contact with the eyes.

➤*Pregnancy: Category: Undetermined.* If pregnant, ask a health care provider before use.

➤*Lactation:* If breast-feeding, ask a health care provider before use.

Drug Interactions

➤*Collagenase:* The enzyme activity of topical collagenase may be inhibited by aluminum acetate solution because of the metal ion and low pH. Cleanse the site of the solution with repeated washings of normal saline before applying the enzyme ointment.

HAMAMELIS WATER (Witch Hazel)

otc	**Witch Hazel** (Various, eg, Humco, Lannett)	**Liquid**	In 120 and 240 mL, pt and gal.
otc	**A•E•R** (Birchwood)	**Pads**: 50%. 12.5% glycerin, methylparaben, benzalkonium chloride	In 40s.

HAMAMELIS WATER — TOPICAL

Indications

➤*Anal/Vaginal irritation:* Temporary relief of anal or vaginal irritation and itching, hemorrhoids, postepisiotomy discomfort, and hemorrhoidectomy discomfort.

Administration and Dosage

➤*Adults:*

Anal/Vaginal irritation – Apply to the affected area up to 6 times daily or after each bowel movement. For vaginal care, cleanse the area by gently wiping, patting, or blotting. Repeat as needed.

➤*Children:*

12 years of age and older – See Adults for dosing.

➤*Administration:* Gently apply to the affected area by patting and then discard. For external use only.

When practical, cleanse the affected area with mild soap and warm water and rinse thoroughly. Gently dry by patting or blotting with toilet tissue or soft cloth before each application of hamamelis water.

➤*Storage/Stability:* Store at 15° to 30°C (59° to 86°F).

Actions

➤*Pharmacology:* Hamamelis water is a mild astringent prepared from twigs of *Hamamelis virginiana*; the distillate is then adjusted with an appropriate amount of alcohol.

Warnings/Precautions

➤*Worsened conditions:* If condition worsens or does not improve within 7 days, consult a physician.

➤*Bleeding:* In case of bleeding, consult a physician promptly.

➤*For external use only:* For external use only. Avoid contact with eyes.

➤*Pregnancy: Category: Undetermined.*

Consult a health care provider before using in pregnant patients.

➤*Lactation:* Consult a health care provider before using in breast-feeding patients.

Patient Information

Consult a doctor if condition worsens or does not improve within 7 days, in case of bleeding, or before exceeding the recommended dosage.

Do not put this product into the rectum using fingers or any mechanical device or applicator.

Keep out of the reach of children. If swallowed, get medical help or contact a poison control center right away.

CAPSAICIN

otc	**Capsin** (Fleming)	**Lotion; topical:** 0.025%	Benzyl alcohol, propylene glycol, denatured alcohol. In 59 mL.
		0.075%	Benzyl alcohol, propylene glycol, denatured alcohol. In 59 mL.
otc	**Capsaicin** (Various, eg, Alpharma, Ivax)	**Cream; topical:** 0.025%	In 45 and 60 g.
otc	**Pain Doctor** (Fougera)		Methyl salicylate 25%, menthol 10%, propylene glycol, parabens. In 60 g.
otc	**Zostrix** (Health Care Products)		In an emollient base. Benzyl alcohol, cetyl alcohol, PEG-100. In 45 and 90 g.
otc	**Capzasin-P** (Chattem)	**Cream; topical:** 0.035%	Alcohols, petrolatum. In 42.5 g.
otc	**Capsaicin** (Various, eg, Alpharma, Ferndale, Ivax)	**Cream; topical:** 0.075%	In 60 g.
otc	**Rid•a•Pain•HP** (Pfeiffer)		Alcohols, parabens. In 45 g.
otc	**Zostrix Maximum Strength** (Health Care Products)		Benzyl alcohol, cetyl alcohol, glyceryl, PEG-100, white petrolatum. In 56.6 g with 25 applicator pads.
otc	**Zostrix Diabetic Foot Pain** (Health Care Products)		Benzyl alcohol, cetyl alcohol, glyceryl, PEG-100, white petrolatum. In 56.6 g with 25 applicator pads.
otc	**Zostrix-HP** (Health Care Products)		In an emollient base. Benzyl alcohol, cetyl alcohol, PEG-100. In 30 and 60 g.
otc	**Capzasin-HP** (Chattem)	**Cream; topical:** 0.1%	Alcohols, petrolatum. In 42.5 g.
otc	**Axsain** (Rodlen Labs)	**Cream; topical:** 0.25%	In an emollient base. Lidocaine, benzyl alcohol, cetyl alcohol, white petrolatum. In 60 g.
otc	**No Pain-HP** (Young Again Products)	**Roll-on; topical:** 0.075%	In 60 mL.
otc	**Icy Hot PM** (Chattem)	**Patch; topical:** 0.025%	Menthol 5%, benzyl alcohol, disodium EDTA. In 6s.
Rx	**Qutenza** (NeurogesX[a])	**Patch; topical:** 8%	In single-use patches with cleansing gel.

[a] NeurogesX, Inc, 2215 Bridgepointe Parkway, Suite 200, San Mateo, CA 94404; 650-358-3300 (phone); 650-649-1798 (fax).

CAPSAICIN — TOPICAL

Indications

➤*OTC:*

Muscle/Joint pain – For the temporary relief of minor aches and pains of muscles and joints associated with backache, strains, sprains, arthritis, rheumatoid arthritis, and osteoarthritis. For use in treating neuralgias, consult a health care provider.

➤*Rx:*

Neuropathic pain – For the management of neuropathic pain associated with postherpetic neuralgia.

➤*Off-label uses:* Capsaicin is being investigated for use in other disorders, including psoriasis, vitiligo, and intractable pruritus, as well as postmastectomy and postamputation neuroma (phantom limb syndrome), vulvar vestibulitis, apocrine chromhidrosis, and reflex sympathetic dystrophy.

Administration and Dosage

➤*General dosing considerations:*

OTC – A burning sensation may occur upon application, but generally disappears with regular use.

Rx – Only physicians, or health care providers under the close supervision of physicians, are to administer capsaicin.

Use only nitrile gloves when handling capsaicin (see Preparation for administration).

➤*Adults:*

OTC –

Muscle/Joint pain: Apply a thin film of capsaicin to affected area 3 to 4 times daily. Application schedules of less than 3 to 4 times a day or for less than 2 weeks may not provide optimum pain relief. Unless treating hands, wash hands thoroughly after each application.

Rx –

Neuropathic pain: Apply a single, 60-minute application of up to 4 patches. May repeat every 3 months or as warranted by the return of pain (not more frequently than every 3 months).

➤*Preparation for administration:*

Rx – Use only nitrile gloves when handling capsaicin and when cleansing capsaicin residue from the skin. Do not use latex gloves because they do not provide adequate protection.

Put on nitrile gloves. Inspect the pouch. Do not use if the pouch has been torn or damaged.

The treatment area (painful area including area of hypersensitivity and allodynia) must be identified by a health care provider and marked on the skin. If necessary, clip hair (do not shave) in and around the identified treatment area to promote patch adherence. Gently wash the treatment area with mild soap and water and dry thoroughly. Use capsaicin only on dry, intact (unbroken) skin.

Pretreat with a topical anesthetic to reduce discomfort associated with the application of capsaicin. Apply topical anesthetic to the entire treatment area and surrounding 1 to 2 cm, and keep the local anesthetic in place until the skin is anesthetized prior to the application of the capsaicin patch. Remove the topical anesthetic with a dry wipe. Gently wash the treatment area with mild soap and water and dry thoroughly.

➤*Administration:*

Rx – Tear open the pouch along the 3 dashed lines and remove the patch. Inspect the capsaicin patch and identify the outer surface backing layer with the printing on one side. The adhesive side of the patch is covered by a clear, unprinted, diagonally cut release liner. Apply the capsaicin patch within 2 hours of opening the pouch. Capsaicin can be cut to match the size and shape of the treatment area. Cut capsaicin before removing the protective release liner. The diagonal cut in the release liner is to aid in its removal. Peel a small section of the release liner back, and place the adhesive side of the patch on the treatment area. While slowly peeling back the release liner from under the patch with one hand, use the other hand to smooth the patch down on to the skin. Once capsaicin is applied, leave in place for 60 minutes. To ensure capsaicin maintains contact with the treatment area, a dressing, such as rolled gauze, may be used. Instruct the patient not to touch the patch or treatment area. Remove capsaicin patches by gently and slowly rolling them inward.

After removal of capsaicin, generously apply cleansing gel to the treatment area and leave on for at least 1 minute. Remove cleansing gel with a dry wipe and gently wash the area with mild soap and water and dry thoroughly.

Inform patients that the treated area may be sensitive to heat for a few days (eg, hot showers/baths, direct sunlight, vigorous exercise).

➤*Storage/Stability:*

OTC – Store at 15° to 30°C (59° to 86°F).

Rx – Store carton between 20° and 25°C (68° and 77°F). Excursions between 15° and 30°C (59° and 86°F) are allowed. Keep the patch in the sealed pouch until immediately before use.

Handling and disposal: The prescription capsaicin patch contains capsaicin capable of producing severe irritation of eyes, skin, respiratory tract, and mucous membranes. Do not dispense the prescription capsaicin patch to patients for self-administration. It is critical that health care providers who administer the prescription capsaicin patch have completely familiarized themselves with proper dosing, handling, and disposal procedures before handling the prescription capsaicin patch to avoid accidental or inadvertent capsaicin exposure to themselves or others.

Do not touch the prescription capsaicin patch, treatment areas, and all supplies or other materials placed in contact with the treatment area without wearing nitrile gloves.

Wear nitrile gloves at all times while handling the prescription capsaicin patch and cleaning treatment areas. Do not use latex gloves.

Do not hold the prescription capsaicin patch near eyes or mucous membranes.

Immediately after use, dispose of used and unused patches, patch clippings, unused cleansing gel, and associated treatment supplies in accordance with local biomedical waste procedures.

Actions

➤*Pharmacology:*

OTC – Capsaicin is a natural chemical derived from plants of the solanaceae family. Although the precise mechanism of action is not fully understood, evidence suggests that the drug renders skin and joints insensitive to pain by depleting and preventing reaccumulation of substance P in peripheral sensory neurons. Substance P is thought to be the principal chemomediator of pain impulses from the periphery to the CNS.

Rx – Capsaicin is an agonist for the transient receptor potential vanilloid 1 receptor (TRPV1), which is an ion channel–receptor complex expressed on

CAPSAICIN — TOPICAL

nociceptive nerve fibers in the skin. Topical administration of capsaicin causes an initial enhanced stimulation of the TRPV1-expressing cutaneous nociceptors that may be associated with painful sensations. This is followed by pain relief thought to be mediated by a reduction in TRPV1-expressing nociceptive nerve endings. Over the course of several months, there may be a gradual re-emergence of painful neuropathy thought to be caused by TRPV1 nerve fiber reinnervation of the treated area.

➤*Pharmacokinetics:*

Absorption –

Rx: Pharmacokinetic data in humans showed transient, low (less than 5 ng/mL) systemic exposure to capsaicin in about one-third of patients with postherpetic neuralgia following 60-minute applications of prescription capsaicin patches. The highest plasma concentration of capsaicin detected was 4.6 ng/mL and occurred immediately after prescription capsaicin patch removal. Most quantifiable levels were observed at the time of prescription capsaicin patch removal and were below the limit of quantitation 3 to 6 hours after prescription capsaicin patch removal. No detectable levels of metabolites were observed in any subject.

Contraindications

None well documented.

Warnings/Precautions

➤*OTC:* OTC capsaicin is for external use only. It should not be applied to wounds or to damaged or irritated skin. It should not be wrapped tightly.

Capsaicin should not come in contact with mucous membranes, eyes, or contact lenses. If this occurs, the affected area should be rinsed thoroughly with water.

This product should be discontinued and a health care provider consulted if condition worsens or does not improve after regular use, if blistering occurs, or if severe burning persists.

Heat should not be applied to the treated area immediately before or after applications, because this may increase the burning sensation.

➤*Rx:*

Eye and mucous membrane exposure – Do not apply prescription capsaicin to the face or scalp to avoid risk of exposure to the eyes or mucous membranes.

Aerosolization – Aerosolization of capsaicin can occur upon rapid removal of prescription capsaicin patches. Therefore, remove capsaicin patches gently and slowly by rolling the adhesive side inward.

If irritation of eyes or airways occurs, remove the affected individual from the vicinity of prescription capsaicin patches. Flush eyes and mucous membranes with cool water.

Inhalation of airborne capsaicin can result in coughing or sneezing. Provide supportive medical care if shortness of breath develops.

Unintended skin exposure – If skin not intended to be treated comes in contact with prescription capsaicin patches, apply cleansing gel for 1 minute and wipe off with dry gauze. After the cleansing gel has been wiped off, wash the area with soap and water.

Application pain – Even following use of a local anesthetic prior to administration of prescription capsaicin patches, patients may experience substantial procedural pain. Prepare to treat acute pain during and following the application procedure with local cooling (such as an ice pack) and/or appropriate analgesic medication (such as opioids). Opioids may affect the ability to perform potentially hazardous activities such as driving or operating machinery.

Hypertension – In clinical trials, increases in blood pressure occurred during or shortly after exposure to prescription capsaicin patches. The changes averaged less than 10 mm Hg, although some patients had greater increases, and these changes lasted for approximately 2 hours after patch removal. Increases in blood pressure were unrelated to the pretreatment blood pressure but were related to treatment-related increases in pain. Monitor blood pressure periodically during treatment and provide adequate support for treatment-related pain.

Patients with unstable or poorly controlled hypertension or a recent history of cardiovascular or cerebrovascular events may be at an increased risk of adverse cardiovascular effects. Consider these factors prior to initiating prescription capsaicin patch treatment.

➤*Hypersensitivity reactions:* If use of this product causes difficulty breathing or swallowing, instruct the patient to consult a health care provider immediately.

➤*Pregnancy: Category C* (OTC); *Category B* (Rx).

There are no adequate and well-controlled studies evaluating prescription capsaicin patches in pregnant women.

➤*Lactation:*

OTC – No data are available on the transfer of OTC capsaicin into human milk. However, topical application to the nipple or areola should be avoided unless it is thoroughly removed prior to breast-feeding.

Rx – There are no adequate and well-controlled studies of prescription capsaicin patches in breast-feeding women. Studies in rats have demonstrated that capsaicin is excreted into breast milk of this species. It is unknown whether capsaicin is excreted in human breast milk. Because prescription capsaicin patches are administered as single 60-minute applications and capsaicin is rapidly cleared from the bloodstream, mothers can reduce infant exposure by not breast-feeding after treatment on the day of treatment.

➤*Children:*

OTC – Consult a health care provider before using in patients younger than 18 years of age.

Rx – The safety and effectiveness of prescription capsaicin patches in patients younger than 18 years of age have not been studied.

➤*Monitoring:*

Rx – Monitor blood pressure periodically during treatment.

Drug Interactions

➤*Angiotensin-converting enzyme inhibitors:* Capsaicin, including topical use, may cause or exacerbate coughing associated with angiotensin-converting enzyme (ACE) inhibitor treatment and vice versa. If a severe cough develops in patients taking an ACE inhibitor and using capsaicin, one or both drugs may need to be discontinued.

Adverse Reactions

➤*OTC:* No systemic adverse reactions have been attributed to OTC capsaicin. A localized burning sensation may be experienced on application. This sensation, typically mild, generally subsides with regular use. Capsaicin should continue to be used consistently as directed, unless the burning sensation becomes too painful to tolerate. Heat and excessive perspiration may intensify the burning sensation; therefore, capsaicin should not be applied immediately before or after activities such as bathing, swimming, sunbathing, or strenuous exercise. Generally, the more capsaicin is used as directed, the more likely it is to obtain maximum relief and minimize the burning sensation. Other adverse reactions include cough, erythema, respiratory tract irritation, and stinging.

➤*Rx:*

Discontinuation – Among patients treated with prescription capsaicin patches, 1% discontinued prematurely because of an adverse reaction.

Common adverse reactions (at least 1%) – The majority of application-site reactions were transient and self-limited. Transient increases in pain were commonly observed on the day of treatment in patients treated with the prescription capsaicin patch. Pain increases occurring during patch application usually began to resolve after patch removal. On average, pain scores returned to baseline by the end of the treatment day and then remained at or below baseline levels. A majority of prescription capsaicin patch–treated patients in clinical studies had adverse reactions with a maximum intensity of mild or moderate.

Capsaicin Adverse Reactions in Postherpetic Neuralgia Patients (≥ 1%)

Adverse reactions	Capsaicin 60 minutes (n = 622)	Control 60 minutes (n = 495)
GI		
Nausea	5%	2%
Vomiting	3%	1%
Local		
Application-site dryness	2%	1%
Application-site edema	4%	1%
Application-site erythema	63%	54%
Application-site pain	42%	21%
Application-site papules	6%	3%
Application-site pruritus	6%	4%
Application-site swelling	2%	1%
Respiratory		
Bronchitis	2%	1%
Nasopharyngitis	4%	2%
Sinusitis	3%	1%
Miscellaneous		
Hypertension	2%	1%
Pruritus	2%	< 1%

Other adverse reactions –

CNS: Burning sensation, dizziness, dysgeusia, headache, hyperesthesia, hypoesthesia, peripheral sensory neuropathy.

Local: Application-site anesthesia, application-site bruising, application-site dermatitis, application-site excoriation, application-site exfoliation, application-site hyperesthesia, application-site inflammation, application-site paresthesia, application-site urticaria, application-site warmth.

Respiratory: Cough, throat irritation.

Miscellaneous: Abnormal skin odor, peripheral edema.

Overdosage

➤*Symptoms:*

Rx – There is no clinical experience with overdose with the prescription capsaicin patch in humans.

➤*Treatment:*

Rx – There is no specific antidote for overdose with capsaicin. In case of suspected overdose, remove patch gently, apply cleansing gel for 1 minute, wipe off with dry gauze, and gently wash the area with soap and water. Use supportive measures and treat symptoms as clinically warranted.

CAPSAICIN — TOPICAL

Patient Information

➤*OTC:* Capsaicin should continue to be used consistently as directed, unless the burning sensation becomes too painful to tolerate.

Heat and excessive perspiration may intensify the burning sensation; therefore, instruct patients that capsaicin should not be applied immediately before or after activities such as bathing, swimming, sunbathing, or strenuous exercise. Generally, the more capsaicin is used as directed, the more likely it is to obtain maximum relief and minimize the burning sensation.

Health care providers prescribe capsaicin for the relief of pain from arthritis and painful neuralgias. For use in painful neuralgias, advise patients to consult a physician.

Regular and frequent application is essential. Proper use of capsaicin is essential for maximum pain relief. Capsaicin must be applied regularly and frequently, as directed, to deplete the supply of substance P in nerve cells and prevent it from building up again. Because it takes time for substance P to be depleted, relief occurs gradually. To achieve optimum pain relief, instruct patients to be sure to apply capsaicin daily as directed. Relief may be delayed or may not occur if cream is applied less often.

Instruct patients to apply capsaicin to the painful area regularly (3 to 4 times a day).

Advise patients not to apply capsaicin to wounds or damaged or irritated skin, not to tightly wrap or bandage the treated area, and not to apply heat to the treated area.

Instruct patients to apply just enough cream to cover the affected area with a thin layer and to gently massage it into the skin until fully absorbed.

Instruct patients to wash their hands thoroughly after use to avoid spreading cream to the eyes, mucous membranes, or other sensitive areas of the body. Because trace amounts of capsaicin may remain on hands even after washing, patients should avoid touching mucous membranes, eyes, or contact lenses after use. If capsaicin gets into the eyes, it will cause a burning sensation, but has not been reported to cause any harm. Eyes should be flushed with water. Exposure of cream to contact lenses should be avoided.

If patients are treating their hands with capsaicin, they should wait 30 minutes after applying before washing hands.

Instruct patients to avoid thick application and to be sure to massage the cream into the skin until no residue remains. Inhaling airborne material from dried residue should be avoided, which can cause coughing, sneezing, tearing, and/or throat or respiratory irritation. If difficulty breathing or swallowing occurs, instruct patients to contact a health care provider.

Advise patients that if the condition worsens or does not improve after 14 to 28 days, the product should be discontinued and they should consult their health care provider.

➤*Rx:* Inform patients that exposure of the skin to the prescription capsaicin patch may result in transient erythema and burning sensation. Instruct patients not to touch the patch and that if they accidentally touch the prescription capsaicin patch it may burn and/or sting.

Instruct patients that if irritation of eyes or airways occurs, or if any of the adverse effects become severe, to notify their health care provider immediately.

Inform patients that the treated area may be sensitive to heat (eg, hot showers/bath, direct sunlight, vigorous exercise) for a few days following treatment.

Inform patients that they may be given medication to treat acute pain during and after the prescription capsaicin patch application procedure. Some of these medications, such as opioids, may affect the ability to perform potentially hazardous activities such as driving or operating machinery.

Inform patients that as a result of treatment-related increases in pain, small transient increases in blood pressure may occur during and shortly after the prescription capsaicin patch treatment and that blood pressure will be monitored during the treatment procedure. Instruct patients to inform their health care provider if they have experienced any recent cardiovascular event.

Instruct patients to notify their health care provider if they are pregnant or breast-feeding.

DESTRUCTIVE AGENTS

Chloroacetic Acids

Indications

➤*Dichloroacetic acid:* Verrucae (warts); calluses; hard and soft corns; xanthoma palpebrarum; seborrheic keratoses; ingrown nails; cysts and benign erosion of the cervix; endocervicitis; epistaxis.

➤*Trichloroacetic acid:* Removal of verrucae.

The CDC recommends trichloroacetic acid as an alternative regimen to cryotherapy for treatment of external genital/perianal warts and vaginal and anal warts.

Actions

➤*Pharmacology:* Rapidly penetrates and cauterizes skin, keratin and other tissues.

Contraindications

Treatment of malignant or premalignant lesions; hypersensitivity to any component.

Warnings/Precautions

➤*Cauterant properties:* These acids are powerful keratolytics and cauterants. Restrict use to areas where these effects are desired. May cause severe burning, inflammation or tenderness of skin.

➤*Cervical lesions:* A careful diagnosis and possibly a biopsy is required to rule out malignancy; treatment is contraindicated in the event of positive findings.

➤*Normal tissue:* Apply only to the lesion being treated. To prevent acid from spreading onto normal skin, apply petrolatum around the area to be treated. If any acid is spilled on normal tissue or if too much acid is applied, remove immediately and wash with water. Sodium bicarbonate may be applied as a local antidote.

MONOCHLOROACETIC ACID

Rx	**Monocete EZ Swabs** (Pedinol)	**Swab; topical:** 80%	PEG 200. In 15s.
Rx	**Mono-Chlor** (Gordon)	**Liquid; topical:** 80%	In 15 mL.

MONOCHLOROACETIC ACID — TOPICAL

For Monochloroacetic Acid prescribing information, see the Chloroacetic Acids group monograph.

Administration and Dosage

Remove callus tissue. Apply to verruca. Apply bandage and allow to remain in place for 5 to 6 days. Remove verruca tissue and reapply as needed. If crystallization of liquid occurs, place capped bottle in hot water to redissolve.

TRICHLOROACETIC ACID

Rx	**Tri-Chlor** (Gordon)	**Liquid:** 80%	In 15 mL.

TRICHLOROACETIC ACID — TOPICAL

Complete prescribing information begins in the Chloroacetic Acids group monograph.

Indications

➤*Condylomata:* To aid in the elimination of condylomata.

The Centers for Disease Control (CDC) recommends trichloroacetic acid as an alternative regimen to cryotherapy for treatment of external genital/perianal warts and vaginal and anal warts.

Administration and Dosage

➤*General dosing considerations:* Debride callous tissue.

➤*Adults:*

Condylomata – Apply to condyloma and cover with suitable dressing for 5 to 6 days. Reapply as needed.

➤*Administration:* For external use only.

If crystallization of liquid occurs, place capped bottle in hot water to redissolve.

Apply only to the lesion being treated. To prevent acid from spreading onto normal skin, apply petrolatum around the area to be treated.

PODOFILOX

Rx	**Condylox** (Watson)	**Gel; topical:** 0.5% podofilox	Alcohol. In 3.5 mL aluminum tubes.
Rx	**Podofilox** (Various, eg, Paddock, Watson)	**Solution; topical:** 0.5% podofilox	95% alcohol. In 3.5 mL.
Rx	**Condylox** (Watson)		Alcohol. In 3.5 mL bottles.

PODOFILOX — TOPICAL

Indications

➤*Warts:* Podofilox gel is indicated for the topical treatment of anogenital warts (external genital warts [condyloma acuminatum]) and perianal warts. It is not indicated for the treatment of mucous membrane warts (see Precautions).

Podofilox topical solution is indicated for the topical treatment of anogenital warts (external genital warts [condyloma acuminatum]). It is not indicated for the treatment of perianal warts or for the treatment of mucous membrane warts (see Precautions).

Administration and Dosage

➤*Adults:*

Genital warts –

Usual dosage: Apply twice daily every 12 hours (eg, morning and evening) for 3 consecutive days, then withhold use for 4 consecutive days.

Maximum dose:

- *Gel* – 0.5 g per day for a maximum of 4 treatment cycles.
- *Solution* – 0.5 mL per day for a maximum of 4 treatment cycles.

Duration of therapy: This 1-week cycle of treatment may be repeated until there is no visible wart tissue for a maximum of 4 cycles.

Discontinuation of therapy: If there is incomplete response after 4 treatment cycles, discontinue treatment and consider alternative treatment.

➤*Preparation for administration:* Podofilox is considered a cytotoxic agent and is also a potential mutagen and potential teratogen. Follow safe handling procedures when preparing, administering, or dispensing podofilox.

➤*Administration:* In order to ensure that the patient is fully aware of the correct method of therapy and to identify which specific warts should be treated, the technique for initial application of the medication should be demonstrated by the prescriber.

Gel – Podofilox gel should be applied to the warts with the applicator tip or finger. Application on the surrounding normal tissue should be minimized. Treatment should be limited to 10 cm^2 or less of wart tissue and to no more than 0.5 g of the gel/day.

Care should be taken to allow the gel to dry before allowing the return of opposing skin surfaces to their normal positions. Patients should be instructed to wash their hands thoroughly before and after each application.

Topical solution – Podofilox solution is applied to the warts with a cotton-tipped applicator supplied with the drug. The drug-dampened applicator should be touched to the wart to be treated, applying the minimum amount of solution necessary to cover the lesion. Treatment should be limited to less than 10 cm^2 of wart tissue, and to no more than 0.5 mL of the solution/day.

Care should be taken to allow the solution to dry before allowing the return of opposing skin surfaces to their normal positions. After each treatment, the used applicator should be carefully disposed of and the patient should wash his or her hands.

➤*Storage/Stability:* Store at controlled room temperature between 15° to 30°C (59° to 86°F). Avoid excessive heat. Do not freeze.

Actions

➤*Pharmacology:* Treatment of genital warts with podofilox results in necrosis of visible wart tissue. The exact mechanism of action is unknown.

➤*Pharmacokinetics:*

Absorption/Distribution – In systemic absorption studies in 52 patients, topical application of 0.05 mL of an ethanolic solution containing 0.5% podofilox to external genitalia did not result in detectable serum levels. Applications of 0.1 to 1.5 mL resulted in peak serum levels of 1 to 17 ng/mL 1 to 2 hours after application.

Excretion – The elimination half-life ranged from 1 to 4.5 hours. The drug was not found to accumulate after multiple treatments.

Contraindications

Hypersensitivity or intolerance to any components of the formulation.

Warnings/Precautions

➤*Cutaneous use only:* Avoid contact with the eyes. If contact with the eyes occurs, patients should immediately flush the eyes with copious quantities of water and seek medical advice.

➤*Flammable:* Drug product is flammable. Keep away from open flame.

➤*Mucous membrane warts:* Data is not available on the safe and effective use of this product for treatment of warts occurring on mucous membranes of the genital area (including the urethra, rectum and vagina). The recommended method of application, frequency of application, and duration of usage should not be exceeded (see Administration and Dosage).

➤*Pregnancy: Category C.* Podofilox was not teratogenic in the rabbit following topical application of up to 0.21/mg/kg (5 times the maximum human dose) once daily for 13 days. The scientific literature contains references that podofilox solution is embryotoxic in rats when administered systemically in a dose ≈ 250 times the recommended maximum human dose.

Teratogenicity and embryotoxicity have not been studied with intravaginal application. Many antimitotic drug products are known to be embryotoxic. There are no adequate and well-controlled studies in pregnant women. Podofilox should be used during pregnancy only if the potential benefit justifies the potential risk to the fetus.

➤*Lactation:* It is not known whether this drug is excreted in human milk. Because of the potential for serious adverse reactions in nursing infants from podofilox, a decision should be made whether to discontinue nursing or to discontinue the drug, taking into account the importance of the drug to the mother.

➤*Children:* Safety and efficacy in pediatric patients have not been established.

Adverse Reactions

➤*Gel:* In clinical trials with podofilox 0.5%, the local adverse reactions listed below were reported during the treatment of anogenital warts. The severity of local adverse reactions were predominantly mild or moderate and did not increase during the treatment period. Severe reactions were most frequent within the first 2 weeks of treatment.

Podofilox Gel Adverse Reactions

Adverse reaction	Mild	Moderate	Severe
Bleeding	19.2%	3%	0.7%
Burning	37.1%	25.9%	11.5%
Erosion	27%	20.8%	8.9%
Inflammation	32.2%	30.4%	9.3%
Itching	32.2%	16%	7.8%
Pain	23.7%	20.4%	11.5%

Local – Other local adverse reactions reported included stinging (7%), and erythema (5%); less commonly reported local adverse events included desquamation, scabbing, discoloration, tenderness, dryness, crusting, fissures, soreness, ulceration, swelling/edema, tingling, rash, and blisters.

Miscellaneous – The most common systemic adverse event reported during the clinical studies was headache (7%).

➤*Topical solution:* In clinical trials, the following local adverse reactions were reported at some point during treatment. Reports of burning and pain were more frequent and of greater severity in women and than in men.

Podofilox Topical Solution Adverse Reactions

Adverse reaction	Males	Females
Burning	64%	78%
Erosion	67%	67%
Inflammation	71%	63%
Itching	50%	65%
Pain	50%	72%

Adverse effects reported in less than 5% of the patients included pain with intercourse, insomnia, tingling, bleeding, tenderness, chafing, malodor, dizziness, scarring, vesicle formation, crusting edema, dryness/peeling, foreskin irretraction, hematuria, vomiting and ulceration.

Overdosage

➤*Symptoms:* Topically applied podofilox may be absorbed systemically (see Pharmacokinetics). Toxicity reported following systemic administration of podofilox in investigational use for cancer treatment included nausea, vomiting, fever, diarrhea, bone marrow depression, and oral ulcers. Following 5 to 10 daily IV doses of 0.5 to 1 mg/kg/day, significant hematological toxicity occurred but was reversible. Other toxicities occurred at lower doses. Toxicity reported following systemic administration of podophyllum resin included nausea, vomiting, fever, diarrhea, peripheral neuropathy, altered mental status, lethargy, coma, tachypnea, respiratory failure, leukocytosis, pancytosis, hematuria, renal failure and seizures.

➤*Treatment:* Treatment of topical overdosage should include washing the skin free of any remaining drug and symptomatic and supportive therapy.

Patient Information

Only use this medication as directed by the health care provider. Instruct patients to wash their hands thoroughly before and after each application. It is for external use only. Avoid contact with the eyes. Advise patients not to use this medication for any disorder other than that for which it was prescribed. Patients should report any signs of adverse reactions to the health care provider. If no improvement is observed after 4 weeks of treatment, discontinue the medication and consult the health care provider.

PODOPHYLLUM RESIN (Podophyllin)

Rx	**Podocon-25** (Paddock)	**Liquid:** 25% podophyllum resin in tincture of benzoin	In 15 mL.
Rx	**Podofin** (Syosset)		In 15 mL.

PODOPHYLLIN — TOPICAL

Indications

➤*Warts:* For the removal of soft genital warts (venereal warts, condylomata acuminata).

Administration and Dosage

➤*General dosing considerations:* Podophyllin is to be applied only by a health care provider. It is not to be dispensed to the patient.

➤*Adults:*

Warts – Thoroughly cleanse affected area. Use supplied applicator to apply podophyllin sparingly to lesion. Allow to dry thoroughly. The first application of podophyllin should be left in contact for only a short time (30 to 40 minutes). After treatment time has elapsed, remove dried podophyllin thoroughly with alcohol or soap and water.

➤*Preparation for administration:* Podophyllum is considered a cytotoxic agent. Follow safe handling procedures when preparing, administering, or dispensing podophyllum.

➤*Administration:* Avoid contact with healthy tissue. Only intact (no bleeding) lesions should be treated. Because podophyllin is a powerful caustic and severe irritant, it is recommended the first application of podophyllin be left in contact for only a short time (30 to 40 minutes) to determine patient's sensitivity. To avoid systemic absorption, time of contact should be minimum time necessary to produce the desired result (1 to 4 hours, depending on condition of lesion and of patient), the health care provider developing his own experience and technique. Large areas or numerous warts should not be treated at once.

➤*Storage/Stability:* Store between 15° and 30°C (59° and 86°F) in tight, light-resistant containers.

Actions

➤*Pharmacology:* Podophyllin resin is a cytotoxic agent that has been used topically in the treatment of genital warts. It arrests mitosis in metaphase, an effect it shares with other cytotoxic agents such as the vinca alkaloids. The active agent is podophyllotoxin, whose concentration varies with the type of podophyllin used; the American source normally containing one-fourth the amount of podophyllotoxin as the Indian source.

Contraindications

In diabetics, patients using steroids, or with poor blood circulation. Do not use podophyllin on bleeding warts, moles, birthmarks or unusual warts with hair growing from them. It is recommended that podophyllin not be used during pregnancy (see Warnings).

Warnings/Precautions

➤*For external use only:* Podophyllin is a powerful caustic and severe irritant. Keep away from the eyes; if eye contact occurs, flush with copious amounts of warm water and consult physician or poison control center immediately for advice.

➤*Irritation/Inflammation:* Do not use podophyllin if wart or surrounding tissue is inflamed or irritated.

➤*Pregnancy: Category C* (per Briggs' *Drugs in Pregnancy and Lactation*). There have been reports of complications associated with the topical use of podophyllin on condylomata of pregnant patients including birth defects, fetal death and stillbirth. In the absence of controlled safety studies, podophyllin remains contraindicated for use on pregnant patients.

➤*Lactation:* It is not known whether podophyllin is excreted in human milk following topical application. In the absence of controlled safety studies, podophyllin remains contraindicated for use on nursing patients.

Adverse Reactions

The use of topical podophyllin has been known to result in paresthesia, polyneuritis, paralytic ileus, pyrexia, leukopenia, thrombocytopenia, coma, and death.

DIAPER RASH PRODUCTS

METHIONINE

Rx[a]	**Methionine** (Various, eg, Mason, Tyson & Assoc.)	**Tablets:** 500 mg	In 30s and 60s.
Rx	**M-Caps** (Pal-Pak)	**Capsules:** 200 mg	In 1000s.
Rx	**Uracid** (Wesley)		In 1000s.
Rx	**Methionine** (Tyson & Assoc.)	**Capsules:** 500 mg	In 30s.

[a] Products available *otc* or *Rx*, depending on product labeling.

METHIONINE — ORAL

Indications

➤*Dermatological conditions:* Treatment of diaper rash in infants and for control of odor; dermatitis and ulceration caused by ammoniacal urine in incontinent adults.

➤*Dietary supplement:* For use as a dietary supplement.

Administration and Dosage

➤*Adults:*

Control of odor in adults with incontinence – 200 to 500 mg, 3 or 4 times daily after meal.

Dietary supplement – 500 mg daily. The recommended daily allowance has not been established.

➤*Administration:* Take with food, milk, or other liquid.

Actions

➤*Pharmacology:* The acid-producing effect of methionine on urine pH creates an ammonia free urine.

Contraindications

A history of liver disease; large doses of methionine may exaggerate the toxemia of the disease.

Warnings/Precautions

➤*Protein intake:* Excessive methionine added alone to the diet over extended periods may result in a less than normal weight gain in infants when protein intake is insufficient. Maintain adequate protein intake during therapy and do not exceed the recommended dosage.

➤*Pregnancy: Category: Undetermined.* There is no information regarding methionine in pregnant women.

➤*Lactation:* There is no information regarding methionine in breast-feeding women.

Patient Information

Take with food, milk or other liquid.

DIAPER RASH PRODUCTS

otc	**Paladin** (Pal Midwest Ltd[a])	**Ointment; topical:** Petrolatum, starch, lanolin, zinc oxide, mineral oil, boric acid, bees wax, vitamin A and D concentrate	In 2 oz.
otc	**Diaper Rash** (Various, eg, Goldline)	**Ointment; topical:** Zinc oxide, cod liver oil, lanolin, methylparaben, petrolatum, talc	In 113 g.
otc	**Desitin Clear** (Pfizer)	**Ointment; topical:** 60.4% white petrolatum, cocoa butter, light mineral oil, mineral oil, modified lanolin, sunflower seed oil, vitamin A, vitamin E	In 50 g and 99 g.
otc	**Benson's Bottom Paint** (Benson's Bottom Paint)	**Ointment; topical:** Cetyl alcohol, emulsifying wax, glycerin, paraffin, petrolatum, stearyl alcohol, triethanolamine, zinc oxide	In 56.7 g.
otc	**Vitamin A & Vitamin D** (Geritrex)	**Ointment; topical:** Vitamin A and vitamin D in a base of lanolin, white petrolatum, paraffin	In 410 g.
otc	**Desitin** (Leeming)	**Ointment; topical:** 40% zinc oxide, cod liver oil, talc, petrolatum, lanolin, methylparaben	In 30, 60, 120, 240, and 270 g.
otc	**Diaper Guard** (Del)	**Ointment; topical:** 1% dimethicone, 66% white petrolatum, cocoa butter, parabens, vitamins A, D_3 and E, zinc oxide	In 49.6 and 99.2 g.

DIAPER RASH PRODUCTS

otc	**Diaparene Diaper Rash** (Lehn & Fink)	**Ointment; topical:** Zinc oxide, petrolatum, parabens, imidazolidinyl urea	In 60 g.
otc	**Flanders Buttocks** (Flanders Inc.)	**Ointment; topical:** Zinc oxide, castor oil, balsam peru	In 60 g.
otc	**Desitin Creamy** (Pfizer)	**Ointment; topical:** 10% zinc oxide, mineral oil, white petrolatum, parabens	In 57 g.
otc	**Lansinoh Diaper Rash** (Lansinoh Labs)	**Ointment; topical:** dimethicone 5%, lanolin 15.5%, zinc oxide 5.5%, beeswax, petrolatum	In 90 g.
otc	**A+D Zinc Oxide** (Schering-Plough)	**Cream; topical:** 1% dimethicone, 10% zinc oxide, aloe, beeswax, benzyl alcohol, coconut oil, cod liver oil, light mineral oil, paraffin	In 113 g.
otc	**Soothe & Cool** (Medline[b])	**Cream; topical:** 5% dimethicone, 5% zinc oxide, lanolin, cetyl alcohol, vitamins A, D, and E	In 118 mL.
otc	**Diaparene Baby** (Lehn & Fink)	**Cream; topical:** Mineral oil, petrolatum, aloe, EDTA, diazolidinyl urea, parabens	In 60 g.
otc	**Amerigel** (Amerx Health Care Corp.)	**Lotion; topical:** Glycerin, lemon oil, parabens, oak extract (oakin).	In 228 g.
otc	**Dyprotex** (Blistex)	**Pads; topical:** 40% micronized zinc oxide, 37.6% petrolatum, 2.5% dimethicone, cod liver oil, aloe	In 3 pads (9 applications) and 8 pads (24 applications).
otc	**Caldesene** (Insight)	**Powder; topical:** 81% talc, 15% zinc oxide	In 142 g.
otc	**Diaparene Cornstarch Baby** (Lehn & Fink)	**Powder; topical:** Corn starch, aloe	In 120, 270, and 420 g.
otc	**Mexsana Medicated** (Schering-Plough)	**Powder; topical:** Kaolin, eucalyptus oil, camphor, corn starch, lemon oil, zinc oxide	In 90, 187.5 and 330 g.
otc	**Desitin with Zinc Oxide** (Pfizer)	**Powder; topical:** 88.2% cornstarch, 10% zinc oxide	In 28 and 397 g.
otc	**Gold Bond Medicated Baby Powder** (Chattem)	**Powder; topical:** Talc, zinc oxide	In 113 and 283 g.
otc	**Gold Bond Cornstarch Plus Medicated Baby Powder** (Chattem)	**Powder; topical:** Cornstarch, zinc oxide, kaolin	In 113 and 283 g.
otc	**Gold Bond Triple Action Medicated Baby Powder** (Chattem)	**Powder; topical:** 89% talc, 10% zinc oxide	In 113 and 283 g.

[a] Pal Midwest Ltd, P.O. Box 624, Rockford, IL 61101; (815) 965-2981; fax (815) 332-3366.

[b] Medline Industries, Inc., One Medline Place, Mundelein, IL, 60060-4486; 1-(800)-MEDLINE; fax 1-(800) 351-1512.

DIAPER RASH PRODUCTS — TOPICAL

Indications

➤*Diaper rash/Ammonia dermatitis:* For use in diaper rash or ammonia dermatitis.

Active Ingredients

The principal active components of these formulations include:

➤*EUCALYPTOL:* Antimicrobial agent. Minimizes bacterial proliferation.

➤*ZINC OXIDE:* For drying.

➤*CAMPHOR:* A local anesthetic. Relieves pain, itching and irritation.

➤*BALSAM PERU:* It is claimed to promote wound healing or tissue repair, but effectiveness has not been conclusively demonstrated.

➤*CALCIUM CARBONATE and KAOLIN:* Used for their moisture absorbing abilities.

➤*PROTECTANTS and LUBRICANTS:* To minimize chafing and irritation.

DIAPER RASH COMBINATIONS

Rx	**Vusion** (GlaxoSmithKline)	**Ointment; topical:** 0.25% miconazole nitrate, 15% zinc oxide, and 81.35% white petrolatum	In 30 g tubes.

MICONAZOLE/ZINC OXIDE — TOPICAL

Indications

➤*Diaper dermatitis:* For the adjunctive treatment of diaper dermatitis only when complicated by documented candidiasis (microscopic evidence of pseudohyphae and/or budding yeast) in immunocompetent children 4 weeks of age and older. A positive fungal culture for *Candida albicans* is not adequate evidence of candidal infection since colonization with *C. albicans* can result in a positive culture. Establish the presence of candidal infection by microscopic evaluation prior to initiating treatment.

See Administration and Dosage for more information.

Administration and Dosage

➤*General dosing considerations:* Use ointment as part of a treatment regimen that includes measures directed at the underlying diaper dermatitis, including gentle cleansing of the diaper area and frequent diaper changes.

Do not use ointment as a substitute for frequent diaper changes or to prevent the occurrence of diaper dermatitis because preventative use may result in the development of drug resistance.

➤*Children:*

Diaper dermatitis –

4 weeks of age and older:

• *Usual dosage –* Apply to the affected area at each diaper change for 7 days.

• *Duration of therapy –* Continue treatment for the full 7 days, even if there is improvement.

➤*Preparation for administration:* Before applying the ointment, gently cleanse the skin with lukewarm water and pat dry with a soft towel. Avoid using any scented soaps, shampoos, or lotions on the diaper area.

➤*Administration:* Gently apply a thin layer of ointment to the diaper area with the fingertips. Do not rub into skin because this may cause additional irritation. Thoroughly wash hands after applying the ointment.

➤*Storage/Stability:* Store at controlled room temperature, between 20° and 25°C (68° and 77°F); excursions are permitted between 15° and 30°C (59° and 86°F).

DRYING AGENTS

ALUMINUM CHLORIDE (HEXAHYDRATE)

Rx	**Aluminum Chloride (Hexahydrate)** (Glades)	**Solution:** 20% in 88.5% SD alcohol 40-2	In 37.5 mL bottle and 35 and 60 mL *Dab-O-Matic* applicator bottle.
Rx	**Drysol** (Person & Covey)	**Solution:** 20% in 93% SD alcohol 40	In 37.5 mL or 35 and 60 mL with *Dab-O-Matic* applicator.

ALUMINUM CHLORIDE (HEXAHYDRATE) — TOPICAL

Indications

➤*Hyperhidrosis:* An astringent used as an aid in the management of hyperhidrosis.

Administration and Dosage

➤*Adults:*

Hyperhidrosis – Aluminum chloride should be applied to the affected area once daily, only at bedtime.

➤*Administration:* To help prevent irritation, the area should be completely dry prior to application. Aluminum chloride (hexahydrate) should not be applied to broken, irritated, or recently shaved skin.

Dab-O-Matic bottle – Solution should be applied from the applicator to the affected area.

Plastic bottle – The solution should be applied with fingers or a moistened cotton ball to the affected area.

For maximum effect – The treated area may be covered with plastic wrap held in place by a snug fitting "T" or body shirt, mitten, or sock. Plastic wrap should not be held in place with tape.

Excessive sweating may be stopped after 2 or more treatments. Thereafter, aluminum chloride (hexahydrate) may be applied once or twice a week or as needed.

The treated area should be washed the following morning.

➤*Storage/Stability:* Store between 15° to 30°C (59° to 86°F). Keep cap tightly closed when not in use to prevent evaporation.

Warnings/Precautions

➤*Sensitivity:* If irritation or sensitization occurs, discontinue use or consult with a health care provider.

➤*For external use only:* Avoid contact with eyes.

➤*Pregnancy: Category: Undetermined.* If pregnant, ask a health care provider before use.

➤*Lactation:* If breast-feeding, ask a health care provider before use.

Adverse Reactions

May produce a burning or prickling sensation.

Patient Information

If irritation or sensitization occurs, discontinue use or consult with a physician.

For external use only. Avoid contact with eyes

Aluminum chloride (hexahydrate) may be harmful to certain metals and fabrics.

Do not use near open flame.

FORMALDEHYDE

Rx	**Formalaz** (River's Edge)	**Liquid**: 10%	In 90 mL roll-on plastic bottle.
Rx	**Formalyde-10** (Pedinol)	**Spray**: 10%	SD-40 alcohol. In 60 mL.
Rx	**Lazer Formalyde** (Pedinol)	**Solution**: 10%	In 90 mL.

FORMALDEHYDE — TOPICAL

Indications

➤*Odor/Perspiration of the feet:* Safeguards against offensive odor and dries excessive moisture of feet. Drying agent for pre- and post-surgical removal of warts or for non-surgical laser treatment of warts where dryness is required.

Administration and Dosage

➤*Adults:*

Odor/Perspiration of the feet – Apply once daily to affected areas, or as directed by a podiatrist, dermatologist, or health care provider.

➤*Administration:*

Liquid – Apply with roll-on applicator. Do not shake the bottle with the cap removed. When not in use, keep cap closed tightly.

Spray – Spray on to affected areas. Keep cap closed tightly. Do not shake the bottle.

Solution – Apply with the roll-on applicator. Do not shake the bottle with the cap removed. Keep cap closed tightly.

➤*Storage/Stability:* Store at 15° to 30°C (59° to 86°F).

Contraindications

Sensitivity to any ingredients in formaldehyde spray or solution.

Warnings/Precautions

➤*For external use only:* Harmful if swallowed. Contact a local poison control center immediately. Avoid contact and keep away from face, eyes, nose and mucous membranes.

➤*Hypersensitivity reactions:* Check skin for sensitivity to formaldehyde prior to application since it may be irritating and sensitizing to the skin of some patients. If redness or irritation persists, consult your podiatrist, dermatologist or physician.

➤*Pregnancy: Category X* (per Hale's *Medications and Mothers' Milk*).

➤*Lactation:* Formaldehyde is rapidly destroyed by plasma and tissue enzymes and it is very unlikely that any would enter human milk following environmental exposures. However, acute intoxications following high oral or inhaled doses could lead to significant levels of maternal plasma formic acid which could enter milk. Hale's *Medications in Mothers' Milk* classifies formaldehyde as possibly hazardous.

➤*Children:* Safety and effectiveness in pediatric patients have not been established.

ENZYME PREPARATIONS

COLLAGENASE

Rx	**Collagenase Santyl** (Ross)	**Ointment**: 250 units collagenase enzyme/g.	White petrolatum. In 15 and 30 g.

COLLAGENASE — TOPICAL

Indications

➤*Dermal ulcers:* For debriding chronic dermal ulcers and severely burned areas.

Administration and Dosage

➤*Adults:*

Dermal ulcers – Apply ointment once daily (or more frequently if the dressing becomes soiled, as from incontinence). When clinically indicated, crosshatching thick eschar with a No. 10 blade allows collagenase ointment more surface contact with necrotic debris. It is also more desirable to remove, with forceps and scissors, as much loosened detritus as can be done readily.

➤*Administration:* For external use only. Avoid contact with the eyes.

Instructions for use

1.) Prior to application the wound should be cleansed of debris and digested material by gently rubbing with a gauze pad saturated with normal saline solution, or with the desired cleansing agent compatible with collagenase ointment, followed by a normal saline solution rinse.
2.) Whenever infection is present, it is desirable to use an appropriate topical antibiotic powder. The antibiotic should be applied to the wound prior to the application of collagenase ointment. Should the infection not respond, therapy with collagenase ointment should be discontinued until remission of the infection.
3.) Collagenase ointment may be applied directly to the wound or to a sterile gauze pad, which is then applied to the wound and properly secured.
4.) Use of the collagenase ointment should be terminated when debridement of necrotic tissue is completed and granulation tissue is well established.

➤*Admixture compatibility:*

Incompatibility – The optimal pH range of collagenase is 6 to 8. Higher or lower pH conditions will decrease the enzyme's activity and appropriate precautions should be taken. The enzymatic activity is also adversely affected by certain detergents, and heavy metal ions such as mercury and silver which are used in some antiseptics. When it is suspected such materials have been used, the site should be carefully cleansed by repeated washing with normal saline before collagenase ointment is applied. Soaks containing metal ions or acidic solutions should be avoided because of the metal ion and low pH.

Compatibility – Cleansing materials such as hydrogen peroxide, Dakin solution, and normal saline are compatible with the collagenase ointment.

➤*Storage/Stability:* Do not store above 25°C (77°F). Sterility is guaranteed until the tube is opened. Collagenase ointment is available in 15 g and 30 g tubes.

Actions

➤*Pharmacology:* Since collagen accounts for 75% of the dry weight of skin tissue, the ability of collagenase to digest collagen in the physiological pH

COLLAGENASE — TOPICAL

and temperature range makes it particularly effective in the removal of detritus. Collagenase thus contributes towards the formation of granulation tissue and subsequent epithelization of dermal ulcers and severely burned areas. Collagen in healthy tissue or in newly formed granulation tissue is not attacked.

Contraindications

Local or systemic hypersensitivity to collagenase.

Warnings/Precautions

➤*External use only:* Avoid contact with the eyes.

➤*Compatible/Incompatible solutions:* The optimal pH range of collagenase is 6 to 8. Higher or lower pH conditions will decrease the enzyme's activity and appropriate precautions should be taken. The enzymatic activity is also adversely affected by certain detergents, and heavy metal ions such as mercury and silver which are used in some antiseptics. When it is suspected such materials have been used, the site should be carefully cleansed by repeated washings with normal saline before collagenase ointment is applied. Soaks containing metal ions or acidic solutions should be avoided because of the metal ion and low pH. Cleansing materials such as hydrogen peroxide, Dakin's solution, and normal saline are compatible with the collagenase ointment.

➤*Erythema:* A slight transient erythema has been noted occasionally in the surrounding tissue, particularly when collagenase ointment was not confined to the wound. Therefore, apply the ointment carefully within the area of the wound.

➤*Children:* Safety and efficacy in pediatric patients have not been established.

➤*Pregnancy: Category: Undetermined.* There is no information regarding collagenase in pregnant women.

➤*Lactation:* There is no information regarding collagenase in breast-feeding women.

➤*Monitoring:* Monitor debilitated patients closely for systematic bacterial infections because of the theoretical possibility that debriding enzymes may increase the risk of bacteremia.

Adverse Reactions

➤*Hypersensitivity:* No allergic sensitivity or toxic reactions have been noted in clinical use when used as directed. However, 1 case of systemic manifestations of hypersensitivity to collagenase in a patient treated for more than 1 year with a combination of collagenase and cortisone has been reported.

Overdosage

➤*Treatment:* If deemed necessary, the enzymes may be inactivated by washing the area with povidone iodine.

ENZYME COMBINATIONS TOPICAL

Rx	**Granulex** (Bertek)	**Aerosol; topical:** 0.12 mg trypsin, 87 mg balsam peru, and 788 mg castor oil per g	In 113.4 g.
Rx	**Vasolex** (Stratus)	**Ointment; topical:** 90 units trypsin, 87 mg balsam peru, 788 mg castor oil	White petrolatum. In 5, 30, and 60 g.
Rx	**Xenaderm** (Healthpoint)		Safflower oil. In 30 and 60 g.
Rx	**Optase** (Onset Therapeutics)	**Gel; topical:** 87 mg balsam peru, 788 mg castor oil, 0.12 mg trypsin	Oleth 10, safflower oil. In 6 and 95 g.

ENZYME COMBINATIONS — TOPICAL

Indications

➤*Topical lesions:* For debridement of necrotic tissue and liquefication of slough in acute and chronic lesions such as pressure ulcers, varicose, diabetic, and decubitus ulcers, burns, postoperative wounds, pilonidal cyst wounds, carbuncles, and miscellaneous traumatic or infected wounds. Also stimulates vascular bed activity to improve epithelization.

Administration and Dosage

➤*General dosing considerations:* Cleanse the wound prior to application with wound cleanser or saline. For products containing papain, avoid cleansing with hydrogen peroxide solution because it may inactivate papain.

➤*Adults:*

Topical lesions –
Aerosol: Apply 2 to 3 times daily, or as often as necessary.
Ointment: Daily or twice daily applications are preferred.

➤*Administration:*

Aerosol – Shake well. Hold upright and approximately 12 inches from the area to be treated. Press the valve and coat the wound rapidly. The wound may be left unbandaged or a wet dressing applied. Apply 2 to 3 times daily or as often as necessary. To remove, wash gently with water.

Ointment – Apply ointment directly to the wound, cover with an appropriate dressing, and secure into place. Daily or twice daily applications are preferred. Irrigate the wound at each redressing to remove any accumulation of liquefied necrotic material.

Longer intervals between redressings (2 or 3 days) have been proven satisfactory, and ointment may be applied under pressure dressings.

➤*Storage/Stability:*

Aerosol – Do not store above 120°F.

Ointment – Store between 15° and 30°C (59° and 86°F).

Contraindications

Sensitivity to papain or any other components of these preparations.

Warnings/Precautions

➤*Arterial clots:* Do not spray aerosol products on fresh arterial clots.

➤*For external use only:* Avoid contact with the eyes.

➤*Transient burning:* Transient burning may occur upon application.

➤*Papain:* Papain may be inactivated by the salts of heavy metals such as lead, silver, and mercury. Avoid contact with medications containing these metals.

➤*Pregnancy: Category: Undetermined.* There is no information regarding these medications in pregnant women.

➤*Lactation:* There is no information regarding these medications in breast-feeding women.

Adverse Reactions

Generally well-tolerated and nonirritating. A transient burning sensation may be experienced by a small percentage of patients upon application. Occasionally, the profuse exudate from enzymatic digestion may irritate the skin. In such cases, more frequent dressing changes will alleviate discomfort until exudate decreases.

Patient Information

Changing the dressing more often may help if irritation occurs.

In sensitive areas, temporary stinging or burning sensation may occur.

Enzyme Combinations, Injectable

COLLAGENASE CLOSTRIDIUM HISTOLYTICUM

Rx	**Xiaflex** (Auxilium)	**Injection, lyophilized powder for solution:** 0.9 mg	Preservative free. Sucrose 18.5 mg. In single-use vials with diluent.[a]

[a] Contains 3 mL of calcium chloride dihydrate 0.3 mg/mL in sodium chloride 0.9%.

COLLAGENASE CLOSTRIDIUM HISTOLYTICUM — INJECTION

Indications

➤*Dupuytren contracture:* For the treatment of adult patients with Dupuytren contracture with a palpable cord.

Administration and Dosage

➤*General dosing considerations:* Inject only one cord at a time. If a patient has other palpable cords with contractures of metacarpophalangeal (MP) or proximal interphalangeal (PIP) joints, these cords may be injected with collagenase *Clostridium histolyticum* in a sequential order.

➤*Adults:*

Dupuytren contracture –
Initial dosage: 0.58 mg per injection into a palpable cord with a contracture of an MP joint or a PIP joint. Approximately 24 hours after injection, perform a finger extension procedure if a contracture persists to facilitate cord disruption.

COLLAGENASE CLOSTRIDIUM HISTOLYTICUM — INJECTION

Volumes Needed for Reconstitution and Administration of Collagenase *Clostridium histolyticum*		
	For cords affecting MP joints	For cords affecting PIP joints
Sterile diluent for reconstitution		
Volume	0.39 mL	0.31 mL
Reconstituted solution to be injected[a]		
Volume	0.25 mL	0.2 mL

[a] The reconstituted collagenase *C. histolyticum* solution to be used in the intralesional injection contains collagenase *C. histolyticum* 0.58 mg. Note: The entire reconstituted collagenase *C. histolyticum* solution contains collagenase *C. histolyticum* 0.9 mg. Reconstituted collagenase *C. histolyticum* solution remaining in the vial after the injection should be discarded.

Repeat dosages: Four weeks after the collagenase *C. histolyticum* injection and finger extension procedure, if an MP or a PIP contracture remains, the cord may be reinjected with a single dose of collagenase *C. histolyticum* 0.58 mg, and the finger extension procedure may be repeated (approximately 24 hours after injection).

Injections and finger extension procedures may be administered up to 3 times per cord at approximately 4-week intervals.

➤*Preparation for administration:* Collagenase *C. histolyticum*, supplied as a lyophilized powder, must be reconstituted with the provided diluent prior to use.

Before use, remove the vial containing the lyophilized powder and the vial containing the diluent for reconstitution from the refrigerator and allow the 2 vials to stand at room temperature for at least 15 minutes and no longer than 60 minutes.

Use only the supplied diluent for reconstitution. The diluent contains calcium, which is required for the activity of collagenase *C. histolyticum*. Using a 1 mL syringe that contains 0.01 mL graduations with a 27-gauge, ½-inch needle (not supplied), withdraw a volume of the diluent supplied as follows: 0.39 mL for cords affecting an MP joint; 0.31 mL for cords affecting a PIP joint. Inject the diluent slowly into the sides of the vial containing the lyophilized powder. Do not invert the vial or shake the solution. Slowly swirl the solution to ensure that all of the lyophilized powder has gone into the solution.

If the reconstituted solution is refrigerated, allow this solution to return to room temperature for approximately 15 minutes before use.

➤*Administration:* Administration of a local anesthetic agent prior to injection is not recommended, because it may interfere with proper placement of the injection.

If injecting into a cord affecting the PIP joint of the fifth finger, care should be taken to inject as close to the palmar digital crease as possible (as far proximal to the digital PIP joint crease); the needle insertion should not be more than 2 to 3 mm in depth. Tendon ruptures have occurred after injections near the digital PIP joint crease.

Reconfirm the cord to be injected. The site chosen for injection should be the area where the contracting cord is maximally separated from the underlying flexor tendons and where the skin is not intimately adhered to the cord.

Injection procedure – Using a new 1 mL hubless syringe that contains 0.01 mL graduations with a permanently fixed, 27-gauge, ½-inch needle (not supplied), withdraw a volume of reconstituted solution (containing collagenase *C. histolyticum* 0.58 mg) as follows: 0.25 mL for cords affecting an MP joint; 0.2 mL for cords affecting a PIP joint. With your nondominant hand, secure the patient's hand to be treated while simultaneously applying tension to the cord. With your dominant hand, place the needle into the cord, using caution to keep the needle within the cord. Avoid having the needle tip pass completely through the cord to help minimize the potential for injection of collagenase *C. histolyticum* into tissues other than the cord. After needle placement, if there is any concern that the needle is in the flexor tendon, apply a small amount of passive motion at the distal interphalangeal (DIP) joint. If insertion of the needle into a tendon is suspected or paresthesia is noted by the patient, withdraw the needle and reposition it into the cord.

If the needle is in the proper location, there will be some resistance noted during the injection procedure. After confirming that the needle is correctly placed in the cord, inject approximately one-third of the dose. Next, withdraw the needle tip from the cord and reposition it in a slightly more distal location (approximately 2 to 3 mm) to the initial injection in the cord and inject another one-third of the dose. Again withdraw the needle tip from the cord and reposition it a third time proximal to the initial injection (approximately 2 to 3 mm) and inject the final portion of the dose into the cord.

Wrap the patient's treated hand with a soft, bulky, gauze dressing. Instruct the patient to limit motion of the treated finger and to keep the injected hand elevated until bedtime. Instruct the patient not to attempt to disrupt the injected cord by self-manipulation and to return to the provider's office the next day for follow-up and a finger extension procedure, if needed.

Discard the unused portion of the reconstituted solution and diluent after injection. Do not store, pool, or use any vials containing unused reconstituted solution or diluent.

Finger extension procedure – At the follow-up visit the day after the injection, if a contracture remains, perform a passive finger extension procedure to facilitate cord disruption. Local anesthesia may be used. Avoid direct pressure on the injection site because it will likely be tender. While the patient's wrist is in the flexed position, apply moderate stretching pressure to the injected cord by extending the finger for approximately 10 to 20 seconds. For cords affecting the PIP joint, perform the finger extension procedure when the MP joint is in the flexed position. If the first finger extension procedure does not result in disruption of the cord, a second and third attempt can be performed at 5- to 10-minute intervals; however, no more than 3 attempts are recommended to disrupt a cord. If the cord has not been disrupted after 3 attempts, a follow-up visit may be scheduled in approximately 4 weeks. If, at that subsequent visit, the contracted cord persists, an additional injection with finger extension procedures may be performed.

Following the finger extension procedure(s), fit patient with a splint and provide instructions for use at bedtime for up to 4 months to maintain finger extension. Also, instruct the patient to perform finger extension and flexion exercises several times a day for several months.

➤*Storage/Stability:* Prior to reconstitution, store the vials and diluent in a refrigerator at 2° to 8°C (36° to 46°F). Do not freeze.

The reconstituted collagenase *C. histolyticum* solution can be kept at room temperature (20° to 25°C [68 ° to 77°F]) for up to 1 hour or refrigerated at 2° to 8°C (36° to 46°F) for up to 4 hours prior to administration.

Actions

➤*Pharmacology:* Collagenases are proteinases that hydrolyze collagen in its native triple helical conformation under physiological conditions, resulting in lysis of collagen deposits. Injection of collagenase *C. histolyticum* into a Dupuytren cord, which is comprised mostly of collagen, may result in enzymatic disruption of the cord.

➤*Pharmacokinetics:*

Absorption – Following administration of a single collagenase *C. histolyticum* dose of 0.58 mg into a Dupuytren cord in 20 patients, no quantifiable levels of collagenase *C. histolyticum* (AUX-I or AUX-II) were detected in plasma up to 30 days postinjection.

Contraindications

None well documented.

Warnings/Precautions

➤*Tendon rupture:* In the controlled and uncontrolled portions of the clinical trials, flexor tendon ruptures occurred after collagenase *C. histolyticum* injection. Injection of collagenase *C. histolyticum* into collagen-containing structures, such as tendons or ligaments of the hand, may result in damage to those structures and possible permanent injury, such as tendon rupture or ligament damage; therefore, only inject collagenase *C. histolyticum* into the collagen cord with an MP or a PIP joint contracture, and take care to avoid injecting into tendons, nerves, blood vessels, or other collagen-containing structures of the hand. When injecting a cord affecting a PIP joint of the fifth finger, insert the needle no more than 2 to 3 mm in depth and avoid injecting more than 4 mm distal to the palmar digital crease.

➤*Local effects:* Other collagenase *C. histolyticum*–associated serious local adverse reactions in the controlled and uncontrolled portions of the studies included complex regional pain syndrome, ligament injury, pulley rupture, and sensory abnormality of the hand.

➤*Coagulation disorders:* In studies 1 and 2, 70% and 38% of collagenase *C. histolyticum*–treated patients developed an ecchymosis/contusion or an injection-site hemorrhage, respectively. The efficacy and safety of collagenase *C. histolyticum* in patients receiving anticoagulant medications (other than low-dose aspirin [eg, up to 150 mg/day]) within 7 days prior to collagenase *C. histolyticum* administration are not known. Therefore, use collagenase *C. histolyticum* with caution in patients with coagulation disorders, including patients receiving concomitant anticoagulants (except for low-dose aspirin).

➤*Immunogenicity:* During clinical studies, patients with Dupuytren contracture were tested at multiple time points for antibodies to the protein components of collagenase *C. histolyticum* (AUX-I and AUX-II). At 30 days after the first injection of collagenase *C. histolyticum* 0.58 mg, 92% of patients had antibodies detected against AUX-I and 86% of patients had antibodies detected against AUX-II. After the fourth injection of collagenase *C. histolyticum*, every collagenase *C. histolyticum*–treated patient developed high titers of antibodies to both AUX-I and AUX-II. Neutralizing antibodies to AUX-I or AUX-II were detected in 10% and 21%, respectively, of patients treated with collagenase *C. histolyticum*. However, there was no apparent correlation of antibody frequency, antibody titers, or neutralizing status to clinical response or adverse reactions.

Because the protein components in collagenase *C. histolyticum* (AUX-I and AUX-II) have some sequence homology with human matrix metalloproteinases (MMPs), anti-product antibodies could theoretically interfere with human MMPs.

➤*Hypersensitivity reactions:* In the controlled portions of the clinical trials (studies 1 and 2), a greater proportion of collagenase *C. histolyticum*–treated patients (15%) compared with placebo-treated patients (1%) had mild allergic reactions (pruritus) after up to 3 injections. The incidence of collagenase *C. histolyticum*–associated pruritus increased after more collagenase *C. histolyticum* injections.

Although there were no severe allergic reactions observed in the collagenase *C. histolyticum* studies (eg, those associated with respiratory compromise, hypotension, or end-organ dysfunction), severe reactions, including anaphylaxis, could occur following collagenase *C. histolyticum* injections. Collagenase *C. histolyticum* contains foreign proteins, and patients developed immunoglobulin E–antidrug antibodies in greater proportions and higher titers with successive collagenase *C. histolyticum* injections. Health care

COLLAGENASE CLOSTRIDIUM HISTOLYTICUM — INJECTION

providers should be prepared to address severe allergic reactions following collagenase *C. histolyticum* injections.

➤*Pregnancy: Category B.* There are no adequate, well-controlled studies of collagenase *C. histolyticum* in pregnant women. Human pharmacokinetic studies showed that collagenase *C. histolyticum* levels were not quantifiable in the systemic circulation following injection into a Dupuytren cord. Almost all patients develop anti-product antibodies (anti–AUX-I and anti–AUX-II) after treatment with collagenase *C. histolyticum*, and the clinical significance of anti-product antibody formation on a developing fetus is not known. Because animal reproduction studies are not always predictive of human response, use collagenase *C. histolyticum* during pregnancy only if clearly needed.

➤*Lactation:* It is not known whether collagenase *C. histolyticum* is excreted in human milk. Because many drugs are excreted in human milk, exercise caution when administering collagenase *C. histolyticum* to a breast-feeding woman.

➤*Children:* The safety and effectiveness of collagenase *C. histolyticum* in children younger than 18 years old have not been established.

➤*Elderly:* No overall differences in safety or effectiveness of collagenase *C. histolyticum* were observed between these patients and younger patients.

Drug Interactions

➤*Anticoagulant drugs (eg, warfarin):* Use collagenase *C. histolyticum* with caution in patients receiving concomitant anticoagulants, except low-dose aspirin (ie, up to 150 mg/day), within 7 days prior to administering collagenase *C. histolyticum*.

Adverse Reactions

➤*Most common adverse reactions:* The most frequently reported adverse drug reactions (at least 25%) in clinical trials included contusion, injection-site reaction, injection-site hemorrhage, pain in the treated extremity, and peripheral edema (mostly swelling of the injected hand).

➤*Adverse reactions (at least 5%):*

Collagenase *C. Histolyticum* Adverse Reactions Through Day 90 After Up to 3 Injections (≥ 5%)		
Adverse reactions	Collagenase *C. histolyticum* (n = 249)	Placebo (n = 125)
All adverse reactions	98%	51%
Dermatologic		
Erythema	6%	0%
Pruritus[a]	15%	1%
Skin laceration	9%	0%
Local		
Injection-site hemorrhage	38%	3%
Injection-site reaction[b]	35%	6%
Injection-site swelling[c]	24%	6%
Tenderness	24%	0%
Miscellaneous		
Axillary pain	6%	0%
Contusion[d]	70%	3%
Lymphadenopathy[e]	13%	0%
Lymph node pain	8%	0%
Pain in extremity	35%	4%
Peripheral edema[f]	73%	5%

[a] Includes the terms pruritus and injection-site pruritus.
[b] Includes the terms injection-site reaction, injection-site erythema, injection-site inflammation, injection-site irritation, injection-site pain, and injection-site warmth.
[c] Includes the terms injection-site swelling and injection-site edema.
[d] Includes the terms contusion (any body system) and ecchymosis.
[e] Includes the terms lymphadenopathy and axillary mass.
[f] Most of these events were swelling of the injected hand.

Some patients developed vasovagal syncope after finger extension procedures.

➤*Tendon rupture:* Out of 1,082 patients who received collagenase *C. histolyticum* 0.58 mg in the controlled and uncontrolled portions of the collagenase *C. histolyticum* studies (2,630 collagenase *C. histolyticum* injections) 0.3% of patients had a flexor tendon rupture of the treated finger within 7 days of the injection.

In the placebo-controlled portions of studies 1 and 2 through day 90, 98% and 51% of collagenase *C. histolyticum*–treated and placebo-treated patients had an adverse reaction after up to 3 injections, respectively. Over 95% of collagenase *C. histolyticum*–treated patients had an adverse reaction of the injected extremity after up to 3 injections. Approximately 81% of these local reactions resolved without intervention within 4 weeks of collagenase *C. histolyticum* injections. The adverse reaction profile was similar for each injection, regardless of the number of injections administered; however, the incidence of pruritus increased with more injections.

Overdosage

➤*Symptoms:* The effects of overdose of collagenase *C. histolyticum* are unknown. It is possible that multiple simultaneous or excessive doses of collagenase *C. histolyticum* may cause more severe local effects, including serious adverse reactions (eg, tendon ruptures), than the recommended doses.

➤*Treatment:* Supportive care and symptomatic treatment are recommended in these circumstances.

Patient Information

Inform patients that serious complications of collagenase *C. histolyticum* injection include tendon rupture or serious ligament damage that may result in the inability to fully bend the finger and may require surgery to correct the complication.

Advise patients that collagenase *C. histolyticum* injection is likely to result in swelling, bruising, bleeding, and/or pain of the injected site and surrounding tissue.

Instruct patients not to flex or extend the fingers of the injected hand to reduce extravasation of collagenase *C. histolyticum* out of the cord and not to attempt to disrupt the injected cord by self-manipulation.

Advise patients to elevate the injected hand until bedtime and to promptly contact their health care provider if there is evidence of infection (eg, fever, chills, increasing redness or edema), sensory changes in the treated finger, or trouble bending the finger after the swelling goes down (symptoms of tendon rupture).

Instruct patients to return to their health care provider's office the next day after injection for an examination of the injected hand and for a possible finger extension procedure to disrupt the cord.

Following the finger extension procedure(s) and fitting patient with a splint, instruct patients as follows: not to perform strenuous activity with the injected hand until advised to do so; to wear the splint at bedtime for up to 4 months; to perform a series of finger flexion and extension exercises each day.

IMMUNOMODULATORS, TOPICAL

IMIQUIMOD

Rx	**Zyclara** (Graceway Pharmaceuticals)	**Cream; topical**: 3.75%	Alcohol, glycerin, parabens, white petrolatum. In boxes containing 28 single-use packets.
Rx	**Imiquimod** (Fougera)	**Cream; topical**: 5%	May contain alcohol, glycerin, parabens, white petrolatum. In boxes containing 24 single-use packets.
Rx	**Aldara** (Graceway Pharmaceuticals)		Alcohol, glycerin, parabens, white petrolatum. In boxes containing 24 single-use packets.

IMIQUIMOD — TOPICAL

Indications

➤*Actinic keratosis:* For the topical treatment of clinically typical, nonhyperkeratotic, nonhypertrophic, visible or palpable actinic keratoses on the face or balding scalp in immunocompetent adults.

➤*Genital and perianal warts:* For the treatment of external genital and perianal warts (condyloma acuminata) in patients 12 years and older.

➤*Superficial basal cell carcinoma (5% cream only):* For the topical treatment of biopsy-confirmed, primary superficial basal cell carcinoma in immunocompetent adults, with a maximum tumor diameter of 2 cm, located on the trunk (excluding anogenital skin), neck, or extremities (excluding hands and feet), only when surgical methods are medically less appropriate and patient follow-up can be reasonably ensured.

Administration and Dosage

➤*Adults:*

Actinic keratosis –

3.75% cream:

• *Usual dosage* – Apply once daily before bedtime to the skin of the affected area (either the face or balding scalp). Leave on the skin for 8 hours, then remove with mild soap and water.

• *Maximum dose* – Up to 2 packets of the cream may be applied to the treatment area at each application.

IMIQUIMOD — TOPICAL

• *Duration of therapy* – Treat for two 2-week treatment cycles separated by a 2-week no-treatment period. Neither 2-week treatment cycle should be extended because of missed doses or rest periods.

A transient increase in actinic keratosis lesion counts may be observed during treatment. Treatment should continue for the full treatment course even if all actinic keratoses appear to be gone. Lesions that do not respond to treatment should be carefully reevaluated and management reconsidered.

5% cream:

• *Usual dosage* – Apply 2 times per week (eg, Monday and Thursday), prior to bedtime, to a defined treatment area on the face or scalp (but not both concurrently). Leave on the skin for approximately 8 hours, then remove with mild soap and water. The treatment area should be one contiguous area of approximately 25 cm^2 (eg, 5 cm × 5 cm) on the face (eg, forehead or one cheek) or scalp.

• *Maximum dose* – No more than 1 packet of cream should be applied to the contiguous treatment area at each application.

• *Duration of therapy* – Continue treatment for the full 16 weeks. However, do not extend the treatment period beyond 16 weeks because of missed doses or rest periods.

Genital and perianal warts –

3.75% cream:

• *Usual dosage* – Apply a thin layer once daily prior to normal sleeping hours and leave on the skin for approximately 8 hours. Remove by washing the area with mild soap and water.

• *Maximum dose* – Up to 1 packet of cream may be applied to the treatment area at each application.

• *Duration of therapy* – Continue treatment until there is total clearance or for up to 8 weeks.

5% cream:

• *Usual dosage* – Apply a thin layer 3 times per week (eg, Monday, Wednesday, Friday) prior to bedtime, and leave on the skin for 6 to 10 hours. Remove by washing with mild soap and water.

• *Duration of therapy* – Continue treatment until there is total clearance of the genital/perianal warts or for a maximum of 16 weeks.

Superficial basal cell carcinoma –

5% cream only:

• *Usual dosage* – Apply once daily 5 times per week, prior to bedtime, and leave on the skin for approximately 8 hours. Remove with mild soap and water. Apply sufficient cream to cover the treatment area, including 1 cm of skin surrounding the tumor.

The target tumor should have a maximum diameter of 2 cm and be located in the trunk (excluding anogenital skin), neck, or extremities (excluding hands and feet).

Amount of Imiquimod for Administration		
Target tumor diameter	Size of cream droplet (diameter)	Approximate amount of cream
0.5 to < 1 cm	4 mm	10 mg
≥ 1 to < 1.5 cm	5 mm	25 mg
≥ 1.5 to 2 cm	7 mm	40 mg

• *Duration of therapy* – Treatment should continue for 6 weeks.

• *Early clinical clearance* – Early clinical clearance cannot be adequately assessed until the resolution of local skin reactions (eg, 12 weeks posttreatment). Local skin reactions or other findings (eg, infection) may require that a patient be seen sooner than the posttreatment assessment for clinical clearance. If there is clinical evidence of persistent tumor at the posttreatment assessment for clinical clearance, consider a biopsy or other alternative intervention.

Lesions that do not respond to therapy should be carefully reevaluated and management reconsidered; the safety and efficacy of a repeat course of treatment have not been established. If any suspicious lesion arises in the treatment area at any time after a determination of clinical clearance, the patient should seek medical evaluation.

➤*Children:*

Genital and perianal warts –

12 years and older:

• *3.75% cream* – See Adults for dosing.

• *5% cream* – See Adults for dosing.

➤*Administration:* For external use only; imiquimod cream is not for ophthalmic, oral, or intravaginal use. Avoid contact with the lips and nostrils and in or near the eyes.

Handwashing before and after cream application is recommended.

Unused packets should be discarded. Partially-used packets should be discarded and not reused.

Actinic keratosis –

3.75% cream: Apply the cream as a thin film to the entire treatment area and rub in until the cream is no longer visible. Leave imiquimod cream on the skin for approximately 8 hours, after which time, remove the cream by washing the area with mild soap and water.

Prescribe patients no more than 56 packets for the total 2-cycle treatment course.

5% cream: Before applying the cream, wash the treatment area with mild soap and water and allow the area to dry thoroughly (at least 10 minutes). Apply the cream to the entire treatment area (eg, forehead, scalp, one cheek) and rub in until the cream is no longer visible. Apply imiquimod cream prior to bedtime and leave on the skin for approximately 8 hours, after which time, remove the cream by washing the area with mild soap and water.

Prescribe patients no more than 36 packets for the 16-week treatment period.

Genital and perianal warts –

3.75% cream: Apply a thin layer of cream to treatment area prior to normal sleeping hours, then remove by washing the area with mild soap and water. Prescribe patients up to 56 packets for the treatment course.

5% cream: Apply a thin layer of cream to the wart area and rub in until the cream is no longer visible. Following the treatment period, remove the cream by washing the treated area with mild soap and water. The application site is not to be occluded. Nonocclusive dressings, such as cotton gauze or cotton underwear, may be used in the management of skin reactions.

Imiquimod 5% cream is packaged in single-use packets that contain sufficient cream to cover a wart area of up to 20 cm^2; avoid use of excessive amounts of cream.

Superficial basal cell carcinoma – Before applying the cream, wash the treatment area with mild soap and water and allow the area to dry thoroughly. Rub the cream into the treatment area until the cream is no longer visible. Following the treatment period, remove the cream by washing the area with mild soap and water.

Prescribe patients no more than 36 packets for the 6-week treatment period.

Local skin reactions: Local skin reactions at the treatment site are common. A rest period of several days may be taken if required by the patient's discomfort or severity of the local skin reaction. Treatment may resume once the reaction subsides.

Response to treatment cannot be adequately assessed until the resolution of local skin reactions. The patient should continue dosing as prescribed. Carefully reevaluate lesions that do not respond to therapy and reconsider management.

➤*Storage/Stability:* Store between 4° and 25°C (39° and 77°F). Avoid freezing.

Actions

➤*Pharmacology:* Imiquimod, an immune response modifier for topical administration, is a Toll-like receptor 7 agonist that activates immune cells. Topical application to the skin is associated with increases in markers for cytokines and immune cells.

The mechanism of action of imiquimod cream in treating actinic keratosis and superficial basal cell carcinoma lesions is unknown.

➤*Pharmacokinetics:*

Absorption –

3.75% cream: Following dosing with 2 packets once daily (imiquimod 18.75 mg/day) for up to 3 weeks, systemic absorption of imiquimod was observed in all subjects when imiquimod 3.75% cream was applied to the face and/or scalp in 17 subjects with at least 10 actinic keratosis lesions. The imiquimod mean peak serum concentration (C_{max}) at the end of the trial was approximately 0.323 ng/mL. The median time to maximal concentrations occurred at 9 hours after dosing. Based on the plasma half-life of imiquimod observed at the end of the study, 29.3±17 hours, steady-state concentrations can be anticipated to occur by day 7 with once-daily dosing.

5% cream: Systemic absorption of imiquimod was observed across the affected skin of 12 patients with genital/perianal warts, with an average dose of 4.6 mg. Mean C_{max} of approximately 0.4 ng/mL was seen during the study.

Systemic absorption of imiquimod across the affected skin of 58 patients with actinic keratosis was observed with a dosing frequency of 3 applications per week for 16 weeks. Mean C_{max} values at the end of week 16 were approximately 0.1, 0.2, and 3.5 ng/mL for the applications to the face (12.5 mg imiquimod, 1 single-use packet), scalp (25 mg, 2 packets), and hands/arms (75 mg, 6 packets), respectively.

The application surface area was not controlled when more than 1 packet was used. Dose proportionality was not observed; however, it appears that systemic exposure may be more dependent on the surface area of application than the amount of applied dose.

Metabolism/Excretion –

5% cream: The apparent half-life was approximately 10 times greater with topical dosing than the 2–hour apparent half-life observed following subcutaneous dosing, suggesting prolonged retention of the drug in the skin. Mean urinary recoveries of imiquimod and metabolites combined were 0.08% and 0.15% of the applied dose in the group using 75 mg (6 packets) for men and women, respectively, following 3 applications per week for 16 weeks.

Mean urinary recoveries of imiquimod and metabolites combined over the whole course of genital/perianal warts treatment, expressed as percent of the estimated applied dose, were 0.11% and 2.41% in the men and women, respectively.

Contraindications

None well documented.

Warnings/Precautions

➤*Local inflammatory reactions:* Intense local inflammatory reactions, including skin weeping or erosion, can occur after few applications of imiquimod and may require an interruption of dosing. Imiquimod has the potential to exacerbate inflammatory conditions of the skin, including chronic graft versus host disease.

➤*Systemic reactions:* Flu-like signs and symptoms may accompany, or even precede, local inflammatory reactions and may include malaise, fever, nausea, myalgias, and rigors. Consider an interruption of dosing and an assessment of the patient.

➤*Previous drug or surgical treatment:* Imiquimod administration is not recommended until the skin is completely healed from any previous drug or surgical treatment.

IMIQUIMOD — TOPICAL

➤*Lymphadenopathy:* Lymphadenopathy occurred in 2% of patients treated with imiquimod 3.75% cream. This reaction resolved in all patients by 4 weeks after completion of treatment.

➤*Actinic keratosis:* Safety and efficacy have not been established for imiquimod 5% cream in the treatment of actinic keratosis with repeated use (ie, more than 1 treatment course) in the same 25 cm^2 area.

The safety of imiquimod 5% cream applied to areas of skin larger than 25 cm^2 (eg, 5 cm × 5 cm) for the treatment of actinic keratosis has not been established.

➤*Other types of basal cell carcinomas:* The safety and efficacy of imiquimod have not been established for other types of basal cell carcinomas, including nodular and morpheaform (fibrosing or sclerosing) types. Imiquimod is not approved for treatment of basal cell carcinoma subtypes other than the superficial variant (ie, superficial basal cell carcinoma). Advise patients with superficial basal cell carcinoma treated with imiquimod to have regular follow up of the treatment site.

The safety and efficacy of treating superficial basal cell carcinoma lesions on the face, head, and anogenital area with imiquimod 5% cream have not been established. The efficacy and safety of imiquimod cream have not been established for patients with basal cell nevus syndrome or xeroderma pigmentosum.

➤*Human papilloma viral disease:* Imiquimod 5% cream has not been evaluated for the treatment of urethral, intravaginal, cervical, rectal, or intra-anal human papilloma viral disease.

➤*Immunosuppressed patients:* The safety and efficacy of imiquimod cream in immunosuppressed patients have not been established; therefore, use with caution in patients with preexisting autoimmune conditions.

➤*Photosensitivity:* Avoid or minimize exposure to sunlight (including sunlamps) during use of imiquimod cream because of concern for heightened sunburn susceptibility. Warn patients to use protective clothing (eg, a hat) when using imiquimod. Advise patients with sunburn not to use imiquimod until fully recovered. Advise patients who may have considerable sun exposure (eg, due to their occupations) and those patients with inherent sensitivity to sunlight to exercise caution when using imiquimod. Imiquimod cream shortened the time to skin tumor formation in an animal photococarcinogenicity study. The enhancement of ultraviolet (UV) carcinogenicity is not necessarily dependent on phototoxic mechanisms; therefore, patients should minimize or avoid natural or artificial sunlight exposure.

➤*Pregnancy: Category C.* There are no adequate and well-controlled studies in pregnant women. Use imiquimod cream during pregnancy only if the potential benefit justifies the potential risk to the fetus.

Systemic embryofetal development studies were conducted in rats and rabbits. Oral dosages of imiquimod 1, 5, and 20 mg/kg/day were administered during the period of organogenesis (gestational days 6 to 15) to pregnant female rats. In the presence of maternal toxicity, fetal effects noted at 20 mg/kg/day (577× and 190× MRHD based on AUC comparisons for the 5% and 3.75% cream, respectively) included increased resorptions, decreased fetal body weights, delays in skeletal ossification, and bent limb bones; 2 fetuses in 1 litter (2 of 1,567 fetuses) demonstrated exencephaly, protruding tongues, and low-set ears. No treatment-related effects on embryofetal toxicity or teratogenicity were noted at 5 mg/kg/day (98× and 32× MRHD based on AUC comparisons for the 5% and 3.75% cream, respectively).

A combined fertility and peri- and postnatal development study was conducted in rats. Oral dosages of imiquimod 1, 1.5, 3, and 6 mg/kg/day were administered to male rats from 70 days prior to mating through the mating period, and to female rats from 14 days prior to mating through parturition and lactation. No effects on growth, fertility, reproduction, or postnatal development were noted at dosages of up to 6 mg/kg/day (87× and 29× MRHD based on AUC comparisons for the 5% and 3.75% cream, respectively), the highest dose evaluated in this study. In the absence of maternal toxicity, bent limb bones were noted in the F1 fetuses at a dosage of 6 mg/kg/day. This fetal effect was also noted in the oral rat embryofetal development study conducted with imiquimod. No treatment-related effects on teratogenicity were noted at 3 mg/kg/day (41× and 14× MRHD based on AUC comparisons for the 5% and 3.75% cream, respectively).

➤*Lactation:* It is not known whether topically applied imiquimod is excreted in breast milk. The relatively low molecular weight (approximately 240) and long elimination half-life (approximately 20 hours) suggest that the drug will be excreted into breast milk. However, the amount absorbed systemically and available for excretion into milk is very low and probably is clinically insignificant. Therefore, although the risk to a breast-feeding infant is unknown, use of imiquimod by the mother appears to be compatible with breast-feeding. Because many drugs are excreted in human milk, exercise caution when imiquimod cream is administered to a breast-feeding woman.

➤*Children:* Safety and efficacy of imiquimod 5% cream in patients younger than 12 years of age with external genital/perianal warts have not been established.

Actinic keratosis and superficial basal cell carcinoma are not conditions generally seen within the pediatric population. The safety and efficacy of imiquimod cream for actinic keratosis or superficial basal cell carcinoma in patients younger than 18 years of age have not been established.

5% cream – Imiquimod was evaluated in 2 randomized, vehicle-controlled, double-blind trials involving 702 children with molluscum contagiosum (MC) (470 exposed to imiquimod 5% cream; median age, 5 years; range, 2 to 12 years of age). Patients applied imiquimod 5% cream or vehicle 3 times weekly for up to 16 weeks. Complete clearance (no MC lesions) was assessed at week 18. In study 1, the complete clearance rate was 24% in the imiquimod group compared with 26% in the vehicle group. In study 2, the clearance rates were 24% in the imiquimod group compared with 28% in the vehicle group. These studies failed to demonstrate efficacy.

Similar to the studies conducted in adults, the most frequently reported adverse reaction from 2 studies in children with MC was application-site reaction. Adverse reactions that occurred more frequently in imiquimod-treated patients compared with vehicle-treated patients generally resembled those seen in studies in indications approved for adults and also included otitis media (5% imiquimod vs 3% vehicle) and conjunctivitis (3% imiquimod vs 2% vehicle).

Erythema was the most frequently reported local skin reaction. Severe local skin reactions reported by imiquimod-treated patients in the pediatric studies included erythema (28%), edema (8%), scabbing/crusting (5%), flaking/scaling (5%), erosion (2%), and weeping/exudate (2%).

Systemic absorption of imiquimod across the affected skin of 22 subjects aged 2 to 12 years of age with extensive MC involving at least 10% of the total body surface area was observed after single and multiple doses at a dosing frequency of 3 applications per week for 4 weeks. The investigator determined the dose applied (1, 2, or 3 packets per dose) based on the size of the treatment area and the subject's weight. The overall median peak serum drug concentrations at the end of week 4 was between 0.26 and 1.06 ng/mL, except in 2-year-old girl who was administered 2 packets of study drug per dose had a C_{max} of 9.66 ng/mL after multiple dosing. Children 2 to 5 years of age received doses of imiquimod 12.5 mg (1 packet) or 25 mg (2 packets) and had median multiple-dose C_{max} of approximately 0.2 or 0.5 ng/mL, respectively. Children 6 to 12 years of age received doses of 12.5, 25, or 37.5 mg (3 packets) and had median multiple dose serum drug levels of approximately 0.1, 0.15, or 0.3 ng/mL, respectively. Among the 20 patients with evaluable laboratory assessments, the median white blood cell (WBC) count decreased by 1.4×10^9/L and the median absolute neutrophil count decreased by 1.42×10^9/L.

➤*Elderly:* No other clinical experience has identified differences in responses between the elderly and younger patients, but greater sensitivity of some older individuals cannot be ruled out.

➤*Monitoring:* Periodically assess response to therapy. Monitor for local skin reactions (eg, erythema, erosion, edema) to the application site and surrounding areas.

Drug Interactions

None well documented.

Adverse Reactions

➤*Actinic keratosis:*

3.75% cream –

Adverse reactions	Imiquimod (n = 160)	Vehicle (n = 159)
Imiquimod 3.75% Cream Adverse Reactions (≥ 2%) in Actinic Keratosis		
CNS		
Dizziness	3%	0%
Fatigue	4%	0%
Headache	6%	3%
GI		
Anorexia	3%	0%
Diarrhea	2%	0%
Nausea	3%	1%
Local		
Application-site irritation	3%	0%
Application-site pain	3%	0%
Application-site pruritus	4%	< 1%
Miscellaneous		
Chest pain	2%	0%
Herpes simplex	3%	< 1%
Lymphadenopathy	2%	0%
Pain	3%	0%
Pyrexia	3%	0%

Local:

Imiquimod 3.75% Cream Local Skin Reactions (%) in Actinic Keratosis	All grades (mild/moderate/severe)		Severe	
Adverse reactions	Imiquimod cream (n = 160)	Vehicle (n = 159)	Imiquimod cream (n = 160)	Vehicle (n = 159)
Edema	75%	19%	6%	0%
Erosion/Ulceration	62%	9%	11%	0%
Erythema	96%	78%	25%	0%
Flaking/Scaling/Dryness	92%	77%	8%	1%
Scabbing/Crusting	93%	45%	14%	0%
Weeping/Exudate	51%	4%	6%	0%

Local skin reactions may extend beyond treatment area.

IMIQUIMOD — TOPICAL

Overall, in the clinical trials, 11% of patients on imiquimod 3.75% cream and 0% on vehicle cream required rest periods because of adverse reactions.

Other adverse reactions: Other adverse reactions observed in patients treated with imiquimod 3.75% cream include application-site bleeding, application-site swelling, arthralgia, cheilitis, chills, dermatitis, herpes zoster, influenza-like illness, insomnia, lethargy, myalgia, pancytopenia, pruritus, squamous cell carcinoma, and vomiting.

5% cream –

Imiquimod 5% Cream Adverse Reactions (> 1%) in Actinic Keratosis		
Adverse reactions	Imiquimod (n = 215)	Vehicle (n = 221)
CNS		
Dizziness	1%	< 1%
Fatigue	1%	1%
Headache	5%	3%
Dermatologic		
Alopecia	1%	0%
Eczema	2%	1%
GI		
Diarrhea	3%	1%
Vomiting	1%	< 1%
Musculoskeletal		
Back pain	1%	1%
Rigors	1%	0%
Respiratory		
Sinusitis	7%	6%
Upper respiratory tract infection	15%	12%
Miscellaneous		
Application-site reaction	33%	14%
Atrial fibrillation	1%	1%
Carcinoma squamous	4%	2%
Fever	1%	0%
Urinary tract infection	1%	< 1%
Viral infection	1%	1%

Local:

Imiquimod 5% Cream Application-Site Adverse Reactions (> 1%) in Actinic Keratosis		
Adverse reactions	Imiquimod (n = 215)	Vehicle (n = 221)
Bleeding	3%	< 1%
Burning	6%	2%
Induration	2%	1%
Irritation	2%	0%
Itching	20%	8%
Pain	3%	1%
Stinging	3%	1%
Tenderness	2%	1%

Local skin reactions were collected independently of the application-site reaction in an effort to provide a better picture of the specific types of local reactions that might be seen. The most frequently reported local skin reactions were erythema, flaking/scaling/dryness, and scabbing/crusting.

Imiquimod 5% Cream Local Skin Reactions (%) in Actinic Keratosis				
	All grades (mild/moderate/severe)		Severe	
Adverse reactions	Imiquimod (n = 215)	Vehicle (n = 220)	Imiquimod (n = 215)	Vehicle (n = 220)
Edema	49%	10%	0%	0%
Erosion/Ulceration	48%	9%	2%	0%
Erythema	97%	93%	18%	2%
Flaking/Scaling/Dryness	93%	91%	7%	3%
Scabbing/Crusting	79%	42%	8%	2%
Vesicles	9%	1%	0%	0%
Weeping/Exudate	22%	1%	0%	0%

The adverse reactions that most frequently resulted in clinical intervention (eg, rest periods, withdrawal from study) were local skin and application-site reactions. Overall, in the clinical studies, 2% of patients discontinued for local skin/application-site reactions. Of the 215 patients treated, 16% of patients on imiquimod cream and 1% of patients on vehicle cream had at least 1 rest period. Of these imiquimod cream–treated patients, 91% resumed therapy after a rest period.

In the actinic keratosis studies, 3.2% of imiquimod-treated patients developed treatment-site infections that required a rest period off imiquimod cream and were treated with antibiotics (19 with oral and 3 with topical). Of the 206 imiquimod cream–treated patients with both baseline and 8-week posttreatment scarring assessments, 2.9% had a greater degree of scarring scores at 8-weeks posttreatment than at baseline.

➤*Superficial basal cell carcinoma:*

5% cream –

Imiquimod 5% Cream Adverse Reactions (> 1%) in Superficial Basal Cell Carcinoma		
Adverse reactions	Imiquimod (n = 185)	Vehicle (n = 179)
CNS		
Anxiety	1%	< 1%
Dizziness	1%	< 1%
Fatigue	2%	1%
Headache	8%	2%
GI		
Dyspepsia	2%	1%
Nausea	1%	0%
Respiratory		
Coughing	2%	< 1%
Pharyngitis	1%	< 1%
Rhinitis	3%	< 1%
Sinusitis	2%	< 1%
Upper respiratory tract infection	3%	1%
Miscellaneous		
Application-site reaction	28%	3%
Back pain	4%	< 1%
Chest pain	1%	0%
Fever	2%	0%
Lymphadenopathy	3%	< 1%

Local: The most frequently reported adverse reactions were local skin and application-site reactions, including burning, edema, erosion, erythema, flaking/scaling, induration, itching, and scabbing/crusting at the application site.

Imiquimod 5% Cream Application-Site Reactions (> 1%) in Superficial Basal Cell Carcinoma		
Adverse reactions	Imiquimod (n = 185)	Vehicle (n = 179)
Bleeding	2%	0%
Burning	6%	1%
Erythema	2%	0%
Infection	1%	0%
Itching	16%	1%
Pain	3%	0%
Papule(s)	2%	0%
Tenderness	1%	0%

Local skin reactions were collected independently of the adverse reaction "application-site reaction" in an effort to provide a better picture of the specific types of local reactions that might be seen.

Imiquimod 5% Cream Local Skin Reactions in Superficial Basal Cell Carcinoma				
	All grades (mild/moderate/severe)		Severe	
Adverse reactions	Imiquimod (n = 184)	Vehicle (n = 178)	Imiquimod (n = 184)	Vehicle (n = 178)
Edema	78%	36%	7%	0%
Erosion	66%	14%	13%	0%
Erythema	100%	97%	31%	2%
Flaking/Scaling	91%	76%	4%	0%
Induration	84%	53%	6%	0%
Scabbing/Crusting	83%	34%	19%	0%
Ulceration	40%	3%	6%	0%
Vesicles	31%	2%	2%	0%

The adverse reactions that most frequently resulted in clinical intervention (eg, rest periods, withdrawal from study) were local skin and application-site reactions; 10% of patients received rest periods. The average number of doses not received per patient because of rest periods was 7 doses, with a

IMIQUIMOD — TOPICAL

range of 2 to 22 doses; 79% of patients resumed therapy after a rest period. Overall, in the clinical studies, 2% of patients discontinued for local skin/application-site reactions.

In the superficial basal cell carcinoma studies, 1.3% of imiquimod-treated patients developed treatment-site infections that required a rest period off imiquimod cream and were treated with antibiotics.

➤*External genital warts:*

5% cream – In controlled clinical trials for genital warts, the most frequently reported adverse reactions were those of local skin and application-site reactions; some patients also reported systemic reactions. Overall, 1.2% of the patients discontinued because of local skin/application-site reactions.

Imiquimod 5% Cream Local Skin Reactions in External Genital Warts

	All grades (mild/moderate/severe)				Severe			
	Women		Men		Women		Men	
Adverse reactions	Imiquimod (n = 114)	Vehicle (n = 99)	Imiquimod (n = 156)	Vehicle (n = 157)	Imiquimod (n = 114)	Vehicle (n = 99)	Imiquimod (n = 156)	Vehicle (n = 157)
Edema	18%	5%	12%	1%	1%	0%	0%	0%
Erosion	31%	8%	30%	6%	1%	0%	1%	0%
Erythema	65%	21%	58%	22%	4%	0%	4%	0%
Excoriation/Flaking	18%	8%	26%	8%	0%	0%	1%	0%
Induration	5%	2%	7%	2%	0%	0%	0%	0%
Scabbing	4%	0%	13%	3%	0%	0%	0%	0%
Ulceration	8%	1%	4%	1%	3%	0%	0%	0%
Vesicles	3%	0%	2%	0%	0%	0%	0%	0%

Remote-site skin reactions were also reported. The severe remote-site skin reactions reported for women were erythema (3%), ulceration (2%), and edema (1%); and for men, erosion (2%), and erythema, edema, induration, and excoriation/flaking (each 1%).

Adverse reactions judged to be probably or possibly related to imiquimod cream are shown in the following table.

Imiquimod 5% Cream Adverse Reactions in External Genital Warts

	Women		Men	
Adverse reactions	Imiquimod (n = 117)	Vehicle (n = 103)	Imiquimod (n = 156)	Vehicle (n = 158)
Application-site disorders/reactions (wart site)				
Burning	26%	12%	9%	5%
Fungal infection[a]	11%	3%	2%	1%
Itching	32%	20%	22%	10%
Pain	8%	2%	2%	1%
Soreness	3%	0%	0%	1%
Systemic reactions				
Headache	4%	3%	5%	2%
Influenza-like symptoms	3%	2%	1%	0%
Myalgia	1%	0%	1%	1%

[a] Incidences reported without regard to causality with imiquimod cream.

Other adverse reactions (greater than 1%):

- *CNS* – Fatigue, headache.
- *Local* –
  - *Wart-site reactions:* Burning, hypopigmentation, irritation, itching, pain, rash, sensitivity, soreness, stinging, tenderness.
  - *Remote-site reactions:* Bleeding, burning, itching, pain, tenderness, tinea cruris.
- *Miscellaneous* – Diarrhea, fever, influenza-like symptoms, myalgia.

➤*Dermatologic:* Provocative repeat-insult patch studies involving induction and challenge phases produced no evidence that imiquimod cream causes photoallergenicity or contact sensitization in healthy skin; however, cumulative irritancy testing revealed the potential for imiquimod 5% cream to cause irritation. Application-site reactions were reported in clinical studies.

➤*Postmarketing:*

5% cream –

Cardiovascular: Arrhythmias (tachycardia, atrial fibrillation, palpitations), capillary leak syndrome, cardiac failure, cardiomyopathy, cerebrovascular accident, chest pain, Henoch-Schonlein purpura syndrome, ischemia, myocardial infarction, pulmonary edema, syncope.

CNS: Agitation, convulsions (including febrile convulsions), depression, insomnia, multiple sclerosis aggravation, paresis, suicide.

Dermatologic: Erythema multiforme, exfoliative dermatitis, hyperpigmentation, hypertrophic scar, tingling at the application site.

GU: Dysuria, proteinuria, urinary retention.

Hematologic: Decreases in red blood cell, WBC, and platelet counts (including idiopathic thrombocytopenic purpura); lymphoma.

Miscellaneous: Abdominal pain, abnormal liver function, angioedema, arthralgia, dyspnea, herpes simplex, thyroiditis.

Overdosage

➤*Symptoms:* Topical overdosing of imiquimod cream could result in severe local skin reactions and may increase the risk of systemic reactions. The most clinically serious adverse reaction reported following multiple oral imiquimod doses of greater than 200 mg (equivalent to imiquimod content of more than 16 packets of 5% cream or more than 21 packets of 3.75% cream) was hypotension, which resolved following oral or IV fluid administration.

Patient Information

This medication is to be used as directed by a health care provider. It is for external use only. Avoid contact with the eyes, lips, and nostrils.

Do not bandage the treatment area or otherwise cover or wrap as to be occlusive.

Advise patients to wash their hands before and after applying imiquimod cream.

Inform patients that localized hypopigmentation and hyperpigmentation following imiquimod use have been reported and that these skin color changes may be permanent in some patients.

Inform patients that it is common to experience local skin reactions (ranging from mild to severe in intensity) during treatment with imiquimod cream, and that these reactions may extend beyond the application site onto the surrounding skin. Inform patients that potential local skin reactions include erythema, edema, vesicles, erosion/ulceration, weeping/exudate, flaking/scaling/dryness, and scabbing/crusting. Patients may also experience application-site reactions such as pain, itching and/or burning. Local skin reactions may be of such an intensity that patients may require rest periods from treatment. Treatment with imiquimod cream can be resumed after the skin reaction has subsided, as determined by the health care provider. Advise patients to contact their health care provider promptly if they experience any sign or symptom at the application site that restricts or prohibits their daily activity or makes continued application of the cream difficult.

Advise patients that because of local skin reactions, during treatment and until healed, the treatment area is likely to appear noticeably different from healthy skin.

Advise patients to use sunscreen and to minimize or avoid exposure to natural or artificial sunlight (tanning beds or UVA/B treatment) while using imiquimod cream.

Inform patients that they may experience flu-like systemic signs and symptoms during treatment with imiquimod cream (even with normal dosing). Systemic signs and symptoms may include malaise, fever, nausea, myalgias, and rigors. Consider an interruption of dosing.

Advise patients to discard and not reuse partially used packets.

➤*Actinic keratosis:* Advise patients to wash the treatment area with mild soap and water 8 hours following imiquimod cream application.

During treatment, subclinical actinic keratosis lesions may become apparent in the treatment area and may subsequently resolve.

Dosing of the 5% cream is twice weekly for the full 16 weeks, unless otherwise directed by the doctor. However, instruct patients not to extend the treatment period beyond 16 weeks due to missed doses or rest periods.

Dosing of the 3.75% cream is once daily before bedtime to the skin of the affected area (entire face or balding scalp) for two 2-week treatment cycles separated by a 2-week no-treatment period. However, instruct patients not to extend the treatment period beyond two 2-week treatment cycles because of missed doses or rest periods. Continue treatment for the full treatment course even if all actinic keratoses appear to be gone.

➤*Superficial basal cell carcinoma:* Advise patients to wash the treatment area with mild soap and water 8 hours after imiquimod cream application.

Inform patients that dosing is 5 times per week for a full 6 weeks, unless otherwise directed by the health care provider. However, instruct patients not to extend the treatment period beyond 6 weeks because of missed doses or rest periods.

Inform patients that the clinical outcome of therapy can be determined after the resolution of application-site reactions and/or local skin reactions.

Advise patients with superficial basal cell carcinoma treated with imiquimod cream to have regular follow-up to reevaluate the treatment site.

➤*External genital warts:* Inform patients to wash the treatment area with mild soap and water 6 to 10 hours following imiquimod cream application.

Advise patients to avoid sexual (genital, anal, oral) contact while the cream is on the skin.

Inform patients that application of imiquimod cream in the vagina is considered internal and should be avoided. Women should take special care if applying the cream at the opening of the vagina because local skin reactions on the delicate moist surfaces can result in pain or swelling, and may cause difficulty in passing urine.

Inform uncircumcised men treating warts under the foreskin to retract the foreskin and clean the area daily.

Advise patients to be aware that new warts may develop during therapy; imiquimod is not a cure. The effect of imiquimod cream on the transmission of genital/perianal warts is unknown.

Inform patients that imiquimod cream may weaken condoms and vaginal diaphragms; therefore, concurrent use is not recommended.

TACROLIMUS

Rx	**Protopic** (Astellas Pharma[a])	**Ointment:** 0.03%	Mineral oil, white petrolatum. In 30, 60, and 100 g.
		0.1%	Mineral oil, white petrolatum. In 30, 60, and 100 g.

[a] Astellas Pharma, 3 Parkway North Center, Deerfield, IL 60016; 800-888-7704; http://www.astellas.com.

TACROLIMUS — TOPICAL

Tacrolimus is also available as a capsule for organ rejection prophylaxis; see the Biologic and Immunologic Agents chapter.

WARNING

Long-term safety of topical calcineurin inhibitors has not been established.

Although a causal relationship has not been established, rare cases of malignancy (ie, skin cancer and lymphoma) have been reported in patients treated with topical calcineurin inhibitors, including tacrolimus ointment.

Therefore:
- Avoid continuous long-term use of topical calcineurin inhibitors, including tacrolimus ointment, in any age group, and limit application to areas of involvement with atopic dermatitis.
- Tacrolimus ointment is not indicated for use in children younger than 2 years of age. Only tacrolimus 0.03% ointment is indicated for use in children 2 to 15 years of age.

Indications

➤*Atopic dermatitis (moderate to severe):* Tacrolimus ointment, both 0.03% and 0.1% for adults, and only 0.03% for children 2 to 15 years of age, is indicated as second-line therapy for the short-term and noncontinuous chronic treatment of moderate to severe atopic dermatitis in nonimmunocompromised adults and children who have failed to respond adequately to other topical prescription treatments for atopic dermatitis, or when those treatments are not advisable.

➤*Off-label uses:*

Cutaneous lupus erythematosus – [4] = Insufficient documentation. Limited evidence suggests topical tacrolimus is effective in treating cutaneous lupus erythematosus. Several different treatment regimens have been explored, including different strengths of tacrolimus ointment and its use in combination with topical clobetasol. Several types of cutaneous lupus erythematosus have been treated with differing results. In general, twice-daily applications of tacrolimus 0.1% were more effective than once daily, and the discoid subtype may be more resistant to tacrolimus treatment than other types of cutaneous lupus erythematosus. Large, randomized trials are needed to determine the safety, efficacy, and optimal dosing regimens for treatment of the various types of cutaneous lupus erythematosus.

Genital lichen planus – [4] = Insufficient documentation. Initial data suggest that topical tacrolimus may be beneficial as a treatment option for women with erosive vulvovaginal lichen planus. Larger controlled trials are needed to further determine efficacy and tolerability.

Oral lichen planus – [3] = Safety concerns. Initial data suggest that topical tacrolimus ointment may be beneficial as a treatment option for patients with oral lichen planus. Additionally, it may be used as an alternative agent for treating patients with symptomatic oral lichen planus who have shown poor results with topical steroid therapy. Larger controlled trials are needed to determine efficacy and tolerability.

Psoriasis – [3] = Safety concerns. Topical tacrolimus was given a level B recommendation for intertriginous or facial psoriasis. The recommendation was based on level II evidence, considered to be limited-quality patient-oriented evidence.

Pyoderma gangrenosum – [2] = Fair documentation. Results of a published trial and several case reports/case series suggest that topical tacrolimus may be beneficial in the treatment of pyoderma gangrenosum.

Vitiligo – [3] = Safety concerns. Published information regarding the use of topical tacrolimus in the treatment of vitiligo suggests that this drug may have therapeutic benefit and was comparable to topical steroid therapy in very small trials (approximately 20 patients).

Administration and Dosage

➤*General dosing considerations:* The safety of tacrolimus ointment under occlusion, which may promote systemic exposure, has not been evaluated. Tacrolimus 0.03% and 0.1% ointment should not be used with occlusive dressings.

➤*Adults:*

Moderate to severe atopic dermatitis –

0.03% and 0.1% ointment: Apply a thin layer to the affected skin twice daily. The minimum amount should be rubbed in gently and completely to control signs and symptoms of atopic dermatitis.

If signs and symptoms (eg, itch, rash, redness) do not improve within 6 weeks, patients should be reexamined to confirm the diagnosis of atopic dermatitis.

- *Duration of therapy* – One source suggests continuing treatment for 1 week after signs and symptoms clear.
- *Discontinuation of therapy* – Stop using when signs and symptoms of atopic dermatitis resolve.

Off-label dosing –

Cutaneous lupus erythematosus: [4] = Insufficient documentation. Tacrolimus 0.1% or 0.3% ointment applied topically once or twice daily from 2 weeks to 6 months, used alone or in a combination formulation with clobetasol.

Genital lichen planus: [4] = Insufficient documentation. Topical tacrolimus 0.1% ointment applied twice daily for up to 3 months. Dose may be tapered down to the lowest effective maintenance dose after 4 weeks. The lowest dosage reported was tacrolimus 0.1% ointment 3 times weekly for 4 weeks.

Oral lichen planus: [3] = Safety concerns. The majority of the studies used topical tacrolimus 0.1% ointment; some used 0.03% and 0.3% as well. Dosing ranged from once daily to up to 4 times per day. The majority of the studies ranged from 4 to 8 weeks (a single study ranged from 2 to 39 months).

Psoriasis: [3] = Safety concerns. A sufficient quantity of 0.1% ointment to cover the affected area, applied twice daily. The maximum appropriate duration of use is not known.

Pyoderma gangrenosum: [2] = Fair documentation. Tacrolimus 0.1%, 0.3%, or 0.5% topical ointment or solution applied once or twice daily to every 3 days from 5 weeks to 12 months. In general, the dosage studied was topical tacrolimus 0.1% ointment once daily for 5 to 12 weeks as monotherapy or adjunctive therapy.

Vitiligo: [3] = Safety concerns. 0.03% to 0.1% ointment applied to lesions twice daily for up to several months.

➤*Children:*

Moderate to severe atopic dermatitis –

0.1% ointment:
- *16 years of age or older* – See Adults for dosing.

0.03% ointment:
- *2 to 15 years of age* – See Adults for dosing.

Off-label dosing –

Psoriasis: [3] = Safety concerns.
- *16 years of age and older* – A sufficient quantity of 0.1% ointment to cover the affected area, applied twice daily. The maximum appropriate duration of use is not known.

Vitiligo: [3] = Safety concerns. 0.03% to 0.1% ointment applied to lesions twice daily for up to several months.

➤*Long-term use:* If signs and symptoms of atopic dermatitis do not improve within 6 weeks, reexamine the patient and confirm the diagnosis. Continuous long-term use of topical calcineurin inhibitors, including tacrolimus ointment, should be avoided, and application should be limited to areas of involvement with atopic dermatitis.

➤*Storage/Stability:* Store at 25°C (77°F); excursions are permitted to 15° to 30°C (59° to 86°F).

Actions

➤*Pharmacology:* The mechanism of action of tacrolimus in atopic dermatitis is not known. While the following have been observed, the clinical significance of these observations in atopic dermatitis is not known. It has been demonstrated that tacrolimus inhibits T-lymphocyte activation by first binding to an intracellular protein, FKBP-12. A complex of tacrolimus-FKBP-12, calcium, calmodulin, and calcineurin is then formed and the phosphatase activity of calcineurin is inhibited. This effect has been shown to prevent the dephosphorylation and translocation of nuclear factor of activated T-cells (NF-AT), a nuclear component thought to initiate gene transcription for the formation of lymphokines (eg, interleukin-2, gamma interferon). Tacrolimus also inhibits the transcription for genes that encode IL-3, IL-4, IL-5, GM-CSF, and TNF-α, all of which are involved in the early stages of T-cell activation. Additionally, tacrolimus has been shown to inhibit the release of pre-formed mediators from skin mast cells and basophils, and to down regulate the expression of FcERI on Langerhans cells.

➤*Pharmacokinetics:*

Absorption –

Adults: The pooled results from 3 pharmacokinetic studies in 88 adult atopic dermatitis patients indicate that tacrolimus is minimally absorbed after the topical application of tacrolimus ointment. Peak tacrolimus blood concentrations ranged from undetectable to 20 ng/mL after single or multiple doses of tacrolimus 0.03% and 0.1% ointment, with 85% (75 of 88) of the patients having peak blood concentrations less than 2 ng/mL. In general, as treatment continued, systemic exposure declined as the skin returned to normal. In clinical studies with periodic blood sampling, a similar distribution of tacrolimus blood levels was also observed in adult patients, with 90% (1,253 of 1,391) of patients having a blood concentration less than 2 ng/mL.

The absolute bioavailability of tacrolimus in atopic dermatitis patients is approximately 0.5%. In adults with an average of 53% body surface area (BSA) treated, exposure area under the curve (AUC) of tacrolimus ointment is approximately 30-fold less than that seen with oral immunosuppressive doses in kidney and liver transplant patients.

Mean peak tacrolimus blood concentrations following oral administration (0.3 mg/kg/day) in adult kidney transplant (n = 26) and liver transplant (n = 17) patients are 24.2 ± 15.8 ng/mL and 68.5 ± 30 ng/mL, respectively. The lowest tacrolimus blood level at which systemic effects (eg, immunosuppression) can be observed is not known.

Children: In a pharmacokinetic study of 14 pediatric atopic dermatitis patients between the ages of 2 and 5 years, peak blood concentrations of tacrolimus ranged from undetectable to 14.8 ng/mL after single or multiple

TACROLIMUS — TOPICAL

doses of tacrolimus 0.03% ointment, with 86% (12 of 14) of patients having peak blood concentrations below 2 ng/mL throughout the study.

The highest peak concentration was observed in 1 patient with 82% BSA involvement on day 1 following application of tacrolimus 0.03% ointment. The peak concentrations for this subject were 14.8 ng/mL on day 1 and 4.1 ng/mL on day 14. Mean peak tacrolimus blood concentrations following oral administration in children with a history of liver transplant (n = 9) were 43.4 ± 27.9 ng/mL.

In a similar pharmacokinetic study with 61 enrolled children (6 to 12 years of age) with atopic dermatitis, peak tacrolimus blood concentrations ranged from undetectable to 5.3 ng/mL after single or multiple doses of tacrolimus 0.1% ointment, with 91% (52 of 57) of evaluable patients having peak blood concentrations below 2 ng/mL throughout the study period. When detected, systemic exposure generally declined as treatment continued.

In clinical studies with periodic blood sampling, a similar distribution of tacrolimus blood levels was also observed, with 98% (509 of 522) of children having a blood concentration below 2 ng/mL.

Distribution – The plasma protein binding of tacrolimus is approximately 99% and is independent of concentration over a range of 5 to 50 ng/mL. Tacrolimus is bound mainly to albumin and alpha-1-acid glycoprotein, and has a high level of association with erythrocytes. The distribution of tacrolimus between whole blood and plasma depends on several factors, such as hematocrit, temperature at the time of plasma separation, drug concentration, and plasma protein concentration. In a US study, the ratio of whole blood concentration to plasma concentration averaged 35 (range, 12 to 67).

There was no evidence based on blood concentrations that tacrolimus accumulates systemically upon intermittent topical application for periods of up to 1 year. As with other topical calcineurin inhibitors, it is not known whether tacrolimus is distributed into the lymphatic system.

Metabolism – Tacrolimus is extensively metabolized by the mixed-function oxidase system, primarily the cytochrome P-450 system (CYP3A). A metabolic pathway leading to the formation of 8 possible metabolites has been proposed. Demethylation and hydroxylation were identified as the primary mechanisms of biotransformation in vitro. The major metabolite identified in incubations with human liver microsomes is 13-demethyl tacrolimus. In in vitro studies, a 31-demethyl metabolite has been reported to have the same activity as tacrolimus.

Excretion – The mean clearance following intravenous (IV) administration of tacrolimus is 0.04, 0.083, and 0.053 L/h/kg in healthy volunteers, adult kidney transplant patients, and adult liver transplant patients, respectively. Less than 1% of the dose administered is excreted unchanged in urine.

In a mass balance study of IV administered radiolabeled tacrolimus to 6 healthy volunteers, the mean recovery of radiolabel was 77.8% ± 12.7%. Fecal elimination accounted for 92.4 ± 1%, and the elimination half-life based on radioactivity was 48.1 ± 15.9 hours, whereas it was 43.5 ± 11.6 hours based on tacrolimus concentrations. The mean clearance of radiolabel was 0.029 ± 0.015 L/h/kg, and the clearance of tacrolimus was 0.029 ± 0.009 L/h/kg.

When administered orally, the mean recovery of the radiolabel was 94.9% ± 30.7%. Fecal elimination accounted for 92.6 ± 30.7%, urinary elimination accounted for 2.3 ± 1.1%, and the elimination half-life based on radioactivity was 31.9 ± 10.5 hours, whereas it was 48.4 ± 12.3 hours based on tacrolimus concentrations. The mean clearance of radiolabel was 0.226 ± 0.116 L/h/kg and clearance of tacrolimus 0.172 ± 0.088 L/h/kg.

Contraindications

History of hypersensitivity to tacrolimus or any other component of the ointment.

Warnings/Precautions

➤*Infections/Lymphomas/Skin Malignancies:* Prolonged systemic use of calcineurin inhibitors for sustained immunosuppression in animal studies and transplant patients following systemic administration has been associated with an increased risk of infections, lymphomas, and skin malignancies. These risks are associated with the intensity and duration of immunosuppression.

Based on the preceding information and the mechanism of action, there is a concern about potential risk with the use of topical calcineurin inhibitors, including tacrolimus ointment. While a causal relationship has not been established, rare cases of skin malignancy and lymphoma have been reported in patients treated with topical calcineurin inhibitors, including tacrolimus ointment.

➤*Immunocompromised patients:* Do not use tacrolimus ointment in immunocompromised adults and children.

➤*Long-term use:* If signs and symptoms of atopic dermatitis do not improve within 6 weeks, reexamine the patient and confirm the diagnosis.

The safety of tacrolimus ointment has not been established beyond 1 year of noncontinuous use.

➤*Renal effects:* Rare postmarketing cases of acute renal failure have been reported in patients treated with tacrolimus ointment. Systemic absorption is more likely to occur in patients with epidermal barrier defects, especially when tacrolimus is applied to large BSAs. Exercise caution in patients predisposed to renal function impairment.

➤*Premalignant/Malignant skin conditions:* Avoid the use of tacrolimus ointment on premalignant and malignant skin conditions. Some malignant skin conditions, such as cutaneous T-cell lymphoma, may mimic atopic dermatitis.

➤*Netherton syndrome:* The use of tacrolimus ointment in patients with Netherton syndrome or other skin diseases in which there is the potential for increased systemic absorption of tacrolimus is not recommended. The safety of tacrolimus ointment has not been established in patients with generalized erythroderma.

➤*Local symptoms:* The use of tacrolimus ointment may cause local symptoms such as skin burning (burning sensation, stinging, soreness) or pruritus. Localized symptoms are most common during the first few days of tacrolimus ointment application and typically improve as the lesions of atopic dermatitis resolve. With tacrolimus 0.1% ointment, 90% of the skin burning events had a duration between 2 minutes and 3 hours (median, 15 minutes). Ninety percent of the pruritus events had a duration between 3 minutes and 10 hours (median, 20 minutes).

➤*Bacterial and viral skin infections:* Before commencing treatment with tacrolimus ointment, cutaneous bacterial or viral infections at treatment sites should be resolved. Studies have not evaluated the safety and efficacy of tacrolimus ointment in the treatment of clinically infected atopic dermatitis.

While patients with atopic dermatitis are predisposed to superficial skin infections, including eczema herpeticum (Kaposi varicelliform eruption), treatment with tacrolimus ointment may be independently associated with an increased risk of varicella zoster virus infection (chickenpox or shingles), herpes simplex virus infection, or eczema herpeticum.

➤*Lymphadenopathy:* In clinical studies, 112 of 13,494 (0.8%) cases of lymphadenopathy were reported and were usually related to infections (particularly of the skin) and noted to resolve upon appropriate antibiotic therapy. Of these 112 cases, the majority had either a clear etiology or were known to resolve. Transplant patients receiving immunosuppressive regimens (eg, systemic tacrolimus) are at increased risk for developing lymphoma; therefore, patients who receive tacrolimus ointment and develop lymphadenopathy should have the etiology of their lymphadenopathy investigated. In the absence of a clear etiology for the lymphadenopathy, or in the presence of acute infectious mononucleosis, discontinue tacrolimus ointment. Monitor patients who develop lymphadenopathy to ensure that the lymphadenopathy resolves.

➤*Photosensitivity:* During the course of treatment, patients should minimize or avoid natural or artificial sunlight exposure, even while tacrolimus is not on the skin. It is not known whether tacrolimus ointment interferes with skin response to UV damage.

➤*Pregnancy:* Category C.

Teratogenic – Reproduction studies were carried out with systemically administered tacrolimus in rats and rabbits. Adverse reactions on the fetus were observed mainly at oral dose levels that were toxic to dams. Tacrolimus at oral doses of 0.32 and 1 mg/kg (0.04 to 0.12 times MRHD based on BSA) during organogenesis in rabbits was associated with maternal toxicity as well as an increase in incidence of abortions. At the higher dose only, an increased incidence of malformations and developmental variations was also seen. Tacrolimus, at oral doses of 3.2 mg/kg during organogenesis in rats, was associated with maternal toxicity and caused an increase in late resorptions, decreased numbers of live births, and decreased pup weight and viability. Tacrolimus, given orally at 1 and 3.2 mg/kg (0.04 to 0.12 times MRHD based on BSA) to pregnant rats after organogenesis and during lactation, was associated with reduced pup weights.

There are no adequate and well-controlled studies of systemically administered tacrolimus in pregnant women. Tacrolimus is transferred across the placenta. The use of systemically administered tacrolimus during pregnancy has been associated with neonatal hyperkalemia and renal dysfunction. Only use tacrolimus ointment during pregnancy if the potential benefit to the mother justifies a potential risk to the fetus.

➤*Lactation:* Although systemic absorption of tacrolimus following topical applications of tacrolimus ointment is minimal relative to systemic administration, it is known that tacrolimus is excreted in human milk. Because of the potential for serious adverse reactions in breast-feeding infants from tacrolimus, decide whether to discontinue breast-feeding or the drug, taking into account the importance of the drug to the mother.

➤*Children:* Tacrolimus ointment is not indicated for children younger than 2 years of age.

Only the lower concentration, 0.03%, of tacrolimus ointment is recommended for use as a second-line therapy for short-term and noncontinuous chronic treatment of moderate to severe atopic dermatitis in nonimmunocompromised children 2 to 15 years of age who have failed to respond adequately to other topical prescription treatments for atopic dermatitis, or when those treatments are not advisable.

The long-term safety and effects of tacrolimus ointment on the developing immune system are unknown.

Four studies were conducted involving a total of about 4,400 patients 2 to 15 years of age: one 12-week, randomized, vehicle-controlled study and 3 open-label safety studies of 1 to 3 years' duration. About 2,500 of these patients were 2 to 6 years of age.

In these studies, the most common adverse reactions associated with tacrolimus ointment application in children were skin burning and pruritus. In addition to skin burning and pruritus, the less common events (less than 5%) of varicella zoster (mostly chickenpox) and vesiculobullous rash were more frequent in patients treated with tacrolimus 0.03% ointment compared with vehicle. In the open-label safety studies, the incidence of adverse reactions, including infections, did not increase with increased duration of study drug exposure or amount of ointment used. In about 4,400 children treated with tacrolimus ointment, 24 (0.5%) were reported with eczema herpeticum. Because the safety and efficacy of tacrolimus ointment have not been established in children younger than 2 years of age, its use in this age group is not recommended.

TACROLIMUS — TOPICAL

In an open-label study, immune response to a 23-valent pneumococcal polysaccharide vaccine was assessed in 23 children 2 to 12 years of age with moderate to severe atopic dermatitis treated with tacrolimus 0.03% ointment. Protective antibody titers developed in all patients. Similarly, in a 7-month, double-blind trial, the vaccination response to meningococcal serogroup C was equivalent in children 2 to 11 years of age with moderate to severe atopic dermatitis treated with tacrolimus 0.03% ointment (n = 121) or a hydrocortisone ointment regimen (n = 111) and in healthy children (n = 44).

➤*Monitoring:* Monitor patients who develop lymphadenopathy to ensure that the lymphadenopathy resolves.

Drug Interactions

➤*QT prolongation:* An additive effect of tacrolimus with other drugs that prolong the QT interval cannot be excluded. The following drugs may prolong the QT interval and increase the risk of life-threatening cardiac arrhythmias, including torsades de pointes: Antiarrhythmic agents (eg, amiodarone, bretylium, disopyramide, dofetilide, procainamide, quinidine, and sotalol), arsenic trioxide, chlorpromazine, cisapride, dolasetron, droperidol, mefloquine, mesoridazine, moxifloxacin, pentamidine, pimozide, tacrolimus, thioridazine, and ziprasidone. For a more complete list of drugs that may prolong the QT interval, see the appendix, Drug-Induced Prolongation of the QT Interval and Torsades de Pointes.

Tacrolimus Topical Drug Interactions

Precipitant drug	Object drug[a]		Description
CYP3A4 inhibitors (eg, calcium channel blockers, cimetidine, erythromycin, itraconazole, ketoconazole, fluconazole)	Tacrolimus	↑	Use with caution.
Tacrolimus	Alcohol	↑	Risk of transient facial flushing may be increased. Avoid alcohol during topical tacrolimus.

[a] ↑ = Object drug increased.

Adverse Reactions

No phototoxicity or photoallergenicity was detected in clinical studies with 12 and 216 healthy volunteers, respectively. One out of 198 healthy volunteers showed evidence of sensitization in a contact sensitization study.

In three 12-week, randomized, vehicle-controlled studies and 4 safety studies, 655 and 9,163 patients, respectively, were treated with tacrolimus ointment. The duration of follow-up for adults and children in the safety studies is tabulated in the following table:

Tacrolimus Topical Duration of Follow-up in 4 Open-Label Safety Studies

Time on study	Adults	Children	Total
< 1 year	4,682	4,481	9,163
≥ 1 year	1,185	1,349	2,534
≥ 2 years	200	275	475
≥ 3 years	118	182	300

The following table depicts the adjusted incidence of adverse reactions pooled across the 3 identically designed 12-week controlled studies for patients in vehicle, tacrolimus 0.03% ointment, and tacrolimus 0.1% ointment treatment groups. The following table also depicts the unadjusted incidence of adverse reactions in 4 safety studies, regardless of relationship to study drug.

Tacrolimus Topical Adverse Reactions

	12-week, randomized, double-blind, phase 3 studies 12-week adjusted incidence rate (%)					Open-label studies (up to 3 years) Tacrolimus 0.1% and 0.03% ointment incidence rate (%)		
	Adults			Children				
Adverse reaction	Vehicle (n = 212)	Tacrolimus 0.03% ointment (n = 210)	Tacrolimus 0.1% ointment (n = 209)	Vehicle (n = 116)	Tacrolimus 0.03% ointment (n = 118)	Adults (n = 4,682)	Children (n = 4,481)	Total (n = 9,163)
Cardiovascular								
Hypertension	0%	0%	1%	0%	0%	2%	0%	1%
CNS								
Asthenia	1%	2%	3%	0%	0 %	1%	0%	1%
Depression	1%	2%	1%	0%	0%	1%	0%	1%
Headache[a]	11%	20%	19%	8%	5%	13%	9%	11%
Hyperesthesia[a]	1%	3%	7%	0%	0%	2%	0 %	1%
Insomnia	3%	4%	3%	1%	1 %	2%	0%	1%
Paresthesia	1%	3%	3%	0%	0%	2%	1%	2%
Dermatologic								
Acne[a]	2%	4%	7%	1%	0%	3%	2%	3%
Alopecia	0%	1%	1%	0%	0%	1%	1%	1%
Cellulitis	1%	1%	1%	0%	0%	1%	1%	1%
Contact dermatitis	1%	3%	3%	3%	4%	2%	2%	2%
Dry skin	7%	3%	3%	0%	1%	1%	1%	1%
Eczema	2%	2%	2%	0%	0%	1%	0%	1%
Eczema herpeticum	0%	1%	1%	0%	2%	0%	0%	0%
Exfoliative dermatitis	3%	3%	1%	0%	0%	0%	1%	0%
Folliculitis[a]	1%	6%	4%	0%	2%	4%	2%	3%
Fungal dermatitis	0%	2%	1%	3%	0%	2%	4%	3%
Maculopapular rash	2%	2%	2%	3%	0%	2%	1%	1%
Pruritus[a]	37%	46%	46%	27%	41%	25%	19%	22%
Pustular rash	2%	3%	4%	3%	2%	2%	7%	5%
Rash[a]	1%	5%	2%	4%	2%	2%	3%	3%
Skin burning[a]	26%	46%	58%	29%	43%	28%	20%	24%
Skin disorder	2%	2%	1%	1%	4%	2%	2%	2%
Skin erythema	20%	25%	28%	13%	12%	12%	7%	9%
Skin infection	11%	12%	5%	14%	10%	9%	16%	12%
Skin neoplasm benign[b]	1%	1%	1%	0%	0%	1%	2%	2%
Skin tingling[a]	2%	3%	8%	1%	2%	2%	1%	1%
Sunburn	1%	2%	1%	0%	0%	2%	1%	1%
Urticaria	3%	3%	6%	1%	1%	3%	4%	4%
Varicella zoster/herpes zoster[c]	0%	1%	0%	0%	5%	1%	2%	2%

TACROLIMUS — TOPICAL

Tacrolimus Topical Adverse Reactions

Adverse reaction	12-week, randomized, double-blind, phase 3 studies 12-week adjusted incidence rate (%)					Open-label studies (up to 3 years) Tacrolimus 0.1% and 0.03% ointment incidence rate (%)		
	Adults			Children				
	Vehicle (n = 212)	Tacrolimus 0.03% ointment (n = 210)	Tacrolimus 0.1% ointment (n = 209)	Vehicle (n = 116)	Tacrolimus 0.03% ointment (n = 118)	Adults (n = 4,682)	Children (n = 4,481)	Total (n = 9,163)
Vesiculobullous rash[a]	3%	3%	2%	0%	4%	2%	1%	1%
GI								
Abdominal pain	3%	1%	1%	2%	3%	1%	3%	2%
Diarrhea	3%	3%	4%	2%	5%	2%	4%	3%
Dyspepsia[a]	1%	1%	4%	0%	0%	2%	2%	2%
Gastroenteritis	1%	2%	2%	3%	0%	2%	4%	3%
Nausea	4%	3%	2%	0%	1%	2%	1%	2%
Periodontal abscess	1%	0%	1%	0%	0%	1%	1%	1%
Tooth disorder	0%	1%	1%	1%	0%	2%	1%	1%
Vomiting	0%	1%	1%	7%	6%	1%	4%	3%
GU								
Dysmenorrhea	2%	4%	4%	0%	0%	2%	1%	1%
Urinary tract infection	0%	0%	1%	0%	0%	2%	1%	2%
Musculoskeletal								
Arthralgia	1%	1%	3%	2%	0%	2%	1%	2%
Back pain[a]	0%	2%	2%	1%	1%	3%	0%	2%
Myalgia[a]	0%	3%	2%	0%	0%	2%	1%	1%
Metabolic								
Face edema	2%	2%	1%	2%	1%	1%	1%	1%
Peripheral edema	2%	4%	3%	0%	0%	2%	0%	1%
Respiratory								
Asthma	4%	6%	4%	6%	6%	4%	13%	8%
Bronchitis	0%	2%	2%	3%	3%	4%	4%	4%
Cough increased	2%	1%	1%	14%	18%	3%	10%	6%
Pharyngitis	3%	3%	4%	11%	6%	4%	12%	8%
Pneumonia	0%	1%	1%	2%	0%	1%	3%	2%
Rhinitis	4%	3%	2%	2%	6%	2%	4%	3%
Sinusitis[a]	1%	4%	2%	8%	3%	6%	7%	6%
Special senses								
Conjunctivitis	0%	2%	2%	2%	1%	3%	3%	3%
Ear pain	1%	0%	1%	0%	1%	0%	1%	1%
Otitis media	4%	0%	1%	6%	12%	2%	11%	6%
Miscellaneous								
Accidental injury	4%	3%	6%	3%	6%	6%	8%	7%
Alcohol intolerance[a]	0%	3%	7%	0%	0%	4%	0%	2%
Allergic reaction	8%	12%	6%	8%	4%	9%	13%	11%
Cyst[a]	0%	1%	3%	0%	0%	1%	0%	1%
Exacerbation of untreated area	1%	0%	1%	1%	0%	1%	1%	1%
Fever	4%	4%	1%	13%	21%	2%	14%	8%
Flu-like symptoms[a]	19%	23%	31%	25%	28%	22%	34%	28%
Herpes simplex	4%	4%	4%	2%	0%	4%	3%	3%
Infection	1%	1%	2%	9%	7%	6%	10%	8%
Lack of drug effect	1%	1%	0%	1%	1%	6%	6%	6%
Lymphadenopathy	2%	2%	1%	0%	3%	1%	2%	1%
Pain	1%	2%	1%	0%	1%	2%	1%	2%
Procedural complication	1%	0%	0%	1%	0%	1%	1%	1%

[a] May be reasonably associated with the use of this drug product.
[b] Generally "warts."
[c] All the herpes zoster cases in the pediatric 12-week study and the majority of cases in the open-label studies in children were reported as chickenpox.

➤*Other adverse reactions (0.2% to less than 1%):*

Cardiovascular – Chest pain, syncope, tachycardia, valvular heart disease, vasodilatation.

CNS – Abnormal thinking, anxiety, chills, dizziness, hypertonia, malaise, migraine, vertigo.

Dermatologic – Cutaneous moniliasis, furunculosis, leukoderma, nail disorder, photosensitivity reaction, seborrhea, skin carcinoma, skin discoloration, skin hypertrophy, skin ulcer, sweating.

GI – Anorexia, colitis, constipation, cramps, gastritis, GI disorder, hernia, mouth ulceration, oral moniliasis, rectal disorder, stomatitis, taste perversion, tooth caries.

GU – Cystitis, moniliasis, vaginal moniliasis, vaginitis.

Hematologic – Anemia, bilirubinemia, ecchymosis, hypercholerestemia.

Metabolic – Dehydration, edema, hypothyroidism.

Musculoskeletal – Arthritis, arthrosis, bone disorder, bursitis, joint disorder, neck pain, tendon disorder.

Respiratory – Dry mouth/nose, dyspnea, epistaxis, laryngitis, lung disorder.

Special senses – Abnormal vision, blepharitis, cataract, conjunctival edema, dry eyes, ear disorder, eye pain, otitis externa.

Miscellaneous – Abscess, anaphylactoid reaction, breast neoplasm benign, neoplasm benign, unintended pregnancy.

➤*Postmarketing:* The following adverse reactions have been identified during postapproval use of tacrolimus ointment. Because these reactions are reported voluntarily from a population of uncertain size, it is not always possible to reliably estimate their frequency or establish a causal relationship to drug exposure.

CNS – Seizures.

Dermatologic – Rosacea.

Renal – Acute renal failure in patients with or without Netherton syndrome, renal function impairment.

TACROLIMUS — TOPICAL

Miscellaneous – Basal cell carcinoma, bullous impetigo, lymphomas, malignant melanoma, osteomyelitis, septicemia, squamous cell carcinoma.

Overdosage

Ointment is not for oral use. Oral ingestion of tacrolimus ointment may lead to adverse reactions associated with systemic administration of tacrolimus. If oral ingestion occurs, patients should seek medical advice.

Patient Information

Tacrolimus ointment should only be used as directed and only for the disorder for which it was prescribed.

Tacrolimus ointment is for external use only.

As with any topical medication, patients or caregivers should wash hands after application if hands are not an area for treatment.

While using tacrolimus ointment, the patient should minimize or avoid exposure to natural or artificial sunlight (tanning beds or UVA/B treatment).

Patients should report any signs of adverse reactions to their physician.

Before applying tacrolimus after a bath or shower, patients should be sure the skin is completely dry.

PIMECROLIMUS

Rx	**Elidel** (Novartis)	**Cream:** 1%	In 30, 60, and 100 g tubes.[a]

[a] With benzyl alcohol, cetyl alcohol, oleyl alcohol, and stearyl alcohol.

PIMECROLIMUS — TOPICAL

WARNING

Long-term safety of topical calcineurin inhibitors has not been established.

Although a causal relationship has not been established, rare cases of malignancy (eg, skin malignancy, lymphoma) have been reported in patients treated with topical calcineurin inhibitors including pimecrolimus.

Therefore,

- Avoid continuous, long-term use of topical calcineurin inhibitors, including pimecrolimus, in any age group, and limit application to areas of involvement with atopic dermatitis.
- Pimecrolimus is not indicated for use in children younger than 2 years of age.

Indications

➤*Atopic dermatitis:* As second-line therapy for short-term and noncontinuous chronic treatment of mild to moderate atopic dermatitis in nonimmunocompromised patients 2 years of age and older who have failed to respond adequately to other topical prescription treatments, or when those treatments are not advisable.

➤*Off-label uses:*

Lichen planus (genital) – [3] = Safety concerns. Preliminary data from a case series suggest that topical pimecrolimus may be useful as second-line treatment of steroid-resistant genital lichen planus.

Lichen planus (oral) – [3] = Safety concerns. Preliminary data from short-term controlled studies and case series suggest that topical pimecrolimus maybe useful as second-line treatment of oral lichen planus.

Psoriasis – [3] = Safety concerns. Topical pimecrolimus was given a level B recommendation. The recommendation was based on level II evidence, considered to be limited-quality patient-oriented evidence.

Vitiligo – [3] = Safety concerns. Published information regarding the use of pimecrolimus in the treatment of vitiligo suggests that it may have therapeutic benefit and is comparable to topical steroid therapy in very small trials (fewer than 15 patients).

Administration and Dosage

➤*General dosing considerations:* The safety of pimecrolimus under occlusion, which may promote systemic exposure, has not been evaluated. Pimecrolimus should not be used with occlusive dressings.

➤*Adults:*

Atopic dermatitis –

Usual dosage: Apply a thin layer of pimecrolimus cream to the affected skin twice daily.

Duration of therapy: Avoid continuous, long-term use of pimecrolimus, and limit application to areas of involvement with atopic dermatitis.

If signs and symptoms persist longer than 6 weeks, patients should be reexamined by their health care provider to confirm the diagnosis of atopic dermatitis.

Discontinuation of therapy: The patient or caregiver should stop using pimecrolimus when signs and symptoms (eg, itch, rash, redness) resolve and should be instructed on what actions to take if symptoms recur.

Off-label dosing –

Lichen planus (genital): [3] = Safety concerns. 1% cream applied twice daily to affected areas for 4 to 6 weeks.

Lichen planus (oral): [3] = Safety concerns. 1% cream applied twice daily to affected areas for 4 weeks and up to 3 months in one case report.

Psoriasis: [3] = Safety concerns. A sufficient quantity of 0.1% cream to cover the affected area, applied twice daily. The maximum appropriate duration of use is not known.

Vitiligo: [3] = Safety concerns. 1% cream applied twice daily for 2 months.

➤*Children:*

Atopic dermatitis –

2 years of age and older: See Adults for dosing.

Off-label dosing –

Vitiligo: [3] = Safety concerns.

- *Adolescents* – 1% cream applied twice daily for 2 months.

➤*Storage/Stability:* Store at 25°C (77°F); excursions are permitted to 15° to 30°C (59° to 86°F). Do not freeze.

Actions

➤*Pharmacology:* The mechanism of action of pimecrolimus in atopic dermatitis is not known. While the following have been observed, the clinical significance of these observations in atopic dermatitis is not known. It has been demonstrated that pimecrolimus binds with high affinity to macrophilin-12 (FKBP-12) and inhibits the calcium-dependent phosphatase, calcineurin. As a consequence, it inhibits T cell activation by blocking the transcription of early cytokines. In particular, pimecrolimus inhibits at nanomolar concentrations interleukin-2 and interferon gamma (Th1-type) and interleukin-4 and interleukin-10 (Th2-type) cytokine synthesis in human T cells. In addition, pimecrolimus prevents the release of inflammatory cytokines and mediators from mast cells in vitro after stimulation by antigen/immunoglobulin E.

➤*Pharmacokinetics:*

Absorption – In adult patients (N = 52) being treated for atopic dermatitis (13% to 62% body surface area [BSA] involvement) for periods up to a year, a maximum pimecrolimus concentration of 1.4 ng/mL was observed among subjects with detectable blood levels. In the majority of samples in adult subjects (91%; 1,244/1,362), blood concentrations of pimecrolimus were less than 0.5 ng/mL.

Distribution – In vitro studies of the protein binding of pimecrolimus indicate that it is 74% to 87% bound to plasma proteins. As with other topical calcineurin inhibitors, it is not known whether pimecrolimus is absorbed into cutaneous lymphatic vessels or in regional lymph nodes.

Metabolism – Following the administration of a single oral radiolabeled dose of pimecrolimus, numerous circulating O-demethylation metabolites were seen. Studies with human liver microsomes indicate that pimecrolimus is metabolized in vitro by the CYP3A subfamily of metabolizing enzymes. No evidence of skin-mediated drug metabolism was identified in vivo using the minipig or in vitro using stripped human skin.

Excretion – Based on the results of the aforementioned radiolabeled study, following a single oral dose of pimecrolimus approximately 81% of the administered radioactivity was recovered, primarily in the feces (78.4%) as metabolites. Less than 1% of the radioactivity found in the feces was caused by unchanged pimecrolimus.

Contraindications

History of hypersensitivity to pimecrolimus or any of the components of the cream.

Warnings/Precautions

➤*Prolonged use:* Prolonged systemic use of calcineurin inhibitors for sustained immunosuppression in animal studies and transplant patients following systemic administration has been associated with an increased risk of infections, lymphomas, and skin malignancies. These risks are associated with the intensity and duration of immunosuppression.

Based on this information and the mechanism of action, there is a concern about a potential risk with the use of topical calcineurin inhibitors, including pimecrolimus. While a causal relationship has not been established, rare cases of skin malignancy and lymphoma have been reported in patients treated with topical calcineurin inhibitors, including pimecrolimus. Therefore, do not use pimecrolimus in immunocompromised adults and children; if signs and symptoms of atopic dermatitis do not improve within 6 weeks, health care providers should reexamine patients and have patients' diagnosis confirmed. The safety of pimecrolimus has not been established beyond 1 year of noncontinuous use.

See the Warning box for more information.

➤*Netherton syndrome:* Do not use pimecrolimus in patients with Netherton syndrome or other skin diseases in which there is the potential of increased systemic absorption of pimecrolimus. The safety of pimecrolimus has not been established in patients with generalized erythroderma.

➤*Local reactions:* The use of pimecrolimus may cause local symptoms such as skin burning (burning sensation, stinging, soreness) or pruritus. Localized symptoms are most common during the first few days of pimecrolimus application and typically improve as the lesions of atopic dermatitis resolve. Most application site reactions lasted no more than 5 days, were mild to moderate in severity, and started within 1 to 5 days of treatment.

➤*Malignant or premalignant skin conditions:* Avoid use of pimecrolimus on malignant or premalignant skin conditions. Malignant or premalignant skin conditions, such as cutaneous T-cell lymphoma, can present as dermatitis.

PIMECROLIMUS — TOPICAL

➤*Lymphadenopathy:* In clinical studies, 14 of 1,544 cases of lymphadenopathy (0.9%) were reported while using pimecrolimus. These cases of lymphadenopathy were usually related to infections and noted to resolve upon appropriate antibiotic therapy. Of these 14 cases, the majority had either a clear etiology or were known to resolve. Patients who receive pimecrolimus and develop lymphadenopathy should have the etiology of their lymphadenopathy investigated. In the absence of a clear etiology for the lymphadenopathy, or in the presence of acute infectious mononucleosis, consider discontinuation of pimecrolimus. Monitor patients who develop lymphadenopathy to ensure that the lymphadenopathy resolves.

➤*Skin disorders:*

Atopic dermatitis – Studies have not evaluated the safety and efficacy of pimecrolimus in the treatment of clinically infected atopic dermatitis. Before commencing treatment with pimecrolimus, resolve bacterial or viral infections at treatment sites. While patients with atopic dermatitis are predisposed to superficial skin infections including eczema herpeticum (Kaposi varicelliform eruption), treatment with pimecrolimus may be associated with an increased risk of varicella-zoster virus infection (chickenpox or shingles), herpes simplex virus infection, or eczema herpeticum. In the presence of these skin infections, evaluate the balance of risks and benefits associated with pimecrolimus use.

Skin papilloma or warts – In clinical studies, 15 of 1,544 cases of skin papilloma or warts (1%) were observed in patients using pimecrolimus. The youngest patient was 2 years of age and the oldest was 12 years of age. In cases in which there is worsening of skin papillomas or they do not respond to conventional therapy, consider discontinuation of pimecrolimus until complete resolution of the warts is achieved.

➤*Photosensitivity:* The enhancement of ultraviolet carcinogenicity is not necessarily dependent on phototoxic mechanisms. Despite the absence of observed phototoxicity in humans, pimecrolimus shortened the time to skin tumor formation in an animal photocarcinogenicity study. Therefore, it is prudent for patients to minimize or avoid natural or artificial sunlight exposure, even while pimecrolimus is not on the skin. The potential reactions of pimecrolimus on skin response to ultraviolet damage are not known.

➤*Pregnancy: Category C.* There are no adequate and well-controlled studies of topically administered pimecrolimus in pregnant women. The experience with pimecrolimus when used by pregnant women is too limited to permit assessment of the safety of its use during pregnancy.

In dermal embryofetal developmental studies, no maternal or fetal toxicity was observed up to the highest practicable dosages tested, 10 mg/kg/day (pimecrolimus 1% cream) in rats (0.14 times the MRHD based on BSA) and 10 mg/kg/day (pimecrolimus 1% cream) in rabbits (0.65 times the MRHD based on AUC comparisons). The pimecrolimus 1% cream was administered topically for 6 hours/day during the period of organogenesis in rats and rabbits (gestational days 6 to 21 in rats and gestational days 6 to 20 in rabbits).

A second dermal embryofetal development study was conducted in rats using pimecrolimus applied dermally to pregnant rats (1 g cream/kg body weight of pimecrolimus 0.2%, 0.6%, and 1% cream) from gestation day 6 to 17 at dosages of 2, 6, and 10 mg/kg/day with daily exposure of approximately 22 hours. No maternal, reproductive, or embryofetal toxicity attributable to pimecrolimus was noted at 10 mg/kg/day (0.66 times the MRHD based on AUC comparisons), the highest dosage evaluated in this study. No teratogenicity was noted in this study at any dosage.

A combined oral fertility and embryofetal developmental study was conducted in rats and an oral embryofetal developmental study was conducted in rabbits. Pimecrolimus was administered during the period of organogenesis (2 weeks prior to mating until gestational day 16 in rats, gestational days 6 to 18 in rabbits) up to dosage levels of 45 mg/kg/day in rats and 20 mg/kg/day in rabbits. In the absence of maternal toxicity, indicators of embryofetal toxicity (postimplantation loss and reduction in litter size) were noted at 45 mg/kg/day (38 times the MRHD based on AUC comparisons) in the oral fertility and embryofetal developmental study conducted in rats. No malformations in the fetuses were noted at 45 mg/kg/day (38 times the MRHD based on AUC comparisons) in this study. No maternal toxicity, embryotoxicity, or teratogenicity were noted in the oral rabbit embryofetal developmental toxicity study at 20 mg/kg/day (3.9 times the MRHD based on AUC comparisons), which was the highest dosage tested in this study.

A second oral embryofetal development study was conducted in rats. Pimecrolimus was administered during the period of organogenesis (gestational days 6 to 17) at dosages of 2, 10, and 45 mg/kg/day. Maternal toxicity, embryolethality, and fetotoxicity were noted at 45 mg/kg/day (271 times the MRHD based on AUC comparisons). A slight increase in skeletal variations that were indicative of delayed skeletal ossification was also noted at this dosage. No maternal toxicity, embryolethality, or fetotoxicity were noted at 10 mg/kg/day (16 times the MRHD based on AUC comparisons). No teratogenicity was noted in this study at any dose.

A second oral embryofetal development study was conducted in rabbits. Pimecrolimus was administered during the period of organogenesis (gestational days 7 to 20) at dosages of 2, 6, and 20 mg/kg/day. Maternal toxicity, embryotoxicity, and fetotoxicity were noted at 20 mg/kg/day (12 times the MRHD based on AUC comparisons). A slight increase in skeletal variations that were indicative of delayed skeletal ossification was also noted at this dosage. No maternal toxicity, embryotoxicity, or fetotoxicity were noted at 6 mg/kg/day (5 times the MRHD based on AUC comparisons. No teratogenicity was noted in this study at any dosage.

An oral peri- and postnatal developmental study was conducted in rats. Pimecrolimus was administered from gestational day 6 through lactational day 21 up to a dosage level of 40 mg/kg/day. Only 2 of 22 females delivered live pups at the highest dosage of 40 mg/kg/day. Postnatal survival, development of the F1 generation, their subsequent maturation and fertility were not affected at 10 mg/kg/day (12 times the MRHD based on AUC comparisons), the highest dosage evaluated in this study.

Pimecrolimus was transferred across the placenta in oral rat and rabbit embryofetal developmental studies.

There are, however, no adequate and well-controlled studies in pregnant women. Because animal reproduction studies are not always predictive of human response, only use this drug if clearly needed during pregnancy.

➤*Lactation:* It is not known whether this drug is excreted in human milk. The molecular weight (about 810) and the long elimination half-life (50 to 100 hours after 28 days of therapy) suggest that if the drug reaches the maternal circulation excretion into breast milk will occur. However, the minimal blood concentrations, high plasma protein binding (99.5%), and extensive metabolism to inactivate metabolites suggest that such excretion will be limited, if it occurs at all. Because of the potential for serious adverse reactions in breast-feeding infants from pimecrolimus, make a decision whether to discontinue breast-feeding or the drug, taking into account the importance of the drug to the mother.

➤*Children:* Pimecrolimus is not indicated for use in children younger than 2 years of age.

The long-term safety and effects of pimecrolimus on the developing immune system in infants are unknown.

The most common local adverse reaction in the short-term studies of pimecrolimus in children 2 to 17 years of age was application site burning (10% vs 13% vehicle); the incidence in the long-term study was 9% pimecrolimus vs 7% vehicle. Adverse reactions that were more frequent (greater than 5%) in patients treated with pimecrolimus compared with vehicle were headache (14% vs 9%) in the short-term trial. Nasopharyngitis (26% vs 21%), influenza (13% vs 4%), pharyngitis (8% vs 3%), viral infection (7% vs 1%), pyrexia (13% vs 5%), cough (16% vs 11%), and headache (25% vs 16%) were increased over vehicle in the 1-year safety study. In 843 patients 2 to 17 years of age treated with pimecrolimus, 9 (0.8%) developed eczema herpeticum (5 on pimecrolimus alone and 4 on pimecrolimus used in sequence with corticosteroids). In 211 patients on vehicle alone, there were no cases of eczema herpeticum. The majority of adverse reactions were mild to moderate in severity.

Two phase 3 studies were conducted involving 436 infants 3 to 23 months of age. One 6-week, randomized, vehicle-controlled study with a 20-week open-label phase and 1 long-term safety study up to 1 year were conducted. In the 6-week study, 11% of pimecrolimus and 48% of vehicle patients did not complete this study; no patient in either group discontinued because of adverse reactions. Infants on pimecrolimus had an increased incidence of some adverse reactions compared with vehicle. In the 6-week vehicle-controlled study these adverse reactions included pyrexia (32% vs 13% vehicle), upper respiratory infection (24% vs 14%), nasopharyngitis (15% vs 8%), gastroenteritis (7% vs 3%), otitis media (4% vs 0%), and diarrhea (8% vs 0%). In the open-label phase of the study, for infants who switched to pimecrolimus from vehicle, the incidence of the above-cited adverse reactions approached or equaled the incidence of those patients who remained on pimecrolimus. In the 6-month safety data, 16% of pimecrolimus and 35% of vehicle patients discontinued early and 1.5% of pimecrolimus and 0% of vehicle patients discontinued because of adverse reactions. Infants on pimecrolimus had a greater incidence of some adverse reactions as compared with vehicle. These included pyrexia (30% vs 20%), upper respiratory tract infection (21% vs 17%), cough (15% vs 9%), hypersensitivity (8% vs 2%), teething (27% vs 22%), vomiting (9% vs 4%), rhinitis (13% vs 9%), viral rash (4% vs 0%), rhinorrhea (4% vs 0%), and wheezing (4% vs 0%).

➤*Monitoring:* Monitor patients who develop lymphadenopathy to ensure that the lymphadenopathy resolves.

Drug Interactions

➤*CYP3A inhibitors:* Use caution when coadministering a known CYP3A family of inhibitors in patients with widespread or erythrodermic disease. Some examples of these drugs are erythromycin, itraconazole, ketoconazole, fluconazole, calcium channel blockers, and cimetidine.

Adverse Reactions

Neither phototoxicity nor photoallergenicity were detected in clinical studies with 24 and 33 healthy volunteers, respectively. In human dermal safety studies, pimecrolimus did not induce contact sensitization or cumulative irritation.

In a 1-year safety study in children 2 to 17 years of age involving sequential use of pimecrolimus and a topical corticosteroid, 43% of pimecrolimus patients and 68% of vehicle patients used corticosteroids during the study. Corticosteroids were used for more than 7 days by 34% of pimecrolimus patients and 54% of vehicle patients. An increased incidence of impetigo, skin infection, superinfection (infected atopic dermatitis), rhinitis, and urticaria were found in the patients who had used pimecrolimus and topical corticosteroid sequentially as compared with pimecrolimus alone.

In 3 randomized, double-blind, vehicle-controlled pediatric studies and 1 active-controlled adult study, 843 and 328 patients, respectively, were treated with pimecrolimus. In these clinical trials, 48 (4%) of the 1,171 pimecrolimus patients and 13 (3%) of 408 vehicle-treated patients discontinued therapy because of adverse reactions. Discontinuations for adverse reactions were primarily due to application site reactions and cutaneous infections. The most common application site reaction was application site burning, which occurred in 8% to 26% of patients treated with pimecrolimus.

The following table depicts the incidence of adverse reactions pooled across the 2 identically designed 6-week studies with their open-label extensions and the 1-year safety study for children 2 to 17 years of age. Data from the adult active-controlled study is also included in this table. Adverse reactions are listed regardless of relationship to study drug.

PIMECROLIMUS — TOPICAL

Pimecrolimus Adverse Reactions (≥ 1%)						
	Pediatric patients[a] vehicle-controlled (6 weeks)		Pediatric patients[a] open-label (20 weeks)	Pediatric patients[a] vehicle-controlled (1 year)		Adult active comparator (1 year)
Adverse reaction	Pimecrolimus cream (n = 267)	Vehicle (n = 136)	Pimecrolimus cream (n = 335)	Pimecrolimus cream (n = 272)	Vehicle (n = 75)	Pimecrolimus cream (n = 328)
At least 1 adverse reaction	68.2%	71.3%	72%	84.6%	74.7%	78%
CNS						
Headache	13.9%	8.8%	11.3%	25.4%	16%	7%
Dermatologic						
Acne NOS[b]	0	0.7%	0.3%	1.5%	< 1%	1.8
Folliculitis	1.1%	0.7%	0.9%	2.2%	4%	6.1%
Herpes simplex, dermatitis	0	0	0.3%	1.5%	0	0.6%
Impetigo	1.9%	2.2%	3.6%	4%	5.3%	2.4%
Molluscum contagiosum	0.7%	0	1.2%	1.8%	0	0
Skin infection NOS	3%	5.1%	5.4%	2.2%	4%	6.4%
Skin papilloma	0.4%	0	0.6%	3.3%	< 1%	0
Urticaria	1.1%	0	0.3%	0.4%	< 1%	0.9%
GI						
Abdominal pain NOS	0.4%	0.7%	1.5%	4.4%	4%	0.3%
Abdominal pain, upper	4.1%	4.4%	3%	5.5%	6.7%	0.3%
Constipation	0.4%	0	0.6%	3.7%	< 1%	0
Diarrhea NOS	1.1%	0.7%	0.6%	7.7%	5.3%	2.1%
Gastroenteritis NOS	0	2.2%	0.6%	7.4%	2.7%	1.8%
Loose stools	0	0.7%	1.2%	< 1%	< 1%	0
Nausea	0.4%	2.2%	1.2%	4%	6.7%	1.8%
Vomiting NOS	3%	4.4%	4.2%	6.6%	8%	0.6%
GU						
Dysmenorrhea	1.1%	0	1.5%	1.1%	1.3%	1.2%
Local						
Application site burning	10.4%	12.5%	1.5%	8.5%	6.7%	25.9%
Application site erythema	0.4%	0	0	2.2%	0	2.1%
Application site irritation	3%	5.9%	0.9%	0.4%	4%	6.4%
Application site pruritus	1.1%	1.5%	0.6%	1.8%	0	5.5%
Application site reaction NOS	3%	5.1%	2.1%	3.3%	2.7%	14.6%
Musculoskeletal						
Arthralgias	0	0	0.3%	1.1%	1.3%	1.5%
Back pain	0.4%	1.5%	0.3%	< 1%	0	1.8%
Ophthalmic						
Conjunctivitis NEC[c]	0.7%	0.7%	2.1%	2.2%	4%	3%
Eye infection NOS	0	0	0	1.1%	< 1%	0.3%
Respiratory						
Asthma aggravated	1.5%	2.2%	3.9%	1.1%	1.3%	0
Asthma NOS	0.7%	0.7%	3.3%	3.7%	2.7%	2.4%
Bronchitis, acute NOS	0	0	0	1.5%	0	0
Bronchitis NOS	0.4%	2.2%	1.2%	10.7%	8%	2.4%
Cough	11.6%	8.1%	9.3%	15.8%	10.7%	2.4%
Dyspnea NOS	0	0	0	1.8%	1.3%	0.6%
Epistaxis	0	0.7%	0	3.3%	1.3%	0.3%
Influenza	3%	0.7%	6.6%	13.2%	4%	9.8%
Nasal congestion	2.6%	1.5%	1.8%	1.5%	1.3%	0.6%
Nasopharyngitis	10.1%	7.4%	19.6%	26.5%	21.3%	7.6%
Pharyngitis NOS	0.7%	1.5%	0.9%	8.1%	2.7%	0.9%
Pharyngitis streptococcal	0.7%	1.5%	3%	0	< 1%	0
Pneumonia NOS	1.1%	0.7%	1.5%	0	1.3%	0.3%
Rhinitis	0.4%	0	1.5%	4.4%	6.7%	2.1%
Rhinorrhea	1.9%	0.7%	0.9%	0.4%	1.3%	0
Sinus congestion	1.1%	0.7%	0.6%	< 1%	< 1%	0.9%
Sinusitis	1.1%	0.7%	3.3%	2.2%	1.3%	0.6%
Tonsillitis, acute NOS	0	0	0	2.6%	0	0
Tonsillitis NOS	0.4%	0	0.9%	6.3%	0	0.6%
Upper respiratory tract infection NOS	14.2%	13.2%	19.4%	4.8%	8%	4.3%
Upper respiratory tract infection, viral NOS	0.4%	0	0.9%	1.5%	0	0.3%
Wheezing	0.4%	0.7%	1.2%	0.7%	< 1%	0
Special senses						
Ear infection NOS	2.2%	1.5%	5.7%	3.3%	1.3%	0.6%
Earache	0.7%	0.7%	0	2.9%	2.7%	0
Otitis media	2.2%	0.7%	3%	2.9%	5.3%	0.6%
Miscellaneous						
Accident NOS	1.1%	0.7%	0.3%	< 1%	1.3%	0
Bacterial infection	1.5%	2.2%	1.2%	1.1%	0	1.8%
Chickenpox	0.7%	0	0.9%	2.9%	4%	0.3%
Herpes simplex	0.4%	0	1.2%	3.3%	2.7%	4%
Hypersensitivity NOS	4.1%	4.4%	4.8%	5.1%	1.3%	3.4%
Influenza-like illness	0.4%	0	0.6%	1.8%	2.7%	1.8%
Laceration	0.7%	0.7%	1.5%	< 1%	< 1%	0
Pyrexia	7.5%	8.8%	12.2%	12.5%	5.3%	1.2%
Sore throat	3.4%	3.7%	5.4%	8.1%	5.3%	3.7%
Staphylococcal infection	0.4%	3.7%	2.1%	0	< 1%	0.9%
Toothache	0.4%	0.7%	0.6%	2.6%	1.3%	0.6%
Viral infection NOS	0.7%	0.7%	0.3%	6.6%	1.3%	0

[a] Two to 17 years of age.
[b] NOS = not otherwise specified.
[c] NEC = not elsewhere classified.

Two cases of septic arthritis have been reported in infants younger than 1 year of age in clinical trials conducted with pimecrolimus (n = 2,443). Causality has not been established.

➤*Postmarketing:*

Hematologic/Lymphatic – Basal cell carcinoma, lymphomas, malignant melanoma, squamous cell carcinoma.

Miscellaneous – Anaphylactic reactions, angioneurotic edema, facial edema, ocular irritation after application of the cream to the eyelids or near the eyes, skin flushing associated with alcohol use.

PIMECROLIMUS — TOPICAL

Overdosage

➤*Symptoms:* There has been no experience of overdose with pimecrolimus. No incidents of accidental ingestion have been reported.

➤*Treatment:* If oral ingestion occurs, seek medical advice.

Patient Information

Instruct caregivers not to not administer pimecrolimus to a child younger than 2 years of age.

Instruct patients and caregivers who are not applying the drug to their hands to wash their hands with soap and water after applying pimecrolimus. This should remove any cream left on the hands.

Instruct patients

- not use pimecrolimus for a long time and to use it exactly as prescribed.
- to use pimecrolimus only on areas of their skin that have eczema.
- to notify their health care provider if they have a skin disease called Netherton syndrome (a rare inherited condition).
- to notify their health care provider if they have any infection on their skin including, chickenpox or herpes.
- to notify their health care provider if they have been told they have a weakened immune system.
- to notify their health care provider if they are pregnant, planning to become pregnant, or breast-feeding.
- to limit sun exposure during treatment with pimecrolimus (even when the medicine is not on their skin) and not to use sunlamps or tanning beds or get treatment with ultraviolet light therapy during treatment with pimecrolimus.
- to contact their health care provider if pimecrolimus is swallowed.
- not to bathe, shower, or swim right after applying pimecrolimus. This could wash off the cream.
- not to cover the skin being treated with bandages, dressings, or wraps. Patients can wear normal clothing.
- not to use pimecrolimus in the eyes; patients should rinse their eyes with cold water if the drug gets in their eyes.

KERATOLYTIC AGENTS

DICLOFENAC SODIUM

Refer to the diclofenac monograph in the Anti-inflammatory Agents section for complete prescribing information.

SALICYLIC ACID

otc	**Panscol** (Baker Cummins)	**Ointment; topical**: 3%	In 90 g.
otc	**MG217 Sal-Acid Ointment** (Triton)	**Ointment; topical**: 3%	Vitamin E. In 2 oz.
otc	**Fostex** (Bristol Products)	**Cream; topical**: 2%	Etetic acid, stearyl alcohol. In 118 g.
Rx	**SA 6%** (River's Edge)	**Cream; topical**: 6%	Alcohol, ammonium lactate, cetyl alcohol, dimethicone, disodium EDTA, glycerin, glyceryl, mineral oil, parabens, PEG-3, PEG-100, trolamine. In 454 g in kits with cleanser.
Rx	**Salacyn** (Stratus)		Cetearyl alcohol, cetyl alcohol, disodium EDTA, glycerin, glyceryl, mineral oil, parabens, PEG-3, PEG-100. In 400 g.
Rx	**Salex** (Coria Laboratories)		Alcohols, glycerin, parabens. In 400 g bottles.
otc	**Panscol** (Baker Cummins)	**Lotion; topical**: 3%	In 120 mL.
Rx	**SA 6%** (River's Edge)	**Lotion; topical**: 6%	Alcohol, disodium EDTA, glycerin, glyceryl, mineral oil, parabens, PEG-100, trolamine. In 237 mL in kits with cleanser.
Rx	**Salacyn** (Stratus)		Cetearyl alcohol, cetyl alcohol, disodium EDTA, glycerin, glyceryl, mineral oil, parabens, PEG-3, PEG-100. In 414 mL.
Rx	**Salex** (Coria Laboratories)		In 414 mL.
otc	**Dr Scholl's Corn/Callus Remover** (Schering-Plough)	**Liquid; topical**: 12.6%	Alcohol 18%, ether 55%, acetone, hydrogenated vegetable oil. In 10 mL with 3 cushions in flexible collodion.
otc	**Freezone** (Whitehall)	**Liquid; topical**: 13.6%	Alcohol 20.5%, ether 64.8%, castor oil. In 9 mL in a collodion-like vehicle.
otc	**Gordofilm** (Gordon)	**Liquid; topical**: 16.7%	In 15 mL with brush applicator in flexible collodion.
otc	**Fung-O** (S.S.S. Company)	**Liquid; topical**: 17%	Alcohol 2%, ether 68%. In 15 mL w/drop applicator.
otc	**Dr Scholl's Wart Remover Kit** (Schering-Plough)		Acetone, alcohol 17%, ether 52%. In 10 mL with brush and cushions in a flexible collodion.
otc	**Occlusal-HP** (Medicis)		Isopropyl alcohol. In 10 mL with brush applicator in a polyacrylic vehicle.
otc	**Compound W** (Medtech)		Alcohol 21.2%, camphor, castor oil, collodion, ether, menthol. In 9 mL.
otc	**DuoFilm** (Schering-Plough)		Alcohol 15.8%, castor oil, ether 42.6%, In 15 mL with brush applicator in flexible collodion.
otc	**Maximum Strength Wart Remover** (Glades)		Alcohol 29%, castor oil. In 13.3 mL with applicator in a flexible collodion.
otc	**Off-Ezy Wart Remover Kit** (Del Pharm)		Acetone, alcohol 21%, ether 65%. In 13.5 mL with skin buffer and applicator in collodion-like vehicle.
otc	**Off-Ezy Corn & Callus Remover Kit** (Del Pharm)		Acetone, alcohol 21%, ether 65%. In 13.5 mL with callus smoother and corn cushions in collodion-like vehicle with.
otc	**Wart-Off** (Pfizer)		Alcohol 26.35%, propylene glycol dipelargonate. In 15 mL with applicator in flexible collodion.
otc	**Salactic Film** (Pedinol)		In 15 mL with brush applicator in collodion-like vehicle.
otc	**Mosco** (Medtech)		Alcohol 33%, ether 65.5%. In 10 mL in a flexible collodion base.
otc	**P & S** (Aero Pharmaceuticals)	**Shampoo; topical**: 2%	Lactic acid, parabens, tetrasodium EDTA, triethanolamine, urea. In 236 mL.
Rx	**Salex** (Coria Laboratories)	**Shampoo; topical**: 6%	Cetearyl alcohol, EDTA, glycerin, parabens. In 177 mL.
otc	**Keralyt** (Summers Labs)	**Gel; topical**: 3%	Alcohol 21%, propylene glycol. In 28.4 g.
otc	**Hydrisalic** (Pedinol)	**Gel; topical**: 6%	Alcohol. In 28.35 g.
otc	**Keralyt** (Summers)		Alcohol SD-40 21%. In 28.4 g.
Rx	**Salicylic Acid** (Kylemore Pharmaceuticals)		EDTA, SD alcohol. In 40 g.

SALICYLIC ACID

otc	**Sal-Plant** (Pedinol)	**Gel; topical:** 17%	In 14 g in collodion-like vehicle.
otc	**Compound W** (Medtech)		Alcohol 67.5%, camphor, castor oil, collodion, colloidal silicon dioxide, hydroxypropyl cellulose, hypophosphorous acid, polysorbate 80. In 7 g.
otc	**DuoPlant** (Schering-Plough)		Alcohol 57.6%, ether 16.42%, ethyl lactate, hydroxypropyl cellulose, polybutene. In 14.2 g in flexible collodion.
Rx	**Salicylic Acid** (Brookstone Pharmaceuticals)	**Aerosol, foam; topical:** 6%	Glycerin, parabens, polysorbate 20, polysorbate 80, propylene glycol, tolamine. In 70 g.
otc	**Salkera** (Onset Therapeutics)		Aloe, edetate disodium dihydrate, cetostearyl alcohol, glycerin, parabens, white petrolatum. In 60 g.
Rx	**Salvax** (Quinnova)		Dimethicone, glycerin, parabens, polysorbate 80, povidone, propylene glycol, trolamine. In 70 and 200 g kits with 150 g *Hydro 35* foam.
otc	**Psor-a-set** (Hogil)	**Soap; topical:** 2%	In 97.5 g.
otc	**DuoFilm** (Schering-Plough)	**Patch:** 40%	In 18s (containing 3 sizes) in a rubber-based vehicle.
otc	**Trans-Ver-Sal PlantarPatch** (Doak)	**Patch; topical:** 15%	Karaya, PEG-300, propylene glycol, quaternium-15. 20 mm patches in 25s with 25 securing tapes and one emery file.
otc	**Trans-Ver-Sal PediaPatch** (Doak)		In 6 mm (20s) with bandage tapes in karaya gum base.
otc	**Trans-Ver-Sal AdultPatch** (Doak)		Karaya, PEG-300, propylene glycol, quaternium-156 or 12 mm patches in 40s with 42 securing tapes and one emery file.
otc	**Mediplast** (Beiersdorf)	**Plaster; topical:** 40%	2″ × 3″ patches in 2s and 25s.
otc	**Dr Scholl's Advanced Pain Relief Corn Removers** (Schering-Plough)	**Disk; topical:** 40%	In 6s with cushions in a rubber-based vehicle.
otc	**Dr Scholl's Callus Removers** (Schering-Plough)		In 4s with 6 pads and 4s with 4 pads (extra-thick).
otc	**Dr Scholl's Clear Away Plantar** (Schering-Plough)		In 24s with cushions.
otc	**Dr Scholl's Clear Away** (Schering-Plough)		In 18s with cover-up disks.
otc	**Dr Scholl's Corn Removers** (Schering-Plough)		In 9s (pads and disks) as regular, extra-thick, soft, small, waterproof and ultra-thin and 6s (pads and disks) as wrap-around.
otc	**Dr Scholl's Moisturizing Corn Remover Kit** (Schering-Plough)		In 6s with moisturizing cream and cushions.
otc	**Dr Scholl's Clear Away OneStep** (Schering-Plough)	**Strips; topical:** 40%	In 14s in a rubber-based vehicle.
otc	**Dr Scholl's OneStep Corn Removers** (Schering-Plough)		In 6s in a rubber-based vehicle.
otc	**Compound W for Kids** (Medtech)	**Pad; topical:** 40%	Lanolin, rubber. In 12s in a plaster vehicle.

SALICYLIC ACID — TOPICAL

Indications

➤*Hyperkeratotic skin disorders:* A topical aid in the removal of excessive keratin in hyperkeratotic skin disorders, including common and plantar warts, psoriasis, calluses and corns.

➤*Off-label uses:* The use of a 40% salicylic acid disk covered with an adhesive strip has been used to aid in the removal of inaccessible splinters in children.

Administration and Dosage

➤*General dosing considerations:* For specific instructions for use of these products, refer to individual product labeling.

➤*Adults:*

Hyperkeratotic skin disorders –

Usual dosage: Apply to affected area. May soak in warm water for 5 minutes prior to use to hydrate skin and enhance the effect. Remove any loose tissue with brush, washcloth, or emery board and dry thoroughly.

Duration of therapy: In general, for treatment of warts, improvement should occur in 1 to 2 weeks; maximum resolution may be expected after 4 to 6 weeks, although application for up to 12 weeks may be necessary. If skin irritation develops or there is no improvement after several weeks, contact a health care provider.

➤*Children:* Prolonged use over large areas, especially in young children, could result in salicylism. Limit use to the area to be treated.

Hyperkeratotic skin disorders – See Adults for dosing.

➤*Storage/Stability:* Some products are flammable; keep away from fire or flame. Keep bottle tightly capped and store at room temperature away from heat.

Actions

➤*Pharmacology:* Salicylic acid is the only *otc* product considered safe and effective by the FDA for use as a keratolytic for corns, calluses and warts. Salicylic acid produces desquamation of the horny layer of skin, while not affecting the structure of the viable epidermis, by dissolving intercellular cement substance. The keratolytic action causes the cornified epithelium to swell, soften, macerate and then desquamate.

Salicylic acid is keratolytic at concentrations of approximately 2% to 6%. These concentrations are generally used for treatment of dandruff, seborrhea and psoriasis. Concentrations of 5% to 17% in collodion are safe and effective for the removal of common and plantar warts; up to 40% in plasters is used to remove warts, corns and calluses.

Salicylic acid preparations, alone or in combination, have also been used to treat dandruff, seborrheic dermatitis, acne, tinea infections and psoriasis.

➤*Pharmacokinetics:*

Absorption/Distribution – In a study of the percutaneous absorption of salicylic acid in four patients with extensive active psoriasis, peak serum salicylate levels never exceeded 5 mg/dl even though more than 60% of the applied salicylic acid was absorbed. Systemic toxic reactions are usually associated with much higher serum levels (30 to 40 mg/dl). Peak serum levels occurred within 5 hours of the topical application under occlusion.

Metabolism/Excretion – The major urinary metabolites identified after topical administration differ from those after oral salicylate administration; those derived from percutaneous absorption contain more salicylate glucuronides (42%) and less salicyluric (52%) and salicylic acid (6%).

Contraindications

Sensitivity to salicylic acid; prolonged use, especially in infants, diabetics, and patients with impaired circulation; use on moles, birthmarks or warts with hair growing from them, genital or facial warts or warts on mucous membranes, irritated skin or any area that is infected or reddened.

Warnings/Precautions

➤*Salicylate toxicity:* Prolonged use over large areas, especially in young children and those patients with significant renal or hepatic impairment, could result in salicylism. Limit the area to be treated and be aware of signs of salicylate toxicity (eg, nausea, vomiting, dizziness, loss of hearing, tinnitus, lethargy, hyperpnea, diarrhea, psychic disturbances). In the event of salicylic acid toxicity, discontinue use.

SALICYLIC ACID — TOPICAL

➤*Special risk patients:* Do not use if diabetic or poor blood circulation exists.

➤*For external use only:* Avoid contact with eyes, mucous membranes and normal skin surrounding warts. If contact with eyes or mucous membranes occurs, immediately flush with water for 15 minutes. Avoid inhaling vapors.

➤*Pregnancy: Category C.* There are no adequate and well controlled studies in pregnant women. Use during pregnancy only if the potential benefit justifies the potential risk to the fetus.

➤*Lactation:* Due to systemic absorption, topical salicylic acid should not be used during breast-feeding. It is known that salicylates are excreted in mother's milk and have been attributed to certain conditions such as Reye syndrome in children.

Drug Interactions

Interactions have been reported with both topical and oral salicylates. Refer to the Salicylates monograph for a complete listing.

Adverse Reactions

Local irritation may occur from contact with normal skin surrounding the affected area. If irritation occurs, temporarily discontinue use and take care to apply only to wart site when treatment is resumed.

Patient Information

For external use only. Avoid contact with eyes, face, genitals, mucous membranes and normal skin surrounding warts.

Medication may cause reddening or scaling of skin when used on open skin lesions.

Contact with clothing, fabrics, plastics, wood, metal or other materials may cause damage; avoid contact.

SULFUR PREPARATIONS

otc	**Sulpho-Lac Acne Medication** (Doak)	**Cream:** 5% sulfur	27% zinc sulfate, 53% Vleminckx's solution base. Greaseless. In 28.35 and 50 g.
otc	**Acne Lotion 10** (C & M)	**Lotion:** 10% colloidal sulfur	22.5% isopropyl alcohol. Tinted. Aqueous. In 60 mL.
otc	**Liquimat** (Galderma)	**Lotion:** 4% sulfur	22% SD alcohol 40, cetyl alcohol. Assorted tints. In 45 mL.
otc	**Sulpho-Lac** (Doak)	**Soap:** 5% sulfur	In a coconut and tallow oil soap base. In 85 g.
otc	**Sulmasque** (C & M)	**Mask:** 6.4% sulfur	With 15% isopropyl alcohol, methylparaben. In 150 g.

SULFUR — TOPICAL

Indications

➤*Dandruff:*

Shampoo – Relieves the itching and scalp flaking associated with dandruff.

For men, women, and children over 2 years of age. Daily shampooing may be helpful if scalp is oily.

➤*Acne:*

Soap – Aids in the treatment of mild acne and oily skin.

Softens the hard shell of acne blemishes, helps dissolve and remove blackheads, washes away excess oils which may cause blackheads, and refreshes skin.

Administration and Dosage

➤*Adults:*

Acne –

Soap: Use twice daily. Work up lather with hands or washcloth and apply to affected areas without scrubbing. Let dry about 1 minute, rinse thoroughly, and pat dry.

Dandruff –

Shampoo: Shake well. Wet hair and vigorously massage a small amount of sulfur topical medicated antidandruff shampoo into hair and scalp, working up a lather. Rinse thoroughly with warm water. Repeat procedure.

➤*Children:*

Acne – See Adults for dosing.

Dandruff –

Shampoo:

- *2 years of age and older* – See Adults for dosing.

Actions

➤*Pharmacology:* Sulfur, a keratolytic, provides peeling and drying actions. Although it may help to resolve comedones, it may also promote the development of new ones by increasing horny cell adhesion.

Warnings/Precautions

➤*Shampoo:* For external use only. Avoid contact with the eyes; if this happens, rinse thoroughly with water. If condition worsens or does not improve after regular use of this product as directed, consult a physician. Do not use on children under 2 years of age except as directed by a physician.

➤*Soap:* Use with other topical acne medications at the same time or immediately following use of this product may increase dryness or irritation of the skin. If this occurs, use only 1 medication unless directed by a doctor. Do not get into eyes.

➤*Pregnancy: Category: Undetermined.* Consult a health care provider before using in pregnant women.

➤*Lactation:* Consult a health care provider before using in breast-feeding women.

Patient Information

Stop use and ask doctor if excessive skin irritation develops or increases.

Keep out of reach of children. If swallowed, get medical help or contact a poison control center immediately.

KERATOLYTIC AGENT COMBINATION

otc	**Gets-It** (Oakhurst)	**Liquid:** Salicylic acid, zinc chloride and collodion in ≈ 35% ether and ≈ 28% alcohol	In 12 mL.
Rx	**Salicylic Acid Shampoo** (Hi-Tech)	**Shampoo:** 6% salicylic acid, edetate disodium, glycerin, parabens	In 177 mL.
otc	**Compound W Freeze Off** (Medtech)	**Aerosol; topical:** Dimethyl ether, isobutane, propane	In 12s.

ACNE PRODUCTS, COMBINATIONS

ACNE PRODUCT COMBINATIONS

otc	**Clearasil Adult Care** (Procter & Gamble)	**Cream; topical:** resorcinol, sulfur	10% alcohol, parabens. In 17 g.
otc	**Acnomel** (Numark)	**Cream; topical:** 2% resorcinol, 8% sulfur	11% alcohol. In 28 g.
otc	**Adult Acnomel** (Numark)		15% alcohol, propylene glycol. Tinted. In 28 g.
otc	**Fostex Acne Cleansing** (Westwood Squibb)	**Cream; topical:** 2% salicylic acid	Stearyl alcohol, EDTA. In 118 g.
otc	**PROPApH Acne Maximum Strength** (Del)		Lanolin alcohol, stearyl alcohol, EDTA, menthol, stearyl alcohol. In 19.5 g.
Rx	**Avar-e LS** (Kylemore)	**Cream; topical:** 10% sodium sulfacetamide, 2% sulfur	Benzyl alcohol, cetyl alcohol, disodium EDTA, glycerin, glyceryl, PEG 100, phenoxyethanol, polawax, zinc oxide. In 45 g.
Rx	**Avar-e Emollient** (Kylemore)	**Cream; topical:** 10% sodium sulfacetamide, 5% sulfur	Glycerin, EDTA, benzyl alcohol, cetyl alcohol. In 45 g.
Rx	**Avar-e Green** (Kylemore)		Glycerin, EDTA, benzyl alcohol, cetyl alcohol. For color correction. In 45 g.
Rx	**Clenia** (Upsher-Smith)		Parabens, EDTA. In 28 g.
Rx	**Plexion SCT** (Medicis)		Witch hazel, benzyl alcohol. In 120 g.

ACNE PRODUCT COMBINATIONS

Rx	**Sulfoxyl Regular** (Stiefel)	**Lotion; topical:** 5% benzoyl peroxide, 2% sulfur	Stearic acid, zinc laurate. In 59 mL.
Rx	**Bencort** (River's Edge)	**Lotion; topical:** 5% benzoyl peroxide, 0.5% hydrocortisone	Acetylated lanolin alcohol, cetyl alcohol, EDTA, lanolin oil, mineral oil, parabens, tetrasodium EDTA. In 25 g.
Rx	**Vanoxide HC** (Summers Labs)		Cetyl alcohol, lanolin oil, mineral oil, parabens, tetrasodium EDTA. In 25 g and in kits with *Benzoyl-Pak* and *ABC Lotion*.
otc	**RA** (Medco Lab)	**Lotion; topical:** 3% resorcinol	43% alcohol. In 120, 240, and 480 mL.
otc	**Rezamid** (Summers)	**Lotion; topical:** 2% resorcinol, 5% sulfur	28% alcohol. In 56.7 mL.
otc	**R/S** (Summers)		28% alcohol. In 56.7 mL.
otc	**Sulforcin** (Galderma)		11.65% SD alcohol 40, methylparaben. In 120 mL.
otc	**Acnotex** (C & M)	**Lotion; topical:** 2% resorcinol, 8% sulfur	20% isopropyl alcohol. In 60 mL.
otc	**PROPApH Cleansing for Normal/ Combination Skin** (Del)	**Lotion; topical:** 0.5% salicylic acid	SD alcohol 40, menthol, EDTA. In 180 mL (lotion) and 45s (pads).
otc	**PROPApH Cleansing for Oily Skin** (Del)	**Lotion; topical:** 0.6% salicylic acid	SD alcohol 40, EDTA, menthol. In 180 mL.
otc	**Oxy Night Watch Sensitive Skin** (SK-Beecham)	**Lotion; topical:** 1% salicylic acid	Cetyl alcohol, EDTA, stearyl alcohol, parabens. In 60 mL.
otc	**Finac** (C & M)	**Lotion; topical:** 2% salicylic acid	22.5% isopropyl alcohol, propylene glycol, acetone. In 60 mL.
otc	**Oxy Night Watch Maximum Strength** (SK-Beecham)		Cetyl alcohol, EDTA, parabens, stearyl alcohol. In 60 mL.
otc	**Sebasorb** (Summers)		10% attapulgite. In 45 mL.
Rx	**Klaron** (Dermik)	**Lotion; topical:** 10% sodium sulfacetamide	Propylene glycol, polyethylene glycol 400, methylparaben, EDTA. In 59 mL.
Rx	**Seb-Prev** (Glades)		Propylene glycol, methylparaben, EDTA. In 118 mL.
Rx	**Sodium Sulfacetamide 10% and Sulfur 5%** (Glades)	**Lotion; topical:** 10% sodium sulfacetamide, 5% sulfur	Cetyl alcohol, benzyl alcohol, EDTA. In 30 mL tube and 25 mL.
Rx	**Sulfacet-R** (Dermik)		Parabens. Tinted. In 25 mL.
Rx	**Vanocin** (Stratus)		Benzyl alcohol, cetyl alcohol, EDTA, parabens, stearyl alcohol. In 30 and 60 g.
Rx	**Sulfacetamide Sodium** (Fougera)	**Suspension;** 10% sodium sulfacetamide	EDTA, methylparaben, sodium metabisulfite. In 118 mL.
Rx	**Plexion TS** (Medicis)	**Suspension; topical:** 10% sodium sulfacetamide, 5% sulfur	Mineral oil, glyceryl stearate, propylene glycol, benzyl alcohol, cetyl alcohol, stearyl alcohol, EDTA, sodium thiosulfate, coco-glycerides. In 30s.
Rx	**Epiduo** (Galderma)	**Gel; topical:** 2.5% benzoyl peroxide, 0.1% adapalene	Edetate disodium, glycerin. In 45 g.
Rx	**Acanya** (Valeant)	**Gel; topical:** 2.5% benzoyl peroxide, 1.2% clindamycin phosphate	In kits with benzoyl peroxide 40 g and clindamycin phosphate 10 g.
Rx	**Clindamycin 1%/Benzoyl Peroxide 5%** (Mylan)	**Gel; topical:** 5% benzoyl peroxide, 1% clindamycin	In 50 g.
Rx	**BenzaClin** (Dermik)		In 25 and 50 g, 35 and 50 g pump, and **BenzaClin Care Kit** with 50 g pump and 20 topical ampules *Viscontour Serum*.
Rx	**Duac CS** (GlaxoSmithKline)		EDTA, glycerin, methylparaben. In 45 g.
Rx	**Benzamycin** (Dermik)	**Gel; topical:** 5% benzoyl peroxide, 3% erythromycin	20% alcohol. In 0.8, 23, and 46 g.
Rx	**Benzamycin Pak** (Dermik)		SD alcohol 40B. In 0.8 g pouches. In 60s.
Rx	**Erythromycin-Benzoyl Peroxide** (Various, eg, Clay-Park)		In 23 and 46 g.
Rx	**BPS** (Breckenridge Pharmaceutical)	**Gel; topical:** 6% benzoyl peroxide, 3% sulfur	Benzyl alcohol, edetate disodium, glycerin. In 43 g.
Rx	**NuOx** (Gentex)		Benzyl alcohol, disodium EDTA, glycerin. In 43 g.
Rx	**Ziana** (Medicis)	**Gel; topical:** clindamycin phosphate 1.2%/ tretinoin 0.025%	EDTA, glycerin, parabens, tromethamine. In 2, 30, and 60 g tubes.
otc	**Sal-Clens Acne Cleanser** (C & M)	**Gel; topical:** 2% salicylic acid	In 240 g.
otc	**Stridex Clear** (Sterling Health)		9.3% SD alcohol. In 30 g.
Rx	**Sodium Sulfacetamide/Sulfur** (River's Edge)	**Gel; topical:** 10% sodium sulfacetamide, 5% sulfur	Benzyl alcohol, cetyl alcohol, dimethicone, disodium EDTA, glyceryl, methylparaben, mineral oil, PEG-100, propylene glycol, stearyl alcohol, urea 10%. In 45 mL.
Rx	**Avar** (Kylemore)		EDTA, benzyl alcohol. In 45 g.
Rx	**Rosula** (Pharmaderm)		Benzyl alcohol, cetyl alcohol, EDTA, mineral oil, PEG 100 stearate, 10% urea. In 45 mL.
Rx	**Rosula** (Pharmaderm)	**Aerosol, foam; topical:** 10% sodium sulfacetamide, 4% sulfur	Cetyl alcohol, lactic acid, parabens, propylene glycol, stearyl alcohol. In 100 g.
Rx	**Sodium Sulfacetamide/Sulfur** (Kylemore)	**Aerosol, foam; topical:** 10% sodium sulfacetamide, 5% sulfur	Cetearyl alcohol, glycerin. In 60 g.
Rx	**Clarifoam EF** (Onset)		Cetyl alcohol, parabens. In 60 g.
Rx	**Clenia** (Upsher-Smith)		Parabens, EDTA. In 170 and 340 mg bottles.
Rx	**Sumaxin TS** (Medimetriks)	**Suspension; topical:** 8% sodium sulfacetamide, 4% sulfur	Aloe, cetyl alcohol, edetate disodium, glyceryl, green tea, parabens, PEG-100, stearyl alcohol. In 473 mL.
Rx	**Sumaxin Wash** (Medimetriks)	**Liquid; topical:** 9% sodium sulfacetamide, 4% sulfur	Aloe, cetyl alcohol, edetate disodium, glyceryl, green tea, parabens, PEG-100, stearyl alcohol. In 473 mL.
Rx	**Rosula Clarifying Wash** (Pharmaderm)	**Liquid; topical:** 10% sodium sulfacetamide, 4% sulfur	EDTA, parabens, PEG-100, stearyl alcohol, 10% urea. In 473 mL.
Rx	**Claris** (Stratus)	**Soap; topical:** 10% sodium sulfacetamide, 1% sulfur	Cetyl alcohol, disodium EDTA, glyceryl stearate, parabens, PEG-100, stearyl alcohol, urea. In 473 mL.

ACNE PRODUCT COMBINATIONS

Rx	**Sodium Sulfacetamide/Sulfur** (Fougera)	**Soap; topical**: 10% sodium sulfacetamide, 4% sulfur	Alcohol, butylated hydroxytoluene, disodium EDTA, glyceryl, parabens, PEG. In 473 mL.
Rx	**BP Cleansing Wash** (Brookstone)		Cetyl alcohol, disodium EDTA, glyceryl stearate, parabens, PEG-100, stearyl alcohol, 10% urea. In 473 mL.
Rx	**Sodium Sulfacetamide/Sulfur** (Acella Pharmaceuticals)	**Soap; topical**: 9% sodium sulfacetamide, 4% sulfur	Aloe, cetyl alcohol, disodium EDTA, glycerol, parabens, PEG-100, stearyl alcohol, white petrolatum. In 473 mL.
Rx	**Zencia** (Stratus)		Aloe, cetyl alcohol, edetate disodium, glyceryl, green tea, parabens, PEG-100, stearyl alcohol. In 473 mL.
Rx	**Sodium Sulfacetamide/Sulfur** (River's Edge)	**Soap; topical**: 10% sodium sulfacetamide, 5% sulfur	Cetyl alcohol, disodium EDTA, glyceryl, parabens, PEG-100, stearyl alcohol, urea 10%. In 355 mL.
Rx	**Cerisa** (Stratus Pharmaceuticals)	**Soap; topical**: 10% sodium sulfacetamide, 1% sulfur	Cetyl alcohol, disodium EDTA, glyceryl stearate, lactic acid, parabens, PEG-100, stearyl alcohol, white petrolatum. In 170.1 g.
Rx	**Sodium Sulfacetamide/Sulfur** (Kylemore)	**Soap; topical**: 10% sodium sulfacetamide, 4% sulfur	Alcohols, BHT, disodium EDTA, parabens, PEG, urea 10%. In 473 mL.
Rx	**Avar LS Cleanser** (Kylemore)	**Soap; topical**: 10% sodium sulfacetamide, 2% sulfur	Benzyl alcohol, cetyl alcohol, phenoxyethanol, propylene glycol, stearyl alcohol. In 226.8 g.
Rx	**Avar** (Kylemore)	**Soap; topical**: 10% sodium sulfacetamide, 5% sulfur	Cetyl alcohol, stearyl alcohol. In 226.8 g.
Rx	**Plexion** (Medicis)		Cetyl alcohol, stearyl alcohol, EDTA, parabens. In 170 and 340 g.
Rx	**Rosaderm** (River's Edge)		Disodium EDTA, mineral oil, parabens. In 170 and 340 g and in kits with RE cleansing lotion.
Rx	**Rosanil** (Galderma)		EDTA, light mineral oil, parabens. In 170 g.
otc	**Medicated Acne** (C & M)	**Soap; topical**: 4% sulfur, 2% resorcinol	In 129 g.
otc	**PROPApH Cleansing** (Del)	**Pads; topical**: 0.5% salicylic acid	SD alcohol 40, EDTA, menthol. In 45s.
otc	**Clearasil Double Clear Regular Strength** (Procter & Gamble)	**Pads; topical**: 1.25% salicylic acid	40% alcohol, witch hazel distillate, menthol. In 32s.
otc	**Clearasil Double Clear Maximum Strength** (Procter & Gamble)	**Pads; topical**: 2% salicylic acid	40% alcohol, witch hazel distillate, menthol. In 32s.
Rx	**Inova 4/1 Acne Control Therapy** (JSJ Pharmaceuticals)	**Pads; topical**: benzoyl peroxide 4%, salicylic acid 1%, tocopherol 5%	Disodium EDTA, glycerin, methylparaben. In kits with 30 benzoyl peroxide pads, 30 salicylic acid pads, and 28 topical tocopherol capsules.
Rx	**Inova 8/2 Acne Control Therapy** (JSJ Pharmaceuticals)	**Pads; topical**: benzoyl peroxide 8%, salicylic acid 2%, tocopherol 5%	Disodium EDTA, glycerin, methylparaben. In kits with 30 benzoyl peroxide pads, 30 salicylic acid pads, and 28 topical tocopherol capsules.
Rx	**Sodium Sulfacetamide Medicated** (A. Aarons)	**Pads; topical**: 10% sodium sulfacetamide	Sodium EDTA, sodium thiosulfate, 10% urea. In 30s.
Rx	**Rosula NS Medicated** (Pharmaderm)		10% urea, sodium EDTA, sodium thiosulfate. In 30s.
Rx	**Sodium Sulfacetamide/Sulfur** (Brookstone Pharmaceuticals)	**Pads; topical**: 10% sodium sulfacetamide, 4% sulfur	Aloe, cetyl alcohol, disodium EDTA, glycerin, green tea, parabens, PEG-100, sodium metabisulfate, sodium thiosulfate, stearyl alcohol. In 60s.
Rx	**Sumaxin** (Medimetriks)		Aloe, cetyl alcohol, edetate disodium, glycerin, glyceryl stearate, green tea, parabens, PEG-100, stearyl alcohol. In 60s.
Rx	**Plexion Cleansing Cloths** (Medicis)	**Pads; topical**: 10% sodium sulfacetamide, 5% sulfur	Glycerine, glyceryl stearate, stearyl alcohol, propylene glycol, propylene glycol oleate, cetyl alcohol, EDTA, parabens, decolorized aloe vera gel. In 30s.
otc	**Clearasil Clearstick Regular Strength** (Procter & Gamble)	**Stick; topical**: 1.25% salicylic acid	39% alcohol, aloe vera gel, menthol, disodium EDTA. In 35 mL.
otc	**Clearasil Clearstick Maximum Strength** (Procter & Gamble)	**Stick; topical**: 2% salicylic acid	39% alcohol, menthol, EDTA. For regular and sensitive skin. In 35 mL.

ACNE PRODUCT COMBINATIONS — TOPICAL

Active Ingredients

These products contain keratolytics and astringents to aid in removing keratin and to dry the skin. Many products also have hydroalcoholic or organic solvent bases to aid in removal of sebum. Individual components include:

➤*ANTIMICROBIAL:* Sodium thiosulfate and sodium sulfacetamide.

➤*ANTISEPTIC:* Ethanol, isopropyl alcohol, phenol, sulfur and acetone.

➤*KERATOLYTICS:* Salicylic acid, resorcinol and sulfur.

➤*PROTECTIVES and ADSORBANTS:* Zinc oxide.

Hydrocortisone-containing acne products are listed under Topical Corticosteroid Combinations.

BENZOYL PEROXIDE COMBINATIONS — TOPICAL

Indications

➤*Acne vulgaris:* Topical treatment of acne vulgaris.

➤*Acne vulgaris, inflamed (Duac only):* Topical treatment of inflammatory acne vulgaris.

Administration and Dosage

➤*Adults:*

Acne vulgaris –

Sulfoxyl lotion, regular and strong: Apply the medication to the affected areas once a day during the first week, and then twice daily thereafter as tolerated. Adjust frequency of use to desired clinical response. Cleanse the affected areas with a nonmedicated soap prior to application. Improvement is typically seen by the third week of therapy. Maximum lesion reduction can be seen in approximately 8 to 12 weeks. Continue use of drug to maintain satisfactory response.

Benzamycin/Benzamycin Pak and *BenzaClin*: Apply twice daily, morning and evening, to affected areas after the skin is thoroughly washed and patted dry.

Acanya gel: Apply a pea-sized amount to the face once daily.

Acne vulgaris, inflamed –

Duac: Apply once daily in the evening to the affected areas after the skin is thoroughly washed and patted dry.

➤*Children:*

12 years of age or older – See Adults for dosing.

➤*Preparation for administration:*

Benzamycin Pak – Instruct patient to mix 2 separate components in foil pouch before applying this medication.

BenzaClin – Prior to dispensing, add purified water to the vial of powder (up to the mark) and shake until contents dissolve. Add this solution to the gel and stir until homogenous.

Benzamycin – Prior to dispensing, add ethyl alcohol 70% to the vial of powder (up to the mark) and shake until contents dissolve. Add this solution to the gel and stir until homogenous.

➤*Storage/Stability:*

Sulfoxyl lotion, regular and strong *–* Store at room temperature, 15° to 30°C (59° to 86°F). Shake well.

Duac – Before dispensing, store in a cold place, preferably a refrigerator, between 2° and 8°C (36° and 46°F). Do not freeze. Once dispensed, store at room temperature, up to 25°C (77°F) with a 2-month expiration date. Discard any unused medication.

Benzamycin Pak – Store at room temperature, 20° to 25°C (68° to 77°F). Keep away from heat and any open flame.

BENZOYL PEROXIDE COMBINATIONS — TOPICAL

Benzamycin and *BenzaClin* – Prior to reconstitution store at room temperature, 20° to 25°C (68° to 77°F). After reconstitution, store refrigerated at 2° to 8°C (36° to 46°F). Do not freeze. Following mixing, *BenzaClin* gel is good for 2 months. *Benzamycin* is good for 3 months. Discard any unused medication after expiration date.

Actions

➤*Pharmacology:*

Benzoyl peroxide – Benzoyl peroxide is an antibacterial agent and has been shown to be effective against *Propionibacterium acnes*, an anaerobe found in sebaceous follicles and comedones. The antibacterial action of benzoyl peroxide is believed to be due to the release of active oxygen, it also has a keratolytic and desquamative effect, which may also contribute to its efficacy. When benzoyl peroxide is applied to the skin, it is absorbed and converted to benzoic acid.

Erythromycin/Clindamycin – Erythromycin and clindamycin are antibiotics that reduce lesions of acne vulgaris in part due to the antibacterial activity; however, the exact mechanism is not fully known. Erythromycin and clindamycin act by inhibition of protein synthesis in susceptible organisms by reversibly binding to 50 S ribosomal subunits, thereby inhibiting translocation of aminoacyl transfer-RNA and inhibiting polypeptide synthesis. Antagonism has been demonstrated in vitro between erythromycin, lincomycin, chloramphenicol, and clindamycin.

➤*Pharmacokinetics:* Benzoyl peroxide has been shown to be absorbed by the skin where it is converted to benzoic acid. Less than 2% of the dose enters systemic circulation as benzoic acid. Mean systemic bioavailability of topical clindamycin is suggested to be less than 1%.

Drug resistance – There are reports of an increase of *Propionibacterium acnes* resistance to clindamycin in the treatment of acne. In patients with *P. acnes* resistant to clindamycin, the clindamycin component may provide no additional benefit beyond benzoyl peroxide alone.

Contraindications

History of hypersensitivity to erythromycin, clindamycin, benzoyl peroxide, sulfur, or to any of its components.

➤*Duac/BenzaClin*: Hypersensitivity to any of its components or to lincomycin; history of regional enteritis, ulcerative colitis, or antibiotic-associated colitis.

Warnings/Precautions

➤*Colitis:* Orally and parenterally administered antibacterial agents, including erythromycin and clindamycin have been associated with severe colitis, which may result in patient death. Use of the topical formulation results in absorption of the antibiotic from the skin surface. Diarrhea, bloody diarrhea, and colitis (including pseudomembranous colitis) have been reported with topical and systemic use of antibiotics. The colitis is characterized by severe persistent diarrhea and severe abdominal cramps and may be associated with the passage of blood and mucus. Endoscopic examination may reveal pseudomembranous colitis, stool culture for *Clostridium difficile* and stool assay for *C. difficile* toxin may be helpful diagnostically. When severe diarrhea occurs, discontinue the drug and institute therapeutic measures. Diarrhea, colitis, and pseudomembranous colitis have been known to occur up to several weeks after cessation of oral and parenteral antibiotic therapy.

Mild cases of pseudomembranous colitis usually respond to drug discontinuation. In moderate to severe cases, consider management with fluids and electrolytes, protein supplementation and treatment with an antibacterial drug clinically effective against *C. difficile* colitis.

➤*Concomitant therapy:* Use concomitant topical acne therapy with caution because a possible cumulative irritancy effect may occur, especially with the use of peeling, desquamating, or abrasive agents. Clindamycin and erythromycin containing products should not be used in combination. In vitro studies have shown antagonism between these 2 antimicrobials. The clinical significance of this is not known.

➤*For external use:* Use externally only. Avoid contact with the eyes, nose, mouth, and mucous membranes. Benzoyl peroxide may cause bleaching when in contact with hair, fabrics, or carpeting.

➤*Superinfection:* The use of antibiotic agents (especially prolonged or repeated therapy) may be associated with the overgrowth of nonsusceptible organisms including fungi. Such overgrowth may lead to a secondary infection. If this occurs, discontinue use and take appropriate measures.

➤*Pregnancy:* *Category C.* There are no adequate and well-controlled trials in pregnant women. Use during pregnancy only if clearly needed.

➤*Lactation:* It is not known whether erythromycin, clindamycin, sulfur, or benzoyl peroxide is excreted in human milk after topical application. However, erythromycin and clindamycin is excreted in human milk following oral and parenteral administration. Because of the potential for serious adverse reactions in nursing infants, a decision should be made whether to discontinue nursing or to discontinue the drug, taking into account the importance of the drug to the mother.

➤*Children:* Safety and efficacy in children younger than 12 years of age have not been established.

Adverse Reactions

Topical Antibiotic and Benzoyl Peroxide Combination Adverse Reactions (%)[a]

Adverse reaction	*BenzaClin* gel (N = 420)	*Benzamycin* gel	*Benzamycin Pak* gel (N = 236)	*Duac* gel (N = 397) (mild to moderate)	Erythromycin-benzoyl peroxide gel	*Sulfoxyl* lotion, Regular and Strong
Application site reaction	3		—	—	—	—
Blepharitis	—		1.7	—	—	—
Burning sensation		✓	2.5	5/< 1	✓	—
Dry skin	12	3	7.6	19/1	3	—
Erythema	1	✓	2.5	26/5		5
Eye inflammation		✓	—		✓	
Eye irritation	—	✓	—		✓	
Face inflammation		✓	—		✓	
Irritation	—	✓	—	—	✓	—
Itching	—	✓	—	—	✓	—
Nose inflammation	—	✓	—		✓	
Oiliness	—	✓	—	—	✓	—
Peeling	2	✓	0.5	17/2	✓	5
Photosensitivity reaction (eg, sunburn, stinging with sun exposure	1	—	1.3	—	—	—
Pruritus	2	—	1.7	—		—
Skin discoloration	—	✓	—	—	✓	—
Stinging	—	—	2.5			
Tenderness	—	✓	—		✓	
Urticarial reaction		3	—	—	3	

[a] All events; data are pooled from separate studies and are not necessarily comparable; — = not applicable; ✓ = incidence not provided.

Patient Information

Benzoyl peroxide may bleach hair, fabrics, or carpets.

Patients should not use any other topical acne preparation unless otherwise directed by a physician.

This medication is to be used externally. Avoid eyes, nose, mouth, and mucous membranes.

Inform patients to mix the *Benzamycin Pak* prior to use. The medication is dispensed in a foil pouch containing medication in 2 separate compartments. Mix contents thoroughly in palm of hand prior to application.

Excessive or prolonged exposure to sunlight should be limited.

After application of medicine, be sure to wash hands.

BenzaClin should be stored in a refrigerator; discard any unused portion after 2 months. *Duac* should be stored at room temperature with a 2 month expiration. *Benzamycin* should be refrigerated and discarded after 3 months.

In addition to the single entity products listed in this section, other products containing topical local anesthetics are listed in other sections, based on their specific uses. These include: Anorectal Preparations and Ophthalmic Local Anesthetics (see individual monographs).

Indications

Because of the diversity of uses of these products, the following is a general discussion. For information on specific applications of individual products, consult the manufacturer's package literature.

➤*Skin disorders:* For topical anesthesia in local skin disorders, including: Pruritus and pain due to minor burns, skin manifestations of systemic disease (eg, chickenpox), prickly heat, abrasions, sunburn, plant poisoning, insect bites, eczema; local analgesia on normal, intact skin (EMLA).

➤*Mucous membranes:* For local anesthesia of accessible mucous membranes, including: Oral, nasal and laryngeal mucous membranes; respiratory or urinary tracts. Also for the treatment of pruritus ani, pruritus vulvae and hemorrhoids.

➤*Off-label uses:*

Migraines –

Lidocaine (intranasal): [2] = Fair documentation.

Administration and Dosage

➤*Topical:* Apply to the affected area as needed. Ointments and creams can be applied to gauze or to a bandage prior to applying to the skin.

➤*Mucous membranes:* Dosage varies and depends upon the area to be anesthetized, vascularity of tissues, individual tolerance and technique of anesthesia. Administer the lowest dose possible that still provides adequate anesthesia. Apply to affected areas using the proper technique (see individual manufacturer inserts).

In debilitated, elderly patients or children, administer lower concentrations.

A combination of tetracaine 0.5%, epinephrine 1:2000 and cocaine 11.8% (also known as TAC) in a liquid topical formulation has been used for minor skin lacerations, especially of the face and scalp. Other preparations include cocaine 11.8% and epinephrine 1:1000, and lidocaine 4%, epinephrine 1:1000 and tetracaine 0.5%, both utilizing methylcellulose for a more viscous gel formulation. Use results in decreased pain on application, allowing for better compliance and tolerance of repair procedure. This may be beneficial in patients who cannot tolerate injection anesthesia or those who are difficult to control (eg, children). A commercial preparation of lidocaine and prilocaine (EMLA) was developed for a similar purpose (increased absorption in children) on intact skin. However, toxic effects are also more likely to occur in infants and children with all of these preparations.

The use of the lidocaine/prilocaine combination appears to be beneficial as a pretreatment in decreasing the pain of DPT vaccinations (and presumably other vaccinations) in infants. The cream is applied at the injection site with occlusive dressing for at least 60 minutes prior to the vaccination.

Actions

➤*Pharmacology:* Local anesthetics inhibit conduction of nerve impulses from sensory nerves. This action results from an alteration of the cell membrane permeability to ions. Although poorly absorbed through the intact epidermis (except for the lidocaine/prilocaine mixture; penetration and subsequent systemic absorption is enhanced over use of each agent alone), these agents are readily absorbed from mucous membranes. When skin permeability has been increased by abrasions or ulcers, the absorption and, subsequently, the efficacy of local anesthetics improves; however, the incidence of side effects also increases. Onset, depth and duration of dermal analgesia provided by the lidocaine/prilocin mixture depends primarily on duration of application.

Topical Local Anesthetics: Indications, Dose, Strength, Peak Effect and Duration

Local anesthetics, topical	Indications: Skin	Indications: Mucous membrane	Maximum adult dose (mg)	Available or recommended strengths (%)	Peak[a] effect (minutes)	Duration[a] of effect (minutes)
Amides	✓		25	0.5-1	< 5	15-45
Dibucaine						
Lidocaine	✓	✓	†[b]	2-5	2-5	15-45
Esters				0.5-20	< 5	15-45
Benzocaine						
Butamben picrate	✓			1		
Cocaine		✓	50-200	4-10	1-5	30-60
Tetracaine	✓	✓	50	0.5-2	3-8	30-60
Miscellaneous		✓	100	0.5-1	< 10	< 60
Dyclonine						
Pramoxine	✓		200	1	3-5	
Lidocaine/Prilocaine	✓			2.5/2.5	60-120	60-120

[a] Based primarily on application to mucous membranes.

[b] Variable depending on doseform.

Contraindications

Hypersensitivity to any component of these products; ophthalmic use.

Warnings/Precautions

➤*Systemic effects:* Use the lowest dose effective for anesthesia to avoid high plasma levels and serious adverse effects. Repeated doses of **lidocaine** and **dyclonine** may cause significant increases in blood levels with each repeated dose because of slow accumulation of the drug or its metabolites. Have resuscitative equipment available for immediate use. Lidocaine/prilocaine is not recommended for use on mucous membranes because of its much greater absorption through this area than through intact skin, potentially resulting in serious adverse effects.

➤*Methomoglobinemia:* **Benzocaine**, **lidocaine** and **prilocaine** should not be used in those rare patients with congenital or idiopathic methemoglobinemia and in infants younger than 12 months of age who are receiving treatment with methemoglobin-inducing agents. Very young patients or patients with glucose-6–phosphate deficiencies are more susceptible to methemoglobinemia.

➤*Ototoxic effects:* **Lidocaine/prilocaine** has an ototoxic effect when instilled into the middle ear of animals, but not when used in the external auditory canal. Do not use this combination in any situation where penetration or migration beyond the tympanic membrane into the middle ear is possible.

➤*For external or mucous membrane use only:* Do not use in the eyes.

➤*Minimal effective dose:* Reactions and complications are best averted by using the minimal effective dose. Not for prolonged use. Give debilitated or elderly patients, acutely ill patients and children dosages commensurate with their age, size and physical condition.

➤*Severe shock / heartblock:* Use **lidocaine** and **dyclonine** with caution.

➤*Traumatized mucosa:* Use cautiously in persons with known drug sensitivities or in patients with severely traumatized mucosa and sepsis in the region of the application. If irritation or rash occurs, discontinue treatment and institute appropriate therapy.

➤*Oral use:* Topical anesthetics may impair swallowing and enhance danger of aspiration. Do not ingest food for 1 hour after anesthetic use in mouth or throat. This is particularly important in children because of their frequency of eating.

➤*Tartrazine sensitivity:* Some of these products contain tartrazine, which may cause allergic-type reactions (including bronchial asthma) in susceptible individuals. Although the incidence of tartrazine sensitivity in the general population is low, it is frequently seen in patients who also have aspirin hypersensitivity. Specific products containing tartrazine are identified in the product listings.

➤*Sulfite sensitivity:* Some of these products contain sulfites which may cause allergic-type reactions including anaphylactic symptoms and life-threatening or less severe asthmatic episodes in certain susceptible persons. The overall prevalence of sulfite sensitivity in the general population is unknown and probably low. Sulfite sensitivity is seen more frequently in asthmatic or atopic non-asthmatic persons. Specific products containing sulfites are identified in the product listings.

➤*Hepatic function impairment:* Patients with severe hepatic disease, because of their inability to metabolize local anesthetics normally, are at greater risk of developing toxic plasma concentrations of lidocaine and prilocaine.

➤*Pregnancy: Category B* (lidocaine); *Category C* (benzocaine, cocaine, dyclonine, tetracaine). Safety for use during pregnancy has not been established. Use in women of childbearing potential, and particularly in early pregnancy, only when the potential benefits outweigh the potential hazards to the fetus.

➤*Lactation:* Lidocaine, and probably prilocaine, are excreted in breast milk. Exercise caution when administering any of these drugs to a nursing woman.

➤*Children:* Safety and efficacy of dyclonine and tetracaine have not been established in children younger than 12 years of age. Do not use benzocaine in infants less than 1 year of age. Dosages in children should be reduced commensurate with age, body weight and physical condition.

Drug Interactions

➤*Class I antiarrhythmic agents:* Use with caution in patients receiving Class I antiarrhythmic drugs (such as tocainide and mexiletine) because the toxic effects are additive and potentially synergistic.

➤*Drug / Lab test interactions:* Dyclonine topical solutions should not be used in cystoscopic procedures following intravenous pyelography because an iodine precipitate occurs which interferes with visualization.

Adverse Reactions

Adverse reactions are, in general, dose-related and may result from high plasma levels due to excessive dosage or rapid absorption, hypersensitivity, idiosyncrasy or diminished tolerance. (See Overdosage.)

➤*Hypersensitivity:* Cutaneous lesions; urticaria; edema; contact dermatitis; bronchospasm; shock; anaphylactoid reactions. The detection of sensitivity by skin testing is of doubtful value.

➤*Local:* Burning; stinging; tenderness; sloughing.

➤*Miscellaneous:* Urethritis with and without bleeding. In a few case reports, methemoglobinemia characterized by cyanosis has followed topical application of **benzocaine** or **lidocaine/prilocaine** and may be more common with prilocaine (see Warnings). Seizures in children have occurred from overuse of **oral lidocaine**.

Overdosage

➤*Symptoms:* Reactions due to overdosage (high plasma levels) are systemic and involve the CNS (convulsions) or the cardiovascular system (hypotension).

CNS – Reactions are excitatory or depressant, and may be characterized by: Nervousness; apprehension; euphoria; confusion; dizziness; lightheadedness; tinnitus; blurred vision; vomiting; sensations of heat, cold or numbness; twitching; tremors; drowsiness; convulsions; unconsciousness; respiratory depression or arrest. Excitatory reactions may be very brief or not occur at all; in this case, first sign of toxicity may be drowsiness, merging into unconsciousness and respiratory arrest.

Cardiovascular – Reactions are depressant, and may be characterized by: Hypotension; myocardial depression; bradycardia; cardiac arrest; cardiovascular collapse.

➤*Treatment:* Maintain airway and support ventilation. Cardiovascular support consists of vasopressors, preferably those that stimulate the myocardium, IV fluids and perhaps blood transfusions. Control convulsions by slow IV of 0.1 mg/kg diazepam or 10 to 50 mg succinylcholine, with continued use of oxygen. Refer to General Management of Acute Overdosage.

Methemoglobinemia – This may be treated with methylene blue 1%, 1 to 2 mg/kg IV over 10 minutes (refer to individual monograph).

Patient Information

Do not ingest food for 1 hour following use of oral topical anesthetic preparations in the mouth or throat. Topical anesthesia may impair swallowing, thus enhancing the danger of aspiration.

Numbness of the tongue or buccal mucosa may increase the danger of biting trauma. Do not eat or chew gum while the mouth or throat area is anesthetized.

When lidocaine/prilocaine is used, the patient should be aware that the production of dermal analgesia may be accompanied by the block of all sensations in the treated skin. For this reason, the patient should avoid inadvertent trauma to the treated area by scratching, rubbing, or exposure to extreme hot or cold temperatures until complete sensation has returned.

Amide Local Anesthetics

DIBUCAINE

otc	**Dibucaine** (Various, eg, IDE, Moore)	**Ointment:** 1%	In 30 g.
otc	**Nupercainal** (Ciba Consumer)		Acetone, sodium bisulfite, lanolin, mineral oil, white petrolatum. In 30 and 60 g.

DIBUCAINE — TOPICAL

Complete prescribing information begins in the Local Anesthetics, Topical group monograph.

Indications

➤*Topical pain:* For prompt, temporary relief of pain, itching and burning due to hemorrhoids or other anorectal disorders. May also be used topically for temporary relief of pain and itching associated with sunburn, minor burns, cuts, scrapes, insect bites or minor skin irritation.

Administration and Dosage

➤*Adults:*

Topical pain – Ointment should be applied externally to the affected area up to 3 or 4 times daily.

➤*Children:*

Topical pain –

12 years of age or older: Ointment should be applied externally to the affected area up to 3 or 4 times daily.

2 to 12 years of age: Advise patients or caregivers not to use this product in this age group except under the advice and supervision of a health care provider.

➤*Preparation for administration:* When practical, affected area should be cleansed with mild soap and warm water and rinsed thoroughly. The area should be gently dried by patting or blotting with toilet tissue or a soft cloth before application of the product. Puncture tube seal with cap or sharp object.

➤*Administration:* For external use only. Product should not be put into the rectum by using fingers or any mechanical device.

➤*Storage/Stability:* Store between 15° to 30°C (59° to 86°F).

LIDOCAINE HYDROCHLORIDE

Rx	**Numby Stuff** (Iomed)	**Solution; topical:** 2% For iontophoretic dermal delivery.	1:100,000 epinephrine per 30 mL multiple-unit fliptop vial.
Rx	**LTA 360 Kit** (Hospira)	**Solution; topical:** 4%	Preservative free. In single use 4 mL prefilled vial.
Rx	**Lidocaine Hydrochloride** (Moore)	**Ointment; topical:** 5%	In 50 g.
otc	**Solarcaine Aloe Extra Burn Relief** (Schering-Plough)	**Cream; topical:** 0.5%	Aloe, lanolin oil, lanolin, camphor, propylparaben, eucalyptus oil, EDTA, menthol, tartrazine. In 120 g.
Rx	**Lidocaine Hydrochloride** (River's Edge)	**Cream; topical:** 3%	Alcohols, aluminum sulfate, glycerin, light mineral oil, parabens, petrolatum. In 28.35 and 85 g.
Rx	**LidaMantle** (Doak Dermatologics)		Cetyl alcohol, stearyl alcohol, glycerin, petrolatum, parabens, light mineral oil. In 28 and 85 g.
Rx	**AneCream** (Focus Health Group)	**Cream; topical:** 4%	Benzyl alcohol, cholesterol, polysorbate 80, propylene glycol, trolamine. In 15 and 30 g and 5 g kits with 5s and 10s *Tegaderm* patches.
otc	**L-M-X4** (Ferndale)		Benzyl alcohol. In 5 and 30 g.
Rx	**Lidocaine Hydrochloride** (River's Edge)	**Lotion; topical:** 3%	Aluminum sulfate, alcohols, glycerin, light mineral oil, parabens, petrolatum. In 177 mL.
otc	**Solarcaine Aloe Extra Burn Relief** (Schering-Plough)	**Gel; topical:** 0.5%	Aloe vera gel, glycerin, EDTA, isopropyl alcohol, menthol, diazolidinyl urea, tartrazine. In 120 and 240 g.
otc	**Burn-O-Jel** (S.S.S. Company)		Aloe vera gel, EDTA, glycerin, ethyl alcohol. In 58 g.
otc	**Regenecare HA** (MPM Medical)	**Gel; topical:** 2%	Glycerin, parabens. In 85 g.
otc	**Regenecare Wound** (MPM Medical)		Aloe, collagen. In 14 g.
otc	**Topicaine** (ESBA Labs)	**Gel; topical** 4%	Aloe vera oil, benzyl alcohol, EDTA, 35% ethanol, glycerin, glyceryl, jojoba oil. In 10, 30, and 113 g.
otc	**Topicaine 5** (ESBA Labs)	**Gel; topical** 5%	Aloe vera oil, benzyl alcohol, EDTA, ethanol, glycerin, glyceryl, jojoba oil, shea butter. In 10, 30, and 113 g.

LIDOCAINE HYDROCHLORIDE

otc	**Solarcaine Aloe Extra Burn Relief** (Schering-Plough)	**Spray; topical:** 0.5%	Aloe vera gel, glycerin, EDTA, diaolidinyl urea, vitamin E, parabens. In 135 mg.
otc	**Anestafoam** (Onset Therapeutics)	**Aerosol foam; topical:** 4%	Benzyl alcohol. In 30 g.
Rx	**Lidocaine Hydrochloride**[a] (Various, eg, Moore, Roxane)	**Solution; topical:** 4% For topical anesthesia of accessible mucous membranes of the oral and nasal cavities and proximal portions of the digestive tract.	In 50 mL.[a]
Rx	**Xylocaine** (APP Pharmaceutical)		Preservative free. Parabens. In 50 mL.
Rx	**Lidocaine 2% Viscous**[b] (Various, eg, Moore, Roxane)	**Solution; topical:** 2% For topical anesthesia of irritated or inflamed mucous membranes of the mouth and pharynx. Also used to reduce gagging during the taking of x-rays or dental impressions.	In 50 and 100 mL and UD 20 mL.[a,b,c]
Rx	**Lidocaine Hydrochloride** (Various, eg, IMS, Teva)	**Jelly; topical:** 2%	Available with or without preservatives. In 30 mL and UD 5, 10, and 20 mL single-use vials.
Rx	**Anestacon** (PolyMedica)		Hydroxypropylmethylcellulose 1%, benzalkonium chloride 0.01%. In 15 and 240 mL disposable units.
Rx	**Xylocaine** (APP Pharmaceutical)		In 5 and 30 mL.
Rx	**Lidoderm** (Endo)	**Patch; topical:** 10 × 14 cm. 5% lidocaine. For relief of pain associated with postherpetic neuralgia.	EDTA, glycerin, parabens, polyvinyl alcohol. In 5s.

[a] May contain parabens.
[b] May contain sodium carboxymethylcellulose.
[c] May contain saccharin.

LIDOCAINE HYDROCHLORIDE — TOPICAL

Complete prescribing information begins in the Local Anesthetics, Topical class monograph.

Indications

➤*Anorectal discomfort:*

Cream 5%, Gel 5% – For the temporary relief of local discomfort, including pain and itching, soreness or burning associated with anorectal disorders.

➤*Anesthetic lubricant for intubation:*

Jelly and ointment – Lidocaine 2% jelly is useful as an anesthetic lubricant for endotracheal intubation (oral and nasal).

Lidocaine 5% ointment is also useful as an anesthetic lubricant for intubation.

➤*Oropharynx anesthetic:*

Ointment – For production of anesthesia of accessible mucous membrane of the oropharynx.

➤*Postherpetic neuralgia:*

Patch – For relief of pain associated with postherpetic neuralgia. Apply only to intact skin.

➤*Skin discomfort/irritation/itching/pain:*

Cream 4% and ointment 2.5% and 5% – For the temporary relief of pain associated with minor cuts and abrasions of the skin, minor burns, including sunburn, minor skin irritation or abrasions of the skin, and insect bites.

Cream 3% – Pruritus, pruritic eczemas, abrasions, minor burns, insect bites, pain, soreness and discomfort due to pruritus ani, pruritus vulvae, hemorrhoids, anal fissures, and similar conditions of the skin and mucous membranes.

Gel 4% – For temporary relief of pain and itching on normal intact skin.

➤*Urethral pain:*

Jelly – For prevention and control of pain in procedures involving the male and female urethra and for topical treatment of painful urethritis.

➤*Off-label uses:*

Migraines – [2] = Fair documentation. Based on the reviewed information, it is not clear if intranasal lidocaine offers a benefit in all migraine patients or which formulation is most effective (eg, gel, solution, spray).

Administration and Dosage

➤*General dosing considerations:* When topical lidocaine formulations are used concomitantly with other products containing lidocaine, the total dose contributed by all formulations must be kept in mind. The amount absorbed is determined by the area over which it is applied and the duration of application.

Although the incidence of systemic adverse reactions is very low, exercise caution, particularly when applying it over large areas and leaving it on for longer than 2 hours. The incidence of systemic adverse reactions can be expected to be directly proportional to the area and time of exposure.

Dosage adjustment may be required for patients with hepatic impairment. (See Hepatic Function Impairment.)

➤*Adults:*

Anesthetic lubricant for intubation –

Jelly 2%:

• *Usual dosage* – Apply a moderate amount to the external surface of the endotracheal tube shortly before use. Care should be taken to avoid introducing the product into the lumen of the tube. Do not use to lubricate endotracheal stylettes. There have been rare reports concerning the inner lumen occlusion.

It is also recommended that use of endotracheal tubes with dried jelly on the external surface be avoided for lack of lubricating effect.

• *Maximum dose* – No more than 600 mg or 30 mL should be given in any 12-hour period.

Ointment 5%:

• *Usual dosage* – Apply to the tube prior to intubation.

• *Maximum dose* – A single application should not exceed 5 g of lidocaine 5% ointment, containing 250 mg of lidocaine base (equivalent chemically to approximately 300 mg of lidocaine hydrochloride). This is roughly equivalent to squeezing a 6 inch length of ointment from the tube. In a 70 kg adult this dose equals 3.6 mg/kg (1.6 mg/lb) lidocaine base. No more than one-half tube, approximately 17 to 20 g of ointment or 850 to 1,000 mg lidocaine base, should be administered in any 1 day.

Anorectal discomfort –

Cream 5%: Apply a thick layer to intact skin.

Oropharynx anesthetic –

Ointment 5%:

• *Usual dosage* – In dentistry, apply to previously dried oral mucosa. Subsequent removal of excess saliva with cotton rolls or saliva ejector minimizes dilution of the ointment, permits maximum penetration, and minimizes the possibility of swallowing the topical ointment.

For use in connection with the insertion of new dentures, apply to all denture surfaces contacting mucosa. Patient should consult a dentist at intervals not exceeding 48 hours throughout the fitting period.

• *Maximum dose* – See Anesthetic Lubricant for Intubation for dosing.

Postherpetic neuralgia –

Patch:

• *Usual dosage* – Apply up to 3 patches, only once for up to 12 hours within a 24-hour period. Apply to intact skin to cover the most painful area.

• *Concomitant therapy* – When used concomitantly with other products containing local anesthetic agents, the amount absorbed from all formulations must be considered.

• *Discontinuation of therapy* – If irritation or a burning sensation occurs during application, remove the patch(es) and do not reapply until the irritation subsides.

Skin discomfort/irritation –

Ointment 5%:

• *Usual dosage* – Apply topically for adequate control of symptoms. The use of a sterile gauze pad is suggested for application to broken skin tissue.

• *Maximum dose* – See Anesthetic Lubricant for Intubation for dosing.

Cream 3%: Apply a thin film to the affected area 2 or 3 times daily.

Cream 4%: Apply a thick layer to intact skin.

Urethral pain –

Jelly 2%:

• *Usual dosage* –

Female patients: Slowly instill 3 to 5 mL (60 to 100 mg of lidocaine) into the urethra. If desired, some jelly may be deposited on a cotton swab and introduced into the urethra. In order to obtain adequate anesthesia, several minutes should be allowed prior to performing urological procedures.

Male patients: Slowly instill approximately 15 mL (300 mg of lidocaine) into the urethra or until the patient has a feeling of tension. A penile clamp is then applied for several minutes at the corona. An additional dose of not more than 15 mL (300 mg) can be instilled for adequate anesthesia.

Amide Local Anesthetics

LIDOCAINE HYDROCHLORIDE — TOPICAL

Prior to sounding or cystoscopy, a penile clamp should be applied for 5 to 10 minutes to obtain adequate anesthesia. A total dose of 30 mL (600 mg) is usually required to fill and dilate the male urethra. Prior to catheterization, smaller volumes of 5 to 10 mL (100 to 200 mg) are usually adequate for lubrication.

- *Maximum dose* – No more than 600 mg or 30 mL should be given in any 12-hour period.

Off-label dosing –

Migraines: [2] = Fair documentation. Dosages of lidocaine 4% solution ranged from 0.4 to 1 mL instilled in 1 or both nostrils. Doses were repeated in 2 to 15 minutes, if needed. Initial doses were administered in a clinical care setting with specific head positioning, and 2 studies provided product for patient use at home.

➤*Children:* Dosages in children should be reduced, commensurate with age, body weight, and physical condition. The maximum dose may be determined by the application of one of the standard pediatric drug formulas (eg, Clark's rule).

Anesthetic lubricant for intubation –

Jelly 2%:
- *Usual dosage* – See Adults for dosing.
- *Maximum dose* – 4.5 mg/kg.

Anorectal discomfort –

12 years of age and older:
- *Cream 5%* – Apply a thick layer to intact skin. A single application in a child weighing less than 10 kg should not be applied over an area greater than 100 cm^2. A single application in children weighing between 10 and 20 kg should not be applied over an area greater than 600 cm^2.

Oropharynx anesthetic –

Ointment 5%: See Adults for dosing.
- *Maximum dose* – 4.5 mg/kg.

Skin discomfort/irritation – A single application in a child weighing less than 10 kg should not be applied over an area greater than 100 cm^2. A single application in children weighing between 10 and 20 kg should not be applied over an area greater than 600 cm^2.

Cream 3%: See Adults for dosing.

Cream 4%:
- *2 years of age and older* – See Adults for dosing.

Urethral pain –

Jelly 2%:
- *Usual dosage* – See Adults for dosing.
- *Maximum dose* – 4.5 mg/kg.

Off-label dosing –

Anesthetic: 3 mg/kg per dose not more often than every 2 hours.

➤*Elderly:* Elderly patients should be given reduced doses commensurate with their age and physical status.

➤*Hepatic function impairment:* Patients with severe hepatic disease, because of their inability to metabolize local anesthetics normally, are at greater risk of developing toxic plasma concentrations of lidocaine. Smaller areas of treatment are recommended.

➤*Debilitated and acutely ill patients:* Debilitated and acutely ill patients should be given reduced doses commensurate with their age and physical status.

➤*Preparation for administration:*

Jelly – When using lidocaine 2% jelly 30 mL tubes, sterilize the plastic cone for 5 minutes in boiling water, cool, and attach to the tube. The cone may be gas sterilized or cold sterilized, as preferred. The lidocaine 2% jelly syringes do not require sterilization. The syringes are prefilled sterile disposable units packaged in presterilized trays.

➤*Administration:* Avoid contact with eyes. Do not apply to irritated skin or if excessive irritation develops. Do not use in large quantities, particularly over raw or blistered area. Application of lidocaine cream to larger area or for longer periods of time than those recommended could result in sufficient absorption of lidocaine resulting in serious adverse effects.

When using in young children, take care to ensure that application of the cream is limited to the intended site.

Cream – Apply topically for adequate control of symptoms. The use of a sterile gauze pad is suggested for application to broken skin tissue.

Jelly 2%, ointment 5% – When indicated for intubation, apply to the tube prior to intubation.

Patch – Patches may be cut into smaller sizes with scissors prior to removal of the release liner. Clothing may be worn over the area of application.

Hands should be washed after the handling of the lidocaine patch and eye contact should be avoided. The used patch should be immediately disposed of in such a way as to prevent access by children or pets.

➤*Storage/Stability:*

Cream and ointment – Store at 15° to 30°C (59° to 86°F). Protect from freezing. Keep container closed tightly at all times when not in use.

Jelly – Store at 20° to 25°C (68° to 77°F).

Patch – Store at 25°C (77°F); excursions are permitted between 15° and 30°C (59° and 86°F).

Ester Local Anesthetics

BENZOCAINE

otc	**Dent's Extra Strength Toothache Gum** (C.S. Dent)	**Gum; dental:** 20%	In 1 g.
otc	**3 in 1 Toothache Relief** (C.S. Dent)	**Gum, Liquid, Lotion/Gel; dental:** Benzocaine	In family first-aid packs.
otc	**Anbesol Cold Sore Therapy** (Wyeth Consumer Health)	**Ointment; dental:** 20%	Allantoin 1%, aloe, benzyl alcohol, camphor 64.9%, menthol, parabens, petrolatum, vitamin E. In 7.1 g.
otc	**Benzodent** (Procter & Gamble)		In 30 g.
otc	**Orajel P.M. Nighttime Formula Toothache Pain Relief** (Del Pharma)	**Cream; dental:** 20%	Menthol, methyl salicylate, saccharin. In 5.4 g.
otc sf	**Babee Teething** (SmithKline Beecham Consumer)	**Lotion; dental:** 2.5%	Dye free, sugar free. Camphor, cetalkonium chloride 0.02%, eucalyptol, menthol. In 15 mL.
otc	**Dent's Lotion-Jel** (C.S. Dent)	**Lotion/Gel; dental:** Benzocaine	In 6 g.
otc	**Double-Action Toothache Kit** (C.S. Dent)	**Liquid; dental:** Benzocaine	Alcohol 74%, chlorobutanol anhydrous 0.09%. Also contains **Maranox Pain Relief Tablets** containing 325 mg acetaminophen. In 8 tablets with 3.7 mL drops.
otc sf	**Tanac Roll-On** (Del Pharm)	**Liquid; dental:** 5%	Benzalkonium chloride 0.12%, saccharin. In 8.8 mL.

BENZOCAINE

otc	**Anbesol** (Wyeth Consumer Health)	**Liquid; dental:** 6.3%	Alcohol 70%, camphor, menthol, phenol 0.5%, povidone-iodine. In 9 and 22 mL.
otc	**Orasol** (Goldline)		Alcohol 70%, camphor, menthol, phenol 0.5%, povidone-iodine. In 14.79 mL.
otc	**Orajel Baby** (Del Pharma)	**Liquid; dental:** 7.5%	Parabens, saccharin, sorbitol. Very berry flavor. In 13.3 mL.
otc	**OraMagic Plus** (MPM Medical)	**Liquid; dental:** 10%	Alcohol free. Aloe vera extract, maltodextrin, xylitol. In 60 mL.
otc	**Tanac** (Del Pharma)		Benzalkonium chloride 0.12%, saccharin. In 13 mL.
otc	**Anbesol Maximum Strength** (Wyeth Consumer Health)	**Liquid; dental:** 20%	Benzyl alcohol, methylparaben, PEG, saccharin. In 9 mL.
otc	**Dent-O-Kain/20** (Geritrex)		Benzyl alcohol, saccharin. In 9 mL.
otc	**Dent's Maximum Strength Toothache Drops** (C.S. Dent)		Alcohol 74%, eugenol, chlorobutanol anhydrous 0.09%. In 3.7 mL.
otc	**Orajel Maximum Strength** (Del Pharm)		Ethyl alcohol 44.2%, phenol, saccharin. In 13.3 mL.
otc	**Orajel Mouth-Aid** (Del)		Cetylpyridinium chloride 0.1%, ethyl alcohol 70%, saccharin. In 13.5 mL.
otc	**Kank-a** (Blistex)	**Liquid/Film; dental:** 20%	Alcohols, benzoin compound tincture, benzyl alcohol, castor oil, saccharin. In 9.9 mL.
otc	**Toothache Gel** (Roberts Med)	**Gel; dental:** Benzocaine	Benzyl alcohol, oil of cloves, propylene glycol. In 15 g.
otc sf	**Anbesol** (Wyeth Consumer)	**Gel; dental:** 6.3%	Sugar free. Alcohol 70%, camphor, phenol 0.5%. In 7.5 g.
otc	**Anbesol Baby** (Pfizer)	**Gel; dental:** 7.5%	Alcohol free. Benzoic acid, edetate disodium, glycerin, parabens, PEG, saccharin. Grape flavor. In 7.1 g.
otc	**Orajel Baby** (Del Pharm)		Alcohol free. Saccharin, sorbitol. In 9.45 g.
otc	**Anbesol Jr.** (Wyeth Consumer Health)	**Gel; dental:** 10%	Acesulfame K, benzyl alcohol, glycerin, methylparaben, PEG. Bubble gum flavor. In 9 g.
otc	**Orajel Baby Nighttime** (Del Pharm)		Alcohol free. Saccharin, sorbitol. Cherry flavor. In 6 g.
otc	**Orajel Regular Strength** (Church Dwight)		PEG, saccharin. In 5.1, 7.1, and 9.4 g.
otc sf	**Orajel/d** (Del Pharm)		Saccharin. In 9.45 g.
otc	**Zilactin-B Medicated** (Zila)		Alcohol 76%. In 7.5 g.
otc	**Benz-O-Sthetic** (Geritrex)	**Gel; dental:** 20%	Benzyl alcohol, PEG. In 29 g.
otc	**Hurricaine** (Beutlich)		Alcohol 60%, saccharin. In 7 g.
otc	**Orajel Maximum Strength** (Del Pharma)		Saccharin. In 9.45 g.
otc sf	**Orajel Mouth-Aid** (Del Pharm)		Sugar free. Benzalkonium chloride 0.02%, saccharin, zinc chloride 0.1%. In 9.45 g.
otc sf	**Orajel Brace-aid** (Del Pharm)		Saccharin. In 14.1 g.
otc	**SensoGARD** (Block)		Parabens. In 0.5 g.
otc	**SensoGARD** (Block)		Parabens. In 0.5 g.
otc	**Orabase** (Colgate)	**Paste; dental:** 20%	In 5 g.
otc	**Orabase-B** (Colgate)		Mineral oil. In 5 and 15 g.

Ester Local Anesthetics

BENZOCAINE

otc	**Hurricaine** (Beutlich)	**Spray; dental**: 20%	Cherry flavor. In 60 mL.
otc	**Hurricaine** (Beutlich)	**Swabs; dental**: 20%	PEG, saccharin. In 72s.
otc	**Foille Medicated First Aid** (Blistex)	**Ointment; topical**: 5%	Benzyl alcohol, chloroxylenol 0.1%, EDTA. In 3.5 and 28 g.
otc	**Boil-Ease** (Del)	**Ointment; topical**: 20%	Camphor, lanolin, eucalyptus oil, menthol, petrolatum, phenol. In 30 g.
otc	**Benzocaine** (Various, eg, IDE)	**Cream; topical**: 5%	In 480 g.
otc	**Bicozene** (Sandoz)	**Cream; topical**: 6%	Castor oil, glycerin, 1.67% resorcinol. In 30 g.
otc	**Lanacane** (Combe)		Alcohol, aloe, benzethonium chloride 0.1%, castor oil, glycerin, parabens. In 28 and 56 g.
otc	**Solarcaine** (Schering-Plough)	**Lotion; topical**: Benzocaine	Alcohol, aloe, camphor, EDTA, menthol, mineral oil, parabens, triclosan. In 120 mL.
otc	**Dermoplast** (Whitehall-Robins)	**Lotion; topical**: 8%	Aloe, glycerin, lanolin. menthol 0.5%, parabens. In 90 mL.
otc	**Chigger-Tox** (Scherer)	**Liquid; topical**: Benzocaine	Benzyl benzoate, green soap. In 30 mL.
otc	**Benz-O-Sthetic** (Geritrex)	**Spray; topical**: 20%	In 56 g.
otc	**Dermoplast** (Medtech)		Aloe, lanolin, menthol 0.5%, methylparaben. In 59 mL.
otc	**Dermoplast Antibacterial** (Medtech)		Aloe, benzethonium chloride 0.2%, lanolin, menthol, methylparaben. In 59 mL.
otc	**Lanacane** (Combe)		Aloe extract, benzethonium chloride 0.1%, ethanol 36%. In 113 mL.
otc	**Solarcaine Medicated First Aid Spray** (Schering-Plough)		Triclosan alcohol 0.13%. In 90 mL.
otc	**Foille Medicated First Aid** (Blistex)	**Aerosol; topical**: 5%	Benzyl alcohol, chloroxylenol 0.6%. In 92 mL.
otc	**Solarcaine** (Schering-Plough)	**Aerosol; topical**: 20%	Alcohols. In 90 and 120 mL.

BENZOCAINE — TOPICAL

Complete prescribing information begins in the Local Anesthetics, Topical group monograph.

Indications

➤*Topical pain:*

Anesthetic lubricant – For general use as a lubricant and topical anesthetic on intratracheal catheters and pharyngeal and nasal airways to obtund the pharyngeal and tracheal reflexes; on nasogastric and endoscopic tubes; urinary catheters; laryngoscopes; proctoscopes; sigmoidoscopes; and vaginal specula.

Cream – For temporary relief of minor skin irritations.

Cream and paste 20% – For temporary pain relief of mouth and gum sores, mouth pain, canker sores, cold sores, fever blisters, minor irritation of the mouth caused by dentures or orthodontic appliances.

Gel – For temporary relief of pain associated with minor dental procedures, canker sores, fever blisters, braces, cold sores, dentures, teething, toothaches, gum pain, minor irritation, sore mouth, and sore throat.

Lubricant 5% or 4% – Helps in temporarily prolonging the time until ejaculation. Safe for use with prophylactics.

➤*Liquid:* For temporary relief of pain associated with:

Medical indications – Minor cuts and burns, nasal packing, nasal biopsies, passing nasogastric tubes, mucositis, stomatitis, thrush, head and neck examinations, condylomata, culdocentesis, proctoscopic exams.

Dental indications – Injections, rubber dams, suture removal, instrumentation, arch bar removal, minor mouth irritation, banding a molar, removal of mobile deciduous teeth, deep scalings, localized gingival curettage, denture discomfort, and post-operation discomfort.

➤*Ointment:* For the temporary relief of local pain, itching, and soreness associated with hemorrhoids and anorectal inflammation.

Anbesol ointment – For temporary relief of pain associated with fever blisters and cold sores.

➤*Spray:* For oral and mucosal anesthesia to control pain and to suppress the gag reflex. For oral or mucosal application.

Administration and Dosage

➤*Adults:* See Indications for specific uses.

Anesthetic lubricant for passage of catheter and instruments – Apply evenly to exterior of tube or instrument prior to use.

Fever blister and cold sores –

Ointment (Anbesol): Apply to the affected area not more than 3 or 4 times daily.

Hemorrhoids –

Ointment: Do not put this product into the rectum by using fingers or any mechanical device or applicator. Do not exceed the recommended dosage unless directed to do so by a health care provider.

Minor skin irritations –

Aerosol, cream, lotion, ointment, spray: Up to 4 times daily or as directed.
• *Liquid* – Apply to area to be anesthetized. Anesthesia is accomplished within 15 to 30 seconds.

Oral and mucosal pain –

Cream, gel, paste: Apply to the affected area, allow to remain in place at least 1 minute, and then spit out. Use up to 4 times daily or as directed by a health care provider or dentist.

Liquid: Apply to area to be anesthetized. Anesthesia is accomplished within 15 to 30 seconds.

Spray: Apply to the affected area. Gargle, swish around mouth, or allow to remain in place no longer than 30 seconds and then spit out. Use up to 4 times daily or as directed by a health care provider or dentist.

Premature ejaculation – Apply a small amount of 4% or 5% lubricant to head and shaft of penis before intercourse, or use as directed by a health care provider. Wash product off after intercourse.

Toothache –

Cream, gel, liquid: Apply to the affected area up to 4 times daily. For cream, squeeze a 1-inch strip onto finger or cotton swab. Apply it to affected cavity and around gum surrounding the teeth before bedtime. The cream will stay in place for extended duration of relief.

BENZOCAINE — TOPICAL

➤*Children:*

Anesthetic lubricant for the passage of catheter and instruments – *1 year and older:* See Adults for dosing.

Fever blister and cold sores – *2 years and older:* See Adults for dosing.

Minor skin irritations – *2 years and older:* See Adults for dosing.

Oral and mucosal pain – Provide adult supervision in the use of this product in children younger than 12 years.

2 years and older:

- *Cream, gel, paste* – See Adults for dosing.
- *Spray* – See Adults for dosing.

Toothache –

Cream, gel, liquid:

- *2 years and older* – See Adults for dosing.

➤*Administration:*

Cream, gel, paste (for oral pain) – To open tube, cut the tip of the tube on the score mark with scissors.

Ointment (for hemorrhoids) – Do not put this product into the rectum by using fingers or any mechanical device or applicator. Do not exceed the recommended dosage unless directed to do so by a health care provider.

Spray – Firmly insert disposable extension tube into hole on side of spray can valve. The extension tube is designed to fit securely. Hold spray extension tube tip 1 to 2 inches away from area to be anesthetized. Spray half a second. Repeat if necessary. Anesthesia is accomplished in 15 to 30 seconds.

20% strengths – Do not use more than 4 times in a 24-hour period unless directed by a health care provider or dentist. Do not use more than directed. Do not use for more than 7 days unless directed by a health care provider or dentist.

➤*Storage/Stability:* Store at room temperature between 20° and 25°C (68° and 77°F).

Lubricant – Store at 15° to 25°C (59° to 77°F).

Spray – Do not store at temperatures above 49°C (120°F).

COCAINE

c-ii	**Cocaine HCl** (Roxane)	**Topical Solution:** 4%	In 10 mL multidose and UD 4 mL.
		10%	In 10 mL multidose and UD 4 mL.
c-ii	**Cocaine Viscous** (Roxane)	**Topical Solution:** 4%	In 10 mL multidose and UD 4 mL.
		10%	In 10 mL multidose bottles and UD 4 mL.
c-ii	**Cocaine HCl** (Mallinckrodt)	**Powder**	In 5 and 25 g.

COCAINE HYDROCHLORIDE — TOPICAL

Indications

➤*Topical anesthesia:* For the introduction of local (topical) anesthesia of accessible mucous membranes of the oral, laryngeal and nasal cavities.

Administration and Dosage

➤*General dosing considerations:* The dosage varies and depends on the area to be anesthetized, vascularity of the tissues, individual tolerance, and the technique of anesthesia.

➤*Adults:*

Topical anesthesia – Apply the lowest dosage needed to provide effective anesthesia.

➤*Children:* Dosages should be reduced for children.

➤*Elderly:* Dosages should be reduced for elderly patients.

➤*Debilitated patients:* Dosages should be reduced for debilitated patients.

➤*Administration:* Cocaine topical solution can be administered by means of cotton applicators or packs, instilled into a cavity, or as a spray.

➤*Storage/Stability:* Store at 15° to 30°C (59° to 86°F).

Actions

➤*Pharmacology:* Cocaine blocks the initiation or conduction of the nerve impulse following local application, thereby effecting local anesthetic action.

➤*Pharmacokinetics:* Cocaine is absorbed from all sites of application, including mucous membranes and the gastrointestinal mucosa. Cocaine is degraded by plasma esterases, with the half-life in the plasma being ≈ 1 hour.

Contraindications

Known history of hypersensitivity to the drug or to the components of the topical solution.

Warnings/Precautions

➤*Resuscitative equipment:* Resuscitative equipment and drugs should be immediately available when any local anesthetic is used.

➤*Special risk:* The lowest dosage that results in effective anesthesia should be used to avoid high plasma levels and serious adverse effects. Debilitated, elderly patients, acutely ill patients, and children should be given reduced doses commensurate with their age and physical status.

Cocaine hydrochloride topical solution should be used with caution in patients with severely traumatized mucosa and sepsis in the region of the proposed application. Use with caution in persons with known drug sensitivities.

➤*Pregnancy: Category C. Category X* (if nonmedical use) (per Briggs' *Drugs in Pregnancy and Lactation*). Animal reproduction studies have not been conducted with cocaine. It is also not known whether cocaine can cause fetal harm when administered to a pregnant woman or can affect reproduction capacity. The low molecular weight (about 340), high water and lipid solubility, and low ionization at physiologic pH indicate cocaine should freely cross to the fetus. Cocaine should be given to a pregnant woman only if needed.

➤*Lactation:* The American Academy of Pediatrics classifies the use of cocaine as contraindicated during breast-feeding.

Adverse Reactions

Adverse reactions may be due to high plasma levels as a result of excessive and rapid absorption of the drug. Reactions are systemic in nature and involve the central nervous system or the cardiovascular system. A small number of reactions may result from hypersensitivity, idiosyncrasy or diminished tolerance on the part of the patient.

➤*Cardiovascular:* Small doses of cocaine slow the heart rate, but after moderate doses, the rate is increased due to central sympathetic stimulation.

➤*CNS:* CNS reactions are excitatory or depressant and may be characterized by nervousness, restlessness and excitement. Tremors and eventually clonicotonic convulsions may result. Emesis may occur. Central stimulation is followed by depression, with death resulting from respiratory failure.

Cocaine is pyrogenic, augmenting heat production in stimulating muscular activity and causing vasoconstriction which decreases heat loss. Cocaine is known to interfere with the uptake of norepinephrine by adrenergic nerve terminals, producing sensitization to catecholamines, causing vasoconstriction and mydriasis.

➤*Ophthalmic:* Cocaine causes sloughing of the corneal epithelium, causing clouding, pitting, and occasionally ulceration of the cornea. The drug is not meant for ophthalmic use.

Overdosage

The fatal dose of cocaine has been approximated at 1.2 g, although severe toxic effects have been reported from doses as low as 20 mg.

➤*Symptoms:* The symptoms of cocaine poisoning are referable to the CNS, namely the patient becomes excited, restless, garrulous, anxious and confused. Enhanced reflexes, headache, rapid pulse, irregular respiration, chills, rise in body temperature, mydriasis, exophthalmos, nausea, vomiting and abdominal pain are noticed. In severe overdoses, delirium, Cheyne-Stokes respiration, convulsions, unconsciousness, and death from respiratory arrest result. Acute poisoning by cocaine is rapid in developing.

➤*Treatment:* The specific treatment of acute cocaine poisoning is the intravenous administration of a short-acting barbiturate or diazepam. Artificial respiration may be necessary. It is important to limit absorption of the drug. If entrance of the drug into circulation can be checked, and respiratory exchange maintained, the prognosis is favorable since cocaine is eliminated fairly rapidly.

PRAMOXINE HYDROCHLORIDE

otc	**Prax** (Ferndale)	**Cream; topical:** 1%	Hydrophilic base with glycerin, cetyl alcohol, white petrolatum. In 30 and 113.4 g and 1 lb.
otc	**Tronothane HCl** (Abbott)		Water miscible base with cetyl alcohol, glycerin, parabens. In 28.4 g.
otc	**Sarna Ultra** (GlaxoSmithKline)		0.5% menthol, 30% petrolatum, benzyl alcohol. In 56.6 g.
otc	**Prax** (Ferndale)	**Lotion; topical:** 1%	Hydrophilic base with mineral oil, cetyl alcohol, glycerin, lanolin, 0.1% potassium sorbate, 0.1% sorbic acid. In 15, 120 and 240 mL.
otc	**Sarna Sensitive Anti-Itch** (Stiefel)		Benzyl alcohol, cetyl alcohol, petrolatum. Fragrance free. In 222 mL.
otc	**PrameGel** (Bioglan)	**Gel; topical:** 1%	Emollient base with 0.5% menthol, benzyl alcohol, SD alcohol 40. In 118 g.
otc	**Itch-X** (Ascher & Co.)		10% benzyl alcohol, aloe vera gel, diazolidinyl urea, SD alcohol 40, parabens. In 35.4 g.
otc	**Itch-X** (Ascher & Co.)	**Spray; topical:** 1%	10% benzyl alcohol, aloe vera gel, SD alcohol 40. In 60 mL.
otc	**Vagisil Maximum Strength** (Combe)	**Wipes; topical:** 1%	Aloe, disodium edetate, glycerin, parabens, PEG-7. In 12s.
otc	**ProctoFoam** (Alaven Pharmaceutical)	**Aerosol, foam; topical:** 1%	Cetyl alcohol, glyceryl, parabens, PEG-100, propylene glycol, trolamine. In 15 g with applicator.

PRAMOXINE HYDROCHLORIDE — TOPICAL

Complete prescribing information begins in the Local Anesthetics, Topical group monograph.

Indications

➤*Topical pain:*

Foam – For temporary relief of pain and itching associated with hemorrhoids.

Gel and spray – For the temporary relief of pain and itching associated with rashes, minor skin irritations, allergic itches, sunburn, hives, minor burns, insect bites, poison ivy, poison oak and poison sumac.

Lotion – Pramoxine lotion is specially formulated to give prompt, temporary relief from dry itching skin and pain due to minor burns, abrasions and other irritated skin conditions, and to use as an anogenital cleansing lotion.

Non-caine and paraben-free, pramoxine lotion is less irritating and can be used on sensitive skin.

Pramoxine lotion is also applied as a rectal wipe for relief from discomfort and pain in hemorrhoids, fissures, anogenital pruritus, bowel movements, and various dermatologic skin disorders. In addition to use for the pain and discomfort associated with hemorrhoids and fissures, pramoxine lotion is also used following rectal surgery.

Administration and Dosage

➤*Adults:*

Anogenital cleansing –
Lotion: For cleansing of anogenital area, spread pramoxine lotion on cotton or a tissue and wipe the affected area.

Discomfort associated with rectal surgery –
Lotion: Apply to the affected area not more than 3 to 4 times daily.

Topical pain associated with hemorrhoids –
Foam: Apply externally to the affected area up to 5 times daily.
Lotion: Apply to the affected area not more than 3 to 4 times daily.

Topical pain associated with minor skin irritations –
Gel and spray: Apply to affected area not more than 3 to 4 times daily.
Lotion: Apply to the affected area not more than 3 to 4 times daily.

➤*Children:*

Discomfort associated with rectal surgery –
Lotion:
- *2 years of age and older* – See Adults for dosing.

Topical pain associated with hemorrhoids –
Foam:
- *12 years of age and older* – See Adults for dosing.

Lotion:
- *2 years of age and older* – See Adults for dosing.

Topical pain associated with minor skin irritations –
Gel and spray:
- *2 years of age and older* – See Adults for dosing.

Lotion:
- *2 years of age and older* – See Adults for dosing.

➤*Administration:*

Foam – When practicable, cleanse the affected area with mild soap and warm water and rinse thoroughly. Gently dry by patting or blotting with toilet tissue or a soft cloth before application of pramoxine foam.

Shake well before use. Dispense pramoxine foam onto a clean tissue or pad and apply externally to the affected area.

➤*Storage/Stability:* Store pramoxine products at controlled room temperature, between 15° and 30°C (59° and 86°F).

Foam – Store upright. Do not refrigerate. Do not store at temperatures above 48.8°C (120°F).

Spray – Flammable. Keep away from fire or flame.

LOCAL ANESTHETICS, TOPICAL COMBINATIONS

otc	**Dendracin Neurodendraxcin** (Physician's Science and Nature)	**Lotion; topical:** 0.0375% capsaicin, 30% methyl salicylate, 10% menthol	Aloe gel, benzocaine, borage oil, cetyl alcohol, parabens, PEG 100. In 60 mL.
otc	**Chigg Away** (Pierson Labs)	**Lotion; topical:** 5% benzocaine, 10% sulfur	Cetyl alcohol, glycerin, glyceryl, isopropyl alcohol, parabens, petrolatum, triethanolamine. In 118 mL.
otc	**Terocin** (Alexso)	**Lotion; topical:** 0.025% capsaicin, 2.5% lidocaine, 10% menthol, 25% methyl salicylate	Aloe, borago seed oil, cetyl alcohol, parabens, PEG, propylene glycol, triethanolamine. In 120 mL.
otc	**Detane** (Del)	**Gel; topical:** 7.5% benzocaine, carbomer 940, PEG 400	In 15 g.
Rx	**Oraqix** (Dentsply Pharmaceutical)	**Gel; topical:** 2.5% lidocaine, 2.5% prilocaine	In 1.7 g single-use glass cartridges with applicator 20s.
otc	**Sting-Kill** (Randob Labs)	**Swabs; topical:** 20% benzocaine, 1% menthol	Isopropyl alcohol 15%. In 0.5 mL.
otc	**Sting-Kill** (Randob Labs)	**Wipes; topical:** 20% benzocaine, 1% menthol	Isopropyl alcohol 15%. In 8s.
Rx	**Cetacaine** (Cetylite)	14% benzocaine, 2% tetracaine HCl, 2% butamben and 0.5% benzalkonium chloride with 0.005% cetyl dimethyl ethyl ammonium bromide in a bland water soluble base	**Gel:** In 29 g.
			Liquid: In 56 mL.
			Ointment: In 37 g.
			Aerosol: In 56 g.
otc	**Anbesol** (Whitehall)	**Liquid; topical:** 6.3% benzocaine with 0.5% phenol, povidone-iodine, 70% alcohol, camphor, menthol	In 9.3 & 22.2 mL.
		Gel; topical: 6.3% benzocaine, 0.5% phenol, 70% alcohol	In 7.5 g.
otc	**StaphAseptic** (Tec Labs)	**Gel; topical:** 0.2% benzethonium chloride, 2.5% lidocaine HCl	Disodium EDTA, glycerine, polyoxyl 35 castor oil, tea tree oil, white thyme oil. In 56.7 g.
Rx	**Lidocaine/Prilocaine** (Various, eg, Hi-Tech, Sandoz)	**Cream; topical:** 2.5% lidocaine, 2.5% prilocaine	In 5, 15, and 30 g.
Rx	**EMLA** (Abraxis Pharm)	**Cream; topical:** 2.5% lidocaine, 2.5% prilocaine	In 5 g with *Tegaderm* dressings and 30 g.

LOCAL ANESTHETICS, TOPICAL COMBINATIONS

Rx	**Pliaglis** (ZARS)	**Cream; topical:** 7% lidocaine, 7% tetracaine	Parabens, petrolatum, polyvinyl alcohol. In 30 g.
otc	**Vagisil** (Combe)	**Cream; topical:** 5% benzocaine, 2% resorcinol	Aloe, cetearyl alcohol, corn oil, lanolin alcohol, methylparaben, mineral oil, PEG-100, triethanolamine, trisodium EDTA, vitamin A, vitamin D_3, vitamin E. In 28 g.
otc	**Unguentine Maximum Strength** (Lee)		Alcohols, methylparaben, mineral oil. In 28.3 g.
otc	**Vagisil Maximum Strength** (Combe)	**Cream; topical:** 20% benzocaine, 3% resorcinol	Aloe, cetearyl alcohol, corn oil, glyceryl, lanolin alcohol, methylparaben, mineral oil, PEG-100, propylene glycol, triethanolamine, trisodium EDTA, vitamin A, vitamin D_3, vitamin E. In 28 g.
otc	**Chiggerex** (Scherer)	**Ointment; topical:** Benzocaine with camphor, menthol	In 50 g.
otc	**Skeeter Stik** (Triton)	**Liquid; topical:** 4% lidocaine with 2% phenol in an isopropyl alcohol base	In 14 mL.
otc	**Bactine Pain Relieving Cleansing Spray** (Bayer Consumer)	**Spray; topical:** 2.5% lidocaine, 0.13% benzalkonium chloride, EDTA	In 150 mL.
otc	**Bactine Antiseptic Anesthetic** (Bayer Consumer)	2.5% lidocaine HCl, 0.13% benzalkonium chloride, EDTA, 3.17% alcohol	**Aerosol:** In 90 g.
			Spray: In 60, 120 and 480 mL.
otc	**Unguentine Plus** (Mentholatum)	**Cream; topical:** 2% lidocaine HCl with 2% chloroxylenol and 0.5% phenol, parabens, mineral oil	In 30 g.
otc	**Medi-Quik** (Mentholatum)	**Aerosol; topical:** Lidocaine HCl and benzalkonium chloride	In 90 mL.
		Spray; topical: 2% lidocaine, 0.13% benzalkonium chloride, 0.2% camphor, benzyl alcohol	In 85 mL.
otc	**Dr. Scholl's Cracked Heel Relief** (Schering-Plough)	**Cream; topical:** 2% lidocaine, 0.13% benzethonium Cl	Aloe. In 89 mL.
otc	**ProTech First-Aid Stik** (Triton)	**Liquid; topical:** 2.5% lidocaine HCl, 10% povidone iodine	In 14 mL dab-on applicator.
Rx	**Synera** (Ferndale Labs)	**Patch; topical:** 70 mg lidocaine, 70 mg tetracaine, polyvinyl alcohol, sorbitan monopalmitate, parabens	In 2s and 10s.
otc	**TheraPatch Cold Sore** (LecTec)	**Patch; topical:** 4% lidocaine HCl, 0.5% camphor, aloe vera, eucalyptus oil, glycerin	In 21s.
otc	**Campho-Phenique Cold Sore Treatment and Scab Relief** (Bayer Consumer)	**Cream; topical:** 1% pramoxine hydrochloride	30% petrolatum, alcohols, EDTA, glycerin, parabens, ureas. Mint flavor. In 6.5 g.
otc	**Gold Bond Intensive Healing** (Chattem)	**Cream; topical:** 6% dimethicone, 1% pramoxine hydrochloride	Aloe, cetearyl alcohol, cetyl alcohol, EDTA, glycerin, glyceryl stearate, parabens, petrolatum, propylene glycol, stearyl alcohol, urea. In 28 g.

Refer to the general discussion of these products beginning in the Local Anesthetics, Topical group monograph.

MISCELLANEOUS TOPICAL ANESTHETICS

Rx	**Ethyl Chloride** (Gebauer)	**Spray:** Chloroethane **Indications:** Topical vapo-coolant to control pain associated with minor surgical procedures (eg, lancing boils, incision and drainage of small abscesses), athletic injuries, injections and for treatment of myofascial pain, restricted motion and muscle spasm	In 100 g metal tubes, 105 mL *Spra-Pak* and 120 mL bottles (fine, medium, and coarse spray).
Rx	**Fluro-Ethyl** (Gebauer)	**Aerosol spray:** 25% ethyl chloride and 75% dichlorotetrafluoroethane **Indications:** Topical refrigerant anesthetic to control pain associated with minor surgical procedures, dermabrasion, injections, contusions and minor strains	In 270 mL.
Rx	**Gebauer's Spray and Stretch** (Gebauer)	**Spray:** Tetrafluoroethane and pentafluoropropane **Indications:** Vapo-coolant for topical application in management of myofascial pain, restricted motion, muscle spasm, and minor sports injuries	In 103.5 mL.
otc	**Aerofreeze** (Graham-Field)	**Spray:** Trichloromonofluoromethane and dichlorodifluoromethane **Indications:** Topical anesthesia for preinjection, skin planing, dermabrasion and minor surgical procedures; for treatment of strains, sprains and muscle spasms	In 240 mL.

Complete prescribing information begins in the Local Anesthetics, Topical group monograph.

MINOXIDIL

MINOXIDIL

otc	**Rogaine** (Pharmacia & Upjohn)	**Solution; topical:** 2%	In 60 mL bottle with multiple applicators.
otc	**Minoxidil Extra Strength for Men** (Apotex USA)	**Solution; topical:** 5%	30% alcohol. In 60 mL bottles (1s and 2s).
otc	**Rogaine Extra Strength for Men** (Pharmacia & Upjohn)		Alcohol. In two 60 mL bottles w/ dropper and sprayer applicators.
otc	**Rogaine Men's Extra Strength** (Pfizer Cons Health)	**Aerosol, foam; topical:** 5%	Cetyl alcohol, SD alcohol, stearyl alcohol. In 60g.

MINOXIDIL — TOPICAL

Indications

➤*Alopecia:* Treatment of androgenetic alopecia, expressed in males as baldness of the vertex of the scalp and in females as diffuse hair loss or thinning of the frontoparietal areas. At least 4 months of twice-daily applications are generally required before evidence of hair growth can be expected.

➤*Off-label uses:* Although further study is needed, topical minoxidil may be useful in the treatment of alopecia areata (a systemic disease in which patches of hair fall out over a period of a few days; any part of the body may be involved).

Administration and Dosage

➤*General dosing considerations:* Do not use in conjunction with other topical agents including topical corticosteroids, retinoids, and petrolatum, or agents that are known to enhance cutaneous drug absorption.

MINOXIDIL — TOPICAL

➤*Adults:*

Alopecia –

Topical solution 2%:

• *Usual dosage* – Advise patients to dry the hair and scalp prior to application. Instruct patients to apply 1 mL to the total affected areas of the scalp twice daily, once in the morning and at night.

• *Maximum dose* – The total daily dosage should not exceed 2 mL.

• *Duration of therapy* – Twice daily application for at least 4 months may be required before evidence of hair regrowth is observed. Onset and degree of hair regrowth may be variable among patients. If hair regrowth is realized, twice daily applications are necessary for additional and continued hair regrowth.

Topical solution 5%:

• *Usual dosage* – Instruct patients to part the hair and apply 1 mL 2 times a day directly onto the scalp in the area of hair thinning/loss, spreading the liquid evenly over the hair loss area. Alert patients that using more or more often will not improve results.

• *Duration of therapy* – Continued use is necessary to increase and keep hair regrowth, or hair loss will begin again.

Foam 5%:

• *Usual dosage* – Instruct patients to apply half a capful 2 times a day to the scalp in the hair loss area; using more or more often will not improve results.

• *Duration of therapy* – Continued use is necessary to increase and keep hair regrowth, or hair loss will begin again.

➤*Administration:* Advise patients that if they use their fingers to wash their hands with soap and warm water immediately after application.

Actions

➤*Pharmacology:* To study the potential for systemic effects of topical minoxidil, 3 concentrations (1%, 2% and 5%) applied twice daily were compared to low oral doses (2.5 and 5 mg given once daily) and placebo in hypertensive patients in a double-blind, controlled trial. The 5 mg oral dose had readily detectable effects, including a fall in diastolic pressure of about 5 mmHg and an increase in heart rate of 7 bpm. No other group had a clear effect, although there was some evidence of a weak and inconsistent effect in the 2.5 mg oral, and possibly the 5% topical, treatments.

➤*Pharmacokinetics:*

Absorption – Topical minoxidil has poor absorption, averaging ≈ 1.4% (range 0.3% to 4.5%) from normal intact scalp, and about 2% in the hypertensive patients, whose scalps were shaved.

In a comparison of topical and oral absorption, peak serum levels of unchanged drug after 1 mL twice a day of 2% solution (the maximum recommended dose) averaged 5.8% (range, 1.4% to 12.7%) of the level observed after 2.5 mg orally twice a day. Similarly, in the hypertension study where patients had shaved scalps, mean concentrations after 1 mL twice a day of 2% topical solution (1.7 ng/mL) were 1⁄20 the concentrations seen after daily oral doses of 2.5 mg (32.8 ng/mL) or 5 mg (59.2 ng/mL). Blood levels obtained in the large controlled hair growth trials averaged less than 2 ng/mL for the 2% solution (range, up to 30 ng/mL). If more than the recommended dose is applied to inflamed skin in an individual with relatively high absorption, blood levels with systemic effects might rarely be obtained.

Serum levels resulting from topical administration are governed by the drug's percutaneous absorption rate. Following cessation of topical dosing, ≈ 95% of systemically absorbed minoxidil is eliminated within 4 days.

Contraindications

Hypersensitivity to any component of the preparation.

Warnings/Precautions

➤*Sensitive surfaces:* This product contains an alcohol base that will cause burning and irritation of the eyes. In the event of accidental contact with sensitive surfaces (eg, eyes, abraded skin, mucous membranes), bathe the area with large amounts of cool tap water.

➤*Inhalation:* Avoid inhaling the spray mist.

➤*For topical use only:* Accidental ingestion could lead to adverse systemic effects.

➤*Pregnancy:* *Category C.* Adequate and well-controlled studies have not been conducted in pregnant women. Do not administer to a pregnant woman.

➤*Lactation:* Because of the potential for adverse effects in nursing infants from minoxidil absorption, do not apply on a nursing woman.

➤*Children:* Safety and efficacy in patients younger than 18 years of age have not been established.

➤*Monitoring:* Give a history and physical examination to patients being considered for topical minoxidil. Advise of the potential risk; the patient and physician should decide that the benefits outweigh the risks.

Monitor patients ≥ 1 month after starting topical minoxidil and ≥ 6 months thereafter. If systemic effects occur, discontinue use.

Adverse Reactions

➤*Cardiovascular:* Edema; chest pain; blood pressure increases/decreases; palpitations; pulse rate increases/decreases (1.5%; placebo, 1.6%).

➤*CNS:* Headache; dizziness; faintness; lightheadedness (3.4%; placebo, 3.5%).

➤*Dermatologic:* Irritant dermatitis; allergic contact dermatitis (7.4%; placebo 5.4%); eczema; hypertrichosis; local erythema; pruritus; dry skin/scalp flaking; exacerbation of hair loss; alopecia.

➤*Endocrine:* Menstrual changes, breast symptoms (0.5%; placebo, 0.5%).

➤*GI:* Diarrhea, nausea, vomiting (4.3%; placebo, 6.6%).

➤*GU:* Urinary tract infections, renal calculi, urethritis, prostatitis, epididymitis, vaginitis, vulvitis, vaginal discharge, itching (0.9%; placebo, 0.8% to 1.1%); sexual dysfunction.

➤*Hematologic:* Lymphadenopathy, thrombocytopenia, anemia (0.3; placebo, 0.6%).

➤*Hypersensitivity:* Nonspecific allergic reactions, hives, allergic rhinitis, facial swelling, sensitivity (1.3%; placebo, 1%).

➤*Metabolic:* Edema, weight gain (1.2%; placebo, 1.3%).

➤*Musculoskeletal:* Fractures, back pain, tendinitis, aches and pains (2.6%; placebo, 2.2%).

➤*Psychiatric:* Anxiety, depression, fatigue (0.4%; placebo, 1%).

➤*Respiratory:* Bronchitis, upper respiratory tract infection, sinusitis (7.2%; placebo, 8.6%).

➤*Special senses:* Conjunctivitis, ear infection, vertigo (1.2%; placebo, 1.2%); visual disturbances, including decreased visual acuity.

Overdosage

Increased systemic absorption of minoxidil topical solution may potentially occur if frequent or larger doses than directed are used or if the drug is applied to large surface areas of the body or areas other than the scalp. There are no known cases of minoxidil overdosage resulting from topical administration.

Patient Information

Evidence of hair growth usually will take ≥ 4 months.

First hair growth may be soft, downy, colorless hair that is barely visible. After further treatment, the new hair should be the same color and thickness as the other hair on the scalp.

If there is no response to treatment after a reasonable period of time (≥ 4 months), consult physician as to whether to discontinue use.

If treatment is stopped, new hair will probably be shed within a few months.

If 1 or 2 daily applications are missed, restart twice-daily application and return to the usual schedule. Do not attempt to make up for missed applications.

More frequent applications or use of larger doses (> 1 mL twice a day) will not speed up the process of hair growth and may increase the possibility of side effects.

Minoxidil topical solution contains alcohol, that could cause burning or irritation of the eyes, mucous membranes, or sensitive skin areas. If accidental contact occurs, bathe the area with large amounts of cool tap water. Consult physician if irritation persists.

Because absorption of minoxidil may be increased and the risk of side effects may become greater, apply only to the scalp; do not use on other parts of the body. Do not use if scalp becomes irritated or is sunburned; do not use along with other topical medications on the scalp.

PHOTOCHEMOTHERAPY

AMINOLEVULINIC ACID HYDROCHLORIDE

Rx	**Levulan Kerastick** (DUSA)	**Solution, topical**: 20% (354 mg aminolevulinic acid HCl)	48% v/v ethanol, isopropyl alcohol. In 4s, 6s, and 12s. Applicator contains 2 glass ampules and an applicator tip. One ampule contains 1.5 mL solution vehicle, the other ampule contains 354 mg aminolevulinic acid HCl.

AMINOLEVULINIC ACID HYDROCHLORIDE — TOPICAL

Indications

➤*Non-hyperkeratotic actinic keratoses:* For the treatment of non-hyperkeratotic actinic keratoses of the face or scalp.

➤*Off-label uses:*

Actinic cheilitis – [4] = Insufficient documentation. One very small study and 4 case reports indicate that topical aminolevulinic acid 20% solution and photodynamic therapy provide total clearance of symptoms in two-thirds to three-fourths of patients with actinic cheilitis, with a follow-up of 1 to 12 months. Aminolevulinic acid and photodynamic therapy were well tolerated; local stinging, burning, and erythema resolved 4 days posttreatment. A larger, controlled study with a long follow-up is needed to establish efficacy, safety, and long-term outcomes.

Other possible off-label uses – (In conjunction with a photodynamic therapy.) Barrett's esophagus; Bowen's disease; epidermodysplasia verruciformis; intraepithelial neoplasma of the lower genital tract; nevus sebaceus; mycosis fungoides; premalignant epithelial lesions of the oral cavity; intraepithelial neoplasia and associated human papillomavirus of the uterine cer-

AMINOLEVULINIC ACID HYDROCHLORIDE — TOPICAL

vix; oral leukoplakia; multifocal superficial transitional cell carcinoma of the upper urinary tract; vulvar lichen sclerosus; advanced-stage esophageal cancer; non-melanoma skin malignanciesof the eyelid; squamous cell carcinoma; Kaposi sarcoma; xeroderma pigmentosum; aids in diagnosis of basal cell carcinomas.

Administration and Dosage

➤*General dosing considerations:* Aminolevulinic acid for topical solution is intended for direct application to individual lesions diagnosed as actinic keratoses, not to perilesional skin.

Each individual aminolevulinic acid should be used for only 1 patient.

The second visit, for illumination, must take place in the 14- to 18-hour window following application.

➤*Adults:*

Non-hyperkeratotic actinic keratoses – Photodynamic therapy for actinic keratoses with aminolevulinic acid for topical solution is a 2-stage process involving application of the product to the target lesions with aminolevulinic acid, followed 14 to 18 hours later by illumination with blue light using the *BLU-U* Blue Light Photodynamic Therapy Illuminator.

Usual dosage:

• *Step A* – Administration of aminolevulinic acid for topical solution application.

• *Step B* – Administration of *BLU-U* treatment 14 to 18 hours after application of aminolevulinic acid HCl topical solution. The recommended treatment frequency is 1 application of the aminolevulinic acid topical solution and 1 dose of illumination per treatment site per 8-week treatment session.

Repeat dosage: Treated lesions that have not completely resolved after 8 weeks may be treated a second time with aminolevulinic acid for topical solution photodynamic therapy. Patients did not receive follow-up past 12 weeks after the initial treatment, so the incidence of recurrence of treated lesions past 12 weeks and the role of further treatment is not known.

Off-label dosing –

Actinic cheilitis: [4] = Insufficient documentation. Apply 20% topical solution. In some cases, aminolevulinic acid 20% cream was applied to the lip lesion and covered with a hydrocolloid dressing. Following an incubation time of 2 to 3 hours, the lips received photodynamic therapy. The process was repeated, as necessary, at 1-month intervals until complete clearing or for up to 3 treatment sessions.

➤*Preparation for administration:*

Aminolevulinic acid preparation – The aminolevulinic acid topical solution should be prepared as follows:

1.) Hold the aminolevulinic acid so that the applicator cap is pointing up.
2.) Crush the bottom ampule containing the solution vehicle by applying finger pressure to Position A on the cardboard sleeve.
3.) Crush the top ampule containing the ALA HCl powder by applying finger pressure to Position B on the cardboard sleeve. Note: To ensure both ampules are crushed, continue crushing the applicator downward, applying finger pressure to Position A.
4.) Holding the *LEVULAN KERASTICK* between the thumb and forefinger, point the applicator cap away from the face, shake the *LEVULAN KERASTICK* gently for at least 3 minutes to completely dissolve the drug powder in the solution vehicle. Do not press on the end cap while shaking.

Following solution admixture, remove the cap from the aminolevulinic acid. The dry applicator tip should be dabbed on a gauze pad until uniformly wet with solution.

➤*Administration:* Application should involve either scalp or face lesions, but not both simultaneously.

Actinic keratoses targeted for treatment should be clean and dry prior to application of aminolevulinic acid topical solution.

Step A –

Aminolevulinic acid solution: Apply the solution directly to the target lesions by dabbing gently with the wet applicator tip. Enough solution should be applied to uniformly wet the lesion surface, including the edges without excess running or dripping. The effect of aminolevulinic acid topical solution on ocular tissues is unknown. Aminolevulinic acid topical solution should not be applied to the periorbital area or allowed to contact ocular or mucosal surfaces. Once the initial application has dried, apply again in the same manner. The aminolevulinic acid topical solution must be used immediately following preparation (dissolution) due to the instability of the activated product. If the solution application is not completed within 2 hours of activation, the applicator should be discarded and new aminolevulinic acid for topical solution used.

Photosensitization of the treated lesions will take place over the next 14 to 18 hours. The actinic keratoses should not be washed during this time. The patient should be advised to wear a wide-brimmed hat or other protective apparel to shade the treated actinic keratosis lesions from sunlight or other bright light sources until *BLU-U* treatment. The patient should be advised to reduce light exposure if the sensations of stinging or burning are experienced.

If for any reason the patient cannot be given *BLU-U* treatment during the prescribed time after aminolevulinic acid topical solution application, he or she may nonetheless experience sensations of stinging or burning if the photosensitized actinic keratoses are exposed to sunlight or prolonged or intense light at that time. The patient should be advised to wear a wide-brimmed hat or other protective apparel to shade the treated actinic keratosis lesions from sunlight or other bright light sources until at least 40 hours after the application of aminolevulinic acid HCl topical solution. The patient should be advised to reduce light exposure if the sensations of stinging or burning are experienced.

Step B –

Administration of BLU-U treatment 14 to 18 hours after application of aminolevulinic acid topical solution: At the visit for light illumination, the actinic keratoses to be treated should be gently rinsed with water and patted dry. Photoactivation of actinic keratoses treated with aminolevulinic acid HCl topical solution is accomplished with *BLU-U* illumination from the *BLU-U* Blue Light Photodynamic Therapy Illuminator. A 1,000-second (16 minutes 40 seconds) exposure is required to provide a 10 J/cm^2 light dose. During light treatment, both patients and medical personnel should be provided with blue blocking protective eyewear, as specified in the *BLU-U* Operating Instructions, to minimize ocular exposure. Please refer to the *BLU-U* Operating Instructions for further information on conducting the light treatment. Patients should be advised that transient stinging or burning at the target lesion sites occurs during the period of light exposure.

If blue light treatment with the *BLU-U* Blue Light Photodynamic Therapy Illuminator is interrupted or stopped for any reason, it should not be restarted, and the patient should be advised to protect the treated lesions from exposure to sunlight or prolonged or intense light for at least 40 hours after application of the aminolevulinic acid HCl topical solution from the first visit.

For patients with facial lesions:

1.) The *BLU-U* Blue Light Photodynamic Therapy Illuminator is positioned so that the base is slightly above the patient's shoulder, parallel to the patient's face.
2.) The *BLU-U* is positioned around the patient's head so the entire surface area to be treated lies between 2 inches and 4 inches from the *BLU-U* surface.
   a.) The patient's nose should be no closer than 2 inches from the surface;
   b.) The patient's forehead and cheeks should be no further than 4 inches from the surface;
   c.) The sides of the patient's face and the patient's ears should be no closer than 2 inches from the *BLU-U* surface.

A chin rest may be used to provide support for the patient's head during treatment.

For patients with scalp lesions –

1.) The knobs on either side of the *BLU-U* are loosened and the *BLU-U* is rotated to a horizontal position.
2.) The *BLU-U* is positioned around the patient's head so the entire surface area to be treated lies between 2 inches and 4 inches from the *BLU-U* surface.
   a.) The patient's scalp should be no closer than 2 inches from the surface;
   b.) The patient's scalp should be no further than 4 inches from the surface;
   c.) The sides of the patient's face and the patient's ears should be no closer than 2 inches from the *BLU-U* surface.

A chin rest may be used to provide support for the patient's head during treatment.

Aminolevulinic acid for topical solution is not intended for use with any device other than the *BLU-U* Blue Light Photodynamic Illuminator. Use of aminolevulinic acid HCl for topical solution without subsequent *BLU-U* illumination is not recommended.

➤*Storage/Stability:* Store at 25°C (77°F); excursions permitted to 15° to 30°C (59° to 86°F). Aminolevulinic acid HCl for topical solution should be used immediately following preparation (dissolution). Solution application must be completed within 2 hours of preparation. An applicator that has been prepared must be discarded 2 hours after mixing (dissolving) and new aminolevulinic acid HCl for topical solution used, if needed.

Actions

➤*Pharmacology:* The metabolism of aminolevulinic acid HCl (ALA) is the first step in the biochemical pathway resulting in heme synthesis. Aminolevulinic acid HCl is not a photosensitizer, but rather a metabolic precursor of protoporphyrin IX (PpIX), which is a photosensitizer. The synthesis of ALA is normally tightly controlled by feedback inhibition of the enzyme, ALA synthetase, presumably by intracellular heme levels. ALA, when provided to the cell, bypasses this control point and results in the accumulation of PpIX, which is converted into heme by ferrochelatase through the addition of iron to the PpIX nucleus.

According to the presumed mechanism of action, photosensitization following application of aminolevulinic acid HCl occurs through the metabolic conversion of ALA to PpIX, which accumulates in the skin to which aminolevulinic acid HCl has been applied. When exposed to light of appropriate wavelength and energy, the accumulated PpIX produces a photodynamic reaction, a cytotoxic process dependent upon the simultaneous presence of light and oxygen. The absorption of light results in an excited state of the porphyrin molecule, and subsequent spin transfer from PpIX to molecular oxygen generates singlet oxygen, which can further react to form superoxide and hydroxyl radicals. Photosensitization of actinic (solar) keratosis lesions using the aminolevulinic acid HCl, plus illumination with the *BLU-U* Blue Light Photodynamic Therapy Illuminator (*BLU-U*), is the basis for aminolevulinic acid HCl photodynamic therapy (PDT).

➤*Pharmacokinetics:* ALA is not indicated for internal use, but has been administered orally for some unlabeled uses.

In a human pharmacokinetic study (n = 6) using a 128 mg dose of sterile intravenous ALA HCl and oral ALA HCl (equivalent to 100 mg ALA) in which plasma ALA and PpIX were measured, the mean half-life of ALA was 0.7 ± 0.18 hours after the oral dose and 0.83 ± 0.05 hours after the intravenous dose. The oral bioavailability of ALA was 50% to 60% with a mean C_{max} of 4.65 ± 0.94 mcg/mL. PpIX concentrations were low and were detectable only in 42% of the plasma samples. PpIX concentrations in plasma were

AMINOLEVULINIC ACID HYDROCHLORIDE — TOPICAL

quite low relative to ALA plasma concentrations, and were below the level of detection (10 ng/mL) after 10 to 12 hours.

ALA does not exhibit fluorescence, while PpIX has a high fluorescence yield. Time-dependent changes in surface fluorescence have been used to determine PpIX accumulation and clearance in actinic keratosis lesions and perilesional skin after application of aminolevulinic acid HCl topical solution in 12 patients. Peak fluorescence intensity was reached in 11 ± 1 hour in actinic keratoses and 12 ± 1 hour in perilesional skin. The mean clearance half-life of fluorescence for lesions was 30 ± 10 hours and 28 ± 6 hours for perilesional skin. The fluorescence in perilesional skin was similar to that in actinic keratoses. Therefore, aminolevulinic acid HCl topical solution should only be applied to the affected skin.

Contraindications

Cutaneous photosensitivity at wavelengths of 400 to 450 nm; porphyria or known allergies to porphyrins; sensitivity to any of the components of the aminolevulinic acid HCl for topical solution.

Warnings/Precautions

➤*For topical use only:* The aminolevulinic acid HCl for topical solution contains alcohol and is intended for topical use only. Do not apply to the eyes or to mucous membranes. Excessive irritation may be experienced if this product is applied under occlusion.

➤*Coagulation disorders:* Aminolevulinic acid HCl for topical solution has not been tested on patients with inherited or acquired coagulation defects.

➤*Photodamaged skin:* Application of aminolevulinic acid HCl topical solution to perilesional areas of photodamaged skin of the face or scalp may result in photosensitization. Upon exposure to activating light from the *BLU-U* Blue Light Photodynamic Therapy Illuminator, such photosensitized skin may produce a stinging or burning sensation and may become erythematous or edematous in a manner similar to that of actinic keratoses treated with aminolevulinic acid HCl. Because of the potential for skin to become photosensitized, aminolevulinic acid HCl for topical solution should be used by a qualified health professional to apply drug only to actinic keratoses and not perilesional skin.

➤*Photosensitivity:* During the time period between the application of aminolevulinic acid HCl topical solution and exposure to activating light from the *BLU-U* Blue Light Photodynamic Therapy Illuminator, the treatment site will become photosensitive. After aminolevulinic acid HCl topical solution application, patients should avoid exposure of the photosensitive treatment sites to sunlight or bright indoor light (eg, examination lamps, operating room lamps, tanning beds, or lights at close proximity) during the period prior to blue light treatment. Exposure may result in a stinging or burning sensation and may cause erythema or edema of the lesions. Before exposure to sunlight, patients should, therefore, protect treated lesions from the sun by wearing a wide-brimmed hat or similar head covering of light-opaque material. Sunscreens will not protect against photosensitivity reactions caused by visible light. It has not been determined if perspiration can spread aminolevulinic acid HCl topical solution outside the treatment site to eye or surrounding skin.

➤*Pregnancy: Category C.* Animal reproduction studies have not been conducted with ALA HCl. It is also not known whether aminolevulinic acid HCl topical solution can cause fetal harm when administered to a pregnant woman or can affect reproductive capacity. Aminolevulinic acid HCl topical solution should be given to a pregnant woman only if clearly needed.

➤*Lactation:* The levels of ALA or its metabolites in the milk of subjects treated with aminolevulinic acid HCl topical solution have not been measured. Because many drugs are excreted in human milk, caution should be exercised when aminolevulinic acid HCl topical solution is administered to a nursing woman.

Drug Interactions

There have been no formal studies of the interaction of aminolevulinic acid HCl for topical solution with any other drugs, and no drug-specific interactions were noted during any of the controlled clinical trials. It is, however, possible that concomitant use of other known photosensitizing agents such as griseofulvin, thiazide diuretics, sulfonylureas, phenothiazines, sulfonamides, and tetracyclines might increase the photosensitivity reaction of actinic keratoses treated with the aminolevulinic acid HCl for topical solution.

Adverse Reactions

In Phase 3 studies, no non-cutaneous adverse events were found to be consistently associated with aminolevulinic acid HCl topical solution application followed by blue light exposure.

Photodynamic therapy response – The constellation of transient local symptoms of stinging or burning, itching, erythema and edema as a result of aminolevulinic acid HCl topical solution plus *BLU-U* treatment was observed in all clinical studies of aminolevulinic acid HCl for topical solution photodynamic therapy for actinic keratoses treatment. Stinging or burning subsided between 1 minute and 24 hours after the *BLU-U* Blue Light Photodynamic Therapy Illuminator was turned off, and appeared qualitatively similar to that perceived by patients with erythropoietic protoporphyria upon exposure to sunlight. There was no clear drug dose or light dose dependent change in the incidence or severity of stinging or burning.

In 2 Phase 3 trials, the sensation of stinging or burning appeared to reach a plateau at 6 minutes into the treatment. Severe stinging or burning at 1 or more lesions being treated was reported by at least 50% of patients at some time during treatment. The majority of patients reported that all lesions treated exhibited at least slight stinging or burning. Less than 3% of patients discontinued light treatment due to stinging or burning.

The most common changes in lesion appearance after aminolevulinic acid HCl for topical solution photodynamic therapy were erythema and edema. In 99% of active treatment patients, some or all lesions were erythematous shortly after treatment, while in 79% of vehicle treatment patients, some or all lesions were erythematous. In 35% of active treatment patients, some or all lesions were edematous, while no vehicle-treated patients had edematous lesions. Both erythema and edema resolved to baseline or improved by 4 weeks after therapy. Aminolevulinic acid HCl topical solution application to photodamaged perilesional skin resulted in photosensitization of photodamaged skin and in a photodynamic response.

➤*Other localized cutaneous adverse experiences:*

Aminolevulinic Acid Post-PDT Cutaneous Adverse Reactions ALA-018/ALA-019								
	Face				Scalp			
	Aminolevulinic acid (n = 139)		Vehicle (n = 41)		Aminolevulinic acid (n = 42)		Vehicle (n = 21)	
Adverse reaction	Mild/ moderate	Severe	Mild/ moderate	Severe	Mild/ moderate	Severe	Mild/ moderate	Severe
Scaling/ crusting	71%	1%	12%	0%	64%	2%	19%	0%
Pain	1%	0%	0%	0%	0%	0%	0%	0%
Tenderness	1%	0%	0%	0%	2%	0%	0%	0%
Itching	25%	1%	7%	0%	14%	7%	19%	0%
Edema	1%	0%	0%	0%	0%	0%	0%	0%
Ulceration	4%	0%	0%	0%	2%	0%	0%	0%
Bleeding/ hemorrhage	4%	0%	0%	0%	2%	0%	0%	0%
Hypo-/hyper-pigmentation	22%		20%		36%		33%	
Vesiculation	4%	0%	0%	0%	5%	0%	0%	0%
Pustules	4%	0%	0%	0%	0%	0%	0%	0%
Oozing	1%	0%	0%	0%	0%	0%	0%	0%
Dysesthesia	2%	0%	0%	0%	0%	0%	0%	0%
Scabbing	2%	1%	0%	0%	0%	0%	0%	0%
Erosion	14%	1%	0%	0%	2%	0%	0%	0%
Excoriation	1%	0%	0%	0%	0%	0%	0%	0%
Wheal/ flare	7%	1%	0%	0%	2%	0%	0%	0%
Skin disorder NOS	5%	0%	0%	0%	12%	0%	5%	0%

➤*Adverse reactions reported by body system:* In the Phase 3 studies, 7 patients experienced a serious adverse event. All were deemed remotely or not related to treatment. No clinically significant patterns of clinical laboratory changes were observed for standard serum chemical or hematologic parameters in any of the controlled clinical trials.

Overdosage

➤*Aminolevulinic acid HCl for topical solution overdose:* Aminolevulinic acid HCl for topical solution overdose have not been reported. In the unlikely event that the drug is ingested, monitoring and supportive care are recommended. The patient should be advised to avoid incidental exposure to intense light sources for at least 40 hours. The consequences of exceeding the recommended topical dosage are unknown.

➤*BLU-U light overdose:* There is no information on overdose of blue light from the *BLU-U* Blue Light Photodynamic Therapy Illuminator following aminolevulinic acid HCl for topical solution application.

Patient Information

➤*Aminolevulinic acid HCl photodynamic therapy for actinic keratoses:* The first step in aminolevulinic acid HCl photodynamic therapy (PDT) for actinic keratoses is application of the aminolevulinic acid HCl for topical solution to actinic keratoses located on the patient's face or scalp. After aminolevulinic acid HCl for topical solution is applied to the actinic keratoses in the doctor's office, the patient will be told to return the next day. During this time the actinic keratoses will become sensitive to light (photosensitive). Care should be taken to keep the treated actinic keratoses dry and out of bright light. After aminolevulinic acid HCl topical solution is applied, it is important for the patient to wear light-protective clothing, such as a wide-brimmed hat, when exposed to sunlight or sources of light. Fourteen to 18 hours after application of aminolevulinic acid HCl topical solution the patient will return to the doctor's office to receive blue light treatment, which is the second and final step in the treatment. Prior to blue light treatment, the actinic keratoses will be rinsed with tap water. The patient will be given goggles to wear as eye protection during the blue light treatment. The blue light is of low intensity and will not heat the skin. However, during the light treatment, which lasts for approximately 17 minutes, the patient will experience sensations of tingling, stinging, prickling or burning of the treated lesions. These feelings of discomfort should improve at the end of the light treatment. Following treatment, the actinic keratoses and, to some degree, the surrounding skin, will redden, and swelling and scaling may also occur. However, these lesion changes are temporary and should completely resolve by 4 weeks after treatment.

➤*Photosensitivity:* After aminolevulinic acid HCl topical solution is applied to the actinic keratoses in the doctor's office, the patient should avoid exposure of the photosensitive actinic keratoses to sunlight or bright indoor light (eg, from examination lamps, operating room lamps, tanning

AMINOLEVULINIC ACID HYDROCHLORIDE — TOPICAL

beds, or lights at close proximity) during the period prior to blue light treatment. If the patient feels stinging or burning on the actinic keratoses, exposure to light should be reduced. Before going into sunlight, the patient should protect treated lesions from the sun by wearing a wide-brimmed hat or similar head covering of light-opaque material. Sunscreens will not protect the patient against photosensitivity reactions.

If for any reason the patient cannot return for blue light treatment during the prescribed period after application of aminolevulinic acid HCl topical solution (14 to 18 hours), the patient should call the doctor. The patient should also continue to avoid exposure of the photosensitized lesions to sunlight or prolonged or intense light for at least 40 hours. If stinging or burning is noted, exposure to light should be reduced.

METHYL AMINOLEVULINATE

Rx	**Metvixia** (PhotoCure ASA)	**Cream; topical:** 16.8%	As methyl aminolevulinate hydrochloride. Almond and peanut oil, edetate disodium, glycerin, parabens, cetostearyl and oleyl alcohol, white petrolatum. In 2 g.

METHYL AMINOLEVULINATE HYDROCHLORIDE — TOPICAL

Indications

➤*Nonhyperkeratotic, nonpigmented actinic keratoses:* For the treatment of thin and moderately thick nonhyperkeratotic, nonpigmented actinic keratoses of the face and scalp in immunocompetent patients in combination with *Aktilite CL128* lamp red light illumination.

➤*Off-label uses:* Nodular basal cell carcinoma; squamous cell carcinoma in situ; Bowen disease.

Administration and Dosage

PDT for nonhyperkeratotic actinic keratoses with methyl aminolevulinate is a multistage process. Two treatment sessions 7 days apart should be conducted.

Nitrile gloves should be worn when applying and removing the cream.

Use of methyl aminolevulinate cream without subsequent red light illumination is not recommended.

➤*Adults:*

Nonhyperkeratotic, nonpigmented actinic keratoses –

Usual dosage: Using a spatula, apply a layer of methyl aminolevulinate cream about 1 mm thick to the lesion and the surrounding 5 mm of normal skin. The area to which the cream has been applied should then be covered with an occlusive, nonabsorbent dressing for 3 hours. Multiple lesions may be treated during the same treatment session using a total of 1 g of cream. Each treatment field is limited to an area of 80 × 180 mm.

Follow application by photoactivation via red light illumination 3 hours later. See Photodynamic Therapy Session.

Two treatment sessions 7 days apart should be conducted. Lesion response should be assessed 3 months after the last treatment session.

Maximum dose: Do not apply more than 1 g (one-half tube) topically per treatment session.

➤*Photodynamic therapy session:* The *Aktilite CL128* lamp, which is equipped with light-emitting diodes (LEDs), emits red light with a narrow spectrum at approximately 630 nm and a half-width of approximately 20 nm. The light dose to be used is 37 J/cm^2, and the lamp should be placed 50 to 80 mm from the skin. The area of skin that can be illuminated is 80 × 180 mm. Calibration by the operator is not needed, and the illumination time is calculated automatically. The LED panel window should be cleaned daily with a slightly moist clean cloth.

If *Aktilite* red light treatment is interrupted or stopped for any reason, it may be restarted. If the patient for any reason cannot have the red light treatment during the prescribed period after application (the 3-hour time span), the cream should be rinsed off and the patient should protect the exposed area from sunlight or prolonged or intense light for at least 48 hours.

Positioning the Aktilite CL128 lamp – See the *Aktilite CL128* operator's manual for specific warnings, cautions, and instructions. If necessary, adjust the dose to 37 J/cm^2. Calibration by the operator is not required. Position the lamp over the area to be illuminated by the use of guide light. The distance between the LED panel and the lesion surface should be 50 to 80 mm (2 to 3.2 inches).

Do not stare into the beam. The patient and operator should wear appropriate eye protection during illumination. Patient protective goggles or eye shields should be dark or metal to block visible light.

Illumination with the Aktilite CL128 lamp red light – The required illumination time (7 to 10 minutes) is calculated automatically, and the remaining time will be displayed at the control panel. The illumination stops automatically. The illumination may be paused and started again.

Patients should be advised that transient pain, burning, or stinging at the target lesion sites may occur during the period of light exposure.

➤*Preparation for administration:*

Lesion debriding – Before applying methyl aminolevulinate cream, the surface of the lesions should be prepared with a small dermal curette to remove scales and crusts and to roughen the surface of the lesion. This is to facilitate access of the cream and light to all parts of the lesion.

➤*Administration:* Methyl aminolevulinate cream is not for ophthalmic, oral, or intravaginal use.

Only nitrile gloves should be worn by the qualified health care provider in order to avoid skin contact with the cream; universal precautions should be taken. Vinyl and latex gloves do not provide adequate protection when using this product.

The area where the cream was applied should be covered with an occlusive, nonabsorbent dressing for 3 hours (at least 2.5 hours but not more than 4 hours). After cream application, advise patients to avoid exposure of the photosensitive treatment sites to sunlight or bright indoor light (eg, examination lamps, lights at close proximity, operating room lamps, tanning beds) during the period prior to *Aktilite* red light treatment. Exposure to light may result in a stinging and/or burning sensation and may cause erythema and/or edema of the lesions. Protect treated areas from the sun by having the patient wear a wide-brimmed hat or similar head covering of light, opaque material. Sunscreens will not protect against photosensitivity reactions caused by visible light. It has not been determined if perspiration can spread the methyl aminolevulinate cream outside the treatment site to the eyes or surrounding skin. The treated site should be protected from extreme cold with adequate clothing or by remaining indoors between application of methyl aminolevulinate cream and *Aktilite* PDT light treatment.

Following removal of the occlusive dressing, clean the area with saline and gauze. Nitrile gloves should be worn at this step by the trained health care provider.

➤*Storage/Stability:* Store at 2° to 8°C (36° to 46°F). Use contents within 1 week of opening. Do not use the product after it has been unrefrigerated for 24 hours.

Actions

➤*Pharmacology:* Photosensitization following application of methyl aminolevulinate cream occurs through the metabolic conversion of methyl aminolevulinate (prodrug) to photoactive porphyrins, which accumulate in the skin lesions where methyl aminolevulinate cream has been applied. When exposed to light of appropriate wavelength and energy, the accumulated photoactive porphyrins produce a photodynamic reaction, resulting in a cytotoxic process dependent on the simultaneous presence of oxygen. The absorption of light results in an excited state of porphyrin molecules, and subsequent spin transfer from photoactive porphyrins to molecular oxygen generates singlet oxygen. Methyl aminolevulinate PDT of actinic (solar) ketatosis lesions is the combination of photosensitization by topical application of methyl aminolevulinate cream to the lesions and subsequent illumination with red light of narrow spectrum using a light dose of 37 J/cm^2 delivered by the *Aktilite CL128* lamp.

➤*Pharmacokinetics:* The time-course of protoporphyrin IX in actinic keratosis lesions and surrounding skin after application of methyl aminolevulinate cream has been monitored by means of fluorescence. The optimal concentration of methyl aminolevulinate cream (16.8%) and duration of application (3 h) were derived from such studies of pharmacokinetics in skin using a range of concentrations (1.6%, 8%, and 16.8%) and cream application times (up to 28 hours). Three hours after the application of methyl aminolevulinate cream fluorescence in the treated lesions was significantly greater than that seen in both treated and untreated normal skin, and after application of vehicle cream (not containing methyl aminolevulinate) to normal skin. In a fluorescence study of 8 patients with actinic keratoses using methyl aminolevulinate cream 16.8% applied for 3 hours and illumination with the *Aktilite CL128* lamp, 88% photodegradation of protoporphyrin IX was observed immediately after illumination, followed by a transient small secondary increase in fluorescence 2 hours after illumination. At 24 and 48 hours, 94% and 96% degradation of protoporphyrin IX, respectively, from baseline, was observed.

Contraindications

Cutaneous photosensitivity or known allergies to porphyrins; known sensitivities to any of the components of methyl aminolevulinate cream, including peanut and almond oil.

Warnings/Precautions

➤*Lesion recurrence:* Methyl aminolevulinate cream has not been studied for more than 1 course, which consists of 2 treatment sessions 1 week apart. There is no information available regarding the recurrence rate for lesions treated with this therapy. Clinical studies did not follow patients beyond 3 months, and the recurrence rate of treated lesions is unknown.

➤*Coagulation defects:* Methyl aminolevulinate has not been tested on patients with inherited or acquired coagulation defects.

➤*Aktilite CL128* lamp: Before operating the *Aktilite CL128* lamp, personnel should refer to the operator's manual for specific warnings, cautions, and instructions. Exercise care when positioning and operating the lamp. During the red light illumination period, the patient, operator, and other persons present should wear protective goggles that sufficiently screen out the appropriate spectrum of red light. The protective goggles or eye shields provided for the patients should be dark or metal to block visible light. The green professional protective glasses provided for the operator screen out the relevant spectrum of red light, and the room will still appear bright for the operator to see. Do not stare into the beam. For lamp assembly, maintenance, service, and technical data, the personnel should refer to the operator's manual.

METHYL AMINOLEVULINATE HYDROCHLORIDE — TOPICAL

➤*Hypersensitivity reactions:* Methyl aminolevulinate cream has demonstrated a high rate of contact sensitization (allergenicity). Take care to avoid inadvertent skin contact when applying methyl aminolevulinate cream. Wear nitrile gloves when applying and removing the cream. Vinyl and latex gloves do not provide adequate protection when using this product.

Methyl aminolevulinate cream is formulated with refined peanut and almond oil. Methyl aminolevulinate cream has not been tested in patients who are allergic to peanuts.

➤*Photosensitivity:* During the time period between the application of methyl aminolevulinate cream and exposure to red light illumination, the treatment site will become photosensitive.

If for any reason the patient cannot have the *Aktilite* red light treatment after application of methyl aminolevulinate cream, the cream should be rinsed off and the patient should protect the treated area from sunlight and prolonged or intense light for 2 days. Avoid prolonged exposure of more than 4 hours to methyl aminolevulinate cream.

See Administration and Dosage for more information.

After illumination of methyl aminolevulinate cream, advise patients to keep the treated area covered and away from light for at least 48 hours.

Because of the potential for skin to become photosensitized, only a trained health care provider should apply methyl aminolevulinate cream to nonhyperkeratotic actinic keratoses and perilesional skin within 5 mm of the lesion. Burning, redness, stinging, and swelling are expected as a result of therapy; however, if these symptoms increase in severity and persist longer than 3 weeks, advise patients to contact their health care provider.

➤*Pregnancy: Category C.*

Teratogenic – There are no adequate and well-controlled studies with methyl aminolevulinate cream in pregnant women. Intravenous (IV) methyl aminolevulinate was teratogenic in rabbits at a high dose. Use methyl aminolevulinate cream during pregnancy only if the potential benefit justifies the potential risk to the fetus.

A maximum topical human dose (MTHD) of 2 g of methyl aminolevulinate cream 16.8% containing methyl aminolevulinate hydrochloride 420 mg corresponding to 7 mg/kg or 259 mg/m^2 for a 60 kg patient and an estimated maximum systemic uptake of 1% was used for the animal multiple of human systemic exposure calculations presented in this monograph.

Development toxicity studies have been performed in pregnant rats with IV dosages of methyl aminolevulinate of up to 700 mg/day on days 6 to 16 of gestation. There were no treatment-related effects on fetal body weight, sex ratio, external malformations and variations, and skeletal abnormalities and ossification extent. Only a slight, nonsignificant increase in early embryonic death was noted in the 700 mg/kg/day group compared with the control group. The fetal No Adverse Effect Level (NOAEL) was methyl aminolevulinate 350 mg/kg/day in pregnant rats (2,100 mg/m^2, 811 times the MTHD based on mg/m^2 comparisons and an estimated maximum systemic uptake of 1%).

In development toxicity studies, pregnant rabbits received IV dosages of methyl aminolevulinate of up to 200 mg/kg/day (up to 926 times the MTHD) on days 6 to 18 of gestation. Slightly lower fetal body weights and increased incidences of fetuses with jugals connected/fused to maxilla, supernumerary ribs, incompletely ossified cranial bones and other ossification irregularities were noted in the high dosage of 200 mg/kg/day (926 times the MTHD) group, compared with the control group. The fetal NOAEL was methyl aminolevulinate 100 mg/kg/day in pregnant rabbits (1,200 mg/m^2, 463 times the MTHD based on mg/m^2 comparisons and an estimated maximum systemic uptake of 1%). The embryofetal effects in the high-dose group were associated with maternal toxicity. These effects did not occur at 463 times the MTHD based on mg/m^2 comparisons and an estimated maximum systemic uptake of 1%. Developmental toxicity studies in rats were negative at daily exposure levels of up to 1,622 times the MTHD on a mg/m^2 basis.

In the prenatal and postnatal development toxicity study, pregnant rats received IV dosages of methyl aminolevulinate of up to 500 mg/kg/day (1,160 × the MTHD) from day 6 of gestation to day 24 of lactation. There were no treatment-related effects on litter size, pup mortality, pup weights, or post-weaning performance in the pups (including development and reproduction). A slightly longer duration of gestation and a slight delay in pup physical development were noted in the 250 and 500 mg/kg/day (580 to 1,160 × the MTHD) groups. The NOAEL was methyl aminolevulinate 125 mg/kg/day (750 mg/m^2, 290 times the MTHD based on mg/m^2 comparisons and an estimated maximum systemic uptake of 1%).

➤*Lactation:* It is not known whether this drug is excreted in human milk. Because many drugs are excreted in human milk, exercise caution when methyl aminolevulinate cream is administered to a breast-feeding woman.

➤*Children:* Actinic keratosis is not a condition generally seen within the pediatric population. The safety and effectiveness in children younger than 18 years of age have not been established.

➤*Elderly:* No overall differences in safety or effectiveness were observed between these subjects and younger subjects, and other reported clinical experience has not identified differences in responses between the elder and younger patients, but greater sensitivity of some older individuals cannot be ruled out.

➤*Monitoring:* Monitor for lesion response at 3 months posttherapy. Monitor for signs and symptoms of local skin reactions (eg, crusting, edema, erythema, pain, severe burning).

Drug Interactions

None well documented.

Adverse Reactions

➤*Dermal safety studies:* Studies in healthy volunteer subjects and subjects with actinic keratoses previously treated with methyl aminolevulinate PDT on at least 4 previous occasions have demonstrated that methyl aminolevulinate cream has the potential to cause irritancy and sensitization. A cumulative irritancy and sensitization (allergenicity) study of methyl aminolevulinate cream with a cross-sensitization challenge with aminolevulinic acid (ALA) was performed in 156 subjects. Methyl aminolevulinate cream was applied 3 times each week for 3 weeks (total of 9 applications), to separate sites on the back of healthy volunteers. After each application, the area was covered by aluminum Finn Chamber. After the 3-week continuous treatment period and a 2-week interval without further applications, subjects were challenged with methyl aminolevulinate cream, methyl aminolevulinate vehicle, ALA, and ALA vehicle creams for 48 hours. Assessment of skin reactions was performed 48, 72, and 96 hours after the start of the challenge cream application. Only 98 of the 156 subjects tested entered the challenge phase because of a high incidence of local irritancy evident as erythema. Of the 58 subjects who were challenged with methyl aminolevulinate cream, 52% showed contact sensitization. Of the 98 subjects who were challenged with ALA, only 2% showed equivocal reactions, the remaining subjects having negative responses.

The potential for sensitization was also assessed by patch testing a total of 21 patients with actinic keratoses previously treated with methyl aminolevulinate PDT on at least 4 previous occasions. Methyl aminolevulinate cream 16.8% and vehicle cream were applied to different sites on the lower back for 48 hours. Three of the 21 patients (14%) showed contact sensitization associated with erythema scores of 4 or higher (strong erythema spreading outside the patch) and edema, vesiculation, papules, and glazing.

➤*Clinical studies:*

Most frequent adverse reactions – The most frequent adverse reactions were associated with phototoxicity at the treatment site. Pain and burning sensation typically began during illumination and generally resolved completely within a few minutes or hours, but may last up to a few days. Erythema and other signs generally resolved within a few days to 3 weeks.

In these 2 studies, out of 126 subjects treated with methyl aminolevulinate cream, 6 methyl aminolevulinate *Aktilite PDT* subjects did not complete the full 2-treatment session regimens because of adverse reactions (eg, headache, pain, burning). These subjects either stopped illumination early or did not have the second treatment. In addition, 12 methyl aminolevulinate PDT subjects paused illumination due to pain, burning, or stinging, but did subsequently complete treatment.

Adverse reactions (1% or more) –

Methyl Aminolevulinate Adverse Reactions (≥ 1%)				
	Methyl aminolevulinate and *Aktilite PDT* (n = 126)		Vehicle and *Aktilite PDT* (n = 105)	
Adverse Reactions	All grades[a]	Severe	All grades[a]	Severe
Any treatment-site adverse reaction	90%	22%	46%	0%
Application-site discharge	2%	0%	0%	0%
Erythema	63%	6%	10%	0%
Pruritus	22%	0%	8%	0%
Scabbing/Crusting/Blister/Erosions	29%	2%	1%	0%
Skin burning/pain/discomfort	86%	20%	36%	0%
Skin exfoliation	14%	3%	3%	0%
Skin hemorrhage	2%	0%	0%	0%
Skin hyperpigmentation	2%	0%	0%	0%
Skin or eyelid edema	18%	2%	1%	0%
Skin tightness	2%	0%	0%	0%
Skin warm	4%	0%	2%	0%

[a] Mild, moderate, or severe.

METHYL AMINOLEVULINATE HYDROCHLORIDE — TOPICAL

➤*Postmarketing:*

Hypersensitivity – Allergic reactions reported include allergic contact dermatitis, eczema, and urticaria. Most cases were localized to the treatment area; rarely, erythema and swelling have been more extensive.

Local – Reports of serious adverse reactions at or near the application site include crusting, edema, erythema, hyperpigmentation, pain, pustules, and scab.

Ophthalmic – There have been occasional reports of eye disorders including edema, eyelid swelling, keratitis, macular edema, and vitreous detachment.

Miscellaneous – At sites distant from the application site, there have been reports of squamous cell carcinoma of the skin, as expected in this population.

Overdosage

➤*Methyl aminolevulinate cream:* Methyl aminolevulinate cream overdose has not been reported. If the patient, for any reason, cannot have the red light treatment during the prescribed period after application (the 3-hour time span), rinse off the cream with saline and water and advise the patient to protect the exposed area from sunlight or prolonged or intense light for 2 days.

➤*Aktilite* red light: Red light overdose (excess illumination time) using *Aktilite CL128* following methyl aminolevulinate cream application has not been reported. If red light overexposure results in a burn, treat the patient in accordance with standard practice for treatment of cutaneous burns.

Patient Information

Advise patients that methyl aminolevulinate is highly allergenic. It contains refined almond oil, peanut oil, and porphyrins, and is contraindicated in patients with sensitivities to these ingredients.

Advise patients that methyl aminolevulinate cream is intended for topical use in a health care provider's office and is for use by trained health care providers only. It is not applied by patients.

Advise patients to avoid exposure to sunlight or bright indoor light during the 3 hours that methyl aminolevulinate cream is on the skin. Instruct patients to wear protective hats and clothing if they are required to be outside in the sun. Advise patients to avoid exposure to cold temperatures during the 3 hours that methyl aminolevulinate cream is on the skin. Instruct patients to wear warm clothing and keep treated skin covered if they are required to be outside in cold temperatures.

Advise patients to tell their health care provider if they experience certain skin reactions after methyl aminolevulinate cream treatment, such as a burning feeling, blistering, bleeding, crusting, infection, itching, pain, peeling, redness, stinging, swelling, and ulcers. If any skin reaction worsens and lasts longer than 3 weeks, instruct the patient to call their health care provider.

Psoralens

METHOXSALEN (8-Methoxypsoralen)

Rx	**8-MOP** (Valeant Pharmaceuticals)	**Capsules; oral:** 10 mg	(ICN 600). Pink. In 50s.
Rx	**Oxsoralen-Ultra** (Valeant Pharmaceuticals)	**Softgel; oral:** 10 mg	(ICN 650). Green. In 50s.
Rx	**Uvadex** (Therakos)	**Solution; extracorporeal:** 20 mcg/mL	Alcohol 0.05 mL. In 10 mL vials.
Rx	**Oxsoralen** (Valeant Pharmaceuticals)	**Lotion; topical:** 1% (10 mg/mL)	Acetone. Alcohol 71%. In 30 mL.

METHOXSALEN — ORAL

WARNING

Only health care providers who have special competence in the diagnosis and treatment of psoriasis and vitiligo (*8-MOP* only) and who have special training and experience in photochemotherapy should use methoxsalen with ultraviolet (UV) radiation. The use of psoralen and UV radiation therapy should be under constant supervision of such a health care provider. For the treatment of patients with psoriasis, restrict photochemotherapy to patients with severe, recalcitrant, disabling psoriasis that is not adequately responsive to other forms of therapy, and only when the diagnosis is certain. Because of the possibility of ocular damage, skin aging, and skin cancer (including melanoma), fully inform the patient of the risks inherent in this therapy.

UVAR system – When methoxsalen (*8-MOP*) is used in combination with photopheresis, refer to the *UVAR* system operator's manual for specific warnings, cautions, indications, and instructions related to photopheresis.

Caution – Do not use *Oxsoralen-Ultra* (methoxsalen soft gelatin capsules) interchangeably with *8-MOP* (methoxsalen hard gelatin capsules). *Oxsoralen-Ultra* soft gelatin capsules exhibit significantly greater bioavailability and earlier photosensitization onset time than previous methoxsalen dosage forms. Treat patients in accordance with the dosimetry specifically recommended for this product. Determine the minimum phototoxic dose and phototoxic peak time after drug administration prior to the onset of photochemotherapy with this dosage form.

8-MOP capsules may not be interchanged with *Oxsoralen-Ultra* capsules without retitration of the patient.

Indications

➤*Cutaneous T-cell lymphoma (8-MOP* only): Photopheresis (methoxsalen with long-wave UV radiation of white blood cells) is indicated for use with the *UVAR* system in the palliative treatment of the skin manifestations of cutaneous T-cell lymphoma in patients who have not been responsive to other forms of treatment.

While *8-MOP* has been approved for use in combination with photopheresis, *Oxsoralen-Ultra* has not been approved for this use.

➤*Psoriasis:* For the symptomatic control of severe, recalcitrant, disabling psoriasis not adequately responsive to other forms of therapy and when the diagnosis has been supported by biopsy. Methoxsalen is intended to be administered only in conjunction with a schedule of controlled doses of long-wave UV radiation.

➤*Vitiligo (8-MOP* only): For the repigmentation of idiopathic vitiligo.

Administration and Dosage

➤*General dosing considerations:* Methoxsalen soft gelatin capsules (*Oxsoralen-Ultra*) represent a new doseform. This new doseform exhibits significantly greater bioavailability and earlier photosensitization onset time than previous methoxsalen dosage forms. Human bioavailability studies have indicated that the following dosage and administration directions are to be used as a guideline only.

➤*Adults:*

Cutaneous T-cell lymphoma –

8-MOP: No FDA-approved dosing is available. For use with the *UVAR* system (see Off-label Uses).

Psoriasis – The number of doses per week of methoxsalen capsules will be determined by the patient's schedule of UVA exposures. Do not give treatments more often than once every other day because the full extent of phototoxic reactions may not be evident until 48 hours after each exposure.

Initial dosage:

Methoxsalen Oral Dosage for Psoriasis

Patient weight (kg)	Patient weight (lbs)	Dose (mg)
< 30	< 66	10
30 to 50	66 to 110	20
51 to 65	112 to 143	30
66 to 80	146 to 176	40
81 to 90	179 to 198	50
91 to 115	201 to 254	60
> 115	> 254	70

Dosage adjustment:

- *Weight change* – In the event that the weight of a patient changes during treatment and the patient falls into an adjacent weight range/dose category, no change in the dose of methoxsalen is usually required. If a weight change is sufficient enough to modify the drug dose, then make an adjustment in the time of exposure to UVA.
- *Dosage increase* – Dosage may be increased by 10 mg after the fifteenth treatment under the proper conditions.

Concomitant therapy: Use in combination with UV radiation.

Determination of minimum toxic dose (Oxsoralen-Ultra only): Evaluate each patient by determining the minimum phototoxic dose and phototoxic peak time after drug administration prior to onset of photochemotherapy with this dosage form.

If the minimal phototoxic dose is used, start at half the minimal phototoxic dose.

Vitiligo –

8-MOP:

- *Usual dosage* – 2 capsules (10 mg each) in 1 dose taken with milk or in food 2 to 4 hours before UV light exposure. Therapy should be on alternate days and never on 2 consecutive days.
- *Concomitant therapy* – Use in conjunction with UV radiation.

Off-label dosing –

Cutaneous T-cell lymphoma (8-MOP only): 0.6 mg/kg administered orally 1 to 2 hours before UVA exposure.

➤*Preparation for administration:* Methoxsalen is considered a potential teratogen. Follow safe handling procedures when preparing, administering, or dispensing methoxsalen.

METHOXSALEN — ORAL

➤*Administration:* Take capsules with food or milk. Nausea also may be minimized or avoided by taking the dose in 2 divided portions, taken approximately 30 minutes apart.

Take the methoxsalen soft gelatin capsules (*Oxsoralen-Ultra*) 1.5 to 2 hours before UVA exposure; take methoxsalen hard gelatin capsules (*8-MOP*) 2 hours before UVA exposure.

➤*Storage/Stability:* Store at 25°C (77°F); excursions are permitted between 15° and 30°C (59° to 86°F).

Actions

➤*Pharmacology:* The exact mechanism of action of methoxsalen with the epidermal melanocytes and keratinocytes is not known. The best known biochemical reaction of methoxsalen is with DNA. Methoxsalen, upon photoactivation, conjugates and forms covalent bonds with DNA, which leads to the formation of monofunctional (addition to a single strand of DNA) and bifunctional (cross-linking of psoralen to both strands of DNA) adducts. Reactions with proteins also have been described.

Methoxsalen acts as a photosensitizer. Administration of the drug and subsequent exposure to UVA can lead to cell injury. Orally administered methoxsalen reaches the skin via the blood, and UVA penetrates well into the skin. If sufficient cell injury occurs in the skin, an inflammatory reaction occurs. The most obvious manifestation of this reaction is delayed erythema, which may not begin for several hours and peaks at 48 to 72 hours. The inflammation is followed over several days to weeks by repair, which is manifested by increased melanization of the epidermis and thickening of the stratum corneum. The mechanisms of therapy are not known.

In the treatment of psoriasis, the mechanism is most often assumed to be DNA photodamage and resulting decrease in cell proliferation, but other vascular, leukocyte, or cell regulatory mechanisms also may be playing some role. Psoriasis is a hyperproliferative disorder, and other agents known to be therapeutic for psoriasis are known to inhibit DNA synthesis.

The combination treatment regimen of psoralen and UV radiation of 320 to 400 nanometer wavelength commonly referred to as UVA is known by the acronym PUVA. Skin reactivity to UVA (320 to 400 nanometers) radiation is markedly enhanced by the ingestion of methoxsalen.

In the treatment of vitiligo, it has been suggested that melanocytes in the hair follicle are stimulated to move up the follicle and to repopulate the epidermis.

➤*Pharmacokinetics:*

Absorption/Distribution – Methoxsalen is reversibly bound to serum albumin and also is preferentially taken up by epidermal cells. At a dose that is 6 times larger than that used in humans, it induces mixed function oxidases in the livers of mice.

Oxsoralen-Ultra: In a well-controlled bioavailability study, these capsules reached peak drug levels in the blood of test subjects between 0.5 and 4 hours (mean, 1.8 hours). Detectable methoxsalen levels were observed up to 12 hours postdose. Photosensitivity studies demonstrated a peak photosensitivity of 1.5 to 2.1 hours.

8-MOP: This drug reaches its maximum bioavailability 1.5 to 3 hours after oral administration and may last for up to 8 hours.

Metabolism – In mice and humans, methoxsalen is rapidly metabolized.

Excretion – Approximately 95% of the drug is excreted as a series of metabolites in the urine within 24 hours.

Oxsoralen-Ultra: Drug half-life is approximately 2 hours.

Contraindications

Methoxsalen is contraindicated in patients exhibiting idiosyncratic reactions to psoralen compounds, and patients with aphakia (because of the significantly increased risk of retinal damage caused by the absence of lenses), invasive squamous cell carcinomas, melanoma, or a history of melanoma. Methoxsalen also is contraindicated in patients possessing a specific history of light-sensitive disease states. These patients should not initiate methoxsalen therapy except under special circumstances. Diseases associated with photosensitivity include lupus erythematosus, porphyria cutanea tarda, erythropoietic protoporphyria, variegate porphyria, xeroderma pigmentosum, and albinism.

Warnings/Precautions

➤*Skin burns/Photosensitivity:* Methoxsalen acts as a photosensitizer. Serious burns from UVA or sunlight (even through window glass) can result if the recommended dosage of the drug and/or exposure schedules are not maintained or exceeded (see also Drug Interactions and Psoriasis Treatment). Patients must avoid sun exposure, even through window glass or cloud cover, for at least 8 hours after methoxsalen ingestion. If sun exposure cannot be avoided, the patient must wear protective devices such as a hat and gloves and/or apply sunscreens that contain ingredients that filter out UVA radiation (eg, sunscreens containing benzophenone and/or para-aminobenzoic acid [PABA] esters that exhibit a sun protective factor of 15 or higher).

➤*Cataracts:*

Human studies – It has been found that the concentration of methoxsalen in the lens is proportional to the serum level. If the lens is exposed to UVA during the time methoxsalen is present in the lens, photochemical action may lead to irreversible binding of methoxsalen to proteins and the DNA components of the lens. However, if the lens is shielded from UVA, the methoxsalen will diffuse out of the lens in a 24-hour period. Emphatically instruct patients to wear UVA absorbing, wrap-around sunglasses for the 24-hour period following ingestion of methoxsalen, whether they are exposed to direct or indirect sunlight in the open or through a window glass.

Among patients using proper eye protection, there is no evidence for a significantly increased risk of cataracts in association with PUVA therapy. Thirty-five of 1,380 patients have developed cataracts in the 5 years since their first PUVA treatment. This incidence is comparable with that expected in a population of this size and age distribution. No relationship between PUVA dose and cataract risk in this group has been noted.

➤*Actinic degeneration:* Exposure to sunlight and/or UV radiation may result in premature aging of the skin.

➤*Basal cell carcinomas:* Diligently observe and treat patients exhibiting multiple basal cell carcinomas or having a history of basal cell carcinomas.

➤*Radiation therapy:* Diligently observe patients who have a history of x-ray therapy or grenz-ray therapy for signs of carcinoma.

➤*Arsenic therapy:* Diligently observe patients having a history of previous arsenic therapy for signs of carcinoma.

➤*Total UVA dosage:* The total cumulative dose of UVA that can be given over long periods of time with safety has not been established.

➤*Vitiligo treatment:* Do not increase the dosage of methoxsalen above 0.6 mg/kg because overdosage may result in serious burning of the skin.

Observe eye and skin protection as described in the following sections.

➤*Psoriasis treatment:*

Before methoxsalen ingestion – Patients must not sunbathe during the 24 hours prior to methoxsalen ingestion and UV exposure. The presence of a sunburn may prevent an accurate evaluation of the patient's response to photochemotherapy.

After methoxsalen ingestion – UVA-absorbing, wrap-around sunglasses must be worn during daylight for 24 hours after methoxsalen ingestion. The protective eyewear must be designed to prevent entry of stray radiation to the eyes, including that which may enter from the sides of the eyewear. The protective eyewear is used to prevent the irreversible binding of methoxsalen to the proteins and DNA components of the lens. Cataracts form when enough of the binding occurs. Permit visual discrimination by the eyewear of patient well-being and comfort.

Patients must avoid sun exposure, even through window glass or cloud cover, for at least 8 hours after methoxsalen ingestion. If sun exposure cannot be avoided, the patient must wear protective devices such as a hat and gloves and/or apply sunscreens that contain ingredients that filter out UVA radiation (eg, sunscreens containing benzophenone and/or PABA esters that exhibit a sun protective factor of 15 or higher). Instruct patients to apply these chemical sunscreens to all areas that might be exposed to the sun (including lips). Do not apply sunscreens to areas affected by psoriasis until after the patient has been treated in the UVA chamber.

During PUVA therapy – Total UVA-absorbing/blocking goggles mechanically designed to give maximal ocular protection must be worn. Failure to do so may increase the risk of cataract formation. A reliable radiometer can be used to verify elimination of UVA transmission through the goggles.

Protect abdominal skin, breasts, genitalia, and other sensitive areas for approximately one-third of the initial exposure time until tanning occurs.

Shield male genitalia, unless it is affected by disease.

After combined methoxsalen/UVA therapy – Wear UVA-absorbing, wrap-around sunglasses during daylight for 24 hours after combined methoxsalen/UVA therapy.

Instruct patients not to sunbathe for 48 hours after therapy. Erythema and/or burning because of photochemotherapy and sunburn because of sun exposure are additive.

➤*Hepatic function impairment:* Treat patients with hepatic function impairment with caution because hepatic biotransformation is necessary for drug urinary excretion.

➤*Special risk:* Do not treat patients with cardiac diseases or others who may be unable to tolerate prolonged standing or exposure to heat stress in a vertical UVA chamber.

➤*Pregnancy: Category C.* According to the manufacturer of *8-MOP* and *Oxsoralen Ultra*, animal reproduction studies have not been conducted with methoxsalen. According to Briggs' *Drugs in Pregnancy and Lactation*, methoxsalen does not appear to be a significant teratogen, and studies evaluating the long-term effects (eg, cancer) of in utero exposure have not been done. However, the manufacturer of *Uvadex* (methoxsalen extracorporeal solution) classifies methoxsalen as Pregnancy Category D and states that methoxsalen may cause fetal harm when given to a pregnant woman. Doses of 80 to 160 mg/kg/day given during organogenesis caused significant fetal toxicity in rats. The lowest of these doses, 80 mg/kg/day, is over 4,000 times more than a single dose of methoxsalen on a mg/m^2 basis. Fetal toxicity was associated with significant maternal weight loss, anorexia, and increased relative liver weight. Signs of fetal toxicity included increased fetal mortality, increased resorptions, late fetal death, fewer fetuses per litter, and decreased fetal weight. Methoxsalen caused an increase in skeletal malformation and variations at doses of 80 mg/kg/day and higher. There are no adequate and well-controlled studies of methoxsalen in pregnant women. If methoxsalen is used during pregnancy, or if the patient becomes pregnant while receiving methoxsalen, apprise the patient of the potential hazard to the fetus. Advise women of childbearing potential to avoid becoming pregnant.

➤*Lactation:* It is not known whether this drug is excreted in human milk. Discontinue either methoxsalen ingestion or breast-feeding. If methoxsalen is given, stop breast-feeding and discard the milk for at least 24 hours because the drug is a photosensitizer.

METHOXSALEN — ORAL

➤*Children:* Safety in children has not been established. Potential hazards of long-term therapy include the possibilities of carcinogenicity and cataractogenicity as described previously, as well as the probability of actinic degeneration, which is also described previously.

➤*Elderly:* Use caution in elderly patients, especially those with a preexisting history of cataracts, cardiovascular conditions, kidney and/or liver dysfunction, or skin cancer.

Clinical studies with *Oxsoralen-Ultra* did not include sufficient numbers of subjects 65 years of age and older to determine whether elderly subjects responded differently from younger subjects. Other reported clinical experience has not identified differences in responses between elderly and younger patients. In general, be cautious about dose selection for an elderly patient, usually starting at the low end of the dosing range, reflecting the greater frequency of hepatic and renal function impairment, decreased cardiac function, and concomitant disease or other drug therapy.

➤*Monitoring:* Instruct patients to have an ophthalmologic examination prior to the start of therapy, and thence yearly.

Instruct patients to have the following tests prior to the start of therapy, and to be retested 6 to 12 months subsequently: complete blood cell count (hemoglobin or hematocrit, white blood cell count [if abnormal, a differential count]); antinuclear antibodies; liver function tests; renal function tests (creatinine or serum urea nitrogen [BUN]). Conduct additional tests at more extended time periods as clinically indicated.

Drug Interactions

➤*Cyclosporine:* Cyclosporine bioavailability may be elevated, increasing the risk of toxicity (eg, nephrotoxicity). Monitor cyclosporine concentrations and for adverse reactions. Adjust cyclosporine dose as needed.

➤*Photosensitivity agents:* Exercise special care in treating patients who are receiving concomitant therapy (either topically or systemically) with known photosensitizing agents such as anthralin, coal tar or coal tar derivatives, griseofulvin, phenothiazines (eg, promethazine), nalidixic acid, halogenated salicylanilides (bacteriostatic soaps), sulfonamides (eg, sulfamethoxazole), tetracyclines (eg, doxycycline), thiazides (eg, hydrochlorothiazide), and certain organic staining dyes such as methylene blue, toluidine blue, rose bengal, and methyl orange.

Adverse Reactions

➤*CNS:* Depression, insomnia, and nervousness.

➤*GI:* The most commonly reported adverse reaction of methoxsalen alone is nausea, which occurs with approximately 10% of all patients. This effect may be minimized or avoided by instructing the patient to take methoxsalen with milk or food, or to divide the dose into 2 portions, taken approximately one-half hour apart.

➤*Combined methoxsalen / UVA therapy:*

Dermatologic –

Pruritus: This adverse reaction occurs with approximately 10% of all patients. In most cases, pruritus can be alleviated with frequent application of bland emollients or other topical agents; severe pruritus may require systemic treatment. If pruritus is unresponsive to these measures, shield pruritic areas from further UVA exposure until the condition resolves. If intractable pruritus is generalized, discontinue UVA treatment until the pruritus disappears.

Erythema: Mild, transient erythema at 24 to 48 hours after PUVA therapy is an expected reaction and indicates that a therapeutic interaction between methoxsalen and UVA occurred. Shield any area showing moderate erythema (higher than grade 2) during subsequent UVA exposures until the erythema has resolved. Erythema higher than grade 2 that appears within 24 hours after UVA treatment may signal a potentially severe burn. Erythema may become progressively worse over the next 24 hours because the peak erythemal reaction characteristically occurs 48 hours or later after methoxsalen ingestion. Protect the patient from further UVA exposures and sunlight, and monitor closely.

Important differences between PUVA erythema and sunburn – PUVA-induced inflammation differs from sunburn or UVB phototherapy in several ways. The in situ depth of photochemistry is deeper within the tissue because UVA is transmitted further into the skin. The percent transmission of UVB varies between 0% to 34% through skin, whereas UVA varies between 1% to 80% transmission; thus, UVA is transmitted to a larger percent through the skin. The DNA lesions induced by PUVA are very different from UV-induced thymine dimers and may lead to a DNA crosslink. This DNA lesion may be more problematic to the cell because crosslinks are more lethal and psoralen-DNA photoproducts may be "new" or unfamiliar substrates for DNA repair enzymes. DNA synthesis is also suppressed longer after PUVA. The time course of delayed erythema is different with PUVA and may not involve the usual mediators seen in sunburn. PUVA-induced redness may be just beginning at 24 hours when UVB erythema has already passed its peak. The erythema dose-response curve is also steeper for PUVA. Compared with equally erythemogenic doses of UVB, the histologic alterations induced by PUVA show more dermal vessel damage and longer duration of epidermal and dermal abnormalities.

Miscellaneous – Other adverse reactions reported include cutaneous tenderness, depression, dizziness, edema, extension of psoriasis, folliculitis, GI disturbances, headache, herpes simplex, hypopigmentation, hypotension, leg cramps, malaise, miliaria, nonspecific rash, urticaria, and vesiculation and bullae formation.

Overdosage

➤*Treatment:* In the event of methoxsalen overdosage, keep the patient in a darkened room for at least 24 hours.

Patient Information

Take capsules with food or milk.

METHOXSALEN — EXTRACORPOREAL

WARNING

Only health care providers who have special competence in the diagnosis and treatment of cutaneous T-cell lymphoma and have special training and experience in the *UVAR* or *UVAR XTS* photopheresis system should use methoxsalen. Consult the appropriate operator's manual before using this product.

Indications

➤*Cutaneous T-cell lymphoma:* For extracorporeal administration with the *UVAR* or *UVAR XTS* photopheresis system in the palliative treatment of skin manifestations of cutaneous T-cell lymphoma that is unresponsive to other forms of treatment.

Administration and Dosage

➤*General dosing considerations:* Each methoxsalen treatment involves collection of leukocytes, photoactivation, and reinfusion of photoactivated cells.

➤*Adults:*

Cutaneous T-cell lymphoma –

Usual dosage: During each photopheresis treatment performed with the *UVAR* system, methoxsalen 10 mL (200 mcg) is injected directly into the photoactivation bag during the first buffy coat collection cycle. At the end of 6 cycles, a total of 740 mL (240 mL of buffy coat, 300 mL of plasma, and 200 mL of normal saline priming fluid) is collected and mixed with the 200 mcg of methoxsalen present in the photoactivation bag.

• *Normal treatment schedule* – Give treatment on 2 consecutive days every 4 weeks for a minimum of 7 treatment cycles (6 months).

• *Accelerated treatment schedule* – If the assessment of the patient during the fourth treatment cycle (approximately 3 months) reveals an increased skin score from the baseline score, the frequency of treatment may be increased to 2 consecutive treatments every 2 weeks. If a 25% improvement in the skin score is attained after 4 consecutive weeks, the regular treatment schedule may resume. Patients who are maintained in the accelerated treatment schedule may receive a maximum of 20 cycles.

Duration of therapy: There is no clinical evidence to show that treatment with methoxsalen for more than 6 months or using a different schedule provides additional benefit.

➤*Preparation for administration:* Methoxsalen is considered a potential teratogen. Follow safe handling procedures when preparing, administering, or dispensing methoxsalen.

➤*Administration:* Not for parenteral administration. For extracorporeal administration with the *UVAR* or *UVAR XTS* photophoresis system.

➤*Storage / Stability:* Store between 15° and 30°C (59° and 86°F).

Actions

➤*Pharmacology:* The exact mechanism of action of methoxsalen is unknown. The best known biochemical reaction of methoxsalen is with DNA. Methoxsalen, upon photoactivation, conjugates and forms covalent bonds with DNA, which leads to the formation of monofunctional (addition to a single strand of DNA) and bifunctional adducts (cross-linking of psoralen to both strands of DNA). Reactions with proteins also have been described.

For the palliative treatment of cutaneous T-cell lymphoma, photopheresis consists of removing a portion of the patient's blood and separating the red blood cells from the white cell layer (buffy coat) by centrifugation. The red cells are returned to the patient and methoxsalen sterile solution is then injected into the instrument and mixed with the buffy coat. The instrument then irradiates this drug-cell mixture with ultraviolet (UVA) light (320 to 400 nm) and returns the treated cells to the patient. See the appropriate operator's manual for details of this process. Although extracorporeal phototherapy exposes less than 10% of the total body burden of malignant cells to methoxsalen plus light, some patients achieve a complete response. Animal studies suggest that the photopheresis may activate an immune-mediated response against the malignant T-cells.

Use of the *UVAR* and *UVAR XTS* systems after oral administration of methoxsalen were previously approved for the treatment of cutaneous T-cell lymphoma. Interpatient variability in peak plasma concentration after an oral dose of methoxsalen ranges from 6- to 15-fold. Methoxsalen is injected directly into the separated buffy coat in the instrument in an attempt to diminish the interpatient variability and to improve the exposure of the cells to the drug.

Systemic administration of methoxsalen followed by UVA exposure leads to cell injury. The most obvious manifestation of this injury after skin exposure is delayed erythema, which may not begin for several hours and peaks at 48 to 72 hours. The inflammation is followed over several days to weeks by repair, which is manifested by increased melanization of the epidermis and thickening of the stratum corneum.

METHOXSALEN — EXTRACORPOREAL

The total dose of methoxsalen delivered in methoxsalen sterile solution is substantially lower (approximately 200 times) than that used with oral administration.

➤*Pharmacokinetics:*

Distribution – Methoxsalen is reversibly bound to serum albumin and is also preferentially taken up by epidermal cells.

Metabolism/Excretion – Methoxsalen is rapidly metabolized in humans, with approximately 95% of the drug excreted as metabolites in the urine within 24 hours.

Contraindications

Patients exhibiting idiosyncratic reactions to psoralen compounds. Do not initiate methoxsalen therapy in patients possessing a specific history of a light-sensitive disease state. Diseases associated with photosensitivity include albinism, erythropoietic protoporphyria, lupus erythematosus, porphyria cutanea tarda, variegate porphyria, and xeroderma pigmentosum.

Patients with aphakia because of the significantly increased risk of retinal damage because of the absence of lenses.

Warnings/Precautions

➤*Actinic degeneration:* After methoxsalen administration, exposure to sunlight and/or UV radiation may result in premature aging of the skin.

➤*Basal cell carcinomas:* Diligently observe and treat patients exhibiting multiple basal cell carcinomas or having a history of basal cell carcinomas.

➤*Skin burns/Photosensitivity:* Serious burns from UVA or sunlight (even through window glass) can result if the recommended dosage of methoxsalen is exceeded or precautions are not followed. Instruct patients to use a sunscreen (SPF 15 or higher) for the 24-hour period following methoxsalen treatment, whether they are exposed to direct or indirect sunlight (see also Drug Interactions).

➤*Cataracts:* Exposure to large doses of UVA light causes cataracts in animals. Oral methoxsalen exacerbates this toxicity. The concentration of methoxsalen in the human lens is proportional to the concentration in serum. Serum methoxsalen concentrations are substantially lower after extracorporeal methoxsalen treatment than after oral methoxsalen treatment. Nevertheless, if the lens is exposed to UVA light while methoxsalen is present, photoactivation of the drug may cause adducts to bind to biomolecules within the lens. If the lens is shielded from UVA light, the methoxsalen will diffuse out of the lens in about 24 hours.

Patients who use proper eye protection after PUVA (oral methoxsalen) therapy appear to have no increased risk of developing cataracts. The incidence of cataracts in these patients 5 years after their first treatment is about the same as that in the general population. Emphatically instruct patients to wear UVA-absorbing, wrap-around sunglasses for 24 hours after methoxsalen extracorporeal solution treatment. Tell patients to wear these glasses any time they are exposed to direct or indirect sunlight, whether they are outdoors or exposed through a window.

➤*Pregnancy: Category D.* Methoxsalen may cause fetal harm when given to a pregnant woman. Doses of 80 to 160 mg/kg/day given during organogenesis caused significant fetal toxicity in rats. The lowest of these doses, 80 mg/kg/day, is over 4,000 times more than a single dose of methoxsalen on a mg/m^2 basis. Fetal toxicity was associated with significant maternal weight loss, anorexia, and increased relative liver weight. Signs of fetal toxicity included increased fetal mortality, increased resorptions, late fetal death, fewer fetuses per litter, and decreased fetal weight. Methoxsalen caused an increase in skeletal malformation and variations at doses of 80 mg/kg/day and higher. There are no adequate and well-controlled studies of methoxsalen in pregnant women. If methoxsalen is used during pregnancy, or if the patient becomes pregnant while receiving methoxsalen, apprise the patient of the potential hazard to the fetus. Advise women of childbearing potential to avoid becoming pregnant.

➤*Lactation:* It is not known whether this drug is excreted in human milk. If methoxsalen is given, stop breast-feeding and discard the milk for at least 24 hours because the drug is a photosensitizer.

➤*Children:* Safety in children has not been established. Potential hazards of long-term therapy include the possibilities of carcinogenicity and cataractogenicity, as well as the probability of actinic degeneration.

Drug Interactions

➤*Cyclosporine:* In a study using methoxsalen capsules, cyclosporine bioavailability was elevated, increasing the risk of toxicity (eg, nephrotoxicity). Monitor cyclosporine concentrations and for adverse reactions. Adjust cyclosporine dose as needed.

➤*Photosensitizing agents:* Exercise special care when treating patients who are receiving concomitant therapy (topically or systemically) with known photosensitizing agents such as anthralin, coal tar or coal tar derivatives, griseofulvin, halogenated salicylamilides (bacteriostatic soaps), nalidoxic acid, phenothiazines (eg, promethazine), sulfonamides (eg, sulfamethoxazole), tetracyclines (eg, doxycycline), thiazides (eg, hydrochlorothiazide), and certain organic staining dyes such as methylene blue, toluidine blue, rose bengal, and methyl orange.

Adverse Reactions

Adverse reactions of photopheresis (methoxsalen used with the *UVAR* photopheresis system) were primarily related to hypotension secondary to changes in extracorporeal volume (more than 1%). In study CTCL 3, 6 serious cardiovascular adverse reactions were reported in 5 patients (5/51; 10%). Five of these 6 reactions were not related to photopheresis and did not interfere with the scheduled photopheresis treatments. One patient (1/51; 2%) with ischemic heart disease had an arrhythmia after the first day of photopheresis that was resolved the next day. Six infections were also reported in 5 patients. Two of the 6 infections were Hickman catheter infections in 1 patient, which did not interrupt the scheduled photopheresis. The other 4 infections were not related to photopheresis and did not interfere with scheduled treatments.

Overdosage

➤*Treatment:* There are no known reports of overdosage with extracorporeal administration of methoxsalen. However, in the event of overdosage, keep the patient in a darkened room for at least 24 hours.

Patient Information

Emphatically instruct patients to wear UVA-absorbing wrap-around sunglasses and cover exposed skin or use a sunscreen (SPF 15 or higher) for the 24-hour period, following treatment with methoxsalen, whether exposed to direct or indirect sunlight in the open or through a window glass.

METHOXSALEN — TOPICAL

WARNING

Methoxsalen lotion is a potent drug capable of producing severe burns if improperly used. It should be applied only by a health care provider under controlled conditions for light exposure and subsequent light shielding. Never dispense this preparation to a patient.

Indications

➤*Vitiligo:* Topical repigmenting agent in vitiligo, used in conjunction with controlled doses of ultraviolet A (UVA) (320 to 400 nm) or sunlight.

Administration and Dosage

➤*General dosing considerations:* Instruct patients to keep the treated areas protected from light by use of protective clothing or sunscreening agents. The area of application may be highly photosensitive for several days and may result in severe burn injury if exposed to additional UV or sunlight.

Individualize treatment. Essentially, idiopathic vitiligo is reversible, but not equally, in every patient. Repigmentation varies in completeness, time of onset, and duration; it occurs more rapidly on fleshy regions, such as the face, abdomen, and buttocks, and less rapidly over less fleshy areas, such as the dorsum of the hands and feet.

➤*Adults:*

Vitiligo –

Usual dosage: Apply lotion to a well-defined area of vitiligo, then expose this area to a suitable source of UVA light. Initial exposure time should be conservative and must not exceed what is predicted to be one-half the minimal erythema dose.

Regulate treatment intervals by erythema response (generally once a week or less, depending on the results).

Duration of therapy: Pigmentation may begin after a few weeks; significant repigmentation may take up to 6 to 9 months of treatment. Periodic re-treatment may be needed to retain the new pigment.

➤*Children:*

Vitiligo –

12 years and older: See Adults for dosing.

➤*Preparation for administration:* Methoxsalen is considered a potential teratogen. Follow safe handling procedures when preparing, administering, or dispensing methoxsalen.

➤*Administration:* Apply topically by a health care provider under controlled conditions for light exposure and subsequent light shielding.

Protect the hands and fingers of the person applying the medication with gloves or finger cots to avoid photosensitization and possible burns.

➤*Storage/Stability:* Store at 25°C (77°F); excursions are permitted between 15° and 30°C (59° and 86°F).

Actions

➤*Pharmacology:* The exact mechanism of action of methoxsalen with the epidermal melanocytes and keratinocytes is not known. Psoralens given orally are preferentially taken up by epidermal cells. The best known biochemical reaction of methoxsalen is with DNA. Methoxsalen, upon photoactivation, conjugates and forms covalent bonds with DNA, which leads to the formation of monofunctional (addition to a single strand of DNA) and bifunctional adducts (cross-linking of psoralen to both strands of DNA). Reactions with proteins have also been described.

Methoxsalen acts as a photosensitizer. Topical application of this drug and subsequent exposure to UVA, whether artificial or sunlight, can cause cell injury. If sufficient cell injury occurs in the skin, an inflammatory reaction will result. The most obvious manifestation of this reaction is delayed erythema, which may not begin for several hours and may not peak for 2 to 3 days or longer. It is crucial to realize that the length of time the skin remains sensitized or when the maximum erythema will occur is quite variable from person to person. The erythematous reaction is followed over several days or weeks by repair, which is manifested by increased melanization of the epidermis and thickening of the stratum corneum. The exact mechanics

METHOXSALEN — TOPICAL

are unknown, but it has been suggested that melanocytes in the hair follicles are stimulated to move up the follicle and to repopulate the epidermis.

Contraindications

Idiosyncratic reactions to psoralen compounds or a history of sensitivity reactions to them; melanoma or a history of melanoma; invasive skin carcinoma, generally; photosensitivity diseases such as porphyria, acute lupus erythematosus, or xeroderma pigmentosum; children younger than 12 years of age because clinical studies to determine the efficacy and safety of treatment in this age group have not been performed.

Warnings/Precautions

➤*Skin burn/photosensitivity:* Serious skin burns from UVA or sunlight (even through window glass) can result if recommended exposure schedule is exceeded and/or protective covering or sunscreens are not used. The blistering of the skin sometimes encountered after UV exposure generally heals without complication or scarring. Suitable covering of the area of application or a topical sunscreen must follow the therapeutic UVA exposure.

Apply this product only in small, well-defined lesions and preferably on lesions that can be protected by clothing or a sunscreen from subsequent exposure to radiant UVA. If this product is used to treat vitiligo of the face or hands, be very emphatic when instructing the patient to keep the treated areas protected from light by use of protective clothing or sunscreening agents. The area of application may be highly photosensitive for several days and may result in severe burn injury if exposed to additional UV or sunlight (see also Drug Interactions).

➤*Pregnancy: Category C.* Animal reproduction studies have not been conducted with topical methoxsalen. It is also not known whether methoxsalen can cause fetal harm when used topically on a pregnant woman or affect reproductive capacity. It is not known to what degree, if any, topical methoxsalen is absorbed systemically. Use topical methoxsalen in women only when clearly indicated.

➤*Lactation:* It is not known whether topical methoxsalen is absorbed or excreted in human milk. Caution is advised when topical methoxsalen is used in a breast-feeding mother.

➤*Children:* Safety and effectiveness in children younger than 12 years of age have not been established.

Drug Interactions

➤*Photosensitivity agents:* Exercise special care in treating patients who are receiving concomitant therapy (topically or systemically) with known photosensitizing agents such as anthralin, coal tar or coal tar derivatives, griseofulvin, phenothiazines (eg, promethazine), nalidixic acid, halogenated salicylanilides (bacteriostatic soaps), sulfonamides (eg, sulfamethoxazole), tetracyclines (eg, doxycycline), thiazides (eg, hydrochlorothiazide), and certain organic staining dyes such as methylene blue, toluidine blue, rose bengal, and methyl orange.

Adverse Reactions

➤*Dermatologic:* The most common adverse reaction is severe burns of the treated area from overexposure to UVA, including sunlight. Treatment must be individualized. Minor blistering of the skin is not a contraindication to further treatment and generally heals without incident. Treatment would be the standard for burn therapy. Since 1953, many studies have demonstrated the safety and effectiveness of topical methoxsalen and UVA for the treatment of vitiligo, when used as directed.

Overdosage

➤*Treatment:* In the unlikely event that the lotion is ingested, follow standard procedures for poisoning. Protection from UVA or daylight for hours or days would also be necessary. Keep the patient in a darkened room.

Patient Information

Instruct the patient to keep the treated areas protected from light by use of protective clothing or sunscreening agents. The area of application may be highly photosensitive for several days and may result in severe burn injury if exposed to additional UV or sunlight.

PIGMENT AGENTS

DIHYDROXYACETONE

otc	**Chromelin Complexion Blender** (Summers)	**Suspension:** 5%	Isopropyl alcohol, propylene glycol. In 30 mL.

DIHYDROXYACETONE — TOPICAL

Indications

➤*Idiopathic vitiligo:* Used to darken light or unpigmented areas of skin affected by vitiligo, scars, and other causes.

Administration and Dosage

➤*Adults:*

Idiopathic vitiligo –

Initial dosage: Suspension should be applied evenly to areas of skin to be darkened and allowed to remain on the skin at least 3 hours before washing. The first effects appear in about 6 hours after initial application. To achieve a darker color, advise patients to repeat application instructions once or twice in 24 hours, more often if darker color is desired.

Maintenance dosage: Maintenance applications of once a day or every other day should be sufficient.

Duration of therapy: The coloration will last 3 to 10 days with gradual and even fading.

➤*Administration:* Applicator top should be used to apply evenly to areas of skin to be darkened.

To prevent darkening of skin surrounding treated areas, advise patients to take a damp tissue and gently wipe off any dihydroxyacetone (DHA) that has overlapped onto normally pigmented skin.

Actions

➤*Pharmacology:* The mechanism of action is not fully understood; however, DHA may involve a reaction (similar to that caused by sun exposure) with amino acids in the stratum corneum of the skin to produce a brownish color. As the concentration of the drug increases, so does the pigmentation.

Warnings/Precautions

➤*For external use only:* Avoid contact with hair, eyes, eyelids, abraded skin, and clothes.

➤*Sun exposure:* Use sunscreen before exposing treated areas to the sun.

➤*Pregnancy: Category: Undetermined.* Consult a health care provider before using in pregnant women.

➤*Lactation:* Consult a health care provider before using in a breast-feeding woman.

Adverse Reactions

➤*Dermatologic:* Rashes with erythemaand allergic dermatitis; skin irritation or sensitivity (rare).

Patient Information

Use sunscreen before exposing treated skin to the sun.

Use applicator to evenly apply to affected areas to be treated; to prevent darkening of skin in surrounding areas, take a damp cloth to wipe off excess.

Do not wash the treated area for 3 hours after application.

First application takes about 6 hours to develop color.

Cosmetics may be applied on treated areas.

May stain clothing; let treated areas dry.

HYDROQUINONE

otc	**Eldopaque** (ICN)	**Cream; topical:** 2%	With sunblock. In 14.2 and 28.4 g.
otc	**Esoterica Facial** (Medicis)		Octyl dimethyl PABA, benzophenone, stearyl alcohol, sodium bisulfite, parabens, EDTA. In 90 g.
otc	**Esoterica Regular** (Medicis)		Light mineral oil, stearyl alcohol, parabens, sodium bisulfite, EDTA. In 90 g.
otc	**Esoterica Sunscreen** (Medicis)		3.3% padimate O, 2.5% oxybenzone, mineral oil, parabens, sodium bisulfite, EDTA. In 85 g.
otc	**Solaquin** (ICN)		With sunscreens. In 28.4 g.

HYDROQUINONE

Rx	**Hydroquinone** (Various, eg, Ethex, Glades)	**Cream; topical:** 4%	May contain EDTA, parabens, mineral oil, sodium metabisulfite. In 28.35 g.
Rx	**Hydroquinone with Sunscreen** (Various, eg, Ethex, Glades)		May contain padimate O, dioxybenzone, oxybenzone, octyl methoxycinnamate, octyl dimethyl-p-aminobenzoate, cetearyl alcohol, vitamin E, parabens, mineral oil, cetearyl alcohol, stearyl alcohol, lactic acid, EDTA, sodium metabisulfite. In 28.35 g.
Rx	**Eldopaque Forte** (ICN)		In a sunblock base. Talc, light mineral oil, EDTA, sodium metabisulfite. In 28.4 g.
Rx	**Eldoquin-Forte** (ICN)		In a vanishing base. Light mineral oil, propylparaben, sodium metabisulfite. In 28.4 g.
Rx	**EpiQuin Micro** (SkinMedica)		Vitamins A, E, and C, cetyl alcohol, benzyl alcohol, EDTA, glycerin, methylparaben, sodium metabisulfite. In 30 g.
Rx	**Glyquin** (ICN)		In a vanishing base. Padimate O, oxybenzone, octyl methoxycinnamate, methylparaben. SPF 15. In 28 g.
Rx	**Glyquin-XM** (ICN)		In a vanishing base. Octocrylene, oxybenzone, avobenzone, vitamin E, methylparaben, EDTA. SPF 15. In 28 g.
Rx	**Solaquin Forte** (ICN)		In a vanishing base. Dioxybenzone, padimate O, oxybenzone, EDTA, sodium metabisulfite, cetearyl alcohol, stearyl alcohol, lactic acid. In 28.4 g.
Rx	**Lustra** (Medicis)		Glycerin, alcohol, cetyl alcohol, cetearyl alcohol, benzyl alcohol, sodium metabisulfite, EDTA. In 28.4 g.
Rx	**Lustra-AF** (Medicis)		Glycerin, alcohol, cetyl alcohol, cetearyl alcohol, benzyl alcohol, sodium metabisulfite, EDTA, octyl methoxycinnamate, avobenzone. In 28.4 g.
Rx	**Nuquin HP** (Stratus)		Octyl methoxycinnamate, glycerin, cetyl alcohol, cetostearyl alcohol, stearyl alcohol, sodium metabisulfite. In 14.2, 28.4, and 56.7 g.
Rx	**Melquin HP** (Stratus)		In a vanishing base. Mineral oil, petrolatum, cetostearyl alcohol, glycerin, sodium metabisulfite. In 14.2 and 28.4 g.
Rx	**Melpaque HP** (Stratus)		In a sunblocking base. Mineral oil, parabens, EDTA, sodium metabisulfite, talc. Tinted. In 14.2 and 28.4 g.
Rx	**Hydroquinone** (Glades)	**Solution; topical:** 3%	SD alcohol 40-B, isopropyl alcohol. In 29 mL with applicator.
otc	**NeoStrata HQ Skin Lightening** (NeoStrata)	**Gel; topical:** 2%	Alcohol, kojic acid 3%, licorice extract, polyhydroxy acids 10%, sodium bisulfite, sodium sulfite, tartrazine. In 28.35 g.
Rx	**Hydroquinone** (Glades)	**Gel; topical:** 3%	Hydroalcoholic base. Padimate O, dioxybenzone, EDTA, sodium metabisulfite. In 30 g.
Rx	**Hydroquinone** (Glades)	**Gel; topical:** 4%	Hydroalcoholic base. Padimate O, dioxybenzone, alcohol, EDTA, sodium metabisulfite. In 28.35 g.
Rx	**Solaquin Forte** (ICN)		Hydroalcoholic base. Padimate O, dioxybenzone, EDTA, alcohol, sodium metabisulfite. In 28.4 g.
Rx	**Hydroquinone** (River's Edge)	**Emulsion; topical:** 4%	Benzyl alcohol, cetyl alcohol, EDTA. In 48 g.
Rx	**Aclaro** (Harmony)		Alcohols, EDTA. In 50 mL spray bottles.

HYDROQUINONE — TOPICAL

Indications

➤*Hyperpigmented skin:* For the gradual temporary bleaching of hyperpigmented skin conditions such as chloasma, melasma, freckles, senile lentigines and other unwanted areas of melanin hyperpigmentation.

Administration and Dosage

➤*General dosing considerations:* Hydroquinone bleaching is faster, more dependable, and easier if the treated area is protected from ultraviolet light.

During the day, an effective broad-spectrum sunscreen should be used and unnecessary solar exposure avoided, or protective clothing should be worn to cover bleached skin in order to prevent repigmentation from occurring.

For best results, use with sunscreen or avoid exposure to sunlight.

➤*Adults:*

Hyperpigmented skin –

Cream, gel, and topical solution: Apply to the affected area(s) and rub in well twice daily or as directed by a health care provider to achieve maximum therapeutic potential. However, *Melpaque HP 4%* should not be rubbed in.

Neostrata HQ gel:

• *Usual dosage* – Apply sparingly to affected areas once or twice daily. Use only as directed by a health care provider. Depigmentation is a gradual process, and results should be expected within 12 weeks of daily use.

• *Maintenance dosage* – To maintain results, use several times a week or as directed by a health care provider.

• *Discontinuation of therapy* – If no improvement is seen within 8 weeks, discontinue use.

➤*Children:*

Hyperpigmented skin –

12 years of age or older: See Adults for dosing.

➤*Storage/Stability:* Keep tube tightly closed to ensure an airtight seal. Note that slight darkening of hydroquinone products is normal and does not affect the potency of the products.

Actions

➤*Pharmacology:* Topical application of hydroquinone produces a reversible depigmentation of the skin by inhibition of the enzymatic oxidation of tyrosine to 3,4-dihydroxyphenylalanine (dopa) and suppression of other melanocyte metabolic processes. Exposure to sunlight or ultraviolet light will cause repigmentation of bleached areas.

In addition to hydroquinone, some products contain sunscreens (eg, octyl dimethyl PABA, ethyl dihydroxypropyl PABA, dioxybenzone, oxybenzone).

Contraindications

Hypersensitivity to hydroquinone or any other ingredients of the products.

Warnings/Precautions

➤*Bleaching:* Hydroquinone is a skin-bleaching agent which may produce unwanted cosmetic effects if not used as directed. The physician should be familiar with the contents of this monograph before prescribing or dispensing this medication.

➤*Irritation:* To evaluate possible susceptibility to irritation, or sensitivity, each patient should begin by applying the medication to a small portion of unbroken skin at or near the pigmented area (approximately 1 cm^2) over a period of several days. If no irritation occurs within 24 hours, begin treatment. Minor redness is not necessarily a contraindication, but treatment should be discontinued if itching, excessive inflammation, or vesicle formation occurs. Use of hydroquinone products in paranasal and infraorbital areas increases the chance of irritation. If no improvement is seen after 2 months of treatment, use of this product should be discontinued.

➤*Sun exposure:* Sunscreen use is an essential aspect of hydroquinone therapy since even minimal sunlight exposure stimulates melanocyte activity. The sunscreens in some hydroquinone products provide the necessary sun protection during skin bleaching activity. During the depigmentation maintenance treatment subsequent to the intensive depigmentation therapy, sun exposure of the bleached skin should be avoided to prevent repigmentation.

➤*For external use only:* Avoid contact with eyes. In case of accidental contact, patient should rinse eyes thoroughly with water and contact physician. A bitter taste and antiseptic effect may occur if applied to the lips.

Do not use near eyes. Use in paranasal and infraorbital areas increases the chance of irritation.

➤*Sensitivity:* This medication is for external use only. A mild, transient stinging may occur in people with sensitive skin. Do not use on broken or

HYDROQUINONE — TOPICAL

irritated skin. Discontinue use if irritation or rash occurs. Avoid contact with eyes and mucous membranes. In case of contact, rinse thoroughly with water.

➤*Peroxide:* Concurrent use of peroxide may result in transient dark staining of skin areas due to oxidation of hydroquinone. Staining can be removed by discontinuing concurrent use and by normal soap cleansing.

➤*Sulfite sensitivity:* Some of these products may contain sodium metabisulfite, a sulfite that may cause serious allergic-type reactions (eg, hives, itching, wheezing, anaphylaxis, serious asthma attacks) in certain susceptible persons. Although the overall prevalence of sulfite sensitivity in the general population is probably low, it is seen more frequently in asthmatics or atopic nonasthmatics.

➤*Pregnancy: Category C.* The safety of topical hydroquinone use during pregnancy has not been established. Animal reproduction studies have not been conducted with topical hydroquinone. It is also not known whether hydroquinone can cause fetal harm when used topically on a pregnant woman or affect reproductive capacity. It is not known to what degree, if any, topical hydroquinone is absorbed systemically. Topical hydroquinone should be used in pregnant women only when clearly indicated. Consult with a physician if you are pregnant or intend to become pregnant within 3 months.

➤*Lactation:* It is not known whether topical hydroquinone is absorbed or excreted in human milk. Caution is advised when topical hydroquinone is used by a nursing mother.

➤*Children:* See Administration and Dosage for more information.

Adverse Reactions

No systemic adverse reactions have been reported. Occasional hypersensitivity (localized contact dermatitis) may occur, in which case the medication should be discontinued and the physician notified immediately.

Overdosage

There have been no systemic reactions from the use of topical hydroquinone. However, treatment should be limited to relatively small areas of the body at one time since some patients experience a transient skin reddening and a mild burning sensation which does not preclude treatment.

Patient Information

For external use only. Avoid contact with eyes.

Do not use on irritated, denuded or damaged skin.

Discontinue use and consult physician if rash or irritation develops.

PIGMENT AGENT COMBINATIONS

Rx	**Tri-Luma** (Galderma)	**Cream; topical**: 0.01% fluocinolone acetonide, 4% hydroquinone, 0.05% tretinoin	Cetyl alcohol, glycerin, parabens, sodium metabisulfite, stearyl alcohol. In 30 g.

PIGMENT AGENT COMBINATIONS — TOPICAL

Indications

➤*Tri-Luma*: Short-term treatment of moderate to severe melasma of the face, in the presence of measures for sun avoidance, including the use of sunscreens.

➤*Solage*: Treatment of solar lentigines as an adjunct to a comprehensive skin care and sun avoidance program. Efficacy of daily use longer than 24 weeks has not been established.

Administration and Dosage

➤*General dosing considerations:*

Tri-Luma – Do not use occlusive dressing. During the day, use a sunscreen of SPF 30 and wear protective clothing. Avoid sunlight exposure. Patients may use moisturizers and/or cosmetics during the day.

Solage – Patients should not shower or bathe the treatment area for at least 6 hours after application.

➤*Adults:*

Melasma of the face, moderate to severe –
Tri-Luma: Apply once daily at night. Apply at least 30 minutes before bedtime. Gently wash the face and neck with a mild cleanser. Rinse and pat the skin dry. Apply a thin film of the cream to the hyperpigmented areas of melasma including about half an inch of healthy-appearing skin surrounding each lesion. Rub lightly and uniformly into the skin.

Solar lentigines –
Solage: Apply using the applicator tip while avoiding application to the surrounding skin. Use twice daily, morning and evening, at least 8 hours apart.

➤*Storage/Stability:* Store at 20° to 25°C (68° to 77°F).

Tri-Luma – Keep tightly closed. Protect from freezing.

Solage – Protect from light by continuing to store in the carton after opening.

Actions

➤*Pharmacology:*

Tri-Luma – One of the components is hydroquinone, a depigmenting agent, which may interrupt 1 or more steps in the tyrosine-tyrosinase pathway of melanin synthesis. However, the mechanism of action of the active ingredients in the treatment of melasma is unknown.

Solage – The mechanism of action of mequinol is unknown. Although mequinol is a substrate for the enzyme tyrosinase and acts as a competitive inhibitor of the formation of melanin precursors, the clinical significance of these findings is unknown. The mechanism of action of tretinoin as a depigmenting agent also is unknown.

➤*Pharmacokinetics:*

Tri-Luma – Percutaneous absorption of unchanged tretinoin, hydroquinone, and fluocinolone acetonide into the systemic circulation of 2 groups of healthy volunteers (n = 59) was found to be minimal following 8 weeks of daily application of 1 or 6 g.

Solage – The percutaneous absorption of tretinoin and the systemic exposure to tretinoin and mequinol were assessed in healthy subjects (n = 8) following 2 weeks of twice daily topical treatment with *Solage*. Approximately 0.8 mL was applied to a 400 cm^2 area of the back, corresponding to a dose of 37.3 mcg/cm^2 for mequinol and 0.23 mcg/cm^2 for tretinoin. The percutaneous absorption of tretinoin was approximately 4.4%, and systemic concentrations did not increase over endogenous levels. The mean C_{max} for mequinol was 9.92 ng/mL and the T_{max} was 2 hours.

Contraindications

Hypersensitivity, allergy or intolerance to the product or any of its components; pregnancy or use in women of childbearing potential (*Solage* only).

Warnings/Precautions

➤*Ochrunosis:* Hydroquinone (contained in *Tri-Luma*) may produce exogenous ochronosis, a gradual blue-black darkening of the skin, whose occurrence should prompt discontinuation of therapy. The majority of patients developing this condition are black, but it may also occur in Caucasians and Hispanics.

➤*Eczema:* Tretinoin has been reported to cause severe irritation on eczematous skin and should be used only with utmost caution in patients with this condition.

➤*Irritation:*

Solage – *Solage* may cause skin irritation, erythema, burning, stinging or tingling, peeling, and pruritus. If the degree of such local irritation warrants, patients should be directed to use less medication, decrease the frequency of application, discontinue use temporarily, or discontinue use altogether.

Tri-Luma – *Tri-Luma* contains hydroquinone and tretinoin that may cause mild to moderate irritation. Local irritation such as skin reddening, peeling, mild burning sensation, dryness, and pruritus may be expected at the site of application. Transient skin reddening or mild burning sensation does not preclude treatment. If a reaction suggests hypersensitivity or chemical irritation, discontinue the medication.

➤*Vitiligo: Solage* should be used with caution by patients with a history or family history of vitiligo.

➤*Adrenal suppression: Tri-Luma* contains the corticosteroid fluocinolone acetonide. Systemic absorption of topical corticosteroids can produce reversible hypothalamic-pituitary-adrenal (HPA) axis suppression with the potential for glucocorticosteroid insufficiency after withdrawal of treatment. Manifestations of Cushing syndrome, hyperglycemia, and glucosuria can also be produced by systemic absorption of topical corticosteroid while on treatment. If HPA axis suppression is noted, the use of *Tri-Luma* should be discontinued. Recovery of HPA axis function generally occurs upon discontinuation of topical corticosteroids.

➤*Weather extremes:* Weather extremes such as wind or cold may be more irritating to patients using *Solage*.

➤*Hypersensitivity reactions:* Cutaneous hypersensitivity to the active ingredients of *Tri-Luma* has been reported in the literature. In a patch test study to determine sensitization potential in 221 healthy volunteers, 3 volunteers developed sensitivity reactions to *Tri-Luma* or its components.

➤*Sulfite sensitivity: Tri-Luma* contains sodium metabisulfite, which may cause allergic-type reactions, including anaphylactic symptoms and life-threatening/less severe asthmatic episodes in susceptible people. The overall prevalence in the general population is unknown and probably low. It is seen more frequently in asthmatic or atopic nonasthmatic people.

➤*Photosensitivity: Solage* should not be administered if the patient is also taking drugs known to be photosensitizers (eg, thiazides, tetracyclines, fluoroquinolones, phenothiazines, sulfonamides) because of the possibility of augmented phototoxicity. Because of heightened burning susceptibility, exposure to sunlight (including sunlamps) to treated areas should be avoided or minimized. Patients must be advised to use protective clothing and comply with a comprehensive sun avoidance program. Patients with sunburn should be advised not to use *Solage* until fully recovered. Patients who may have considerable sun exposure because of their occupation and those patients with inherent sensitivity to sunlight should exercise particular caution.

PIGMENT AGENT COMBINATIONS — TOPICAL

➤*Pregnancy:* Category C (*Tri-Luma*), Category X (*Solage*).

Tri-Luma – *Tri-Luma* contains the teratogen tretinoin, which may cause embryofetal death, altered fetal growth, congenital malformations, and potential neurologic deficits. There are no adequate and well-controlled studies in pregnant women. *Tri-Luma* should be used during pregnancy only if the potential benefit justifies the potential risk to the fetus.

Solage – The combination of mequinol and tretinoin may cause fetal harm when administered to a pregnant woman. Due to the known effects of these active ingredients, *Solage* should not be used in women of childbearing potential. No adequate or well-controlled trials have been conducted with *Solage* in pregnant women.

➤*Lactation:* Corticosteroids (contained in *Tri-Luma*), when systemically administered, appear in human milk. It is not known if the other ingredients in *Tri-Luma* or *Solage* are excreted in human milk. Exercise caution when administering to a nursing woman.

➤*Children:* Safety and efficacy in pediatric patients have not been established. *Solage* should not be used on children.

Drug Interactions

➤*Topical preparations:* Concomitant topical products with a strong skin drying effect, products with high concentrations of alcohol, astringents, spices or lime, medicated soaps or shampoos, permanent wave solutions, electrolysis, hair depilatories or waxes, or other preparations that might dry or irritate the skin should be used with caution in patients being treated with *Solage* because they may increase irritation.

➤*Photosensitizers:* Avoid drugs known to be photosensitizers (eg, thiazides, tetracyclines, fluoroquinolones, phenothiazines, sulfonamides) because of the possibility of augmented phototoxicity.

Adverse Reactions

➤*Tri-Luma*: The most frequently reported events were erythema, desquamation, burning, dryness, and pruritus at the site of application. The majority of these events were mild to moderate in severity.

***Tri-Luma* Adverse Reactions (≥ 1%)**

Adverse reaction	Incidence (n = 161)
Erythema	41%
Desquamation	38%
Burning	18%
Dryness	14%
Pruritus	11%
Acne	5%
Paresthesia	3%
Telangiectasia	3%
Hyperesthesia	2%
Pigmentary changes	2%
Irritation	2%
Papules	1%
Acne-like rash	1%
Rosacea	1%
Dry mouth	1%
Rash	1%
Vesicles	1%

The following local adverse reactions have been reported infrequently with topical corticosteroids. They may occur more frequently with the use of occlusive dressings, especially with higher potency corticosteroids. These reactions are listed in an approximate decreasing order of occurrence: Burning, itching, irritation, dryness, folliculitis, acneiform eruptions, hypopigmentation, perioral dermatitis, allergic contact dermatitis, secondary infection, skin atrophy, striae, miliaria.

Tri-Luma contains hydroquinone, which may produce exogenous ochronosis, a gradual blue-black darkening of the skin, whose occurrence should prompt discontinuation of therapy.

Cutaneous hypersensitivity to the active ingredients of *Tri-Luma* has been reported in the literature. In a patch test study to determine sensitization potential in 221 healthy volunteers, 3 volunteers developed sensitivity reactions to *Tri-Luma* or its components.

➤*Solage*: The most frequent adverse reactions were erythema (49%); burning, stinging, or tingling (26%); desquamation (14%); pruritus (12%); skin irritation (5%).

Some patients experienced temporary hypopigmentation of treated lesions (5%) or of the skin surrounding treated lesions (7%); 89% had resolution of hypopigmentation upon discontinuation of treatment to the lesion, and/or re-instruction on proper application to the lesion only. Another 8% of patients with hypopigmentation events had resolution within 120 days after the end of treatment, and 2.8% had persistence of hypopigmentation beyond 120 days. Approximately 6% of patients discontinued study participation with *Solage* because of adverse reactions. These discontinuations were due primarily to skin redness (erythema) or related cutaneous adverse reactions.

***Solage* Adverse Events (> 1%)**

Adverse event	Incidence
Erythema	44.6%
Burning/Stinging/Tingling	21.9%
Desquamation	12.6%
Pruritus	11%
Skin irritation	7.3%
Halo hypopigmentation	6.2%
Hypopigmentation	4.1%
Dry skin	3.1%
Rash	2.5%
Crusting	2.4%
Rash vesicular bullae	2.1%
Dermatitis	2%

Overdosage

If applied excessively, no more rapid or better results will be obtained and marked redness, peeling, discomfort, or hypopigmentation may occur. Oral ingestion of *Solage* may lead to the same adverse effects as those associated with excessive oral intake of vitamin A (hypervitaminosis A). If oral ingestion occurs, the patient should be monitored, and appropriate supportive measures administered as necessary. The maximal no-effect level for oral administration of *Solage* in rats was 5 mL/kg (30 mg/m^2). Clinical signs observed were attributed to the high alcohol content (77%) of the drug formulation.

Patient Information

Solage should not be used in women of childbearing potential or in pregnant women.

Exposure to sunlight, sunlamp, or UV light should be avoided. Patients who are consistently exposed to sunlight or skin irritants either through their work environment or habits should exercise particular caution. Sunscreen and protective covering (such as the use of a hat) over the treated areas should be used.

Sunscreen use is an essential aspect of melasma therapy, as even minimal sunlight sustains melanocytic activity.

Weather extremes such as heat or cold may be irritating to patients. Because of the drying effect of *Tri-Luma*, a moisturizer may be applied to the face in the morning after washing.

Application should be kept away from the eyes, nose, or angles of the mouth because the mucosa is much more sensitive than the skin to the irritant effect. If local irritation persists or becomes severe, application of the medication should be discontinued and the health care provider consulted. Allergic contact dermatitis, blistering, crusting, and severe burning or swelling of the skin, and irritation of the mucous membranes of the eyes, nose, and mouth require medical attention. If the medication is applied excessively, marked redness, peeling, or discomfort may occur.

POISON IVY TREATMENT PRODUCTS

otc	**Maximum Strength Ivarest** (Blistex)	**Cream; topical:** 14% calamine and 2% diphenhydramine HCl[a]	Lanolin oil, petrolatum, propylene glycol. In 56 g.
otc	**Zanfel** (Zanfel Labs)	**Cream; topical:** Polyethylene granules, nonoxynol-9, disodium EDTA, triethanolamine	In 30 g.
otc	**Aveeno Anti-Itch** (Johnson & Johnson)	**Cream; topical:** 3% calamine and 1% pramoxine HCl	Camphor, cetyl alcohol, petrolatum. In 28 g.
otc	**Calamine** (Various, eg, Goldline, Major, Moore)	**Lotion; topical:** 6.97% calamine, 6.97% zinc oxide	Glycerin. In 118, 240, and 480 mL.
otc	**Phenolated Calamine** (Humco)	**Lotion; topical:** Calamine, zinc oxide	Glycerin, 1% liquefied phenol. In 177 mL.
otc	**Caladryl** (Pfizer)	**Lotion; topical:** 8% calamine, 1% pramoxine HCl	Alcohol, camphor, diazolidinyl urea, parabens. In 177 mL.
otc	**Ivy Super Dry** (Ivy Corp)	**Liquid; topical:** 2% zinc acetate, 10% benzyl alcohol, 35% isopropanol, menthol, camphor	Glycerin, parabens. In 177 mL.

POISON IVY TREATMENT PRODUCTS

otc	**Ivy-Dry** (Ivy Corp)	**Lotion; topical:** 2% zinc acetate, 12.5% isopropanol	Glycerin, methylparaben. In 118 mL.
otc	**Caladryl Clear** (Pfizer)	**Lotion; topical:** 1% pramoxine HCl, 0.1% zinc acetate	Alcohol, camphor, diazolidinyl urea, parabens. In 177 mL.
otc	**Itch Relief Gel Spritz** (Band-Aid)	**Spray; topical:** 0.5% camphor	Benzyl alcohol, glycerin, SD alcohol 40 B (43%). In 56 g.
otc	**Ivy Soothe** (Enviroderm)	**Cream; topical:** 1% hydrocortisone	Parabens, cetyl alcohol, glycerin, white petrolatum. In 28 g.
otc	**Zanfel** (Zanfel Labs)	**Wash; topical:** Polyethylene granules, sodium lauroyl sarcosinate, nonoxynol-9, EDTA, triethanolamine	In 30 mL.

[a] Do not use with other products that contain diphenhydramine.

POISON IVY TREATMENT PRODUCTS — TOPICAL

For other products used for relief of symptoms associated with contact dermatoses, see also: Antihistamine-Containing Preparations, Topical; Local Anesthetics, Topical; Corticosteroids, Topical.

Indications

➤*Ivy, oak, sumac poisoning:* For the relief of itching, pain, and discomfort of ivy, oak, sumac poisoning. Some products are also recommended for insect bites and other minor skin irritations.

Administration and Dosage

➤*General dosing considerations:* Please refer to individual product labeling for specific information.

➤*Adults:*

Ivy, oak, sumac poisoning – Apply to affected area 3 to 4 times daily as needed.

➤*Children:* *Ivy Super Dry* is not recommended for use in children younger than 6 years of age.

2 years of age and older –

Ivy, oak, sumac poisoning: Apply to affected area 3 to 4 times daily as needed.

➤*Administration:* Shake calamine lotions well before using.

Active Ingredients

The principal active components of these products include:

➤*Antimicrobial:* Benzyl alcohol.

➤*Antiseptic:* Phenol, isopropyl alcohol, benzalkonium chloride, camphor, menthol, zinc oxide.

➤*Protectants/Astringents:* Calamine, zinc oxide.

➤*Local anesthetics/Analgesics:* Benzocaine, camphor, pramoxine, menthol, phenylcarbinol (benzyl alcohol), methyl salicylate.

➤*Antipruritics:* Benzyl alcohol, camphor.

➤*Antihistamines:* Diphenhydramine.

Warnings/Precautions

➤*For external use only:* Do not use in the eyes. If the condition for which these preparations are used persists or recurs, or if rash, irritation or sensitivity develops, discontinue use and consult physician.

➤*Irritation:* Do not use on blistered or broken skin.

➤*Application considerations:* Do not use on large areas of the body.

➤*Children:* Most of these products are not recommended for use on children younger than 2 years of age.

Ivy Super Dry is not recommended for use in children younger than 6 years of age.

➤*Sulfite sensitivity:* Some of these products contain sulfites that may cause allergic-type reactions, including anaphylactic symptoms and life-threatening/less severe asthmatic episodes in susceptible persons. The overall prevalence in the general population is unknown and probably low. It is seen more frequently in asthmatic or atopic nonasthmatic persons.

➤*Pregnancy: Category: Undetermined.* Consult a health care provider before using in pregnant women.

➤*Lactation:* Consult a health care provider before using in breast-feeding women.

POISON IVY PREVENTATIVES

otc	**Tecnu Outdoor Skin Cleanser** (Tec Labs)	**Lotion:** Deodorized mineral spirits, propylene glycol, octylphenoxypolyethoxyethanol, mixed fatty acid soap	In 118 and 355 mL.
otc	**Ivy Stat** (Tec Labs)	**Gel:** 1% hydrocortisone	Propylene glycol, menthol, SD alcohol 40-B. In 89 mL.
otc	**Ivy Block** (EnviroDerm)	**Lotion:** 5% bentoquatam	Benzyl alcohol, methylparaben, SDA 40 denatured alcohol. In 118 mL.
otc	**Ivy Cleanse** (EnviroDerm)	**Wipes:** Isopropyl and cetyl alcohol	In packet of 12 individually wrapped towelettes.

POISON IVY PREVENTATIVES — TOPICAL

Indications

➤*Poison ivy, oak, and sumac:* For the removal of the toxic oils that cause rash and itching of poison ivy, oak, and sumac from affected skin; and to stop the irritant from spreading.

Administration and Dosage

➤*Adults:*

Poison ivy, oak, and sumac – Please refer to individual product labeling for more specific information.

Ivy Block: Shake well before use. Apply 15 minutes before risk of exposure to poison plants. Avoid contact with poison ivy, oak, and sumac. Apply every 4 hours for continued protection or sooner if needed. Remove with soap and water after risk of exposure.

Ivy Cleanse: Immediately wipe exposed skin areas with towelette; discard. Avoid contaminating cleansed areas. Clean hands with a fresh towelette.

Ivy Stat:

• *Step 1* – Cleanse affected skin with exfoliate. Rub gently for 15 to 30 seconds. Rinse off with running water and towel dry gently. Repeat as needed and before bedtime.

• *Step 2* – Apply hydrocortisone 1% gel and rub thoroughly into skin 3 to 4 times per day as needed. If itching recurs, repeat steps 1 and 2.

Tecnu: Use within the first few hours after exposure or as soon as the rash appears. Use before smoking, going to the bathroom, and at day's end to minimize spreading oils.

• *Before rash has started* – Apply to exposed, dry skin within 2 to 8 hours after exposure to poison plant. Rub vigorously for 2 minutes to remove oils. If the patient is hypersensitive to poison plants, instruct him or her wash the entire body. Rinse skin clean with cool running water or wipe off with a cloth; repeat.

• *As soon as rash appears* – Rub on affected skin and surrounding areas or to entire body for 2 minutes for best results. Avoid breaking the skin. Rinse off with cool running water to remove cleanser and oils. If itching persists, reapply and rinse in a very warm shower (not a bath). Towel dry gently. Repeat as needed and before bedtime.

• *To clean clothing and equipment* – Saturate contaminated, dry clothing. Let soak for several minutes. Launder clothing by itself with detergent and hot water. Wipe off equipment and tools with a clean cloth saturated with the cleanser and then wipe off or rinse with running water. Clean hands with cleanser after handling contaminated items.

➤*Children:*

Poison ivy, oak, and sumac –

Ivy Block:

• *6 years of age and older* – See Adults for dosing.

Ivy Cleanse: See Adults for dosing.

Ivy Stat:

• *2 years of age and older* – See Adults for dosing.

Tecnu: See Adults for dosing.

➤*Administration:* Do not apply to deep puncture wounds, burns, or oozing areas of skin. May irritate sensitive skin.

For external use only. Do not use in eyes or near other mucous membranes.

Warnings/Precautions

➤*Irritation:* Do not apply to deep puncture wounds, burns, or oozing areas of skin. May irritate sensitive skin.

POISON IVY PREVENTATIVES — TOPICAL

➤*For external use only:* Do not use in eyes or near other mucous membranes.

➤*Hydrocortisone:* Do not use within 3 days of using hydrocortisone ointments on affected areas.

➤*Colorfastness:* May cause colorfastness when used on clothing. Check for colorfastness of fabric first by testing a corner of the fabric.

➤*Pregnancy: Category: Undetermined.* Consult a health care provider before using in pregnant women.

➤*Lactation:* Consult a health care provider before using in breast-feeding women.

Adverse Reactions

➤*Dermatologic:* Rash; may irritate sensitive skin.

Patient Information

Advise patient to discontinue use and consult doctor if symptoms persist for more than 7 days or if redness, irritation, increased itching, or infection occurs.

Advise patient that this product is for external use only.

Advise patient to launder clothing and decontaminate exposed pets, tools, etc.

PYRIMIDINE ANTAGONIST, TOPICAL

FLUOROURACIL

Rx	**Carac** (Dermik)	**Cream; topical:** 0.5%	Glycerin, parabens. In 30 g.
Rx	**Fluoroplex** (Allergan)	**Cream; topical:** 1%	Benzyl alcohol, emulsifying wax, mineral oil. In 30 g.
Rx	**Fluorouracil** (Oceanside Pharmaceuticals)	**Cream; topical:** 5%	Parabens, white petrolatum, stearyl alcohol. In 40 g.
Rx	**Efudex** (Valeant Pharmaceuticals)		Parabens, white petrolatum, stearyl alcohol. In 40 g.
Rx	**Fluorouracil** (Taro)	**Solution; topical:** 2%	In 10 mL dropper bottle.
Rx	**Fluorouracil** (Taro)	**Solution; topical:** 5%	In 10 mL dropper bottle.

FLUOROURACIL — TOPICAL

Indications

➤*Actinic or solar keratoses:* For the topical treatment of multiple actinic or solar keratoses.

➤*Superficial basal cell carcinomas (5% strength):* For the treatment of superficial basal cell carcinomas when conventional methods are impractical, such as with multiple lesion sites.

➤*Off-label uses:* Condylomata acuminata.

Administration and Dosage

➤*Adults:*

Actinic or solar keratoses –

0.5% cream:

• *Usual dosage* – Apply once a day to the skin where actinic keratosis lesions appear, using enough to cover the entire area with a thin film.

• *Duration of therapy* – Fluorouracil should be applied for up to 4 weeks as tolerated. Continued treatment for up to 4 weeks results in greater lesion reduction. Local irritation is not markedly increased by extending treatment from 2 to 4 weeks and is generally resolved within 2 weeks of cessation of treatment.

1% cream:

• *Usual dosage* – Apply sufficient medication to cover the entire face or other affected areas twice daily.

• *Duration of therapy* – A treatment period of 2 to 6 weeks is usually required. Increased frequency of application and a longer period of administration with fluorouracil cream may be required on areas other than the head and neck.

• *Discontinuation of therapy* – When the inflammatory reaction reaches the erosion, ulceration, and necrosis stages, the use of the drug should be terminated. Responses may sometimes occur in areas that appear clinically normal. These may be sites of subclinical actinic (solar) keratosis that the medication is affecting.

5% cream and 2% and 5% solutions:

• *Usual dosage* – Apply cream or solution twice daily in an amount sufficient to cover the lesions.

When fluorouracil is applied to a lesion, a response occurs with the following sequence: erythema, usually followed by vesiculation, desquamation, erosion, and reepithelialization.

• *Duration of therapy* – The usual duration of therapy is from 2 to 4 weeks.

• *Discontinuation of therapy* – Medication should be continued until the inflammatory response reaches the erosion stage, at which time use of the drug should be terminated.

Complete healing of the lesions may not be evident for 1 to 2 months following cessation of fluorouracil therapy.

Superficial basal cell carcinomas –

5% strengths:

• *Usual dosage* – Apply cream or solution twice daily in an amount sufficient to cover the lesions.

• *Duration of therapy* – Treatment should be continued for at least 3 to 6 weeks. Therapy may be required for as long as 10 to 12 weeks before the lesions are obliterated. As in any neoplastic condition, the patient should be followed for a reasonable period of time to determine if a cure has been obtained.

➤*Administration:*

0.5% cream – Fluorouracil should not be applied near the eyes, mouth, or nostrils. Fluorouracil should be applied 10 minutes after thoroughly washing, rinsing, and drying the entire area. Fluorouracil cream may be applied using the fingertips. Immediately after application, the hands should be thoroughly washed.

1% cream – Patients should be instructed to apply sufficient medication to cover the entire face or other affected areas twice daily with nonmetallic applicator or fingertips and to wash their hands afterwards.

5% cream and 2% and 5% solutions – Fluorouracil preferably should be applied with a nonmetal applicator or suitable glove. If fluorouracil is applied with the fingers, the hands should be washed immediately afterward.

➤*Storage/Stability:*

0.5% cream – Store at 20° to 25°C (68° to 77°F).

1% cream – Store at 15° to 30°C (59° to 86°F) in tight containers. Avoid freezing.

5% cream and 2% and 5% solution – Store at 25°C (77°F); excursions are permitted to between 15° and 30°C (59° and 86°F).

Actions

➤*Pharmacology:* There is evidence that the metabolism of the fluorinated pyrimidine fluorouracil, an antineoplastic antimetabolite in the anabolic pathway, blocks the methylation reaction of deoxyuridylic acid to thymidylic acid. In this manner, fluorouracil interferes with the synthesis of DNA and, to a lesser extent, inhibits the formation of RNA. Because DNA and RNA are essential for cell division and growth, the effect of fluorouracil may be to create a thymine deficiency that provokes unbalanced growth and death of the cell. The effects of DNA and RNA deprivation are most marked on those cells that grow more rapidly and take up fluorouracil at a more rapid rate.

➤*Pharmacokinetics:*

Absorption – Systemic absorption studies of topically applied fluorouracil have been performed on patients with actinic keratoses using tracer amounts of ^{14}C-labeled fluorouracil added to a 5% preparation. All patients had been receiving nonlabeled fluorouracil until the peak of the inflammatory reaction occurred (2 to 3 weeks), ensuring that the time of maximum absorption was used for measurement. One gram of labeled preparation was applied to the entire face and neck and left in place for 12 hours. Urine samples were then collected. At the end of 3 days, the total recovery ranged between 0.48% and 0.94%, with an average of 0.76%, indicating that approximately 5.98% of the topical dose was absorbed systemically. If applied twice daily, this would indicate systemic absorption of topical fluorouracil to be in the range of 5 to 6 mg per daily dose of 100 mg. In an additional study, negligible amounts of labeled material were found in plasma, urine, and expired carbon dioxide after 3 days of treatment with topically applied ^{14}C-labeled fluorouracil.

Fluorouracil Plasma Pharmacokinetic Summary[a]

Pharmacokinetic parameter	*Carac* cream (n = 1)	*Efudex* (mean ± SD) (n = 6)
C_{max}	0.77 ng/mL	11.49 ± 8.24 ng/mL
T_{max}	1 h	1.03 ± 0.028 h
AUC (0-24)	2.8 ng•h/mL	22.39 ± 7.89 ng•h/mL

[a] SD = standard deviation; C_{max} = maximal drug concentration; T_{max} = time of maximal concentration; AUC (0-24) = area under the curve.

Excretion –

Fluorouracil Urine Pharmacokinetic Summary

Pharmacokinetic parameter	*Carac* (mean ± SD) (n = 10)	*Efudex* (mean ± SD) (n = 10)
Cumulative urinary excretion (min-max)	2.74 ± 5.22 mcg (range, 0 to 15.02)	119.83 ± 94.8 mcg (range, 0 to 329.87)

FLUOROURACIL — TOPICAL

Fluorouracil Urine Pharmacokinetic Summary		
Pharmacokinetic parameter	*Carac* (mean ± SD) (n = 10)	*Efudex* (mean ± SD) (n = 10)
Max excretion rate (min-max)	0.19 ± 0.52 mcg/h (range, 0 to 1.67)	40.27 ± 47.14 mcg/h (range, 0 to 164.5)

Contraindications

Women who are or may become pregnant; known hypersensitivity to any of fluorouracil's components.

Do not use fluorouracil in patients with dihydropyrimidine dehydrogenase (DPD) enzyme deficiency. A large percentage of fluorouracil is catabolized by the enzyme DPD. DPD enzyme deficiency can result in shunting of fluorouracil to the anabolic pathway, leading to cytotoxic activity and potential toxicities.

Warnings/Precautions

➤*DPD enzyme deficiency:* See Contraindications for more information.

Rarely, life-threatening toxicities such as diarrhea, neutropenia, neurotoxicity, and stomatitis have been reported with intravenous (IV) administration of fluorouracil in patients with DPD enzyme deficiency.

A case of life-threatening systemic toxicity has been reported with the topical use of fluorouracil 5% in a patient with DPD enzyme deficiency. Symptoms included bloody diarrhea, chills, fever, severe abdominal pain, and vomiting. Physical examination revealed erythematous skin rash; inflammation of the esophagus, stomach, and small bowel; neutropenia; stomatitis; and thrombocytopenia. Although this case was observed with fluorouracil 5% cream, it is unknown whether patients with profound DPD enzyme deficiency would develop systemic toxicity with lower concentrations of topically applied fluorouracil.

➤*Mucous membranes:* Avoid applications to mucous membranes because of the possibility of local inflammation and ulceration. Additionally, cases of miscarriage and a birth defect (ventricular septal defect) have been reported when fluorouracil was applied to mucus membrane areas during pregnancy.

➤*Occlusive dressing:* Occlusion of the skin with resultant hydration has been shown to increase percutaneous penetration of several topical preparations. If an occlusive dressing is used, there may be an increase in the incidence of inflammatory reactions in the adjacent healthy skin. A porous gauze dressing may be applied for cosmetic reasons without increase in reaction.

➤*Ulcerated/Inflamed skin:* There is a possibility of increased absorption through ulcerated or inflamed skin.

➤*Hypersensitivity reactions:* The potential for a delayed hypersensitivity reaction to fluorouracil exists. Patch testing to prove hypersensitivity may be inconclusive.

➤*Photosensitivity:* Advise the patient to avoid prolonged exposure to sunlight or other forms of ultraviolet irradiation during treatment with fluorouracil because the intensity of the reaction may be increased.

➤*Pregnancy: Category X* per manufacturer's prescribing information. *Category X* per Briggs' *Drugs in Pregnancy and Lactation*.

Fluorouracil may cause fetal harm when administered to a pregnant woman.

Teratogenic – There are no adequate and well-controlled studies in pregnant women with either topical or parenteral forms of fluorouracil. One birth defect (cleft lip and palate) has been reported in the newborn of a patient using fluorouracil as recommended. One birth defect (ventricular septal defect) and cases of miscarriage have been reported when fluorouracil was applied to mucous membrane areas. Multiple birth defects have been reported in the fetus of a patient treated with IV fluorouracil.

Fluorouracil administered parenterally has been shown to be teratogenic in hamsters, mice, and rats, and when given at doses equivalent to the usual human IV dose; however, the amount of fluorouracil absorbed systemically after topical administration of actinic keratoses is minimal. Fluorouracil exhibited maximum teratogenicity when given to mice as single intraperitoneal injections of 10 to 40 mg/kg on day 10 or 12 of gestation. Similarly, intraperitoneal doses of 12 to 37 mg/kg given to rats between days 9 and 12 of gestation, and intramuscular doses of 3 to 9 mg/kg given to hamsters between days 8 and 11 of gestation were teratogenic and/or embryotoxic (ie, resulted in increased resorptions or embryolethality). In monkeys, divided doses of 40 mg/kg given between days 20 and 24 of gestation were not teratogenic. Doses of more than 40 mg/kg resulted in abortion. If this drug is used during pregnancy or if the patient becomes pregnant while taking this drug, apprise the patient of the potential hazard to the fetus.

➤*Lactation:* It is not known whether fluorouracil is excreted in human milk. Because there is some systemic absorption of fluorouracil after topical administration, because many drugs are excreted in human milk, and because of the potential for serious adverse reactions in breast-feeding infants from fluorouracil, decide whether to discontinue breast-feeding or the drug, taking into account the importance of the drug to the mother.

➤*Children:* Safety and effectiveness have not been established in patients younger than 18 years of age.

➤*Monitoring:* Solar keratoses that do not respond should be biopsied to confirm the diagnosis. Perform follow-up biopsies as indicated in the management of superficial basal cell carcinoma.

Drug Interactions

None known.

Adverse Reactions

➤*0.5% cream:* The following were adverse reactions considered to be drug related and occurring with a frequency of 1% or more with fluorouracil: application-site reaction (94.6%) and eye irritation (5.4%).

Fluorouracil Facial Irritation Signs and Symptoms (> 1%)					
Adverse reaction	Active 1 week (n = 85)	Active 2 week (n = 87)	Active 4 week (n = 85)	All active treatments (n = 257)	Vehicle treatments (n = 127)
Burning	60%	80.5%	83.5%	74.7%	22%
Dryness	69.4%	87.4%	92.9%	83.3%	47.2%
Edema	14.1%	32.2%	60%	35.4%	4.7%
Erosion	24.7%	43.7%	63.5%	44%	13.4%
Erythema	89.4%	94.3%	96.5%	93.4%	59.8%
Pain	30.6%	39.1%	61.2%	43.6%	5.5%

During clinical trials, irritation generally began on day 4 and persisted for the remainder of treatment. Severity of facial irritation at the last treatment visit was slightly below baseline for the vehicle group, mild to moderate for the 1-week active treatment group, and moderate for the 2- and 4-week active treatment groups. Mean severity declined rapidly for each active group after completion of treatment and was below baseline for each group at the week-2 posttreatment follow-up visit.

Thirty-one patients (12% of those treated with fluorouracil in the phase 3 clinical studies) discontinued study treatment early because of facial irritation. Except for 3 patients, discontinuation of treatment occurred on or after day 11 of treatment.

Eye irritation adverse reactions, described as mild to moderate in intensity, were characterized as burning, watering, sensitivity, stinging, and itching. These adverse reactions occurred across all treatment arms in 1 of the 2 phase 3 studies.

Fluorouracil Adverse Reactions (≥ 1%)					
Adverse reaction	Active 1 week (n = 85)	Active 2 week (n = 87)	Active 4 week (n = 85)	All active treatments (n = 257)	Vehicle treatments (n = 127)
Dermatologic	91.8%	95.4%	96.5%	94.6%	66.9%
Application-site reaction	91.8%	95.4%	96.5%	94.6%	65.4%
Skin irritation	1.2%	0%	2.4%	1.2%	0%
Musculoskeletal	1.2%	1.1%	1.2%	1.2%	3.9%
Muscle soreness	0%	0%	0%	0%	1.6%
Ophthalmic	7.1%	4.6%	7.1%	6.2%	4.7%
Eye irritation	5.9%	3.4%	7.1%	5.4%	2.4%
Respiratory	5.9%	0%	1.2%	2.3%	4.7%
Sinusitis	4.7%	0%	0%	1.6%	1.6%
Miscellaneous	8.2%	6.9%	14.1%	9.7%	11.8%
Allergy	0%	2.3%	1.2%	1.2%	1.6%
Common cold	4.7%	0%	2.4%	2.3%	2.4%
Headache	3.5%	2.3%	3.5%	3.1%	2.4%
Upper respiratory tract infection	0%	0%	0%	0%	1.6%

➤*Serious adverse reactions:* In the phase 3 studies, no serious adverse reaction was considered related to study drug. A total of 5 patients, 3 in the active treatment groups and 2 in the vehicle group, experienced at least 1 serious adverse reaction. Three patients died as a result of adverse reaction(s) considered unrelated to study drug (ie, cardiac failure, myocardial infarction, stomach cancer).

➤*1% cream:* Allergic contact dermatitis, burning, inflammation, irritation, pain, pruritus, and telangiectasia have been reported. Occasionally, hyperpigmentation and scarring have also been reported.

➤*5% cream and 2% and 5% solutions:*

Most frequent adverse reactions –

Dermatologic: Allergic contact dermatitis, burning, crusting, erosions, erythema, hyperpigmentation, irritation, pain, photosensitivity, pruritus, rash, scarring, soreness, and ulceration. Ulcerations, other local reactions, cases of miscarriage, and a birth defect (ventricular septal defect) have been reported when fluorouracil was applied to mucous membrane areas.

Hematologic/Lymphatic: Leukocytosis.

Other adverse reactions –

CNS: Emotional upset, insomnia, irritability.

Dermatologic: Alopecia, blistering, bullous pemphigoid, discomfort, ichthyosis, scaling, skin rash, suppuration, swelling, telangiectasia, tenderness, urticaria.

GI: Medicinal taste, stomatitis.

Hematologic: Eosinophilia, thrombocytopenia, toxic granulation.

Special senses: Conjunctival reaction, corneal reaction, lacrimation, nasal irritation.

Miscellaneous: Herpes simplex.

FLUOROURACIL — TOPICAL

Overdosage

➤*Symptoms:* There have been no reports of overdosage with fluorouracil. Ordinarily, topical overdosage will not cause acute problems.

➤*Treatment:* If fluorouracil is accidentally ingested, induce gastric lavage. Administer symptomatic and supportive care as needed. If contact is made with the eye, flush with copious amounts of water or isotonic sodium chloride solution.

Patient Information

Advise patient to cleanse the affected area and wait 10 minutes before applying fluorouracil.

If the patient develops abdominal pain, bloody diarrhea, chills, fever, or vomiting while on fluorouracil therapy, advise the patient to stop the medication and contact the health care provider.

Forewarn patients that the reaction in the treated areas may be unsightly during therapy and, usually, for several weeks following cessation of therapy. Instruct patients to avoid exposure to ultraviolet rays during and immediately following treatment with fluorouracil because the intensity of the reaction may be increased. If fluorouracil is applied with the fingers, wash the hands immediately afterward. Instruct patients to avoid applying fluorouracil on the eyelids or directly into the eyes, nose, or mouth because irritation may occur.

PYRITHIONE ZINC

PYRITHIONE ZINC

otc	**Noble Formula** (Ontos)	**Cream; topical:** 0.25%	Alcohol, almond oil, rose hip oil, vitamin E. In 120 mL.
otc	**Dermazinc** (Dermalogix)	**Shampoo; topical:** 0.25%	Parabens. In 240 mL.
otc	**Zincon** (Medtech)	**Shampoo; topical:** 1%	Propylene glycol. In 118 and 240 mL.
otc	**Head & Shoulders** (Procter & Gamble)		Cetyl and benzyl alcohol. In "normal to oily" and "normal to dry" formulas. In 200, 400, and 750 mL.
otc	**Head & Shoulders Dry Scalp** (Procter & Gamble)		Cetyl and benzyl alcohol. In regular and conditioning formulas. In 200, 400, 750, and 1000 mL.
otc	**DHS Zinc** (Person & Covey)	**Shampoo; topical:** 2%	In 240 and 360 mL.
otc	**Denorex Everyday Dandruff** (Medtech)		Propylene glycol, menthol. In 118 and 240 mL.
otc	**Noble Formula** (Ontos)	**Spray; topical:** 0.25%	Alcohol. In 120 mL.
otc	**ZNP Bar** (Stiefel)	**Soap; topical:** 2%	Alcohol, castor oil, cetearyl alcohol, glycerin, lactic acid, mineral oil, PEG, titanium dioxide, trisodium EDTA. In 119 g.

[a] Also contains corn starch, glycerin, hydrogenated castor oil, and mineral oil.

PYRITHIONE ZINC — TOPICAL

Indications

➤*Hyperkeratotic skin conditions:* Pyrithione zinc products relieve the symptoms of itching, flaking, and inflammation caused by psoriasis, eczema, dandruff, lichen planus, seborrheic dermatitis, and other hyperkeratotic skin conditions of the face, body, and scalp. It also may help prevent recurrence of symptoms.

Administration and Dosage

➤*Adults:*

Hyperkeratotic skin conditions –

Shampoo: Shake well. Apply shampoo; lather, rinse, and repeat. Use at least twice weekly for best results.

Soap: Use on affected areas in place of regular soap. Work up a rich lather using warm water and massage into affected areas; rinse well, then repeat. Use twice weekly for best results. May be used as a shampoo.

➤*Children:*

Hyperkeratotic skin conditions –

2 years of age and older: See Adults for dosing.

➤*Storage/Stability:* Store at 20° to 25°C (68° to 77°F).

Actions

➤*Pharmacology:* Pyrithione zinc, a cytostatic agent, reduces cell turnover rate. Its action is thought to be due to a nonspecific toxicity for epidermal cells. The compound strongly binds to hair and external skin layers.

Warnings/Precautions

➤*For external use only:* Keep out of eyes; if contact occurs, rinse thoroughly with water.

➤*Pregnancy: Category: Undetermined.* Consult a health care provider before using in pregnant women.

➤*Lactation:* Consult a health care provider before using in breast-feeding women.

➤*Children:* Do not use on children younger than 2 years of age unless directed by a doctor.

Adverse Reactions

Irritation of the skin (rare).

Patient Information

For external use only.

Ask a doctor before use if you have a condition that covers a large area of the body.

When using this product, avoid contact with the eyes. If contact occurs, rinse eyes thoroughly with water.

Stop use and ask a doctor if:
- Condition worsens.
- Condition does not improve after regular use of this product as directed.

Keep out of the reach of children. If swallowed, get medical help or contact a poison control center right away.

RETINOIDS (DERMATOLOGIC)

ADAPALENE

Rx	**Adapalene** (Fougera)	**Cream; topical:** 0.1%	Edetate disodium, glycerin, parabens, PEG-20, phenoxyethanol, squalane, trolamine. In 45 g.
Rx	**Differin** (Galderma)		EDTA, parabens, glycerin. In 45 g.
Rx	**Differin** (Galderma)	**Lotion; topical:** 0.1%	EDTA, parabens, phenoxyethanol, propylene glycol, stearyl alcohol, triglycerides. In 56.6 g.
Rx	**Adapalene** (Teva)	**Gel; topical:** 0.1%	Disodium edetate, methylparaben, propylene glycol. In 45 g.
Rx	**Differin** (Galderma)		EDTA, methylparaben. In 45 g.
Rx	**Differin** (Galderma)	**Gel; topical:** 0.3%	EDTA, methylparaben. In 45 g.

ADAPALENE — TOPICAL

Indications

➤*Acne vulgaris:* For the topical treatment of acne vulgaris.

Administration and Dosage

➤*General dosing considerations:* During the early weeks of therapy, an apparent exacerbation of acne may occur. This is due to the action of the medication on previously unseen lesions and should not be considered a reason to discontinue therapy.

ADAPALENE — TOPICAL

Therapeutic results should be noticed after 8 to 12 weeks of treatment.

➤*Adults:*

Acne vulgaris – Apply once a day to affected areas after washing in the evening and before retiring. A mild, transitory sensation of warmth or slight stinging may occur shortly after application.

Differin Lotion: Apply a thin film of lotion to the entire face and other affected areas of the skin once daily, after washing gently with a mild soapless cleanser. Dispense a nickel size amount of lotion (3 to 4 actuations of the pump) to cover the entire face.

➤*Children:*

Acne vulgaris –

12 years of age or older: See Adults for dosing.

➤*Administration:* A thin film should be applied; avoid eyes, lips, and mucous membranes.

➤*Storage/Stability:* Store between 20° and 25°C (68° and 77°F). Protect from freezing.

Actions

➤*Pharmacology:* Adapalene is a chemically stable, retinoid-like compound.

Biochemical and pharmacological profile studies have demonstrated that adapalene is a modulator of cellular differentiation, keratinization, and inflammatory processes all of which represent important features in the pathology of acne vulgaris.

Mechanistically, adapalene binds to specific retinoic acid nuclear receptors but does not bind to the cytosolic receptor protein. Although the exact mode of action of adapalene is unknown, it is suggested that topical adapalene may normalize the differentiation of follicular epithelial cells resulting in decreased microcomedone formation.

➤*Pharmacokinetics:*

Absorption/Distribution – Absorption of adapalene through human skin is low.

Only trace amounts (less than 0.25 ng/mL) of parent substance have been found in the plasma of acne patients following chronic topical application of adapalene in controlled clinical trials.

Cream: In a pharmacokinetic study with 6 acne patients treated once daily for 5 days with 2 g of adapalene cream applied to 1000 cm^2 of acne-involved skin, there were no quantifiable amounts (limit of quantification = 1.35 ng/mL) of adapalene in the plasma samples from any patient.

Excretion – Excretion appears to be primarily by the biliary route.

Contraindications

Hypersensitivity to adapalene or any of the components in the vehicle.

Warnings/Precautions

➤*For external use only:* Avoid contact with the eyes, lips, angles of the nose, and mucous membranes. The product should not be applied to cuts, abrasions, eczematous skin, or sunburned skin.

As with other retinoids, use of "waxing" as a depilatory method should be avoided on skin treated with adapalene.

➤*Local adverse reactions:* Certain cutaneous signs and symptoms such as erythema, dryness, scaling, burning or pruritus may be experienced during treatment. These are most likely to occur during the first 2 to 4 weeks; with the cream they are mostly mild to moderate in intensity and will usually lessen with continued use of the medication. Depending upon the severity of adverse events, patients should be instructed to reduce the frequency of application or discontinue use.

➤*Hypersensitivity reactions:* Use of adapalene should be discontinued if hypersensitivity to any of the ingredients is noted.

➤*Photosensitivity:* Patients with sunburn should be advised not to use the product until fully recovered. If a reaction suggesting sensitivity or chemical irritation occurs, use of the medication should be discontinued. Exposure to sunlight, including sunlamps, should be minimized during the use of adapalene. Patients who normally experience high levels of sun exposure, and those with inherent sensitivity to sun, should be warned to exercise caution. Use of sunscreen products and protective clothing over treated areas is recommended when exposure cannot be avoided. Weather extremes, such as wind or cold, also may be irritating to patients under treatment with adapalene.

➤*Pregnancy:* Category C.

Teratogenic – No teratogenic effects were seen in rats at oral doses of adapalene 0.15 to 5 mg/kg/day, up to 120 times the maximal daily human topical dose (for adapalene cream up to 20 times the MRHD based on mg/m^2 comparisons). However, adapalene administered orally at doses of ≥ 25 mg/kg, (100 times the MRHD for rats or 200 times MRHD for rabbits) has been shown to be teratogenic. Cutaneous route teratology studies conducted in rats and rabbits at doses of 0.6, 2, and 6 mg/kg/day, up to 150 times the maximal daily human topical dose; for adapalene cream, 24 times the MRHD for rats, or 48 times the MRHD for rabbits, exhibited no fetotoxicity and only minimal increases in supernumerary ribs in rats. There are no adequate and well-controlled studies in pregnant women. Adapalene should be used during pregnancy only if the potential benefit justifies the potential risk to the fetus.

➤*Lactation:* It is not known whether this drug is excreted in human milk. Because many drugs are excreted in human milk, caution should be exercised when adapalene is administered to a nursing woman.

➤*Children:* Safety and efficacy in pediatric patients below the age of 12 have not been established.

Drug Interactions

As adapalene has the potential to produce local irritation in some patients, concomitant use of other potentially irritating topical products (medicated or abrasive soaps and cleansers, soaps and cosmetics that have a strong drying effect, and products with high concentrations of alcohol, astringents, spices, or lime) should be approached with caution.

Particular caution should be exercised in using preparations containing sulfur, resorcinol, or salicylic acid in combination with adapalene. If these preparations have been used, it is advisable not to start therapy with adapalene until the effects of such preparations in the skin have subsided.

Adverse Reactions

➤*Gel:* Some adverse effects such as erythema, scaling, dryness, pruritus, and burning will occur in 10% to 40% of patients with adapalene gel. Pruritus or burning immediately after application also occurs in ≈ 20% of patients with adapalene gel. The following additional adverse experiences were reported in ≈ 1% or less of patients: Skin irritation, burning/stinging, erythema, sunburn, and acne flares. These are most commonly seen during the first month of therapy and decrease in frequency and severity thereafter. All adverse effects with use of adapalene during clinical trials were reversible upon discontinuation of therapy.

➤*Cream:* In controlled clinical trials, local cutaneous irritation was monitored in 285 acne patients who used adapalene cream once daily for 12 weeks. The frequency and severity of erythema, scaling, dryness, pruritus, and burning were assessed during these studies. The incidence of local cutaneous irritation with adapalene cream from the controlled clinical studies is provided in the following table.

Incidence of Local Cutaneous Irritation With Adapalene Cream From Controlled Clinical Studies (N = 285)

	None	Mild	Moderate	Severe
Erythema	52% (148)	38% (108)	10% (28)	< 1% (1)
Scaling	58% (166)	35% (100)	6% (18)	< 1% (1)
Dryness	48% (136)	42% (121)	9% (26)	< 1 (2)
Pruritus (persistent)	74% (211)	21% (61)	4% (12)	< 1% (1)
Burning/ stinging	71% (202)	24% (69)	4% (12)	< 1% (2)

Other reported local cutaneous adverse events in patients who used adapalene cream once daily included: Sunburn (2%), skin discomfort-burning and stinging (1%), and skin irritation (1%). Events occurring in less than 1% of patients treated with adapalene cream included: Acne flare, dermatitis and contact dermatitis, eyelid edema, conjunctivitis, erythema, pruritus, skin discoloration, rash, and eczema.

Overdosage

Adapalene is intended for cutaneous use only. If the medication is applied excessively, no more rapid or better results will be obtained and marked redness, peeling, or discomfort may occur. The acute oral toxicity of adapalene in mice and rats is greater than 10 mL/kg. Chronic ingestion of the drug may lead to the same side effects as those associated with excessive oral intake of vitamin A.

Patient Information

This medication is to be used only as directed by the physician.

It is for external use only.

Avoid contact with the eyes, lips, angles of the nose, and mucous membranes.

Cleanse area with a mild or soapless cleanser before applying this medication.

Moisturizers may be used if necessary; however, products containing alpha hydroxy or glycolic acids should be avoided.

Exposure of the eye to this medication may result in reactions such as swelling, conjunctivitis, and eye irritation.

This medication should not be applied to cuts, abrasions, eczematous or sunburned skin.

Wax epilation should not be performed on treated skin due to the potential for skin erosions.

During the early weeks of therapy, an apparent exacerbation of acne may occur. This is due to the action of this medication on previously unseen lesions and should not be considered a reason to discontinue therapy. Overall clinical benefit may be noticed after 2 weeks of therapy, but at least 8 weeks are required to obtain consistent beneficial effects.

First Generation Retinoids

TRETINOIN (trans-Retinoic Acid; Vitamin A Acid)

Rx	**Renova** (Ortho Dermatological)	**Cream; topical:** 0.02%	Parabens, benzyl alcohol, cetyl alcohol, stearyl alcohol, EDTA. In 40 g.
Rx	**Tretinoin** (Alpharma, Spear Dermatology)	**Cream; topical:** 0.025%	May contain stearyl alcohol. In 20 and 45 g.
Rx	**Altinac** (Upsher-Smith)		Stearyl alcohol. In 20 and 45 g.
Rx	**Avita** (Bertek)		Stearyl alcohol. In 20 and 45 g.
Rx	**Retin-A** (Ortho)		Hydrophilic vehicle. In 20 and 45 g.
Rx	**Tretin X** (Triax Pharmaceuticals)		Stearyl alcohol. In 35 g.
Rx	**Tretinoin** (Spear Dermatology)	**Cream; topical:** 0.05%	Stearyl alcohol. In 20 and 45 g.
Rx	**Altinac** (Upsher-Smith)		Stearyl alcohol. In 20 and 45 g.
Rx	**Renova** (Ortho Dermatological)		Methylparaben, stearyl alcohol, EDTA. In 20, 40, and 60 g.
Rx	**Retin-A** (Ortho)		Hydrophilic vehicle. In 20 and 45 g.
Rx	**Tretin X** (Triax Pharmaceuticals)		Stearyl alcohol. In 35 g.
Rx	**Tretinoin** (Spear Dermatology)	**Cream; topical:** 0.1%	Stearyl alcohol. In 20 and 45 g.
Rx	**Altinac** (Upsher-Smith)		Stearyl alcohol. In 20 and 45 g.
Rx	**Retin-A** (Ortho)		Stearyl alcohol. In 20 and 45 g.
Rx	**Tretin X** (Triax Pharmaceuticals)		Stearyl alcohol. In 35 g.
Rx	**Tretinoin** (Spear Dermatology)	**Gel; topical:** 0.01%	Alcohol. In 15 and 45 g.
Rx	**Retin-A** (Ortho)		90% alcohol. In 15 and 45 g.
Rx	**Tretin X** (Triax Pharmaceuticals)		90% alcohol. In 35 g.
Rx	**Tretinoin** (Spear Dermatology)	**Gel; topical:** 0.025%	Alcohol. In 15 and 45 g.
Rx	**Avita** (Bertek)		83% ethanol. In 20 and 45 g.
Rx	**Retin-A** (Ortho)		90% alcohol. In 15 and 45 g.
Rx	**Tretin X** (Triax Pharmaceuticals)		90% alcohol. In 35 g.
Rx	**Retin-A Micro** (Ortho)	**Gel; topical:** 0.04%	Glycerin, EDTA, propylene glycol, benzyl alcohol. In 20 and 45 g.
Rx	**Atralin** (Coria Laboratories)	**Gel; topical:** 0.05%	Benzyl alcohol, glycerin, parabens. In 45 g.
Rx	**Retin-A Micro** (Ortho)	**Gel; topical:** 0.1%	Glycerin, EDTA, propylene glycol, benzyl alcohol. In 20 and 45 g.

TRETINOIN — TOPICAL

Indications

➤*Acne (except Renova):* Topical treatment of acne vulgaris.

➤*Renova:*

Dermatologic conditions –

0.02% cream: Adjunctive agent for use in the mitigation (palliation) of fine wrinkles in patients who use comprehensive skin care and sun avoidance programs.

0.05% cream: Adjunctive agent for use in the mitigation (palliation) of fine wrinkles, mottled hyperpigmentation, and tactile roughness of facial skin in patients who do not achieve such palliation using comprehensive skin care and sun avoidance programs alone.

➤*Off-label uses:* Treatment of hyperpigmentation of photoaged skin, postinflammatory, hyperpigmentation, melasma, and facial actinic keratoses.

Administration and Dosage

➤*General dosing considerations:* Closely monitor alterations of vehicle, drug concentration, or dose frequency. During the early weeks of therapy, an apparent exacerbation of inflammatory lesions may occur due to the action of the medication on deep, previously undetected lesions; this is not a reason to discontinue therapy.

Therapeutic results should be seen after 2 to 3 weeks, but may not be optimal until after 6 weeks. Once lesions have responded satisfactorily, maintain therapy with less frequent applications or other dosage forms.

Renova – Mitigation (palliation) of fine facial wrinkling, mottled hyperpigmentation, and tactile roughness may occur gradually over the course of therapy. Up to 6 months of therapy may be required before the effects are seen. Most of the improvement noted with tretinoin is seen during the first 24 weeks of therapy. Thereafter, therapy primarily maintains the improvement noticed during the first 24 weeks.

➤*Adults:*

Acne treatment (except Renova) – Apply once a day before bedtime or in the evening. Cover the entire affected area lightly.

Dermatologic conditions (Renova only*)* – Gently wash face with a mild soap, pat the skin dry, and wait 20 to 30 minutes before applying. Apply a pea-sized amount of cream to cover the entire face. Apply to the face once a day in the evening, using only enough to cover the entire affected area lightly. Take caution to avoid contact with eyes, ears, nostrils, and mouth.

➤*Children:*

Acne treatment (except Renova) –

12 years of age and older (Retin-A Micro): Apply once a day before bedtime or in the evening. Cover the entire affected area lightly.

10 years of age and older (Atralin): Apply once a day before bedtime or in the evening. Cover the entire affected area lightly.

➤*Administration:* For external use only. Keep away from the eyes, mouth, angles of the nose, and mucous membranes.

Patients may use cosmetics, but thoroughly cleanse area to be treated before applying medication.

Liquid – Apply with fingertip, gauze pad, or cotton swab. Do not oversaturate gauze or cotton to the extent that liquid will run into unaffected areas.

Gel – Excessive application results in pilling of the gel, which minimizes the likelihood of overapplication by the patient.

Renova – For best results, do not apply another skin care product or cosmetic or wash face for at least 1 hour after applying tretinoin. Application of tretinoin may cause a transitory feeling of warmth or slight stinging.

➤*Storage / Stability:* Store between 15° to 25°C (59° to 77°F).

Actions

➤*Pharmacology:* Tretinoin is a retinoid metabolite of vitamin A. Although the exact mode of action of tretinoin is unknown, current evidence suggests that topical tretinoin decreases cohesiveness of follicular epithelial cells with decreased microcomedo formation. Additionally, tretinoin stimulates mitotic activity and increases turnover of follicular epithelial cells, causing extrusion of the comedones.

➤*Pharmacokinetics:*

Absorption – The transdermal absorption of tretinoin from various topical formulations ranged from 1% to 31% of applied dose, depending on whether it was applied to healthy or dermatitic skin.

In vitro and in vivo pharmacokinetic studies with tretinoin cream and gel indicated that less than 0.3% of the topically applied dose is bioavailable. Circulating plasma levels of tretinoin are only slightly elevated above those found in healthy normal controls. Estimates of in vivo bioavailability of *Retin-A Micro* following single and multiple daily applications, for a period of 28 days with the 0.1% gel, were approximately 0.82% and 1.41%, respectively. When percutaneous absorption of *Renova* was assessed in healthy male subjects (n = 14) after a single application, as well as after repeated daily applications for 28 days, the absorption of tretinoin was less than 2% and endogenous concentrations of tretinoin and its major metabolites were unaltered.

Contraindications

Hypersensitivity to any component of the product; discontinue if hypersensitivity to any ingredient is noted.

Warnings/Precautions

➤*For external use only:* Keep tretinoin away from the eyes, mouth, angles of the nose, and mucous membranes.

➤*Renova:*

Mitigating effects – Tretinoin has shown no mitigating effects on significant signs of chronic sun exposure (eg, coarse or deep wrinkling, skin yellowing, lentigines, telangiectasia, skin laxity, keratinocytic atypia, melanocytic atypia, dermal elastosis).

Tretinoin 0.02% cream has shown no mitigating effects on tactile roughness or mottled hyperpigmentation.

Tretinoin does not eliminate wrinkles, repair sun damaged skin, reverse photoaging, or restore a more youthful or younger dermal histologic pattern.

TRETINOIN — TOPICAL

Many patients achieve desired palliative effect on fine wrinkling, mottled hyperpigmentation, and tactile roughness of facial skin with the use of comprehensive skin care and sun avoidance programs including sunscreens, protective clothing, and nonprescription emollient creams.

Long-term use – Tretinoin is a dermal irritant, and the results of continued irritation of the skin for greater than 48 weeks are not known. There is evidence of atypical changes in melanocytes and keratinocytes and of increased dermal elastosis in some patients treated with tretinoin 0.05% for longer than 52 weeks.

➤*Irritation:* Tretinoin may induce severe local erythema, pruritus, burning, stinging, and peeling at the application site. If the degree of local irritation warrants, use medication less frequently or discontinue use temporarily or completely. Tretinoin may cause severe irritation to eczematous skin; use with caution in patients with this condition.

➤*Photosensitivity:* It is advisable to "rest" a patient's skin until effects of keratolytic agents subside before beginning tretinoin. Minimize exposure to sunlight and sunlamps, and advise patients with sunburn not to use tretinoin until fully recovered because of heightened susceptibility to sunlight as a result of tretinoin use. Patients who undergo considerable sun exposure due to occupation and those with inherent sun sensitivity should exercise particular caution. Use sunscreen products and wear protective clothing over treated areas. Weather extremes, such as wind and cold, also may irritate treated areas.

➤*Pregnancy: Category C.* Oral tretinoin is teratogenic. There are no adequate and well-controlled studies in pregnant women. Use during pregnancy only if the potential benefit justifies the potential risk. Do not use *Renova* and *Avita* during pregnancy.

Topical tretinoin in animal teratogenicity tests has generated equivocal results. There is evidence of teratogenicity (shortened or kinked tail) of topical tretinoin in Wistar rats at doses greater than 1 mg/kg/day (200 times the recommended human topical clinical dose) Anomalies (humerus: short 13%, bent 6%; os parietal incompletely ossified 14%) also have been reported in rats when 10 mg/kg/day was dermally applied.

There are other reports in New Zealand White rabbits with doses of approximately 80 times the recommended human topical clinical dose of an increased incidence of domed head and hydrocephaly, typical of retinoid-induced fetal malformations in this species.

In contrast, several well-controlled animal studies have shown that dermally applied tretinoin was not teratogenic at doses of 100 and 200 times the recommended human topical clinical dose in rats and rabbits, respectively.

Dermal tretinoin has been shown to be fetotoxic in rabbits when administered in doses 100 times the recommended topical human clinical dose.

Thirty cases of temporally associated congenital malformations have been reported during 2 decades of clinical use of another formulation of topical tretinoin (acne preparation). Although no definite pattern of teratogenicity and no causal association has been established from these cases, 5 of the reports describe the rare birth defect category holoprosencephaly (defects associated with incomplete midline development of the forebrain). The significance of these spontaneous reports in terms of risk to the fetus is unknown.

➤*Lactation:* It is not known whether this drug is excreted in breast milk. Exercise caution when tretinoin is administered to a nursing mother.

➤*Children:*

Renova – Safety and efficacy in patients less than 18 years of age have not been established.

Drug Interactions

➤*Sulfur, resorcinol, benzoyl peroxide, or salicylic acid:* Cautiously use concomitant topical medications because of possible interactions with tretinoin. Significant skin irritation may result. It also is advisable to "rest" a patient's skin until the effects of such preparations subside before use of tretinoin is begun.

➤*Topical preparations:* Cautiously use medicated or abrasive soaps and cleansers, soaps and cosmetics that have a strong drying effect, and products with high concentrations of alcohol, astringents, spices, or lime, permanent wave solutions, electrolysis, hair depilatories or waxes, and products that may irritate the skin in patients being treated with tretinoin because they may increase irritation.

➤*Photosensitizers:* Do not use tretinoin if the patient also is taking drugs known to be photosensitizers (eg, thiazides, tetracyclines, fluoroquinolones, phenothiazines, sulfonamides) because of the possibility of augmented phototoxicity.

Adverse Reactions

Almost all patients reported 1 or more local reactions such as peeling, dry skin, burning, stinging, erythema, and pruritus during therapy with tretinoin.

Sensitive skin may become excessively red, edematous, blistered, or crusted. If these effects occur, discontinue medication until skin integrity is restored or adjust to a tolerable level. True contact allergy is rare.

Temporary hyperpigmentation or hypopigmentation has been reported with repeated application. Some individuals have a heightened susceptibility to sunlight while under treatment.

All adverse effects have been reversible upon discontinuation.

Overdosage

➤*Symptoms:* Application of larger amounts of medication than recommended has not been shown to lead to more rapid or better results, and marked redness, peeling, or discomfort may occur. Oral ingestion of the drug may lead to the same side effects as those associated with excessive oral intake of vitamin A.

Patient Information

➤*Renova*: Apply only as an adjunct to a comprehensive skin care and sun avoidance program. Apply a moisturizing sunscreen with a minimum SPF of 15 every morning when being treated with tretinoin. Avoid direct sun exposure as much as possible and totally avoid sunlamps while using tretinoin. Do not use if sunburned or if eczema or other chronic skin conditions exist. Do not use if inherently sensitive to sunlight or if also taking other drugs that increase sensitivity to sunlight.

Do not use if pregnant, attempting to become pregnant, or at high risk of pregnancy.

A majority of patients will lose most mitigating effects on fine wrinkles, mottled hyperpigmentation, and tactile roughness of facial skin with discontinuation of a comprehensive skin care and sun avoidance program including tretinoin; however, the safety and efficacy of tretinoin daily use for greater than 48 weeks have not been established.

ISOTRETINOIN (13-cis-Retinoic Acid)

Rx	**Amnesteem** (Mylan)	**Capsules; oral:** 10 mg	EDTA. (I10). Reddish brown. In UD 30s and UD 100s.
Rx	**Claravis** (Teva)		Edetate disodium. (barr 934). Lt. gray. In UD 30s and UD 100s.
Rx	**Amnesteem** (Mylan)	**Capsules; oral:** 20 mg	EDTA. (I20). Reddish brown and cream. In 30s and 100s.
Rx	**Claravis** (Teva)		Edetate disodium. (barr 935). Brown. In UD 30s and UD 100s.
Rx	**Claravis** (Teva)	**Capsules; oral:** 30 mg	Edetate disodium. (barr 454). Orange. In UD 30s.
Rx	**Amnesteem** (Mylan)	**Capsules; oral:** 40 mg	EDTA. (I40). Orange brown. In 30s and 100s.
Rx	**Claravis** (Teva)		Edetate disodium. (barr 936). Lt. orange. In UD 30s and UD 100s.
Rx	**Sotret** (Ranbaxy)	**Capsules, softgel; oral:** 10 mg	Parabens. (5R). EDTA Lt. pink. In 30s and 100s.
		20 mg	EDTA, parabens. (6R). Maroon. In 30s and 100s.
		30 mg	EDTA, parabens. (8R). Golden yellow. In 30s and 100s.
		40 mg	EDTA, parabens. (7R). Yellow. In 30s and 100s.

[a] Capsule contains suspension of drug in soybean oil; also contains parabens and EDTA.

ISOTRETINOIN — ORAL

WARNING

Isotretinoin must not be used by women and adolescents who are pregnant or who may become pregnant. There is an extremely high risk that severe birth defects can result if pregnancy occurs while taking isotretinoin in any amount, even for short periods of time. Potentially, any fetus exposed during pregnancy can be affected. There are no accurate means of determining whether an exposed fetus has been affected.

Birth defects that have been documented following isotretinoin exposure include abnormalities of the face, eyes, ears, skull, CNS, cardiovascular system, and thymus and parathyroid glands. Cases of intelligence quotient (IQ) scores less than 85 with or without other abnormalities have been reported. There is an increased risk of spontaneous abortion, and premature births have been reported.

Documented external abnormalities include skull abnormality; ear abnormalities (including anotia, micropinna, small or absent external auditory canals); eye abnormalities (including microphthalmia); facial dysmorphia; cleft palate. Documented internal abnormalities include CNS abnormalities (including cerebral abnormalities, cerebellar malformation, hydrocephalus, microcephaly, cranial nerve deficit); cardiovascular abnormalities; thymus gland abnormality; parathyroid hormone deficiency. In some cases, death has occurred with some of the abnormalities previously noted.

If pregnancy does occur during treatment of a female patient who is taking isotretinoin, isotretinoin must be discontinued immediately and she should be referred to an obstetrician-gynecologist experienced in reproductive toxicity for further evaluation and counseling.

Special prescribing requirements – Because of isotretinoin's teratogenicity and to minimize fetal exposure, isotretinoin is approved for marketing only under a special restricted distribution program approved by the Food and Drug Administration. This program is called iPLEDGE. Isotretinoin must only be prescribed by prescribers who are registered and activated with the iPLEDGE program. Isotretinoin must only be dispensed by a pharmacy registered and activated with iPLEDGE, and must only be dispensed to patients who are registered and meet all the requirements of iPLEDGE.

Information for pharmacist – Access the iPLEDGE system via the internet (http://www.ipledgeprogram.com) or telephone (1-866-495-0654) to obtain an authorization and the "do not dispense to patient after" date. Isotretinoin must only be dispensed in no more than a 30-day supply.

Refills require a new prescription and a new authorization from the iPLEDGE system.

An isotretinoin Medication Guide must be given to the patient each time isotretinoin is dispensed, as required by law. This isotretinoin Medication Guide is an important part of the risk management program for the patient.

Indications

➤*Severe recalcitrant nodular acne:* For the treatment of severe recalcitrant nodular acne. Nodules are inflammatory lesions with a diameter of 5 mm or more. The nodules may become suppurative or hemorrhagic. "Severe," by definition, means "many" as opposed to "few or several" nodules. Because of significant adverse effects associated with its use, reserve isotretinoin for patients with severe nodular acne who are unresponsive to conventional therapy, including systemic antibiotics. In addition, isotretinoin is indicated only for those females who are not pregnant because isotretinoin can cause severe birth defects.

➤*Off-label uses:* Pityriasis rubra pilaris, rosacea, psoriasis; prevention and treatment of basal cell carcinoma; adjunctive treatment of inoperable neoplasms such as squamous cell carcinoma of the lung; treatment of advanced squamous cell carcinoma of the skin; keratoacanthomas; cutaneous T-cell lymphomas.

A combination of systemic isotretinoin and interferon alpha-2a may provide a more potent effect than isotretinoin alone in prevention and treatment of skin cancers.

Administration and Dosage

➤*General dosing considerations:* Isotretinoin must only be prescribed by health care providers who are registered and activated with the iPLEDGE program. Isotretinoin must only be dispensed by a pharmacy registered and activated with iPLEDGE and must only be dispensed to patients who are registered and meet all the requirements of iPLEDGE. Registered and activated pharmacies must receive isotretinoin only from wholesalers registered with iPLEDGE.

➤*Adults:*

Severe recalcitrant nodular acne –

Usual dosage: 0.5 to 1 mg/kg/day given in 2 divided doses with food daily for 15 to 20 weeks. Once-daily dosing is not recommended.

Dosage adjustment: During treatment, the dose may be adjusted according to response of the disease and/or the appearance of clinical side effects, some of which may be dose related.

Adult patients whose disease is very severe with scarring or is primarily manifested on the trunk may require dose adjustments of 2 mg/kg/day or less, as tolerated. Failure to take isotretinoin with food will significantly decrease absorption. Before upward dose adjustments are made, the patients should be questioned about their compliance with food instructions.

Discontinuation of therapy: If the total nodule count has been reduced by more than 70% prior to completing 15 to 20 weeks of treatment, the drug may be discontinued.

Long-term use: Long-term use of isotretinoin, even in low doses, has not been studied, and is not recommended. It is important that isotretinoin be given at the recommended doses for no longer than the recommended duration. The effect of long-term use of isotretinoin on bone loss is unknown. Isotretinoin has been shown to decrease bone mineral density (BMD) and to cause hyperostosis and premature epiphyseal closure.

Re-treatment: In studies comparing 0.1, 0.5, and 1 mg/kg/day, it was found that all dosages provided initial clearing of disease, but there was a greater need for retreatment with the lower dosages.

After a period of 2 months or more off therapy, and if warranted by persistent or recurring severe nodular acne, a second course of therapy may be initiated. The optimal interval before re-treatment has not been defined for patients who have not completed skeletal growth. Contraceptive measures must be followed for any subsequent course of therapy.

➤*Children:*

Severe recalcitrant acne –

12 to 17 years of age: See Adults for dosing.

➤*Monthly required iPLEDGE interactions:*

Monthly Required iPLEDGE Interactions

	Female patients of childbearing potential	Male and female patients not of childbearing potential
Prescriber		
Confirms patient counseling	X	X
Enters the 2 contraception methods chosen by the patient	X	
Enters pregnancy test results	X	
Patient		
Answers educational questions before every prescription	X	
Enters 2 forms of contraception	X	
Pharmacist		
Calls system to get an authorization	X	X

➤*Administration:* Isotretinoin should be administered with a meal.

Isotretinoin is considered a teratogen. Follow safe handling procedures when preparing, administering, or dispensing isotretinoin.

➤*Storage/Stability:*

Amnesteem – Store at controlled room temperature, 15° to 30°C (59° to 86°F). Protect from light.

Claravis and *Sotret* – Store at 20° to 25°C (68° to 77°F). Protect from light.

Actions

➤*Pharmacology:* Isotretinoin is a retinoid, which, when administered in pharmacologic doses of 0.5 to 1 mg/kg/day, inhibits sebaceous gland function and keratinization. The exact mechanism of action of isotretinoin is unknown.

Clinical improvement in nodular acne patients occurs in association with a reduction in sebum secretion. The decrease in sebum secretion is temporary and is related to the dose and duration of treatment with isotretinoin. It reflects a reduction in sebaceous gland size and an inhibition of sebaceous gland differentiation.

➤*Pharmacokinetics:*

Absorption – Because of its high lipophilicity, oral absorption of isotretinoin is enhanced when given with a high-fat meal. In a crossover study, 74 healthy adult subjects received a single 80 mg oral dose (2 times 40 mg capsules) of isotretinoin under fasted and fed conditions. Both peak plasma concentration (C_{max}) and the total exposure (area under the curve [AUC]) of isotretinoin were more than doubled following a standardized high-fat meal when compared with isotretinoin given under fasted conditions. The observed elimination half-life was unchanged. This lack of change in half-life suggests that food increases the bioavailability of isotretinoin without altering its disposition. The time to peak concentration (T_{max}) was also increased with food and may be related to a longer absorption phase. Therefore, isotretinoin should always be taken with food. Clinical studies have shown that there is no difference in the pharmacokinetics of isotretinoin between patients with nodular acne and healthy subjects with normal skin.

ISOTRETINOIN — ORAL

Pharmacokinetic Parameters of Isotretinoin Mean (%CV[a]) (N = 74)				
Isotretinoin 2 × 40 mg capsules	$AUC_{0-\infty}$ (ng•h/mL)	C_{max} (ng/mL)	T_{max} (h)	t½[b] (h)
Fed[c]	10,004 (22%)	862 (22%)	5.3 (77%)	21 (39%)
Fasted	3,703 (46%)	301 (63%)	3.2 (56%)	21 (30%)

[a] CV = coefficient of variation.
[b] t½ = half-life.
[c] Eating a standardized high-fat meal.

Distribution – Isotretinoin is more than 99.9% bound to plasma proteins, primarily albumin.

Metabolism – Following oral administration of isotretinoin, at least 3 metabolites have been identified in human plasma: 4-oxo-isotretinoin, retinoic acid (tretinoin), and 4-oxo-retinoic acid (4-oxo-tretinoin). Retinoic acid and 13-cis-retinoic acid are geometric isomers and show reversible interconversion. The administration of one isomer will give rise to the other. Isotretinoin is also irreversibly oxidized to 4-oxo-isotretinoin, which forms its geometric isomer 4-oxo-tretinoin.

After a single oral dose of isotretinoin 80 mg to 74 healthy adult subjects, coadministration of food increased the extent of formation of all metabolites in plasma when compared with the extent of formation under fasted conditions.

All of these metabolites possess retinoid activity that is in some in vitro models more than that of the parent isotretinoin. However, the clinical significance of these models is unknown. After multiple oral dose administration of isotretinoin to adult cystic acne patients (18 years of age and older), the exposure of patients to 4-oxo-isotretinoin at steady state under fasted and fed conditions was approximately 3.4 times higher than that of isotretinoin.

In vitro studies indicate that the primary P-450 isoforms involved in isotretinoin metabolism are 2C8, 2C9, 3A4, and 2B6. Isotretinoin and its metabolites are further metabolized into conjugates, which are then excreted in urine and feces.

Excretion – Following oral administration of an 80 mg dose of ^{14}C-isotretinoin as a liquid suspension, ^{14}C activity in blood declined, with a half-life of 90 hours. The metabolites of isotretinoin and any conjugates are ultimately excreted in the feces and urine in relatively equal amounts (total of 65% to 83%). After a single 80 mg oral dose of isotretinoin to 74 healthy adult subjects under fed conditions, the mean ± standard deviation (SD) elimination half-lives of isotretinoin and 4-oxo-isotretinoin were 21 ± 8.2 hours and 24 ± 5.3 hours, respectively. After both single and multiple doses, the observed accumulation ratios of isotretinoin ranged from 0.9 to 5.43 in patients with cystic acne.

Contraindications

Pregnancy (see Warning Box); hypersensitivity to this medication or to any of its components; hypersensitivity to parabens, which are used as a preservative in the gelatin capsule (*Sotret*).

Warnings/Precautions

➤*Psychiatric disorders:* Isotretinoin may cause depression, psychosis, and, rarely, suicidal ideation, suicide attempts, suicide, and aggressive and/or violent behaviors. No mechanism of action has been established for these events.

Health care providers should read the brochure, *Recognizing Psychiatric Disorders in Adolescents and Young Adults: A Guide for Prescribers of Isotretinoin*. Health care providers should be alert to the warning signs of psychiatric disorders to guide patients to receive the help they need. Therefore, prior to initiation of isotretinoin therapy, ask patients and family members about any history of psychiatric disorder, and at each visit during therapy, assess patients for symptoms of depression, mood disturbance, psychosis, or aggression to determine if further evaluation may be necessary. Signs and symptoms of depression, as described in the brochure (*"Recognizing Psychiatric Disorders in Adolescents and Young Adults"*), include sad mood; hopelessness; feelings of guilt, worthlessness, or helplessness; loss of pleasure or interest in activities; fatigue; difficulty concentrating; change in sleep pattern; change in weight or appetite; suicidal thoughts or attempts; restlessness; irritability; acting on dangerous impulses; and persistent physical symptoms unresponsive to treatment. Patients should stop isotretinoin and the patient or a family member should promptly contact their health care provider without waiting until the next visit if depression, mood disturbance, psychosis, or aggression develops. Discontinuation of isotretinoin therapy my be insufficient; further evaluation may be necessary. While such monitoring may be helpful, it may not detect all patients at risk. Patients may report mental health problems or family history of psychiatric disorders. These reports should be discussed with the patient and/or the patient's family. A referral to a mental health professional may be necessary. The health care provider should consider whether isotretinoin therapy is appropriate in this setting; for some patients, the risks may outweigh the benefits of isotretinoin therapy.

➤*Pseudotumor cerebri:* Isotretinoin use has been associated with a number of cases of pseudotumor cerebri (benign intracranial hypertension), some of which involved concomitant use of tetracyclines. Therefore, avoid concomitant treatment with tetracyclines. Early signs and symptoms of pseudotumor cerebri include papilledema, headache, nausea and vomiting, and visual disturbances. Screen patients with these symptoms for papilledema, and, if present, tell them to discontinue isotretinoin immediately and refer them to a neurologist for further diagnosis and care.

➤*Pancreatitis:* Acute pancreatitis has been reported in patients with either elevated or normal serum triglyceride levels. In rare instances, fatal hemorrhagic pancreatitis has been reported. Discontinue isotretinoin if hypertriglyceridemia cannot be controlled at an acceptable level or if symptoms of pancreatitis occur.

➤*Hypertriglyceridemia:* Elevations of serum triglycerides in excess of 800 mg/dL have been reported in patients treated with isotretinoin. Marked elevations of serum triglycerides were reported in approximately 25% of patients receiving isotretinoin in clinical trials. In addition, approximately 15% developed a decrease in high-density lipoprotein (HDL), and approximately 7% showed an increase in cholesterol levels. In clinical trials, these effects on triglycerides, HDL, and cholesterol were reversible upon cessation of isotretinoin therapy. Some patients have been able to reverse triglyceride elevation by reduction in weight, restriction of dietary fat and alcohol, and reduction in dose while continuing isotretinoin.

Perform blood lipid determinations before isotretinoin is given and then at intervals until the lipid response to isotretinoin is established, which usually occurs within 4 weeks. Especially careful consideration must be given to risk/benefit for patients who may be at high risk during isotretinoin therapy (eg, patients with diabetes, obesity, increased alcohol intake, lipid metabolism disorder or familial history of lipid metabolism disorder). If isotretinoin therapy is instituted, more frequent checks of serum values for lipids and/or blood sugar are recommended.

The cardiovascular consequences of hypertriglyceridemia associated with isotretinoin are unknown.

➤*Hearing impairment:* Hearing impairment has been reported in patients taking isotretinoin; in some cases, the hearing impairment has been reported to persist after therapy has been discontinued. Mechanism(s) and causality for this event have not been established. Patients who experience tinnitus or hearing impairment should discontinue isotretinoin treatment and be referred to specialized care for further evaluation.

➤*Hepatotoxicity:* Clinical hepatitis considered to be possibly or probably related to isotretinoin therapy has been reported. Additionally, mild to moderate elevations of liver enzymes have been observed in approximately 15% of individuals treated during clinical trials, some of which normalized with dosage reduction or continued administration of the drug. If normalization does not readily occur or if hepatitis is suspected during treatment with isotretinoin, discontinue the drug and investigate the etiology further.

➤*Inflammatory bowel disease:* Isotretinoin has been associated with inflammatory bowel disease (including regional ileitis) in patients without a history of intestinal disorders. In some instances, symptoms have been reported to persist after isotretinoin treatment has been stopped. Immediately discontinue isotretinoin in patients experiencing abdominal pain, rectal bleeding, or severe diarrhea.

➤*Musculoskeletal effects:*

BMD – Effects of multiple courses of isotretinoin on the developing musculoskeletal system are unknown. There is some evidence that long-term, high-dose, or multiple courses of therapy with isotretinoin have more of an effect than a single course of therapy on the musculoskeletal system. In an open-label clinical trial (n = 217) of a single course of therapy with isotretinoin for severe recalcitrant nodular acne, bone density measurements at several skeletal sites were not significantly decreased (lumbar spine change more than −4% and total hip change more than −5%) or were increased in the majority of patients. One patient had a decrease in lumbar spine BMD more than 4% based on unadjusted data. Sixteen (7.9%) patients had decreases in lumbar spine BMD more than 4%, and all the other patients (92%) did not have significant decreases or had increases (adjusted for body mass index [BMI]). Nine (4.5%) patients had a decrease in total hip BMD more than 5% based on unadjusted data. Twenty-one (10.6%) patients had decreases in total hip BMD more than 5%, and all the other patients (89%) did not have significant decreases or had increases (adjusted for BMI). Follow-up studies performed in 8 of the patients with decreased BMD for up to 11 months thereafter demonstrated increasing bone density in 5 patients at the lumbar spine, while the other 3 patients had lumbar spine bone density measurements below baseline values. Total hip BMDs remained below baseline (range, −1.6% to −7.6%) in 5 of 8 (62.5%) patients.

In a separate open-label extension study of 10 patients, ages 13 to 18 years, who started a second course of isotretinoin 4 months after the first course, 2 patients showed a decrease in mean lumbar spine BMD of 3.25% or less.

Spontaneous reports of osteoporosis, osteopenia, bone fractures, and delayed healing of bone fractures have been seen in the isotretinoin population. While causality to isotretinoin has not been established, an effect cannot be ruled out. Longer-term effects have not been studied. It is important that isotretinoin be given at the recommended doses for no longer than the recommended duration.

Hyperostosis: A high prevalence of skeletal hyperostosis was noted in clinical trials for disorders of keratinization with a mean dose of 2.24 mg/kg/day. Additionally, skeletal hyperostosis was noted in 6 of 8 patients in a prospective study of disorders of keratinization. Minimal skeletal hyperostosis and calcification of ligaments and tendons have also been observed by x-rays in prospective studies of nodular acne patients treated with a single course of therapy at recommended doses. The skeletal effects of multiple isotretinoin treatment courses for acne are unknown.

In a clinical study of 217 children (12 to 17 years of age) with severe recalcitrant nodular acne, hyperostosis was not observed after 16 to 20 weeks of treatment with approximately 1 mg/kg/day of isotretinoin given in 2 divided doses. Hyperostosis may require a longer time frame to appear. The clinical course and significance remain unknown.

ISOTRETINOIN — ORAL

Premature epiphyseal closure – There are spontaneous reports of premature epiphyseal closure in acne patients receiving recommended doses of isotretinoin. The effect of multiple courses of isotretinoin on epiphyseal closure is unknown.

➤*Ophthalmologic effects:*

Vision impairment – Carefully monitor visual problems. All isotretinoin patients experiencing visual difficulties should discontinue isotretinoin treatment and have an ophthalmological examination.

Corneal opacities – Corneal opacities have occurred in patients receiving isotretinoin for acne and have occurred more frequently when higher drug dosages were used in patients with disorders of keratinization. The corneal opacities that have been observed in clinical trial patients treated with isotretinoin have either completely resolved or were resolving at follow-up 6 to 7 weeks after discontinuation of the drug.

Decreased night vision – A number of cases of decreased night vision have occurred during isotretinoin therapy and in some instances the event has persisted after therapy was discontinued. Because the onset in some patients was sudden, advise patients of this potential problem and warn them to be cautious when driving or operating any vehicle at night. Carefully monitor visual problems.

➤*iPLEDGE program:* Isotretinoin must only be prescribed by health care providers who are registered and activated with the iPLEDGE program. Isotretinoin must only be dispensed by a pharmacy registered and activated with iPLEDGE and must only be dispensed to patients who are registered and meet all the requirements of iPLEDGE. Registered and activated pharmacies must receive isotretinoin only from wholesalers registered with iPLEDGE.

Prescribers –

To prescribe isotretinoin, the health care provider must access the iPLEDGE system via the internet (http://www.ipledgeprogram.com) or telephone (1-866-495-0654) to:

1.) Register each patient in the iPLEDGE program.
2.) Confirm monthly that each patient has received counseling and education.

For female patients of childbearing potential:

- Enter patient's 2 chosen forms of contraception each month.
- Enter monthly result from CLIA-certified laboratory conducted pregnancy test.

Pharmacists –

To dispense isotretinoin, the pharmacist must:

1.) Be trained by the responsible site pharmacist concerning the iPLEDGE program requirements.
2.) Obtain authorization from the iPLEDGE program via the internet (http://www.ipledgeprogram.com) or telephone (1-866-495-0654) for every isotretinoin prescription. Authorization signifies that the patient has met all program requirements and is qualified to receive isotretinoin.
3.) Write the Risk Management Authorization (RMA) number on the prescription.

Isotretinoin must be dispensed only:

- in no more than a 30-day supply
- with an isotretinoin Medication Guide
- after authorization from the iPLEDGE program
- prior to the "do not dispense to patient after" date provided by the iPLEDGE system (within 7 days of the office visit)
- with a new prescription for refills and another authorization from the iPLEDGE program (no automatic refills allowed).

➤*Elevated creatine phosphokinase (CPK):* Some patients undergoing vigorous physical activity while on isotretinoin therapy have experienced elevated CPK levels; however, the clinical significance is unknown. There have been rare postmarketing reports of rhabdomyolysis, some associated with strenuous physical activity. In a clinical trial of 217 children (12 to 17 years of age) with severe recalcitrant nodular acne, transient elevations in CPK were observed in 12% of patients, including those undergoing strenuous physical activity in association with reported musculoskeletal adverse reactions such as back pain, arthralgia, limb injury, or muscle sprain. In these patients, approximately half of the CPK elevations returned to normal within 2 weeks, and half returned to normal within 4 weeks. No cases of rhabdomyolysis were reported in this trial.

➤*Elevated glucose:* Some patients receiving isotretinoin have experienced problems in the control of their blood sugar. In addition, new cases of diabetes have been diagnosed during isotretinoin therapy, although no causal relationship has been established.

➤*Hypersensitivity reactions:* Anaphylactic reactions and other allergic reactions have been reported. Cutaneous allergic reactions and serious cases of allergic vasculitis, often with purpura (bruises and red patches) of the extremities and extracutaneous involvement (including renal), have been reported. Severe allergic reaction necessitates discontinuation of therapy and appropriate medical management.

➤*Special risk:* Although an effect of isotretinoin on bone loss is not established, use caution when prescribing isotretinoin to patients with a genetic predisposition for age-related osteoporosis, a history of childhood osteoporosis conditions, osteomalacia, or other disorders of bone metabolism. This would include patients diagnosed with anorexia nervosa and those who are on chronic drug therapy that causes drug-induced osteoporosis/osteomalacia and/or affects vitamin D metabolism, such as systemic corticosteroids and any anticonvulsant.

Patients may be at increased risk when participating in sports with repetitive impact where the risks of spondylolisthesis with and without pars fractures and hip growth plate injuries in early and late adolescence are known. There are spontaneous reports of fractures or delayed healing in patients while on treatment with isotretinoin or following cessation of treatment with isotretinoin while involved in these activities. While causality to isotretinoin has not been established, an effect cannot be ruled out.

➤*Pregnancy: Category X.* See the Warning box for more information.

➤*Lactation:* It is not known whether this drug is excreted in human milk. Because of the potential for adverse reactions, breast-feeding mothers should not receive isotretinoin.

➤*Children:* The use of isotretinoin in children younger than 12 years of age has not been studied. Carefully consider the use of isotretinoin for the treatment of severe recalcitrant nodular acne in children 12 to 17 years of age, especially for those patients in whom a known metabolic or structural bone disease exists.

In studies with isotretinoin, adverse reactions reported in children were similar to those described in adults except for the increased incidence of back pain and arthralgia (both of which were sometimes severe) and myalgia in children.

➤*Elderly:* Although reported clinical experience has not identified differences in responses between elderly and younger patients, effects of aging might be expected to increase some risks associated with isotretinoin therapy.

➤*Monitoring:*

Vision impairment – Carefully monitor visual problems. All isotretinoin patients experiencing visual difficulties should discontinue isotretinoin treatment and have an ophthalmological examination.

Lipids – Obtain pretreatment and follow-up blood lipids under fasting conditions. After consumption of alcohol, at least 36 hours should elapse before these determinations are made. It is recommended that these tests be performed at weekly or biweekly intervals until the lipid response to isotretinoin is established. The incidence of hypertriglyceridemia is 1 patient in 4 on isotretinoin therapy.

Liver function tests – Because elevations of liver enzymes have been observed during clinical trials, and hepatitis has been reported, perform pretreatment and follow-up liver function tests at weekly or biweekly intervals until the response to isotretinoin has been established.

Pregnancy test – Female patients of childbearing potential must have negative results from 2 urine or serum pregnancy tests with a sensitivity of at least 25 milliunit/mL before receiving the initial isotretinoin prescription. The first test is obtained by the prescriber when the decision is made to pursue qualification of the patient for isotretinoin (a screening test). The second pregnancy test (a confirmation test) must be done in a CLIA-certified laboratory. The interval between the 2 tests must be at least 19 days.

For patients with regular menstrual cycles, the second pregnancy test must be done during the first 5 days of the menstrual period and within 7 days following the office visit, immediately preceding the beginning of isotretinoin therapy, and after the patient has used 2 forms of contraception for 1 month.

For patients with amenorrhea or irregular cycles, or for those using a contraceptive method that precludes withdrawal bleeding, the second pregnancy test must be done within 7 days following the office visit, immediately preceding the beginning of isotretinoin therapy, and after the patient has used 2 forms of contraception for 1 month.

Each month of therapy, the patient must have a negative result from a urine or serum pregnancy test. A pregnancy test must be repeated each month, in a CLIA-certified laboratory, prior to the female patient receiving each prescription.

Drug Interactions

Isotretinoin Drug Interactions

Precipitant drug	Object drug[a]		Description
Corticosteroids, systemic	Isotretinoin	↑	Systemic corticosteroids are known to cause osteoporosis. There have been spontaneous reports of osteoporosis (eg, bone fractures, osteopenia) seen with isotretinoin use. There may be an interactive effect on bone loss between systemic corticosteroids and isotretinoin. Use with caution.
Isotretinoin	Corticosteroids, systemic		
Phenytoin	Isotretinoin	↑	Phenytoin is known to cause osteomalacia. There have been spontaneous reports of osteoporosis (eg, bone fractures, osteopenia) with isotretinoin use. There may be an interactive effect on bone loss between phenytoin and isotretinoin. Use with caution.
Isotretinoin	Phenytoin		
Tetracyclines	Isotretinoin	↑	Isotretinoin use has been associated with a number of cases of pseudotumor cerebri (benign intracranial hypertension), some of which involved concomitant use of tetracyclines. Avoid concomitant use.

First Generation Retinoids

ISOTRETINOIN — ORAL

Isotretinoin Drug Interactions			
Precipitant drug	Object drug[a]		Description
Vitamin A	Isotretinoin	↑	Because of the relationship of isotretinoin to vitamin A, concomitant use may cause additive toxic reactions.
Isotretinoin	Vitamin A		

[a] ↑ = object drug increased.

➤*Drug/Food interactions:* Because of its high lipophilicity, oral absorption of isotretinoin is enhanced when given with a high-fat meal. In a crossover study, 74 healthy adult subjects received a single 80 mg oral dose (2 times 40 mg capsules) of isotretinoin under fasted and fed conditions. Both peak plasma concentration (C_{max}) and the total exposure (AUC) of isotretinoin were more than doubled following a standardized high-fat meal when compared with isotretinoin given under fasted conditions.

Adverse Reactions

➤*Dose relationship:* Cheilitis and hypertriglyceridemia are usually dose related. Most adverse reactions reported in clinical trials were reversible when therapy was discontinued; however, some persisted after cessation of therapy.

Cardiovascular – Palpitation, stroke, tachycardia, vascular thrombotic disease.

CNS – Aggression, depression, dizziness, drowsiness, emotional instability, headache, insomnia, lethargy, malaise, nervousness, paresthesias, pseudotumor cerebri, psychosis, seizures, stroke, suicidal ideation, suicide, suicide attempts, syncope, violent behaviors, weakness.

Of the patients reporting depression, some reported that the depression subsided with discontinuation of therapy and recurred with reinstitution of therapy.

Dermatologic – Abnormal wound healing (delayed healing or exuberant granulation tissue with crusting), acne fulminans, alopecia (which in some cases persists), bruising, cheilitis (dry lips), dry mouth, dry nose, dry skin, epistaxis, eruptive xanthomas, flushing, fragility of skin, hair abnormalities, hirsutism, hyperpigmentation and hypopigmentation, infections (including disseminated herpes simplex), nail dystrophy, paronychia, peeling of palms and soles, photoallergic/photosensitizing reactions, pruritus, pyogenic granuloma, rash (including eczema, facial erythema, and seborrhea), sunburn susceptibility increased, sweating, urticaria, vasculitis (including Wegener granulomatosis).

Endocrine – Alterations in blood sugar levels, hypertriglyceridemia.

GI – Bleeding and inflammation of the gums, colitis, esophageal ulceration, esophagitis, hepatitis, ileitis, inflammatory bowel disease, nausea, pancreatitis, other nonspecific GI symptoms.

GU – Abnormal menses, glomerulonephritis, microscopic or gross hematuria, nonspecific urogenital findings, proteinuria, white cells in the urine.

Lab test abnormalities – Decrease in serum HDL levels, elevation of plasma triglycerides, elevations of serum cholesterol during treatment.

Increased alkaline phosphatase, ALT, AST, gamma-glutamyl transpeptidase (GGTP), or lactate dehydrogenase (LDH).

Elevation of CPK, elevations of fasting blood sugar, hyperuricemia.

Decreases in red blood cell parameters, decreases in white blood cell counts (including severe neutropenia and rare reports of agranulocytosis), elevated platelet counts, elevated sedimentation rates, thrombocytopenia.

Microscopic or gross hematuria, proteinuria, white cells in the urine.

Musculoskeletal – Arthritis, calcification of tendons and ligaments, decreases in BMD, elevations of CPK/rare reports of rhabdomyolysis, musculoskeletal symptoms (sometimes severe) including arthralgia, back pain, and myalgia, other types of bone abnormalities, premature epiphyseal closure, skeletal hyperostosis, tendonitis, transient pain in the chest.

Ophthalmic – Cataracts, color vision disorder, conjunctivitis, corneal opacities, decreased night vision that may persist, dry eyes, eyelid inflammation, keratitis, optic neuritis, photophobia, visual disturbances.

Respiratory – Bronchospasms (with or without a history of asthma), respiratory tract infection, voice alteration.

Special senses – Hearing impairment, tinnitus.

Miscellaneous – Allergic reactions including systemic hypersensitivity and vasculitis, edema, fatigue, lymphadenopathy, weight loss.

Overdosage

Isotretinoin causes serious birth defects at any dosage. Female patients of childbearing potential who present with isotretinoin overdose must be evaluated for pregnancy. Patients who are pregnant should receive counseling about the risks to the fetus, as described in the Warning Box and Contraindications sections. Nonpregnant patients must be warned to avoid pregnancy for at least 1 month and receive contraceptive counseling as described in the Warnings section. Educational materials for such patients can be obtained by calling the manufacturer.

Because an overdose would be expected to result in higher levels of isotretinoin in semen than found during a normal treatment course, men should use a condom, or avoid reproductive sexual activity with a female patient who is or might become pregnant, for 1 month after the overdose. All patients with isotretinoin overdose should not donate blood for at least 1 month.

➤*Symptoms:* In humans, overdose has been associated with vomiting, facial flushing, cheilosis, abdominal pain, headache, dizziness, and ataxia. All symptoms quickly resolved without apparent residual effects.

Patient Information

Instruct women of childbearing potential that they must not be pregnant when isotretinoin therapy is initiated, and that they should use 2 forms of effective contraception 1 month before starting isotretinoin, while taking isotretinoin, and for 1 month after isotretinoin has been stopped, unless they commit to continuous abstinence from heterosexual intercourse. Have them also sign a second Patient Information/Informed Consent About Birth Defects (for female patients who can get pregnant) form prior to beginning isotretinoin therapy. Give them an opportunity to enroll in the isotretinoin survey and to review the patient DVD provided by the manufacturer to the prescriber. The DVD includes information about contraception, the most common reasons that contraception fails, and the importance of using 2 forms of effective contraception when taking teratogenic drugs and comprehensive information about types of potential birth defects which could occur if a woman who is pregnant takes isotretinoin at any time during pregnancy. Have female patients see their prescribers monthly and have a urine or serum pregnancy test performed each month during treatment to confirm negative pregnancy status before another isotretinoin prescription is written.

Inform patients that they must not share isotretinoin with anyone else because of the risk of birth defects and other serious adverse reactions.

Inform patients not to donate blood during therapy and for 1 month following discontinuation of the drug because the blood might be given to a pregnant woman whose fetus must not be exposed to isotretinoin.

Remind patients to take isotretinoin with a meal. To decrease the risk of esophageal irritation, have patients swallow the capsules with a full glass of liquid.

Instruct patients to immediately report abdominal pain, depression, difficulty in controlling blood sugar, rectal bleeding, severe diarrhea, or visual disturbances to a health care provider.

Inform patients that transient exacerbation (flare) of acne has been seen, generally during the initial period of therapy.

Patients should avoid wax epilation and skin resurfacing procedures (such as dermabrasion, laser) during isotretinoin therapy and for at least 6 months thereafter because of the possibility of scarring. Isotretinoin may cause abnormal wound healing.

Advise patients to avoid prolonged exposure to ultraviolet rays or sunlight.

Inform patients that they may experience decreased tolerance to contact lenses during and after therapy.

Inform patients that approximately 16% of patients treated with isotretinoin in a clinical trial developed musculoskeletal symptoms (including arthralgia) during treatment. In general, these symptoms were mild to moderate, but occasionally required discontinuation of the drug. Transient pain in the chest has been reported less frequently. In the clinical trial, these symptoms generally cleared rapidly after discontinuation of isotretinoin, but in some cases persisted. There have been rare postmarketing reports of elevated CPK levels/rhabdomyolysis, some associated with strenuous physical activity.

Second Generation Retinoids

ACITRETIN

Rx	**Soriatane** (GlaxoSmithKline)	**Capsules; oral**[a]: 10 mg	(A-10 mg). Brown/white. In 30s.
		17.5 mg	(A-17.5 mg). Yellow. In 30s.
		22.5 mg	(A-22.5 mg). Brown. In 30s.
		25 mg	(A-25 mg). Brown/yellow. In 30s.
Rx	**Soriatane CK** (GlaxoSmithKline)	**Capsules; oral**[a]: 10 mg	**Capsule:** Maltodextrin. (SORIATANE 10 mg). Brown/white. In 30s. **Foam:** Cetyl alcohol, mineral oil, petrolatum. In 94 g.

[a] Capsule shells contain gelatin, iron oxide, titanium dioxide, and may also contain benzyl alcohol.

ACITRETIN — ORAL

WARNING

Acitretin causes birth defects. Female patients must not get pregnant.

Acitretin must not be used by females who are pregnant, or who intend to become pregnant during therapy or at any time for at least 3 years following discontinuation of therapy. Acitretin also must not be used by females who may not use reliable contraception while undergoing treatment or for at least 3 years following discontinuation of treatment. Acitretin is a metabolite of etretinate, and major human fetal abnormalities have been reported with the administration of etretinate and acitretin. Potentially, any fetus exposed can be affected.

Clinical evidence has shown that concurrent ingestion of acitretin and ethanol has been associated with the formation of etretinate, which has a longer elimination half-life than acitretin. Because the longer elimination half-life of etretinate would increase the duration of teratogenic potential for female patients, ethanol must not be ingested by female patients either during treatment with acitretin or for 2 months after cessation of therapy. This allows for elimination of acitretin, thus removing the substrate for transesterification to etretinate. The mechanism of the metabolic process for conversion of acitretin to etretinate has not been fully defined. It is not known whether substances other than ethanol are associated with transesterification.

Acitretin has been shown to be embryotoxic or teratogenic in rabbits, mice, and rats at doses of 0.6, 3, and 15 mg/kg, respectively. These doses are approximately 0.2, 0.3, and 3 times the maximum recommended therapeutic dose, respectively, based on a mg/m^2 comparison.

Major human fetal abnormalities associated with acitretin or etretinate administration have been reported including meningomyelocele, meningoencephalocele, multiple synostoses, facial dysmorphia, syndactylies, absence of terminal phalanges, malformations of hip, ankle and forearm, low set ears, high palate, decreased cranial volume, cardiovascular malformation, and alterations of the skull and cervical vertebrae.

Acitretin should be prescribed only by those who have special competence in the diagnosis and treatment of severe psoriasis, are experienced in the use of systemic retinoids, and understand the risk of teratogenicity.

Important information for women of childbearing potential – Acitretin should be considered only for women with severe psoriasis unresponsive to other therapies or whose clinical condition contraindicates the use of other treatments.

Females of reproductive potential must not be given a prescription for acitretin until pregnancy is excluded. Acitretin is contraindicated in females of reproductive potential unless the patient meets all of the following conditions:

- Must have had 2 negative urine or serum pregnancy tests with a sensitivity of at least 25 mIU/mL before receiving the initial acitretin prescription. The first test (a screening test) is obtained by the prescriber when the decision is made to pursue acitretin therapy. The second pregnancy test (a confirmation test) should be done during the first 5 days of the menstrual period immediately preceding the beginning of acitretin therapy. For patients with amenorrhea, the second test should be done at least 11 days after the last act of unprotected sexual intercourse (without using 2 effective forms of contraception [birth control] simultaneously). Timing of pregnancy testing throughout the treatment course should be monthly or individualized based on the prescriber's clinical judgment.
- Must have selected and have committed to use 2 effective forms of contraception (birth control) simultaneously, at least 1 of which must be a primary form, unless absolute abstinence is the chosen method, or the patient has undergone a hysterectomy or is clearly postmenopausal.

WARNING (cont.)

- Patients must use 2 effective forms of contraception (birth control) simultaneously for at least 1 month prior to initiation of acitretin therapy, during acitretin therapy, and for at least 3 years after discontinuing acitretin therapy. An acitretin patient referral form is available so that patients can receive an initial free contraceptive counseling session and pregnancy testing. Counseling about contraception and behaviors associated with an increased risk of pregnancy must be repeated on a regular basis by the prescriber. To encourage compliance with this recommendation, a limited supply of the drug should be prescribed. Effective forms of contraception include both primary and secondary forms of contraception. Primary forms of contraception include the following: Tubal ligation, partner's vasectomy, intrauterine devices, birth control pills, and injectable/implantable/insertable/topical hormonal birth control products. Secondary forms of contraception include diaphragms, latex condoms, and cervical caps; each secondary form must be used with a spermicide. Any birth control method can fail. Therefore, it is critically important that women of childbearing potential use 2 effective forms of contraception (birth control) simultaneously. It has not been established if there is a pharmacokinetic interaction between acitretin and combined oral contraceptives. However, it has been established that acitretin interferes with the contraceptive effect of microdosed progestin preparations. Microdosed "minipill" progestin preparations are not recommended for use with acitretin. It is not known whether other progestational contraceptives, such as implants and injectables, are adequate methods of contraception during acitretin therapy. Prescribers are advised to consult the package insert of any medication administered concomitantly with hormonal contraceptives, since some medications may decrease the effectiveness of these birth control products. Patients should be prospectively cautioned not to self-medicate with the herbal supplement St. John's wort because a possible interaction has been suggested with hormonal contraceptives based on reports of breakthrough bleeding on oral contraceptives shortly after starting St. John's wort. Pregnancies have been reported by users of combined hormonal contraceptives who also used some form of St. John's wort.
- Must have signed a Patient Agreement/Informed Consent for Female Patients that contains warnings about the risk of potential birth defects if the fetus is exposed to acitretin, about contraceptive failure, and about the fact that they must not ingest beverages or products containing ethanol while taking acitretin and for 2 months after acitretin treatment has been discontinued.

If pregnancy does occur during acitretin therapy or at any time for at least 3 years following discontinuation of acitretin therapy, the prescriber and patient should discuss the possible effects on the pregnancy. The available information is as follows:

Acitretin, the active metabolite of etretinate, is teratogenic and is contraindicated during pregnancy. The risk of severe fetal malformations is well established when systemic retinoids are taken during pregnancy. Pregnancy must also be prevented after stopping acitretin therapy, while the drug is being eliminated to below a threshold blood concentration that would be associated with an increased incidence of birth defects. Because this threshold has not been established for acitretin in humans and because elimination rates vary among patients, the duration of posttherapy contraception to achieve adequate elimination cannot be calculated precisely. It is strongly recommended that contraception be continued for at least 3 years after stopping treatment with acitretin, based on the following considerations:

- In the absence of transesterification to form etretinate, greater than 98% of the acitretin would be eliminated within 2 months, assuming a mean elimination half-life of 49 hours.
- In cases where etretinate is formed, as has been demonstrated with concomitant administration of acitretin and ethanol, greater than 98% of the etretinate formed would be eliminated in 2 years, assuming a mean elimination half-life of 120 days, and greater than 98% of the etretinate formed would be eliminated in 3 years, based on the longest demonstrated elimination half-life of 168 days. However, etretinate was found in plasma and subcutaneous fat in 1 patient reported to have had sporadic alcohol intake, 52 months after she stopped acitretin therapy.
- Severe birth defects have been reported where conception occurred during the time interval when the patient was being treated with acitretin and/or etretinate. In addition, severe birth defects have also been reported when conception occurred after the mother completed therapy. These cases have been reported both prospectively (before the outcome was known) and retrospectively (after the outcome was known). The events below are listed without distinction as to whether the reported birth defects are consistent with retinoid-induced embryopathy or not.

ACITRETIN — ORAL

WARNING (cont.)

- There have been 318 prospectively reported cases involving pregnancies and the use of etretinate, acitretin or both. In 238 of these cases, the conception occurred after the last dose of etretinate (103 cases), acitretin (126) or both (9). Fetal outcome remained unknown in approximately one-half of these cases, of which 62 were terminated and 14 were spontaneous abortions. Fetal outcome is known for the other 118 cases and 15 of the outcomes were abnormal (including cases of absent hand/wrist, clubfoot, GI malformation, hypocalcemia, hypotonia, limb malformation, neonatal apnea/anemia, neonatal ichthyosis, placental disorder/death, undescended testicle and 5 cases of premature birth). In the 126 prospectively reported cases where conception occurred after the last dose of acitretin only, 43 cases involved conception at least 1 year but less than 2 years after the last dose. There were 3 reports of abnormal outcomes out of these 43 cases (involving limb malformation, GI tract malformations and premature birth). There were only 4 cases where conception occurred at least 2 years after the last dose but there were no reports of birth defects in these cases.
- There is also a total of 35 retrospectively reported cases where conception occurred at least 1 year after the last dose of etretinate, acitretin or both. From these cases there are 3 reports of birth defects when the conception occurred at least 1 year but less than 2 years after the last dose of acitretin (including heart malformations, Turner's Syndrome, and unspecified congenital malformations) and 4 reports of birth defects when conception occurred 2 or more years after the last dose of acitretin (including foot malformation, cardiac malformations [2 cases] and unspecified neonatal and infancy disorder). There were 3 additional abnormal outcomes in cases where conception occurred 2 or more years after the last dose of etretinate (including chromosome disorder, forearm aplasia, and stillbirth).
- Females who have taken etretinate must continue to follow the contraceptive recommendations for etretinate. Etretinate is no longer marketed in the US; for information, call the manufacturer at 1-800-526-6367.
- Patients should not donate blood during and for at least 3 years following the completion of acitretin therapy because women of childbearing potential must not receive blood from patients being treated with acitretin.

Important information for males taking acitretin – Patients should not donate blood during and for at least 3 years following acitretin therapy because women of childbearing potential must not receive blood from patients being treated with acitretin.

Samples of seminal fluid from 3 male patients treated with acitretin and 6 male patients treated with etretinate have been assayed for the presence of acitretin. The maximum concentration of acitretin observed in the seminal fluid of these men was 12.5 ng/mL. Assuming an ejaculate volume of 10 mL, the amount of drug transferred in semen would be 125 ng, which is 1/200,000 of a single 25 mg capsule. Thus, although it appears that residual acitretin in seminal fluid poses little, if any, risk to a fetus while a male patient is taking the drug or after it is discontinued, the no-effect limit for teratogenicity is unknown and there is no registry for birth defects associated with acitretin. The available data are as follows:

There have been 25 cases of reported conception when the male partner was taking acitretin. The pregnancy outcome is known in 13 of these 25 cases. Of these, 9 reports were retrospective and 4 were prospective (meaning the pregnancy was reported prior to knowledge of the outcome).

- When acitretin treatment was given at time of conception, there were 5 deliveries of healthy neonates (4 of 5 cases were prospective), 5 spontaneous abortions, and 1 induced abortion.
- When acitretin was discontinued approximately 4 weeks prior to conception, there was 1 induced abortion (with malformation pattern not typical of retinoid embryopathy [bilateral cystic hygromas of neck, hypoplasia of lungs bilateral, pulmonary atresia, VSD with overriding truncus arteriosus]).
- When acitretin was discontinued approximately 6 to 8 months prior to conception, there was 1 spontaneous abortion.

For all patients – An acitretin medication guide must be given to the patient each time acitretin is dispensed, as required by law.

WARNING (cont.)

Hepatotoxicity – Of the 525 patients treated in US clinical trials, 2 had clinical jaundice with elevated serum bilirubin and transaminases considered related to acitretin treatment. Liver function test results in these patients returned to normal after acitretin was discontinued. Two of the 1289 patients treated in European clinical trials developed biopsy-confirmed toxic hepatitis. A second biopsy in one of these patients revealed nodule formation suggestive of cirrhosis. One patient in a Canadian clinical trial of 63 patients developed a 3-fold increase of transaminases. A liver biopsy of this patient showed mild lobular disarray, multifocal hepatocyte loss and mild triaditis of the portal tracts compatible with acute reversible hepatic injury. The patient's transaminase levels returned to normal 2 months after acitretin was discontinued.

The potential of acitretin therapy to induce hepatotoxicity was prospectively evaluated using liver biopsies in an open-label study of 128 patients. Pretreatment and posttreatment biopsies were available for 87 patients. A comparison of liver biopsy findings before and after therapy revealed 49 (58%) patients showed no change, 21 (25%) improved and 14 (17%) patients had a worsening of their liver biopsy status. For 6 patients, the classification changed from class 0 (no pathology) to class I (normal fatty infiltration; nuclear variability and portal inflammation; both mild); for 7 patients, the change was from class I to class II (fatty infiltration, nuclear variability, portal inflammation and focal necrosis; all moderate to severe); and for 1 patient, the change was from class II to class IIIb (fibrosis, moderate to severe). No correlation could be found between liver function test result abnormalities and the change in liver biopsy status, and no cumulative dose relationship was found.

Elevations of AST, ALT, GGT (GGTP) or LDH have occurred in approximately 1 in 3 patients treated with acitretin. Of the 525 patients treated in clinical trials in the US, treatment was discontinued in 20 (3.8%) due to elevated liver function test results. If hepatotoxicity is suspected during treatment with acitretin, the drug should be discontinued and the etiology further investigated.

Ten of 652 patients treated in US clinical trials of etretinate, of which acitretin is the active metabolite, had clinical or histologic hepatitis considered to be possibly or probably related to etretinate treatment. There have been reports of hepatitis-related deaths worldwide; a few of these patients had received etretinate for 1 month or less before presenting with hepatic symptoms or signs.

Indications

➤*Psoriasis:* For the treatment of severe psoriasis in adults. Because of significant adverse effects associated with its use, acitretin should be prescribed only by physicians knowledgeable in the systemic use of retinoids. In females of reproductive potential, acitretin should be reserved for nonpregnant patients who are unresponsive to other therapies or whose clinical condition contraindicates the use of other treatments.

Most patients experience relapse of psoriasis after discontinuing therapy. Subsequent courses, when clinically indicated, have produced results similar to the initial course of therapy.

➤*Off-label uses:* Darier's disease, palmoplantar pustulosis, lichen planus (30 mg/day for 4 weeks, titrated to 10 to 50 mg/day for 12 weeks total); children with lamellar ichthyosis, non-bullous, and bullous ichthyosiform erythroderma, Sjogren-Larsson syndrome (0.47 mg/kg/day); additional studies indicate mild to marked improvement in lichen sclerosus et atrophicus of the vulva and palmoplantar lichen nitidus.

Administration and Dosage

➤*General dosing considerations:* Individualization of dosage is required to achieve maximum therapeutic response while minimizing adverse reactions.

➤*Adults:*

Psoriasis –

Initial dosage: 25 or 50 mg/day, given as a single dose with the main meal.

Maintenance dosage: 25 to 50 mg/day may be given dependent upon an individual patient's response to initial treatment. Relapses may be treated as outlined for initial therapy.

Concomitant therapy: When acitretin is used with phototherapy, the prescriber should decrease the phototherapy dose, dependent on the patient's individual response.

Females who have taken etretinate (*Tegison*) must continue to follow the contraceptive recommendations for etretinate.

➤*Renal function impairment:* Acitretin is contraindicated in patients with severely impaired kidney function.

➤*Hepatic function impairment:* Acitretin is contraindicated in patients with severely impaired liver function.

➤*Administration:* Give as a single dose with the main meal.

➤*Storage/Stability:* Store between 15° and 25°C (59° and 77°F). Protect from light. Avoid exposure to high temperatures and humidity after the bottle is opened.

Actions

➤*Pharmacology:* The mechanism of action of acitretin is unknown.

➤*Pharmacokinetics:*

Absorption – Oral absorption of acitretin is optimal when given with food. For this reason, acitretin was given with food in all of the following studies. After administration of a single 50 mg oral dose of acitretin to 18 healthy

ACITRETIN — ORAL

subjects, maximum plasma concentrations ranged from 196 to 728 ng/mL (mean: 416 ng/mL) and were achieved in 2 to 5 hours (mean: 2.7 hours). The oral absorption of acitretin is linear and proportional with increasing doses from 25 to 100 mg. Approximately 72% (range: 47% to 109%) of the administered dose was absorbed after a single 50 mg dose of acitretin was given to 12 healthy subjects.

Distribution – Acitretin is more than 99.9% bound to plasma proteins, primarily albumin.

Metabolism – Following oral absorption, acitretin undergoes extensive metabolism and interconversion by simple isomerization to its 13-cis form (cis-acitretin). The formation of cis-acitretin relative to parent compound is not altered by dose or fed/fast conditions of oral administration of acitretin. Both parent compound and isomer are further metabolized into chain-shortened breakdown products and conjugates which are excreted. Following multiple-dose administration of acitretin, steady-state concentrations of acitretin and cis-acitretin in plasma are achieved within approximately 3 weeks.

Excretion – The chain-shortened metabolites and conjugates of acitretin and cis-acitretin are ultimately excreted in the feces (34% to 54%) and urine (16% to 53%). The terminal elimination half-life of acitretin following multiple-dose administration is 49 hours (range 33 to 96 hours), and that of cis-acitretin under the same conditions is 63 hours (range 28 to 157 hours). The accumulation ratio of the parent compound is 1.2; that of cis-acitretin is 6.6.

Special populations –

Renal function impairment: Plasma concentrations of acitretin were significantly lower (59.3%) in end-stage renal failure subjects (n = 6) when compared to age-matched controls, following single 50 mg oral doses. Acitretin was not removed by hemodialysis in these subjects.

Elderly: In a multiple-dose study in healthy young (n = 6) and elderly (n = 8) subjects, a 2-fold increase in acitretin plasma concentrations were seen in elderly subjects, although the elimination half-life did not change.

Psoriasis: In an 8-week study of acitretin pharmacokinetics in patients with psoriasis, mean steady-state trough concentrations of acitretin increased in a dose proportional manner with dosages ranging from 10 to 50 mg daily. Acitretin plasma concentrations were nonmeasurable (less than 4 ng/mL) in all patients 3 weeks after cessation of therapy.

Contraindications

Pregnancy *Category X.* Severely impaired liver or kidney function; chronic abnormally elevated blood lipid values.

An increased risk of hepatitis has been reported to result from combined use of methotrexate and etretinate. Consequently, the combination of methotrexate with acitretin is also contraindicated.

Since both acitretin and tetracyclines can cause increased intracranial pressure, their combined use is contraindicated.

Acitretin is contraindicated in cases of hypersensitivity to the preparation (acitretin or excipients) or to other retinoids.

Warnings/Precautions

➤*Pancreatitis:* Lipid elevations occur in 25% to 50% of patients treated with acitretin. Triglyceride increases sufficient to be associated with pancreatitis are much less common, although fatal fulminant pancreatitis has been reported. There have been rare reports of pancreatitis during acitretin therapy in the absence of hypertriglyceridemia.

➤*Pseudotumor cerebri:* Acitretin and other retinoids administered orally have been associated with cases of pseudotumor cerebri (benign intracranial hypertension). Some of these events involved concomitant use of isotretinoin and tetracyclines. However, the event seen in a single acitretin patient was not associated with tetracycline use. Early signs and symptoms include papilledema, headache, nausea and vomiting and visual disturbances. Patients with these signs and symptoms should be examined for papilledema and, if present, should discontinue acitretin immediately and be referred for neurological evaluation and care. Since both acitretin and tetracyclines can cause increased intracranial pressure, their combined use is contraindicated.

➤*Ophthalmologic effects:* The eyes and vision of 329 patients treated with acitretin were examined by ophthalmologists. The findings included dry eyes (23%), irritation of eyes (9%) and brow and lash loss (5%). The following were reported in less than 5% of patients: Bell's palsy, blepharitis and/or crusting of lids, blurred vision, conjunctivitis, corneal epithelial abnormality, cortical cataract, decreased night vision, diplopia, itchy eyes or eyelids, nuclear cataract, pannus, papilledema, photophobia, posterior subcapsular cataract, recurrent sties and subepithelial corneal lesions.

Any patient treated with acitretin who is experiencing visual difficulties should discontinue the drug and undergo ophthalmologic evaluation.

➤*Hyperostosis:* In adults receiving long-term treatment with acitretin, appropriate examinations should be periodically performed in view of possible ossification abnormalities. Because the frequency and severity of iatrogenic bony abnormality in adults is low, periodic radiography is only warranted in the presence of symptoms or long-term use of acitretin. If such disorders arise, the continuation of therapy should be discussed with the patient on the basis of a careful risk/benefit analysis. In clinical trials with acitretin, patients were prospectively evaluated for evidence of development or change in bony abnormalities of the vertebral column, knees, and ankles.

➤*Vertebral results:* Of 380 patients treated with acitretin, 15% had preexisting abnormalities of the spine which showed new changes or progression of preexisting findings. Changes included degenerative spurs, anterior bridging of spinal vertebrae, diffuse idiopathic skeletal hyperostosis, ligament calcification and narrowing and destruction of a cervical disc space.

De novo changes (formation of small spurs) were seen in 3 patients after 1½ to 2½ years.

➤*Skeletal appendicular results:* Six of 128 patients treated with acitretin showed abnormalities in the knees and ankles before treatment that progressed during treatment. In 5 patients, these changes involved the formation of additional spurs or enlargement of existing spurs. The sixth patient had degenerative joint disease which worsened. No patients developed spurs de novo. Clinical complaints did not predict radiographic changes.

➤*Lipids and possible cardiovascular effects:* Blood lipid determinations should be performed before acitretin is administered and again at intervals of 1 to 2 weeks until the lipid response to the drug is established, usually within 4 to 8 weeks. In patients receiving acitretin during clinical trials, 66% and 33% experienced elevation in triglycerides and cholesterol, respectively. Decreased high density lipoproteins (HDL) occurred in 40% of patients. These effects of acitretin were generally reversible upon cessation of therapy.

Patients with an increased tendency to develop hypertriglyceridemia included those with disturbances of lipid metabolism, diabetes mellitus, obesity, increased alcohol intake, or a familial history of these conditions. Because of the risk of hypertriglyceridemia, serum lipids must be more closely monitored in high-risk patients and during long-term treatment.

Hypertriglyceridemia and lowered HDL may increase a patient's cardiovascular risk status. Although no causal relationship has been established, there have been postmarketing reports of acute MI or thromboembolic events in patients on acitretin therapy. In addition, elevation of serum triglycerides to greater than 800 mg/dL has been associated with fatal fulminant pancreatitis. Therefore, dietary modifications, reduction in acitretin dose, or drug therapy should be employed to control significant elevations of triglycerides. If, despite these measures, hypertriglyceridemia and low HDL levels persist, the discontinuation of acitretin should be considered.

➤*Hepatotoxicity:* See the Warning box for more information.

➤*Females of reproductive potential:* See the Warning box for more information.

➤*Psychiatric symptoms:* Depression or other psychiatric symptoms such as aggressive feelings or thoughts of self-harm have been reported. These events, including self-injurious behavior, have been reported in patients taking other systemically administered retinoids, as well as in patients taking acitretin. Since other factors may have contributed to these events, it is not known if they are related to acitretin. Patients should be counseled to stop taking acitretin and notify their prescriber immediately if they experience psychiatric symptoms.

➤*Worsening symptoms:* Patients should be advised that a transient worsening of psoriasis is sometimes seen during the initial treatment period. Patients should be advised that they may have to wait 2 to 3 months before they get the full benefit of acitretin, although some patients may achieve significant improvements within the first 8 weeks of treatment as demonstrated in clinical trials.

➤*Contact lenses:* Patients should be advised that they may experience decreased tolerance to contact lenses during the treatment period and sometimes after treatment has stopped.

➤*Blood donation:* Patients should not donate blood during and for at least 3 years following therapy because acitretin can cause birth defects and women of childbearing potential must not receive blood from patients being treated with acitretin.

➤*Photosensitivity:* Patients should avoid the use of sun lamps and excessive exposure to sunlight (nonmedical UV exposure) because the effects of UV light are enhanced by retinoids.

➤*Phototherapy:* Significantly lower doses of phototherapy are required when acitretin is used because acitretin-induced effects on the stratum corneum can increase the risk of erythema (burning).

➤*Special risk:* Caution is advised in patients with severely impaired liver or kidney function.

➤*Hazardous tasks:* Decreased night vision has been reported with acitretin therapy. Patients should be advised of this potential problem and warned to be cautious when driving or operating any vehicle at night. Visual problems should be carefully monitored.

➤*Pregnancy: Category X.*

Teratogenic – See the Warning box for more information.

Nonteratogenic – In rats dosed at 3 mg/kg/day (approximately one-half the maximum recommended therapeutic dose based on a mg/m^2 comparison), slightly decreased pup survival and delayed incisor eruption were noted. At the next lowest dose tested, 1 mg/kg/day, no treatment-related adverse effects were observed.

➤*Lactation:* Studies on lactating rats have shown that etretinate is excreted in the milk. There is 1 prospective case report where acitretin is reported to be excreted in human milk. Therefore, nursing mothers should not receive acitretin prior to or during nursing because of the potential for serious adverse reactions in nursing infants.

➤*Children:* Safety and efficacy in pediatric patients have not been established. No clinical studies have been conducted in pediatric patients. Ossification of interosseous ligaments and tendons of the extremities, skeletal hyperostoses, decreases in bone mineral density, and premature epiphyseal

ACITRETIN — ORAL

closure have been reported in children taking other systemic retinoids, including etretinate, a metabolite of acitretin. A causal relationship between these effects and acitretin has not been established. While it is not known that these occurrences are more severe or more frequent in children, there is concern in pediatric patients because of the implications for growth potential.

➤*Elderly:* Clinical studies of acitretin did not include sufficient numbers of subjects aged 65 and older to determine whether they respond differently than younger subjects. Other reported clinical experience has not identified differences in responses between the elderly and younger patients. In general, dose selection for an elderly patient should be cautious, usually starting at the low end of the dosing range, reflecting the greater frequency of decreased hepatic, renal, or cardiac function, and of concomitant disease or other drug therapy. A 2-fold increase in acitretin plasma concentrations was seen in healthy elderly subjects compared with young subjects, although the elimination half-life did not change.

➤*Monitoring:* If significant abnormal laboratory results are obtained, either dosage reduction with careful monitoring or treatment discontinuation is recommended, depending on clinical judgment.

Blood sugar – Some patients receiving retinoids have experienced problems in the control of their blood sugar. In addition, new cases of diabetes have been diagnosed during retinoid therapy, including diabetic ketoacidosis. In diabetics, blood sugar levels should be monitored very carefully.

Lipids – In clinical studies, the incidence of hypertriglyceridemia was 66%, hypercholesterolemia was 33% and that of decreased HDL was 40%. Pretreatment and follow-up measurements should be obtained under fasting conditions. It is recommended that these tests be performed weekly or every other week until the lipid response to acitretin has stabilized.

Liver function tests – Elevations of AST, ALT, or LDH were experienced by approximately 1 in 3 patients treated with acitretin. It is recommended that these tests be performed prior to initiation of acitretin therapy, at 1- to 2-week intervals until stable and thereafter at intervals as clinically indicated. Acitretin is contraindicated in patients with severely impaired liver or kidney function and in patients with chronic abnormally elevated blood lipid values.

Drug Interactions

Acitretin Drug Interactions

Precipitant drug	Object drug[a]		Description
Acitretin	Glyburide	↔	Possible potentiation of blood glucose lowering effect of glyburide in 3 of 7 subjects. Careful supervision is recommended.
Acitretin	Methotrexate	⬆	Increased risk of hepatitis with combined use. Concomitant use is contraindicated.
Acitretin	Oral contraceptives (progestin only)	⬇	It has been established that acitretin interferes with the contraceptive effect of microdosed progestin "minipill" preparations. It is not known if there is an interaction with combined oral contraceptives.
Acitretin	Phenytoin	⬆	The protein binding of phenytoin may be decreased.
Ethanol	Acitretin		Etretinate formation has occurred with concomitant ingestion of alcohol and acitretin. Etretinate has a much longer half-life than acitretin (≈ 120 days) which appears to be a result of storage in adipose tissue (see Pharmacokinetics).
Acitretin	Tetracyclines	⬆	Concomitant use is contraindicated due to the increased risk for increased intracranial pressure.
Tetracyclines	Acitretin		
Acitretin	Vitamin A and oral retinoids	⬆	Avoid coadministration because of the increased risk of hypervitaminosis A.
Vitamin A and oral retinoids	Acitretin		

[a] ⬆ = Object drug increased. ⬇ = Object drug decreased. ↔ = Undetermined clinical effect.

Adverse Reactions

Hypervitaminosis A produces a wide spectrum of signs and symptoms primarily of the mucocutaneous, musculoskeletal, hepatic, neuropsychiatric, and central nervous systems. Many of the clinical adverse reactions reported to date with acitretin administration resemble those of the hypervitaminosis A syndrome.

➤*Adverse events/postmarketing reports:* In addition to the events listed in the tables for the clinical trials, the following adverse events have been identified during postapproval use of acitretin. Because these events are reported voluntarily from a population of uncertain size, it is not always possible to reliably estimate their frequency or establish a causal relationship to drug exposure.

Cardiovascular – Acute myocardial infarction, thromboembolism, stroke

CNS – Myopathy with peripheral neuropathy has been reported during acitretin therapy. Both conditions improved with discontinuation of the drug.

Dermatologic – Thinning of the skin, skin fragility and scaling may occur all over the body, particularly on the palms and soles; nail fragility is frequently observed.

GU – Vulvo-vaginitis due to *Candida albicans*.

Psychiatric – Aggressive feelings or suicidal thoughts have been reported. These events, including self-injurious behavior, have been reported in patients taking other systemically administered retinoids, as well as in patients taking acitretin. Since other factors may have contributed to these events, it is not known if they are related to acitretin.

➤*Clinical trials:* During clinical trials with acitretin, 513/525 (98%) of patients reported a total of 3545 adverse events. One-hundred sixteen (22%) patients left studies prematurely, primarily because of adverse experiences involving the mucous membranes and skin. Three (3) patients died. Two of the deaths were not drug related (pancreatic adenocarcinoma and lung cancer); the other patient died of an acute MI, considered remotely related to drug therapy.

In clinical trials, acitretin has been associated with elevations in liver function test results or triglyceride levels and hepatitis.

Frequently Reported Adverse Events During Clinical Trials With Acitretin (N = 525)

Adverse reaction	> 75%	50% to 75%	25% to 50%	10% to 25%
CNS				
Rigors				✓
Dermatologic				
Alopecia		✓		
Dry skin			✓	
Erythematous rash				✓
Hyperesthesia				✓
Nail disorder			✓	
Paresthesia				✓
Paronychia				✓
Pruritus			✓	
Skin atrophy				✓
Skin peeling		✓		
Sticky skin				✓
Mucous membranes				
Cheilitis	✓			
Dry mouth				✓
Epistaxis				✓
Rhinitis			✓	
Musculoskeletal				
Arthralgia				✓
Spinal hyperostosis (progression of existing lesions)				✓
Ophthalmic				
Xerophthalmia				✓

Less Frequent Adverse Events During Clinical Trials with Acitretin (Some Bear No Relationship to Therapy) (N = 525)

Adverse reaction	1% to 10%	< 1%
Cardiovascular		
Chest pain		✓
Cyanosis		✓
Flushing	✓	
Increased bleeding time		✓
Intermittent claudication		✓
Peripheral ischemia		✓
CNS (also see psychiatric)		
Abnormal gait		✓
Headache	✓	
Migraine		✓
Neuritis		✓
Pseudotumor cerebri (intracranial hypertension)		✓
Pain	✓	

ACITRETIN — ORAL

Less Frequent Adverse Events During Clinical Trials with Acitretin (Some Bear No Relationship to Therapy) (N = 525)		
Adverse reaction	1% to 10%	< 1%
Dermatologic		
Abnormal skin odor	✓	
Acne		✓
Abnormal hair texture	✓	
Breast pain		✓
Bullous eruption	✓	
Cyst		✓
Cold/clammy skin	✓	
Dermatitis	✓	
Eczema		✓
Fungal infection		✓
Furunculosis		✓
Hair discoloration		✓
Herpes simplex		✓
Hyperkeratosis		✓
Hypertrichosis		✓
Hypoesthesia		✓
Impaired healing		✓
Increased sweating	✓	
Infection	✓	
Otitis externa		✓
Otitis media		✓
Photosensitivity reaction		✓
Psoriasis aggravated		✓
Psoriasiform rash	✓	
Purpura	✓	
Pyogenic granuloma	✓	
Rash	✓	
Seborrhea	✓	
Skin fissures	✓	
Skin ulceration	✓	
Sunburn	✓	
Scleroderma		✓
Skin nodule		✓
Skin hypertrophy		✓
Skin disorder		✓
Skin irritation		✓
Sweat gland disorder		✓
Urticaria		✓
Verrucae		✓
GI		
Abdominal pain	✓	
Constipation		✓
Diarrhea	✓	
Dyspepsia		✓
Esophagitis		✓
Gastritis		✓
Gastroenteritis		✓
Glossitis		✓
Hemorrhoids		✓
Melena		✓
Nausea		✓
Tenesmus		✓
Tongue disorder		✓
Tongue ulceration		✓
GU		
Abnormal urine		✓
Dysuria		✓
Penis disorder		✓
Hepatic		
Hepatic function abnormal		✓
Hepatitis		✓
Jaundice		✓
Mucous membranes		
Altered saliva		✓
Anal disorder		✓
Gingival bleeding	✓	
Gingivitis	✓	
Gum hyperplasia		✓
Hemorrhage		✓
Increased saliva		✓
Pharyngitis		✓
Stomatitis	✓	
Thirst	✓	
Ulcerative stomatitis	✓	
Musculoskeletal		
Arthritis	✓	
Arthrosis	✓	
Back pain	✓	
Bone disorder		✓
Hypertonia	✓	
Myalgia	✓	
Olecranon bursitis		✓
Osteodynia	✓	
Peripheral joint hyperostosis (progression of existing lesions)	✓	
Spinal hyperostosis (new lesions)		✓
Tendonitis		✓
Ophthalmic		
Abnormal/blurred vision		✓
Abnormal lacrimation		✓
Blepharitis	✓	
Chalazion		✓
Conjunctival hemorrhage		✓
Conjunctivitis/irritation	✓	
Corneal epithelial abnormality	✓	
Corneal ulceration		✓
Decreased night vision/night blindness	✓	
Diplopia		✓
Ectropion		✓
Eye abnormality	✓	
Eye pain	✓	
Itchy eyes and lids		✓
Papilledema		✓
Photophobia	✓	
Recurrent sties		✓
Subepithelial corneal lesions		✓
Psychiatric		
Anxiety		✓
Depression	✓	
Dysphonia		✓
Insomnia	✓	
Libido decreased		✓
Nervousness		✓
Somnolence		✓
Reproductive		
Atrophic vaginitis		✓
Leukorrhea		✓
Respiratory		
Coughing		✓
Increased sputum	✓	
Laryngitis		✓
Sinusitis		✓
Special senses		
Ceruminosis		✓
Deafness		✓
Earache		✓
Taste loss		✓
Taste perversion		✓
Tinnitus		✓
Miscellaneous		
Alcohol tolerance		✓
Anorexia	✓	
Dizziness		✓
Edema	✓	
Fatigue	✓	
Fever		✓
Hot flashes	✓	
Increased appetite	✓	
Influenza-like symptoms		✓
Malaise		✓
Moniliasis		✓
Muscle weakness		✓
Weight increase		✓

Lab test abnormalities – Acitretin therapy induces changes in liver function tests in a significant number of patients. Elevations of AST, ALT or LDH were experienced by approximately 1 in 3 patients treated with acitretin. In most patients, elevations were slight to moderate and returned to

ACITRETIN — ORAL

normal either during continuation of therapy or after cessation of treatment. In patients receiving acitretin during clinical trials, 66% and 33% experienced elevation in triglycerides and cholesterol, respectively. Decreased high density lipoproteins (HDL) occurred in 40%. Transient, usually reversible elevations of alkaline phosphatase have been observed.

Abnormal Laboratory Test Results With Acitretin Use During Clinical Trials

Adverse reaction	50% to 75%	25% to 50%	10% to 25%	1% to 10%
Electrolytes				
Increased phosphorus			✓	
Decreased phosphorus				✓
Increased potassium			✓	
Decreased potassium				✓
Increased sodium				✓
Decreased sodium				✓
Increased and decreased magnesium			✓	
Increased and decreased calcium				✓
Increased and decreased chloride				✓
GU				
Acetonuria			✓	
Glycosuria				✓
Hematuria			✓	
Proteinuria				✓
RBC in urine				✓
WBC in urine		✓		
Hematologic				
Increased reticulocytes		✓		
Decreased hematocrit			✓	
Increased bands				✓
Increased basophils				✓
Decreased hemoglobin				✓
Increased eosinophils				✓
Decreased WBC			✓	
Increased haptoglobin			✓	
Increased hematocrit				✓
Increased hemoglobin				✓
Increased neutrophils				✓
Increased WBC			✓	
Increased lymphocytes				✓
Increased monocytes				✓
Decreased haptoglobin				✓
Decreased lymphocytes				✓
Decreased neutrophils				✓
Decreased reticulocytes				✓
Increased or decreased platelets				✓
Increased or decreased RBC				✓
Hepatic				
Increased alkaline phosphatase			✓	
Increased cholesterol		✓		
Increased globulin				✓
Increased direct bilirubin			✓	
Increased total bilirubin				✓
Increased LDH		✓		
Increased AST		✓		
Increased GGTP			✓	
Increased total protein				✓
Increased ALT		✓		
Increased and decreased serum albumin				✓
Decreased HDL cholesterol		✓		
Renal				
Increased BUN				✓
Increased creatinine				✓
Increased uric acid			✓	
Miscellaneous				
Increased CPK		✓		
Decreased fasting blood sugar			✓	
Increased and decreased iron				✓
Increased triglycerides	✓			
Increased fasting blood sugar		✓		
Increased high occult blood			✓	

Overdosage

➤*Symptoms:* Symptoms of overdose are identical to acute hypervitaminosis A (ie, headache and vertigo). The acute oral toxicity (LD_{50}) of acitretin in both mice and rats was greater than 4000 mg/kg.

In one reported case of overdose, a 32-year-old male with Darier's disease took 21 × 25 mg capsules (525 mg single dose). He vomited several hours later but experienced no other ill effects.

➤*Treatment:* In the event of acute overdosage, acitretin must be withdrawn at once.

All female patients of childbearing potential who have taken an overdose of acitretin must have a pregnancy test at the time of overdose and be counseled regarding birth defects and contraceptive use for at least 3 years' duration after the overdose.

Patient Information

➤*Females of reproductive potential:* Acitretin can cause severe birth defects. Female patients must not be pregnant when acitretin therapy is initiated, they must not become pregnant while taking acitretin, and for at least 3 years after stopping acitretin, so that the drug can be eliminated to below a blood concentration that would be associated with an increased incidence of birth defects. Because this threshold has not been established for acitretin in humans and because elimination rates vary among patients, the duration of posttherapy contraception to achieve adequate elimination cannot be calculated precisely.

Females of reproductive potential should also be advised that they must not ingest beverages or products containing ethanol while taking acitretin and for 2 months after acitretin treatment has been discontinued. This allows for elimination of the acitretin which can be converted to etretinate in the presence of alcohol.

Female patients should be advised that any method of birth control can fail, including tubal ligation, and that microdosed progestin "minipill" preparations are not recommended for use with acitretin. Data from 1 patient who received a very low-dosed progestin contraceptive (levonorgestrel 0.03 mg) had a significant increase of the progesterone level after 3 menstrual cycles during acitretin treatment.

Female patients should sign a consent form prior to beginning acitretin therapy.

➤*All patients:* Depression or other psychiatric symptoms such as aggressive feelings or thoughts of self-harm have been reported. These events, including self-injurious behavior, have been reported in patients taking other systemically administered retinoids, as well as in patients taking acitretin. Since other factors may have contributed to these events, it is not known if they are related to acitretin. Patients should be counseled to stop taking acitretin and notify their prescriber immediately if they experience psychiatric symptoms.

Patients should be advised that a transient worsening of psoriasis is sometimes seen during the initial treatment period. Patients should be advised that they may have to wait 2 to 3 months before they get the full benefit of acitretin, although some patients may achieve significant improvements within the first 8 weeks of treatment as demonstrated in clinical trials.

Patients should be advised that they may experience decreased tolerance to contact lenses during the treatment period and sometimes after treatment has stopped.

Patients should not donate blood during and for at least 3 years following therapy because acitretin can cause birth defects and women of childbearing potential must not receive blood from patients being treated with acitretin.

Because of the relationship of acitretin to vitamin A, patients should be advised against taking vitamin A supplements in excess of minimum recommended daily allowances to avoid possible additive toxic effects.

Patients should avoid the use of sun lamps and excessive exposure to sunlight (nonmedical UV exposure) because the effects of UV light are enhanced by retinoids.

Patients should be advised that they must not give their acitretin capsules to any other person.

Second Generation Retinoids

ALITRETINOIN

Rx	**Panretin** (Ligand)	**Gel:** 0.1%	Dehydrated alcohol. In 60 g tubes.

ALITRETINOIN — TOPICAL

Indications

➤*Kaposi sarcoma (KS) cutaneous lesions:* Topical treatment of cutaneous lesions in patients with AIDS-related KS.

➤*Off-label uses:* Treatment of refractory cutaneous T-cell lymphoma.

Administration and Dosage

➤*General dosing considerations:* Do not use occlusive dressings with alitretinoin gel.

➤*Adults:*

Kaposi sarcoma cutaneous lesions –

Initial dosage: Initially apply 2 times per day to cutaneous KS lesions.

Dosage adjustment: The application frequency can be gradually increased to 3 or 4 times/day according to individual lesion tolerance. If application site toxicity occurs, the application frequency can be reduced.

Duration of therapy: A response of KS lesions may be seen as soon as 2 weeks after initiation of therapy, but most patients require longer application. With continued application, further benefit may be attained. Some patients have required over 14 weeks to respond. In clinical trials, alitretinoin gel was applied for up to 96 weeks. Continue alitretinoin gel as long as the patient is deriving benefit.

Discontinuation of therapy: If severe irritation occurs, application of drug can be discontinued for a few days until the symptoms subside.

➤*Preparation for administration:* Alitretinoin is considered a potential teratogen. Follow safe handling procedures when preparing, administering, or dispensing alitretinoin.

➤*Administration:* Apply sufficient gel to cover the lesion with a generous coating. Allow the gel to dry for 3 to 5 minutes before covering with clothing. Because unaffected skin may become irritated, avoid application of the gel to healthy skin surrounding the lesions. In addition, do not apply the gel on or near mucosal surfaces of the body.

Actions

➤*Pharmacology:* Alitretinoin (9-cis-retinoic acid) is a naturally occurring endogenous retinoid that binds to and activates all known intracellular retinoid receptor subtypes (RARα, RARβ, RARγ, RXRα, RXRβ, and RXRγ). Once activated, these receptors function as transcription factors that regulate the expression of genes that control the process of cellular differentiation and proliferation in healthy and neoplastic cells. Alitretinoin inhibits the growth of KS cells in vitro.

➤*Pharmacokinetics:* There is indirect evidence that absorption of 9-cis-retinoic acid is not extensive. Plasma concentrations were evaluated during clinical studies in patients with cutaneous lesions of AIDS-related KS after repeated multiple daily dose application of alitretinoin gel for up to 60 weeks. The range of 9-cis-retinoic acid plasma concentrations in these patients was similar to the range of circulating, naturally occurring 9-cis-retinoic acid plasma concentrations in untreated healthy volunteers.

Although there are no detectable plasma concentrations of 9-cis-retinoic acid metabolites after topical application of alitretinoin gel, in vitro studies indicate that the drug is metabolized to 4-hydroxy-9-cis-retinoic acid and 4-oxo-9-cis-retinoic acid by CYP 2C9, 3A4, 1A1, and 1A2 enzymes. In vivo, 4-oxo-9-cis-retinoic acid is the major circulating metabolite following oral administration of 9-cis-retinoic acid.

Contraindications

Hypersensitivity to retinoids or to any of the ingredients of the product; when systemic anti-KS therapy is required (eg, more than 10 new KS lesions in the prior month, symptomatic lymphedema, symptomatic pulmonary KS, symptomatic visceral involvement).

Warnings/Precautions

➤*Systemic therapy:* Alitretinoin gel is not a systemic therapy; therefore, it cannot treat visceral KS, nor prevent the development of new KS lesions where it has not been applied. Alitretinoin is not indicated when systemic anti-KS therapy is required (see Contraindications). There is no experience to date using alitretinoin gel with systemic anti-KS treatment.

➤*Response:* In the clinical trials, responses were seen as early as 2 weeks; however, most patients required 4 to 8 weeks of treatment, and some patients did not experience significant improvement until 14 weeks or more of treatment. The cumulative percentage of patients who achieved a response was less than 1% at 2 weeks, 10% at 4 weeks, and 28% at 8 weeks.

➤*Cutaneous T-cell lymphoma:* Alitretinoin gel is indicated for topical treatment of KS. Patients with cutaneous T-cell lymphoma were less tolerant of topical alitretinoin gel; 5 of 7 patients had 6 episodes of treatment-limiting toxicities (grade 3 dermal irritation) with alitretinoin gel (0.01% or 0.05%).

➤*Photosensitivity:* Retinoids as a class have been associated with photosensitivity. There were no reports of photosensitivity associated with the use of alitretinoin gel in clinical studies. Nonetheless, because in vitro data indicate that 9-cis-retinoic acid may have a weak photosensitizing effect, advise patients to minimize exposure of treated areas to sunlight and sunlamps during the use of alitretinoin gel.

➤*Pregnancy: Category D.* Alitretinoin gel could cause fetal harm if significant absorption were to occur in a pregnant woman. 9-cis-retinoic-acid is teratogenic in rabbits and mice. An increased incidence of fused sternebrae, and limb and craniofacial defects occurred in rabbits given oral doses of 0.5 mg/kg/day (about 5 times the estimated daily human topical dose on a mg/m^2 basis) during the period of organogenesis. Oral 9-cis-retinoic acid also was embryocidal, as indicated by early resorptions and postimplantation loss when it was given to rabbits during the period of organogenesis at doses of 1.5 mg/kg/day and to rats at doses of 5 mg/kg/day. It is not known whether topical alitretinoin gel can modulate endogenous 9-cis-retinoic acid levels in a pregnant woman nor whether systemic exposure is increased by application to ulcerated lesions or by duration of treatment. There are no adequate and well-controlled studies in pregnant women. If alitretinoin gel is used during pregnancy, or if the patient becomes pregnant while taking the drug, apprise the patient of the potential hazard to the fetus. Advise women of childbearing potential to avoid becoming pregnant.

➤*Lactation:* It is not known whether alitretinoin or its metabolites are excreted in breast milk. Because of the potential for adverse reactions from alitretinoin gel in nursing infants, mothers should discontinue nursing prior to using the drug.

➤*Children:* Safety and efficacy in children have not been established.

Drug Interactions

➤*DEET:* Do not use products that contain DEET (N,N-diethyl-m-toluamide), a common component of insect repellent products, while using alitretinoin gel. Animal toxicology studies showed increased DEET toxicity when DEET was included as part of the formulation.

Adverse Reactions

Adverse events associated with the use of alitretinoin gel in patients with AIDS-related KS occurred almost exclusively at the site of application. The dermal toxicity begins as erythema; with continued application, erythema may increase and edema may develop. Dermal toxicity may become treatment-limiting, with intense erythema, edema, and vesiculation. Adverse events are usually mild to moderate in severity; they led to withdrawal from the study in only 7% of the patients. Severe local (application site) skin adverse events occurred in about 10% of patients in the US study (vs 0% in the control group).

Alitretinoin Application Site Reactions (≥ 5%)

Adverse reaction	Study 1		Study 2	
	Alitretinoin gel (n = 134)	Vehicle gel (n = 134)	Alitretinoin gel (n = 36)	Vehicle gel (n = 46)
Rash (eg, erythema, scaling, irritation, redness, rash, dermatitis)	77	11	25	4
Pain (eg, burning, pain)	34	7	0	4
Pruritus (eg, itching)	11	4	8	4
Exfoliative dermatitis (eg, flaking, peeling, desquamation, exfoliation)	9	2	3	0
Skin disorder (eg, excoriation, cracking, scabbing, crusting, drainage, eschar, fissure, oozing)	8	1	0	0
Paresthesia (eg, stinging, tingling)	3	0	22	7
Edema (eg, swelling, inflammation)	8	3	3	0

Overdosage

Systemic toxicity following acute overdosage with topical application of alitretinoin gel is unlikely because of limited systemic plasma levels observed with normal therapeutic doses. There is no specific antidote for overdosage.

Patient Information

Advise patients against applying gel on or near mucosal surfaces of the body such as eyes, nostrils, mouth, lips, vagina, tip of the penis, rectum, or anus.

Advise patients against using insect repellents containing DEET or other products containing DEET while using alitretinoin.

Instruct patients to keep out of reach of children.

Product contains alcohol; keep away from open flame.

Do not administer to patients who are pregnant or breastfeeding. Instruct patients to take precautions to avoid becoming pregnant while using altretinoin. If the patient is pregant, thinking of becoming pregnant, or breastfeeding, advise them to speak with their health care provider for more information.

Inform patients that KS lesions can appear and affect other parts of their body, including internal organs (eg, lungs and intestines). Advise patients to

ALITRETINOIN — TOPICAL

regularly consult their health care provider about the status of their KS disease, especially if they note changes.

Alitretinoin does not treat lung or intestinal KS.

Alitretinoin does not prevent the appearance of new KS lesions or the increased growth of KS lesions not treated with alitretinoin.

Alitretinoin does not treat extremity swelling associated with KS.

Instruct patients to avoid applying the gel to areas of healthy skin around a KS lesion. Exposure of healthy skin to alitretinoin may cause unnecessary irritation or redness.

Instruct patients to avoid showering, bathing, or swimming for at least 3 hours after any application, if possible.

Instruct patients to avoid covering the KS lesions treated with gel with any bandage or material other than loose clothing.

Instruct patients to avoid prolonged exposure of the treated area to sunlight or other ultraviolet light (eg, tanning lamps).

Instruct patients to avoid the use of other topical products on treated KS lesions. Mineral oil may be used between alitretinoin applications in order to help prevent excessive dryness or itching. Mineral oil should not be applied for at least 2 hours before or after the application of alitretinoin.

Instruct patients to avoid scratching the treated areas.

Instruct patients to always use the cap to close the tube tightly after each use.

TAZAROTENE

Rx	**Tazorac** (Allergan)	**Cream:** 0.05%	1% benzyl alcohol, EDTA, medium chain triglycerides, mineral oil. In 15, 30, and 60 g.
Rx	**Avage** (Allergan)	**Cream:** 0.1%	1% benzyl alcohol, EDTA, medium chain triglycerides, mineral oil. In 15 and 30 g.
Rx	**Tazorac** (Allergan)		1% benzyl alcohol, EDTA, medium chain triglycerides, mineral oil. In 15, 30, and 60 g.
Rx	**Tazorac** (Allergan)	**Gel:** 0.05%	1% benzyl alcohol, EDTA. In 30 and 100 g.
		0.1%	1% benzyl alcohol, EDTA. In 30 and 100 g.

TAZAROTENE — TOPICAL

Indications

➤*Tazorac cream:*

Acne – Topical treatment of patients with acne vulgaris (0.1% only).

Psoriasis – For the topical treatment of patients with plaque psoriasis.

➤*Tazorac gel:*

Acne – Topical treatment of patients with facial acne vulgaris of mild to moderate severity (0.1% only).

The efficacy of tazarotene in the treatment of acne previously treated with other retinoids or resistant to oral antibiotics has not been established.

Psoriasis – Topical treatment of patients with stable plaque psoriasis of up to 20% body surface area involvement.

➤*Avage:*

Wrinkling, hyper- and hypopigmentation, lentigines – As an adjunctive agent for use in the mitigation (palliation) of facial fine wrinkling, facial mottled hyper- and hypopigmentation, and benign facial lentigines in patients who use comprehensive skin care and sunlight avoidance programs. This product does not eliminate or prevent wrinkles, repair sun-damaged skin, reverse photoaging, or restore more youthful or younger skin.

- *Avage* has not demonstrated a mitigating effect on significant signs of chronic sunlight exposure such as coarse or deep wrinkling, tactile roughness, telangiectasia, skin laxity, keratinocytic atypia, melanocytic atypia, or dermal elastosis.
- *Avage* should be used under medical supervision as an adjunct to a comprehensive skin care and sunlight avoidance program that includes the use of effective sunscreens (minimum SPF 15) and protective clothing.
- Neither the safety nor the effectiveness of *Avage* for the prevention or treatment of actinic keratoses, skin neoplasms, or lentigo maligna has been established.
- Neither the safety nor the efficacy of using *Avage* daily for greater than 52 weeks has been established, and daily use beyond 52 weeks has not been systematically and histologically investigated in adequate and well-controlled trials.

Administration and Dosage

➤*Adults:*

Acne –

Cream and gel (Tazorac): Cleanse the face gently. After the skin is dry, apply a thin film of tazarotene (2 mg/cm²) once a day in the evening to the skin where acne lesions appear. Use enough to cover the entire affected area.

Psoriasis –

Cream and gel (Tazorac): Apply tazarotene once a day in the evening to psoriatic lesions, using enough (2 mg/cm²) to cover only the lesion with a thin film. The gel should cover no more than 20% of body surface area. If a bath or shower is taken prior to application, dry the skin before applying. If emollients are used, apply them at least 1 hour before *Tazorac* cream. Because unaffected skin may be more susceptible to irritation, carefully avoid application of tazarotene to these areas. It is recommended that treatment start with the 0.05% cream with strength increase to 0.1% if tolerated and medically indicated.

Wrinkling, hyper- and hypopigmentation, lentigines –

Cream (Avage): Apply a pea-sized amount once a day at bedtime to lightly cover the entire face including the eyelids if desired. Facial moisturizers may be used as frequently as desired. Remove any makeup before applying the cream to the face. If the face is washed or a bath or shower is taken prior to application, the skin should be dry before applying the cream. If emollients or moisturizers are used, they can be applied before or after application of tazarotene cream, ensuring that the first cream or lotion has absorbed into the skin and has dried completely.

➤*Children:*

Acne

Cream and Gel (Tazorac):

- *12 years of age or older* – See Adults for dosing.

Psoriasis –

Gel (Tazorac):

- *12 years of age or older* – Apply tazarotene once a day in the evening to psoriatic lesions, using enough (2 mg/cm²) to cover only the lesion with a thin film. The gel should cover no more than 20% of body surface area. If a bath or shower is taken prior to application, dry the skin before applying. Because unaffected skin may be more susceptible to irritation, carefully avoid application of tazarotene to these areas.

➤*Administration:* For topical use only. Not for ophthalmic, oral, or intravaginal use.

Application may cause excessive irritation in the skin of certain sensitive individuals. In cases where it has been necessary to temporarily discontinue therapy or where the dosing has been reduced to a lower concentration (in patients with psoriasis) or to an interval the patient can tolerate, therapy can be resumed, or the drug concentration or frequency of application can be increased as the patient becomes able to tolerate the treatment.

Efficacy has not been established for less than once daily dosing frequencies.

➤*Storage/Stability:*

Tazorac and Avage cream – Store at 25°C (77°F). Excursions are permitted from -5° to 30°C (23° to 86°F).

Gel – Store at 25°C (77°F). Excursion are permitted to 15° to 30°C (59° to 86°F).

Actions

➤*Pharmacology:* Tazarotene is a retinoid prodrug that is converted to its active form, tazarotenic acid, by rapid de-esterification in most biological systems. Tazarotenic acid binds to all 3 members of the retinoic acid receptor (RAR) family (RARα, RARβ and RARγ), but shows relative selectivity for RARβ and RARγ and may modify gene expression. The clinical significance of these findings is unknown.

The mechanism of tazarotene action is not defined. Tazarotene inhibited corneocyte accumulation in rhino mouse skin and cross-linked envelope formation in cultured human keratinocytes. Topical tazarotene blocks induction of mouse epidermal ornithine decarboxylase (ODC) activity, which is associated with cell proliferation and hyperplasia. In cell culture and in vitro models of skin, tazarotene suppresses expression of MRP8, a marker of inflammation present in the epidermis of psoriasis subjects at high levels. In human keratinocyte cultures, it inhibits cornified envelope formation, whose build-up is an element of psoriatic scale. Tazarotene also induces the expression of a gene that may be a growth suppressor in human keratinocytes and that may inhibit epidermal hyperproliferation in treated plaques. The clinical significance of these findings is unknown.

➤*Pharmacokinetics:*

Absorption/Distribution – Following topical application, tazarotene undergoes esterase hydrolysis to form its active metabolite, tazarotinic acid. Little parent compound can be detected in the plasma. Tazarotenic acid is highly bound to plasma proteins (more than 99%).

Cream: In a multiple dose study with a once-daily dose for 14 consecutive days in 9 psoriatic patients, measured doses of tazarotene 0.1% cream were applied to involved skin without occlusion. The C_{max} of tazarotenic acid was

TAZAROTENE — TOPICAL

2.31 ng/mL occurring 8 hours after the final dose, and the AUC_{0-24h} was 31.2 ng•h/mL on day 15 in the 5 patients who were administered clinical doses of 2 mg cream/cm^2.

Tazarotene cream 0.1% was applied once daily to the face (N = 8) or to 15% of body surface area (N = 10) of female patients with moderate to severe acne vulgaris. The mean C_{max} and AUC values of tazarotenic acid peaked at day 15 for both dosing groups during a 29-day treatment period. Mean C_{max} and AUC_{0-24h} values of tazarotenic acid from patients in the 15% body surface area dosing group were more than 10 times higher than those from patients in the face-only dosing group. In the face-only group, the C_{max} and AUC_{0-24h} of tazarotenic acid on day 15 were 0.1 ng/mL and 1.54 ng•h/mL, respectively, whereas in the 15% body surface area dosing group, the C_{max} and AUC_{0-24h} of tazarotenic acid on day 15 were 1.2 ng/mL and 17.01 ng•h/mL, respectively. The steady state pharmacokinetics of tazarotenic acid had been reached by day 8 in the face-only and by day 15 in the 15% body surface area dosing groups.

Tazarotene cream 0.1% was topically applied once daily to the face or to 15% of body surface area over 4 weeks in patients with fine wrinkling and mottled hyperpigmentation. In the "face-only" dosing group, the maximum average C_{max} and AUC_{0-24h} values of tazarotenic acid occurred on day 15 with C_{max} and AUC_{0-24h} of tazarotenic acid being 0.236 ng/mL and 2.44 ng•h/mL, respectively. The mean C_{max} and AUC_{0-24h} values of tazarotenic acid from patients in the 15% body surface area dosing group were approximately 10 times higher than those from patients in the face-only dosing group. The single highest C_{max} throughout the study period was 3.43 ng/mL on day 29 from patients in the 15% body surface area dosing group.

Gel: Studies following a single, topical dose of tazarotene determined that systemic absorption of the total dose was less than 1% without occlusion in psoriatic patients and approximately 5% under occlusion in healthy patients. Another study found the C_{max} and AUC for the 0.1% gel to be 40% higher than the 0.05% gel. Systemic absorption of 2 mg/cm^2 doses of 0.1% gel applied topically without occlusion was less than 1% after 7 days of therapy when applied to 20% of the total body surface area (BSA) of healthy patients and was about 15% after 14 days when applied to approximately 13% of total BSA in psoriatic patients. The results of these in vivo studies refer to the active metabolite only.

An in vitro percutaneous absorption study indicated that about 4% to 5% of the applied dose was in the stratum corneum (tazarotene:metabolite, 5:1) and 2% to 4% was in the viable epidermis-dermis layer (tazarotene:metabolite, 2:1) 24 hours after topical application of the gel.

Metabolism / Excretion – The half-life of the metabolite following topical application of tazarotene is approximately 18 hours and is similar among healthy and psoriatic patients. The parent drug and metabolite are further metabolized and eliminated through urinary and fecal pathways.

Contraindications

Pregnancy; hypersensitivity to any components of the product.

Warnings/Precautions

➤*For external use only:* Apply only to the affected areas. Avoid contact with eyes, eyelids (*Tazorac* only), and mouth. If contact with the eyes occurs, rinse thoroughly with water. The safety of use of tazarotene gel over more than 20% of body surface area has not been established in psoriasis or acne.

➤*Eczematous skin:* Do not use retinoids on eczematous skin, as they may cause severe irritation.

➤*Dermatologic medications and cosmetics:* Avoid those medications and cosmetics that have a strong drying effect. It also is advisable to "rest" a patient's skin until the effects of such preparations subside before use of tazarotene is begun

➤*Photosensitizers (eg, thiazides, tetracyclines, fluoroquinolones, phenothiazines, sulfonamides):* Administer with caution if the patient is also taking drugs known to be photosensitizers because of the increased possibility of augmented photosensitivity.

➤*Discontinue:* If pruritus, burning, skin redness, or peeling is excessive, discontinue until the integrity of the skin is restored, or reduce the dosing to an interval the patient can tolerate. However, efficacy at reduced frequency of application has not been established. Alternatively, patients with psoriasis who are being treated with *Tazorac* 1% cream can be switched to the lower concentration (0.05%).

➤*Weather extremes:* Wind or cold may be more irritating to patients using tazarotene.

➤*Lentigo maligna:* Some facial pigmented lesions are not lentigines, but rather lentigo maligna, a type of melanoma. Facial pigmented lesions of concern should be carefully assessed by a qualified physician (eg, dermatologist) before application of *Avage*. Do not treat lentigo maligna with *Avage*.

➤*Photosensitivity:* Photosensitization (photoallergy or phototoxicity) may occur; therefore, caution patients to take protective measures (ie, sunscreens, protective clothing) against exposure to sunlight or ultraviolet light (eg, tanning beds) until tolerance is determined.

Because of heightened burning susceptibility, avoid exposure to sunlight (including sunlamps) unless deemed medically necessary; in such cases, minimize exposure during the use of tazarotene. Warn patients to use sunscreens (minimum SPF 15) and protective clothing when using tazarotene. Advise patients with sunburn not to use tazarotene until fully recovered. Patients who may have considerable sun exposure because of their occupation and those patients with inherent sensitivity to sunlight should exercise particular caution when using tazarotene.

In human dermal safety studies, tazarotene did not induce allergic contact sensitization, phototoxicity, or photoallergy.

➤*Pregnancy: Category X.* In rabbits, topical tazarotene caused retinoid malformations, including spina bifida, hydrocephaly, and heart anomalies.

As with other retinoids, when tazarotene was given orally to experimental animals, developmental delays were seen in rats, and teratogenic effects and postimplantation loss were observed in rats and rabbits at doses producing 2.1 and 52 times, respectively, the maximum AUC_{0-24h} in patients treated with 2 mg/cm^2 of tazarotene cream 0.1% over 15% body surface area for fine wrinkling and mottled hyperpigmentation.

In a study of the effect of oral tazarotene on fertility and early embryonic development in rats, decreased number of implantation sites, decreased litter size, decreased number of live fetuses, and decreased fetal body weights, all classic developmental effects of retinoids, were observed when female rats were administered 2 mg/kg/day from 15 days before mating through gestation day 7. A low incidence of retinoid-related malformations at that dose were reported to be related to treatment. That dose produced an AUC_{0-24h} that was 6.7 times the maximum AUC_{0-24h} in patients treated with 2 mg/cm^2 of tazarotene cream 0.1% over 15% body surface area for signs of fine wrinkling and mottled hyperpigmentation.

Tazarotene is contraindicated in women who are or may become pregnant. If this drug is used during pregnancy or if the patient becomes pregnant while taking this drug, discontinue treatment and apprise the patient of the potential hazard to the fetus. Warn women of childbearing potential of the potential risk and to use adequate birth-control measures when using tazarotene. Consider the possibility that a woman of childbearing potential is pregnant at the time of institution of therapy. Obtain a negative result for a pregnancy test having a sensitivity down to at least 50 mIU/mL for human chorionic gonadotropin (hCG) within 2 weeks prior to tazarotene therapy, which should begin during a normal menstrual period.

Fertility impairment – There was a significant decrease in the number of estrous stages and an increase in developmental effects at oral doses up to 2 mg/kg/day. That dose produced an AUC_{0-24h} that was 6.7 times the maximum AUC_{0-24h} in patients treated with 2 mg/cm^2 of tazarotene cream 0.1% over 15% body surface area for signs of fine wrinkling and mottled hyperpigmentation.

➤*Lactation:* Tazarotene is excreted in breast milk of rats. It is not known whether this drug is excreted in human milk. Exercise caution when tazarotene is administered to a breast-feeding woman.

➤*Children:*

Tazorac – The safety and efficacy of tazarotene cream have not been established in patients with psoriasis under the age of 18 years or in patients with acne under the age of 12 years.

Avage – The safety and efficacy of tazarotene cream have not been established in patients under the age of 17 years with facial fine wrinkling, facial mottled hypo- and hyperpigmentation, and benign facial lentigines.

Gel – The safety and efficacy of tazarotene have not been established in pediatric patients under the age of 12 years.

Drug Interactions

Concomitant dermatologic medications and cosmetics that have a strong drying effect should be avoided. It is also advisable to "rest" a patient's skin until the effects of such preparations subside before use of tazarotene is begun.

Adverse Reactions

The most frequent adverse events with tazarotene are limited to the skin and include the following:

➤*Gel:*

Acne – Desquamation, burning/stinging, dry skin, erythema, pruritus (10% to 30%); irritation, skin pain, fissuring, localized edema, skin discoloration (1% to 10%).

Psoriasis – Pruritus, burning/stinging, erythema, worsening of psoriasis, irritation, skin pain (10% to 30%); rash, desquamation, irritant contact dermatitis, skin inflammation, fissuring, bleeding, dry skin (1% to 10%). In general, the incidence of adverse events with 0.05% gel was 2% to 5% lower than that seen with 0.1% gel.

Increases in psoriasis worsening and sun-induced erythema were noted in some patients over months 4 to 12, as compared with the first 3 months of a 1-year study.

➤*Tazorac cream:*

Acne – Desquamation, dry skin, erythema, burning sensation (10% to 30%); pruritus, irritation, face pain, stinging (1% to 5%).

Psoriasis – Pruritus, erythema, burning (10% to 23%); irritation, desquamation, stinging, contact dermatitis, dermatitis, eczema, worsening of psoriasis, skin pain, rash, hypertriglyceridemia, dry skin, skin inflammation, peripheral edema (more than 1% to less than 10%).

Tazorac 0.1% cream was associated with a somewhat greater degree of local irritation than the 0.05% cream. In general, the rates of irritation adverse events reported during psoriasis studies with 0.1% cream were 1% to 4% higher than those reported for the 0.05% cream.

➤*Avage* cream: Desquamation (40%); erythema (34%); burning sensation (26%); dry skin (16%); skin irritation, pruritus (10%); irritant contact dermatitis (8%); stinging, acne, rash (3%); cheilitis (1%). A few patients reported adverse events at week 0; however, for patients who were treated with *Avage*, the highest number of new reports for each adverse event was at week 2. When combining data from the 2 pivotal studies, 5.3% of patients in the tazarotene group and 0.9% of patients in the vehicle group discontinued because of adverse events. Overall, 3.5% of patients in the tazarotene group

TAZAROTENE — TOPICAL

and 2.8% of patients in the vehicle group reported adverse events (including edema, irritation, and inflammation) directly related to the eye or eyelid. The majority of these conditions were mild.

Overdosage

➤*Symptoms:* Excessive topical use of tazarotene may lead to marked redness, peeling, or discomfort.

Oral ingestion of the drug may lead to the same adverse effects as those associated with excessive oral intake of vitamin A (hypervitaminosis A) or other retinoids.

➤*Treatment:* If oral ingestion occurs, monitor the patient and administer appropriate supportive measures as necessary. Refer to General Management of Acute Overdosage.

Patient Information

Do not use tazarotene if you are pregnant, plan to become pregnant, or may become pregnant because of the potential harm to the unborn child. Talk with your doctor about effective birth control if you are a woman who is able to become pregnant. If you become pregnant while using tazarotene, contact your physician immediately.

Do not use tazarotene if you have a sunburn, eczema, or other continuing skin conditions.

Do not use tazarotene if you are sensitive to sunlight.

For best results, if emollients or moisturizers are used, they can be applied before or after tazarotene cream, ensuring that the first cream or lotion has absorbed into the skin and dried completely.

Avoid sunlight and other medicines that may increase your sensitivity to sunlight. Avoidance of excessive sun exposure and the use of sunscreens with protective measures (hat, visor) are recommended. In the morning, apply a moisturizing sunscreen SPF 15 or greater.

Refer to patient package insert for additional patient information.

➤*Avage:* Apply only a small, pea-sized amount (about ¼ inch or 5 mm diameter) of *Avage* to your face at one time.

Avage does not remove or prevent wrinkles or repair sun-damaged skin.

➤*Tazorac:* Apply a thin film to your psoriasis areas once a day in the evening.

Usually your acne will begin to improve in about 4 weeks. Continue to use *Tazorac* for up to 12 weeks as directed by your doctor.

REXINOIDS

BEXAROTENE

Rx	**Targretin** (Eisai Inc.)	**Gel; topical:** 1%	Dehydrated alcohol. In 60 g.

BEXAROTENE — TOPICAL

Indications

➤*Cutaneous T-cell lymphoma:* For the topical treatment of cutaneous lesions in patients with cutaneous T-cell lymphoma (CTCL) (Stage IA and IB) who have refractory or persistent disease after other therapies or who have not tolerated other therapies.

Administration and Dosage

➤*General dosing considerations:* Do not use occlusive dressings with bexarotene.

➤*Adults:*

Cutaneous T-cell lymphoma –

Initial dosage: Initially apply once every other day for the first week.

Dosage titration: Increase the application frequency at weekly intervals to once daily, then twice daily, then 3 times daily and finally 4 times daily according to individual lesion tolerance.

Maintenance dosage: Generally, patients were able to maintain a dosing frequency of 2 to 4 times/day. Most responses were seen at dosing frequencies of 2 times/day and higher.

Dosage adjustment: If application site toxicity occurs, the application frequency can be reduced.

Duration of therapy: A response may be seen as soon as 4 weeks after initiation of therapy, but most patients require longer application. Continue bexarotene as long as the patient is deriving benefit.

Discontinuation of therapy: If severe irritation occurs, application of drug can be temporarily discontinued for a few days until the symptoms subside.

➤*Administration:* Bexarotene is a topical therapy and is not intended for systemic use.

Apply sufficient gel to cover the lesion with a generous coating. Allow the gel to dry before covering with clothing. Because unaffected skin may become irritated, avoid application of the gel to normal skin surrounding the lesions. In addition, do not apply the gel near mucosal surfaces of the body.

➤*Storage/Stability:* Store at 25°C (77°F); excursions are permitted to 15° to 30°C (59° to 86°F) (see USP). Avoid exposing to high temperatures and humidity after the tube is opened. Protect from light.

Actions

➤*Pharmacology:* Bexarotene selectively binds and activates retinoid X receptor subtypes (RXRα, RXRβ, RXRγ). RXRs can form heterodimers with various receptor partners such as retinoic acid receptors (RARs), vitamin D receptor, thyroid receptor, and peroxisome proliferator activator receptors (PPARs). Once activated, these receptors function as transcription factors that regulate the expression of genes that control cellular differentiation and proliferation. Bexarotene inhibits the growth in vitro of some tumor cell lines of hematopoietic and squamous cell origin. It also induces tumor regression in vivo in some animal models. The exact mechanism of action of bexarotene in the treatment of CTCL is unknown.

➤*Pharmacokinetics:*

Absorption/Distribution – Plasma concentrations of bexarotene were determined during clinical studies in patients with CTCL or following repeated single or multiple-daily dose applications of bexarotene 1% for up to 132 weeks. Plasma bexarotene concentrations were generally less than 5 ng/mL and did not exceed 55 ng/mL. However, only 2 patients with very intense dosing regimens (greater than 40% BSA lesions and 4 times daily dosing) were sampled. Plasma bexarotene concentrations and the frequency of detecting quantifiable plasma bexarotene concentrations increased with increasing percent body surface area treated and increasing quantity of bexarotene applied. The sporadically observed and generally low plasma bexarotene concentrations indicated that, in patients receiving doses of low-to-moderate intensity, there is a low potential for significant plasma concentrations following repeated application of bexarotene. Bexarotene is highly bound (greater than 99%) to plasma proteins. The plasma proteins to which bexarotene binds have not been elucidated, and the ability of bexarotene to displace drugs bound to plasma proteins and the ability of drugs to displace bexarotene binding have not been studied (see Precautions). The uptake of bexarotene by organs or tissues has not been evaluated.

Metabolism – Four bexarotene metabolites have been identified in plasma following oral administration of bexarotene: 6- and 7-hydroxy-bexarotene and 6- and 7-oxo-bexarotene. In vitro studies suggest that cytochrome P450 3A4 is the major cytochrome P450 responsible for formation of the oxidative metabolites and that the oxidative metabolites may be glucuronidated. The oxidative metabolites are active in in vitro assays of retinoid receptor activation, but the relative contribution of the parent and any metabolites to the efficacy and safety of bexarotene gel is unknown.

Excretion – The renal elimination of bexarotene and its metabolites was examined in patients with type 2 diabetes mellitus following oral administration of bexarotene. Neither bexarotene nor its metabolites were excreted in urine in appreciable amounts.

Contraindications

Hypersensitivity to bexarotene or other components of the product.

Warnings/Precautions

➤*Protein binding:* Bexarotene is highly bound (greater than 99%) to plasma proteins. The plasma proteins to which bexarotene binds have not been elucidated, and the ability of bexarotene to displace drugs bound to plasma proteins and the ability of drugs to displace bexarotene binding have not been studied.

➤*Renal function impairment:* No formal studies have been conducted with bexarotene in patients with renal insufficiency. Urinary elimination of bexarotene and its known metabolites is a minor excretory pathway for bexarotene (less than 1% of an orally administered dose), but because renal insufficiency can result in significant protein binding changes, and bexarotene is more than 99% protein bound, pharmacokinetics may be altered in patients with renal insufficiency.

➤*Hepatic function impairment:* No specific studies have been conducted with bexarotene in patients with hepatic insufficiency. Because less than 1% of the dose of oral bexarotene is excreted in the urine unchanged and there is in vitro evidence of extensive hepatic contribution to bexarotene elimination, hepatic impairment would be expected to lead to greatly decreased clearance.

➤*Special risk:* Bexarotene should be used with caution in patients with a known hypersensitivity to other retinoids. No clinical instances of cross-reactivity have been noted.

➤*Photosensitivity:* Retinoids as a class have been associated with photosensitivity. In vitro assays indicate that bexarotene is a potential photosensitizing agent. There were no reports of photosensitivity in patients in the clinical studies. Patients should be advised to minimize exposure to sunlight and artificial ultraviolet light during the use of bexarotene.

➤*Pregnancy: Category X.* Bexarotene 1% may cause fetal harm when administered to a pregnant woman.

Bexarotene must not be given to a pregnant woman or a woman who intends to become pregnant. If a woman becomes pregnant while taking bexarotene, bexarotene must be stopped immediately and the woman given appropriate counseling.

Bexarotene caused malformations when administered orally to pregnant rats during days 7 to 17 of gestation. Developmental abnormalities included incomplete ossification at 4 mg/kg/day and cleft palate, depressed eye bulge/microphthalmia, and small ears at 16 mg/kg/day. At doses greater than 10 mg/kg/day, bexarotene caused developmental mortality. The no-effect oral dose in rats was 1 mg/kg/day. Plasma bexarotene concentrations in patients

BEXAROTENE — TOPICAL

with CTCL applying bexarotene 1% were generally less than one hundredth the C_{max} associated with dysmorphogenesis in rats, although some patients had C_{max} levels that were approximately one-eighth the concentration associated with dysmorphogenesis in rats.

Women of childbearing potential should be advised to avoid becoming pregnant when bexarotene is used. The possibility that a woman of childbearing potential is pregnant at the time therapy is instituted should be considered. A negative pregnancy test (eg, serum beta-human chorionic gonadotropin, beta-HCG) with a sensitivity of at least 50 mIU/L should be obtained within 1 week prior to bexarotene therapy, and the pregnancy test must be repeated at monthly intervals while the patient remains on bexarotene. Effective contraception must be used for 1 month prior to the initiation of therapy, during therapy and for at least 1 month following discontinuation of therapy; it is recommended that 2 reliable forms of contraception be used simultaneously unless abstinence is the chosen method. Male patients with sexual partners who are pregnant, possibly pregnant, or who could become pregnant must use condoms during sexual intercourse while applying bexarotene and for at least 1 month after the last dose of drug. Bexarotene therapy should be initiated on the second or third day of a normal menstrual period. No more than a 1 month supply of bexarotene should be given to the patient so that the results of pregnancy testing can be assessed and counseling regarding avoidance of pregnancy and birth defects can be reinforced.

➤*Lactation:* It is not known whether bexarotene is excreted in human milk. Because many drugs are excreted in human milk and because of the potential for serious adverse reactions in nursing infants from bexarotene, a decision should be made whether to discontinue nursing or to discontinue the drug, taking into account the importance of the drug to the mother.

➤*Children:* Safety and effectiveness in pediatric patients have not been established.

➤*Elderly:* Of the total patients with CTCL in clinical studies of bexarotene, 62% were younger than 65 years of age, and 38% were ≥ 65 years of age. No overall differences in safety were observed between patients ≥ 65 years and younger patients, but greater sensitivity of some older individuals to bexarotene cannot be ruled out. Responses to bexarotene were observed across all age group decades, without preference for any individual age group decade.

Drug Interactions

➤*Vitamin A:* In clinical studies, patients were advised to limit vitamin A intake to ≤ 15,000 IU/day. Because of the relationship of bexarotene to vitamin A, patients should be advised to limit vitamin A supplements to avoid potential additive toxic effects.

➤*DEET:* Patients who are applying bexarotene should not concurrently use products that contain DEET (N,N-diethyl-m-toluamide), a common component of insect repellent products. An animal toxicology study showed increased DEET toxicity when DEET was included as part of the formulation.

➤*CYP-450 system:* On the basis of the metabolism of bexarotene by cytochrome P450 3A4, concomitant ketoconazole, itraconazole, erythromycin and grapefruit juice could increase bexarotene plasma concentrations. Similarly, based on data that gemfibrozil increases bexarotene concentrations following oral bexarotene administration, concomitant gemfibrozil could increase bexarotene plasma concentrations. However, due to the low systemic exposure to bexarotene after low to moderately intense gel regimens (see Pharmacokinetics), increases that occur are unlikely to be of sufficient magnitude to result in adverse effects.

Adverse Reactions

The safety of bexarotene has been assessed in clinical studies of 117 patients with CTCL who received bexarotene for up to 172 weeks. In the multicenter open-label study, 50 patients with CTCL received bexarotene for up to 98 weeks. The mean duration of therapy for these 50 patients was 199 days. The most common adverse events reported with an incidence at the application site of at least 10% in patients with CTCL were rash, pruritus, skin disorder, and pain.

Adverse events leading to dose reduction or study drug discontinuation in at least 2 patients were rash, contact dermatitis, and pruritus.

Of the 49 patients (98%) who experienced any adverse event, most experienced events categorized as mild (9 patients, 18%) or moderate (27 patients, 54%). There were 12 patients (24%) who experienced at least 1 moderately severe adverse event. The most common moderately severe events were rash (7 patients, 14%) and pruritus (3 patients, 6%). Only 1 patient (2%) experienced a severe adverse event (rash).

In the patients with CTCL receiving bexarotene, adverse events reported regardless of relationship to study drug at an incidence of ≥ 5% are presented below.

A similar safety profile for bexarotene was demonstrated in the Phase I to II program. For the 67 patients enrolled in the Phase I to II program, the mean duration of treatment was 436 days (range 12 to 1203 days). As in the multicenter study, the most common adverse events regardless of relationship to study drug in the Phase I to II program were rash (78%), pain (40%), and pruritus (40%).

Adverse Reactions[a] for All Application Frequencies of Bexarotene Topical Gel in The Multicenter CTCL Study (≥ 5%)

Adverse reaction	All adverse reactions (n = 50)	Application site adverse reactions (n = 50)
Cardiovascular		
Edema	5 (10%)	0
Peripheral edema	3 (6%)	0
CNS		
Paresthesia	3 (6%)	3 (6%)
Dermatologic		
Contact dermatitis[b]	7 (14%)	4 (8%)
Exfoliative dermatitis	3 (6%)	0
Pruritus[c]	18 (36%)	9 (18%)
Rash[d]	36 (72%)	28 (56%)
Maculopapular rash	3 (6%)	0
Skin disorder (NOS)[e]	13 (26%)	9 (18%)
Sweating	3 (6%)	0
Hematologic/Lymphatic		
Leukopenia	3 (6%)	0
Lymphadenopathy	3 (6%)	0
WBC abnormal	3 (6%)	0
Metabolic/Nutritional		
Hyperlipemia	5 (10%)	0
Respiratory		
Cough increased	3 (6%)	0
Pharyngitis	3 (6%)	0
Miscellaneous		
Asthenia	3 (6%)	0
Headache	7 (14%)	0
Infection	9 (18%)	0
Pain	15 (30%)	9 (18%)

[a] Regardless of association with treatment.
[b] Includes investigator terms such as contact dermatitis, irritant contact dermatitis, irritant dermatitis.
[c] Includes investigator terms such as pruritus, itching, itching of lesion.
[d] Includes investigator terms such as erythema, scaling, irritation, redness, rash, dermatitis.
[e] Includes investigator terms such as skin inflammation, excoriation, sticky or tacky sensation of skin; NOS = Not Otherwise Specified.

Overdosage

➤*Symptoms:* Systemic toxicity following acute overdosage with topical application of bexarotene is unlikely because of low systemic plasma levels observed with normal therapeutic doses.

➤*Treatment:* There is no specific antidote for overdosage.

There has been no experience with acute overdose of bexarotene in humans. Any overdose with bexarotene should be treated with supportive care for the signs and symptoms exhibited by the patient.

SCABICIDES/PEDICULICIDES

CROTAMITON

Rx	**Eurax** (Bristol-Myers Squibb)	**Cream:** 10%	Vanishing base. Cetyl alcohol. In 60 g.
		Lotion: 10%	Emollient base. Cetyl alcohol. In 60 and 454 g.

CROTAMITON — TOPICAL

Indications

➤*Scabies/Pruritus:* For eradication of scabies (*Sarcoptes scabiei*) and for symptomatic treatment of pruritic skin.

Administration and Dosage

➤*Adults:*

Scabies – Thoroughly massage into the skin of the whole body from the chin down, paying particular attention to all folds and creases. A second application is advisable 24 hours later.

Clothing and bed linen should be changed the next morning. A cleansing bath should be taken 48 hours after the last application.

CROTAMITON — TOPICAL

Pruritus – Massage gently into affected areas until medication is completely absorbed. Repeat as needed.

➤*Discontinuation of therapy:* If severe irritation or sensitization develops, treatment with this product should be discontinued and appropriate therapy instituted.

➤*Administration:* Shake lotion well before using.

➤*Storage/Stability:* Store at room temperature.

Actions

➤*Pharmacology:* Crotamiton has scabicidal and antipruritic actions. The mechanisms of these actions are not known.

Contraindications

Crotamiton should not be applied topically to patients who develop a sensitivity or are allergic to it or who manifest a primary irritation response to topical medications.

Warnings/Precautions

➤*Irritation:* If severe irritation or sensitization develops, treatment with this product should be discontinued and appropriate therapy instituted.

➤*General:* Crotamiton should not be applied in the eyes or mouth because it may cause irritation. It should not be applied to acutely inflamed skin or raw or weeping surfaces until the acute inflammation has subsided.

➤*Pregnancy: Category C* per manufacturer's prescribing information. *Category D* per Briggs' *Drugs in Pregnancy and Lactation*. Animal reproduction studies have not been conducted with crotamiton. It is also not known whether crotamiton can cause fetal harm when applied topically to a pregnant woman or can affect reproduction capacity. Crotamiton should be given to a pregnant woman only if clearly needed.

➤*Lactation:* There are no data regarding the use of crotamiton in breast-feeding women.

➤*Children:* Safety and effectiveness in children have not been established.

Adverse Reactions

Allergic sensitivity or primary irritation reactions may occur in some patients.

Overdosage

➤*Acute toxicity (after accidental oral administration in children): Highest known doses ingested* –

Cream: Children — 2 g (age 1½ years).

Lotion: 1 ounce (age 2 years.) A death was reported but cause was not confirmed.

Oral LD $_{50}$ in animals (mg/kg); rats, 2212; mice, 2011.

➤*Symptoms:*

Oral ingestion – Burning sensation in the mouth, irritation of the buccal, esophageal and gastric mucosa, nausea, vomiting, abdominal pain.

➤*Treatment:* There is no specific antidote if taken orally. General measures to eliminate the drug and reduce its absorption, combined with symptomatic treatment, are recommended.

Patient Information

Take a routine bath or shower. Thoroughly massage crotamiton cream or lotion into the skin from the chin to the toes including folds and creases.

A second application is advisable 24 hours later.

This 60 gram tube or bottle is sufficient for two applications.

Clothing and bed linen should be changed the next day. Contaminated clothing and bed linen may be dry-cleaned, or washed in the hot cycle of the washing machine.

A cleansing bath should be taken 48 hours after the last application.

LINDANE (Gamma Benzene Hexachloride)

Rx	**Lindane** (Various, eg, Alpharma, Major)	**Lotion:** 1%	In 30 and 59 mL, and pharmacy-size only pint.
		Shampoo: 1%	In 30 and 59 mL, and pharmacy-size only pint.

LINDANE — TOPICAL

WARNING

Only use lindane in patients who cannot tolerate or have failed first-line treatment with safer medications for the treatment of scabies.

Neurologic toxicity – Seizures and deaths have been reported following lindane use with repeat or prolonged application, but also in rare cases following a single application used according to directions. Exercise caution when using lindane in infants, children, the elderly, and individuals with other skin conditions (eg, atopic dermatitis, psoriasis) and in those who weigh less than 110 lbs (50 kg) as they may be at risk of serious neurotoxicity.

Contraindications – See Contraindications for more information.

Proper use – Instruct patients on the proper use of lindane, the amount to apply, how long to leave it on, and avoiding retreatment. Inform patients that itching occurs after the successful killing of scabies and is not necessarily an indication for retreatment with lindane.

Indications

➤*Lotion:* For the treatment of scabies (*Sarcoptes scabiei*) **only in patients** who cannot tolerate or who have failed other treatments.

➤*Shampoo:* For the treatment of head lice (*Pediculosis humanis capitis*), crab lice (*Pthirus pubis*), and their ova only in patients who cannot tolerate or who have failed other treatments.

Administration and Dosage

➤*General dosing considerations:* Lindane does not prevent infestation or reinfestation and should not be used to ward off a possible infestation.

One ounce (30 mL) is sufficient for an average adult. Do not prescribe more than 2 ounces (60 mL) for larger adults.

Washing of all recently worn clothing, underwear, pajamas, sheets, pillows, and towels is very important.

Treat sexual contacts concurrently.

➤*Adults:*

Head lice/crab lice –

Shampoo: Apply shampoo directly to dry hair without adding water. Work thoroughly into the hair and allow to remain in place for 4 minutes only. Give special attention to the fine hairs along the neck. After 4 minutes, add small quantities of water to hair until a good lather forms. Immediately rinse all lather away. Towel briskly and then remove nits with nit comb or tweezers. Do not cover the hair with shower cap or towel. Avoid unnecessary contact of lather with other body surfaces. Do not re-treat or use as a routine shampoo.

Scabies –

Lotion: Apply a thin layer of lotion over all skin (ie, entire trunk, extremities, soles of feet, underneath finger nails) from the neck down.

Apply once and wash off in 8 to 12 hours. Do not re-treat unless instructed to do so by a health care provider; 1 application of lindane is generally successful. Do not cover areas where medication is applied.

Patient may bathe prior to application; however, wait at least 1 hour after bathing before applying lindane to skin. Wet and warm skin may increase absorption, leading to toxicity (eg, seizures).

➤*Children:* Children have a higher surface-to-volume ratio and may be at risk of greater systemic exposure when lindane is applied to the body. Use lindane with extreme caution in patients who weigh less than approximately 110 lbs (50 kg), and especially in infants.

Head lice/crab lice – See Adults for dosing.

Scabies – See Adults for dosing.

➤*Administration:* Do not administer orally.

Instruct caregivers to wear gloves or wash hands immediately after applying the lotion or shampoo.

Inform patient that itching occurs after the successful killing of scabies or lice and it is not necessarily an indication for retreatment with lindane.

Actions

➤*Pharmacology:* An ectoparasiticide and ovicide effective against *Sarcoptes scabiei* (scabies). Parasiticidal action is exerted direct absorbtion into the parasites and their ova.

➤*Pharmacokinetics:* Approximately 10% systemic absorption of a lindane acetone solution was reported when applied to the forearm of human subjects and left in place for 24 hours. A blood level of 290 ng/mL was associated with convulsions following the accidental ingestion of a lindane-containing product. It was found that the greatest peak blood level of 64 ng/mL occurred 6 hours after total body application of lindane in 1 of 8 nonscabietic pediatric patients. The half-life in blood was determined to be approximately 18 hours. Data available suggest that lindane has a rapid distribution phase followed by a longer β-elimination phase.

Contraindications

Premature neonates, because their skin may be more permeable than that of full-term infants and their liver enzymes may not be sufficiently developed; patients with known seizure disorders; hypersensitivity to lindane or any component of the products; crusted (Norwegian) scabies and other skin conditions (eg, atopic dermatitis, psoriasis) that may increase systemic absorption.

Warnings/Precautions

➤*Absorption:* Simultaneous application of creams, ointments, or oils may enhance absorption.

➤*Neurotoxicity:* Seizures and deaths have been reported following lindane use with repeat or prolonged application, but also in rare cases following a single application. Infants, children, the elderly, individuals with other skin conditions, and those who weigh less than 110 lbs (50 kg) may be at greater risk of serious neurotoxicity. Give careful consideration before prescribing lindane to patients with conditions that may increase the risk of seizure, such as HIV infection, history of head trauma or a prior seizure, CNS tumor, the presence of severe hepatic cirrhosis, excessive use of alcohol, abrupt

LINDANE — TOPICAL

withdrawal from alcohol or sedatives, as well as concomitant use of medications known to lower seizure threshold.

➤*Deaths:* Serious outcomes such as hospitalization and disability or death has occurred. In approximately 20% of the total reported cases, lindane was reported to have been used according to the labeled directions. Of these cases, 13 deaths were reported, many cases of which were remote from the time of actual lindane use. Lindane toxicity, verified by autopsy, was the cause of 1 infant's death and was the cause of death reported for an adult who ingested it orally in a successful suicide. The direct causes of death for the other cases were attributed to reasons other than lindane. Most of these adverse events occurred with lindane lotion.

➤*For external use only:* Avoid contact with eyes; if this occurs, immediately flush eyes with water.

➤*Oils:* Oils may enhance absorption of lindane. Avoid using oil treatment, oil-based hair dressings, or conditioners before and after applying lindane.

➤*Pregnancy: Category C* per manufacturer's prescribing information. *Category B* per Briggs' *Drugs in Pregnancy and Lactation*. Give lindane to pregnant women only if clearly needed. There are no adequate and well-controlled studies in pregnant women. There are no known maternal or fetal health risks if the scabies is not treated. Lindane is lipophilic and may accumulate in the placenta. There has been a single case report of a stillborn infant following multiple maternal exposures to lindane during pregnancy. The relationship of the maternal exposures to the fetal outcome is unknown.

Animal data suggest that lindane exposure of the fetus may increase the likelihood of neurologic developmental abnormalities. The immature central nervous system (as in the fetus) may have increased susceptibility to the effects of the drug.

When rats received lindane in the diet from day 6 of gestation through day 10 of lactation, reduced pup survival, decreased pup weight and decreased weight gains during lactation, increased motor activity, and decreased motor activity habituation were seen in pups at 5.6 mg/kg. An increased number of stillborn pups was seen at 8 mg/kg, and increased pup mortality was seen at 5.6 mg/kg.

➤*Lactation:* Lindane is lipophilic and is present in human breast milk, but exact quantities are not known. There may be a risk of central nervous system stimulation, ranging from dizziness to seizures, if lindane is ingested from breast milk, or from skin absorption from mother to baby in the course of breastfeeding when lindane is applied topically to the chest area. Advise nursing mothers who require treatment with lindane of the potential risks. Counsel them to avoid large areas of skin-to-skin contact with the infant while lindane is applied, as well as to interrupt breastfeeding, with expression and discarding of milk, for at least 24 hours following use.

➤*Children:* Animal data demonstrated increased risk of adverse events in the young across species. Pediatric patients have a higher surface to volume ratio and may be at risk of greater systemic exposure when lindane is applied to the body. Infants and children may be at an even higher risk due to immaturity of organ systems such as skin and liver. Use lindane with extreme caution in patients who weigh less than approximately 110 lbs (50 kg) and especially in infants.

➤*Elderly:* There have been no studies of lindane in the elderly. There are 4 postmarketing reports of deaths in elderly patients who were treated for scabies with lindane. Two patients died within 24 hours of lindane application, and the third patient died 41 days after application of lindane, having suffered a seizure on the day of death. A fourth patient died of an unreported cause of death on the same day that lindane treatment for scabies was administered.

Drug Interactions

Use lindane with caution with drugs that lower seizure threshold. These drugs may include the following: Antipsychotics, antidepressants, theophylline, cyclosporine, mycophenolate mofetil, tacrolimus capsules, penicillins, imipenem, quinolone antibiotics, chloroquine sulfate, pyrimethamine, isoniazid, meperidine, radiographic contrast agents, centrally active anticholinesterases, methocarbamol.

Adverse Reactions

Lindane has been reported to cause CNS stimulation ranging from dizziness to seizures. Although seizures were almost always associated with ingestion or misuse of the product (to include repeat treatment), seizures and deaths have been reported when lindane was used according to directions. Irritant dermatitis from contact with this product has also been reported.

➤*Postmarketing experience:* Alopecia, dermatitis, headache, pain, paresthesia, pruritus, and urticaria. The relationship of some of these events to lindane therapy is unknown.

Overdosage

➤*Symptoms:* Overdosage or oral ingestion can cause CNS excitation and, if taken in sufficient quantities, seizures may occur. A blood level of 290 ng/mL was associated with convulsions following the accidental ingestion of a lindane-containing product.

➤*Treatment:* If accidental ingestion occurs, institute prompt gastric emptying. However, because oils favor absorption, give saline cathartics for intestinal evacuation rather than oil laxatives. If CNS manifestations occur, administer pentobarbital, phenobarbital, or diazepam. Refer to General Management of Acute Overdosage.

Patient Information

The skin should be clean and without any other lotion, cream, or oil on it. Oils can make lindane go through the skin faster and possibly increase the risk of neurotoxicity (eg, seizures).

Wait at least 1 hour after bathing or showering before putting lindane on the skin.

Wet or warm skin can make lindane go through skin faster; make sure skin is dry and cool before application.

Put lotion under fingernails after trimming the fingernails short, because scabies are very likely to remain there. A toothbrush can be used to apply the lotion under the fingernails. Immediately after use, wrap the toothbrush in paper and throw away.

Use only a single application, applied as a very thin layer over all skin from the neck down.

Do not use any covering over the applied lindane that does not breathe (eg, diapers with plastic lining, plastic clothes, tight clothes, or blankets).

Wash the lindane completely off after 8 to 12 hours. Never leave lindane on the skin for more than 12 hours. Warm, but not hot water can be used.

Wash all recently worn clothing, underwear, pajamas, used sheets, pillow cases, and towels in very hot water or dry-clean.

The patient may still itch after using lindane, even after all the scabies (insects) are dead.

For external use only (oral ingestion can lead to serious CNS toxicity). Do not apply to face. Avoid eyes; if there is contact, flush well with water for several minutes. Avoid unnecessary skin contact or contact with mucous membranes (eg, nose, mouth). Wear rubber gloves, particularly when applying to more than 1 person.

Notify physician if condition worsens or if itching, redness, swelling, burning, or skin rash occurs.

Avoid use on open cuts and extensive excoriations.

Treat sexual contacts simultaneously.

Lindane does not prevent infestation or reinfestation and should not be used to ward off a possible infestation.

A lindane medication guide must be given to the patient each time lindane is dispensed.

MALATHION

Rx	**Malathion** (Various, eg, Karalex Pharma, Taro)	**Lotion; topical:** 0.5%[a]	In 59 mL.
Rx	**Ovide** (Taro)		In 59 mL.

[a] In a vehicle of isopropyl alcohol 78%, terpineol, dipentene, and pine needle oil.

MALATHION — TOPICAL

Indications

➤*Head lice:* For patients infected with *Pediculus humanus capitis* (head lice and their ova) of the scalp hair.

Administration and Dosage

➤*General dosing considerations:* Further treatment is generally not necessary. Other family members should be evaluated by a health care provider to determine if infested, and if so, receive treatment.

➤*Adults:*

Head lice – Apply lotion on dry hair in an amount just sufficient to thoroughly wet the hair and scalp. Pay particular attention to the back of the head and neck while applying malathion. Wash hands after applying to scalp.

Allow hair to dry naturally; use no electric heat source, and allow hair to remain uncovered. After 8 to 12 hours, the hair should be shampooed. Rinse and use a fine-toothed (nit) comb to remove dead lice and eggs. If lice are still present after 7 to 9 days, repeat with a second application of malathion.

➤*Children:* Malathion lotion should only be used on children under the direct supervision of an adult.

Head lice –

6 years of age or older: See Adults for dosing.

➤*Administration:* Close eyes tightly during product application. If accidentally placed in the eye, flush immediately with water. Use only on scalp hair.

➤*Storage/Stability:* Store at 20° to 25°C (68° to 77°F). Flammable, keep away from heat and open flame.

Actions

➤*Pharmacology:* Malathion is an organophosphate agent which acts as a pediculicide by inhibiting cholinesterase activity in vivo. Inadvertent transdermal absorption of malathion has occurred from its agricultural use. In such cases, acute toxicity was manifested by excessive cholinergic activity (ie, increased sweating, salivary and gastric secretion, GI and uterine motility, and bradycardia). Because the potential for transdermal absorption of malathion from malathion lotion is not known at this time, strict adherence

MALATHION — TOPICAL

to the dosing instructions regarding its use in children, method of application, duration of exposure, and frequency of application is required.

Contraindications

In neonates and infants because their scalps are more permeable and may have increased absorption of malathion; do not use on individuals known to be sensitive to malathion or to any of the ingredients in the vehicle.

Warnings/Precautions

➤*Flammable:* Malathion lotion is flammable. The lotion and wet hair should not be exposed to open flames or electric heat sources, including hair dryers and electric curlers. Do not smoke while applying lotion or while hair is wet. Allow hair to dry naturally and to remain uncovered after application of malathion lotion.

➤*Irritation:* If malathion comes into contact with the eyes, flush immediately with water. Consult a physician if eye irritation persists.

If skin irritation occurs, discontinue use of product until irritation clears. Reapply the malathion, and if irritation reoccurs, consult a physician.

Slight stinging sensations may occur with the use of malathion.

Close eyes tightly during product application. If accidentally placed in the eye, flush immediately with water. Use only on scalp hair.

➤*Pregnancy: Category B.* There was no evidence of teratogenicity in studies in rats and rabbits at doses up to 900 mg/kg/day and 100 mg/kg/day malathion, respectively. A study in rats failed to show any gross fetal abnormalities attributable to feeding malathion up to 2500 ppm (approximately 200 mg/kg/day) in the diet during a 3-generation evaluation period. These doses were approximately 2 to 10 times higher than the anticipated human dose (based on body surface area and assuming 100% bioavailability). Because animal reproduction studies are not always predictive of human responses, this drug should be used (or handled) during pregnancy only if clearly needed.

➤*Lactation:* Malathion in an acetone vehicle has been reported to be absorbed through human skin to the extent of 8% of the applied dose. However, percutaneous absorption from the malathion, 0.5% formulation has not been studied, and it is not known whether malathion is excreted in human milk. Because many drugs are excreted in human milk, caution should be exercised when malathion is administered to (or handled by) a nursing mother.

➤*Children:* The safety and efficacy of malathion in children younger than 6 years of age have not been established via well controlled trials. Malathion lotion should only be used on children under the direct supervision of an adult.

➤*Monitoring:* There are no special laboratory tests needed in order to use this medication.

Adverse Reactions

➤*Dermatologic:* Malathion has been shown to be irritating to the skin and scalp. Accidental contact with the eyes can result in mild conjunctivitis. It is not known if malathion has the potential to cause contact allergic sensitization.

Overdosage

➤*Symptoms:* Malathion, although a weaker cholinesterase inhibitor than some other organophosphates, may be expected to exhibit the same symptoms of cholinesterase depletion after accidental ingestion orally.

Severe respiratory distress is the major and most serious symptom of organophosphate poisoning.

➤*Treatment:* Severe respiratory distress may require artificial respiration, and atropine may be needed to counteract the symptoms of cholinesterase depletion.

Consideration should be given, as part of the treatment program, to the high concentration of isopropyl alcohol in the vehicle.

If accidentally swallowed, vomiting should be induced promptly or the stomach lavaged with 5% sodium bicarbonate solution.

Repeat analyses of serum and RBC cholinesterase may assist in establishing the diagnosis and formulating a long-range prognosis.

Patient Information

Malathion is flammable. The lotion and hair wet with lotion should not be exposed to open flames or electric heat sources, including hair dryers and electric curlers. Do not smoke while applying lotion or while hair is wet. The person applying malathion lotion should wash hands after application. Allow hair to dry naturally and to remain uncovered after application of malathion lotion.

Malathion should only be used on children under the direct supervision of an adult. Children should be warned to stay away from lighted cigarettes, open flames, and electric heat sources while the hair is wet.

In case of accidental ingestion of malathion lotion by mouth, seek medical attention immediately.

If you are pregnant or nursing, contact your physician before using malathion.

If malathion comes into contact with the eyes, flush immediately with water. Consult a physician if eye irritation persists or if visual changes occur.

If skin irritation occurs, wash scalp and hair immediately. If the irritation clears, malathion lotion may be reapplied. If irritation reoccurs, consult a physician.

Slight stinging sensations may be produced when using malathion lotion.

Apply malathion on the scalp hair in an amount just sufficient to thoroughly wet hair and scalp. Pay particular attention to the back of the head and neck when applying malathion. Anyone applying malathion should wash hands immediately after the application process is complete.

Allow hair to dry naturally and to remain uncovered. Shampoo hair after 8 to 12 hours, again paying attention to the back of the head and neck while shampooing.

Rinse hair and use a fine-toothed (nit) comb to remove dead lice and eggs.

If lice are still present after 7 to 9 days, repeat with a second application of malathion.

Further treatment is generally not necessary. Other family members should be evaluated by a physician to determine if infested, and if so, receive treatment.

PERMETHRIN

Rx	**Permethrin** (Various, eg, Clay-Park)	**Cream:** 5%	In 60 g tubes.
Rx	**Elimite** (Allergen)		Lanolin alcohols, coconut oil, mineral oil. In 60 g tubes.
Rx	**Acticin** (Bertek)		Coconut oil, lanolin alcohols, light mineral oil. In 60 g tubes.
otc	**Nix** (Insight Pharmaceuticals)	**Cream:** 1%	Cetyl alcohol, isopropyl alcohol, parabens. In 60 mL with comb.
otc	**Permethrin** (Various, eg, Alpharma)	**Lotion:** 1%	In 60 mL with comb.
otc	**Nix Complete Lice Treatment System** (Insight)	**Liquid; topical:** 1%	Cetyl alcohol, isopropyl alcohol 20%, parabens. In 59 mL with comb, gloves, cape, and drop cloth.

PERMETHRIN — TOPICAL

Indications

➤*Cream:* For the treatment of scabies (*Sarcoptes scabiei*) infestation.

➤*Lotion/Cream rinse:* For the treatment of head lice (*Pediculus humanus capitis*) and its nits (eggs).

➤*Liquid:* For the treatment of infestation with *Pediculus humanus* var. *capitis* (the head louse) and its nits (eggs). Treatment for recurrences is required in less than 1% of patients since the ovicidal activity may be supplemented by residual persistence in the hair. If live lice are observed 7 or more days following the initial application, give a second application.

➤*Off-label uses:* Permethrin appears to be effective for the topical treatment of papulopustular rosacea.

Administration and Dosage

➤*General dosing considerations:* Usually 30 g is sufficient to treat an average adult for scabies.

➤*Adults:*

Head lice –

Lotion/cream rinse: Apply to hair after washing with shampoo; rinse with water and towel dry. Apply a sufficient amount to saturate hair and scalp (especially behind the ears and nape of neck). Leave on hair for no longer than 10 minutes, then rinse with water. A single application is generally sufficient; however, if lice are observed within 7 days after application, apply a second treatment. Remove any remaining nits with the nit comb provided.

Scabies –

Cream:

• *Usual dosage* – Thoroughly massage cream into the skin from the head to the soles of the feet. Scabies rarely infest the scalp of adults, although the hairline, neck, temple, and forehead may be infested in geriatric patients. Remove the cream by washing (shower or bath) after 8 to 14 hours. Treat infants on the scalp, temple, and forehead. One application is generally curative.

PERMETHRIN — TOPICAL

• *Retreatment* – Patients often experience pruritus after treatment. This is rarely a sign of treatment failure and is not an indication for retreatment. Demonstrable living mites after 14 days indicate that retreatment is necessary.

➤*Children:*

2 months of age and older –

Head lice: See Adults for dosing.

Scabies:

• *Cream* –

Usual dosage: Thoroughly massage cream into the skin from the head to the soles of the feet. For infants, also apply on the scalp, hairline, neck, temple, and forehead. Remove the cream by washing (shower or bath) after 8 to 14 hours. Treat infants on the scalp, temple, and forehead. One application is generally curative.

Retreatment: Patients often experience pruritus after treatment. This is rarely a sign of treatment failure and is not an indication for retreatment. Demonstrable living mites after 14 days indicate that retreatment is necessary.

➤*Storage/Stability:* Store at 15° to 25°C (59° to 77°F).

Actions

➤*Pharmacology:* Permethrin is a pyrethroid active against lice, ticks, mites, and fleas. It acts on the parasites' nerve cell membranes to disrupt the sodium channel current, resulting in delayed repolarization and paralysis of the pests.

➤*Pharmacokinetics:* Permethrin is rapidly metabolized by ester hydrolysis to inactive metabolites that are excreted primarily in the urine. Although the amount of permethrin absorbed after a single application of the 5% cream has not been determined precisely, preliminary data suggest it is 2% or less of the amount applied. Residual persistence is detectable on the hair for at least 10 days following a single application.

Contraindications

Hypersensitivity to any synthetic pyrethroid or pyrethrin, or to any component of the product. If hypersensitivity develops, discontinue use.

Warnings/Precautions

➤*For external use only:* Do not use near eyes, mucous membranes (ie, nose, mouth, vagina), or ingest orally. If infestation of eyelashes or eyebrows occurs, consult physician.

➤*Asthmatics:* Permethrin may cause breathing difficulties or exacerbate asthmatic episodes.

➤*Pruritus, erythema, and edema:* These often accompany scabies and head lice infestation. Treatment with permethrin may temporarily exacerbate these conditions.

➤*Pregnancy: Category B.* There are no adequate and well-controlled studies in pregnant women. Use during pregnancy only if clearly needed.

➤*Lactation:* It is not known whether this drug is excreted in breast milk. Because of the evidence for tumorigenic potential of permethrin in animal studies, consider discontinuing nursing temporarily or withholding the drug while the mother is nursing.

➤*Children:* Safety and efficacy for use in children younger than 2 months of age have not been established.

Adverse Reactions

The most frequent adverse reaction is pruritus. Usually a consequence of scabies or head lice infestation itself, it may be temporarily aggravated following treatment.

➤*Cream:* Mild transient burning/stinging (10%); itching (7%); tingling, numbness, erythema, or rash (2% or less).

Postmarketing reactions – Headache, fever, dizziness, abdominal pain, diarrhea, nausea, vomiting (5%); seizure (rare).

➤*Lotion/Cream rinse:* Itching, redness, swelling of scalp.

Overdosage

If ingested, perform gastric lavage and employ general supportive measures. Excessive topical use may result in increased irritation and erythema.

Patient Information

For external use only. Avoid contact with the mucous membranes (eg, nose, mouth, vagina). May be irritating to the eyes. Avoid contact with the eyes; flush with water immediately if eye contact with the drug occurs.

Itching, redness, or swelling of the scalp may occur; notify physician if irritation persists.

Patient instructions and information are available with the product. Do not exceed the prescribed dosage.

Inform patients that they may still experience pruritus after treatment. This is rarely a sign of treatment failure or an indication for retreatment.

Inform patients on the importance of washing in hot water all personal articles susceptible to infestation (eg, sheets, pillows, clothing, combs, brushes). It is recommended to thoroughly vacuum rooms.

SPINOSAD

Rx	**Natroba** (ParaPRO[a]/Pernix Therapeutics[b])	**Suspension; topical:** 0.9%	Alcohols, butylated hydroxytoluene, propylene glycol. In 120 mL.

[a] ParaPRO LLC, 11550 North Meridian Street, Suite 600, Carmel, IN 46032; fax: 317-580-8296; http://www.parapro.com.

[b] Pernix Therapeutics Inc, 33219 Forest West Dr, Magnolia, TX 77354; 800-793-2145; http://www.pernixtx.com.

SPINOSAD — TOPICAL

Indications

➤*Head lice:* For the topical treatment of head lice infestation in patients 4 years of age and older.

Administration and Dosage

➤*General dosing considerations:* Spinosad should be used in the context of an overall lice management program that includes washing (in hot water) or dry-cleaning all recently worn clothing, hats, used bedding and towels; washing personal care items, such as combs, brushes, and hair clips in hot water; and using a fine-tooth comb or special nit comb to remove dead lice and nits.

➤*Adults:*

Head lice –

Usual dosage: Depending on hair length, apply up to 120 mL (1 bottle) to adequately cover the scalp and hair.

Repeat dosage: If live lice are seen 7 days after the first treatment, a second treatment should be applied.

➤*Children:*

Head lice –

4 years of age and older: See Adults for dosing.

➤*Administration:* For topical use only; not for oral, ophthalmic, or intravaginal use. Avoid contact with eyes.

Shake the bottle well. Apply sufficient spinosad topical suspension to cover the dry scalp, then apply to dry hair. Leave on for 10 minutes, then thoroughly rinse off suspension with warm water.

➤*Storage/Stability:* Store at 25°C (77°F); excursions are permitted between 15° and 30°C (59° and 86°F).

Actions

➤*Pharmacology:* Spinosad causes neuronal excitation in insects. After periods of hyperexcitation, lice become paralyzed and die.

➤*Pharmacokinetics:* An open-label, single-center study was conducted over a period of 7 days to determine the pharmacokinetic profile of spinosad 1.8% in children with head lice infestation. Fourteen subjects, 4 to 15 years of age, with head lice were enrolled in the study. All subjects applied a single topical (scalp) treatment of spinosad 1.8% for 10 minutes, after which the test article was washed off, and subjects underwent plasma sampling. Plasma samples were analyzed by a validated LC/MS/MS method. Results demonstrated that spinosad was below the limit of quantitation (3 ng/mL) in all samples.

Contraindications

None well documented.

Warnings/Precautions

➤*Benzyl alcohol:* Spinosad contains benzyl alcohol and is not recommended for use in neonates and infants younger than 6 months of age. Systemic exposure to benzyl alcohol has been associated with serious adverse reactions and death in neonates and low birth-weight infants.

The "gasping syndrome" (characterized by central nervous system depression, metabolic acidosis, gasping respirations, and high levels of benzyl alcohol and its metabolites found in the blood and urine) has been associated with benzyl alcohol dosages greater than 99 mg/kg/day in neonates and low birth-weight infants. Additional symptoms may include gradual neurological deterioration, seizures, intracranial hemorrhage, hematologic abnormalities, skin breakdown, hepatic and renal failure, hypotension, bradycardia, and cardiovascular collapse.

The minimum amount of benzyl alcohol at which toxicity may occur is not known. Premature and low birth-weight infants, as well as patients receiving high dosages, may be more likely to develop toxicity.

➤*Pregnancy: Category B.* There are no adequate and well-controlled studies with spinosad in pregnant women. Studies in humans did not assess for the absorption of benzyl alcohol contained in spinosad topical suspension. Reproduction studies conducted in rats and rabbits were negative for teratogenic effects. Because animal reproduction studies are not always predictive of human response, use this drug during pregnancy only if clearly needed.

In the presence of maternal toxicity, increased dystocia in parturition, decreased gestation survival, decreased litter size, decreased pup body weight, and decreased neonatal survival occurred at a dosage of 100 mg/kg/day.

➤*Lactation:* Spinosad is not systemically absorbed; therefore, it will not be present in human milk. However, spinosad topical suspension contains benzyl alcohol, which may be systemically absorbed through the skin; the amount of benzyl alcohol excreted in human milk with use of spinosad topical suspension is unknown. Exercise caution when spinosad is administered

SPINOSAD — TOPICAL

to a breast-feeding woman. A breast-feeding woman may choose to pump and discard breast milk for 8 hours (5 half-lives of benzyl alcohol) after use to avoid infant ingestion of benzyl alcohol.

➤*Children:* The safety and effectiveness of spinosad have been established in children 4 years of age and older with active head lice infestation.

Safety in children younger than 4 years of age has not been established. Spinosad is not recommended in children younger than 6 months of age because of the potential for increased systemic absorption due to a high ratio of skin surface area to body mass and the potential for an immature skin barrier.

Drug Interactions

None well documented.

Adverse Reactions

➤*Adverse reactions (1% or more):*

Spinosad Adverse Reactions (≥ 1%)		
Adverse reactions	Spinosad (n = 552)	Permethrin 1% (n = 457)
Local		
Application-site erythema	3%	7%
Application-site irritation	1%	2%
Special senses		
Ocular erythema	2%	3%

➤*Other adverse reactions:* Other less common reactions (less than 1% but more than 0.1%) were alopecia, application-site dryness, application-site exfoliation, and dry skin.

Overdosage

➤*Treatment:* If oral ingestion occurs, seek medical advice immediately.

Patient Information

Instruct patients to shake the bottle well immediately prior to use.

Advise patients to use spinosad topical suspension only on dry scalp and dry scalp hair.

Instruct patients to avoid contact with eyes. If spinosad topical suspension gets in or near the eyes, rinse thoroughly with water.

Instruct patients to wash hands after applying spinosad topical suspension.

Advise patients that spinosad topical suspension for use on children should only be applied under direct supervision of an adult.

Advise patients that if they are pregnant or breast-feeding to consult a health care provider before use.

Educate patients that spinosad is not for oral use and should not be swallowed.

MISCELLANEOUS PEDICULICIDES

otc	**Tisit**[a] (Pfeiffer)	**Lotion:** 0.3% pyrethrins, 2% piperonyl butoxide	In 59 and 118 mL.
otc	**Tisit** (Pfeiffer)	**Gel:** 0.3% pyrethrins, 3% piperonyl butoxide	In 30 mL.
otc	**Klout** (PediaMed)	**Shampoo:** Acetic acid, isopropanol, sodium laureth sulfate	Parabens. In 118.3 mL with comb.
otc	**Licide Complete Lice Treatment Kit** (Reese Chemical)	**Shampoo:** 0.33% pyrethrins, 4% piperonyl butoxide	*Shampoo*: castor oil, PEG-25, SD alcohol. *Gel*: disodium EDTA, glycerin. In 118 mL kits containing gel, comb, and lice control spray.
otc	**Pronto** (Del)		Benzyl alcohol, decyl alcohol, isopropyl alcohol. In 60 and 120 mL with comb.
otc	**Pyrinyl Plus** (Rugby)		Benzyl alcohol. In 59 mL.
otc	**RID** (Bayer Consumer)		SD alcohol. In 60, 120, and 240 mL, and 120 mL kits containing gel, comb, and lice control spray.
otc	**Tisit** (Pfeiffer)		In 59 and 118 mL with comb.
otc	**Lice Treatment** (Goldline)		Benzyl alcohol. In 59 and 118 mL with comb.
otc	**RID** (Bayer Consumer)	**Mousse:** 0.33% pyrethrins, 4% piperonyl butoxide	Cetearyl alcohol, SD alcohol, isobutane. In 165 mL with comb.

[a] Contains petroleum distillate and piperonyl butoxide equivalent to 1.6% ether.

MISCELLANEOUS PEDICULICIDES — TOPICAL

Indications

➤*Lice:* Treatment of infestations of head lice, body lice, and pubic (crab) lice and their eggs.

Administration and Dosage

➤*Adults:*

Lice – Administration and dosage varies. Refer to individual package inserts for information.

➤*Children:*

Lice – Administration and dosage varies. Refer to individual package inserts for information.

Contraindications

Hypersensitivity to ingredients; ragweed sensitized persons (pyrethrins and permethrins).

Warnings/Precautions

➤*For external use only:* Harmful if swallowed or inhaled. May be irritating to the eyes and mucous membranes (eg, nose, mouth, vagina). In case of contact with eyes, flush with water. Discontinue use and notify physician if irritation or infection occurs.

➤*Infestation of eyelashes or eyebrows:* Do not use in these areas; consult physician.

➤*Reinfestation:* To prevent reinfestation, sterilize or treat all brushes/combs, towels, clothing, and bedding concurrently. It is recommended that all rooms inhabited by infected patients be thoroughly vacuumed. A second treatment may need to be repeated in 7 to 10 days to kill any newly hatched lice.

➤*Pubic lice:* May be transmitted by sexual contact. Treat sexual partners simultaneously.

➤*Pregnancy: Category C* (per Briggs' *Drugs in Pregnancy and Lactation*). Topical absorption is poor.

➤*Lactation:* There are no data available in breast-feeding women.

FIBRIN AGENTS

FIBRIN SEALANT (HUMAN)

Rx	**Artiss**[a] (Baxter)	**Powder for solution; topical:** total protein 96 to 125 mg/mL, fibrinogen 67 to 106 mg/mL, fibrinolysis inhibitor (synthetic) 2,250 to 3,750 kallikrein-inhibiting units/mL, thrombin (human) 2.5 to 6.5 units/mL, calcium chloride 36 to 44 mcmol/mL (when reconstituted)	In 2, 4, and 10 mL single-use vials with or without *Duploject* system.
Rx	**Tisseel**[a] (Baxter)	**Powder for solution; topical:** total protein 96 to 125 mg/mL, fibrinogen 67 to 106 mg/mL, fibrinolysis inhibitor (synthetic) 2,250 to 3,750 kallikrein-inhibiting units/mL, thrombin (human) 400 to 625 units/mL, calcium chloride 36 to 44 mcmol/mL (when reconstituted)	In 2, 4, and 10 mL single-use vials with or without *Duploject* system.
Rx	**Artiss** (Baxter)	**Solution; topical:** total protein 96 to 125 mg/mL, fibrinogen 67 to 106 mg/mL, fibrinolysis inhibitor (synthetic) 2,250 to 3,750 kallikrein-inhibiting units/mL, thrombin (human) 2.5 to 6.5 units/mL, calcium chloride 36 to 44 mcmol/mL	In 2, 4, and 10 mL single-use prefilled (frozen) syringe with *DUO Set*.

FIBRIN SEALANT (HUMAN)

Rx	**Tisseel** (Baxter)	**Solution; topical:** total protein 96 to 125 mg/mL, fibrinogen 67 to 106 mg/mL, fibrinolysis inhibitor (synthetic) 2,250 to 3,750 kallikrein-inhibiting units/mL, thrombin (human) 400 to 625 units/mL, calcium chloride 36 to 44 mcmol/mL (when reconstituted)	In 2, 4, and 10 mL single-use prefilled (frozen) syringe with *DUO Set.*
Rx	**TachoSil** (Baxter)	**Patch; topical:** human fibrinogen 3.6 to 7.4 mg (5.5 mg) and human thrombin 1.3 to 2.7 units (2 units) per cm^2	In package of 1s, 2s, and 5s.[a]

[a] Kits contains the following substances in 4 separate vials: sealer protein concentrate (human), fibrinolysis inhibitor solution (synthetic), thrombin (human), and calcium chloride solution.

[b] Patch sizes are available as follows: packages of 1 in 3 cm × 2.5 cm and 9.5 cm × 4.8 cm, package of 2s in 4.8 cm × 4.8 cm, and package of 5s in 3 cm × 2.5 cm.

FIBRIN SEALANT (HUMAN) — TOPICAL

Indications

➤*Hemostasis:*

TachoSil – As an adjunct to hemostasis for use in cardiovascular surgery when control of bleeding by standard surgical techniques (such as suture, ligature, or cautery) is ineffective or impractical.

Tisseel – As an adjunct to hemostasis in surgeries involving cardiopulmonary bypass and treatment of splenic injuries due to blunt or penetrating trauma to the abdomen, when control of bleeding by conventional surgical techniques, including suture, ligature, and cautery, is ineffective or impractical.

➤*Sealing (Tisseel):* As an adjunct to prevent leakage from colonic anastomoses following the reversal of temporary colostomies.

➤*Skin graft adhesion (Artiss):* To adhere autologous skin grafts to surgically prepared wound beds resulting from burns in adults and children.

Administration and Dosage

➤*Dosage:*

Artiss –

Artiss Dosage Recommendations

Approximate area requiring skin graft fixation	Required package size of *Artiss*
100 cm^2	2 mL
200 cm^2	4 mL
500 cm^2	10 mL

It is recommended that every time a patient receives a dose fibrin sealant, the name and lot number (batch number) of the product are documented in order to maintain a record of the batches used.

Tisseel –

Tisseel Dosage Recommendation

Maximum size of the area to be sealed using cannula	Maximum size of the area to be sealed using compressed gas	Required package size of *Tisseel*
8 cm^2	100 cm^2	2 mL
16 cm^2	200 cm^2	4 mL
40 cm^2	500 cm^2	10 mL

TachoSil – Apply on the surface of tissue only. Do not use intravascularly.

The number of patches to be applied should be determined by the size of the bleeding area to be treated.

Apply the yellow, active side of the patch to the bleeding area.

For record-keeping purposes, record patient name and *TachoSil* batch number every time that *TachoSil* is administered to a patient.

When applying, do not exceed the maximum number of patches, as shown in the following table.

Amount of Fibrinogen and Thrombin Per Total Patch Size and Maximum Number of Patches to Be Applied

TachoSil	Amount of human fibrinogen/ total patch size	Amount of human thrombin/ total patch size	Maximum number of *TachoSil* patches to be applied
9.5 cm × 4.8 cm	337.4 mg	123.1 units	7
4.8 cm × 4.8 cm	170.5 mg	62.2 units	14
3 cm × 2.5 cm	55.5 mg	20.3 units	42

➤*Preparation for administration:*

Artiss –

Vials: During preparation of fibrin sealant kit, do not expose to temperatures above 37°C (98.6°F) and do not refrigerate after reconstitution. After reconstitution, the product must be used within 4 hours.

Do not use iodine or heavy metal containing preparations such as betadine for disinfection of vial stoppers. Allow alcohol-based disinfectants to evaporate before puncturing stopper.

Use separate syringes for reconstituting sealer protein and thrombin solutions and for application to prevent premature clotting.

Freeze-dried sealer protein concentrate and thrombin are reconstituted in fibrinolysis inhibitor solution and calcium chloride solution, respectively. The sealer protein solution and thrombin solution are then combined using the *Duploject* preparation and application system or an equivalent delivery device cleared by the Food and Drug Administration (FDA) for use with fibrin sealant to form the fibrin sealant.

• *Prewarming fibrin sealant kit with Fibrinotherm* – If a *Fibrinotherm* device is not available, contact the manufacturer for assistance. See *Fibrinotherm* manual for complete operating instructions.

Plug the *Fibrinotherm* heating and stirring device into an electrical socket and activate the warmer (amber switch). Ensure that the stirring mechanism of the *Fibrinotherm* device is initially switched off (green switch).

Place all 4 vials from the fibrin sealant kit into the prewarmed wells of the *Fibrinotherm*, using the appropriately sized adapter rings, and allow the vials to warm for up to 5 minutes (room temperature product may take less time).

• *Preparation of sealer protein solution with Fibrinotherm* – Remove the flip-off caps from the vial containing the sealer protein concentrate and the vial containing the fibrinolysis inhibitor solution; disinfect the rubber stoppers of both vials with a germicidal solution and allow to dry.

Transfer the fibrinolysis inhibitor solution into the vial containing the freeze-dried sealer protein concentrate using the sterile reconstitution components provided with the *Duploject* preparation and application system or an equivalent device cleared by the FDA for use with fibrin sealant (see directions provided with the device system for specific reconstitution instructions). Gently swirl the vial to ensure that the freeze-dried material is completely soaked.

Place the vial into the largest opening of the *Fibrinotherm* device with the appropriate adaptor. Switch on the stirrer (green switch) and allow the vial contents to stir until all sealer protein concentrate is dissolved.

Reconstitution of the freeze-dried sealer protein concentrate is complete as soon as no undissolved particles are visible. Otherwise, return the vial to the *Fibrinotherm* device and agitate for a few more minutes until the solution appears homogeneous.

Do not use the sealer protein concentrate until it has fully dissolved. If the sealer protein concentrate has not dissolved within 20 minutes using the *Fibrinotherm* device, discard the vial and prepare a fresh kit. Excessive stirring (20 minutes or more) may compromise product quality.

If not used promptly, keep the sealer protein solution at 37°C without stirring. To ensure homogeneity, switch on the stirrer of the *Fibrinotherm* device shortly before drawing up the solution.

• *Preparation of thrombin solution with Fibrinotherm* – Remove the flip-off caps from the vial containing thrombin and the vial containing calcium chloride solution; disinfect the rubber stoppers of both vials with a germicidal solution and allow to dry.

Transfer the contents of the vial with calcium chloride solution into the vial containing the freeze-dried thrombin using the sterile reconstitution components provided with the *Duploject* preparation and application system or an equivalent device cleared by the FDA for use with fibrin sealant (see directions provided with the device system for specific reconstitution instructions).

Swirl briefly. Place the vial into the adapted opening of the *Fibrinotherm* device. Reconstitution of thrombin is complete when all of the thrombin concentrate is dissolved. Keep the thrombin solution at 37°C until used.

• *Transferring to the sterile field* – For transfer of the sealer protein solution and the thrombin solution to the sterile field, the scrub nurse should withdraw the solutions while the circulating nurse holds the nonsterile vials. The solutions should be withdrawn slowly by firm, constant aspiration to reduce the risk of large air bubbles.

Prefilled syringe: During preparation of fibrin sealant (frozen), do not expose to temperatures above 37°C, do not microwave, and do not refrigerate or refreeze after thawing.

Do not use fibrin sealant (frozen) unless it is completely thawed and warmed (liquid consistency). Do not remove the protective syringe cap until thawing is complete and the application tip is ready to be attached.

Fibrin sealant (frozen) can be prepared (thawed) using either the room temperature thawing method or quick thawing method.

• *Room temperature thawing* –

Artiss Room Temperature Thawing Recommendations

Pack size	Room temperature (in pouches)
2 mL	60 minutes
4 mL	110 minutes
10 mL	160 minutes

Unopened pouches, thawed at room temperature, may be stored for up to 14 days at 15° to 25°C (59° to 77°F).

Prior to use, the product should be warmed to 33° to 37°C (91.4° to 98.6°F).

FIBRIN SEALANT (HUMAN) — TOPICAL

Artiss Warming Recommendations Prior to Use	
Pack size	33° to 37°C incubator (in pouches)
2 mL	15 minutes
4 mL	25 minutes
10 mL	35 minutes

• *Quick thawing –*

Thawing on the sterile field using a water bath: 33° to 37°C sterile water bath: Transfer the inner pouch to the sterile field, remove prefilled syringe from inner pouch, and place directly into sterile water bath. Ensure the contents of the prefilled syringe are completely immersed under the water.

Artiss Sterile Water Bath Quick Thawing	
Pack size	33° to 37°C sterile water bath (pouches removed)
2 mL	5 minutes
4 mL	5 minutes
10 mL	12 minutes

Thawing off the sterile field using a water bath: 33° to 37°C nonsterile water bath in 2 pouches: Maintain the prefilled syringe in both pouches and place into a water bath off the sterile field for appropriate time. Ensure the pouches remain submerged throughout thawing. Remove from the water bath after thawing, dry external pouch, and transfer inner pouch with prefilled syringe onto the sterile field.

Artiss Nonsterile Water Bath Quick Thawing	
Pack size	33° to 37°C nonsterile water bath (in pouches)
2 mL	30 minutes
4 mL	40 minutes
10 mL	80 minutes

Thawing off the sterile field using an incubator: 33° to 37°C incubator in pouches: Maintain the prefilled syringe in both pouches and place into an incubator for appropriate time. Remove from incubator after thawing and transfer inner pouch with prefilled syringe onto the sterile field.

Artiss Quick Thawing With an Incubator	
Pack size	33° to 37°C incubator (in pouches)
2 mL	40 minutes
4 mL	85 minutes
10 mL	105 minutes

Maintain the product at 33° to 37°C until use. If product is removed from original pouch or warmed to 33° to 37°C, it must be used within 12 hours.

Tisseel –

Vials: During preparation of fibrin sealant kit, do not expose to temperatures above 37°C and do not refrigerate after reconstitution. After reconstitution, the product must be used within 4 hours.

Do not use iodine or heavy metal containing preparations such as betadine for disinfection of vial stoppers. Allow alcohol-based disinfectants to evaporate before puncturing stopper.

Use separate syringes for reconstituting sealer protein and thrombin solutions and for application to prevent premature clotting.

Freeze-dried sealer protein concentrate and thrombin are reconstituted in fibrinolysis inhibitor solution and calcium chloride solution, respectively. The sealer protein solution and thrombin solution are then combined using the *Duploject* preparation and application system or an equivalent delivery device cleared by the FDA for use with fibrin sealant to form the fibrin sealant.

• *Prewarming fibrin sealant kit with Fibrinotherm* – If a *Fibrinotherm* device is not available, contact the manufacturer for assistance. See *Fibrinotherm* manual for complete operating instructions.

Plug the *Fibrinotherm* heating and stirring device into an electrical socket and activate the warmer (amber switch). Ensure that the stirring mechanism of the *Fibrinotherm* device is initially switched off (green switch).

Place all 4 vials from the fibrin sealant kit into the prewarmed wells of the *Fibrinotherm*, using the appropriately sized adapter rings, and allow the vials to warm for up to 5 minutes (room temperature product may take less time).

• *Preparation of sealer protein solution with Fibrinotherm* – Remove the flip-off caps from the vial containing the sealer protein concentrate and the vial containing the fibrinolysis inhibitor solution; disinfect the rubber stoppers of both vials with a germicidal solution and allow to dry.

Transfer the fibrinolysis inhibitor solution into the vial containing the freeze-dried sealer protein concentrate using the sterile reconstitution components provided with the *Duploject* preparation and application system or an equivalent device cleared by the FDA for use with fibrin sealant (see directions provided with the device system for specific reconstitution instructions). Gently swirl the vial to ensure that the freeze-dried material is completely soaked.

Place the vial into the largest opening of the *Fibrinotherm* device with the appropriate adaptor. Switch on the stirrer (green switch) and allow the vial contents to stir until all sealer protein concentrate is dissolved.

Reconstitution of the freeze-dried sealer protein concentrate is complete as soon as no undissolved particles are visible. Otherwise, return the vial to the *Fibrinotherm* device and agitate for a few more minutes until the solution appears homogeneous.

Do not use the sealer protein concentrate until it has fully dissolved. If the sealer protein concentrate has not dissolved within 20 minutes using the *Fibrinotherm* device, discard the vial and prepare a fresh kit.

If not used promptly, keep the sealer protein solution at 37°C without stirring. To ensure homogeneity, switch on the stirrer of the *Fibrinotherm* device shortly before drawing up the solution.

• *Preparation of thrombin solution with Fibrinotherm* – Remove the flip-off caps from the vial containing thrombin and the vial containing calcium chloride solution; disinfect the rubber stoppers of both vials with a germicidal solution and allow to dry.

Transfer the contents of the vial with calcium chloride solution into the vial containing the freeze-dried thrombin using the sterile reconstitution components provided with the *Duploject* preparation and application system or an equivalent device cleared by the FDA for use with fibrin sealant (see directions provided with the device system for specific reconstitution instructions).

Swirl briefly. Place the vial into the adapted opening of the *Fibrinotherm* device. Reconstitution of thrombin is complete when all of the thrombin concentrate is dissolved. Keep the thrombin solution at 37°C until used.

• *Transferring to the sterile field* – For transfer of the sealer protein solution and the thrombin solution to the sterile field, the scrub nurse should withdraw the solutions while the circulating nurse holds the non-sterile vials. The solutions should be withdrawn slowly by firm, constant aspiration to reduce the risk of large air bubbles.

Prefilled syringe: During preparation of fibrin sealant (frozen), do not expose to temperatures above 37°C, do not microwave, and do not refrigerate or refreeze. After thawing, the product must be stored between 15° and 37°C (room temperature and 37°C).

Do not use fibrin sealant (frozen) unless it is completely thawed and warmed (liquid consistency). Do not remove the protective syringe cap until use.

Thaw prefilled syringes in 1 of the 3 following options:

• *Thawing on the sterile field using a water bath* – 33° to 37°C sterile water bath: transfer *DUO* set and the inner pouch to the sterile field, remove prefilled syringe from inner pouch and place directly into sterile water bath. Ensure the contents of the prefilled syringe are completely immersed under the water.

Tisseel Thawing on the Sterile Field (Water Bath)	
Pack size	Thawing/warming times 33° to 37°C sterile water bath (pouches removed)
2 mL	5 minutes
4 mL	5 minutes
10 mL	12 minutes

Thawing off the sterile field using a water bath: 33° to 37°C nonsterile water bath in 2 pouches: Maintain the prefilled syringe in both pouches and place into a water bath off the sterile field for appropriate time. Ensure the pouches remain submerged throughout thawing. Remove from the water bath after thawing, dry external pouch, and transfer inner pouch with prefilled syringe onto the sterile field.

Tisseel Thawing Off the Sterile Field (Water Bath)	
Pack size	Thawing/warming times 33° to 37°C nonsterile water bath (in pouches)
2 mL	30 minutes
4 mL	40 minutes
10 mL	80 minutes

Thawing off the sterile field using an incubator: 33° to 37°C incubator in pouches: Maintain the prefilled syringe in both pouches and place into an incubator for appropriate time. Remove from incubator after thawing and transfer inner pouch with prefilled syringe onto the sterile field.

Tisseel Thawing off the Sterile Field (With an Incubator)	
Pack size	33° to 37°C incubator (in pouches)
2 mL	40 minutes
4 mL	85 minutes
10 mL	105 minutes

Maintain the product at 33° to 37°C until use.

TachoSil – Packages come ready to use and must be handled accordingly. Use only undamaged packages as resterilization is not possible.

When in the operating room, the outer aluminum foil pouch may be opened in a nonsterile environment. The inner sterile blister must be opened in a sterile environment.

Remove the patch from the blister, which can be used as a container for premoistening of the patch, if needed.

Tailor the selection and application according to the size of the bleeding area. Select the appropriate patch so that it extends 1 to 2 cm beyond the margins of the wound. The patch can be cut to the correct size and shape if desired. If more than one patch is used, overlap patches by at least 1 cm.

➤*Administration:* For topical use only. Do not inject.

FIBRIN SEALANT (HUMAN) — TOPICAL

Artiss – Apply fibrin sealant using the *Easyspray* and *Spray Set* or an equivalent device cleared by the FDA for application of fibrin sealant. See additional instructions for use provided with the spray set.

The wound surface should be as dry as possible before application.

Apply fibrin sealant as a thin layer to avoid the formation of excess granulation tissue and to ensure gradual absorption of the polymerized fibrin sealant. The aerosolized sealant should be applied to the wound in a painting motion from side to side to achieve a single thin application. The wound bed will glisten in the area to which fibrin sealant has been applied. Any areas not covered by fibrin sealant will be clearly visible. The skin graft should be attached to the wound bed immediately after fibrin sealant has been sprayed. The surgeon has approximately 60 seconds to manipulate and position the graft prior to polymerization. To prevent adherence, wet gloves with normal saline before product contact.

After the graft has been applied, hold in the desired position by gentle compression for at least 3 minutes to ensure fibrin sealant sets properly and adheres firmly to the surrounding tissue. The solidified fibrin sealant reaches its final strength approximately 2 hours after application.

The cannulas included with the *Duploject* preparation and application system or *DUO Set* may be used for small wounds or for edges of a skin graft that did not adhere to the wound bed. Immediately before application, expel and discard the first several drops from the application cannula to ensure adequate mixing of the sealer protein and thrombin solutions.

Vials and prefilled syringes are for single use only. Discard unused contents.

Vials: Refer to instructions for use provided with the *Duploject* preparation and application system.

Prefilled syringe:

• *DUO Set* instructions –

1.) Insert plunger into syringe barrel.
2.) Firmly connect the 2 syringe nozzles to the joining piece and secure it by fastening the tether strap to the syringe.
3.) Fit an application cannula to the joining piece.

If application of fibrin sealant in interrupted, replace the cannula immediately before application is resumed.

Tisseel – Application must be completed within 4 hours after reconstitution of the freeze-dried kit or opening the prefilled frozen syringes. Ensure fibrin sealant is warmed to 33° to 37°C prior to application.

Vials and prefilled syringes are for single use only. Discard any unused product.

The wound surface should be as dry as possible before application.

Immediately before application, expel and discard the first several drops from the application cannula to ensure adequate mixing of the sealer protein and thrombin solutions in cases where very small volumes (1 to 2 drops) of product are administered.

To prevent adherence, wet gloves with normal saline before product contact.

Apply as a thin layer. The initial amount of the product to be applied should be sufficient to entirely cover the intended application area. The application can be repeated, if necessary.

After the 2 components have been applied, fix or hold the sealed parts in the desired position for at least 3 to 5 minutes to ensure the setting adheres firmly to the surrounding tissue.

Vials: Apply using the *Duploject* fibrin sealant preparation and application system or an equivalent delivery device cleared by the FDA for use with the fibrin sealant. Specific instructions for use in conjunction with each cleared delivery device are provided with the device.

Prefilled syringe: Apply prefilled syringe using the *DUO* set accessory devices provided with the product or an equivalent delivery device cleared by the FDA for use with the product.

• *DUO* set instructions – Insert plunger into syringe barrel.

Firmly connect the 2 syringe nozzles to the joining piece and secure it by fastening the tether strap to the syringe.

Fit an application cannula to the joining piece. If application is interrupted, replace the cannula immediately before application is resumed.

TachoSil – Prior to application, cleanse the area to be treated to remove disinfectants and other fluids. The fibrinogen and thrombin proteins can be denatured by alcohol, iodine, or heavy metal ions. If any of these substances have been used to clean the wound area, thoroughly irrigate the area before applying *TachoSil*.

Apply *TachoSil* directly to the bleeding area either wet or dry. If applied wet, premoisten *TachoSil* in 0.9% saline solution for no more than 1 minute and then apply immediately. In the case of a wet tissue surface (eg, oozing bleeding) *TachoSil* may be applied without premoistening.

Apply the yellow, active side of the patch to the bleeding areaand hold in place with gentle pressure applied through moistened gloves or a moist pad for at least 3 minutes.

When applying *TachoSil*, use precaution because the white, inactive side may also adhere to surgical instruments (eg, forceps) or gloves covered with blood due to the affinity of collagen to blood. Premoisten surgical instruments and gloves with saline solution to reduce the adherence.

After gently holding *TachoSil* to the bleeding area for at least 3 minutes, remove the gloved hand or moistened pad carefully from the patch. To avoid pulling the patch loose, first place a premoistened surgical instrument at one end of the patch before relieving the pressure.Gentle irrigation may also aid in removing the premoistened pad or glove hand without removing *TachoSil* from the bleeding area.

Leave *TachoSil* in place once it adheres to organ tissue. Remove unattached *TachoSil* patches (or part of) and replace with new patches.

TachoSil cannot be resterilized once removed from inner pouch. Discard unused, open packages of *TachoSil*.

For record-keeping purposes, record patient name and batch number every time that the patch is administered to a patient.

➤*Storage / Stability:*

Artiss –

Vial: Store at 2° to 25°C (35.6° to 77°F). Avoid freezing. After reconstitution, the product must be used within 4 hours. Reconstituted solutions must not be refrigerated or frozen.

Prefilled syringe:

• *Long term* – Store at −20°C (−68°F) or colder.
• *Short term* –

Room temperature thawing: Unopened pouches thawed at room temperature may be stored for up to 14 days at 15° to 25°C after removal from the freezer.

Quick thawing: Maintain the product at 33° to 37°C until use. If the product is removed from original pouch or warmed to 33° to 37°C, it must be used within 12 hours.

Do not refrigerate or refreeze after thawing. Do not microwave.

Tisseel – Thawed, unopened pouches may be stored for up to 48 hours at 15° to 25°C after removal from the freezer. Do not refrigerate or refreeze. After reconstitution of the solutions of the kit and after opening the frozen package, the fibrin sealant must be used within 4 hours. Discard if packaging of any component is damaged. Do not expose to temperatures above 37°C.

TachoSil – Store between 2° and 25°C. Refrigeration is not required. Do not freeze. Discard if packaging of any components is damaged.

Actions

➤*Pharmacology:* Fibrin sealant mimics the final stage of the blood coagulation cascade. Upon mixing sealer protein (human) and thrombin (human), soluble fibrinogen is transformed into fibrin that adheres to the wound surface and to the skin graft to be affixed. Because of the low thrombin concentration, polymerization of fibrin sealant will take approximately 60 seconds.

➤*Pharmacokinetics:*

Absorption / Distribution – Because fibrin sealant is applied only topically, systemic exposure or distribution to other organs or tissues is not expected.

Excretion – Free aprotinin and its metabolites have a half-life of 30 to 60 minutes and are eliminated by the kidney.

Contraindications

Known hypersensitivity to aprotinin, human blood products, horse proteins, or any active substances or excipients of the drug; severe or brisk arterial bleeding; intravascular application (do not inject fibrin sealant directly into blood vessels. Intravascular application of fibrin sealant may result in life-threatening thromboembolic events).

Warnings/Precautions

➤*Infection risk:* Fibrin sealant is made from human plasma. Products made from human plasma may contain infectious agents, such as viruses, that can cause disease. The risk that such products will transmit an infectious agent has been reduced by screening plasma donors for prior exposure to certain viruses, testing for the presence of certain current virus infections, and inactivating and removing certain viruses. Despite these measures, such products can still potentially transmit disease. Because this product is made from human blood, it may carry a risk of transmitting infectious agents (eg, viruses) and theoretically, the Creutzfeldt-Jakob disease agent. Report all infections thought by a health care provider possibly to have been transmitted by this product to the manufacturer (1-866-888-2472).

➤*Application precautions:* Apply fibrin sealant as a thin layer. Excessive clot thickness may negatively interfere with the product's efficacy and the wound healing process.

Caution must be used when applying fibrin sealant using pressurized gas. Any application of pressurized gas may be associated with a potential risk of air embolism, tissue rupture, or gas entrapment with compression, which may be life-threatening.

The sealer protein and thrombin solutions can be denatured by alcohol, iodine, or heavy metal ions. If any of these substances have been used to clean the wound area, the area must be thoroughly rinsed before application of fibrin sealant and made as dry as possible.

➤*Hypersensitivity reactions:* Hypersensitivity or allergic/anaphylactoid reactions may occur with the use of fibrin sealant. Cases (less than 0.01%) have been reported in postmarketing experience with fibrin sealant. In specific cases, these reactions have progressed to severe anaphylaxis. Such reactions may especially be seen if fibrin sealant is applied repeatedly over time or in the same setting, or if systemic aprotinin has been administered previously. Even if the first treatment was well tolerated, a subsequent administration of fibrin sealant or systemic aprotinin may not exclude the occurrence of an allergic reaction. Such reactions may also occur in patients receiving fibrin sealant for the first time.

Discontinue administration of fibrin sealant in the event of hypersensitivity reactions. Remove the already applied, polymerized product from the surgical field. Mild reactions can be managed with antihistamines. Severe hypotensive reactions require immediate intervention using current principles of shock therapy.

➤*Pregnancy: Category C.* Some viruses, such as parvovirus B19, are particularly difficult to remove or inactivate at this time. Parvovirus B19 most seriously affects pregnant women (fetal infection). Give fibrin sealant to a pregnant woman only if deemed medically necessary.

FIBRIN SEALANT (HUMAN) — TOPICAL

➤*Lactation:* It is not known whether this drug is excreted in human milk. Because many drugs are excreted in human milk, exercise caution when administering fibrin sealant to a lactating woman.

Drug Interactions

None known.

Adverse Reactions

Adverse reactions occurring in more than 1% of patients treated with fibrin sealant were skin graft failure and pruritus.

➤*Hypersensitivity:* Hypersensitivity or allergic/anaphylactoid reactions may occur. No adverse reactions of this type were reported during clinical trials.

➤*Clinical trials experience:* The following adverse reactions have been reported from a clinical trial in which fibrin sealant was used to affix split thickness sheet skin grafts to excised burn wounds. A total of 8 nonserious adverse reactions were deemed related to the use of fibrin sealant by the investigator. Of the 8 related nonserious adverse reactions, 5 were incidences of skin graft failure: 4 were graft detachment/nonadherence and 1 was graft necrosis. The graft detachment in 2 patients may have been related to the maximum thawing temperature (40°C) being exceeded during study product preparation. The 3 other nonserious adverse reactions considered related to fibrin sealant were 2 incidences of pruritus and 1 incidence of dermal cyst. The graft necrosis and the 2 cases of pruritus considered related to fibrin sealant each had an equivalent adverse reaction with the exact start date and severity reported at a control wound where skin grafts were affixed with staples. Therefore, these reactions are most likely not related to fibrin sealant, but instead are expected outcomes for any grafted wound regardless of the method of attachment.

Overall, the data collected and analyzed during this study demonstrated that fibrin sealant is safe for the attachment of sheet skin grafts in subjects with deep partial thickness or full thickness burn wounds.

Fibrin Sealant Adverse Reactions

Adverse reactions	Number of reactions (N = 138)
Dermatological	
Dermal cyst	1
Pruritus	2
Skin graft failure	5

➤*Postmarketing:*

Cardiovascular – Bradycardia, tachycardia.

Dermatologic – Urticaria.

GI – Nausea.

Hypersensitivity – Anaphylactic responses, hypersensitivity.

Respiratory – Dyspnea.

Miscellaneous – Edema, flushing, impaired healing, pyrexia, seroma.

Patient Information

Because this product is made from human plasma, discuss the risks and benefits with the patient.

Instruct patients to consult their health care provider if symptoms of B19 virus infection appear (fever, drowsiness, chills, and runny nose followed about 2 weeks later by a rash and joint pain).

WOUND HEALING AGENTS

SILVER

otc	**Elta SilverGel** (Swiss-American)	**Gel; topical:** 55 ppm[a]	In 30, 45, 236, and 473 mL and in 2" × 2" and 4" × 4" dressings in 10s.

[a] Parts per million.

SILVER — TOPICAL

Indications

➤*Topical wounds:* For nonprescription use for the management of minor burns, superficial cuts, lacerations, abrasions, and minor irritation of the skin.

May be used under the supervision of a health care provider for partial and full thickness wounds, including pressure ulcers, venous stasis ulcers, diabetic ulcers, first and second degree burns, skin tears, grafted wounds, donor sites, and surgical wounds where infection exists or threatens.

Administration and Dosage

➤*Adults:*

Topical wounds – Evenly apply a generous amount of silver gel approximately ⅛- to ¼-inch thick onto the burn or wound area. Cover wound with appropriate dressing. Repeat as necessary to keep wound moist.

➤*Children:* See Adults for dosing.

➤*Elderly:* See Adults for dosing.

➤*Dressing changes:* Dressing should be changed if excessive exudate begins forming or if secondary dressings become soaked with exudate. Remove secondary dressing. Cleanse the wound bed, removing any remaining silver gel. Reapply following application directions.

Silver gel may be left in a wound for up to 3 days. Dressing should be changed as recommended by an appropriate clinical authority.

➤*Preparation for administration:* Cleanse wound with cleansing liquid, such as *Elta Wound Cleanser*.

➤*Storage / Stability:* Store at 75°F (24°C). Avoid storing in light. Although potency is unaffected by light exposure, silver gel can darken slightly with extensive exposure to light.

Actions

➤*Pharmacology:* Silver gel is a broad spectrum amorphous antimicrobial wound gel. The amorphous gel provides for antimicrobial contact with entire wound bed. Silver gel is noncytotoxic. Silver gel is designed to provide a moist healing environment and to help control bioburden.

➤*Pharmacokinetics:*

Absorption – Silver is not absorbed through the skin

Silver gel has sustained and effective silver ion release for at least 3 days.

➤*Microbiology:* Silver gel has been shown to inhibit the growth of *Escherichia coli*, *Staphylococcus aureus*, methicillin-resistant *S. aureus* (MRSA), *Pseudomonas aeruginosa*, *Candida albicans*, *Aspergillus niger*, and others.

Contraindications

None known.

Warnings/Precautions

➤*Pregnancy:* Category undetermined. Silver is not absorbed through the skin.

➤*Lactation:* Silver is not absorbed through the skin.

Drug Interactions

None known.

Patient Information

If condition worsens or does not improve within 10 to 14 days, consult a health care provider. Keep this and all similar products out of the reach of children.

Advise patient that silver gel will not discolor or stain tissues.

Inform patients that silver gel may be left in the wound for up to 3 days.

BECAPLERMIN

Rx	**Regranex** (Ortho-McNeil)	**Gel; topical:** 0.01%	Parabens. In 2 and 15 g tubes.

BECAPLERMIN — TOPICAL

WARNING

An increased rate of mortality secondary to malignancy was observed in patients treated with 3 or more tubes of becaplermin in a postmarketing retrospective cohort study. Use becaplermin only when the benefits can be expected to outweigh the risks. Use becaplermin with caution in patients with known malignancy.

Indications

➤*Diabetic neuropathic ulcers:* For the treatment of lower extremity diabetic neuropathic ulcers that extend into the subcutaneous tissue or beyond and have an adequate blood supply.

Administration and Dosage

➤*General dosing considerations:* The weight of becaplermin from a 15 g tube is 0.65 g per inch length and 0.25 g per cm length.

➤*Adults:*

Diabetic neuropathic ulcers –

Usual dosage: The amount of becaplermin to be applied will vary depending upon the size of the ulcer area.

To calculate the length of gel to apply to the ulcer, measure the greatest length by the greatest width of the ulcer in either inches or centimeters. To calculate the length of gel in inches and centimeters, use the formulas in the following table.

BECAPLERMIN — TOPICAL

Formulas to Calculate the Length of Becaplermin Gel to be Applied Daily		
Tube size	Inches formula	Centimeters formula
15 g	length × width × 0.6	length × width ÷ 4
2 g	length × width × 1.3	length × width ÷ 2

Recalculating dose: The amount of becaplermin to be applied should be recalculated by the health care provider or wound care giver at weekly or biweekly intervals, depending on the rate of change in ulcer area.

➤*Children:*

16 years of age and older – See Adults for dosing.

➤*Administration:* For external use only.

To apply becaplermin, the calculated length of gel should be squeezed on to a clean measuring surface (eg, wax paper). The measured becaplermin is transferred from the clean measuring surface using an application aid and then spread over the entire ulcer area to yield a thin continuous layer of approximately 1/16 of an inch thickness. The site(s) of application should then be covered by a saline-moistened dressing and left in place for approximately 12 hours. The dressing should then be removed and the ulcer rinsed with saline or water to remove residual gel and covered again with a second moist dressing (without becaplermin) for the remainder of the day.

Becaplermin should be applied once daily to the ulcer until complete healing has occurred. If the ulcer does not decrease in size by approximately 30% after 10 weeks of treatment or complete healing has not occurred in 20 weeks, continued treatment with becaplermin should be reassessed.

➤*Storage/Stability:* Store refrigerated at 2° to 8°C (36° to 46°F). Do not freeze. Do not use the gel after the expiration date at the bottom of the tube.

Actions

➤*Pharmacology:* Becaplermin has biological activity similar to that of endogenous platelet-derived growth factor (PDGF), which includes promoting the chemotactic recruitment and proliferation of cells involved in wound repair and enhancing the formation of granulation tissue.

➤*Pharmacokinetics:*

Absorption – Ten patients with stage III or IV (as defined in the International Association of Enterostomal Therapy [IAET] guide to chronic wound staging) lower extremity diabetic ulcers received topical applications of becaplermin 0.01% at a dose range of 0.32 to 2.95 mcg/kg (7 mcg/cm^2) daily for 14 days. Six patients had nonquantifiable PDGF levels at baseline and throughout the study, 2 patients had PDGF levels at baseline which did not increase substantially, and 2 patients had PDGF levels that increased sporadically above their baseline values during the 14-day study period.

Systemic bioavailability of becaplermin was less than 3% in rats with full thickness wounds receiving single or multiple (5 days) topical applications of 127 mcg/kg (20.1 mcg/cm^2 of wound area) of becaplermin.

Contraindications

Known hypersensitivity to any component of this product (eg, parabens); known neoplasm(s) at the site(s) of application.

Warnings/Precautions

➤*Malignancy:* Becaplermin, a rhPDGF, promotes cellular proliferation and angiogenesis. Carefully evaluate the benefits and risks of becaplermin treatment before prescribing. Use becaplermin with caution in patients with a known malignancy.

Malignancies distant from the site of application have occurred in becaplermin users in a clinical study and postmarketing use, and an increased rate of death from systemic malignancies was seen in patients who have received 3 or more tubes of becaplermin.

➤*Other wounds:* Becaplermin is a nonsterile, low bioburden preserved product; therefore, do not use it in wounds that close by primary intention.

➤*Exposed joints, tendons, ligaments, and bone:* The effects of becaplermin on exposed joints, tendons, ligaments, and bone have not been established in humans. In preclinical studies, rats injected at the metatarsals with 3 or 10 mcg/site (approximately 60 or 200 mcg/kg) of becaplermin every other day for 13 days displayed histological changes indicative of accelerated bone remodeling consisting of periosteal hyperplasia and subperiosteal bone resorption and exostosis. The soft tissue adjacent to the injection site had fibroplasia with accompanying mononuclear cell infiltration reflective of the ability of PDGF to stimulate connective tissue growth.

➤*Hypersensitivity reactions:* If application site reactions occur, consider the possibility of sensitization or irritation caused by parabens or m-cresol.

➤*Pregnancy: Category C.* Animal reproduction studies have not been conducted with becaplermin. It is also not known whether becaplermin can cause fetal harm when administered to a pregnant woman or can affect reproductive capacity. Give becaplermin to pregnant women only if clearly needed.

➤*Lactation:* It is not known whether becaplermin is excreted in human milk. Because many drugs are secreted in human milk, exercise caution when becaplermin is administered to breast-feeding women.

➤*Children:* Safety and efficacy of becaplermin in children and adolescents younger than 16 years of age have not been established.

➤*Elderly:* Among patients receiving any dose of becaplermin in clinical studies of diabetic lower extremity ulcers, 150 patients were 65 years of age and older. No overall differences in safety or effectiveness were observed between patients younger than 65 years of age and patients 65 years of age and older. There was an insufficient number (n = 34) of subjects 75 years of age and older to determine whether they respond differently than younger patients.

➤*Monitoring:* Monitor patients for evidence of reduced ulcer.

Adverse Reactions

Patients receiving becaplermin, placebo, and good ulcer care alone had a similar incidence of ulcer-related adverse reactions, such as infection, cellulitis, or osteomyelitis. However, erythematous rashes occurred in 2% of becaplermin- and placebo-treated patients and in none of the patients receiving good ulcer care alone. The incidence of cardiovascular, respiratory, musculoskeletal, and central and peripheral nervous system disorders was not different across all treatment groups. Patients treated with becaplermin did not develop neutralizing antibodies against becaplermin.

Patient Information

Advise patients to thoroughly wash hands before applying becaplermin.

The tip of the tube should not come into contact with the ulcer or any other surface; tightly recap the tube after each use.

Use a cotton swab, tongue depressor, or other application aid to apply becaplermin.

Only apply becaplermin once a day in a carefully measured quantity. Evenly spread the measured quantity of gel over the ulcerated area to yield a thin continuous layer of approximately 1⁄16 of an inch thickness. Adjust the measured length of the gel to be squeezed from the tube according to the size of the ulcer. Recalculate the amount of becaplermin to be applied daily at weekly or biweekly intervals by the health care provider or wound caregiver.

➤*Step-by-step instructions for application of becaplermin:*

- Squeeze the calculated length of gel on to a clean, firm, nonabsorbable surface (eg, wax paper).
- With a clean cotton swab, tongue depressor, or similar application aid, spread the measured becaplermin over the ulcer surface to obtain an even layer.
- Cover with a saline-moistened gauze dressing.

After approximately 12 hours, gently rinse the ulcer with saline or water to remove residual gel and cover with a saline-moistened gauze dressing (without becaplermin).

It is important to use becaplermin together with a good ulcer care program, including a strict nonweight-bearing program.

Excess application of becaplermin has not been shown to be beneficial.

Store becaplermin in the refrigerator. Do not freeze becaplermin.

Do not use becaplermin after the expiration date on the bottom, crimped end of the tube.

CHLOROPHYLL DERIVATIVES

otc	**Chloresium** (Rystan)	**Ointment:** 0.5% chlorophyllin copper complex in a hydrophilic base	In 30 and 120 g and lb.
		Solution: 0.2% chlorophyllin copper complex in isotonic saline	In 240 and 960 mL.

CHLOROPHYLL DERIVATIVES — TOPICAL

Refer to the Gastrointestinal Agents chapter for additional information.

Indications

➤*Dermatoses:* Arteriosclerotic, diabetic and varicose ulcers; trophic decubitus ulcers and chronic ulcers of nonspecific origin; malignant lesions (where deodorization is desired); traumatic injuries; skin grafting and skin defects; thermal, chemical and irradiation injuries; a wide variety of dermatoses.

Administration and Dosage

➤*Adults:*

Dermatoses –

Ointment: Apply generously and cover with gauze, linen, or another appropriate dressing. For best results, do not change dressings more than every 48 to 72 hours.

Solution: Apply full strength as a continuous wet dressing or instill directly into sinus tracts, fistulae, deep ulcers, or cavities.

Actions

➤*Pharmacology:* Aids wound healing by helping to produce a clean, granulating wound base for epithelialization or skin grafting. It also soothes inflamed, painful tissues and controls wound odor, even in malignant lesions. This is a true deodorizing, not a masking, action.

Warnings/Precautions

➤*Pregnancy: Category: Undetermined.* Consult a health care provider before using in pregnant women.

➤*Lactation:* Consult a health care provider before using in breast-feeding women.

Adverse Reactions

Sensitivity reactions (rare); itching; irritation.

SINECATECHINS

Rx	**Veregen** (Doak Dermatologics)	**Ointment:** 15%	Gallic acid, caffeine, theobromine, isopropyl myristate, oleyl alcohol.[a] In 15 g tube.

[a] Gallic acid, caffeine, and theobromine constitute approximately 2.5% of the product.

SINECATECHINS — TOPICAL

Indications

➤*External genital and perianal warts:* For the topical treatment of external genital and perianal warts (*Condyloma acuminatum*) in immunocompetent patients 18 years of age and older.

Administration and Dosage

➤*Adults:*

External genital and perianal warts –

Usual dosage: Apply a thin layer (approximately a 0.5 cm strand) 3 times per day to all external genital and perianal warts.

Duration of therapy: Treatment should be continued until complete clearance of all warts; however, treatment should not last longer than 16 weeks. Local skin reactions (eg, erythema) at the treatment site are frequent. Nevertheless, treatment should be continued when the severity of the local skin reaction is acceptable.

➤*Administration:* Approximately a 0.5 cm strand of the ointment should be applied to each wart using the fingers, dabbing it on to ensure complete coverage and leaving a thin layer of the ointment on the warts.

It is recommended to wash the hands before and after application. It is not necessary to wash off the ointment from the treated area prior to the next application.

➤*Storage/Stability:* Prior to dispensing to the patient, store refrigerated at 2° to 8°C (36° to 46°F). After dispensing, store refrigerated or at a temperature of up to 25°C (77°F). Do not freeze.

Actions

➤*Pharmacology:* The mode of action of sinecatechins ointment involved in the clearance of genital and perianal warts is unknown. In vitro, sinecatechins had antioxidative activity; the clinical significance of this finding is unknown.

➤*Pharmacokinetics:* The pharmacokinetics of topically applied sinecatechins has not been sufficiently characterized at this time. However, data suggest that systemic exposure to catechins after repeated topical application of sinecatechins is likely to be less than that observed after a single oral intake of green tea 400 mL.

Contraindications

History of sensitivity reactions to any of the components of the ointment. In case of hypersensitivity, discontinue treatment.

Warnings/Precautions

➤*Human papilloma viral disease:* Sinecatechins has not been evaluated for the treatment of urethral, intravaginal, cervical, rectal, or intra-anal human papilloma viral disease; do not use it for the treatment of these conditions.

➤*Open wounds:* Avoid using sinecatechins on open wounds.

➤*Immunosuppressed patients:* The safety and efficacy in immunosuppressed patients have not been established.

➤*Photosensitivity:* Advise patients to avoid exposure of the genital and perianal area to sunlight and ultraviolet (UV) light; sinecatechins has not been tested under these circumstances.

➤*Pregnancy: Category C.* In the presence of maternal toxicity (characterized by marked local irritation at the administration sites, and decreased body weight and food consumption) in pregnant female rabbits, subcutaneous doses of sinecatechins 12 and 36 mg/kg/day during the period of organogenesis (gestational days 6 to 19) resulted in corresponding influences on fetal development including reduced fetal body weights and delays in skeletal ossification. No treatment-related effects on embryofetal development were noted at 4 mg/kg/day (0.7-fold maximum recommended human dose [MRHD]). There was no evidence of teratogenic effects at any of the doses evaluated in this study.

A pre- and postnatal development study was conducted in rats using vaginal administration of sinecatechins at doses of 0.05, 0.1, and 0.15 mL/rat/day from day 6 of gestation through parturition and lactation. The high and intermediate dose levels of 0.15 (8-fold MRHD) and 0.1 mL/rat/day resulted in an increased mortality of the F_0 dams, associated with indications of parturition complications. The high dose level of 0.15 mL/rat/day also resulted in an increased incidence of stillbirths. There were no other treatment-related effects on pre- and postnatal development, growth, reproduction, and fertility at any dose tested.

There are no adequate and well-controlled studies in pregnant women. Use sinecatechins during pregnancy only if the potential benefit justifies the potential risk to the fetus.

➤*Lactation:* It is not known whether topically applied sinecatechins is excreted in breast milk.

➤*Children:* Safety and efficacy in children have not been established.

Drug Interactions

None known.

Adverse Reactions

Serious local adverse reactions of pain and inflammation were reported in 2 (0.5%) subjects, both women.

In clinical trials, the incidence of local adverse reactions leading to discontinuation or dose interruption (reduction) was 5% (19 of 397 subjects). These included application-site reactions (eg, erythema, local pain, skin erosion/ulceration, vesicles), dysuria, erosions in the urethral meatus, genital herpes simplex, hypersensitivity, inguinal lymphadenitis, phimosis, pruritus, pyodermitis, skin ulcer, superinfection of warts and ulcers, urethral meatal stenosis, and vulvitis.

Sinecatechins Adverse Reactions (> 1%)

Adverse reaction	Sinecatechins (n = 397)	Vehicle (n = 207)
Dermatologic		
Bleeding	2%	< 1%
Burning	67%	31%
Desquamation	5%	< 1%
Discharge	3%	< 1%
Erosion/Ulceration	49%	10%
Erythema	70%	32%
Irritation	1%	0%
Pruritus	69%	45%
Rash	1%	0%
Rash vesicular	20%	6%
Regional lymphadenitis	3%	1%
Scar	1%	0%
Miscellaneous		
Edema	45%	11%
Induration	35%	11%
Pain/Discomfort	56%	14%
Reaction	2%	0%

A total of 67% (266 of 397) subjects in the sinecatechins group had either a moderate or a severe reaction that was considered probably related and, of these subjects, 120 (30%) had a severe reaction. Severe reactions occurred in 37% (71 of 192) of women and 24% (49 of 205) of men. The percentage of subjects with at least 1 severe, related adverse reaction was 26% (86 of 328) in subjects with genital warts only, 42% (19 of 45) in subjects with both genital and perianal warts, and 48% (11 of 23) in subjects with perianal warts only.

Phimosis occurred in 3% (5 of 174) of uncircumcised male subjects treated with sinecatechins and in 1% (1 of 99) in vehicle.

The maximum mean severity of edema, erosion, erythema, and induration was observed by week 2 of treatment.

Less common local adverse reactions included discoloration, dryness, eczema, hyperesthesia, necrosis, papules, perianal infection, pigmentation changes, and urethritis. Other less common adverse reactions included cervical dysplasia, cutaneous facial rash, pelvic pain, and staphylococcemia.

In a dermal sensitization study of sinecatechins in healthy volunteers, hypersensitivity (type IV) was observed in 2.4% (5 of 209) subjects under occlusive conditions.

Overdosage

Overdosage with sinecatechins has not been reported.

Patient Information

Advise patients that this medication is only to be used as directed by a health care provider. It is for external use only. Avoid eye contact, as well as application into the vagina or anus.

Advise patients that it is not necessary to wash off sinecatechins prior to the next application. When the treatment area is washed or a bath is taken, apply the ointment afterwards.

Advise patients that it is common to experience local skin reactions, such as erythema, erosion, edema, itching, and burning, at the site of application. Severe skin reactions can occur; instruct patients to promptly report such

SINECATECHINS — TOPICAL

reactions to their health care provider. If severe local skin reactions occur, instruct patients to remove the ointment by washing the treatment area with mild soap and water; hold further doses.

Instruct patients to avoid sexual (genital, anal, or oral) contact while the ointment is on the skin, or to wash off the ointment prior to these activities. Sinecatechins ointment may weaken condoms and vaginal diaphragms; therefore, the use in combination with sinecatechins ointment is not recommended.

Instruct women using tampons to insert the tampon before applying the ointment. If the tampon is changed while the ointment is on the skin, instruct the patient to avoid accidental application of the ointment into the vagina.

Advise patients that sinecatechins may stain clothing and bedding.

Advise patients that sinecatechins is not a cure and new warts might develop during or after a course of therapy. If new warts develop during the 16-week treatment period, treat with sinecatechins ointment.

Advise patients that the effect of sinecatechins on the transmission of genital/perianal warts is unknown.

Advise patients to avoid exposure of the genital and perianal area to sunlight or UV light; sinecatechins has not been tested under these circumstances.

Instruct patients not to bandage or otherwise cover or wrap the treatment area in such a way as to be occlusive.

Instruct uncircumcised men treating warts under the foreskin to retract the foreskin and clean the area daily.

EFLORNITHINE HYDROCHLORIDE

EFLORNITHINE HYDROCHLORIDE

Rx	Vaniqa (SkinMedica)	Cream: 13.9%	Parabens, mineral oil, alcohols. In 30 g.

EFLORNITHINE HYDROCHLORIDE — TOPICAL

Indications

➤*Reduction of facial hair:* For the reduction of unwanted facial hair in women.

Administration and Dosage

➤*General dosing considerations:* Cosmetics or sunscreens may be applied over treated areas after cream has dried.

The patient should continue to use hair removal techniques as needed in conjunction with eflornithine. Eflornithine should be applied at least 5 minutes after hair removal.

➤*Adults:*

Reduction of facial hair – Apply a thin layer of eflornithine HCl to affected areas of the face and adjacent involved areas under the chin and rub in thoroughly. Do not wash treated area for at least 4 hours. Use twice daily at least 8 hours apart or as directed by a health care provider.

➤*Children:*

Reduction of facial hair –

12 years of age or older: See Adults for dosing.

➤*Storage/Stability:* Store at 25°C (77°F); excursions permitted to 15° to 30°C (59° to 86°F). Do not freeze.

Actions

➤*Pharmacology:* There are no studies examining the inhibition of the enzyme ornithine decarboxylase (ODC) in human skin following the application of topical eflornithine. However, there are studies in the literature that report the inhibition of ODC activity in skin following oral eflornithine. It is postulated that topical eflornithine HCl irreversibly inhibits skin ODC activity. This enzyme is necessary in the synthesis of polyamines. Animal data indicate that inhibition of ornithine decarboxylase inhibits cell division and synthetic functions, which affect the rate of hair growth. Eflornithine HCl cream has been shown to retard the rate of hair growth in nonclinical and clinical studies.

➤*Pharmacokinetics:*

Absorption/Distribution – The mean percutaneous absorption of eflornithine in women with unwanted facial hair, from a 13.9% w/w cream formulation, is less than 1% of the radioactive dose, following either single or multiple doses under conditions of clinical use, that included shaving within 2 hours before radiolabeled dose application in addition to other forms of cutting or plucking and tweezing to remove facial hair. Steady state was reached within 4 days of twice daily application. The apparent steady-state plasma $t_{½}$ of eflornithine was ≈ 8 hours. Following twice-daily application of 0.5 g of the cream (total dose 1 g/day; 139 mg as anhydrous eflornithine HCl), under conditions of clinical use in women with unwanted facial hair (n = 10), the steady-state C_{max}, C_{trough} and area under the plasma concentration curve (AUC_{12hr}) were ≈ 10 ng/mL, 5 ng/mL, and 92 ng•hr/mL, respectively, expressed in terms of the anhydrous free base of eflornithine HCl. At steady state, the dose-normalized peak concentrations (C_{max}) and the extent of daily systemic exposure (AUC) of eflornithine following twice-daily application of 0.5 g of the cream (total dose 1 g/day) is estimated to be ≈ 100- and 60-fold lower, respectively, when compared to 370 mg/day once daily oral doses.

Metabolism/Excretion – This compound is not known to be metabolized and is primarily excreted unchanged in the urine.

Contraindications

Sensitivity to any components of the preparation.

Warnings/Precautions

➤*Usage:* For external use only. Transient stinging or burning may occur when applied to abraded or broken skin.

➤*Hypersensitivity reactions:* Discontinue use if hypersensitivity occurs.

➤*Pregnancy: Category C.* In the first dermal embryo-fetal development study in rats treated with eflornithine HCl cream, 13.9% (in which no precautions were taken to prevent ingestion of drug from application sites), maternal toxicity and fetal effects including reduced numbers of live fetuses, decreased fetal weights, and delayed ossification and development of the viscera were observed at doses of 225 and 450 mg/kg (15 × and 29 × the MRHD based on BSA, respectively). When the study was repeated under conditions that avoided ingestion from application sites, no maternal, fetal or teratogenic effects were observed at doses up to 450 mg/kg (29 × the MRHD based on BSA). In the first study in which no precautions were taken to prevent ingestion, circulating plasma levels were 11- to 14- fold higher than in the second study in which ingestion was prevented. In a dermal embryo-fetal development study in rabbits treated with eflornithine HCl cream no adverse maternal or fetal effects occurred at doses up to 90 mg/kg (11 × the MRHD based on BSA). Significant dermal irritation, as well as possible ingestion of eflornithine HCl cream occurred at 300 mg/kg/day (36 × the MRHD based on BSA) and was associated with maternal deaths, abortions, increased fetal resorptions, and reduced fetal weights. Fetotoxicity in the absence of maternal toxicity has been reported in oral studies with eflornithine with fetal no-effect doses of 80 mg/kg in rats and 45 mg/kg in rabbits. In these studies, no evidence of teratogenicity was observed in rats given up to 200 mg/kg or in rabbits given up to 135 mg/kg.

Although eflornithine HCl cream was not formally studied in pregnant patients, 22 pregnancies occurred during the trials. Nineteen of these pregnancies occurred while patients were using eflornithine HCl. Of the 19 pregnancies, there were 9 healthy infants, 4 spontaneous abortions, 5 induced/elective abortions, and 1 birth defect (Down's syndrome to a 35 year-old). Because there are no adequate and well-controlled studies in pregnant women, the risk/benefit ratio of using eflornithine HCl in women with unwanted facial hair who are pregnant should be weighed carefully with serious consideration for either not implementing or discontinuing use of eflornithine HCl cream.

➤*Lactation:* It is not known whether or not eflornithine HCl is excreted in human milk. Caution should be exercised when eflornithine HCl is administered to a nursing woman.

➤*Children:* The safety and effectiveness of this product have not been established in pediatric patients younger than 12 years of age.

Adverse Reactions

Eflornithine Adverse Reactions (> 1%)

Adverse Reaction	Vehicle-controlled studies: Eflornithine HCl cream (n = 393)	Vehicle-controlled studies: Vehicle (n = 201)%	Vehicle-controlled and open-label studies: Eflornithine HCl cream (n = 1373)
Acne	21.3%	21.4%	10.8%
Alopecia	1.5%	2.5%	1.3%
Anorexia	1%	2%	0.7%
Asthenia	0%	1%	0.3%
Burning skin	4.3%	2%	3.5%
Dizziness	1.5%	1.5%	1.3%
Dry skin	1.8%	3%	3.3%
Dyspepsia	2.5%	2%	1.9%
Erythema (redness)	1.3%	0%	2.5%
Facial edema	0.3%	3%	0.7%
Folliculitis	0.5%	0%	1%
Hair ingrown	0.3%	2%	0.9%
Headache	3.8%	5%	4%
Nausea	0.5%	1%	0.7%
Pruritus (itching)	3.8%	4%	3.1%
Pseudofolliculitis barbae	16.3%	15.4%	4.9%
Rash	2.8%	0%	1.5%
Skin irritation	1%	1%	1.8%
Stinging skin	7.9%	2.5%	4.1%

EFLORNITHINE HYDROCHLORIDE — TOPICAL

Eflornithine Adverse Reactions (> 1%)			
	Vehicle-controlled studies		Vehicle-controlled and open-label studies
Adverse Reaction	Eflornithine HCl cream (n = 393)	Vehicle (n = 201)%	Eflornithine HCl cream (n = 1373)
Tingling skin	3.6%	1.5%	2.2%
Vertigo	0.3%	1%	0.1%

➤*Dermatologic:* Treatment-related skin adverse events that occurred in less than 1% of the subjects treated with eflornithine HCl are the following: Bleeding skin, cheilitis, contact dermatitis, swelling of lips, herpes simplex, numbness and rosacea.

➤*Lab test abnormalities:* No laboratory test abnormalities have been consistently found to be associated with eflornithine HCl cream. In an open-labeled study, some patients showed an increase in their transaminases; however, the clinical significance of these findings is not known.

Overdosage

Overdosage information with eflornithine HCl cream is unavailable. Given the low percutaneous penetration of this drug, overdosage via the topical route is not expected (see Pharmacokinetics).

➤*Treatment:* However, should very high topical doses (eg, multiple tubes per day) or oral ingestion be encountered (a 30 g tube contains 4.2 g of eflornithine HCl), the patient should be monitored, and appropriate supportive measures administered as necessary.

Patient Information

➤*Who should not use eflornithine HCl cream?:* You should not use eflornithine HCl cream if you are allergic to any of the ingredients in the cream. All ingredients are listed on the tube and at the beginning of this leaflet.

You should not use eflornithine HCl cream if you are younger than 12 years of age.

➤*What should you tell your doctor before using eflornithine HCl cream?:* If you are allergic to any of the ingredients, tell your doctor.

If you are pregnant or plan to become pregnant, discuss with your doctor whether you should use eflornithine HCl cream during pregnancy. No clinical studies have been performed in pregnant women.

If you are breastfeeding, consult your doctor before using eflornithine HCl cream. It is not known if eflornithine HCl cream is passed to infants through breast milk.

If you are taking any prescription medicines, nonprescription medicines or using any facial or skin creams, check with your physician before use of eflornithine HCl cream.

➤*What are the possible side effects of eflornithine HCl cream?:* Eflornithine HCl cream may cause temporary redness, stinging, burning, tingling or rash on areas of the skin where it is applied. Folliculitis (hair bumps) may also occur. If these persist, consult your doctor.

EMOLLIENTS

DEXPANTHENOL

otc	**Panthoderm** (Jones Medical)	**Cream; topical**: 2% in a water miscible base	In 30 and 60 g.

DEXPANTHENOL — TOPICAL

Indications

➤*Dermatological conditions:* Relieves itching and aids healing of skin in mild eczemas and dermatoses; itching skin, minor wounds, stings, bites, poison ivy, poison oak (dry stage) and minor skin irritations. Also used in infants and children for diaper rash, chafing and mild skin irritations.

Administration and Dosage

➤*Adults:*

Dermatological conditions – Apply to affected areas once or twice daily.

➤*Children:*

Dermatological conditions – Apply to affected areas once or twice daily.

➤*Administration:* For external use only. Avoid contact with the eyes.

UREA (Carbamide)

Rx	**Urea 50%** (E. Fougera)	**Ointment; topical**: 50%	Cetyl alcohol, disodium EDTA, glycerin, lactic acid, PEG 6, vitamin E, zinc pyrithione. In 45 g.
Rx	**Keralac** (Pharmaderm)		Vitamin E, lactic acid, zinc pyrithione, glycerin, EDTA, cetyl alcohol. In 45 g.
otc	**Urea 10%** (Stratus)	**Cream; topical**: 10%	Propylene glycol, trolamine. In 85 g.
otc	**Aquacare** (Numark Labs)		Petrolatum, glycerin, lanolin oil, mineral oil, lanolin alcohol, benzyl alcohol. In 75 g.
otc	**Carmol 20** (Pharmaderm)	**Cream; topical**: 20%	Nonlipid vanishing cream base. In 85 g.
otc	**Gormel Creme** (Gordon)		Mineral oil, parabens. In 75 and 120 g.
otc	**Lanaphilic** (Medco)		Petrolatum, lanolin oil, PPG, lactic acid, parabens. In 150 and 454 g.
otc	**Ureacin-20** (Pedinol)		Lactic acid, glycerin, mineral oil, parabens, EDTA. In 75 g.
Rx	**Urea** (Various, eg, Clay Park, Hi-Tech)	**Cream; topical**: 40%	Mineral oil, petrolatum, cetyl alcohol. In 28.35 and 198.6 g.
Rx	**Aluvea** (Merz Pharmaceutical)		Emulsifying wax, glycerin 99.7%. In 237 mL.
Rx	**Carmol 40** (Pharmaderm)		Mineral oil, petrolatum, cetyl alcohol. In 28.35 and 85 g.
Rx	**Gordon's Urea 40%** (Gordon)		Petrolatum base. In 30 g.
Rx	**Vanamide** (Dermik)		Light mineral oil, cetyl alcohol, petrolatum. In 85 and 199 g.
Rx	**Urea** (River's Edge)	**Cream; topical**: 45%	Camphor, edetate disodium, ethyl alcohol, eucalyptus oil, menthol, titanium dioxide. In 255 g.
Rx	**Uramaxin** (Medimetriks Pharmaceuticals)		Camphor, edetate disodium, eucalyptus oil, menthol. In 255 g.
Rx	**Keralac** (Pharmaderm)	**Cream; topical**: 50%	Cetyl alcohol, EDTA, lactic acid. In 142 and 255 g.
otc	**Urea 10%** (Stratus)	**Lotion; topical**: 10%	Propylene glycol, trolamine. In 473, 236, and 177 mL.
otc	**Aquacare** (Numark Labs)		Mineral oil, petrolatum, parabens. In 240 mL.
otc	**Carmol 10** (Pharmaderm)		In 180 mL.
otc	**Ureacin-10** (Pedinol)		EDTA, parabens, lactic acid. In 240 mL.
otc	**Dermal Therapy Finger Care** (Bayer)	**Lotion; topical**: 20%	Beeswax, cetyl alcohol, disodium EDTA, emulsifying wax, parabens, PEG, petrolatum, lactic acid, triethanolamine. In 18 mL.
otc	**Ultra Mide 25** (Ivax)	**Lotion; topical**: 25%	Mineral oil, glycerin, lanolin, EDTA. In 240 mL.
Rx	**Urea** (River's Edge)	**Lotion; topical**: 35%	Cetyl alcohol, EDTA, lactic acid. In 207 and 325 mL.
Rx	**Keralac** (Pharmaderm)		Cetyl alcohol, EDTA, lactic acid. In 207 and 325 mL.
Rx	**Urealac** (Hi-Tech)		Cetyl alcohol, edetate disodium, lactic acid, mineral oil, vitamin E. In 207 and 325 mL.
Rx	**Urea** (Various, eg, Clay Park, Hi-Tech)	**Lotion; topical**: 40%	Mineral oil, petrolatum, cetyl alcohol. In 236.6 mL.

UREA (Carbamide)

Rx	**TL 45%** (Trigen Laboratories)	**Lotion; topical:** 45%	Camphor, disodium EDTA, ethyl alcohol, eucalyptus oil, menthol. In 473 g.
Rx	**Uramaxin** (Medimetriks Pharmaceuticals)		Camphor, edetate disodium, ethyl alcohol, eucalyptus oil, menthol, titanium dioxide. In 473 g.
Rx	**Urea** (Various, eg, Clay Park, Hi-Tech)	**Gel; topical:** 40%	Glycerin, EDTA. In 15 mL.
Rx	**Carmol 40** (Pharmaderm)		Glycerin, EDTA. In 15 mL.
Rx	**Urea 40** (Kylemore)		Disodium EDTA, glycerin, PEG. In 15 mL w/ applicator brush.
Rx	**Urea Nail Gel** (Kylemore Pharmaceuticals)	**Gel; topical:** 45%	Camphor, disodium EDTA, eucalyptus oil, menthol. In 28 mL.
Rx	**Urea Nail Gel** (A. Aarons)	**Gel; topical:** 50%	EDTA. In 18 mL.
Rx	**Keralac** (Pharmaderm)		EDTA, lactic acid. In 18 mL.
Rx	**Urea** (Prasco)	**Suspension; topical:** 40%	EDTA, glycerin, shea butter, sunflower oil. In 300 mL.
Rx	**Umecta** (JSJ)		*Helianthus annuus* oil, EDTA. In 283.4 g.
Rx	**Umecta Nail Film** (JSJ)		EDTA, glycerin. In 18 mL with applicator.
Rx	**Umecta PD** (JSJ)	**Suspension, bioadhesive; topical:** 40%	0.3% sodium hyaluronate. *Helianthus annuus* oil, EDTA. In 283.4 g.
Rx	**Urea** (Various, eg, A. Aarons, Fougera)	**Suspension; topical:** 50%	May contain Caprylic/capric triglyceride, cetyl alcohol, edetate disodium, glycerin, lactic acid, linoleic acid, PEG-6, propylene glycol, salicylic acid, titanium dioxide, triethanolamine, vitamin E. In 284 g tubes.
Rx	**Kerol** (Doak)		Cetyl alcohol, lactic acid, PEG-6, titanium dioxide. In 284 g tubes.
Rx	**Urea** (Prasco)	**Emulsion; topical:** 40%	EDTA, glycerin, shea butter, sunflower oil. In 120 and 240 g.
Rx	**Umecta** (JSJ)		*Helianthus annuus* oil, EDTA. In 113.5 g.
Rx	**Kerol AD** (Pharmaderm)	**Emulsion; topical:** 45%	Cetyl alcohol, EDTA disodium, glycerin, lactic acid, PEG, titanium dioxide. In 240 mL.
Rx	**Latrix XM** (Stratus)		Caprylic/Capric triglycerides, cetyl alcohol, EDTA disodium, glycerin, lactic acid, linoleic acid, PEG 300, titanium dioxide. In 240 mL.
Rx	**Urea** (Fougera)	**Emulsion; topical:** 50%	Cetyl alcohol, disodium EDTA, glycerin, lactic acid, PEG-6, titanium dioxide, vitamin E. In 284 g.
Rx	**BP-50** (Brookstone)		Cetyl alcohol, disodium EDTA, glycerin, lactic acid, PEG-6, titanium dioxide, vitamin E. In 284 g.
Rx	**Kerol** (PharmaDerm)		Cetyl alcohol, disodium EDTA, glycerin, lactic acid, PEG-6, vitamin E. In 284 g.
Rx	**Uramaxin GT** (Medimetriks)	**Solution; topical:** 45%	Camphor, edetate disodium, eucalyptus oil, menthol, propylene glycol. In 20 mL prefilled applicator.
Rx	**Keralac Nailstik** (Pharmaderm)	**Solution; topical:** 50%	EDTA. In carton of 6 nailsticks, each containing 2.4 mL.
Rx	**Kerol ZX** (PharmaDerm)		Disodium EDTA, lactic acid, PEG-6, vitamin E. In 12 mL prefilled applicator.
Rx	**RE Urea 50** (River's Edge)		Cetyl alcohol, disodium EDTA, glycerin, lactic acid, mineral oil, PEG-6, titanium dioxide. In 4 mL prefilled applicators.
Rx	**Urea Nailstick 50%** (Fougera)		Disodium EDTA, lactic acid, PEG-6, propylene glycol, triethanolamine, zinc pyrithione. In 2.4 mL.
Rx	**Uramaxin** (Medimetriks)	**Foam; topical:** 20%	Cetearyl alcohol, cetyl alcohol, PEG-100, white petrolatum. In 100 g.
Rx	**Kerafoam** (Onset Therapeutics)	**Foam; topical:** 30%	Cetyl alcohol, parabens. In 60 g.
Rx	**Urea 35%** (Acella)	**Aerosol, foam; topical:** 35%	Dimethicone, glycerin, lactic acid, parabens, propylene glycol, trolamine. In 150 g.
Rx	**Hydro 35** (Quinnova)		Dimethicone, glycerin, lactic acid, parabens. In 150 g.
Rx	**Hydro 40** (Quinnova)	**Aerosol, foam; topical:** 40%	Colloidal oatmeal, glycerin, parabens. In 70 g aerosolized canister.
Rx	**RE-U40** (River's Edge)		Colloidal oatmeal, glycerin, parabens. In 70 g aerosolized canister.
Rx	**Kerafoam 42** (Onset Therapeutics)	**Aerosol, foam; topical:** 42%	Cetearyl alcohol, edetate disodium, parabens. In 60 g.
Rx	**Umecta** (JSJ Pharmaceuticals)	**Foam, topical:** 40%	Shea butter, sunflower oil. In 120 mL.
Rx	**Urea 42%** (River's Edge)	**Cloths, topical:** 42%	Disodium EDTA, glycerine, lactic acid. In 30s.
Rx	**Rinnovi Nail System** (Quinnova)	**Stick; topical:** 50%	EDTA. In 6s with nail stick, cuticle cleanser and protectant spray.

UREA — TOPICAL

Indications

➤*Urea 42%:* For softening, smoothing and removing rough scaling hyperkeratotic skin in conditions such as xerosis, ichthyosis, skin cracks and fissures, dermatitis, eczema, psoriasis, keratosis and calluses.

➤*Urea 40%, 40% (foam), 35% (foam), 45% (cream), and 50%:* For debridement and promotion of normal healing of hyperkeratotic surface lesions, particularly where healing is retarded by local infection, necrotic tissue, fibrinous or purulent debris, or eschar. Urea is useful for the treatment of hyperkeratotic conditions, such as dry, rough skin; dermatitis; psoriasis; xerosis; ichthyosis; eczema; keratosis; keratoderma; and corns and calluses; as well as damaged, ingrown, and devitalized nails.

➤*Urea 10% and 20%:* For moisturizing and softening dry, cracked, calloused rough and hardened skin of feet, hands, or elbows.

➤*Urea 30% (foam):* For softening, smoothing, and removing rough scaling hyperkeratotic skin in conditions such as xerosis, ichthyosis, skin cracks and fissures, dermatitis, eczema, psoriasis, keratoses, and calluses.

Administration and Dosage

➤*Urea 40% and 50%:* Apply urea cream, lotion, ointment, stick, or gel to affected areas twice per day, or as directed by a health care provider. Rub in until completely absorbed. Protect surrounding tissue.

Apply to diseased or damaged nail tissue twice per day, or as directed by a health care provider. If desired, cover with an adhesive bandage or gauze and secure with adhesive tape.

When applying to diseased or damaged nail surfaces, use an ample amount. Cover as previously described. You can also remove a "finger" from a plastic or vinyl glove and slip over the bandage-covered site. Secure glove finger with additional adhesive tape. Keep dry and occlusive for 3 to 7 days.

➤*Urea 45%:* Apply to affected skin twice per day, or damaged nails twice per day, or as directed by a physician.

➤*Urea 10% and 20%:* Massage into dry skin areas once daily or as prescribed by a health care provider.

➤*Urea 30% (foam):* Shake well before use.

Upon initial use only, prime the aerosol can by holding it upright, direct away from the patient, and depress the actuator for 3 to 5 seconds or until foam begins to dispense.

Holding can upright, dispense and apply to affected area twice per day, or as directed by a health care provider. Rub in until completely absorbed. Wipe off any excess foam from actuator after use.

➤*Urea 40% (foam):* Unless otherwise directed by a prescribing health care provider, urea 40% should be applied to the affected area twice a day. Urea 40% should be rubbed into the skin until it is completely absorbed.

UREA — TOPICAL

➤*Urea 42% (foam):* Upon initial use only, prime the aerosol can by gently tapping the bottom of the can onto palm of other hand or a solid surface at least 3 times. Hold the can upright, away from the patient, and firmly depress the actuator for 1 to 3 seconds or until foam begins to dispense. Shake vigorously and gently tap bottom of can onto palm of other hand or a solid surface at least 3 times. Holding can upright, dispense foam into palm of hand and apply to affected area twice per day, or as directed by a physician. Rub in until completely absorbed. Wipe off any excess foam from actuator after use.

➤*Urea 50% (emulsion):* Apply *Kerol* Emulsion to affected skin twice per day, or as directed by a physician. Rub until completely absorbed.

➤*Urea 42% (cloths):* Apply Urea 42% Cloths to affected skin twice per day, or as directed by a physician.

➤*Storage/Stability:* Store at controlled room temperature, 15° to 30°C (59° to 86°F).

Store foam at 15° to 25°C (59° to 77°F).

Protect from freezing. Keep this and all medications out of the reach of children.

VITAMIN E TOPICAL

otc	**Chantel Vitamin E** (National Vitamin)	**Cream; topical**: dl-alpha tocopheryl acetate, ergocalciferol, cetyl alcohol, panthenol, parabens, safflower oil, urea, vegetable oil	In 454 g.
otc	**Vitamin E** (Various, eg, Nature's Bounty)	**Cream; topical**	In 60 g.
otc	**Vitec** (Pharmaceutical Specialities)	**Cream; topical**: dl-alpha tocopheryl acetate in a vanishing cream base, cetearyl alcohol, sorbitol, propylene glycol, simethicone, glyceryl monostearate, PEG monostearate	In 120 g.
otc	**Vite E Creme** (Gordon)	**Cream; topical**: 50 mg dl-alpha tocopheryl acetate per g	In lb.
otc	**Vitamin E** (Various, eg, Nature's Bounty)	**Lotion; topical**	In 120 mL.
otc	**Palomar "E"** (Pal Midwest)	**Ointment; topical**: Vitamin E, boric acid, beeswax, lanolin, mineral oil, petroleum, starch, zinc oxide	In 2 oz.
otc	**Coppertone Aloe Aftersun Lotion** (Schering-Plough)	**Lotion; topical**: Vitamin E, aloe, glyceryl, lanolin, paraben, EDTA, jojoba oil, cocoa butter, mineral oil	In 473 mL.
otc	**E-Oil** (Nature's Bounty)	**Oil; topical**: Vitamin E, corn oil, lemon oil, sesame oil, soybean oil, wheat germ oil	In 74 mL.
otc	**Vitamin E** (Various, eg, Mission, Nature's Bounty)	**Oil; topical**	In 30 and 60 mL.[a]

[a] May or may not contain aloe.

VITAMIN E — TOPICAL

Indications

➤*Dermatological conditions:* Temporary relief of minor skin disorders such as diaper rash, burns, sunburn and chapped or dry skin.

Administration and Dosage

➤*Adults:*

Dermatological conditions – Apply a thin layer over affected area.

➤*Children:*

Dermatological conditions – Apply a thin layer over affected area.

➤*Administration:* For external use only. Avoid contact with the eyes.

VITAMINS A, D and E

otc	**Vitamin A & D** (Various, eg, Goldline)	**Ointment; topical**	In 60 g and lb.
otc	**A and D** (Schering-Plough)	**Ointment; topical**: Fish liver oil, cholecalciferol, lanolin, petrolatum, mineral oil	In 45, 120, 480 g, 75 g pump dispenser.
otc	**Caldesene** (Insight)	**Ointment; topical**: Cod liver oil (vitamins A and D), 15% zinc oxide, lanolin oil, 54% petrolatum, parabens, talc	In 37.5 g.
otc	**Comfortine** (Dermik)	**Ointment; topical**: Vitamins A and D, lanolin, zinc oxide, chloroxylenol, iron oxides, lanolin alcohol, mineral oil, triethanolamine, vegetable oil	In 45 and 120 g.
otc	**Desitin** (Pfizer)	**Ointment; topical**: Cod liver oil (vit A & D), 40% zinc oxide, talc, petrolatum-lanolin base	In 30, 60, 120, 240, 270 g.
otc	**Lobana Peri-Garde** (Ulmer)	**Ointment; topical**: Vitamins A, D and E and chloroxylenol in an emollient base	In 240 g.
otc	**Clocream** (Roberts)	**Cream; topical**: Cod liver oil (vitamins A and D), cholecalciferol, vitamin A palmitate, cottonseed oil, glycerin, parabens, mineral oil	Vanishing base. In 30 g.
otc	**Lazer Creme** (Pedinol)	**Cream; topical**: Vitamins A (3333.3 units/g) and E (116.67 units/g)	In 60 g.
otc	**Lobana Derm-Ade** (Ulmer)	**Cream; topical**: Vitamins A, D and E, moisturizers, emollients, silicone	Vanishing base. In 270 g.
otc	**Retinol** (Nature's Bounty)	**Cream; topical**: 100,000 IU vitamin A, glycol stearate, mineral oil, propylene glycol, lanolin oil, propylene glycol stearate SE, lanolin alcohol, retinol, parabens, EDTA	In 60 g.
otc	**Retinol-A** (Young Again Products)	**Cream; topical**: 300,000 IU vitamin A palmitate per 30 g.	In 60 g.
otc	**Sween Cream** (Coloplast)	**Cream; topical**: Beeswax, benzethonium chloride, cetyl alcohol, cod liver oil (vitamins A and D), lanolin oil, stearyl alcohol	In 340 g.
otc	**Aloe Grande** (Gordon)	**Lotion; topical**: Vitamins A (3333.3 units/g) and E (50 units/g), petrolatum, mineral oil, sodium lauryl sulfate, oleic acid, parabens, triethanolamine, aloe	In 240 mL.
otc	**Coppertone Cool Beads** (Schering-Plough)	**Lotion; topical**: Vitamins A and E, aloe vera, glycol, EDTA, lactose	In 340 g.

VITAMINS A, D and E — TOPICAL

Indications

➤*Dermatological conditions:* For temporary relief of discomfort due to minor burns, sunburn, windburn, abrasions, chapped or chafed skin and other minor non-infected skin irritations including diaper rash and irritations associated with ileostomy and colostomy skin drainage.

Administration and Dosage

➤*Adults:*

Dermatological conditions – Apply locally to affected skin with gentle massage.

➤*Children:*

Dermatological conditions – Apply locally to affected skin with gentle massage.

➤*Administration:* For external use only; avoid contact with the eyes.

Warnings/Precautions

➤*For external use only:* Avoid contact with the eyes.

➤*Worsened condition:* If the condition for which these preparations is used worsens or does not improve within 7 days, consult a physician.

VITAMINS A, D and E — TOPICAL

➤*Pregnancy: Category: Undetermined.* Consult a health care provider before administering to a pregnant woman.

➤*Lactation:* Consult a health care provider before administering to a breast-feeding woman.

EMOLLIENTS, MISCELLANEOUS

otc	**Balmex** (Chattem)	**Ointment; topical:** 11.3% zinc oxide, aloe vera gel, parabens, mineral oil	In 30, 60, 120, and 454 g.
otc	**Lanaphilic** (Medco Lab)	**Ointment; topical:** Lanolin oil, parabens, stearyl alcohol, white petrolatum	In 454 g.
otc	**Lan-O-Soothe** (Geritrex)	**Ointment; topical:** 100% lanolin	In 56 g.
otc	**Lansinoh** (Lansinoh Labs)		In 59 g.
Rx	**Venelex** (Stratus)	**Ointment; topical:** 87 mg balsam peru, 788 mg castor oil, white petrolatum	In 60 g.
otc	**DermaPhor** (DermaRite)	**Ointment; topical:** 44% petrolatum, lanolin alcohol, mineral oil, paraffin wax	In 228 g.
otc	**Balmex** (Chattem)	**Cream; topical:** 11.3% zinc oxide, dimethicone, soybean oil, parabens, mineral oil, propylene glycol, tocopherol	In 113 g.
otc	**Allercreme Ultra Emollient** (Carme)	**Cream; topical:** Mineral oil, petrolatum, lanolin, lanolin alcohol, lanolin oil, glycerin, glyceryl stearate, PEG-100 stearate, squalane, parabens	Unscented. In 60 g.
Rx	**Atopiclair** (Graceway Pharmaceuticals)	**Cream; topical:** Arachidyl alcohol, behenyl alcohol, disodium EDTA, PEG-100 stearate, tocopheryl acetate, sodium hyaluronate	In 100 g.
otc	**AmLactin** (Upsher-Smith)	**Cream; topical:** 12% ammonium lactate	In 140, 225, and 400 g.
otc	**Geri-Hydrolac** (Geritrex)		Mineral oil, petrolatum, parabens. In 140 g.
Rx	**Lac-Hydrin** (Ranbaxy)		Cetyl alcohol, glycerin, glyceryl stearate, lt. mineral oil, parabens. In 280 and 385 g.
Rx	**LAC-Lotion** (Paddock)	**Cream; topical:** 12% ammonium lactate (12% lactic acid neutralized with ammonium hydroxide), light mineral oil, cetyl alcohol, parabens, glycerin	In 225 and 400 g.
otc	**AmLactin Foot Cream Therapy** (Upsher-Smith)	**Cream; topical:** Ammonium lactate, emulsifying wax, glycerin, light mineral oil, parabens, potassium lactate, white petrolatum	In 85 g.
otc	**Aqua Glycolic Face** (Merz)	**Cream; topical:** Cetyl ricinoleate, C12-15 alkyl benzoate, glycolic acid, hyaluronic acid, ceresin, ammonium glycolate, glyceryl stearate, PEG-100 stearate, sorbitan stearate, sorbitol, propylene glycol, diazolidinyl urea, parabens, magnesium aluminum silicate, dimethicone, xanthan gum, trisodium EDTA	In 50 mL.
otc	**Aveeno Moisturizing** (Johnson & Johnson Consumer)	**Cream; topical:** 1% colloidal oatmeal, glycerin, petrolatum, dimethicone, phenylcarbinol	In 120 g.
otc	**Beta XMA** (Beta Dermaceuticals)	**Cream; topical:** Aloe, C14-22 alcohols, castor oil, cetyl alcohol, *butyrospermum parkii*, dimethicone, emu oil, methylparaben, PEG-40, PEG-100, triethanolamine	In 118 g.
otc	**Catrix Correction** (Donell DerMedex)	**Cream; topical:** Dipentaerythrityl, hexacaprylate/hexacaprate, sesame oil, **Catrix** (bovine-derived complex mucopolysaccharide), ceteareth-20, glycerin, caprylic/capric triglyceride, glycereth-7, dimethicone, xanthan gum, tocopheryl linoleate, alanine, glycine, urea, EDTA, imidazolidinyl urea, parabens, phenoxyethanol, orange oil, cardamon oil, titanium dioxide	In 36.9 g.
otc	**CeraVe** (Coria)	**Cream; topical:** Caprylic/capric triglyceride, cetyl alcohol, cetearyl alcohol, dimethicone, disodium EDTA, glycerin, parabens, petrolatum	In 453 g.
otc	**Complex 15 Face** (Schering-Plough)	**Cream; topical:** Caprylic/capric triglyceride, squalane, glycerin, glyceryl stearate, lecithin, PEG-50 stearate, propylene glycol, dimethicone, diazolidinyl urea, carbomer-934P, EDTA	In 75 g.
otc	**Complex 15 Hand & Body** (Schering-Plough)	**Cream; topical:** Mineral oil, glycerin, squalane, caprylic/capric triglyceride, glycol stearate, PEG-50, carboxylic acid sterol ester, glyceryl stearate, lecithin, dimethicone, diazolidinyl urea, carbomer-934, EDTA	In 120 g.
otc	**Curel Moisturizing** (Bausch & Lomb Personal Products)	**Cream; topical:** Glycerin, petrolatum, dimethicone, parabens	In 90 g.
otc	**Cutemol** (Summers)	**Cream; topical:** Allantoin, mineral oil, acetylated lanolin, lanolin alcohols extract, mineral wax, beeswax, sorbitan sesquioleate, parabens	In 60 and 240 g.
otc	**DML Forte** (Person & Covey)	**Cream; topical:** Petrolatum, PPG-2 myristyl ether propionate, glyceryl stearate, glycerin, simethicone, benzyl alcohol, silica, EDTA, sodium carbomer 1342	In 113 g.
otc	**Formula 405 Enriched Face Cream** (Doak)	**Cream; topical:** Acetylated lanolin, coconut oil, imidazolidinyl urea, PEG-40 stearate, lanolin alcohol, mineral oil, parabens, petrolatum, stearyl alcohol, sweet almond oil, vitamin E acetate	In 56.7 g.
otc	**Geri-Hydrolac** (Geritrex)	**Cream; topical:** Ammonium lactate (equivalent to 12% lactic acid), light mineral oil, petrolatum, propylene glycol, glycerin, cetyl alcohol, parabens	In 140 g.
otc	**Hydrisinol** (Pedinol)	**Cream; topical:** Sulfonated hydrogenated castor oil, hydrogenated vegetable oil	In 120 g and lb.
otc	**Hydrocerin** (Geritrex)	**Cream; topical:** Petrolatum, mineral oil, mineral wax, ceresin lanolin alcohol, parabens	In 480 g.
otc	**Kerasal AL** (Taro Consumer)	**Cream; topical:** Ammonium lactate, lt. mineral oil, glycerin, propylene glycol, cetyl alcohol, glyceryl monostearate, polyoxyethylene 100 stearate, magnesium aluminum silicate, methylcellulose, polyoxyl 40 stearate, laureth-4, parabens	May contain ammonium hydroxide and lactic acid. In 42 g.
otc	**Keri Creme** (Westwood Squibb)	**Cream; topical:** Mineral oil, lanolin alcohol, talc, sorbitol, ceresin, propylene glycol, magnesium stearate, glyceryl oleate, parabens	In 75 g.
otc	**Keri Long Lasting Hand Cream** (Novartis Consumer Health)	**Cream; topical:** Cetearyl alcohol, cetyl alcohol, dimethicone, disodium EDTA, mineral oil, parabens, tocopheryl acetate	In 113 g.
otc	**Kinerase** (Valeant)	**Cream; topical:** 0.1% N^6-furfuryladenine, stearic acid, cetyl alcohol, safflower oil, stearyl alcohol, aloe vera, parabens, imidazolidinyl urea, ascorbic acid	In 40 and 80 g.
otc	**Kinerase Intensive Eye Cream** (ICN Pharm)	**Cream; topical:** 0.125% kinetin, safflower seed oil, cetyl alcohol, urea, parabens	In 20 g.
otc	**Lanolor** (Westwood Squibb)	**Cream; topical:** Lanolin oil, glyceryl stearates, propylene glycol, sodium lauryl sulfate, simethicone, polyoxyl 40 stearate, cetyl esters wax, methylparaben	In 60 and 240 g.
otc	**Lubriderm** (Warner-Lambert)	**Cream; topical:** Mineral oil, petrolatum, lanolin, lanolin alcohol, lanolin oil, glycerin, glyceryl stearate, PEG-100 stearate, sorbitan laurate, parabens	Scented and unscented. In 81 g.

EMOLLIENTS, MISCELLANEOUS

otc	**Neutrogena Norwegian Formula Hand** (Neutrogena)	**Cream; topical**: Glycerin, sodium cetearyl sulfate, sodium sulfate, parabens	Scented and unscented. In 56.7 g.
Rx	**Lactic Acid E** (Stratus Pharmaceutical)	**Cream; topical**: 10% lactic acid, vitamin E, cetyl alcohol, disodium EDTA, glycerin, glyceryl, PEG-40, PEG-100, parabens	In 113.4 g.
otc	**Lady Esther** (Menley & James)	**Cream; topical**: Mineral oil	In 120 g
Rx	**Neosalus** (Quinnova)	**Cream; topical**: Dimethicone, glycerin, parabens, trolamine	In 60 and 100 g.
otc	**Nouriva Repair** (Ferndale)	**Cream; topical**: Petrolatum, paraffin, mineral oil, sorbitan oleate, carnauba wax, ceramide 3, cholesterol, glycerin, oleic acid, palmitic acid, acrylates/C 10-30 albyl acrylate crosspolymer, tromethamine	In 30 g.
otc	**Nutraderm** (Owen/Galderma)	**Cream; topical**: Mineral oil, sorbitan stearate, stearyl alcohol, sorbitol, citric acid, cetyl esters wax, sodium lauryl sulfate, dimethicone, parabens, diazolidinyl urea	In 90, 240, and 480 g.
otc	**Pacquin Medicated** (Pfizer)	**Cream; topical**: Dimethicone, glycerin, cetyl alcohol, parabens	In 227 g.
otc	**Pacquin Dry Skin** (Pfizer)	**Cream; topical**: Glycerin, cetyl alcohol, parabens	In 227 g.
otc	**Pacquin Plus** (Pfizer)	**Cream; topical**: Glycerin, lanolin, cetyl alcohol, parabens	In 227 g.
otc	**Pacquin Plus with Aloe** (Pfizer)	**Cream; topical**: Aloe vera gel, mineral oil, petrolatum, synthetic beeswax, cetyl alcohol, lanolin, dimethicone, stearic acid, methylparaben	In 227 g.
otc	**Pacquin Skin Cream with Aloe** (Pfizer)	**Cream; topical**: Aloe vera gel, mineral oil, petrolatum, synthetic beeswax, cetyl alcohol, methylparaben	In 227 g.
otc	**Penecare** (Reed & Carnrick)	**Cream; topical**: Lactic acid, mineral oil, imidurea	In 120 g.
otc	**Pedi-Vit-A Creme** (Pedinol)	**Cream; topical**: 100,000 units vitamin A per 30 g	In 60 g.
otc	**Pen•Kera** (B.F. Ascher)	**Cream; topical**: Glycerin, mineral oil, sorbitan stearate, urea, wheat germ glycerides, carbomer 940, triethanolamine, DMDM hydantoin, diazolidinyl urea	Dye and fragrance free. In 237 mL.
otc	**Phicon** (T.E. Williams)	**Cream; topical**: 250 units vitamin A and 66.7 units E per g, aloe vera, 5% pramoxine hydrochloride	In 60 g.
Rx	**PR** (PruGen)	**Cream; topical**: Cyclomethicone, dimethicone, hexyl laurate, polyglyceryl-4-isostearate, propylparaben	Dye free. In 56.7 g kits with *PruDrate* moisturizing cream.
otc	**Pretty Feet and Hands** (B.F. Ascher)	**Cream; topical**: Mineral oil, glyceryl stearate, stearyl alcohol, cetyl alcohol, aloe vera gel, parabens	In 88.7 mL.
otc	**Triple Cream** (Summers Labs)	**Cream; topical**: Avena sativa, beeswax, benzyl alcohol, white petrolatum	In 114 g.
Rx	**Promiseb** (Promius Pharma)	**Cream; topical**: Castor oil, disodium EDTA, PEG-30	In 30 g.
otc	**Udderly Smooth** (Redex)	**Cream; topical**: Dimethicone, isopropyl myristate, lanolin oil, mineral oil, parabens, PEG-2, urea	In 227 g.
otc	**Sensi-Care Moisturizing Body Cream** (ConvaTec)	**Cream; topical**: 1% dimethicone, 30% petrolatum, cetyl alcohol, glycerin, urea	In 85 g.
otc	**Impruv Natural Repair** (GlaxoSmithKline)	**Cream; topical**: Caprylic/capric triglyceride, glycerin, *butyrispermum parkii*, cocos nucifera	In 156 g.
otc	**DermaZinc** (Dermalogix)	**Cream; topical**: 0.25% zinc pyrithione, aloe vera, cetyl alcohol, dimethicone, lanolin, methylparaben, mineral oil, PEG-75	In 114 g.
otc	**Kerasal Ultra 20** (Alterna)	**Cream; topical**: 5% ammonium lactate, 20% urea, cetyl alcohol, disodium EDTA, glycerin, glyceryl, mineral oil, parabens, PEG-100, petrolatum, propylene glycol	In 56.8 g.
otc	**Carb-O-Lac HP Cream** (Geritrex)	**Cream; topical**: 10% ammonium lactate, 20% urea, lactic acid, petrolatum, propylene glycol, stearyl alcohol	In 277 g.
otc	**Lantiseptic Therapeutic Cream** (Summit)	**Cream; topical**: 37% lanolin, beeswax, HEEDTA, lanolin alcohol, mineral oil, petrolatum	In 113 g.
otc	**Carb-O-Philic/10** (Geritrex)	**Cream; topical**: DMDM hydantoin, lactic acid, lemon oil, petrolatum, propylene gylcol, urea	In 454 g.
otc	**Carb-O-Philic/20** (Geritrex)	**Cream; topical**: DMDM hydantoin, lactic acid, lemon oil, petrolatum, propylene glycol, urea	In 454 g.
otc	**Penecare** (Reed & Carnrick)	**Lotion; topical**: Lactic acid, imidurea	In 240 mL.
otc	**al12** (JSJ Pharmaceuticals)	**Lotion; topical**: 12% ammonium lactate, cetyl alcohol, glycerin, mineral oil, PEG-40, PEG-100, parabens	In 423 mL.
otc	**Allercreme Skin** (Carme)	**Lotion; topical**: Mineral oil, sorbitol, triethanolamine, parabens	In 240 mL.
otc	**Aloe Vesta** (ConvaTec)	**Lotion; topical**: 3% dimethicone	Alcohols, aloe, glycerin, petrolatum. In 60 mL.
otc	**AmLactin** (Upsher-Smith)	**Lotion; topical**: 12% ammonium lactate, parabens, light mineral oil	In 225 and 400 g.
Rx	**Ammonium Lactate** (Glades)	**Lotion; topical**: Ammonium lactate (equiv. to 12% lactic acid), light mineral oil, glyceryl stearate, glycerin, cetyl alcohol, parabens	In 225 and 400 g.
otc	**Aqua Glycolic Hand & Body** (Merz)	**Lotion; topical**: Glycolic acid, ammonium glycolate, cetyl alcohol, glyceryl stearate, PEG-100 stearate, C12-15 alkyl benzoate, mineral oil, stearyl alcohol, magnesium aluminum silicate, xanthan gum, parabens, disodium EDTA	In 177 mL.
otc	**Aquanil** (Person & Covey)	**Lotion; topical**: Glycerin, benzyl alcohol, sodium laureth sulfate, stearyl alcohol, xanthan gum	In 240 and 480 mL.
otc	**Aveeno** (Johnson & Johnson Consumer)	**Lotion; topical**: 1% colloidal oatmeal, glycerin, phenylcarbinol, petrolatum, dimethicone, benzyl alcohol	In 240 mL.
otc	**Aveeno Baby** (J & J Consumer)	**Lotion; topical**: Benzyl alcohol, cetyl alcohol, 1.2% dimethicone, glycerin, petrolatum	In 227 mL.
otc	**Aveeno Daily Moisturizing Lotion** (J & J Consumer)	**Lotion; topical**: Benzyl alcohol, cetyl alcohol, 1.25% dimethicone, glycerin, petrolatum	In 354 mL.
otc	**Balmex Emollient** (Macsil)	**Lotion; topical**: Lanolin oil, silicone, Balsam Peru, glycerol monostearate	In 180 mL.

EMOLLIENTS, MISCELLANEOUS

otc	**Cetaphil Daily Advance** (Galderma)	**Lotion; topical:** Benzyl alcohol, butyrospermum parkii, cetearyl alcohol, glycerin, macadamia seed oil, stearyl alcohol	In 226 g.
otc	**Choice DM Daily Moisturizing** (Bristol-Myers Squibb)	**Lotion; topical:** Petrolatum, glycerin, dimethicone, steareth-2, cetyl alcohol, benzyl alcohol, laureth-23, magnesium aluminum silicate, carbomer, potassium sorbate, sodium hydroxide, aloe	Fragrance free. In 226.8 g.
otc	**Complex 15 Hand & Body** (Schering-Plough)	**Lotion; topical:** Caprylic/capric triglyceride, PEG-50 stearate, squalane, carboxylic acid sterol ester, diazolidinyl urea, glycerin, glyceryl stearate, lecithin, dimethicone, glycol stearate, carbomer-934P, EDTA	Unscented. In 30 mL.
otc	**Corn Huskers** (Warner-Lambert)	**Lotion; topical:** 6.7% glycerin, 5.7% SD alcohol 40, algin, guar gum, methylparaben	In 120 and 210 mL.
otc	**Dermasil** (Unilever)	**Lotion; topical:** Dimethicone, mineral oil, glycerin, sunflower seed oil, borage seed oil, cetyl alcohol, lanolin alcohol, sweet almond oil, rose extract, sandalwood oil, EDTA, parabens	In 472 mL.
otc	**Derma Viva** (Rugby)	**Lotion; topical:** Mineral oil, glyceryl stearate, laureth-4, lanolin oil, PEG-100 stearate, PEG-40 stearate, PEG-4 dilaurate, trolamine, DSS, parabens	In 237 mL.
otc	**DML** (Person & Covey)	**Lotion; topical:** Petrolatum, glycerin, dimethicone, benzyl alcohol, volatile silicone, glyceryl stearate, palmitic acid, carbomer 941, xanthan gum	Unscented. In 240 and 480 mL.
otc	**Emollia** (Gordon Labs)	**Lotion; topical:** Mineral oil, propylene glycol, white wax, sodium lauryl sulfate, oleic acid, parabens	In 120 and 240 mL and gal.
otc	**Epilyt** (GlaxoSmithKline)	**Lotion, concentrate; topical:** Propylene glycol, glycerin, oleic acid, lactic acid	In 118 mL.
otc	**Esotérica Dry Skin Treatment** (SK-Beecham)	**Lotion; topical:** Propylene glycol, dicaprylate/dicaprate, mineral oil, glyceryl stearate, cetyl esters wax, hydrolyzed animal protein, dimethicone, TEA-carbomer-941, parabens	In 37.5 mL.
otc	**Eucerin Moisturizing** (Beiersdorf)	**Lotion; topical:** Mineral oil, PEG-40 sorbitan peroleate, lanolin acid glycerin ester, sorbitol, propylene glycol, cetyl palmitate, lanolin alcohol	Unscented. In 52.5, 120, and 240 mL, pt and gal.
otc	**Geri-Hydrolac 5%** (Geritrex)	**Lotion; topical:** 5% lactic acid buffered with ammonium hydroxide, cetyl alcohol, dimethicone, EDTA, glycerin, parabens, petrolatum	In 237 mL.
otc	**Geri SS** (Geritrex)	**Lotion; topical:** Mineral oil, propylene glycol, cetearyl alcohol, petrolatum, glycerin, dimethicone, colloidal oatmeal, hydrogenated castor oil, parabens, stearyl alcohol, EDTA, lemon oil, tocopheryl acetate	In 240 g.
otc	**Geri-Soft** (Geritrex)	**Lotion; topical:** Mineral oil, propylene glycol, cetearyl alcohol, sorbitol, petrolatum, dimethicone, lanolin, castor oil, stearic acid, parabens, stearyl alcohol, EDTA, lemon oil	In 240 g.
otc	**Gold Bond Medicated Triple Action Relief** (Chattem)	**Lotion; topical:** 5% dimethicone, 0.15% menthol	Aloe, cetyl alcohol, EDTA, glycerin, parabens, petrolatum, stearyl alcohol. In 236 mL.
otc	**Hydrisea** (Pedinol)	**Lotion; topical:** 8% Dead Sea salts concentrate, NaCl, MgCl, KCl, CaCl, mineral oil, propylene glycol, sorbitan stearate, glyceryl stearate, PEG-75 lanolin, EDTA, imidazolidinyl urea, tartrazine, parabens	In 120 mL.
otc	**Hydrisinol** (Pedinol)	**Lotion; topical:** Sulfonated castor oil, hydrogenated vegetable oil, propylene glycol stearate SE, mineral oil, lanolin, lanolin alcohol, sesame oil, sunflower oil, aloe, triethanolamine, sorbitan stearate, parabens, hydroxyethyl cellulose	In 240 mL.
otc	**Hydrocerin** (Geritrex)	**Lotion; topical:** EDTA, lanolin, parabens, mineral oil, PEG-40 sorbitan, peroleate, propylene glycol, sorbitol, water	In 240 g.
otc	**Johnson's Shea & Cocoa Butter Baby Lotion** (J & J Consumer)	**Lotion; topical:** *Butyrospermum parkii*, glycerin, mineral oil, parabens, stearyl alcohol, theobroma cacao	In 798 mL.
otc	**Keri Original** (Novartis Consumer Health)	**Lotion; topical:** Mineral oil, glycerin, PEG-40 stearate, glyceryl stearate, PEG-100 stearate, PEG-4 dilaurate, laureth-4, aloe, sunflower seed oil, tocopheryl acetate, parabens, fragrance, DMDM hydantoin, EDTA	Scented and unscented. In 241 g.
otc	**Keri Advanced** (Novartis Consumer Health)	**Lotion; topical:** Glycerin, stearic acid, hydrogenated polyisobutene, petrolatum, cetyl alcohol, aloe, tocopheryl acetate, dimethicone, PEG-100 stearate, parabens, PEG-5 soya sterol, magnesium aluminum silicate, phenoxyethanol, EDTA, diazolidinyl urea, fragrance	Oil free. In 241 g.
otc	**Keri Age Defy & Protect** (Novartis Consumer Health)	**Lotion; topical:** 7.5% octinoxate, 2% oxybenzone, cetearyl alcohol, glycerin, ammonium lactate, dimethicone, tocopheryl, EDTA	With alpha hydroxy and SPF +15. In 425 g.
otc	**Keri Deep Conditioning Overnight** (Novartis Consumer Health)	**Lotion; topical:** Castor oil, cetearyl alcohol, cetyl alcohol, disodium EDTA, glycerin, glyceryl, parabens, PEG-8, shea butter, vitamins A, C, and E	In 425 g.
otc	**Keri Light** (Bristol Myers Squibb)	**Lotion; topical:** Glycerin, stearyl alcohol, ceteareth–20, cetearyl octanoate, stearyl heptanoate, squalane, parabens, carbomer-934	In 195 and 390 mL.
otc	**Keri Nourishing Shea Butter** (Novartis Consumer Health)	**Lotion; topical:** Mineral oil, glycerin, shea butter, vitamin E acetate, parabens, sunflower seed oil, EDTA, aloe	In 425 g.
otc	**Keri Renewal Milk Body** (Novartis Consumer Health)	**Lotion; topical:** Borage oil, disodium EDTA, glyceryl oleate, glyceryl stearate, lactic acid, parabens, PEG-20, sunflower oil	In 241 g.
otc	**Keri Renewal Skin Firming** (Novartis Consumer Health)	**Lotion; topical:** Cetyl alcohol, dimethicone, glyceryl stearate, PEG-6, parabens	In 119 g.
otc	**Keri Sensitive Skin** (Novartis Consumer Health)	**Lotion; topical:** Glycerin, hydrogenated polyisobutane, petrolatum, cetyl alcohol, aloe barbadensis gel, vitamin E acetate, EDTA, parabens	In 241 g.
otc	**Keri Shave Minimizing** (Bristol-Myers Squibb)	**Lotion; topical:** Glycerin, cetearyl alcohol, mineral oil, petrolatum, SD alcohol 40-B, DMDM hydantoin, glyceryl dilaurate, dimethicone, aluminum starch octenyl-succinate, fragrance, parabens, cyclomethicone, sangulsorba officinalis root extract, hydrolyzed soy protein	In 425 g.
otc	**Kinerase** (Valeant)	**Lotion; topical:** 0.1% N^6-furfuryladenine, glycerin, stearyl alcohol, safflower oil, cetyl alcohol, aloe, parabens, corn oil, vitamin E acetate, ascorbic acid, retinyl palmitate	In 40 and 80 mL.
otc	**Geri-Hydrolac 12** (Geritrex Corp)	**Lotion; topical:** 12% ammonium lactate, mineral oil, cetyl alcohol, parabens, PEG-100, propylene glycol, glycerin	In 225 and 400 g.

EMOLLIENTS, MISCELLANEOUS

Rx	**Lac-Hydrin** (Ranbaxy)	**Lotion; topical:** 12% ammonium lactate (12% lactic acid neutralized with ammonium hydroxide), light mineral oil, cetyl alcohol, parabens	In 150 and 360 mL.
otc	**Lac-Hydrin Five** (Ranbaxy)	**Lotion; topical:** Lactic acid, glycerin, petrolatum, squalane, steareth-2, PCE-21-stearyl ether, propylene glycol dioctanoate, dimethicone, cetyl palmitate, diazolidinyl urea	Unscented. In 120 and 240 mL.
otc	**LactiCare** (GlaxoSmith-Kline)	**Lotion; topical:** Lactic acid, mineral oil, sodium hydroxide, glyceryl stearate, PEG-100 stearate, carbomer-940, DMDM hydantoin	In 222 and 345 mL.
otc	**Lobana Body** (Ulmer)	**Lotion; topical:** Mineral oil, triethanolamine stearate, lanolin, propylene glycol, and parabens	In 120 and 240 mL and gal.
otc	**Lubriderm** (Warner-Lambert)	**Lotion; topical:** Mineral oil, petrolatum, sorbitol, lanolin, lanolin alcohol, triethanolamine, and parabens	Scented and unscented. In 75, 120, 240, 360, 480 mL.
otc	**Lubriderm Daily Moisture with SPF 15** (Pfizer Consumer Health)	**Lotion; topical:** 7.5% octinoxate, 4% octisalate, 3% oxybenzone	In 100, 177, 296, and 473 mL.
otc	**Lubriderm Skin Nourishing with Sea Kelp Extract** (Pfizer Consumer)	**Lotion; topical:** Glycerin, glyceryl stearate SE, cetyl alcohol, emulsifying wax, petrolatum, caprylic/capric triglyceride, castor oil, octyldodecanol, dimethicone, diazolidinyl urea, propylene glycol, xanthan gum, disodium EDTA, fragrance, giant kelp leaf extract, iodopropynyl butylcarbamate	In 100, 177, and 473 mL.
otc	**Lubriskin** (Geritrex)	**Lotion; topical:** Mineral oil, petrolatum, lanolin, lanolin alcohol, cetearyl alcohol, castor oil, triethanolamine, stearyl alcohol, propylene glycol, parabens, EDTA	In 240 g.
otc	**Neutrogena Body** (Neutrogena)	**Lotion; topical:** Glyceryl stearate, PEG-100 stearate, imidazolidinyl urea, carbomer-954, parabens, sodium lauryl sulfate, triethanolamine	Scented and unscented. In 240 mL.
otc	**Nivea After Tan** (Beiersdorf)	**Lotion; topical:** SD alcohol 40B, mineral oil, PEG-40 castor oil, glyceryl stearate, parabens, aloe extract, lanolin alcohol, imidazolidinyl urea, phenoxyethanol, triethanolamine, chamomile extract, carbomer, simethicone	In 120 mL.
otc	**Nivea Moisturizing Extra Enriched** (Beiersdorf)	**Lotion; topical:** Mineral oil, PEG-40 sorbitan peroleate, glycerin, polyglyceryl-3 diisostearate, petrolatum, glyceryl lanolate, lanolin alcohol, phenoxyethanol	In 120, 240, and 360 mL.
otc	**Nutraderm** (Owen/Galderma)	**Lotion; topical:** Mineral oil, sorbitan stearate, stearyl alcohol, sodium lauryl sulfate, carbomer 940, diazolidinyl urea, parabens, triethanolamine	In 240 and 480 mL.
otc	**Shepard's Cream** (Dermik)	**Lotion; topical:** Glycerin, sesame oil, vegetable oil, SD alcohol 40-B, propylene glycol, ethoxydiglycol, triethanolamine, glyceryl stearate, simethicone, monoglyceride citrate, parabens	Unscented. In 240 and 480 mL.
otc	**Therapeutic Bath** (Goldline)	**Lotion; topical:** Mineral oil, glyceryl stearate, PEG-100 stearate, propylene glycol, PEG-40 stearate, laureth-4, PEG-4 dilaurate, lanolin oil, parabens, carbomer 934, trolamine, DSS	In 236 mL.
otc	**Ultra Derm** (Baker Cummins)	**Lotion; topical:** Mineral oil, petrolatum, lanolin oil, glycerin, propylene glycol, glyceryl stearate, PEG-50 stearate, propylene glycol stearate SE, sorbitan laurate, potassium sorbate, phosphoric acid, EDTA	In 240 mL.
otc	**Vaseline Intensive Care** (Unilever)	**Lotion; topical:** Ethylhexyl p-methoxycinnamate, (SPF5). Glycerin, sunflower seed oil, cetyl alcohol, corn oil, methylparaben, EDTA	In 325 mL.
otc	**Wibi** (Owen/Galderma)	**Lotion; topical:** Glycerin, SD alcohol 40, PEG-4, PEG-6-32 stearate, PEG-6-32, carbomer-940, PEG-75, parabens, triethanolamine, menthol	In 240 and 480 mL.
otc	**Wondra** (Richardson-Vicks)	**Lotion; topical:** Petrolatum, lanolin acid, glycerin, EDTA, hydrogenated vegetable glycerides phosphate, carbomer, dimethicone, imidazolidinyl urea, EDTA, titanium dioxide, parabens	Scented and unscented. In 300 mL.
otc	**Collastin Oil Free Moisturizer** (Dermol)	**Lotion; topical:** Soluble collagen, hydrolyzed elastin	In 60 mL.
otc	**Eucerin Plus** (Beiersdorf)	**Lotion; topical:** Mineral oil, hydrogenated castor oil, 5% sodium lactate, 5% urea, glycerin, lanolin alcohol	In 177 mL.
Rx	**Lactinol** (Pedinol)	**Lotion; topical:** 10% lactic acid	In 237 mL.
otc	**Impruv Deep Moisturizing** (GlaxoSmithKline)	**Lotion; topical:** Cetyl alcohol, glyceryl, lactic acid, mineral oil, myristyl alcohol, parabens, PEG-100, stearyl alcohol	In 200 mL.
otc	**CeraVe PM** (Coria Labs)	**Lotion, controlled-release; topical:** Caprylic/capric triglyceride, ceramide, cetearyl alcohol, cholesterol, dimethicone, disodium EDTA, glycerin, glyceryl, hyaluronic acid, niacinamide, methosulfate, parabens	In 89 mL.
Rx	**Zenieva** (River's Edge)	**Emulsion; topical:** Glycerin, olive oil, squalane, vegetable oil	Fragrance free. In kits 70 g in kits with *Pure* cleanser.
otc	**Hawaiian Tropic Cool Aloe With I.C.E.** (Tanning Research)	**Gel; topical:** Lidocaine, menthol, aloe, SD alcohol 40, diazolidinyl urea, EDTA, vitamins A and E, tartrazine	In 360 g.
otc	**Coppertone Aloe Vera Gel** (Schering-Plough)	**Gel; topical:** Aloe vera, glycerin, parabens, EDTA	Alcohol free. In 454 g.
otc	**Neutrogena Body** (Neutrogena)	**Oil; topical:** Sesame oil, PEG-40 sorbitan peroleate	In 240 mL.
otc	**Nivea Skin** (Beiersdorf)	**Oil; topical:** Mineral oil, lanolin, petrolatum, glyceryl lanolate, lanolin alcohol	In 240 mL.
otc	**Eucerin Itch-Relief Moisturizing Spray** (Beiersdorf)	**Spray; topical:** 0.15% menthol, glycerin, mineral oil, cetyl alcohol, *Oenothera biennis* (evening primrose oil)	In 200 mL.
otc	**Aloe Vesta** (ConvaTec)	**Spray; topical:** 36% petrolatum, hexamethyldisiloxane, *Softisan* 649, mineral oil, aloe extract	In 60 g.
otc	**AL12** (JSJ Pharmaceutical)	**Aerosol, foam; topical:** 12% ammonium lactate, butyrospermum parkii, cetyl alcohol, helianthus annuus seed oil	In 113.4 g
Rx	**Neosalus** (Quinnova)	**Aerosol, foam; topical:** Dimethicone, glycerin, parabens	In 70 and 200 g.
Rx	**Hylatopic** (Onset Therapeutics)	**Foam; topical:** Cetearyl alcohol, disodium EDTA, glycerin, petrolatum, parabens, theobroma grandiflorum seed butter	In 100 g.
otc	**Sardoettes** (Schering-Plough)	**Towelettes; topical:** Mineral oil, tocopherol, beta-carotene	In 25s.
otc	**Albolene** (DSE Healthcare)	**Soap; topical:** Mineral oil, petrolatum	Fragrance free. In 340 g.

EMOLLIENTS, MISCELLANEOUS — TOPICAL

Indications

➤*Dry, itchy skin:* These preparations lubricate and moisturize the skin, counteracting dryness and itching.

EMOLLIENT BATH PREPARATIONS

otc	**ActiBath Effervescent Tablets** (Jergens)	20% colloidal oatmeal	In 4s.
otc	**Aveeno Shave Gel** (Johnson & Johnson Consumer)	Oatmeal flour	In 210 g.
otc	**Nutra•Soothe** (Pertussin)	Colloidal oatmeal, light mineral oil	In individual oil (9) and oatmeal powder packets (9).
otc	**Nutraderm Bath Oil** (Owen/Galderma)	Mineral oil, lanolin oil, PEG-4 dilaurate, benzophenone-3, butylparaben	In 240 mL.
otc	**Sardo Bath & Shower Oil** (Schering-Plough)	Mineral oil, tocopherol	In 112.5 mL.
otc	**Ultra Derm Bath Oil** (Baker Cummins)	Mineral oil, lanolin oil, octoxynol-3	In 240 mL.
otc	**Alpha Keri Shower & Bath Oil** (Novartis Consumer Health)	Mineral oil, lanolin oil, PEG-4 dilaurate, benzophenone-3	In 236.6 and 473.2 mL.
otc	**Therapeutic Bath Oil** (Goldline)		In 473 mL.
otc	**Geri-Silk Bath Oil** (Geritrex)	Mineral oil, PEG-4 dilaurate, lanolin oil, D&C Green #6, fragrance	In 237 mL.
otc	**LubraSol Bath Oil** (Pharmaceutical Specialties)	Mineral oil, lanolin oil, PEG-200 dilaurate, oxybenzone	In 240 mL.
otc	**Domol Bath & Shower Oil** (Miles)	Di-isopropyl sebacate, mineral oil	In 240 mL.
otc	**Cameo Oil** (Medco)	Mineral oil, PEG-8 dioleate, lanolin oil	Unscented. In 240, 480, and 960 mL.
otc	**RoBathol Bath Oil** (Pharmaceutical Specialties)	Cottonseed oil, alkyl aryl polyether alcohol	Lanolin free. Dye free. In 240 mL, pt, and gal.
otc	**Esoterica Soap** (Medicis)	Sodium tallowate, sodium cocoate, mineral oil, acacia, sodium cocoyl isethionate, lauramide DEA, potassium oleate, titanium dioxide, pentasodium pentetate, tetra sodium etidronate	In 85 g.
otc	**Dermasil Lotion** (Chesebrough-Ponds)	Glycerin, dimethicone, sunflower seed oil, petrolatum, borage seed oil, vitamin E acetate, vitamin A palmitate, vitamin D_3, corn oil, EDTA, methylparaben	In 120 and 240 mL.
otc	**Aveeno Shower & Bath Oil** (Johnson & Johnson Consumer)	5% colloidal oatmeal, mineral oil, glyceryl stearate, PEG 100 stearate, laureth-4, benzyl alcohol, silica benzaldehyde	In 240 mL.

EMOLLIENT BATH PREPARATIONS — TOPICAL

Indications

➤*Dermatoses:* These products contain colloidal solids and various oils which act as emollients. They are recommended for relief of minor skin irritations and pruritus associated with common dermatoses and dry skin conditions.

Warnings/Precautions

➤*For external use only:* Avoid contact with the eyes; if this occurs, flush with clear water.

Use caution – To avoid slipping in tub when using bath oils.

Do not use – On acutely inflamed areas.

➤*Pregnancy: Category: Undetermined.* There is no information in pregnant women.

➤*Lactation:* There is no information in breast-feeding women.

PROTECTANTS

ZINC OXIDE

otc	**Dr. Smith's Adult Care** (Beta Dermaceuticals)	**Ointment; topical:** 10%	Petrolatum, lanolin, mineral oil, olive oil. In 85 g.
otc	**Dr. Smith's Diaper Ointment** (Beta Dermaceuticals)		Petrolatum, lanolin, mineral oil, olive oil. In 85 g.
otc	**Zinc Oxide** (Various, eg, Moore, Paddock)	**Ointment; topical:** 20%	In 30 and 60 g and lb.
otc	**Delazinc** (Mericon)	**Ointment; topical:** 25%	Mineral oil, petrolatum. In 454 g.
otc	**Zinc Oxide** (Gallipot)	**Paste; topical:** 25%	Petrolatum. In 454 g.

ZINC OXIDE — TOPICAL

Indications

➤*Diaper rash:* Zinc oxide diaper rash ointment promotes healing, protects skin and relieves chafing.

➤*Other dermatologic conditions:* In addition to healing diaper rash, zinc oxide ointment is indicated for treating many everyday skin problems. It promotes healing, protects, and helps seal out wetness. Use for minor burns, cuts, and scrapes.

Administration and Dosage

➤*Adults:*

Dermatologic conditions – Apply a thin layer of zinc oxide to superficial non-infected wounds and burns using a gauze dressing if necessary.

➤*Children:*

Dermatologic conditions – See Adults for dosing.

Diaper rash – Apply ointment 3 or more times daily as needed if diaper rash is present or at the first sign of redness, chafing, or minor skin irritation. To help prevent diaper rash, instruct individuals to apply the ointment to the diaper area before it is necessary, especially at bedtime when exposure to wet diapers may be prolonged.

➤*Storage/Stability:* Store between 15° and 30°C (59° and 86°F).

PROTECTANTS, MISCELLANEOUS

otc	**PeriGuard** (Dermarite)	**Ointment; topical**: aloe vera gel, lanolin, mineral oil, parabens, vitamin A, vitamin D, vitamin E	In 100 g.
otc	**Calmoseptine** (Calmoseptine)	**Ointment; topical**: 20.625% zinc oxide, 0.44% menthol, glycerin, lanolin	In 120 g.
otc	**Hydropel** (C & M)	**Ointment; topical**: 30% silicone, 10% hydrophobic starch derivative, petrolatum	In 60 g and lb.
otc	**Silicone No. 2** (C & M)	**Ointment; topical**: 10% silicone in petrolatum, hydrophobic starch derivative, methylparaben	In 30 and 480 g.
otc	**White Cloverine Salve** (Medtech)	**Ointment; topical**: 97% white petrolatum, rectified turpentine oil, white wax	In 30 g.
otc	**Remedy Calazime** (Medline)	**Ointment; topical**: 0.2% menthol, 20% zinc oxide, beeswax, *Carthamus tinctorious* seed oil, citrus aurantium dulcis peel oil, citrus grands peel oil, citrus tangerina peel oil, glycerin, glycine, methylparaben, olea europaea fruit oil, PEG-8, white petrolatum, zea mays oil	In 113 g.
otc	**ARC** (Xttrium Labs)	**Ointment; topical**: 28.5% petrolatum, 9.14% zinc oxide, beeswax, lanolin, mineral oil, parabens	In 113 g.
otc	**PeleVerus Clear** (LTC Products)	**Ointment; topical**: 0.9% zinc acetate, beeswax, panthenol, petrolatum, vitamin E	In 100 g.
otc	**4-N-1** (DermaRite)	**Cream; topical**: 1% dimethicone, alcohols, parabens, PEG	Latex free. In 114 g.
otc	**Kerodex** (Whitehall)	**Cream; topical**: #51-Bentonite, calcium carbonate, cellulose gum, chloroxylenol, glycerin, iron oxides, isopropyl alcohol, kaolin, parabens, petrolatum, sodium lauryl sulfate, spermaceti. Nongreasy invisible barrier for dry or oily work	In 113 g.
		Cream; topical: #71-Calcium carbonate, cetrimonium bromide, iron oxide, isopropyl alcohol, kaolin, parabens, mineral oil, paraffin, petrolatum, sodium hexametaphosphate, sodium lauryl sulfate, zinc oxide. Nongreasy invisible water repellent barrier for wet work	In 113 g.
otc	**Elon Barrier Protectant** (Dartmouth)	**Liquid; topical**: Paraffinum, liquidum, isopropyl palmitate, cetearyl alcohol, polyglyceryl-2 dipolyhydroxystearate, propylene glycol, cetearyl glucoside, C12-15 alkyl benzoate, stearic acid, bisabolol, petrolatum, phenoxyethanol, PEG-30 dipolyhydroxystearate, PEG-40 stearate, parabens, hamamelis virginiana, denatured alcohol.	In 28 g.
otc	**BlisterGard** (Medtech)	**Liquid; topical**: 6.7% alcohol, pyroxylin solution, oil of cloves, 8-hydroxyquinoline	In 30 mL.
otc	**New-Skin** (Medtech)		In 10 and 30 mL bottle and 3.5 mL tube.
otc	**Skin Shield** (Del)	**Liquid; topical**: 0.75% dyclonine HCl, 0.2% benzethonium chloride, acetone, castor oil, 10% SD alcohol 40. Waterproof.	In 13.3 mL.
otc	**New-Skin Antiseptic** (Medtech)	**Spray Liquid; topical**: Pyroxylin solution, acetone ACS, oil of cloves, 8-hydroxyquinoline, 4.2% alcohol	In 28.5 g.
otc	**Sprayzoin** (Geritrex)	**Spray; topical**: Benzoin compound, ethyl alcohol	In 118 mL.
otc	**Aerozoin** (Graham Field)	**Spray**: 30% tincture of benzoin compound, 44.8% isopropyl alcohol	In 105 mL.
otc	**Benzoin** (Various, eg, Humco, Lannett)	**Tincture**	In 60 and 120 mL, pt and gal.
otc	**Benzoin Compound** (Various, eg, Century, Geritrex. Humco, Lannett, Paddock, Purepac)	**Tincture**: Benzoin, aloe, storax, tolu balsam, 74% to 80% alcohol	In 30, 60 and 120 mL, pt and gal.
otc	**TinBen** (Ferndale)	**Tincture**: Benzoin, 75% to 83% alcohol	In 120 mL.
otc	**TinCoBen** (Ferndale)	**Tincture**: Benzoin, aloe, tolu balsam, storax, 77% alcohol	In 120 mL.
otc	**Pro-Q** (CollaGenex)	**Foam**: Dimethicone, glycerin, parabens	In 75 and 161 mL.

PROTECTANTS, MISCELLANEOUS — TOPICAL

Indications

➤*Dermatological conditions:* To protect skin against contact irritants.

Contraindications

Do not use silicone on wet, exudative lesions or inflamed or abraded skin.

Warnings/Precautions

➤*Pregnancy: Category: Undetermined.* Consult a health care provider before administering to a pregnant woman.

➤*Lactation:* Consult a health care provider before administering to a breast-feeding woman.

SUNSCREENS

SUNSCREENS

		SPF		
otc	**Neutrogena Ultra Sheer Dry-Touch Sunblock** (Neutrogena Corporation)	70	**Lotion**: Avobenzone, homosalate, glyceryl, PEG-100, octisalate, octocrylene, oxybenzone	PABA free. Waterproof. In 88 mL.
otc	**Bull Frog Quik Gel With UV Extender** (Chattem)	50	**Gel**: Avobenzone 3%, homosalate 15%, octisalate 5%, octocrylene 10%, oxybenzone 6%. Aloe, glycerin, propylene glycol, SD alcohol	In 147 mL.
otc	**Bull Frog Marathon Mist With UV Extender** (Chattem)	50	**Spray**: Avobenzone 3%, homosalate 15%, octisalate 5%, octocrylene 10%, oxybenzone 6%. Aloe, glycerin, propylene glycol, SD alcohol	In 177 mL.
otc	**Anthelios 40** (La Roche-Posay)	40	**Cream**: 2% avobenzone, 3% *Mexoryl SX*, 10% octocrylene, 5% titanium dioxide	PABA free. In 50 g.
otc	**Vanicream Sunscreen** (Pharmaceutical Specialties, Inc)	35	**Cream**: 7.5% octinoxate, 8% zinc oxide, glycerin, PEG-30, castor oil, vitamin E	PABA free. In 113 g.
otc	**Hawaiian Tropic Baby Faces Sunblock** (Tanning Research)	30+	**Lotion**: Titanium dioxide, octyl methoxycinnamate, octocrylene, benzophenone-3, octyl salicylate	PABA free. Waterproof. In 120 mL.
otc	**SolBar PF** (Person & Covey)	30+	**Cream**: Oxybenzone, octyl methoxycinnamate, octocrylene	PABA free. Waterproof. In 120 g.
otc	**Coppertone Sport** (Schering-Plough)	30+	**Lotion**: Ethylhexyl, p-methoxycinnamate, oxybenzone, 2-ethylhexyl salicylate, homosalate. Parabens, aloe	PABA free. Waterproof. In 118 mL.
otc	**Hawaiian Tropic Sunblock** (Tanning Research)	30+	**Lotion**: Titanium dioxide, octyl methoxycinnamate, benzophenone-3, octyl salicylate, octocrylene	PABA free. Waterproof. In 120 and 300 mL.
otc	**Coppertone Moisturizing Sunblock** (Schering-Plough)	30+	**Lotion**: Ethylhexyl p-methoxycinnamate, 2-ethylhexyl salicylate, octocrylene, oxybenzone	PABA free. Waterproof. In 120 and 300 mL.

SUNSCREENS

		SPF		
otc	**Coppertone Shade Sunblock** (Schering-Plough)	30+	**Lotion**: Ethylhexyl p-methoxycinnamate, 2-ethylhexyl salicylate, oxybenzone, homosalate. Sorbitol, benzyl alcohol, aloe, vitamin E, parabens, jojoba oil, EDTA, phenethyl alcohol	PABA free. Waterproof. In 118 mL.
otc	**Coppertone Water Babies** (Schering-Plough)	30+	**Lotion**: Ethylhexyl p-methoxycinnamate, 2-ethylhexyl salicylate, oxybenzone, homosalate. Alcohol, aloe, parabens	PABA free. Waterproof. In 118 mL.
otc	**Water Babies UVA/UVB Sunblock** (Schering-Plough)	30+	**Lotion**: Ethylhexyl p-methoxycinnamate, 2-ethylhexyl salicylate, octocrylene, oxybenzone	PABA free. Waterproof. In 120 mL.
otc	**Hawaiian Tropic Just For Kids Sunblock** (Tanning Research)	30+	**Lotion**: Octyl methoxycinnamate, benzophenone-3, octyl salicylate, octocrylene, titanium dioxide	PABA free. Waterproof, all day protection. In 88.7 mL.
otc	**Coppertone Kids** (Schering-Plough)	30+	**Lotion**: Ethylhexyl p-methoxycinnamate, 2-ethylhexyl salicylate, oxybenzone, homosalate. Sorbitol, benzyl alcohol, aloe, jojoba oil, parabens	PABA free. Waterproof. In 237 mL.
otc	**Vaseline Intensive Care Blockout** (Chesebrough Ponds)	30+	**Lotion**: Padimate, ethylhexyl p-methoxycinnamate, oxybenzone, 2-ethylhexyl salicylate, titanium dioxide	Waterproof. In 120 mL.
otc	**Bullfrog Sunblock** (Chattem)	30+	**Gel**: Benzophenone-3, octocrylene, octyl methoxycinnamate. Aloe, vitamin E, isostearyl alcohol	PABA free. Waterproof, all day protection. In 120 g.
otc	**Hawaiian Tropic Baby Faces Sunblock** (Tanning Research)	30+	**Lotion; topical**: Octyl methoxycinnamate, benzophenone-3, octyl salicylate, titanium dioxide, octocrylene	PABA free. Waterproof, all day protection. In 60, 120 and 300 mL.
otc	**Hawaiian Tropic Sunblock** (Tanning Research)	30+	**Lotion; topical**: Homosalate, octyl methoxycinnamate, benzophenone-3, menthyl anthranilate, octyl salicylate	PABA free. Waterproof, all day protection. In 120 mL.
otc	**CeraVe AM** (Coria Labs)	30	**Lotion**: Homosalate 12%, octinoxate 7.5%, octocrylene 2%, zinc oxide 3.5%, cetearyl alcohol, dimethicone, disodium EDTA, glycerin, hyaluronic acid, parabens	In 89 mL.
otc	**Coppertone Oil Free** (Schering-Plough)	30	**Lotion**: Ethylhexyl p-methoxycinnamate, oxybenzone, 2-ethylhexyl salicylate, homosalate. Parabens, EDTA, glyceryl	PABA free. Waterproof. In 118 mL.
otc	**Coppertone Water Babies** (Schering-Plough)	30	**Lotion**: Ethylhexyl p-methoxycinnamate, oxybenzone, 2-ethylhexyl salicylate, homosalate. Glyceryl, alcohol, parabens	PABA free. Waterproof. In 118 mL.
otc	**Neutrogena No-Stick Sunscreen** (Neutrogena)	30	**Cream**: 7.5% octyl methoxycinnamate, 15% homosalate, 6% benzophenone-3, 5% octyl salicylate	EDTA, parabens, diazolidinyl urea. In 118 g.
otc	**Vanicream Sunscreen** (Pharmaceutical Specialties, Inc)	30	**Cream**: 5% titanium dioxide, 5% zinc oxide, caprylic/capric triglyceride, cetyl alcohol, PEG-12, PEG-30, etrasodium EDTA, vitamin E	PABA free. In 113 g.
otc	**PreSun Active** (Bristol-Myers)	30	**Gel**: Octyl methoxycinnamate, oxybenzone, octyl salicylate. 69% SD alcohol 40	PABA free. Waterproof, non-greasy. In 120 mL.
otc	**PreSun Ultra** (Westwood Squibb)	30	**Lotion**: 7.5% octyl methoxycinnamate, 5% octyl salicylate, 3% oxybenzone, 3% avobenzone	In 120 mL.
otc	**PreSun Ultra** (Westwood Squibb)	30	**Gel**: 7.5% octyl methoxycinnamate, 5% octyl salicylate, 6% oxybenzone, 3% avobenzone	65.5% SD alcohol 40. In 120 mL.
otc	**Sundown Sunblock** (Johnson & Johnson)	30	**Lotion**: Octyl methoxycinnamate, octyl salicylate, oxybenzone, titanium dioxide	PABA free. Waterproof, non-greasy. In 120 mL.
otc	**Bain de Soleil All Day for Kids** (Procter & Gamble)	30	**Lotion**: Ethylhexyl p-methoxycinnamate, 2-ethylhexyl 2-cyano-3, 3-diphenylacrylate, oxybenzone, titanium dioxide. Stearyl alcohol, vitamin E, EDTA	PABA free. Waterproof. In 120 mL.
otc	**Bain de Soleil All Day Waterproof Sunblock** (Procter & Gamble)	30	**Lotion**: Ethylhexyl p-methoxycinnamate, 2-ethylhexyl 2-cyano-3, 3-diphenylacrylate, oxybenzone, titanium dioxide. Stearyl alcohol, vitamin E, EDTA	PABA free. Waterproof, non-greasy, all day protection. In 120 mL.
otc	**Coppertone Moisturizing Sunblock** (Schering-Plough)	30	**Lotion**: Ethylhexyl p-methoxycinnamate, oxybenzone, 2-ethylhexyl salicylate, homosalate	PABA free. Waterproof. In 120 and 240 mL.
otc	**Coppertone Sport** (Schering-Plough)	30	**Lotion**: Ethylhexyl p-methoxycinnamate, oxybenzone, 2-ethylhexyl salicylate	PABA free. Waterproof. In 120 mL.
otc	**Shade Sunblock** (Schering-Plough)	30	**Stick**: Ethylhexyl p-methoxycinnamate, oxybenzone, 2-ethylhexyl salicylate, homosalate	Waterproof. In 18 g.
otc	**Shade Sunblock** (Schering-Plough)	30	**Lotion**: Ethylhexyl p-methoxycinnamate, 2-ethylhexyl salicylate, homosalate, oxybenzone	Waterproof. In 120 mL.
otc	**Shade Sunblock** (Schering-Plough)	30	**Gel**: Ethylhexyl p-methoxycinnamate, homosalate, oxybenzone. 73% SD alcohol 40	Waterproof. Oil free. In 120 g.
otc	**Water Babies UVA/UVB Sunblock** (Schering-Plough)	30	**Lotion**: Ethylhexyl p-methoxycinnamate, 2-ethylhexyl salicylate, homosalate, oxybenzone	PABA free. Waterproof. In 120 and 240 mL.
otc	**Hawaiian Tropic Just For Kids Sunblock** (Tanning Research)	30	**Lotion**: Homosalate, octyl methoxycinnamate, benzophenone-3, menthyl anthranilate, octyl salicylate	PABA free. Waterproof, all day protection. In 88.7 mL.
otc	**Hawaiian Tropic Sport Sunblock** (Tanning Research)	30	**Lotion**: Octyl methoxycinnamate, octocrylene, benzophenone-3, octyl salicylate, titanium dioxide	PABA free. Waterproof, all day protection. In 88.7 mL.
otc	**SolBar PF** (Person & Covey)	30	**Liquid**: 10% octocrylene, 7.5% octyl methoxycinnamate, 6% oxybenzone. 77% SD alcohol 40	PABA free. In 114 mL.
otc	**Bain de Soleil SPF 30 + Color** (Procter & Gamble)	30	**Lotion**: Octocrylene, octyl methoxycinnamate, oxybenzone. Mineral oil, cetyl alcohol, EDTA	Waterproof. In 118 mL.
otc	**Coppertone Kids Sunblock** (Schering-Plough)	30	**Lotion**: Octocrylene, ethylhexyl p-methoxycinnamate, oxybenzone, 2-ethylhexyl salicylate	PABA free. Waterproof. In 120 and 240 mL.
otc	**Tréo** (Biopharm Lab)	30	**Lotion**: Octocrylene, octyl methoxycinnamate, benzophenone-3, octyl salicylate. Isostearyl alcohol, diazolidinyl urea, propylparabens. Also contains 0.05% citronella oil as an insect repellent	PABA free. Waterproof. In 118 mL.
otc	**Coppertone Kids Spray 'n Splash** (Schering-Plough)	30	**Spray**: Ethylhexyl p-methoxycinnamate, oxybenzone, 2-ethylhexyl salicylate, homosalate. Parabens, EDTA	PABA free. Waterproof. In 236 mL.
otc	**Coppertone To Go Sunblock** (Schering-Plough)	30	**Spray**: Ethylhexyl p-methoxycinnamate, oxybenzone, 2-ethylhexyl salicylate, homosalate. Alcohol	PABA free. Waterproof. In 112 mL.

SUNSCREENS

		SPF		
otc	**Coppertone Sport Sunblock Spray** (Schering-Plough)	30	**Spray**: Ethylhexyl p-methoxycinnamate, oxybenzone, 2-ethylhexyl salicylate, homosalate. Alcohol	PABA free. Waterproof. In 112 mL.
otc	**Coppertone Moisturizing Sunblock** (Schering-Plough)	25	**Lotion**: Ethylhexyl p-methoxycinnamate, oxybenzone, 2-ethylhexyl salicylate, homosalate	PABA free, Waterproof. In 120 mL.
otc	**Vaseline Intensive Care Moisturizing Sunblock** (Chesebrough Ponds)	25	**Lotion**: Ethylhexyl p-methoxycinnamate, oxybenzone, 2-ethylhexyl salicylate. Glycerin, aloe vera gel, C12-15 alkyl benzoate, cetyl alcohol, petrolatum, vitamin E, parabens, EDTA	PABA free. Waterproof. In 118 mL.
otc	**Neutrogena Sunblock Stick** (Neutrogena)	25	**Stick**: Octyl methoxycinnamate, benzophenone-3, octyl salicylate. Castor oil, cetearyl alcohol, propylparaben, shea butter	PABA free. Waterproof. In 12.6 g.
otc	**PreSun Moisturizing Sunscreen with Keri** (Bristol-Myers)	25	**Lotion**: Octyl methoxycinnamate, oxybenzone, octyl salicylate. Petrolatum, cetyl alcohol, diazolidinyl urea	Waterproof. In 120 mL.
otc	**PreSun for Kids Spray Mist** (Bristol-Myers)	23	Waterproof. In 105 mL.	
otc	**Eucerin Dry Skin Care Daily Facial** (Beiersdorf)	20	**Lotion**: Ethylhexyl p-methoxycinnamate, titanium dioxide, 2-phenylbenzimidazole-5-sulfonic acid, 2-ethylhexyl salicylate. Mineral oil, cetearyl alcohol, castor oil, lanolin alcohol, EDTA	In 120 mL.
otc	**Hawaiian Tropic Baby Faces** (Tanning Research)	20	**Gel**: Octyl methoxycinnamate, octocrylene, benzophenone-3, menthyl anthranilate	PABA free. Waterproof. In 120 g.
otc	**TI•Screen Sports** (Pedinol)	20	**Gel**: 7.5% octinoxate, 6% oxybenzone, 5% octisalate, 2% avobenzone	70% alcohol. In 120 mL.
otc	**Capital Soleil 20** (Vichy)	20	**Cream**: 2% avobenzone, 2% ecamsule, 10% octocrylene, 2% titanium dioxide	In 100 g.
otc	**Bullfrog Sunblock** (Chattem)	18	**Gel**: Octocrylene, benzophenone-3, octyl methoxycinnamate. Isostearyl alcohol, vitamin E, aloe	PABA free. Waterproof, all day protection. In 120 g.
otc	**Bullfrog** (Chattem)	18	**Stick**: Benzophenone-3, octyl methoxycinnamate. Isostearyl alcohol, aloe, hydrogenated vegetable oil, vitamin E	Waterproof. In 16.5 g.
otc	**Bullfrog Extra Moisturizing Gel** (Chattem)	18	**Gel**: Benzophenone-3, octocrylene, octyl methoxycinnamate. Vitamin E, aloe	PABA free. Waterproof, all day protection. In 90 g.
otc	**Bullfrog Sport Lotion** (Chattem)	18	**Lotion**: Benzophenone-3, octocrylene, octyl methoxycinnamate, octyl salicylate, titanium dioxide. Diazolidinyl urea, EDTA, parabens, vitamin E, aloe	Waterproof, all day protection. In 120 mL.
otc	**Bullfrog for Kids** (Chattem)	18	**Gel**: Octocrylene, octyl methoxycinnamate, octyl salicylate. Vitamin E, aloe, C12-15 alcohols benzoate	Waterproof, non-greasy, all day protection. In 60 g.
otc	**Neutrogena Chemical-Free Sunblocker** (Neutrogena)	17	**Lotion**: Titanium dioxide. Parabens, diazolidinyl urea, shea butter	PABA free. In 120 mL.
otc	**SUNPRuF 17** (C & M)	17	**Gel**: 7.8% octyl methoxycinnamate, 5.2% octyl salicylate	Oil free, water-resistant. In 120 g.
otc	**TI•Screen Sunless** (Pedinol)	17	**Creme**: 7.5% octyl methoxycinnamate, 3% benzophenone-3. Mineral oil, alcohols, PEG-100, parabens	In 118 mL.
otc	**TI•Baby Natural** (Pedinol)	16	**Lotion**: 5% titanium dioxide	PABA free. Waterproof. In 120 mL.
otc	**TI•Screen Natural** (Pedinol)	16	**Lotion**: 5% titanium dioxide	PABA free. Waterproof. In 120 mL.
otc	**Hawaiian Tropic 15 Plus Sunblock** (Tanning Research)	15+	**Lotion**: Menthyl anthranilate, octyl methoxycinnamate, benzophenone-3	PABA free. Waterproof, all day protection. In 7.5, 15, 60, 120, 240 and 300 mL.
otc	**Hawaiian Tropic 15 Plus** (Tanning Research)	15+	**Gel**: Octyl methoxycinnamate, octocrylene, benzophenone-3, menthyl anthranilate	PABA free. Waterproof, all day protection. In 120 g.
otc	**Anthelios SX** (La Roche-Posay)	15	**Cream**: 2% avobenzone, 2% ecamsule, 10% octocrylene	EDTA, glycerin, parabens, stearyl alcohol. In 100 g.
otc	**UV Protective** (Kiehl's)	15	**Cream**: 2% avobenzone, 2% ecamsule, 10% octocrylene	EDTA, glycerin, parabens, stearyl alcohol. Fragrance free. In 100 g.
otc	**TI•Lite** (Pedinol)	15	**Cream**: 7.5% ethylhexyl p-methoxycinnamate, 2% titanium dioxide. Cetyl alcohol, phenethyl alcohol, parabens, EDTA	In 60 g.
otc	**Aquaderm** (Baker Cummins)	15	**Cream**: 7.5% octyl methoxycinnamate, 6% oxybenzone	In 105 g.
otc	**SolBar PF Sunscreen** (Person & Covey)	15	**Liquid**: 7.5% octyl methoxycinnamate, 5% oxybenzone. 76% SD alcohol 40	PABA free. In 120 mL.
otc	**SUNPRuF 15** (C & M)	15	**Lotion**: 7.5% octyl methoxycinnamate, 5% benzophenone-3	PABA free. Water-resistant. In 240 mL.
otc	**Bain de Soleil SPF 15 + Color** (Procter & Gamble)	15	**Lotion**: Octyl methoxycinnamate, octocrylene, oxybenzone. Mineral oil, cetyl alcohol, EDTA	Waterproof. In 118 mL.
otc	**Catrix Correction** (Donell DerMedex)	15	**Cream**: Octyl methoxycinnamate, menthyl anthranilate, benzophenone 3, titanium dioxide. Sesame oil, cetearyl alcohol, urea, EDTA, imidazolidinyl urea, parabens	PABA free. In 39 g.
otc	**Oil of Olay Daily UV Protectant** (Procter & Gamble)	15	**Cream**: Octyl methoxycinnamate, titanium dioxide. Phenylbenzimidazole sulfonic acid, glycerin, cetyl alcohol, imidazolidinyl urea, parabens, EDTA, castor oil	Scented or unscented. In 51 g.
otc	**Bain de Soleil All Day Waterproof Sunblock** (Procter & Gamble)	15	**Lotion**: Ethylhexyl p-methoxycinnamate, 2-ethylhexyl 2-cyano-3, 3-diphenylacrylate, oxybenzone, titanium dioxide. Stearyl alcohol, vitamin E, EDTA	PABA free. Waterproof, non-greasy, all day protection. In 120 mL.
otc	**Coppertone Sport** (Schering-Plough)	15	**Lotion**: Ethylhexyl p-methoxycinnamate, oxybenzone	PABA free. Waterproof. In 120 mL.
otc	**Shade Sunblock** (Schering-Plough)	15	**Gel**: Ethylhexyl p-methoxycinnamate, oxybenzone. 75% SD alcohol 40	Waterproof. Oil free. In 120 g.
otc	**Vaseline Intensive Care Sport Sunblock** (Chesebrough Ponds)	15	**Lotion**: Ethylhexyl p-methoxycinnamate, oxybenzone, C12-15 alkyl benzoate. Aloe vera gel, vitamin E, EDTA	PABA free. Waterproof, non-greasy. In 118 mL.
otc	**Coppertone Kids Sunblock** (Schering-Plough)	15	**Lotion**: Ethylhexyl p-methoxycinnamate, oxybenzone, 2-ethylhexyl salicylate, homosalate	PABA free. Waterproof. In 120 and 240 mL.

SUNSCREENS

		SPF		
otc	**Coppertone Moisturizing Sunblock** (Schering-Plough)	15	**Lotion:** Ethylhexyl p-methoxycinnamate, oxybenzone	PABA free. Waterproof. In 120, 240 and 300 mL.
otc	**Faces Only Moisturizing Sunblock by Coppertone** (Schering-Plough)	15	**Lotion:** Ethylhexyl p-methoxycinnamate, oxybenzone	PABA free. In 55.5 mL.
otc	**Oil of Olay Daily UV Protectant** (Procter & Gamble)	15	**Lotion:** Ethylhexyl p-methoxycinnamate, 2-phenylbenzimidazole-5-sulfonic acid, titanium dioxide. Cetyl alcohol, imidazolidinyl urea, parabens, EDTA, castor oil, tartrazine	PABA free. Greaseless. Scented or unscented. In 105 and 157.7 mL.
otc	**Vaseline Intensive Care Ultra Violet Daily Defense** (Chesebrough Ponds)	15	**Lotion:** Ethylhexyl p-methoxycinnamate, oxybenzone. Vitamin E, cetyl alcohol, acetylated lanolin alcohol, parabens, EDTA	PABA free. Non-greasy. In 120 and 300 mL.
otc	**Hawaiian Tropic Sport Sunblock** (Tanning Research)	15	**Lotion:** Octyl methoxycinnamate, benzophenone-3, octocrylene	PABA free. Waterproof, all day protection. In 88.7 mL.
otc	**Neutrogena Intensified Day Moisture** (Neutrogena)	15	**Cream:** Octyl methoxycinnamate, 2-phenylbenzimidazole sulfonic acid, titanium dioxide. Cetyl alcohol, diazolidinyl urea, parabens, EDTA	PABA free. In 67.5 g.
otc	**Ray Block** (Del Ray)	15	**Lotion:** 5% octyl dimethyl PABA, 3% benzophenone-3. SD alcohol	In 118.3 mL.
otc	**Johnson's Baby Sunblock** (Johnson & Johnson)	15	**Lotion:** Titanium dioxide. Hydrogenated castor oil, EDTA, hydroxylated lanolin, zinc oxide, mineral oil	PABA free. Waterproof. In 120 mL.
otc	**Total Eclipse Oily and Acne Prone Skin Sunscreen** (Triangle Labs)	15	**Lotion:** Padimate O, oxybenzone, glyceryl PABA. 77% alcohol	In 120 mL.
otc	**Total Eclipse Moisturizing** (Triangle Labs)	15	**Lotion:** Padimate O, oxybenzone, octyl salicylate	In 120 mL.
otc	**Shade UVAGuard** (Schering-Plough)	15	**Lotion:** 7.5% octyl methoxycinnamate, 3% avobenzone, 3% oxybenzone	Waterproof. In 120 mL.
otc	**SolBar Plus 15** (Person & Covey)	15	**Cream:** 4% oxybenzone, 2% dioxybenzone, 6% octyl dimethyl PABA	In 113 g.
otc	**PreSun Moisturizing Sunscreen with Keri** (Bristol-Myers)	15	**Lotion:** Octyl dimethyl PABA, oxybenzone. Cetyl alcohol, diazolidinyl urea	Waterproof. In 120 mL.
otc	**SolBar PF** (Person & Covey)	15	**Cream:** 7.5% octyl methoxycinnamate, 5% oxybenzone	PABA free. In 222 g.
otc	**Sundown Sunblock** (Johnson & Johnson)	15	**Lotion:** Octyl methoxycinnamate, oxybenzone, octyl salicylate, titanium dioxide	PABA free. Waterproof, non-greasy. In 120 mL.
otc	**Water Babies UVA/UVB Sunblock** (Schering-Plough)	15	**Lotion:** Ethylhexyl p-methoxycinnamate, oxybenzone	PABA free. Waterproof. In 120 mL.
otc	**DML Facial Moisturizer** (Person & Covey)	15	**Cream:** 8% octyl methoxycinnamate, 4% oxybenzone. Benzyl alcohol, petrolatum, EDTA	In 45 g.
otc	**Hawaiian Tropic Self Tanning Sunblock** (Tanning Research)	15	**Cream:** Octyl methoxycinnamate, benzophenone-3. Aloe, cetyl alcohol, stearyl alcohol, cocoa butter, parabens, vitamin E	PABA free. In 93.75 mL.
otc	**Nivea Sun** (Beiersdorf)	15	**Lotion:** Octyl methoxycinnamate, octyl salicylate, benzophenone-3, 2-phenylbenzimidazole-5-sulfonic acid	PABA free. Waterproof. In 120 mL.
otc	**Neutrogena Moisture** (Neutrogena)	15	**Lotion:** Octyl methoxycinnamate, benzophenone-3. Parabens, diazolidinyl urea	PABA free. In sheer tint and untinted. In 120 mL.
otc	**Neutrogena Sunblock** (Neutrogena)	15	**Cream:** Octyl methoxycinnamate, octyl salicylate, menthyl anthranilate, titanium dioxide. Mineral oil, propylparaben	PABA free. Waterproof. In 67.5 g.
otc	**Tréo** (Biopharm Lab)	15	**Lotion:** Octocrylene, octyl methoxycinnamate, benzophenone-3, octyl salicylate. Isostearyl alcohol, diazolidinyl urea, propylparabens. Also contains 0.05% citronella oil as an insect repellent	PABA free. Waterproof. In 118 mL.
otc	**Coppertone Oil Free** (Schering-Plough)	15	**Lotion:** Ethylhexyl p-methoxycinnamate, oxybenzone. Aloe, parabens, EDTA	PABA free. Waterproof. In 118 and 237 mL.
otc	**Coppertone Sport Sunblock Spray** (Schering-Plough)	15	**Spray:** Ethylhexyl p-methoxycinnamate, 2-ethylhexyl salicylate, homosalate, oxybenzone. Alcohol	PABA free. Waterproof. In 112 mL.
otc	**Hawaiian Tropic 10 Plus** (Tanning Research)	10+	**Lotion:** Octyl methoxycinnamate, benzophenone-3, menthyl anthranilate	PABA free. Waterproof, all day protection. In 120 mL.
otc	**Original Eclipse Sunscreen** (Triangle Labs)	10	**Lotion:** Padimate O, glyceryl PABA	In 120 mL.
otc	**Scar Cream Maximum Strength** (Clay-Park Labs)	10	**Cream:** 7.5% octyl methoxycinnamate, 5% octyl salicylate.	Alcohols, mineral oil, parabens, urea. In 28 g.
otc	**Hawaiian Tropic 8 Plus** (Tanning Research)	8+	**Gel:** Octyl methoxycinnamate, benzophenone-3, menthyl anthranilate	PABA free. Waterproof, all day protection. In 120 g.
otc	**Vaseline Intensive Care No Burn No Bite** (Chesebrough Ponds)	8	**Lotion:** Ethylhexyl p-methoxycinnamate, oxybenzone	PABA free. Waterproof. In 180 mL.
otc	**TI•Screen** (Pedinol)	8	**Lotion:** 6% ethylhexyl p-methoxycinnamate, 2% oxybenzone	PABA free. Water resistant. In 120 mL.
otc	**Bain de Soleil All Day Waterproof Sunfilter** (Procter & Gamble)	8	**Lotion:** 2-ethylhexyl 2-cyano-3, 3-diphenylacrylate, ethylhexyl p-methoxycinnamate, titanium dioxide. Stearyl alcohol, vitamin E, EDTA	PABA free. Waterproof, non-greasy, all day protection. In 120 mL.
otc	**Coppertone Moisturizing Sunscreen** (Schering-Plough)	8	**Lotion:** Ethylhexyl p-methoxycinnamate, oxybenzone	PABA free. Waterproof. In 120 and 240 mL.
otc	**Coppertone Oil Free** (Schering-Plough)	8	**Lotion:** Ethylhexyl p-methoxycinnamate, oxybenzone. Aloe, parabens, vitamin E, EDTA	PABA free. Waterproof. In 118 mL.
otc	**Coppertone Sport** (Schering-Plough)	8	**Lotion:** Ethylhexyl p-methoxycinnamate, oxybenzone	PABA free. Waterproof. In 120 mL.
otc	**Bain de Soleil SPF 8 + Color** (Procter & Gamble)	8	**Lotion:** Octyl methoxycinnamate, octocrylene. Mineral oil, cetyl alcohol, EDTA	Waterproof. In 118 mL.
otc	**Neutrogena Glow Sunless Tanning** (Neutrogena)	8	**Lotion:** Octyl methoxycinnamate. Cetyl alcohol, diazolidinyl urea, parabens, EDTA	PABA free. In 120 mL.
otc	**Neutrogena Sunblock** (Neutrogena)	8	**Cream:** Octyl methoxycinnamate, menthyl anthranilate, titanium dioxide. Mineral oil	PABA free. Waterproof. In 67.5 g.
otc	**Sundown Sunscreen** (Johnson & Johnson)	8	**Lotion:** Octyl methoxycinnamate, octyl salicylate, oxybenzone, titanium dioxide	PABA free. Waterproof. In 120 mL.

SUNSCREENS

		SPF		
otc	**Tréo** (Biopharm Lab)	8	**Lotion:** Octocrylene, octyl methoxycinnamate, benzophenone-3, octyl salicylate. Isostearyl alcohol, diazolidinyl urea, propylparabens. Also contains 0.05% citronella oil as an insect repellent	PABA free. Waterproof. In 118 mL.
otc	**Hawaiian Tropic Protective Tanning** (Tanning Research)	6	**Lotion:** Titanium dioxide	PABA free. Waterproof. In 240 mL.
otc	**Coppertone Moisturizing Sunscreen** (Schering-Plough)	6	**Lotion:** Ethylhexyl p-methoxycinnamate, oxybenzone	PABA free. Waterproof. In 120 mL.
otc	**Faces Only Clear Sunscreen by Coppertone** (Schering-Plough)	6	**Gel:** Ethylhexyl p-methoxycinnamate, oxybenzone	PABA free. In 55.5 g.
otc	**Hawaiian Tropic Protective Tanning Dry** (Tanning Research)	6	**Oil:** 2-ethylhexyl p-methoxycinnamate, homosalate, menthyl anthranilate	Waterproof. In 180 mL.
			Gel: Phenylbenzimidazole, sulfonic acid, benzophenone-4	In 180 g.
otc	**Neutrogena Moisture** (Neutrogena)	5	**Lotion:** Octyl methoxycinnamate. Petrolatum, cetyl alcohol, parabens, diazolidinyl urea, EDTA, cetyl alcohol	PABA free. In 60 and 120 mL.
otc	**Bain de Soleil Mega Tan** (Procter & Gamble)	4	**Lotion:** Ethylhexyl p-methoxycinnamate, 2-ethylhexyl salicylate. Lanolin, cocoa butter, palm oil, aloe, DMDM hydantoin, xanthan gum, shea butter, EDTA	Waterproof. In 120 mL.
otc	**Bain de Soleil Orange Gelée** (Procter & Gamble)	4	**Gel:** Ethylhexyl p-methoxycinnamate, 2-ethylhexyl salicylate	PABA free. In 93.75 g.
otc	**Bain de Soleil Tropical Deluxe** (Procter & Gamble)	4	**Lotion:** Ethylhexyl p-methoxycinnamate, 2-ethylhexyl salicylate. Cetyl alcohol, EDTA	PABA free. Waterproof. In 240 mL.
otc	**Coppertone Moisturizing Suntan** (Schering-Plough)	4	**Lotion:** Ethylhexyl p-methoxycinnamate, oxybenzone	PABA free. Waterproof. In 120 and 240 mL.
otc	**Hawaiian Tropic Dark Tanning with Sunscreen** (Tanning Research)	4	**Oil:** Ethylhexyl p-methoxycinnamate, octyl dimethyl PABA	Waterproof. In 240 mL.
			Gel: Phenylbenzimidazole, sulfonic acid	PABA free. In 240 g.
otc	**Tropical Blend Dark Tanning** (Schering-Plough)	4	**Lotion:** Ethylhexyl p-methoxycinnamate, oxybenzone	Waterproof. In 240 mL.
			Oil: Padimate O, oxybenzone	Waterproof. In 240 mL.
otc	**Coppertone Sport** (Schering-Plough)	4	**Lotion:** Ethylhexyl p-methoxycinnamate, oxybenzone	PABA free. Waterproof. In 120 mL.
otc	**Coppertone Tan Magnifier Suntan** (Schering-Plough)	4	**Lotion:** Ethylhexyl p-methoxycinnamate	PABA free. In 120 mL.
			Gel: 2-phenylbenzimidazole-5-sulfonic acid	PABA free. In 120 g.
otc	**Bain de Soleil All Day** (Procter & Gamble)	4	**Lotion:** 2-ethylhexyl 2-cyano-3, 3-diphenylacrylate, ethylhexyl p-methoxycinnamate, titanium dioxide. Stearyl alcohol, vitamin E, EDTA	PABA free. Waterproof. In 120 mL.
otc	**Tropical Blend Dry Oil** (Schering-Plough)	4	**Oil:** Homosalate, oxybenzone	Non-greasy. In 180 mL.
otc	**Tropical Blend Tan Magnifier** (Schering-Plough)	4	**Oil:** Triethanolmine salicylate	Waterproof. In 240 mL.
otc	**Coppertone Gold Dark Tanning Oil** (Schering Plough)	4	**Spray:** Homosalate, oxybenzone. Aloe, vitamin E, mineral oil, paraben	In 236 mL.
otc	**Coppertone Gold Dark Tanning Exotic Oil** (Schering-Plough)	*	**Spray:** Homosalate. Mineral oil, coconut oil, olive oil, macadamia nut oil, cocoa butter, vitamin E, lanolin oil, sweet almond oil, jojoba oil, aloe	In 236 mL.
otc	**Q.T. Quick Tanning Suntan by Coppertone** (Schering-Plough)	2	**Lotion:** Ethylhexyl p-methoxycinnamate, dihydroxyacetone	PABA free. In 120 mL.
otc	**Coppertone Moisturizing Suntan** (Schering-Plough)	2	**Oil:** Homosalate	PABA free. Waterproof. In 120 mL.
otc	**Tropical Blend Dark Tanning** (Schering-Plough)	2	**Lotion/Oil:** Homosalate	Waterproof. In 240 mL.
otc	**Tropical Blend Dry Oil** (Schering-Plough)	2	**Oil:** Homosalate	Non-greasy. In 180 mL.
otc	**Hawaiian Tropic Dark Tanning** (Tanning Research)	2	**Gel:** Phenylbenzimidazole sulfonic acid	In 240 mL.
			Oil: 2-ethylhexyl methoxycinnamate, octyl dimethyl PABA	Waterproof. In 240 mL.
otc	**Coppertone Tan Magnifier Suntan** (Schering-Plough)	2	**Oil:** Triethanolamine salicylate	PABA free. In 120 mL.
otc	**Tropical Blend Tan Magnifier** (Schering-Plough)	2	**Oil:** Triethanolamine salicylate	Waterproof. In 240 mL.
otc	**Coppertone Gold Tan Magnifier Oil** (Schering-Plough)	2	**Oil:** Triethanolamine salicylate. Glycerin, aloe, lanolin oil, cocoa butter, macadamia nut oil, olive oil, sweet almond oil, vitamin E, jojoba oil, coconut oil, parabens	In 236 mL.
otc	**Coppertone Gold Dark Tanning Sandproof Dry Oil** (Schering-Plough)	2	**Spray:** Homosalate. Aloe, vitamin E, mineral oil, paraben	In 236 mL.
otc	**A-Fil** (PharmaDerm)	*	**Cream:** 5% menthyl anthranilate, 5% titanium dioxide	In 45 g.
otc	**RVPaque** (ICN)	*	**Cream:** Red petrolatum, zinc oxide, cinoxate	Water resistant. Greaseless. Tinted. In 15 and 37.5 g.
otc	**Coppertone Sunless Tanner Spray** (Schering-Plough)	*	**Spray, non-aerosol:** Aloe vera, vitamin E, glycerin	In 118 mL.
otc	**Hawaiian Tropic 45 Plus Sunblock Lip Balm** (Tanning Research)	30+	**Lip balm:** Octyl methoxycinnamate, benzophenone-3, octyl salicylate, titanium dioxide, menthyl anthranilate	PABA free. Waterproof. Tropical, mint and cherry flavors. In 4.2 g.
otc	**Herpecin-L** (Chattem)	30+ 30	**Lip balm:** 7.5% octyl methoxycycinnamate, 6% oxybenzone, 5% octyl salicylate, 1% dimethicone. Beeswax, petrolatum, zinc oxide	In 2.8 g.
otc	**Blistex Ultra Protection** (Blistex)	30	**Lip balm:** Octyl methoxycinnamate, oxybenzone, octyl salicylate, menthyl anthranilate, homosalate, dimethicone	PABA free. Water resistant. In 4.2 g.
otc	**Coppertone Little Licks** (Schering-Plough)	30	**Lip balm:** Ethylhexyl p-methoxycinnamate, oxybenzone, 2-ethylhexyl salicylate. Paraben, aloe, saccharin	Waterproof. Cherry flavor. In 4.2 g.

SUNSCREENS

		SPF		
otc	**Water Babies Little Licks by Coppertone** (Schering-Plough)	30	**Lip Balm:** Ethylhexyl p-methoxycinnamate, oxybenzone, 2-ethylhexyl salicylate	PABA free. Waterproof. In 4.5 g.
otc	**Stay Moist Lip Conditioner** (Stanback)	15+	**Lip balm:** Padimate O, oxybenzone. Aloe vera, vitamin E	Tropical fruit flavor. In 4.8 g.
otc	**TI·Screen** (Pedinol)	15+	**Lip balm:** 7.5% ethylhexyl p-methoxycinnamate, 5% oxybenzone. Petrolatum	PABA free. In 4.5 g.
otc	**Catrix Lip Saver** (Donell DerMedex)	15	**Lip Balm:** Allantoin, ethylhexyl p-methoxycinnamate, oxybenzone. Mineral oil, castor oil, petrolatum, vitamin E, propylparaben	PABA free. In 4.5 g.
otc	**ChapStick Sunblock 15 Petroleum Jelly Plus** (Robins)	15	**Ointment:** 89% white petrolatum, 7% padimate O, 3% oxybenzone. Aloe, lanolin	In 10 g.
otc	**Chapstick Sunblock 15** (Robins)	15	**Lip balm:** 7% padimate O, 3% oxybenzone. 0.5% cetyl alcohol, 44% petrolatums, 0.5% lanolin, 0.5% isopropyl myristate, parabens, mineral oil, titanium dioxide	In 4.25 g.
otc	**Eclipse Lip and Face Protectant** (Triangle Labs)	15	**Stick:** Padimate O, oxybenzone	In 4.5 g.
otc	**Neutrogena Lip Moisturizer** (Neutrogena)	15	**Lip balm:** Octyl methoxycinnamate, benzophenone-3. Corn oil, castor oil, mineral oil, lanolin oil, petrolatum, lanolin, stearyl alcohol	PABA free. In 4.5 g.
otc	**Daily Conditioning Treatment** (Blistex)	15	**Lip balm:** 7.5% padimate O, 3.5% oxybenzone, cetyl alcohol, aloe, cocoa butter, lanolin, vitamins A and E, petrolatum	In 7 g.
otc	**Blistex** (Blistex)	10	**Lip balm:** 6.6% padimate O, 2.5% oxybenzone. 2% dimethicone, cocoa butter, lanolin, parabens, mineral oil, petrolatum	Regular, mint, berry flavors. In 4.5 g.

SUNSCREENS — TOPICAL

Indications

➤*Sunburn prevention:* Overexposure to the sun may cause premature skin aging and skin cancer. The liberal and regular use of these products may help reduce the occurrence of these harmful effects.

➤*Sunburn prevention:* For persons with conditions such as systemic lupus erythematosus, solar urticaria, erythropoietic protoporphyria or those taking photosensitizing drugs. Following is a partial list of drugs that may cause photosensitivity:

- Antihistamines (eg, cyproheptadine, diphenhydramine)
- Anti-infectives (eg, tetracyclines, nalidixic acid, sulfonamides)
- Antineoplastic agents (eg, fluorouracil, methotrexate, procarbazine)
- Antipsychotic agents (eg, phenothiazines, haloperidol)
- Diuretics (eg, thiazides, acetazolamide, amiloride)
- Hypoglycemic agents (eg, sulfonylureas)
- Nonsteroidal anti-inflammatory drugs (eg, phenylbutazone, ketoprofen, naproxen)
- Miscellaneous (eg, bergamot oils, etc, used in cosmetics; coal tar; psoralens; amiodarone; oral contraceptives; quinidine; disopyramide; gold salts; isotretinoin; captopril; carbamazepine)

Administration and Dosage

➤*General dosing considerations:* SPFs greater than 15 were not recommended by the 1978 FDA advisory panel on sunscreens. However, the agency issued a tentative final monograph on this product class in May 1993, and is proposing an upper limit for SPF values of 30. Scientific evidence shows a point of diminishing returns at levels above SPF 30; any benefits that might be derived from using sunscreens with SPFs greater than 30 are negligible. An SPF of at least 15 for most individuals is recommended by the Skin Cancer Foundation.

➤*Adults:*

Sunburn prevention – Apply liberally to all exposed areas (2 mg/cm^2 is recommended) at least 30 minutes prior to sun exposure (up to 2 hours for aminobenzoic acid and its esters) to allow for penetration and binding to the skin. Reapply after swimming or excessive sweating.

➤*Children:* Do not use SPFs as low as 2 or 3 on children younger than 2 years of age.

6 months of age and older – See Adults.

➤*Sun protection factor (SPF):* Sunscreen products include SPF ratings. This factor indicates the amount of increased resistance to sunburning the product provides, relative to unprotected skin. The SPF value is based on a numerical index designed to tell how much protection from the sun a product will provide. The SPF value is defined as the ratio of the amount of energy required to produce a minimal erythema dose (MED) or minimal sunburn through a film of a sunscreen drug product to the amount of energy required to produce the same MED without any treatment. (Example: Using a product with an SPF value of 6 would permit 6 times as much sun exposure.) Base product selection on the patient's history of response to sun exposure.

Recommended Sunscreen Product Guide[a]

Skin type	Patient characteristics[b]	Suggested product SPF
I	Always burns easily; rarely tans	20 to 30
II	Always burns easily; tans minimally	12 to < 20
III	Burns moderately; tans gradually	8 to < 12
IV	Burns minimally; always tans well	4 to < 8
V	Rarely burns; tans profusely	2 to < 4
VI[c]	Never burns; deeply pigmented (insensitive)	None indicated

[a] Based on the FDA's tentative final monograph (TFM) for sunscreen products.
[b] Based on first 45 to 60 minutes sun exposure after winter season or no sun exposure.
[c] This skin type not included in TFM.

➤*Administration:*

Waterproof formulas – Maintain sunburn protection after being in the water up to 80 minutes.

Water-resistant formulas – Maintain sunburn protection after being in the water up to 40 minutes.

Sweat-resistant formulas – Maintain protection after 30 minutes or less of continuous heavy perspiration.

Actions

➤*Pharmacology:* Sunscreens provide either a chemical or a physical barrier to sunlight. These agents help to prevent sunburn, actinic keratosis, premature aging, photosensitivity reactions, and to reduce incidences of skin cancer. Chemical sunscreens act by absorbing ultraviolet (UV) radiation in the medium wavelength range of 290 to 320 nm (UVB range). This is the spectrum of UV radiation primarily responsible for sunburning and inducing skin cancer. UVA may augment the carcinogenic effects of UVB. Long wavelength UV radiation in the 320 to 400 nm (UVA range) can cause tanning and is responsible for most photosensitivity reactions that occur with many drugs, plants, soaps and cosmetics; it is also a major risk factor for serious skin damage. UVA irradiation can exceed that of UVB by 10- to 1,000-fold. UVA deeply penetrates into the dermis; UVB is primarily absorbed in the epidermis. There has been discussion of dividing UVA into UVA I (340 to 400 nm) and UVA II (320 to 340 nm); besides UVB, UVA II may cause the most skin damage. Physical sunscreens reflect or scatter light in both the visible and UV spectrum (290 to 700 nm), preventing penetration of the skin.

UV radiation in the 200 to 290 nm band is known as UVC; although little reaches the earth from the sun, some artificial sources emit UVC. UVC is thought to cause some erythema of the skin.

Sunscreen effectiveness is dependent on UV absorption spectrum, concentration, vehicle and ability to withstand swimming or sweating.

SUNSCREENS — TOPICAL

	Sunscreens	UV spectrum (nm)	Concentrations (%)
	Sunscreen Ingredients		
Chemical	*Benzophenones*	UVA and UVB	
	Oxybenzone	270 to 350	2 to 6
	Dioxybenzone	260 to 380[a]	3
	PABA and PABA esters	UVB	
	p-aminobenzoic acid	260 to 313	5 to 15
	Ethyl dihydroxy propyl PABA	280 to 330	1 to 5
	Padimate O (octyl dimethyl PABA)	290 to 315	1.4 to 8
	Glyceryl PABA	264 to 315	2 to 3
	Cinnamates	UVB[b]	
	Cinoxate	270 to 328	1 to 3
	Ethylhexyl p-methoxycinnamate	290 to 320	2 to 7.5
	Octocrylene	250 to 360	7 to 10
	Octyl methoxycinnamate	290-320	—
	Salicylates	UVB[c]	
	Ethylhexyl salicylate	280 to 320	3 to 5
	Homosalate	295 to 315	4 to 15
	Octyl salicylate	280 to 320	3 to 5
	Miscellaneous	UVB	
	Menthyl anthranilate	260 to 380[d]	3.5 to 5
	Digalloyl trioleate	270 to 320	2 to 5
	Avobenzone (butyl-methoxy-dibenzoylmethane; Parsol 1789)	UVA 320 to 400	3
Physical	Titanium dioxide	290 to 700	2 to 25
	Red petrolatum	290 to 365[e]	30 to 100
	Zinc oxide	290 to 700	—

[a] Values available when used in combination with other screens.
[b] Some UVA spectrum.
[c] Primarily UVB, but has about ⅓ the absorbency of PABA.
[d] Values are for concentrations higher than normally found in nonprescription drugs.
[e] At 334 nm, 16% UV radiation is transmitted; at 365 nm, 58% is transmitted.

Warnings/Precautions

➤*Sensitivity:* Avoid prolonged exposure to sun and to tanning lamps. Sun-sensitive persons particularly should exercise caution. If irritation or sensitization occurs, discontinue use.

Do not use sunscreens containing PABA or its derivatives if sensitive to benzocaine, procaine, sulfonamides, thiazides, PABA or PABA esters.

➤*For external use only:* Avoid contact with eyes.

➤*Vehicle:* Do not use sunscreens in highly alcoholic vehicles on eczematous or inflamed skin.

➤*PABA:* May cause a permanent yellow stain on clothing.

➤*Vitamin D deficiency:* May occur in elderly patients; sunscreens that block UV-B may block cutaneous vitamin D synthesis.

➤*UV exposure:* The amount of UV exposure is influenced by many factors (eg, time of day, season, latitude, altitude, atmospheric conditions). UVB radiation is strongest between 10 am and 2 pm; UVA is relatively constant. Each 1,000 foot increase in altitude adds 4% to UV light intensity. Reflectance from water depends on the angle of exposure, with almost 100% when the sun is directly overhead. Fresh snow reflects approximately 85% to 100% of UV light, and sand reflects 20% to 25%.

➤*Pregnancy: Category: Undetermined*. Consult a health care provider before using in pregnant women.

➤*Lactation:* Consult a health care provider before using in breast-feeding women.

Adverse Reactions

Contact dermatitis may develop with PABA or its esters (especially glyceryl PABA), benzophenones and cinnamates. Physical sunscreens are occlusive; miliaria or folliculitis may occur.

Patient Information

Follow directions on product container concerning frequency of application; reapply after swimming or sweating. Reapplication does not extend the protection period.

➤*For external use only:* Do not swallow. Avoid contact with the eyes.

Discontinue use if signs of irritation or rash appear.

PABA may permanently stain clothing yellow.

Wear protective eye coverings or sunglasses; UV light can cause corneal damage.

OINTMENT AND LOTION BASES

otc	**Lanaphilic** (Medco)	**Ointment; topical**: Stearyl alcohol, white petrolatum, isopropyl palmitate, lanolin oil, propylene glycol, sorbitol, sodium lauryl sulfate, parabens	In lb.
otc	**Lanaphilic w/Urea 10%** (Medco)	**Ointment; topical**: Urea, stearyl alcohol, white petrolatum, isopropyl palmitate, lanolin oil, sorbitol, propylene glycol, sodium lauryl sulfate, lactic acid, parabens	In lb.
otc	**Petrolatum** (Carolina Medical)	**Ointment; topical**: Petrolatum, mineral oil, ceresin wax, woolwax alcohol	In 430 g.
otc	**Absorbase** (Carolina Medical)	**Ointment; topical**: Petrolatum, mineral oil, ceresin wax, woolwax alcohol, potassium sorbate	Unscented. In 114 and 454 g.
otc	**Hydrophilic** (Rugby)	**Ointment; topical**: White petrolatum, stearyl alcohol, propylene glycol, sodium lauryl sulfate, parabens	In 454 g.
otc	**Aquabase** (Paddock)	**Ointment; topical**: Petrolatum, mineral oil, mineral wax, woolwax alcohol, sorbitan sesquioleate	Unscented. Dye free. In 454 g.
otc	**Aquaphilic** (Medco)	**Ointment; topical**: Stearyl alcohol, white petrolatum, isopropyl palmitate, sorbitol, propylene glycol, sodium lauryl sulfate, parabens	In lb.
otc	**Aquaphilic w/Carbamide 10% and 20%** (Medco)	**Ointment; topical**: Urea, stearyl alcohol, white petrolatum, isopropyl palmitate, propylene glycol, sorbitol, sodium lauryl sulfate, lactic acid, parabens	In lb.
otc	**Aquaphor** (Beiersdorf)	**Ointment; topical**: Petrolatum, mineral oil, lanolin, alcohol, panthenol, glycerin.	In 10 and 50 g tubes and 99 and 396 g jars.
otc	**Polyethylene Glycol** (Medco)	**Ointment; topical**: Water soluble greaseless base with PEG-8 and PEG-75	In lb.
otc	**Solumol** (C & M)	**Ointment; topical**: Petrolatum, mineral oil, cetearyl alcohol, sodium lauryl sulfate, glycerin, propylene glycol	In lb.
otc	**A-Mantle** (Doak)	**Cream; topical**: Cetearyl alcohol, glycerin, petrolatum, synthetic beeswax, mineral oil, methylparaben, white potato dextrin	In 30 g.
otc	**Velvachol** (Owen/Galderma)	**Cream; topical**: Water miscible vehicle containing petrolatum, mineral oil, stearyl alcohol, sodium lauryl sulfate, cholesterol, parabens	In lb.
otc	**Dermabase** (Paddock)	**Cream; topical**: Mineral oil, petrolatum, cetostearyl alcohol, propylene glycol, sodium lauryl sulfate, isopropyl palmitate, imidazolidinyl urea, parabens	In 454 g.
otc	**Dermovan** (Owen/Galderma)	**Cream; topical**: Nonionic, water miscible vanishing cream vehicle containing glyceryl stearate, stearamidoethyl diethylamine, glycerin, mineral oil, cetyl esters, parabens	In lb.
otc	**Hydrocream Base** (Paddock)	**Cream; topical**: Petrolatum, mineral oil, mineral wax, woolwax alcohol, cholesterol, imidazolidinyl urea, parabens	In 454 g.
otc	**Eucerin** (Beiersdorf)	**Cream; topical**: Petrolatum, mineral oil, mineral wax, woolwax alcohol	In 60, 120, 240 and 480 g.
otc	**Hydrocerin** (Geritrex)	**Cream; topical**: Petrolatum, mineral oil, lanolin alcohol, parabens	In 120 g.
otc	**PENcream** (Humco)	**Cream; topical**: Caprylic/capric triglyceride, ceteareth 20, cetearyl alcohol, ethylhextlglycerin, glyceryl stearate, isopropyl palmitate, lecithin, octyldodecanol, PEG 100, phenoxyethanol, propylene glycol	In 45 g.

OINTMENT AND LOTION BASES

otc	**Vanicream** (Pharmaceutical Specialties)	**Cream; topical**: White petrolatum, cetearyl alcohol, ceteareth-20, sorbitol solution, propylene glycol, simethicone, glyceryl monostearate, polyethylene glycol monostearate	In 120 g and lb.
otc	**Versa HRT Base Botanical** (Humco)	**Cream; topical**: Almond, aloe, carbomer, cetyl alcohol, folic acid, glycerin, glyceryl stearate, grape, MSM, PEG-100 stearate, phenoxyethanol, primrose, red clover, salicylic acid, selenium, stearic acid, triethanolamine, wheat, and vitamins A, C, D, and E	In 1, 10, 20, and 40 lb.
otc	**Versa HRT Base Heavy** (Humco)	**Cream; topical**: Almond, C12–15 alkyl benzoate, caprylic/capric triglyceride, carbomer, cetyl alcohol, dimethicone, glyceryl stearate, olive, PEG-100 stearate, propylene glycol, stearic acid, triethanolamine, wheat, and vitamins A and E	In 1, 10, 20, and 40 lb.
otc	**Versa HRT Base Natural** (Humco)	**Cream; topical**: Almond, carbomer, cetyl alcohol, glycerin, glyceryl stearate, PEG-100 stearate, phenoxyethanol, salicylic acid, stearic acid, triethanolamine, wheat, and vitamins A, C, and E	In 1, 10, 20, and 40 lb.
otc	**Versa LipoBase Heavy** (Humco)	**Cream; topical**: Ceteareth-12, ceteareth-20, cetearyl alcohol, cetearyl isononanoate, cetyl palmitate, glycerin, glyceryl stearate, lecithin, honeysuckle, perilla, polyquaternium-37, PPG-1 trideceth-7, propylene glycol dicaprylate/dicaprate, tea tree, vitamin E	Water and oil soluble. In 1, 10, 20, and 40 lb.
otc	**Versa LipoBase Regular** (Humco)	**Cream; topical**: Almond, aloe, C12–15 alkyl benzoate, cetearyl alcohol, cetearyl glucoside, cetyl alcohol, dimethicone, glycerin, glyceryl stearate, grape, hydroxymethylglycinate, lecithin, perilla, phenoxyethanol, polyacrylamide, silicate, wheat, xanthan, and vitamins A, C, and E	Water and oil soluble. In 1, 10, 20, and 40 lb.
otc	**Versa VaniBase** (Humco)	**Cream; topical**: Caprylic/Capric triglyceride, ceteareth-20, cetearyl alcohol, dimethicone, ethylhexylglycerine, glyceryl stearate, isopropyl palmitate, octyldodecanol, PEG-100 stearate, phenoxyethanol, propylene glycol, triethanolamine	Fragrance and dye free. In 1 lb.
otc	**Versabase** (PCCA)	**Cream; topical**: Aloe, cyclopentasiloxane, disodium EDTA, octylstearate, vitamin E	In
otc	**Nutraderm** (Owen/Galderma)	**Lotion; topical**: Mineral oil, sorbitan stearate, stearyl alcohol, sodium lauryl sulfate, cetyl alcohol, carbomer-940, parabens, triethanolamine	In 240 and 480 mL.
otc	**Hydrocerin** (Geritrex)	**Lotion; topical**: Mineral oil, lanolin alcohol, parabens	In 473 mL.
otc	**Vehicle/N** (Neutrogena)	**Solution; topical**: 45% SD alcohol 40, laureth-4, propylene glycol, 4% isopropyl alcohol	In 50 mL with applicator.
otc	**Vehicle/N Mild** (Neutrogena)	**Solution; topical**: 37.5% SD alcohol 40, laureth-4, 5% isopropyl alcohol	In 50 mL with applicator.
otc	**Solvent-G** (Syosset)	**Liquid; topical**: 55% SD alcohol 40B, laureth-4, isopropyl alcohol, propylene glycol	In 50 mL.
otc	**Versa Alcohol Base** (Humco)	**Gel; topical**: Aloe, ethylhexylglycerin, SD alcohol 40, polyacrylamide, laureth-7, phenoxyethanol	Fragrance, oil, and dye free. In 1, 10, 20, and 40 lb.
otc	**Versa Aqua Base** (Humco)	**Gel; topical**: DMDM hydantoin, iodopropyl butylcarbamate, PEG-18 palmitate, PPG-18 butyl ether, propylene glycol, SD alcohol 40, triethanolamine	Fragrance and dye free. In 1, 10, 20, and 40 lb.
otc	**Versa PLO20** (Humco)	**Gel; topical**: Isopropyl palmitate, lecithin, poloxamer 407	In flowable (with SD alcohol 40) and regular. In 1 lb.

OINTMENT AND LOTION BASES — TOPICAL

Indications

➤*Bases:* These products are used as bases for incorporation of various active ingredients in extemporaneously compounded dermatological prescriptions.

RUBS AND LINIMENTS

Indications

➤*Topical pain:* These products are used for relief of pain of muscular aches, neuralgia, rheumatism, arthritis, sprains and like conditions, when skin is intact.

Contraindications

Allergy to components of any formulation or to salicylates.

Warnings/Precautions

➤*For external use only:* Avoid contact with eyes and mucous membranes.

➤*Apply to affected parts only:* Do not apply to irritated skin; if excessive irritation develops, discontinue use. If pain persists for more than 7 to 10 days, or if redness is present, or in conditions affecting children younger than 10 years of age, consult a physician.

➤*Heat therapy:* Do not use an external source of heat (eg, heating pad) with these agents since irritation or burning of the skin may occur.

➤*Protective covering:* Applying a tight bandage or wrap over these agents is not recommended since increased absorption may occur.

Drug Interactions

➤*Anticoagulants:* An enhanced anticoagulant effect (eg, increased prothrombin time) occurred in several patients receiving an anticoagulant and using topical methylsalicylate concurrently.

Adverse Reactions

If applied to large skin areas, salicylate side effects may occur, such as tinnitus, nausea or vomiting. Toxic if ingested.

Counterirritants may cause local irritation, especially in patients with sensitive skin.

GELS, CREAMS AND OINTMENTS

otc	**Aspercreme Cream** (Chattem)	10% trolamine salicylate	In 37.5, 90, and 150 g.
otc	**Mobisyl Creme** (Ascher)		In 35.4, 100, and 227 g.
otc	**Myoflex Creme** (Novartis Consumer)		In 60, 120, and 240 g and lb.
otc	**Sportscreme** (Chattem)		In 37.5 and 90 g.
otc	**Analgesic Creme Rub** (Major)	10% trolamine salicylate, aloe vera, cetyl alcohol, glycerin, mineral oil, parabens, triethanolamine	In 85 g.
otc	**Flex-Power Performance Sports** (Flex-Power)	10% trolamine salicylate, cetyl alcohol, EDTA, parabens, glycerols, stearyl alcohol, sodium metabisulfite	Citrus light and clean scents. In 120 g.
otc	**Icy Hot Cream** (Chattem)	30% methyl salicylate, 10% menthol, carbomer, cetyl esters wax, emulsifying wax, trolamine	In 37.5 and 90 g.
otc	**Musterole Deep Strength Rub** (Schering-Plough)	30% methyl salicylate, 0.5% methyl nicotinate and 3% menthol	In 37 and 90 g.
otc	**Bengay Ultra Strength Cream** (Pfizer)	30% methyl salicylate, 10% menthol, 4% camphor, EDTA, glyceryl stearate SE, anhydrous lanolin, polysorbate 80, potassium carbomer and stearate, triethanolamine carbomer and stearate	In 35 g.

GELS, CREAMS AND OINTMENTS

otc	**Arthritis Formula Bengay** (Pfizer)	30% methyl salicylate, 8% menthol, glyceryl stearate SE, anhydrous lanolin, polysorbate 85, potassium stearate, sorbitan tristearate, xanthan gum	In 35 g.
otc	**Icy Hot Chill Stick** (Chattem)	30% methyl salicylate, 10% menthol	Hydrogenated castor oil, stearyl alcohol. In 49 g.
otc	**Icy Hot Balm** (Chattem)	29% methyl salicylate, 7.6% menthol, paraffin, white petrolatum	In 105 g.
otc	**Bengay Original Ointment** (Pfizer)	18.3% methyl salicylate, 16% menthol, anhydrous lanolin, microcrystalline wax, synthetic bees wax	In 35 and 90 g.
otc	**Pain Bust•RII** (Continental)	17% methyl salicylate, 12% menthol	In 90 g.
otc	**Arthritis Hot Creme** (Chattem)	15% methyl salicylate, 10% menthol, glyceryl stearate, carbomer 934, lanolin, PEG-100 stearate, propylene glycol, trolamine, parabens	In 90 g.
otc	**Menthoderm Ointment** (Pharmaceutica North America)	15% methyl salicylate, 10% menthol, glycerin, parabens, polysorbate 20, propylene glycol, tartrazine, triethanolamine, SD-alcohol, urea	In 60 and 120 g.
otc	**Icy Hot Arthritis Therapy Gel** (Chattem)	0.025% capsaicin, parabens, aloe vera, alcohol, wax, soybean oil	In 70.8 g.
otc	**Deep-Down Rub** (SK-Beecham)	15% methyl salicylate, 5% menthol, 0.5% camphor, 40.5% SD alcohol	In 37.5 and 90 g.
otc	**Minit-Rub** (Bristol-Myers Products)	15% methyl salicylate, 3.5% menthol, 2.3% camphor, anhydrous lanolin	In 45 and 90 g.
otc	**Thera-gesic Cream** (Mission)	15% methyl salicylate, menthol, dimethylpolysiloxane, glycerin, carbopol, triethanolamine, parabens	In 90 and 150 g.
otc	**Ziks Cream** (Nodum)	12% methyl salicylate, 1% menthol, 0.025% capsaicin, cetyl alcohol	In 60 g.
otc	**Gordogesic Creme** (Gordon)	10% methyl salicylate, propylene glycol, mineral oil, white wax, triethanolamine, parabens	In 75 g and lb.
otc	**Methagual** (Gordon)	8% methyl salicylate, 2% guaiacol, petrolatum, white wax, parabens	In 60 g and lb.
otc	**Iodex Ointment** (Lee Pharmaceutical)	4.8% methyl salicylate, 4.7% iodine, oleic acid, paraffin, petrolatum	In 28.35 g.
otc	**Blue Gel Muscular Pain Reliever** (Rugby)	Menthol	In 240 g.
otc	**Gold Bond Foot Pain Relieving Cream** (Chattem)	16% menthol, aloe, benzyl alcohol, cetyl alcohol, capsaicin, cetearyl alcohol, disodium EDTA, 2% SD alcohol, stearyl alcohol, urea	In 113 g.
otc	**Eucalyptamint Maximum Strength Ointment** (Ciba)	16% menthol, lanolin, eucalyptus oil	In 60 mL.
otc	**Flexall Ultra Plus** (Chattem)	16% menthol, 10% methyl salicylate, 3.1% camphor in aloe vera gel base, eucalyptus oil, glycerin, peppermint oil, alcohol	In 70.8 g.
otc	**Maximum Strength Flexall 454** (Chattem)	16% menthol, aloe vera gel, eucalyptus oil, methyl salicylate, peppermint oil, SD alcohol 38-B, thyme oil	In 90 g.
otc	**Bayer Muscle and Joint Cream** (Bayer)	10% menthol, 4% camphor, 30% methyl salicylate, EDTA, glyceryl, lanolin, stearyl alcohol	In 56 and 114 g.
otc	**Eucalyptamint Gel** (Ciba Consumer)	8% menthol, eucalyptus oil, SD 3A alcohol	In 60 g.
otc	**Flexall Gel** (Chattem)	7% menthol, aloe leaf juice, eucalyptus oil, glycerin, peppermint oil, methyl salicylate, SD-alcohol, thyme oil, thriethanolamine, tocopherol	In 113.3 g.
otc	**Icy Hot Pro-Therapy Medicated Foam Pad** (Chattem)	5% menthol, parabens, tartrazine, urea	In 4s with knee wrap.
otc	**Wonder Ice Gel** (Pedinol)	5.25% menthol	In 113 and 473 g.
otc	**Berri-Freez** (Geritrex)	3.5% menthol, camphor, glycerin, isopropyl alcohol, parabens, triethanolamine	In 473 g.
otc	**Mineral Freez Gel** (Geritrex)	2% menthol	Alcohol. In 226.8 g.
otc	**Pain Gel Plus** (Mentholatum Co.)	4% menthol, aloe, vitamin E	In 57 g.
otc	**Vanishing Scent Bengay** (Pfizer)	2.5% menthol, alcohol, camphor	In 120 g.
otc	**Tiger Balm Ointment** (Prince of Peace)	8% menthol, 11% camphor, cajuput oil, clove oil, mint oil, petrolatum	In 18 g.
otc	**Sōltice Quick-Rub** (Oakhurst)	5.1% menthol, 5.1% camphor	Eucalyptus oil, glycerin, methyl salicylate. In 37 and 85 g.
otc	**Analgesic Balm** (Various, eg, URL)	Methyl salicylate, menthol	In 30 and 454 g.
otc	**Analgesic Balm-GRX** (Geritrex)	14% methyl salicylate, 6% menthol	In 28 g.
otc	**Medrox Ointment** (Pharmaceutica North America)	20% methyl salicylate, 5% menthol, 0.0375% capsaicin, urea	Cetyl alcohol, glycerin, parabens, PEG-150. In 60 and 120 g.
otc	**TheraFlu Vapor Stick Cough & Muscle Aches** (Novartis)	4.8% camphor, 2.6% menthol, cetyl alcohol, eucalyptus oil, parabens	In 51 g.
otc	**Vicks VapoRub Ointment** (Procter & Gamble Co.)	4.8% camphor, 1.2% eucalyptus oil, 2.6% menthol, cedarleaf oil, nutmeg oil, petrolatum, turpentine oil	In 50 g.
otc	**Vicks VapoRub Cream** (Procter & Gamble Co.)	4.7% camphor, 2.6% menthol, 1.2% eucalyptus oil, cedarleaf oil, EDTA, glycerin, imidazolidinyl urea, cetyl and stearyl alcohols, parabens, nutmeg oil, titanium dioxide, spirits of turpentine	In 45, 60, 90 and 180 g.

GELS, CREAMS AND OINTMENTS

otc	**Therapeutic Mineral Ice Exercise Formula Gel** (Novartis Consumer Health)	4% menthol, ammonium hydroxide, carbomer 934P or 934, cupric sulfate, isopropyl alcohol, thymol	In 90 g.
otc	**Bengay Vanishing Scent Gel** (Pfizer)	3% menthol, benzophenone-4, camphor, diazolidinyl urea, EDTA, isopropyl alcohol, potassium carbomer 940	In 35 g.
otc	**Blue Ice Gel** (Geritrex)	2% menthol	Isopropyl alcohol. In 227 g.
otc	**Therapy Ice Gel** (Major)	2% menthol	Isopropyl alcohol. In 226.8 g.
otc	**Icy Hot Pain Relieving Gel** (Chattem)	2.5% menthol	Alcohol 15%, aloe, parabens, triethanolamine. In 70.8 g.
otc	**Sportscreme Ice Gel** (Thompson)	2% menthol, carbomer 934, styrene/acrylate copolymer, triethanolamine, 38% SD alcohol 40	In 227 g.
otc	**Mineral Ice Gel Therapeutic** (Novartis Consumer Health)	2% menthol, cupric sulfate, isopropyl alcohol	In 99.2, 226.8, and 453.6 g.
otc	**Flex-all 454 Gel** (Chattem)	Menthol in an aloe vera gel, methyl salicylate, alcohol, allantoin, boric acid, carbomer 940, diazolidinyl urea, iodine, polysorbate 60, propylene glycol, potassium iodide, triethanolamine, eucalyptus oil, glycerin, parabens	In 60, 120, and 240 g.
otc	**Eucalyptamint Gel**(Ciba Consumer)	8% menthol	
otc	**Duraflex Comfort Gel** (Trimarc Labs)	Aloe, capsicum, glucosamine, menthol, methyl salicylate, methyl sulfonyl methane, methylparaben, sorbitol, urea	In 59.14 g.
otc	**Pain Relieving Rub Cream** (G & W Labs)	Menthol 10%, methyl salicylate 15%. Cetyl alcohol, glycerin, glyceryl, triethanolamine	In 114 g.

LIQUIDS

otc	**Maximum Strength Blue-Emu** (NFI Consumer Products)	**Spray; topical**: 2.5% menthol, aloe vera gel, balm mint extract, boswellia extract, citrus extract, emu oil, eucalyptus oil, ginger extract, isopropyl alcohol, peppermint extract, rosemary oil, urea	In 59.15 mL.
otc	**Absorbine Jr** (W.F. Young)	**Liquid; topical**: 1.27% menthol, absinthium oil, echinacea, iodine, plant extracts of calendula, potassium iodide, thymol, wormwood	In 118 mL w/ applicator.
otc	**Extra Strength Absorbine Jr. Liquid** (W.F. Young)	**Liquid; topical**: 4% menthol	In 59 and 118 mL.
otc	**Aspercreme Max Roll-On** (Chattem)	**Liquid; topical**: 16% menthol, capsaicin, glycerin, propylene glycol, SD alcohol, triethanolamine	In 73 mL.
otc	**Gold Bond Pain Relieving Foot Roll-On** (Chattem)		In 73 mL.

LOTIONS AND LINIMENTS

otc	**Aspercreme Rub Lotion** (Thompson)	10% trolamine salicylate, cetyl alcohol, glyceryl stearate, lanolin, parabens, potassium phosphate, propylene glycol, sodium lauryl sulfate, stearic acid	In 180 mL.
otc	**Panalgesic Gold Liniment** (ECR Pharm)	55% methyl salicylate, 3.1% camphor, 1.25% menthol, 18.6% emollient oils, 22% alcohol	In 120 mL.
otc	**Gordobalm** (Gordon)	Menthol, camphor, methyl salicylate, 16% isopropyl alcohol, tragacanth, thymol, acetone, eucalyptus oil, tartrazine	In 120 mL and gal.
otc	**Heet Liniment** (Whitehall)	15% methyl salicylate, 3.6% camphor, capsicum oleoresin (as 0.025% capsaicin), acetone, 70% alcohol	In 68.5 and 150 mL.
otc	**Banalg Hospital Strength Lotion** (Forest)	14% methyl salicylate, 3% menthol	In 60 mL.
otc	**Banalg Lotion** (Forest)	4.9% methyl salicylate, 2% camphor, 1% menthol	In 60 and 480 mL.
otc	**Extra Strength Absorbine Jr.** (W.F. Young)	4% natural menthol	In 60 mL.
otc	**Absorbine Jr. Liniment** (W.F. Young)	1.27% menthol, plant extracts of calendula, echinacea and wormwood, iodine, potassium iodide, thymol, acetone, chloroxylenol	In 60 and 120 mL.
otc	**Icy Hot PM Medicated Lotion** (Chattem)	Aloe, benzyl alcohol, capsaicin, cetearyl alcohol, cetyl alcohol, disodium EDTA, ethanol, 7.5% menthol, PEG-2, stearyl alcohol	In 113 g.
otc	**Arth-Rx Topical Analgesic Lotion** (Phillips Gulf)	0.5% methyl nicotinate, 0.025% capsaicin, aloe vera gel, extracts of arnica, rue, chamomile, boswellia	In 90 mL roll-on applicator.
otc	**Yager's Liniment** (Oakhurst Company)	3.1% camphor, 8.3% turpentine, clove oil	In 120 and 240 mL.

SPRAYS

otc	**Absorbine Jr Ultra Strength** (W.F. Young)	**Spray; topical**: 12% menthol, alcohol, echinacea, plant extracts of calendula, spearmint oil, wormwood	In 118 mL.
otc	**Sports Spray** (Mentholatum)	**Spray; topical**: 35% methyl salicylate, 10% menthol, 5% camphor, 58% alcohol	In 85 g.

PATCHES

otc	**Bengay** (Pfizer)	**Patch; topical:** 1.4% menthol	Glycerin. In regular and large sizes. In 1s.
otc	**Absorbine Jr Back Patch** (W. F. Young)	**Patch; topical:** 5% menthol	Aloe barbadensis, camphor, lanolin, zinc oxide. 22 x 10 cm. In 4s.
otc	**Cold & Hot Pain Relief Therapy Patch** (Major Pharmaceuticals)		Aloe vera, disodium EDTA, methylparaben. 8 x 12 cm. In 5s.
otc	**Icy Hot Back Pain Relief** (Chattem)		Glycerin. In 5s.
otc	**Icy Hot Pop & Peel** (Chattem)		Glycerin. In 5s.
otc	**Absorbine Jr Ultra Strength** (W.F. Young)	**Patch; topical:** 6.5% menthol	Alcohol, camphor, eucalyptus, glycerin, kaolin, leaf oil, polysorbate 80, titanium dioxide. In 6s.
otc	**Icy Hot Roll** (Chattem)	**Patch; topical:** 7.5% menthol	Mineral oil. In 3s.
otc	**DuraProxin** (Pharmaceutica North America)	**Patch; topical:** 3% camphor, 1.25% menthol	Disodium ethylenediaminetertraacetate, glycerin, polysorbate 80. In 30s.
otc	**DuraProxin ES** (Pharmaceutica North America)	**Patch; topical:** 3% camphor, 1.25% menthol, 10% methyl salicylate	Disodium ethylenediaminetertraacetate, glycerin, polysorbate 80. In 30s.

TOPICAL COMBINATIONS, MISCELLANEOUS

TOPICAL COMBINATIONS, MISCELLANEOUS

otc	**Boyol Salve** (Pfeiffer)	**Salve; topical:** 10% ichthammol, benzocaine, lanolin, petrolatum	In 30 g.
otc	**Dermadrox** (Geritrex)	**Ointment; topical:** Aluminum hydroxide gel, zinc chloride, lanolin, calcium carbonate, vitamin A in a hydrophilic ointment base *For relief of minor skin irritations such as chafing, interico and galling.*	In 113 g.
otc	**Wonderful Dream** (Wonderful Dream Salve Corp.)	**Salve; topical:** Phenyl mercury nitrate 1:5000, oil of tar, turpentine, olive oil, linseed oil, posin, burgundy pitch, camphor, beeswax, mutton tallow	In 34 g.
otc	**Dr. Dermi-Heal** (Quality)	**Ointment; topical:** 1% allantoin, zinc oxide, Balsam Peru, castor oil, petrolatum *For relief of diaper rash, chafing, minor burns, bed sores, external vaginal itching and irritation, ostomy irritation and heat rash.*	In 75 g.
otc	**Saratoga** (Blair)	**Ointment; topical:** Zinc oxide, boric acid, eucalyptol, acetylated lanolin alcohols, white petrolatum, white beeswax *For temporary relief of itching and minor skin irritations, chapped and chafed skin, diaper rash, bed sores, mild burns.*	In 28 and 60 g.
otc	**Unguentine** (Mentholatum)	**Ointment; topical:** 1% phenol, petrolatum, oleostearine, zinc oxide, eucalyptus oil, thyme oil *For pain relief in minor burns.*	In 30 g.
otc	**Amerigel** (Amerx Health Care Corp.)	**Ointment; topical:** Meadowsweet extract, oakbark extract, polyethylene glycol 400, polyethylene glycol 3350, zinc acetate. *For stage I-IV pressure ulcers, stasis ulcers, diabetic skin ulcers, post-surgical incisions, 1st and 2nd degree burns, cuts, and abrasions.*	In 28.3 g.
otc	**Ichthammol** (Allan)	**Ointment; topical:** 20% ichthammol	Lanolin, mineral oil, petrolatum. In 30 g.
Rx	**Mimyx** (GlaxoSmithKline)	**Cream; topical:** Betaine, olive oil, glycerin, pentylene glycol, palm glycerides, vegetable oil, squalane, hydroxyethyl cellulose, carbomer, xanthan gum. *To manage and relieve the burning and itching experienced with various types of dermatoses, including atopic dermatitis, allergic contact dermatitis, and radiation dermatitis.*	Preservative-free. In 70 g.
Rx	**Xclair** (Align)	**Cream; topical:** Isohexadecane, butyrospermum parkii, ethylhexyl palmitate, glycyrrhetinic acid, cera alba, peg-30 dipolyhydroxystearate, bisabolol, polyglyceryl-6, polyricinoleate, tocopheryl acetate (antioxidant), castor oil, sodium hyaluronate nylon 12, butylene glycol, magnesium sulfate, piroctone olamine, allantoin, magnesium stearate, disodium EDTA, vitis vinifera, ascorbyl tetraisopalmitate, propyl gallate, telmesteine	In 75 mL.
Rx	**PruMyx** (PruGen)	**Cream; topical:** Olive oil, glycerin, palm glycerides, vegatable oil, lecithin, squalane, betaine, palmitamide MEA, sarcosine, acetamide MEA, hydroxyethyl cellulose, sodium carbomer, xanthan gum. Preservative free, fragrance free.	In 140 g.
Rx	**Tetrix** (Coria)	**Cream; topical:** Aluminum magnesium hydroxide stearate, cetyl dimethicone copolyol, cyclomethicone, dimethicone, hexyl laurate, polyglyceryl-4 isostearate, and sodium chloride.	Propylparabens. In kits with two 56.7 g tubes and two 56.7 tubes of **Cara Ve** moisturizing cream.
otc	**Ostiderm** (Pedinol)	**Lotion; topical:** Aluminum sulfate, zinc oxide *For foot odor/excessive moisture.*	In 42.5 mL.
		Roll-On; topical: Aluminum chlorohydrate, camphor, alcohol, EDTA, diazolidinyl urea, *Safeguards against offensive odor and dries excessive moisture of the feet.*	In 88.7 mL.
otc	**Men-Phor** (Geritrex Corp.)	**Lotion; topical:** 0.5% camphor, 0.5% menthol, carbopol, cetearyl alcohol, cetyl alcohol, hydantoin, castor oil, petrolatum. *To provide temporary relief for dry itching skin, sunburn, insect bites, and pruritus.*	In 222 mL.
otc	**Sarna Anti-Itch** (GlaxoSmithKline)	**Lotion; topical:** 0.5% camphor, 0.5% menthol, carbomer 940, DMDM hydantoin, glyceryl stearate, PEG-8 stearate, PEG-100 stearate, petrolatum *For relief of dry, itching skin, sunburn, poison ivy and poison oak.*	In 222 mL.
otc	**Schamberg's** (C & M)	**Lotion; topical:** Zinc oxide, 0.15% menthol, 1% phenol, peanut oil and lime water *For the temporary relief of itching.*	In 480 mL.
otc	**Soothaderm** (Pharmakon)	**Lotion; topical:** 2.07 mg pyrilamine maleate, 2.08 mg benzocaine and 41.35 mg zinc oxide per mL, simethicone, parabens, propylene glycol, camphor, menthol *For relief of itching due to chickenpox, diaper rash, insect bites, poison ivy/oak, prickly heat and sunburn.*	In 118 mL.
otc	**Florida Sunburn Relief** (Pharmacel)	**Lotion; topical:** 3% benzyl alcohol, 0.4% phenol, 0.2% camphor, 0.15% menthol *For relief of pain due to sunburn.*	In 60 mL.
otc	**Outgro** (Whitehall)	**Solution; topical:** 25% tannic acid, 5% chlorobutanol, 83% isopropyl alcohol *For temporary pain relief of ingrown toenails.*	In 9.3 mL.

TOPICAL COMBINATIONS, MISCELLANEOUS

otc	**Stypto-Caine** (Pedinol)	**Solution; topical:** 250 mg aluminum chloride, 2.5 mg tetracaine HCl, 1 mg oxyquinoline sulfate per g with glycerin *To stop bleeding in minor cuts.*	In 59 mL.
otc	**Campho-Phenique** (Sterling Health)	**Liquid; topical:** 10.8% camphor, 4.7% phenol, eucalyptus oil, light mineral oil *To relieve pain and combat infections.*	In 22.5, 45 and 120 mL.
otc	**Oxyzal Wet Dressing** (Gordon)	**Liquid; topical:** Oxyquinoline sulfate, benzalkonium Cl 1:2000 *For minor infections.*	In 30, 120 and 480 mL.
Rx	**EpiCream** (Promius Pharma)	**Emulsion; topical:** Disodium EDTA, glycerin, glyceryl stearate, hydroxypropyl bispalmitamide MEA (ceramide), PEG-100, petrolatum. *To manage and relieve the burning and itching experienced with various types of dermatoses, including atopic dermatitis, irritant contact dermatitis, and radiation dermatitis.*	In 90 g.
Rx	**Aloquin** (Primus Pharma)	**Gel; topical:** 1% aloe polysaccharides, 1.25% iodoquinol, benzyl alcohol, PEG-20, SDA alcohol 40 B	In 60 g.
otc	**Campho-Phenique** (Sterling Health)	**Gel; topical:** 4.7% phenol, 10.8% camphor, colloidal silicon dioxide, eucalyptus oil, glycerin, light mineral oil *Pain relief in cold sores, fever blisters, cuts, scrapes, burns and insect bites.*	In 6.9 and 15 g.
otc	**Topic** (Syntex)	**Gel; topical:** 5% benzyl alcohol, camphor, menthol, 30% isopropyl alcohol *For temporary relief of itching from poison oak/ivy, insect bites, eczema, minor skin allergies and heat rash.*	In 60 g.
otc	**Mederma** (Merz)	**Gel; topical:** Water (purified), PEG-4, onion (allium cepa) extract, xanthan gum, allantoin, fragrance, methylparaben, sorbic acid. *Helps scars appear softer and smoother.*	In 50g.
otc	**Benadryl Children's Anti-Itch** (J&J Consumer)	**Gel; topical:** Camphor 0.45%. Benzyl alcohol, EDTA, menthol, SD alcohol.	In 85 g.
otc	**Aluminum Paste** (Paddock)	**Ointment; topical:** 10% metallic aluminum *An occlusive skin protectant.*	White petrolatum base. In lb.
Rx	**Salvax Duo** (Quinnova)	**Foam; topical:** 6% salicylic acid, 40% urea, glycerin, parabens *For the removal of excessive keratin in hyperkeratotic skin disorders.*	In 70 g.
otc	**Sarna Anti-Itch** (GlaxoSmithKline)	**Foam; topical:** 0.5% camphor, 0.5% menthol, carbomer 940, DMDM hydantoin, glyceryl stearate, PEG-8 and PEG-100 stearate, petrolatum *For relief of dry, itching skin.*	In 99 g.
otc	**ProTech First-Aid Stik** (Triton)	**Liquid; topical:** 10% povidone-iodine, 2.5% lidocaine HCl *For cleaning and pain relief of cuts, scrapes and burns.*	In 14 mL.
otc	**Proderm Topical** (Dow B. Hickam)	**Dressing; topical:** 650 mg castor oil and 72.5 mg Balsam Peru per 0.82 mL *For prevention and management of decubitus ulcers.*	In 113.4 g.
otc	**Dome-Paste** (Miles)	**Wound dressing; topical:** Zinc oxide, calamine, gelatin *For conditions of extremities (eg, varicose ulcers) requiring protection.*	3″ by 10 yd or 4″ by 10 yd bandages.
otc	**Breezee Mist Foot Powder** (Pedinol)	**Powder; topical:** Isobutane, talc, aluminum chlorohydrate, cyclomethicone, isopropyl myristate. propylene carbonate, stearalkonium hectorite, undecylenic acid, fragrance, menthol *Cooling formula soothes and helps keep feet dry and odor free.*	In 113 g aerosol can.
otc	**Columbia Antiseptic Powder** (F.C. Sturtevant[a])	**Powder; topical:** Zinc oxide, talc, carbolic acid, boric acid.	In 30 and 420 g.
Rx	**Scarlet Red Ointment Dressings** (Sherwood Medical)	**Wound dressings; topical:** 5% scarlet red, lanolin, olive oil and petrolatum in fine mesh absorbent gauze *For epithelialization of donor sites, burns and wounds.*	In 5″ x 9″ strips.

[a] The F.C. Sturtevant Company, P.O. Box 607, Bronxville, NY 10708; 914-337-5131, 888-871-5661; fax 914-337-5309; http://www.columbiapowder.com.

TOPICAL COMBINATIONS, MISCELLANEOUS

Active Ingredients

Principal active ingredients of these formulations include:

➤*BORIC ACID, OXYQUINOLINE and BENZALKONIUM Cl:* Used as antiseptics.

➤*ZINC OXIDE and ALUMINUM:* Provide astringent and topical protectant actions.

➤*CAMPHOR, EUCALYPTOL, MENTHOL and PHENOL:* Used as antipruritics, mild local anesthetics and counterirritants.

➤*BENZOCAINE and LIDOCAINE:* Local anesthetics.

➤*PYRILAMINE MALEATE:* An antihistamine.

➤*CASTOR OIL (RICINUS OIL), GLYCERIN and MINERAL OIL:* Used as emollients.

➤*BENZYL ALCOHOL:* Used as an antipruritic.

➤*BISMUTH SUBNITRATE:* Used as a skin protectant.

➤*BALSAM PERU:* Used to stimulate tissue growth.

➤*BIEBRICH SCARLET RED:* Used to promote wound healing.

➤*ICHTHAMMOL:* Used as an anti-infective.

DRESSINGS AND GRANULES

FLEXIBLE HYDROACTIVE DRESSINGS AND GRANULES

Rx	**Biafine** (OrthoNeutrogena)	**Emulsion; topical**	Avocado oil, parabens. In 45 and 90 g tubes.
otc	**IntraSite** (Smith & Nephew)	**Gel; topical:** 2% graft T starch copolymer, 78% water, 20% propylene glycol. Sterile amorphous hydrogel dressing	In UD 25 g (10s).
otc	**Shur-Clens** (Calgon Vestal)	**Solution; topical:** 20% poloxamer 188	In UD 100 and 200 mL.
otc	**FlexiGel Strands** (Smith-Nephew)	**Absorbent wound dressing; topical**	Single-use absorbent matrix. 6 g unit. In 10s.
otc	**DuoDerm** (ConvaTec)	**Dressings, sterile; topical:** 4″ x 4″, 6″ x 8″, 8″ x 8″ and 8″ x 12″	In 3s (8″ x 12″ only), 5s and 20s
		Dressing, adhesive border; topical: 4″ x 4″ 8″ x 8″	In 5s. In 3s.
		Granules, sterile; topical: 5 g per tube	In 5s.
		Paste, sterile	In 30 g tube.

FLEXIBLE HYDROACTIVE DRESSINGS AND GRANULES

Rx	**RadiaPlexRx** (MPM Medical)	**Gel; topical**: Acrylates, allantoin, aloe vera extract complex carbohydrates, carbomer, diazolidinyl urea and iodopropynyl butylcarbamate, disodium EDTA, glycerin, glyceryl stearate, isopropyl palmitate, lipowax, mineral oil, myritol, phenoxyethanol, polymethylsiloxane fluid, propylene glycol, sodium hyaluronate, triethanolamine	In 170 g.
otc	**DuoDerm CGF** (ConvaTec)	**Control gel formula dressing, sterile; topical**: 4" x 4", 6" x 6", 8" x 8"	In 5s.
		Control gel formula border dressing, sterile; topical: 2.5" x 2.5", 4" x 4", 6" x 6", 4" x 5", 6" x 7" with adhesive borders	In 5s.
otc	**DuoDerm Extra Thin** (ConvaTec)	**Control gel formula dressing, extra thin, sterile; topical**: 4" x 4", 6" x 6"	In 10s.
otc	**Sorbsan** (Dow B. Hickam)	**Pads, sterile; topical**: Calcium alginate fiber 2" x 2", 3" x 3", 4" x 4" and 4" x 8"	In 1s.
		Wound packing fibers, sterile; topical: Calcium alginate fiber. 12" (2 g)	In 1s.

FLEXIBLE HYDROACTIVE DRESSINGS AND GRANULES — TOPICAL

Indications

➤*Dressings:* For the local management of: Dermal ulcers; pressure ulcers; leg ulcers; superficial wounds (eg, minor abrasions, donor sites, second-degree burns); protective dressings; postoperative wounds.

➤*Granules:* For use in the local management of exudating dermal ulcers in association with the dressings.

➤*Paste:* For use in association with *DuoDerm* dressings for local management of exudating dermal ulcers.

Administration and Dosage

➤*Adults:*

Dermal ulcers –

Dressings, granules, and paste: Clean and prepare the wound site before application. See package labeling for wound management and application/removal instructions for the dressing and granules. Dressings are designed to remain in place from 1 to 7 days.

Actions

➤*Pharmacology:* The dressings interact with wound exudate producing a soft moist gel at the wound surface enabling removal of the dressing with little or no damage to newly formed tissues. They are designed to remain in place from 1 to 7 days.

Contraindications

Dermal ulcers involving muscle, tendon or bone; ulcers resulting from infection, such as tuberculosis, syphilis and deep fungal infections; lesions in patients with active vasculitis, such as periarteritis nodosa, systemic lupus erythematosus and cryoglobulinemia; third-degree burns; clinically infected wounds.

Warnings/Precautions

➤*Excess exudate:* In the presence of excess exudate, the ability of the dressings to remain in place with less frequent leakage may be improved by applying the granules directly into the wound site. Used in this way, with the dressings, the granules may reduce the frequency of dressing change.

➤*Odor:* Wounds often have a characteristic disagreeable odor. The odor usually disappears following wound cleansing.

➤*Wound deterioration:* When using any occlusive dressing, the wound will increase in size and depth during the initial phase as the necrotic debris is cleaned away.

➤*Infection:* If clinical infection develops, discontinue *DuoDerm* and institute appropriate treatment. Restart *DuoDerm* when the infection has been eradicated.

➤*Pregnancy: Category: Undetermined.* There is no information in pregnant women.

➤*Lactation:* There is no information in breast-feeding women.

IRRIGATING SOLUTIONS

PHYSIOLOGICAL IRRIGATING SOLUTIONS

Rx	**0.45% Sodium Chloride Irrigation** (Abbott)	**Solution**: 450 mg sodium chloride per 100 mL	In 250 and 500 mL and 1, 1.5, 2 and 3 L.
Rx	**0.9% Sodium Chloride Irrigation** (Abbott)	**Solution**: 900 mg sodium chloride per 100 mL	In 100, 250 and 500 mL and 1, 1.5, 2 and 3 L.
Rx	**Ringer's Irrigation** (Various, eg, McGaw)	**Solution**: 860 mg sodium chloride, 30 mg potassium chloride, 33 mg calcium chloride per 100 mL	In 1 L.
Rx	**Tis-U-Sol** (Baxter)	**Solution**: 800 mg NaCl, 40 mg KCl, 20 mg magnesium sulfate, 8.75 mg dibasic sodium phosphate heptahydrate and 6.25 mg monobasic potassium phosphate per 100 mL	In 1 L.
Rx	**Lactated Ringer's Irrigation** (Hospira)	**Solution**: 600 mg sodium chloride, 310 mg sodium lactate, anhydrous, 30 mg potassium chloride, 20 mg calcium chloride, dihydrate per 100 mL	In 300 mL.
Rx	**Physiolyte** (B. Braun/McGaw)	**Solution**: 530 mg NaCl, 370 mg sodium acetate, 500 mg sodium gluconate, 37 mg KCl and 30 mg magnesium Cl per 100 mL	In 1 L.
Rx	**PhysioSol** (Hospira)	**Solution**: 526 mg NaCl, 222 mg sodium acetate, 502 mg sodium gluconate, 37 mg KCl and 30 mg magnesium chloride hexahydrate per 100 mL	In 250 and 500 mL and 1 L.
Rx	**Cytosol** (Cytosol Ophthalmics)	**Solution**: 48 mg calcium chloride, 30 mg magnesium chloride, 75 mg potassium chloride, 390 mg sodium acetate, 640 mg sodium chloride, 170 mg sodium citrate per 100 mL	In 200 and 500 mL.
Rx	**Saf-Clens** (Calgon Vestal)	**Spray**: Meroxapol 105, NaCl, potassium sorbate NF, DMDM hydantoin	In 177 mL.

PHYSIOLOGICAL IRRIGATING SOLUTIONS — TOPICAL

Indications

➤*Irrigation:* For general irrigation, washing and rinsing purposes which permit use of a sterile, nonpyrogenic electrolyte solution.

Administration and Dosage

➤*Adults:*

Irrigation – The dose depends on the capacity or surface area of the structure to be irrigated and the nature of the procedure. When used as a vehicle for other drugs, follow manufacturer's recommendations.

➤*Children:*

Irrigation – See Adults.

➤*Storage/Stability:* Avoid excessive heat. Do not freeze. Store at 25°C (77°F); however, brief exposure to 40°C (104°F) does not cause adverse effects.

Contraindications

Irrigation during electrosurgical procedures.

Warnings/Precautions

➤*For irrigation only:* Not for injection.

➤*Absorption:* Irrigating fluids enter the systemic circulation in relatively large volumes and must be regarded as a systemic drug. Absorption of large amounts can cause fluid or solute overloading resulting in dilution of serum electrolyte concentrations, overhydration, congested states or pulmonary edema.

➤*Dilutional states:* The risk of dilutional states is inversely proportional to the electrolyte concentrations of administered parenteral solutions. The risk of solute overload causing congested states with peripheral and pulmonary edema is directly proportional to the electrolyte concentrations of such solutions.

➤*Do not heat:* Do not heat to higher than 66°C (higher than 150°F).

➤*Continuous irrigation:* Observe caution when solution is used for continuous irrigation or allowed to "dwell" inside body cavities because of possible absorption into the blood stream and circulatory overload.

PHYSIOLOGICAL IRRIGATING SOLUTIONS — TOPICAL

➤*Aseptic technique:* This is essential for irrigation of body cavities, wounds and urethral catheters or for wetting dressings that come in contact with body tissues.

➤*Accidental contamination:* Careless technique may transmit infection.

➤*Containers:* When used as a "pour" irrigation, do not allow any part of the contents to contact the surface below the outer protected thread area of the semi-rigid wide mouth container. When used via irrigation equipment, attach the administration set promptly. Discard unused portions and use a fresh container for the start-up of each cycle or repeat procedure. For repeated irrigations of urethral catheters, use a separate container for each patient.

➤*Displaced catheters/drainage tubes:* This can lead to irrigation or infiltration of unintended structures or cavities.

➤*Additives:* May be incompatible. When introducing additives, use aseptic technique, mix thoroughly and do not store.

➤*Tissue distention/disruption:* Excessive volume or pressure during irrigation of closed cavities may cause undue distention or disruption of tissues.

➤*Pregnancy: Category C.* It is not known whether these solutions can cause fetal harm when administered to a pregnant woman or can affect reproduction capacity. Give to a pregnant woman only if clearly needed.

➤*Lactation:* It is not known whether this drug is excreted in human milk. Because many drugs are excreted in human milk, exercise caution when administering to a breast-feeding woman.

Adverse Reactions

Should any adverse reaction occur, discontinue the irrigant, evaluate the patient, institute appropriate countermeasures and save the remainder of the fluid for examination.

Overdosage

In overhydration or solute overload, reevaluate and institute corrective measures.

➤*General Considerations in Topical Ophthalmic Drug Therapy:* Proper administration is essential to optimal therapeutic response. In many instances, health professionals may be too casual when instructing patients on proper use of ophthalmics. The administration technique used often determines drug safety and efficacy.

- The normal eye retains approximately 10 mcL of fluid (adjusted for blinking). The average dropper delivers 25 to 50 mcL/drop. The value of more than one drop is questionable.
- Minimize systemic absorption of ophthalmic drops by compressing lacrimal sac for 3 to 5 minutes after instillation. This retards passage of drops via nasolacrimal duct into areas of potential absorption such as nasal and pharyngeal mucosa.
- Because of rapid lacrimal drainage and limited eye capacity, if multiple drop therapy is indicated, the best interval between drops is 5 minutes. This ensures that the first drop is not flushed away by the second or that the second is not diluted by the first.
- Topical anesthesia will increase the bioavailability of ophthalmic agents by decreasing the blink reflex and the production and turnover of tears.
- Factors that may increase absorption from ophthalmics include lax eyelids of some patients, usually the elderly, which creates a greater reservoir for retention of drops, and hyperemic or diseased eyes.
- Eyecup use is discouraged due to risk of contamination.
- Ophthalmic suspensions mix with tears less rapidly and remain in the cul-de-sac longer than solutions.
- Ophthalmic ointments maintain contact between the drug and ocular tissues by slowing the clearance rate to as little as 0.5% per minute. Ophthalmic ointments provide maximum contact between drug and external ocular tissues.
- Ophthalmic ointments may impede delivery of other ophthalmic drugs to the affected side by serving as a barrier to contact.
- Ointments may blur vision during the waking hours. Use with caution in conditions where visual clarity is critical (eg, operating motor equipment, reading) or use at bedtime.
- Monitor expiration dates closely. Do not use outdated medication.
- Solutions and ointments are frequently misused. Do not assume that patients know how to maximize safe and effective use of these agents. Combine appropriate patient education and counseling with prescribing and dispensing of ophthalmics.

Topical application is the most common route of administration for ophthalmic drugs. Advantages include convenience, simplicity, noninvasive nature and the ability of the patient to self-administer. Because of blood and aqueous losses of drug, topical medications do not typically penetrate in useful concentrations to posterior ocular structures and therefore are of no therapeutic benefit for diseases of retina, optic nerve and other posterior segment structures.

➤*Ingredients:* The following inactive agents may be present in ophthalmic products:

PRESERVATIVES – Preservatives destroy or inhibit multiplication of microorganisms introduced into the product by accident and are as follows:

Benzalkonium Cl, benzethonium Cl, cetylpyridinium Cl, chlorobutanol, EDTA, mercurial preservatives (phenylmercuric nitrate, phenyl mercuric acetate, thimerosal), methyl/propylparabens, phenylethyl alcohol, sodium benzoate, sodium propionate, sorbic acid.

VISCOSITY-INCREASING AGENTS – Viscosity-increasing agents slow drainage of the product from the eye, thus increasing retention time of the active drug. Increased bioavailability may result. Viscosity-increasing agents are as follows:

Carboxymethylcellulose sodium, dextran 70, gelatin, glycerin, hydroxyethylcellulose, hydroxypropyl methylcellulose, methylcellulose, PEG, poloxamer 407, polysorbate 80, propylene glycol, polyvinyl alcohol, polyvinylpyrrolidone (povidone).

ANTIOXIDANTS – Antioxidants prevent or delay deterioration of products by oxygen in the air and are as follows:

EDTA, sodium bisulfite, sodium metabisulfite, sodium thiosulfate, thiourea.

WETTING AGENTS – Wetting agents reduce surface tension, allowing drug solution to spread over eye and are as follows:

Polysorbate 20 and 80, poloxamer 282, tyloxapol.

BUFFERS – Buffers help maintain ophthalmic products in the range of pH 6 to 8, which is the comfortable range for ophthalmic instillation and are as follows:

Acetic acid, boric acid, phosphoric acid, potassium bicarbonate, potassium borate and tetraborate, potassium carbonate, potassium citrate, potassium phosphates, sodium acetate, sodium bicarbonate, sodium biphosphate, sodium borate, sodium carbonate, sodium citrate, sodium hydroxide, sodium phosphate, hydrochloric acid.

TONICITY AGENTS – Tonicity agents help the ophthalmic product solutions to be isotonic with natural tears. Products in the sodium chloride equivalence range of 0.9% ± 0.2% are considered isotonic and will help prevent ocular pain and tissue damage. A range of 0.6% to 1.8% is usually comfortable for ophthalmic use. Tonicity agents are as follows:

Buffers, dextran 40 and 70, dextrose, glycerin, potassium Cl, propylene glycol, sodium Cl.

➤*Packaging Standards:* To help reduce confusion in labeling and identification of various topical ocular medications, drug packaging standards have been proposed. When fully implemented by the ophthalmic drug industry, the standard colors for drug labels and bottle caps will include the following:

Ophthalmic Drug Packaging Standards

Therapeutic class	Proposed color
Beta blockers	Yellow, blue or both
Mydriatics and cycloplegics	Red
Miotics	Green
Nonsteroidal anti-inflammatory agents	Grey
Anti-infectives	Brown, tan

➤*Medications:*

Solutions and suspensions – Most topical ocular preparations are commercially available as solutions or suspensions that are applied directly to the eye from the bottle, which serves as the eye dropper. Avoid touching the dropper tip to the eye because this can lead to contamination of the medication and may also cause ocular injury. Resuspend suspensions (notably, many ocular steroids) by shaking to provide an accurate dosage of drug.

Recommended procedures for administration of solutions or suspensions –

- Wash hands thoroughly before administration.
- Tilt head backward or lie down and gaze upward.
- Gently grasp lower eyelid below eyelashes and pull the eyelid away from the eye to form a pouch.
- Place dropper directly over eye. Avoid contact of the dropper with the eye, finger or any surface.
- Look upward just before applying a drop.
- After instilling the drop, look downward for several seconds.
- Release the lid slowly and close eyes gently.
- With eyes closed, apply gentle pressure with fingers to the inside corner of eye for 3 to 5 min. This retards drainage of solution from intended solution.
- Do not rub the eye or squeeze the eyelid. Minimize blinking.
- Do not rinse the dropper.
- Do not use eye drops that have changed color or contain a precipitate.
- If more than one type of ophthalmic drop is used, wait 5 minutes or longer before administering the second agent.
- When the instillation of eye drops is difficult (eg, pediatric patients, adults with particularly strong blink reflex), the close-eye method may be used. This involves lying down, placing the prescribed number of drops on the eyelid in the inner corner of the eye, then opening eye so that drops will fall into the eye by gravity.

Ointments – The primary purpose for an ophthalmic ointment vehicle is to prolong drug contact time with the external ocular surface. This is particularly useful for treating children, who may "cry out" topically applied solutions, and for medicating ocular injuries, such as corneal abrasions, when the eye is to be patched. Administer solutions before ointments. Ointments preclude entry of subsequent drops.

Recommended procedures for administration of ointments –

- Wash hands thoroughly before administration.
- Holding the ointment tube in the hand for a few minutes will warm the ointment and facilitate flow.
- When opening the ointment tube for the first time, squeeze out and discard the first 0.25 inch of ointment as it may be too dry.
- Tilt head backward or lie down and gaze upward.
- Gently pull down the lower eyelid to form a pouch.
- Place 0.25 to 0.5 inch of ointment with a sweeping motion inside the lower eyelid by squeezing the tube gently and slowly release the eyelid.
- Close the eye for 1 to 2 minutes and roll the eyeball in all directions.
- Temporary blurring of vision may occur. Avoid activities requiring visual acuity until blurring clears.
- Remove excessive ointment around the eye or ointment tube tip with a tissue.
- If using more than one kind of ointment, wait about 10 minutes before applying the second drug.

Gels – Ophthalmic gels are similar in viscosity and clinical usage to ophthalmic ointments. Pilocarpine (*Pilopine HS*) is currently the only ophthalmic preparation available in gel form, and it is intended to serve as a "sustained-release" pilocarpine, requiring only once-daily administration (at bedtime).

Sprays – Although not commercially available, some practitioners use mydriatics or cycloplegics, alone or in combination, administered as a spray to the eye to dilate the pupil or for cycloplegic examination. This is most often used for pediatric patients, and the solution is administered using a sterile perfume atomizer.

Lid scrubs – Commercially available eyelid cleansers or antibiotic solutions or ointments can be applied directly to the lid margin for the treatment of noninfectious blepharitis. This is best accomplished by applying the medication to the end of a cotton-tipped applicator and then scrubbing the eyelid margin several times daily. The gauze pads supplied with commercially available eyelid cleansers are also convenient.

➤*Devices:*

Contact lenses – Soft contact lenses can absorb water-soluble drugs and release them over prolonged periods of time. This has the clinical advantage of promoting sustained-release solutions or suspensions that would otherwise be removed quickly from the external ocular tissues. Soft contact lenses as delivery devices are most often used in the management of dry eye disorders, but the technique is occasionally used for the treatment of ocular infections, including corneal ulcers.

Corneal shields – A non-cross-linked, homogenized, porcine scleral collagen shield is available (*Bio-Cor Fyodoror Collagen Corneal Shield*). This is placed as a bandage on the cornea following surgery or injury, protecting and lubricating the cornea. Topical antibiotics have been used with the shield to promote healing of corneal ulcers.

Cotton pledgets – Small pieces of cotton can be saturated with ophthalmic solutions and placed in the conjunctival sac. These devices allow a prolonged ocular contact time with solutions that are normally administered topically into the eye. The clinical use of pledgets is usually reserved for mydriatic solutions such as cocaine or phenylephrine. This drug delivery method promotes maximum mydriasis in an attempt to break posterior synechiae or to dilate sluggish pupils.

Filter paper strips – Sodium fluorescein and rose bengal dyes are commercially available as drug-impregnated filter paper strips. The strips help ensure sterility of sodium fluorescein which, when prepared in solution, can become easily contaminated with Pseudomonas aeruginosa. These dyes are used diagnostically to disclose corneal injuries, infections such as herpes simplex, and dry eye disorders.

Artificial tear inserts – A rod-shaped pellet of hydroxypropyl cellulose without preservative (*Lacrisert*), is inserted into the inferior conjunctival sac with a specially designed applicator. Following placement, the device absorbs fluid, swells and then releases the nonmedicated polymer to the eye for up to 24 hours. The device is designed as a sustained-release artificial tear for the treatment of dry eye disorders.

Membrane-bound inserts – A membrane-controlled drug delivery system (*Ocusert*) delivers a constant quantity of pilocarpine to the eye for up to 1 week. Placed onto the bulbar conjunctiva under the upper or lower eyelid, it is a useful substitute for pilocarpine drops or gel in glaucoma patients who cannot comply with more frequent instillation or in those with ocular or visual side effects from pilocarpine solutions.

AGENTS FOR GLAUCOMA

Glaucoma is a condition of the eye in which there is progressive cupping and atrophy of the optic nerve head, and deterioration of the visual fields. *Primary open-angle glaucoma* is the most common type of glaucoma. *Angle-closure glaucoma* and *congenital glaucoma* are treated primarily by surgical methods, although short-term drug therapy is used to decrease intraocular pressure (IOP) prior to surgery.

Drugs used in the therapy of primary open-angle glaucoma include a variety of agents with different mechanisms of action. The therapeutic goal in treating glaucoma is reducing the IOP, a major risk factor in the pathogenesis of glaucomatous visual field loss. The higher the level of IOP, the greater the likelihood of optic nerve damage and glaucomatous visual field loss. Reduction of IOP may be accomplished by: 1) decreasing the rate of production of aqueous humor or 2) increasing the rate of outflow (drainage) of aqueous humor from the eye.

The seven groups of agents used in the therapy of primary open-angle glaucoma are listed in Table 1: Agents for Glaucoma, which summarizes their mechanism of decreasing IOP, effects on pupil size and ciliary muscle, and duration of action.

➤*ALPHA-2 ADRENERGIC AGONISTS:* Alpha-2 adrenergic agonists (apraclonidine [*Iopidine*] and brimonidine [*Alphagan*]) are relatively new to the treatment of glaucoma. Apraclonidine is used primarily before or after laser surgery to control or prevent postsurgical elevations of IOP and as short-term adjunctive therapy for patients requiring additional IOP reduction. Approximately 30% of patients on apraclonidine developed an allergic response. Also, the drug loses its effectiveness in approximately 40% of patients after 2 to 3 months of chronic use. Brimonidine, the newer alpha-2 agonist, seems to have a much lower allergic response associated with it and is much more effective as chronic therapy for most patients. Brimonidine-P 0.15% and 0.1% in lower concentrations and neutral pH contains a different preservative (*Purite*) and has similar IOP lowering efficacy to the 0.2% formulation, but with less incidence of allergy.

➤*BETA-ADRENERGIC BLOCKING AGENTS:* Beta-adrenergic blocking agents (eg, betaxolol [*Betoptic*], carteolol [*Ocupress*], levobunolol [eg, *Betagan*], metipranolol [*OptiPranolol*], timolol [eg, *Betimol, Timoptic*]) may be used alone or in conjunction with other agents. They may be more effective than either pilocarpine or epinephrine alone and have the advantage of not affecting either pupil size or accommodation. They lower IOP by decreasing the rate of aqueous production.

➤*DIRECT-ACTING MIOTICS:* Direct-acting miotics, (eg, carbachol [eg, *Isopto Carbachol*], pilocarpine [eg, *Isopto Carpine*]) were once considered the first step in glaucoma therapy before the beta-blocker era began in the late 1970s. They are now useful adjunctive agents that are additive to beta-blockers, carbonic anhydrase inhibitors, or sympathomimetics. Additivity to first-line prostaglandin therapy is less well established. Dosage and frequency of administration must be individualized. Study data indicate pilocarpine 2% and carbachol 1.5% every 12 hours with nasolacrimal occlusion (NLO) provide maximum effect. Increasing the concentration and dosage intervals may correct an inadequate response. Concentrations greater than pilocarpine 4% or carbachol 3% are occasionally required in patients with darkly pigmented irides.

➤*CHOLINESTERASE INHIBITOR MIOTICS:* Cholinesterase inhibitor miotics include both reversible/short-acting (physostigmine, demecarium [*Humorsol*]), and irreversible/long-acting (echothiophate [*Phospholine Iodide*]) agents, which enhance the effects of endogenous acetylcholine by inactivation of the enzyme acetylcholinesterase. These agents are more potent and longer acting than the direct-acting miotics. Side effects and systemic toxicity are more common and of greater significance than the direct-acting miotics. Using a direct-acting cholinergic and a cholinesterase inhibitor provides no improvement in response.

➤*CARBONIC ANHYDRASE INHIBITORS:* Carbonic anhydrase inhibitors (eg, acetazolamide [eg, *Diamox*], dichlorphenamide [*Daranide*], methazolamide) are administered systemically. Dorzolamide (*Trusopt*) and brinzolamide (*Azopt*) are administered topically. IOP is lowered by a direct action on the ciliary epithelium to suppress the secretion of aqueous humor (inflow). Carbonic anhydrase inhibitors are often used as adjunctive therapy.

➤*PROSTAGLANDINS:* Although it has been long recognized that prostaglandins have IOP-lowering effects, side effects such as ocular redness, stinging, and burning long delayed the development of this drug class as an acceptable chronic treatment for glaucoma. The major prostaglandin analogs latanoprost (*Xalatan*), travoprost (*Travatan*) and bimatoprost (*Lumigan*) are very well tolerated although they are associated with a greater incidence of mild cosmetic and tolerability issues such as ocular redness, lash growth, and periocular hyperpigmentation. The prostaglandin analogs can darken the iris color in some patients after chronic use, but after 5 years of study, this appears to be only cosmetic and quite uncommon. Green and mized hazel-colored irides appear to be most susceptible to color change.

The prostaglandin analogs are currently the most used glaucoma drugs world-wide. They are more effective than the beta-blockers for lowering IOP and are additive to most ocular hypotensive agents. These drugs have replaced timolol as the new "gold standard" because of their superior therapeutic index. Recently, a formulation of travoprost (*Travatan Z*) was introduced using a new ocular drop preservative instead of the more common BAK (benzalkonium chloride). The therapeutic profile of *Travatan Z* is similar to *Travatan*, and can be used in patients who are sensitive to BAK.

➤*EPINEPHRINES:* Epinephrine (eg, *Epifrin*) and dipivefrin (*Propine*) have both alpha and beta activity. They lower IOP mainly by increasing aqueous outflow. Epinephrine, usually used as an adjunct to miotic or beta-blocker therapy, may also be used as primary therapy. The combination of a miotic and a sympathomimetic (eg, epinephrine) will have additive effects in lowering IOP. However, epinephrine is no longer commercially available.

Dipivefrin hydrochloride is a prodrug with enhanced corneal penetration compared to epinephrine and is metabolized to epinephrine in vivo. The IOP-lowering and intraocular effects are qualitatively and quantitatively similar to epinephrine; however, dipivefrin may be better tolerated and have a lower incidence of adverse effects because of its lower concentration.

Table 1: Agents for Glaucoma

Drug	Strength	Duration (hrs)	Decrease aqueous production	Increase aqueous outflow
Epinephrines				
Dipivefrin	0.1%	12	+	++
Alpha-2 Adrenergic Agonists				
Apraclonidine	0.5%-1%	7-12	+++	NR
Brimonidine	0.15%	6-8	++	++
Beta-Blockers				
Betaxolol	0.25%	12	+++	NR
Carteolol	1%	12	+++	nd
Levobunolol	0.25%-0.5%	12-24	+++	NR
Metipranolol	0.3%	12-24	+++	NR
Timolol	0.25%-0.5%	12-24	+++	NR
Miotics, Direct-Acting				
Carbachol[a]	0.75%-3%	6-8	NR	+++
Pilocarpine[b]	0.25%-10%	4-8	NR	+++
Miotics, Cholinesterase Inhibitors				
Physostigmine	0.25%-0.5%	12-36	NR	+++
Echothiophate	0.125%	days/wks	NR	+++
Carbonic Anhydrase Inhibitors				
Acetazolamide[c]	125-500 mg	8-12	+++	NR
Brinzolamide [d]	1%	≈ 8	+++	NR
Dorzolamide[d]	2%	≈ 8	+++	NR
Methazolamide[c]	25-50 mg	10-18	+++	NR
Prostaglandins and Prostamides				
Latanoprost	0.005%	24	NR	+++
Bimatoprost	0.03%	24	NR	+++
Travoprost	0.004%	24	NR	+++

+++ = Significant activity.
++ = Moderate activity.
+ = Some activity.
NR = No activity reported.
nd = No data available.
[a] Available as intraocular administration during surgery; carbachol also available as a topical agent.
[b] Also available as a gel and an insert; the duration of these dosage forms is longer (18 to 24 hours and 1 week, respectively) than the solution.
[c] Systemic agents.
[d] Topical ophthalmic agent.

➤*HYPEROSMOTIC AGENTS:* Hyperosmotic agents (eg, mannitol [eg, *Osmitrol*]), glycerin [*Osmoglyn*], isosorbide [eg, *Ismotic*]) are useful in lowering IOP in acute situations (see the Hyperosmotic Agents chapter). These agents lower IOP by creating an osmotic gradient between the ocular fluids and plasma. These agents are not for chronic use.

Ophthalmic Alpha Adrenergic Agonists

BRIMONIDINE TARTRATE

Rx	**Brimonidine Tartrate** (Various, eg, Bausch & Lomb, Falcon)	**Solution:** 0.2%	In 5, 10, 15 mL.
Rx	**Alphagan P** (Allergan)	**Solution:** 0.1%	In 5, 10, and 15 mL bottles.[a]
		0.15%	In 5, 10, and 15 mL bottles.[a]

[a] With 0.005% *Purite*; boric acid; potassium chloride; sodium borate; sodium chloride; hydrochloric acid and/or sodium hydroxide to adjust pH.

BRIMONIDINE TARTRATE — OPHTHALMIC

Refer to Topical Ophthalmic Drugs introduction for complete and comparative prescribing information.

Indications

➤*Intraocular pressure (IOP):* For lowering intraocular pressure in patients with open-angle glaucoma or ocular hypertension. The IOP-lowering efficacy of brimonidine tartrate ophthalmic solution diminishes over time in some patients. This loss of effect appears with a variable time of onset in each patient and should be closely monitored.

Administration and Dosage

➤*Adults:*

Increased intraocular pressure –

Usual dosage: Instill 1 drop in the affected eye(s) 3 times daily, approximately 8 hours apart.

Concomitant therapy: May be used concomitantly with other topical ophthalmic drug products to lower intraocular pressure.

➤*Children:*

Increased intraocular pressure –

2 years of age and older: See adults for dosing.

• *Usual dosage –* Instill 1 drop in the affected eye(s) 3 times daily, approximately 8 hours apart.

• *Concomitant therapy –* May be used concomitantly with other topical ophthalmic drug products to lower intraocular pressure.

➤*Administration:* If more than 1 topical ophthalmic product is being used, the products should be administered at least 5 minutes apart.

➤*Storage/Stability:* Store between 15° and 25°C (59° to 77°F).

Actions

➤*Pharmacology:* Brimonidine tartrate is an alpha adrenergic receptor agonist. It has a peak ocular hypotensive effect occurring at 2 hours post-dosing. Fluorophotometric studies in animals and humans suggest that brimonidine tartrate has a dual mechanism of action by reducing aqueous humor production and increasing uveoscleral outflow.

➤*Pharmacokinetics:*

Absorption/Distribution – After ocular administration of either a 0.1% or 0.2% solution, plasma concentrations peaked within 0.5 to 2.5 hours and declined with a systemic half-life of approximately 2 hours.

Metabolism/Excretion – In humans, systemic metabolism of brimonidine is extensive. It is metabolized primarily by the liver. Urinary excretion is the major route of elimination of the drug and its metabolites. Approximately 87% of an orally administered radioactive dose was eliminated within 120 hours, with 74% found in the urine.

Contraindications

Hypersensitivity to brimonidine tartrate or any component of this medication; patients receiving monoamine oxidase (MAO) inhibitor therapy.

Warnings/Precautions

➤*Renal/Hepatic function impairment:* Brimonidine tartrate has not been studied in patients with hepatic or renal impairment; caution should be used in treating such patients.

➤*Special risk:* Although brimonidine tartrate had minimal effect on blood pressure of patients in clinical studies, caution should be exercised in treating patients with severe cardiovascular disease.

Brimonidine tartrate should be used with caution in patients with depression, cerebral or coronary insufficiency, Raynaud's phenomenon, orthostatic hypotension or thromboangiitis obliterans. During the studies there was a loss of effect in some patients. The IOP-lowering efficacy observed with brimonidine tartrate ophthalmic solution during the first month of therapy may not always reflect the long-term level of IOP reduction.

➤*Hazardous tasks:* As with other drugs in this class, brimonidine tartrate may cause fatigue or drowsiness in some patients. Patients who engage in hazardous activities should be cautioned of the potential for a decrease in mental alertness.

➤*Pregnancy: Category B.*

Teratogenic – There are no adequate and well-controlled studies of brimonidine tartrate in pregnant women; however in animal studies, brimonidine crossed the placenta and entered into the fetal circulation to a limited extent. Brimonidine tartrate should be used during pregnancy only if the potential benefit to the mother justifies the potential risk to the fetus.

➤*Lactation:* It is not known whether brimonidine tartrate is excreted in human milk, although in animal studies, brimonidine tartrate has been shown to be excreted in breast milk. A decision should be made whether to discontinue nursing or to discontinue the drug, taking into account the importance of the drug to the mother.

➤*Children:* In a well-controlled clinical study in pediatric glaucoma patients (ages 2 to 7 years), the most commonly observed adverse reactions with brimonidine tartrate ophthalmic 0.2% dosed 3 times daily were somnolence (50% to 83% in patients ages 2 to 6 years) and decreased alertness. In pediatric patients 7 years of age or older (greater than 20 kg), somnolence appears to occur less frequently (25%). Approximately 16% of patients on brimonidine tartrate ophthalmic solution discontinued from the study due to somnolence.

The safety and efficacy of brimonidine tartrate ophthalmic solution have not been studied in pediatric patients below the age of 2 years. Brimonidine tartrate ophthalmic solution is not recommended for use in pediatric patients under the age of 2 years.

➤*Monitoring:* Patients prescribed IOP-lowering medication should be routinely monitored for IOP.

Drug Interactions

Brimonidine Drug Interactions

Precipitant Drug	Object Drug[a]		Description
Brimonidine	Beta blockers, antihypertensives, cardiac glycosides	⬆	Because alpha-agonists, as a class, may reduce pulse and blood pressure, use caution with concomitant drugs such as beta-blockers (ophthalmic and systemic), antihypertensives, and/or cardiac glycosides.
Brimonidine	CNS depressants (eg, alcohol, barbiturates, opiates, sedatives or anesthetics)	⬆	Consider the possibility of an additive or potentiating effect with CNS depressants.
Brimonidine	MAOIs	⬆	Coadministration is contraindicated.
Tricyclic antidepressants	Brimonidine	⬇	Tricyclic antidepressants can affect the metabolism and uptake of circulating amines.

[a] ⬆ = Object drug increased. ⬇ = Object drug decreased.

Adverse Reactions

➤*0.1% and 0.15% ophthalmic solution:*

Adverse reactions occurring in approximately 10% to 20% of subjects – Allergic conjunctivitis, conjunctival hyperemia, and eye pruritus.

Adverse reactions occurring in approximately 5% to 9% of subjects – Burning sensation, conjunctival folliculosis, hypertension, oral dryness, and visual disturbance.

Reactions occurring in approximately 1% to 4% of subjects – Allergic reaction, asthenia, blepharitis, bronchitis, conjunctival edema, conjunctival hemorrhage, conjunctivitis, cough, dizziness, dyspepsia, dyspnea, epiphora, eye discharge, eye dryness, eye irritation, eye pain, eyelid edema, eyelid erythema, flu syndrome, follicular conjunctivitis, foreign body sensation, headache, pharyngitis, photophobia, rash, rhinitis, sinus infection, sinusitis, superficial punctate keratopathy, visual field defect, vitreous floaters, and worsened visual acuity.

The following reactions were reported in less than 1% of subjects – Corneal erosion, insomnia, nasal dryness, somnolence, and taste perversion.

➤*0.2% ophthalmic solution:*

Adverse events occurring in approximately 10% to 30% – In descending order of incidence, adverse events included oral dryness, ocular hyperemia, burning and stinging, headache, blurring, foreign body sensation, fatigue/drowsiness, conjunctival follicles, ocular allergic reactions, and ocular pruritus.

Reactions occurring in approximately 3% to 9% – In descending order, adverse events included corneal staining/erosion, photophobia, eyelid erythema, ocular ache/pain, ocular dryness, tearing, upper respiratory tract symptoms, eyelid edema, conjunctival edema, dizziness, blepharitis, ocular irritation, gastrointestinal symptoms, asthenia, conjunctival blanching, abnormal vision and muscular pain.

BRIMONIDINE TARTRATE — OPHTHALMIC

Adverse reactions reported in less than 3% – Lid crusting, conjunctival hemorrhage, abnormal taste, insomnia, conjunctival discharge, depression, hypertension, anxiety, palpitations, nasal dryness, and syncope.

Postmarketing – The following reactions have been identified during postmarketing use of brimonidine tartrate 0.2% in clinical practice. Because they are reported voluntarily from a population of unknown size, estimates of the frequency cannot be made. The reactions, which have been chosen for inclusion due to either their seriousness, frequency of reporting, possible causal connection to brimonidine tartrate, or a combination of these factors, include: Bradycardia; hypotension; iritis; miosis; skin reactions (including erythema, eyelid pruritus, rash, and vasodilation); and tachycardia. Apnea, bradycardia, hypotension, hypothermia, hypotonia, and somnolence have been reported in infants receiving brimonidine tartrate.

Overdosage

No information is available on overdosage in humans. Treatment of an oral overdose includes supportive and symptomatic therapy; a patent airway should be maintained.

Patient Information

The preservative in brimonidine tartrate 0.2%, benzalkonium chloride, may be absorbed by soft contact lenses. Patients wearing soft contact lenses should be instructed to wait at least 15 minutes after instilling brimonidine tartrate to insert soft contact lenses.

As with other drugs in this class, brimonidine tartrate may cause fatigue or drowsiness in some patients. Patients who engage in hazardous activities should be cautioned of the potential for a decrease in mental alertness.

APRACLONIDINE HYDROCHLORIDE

Rx	**Iopidine** (Alcon)	**Solution:** 1%	0.01% benzalkonium chloride. In 0.1 mL (2s).
		Solution: 0.5%	0.01% benzalkonium chloride. In 5 mL and 10 mL *Drop-Tainers*.

APRACLONIDINE HYDROCHLORIDE — OPHTHALMIC

Refer to Topical Ophthalmic Drugs introduction for complete and comparative prescribing information.

Indications

➤*0.5% solution:* For short-term adjunctive therapy in patients on maximally tolerated medical therapy who require additional IOP reduction. Patients on maximally tolerated medical therapy who are treated with apraclonidine ophthalmic solution to delay surgery should have frequent follow-up examinations and treatment should be discontinued if the IOP rises significantly.

The addition of apraclonidine ophthalmic solution to patients already using 2 aqueous suppressing drugs (ie, beta blocker plus carbonic anhydrase inhibitor) as part of their maximally tolerated medical therapy may not provide additional benefit. This is because apraclonidine ophthalmic solution is an aqueous suppressing drug and the addition of a third aqueous suppressant may not significantly reduce IOP.

The IOP-lowering efficacy of apraclonidine ophthalmic solution diminishes over time in some patients. This loss of effect, or tachyphylaxis, appears to be an individual occurrence with a variable time of onset and should be closely monitored. The benefit for most patients is less than 1 month.

➤*1% solution:* To control or prevent post-surgical elevations in intraocular pressure (IOP) that occur in patients after argon laser trabeculoplasty, argon laser iridotomy, or Nd:YAG posterior capsulotomy.

Administration and Dosage

➤*Adults:*

Intraocular pressure reduction –

0.5% solution: Instill 1 to 2 drops in the affected eye(s) 3 times daily.

1% solution: Instill 1 drop in the scheduled operative eye 1 hour before initiating anterior segment laser surgery and instill a second drop to the same eye immediately upon completion of the laser surgical procedure.

➤*Administration:* Not for injection into the eye. Not for oral ingestion. Do not touch dropper tip to any surface as this may contaminate the contents.

0.5% solution – Because apraclonidine will be used with other ocular glaucoma therapies, practice an approximate 5-minute interval between instillation of each medication to prevent washout of the previous dose.

1% solution – Use a separate container for each single-drop dose, and discard each container after use.

➤*Storage/Stability:* Store between 2° to 25°C (36° to 77°F). Protect from freezing and light.

Actions

➤*Pharmacology:* Apraclonidine is a relatively selective alpha-2-adrenergic agonist and does not have significant membrane stabilizing (local anesthetic) activity. When instilled in the eye, apraclonidine ophthalmic solution, has the action of reducing elevated, as well as normal IOP, whether or not accompanied by glaucoma. Ophthalmic apraclonidine has minimal effect on cardiovascular parameters.

➤*Pharmacokinetics:*

Absorption –

0.5%: The onset of action of apraclonidine can usually be noted within 1 hour, and maximum IOP reduction occurs about 3 hours after instillation.

Topical use of apraclonidine ophthalmic solution leads to systemic absorption. Studies of apraclonidine 0.5% ophthalmic solution dosed 1 drop 3 times a day in both eyes for 10 days in healthy volunteers yielded mean peak and trough concentrations of 0.9 ng/mL and 0.5 ng/mL, respectively.

1%: The onset of action with apraclonidine 1% can usually be noted within 1 hour and the maximum IOP reduction usually occurs 3 to 5 hours after application of a single dose.

Metabolism – The half-life of apraclonidine 0.5% ophthalmic solution was calculated to be 8 hours.

Contraindications

Hypersensitivity to apraclonidine or any other component of this medication, as well as systemic clonidine; patients receiving monoamine oxidase (MAO) inhibitors.

Warnings/Precautions

➤*Corneal edema:* Topical ocular administration of 2 drops of 0.5%, 1% and 1.5% apraclonidine ophthalmic solution to New Zealand albino rabbits 3 times daily for 1 month resulted in sporadic and transient instances of minimal corneal edema in the 1.5% group only; no histopathological changes were noted in those eyes.

➤*Hypersensitivity reactions:* Use of apraclonidine ophthalmic solution can lead to an allergic-like reaction characterized wholly or in part by the symptoms of hyperemia, pruritus, discomfort, tearing, foreign body sensation, and edema of the lids and conjunctiva. Discontinue apraclonidine ophthalmic solution therapy if ocular allergic-like symptoms occur.

➤*Renal function impairment:* Although the topical use of apraclonidine ophthalmic solution has not been studied in renal failure patients, structurally related clonidine undergoes a significant increase in half-life in patients with severe renal impairment. Close monitoring of cardiovascular parameters in patients with impaired renal function is advised if they are candidates for topical apraclonidine therapy. Close monitoring of cardiovascular parameters in patients with impaired liver function is also advised as the systemic dosage form of clonidine is partly metabolized in the liver.

➤*Special risk:* Use apraclonidine ophthalmic solution with caution in patients with coronary insufficiency, recent myocardial infarction, cerebrovascular disease, chronic renal failure, Raynaud's disease, or thromboangiitis obliterans. Caution and monitoring of depressed patients are advised since apraclonidine has been infrequently associated with depression.

While the topical administration of apraclonidine ophthalmic solution had minimal effect on heart rate or blood pressure in clinical studies evaluating glaucoma patients and patients undergoing anterior segment laser surgery, the preclinical pharmacology profile of this drug suggests that caution should be observed in treating patients with severe cardiovascular disease, including hypertension.

1% – Consider the possibility of a vasovagal attack occurring during laser surgery and use caution in patients with a history of such episodes.

➤*Hazardous tasks:* Apraclonidine can cause dizziness and somnolence. Warn patients who engage in hazardous activities requiring mental alertness of the potential for a decrease in mental alertness while using apraclonidine.

➤*Pregnancy: Category C.* Apraclonidine has been shown to have an embryocidal effect in rabbits when given in an oral dose of 3 mg/kg (60 and 150 times the maximum recommended human dose for 0.5% and 1% solutions, respectively). Dose related maternal toxicity was observed in pregnant rats at 0.3 mg/kg (6 and 15 times the maximum recommended human dose for 0.5% and 1% solutions, respectively). There are no adequate and well controlled studies in pregnant women. Use apraclonidine ophthalmic solution during pregnancy only if the potential benefit justifies the potential risk to the fetus.

➤*Lactation:* It is not known whether this drug is excreted in human milk. Because many drugs are excreted in human milk, exercise caution when apraclonidine ophthalmic solution is administered to a nursing woman.

➤*Children:* Safety and effectiveness in pediatric patients have not been established.

➤*Elderly:* No overall differences in safety and effectiveness have been observed between elderly and younger patients.

➤*Monitoring:* Periodically monitor the visual fields of glaucoma patients on maximally tolerated medical therapy who are treated with apraclonidine ophthalmic solution to delay surgery.

Since apraclonidine is a potent depressor of IOP, closely monitor patients who develop exaggerated reduction in IOP.

Ophthalmic Alpha Adrenergic Agonists

APRACLONIDINE HYDROCHLORIDE — OPHTHALMIC

Drug Interactions

Apraclonidine Drug Interactions

Precipitant drug	Object drug[a]		Description
Apraclonidine	Cardiovascular agents	⬇	Since apraclonidine may reduce pulse and blood pressure, caution in using cardiovascular drugs is advised. Patients using cardiovascular drugs concurrently with apraclonidine 0.5% should have pulse and blood pressures frequently monitored.
Apraclonidine	MAO inhibitors	⬆	Apraclonidine should not be used in patients receiving MAO inhibitors (see Contraindications).

[a] ⬆ = Object drug increased. ⬇ = Object drug decreased.

Do not use apraclonidine in patients receiving MAO inhibitors. Although no specific drug interactions with topical glaucoma drugs or systemic medications were identified in clinical studies of apraclonidine 0.5% ophthalmic solution, consider the possibility of an additive or potentiating effect with CNS depressants (alcohol, barbiturates, opiates, sedatives, anesthetics). Tricyclic antidepressants have been reported to blunt the hypotensive effect of systemic clonidine. It is not known whether the concurrent use of these agents with apraclonidine can lead to a reduction in IOP-lowering effect. No data on the level of circulating catecholamines after apraclonidine withdrawal are available. Caution, however, is advised in patients taking tricyclic antidepressants which can affect the metabolism and uptake of circulating amines. Exercise caution with simultaneous use of clonidine and other similar pharmacologic agents.

An additive hypotensive effect has been reported with the combination of systemic clonidine and neuroleptic therapy. Systemic clonidine may inhibit the production of catecholamines in response to insulin-induced hypoglycemia and mask the signs and symptoms of hypoglycemia.

Adverse Reactions

➤*0.5% solution:* In clinical studies the overall discontinuation rate related to apraclonidine 0.5% ophthalmic solution was 15%. The most commonly reported events leading to discontinuation included (in decreasing order of frequency) hyperemia, pruritus, tearing, discomfort, lid edema, dry mouth, and foreign body sensation.

The following adverse reactions (incidences) were reported in clinical studies of apraclonidine 0.5% ophthalmic solution as being possibly, probably, or definitely related to therapy:

Ophthalmic –
The following adverse reactions were reported in 5% to 15% of patients: Discomfort, hyperemia, and pruritus.

The following adverse reactions were reported in 1% to 5% of patients: Blanching, blurred vision, conjunctivitis, discharge, dry eye, foreign body sensation, lid edema, and tearing.

The following adverse reactions were reported in less than 1% of patients: Abnormal vision, blepharitis, blepharoconjunctivitis, conjunctival edema, conjunctival follicles, corneal erosion, corneal infiltrate, corneal staining, edema, irritation, keratitis, keratopathy, lid disorder, lid erythema, lid margin crusting, lid retraction, lid scales, pain, photophobia.

Miscellaneous – Dry mouth occurred in approximately 10% of the patients.

The following adverse reactions were reported in less than 3% of patients: Abnormal coordination, asthenia, arrhythmia, asthma, chest pain, constipation, contact dermatitis, depression, dermatitis, dizziness, dry nose, dyspnea, facial edema, headache, insomnia, malaise, myalgia, nausea, nervousness, paresthesia, parosmia, peripheral edema, pharyngitis, rhinitis, somnolence, and taste perversion.

Postmarketing – The following events have been identified during postmarketing use of apraclonidine 0.5% ophthalmic solution in clinical practice. Because they are reported voluntarily from a population of unknown size, estimates of frequency cannot be made. The events, which have been chose for inclusion due to either their seriousness, frequency of reporting, possible causal connection to apraclonidine 0.5% ophthalmic solution, or a combination of these factors, include bradycardia.

➤*1% solution:* The following adverse events, occurring in less than 2% of patients, were reported in association with the use of apraclonidine ophthalmic solution in laser surgery: conjunctival blanching, irregular heart rate, mydriasis, nasal decongestion, ocular inflammation, ocular injection, and upper lid elevation.

The following adverse events were observed in investigational studies dosing apraclonidine ophthalmic solution once or twice daily for up to 28 days in nonlaser studies:

CNS – Decreased libido, dream disturbances, insomnia, irritability.

GI – Abdominal pain, diarrhea, emesis, stomach discomfort.

Ophthalmic – Allergic response, blurred or dimmed vision, burning, conjunctival blanching, conjunctival microhemorrhage, discomfort, dryness, foreign body sensation, hypotony, itching, mydriasis, upper lid elevation.

Miscellaneous – Body heat sensation, chest heaviness or burning, clammy or sweaty palms, dry mouth, extremity pain or numbness, fatigue, head cold sensation, headache, increased pharyngeal secretion, nasal burning or dryness, paresthesia, pruritus not associated with rash, shortness of breath, taste abnormalities.

Overdosage

➤*Symptoms:* Ingestion of apraclonidine 0.5% ophthalmic solution has been reported to cause bradycardia, drowsiness, and hypothermia.

Accidental or intentional ingestion of oral clonidine has been reported to cause apnea, arrhythmias, asthenia, bradycardia, conduction defects, diminished or absent reflexes, dryness of the mouth, hypotension, hypothermia, hypoventilation, irritability, lethargy, miosis, pallor, respiratory depression, sedation or coma, seizure, somnolence, transient hypertension, and vomiting.

➤*Treatment:* Treatment of an oral overdose includes supportive and symptomatic therapy; maintain a patent airway. Hemodialysis is of limited value, since a maximum of 5% of circulating drug is removed.

Patient Information

Do not touch dropper tip to any surface as this may contaminate the contents.

Apraclonidine can cause dizziness and somnolence. Warn patients who engage in hazardous activities requiring mental alertness of the potential for a decrease in mental alertness, physical dexterity, or coordination while using apraclonidine.

Ophthalmic Beta-Adrenergic Blocking Agents (Beta Blockers)

Refer to the general discussion of these products in the Topical Ophthalmic Introduction for more complete and comparative information.

Indications

➤*Glaucoma:* Lowering intraocular pressure (IOP) in patients with chronic open-angle glaucoma.

For specific approved indications, refer to individual drug monographs.

Administration and Dosage

➤*Concomitant therapy:* If IOP is not controlled with these agents, institute concomitant pilocarpine, other miotics, dipivefrin or systemic carbonic anhydrase inhibitors.

Use of epinephrine with topical β-blockers is controversial. Some reports indicate initial effectiveness of the combination decreases over time (see Drug Interactions).

➤*Monitoring:* The IOP-lowering response to betaxolol and timolol may require a few weeks to stabilize.

Because of diurnal IOP variations in individual patients, satisfactory response to once-a-day therapy is best determined by measuring IOP at different times during the day.

Actions

➤*Pharmacology:* Timolol, levobunolol, carteolol and metipranolol are noncardioselective (β_1 and β_2) β-blockers; betaxolol is a cardioselective (β_1) β-blocker. Topical β-blockers do not have significant membrane-stabilizing (local anesthetic) actions or intrinsic sympathomimetic activity. They reduce elevated and normal IOP, with or without glaucoma.

The exact mechanism of ocular antihypertensive action is not established, but it appears to be a reduction of aqueous production. However, some studies show a slight increase in outflow facility with timolol and metipranolol.

These agents reduce IOP with little or no effect on pupil size or accommodation. Blurred vision and night blindness often associated with miotics are not associated with these agents. The inability to see around lenticular opacities when the pupil is constricted is avoided. These agents may be absorbed systemically (see Warnings).

➤*Pharmacokinetics:*

Pharmacokinetics of Ophthalmic Beta-Adrenergic Blocking Agents

Drug	β-receptor selectivity	Onset (min)	Maximum effect (hr)	Duration (hr)
Carteolol	β_1 and β_2	nd[a]	2	12
Betaxolol	β_1	≤ 30	2	12
Levobunolol	β_1 and β_2	less than 60	2 to 6	≤ 24
Metipranolol	β_1 and β_2	≤ 30	≈ 2	24
Timolol	β_1 and β_2	≤ 30	1 to 2	≤ 24

[a] nd = No data

Contraindications

Bronchial asthma, a history of bronchial asthma or severe chronic obstructive pulmonary disease; sinus bradycardia; second-degree and third-degree AV block; overt cardiac failure; cardiogenic shock; hypersensitivity to any component of the products.

Ophthalmic Beta-Adrenergic Blocking Agents (Beta Blockers)

Warnings/Precautions

➤*Systemic absorption:* These agents may be absorbed systemically. The same adverse reactions found with systemic β-blockers (see group monograph in Cardiovascular section) may occur with topical use. For example, severe respiratory reactions and cardiac reactions, including death due to bronchospasm in asthmatics, and rarely, death associated with cardiac failure, have been reported with topical β-blockers.

➤*Cardiovascular:* Timolol may decrease resting and maximal exercise heart rate even in healthy subjects.

Cardiac failure – Sympathetic stimulation may be essential for circulation support in diminished myocardial contractility; its inhibition by β-receptor blockade may precipitate more severe failure.

In patients without history of cardiac failure, continued depression of myocardium with β-blockers may lead to cardiac failure. Discontinue at the first sign or symptom of cardiac failure.

➤*Non-allergic bronchospasm:* Patients with a history of chronic bronchitis, emphysema, etc, should receive β-blockers with caution; they may block bronchodilation produced by catecholamine stimulation of β_2-receptors.

➤*Major surgery:* Withdrawing β-blockers before major surgery is controversial. Beta-receptor blockade impairs the heart's ability to respond to β-adrenergically mediated reflex stimuli. This may augment the risk of general anesthesia. Some patients on β-blockers have had protracted severe hypotension during anesthesia. Difficulty restarting and maintaining heartbeat has been reported. In elective surgery, gradual withdrawal of β-blockers may be appropriate.

The effects of β-blocking agents may be reversed by β-agonists such as isoproterenol, dopamine, dobutamine, or levarterenol.

➤*Diabetes mellitus:* Administer with caution to patients subject to spontaneous hypoglycemia or to diabetic patients (especially labile diabetics). Beta-blocking agents may mask signs and symptoms of acute hypoglycemia.

➤*Thyroid:* Beta-adrenergic blocking agents may mask clinical signs of hyperthyroidism (eg, tachycardia). Manage patients suspected of developing thyrotoxicosis carefully to avoid abrupt withdrawal of β-blockers, which might precipitate thyroid storm.

➤*Cerebrovascular insufficiency:* Because of potential effects of β-blockers on blood pressure and pulse, use with caution in patients with cerebrovascular insufficiency. If signs or symptoms suggesting reduced cerebral blood flow develop, consider alternative therapy.

➤*Angle-closure glaucoma:* The immediate objective is to reopen the angle, requiring constriction of the pupil with a miotic. These agents have little or no effect on the pupil. When they are used to reduce elevated IOP in angle-closure glaucoma, use with a miotic.

➤*Muscle weakness:* Beta-blockade may potentiate muscle weakness consistent with certain myasthenic symptoms (eg, diplopia, ptosis, generalized weakness). Timolol has increased muscle weakness in some patients with myasthenic symptoms or myasthenia gravis.

➤*Long-term therapy:* In long-term studies (2 and 3 years), no significant differences in mean IOP were observed after initial stabilization.

➤*Sulfite sensitivity:* Some of these products contain sulfites which may cause allergic-type reactions (eg, hives, itching, wheezing, anaphylaxis) in certain susceptible persons. Although the overall prevalence of sulfite sensitivity in the general population is probably low, it is seen more frequently in asthmatics or atopic nonasthmatics.

➤*Pregnancy: Category C.* There have been no adequate and well controlled studies in pregnant women. Use during pregnancy only if the potential benefits outweigh potential hazards to the fetus.

Carteolol – Increased resorptions and decreased fetal weights occurred in rabbits and rats at maternal doses approximately 1052 and 5264 times the maximum human dose, respectively. A dose-related increase in wavy ribs was noted in the developing rat fetus when pregnant rats received doses approximately 212 times the maximum human dose.

Betaxolol – In oral studies with rats and rabbits, evidence of post-implantation loss was seen at dose levels above 12 mg/kg and 128 mg/kg, respectively. Betaxolol was not teratogenic, however, and there were no other adverse effects on reproduction at subtoxic dose levels.

Levobunolol – Fetotoxicity was observed in rabbits at doses 200 and 700 times the glaucoma dose.

Metipranolol – Increased fetal resorption, fetal death and delayed development occurred in rabbits receiving 50 mg/kg orally during organogenesis.

Timolol – Doses of 1000 mg/kg/day (142,000 times the maximum recommended human ophthalmic dose) were maternotoxic in mice and resulted in increased fetal resorptions. Increased fetal resorptions were also seen in rabbits at 14,000 times the systemic exposure following the maximum recommended human ophthalmic dose, in this case without apparent maternotoxicity.

➤*Lactation:* It is not known whether betaxolol, levobunolol or metipranolol are excreted in breast milk. Systemic β-blockers and topical and ophthalmic timolol maleate are excreted in milk. Carteolol is excreted in breast milk of animals. Exercise caution when administering to a nursing mother.

Because of the potential for serious adverse reactions from timolol in nursing infants, decide whether to discontinue nursing or discontinue the drug taking into account the importance of the drug to the mother.

➤*Children:* Safety and efficacy for use in children have not been established.

Drug Interactions

Ophthalmic Beta Blocker Drug Interactions

Precipitant drug	Object drug[a]		Description
Beta blockers, ophthalmic	Beta blockers, oral	↑	Use topical beta blockers with caution because of the potential for additive effects on systemic and ophthalmic beta-blockade.
Beta blockers, ophthalmic	Calcium antagonists	↑	Possible cases of hypotension, left ventricular failure, and atrioventricular conduction disturbances may occur from coadministration of timolol maleate and calcium antagonists. Avoid use in patients with impaired cardiac function.
Beta blockers, ophthalmic	Catecholamine-depleting drugs (eg, reserpine)	↑	Use of reserpine with ophthalmic beta blockers can cause additive effects and the production of hypotension or marked bradycardia, which may result in syncope, vertigo, or postural hypotension. Close observation is recommended.
Catecholamine-depleting drugs (eg, reserpine)	Beta blockers, ophthalmic		
Beta blockers, ophthalmic	Digitalis	↑	Coadministration of ophthalmic beta blockers with digitalis and calcium antagonists may have additive effects in prolonging atrioventricular conduction time.
Digitalis	Beta blockers, ophthalmic		
Quinidine	Beta blockers, ophthalmic	↑	Decreased heart rate has been reported during combined treatment with timolol maleate and quinidine, possibly because quinidine inhibits the metabolism of timolol maleate via the P450 enzyme, CYP2D6.
Beta blockers	Phenothiazine compounds	↑	Potential additive hypotensive effects due to mutual inhibition of metabolism.

[a] ↑ = Object drug increased.

Other drugs that may interact with systemic β-adrenergic blocking agents may also interact with ophthalmic agents. For further information, refer to the β-blocker group monograph in the Cardiovasculars chapter.

Adverse Reactions

➤*The following have occurred with ophthalmic β_1 and β_2 (nonselective) blockers:*

Cardiovascular – Arrhythmia; syncope; heart block; cerebral vascular accident; cerebral ischemia; congestive heart failure; palpitation.

CNS – Headache; depression.

Dermatologic – Hypersensitivity, including localized and generalized rash.

Endocrine – Masked symptoms of hypoglycemia in insulin-dependent diabetics (see Warnings).

GI – Nausea.

Ophthalmic – Keratitis; blepharoptosis; visual disturbances including refractive changes (due to withdrawal of miotic therapy in some cases); diplopia; ptosis.

Respiratory – Bronchospasm (predominantly in patients with preexisting bronchospastic disease); respiratory failure.

➤*Carteolol:*

Ophthalmic – Transient irritation, burning, tearing, conjunctival hyperemia, edema (approximately 25%); blurred/cloudy vision; photophobia; decreased night vision; ptosis; blepharoconjunctivitis; abnormal corneal staining; corneal sensitivity.

Systemic – Bradycardia; decreased blood pressure; arrhythmia; heart palpitation; dyspnea; asthenia; headache; dizziness; insomnia; sinusitis; taste perversion.

➤*Betaxolol:*

Cardiovascular – Bradycardia; heart block; CHF.

CNS – Dizziness; vertigo; headaches; depression; lethargy; increase in signs and symptoms of myasthenia gravis.

Ophthalmic – Brief discomfort (25%); occasional tearing (5%). Rare: Decreased corneal sensitivity; erythema; itching; corneal punctate staining; keratitis, anisocoria; photophobia; edema.

Pulmonary – Pulmonary distress characterized by dyspnea, bronchospasm, thickened bronchial secretions, asthma, and respiratory failure.

Miscellaneous – Taste and smell perversions; hives; toxic epidermal necrolysis; hair loss; glossitis; insomnia.

Ophthalmic Beta-Adrenergic Blocking Agents (Beta Blockers)

➤*Metipranolol:*
Ophthalmic – Transient local discomfort; conjunctivitis; eyelid dermatitis; blepharitis; blurred vision; tearing; browache; abnormal vision; photophobia; edema; uveitis.

Systemic – Allergic reaction; headache; asthenia; hypertension; MI; atrial fibrillation; angina; palpitation; bradycardia; nausea; rhinitis; dyspnea; epistaxis; bronchitis; coughing; dizziness; anxiety; depression; somnolence; nervousness; arthritis; myalgia; rash.

➤*Levobunolol:*
Cardiovascular – Effects may resemble timolol.

CNS – Ataxia, dizziness, headache, lethargy (rare).

Dermatologic – Urticaria, pruritus (rare).

Ophthalmic – Transient burning/stinging (up to 33%); blepharoconjunctivitis (up to 5%); iridocyclitis (rare); decreased corneal sensitivity.

➤*Timolol:*
Cardiovascular – Bradycardia; arrhythmia; hypotension; syncope; heart block; cerebral vascular accident; cerebral ischemia; heart failure; palpitation; cardiac arrest.

CNS – Dizziness; depression; fatigue; lethargy; hallucinations; confusion.

Ophthalmic – Ocular irritation including conjunctivitis; blepharitis; keratitis; blepharoptosis; decreased corneal sensitivity; visual disturbances including refractive changes; diplopia; ptosis.

Respiratory – Bronchospasm (mainly in patients with preexisting bronchospastic disease); respiratory failure; dyspnea.

Miscellaneous – Aggravation of myasthenia gravis; alopecia; nausea; localized and generalized rash; urticaria; impotence; decreased libido; masked symptoms of hypoglycemia in diabetics; diarrhea.

➤*Systemic β-adrenergic blocker-associated reactions:* Consider potential effects with ophthalmic use (see Warnings).

Overdosage

If ocular overdosage occurs, flush eye(s) with water or normal saline. If accidentally ingested, efforts to decrease further absorption may be appropriate (gastric lavage).

The most common signs and symptoms of overdosage from systemic β-blockers are bradycardia, hypotension, bronchospasm and acute cardiac failure. If these occur, discontinue therapy and initiate appropriate supportive therapy.

Patient Information

Transient stinging/discomfort is relatively common; notify physician if severe.

Do not touch dropper tip to any surface; do not use with contact lenses in eyes.

LEVOBUNOLOL HYDROCHLORIDE

Rx	**Levobunolol** (Various, eg, Bausch & Lomb)	**Solution:** 0.25%	In 5 and 10 mL.
Rx	**Betagan Liquifilm** (Allergan)		In 5 and 10 mL dropper bottles with B.I.D. *C Cap*.[a]
Rx	**Levobunolol** (Various, eg, Bausch & Lomb, Falcon)	**Solution:** 0.5%	In 5, 10, and 15 mL.
Rx	**Betagan Liquifilm** (Allergan)		In 2 mL bottles with standard cap and 5, 10, and 15 mL with B.I.D. and Q.D. *C Cap*.[a]

[a] With 1.4% polyvinyl alcohol; 0.004% benzalkonium chloride; sodium metabisulfite; EDTA; sodium phosphate, dibasic; potassium phosphate, monobasic; NaCl; hydrochloric acid; sodium hydroxide.

LEVOBUNOLOL HYDROCHLORIDE — OPHTHALMIC

For complete and comparative prescribing information, refer to the Ophthalmic Beta-Adrenergic Blocking Agents group monograph.

Indications

➤*Elevated IOP:* Lowering IOP in chronic open-angle glaucoma or ocular hypertension.

Administration and Dosage

➤*Adults:*
Elevated intraocular pressure –
0.25% solution: 1 to 2 drops in the affected eye(s) twice daily.
0.5% solution: 1 to 2 drops in the affected eye(s) once a day. In patients with more severe or uncontrolled glaucoma, the 0.5% solution can be administered twice a day.
Dosages greater than 1 drop of 0.5% levobunolol twice daily are not generally more effective. If IOP is not at a satisfactory level on this regimen, concomitant therapy can be instituted.

➤*Concomitant therapy:* Do not administer 2 or more ophthalmic beta-adrenergic blocking agents simultaneously.

➤*Storage/Stability:* Store at 15° to 30°C (59° to 86°F). Protect from light.

BETAXOLOL HYDROCHLORIDE

Rx	**Betaxolol HCl** (Various, Akorn, Falcon)	**Solution:** 5.6 mg (equiv. to 5 mg base) per mL (0.5%)	In 2.5, 5, 10, and 15 mL.
Rx	**Betoptic S** (Alcon)	**Suspension:** 2.8 mg (equiv. to 2.5 mg base) per mL (0.25%)	In 2.5, 5, 10, and 15 mL *Drop-Tainer* dispensers.[b]

[a] With 0.01% benzalkonium chloride, NaCl, hydrochloric acid and/or sodium hydroxide, EDTA.
[b] With 0.01% benzalkonium chloride, mannitol, poly sulfonic acid, hydrochloric acid or sodium hydroxide, EDTA.

BETAXOLOL HYDROCHLORIDE — OPHTHALMIC

For complete and comparative prescribing information, refer to the Ophthalmic Beta-Adrenergic Blocking Agents group monograph.

Indications

➤*Elevated intraocular pressure:* Treatment of ocular hypertension and chronic open-angle glaucoma. May be used alone or in combination with other antiglaucoma drugs.

Administration and Dosage

➤*General dosing considerations:* In some patients, the intraocular pressure-lowering responses to betaxolol may require a few weeks to stabilize.

➤*Adults:*
Elevated intraocular pressure –
Usual dosage: 1 to 2 drops in the affected eye(s) twice daily.
Concomitant therapy: If the intraocular pressure of the patient is not adequately controlled on this regimen, concomitant therapy with pilocarpine and other miotics, or epinephrine or carbonic anhydrase inhibitors can be instituted.

➤*Administration:* Shake suspension well before using. Do not touch dropper tip to any surface as this may contaminate the solution.

➤*Storage/Stability:* Store at room temperature.

METIPRANOLOL

Rx	**Metipranolol** (Falcon)	**Solution:** 0.3%	In 5 and 10 mL.[a]
Rx	**OptiPranolol** (Bausch & Lomb)		In 5 and 10 mL dropper bottles.[b]

[a] With 0.004% benzalkonium chloride, povidone, hydrochloric acid, NaCl, EDTA.
[b] With 0.004% benzalkonium chloride, glycerin, povidone, hydrochloric acid, NaCl, sodium hydroxide and/or hydrochloric acid, EDTA.

METIPRANOLOL — OPHTHALMIC

For complete and comparative prescribing information, refer to the Ophthalmic Beta-Adrenergic Blocking Agents group monograph.

Indications

➤*Elevated intraocular pressure:* Treatment of elevated intraocular pressure (IOP) in patients with ocular hypertension or open-angle glaucoma.

Administration and Dosage

➤*Adults:*
Elevated intraocular pressure –
Usual dosage: 1 drop in the affected eye(s) twice daily.
Concomitant therapy: Concomitant therapy to lower IOP can be instituted.

➤*Storage/Stability:* Store between 15° to 30°C (59° to 86°F). Replace cap immediately after use.

Ophthalmic Beta-Adrenergic Blocking Agents (Beta Blockers)

CARTEOLOL HYDROCHLORIDE

Rx	Carteolol HCl (Various, eg, Akorn, Falcon)	Solution: 1%	In 5, 10, and 15 mL.[a]

[a] With 0.005% benzalkonium chloride; NaCl; sodium phosphate, dibasic and monobasic.

CARTEOLOL HYDROCHLORIDE — OPHTHALMIC

For complete and comparative prescribing information, refer to the Ophthalmic Beta-Adrenergic Blocking Agents group monograph.

Indications

➤*Elevated IOP:* Lowering of IOP in chronic open-angle glaucoma and intraocular hypertension.

Administration and Dosage

➤*Adults:*

Elevated IOP – Instill 1 drop in affected eye(s) twice daily. If the patient's IOP is not at a satisfactory level on this regimen, concomitant therapy can be instituted.

➤*Storage/Stability:* Store at 15° to 25°C (59° to 77°F) and protect from light.

TIMOLOL MALEATE

Rx	**Timolol Maleate** (Various, eg, Akorn, Bausch & Lomb, Falcon, Fougera)	**Solution:** 0.25%	In 2.5, 5, 10, and 15 mL.
Rx	**Betimol**[a] (Vistakon[b])		In 5, 10, and 15 mL.[c]
Rx	**Timoptic**[d] (Aton Pharma)		Preservative free. In UD 60s *Ocudose*.[e]
Rx	**Timoptic**[d] (Aton Pharma)		In 5 and 10 mL *Ocumeters*.[f]
Rx	**Timolol Maleate** (Various, eg, Akorn, Bausch & Lomb, Falcon, Fougera)	**Solution:** 0.5%	In 2.5, 5, 10, and 15 mL.
Rx	**Betimol**[a] (Vistakon[b])		In 5, 10, and 15 mL.[c]
Rx	**Istalol**[d] (Ista Pharm)		In 5 mL.[g]
Rx	**Timoptic**[d] (Aton Pharma)		Preservative free. In UD 60s *Ocudose*.[e]
Rx	**Timoptic**[d] (Aton Pharma)		In 5 and 10 mL *Ocumeters*.[g]
Rx	**Timolol GFS**[d] (Falcon)	**Solution, gel-forming:** 0.25%	In 2.5 and 5 mL.[h]
Rx	**Timoptic-XE**[d] (Aton Pharma)		In 5 mL *Ocumeters*.[h]
Rx	**Timolol GFS**[d] (Falcon)	**Solution, gel-forming:** 0.5%	In 2.5 and 5 mL.[h]
Rx	**Timoptic-XE**[d] (Aton Pharma)		In 5 mL *Ocumeters*.[h]

[a] As hemihydrate.
[b] Vistakon Pharmaceuticals, Jacksonville, FL 32256.
[c] With 0.01% benzalkonium chloride and monosodium and disodium phosphate dihydrate.
[d] As maleate.
[e] Preservative free; use immediately after opening; discard remaining contents. With monobasic and dibasic sodium phosphate and sodium hydroxide.
[f] With 0.01% benzalkonium chloride, sodium hydroxide, and monobasic and dibasic sodium phosphate.
[g] With 0.005% benzalkonium chloride, monobasic sodium phosphate monohydrate, 0.47% potassium sorbate, and sodium hydroxide.
[h] With 0.012% benzododecinium bromide.

TIMOLOL — OPHTHALMIC

For complete and comparative prescribing information, refer to the Ophthalmic Beta-Adrenergic Blocking Agents group monograph.

Indications

➤*Elevated intraocular pressure (IOP):* Treatment of elevated IOP in patients with ocular hypertension or open-angle glaucoma.

Administration and Dosage

➤*General dosing considerations:* Since in some patients the pressure-lowering response to timolol may require a few weeks to stabilize, evaluation should include a determination of intraocular pressure after approximately 4 weeks of treatment with timolol.

➤*Adults:*

Elevated intraocular pressure –

Timoptic-XE:

• *Usual dosage* – 1 drop of 0.25% or 0.5% in the affected eye(s) once daily.

• *Concomitant therapy* – If the intraocular pressure (IOP) is still not at a satisfactory level on 1 drop of 0.5% once daily, concomitant therapy may be considered. The concomitant use of 2 topical beta-adrenergic blocking agents is not recommended.

• *Conversion* – When patients have been switched from timolol administered twice daily to timolol gel-forming administered once daily, the ocular hypotensive effect has remained consistent.

Timoptic and *Timoptic in Ocudose*:

• *Initial dosage* – 1 drop of 0.25% in the affected eye(s) twice daily.

• *Dosage titration* – If the clinical response is not adequate, the dosage may be changed to 1 drop of 0.5% solution in the affected eye(s) twice daily.

• *Maintenance dosage* – If the IOP is maintained at satisfactory levels, the dosage schedule may be changed to 1 drop once daily in the affected eye(s).

• *Concomitant therapy* – Dosages above 1 drop of 0.5% twice daily generally have not been shown to produce further reduction in IOP. If the IOP is still not at a satisfactory level on this regimen, concomitant therapy with other agent(s) can be instituted. The concomitant use of 2 topical beta-adrenergic blocking agents is not recommended.

Istalol:

• *Initial dosage* – 1 drop of 0.5% in the affected eye(s) once daily in the morning.

• *Concomitant therapy* – If the IOP is not at a satisfactory level on this regimen, concomitant therapy with other agent(s) can be instituted. The concomitant use of 2 topical beta-adrenergic blocking agents is not recommended.

➤*Administration:*

Timolol gel-forming solution – Invert the closed container and shake once before each use. It is not necessary to shake the container more than once. Administer other topically applied ophthalmic medications at least 10 minutes before timolol gel-forming solution.

Timolol preservative-free solution – Apply enough gentle pressure on the individual container to obtain a single drop of solution. *Timoptic in Ocudose* does not contain a preservative. The solution from 1 individual unit is to be used immediately after opening for administration to 1 or both eyes. Because sterility cannot be guaranteed after the individual unit is opened, discard the remaining contents immediately after administration.

➤*Storage/Stability:*

Timoptic products – Store between 15° and 30°C (59° and 86°F). Protect from freezing. Protect from light. Because evaporation can occur through the unprotected polyethylene unit dose container of the preservative-free solution and prolonged exposure to direct light can modify the product, keep the unit dose container in the protective foil overwrap and use within 1 month after the foil package has been opened.

Istalol – Store between 15° and 25°C (59° and 77°F).

Refer to the Topical Ophthalmic Drugs introduction and Agents for Glaucoma introduction for a general discussion of these products. For information on the oral use of pilocarpine, refer to the monograph in the Mouth and Throat Products section.

Indications

➤*Carbachol, topical; pilocarpine:*

Glaucoma – To decrease elevated IOP in glaucoma.

➤*Acetylcholine; carbachol, intraocular:*

Miosis – To induce miosis during surgery.

Actions

➤*Pharmacology:* The direct-acting miotics are parasympathomimetic (cholinergic) drugs which duplicate the muscarinic effects of acetylcholine. When applied topically, these drugs produce pupillary constriction, stimulate the ciliary muscles and increase aqueous humor outflow facility. Miosis, produced through contraction of the iris sphincter, causes increased tension on the scleral spur (reducing outflow resistance) and opening of the trabecular meshwork spaces facilitating outflow. With the increase in outflow facility, there is a decrease in intraocular pressure (IOP). Topical ophthalmic instillation of acetylcholine causes no discernible response as cholinesterase destroys the molecule more rapidly than it can penetrate the cornea; therefore, acetylcholine is only used intraocularly.

Miosis Induction of Direct-Acting Miotics

Miotic	Onset	Peak	Duration
Acetylcholine, intraocular	seconds	—	10 min
Carbachol			
Intraocular	seconds	2 to 5 min	1 to 2 days
Topical	10 to 20 min	—	4 to 8 hours
Pilocarpine, topical	10 to 30 min	—	4 to 8 hours

Contraindications

Hypersensitivity to any component of the formulation; where constriction is undesirable (eg, acute iritis, acute or anterior uveitis, some forms of secondary glaucoma, pupillary block glaucoma, acute inflammatory disease of the anterior chamber).

Warnings/Precautions

➤*Corneal abrasion:* Use carbachol with caution in the presence of corneal abrasion to avoid excessive penetration.

➤*Systemic reactions:* Caution is advised in patients with acute cardiac failure, bronchial asthma, peptic ulcer, hyperthyroidism, GI spasm, urinary tract obstruction, Parkinson's disease, recent MI, hypertension or hypotension.

➤*Retinal detachment:* Retinal detachment has been caused by miotics in susceptible individuals, in individuals with preexisting retinal disease or in those who are predisposed to retinal tears. Fundus examination is advised for all patients prior to initiation of therapy.

➤*Miosis:* Miosis usually causes difficulty in dark adaptation. Advise patients to use caution while night driving or performing hazardous tasks in poor light.

➤*Angle-closure:* Although withdrawal of the peripheral iris from the anterior chamber angle by miosis may reduce the tendency for narrow-angle closure, miotics can occasionally precipitate angle closure by increasing resistance to aqueous flow from posterior to anterior chamber.

➤*Pilocarpine ocular system (Ocusert):* Carefully consider and evaluate patients with acute infectious conjunctivitis or keratitis prior to use.

➤*Pregnancy: Category C* (carbachol, pilocarpine, acetyl choline [per Briggs' *Drugs in Pregnancy and Lactation*]). Safety for use during pregnancy has not been established. Use only when clearly needed.

➤*Lactation:* It is not known whether these drugs are excreted in breast milk; exercise caution when administering to a breast-feeding woman.

➤*Children:* Safety and efficacy for use in children have not been established.

Drug Interactions

➤*Nonsteroidal anti-inflammatory agents (NSAIDs), topical:* Although studies with acetylcholine chloride or carbachol revealed no interference, and there is no known pharmacological basis for an interaction, there have been reports that these drugs have been ineffective when used in patients treated with topical NSAIDs.

Adverse Reactions

➤*Acetylcholine:*

Ophthalmic – Corneal edema, clouding, and decompensation.

Systemic – Bradycardia; hypotension; flushing; breathing difficulties; sweating.

➤*Carbachol:*

Ophthalmic – Transient stinging and burning; corneal clouding; persistent bullous keratopathy; postoperative iritis following cataract extraction with intraocular use; retinal detachment; transient ciliary and conjunctival injection; ciliary spasm with resultant temporary decrease of visual acuity.

Systemic – Headache; salivation; GI cramps; vomiting; diarrhea; asthma; syncope; cardiac arrhythmia; flushing; sweating; epigastric distress; tightness in bladder; hypotension; frequent urge to urinate.

➤*Pilocarpine:*

Ophthalmic – Transient stinging and burning; tearing; ciliary spasm; conjunctival vascular congestion; temporal, peri- or supra-orbital headache; superficial keratitis; induced myopia (especially in younger individuals who have recently started administration); blurred vision; poor dark adaptation; reduced visual acuity in poor illumination in older individuals and in individuals with lens opacity. A subtle corneal granularity has occurred with pilocarpine gel. Lens opacity (prolonged use), retinal detachment (rare; see Precautions).

Systemic – Hypertension, tachycardia, bronchiolar spasm, pulmonary edema, salivation, sweating, nausea, vomiting, diarrhea (rare).

Pilocarpine ocular system (Ocusert): Conjunctival irritation, including mild erythema with or without a slight increase in mucus secretion with first use. These symptoms tend to lessen or disappear after the first week of therapy. Ciliary spasm may occur with pilocarpine usage but is not a contraindication to continued therapy unless the induced myopia is debilitating to the patient. Rarely, a sudden increase in pilocarpine effects has been reported during use.

Irritation from pilocarpine has been infrequently encountered and may require cessation of therapy. True allergic reactions are uncommon, but require discontinuation of therapy. Corneal abrasion and visual impairment have been reported.

Overdosage

Should accidental overdosage in the eye(s) occur, flush with water.

➤*Treatment:* Treatment includes usual supportive measures. Refer to General Management of Acute Overdosage. Observe patients for signs of toxicity (eg, salivation, lacrimation, sweating, nausea, vomiting, diarrhea). If these occur, anticholinergics (atropine) may be necessary. Bronchial constriction may be a problem in asthmatic patients.

Patient Information

May sting upon instillation, especially first few doses.

May cause headache, browache and decreased night vision. Use caution while night driving or performing hazardous tasks in poor light.

To avoid contamination, do not touch tip of container to any surface. Replace cap after using. Keep bottle tightly closed when not in use. Discard solution after expiration date.

ACETYLCHOLINE CHLORIDE

Rx	**Miochol-E** (Novartis Pharm)	**Solution:** 1:100 acetylcholine chloride when reconstituted	In 2 mL dual chamber univial (lower chamber 20 mg lyophilized acetylcholine chloride and 56 mg mannitol; upper chamber 2 mL electrolyte diluent[a] and sterile water for injection).

[a] Sodium chloride, potassium chloride, magnesium chloride hexahydrate, calcium chloride dihydrate.

ACETYLCHOLINE CHLORIDE — INTRAOCULAR

For complete and comparative prescribing information, refer to the Miotics, Direct-Acting group monograph.

Indications

➤*Miosis:* To obtain miosis of the iris in seconds after delivery of the lens in cataract surgery, in penetrating keratoplasty, iridectomy and other anterior segment surgery where rapid miosis may be required.

Administration and Dosage

➤*Adults:*

Miosis – In most cases, 0.5 to 2 mL produces satisfactory miosis.

➤*Preparation for administration:* Prepare solution immediately before use. In the reconstitution of the solution, if the center rubber plug seal in the univial does not go down or is down, do not use the vial. Inspect univial while inside unopened blister. Diluent must be in upper chamber. Open under aseptic conditions only. Peel open blister. Aseptically transfer univial to sterile field. Maintain sterility of outer container during preparation of solution. Immediately before use, give plunger-stopper a quarter turn and press to force diluent and center plug into lower chamber. Shake gently to dissolve drug. With a new needle of sturdy gauge, 18 to 20, draw all the solution into a dry, sterile syringe. Replace needle with a suitable atraumatic cannulae for intraocular irrigation.

➤*Administration:* The acetylcholine is instilled into the anterior chamber before or after securing one or more sutures. Instillation should be gentle and parallel to the iris face and tangential to pupil border. In cataract surgery, use acetylcholine only after delivery of the lens.

If there are no mechanical hindrances, the pupil starts to constrict in seconds and the peripheral iris is drawn away from the angle of the anterior chamber. Any anatomical hindrance to miosis must be released to permit the desired effect of the drug.

➤*Storage/Stability:* Keep from freezing. Store at 4° to 25°C (39° to 77°F).

Miotics, Direct-Acting

CARBACHOL

Rx	**Miostat** (Alcon)	**Solution; intraocular:** 0.01%	In 1.5 mL vials.[a]
Rx	**Isopto Carbachol** (Alcon)	**Solution; topical:** 1.5%	In 15 and 30 mL *Drop-Tainers*.[b]
		3%	In 15 and 30 mL *Drop-Tainers*.[b]

[a] With 0.64% sodium chloride, 0.075% potassium chloride, 0.048% calcium chloride dihydrate, 0.03% magnesium chloride hexahydrate, 0.39% sodium acetate trihydrate, 0.17% sodium citrate dihydrate, sodium hydroxide, hydrochloric acid.

[b] With 0.005% benzalkonium chloride, 1% hydroxypropyl methylcellulose, sodium chloride, boric acid and sodium borate.

CARBACHOL — INTRAOCULAR

For complete and comparative prescribing information, refer to the Miotics, Direct-Acting group monograph.

Indications

➤*Miosis:* Intraocular use for miosis during surgery.

Administration and Dosage

➤*Adults:*

Miosis –

Usual dosage: Gently instill no more than 0.5 mL into the anterior chamber before or after securing sutures.

➤*Administration:* For single-dose intraocular use only. Open under aseptic conditions only. Discard unused portion.

➤*Storage/Stability:* Store at 15° to 30°C (59° to 86°F).

CARBACHOL — OPHTHALMIC

For complete prescribing information, refer to the Miotics, Direct-Acting class monograph.

Indications

➤*Glaucoma:* For lowering intraocular pressure in the treatment of glaucoma.

Administration and Dosage

➤*Adults:*

Glaucoma – Instill 2 drops into eye(s) up to 3 times daily.

➤*Storage/Stability:* Store at 8° to 27°C (46° to 80°F).

PILOCARPINE HYDROCHLORIDE

Rx	**Pilocarpine Hydrochloride** (Various)	**Solution:** 0.5%	In 15 and 30 mL.
Rx	**Pilocarpine Hydrochloride** (Various, eg, Alcon, Goldline)	**Solution:** 1%	In 2, 15 and 30 mL and UD 1 mL.
Rx	**Isopto Carpine** (Alcon)		In 15 and 30 mL.[a]
Rx	**Pilocarpine Hydrochloride** (Various eg, Alcon, Goldline)	**Solution:** 2%	In 2, 15, and 30 mL.
Rx	**Isopto Carpine** (Alcon)		In 15 and 30 mL.[a]
Rx	**Pilocarpine Hydrochloride** (Various, eg, Alcon, Goldline)	**Solution:** 4%	In 2, 15 and 30 mL.
Rx	**Isopto Carpine** (Alcon)		In 15 and 30 mL.[a]
Rx	**Pilocarpine Hydrochloride** (Various)	**Solution:** 6%	In 15 mL.
Rx	**Pilopine HS** (Alcon)	**Gel:** 4%	In 3.5 g.[d]

[a] With 0.5% hydroxypropyl methylcellulose and 0.01% benzalkonium chloride.
[b] With dydroxypropyl methylcellulose, benzalkonium chloride and EDTA.
[c] With polyvinyl alcohol, benzalkonium chloride and EDTA.
[d] With 0.008% benzalkonium chloride, carbopol 940 and EDTA.

PILOCARPINE HYDROCHLORIDE — Ophthalmic Gel

Indications

➤*Intraocular pressure:* To control intraocular pressure. May be used in combination with other miotics, beta-blockers, carbonic anhydrase inhibitors, sympathomimetics, or hyperosmotic agents.

Administration and Dosage

➤*Adults:*

Intraocular pressure –

Usual dosage: Apply a ½-inch ribbon in the lower conjunctival sac of the affected eye(s) once daily at bedtime.

Concomitant therapy: May be used in combination with other miotics, beta-blockers, carbonic anhydrase inhibitors, sympathomimetics, or hyperosmotic agents.

➤*Administration:* For topical use only.

➤*Storage/Stability:* Store between 2° and 27°C (36° and 80°F). Avoid excessive heat. Do not freeze. Pilocarpine does not need to be refrigerated.

PILOCARPINE HYDROCHLORIDE — Ophthalmic Solution

Indications

➤*Glaucoma:* For the management of glaucoma, especially open-angle glaucoma. Patients may be maintained on pilocarpine as long as intraocular pressure (IOP) is controlled and there is no deterioration in the visual fields. May be used alone or in combination with other miotics, beta-adrenergic blocking agents, epinephrine, carbonic anhydrase inhibitors, or hyperosmotic agents to decrease IOP prior to surgery.

➤*Miosis:* To counter the effects of mydriatic or cycloplegic agents.

Administration and Dosage

➤*General dosing considerations:* The frequency of instillation and the concentration are determined by patient response.

Individuals with heavily pigmented irides may require higher strengths.

➤*Adults:*

Glaucoma –

Usual dosage: 1 or 2 drops 3 to 4 times a daily. During acute phase, the mitotic agent must be instilled into the unaffected eye to prevent an attack of angle-closure glaucoma.

Concomitant therapy: May be used in combination with other miotics, beta-adrenergic blocking agents, epinephrine, carbonic anhydrase inhibitors, or hyperosmotic agents to decrease IOP prior to surgery in patients with acute (angle-dose) glaucoma.

➤*Administration:* To avoid contamination, do not touch tip of container to any surface. Replace cap after administration.

➤*Storage/Stability:* Store between 59° and 86°F. Do not freeze.

ECHOTHIOPHATE IODIDE

Rx	**Phospholine Iodide** (Wyeth-Ayerst)	**Powder for reconstitution:** 6.25 mg to make 0.125%	With 5 mL diluent.[a]

[a] With potassium acetate, 0.55% chlorobutanol and 1.2% mannitol.

ECHOTHIOPHATE IODIDE — OPHTHALMIC

Indications

➤*Glaucoma:* Chronic open-angle glaucoma; subacute or chronic angle-closure glaucoma after iridectomy or where surgery is refused or contraindicated; certain nonuveitic secondary types of glaucoma, especially glaucoma following cataract surgery.

➤*Accommodative esotropia:* For concomitant esotropias with a significant accommodative component.

Administration and Dosage

➤*Adults:*

Advanced chronic simple glaucoma – 0.03% twice a day. When the patient is being transferred to echothiophate iodide because of unsatisfactory control with pilocarpine, carbachol, epinephrine, etc, one of the higher strengths, 0.06%, 0.125%, or 0.25%, will usually be needed. In this case, a brief trial with the 0.03% eye drops will be advantageous because the higher strengths will then be more easily tolerated.

Glaucoma secondary to cataract surgery – See Advanced chronic simple glaucoma.

Early chronic simple glaucoma – 0.03% twice a day. If this dosage is inadequate, epinephrine and a carbonic anhydrase inhibitor may be added to the regimen. When still more effective medication is required, the higher strengths of echothiophate iodide may be prescribed with the recognition that the control of the intraocular pressure should have priority regardless of potential side effects. A change in therapy is indicated if, at any time, the tension fails to remain at an acceptable level on this regimen.

➤*Children:*

Diagnosis of accommodative esotropia –

Usual dosage: One drop of 0.125% once a day in both eyes on retiring for a period of 2 or 3 weeks.

Duration of therapy: Only a short period is required and little time will be lost in instituting other procedures if the esotropia proves to be unresponsive.

Treatment of accommodative esotropia –

Usual dosage: After the initial period of treatment for diagnostic purposes, the schedule may be reduced to 0.125% every other day or 0.06% every day. These dosages can often be gradually lowered as treatment progresses. The 0.03% strength has proven to be effective in some cases. The maximum recommended dosage is usually 0.125% once a day, although more intensive therapy has been used for short periods.

Duration of therapy: There is no definite limit so long as the drug is well tolerated. However, if the eye drops, with or without eyeglasses, are gradually withdrawn after about a year or 2 and deviation recurs, surgery should be considered. As with other miotics, tolerance may occasionally develop after prolonged use. In such cases, a rest period will restore the original activity of the drug.

➤*Concomitant therapy:* May be used concomitantly with epinephrine, a carbonic anhydrase inhibitor, or both.

➤*Preparation for administration:* Tear off aluminum seals and remove and discard rubber plugs from both drug and diluent containers. Pour diluent into drug container. Remove dropper assembly from its sterile wrapping. Holding dropper assembly by the screw cap and, without compressing rubber bulb, insert into drug container and screw down tightly. Shake for several seconds to ensure mixing. Do not cover nor obliterate instructions to patient regarding storage of eye drops.

➤*Administration:* The daily dose or 1 of the 2 daily doses should always be instilled just before retiring to avoid inconvenience caused by the miosis. Two doses a day are preferred to 1 in order to maintain as smooth a diurnal tension curve as possible, although a single dose per day or every other day has been used with satisfactory results. Because of prolonged action, control during the night and early morning hours may then sometimes be obtained.

Good technique in the administration of echothiophate requires that finger pressure at the inner canthus be exerted for a minute or 2 following instillation of the eye drops to minimize drainage into the nose and throat. Excess solution around the eye should be removed with tissue, and any medication on the hands should be rinsed off.

➤*Storage/Stability:* Store under refrigeration (2° to 8°C). Reconstituted product may be stored at room temperature (approximately 25°C) for up to 4 weeks.

Actions

➤*Pharmacology:* Echothiophate iodide is a long-acting cholinesterase inhibitor for topical use which enhances the effect of endogenously liberated acetylcholine in iris, ciliary muscle, and other parasympathetically innervated structures of the eye. It thereby causes miosis, increase in facility of outflow of aqueous humor, fall in intraocular pressure, and potentiation of accommodation.

Echothiophate iodide will depress both plasma and erythrocyte cholinesterase levels in most patients after a few weeks of eyedrop therapy.

Contraindications

Active uveal inflammation; most cases of angle-closure glaucoma, due to the possibility of increasing angle block; hypersensitivity to the active or inactive ingredients.

Warnings/Precautions

➤*Systemic effects:* While systemic effects are infrequent, proper use of the drug requires digital compression of the nasolacrimal ducts for a minute or two following instillation to minimize drainage into the nasal chamber with its extensive absorption area. To prevent possible skin absorption, hands should be washed following instillation.

Temporary discontinuance of medication is necessary if cardiac irregularities occur.

Temporary discontinuance of medication is necessary if salivation, urinary incontinence, diarrhea, profuse sweating, muscle weakness, or respiratory difficulties occur.

➤*Insecticides/Pesticides:* Patients receiving echothiophate iodide who are exposed to carbamateor organophosphate-type insecticides and pesticides (eg, professional gardeners, farmers, workers in plants manufacturing or formulating such products) should be warned of the additive systemic effects possible from absorption of the pesticide through the respiratory tract or skin. During periods of exposure to such pesticides, the wearing of respiratory masks, and frequent washing and clothing changes may be advisable.

➤*Special risk:* Where there is a quiescent uveitis or a history of this condition, anticholinesterase therapy should be avoided or used cautiously because of the intense and persistent miosis and ciliary muscle contraction that may occur.

Anticholinesterase drugs should be used with extreme caution, if at all, in patients with marked vagotonia, bronchial asthma, spastic GI disturbances, peptic ulcer, pronounced bradycardia and hypotension, recent MI, epilepsy, parkinsonism, and other disorders that may respond adversely to vagotonic effects.

Anticholinesterase drugs should be employed prior to ophthalmic surgery only as a considered risk because of the possible occurrence of hyphemia.

Echothiophate iodide should be used with great caution, if at all, where there is a prior history of retinal detachment.

➤*Pregnancy: Category C.* Animal reproduction studies have not been conducted with echothiophate iodide. It is also not known whether echothiophate iodide can cause fetal harm when administered to a pregnant woman or can affect reproduction capacity. Echothiophate iodide should be given to a pregnant woman only if clearly needed.

➤*Lactation:* Because of the potential for serious adverse reactions in nursing infants from echothiophate iodide, a decision should be made whether to discontinue nursing or to discontinue the drug, taking into account the importance of the drug to the mother.

➤*Monitoring:* Gonioscopy is recommended prior to initiation of therapy. Routine examinations to detect lens opacity should accompany clinical use of echothiophate iodide solution.

Drug Interactions

Echothiophate iodide solution potentiates other cholinesterase inhibitors such as succinylcholine or organophosphate and carbamate insecticides. Patients undergoing systemic anticholinesterase treatment should be warned of the possible additive effects of echothiophate iodide.

Succinylcholine should be administered only with great caution, if at all, prior to or during general anesthesia to patients receiving anticholinesterase medication because of possible respiratory or cardiovascular collapse.

Caution should be observed in treating glaucoma with echothiophate iodide in patients who are at the same time undergoing treatment with systemic anticholinesterase medications for myasthenia gravis, because of possible adverse additive effects.

Adverse Reactions

➤*Cardiovascular:* Cardiac irregularities.

➤*Ophthalmic:* Although the relationship, if any, of retinal detachment to the administration of echothiophate iodide has not been established, retinal detachment has been reported in a few cases during the use of echothiophate iodide in adult patients without a history of this disorder.

Stinging, burning, lacrimation, lid muscle twitching, conjunctival and ciliary redness, browache, induced myopia with visual blurring may occur.

Activation of latent iritis or uveitis may occur.

Iris cysts may form, and if treatment is continued, may enlarge and obscure vision. This occurrence is more frequent in children. The cysts usually shrink upon discontinuance of the medication, reduction in strength of the drops or frequency of instillation. Rarely, they may rupture or break free into the aqueous. Regular examinations are advisable when the drug is being prescribed for the treatment of accommodative esotropia.

ECHOTHIOPHATE IODIDE — OPHTHALMIC

Prolonged use may cause conjunctival thickening, obstruction of nasolacrimal canals.

Lens opacities occurring in patients under treatment for glaucoma with echothiophate iodide solution have been reported and similar changes have been produced experimentally in healthy monkeys. Routine examinations should accompany clinical use of the drug.

Paradoxical increase in intraocular pressure may follow anticholinesterase instillation. This may be alleviated by prescribing a sympathomimetic mydriatic such as phenylephrine.

Ophthalmic Carbonic Anhydrase Inhibitors

Refer to the Topical Ophthalmic Drugs introduction for more complete information.

Indications

➤*Elevated intraocular pressure (IOP):* Treatment of elevated IOP in patients with ocular hypertension or open-angle glaucoma.

Actions

➤*Pharmacology:* Dorzolamide and brinzolamide are carbonic anhydrase inhibitors for ophthalmic use. Carbonic anhydrase (CA) is an enzyme found in many tissues of the body, including the eye. It catalyzes the reversible reaction involving the hydration of carbon dioxide and the dehydration of carbonic acid. In humans, CA exists as a number of isoenzymes, the most active being CA-II, found primarily in red blood cells (RBCs), but also in other tissues. Inhibition of CA in the ciliary processes of the eye decreases aqueous humor secretion, presumably by slowing the formation of bicarbonate ions with subsequent reduction in sodium and fluid transport. The result is a reduction in intraocular pressure (IOP). Dorzolamide and brinzolamide reduce elevated IOP by inhibiting CA-II. Elevated IOP is a major risk factor in the pathogenesis of optic nerve damage and glaucomatous visual field loss.

➤*Pharmacokinetics:* When topically applied, dorzolamide and brinzolamide reach the systemic circulation and accumulate in RBCs during chronic dosing as a result of binding to CA-II. Extensive distribution into RBCs yields a long half-life, approximately 3.5 to 4 months. The parent drugs form a single N-desethyl metabolite that inhibits CA-II less potently than the parent drug, but also inhibits CA-I. The metabolite also accumulates in RBCs, where it binds primarily to CA-I. Plasma concentrations of parent and metabolite are generally below the assay limit of quantitation. Plasma protein binding is moderate (approximately 33%) for dorzolamide and approximately 60% for brinzolamide. These agents are primarily excreted unchanged in the urine, and the metabolite also is excreted in urine.

Contraindications

Hypersensitivity to any component of these products.

Warnings/Precautions

➤*Systemic effects:* Dorzolamide and brinzolamide are sulfonamides and, although administered topically, are absorbed systemically. Therefore, the same types of adverse reactions attributable to systemic sulfonamides may occur with topical administration of these agents (refer to the systemic Sulfonamides monograph in the Anti-Infectives chapter). Fatalities have occurred, although rarely, because of severe reactions to sulfonamides including Stevens-Johnson syndrome, toxic epidermal necrolysis, fulminant hepatic necrosis, agranulocytosis, aplastic anemia, and other blood dyscrasias. Sensitization may recur when a sulfonamide is readministered regardless of the route of administration. If signs of serious reactions or hypersensitivity occur, discontinue the use of this preparation.

➤*Corneal endothelium effects:* Carbonic anhydrase activity has been observed in both the cytoplasm and around the plasma membranes of the corneal endothelium. The effect of continued administration of dorzolamide or brinzolamide on the corneal endothelium has not been fully evaluated.

➤*Acute angle-closure glaucoma:* The management of patients with acute angle-closure glaucoma requires therapeutic interventions in addition to ocular hypotensive agents. Dorzolamide and brinzolamide have not been studied in patients with acute angle-closure glaucoma.

➤*Ocular effects:* Local ocular adverse effects, primarily conjunctivitis and lid reactions, were reported with chronic administration of dorzolamide. Many of these reactions had the clinical appearance and course of an allergic-type reaction that resolved upon discontinuation of drug therapy. If such reactions are observed, discontinue the drug and evaluate the patient before considering restarting the drug.

➤*Concomitant oral CA inhibitors:* There is a potential for an additive effect on the known systemic effects of CA inhibition in patients receiving an oral CA inhibitor and dorzolamide or brinzolamide. Concomitant administration of ophthalmic and oral CA inhibitors is not recommended.

➤*Bacterial keratitis:* There have been reports of bacterial keratitis associated with the use of topical ophthalmic products in multiple-dose containers. These containers had been inadvertently contaminated by patients who, in most cases, had a concurrent corneal disease or a disruption of the ocular epithelial surface. Serious damage to the eye and subsequent loss of vision may result from using contaminated solutions.

➤*Contact lenses:* The preservative used in these products, benzalkonium chloride, may be absorbed by soft contact lenses. Do not administer these agents while wearing soft contact lenses; reinsert lenses 15 minutes or longer after drug administration.

➤*Renal/Hepatic function impairment:* These agents have not been studied in patients with severe renal impairment (Ccr less than 30 mL/min). However, because dorzolamide, brinzolamide, and their metabolites are excreted predominantly by the kidney, these agents are not recommended in such patients.

Dorzolamide and brinzolamide have not been studied in patients with hepatic impairment and should be used with caution in such patients.

➤*Pregnancy: Category C.* Maternal toxicity and a significant increase in the number of fetal variations (eg, malformations of the vertebral bodies) was seen in animals at doses greater than 20 times the recommended human ophthalmic dose. These malformations occurred at doses that caused metabolic acidosis with decreased body weight gain in dams and decreased fetal weights. There are no adequate and well controlled studies in pregnant women. Use during pregnancy only if the potential benefit justifies the risk to the fetus.

➤*Lactation:* In lactating rats, decreases in body weight gain were seen in offspring with these agents at oral doses greater than 94 times the recommended human ophthalmic dose. A slight delay in postnatal development (incisor eruption, vaginal canalization, and eye openings), secondary to lower fetal body weight, also was noted with dorzolamide.

It is not known whether this drug is excreted in breast milk. Because of the potential for serious adverse reactions in nursing infants, decide whether to discontinue nursing or to discontinue the drug, taking into account the importance of the drug to the mother.

➤*Children:* Safety and efficacy in children have not been established.

➤*Elderly:* Of all the patients in dorzolamide clinical studies, 44% were 65 years of age or older, and 10% were 75 years of age or older. No overall differences in efficacy or safety were observed between these patients and younger patients, but greater sensitivity of some older individuals to the product cannot be ruled out.

Drug Interactions

Although acid-base and electrolyte disturbances were not reported in the clinical trials with dorzolamide and brinzolamide, these disturbances have been reported with oral CA inhibitors and have, in some instances, resulted in drug interactions (eg, toxicity associated with high-dose salicylate therapy). Therefore, consider the potential for such drug interactions in patients receiving either of these agents.

Adverse Reactions

➤*Dorzolamide:*

Miscellaneous – Ocular burning, stinging or discomfort immediately following administration (approximately 33%); bitter taste following administration (approximately 25%); superficial punctate keratitis (10% to 15%); signs and symptoms of ocular allergic reaction (approximately 10%); blurred vision, tearing, dryness, photophobia (approximately 1% to 5%); headache, nausea, asthenia/fatigue (infrequent); skin rashes, urolithiasis, iridocyclitis (rare).

➤*Brinzolamide:*

Miscellaneous – Blurred vision, bitter, sour, or unusual taste (approximately 5% to 10%); blepharitis, dermatitis, dry eye, foreign body sensation, headache, hyperemia, ocular discharge, ocular discomfort, ocular keratitis, ocular pain, ocular pruritus, rhinitis (1% to 5%); allergic reactions, alopecia, chest pain, conjunctivitis, diarrhea, diplopia, dizziness, dry mouth, dyspnea, dyspepsia, eye fatigue, hypertonia, keratoconjunctivitis, keratopathy, kidney pain, lid margin crusting or sticky sensation, nausea, pharyngitis, tearing, urticaria (less than 1%).

Overdosage

Electrolyte imbalance, development of an acidotic state and possible CNS effects may occur. Monitor serum electrolyte levels (particularly potassium) and blood pH levels. Significant lethality was observed in female rats and mice after single oral doses of 1927 and 1320 mg/kg of dorzolamide, respectively.

Patient Information

Dorzolamide and brinzolamide are sulfonamides and, although administered topically, are absorbed systemically. Therefore, the same types of adverse reactions that are attributable to systemic sulfonamides may occur with topical administration. Advise patients that if serious or unusual reactions or signs of hypersensitivity occur, they should discontinue use of the product and consult their physician.

Vision may be temporarily blurred. Instruct patients to exercise care in operating machinery or driving a motor vehicle.

Advise patients that if they develop any ocular reactions, particularly conjunctivitis and lid reactions, they should discontinue medication use and seek their physician's advice.

Instruct patients to avoid allowing the tip of the dispensing container to contact the eye or surrounding structures. Ocular solutions, if handled improperly or if the tip of the dispensing container contacts the eye or surrounding structures, can become contaminated by common bacteria known to cause ocular infections. Serious damage to the eye and subsequent loss of vision may result from using contaminated solutions.

Advise patients that if they develop an intercurrent ocular condition (eg, trauma, ocular surgery, infection), they should immediately seek their physician's advice concerning the continued use of the present multidose container.

If more than one topical ophthalmic drug is being used, administer the drugs at least 10 minutes apart.

Ophthalmic Carbonic Anhydrase Inhibitors

DORZOLAMIDE

Rx	Dorzolamide (Prasco Labs)	Solution; ophthalmic: 2%	As dorzolamide hydrochloride. In 10 mL *Ocumeter Plus*.[a]
Rx	Trusopt (Merck)		As dorzolamide hydrochloride. In 5 and 10 mL *Ocumeters*.[a]

[a] With benzalkonium chloride 0.0075%, hydroxyethyl cellulose, sodium hydroxide, and sodium citrate.

DORZOLAMIDE HYDROCHLORIDE — OPHTHALMIC

For complete and comparative prescribing information, refer to the Ophthalmic Carbonic Anhydrase Inhibitors group monograph.

Indications

➤*Elevated intraocular pressure (IOP):* For the treatment of elevated IOP in patients with ocular hypertension or open-angle glaucoma.

Administration and Dosage

➤*Adults:*

Elevated intraocular pressure –

Usual dosage: One drop in the affected eye(s) 3 times daily.

Concomitant therapy: May be used concomitantly with other topical ophthalmic drug products to lower IOP.

➤*Children:*

Elevated intraocular pressure – See Adults for dosing.

➤*Renal function impairment:* Not recommended in patients with severe renal function impairment (creatinine clearance less than 30 mL/min).

➤*Administration:* If more than 1 ophthalmic drug is being used, administer the drugs at least 10 minutes apart.

➤*Storage/Stability:* Store at 15° to 30°C (59° to 86°F). Protect from light.

BRINZOLAMIDE

Rx	Azopt (Alcon)	Suspension: 1%	In 2.5, 5, 10, and 15 mL *Drop-Tainers*.[a]

[a] With 0.01% benzalkonium chloride, mannitol, carbomer 974P, tyloxapol, sodium chloride, hydrochloric acid and/or sodium hydroxide, and EDTA.

BRINZOLAMIDE — OPHTHALMIC

For complete and comparative prescribing information, refer to the Ophthalmic Carbonic Anhydrase Inhibitors group monograph.

Indications

➤*Elevated intraocular pressure (IOP):* Treatment of elevated IOP in patients with ocular hypertension or open-angle glaucoma.

Administration and Dosage

➤*Adults:*

Increased intraocular pressure –

Usual dosage: One drop in the affected eye(s) 3 times daily.

Concomitant therapy: May be used concomitantly with other topical ophthalmic drug products to lower intraocular pressure.

➤*Renal function impairment:* Not recommended in patients with severe renal impairment.

➤*Administration:* Shake well before use. If more than one topical ophthalmic drug is being used, administer the drugs at least 10 minutes apart.

➤*Storage/Stability:* Store at 4° to 30°C (39° to 86°F).

Prostaglandin Agonists

LATANOPROST

Rx	Xalatan (Pfizer)	Solution: 0.005%	Benzalkonium chloride 0.02%, sodium chloride. In 2.5 mL fill dropper bottles.

LATANOPROST OPHTHALMIC

Refer to the Topical Ophthalmic Drugs introduction for more complete and comparative information.

Indications

➤*Elevated intraocular pressure:* For the reduction of elevated intraocular pressure in patients with open-angle glaucoma and ocular hypertension who are intolerant of other intraocular pressure lowering medications or insufficiently responsive (failed to achieve target IOP determined after multiple measurements over time) to another intraocular pressure lowering medication.

Administration and Dosage

➤*Adults:*

Elevated intraocular pressure –

Usual dosage: 1 drop in the affected eye(s) once daily in the evening.

Maximum dose: 1 drop once daily.

Concomitant therapy: May be used concomitantly with other topical ophthalmic drug products to lower intraocular pressure.

➤*Administration:* If more than 1 ophthalmic drug is being used, the drugs should be administered at least 5 minutes apart.

➤*Storage/Stability:* Store unopened bottle under refrigeration at 2° to 8°C (36° to 46°F). During shipment to the patient, the bottle may be maintained at temperatures up to 40°C (104°F) for a period not exceeding 8 days. Once a bottle is opened for use, it may be stored at room temperature, up to 25°C (77°F) for 6 weeks. Protect from light.

Actions

➤*Pharmacology:* Latanoprost is a prostanoid selective FP receptor agonist which is believed to reduce the intraocular pressure by increasing the outflow of aqueous humor. Studies in animals and man suggest that the main mechanism of action is increased uveoscleral outflow. Elevated IOP represents a major risk factor for glaucomatous field loss. The higher the level of IOP, the greater the likelihood of optic nerve damage and visual field loss.

➤*Pharmacokinetics:*

Absorption – Latanoprost is absorbed through the cornea where the isopropyl ester prodrug is hydrolyzed to the acid form to become biologically active. Studies in man indicate that the peak concentration in the aqueous humor is reached about 2 hours after topical administration.

Distribution – The distribution volume in humans is 0.16 ± 0.02 L/kg. The acid of latanoprost could be measured in aqueous humor during the first 4 hours, and in plasma only during the first hour after local administration.

Metabolism – Latanoprost, an isopropyl ester prodrug, is hydrolyzed by esterases in the cornea to the biologically active acid. The active acid of latanoprost reaching the systemic circulation is primarily metabolized by the liver to the 1,2-dinor and 1,2,3,4-tetranor metabolites via fatty acid β-oxidation.

Excretion – The elimination of the acid of latanoprost from human plasma was rapid ($t_{1/2}$ = 17 minutes) after both intravenous and topical administration. Systemic clearance is approximately 7 mL/min/kg. Following hepatic β-oxidation, the metabolites are mainly eliminated via the kidneys. Approximately 88% and 98% of the administered dose is recovered in the urine after topical and intravenous dosing, respectively.

Contraindications

Known hypersensitivity to latanoprost, benzalkonium chloride or any other ingredients in this product.

Warnings/Precautions

➤*Ocular pigment changes:* Latanoprost has been reported to cause changes to pigmented tissues. The most frequently reported changes have been increased pigmentation of the iris and periorbital tissue (eyelid) and increased pigmentation and growth of eyelashes. These changes may be permanent. Pigmentation is expected to increase as long as latanoprost is administered. After discontinuation of latanoprost, pigmentation of the iris is likely to be permanent while pigmentation of the periorbital tissue and eyelash changes have been reported to be reversible in some patients. Patients who receive treatment should be informed of the possibility of increased pigmentation. The effects of increased pigmentation beyond 5 years are not known.

Latanoprost sterile ophthalmic solution may gradually change eye color, increasing the amount of brown pigment in the iris by increasing the number of melanosomes (pigment granules) in melanocytes. The long-term effects on the melanocytes and the consequences of potential injury to the melanocytes or deposition of pigment granules to other areas of the eye are currently unknown. The change in iris color occurs slowly and may not be noticeable for several months to years. Patients should be informed of the possibility of iris color change.

Eyelid skin darkening has also been reported in association with the use of latanoprost.

LATANOPROST — OPHTHALMIC

Latanoprost may gradually change eyelashes and vellus hair; these changes include increased length, thickness, pigmentation, and number of lashes or hairs, and misdirected growth of eyelashes. Eyelash changes are usually reversible upon discontinuation of treatment.

Patients who are expected to receive treatment in only 1 eye should be informed about the potential for increased brown pigmentation of the iris, periorbital tissue, and eyelashes in the treated eye and thus, heterochromia between the eyes. They should also be advised of the potential for a disparity between the eyes in length, thickness, or number of eyelashes. These changes in pigmentation and lash growth may be permanent.

➤*Other forms of glaucoma:* There is limited experience with latanoprost in the treatment of angle closure, inflammatory or neovascular glaucoma.

➤*Infections:* There have been reports of bacterial keratitis associated with the use of multiple-dose containers of topical ophthalmic products. These containers had been inadvertently contaminated by patients who, in most cases, had a concurrent corneal disease or a disruption of the ocular epithelial surface.

➤*Contact lenses:* Contact lenses should be removed prior to the administration of latanoprost, and may be reinserted 15 minutes after administration.

➤*Renal/Hepatic function impairment:* Latanoprost has not been studied in patients with renal or hepatic impairment and should therefore be used with caution in such patients.

➤*Special risk:*

Active intraocular inflammation (iritis/uveitis) – Latanoprost should be used with caution in patients with a history of intraocular inflammation (iritis/uveitis) and should generally not be used in patients with active intraocular inflammation.

Macular edema, including cystoid macular edema – Macular edema, including cystoid macular edema, has been reported during treatment with latanoprost. These reports have mainly occurred in aphakic patients, in pseudophakic patients with a torn posterior lens capsule, or in patients with known risk factors for macular edema. Latanoprost should be used with caution in patients who do not have an intact posterior capsule or who have known risk factors for macular edema.

➤*Pregnancy: Category C.* Reproduction studies have been performed in rats and rabbits. In rabbits an incidence of 4 of 16 dams had no viable fetuses at a dose that was approximately 80 times the maximum human dose, and the highest nonembryocidal dose in rabbits was approximately 15 times the maximum human dose.

There are no adequate and well-controlled studies in pregnant women. Latanoprost should be used during pregnancy only if the potential benefit justifies the potential risk to the fetus.

➤*Lactation:* It is not known whether this drug or its metabolites are excreted in human milk. Because many drugs are excreted in human milk, caution should be exercised when latanoprost is administered to a nursing woman.

➤*Children:* Safety and effectiveness in pediatric patients have not been established.

➤*Monitoring:* Latanoprost is hydrolyzed in the cornea. The effect of continued administration of latanoprost sterile ophthalmic solution on the corneal endothelium has not been fully evaluated. Latanoprost sterile ophthalmic solution may gradually increase the pigmentation of the iris. The eye color change is due to increased melanin content in the stromal melanocytes of the iris rather than to an increase in the number of melanocytes. This change may not be noticeable for several months to years. Typically the brown pigmentation around the pupil spreads concentrically towards the periphery of the iris and the entire iris or parts of the iris become more brownish. Neither nevi nor freckles of the iris appear to be affected by treatment. While treatment with latanoprost can be continued in patients who develop noticeably increased iris pigmentation, these patients should be examined regularly and, depending on the clinical situation, treatment may be stopped if increased pigmentation ensues.

During clinical trials, the increase in brown iris pigment has not been shown to progress further upon discontinuation of treatment, but the resultant color change may be permanent.

Drug Interactions

In vitro studies have shown that precipitation occurs when eye drops containing thimerosal are mixed with latanoprost. If such drugs are used they should be administered with an interval of at least 5 minutes between applications.

Adverse Reactions

➤*Adverse reactions referred to in other sections:* Eyelash changes (increased length, thickness, pigmentation, and number of lashes); eyelid skin darkening; intraocular inflammation (iritis/uveitis); iris pigmentation changes; and macular edema, including cystoid macular edema.

➤*Adverse reactions in controlled clinical trials:* Local conjunctival hyperemia was observed; however, less than 1% of the patients treated with latanoprost required discontinuation of therapy because of intolerance to conjunctival hyperemia.

Ophthalmic – The ocular adverse reactions and ocular signs and symptoms reported in 5% to 15% of the patients on latanoprost sterile ophthalmic solution in the 6-month, multicenter, double-masked, active-controlled trials were blurred vision, burning and stinging, conjunctival hyperemia, foreign body sensation, itching, increased pigmentation of the iris, and punctate epithelial keratopathy.

In addition to the above listed ocular reactions/signs and symptoms, the following were reported in 1% to 4% of the patients: Dry eye, excessive tearing, eye pain, lid crusting, lid discomfort/pain, lid edema, lid erythema, and photophobia.

The following events were reported in less than 1% of the patients: Conjunctivitis, diplopia and discharge from the eye. During clinical studies, there were extremely rare reports of the following: Retinal artery embolus, retinal detachment, and vitreous hemorrhage from diabetic retinopathy.

Systemic – The most common systemic adverse reactions seen with latanoprost were upper respiratory tract infection/cold/flu which occurred at a rate of approximately 4%. Chest pain/angina pectoris, muscle/joint/back pain, and rash/allergic skin reaction each occurred at a rate of 1% to 2%.

➤*Postmarketing:* The following reactions have been identified during postmarketing use of latanoprost in clinical practice. Because they are reported voluntarily from a population of unknown size, estimates of frequency cannot be made. The reactions, which have been chosen for inclusion due to either their seriousness, frequency of reporting, possible causal connection to latanoprost, or a combination of these factors, include the following: Asthma and exacerbation of asthma; corneal edema and erosions; dyspnea; eyelash changes (increased length, thickness, pigmentation, and number); vellus hair changes (increased length, thickness, pigmentation, and number); eyelid skin darkening; herpes keratitis; intraocular inflammation (iritis/uveitis); keratitis; macular edema, including cystoid macular edema; misdirected eyelashes sometimes resulting in eye irritation; and toxic epidermal necrolysis.

Overdosage

➤*Symptoms:* Apart from ocular irritation and conjunctival or episcleral hyperemia, the ocular effects of latanoprost administered at high doses are not known. Intravenous administration of large doses of latanoprost in monkeys has been associated with transient bronchoconstriction; however, in 11 patients with bronchial asthma treated with latanoprost, bronchoconstriction was not induced. Intravenous infusion of up to 3 mcg/kg in healthy volunteers produced mean plasma concentrations 200 times higher than during clinical treatment and no adverse reactions were observed. Intravenous dosages of 5.5 to 10 mcg/kg caused abdominal pain, dizziness, fatigue, hot flushes, nausea and sweating.

➤*Treatment:* If overdosage with latanoprost sterile ophthalmic solution occurs, treatment should be symptomatic.

Patient Information

Patients should be advised about the potential for increased brown pigmentation of the iris, which may be permanent. Patients should also be informed about the possibility of eyelid skin darkening, which may be reversible after discontinuation of latanoprost.

Patients should also be informed of the possibility of eyelash and vellus hair changes in the treated eye during treatment with latanoprost. These changes may result in a disparity between eyes in length, thickness, pigmentation, number of eyelashes or vellus hairs, or direction of eyelash growth. Eyelash changes are usually reversible upon discontinuation of treatment.

The increased pigmentation to the iris and eyelid, as well as the changes to the eyelashes, may be permanent.

Patients should be instructed to avoid allowing the tip of the dispensing container to contact the eye or surrounding structures because this could cause the tip to become contaminated by common bacteria known to cause ocular infections. Serious damage to the eye and subsequent loss of vision may result from using contaminated solutions.

Patients also should be advised that if they develop an intercurrent ocular condition (eg, trauma, or infection) or have ocular surgery, they should immediately seek their physician's advice concerning the continued use of the multidose container.

Patients should be advised that if they develop any ocular reactions, particularly conjunctivitis and lid reactions, they should immediately seek their physician's advice.

Patients should also be advised that latanoprost contains benzalkonium chloride which may be absorbed by contact lenses. Contact lenses should be removed prior to administration of the solution. Lenses may be reinserted 15 minutes following administration of latanoprost. If more than 1 topical ophthalmic drug is being used, the drugs should be administered at least 5 minutes apart.

TRAVOPROST

Rx	Travatan Z (Alcon)	Solution: 0.004%	Polyoxyl 40 hydrogenated castor oil, *sofZia*[a] as a preservative. In 2.5 and 5 mL *Drop-Tainers.*

[a] Boric acid, propylene glycol, sorbitol, zinc chloride.

TRAVOPROST — OPHTHALMIC

Indications

➤*Elevated intraocular pressure:* For the reduction of elevated intraocular pressure in patients with open-angle glaucoma or ocular hypertension who are intolerant of other intraocular pressure-lowering medications or insufficiently responsive (failed to achieve target IOP determined after multiple measurements over time) to another intraocular pressure-lowering medication.

Administration and Dosage

➤*Adults:*

Elevated intraocular pressure –

Usual dosage: 1 drop in the affected eye(s) once daily in the evening.

Maximum dose: The dosage should not exceed once daily because it has been shown that more frequent administration may decrease the intraocular pressure–lowering effect.

Concomitant therapy: May be used concomitantly with other topical ophthalmic drug products to lower intraocular pressure.

➤*Administration:* If more than 1 topical ophthalmic drug is being used, the drugs should be administered at least 5 minutes apart. Travoprost should not be administered while wearing contact lenses. Remove contact lenses prior to and for 15 minutes following administration.

➤*Storage/Stability:* Store at 2° to 25°C (36° to 77°F).

Actions

➤*Pharmacology:* Travoprost free acid is a selective FP prostanoid receptor agonist which is believed to reduce intraocular pressure by increasing uveoscleral outflow. The exact mechanism of action is unknown at this time.

➤*Pharmacokinetics:*

Absorption – Travoprost is absorbed through the cornea and is hydrolyzed to the active free acid. Data from 4 multiple-dose pharmacokinetic studies (totaling 107 subjects) have shown that plasma concentrations of the free acid are below 0.01 ng/mL (the quantitation limit of the assay) in two-thirds of the subjects. In those individuals with quantifiable plasma concentrations (n = 38), the mean plasma C_{max} was 0.018 ± 007 ng/mL (ranged 0.01 to 0.052 ng/mL) and was reached within 30 minutes. From these studies, travoprost is estimated to have a plasma half-life of 45 minutes. There was no difference in plasma concentrations between days 1 and 7, indicating steady-state was reached early and that there was no significant accumulation.

Metabolism – Travoprost, an isopropyl ester prodrug, is hydrolyzed by esterases in the cornea to its biologically active free acid. Systemically, travoprost free acid is metabolized to inactive metabolites via beta-oxidation of the α(carboxylic acid) chain to give the 1,2-dinor and 1,2,3,4-tetranor analogs, via oxidation of the 15-hydroxyl moiety, as well as via reduction of the 13, 14 double bond.

Excretion – Elimination of travoprost free acid from human plasma was rapid and levels were generally below the limit of quantification within 1 hour after dosing. The terminal elimination half-life of travoprost free acid was estimated from 14 subjects and ranged from 17 minutes to 86 minutes with the mean half-life of 45 minutes. Less than 2% of the topical ocular dose of travoprost was excreted in the urine within 4 hours as the travoprost free acid.

Contraindications

Known hypersensitivity to travoprost, benzalkonium chloride, or any other ingredients in this product. Travoprost may interfere with the maintenance of pregnancy and should not be used by women during pregnancy or by women attempting to become pregnant.

Warnings/Precautions

➤*Ocular pigment changes:* Travoprost has been reported to cause changes to pigmented tissues. The most frequently reported changes have been increased pigmentation of the iris and periorbital tissue (eyelid) and increased pigmentation and growth of eyelashes. These changes may be permanent.

Travoprost may gradually change eye color, increasing the amount of brown pigmentation in the iris by increasing the number of melanosomes (pigment granules) in melanocytes. The long-term effects on the melanocytes and the consequences of potential injury to the melanocytes or deposition of pigment granules to other areas of the eye are currently unknown. The change in iris color occurs slowly and may not be noticeable for months to years. Patients should be informed of the possibility of iris color change.

Eyelid skin darkening has been reported in association with the use of travoprost.

Travoprost may gradually change eyelashes in the treated eye; these changes include increased length, thickness, pigmentation, or number of lashes. Patients who are expected to receive treatment in only 1 eye should be informed about the potential for increased brown pigmentation of the iris, periorbital or eyelid tissue, and eyelashes in the treated eye and thus heterochromia between the eyes. They should also be advised of the potential for a disparity between the eyes in length, thickness, or number of eyelashes.

➤*Infections:* There have been reports of bacterial keratitis associated with the use of multiple-dose containers of topical ophthalmic products. These containers had been inadvertently contaminated by patients who, in most cases, had a concurrent corneal disease or a disruption of the epithelial surface.

➤*Other forms of glaucoma:* Travoprost has not been evaluated for the treatment of angle closure, inflammatory or neovascular glaucoma.

➤*Contact lenses:* Travoprost should not be administered while wearing contact lenses.

Patients should be advised that travoprost contains benzalkonium chloride which may be absorbed by contact lenses. Contact lenses should be removed prior to the administration of the solution. Lenses may be reinserted 15 minutes following administration of travoprost.

➤*Special risk:* Travoprost should be used with caution in patients with a history of intraocular inflammation (iritis/uveitis) and should generally not be used in patients with active intraocular inflammation.

Macular edema, including cystoid macular edema, has been reported during treatment with prostaglandin $F_{2\alpha}$ analogues. These reports have mainly occurred in aphakic patients, pseudophakic patients with a torn posterior lens capsule, or in patients with known risk factors for macular edema. Travoprost should be used with caution in these patients.

➤*Pregnancy: Category C.*

Teratogenic – Travoprost was teratogenic in rats, at an IV dose up to 10 mcg/kg/day (250 times the MRHOD), evidenced by an increase in the incidence of skeletal malformations as well as external and visceral malformations, such as fused sternebrae, domed head and hydrocephaly. Travoprost was not teratogenic in rats at IV doses up to 3 mcg/kg/day (75 times the MRHOD), and in mice at subcutaneous doses up to 1 mcg/kg/day (25 times the MRHOD). Travoprost produced an increase in post-implantation losses and a decrease in fetal viability in rats at IV doses greater than 3 mcg/kg/day (75 times the MRHOD) and in mice at subcutaneous doses greater than 0.3 mcg/kg/day (7.5 times the MRHOD).

In the offspring of female rats that received travoprost subcutaneously from day 7 of pregnancy to lactation day 21 at the doses of greater than or equal to 0.12 mcg/kg/day (3 times the MRHOD), the incidence of postnatal mortality was increased, and neonatal body weight gain was decreased. Neonatal development was also affected, evidenced by delayed eye opening, pinna detachment and preputial separation, and by decreased motor activity.

No adequate and well-controlled studies have been performed in pregnant women. Travoprost may interfere with the maintenance of pregnancy and should not be used by women during pregnancy or by women attempting to become pregnant.

Since prostaglandins are biologically active and may be absorbed through the skin, women who are pregnant or attempting to become pregnant should exercise appropriate precautions to avoid direct exposure to the contents of the bottle. In case of accidental contact with the contents of the bottle, thoroughly cleanse the exposed area with soap and water immediately.

➤*Lactation:* A study in lactating rats demonstrated that radiolabeled travoprost or its metabolites were excreted in milk. It is not known whether this drug or its metabolites are excreted in human milk. Because many drugs are excreted in human milk, caution should be exercised when travoprost is administered to a nursing woman.

➤*Children:* Safety and efficacy in pediatric patients have not been established.

➤*Monitoring:* Patients may slowly develop increased brown pigmentation of the iris. This change may not be noticeable for months to years. Iris pigmentation changes may be more noticeable in patients with mixed colored irides (ie, blue-brown, grey-brown, yellow-brown, and green-brown); however, it has also been observed in patients with brown eyes. The color change is believed to be due to increased melanin content in the stromal melanocytes of the iris. The exact mechanism of action is unknown at this time. Typically, the brown pigmentation around the pupil spreads concentrically towards the periphery in affected eyes, but the entire iris or parts of it may become more brownish. Until more information about increased brown pigmentation is available, patients should be examined regularly and, depending on the situation, treatment may be stopped if increased pigmentation ensues.

Adverse Reactions

The most common ocular adverse event observed in controlled clinical studies with travoprost 0.004% was ocular hyperemia which was reported in 35% to 50% of patients. Approximately 3% of patients discontinued therapy due to conjunctival hyperemia.

Ocular adverse events reported at an incidence of 5% to 10% included decreased visual acuity, eye discomfort, foreign body sensation, pain, and pruritus.

Ocular adverse events reported at an incidence of 1% to 4% included, abnormal vision, blepharitis, blurred vision, cataract, cells, conjunctivitis, dry eye, eye disorder, flare, iris discoloration, keratitis, lid margin crusting, photophobia, subconjunctival hemorrhage, and tearing.

TRAVOPROST — OPHTHALMIC

Nonocular adverse events reported at a rate of 1% to 5% were accidental injury, angina pectoris, anxiety, arthritis, back pain, bradycardia, bronchitis, chest pain, cold syndrome, depression, dyspepsia, gastrointestinal disorder, headache, hypercholesterolemia, hypertension, hypotension, infection, pain, prostate disorder, sinusitis, urinary incontinence, and urinary tract infection.

Patient Information

Patients should also be instructed to avoid allowing the tip of the dispensing container to contact the eye or surrounding structures because this could cause the tip to become contaminated by common bacteria known to cause ocular infections. Serious damage to the eye and subsequent loss of vision may result from using contaminated solutions.

Patients also should be advised that if they develop an intercurrent ocular condition (eg, trauma, infection) or have ocular surgery, they should immediately seek their physician's advice concerning the continued use of the multi-dose container.

Patients should be advised that if they develop any ocular reactions, particularly conjunctivitis and lid reactions, they should immediately seek their physician's advice.

If more than 1 topical ophthalmic drug is being used, the drugs should be administered at least 5 minutes apart.

Travoprost has been reported to cause changes to pigmented tissues. The most frequently reported changes have been increased pigmentation of the iris and periorbital tissue (eyelid) and increased pigmentation and growth of eyelashes. These changes may be permanent.

Travoprost should not be administered while wearing contact lenses.

Travoprost should be used with caution in patients with a history of intraocular inflammation (iritis/uveitis) and should generally not be used in patients with active intraocular inflammation.

BIMATOPROST

Rx	**Lumigan** (Allergan)	**Solution; ophthalmic:** 0.03%	Benzalkonium chloride. In 2.5, 5, and 7.5 mL.
Rx	**Latisse** (Allergan)		Benzalkonium chloride. In 3 mL with 60 disposable applicators.

BIMATOPROST — OPHTHALMIC

Indications

➤*Elevated intraocular pressure (Lumigan)*: For the reduction of elevated intraocular pressure (IOP) in patients with open-angle glaucoma or ocular hypertension.

➤*Hypotrichosis of the eyelashes (Latisse)*: For the treatment of hypotrichosis of the eyelashes by increasing their growth, including length, thickness, and darkness.

Administration and Dosage

➤*Adults:*

Elevated intraocular pressure –

Usual dosage: 1 drop in the affected eye(s) once daily in the evening. Reduction of the IOP starts approximately 4 hours after the first administration, with maximum effect reached within approximately 8 to 12 hours.

Maximum dose: Do not exceed once-daily dosing because it has been shown that more frequent administration may decrease the IOP-lowering effect.

Concomitant therapy: Bimatoprost may be used concomitantly with other topical ophthalmic drug products to lower IOP. If more than 1 topical ophthalmic drug is being used, the drugs should be administered at least 5 minutes apart.

Hypotrichosis of the eyelashes – Advise patients to ensure their face is clean and that makeup and contact lenses are removed. Once nightly, patients should place 1 drop of bimatoprost 0.03% ophthalmic solution on the disposable sterile applicator supplied with the package and apply evenly along the skin of the upper eyelid margin at the base of the eyelashes. Bimatoprost should not be applied to the lower eyelash line. The upper lid margin in the area of lash growth should feel lightly moist without runoff. Any excess solution runoff outside the upper eyelid margin should be blotted with a tissue or other absorbent cloth. The applicator should be disposed of after one use. This procedure should be repeated for the opposite eyelid margin using a new sterile applicator.

➤*Administration:*

Hypotrichosis of the eyelashes – Applicators should not be reused and other brushes/applicators should not be used to apply bimatoprost.

➤*Storage/Stability:* Store in the original container at 2° to 25°C (36° to 77°F).

Actions

➤*Pharmacology:* Bimatoprost is a prostamide, a synthetic structural analog of prostaglandin with ocular hypotensive activity. It selectively mimics the effects of naturally occurring substances, prostamides. Bimatoprost is believed to lower IOP in humans by increasing outflow of aqueous humor through the trabecular meshwork and uveoscleral routes. Elevated IOP presents a major risk factor for glaucomatous field loss. The higher the level of IOP, the greater the likelihood of optic nerve damage and visual field loss. The precise mechanism of action in hypotrichosis of the eyelashes is unknown, but the growth of eyelashes is believed to occur by increasing the percent of hairs in, and the duration of, the anagen or growth phase.

➤*Pharmacokinetics:*

Absorption – After 1 drop of bimatoprost was administered once daily to both eyes (cornea and/or conjunctival sac) of 15 healthy subjects for 2 weeks, blood concentrations peaked within 10 minutes after dosing and were below the lower limit of detection (0.025 ng/mL) in most subjects within 1.5 hours after dosing. Mean maximum plasma concentrations (C_{max}) and area under the curve ($AUC_{0\text{-}24h}$) values were similar on days 7 and 14 at approximately 0.08 ng/mL and 0.09 ng•h/mL, respectively, indicating that steady state was reached during the first week of ocular dosing. There was no significant systemic drug accumulation over time.

Distribution – Bimatoprost is moderately distributed into body tissues with a steady-state volume of distribution of 0.67 L/kg. In human blood, bimatoprost resides mainly in the plasma. Approximately 12% of bimatoprost remains unbound in human plasma.

Metabolism – Bimatoprost is the major circulating species in the blood once it reaches the systemic circulation following ocular dosing. Bimatoprost then undergoes oxidation, N-deethylation, and glucuronidation to form a diverse variety of metabolites.

Excretion – Following an intravenous dose of radiolabeled bimatoprost (3.12 mcg/kg) to 6 healthy subjects, the C_{max} of unchanged drug was 12.2 ng/mL and decreased rapidly, with an elimination half-life of approximately 45 minutes. The total blood clearance of bimatoprost was 1.5 L/h/kg. Up to 67% of the administered dose was excreted in the urine, while 25% of the dose was recovered in the feces.

Contraindications

Hypersensitivity to bimatoprost or any other ingredient in this product.

Warnings/Precautions

➤*Ocular pigment changes:* Bimatoprost has been reported to cause changes to pigmented tissues. The most frequently reported changes have been increased pigmentation of the iris, periorbital tissue (eyelid), and eyelashes, as well as increased growth of eyelashes. Pigmentation is expected to increase as long as bimatoprost is administered. After discontinuation of bimatoprost, pigmentation of the iris is likely to be permanent, while pigmentation of the periorbital tissue and eyelash changes have been reported to be reversible in some patients. Inform patients who receive treatment of the possibility of increased pigmentation. The effects of pigmentation beyond 5 years are not known.

➤*Eye color changes:* Bimatoprost may gradually increase the pigmentation of the iris. The eye color change is due to increased melanin content in the stromal melanocytes of the iris, rather than to an increase in the number of melanocytes. This change may not be noticeable for several months to years. Typically, the brown pigmentation around the pupil spreads concentrically toward the periphery of the iris and the entire iris or parts of the iris become more brownish. Neither nevi nor freckles of the iris appear to be affected by treatment. While treatment with bimatoprost can be continued in patients who develop increased iris pigmentation, examine these patients regularly.

During clinical trials, the increase in brown iris pigment has not been shown to progress further upon discontinuation of treatment, but the resultant color change may be permanent.

➤*Eyelid skin darkening:* Eyelid skin darkening, which may be reversible upon discontinuation of treatment, has been reported in association with the use of bimatoprost.

Bimatoprost may gradually change eyelashes and vellus hair in the treated eye; these changes include increased length, thickness, and number of lashes. Eyelash changes are usually reversible upon discontinuation of treatment.

➤*Hair growth:* There is a potential for hair growth to occur in areas where bimatoprost solution comes in repeated contact with the skin surface. It is important to apply bimatoprost for hypotrichosis of the eyelashes only to the skin of the upper eyelid margin at the base of the eyelashes using the accompanying sterile applicators, and to carefully blot any excess solution from the eyelid margin to avoid it running onto the cheek or other skin areas.

➤*Active intraocular inflammation:* Use bimatoprost with caution in patients with active intraocular inflammation (eg, uveitis) because the inflammation may be exacerbated.

➤*Macular edema:* Macular edema, including cystoid macular edema, has been reported during treatment with bimatoprost for elevated IOP. Use bimatoprost with caution in aphakic patients, pseudophakic patients with a torn posterior lens capsule, and patients with known risk factors for macular edema.

➤*Contact lenses:* These products contain benzalkonium chloride, which may be absorbed by soft contact lenses. Contact lenses should be removed prior to instillation of bimatoprost; they may be reinserted 15 minutes following its administration.

➤*Pregnancy: Category C.* In embryo/fetal developmental studies in pregnant mice and rats, abortion was observed at oral doses of bimatoprost that

BIMATOPROST — OPHTHALMIC

achieved at least 33 or 97 times, respectively, the intended human exposure based on blood AUC levels after topical ophthalmic administration to the cornea or conjunctival sac.

At doses 41 times the intended human exposure based on blood AUC levels, the gestation length was reduced in dams; the incidence of dead fetuses, late resorptions, and peri- and postnatal pup mortality were increased; and pup body weights were reduced.

There are no adequate and well-controlled studies of bimatoprost in pregnant women. Because animal reproductive studies are not always predictive of human response, administer bimatoprost during pregnancy only if the potential benefit justifies the potential risk to the fetus.

➤*Lactation:* It is not known whether bimatoprost is excreted in human milk, although in animal studies, bimatoprost has been shown to be excreted in breast milk. Because many drugs are excreted in human milk, exercise caution when bimatoprost is administered to a breast-feeding woman.

➤*Children:* Safety and efficacy in children have not been established.

Drug Interactions

➤*Prostaglandin analogs:* In ocular hypertension studies with *Lumigan*, it has been shown that exposure of the eye to more than 1 dose of bimatoprost daily may decrease the IOP-lowering effect. In patients using *Lumigan* or other prostaglandin analogs for the treatment of elevated IOP, the concomitant use of *Latisse* may interfere with the desired reduction in IOP. Patients using prostaglandin analogs, including *Lumigan*, for IOP reduction should only use *Latisse* after consulting with their health care provider and should be monitored for changes to their IOP.

Adverse Reactions

➤*Lumigan:*

Most frequent ophthalmic adverse reactions – Conjunctival hyperemia, growth of eyelashes, ocular pruritus (15% to 45%).

Discontinuation: Approximately 3% of patients discontinued therapy because of conjunctival hyperemia.

Other ophthalmic adverse reactions: Blepharitis, cataract, eye pain, eyelash darkening, eyelid erythema, foreign body sensation, ocular burning, ocular dryness, ocular irritation, pigmentation of the periocular skin, superficial punctate keratitis, visual disturbance (3% to 10%); allergic conjunctivitis, asthenopia, conjunctival edema, eye discharge, increases in iris pigmentation, photophobia, tearing (1% to 3%); intraocular inflammation reported as iritis (less than 1%).

Systemic adverse reactions – Infections (primarily colds and upper respiratory tract infections) (10%); abnormal liver function tests, asthenia, headaches, hirsutism (1% to 5%).

➤*Latisse:*

Most frequent adverse reactions: Conjunctival hyperemia, dry eye symptoms, erythema of the eyelid, eye pruritis, ocular irritation, skin hyperpigmentation (less than 4%).

Patient Information

Advise patients about the potential for increased brown pigmentation of the iris, which may be permanent. Inform patients about the possibility of eyelid skin darkening, which may be reversible after discontinuation of bimatoprost.

Inform patients of the possibility of eyelash and vellus hair changes in the treated eye during treatment with bimatoprost. These changes may result in a disparity between eyes in length, thickness, pigmentation, number of eyelashes or vellus hairs, and/or direction of eyelash growth. Eyelash changes are usually reversible upon discontinuation of treatment.

Instruct patients to avoid allowing the tip of the dispensing container to contact the eye, surrounding structures, fingers, or any other surface in order to avoid contamination of the solution by common bacteria known to cause ocular infections. Serious damage to the eye and subsequent loss of vision may result from using contaminated solutions.

Advise patients to immediately seek their health care provider's advice concerning the continued use of the multidose container if they develop an intercurrent ocular condition (eg, trauma, infection), have ocular surgery, experience a sudden decrease in visual acuity, or develop any ocular reactions, particularly conjunctivitis and eyelid reactions.

Advise patients to immediately seek their health care provider's advice if they develop any ocular reactions, particularly conjunctivitis and eyelid reactions.

Advise patients that bimatoprost contains benzalkonium chloride, which may be absorbed by soft contact lenses. Instruct patients to remove contact lenses prior to instillation of bimatoprost; they may be reinserted 15 minutes following its administration.

If more than 1 topical ophthalmic drug is being used, instruct the patient to wait at least 5 minutes between the administration of each drug.

Inform patients that additional applications of bimatoprost for hypotrichosis of the eyelashes will not increase the growth of eyelashes.

When using bimatoprost for hypotrichosis of the eyelashes, the onset of effect is gradual but is not significant in the majority of patients until 2 months. Counsel patients that the effect is not permanent and can be expected to gradually return to the original level upon discontinuation of treatment with bimatoprost.

Instruct patients using bimatoprost for hypotrichosis of the eyelashes to only use the applicator supplied with the product once and then discard because reuse could result in using a contaminated applicator. Serious infections may result from using contaminated solutions or applicators.

Latisse may lower IOP, although not to a level that will cause clinical harm.

In patients using *Lumigan* or other prostaglandin analogs for the treatment of elevated IOP, the concomitant use of *Latisse* may interfere with the desired reduction in IOP. Patients using prostaglandin analogs for IOP reduction should only use *Latisse* after consulting with their health care provider.

Patients on IOP-lowering medications should not use *Latisse* without prior consultation with their health care provider.

Combinations

DORZOLAMIDE HYDROCHLORIDE/TIMOLOL MALEATE

Rx	**Dorzolamide HCl/Timolol Maleate** (Various, eg, Hi-Tech, Prasco Labs)	**Solution; ophthalmic:** 2% dorzolamide/0.5% timolol	In 5 and 10 mL.[a]
Rx	**Cosopt** (Merck)		In 5 and 10 mL *Ocumeters*.[a]

[a] With 0.0075% benzalkonium chloride and mannitol.

DORZOLAMIDE HYDROCHLORIDE/TIMOLOL MALEATE — OPHTHALMIC

Refer to the general discussion of Carbonic Anhydrase Inhibitors and Beta-adrenergic Blocking Agents.

Indications

➤*Elevated intraocular pressure (IOP):* Treatment of elevated IOP in patients with ocular hypertension or open-angle glaucoma.

Administration and Dosage

➤*Adults:*

Elevated intraocular pressure – Instill one drop into the affected eye(s) 2 times daily.

➤*Administration:* If more than one topical ophthalmic drug is being used, the drugs should be administered at least 10 minutes apart.

➤*Storage/Stability:* Store between 15° and 25°C (59° and 77°F). Protect from light.

Warnings/Precautions

➤*Pregnancy: Category C.* Developmental studies with dorzolamide hydrochloride in rabbits at oral dosages of at least 2.5 mg/kg/day (31 times the recommended human ophthalmic dose) revealed malformations of the vertebral bodies. These malformations occurred at doses that caused metabolic acidosis with decreased body weight gain in dams and decreased fetal weights. No treatment-related malformations were seen at 1 mg/kg/day (13 times the recommended human ophthalmic dose).

Teratogenicity studies with timolol in mice, rats, and rabbits at oral doses of up to 50 mg/kg/day (7,000 times the systemic exposure following the maximum recommended human ophthalmic dose) demonstrated no evidence of fetal malformations. Although delayed fetal ossification was observed at this dose in rats, there were no adverse effects on postnatal development of offspring. Doses of 1,000 mg/kg/day (142,000 times the systemic exposure following the maximum recommended human ophthalmic dose) were maternotoxic in mice and resulted in an increased number of fetal resorption. Increased fetal resorption was also seen in rabbits at doses of 14,000 times the systemic exposure following the maximum recommended human ophthalmic dose, in this case without apparent maternal toxicity.

There are no adequate and well-controlled studies in pregnant women. Use during pregnancy only if the potential benefit justifies the potential risk to the fetus.

➤*Lactation:* It is not known whether dorzolamide is excreted in human milk. Timolol has been detected in human milk following oral and ophthalmic drug administration. Because of the potential for serious adverse reactions in breast-feeding infants, a decision should be made whether to discontinue the drug, taking into account the importance of the drug to the mother.

BRIMONIDINE TARTRATE/TIMOLOL

Rx	**Combigan** (Allergan Inc.)	**Solution; ophthalmic**: brimonidine tartrate 0.2%/timolol 0.5%	As timolol maleate 6.8 mg per mL. Benzalkonium chloride 0.005%. In 5, 10, and 15 mL bottles.

BRIMONIDINE TARTRATE/TIMOLOL MALEATE — OPHTHALMIC

Indications

➤*Elevated intraocular pressure (IOP):* For the reduction of elevated IOP in patients with glaucoma or ocular hypertension who require adjunctive or replacement therapy because of inadequately controlled IOP.

The IOP-lowering effect of brimonidine/timolol dosed twice daily was slightly less than that seen with the coadministration of timolol 0.5% dosed twice daily and brimonidine 0.2% dosed 3 times daily.

Administration and Dosage

➤*Adults:*

Elevated intraocular pressure – 1 drop in the affected eye(s) twice daily approximately every 12 hours.

➤*Children:*

Elevated intraocular pressure –

2 years of age and older: See Adults for dosing.

➤*Administration:* Benzalkonium chloride is a preservative in this product that may be absorbed by soft contact lenses. Advise patients wearing soft contact lenses to wait at least 15 minutes after instilling this medication before reinserting their lenses.

If more than 1 topical ophthalmic drug is being used, advise patients to administer the drugs at least 5 minutes apart.

➤*Storage/Stability:* Store between 15° and 25°C (59° and 77°F). Protect from light.

Actions

➤*Pharmacology:* Brimonidine/timolol ophthalmic solution is a selective alpha-2 adrenergic receptor agonist with a nonselective beta-adrenergic receptor inhibitor. Each of these 2 components decreases elevated IOP, whether or not associated with glaucoma. Elevated IOP is a major risk factor in the pathogenesis of optic nerve damage and glaucomatous visual field loss. The higher the level of IOP, the greater the likelihood of glaucomatous field loss and optic nerve damage.

Both brimonidine and timolol have a rapid onset of action, with peak ocular hypotensive effect seen at 2 hours postdosing for brimonidine and 1 to 2 hours for timolol.

Fluorophotometric studies in animals and humans suggest that brimonidine has a dual mechanism of action by reducing aqueous humor production and increasing nonpressure-dependent uveoscleral outflow.

Timolol is a beta-1 and beta-2 adrenergic receptor inhibitor that does not have significant intrinsic sympathomimetic, direct myocardial depressant, or local anesthetic (membrane-stabilizing) activity.

➤*Pharmacokinetics:*

Absorption – Systemic absorption of brimonidine and timolol was assessed in healthy volunteers and patients following topical dosing with brimonidine/timolol. Healthy volunteers dosed with 1 drop of brimonidine/timolol twice daily in both eyes for 7 days showed peak plasma brimonidine and timolol concentrations of 30 pg/mL and 400 pg/mL, respectively. Plasma concentrations of brimonidine peaked at 1 to 4 hours after ocular dosing. Peak plasma concentrations of timolol occurred approximately 1 to 3 hours postdose. In a crossover study of brimonidine/timolol, brimonidine 0.2%, and timolol 0.5% administered twice daily for 7 days in healthy volunteers, the mean brimonidine area under the curve (AUC) for brimonidine/timolol was 128 ± 61 pg•h/mL versus 141 ± 106 pg•h/mL for the respective monotherapy treatments; mean maximal drug concentration (C_{max}) values of brimonidine were comparable following brimonidine/timolol treatment versus monotherapy (32.7 ±15 pg/mL vs 34.7 ± 22.6 pg/mL, respectively). Mean timolol AUC for brimonidine/timolol was similar to that of the respective monotherapy treatment (2,919 ± 1,679 pg•h/mL vs 2,909 ± 1,231 pg•h/mL, respectively); mean C_{max} of timolol was approximately 20% lower following brimonidine/timolol treatment versus monotherapy.

In a parallel study in patients dosed twice daily with brimonidine/timolol, twice daily with timolol 0.5%, or 3 times daily with brimonidine 0.2%, 1-hour postdose plasma concentrations of timolol and brimonidine were approximately 30% to 40% lower with brimonidine/timolol than their respective monotherapy values. The lower plasma brimonidine concentrations with brimonidine/timolol appear to be because of twice-daily dosing for brimonidine/timolol versus 3-times-daily dosing with brimonidine 0.2%.

Distribution – The protein binding of timolol is approximately 60%. The protein binding of brimonidine has not been studied.

Metabolism – In humans, brimonidine is extensively metabolized by the liver. Timolol is partially metabolized by the liver.

Excretion – In the crossover study in healthy volunteers, the plasma concentration of brimonidine declined with a systemic half-life of approximately 3 hours. The apparent systemic half-life of timolol was about 7 hours after ocular administration.

Urinary excretion is the major route of elimination of brimonidine and its metabolites. Approximately 87% of an orally administered radioactive dose of brimonidine was eliminated within 120 hours, with 74% found in the urine. Unchanged timolol and its metabolites are excreted by the kidney.

Special populations –

Renal function impairment: A study of patients with renal failure showed that timolol was not readily removed by dialysis. The effect of dialysis on brimonidine pharmacokinetics in patients with renal failure is not known.

Contraindications

Bronchial asthma, a history of bronchial asthma, and/or severe chronic obstructive pulmonary disease (COPD); sinus bradycardia, second- or third-degree atrioventricular block, overt cardiac failure, and/or cardiogenic shock; known hypersensitivity reaction to any component of this medication.

Warnings/Precautions

➤*Respiratory reactions, including asthma:* Brimonidine/timolol contains timolol and, although administered topically, can be absorbed systemically. Therefore, the same types of adverse reactions found with systemic administration of beta-adrenergic blocking agents may occur with topical administration. For example, severe respiratory reactions, including death due to bronchospasm in patients with asthma, have been reported following systemic or ophthalmic administration of timolol.

➤*Cardiac failure:* Sympathetic stimulation may be essential for support of the circulation in individuals with diminished myocardial contractility; its inhibition by beta-adrenergic receptor blockage may precipitate more severe failure.

In patients without a history of cardiac failure, continued depression of the myocardium with beta-blocking agents over a period of time can, in some cases, lead to cardiac failure. At the first sign or symptom of cardiac failure, discontinue brimonidine/timolol.

➤*Obstructive pulmonary disease:* Patients with COPD (eg, chronic bronchitis, emphysema) of mild or moderate severity, bronchospastic disease, or a history of bronchospastic disease (other than bronchial asthma or a history of bronchial asthma in which brimonidine/timolol is contraindicated) should, in general, not receive beta-blocking agents, including brimonidine/timolol ophthalmic solution.

➤*Vascular insufficiency:* Brimonidine/timolol may potentiate syndromes associated with vascular insufficiency. Use brimonidine/timolol with caution in patients with depression, cerebral or coronary insufficiency, Raynaud phenomenon, orthostatic hypotension, or thromboangiitis obliterans.

➤*Increased reactivity to allergens:* While taking beta-blockers, patients with a history of atopy or a history of severe anaphylactic reactions to a variety of allergens may be more reactive to repeated accidental, diagnostic, or therapeutic challenge with such allergens. Such patients may be unresponsive to the usual doses of epinephrine used to treat anaphylactic reactions.

➤*Muscle weakness:* Beta-adrenergic blockade has been reported to potentiate muscle weakness consistent with certain myasthenic symptoms (eg, diplopia, generalized weakness, ptosis). Timolol has been reported rarely to increase muscle weakness in some patients with myasthenia gravis or myasthenic symptoms.

➤*Diabetes mellitus:* Administer beta-adrenergic blocking agents with caution in patients subject to spontaneous hypoglycemia or to diabetic patients (especially those with labile diabetes) who are receiving insulin or oral hypoglycemic agents. Beta-adrenergic receptor blocking agents may mask the signs and symptoms of acute hypoglycemia.

➤*Thyrotoxicosis:* Beta-adrenergic blocking agents may mask certain clinical signs (eg, tachycardia) of hyperthyroidism. Carefully manage patients suspected of developing thyrotoxicosis to avoid abrupt withdrawal of beta-adrenergic blocking agents that might precipitate a thyroid storm.

➤*Bacterial keratitis:* There have been reports of bacterial keratitis associated with the use of multidose containers of topical ophthalmic products. These containers had been inadvertently contaminated by patients who, in most cases, had a concurrent corneal disease or a disruption of the ocular epithelial surface.

➤*Benzalkonium chloride:* Benzalkonium chloride is a preservative in this product that may be absorbed by soft contact lenses. Advise patients wearing soft contact lenses to wait at least 15 minutes after instilling this medication before reinserting their lenses.

➤*Major surgery:* The necessity or desirability of withdrawal of beta-adrenergic blocking agents prior to major surgery is controversial. Beta-adrenergic receptor blockade impairs the ability of the heart to respond to beta-adrenergically mediated reflex stimuli. This may augment the risk of general anesthesia in surgical procedures. Some patients receiving beta-adrenergic receptor blocking agents have experienced protracted severe hypotension during anesthesia. Difficulty in restarting and maintaining the heartbeat has also been reported. For these reasons, in patients undergoing elective surgery, some authorities recommend gradual withdrawal of beta-adrenergic receptor blocking agents.

If necessary during surgery, the effects of beta-adrenergic blocking agents may be reversed by sufficient doses of adrenergic agonists.

➤*Pregnancy: Category C.* Teratogenicity studies have been performed in animals.

Brimonidine was not teratogenic when given orally during gestation days 6 through 15 in rats and days 6 through 18 in rabbits. The highest doses of brimonidine in rats (1.65 mg/kg/day) and rabbits (3.33 mg/kg/day) achieved

BRIMONIDINE TARTRATE/TIMOLOL MALEATE — OPHTHALMIC

AUC exposure values 580- and 37-fold higher, respectively, than similar values estimated in humans treated with brimonidine/timolol (1 drop in both eyes twice daily).

Teratogenicity studies with timolol in mice, rats, and rabbits at oral doses up to 50 mg/kg/day (4,200 times the maximum recommended human ocular dose of 0.012 mg/kg/day on a mg/kg basis) demonstrated no evidence of fetal malformations. Although delayed fetal ossification was observed at this dose in rats, there were no adverse effects on postnatal development of offspring. Doses of 1,000 mg/kg/day (83,000 times the maximum recommended human ocular dose) were maternotoxic in mice and resulted in an increased number of fetal resorptions. Increased fetal resorptions were also seen in rabbits at doses 8,300 times the maximum recommended human ocular dose without apparent maternotoxicity.

There are no adequate and well-controlled studies in pregnant women; however, in animal studies, brimonidine crossed the placenta and entered into the fetal circulation to a limited extent. Because animal reproduction studies are not always predictive of human response, use brimonidine/timolol during pregnancy only if the potential benefit to the mother justifies the potential risk to the fetus.

➤*Lactation:* Timolol has been detected in human milk following oral and ophthalmic drug administration. It is not known whether brimonidine is excreted in human milk; however, in animal studies, brimonidine has been shown to be excreted in breast milk. Because of the potential for serious adverse reactions from brimonidine/timolol in breast-feeding infants, decide whether to discontinue breast-feeding or to discontinue the drug, taking into account the importance of the drug to the mother.

➤*Children:* Brimonidine/timolol is not recommended for use in children younger than 2 years of age. During postmarketing surveillance, apnea, bradycardia, hypotension, hypothermia, hypotonia, and somnolence have been reported in infants receiving brimonidine. The safety and effectiveness of brimonidine and timolol have not been studied in children younger than 2 years of age.

The safety and effectiveness of brimonidine/timolol have been established in children 2 to 16 years of age. Use of brimonidine/timolol in these age groups is supported by evidence from adequate and well-controlled studies of brimonidine/timolol in adults with additional data from a study of the concomitant use of brimonidine tartrate 0.2% ophthalmic solution and timolol ophthalmic solution in pediatric glaucoma patients (2 to 7 years of age). In this study, brimonidine 0.2% ophthalmic solution was dosed 3 times daily as adjunctive therapy to beta-blockers. The most commonly observed adverse reactions were somnolence (50% to 83% in patients 2 to 6 years of age) and decreased alertness. In children 7 years of age or older (weighing more than 20 kg), somnolence appears to occur less frequently (25%). Approximately 16% of patients on brimonidine discontinued from the study because of somnolence.

Drug Interactions

Brimonidine/Timolol Drug Interactions[a]

Precipitant drug	Object drug		Description
Antihypertensives, cardiac glycosides	Brimonidine/timolol, ophthalmic	↑	Because brimonidine/timolol ophthalmic may reduce blood pressure, caution is advised in using drugs such as antihypertensives and/or cardiac glycosides with brimonidine/timolol ophthalmic solution.
MAOIs[b]	Brimonidine/timolol, ophthalmic	↑	MAOIs may interfere with the metabolism of brimonidine and potentially result in an increased systemic adverse reaction such as hypotension. Use with caution.
Quinidine	Brimonidine/timolol, ophthalmic	↑	Decreased heart rate and depression have been reported during combined treatment with timolol and quinidine, possibly because quinidine inhibits the metabolism of timolol with the P450 enzyme CYP2D6.
SSRIs[b]	Brimonidine/timolol, ophthalmic	↑	Decreased heart rate and depression have been reported during combined treatment with timolol and SSRIs, possibly because SSRIs inhibit the metabolism of timolol with the P450 enzyme CYP2D6.
Tricyclic antidepressants	Brimonidine/timolol, ophthalmic	↓	Tricyclic antidepressants can affect the metabolism and uptake of circulating amines. Coadministration may result in interference with IOP-lowering effect. Use with caution.
Brimonidine/timolol, ophthalmic	Beta-blockers, oral	↑	Potential additive effects of beta blockade, both systemic and on IOP, may occur during coadministration of oral beta-blockers and brimonidine/timolol ophthalmic. Concurrent use is not recommended.
Beta-blockers, oral	Brimonidine/timolol, ophthalmic		
Brimonidine/timolol, ophthalmic	Calcium antagonists	↑	Use caution in the coadministration of beta-blocking agents such as brimonidine/timolol ophthalmic and oral or intravenous calcium antagonists because of possible atrioventricular conduction disturbances, left ventricular failure, and hypotension. In patients with impaired cardiac function, avoid coadministration.
Brimonidine/timolol, ophthalmic	Catecholamine-depleting drugs (eg, reserpine)	↑	Coadministration of brimonidine/timolol ophthalmic with catecholamine-depleting drugs can cause additive effects and the production of hypotension and/or marked bradycardia, which may result in vertigo, syncope, or postural hypotension.
Catecholamine-depleting drugs (eg, reserpine)	Brimonidine/timolol, ophthalmic		
Brimonidine/timolol, ophthalmic	CNS depressants (eg, alcohol, anesthetics, barbiturates, opiates, sedatives)	↑	Consider the possibility of an additive or potentiating effect with CNS depressants.
Brimonidine/timolol, ophthalmic	Digitalis	↑	Coadministration of brimonidine/timolol ophthalmic with digitalis may have additive effects in prolonging atrioventricular conduction time.
Digitalis	Brimonidine/timolol, ophthalmic		

[a] ↑ = object drug increased; ↓ = object drug decreased.
[b] MAOIs = monoamine oxidase inhibitors; SSRIs = selective serotonin reuptake inhibitors.

Adverse Reactions

➤*Brimonidine/Timolol:* In clinical trials of 12 months' duration with brimonidine/timolol, the most frequent reactions associated with its use included the following:

Cardiovascular – Hypertension (1% to 5%).

CNS – Asthenia, depression, headache, somnolence (1% to 5%).

GI – Oral dryness (1% to 5%).

Ophthalmic – Allergic conjunctivitis, conjunctival folliculosis, conjunctival hyperemia, eye pruritus, ocular burning and stinging (5% to 15%); blepharitis, corneal erosion, epiphora, eye discharge, eye dryness, eye irritation, eye pain, eyelid edema, eyelid erythema, eyelid pruritus, foreign body sensation, superficial punctate keratitis, visual disturbance (1% to 5%).

Other adverse reactions that have been reported with the individual components of brimonidine/timolol are listed in the following sections.

➤*Brimonidine (0.1% to 0.2%):*

CNS – Dizziness, fatigue, insomnia.

GI – Abnormal taste, dyspepsia, GI disorder, taste perversion.

Hypersensitivity – Allergic reaction, ocular allergic reaction.

Ophthalmic – Blepharoconjunctivitis, blurred vision, cataract, conjunctival edema, conjunctival hemorrhage, conjunctivitis, follicular conjunctivitis, hordeolum, keratitis, lid disorder, photophobia, tearing, visual field defect, vitreous detachment, vitreous disorder, vitreous floaters, worsened visual acuity.

Respiratory – Bronchitis, cough, dyspnea, infection (primarily colds and respiratory infections), nasal dryness, pharyngitis, rhinitis, sinus infection, sinusitis.

Miscellaneous – Flu syndrome, hypercholesterolemia, hypotension, rash.

BRIMONIDINE TARTRATE/TIMOLOL MALEATE — OPHTHALMIC

➤*Timolol (ocular administration):*

Cardiovascular – Arrhythmia, bradycardia, cardiac arrest, cardiac failure, cerebral ischemia, cerebral vascular accident, claudication, heart block, palpitation, pulmonary edema, Raynaud phenomenon, syncope, worsening of angina pectoris.

CNS – Behavioral changes and psychic disturbances, including anxiety, confusion, disorientation, hallucinations, memory loss, and nervousness; increase in signs and symptoms of myasthenia gravis; insomnia; nightmares; paresthesia.

Dermatologic – Alopecia, psoriasiform rash or exacerbation of psoriasis.

Endocrine – Masked symptoms of hypoglycemia in diabetes patients.

GI – Anorexia, diarrhea, nausea.

GU – Decreased libido, impotence, Peyronie disease, retroperitoneal fibrosis.

Hypersensitivity – Signs and symptoms of systemic allergic reactions, including anaphylaxis, angioedema, generalized and localized rash, and urticaria.

Respiratory – Bronchospasm (predominantly in patients with pre-existing bronchospastic disease), dyspnea, nasal congestion, respiratory failure.

Special senses – Choroidal detachment following filtration surgery, cystoid macular edema, decreased corneal sensitivity, diplopia, pseudophemphigoid, ptosis, refractive changes, tinnitus.

Miscellaneous – Chest pain, cold hands and feet, edema, systemic lupus erythematosus.

➤*Postmarketing:*

Brimonidine (ophthalmic) – The reactions, which have been chosen for inclusion because of either their seriousness, frequency of reporting, possible causal connection to brimonidine ophthalmic solutions, or a combination of these factors, include:

Cardiovascular – Bradycardia, tachycardia; bradycardia, hypotension (infants).

CNS – Depression; hypothermia, hypotonia, somnolence (infants).

Dermatologic – Skin reactions (including erythema, eyelid pruritus, rash, and vasodilation).

GI – Nausea.

Ophthalmic – Iritis, keratoconjunctivitis sicca, miosis.

Respiratory – Apnea (infants).

Overdosage

➤*Symptoms:* No information is available on overdosage with brimonidine/timolol ophthalmic solution in humans. There have been reports of inadvertant overdosage with timolol ophthalmic solution resulting in systemic effects similar to those seen with systemic beta-adrenergic blocking agents such as dizziness, headache, shortness of breath, bradycardia, bronchospasm, and cardiac arrest.

➤*Treatment:* Treatment of an oral overdose includes supportive and symptomatic therapy; maintain a patent airway.

Patient Information

Advise patients with bronchial asthma, a history of bronchial asthma, severe COPD, sinus bradycardia, second- or third-degree atrioventricular block, or cardiac failure not to take this product.

Instruct patients that ocular solutions, if handled improperly or if the tip of the dispensing container contacts the eye or surrounding structures, can become contaminated by common bacteria known to cause ocular infections. Serious damage to the eye and subsequent loss of vision may result from using contaminated solutions.

Advise patients that if they have ocular surgery or develop an intercurrent ocular condition (eg, trauma, infection) to immediately seek their health care provider's advice concerning the continued use of the present multidose container.

If more than 1 topical ophthalmic drug is being used, advise patients to administer the drugs at least 5 minutes apart.

Advise patients that brimonidine/timolol contains benzalkonium chloride, which may be absorbed by soft contact lenses. Instruct patients to remove contact lenses prior to administration of the solution. Lenses may be reinserted 15 minutes following administration of brimonidine/timolol.

As with other similar medications, brimonidine/timolol may cause fatigue and/or drowsiness in some patients. Caution patients who engage in hazardous activities of the potential for a decrease in mental alertness.

Refer to the Topical Ophthalmic Drugs introduction for complete and comparative information.

Indications

➤*Bromfenac:* For the treatment of postoperative ocular inflammation and the reduction of ocular pain in patients who have undergone cataract extraction.

➤*Diclofenac:* For the treatment of postoperative ocular inflammation in patients who have undergone cataract extraction; for the temporary relief of pain and photophobia in patients undergoing corneal refractive surgery.

➤*Flurbiprofen:* For the inhibition of intraoperative miosis.

➤*Ketorolac:* For the reduction of ocular pain and burning/stinging following corneal refractive surgery (0.4% solution); for the temporary relief of ocular itching caused by seasonal conjunctivitis (0.5% solution); for the treatment of postoperative inflammation in patients who have undergone cataract extraction (0.5% solution); for the treatment of pain and inflammation following cataract surgery (0.45% solution).

➤*Nepafenac:* For the treatment of inflammation and pain associated with cataract surgery.

➤*Off-label uses:* For topical treatment of cystoid macular edema after cataract surgery (diclofenac and ketorolac).

Actions

➤*Pharmacology:* Flurbiprofen, bromfenac, nepafenac, diclofenac, and ketorolac are NSAIDs available as ophthalmic solutions. Flurbiprofen is a phenylalkanoic acid, diclofenac is a phenylacetic acid, and ketorolac tromethamine is a member of the pyrrolo-pyrrole group (eg, analgesic, antipyretic, anti-inflammatory activity). Their mechanism of action is believed to be through inhibition of the prostaglandin H synthase (cyclooxygenase enzyme), which is essential in the biosynthesis of prostaglandins. Nepafenac is a nonsteroidal anti-inflammatory and analgesic prodrug. After topical ocular dosing, nepafenec penetrates the cornea and is converted by ocular tissue hydrolases to amfenac, which is thought to inhibit the action of cyclooxygenase, an enzyme required for prostaglandin production.

In animals, prostaglandins are mediators of certain kinds of intraocular inflammation. Prostaglandins produce disruption of the blood-aqueous humor barrier, vasodilation, increased vascular permeability, leukocytosis, and increased intraocular pressure (IOP). These agents have no significant effect on IOP.

Prostaglandins also appear to play a role in the miotic response produced during ocular surgery by constricting the iris sphincter independently of cholinergic mechanisms. These agents inhibit the miosis induced during the course of cataract surgery.

➤*Pharmacokinetics:*

Bromfenac – Based on the maximum proposed dose of 1 drop (0.09 mg) to each eye, the systemic concentration is estimated to be below the limit of quantification (50 ng/mL) at steady state in humans.

Diclofenac – Results from a bioavailability study established that plasma levels following ocular instillation of 2 drops of diclofenac to each eye were below the limit of quantification (10 ng/mL) over a 4-hour period. This study suggests that limited, if any, systemic absorption occurs.

Ketorolac – When ketorolac 10 mg is administered systemically every 6 hours, peak plasma levels at steady state are around 960 ng/mL. After 1 drop (0.05 mL) of 0.5% ophthalmic solution was instilled, only 5 of 26 subjects had a detectable amount of ketorolac in plasma (range, 10.7 to 22.5 ng/mL) at day 10 during topical ocular treatment. Two drops (0.1 mL) of ketorolac 0.5% instilled into the eyes of patients 12 hours and 1 hour prior to cataract extraction achieved measurable levels in 8 of 9 patients' eyes (mean ketorolac concentration 95 ng/mL aqueous humor; range, 40 to 170 ng/mL) and the mean concentration of prostaglandin E2 was 28 pg/mL.

Nepafenac – Low but quantifiable plasma concentrations of nepafenac and amfenac were observed in the majority of subjects 2 and 3 hours postdose, respectively, following bilateral topical ocular 3 times daily dosing. The mean steady-state C_{max} for nepafenac and amfenac were 0.3 ± 0.104 mg/mL and 0.422 ± 0.121 ng/mL, respectively, following ocular administration.

Contraindications

Hypersensitivity to the drugs or any component of the products.

Warnings/Precautions

➤*Bleeding tendencies:* With some NSAIDs, there exists the potential for increased bleeding time caused by interference with thrombocyte aggregation. There have been reports that ocularly applied NSAIDs may cause increased bleeding of ocular tissues (including hyphemas) in conjunction with ocular surgery. Use with caution in surgical patients with known bleeding tendencies or in patients taking drugs known to cause bleeding (eg, anticoagulants).

➤*Cross-sensitivity:* The potential for cross-sensitivity to acetylsalicylic acid, phenylacetic acid derivatives, and other NSAIDs exists. Use caution when treating individuals who have previously exhibited sensitivities to these drugs.

➤*IOP:* Results from clinical studies indicate that topical NSAIDs have no significant effect upon ocular pressure. However, elevations in IOP may occur following cataract surgery.

➤*Duration of therapy:* Postmarketing experience with topical NSAIDs suggests that use more than 24 hours prior to surgery or beyond 14 days postsurgery may increase patient risk for the occurrence and severity of corneal adverse reactions.

➤*Wound healing:* Topical NSAIDs may slow or delay healing. Topical corticosteroids also are known to slow or delay healing. Concomitant use of topical NSAIDs and topical steroids may increase the potential for healing problems.

➤*Keratitis:* Use of topical NSAIDs may result in keratitis. In some susceptible patients, continued use of topical NSAIDs may result in epithelial breakdown, corneal thinning, corneal erosion, corneal ulceration, or corneal perforation. These events may be sight-threatening. If evidence of corneal epithelial breakdown appears, discontinue the drug immediately and closely monitor for corneal health.

➤*Contact lenses:* Do not administer medication while patients are wearing contact lenses.

➤*Sulfite sensitivity:* Bromfenac contains sodium sulfite, a sulfite that may cause allergic-type reactions, including anaphylactic symptoms and life-threatening or less severe asthmatic episodes, in certain susceptible people. The overall prevalence of sulfite sensitivity in the general population is unknown and probably low. Sulfite sensitivity is seen more frequently in asthmatic than in nonasthmatic people.

➤*Special risk:* Postmarketing experience with topical NSAIDs suggests that patients with complicated ocular surgeries, corneal denervation, corneal epithelial defects, diabetes mellitus, ocular surface diseases (eg, dry eye syndrome), rheumatoid arthritis, or repeat ocular surgeries within a short period of time may be at increased risk for corneal adverse reactions, which may become sight-threatening. Use topical NSAIDs with caution in these patients.

➤*Pregnancy:* *Category C.* **Flurbiprofen** is embryocidal, delays parturition, prolongs gestation, reduces weight, and/or slightly retards fetal growth in rats at daily oral doses of at least 0.4 mg/kg (approximately 300 times the human daily topical dose).

Oral dosages of **bromfenac** 0.9 mg/kg/day in rats caused embryofetal lethality, increased neonatal mortality, and reduced postnatal growth. Pregnant rabbits treated with 7.5 mg/kg/day had increased postimplantation loss.

Oral dosages of **nepafenac** of 10 mg/kg or more in rats were associated with dystocia, increased postimplantation loss, reduced fetal weights and growth, and reduced fetal survival. Nepafenac has been shown to cross the placental barrier in rats.

Oral dosages of **ketorolac** up to 45 times the maximum recommended human topical ophthalmic dose on a mg/kg basis administered after gestation day 17 caused dystocia and higher pup mortality in rats.

Oral **diclofenac** in mice and rats crosses the placental barrier. In rats, maternally toxic doses were associated with dystocia, prolonged gestation, and reduced fetal weights, growth, and survival.

There are no adequate and well-controlled studies in pregnant women. Use during pregnancy only if the potential benefits outweigh the potential hazards to the fetus.

Because of the known effects of prostaglandin biosynthesis–inhibiting drugs on the fetal cardiovascular system (closure of ductus arteriosis), avoid the use of ophthalmic NSAIDs during late pregnancy.

➤*Lactation:* It is not known whether **flurbiprofen** or **diclofenac** is excreted in breast milk. Because of the potential for serious adverse reactions in breast-fed infants, decide whether to discontinue breast-feeding or the drug, taking into account the importance of the drug to the mother.

Nepafenac is excreted in the milk of pregnant rats. It is not known whether this drug is excreted in human milk. Exercise caution when nepafenac is administered to a breast-feeding woman.

Exercise caution while **ketorolac** and/or **bromfenac** is administered to a breast-feeding woman.

➤*Children:* Safety and efficacy for use in children have not been established (**bromfenac**, **diclofenac**, **flurbiprofen**, **ketorolac** 0.45% solution). Safety and efficacy in children younger than 3 years of age (**ketorolac** 0.4% and 0.5% solution), and younger than 10 years of age (**nepafenac**), have not been established

➤*Monitoring:* The refractive stability of patients undergoing corneal refractive procedures who are treated with diclofenac has not been established. Monitor patients for a year following use in this setting.

Drug Interactions

➤*Acetylcholine and carbachol:* Although clinical and animal studies revealed no interference, and there is no known pharmacological basis for an interaction, acetylcholine and carbachol have reportedly been ineffective when used in patients treated with **flurbiprofen**.

Adverse Reactions

Bromfenac – Abnormal sensation in eye, conjunctival hyperemia, eye irritation (including burning/stinging), eye pain, eye pruritus, eye redness, headache, iritis (2% to 7%).

Diclofenac – Lacrimation (30%, cases undergoing incisional refractive surgery); keratitis (28%, although most cases occurred in cataract studies prior to drug therapy); elevated IOP (most cases occurred postsurgery and prior to drug therapy), stinging, transient burning (15%); abnormal vision, acute elevated IOP, blurred vision, conjunctivitis, corneal deposits, corneal edema, corneal opacity, corneal lesions, discharge, eyelid swelling, iritis, irritation, itching, lacrimation disorder, ocular allergy (5%); abdominal pain, asthenia, chills, dizziness, facial edema, fever, headache, insomnia, nausea, pain, rhinitis, viral infection, vomiting (no more than 3%).

Flurbiprofen – Fibrosis, increased bleeding tendency of ocular tissues in conjunction with ocular surgery, miosis, mydriasis, stinging upon instillation, transient burning.

Ketorolac – Stinging upon instillation, transient burning (20% to 40%); allergic reactions, corneal edema, iritis, ocular inflammation, ocular irritation, ocular pain, superficial keratitis, superficial ocular infections (1% to 10%); blurred vision, conjunctival hyperemia and/or hemorrhage, corneal edema, headache, increased intraocular pressure, ocular pain, tearing (1% to 6%, 0.45% solution); conjunctival hyperemia, corneal infiltrates, headache, ocular edema, ocular pain (1% to 5%, 0.4% solution); corneal ulcer, eye dryness, headache, visual disturbance such as blurry vision (rare, 0.5% solution).

Nepafenac – Capsular opacity, decreased visual acuity, foreign body sensation, increased IOP, sticky sensation (5% to 10%); conjunctival edema, corneal edema, dry eye, lid-margin crusting, ocular discomfort, ocular hyperemia, ocular pain, ocular pruritus, photophobia, tearing, vitreous detachment (1% to 5%); headache, hypertension, nausea, sinusitis, vomiting (1% to 4%).

➤*Postmarketing:*

Bromfenac, ketorolac – Corneal erosion, corneal perforation, corneal thinning, epithelial breakdown.

Diclofenac – Corneal erosion, corneal infiltrates, corneal perforation, corneal thinning, corneal ulceration, epithelial breakdown, superficial punctate keratitis.

Overdosage

Overdosage will not ordinarily cause acute problems. If accidentally ingested, instruct patient to drink fluids to dilute.

Patient Information

Instruct patients not to administer medication while wearing contact lenses.

If more than 1 topical ophthalmic medication is being used, administer the medicines at least 5 minutes apart.

Except for the use of a bandage hydrogel soft contact lens during the first 3 days following refractive surgery, **diclofenac** should not be used in patients currently wearing soft contact lenses.

Instruct patients to use the solution from 1 individual single-use **ketorolac** 0.45% vial immediately after opening for administration and inform the patients to discard the remaining contents immediately after administration.

Inform patients that slow or delayed healing may occur while using NSAIDs.

Inform patients that use of contaminated ocular solutions can cause ocular infection and serious damage to the eye with subsequent loss of vision. To avoid contamination, do not touch the tip of the dropper bottle to the eye or any other surface.

FLURBIPROFEN SODIUM

Rx	**Flurbiprofen Sodium** (Various, eg, Bausch & Lomb)	**Solution, ophthalmic:** 0.03%	In 2.5 mL.[a]
Rx	**Ocufen** (Allergan)		In 2.5 mL dropper bottles.[a]

[a] With polyvinyl alcohol 1.4%, thimerosal 0.005%, and EDTA.

FLURBIPROFEN SODIUM — OPHTHALMIC

For complete and comparative prescribing information, refer to the Ophthalmic NSAIDs group monograph.

Indications

➤*Intraoperative miosis:* For the inhibition of intraoperative miosis.

Administration and Dosage

➤*Adults:*

Intraoperative miosis – A total of 4 drops should be administered by instilling 1 drop approximately every 30 minutes beginning 2 hours before surgery.

➤*Storage/Stability:* Store between 15° and 25°C (59° and 79°F).

DICLOFENAC SODIUM

Rx	**Diclofenac Sodium** (Akorn)	**Solution; ophthalmic:** 0.1%	In 2.5 and 5 mL bottles with dropper.[a]
Rx	**Voltaren** (Novartis Pharmaceuticals)		In 2.5 and 5 mL dropper bottles.[a]

[a] With EDTA 1 mg/mL, boric acid, polyoxyl 35 castor oil, sorbic acid 2 mg/mL, and tromethamine.

DICLOFENAC SODIUM — OPHTHALMIC

For complete and comparative prescribing information, refer to the Ophthalmic NSAIDs group monograph.

Indications

➤*Postoperative ocular inflammation:* For the treatment of postoperative inflammation in patients who have undergone cataract extraction.

➤*Ocular pain/photophobia:* For the temporary relief of pain and photophobia in patients undergoing corneal refractive surgery.

Administration and Dosage

➤*Adults:*

Ocular pain/photophobia – Instill 1 or 2 drops of solution to the operative eye within the hour prior to corneal refractive surgery. Within 15 minutes after surgery, instill 1 or 2 drops to the operative eye and continue 4 times daily for up to 3 days.

Postoperative ocular inflammation – Instill 1 drop of solution to the affected eye 4 times daily beginning 24 hours after cataract surgery and continuing throughout the first 2 weeks of the postoperative period.

➤*Storage/Stability:* Store between 15° and 30°C (59° and 86°F). Protect from light. Dispense in original, unopened container only.

KETOROLAC TROMETHAMINE

Rx	**Ketorolac Tromethamine** (Apotex)	**Solution; ophthalmic:** 0.4%	May contain benzalkonium chloride, edetate disodium. In 5 and 10 mL dropper bottles.
Rx	**Acular LS** (Allergan)		In 5 mL dropper bottles.[a]
Rx	**Acuvail** (Allergan)	**Solution; ophthalmic:** 0.45%	Preservative free. In 0.4 mL single-use vials.[b]
Rx	**Ketorolac Tromethamine** (Apotex)	**Solution; ophthalmic:** 0.5%	May contain benzalkonium chloride, edetate disodium. In 3, 5, and 10 mL.
Rx	**Acular** (Allergan)		In 3, 5, and 10 mL dropper bottles.[c]

[a] With edetate disodium 0.015%, benzalkonium chloride 0.006%, sodium chloride, octoxynol 40, hydrochloric acid, and/or sodium hydroxide.
[b] With carboxymethylcellulose, sodium chloride, sodium citrate, and sodium hydroxide and/or hydrochloric acid.
[c] With benzalkonium chloride 0.01%, edetate disodium 0.1%, octoxynol 40, sodium chloride, hydrochloric acid, and/or sodium hydroxide.

KETOROLAC TROMETHAMINE — OPHTHALMIC

For complete and comparative prescribing information, refer to the Ophthalmic NSAIDs class monograph.

Indications

➤*Postoperative ocular inflammation following cataract extraction (0.5% solution):* For the treatment of postoperative inflammation in patients who have undergone cataract extraction.

➤*Postoperative ocular pain following corneal refractive surgery (0.4% solution):* For the reduction of ocular pain and burning/stinging following corneal refractive surgery.

➤*Postoperative ocular pain/inflammation following cataract surgery (0.45% solution):* For the treatment of pain and inflammation following cataract surgery.

➤*Seasonal allergic conjunctivitis (ocular itching) (0.5% solution):* For the temporary relief of ocular itching caused by seasonal allergic conjunctivitis.

Administration and Dosage

➤*General dosing considerations:* Postmarketing experience with topical nonsteroidal anti-inflammatory drugs (NSAIDs) suggests that use more than 24 hours prior to surgery or use beyond 14 days postsurgery may increase patient risk for the occurrence and severity of corneal adverse reactions.

KETOROLAC TROMETHAMINE — OPHTHALMIC

➤*Adults:*

0.4% solution –

Postoperative ocular pain following corneal refractive surgery:

• *Usual dosage* – Instill 1 drop 4 times daily in the operated eye as needed for up to 4 days following surgery.

• *Concomitant therapy* – May be administered in conjunction with other ophthalmic medications, such as antibiotics, beta-blockers, carbonic anhydrase inhibitors, cycloplegics, and mydriatics.

0.45% solution –

Postoperative ocular pain/inflammation following cataract surgery:

• *Usual dosage* – Instill 1 drop to the affected eye twice daily beginning 1 day prior to cataract surgery, continuing on the day of surgery and through the first 2 weeks of the postoperative period.

• *Concomitant therapy* – May be administered in conjunction with other topical ophthalmic medications, such as alpha-agonists, beta-blockers, cycloplegics, and mydriatics.

0.5% solution –

Postoperative ocular inflammation following cataract extraction: Instill 1 drop to the affected eye(s) 4 times daily beginning 24 hours after cataract surgery and continuing through the first 2 weeks of the postoperative period.

Seasonal allergic conjunctivitis (ocular itching): Instill 1 drop 4 times daily.

Concomitant therapy: May be administered in conjunction with other ophthalmic medications, such as antibiotics, beta-blockers, carbonic anhydrase inhibitors, cycloplegics, and mydriatics.

➤*Children:*

3 years of age and older –

0.4% solution: See Adults for dosing.

0.5% solution: See Adults for dosing.

➤*Administration:* For ophthalmic use only. If administering other ophthalmic products in conjunction with ketorolac, administer at least 5 minutes apart. Do not administer while wearing contact lenses.

➤*Storage/Stability:*

0.4% and 0.5% solutions – Store between 15° and 25°C (59° and 77°F). Protect from light.

0.45% solution – Store between 15° and 30°C (59° and 86°F). Store the vials in the pouch, protected from light. Fold pouch ends closed.

BROMFENAC

Rx	**Xibrom** (Ista Pharm)	**Solution, ophthalmic:** 0.09%	In 5 mL dropper bottles.[a]

[a] With benzalkonium chloride 0.05 mg/mL, EDTA 0.2 mg/mL, povidone 20 mg/mL, sodium sulfite 0.2 mg/mL, boric acid, sodium borate, and sodium hydroxide.

BROMFENAC — OPHTHALMIC

For complete and comparative prescribing information, refer to the Ophthalmic NSAIDs group monograph.

Indications

➤*Postoperative ocular inflammation/pain:* For the treatment of postoperative inflammation and the reduction of ocular pain in patients who have undergone cataract extraction.

Administration and Dosage

➤*Adults:*

Postoperative ocular inflammation/pain – Instill 1 drop to the affected eye(s) 2 times daily beginning 24 hours after cataract surgery and continuing through the first 2 weeks of the postoperative period.

➤*Storage/Stability:* Store at 15° to 25°C (59° to 77°F).

NEPAFENAC

Rx	**Nevanac** (Alcon)	**Suspension, ophthalmic:** 0.1%	In 3 mL dropper bottles.[a]

[a] With benzalkonium chloride 0.005%, EDTA, sodium chloride, tyloxapol, sodium hydroxide, and or hydrochloric acid.

NEPAFENAC — OPHTHALMIC

Indications

➤*Postoperative ocular inflammation/pain:* For the treatment of pain and inflammation associated with cataract surgery.

Administration and Dosage

➤*Adults:*

Postoperative ocular inflammation/pain – Instill 1 drop to the affected eye(s) 3 times daily beginning 1 day prior to cataract surgery; continue on the day of surgery, and through the first 2 weeks of the postoperative period.

➤*Children:*

Postoperative ocular inflammation/pain –

10 years of age and older: See Adults for dosing.

➤*Administration:* Shake well before use.

➤*Storage/Stability:* Store at 2° to 25°C (36° to 77°F).

OPHTHALMIC CORTICOSTEROIDS

Refer to the Topical Ophthalmics introduction for complete and comparative information on administration and use.

Indications

➤*General information:* See individual monographs for specific indications and administration and dosage.

➤*Corneal injury:* For the treatment of corneal injury from chemical, radiation, or thermal burns, or penetration of foreign bodies.

➤*Ophthalmic inflammatory conditions:* For the treatment of steroid-responsive inflammatory conditions of the palpebral and bulbar conjunctiva, cornea, and anterior segment of the globe such as allergic conjunctivitis, acne rosacea, cyclitis, superficial punctate keratitis, herpes zoster keratitis, iritis, and selected infective conjunctivitis; noninfectious uveitis affecting the posterior segment of the eye; and postoperative inflammation following ocular surgery.

➤*Otic inflammatory conditions:* Dexamethasone sodium phosphate solution is also approved for otic use. Refer to Dexamethasone Sodium Phosphate in Otic Corticosteroids for specific indications and administration and dosage.

Actions

➤*Pharmacology:* Ocular corticosteroids are thought to act by the induction of phospholipase A_2 inhibitory proteins, collectively called lipocortins. It is postulated that these proteins control the biosynthesis of potent mediators of inflammation such as prostaglandins and leukotrienes by inhibiting the release of their common precursor arachidonic acid. Arachidonic acid is released from membrane phospholipids by phospholipase A_2. Corticosteroids inhibit the inflammatory response to a variety of inciting agents that may delay or slow healing. They inhibit edema, fibrin deposition, capillary dilation, leukocyte migration, capillary proliferation, fibroblast proliferation, deposition of collagen, and scar formation associated with inflammation. Ocular corticosteroids are capable of producing a rise in intraocular pressure.

➤*Pharmacokinetics:*

Fluocinolone – Aqueous and vitreous humor samples were assayed for fluocinolone in a subset of patients. While detectable concentrations of fluocinolone were seen throughout the observation interval (up to 34 months), the concentrations were highly variable, ranging from below the limit of detection (0.2 ng/mL) to 589 ng/mL.

Rimexolone – Half-life is 1 to 2 hours.

Contraindications

Most viral diseases of the cornea and conjunctiva, including acute epithelial herpes simplex keratitis (dendritic keratitis), vaccinia, and varicella; mycobacterial infections of the eye and fungal disease of ocular structures; tuberculosis of the eye; acute, purulent untreated eye infections; known or suspected hypersensitivity to any of the ingredients in these preparations or to other corticosteroids.

The use of **prednisolone sodium phosphate** is contraindicated after uncomplicated removal of a superficial corneal foreign body.

Warnings/Precautions

➤*Prolonged use:* Prolonged use may result in glaucoma with damage to the optic nerve, defects in visual acuity and fields of vision, corneal and scleral thinning, and posterior subcapsular cataract formation. Prolonged use may suppress the host response and thus increase the hazard of secondary ocular infections.

➤*Glaucoma:* Use with caution in the presence of glaucoma.

➤*Visual acuity:* Following the implantation of **fluocinolone**, nearly all patients will experience an immediate and temporary decrease in visual acuity in the implanted eye, which lasts for approximately 1 to 4 weeks post-operatively.

➤*Cataract surgery:* Nearly all phakic eyes are expected to develop cataracts and require cataract surgery. The use of topical steroids after cataract surgery may delay healing and increase the incidence of bleb formation.

➤*Perforation:* In those diseases causing thinning of the cornea or sclera, perforations have been known to occur with the use of topical steroids.

➤*Infections:* Use of ocular steroids may prolong the course and exacerbate the severity of many viral infections of the eye (including herpes simplex). Employment of a corticosteroid in the treatment of patients with a history of herpes simplex requires great caution and frequent slit-lamp examinations. In acute purulent conditions of the eye, steroids may mask infection or enhance existing infection.

➤*Administration:* For topical ophthalmic use only; not for injection. Dexamethasone sodium phosphate solution is also approved for otic use.

➤*Fungal infection:* Fungal infections of the cornea are particularly prone to develop coincidentally with long-term local steroid application. Consider fungal invasion in any persistent corneal ulceration where a steroid has been or is currently used. Take fungal cultures when appropriate.

➤*Corneal healing:* Ophthalmic ointments may retard corneal healing.

➤*Bilateral implantation:* In order to limit the potential for bilateral post-operative infection, do not carry out simultaneous bilateral implantation.

➤*Benzalkonium chloride:* Benzalkonium chloride is a preservative that can be absorbed by soft contact lenses and is used in some of the products.

➤*Sulfite sensitivity:* **Dexamethasone sodium phosphate** and **prednisolone acetate** contain sodium bisulfite that may cause allergic type reactions in susceptible people.

➤*Pregnancy: Category C.* Corticosteroids are generally teratogenic in laboratory animals when administered systemically at relatively low dosage levels. There are no adequate and well-controlled studies in pregnant women. Use during pregnancy only if the potential benefit justifies the potential risk to the fetus. Carefully observe infants born to mothers who have received substantial doses of corticosteroids during pregnancy for signs of hypoadrenalism.

➤*Lactation:* It is not known whether topical ophthalmic administration of corticosteroids could result in sufficient systemic absorption to produce detectable quantities in human milk. Exercise caution when administering these drugs to a breast-feeding woman.

Because of the potential for serious adverse reactions in breast-feeding infants from **fluorometholone**, decide whether to discontinue breast-feeding or the drug, taking into account the importance of the drug to the mother.

➤*Children:* Safety and efficacy in children have not been established. Safety and efficacy of **fluocinolone** in children younger than 12 years of age have not been established. Safety and efficacy of **fluorometholone** in infants younger than 2 years of age have not been established.

➤*Monitoring:* Monitor patients for increased intraocular pressure. Make the initial prescription and renewal of the medication order only after examination of the patient with the aid of magnification, such as slit lamp biomicroscopy and, where appropriate, fluorescein staining. If signs and symptoms fail to improve after 2 days, reevaluate the patient.

Adverse Reactions

➤*Ophthalmic:* Elevated intraocular pressure with possible development of glaucoma, optic nerve damage, and visual acuity and field defects; posterior subcapsular cataract formation; delayed wound healing; acute anterior uveitis; keratitis; conjunctivitis; corneal ulcers; mydriasis; conjunctival hyperemia; loss of accommodation; ptosis; perforation of the globe where there is thinning of the sclera. Rarely, filtering blebs have been reported when topical steroids have been used following cataract surgery. Transient stinging or burning upon installation, ocular irritation, foreign body sensation, and visual disturbances (blurry vision) may also occur.

The development of secondary ocular infection (bacterial, fungal, and viral) has occurred. Fungal and viral infections of the cornea are particularly prone to develop coincidentally with long-term applications of steroids. Consider the possibility of fungal invasion in any persistent corneal ulceration where steroid treatment has been used.

➤*Miscellaneous:* Allergic reactions, hypercorticoidism (rare), taste perversion. There have been rare occurrences of systemic hypercorticoidism.

➤*Difluprednate:*

Ophthalmic – Anterior chamber cells, anterior chamber flare, blepharitis, ciliary and conjunctival hyperemia, conjunctival edema, corneal edema, eye pain, photophobia, posterior capsule opacification (5% to 15%); eye inflammation, iritis, punctate keratitis, reduced visual acuity (1% to 5%); application-site discomfort or irritation, corneal pigmentation and striae, episcleritis, eye pruritus, eyelid irritation and crusting, foreign body sensation, increased lacrimation, macular edema, scleral hyperemia, uveitis (less than 1%).

➤*Fluocinolone:*

Ophthalmic – Cataract, eye pain, increased intraocular pressure, procedural complication (eg, cataract fragments in the eye post-op, implant expulsion, injury, mechanical complication of implant, migration of implant, post-op complications, post-op wound complications, wound dehiscence) (50% to 90%); abnormal sensation in the eye, blurred vision, conjunctival hemorrhage, conjunctival hyperemie, dry eye, eye inflammation, eye irritation, eyelid edema, glaucoma, hypotony, increased tearing, maculopathy, pruritus, ptosis, reduced visual acuity, vitreous floaters, vitreous hemorrhage (10% to 35%); blepharitis, choroidal detachment, conjunctival edema/chemosis, corneal edema, eye discharge, eye swelling, macular edema, photophobia, photopsia, retinal hemorrhage, visual disturbance, vitreous opacities (5% to 9%).

Miscellaneous – Headache (31%); arthralgia, back pain, cough, dizziness, influenza, limb pain, nasopharyngitis, nausea, pain, pyrexia, rash, sinusitis, upper respiratory tract infection, vomiting (5% to 15%).

➤*Loteprednol:*

Ophthalmic – Abnormal vision/blurring, burning on installation, chemosis, discharge, dry eyes, epiphora, foreign body sensation, infection, itching, photophobia (5% to 15%); conjunctivitis, corneal abnormalities, eyelid erythema, keratoconjunctivitis, ocular irritation/pain/discomfort, papillae, uveitis (less than 5%).

Miscellaneous – Headache, pharyngitis, rhinitis (less than 15%).

➤*Rimexolone:*

Ophthalmic – Blurred vision, discharge, discomfort, foreign body sensation, hyperemia, increased intraocular pressure, ocular pain, pruritus (1% to 5%); brow ache, conjunctival edema, corneal edema, corneal erosion, corneal staining, corneal ulcer, dry eye, edema, increased fibrin, infiltrate, irritation, keratitis, lid margin crusting, photophobia, sticky sensation, tearing (less than 1%).

Miscellaneous – Headache, hypotension, pharyngitis, rhinitis, taste perversion (less than 2%).

Overdosage

➤*Treatment:* If accidently ingested, drink fluids to dilute.

Patient Information

Advise patients not to allow the dropper tip to touch any surface and to replace the cap after using.

Advise patients to consult their health care provider if pain, redness, itching, or inflammation becomes aggravated or persists longer than 48 hours.

Advise patients not to wear soft contact lenses when using these products.

Advise patient not to discontinue therapy prematurely.

➤*Fluocinolone:* Advise patients to have ophthalmic follow-up examinations of both eyes at appropriate intervals following implantation of fluocinolone.

Advise patients that the potential complications that may accompany intraocular surgery to place fluocinolone into the vitreous cavity may include cataract formation, choroidal detachment, temporary decreased visual acuity, endophthalmitis, hypotony, increased intraocular pressure, exacerbation of intraocular inflammation, retinal detachment, vitreous hemorrhage, vitreous loss, and wound dehiscence.

Advise patients that nearly all patients will experience an immediate and temporary decrease in visual acuity in the implanted eye, which lasts for 1 to 4 weeks postoperatively.

DEXAMETHASONE

Rx	**Dexamethasone Sodium Phosphate** (Various, eg, Bausch & Lomb, Falcon)	**Solution; ophthalmic:** 0.1% (as phosphate)	In 5 mL.
Rx	**Maxidex** (Alcon)	**Suspension; ophthalmic:** 0.1%	In 5 and 15 mL *Drop-Tainers.*[a]
Rx	**Ozurdex** (Allergan)	**Implant; intravitreal:** 0.7 mg	Preservative free. In a foil pouch with a single-use applicator.

[a] With benzalkonium chloride 0.01%, EDTA, hypromellose 0.5%, polysorbate 80, sodium chloride, and dibasic sodium phosphate.

DEXAMETHASONE — OPHTHALMIC

Complete and comparative prescribing information begins in the Ophthalmic Corticosteroids group monograph.

Indications

➤*Corneal injury:* For the treatment of corneal injury from chemical, radiation, or thermal burns, or penetration of foreign bodies.

➤*Ophthalmic inflammatory conditions:* For the treatment of steroid-responsive inflammatory conditions of the palpebral and bulbar conjunctiva, cornea, and anterior segment of the globe, such as allergic conjunctivitis, acne rosacea, superficial punctate keratitis, cyclitis, herpes zoster keratitis, iritis, and selected infective conjunctivitis when the inherent hazard of steroid use is accepted to obtain advisable edema and inflammation diminution.

➤*Otic inflammatory conditions:* Dexamethasone sodium phosphate solution is also approved for otic use. Refer to Dexamethasone Sodium Phosphate in Otic Corticosteroids for specific indications and administration and dosage.

DEXAMETHASONE — OPHTHALMIC

Administration and Dosage

➤*Adults:*

Corneal injury –

Solution:

• *Usual dosage* – Instill 1 to 2 drops into the conjunctival sac every hour during the day and every 2 hours during the night as initial therapy. When a favorable response is observed, reduce dosage to 1 drop every 4 hours. Further reduction in dosage to 1 drop 3 or 4 times daily may suffice to control symptoms.

• *Duration of therapy* – The duration of treatment will vary with the type of lesion and may extend from a few days to several weeks, according to therapeutic response. Relapses, more common in chronic active lesions than in self-limited conditions, usually respond to re-treatment.

Suspension: Instill 1 or 2 drops in the conjunctival sac(s). In severe disease, drops may be used hourly, being tapered to discontinuation as inflammation subsides. In mild disease, drops may be used up to 4 to 6 times daily.

Ophthalmic inflammatory conditions – See Corneal Injury for dosing.

➤*Administration:* Shake suspension well before using.

➤*Storage / Stability:*

Solution – Store at 15° to 30°C (59° to 86°F).

Suspension – Store upright at 8° to 27°C (46° to 80°F).

DEXAMETHASONE — OPHTHALMIC IMPLANT

Indications

➤*Macular edema:* For the treatment of macular edema following branch retinal vein occlusion or central retinal vein occlusion.

➤*Posterior segment uveitis:* For the treatment of noninfectious uveitis affecting the posterior segment of the eye.

Administration and Dosage

➤*Adults:*

Macular edema – 1 implant (0.7 mg) injected intravitreally into each affected eye.

Posterior segment uveitis – See Macular Edema for dosing.

➤*Monitoring:* Following intravitreal injection, patients should be monitored for elevation in intraocular pressure (IOP) and for endophthalmitis. Monitoring may consist of a check for perfusion of the optic nerve head immediately after the injection, tonometry within 30 minutes following the injection, and biomicroscopy between 2 and 7 days following the injection. Patients should be instructed to immediately report any symptoms suggestive of endophthalmitis.

➤*Preparation for administration:* The intravitreal injection procedure should be performed under controlled aseptic conditions that include the use of sterile gloves, a sterile drape, and a sterile eyelid speculum (or equivalent). Administration of adequate anesthesia and a broad-spectrum microbicide are recommended prior to the injection.

➤*Administration:* Remove the foil pouch from the carton and examine for damage. Then, in a sterile field, open the foil pouch and gently place the applicator on a sterile tray. Carefully remove the cap from the applicator. Hold the applicator in one hand and pull the safety tab straight off the applicator. Do not twist or flex the tab. The long axis of the applicator should be held parallel to the limbus, and the sclera should be engaged at an oblique angle with the bevel of the needle up (away from the sclera) to create a shelved scleral path. The tip of the needle is advanced within the sclera for about 1 mm (parallel to the limbus), then redirected toward the center of the eye and advanced until penetration of the sclera is completed and the vitreous cavity is entered. The needle should not be advanced past the point where the sleeve touches the conjunctiva.

Slowly depress the actuator button until an audible click is noted. Before withdrawing the applicator from the eye, make sure that the actuator button is fully depressed and has locked flush with the applicator surface. Remove the needle in the same direction as used to enter the vitreous.

Each applicator can only be used for the treatment of a single eye. If the contralateral eye requires treatment, a new applicator must be used, and the sterile field, syringe, gloves, drapes, and eyelid speculum should be changed before the intravitreal implant is administered to the other eye.

➤*Storage / Stability:* Store at 15° to 30°C (59° to 86°F).

DIFLUPREDNATE

Rx	**Durezol** (Sirion Therapeutics)	**Emulsion; ophthalmic:** 0.05%	Sodium EDTA, boric acid, castor oil, glycerin, polysorbate 80, sodium acetate, sodium hydroxide, sorbic acid 0.1%. In 2.5 and 5 mL.

DIFLUPREDNATE — OPHTHALMIC

Indications

➤*Ocular inflammation and pain:* For the treatment of inflammation and pain associated with ocular surgery.

Administration and Dosage

➤*Adults:*

Ocular inflammation and pain – Instill 1 drop into the conjunctival sac of the affected eye(s) 4 times daily beginning 24 hours after surgery and continuing throughout the first 2 weeks of the postoperative period, followed by 2 times daily for 1 week and then a taper based on the response.

➤*Administration:* For topical ophthalmic use only.

➤*Storage / Stability:* Store at 15° to 25°C (59° to 77°F). Do not freeze. Protect from light.

FLUOCINOLONE ACETONIDE

Rx	**Retisert** (Bausch & Lomb)	**Implant, ophthalmic:** 0.59 mg	In individual cartons.

FLUOCINOLONE ACETONIDE — OPHTHALMIC

Complete and comparative prescribing information begins in the Ophthalmic Corticosteroids group monograph.

Indications

➤*Uveitis:* For the treatment of chronic, noninfectious uveitis affecting the posterior segment of the eye.

Administration and Dosage

➤*General dosing considerations:* The implant contains 1 tablet of fluocinolone 0.59 mg.

Following depletion of fluocinolone from the implant as evidenced by recurrence of uveitis, the fluocinolone implant may be replaced.

➤*Adults:*

Uveitis – The implant is designed to release fluocinolone at a nominal initial rate 0.6 mcg/day, decreasing over the first month to a steady state between 0.3 to 0.4 mcg/day within approximately 30 months.

➤*Children:*

12 years of age and older –

Uveitis: See Adults for dosing.

➤*Elderly:* See Adults for dosing.

➤*Administration:* Fluocinolone is implanted surgically into the posterior segment of the affected eye through a pars plana incision.

Handling and disposal – Caution should be exercised in handling fluocinolone in order to avoid damage to the implant, which may result in an increased rate of drug release from the implant. Thus, fluocinolone should be handled only by the suture tab. Care should be taken during implantation and explantation to avoid sheer forces on the implant that could disengage the silicone cup reservoir (which contains a fluocinolone tablet) from the suture tab. Aseptic technique should be maintained at all times prior to and during the surgical implantation procedure. Fluocinolone should not be resterilized by any method.

➤*Storage / Stability:* Store in the original container at 15° to 25°C (59° to 77°F). Protect from freezing.

FLUOROMETHOLONE

Rx	**FML S.O.P.** (Allergan)	**Ointment, ophthalmic:** 0.1%	In 3.5 g.[a]
Rx	**FML Forte** (Allergan)	**Suspension, ophthalmic:** 0.25%	In 5, 10, and 15 mL.[b]
Rx	**Fluorometholone** (Various, eg, Falcon)	**Suspension, ophthalmic:** 0.1%	In 5, 10, and 15 mL.[c]
Rx	**FML** (Allergan)		In 5, 10, and 15 mL.[d]
Rx	**Flarex** (Alcon)	**Suspension, ophthalmic:** 0.1% (as acetate)	In 2.5, 5, and 10 mL *Drop-Tainers*.[e]

[a] With 0.0008% phenylmercuric acetate, white petrolatum, mineral oil, and lanolin alcohol.
[b] With 0.005% benzalkonium chloride, EDTA, polysorbate 80, 1.4% polyvinyl alcohol, sodium chloride, and sodium phosphate.
[c] With 0.004% benzalkonium chloride, EDTA, polysorbate 80, and 1.4% polyvinyl alcohol.
[d] With 0.004% benzalkonium chloride, EDTA, polysorbate 80, 1.4% polyvinyl alcohol, sodium chloride, and sodium phosphate.
[e] With 0.01% benzalkonium chloride, EDTA, hydroxyethylcellulose, tyloxapol, sodium chloride, and monobasic sodium phosphate.

FLUOROMETHOLONE — OPHTHALMIC

Complete and comparative prescribing information begins in the Ophthalmic Corticosteroids group monograph.

Indications

➤*Ophthalmic inflammatory conditions:* For the treatment of steroid-responsive inflammation of the palpebral and bulbar conjunctiva, cornea, and anterior segment of the globe.

Administration and Dosage

➤*General dosing considerations:* If signs and symptoms fail to improve after 2 days, the patient should be reevaluated.

➤*Adults:*

Ophthalmic inflammatory conditions –

Usual dosage:

• *Ointment* – A small amount (approximately ½-inch ribbon) of ointment should be applied to the conjunctival sac 1 to 3 times daily. During the initial 24 to 48 hours, the frequency of dosing may be increased to 1 application every 4 hours.

• *Suspension* – Instill 1 drop into the conjunctival sac 2 to 4 times daily. During the initial 24 to 48 hours, the dosage may be increased to 1 drop every 4 hours.

Dosage adjustment: The dosing may be reduced, but care should be taken not to discontinue therapy prematurely.

Discontinuation of therapy: Care should be taken not to discontinue therapy prematurely.

In chronic conditions, withdrawal of treatment should be carried out by gradually decreasing the frequency of applications.

➤*Children:*

Ophthalmic inflammatory conditions –

2 years of age and older: See Adults for dosing.

➤*Storage/Stability:*

Ointment – Store at or below 25°C (77°F). Avoid exposure to temperatures above 40°C (104°F).

Suspension – Shake well before using. Keep bottle tightly closed when not in use. Store at or below 25°C (77°F). Protect from freezing.

FLUOROMETHOLONE ACETATE — OPHTHALMIC

Complete and comparative prescribing information begins in the Ophthalmic Corticosteroids group monograph.

Indications

➤*Ophthalmic inflammatory conditions:* For use in the treatment of steroid-responsive inflammatory conditions of the palpebral and bulbar conjunctiva, cornea, and anterior segment of the eye.

Administration and Dosage

➤*General dosing considerations:* If there is no improvement after 2 weeks, advise patients to consult their health care provider.

➤*Adults:*

Ophthalmic inflammatory conditions – One to 2 drops should be instilled into the conjunctival sac(s) 4 times daily. During the initial 24 to 48 hours, the dosage may be safely increased to 2 drops every 2 hours.

➤*Administration:* Shake well before using.

➤*Storage/Stability:* Store at 2° to 27°C (36° to 80°F) in an upright position. Protect from freezing.

LOTEPREDNOL ETABONATE

Rx	**Alrex** (Bausch & Lomb)	**Suspension, ophthalmic:** 0.2%	In 5 and 10 mL.[a]
Rx	**Lotemax** (Bausch & Lomb)	**Suspension, ophthalmic:** 0.5%	In 2.5, 5, 10, and 15 mL.[a]

[a] With 0.01% benzalkonium chloride, EDTA, glycerin, and povidone.

LOTEPREDNOL ETABONATE — OPHTHALMIC

Complete and comparative prescribing information begins in the Ophthalmic Corticosteroids group monograph.

Indications

➤*Ophthalmic inflammatory conditions (Lotemax)*: For the treatment of steroid-responsive inflammatory conditions of the palpebral and bulbar conjunctiva, cornea, and anterior segment of the globe such as allergic conjunctivitis, acne rosacea, superficial punctate keratitis, herpes zoster keratitis, iritis, cyclitis, and selected infective conjunctivitides when the inherent hazard of steroid use is accepted to obtain an advisable diminution in edema and inflammation; for the treatment of postoperative inflammation following ocular surgery.

➤*Seasonal allergic conjunctivitis (Alrex)*: For the temporary relief of the signs and symptoms of seasonal allergic conjunctivitis.

Administration and Dosage

➤*General dosing considerations:* If signs and symptoms fail to improve after 2 days, the patient should be reevaluated.

➤*Adults:*

Postoperative inflammation (Lotemax) – Instill 1 to 2 drops into the conjunctival sac of the operated eye(s) 4 times daily beginning 24 hours after surgery and continuing throughout the first 2 weeks of the postoperative period.

Seasonal allergic conjunctivitis (Alrex) – Instill 1 drop into the affected eye(s) 4 times daily.

Steroid-responsive inflammatory conditions (Lotemax) –

Usual dosage: Instill 1 to 2 drops into the conjunctival sac of the affected eye(s) 4 times daily.

Dosage adjustment: During the initial treatment within the first week, the dosing may be increased up to 1 drop every hour, if necessary.

Discontinuation of therapy: Care should be taken not to discontinue therapy prematurely.

➤*Administration:* Shake vigorously before using. Apply into the conjunctival sac of the involved eye(s).

➤*Storage/Stability:* Store upright at 15° to 25°C (59° to 77°F). Do not freeze.

PREDNISOLONE

Rx	**Prednisolone Sodium Phosphate** (Bausch & Lomb)	**Solution, ophthalmic:** 1% (as sodium phosphate)	In 5, 10, and 15 mL.[a]
Rx	**Pred Mild** (Allergan)	**Suspension, ophthalmic:** 0.12% (as acetate)	In 5 and 10 mL.[c]
Rx	**Prednisolone Acetate** (Various, eg, Falcon, Pacific Pharma)	**Suspension, ophthalmic:** 1% (as acetate)	In 5, 10, and 15 mL.[d]
Rx	**Omnipred** (Alcon)		In 5 and 10 mL *Drop-Tainers*.[e]
Rx	**Pred Forte** (Allergan)		In 1, 5, 10, and 15 mL.[c]

[a] With hypromellose, monobasic and dibasic sodium phosphate, sodium chloride, EDTA, and 0.01% benzalkonium chloride.
[c] With benzalkonium chloride, EDTA, polysorbate 80, hydroxypropyl methylcellulose, sodium bisulfite, boric acid, sodium chloride, and sodium citrate.
[d] With 0.01% benzalkonium chloride, EDTA, polysorbate 80, glycerin, hypromellose, and dibasic sodium phosphate.
[e] With 0.01% benzalkonium chloride, EDTA, polysorbate 80, glycerin, hydroxypropyl methylcellulose.

PREDNISOLONE ACETATE — OPHTHALMIC

Complete and comparative prescribing information begins in the Ophthalmic Corticosteroids group monograph.

Indications

➤*Corneal injury:* For the treatment of corneal injury from chemical, radiation, or thermal burns, or penetration of foreign bodies.

➤*Ophthalmic inflammatory conditions:* For the treatment of steroid-responsive inflammatory conditions of the palpebral and bulbar conjunctiva, cornea, and anterior segment of the globe such as acne rosacea, allergic conjunctivitis, cyclitis, herpes zoster keratitis, iritis, superficial punctate keratitis, and selected infective conjunctivitis when the inherent hazard of steroid use is accepted to obtain an advisable edema and inflammation diminution.

Administration and Dosage

➤*Adults:*

Corneal injury –

Usual dosage: Instill 2 drops in the eye(s) 4 times daily. If signs and symptoms fail to improve after 2 days, the patient should be reevaluated.

• *Pred Mild/Pred Forte –* Instill 1 to 2 drops in the conjunctival sac 2 to 4 times daily; during the initial 24 to 48 hours, the dosing frequency may be increased if necessary.

Concomitant therapy: In cases of bacterial infections, concomitant use of anti-infective agents is mandatory.

Discontinuation of therapy: The dosing of the suspension may be reduced, but take care not to discontinue therapy prematurely. In chronic conditions, carry out treatment withdrawal by gradually decreasing the frequency of applications.

Ophthalmic inflammatory conditions – See Corneal injury for dosing.

➤*Children:*

Off-label dosing –

Ophthalmic disorders:

• *Initial dosage –* 1 to 2 drops every hour during the day and every 2 hours during the night.

• *Dosage reduction –* After a favorable response is obtained, reduce dose to 1 drop every 4 hours; dose may be reduced further to 1 drop 3 to 4 times daily.

➤*Administration:* Shake well before using.

➤*Storage/Stability:* Store at 8° to 24°C (46° to 75°F) in an upright position.

Pred Mild – Store at 15° to 30°C (59° to 86°F). Protect from freezing.

Pred Forte – Store up to 25°C (77°F).

PREDNISOLONE SODIUM PHOSPHATE — OPHTHALMIC

Complete and comparative prescribing information begins in the Ophthalmic Corticosteroids group monograph.

Indications

➤*Ophthalmic inflammatory conditions:* For the treatment of steroid-responsive inflammatory conditions of the palpebral and bulbar conjunctiva, cornea, and anterior segment of the globe, such as allergic conjunctivitis, acne rosacea, superficial punctate keratitis, herpes zoster keratitis, iritis, cyclitis, and selected infective conjunctivitis when the inherent hazard of steroid use is accepted to obtain an advisable edema and inflammation diminution; corneal injury from chemical, radiation, or thermal burns, or penetration of foreign bodies.

Moderate to severe – Prednisolone 1% solution is recommended for moderate to severe inflammations, particularly when unusually rapid control is desired. In stubborn cases of anterior segment eye disease, systemic adrenocortical hormone therapy may be required. When the deeper ocular structures are involved, systemic therapy is necessary.

Administration and Dosage

➤*Adults:*

Ophthalmic inflammatory conditions –

Initial dosage: Depending on the severity of inflammation, instill 1 or 2 drops of solution into the conjunctival sac up to every hour during the day and every 2 hours during the night as necessary as initial therapy.

Dosage adjustment: When a favorable response is observed, reduce dosage to 1 drop every 4 hours. Later, further reduction in dosage to 1 drop 3 to 4 times daily may suffice to control symptoms.

Duration of therapy: The duration of treatment will vary with the type of lesion and may extend from a few days to several weeks, according to therapeutic response. Relapses, more common in chronic active lesions than in self-limiting conditions, usually respond to re-treatment.

➤*Children:*

Off-label dosing –

Ophthalmic disorders:

• *Initial dosage –* 1 to 2 drops every hour during the day and every 2 hours during the night.

• *Dosage reduction –* After a favorable response is obtained, reduce dose to 1 drop every 4 hours; dose may be reduced further to 1 drop 3 to 4 times daily.

➤*Administration:* Not for injection into the eye. For topical use only.

➤*Storage/Stability:* Store at 15° and 30°C (59° to 86°F). Protect from light. Keep tightly closed.

RIMEXOLONE

Rx	**Vexol** (Alcon)	**Suspension, ophthalmic:** 1%	In 5 and 10 mL *Drop-Tainers*.[a]

[a] With 0.01% benzalkonium chloride, polysorbate 80, EDTA, and sodium chloride.

RIMEXOLONE — OPHTHALMIC

Complete and comparative prescribing information begins in the Ophthalmic Corticosteroids group monograph.

Indications

➤*Ophthalmic inflammatory conditions:* For the treatment of postoperative inflammation following ocular surgery; for the treatment of anterior uveitis.

Administration and Dosage

➤*Adults:*

Ophthalmic inflammatory conditions –

Postoperative inflammation: Instill 1 to 2 drops into the conjunctival sac of the affected eye 4 times daily beginning 24 hours after surgery and continuing throughout the first 2 weeks of the postoperative period.

Anterior uveitis: Instill 1 to 2 drops into the conjunctival sac of the affected eye every hour during waking hours for the first week, 1 drop every 2 hours during waking hours of the second week, and then taper until uveitis is resolved.

➤*Storage/Stability:* Store upright at 2° to 25°C (36° to 77°F). Shake well before using. Do not freeze.

TRIAMCINOLONE ACETONIDE

Rx	**Triesence** (Alcon)	**Injection, suspension; intravitreal:** 40 mg/mL	In 1 mL single-use vials.
Rx	**Trivaris** (Allergan)	**Injection, gel suspension; intravitreal:** 80 mg/mL	Preservative free. Sodium hyaluronate 2.3%. In blister packs with 1 single-use glass syringe.

TRIAMCINOLONE ACETONIDE — INTRAVITREAL INJECTION

Indications

➤*Ophthalmic diseases:* For sympathetic ophthalmia, temporal arteritis, uveitis, and ocular inflammatory conditions unresponsive to topical corticosteroids.

➤*Vitrectomy (Triesence* only): For visualization during vitrectomy.

Administration and Dosage

➤*General dosing considerations:* Strict aseptic technique is mandatory.

➤*Adults:*

Ophthalmic disease –

Triesence: The initial recommended dose is 4 mg per 0.1 mL (100 mcL of 40 mg/mL suspension) with subsequent dosage as needed throughout the course of treatment.

Trivaris: The recommended intravitreal dose is a single injection of 4 mg per 0.05 mL (50 mcL of 80 mg/mL suspension).

Vitrectomy (Triesence only) – 1 to 4 mg (25 to 100 mcL of 40 mg/mL suspension) administered intravitreally.

➤*Children:* See Adults for dosing.

TRIAMCINOLONE ACETONIDE — INTRAVITREAL INJECTION

➤*Preparation for administration:*

Triesence – The vial should be shaken vigorously for 10 seconds before use to ensure a uniform suspension. Prior to withdrawal, the suspension should be inspected for clumping or granular appearance (agglomeration). An agglomerated product results from exposure to freezing temperatures and should not be used. After withdrawal, triamcinolone should be injected without delay to prevent settling in the syringe.

Trivaris – Always allow the prefilled glass syringe to sit at room temperature for at least 30 minutes before the procedure.

The product is supplied without an attached needle; therefore, it is necessary to firmly attach a desired needle to the syringe. A 27-gauge, ½-inch needle is suggested. Prepare the proper volume to be injected by advancing the plunger to the single line marked on the prefilled glass syringe shaft. Hold the syringe and needle at an angle and express excess gel suspension over a sterile surface. The plunger is correctly positioned when white compound is no longer visible between the plunger and the fill line on the syringe. This will provide the recommended dose of 4 mg per 0.05 mL. Always check the needle to ensure it is firmly attached to the syringe before injecting the patient.

➤*Administration:* The injection procedure should be carried out under controlled aseptic conditions, which include the use of sterile gloves, a sterile drape, and a sterile eyelid speculum (or equivalent). Adequate anesthesia and a broad-spectrum microbicide should be given prior to the injection.

Each vial or syringe should only be used for the treatment of a single eye. If the contralateral eye requires treatment, a new vial should be used and the sterile field, syringe, gloves, drapes, eyelid speculum, filter, and injection needles should be changed before triamcinolone is administered to the other eye.

Careful technique should be employed to avoid the possibility of entering a blood vessel or introducing organisms that can cause infection. Strict aseptic technique is mandatory.

➤*Storage/Stability:*

Triesence – Store between 4° and 25°C (39° and 77°F). Do not freeze. Protect from light by storing in carton.

Trivaris – Keep refrigerated between 2° and 8°C (36° and 46°F) until use. Avoid freezing and protect from light.

OPHTHALMIC MAST CELL STABILIZERS

PEMIROLAST POTASSIUM

Rx	**Alamast** (Vistakon)	**Solution, ophthalmic:** 0.1% (1 mg/mL)	0.005% lauralkonium chloride, glycerin, dibasic and monobasic sodium phosphate, phosphoric acid, and/or sodium hydroxide. In 10 mL.

PEMIROLAST POTASSIUM — OPHTHALMIC

Indications

➤*Allergic conjunctivitis:* For the prevention of itching of the eye due to allergic conjunctivitis.

Administration and Dosage

➤*Adults:*

Allergic conjunctivitis –

Usual dosage: 1 to 2 drops in each affected eye 4 times daily.

Duration of therapy: Symptomatic response to therapy (decreased itching) may be evident within a few days, but frequently requires longer treatment (up to 4 weeks).

➤*Children:*

3 years of age and older – See Adults for dosing.

➤*Administration:* For topical ophthalmic use only. Not for injection or oral use.

➤*Storage/Stability:* Store at 15° to 25°C (59° to 77°F).

Actions

➤*Pharmacology:* Pemirolast potassium is a mast cell stabilizer that inhibits the in vivo type I immediate hypersensitivity reaction.

In vitro and in vivo studies have demonstrated that pemirolast potassium inhibits the antigen-induced release of inflammatory mediators (eg, histamine, leukotriene C_4, D_4, E_4) from human mast cells.

In addition, pemirolast potassium inhibits the chemotaxis of eosinophils into ocular tissue and blocks the release of mediators from human eosinophils.

Although the precise mechanism of action is unknown, the drug has been reported to prevent calcium influx into mast cells upon antigen stimulation.

➤*Pharmacokinetics:*

Absorption/Distribution – Topical ocular administration of 1 to 2 drops of pemirolast potassium ophthalmic solution in each eye 4 times daily in 16 healthy volunteers for 2 weeks resulted in detectable concentrations in the plasma. The mean (± SE) peak plasma level of 4.7 ± 0.8 ng/mL occurred at 0.42 ± 0.05 hours and the mean $t_{1/2}$ was 4.5 ± 0.2 hours. When a single 10 mg pemirolast potassium dose was taken orally, a peak plasma concentration of 0.723 mcg/mL was reached.

Excretion – Following topical administration, about 10% to 15% of the dose was excreted unchanged in the urine.

Contraindications

Hypersensitivity to any of the ingredients of this product.

Warnings/Precautions

➤*Administration:* For topical ophthalmic use only. Not for injection or oral use.

➤*Pregnancy:* Category C.

Teratogenic – Pemirolast potassium caused an increased incidence of thymic remnant in the neck, interventricular septal defect, fetuses with wavy rib, splitting of thoracic vertebral body, and reduced numbers of ossified sternebrae, sacral and caudal vertebrae, and metatarsi when rats were given oral doses greater than or equal to 250 mg/kg (approximately 20,000-fold the human dose at 2 drops/eye, 40 mcL/drop, 4 times a day for a 50 kg adult) during organogenesis. Increased incidence of dilation of renal pelvis/ureter in the fetuses and neonates was also noted when rats were given an oral dose of 400 mg/kg pemirolast potassium (approximately 30,000-fold the human dose). Pemirolast potassium was not teratogenic in rabbits given oral doses up to 150 mg/kg (approximately 12,000-fold the human dose) during the same time period. There are no adequate and well-controlled studies in pregnant women. Because animal reproductive studies are not always predictive of human response, pemirolast potassium ophthalmic solution should be used during pregnancy only if the benefit outweighs the risk.

Nonteratogenic – Pemirolast potassium produced increased pre- and post-implantation losses, reduced embryo/fetal and neonatal survival, decreased neonatal body weight, and delayed neonatal development in rats receiving an oral dose at 400 mg/kg (approximately 30,000-fold the human dose). Pemirolast potassium also caused a reduction in the number of corpus lutea, the number of implantations, and number of live fetuses in the F_1 generation in rats when F_0 dams were given oral dosages greater than or equal to 250 mg/kg (approximately 20,000-fold the human dose) during late gestation and the lactation period.

➤*Lactation:* Pemirolast potassium is excreted in the milk of lactating rats at concentrations higher than those in plasma. It is not known whether pemirolast potassium is excreted in human milk. Because many drugs are excreted in human milk, caution should be exercised when pemirolast potassium ophthalmic solution is administered to a nursing woman.

➤*Children:* Safety and effectiveness in pediatric patients below the age of 3 years have not been established.

Adverse Reactions

➤*Less than 5%:* The following ocular and non-ocular adverse reactions were reported at an incidence of less than 5%:

Ophthalmic – Burning, dry eye, foreign body sensation, and ocular discomfort.

Miscellaneous – Allergy, back pain, bronchitis, cough, dysmenorrhea, fever, sinusitis, and sneezing/nasal congestion.

➤*Miscellaneous:* In clinical studies lasting up to 17 weeks with pemirolast potassium ophthalmic solution, headache, rhinitis, and cold/flu symptoms were reported at an incidence of 10% to 25%. The occurrence of these side effects was generally mild. Some of these events were similar to the underlying ocular disease being studied.

Overdosage

No accounts of pemirolast potassium ophthalmic solution overdose were reported following topical ocular application.

Oral ingestion of the contents of a 10 mL bottle would be equivalent to 10 mg of pemirolast potassium.

Patient Information

For topical ophthalmic use only. Not for injection or oral use.

To prevent contaminating the dropper tip and solution, do not touch the eyelids or surrounding areas with the dropper tip. Keep the bottle tightly closed when not in use.

Patients should be advised not to wear contact lenses if their eyes are red. Pemirolast potassium ophthalmic solution should not be used to treat contact lens related irritation. The preservative in pemirolast potassium ophthalmic solution, lauralkonium chloride, may be absorbed by soft contact lenses. Patients who wear soft contact lenses and whose eyes are not red should be instructed to wait at least 10 minutes after instilling pemirolast potassium before they insert their contact lenses.

NEDOCROMIL SODIUM

Rx	**Alocril** (Allergan)	**Solution, ophthalmic:** 2% (20 mg/mL)	0.01% benzalkonium Cl, 0.5% NaCl, 0.05% EDTA. In 5 mL w/ dropper tip.

NEDOCROMIL SODIUM — OPHTHALMIC

Indications

➤*Allergic conjunctivitis:* For the treatment of itching associated with allergic conjunctivitis.

Administration and Dosage

➤*Adults:*

Allergic conjunctivitis –

Usual dosage: 1 or 2 drops in each eye twice a day. Use at regular intervals.

Duration of therapy: Continue treatment throughout the period of exposure (ie, until the pollen season is over or until exposure to the offending allergen is terminated), even when symptoms are absent.

➤*Children:*

3 years of age and older – See Adults for dosing.

➤*Storage/Stability:* Store between 2° and 25°C (36° and 77°F). Keep tightly closed and out of the reach of children.

Actions

➤*Pharmacology:* Nedocromil sodium is a mast cell stabilizer. It inhibits the release of mediators from cells involved in hypersensitivity reactions. Decreased chemotaxis and decreased activation of eosinophils have also been demonstrated.

In vitro studies with adult human bronchoalveolar cells showed that nedocromil sodium inhibits histamine release from a population of mast cells as belonging to the mucosal subtype and beta-glucuronidase release from macrophages.

➤*Pharmacokinetics:* Nedocromil sodium exhibits low systemic absorption, with less than 4% of the total dose systemically absorbed following multiple dosing. Absorption is mainly through the nasolacrimal duct rather than through the conjunctiva. It is not metabolized and is eliminated primarily unchanged in urine (70%) and feces (30%).

Contraindications

Hypersensitivity to nedocromil sodium or to any of the other ingredients.

Warnings/Precautions

➤*Pregnancy: Category B.* Reproduction studies performed in mice, rats, and rabbits using a subcutaneous dose of 100 mg/kg/day (greater than 1,600 times the maximum recommended human daily ocular dose on a mg/kg basis) revealed no evidence of teratogenicity or harm to the fetus caused by nedocromil sodium. However there are no adequate and well-controlled studies in pregnant women. Because animal reproduction studies are not always predictive of human response, use nedocromil sodium during pregnancy only if clearly needed.

➤*Lactation:* After IV administration to lactating rats, nedocromil was excreted in milk. It is not known whether this drug is excreted in human milk. Exercise caution when nedocromil sodium is administered to nursing women.

➤*Children:* Safety and efficacy in children younger than 3 years of age have not been established.

Adverse Reactions

The most frequently reported adverse experience was headache (approximately 40%). Ocular burning, irritation and stinging, unpleasant taste, nasal congestion (10% to 30%); asthma, conjunctivitis, eye redness, photophobia, rhinitis (1% to 10%).

Patient Information

Instruct patients to refrain from wearing contact lenses while exhibiting the signs and symptoms of allergic conjunctivitis.

LODOXAMIDE TROMETHAMINE

Rx	**Alomide** (Alcon)	**Solution:** 0.1%	In 10 mL *Drop-Tainers.*

LODOXAMIDE TROMETHAMINE — OPHTHALMIC

Indications

➤*Ocular disorders:* Treatment of the ocular disorders referred to by the terms vernal keratoconjunctivitis, vernal conjunctivitis, and vernal keratitis.

Administration and Dosage

➤*Adults:*

Vernal keratoconjunctivitis/vernal conjunctivitis/vernal keratitis – 1 to 2 drops in each affected eye 4 times daily for up to 3 months.

➤*Children:*

2 years of age and older – See Adults for dosing.

➤*Storage/Stability:* Store at 15° to 27°C (59° to 80°F).

Actions

➤*Pharmacology:* Lodoxamide tromethamine is a mast cell stabilizer that inhibits the in vivo Type I immediate hypersensitivity reaction. Lodoxamide therapy inhibits the increases in cutaneous vascular permeability that are associated with reagin or IgE and antigen-mediated reactions.

In vitro studies have demonstrated the ability of lodoxamide to stabilize rodent mast cells and prevent antigen-stimulated release of histamine. In addition, lodoxamide prevents the release of other mast cell inflammatory mediators (ie, SRS-A, slow-reacting substances of anaphylaxis, also known as the peptido-leukotrienes) and inhibits eosinophil chemotaxis. Although lodoxamide's precise mechanism of action is unknown, the drug has been reported to prevent calcium influx into mast cells upon antigen stimulation.

➤*Pharmacokinetics:* The disposition of 14C-lodoxamide was studied in six healthy adult volunteers receiving a 3 mg (50 mCi) oral dose of lodoxamide. Urinary excretion was the major route of elimination. The elimination half-life of 14C-lodoxamide was 8.5 hours in urine. In a study conducted in twelve healthy adult volunteers, topical administration of lodoxamide tromethamine ophthalmic solution 0.1%, one drop in each eye four times per day for ten days, did not result in any measurable lodoxamide plasma levels at a detection limit of 2.5 ng/mL.

Contraindications

Hypersensitivity to any component of this product.

Warnings/Precautions

➤*Contact lenses:* As with all ophthalmic preparations containing benzalkonium chloride, patients should be instructed not to wear soft contact lenses during treatment with lodoxamide tromethamine ophthalmic solution.

➤*Ocular effects:* Patients may experience a transient burning or stinging upon instillation of lodoxamide tromethamine ophthalmic solution. Should these symptoms persist, the patient should be advised to contact the prescribing physician.

➤*Pregnancy: Category B.* Reproduction studies with lodoxamide tromethamine administered orally to rats and rabbits in doses of 100 mg/kg/day (more than 5000 times the proposed human clinical dose) produced no evidence of developmental toxicity. There are, however, no adequate and well-controlled studies in pregnant women. Because animal reproduction studies are not always predictive of human response, lodoxamide tromethamine ophthalmic solution 0.1% should be used during pregnancy only if clearly needed.

➤*Lactation:* It is not known whether lodoxamide tromethamine is excreted in human milk. Because many drugs are excreted in human milk, caution should be exercised when lodoxamide tromethamine ophthalmic solution 0.1% is administered to nursing women.

➤*Children:* Safety and effectiveness in pediatric patients below the age of 2 have not been established.

Adverse Reactions

During clinical studies of lodoxamide tromethamine ophthalmic solution 0.1%, the most frequently reported ocular adverse experiences were transient burning, stinging, or discomfort upon instillation, which occurred in approximately 15% of the subjects. Other ocular events occurring in 1% to 5% of the subjects included ocular itching/pruritus, blurred vision, dry eye, tearing/discharge, hyperemia, crystalline deposits, and foreign body sensation. Events that occurred in less than 1% of the subjects included corneal erosion/ulcer, scales on lid/lash, eye pain, ocular edema/swelling, ocular warming sensation, ocular fatigue, chemosis, corneal abrasion, anterior chamber cells, keratopathy/keratitis, blepharitis, allergy, sticky sensation, and epitheliopathy.

Nonocular events reported were headache (1.5%) and (at less than 1%) heat sensation, dizziness, somnolence, nausea, stomach discomfort, sneezing, dry nose, and rash.

Overdosage

➤*Symptoms:* There have been no reports of lodoxamide tromethamine opthalmic solution 0.1% overdose following topical ocular application. Accidental overdose of an oral preparation of 120 to 180 mg of lodoxamide resulted in a temporary sensation of warmth, profuse sweating, diarrhea, lightheadedness, and a feeling of stomach distension; no permanent adverse effects were observed. Side effects reported following systemic oral administration of 0.1 mg to 10 mg of lodoxamide include a feeling of warmth or flushing, headache, dizziness, fatigue, sweating, nausea, loose stools, and urinary frequency/urgency.

➤*Treatment:* The physician may consider emesis in the event of accidental ingestion.

Patient Information

As with all ophthalmic preparations containing benzalkonium chloride, patients should be instructed not to wear soft contact lenses during treatment with lodoxamide.

CROMOLYN SODIUM

Rx	**Cromolyn Sodium** (Various, eg, Akorn, Falcon, Teva)	**Solution:** 4%	In 10 mL and 15 mL.

CROMOLYN SODIUM — OPHTHALMIC

Indications

➤*Ocular disorders:* Treatment of vernal keratoconjunctivitis, vernal conjunctivitis, and vernal keratitis.

Administration and Dosage

➤*General dosing considerations:* Patients should be advised that the effect of cromolyn sodium ophthalmic solution therapy is dependent upon its administration at regular intervals, as directed.

One drop contains cromolyn sodium approximately 1.6 mg.

Do not exceed the recommended frequency of administration.

➤*Adults:*

Vernal conjunctivitis –

Usual dosage: Instill 1 to 2 drops in each eye 4 to 6 times a day at regular intervals.

Duration of therapy: Symptomatic response to therapy (decreased itching, tearing, redness, and discharge) is usually evident within a few days, but longer treatment for up to 6 weeks is sometimes required. Once symptomatic improvement has been established, therapy should be continued for as long as needed to sustain improvement.

Concomitant therapy: If required, corticosteroids may be used concomitantly with cromolyn sodium ophthalmic solution.

Vernal keratoconjunctivitis – See Vernal conjunctivitis for dosing.

Vernal keratitis – See Vernal conjunctivitis for dosing.

➤*Children:*

4 years of age and older – See Adults for dosing.

➤*Storage/Stability:* Store between 15° to 30°C (59° to 86°F). Protect from light. Store in original carton. Keep tightly closed.

Actions

➤*Pharmacology:* In vitro and in vivo animal studies have shown that cromolyn sodium inhibits the degranulation of sensitized mast cells which occurs after exposure to specific antigens. Cromolyn sodium acts by inhibiting the release of histamine and SRS-A (slow-reacting substance of anaphylaxis) from the mast cell.

Another activity demonstrated in vitro is the capacity of cromolyn sodium to inhibit the degranulation of non-sensitized rat mast cells by phospholipase A and the subsequent release of chemical mediators. Another study showed that cromolyn sodium did not inhibit the enzymatic activity of released phospholipase A on its specific substrate.

➤*Pharmacokinetics:*

Absorption/Distribution – Cromolyn sodium is poorly absorbed. When multiple doses of cromolyn sodium ophthalmic solution are instilled into healthy rabbit eyes, less than 0.07% of the administered dose of cromolyn sodium is absorbed into the systemic circulation (presumably by way of the eye, nasal passages, buccal cavity and gastrointestinal tract). Trace amounts (less than 0.01%) of the cromolyn sodium dose penetrate into the aqueous humor and clearance from this chamber is virtually complete within 24 hours after treatment is stopped.

Excretion – In healthy volunteers, analysis of drug excretion indicates that approximately 0.03% of cromolyn sodium is absorbed following administration to the eye.

Contraindications

Hypersensitivity to cromolyn sodium or to any of the other ingredients.

Warnings/Precautions

➤*Ocular effects:* Patients may experience a transient stinging or burning sensation following application of cromolyn sodium ophthalmic solution.

➤*Usage:* Do not exceed the recommended frequency of administration. Advise patients that the effect of cromolyn sodium ophthalmic solution therapy is dependent upon its administration at regular intervals, as directed.

➤*Pregnancy: Category B.*

Teratogenic – Reproduction studies with cromolyn sodium administered subcutaneously to pregnant mice and rats at maximum daily doses of 540 mg/kg (1620 mg/m^2) and 164 mg/kg (984 mg/m^2), respectively, and intravenously to rabbits at a maximum daily dose of 485 mg/kg (5820 mg/m^2) produced no evidence of fetal malformation. These doses represent approximately 57, 35, and 205 times the maximum daily human dose, respectively, on a mg/m^2 basis. Adverse fetal effects (increased resorption and decreased fetal weight) were noted only at the very high parenteral doses that produced maternal toxicity. There are, however, no adequate and well-controlled studies in pregnant women. Because animal reproduction studies are not always predictive of human response, this drug should be used during pregnancy only if clearly needed.

➤*Lactation:* It is not known whether this drug is excreted in human milk. Because many drugs are excreted in human milk, caution should be exercised when cromolyn sodium ophthalmic solution is administered to a nursing woman.

➤*Children:* Safety and effectiveness in pediatric patients below the age of 4 years have not been established.

Adverse Reactions

➤*Hypersensitivity:* Immediate hypersensitivity reactions have been reported rarely and include dyspnea, edema, and rash.

➤*Ophthalmic:* The most frequently reported adverse reaction attributed to the use of cromolyn sodium ophthalmic solution, on the basis of recurrence following readministration, is transient ocular stinging or burning upon instillation.

The following adverse reactions have been reported as infrequent events. It is unclear whether they are attributed to the drug: Conjunctival injection; watery eyes; itchy eyes; dryness around the eye; puffy eyes; eye irritation; styes.

Patient Information

Users of contact lenses should refrain from wearing lenses while exhibiting the signs and symptoms of vernal keratoconjunctivitis, vernal conjunctivitis, or vernal keratitis. Do not wear contact lenses during treatment with cromolyn sodium ophthalmic solution.

➤*Special tips:*

1.) Avoid placing cromolyn sodium ophthalmic solution directly on the cornea (the area just over the pupil), because it is especially sensitive. You will find the administration of the eye drops more comfortable if you place the drops just inside the lower eyelid.
2.) To avoid contamination of the solution, do not touch the dropper tip to the eye, fingers, or any other surface. Replace cap after use. It is recommended that any remaining contents be discarded after the treatment period described by your physician.
3.) Store between 15° to 30°C (59° to 86°F). Protect from light; store in original carton.
4.) Keep tightly closed and out of the reach of children.
5.) Do not use with any other ocular medication unless directed by your physician. Do not wear contact lenses during treatment with cromolyn sodium ophthalmic solution.

BEPOTASTINE BESILATE

Rx	**Bepreve** (ISTA Pharmaceuticals)	**Solution; ophthalmic:** 1.5%	Equiv. to bepotastine 10.7 mg base. In 10 mL bottles.[a]

[a] With benzalkonium chloride 0.005%, monobasic sodium phosphate dihydrate, sodium chloride, and sodium hydroxide.

BEPOTASTINE BESILATE — OPHTHALMIC

Indications

➤*Allergic conjunctivitis:* For the treatment of itching associated with signs and symptoms of allergic conjunctivitis.

Administration and Dosage

➤*Adults:*

Allergic conjunctivitis – Instill 1 drop into the affected eye(s) twice a day.

➤*Children:*

Allergic conjunctivitis – See Adults for dosing for children 2 years of age and older.

➤*Storage/Stability:* Store at 15° to 30°C (59° to 77°F).

Actions

➤*Pharmacology:* Bepotastine is a topically active, direct H_1-receptor antagonist and an inhibitor of the release of histamine from mast cells.

➤*Pharmacokinetics:*

Absorption – The extent of systemic exposure to bepotastine following topical ophthalmic administration of bepotastine besilate 1% and 1.5% ophthalmic solutions was evaluated in 12 healthy adults. Following 1 drop of bepotastine besilate 1% or 1.5% ophthalmic solution to both eyes 4 times daily for 7 days, bepotastine plasma concentrations peaked at approximately 1 to 2 hours postinstillation. Maximum plasma concentration for the 1% and 1.5% strengths were 5.1 ± 2.5 ng/mL and 7.3 ± 1.9 ng/mL, respectively. Plasma concentration at 24 hours postinstillation were below the quantifiable limit (2 ng/mL) in 11 of 12 subjects in the 2 dose groups.

Distribution – The extent of protein binding of bepotastine is approximately 55% and independent of bepotastine concentration.

Metabolism – In vitro metabolism studies with human liver microsomes demonstrated that bepotastine is minimally metabolized by cytochrome P-450 isozymes.

BEPOTASTINE BESILATE — OPHTHALMIC

In vitro studies demonstrated that bepotastine does not inhibit the metabolism of various CYP-450 substrates via inhibition of CYP3A4, CYP2C9, and CYP2C19. Bepotastine has a low potential for drug interaction via inhibition of CYP3A4, CYP2C9, and CYP2C19.

Excretion – The main route of elimination of bepotastine is urinary excretion (with approximately 75% to 90% excreted unchanged in urine).

Contraindications

None known.

Warnings/Precautions

➤*Contamination:* To minimize contamination of the dropper tip and solution, patients should take care not to touch the eyelids or surrounding areas with the dropper tip of the bottle. Advise patients to keep bottle tightly closed when not in use.

➤*Contact lens use:* Advise patients not to wear a contact lens if their eye is red and not to use bepotastine to treat contact lens–related irritation. Advise patients not to instill bepotastine while wearing contact lenses and to remove contact lenses prior to instillation of bepotastine. The preservative in bepotastine, benzalkonium chloride, may be absorbed by soft contact lenses. Lenses may be reinserted after 10 minutes following administration of bepotastine.

➤*Pregnancy: Category C.* There are no adequate and well-controlled studies of bepotastine in pregnant women. Because animal reproduction studies are not always predictive of human response, bepotastine besilate 1.5% ophthalmic solution should be used during pregnancy only if the potential benefit justifies the potential risk to the fetus.

Teratogenicity studies have been performed in animals. Bepotastine was not found to be teratogenic in rats during organogenesis and fetal development at oral dosages of up to 200 mg/kg/day (representing a systemic concentration approximately 3,300 times that anticipated for topical ocular use in humans) but did show some potential for causing skeletal abnormalities at 1,000 mg/kg/day. Evidence of infertility was seen in rats given oral bepotastine 1,000 mg/kg/day; however, no evidence of infertility was observed in rats given 200 mg/kg/day (approximately 3,300 times the topical ocular use in humans). The concentration of radiolabeled bepotastine was similar in fetal liver and maternal blood plasma following a single 3 mg/kg oral dose. The concentration in other fetal tissues was one-third to one-tenth the concentration in maternal blood plasma.

An increase in stillborns and decreased growth and development were observed in pups born from rats given oral dosages of 1,000 mg/kg/day during perinatal and lactation periods. There were no observed effects in rats treated with 100 mg/kg/day.

➤*Lactation:* Following a single 3 mg/kg oral dose of radiolabeled bepotastine to nursing rats 11 days after delivery, the maximum concentration of radioactivity in milk was 0.4 mcg-eq/mL 1 hour after administration; at 48 hours after administration, the concentration was below detection limits. The milk concentration was higher than the maternal blood plasma concentration at each time of measurement.

It is not known if bepotastine is excreted in human milk. Exercise caution when bepotastine besilate 1.5% ophthalmic solution is administered to a breast-feeding woman.

➤*Children:* Safety and efficacy of bepotastine have not been established in children younger than 2 years of age. Efficacy in children younger than 10 years of age was extrapolated from clinical trials conducted in children older than 10 years of age and from adults.

➤*Elderly:* No overall difference in safety or effectiveness has been observed between elderly and younger patients.

Drug Interactions

None known.

Adverse Reactions

The most common reported adverse reaction occurring in approximately 25% of subjects was a mild taste following instillation.

Other adverse reactions occurring in 2% to 5% of subjects were eye irritation, headache, and nasopharyngitis.

Patient Information

Counsel patients that this medication is for topical ophthalmic administration only.

Advise patients not to touch dropper tip to any surface, as this may contaminate the contents.

Advise patients not to wear a contact lens if their eye is red. Advise patients not to use bepotastine to treat contact lens–related irritation.

Advise patients to remove contact lenses prior to instillation of bepotastine. The preservative in bepotastine, benzalkonium chloride, may be absorbed by soft contact lenses. Lenses may be reinserted after 10 minutes following administration of bepotastine.

OPHTHALMIC DECONGESTANTS

Refer to the Topical Ophthalmic Drugs introduction for more complete information.

Indications

➤*General information:* Refer to individual monographs for further information.

➤*Ocular vasoconstrictor / decongestant:* For use as a topical vasoconstrictor and for the temporary relief of redness due to minor eye irritation, for protection against further irritation, and for the temporary relief of burning and irritation due to dryness of the eye.

➤*Ocular mydriatic (phenylephrine only):* For refraction without cycloplegia, use in diagnostic procedures (eg, provocative test for angle closure glaucoma, retinoscopy, blanching test), ophthalmoscopic examination (2.5% solution only), pupillary dilation in uveitis (to prevent or aid in the disruption of posterior synechia formation), and wide dilation of the pupil before intraocular surgical procedures (2.5% and 10% solution only).

Actions

➤*Pharmacology:* The effects of sympathomimetic agents on the eye include pupil dilation, increase in outflow of aqueous humor and vasoconstriction (alpha-adrenergic effects); relaxation of the ciliary muscle, and a decrease in the formation of aqueous humor (beta-adrenergic effects).

Strong (alpha) vasoconstriction preparations (phenylephrine 2.5% and 10%) cause vasoconstriction and pupillary dilation for diagnostic eye exams, during surgery, and to prevent synechiae formation in uveitis. Weak sympathomimetic solutions (phenylephrine 0.12%; oxymetazoline; naphazoline; tetrahydrozoline) are used as ophthalmic decongestants (vasoconstriction of conjunctival blood vessels) for symptomatic relief of minor eye irritations.

Phenylephrine 2.5% and 10% exhibit rapid and moderately prolonged action and produce little rebound vasodilation. Systemic side effects are uncommon, although rare systemic absorption of sufficient quantities may lead to systemic alpha-adrenergic affects, such as a rise in blood pressure, which may be accompanied by a reflex atropine-sensitive bradycardia.

Ophthalmic Vasoconstrictors/Mydriatics

Vasoconstrictor/ mydriatic	Duration of action (h)	Available concentration	Prescription status
Naphazoline	4 to 6	0.012%	otc
		0.02%	otc
		0.03%	otc
		0.1%	Rx
Oxymetazoline	Up to 12	0.025%	otc
Phenylephrine	Up to 4	0.12%	otc
		2.5%	Rx
		10%	Rx
Tetrahydrozoline	4 to 6	0.05%	otc

Contraindications

Known hypersensitivity to any of these agents; patients with anatomically narrow angles or narrow-angle glaucoma (phenylephrine and naphazoline only).

➤*Phenylephrine:* Infants (10% solution) and low–birth-weight infants (2.5% solution); elderly with severe arteriosclerotic, cardiovascular, or cerebrovascular disease; use during intraocular operative procedures when the corneal epithelial barrier has been disturbed.

Warnings/Precautions

➤*Anesthetics:* Use of a local anesthetic prior to phenylephrine 2.5% or 10% may help prevent pain.

➤*Cardiovascular effects:* There have been rare reports associating the use of **phenylephrine** 10% solution with the development of serious cardiovascular reactions, including ventricular arrhythmia and myocardial infarction. These episodes, some ending fatally, have usually occurred in elderly patients with preexisting cardiovascular diseases.

The hypertensive effects of phenylephrine may be treated with an alpha-adrenergic blocking agent, such as phentolamine 5 to 10 mg intravenously (IV), repeated as necessary.

➤*Narrow-angle glaucoma:* Ordinarily, any mydriatic is contraindicated in patients with glaucoma because it may occasionally raise intraocular pressure. However, when temporary pupil dilation may free adhesions or vasoconstriction of intrinsic vessels may lower intraocular tension, these advantages may temporarily outweigh danger from coincident pupil dilation.

➤*Rebound congestion hyperemia:* Rebound congestion may occur with frequent or extended use of ophthalmic vasoconstrictors.

➤*Rebound miosis:* Rebound miosis has occurred in older persons 1 day after receiving phenylephrine; reinstillation produced a reduction in mydriasis. This may be of importance when prior to cataract surgery or there is retinal detachment.

➤*Systemic absorption:* Exceeding recommended dosages of these agents or applying **phenylephrine** 2.5% or 10% solutions to the instrumented, traumatized, diseased, or postsurgical eye or adnexa, or to patients with suppressed lacrimation, as during anesthesia, may result in the absorption of sufficient quantities to produce a systemic vasopressor response. The lacrimal sac should be compressed by digital pressure for 2 to 3 minutes after instillation to avoid excessive systemic absorption.

➤*Contact lenses:* Remove contact lenses before using ophthalmic decongestant.

➤*Pigment floaters:* Older individuals may develop transient pigment floaters in the aqueous humor 30 to 45 minutes after instillation of **phenylephrine**. The appearance may be similar to anterior uveitis or a microscopic hyphema.

➤*Hazardous tasks:* **Phenylephrine** may cause temporary blurred or unstable vision; observe caution while driving or performing other hazardous tasks.

➤*Sulfite sensitivity:* Some of these products contain sulfites that may cause allergic-type reactions (eg, hives, itching, wheezing, anaphylaxis) in certain susceptible persons. Although the overall prevalence of sulfite sensitivity in the general population is probably low, it is seen more frequently in asthmatics or in atopic nonasthmatic persons.

➤*Special risk:* Use with caution in the presence of hypertension, diabetes, hyperthyroidism, cardiovascular abnormalities, infection, or injury.

➤*Pregnancy: Category C.* Safety for use during pregnancy is not established. Use only if clearly needed and if the potential benefits outweigh potential hazards to the fetus.

➤*Lactation:* Safety for use during breast-feeding has not been established. Because many drugs are distributed into milk, use caution when administering to a breast-feeding woman.

➤*Children:* Safety and efficacy have not been established for **naphazoline**; however, use of naphazoline 0.1% solution in children, especially infants, may result in CNS depression, leading to coma and marked reduction in body temperature. **Oxymetazoline** and **tetrahydrozoline** may be used in children 6 years of age and older. **Phenylephrine** 10% is contraindicated in infants and the 2.5% solution is contraindicated in low–birth-weight neonates and infants.

➤*Monitoring:* Monitor blood pressure in elderly patients with known cardiac disease.

Drug Interactions

Ophthalmic Sympathomimetic Drug Interactions

Precipitant drug	Object drug[a]		Description
Atropine	Ophthalmic sympathomimetics (eg, phenylephrine)	↑	Concomitant use of phenylephrine and atropine may enhance the pressor effects of phenylephrine and induce tachycardia in some patients, especially infants.
Atropine-like drugs Guanethidine Methyldopa Reserpine	Ophthalmic sympathomimetics Phenylephrine	↑	Coadministration may potentiate the pressor effects of phenylephrine.
Beta-blockers Propranolol	Ophthalmic sympathomimetics	↑	Systemic adverse reactions may occur more readily in patients taking these drugs.
MAOIs[b]	Ophthalmic sympathomimetics	↑	When given with, or up to 21 days after discontinuation of, MAOIs, exaggerated adrenergic effects or a severe hypertensive crisis may occur. Careful supervision and adjustment of doses are required.
Maprotiline	Ophthalmic sympathomimetics (eg, naphazoline)	↑	Coadministration of maprotiline and naphazoline may potentiate the pressor effects of naphazoline.
Ophthalmic sympathomimetics Phenylephrine	Anesthetics	↑	Phenylephrine may potentiate the cardiovascular depressant effects of potent inhalation anesthetic agents.
Tricyclic antidepressants	Ophthalmic sympathomimetics	↑	The pressor response of adrenergic agents may be potentiated.

[a] ↑ = object drug increased.
[b] MAOI = monoamine oxidase inhibitor.

Also consider drug interactions that may occur with systemic use of the sympathomimetics (see Vasopressors Used in Shock).

Adverse Reactions

➤*Ophthalmic:* Blurring of vision; discomfort; increased intraocular pressure; increased redness; irritation; lacrimation; mydriasis; punctate keratitis; transitory stinging on initial instillation.

Phenylephrine – Phenylephrine may cause rebound miosis and decreased mydriatic response to therapy in older persons.

➤*Cardiovascular:* Cardiac irregularities.

Phenylephrine 10% – A marked increase in blood pressure has been reported in low-weight premature neonates, infants, and adult patients with idiopathic orthostatic hypotension. Cardiovascular reactions occurring primarily in elderly patients include marked increase in blood pressure, syncope, myocardial infarction, tachycardia, arrhythmia, and fatal subarachnoid hemorrhage. Other reactions have included bradycardia.

➤*Miscellaneous:* Dizziness; drowsiness; excitability; headache; hyperglycemia; nausea; nervousness; sweating; weakness.

Patient Information

Advise patients not to use beyond 48 to 72 hours without consulting a health care provider.

Advise patients to discontinue use and consult a health care provider if irritation, blurring, or redness persists, or if severe eye pain, headache, vision changes, floating spots, dizziness, decrease in body temperature, drowsiness, acute eye redness or pain with light exposure occur.

Advise patients with glaucoma not to use this medicine, except under the advice of a health care provider.

Advise patients to remove contact lenses before using ophthalmic decongestant.

Inform patients that overuse may produce increased redness of the eye.

Tell patients not to touch the dropper tip to any surface because this may contaminate the solution.

Tell patients not to use if ophthalmic solution is brown or contains a precipitate.

Advise patients to compress the lacrimal sac by applying pressure with a finger for 2 to 3 minutes after instillation to avoid excessive systemic absorption.

Phenylephrine may cause temporary blurred or unstable vision; tell patients to observe caution while driving or performing other hazardous tasks.

TETRAHYDROZOLINE HYDROCHLORIDE

otc	**Tetrahydrozoline Hydrochloride** (Various)	**Solution; ophthalmic:** 0.05%	In 15 mL.
otc	**Altazine Irritation Relief** (Altaire)		In 15 mL.[a]
otc	**Altazine Moisture Relief** (Altaire)		In 15 mL.[b]
otc	**Murine Plus** (MedTech)		In 15 mL.[e]
otc	**Opti-Clear** (Major)		In 15 mL.[f]
otc	**Optigene 3** (Pfeiffer)		In 15 mL.[d]
otc	**Visine** (J & J Healthcare)		In 15 and 30 mL.[c]
otc	**Visine A.C.** (J & J Healthcare)		In 15 and 30 mL.[h]
otc	**Visine Advanced Relief** (J & J Healthcare)		In 30 mL.[g]
otc	**Visine Maximum Redness Relief** (J & J Healthcare)		In 15 mL.[i]
otc	**Visine Totality Multi-Symptom Relief** (J & J Healthcare)		In 15 mL.[j]

[a] With 0.25% zinc sulfate.
[b] With 1% dextran, 1% polyethylene glycol 400, and 1% povidone.
[c] With benzalkonium chloride, boric acid, EDTA, and sodium borate.
[d] With 0.01% benzalkonium chloride, boric acid, 0.1% EDTA, and sodium borate.
[e] With 0.5% polyvinyl alcohol, 0.6% povidone, benzalkonium chloride, dextrose, EDTA, sodium bicarbonate, sodium chloride, sodium citrate, sodium phosphate mono- and dibasic.
[f] With 0.01% benzalkonium chloride, boric acid, EDTA, sodium borate, and sodium chloride.
[g] With 0.1% dextran 70, 1% polyethylene glycol 400, 1% povidone, benzalkonium chloride, boric acid, EDTA, and sodium borate.
[h] With benzalkonium chloride, boric acid, edetate disodium, sodium chloride, sodium citrate, 0.25% zinc.
[i] With benzalkonium chloride, boric acid, edetate disodium, glycerin, hypromellose 0.36%, PEG, sodium chloride, sodium citrate.
[j] With benzalkonium chloride, boric acid, edetate disodium, glycerin, hypromellose 0.36%, PEG, sodium chloride, sodium citrate, zinc sulfate 0.25%.

TETRAHYDROZOLINE HYDROCHLORIDE — OPHTHALMIC SOLUTION

For complete and comparative prescribing information, refer to the Ophthalmic Decongestants class monograph.

Indications

➤*Ocular decongestant:* Relieves redness of the eye due to minor eye irritation.

Administration and Dosage

➤*Adults:*

Ocular decongestant – Instill 1 to 2 drops in the affected eye(s) up to 4 times daily.

➤*Storage/Stability:* Store at room temperature, 15° to 30°C (59° to 86°F). If the solution changes color or becomes cloudy, do not use. Replace cap after use and keep tightly closed.

PHENYLEPHRINE HYDROCHLORIDE

otc	**Refresh Redness Relief** (Allergan)	**Solution; ophthalmic:** 0.12%	In 15 mL.
Rx	**Phenylephrine hydrochloride** (Various, eg, Falcon, Deca Pharmaceuticals, LLC)	**Solution; ophthalmic:** 2.5%	In 15 mL.
Rx	**AK-Dilate** (Akorn)		In 2 and 15 mL.[a]
Rx	**Altafrin** (Altaire)		In 5 and 15 mL.[b]
Rx	**Mydfrin 2.5%** (Alcon)		In 3 and 5 mL *Drop-Tainers*.[c]
Rx	**Neofrin** (Ocusoft)		In 15 mL.[d]
Rx	**Phenylephrine hydrochloride** (Various, eg, Deca Pharmaceuticals, LLC)	**Solution; ophthalmic:** 10%	In 2 and 5 mL.
Rx	**AK-Dilate** (Akorn)		In 5 mL.[c]
Rx	**Altafrin** (Altaire)		In 5 mL.[e]
Rx	**Neofrin** (Ocusoft)		In 15 mL.[e]

[a] With 0.01% benzalkonium chloride and sodium phosphate mono- and dibasic.
[b] With benzalkonium chloride, boric acid, and sodium phosphate mono- and dibasic.
[c] With 0.01% benzalkonium chloride, EDTA, sodium bisulfite, and boric acid.
[d] With 0.01% benzalkonium chloride, boric acid, EDTA, sodium borate, and sodium bisulfite.
[e] With benzalkonium chloride and sodium phosphate mono- and dibasic.

PHENYLEPHRINE HYDROCHLORIDE — OPHTHALMIC SOLUTION

For complete and comparative prescribing information, refer to the Ophthalmic Decongestants group monograph.

Indications

➤*2.5% and 10% solutions:* For use as a vasoconstrictor, decongestant, and mydriatic in a variety of ophthalmic conditions and procedures. Some of its uses are for pupillary dilation in uveitis (to prevent or aid in the disruption of posterior synechia formation) and for many ophthalmic surgical procedures. The 2.5% solution may also be used for refraction without cycloplegia and for funduscopy and other diagnostic procedures.

➤*0.12% solution:* Used to relieve redness of the eye due to minor eye irritations and as a lubricant to prevent further irritation or to relieve dryness of the eye.

Administration and Dosage

➤*Adults:*

Diagnostic procedures –

Blanching test:

• *2.5% solution* – Instill 1 or 2 drops of phenylephrine 2.5% ophthalmic solution into the injected eye. After 5 minutes, examine for perilimbal blanching. If blanching occurs, the congestion is superficial and probably does not indicate iridocyclitis.

Provocative test for angle closure glaucoma:

• *2.5% solution* – Phenylephrine 2.5% may be used cautiously as a provocative test when intermittent narrow-angle closure glaucoma is suspected. Intraocular tension and gonioscopy are performed before and after dilation of the pupil with phenylephrine. A significant intraocular pressure rise, combined with gonioscopic evidence of angle closure, indicates an anterior segment anatomy capable of angle closure. A negative test does not rule this out. This pharmacologically induced angle closure glaucoma may not simulate real life conditions and other causes for transient elevations of intraocular pressure should be excluded.

Retinoscopy:

• *2.5% solution* – When dilation of the pupil without cycloplegic action is desired for retinoscopy, phenylephrine 2.5% ophthalmic solution may be used alone.

Glaucoma – Phenylephrine 2.5% and 10% ophthalmic solutions may be used with miotics in patients with open-angle glaucoma. It reduces the difficulties experienced by the patient because of the small field produced by miosis, and still it permits and often supports the effect of the miotic in lowering the intraocular pressure. Hence, there may be marked improvement in visual acuity after using phenylephrine ophthalmic solutions in conjunction with miotic drugs.

10% solution: In certain patients with glaucoma, temporary reduction of intraocular tension may be attained by producing vasoconstriction of the intraocular vessels. This treatment may be repeated as often as necessary.

Ophthalmoscopic examination –

2.5% solution: Instill one drop in each eye. Sufficient mydriasis to permit examination is produced in 15 to 30 minutes. Dilation lasts from 4 to 6 hours.

Ophthalmic redness/lubricant –

0.12% solution: Instill 1 or 2 drops in the affected eye up to 4 times daily.

Refraction –

2.5 % solution:

• *Usual dosage* – One drop of the preferred cycloplegic is placed in each eye, followed in 5 minutes by 1 drop of phenylephrine 2.5% ophthalmic solution. Because adequate cycloplegia is achieved at different time intervals after the instillation of the necessary number of drops, different cycloplegics will require different waiting periods to achieve adequate cycloplegia.

• *Concomitant therapy* – May be used effectively to increase mydriasis with homatropine, atropine, cyclopentolate, and tropicamide.

Surgery –

2.5% and 10% solution: When a short-acting mydriatic is needed for wide dilation of the pupil before intraocular surgery, phenylephrine 2.5% and 10% ophthalmic solutions may be applied topically 30 to 60 minutes before the operation.

Uveitis –

Posterior synechiae:

• *2.5% and 10% solution* – To free recently formed posterior synechiae, 1 drop of phenylephrine ophthalmic solution may be applied and be repeated as necessary, not to exceed 3 times. Treatment may be continued the following day if necessary. In the interim, hot compresses should be applied for 5 or 10 minutes 3 times a day, with 1 drop of a 1% or 2% solution of atropine sulfate before and after each series of compresses.

Phenylephrine 2.5% and 10% ophthalmic solutions may be used in patients with uveitis when synechiae are present or may develop. The formation of synechiae may be prevented by the use of these solutions and atropine or other cycloplegics to produce wide dilation of the pupil. It should be emphasized, however, that the vasoconstrictor effect of phenylephrine may be antagonistic to the increase of local blood flow in uveal infection.

Vasoconstriction and pupil dilation –

2.5% and 10% solution: A drop of a suitable topical anesthetic may be applied, followed by 1 drop of phenylephrine ophthalmic solution on the upper limbus. The anesthetic prevents stinging and consequent dilution of the solution by lacrimation. It may occasionally be necessary to repeat the instillation after 1 hour, again preceded by the use of the topical anesthetic.

➤*Children:*

Refraction – For a one-application method, phenylephrine 2.5% may be combined with one of the preferred rapid-acting cycloplegics to produce adequate cycloplegia.

➤*Administration:* Do not touch the dropper tip to any surface because this may contaminate the solution.

➤*Storage/Stability:* Store at 20° to 25°C (68° to 77°F). Keep the container tightly closed. Protect from light and excessive heat. Prolonged exposure to air or strong light may cause oxidation and discoloration. Do not use if solution is brown or contains a precipitate.

Neofrin – Store in a refrigerator at 2° to 8°C (36° to 46°F). Keep tightly closed.

OXYMETAZOLINE HYDROCHLORIDE

otc	**Visine LR** (J & J Healthcare)	**Solution, ophthalmic:** 0.025%	In 15 and 30 mL.[a]

[a] With benzalkonium chloride, boric acid, sodium borate, sodium chloride, and EDTA.

OXYMETAZOLINE HYDROCHLORIDE — OPHTHALMIC SOLUTION

For complete and comparative prescribing information, refer to the Ophthalmic Decongestants group monograph.

Indications

➤*Ocular decongestant:* For relief of redness of the eye due to minor eye irritation.

Administration and Dosage

➤*Adults:*

Ocular decongestant – Instill 1 or 2 drops in the affected eye(s) every 6 hours.

➤*Children:*

6 years of age and older – See Adults for dosing.

➤*Storage/Stability:* Store at 15° to 25°C (59° to 77°F).

NAPHAZOLINE HYDROCHLORIDE

otc	**20/20 Eye Drops** (S.S.S. Company)	**Drops, ophthalmic:** 0.012%	In 15 mL.[a]
otc	**Advanced Eye Relief, Redness Instant Relief** (Bausch & Lomb Personal Products)	**Solution, ophthalmic:** 0.012%	In 15 mL.[b]
otc	**Clear Eyes ACR Seasonal Relief** (Medtech)		In 15 mL.[c]
otc	**Clear Eyes for Dry Eyes Plus Redness Relief** (Medtech)		In 15 mL.[d]
otc	**Clear Eyes for Redness Relief** (Medtech)		In 6, 15, and 30 mL.[e]
otc	**Naphcon** (Alcon)		In 15 mL.[f]
otc	**Advanced Eye Relief, Redness Maximum Relief** (Bausch & Lomb Personal Products)	**Solution, ophthalmic:** 0.03%	In 15 mL.[g]
Rx	**Naphazoline** (Various, eg, Goldline)	**Solution, ophthalmic:** 0.1%	In 15 mL.
Rx	**AK-Con** (Akorn)		In 15 mL.[f]

[a] With benzalkonium chloride, EDTA, and 0.2% glycerin.
[b] With 0.2% polyethylene 300, 0.01% benzalkonium chloride, boric acid, sodium borate, sodium chloride, and EDTA.
[c] With benzalkonium chloride, EDTA, 0.25% zinc sulfate, 0.2% glycerin, boric acid, sodium citrate, and sodium chloride.
[d] With 0.8% hypromellose, 0.25% glycerin, benzalkonium chloride, boric acid, calcium chloride, magnesium chloride, potassium chloride, sodium borate, sodium chloride, and EDTA.
[e] With 0.2% glycerin, benzalkonium chloride, boric acid, EDTA, and sodium borate.
[f] With 0.01% benzalkonium chloride, and EDTA.
[g] With 0.01% benzalkonium chloride, 0.5% hydroxypropyl methylcellulose, boric acid, sodium borate, sodium chloride, and EDTA.

NAPHAZOLINE HYDROCHLORIDE — OPHTHALMIC SOLUTION

For complete and comparative prescribing information, refer to the Ophthalmic Decongestants class monograph.

Indications

➤*Ocular vasoconstrictor/decongestant:* For use as a topical ocular vasoconstrictor; for the temporary relief of redness due to minor eye irritation, protection against further irritation, and temporary relief of burning and irritation due to dryness of the eye.

Administration and Dosage

➤*Adults:*

Ocular vasoconstrictor/decongestant – Instill 1 or 2 drops into the conjunctival sac of affected eye(s) every 3 to 4 hours, up to 4 times daily.

➤*Storage/Stability:* Store at 20° to 25°C (68° to 77°F). Keep the container tightly closed.

Warnings/Precautions

➤*Pregnancy: Category C.* Animal reproduction studies have not been conducted with naphazoline. It is also not known whether naphazoline can cause harm when administered to a pregnant woman or can affect reproduction capacity. Give naphazoline to pregnant women only if clearly needed.

➤*Lactation:* It is not known whether naphazoline is excreted in human milk. Because many drugs are excreted in human milk, exercise caution when naphazoline is administered to a breast-feeding woman.

OPHTHALMIC ANTIHISTAMINES

OLOPATADINE HYDROCHLORIDE

Rx	**Patanol** (Alcon)	**Solution; ophthalmic:** 0.1%	In 5 mL *Drop-Tainer* dispenser.[a]
Rx	**Olopatadine Hydrochloride** (Alcon)	**Solution; ophthalmic:** 0.2%	In 2.5 mL fill in 4 mL bottle.[b]
Rx	**Pataday** (Alcon)		In 2.5 mL *Drop-Tainer* dispenser.[a]

[a] With benzalkonium chloride.
[b] With benzalkonium chloride 0.01%, EDTA, povidone, dibasic sodium phosphate, sodium chloride, hydrochloric acid/sodium hydroxide.

OLOPATADINE HYDROCHLORIDE — OPHTHALMIC

Indications

➤*Allergic conjunctivitis:* For temporary prevention of itching of the eye due to allergic conjunctivitis.

Administration and Dosage

➤*Adults:*

Allergic conjunctivitis –

Usual dosage:

- *0.1% solution* – 1 to 2 drops in each affected eye 2 times per day at an interval of 6 to 8 hours.
- *0.2% solution* – 1 drop in each affected eye once a day.

➤*Children:*

3 years of age and older –

Allergic conjunctivitis: See Adults for dosing.

➤*Administration:* Not for injection. Do not instill while wearing contact lenses.

➤*Storage/Stability:* Store at 2° to 25°C (36° to 77°F).

Actions

➤*Pharmacology:* Olopatadine is an inhibitor of histamine release from the mast cell and a relatively selective histamine H_1-antagonist that inhibits the in vivo and in vitro type 1 immediate hypersensitivity reaction. Olopatadine is devoid of effects on alpha-adrenergic, dopamine, muscarinic type 1 and 2, and serotonin receptors.

➤*Pharmacokinetics:* Olopatadine has low systemic exposure. Plasma concentrations are generally below the quantitation limit of the assay (less than 0.5 ng/mL). Samples in which olopatadine is quantifiable are typically found within 2 hours of dosing and range from 0.5 to 1.3 ng/mL. The half-life in plasma is approximately 3 hours, and elimination is predominantly through renal excretion. Approximately 60% to 70% of the dose is recovered in the urine as parent drug. Two metabolites, the mono-desmethyl and the N-oxide, were detected at low concentrations in the urine.

Contraindications

Hypersensitivity to any component of this product.

Warnings/Precautions

➤*Administration:* Not for injection. Do not instill olopatadine while wearing contact lenses.

➤*Pregnancy: Category C.* Olopatadine was not found to be teratogenic in rats and rabbits. There are no adequate and well controlled studies in pregnant women. Use this drug in pregnant women only if the potential benefit to the mother justifies the potential risk to the embryo or fetus.

OLOPATADINE HYDROCHLORIDE — OPHTHALMIC

➤*Lactation:* Olopatadine has been identified in the milk of nursing rats following oral administration. It is not known whether topical ocular administration could result in sufficient systemic absorption to produce detectable quantities in breast milk. Exercise caution when olopatadine is administered to a nursing mother.

➤*Children:* Safety and effectiveness in pediatric patients younger than 3 years of age have not been established.

Adverse Reactions

➤*Ophthalmic:* Burning or stinging, dry eye, foreign body sensation, hyperemia, keratitis, lid edema, pruritus (less than 5%).

➤*Miscellaneous:* Headache (7%); asthenia, cold syndrome, pharyngitis, rhinitis, sinusitis, taste perversion (less than 5%).

Patient Information

To prevent contaminating the dropper tip and solution, do not touch the eyelids and surrounding areas with the dropper tip of the bottle.

Keep bottle tightly closed when not in use.

EMEDASTINE DIFUMARATE

Rx	Emadine (Alcon)	**Solution:** 0.05%	Benzalkonium chloride. In 5 mL.

EMEDASTINE DIFUMARATE — OPHTHALMIC

Indications

➤*Allergic conjunctivitis:* For the temporary relief of the signs and symptoms of allergic conjunctivitis.

Administration and Dosage

➤*Adults:*

Allergic conjunctivitis – Instill 1 drop in the affected eye up to 4 times daily.

➤*Children:*

3 years of age and older – See Adults for dosing.

➤*Storage/Stability:* Store at 4° to 30°C (39° to 86°F).

Actions

➤*Pharmacology:* Emedastine is a relatively selective, histamine H_1 antagonist. In vitro examinations of emedastine's affinity for histamine receptors (H_1: Ki = 1.3 nM, H_2: Ki = 49,067 nM, and H_3: Ki = 12,430 nM) demonstrate relative selectivity for the H_1 histamine receptor. In vivo studies have shown concentration-dependent inhibition of histamine-stimulated vascular permeability in the conjunctiva following topical ocular administration. Emedastine appears to be devoid of effects on adrenergic, dopaminergic and serotonin receptors.

➤*Pharmacokinetics:*

Absorption – Following topical administration in man, emedastine was shown to have low systemic exposure. In a study involving 10 healthy volunteers dosed bilaterally twice daily for 15 days with emedastine difumarate, plasma concentrations of the parent compound were generally below the quantitation limit of the assay (less than 0.3 ng/mL). Samples in which emedastine was quantifiable ranged from 0.3 to 0.49 ng/mL.

Metabolism/Excretion – The elimination half-life of oral emedastine in plasma is 3 to 4 hours. Approximately 44% of the oral dose is recovered in the urine over 24 hours with only 3.6% of the dose excreted as parent drug. Two primary metabolites, 5- and 6-hydroxyemedastine, are excreted in the urine as both free and conjugated forms. The 5'-oxoanalogs of 5- and 6-hydroxyemedastine and the N-oxide are also formed as minor metabolites.

Contraindications

Hypersensitivity to the solution or any of its components.

Warnings/Precautions

➤*Administration:* Emedastine difumarate is for topical use only and not for injection or oral use.

➤*Pregnancy: Category B.* Teratology and perinatal and postnatal studies have been conducted with emedastine difumarate in rats and rabbits. At 15,000 times the maximum recommended ocular human use level, emedastine difumarate was shown not to be teratogenic in rats and rabbits and no effects on peri/postnatal development were observed in rats. However, at 70,000 times the maximum recommended ocular human use level, emedastine difumarate was shown to increase the incidence of external, visceral and skeletal anomalies in rats. There are, however, no adequate and well-controlled studies in pregnant women. Because animal studies are not always predictive of human response, this drug should be used during pregnancy only if clearly needed.

➤*Lactation:* Emedastine has been identified in breast milk in rats following oral administration. It is not known whether topical ocular administration could result in sufficient systemic absorption to produce detectable quantities in breast milk. Nevertheless, caution should be exercised when emedastine difumarate is administered to a nursing mother.

➤*Children:* Safety and effectiveness in pediatric patients less than 3 years of age have not been established.

Adverse Reactions

In controlled clinical studies of emedastine difumarate ophthalmic solution 0.05% lasting for 42 days, the most frequent adverse reaction was headache (11%).

➤*Adverse reactions reported in less than 5% of patients:* The following adverse reactions were reported in less than 5% of patients: Abnormal dreams, asthenia, bad taste in the mouth, blurred vision, burning or stinging, corneal infiltrates, corneal staining, dermatitis, discomfort, dry eye, foreign body sensation, hyperemia, keratitis, pruritus, rhinitis, sinusitis and tearing. Some of these events were similar to the underlying disease being studied.

Overdosage

➤*Symptoms:* Somnolence and malaise have been reported following daily oral administration. Oral ingestion of the contents of a 15 mL dispenser would be equivalent to 7.5 mg.

➤*Treatment:* In case of overdosage, treatment is symptomatic and supportive.

Patient Information

To prevent contaminating the dropper tip and solution, care should be taken not to touch the eyelids or surrounding areas with the dropper tip of the bottle. Keep the bottle tightly closed when not in use. Do not use if the solution has become discolored.

Patients should be advised not to wear a contact lens if their eye is red. Emedastine difumarate should not be used to treat contact lens-related irritation. The preservative in emedastine difumarate, benzalkonium chloride, may be absorbed by soft contact lenses. Patients who wear soft contact lenses, and whose eyes are not red, should be instructed to wait at least 10 minutes after instilling emedastine difumarate before they insert their contact lenses.

AZELASTINE HYDROCHLORIDE

Rx	Azelastine (Various, eg, Apotex, Sun Pharmaceutical)	**Solution; ophthalmic:** 0.05%	Equiv. to 0.457 mg azelastine. Benzalkonium chloride 0.25 mg, disodium edetate dihydrate, hydroxypropylmethylcellulose, sodium hydroxide. In 6 mL with dropper.
Rx	Optivar (MedPointe Healthcare[a])		Equiv. to 0.457 mg azelastine. Benzalkonium chloride 0.125 mg, disodium edetate dihydrate, hydroxypropylmethylcellulose, sodium hydroxide. In 6 mL with dropper.

[a] MedPointe Healthcare Inc, 265 Davidson Avenue, Suite 300, Somerset, NJ 08873–4120; (732) 564–2200; http://www.medpointeinc.com.

AZELASTINE HYDROCHLORIDE — OPHTHALMIC

For more comparative information, see Azelastine HCl in the Antihistamines group monograph.

Indications

➤*Allergic conjunctivitis:* For the treatment of itching of the eye associated with allergic conjunctivitis.

Administration and Dosage

➤*Adults:*

Allergic conjunctivitis – 1 drop instilled into each affected eye twice a day.

➤*Children:*

Allergic conjunctivitis –

3 years of age and older: See Adults for dosing.

➤*Administration:* Azelastine is for ocular use only and not for injection or oral use.

➤*Storage/Stability:* Store upright between 2° and 25°C (36° and 77°F).

Actions

➤*Pharmacology:* Azelastine hydrochloride is a relatively selective histamine H_1 antagonist and an inhibitor of the release of histamine and other mediators from cells (eg, mast cells) involved in the allergic response. Based on in vitro studies using human cell lines, inhibition of other mediators involved in allergic reactions (eg, leukotrienes, PAF) has been demonstrated with azelastine hydrochloride. Decreased chemotaxis and activation of eosinophils has also been demonstrated.

AZELASTINE HYDROCHLORIDE — OPHTHALMIC

➤*Pharmacokinetics:*

Absorption – Absorption of azelastine following ocular administration was relatively low. A study in symptomatic patients receiving 1 drop of azelastine hydrochloride in each eye 2 to 4 times a day (0.06 to 0.12 mg azelastine hydrochloride) demonstrated plasma concentrations of azelastine hydrochloride to generally be between 0.02 and 0.25 ng/mL after 56 days of treatment. Three of 19 patients had quantifiable amounts of N-desmethylazelastine that ranged from 0.25 to 0.87 ng/mL at day 56.

Metabolism/Excretion – Based on IV and oral administration, the elimination half-life, steady-state volume of distribution and plasma clearance were 22 hours, 14.5 L/kg and 0.5 L/hr/kg, respectively. Approximately 75% of an oral dose of radiolabeled azelastine hydrochloride was excreted in the feces with less than 10% as unchanged azelastine. Azelastine hydrochloride is oxidatively metabolized to the principal metabolite, N-desmethylazelastine, by the cytochrome P450 enzyme system. In vitro studies in human plasma indicate that the plasma protein binding of azelastine and N-desmethylazelastine are approximately 88% and 97%, respectively.

Contraindications

Hypersensitivity to any of its components.

Warnings/Precautions

➤*Administration:* Azelastine hydrochloride is for ocular use only and not for injection or oral use.

➤*Pregnancy: Category C.*

Teratogenic – Azelastine hydrochloride has been shown to be embryotoxic, fetotoxic, and teratogenic (external and skeletal abnormalities) in mice at an oral dose of 68.6 mg/kg/day (57,000 times the recommended ocular human use level). At an oral dose of 30 mg/kg/day (25,000 times the recommended ocular human use level), delayed ossification (undeveloped metacarpus) and the incidence of 14th rib were increased in rats. At 68.6 mg/kg/day (57,000 times the maximum recommended ocular human use level) azelastine hydrochloride caused resorption and fetotoxic effects in rats. The relevance to humans of these skeletal findings noted at only high drug exposure levels is unknown.

There are no adequate and well-controlled studies in pregnant women. Only use azelastine hydrochloride during pregnancy if the potential benefit justifies the potential risk to the fetus.

➤*Lactation:* It is not known whether azelastine hydrochloride is excreted in human milk. Because many drugs are excreted in human milk, exercise caution when administering azelastine hydrochloride to a nursing woman.

➤*Children:* Safety and efficacy in pediatric patients below the age of 3 years have not been established.

➤*Elderly:* No overall differences in safety or efficacy have been observed between elderly and younger adult patients.

Adverse Reactions

In controlled multiple-dose studies where patients were treated for up to 56 days, the most frequently reported adverse reactions were transient eye burning/stinging (approximately 30%), headaches (approximately 15%) and bitter taste (approximately 10%). The occurrence of these events was generally mild.

The following events were reported in 1% to 10% of patients: Asthma, conjunctivitis, dyspnea, eye pain, fatigue, influenza-like symptoms, pharyngitis, pruritus, rhinitis and temporary blurring. Some of these events were similar to the underlying disease being studied.

Patient Information

To prevent contaminating the dropper tip and solution, take care not to touch any surface, the eyelids or surrounding areas with the dropper tip of the bottle. Keep bottle tightly closed when not in use. This product is sterile when packaged.

Advise patients not to wear a contact lens if their eyes are red. Azelastine hydrochloride should not be used to treat contact lens-related irritation. The preservative in azelastine hydrochloride, benzalkonium chloride, may be absorbed by soft contact lenses. Instruct patients who wear soft contact lenses, and whose eyes are not red, to wait at least 10 minutes after instilling azelastine hydrochloride before they insert their contact lenses.

KETOTIFEN

otc	**Ketotifen Fumarate** (Various, eg, Akorn)	**Solution; ophthalmic:** 0.025%	As ketotifen fumarate. In 5 mL.[a]
otc	**Alaway** (Bausch & Lomb)		As ketotifen fumarate. In 10 mL.[b]
otc	**Claritin Eye** (Schering-Plough)		As ketotifen fumarate. In 5 mL.[c]
otc	**Itchy Eye Drops** (Major)		As ketotifen fumarate. In 5 mL.[b]
otc	**Visine All Day Eye Itch Relief** (Johnson & Johnson)		As ketotifen fumarate. In 5 mL.[a]
otc	**Zaditor** (Novartis Pharmaceuticals)		As ketotifen fumarate. In 1 and 5 mL.[c]
otc	**Zyrtec Itchy Eye Drops** (McNeil)		As ketotifen fumarate. In 5 mL.[a]

[a] May contain glycerol, sodium hydroxide and/or hydrochloric acid, and benzalkonium chloride 0.01%.
[b] With 0.01% benzalkonium chloride, glycerin, sodium hydroxide, and/or hydrochloric acid.
[c] With glycerol, sodium hydroxide and/or hydrochloric acid, and benzalkonium chloride 0.01%.

KETOTIFEN FUMARATE — OPHTHALMIC

Indications

➤*Rx:* For the temporary prevention of itching of the eye due to allergic conjunctivitis.

➤*OTC:* For the temporary relief of itchy eyes due to pollen, ragweed, grass, animal hair, and dander.

Administration and Dosage

➤*Adults:*

Ocular pruritus due to allergic conjunctivitis (Rx) – 1 drop in the affected eye(s) every 8 to 12 hours.

Allergic conditions due to pollen, ragweed, grass, animal hair, and dander (OTC) – 1 drop in the affected eye(s) every 8 to 12 hours.

➤*Children:*

3 years of age and older – See Adults for dosing.

➤*Administration:* For topical ophthalmic use only. Not for injection or oral use.

➤*Storage/Stability:* Store at 4° to 25°C (39° to 77°F).

Actions

➤*Pharmacology:* Ketotifen is a relatively selective, noncompetitive histamine antagonist (H_1-receptor) and mast cell stabilizer. Ketotifen inhibits the release of mediators from cells involved in hypersensitivity reactions. Decreased chemotaxis and activation of eosinophils have also been demonstrated.

In human conjunctival allergen-challenge studies, ketotifen fumarate was significantly more effective than placebo in preventing ocular itching associated with allergic conjunctivitis. The action of ketotifen occurs rapidly with an effect seen within minutes after administration.

Contraindications

Hypersensitivity to any component of this product.

Warnings/Precautions

➤*Administration:* For topical ophthalmic use only. Not for injection or oral use.

➤*Pregnancy: Category C.* Oral treatment of pregnant rabbits during organogenesis with 45 mg/kg/day of ketotifen (30,000 times the MRHOD) resulted in an increased incidence of retarded ossification of the sternebrae. However, no effects were observed in rabbits treated with up to 15 mg/kg/day (10,000 times the MRHOD). Similar treatment of rats during organogenesis with 100 mg/kg/day of ketotifen (66,667 times the MRHOD) did not reveal any biologically relevant effects.

Oral treatment of pregnant rats (up to 100 mg/kg/day or 66,667 times the MRHOD) and rabbits (up to 45 mg/kg/day or 30,000 times the MRHOD) during organogenesis did not result in any biologically relevant embryofetal toxicity. In the offspring of the rats that received ketotifen orally from day 15 of pregnancy to day 21 postpartum at 50 mg/kg/day (33,333 times the MRHOD), a maternally toxic treatment protocol, the incidence of postnatal mortality was slightly increased, and body weight gain during the first 4 days postpartum was slightly decreased.

There are no adequate and well-controlled studies in pregnant women. Use during pregnancy only if the potential benefits outweigh the potential hazards to the fetus.

➤*Lactation:* Ketotifen fumarate has been identified in breast milk in rats following oral administration. It is not known whether topical ocular administration could result in sufficient systemic absorption to produce detectable quantities in breast milk. Nevertheless, caution should be exercised when ketotifen fumarate is administered to a nursing mother.

➤*Children:* Safety and efficacy in pediatric patients under the age of 3 years have not been established.

Adverse Reactions

In controlled clinical studies, conjunctival injection, headaches, and rhinitis were reported at an incidence of 10% to 25%. The occurrence of these side effects was generally mild. Some of these events were similar to the underlying ocular disease being studied.

KETOTIFEN FUMARATE — OPHTHALMIC

The following ocular and nonocular adverse reactions were reported at an incidence of less than 5%:

➤*Ophthalmic:* Allergic reactions, burning or stinging, conjunctivitis, discharge, dry eyes, eye pain, eyelid disorder, itching, keratitis, lacrimation disorder, mydriasis, photophobia, and rash.

➤*Miscellaneous:* Flu syndrome, pharyngitis.

Overdosage

➤*Symptoms:* Oral ingestion of the contents of a 5 mL bottle would be equivalent to 1.725 mg of ketotifen fumarate. Clinical results have shown no serious signs or symptoms after the ingestion of up to 20 mg of ketotifen fumarate.

Patient Information

To prevent contaminating the dropper tip and solution, care should be taken not to touch the eyelids or surrounding areas with the dropper tip of the bottle. Keep the bottle tightly closed when not in use. Patients should be advised not to wear a contact lens if their eye is red. Ketotifen fumarate ophthalmic solution should not be used to treat contact lens-related irritation. The preservative in ketotifen fumarate ophthalmic solution, benzalkonium chloride, may be absorbed by soft contact lenses. Patients who wear soft contact lenses and whose eyes are not red, should be instructed to wait at least 10 minutes after instilling ketotifen fumarate ophthalmic solution before they insert their contact lenses.

EPINASTINE HYDROCHLORIDE

Rx	Elestat (Allergan)	Solution, ophthalmic: 0.05%	0.01% benzalkonium chloride, EDTA. In 8 and 15 mL.

EPINASTINE HYDROCHLORIDE — OPHTHALMIC

Indications

➤*Allergic conjunctivitis:* For the prevention of itching associated with allergic conjunctivitis.

Administration and Dosage

➤*Adults:*

Allergic conjunctivitis –

Usual dosage: Instill 1 drop in each eye twice a day.

Duration of therapy: Continue treatment throughout the period of exposure (ie, until the pollen season is over or until exposure to the offending allergen is terminated), even when symptoms are absent.

➤*Children:*

Allergic conjunctivitis –

3 years of age and older: See Adults for dosing.

➤*Administration:* Epinastine is for topical ophthalmic use only and not for injection or oral use.

➤*Storage/Stability:* Store at 15° to 25°C (59° to 77°F). Keep bottle tightly closed.

Actions

➤*Pharmacology:* Epinastine is a topically active, direct H_1-receptor antagonist and an inhibitor of the release of histamine from the mast cell. Epinastine is selective for the histamine H_1-receptor and has affinity for the histamine H_2 receptor. Epinastine also possesses affinity for the α_1-, α_2-, and 5- HT_2-receptors. Epinastine does not penetrate the blood/brain barrier and, therefore, is not expected to induce side effects of the central nervous system.

➤*Pharmacokinetics:*

Absorption/Distribution – Fourteen subjects, with allergic conjunctivitis, received 1 drop of epinastine in each eye twice daily for 7 days. On day 7, average maximum epinastine plasma concentrations of 0.04 ± 0.014 ng/mL were reached after about 2 hours, indicating low systemic exposure. While these concentrations represented an increase over those seen following a single dose, the day 1 and day 7 area under the curve (AUC) values were unchanged, indicating that there is no increase in systemic absorption with multiple dosing. Epinastine is 64% bound to plasma proteins.

Metabolism/Excretion – The total systemic clearance is approximately 56 L/hr and the terminal plasma elimination half-life is about 12 hours. Epinastine is mainly excreted unchanged. About 55% of an intravenous dose is recovered unchanged in the urine with about 30% in feces. Less than 10% is metabolized. The renal elimination is mainly via active tubular secretion.

Contraindications

Hypersensitivity to epinastine or to any of the other ingredients.

Warnings/Precautions

➤*Administration:* Epinastine hydrochloride is for topical ophthalmic use only and not for injection or oral use.

➤*Contact lenses:* Advise patients not to wear a contact lenses if their eyes are red. Do not use epinastine to treat contact-lens-related irritation. The preservative in epinastine, benzalkonium chloride, may be absorbed by soft contact lenses. Contact lenses should be removed prior to instillation of epinastine and may be reinserted after 10 minutes following its administration.

➤*Administration:* Instruct patients to avoid allowing the tip of the dispensing container to contact the eye, surrounding structures, fingers, or any other surface in order to avoid contamination of the solution by common bacteria known to cause ocular infections. Serious damage to the eye and subsequent loss of vision may result from using contaminated solutions. Keep bottle tightly closed when not in use.

➤*Pregnancy: Category C.* There are, however, no adequate and well-controlled studies in pregnant women. Because animal reproduction studies are not always predictive of human response, epinastine ophthalmic solution should be used during pregnancy only if the potential benefit justifies the potential risk to the fetus.

Teratogenic – In an embryofetal developmental study in pregnant rats, maternal toxicity with no embryofetal effects was observed at an oral dose that was approximately 150,000 times the MROHD. Total resorptions and abortion were observed in an embryofetal study in pregnant rabbits at an oral dose that was approximately 55,000 times the MROHD. In both studies, no drug-induced teratogenic effects were noted.

Epinastine reduced pup body weight gain following an oral dose to pregnant rats that was approximately 90,000 times the MROHD.

➤*Lactation:* A study in lactating rats revealed excretion of epinastine in the breast milk. It is not known whether this drug is excreted in human milk. Because many drugs are excreted in human milk, caution should be exercised when epinastine ophthalmic solution is administered to a nursing woman.

➤*Children:* Safety and effectiveness in pediatric patients younger than the age of 3 years have not been established.

➤*Elderly:* No overall differences in safety or effectiveness have been observed between elderly and younger patients.

Adverse Reactions

The most frequently reported ocular adverse events occurring in approximately 1% to 10% of patients were burning sensation in the eye, folliculosis, hyperemia, and pruritus.

The most frequently reported non-ocular adverse events were infection (cold symptoms and upper respiratory tract infections) seen in approximately 10% of patients, and headache, rhinitis, sinusitis, increased cough, and pharyngitis seen in approximately 1% to 3% of patients.

Some of these events were similar to the underlying disease being studied.

Patient Information

Advise patients not to wear a contact lenses if their eyes are red. Do not use epinastine hydrochloride ophthalmic solution to treat contact-lens-related irritation. The preservative in epinastine, benzalkonium chloride, may be absorbed by soft contact lenses. Contact lenses should be removed prior to instillation of epinastine and may be reinserted after 10 minutes following its administration.

Instruct patients to avoid allowing the tip of the dispensing container to contact the eye, surrounding structures, fingers, or any other surface in order to avoid contamination of the solution by common bacteria known to cause ocular infections. Serious damage to the eye and subsequent loss of vision may result from using contaminated solutions.

Keep bottle closed tightly when not in use.

ALCAFTADINE

Rx	Lastacaft (Vistakon Pharmaceuticals)	Solution; ophthalmic: 0.25%	Benzalkonium chloride 0.005%, edetate disodium. In 3 mL bottle.

ALCAFTADINE — OPHTHALMIC

Indications

➤*Allergic conjunctivitis:* For the prevention of itching associated with allergic conjunctivitis.

Administration and Dosage

➤*Adults:*

Allergic conjunctivitis – Instill 1 drop in each eye once daily.

➤*Children:*

2 years of age and older – See Adults for dosing.

➤*Administration:* For topical ophthalmic use only.

To minimize contamination of the dropper tip and solution, care should be taken not to touch the eyelids or surrounding areas with the dropper tip of the bottle. Keep bottle tightly closed when not in use.

➤*Storage/Stability:* Store at 15° to 25°C (59° to 77°F).

ALCAFTADINE — OPHTHALMIC

Actions

➤*Pharmacology:* Alcaftadine is a histamine 1 receptor antagonist and inhibits the release of histamine from mast cells. Decreased chemotaxis and inhibition of eosinophil activation has also been demonstrated.

➤*Pharmacokinetics:*

Absorption – Following bilateral topical ocular administration of alcaftadine 0.25% ophthalmic solution, the mean peak plasma concentration (C_{max}) of alcaftadine was approximately 60 pg/mL and the median time to peak plasma concentration occurred at 15 minutes. Plasma concentrations of alcaftadine were below the lower limit of quantification (10 pg/mL) by 3 hours after dosing. The mean C_{max} of the active carboxylic acid metabolite was approximately 3 ng/mL and occurred at 1 hour after dosing. Plasma concentrations of the carboxylic acid metabolite were below the lower limit of quantification (100 pg/mL) by 12 hours after dosing. There was no indication of systemic accumulation or changes in plasma exposure of alcaftadine or the active metabolite following daily topical ocular administration.

Distribution – The protein binding of alcaftadine and the active metabolite are 39.2% and 62.7%, respectively.

Metabolism – The metabolism of alcaftadine is mediated by non–cytochrome P450 (CYP-450) cytosolic enzymes to the active carboxylic acid metabolite.

Excretion – The elimination half-life of the carboxylic acid metabolite is approximately 2 hours following topical ocular administration. Based on data following oral administration of alcaftadine, the carboxylic acid metabolite is primarily eliminated unchanged in the urine.

Contraindications

None well documented.

Warnings/Precautions

➤*Contact lens use:* Patients should be advised not to wear a contact lens if their eye is red.

Alcaftadine should not be used to treat contact lens-related irritation.

Alcaftadine should not be instilled while the patient is wearing contact lenses. Advise patients to remove contact lenses prior to instillation of alcaftadine. The preservative in alcaftadine, benzalkonium chloride, may be absorbed by soft contact lenses. Lenses may be reinserted 10 minutes after administration of alcaftadine.

➤*Pregnancy: Category B.* There are no adequate and well-controlled studies in pregnant women. Because animal reproduction studies are not always predictive of human response, only use this drug during pregnancy if clearly needed.

➤*Lactation:* It is not known whether this drug is excreted in human milk. Because many drugs are excreted in human milk, exercise caution when administering alcaftadine to a breast-feeding woman.

➤*Children:* Safety and effectiveness in children younger than 2 years of age have not been established.

➤*Elderly:* No overall differences in safety or effectiveness were observed between elderly and younger subjects.

Drug Interactions

None well documented.

Adverse Reactions

➤*Ophthalmic:* The most frequent ocular adverse reactions, occurring in less than 4% of alcaftadine-treated eyes, were eye irritation, burning and/or stinging upon instillation, eye redness, and eye pruritus.

➤*Systemic:* The most frequent nonocular adverse reactions, occurring in less than 3% of subjects with alcaftadine-treated eyes, were nasopharyngitis, headache, and influenza. Some of these events were similar to the underlying disease being studied.

Patient Information

Advise patients not to touch dropper tip to any surface because this may contaminate the contents.

Advise patients not to wear a contact lens if their eye is red. Inform patients not to use alcaftadine to treat contact lens–related irritation. Also inform patients to remove contact lenses prior to instillation of alcaftadine. The preservative in alcaftadine, benzalkonium chloride, may be absorbed by soft contact lenses. Lenses may be reinserted 10 minutes after administration of alcaftadine.

OPHTHALMIC DECONGESTANT/ANTIHISTAMINE COMBINATIONS

OPHTHALMIC DECONGESTANT/ANTIHISTAMINE COMBINATIONS

	Product & Distributor	Decongestant	Antihistamine	How Supplied
otc	**Naphazoline HCl & Pheniramine Maleate** Solution (Various, eg, Moore)	naphazoline HCl 0.025%	pheniramine maleate 0.3%	In 15 mL.
otc	**Naphcon-A Solution** (Alcon)			In 15 mL *Drop-Tainers*.[b]
otc	**Visine-A** (J & J Healthcare)			EDTA. In 15 mL.
otc	**Opcon-A Solution** (Bausch & Lomb Personal Products)	naphazoline HCl 0.027%	pheniramine maleate 0.315%	In 15 mL.[c]

[a] With 0.01% benzalkonium Cl, polysorbate 80, 0.25% zinc sulfate.
[b] With 0.01% benzalkonium Cl, EDTA.
[c] With 0.5% hydroxypropyl methylcellulose, 0.01% benzalkonium CL, 0.1% EDTA, boric acid.

OPHTHALMIC DECONGESTANT/ANTIHISTAMINE COMBINATIONS — OPHTHALMIC

Indications

➤*Itching/Redness:* Temporary relief of the minor eye symptoms of itching and redness caused by pollen, animal hair, etc.

Administration and Dosage

➤*Adults:*

Itching/Redness – Recommendations vary. Refer to manufacturer package insert for instructions.

Warnings/Precautions

➤*Antihistamines:* Topical antihistamines are potential sensitizers and may produce a local sensitivity reaction. Because they may produce angle closure, use with caution in persons with a narrow angle or a history of glaucoma.

➤*Pregnancy: Category C* (tetrahydrozoline, naphazoline [per manufacturer's prescribing information]) (pheniramine, antazoline [per Briggs' *Drugs in Pregnancy and Lactation*]). Give to a pregnant woman only if clearly needed.

➤*Lactation:* Because many drugs are excreted in human milk, caution should be exercised when administered to a breast-feeding woman.

CYCLOPLEGIC MYDRIATICS

Refer to the Topical Ophthalmic Drugs introduction for more complete and comparative information.

Indications

➤*Mydriasis/Cycloplegia:* For cycloplegic refraction and for pre- and postoperative states when mydriasis is required. See individual monographs for specific indications.

➤*Uveitis:* For dilating the pupil and for the treatment of inflammatory condition of the iris and uveal tract.

Actions

➤*Pharmacology:* Anticholinergic agents block the responses of the sphincter muscle of the iris and the muscle of the ciliary body to cholinergic stimulation, producing pupillary dilation (mydriasis) and paralysis of accommodation (cycloplegia).

Cycloplegic Mydriatics

Drug	Mydriasis Peak (min)	Mydriasis Recovery (days)	Cycloplegia Peak (min)	Cycloplegia Recovery (days)	Solution available
Atropine	30 - 40	7 - 10	60 - 180	6 - 12	0.5% - 2%
Homatropine	30 - 60	1 - 3	30 - 60	1 - 3	2% - 5%
Scopolamine	20 - 30	3 - 7	30 - 60	3 - 7	0.25%
Cyclopentolate	30 - 60	1	25 - 75	.25 - 1	0.5% - 2%
Tropicamide	20 - 40	0.25	20 - 35	< 0.25	0.5% - 1%

Contraindications

Primary glaucoma or a tendency toward glaucoma (eg, narrow anterior chamber angle); hypersensitivity to belladonna alkaloids or any component of the products; adhesions (synechiae) between the iris and the lens (excluding homatropine); children who have previously had a severe systemic reaction to atropine.

Warnings/Precautions

➤*Topical ophthalmic use only:* For topical ophthalmic use only. Not for injection.

➤*Glaucoma:* Determine the intraocular tension and the depth of the angle of the anterior chamber before and during use to avoid glaucoma attacks.

➤*Systemic effects:* Avoid excessive systemic absorption by compressing the lacrimal sac by digital pressure for 1 to 3 minutes after instillation.

Excessive topical use of homatropine can potentially lead to a confusional state characterized by delirium, agitation, and, rarely, coma. This state is more apt to occur in children and elderly patients.

➤*Sulfite sensitivity:* Some of these products contain sulfites which may cause allergic-type reactions (eg, hives, itching, wheezing, anaphylaxis) in certain susceptible persons. Although the overall prevalence of sulfite sensitivity in the general population is probably low, it is seen more frequently in asthmatics or in atopic nonasthmatic persons. Specific products containing sulfites are identified in the product listings.

➤*Special risk:* Risk-benefit should be considered when the following medical conditions exist: keratoconus (homatropine may produce fixed dilated pupil); Down syndrome, children with brain damage, and elderly patients (increased susceptibility).

➤*Hazardous tasks:* May produce drowsiness, blurred vision or sensitivity to light (due to dilated pupils); observe caution while driving or performing other tasks requiring alertness, coordination or physical dexterity.

➤*Pregnancy: Category C* (atropine, homatropine). Safety for use during pregnancy has not been established. Give to a pregnant woman only if clearly needed.

➤*Lactation:* Atropine and homatropine may be detectable, in very small amounts, in breast milk. Although this is controversial, according to the American Academy of Pediatrics, these agents are compatible with breast-feeding. It is not known if cyclopentolate is excreted in breast milk. Exercise caution when administering to a nursing woman.

➤*Children:* Excessive use in children and in certain susceptible individuals may product systemic toxic symptoms. Use with extreme caution in infants and small children.

Tropicamide and cyclopentolate may cause CNS disturbances, which may be dangerous in infants and children. Keep in mind the possibility of occurrence of psychotic reaction and behavioral disturbance due to hypersensitivity to anticholinergic drugs. Use with extreme caution. Increased susceptibility to cyclopentolate has been reported in infants, young children and in children with spastic paralysis or brain damage. Feeding intolerance may follow ophthalmic use of this product in neonates. It is recommended that feeding be withheld for 4 hours after examination. Do not use in concentrations greater than 0.5% in small infants.

Safety and effectiveness of homatropine 5% solution in children have not been established; only the 2% solution should be used.

➤*Elderly:* Use these products with caution in the elderly and others where increased IOP may be encountered.

Adverse Reactions

➤*Local:* Increased intraocular pressure; transient stinging/burning; irritation with prolonged use (eg, allergic lid reactions, hyperemia, follicular conjunctivitis, blepharoconjunctivitis, vascular congestion, edema, exudate, eczematoid dermatitis).

➤*Systemic:* Dryness of the mouth and skin; blurred vision; photophobia with or without corneal staining; tachycardia; headache; parasympathetic stimulation; somnolence; visual hallucinations.

Other toxic manifestations of anticholinergic drugs include: Skin rash; abdominal distention in infants; unusual drowsiness; hyperpyrexia; vasodilation; urinary retention; diminished GI motility; decreased secretion in salivary and sweat glands, pharynx, bronchii and nasal passages. Severe manifestations of toxicity include: Coma; medullary paralysis; death. Severe reactions are manifested by hypotension with progressive respiratory depression.

Cyclopentolate and tropicamide have been associated with psychotic reactions and behavioral disturbances in children. CNS disturbances have occurred in children on tropicamide. Ataxia, incoherent speech, restlessness, hallucinations, hyperactivity, seizures, disorientation as to time and place, and failure to recognize people have occurred with cyclopentolate.

Overdosage

➤*Ocular:* If ocular overdosage occurs, flush eye(s) with water or normal saline. Use of a topical miotic may be required. If accidentally ingested, induce emesis or gastric lavage.

➤*Systemic:* If symptoms develop (see Adverse Reactions), patients usually recover spontaneously when the drug is discontinued. In cases of severe toxicity, give physostigmine salicylate (see individual monograph). Have atropine (1 mg) available for immediate injection if physostigmine causes bradycardia, convulsions or bronchoconstriction.

➤*Cyclopentolate toxicity:* Cyclopentolate toxicity may cause exaggerated symptoms (see Adverse Reactions). When administration of the drug product is discontinued, the patient usually recovers spontaneously. In case of severe manifestation of toxicity, the antidote of choice is physostigmine salicylate.

Children – Slowly inject 0.5 mg physostigmine salicylate IV. If toxic symptoms persist and no cholinergic symptoms are produced, repeat at 5 minute intervals to a maximum cumulative dose of 2 mg.

Adults and adolescents – Slowly inject 2 mg physostigmine salicylate IV. A second dose of 1 to 2 mg may be given after 20 minutes if no reversal of toxic manifestations has occurred.

Patient Information

To avoid contamination, advise the patient to not touch dropper tip to any surface. Replace cap after using.

Advise patients that the product may cause blurred vision. Inform patients not to drive or engage in any hazardous activities while the pupils are dilated.

Advise patients that products may cause sensitivity to light and to protect eyes in bright illumination during dilation.

Inform patients to keep out of the reach of children. Inform patients that these drugs should not be taken orally. Advise patients to wash their own hands and the child's following administration.

If eye pain occurs, advise patients to discontinue use and consult a health care provider immediately.

Refer to the Topical Ophthalmics Introduction for more complete information on administration and use.

ATROPINE SULFATE

Rx	**Atropine Sulfate Ophthalmic** (Various, eg, Bausch & Lomb, Goldline)	**Ointment:** 1%	In 3.5 and UD 1 g.
Rx	**Atropine Sulfate** (Various, eg, Alcon)	**Solution:** 1%	In 2, 5 and 15 mL and UD 1 mL.
Rx	**Isopto Atropine** (Alcon)		In 5 and 15 mL Drop-Tainers.[a]

[a] With 0.01% benzalkonium chloride, 0.5% hypromellose 2910, and boric acid.

ATROPINE SULFATE — OPHTHALMIC

For complete and comparative prescribing information, refer to the Cycloplegic Mydriatics group monograph.

Indications

➤*Mydriasis/Cycloplegia:* For mydriasis or cycloplegia. For cycloplegic refraction, for pupillary dilation desired in inflammatory conditions of the iris and uveal tract.

➤*Off-label uses:*

Other possible off-label uses – Atropine has been used for uveitis in children. (See also Administration and Dosage.)

Administration and Dosage

➤*Adults:*

Mydriasis/Cycloplegia –

Solution: 1 or 2 drops in the eye(s) 3 times daily, or as directed by a health care provider.

Ointment: A small amount in the conjunctival sac once or twice daily, or as directed by a health care provider.

➤*Children:* In children, use with extreme caution. This product should not be used in children who have previously had a severe systemic reaction to atropine.

Off-label dosing –

Uveitis: 1 to 2 drops of 0.5% solution in both eyes 1 to 3 times a day.

➤*Administration:* For topical use only; not for injection. Do not touch dropper tip to any surface because this may contaminate the solution.

To avoid excessive systemic absorption, the lacrimal sac should be compressed by digital pressure for 2 to 3 minutes after instillation.

➤*Storage/Stability:* Store between 15° and 30°C (59° and 86°F). Use solution only if imprinted neckband is intact. Use ointment only if bottom ridge of tube cap is not exposed.

SCOPOLAMINE HYDROBROMIDE (Hyoscine Hydrobromide)

Rx	**Isopto Hyoscine** (Alcon)	**Solution; ophthalmic:** 0.25%	In 5 and 15 mL *Drop-Tainers*.[a]

[a] With benzalkonium chloride 0.01% and hypromellose 0.5%.

SCOPOLAMINE HYDROBROMIDE (Hyoscine Hydrobromide) — OPHTHALMIC

For complete and comparative prescribing information, refer to the Cycloplegic Mydriatics class monograph.

Indications

➤*Iridocyclitis:* For some preoperative and postoperative states in the treatment of iridocyclitis.

➤*Mydriasis/Cycloplegia:* For cycloplegia and mydriasis in diagnostic procedures.

Administration and Dosage

➤*Adults:*

Iridocyclitis – Instill 1 or 2 drops into the eye(s) up to 4 times daily.

Mydriasis/Cycloplegia – Instill 1 or 2 drops into the eye(s) 1 hour before refracting.

➤*Administration:* For topical ophthalmic use only; not for injection.

Compress the lacrimal sac by digital pressure for several minutes after instillation.

➤*Storage/Stability:* Store at 8° to 27°C (46° to 80°F). Protect from light.

Actions

➤*Pharmacology:* This anticholinergic preparation blocks the responses of the sphincter muscle of the iris and the accommodative muscle of the ciliary body to cholinergic stimulation, producing pupillary dilation (mydriasis) and paralysis of accommodation (cycloplegia).

Contraindications

Primary glaucoma or a tendency toward glaucoma (eg, narrow anterior chamber angle); hypersensitivity to any component of this preparation.

Warnings/Precautions

➤*Contamination:* Do not touch dropper tip to any surface, as this may contaminate the solution.

➤*Angle-closure glaucoma:* To avoid inducing angle-closure glaucoma, make an estimation of the depth of the angle of the anterior chamber.

➤*Pregnancy: Category C.* Scopolamine readily crosses the placenta.

➤*Lactation:* Scopolamine is excreted in human milk. The American Academy of Pediatrics classifies scopolamine as compatible with breast-feeding.

➤*Children:* Safety and effectiveness in children have not been established.

Drug Interactions

None well documented.

Adverse Reactions

➤*Ophthalmic:* Prolonged use may produce local irritation, characterized by follicular conjunctivitis, vascular congestion, edema, exudate, and an eczematoid dermatitis.

➤*Miscellaneous:* Somnolence, dryness of the mouth, or visual hallucinations may occur.

Overdosage

None well documented.

Patient Information

Advise patient not to drive or engage in other hazardous activities when drowsy or while pupils are dilated.

Patients may experience sensitivity to light; instruct them to protect eyes in bright illumination during dilation.

Warn parents not to get this preparation in their child's mouth and to wash their own hands and the child's hands following administration.

HOMATROPINE HYDROBROMIDE

Rx	**Isopto Homatropine** (Alcon)	**Solution; ophthalmic:** 2%	In 5 mL *Drop-Tainers*.[a]
Rx	**Homatropine Hydrobromide** (Various, eg, Alcon, Novartis Ophthalmics, OcuSoft)	**Solution; ophthalmic:** 5%	In 5 mL.
Rx	**Isopto Homatropine** (Alcon)		In 5 mL *Drop-Tainers*.[b]

[a] With benzalkonium chloride 0.01%, hypromellose 0.5%, polysorbate 80.

[b] With benzethonium chloride 0.005%, hypromellose 0.5%, polysorbate 80.

HOMATROPINE HYDROBROMIDE — OPHTHALMIC

For complete and comparative prescribing information, refer to the Cycloplegic Mydriatics class monograph.

Indications

➤*Mydriasis and cycloplegia for refraction:* A moderately long-acting mydriatic and cycloplegic for cycloplegic refraction. For pre- and postoperative states when mydriasis is required.

➤*Optical aid:* For use as an optical aid in some cases of axial lens opacities.

➤*Uveitis:* For the treatment of inflammatory conditions of the uveal tract.

Administration and Dosage

➤*General dosing considerations:* Individuals with heavily pigmented irides may require larger doses.

➤*Adults:*

Mydriasis and cycloplegia for refraction – For refraction, instill 1 or 2 drops of the 2% or 5% solution in the affected eye(s). May be repeated in 5 or 10 minutes if necessary.

Uveitis – Instill 1 or 2 drops of the 2% or 5% solution into the affected eye(s) up to every 3 or 4 hours.

➤*Children:*

Mydriasis and cycloplegia for refraction – For refraction, instill 1 or 2 drops of the 2% solution only in the affected eye(s). May be repeated in 5 or 10 minutes if necessary.

Uveitis – Instill 1 or 2 drops of the 2% solution only into the affected eye(s) up to every 3 or 4 hours.

➤*Administration:* For topical ophthalmic use only.

To avoid excessive systemic absorption, the lacrimal sac should be compressed by digital pressure for 1 minute after instillation.

➤*Storage/Stability:* Store at 8° to 24°C (46° to 75°F).

TROPICAMIDE

Rx	**Tropicamide** (Various, eg, Bausch & Lomb)	**Solution:** 0.5%	In 2 and 15 mL.
Rx	**Mydral** (OcuSoft)		In 15 mL.[a]
Rx	**Tropicacyl** (Akorn)		In 15 mL.[b]
Rx	**Tropicamide** (Various, eg, Bausch & Lomb)	**Solution:** 1%	In 15 mL.
Rx	**Mydral** (OcuSoft)		In 2 and 15 mL.[a]
Rx	**Mydriacyl** (Alcon)		In 3 and 15 mL *Drop-Tainers*.[a]
Rx	**Tropicacyl** (Akorn)		In 2 and 15 mL.[b]

[a] With 0.01% benzalkonium chloride and EDTA.

[b] With 0.1% benzalkonium chloride and EDTA.

TROPICAMIDE — OPHTHALMIC

For complete and comparative prescribing information, refer to the Cycloplegic Mydriatics group monograph.

Indications

➤*Mydriasis/Cycloplegia:* For mydriasis and cycloplegia for diagnostic procedures.

Administration and Dosage

➤*General dosing considerations:* Individuals with heavily pigmented irides may require higher strength or more doses.

Mydriasis will reverse spontaneously with time, typically in 4 to 8 hours. However, in some cases, complete recovery may take up to 24 hours.

TROPICAMIDE — OPHTHALMIC

➤*Adults:*

Cycloplegia – For refraction, instill 1 or 2 drops of 1% solution in the eye(s); repeat in 5 minutes. If the patient is not seen within 20 to 30 minutes, an additional drop may be instilled to prolong mydriatic effect.

Mydriasis – For examination of fundus, instill 1 or 2 drops of 0.5% solution 15 or 20 minutes prior to examination.

➤*Administration:* For topical ophthalmic use only.

Remove contact lenses before using.

To avoid inducing angle closure glaucoma, an estimation of the depth of the angle of the anterior chamber should be made. The lacrimal sac should be compressed by digital pressure for 2 to 3 minutes after instillation to reduce excessive systemic absorption.

➤*Storage/Stability:* Store between 15° to 30°C (59° to 86°F). Do not refrigerate or store at high temperatures. Keep container closed tightly.

CYCLOPENTOLATE HYDROCHLORIDE

Rx	**Cyclogyl** (Alcon)	**Solution:** 0.5%	In 2, 5 and 15 mL *Drop-Tainers*.[a]
Rx	**Cyclopentolate HCl** (Various, eg, Steris)	**Solution:** 1%	In 2, 5 and 15 mL.
Rx	**AK-Pentolate** (Akorn)		In 1 and 15 mL.[a]
Rx	**Cyclogyl** (Alcon)		In 2, 5 and 15 mL.[a]
Rx	**Cyclogyl** (Alcon)	**Solution:** 2%	In 2, 5 and 15 mL *Drop-Tainers*.[a]

[a] With 0.01% benzalkonium chloride, EDTA and boric acid.

CYCLOPENTOLATE HYDROCHLORIDE — OPHTHALMIC

For complete and comparative prescribing information, refer to the Cycloplegic Mydriatics group monograph.

Indications

➤*Mydriasis/Cycloplegia:* Used to produce mydriasis and cycloplegia in diagnostic procedures.

Administration and Dosage

➤*General dosing considerations:* Use of cyclopentolate has been associated with psychotic reactions and behavioral disturbances in children. Observe infants closely for at least 30 minutes following instillation.

Individuals with heavily pigmented irides may require higher strengths.

➤*Adults:*

Mydriasis/Cycloplegia – Instill 1 or 2 drops of 0.5%, 1% or 2% solution in the eye, which may be repeated in 5 to 10 minutes if necessary. Complete recovery usually occurs in 24 hours. Complete recovery from mydriasis in some individuals may require several days.

➤*Children:*

Mydriasis/Cycloplegia –

12 months of age and older: Instill 1 or 2 drops of 0.5%, 1% or 2% solution in the eye, which may be repeated 5 to 10 minutes later by a second application of 0.5% or 1% solution if necessary.

11 months of age and younger: A single instillation of 1 drop of 0.5% cyclopentolate in the eye. To minimize absorption, apply pressure over the nasolacrimal sac for 2 to 3 minutes. Observe infant closely for at least 30 minutes following instillation.

➤*Administration:* To minimize absorption, use only 1 drop of 0.5% cyclopentolate solution per eye, followed by pressure applied over the nasolacrimal sac for 2 to 3 minutes.

For topical ophthalmic use only.

➤*Storage/Stability:* Store at 8° to 27°C (46° to 80°F).

Mydriatic Combinations

Rx	**Cyclomydril** (Alcon)	**Solution; ophthalmic:** cyclopentolate hydrochloride 0.2%/phenylephrine hydrochloride 1%	In 2 and 5 mL *Drop-Tainers*.[a]
Rx	**Paremyd** (Akorn)	**Solution; ophthalmic:** hydroxyamphetamine hydrobromide 1%/tropicamide 0.25%	In 15 mL.[b]

[a] With benzalkonium chloride 0.01%, edetate disodium, and boric acid.

[b] With benzalkonium chloride 0.005% and edetate disodium 0.015%.

These combinations induce mydriasis that is considerably greater than either drug alone. See individual monographs for complete prescribing information.

OPHTHALMIC ANTIBIOTICS

Refer to the Topical Ophthalmic Drugs introduction for more complete information.

Indications

➤*General information:* For a list of microorganisms usually susceptible to these agents, refer to systemic monographs in the Anti-infectives chapter.

➤*Ocular infections:* Treatment of superficial ocular infections involving the conjunctiva or cornea (eg, conjunctivitis, keratitis, keratoconjunctivitis, corneal ulcers, blepharitis, blepharoconjunctivitis, acute meibomianitis and dacryocystitis) caused by strains of microorganisms susceptible to antibiotics.

➤*Erythromycin:* Prophylaxis of ophthalmia neonatorum due to *Neisseria gonorrhoeae* or *Chlamydia trachomatis*.

➤*Chloramphenicol:* Use only in those serious infections for which less potentially dangerous drugs are ineffective or contraindicated (see Warnings).

Topical Ophthalmic Antibiotic Preparations

		Miscellaneous							Quinolones				Aminoglycosides			Sulfonamides	
	Organism/Infection	Bacitracin	Gramicidin	Polymyxin B	Erythromycin	Chloramphenicol	Trimethoprim	Oxytetracycline	Ciprofloxacin	Levofloxacin	Moxifloxacin	Ofloxacin	Neomycin	Gentamicin	Tobramycin	Sodium Sulfacetamide	Sulfisoxazole
Gram-positive	*Staphylococcus sp.*	✓	✓						✓			✓		✓	✓		
	S. aureus	✓	✓		✓	✓	✓		✓	✓	✓	✓	✓	✓[a]	✓	✓	✓
	S. epidermis									✓	✓						
	Streptococcus sp.	✓	✓			✓			✓	✓		✓			✓	✓	✓
	S. pneumoniae	✓	✓		✓	✓	✓		✓	✓	✓	✓		✓[a]	✓	✓	✓
	α-hemolytic streptococci (viridans group)				✓					✓	✓					✓	✓
	β-hemolytic streptococci	✓												✓[a]	✓		
	S. pyogenes	✓			✓		✓		✓			✓		✓		✓	✓
	S warneri										✓						
	S. haemolyticus										✓						
	S. hominis										✓						
	Corynebacterium sp.	✓	✓		✓					✓	✓		✓	✓	✓		
	Micrococcus luteus				✓						✓						

Topical Ophthalmic Antibiotic Preparations

		Miscellaneous							Quinolones				Aminoglycosides			Sulfonamides	
	Organism/Infection	Bacitracin	Gramicidin	Polymyxin B	Erythromycin	Chloramphenicol	Trimethoprim	Oxytetracycline	Ciprofloxacin	Levofloxacin	Moxifloxacin	Ofloxacin	Neomycin	Gentamicin	Tobramycin	Sodium Sulfacetamide	Sulfisoxazole
Gram-negative	*Escherichia coli*			✓		✓	✓	✓	✓			✓	✓	✓	✓	✓	✓
	Haemophilus aegyptius					✓	✓							✓	✓	✓	✓
	H. ducreyi					✓		✓	✓					✓	✓		
	H. influenzae or parainfluenzae			✓	✓	✓	✓	✓	✓	✓	✓	✓	✓	✓	✓		
	Klebsiella sp					✓		✓	✓			✓				✓	✓
	K. pneumoniae			✓			✓		✓			✓		✓	✓		
	Neisseria sp	✓				✓			✓				✓	✓	✓		
	N. gonorrhoeae	✓			✓[b]				✓			✓		✓		✓	
	Proteus sp.						✓		✓			✓	✓	✓	✓	✓	✓
	Acinetobacter calcoaceticus								✓			✓		✓	✓		
	Enterobacter aerogenes			✓			✓	✓	✓			✓	✓	✓	✓		
	Enterobacter sp.					✓			✓			✓	✓	✓	✓	✓	✓
	Serratia marcescens						✓		✓	✓		✓		✓	✓		
	Moraxella sp.					✓						✓		✓	✓		
	Chlamydia trachomatis				✓[b]				✓		✓	✓				✓	✓
	Pasteurella tularensis							✓									
	Pseudomonas aeruginosa			✓					✓	✓		✓		✓[a]	✓		
	Bartonella bacilliformis							✓									
	Bacteroides sp.							✓									
	Vibrio sp					✓		✓	✓					✓	✓		
	Providencia sp.								✓								
	Acinebacter lwoffi									✓	✓						

[a] Increasing resistance has been seen.

[b] For prophylaxis.

Administration and Dosage

Administration and dosage varies for the individual products. Refer to the individual monographs for specific dosing information.

Contraindications

Hypersensitivity to any component of these products; epithelial herpes simplex keratitis (dendritic keratitis); vaccinia; varicella; mycobacterial infections of the eye; fungal diseases of the ocular structure; use of steroid combinations after uncomplicated removal of a corneal foreign body.

Warnings/Precautions

➤*Sensitization:* Sensitization from the topical use of an antibiotic may contraindicate the drug's later systemic use in serious infections. For this reason, topical preparations containing antibiotics not ordinarily administered systemically are preferable.

Products with neomycin sulfate may cause cutaneous/conjunctival sensitization.

➤*Cross-sensitivity:* Allergic cross-reactions may occur that could prevent future use of any or all of the following antibiotics: kanamycin, neomycin, paromomycin, streptomycin, and possibly, gentamicin.

➤*Hematopoietic toxicity:* Hematopoietic toxicity has occurred occasionally with the systemic use of **chloramphenicol** and rarely with topical administration. It generally is a dose-related toxic effect on bone marrow, and usually is reversible on cessation of therapy. Rare cases of aplastic anemia, bone marrow hypoplasia, and death have been reported with prolonged (months to years) or frequent intermittent (over months and years) use of ocular chloramphenicol.

➤*Contact lenses:* Advise patients not to wear contact lenses if they have signs and symptoms of bacterial conjunctivitis.

➤*Corneal healing:* Ophthalmic ointments may retard corneal epithelial healing.

➤*Systemic antibiotics:* In all except very superficial infections, supplement the topical use of antibiotics with appropriate systemic medication. Systemic aminoglycoside antibiotics require monitoring the total serum concentration (peak and trough).

➤*Crystalline precipitate:* A white crystalline precipitate located in the superficial portion of the corneal defect was observed in approximately 17% of patients on **ciprofloxacin**. Onset was within 1 to 7 days after starting therapy. The precipitate resolved in most patients within 2 weeks, and did not preclude continued use or adversely affect the clinical course or outcome.

➤*Sulfite sensitivity:* Some of these products contain sulfites that may cause allergic-type reactions (eg, hives, itching, wheezing, anaphylaxis) in certain susceptible people. Although the overall prevalence of sulfite sensitivity in the general population is probably low, it is seen more frequently in asthmatics or in atopic nonasthmatic people. Specific products containing sulfites are identified in the product listings.

➤*Superinfection:* Do not use topical antibiotics in deep-seated ocular infections or in those that are likely to become systemic. Use of antibiotics (especially prolonged or repeated therapy) may result in bacterial or fungal overgrowth of nonsusceptible organisms. Such overgrowth may lead to a secondary infection. Take appropriate measures if superinfection occurs.

➤*Pregnancy: Category B* (erythromycin, tobramycin), *Category C* (gentamicin, levofloxacin, moxifloxacin, ciprofloxacin, ofloxacin, polymyxin B). Safety for use during pregnancy has not been established. Use only when clearly needed and when the potential benefits outweigh the potential hazards to the fetus.

➤*Lactation:* It is not known whether **ciprofloxacin**, **levofloxacin**, **moxifloxacin**, or **ofloxacin** appears in breast milk following ophthalmic use. Exercise caution when administering **ciprofloxacin**, **levofloxacin**, and **moxifloxacin** to a breast-feeding mother. Because of the potential for adverse reactions in breast-feeding infants from **ofloxacin**, **chloramphenicol**, and **tobramycin**, decide whether to discontinue breast-feeding or discontinue the drug, taking into account the importance of the drug to the mother.

➤*Children:* **Tobramycin** is safe and effective in children. Safety and efficacy of **fluoroquinolones** in infants younger than 1 year of age, and **polymyxin B/trimethoprim** in infants younger than 2 months have not been established. Safety and effectiveness in children younger than 6 years of age for levofloxacin 1.5% solution strength have not been established.

➤*Monitoring:* Perform culture and susceptibility testing during treatment.

Drug Interactions

None known.

Adverse Reactions

Sensitivity reactions such as transient irritation, burning, stinging, itching, inflammation, angioneurotic edema, urticaria, and vesicular and maculopapular dermatitis have occurred in some patients.

➤*Chloramphenicol:* Hematological reactions (including aplastic anemia) have been reported (see Warnings).

➤*Fluoroquinolones:* White crystalline precipitates; lid margin crusting; crystals/scales; foreign body sensation; conjunctival hyperemia; bad/bitter taste in mouth; corneal staining; keratopathy/keratitis; allergic reactions; lid edema; tearing; photophobia; corneal infiltrates; nausea; decreased vision; chemosis; fever; increased cough; infection; otitis media; pharyngitis; rhinitis; subconjunctival hemorrhage; corneal erosion; corneal ulcer; diplopia; floaters; headache.

➤*Aminoglycosides:* Localized ocular toxicity and hypersensitivity, lid itching, lid swelling, and conjunctival erythema (less than 3% with tobramycin); bacterial/fungal corneal ulcers; nonspecific conjunctivitis; conjunctival epithelial defects; conjunctival hyperemia (gentamicin). Similar reactions may occur with the topical use of other aminoglycoside antibiotics.

Overdosage

➤*Symptoms:* Symptoms of tobramycin overdose include punctate keratitis, erythema, increased lacrimation, edema, and lid itching. These may be similar to adverse reactions.

➤*Treatment:* A topical overdose of **ciprofloxacin** may be flushed from the eyes with warm tap water.

Patient Information

Instruct patient to tilt head back, place medication in conjunctival sac, and close eyes. Patients should apply light finger pressure on lacrimal sac for 1 minute following instillation.

May cause temporary blurring of vision or stinging following administration. Advise patient to notify health care provider if stinging, burning, or itching becomes pronounced or if redness, irritation, swelling, decreasing vision, or pain persists or worsens.

To avoid contamination, instruct patient to not touch tip of container to any surface and replace cap after using.

In general, patients being treated for bacterial conjunctivitis should not wear contact lenses; however, if the health care provider considers contact lens use appropriate, wait at least 15 minutes after using any solutions containing benzalkonium chloride before inserting the lens, as it may be absorbed by the lens.

➤*Quinolones:* Advise patient to discontinue and to notify health care provider at the first sign of a skin rash or other allergic reaction.

ERYTHROMYCIN

Rx	**Erythromycin** (Various, eg, Akorn, Goldline)	**Ointment; ophthalmic:** 0.5%	In 3.5 g.
Rx	**Ilotycin** (Fera Pharmaceuticals)		Mineral oil, white petrolatum. In 1 g.

ERYTHROMYCIN — OPHTHALMIC

Complete and comparative prescribing information begins in the Ophthalmic Antibiotics class monograph.

Indications

➤*Ocular infections:* For the treatment of superficial ocular infections involving the conjunctiva or cornea caused by organisms susceptible to erythromycin ophthalmic ointment.

For prophylaxis of ophthalmia neonatorum due to *N. gonorrhoeae* or *C. trachomatis*.

The effectiveness of erythromycin in the prevention of ophthalmia caused by *penicillinase-producing N. gonorrhoeae* is not established.

For infants born to mothers with clinically apparent gonorrhea, intravenous or intramuscular injections of aqueous crystalline penicillin G should be given; a single dose of 50,000 units for term infants or 20,000 units for infants of low birth weight. Topical prophylaxis alone is inadequate for these infants.

Administration and Dosage

➤*Adults:*

Ocular infections (superficial) – Approximately 1 cm in length should be applied directly to the infected eye(s) up to 6 times daily, depending on the severity of the infection.

➤*Children:*

Ocular infections (superficial) – See Adults for dosing.

Prophylaxis of neonatal gonococcal or chlamydial ophthalmia – A ribbon of ointment approximately 1 cm in length should be instilled into each lower conjunctival sac. The ointment should not be flushed from the eye following instillation. A new tube should be used for each infant.

➤*Storage/Stability:* Store between 15° to 30°C (59° to 86°F).

AZITHROMYCIN

Rx	**AzaSite** (Inspire Pharmaceuticals)	**Solution; ophthalmic:** 1%	Edetate disodium, mannitol.[a] In 2.5 mL.

[a] Also contains benzalkonium chloride 0.003%, citric acid, sodium chloride, sodium citrate, poloxamer 407, and polycarbophil.

AZITHROMYCIN — OPHTHALMIC

Complete prescribing information begins in the Ophthalmic Antibiotics class monograph.

Indications

➤*Bacterial conjunctivitis:* For the treatment of bacterial conjunctivitis caused by susceptible isolates of the following microorganisms: Centers for Disease Control and Prevention (CDC) coryneform group G (efficacy studied in fewer than 10 infections), *Haemophilus influenzae*, *Staphylococcus aureus*, *Streptococcus mitis* group, and *Streptococcus pneumoniae*.

Administration and Dosage

➤*Adults:*

Bacterial conjunctivitis – Instill 1 drop in the affected eye(s) twice daily, 8 to 12 hours apart for the first 2 days, and then instill 1 drop in the affected eye(s) once daily for the next 5 days.

➤*Children:* See Adults for dosing for children 1 year of age and older.

➤*Administration:* Azithromycin is indicated for topical ophthalmic use only and should not be administered systemically, injected subconjunctivally, or introduced directly into the anterior chamber of the eye.

➤*Storage/Stability:* Store unopened bottle under refrigeration at 2° to 8°C (36° to 46°F). Once the bottle is opened, store at 2° to 25°C (36° to 77°F) for up to 14 days. Discard after 14 days.

GENTAMICIN SULFATE

Rx	**Gentamicin Ophthalmic** (Various, eg, Goldline, Schein)	**Solution; ophthalmic:** 0.3%	In 5 and 15 mL.
Rx	**Gentak** (Akorn)		Benzalkonium chloride. In 5 mL dropper bottles.
Rx	**Gentamicin Sulfate Ophthalmic** (E. Fougera)	**Ointment; ophthalmic:** 0.3%	In 3.5 g.[a]
Rx	**Gentak** (Akorn)		In 3.5 g.[b]

[a] In a base of white petrolatum and mineral oil.

[b] With white petrolatum and parabens.

GENTAMICIN SULFATE — OPHTHALMIC

Complete and comparative prescribing information begins in the Ophthalmic Antibiotics group monograph.

Indications

➤*Ocular infections:* For the topical treatment of ocular bacterial infections, including conjunctivitis, keratitis, keratoconjunctivitis, corneal ulcers, blepharitis, blepharoconjunctivitis, acute meibomianitis, and dacryocystitis caused by susceptible strains of the following microorganisms: *Staphylococcus aureus*, *Staphylococcus epidermidis*, *Streptococcus pyogenes*, *Streptococcus pneumoniae*, *Enterobacter aerogenes*, *Escherichia coli*, *Haemophilus influenzae*, *Klebsiella pneumoniae*, *Neisseria gonorrhoeae*, *Pseudomonas aeruginosa*, and *Serratia marcescens*.

Administration and Dosage

➤*Adults:*

Ocular infections –

Solution: Instill 1 or 2 drops into the affected eye every 4 hours. In severe infections, dosage may be increased to as much as 2 drops once every hour.

Ointment: Apply a small amount (about ½ inch) to the affected eye 2 to 3 times daily.

➤*Children:*

Ocular infections –

Children 1 month of age and older:

• *Solution* – Instill 1 or 2 drops into the affected eye every 4 hours. Gentamicin has also been given every 2 to 4 hours. In severe infections, dosage may be increased to as much as 2 drops once every hour.

• *Ointment* – Apply a small amount (about ½ inch) to the affected eye 2 to 3 times daily.

➤*Administration:* Gentamicin ophthalmic solution and ointment are not for injection into the eye. They should never be injected subconjunctivally, nor should they be directly introduced into the anterior chamber of the eye.

➤*Storage/Stability:* Store gentamicin sulfate ophthalmic ointment and solution between 2° and 30°C (36° and 86°F).

TOBRAMYCIN

Rx	**Tobramycin** (Various, eg, Bausch & Lomb)	**Solution**: 0.3% tobramycin	In 5 mL bottle.[a]
Rx	**AKTob** (Akorn)		In 5 mL.[b]
Rx	**Tobrasol** (OcuSoft)		In 5 mL.[e]
Rx	**Tobrex** (Alcon)		In 5 mL *Drop-Tainers*.[c]
Rx	**Tobrex** (Alcon)	**Ointment**: 3 mg tobramycin per g	In 3.5 g.[d]

[a] With 0.01% benzalkonium Cl and boric acid.
[b] With 0.01% benzalkonium chloride, boric acid and sodium sulfate.
[c] With 0.01% benzalkonium chloride, tyloxapol and boric acid.
[d] With white petrolatum, mineral oil and 0.5% chlorobutanol.
[e] With 0.01% benzalkonium chloride, boric acid, sodium sulfate, sodium chloride, tyloxapol.

TOBRAMYCIN — OPHTHALMIC

Complete and comparative prescribing information begins in the Ophthalmic Antibiotics group monograph.

Indications

➤*Ocular infections:* For the treatment of external infections of the eye and its adnexa caused by susceptible bacteria.

Administration and Dosage

➤*Adults:*

Bacterial ocular infections –

Solution:

• *Mild to moderate infections* – Instill 1 or 2 drops into the affected eye(s) every 4 hours.

• *Severe infections* – Instill 2 drops into the eye(s) hourly until improvement, following which treatment should be reduced prior to discontinuation.

Ointment:

• *Mild to moderate infections* – Apply a half-inch ribbon into the affected eye(s) 2 or 3 times a day.

• *Severe infections* – Instill a half-inch ribbon into the affected eye(s) every 3 to 4 hours until improvement, following which treatment should be reduced prior to discontinuation.

➤*Children:* Safety and efficacy in pediatric patients younger than 2 months of age have not been established. See Adults for dosing for children 2 months of age and older.

➤*Administration:*

Ointment –

1.) Tilt head back.
2.) Place a finger on the cheek just under the eye and gently pull down until a "V" pocket is formed between the eyeball and the lower lid.
3.) Place a small amount (about ½ inch) of ointment in the "V" pocket. Do not let the tube touch the eye.
4.) Instruct the patient to look downward before closing the eye.

➤*Storage/Stability:* Store at 8° to 27°C (46° to 80°F).

BACITRACIN

Rx	**Bacitracin** (Various, eg, Fera, Goldline, Major, Schein, URL)	**Ointment; ophthalmic**: 500 units/g	In 3.5 and 3.75 g.

[a] With white petrolatum and mineral oil.

BACITRACIN — OPHTHALMIC

Complete and comparative prescribing information begins in the Ophthalmic Antibiotics class monograph.

Indications

➤*General information:* For a list of microorganisms usually susceptible to these agents, refer to systemic monographs in the Anti-infectives chapter.

➤*Ocular infections:* Treatment of superficial ocular infections involving the conjunctiva or cornea (eg, conjunctivitis, keratitis, keratoconjunctivitis, corneal ulcers, blepharitis, blepharoconjunctivitis, acute meibomianitis and dacryocystitis) due to strains of microorganisms susceptible to antibiotics.

Administration and Dosage

➤*Adults:*

Ocular infections – Administration and dosage varies for the individual products. Refer to the individual manufacturer inserts.

➤*Children:*

Off-label dosing –

Ocular infections: Apply ¼ to ½ inch ribbon into the conjunctival sac of affected eye(s) every 3 to 12 hours.

CIPROFLOXACIN HYDROCHLORIDE

Rx	**Ciprofloxacin** (Various, eg, Bausch & Lomb, Novax)	**Solution**: 3.5 mg/mL (equivalent to 3 mg base)	In 2.5, 5, and 10 mL dropper bottles.[a]
Rx	**Ciloxan** (Alcon)		In 2.5 and 5 mL *Drop-Tainers*.[b]
Rx	**Ciloxan** (Alcon)	**Ointment**: 3.33 mg/g (equivalent to 3 mg base)	Mineral oil, white petrolatum. In 3.5 g.

[a] With 0.006% benzalkonium chloride, mannitol, and EDTA.
[b] With 0.006% benzalkonium chloride, 4.6% mannitol, and 0.05% EDTA.

CIPROFLOXACIN HYDROCHLORIDE — OPHTHALMIC

Complete and comparative prescribing information begins in the Ophthalmic Antibiotics group monograph.

Indications

➤*Ocular infections:* For the treatment of superficial ocular infections involving the conjunctiva or cornea (eg, conjunctivitis, keratitis, keratoconjunctivitis, corneal ulcers, blepharitis, blepharoconjunctivitis, acute meibomianitis, dacryocystitis) due to strains of microorganisms susceptible to antibiotics.

➤*Ophthalmic ointment:* For the treatment of bacterial conjunctivitis caused by susceptible strains of the following microorganisms:

Gram-positive – *Staphylococcus aureus*; *Staphylococcus epidermidis*; *Streptococcus pneumoniae*; *Streptococcus (viridans group).*

Gram-negative – *Haemophilus influenzae.*

➤*Ophthalmic solution:* For the treatment of infections caused by susceptible strains of the designated microorganisms in the conditions listed below:

Corneal ulcers – *Pseudomonas aeruginosa*, *Serratia marcescens* (efficacy for this organism was studied in fewer than 10 infections), *Staphylococcus aureus*, *Staphylococcus epidermidis*, *Streptococcus pneumoniae*, *Streptococcus* (viridans group) (efficacy for this organism was studied in fewer than 10 infections).

Conjunctivitis – *Haemophilus influenzae*, *Staphylococcus aureus*, *Staphylococcus epidermidis*, *Streptococcus pneumoniae*.

Administration and Dosage

➤*Adults:*

Bacterial conjunctivitis –

Ophthalmic ointment: Apply a ½ inch ribbon into the conjunctival sac 3 times a day on the first 2 days, then apply a ½ inch ribbon 2 times a day for the next 5 days.

Ophthalmic solution: Instill 1 or 2 drops into the conjunctival sac(s) every 2 hours while awake for 2 days and 1 or 2 drops every 4 hours while awake for the next 5 days.

Corneal ulcers –

Ophthalmic solution: Instill 2 drops into the affected eye every 15 minutes for the first 6 hours and then 2 drops into the affected eye every 30 minutes for the remainder of the first day. On the second day, instill 2 drops in the affected eye hourly. On the third through the fourteenth day, place 2 drops in the affected eye every 4 hours. Treatment may be continued after 14 days if corneal re-epithelialization has not occurred.

➤*Children:*

Ophthalmic ointment – Safety and efficacy of ciprofloxacin ophthalmic ointment 0.3% in pediatric patients younger than 2 years of age have not been established. See Adults for dosing.

Ophthalmic solution – Safety and efficacy in pediatric patients younger than 1 year of age have not been established. See Adults for dosing.

➤*Storage/Stability:*

Ophthalmic ointment – Store at 2° to 25°C (36° to 77°F).

Ophthalmic solution – Store at 2° to 30°C (36° to 86°F). Protect from light.

GATIFLOXACIN

Rx	**Zymar** (Allergan)	**Solution; ophthalmic:** 0.3%	In 2.5 and 5 mL dropper bottles.[a]
Rx	**Zymaxid** (Allergan)	**Solution; ophthalmic:** 0.5%	In 2.5 mL in 5 mL bottle.[a]

[a] With 0.005% benzalkonium chloride and EDTA.

GATIFLOXACIN — OPHTHALMIC

Complete and comparative prescribing information begins in the Ophthalmic Antibiotics group monograph.

Indications

➤*Bacterial conjunctivitis:* Treatment of bacterial conjunctivitis caused by susceptible strains of the following organisms listed below:

Gram positive bacteria – *Cornyebacterium propinquum*, *Streptococcus mitis*, *Streptococcus oralis* (efficacy for these organisms was studied in fewer than 10 infections); *Staphylococcus aureus*; *Staphylococcus epidermidis*; *Streptococcus pneumoniae*.

Gram negative bacteria – *Haemophilus influenzae*.

Administration and Dosage

➤*Adults:*

Bacterial conjunctivitis –

Usual dosage:

- *Zymar* –
  - *Days 1 and 2:* Instill 1 drop in affected eye(s) every 2 hours while awake, up to 8 times/day.
  - *Days 3 through 7:* Instill 1 drop up to 4 times/day while awake.
- *Zymaxid* –
  - *Day 1:* Instill 1 drop in affected eye(s) every 2 hours while awake, up to 8 times/day.
  - *Days 2 through 7:* Instill 1 drop up to 4 times/day while awake.

➤*Children:*

Bacterial conjunctivitis –

1 year of age and older: See Adults for dosing.

➤*Administration:* Gatifloxacin ophthalmic solution should not be injected subconjunctivally, nor should it be introduced directly into the anterior chamber of the eye.

➤*Storage / Stability:* Store between 15° and 25°C (59° and 77°F). Protect from freezing.

MOXIFLOXACIN HYDROCHLORIDE

Rx	**Vigamox** (Alcon)	**Solution:** 0.5% (5 mg/mL)	In 3 mL *Drop-Tainer*.[a]

[a] With boric acid, sodium chloride, and purified water.

MOXIFLOXACIN HYDROCHLORIDE — OPHTHALMIC

Complete and comparative prescribing information begins in the Ophthalmic Antibiotics group monograph.

Indications

➤*Bacterial conjunctivitis:* For the treatment of bacterial conjunctivitis caused by susceptible strains of the following organisms:

Aerobic gram-positive microorganisms – *Corynebacterium* species, *Micrococcus luteus*, *Staphylococcus warneri* (efficacy for these organisms was studied in fewer than 10 infections); *Staphylococcus aureus*; *Staphylococcus epidermidis*; *Staphylococcus haemolyticus*; *Staphylococcus hominis*; *Streptococcus pneumoniae*; *Streptococcus* viridans group.

Aerobic gram-negative microorganisms – *Acinetobacter lwoffii*, *Haemophilus parainfluenzae* (efficacy for these organisms was studied in fewer than 10 infections); *Haemophilus influenzae*.

Other microorganisms – *Chlamydia trachomatis*.

Administration and Dosage

➤*Adults:*

Bacterial conjunctivitis – Instill 1 drop in the affected eye 3 times a day for 7 days.

➤*Children:* The safety and efficacy in infants below 1 year of age have not been established. See Adults for dosing for children 1 year of age and older.

➤*Storage / Stability:* Store at 2° to 25°C (36° to 77°F).

BESIFLOXACIN

Rx	**Besivance** (Bausch & Lomb)	**Suspension; ophthalmic:** 0.6%	Besifloxacin hydrochloride 6.63 mg equivalent to 6 mg base. In 5 mL bottle.[a]

[a] With benzalkonium chloride 0.01% and edetate disodium dihydrate.

BESIFLOXACIN HYDROCHLORIDE — OPHTHALMIC

Indications

➤*Bacterial conjunctivitis:* For the treatment of bacterial conjunctivitis caused by susceptible isolates of the following bacteria: Centers for Disease Control and Prevention (CDC) coryneform group G, *Haemophilus influenzae*, *Staphylococcus aureus*, *Staphylococcus epidermidis*, *Streptococcus mitis* group, *Streptococcus oralis*, *Streptococcus pneumoniae*, *Corynebacterium pseudodiphtheriticum* (efficacy for this organism was studied in fewer than 10 infections), *Corynebacterium striatum* (efficacy for this organism was studied in fewer than 10 infections), *Moraxella lucunata* (efficacy for this organism was studied in fewer than 10 infections), *Staphylococcus hominis* (efficacy for this organism was studied in fewer than 10 infections), *Staphylococcus lugdunensis* (efficacy for this organism was studied in fewer than 10 infections), *Streptococcus salivarius* (efficacy for this organism was studied in fewer than 10 infections).

Administration and Dosage

➤*Adults:*

Bacterial conjunctivitis – Instill 1 drop in the affected eye(s) 3 times per day, 4 to 12 hours apart for 7 days.

➤*Elderly:* See Adults for dosing.

➤*Administration:* Administer ophthalmic suspension 3 times per day.

Invert closed bottle and shake once before use.

➤*Storage / Stability:* Store at 15° to 25°C (59° to 77°F). Protect from light.

OFLOXACIN

Rx	**Ofloxacin** (Pacific Pharma)	**Solution:** 0.3% (3 mg/mL)	In 5 and 10 mL.[a]
Rx	**Ocuflox** (Allergan)		In 1, 5, and 10 mL.[a]

[a] With 0.005% benzalkonium chloride.

OFLOXACIN — OPHTHALMIC

Complete and comparative prescribing information begins in the Ophthalmic Antibiotics group monograph.

Indications

➤*Conjunctivitis:* For the treatment of conjunctivitis caused by susceptible strains of the following bacteria in the conditions listed below:

Gram-positive bacteria – *Staphylococcus aureus*; *Staphylococcus epidermidis*; *Streptococcus pneumoniae*.

Gram-negative bacteria – *Enterobacter cloacae*; *Haemophilus influenzae*; *Proteus mirabilis*; *Pseudomonas aeruginosa*.

➤*Corneal ulcers:* For the treatment of corneal ulcers caused by susceptible strains of the following bacteria in the conditions listed below:

Gram-positive bacteria – *Staphylococcus aureus*; *Staphylococcus epidermidis*; *Streptococcus pneumoniae*.

Gram-negative bacteria – *Pseudomonas aeruginosa*; *Serratia marcescens* (efficacy for this organism was studied in fewer than 10 infections).

Anaerobic species – *Propionibacterium acnes*.

Administration and Dosage

➤*Adults:*

Ofloxacin Ophthalmic Dosage Regimens		
Bacterial conjunctivitis	Days 1 and 2	Instill 1 to 2 drops every 2 to 4 hours in the affected eye(s).
	Days 3 through 7	Instill 1 to 2 drops 4 times daily.
Bacterial corneal ulcer	Days 1 and 2	Instill 1 to 2 drops into the affected eye every 30 minutes while awake. Awaken at approximately 4 and 6 hours after retiring and instill 1 to 2 drops.
	Days 3 through 7 to 9	Instill 1 to 2 drops hourly while awake.
	Days 7 to 9 through treatment completion	Instill 1 to 2 drops 4 times daily.

➤*Children:*

1 year of age and older – See Adults for dosing.

➤*Storage/Stability:* Store at 15° to 25°C (59° to 77°F).

LEVOFLOXACIN

Rx	**Levofloxacin** (Pack Pharmaceuticals)	**Solution; ophthalmic:** 0.5%	In 5 mL.[a]
Rx	**Quixin** (Vistakon Pharmaceuticals)		In 5 mL.[a]
Rx	**Iquix** (Vistakon Pharmaceuticals)	**Solution; ophthalmic:** 1.5%	In 5 mL.

[a] With benzalkonium chloride 0.005%.

LEVOFLOXACIN — OPHTHALMIC

Complete and comparative prescribing information begins in the Ophthalmic Antibiotics group monograph.

Indications

➤*Conjunctivitis (0.5% solution):* For the treatment of bacterial conjunctivitis caused by susceptible strains of the following organisms:

Gram-positive microorganisms – *Corynebacterium* species (efficacy for this organism was studied in fewer than 10 infections); *Staphylococcus aureus*; *Staphylococcus epidermidis*; *Streptococcus pneumoniae*; *Streptococcus* (groups C/F); *Streptococcus* (group G); *Viridans* group streptococci.

Gram-negative microorganisms – *Acinetobacter lwoffii* (efficacy for this organism was studied in fewer than 10 infections); *Haemophilus influenzae*; *Serratia marcescens* (efficacy for this organism was studied in fewer than 10 infections).

➤*Corneal ulcer (1.5% solution):* For the treatment of corneal ulcer caused by susceptible strains of the following bacteria:

Gram-positive microorganisms – *Corynebacterium* species (efficacy for this organism was studied in fewer than 10 infections); *S. aureus*; *S. epidermidis*; *S. pneumoniae*; *Viridans* group streptococci (efficacy for this organism was studied in fewer than 10 infections).

Gram-negative microorganisms – *Pseudomonas aeruginosa*; *S. marcescens* (efficacy for this organism was studied in fewer than 10 infections).

Administration and Dosage

➤*Adults:*

Bacterial conjunctivitis –

0.5% solution:

• *Days 1 and 2* – Instill 1 to 2 drops in the affected eye(s) every 2 hours while awake, up to 8 times per day.

• *Days 3 through 7* – Instill 1 to 2 drops in the affected eye(s) every 4 hours while awake, up to 4 times per day.

Corneal ulcer –

1.5% solution:

• *Days 1 through 3* – Instill 1 to 2 drops in the affected eye(s) every 30 to 2 hours while awake and approximately 4 and 6 hours after retiring.

• *Day 4 through treatment completion* – Instill 1 to 2 drops in the affected eye(s) every 1 to 4 hours while awake.

➤*Children:* Safety and effectiveness in children younger than 1 year of age for the 0.5% solution or in children younger than 6 years of age for the 1.5% solution have not been established. See Adults for dosing for children 1 year of age and older for the 0.5% solution and for children 6 years of age and older for the 1.5% solution.

➤*Storage/Stability:* Store at 15° to 25°C (59° to 77°F).

SULFACETAMIDE SODIUM

Rx	**Sulster** (Akorn)	**Solution:** 1%	In 5 and 10 mL.
Rx	**Sulfacetamide Sodium** (Various, eg, Fougera, Goldline, Moore, Optopics, Steris)	**Solution:** 10%	In 15 mL.
Rx	**AK-Sulf** (Akorn)		In 2, 5 and 15 mL.[a]
Rx	**Bleph-10** (Allergan)		In 2.5, 5 and 15 mL.[b]
Rx	**AK-Sulf** (Akorn)	**Ointment:** 10%	In 3.5 g.[c]

[a] 3.1 mg sodium thiosulfate pentahydrate, 5 mg methylcellulose, 0.5 mg methylparaben and 0.1 mg propylparaben per mL.
[b] With 1.4% polyvinyl alcohol, 0.005% benzalkonium chloride, polysorbate 80, sodium thiosulfate and EDTA.
[c] With 0.5 mg methylparaben, 0.1 mg propylparaben, 0.25 mg benzalkonium chloride and petrolatum base per g.

SULFACETAMIDE SODIUM — OPHTHALMIC

Complete and comparative prescribing information begins in the Sulfonamides group monograph.

Indications

➤*Ocular infections:* For the treatment of conjunctivitis and other superficial ocular infections due to susceptible microorganisms, and as an adjunctive in systemic sulfonamide therapy of trachoma: *Escherichia coli*, *Staphylococcus aureus*, *Streptococcus pneumoniae*, *Streptococcus* (viridans group), *Haemophilus influenzae*, *Klebsiella* species, and *Enterobacter* species.

Topically applied sulfonamides do not provide adequate coverage against *Neisseria* species, *Serratia marcescens* and *Pseudomonas aeruginosa*. A significant percentage of staphylococcal isolates are completely resistant to sulfa drugs.

Administration and Dosage

➤*Adults:*

Conjunctivitis and other superficial ocular infections –

Usual dosage: Instill 1 or 2 drops into the conjunctival sac(s) of the affected eye(s) every 2 to 3 hours initially.

Duration of therapy: 7 to 10 days.

Tapering: Dosages may be tapered by increasing the time interval between doses as the condition responds.

Trachoma –

Usual dosage: Instill 2 drops into the conjunctival sac(s) of the affected eye(s) every 2 hours.

Concomitant therapy: Topical administration must be accompanied by systemic administration.

➤*Children:*

2 months of age and older – See Adults for dosing.

➤*Administration:* For topical eye use only. Not for injection.

➤*Storage/Stability:* Store between 8° and 25°C (46° to 77°F). Sulfonamide solutions, on long standing, will darken in color and should be discarded. Protect from light.

OPHTHALMIC COMBINATION ANTIBIOTIC PRODUCTS

	Product and Distributor	Polymyxin B Sulfate (units/g or mL)	Neomycin (mg/g or mL)	Bacitracin Zinc (units/g)	Other Antibiotics	How Supplied
Rx	**Neomycin/Polymyxin B Sulfates/Bacitracin Zinc Ophthalmic Ointment** (Various, eg, Bausch & Lomb, Fougera)	10,000	3.5[a]	400		White petrolatum, mineral oil. In 3.5 g.
Rx	**Neomycin/Polymyxin B Sulfates/Gramicidin Ophthalmic Solution** (Various, eg, Bausch & Lomb, URL, Zenith Goldline)	10,000	1.75		0.025 mg/mL gramicidin	Sodium chloride, 0.5% alcohol, propylene glycol, hydrochloric acid, 0.001% thimerosal, poloxamer 188, ammonium hydroxide. In 10 mL.
Rx	**Neosporin Ophthalmic Solution** (Monarch)					Alcohol 0.5%, 0.001% thimerosal, propylene glycol, sodium chloride. In 10 mL *Drop Dose*.
Rx	**Bacitracin Zinc/Polymyxin B Sulfate Ophthalmic Ointment** (Bausch & Lomb)	10,000		500		White petrolatum, mineral oil. In 3.5 g.
Rx	**AK-Poly-Bac** Ophthalmic **Ointment** (Akorn)					White petrolatum, mineral oil. In 3.5 g.
Rx	**Trimethoprim Sulfate/Polymyxin B Sulfate Ophthalmic Solution** (Various, eg, Bausch and Lomb, Falcon)	10,000			1 mg/mL trimethoprim sulfate	In 10 mL.
Rx	**Polytrim Ophthalmic Solution** (Allergan)					0.04 mg/mL benzalkonium chloride, sodium chloride, sodium hydroxide. In 5 and 10 mL.

[a] Equivalent to 5 g neomycin sulfate.

STEROID AND ANTIBIOTIC SOLUTIONS AND SUSPENSIONS

	Product & Distributor	Steroid (per mL)	Antibiotic (per mL)	Other Content	How Supplied
Rx	**Poly-Pred Ophthalmic Suspension** (Allergan)	Prednisolone acetate 0.5%	Neomycin 3.5 mg polymyxin B sulfate 10,000 units	Thimerosal 0.001%, polyvinyl alcohol, polysorbate 80, propylene glycol, sodium acetate	In 5 mL.
Rx	**Pred-G Ophthalmic Suspension** (Allergan)	Prednisolone acetate 1%	Gentamicin 0.3%	Benzalkonium chloride 0.005%, polyvinyl alcohol 1.4%, edetate disodium, polysorbate 80, sodium chloride, sodium citrate, hypromellose	In 5 and 10 mL.
Rx	**Tobramycin and Dexamethasone Ophthalmic Suspension** (Various, eg, Alcon Labs, Bausch and Lomb)	Dexamethasone 0.1%	Tobramycin 0.3%	Benzalkonium chloride 0.01%, edetate disodium	In 2.5, 5, and 10 mL.
Rx	**TobraDex Ophthalmic Suspension** (Alcon Pharmaceuticals)			Benzalkonium chloride 0.01%, edetate disodium, sodium chloride, tyloxapol	In 3.5 mL.
Rx	**TobraDex ST Ophthalmic Suspension** (Alcon)	Dexamethasone 0.05%	Tobramycin 0.3%	Benzalkonium chloride 0.1 mg, edetate disodium, xanthan gum, sodium chloride, tyloxapol, propylene glycol	In 2.5, 5 and 10 mL *Drop-Tainers*
Rx	**Neomycin/Polymyxin B Sulfate and Dexamethasone Ophthalmic Suspension** (Various, eg, Falcon)	Dexamethasone 0.1%	Neomycin 3.5 mg, polymyxin B sulfate 10,000 units	Benzalkonium chloride 0.004%, hypromellose, sodium chloride, polysorbate 20	In 5 mL.
Rx	**Methadex Ophthalmic Suspension** (Major)				In 5 mL.
Rx	**Maxitrol Ophthalmic Suspension** (Alcon)				In 5 mL *Drop-Tainers.*
Rx	**Poly–Dex Ophthalmic Suspension** (OcuSoft)			Benzalkonium chloride 0.004%, sodium chloride, hypromellose, polysorbate 80	In 5 mL.
Rx	**Neomycin/Polymyxin B Sulfates/ Hydrocortisone Ophthalmic Suspension** (Various, eg, Falcon)	Hydrocortisone 1%	Neomycin 3.5 mg, polymyxin B sulfate 10,000 units	Thimerosal 0.001%, cetyl alcohol, glyceryl monostearate, mineral oil, polyoxyl 40 stearate, propylene glycol	In 7.5 mL *Drop-Tainers.*
Rx	**Zylet Ophthalmic Suspension** (Bausch & Lomb)	Loteprednol 0.5%	Tobramycin 0.3%	Benzalkonium chloride 0.01%, edetate disodium, glycerin, povidone, tyloxapol	In 2.5, 5, and 10 mL.

STEROID AND ANTIBIOTIC SOLUTIONS AND SUSPENSIONS — OPHTHALMIC

Indications

➤*Ocular inflammation/infection:* For steroid-responsive inflammatory ocular conditions in which a corticosteroid is indicated and in which superficial bacterial infection or risk of infection exists.

For inflammatory conditions of the palpebral and bulbar conjunctiva, cornea and anterior segment of the globe in which the inherent risk of corticosteroid use in certain infective conjunctivitis is accepted to obtain a diminution in edema and inflammation. For chronic anterior uveitis and corneal injury from chemical, radiation or thermal burns, or penetration of foreign bodies.

The use of a combination drug with an anti-infective component is indicated when the risk of infection is high or when there is an expectation that potentially dangerous numbers of bacteria will be present in the eye.

Administration and Dosage

➤*General dosing considerations:* Do not prescribe more than 20 mL initially; do not refill without further evaluation.

➤*Adults:*

Ocular inflammation/infection –

Usual dosage: For complete dosage instructions, see individual manufacturer inserts.

Dosage adjustment: Reduce dose frequency as inflammation is brought under control.

Discontinuation of therapy: Decrease gradually as warranted by improvement in clinical signs. Take care not to discontinue therapy prematurely.

➤*Children:*

Ocular inflammation/infection –

Gentamicin/Prednisolone: Safety and efficacy have not been established.

Neomycin/Polymyxin B sulfate/Dexamethasone: Safety and efficacy have not been established.

Neomycin/Polymyxin B sulfate/Hydrocortisone: Safety and efficacy have not been established.

Neomycin/Polymyxin B sulfate/Prednisolone: Safety and efficacy have not been established.

Tobramycin/Dexamethasone: Refer to Adults for dosing for children 2 years of age and older.

Tobramycin/Loteprednol: Safety and efficacy have not been established.

➤*Storage/Stability:* Store between 15° to 25°C (59° and 77°F). Protect from freezing. Store suspensions upright and shake well before using.

Warnings/Precautions

➤*Pregnancy: Category C.* There are no adequate or well-controlled studies in pregnant women. These drugs should be used during pregnancy only if the potential benefit to the mother justifies the potential risk to the embryo or fetus.

➤*Lactation:* Systemically administered corticosteroids appear in human milk and could suppress growth, interfere with endogenous corticosteroid production, or cause other untoward effects. It is not known whether topical administration of corticosteroids could result in sufficient systemic absorption to produce detectable quantities in human milk. Because many drugs are excreted in human milk, exercise caution when administering to a breast-feeding woman.

Neomycin/Polymyxin B sulfate/prednisolone – This drug combination is excreted in breast milk.

STEROID AND ANTIBIOTIC OINTMENTS

	Product & Distributor	Steroid (per g)	Antibiotic (per g)	Other Content	How Supplied
Rx	**Neomycin/Polymyxin B Sulfate/Bacitracin Zinc/ Hydrocortisone** (Various, eg, Fougera)	Hydrocortisone 1%	Neomycin 3.5 mg, polymyxin B 10,000 units, bacitracin 400 units	White petrolatum, mineral oil	In 3.5 g.
Rx	**Pred-G** (Allergan)	Prednisolone acetate 0.6%	Gentamicin 0.3%	Chlorobutanol 0.5%, mineral oil, petrolatum, lanolin alcohol	In 3.5 g.
Rx	**TobraDex** (Alcon)	Dexamethasone 0.1%	Tobramycin 0.3%	Chlorobutanol 0.5%, white petrolatum, mineral oil	In 3.5 g.
Rx	**Neomycin/Polymyxin B Sulfate/Dexamethasone** (Various, eg, Fougera)	Dexamethasone 0.1%	Neomycin 3.5 mg, polymyxin B sulfate 10,000 units	Lanolin, white petrolatum	In 3.5 g.
Rx	**Maxitrol** (Alcon)			Parabens, white petrolatum, lanolin	In 3.5 g.

STEROID AND ANTIBIOTIC OINTMENTS — OPHTHALMIC

Indications

➤*Ocular inflammation/infection:* For steroid-responsive inflammatory ocular conditions in which a corticosteroid is indicated and in which bacterial infection or risk of infection exists.

For inflammatory conditions of the palpebral and bulbar conjunctiva, cornea and anterior segment of the globe in which the inherent risk of steroid use in certain infective conjunctivitis is accepted to obtain a diminution in edema and inflammation. For chronic anterior uveitis and corneal injury from chemical, radiation or thermal burns, or penetration of foreign bodies.

Administration and Dosage

➤*General dosing considerations:* Do not prescribe more than 8 g initially, and the prescription should not be refilled until further evaluation. For complete dosage instructions, see individual manufacturer inserts.

➤*Adults:*

Ocular inflammation/infection – Apply ointment to the affected eye(s) every 3 or 4 hours, depending on the severity of the condition.

➤*Storage/Stability:* Store between 15° and 25°C (59° and 77°F).

Warnings/Precautions

➤*Pregnancy: Category C.* There are no adequate or well-controlled studies in pregnant women. These drugs should be used during pregnancy only if the potential benefit to the mother justifies the potential risk to the embryo or fetus. Infants born to mothers who have received substantial doses of corticosteroids during pregnancy should be observed carefully for signs of hypoadrenalism.

➤*Lactation:* Systemically administered corticosteroids appear in human milk and could suppress growth, interfere with endogenous corticosteroid production, or cause other untoward effects. It is not known whether topical administration of corticosteroids could result in sufficient systemic absorption to produce detectable quantities in human milk. Because many drugs are excreted in human milk, exercise caution when administering to a breast-feeding woman.

Steroid Sulfonamide Combinations

STEROID AND SULFONAMIDE COMBINATIONS, SUSPENSIONS AND SOLUTIONS

	Product & Distributor	Steroid	Sulfonamide	Other Content	How Supplied
Rx	**FML-S Suspension** (Allergan)	Fluorometholone 0.1%	Sodium sulfacetamide 10%	EDTA, polyvinyl alcohol 1.4%, benzalkonium chloride 0.006% , polysorbate 80, povidone, sodium thiosulfate, sodium chloride	In 5 and 10 mL.
Rx	**Blephamide Suspension** (Allergan)	Prednisolone acetate 0.2%	Sodium sulfacetamide 10%	EDTA, polyvinyl alcohol 1.4%, polysorbate 80, sodium thiosulfate, benzalkonium chloride	In 2.5, 5, and 10 mL.
Rx	**Sulfacetamide Sodium and Prednisolone Sodium Phosphate** (Schein)	Prednisolone sodium 0.25% phosphate	Sodium sulfacetamide 10%	Thimerosal 0.01% mg , EDTA, boric acid	In 5 and 10 mL
Rx	**Vasocidin Solution** (Novartis)			EDTA, thimerosal 0.01%, poloxamer 407	In 5 and 10 mL.

STEROID AND SULFONAMIDE COMBINATIONS, SUSPENSIONS AND SOLUTIONS — OPHTHALMIC

The information for steroid preparations and sulfonamide preparations must be considered when using these products. See individual monographs.

Indications

➤*Inflammation/Infection:* For corticosteroid-responsive inflammatory ocular conditions for which a corticosteroid is indicated and where superficial bacterial ocular infection or a risk of infection exists.

Administration and Dosage

➤*General dosing considerations:* Do not prescribe more than 20 mL initially or refill prescription without further evaluation.

➤*Adults:*

Ophthalmic Inflammation/Infection – Instill 1 to 3 drops into the conjunctival sac(s) every 1 to 4 hours during the day and at bedtime until a favorable response is obtained.

For complete dosage instructions, see individual manufacturer inserts.

➤*Storage/Stability:* Protect from light. Do not freeze. Shake well before using. Do not use if solution or suspension has darkened. Clumping may occur on long standing at high temperatures.

STEROID AND SULFONAMIDE COMBINATIONS, OINTMENTS

	Product & Distributor	Steroid	Sulfonamide	Other Content	How Supplied
Rx	**Blephamide** (Allergan)	0.2% prednisolone acetate	10% sodium sulfacetamide	0.0008% phenylmercuric acetate, mineral oil, white petrolatum, lanolin alcohol	In 3.5 g.

STEROID AND SULFONAMIDE COMBINATIONS, OINTMENTS — OPHTHALMIC

The information for steroid preparations and sulfonamide preparations must be considered when using these products. See individual monographs.

Indications

➤*Inflammation/Infection:* For corticosteroid-responsive inflammatory ocular conditions for which a corticosteroid is indicated and where superficial bacterial ocular infection or a risk of infection exists.

Administration and Dosage

Apply a small amount (approximately ½ inch ribbon) into the conjunctival sac(s) 3 or 4 times daily and once at bedtime (or once or twice at night) until a favorable response is obtained.

Do not prescribe more than 8 g initially, and the prescription should not be refilled without further evaluation.

For complete dosage instructions, see individual manufacturer inserts.

➤*Storage/Stability:* Keep tightly closed. Store away from heat.

POVIDONE IODINE

Rx	**Betadine 5% Sterile Ophthalmic Prep Solution** (Alcon)	**Solution:** 5% povidone iodine	In 50 mL.[a]

[a] Glycerin, sodium chloride, sodium hydroxide and sodium phosphate.

POVIDONE IODINE — OPHTHALMIC

Indications

➤*Ophthalmic preoperative prep:* Used prior to eye surgery to prep the periocular region (lids, brow and cheek) and irrigate the ocular surface (cornea, conjunctiva and palpebral fornices).

Administration and Dosage

➤*Adults:*

Ophthalmic preoperative prep – Transfer solution to a sterile prep cup. Apply to lashes and lid margins with sterile applicator, repeat once. Apply to lids, brow, and cheek with sterile applicator, repeat 3 times. Irrigate cornea, conjunctiva, and palpebral fornices with solution and leave in for 2 minutes; flush with sterile saline solution.

➤*Administration:* For external use only. Not for intraocular injection or irrigation.

Actions

➤*Pharmacology:* Povidone iodine has broad-spectrum antimicrobial action.

Contraindications

Hypersensitivity to iodine.

Warnings/Precautions

➤*For external use only:* Not for intraocular injection or irrigation.

➤*Thyroid disorders:* Use caution in patients with thyroid disorders due to the possibility of iodine absorption.

➤*Pregnancy: Category C.* Safety for use during pregnancy has not been established. Use only when clearly needed.

➤*Lactation:* Because of the potential for adverse reactions in nursing infants, decide whether to discontinue nursing or discontinue the drug, taking into account the importance of the drug to the mother.

➤*Children:* Safety and efficacy have not been established.

Adverse Reactions

Local sensitivity has been exhibited by some individuals.

OPHTHALMIC ANTIFUNGALS

NATAMYCIN — OPHTHALMIC

Rx	**Natacyn** (Alcon)	**Suspension:** 5%	With 0.02% benzalkonium chloride. In 15 mL.

NATAMYCIN — OPHTHALMIC

Indications

➤*Ocular fungal infections:* For the treatment of fungal blepharitis, conjunctivitis, and keratitis caused by susceptible organisms including *Fusarium solani* keratitis. As in other forms of suppurative keratitis, initial and sustained therapy of fungal keratitis should be determined by the clinical diagnosis, laboratory diagnosis by smear and culture of corneal scrapings and drug response. Whenever possible the in vitro activity of natamycin against the responsible fungus should be determined. The effectiveness of natamycin as a single agent in fungal endophthalmitis has not been established.

Administration and Dosage

➤*General dosing considerations:* Failure of improvement of keratitis following 7 to 10 days of administration of the drug suggests that the infection may be caused by a microorganism not susceptible to natamycin.

➤*Adults:*

Ocular fungal infections –

Initial dosage: The preferred initial dosage in fungal keratitis is one drop instilled in the conjunctival sac at hourly or 2-hour intervals. Less frequent initial dosage (4 to 6 daily applications) may be sufficient in fungal blepharitis and conjunctivitis.

Dosage adjustment: The frequency of application can usually be reduced to 1 drop 6 to 8 times daily after the first 3 to 4 days.

Duration of therapy: Therapy should generally be continued for 14 to 21 days or until there is resolution of active fungal keratitis. In many cases, it may be helpful to reduce the dosage gradually at 4 to 7 day intervals to assure that the replicating organism has been eliminated.

➤*Administration:* Shake well before using. For topical eye use only; not for injection.

➤*Storage/Stability:* Store in refrigerator at 2° to 8°C (36° to 46°F) or at room temperature 8° to 24°C (46° to 75°F). Do not freeze. Avoid exposure to light and excessive heat.

Actions

➤*Pharmacology:* Natamycin is a tetraene polyene antibiotic derived from *Streptomyces natalensis*. It possesses in vitro activity against a variety of yeast and filamentous fungi, including *Candida*, *Aspergillus*, *Cephalosporium*, *Fusarium* and *Penicillium*. The mechanism of action appears to be through binding of the molecule to the sterol moiety of the fungal cell membrane. The polyenesterol complex alters the permeability of the membrane to produce depletion of essential cellular constituents. Although the activity against fungi is dose-related, natamycin is predominantly fungicidal. Natamycin is not effective in vitro against gram-positive or gram-negative bacteria. Topical administration appears to produce effective concentrations of natamycin within the corneal stroma but not in intraocular fluid. Systemic absorption should not be expected following topical administration of natamycin ophthalmic suspension, USP 5%. As with other polyene antibiotics, absorption from the gastrointestinal tract is very poor. Studies in rabbits receiving topical natamycin revealed no measurable compound in the aqueous humor or sera, but the sensitivity of the measurement was no greater than 2 mg/mL.

Contraindications

Hypersensitivity to any of its components.

Warnings/Precautions

➤*Usage:* Failure of improvement of keratitis following 7 to 10 days of administration of the drug suggests that the infection may be caused by a microorganism not susceptible to natamycin. For topical eye use only; not for injection.

Continuation of therapy should be based on clinical re-evaluation and additional laboratory studies.

➤*Toxicity:* Adherence of the suspension to areas of epithelial ulceration or retention of the suspension in the fornices occurs regularly. There have only been a limited number of cases in which natamycin has been used; therefore, it is possible that adverse reactions of which we have no knowledge at present may occur. For this reason, patients on this drug should be monitored at least twice weekly. Should suspicion of drug toxicity occur, the drug should be discontinued.

➤*Pregnancy: Category C.* Animal reproduction studies have not been conducted with natamycin. It is also not known whether natamycin can cause fetal harm when administered to a pregnant woman or can affect reproduction capacity. Natamycin ophthalmic suspension, USP 5% should be given to a pregnant woman only if clearly needed.

➤*Lactation:* It is not known whether these drugs are excreted in human milk. Because many drugs are excreted in human milk, caution should be exercised when natamycin is administered to a nursing woman.

➤*Children:* Safety and effectiveness in pediatric patients have not been established.

Adverse Reactions

One case of conjunctival chemosis and hyperemia, thought to be allergic in nature, has been reported.

Patient Information

Do not touch dropper tip to any surface, as this may contaminate the suspension.

TRIFLURIDINE OPHTHALMIC

Rx	**Trifluridine** (Falcon)	**Solution:** 1%	In aqueous solution with NaCl, 0.001% thimerosal. In 7.5 mL.
Rx	**Viroptic** (Monarch)		In aqueous solution with NaCl and 0.001% thimerosal. In 7.5 mL *Drop-Dose*.

TRIFLURIDINE — OPHTHALMIC

Indications

➤*Ocular viral infections:* For the treatment of primary keratoconjunctivitis and recurrent epithelial keratitis due to herpes simplex virus, types 1 and 2.

Administration and Dosage

➤*Adults:*

Ocular viral infections –

Usual dosage: Instill 1 drop onto the cornea of the affected eye every 2 hours while awake for a maximum daily dosage of 9 drops until the corneal ulcer has completely re-epithelialized.

Following re-epithelialization, treatment for an additional 7 days of 1 drop every 4 hours while awake for a minimum daily dosage of 5 drops is recommended. If there are no signs of improvement after 7 days of therapy or complete re-epithelialization has not occurred after 14 days of therapy, consider other forms of therapy.

Maximum dose: 9 drops per day to affected eye(s).

Duration of therapy: Avoid continuous administration of trifluridine for periods exceeding 21 days because of potential ocular toxicity.

➤*Children:*

6 years of age and older – See Adults for dosing.

➤*Storage/Stability:* Store under refrigeration 2° to 8°C (36° to 46°F).

Actions

➤*Pharmacology:* Trifluridine is a fluorinated pyrimidine nucleoside with in vitro and in vivo activity against herpes simplex virus, types 1 and 2 and vacciniavirus. Some strains of adenovirus are also inhibited in vitro.

Trifluridine is also effective in the treatment of epithelial keratitis that has not responded clinically to the topical adminstration of idoxuridine or when ocular toxicity or hypersensitivity to idoxuridine has occurred. In a smaller number of patients found to be resistant to topical vidarabine, trifluridine was also effective.

Trifluridine interferes with DNA synthesis in cultured mammalian cells. However, its antiviral mechanism of action is not completely known.

➤*Pharmacokinetics:*

Absorption – Systemic absorption of trifluridine following therapeutic dosing with trifluridine appears to be negligible. No detectable concentrations of trifluridine or 5-carboxy-2′-deoxyuridine were found in the sera of adult healthy subjects who had trifluridine instilled into their eyes 7 times daily for 14 consecutive days.

Contraindications

Hypersensitivity reactions or chemical intolerance to trifluridine.

Warnings/Precautions

➤*Animal pharmacology and animal toxicology:* Corneal wound-healing studies in rabbits showed that trifluridine did not significantly retard closure of epithelial wounds. However, mild toxic changes such as intracellular edema of the basal cell layer, mild thinning of the overlying epithelium and reduced strength of stromal wounds were observed.

Whereas instillation of trifluridine into rabbit eyes during a subchronic toxicity study produced some degree of corneal epithelial thinning, a 12-month chronic toxicity study in rabbits in which trifluridine was instilled into eyes in intermittent, multiple, full-therapy courses showed no drug-related changes in the cornea.

➤*Diagnosis:* Only prescribe trifluridine ophthalmic solution for patients who have a clinical diagnosis of herpetic keratitis.

➤*Irritation:* Trifluridine may cause mild local irritation of the conjunctiva and cornea when instilled, but these effects are usually transient.

➤*Resistance:* Although documented in vitro viral resistance to trifluridine has not been reported following multiple exposures to trifluridine, the possibility of the development of viral resistance exists.

➤*Pregnancy:* Category C.

Teratogenic – Trifluridine was not teratogenic at doses up to 5 mg/kg/day (23 times the estimated human exposure) when given SC to rats and rabbits. However, fetal toxicity consisting of delayed ossification of portions of the skeleton occurred at dose levels of 2.5 and 5 mg/kg/day in rats and at 2.5 mg/kg/day in rabbits. In addition, both 2.5 and 5 mg/kg/day produced fetal death and resorption in rabbits. In both rats and rabbits, 1 mg/kg/day (5 times the estimated human exposure) was a no-effect level. There were no teratogenic or fetotoxic effects after topical application of trifluridine ophthalmic solution (≈ 5 times the estimated human exposure) to the eyes of rabbits on the sixth through the 18th days of pregnancy. In a nonstandard test, trifluridine solution has been shown to be teratogenic when injected directly into the yolk sac of chicken eggs. There are no adequate and well-controlled studies in pregnant women. Trifluridine ophthalmic solution should be used during pregnancy only if the potential benefit justifies the potential risk to the fetus.

➤*Lactation:* It is unlikely that trifluridine is excreted in human milk after ophthalmic instillation of trifluridine because of the relatively small dosage (≤ 5 mg/day), its dilution in body fluids and its extremely short half-life (≈ 12 minutes). The drug should not be prescribed for nursing mothers unless the potential benefits outweigh the potential risks.

➤*Children:* Safety and efficacy in pediatric patients below 6 years of age have not been established.

Adverse Reactions

The most frequent adverse reactions reported during controlled clinical trials were mild, transient burning or stinging upon instillation (4.6%) and palpebral edema (2.8%). Other adverse reactions in decreasing order of reported frequency were superficial punctate keratopathy, epithelial keratopathy, hypersensitivity reaction, stromal edema, irritation, keratitis sicca, hyperemia, and increased intraocular pressure.

Overdosage

➤*Symptoms:* Overdosage by ocular instillation is unlikely because any excess solution should be quickly expelled from the conjunctival sac.

Acute overdosage by accidental oral ingestion of trifluridine has not occurred. However, should such ingestion occur, the 75 mg dosage of trifluridine in a 7.5 mL bottle of trifluridine is not likely to produce adverse effects. Single IV doses of 1.5 to 30 mg/kg/day in children and adults with neoplastic disease produce reversible bone marrow depression as the only potentially serious toxic effect and only after 3 to 5 courses of therapy. The acute oral LD_{50} in the mouse and rat was greater than or equal to 4379 mg/kg.

GANCICLOVIR

Rx	**Vitrasert** (Bausch & Lomb Inc)	**Implant; intravitreal:** 4.5 mg	In individual unit boxes.

GANCICLOVIR — OPHTHALMIC IMPLANT

Indications

➤*Cytomegalovirus (CMV) retinitis:* For the treatment of CMV retinitis in patients with acquired immune deficiency syndrome (AIDS).

Administration and Dosage

➤*Adults:*

Cytomegalovirus retinitis –

Usual dosage: 1 implant inserted into each affected eye by intravitreal implantation.

Duration of therapy: Each ganciclovir implant is designed to release the drug over a 5- to 8-month period of time. Following depletion of ganciclovir from the ganciclovir implant, as evidenced by progression of retinitis, the ganciclovir implant may be removed or replaced.

➤*Children:* Safety and efficacy in patients younger than 9 years of age have not been established.

See Adults for dosing for patients 9 years of age and older.

➤*Administration:* The ganciclovir implant is for intravitreal implantation only.

Caution should be exercised in handling the ganciclovir implant in order to avoid damage to the polymer coating on the implant, which may result in an increased rate of drug release. Thus, the ganciclovir implant should be handled only by the suture tab. Aseptic technique should be maintained at all times prior to and during the surgical implantation procedure.

➤*Storage/Stability:* Store at controlled room temperature, 15° to 30°C (59° to 86°F). Protect from freezing, excessive heat, and light.

Because the ganciclovir implant contains ganciclovir, which shares some of the properties of antitumor agents (ie, carcinogenicity, mutagenicity), consideration should be given to handling and disposal of the ganciclovir implant according to guidelines issued for antineoplastic drugs.

Actions

➤*Pharmacology:* Ganciclovir is a synthetic nucleoside analog of 2′-deoxyguanosine that inhibits replication of herpes viruses both in vitro and in vivo. Sensitive human viruses include CMV, herpes simplex virus (types 1 and 2), Epstein-Barr virus, and varicella zoster virus. Clinical studies have been limited to assessment of efficacy in patients with CMV infection.

Median effective inhibitory doses (ED_{50}) of ganciclovir for human CMV isolates tested in vitro in several cell lines ranged from 0.2 to 3 mcg/mL. The relationship between in vitro sensitivity of CMV to ganciclovir and clinical response has not been established. Ganciclovir inhibits mammalian cell proliferation in vitro at higher concentrations (10 to 60 mcg/mL) with bone marrow colony forming cells being the most sensitive (ID_{50} greater than 10 mcg/mL) of those cell types tested.

Emergence of viral resistance has been reported based on in vitro sensitivity testing of CMV isolates from patients receiving intravenous (IV) ganciclovir treatment. The prevalence of resistant isolates is unknown, and there is a possibility that some patients may be infected with strains of CMV resistant

GANCICLOVIR — OPHTHALMIC IMPLANT

to ganciclovir. Therefore, consider the possibility of viral resistance in patients who show poor clinical response.

➤*Pharmacokinetics:*

Absorption / Distribution – In a clinical trial of ganciclovir implants, 26 patients (30 eyes) received a total of 39 primary implants and 12 exchange implants (performed 32 weeks after the implant was inserted or earlier if progression of CMV retinitis occurred). Because most of the exchanged implants were empty, the time the implant actually ran out of drug was unknown, and a precise in vivo release rate could not be calculated. However, approximate in vivo release rates could be determined for the exchanged implants, which ranged from 1 mcg/h to more than 1.62 mcg/h.

In 14 implants (3 exchanged, 11 autopsy) in which the in vivo release rate could accurately be calculated, the mean release rate was 1.4 mcg/h, with a range from 0.5 to 2.88 mcg/h. The mean vitreous drug levels in 8 eyes (4 collected at the time of retinal detachment surgery; 2 collected from autopsy eyes within 6 hours of death and prior to fixation; 2 collected from implant exchanges) was 4.1 mcg/mL.

Contraindications

Hypersensitivity to ganciclovir or acyclovir, and in patients with any contraindications for intraocular surgery, (eg, external infection, severe thrombocytopenia).

Warnings/Precautions

➤*Extraocular CMV disease:* CMV retinitis may be associated with CMV elsewhere in the body. The ganciclovir implant provides localized therapy limited to the implanted eye. The ganciclovir implant does not provide treatment for systemic CMV disease. Monitor patients for extraocular CMV disease.

➤*Surgical risk:* As with any surgical procedure, there is risk involved. Potential complications accompanying intraocular surgery to place the ganciclovir implant into the vitreous cavity may include, but are not limited to, the following: vitreous loss, vitreous hemorrhage, cataract formation, retinal detachment, uveitis, endophthalmitis, and disease in visual acuity.

➤*Visual acuity:* Following implantation of the ganciclovir implant, nearly all patients will experience an immediate and temporary decrease in visual acuity in the implanted eye which lasts for approximately 2 to 4 weeks postoperatively. The decrease in visual acuity is likely a result of the surgical implant procedure.

➤*Handling:* As with all intraocular surgery, rigorously maintain sterility of the surgical field and the ganciclovir implant. maintained. Handle the ganciclovir implant only by the suture tab in order to avoid damaging the polymer coatings because this could affect release rate of ganciclovir inside the eye. Do not resterilize the ganciclovir implant by any method.

➤*Experienced surgeons:* A high level of surgical skill is required for implantation of the ganciclovir implant. A surgeon should have observed or assisted in surgical implantation of the ganciclovir implant prior to attempting the procedure.

➤*Retinal tamponade:* There is limited experience with retinal tamponade in conjunction with the ganciclovir implant.

➤*Pregnancy: Category C.* Ganciclovir has been shown to be teratogenic in rabbits and embryotoxic in rabbits and mice following IV administration. Fetal reabsorption was present in at least 85% of rabbits and mice administered 60 and 108 mg/kg/day, respectively. Effects observed in rabbits included: fetal growth retardation, embryolethality, teratogenicity, and/or maternal toxicity. Teratogenic changes included cleft palate, anophthalmia/microphthalmia, aplastic organs (kidney and pancreas), hydrocephaly, and brachygnathia. In mice, effects observed were maternal/fetal toxicity and embryolethality.

Daily IV doses of 90 mg/kg administered to female mice prior to mating, during gestation, and during lactation caused hypoplasia of the testes and seminal vesicles in the month-old male offspring, as well as pathologic changes in the nonglandular region of the stomach.

Although each ganciclovir implant contains 4.5 to 6.4 mg of ganciclovir, which is released locally in the vitreous, there are no adequate and well-controlled studies in pregnant women on the effects of the ganciclovir implant. Therefore, only use ganciclovir implant used during pregnancy if the potential benefit justifies the potential risk to the fetus.

➤*Lactation:* It is not known whether ganciclovir from the ganciclovir implant is excreted in human milk. Daily IV doses of 90 mg/kg administered to female mice prior to mating, during gestation, and during lactation caused hypoplasia of the testes and seminal vesicles in the month-old male offspring, as well as pathologic changes in the nonglandular region of the stomach. Because many drugs are excreted in human milk, and because carcinogenicity and teratogenicity effects occurred in animals treated with ganciclovir, instruct mothers to discontinue breast-feeding if they have the ganciclovir implant.

➤*Children:* Safety and efficacy in patients younger than below 9 years of age have not been established.

➤*Monitoring:* Monitor patients for extraocular CMV disease.

Drug Interactions

No drug interactions have been observed with the ganciclovir implant.

Adverse Reactions

➤*Ophthalmic:* During clinical trials, the most frequent adverse reactions seen in patients treated with the ganciclovir implant involved the eye.

During the first 2 months following implantation, visual acuity loss of 3 lines or more, vitreous hemorrhage, and retinal detachments occurred in approximately 10% to 20% of patients. Cataract formation/lens opacities, macular abnormalities, intraocular pressure spikes, optic disk/nerve changes, hyphemas, and uveitis occurred in approximately 1% to 5%.

Adverse reactions with an incidence of less than 1% were: angle closure glaucoma with anterior chamber shallowing, anterior chamber cell and flare, astigmatism, chemosis, choroidal folds, choroiditis, corneal dellen, cotton wool spots, endophthalmitis, gliosis, hemorrhage (other than vitreous), hypotony, keratopathy, microangiopathy, pellet extrusion from scleral wound, phthisis bulbi, retinal hole, retinal tear, retinopathy, sclerosis, severe postoperative inflammation, synechia, vitreous detachment, and vitreous traction.

Patient Information

Advise the patient that the ganciclovir implant is not a cure for CMV retinitis, and some immunocompromised patients may continue to experience progression of retinitis with the ganciclovir implant. Advise patients to have ophthalmologic follow-up examinations of both eyes at appropriate intervals following implantation of the ganciclovir implant.

As with any surgical procedure, there is risk involved. Potential complications accompanying intraocular surgery to place the ganciclovir implant into the vitreous cavity may include, but are not limited to, the following: intraocular infection or inflammation, detachment of the retina, and formation of cataract in the natural crystalline lens.

Following implantation of the ganciclovir implant, nearly all patients will experience an immediate and temporary decrease in visual acuity in the implanted eye which lasts for approximately 2 to 4 weeks. This decrease in visual acuity is likely a result of the surgical implant procedure.

The ganciclovir implant only treats eyes in which it has been implanted. Additionally, because CMV is a systemic disease, monitor patients for extraocular CMV infections (eg, pneumonitis, colitis) in the body.

Advise patients that ganciclovir has caused decreased sperm production in animals and may cause infertility in humans. Advise women of childbearing potential that ganciclovir causes birth defects in animals and should not be used during pregnancy. Also advise patients that ganciclovir has caused tumors in animals. Although there is no information from human studies, consider ganciclovir a potential carcinogen.

GANCICLOVIR

Rx	**Zirgan** (Sirion Therapeutics Inc)	**Gel; ophthalmic:** 0.15%	Benzalkonium chloride 0.075 mg. In 5 g tubes.

GANCICLOVIR — OPHTHALMIC GEL

Indications

➤*Herpetic keratitis:* For the treatment of acute herpetic keratitis (dendritic ulcers).

Administration and Dosage

➤*Adults:*

Herpetic keratitis –

Initial dosage: 1 drop in the affected eye 5 times per day (approximately every 3 hours while awake) until the corneal ulcer heals.

Maintenance dosage: 1 drop 3 times per day for 7 days.

➤*Children:*

Herpetic keratitis – See Adults for dosing for children 2 years of age and older.

➤*Administration:* For topical ophthalmic use only.

➤*Storage / Stability:* Store at 15° to 25°C (59° to 77°F). Do not freeze.

Actions

➤*Pharmacology:* Ganciclovir is a guanosine derivative that, upon phosphorylation, inhibits DNA replication by herpes simplex viruses (HSV). Ganciclovir is transformed by viral and cellular thymidine kinases (TK) to ganciclovir triphosphate, which works as an antiviral agent by inhibiting the synthesis of viral DNA in 2 ways, competitive inhibition of viral DNA-polymerase and direct incorporation into viral primer strand DNA, which results in DNA chain termination and prevention of replication.

➤*Pharmacokinetics:* The estimated maximum daily dose of ganciclovir administered as 1 drop, 5 times per day is 0.375 mg. Compared with maintenance doses of systemically administered ganciclovir 900 mg (oral valganciclovir) and 5 mg/kg (IV ganciclovir), the ophthalmically administered daily dose is approximately 0.04% and 0.1% of the oral dose and IV doses, respectively; thus, minimal systemic exposure is expected.

Contraindications

None known.

Warnings/Precautions

➤*Contact lenses:* Instruct patients not to wear contact lenses if they have signs or symptoms of herpetic keratitis or during the course of therapy with ganciclovir.

GANCICLOVIR — OPHTHALMIC GEL

➤*Pregnancy: Category C.*

Teratogenic – Ganciclovir has been shown to be embryotoxic in rabbits and mice following IV administration and teratogenic in rabbits. Fetal resorptions were present in at least 85% of rabbits and mice administered 60 and 108 mg/kg/day (approximately 10,000 and 17,000 times the human ocular dosage of 6.25 mcg/kg/day), respectively, assuming complete absorption. Effects observed in rabbits included fetal growth retardation, embryolethality, teratogenicity, and/or maternal toxicity. Teratogenic changes included cleft palate, anophthalmia/microphthalmia, aplastic organs (kidney and pancreas), hydrocephaly, and brachygnathia. In mice, effects observed were maternal/fetal toxicity and embryolethality. Daily IV dosages of 90 mg/kg/day (14,000 times the human ocular dose) administered to female mice prior to mating, during gestation, and during lactation caused hypoplasia of the testes and seminal vesicles in the month-old male offspring, as well as pathologic changes in the nonglandular region of the stomach.

There are no adequate and well-controlled studies in pregnant women. Use during pregnancy only if the potential benefit justifies the potential risk to the fetus.

➤*Lactation:* It is not known whether topical ophthalmic ganciclovir administration could result in sufficient systemic absorption to produce detectable quantities in breast milk. Exercise caution when ganciclovir is administered to breast-feeding mothers.

➤*Children:* Safety and efficacy in children younger than 2 years of age have not been established.

Drug Interactions

None known.

Adverse Reactions

➤*Common adverse reactions:* Most common adverse reactions reported in patients were blurred vision (60%), eye irritation (20%), punctate keratitis (5%), and conjunctival hyperemia (5%).

Patient Information

Advise patients that this product is sterile when packaged. Advise patients not to allow the dropper tip to touch any surface, because this may contaminate the gel.

Advise patients to consult their health care provider if pain develops, or if redness, itching, or inflammation becomes aggravated.

Advise patients not to wear contact lenses if they have signs and symptoms of herpetic keratitis or when using ganciclovir gel.

OPHTHALMIC IMMUNOLOGIC AGENTS

CYCLOSPORINE

Rx	**Restasis** (Allergan)	**Emulsion, ophthalmic:** 0.05%[a]	Preservative-free. In 0.4 mL single-use vials.

[a] With glycerin, castor oil, and polysorbate 80.

CYCLOSPORINE — OPHTHALMIC

Indications

➤*Increased tear production:* To increase tear production in patients whose tear production is presumed to be suppressed due to ocular inflammation associated with keratoconjunctivitis sicca. Increased tear production was not seen in patients currently taking topical anti-inflammatory drugs or using punctal plugs.

Administration and Dosage

➤*General dosing considerations:* Invert the unit dose vial a few times to obtain a uniform, white, opaque emulsion before using.

➤*Adults:*

Increased tear production –

Usual dosage: Instill 1 drop of cyclosporine ophthalmic emulsion twice a day in each eye, approximately 12 hours apart.

Concomitant therapy: Cyclosporine can be used concomitantly with artificial tears; allow a 15-minute interval between products.

➤*Children:*

16 years of age and older – See Adults for dosing.

➤*Preparation for administration:* Cyclosporine is an immunosuppressant and is also considered a potential teratogen and potential mutagen. Follow safe handling procedures when preparing, administering, or dispensing cyclosporine.

A 10% (100 mg/mL) solution is prepared by the addition of 10 mL of an aqueous diluent such as water for injection or dextrose 5% injection.

➤*Administration:* Cyclosporine ophthalmic emulsion is for ophthalmic use only.

➤*Storage/Stability:* Store cyclosporine ophthalmic emulsion between 15° and 25°C (59° and 77°F). Keep out of the reach of children. Discard vial immediately after use.

Actions

➤*Pharmacology:* Cyclosporine is an immunosuppressive agent when administered systemically.

In patients whose tear production is presumed to be suppressed due to ocular inflammation associated with keratoconjunctivitis sicca, cyclosporine emulsion is thought to act as a partial immunomodulator. The exact mechanism of action is not known.

➤*Pharmacokinetics:*

Absorption – Blood cyclosporin A concentrations were measured using a specific high-pressure liquid chromatography-mass spectrometry assay. Blood concentrations of cyclosporine, in all the samples collected, after topical administration of cyclosporine ophthalmic suspension 0.05%, twice daily, in humans for up to 12 months, were below the quantitation limit of 0.1 ng/mL. There was no detectable accumulation in blood during 12 months of treatment with cyclosporine ophthalmic emulsion.

Contraindications

In patients with active ocular infections; in patients with known or suspected hypersensitivity to any of the ingredients in the formulation.

Warnings/Precautions

➤*Herpes keratitis:* Cyclosporine ophthalmic emulsion has not been studied in patients with a history of herpes keratitis.

➤*Administration:* Cyclosporine ophthalmic emulsion is for ophthalmic use only.

➤*Pregnancy: Category C.* There are no adequate and well-controlled studies of cyclosporine ophthalmic emulsion in pregnant women. Only administer cyclosporine ophthalmic emulsion to a pregnant woman if clearly needed.

Nonteratogenic – Adverse reactions were seen in reproduction in rats and rabbits only at dose levels toxic to dams. At toxic doses (rats at 30 mg/kg/day and rabbits at 100 mg/kg/day), cyclosporine oral solution was embryo- and fetotoxic as indicated by increased pre- and postnatal mortality and reduced fetal weight together with related skeletal retardations. These doses are 30,000 and 100,000 times greater, respectively, than the daily human dose of 1 drop (28 mcL) of 0.05% cyclosporine ophthalmic emulsion twice daily into each eye of a 60 kg person (0.001 mg/kg/day), assuming that the entire dose is absorbed.

No evidence of embryofetal toxicity was observed in rats or rabbits receiving cyclosporine at oral doses up to 17/mg/kg/day or 30 mg/kg/day, respectively, during organogenesis. These doses in rats and rabbits are approximately 17,000 and 30,000 times greater, respectively, than the daily human dose.

Offspring of rats receiving a 45 mg/kg/day oral dose of cyclosporine from day 15 of pregnancy until day 21 postpartum, a maternally toxic level, exhibited an increase in postnatal mortality; this dose is 45,000 times greater than the daily human topical dose, 0.001 mg/kg/day, assuming that the entire dose is absorbed. No adverse events were observed at oral doses up to 15 mg/kg/day (15,000 times greater than the daily human dose).

➤*Lactation:* Cyclosporine is known to be excreted in human milk following systemic administration, but excretion in human milk after topical treatment has not been investigated. Although blood concentrations are undetectable after topical administration of cyclosporine ophthalmic emulsion, caution should be exercised when cyclosporine ophthalmic emulsion is administered to a nursing woman.

➤*Children:* The safety and efficacy of cyclosporine ophthalmic emulsion have not been established in pediatric patients below 16 years of age.

Adverse Reactions

The most common adverse reaction following the use of cyclosporine ophthalmic emulsion was ocular burning (17%).

Other events reported in 1% to 5% of patients included conjunctival hyperemia, discharge, epiphora, eye pain, foreign body sensation, pruritus, stinging, and visual disturbance (most often blurring).

Patient Information

The emulsion from 1 individual single-use vial is to be used immediately after opening for administration to 1 or both eyes, and the remaining contents should be discarded immediately after administration.

Do not allow the tip of the vial to touch the eye or any surface, as this may contaminate the emulsion.

Cyclosporine ophthalmic emulsion should not be administered while wearing contact lenses. Patients with decreased tear production typically should not wear contact lenses. If contact lenses are worn, they should be removed prior to the administration of the emulsion. Lenses may be reinserted 15 minutes following administration of cyclosporine ophthalmic emulsion.

PEGAPTANIB SODIUM

Rx	Macugen (Eyetech)	Injection: 0.3 mg[a]	In 1 mL glass syringe. With 27-gauge needle and shield.

[a] Equivalent to 1.6 mg pegaptanib sodium (pegylated oligonucleotide) or 3.2 mg when expressed as the sodium salt form of the oligonucleotide moiety.

PEGAPTANIB SODIUM — OPHTHALMIC INJECTION

Indications

➤*Neovascular age-related macular degeneration (AMD):* For the treatment of neovascular (wet) AMD.

➤*Off-label uses:* Treatment of diabetic macular edema.

Administration and Dosage

➤*General dosing considerations:* The patient's medical history of hypersensitivity reactions should be evaluated prior to performing the intravitreal procedure.

Adequate anesthesia and a broad-spectrum microbicide should be given prior to the injection.

Following the injection, monitor the patient for elevation in intraocular pressure and for endophthalmitis. Monitoring may consist of a check for perfusion of the optic nerve head immediately after the injection, tonometry within 30 minutes following the injection, and biomicroscopy between 2 and 7 days following the injection. Instruct patients to report any symptoms suggestive of endophthalmitis immediately.

➤*Adults:*

Neovascular age-related macular degeneration (AMD) – 0.3 mg once every 6 weeks by intravitreous injection into the eye to be treated.

➤*Preparation for administration:* Administration of the syringe contents involves attaching the threaded plastic plunger rod to the rubber stopper inside the barrel of the syringe. Do not pull back on the plunger. Remove the syringe needle cap. Holding the syringe with the needle pointing up, check the syringe for bubbles. If there are bubbles, gently tap the syringe with your finger until the bubbles rise to the top of the syringe. Slowly push the plunger up to force all the bubbles out of the syringe.

➤*Administration:* For ophthalmic intravitreal injection only.

➤*Storage/Stability:* Refrigerate at 2° to 8°C (36° to 46°F). Do not freeze or shake vigorously.

Actions

➤*Pharmacology:* Pegaptanib is a selective vascular endothelial growth factor (VEGF) antagonist. VEGF is a secreted protein that selectively binds and activates its receptors, which are located primarily on the surface of vascular endothelial cells. VEGF induces angiogenesis and increases vascular permeability and inflammation, all of which are thought to contribute to the progression of the neovascular (wet) form of AMD, a leading cause of blindness. VEGF has been implicated in blood retinal barrier breakdown and pathological ocular neovascularization.

Pegaptanib is an aptamer, a pegylated modified oligonucleotide that adopts a 3-dimensional conformation that enables it to bind to extracellular VEGF. Under in vitro testing conditions, pegaptanib binds to the major pathological VEGF isoform, extracellular $VEGF_{165}$, thereby inhibiting $VEGF_{165}$ binding to its VEGF receptors. The inhibition of $VEGF_{164}$, the rodent counterpart of human $VEGF_{165}$, was effective at suppressing pathological neovascularization.

➤*Pharmacokinetics:*

Absorption – In animals, pegaptanib is slowly absorbed into the systemic circulation from the eye after intravitreous administration. The rate of absorption from the eye is the rate-limiting step in the disposition of pegaptanib in animals and is likely to be the rate-limiting step in humans.

In humans, a mean maximum plasma concentration (C_{max}) of approximately 80 ng/mL occurs within 1 to 4 days after a 3 mg monocular dose (10 times the recommended dose). The mean area under the plasma concentration-time curve (AUC) is approximately 25 mcg•h/mL at this dose.

Distribution – Twenty-four hours after intravitreous administration of a radiolabeled dose of pegaptanib to both eyes of rabbits, radioactivity was mainly distributed in vitreous fluid, retina, and aqueous fluid. After intravitreous and intravenous administrations of radiolabeled pegaptanib to rabbits, the highest concentrations of radioactivity (excluding the eye for the intravitreous dose) were obtained in the kidney.

Metabolism/Excretion – In rabbits, the component nucleotide, 2-fluorouridine, is found in plasma and urine after single radiolabeled pegaptanib IV and intravitreous doses. In rabbits, pegaptanib is eliminated as parent drug and metabolites primarily in the urine.

Based on preclinical data, pegaptanib is metabolized by endo- and exonucleases.

In humans, after a 3 mg monocular dose (10 times the recommended dose), the average (± standard deviation) apparent plasma half-life of pegaptanib is 10 (± 4) days.

Special populations –

Renal function impairment: Dose adjustment for patients with renal function impairment is not needed when administering the 0.3 mg dose.

Following a single 3 mg dose (10 times the recommended dose) in patients with severe (n = 7), moderate (n = 18), and mild (n = 10) renal function impairment, the mean coefficient of variation pegaptanib AUC values were 37.8 (17%), 26.7 (31%), and 23.6 (21%) mcg•h/mL, respectively. The corresponding C_{max} values were 96.8 (23%), 81.6 (29.2%), and 66.5 (47%) ng/mL, respectively.

In patients with renal function impairment, following administration of pegaptanib 3 mg doses every 6 weeks, the last detectable pegaptanib concentrations in plasma after the fourth dose were highly variable (ranging from 8 to 66 ng/mL), and the variability was more pronounced in patients with severe renal function impairment.

Contraindications

Ocular or periocular infections; known hypersensitivity to pegaptanib or any other excipient in this product.

Warnings/Precautions

➤*Endophthalmitis:* Intravitreous injections, including those with pegaptanib, have been associated with endophthalmitis. Use proper aseptic injection technique when administering pegaptanib. In addition, monitor patients during the week following the injection to permit early treatment if an infection occurs.

➤*Increased intraocular pressure:* Increases in intraocular pressure have been seen within 30 minutes of injection with pegaptanib. Therefore, monitor and manage intraocular pressure, as well as the perfusion of the optic nerve head.

➤*Administration:* For ophthalmic intravitreal injection only.

➤*Hypersensitivity reactions:* Rare cases of anaphylaxis/anaphylactoid reactions, including angioedema, have been reported in the postmarketing experience following the pegaptanib intravitreal administration procedure.

➤*Pregnancy: Category B.* There are no studies in pregnant women. The potential risk to humans is unknown. Use pegaptanib during pregnancy only if the potential benefit to the mother justifies the potential risk to the fetus.

➤*Lactation:* It is not known whether pegaptanib is excreted in human milk. Because many drugs are excreted in human milk, exercise caution when pegaptanib is administered to a breast-feeding woman.

➤*Children:* Safety and efficacy of pegaptanib in children have not been studied.

➤*Monitoring:* Following the injection, monitor the patient for elevation in intraocular pressure and for endophthalmitis. Monitoring may consist of a check for perfusion of the optic nerve head immediately after the injection, tonometry within 30 minutes following the injection, and biomicroscopy between 2 and 7 days following the injection. Instruct patients to report any symptoms suggestive of endophthalmitis immediately.

Drug Interactions

None known.

Adverse Reactions

Serious adverse reactions related to the injection procedure occurring in less than 1% of intravitreous injections included endophthalmitis, retinal detachment, and iatrogenic traumatic cataract.

The most frequently reported adverse reactions in patients treated with pegaptanib 0.3 mg for up to 2 years were anterior chamber inflammation, blurred vision, cataract, conjunctival hemorrhage, corneal edema, eye discharge, eye irritation, eye pain, hypertension, increased intraocular pressure, ocular discomfort, punctate keratitis, reduced visual acuity, visual disturbance, vitreous floaters, and vitreous opacities. These reactions occurred in approximately 10% to 40% of patients.

➤*Reactions reported in 6% to 10% of patients receiving pegaptanib 0.3 mg therapy:*

CNS – Dizziness, headache.

GI – Diarrhea, nausea.

Special senses – Blepharitis, conjunctivitis, photopsia, vitreous disorder.

Miscellaneous – Bronchitis, urinary tract infection.

➤*Reactions reported in 1% to 5% of patients receiving pegaptanib 0.3 mg therapy:*

Cardiovascular – Carotid artery occlusion, cerebrovascular accident, transient ischemic attack.

GI – Dyspepsia, vomiting.

Musculoskeletal – Arthritis, bone spur.

Special senses – Allergic conjunctivitis, conjunctival edema, corneal abrasion, corneal deposits, corneal epithelium disorder, endophthalmitis, eye inflammation, eye swelling, eyelid irritation, hearing loss, meibomianitis, mydriasis, periorbital hematoma, retinal edema, vitreous hemorrhage.

Miscellaneous – Chest pain, contact dermatitis, contusion, diabetes mellitus, pleural effusion, urinary retention, vertigo.

➤*Postmarketing experience:*

Hypersensitivity – See Warnings/Precautions for more information.

Overdosage

Doses of pegaptanib up to 10 times the recommended dose of 0.3 mg have been studied. No additional adverse reactions have been noted, but there is decreased efficacy with doses greater than 1 mg.

PEGAPTANIB SODIUM — OPHTHALMIC INJECTION

Patient Information

In the days following pegaptanib administration, patients are at risk for the development of endophthalmitis. If the eye becomes red, sensitive to light, painful, or develops a change in vision, the patient should seek immediate care from an ophthalmologist.

RANIBIZUMAB

Rx	**Lucentis** (Genentech)	**Injection, solution; intravitreal:** 10 mg/mL	Preservative free. In single-use vials.[a]

[a] Designed to deliver 0.05 mL of ranibizumab 10 mg/mL solution.

RANIBIZUMAB — INTRAVITREAL

Indications

➤*Macular degeneration:* For the treatment of patients with neovascular (wet) age-related macular degeneration (AMD).

➤*Macular edema:* For the treatment of patients with macular edema following retinal vein occlusion.

Administration and Dosage

➤*Adults:*

Macular degeneration –

Usual dosage: Administer 0.5 mg (0.05 mL) by intravitreal injection once a month (approximately every 28 days).

Alternative dosage: Although less effective, treatment may be reduced to 1 injection every 3 months after the first 4 injections if monthly injections are not feasible. Compared with continued monthly dosing, dosing every 3 months will lead to an approximate 5-letter (1-line) loss of visual acuity benefit, on average, over the following 9 months. Patients should be treated regularly.

Macular edema – Administer 0.5 mg (0.05 mL) by intravitreal injection once a month (approximately every 28 days).

➤*Preparation for administration:* Using aseptic technique, all (0.2 mL) of the ranibizumab vial contents are withdrawn through a 5-micron, 19-gauge filter needle attached to a 1 mL tuberculin syringe. The filter needle should be discarded after withdrawal of the vial contents and should not be used for intravitreal injection. The filter needle should be replaced with a sterile 30-gauge × ½-needle for the intravitreal injection. The contents should be expelled until the plunger tip is aligned with the line that marks 0.05 mL on the syringe.

➤*Administration:* For ophthalmic intravitreal injection only.

Each vial should only be used for the treatment of a single eye. If the contralateral eye requires treatment, a new vial should be used and the sterile field, syringe, gloves, drapes, eyelid speculum, filter, and injection needles should be changed before ranibizumab is administered to the other eye.

➤*Storage / Stability:* Refrigerate at 2° to 8°C (36° to 46°F). Do not freeze. Protect from light. Store in the original carton until time of use.

Actions

➤*Pharmacology:* Ranibizumab binds to the receptor-binding site of active forms of vascular endothelial growth factor A (VEGF-A), including the biologically active, cleaved form of this molecule, $VEGF_{110}$. VEGF-A has been shown to cause neovascularization and leakage in models of ocular angiogenesis and vascular occlusion and is thought to contribute to the progression of neovascular AMD and macular edema following retinal vein occlusion (RVO). The binding of ranibizumab to VEGF-A prevents the interaction of VEGF-A with its receptors (VEGFR1 and VEGFR2) on the surface of endothelial cells, reducing endothelial cell proliferation, vascular leakage, and new blood vessel formation.

➤*Pharmacokinetics:*

Absorption / Distribution – In patients with neovascular AMD following monthly intravitreal administration, maximum ranibizumab serum concentrations were low (0.3 to 2.36 ng/mL). These levels were below the concentration of ranibizumab (11 to 27 ng/mL) thought to be necessary to inhibit the biological activity of VEGF-A by 50%, as measured in an in vitro cellular proliferation assay. The maximum observed serum concentration was dose proportional over the dose range of 0.05 to 1 mg/eye. Serum ranibizumab concentrations in RVO patients were similar to those observed in neovascular AMD patients.

Based on a neovascular AMD population pharmacokinetic analysis, maximum serum concentrations of 1.5 ng/mL are predicted to be reached at approximately 1 day after monthly intravitreal administration of ranibizumab 0.5 mg/eye. Steady-state minimum concentration is predicted to be 0.22 ng/mL with a monthly dosing regimen. In humans, serum ranibizumab concentrations are predicted to be approximately 90,000-fold lower than vitreal concentrations. In animal studies, systemic exposure of ranibizumab is more than 2,000-fold lower than in the vitreous.

Excretion – In patients with neovascular AMD, based on the disappearance of ranibizumab from serum, the estimated average vitreous elimination half-life was approximately 9 days. In animal studies, following intravitreal injection, ranibizumab was cleared from the vitreous with a half-life of approximately 3 days. After reaching a maximum at approximately 1 day, the serum concentration of ranibizumab declined in parallel with the vitreous concentration.

Contraindications

Ocular or periocular infections; known hypersensitivity to ranibizumab or any of its excipients.

Warnings/Precautions

➤*Endophthalmitis and retinal detachments:* Intravitreal injections, including those with ranibizumab, have been associated with endophthalmitis and retinal detachments. Use proper aseptic injection technique when administering ranibizumab. Monitor patients during the week following the injection to permit early treatment in case an infection occurs.

➤*Increased intraocular pressure:* Increases in intraocular pressure have been noted within 60 minutes of intravitreal injection with ranibizumab. Therefore, monitor and appropriately manage intraocular pressure, as well as the perfusion of the optic nerve head.

➤*Thromboembolic events:* Although there was a low rate of arterial thromboembolic events observed in the ranibizumab clinical trials, there is a potential risk of arterial thromboembolic events following intravitreal use of VEGF inhibitors. Arterial thromboembolic events are defined as nonfatal stroke, nonfatal myocardial infarction, or vascular death (including deaths of unknown cause).

Macular degeneration – The arterial thromboembolic event rate in the 3 controlled neovascular AMD studies during the first year was 1.9% in the combined group of patients treated with ranibizumab 0.3 or 0.5 mg compared with 1.1% in patients from the control arms. In the second year of studies AMD-1 and AMD-2, the arterial thromboembolic event rate was 2.6% in the combined group of ranibizumb-treated patients compared with 2.9% in patients from the control arms.

In a pooled analysis of 2-year controlled studies (AMD-1, AMD-2, and a study of ranibizumab used adjunctively with verteporfin photodynamic therapy), the stroke rate (including ischemic and hemorrhagic stroke) was 2.7% in patients treated with ranibizumab 0.5 mg compared with 1.1% in patients in the control arms (odds ratio, 2.2 [95% confidence interval, 0.8 to 7.1]).

Macular edema – The arterial thromboembolic event rate in the 2 controlled RVO studies during the first 6 months was 0.8% in both the ranibizumab and control arms of the studies (4 of 525 in the combined group of patients treated with ranibizumab 0.3 or 0.5 mg and 2 of 260 in the control arms). The stroke rate was 0.2% in the combined group of ranibizumab-treated patients compared with 0.4% in the control arms.

➤*Immunogenicity:* As with all therapeutic proteins, there is the potential for an immune response in patients treated with ranibizumab. The immunogenicity data reflect the percentage of patients whose test results were considered positive for antibodies to ranibizumab in immunoassays and are highly dependent on the sensitivity and specificity of the assays.

The pretreatment incidence of immunoreactivity to ranibizumab was 0% to 5% across treatment groups. After monthly dosing with ranibizumab for 6 to 24 months, antibodies to ranibizumab were detected in approximately 1% to 8% of patients.

The clinical significance of immunoreactivity to ranibizumab is unclear at this time. Among neovascular AMD patients with the highest levels of immunoreactivity, some were noted to have iritis or vitritis. Intraocular inflammation was not observed in the RVO patients with the highest levels of immunoreactivity.

➤*Hypersensitivity reactions:* Hypersensitivity reactions may manifest as intraocular inflammation.

➤*Pregnancy: Category C.* Animal reproduction studies have not been conducted with ranibizumab. The high molecular weight (48,000) and very low concentrations in the systemic circulation suggest that the antibody will not cross to the embryo or fetus. However, immunoglobulin G crosses the placenta, and, therefore, ranibizumab may cross as well. It also is not known whether ranibizumab can cause fetal harm when administered to a pregnant woman or can affect reproduction capacity. Give ranibizumab to a pregnant woman only if clearly needed.

➤*Lactation:* It is not known whether ranibizumab is excreted in human milk. Although the long plasma elimination half-life (about 9 days) favors excretion, the molecular weight (48,000) and very low plasma concentrations suggest that the antibody will not be detected in milk. However, immunoglobulin G is excreted into milk. Nevertheless, even if excretion does occur, it should be in clinically insignificant amounts. Because many drugs are excreted in human milk, and because the potential for absorption and harm to infant growth and development exists, exercise caution when ranibizumab is administered to a breast-feeding woman.

➤*Children:* The safety and effectiveness of ranibizumab in children have not been established.

➤*Monitoring:* Following the intravitreal injection, monitor patients for elevation in intraocular pressure and for endophthalmitis. Monitoring may consist of a check for perfusion of the optic nerve head immediately after the injection and tonometry within 30 minutes following the injection. Instruct patients to report any symptoms suggestive of endophthalmitis without delay. Monitor patients during the week following the injection to permit

RANIBIZUMAB — INTRAVITREAL

early treatment in case an infection occurs. Monitor and appropriately manage intraocular pressure, as well as the perfusion of the optic nerve head.

Drug Interactions

➤*Verteporfin photodynamic therapy:* Ranibizumab has been used adjunctively with verteporfin photodynamic therapy (PDT). Eleven percent of patients with neovascular AMD developed serious intraocular inflammation; in 83% of these patients, this occurred when ranibizumab was administered 7 days (± 2 days) after verteporfin PDT.

Adverse Reactions

➤*Injection procedure:* Serious adverse reactions related to the injection procedure have occurred in less than 0.1% of intravitreal injections, including endophthalmitis, iatrogenic traumatic cataracts, and rhegmatogenous retinal detachments.

➤*Adverse reactions:*

Ranibizumab Adverse Reactions

Adverse reactions	AMD 2-year Ranibizumab (n = 379)	AMD 2-year Control (n = 379)	AMD 1-year Ranibizumab (n = 440)	AMD 1-year Control (n = 441)	RVO 6-month Ranibizumab (n = 259)	RVO 6-month Control (n = 260)
CNS						
Anxiety	4%	4%	3%	2%	1%	2%
Headache	12%	9%	6%	5%	3%	3%
Insomnia	5%	5%	3%	2%	1%	1%
GI						
Gastroenteritis viral	4%	1%	3%	1%	1%	0%
Nausea	9%	6%	5%	5%	1%	2%
Musculoskeletal						
Arthralgia	11%	9%	5%	5%	2%	1%
Pain in extremity	5%	6%	3%	2%	1%	1%
Respiratory						
Bronchitis	11%	9%	6%	5%	0%	2%
Chronic obstructive pulmonary disease	6%	3%	1%	0%	0%	0%
Cough	9%	8%	5%	4%	2%	2%
Dyspnea	4%	3%	2%	2%	0%	0%
Nasopharyngitis	16%	13%	8%	9%	5%	4%
Sinusitis	8%	7%	5%	5%	3%	2%
Upper respiratory tract infection	9%	8%	5%	5%	2%	2%
Special senses						
Blepharitis	12%	8%	8%	5%	0%	1%
Cataract	17%	14%	11%	9%	2%	2%
Conjunctival hemorrhage	74%	60%	64%	50%	48%	37%
Conjunctival hyperemia	7%	6%	5%	4%	0%	0%
Dry eye	12%	7%	7%	7%	3%	3%
Eye irritation	15%	15%	13%	12%	7%	6%
Eye pain	35%	30%	26%	20%	17%	12%
Eye pruritus	12%	11%	9%	7%	1%	2%
Foreign body sensation in eyes	16%	14%	13%	10%	7%	5%
Injection-site hemorrhage	5%	2%	3%	1%	0%	0%
Intraocular inflammation	18%	8%	13%	7%	1%	3%
Intraocular pressure increased	24%	7%	17%	5%	7%	2%
Lacrimation increased	14%	12%	8%	8%	2%	3%
Maculopathy	9%	9%	6%	6%	11%	7%
Ocular discomfort	7%	4%	5%	2%	2%	2%
Ocular hyperemia	11%	8%	7%	4%	5%	3%
Posterior capsule opacification	7%	4%	2%	2%	0%	1%
Retinal degeneration	8%	6%	5%	3%	1%	0%
Retinal disorder	10%	7%	8%	4%	2%	1%
Visual disturbance or vision blurred	18%	15%	13%	10%	5%	3%
Vitreous detachment	21%	19%	15%	15%	4%	2%
Vitreous floaters	27%	8%	19%	5%	7%	2%
Miscellaneous						
Anemia	8%	7%	4%	3%	1%	1%
Atrial fibrillation	5%	4%	2%	2%	1%	0%
Hypercholesterolemia	5%	5%	3%	2%	1%	1%
Influenza	7%	5%	3%	2%	3%	2%
Urinary tract infection	9%	9%	5%	5%	1%	2%

Overdosage

➤*Symptoms:* Planned initial single doses of ranibizumab 1 mg injection were associated with clinically significant intraocular inflammation in 2 of 2 neovascular AMD patients injected. With an escalating regimen of doses beginning with initial doses of ranibizumab 0.3 mg injection, doses as high as 2 mg were tolerated in 15 of 20 neovascular AMD patients.

Patient Information

Advise patients that they are at risk of developing endophthalmitis in the days following ranibizumab administration. If the eye becomes red, sensitive to light, painful, or develops a change in vision, advise patients to seek immediate care from an ophthalmologist.

VERTEPORFIN

Rx	**Visudyne** (QLT PhotoTherapeutics)	**Lyophilized cake for injection:** 15 mg (reconstituted to 2 mg/mL)	Egg phosphatidylglycerol. In single-use vials.

VERTEPORFIN — INJECTION

Indications

➤*Subfoveal choroidal neovascularization:* For the treatment of patients with predominantly classic subfoveal choroidal neovascularization due to age-related macular degeneration, pathologic myopia or presumed ocular histoplasmosis.

There is insufficient evidence to indicate verteporfin for the treatment of predominately occult subfoveal choroidal neovascularization.

➤*Off-label uses:*

Plaque psoriasis – [4] = Insufficient documentation. Data from a small, noncontrolled study suggest that verteporfin may be beneficial in the treatment of plaque-stage psoriasis in patients who do not respond to topical agents. Larger, controlled trials with longer follow-up periods that assess adverse effects, including carcinogenicity, are needed.

Psoriatic arthritis – [4] = Insufficient documentation. Preliminary data from a noncontrolled, unpublished trial suggest that verteporfin may have some benefit for patients with psoriatic arthritis. (See Administration and Dosage.)

Rheumatoid arthritis – [4] = Insufficient documentation. Conclusions about the efficacy of verteporfin for the treatment of rheumatoid arthritis are not possible because the results of a phase 1 trial are not available.

Other possible off-label uses – Treatment of nonmelanoma skin cancers; circumscribed choroidal hemangioma.

Administration and Dosage

➤*General dosing considerations:* A course of verteporfin therapy is a 2-step process requiring administration of both drug and light. The first step is the intravenous (IV) infusion of verteporfin. The second step is the activation of verteporfin with light from a nonthermal diode laser.

➤*Adults:*

Classic subfoveal choroidal neovascularization –

Usual dosage:

• *IV Infusion* – 6 mg/m^2 body surface area (BSA) administered IV over 10 minutes at a rate of 3 mL/min.

• *Light* – 50 J/cm^2 of neovascular lesion administered at an intensity of 600 mW/cm^2. This dose is administered over 83 seconds.

Duration of therapy: The health care provider should re-evaluate the patient every 3 months and if choroidal neovascular leakage is detected on fluorescein angiography, therapy should be repeated.

Off-label dosing –

Plaque psoriasis: [4] = Insufficient documentation. 8 mg/m^2 of body surface injected IV with 3 hours of irradiation with 600 to 700 nm light weekly for up to 5 weeks.

Psoriatic arthritis: [4] = Insufficient documentation. 8 mg/m^2 and subsequent half- or whole-body light irradiation 3 hours later (ultraviolet A) for 4 weekly treatments.

Rheumatoid arthritis: [4] = Insufficient documentation. 8 mg/m^2 and subsequent whole-body blue light irradiation.

➤*Concurrent bilateral treatment:* The controlled trials only allowed treatment of one eye per patient. In patients who present with eligible lesions in both eyes, physicians should evaluate the potential benefits and risks of treating both eyes concurrently. If the patient has already received previous verteporfin therapy in one eye with an acceptable safety profile, both eyes can be treated concurrently after a single administration of verteporfin. The more aggressive lesion should be treated first, at 15 minutes after the start of infusion. Immediately at the end of light application to the first eye, the laser settings should be adjusted to introduce the treatment parameters for the second eye, with the same light dose and intensity as for the first eye, starting no later than 20 minutes from the start of infusion.

In patients who present for the first time with eligible lesions in both eyes without prior verteporfin therapy, it is prudent to treat only one eye (the most aggressive lesion) at the first course. One week after the first course, if no significant safety issues are identified, the second eye can be treated using the same treatment regimen after a second verteporfin infusion. Approximately 3 months later, both eyes can be evaluated and concurrent treatment following a new verteporfin infusion can be started if both lesions still show evidence of leakage.

➤*Lesion size determination:* The greatest linear dimension (GLD) of the lesion is estimated by fluorescein angiography and color fundus photography. All classic and occult choroidal neovascularization (CNV), blood and/or blocked fluorescence, and any serous detachments of the retinal pigment epithelium should be included for this measurement. Fundus cameras with magnification within the range of 2.4 to 2.6X are recommended. The GLD of the lesion on the fluorescein angiogram must be corrected for the magnification of the fundus camera to obtain the GLD of the lesion on the retina.

➤*Spot size determination:* The treatment spot size should be 1,000 microns larger than the GLD of the lesion on the retina to allow a 500 micron border, ensuring full coverage of the lesion. The maximum spot size used in the clinical trials was 6,400 microns.

The nasal edge of the treatment spot must be positioned at least 200 microns from the temporal edge of the optic disc, even if this will result in lack of photoactivation of CNV within 200 microns of the optic nerve.

➤*Preparation for administration:*

Reconstitution – Reconstitute each vial of verteporfin with 7 mL of sterile water for injection to provide 7.5 mL containing 2 mg/mL. Reconstituted verteporfin must be protected from light and used within 4 hours. It is recommended that reconstituted verteporfin be inspected visually for particulate matter and discoloration prior to administration. Reconstituted verteporfin is an opaque dark green solution.

The volume of reconstituted verteporfin required to achieve the desired dose of 6 mg/m^2 body surface area is withdrawn from the vial and diluted with 5% dextrose for injection to a total infusion volume of 30 mL.

Safe handling/disposal – Verteporfin is considered a cytotoxic agent and a photosensitizer. Follow safe handling procedures when preparing, administering, or dispensing verteporfin.

Spills of verteporfin should be wiped up with a damp cloth. Skin and eye contact should be avoided due to the potential for photosensitivity reactions upon exposure to light. Use of rubber gloves and eye protection is recommended. All materials should be disposed of properly.

Because of the potential to induce photosensitivity reactions, it is important to avoid contact with the eyes and skin during preparation and administration of verteporfin. Any exposed person must be protected from bright light.

➤*Administration:*

IV infusion – The full infusion volume is administered intravenously over 10 minutes at a rate of 3 mL/min, using an appropriate syringe pump and in-line filter. The clinical studies were conducted using a standard infusion line filter of 1.2 microns.

Following injection with verteporfin, care should be taken to avoid exposure of skin or eyes to direct sunlight or bright indoor light for 5 days.

Extravasation – Precautions should be taken to prevent extravasation at the injection site. In the event of extravasation during infusion, the extravasation area must be thoroughly protected from direct light until the swelling and discoloration have faded in order to prevent the occurrence of a local burn which could be severe. If emergency surgery is necessary within 48 hours after treatment, as much of the internal tissue as possible should be protected from intense light.

Light – Initiate 689 nm wavelength laser light delivery to the patient 15 minutes after the start of the 10-minute infusion with verteporfin.

Photoactivation of verteporfin is controlled by the total light dose delivered.

Light dose, light intensity, ophthalmic lens magnification factor and zoom lens setting are important parameters for the appropriate delivery of light to the predetermined treatment spot. Follow the laser system manuals for procedure set up and operation.

The laser system must deliver a stable power output at a wavelength of 689 ± 3 nm. Light is delivered to the retina as a single circular spot via a fiber optic and a slit lamp, using a suitable ophthalmic magnification lens.

➤*Extravasation:* Standard precautions should be taken during infusion of verteporfin to avoid extravasation. Examples of standard precautions include, but are not limited to:

- A free-flowing intravenous (IV) line should be established before starting verteporfin infusion and the line should be carefully monitored.
- Due to the possible fragility of vein walls of some elderly patients, it is strongly recommended that the largest arm vein possible, preferably antecubital, be used for injection.
- Small veins in the back of the hand should be avoided.

If signs or symptoms of extravasation occur, stop the infusion immediately. If possible, withdraw 3 to 5 mL of blood to remove some of the drug. Remove the infusion needle. Delineate the infiltrated area on the patient's skin with a felt-tip marker. To prevent severe local burns, protect the extravasation site from direct light (eg, sunlight, bright indoor light) until swelling and discoloration fade. If possible, avoid surgery within 48 hours after extravasation. If surgery is needed during this period, protect internal tissue from intense light. May apply ice compresses for 15 minutes every 6 hours for 48 hours. Elevate for 48 hours above heart level using a sling or stockinette dressing with an observation window cut in the dressing. Avoid pressure or friction. Do not rub the area. Observe for signs of increased erythema, pain, or skin necrosis. If increased symptoms occur, consult a plastic surgeon. Ensure that no medication is given distally to the extravasation site. After 48 hours, encourage the patient to use the extremity normally to promote full range of motion.

➤*Storage/Stability:* Store verteporfin between 20° and 25°C (68° to 77°F).

Actions

➤*Pharmacology:* Verteporfin therapy is a 2-stage process requiring administration of both verteporfin for injection and nonthermal red light.

Verteporfin is transported in the plasma primarily by lipoproteins. Once verteporfin is activated by light in the presence of oxygen, highly reactive, short-lived singlet oxygen and reactive oxygen radicals are generated. Light activation of verteporfin results in local damage to neovascular endothelium, resulting in vessel occlusion. Damaged endothelium is known to release procoagulant and vasoactive factors through the lipo-oxygenase (leukotriene) and cyclo-oxygenase (eicosanoids such as thromboxane) pathways, resulting in platelet aggregation, fibrin clot formation and vasoconstriction. Vertepor-

VERTEPORFIN — INJECTION

fin appears to somewhat preferentially accumulate in neovasculature, including choroidal neovasculature. However, animal models indicate that the drug is also present in the retina. Therefore, there may be collateral damage to retinal structures following photoactivation including the retinal pigmented epithelium and outer nuclear layer of the retina. The temporary occlusion of CNV following verteporfin therapy has been confirmed in humans by fluorescein angiography.

➤*Pharmacokinetics:*

Metabolism/Excretion – Following intravenous infusion, verteporfin exhibits a bi-exponential elimination with a terminal elimination half-life of approximately 5 to 6 hours. The extent of exposure and the maximal plasma concentration are proportional to the dose between 6 and 20 mg/m². At the intended dose, pharmacokinetic parameters are not significantly affected by gender.

Verteporfin is metabolized to a small extent to its diacid metabolite by liver and plasma esterases. NADPH-dependent liver enzyme systems (including the cytochrome P450 isozymes) do not appear to play a role in the metabolism of verteporfin. Elimination is by the fecal route, with less than 0.01% of the dose recovered in urine.

Special populations –

Hepatic function impairment: In a study of patients with mild hepatic insufficiency (defined as having two abnormal hepatic function tests at enrollment), AUC and C_{max} were not significantly different from the control group, half-life however was significantly increased by approximately 20%.

Contraindications

Porphyria or a known hypersensitivity to any component of this preparation.

Warnings/Precautions

➤*Light exposure:* Following injection with verteporfin, care should be taken to avoid exposure of skin or eyes to direct sunlight or bright indoor light for 5 days. In the event of extravasation during infusion, the extravasation area must be thoroughly protected from direct light until the swelling and discoloration have faded in order to prevent the occurrence of a local burn which could be severe. If emergency surgery is necessary within 48 hours after treatment, as much of the internal tissue as possible should be protected from intense light.

➤*Decrease in vision:* Patients who experience severe decrease of vision of 4 lines or more within 1 week after treatment should not be retreated, at least until their vision completely recovers to pretreatment levels and the potential benefits and risks of subsequent treatment are carefully considered by the treating physician.

➤*Lasers:* Use of incompatible lasers that do not provide the required characteristics of light for the photoactivation of verteporfin could result in incomplete treatment due to partial photoactivation of verteporfin, overtreatment due to overactivation of verteporfin, or damage to surrounding normal tissue.

➤*Anesthesia:* There is no clinical data related to the use of verteporfin in anesthetized patients. At a greater than 10-fold higher dose given by bolus injection to anesthetized pigs, verteporfin caused severe hemodynamic effects, including death, probably as a result of complement activation. These effects were diminished or abolished by pretreatment with antihistamine, and they were not seen in conscious nonsedated pigs. Verteporfin resulted in a concentration-dependent increase in complement activation in human blood in vitro. At 10 mcg/mL (approximately 5 times the expected plasma concentration in human patients), there was mild to moderate complement activation. At greater than or equal to 100 mcg/mL, there was significant complement activation. Signs (chest pain, syncope, dyspnea, and flushing) consistent with complement activation have been observed in less than 1% of patients administered verteporfin. Patients should be supervised during verteporfin infusion.

➤*Extravasation:* See Administration and Dosage for more information.

➤*Hepatic function impairment:* Verteporfin therapy should be considered carefully in patients with moderate to severe hepatic impairment or biliary obstruction since there is no clinical experience with verteporfin in such patients.

➤*Pregnancy: Category C.* There are no adequate and well-controlled studies in pregnant women. Only use verteporfin during pregnancy if the benefit justifies the potential risk to the fetus.

Teratogenic – Rat fetuses of dams administered verteporfin for injection intravenously at greater than or equal to 10 mg/kg/day during organogenesis (approximately 40-fold human exposure at 6 mg/m² based on AUC_{inf} in female rats) exhibited an increase in the incidence of anophthalmia/microphthalmia. Rat fetuses of dams administered 25 mg/kg/day (approximately 125-fold the human exposure at 6 mg/m² based on AUC_{inf} in female rats) had an increased incidence of wavy ribs and anophthalmia/microphthalmia.

In pregnant rabbits, a decrease in body weight gain and food consumption was observed in animals that received verteporfin for injection intravenously at greater than or equal to 10 mg/kg/day during organogenesis. The no observed adverse effect level (NOAEL) for maternal toxicity was 3 mg/kg/day (approximately 7-fold human exposure at 6 mg/m² based on body surface area). There were no teratogenic effects observed in rabbits at doses up to 10 mg/kg/day.

➤*Lactation:* It is not known whether verteporfin for injection is excreted in human milk. Because many drugs are excreted in human milk, caution should be exercised when verteporfin is administered to a woman who is nursing.

➤*Children:* Safety and effectiveness in pediatric patients have not been established.

➤*Elderly:* Approximately 90% of the patients treated with verteporfin in the clinical efficacy trials were greater than 65 years of age. A reduced treatment effect was seen with increasing age.

Drug Interactions

Based on the mechanism of action of verteporfin, many drugs used concomitantly could influence the effect of verteporfin therapy. Possible examples include the following:

Calcium channel blockers, polymyxin B or radiation therapy could enhance the rate of verteporfin uptake by the vascular endothelium. Other photosensitizing agents (eg, tetracyclines, sulfonamides, phenothiazines, sulfonylurea hypoglycemic agents, thiazide diuretics and griseofulvin) could increase the potential for skin photosensitivity reactions. Compounds that quench active oxygen species or scavenge radicals, such as dimethyl sulfoxide, β-carotene, ethanol, formate and mannitol, would be expected to decrease verteporfin activity. Drugs that decrease clotting, vasoconstriction or platelet aggregation (eg, thromboxane A_2 inhibitors) could also decrease the efficacy of verteporfin therapy.

Adverse Reactions

The most frequently reported adverse events to verteporfin are injection site reactions (including extravasation and rashes) and visual disturbances (including blurred vision, decreased visual acuity and visual field defects). These events occurred in approximately 10% to 30% of patients. The following events, listed by body system, were reported more frequently with verteporfin therapy than with placebo therapy and occurred in 1% to 10% of patients.

➤*Cardiovascular:* Atrial fibrillation, hypertension, peripheral vascular disorder, varicose veins.

➤*CNS:* Hypesthesia, sleep disorder, vertigo.

➤*Dermatologic:* Eczema.

➤*GI:* Constipation, gastrointestinal cancers, nausea.

➤*GU:* Prostatic disorder.

➤*Hematologic/Lymphatic:* Anemia, white blood cell count decreased, white blood cell count increased.

➤*Hepatic:* Elevated liver function tests.

➤*Metabolic/Nutritional:* Albuminuria, creatinine increased.

➤*Musculoskeletal:* Arthralgia, arthrosis, myasthenia.

➤*Ophthalmic:* Blepharitis, cataracts, conjunctivitis/conjunctival injection, dry eyes, ocular itching, severe vision loss with or without subretinal or vitreous hemorrhage.

Severe vision decrease, equivalent of 4 lines or more, within 7 days after treatment has been reported in 1% to 5% of patients. Partial recovery of vision was observed in some patients.

➤*Respiratory:* Cough, pharyngitis, pneumonia.

➤*Special senses:* Decreased hearing, diplopia, lacrimation disorder.

➤*Miscellaneous:* Asthenia, back pain, fever, flu syndrome, photosensitivity reactions.

Photosensitivity reactions usually occurred in the form of skin sunburn following exposure to sunlight.

The higher incidence of back pain in the verteporfin group occurred primarily during infusion.

➤*Other adverse events:* The following adverse events have occurred either at low incidence (less than 1%) during clinical trials or have been reported during the use of verteporfin in clinical practice where these events were reported voluntarily from a population of unknown size and frequency of occurrence cannot be determined precisely. They have been chosen for inclusion based on factors such as seriousness, frequency of reporting, possible causal connection to verteporfin, or a combination of these factors:

Ophthalmic – Retinal detachment (nonrhegmatogenous), retinal or choroidal vessel nonperfusion.

Miscellaneous – Chest pain and other musculoskeletal pain during infusion, hypersensitivity reactions (which can be severe), syncope, severe allergic reactions with dyspnea and flushing, and vaso-vagal reactions.

Overdosage

Overdose of drug and/or light in the treated eye may result in nonperfusion of normal retinal vessels with the possibility of severe decrease in vision that could be permanent. An overdose of drug will also result in the prolongation of the period during which the patient remains photosensitive to bright light. In such cases, it is recommended to extend the photosensitivity precautions for a time proportional to the overdose.

Patient Information

Patients who receive verteporfin will become temporarily photosensitive after the infusion. Patients should wear a wrist band to remind them to avoid direct sunlight for 5 days. During that period, patients should avoid exposure of unprotected skin, eyes or other body organs to direct sunlight or bright indoor light. Sources of bright light include, but are not limited to, tanning salons, bright halogen lighting and high power lighting used in surgical operating rooms or dental offices. Prolonged exposure to light from light-emitting medical devices such as pulse oximeters should also be avoided for 5 days following verteporfin administration.

VERTEPORFIN — INJECTION

If treated patients must go outdoors in daylight during the first 5 days after treatment, they should protect all parts of their skin and their eyes by wearing protective clothing and dark sunglasses. UV sunscreens are not effective in protecting against photosensitivity reactions because photoactivation of the residual drug in the skin can be caused by visible light.

Patients should not stay in the dark and should be encouraged to expose their skin to ambient indoor light, as it will help inactivate the drug in the skin through a process called photobleaching.

OCULAR LUBRICANTS

OCULAR LUBRICANTS

otc	**Dry Eyes** (Bausch & Lomb)	**Ointment; ophthalmic:** 94% white petrolatum, 3% mineral oil, lanolin	Preservative free. In 3.5 g.
otc	**Systane Nighttime** (Alcon)		Preservative free. In 3.5 g.
otc	**Tears Naturale P.M.** (Alcon)		Preservative free. In 3.5 g.
otc	**Puralube** (Fera Pharmaceuticals)	**Ointment; ophthalmic:** 85% white petrolatum, 15% mineral oil	In 3.5 g and UD 1 g (20s).
otc	**Artificial Tears** (Rugby)	**Ointment; ophthalmic:** White petrolatum, anhydrous liquid lanolin, mineral oil	In 3.5 g.
otc	**Duratears Naturale** (Alcon)		Preservative free. In 3.5 g.
otc	**Tears Again** (Altaire)	**Ointment; ophthalmic:** White petrolatum, mineral oil	In 3.5 g.
otc	**HypoTears** (Novartis Ophthalmics)	**Ointment; ophthalmic:** White petrolatum, light mineral oil	Preservative and lanolin free. In 3.5 g.
otc	**Tears Renewed** (Akorn)		Preservative and lanolin free. In 3.5 g.
otc	**Stye** (Del Pharm)	**Ointment; ophthalmic:** 57.7% white petrolatum, 31.9% mineral oil	In 3.5 g.
otc	**Lacri-Lube NP** (Allergan)	**Ointment; ophthalmic:** 55.5% white petrolatum, 42.5% mineral oil, 2% petrolatum/lanolin alcohol	Preservative free. In 0.7 g (UD 24s).
otc	**Refresh PM** (Allergan)	**Ointment; ophthalmic:** 56.8% white petrolatum, 41.5% mineral oil, lanolin alcohols, sodium chloride	Preservative free. In 3.5 g.
otc	**Lacri-Lube S.O.P.** (Allergan)	**Ointment; ophthalmic:** 56.8% white petrolatum, 42.5% mineral oil, chlorobutanol, lanolin alcohols	In 3.5 and 7 g.
otc	**Advanced Eye Relief Night Time** (Bausch & Lomb Personal Products)	**Ointment; ophthalmic:** 80% white petrolatum, 20% mineral oil	Preservative free. In 3.5 g.
otc	**LubriFresh P.M.** (Major)	**Ointment; ophthalmic:** 83% white petrolatum, 15% mineral oil	Preservative free. Lanolin oil. In 3.5 g.
otc	**GenTeal PM** (Novartis)	**Ointment; ophthalmic:** 15% mineral oil, 85% white petrolatum	In 3.5 mL.
otc	**GenTeal Severe Eye Relief** (Novartis)	**Gel; ophthalmic:** 0.3% hypromellose, phosphonic acid, sodium hydroxide, sodium perborate	Preservative free. In 10 g.
otc	**Tears Again Night & Day** (OcuSoft)	**Gel; ophthalmic:** 1.5% carboxymethylcellulose sodium, 0.1% polyvinylpyrrolidone	In 3.5 g.
otc	**Tears Again Advanced** (OcuSoft)	**Spray, solution; ophthalmic:** retinyl palmitate, tocopheryl acetate, magnesium ascorbyl phosphate, polysorbate 80, sodium chloride, sodium hydroxide, phenoxyethanol, alcohol, disodium EDTA, PEG-12, glyceryl	In 15 mL.

OCULAR LUBRICANTS — OPHTHALMIC

Refer to the Topical Ophthalmics introduction for more complete and comparative information.

Indications

➤*Ophthalmic lubrication:* Protection and lubrication of the eye.

Administration and Dosage

➤*Adults:*

Ointment – Pull down the lower lid of affected eye(s) and apply a small amount (0.25 inch) of ointment to the inside of the eyelid.

Spray – Use 3 to 4 times daily as needed.

➤*Administration:* Do not touch tube tip to any surface because this may contaminate the product.

Do not use with contact lenses.

Spray – Holding the spray tip approximately 4 to 6 inches away and with the eye closed, spray directly onto the surface of the eyelid. Gently massage into the eyelid, extending to the lashes. Repeat procedure with the other eye. If you prefer, you may spray onto the inner side of the finger and then gently massage onto the eyelids and lashes.

➤*Storage/Stability:* Store at room temperature, between 15° to 30°C (59° to 8°F). Store away from heat.

Actions

➤*Pharmacology:* These products serve as lubricants and emollients.

Contraindications

Hypersensitivity to any component of the products.

Warnings/Precautions

➤*Pregnancy:* Category: *Undetermined.* Consult a health care provider before using in pregnant women.

➤*Lactation:* Consult a health care provider before using in breast-feeding women.

Patient Information

Do not touch tube tip to any surface since this may contaminate the product.

Do not use with contact lenses.

If eye pain, vision changes or continued redness or irritation occurs, or if the condition worsens or persists for greater than 72 hours, discontinue use and contact a physician.

TYLOXAPOL

otc	**Enuclene** (Alcon)	**Solution:** 0.25%	0.02% benzalkonium Cl. In 15 mL *Drop-Tainers.*

TYLOXAPOL — OPHTHALMIC

Indications

➤*Ocular lubrication:* Tyloxapol solution is recommended for wearers of artificial eyes. Tyloxapol solution lubricates, cleans, and wets the artificial eye, thereby increasing the wearing comfort to the patient.

Administration and Dosage

➤*Adults:*

Artificial eye wearers – The drops should be used just as ordinary eye drops are used. With the artificial eye in place, drop 1 or 2 drops onto it, 3 or 4 times daily. The artificial eye may be removed periodically if advised by the physician and 2 or 3 drops applied to remove oily or mucous materials.

TYLOXAPOL — OPHTHALMIC

The artificial eye is then rubbed between the fingers and rinsed with tap water. Then 1 or 2 drops may be applied to the artificial eye, either prior to or after reinsertion.

➤*Storage / Stability:* Store at 8° to 27°C (46° to 80°F).

Contraindications

Contraindicated in those persons who have shown hypersensitivity to any component of this preparation.

Warnings/Precautions

➤*Pregnancy: Category: Undetermined.* Consult a health care provider before administering to a pregnant woman.

➤*Lactation:* Consult a health care provider before administering to a breast-feeding woman.

Patient Information

Do not touch dropper tip to any surface as this may contaminate the solution.

If irritation persists or increases, discontinue use and consult physician.

Keep container tightly closed.

Keep out of reach of children.

ARTIFICIAL TEARS

ARTIFICIAL TEAR SOLUTIONS

otc	**20/20 Tears** (S.S.S. Co.)	**Solution; ophthalmic:** 1.4% PVA, NaCl, KCl, 0.05% EDTA, 0.01% benzalkonium Cl	In 0.5 fl oz.
otc	**Advanced Eye Relief** (Bausch & Lomb)	**Solution; ophthalmic:** 0.3% glycerin, 1% propylene glycol, 0.01% benzalkonium chloride, boric acid, edetate disodium, potassium chloride, sodium borate, sodium chloride	In 30 mL.
otc	**Advanced Eye Relief Preservative Free** (Bausch & Lomb)	**Solution; ophthalmic:** 0.95% propylene glycol, boric acid, edetate disodium, sodium borate, sodium chloride	Preservative free. In single-use containers.
otc	**AquaSite** (Novartis Ophthalmics)	**Solution; ophthalmic:** 0.2% PEG-400, 0.1% dextran 70, polycarbophil, NaCl, EDTA, sodium hydroxide	Preservative free. In 24 × 1 single dose and 15 mL multidose.
otc	**Artificial Tears** (Various, eg, URL)	**Solution; ophthalmic:** 0.01% benzalkonium chloride. May also contain EDTA, NaCl, polyvinyl alcohol, hydroxypropyl methylcellulose	In 15 and 30 mL.
otc	**Artificial Tears Plus** (Various)	**Solution; ophthalmic:** 1.4% polyvinyl alcohol, 0.6% povidone, 0.5% chlorobutanol, NaCl	In 15 mL.
otc	**Bion Tears** (Alcon)	**Solution; ophthalmic:** 0.1% dextran 70, 0.3% hydroxypropyl methylcellulose 2910, NaCl, KCl, sodium bicarbonate	Preservative free. In single-use 0.45 mL containers (28s).
otc	**Blink Tears** (Abbott Medical Optics)	**Solution; ophthalmic:** 0.25% polyethylene glycol 400	In 15 mL.
otc	**Blink Tears Preservative Free** (Abbott Medical Optics)	**Solution; ophthalmic:** 0.25% polyethylene glycol 400	Preservative free. In single-use 0.4 mL containers (25s).
otc	**Celluvisc** (Allergan)	**Solution; ophthalmic:** 1% carboxymethylcellulose, NaCl, KCl, sodium lactate	Preservative free. In 0.3 mL (UD 30s).
otc	**Clear Eyes Contact Lens Relief** (Medtech)	**Solution; ophthalmic:** 0.25% sorbic acid, 0.1% EDTA, sodium chloride, hypromellose, glycerin	In 15 mL.
otc	**Clear Eyes for Dry Eyes** (Medtech)	**Solution; ophthalmic:** 1% carboxymethylcellulose sodium, 0.25% glycerin	Boric acid, EDTA. In 15 mL.
otc	**Comfort Tears** (Allergan)	**Solution; ophthalmic:** Hydroxyethylcellulose, 0.005% benzalkonium chloride, 0.02% EDTA	In 15 mL.
Rx	**FreshKote** (Focus Labs)	**Solution; ophthalmic:** 2.7% polyvinyl alcohol, 2% polyvinyl pyrrolidone, boric acid, disodium EDTA, polixetonium, potassium chloride, sodium chloride	In 15 mL.
otc	**GenTeal** (Novartis Ophthalmics)	**Solution; ophthalmic:** 0.3% hydroxypropyl methylcellulose, boric acid, phosphone acid, sodium chloride, sodium perborate	In 15 and 25 mL.
otc	**GenTeal Mild** (Novartis)	**Solution; ophthalmic:** 0.2% hypromellose, boric acid, phosphonic acid, potassium chloride, sodium chloride, sodium perborate	Preservative free. In 25 mL.
otc	**GenTeal Mild to Moderate** (Novartis)	**Solution; ophthalmic:** 0.3% hypromellose, boric acid, phosphonic acid, potassium chloride, sodium chloride, sodium perborate	Preservative free. In 25 mL.
otc	**HypoTears** (Novartis Ophthalmics)	**Solution; ophthalmic:** 1% polyvinyl alcohol, PEG-400, 1% dextrose, 0.01% benzalkonium Cl, EDTA	In 15 and 30 mL.
otc	**Isopto Plain** (Alcon)	**Solution; ophthalmic:** 0.5% hydroxypropyl methylcellulose 2910, 0.01% benzalkonium chloride, NaCl, sodium phosphate, sodium citrate	In 15 mL *Drop-Tainers.*
otc	**Isopto Tears** (Alcon)		In 15 and 30 mL.
otc	**Moisture Eyes Preservative Free** (Bausch & Lomb)	**Solution; ophthalmic:** 0.95% propylene glycol, boric acid, NaCl, KCl, sodium borate, edetate disodium	Preservative free. In 0.6 mL (UD 32s).
otc	**Murine Tears for Dry Eyes** (Prestige/Medtech)	**Solution; ophthalmic:** 0.6% PVP, 0.5% PVA, benzalkonium chloride, dextrose, EDTA, KCl, NaCl, sodium bicarbonate, sodium citrate, sodium phosphate	In 15 and 30 mL.
otc	**Murocel** (Bausch & Lomb)	**Solution; ophthalmic:** 1% methylcellulose, propylene glycol, NaCl, 0.046% methylparaben, 0.02% propylparaben, boric acid, sodium borate	In 15 mL.
otc	**Nu-Tears** (Optopics)	**Solution; ophthalmic:** 1.4% polyvinyl alcohol, EDTA, sodium chloride, benzalkonium chloride, KCl	In 15 mL.
otc	**Nu-Tears II** (Optopics)	**Solution; ophthalmic:** 1% polyvinyl alcohol, 1% PEG-400, EDTA, benzalkonium chloride	In 15 mL.
otc	**Optive** (Allergan)	**Solution; ophthalmic:** 0.5% carboxymethylcellulose, 0.9% glycerin	In 15 mL.
otc	**OptiZen** (InnoZen)	**Solution; ophthalmic:** 0.5% polysorbate 80	EDTA, NaCl, sodium phosphate, sorbic acid. In 10 mL.
otc	**Puralube Tears** (Fougera)	**Solution; ophthalmic:** 1% polyvinyl alcohol, 1% PEG 400, EDTA, benzalkonium Cl	In 15 mL.
otc	**Refresh Classic** (Allergan)	**Solution; ophthalmic:** 1.4% polyvinyl alcohol, 0.6% povidone, sodium chloride	Preservative free. In 0.4 mL single-use containers.
otc	**Refresh Dry Eye Therapy** (Allergan Optical)	**Solution; ophthalmic:** 1% glycerin, 1% polysorbate 80, castor oil	Preservative free. In 0.4 mL single-use containers.

ARTIFICIAL TEAR SOLUTIONS

otc	**Refresh Liquigel** (Allergan)	**Solution; ophthalmic:** 1% carboxymethylcellulose sodium, boric acid, calcium chloride, magnesium chloride, potassium chloride, sodium borate, sodium chloride	In 15 and 30 mL.
otc	**Refresh Plus** (Allergan)	**Solution; ophthalmic:** 0.5% carboxymethylcellulose sodium, KCl, NaCl	Preservative free. In 0.3 mL single-use containers (30s and 50s).
otc	**Refresh Tears** (Allergan)	**Solution; ophthalmic:** 0.5% carboxymethylcellulose sodium	In 15 mL dropper bottles.
otc	**Soothe XP** (Bausch & Lomb)	**Solution; ophthalmic:** 1% light mineral oil, 4.5% mineral oil, edetate disodium, octoxynol-40, polyhexamethylene biguanide, polysorbate-80, NaCl, sodium phosphate dibasic, sodium phosphate monobasic	In 15 mL.
otc	**Systane** (Alcon)	**Solution; ophthalmic:** 0.3% propylene glycol, 0.4% PEG-400	In 20 mL.
otc	**Tearisol** (Novartis Ophthalmics)	**Solution; ophthalmic:** 0.5% hydroxypropyl methylcellulose, 0.01% benzalkonium chloride, EDTA, boric acid, KCl	In 15 mL.
otc	**Tears Again** (OcuSOFT Inc.)[a]	**Solution; ophthalmic:** 0.3% hydroxypropyl methylcellulose, boric acid, phosphoric acid, potassium chloride, sodium chloride *Dissipate* as a preservative	In 15 mL.
otc	**Tears Naturale** (Alcon)	**Solution; ophthalmic:** 0.1% dextran 70, 0.01% benzalkonium chloride, 0.3% hydroxypropyl methylcellulose, NaCl, EDTA, hydrochloric acid, sodium hydroxide, KCl	In 15 and 30 mL.
otc	**Tears Naturale II** (Alcon)	**Solution; ophthalmic:** 0.1% dextran 70, 0.3% hydroxypropyl methylcellulose 2910, 0.001% polyquaternium-1, NaCl, KCl, sodium borate	In 15 and 30 mL *Drop-Tainers.*
otc	**Tears Naturale Free** (Alcon)	**Solution; ophthalmic:** 0.3% hydroxypropyl methylcellulose 2910, 0.1% dextran 70, NaCl, KCl, sodium borate	Preservative free. In 0.6 mL single-use containers.
otc	**Tears Naturale Forte** (Alcon)	**Solution; ophthalmic:** 0.1% dextran 70, 0.3% hydroxypropyl methylcellulose, 0.2% glycerin, 0.001% polyquaternium-1, NaCl, KCl, sodium borate	In 15 and 30 mL.
otc	**Tears Plus** (Allergan)	**Solution; ophthalmic:** 1.4% polyvinyl alcohol, NaCl, 0.6% povidone, 0.5% chlorobutanol	In 15 and 30 mL.
otc	**TheraTears** (Advanced Vision)	**Solution; ophthalmic:** 0.25% sodium carboxymethylcellulose, borate buffers, calcium chloride, KCl, magnesium chloride, NaCl, sodium bicarbonate, sodium phosphate	Preservative free. In 15 and 30 mL.
otc	**Visine for Contacts** (J & J Healthcare)	**Solution; ophthalmic:** sterile isotonic solution with borate buffer system, hypromellose, glycerin	EDTA. In 15 and 30 mL.
otc	**Visine Tears** (J & J Healthcare)	**Solution; ophthalmic:** 0.2% glycerin, 0.2% hypromellose, 1% polyethylene glycol 400	In 15 and 30 mL.
otc	**Visine Tears Preservative Free** (J & J Healthcare)		Preservative-free. In 0.4 mL single-use containers.
otc	**Visine Pure Tears** (J & J Healthcare)		In 9.5 mL single-drop dispenser.
otc	**Viva-Drops** (Vision Pharm)	**Solution; ophthalmic:** Polysorbate 80, sodium chloride, EDTA, retinyl palmitate, mannitol, sodium citrate, pyruvate	Preservative free. In 10 and 15 mL.
otc	**GenTeal Moderate to Severe** (Novartis)	**Solution, gel forming; ophthalmic:** 0.25% carboxymethylcellulose sodium, 0.3% hypromellose, boric acid, sodium perborate, magnesium chloride, phosphonic acid, potassium chloride, sodium chloride	Preservative free. In 25 mL.
otc	**Tears Again** (OcuSoft)	**Solution, gel forming; ophthalmic:** 0.7% carboxymethyl cellulose sodium, boric acid, phosphoric acid, potassium chloride, sodium chloride	In 15 mL.
otc	**TheraTears** (Advanced Vision Research)	**Gel; ophthalmic:** 1% carboxymethylcellulose sodium, KCl, sodium bicarbonate, NaCl, sodium phosphate	In UD 28s.

[a] OcuSOFT Inc., P.O. Box 429, Richmond, TX 77406; (281) 342-3350.

[b] Alimera Sciences, 6120 Windward Parkway, Alpharetta, GA 30005; (678) 990-5740.

ARTIFICIAL TEAR SOLUTIONS

Indications

➤*Ophthalmic lubricants:* These products offer tear-like lubrication for the relief of dry eyes and eye irritation associated with deficient tear production. Also used as ocular lubricants for artificial eyes.

Administration and Dosage

➤*Adults:*

Ophthalmic lubricants – Instill 1 to 2 drops into eye(s) 3 or 4 times daily, as needed.

Actions

➤*Pharmacology:* These products contain balanced amounts of salts to maintain ocular tonicity (0.9% NaCl equivalent), buffers to adjust pH, viscosity agents to prolong eye contact time, and preservatives for sterility. See the Topical Ophthalmics introduction for a description and listing of these ingredients.

Warnings/Precautions

➤*Pregnancy: Category: Undetermined.* Consult a health care provider before administering to a pregnant woman.

➤*Lactation:* Consult a health care provider before administering to a breast-feeding woman.

Patient Information

Do not touch the tip of the container or dropper to any surface. Close container immediately after use.

If headache, eye pain, vision changes, continued redness or irritation occurs, or if condition worsens or persists for longer than 3 days, discontinue use and consult a physician.

May cause mild stinging or temporary blurred vision.

Some of these products should not be used with soft contact lenses.

HYDROXYPROPYL CELLULOSE

Rx	**Lacrisert** (Aton Pharma)	**Insert; ophthalmic:** 5 mg hydroxypropyl cellulose	Preservative free. In 60s with applicator.

HYDROXYPROPYL CELLULOSE — INSERT

Indications

➤*Dry eye syndromes, moderate to severe:* Keratoconjunctivitis sicca (especially in patients who remain symptomatic after an adequate trial of artificial tear solutions); exposure keratitis; decreased corneal sensitivity; recurrent corneal erosions.

Administration and Dosage

➤*General dosing considerations:* Occasionally, the insert is inadvertently expelled from the eye, especially in patients with shallow conjunctival fornices.

Caution the patient against rubbing the eyelid(s), especially upon awakening, so as not to dislodge or expel the insert. If required, another insert may be used.

HYDROXYPROPYL CELLULOSE — INSERT

If transient blurred vision develops, the patient may want to remove the insert a few hours after insertion to avoid this.

➤*Adults:*

Dry eye syndromes, moderate to severe – One insert in each eye once daily. Individual patients may require twice-daily use for optimal results.

➤*Administration:* Once daily, inserted into inferior cul-de-sac beneath the base of the tarsus, not in apposition to the cornea nor beneath the eyelid at the level of the tarsal plate.

If not properly positioned, the insert will be expelled into the interpalpebral fissure, and may cause symptoms of a foreign body.

➤*Storage/Stability:* Store below 30°C (86°F).

Actions

➤*Pharmacology:* The hydroxypropyl cellulose insert acts to stabilize and thicken the precorneal tear film and prolong tear film breakup time, which is usually accelerated in patients with dry eye states. The insert also acts to lubricate and protect the eye.

Signs and symptoms resulting from moderate to severe dry eye syndromes, such as conjunctival hyperemia, corneal and conjunctival staining with rose bengal, exudation, itching, burning, foreign body sensation, smarting, photophobia, dryness and blurred or cloudy vision are reduced. Progressive visual deterioration may be retarded, halted or sometimes reversed.

➤*Pharmacokinetics:* Hydroxypropyl cellulose is a physiologically inert substance. Dissolution studies in rabbits showed that the inserts became softer within 1 hour after they were placed in the conjunctival sac. Most dissolved completely in 14 to 18 hours; with a single exception, all had disappeared by 24 hours after insertion. Similar dissolution of inserts was observed during prolonged use (up to 54 weeks).

Contraindications

Hypersensitivity to hydroxypropyl cellulose.

Warnings/Precautions

➤*Corneal abrasion:* Corneal abrasion may result if insert is improperly placed.

➤*Pregnancy: Category: Undetermined.* There are no information regarding hydroxypropyl cellulose in pregnant patients.

➤*Lactation:* There are no information regarding hydroxypropyl cellulose in breast-feeding patients.

➤*Children:* Safety and effectiveness are not established in children.

Adverse Reactions

The following have occurred, but in most instances were mild and transient: Transient blurring of vision; ocular discomfort or irritation; matting or stickiness of eyelashes; photophobia; hypersensitivity; edema of the eyelids; hyperemia.

Patient Information

May produce transient blurring of vision; exercise caution while operating hazardous machinery or driving a motor vehicle.

If improperly placed in the inferior cul-de-sac, corneal abrasion may result. Patient should practice insertion and removal in physician's office until proficiency is achieved.

Illustrated instructions are included in each package.

If symptoms worsen, remove insert and notify physician.

OPHTHALMIC PUNCTAL PLUGS

PUNCTAL PLUGS

Rx	**Herrick Lacrimal Plug** (Lacrimedics)	**Plug**: Silicone plug	In 0.3 and 0.5 mm sizes (packs of 2 plugs).
Rx	**Punctum Plug** (Eagle Vision)		In 0.5, 0.6, 0.7 and 0.8 mm sizes (packs of 2 plugs). Contains one inserter tool.

PUNCTAL PLUGS — OPHTHALMIC

Indications

➤*Keratitis sicca (dry eye):* Treatment of symptoms of dry eye (eg, redness, burning, reflex tearing, itching, foreign body sensation); after eye surgery to prevent complications due to dry eye; to enhance the efficacy of ocular medications; for patients experiencing dry eye-related contact lens problems.

Administration and Dosage

➤*General dosing considerations:* Do not dilate punctal opening greater than 1.2 mm.

If irritation caused by plug insertion persists longer than several days, re-examine the patient and consider plug removal.

➤*Adults:*

Keratitis sicca (dry eye) – Plugs must be inserted by a physician or doctor of optometry.

Actions

➤*Pharmacology:* These flexible silicone plugs partially block the puncta and horizontal canaliculus and eliminate tear loss by this route.

Contraindications

Hypersensitivity to silicone; eye infection.

Warnings/Precautions

➤*Injection path:* If injecting an anesthetic agent in the region of the canaliculus, maintain approximately a 5 mm distance between the injection path and the angular vessels.

➤*Dilation:* Do not dilate punctal opening greater than 1.2 mm.

➤*Irritation:* If irritation caused by plug insertion persists longer than several days, reexamine the patient and consider plug removal.

➤*Pregnancy: Category: Undetermined.* There is no information regarding punctal plugs in pregnant women.

➤*Lactation:* There is no information regarding punctal plugs in breast-feeding women.

Patient Information

Do not press fingers on or near the eyelid. Use a cotton-tipped swab to remove "sleep" from the corner of eyes.

Do not attempt to replace a plug that has fallen out.

Relief may not occur immediately after insertion; some discomfort and tearing may occur for a few days.

OPHTHALMIC COLLAGEN IMPLANTS

COLLAGEN IMPLANTS

Rx	**Collagen Implant** (Lacrimedics)	**Implant**: Collagen implant	In 0.2, 0.3, 0.4, 0.5 and 0.6 mm sizes (72s).
Rx	**TearSaver** (FCI)		In 0.2, 0.3, and 0.4 mm sizes.
Rx	**Temporary Punctal/Canalicular Collagen Implant** (Eagle Vision)		In 0.2, 0.3, 0.4, 0.5 and 0.6 mm sizes (72s).

COLLAGEN — IMPLANTS

Indications

➤*Dry eyes:* For the relief of dry eyes and secondary abnormalities such as conjunctivitis, corneal ulcer, pterygium, blepharitis, keratitis, red lid margins, recurrent chalazion, recurrent corneal erosion, filamentary keratitis and other noninfectious external eye diseases; to enhance the effect of ocular medications; treatment of symptoms of dry eye (eg, redness, burning, reflex tearing, itching, foreign body sensation); after eye surgery to prevent complications; for patients experiencing dry eye-related contact lens problems.

Administration and Dosage

➤*Adults:*

Dry eyes – Implants must be inserted by a physician or doctor of optometry. Placement of implants in all 4 canaliculi is recommended to prevent a false-negative response.

Actions

➤*Pharmacology:* These absorbable implants partially block the puncta and horizontal canaliculus, eliminating tear loss by this route.

Contraindications

Tearing secondary to chronic dacryocystitis with mucopurulent discharge; allergy to bovine collagen; inflammation of eyelid; epiphora.

Warnings/Precautions

➤*Pregnancy: Category: Undetermined.* There is no information regarding collagen implants in pregnant women.

➤*Lactation:* There is no information regarding collagen implants in breast-feeding women.

COLLAGEN — IMPLANTS

Patient Information

Relief may not occur immediately after insertion.

No removal is necessary; implants dissolve within 7 to 10 days.

Reexamination is usually required within 14 days.

Successful treatment may indicate a need for permanent treatment (eg, nondissolvable silicone plugs).

HYPEROSMOTIC AGENTS

SODIUM CHLORIDE, HYPERTONIC

otc	**Muro 128** (Bausch & L omb)	**Solution:** 2%	In 15 mL.[a]
otc	**AK-NaCl** (Akorn)	**Solution:** 5%	In 15 mL.[b]
otc	**Muro 128** (Bausch & Lomb)		In 15 and 30 mL.[c]
otc	**Sochlor** (OcuSoft)		In 15 mL.[d]
otc	**AK-NaCl** (Akorn)	**Ointment:** 5%	Preservative free. In 3.5 g.[e]
otc	**Muro 128** (Bausch & Lomb)		In 3.5 g single and twin packs.[f]
otc	**Sochlor** (OcuSoft)		In 3.5 g.[e]

[a] With hydroxypropyl methylcellulose 2906, 0.046% methylparaben, 0.02% propylparaben, propylene glycol, boric acid.
[b] With hydroxypropyl methylcellulose, propylene glycol, 0.023% methylparaben, 0.01% propylparaben, boric acid.
[c] Boric acid, hydroxypropyl methylcellulose 2910, propylene glycol, 0.023% methylparaben, 0.01% propylparaben.
[d] With hydroxypropyl methylcellulose 2906, propylene glycol, 0.023% methylparaben, 0.01% propylparaben, boric acid.
[e] With mineral oil, white petrolatum, lanolin oil.
[f] With mineral oil, white petrolatum, lanolin.

SODIUM CHLORIDE, HYPERTONIC — OPHTHALMIC

Indications

For ophthalmic use only.

➤*Corneal edema:* For the temporary relief of corneal edema.

Administration and Dosage

➤*Adults:*

Corneal edema relief –

Ointment: Pull down lower lid of the affected eye(s) and apply a small amount (approximately ¼ inch) of the ointment to the inside of the eyelid every 3 or 4 hours, or as directed by a health care provider.

Solution: Instill 1 or 2 drops in the affected eye(s) every 3 or 4 hours, or as directed by a health care provider.

➤*Administration:* For ophthalmic use only.

➤*Storage/Stability:* Store between 15° and 30°C (59° and 86°F). Do not freeze. Keep tightly closed and protect from light.

Ointment – Do not use if bottom ridge of tube cap is exposed and imprinted seal on box is broken or missing. Note: Tubes are filled by weight (⅛ oz/3.5 g), not volume.

Sodium chloride ophthalmic solution – Store upright and immediately replace cap after use. Do not use if imprinted neckband is not intact.

Actions

➤*Pharmacology:* A hypertonic (hyperosmolar) solution exerts an osmotic gradient greater than that present in the body tissues and fluids, so that water is drawn from the body tissues and fluids across semipermeable membranes. Applied topically to the eye, a hypertonicity agent creates an osmotic gradient which draws water out of the cornea.

Contraindications

Hypersensitivity to any component of the product.

Warnings/Precautions

➤*Usage:* Do not use this product except under the advice and supervision of a doctor.

If you experience eye pain, changes in vision, continued redness or irritation of the eye, or if the condition worsens or persists, consult a doctor.

➤*Sodium chloride ophthalmic solution:* If the solution changes color or becomes cloudy, do not use.

➤*Pregnancy:* Category: *Undetermined*. Consult a health care provider before using in pregnant women.

➤*Lactation:* Consult a health care provider before using in breast-feeding women.

Adverse Reactions

May cause temporary burning and irritation upon instillation.

Patient Information

To avoid contamination, do not touch tip of container to any surface. Replace cap after using.

Do not use this product except under the advice and supervision of a physician. If you experience eye pain, changes in vision, continued redness or irritation of the eye or if the condition worsens or persists, discontinue use and consult a physician.

Product may cause temporary burning and irritation when instilled into the eye.

CONTACT LENS CARE

➤*Contact lens guidelines:* Inadequate cleaning can lead to lens discoloration and lens surface buildup of protein, lipids, minerals and other environmental contaminants, which can contribute to giant papillary conjunctivitis (GPC), superficial punctate keratitis (SPK) and corneal abrasion. Irregular contact lens disinfection can cause severe ocular infection.

Contact Lens Guidelines

- Proper contact lens care will increase success and decrease complications.
- Cleaning does not disinfect lenses.
- Disinfecting does not clean lenses.
- Enzyme solutions are not a substitute for disinfection.
- Wash and rinse hands thoroughly before handling contact lenses.
- Do not insert contact lenses if eyes are red or irritated. If eyes become painful or vision worsens while wearing lenses, remove lenses and consult an eye-care practitioner immediately.
- Do not wear contact lenses while sleeping unless they have been prescribed for extended wear.
- For soft lens care, use only products designed for soft lenses.
- For rigid lens care, use only products designed for rigid lenses.
- Do not change or substitute products from a different manufacturer without consulting a doctor.
- Do not use non-sterile, home-prepared saline solutions unless recommended by your eye-care practitioner.
- Always follow label directions or doctor's recommendations.
- Do not store lenses in tap water.
- After removal, lenses must be cleaned, rinsed and disinfected before wearing again.
- Lenses that are stored greather than 12 hours may again require cleaning, rinsing and disinfection; consult package insert or eye care practitioner.

Contact Lens Guidelines

- Never use saliva to wet contact lenses.
- Keep lens care products out of the reach of children.
- Do not instill topical medications while contact lenses are being worn unless directed by a doctor.
- Do not get cosmetic lotions, creams or sprays in your eyes or on lenses. It is best to put on lenses before putting on makeup and remove them before removing makeup. Water-based cosmetics are less likely to damage lenses than oil-based products.
- Schedule and keep follow-up appointments with your eye-care practitioner (approximately every 6 to 12 months or as recommended).
- Contact lenses wear out with time and should be replaced regularly. Throw away disposable lenses after the recommended wearing period.
- Check with your eye-care practitioner regarding wearing lenses during sports activities.

➤*Contact lens materials:* Three types of contact lenses are manufactured: Hard, rigid gas permeable and soft.

➤*Hard contact lenses:* Hard contact lenses are made from polymethylmethacrylate (PMMA). PMMA does not transmit the oxygen needed for normal corneal integrity. Hard contact lenses have caused chronic corneal edema, corneal distortion, edematous corneal formations, spectacle blur, polymegathism and corneal abrasions. Because of these ocular complications, hard lenses are seldom the lens of choice for a new contact lens patient. Less than 1% of the contact lens population wear hard contact lenses.

➤*Rigid gas permeable lenses:* Approximately 20% of contact lens patients wear rigid gas permeable (RGP) lenses. These lenses are oxygen permeable; therefore, the RGP patient does not have the severe physiological complications of the hard lens patient. Several lens polymers with a high degree of oxygen permeability have been approved by the FDA for extended wear. RGP lenses provide the patient with good vision, durability and easy care.

➤*Soft contact lenses:* Soft contact lenses are made of hydroxyethylmethacrylate (HEMA), a plastic compound. The first soft lens was marketed in the US in 1971. Today, most soft lenses manufactured from HEMA contain 30% to 50% water.

Daily wear soft contact lenses are designed to be worn all day (12 to 14 hours), but must be removed nightly to be cleaned and disinfected. Extended wear soft lenses can be worn for greather than or equal to 24 hours. The FDA and most eye care practitioners recommend a maximum wearing period of 7 days. The lenses must then be removed overnight for cleaning and disinfection. The major advantage of extended wear lenses is convenience. Daily wear soft lenses provide the same level of comfort and vision as extended wear soft lenses. The popularity of extended wear soft lenses has decreased due to the increased risk of infection.

➤*Disposable soft lenses:* Disposable soft lenses are designed to eliminate the complications of lens deposits by planned lens replacement. Lens deposits can interfere with vision, cause corneal irritation and contribute to ocular infection. In addition, disposable lenses offer the patient the convenience of reduced lens care.

Disposable lenses are approved for daily wear and extended wear. It is recommended that the lenses be discarded after a specified length of time; the physician will prescribe the replacement schedule for each patient. If a disposable lens is not discarded immediately after lens removal, it should be cleaned with a surfactant cleaner and stored in a disinfection solution.

➤*Contact Lens Care Products:* Products for use with contact lenses possess the same general characteristics of all ophthalmic products (eg, sterile, isotonic, free of particulate matter). Additionally, product formulations contain various components to achieve specific goals of contact lens care.

Although all contact lenses serve similar functions in correcting visual defects, each distinct type of lens material requires a unique lens care program. In selecting appropriate lens care solutions, it is essential to correctly identify the type of lens the patient is using.

➤*Hard and rigid gas permeable lenses:* Similar lens care is used for the hard and RGP lenses. Products include *wetting/soaking/disinfecting solutions,* cleaning agents and rewetting solutions.

When a rigid contact lens is removed from the eye, it may be covered with lipids, proteins, eye makeup and other debris. After removal, immediately clean the lens with a *surfactant cleaner*. Improper cleaning can contribute to a lens surface buildup that can interfere with vision and potentially cause corneal irritation.

Soak rigid lenses overnight in a *wetting/soaking/disinfecting solution*. This solution has four major functions:

1.) To enhance the lens surface wettability
2.) To maintain the lens hydration similar to that achieved during daily contact lens wear
3.) To disinfect the lens
4.) To act as a mechanical buffer between the lens and the cornea

It is not uncommon for a rigid lens patient to experience dryness after several hours of wear. This is especially true with RGP lens patients because of the hydrophobic nature of the lens material. *Rewetting drops* can provide temporary relief by rinsing some debris off the lens surface and rewetting the eye and the lens.

Many clinicians recommend the weekly use of an enzyme (papain) cleaner with RGP lenses. This weekly cleaning process is very effective in removing protein deposits from the lens surface. A protein film on an RGP lens can decrease vision and cause giant papillary conjunctivitis.

➤*Soft contact lenses:* Soft contact lens care systems are designed to clean, disinfect and rewet the lenses. The first step is cleaning. Cleaning the lens gently in the palm of the hand with a *daily surfactant cleaner* will remove fresh lipids, oils and other debris. Clean soft lenses thoroughly with a surfactant cleaner each time a lens is removed. After cleaning the lens, thoroughly rinse with a soft lens *rinsing/storage solution*. All *rinsing/storage solutions* contain 0.9% saline. Some are available with no preservatives in unit-dose vials or aerosol containers. Other saline solutions contain preservatives to decrease microorganism growth. Discourage use of saline made with salt tablets because of risk of contamination and infection (see Precautions).

Enzymatic cleaners – Enzymatic cleaners are generally used on a weekly basis. They more effectively remove protein deposits than surfactant cleaners because they contain proteolytic enzymes (papain, pancreatin or subtilisin). Most enzymes are dissolved directly in saline, but the subtilisin enzyme tablet can be dissolved in a hydrogen peroxide disinfection solution.

Disinfection – Disinfection is the most important step in soft lens care. Disinfection is achieved by using a thermal (heat) or chemical (cold) system.

Thermal disinfection: Thermal disinfection was the first system approved for soft contact lenses. A heat unit designed for soft lenses is used for 10 min at 80°C (176°F). This procedure will kill most microorganisms that are dangerous to the eye. Recently, Acanthamoeba keratitis has become a concern to many clinicians. Heat disinfection is the most effective procedure to successfully kill Acanthamoeba; however, heat disinfection cannot be used with all soft lens material. Also, continued use of heat can shorten soft lens life.

Chemical disinfection: The original chemical soft lens disinfection systems used thimerosal with either chlorhexidine or a quaternary ammonium compound. These systems had a high incidence of sensitivity reactions. Various hydrogen peroxide care systems are currently available in the US. Most systems require two steps to achieve disinfection and hydrogen peroxide neutralization; one other system combines disinfection and neutralization in a single step. Hydrogen peroxide (3%) is very effective and can be used with all soft lens polymers. However, hydrogen peroxide care systems can be complex and expensive. Do not substitute generic peroxide solutions for solutions formulated for contact lenses. They may be contaminated with heavy metals, have different concentrations of hydrogen peroxide or use stabilizers that may discolor soft lenses.

The two newest chemical soft lens care systems introduced into the US marketplace include *Opti-Free* by Alcon and *ReNu* by Bausch & Lomb. Polyquad (polyquaternium-1) and Dymed (polyammopropylbiguamide) are the disinfection agents utilized in these care systems. Both are simple to use and may therefore increase patient compliance. These two chemical systems have become the care system of choice for the majority of soft lens patients.

Recommended Disinfection Times For Soft Lenses by Product

System	Manufacturer	Disinfection time (minimum)	Neutralization time (minimum)
AOSEPT	Novartis Ophthalmics	6 hrs[a]	6 hrs[a]
Disinfecting Solution	Bausch & Lomb	4 hrs	none
Flex-Care	Alcon	4 hrs	none
MiraSept System	Alcon	10 min	10 min
Opti-Free	Alcon	4 hrs	none
Opti-Soft	Alcon	4 hrs	none
ReNu Multi-Purpose	Bausch & Lomb	4 hrs	none
Soft Mate Consept	Pilkington Barnes Hind	10 min	10 min

[a] One-step method: Disinfection and neutralization occur together for a total of 6 hours.

Soft lens rewetting solutions – Soft lens rewetting solutions permit the lubrication of the soft lens while it is on the eye. Most patients find these rewetting drops minimally effective in reducing the symptoms of dryness. Maximum relief can be achieved by removing the lens, cleaning it with a daily surfactant cleaner and thoroughly rinsing it with a rinsing/storage saline solution.

➤*Precautions:*

Acanthamoeba keratitis – Soft contact lens wearers who use homemade saline solution are at risk of developing Acanthamoebakeratitis, a serious and painful corneal infection that may cause blindness or impaired vision. Homemade saline solutions (nonsterile) may be used during thermal disinfection but NOT after.

Drug interference with contact lens use – Systemic medications may affect the physiology of the cornea, lids and tear system. In addition, many drugs may discolor soft contact lenses. Pharmacists and eye-care practitioners should be aware of the interaction of systemic medications and contact lenses.

Drug Interference With Contact Lens Use

Drug	RGP/Hard/Soft Lens	Action
Anticholinergics	RGP, hard, soft	Tear volume decreased
Antihistamines, sympathomimetics	RGP, hard, soft	Tear volume decreased, blink rate decreased
Chlorthalidone	RGP, hard, soft	Causes lid or corneal edema
Clomiphene	RGP, hard, soft	Causes lid or corneal edema
Diuretics, thiazide	RGP, hard, soft	Tear volume decreased
Dopamine	soft	Discoloration of contact lenses
Epinephrine, topical	soft	Discoloration of contact lenses
Fluorescein, topical	soft	Lens absorbs the yellow dye
Hypnotics, sedatives, muscle relaxants	RGP, hard, soft	Blink rate decreased
Iodine groups	soft	Discoloration of contact lenses
Nitrofurantoin	soft	Discoloration of contact lenses
Oral contraceptives	RGP, hard, soft	Increased stickiness of mucus; corneal lid edema due to fluid retention properties of estrogens
Phenazopyridine	soft	Discoloration of contact lenses
Phenolphthalein	soft	Discoloration of contact lenses
Phenylephrine	soft	Discoloration of contact lenses
Primidone	RGP, hard, soft	Causes lid or corneal edema
Rifampin	soft	Lens absorbs drug, causing orange discoloration
Sulfasalazine	soft	Yellow staining
Tetracycline	soft	Discoloration of contact lenses
Tricyclic antidepressants	RGP, hard, soft	Tear volume decreased

Products are listed on the following pages and are grouped as follows:

Contact Lens Solutions

Type of lens	Type of solution
Hard	Wetting Cleaning Cleaning/Soaking Wetting/Soaking Cleaning/Soaking/Wetting Rewetting
RGP	Disinfecting/Wetting/Soaking Cleaning Enzymatic Cleaners Cleaning/Disinfecting/Soaking Rewetting

Contact Lens Solutions

Type of lens	Type of solution
Soft	Rinsing/Storage Chemical Disinfection Surfactant Cleaning Enzymatic Cleaners Rewetting

Rigid Gas Permeable Contact Lens Products

Refer to the general discussion of these products in Contact Lens Products monograph.

Actions

➤*Pharmacology:*

Gas permeable hard lenses – Silicone/acrylate and fluoropolymers are used in rigid gas permeable (RGP) contact lenses. Lens care regimens include the use of a surfactant cleaner, enzyme cleaner and storage in a chemical disinfecting solution. Advise patients to follow the lens care protocol provided by the lens manufacturer or the instructions of their doctor.

DISINFECTING/WETTING/SOAKING/CLEANING SOLUTIONS, RGP LENSES

otc	**Bausch & Lomb Wetting and Soaking for RGP & Hard Lenses** (Bausch & Lomb)	**Solution**: Buffered, slightly hypertonic, low viscosity. 0.05% EDTA, 0.006% chlorhexidine gluconate. Cationic cellulose derivative polymer.	In 120 mL.
otc	**Boston Conditioning Solution** (Bausch & Lomb/ Boston)	**Solution**: Buffered, slightly hypertonic. 0.05% EDTA, 0.006% chlorhexidine gluconate. Cationic cellulose derivative polymer, polyvinyl alcohol, PEG, cellulosic viscosifier.	In 120 mL.
otc	**Boston Simplus** (Bausch & Lomb/Boston)	**Solution**: Buffered. Chlorhexidine gluconate, polyaminopropyl biguanide. Poloxamine, hydroxyalkylphosphonate, Glucam-20.	In 105 mL.
otc	**Improved Formula Boston Conditioning Solution** (Bausch & Lomb)	**Solution**: Buffered. Chlorhexidine gluconate .006%, disodium edetate .05%. Poloxamer 407, hydroxyethylcellulose, polyquaternium 10, polyvinylalcohol.	In 105 mL.
otc	**Opti-Free GP Multi-Purpose Solution** (Alcon)	**Solution**: Buffered, 0.0011% polyquad and 0.01% EDTA. Hydroxypropyl guar, polyethylene glycol, Tetronic, boric acid, propylene glycol.	In 90 mL.
otc	**Optimum by Lobob Cleaning, Disinfecting and Storage Solution** (Lobob)	**Solution**: Lauryl salt of imidazoline, octylphenoxypolyethoxyethanol, and preserved with benzyl alcohol 0.3% and disodium edetate 0.5%.	In 118 mL.
otc	**Sereine Wetting & Soaking Solution** (Optikem)	**Solution**: Buffered, isotonic, 0.1% EDTA, 0.01% benzalkonium chloride, sodium chloride, polyoxypropylene polyoxyethylene copolymer.	In 120 mL.

DISINFECTING/WETTING/SOAKING/CLEANING SOLUTIONS, RGP LENSES — OPHTHALMIC

Indications

These solutions are used for both insertion and soaking/disinfection of GP lenses. They enhance lens surface wettability, maintain lens hydration similar to that achieved during contact lens wear, disinfect the lens, and act as a mechanical buffer between the lens and the cornea.

Actions

➤*Pharmacology:* These solutions are formulated for comfort and compatibility with ocular tissues. Therefore, the pH of the solution should be near physiologic pH, or only slightly buffered to allow the pH to rapidly adjust to that of tear film. A wetting agent such as PVA and possibly a viscosity-building agent such as methylcellulose will be used to enhance the tear spreading properties over the surface of the lens. Preservative use is such to disinfect the lens while not being toxic to the eye.

Warnings/Precautions

These solutions are not compatible with soft lens material.

CLEANING SOLUTIONS, RGP LENSES

otc	**AOSept Clear Care** (Ciba Vision)	**Solution**: Buffered. 3% hydrogen peroxide, 0.79% sodium chloride, phosphonic acid, pluronic 17R4.	In 120, 237, and 355 mL.
otc	**Bausch & Lomb Concentrated Cleaner for RGP & Hard Lenses** (Bausch & Lomb)	**Solution**: Concentrated homogenous surfactant. Alkyl ether sulfate, ethoxylated alkyl phenol, triquaternary cocoa-based phospholipid, silica gel	In 30 mL.
otc	**Bausch & Lomb Boston Advance Cleaner** (Bausch & Lomb)	**Solution**: Concentrated homogenous surfactant. Alkyl ether sulfate, ethoxylated alkyl phenol, triquaternary cocoa-based phospholipid, titanium dioxide, silica gel	In 30 mL.
otc	**Boston Original Formula Cleaner** (Bausch & Lomb)	**Solution**: Concentrated homogenous surfactant. Alkyl ether sulfate, titanium dioxide, silica gel	In 30 mL.
otc	**Clear Clean** (Contex)	**Solution**: Preservative-free. Distilled water, euphrasi	In 120 mL.
otc	**MeniCare GP CDS Cleaning, Disinfecting and Storage Solution** (Menicon)	**Solution**: Lauryl salt of imidazoline, octylphenoxypolyethoxyethanol, and preserved with benzyl alcohol 0.3% and disodium edetate 0.5%	In 118 mL.
otc	**Opti-Free Daily Cleaner** (Alcon)	**Solution**: Buffered, isotonic. 0.1% EDTA, 0.001% polyquad. Polysorbate 21, polymeric cleaning agents	In 12 and 20 mL.
otc	**Optimum by Lobob Extra Strength Cleaner** (Lobob)	**Solution**: Slightly alkaline, aqueous with cocoamphodiacetate and glycols	Preservative-free. In 60 mL.

Rigid Gas Permeable Contact Lens Products

CLEANING SOLUTIONS, RGP LENSES

otc	**Sereine Cleaner** (Optikem)	**Solution:** Amphoteric surfactants, edetate disodium 0.1%, 0.01% benzalkonium chloride	In 120 mL

CLEANING SOLUTIONS, RGP LENSES — OPHTHALMIC

Indications

All GP wearing patients should use some type of cleaning solution upon lens removal because lipids, mucus, proteins, and other substances such as cosmetics and hand creams can adhere to the lens surface resulting in blurred vision and possibly reduced wearing time. These solutions help maintain a clean, wettable surface and good optics. If an abrasive cleaner is used, do not clean the lens forcefully between the fingers, because increases in minus power and warpage have been reported over time.

Actions

➤*Pharmacology:* These solutions use cleaners that typically consist of nonionic surfactant (detergents). Mild abrasive particles are added in some formulations for greater effect against bound muco-protein deposit complexes.

Warnings/Precautions

Solutions used strictly for cleaning should never be used for wetting/rewetting GP lenses or chemical keratitis may result.

SURFACTANT CLEANERS, RGP LENSES

otc	**Bausch & Lomb Concentrated Cleaner for RGP & Hard Lenses** (Bausch & Lomb)	**Solution:** Concentrated homogenous surfactant. Alkyl ether sulfate, ethoxylated alkyl phenol, triquaternary cocoa-based phospholipid, silica gel.	In 30 mL.
otc	**Bausch & Lomb Boston Advance Cleaner Solution** (Bausch & Lomb)	**Solution:** Concentrated homogenous surfactant. Alkyl ether sulfate, ethoxylated alkyl phenol, triquaternary cocoa-based phospholipid, titanium dioxide, silica gel.	In 30 mL.
otc	**Boston Cleaner Solution** (Bausch & Lomb)	**Solution:** Concentrated homogenous surfactant. Alkyl ether sulfate, silica gel, titanium dioxide.	In 30 mL.
otc	**Opti-Clean II Daily Cleaner Especially for Sensitive Eyes Solution** (Alcon)	**Solution:** Buffered, isotonic. 0.1% EDTA, 0.001% polyquad. Polysorbate 21, polymeric cleaning agents.	Thimerosal free. In 15 and 30 mL.
otc	**Opti-Free Daily Cleaner** (Alcon)	**Solution:** Buffered, isotonic with polymeric beads (25 mg) with polyquaternium-1 (0.001% and edetate disodium 0.1%.	In 15 and 30mL.
otc	**Optimum by Lobob Extra Strength Cleaner** (Lobob)	**Solution:** Slightly alkaline, aqueous solution with cocoamphodiacetate and glycols.	Preservative free. In 60 mL.
otc	**Resolve/GP Daily Cleaner Solution** (Advanced Medical Optics)	**Solution:** Buffered. Cocoamphocarboxyglycinate, sodium lauryl sulfate, hexylene glycol, alkyl ether sulfate, fatty acid amide surfactants.	Preservative free. In 30 mL.
otc	**Sereine Cleaner** (Optikem)	**Solution:** Amphoteric surfactants, edetate disodium 0.1%, benzalkonium chloride 0.01%.	In 60 mL.
otc	**Sereine Soaking & Cleaning Solution** (Optikem)	**Solution:** 0.25% EDTA, 0.01% benzalkonium chloride.	In 120 mL.

SURFACTANT CLEANERS, RGP LENSES — OPHTHALMIC

Indications

All GP wearing patients should use some type of cleaning solution upon lens removal because lipids, mucus, proteins, and other substances such as cosmetics and hand creams can adhere to the lens surface resulting in blurred vision and possibly reduced wearing time. These solutions help maintain a clean, wettable surface and good optics. If an abrasive cleaner is used, do not clean the lens forcefully between the fingers, because increases in minus power and warpage have been reported over time.

Actions

➤*Pharmacology:* These solutions use cleaners that typically consist of nonionic surfactant (detergents). Mild abrasive particles are added in some formulations for greater effect against bound muco-protein deposit complexes.

Warnings/Precautions

Solutions used strictly for cleaning should never be used for wetting/rewetting GP lenses or chemical keratitis may result.

ENZYMATIC CLEANERS, RGP LENSES

otc	**Boston One-Step Liquid Enzymatic Cleaner** (Bausch & Lomb/Boston)	**Solution:** Subtilisin. Glycerol.	Preservative free. In 1 and 2.4 mL.
otc	**Opti-Free Supra Clens Daily Protein Remover** (Alcon)	**Solution:** Propylene glycol, sodium borate, highly purified porcine pancreatin enzymes.	Preservative free. In 3 mL.

ENZYMATIC CLEANERS, RGP LENSES — OPHTHALMIC

Indications

Enzyme cleaners are used as an adjunct to surfactant cleaning for the removal of adherent deposits. They are especially beneficial in dry eye patients who are more prone to deposit formation and for individuals who are not compliant with regular surfactant cleaning. Commonly available in tablet form, which dissolves in saline, they are currently available in a liquid form as marketed by 2 companies (*Boston One-Step Liquid Enzyme Cleaner* for weekly use from Bausch & Lomb/Boston ; *Opti-Free Supra-Clens Daily Protein Removal* for daily use from Alcon). The liquid enzyme has the benefit of promoting patient compliance via the simplicity of adding a drop of the enzyme solution to the disinfecting solution in each case well for overnight use.

Actions

➤*Pharmacology:* An enzymatic cleaner acts chemically to dissolve adherent muco-protein complexes on the surface of the lens. Specific enzymes currently in use include papain (from papaya fruit), pancreatin (from hog pancreas), and Subtilisin A and B (produced by microorganisms).

Warnings/Precautions

Enzyme solutions are not to be used for wetting or rewetting of GP lenses or chemical keratitis may result.

REWETTING SOLUTIONS, RGP LENSES

otc	**Aquify Long Lasting Comfort Drops** (Ciba Vision)	Sodium perborate stabilized with perborate acid.	In 10 mL.
otc	**blink Contacts Lubricant Eye Drops** (Advanced Medical Optics)	**Solution:** Buffered, isotonic with sodium hyaluronate, sodium chloride, potassium chloride, calcium chloride, magnesium chloride, boric acid, and *OcuPure* (stabilized oxychloro complex) 0.005% as the preservative.	In 10 mL.
otc	**Boston Rewetting Drops** (Bausch & Lomb /Boston)	**Solution:** Buffered, slightly hypertonic. 0.05% EDTA, 0.006% chlorhexidine gluconate. Cationic cellulose derivative polymer, polyvinyl alcohol, hydroxyethyl cellulose.	In 10 mL.

Rigid Gas Permeable Contact Lens Products

REWETTING SOLUTIONS, RGP LENSES

otc	**Complete Blink-N-Clean Lens Drops** (Advanced Medical Optics)	**Solution**: Buffered, isotonic. 0.0001% polyhexamethylene biguanide, tromethamine, hydroxypropyl methylcellulose, tyloxapol, EDTA, sodium chloride.	Thimerosal free. In 20 mL.
otc	**Menicare GP WRW** (Menicon)	**Solution**: Sodium and potassium salts, polyvinylpyrrolidone, polyvinyl alcohol, hydroxyethyl cellulose, sodium bisulfite 0.02% with benzyl alcohol 0.1%, sorbic acid 0.05% and disodium edetate 0.1%.	In 118 mL
otc	**Opti-Free RepleniSH Rewetting Drops** (Alcon)	**Solution**: Buffered, Isotonic, aqueous solution with a citrate/borate buffer and sodium chloride, with edetate disodium 0.05% and *Polyquad* (polyquaternium-1) 0.001% as preservatives and RLM-100 (PEG-11 lauryl ether carboxylic acid) and *Tetronic* 1304.	In 10 mL.
otc	**Optimum Wetting and Rewetting Drops** (Lobob)	**Solution**: Sodium and potassium chloride salts, polyvinylpyrrolidone, polyvinyl alcohol, hydroxyethyl cellulose, 0.02% sodium bisulfite. 0.1% benzyl alcohol, 0.5% sorbic acid, 0.1% EDTA.	In 30 mL.
otc	**Sereine Wetting Solution** (Optikem)	**Solution**: Buffered. 0.1% EDTA, 0.01% benzalkonium chloride.	In 60 mL.
otc	**TheraTears Contact Lens Comfort Drops** (Advanced Vision Research)	**Solution**: Sodium carbo methyl cellulose (0.25%), sodium perborate as preservative.	In 15 mL.

REWETTING SOLUTIONS, RGP LENSES — OPHTHALMIC

Indications

Rewetting solutions are needed when an GP wearing patient experiences dryness or redness. These solutions rewet the lens surface, rinse away trapped debris, and break up loosely-adherent deposits.

Actions

➤*Pharmacology:* Rewetting drops are usually isotonic or slightly hypertonic. They typically contain a viscosity agent or wetting agent to enhance surface wettability.

Warnings/Precautions

Several formulations are not compatible for use with soft lenses.

Soft (Hydrogel) Contact Lens Products

Refer to the general discussion of these products in the Contact Lens Products monograph.

> **WARNING**
>
> Do NOT use conventional (hard) lens solutions on soft contact lenses. Use caution in product selection. Not all products are intended for use on all types of soft lenses.

Indications

Soft contact lens care systems are designed to clean, disinfect, and rewet the lenses. Lenses are cleaned gently in the palm of the hand prior to disinfection. Disinfection of hydrogel lenses is the most important step in the care process. Disinfection is achieved by using a thermal (heat), chemical (non-hydrogen peroxide), or hydrogen peroxide (oxidative) system. Heat is rarely used today and, in fact, in the United States today approximately 80% of disinfection is performed via chemical disinfection and 20% via hydrogen peroxide systems.

Actions

➤*Pharmacology:* Soft (hydrogel) contact lenses are made of hydrophilic polymers. Hydrogel lenses must be maintained in a hydrated state in physiological saline to prevent them from becoming brittle. Hydrogel lenses will absorb many substances; therefore, use only solutions specifically formulated for hydrogel lenses. In addition, these lenses must be disinfected either by heating in saline solution or by soaking in a chemical solution. Heating a lens in solutions used for chemical disinfection only may cause the lens to become opaque.

Soft lens solutions are especially formulated to be compatible with, and to meet the particular needs of, soft contact lenses. Of particular importance to soft lens care is the need for thorough cleaning to remove deposits which coat and may discolor the lens, especially when subjected to asepticizing by heating.

CHEMICAL DISINFECTION SYSTEMS

Actions

➤*Pharmacology:* Chemical disinfection is an alternative to heat. Two-solution systems use separate disinfecting and rinsing solutions. One-solution systems use the same solution for rinsing and storage.

Warnings/Precautions

➤*Heat disinfection:* Lenses must NOT be disinfected by heating when using these solutions.

HYDROGEN PEROXIDE-CONTAINING SYSTEMS, SOFT LENSES

otc	**AOSept** (Ciba Vision)	**Disinfecting solution**: Buffered. 3% hydrogen peroxide, 0.85% NaCl, phosphoric acid, phosphates.	Thimerosal free. In 118, 237, 355, and 473 mL.
		AODISC neutralizer: Platinum-coated disc.	Disc good for 100 uses or 3 months of daily use.[a]
otc	**AOSept Clear Care** (Ciba Vision)	**Solution**: Buffered. 3% hydrogen peroxide, 0.79% sodium chloride, phosphonic acid, pluronic 17R4.	In 120, 237, and 355 mL.
otc	**Oxysept UltraCare** (Abbott Medical Optics)	**Disinfecting solution**: Buffered. 3% hydrogen peroxide, sodium stannate, sodium nitrate, phosphates.	In 360 mL.
		Neutralizing tablets: Catalase, hydroxypropyl methylcellulose, cyanocobalamin, buffering and tableting agents.	Beige/pink. In 36s with cup.
otc	**Sauflon One Step Hydrogen Peroxide Cleaning and Disinfecting System** (Sauflon Pharmaceuticals)	**Solution**: Hydrogen peroxide 3% buffered (with phosphates), stabilized (with phosphonic acid), poloxamer.	In 360 mL.

[a] For use only with the AOSEPT system.

HYDROGEN PEROXIDE-CONTAINING SYSTEMS, SOFT LENSES — OPHTHALMIC

Indications

For the disinfection of hydrogel lenses. It offers many advantages over other chemical systems. It is safe, very effective, and does not contain sensitizing ingredients. Hydrogen peroxide penetrates into hydrogel lenses and is reported to provide deep-cleaning action by expanding the lens matrix and oxidizing foreign matter.

Actions

➤*Pharmacology:* Oxidative disinfection consists of a 3% hydrogen peroxide solution; neutralizing solution, tablet, or disc; saline; and cleaner. Hydrogen peroxide does not result in clinically significant sensitivity problems when used properly because it breaks down into water and oxygen. Hydrogen peroxide usually is hypotonic and has an approximate pH of 4. It is important that some method of neutralization is present to prevent this acidic solution from direct contact with the eye. Present formulations are stable and newer systems appear to be less complex and more patient-friendly. These chemical properties result in lens expansion and contraction, which is believed to break protein and lipid bonds.

Warnings/Precautions

➤*Punctate keratitis:* Hydrogen peroxide will produce a mild to moderate punctate keratitis if not neutralized prior to instillation into the eye. To minimize this problem, many of the hydrogen peroxide solutions are currently packaged in bottles with red tips and warning labels on the bottles that direct the patient not to use the solution directly on the eye.

Soft (Hydrogel) Contact Lens Products

HYDROGEN PEROXIDE-CONTAINING SYSTEMS, SOFT LENSES — OPHTHALMIC

➤*Discoloration:* Use of an *OTC* hydrogen peroxide not formulated for contact lens use may result in discoloration and patient sensitivity because of colorants, incompatible stabilizers, and lack of salts necessary to provide satisfactory saline following neutralization.

NON-HYDROGEN PEROXIDE-CONTAINING SYSTEMS, SOFT LENSES

otc	**All in One Lite No Rub Multipurpose Solution** (Sauflon Pharmaceuticals)	**Solution**: Buffered, isotonic, poloxamer, sodium chloride buffer, sodium chloride with polyhexanide .0001%, and disodium edetate.	In 270 mL.
otc	**Aquify MPS** (Ciba Vision)	**Solution**: Sterile aqueous solution with sorbitol, tromethamine, pluronic F127, sodium phosphate dihydrogen, Dexpant-5, edetate disodium dehydrate with polyhexanide 0.0001%.	In 118 and 355 mL.
otc	**Biotrue Multi-Purpose Solution** (Bausch & Lomb)	**Solution**: Sterile, isotonic. Hyaluronan, sulfobetaine, poloxamine, boric acid, sodium borate, edetate disodium, sodium chloride, polyaminopropyl biguanide 0.00013%, polyquaternium 0.0001%	In 60, 118, 296, and 473 mL.
otc	**Complete Multi-Purpose Solution — No Rub** (Advanced Medical Optics)	**Solution**: Buffered, isotonic. Polyhexamethylene biguanide 0.0001%, edetate disodium, hydroxypropyl methylcellulose, propylene glycol, taurine, phosphate buffers, poloxamer 237, NaCl.	In 118, 355, and 473 mL.
otc	**Naturalens RDS Contact Lens Solution** (Advanced Vision Technologies)	**Solution**: Buffered. Polyhexanide 0.0001%, edetate disodium dehydrate 0.025%. Bis-tris propane, pluronic F127, cremophor RH40	In 360 mL
otc	**Opti-Free Express Multi-Purpose Disinfecting No Rub Formula** (Alcon)	**Solution**: Buffered, isotonic. EDTA, 0.001% polyquad, 0.0005% myristamidopropyl dimethylamine. Citrate, NaCl, boric acid, sorbitol, AMP-95, *Tetronic* 1304.	In 118, 355, and 473 mL.
otc	**Opti-Free RepleniSH** (Alcon)	**Solution**: Buffered, isotonic, aqueous solution with sodium citrates, sodium chloride. Sodium borate, propylene glycol, *Tearglyde* (*Tetronic* 1304, nonanoyl ethylenediametriacetic acid) with *Polyquad* (polyquaternium) 0.001% and *Aldox* (myristamidopropyl dimethylamine) 0.0005% as preservatives.	In 118 and 300 mL.
otc	**Purilens UV Disinfection System** (Purilens)	**Solution**: Uses cleaning unit with UV-C radiation to disinfect lenses.	
otc	**ReNu MultiPlus Multi-Purpose Solution** (Bausch & Lomb)	**Solution**: Isotonic. 0.0001% polyaminopropyl biguanide (DYMED). Hydroxyalkylphosphonate, boric acid, EDTA, poloxamine, sodium borate, NaCl.	Thimerosal free. In 60, 118, 237, and 355 mL.
otc	**ReNu Multi-Purpose Solution** (Bausch & Lomb)	**Solution**: Isotonic, 0.00005% polyaminopropyl biguanide (DYMED). Boric acid, EDTA, sodium borate, NaCl.	In 118, 237, and 355 mL.

NON-HYDROGEN PEROXIDE-CONTAINING SYSTEMS, SOFT LENSES — OPHTHALMIC

Indications

For disinfection of hydrogel lenses. Other functions—including wetting, rinsing, and cleaning—may be present as well.

Actions

➤*Pharmacology:* Disinfection is defined as the process whereby vegetative or living microorganisms are completely killed or inactivated. This involves the destruction of microorganisms by attacking the cell wall or membrane, the inhibition of protein synthesis, or both. Current disinfecting products must pass specific FDA and International Organization for Standardization (ISO) microbiological and cleaning efficacy tests in order to gain approval to use particular labeling. Upon passing the appropriate test, a solution may be designated a "multipurpose" solution (MPS), a "multipurpose disinfecting"solution (MPDS), or a "no-rub required" disinfecting solution.

These solutions disinfect via the use of preservatives compatible with hydrogel lens materials. Because many of these solutions combine wetting and, in a few cases, cleaning, they incorporate buffers and a mild surfactant. Typically, a minimum of 4 hours is recommended for disinfection. One faster system, *Quick Care* (Ciba Vision), allows for disinfection and cleaning in a 5-minute period. The starting solution is hypertonic with a surfactant and isopropyl alcohol. Then it is stored for 1 minute in a saline solution with a trace amount of hydrogen peroxide.

Warnings/Precautions

Some patients may exhibit a sensitivity to the preservatives in a given system.

THERMAL DISINFECTION, SOFT CONTACT LENSES

Indications

Heat disinfection is recommended when the other systems are not effective. Lens life is reduced because it heats deposits directly on the lens surface, resulting in discoloration. It is limited to lower water content lens materials.

Actions

➤*Pharmacology:* Heat disinfection avoids the use of preservatives and their corresponding potential for sensitivity. Heat is the most effective disinfection method, often killing organisms within 15 to 20 minutes compared with several hours with many chemical systems. Most of the units have temperatures reaching a maximum of 80° to 90°C.

Warnings/Precautions

Heat disinfection should not be used with Group 2 or Group 4 lenses.

PRESERVED SALINE SOLUTIONS, SOFT CONTACT LENSES

otc	**Sensitive Eyes Plus Saline Solution** (Bausch & Lomb)	**Solution**: Buffered, isotonic. 0.025% EDTA, 0.00003% polyaminopropyl biguanide. Boric acid, sodium borate, potassium chloride, NaCl.	In 118 and 355 mL.
otc	**Sensitive Eyes Saline Solution** (Bausch & Lomb)	**Solution**: Buffered, isotonic. 0.1% sorbic acid, 0.025% EDTA. Boric acid, sodium borate, NaCl.	Thimerosal free. In 118, 237, and 355 mL.

PRESERVATIVE FREE SALINE SOLUTIONS, SOFT CONTACT LENSES

otc	**Blairex Sterile Saline Solution** (Blairex)	**Solution**: Buffered, isotonic. NaCl, boric acid, sodium borate.	Preservative free. In 90, 240, and 360 mL aerosol.
otc	**Unisol 4 Solution** (Alcon)	**Solution**: Buffered, isotonic. NaCl, boric acid, sodium borate.	Preservative free. Thimerosal free. In 120 mL.

SURFACTANT CLEANING SOLUTIONS, SOFT CONTACT LENSES

otc	**MiraFlow Extra-Strength Daily Cleaner** (Ciba Vision)	**Solution**: 15.7% isopropyl alcohol, poloxamer 407, amphoteric 10.	Preservative free. Thimerosal free. In 12 and 20 mL.
otc	**Opti-Free Daily Cleaner** (Alcon)	**Solution**: Buffered, isotonic. 0.1% EDTA, 0.001% polyquad. Polysorbate 21, polymeric cleaning agents.	In 12 and 20 mL.

Soft (Hydrogel) Contact Lens Products

SURFACTANT CLEANING SOLUTIONS, SOFT CONTACT LENSES

otc	**Opti-Free Supra Clens Daily Protein Remover** (Alcon)	**Solution:** Propylene glycol, sodium borate, highly purified porcine pancreatin enzymes.	Preservative free. In 3 mL.
otc	**Sensitive Eyes Daily Cleaner Solution** (Bausch & Lomb)	**Solution:** Buffered, isotonic. 0.5% EDTA, 0.25% sorbic acid. Hydroxypropyl methylcellulose, poloxamine, sodium borate, NaCl.	In 20 mL.
otc	**Sereine Extra-Strength Daily Cleaner** (Optikem, Inc.)	**Solution:** Amphoteric surfactant, poloxamer 407, isopropyl alcohol.	In 30 mL.
otc	**SOF/PRO-CLEAN (Lobob) Sterile Extra Strength Cleaner** (Lobob)	**Solution:** Sorbic acid 0.1%, edetate trisodium 0.25.	In 60 mL.

SURFACTANT CLEANING SOLUTIONS, SOFT CONTACT LENSES — OPHTHALMIC

Indications

Similar to GP lens solutions. These solutions help to maintain a clean, wettable surface with good optics. They are typically recommended for use after lens removal.

Actions

➤*Pharmacology:* Similar to GP lens solutions. The purpose of surfactants is to remove loosely adherent deposits and debris, including microorganisms. They act to break up the deposits through the formation of micelles. Most cleaners contain nonionic or ionic detergents, wetting agents, chelating agents, buffers, and preservatives.

Warnings/Precautions

Same as GP lens solutions.

ENZYMATIC CLEANERS, SOFT CONTACT LENSES

otc	**Opti-Free Supra Clens Daily Protein Remover** (Alcon)	**Solution:** Propylene glycol, sodium borate, highly purified porcine pancreatin enzymes.	Preservative free. In 5 mL.
otc	**ReNu 1 Step Daily Liquid Protein Remover** (Bausch & Lomb)	**Liquid:** Proteolytic enzyme (subtilisin) glycerin and borate buffer.	In 7.5 mL.
otc	**Ultrazyme Enzymatic Cleaner** (American Medical Optics)	**Tablets:** Subtilisin A. Effervescing, buffering, and tableting agents. *To make solution for soaking, dilute in 3% hydrogen peroxide disinfecting solution.*	In 5s, 10s, and 20s.
otc	**Unizyme Enzymatic Cleaner** (Ciba Vision)	**Tablets:** Subtilisin A. Potassium carbonate, citric acid, polyethylene glycol, sodium benzoate. *For use with all Ciba Vision disinfection systems.*	In 12s.

ENZYMATIC CLEANERS/DAILY PROTEIN REMOVERS, SOFT CONTACT LENSES — OPHTHALMIC

Indications

➤*Enzymatic cleaning:* Similar to GP lens solutions. It has been estimated that 80% of all clinical complications related to contact lens wear may be attributed to deposits, most often protein deposits. Enzymatic cleaners are most effective against bound tear protein, notably lysozyme. The level of protein deposition on a hydrogel lens surface appears to be directly related to the water content and the ionic nature of the lens.

Administration and Dosage

➤*Dosage:* Soak in a solution prepared from enzyme tablets once weekly.

Actions

➤*Pharmacology:* Similar to GP lens solutions. As subtilisin is not deactivated quickly in hydrogen peroxide, it has been incorporated in several systems for use during hydrogen peroxide disinfection, decreasing the number of steps necessary for care and potentially increasing patient compliance. Likewise, commonly used chemical disinfection solutions (eg, *ReNu One-Step*) combine enzymatic cleaning with disinfection. Several daily protein removers are available that use either an enzyme or a surfactant to remove adherent mucoprotein complexes. Several systems have been discontinued in the past year due to the increasing popularity of disposable lenses.

Warnings/Precautions

Same as GP lens solutions.

DISINFECTING/WETTING/SOAKING SOLUTIONS, SOFT CONTACT LENSES

otc	**ReNu MultiPlus Multi-Purpose Solution** (Bausch & Lomb)	**Solution:** Isotonic. 0.0001% polyaminopropyl biguanide. Hydroxyalkylphosphonate, boric acid, EDTA, poloxamine, sodium borate, NaCl.	Thimerosal free. In 60, 118, 237, and 355 mL.

REWETTING SOLUTIONS, SOFT CONTACT LENSES

otc	**Aquify Long Lasting Comfort Drops** (Ciba Vision)	**Solution:** Sodium perborate stabilized with perborate acid.	In 10 mL.
otc	**blink Contacts Lubricant Eye Drops** (Advanced Medical Optics)	**Solution:** Buffered, isotonic with sodium hyaluronate, sodium chloride, potassium chloride, calcium chloride, magnesium chloride, boric acid, and *OcuPure* (stabilized oxychloro complex) 0.005% as the preservative.	In 10 mL.
otc	**Clerz Plus Lens Drops** (Alcon)	**Solution:** Sterile, buffered, isotonic, aqueous solution. Citrate buffer, sodium chloride, edetate disodium 0.05%, polyquaternium-1 0.001%, PEG-11 lauryl ether carboxylic acid, tetronic 1304	In 5 and 8 mL.
otc	**Complete Blink-N-Clean Lens Drops** (Advanced Medical Optics)	**Solution:** Buffered, isotonic. 0.0001% polyhexamethylene biguanide, tromethamine, hydroxypropyl methylcellulose, tyloxapol, EDTA, sodium chloride.	Thimerosal free. In 20 mL.
otc	**Opti-Free RepleniSH Rewetting Drops** (Alcon)	**Solution:** Buffered, isotonic, aqueous solution with a citrate/borate buffer and sodium chloride, with edetate disodium 0.05% and *Polyquad* (polyquaternium-1) 0.001% as preservatives and RLM-100 (PEG-11 lauryl ether carboxylic acid) and *Tetronic* 1304.	In 10 mL.
otc	**Refresh Contacts, Contact Lens Comfort Drops** (Allergan)	**Solution:** Buffered, isotonic. 0.005% purite. Carboxymethylcellulose sodium, sodium chloride, boric acid, potassium chloride, calcium chloride, magnesium chloride.	Thimerosal free. In 12 mL.
otc	**ReNu Rewetting Drops** (Bausch & Lomb)	**Solution:** Isotonic. 0.15% sorbic acid, 0.1% EDTA. Boric acid, poloxamine, sodium borate, NaCl.	In 15 mL.
otc	**ReNu MultiPlus Lubricating & Rewetting Drops** (Bausch & Lomb)	**Solution:** Isotonic. 0.1% EDTA, 0.1% sorbic acid. Povidone, boric acid, potassium chloride, sodium borate, NaCl.	In 8 mL.

Soft (Hydrogel) Contact Lens Products

REWETTING SOLUTIONS, SOFT CONTACT LENSES

otc	**Sensitive Eyes Drops** (Bausch & Lomb)	**Solution:** Buffered. 0.1% sorbic acid, 0.025% EDTA. Boric acid, sodium borate, NaCl.	Thimerosal free. In 15 and 30 mL.
otc	**TheraTears Contact Lens Comfort Drops** (Advanced Vision Research)	**Solution:** Sodium carbo methyl cellulose (0.25%), sodium perborate as preservative.	In 15 mL.
otc	**Viva-Drops** (Amcon)	**Solution:** Sorbic acid 0.25%, EDTA 0.10%	In 15 mL.

REWETTING SOLUTIONS, SOFT CONTACT LENSES — OPHTHALMIC

Indications

Similar to GP lenses with the additional benefit of rehydrating the lens for additional comfort and increased wearing time.

Actions

➤*Pharmacology:* Similar to GP lens solutions. Typically, these products contain a low concentration of a nonionic surfactant to promote cleaning, a polymer to lubricate the lens, buffering agents, and preservatives.

May be used directly in the eye to rehydrate and improve comfort of hydrogel lenses.

OPHTHALMIC LOCAL ANESTHETICS

Refer to the Topical Ophthalmic Drugs introduction for more complete information.

Indications

➤*Ophthalmic anesthesia:* For corneal anesthesia of short duration (eg, tonometry, gonioscopy, removal of foreign bodies and sutures); short corneal and conjunctival procedures; conjunctival and corneal scraping for diagnostic purposes.

Actions

➤*Pharmacology:* Topical anesthetics stabilize the neuronal membrane so the neuron is less permeable to ions. This prevents the initiation and transmission of nerve impulses, thereby producing the local anesthetic action.

Studies indicate that local anesthetics influence the permeability of the nerve membrane by limiting sodium ion permeability by closing the pores through which the ions migrate in the lipid layer of the nerve cell membrane. This limitation prevents the fundamental change necessary for the generation of the action potential.

➤*Pharmacokinetics:* Onset, 30 seconds; duration, 10 to 20 minutes.

Contraindications

Hypersensitivity to similar drugs and to any other ingredients in these preparations; self-medication.

Warnings/Precautions

➤*For ophthalmic use only:* Not for injection.

➤*Prolonged use:* Prolonged use is not recommended. Prolonged use may diminish duration of anesthesia, retard wound healing, and cause corneal infection and/or opacification with accompanying permanent visual loss or corneal perforation.

➤*Systemic toxicity:* Systemic toxicity (CNS stimulation followed by CNS and cardiovascular depression) is rare with topical ophthalmic application of local anesthetics.

➤*Protection of the eye:* Protection of the eye from other irritating chemicals, foreign bodies, and rubbing during the period of anesthesia is very important. Thoroughly rinse tonometers soaked in sterilizing or detergent solutions with sterile distilled water before use and avoid touching the eye until anesthesia has worn off.

➤*Special risk:* Use cautiously and sparingly in patients with known allergies, cardiac disease, or hyperthyroidism.

➤*Pregnancy: Category C.* Animal reproduction studies have not been conducted. It is also not known whether these drugs can cause fetal harm when administered to a pregnant woman or affect reproduction capacity. Administer these drugs to a pregnant woman only if clearly needed.

➤*Lactation:* It is not known whether these drugs are excreted in human milk. Because many drugs are excreted in human milk, exercise caution when these drugs are administered to a breast-feeding woman.

➤*Children:* Safety and efficacy of proparacaine in children have been established. Safety and efficacy of the anesthetic combination products and tetracaine in children have not been established.

Adverse Reactions

➤*Ophthalmic:* Transient stinging, burning, and conjunctival redness may occur. A rare, severe, immediate type of allergic corneal reaction has been reported, characterized by acute, intense diffuse epithelial keratitis with filament formation and/or sloughing of large areas of necrotic epithelium; diffuse stromal edema; a gray, ground glass appearance; descemetitis; and iritis.

Allergic contact dermatitis with drying and fissuring of the fingertips and softening and erosion of the corneal epithelium, and conjunctival congestion and hemorrhage have been reported.

Patient Information

Advise patients to avoid touching or rubbing the eye until the anesthesia has worn off because inadvertent damage may be done to the anesthetized cornea and conjunctiva.

TETRACAINE HYDROCHLORIDE

Rx	**Tetracaine Hydrochloride** (Various, eg, Alcon, Bausch & Lomb)	**Solution:** 0.5%	In 1, 2, and 15 mL.
Rx	**Tetcaine** (Ocusoft)		In 15 mL.[a]
Rx	**Altacaine** (Altaire)		In 15 and 30 mL.[b]

[a] With 0.4% chlorobutanol and 0.75% sodium chloride.

[b] With chlorobutanol, boric acid, potassium chloride, and hydrochloric acid and/or sodium hydroxide.

TETRACAINE HYDROCHLORIDE — OPHTHALMIC

For complete and comparative prescribing information, refer to the Local Anesthetics, Topical class monograph.

Indications

➤*Ophthalmic anesthesia:* For procedures in which a rapid and short-acting topical ophthalmic anesthetic is indicated, such as in tonometry, gonioscopy, removal of corneal foreign bodies and sutures, conjunctival scraping for diagnostic procedures, and other short corneal and conjunctival procedures.

Administration and Dosage

➤*Adults:*

Ophthalmic anesthesia –

Cataract extraction: 1 or 2 drops in the eye(s) every 5 to 10 minutes for 3 to 5 doses.

Foreign body / suture removal: 1 to 2 drops every 5 to 10 minutes for 1 to 3 instillations.

Tonometry: 1 or 2 drops just prior to evaluation.

➤*Storage / Stability:* Store at 15° to 30°C (59° to 86°F). Keep tightly closed.

PROPARACAINE HYDROCHLORIDE

Rx	**Proparacaine Hydrochloride** (Various, eg, Akorn, Falcon)	**Solution:** 0.5%	In 15 mL.
Rx	**Alcaine** (Alcon)		In 15 mL *Drop-Tainers*.[a]
Rx	**Ophthetic** (Allergan)		In 15 mL.[b]
Rx	**Parcaine** (Ocusoft)		In 15 mL.

[a] With glycerin and 0.01% benzalkonium chloride.

[b] With 0.01% benzalkonium chloride, glycerin, sodium chloride, and hydrochloric acid and/or sodium hydroxide.

PROPARACAINE HYDROCHLORIDE — OPHTHALMIC

For complete and comparative prescribing information, refer to the Local Anesthetics, Topical group monograph.

Indications

➤*Ophthalmic anesthesia:* For procedures in which a topical ophthalmic anesthetic is indicated, such as corneal anesthesia of short duration (eg, tonometry, gonioscopy, removal of foreign bodies) and short corneal and conjunctival procedures.

Administration and Dosage

➤*Adults:*

Ophthalmic anesthesia –

Foreign body removal: Instill 1 or 2 drops prior to operating.

Short corneal and conjunctival procedures: Instill 1 drop every 5 to 10 minutes for 5 to 7 doses.

Suture removal: Instill 1 or 2 drops 2 or 3 minutes before removal of stitches.

Tonometry: Instill 1 or 2 drops immediately before measurement.

➤*Children:* Controlled clinical studies have not been performed with proparacaine to establish safety and efficacy in children; however, the literature cites the use of proparacaine as a topical ophthalmic anesthetic agent in children.

➤*Administration:* For topical ophthalmic use only.

➤*Storage/Stability:* Store at 2° to 8°C (36° to 46°F). Store in unit carton to protect from light.

Note – Proparacaine should be straw colored. Discard the solution if it becomes darker.

LIDOCAINE HYDROCHLORIDE

Rx	**Akten** (Akorn)	**Gel; ophthalmic:** 3.5%	Preservative free. In 5 mL single-use dropper bottle.

LIDOCAINE HYDROCHLORIDE — OPHTHALMIC

For complete and comparative prescribing information, refer to the ophthalmic and otic class monograph and ophthalmic local anesthetics class monographs. Refer to the Topical Ophthalmic Drugs introduction for more complete information.

Indications

➤*Ophthalmic anesthesia:* For ocular surface anesthesia during ophthalmic procedures.

Administration and Dosage

➤*Adults:*

Ophthalmic anesthesia – Two drops applied to the ocular surface in the area of the planned procedure. It may be reapplied to maintain anesthetic effect.

➤*Children:* See Adults for more information.

➤*Storage/Stability:* Store at 15° to 25°C (59° to 77°F). Keep container closed and protected from light in the original carton until use. Discard after use.

MISCELLANEOUS LOCAL ANESTHETIC COMBINATIONS

Rx	**Fluorescein Sodium with Proparacaine Hydrochloride** (Various, eg, Altaire, Deca Pharm)	**Solution; ophthalmic:** proparacaine hydrochloride 0.5% and fluorescein sodium 0.25%	In 5 mL with dropper.[a]
Rx	**Flucaine** (OcuSoft)		In 5 mL.
Rx	**Fluoracaine** (Akorn)		In 5 mL.[b]
Rx	**Fluorescein Sodium/Benoxinate Hydrochloride** (Bausch & Lomb)	**Solution; ophthalmic:** benoxinate hydrochloride 0.4% and fluorescein sodium 0.25%	In 5 mL with dropper.[c]
Rx	**Altafluor** (Altaire)		In 5 mL with dropper.[c]
Rx	**Fluress** (Akorn)		In 5 mL with dropper.[d]
Rx	**Flurox** (Ocusoft)		In 5 mL.
Rx	**FluraSafe** (Altaire)	**Solution; ophthalmic:** benoxinate hydrochloride 0.4% and fluorexon disodium 0.35%	In 6 mL with dropper.[e]

[a] With povidone, glycerin, EDTA, and thimerosal 0.01%.
[b] With glycerin, povidone, polysorbate 80, thimerosal 0.01%, boric acid, and with sodium hydroxide and/or hydrochloric acid.
[c] With povidone, boric acid, chlorobutanol 1%.
[d] With povidone, boric acid, chlorobutanol 1%, and sodium hydroxide and/or hydrochloric acid.
[e] With povidone, boric acid, chlorobutanol 0.5%, polysorbate 80, PEG-400.

MISCELLANEOUS LOCAL ANESTHETIC COMBINATIONS — OPHTHALMIC

For complete and comparative prescribing information, refer to the Local Anesthetics, Topical group monograph.

Indications

➤*Ophthalmic anesthesia:* For procedures in which a topical ophthalmic anesthetic agent in conjunction with a disclosing agent is indicated, such as corneal anesthesia of short duration (eg, tonometry, gonioscopy, removal of foreign bodies) and short corneal and conjunctival procedures.

Administration and Dosage

➤*General dosing considerations:* The use of an eye patch is recommended.

➤*Adults:*

Ophthalmic anesthesia –

Benoxinate/fluorescein: Instill 2 drops into each eye at 90-second intervals for 3 instillations.

Proparacaine/fluorescein: Instill 1 drop in each eye every 5 to 10 minutes for 5 to 7 doses.

Benoxinate/fluorexon: 1 to 2 drops (in single instillations) in each eye before operating.

➤*Storage/Stability:* Refrigerate at 2° to 8°C (36° to 46°F). May store benoxinate/fluorescein and benoxinate/fluorexon at room temperature for up to 1 month. Keep tightly closed. Store in carton to protect from light.

OPHTHALMIC DIAGNOSTIC PRODUCTS

In addition to the following products, the ophthalmic vasoconstrictors, cycloplegic mydriatics and topical local anesthetics are used in diagnostic procedures (see individual monographs).

➤*Vasoconstrictors/Mydriatics:* With α-sympathomimetic activity cause dilation of the pupil and are used to facilitate ophthalmoscopic examination and other diagnostic procedures.

➤*Cycloplegic Mydriatics:* Cycloplegic Mydriatics (anticholinergics) cause both dilation of the pupil and paralysis of accommodation. These agents are used to facilitate refraction.

➤*Local Anesthetics:* Used to facilitate gonioscopy, tonometry and other procedures.

FLUORESCEIN SODIUM

Rx	**Fluorescein Lite** (HUB Pharmaceuticals)	**Injection, solution:** 10%	In 5 mL single dose vials.
Rx	**AK-Fluor** (Akorn)		In 5 mL amps and vials.
Rx	**Angiofluor** (Alliance)		In 5 mL single-dose vials and boxes of 12 vials.
Rx	**Angiofluor Lite** (Alliance)		In 5 mL single-dose vials and boxes of 12 vials.
Rx	**Fluorescite** (Alcon)		In 5 mL amps with syringes.
Rx	**AK-Fluor** (Akorn)	**Injection, solution:** 25%	In 2 mL amps and vials.
Rx	**Angiofluor** (Alliance)		In 2 mL single-dose vials and boxes of 12 vials.
Rx	**Angiofluor Lite** (Alliance)		In 2 mL single-dose vials and boxes of 12 vials.
otc	**Ful-Glo** (Akorn)	**Strips; ophthalmic:** 0.6 mg	In 300s.
otc	**BioGlo** (Hub Pharmaceuticals)	**Strips; ophthalmic:** 1 mg	In 100s.
otc	**Fluorets** (Bausch & Lomb)		In 100s.

FLUORESCEIN SODIUM — INJECTION

Indications

➤*Angiography/Angioscopy:* Indicated in diagnostic fluorescein angiography or angioscopy of the fundus and of the iris vasculature.

Administration and Dosage

➤*Adults:*

Diagnostic angiography/angioscopy –

Usual dosage: Inject the contents of the ampul or vial rapidly into the antecubital vein, after taking precautions to avoid extravasation. (See Administration.)

Test dose: If potential allergy is suspected, an intradermal skin test may be performed prior to intravenous (IV) administration (ie, 0.05 mL injected intradermally to be evaluated 30 to 60 minutes following injection).

➤*Children:* Safety and efficacy in children have not been established. However, if used in children, the dose is calculated on the basis of 35 mg per 10 pounds of body weight.

➤*Administration:* Administer IV.

A syringe filled with fluorescein is attached to transparent tubing and a 25-gauge scalp vein needle for injection. Insert the needle and draw the patient's blood to the hub of the syringe so that a small air bubble separates the patient's blood in the tubing from the fluorescein. With the room lights on, slowly inject the blood back into the vein while watching the skin over the needle tip. If the needle has extravasated, the patient's blood will be seen to bulge the skin; stop the injection before any fluorescein is injected. When assured that extravasation has not occurred, the room light may be turned off and the fluorescein injection completed. Luminescence appears in the retina and choroidal vessels in 9 to 14 seconds and can be observed by standard viewing equipment.

➤*Extravasation:* Care must be taken to avoid extravasation during injection because the high pH of fluorescein solution can result in severe local tissue damage. The following complications resulting from extravasation of fluorescein have been noted to occur: sloughing of the skin, superficial phlebitis, subcutaneous granuloma, and toxic neuritis along the median curve in the antecubital area. Complications resulting from extravasation can cause severe pain in the arm for up to several hours. When significant extravasation occurs, discontinue the injection and implement conservative measures to treat damaged tissues and relieve pain.

If signs or symptoms of extravasation occur, stop the infusion immediately. If possible, withdraw 3 to 5 mL of blood to remove some of the drug. Remove the infusion needle. Delineate the infiltrated area on the patient's skin with a felt-tip marker. There is no information on the use of hyaluronidase to treat reactions, but it is well tolerated and might be used empirically. If hyaluronidase is to be used, administer promptly within the first few minutes to 1 hour after extravasation. Higher doses (150 units) have primarily been used in adults while lower doses (15 units) have been used in children. Administer hyaluronidase according to the following steps. Dilute hyaluronidase to desired concentration, depending on the dose and product used. (Note: Some products do not require dilution.) For example, if the total dose is 15 units, make 15 units/mL dilution. If the total dose is 150 units, make 150 units/mL dilution. Cleanse area with povidone-iodine. Inject hyaluronidase locally, subcutaneously or intradermally, using a 25-gauge needle or smaller. The dose is given as five 0.2 mL injections at the leading edge of the extravasation site. Change needle after each injection. Elevate for 48 hours above heart level using a sling or stockinette dressing with an observation window cut in the dressing. Avoid pressure or friction. Do not rub area. Observe for signs of increased erythema, pain, or skin necrosis. If increased symptoms occur, consult a plastic surgeon. Ensure that no medication is given distally to extravasation site. After 48 hours, encourage the patient to use the extremity normally to promote full range of motion.

➤*Storage/Stability:* Store at 15° to 25°C (59° to 77°F); protect from freezing.

Actions

➤*Pharmacology:* The yellowish green fluorescence of the product demarcates the vascular area under observation, distinguishing it from adjacent areas.

Contraindications

Hypersensitivity to any component of this preparation.

Warnings/Precautions

➤*Extravasation:* See Administration and Dosage for more information.

➤*Special risk:* Exercise caution in patients with a history of allergy or bronchial asthma. An emergency tray including such items as 0.1% epinephrine for IV or IM use; an antihistamine, soluble steroid, and aminophylline for IV use; and oxygen should always be available in the event of possible reaction to fluorescein injection.

➤*Pregnancy: Category C.* Avoid angiography on patients who are pregnant, especially those in first trimester. There have been no reports of fetal complications from fluorescein injection during pregnancy.

➤*Lactation:* Exercise caution when fluorescein injection is administered to a nursing woman.

➤*Children:* Safety and efficacy in children have not been established.

Adverse Reactions

Nausea and headache, GI distress, syncope, vomiting, hypotension, and other symptoms and signs of hypersensitivity have occurred. Cardiac arrest, basilar artery ischemia, severe shock, convulsions, thrombophlebitis at the injection site and rare cases of death have been reported. Extravasation of the solution at the injection site causes intense pain at the site and a dull aching pain in the injected arm. Generalized hives and itching, bronchospasm, and anaphylaxis have been reported. A strong taste may develop after injection.

The most common reaction is nausea.

Patient Information

Skin will attain a temporary yellowish discoloration. Urine attains a bright yellow color. Discoloration of the skin fades in 6 to 12 hours; urine fluorescence in 24 to 36 hours.

FLUORESCEIN SODIUM — OPHTHALMIC

Indications

➤*Ophthalmic solution:* Fluorescein ophthalmic solution is indicated for the detection of corneal stippling, abrasions and ulcerations. Fluorescein ophthalmic solution is also indicated for detecting pressure points from contact lenses. Fluorescein ophthalmic solution is indicated for use in conjunction with certain applanation tonometers for measurement of intraocular pressure. This medication is also indicated for use in testing wound leakage (Seidel test).

➤*Ophthalmic strips:* Fluorescein sodium ophthalmic strips are indicated for staining the anterior segment of the eye when:

- Delineating a corneal injury, herpetic lesion or foreign body.
- Determining the site of an intraocular injury.
- Fitting contact lenses.
- Making the fluorescein test to ascertain postoperative closure of the sclerocorneal (also referred to as cornecoscleral) wound in delayed anterior chamber reformation.
- Making the lacrimal drainage test.
- In applanation tonometry.

Administration and Dosage

➤*Adults:*

Detection of corneal stippling, abrasions, and ulcerations –

Ophthalmic solution: One drop topically in the eye(s) followed by irrigation of excess as needed. Additional drops may be instilled if needed.

Detection of pressure points from contact lenses – See Detection of corneal stippling, abrasions, and ulcerations for dosing.

Measurement of intraocular pressure – See Detection of corneal stippling, abrasions, and ulcerations for dosing.

Testing wound leakage (Seidel test) – See Detection of corneal stippling, abrasions, and ulcerations for dosing.

Staining the anterior segment of the eye –

Ophthalmic strips: Apply 1 strip per eye. See Administration.

➤*Administration:* Fluorescein is for topical ophthalmic external use only; it is not for injection.

Strips – To open the envelope, grasp pull tabs firmly and separate slowly. Separate the 2 strips by tearing off the white tab end. To ensure full fluorescence and patient comfort, the fluorescein sodium ophthalmic strip impregnated tip should be moistened before application. One or 2 drops of sterile, isotonic irrigation solution, sterile water, or other ophthalmic solution should be used for this purpose. While the patient looks down, stroke the tip across the bulbar conjunctiva or fornix. The patient should then blink several times after application to obtain the best results. For best results, patient should close lid tightly over strip until desired amount of staining is obtained. Another method is to retract upper lid and touch tip of strip to the bulbar conjunctiva on the temporal side until an adequate amount of stain is available for a clearly defined end point reading.

Never use fluorescein while the patient is wearing soft contact lenses because the lenses may become stained. Whenever fluorescein is used, flush the eyes with sterile, normal saline solution, and wait at least 1 hour before replacing the lenses.

➤*Storage/Stability:*

Ophthalmic solution – Store at 8° to 30°C (46° to 80°F).

9 mg strips – Store at room temperature (approximately 25°C [77°F]). Contents may not be sterile if individual strip package has been damaged or previously opened.

Actions

Contraindications

Hypersensitivity to any component of this preparation; hypersensitivity to mercury-containing compounds.

Warnings/Precautions

➤*Administration:* Fluorescein sodium is for topical ophthalmic external use only; it is not for injection.

➤*9 mg strips:* Never use fluorescein while the patient is wearing soft contact lenses because the lenses may become stained. Whenever fluorescein is used, flush the eyes with sterile, normal saline solution, and wait at least 1 hour before replacing the lenses. Do not touch dropper tip to any surface, as this may contaminate the solution.

FLUORESCEIN SODIUM — OPHTHALMIC

➤*Usage:* This medication may stain soft contact lenses. Do not touch dropper tip to any surface, as this may contaminate the solution.

➤*Hypersensitivity reactions:* Discontinue if sensitivity develops.

➤*Pregnancy: Category B* (per Briggs' *Drugs in Pregnancy and Lactation*). Use of fluorescein in the eye produces measurable concentrations of dye in the systemic circulation; expect passage to the fetus.

➤*Lactation:* Fluorescein has been demonstrated to be excreted in human milk. Exercise caution when fluorescein is administered to a breast-feeding woman. The American Academy of Pediatrics classifies fluorescein as compatible with breast-feeding.

Patient Information

This medication may cause strong taste with use.

This medication may cause temporary yellowish discoloration of the skin. Urine will turn bright yellow. Discoloration of skin fades in 6 to 12 hours; urine, in 24 to 36 hours.

Soft contact lenses may become stained. Do not wear lenses while fluorescein is being used. Whenever fluorescein is used, flush the eyes with sterile normal solution and wait at least 1 hour before replacing the lenses.

FLUOREXON

otc	**Fluoresoft-0.35%** (Various, eg, Amcon, Con-cise Lens, Eye Care and Cure, Holles, Ocusoft)	**Solution:** 0.35%	Preservative-free. In 0.35 mL ampules. In 20s.

FLUOREXON — OPHTHALMIC

Indications

➤*Applanation tonometry:* For conducting the applanation tonometry procedure without removing the lens.

➤*Contact lens fitting aid:* For the assessment of proper fitting characteristics of hydrogel lenses. For quickly and accurately locating the optic zone in aphakic or low-plus lenses.

For the evaluation of corneal integrity of patients wearing hydrogel contact lenses. In many instances, arcuate staining will show definite correlation with the edge of the optic zone, indicating improper bearing surfaces.

➤*Tear break-up time test:* For use in place of sodium fluorescein when conducting the tear breakup time test.

➤*Toric lenses:* For locating the lathe-cut index markings (toric lenses). Use as directed for fitting contact lenses.

Administration and Dosage

➤*Adults:*

Applanation tonometry – After seating the patient at the slit lamp and either removing the contact lens or displacing it to the side, instill a drop of proparacaine or similar topical anesthetic, followed 1 to 2 minutes later by a drop of fluorexon. Take the reading immediately after, followed by rinsing out the eye and replacing the contact lens.

Contact lens fitting aid –

Usual dosage: Place 1 drop on the concave surface of the lens and place the lens immediately on the eye.

As the dye passes under the lens, observe a central dark zone of 6 to 9 mm in diameter (ie, a limbal fluorescent ring about 2 mm wide) that forms after each blink. If such staining pattern cannot be observed immediately, slide the lens upward by gently pushing it with a finger, causing the dye to penetrate under the lens as it slides back into normal position. Additional drops may be used if the fluorescence starts to dissipate after prolonged examination.

Begin the examination immediately after instillation of fluorexon drops. The material tends to dissipate readily with the tear flow, leading to a progressive reduction in fluorescence. Prolonged examination may require sequential application of drops.

When the examination is completed, rinse the eye and lens with saline. The lens may be reinserted immediately, as opposed to the long waiting period required after the use of fluorescein.

Alternative dosage: Alternately, place 1 or 2 drops in the lower cul-de-sac and have the patient blink several times.

Tear break-up time test – See Contact lens fitting aid for dosing.

Toric lenses – See Contact lens fitting aid for dosing.

➤*Storage/Stability:* Store below 24°C (75°F). Avoid direct sunlight. For one-time use only; discard ampule after use.

Actions

➤*Pharmacology:* Fluorexon is a large molecular weight fluorescent solution for use as a diagnostic and fitting aid for patients with hydrogel contact lenses. Fluorexon is used, with or without lens in place (when fluorescein is contraindicated), most commonly to avoid staining lenses. It may be used for soft and hard lenses.

Contraindications

Hypersensitivity to sodium fluorescein.

Warnings/Precautions

➤*Contact lenses:* When used with lenses of greater than 55% hydration, some color may remain on lens. Remove by washing repeatedly with washing solution approved for the lens. Rinse with saline or water. Any residual coloring will wash out with the tear flow when the lens is reinserted in the eye. With highly hydrated lenses, the amount of coloring picked up will vary with exposure. Avoid unnecessary delays in examination procedure.

➤*Hydrogen peroxide:* Do not use hydrogen peroxide solutions to clean or sterilize lenses until all traces of fluorexon are removed because this oxidizing agent can bind fluorexon molecules to the lens.

➤*Pregnancy: Category: Undetermined.* There is no information regarding fluorexon in pregnant women.

➤*Lactation:* There is no information regarding fluorexon in breast-feeding women.

ROSE BENGAL

otc	**Rose Bengal** (Akorn)	**Strips:** 1.3 mg per strip	In 100s.

ROSE BENGAL — OPHTHALMIC

Indications

➤*Suspected corneal/conjunctival damage:* A diagnostic agent in routine ocular examinations or when superficial corneal or conjunctival tissue damage is suspected. Effective aid for diagnosis of keratitis, keratoconjunctivitis sicca, corrosions or abrasions, and for the detection of foreign bodies.

Administration and Dosage

➤*Adults:*

Suspected corneal/conjunctival damage – Thoroughly saturate tip of strip with 2 or 3 drops of sterile ophthalmic solution. Touch bulbar conjunctiva or lower fornix with moistened strip. The patient should blink several times after application.

Actions

➤*Pharmacology:* Rose bengal is an iodine derivative of fluorescein and stains dead or degenerated epithelial cells (corneal and conjunctival) and the mucus of the precorneal tear film.

Contraindications

Hypersensitivity to rose bengal or any component of the formulation.

Warnings/Precautions

➤*Irritation:* The solution may be irritating.

➤*Staining:* Rose bengal can stain eyelids, cheeks, fingers, and clothing in a concentration-dependent manner. Keeping the amount of dye at a minimum and irrigating the eye can help circumvent this problem.

➤*Pregnancy: Category: Undetermined.* Consult a health care provider before using in pregnant women.

➤*Lactation:* Consult a health care provider before using in breast-feeding women.

Adverse Reactions

➤*Ophthalmic:* Irritation and discomfort.

INDOCYANINE GREEN

See the Indocyanine green monograph in the Diagnostic Aids chapter.

LISSAMINE GREEN

Rx	**Lissamine Green** (Rose Stone Enterprises)	**Strip; ophthalmic:** 1.5 mg	In 100s.
Rx	**Green Glo** (beHub Pharmaceuticals)		In 100s.

LISSAMINE GREEN — OPHTHALMIC

Indications

➤*Diagnostic agent for corneal abnormality:* As an aid in disclosing corneal abnormality.

Administration and Dosage

➤*Adults:*

Diagnostic agent for corneal abnormality – Moisten the impregnated part of the strip with sterile normal saline. While the patient looks up, stroke the moistened tip along the bulbar conjunctiva. The patient should blink several times for best results.

➤*Elderly:* See Adults for dosing.

➤*Administration:* Directions for use:

1.) Hold the pouch in the middle and tear towards the sterile strip.
2.) Flip over and tear from the other side, taking care not to tear sterile strip.
3.) Grasp each end of the pouch without grasping the strip within and pull apart.
4.) Handle the exposed strip by holding the white holding paper.
5.) Alternately, tear fluid from the lower fornix may be used. While the patient looks up, stroke the moistened tip along the bulbar conjunctiva. The patient should then blink several times to obtain best results.
6.) Observe under slit lamp for stained cells. The extent of staining is indicative of corneal epithelial cell damage.

➤*Storage/Stability:* The expiration date should be verified before using the product; do not use after the expiration date indicated on the package. Do not store in a moist environment. Do not use the strip if the sterile packing has been damaged (traces of leakage).

Actions

➤*Pharmacology:* Each sterile strip is impregnated with lissamine green 1.5 mg. The strip is made of an absorbent paper that is impregnated with the dye. It aids in staining and detecting cells that are dead or degenerated where the cell wall is not broken. It stains mucous fibrils. The cell nucleus is stained more intensely with a bluish green color, than the cytoplasm.

Contraindications

Use with gas permeable lenses or soft contact lenses as these will stain the lenses.

Warnings/Precautions

➤*Administration:* For external use only. The product is meant for professional use only.

➤*Discontinuation of therapy:* Discontinue use in case of persistent irritation or burning sensation.

Drug Interactions

None known.

Adverse Reactions

➤*Ophthalmic:* Irritation or burning sensation.

Patient Information

Do not wear contact lenses while lissamine green strips are being used; contact lenses may become stained.

TEAR TEST STRIPS

Rx	**Schirmer Tear Test** (Various, eg, Alcon)	**Strips:** Sterile tear flow test strips	In 250s.

TEAR TEST STRIPS — OPHTHALMIC

Indications

➤*Schirmer Tear Test:*

Test I – To diagnose dry eye syndrome, to evaluate lacrimal gland function in contact lens wearers, to check tear production prior to eyelid surgery and prior to corneal transplantation and cataract surgery.

Test II – To assess the adequacy of reflex lacrimation.

➤*Sno-Strips:* To assess tear secretion.

Administration and Dosage

➤*General dosing considerations:* Perform test on eye before any topical medication (especially anesthetic) is administered or other procedures are carried out (eg, manipulation of eyelids).

➤*Adults:*

Schirmer Tear Test –

Test I: Strips are placed at the junction of the middle and temporal one third of the eyelid margin. To avoid increased reflex lacrimation and pain, do not touch the cornea. After 5 minutes, remove the strips and measure the length of the moistened area. A value of less than 5 mm is very suggestive of a true dry eye state.

Test II: For the Schirmer II Tear Test, insert the strips in the usual manner. Gently irritate the nasal mucosa with a cotton-tip applicator to provoke reflex lacrimation. Remove the strips after 5 minutes. A value of less than 10 mm suggests that the patient is unable to produce reflex lacrimation and has demonstrated reflex secretion failure.

Sno-Strips – Apply to lower temporal lid margin of eye. The distance between the notch and shoulder of strip is 10 mm, which should be wetted in approximately 3 minutes. Repeat if greater than 5 minutes; greater than 10 minutes indicates reduced tear secretion.

OPHTHALMIC SURGICAL ADJUNCTS

TRYPAN BLUE

Rx	**VisionBlue** (Dutch Ophthalmic USA[a])	**Solution; ophthalmic:** 0.06%	0.5 mL in single-use *Luer Lok* syringe.
Rx	**MembraneBlue** (Dutch Ophthalmic USA)	**Solution; ophthalmic:** 0.15%	0.5 mL single-use *Luer Lok* syringe.

[a] Dutch Ophthalmic USA; 10 Continental Drive, Bldg 1; Exeter, NH 03833; 800-753-8824 or 603-778-6929; fax: 603-778-0911; http://www.dorc.nl.

TRYPAN BLUE — OPHTHALMIC

Indications

➤*Surgical aid:*

VisionBlue – Aids in ophthalmic surgery by staining the anterior capsule of the lens.

MembraneBlue – Aids in ophthalmic surgery by staining the epiretinal membranes during ophthalmic surgical vitrectomy procedures, facilitating removal of the tissue.

Administration and Dosage

➤*Adults:*

Surgical aid – One syringe per procedure.

➤*Children:*

Surgical aid – One syringe per procedure.

➤*Administration:*

VisionBlue – After opening the eye, inject an air bubble into the anterior chamber of the eye to minimize dilution of trypan blue by the aqueous humor. Carefully apply trypan blue onto the anterior lens capsule using a blunt cannula. Sufficient staining is achieved as soon as the dye has contacted the capsule. Then irrigate the anterior chamber with balanced salt solution to remove all excess dye. An anterior capsulotomy can then be performed.

MembraneBlue – Before injection of trypan blue, perform a "fluid-air exchange" (ie, filling the entire vitreous cavity with air to prevent aqueous dilution of trypan blue). Trypan blue is carefully applied to the retinal membrane using a blunt cannula attached to the trypan blue syringe, without allowing the cannula to contact or damage the retina. Sufficient staining is expected on contact with the membrane. All excess dye should be removed from the vitreous cavity before performing an air-fluid exchange to prevent unnecessary spreading of the dye. Trypan blue can also be injected directly in a buffered saline solution–filled vitreous cavity (instead of injecting under air). Clinical use demonstrated that, after complete vitreous and posterior hyaloid removal, sufficient staining is achieved after 30 seconds of application under buffered saline solution.

Trypan blue is intended to be applied directly on the areas where membranes could be present, staining any portion of the membrane that comes in contact with the dye. The dye does not penetrate the membrane.

➤*Storage/Stability:* Store at 15° to 25°C (59° to 77°F). Protect from direct sunlight.

TRYPAN BLUE — OPHTHALMIC

Actions

➤*Pharmacology:*

VisionBlue – Trypan blue selectively stains connective tissue structures in the human eye, such as the anterior lens capsule of the human crystalline lens.

Trypan blue is intended to be applied directly onto the anterior lens capsule, staining any portion of the capsule that comes in contact with the dye. Excess dye is washed out of the anterior chamber. The dye does not penetrate the capsule, permitting visualization of the anterior capsule in contrast to the nonstained lens cortex and inner lens material.

MembraneBlue – Trypan blue selectively stains membranes in the human eye during posterior surgery, such as epiretinal membranes and internal limiting membranes.

Contraindications

When a nonhydrated (dry state), hydrophilic acrylic intraocular lens is planned to be inserted into the eye because the dye may be absorbed by and stain the intraocular lens.

Warnings/Precautions

➤*Irrigation:* After injection, immediately remove all excess trypan blue from the eye by thorough irrigation of the anterior chamber.

➤*Pregnancy: Category C.* There are no adequate and well-controlled studies in pregnant women. Give trypan blue to a pregnant woman only if the potential benefit justifies the potential risk to the fetus. Trypan blue is teratogenic in rats, mice, rabbits, hamsters, dogs, guinea pigs, pigs, and chickens. The majority of teratogenicity studies performed involve intravenous, intraperitoneal, or subcutaneous administration in the rat. The teratogenic dose is 50 mg/kg as a single dose or 25 mg/kg/day during embryogenesis in the rat. In *VisionBlue*, these doses are approximately 50,000- and 25,000-fold the maximum recommended human dose of 0.06 mg per injection in a 60 kg person, assuming total absorption. In *MembraneBlue*, these doses are approximately 4,000- and 2,000-fold the maximum recommended human dose of 0.75 mg per injection based in a 60 kg person, assuming total absorption. Characteristic anomalies included neural tube, cardiovascular, vertebral, tail, and eye defects. Trypan blue also caused an increase in postimplantation mortality and decreased fetal weight.

In the monkey, trypan blue caused abortions with 1 or 2 daily doses of 50 mg/kg between the 20th through 25th days of pregnancy, but no apparent increase in birth defects (for *VisionBlue*, approximately 50,000-fold maximum recommended human dose of 0.06 mg per injection, assuming total absorption; for *MembraneBlue*, approximately 4,000-fold maximum recommended human dose of 0.75 mg per injection, assuming total absorption).

➤*Lactation:* It is not known whether this drug is excreted in human milk. Because many drugs are excreted in human milk, exercise caution when trypan blue is administered to a breast-feeding woman.

Drug Interactions

None known.

Adverse Reactions

➤*Ophthalmic:* Discoloration of high water content hydrogen intraocular lenses and inadvertent staining of the posterior lens capsule and vitreous face. Staining of the posterior lens capsule or the vitreous face is generally self limited, lasting up to 1 week.

Patient Information

Advise patients that staining of the posterior lens capsule or the vitreous face will last for up to 1 week.

SODIUM HYALURONATE

Rx	**Healon** (Abbott)	**Injection:** 10 mg/mL	In 0.4, 0.55, 0.85 and 2 mL disp. syringes.[a]
Rx	**ProVisc** (Alcon)		In 0.4, 0.55, and 0.85 mL disposable syringes.[b]
Rx	**Amvisc** (Chiron)	**Injection:** 12 mg/mL[c]	In 0.5 or 0.8 mL disp. syringe.
Rx	**Coease** (Advance Medical)		In 0.5 or 0.8 mL disposable syringes.
Rx	**Shellgel** (Cytosol Ophthalmics)		In 0.8 mL disposable syringes.
Rx	**Healon GV** (Abbott)	**Injection:** 14 mg/mL[a]	In 0.55 and 0.85 mL disp. syringes.
Rx	**Amvisc Plus** (Bausch & Lomb Surgical)	**Injection:** 16 mg/mL[c]	In 0.5 or 8 mL disp. syringe.
Rx	**Healon5** (Advanced Medical Optics)	**Injection:** 23 mg/mL[a]	In 0.6 mLdisposable syringe.

[a] With 8.5 mg NaCl per mL.
[b] With 8.4 mg NaCl per mL.
[c] With 9 mg NaCl per mL.

SODIUM HYALURONATE — OPHTHALMIC

Indications

➤*Surgical aid:* For use as a surgical aid to protect corneal endothelium during cataract extraction (extracapsular) procedures, intraocular lens (IOL) implantation and anterior segment surgery. When introduced in the anterior segment of the eye during these surgical procedures, sodium hyaluronate viscoelastic preparation serves to maintain a deep anterior chamber.

In addition, sodium hyaluronate viscoelastic preparation helps to push back the vitreous face and prevent formation of a postoperative flat chamber.

Administration and Dosage

➤*General dosing considerations:* Additional sodium hyaluronate viscoelastic preparation can be injected during surgery to replace any sodium hyaluronate viscoelastic preparation lost during surgical manipulation.

➤*Adults:*

Surgical aid – Sodium hyaluronate viscoelastic preparation should be slowly and carefully introduced into the anterior segment of the eye using a cannula or needle.

➤*Administration:* Refrigerated sodium hyaluronate viscoelastic preparation should be allowed to attain room temperature (approximately 20 to 30 minutes) prior to use.

Injection of sodium hyaluronate viscoelastic preparation can be performed either before or after delivery of the lens. Sodium hyaluronate viscoelastic preparation may also be used to coat surgical instruments and the intraocular lenses prior to insertion.

Cannulas are intended for single patient use only. If reuse becomes necessary on the same patient during the surgical procedures, rinse the cannula thoroughly with sterile distilled water to remove all traces of residual material.

➤*Admixture compatibility:* Mixing of quaternary ammonium salts, such as benzalkonium chloride with sodium hyaluronate, results in the formation of a precipitate. The eye should not be irrigated with any solution containing benzalkonium chloride if sodium hyaluronate viscoelastic preparation is to be used during surgery.

➤*Storage/Stability:* Store in refrigerator 2° to 8°C (36° to 46°F). Protect from freezing. Protect from light. Bring to room temperature prior to use (approximately 20 to 40 minutes).

Actions

➤*Pharmacology:* Sodium hyaluronate is a high molecular weight polysaccharide, composed of sodium glucuronate and N-acetyl-glucosamine which forms a repeating disaccharide unit by linking alternately beta 1-3 and beta 1-4 glycosidic bonds. The 1% viscous and transparent material, sodium hyaluronate, is a specific fraction of sodium hyaluronate, developed as an aid in ophthalmic surgery. It acts as a space occupying fluid that is replaced by the body's natural fluids.

Sodium hyaluronate is a physiological material that is widely distributed in the connective tissues of both animals and man. Chemically identical in all species, hyaluronate can be found in the vitreous and aqueous humor of the eye, the synovial fluid, the skin and the umbilical cord.

Sodium hyaluronate viscoelastic preparation has the following properties:

- High molecular weight (mass average molecular weight approximately 3 million daltons)
- High viscosity

Contraindications

At present there are no known contraindications to the use of sodium hyaluronate viscoelastic material when used as recommended; care should be used in patients with hypersensitivity to any components in this material (see Precautions).

Warnings/Precautions

➤*Compatibility:* Mixing of quaternary ammonium salts such as benzalkonium chloride with sodium hyaluronate results in the formation of a precipitate. The eye should not be irrigated with any solution containing benzalkonium chloride if sodium hyaluronate viscoelastic preparation is to be used during surgery.

➤*Usage:* Precautions normally associated with anterior segment surgical procedures should be observed.

Cannulas are intended for single patient use only. If reuse becomes necessary on the same patient during the surgical procedures, rinse the cannula thoroughly with sterile distilled water to remove all traces of residual material.

On rare occasions, viscoelastic products containing sodium hyaluronate have been observed to become slightly opaque or to form a slight precipitate upon instillation into the eye. The clinical significance, if any, of this phenomenon is not known. The physician should, however, be aware of this possibility, and, should it be observed, the cloudy or precipitated material should be removed by irrigation and/or aspiration.

➤*Intraocular pressure:* Preexisting glaucoma or compromised outflow and operative procedures and sequelae thereto, including enzymatic zonulysis, absence of an iridectomy, trauma to filtration structures, and by blood and lenticular remnants in the anterior chamber may increase postoperative intraocular pressure. Therefore, do not overfill the eye chamber with sodium hyaluronate viscoelastic preparation; remove all remaining sodium hyaluronate viscoelastic preparation by irrigation and/or aspiration at the close of surgery; and carefully monitor the intraocular pressure, espe-

SODIUM HYALURONATE — OPHTHALMIC

cially during the immediate postoperative period. If a significant rise is observed, treat appropriately.

Instilling excessive amounts of sodium hyaluronate viscoelastic preparation into the anterior segment of the eye may cause increased intraocular pressure.

➤*Hypersensitivity reactions:* Sodium hyaluronate material is obtained from microbial fermentation by a purified proprietary process. Although precautions have been taken to make this device protein-free and it has been tested in animals for allergenic response, this device, used in susceptible persons, may produce allergenic responses

Sodium hyaluronate viscoelastic preparation is a highly purified substance extracted from bacterial cells. However, physicians should be aware of immunological, allergic and other potential risks of the type that can occur from the injection of any biological substance since the presence of minute quantities of impurities (eg, proteins) cannot be totally excluded.

ProVisc contains dry natural rubber; use with caution in patients with latex sensitivity.

➤*Pregnancy: Undetermined.* There is no information regarding sodium hyaluronate in pregnant women.

➤*Lactation:* There is no information regarding sodium hyaluronate in breast-feeding women.

Adverse Reactions

Sodium hyaluronate viscoelastic preparation is tolerated after injection into human eyes during ophthalmic surgical procedures. As with most viscoelastic ophthalmic materials, a transient rise in intraocular pressure has been reported in some cases.

Postoperative inflammatory reactions such as hypopyon and iritis have been reported with the use of ophthalmic viscoelastic materials, as well as incidents of corneal edema and corneal decompensation. Their relationship to the use of sodium hyaluronate has not been established.

In clinical trials, 298 patients were treated with sodium hyaluronate viscoelastic preparation and 224 patients were treated with sodium hyaluronate, an approved comparative device on the US market for more than 5 years. The incidences of adverse experiences that were reported in greater than 1% of the patients are shown in the table below.

Sodium Hyaluronate Viscoelastic Preparation Adverse Reactions Reported in > 1% of Patients

Adverse Reaction	Sodium hyaluronate viscoelastic preparation[a] n = 298 (%)	Control[a] n = 224 (%)
Increased intraocular pressure requiring treatment[b]	22 (7.4%)	17 (7.6%)
Superficial and conjunctival punctate keratitis	12 (4%)	5 (2.2%)
Cystoid macular edema	8 (2.7%)	2 (0.9%)
Posterior capsule opacity	8 (2.7%)	10 (4.5%)
Seidel phenomenon	4 (1.3%)	4 (1.8%)
Conjunctivitis	3 (1%)	3 (1.3%)
Corneal edema	3(1%)	0
Corneal erosion	3 (1%)	0
Sphincter damage	3 (1%)	1 (0.4%)
Uveitis	3 (1%)	3 (1.3%)

[a] There is no statistically significant difference in the number of adverse events between the 2 treatment groups.
[b] Mean IOP sodium hyaluronate viscoelastic preparation = 36.7 mmHg (30 mmHg to 52 mmHg). Mean IOP control = 33.6 mmHg (28 mmHg to 48 mmHg).

Adverse reactions that occurred in less than 1% and in at least 2 patients include: Ocular hemorrhage, corneoscleral leak, suture related adverse reactions, vitreous in anterior chamber, hyphema and hematic Tyndall, synechiae, capsule rupture, and cyclytic membrane.

SODIUM HYALURONATE/CHONDROITIN SULFATE

Rx	**Viscoat** (Alcon)	**Solution:** ≤ 40 mg sodium chondroitin sulfate, 30 mg sodium hyaluronate per mL	0.45 mg sodium dihydrogen phosphate hydrate, 2 mg disodium hydrogen phosphate, 4.3 mg sodium chloride per mL. In 0.5 mL disposable syringes.

SODIUM HYALURONATE/CHONDROITIN SULFATE

Refer to the Sodium Hyaluronate monograph for more and comparative complete information.

HYDROXYPROPYL METHYLCELLULOSE

Rx	**OcuCoat** (Storz)	**Solution:** 2%	In a balanced salt solution. In 1 mL syringe with cannula.
otc	**Gonak** (Akorn)	**Solution:** 2.5%	In 15 mL.[a]
otc	**Goniosoft** (Ocusoft)		In 15 mL.[a]
otc	**Goniosol** (Novartis Ophthalmics)		In 15 mL.[a]

[a] With 0.01% benzalkonium chloride and EDTA.

BOTULINUM TOXIN TYPE A

For prescribing information, refer to the Botulinum Toxin monographs in the CNS chapter.

POLYDIMETHYLSILOXANE (Silicone Oil)

Rx	**AdatoSil 5000** (Escalon Ophthalmics)	**Injection:** Polydimethylsiloxane oil	In single-use 10 and 15 mL vials.

INTRAOCULAR IRRIGATING SOLUTIONS

Rx	**Balanced Salt Solution** (Various, eg, Akorn)	**Solution; intraocular:** 0.64% NaCl, 0.075% KCl, 0.03% magnesium chloride, 0.048% calcium chloride, 0.39% sodium acetate, 0.17% sodium citrate and sodium hydroxide or hydrochloric acid	In 18 and 500 mL.
Rx	**BSS** (Alcon)		Preservative free. In 15, 30, 250 and 500 mL.
Rx	**BSS Plus** (Alcon)	**Solution; intraocular:** 0.0154% calcium chloride, 0.714% sodium chloride, 0.038% potassium chloride, 0.02% magnesium chloride, 0.42% sodium phosphate, 0.2% sodium bicarbonate, 0.092% dextrose, 0.0184% glutathione disulfide	Preservative free. In 10 mL (Part 1) and in 240 mL fill in 250 mL bottle (Part 2).

OPHTHALMIC NON-SURGICAL ADJUNCTS

LID SCRUBS

otc	**Eye Scrub** (Novartis Ophthalmics)	**Solution:** PEG-200 glyceryl monotallowate, disodium laureth sulfosuccinate, cocoamidopropylamine oxide, PEG-78 glyceryl monococoate, benzyl alcohol, EDTA	In 240 mL.
otc	**OCuSOFT** (OCuSOFT)	**Solution:** PEG-80 sorbitan laurate, sodium trideceth sulfate, PEG-150 distearate, cocoamidopropyl hydroxysultaine, lauroamphocarboxyglycinate, sodium laureth-13 carboxylate, PEG-15 tallow polyamine, quaternium-15	Alcohol and dye free. In UD 30s (pads), 30, 120 and 240 mL and compliance kit (120 mL and 100 pads).

EXTRAOCULAR IRRIGATING SOLUTIONS

otc	**Collyrium for Fresh Eyes Wash** (Wyeth-Ayerst)	**Solution:** Boric acid, sodium borate, benzalkonium Cl	In 120 mL.
otc	**Eye Stream** (Alcon)	**Solution:** 0.64% NaCl, 0.075% KCl, 0.03% magnesium Cl hexahydrate, 0.048% calcium Cl dihydrate, 0.39% sodium acetate trihydrate, 0.17% sodium citrate dihydrate, 0.013% benzalkonium Cl	In 30 and 118 mL.
otc	**Eye Wash** (Goldline)	**Solution:** Boric acid, KCl, EDTA, anhydrous sodium carbonate, 0.01% benzalkonium Cl	In 118 mL.
otc	**Eye Irrigating Solution** (Rugby)	**Solution:** NaCl, mono- and dibasic sodium phosphate, benzalkonium Cl, EDTA	In 118 mL.
otc	**OCuSOFT** (OCuSOFT)	**Solution:** Benzalkonium chloride, edetate disodium, NaCl, sodium phosphate dibasic, sodium phosphate monobasic	In 30 mL.

OTIC PREPARATIONS

The otic preparations on the following pages are divided into groups as follows:

Steroid and Antibiotic Combinations
Miscellaneous Preparations
Antibiotics

➤*Patient Information:* For use in the ear only. Avoid contact with the eyes.

Notify physician if burning or itching occurs or if condition persists.

Perforated tympanic membrane is considered a contraindication to the use of any medication in the external ear canal.

Proper use of ear drops –
- Wash hands thoroughly.
- Avoid touching the dropper to the ear or any other surface. For accuracy and to avoid contamination, have another person insert the ear drops when possible.
- Hold container in the hand for a few minutes to warm to near body temperature if it has been refrigerated.
- If the drops are in a suspension form, shake well for 10 seconds before using.
- Lie on your side or tilt the affected ear up for ease of administration. To allow the drops to run in:
  Adults-Hold the earlobe up and back.
  Children-Hold the earlobe down and back.
- Instill the prescribed number of drops in the ear.
- Do not insert the dropper into the ear.
- Keep the ear tilted for about 2 minutes, or insert a soft cotton plug, whichever is recommended.

Products used to soften, loosen and remove earwax –
- Do not use if ear drainage, discharge, pain, irritation or rash occurs.
- If you become dizzy, consult a physician.
- Do not use if injury or perforation of the ear drum exists or after ear surgery unless directed otherwise.
- Do not use for greater than 4 days; if excessive earwax remains after use of this product, consult a physician.
- Any wax remaining after treatment may be removed by gently flushing with warm water using a soft rubber bulb ear syringe.

Otic Corticosteroids

DEXAMETHASONE SODIUM PHOSPHATE

Rx	**Dexamethasone Sodium Phosphate** (Bausch & Lomb)	**Solution, otic:** 0.1% (as phosphate)	In 5 mL.[a]

[a] With sodium citrate, sodium borate, polysorbate 80, edetate disodium dihydrate, sodium bisulfite 0.1%, phenylethyl alcohol 0.25%, and benzalkonium chloride 0.02%.

DEXAMETHASONE SODIUM PHOSPHATE — OTIC

Indications

➤*Otic inflammatory conditions:* For the treatment of steroid-responsive inflammatory conditions of the external auditory meatus, such as allergic otitis externa and selected purulent and nonpurulent infective otitis externa, when the hazard of steroid use is accepted to obtain an advisable diminution in edema and inflammation.

➤*Ophthalmic inflammatory conditions:* Dexamethasone sodium phosphate is also approved for ophthalmic inflammatory conditions. Refer to the monograph in Corticosteroids for specific indications and administration and dosage.

Administration and Dosage

➤*Adults:*

Otic inflammatory conditions –

Usual dosage: A suggested initial dosage is 3 or 4 drops 2 or 3 times daily. When a favorable response is obtained, reduce dosage gradually and eventually discontinue.

Duration of therapy: The duration of treatment will vary with the type of lesion and may extend from a few days to several weeks, according to therapeutic response. Relapses, more common in chronic active lesions than in self-limited conditions, usually respond to retreatment.

➤*Administration:* Clean the aural canal thoroughly and sponge dry. Instill the solution directly into the aural canal.

If preferred, the aural canal may be packed with a gauze wick saturated with solution. Keep the wick moist with the preparation and remove from the ear after 12 to 24 hours. Treatment may be repeated as often as necessary at the discretion of the health care provider.

➤*Storage/Stability:* Store between 15° and 30°C (59° and 86°F).

Actions

➤*Pharmacology:* Dexamethasone sodium phosphate suppresses the inflammatory response to a variety of agents and it probably delays or slows healing. No generally accepted explanation of these steroid properties has been advanced.

Contraindications

Hypersensitivity to any component of the product, including sulfites; perforation of a drum membrane.

Warnings/Precautions

➤*Mask/enhance infection:* In acute purulent conditions of the eye or ear, corticosteroids may mask infection or enhance existing infection.

➤*Caution in herpes simplex treatment:* Employment of corticosteroid medication in the treatment of herpes simplex other than epithelial herpes simplex keratitis, in which it is contraindicated, requires great caution; periodic slit-lamp microscopy is essential.

➤*Sulfite sensitivity:* This product contains sodium bisulfite, a sulfite that may cause allergic-type reactions including anaphylactic symptoms and life-threatening or less severe asthmatic episodes in certain susceptible people. The overall prevalence of sulfite sensitivity in the general population is unknown and probably low. Sulfite sensitivity is seen more frequently in patients with asthma than patients without asthma.

➤*Pregnancy: Category C.* Following topical ophthalmic application in multiples of the therapeutic dose in mice and rabbits, dexamethasone has been shown to be teratogenic.

In the mouse, corticosteroids produce fetal resorptions and a specific abnormality, cleft palate. In the rabbit, corticosteroids have produced fetal resorptions and multiple abnormalities involving the head, ears, limbs, palate, etc.

There are no adequate and well-controlled studies in pregnant women. Only use dexamethasone sodium phosphate solution during pregnancy if the potential benefit to the mother justifies the potential risk to the embryo or fetus. Carefully observe infants born to mothers who have received substantial doses of corticosteroids during pregnancy for signs of hypoadrenalism.

➤*Lactation:* Topically applied steroids are absorbed systemically; therefore, because of the potential for serious adverse reactions in breast-feeding infants from dexamethasone sodium phosphate, decide whether to discontinue breast-feeding or the drug, taking into account the importance of the drug to the mother.

➤*Children:* Safety and efficacy in children have not been established.

Adverse Reactions

Rarely, stinging or burning may occur.

Patient Information

Tell patients to notify their health care provider if burning or itching occurs or if the condition persists.

➤*Teach patients how to properly use ear drops:*
- Wash hands thoroughly.
- Lie on your side or tilt the affected ear up for ease of administration.
- Instill the prescribed number of drops in the ear.
- Do not insert the dropper into the ear.
- Keep the ear tilted for about 2 minutes or insert a soft cotton plug, whichever is recommended.

FLUOCINOLONE ACETONIDE

Rx	**DermOtic** (Hill)	**Oil; otic:** 0.01%	Isopropyl alcohol, light mineral oil, peanut oil. In 20 mL.

FLUOCINOLONE ACETONIDE — OTIC

Indications

➤*Eczematous external otitis:* For the treatment of chronic eczematous external otitis in adults and children 2 years of age and older.

Administration and Dosage

➤*Adults:*

Eczematous external otitis –

Usual dosage: Apply 5 drops of fluocinolone oil into the affected ear twice each day.

Duration of therapy: 7 to 14 days.

➤*Children:*

2 years of age and older –

Eczematous external otitis: See Adults for dosing.

➤*Administration:* Fluocinolone oil is for otic use only; not for ophthalmic use. It is not recommended for use on the face.

To apply, tilt head to one side so that the ear is facing up. Then gently pull the ear lobe backward and upward and apply 5 drops of fluocinolone oil into the ear. Keep head tilted for about a minute to allow fluocinolone oil to penetrate lower into the ear canal. Gently pat excess material dripping out of the ear using a clean cotton ball.

➤*Storage/Stability:* Keep tightly closed. Store at 20° to 25°C (68° to 77°F); excursions are permitted to 15° to 30°C (59° to 86°F).

Actions

➤*Pharmacology:* Fluocinolone acetonide oil is a low to medium potency corticosteroid.

Like other topical corticosteroids, fluocinolone has anti-inflammatory, antipruritic, and vasoconstrictive properties. The mechanism of the anti-inflammatory activity of the topical steroids, in general, is unclear. However, corticosteroids are thought to act by the induction of phospholipase A_2 inhibitory proteins, collectively called lipocortins. It is postulated that these proteins control the biosynthesis of potent mediators of inflammation, such as prostaglandins and leukotrienes, by inhibiting the release of their common precursor arachidonic acid. Arachidonic acid is released from membrane phospholipids by phospholipase A_2.

➤*Pharmacokinetics:*

Absorption – The extent of percutaneous absorption of topical corticosteroids is determined by many factors including the vehicle and the integrity of the epidermal barrier. Occlusion of topical corticosteroids can enhance penetration. Topical corticosteroids can be absorbed from normal intact skin. Also, inflammation and/or other disease processes in the skin can increase percutaneous absorption.

Contraindications

History of hypersensitivity to any of the components of the preparation. This product contains refined peanut oil.

Warnings/Precautions

➤*Hypothalamic-pituitary-adrenal (HPA) axis suppression:* Systemic absorption of topical corticosteroids can produce reversible HPA axis suppression with the potential for glucocorticosteroid insufficiency after withdrawal of treatment. Manifestations of Cushing syndrome, hyperglycemia, and glucosuria can also be produced in some patients by systemic absorption of topical corticosteroids while on treatment.

If HPA axis suppression is noted, an attempt should be made to withdraw the drug, to reduce the frequency of application, or to substitute a less potent corticosteroid. Infrequently, signs and symptoms of glucocorticoid insufficiency may occur, requiring supplemental systemic corticosteroids. For information on systemic supplementation, see the monographs for those products.

➤*Infection:* If concomitant skin infections are present or develop, use an appropriate antifungal or antibacterial agent. If a favorable response does not occur promptly, discontinue use of fluocinolone oil until the infection has been adequately controlled.

➤*Otic use only:* Fluocinolone oil is for otic use only; not for ophthalmic use. It is not recommended for use on the face.

➤*Hypersensitivity reactions:* Allergic contact dermatitis to any component of topical corticosteroids is usually diagnosed by a failure to heal rather than noting a clinical exacerbation, which may occur with most topical products not containing corticosteroids. Such an observation should be corroborated with appropriate diagnostic testing. One peanut-sensitive child experienced a flare of his atopic dermatitis after 5 days of twice daily treatment with fluocinolone topical oil. If wheal and flare–type reactions (which may be limited to pruritus) or other manifestations of hypersensitivity develop, fluocinolone oil should be discontinued immediately and appropriate therapy instituted.

Peanut oil – Fluocinolone oil is formulated with 48% refined peanut oil. Peanut oil used in this product is routinely tested for peanut proteins through amino acid analysis; the quantity of amino acids is below 0.5 parts per million (ppm). Use caution in prescribing fluocinolone oil for peanut-sensitive individuals.

➤*Pregnancy: Category C.* There are no adequate and well-controlled studies in pregnant women on teratogenic effects from fluocinolone oil. Therefore, give fluocinolone oil during pregnancy only if the potential benefit justifies the potential risk to the fetus.

Teratogenic – Corticosteroids have been shown to be teratogenic in laboratory animals when administered systemically at relatively low dosage levels. Some corticosteroids have been shown to be teratogenic after dermal application in laboratory animals.

➤*Lactation:* Systemically administered corticosteroids appear in human milk and could suppress growth, interfere with endogenous corticosteroid production, or cause other untoward effects. It is not known whether topical administration of corticosteroids could result in sufficient systemic absorption to produce detectable quantities in human milk. Because many drugs are excreted in human milk, exercise caution when fluocinolone oil is administered to a breast-feeding woman.

➤*Children:* Fluocinolone oil may be used twice daily for up to 2 weeks in children 2 years of age and older with chronic eczematous external otitis.

Because of a higher ratio of skin surface area to body mass, children are at a greater risk than adults of HPA axis suppression when they are treated with topical corticosteroids. They are, therefore, also at greater risk of glucocorticosteroid insufficiency after withdrawal of treatment and of Cushing syndrome while on treatment. Adverse reactions, including striae, have been reported with inappropriate use of topical corticosteroids in infants and children.

HPA axis suppression, Cushing syndrome, and intracranial hypertension have been reported in children receiving topical corticosteroids. Children may be more susceptible to systemic toxicity from equivalent doses because of their larger skin surface to body mass ratios. Manifestations of adrenal suppression in children include linear growth retardation, delayed weight gain, low plasma cortisol levels, and absence of response to adrenocorticotropic hormone (ACTH) stimulation. Manifestations of intracranial hypertension include bulging fontanelles, headaches, and bilateral papilledema.

Peanut oil – See Hypersensitivity reactions.

➤*Monitoring:* Patients applying a topical steroid to a large surface area or to areas under occlusion should be evaluated periodically for evidence of HPA axis suppression. This may be done by using the ACTH stimulation, AM plasma cortisol, and urinary-free cortisol tests.

Drug Interactions

None known.

Adverse Reactions

➤*Dermatologic:* The following local adverse reactions have been reported infrequently with topical corticosteroids. They may occur more frequently with the use of occlusive dressings, especially with higher potency corticosteroids. These reactions are listed in an approximate decreasing order of occurrence: burning, itching, irritation, dryness, folliculitis, acneiform eruptions, hypopigmentation, perioral dermatitis, allergic contact dermatitis, secondary infection, skin atrophy, striae, and miliaria. One peanut-sensitive child experienced a flare of his atopic dermatitis after 5 days of twice-daily treatment with fluocinolone topical oil.

Overdosage

➤*Symptoms:* Topically applied fluocinolone oil can be absorbed in sufficient amounts to produce systemic effects.

Patient Information

This medication is to be used as directed by the health care provider. It is for external ear use only. Do not use occlusive dressings.

Avoid contact with the eyes. In case of contact, wash eyes liberally with water.

Patients should promptly report any worsening of their skin condition to their health care provider.

As with other corticosteroids, discontinue therapy when control is achieved. If no improvement is seen within 2 weeks, instruct patients to contact their health care provider.

This product contains peanut oil. Use with caution in peanut-sensitive patients.

Steroid and Antibiotic Combinations

Refer also to Patient Information in the Otic Product Preparations introduction for instructions on the use of these products.

Indications

➤*Otic bacterial infections:* Treatment of superficial bacterial infections of the external auditory canal.

➤*Suspension:* Also used to treat infections of mastoidectomy and fenestration cavities.

Administration and Dosage

The usual adult dose is 4 drops instilled 3 or 4 times daily.

Actions

➤*Pharmacology:*

In these combinations –

HYDROCORTISONE: Hydrocortisone is used for its antiallergic, antipruritic and anti-inflammatory effects.

ANTIBIOTICS: Antibiotics are used for their antibacterial actions.

Contraindications

Hypersensitivity to any component.

Warnings/Precautions

➤*Superinfection:* Prolonged treatment may result in overgrowth of nonsusceptible organisms and fungi (eg, herpes simplex, vaccinia, varicella).

STEROID AND ANTIBIOTIC COMBINATIONS, SOLUTIONS

Rx	**Antibiotic Ear Solution** (Various, eg, Geneva)	**Solution**: 1% hydrocortisone, 5 mg neomycin sulfate[a], 10,000 units polymyxin B	In 10 mL.
Rx	**AntibiOtic** (Parnell)		In 10 mL.[b]
Rx	**LazerSporin-C** (Pedinol)		In 10 mL with dropper.
Rx	**Otosporin** (Bristol-Myers Squibb Company)		In 10 mL with dropper.

[a] 5 mg neomycin sulfate is equivalent to 3.5 mg neomycin base.
[b] With propylene glycol, glycerin and potassium metabisulfite.
[c] With cupric sulfate, propylene glycol, glycerin and potassium metabisulfite.

STEROID AND ANTIBIOTIC COMBINATIONS, SOLUTIONS — OTIC

Complete and comparative prescribing information begins in the Steroid and Antibiotic Combinations monograph.

STEROID AND ANTIBIOTIC COMBINATIONS, SUSPENSIONS

Rx	**Antibiotic Ear Suspension** (Various, eg, Geneva)	**Suspension; otic**: 1% hydrocortisone, 5 mg neomycin sulfate[a], 10,000 units polymyxin B	In 10 mL with dropper.
Rx	**Neomycin/Polymyxin B Sulfates/ Hydrocortisone Otic** (Steris)		In 10 mL with dropper.[b]
Rx	**Coly-Mycin S Otic** (JHP Pharm)	**Suspension; otic**: 1% hydrocortisone, 4.71 mg neomycin sulfate[d]	With 3 mg colistin (as sulfate) and 0.05% thonzonium Br/mL. In 5 and 10 mL with dropper.[e]
Rx	**Cortisporin-TC Otic** (Monarch)	**Suspension; otic**: 1% hydrocortisone, 3.3 mg neomycin sulfate	With 3 mg colistin (as sulfate) and 0.5 mg thonzonium bromide. In 10 mL with dropper
Rx	**Cipro HC Otic** (Alcon)	**Suspension; otic**: 0.2% ciprofloxacin, 1% hydrocortisone per mL	Benzyl alcohol. In 10 mL.
Rx	**Ciprodex** (Alcon)	**Suspension; otic**: 0.3% ciprofloxacin, 0.1% dexamethasone	Benzalkonium chloride, boric acid, EDTA. In 5 and 7.5 mL *Drop-Tainer*.

[a] 5 mg neomycin sulfate is equivalent to 3.5 mg neomycin base.
[b] With cetyl alcohol, propylene glycol, polysorbate 80 and thimerosal.
[c] With thimerosal, cetyl alcohol, glyceryl monostearate, mineral oil, polyoxyl 40 stearate and propylene glycol.
[d] 4.71 mg neomycin sulfate is equivalent to 3.3 mg neomycin base.
[e] With polysorbate 80, acetic acid, sodium acetate and thimerosal.

STEROID AND ANTIBIOTIC COMBINATIONS, SUSPENSIONS — OTIC

Complete and comparative prescribing information begins in the Steroid and Antibiotic Combinations group monograph.

MISCELLANEOUS OTIC PREPARATIONS

Rx	**Acetasol HC** (Actavis Mid Atlantic)	**Solution; otic**: 1% hydrocortisone, 2% acetic acid, 3% propylene glycol diacetate, 0.015% sodium acetate and 0.02% benzethonium chloride *Dose:* Insert saturated wick into ear; leave in for 24 hours, keeping moist with 3 to 5 drops every 4 to 6 hours. Keep moist for 24 hours. Remove wick and instill 5 drops 3 or 4 times daily	With 0.05% citric acid. In 10 mL with dropper.
Rx	**Hydrocortisone and Acetic Acid** (Taro)	**Solution; otic**: 1% hydrocortisone, 2% acetic acid, 3% propylene glycol diacetate, 0.015% sodium acetate and 0.02% benzethonium chloride *Dose:* Adults – Insert saturated wick into ear; leave in for at least 24 hours, keeping moist with 3 to 5 drops every 4 to 6 hours. Wick may be removed after 24 hours, but continue to instill 5 drops 3 or 4 times daily as indicated. Children – 3 to 4 drops may be sufficient because of smaller ear canal capacity.	With 0.2% citric acid. In 10 mL dropper tip bottle.
otc	**EarSol-HC** (Parnell)	**Solution; otic**: 1% hydrocortisone, 44% alcohol, propylene glycol, *Dermprotective Factor* yerba santa, benzyl benzoate *Dose:* Insert 4 to 6 drops into ear ≤ 3 to 4 times/day	In 30 mL.
otc	**VōSoL HC** (ECR Pharmaceuticals)	**Solution; otic**: 1% hydrocortisone, 2% acetic acid, 0.02% benzethonium chloride, 3% propylene glycol diacetate *Dose:* Insert saturated wick into ear; leave in for 24 hours, keeping moist with 3 to 5 drops every 4 to 6 hours. Remove wick and instill 5 drops 3 or 4 times daily	In 10 mL.
otc	**Min-O-Ear** (Geritrex)	**Drops; otic**: mineral oil *Dose:* Insert 2 to 6 drops and avoid pushing dropper into ear canal. Remain in position 10 to 15 minutes to allow the water to penetrate.	In 22 mL.
Rx	**Cortic** (Everett)	**Drops; otic**: 1% hydrocortisone, 1% pramoxine HCl, 0.1% chloroxylenol, 3% propylene glycol diacetate and benzalkonium chloride *Dose:* Insert saturated wick into ear; leave in for 24 hours, keeping moist with 3 to 5 drops every 4 to 6 hours. Remove wick and instill 5 drops 3 or 4 times daily	In 10 mL.
Rx	**Cortic-ND** (Everett)	**Drops; otic**: 1% hydrocortisone, 1% pramoxine HCl, 0.1% chloroxylenol, and benzalkonium chloride *Dose:* Adults - 4 to 5 drops into affected ear tid or qid; infants and small children - 3 drops.	In 15 mL.
Rx	**Cortane-B Aqueous** (Blansett)	**Drops; otic**: 1% hydrocortisone, 1% pramoxine HCl, 0.1% chloroxylenol *Dose:* 4 to 5 drops into affected ear tid or qid; infants and small children - 3 drops.	In 10 mL.
Rx	**Cortane-B** Otic (Blansett)	**Drops; otic**: 1% hydrocortisone, 1% pramoxine HCl, 0.1% chloroxylenol *Dose:* 4 to 5 drops into affected ear tid or qid; infants and small children - 3 drops.	In 10 mL.
Rx	**Neotic** (Arbor)	**Drops; otic**: 1% benzocaine, 5.4% antipyrine, 2% glycerin, 1% zinc acetate dihydrate *Dose:* Instill 3 times daily for 2 or 3 days. Before and after removal of cerumen a cotton pledget moistened with product should be inserted.	In 10 mL with dropper.

MISCELLANEOUS OTIC PREPARATIONS

Rx	**Allergen Ear Drops** (Goldline)	**Solution; otic**: 1.4% benzocaine, 5.4% antipyrine, glycerin *Dose:* Fill ear canal with 2 to 4 drops; insert saturated cotton pledget. Repeat 3 or 4 times daily, or up to once every 1 to 2 hours	In 15 mL with dropper.[a]
Rx	**Antipyrine/Benzocaine** Otic (URL)		In 15 mL with dropper.
Rx	**Auralgan** (Deston Therapeutics)	**Solution; otic**: 1.4% benzocaine, 5.4% antipyrine, 0.0097% u-polycosanol 410 alcohol, acetic acid, glycerin *Dose: Acute otitis media* - Fill ear canal, insert saturated cotton pledget. Repeat every 1 to 2 hours until pain and congestion are relieved. *Removal of cerumen*- Instill 3 times daily for 2 to 3 days. Insert saturated cotton pledget after administration.	In 14 mL with dropper.
Rx	**Otic Edge** (River's Edge)	**Solution; otic**: Antipyrine 5.4%, benzocaine 1.4%, policosanol 0.0097%, acetic acid, glycerin *Dose: Acute otitis media* - Fill ear canal, insert saturated cotton pledget. Repeat every 1 to 2 hours until pain and congestion are relieved. *Removal of cerumen*- Instill 3 times daily for 2 to 3 days. Insert saturated cotton pledget after administration.	In 14 mL with dropper.
Rx	**Treagan** (Trigen Labs)	**Solution; otic**: Antipyrine 5.4%, benzocaine 1.4%, u-polycosanol 410 0.0097%, acetic acid, glycerin *Dose: Acute otitis media* - Instill the product, permitting the solution to run along the wall of the canal until it is filled. Avoid touching the ear with dropper. Then moisten a cotton pledget with the product and insert into meatus. Repeat every 1 to 2 hours until pain and congestion are relieved. *Removal of cerumen* - Instill 3 times daily for 2 to 3 days. Insert saturated cotton pledget after administration.	In 15 mL with dropper.
Rx	**Auroguard Otic** (SDA)	**Solution; otic**: 1.4% benzocaine, 5.4% antipyrine, glycerin, oxyquinoline sulfate *Dose:* Instill 2 to 4 drops into affected ear. Moisten cotton pledget with solution and gently insert into ear canal. Repeat 3 or 4 times daily.	In 15 mL.
Rx	**Acetic Acid/Antipyrine/ Benzocaine/Polycosanol 410** (Brookstone)	**Solution; otic**: 0.01% acetic acid, 5.4% antipyrine, 1.4% benzocaine, 0.01% polycosanol 410, glycerin *Dose:* Instill permitting the solution to run along the wall of the canal until it is filled. Moisten a cotton pledget with the product and insert into meatus. Repeat every 1 to 2 hours until pain and congestion are relieved.	In 15 mL with dropper.
Rx	**AABP** (Brookstone)		In 15 mL with dropper.
Rx	**Auralgan** (Deston Therapeutics)		In 14 mL with dropper.
Rx	**Ear-Gesic** (Qualitest)	**Solution; otic**: 5% benzocaine, 5% antipyrine, 0.25% phenylephrine HCl, sodium metabisulfite	In 15 mL.
Rx	**Otocain** (Abana)	**Solution; otic**: 20% benzocaine, 0.1% benzethonium chloride, 1% glycerin, PEG 300 *Dose:* Instill 4 or 5 drops. Insert cotton pledget. Repeat every 1 to 2 hours	In 15 mL.
Rx	**Cresylate** (Recsei)	**Solution; otic**: 25% m-cresyl acetate, 25% isopropanol, 1% chlorobutanol, 1% benzyl alcohol, 5% castor oil, propylene glycol *Dose:* 2 to 4 drops as required	In 15 mL with dropper and pt.
Rx	**Acetic Acid** Otic (Various)	**Solution; otic**: 2% acetic acid with 3% propylene glycol diacetate, 0.02% benzethonium chloride, 0.015% sodium acetate *Dose:* Insert saturated wick; keep moist 24 hours. Remove wick and instill 5 drops 3 or 4 times daily	In 15 mL.
Rx	**Acetasol** (Actavis Mid Atlantic)		In 15 mL.
Rx	**Acetic Acid 2% and Aluminum Acetate Otic Solution** (Bausch & Lomb)	**Solution; otic**: 2% acetic acid in aluminum acetate solution *Dose:* Insert saturated wick; keep moist for 24 hours. Instill 4 to 6 drops every 2 to 3 hours	In 60 mL.
Rx	**Burow's Otic** (Rugby)		In 60 mL.
Rx	**Otic Domeboro** (Bayer Pharmaceutical)		In 60 mL with dropper.
Rx	**Borofair** (Major)	**Solution; otic**: 2% acetic acid, aluminum acetate	In 60 mL.
Rx	**Zoto-HC** (Horizon)	**Drops; otic**:1 mg chloroxylenol, 10 mg pramoxine HCl, 10 mg hydrocortisone, 3% propylene glycol diacetate, benzalkonium chloride. *Dose:* Instill 4 to 5 drops into affected ear 3 or 4 times daily	In 10 mL plastic dropper vials.
Rx	**Oto-End 10** (Larken Labs)	**Drops; otic**: 0.1 % chloroxylenol, 1% pramoxine HCl, 1% hydrocortisone, edetate disodium. *Dose:* Instill 4 to 5 drops into affected ear 3 or 4 times daily. For infants and small children, 3 drops are suggested because of the smaller capacity of the ear canal.	In 10 mL with dropper.
Rx	**Mediotic-HC** (Dayton)	**Drops; otic**: 0.1 % chloroxylenol, 1% pramoxine HCl, 1% hydrocortisone, 0.01% benzalkonium chloride. *Dose:* Adults and children over 12 yr of age: Instill 4 to 5 drops into affected ear 3 or 4 times daily. Infants and children under 12 yr of age - Instill 3 drops in affected ear 3 or 4 times daily.	In 15 mL with dropper.
Rx	**Zinotic** (Arbor)	**Drops; otic**: 0.1% chloroxylenol, 0.5% pramoxine HCl, 1% glycerin, 0.1% zinc acetate dihydrate. *Dose: Adults:* Instill 4 to 5 drops into the infected ear 3 times daily but not more than 4 times daily. *Children 2 years of age and older* - Instill 3 drops into the infected ear 3 times daily but not more than 4 times daily.	In 2 and 15 mL with dropper.
Rx	**Zinotic ES** (Arbor)	**Drops; otic**: 0.1 % chloroxylenol, 1% pramoxine HCl, 1 % glycerin, 1% zinc acetate dihydrate. *Dose: Adults:* Instill 4 to 5 drops into the infected ear 3 times daily but not more than 4 times daily. *Children 2 years of age and older* - Instill 3 drops into the infected ear 3 times daily but not more than 4 times daily.	In 1 and 15 mL with dropper.
Rx	**Otomar-HC** (Marnel)	**Solution; otic**: 1 mg chloroxylenol, 10 mg hydrocortisone, 10 mg pramoxine HCl per mL. *Dose:* Instill 5 drops into affected ear 3 or 4 times daily.	In 10 mL plastic dropper vials.
otc	**Auro-Dri** (Del Pharmaceuticals)	**Solution; otic**: 2.75% boric acid, isopropyl alcohol *Dose:* Instill 3 to 8 drops in each ear	In 30 mL with dropper.
otc	**Ear-Dry** (Scherer)		In 30 mL with dropper.
otc	**Star-Otic** (Stellar)	**Solution; otic**: Nonaqueous acetic acid, Burow's solution, boric acid, propylene glycol *Dose:* Instill 2 to 3 drops before and after swimming or showering	In 15 mL with dropper.
otc	**Debrox** (Glaxo Consumer Health)	**Drops; otic**: 6.5% carbamide peroxide, glycerin, propylene glycol *Dose:* Instill 5 to 10 drops twice daily for up to 4 days	In 15mL with dropper.
otc	**Murine Ear** (Ross)	**Drops; otic**: 6.5% carbamide peroxide, 6.3% alcohol, glycerin, polysorbate 20 *Dose:* Instill 5 to 10 drops twice daily for up to 4 days	In 15 mL.
otc	**Auro Ear Drops** (Del Pharmaceuticals)	**Solution; otic**: 6.5% carbamide peroxide in an anhydrous glycerine base *Dose:* Instill 5 to 10 drops twice daily for up to 4 days	In 15 mL.

Steroid and Antibiotic Combinations

MISCELLANEOUS OTIC PREPARATIONS

otc	**Ear-Gesic** (Qualitest)	**Solution; otic:** 5% antipyrine, 5% benzocaine, .25% phenylephrine HCl *Dose:* Instill solution in the external ear canal allowing the solution to run into the canal until filled. Insert a cotton pledget into the meatus after moistening with the otic solution. Repeat every 2 to 4 hours, until pain is relieved.	In 15 mL.
otc	**E•R•O Ear** (Scherer)	**Drops; otic** 6.5% carbamide peroxide, anhydrous glycerin *Dose:* Instill 5 to 10 drops twice daily for up to 4 days	In 15 mL.
otc	**Mollifene Ear Wax Removing Formula** (Pfeiffer)		With propylene glycol and sodium stannate. In 15 mL with dropper.
Rx	**Oticin** (Teral)	**Drops; otic:** parachlormetaxylenol 0.01 g, proxazocaine HCl 0.1 g *Dose:* Instill 4 to 5 drops into the affected ear 3 to 4 times/day. For infants and small children, 3 drops are suggested because of the smaller capacity of the ear canal.	In 10 mL with dropper.
Rx	**Oticin HC** (Teral)	**Drops; otic:** hydrocortisone .1 g, parachlormetaxylenol 0.01 g, proxazocaine HCl 0.1 g *Dose:* Instill 4 to 5 drops into the affected ear 3 to 4 times/day. For infants and small children, 3 drops are suggested because of the smaller capacity of the ear canal.	Edetate disodium. In 10 mL with dropper.
Rx	**TriOxin** (Vertical Pharmaceuticals)	**Suspension; otic:** 15 mg benzocaine, 1 mg chloroxylenol, 10 mg hydrocortisone acetate per mL	Isopropyl alcohol, PEG-12, PEG-40. In 15 mL.
otc	**Dri/Ear** (Pfeiffer)	**Liquid; otic:** 95% isopropyl alcohol, 5% glycerin *Dose:* Instill 4 or 5 drops in affected ear	In 30 mL.
Rx	**Aurodex** (Major)	**Solution; otic:** Antipyrine 5.4%, benzocaine 1.4% *Dose: Acute otitis media* - Instill solution into ear, permitting solution to run along the wall of the canal until it is filled. Insert a cotton pledget moistened with solution into meatus. Repeat every 1 to 2 hours until pain and congestion are relieved. *Removal of cerumen* - Instill solution 3 times daily for 2 to 3 days to help detach cerumen from canal wall. After instillation, insert cotton pledget moistened with solution into meatus.	Glycerin. In 15 mL.
Rx	**VōSol** (ECR Pharmaceuticals)	**Solution; otic:** Acetic acid 2%, propylene glycol diacetate 3%, benzethonium chloride 0.02%, sodium acetate 0.015% *Dose:* Insert a wick of saturated cotton into the ear canal; the wick may also be saturated after insertion. Keep the wick in for at least 24 hours and keep it moist by adding 3 to 5 drops every 4 to 6 hours. The wick may be removed after 24 hours but continue to instill 5 drops 3 or 4 times daily thereafter, as long as indicated. In children, 3 to 4 drops may be sufficient.	In 15 mL with dropper.

[a] With oxyquinoline sulfate.

MISCELLANEOUS OTIC PREPARATIONS — OTIC

Indications

➤*In these combinations:*

HYDROCORTISONE and DESONIDE – Hydrocortisone and desonide are steroids used for their anti-inflammatory and antipruritic effects.

PHENYLEPHRINE – Phenylephrine is a vasoconstrictor which may be a decongestant.

ACETIC ACID, M-CRESYL ACETATE, BORIC ACID, BENZALKONIUM CHLORIDE, BENZETHONIUM CHLORIDE and ALUMINUM ACETATE (BUROW'S SOLUTION) – Acetic acid, M-cresyl acetate, boric acid, benzalkonium chloride, benzethonium chloride and aluminum acetate (Burow's Solution) provide antibacterial or antifungal action.

CARBAMIDE PEROXIDE and TRIETHANOLAMINE – Carbamide peroxide and triethanolamine emulsify and disperse ear wax.

GLYCERIN – Glycerin is a solvent and vehicle; it has emollient, hygroscopic and humectant properties.

BENZOCAINE – Benzocaine is a local anesthetic.

ANTIPYRINE – Antipyrine is an analgesic.

Otic Antibiotics

OFLOXACIN — OTIC

Rx	**Ofloxacin** (Various, eg, Allergan, Apotex USA, Falcon)	**Solution; otic:** 0.3% (3 mg/mL)	In 5 and 10 mL dropper bottles.[a]
Rx	**Floxin Otic** (Daiichi)		In 5 and 10 mL dropper bottles.[b]

[a] With 0.005% benzalkonium chloride. [b] With 0.0025% benzalkonium chloride.

OFLOXACIN — OTIC

Indications

➤*General information:* For the treatment of infections caused by susceptible isolates of the designated microorganisms in the following specific conditions:

➤*Acute otitis media:* In children 1 year of age and older with tympanostomy tubes due to *Staphylococcus aureus*, *Streptococcus pneumoniae*, *Haemophilus influenzae*, *Moraxella catarrhalis*, and *Pseudomonas aeruginosa*.

➤*Chronic suppurative otitis media:* In patients 12 years of age and older with perforated tympanic membranes caused by *Proteus mirabilis*, *P. aeruginosa*, and *S. aureus*.

➤*Otitis externa:* In adults and children 6 months of age and older, caused by *Escherichia coli*, *P. aeruginosa*, and *S. aureus*.

Administration and Dosage

➤*Adults:*

Chronic suppurative otitis media with perforated tympanic membranes – 10 drops (0.5 mL, ofloxacin 1.5 mg) instilled into the affected ear twice daily for 14 days.

Otitis externa – 10 drops (0.5 mL, ofloxacin 1.5 mg) instilled into the affected ear once daily for 7 days.

➤*Children:*

Acute otitis media in children with tympanostomy tubes –

1 to 12 years of age: 5 drops instilled into the affected ear twice daily for 10 days.

Chronic suppurative otitis media with perforated tympanic membranes –

12 years of age and older: 10 drops instilled into the affected ear twice daily for 14 days.

Otitis externa – (See also Off-label dosing.)

13 years of age and older: 10 drops instilled into the affected ear once daily for 7 days.

6 months to 13 years of age: 5 drops instilled into the affected ear once daily for 7 days.

Off-label dosing –

Otis externa:

- *12 years of age and older* – Instill 10 drops into affected ear twice a day for 10 days.
- *1 to 12 years of age* – Instill 5 drops into affected ear twice a day for 10 days.

➤*Administration:* The solution should be warmed by holding the bottle in the hand for 1 or 2 minutes to avoid dizziness that may result from the instillation of a cold solution. The patient should lie with the affected ear upward, and then the drops should be instilled. This position should be maintained for 5 minutes to facilitate penetration of the drops into the ear canal. Repeat, if necessary, for the opposite ear.

OFLOXACIN — OTIC

Acute otitis media and chronic suppurative otitis media – After instillation, the tragus should then be pumped 4 times by pushing inward to facilitate penetration of the drops into the middle ear.

➤*Storage/Stability:* Store at 25°C (77°F); excursions are permitted to 15° to 30°C (59° to 86°F). Protect from light.

Actions

➤*Pharmacology:* Ofloxacin has in vitro activity against a wide range of gram-negative and gram-positive microorganisms. Ofloxacin exerts its antibacterial activity by inhibiting DNA gyrase, a bacterial topoisomerase. DNA gyrase is an essential enzyme, which controls DNA topology and assists in DNA replication, repair, deactivation, and transcription. Cross-resistance has been observed between ofloxacin and other fluoroquinolones. There is generally no cross-resistance between ofloxacin and other classes of antibacterial agents such as beta-lactams or aminoglycosides.

➤*Pharmacokinetics:* Drug concentrations in serum (in subjects with tympanostomy tubes and perforated tympanic membranes), in otorrhea, and in mucosa of the middle ear (in subjects with perforated tympanic membranes) were determined following otic administration of ofloxacin solution. In 2 single-dose studies, mean ofloxacin serum concentrations were low in adult patients with tympanostomy tubes, with and without otorrhea, after otic administration of a 0.3% solution (4.1 ng/mL (n = 3) and 5.4 ng/mL (n = 5), respectively). In adults with perforated tympanic membranes, the maximum serum drug level of ofloxacin detected was 10 ng/mL after administration of a 0.3% solution.

Ofloxacin was detectable in the middle ear mucosa of some adult subjects with perforated tympanic membranes (11 of 16 subjects). The variability of ofloxacin concentration in middle ear mucosa was high. The concentrations ranged from 1.2 to 602 mcg/g after otic administration of a 0.3% solution. Ofloxacin was present in high concentrations in otorrhea (389 to 2850 mcg/g, n = 13) 30 minutes after otic administration of a 0.3% solution in subjects with chronic suppurative otitis media and perforated tympanic membranes. However, the measurement of ofloxacin in the otorrhea does not necessarily reflect the exposure of the middle ear to ofloxacin.

➤*Microbiology:* Ofloxacin has been shown to be active against most strains of the following microorganisms, both in vitro and clinically in otic infections.

Aerobes, gram-positive – *Staphylococcus aureus* and *Streptococcus pneumoniae*.

Aerobes, gram-negative – *Haemophilus influenzae, Moraxella catarrhalis, Proteus mirabilis*, and *Pseudomonas aeruginosa*.

Contraindications

Hypersensitivity to ofloxacin, to other quinolones, or to any of the components in this medication.

Warnings/Precautions

➤*Administration:* Ofloxacin otic solution is not for ophthalmic use or for injection.

➤*Arthropathy:* The systemic administration of quinolones, including ofloxacin at doses much higher than given or absorbed by the otic route, has led to lesions or erosions of the cartilage in weight-bearing joints and other signs of arthropathy in immature animals of various species.

Young growing guinea pigs dosed in the middle ear with 0.3% ofloxacin otic solution showed no systemic effects, lesions, or erosions of the cartilage in weight-bearing joints, or other signs of arthropathy. No drug-related structural or functional changes of the cochlea and no lesions in the ossicles were noted in the guinea pig following otic administration of 0.3% ofloxacin for 1 month.

➤*Hypersensitivity reactions:* Serious and occasionally fatal hypersensitivity (anaphylactic) reactions, some following the first dose, have been reported in patients receiving systemic quinolones, including ofloxacin. Some reactions were accompanied by cardiovascular collapse, loss of consciousness, angioedema (including laryngeal, pharyngeal or facial edema), airway obstruction, dyspnea, urticaria, and itching. If an allergic reaction to ofloxacin is suspected, stop the drug. Serious acute hypersensitivity reactions may require immediate emergency treatment. Oxygen and airway management, including intubation, should be administered as clinically indicated.

➤*Superinfection:* As with other anti-infective preparations, prolonged use may result in overgrowth of nonsusceptible organisms, including fungi. If the infection is not improved after 1 week, cultures should be obtained to guide further treatment. If otorrhea persists after a full course of therapy, or if 2 or more episodes of otorrhea occur within 6 months, further evaluation is recommended to exclude an underlying condition such as cholesteatoma, foreign body, or a tumor.

➤*Pregnancy: Category C.*

Teratogenic – Ofloxacin has been shown to have an embryocidal effect in rats at a dose of 810 mg/kg/day and in rabbits at 160 mg/kg/day.

These dosages resulted in decreased fetal body weights and increased fetal mortality in rats and rabbits, respectively. Minor fetal skeletal variations were reported in rats receiving doses of 810 mg/kg/day. Ofloxacin has not been shown to be teratogenic at doses as high as 810 mg/kg/day and 160 mg/kg/day when administered to pregnant rats and rabbits, respectively.

Ofloxacin has not been shown to have any adverse effects on the developing embryo or fetus at doses relevant to the amount of ofloxacin that will be delivered ototopically at the recommended clinical doses.

Nonteratogenic – Additional studies in the rat demonstrated that doses up to 360 mg/kg/day during late gestation had no adverse effects on late fetal development, labor, delivery, lactation, neonatal viability, or growth of the newborn. There are, however, no adequate and well-controlled studies in pregnant women. Ofloxacin otic should be used during pregnancy only if the potential benefit justifies the potential risk to the fetus.

➤*Lactation:* In nursing women, a single 200 mg oral dose resulted in concentrations of ofloxacin in milk, which were similar to those found in plasma. It is not known whether ofloxacin is excreted in human milk following topical otic administration. Because of the potential for serious adverse reactions from ofloxacin in nursing infants, a decision should be made whether to discontinue nursing or to discontinue the drug, taking into account the importance of the drug to the mother.

➤*Children:* No changes in hearing function occurred in 30 children treated with ofloxacin otic and tested for audiometric parameters. Although safety and efficacy have been demonstrated in children greater than or equal to 1 year of age, safety and efficacy in infants younger than 1 year of age have not been established. Although quinolones, including ofloxacin, have been shown to cause arthropathy in immature animals after systemic administration, young growing guinea pigs dosed in the middle ear with 0.3% ofloxacin otic solution for 1 month showed no systemic effects, quinolone-induced lesions, erosions of the cartilage in weight-bearing joints, or other signs of arthropathy.

Drug Interactions

Specific drug interaction studies have not been conducted with ofloxacin otic.

Adverse Reactions

➤*Subjects with otitis externa:* The following treatment-related adverse reactions occurred in greater than or equal to 1% of the subjects with intact tympanic membranes

Ofloxacin Otic Adverse Reactions in Otitis Externa Patients with Intact Tympanic Membranes (≥ 1%)

Adverse reaction	Frequency (n = 229)
Application site reaction	3%
Dizziness	1%
Earache	1%
Pruritus	4%
Vertigo	1%

The following treatment-related adverse reactions were each reported in a single subject: Dermatitis; eczema; erythematous rash; follicular rash; rash; hypoaesthesia; tinnitus; dyspepsia; hot flushes; flushing; otorrhagia.

➤*Subjects with acute otitis media with tympanostomy tubes and subjects with chronic suppurative otitis media with perforated tympanic membranes:* The following treatment-related adverse reactions occurred in greater than or equal to 1% of the subjects with nonintact tympanic membranes.

Ofloxacin Otic Adverse Reactions in Patients with Acute Otitis Media with Tympanostomy Tubes and Patients with Chronic Suppurative Otitis Media with Perforated Tympanic Membranes (≥ 1%)

Adverse reaction	Frequency (n = 656)
Dizziness	1%
Earache	1%
Paraesthesia	1%
Pruritus	1%
Rash	1%
Taste perversion	7%

Other treatment-related adverse reactions reported in subjects with nonintact tympanic membranes included the following: Diarrhea (0.6%); nausea (0.3%); vomiting (0.3%); dry mouth (0.5%); headache (0.3%); vertigo (0.5%); otorrhagia (0.6%); tinnitus (0.3%); fever (0.3%). The following treatment-related adverse reactions were each reported in a single subject: Application site reaction; otitis externa; urticaria; abdominal pain; dysaesthesia; hyperkinesia; halitosis; inflammation; pain; insomnia; coughing; pharyngitis; rhinitis; sinusitis; tachycardia.

Patient Information

Avoid contaminating the applicator tip with material from the fingers or other sources. This precaution is necessary if the sterility of the drops is to be preserved. Systemic quinolones, including ofloxacin, have been associated with hypersensitivity reactions, even following a single dose. Discontinue use immediately and contact your physician at the first sign of a rash or allergic reaction.

➤*Otitis externa:* Prior to administration of ofloxacin otic in patients with otitis externa, the solution should be warmed by holding the bottle in the hand for 1 or 2 minutes to avoid dizziness which may result from the instillation of a cold solution. The patient should lie with the affected ear upward, and then the drops should be instilled. This position should be maintained for 5 minutes to facilitate penetration of the drops into the ear canal. Repeat, if necessary, for the opposite ear (see Administration and Dosage).

➤*Acute otitis media and chronic suppurative otitis media:* In children 1 to 12 years of age with acute otitis media with tympanostomy tubes and in patients with chronic suppurative otitis media with perforated tym-

OFLOXACIN — OTIC

panic membranes, prior to administration, the solution should be warmed by holding the bottle in the hand for 1 or 2 minutes to avoid dizziness which may result from the instillation of a cold solution. The patient should lie with the affected ear upward, and then the drops should be instilled. The tragus should then be pumped 4 times by pushing inward to facilitate penetration of the drops into the middle ear. This position should be maintained for 5 minutes. Repeat, if necessary, for the opposite ear (see Administration and Dosage).

CIPROFLOXACIN

Rx	Cetraxal (WraSer Pharmaceuticals)	Solution; otic: 0.2%	As ciprofloxacin hydrochloride. Preservative free. In 14 single-use containers.

CIPROFLOXACIN HYDROCHLORIDE — OTIC

Indications

➤*Otitis externa:* For the treatment of acute otitis externa caused by susceptible isolates of *Pseudomonas aeruginosa* or *Staphylococcus aureus*.

Administration and Dosage

➤*Adults:*

Otitis externa – Instill the contents of 1 single-use container (deliverable volume: 0.25 mL) into the affected ear twice daily (approximately 12 hours apart) for 7 days.

➤*Children:*

Otitis externa –

1 year of age and older: See Adults for dosing.

➤*Administration:* Wash hands before use. The solution should be warmed by holding the container in the hands for at least 1 minute to minimize the dizziness that may result from the instillation of a cold solution into the ear canal. The patient should lie with the affected ear upward and then the solution should be instilled. This position should be maintained for at least 1 minute to facilitate penetration of the drops into the ear. Repeat, if necessary, for the opposite ear.

➤*Storage/Stability:* Store at 15° to 25°C (59° to 77°F). Discard used containers. Store unused containers in pouch to protect from light.

Actions

➤*Pharmacology:* Ciprofloxacin is a fluoroquinolone antimicrobial. The bactericidal action of ciprofloxacin results from interference with the enzyme DNA gyrase, which is needed for the synthesis of bacterial DNA. Bacterial resistance to quinolones can develop through chromosomally or plasmid-mediated mechanisms.

➤*Pharmacokinetics:*

Absorption – The maximum plasma concentration of ciprofloxacin is anticipated to be less than 5 ng/mL.

➤*Microbiology:* Ciprofloxacin has been shown to be active against most isolates of the following bacteria, both in vitro and in clinical infections of acute otitis externa.

Aerobes, gram-positive – *S. aureus*.

Aerobes, gram-negative – *P. aeruginosa*.

Contraindications

Hypersensitivity to ciprofloxacin.

Warnings/Precautions

➤*Administration:* Ciprofloxacin is for otic use only. It should not be used for injection, for inhalation, or for topical ophthalmic use.

➤*Arthropathy:* There is no evidence that the otic administration of quinolones has any effect on weight bearing joints, even though systemic administration of some quinolones has been shown to cause arthropathy in immature animals.

➤*Lack of clinical response:* If the infection is not improved after one week of therapy, cultures may help guide further treatment.

➤*Hypersensitivity reactions:* Discontinue ciprofloxacin at the first appearance of a skin rash or any other sign of hypersensitivity.

➤*Superinfection:* As with other anti-infectives, use of ciprofloxacin may result in overgrowth of nonsusceptible organisms, including yeast and fungi. If super-infection occurs, discontinue use and institute alternative therapy.

➤*Pregnancy: Category C.*

In rabbits, ciprofloxacin (30 and 100 mg/kg orally) produced GI disturbances resulting in maternal weight loss and an increased incidence of abortion, but no teratogenicity was observed at either dose.

Animal reproduction studies have not been conducted with ciprofloxacin. No adequate and well-controlled studies have been performed in pregnant women. The use of ciprofloxacin during human gestation does not appear to be associated with an increased risk of major congenital malformations. Exercise caution when ciprofloxacin is used by a pregnant woman.

➤*Lactation:* Ciprofloxacin is excreted in human milk with systemic use. It is not known whether ciprofloxacin is excreted in human milk following otic use. Because of the potential for serious adverse reactions in breast-feeding infants, decide whether to discontinue breast-feeding or the drug, taking into account the importance of the drug to the mother. The American Academy of Pediatrics classifies ciprofloxacin as compatible with breast-feeding.

➤*Children:* The safety and effectiveness of ciprofloxacin in infants younger than 1 year of age have not been established.

Adverse Reactions

➤*Most frequent:*

Special senses – Ear pruritus, fungal ear superinfection (2% to 3%).

Miscellaneous – Application site pain, headache (2% to 3%).

Patient Information

Advise patients that ciprofloxacin is for otic use only; not for ophthalmic, injection, or inhalation use.

Advise patients that ciprofloxacin is administered 2 times each day (about 12 hours apart) in each infected ear.

Advise patients to use ciprofloxacin for as long as it is prescribed, even if the symptoms improve. Advise patients to wash their hands before use and warm the container in their hands for at least 1 minute prior to use to minimize dizziness that may result from the instillation of a cold solution into the ear canal.

Advise patients to lie with the affected ear upward and instill the contents of 1 container into the ear; maintain this position for at least 1 minute to facilitate penetration of the drops into the ear and repeat, if necessary, for the opposite ear.

Advise patients to discard used container and store unused containers in pouch to protect from light.

Advise patients to immediately discontinue ciprofloxacin at the first appearance of a skin rash or any other sign of hypersensitivity.

The chemotherapeutic agents include a wide range of compounds that work by various mechanisms. Although development has been directed toward agents capable of selective actions on neoplastic tissues, those presently available manifest significant toxicity on normal tissues as a major complication of therapy. Thoroughly consider the risks vs benefits of therapy when using these agents.

Because of the complexities and dangers in cancer chemotherapy, use should be restricted to, or under the direct supervision of, physicians experienced in its use. In addition to drug therapy, surgical excision and radiation therapy also are employed when appropriate.

➤*Handling of cytotoxic agents:* Most antineoplastics are toxic compounds known to be carcinogenic, mutagenic, or teratogenic. Direct contact may cause irritation of the skin, eyes, and mucous membranes. Safe and aseptic handling of parenteral chemotherapeutic drugs by medical personnel involved in preparation and administration of these agents is mandatory. Potential risks from repeated contact with parenteral antineoplastics can be controlled by a combination of specific containment equipment and proper work techniques. The NIH Division of Safety brochure outlines recommendations for safe handling of these agents.

➤*Mechanisms of action:* The mechanism of action by which these agents suppress proliferation of neoplasms is not fully understood. Generally, they affect at least 1 stage of cell growth or replication. Those more active at 1 specific phase of cellular growth are referred to as *cell cycle specific* agents; those that are active on both proliferating and resting cells are *cell cycle nonspecific* agents. The selectivity of cytotoxic agents inversely follows cell cycle specificity. Rapidly dividing normal tissues including bone marrow, blood components, hair follicles, and mucous membranes of the GI tract may also experience major adverse effects.

➤*Alkylating agents:* These agents form highly reactive carbonium ions that react with essential cellular components, thereby altering normal biological function. Alkylating agents replace hydrogen atoms with an alkyl radical causing cross-linking and abnormal base pairing in deoxyribonucleic acid (DNA) molecules. They also react with sulfhydryl, phosphate, and amine groups resulting in multiple lesions in both dividing and nondividing cells. The resultant defective DNA molecules are unable to carry out normal cellular reproductive functions. Examples of alkylating agents include the following:

busulfan
carboplatin
carmustine
chlorambucil
cisplatin
cyclophosphamide
dacarbazine
estramustine
ifosfamide
lomustine
mechlorethamine
melphalan
pipobroman
streptozocin
thiotepa
uracil mustard

➤*Antimetabolites:* Antimetabolites include a diverse group of compounds that interfere with various metabolic processes, thereby disrupting normal cellular functions. These agents may act by 2 general mechanisms: By incorporating the drug, rather than a normal cellular constituent, into an essential chemical compound; or by inhibiting a key enzyme from functioning normally. Their primary benefit is the ability to disrupt nucleic acid synthesis. These agents work only on dividing cells during the S phase of nucleic acid synthesis and are most effective on rapidly proliferating neoplasms. Examples of antimetabolites include the following:

cytarabine
floxuridine
5-fluorouracil
fludarabine
gemcitabine
hydroxyurea
mercaptopurine
methotrexate
thioguanine

➤*Hormones:* These have been used to treat several types of neoplasms. Hormonal therapy interferes at the cellular membrane level with growth stimulatory receptor proteins. The mechanism of action, however, is still unclear. Adrenocortical steroids are used primarily for their suppressant effect on lymphocytes in leukemias and lymphomas and as a component in many combination regimens. The counterbalancing effect of androgens, estrogens, and progestins has been used to advantage in the therapy of malignancies of tissues dependent upon these sex-related hormones (eg, tumors of the breast, endometrium, prostate). These agents have the advantage of greater specificity for tissues responsive to their effects, thus inhibiting proliferation without a direct cytotoxic action.

Examples of hormone agents include the following:

aminoglutethimide
anastrozole
bicalutamide
diethylstilbestrol
estramustine
flutamide
goserelin
leuprolide
medroxyprogesterone
megestrol
mitotane
polyestradiol
tamoxifen
testolactone

➤*Antibiotic:* Antibiotic-type agents, unlike their anti-infective relatives, are capable of disrupting cellular functions of host (mammalian) tissues. Their primary mechanisms of action are to inhibit DNA-dependent RNA synthesis and to delay or inhibit mitosis. The antibiotics are cell cycle nonspecific. Examples of antineoplastic antibiotics include the following:

bleomycin
dactinomycin
daunorubicin
doxorubicin
idarubicin
mitomycin
mitoxantrone
pentostatin
plicamycin

➤*Mitotic inhibitors:* Mitotic inhibitor mechanisms that are not fully understood. Podophyllotoxin derivatives inhibit DNA synthesis at specific phases of the cell cycle. Vinca alkaloids bind to tubulin, the subunits of the microtubules that form the mitotic spindle. This complex inhibits microtubule assembly, causing metaphase arrest. In contrast, paclitaxel enhances the polymerization of tubulin and induces the production of stable, nonfunctional microtubules, thus inhibiting cell replication. Podophyllotoxin derivatives include etoposide and teniposide. Vinca alkaloids include vinblastine, vincristine, and vinorelbine. A new class of agents called taxanes includes paclitaxel and docetaxel.

➤*Radiopharmaceuticals:* Radiopharmaceuticals exert direct toxic effects on exposed tissue via radiation emission. Primary activity is against metastatic disease. Examples include strontium-89, sodium iodide I 131, and chromic phosphate P 32.

➤*Biological response modifiers:* Biological response modifiers have complex antineoplastic, antiviral, and immunomodulating activities. It is believed that the antitumor activity of interferons is a result of a direct antiproliferative action against tumor cells and modulation of the host immune response. Examples of biological agents include the following:

aldesleukin (human interleukin-2)
interferon alfa-2a (recombinant DNA)
interferon alfa-2b (recombinant DNA)
interferon alfa-n3 (human leukocyte)
interferon gamma-1B (recombinant DNA)

➤*Miscellaneous:* Metabolism of altretamine is required for cytotoxicity, although the mechanisms are not clear. Asparaginase is an enzyme that inhibits protein synthesis of malignant cells by inhibiting asparagine, which is required for protein synthesis. Intravesical BCG is a suspension of *Mycobacterium bovis* that promotes a local inflammatory reaction in the urinary bladder and reduces cancerous lesions. Cladribine inhibits DNA synthesis and repair through a complex mechanism. Levamisole is an immunomodulator with complex effects. Procarbazine produces toxic metabolites, which induce chromosomal breakage. Tretinoin is a retinoid related to retinol (vitamin A), which induces cytodifferentiation. Porfimer is a photosensitivity agent. Topotecan and irinotecan are topoisomerase I inhibitors.

➤*Extravasation:* This occurs when IV fluid and medication leak into interstitial tissue. Damage resulting from extravasation of certain antineoplastic agents can range from painful erythematous swelling to full-thickness injury with deep necrotic lesions requiring surgical debridement and skin grafting.

Prevention of extravasation injury – This is based on careful, accurate IV drug administration. Avoid areas of previous irradiation and extremities with poor venous circulation for IV cannula placement. Dilute drugs properly and give at an appropriate rate.

Treatment – Treatment of extravasation includes immediate discontinuation of infusion and appropriate antidote administration. Goals of treatment are palliation and prevention of severe tissue damage. For further information regarding the instillation of a specific antidote, refer to individual product monographs. Consider surgical evaluation if an open wound occurs. Some practitioners recommend leaving the IV cannula in place to aspirate some of the chemotherapeutic agent and administering an antidote to the injured site. Others recommend immediate removal of the cannula and administration of the antidote by intradermal or SC injections. Immediate removal of the cannula followed by application of ice has also been recommended for all agents except etoposide, vinblastine, and vincristine (warm compresses are recommended for these agents). Apply the ice for 15 to 20 minutes every 4 to 6 hours for the first 72 hours. Elevate the affected area.

Hydrocortisone sodium succinate or dexamethasone sodium phosphate have been used on the extravasated site for their anti-inflammatory activity. However, these agents as well as other drugs (sodium bicarbonate, DMSO) are unproven for antidote use. Specific antidotes that are recommended include sodium thiosulfate for mechlorethamine and hyaluronidase for vincristine and vinblastine.

Drugs associated with severe local necrosis (vesicants) include the following –

dacarbazine
dactinomycin
daunorubicin
doxorubicin
epirubicin
idarubicin
mechlorethamine
mitomycin
streptozocin

vinblastine
vincristine
vinorelbine

➤*Nausea and vomiting:* These may be the most prominent adverse reactions of cancer chemotherapy from the patient's perspective. In clinical trials, 17% to 98% of patients reported emesis. At least 30% of patients experience acute emesis despite antiemetic therapy. Uncontrolled emesis may cause serious complications, including dehydration, malnutrition, metabolic disorders, esophageal injury, and aspiration. In addition, the patient's quality of life may be reduced significantly. Prevention and management of nausea and vomiting is an important aspect of cancer treatment.

Antineoplastics can be categorized according to their emetogenic potential based on the frequency of emesis. Level 1 is the least emetogenic, while Level 5 is the most emetogenic. Combining antineoplastic agents may increase the overall risk for emesis. For example, a combination of drugs with the risks factors of 2 + 2 + 2 may give a combined emetogenic risk of Level 3 (or 2 + 2 + 3 = 4 and 3 + 3 + 3 = 5).

Emetogenic Potential of Antineoplastics

Level	Frequency of emesis	Chemotherapeutic agent	
1	< 10%	Bleomycin Busulfan (oral, < 4 mg/kg/day) Chlorambucil (oral) Cladribine Doxorubicin, liposomal Estramustine Floxuridine Fludarabine Hydroxyurea	Interferon alfa Melphalan (oral) Mercaptopurine Methotrexate ≤ 50 mg/m^2 Pentostatin Thioguanine (oral) Tretinoin Vinblastine Vincristine Vinorelbine
2	10% to 30%	Asparaginase Cytarabine (< 1000 mg/m^2) Daunorubicin, liposomal Docetaxel Doxorubicin HCl (< 20 mg/m^2) Etoposide Fluorouracil (< 1000 mg/m^2) Denileukin diftitox	Gemcitabine Methotrexate (50 to 250 mg/m^2) Mitomycin Paclitaxel Pegaspargase Teniposide Thiotepa Topotecan
3	30% to 60%	Aldesleukin Altretamine (oral) Capecitabine (oral) Cyclophosphamide (≤ 750 mg/m^2) Cyclophosphamide (oral) Dactinomycin (≤ 1.5 mg/m^2) Daunorubicin (≤ 50 mg/m^2)	Doxorubicin HCl (20 to 60 mg/m^2) Epirubicin Idarubicin Ifosfamide (≤ 1500 mg/m^2) Methotrexate (250 to 1000 mg/m^2) Mitoxantrone (< 15 mg/m^2) Temozolomide
4	60% to 90%	Carboplatin Carmustine (≤ 250 mg/m^2) Cisplatin (< 50 mg/m^2) Cyclophosphamide (750 to 1500 mg/m^2) Cytarabine (≥ 1000 mg/m^2) Dactinomycin (> 1.5 mg/m^2) Daunorubicin (> 50 mg/m^2)	Doxorubicin HCl (> 60 mg/m^2) Irinotecan Lomustine (≤ 60 mg/m^2) Melphalan (IV) Methotrexate (≥ 1000 mg/m^2) Mitoxantrone (≥ 15 mg/m^2) Procarbazine
5	> 90%	Carmustine (> 250 mg/m^2) Cisplatin (≥ 50 mg/m^2) Cyclophosphamide (> 1500 mg/m^2) Dacarbazine	Ifosfamide (> 1500 mg/m^2) Lomustine (> 60 mg/m^2) Mechlorethamine Streptozocin

The incidence of emesis with these and other agents varies greatly among individuals. Dose, schedule, concomitant therapy, other medical complications, and psychologic parameters may affect the incidence, as well.

Prevention and treatment – Prevention and treatment of nausea and vomiting should include measures such as dietary adjustment, restriction of activity, and positive support. However, if pharmacologic management is necessary, several agents or groups of agents may prove useful. Some drugs that have been used with varying degrees of success, either alone or in combination, include 5-HT_3 receptor antagonists (such as ondansetron, dolasetron, and granisetron), phenothiazines, butyrophenones, cannabinoids, corticosteroids, antihistamines, benzodiazepines, metoclopramide, and scopolamine.

Combinations of antineoplastic agents are frequently superior to single-drug therapy in the management of many diseases, leading to higher response rates and increased duration of remissions. Using agents that work by differing mechanisms may improve antineoplastic efficacy. Neoplastic cells that acquire rapid resistance to a single agent by random mutation develop resistance less rapidly when treated with a combination of agents.

The selection of agents for combination chemotherapeutic regimens is based on mechanism of drug action, cell-cycle specificity of action, responsiveness to dosage schedules, and drug toxicity.

Many lists of chemotherapy regimens have been published; most sort the regimens by the malignancy treated. Acronyms and abbreviations used to describe chemotherapy regimens can be a source of confusion and inaccuracy. Practitioners should be cautious for several reasons, including the following:

1.) a given acronym may refer to several different regimens,
2.) different acronyms may be used for the same regimen,
3.) abbreviations are frequently cited inconsistently in the literature, and
4.) inaccuracies have been propagated in the literature when regimens were cited incorrectly.

Referring to a regimen by an acronym or abbreviation may cause misunderstandings and misinterpretations, with potentially serious consequences. Whenever possible, acronyms and abbreviations should not be used to order drug regimens for patients. Use of abbreviations sacrifices clarity.

This section provides abbreviations to aid the reader when they are encountered. Please keep in mind that the interpretations listed here may not be what the original author intended. If abbreviations are used when writing drug orders, the physician should be called and the orders clarified. Avoid perpetuating erroneous or unclear information caused by using abbreviations.

This is only a summary and is not an exhaustive review. Please consult the primary literature for additional information. Dosage adjustments for renal insufficiency, liver disease, or organ toxicity (eg, decreased granulocyte count) are not included.

Patients may also require additional medications with specific chemotherapy agents, including premedication regimens (eg, antihistamines and corticosteroids prior to paclitaxel), antiemetics, or allopurinol (eg, for patients being treated for leukemia). Consult the prescribing information for specific antineoplastic agents for such recommendations.

As a guide, a number of commonly used combination chemotherapeutic regimens are listed on the following pages. We consistently refer to the first day of chemotherapy as day 1; we renumbered dates for references reporting the first day of chemotherapy as day 0. We specified the number of cycles to be given or the recommended duration of therapy whenever this information was reported in the primary literature references. Older regimens are included for historical reference.

COMMON ABBREVIATIONS OF CHEMOTHERAPY REGIMENS

5 + 2

Use: Acute myelocytic leukemia (AML; reinduction).
Cycle: 7 days. Regimen given once after an induction regimen has been used.

Regimen: Cytarabine 100 to 200 mg/m²/day continuous IV infusion, days 1 through 5
with
Daunorubicin 45 mg/m²/day IV, days 1 and 2
or
Mitoxantrone 12 mg/m²/day IV, days 1 and 2

7 + 3

Use: Acute myelocytic leukemia (AML; induction).
Cycle: 7 days. Give 1 cycle only.

Regimen: Cytarabine 100 to 200 mg/m²/day continuous IV infusion, days 1 through 7
with
Daunorubicin 30 or 45 mg/m²/day IV, days 1 through 3
or
Idarubicin 12 mg/m²/day IV, days 1 through 3
or
Mitoxantrone 12 mg/m²/day IV, days 1 through 3

7 + 3 + 7

Use: Acute myelocytic leukemia (AML; induction—adults).
Cycle: 21 days. Give 1 cycle. If patient has persistent leukemia at day 21, give 1 to 2 additional cycles.

Regimen: Cytarabine 100 mg/m²/day continuous IV infusion, days 1 through 7
Daunorubicin 50 mg/m²/day IV, days 1 through 3
Etoposide 75 mg/m²/day IV, days 1 through 7

"8 in 1"

Use: Brain tumors (pediatrics).
Cycle: 14 days

Regimen: Methylprednisolone 300 mg/m²/dose PO every 6 hours for 3 doses, day 1, starting at hour 0
Vincristine 1.5 mg/m² (2 mg maximum dose) IV, day 1, hour 0
Lomustine 100 mg/m² PO, day 1, hour 0
Procarbazine 75 mg/m² PO, day 1, hour 1
Hydroxyurea 3,000 mg/m² PO, day 1, hour 2
Cisplatin 90 mg/m² IV, day 1, starting at hour 3 (6-hour infusion)
Cytarabine 300 mg/m² IV, day 1, hour 9
Dacarbazine 150 mg/m² IV, day 1, hour 12

ABV

Use: Kaposi sarcoma.
Cycle: 28 days

Regimen: Doxorubicin 40 mg/m² IV, day 1
Bleomycin 15 units IV, days 1 and 15
Vinblastine 6 mg/m² IV, day 1

Use: Kaposi sarcoma.
Cycle: 28 days, continue until disease progression or intolerable toxicity

Regimen: Doxorubicin 10 mg/m² IV, days 1 and 15
Bleomycin 15 units IV, days 1 and 15
Vincristine 1 mg (dose is not in mg/m²) IV, days 1 and 15

Use: Kaposi sarcoma.
Cycle: 28 days for up to 6 cycles

Regimen: Doxorubicin 20 mg/m^2 IV, days 1 and 15
Bleomycin 10 units/m^2 IV, days 1 and 15
Vincristine 1 mg (dose is not in mg/m^2) IV, days 1 and 15

ABVD

Use: Lymphoma (Hodgkin).
Cycle: 28 days for up to 6 cycles

Regimen: Doxorubicin 25 mg/m^2 IV, days 1 and 15
Bleomycin 10 units/m^2 IV, days 1 and 15
Vinblastine 6 mg/m^2 IV, days 1 and 15
with
Dacarbazine 375 mg/m^2 IV, days 1 and 15
or
Dacarbazine 150 mg/m^2/day IV, days 1 through 5

AC (CY/A)

Use: Breast cancer.
Cycle: 21 days for up to 4 cycles

Regimen: Doxorubicin 60 mg/m^2 IV, day 1
Cyclophosphamide 600 mg/m^2 IV, day 1

Use: Sarcoma (bone).
Cycle: 21 to 28 days for up to 6 cycles

Regimen: Doxorubicin 30 mg/m^2/day continuous IV infusion, days 1 through 3
Cisplatin 100 mg/m^2 IV, day 4

Use: Sarcoma (bone).
Cycle: 21 days for 6 cycles

Regimen: Doxorubicin 25 mg/m^2/day IV, days 1 through 3
Cisplatin 100 mg/m^2 IV, day 1

Use: Neuroblastoma (pediatrics).
Cycle: 21 to 28 days for up to 5 cycles

Regimen: Cyclophosphamide 150 mg/m^2/day PO, days 1 through 7
Doxorubicin 35 mg/m^2 IV, day 8

Use: Endometrial cancer.
Cycle: 21 days for up to 8 cycles

Regimen: Doxorubicin 60 mg/m^2 IV, day 1
Cyclophosphamide 500 mg/m^2 IV, day 1

AC/Docetaxel, Dose Dense

Use: Breast cancer.
Cycle: 14 days. Give 4 cycles of AC, followed by 4 cycles of Docetaxel alone.*

Regimen: **Dose Dense AC** (cycles 1 through 4)
Doxorubicin 60 mg/m^2 IV, day 1
Cyclophosphamide 600 mg/m^2 IV, day 1
Pegfilgrastim 6 mg subcutaneously, day 2
followed by
Docetaxel alone (cycles 5 through 8)
Docetaxel 75 mg/m^2 IV, day 1 for 4 cycles
Pegfilgrastim 6 mg subcutaneously, day 2

*Note: Two different therapy sequences (Dose Dense AC followed by Docetaxel versus Dose Dense Docetaxel followed by AC) were compared; the best results are seen when Dose Dense Docetaxel is followed by AC, rather than the converse.

AC/Docetaxel, Sequential

Use: Breast cancer.
Cycle: 21 days

Regimen: Give 4 cycles of AC regimen for breast cancer
followed by
Docetaxel 100 mg/m^2 IV, day 1 for 4 cycles

AC/Paclitaxel, Dose Dense

Use: Breast cancer.
Cycle: 14 days. Give 4 cycles of Dose Dense AC, followed by 4 cycles of Paclitaxel alone.

Regimen: **Dose Dense AC** (cycles 1 through 4)
Doxorubicin 60 mg/m^2 IV, day 1
Cyclophosphamide 600 mg/m^2 IV, day 1
Filgrastim 5 mcg/kg/day subcutaneously (rounded to 300 or 480 mcg), days 3 through 10
Paclitaxel alone (cycles 5 through 8)
Paclitaxel 175 mg/m^2 IV over 3 hours, day 1 for 4 cycles
Filgrastim 5 mcg/kg/day subcutaneously (rounded to 300 or 480 mcg), days 3 through 10

AC/Paclitaxel, Sequential

Use: Breast cancer.
Cycle: 21 days

Regimen: Give 4 cycles of AC regimen for breast cancer
followed by
Paclitaxel 175 or 225 mg/m^2 IV over 3 hours, day 1 for 4 cycles

AC/Paclitaxel-Weekly, Sequential

Use: Breast cancer.
Cycle: 21 days

Regimen: Give 4 cycles of AC regimen for breast cancer
followed by
Paclitaxel 80 mg/m^2 IV over 1 hour, day 1 of each week for 12 weeks

AC/Paclitaxel + Trastuzumab, Dose Dense

Use: Breast cancer.
Cycle: See below, cycle length varies throughout protocol. Give 4 cycles of Dose Dense AC, followed by 4 cycles of Paclitaxel + Trastuzumab, followed by Trastuzumab maintenance.

Regimen: **Dose Dense AC (cycles 1 through 4).** *Cycle:* 14 days for 4 cycles
Doxorubicin 60 mg/m^2 IV, day 1
Cyclophosphamide 600 mg/m^2 IV, day 1
Paclitaxel + Trastuzumab (cycles 5 through 8). *Cycle:* 14 days for 4 cycles
Paclitaxel 175 mg/m^2 IV over 3 hours, day 1
Trastuzumab 4 mg/kg IV, day 1 of first cycle only (loading dose)
Trastuzumab 2 mg/kg IV weekly, days 1 and 8, except for day 1 of first cycle
Pegfilgrastim 6 mg subcutaneously, day 2
Trastuzumab maintenance (cycles 9 through 21). *Cycle:* 21 days for 13 cycles
Trastuzumab 6 mg/kg IV, day 1 (for a total of 52 weeks of trastuzumab throughout protocol)

AC/Paclitaxel + Trastuzumab, Sequential

Use: Breast cancer.
Cycle: 21 days

Regimen: Give 4 cycles of AC regimen for breast cancer
followed by
Trastuzumab 4 mg/kg IV, day 1 for first week only (loading dose); then trastuzumab 2 mg/kg IV, day 1 of each week for 51 weeks (52 weeks total)
with
Paclitaxel 175 mg/m^2 IV over 3 hours, every 3 weeks for 12 weeks
or
Paclitaxel 80 mg/m^2 IV, day 1 of each week for 12 weeks

ACE (CAE)

Use: Lung cancer (small cell).
Cycle: 21 to 28 days

Regimen: Doxorubicin 45 mg/m^2 IV, day 1
Cyclophosphamide 1,000 mg/m^2 IV, day 1
Etoposide 50 mg/m^2/day IV, days 1 through 5

ACe

Use: Breast cancer.
Cycle: 21 to 28 days

Regimen: Doxorubicin 40 mg/m^2 IV, day 1
Cyclophosphamide 200 mg/m^2/day PO, days 3 through 6

AD

Use: Sarcoma (bone, soft tissue).
Cycle: 21 days

Regimen 1: **Patients younger than 65 years of age, or patients without extensive prior radiation therapy:**
Doxorubicin 60 mg/m^2 IV, day 1
Dacarbazine 250 mg/m^2/day IV, days 1 through 5

Regimen 2: **Patients 65 years of age and older, or patients with extensive prior radiation therapy:**
Doxorubicin 45 mg/m^2 IV, day 1
Dacarbazine 200 mg/m^2/day IV, days 1 through 5

Use: Sarcoma (bone, soft tissue).
Cycle: 21 days

Regimen: Doxorubicin 15 mg/m^2/day continuous IV infusion, days 1 through 4
Dacarbazine 250 mg/m^2/day continuous IV infusion, days 1 through 4

ADE

Use: Acute myelocytic leukemia (AML; induction).
Cycle: 21 to 28 days for 2 cycles

Regimen: Cytarabine 100 mg/m^2/dose IV every 12 hours for 16 doses, days 1 through 8 of both cycles
Cytarabine 100 mg/m^2/dose IV every 12 hours for 4 doses, days 9 and 10 of first cycle only (ie, a total of 20 doses are given during the first cycle)
Daunorubicin 50 mg/m^2 IV, days 1, 3, and 5
Etoposide 100 mg/m^2/day IV, days 1 through 5

ADOC

Use: Thymoma.
Cycle: 21 to 28 days, delay subsequent cycles until hematologic recovery

Regimen: Doxorubicin 40 mg/m^2 IV, day 1
Cisplatin 50 mg/m^2 IV, day 1
Vincristine 0.6 mg/m^2 IV, day 3
Cyclophosphamide 700 mg/m^2 IV, day 4

Advanced Stage Burkitt or B-Cell ALL Pediatric Protocol (SNCCL/B-ALL)

Use: Lymphoma (Burkitt or B-cell ALL—pediatrics).
Cycle: 18 to 25 days, based on hematologic recovery. Give Treatment A, then follow with Treatment B after hematologic recovery; repeat alternating treatments a total of 4 times over 5 to 6 months.

Regimen: **Treatment A**
Methotrexate 10 mg/m^2 intrathecal, hours 0 and 72 for first cycle; then hour 0 only of subsequent cycles
Cytarabine 50 mg/m^2 intrathecal, hours 0 and 72 for first cycle; then hour 0 only of subsequent cycles
Cyclophosphamide 300 mg/m^2/dose IV, every 12 hours for 6 doses, given at hours 0, 12, 24, 36, 48, and 60
Vincristine 1.5 mg/m^2 IV, hour 72 (first cycle only: give an additional dose at day 11)
Doxorubicin 50 mg/m^2 IV, hour 72

Treatment B (give after hematologic recovery)
Methotrexate 12 mg/m^2 intrathecal, hour 0
Methotrexate 200 mg/m^2 IV, hour 0 (on day 1)
then
Methotrexate 800 mg/m^2/day continuous IV infusion over 24 hours, begin hour 0 (on day 1)
Cytarabine 50 mg/m^2 intrathecal, hour 24 (on day 2, give at end of methotrexate infusion)
Cytarabine 200 mg/m^2/day continuous IV infusion, days 2 and 3 for first cycle. Increase to 400 mg/m^2/day continuous IV infusion, days 2 and 3 for second cycle; 800 mg/m^2/day continuous IV infusion, days 2 and 3 for third cycle; and 1,600 mg/m^2/day continuous IV infusion, days 2 and 3 for final cycle.

Leucovorin 30 mg/m^2/dose IV, every 6 hours for 2 doses at hours 36 and 42
then
Leucovorin 3 mg/m^2/dose IV, every 12 hours for 3 doses at hours 54, 66, and 78

Use: Lymphoma (Burkitt or B-cell ALL—pediatrics).
Cycle: Repeat based on hematologic recovery. Give Treatment A, then follow with Treatment B after hematologic recovery; repeat alternating treatments a total of 3 times over 4 to 6 months.

Regimen: **Treatment A**
Cyclophosphamide 300 mg/m^2/dose IV, every 12 hours for 6 doses, given at hours 0, 12, 24, 36, 48, and 60
Cytarabine 50 mg/m^2 (50 mg maximum dose) intrathecal, days 1, 2, and 11
Doxorubicin 50 mg/m^2 IV, day 4
Vincristine 1.5 mg/m^2 (2 mg maximum dose) IV, days 4 and 11
Methotrexate 12 mg/m^2 (12 mg maximum dose) intrathecal, days 4 and 11
Filgrastim 10 mcg/kg/day IV or subcutaneously, from day 5 until the absolute neutrophil count (ANC) is at least 1,500 cells/mm^3 for at least 2 consecutive days

(continued on next page)

Advanced Stage Burkitt or B-Cell ALL Pediatric Protocol (SNCCL/B-ALL) (cont.)

Treatment B (give after hematologic recovery)
Methotrexate 12 mg/m² (12 mg maximum dose) intrathecal, hour 0
Methotrexate 200 mg/m² IV, hour 0 (on day 1)
then
Methotrexate 800 mg/m²/day continuous IV infusion over 24 hours, begin hour 0 (on day 1)
Cytarabine 3,000 mg/m²/dose IV, every 12 hours for 4 doses, days 2 and 3
Leucovorin 30 mg/m² IV for 1 dose, hour 42
then
Leucovorin 3 mg/m²/dose IV, every 12 hours for 3 doses at hours 54, 66, and 78
Filgrastim 10 mcg/kg/day IV or subcutaneously, from day 5 until the ANC is at least 1,500 cells/mm³ for at least 2 consecutive days

AI—see DI

AIDA

Use: Acute promyelocytic leukemia (APL; induction).
Cycle: Give a single induction cycle

Regimen 1: Patients 20 years of age and younger:
Tretinoin 25 mg/m²/day PO, days 1 through 90, or until complete remission, whichever occurs earlier
Idarubicin 12 mg/m² IV, days 2, 4, 6, and 8

Regimen 2: Patients older than 20 years of age:
Tretinoin 45 mg/m²/day PO, days 1 through 90, or until complete remission, whichever occurs earlier
Idarubicin 12 mg/m² IV, days 2, 4, 6, and 8

Anastrozole-Goserelin

Use: Breast cancer
Cycle: Ongoing for 3 years

Regimen: Anastrozole 1 mg PO daily, continuously
Goserelin acetate 3.6 mg/dose implant subcutaneously, every 28 days

Anastrozole-Goserelin-Zoledronic Acid

Use: Breast cancer.
Cycle: Ongoing for 3 years

Regimen: Anastrozole 1 mg PO daily, continuously
Goserelin acetate 3.6 mg/dose implant subcutaneously, every 28 days
Zoledronic acid 4 mg IV, every 6 months

AP

Use: Ovarian cancer, endometrial cancer.
Cycle: 21 to 28 days for up to 8 cycles

Regimen: Doxorubicin 50 to 60 mg/m² IV, day 1; consider decreasing initial dose by 25% in patients with radiation therapy during 6 months prior to chemotherapy
Cisplatin 50 to 60 mg/m² IV, day 1

Use: Mesothelioma.
Cycle: 21 to 28 days for up to 8 cycles

Regimen: Doxorubicin 60 mg/m² IV, day 1
Cisplatin 60 mg/m² IV, day 1

Use: Thyroid cancer.
Cycle: 21 days

Regimen 1: Patients without extensive prior radiation therapy:
Doxorubicin 60 mg/m² IV, day 1
Cisplatin 40 mg/m² IV, day 1

Regimen 2: Patients with extensive prior radiation therapy:
Doxorubicin 45 mg/m² IV, day 1
Cisplatin 40 mg/m² IV, day 1

Ara-C-Clofarabine

Use: Acute myelocytic leukemia (AML; induction).
Cycle: 28 to 42 days, based on hematologic recovery. Give up to 3 cycles.

Regimen: Clofarabine 40 mg/m²/day IV, days 1 through 5, except for day 1 of first cycle
Clofarabine 40 mg/m²/day IV, day 6 of first cycle only
Cytarabine 1,000 mg/m²/day IV, days 1 through 5 (give after clofarabine)

Ara-C-DNR (also see DA)

Use: Acute myelocytic leukemia (AML).

Cycle: 14 days. Give 1 cycle. If patient has persistent leukemia on day 14, give 1 to 2 additional cycles as described below.

Regimen: Cytarabine 100 mg/m^2/day continuous IV infusion, days 1 through 7

Daunorubicin 30 or 45 mg/m^2/day IV, days 1 through 3

If leukemia is persistent on day 14, additional doses are given: cytarabine on days 1 through 5 and daunorubicin on days 1 and 2, both at same dose as previous cycle.

Ara-C-DNR, Ambulatory

Use: Acute myelocytic leukemia (AML; consolidation)

Cycle: 28 days for 6 cycles

Regimen: Cytarabine 120 mg/m^2/day continuous subcutaneous infusion (60 mg/m^2/dose every 12 hours for 10 doses), days 1 through 5

Daunorubicin 45 mg/m^2 IV, day 1

Ara-C-Doxorubicin

Use: Acute myelocytic leukemia (AML; induction).

Cycle: 14 days. Give 1 cycle. If patient has persistent leukemia on day 14, give 1 to 2 additional cycles as described below.

Regimen: Cytarabine 100 mg/m^2/day continuous IV infusion, days 1 through 7

Doxorubicin 30 mg/m^2/day IV, days 1 through 3

If leukemia is persistent on day 14, additional doses are given: cytarabine on days 1 through 5 and doxorubicin on days 1 and 2, both at same dose as previous cycle.

Ara-C-Idarubicin

Use: Acute myelocytic leukemia (AML).

Regimen: **Remission induction.** *Cycle:* Give 1 cycle. May be given a second time based on individual response. Time between cycles not specified.

Cytarabine 100 mg/m^2/day continuous IV infusion, days 1 through 7

Idarubicin 13 mg/m^2/day IV, days 1 through 3

Consolidation therapy. *Cycle:* Give 2 cycles. Time between cycles not specified.

Cytarabine 100 mg/m^2/day continuous IV infusion, days 1 through 5

Idarubicin 13 mg/m^2/day IV, days 1 and 2

Use: Acute lymphocytic leukemia (ALL; induction—adults).

Cycle: Give a single cycle.

Regimen: Cytarabine 3,000 mg/m^2/day IV, days 1 through 5

Methotrexate 6 mg/m^2 intrathecally, days 2 and 4

Idarubicin 40 mg/m^2 IV, day 3

Filgrastim 5 mcg/kg/day subcutaneously, starting on day 7 and continued until the absolute neutrophil count (ANC) exceeds 5,000 cells/mm^3

Ara-C-Idarubicin, Ambulatory

Use: Acute myelocytic leukemia (AML; consolidation).

Cycle: 28 days for 6 cycles

Regimen: Cytarabine 120 mg/m^2/day continuous subcutaneous infusion (60 mg/m^2/dose every 12 hours for 10 doses), days 1 through 5

Idarubicin 9 mg/m^2 IV, day 1

Ara-C-Mitoxantrone

Use: Acute myelocytic leukemia (AML).

Cycle: Give 1 cycle. May be given a second time after 28 days based on individual response.

Regimen: Cytarabine 500 mg/m^2/dose IV every 12 hours for 12 doses, days 1 through 6

Mitoxantrone 5 mg/m^2 IV, days 1 through 5

AT (also see Docetaxel-Doxorubicin)

Use: Breast cancer.

Cycle: 21 days for up to 8 cycles

Regimen: Doxorubicin 50 mg/m^2 IV, day 1

Paclitaxel 200 to 220 mg/m^2 IV over 3 hours, day 2 (given 24 hours after doxorubicin)

Use: Breast cancer.

Cycle: 21 days for up to 8 cycles

Regimen: Doxorubicin 50 mg/m^2 IV, day 1

Paclitaxel 150 mg/m^2 continuous IV infusion over 24 hours, day 1 (start 3 hours after doxorubicin)

Filgrastim 5 mcg/kg/day subcutaneously, from day 3 until neutropenia resolves (start 24 hours after completing paclitaxel infusion)

AT (also see Docetaxel-Doxorubicin) (cont.)

Use: Endometrial cancer.
Cycle: 21 days for up to 7 cycles

Regimen 1: Patients aged 65 years and younger, or patients with no prior pelvic radiation therapy:
- Doxorubicin 50 mg/m² IV, day 1
- Paclitaxel 150 mg/m² continuous IV infusion over 24 hours, day 1 (start 4 hours after doxorubicin)
- Filgrastim 5 mcg/kg/day subcutaneously, days 3 through 12 or until white blood cell count (WBC) is at least 10,000 cells/mm³

Regimen 2: Patients older than 65 years of age, or patients with prior pelvic radiation therapy:
- Doxorubicin 40 mg/m² IV, day 1
- Paclitaxel 120 mg/m² continuous IV infusion over 24 hours, day 1 (start 4 hours after doxorubicin)
- Filgrastim 5 mcg/kg/day subcutaneously, days 3 through 12 or until WBC is at least 10,000 cells/mm³

AT ➡ T, Sequential

Use: Breast cancer.
Cycle: 21 days. Give 4 cycles of AT, followed by 4 cycles of Paclitaxel maintenance.

Regimen: **AT** (cycles 1 through 4)
- Doxorubicin 50 mg/m² IV, day 1
- Paclitaxel 200 mg/m² IV (infusion duration not specified), day 1

Paclitaxel maintenance (cycles 5 through 8)
- Paclitaxel 80 mg/m² IV (infusion duration not specified), weekly, days 1, 8, and 15

ATC, Sequential, Dose Dense

Use: Breast cancer.
Cycle: 14 days. Give 4 cycles of Treatment A, followed by 4 cycles of Treatment B, followed by 4 cycles of Treatment C.

Regimen: **Treatment A** (cycles 1 through 4)
- Doxorubicin 60 mg/m² IV, day 1
- Filgrastim 5 mcg/kg/day subcutaneously (rounded to 300 or 480 mcg), days 3 through 10

Treatment B (cycles 5 through 8)
- Paclitaxel 175 mg/m² IV, over 3 hours, day 1 for 4 cycles
- Filgrastim 5 mcg/kg/day subcutaneously (rounded to 300 or 480 mcg), days 3 through 10

Treatment C (cycles 9 through 10)
- Cyclophosphamide 600 mg/m² IV, day 1
- Filgrastim 5 mcg/kg/day subcutaneously (rounded to 300 or 480 mcg), days 3 through 10

ATRA-Arsenic

Use: Acute promyelocytic leukemia (APL; induction and consolidation).
Cycle: Give 1 induction cycle followed by 1 consolidation cycle after hematologic recovery

Regimen: **Induction.** *Cycle:* 85 days. Give 1 cycle.
- Tretinoin 22.5 mg/m²/dose (45 mg/m²/day) PO twice daily, days 1 through 85, or until complete remission, whichever occurs earlier
- Arsenic trioxide 0.15 mg/kg/day IV, days 10 through 85

Consolidation. *Cycle:* 28 weeks. Give 1 cycle.
- Tretinoin 22.5 mg/m²/dose (45 mg/m²/day) PO twice daily, give for 2 weeks followed by 2 weeks of rest; administer on days 1 through 14, days 29 through 42, days 57 through 70, days 85 through 98, days 113 through 126, days 141 through 154, and days 169 through 182
- Arsenic trioxide 0.15 mg/kg/day IV, for 5 days each week (ie, Monday through Friday), give every other month through week 28, on days 1 through 28, days 57 through 84, days 113 through 140, and days 169 through 196

ATRA + CT—see DA + ATRA

Augmented BFM

Use: Acute lymphocytic leukemia (ALL; consolidation and intensification—pediatrics).

Regimen: **Consolidation.** *Cycle:* 9 weeks. Give a single cycle.
- Cyclophosphamide 1,000 mg/m²/day IV, days 1 and 29
- Cytarabine 75 mg/m²/day IV or subcutaneously, days 2 through 5, days 9 through 12, days 30 through 33, and days 37 through 40
- Mercaptopurine 60 mg/m²/day PO, days 1 through 14 and days 29 through 42
- Vincristine* 1.5 mg/m² IV, days 15, 22, 43, and 50
- Asparaginase 6,000 units/m²/dose IM, days 15, 17, 19, 22, 24, 26, 43, 45, 47, 50, 52, and 54
- Methotrexate intrathecal (dose is based on patient's age, as shown below)†:
  - Patients without CNS involvement at diagnosis: Give on days 2, 9, 16, and 23
  - Patients with CNS involvement at diagnosis: Give on days 2 and 9

used in conjunction with
Radiation therapy

Interim Maintenance I. *Cycle:* 8 weeks. Give a single cycle.
- Vincristine* 1.5 mg/m² IV, days 1, 11, 21, 31, and 41
- Methotrexate 100 mg/m² IV, day 1
- Methotrexate 150 mg/m² IV, day 11
- Methotrexate 200 mg/m² IV, day 21
- Methotrexate 250 mg/m² IV, day 31
- Methotrexate 300 mg/m² IV, day 41
- Asparaginase 15,000 units/m²/dose IM, days 2, 12, 22, 32, and 42

(continued on next page)

Augmented BFM (cont.)

Delayed Intensification I. *Cycle:* 8 weeks. Give a single cycle.
Dexamethasone 10 mg/m^2/day PO, days 1 through 21, then taper off over next 7 days
Vincristine* 1.5 mg/m^2 IV, days 1, 15, 22, 43, and 50
Doxorubicin 25 mg/m^2 IV, days 1, 8, and 15
Asparaginase 6,000 units/m^2/dose IM for 6 doses each month, days 4, 6, 8, 11, 13, 15, 43, 45, 47, 50, 52, and 54
Cyclophosphamide 1,000 mg/m^2 IV, day 29
Thioguanine 60 mg/m^2/day PO, days 29 through 42
Cytarabine 75 mg/m^2/day IV or subcutaneously, days 30 through 33 and days 37 through 40
Methotrexate intrathecal (dose is based on patient's age, as shown below),† days 30 and 37

Interim Maintenance II. *Cycle:* 8 weeks. Give a single cycle.
Vincristine* 1.5 mg/m^2 IV, days 1, 11, 21, 31, and 41
Methotrexate 100 mg/m^2 IV, day 1
Methotrexate 150 mg/m^2 IV, day 11
Methotrexate 200 mg/m^2 IV, day 21
Methotrexate 250 mg/m^2 IV, day 31
Methotrexate 300 mg/m^2 IV, day 41
Asparaginase 15,000 units/m^2/dose IM, days 2, 12, 22, 32, and 42
Methotrexate intrathecal (dose is based on patient's age, as shown below),† days 1, 21, and 41

Delayed Intensification II (same as Delayed Intensification I; doses shown below). *Cycle:* 8 weeks. Give a single cycle.
Dexamethasone 10 mg/m^2/day PO, days 1 through 21, then taper off over next 7 days
Vincristine* 1.5 mg/m^2 IV, days 1, 15, 22, 43, and 50
Doxorubicin 25 mg/m^2 IV, days 1, 8, and 15
Asparaginase 6,000 units/m^2/dose IM, days 4, 6, 8, 11, 13, 15, 43, 45, 47, 50, 52, and 54
Cyclophosphamide 1,000 mg/m^2 IV, day 29
Thioguanine 60 mg/m^2/day PO, days 29 through 42
Cytarabine 75 mg/m^2/day IV or subcutaneously, days 30 through 33 and days 37 through 40
Methotrexate intrathecal (dose is based on patient's age, as shown below),† days 30 and 37

Maintenance. *Cycle:* 84 days, continue until 24 months after first interim maintenance in females and until 36 months after first interim maintenance in males.
Vincristine* 1.5 mg/m^2 IV, days 1, 29, and 57
Prednisone 60 mg/m^2/day PO, days 1 through 5, days 29 through 33, and days 57 through 61
Mercaptopurine 75 mg/m^2/day IM, days 1 through 84
Methotrexate 20 mg/m^2/dose PO weekly except for first week, days 8, 15, 22, 29, 36, 43, 50, 57, 64, 71, and 78
Methotrexate intrathecal (dose is based on patient's age, as shown below),† day 1

*Note: The vincristine dose is not capped in this protocol. Consult the prescriber if there is any question about the intended vincristine dose.

†Note: Dose of intrathecal methotrexate is based on patient's age as follows:
Age 1 to 2 years: Methotrexate 8 mg
Age 2 to 3 years: Methotrexate 10 mg
Age 3 years and older: Methotrexate 12 mg

B-CAVe

Use: Lymphoma (Hodgkin).
Cycle: 28 days

Regimen:
Bleomycin 5 units/m^2 IV, days 1, 28, and 35
Lomustine 100 mg/m^2 PO, day 1
Doxorubicin 60 mg/m^2 IV, day 1
Vinblastine 5 mg/m^2 IV, day 1

BCVPP

Use: Lymphoma (Hodgkin).
Cycle: 28 days for at least 6 cycles

Regimen:
Carmustine 100 mg/m^2 IV, day 1
Cyclophosphamide 600 mg/m^2 IV, day 1
Vinblastine 5 mg/m^2 IV, day 1
Procarbazine 50 mg/m^2 PO, day 1
Procarbazine 100 mg/m^2/day PO, days 2 through 10
Prednisone 60 mg/m^2/day PO, days 1 through 10

BEACOPP

Use: Lymphoma (Hodgkin).
Cycle: 21 days for up to 8 cycles

Regimen:
Etoposide 100 mg/m^2/day IV, days 1 through 3
Doxorubicin 25 mg/m^2 IV, day 1
Cyclophosphamide 650 mg/m^2 IV, day 1
Vincristine 1.4 mg/m^2 (2 mg maximum dose) IV, day 1 or 8
Procarbazine 100 mg/m^2/day PO, days 1 through 7
Prednisone 40 mg/m^2/day PO, days 1 through 14
Bleomycin 10 units/m^2 IV, day 8
Filgrastim 300 mcg/day (patients weighing less than 70 kg) to 480 mcg/day (patients weighing 70 kg or more) subcutaneously, starting on day 8, give for at least 3 days or until leukocytes exceed 2,000 cells/mm^3 for 3 days

BEACOPP-14

Use: Lymphoma (Hodgkin).

Cycle: 14 days for up to 8 cycles. Delay subsequent cycles until leukocyte count is greater than 2,500 cells/mm^3 post-nadir and platelet count is greater than 80,000 cells/mm^3 post-nadir.

Regimen:
Etoposide 100 mg/m^2/day IV, days 1 through 3
Doxorubicin 25 mg/m^2 IV, day 1
Cyclophosphamide 650 mg/m^2 IV, day 1
Procarbazine 100 mg/m^2/day PO, days 1 through 7
Prednisone 80 mg/m^2/day PO, days 1 through 7
Vincristine 1.4 mg/m^2 (2 mg maximum dose) IV, day 8
Bleomycin 10 units/m^2 IV, day 8
with
Filgrastim 300 mcg/day (patients weighing less than 75 kg) to 480 mcg/day (patients weighing 75 kg or more) subcutaneously, days 8 through 13
or
Pegfilgrastim 6 mg subcutaneously, day 4*
*Note: A phase 2 study states that a single dose of pegfilgrastim may be given on day 4 or 8 of each cycle. However, the best results were seen when pegfilgrastim was given on day 4.

BEACOPP Escalated

Use: Lymphoma (Hodgkin).

Cycle: 21 days for up to 8 cycles

Regimen:
Etoposide 200 mg/m^2/day IV, days 1 through 3
Doxorubicin 35 mg/m^2 IV, day 1
Cyclophosphamide 1,200 to 1,250 mg/m^2 IV, day 1
Vincristine 1.4 or 2 mg/m^2 (2 mg maximum dose) IV, day 1 or 8
Procarbazine 100 mg/m^2/day PO, days 1 through 7
Prednisone 40 mg/m^2/day PO, days 1 through 14
Bleomycin 10 units/m^2 IV, day 8
Filgrastim 300 mcg/day (patients weighing less than 70 kg) to 480 mcg/day (patients weighing 70 kg or more) subcutaneously, starting on day 8, give for at least 3 days or until leukocytes exceed 2,000 cells/mm^3 for 3 days

BEP (PEB)

Use: Testicular cancer, germ cell tumors.

Cycle: 21 days for up to 4 cycles

Regimen:
Etoposide 100 mg/m^2/day IV, days 1 through 5
Cisplatin 20 mg/m^2/day IV, days 1 through 5
Bleomycin 30 units IV, days 2, 9, and 16

Use: Testicular cancer, germ cell tumors.

Cycle: 21 days for 3 to 4 cycles

Regimen:
Etoposide 165 mg/m^2/day IV, days 1 through 3
Cisplatin 50 mg/m^2/day IV, days 1 and 2
Bleomycin 30 units IV, days 1, 8, and 15, of cycles 1 through 3

Use: Adenocarcinoma (unknown primary).

Cycle: 21 days for up to 4 cycles

Regimen:
Bleomycin 30 units IV, days 1, 8, and 15
Etoposide 100 mg/m^2/day IV, days 1 through 5
Cisplatin 20 mg/m^2/day IV, days 1 through 5

Bevacizumab-Erlotinib

Use: Adenocarcinoma (unknown primary).

Cycle: 14 days, continue until disease progression or intolerable toxicity

Regimen:
Bevacizumab 10 mg/kg IV, day 1
Erlotinib 150 mg/day PO, throughout entire course

Bevacizumab-Interferon alfa

Use: Renal cell carcinoma.

Cycle: 14 days, continue until disease progression or intolerable toxicity

Regimen:
Bevacizumab 10 mg/kg IV, day 1
Interferon alfa-2a* 9 million units/dose subcutaneously 3 times weekly, throughout entire course
*Note: Interferon alfa-2a is no longer available in the United States. The manufacturer discontinued this product in October 2007 for commercial reasons, not for safety or efficacy reasons.

Bevacizumab-Irinotecan

Use: Brain tumor.
Cycle: 14 days, continue until disease progression or intolerable toxicity

Regimen 1: Patients not taking enzyme-inducing antiepileptic drugs:
Irinotecan 125 mg/m^2 IV, day 1 (give before bevacizumab)
Bevacizumab 10 mg/kg IV, day 1

Regimen 2: Patients taking enzyme-inducing antiepileptic drugs:
Irinotecan 340 mg/m^2 IV, day 1 (give before bevacizumab)
Bevacizumab 10 mg/kg IV, day 1

BIC

Use: Cervical cancer.
Cycle: 28 days for up to 6 cycles

Regimen: Bleomycin 30 units IV, day 1
Ifosfamide 2,000 mg/m^2/day IV, days 1 through 3
Carboplatin 200 mg/m^2 IV, day 1
Mesna 400 mg/m^2/dose IV, given 15 minutes before and 4 hours after ifosfamide, days 1 through 3
Mesna 800 mg/m^2/dose PO, given 8 hours after ifosfamide, days 1 through 3

Bicalutamide + LHRH-A

Use: Prostate cancer.
Cycle: Ongoing

Regimen: Bicalutamide 50 mg PO daily
with
Goserelin acetate 3.6 mg/dose implant subcutaneously, every 28 days
or
Leuprolide depot 7.5 mg/dose IM, every 28 days

Bio-Chemotherapy—see Interleukin 2-Interferon alfa 2

BIP

Use: Cervical cancer.
Cycle: 21 days

Regimen: Bleomycin 30 units/day continuous IV infusion over 24 hours, day 1
Cisplatin 50 mg/m^2 IV, day 2
Ifosfamide 5,000 mg/m^2/day continuous IV infusion over 24 hours, day 2
Mesna 6,000 mg/m^2/cycle continuous IV infusion over 36 hours, day 2 (start with ifosfamide)

BiRD

Use: Multiple myeloma.
Cycle: 28 days

Regimen: Cycle 1: Dexamethasone 40 mg/day PO, days 1, 2, 3, 8, 15, and 22
Clarithromycin 500 mg PO twice daily, days 2 through 28
Lenalidomide 25 mg/day PO, days 3 through 21
All subsequent cycles: Dexamethasone 40 mg/day PO, once weekly, on days 1, 8, 15, and 22
Clarithromycin 500 mg PO twice daily, days 1 through 28
Lenalidomide 25 mg/day PO, days 1 through 21
used in conjunction with antithrombotic prophylaxis
Aspirin 81 mg PO once daily, throughout entire course
used in conjunction with other prophylaxis
Omeprazole 20 mg PO daily, throughout entire course
Cotrimoxazole double-strength (160/800) 1 tablet PO twice daily, given 3 times weekly (eg, Monday, Wednesday, Friday), throughout entire course

BOMP

Use: Cervical cancer.
Cycle: 6 weeks

Regimen: Bleomycin 10 units IM weekly, days 1, 8, 15, 22, 29, and 36
Vincristine 1 mg/m^2 (2 mg maximum dose) IV, days 1, 8, 22, and 29
Mitomycin 10 mg/m^2 IV, day 1
Cisplatin 50 mg/m^2 IV, days 1 and 22

Bortezomib + Liposomal Doxorubicin

Use: Multiple myeloma.
Cycle: 21 days for up to 8 cycles

Regimen: Bortezomib 1.3 mg/m^2 IV, days 1, 4, 8, and 11
Liposomal doxorubicin 30 mg/m^2 IV, day 4 (give after bortezomib)

Bortezomib-Melphalan

Use: Multiple myeloma.
Cycle: 28 days for up to 8 cycles

Regimen: Bortezomib 1 mg/m^2 IV, days 1, 4, 8, and 11
Melphalan 0.1 mg/kg/day PO, days 1 through 4

BV

Use: Kaposi sarcoma.
Cycle: 14 days, continue for 2 cycles after maximal response

Regimen: Bleomycin 10 units/m^2 IV, day 1
Vincristine 1.4 mg/m^2 (2 mg maximum dose) IV, day 1

Use: Kaposi sarcoma.
Cycle: 21 days for 6 cycles

Regimen: Bleomycin 15 units/m^2 IV, day 1
Vincristine 1.4 mg/m^2 (2 mg maximum dose) IV, day 1

C-MOPP—see COPP

CA

Use: Acute myelocytic leukemia (AML; induction—pediatrics).
Cycle: 7 days. Give 2 cycles. If patient has persistent blasts at day 15, give a third cycle.

Regimen: Cytarabine 3,000 mg/m^2/dose IV every 12 hours for 4 doses, days 1 and 2
Asparaginase 6,000 units/m^2 IM, at hour 42

CA-VP16

Use: Lung cancer (small cell).
Cycle: 21 days for up to 10 cycles

Regimen: Cyclophosphamide 1,000 mg/m^2 IV, day 1
Doxorubicin 45 mg/m^2 IV, day 1
Etoposide 80 mg/m^2/day IV, days 1 through 3

CABO

Use: Head and neck cancer.
Cycle: 21 days for up to 3 cycles

Regimen: Methotrexate 40 mg/m^2 IV, days 1 and 15
Bleomycin 10 units/dose IV, days 1, 8, and 15
Vincristine 2 mg/dose (dose is not in mg/m^2) IV, days 1, 8, and 15 of first 2 cycles
Cisplatin 50 mg/m^2 IV, day 4

CAE—see ACE

CAF

Use: Breast cancer.
Cycle: 28 days

Regimen: Cyclophosphamide 100 mg/m^2/day PO, days 1 through 14
Doxorubicin 30 mg/m^2 IV, days 1 and 8
Fluorouracil 500 mg/m^2 IV, days 1 and 8

Use: Breast cancer.
Cycle: 21 days for 9 to 10 cycles

Regimen: Cyclophosphamide 500 mg/m^2 IV, day 1
Doxorubicin 50 mg/m^2 IV, day 1
Fluorouracil 500 mg/m^2 IV, day 1

CAF, Dose Dense

Use: Breast cancer.
Cycle: 28 days for up to 4 cycles

Regimen: Cyclophosphamide 600 mg/m^2 IV, day 1
Doxorubicin 60 mg/m^2 IV, day 1
Fluorouracil 600 mg/m^2 IV, day 1

CAL-G—see Larson Regimen

CALGB 8811—see Larson Regimen

CALGB 9111—see Larson Regimen

CALGB 9251

Use: Lymphoma (Burkitt).

Cycle: See below, cycle length varies throughout protocol. Give a single cycle of Treatment A, followed by 6 cycles of Treatment B alternating with Treatment C (ie, 3 cycles of Treatment B and 3 cycles of Treatment C).

Regimen: **Treatment A (cycle 1).** *Cycle*: Give a single cycle
- Cyclophosphamide 200 mg/m^2/day IV, days 1 through 5
- Prednisone 60 mg/m^2/day PO, days 1 through 7

followed immediately by

Treatment B (cycles 2, 4, and 6). *Cycle*: 21 days for 3 cycles
- Ifosfamide 800 mg/m^2/day IV, days 1 through 5
- Mesna 200 mg/m^2/dose IV before, then 4 and 8 hours after each ifosfamide infusion, days 1 through 5
- Dexamethasone 10 mg/m^2/day PO, days 1 through 5
- Vincristine 2 mg (dose is not in mg/m^2) IV, day 1
- Methotrexate 150 mg/m^2 IV over 30 minutes, day 1
- Methotrexate 1,350 mg/m^2/day continuous IV infusion over 23.5 hours, day 1 (begin after 150 mg/m^2 dose)
- Leucovorin 50 mg/m^2 IV, day 2, given 36 hours after the start of the methotrexate infusion
- Leucovorin 15 mg/m^2/dose IV every 6 hours, beginning 42 hours after the start of the methotrexate infusion and continued until the methotrexate concentration is below 0.05 microMol/L
- Cytarabine 150 mg/m^2/day continuous IV infusion, days 4 and 5
- Etoposide 80 mg/m^2/day IV, days 4 and 5
- Methotrexate 15 mg intrathecal, day 1
- Cytarabine 40 mg intrathecal, day 1
- Hydrocortisone 50 mg intrathecal, day 1

Treatment C (cycles 3, 5, and 7). *Cycle*: 21 days for 3 cycles
- Cyclophosphamide 200 mg/m^2/day IV, days 1 through 5
- Dexamethasone 10 mg/m^2/day PO, days 1 through 5
- Vincristine 2 mg (dose is not in mg/m^2) IV, day 1
- Methotrexate 150 mg/m^2 IV over 30 minutes, day 1
- Methotrexate 1,350 mg/m^2/day continuous IV infusion over 23.5 hours, day 1 (begin after 150 mg/m^2 dose)
- Leucovorin 50 mg/m^2 IV, day 2, given 36 hours after the start of the methotrexate infusion
- Leucovorin 15 mg/m^2/dose IV every 6 hours, beginning 42 hours after the start of the methotrexate infusion and continued until the methotrexate concentration is below 0.05 microMol/L
- Doxorubicin 25 mg/m^2/day IV, days 4 and 5
- Methotrexate 15 mg intrathecal, day 1
- Cytarabine 40 mg intrathecal, day 1
- Hydrocortisone 50 mg intrathecal, day 1

CAMP

Use: Lung cancer (non-small cell).

Cycle: 28 days

Regimen:
- Cyclophosphamide 300 mg/m^2 IV, days 1 and 8
- Doxorubicin 20 mg/m^2 IV, days 1 and 8
- Methotrexate 15 mg/m^2 IV, days 1 and 8
- Procarbazine 100 mg/m^2/day PO, days 1 through 10

CAP

Use: Lung cancer (non-small cell).

Cycle: 28 days

Regimen:
- Cyclophosphamide 400 mg/m^2 IV, day 1
- Doxorubicin 40 mg/m^2 IV, day 1
- Cisplatin 60 mg/m^2 IV, day 1

Use: Mesothelioma.

Cycle: 21 days, continue until disease progression or intolerable toxicity

Regimen:
- Cyclophosphamide 500 mg/m^2 IV, day 1
- Doxorubicin 50 mg/m^2 IV, day 1
- Cisplatin 80 mg/m^2 IV, day 1 for first 3 cycles; decrease to cisplatin 50 mg/m^2 IV, day 1 for subsequent cycles

Capecitabine-Bevacizumab

Use: Breast cancer.

Cycle: 21 days for up to 35 cycles, or until disease progression or intolerable toxicity

Regimen 1: Patients with creatinine clearance greater than 50 mL/min:
- Capecitabine 1,250 mg/m^2/dose PO twice daily, days 1 through 14
- Bevacizumab 15 mg/kg IV, day 1

Regimen 2: Patients with creatinine clearance between 30 and 50 mL/min:
- Capecitabine 937.5 mg/m^2/dose PO twice daily, days 1 through 14
- Bevacizumab 15 mg/kg IV, day 1

Capecitabine-Cisplatin (XP)

Use:	Head and neck cancer. *Cycle:* 21 days for up to 6 cycles
Regimen:	Capecitabine 1,000 mg/m²/dose PO twice daily, days 1 through 14 Cisplatin 75 mg/m² IV, day 1
Use:	Gastric cancer. *Cycle:* 21 days, continue until disease progression or intolerable toxicity
Regimen:	Capecitabine 1,000 mg/m²/dose PO twice daily, days 1 through 14 Cisplatin 80 mg/m² IV, day 1
Use:	Biliary tract cancer *Cycle:* 21 days, continue until disease progression or intolerable toxicity
Regimen:	Capecitabine 1,250 mg/m²/dose PO twice daily, days 1 through 14 Cisplatin 60 mg/m² IV, day 1

Capecitabine-Docetaxel (X + T)

Use:	Breast cancer. *Cycle:* 21 days, continue until disease progression or intolerable toxicity
Regimen:	Capecitabine 1,250 mg/m²/dose PO twice daily, days 1 through 14 Docetaxel 75 mg/m² IV, day 1

Capecitabine-Docetaxel-Trastuzumab (XTH)

Use:	Breast cancer. *Cycle:* 21 days for up to 4 cycles
Regimen:	Capecitabine 825 mg/m²/dose PO twice daily, days 1 through 14 Docetaxel 75 mg/m² IV, day 1 Trastuzumab 4 mg/kg IV, day 1 of first cycle only (loading dose) Trastuzumab 2 mg/kg IV weekly, days 1, 8, and 15, except for day 1 of first cycle

Capecitabine-Erlotinib

Use:	Pancreatic cancer. *Cycle:* 21 days, continue until disease progression or intolerable toxicity
Regimen:	Capecitabine 1,000 mg/m²/dose PO twice daily, days 1 through 14 Erlotinib 150 mg/day PO, throughout entire course

Capecitabine-Trastuzumab

Use:	Breast cancer *Cycle:* 21 days, continue until disease progression or intolerable toxicity
Regimen:	Capecitabine 1,250 mg/m²/dose PO twice daily, days 1 through 14 *with* Trastuzumab 4 mg/kg IV, day 1 of first cycle only (loading dose); then trastuzumab 2 mg/kg IV weekly, days 1, 8, and 15, except for day 1 of first cycle *or* Trastuzumab 8 mg/kg IV, day 1 of first cycle only (loading dose); then trastuzumab 6 mg/kg IV, day 1 of subsequent cycles

CapeOx-B, Modified (also see XELOX + Bevacizumab)

Use:	Colorectal cancer. *Cycle:* 21 days, continue until disease progression or intolerable toxicity
Regimen 1:	Patients with creatinine clearance greater than 50 mL/min: Capecitabine 850 mg/m²/dose PO twice daily, days 1 through 14 Bevacizumab 7.5 mg/kg IV, day 1 (give before oxaliplatin) Oxaliplatin 130 mg/m² IV, day 1
Regimen 2:	Patients with creatinine clearance between 30 and 50 mL/min: Capecitabine 650 mg/m²/dose PO twice daily, days 1 through 14 Bevacizumab 7.5 mg/kg IV, day 1 (give before oxaliplatin) Oxaliplatin 130 mg/m² IV, day 1

CAPIRI (also see XELIRI)

Use:	Colorectal cancer. *Cycle:* 21 days
Regimen:	Capecitabine 1,000 mg/m²/dose PO twice daily, days 1 through 14 Irinotecan 80 to 100 mg/m² IV, days 1 and 8

Carbo-Tax (also see CaT; also see CT; also see Paclitaxel-Carboplatin; also see PC)

Use: Ovarian cancer.
Cycle: 21 days for up to 8 cycles

Regimen: Paclitaxel 175 mg/m^2 IV over 3 hours, day 1
Carboplatin IV dose by Calvert equation to AUC 5 to 7.5 mg/mL/min, day 1 (give after paclitaxel)

Use: Ovarian cancer.
Cycle: 21 days

Regimen: Paclitaxel 185 mg/m^2 IV over 3 hours, day 1
Carboplatin IV dose by Calvert equation to AUC 6 mg/mL/min, day 1 (give after paclitaxel)

Use: Adenocarcinoma (unknown primary).
Cycle: 21 days for up to 8 cycles

Regimen: Carboplatin IV dose by Calvert equation to AUC 6 mg/mL/min, day 1
Paclitaxel 200 mg/m^2 IV over 3 hours, day 1 (give after carboplatin)
Filgrastim 300 mcg/day subcutaneously, days 5 through 12

Use: Breast cancer.
Cycle: 21 days, continue until disease progression or intolerable toxicity

Regimen: Paclitaxel 200 mg/m^2 IV over 3 hours, day 1
Carboplatin IV dose by Calvert equation to AUC 6 mg/mL/min, day 1 (after paclitaxel)

Carboplatin-Docetaxel

Use: Breast cancer, lung cancer (non-small cell).
Cycle: 21 days for up to 6 cycles or until disease progression or intolerable toxicity

Regimen: Docetaxel 75 mg/m^2 IV, day 1
Carboplatin IV dose by Calvert equation to AUC 6 mg/mL/min, day 1 (give after docetaxel)

Use: Lung cancer (non-small cell).
Cycle: 21 to 28 days, continue until disease progression or intolerable toxicity.

Regimen: Carboplatin IV dose by Calvert equation to AUC 6 mg/mL/min, day 1
Docetaxel 60 to 70 mg/m^2 IV, day 1 (give after carboplatin)

Carboplatin-Fluorouracil—see CF

Carboplatin-Irinotecan

Use: Lung cancer (small cell).
Cycle: 28 days for up to 6 cycles

Regimen: Irinotecan 50 mg/m^2 IV, days 1, 8, and 15
Carboplatin IV dose by Calvert equation to AUC 5 mg/mL/min, day 1

Use: Lung cancer (small cell).
Cycle: 21 days for up to 4 cycles

Regimen: Irinotecan 175 mg/m^2 IV, day 1
Carboplatin IV dose by Calvert equation to AUC 4 mg/mL/min, day 1

Carboplatin-Weekly Paclitaxel + Maintenance Paclitaxel

Use: Lung cancer (non-small cell).
Cycle: 28 days. Give 4 cycles of Carboplatin-Paclitaxel, followed by maintenance paclitaxel.

Regimen: **Carboplatin-Paclitaxel** (cycles 1 through 4)
Paclitaxel 100 mg/m^2 IV over 3 hours, days 1, 8, and 15
Carboplatin IV dose by Calvert equation to AUC 6 mg/mL/min, day 1 (give after paclitaxel)
followed by
Maintenance Paclitaxel. *Cycle:* 28 days, continue until disease progression or intolerable toxicity
Paclitaxel 70 mg/m^2 IV over 3 hours, weekly for 3 weeks, followed by 1 week of rest; administer on days 1, 8, and 15

CaT (also see Carbo-Tax; also see CT; also see Paclitaxel-Carboplatin; also see PC)

Use: Adenocarcinoma (unknown primary), lung cancer (non-small cell), ovarian cancer.
Cycle: 21 days for up to 6 cycles

Regimen: Paclitaxel 175 mg/m^2 IV over 3 hours, day 1
or
Paclitaxel 135 mg/m^2/day continuous IV infusion over 24 hours, day 1
with
Carboplatin IV dose by Calvert equation to AUC 7.5 mg/mL/min, day 1 or 2 (give after paclitaxel infusion)

Use: Lung cancer (non-small cell).
Cycle: 21 days for 4 to 9 cycles, or until disease progression or intolerable toxicity

Regimen: Paclitaxel 175 to 225 mg/m^2 IV over 3 hours, day 1
Carboplatin IV dose by Calvert equation to AUC 6 mg/mL/min, day 1 (give after paclitaxel)

(continued on next page)

CaT (also see Carbo-Tax; also see CT; also see Paclitaxel-Carboplatin; also see PC) (cont.)

Use:	Lung cancer (non-small cell). *Cycle:* 7 days for 7 cycles
Regimen:	Carboplatin IV dose by Calvert equation to AUC 2 mg/mL/min, day 1 (sequence of administration not specified) Paclitaxel 50 mg/m^2 IV over 1 hour, day 1 *used in conjunction with* Radiation therapy, days 1 through 48 *followed by 1 additional day of chemotherapy given 3 weeks after the end of radiation therapy* Paclitaxel 200 mg/m^2 IV over 3 hours, day 1 Carboplatin IV dose by Calvert equation to AUC 6 mg/mL/min, day 1 (give after paclitaxel)
Use:	Lung cancer (small cell). *Cycle:* 28 days for 6 cycles
Regimen:	Carboplatin IV dose by Calvert equation to AUC 2 mg/mL/min, days 1, 8, and 15 (sequence of administration not specified) Paclitaxel 80 mg/m^2 IV over 1 hour, days 1, 8, and 15

CAV (VAC)

Use:	Lung cancer (small cell). *Cycle:* 21 days for up to 6 cycles
Regimen:	Cyclophosphamide 1,000 mg/m^2 IV, day 1 Doxorubicin 40 to 50 mg/m^2 IV, day 1 Vincristine 1 to 1.4 mg/m^2 (2 mg maximum dose) IV, day 1
Use:	Sarcoma (bone). *Cycle:* 21 days for up to 1 year
Regimen:	Cyclophosphamide 1,200 mg/m^2 IV, day 1 *with* Doxorubicin 75 mg/m^2 IV, day 1 for first 5 to 6 cycles (up to maximum cumulative dose of doxorubicin 375 to 450 mg/m^2) *or* Dactinomycin 1.25 mg/m^2 IV, day 1 for subsequent cycles after maximum cumulative doxorubicin dose is reached *with* Vincristine 1.4 or 2 mg/m^2 (2 mg maximum dose) IV, day 1 Mesna 240 mg/m^2/dose IV, given before and 4 and 8 hours after cyclophosphamide, day 1
Use:	Merkel cell carcinoma. *Cycle:* 21 days, continue until maximal response
Regimen:	Cyclophosphamide 1,000 mg/m^2 IV, day 1 Doxorubicin 45 mg/m^2 IV, day 1 Vincristine 2 mg (dose is not in mg/m^2) IV, day 1

CAV/EP

Use:	Lung cancer (small cell). *Cycle:* 42 days for 3 cycles
Regimen:	Cyclophosphamide 1,000 mg/m^2 IV, day 1 Doxorubicin 50 mg/m^2 IV, day 1 Vincristine* 1.2 mg/m^2 IV, day 1 Etoposide 100 mg/m^2/day IV, days 22 through 24 Cisplatin 25 mg/m^2/day IV, days 22 through 24 *Note: The vincristine dose is not capped in this protocol. Consult the prescriber if there is any question about the intended vincristine dose.

CAV/IE

Use:	Sarcoma (bone). *Cycle:* 21 days for up to 1 year
Regimen:	Alternate CAV and IE regimens every 21 days

CAV + P/VP

Use: Neuroblastoma (pediatrics).

Cycle: Repeat based on hematologic recovery, usually every 20 to 31 days for 7 cycles. Delay subsequent cycles until hematologic recovery.

Regimen: **CAV** (cycles 1, 2, 4, and 6)

Cyclophosphamide 70 mg/kg/day IV, days 1 and 2
Doxorubicin 25 mg/m^2/day continuous IV infusion, days 1 through 3
Vincristine* 0.033 mg/kg/day (dose is not in mg/m^2) continuous IV infusion, days 1 through 3
Vincristine* 1.5 mg/m^2 IV, day 9

P/VP (cycles 3, 5, and 7)

Cisplatin 50 mg/m^2/day IV, days 1 through 4
Etoposide 200 mg/m^2/day IV, days 1 through 3

used in conjunction with antimicrobial prophylaxis†

Cotrimoxazole (either 80/400 or 160/800 strength) 1 tablet PO daily, throughout entire course

*Note: The vincristine dose is not capped in this protocol. Consult the prescriber if there is any question about the intended vincristine dose.

†Note: Antimicrobial prophylaxis doses not specified in original article; the dose given here is derived from the Aberg *Infectious Diseases Handbook,* 6th edition, a tertiary resource.

CAVE

Use: Lung cancer (small cell).

Cycle: 21 days for up to 5 cycles

Regimen:

Cyclophosphamide 1,000 mg/m^2 IV, day 1
Doxorubicin 50 mg/m^2 IV, day 1
Vincristine 2 mg (dose is not in mg/m^2) IV, day 1
Etoposide 100 mg/m^2/day IV, days 2 through 4

CC

Use: Ovarian cancer.

Cycle: 28 days for up to 6 cycles

Regimen:

Cyclophosphamide 600 mg/m^2 IV, day 1
Carboplatin 300 to 350 mg/m^2 IV, day 1

CCG 1891 – Double-Delayed Intensification

Use: Acute lymphocytic leukemia (ALL; consolidation, intensification, and maintenance—pediatrics).

Regimen: **Consolidation.** *Cycle:* 4 weeks. Give a single cycle.

Mercaptopurine 75 mg/m^2/day PO, days 1 through 28
Vincristine* 1.5 mg/m^2 IV, day 1
Methotrexate intrathecal (dose is based on patient's age, as shown below) weekly,† days 1, 8, 15, and 22
may be used in conjunction with
Radiation therapy

Interim Maintenance and Delayed Intensification. *Cycle:* 8 weeks. Repeat cycles ABAB for 4 cycles total.

Treatment A: Interim Maintenance (cycles 1 and 3)

Prednisone 40 mg/m^2/day PO, days 1 through 5 and days 29 through 33
Mercaptopurine 75 mg/m^2/day PO, days 1 through 56
Methotrexate 20 mg/m^2/dose PO weekly, days 1, 8, 15, 22, 29, 36, 43, and 50
Vincristine* 1.5 mg/m^2 IV, days 1 and 29
Methotrexate intrathecal (dose is based on patient's age as shown below),† day 1

Treatment B: Delayed Intensification (cycles 2 and 4)

Dexamethasone 10 mg/m^2/day IV or PO, days 1 through 21, then taper off over next 7 days
Vincristine* 1.5 mg/m^2 IV, days 1, 8, and 15
Doxorubicin 25 mg/m^2 IV, days 1, 8, and 15
Asparaginase 6,000 units/m^2/dose IM 3 times weekly for 6 doses (eg, days 2, 5, 7, 9, 12, and 14)
Cyclophosphamide 1,000 mg/m^2 IV, day 29
Cytarabine 75 mg/m^2/day IV or subcutaneously, days 30 through 33 and days 37 through 40
Thioguanine 60 mg/m^2/day PO, days 29 through 42
Methotrexate intrathecal (dose is based on patient's age as shown below),† days 29 and 36

Maintenance. *Cycle:* 84 days, continue until 24 months after first interim maintenance in females and until 36 months after first interim maintenance in males.

Prednisone 40 mg/m^2/day PO, days 1 through 5, days 29 through 33, and days 57 through 61
Vincristine* 1.5 mg/m^2 IV, days 1, 29, and 57
Mercaptopurine 75 mg/m^2/day PO, days 1 through 84
Methotrexate 20 mg/m^2/dose PO weekly, days 1, 8, 15, 22, 29, 36, 43, 50, 57, 64, 71, and 78
Methotrexate intrathecal (dose is based on patient's age as shown below),† day 1

*Note: The vincristine dose is not capped in this protocol. Consult the prescriber if there is any question about the intended vincristine dose.

†Note: Dose of intrathecal methotrexate is based on patient's age as follows:

Age 1 to 2 years: Methotrexate 8 mg
Age 2 to 3 years: Methotrexate 10 mg
Age 3 years and older: Methotrexate 12 mg

CCG 1922 – OD, Induction

Use: Acute lymphocytic leukemia (ALL—pediatrics).

Regimen: **Induction.** *Cycle:* 28 days. Give a single cycle.

Dexamethasone 2 mg/m^2/dose (6 mg/m^2/day) PO 3 times daily, days 1 through 28
Vincristine* 1.5 mg/m^2 IV weekly, days 1, 8, 15, and 22
Asparaginase 6,000 units/m^2/dose IM 3 times weekly for 9 doses, starting between days 2 and 4 (eg, days 3, 5, 7, 10, 12, 14, 17, 19, and 21)
Methotrexate intrathecal (dose is based on patient's age, as shown below):†
Patients without CNS involvement at diagnosis: Give on days 1 and 15
Patients with CNS involvement at diagnosis: Give once weekly on days 1, 8, 15, and 22

Consolidation. *Cycle:* 84 days. Give a single cycle.

Dexamethasone 2 mg/m^2/dose (6 mg/m^2/day) PO 3 times daily, days 29 through 33 and days 57 through 61
Vincristine* 1.5 mg/m^2 IV, days 1, 29, and 57
Mercaptopurine 75 mg/m^2/day PO, days 1 through 71
Methotrexate 20 mg/m^2/dose PO, days 29, 36, 43, 50, 57, 64, and 71
Methotrexate intrathecal (dose is based on patient's age, as shown below):†
Patients without CNS involvement at diagnosis: Give once weekly on days 1, 8, 15, and 22
Patients with CNS involvement at diagnosis: Give on days 1 and 15

Delayed Intensification. *Cycle:* 56 days. Give a single cycle.

Dexamethasone 10 mg/m^2/day PO, days 1 through 21, then taper off over next 7 days
Vincristine* 1.5 mg/m^2 IV, days 1, 8, and 15
Asparaginase 6,000 units/m^2/dose IM 3 times weekly for 6 doses total, given between days 3 and 17 (eg, days 3, 6, 8, 10, 13, and 15)
Doxorubicin 25 mg/m^2 IV, days 1, 8, and 15
Cyclophosphamide 1,000 mg/m^2 IV, day 29
Thioguanine 60 mg/m^2/day PO, days 29 through 42
Cytarabine 75 mg/m^2/day IV, days 30 through 33 and days 37 through 40
Methotrexate intrathecal (dose is based on patient's age, as shown below)†, day 29

Maintenance. *Cycle:* 84 days, continue until 26 months after diagnosis in females and until 38 months after diagnosis in males.

Dexamethasone 6 mg/m^2/day PO for 5 days each month, days 1 through 5, days 29 through 33, and days 57 through 61
Mercaptopurine 75 mg/m^2/day PO, days 1 through 84
Vincristine* 1.5 mg/m^2 IV, days 1, 29, and 57
Methotrexate 20 mg/m^2/dose PO weekly except for first week, days 8, 15, 22, 29, 36, 43, 50, 57, 64, 71, and 78
Methotrexate intrathecal (dose is based on patient's age, as shown below),† day 1

*Note: The vincristine dose is not capped in this protocol. Consult the prescriber if there is any question about the intended vincristine dose.

†Note: Dose of intrathecal methotrexate is based on patient's age as follows:
Age 1 to 2 years: Methotrexate 8 mg
Age 2 to 3 years: Methotrexate 10 mg
Age 3 years and older: Methotrexate 12 mg

CCG 1962, Induction

Use: Acute lymphocytic leukemia (ALL; induction—pediatrics).
Cycle: 28 days. Give a single cycle.

Regimen: Vincristine* 1.5 mg/m^2 IV weekly, days 1, 8, 15, and 22
Prednisone 40 mg/m^2/day PO daily, days 1 through 28, then taper off over next 10 days
with
Pegaspargase 2,500 units/m^2 IM, day 4
or
Asparaginase 6,000 units/m^2/dose IM for 9 doses, days 4, 6, 9, 11, 13, 16, 18, 20, and 23
used in conjunction with
Intrathecal chemotherapy
*Note: The vincristine dose is not capped in this protocol. Consult the prescriber if there is any question about the intended vincristine dose.

CD

Use: Hepatoblastoma (pediatrics).
Cycle: 21 days for up to 6 cycles

Regimen 1: Patients weighing less than 10 kg:
Cisplatin 2.67 mg/kg IV, day 1
Doxorubicin 1 mg/kg/day continuous IV infusion, days 2 through 3

Regimen 2: Patients weighing at least 10 kg:
Cisplatin 80 mg/m^2/day continuous IV infusion, day 1
Doxorubicin 30 mg/m^2/day continuous IV infusion, days 2 through 3

CDB

Use: Melanoma.
Cycle: 21 days, continue until disease progression or intolerable toxicity

Regimen: Cisplatin 25 mg/m^2/day IV, days 1 through 3
Dacarbazine 220 mg/m^2/day IV, days 1 through 3
Carmustine 150 mg/m^2 IV, day 1 of odd-numbered cycles only (eg, cycle 1, 3, 5)

CDB + Tamoxifen (Dartmouth Regimen)

Use: Melanoma.
Cycle: 21 days, continue until disease progression or intolerable toxicity

Regimen: Tamoxifen 10 mg PO twice daily, throughout entire course, started 1 week prior to cytotoxic chemotherapy
Carmustine 150 mg/m^2 IV, day 1 of odd-numbered cycles only (eg, cycle 1, 3, 5), given before cisplatin and dacarbazine
Cisplatin 25 mg/m^2/day IV, days 1 through 3
Dacarbazine 220 mg/m^2/day IV, days 1 through 3

CDDP/VP-16

Use: Brain tumors (pediatrics).
Cycle: 21 days for up to 4 cycles

Regimen: Cisplatin 90 mg/m^2 IV, day 1
Etoposide 150 mg/m^2/day IV, days 3 and 4

CDE

Use: Lymphoma (HIV-related, non-Hodgkin—adults).
Cycle: 28 days for up to 6 cycles

Regimen: Cyclophosphamide 200 mg/m^2/day continuous IV infusion, days 1 through 4
Doxorubicin 12.5 mg/m^2/day continuous IV infusion, days 1 through 4
Etoposide 60 mg/m^2/day continuous IV infusion, days 1 through 4
Filgrastim 5 mcg/kg/day subcutaneously starting on day 6, at least 24 hours after the end of the continuous infusions, and ending when the absolute neutrophil count (ANC) is 10,000 cells/mm^3 or higher

CEF (also see FEC)

Use: Breast cancer.
Cycle: 28 days for up to 6 cycles

Regimen: Cyclophosphamide 75 mg/m^2/day PO, days 1 through 14
Epirubicin 60 mg/m^2 IV, days 1 and 8
Fluorouracil 500 mg/m^2 IV, days 1 and 8
Cotrimoxazole 2 tablets (strength not specified) PO twice daily, days 1 through 28

CEPP(B)

Use: Lymphoma (non-Hodgkin).
Cycle: 28 days

Regimen: Cyclophosphamide 600 to 650 mg/m^2 IV, days 1 and 8
Etoposide 70 to 85 mg/m^2/day IV, days 1 through 3
Prednisone 60 mg/m^2/day PO, days 1 through 10
Procarbazine 60 mg/m^2/day PO, days 1 through 10
may or may not give with
Bleomycin 15 units/m^2 IV, days 1 and 15

CetIri—see Cetuximab-Irinotecan

Cetuximab-Bevacizumab

Use: Colorectal cancer.
Cycle: 14 days, continue until disease progression or intolerable toxicity

Regimen: Cetuximab 400 mg/m^2 IV, day 1 of first cycle only (loading dose)
Cetuximab 250 mg/m^2 IV weekly, days 1 and 8, except for day 1 of first cycle
Bevacizumab 5 mg/kg IV, day 1 (after cetuximab), except for day 1 of first cycle
Bevacizumab 5 mg/kg IV, day 2 of first cycle only

Cetuximab-Carboplatin

Use: Head and neck cancer.
Cycle: 21 to 28 days for up to 8 cycles or until disease progression or intolerable toxicity

Regimen: Cetuximab 400 mg/m^2 IV, day 1 of first cycle only (loading dose)
Cetuximab 250 mg/m^2 IV weekly, except for day 1 of first cycle
Carboplatin IV dose by Calvert equation to AUC 5 mg/mL/min, day 1

Cetuximab-Carboplatin-Fluorouracil

Use: Head and neck cancer.
Cycle: 21 days for up to 6 cycles

Regimen: Cetuximab 400 mg/m^2 IV, day 1 of first cycle only (loading dose)
Cetuximab 250 mg/m^2 IV weekly, days 1, 8, and 15, except for day 1 of first cycle
Carboplatin IV dose by Calvert equation to AUC 5 mg/mL/min, day 1
Fluorouracil 1,000 mg/m^2/day continuous IV infusion, days 1 through 4
followed by
Cetuximab 250 mg/m^2 IV weekly until disease progression or intolerable toxicity

Cetuximab-Cisplatin

Use: Head and neck cancer.
Cycle: 21 to 28 days for up to 6 to 8 cycles or until disease progression or intolerable toxicity

Regimen: Cetuximab 400 mg/m^2 IV, day 1 of first cycle only (loading dose)
Cetuximab 250 mg/m^2 IV weekly, except for day 1 of first cycle
Cisplatin 75 or 100 mg/m^2 IV, day 1

Cetuximab-Cisplatin-Fluorouracil

Use: Head and neck cancer.
Cycle: 21 days for up to 6 cycles

Regimen: Cetuximab 400 mg/m^2 IV, day 1 of first cycle only (loading dose)
Cetuximab 250 mg/m^2 IV weekly, days 1, 8, and 15, except for day 1 of first cycle
Cisplatin 100 mg/m^2 IV, day 1
Fluorouracil 1,000 mg/m^2/day continuous IV infusion, days 1 through 4
followed by
Cetuximab 250 mg/m^2 IV weekly until disease progression or intolerable toxicity

Cetuximab-Cisplatin-Vinorelbine

Use: Lung cancer (non-small cell).
Cycle: 21 days for up to 6 cycles

Regimen: Cetuximab 400 mg/m^2 IV, day 1 of first cycle only (loading dose)
Cetuximab 250 mg/m^2 IV weekly, days 1, 8, and 15, except for day 1 of first cycle
Cisplatin 80 mg/m^2 IV, day 1
Vinorelbine 25 mg/m^2 IV, days 1 and 8
followed by
Cetuximab 250 mg/m^2 IV weekly until disease progression or intolerable toxicity

Cetuximab-Gemcitabine

Use: Pancreatic cancer.
Cycle: 56 days, continue until disease progression or intolerable toxicity

Regimen: Cetuximab 400 mg/m^2 IV, day 1 of first cycle only (loading dose)
Cetuximab 250 mg/m^2 IV weekly, on days 1, 8, 15, 22, 29, 36, 43, and 50, except for day 1 of first cycle
Gemcitabine 1,000 mg/m^2 IV, weekly for 7 weeks for first cycle. During subsequent cycles, give weekly for 3 weeks followed by 1 week of rest; administer on days 1, 8, 15, 29, 36, and 43

Cetuximab-Irinotecan (CetIri)

Use: Colorectal cancer.
Cycle: 42 days, continue until disease progression or intolerable toxicity

Regimen: Cetuximab 400 mg/m^2 IV, day 1 of first cycle only (loading dose)
Cetuximab 250 mg/m^2 IV weekly, days 1, 8, 15, 22, 29, and 36, except for day 1 of first cycle
with
Irinotecan 125 mg/m^2 IV, weekly for 4 weeks, followed by 2 weeks of rest; administer on days 1, 8, 15, and 22
or
Irinotecan 180 mg/m^2 IV, days 1, 15, and 29
or
Irinotecan 350 mg/m^2 IV, days 1 and 22; reduce each dose to irinotecan 300 mg/m^2 IV in patients 70 years of age and older

Use: Colorectal cancer.
Cycle: 14 days, continue until disease progression or intolerable toxicity

Regimen: Cetuximab 500 mg/m^2 IV, day 1
Irinotecan 180 mg/m^2 IV, day 1

CEV

Use: Lung cancer (small cell).
Cycle: 21 days, continue until disease progression or intolerable toxicity

Regimen: Cyclophosphamide 1,000 mg/m^2 IV, day 1
Vincristine 1.4 mg/m^2 (2 mg maximum dose) IV, day 1
Etoposide 50 mg/m^2 IV, day 1
Etoposide 100 mg/m^2/day PO, days 2 through 5

CF (also see Cisplatin-Fluorouracil; also see FUP)

Use: Adenocarcinoma, head and neck cancer.
Cycle: 21 to 28 days for up to 3 cycles or until disease progression or intolerable toxicity

Regimen: Cisplatin 100 mg/m^2 IV, day 1
Fluorouracil 1,000 mg/m^2/day continuous IV infusion, days 1 through 4 or days 1 through 5
may be used in conjunction with
Radiation therapy

(continued on next page)

CF (also see Cisplatin-Fluorouracil; also see FUP) (cont.)

Use: Head and neck cancer.
Cycle: 21 to 28 days for up to 3 cycles or until disease progression or intolerable toxicity

Regimen: Carboplatin 300 or 400 mg/m^2 IV, day 1
Fluorouracil 1,000 mg/m^2/day continuous IV infusion, days 1 through 4 or days 1 through 5

Use: Head and neck cancer.
Cycle: 21 days for 3 cycles

Regimen: Carboplatin 70 mg/m^2/day continuous IV infusion, days 1 through 4
Fluorouracil 600 mg/m^2/day continuous IV infusion, days 1 through 4
used in conjunction with
Radiation therapy

Use: Gastric cancer.
Cycle: 28 days

Regimen: Cisplatin 100 mg/m^2 IV, day 1
Fluorouracil 1,000 mg/m^2/day continuous IV infusion, days 1 through 5

Use: Anal cancer.
Cycle: 28 days

Regimen: Fluorouracil 1,000 mg/m^2/day continuous IV infusion, days 1 through 4 (for 96 hours total)
Cisplatin 100 mg/m^2 IV, day 2

CFAR

Use: Chronic lymphocytic leukemia (CLL).
Cycle: 28 days for up to 6 cycles

Regimen: Alemtuzumab 30 mg IV, days 1, 3, and 5
Fludarabine 25 mg/m^2/day IV, days 3 through 5
Cyclophosphamide 250 mg/m^2/day IV, days 3 through 5
Rituximab 375 to 500 mg/m^2 IV, day 2
Pegfilgrastim 6 mg subcutaneously, day 6
used in conjunction with antimicrobial prophylaxis
Cotrimoxazole double-strength (160/800) 1 tablet PO twice daily, given 2 to 3 times weekly, throughout entire course and continued for 2 months after chemotherapy
plus
Valacyclovir 500 mg/day PO, throughout entire course and continued for 2 months after chemotherapy
or
Valganciclovir 900 mg/day PO, throughout entire course and continued for 2 months after chemotherapy*
*Note: Valganciclovir CMV prophylaxis dose not specified in original articles; the dose given here is derived from *AHFS 2009 Drug Information,* a tertiary resource.

CFM—see CNF

CHAMOCA (Modified Bagshawe)

Use: Gestational trophoblastic neoplasm.
Cycle: 18 days or longer, as toxicity permits

Regimen: Hydroxyurea 500 mg/dose PO every 6 hours for 4 doses, day 1 (start at 6 am)
Dactinomycin 0.2 mg/day (dose is not in mg/m^2) IV, days 1 through 3 (give at 7 pm)
Vincristine 1 mg/m^2 (2 mg maximum dose) IV, day 2 (give at 7 am)
Methotrexate 100 mg/m^2 IV push, day 2 (give at 7 pm)
Methotrexate 200 mg/m^2 IV over 12 hours, day 2 (give after IV push dose)
Leucovorin 14 mg/dose IM every 6 hours for 6 doses, days 3 through 5 (begin at 7 pm on day 3)
Cyclophosphamide 500 mg/m^2 IV, days 3 and 8 (give at 7 pm)
Dactinomycin 0.5 mg/day (dose is not in mg/m^2) IV, days 4 and 5 (give at 7 pm)
Doxorubicin 30 mg/m^2 IV, day 8 (give at 7 pm)

CHAP

Use: Ovarian cancer.
Cycle: 28 days for up to 12 cycles

Regimen: Cyclophosphamide 400 mg/m^2 IV, day 1
or
Cyclophosphamide 150 mg/m^2/day PO, days 2 through 8
with
Doxorubicin 30 mg/m^2 IV, day 1
Cisplatin 50 to 60 mg/m^2 IV, day 1
Altretamine 150 mg/m^2/day PO, days 2 through 8

ChlVPP

Use: Lymphoma (Hodgkin).
Cycle: 28 days, continue for 2 cycles after achieving remission

Regimen:
Chlorambucil 6 mg/m²/day (10 mg/day maximum dose) PO, days 1 through 14
Vinblastine 6 mg/m² (10 mg/day maximum dose) IV, days 1 and 8
Procarbazine 100 mg/m²/day (150 mg/day maximum dose) PO, days 1 through 14
Prednisone 40 to 50 mg/day PO, days 1 through 14*
*Note: Prednisolone is recommended in the British literature. In the United States, prednisone is the preferred corticosteroid. The doses of these 2 corticosteroids are equivalent (ie, prednisone 40 mg PO = prednisolone 40 mg PO).

ChlVPP/EVA

Use: Lymphoma (Hodgkin).
Cycle: 28 days for up to 8 cycles

Regimen:
Chlorambucil 10 mg/day PO, days 1 through 7
Vinblastine 10 mg (dose is not in mg/m²) IV, day 1
Procarbazine 150 mg/day PO, days 1 through 7
Prednisone 50 mg/day PO, days 1 through 7*
with
Etoposide 200 mg/m² IV, day 8
Vincristine 2 mg (dose is not in mg/m²) IV, day 8
Doxorubicin 50 mg/m² IV, day 8
*Note: Prednisolone is recommended in the British literature. In the United States, prednisone is the preferred corticosteroid. The doses of these 2 corticosteroids are equivalent (ie, prednisone 40 mg PO = prednisolone 40 mg PO).

CHOP

Use: Lymphoma (non-Hodgkin, HIV-related).
Cycle: 21 to 28 days for 4 to 6 cycles, or for 3 cycles after achieving remission

Regimen:
Cyclophosphamide 750 mg/m² IV, day 1
Doxorubicin 50 mg/m² IV, day 1
Vincristine 1.4 mg/m² (2 mg maximum dose) IV, day 1
Prednisone 100 mg/day PO, days 1 through 5

Use: Lymphoma (non-Hodgkin; induction and consolidation—pediatrics)

Regimen:
Induction. *Cycle:* Give 1 cycle only (6 weeks)
Cyclophosphamide 750 mg/m² IV, days 1 and 22
Doxorubicin 40 mg/m² IV, days 1 and 22
Vincristine 1.5 mg/m² (2 mg maximum dose) IV weekly, weeks 1 through 6
Prednisone 40 mg/m²/day PO, days 1 through 28
may be used in conjunction with
Radiation therapy
Consolidation therapy. *Cycle:* 21 days
Cyclophosphamide 750 mg/m² IV, day 1
Doxorubicin 40 mg/m² IV, day 1
Vincristine 1.5 mg/m² (2 mg maximum dose) IV, day 1
Prednisone 40 mg/m²/day PO, days 1 through 5
Note: CHOP refers to induction and consolidation phase. Protocol also includes maintenance and central nervous system prophylaxis.

CHOP-14

Use: Lymphoma (non-Hodgkin).
Cycle: 14 days for up to 6 cycles

Regimen:
Cyclophosphamide 750 mg/m² IV, day 1
Doxorubicin 50 mg/m² IV, day 1
Vincristine 2 mg (dose is not in mg/m²) IV, day 1
Prednisone 100 mg/day PO, days 1 through 5
Filgrastim 300 mcg/day (patients weighing less than 75 kg) to 480 mcg/day (patients weighing 75 kg or more) subcutaneously, days 4 through 13

CHOP-14 + Rituximab (R-CHOP-14)

Use: Lymphoma (B-cell).
Cycle: 14 days for up to 6 to 8 cycles

Regimen:
Rituximab 375 mg/m² IV, day 1
Cyclophosphamide 750 mg/m² IV, day 1
Doxorubicin 50 mg/m² IV, day 1
Vincristine 1.4 mg/m² (2 mg maximum dose) IV, day 1
Prednisone 100 mg/day PO, days 1 through 5*
Filgrastim 5 mcg/kg/day subcutaneously (rounded to 300 or 480 mcg), days 4 through 10, or until the white blood cell count (WBC) is at least 2,500 cells/mm³ (whichever occurs earlier)
*Note: Prednisolone is recommended in the European literature. In the United States, prednisone is the preferred corticosteroid. The doses of these 2 corticosteroids are equivalent (ie, prednisone 40 mg PO = prednisolone 40 mg PO).

CHOP-Bleo

Use: Lymphoma (non-Hodgkin).
Cycle: 21 to 28 days for at least 2 cycles

Regimen: **Add to CHOP:** Bleomycin 15 units/day IV, days 1 through 5

CHOP + High-Dose Methotrexate

Use: Lymphoma (non-Hodgkin).
Cycle: 21 days for 6 to 9 cycles

Regimen:
Cyclophosphamide 1,200 mg/m^2 IV, day 1
Doxorubicin 40 mg/m^2 IV, day 1
Vincristine 1.4 mg/m^2 (2 mg maximum dose) IV, day 1
Prednisone 40 mg/m^2/day IV or PO, days 1 through 5
Methotrexate 3,000 mg/m^2 IV, day 10, cycles 1 through 5 only
Leucovorin 25 mg/m^2/dose IV or PO every 6 hours for 12 doses, begin 24 hours after each methotrexate dose, cycles 1 through 5 only
Methotrexate 12 mg intrathecal, days 1 and 10

CHOP + Rituximab (R-CHOP)

Use: Lymphoma (B-cell).
Cycle: 21 days for up to 8 cycles

Regimen: **Add to CHOP:** Rituximab 375 mg/m^2 IV, day 1

Use: Lymphoma (B-cell).
Cycle: 21 days for up to 8 cycles

Regimen:
Rituximab 375 mg/m^2 IV, day 1
Cyclophosphamide 750 mg/m^2 IV, day 3
Doxorubicin 50 mg/m^2 IV, day 3
Vincristine 1.4 mg/m^2 (2 mg maximum dose) IV, day 3
Prednisone 100 mg/day PO, days 3 through 7

Use: Lymphoma (mantle cell).
Cycle: 21 days for up to 6 cycles

Regimen:
Rituximab 375 mg/m^2 IV, day 1
Cyclophosphamide 750 mg/m^2 IV, day 2
Doxorubicin 50 mg/m^2 IV, day 2
Vincristine 1.4 mg/m^2 (2 mg maximum dose) IV, day 2
Prednisone 100 mg/day PO, days 2 through 6

CIM

Use: Endometrial cancer.
Cycle: 21 days for up to 3 cycles

Regimen:
Cisplatin 20 mg/m^2/day IV, days 1 through 4
Ifosfamide 1,500 mg/m^2/day IV, days 1 through 4
Mesna 120 mg/m^2/day IV given before ifosfamide, days 1 through 4
Mesna 1,500 mg/m^2/day continuous IV infusion, days 1 through 4 (give after mesna bolus)

CISCA

Use: Bladder cancer.
Cycle: 21 to 28 days

Regimen 1: Patients without extensive prior radiation therapy, or patients without tumor in bone marrow:
Cyclophosphamide 650 mg/m^2 IV, day 1
Doxorubicin 50 mg/m^2 IV, day 1
Cisplatin 100 mg/m^2 IV, day 2

Regimen 2: Patients with extensive prior radiation therapy, or patients with tumor in bone marrow:
Cyclophosphamide 550 mg/m^2 IV, day 1, of first cycle only
Cyclophosphamide 650 mg/m^2 IV, day 1, except for first cycle
Doxorubicin 40 mg/m^2 IV, day 1, of first cycle only
Doxorubicin 50 mg/m^2 IV, day 1, except for first cycle
Cisplatin 100 mg/m^2 IV, day 2

CISCA II/VB IV

Use: Germ cell tumors.
Cycle: Individualized based on duration of myelosuppression, continue for 2 cycles after response or remission

Regimen:
Cyclophosphamide 500 mg/m^2/day IV, days 1 and 2
Doxorubicin 40 to 45 mg/m^2/day IV, days 1 and 2
Cisplatin 100 to 120 mg/m^2 IV, day 3
alternating with
Vinblastine 3 mg/m^2/day continuous IV infusion, days 1 through 5
Bleomycin 30 units/day continuous IV infusion, days 1 through 5

Cisplatin-Docetaxel (also see Docetaxel-Cisplatin; also see TC)

Use:	Bladder cancer. *Cycle:* Every 7 days for 8 weeks
Regimen:	Cisplatin 30 mg/m² IV, day 1 Docetaxel 40 mg/m² IV, day 4 *used in conjunction with* Radiation therapy

Use:	Bladder cancer. *Cycle:* 21 days for up to 8 cycles
Regimen:	Cisplatin 75 mg/m² IV, day 1 Docetaxel 75 mg/m² IV, day 1

Use:	Head and neck cancer. *Cycle:* 21 days for up to 12 months, or until disease progression or intolerable toxicity
Regimen:	Docetaxel 75 mg/m² IV, day 1 Cisplatin 75 mg/m² IV, day 1

Cisplatin-Doxorubicin-Etoposide-Cyclophosphamide, High Risk Neuroblastoma

Use:	High-risk neuroblastoma (pediatrics). *Cycle:* 28 days for 5 cycles
Regimen:	Cisplatin 60 mg/m² IV, day 1 Doxorubicin 30 mg/m² IV, day 3 Etoposide 100 mg/m² IV, days 3 and 6 Cyclophosphamide 1,000 mg/m²/day IV, days 4 and 5

Cisplatin-Doxorubicin-Mitomycin, Chemoembolization Protocol

Use:	Hepatocellular cancer, hepatic metastases. *Cycle:* May give a single cycle, or repeat every 4 to 8 weeks, depending on the protocol
Regimen:	Cisplatin 50 to 100 mg intraarterially, day 1* Doxorubicin 50 mg intraarterially, day 1* Mitomycin 10 mg intraarterially, day 1* *all mixed in same infusion bag to a total volume of 10 to 20 mL with* Radiopaque contrast media, quantity sufficient to provide final volume of 10 to 20 mL *either of the following may be mixed with the other agents or given subsequently as a separate injection, depending on the protocol* Gelfoam powder, mixed to 25 to 30 mg/mL, and given intraarterially, day 1 *or* Polyvinyl alcohol *Note: All agents are mixed together in the same infusion bag. This regimen is usually administered by the Interventional Radiology staff to ensure delivery into the hepatic artery.

Cisplatin-Epirubicin

Use:	Testicular cancer, germ cell tumors. *Cycle:* 21 days for up to 4 cycles
Regimen:	Cisplatin 20 mg/m² IV, days 1 through 5 Epirubicin 90 mg/m² IV, day 1 *with* Filgrastim 5 mcg/kg/day subcutaneously, days 7 through 16 *or* Pegfilgrastim 6 mg subcutaneously, day 6 or 7

Cisplatin-Erlotinib

Use:	Head and neck cancer. *Cycle:* 21 days for up to 6 cycles
Regimen:	Erlotinib 100 mg/day PO, throughout entire course, starting 7 days before first cisplatin dose. Cisplatin 75 mg/m² IV, day 1 *followed by* Erlotinib 100 mg/day PO until disease progression or intolerable toxicity

Cisplatin-Fluorouracil (also see CF; also see FUP)

Use:	Cervical cancer. *Cycle:* 21 days for up to 3 cycles
Regimen:	Cisplatin 75 mg/m² IV, day 1 *followed by* Fluorouracil 1,000 mg/m²/day continuous IV infusion, days 1 through 4 (for 96 hours total) *used in conjunction with* Radiation therapy

(continued on next page)

Cisplatin-Fluorouracil (also see CF; also see FUP) (cont.)

Use:	Cervical cancer. *Cycle:* 28 days for up to 2 cycles
Regimen:	Cisplatin 50 mg/m² IV, day 1 starting 4 hours *before* external beam radiotherapy Fluorouracil 1,000 mg/m²/day continuous IV infusion, days 2 through 5 *used in conjunction with* Radiation therapy
Use:	Cervical cancer. *Cycle:* 21 days for 4 cycles
Regimen:	Cisplatin 70 mg/m² IV, day 1 Fluorouracil 1,000 mg/m²/day continuous IV infusion, days 1 through 4 *used in conjunction with* Radiation therapy, during first 2 cycles only
Use:	Head and neck cancer, esophageal cancer. *Cycle:* 21 days for 3 cycles
Regimen:	Cisplatin 100 mg/m² IV, day 1 Fluorouracil 1,000 mg/m²/day continuous IV infusion, days 1 through 5 (for 120 hours total)
Use:	Bladder cancer. *Cycle:* 63 days for up to 2 cycles
Regimen:	Cisplatin 15 mg/m²/day IV, days 1 through 3 and days 15 through 17 Fluorouracil 400 mg/m²/day IV, days 1 through 3 and days 15 through 17 *used in conjunction with* Radiation therapy
Use:	Esophageal cancer. *Cycle:* 32 days. Give a single cycle prior to surgery.
Regimen:	Cisplatin 100 mg/m² IV, day 1 Fluorouracil 1,000 mg/m²/day continuous IV infusion, days 1 through 4 and days 29 through 32 *used in conjunction with* Radiation therapy
Use:	Esophageal cancer. *Cycle:* 28 days for 1 to 2 cycles
Regimen:	Cisplatin 75 mg/m² IV, day 1 Fluorouracil 1,000 mg/m²/day continuous IV infusion, days 1 through 4 (for 96 hours total) *used in conjunction with* Radiation therapy *followed by 4 to 6 weeks of rest then* Repeat chemotherapy for an additional 2 cycles
Use:	Esophageal cancer. *Cycle:* 21 days for up to 5 cycles
Regimen:	Cisplatin 15 mg/m²/day IV, days 1 through 5 Fluorouracil 800 mg/m²/day continuous IV infusion, days 1 through 5 (for 120 hours total) *used in conjunction with* Radiation therapy
Use:	Head and neck cancer. *Cycle:* 21 days for 2 cycles prior to surgery
Regimen:	Cisplatin 20 mg/m²/day continuous IV infusion, days 1 through 4 Fluorouracil 1,000 mg/m²/day continuous IV infusion, days 1 through 4 *used in conjunction with* Radiation therapy
Use:	Anal cancer. *Cycle:* 7 days for 6 cycles
Regimen:	Cisplatin 4 mg/m²/day continuous IV infusion, days 1 through 5 Fluorouracil 250 mg/m²/day continuous IV infusion, days 1 through 5 *used in conjunction with* Radiation therapy

Cisplatin-Fluorouracil-Leucovorin

Use: Biliary tract cancer.
Cycle: 14 days for at least 6 months, or until disease progression or intolerable toxicity

Regimen: Leucovorin 200 mg/m²/day IV, days 1 and 2
Fluorouracil 400 mg/m²/day IV bolus, days 1 and 2 (after starting leucovorin)
then
Fluorouracil 600 mg/m²/dose continuous IV infusion for 22 hours, days 1 and 2
Cisplatin 50 mg/m² IV, day 2

Cisplatin-Fluorouracil + Radiation + Surgery ➡ CT

Use: Esophageal cancer.
Cycle: see below, cycle length varies throughout protocol. Give a single cycle of Cisplatin-Fluorouracil + Radiation, followed by surgical resection, followed by 3 cycles of CT.

Regimen: **Cisplatin-Fluorouracil + Radiation.** *Cycle*: 30 days. Give a single cycle prior to surgery.
Cisplatin 20 mg/m²/day IV, days 1 through 5 and days 26 through 30
Fluorouracil 225 mg/m²/day continuous IV infusion, days 1 through 30
used in conjunction with
Radiation therapy
followed after 4 weeks by
Surgical resection
followed after 8 to 12 weeks by
CT. *Cycle*: 21 days for 3 cycles
Paclitaxel 135 mg/m²/day continuous IV infusion over 24 hours, day 1
Cisplatin 75 mg/m² IV, day 2 (given after paclitaxel)
Filgrastim 300 mcg/day subcutaneously, starting on day 3 and continuing until the neutrophil count is above 10,000 cells/mm³

Cisplatin-Fluorouracil-Vinblastine + Radiation + Surgery

Use: Esophageal cancer.
Cycle: 21 days. Give a single cycle prior to surgery.

Regimen: Cisplatin 20 mg/m²/day continuous IV infusion, days 1 through 5 and days 17 through 21
Fluorouracil 300 mg/m²/day continuous IV infusion, days 1 through 21
Vinblastine 1 mg/m²/day IV, days 1 through 4 and days 17 through 20
used in conjunction with
Radiation therapy
followed after 3 weeks by
Surgical resection

Cisplatin-Irinotecan

Use: Cervical cancer, lung cancer (small cell).
Cycle: 28 days for up to 4 to 6 cycles

Regimen: Irinotecan 60 mg/m² IV, days 1, 8, and 15
Cisplatin 60 mg/m² IV, day 1 (give after irinotecan)

Use: Lung cancer (small cell).
Cycle: 21 days for at least 4 cycles or until disease progression or intolerable toxicity

Regimen: Cisplatin 30 mg/m² IV, days 1 and 8
Irinotecan 65 mg/m² IV, days 1 and 8

Use: Esophageal cancer, gastric cancer.
Cycle: 42 days for at least 3 cycles or until disease progression or intolerable toxicity

Regimen: Cisplatin 30 mg/m² IV, weekly for 4 weeks, followed by 2 weeks of rest; administer on days 1, 8, 15, and 22.
Irinotecan 65 mg/m² IV, weekly for 4 weeks, followed by 2 weeks of rest; administer on days 1, 8, 15, and 22

Use: Gastric cancer.
Cycle: 28 days, continue until disease progression or intolerable toxicity

Regimen: Cisplatin 80 mg/m² IV, day 1
Irinotecan 70 mg/m² IV, days 1 and 15

Cisplatin-Irinotecan-Bevacizumab—see IPB

Cisplatin-Mitotane

Use: Adrenal cancer.
Cycle: 21 days for 18 months or until disease progression or intolerable toxicity

Regimen 1: Patients younger than 65 years of age, patients without intolerable adverse effects from prior chemotherapy, or patients without extensive prior radiation therapy:
Cisplatin 100 mg/m² IV, day 1
Mitotane 1,000 mg/dose (4,000 mg/day) PO 4 times daily, throughout entire course
used in conjunction with mineralocorticoid and glucocorticoid supplementation
Hydrocortisone 10 to 30 mg/day PO in divided doses, throughout entire course*
Fludrocortisone 0.1 mg/day PO, throughout entire course*

(continued on next page)

Cisplatin-Mitotane (cont.)

Regimen 2: Patients 65 years of age and older, patients with intolerable adverse effects from prior chemotherapy, or patients with extensive prior radiation therapy:
Cisplatin 75 mg/m² IV, day 1
Mitotane 1,000 mg/dose (4,000 mg/day) PO 4 times daily, throughout entire course
used in conjunction with mineralocorticoid and glucocorticoid supplementation
Hydrocortisone 10 to 30 mg/day PO in divided doses, throughout entire course*
Fludrocortisone 0.1 mg/day PO, throughout entire course*
*Note: Mineralocorticoid and glucocorticoid doses not specified in original article; the dose given here is derived from *AHFS 2008 Drug Information,* a tertiary resource.

Cisplatin + Radiation ➡ Cisplatin-Fluorouracil

Use: Head and neck cancer (nasopharyngeal).
Cycle: See below, cycle length varies throughout protocol. Give 3 cycles of Cisplatin + Radiation, followed by 3 cycles of Cisplatin-Fluorouracil.

Regimen: **Cisplatin + Radiation.** *Cycle*: 21 days for 3 cycles
Cisplatin 100 mg/m² IV, day 1
used in conjunction with
Radiation therapy
followed after 4 weeks by
Cisplatin-Fluorouracil. *Cycle*: 28 days for 3 cycles
Cisplatin 80 mg/m² IV, day 1
Fluorouracil 1,000 mg/m²/day continuous IV infusion, days 1 through 4

Cisplatin-Topotecan

Use: Cervical cancer.
Cycle: 21 days for 6 cycles or until disease progression or intolerable toxicity

Regimen: Cisplatin 50 mg/m² IV, day 1
Topotecan 0.75 mg/m²/day IV, days 1 through 3

Use: Lung cancer (small cell).
Cycle: 21 days for up to 4 cycles, or for 2 cycles after maximal response

Regimen: Topotecan 1.7 mg/m²/day PO, days 1 through 5 for first cycle; may increase dose in increments of 0.3 mg/m² (to maximum of topotecan 2.3 mg/m² PO, day 1) for subsequent cycles if tolerated
Cisplatin 60 mg/m² IV, day 5 for first 3 cycles; may increase dose to maximum of cisplatin 75 mg/m² IV, day 5) for subsequent cycles if maximum topotecan dose tolerated for at least 2 cycles

Cisplatin-Vincristine-Cyclophosphamide

Use: Brain tumor (pediatrics).
Cycle: 6 weeks for up to 8 cycles

Regimen: Cisplatin 75 mg/m² IV, day 1
Vincristine 1.5 mg/m² (2 mg maximum dose) IV, days 2, 8, and 15
Cyclophosphamide 1,000 mg/m² IV, days 22 and 23

Cisplatin-Vinorelbine (also see Vinorelbine-Cisplatin)

Use: Cervical cancer, head and neck cancer.
Cycle: 21 days for up to 6 to 8 cycles

Regimen: Cisplatin 80 mg/m² IV, day 1
Vinorelbine 25 mg/m² IV, days 1 and 8

Use: Lung cancer (non-small cell).
Cycle: 28 days for 4 cycles

Regimen: Cisplatin 50 mg/m² IV, days 1 and 8
Vinorelbine 25 mg/m² IV weekly, days 1, 8, 15, and 22

CLAG

Use: Acute myelocytic leukemia (AML; reinduction).
Cycle: 27 to 34 days. Give 1 cycle. If patient has persistent leukemia between days 27 and 34, give 1 additional cycle.

Regimen: Filgrastim 300 mcg/day subcutaneously, from days 1 through 6
Cladribine 5 mg/m²/day IV, days 2 through 6
Cytarabine 2,000 mg/m²/day IV, days 2 through 6 (begin 2 hours after starting cladribine)

CLAG-M

Use: Acute myelocytic leukemia (AML; reinduction).
Cycle: Give 1 induction cycle, followed by 1 consolidation cycle. May give 1 additional induction cycle if complete response not achieved (eg, persistent blasts). Time between cycles not specified.

Regimen: Filgrastim 300 mcg/day subcutaneously, days 1 through 6
Cladribine 5 mg/m²/day IV, days 2 through 6
Cytarabine 2,000 mg/m²/day IV, days 2 through 6 (begin 2 hours after starting cladribine)
Mitoxantrone 10 mg/m² IV, days 2 through 4

CLD-BOMP

Use: Cervical cancer.
Cycle: 21 days, continue until disease progression or intolerable toxicity

Regimen:
Bleomycin 5 units/day continuous IV infusion, days 1 through 7
Cisplatin 10 $mg/m^2/day$ IV, days 1 through 7
Vincristine* 0.7 mg/m^2 IV, day 7
Mitomycin 7 mg/m^2 IV, day 7
*Note: The vincristine dose is not capped in this protocol. Consult the prescriber if there is any question about the intended vincristine dose.

CMC

Use: Chronic lymphocytic leukemia (CLL, B-cell), lymphoma (non-Hodgkin).
Cycle: 28 days for up to 3 cycles or until disease progression or intolerable toxicity

Regimen:
Cladribine 0.12 mg/kg/day IV, days 1 through 3*
Mitoxantrone 10 mg/m^2 IV, day 1
Cyclophosphamide 650 mg/m^2 IV, day 1
*Note: In 2 studies, investigators compared cladribine for 3 days with cladribine for 5 days at the same daily dose. Response rates were similar with both regimens. Because toxicity increased with cladribine for 5 days, the 3-day cladribine regimen is recommended.

CMF

Use: Breast cancer.
Cycle: 28 days for up to 12 cycles

Regimen 1: Patients 65 years of age and younger:
- Methotrexate 40 mg/m^2 IV, days 1 and 8
- Fluorouracil 600 mg/m^2 IV, days 1 and 8
- *with*
- Cyclophosphamide 100 $mg/m^2/day$ PO, days 1 through 14
- *or*
- Cyclophosphamide 750 mg/m^2 IV, day 1

Regimen 2: Patients older than 65 years of age:
- Methotrexate 30 mg/m^2 IV, days 1 and 8
- Fluorouracil 400 mg/m^2 IV, days 1 and 8
- Cyclophosphamide 100 $mg/m^2/day$ PO, days 1 through 14

CMF-IV

Use: Breast cancer.
Cycle: 21 days for up to 12 cycles

Regimen:
Cyclophosphamide 600 mg/m^2 IV, day 1
Methotrexate 40 mg/m^2 IV, day 1
Fluorouracil 600 mg/m^2 IV, day 1

CMFP

Use: Breast cancer.
Cycle: 28 days

Regimen:
Cyclophosphamide 100 $mg/m^2/day$ PO, days 1 through 14
Methotrexate 30 to 40 mg/m^2 IV, days 1 and 8
Fluorouracil 400 to 600 mg/m^2 IV, days 1 and 8
Prednisone 40 $mg/m^2/day$ PO, days 1 through 14

CMFVP

Use: Breast cancer.
Cycle: 28 days for up to 6 cycles

Regimen:
Cyclophosphamide 400 mg/m^2 IV, day 1
Methotrexate 30 mg/m^2 IV, days 1 and 8
Fluorouracil 400 mg/m^2 IV, days 1 and 8
Vincristine 1 mg (dose is not in mg/m^2) IV, days 1 and 8
Prednisone 20 mg/dose PO, given 4 times daily, days 1 through 7

CMV

Use: Bladder cancer.
Cycle: 21 days for at least 2 cycles

Regimen:
Methotrexate 30 mg/m^2 IV, days 1 and 8
Vinblastine 4 mg/m^2 IV, days 1 and 8
Cisplatin 100 mg/m^2 IV, day 2 (at least 12 hours after methotrexate and vinblastine)

(continued on next page)

CMV (cont.)

Use: Bladder cancer.
Cycle: 28 days for 2 cycles prior to radiation therapy

Regimen:
Methotrexate 30 mg/m² IV, days 1, 15, and 22
Cisplatin 70 mg/m² IV, day 2
Vinblastine 3 mg/m² IV, days 2, 15, and 22

CNF (CFM, FNC)

Use: Breast cancer.
Cycle: 21 days, continue until disease progression or intolerable toxicity

Regimen:
Cyclophosphamide 500 mg/m² IV, day 1
Mitoxantrone 10 mg/m² IV, day 1
Fluorouracil 500 mg/m² IV, day 1

Use: Breast cancer.
Cycle: 21 days for up to 10 cycles

Regimen:
Cyclophosphamide 600 mg/m² IV, day 1
Mitoxantrone 12 mg/m² IV, day 1
Fluorouracil 600 mg/m² IV, day 1

CNOP

Use: Lymphoma (non-Hodgkin).
Cycle: 21 to 28 days for up to 8 cycles

Regimen:
Cyclophosphamide 750 mg/m² IV, day 1
Mitoxantrone 10 or 12 mg/m² IV, day 1
Vincristine 1.4 mg/m² (2 mg maximum dose) IV, day 1
Prednisone 50 mg/m²/day (or 100 mg/day) PO, days 1 through 5

COB

Use: Head and neck cancer.
Cycle: 21 days for 2 to 3 cycles

Regimen:
Cisplatin 100 mg/m² IV, day 1
Vincristine 1 mg (dose is not in mg/m²) IV, days 2 and 5
Bleomycin 30 units/day continuous IV infusion, days 2 through 5

CODE

Use: Lung cancer (small cell).
Cycle: 9-week regimen (give a single cycle)

Regimen:
Cisplatin 25 mg/m² IV, every week for 9 weeks
Vincristine* 1 mg/m² IV weekly, weeks 1, 2, 4, 6, and 8
Doxorubicin 40 mg/m² IV weekly, weeks 1, 3, 5, 7, and 9
Etoposide 80 mg/m² IV, day 1 of weeks 1, 3, 5, 7, and 9
Etoposide 80 mg/m²/day PO, days 2 and 3 of weeks 1, 3, 5, 7, and 9
used in conjunction with
Prednisone 50 mg PO daily for 5 weeks, then alternate days until chemotherapy completion, then taper off over 2 weeks
used in conjunction with antimicrobial prophylaxis
Cotrimoxazole double-strength (160/800) 1 tablet PO twice daily, starting on day 8 and continued throughout chemotherapy
Ketoconazole 200 mg PO daily, starting on day 8 and continued throughout chemotherapy
*Note: The vincristine dose is not capped in this protocol. Consult the prescriber if there is any question about the intended vincristine dose.

CODOX-M, Modified

Use: Lymphoma (B-cell, Burkitt).
Cycle: Give 3 cycles as myelosuppression permits. Give next cycle when granulocyte count is above 1,000 cells/mm³ and platelet count is above 50,000 cells/mm³.

Regimen:
Cyclophosphamide 800 mg/m² IV, day 1
Cyclophosphamide 200 mg/m²/day IV, days 2 through 5
Vincristine 1.5 mg/m² (2 mg maximum dose) IV, days 1 and 8
Doxorubicin 40 mg/m² IV, day 1
Methotrexate 1,200 mg/m² IV over 1 hour, day 10
Methotrexate 240 mg/m²/hour continuous IV infusion over 23 hours, day 10 (begin after 1,200 mg/m² dose)
Leucovorin 192 mg/m² IV, day 11, given 36 hours after the start of the methotrexate infusion
Leucovorin 12 mg/m²/dose IV every 6 hours, day 11, beginning 42 hours after the start of the methotrexate infusion and continued until the methotrexate concentration is below 0.05 microMol/L
Cytarabine 70 mg intrathecal, day 1
Methotrexate 12 mg intrathecal, day 3 or 15
Patients with malignant pleocytosis receive additional intrathecal drugs during each cycle:
Cytarabine 70 mg intrathecal, days 3 and 5
Methotrexate 12 mg intrathecal, day 17
Filgrastim 5 mcg/kg/day subcutaneously, starting on day 13 and continuing until granulocyte count is above 1,000 cells/mm³

CODOX-M/IVAC*

Use: Lymphoma (advanced B-cell).

Cycle: Give 4 cycles as myelosuppression permits. Give next cycle when granulocyte count is above 1,000 cells/mm^3 and platelet count is above 50,000 cells/mm^3.

Regimen: **CODOX-M** (cycles 1 and 3)

- Cyclophosphamide 800 mg/m^2 IV, day 1
- Cyclophosphamide 200 mg/m^2/day IV, days 2 through 5
- Vincristine 1.5 mg/m^2 (2 mg maximum dose) IV, days 1 and 8 of all cycles
- Vincristine 1.5 mg/m^2 (2 mg maximum dose) IV, day 15 of cycle 3 only
- Doxorubicin 40 mg/m^2 IV, day 1
- Methotrexate 1,200 mg/m^2 IV over 1 hour, day 10
- Methotrexate 240 mg/m^2/hour continuous IV infusion over 23 hours, day 10 (begin after 1,200 mg/m^2 dose)
- Leucovorin 192 mg/m^2 IV, day 11, given 36 hours after the start of the methotrexate infusion
- Leucovorin 12 mg/m^2/dose IV every 6 hours, day 11, beginning 42 hours after the start of the methotrexate infusion and continued until the methotrexate concentration is below 0.05 microMol/L
- Cytarabine 70 mg intrathecal, days 1 and 3
- Methotrexate 12 mg intrathecal, day 15
- Filgrastim 5 mcg/kg/day subcutaneously, starting on day 13 and continuing until granulocyte count is above 1,000 cells/mm^3

IVAC (cycles 2 and 4)

- Ifosfamide 1,500 mg/m^2/day IV, days 1 through 5
- Mesna 1,500 mg/m^2/day continuous IV infusion, days 1 through 5
- Etoposide 60 mg/m^2/day IV, days 1 through 5
- Cytarabine 2,000 mg/m^2/dose IV every 12 hours for 4 doses, days 1 and 2
- Methotrexate 12 mg intrathecal, day 5
- Filgrastim 5 mcg/kg/day subcutaneously, starting on day 7 and continuing until granulocyte count is above 1,000 cells/mm^3

*Note: These 2 regimens are normally used in combination with each other and are rarely given alone.

Patients with malignant pleocytosis receive additional intrathecal drugs:

Cycle 1 (CODOX-M): Cytarabine 70 mg intrathecal on day 5 and methotrexate 12 mg intrathecal on day 17

Cycle 2 (IVAC): Cytarabine 70 mg intrathecal on days 7 and 9

COI

Use: Colorectal cancer.

Cycle: 14 days for at least 6 cycles, or until disease progression or intolerable toxicity

Regimen:

- Irinotecan 180 mg/m^2 IV, day 1
- Oxaliplatin 85 mg/m^2 IV, day 2
- Capecitabine 1,000 mg/m^2/dose PO twice daily, days 2 through 6

COMLA

Use: Lymphoma (non-Hodgkin).

Cycle: 78 to 85 days for up to 3 cycles

Regimen:

- Cyclophosphamide 1,500 mg/m^2 IV, day 1
- Vincristine 1.4 mg/m^2 (2 mg maximum dose) IV, days 1, 8, and 15
- Methotrexate 120 mg/m^2 IV, days 22, 29, 36, 43, 50, 57, 64, and 71
- Leucovorin 25 mg/m^2/dose PO every 6 hours for 4 doses, beginning 24 hours after each methotrexate dose, days 23, 30, 37, 44, 51, 58, 65, and 72
- Cytarabine 300 mg/m^2 IV, days 22, 29, 36, 43, 50, 57, 64, and 71

COMP

Use: Lymphoma (non-Hodgkin—pediatrics).

Regimen: **Induction.** *Cycle:* Give 1 cycle only

- Cyclophosphamide 1,200 mg/m^2 IV, day 1
- Vincristine 2 mg/m^2 (2 mg maximum dose) IV, days 3, 10, 17, and 24
- Prednisone 15 mg/m^2/dose (60 mg/day maximum dose) PO 4 times daily, days 3 through 30, then taper for 7 to 10 days
- Methotrexate 300 mg/m^2 IV, day 12 or 17

used in conjunction with

Intrathecal chemotherapy

Maintenance therapy. *Cycle:* 28 days for 15 cycles

- Cyclophosphamide 1,000 mg/m^2 IV, day 1
- Vincristine 1.5 mg/m^2 (2 mg maximum dose) IV, days 1 and 15
- Prednisone 15 mg/m^2/dose (60 mg/day maximum dose) PO 4 times daily, days 1 through 5, cycles 2 through 15
- Methotrexate 300 mg/m^2 IV, day 15

used in conjunction with

Intrathecal chemotherapy

Cooper Regimen

Use: Breast cancer.
Cycle: 36 weeks (give a single cycle)

Regimen:
Cyclophosphamide 2 mg/kg/day PO, weeks 1 through 36
Methotrexate 0.7 mg/kg IV weekly, weeks 1 through 8
Methotrexate 0.7 mg/kg IV every other week, weeks 10, 12, 14, 16, 18, 20, 22, 24, 26, 28, 30, 32, 34, and 36
Fluorouracil 12 mg/kg IV weekly, weeks 1 through 8
Fluorouracil 12 mg/kg IV every other week, weeks 10, 12, 14, 16, 18, 20, 22, 24, 26, 28, 30, 32, 34, and 36
Vincristine* 0.035 mg/kg IV weekly, weeks 1 through 5
Vincristine* 0.035 mg/kg IV monthly, weeks 8, 12, 16, 20, 24, 28, 32, and 36
Prednisone 0.75 mg/kg/day PO, days 1 through 10, then taper off over next 40 days
*Note: The vincristine dose is not capped in this protocol. Consult the prescriber if there is any question about the intended vincristine dose.

COP

Use: Lymphoma (non-Hodgkin).
Cycle: 14 to 28 days for up to 12 cycles

Regimen:
Cyclophosphamide 800 to 1,000 mg/m^2 IV, day 1
Vincristine 2 mg (dose is not in mg/m^2) IV, day 1
Prednisone 60 mg/m^2/day (or 100 mg/day) PO, days 1 through 5, then taper off over next 3 days

COPE

Use: Lung cancer (small cell).
Cycle: 21 days for up to 4 cycles

Regimen:
Cyclophosphamide 750 mg/m^2 IV, day 1
Etoposide 100 mg/m^2/day IV, days 1 through 3
Cisplatin 50 mg/m^2 IV, day 2
Vincristine 2 mg (dose is not in mg/m^2) IV, day 14

COPE (Baby Brain I)

Use: Brain tumors (pediatrics).
Cycle: 28 days for up to 24 months

Regimen:
Alternate cycles AABAAB.
Cycle A: Vincristine 0.065 mg/kg (1.5 mg maximum dose) IV, days 1 and 8
Cyclophosphamide 65 mg/kg IV, day 1
Cycle B: Cisplatin 4 mg/kg IV, day 1
Etoposide 6.5 mg/kg/day IV, days 3 and 4

COPP (C-MOPP)

Use: Lymphoma (non-Hodgkin or Hodgkin).
Cycle: 28 days for up to 6 cycles

Regimen:
Cyclophosphamide 450 to 650 mg/m^2 IV, days 1 and 8
Vincristine 1.4 to 2 mg/m^2 (2 mg maximum dose) IV, days 1 and 8
Procarbazine 100 mg/m^2/day PO, days 1 through 14
Prednisone 40 mg/m^2/day PO, cycles 1 and 4,* days 1 through 14
*Note: Some clinicians give prednisone with every cycle of COPP. The original clinical trials gave prednisone only with the first and fourth cycles.

CP

Use: Chronic lymphocytic leukemia (CLL).
Cycle: 14 days for up to 18 months

Regimen:
Chlorambucil 30 mg/m^2 PO, day 1
Prednisone 80 mg/day PO, days 1 through 5

Use: Ovarian cancer.
Cycle: 21 to 28 days for 6 to 12 cycles

Regimen:
Cyclophosphamide 600 to 1,000 mg/m^2 IV, day 1
Cisplatin 60 to 80 mg/m^2 IV, day 1

Use: Ovarian cancer.
Cycle: 28 days for up to 6 cycles

Regimen:
Cyclophosphamide 600 mg/m^2 IV, day 1
Cisplatin 100 mg/m^2 IV, day 1

CT

Use:	Ovarian cancer. *Cycle:* 21 days for at least 6 cycles
Regimen:	Paclitaxel 175 mg/m^2 IV over 3 hours, day 1 *or* Paclitaxel 135 mg/m^2/day continuous IV infusion over 24 hours, day 1 *with* Cisplatin 75 mg/m^2 IV, day 1 or 2 (give immediately after paclitaxel infusion)

Use:	Ovarian cancer. *Cycle:* 21 days for 3 to 8 cycles
Regimen:	Paclitaxel 175 mg/m^2 IV over 3 hours, day 1 Cisplatin 50 mg/m^2 IV, day 1 (give after paclitaxel)

Use:	Cervical cancer. *Cycle:* 21 days for up to 6 cycles
Regimen:	Paclitaxel 135 mg/m^2/day continuous IV infusion over 24 hours, day 1 Cisplatin 50 mg/m^2 IV, day 2 (give immediately after paclitaxel infusion)

Use:	Cervical cancer. *Cycle:* 10 days. Give 3 cycles prior to surgery or radiation therapy.
Regimen:	Paclitaxel 60 mg/m^2 IV over 3 hours, day 1 Cisplatin 60 mg/m^2 IV, day 1 (give after paclitaxel)

Use:	Lung cancer (non-small cell), head and neck cancer. *Cycle:* 21 days, until disease progression or intolerable toxicity
Regimen:	Paclitaxel 135 mg/m^2/day continuous IV infusion over 24 hours, day 1 Cisplatin 75 mg/m^2 IV, day 2 (give after paclitaxel infusion)

Use:	Esophageal cancer. *Cycle:* 21 days for at least 2 cycles, continue until disease progression or intolerable toxicity
Regimen:	Paclitaxel 200 mg/m^2/day continuous IV infusion over 24 hours, day 1 Cisplatin 75 mg/m^2 IV, day 2 (give after paclitaxel infusion) Filgrastim 5 mcg/kg/day subcutaneously (rounded to 300 or 480 mcg), from day 3 until the absolute neutrophil count (ANC) is at least 10,000 cells/mm^3 (start at least 24 hours after completion of chemotherapy infusions)

Use:	Gastric cancer. *Cycle:* 14 days for up to 12 cycles
Regimen:	Paclitaxel 160 mg/m^2 IV over 3 hours, day 1 Cisplatin 60 mg/m^2 IV, day 1 (sequence of administration not specified)

CT - Intraperitoneal

Use:	Ovarian cancer. *Cycle:* 21 days for 6 cycles
Regimen:	Paclitaxel 135 mg/m^2/day continuous IV infusion over 24 hours, day 1 Cisplatin 100 mg/m^2 intraperitoneal, day 2 (give after paclitaxel infusion) Paclitaxel 60 mg/m^2 intraperitoneal, day 8

CVD

Use:	Malignant melanoma. *Cycle:* 21 days for at least 2 cycles
Regimen:	Vinblastine 1.6 mg/m^2/day IV, days 1 through 5 Dacarbazine 800 mg/m^2 IV, day 1 Cisplatin 20 mg/m^2/day IV, days 2 through 5

Use:	Malignant melanoma. *Cycle:* 21 days for at least 2 cycles
Regimen:	Cisplatin 20 mg/m^2/day IV, days 1 through 4 Vinblastine 2 mg/m^2/day IV, days 1 through 4 Dacarbazine 800 mg/m^2 IV, day 1

CVD + IL-2I

Use:	Malignant melanoma. *Cycle:* 21 days for 6 to 7 cycles
Regimen:	Cisplatin 20 mg/m^2/day IV, days 1 through 4 Vinblastine 1.6 mg/m^2/day IV, days 1 through 4 Dacarbazine 800 mg/m^2 IV, day 1 Aldesleukin 9 million units/m^2/day continuous IV infusion, days 1 through 4 Interferon alfa 5 million units/m^2/day subcutaneously, days 1 through 5, and days 7, 9, 11, and 13

(continued on next page)

CVD + IL-2I (cont.)

Use: Malignant melanoma.
Cycle: 42 days for up to 3 cycles

Regimen:
Cisplatin 20 mg/m²/day IV, days 1 through 4 and days 22 through 25
Vinblastine 1.5 mg/m²/day IV, days 1 through 4 and days 22 through 25
Dacarbazine 800 mg/m² IV, days 1 and 22
Aldesleukin 9 million units/m²/day continuous IV infusion, days 5 through 8, days 17 through 20, and days 26 through 29
Interferon alfa-2b 5 million units/m²/day subcutaneously, days 5 through 9, days 17 through 21, and days 26 through 30

CVD + IL-2I, Modified

Use: Malignant melanoma.
Cycle: 21 days for up to 4 cycles

Regimen:
Cisplatin 20 mg/m²/day IV, days 1 through 4
Vinblastine 1.2 mg/m²/day IV, days 1 through 4
Dacarbazine 800 mg/m² IV, day 1
Aldesleukin 9 million units/m²/day continuous IV infusion, days 1 through 4
Interferon alfa-2b 5 million units/m²/day subcutaneously, days 1 through 5, and days 8, 10, and 12
Filgrastim 5 mcg/kg/day subcutaneously (rounded to 300 or 480 mcg), days 7 through 16
*used in conjunction with antimicrobial prophylaxis**
Ciprofloxacin 500 mg PO twice daily, days 1 through 14
or
Cephalexin 500 mg PO twice daily, days 1 through 14
*Note: Antimicrobial prophylaxis doses not specified in original article; the dose given here is derived from *AHFS 2008 Drug Information,* a tertiary resource.

CVI (VIC)

Use: Lung cancer (non-small cell).
Cycle: 28 days for up to 6 cycles

Regimen:
Carboplatin 300 to 350 mg/m² IV, day 1
Etoposide 60 to 100 mg/m² IV, days 1, 3, and 5
Ifosfamide 1,500 mg/m² IV, days 1, 3, and 5
Mesna 400 mg/m² IV, given before ifosfamide, days 1, 3, and 5
Mesna 1,600 mg/m²/day continuous IV infusion, days 1, 3, and 5 (give after mesna bolus)

CVP

Use: Lymphoma (non-Hodgkin), chronic lymphocytic leukemia (CLL).
Cycle: 21 days

Regimen:
Cyclophosphamide 300 to 400 mg/m²/day PO, days 1 through 5
Vincristine 1.2 to 1.4 mg/m² (2 mg maximum dose) IV, day 1
Prednisone 40 to 100 mg/m²/day PO, days 1 through 5

Use: Lymphoma (non-Hodgkin).
Cycle: 21 days for up to 8 cycles

Regimen:
Cyclophosphamide 750 to 1,000 mg/m²/day IV, day 1
Vincristine 1.4 mg/m² (2 mg maximum dose) IV, day 1
Prednisone 40 to 100 mg/m²/day PO, days 1 through 5

CVP + Maintenance Rituximab

Use: Lymphoma (non-Hodgkin).
Cycle: See below, cycle length varies throughout protocol. Give 6 to 8 cycles of CVP, followed by 4 cycles (ie, 24 months) of maintenance rituximab.

Regimen:
CVP. *Cycle*: 21 days for 6 to 8 cycles
Cyclophosphamide 1,000 mg/m²/day IV, day 1
Vincristine 1.4 mg/m² (2 mg maximum dose) IV, day 1
Prednisone 100 mg/m²/day PO, days 1 through 5
followed by 4 weeks of rest then
Maintenance Rituximab. *Cycle*: 6 months for 4 cycles
Rituximab 375 mg/m² IV weekly for 4 weeks

CVP + Rituximab (R-CVP)

Use: Lymphoma (non-Hodgkin).
Cycle: 21 days for up to 8 cycles

Regimen:
Cyclophosphamide 750 mg/m² IV, day 1
Vincristine 1.4 mg/m² (2 mg maximum dose) IV, day 1
Prednisone 40 mg/m²/day PO, days 1 through 5
Rituximab 375 mg/m² IV, day 1

CVPP

Use: Lymphoma (Hodgkin).
Cycle: 28 days for up to 6 cycles

Regimen: Lomustine 75 mg/m² PO, day 1
Vinblastine 4 mg/m² IV, days 1 and 8
Procarbazine 100 mg/m²/day PO, days 1 through 14
Prednisone 40 mg/m²/day PO, cycles 1 and 4, days 1 through 14

CY/A—see AC

Cyclophosphamide-Bevacizumab

Use: Ovarian cancer.
Cycle: 14 days, continue until disease progression or intolerable toxicity

Regimen: Cyclophosphamide 50 mg PO once daily, throughout entire course
Bevacizumab 10 mg/kg IV, day 1
Bevacizumab 10 mg/kg IV, day 8 of first cycle only (loading dose)

Cyclophosphamide-Fludarabine

Use: Chronic lymphocytic leukemia (CLL).
Cycle: 28 days for up to 6 cycles

Regimen: Cyclophosphamide 250 mg/m²/day IV, days 1 through 3
Fludarabine 25 to 30 mg/m²/day IV, days 1 through 3

Cyclophosphamide-Topotecan—see Topo/CTX

CYVADIC

Use: Sarcoma (bone, soft tissue).
Cycle: 21 days for up to 8 cycles

Regimen: Cyclophosphamide 500 mg/m² IV, day 1
Vincristine 1 mg/m² (2 mg maximum dose) IV, days 1 and 5
Doxorubicin 50 mg/m² IV, day 1
Dacarbazine 250 mg/m²/day IV, days 1 through 5

Use: Sarcoma (bone, soft tissue).
Cycle: 21 days

Regimen: Cyclophosphamide 500 mg/m² IV, day 1
Vincristine 1.5 mg/m² (2 mg maximum dose) IV, day 1
Doxorubicin 50 mg/m² IV, day 1 (total cumulative dose 550 mg/m²)
Dacarbazine 750 mg/m²/day IV, day 1

CYVE + Autologous Stem Cell Transplantation

Use: Lymphoma (central nervous system).
Cycle: 28 days for 2 cycles, then followed by autologous stem cell transplantation

Regimen 1: Patients younger than 60 years of age:
Cytarabine 50 mg/m²/day continuous IV infusion over 12 hours, days 1 through 5
Cytarabine 2,000 mg/m²/day IV over 3 hours, days 2 through 5
Etoposide 200 mg/m²/day IV, days 2 through 5
used in conjunction with
Autologous stem cell transplantation

Regimen 2: Patients 60 years of age and older:
Cytarabine 50 mg/m²/day continuous IV infusion over 12 hours, days 1 through 5
Cytarabine 2,000 mg/m²/day IV over 3 hours, days 2 through 4
Etoposide 150 mg/m²/day IV, days 2 through 5
used in conjunction with
Autologous stem cell transplantation

D + P—see Docetaxel-Prednisone

DA (also see Ara-C-DNR)

Use: Acute myelocytic leukemia (AML; induction—pediatrics).
Cycle: 14 days. Give 1 cycle. If patient has persistent leukemia on day 14, give 1 to 2 additional cycles as described below.

Regimen: Daunorubicin 45 to 60 mg/m²/day IV, days 1 through 3
Cytarabine 100 mg/m²/day continuous IV infusion, days 1 through 7
If leukemia is persistent on day 14, additional doses are given: cytarabine on days 1 through 5 and daunorubicin on days 1 and 2, both at same dose as previous cycle.

DA + ATRA (ATRA + CT)

Use: Acute promyelocytic leukemia (APL; induction and consolidation).

Regimen: Tretinoin 45 mg/m²/day PO, days 1 through 90, or until complete remission, whichever occurs earlier

Induction. *Cycle:* Give 1 induction cycle followed by 2 consolidation cycles after hematologic recovery.
Daunorubicin 60 mg/m²/day IV, days 3 through 5
Cytarabine 200 mg/m²/day continuous IV infusion, days 3 through 9

First consolidation. *Cycle:* Give 1 cycle.
Daunorubicin 60 mg/m²/day IV, days 1 through 3
Cytarabine 200 mg/m²/day continuous IV infusion, days 1 through 7

Second consolidation. *Cycle:* Give 1 cycle. Do not give to patients older than 65 years of age.
Daunorubicin 45 mg/m²/day IV, days 1 through 3
Cytarabine 1,000 mg/m²/dose IV every 12 hours for 8 doses, days 1 through 4

Dartmouth Regimen—see CDB + Tamoxifen

DAT

Use: Acute myelocytic leukemia (AML; induction—pediatrics).
Cycle: 14 to 21 days for up to 3 cycles

Regimen:
Cytarabine 100 mg/m²/dose IV every 12 hours for 14 doses, days 1 through 7
Thioguanine 100 mg/m²/dose PO every 12 hours for 14 doses, days 1 through 7
Daunorubicin 60 mg/m²/day continuous IV infusion, days 5 through 7

Use: Acute myelocytic leukemia (AML; induction—pediatrics).

Regimen:
Remission induction. *Cycle:* Give 1 cycle only
Daunorubicin 45 mg/m²/day IV, days 1 through 3
Cytarabine 100 mg/m²/day continuous IV infusion, days 1 through 7
Thioguanine 100 mg/m²/day PO, days 1 through 7

Second induction. *Cycle*: Give a single cycle 14 days after initial remission induction course; delay until hematologic recovery in patients with remission or with hypoplastic marrow.
Daunorubicin 45 mg/m²/day IV, days 1 and 2
Cytarabine 100 mg/m²/day continuous IV infusion, days 1 through 5
Thioguanine 100 mg/m²/day PO, days 1 through 5

used in conjunction with
Intrathecal chemotherapy

DAV

Use: Acute myelocytic leukemia (AML; induction—pediatrics).
Cycle: Give a single cycle

Regimen:
Cytarabine 100 mg/m²/day continuous IV infusion, days 1 through 2
Cytarabine 100 mg/m²/dose IV every 12 hours for 12 doses, days 3 through 8
Daunorubicin 60 mg/m²/day IV, days 3 through 5
Etoposide 150 mg/m²/day IV, days 6 through 8

DCF (also see TPF)

Use: Gastric cancer.
Cycle: 21 days, continue until disease progression or intolerable toxicity

Regimen:
Docetaxel 75 mg/m² IV, day 1
Cisplatin 75 mg/m² IV, day 1
Fluorouracil 750 mg/m²/day continuous IV infusion, days 1 through 5 (for 120 hours total)

DCT

Use: Acute myelocytic leukemia (AML; induction—adults).
Cycle: 7 days. Give once. May be given a second time based on individual response. Time between cycles not specified.

Regimen:
Daunorubicin 40 mg/m²/day IV, days 1 through 3
Cytarabine 100 mg/m²/dose IV every 12 hours for 14 doses, days 1 through 7
Thioguanine 100 mg/m²/dose PO every 12 hours for 14 doses, days 1 through 7

DCTER

Use: Acute myelocytic leukemia (AML; induction and consolidation—pediatrics).
Cycle: 10 to 14 days. Give 4 cycles.

Regimen 1: Patients younger than 3 years of age:
Dexamethasone 0.067 mg/kg/dose (0.2 mg/kg/day) PO given 3 times daily, days 1 through 4
Cytarabine 6.7 mg/kg/day continuous IV infusion, days 1 through 4*
Thioguanine 1.65 mg/kg/dose (3.3 mg/kg/day) PO given twice daily, days 1 through 4
Etoposide 3.3 mg/kg/day continuous IV infusion, days 1 through 4*
Daunorubicin 0.67 mg/kg/day continuous IV infusion, days 1 through 4*

used in conjunction with
Cytarabine intrathecal, day 1 (dose is based on patient's age):
Age up to 1 year: Cytarabine 20 mg
Age 1 to 2 years: Cytarabine 30 mg
Age 2 to 3 years: Cytarabine 50 mg

(continued on next page)

DCTER (cont.)

Regimen 2: Patients 3 years of age and older:
- Dexamethasone 2 mg/m²/dose (6 mg/m²/day) PO given 3 times daily, days 1 through 4
- Cytarabine 200 mg/m²/day continuous IV infusion, days 1 through 4*
- Thioguanine 50 mg/m²/dose (100 mg/m²/day) PO given twice daily, days 1 through 4
- Etoposide 100 mg/m²/day continuous IV infusion, days 1 through 4*
- Daunorubicin 20 mg/m²/day continuous IV infusion, days 1 through 4*

used in conjunction with

Cytarabine 70 mg intrathecal, day 1

*Note: Cytarabine, etoposide, and daunorubicin may be mixed and administered in the same infusion bag.

Decitabine-Valproic Acid

Use: Acute myelocytic leukemia (AML—elderly patients).
Cycle: 28 days for up to 24 cycles

Regimen:
Decitabine 15 mg/m²/day IV, days 1 through 10
Valproic acid 50 mg/kg/day PO in 2 to 3 divided doses, days 1 through 10

DHAOx

Use: Lymphoma (non-Hodgkin).
Cycle: 21 days

Regimen:
Oxaliplatin 130 mg/m² IV, day 1
Dexamethasone 40 mg/day IV or PO, days 1 through 4
Cytarabine 2,000 mg/m²/dose IV every 12 hours for 2 doses (total dose 4,000 mg/m²), day 2
Filgrastim 5 mcg/kg/day subcutaneously, starting on day 3 and continued until granulocyte count is above 500 cells/mm³

DHAP

Use: Lymphoma (non-Hodgkin).
Cycle: 21 to 28 days for 6 to 10 cycles

Regimen:
Cisplatin 100 mg/m²/day continuous IV infusion, day 1
Dexamethasone 40 mg/day IV or PO, days 1 through 4
Cytarabine 2,000 mg/m²/dose IV every 12 hours for 2 doses (total dose 4,000 mg/m²), day 2

DI (AI)

Use: Sarcoma (soft tissue).
Cycle: 21 days, continue until disease progression or intolerable toxicity

Regimen:
Doxorubicin 50 mg/m² IV, day 1
Ifosfamide 5,000 mg/m²/day continuous IV infusion, day 1 (after doxorubicin)
Mesna 600 mg/m² IV bolus infusion, day 1 (before ifosfamide)
Mesna 2,500 mg/m²/day continuous IV infusion over 36 hours, day 1 (give after mesna bolus)

Use: Sarcoma.
Cycle: 21 days

Regimen:
Doxorubicin 25 mg/m²/day continuous IV infusion, days 1 through 3
Ifosfamide 2,000 mg/m²/day IV, days 1 through 5
Mesna 400 mg/m² IV bolus at same time as first ifosfamide dose, day 1
Mesna 1,200 mg/m²/day continuous IV infusion, days 1 through 5 (start after mesna bolus on day 1)

Use: Sarcoma.
Cycle: 21 days

Regimen:
Doxorubicin 30 mg/m²/day continuous IV infusion, days 1 through 3
Ifosfamide 2,500 mg/m²/day IV, days 1 through 4
Mesna 500 mg/m² IV bolus at same time as first ifosfamide dose, day 1
Mesna 1,500 mg/m²/day continuous IV infusion, days 1 through 4 (start after mesna bolus on day 1)
Filgrastim 5 mcg/kg/day subcutaneously (rounded to 300 or 480 mcg), starting on day 5, continued until absolute neutrophil count (ANC) is at least 10,000 cells/mm³

Use: Sarcoma (soft-tissue).
Cycle: 21 days for up to 6 cycles, or until disease progression or intolerable toxicity

Regimen:
Doxorubicin 20 mg/m²/day continuous IV infusion, days 1 through 3
Ifosfamide 1,500 mg/m²/day IV, days 1 through 4
Mesna 225 mg/m² IV before, then 4 and 8 hours after each ifosfamide infusion, days 1 through 4
Filgrastim 5 mcg/kg/day subcutaneously (rounded to 300 or 480 mcg), starting on day 5, continued for 10 days

Docetaxel/AC, Dose Dense

Use: Breast cancer.
Cycle: 14 days. Give 4 cycles of Docetaxel alone, followed by 4 cycles of Dose Dense AC.*

Regimen:
Docetaxel alone (cycles 1 through 4)
Docetaxel 75 mg/m^2 IV, day 1 for 4 cycles
Pegfilgrastim 6 mg subcutaneously, day 2
followed by
Dose Dense AC (cycles 5 through 8)
Doxorubicin 60 mg/m^2 IV, day 1
Cyclophosphamide 600 mg/m^2 IV, day 1
Pegfilgrastim 6 mg subcutaneously, day 2

*Note: A phase 2 trial compared 2 different therapy sequences (Dose Dense AC followed by Docetaxel versus Dose Dense Docetaxel followed by AC). The best results are seen when Dose Dense Docetaxel is followed by AC, rather than the converse.

Docetaxel-Bevacizumab

Use: Lung cancer (non-small cell).
Cycle: 21 days for up to 52 weeks, or until disease progression or intolerable toxicity

Regimen:
Docetaxel 75 mg/m^2 IV, day 1
Bevacizumab 15 mg/kg IV, day 1

Use: Breast cancer.
Cycle: 21 days for up to 9 cycles

Regimen:
Docetaxel 100 mg/m^2 IV, day 1
Bevacizumab 7.5 or 15 mg/kg IV, day 1
followed by
Bevacizumab 7.5 or 15 mg/kg IV, every 3 weeks until disease progression or intolerable toxicity

Docetaxel-Carboplatin

Use: Ovarian cancer.
Cycle: 21 days for up to 6 cycles

Regimen:
Docetaxel 75 mg/m^2 IV, day 1
Carboplatin IV dose by Calvert equation to AUC 5 mg/mL/min, day 1 (give after docetaxel)

Use: Ovarian cancer, cervical cancer.
Cycle: 21 days for up to 6 cycles

Regimen:
Docetaxel 60 mg/m^2 IV, day 1
Carboplatin IV dose by Calvert equation to AUC 6 mg/mL/min, day 1 (give after docetaxel)

Docetaxel-Cisplatin (also see Cisplatin-Docetaxel; also see TC)

Use: Lung cancer (non-small cell).
Cycle: 21 days for up to 6 cycles

Regimen:
Docetaxel 75 mg/m^2 IV, day 1
Cisplatin 75 mg/m^2 IV, day 1 (give after docetaxel)

Docetaxel-Cyclophosphamide

Use: Breast cancer.
Cycle: 21 days for up to 4 cycles

Regimen:
Docetaxel 75 mg/m^2 IV, day 1
Cyclophosphamide 600 mg/m^2 IV, day 1

Docetaxel-Doxorubicin

Use: Breast cancer.
Cycle: 21 days

Regimen:
Doxorubicin 50 mg/m^2 IV, day 1
Docetaxel 75 mg/m^2 IV, day 1 (give after doxorubicin)
used in conjunction with antimicrobial prophylaxis
Ciprofloxacin 500 mg PO twice daily, days 5 through 14 (10 days total)

Docetaxel-Estramustine

Use: Prostate cancer.
Cycle: 21 days for up to 6 cycles

Regimen:
Estramustine 280 mg/dose (1,120 mg/day) PO every 6 hours for 5 doses, day 1
Docetaxel 70 mg/m^2 IV, day 1 (given 12 hours after first estramustine dose)
used in conjunction with antithrombotic prophylaxis
Warfarin 2 mg PO once daily, throughout entire course

(continued on next page)

Docetaxel-Estramustine (cont.)

Use: Prostate cancer.
Cycle: 21 days for up to 12 cycles

Regimen: Estramustine 280 mg/dose (840 mg/day) PO 3 times daily, days 1 through 5
Docetaxel 60 mg/m^2 IV, day 2 for first cycle; may increase to docetaxel 70 mg/m^2 IV day 1 for subsequent cycles if tolerated
used in conjunction with antithrombotic prophylaxis
Warfarin 2 mg PO once daily, throughout entire course
Aspirin 325 mg PO once daily, throughout entire course

Use: Prostate cancer.
Cycle: 21 days, continue until disease progression or intolerable toxicity

Regimen: Estramustine 420 mg/dose (1,260 mg/day) PO 3 times daily for 4 doses, on days 1 (give in morning, afternoon, and evening) and 2 (give in morning only)
Estramustine 280 mg/dose (840 mg/day) PO 3 times daily for 5 doses, days 2 (give in afternoon and evening) and 3 (give in morning afternoon, and evening)
Docetaxel 35 mg/m^2 IV, days 2 and 9
Estramustine 420 mg/dose (1,260 mg/day) PO 3 times daily for 4 doses, on days 8 (give in morning, afternoon, and evening) and 9 (give in morning only)
Estramustine 280 mg/dose (840 mg/day) PO 3 times daily for 5 doses, days 9 (give in afternoon and evening) and 10 (give in morning afternoon, and evening)

Docetaxel-Estramustine ➡ Goserelin-Bicalutamide

Use: Prostate cancer.
Cycle: See below, cycle length varies throughout protocol. Give 4 cycles of Docetaxel-Estramustine, followed by 5 cycles (ie, 15 months) of hormone therapy.

Regimen: **Docetaxel-Estramustine.** *Cycle*: 21 days for 4 cycles
Estramustine 3.33 mg/kg/dose (rounded to nearest 140 mg) (10 mg/kg/day) PO 3 times daily, days 1 through 5
Docetaxel 70 mg/m^2 IV, day 2
used in conjunction with antithrombotic prophylaxis
Warfarin 1 mg PO once daily, throughout entire course
followed by
Hormone Therapy. *Cycle:* 3 months for 5 cycles
Bicalutamide 50 mg PO daily, throughout entire course
Goserelin acetate 10.8 mg/dose implant subcutaneously, day 1

Docetaxel-Liposomal Doxorubicin

Use: Breast cancer.
Cycle: 21 days for up to 6 cycles

Regimen: Liposomal doxorubicin 30 mg/m^2 IV, day 1
with
Docetaxel 60 mg/m^2 IV, day 1 (give after liposomal doxorubicin)
or
Docetaxel 75 mg/m^2 IV, day 2

Docetaxel-Prednisone (D + P)

Use: Prostate cancer.
Cycle: 21 days for up to 10 cycles

Regimen: Docetaxel 75 mg/m^2 IV, day 1
Prednisone 5 mg/dose PO twice daily, throughout entire course

---

Use: Prostate cancer.
Cycle: 42 days for up to 5 cycles

Regimen: Docetaxel 30 mg/m^2 IV, weekly for 5 weeks, followed by 1 week of rest; administer on days 1, 8, 15, 22, and 29
Prednisone 5 mg/dose PO twice daily, throughout entire course

---

Docetaxel + Trastuzumab ➡ FEC

Use: Breast cancer.
Cycle: 21 days. Give 3 cycles of Docetaxel + Trastuzumab, followed by 3 cycles of FEC.

Regimen: **Docetaxel + Trastuzumab** (cycles 1 through 3)
Trastuzumab 4 mg/kg IV, day 1 of first cycle only (loading dose)
Trastuzumab 2 mg/kg IV weekly, days 1, 8, and 15, except for day 1 of first cycle
Docetaxel 100 mg/m^2 IV, day 1 (give after trastuzumab)
followed by
FEC (cycles 4 through 6)
Fluorouracil 600 mg/m^2 IV, day 1
Epirubicin 60 mg/m^2 IV, day 1
Cyclophosphamide 600 mg/m^2 IV, day 1

Dox → CMF, Sequential

Use: Breast cancer.
Cycle: 21 days

Regimen: Doxorubicin 75 mg/m² IV, day 1 for 4 cycles
followed by
CMF-IV for 8 cycles

Doxorubicin-Streptozocin

Use: Islet-cell carcinoma.
Cycle: 42 days, continue until disease progression or intolerable toxicity

Regimen: Doxorubicin 50 mg/m² IV, days 1 and 22
Streptozocin 500 mg/m²/day IV, days 1 through 5

DTIC/Tamoxifen

Use: Malignant melanoma.
Cycle: 21 days, continue until disease progression or intolerable toxicity

Regimen: Dacarbazine 250 mg/m²/day IV, days 1 through 5
Tamoxifen 20 mg/m²/day PO, days 1 through 5

DTPACE

Use: Multiple myeloma.
Cycle: 28 to 42 days for up to 6 cycles, delay each subsequent cycle until hematologic recovery

Regimen: Dexamethasone 40 mg/day PO, days 1 through 4
Thalidomide 400 mg/day PO, throughout entire course
Cisplatin 10 mg/m²/day continuous IV infusion, days 1 through 4*
Doxorubicin 10 mg/m²/day continuous IV infusion, days 1 through 4
Cyclophosphamide 400 mg/m²/day continuous IV infusion, days 1 through 4*
Etoposide 40 mg/m²/day continuous IV infusion, days 1 through 4*
Filgrastim 300 mcg/day subcutaneously, from day 5 until the absolute neutrophil count (ANC) is at least 1,000 cells/mm³ for 2 consecutive days; increase dose to filgrastim 10 mcg/kg/day subcutaneously during first cycle in patients undergoing peripheral blood stem cell mobilization
used in conjunction with antimicrobial prophylaxis
Fluconazole 200 mg/dose PO 4 times daily, from day 1 until neutropenia resolves
Levofloxacin 250 mg/dose PO 4 times daily, from day 1 until neutropenia resolves
Acyclovir 400 mg PO twice daily, from day 1 until neutropenia resolves
Cotrimoxazole double-strength (160/800) 1 tablet PO twice daily, from day 1 until neutropenia resolves
*Note: Cisplatin, cyclophosphamide, and etoposide may be mixed and administered in the same infusion bag.

DVd

Use: Multiple myeloma.
Cycle: 28 days, continue until complete remission, disease progression, or intolerable toxicity

Regimen: Liposomal doxorubicin 40 mg/m² IV, day 1
Vincristine 1.4 mg/m² (2 mg maximum dose) IV, day 1
Dexamethasone 40 mg/day PO, days 1 through 4

DVP

Use: Acute lymphocytic leukemia (ALL; induction—pediatrics).
Cycle: 35 days. Give a single cycle.

Regimen: Daunorubicin 25 mg/m² IV, days 1, 8, and 15
Vincristine 1.5 mg/m² (2 mg maximum dose) IV, weekly for 4 weeks, followed by 1 week of rest; administer on days 1, 8, 15, and 22
Prednisone 60 mg/m²/day PO, days 1 through 28, then taper off over next 14 days
used in conjunction with
Intrathecal chemotherapy

EAP

Use: Gastric cancer, small bowel cancer.
Cycle: 21 to 28 days for up to 6 cycles

Regimen: Doxorubicin 20 mg/m² IV, days 1 and 7
Cisplatin 40 mg/m² IV, days 2 and 8
Etoposide 100 to 120 mg/m²/day IV, days 4 through 6

EC

Use: Lung cancer (small cell).
Cycle: 21 to 28 days for up to 4 to 6 cycles

Regimen: Etoposide 100 to 120 mg/m^2/day IV, days 1 through 3
with
Carboplatin 300 mg/m^2 IV, day 1
or
Carboplatin IV dose by Calvert equation to AUC 5 to 6 mg/mL/min, day 1
may be used in conjunction with
Radiation therapy

Use: Lung cancer (non-small cell).
Cycle: 21 to 28 days for up to 4 to 6 cycles

Regimen: Etoposide 100 to 120 mg/m^2/day IV, days 1 through 3
with
Carboplatin 300 to 350 mg/m^2 IV, day 1
may be used in conjunction with
Radiation therapy

Use: Lung cancer (small cell).
Cycle: 21 to 28 days for up to 4 cycles

Regimen: Etoposide 80 mg/m^2/day IV, days 1 through 3
Carboplatin IV dose by Calvert equation to AUC 5 mg/mL/min, day 1
may be used in conjunction with
Filgrastim 5 mcg/kg/day subcutaneously, from day 4 until the leukocyte count is greater than 10,000 cells/mm^3*
*Note: Filgrastim dose not specified in original article; the doses given here are derived from *AHFS 2009 Drug Information,* a tertiary resource.

Use: Prostate cancer.
Cycle: 21 days, continue until disease progression or intolerable toxicity

Regimen: Etoposide 80 mg/m^2/day IV, day 1
Carboplatin IV dose by Calvert equation to AUC 5 mg/mL/min, day 1
Etoposide 80 mg/m^2/day PO, days 2 and 3

Use: Merkel cell carcinoma.
Cycle: 21 days for up to 6 cycles

Regimen: Etoposide 100 mg/m^2/day IV, days 1 through 3
with
Carboplatin 300 mg/m^2 IV, day 1
or
Carboplatin IV dose by Calvert equation to AUC 5 mg/mL/min, day 1

ECF

Use: Gastric cancer, esophageal cancer.
Cycle: 21 days for up to 8 cycles

Regimen: Epirubicin 50 mg/m^2 IV, day 1
Cisplatin 60 mg/m^2 IV, day 1
Fluorouracil 200 mg/m^2/day continuous IV infusion, days 1 through 180
may be used in conjunction with antithrombotic prophylaxis
Warfarin 1 mg PO once daily, throughout entire course

ECF + Surgery ➜ ECF

Use: Esophageal cancer.
Cycle: 21 days. Give 3 cycles of ECF, followed by surgery, then 3 additional cycles of ECF.

Regimen: **ECF** (cycles 1 through 3)
Epirubicin 50 mg/m^2 IV, day 1
Cisplatin 60 mg/m^2 IV, day 1
Fluorouracil 200 mg/m^2/day continuous IV infusion, days 1 through 21
used in conjunction with antithrombotic prophylaxis
Warfarin 1 mg PO once daily, throughout entire course
followed after 3 to 6 weeks by
Surgical resection
followed after 6 to 12 weeks by
Repeat ECF chemotherapy (cycles 4 through 6)

ECX

Use: Gastric cancer, esophageal cancer.
Cycle: 21 days for up to 8 cycles

Regimen: Epirubicin 50 mg/m^2 IV, day 1
Cisplatin 60 mg/m^2 IV, day 1
Capecitabine 625 mg/m^2/dose PO twice daily, throughout entire course

EDP-Mitotane

Use: Adrenal cancer.
Cycle: 28 days for up to 6 cycles

Regimen:
Doxorubicin 20 mg/m^2 IV, days 1 and 8
Cisplatin 40 mg/m^2 IV, days 1 and 9
Etoposide 100 mg/m^2/day IV, days 5 through 7
Mitotane 1,000 mg/dose (4,000 mg/day) PO 4 times daily, throughout entire course
some patients may require mineralocorticoid or glucocorticoid supplementation
Hydrocortisone 10 to 30 mg/day PO in divided doses, throughout entire course*
Fludrocortisone 0.1 mg/day PO, throughout entire course*
*Note: Mineralocorticoid and glucocorticoid doses not specified in original article; the dose given here is derived from *AHFS 2008 Drug Information,* a tertiary resource.

EFP

Use: Gastric cancer, small bowel cancer.
Cycle: 21 to 28 days

Regimen:
Etoposide 80 to 100 mg/m^2 IV, days 1, 3, and 5
Fluorouracil 800 to 900 mg/m^2/day continuous IV infusion, days 1 through 5
Cisplatin 20 mg/m^2/day IV, days 1 through 5

ELF

Use: Gastric cancer.
Cycle: 21 to 28 days for up to 9 cycles

Regimen:
Etoposide 120 mg/m^2/day IV, days 1 through 3
with
Leucovorin 300 mg/m^2/day IV, days 1 through 3
or
Levoleucovorin 150 mg/m^2/day IV, days 1 through 3
plus
Fluorouracil 500 mg/m^2/day IV, days 1 through 3 (give after leucovorin or levoleucovorin)

EM-V—see Estramustine/Vinblastine

EMA 86

Use: Acute myelocytic leukemia (AML; induction—adults).
Cycle: Give a single cycle

Regimen:
Mitoxantrone 12 mg/m^2/day IV, days 1 through 3
Cytarabine 500 mg/m^2/day continuous IV infusion, days 1 through 3 and days 8 through 10
Etoposide 200 mg/m^2/day continuous IV infusion, days 8 through 10

EOF

Use: Gastric cancer, esophageal cancer.
Cycle: 21 days for up to 8 cycles

Regimen:
Epirubicin 50 mg/m^2 IV, day 1
Oxaliplatin 130 mg/m^2 IV, day 1
Fluorouracil 200 mg/m^2/day continuous IV infusion, throughout entire course
used in conjunction with antithrombotic prophylaxis
Warfarin 1 mg PO once daily, throughout entire course

EOX

Use: Gastric cancer, esophageal cancer.
Cycle: 21 days for up to 8 cycles

Regimen:
Epirubicin 50 mg/m^2 IV, day 1
Oxaliplatin 130 mg/m^2 IV, day 1
Capecitabine 625 mg/m^2/dose PO twice daily, throughout entire course

EP

Use: Testicular cancer.
Cycle: 21 days for 2 to 4 cycles

Regimen:
Etoposide 100 mg/m^2/day IV, days 1 through 5
Cisplatin 20 mg/m^2/day IV, days 1 through 5

Use: Thymoma.
Cycle: 21 days for up to 8 cycles

Regimen:
Etoposide 120 mg/m^2/day IV, days 1 through 3
Cisplatin 60 mg/m^2 IV, day 1

(continued on next page)

EP (cont.)

Use: Lung cancer (non-small cell), adenocarcinoma (unknown primary).
Cycle: 21 to 28 days for 2 to 6 cycles

Regimen: Etoposide 80 to 100 mg/m^2/day IV, days 1 through 3
Cisplatin 80 to 100 mg/m^2 IV, day 1

Use: Lung cancer (small cell).
Cycle: 21 days for 4 to 8 cycles

Regimen: Etoposide 80 to 120 mg/m^2/day IV, days 1 through 3
Cisplatin 60 to 80 mg/m^2 IV, day 1
may be used in conjunction with
Radiation therapy

Use: Lung cancer (small cell).
Cycle: 21 to 28 days for 4 to 6 cycles

Regimen: Etoposide 80 to 100 mg/m^2/day IV, days 1 through 3
Cisplatin 25 mg/m^2/day IV, days 1 through 3
may be used in conjunction with
Filgrastim 5 mcg/kg/day subcutaneously, from day 4 until the leukocyte count is greater than 10,000 cells/mm^3*
may be used in conjunction with
Radiation therapy
*Note: Filgrastim dose not specified in the original article; the doses given here are derived from *AHFS 2009 Drug Information,* a tertiary resource.

Use: Neuroendocrine tumor.
Cycle: 28 days, continue until disease progression or intolerable toxicity

Regimen: Etoposide 130 mg/m^2/day continuous IV infusion, days 1 through 3
Cisplatin 45 mg/m^2/day continuous IV infusion, days 2 through 3

EP + Docetaxel, Sequential

Use: Lung cancer (non-small cell).
Cycle: See below, cycle length varies throughout protocol. Give 2 cycles of EP + Radiation, followed by 3 cycles of Docetaxel alone.

Regimen: **EP + Radiation.** *Cycle*: 28 days for 2 cycles
Etoposide 50 mg/m^2/day IV, days 1 through 5
Cisplatin 50 mg/m^2 IV, days 1 and 8
used in conjunction with
Radiation therapy
followed after 4 to 6 weeks by
Docetaxel alone. *Cycle:* 21 days for 3 cycles
Docetaxel 75 mg/m^2 IV, day 1 for the first cycle; may increase to docetaxel 100 mg/m^2 IV, day 1 for subsequent cycles if tolerated

EP + EP, Sequential (Intergroup 0160, SWOG 9416)

Use: Lung cancer (non-small cell).
Cycle: 28 days. Give 2 cycles of EP + Radiation, followed by surgical resection, followed by 2 additional cycles of EP.

Regimen: **EP + Radiation** (cycles 1 and 2, given prior to surgery)
Etoposide 50 mg/m^2/day IV, days 1 through 5
Cisplatin 50 mg/m^2 IV, days 1 and 8
used in conjunction with
Radiation therapy
followed after 3 to 5 weeks by
Surgical resection
followed by
EP (cycles 3 and 4)
Etoposide 50 mg/m^2/day IV, days 1 through 5
Cisplatin 50 mg/m^2 IV, days 1 and 8

EP + Radiation

Use: Lung cancer (non-small cell).
Cycle: 28 days for 2 cycles

Regimen: Etoposide 50 mg/m^2/day IV, days 1 through 5
Cisplatin 50 mg/m^2 IV, days 1 and 8
used in conjunction with
Radiation therapy

EP + Radiation ➡ Cisplatin-Irinotecan

Use: Lung cancer (small cell).

Cycle: See below, cycle length varies throughout protocol. Give 1 cycle of EP + Radiation, followed by 3 cycles of Cisplatin-Irinotecan.

Regimen: **EP + Radiation.** *Cycle*: 21 days. Give a single cycle.

Etoposide 100 mg/m²/day IV, days 1 through 3
Cisplatin 80 mg/m² IV, day 1
used in conjunction with
Radiation therapy

followed after 4 weeks by

Cisplatin-Irinotecan. *Cycle*: 28 days for 3 cycles

Irinotecan 60 mg/m² IV, days 1, 8, and 15
Cisplatin 60 mg/m² IV, day 1 (give after irinotecan)

Epirubicin ➡ CMF

Use: Breast cancer.

Cycle: See below, cycle length varies throughout protocol. Give 4 cycles of Epirubicin alone, followed by 4 cycles of CMF.

Regimen: **Epirubicin alone.** *Cycle:* 21 days for 4 cycles

Epirubicin 100 mg/m² IV, day 1

followed by

CMF. *Cycle:* 28 days for 4 cycles

Methotrexate 40 mg/m² IV, days 1 and 8
Fluorouracil 600 mg/m² IV, days 1 and 8
with
Cyclophosphamide 100 mg/m²/day PO, days 1 through 14
or
Cyclophosphamide 600 mg/m² IV, days 1 and 8

Epirubicin ➡ CMF-IV

Use: Breast cancer.

Cycle: 21 days. Give 4 cycles of Epirubicin alone, followed by 4 cycles of CMF-IV.

Regimen: **Epirubicin alone** (cycles 1 through 4)

Epirubicin 100 mg/m² IV, day 1

followed by

CMF-IV (cycles 5 through 8)

Cyclophosphamide 750 mg/m² IV, day 1
Methotrexate 50 mg/m² IV, day 1
Fluorouracil 600 mg/m² IV, day 1

Epirubicin-Cyclophosphamide (also see HEC)

Use: Breast cancer.

Cycle: 21 days for 6 cycles

Regimen: Epirubicin 75 mg/m² IV, day 1
Cyclophosphamide 600 mg/m² IV, day 1

Epirubicin-Cyclophosphamide/Paclitaxel, Dose Dense

Use: Breast cancer.

Cycle: See below, cycle length varies throughout protocol. Give 6 cycles of Dose Dense Epirubicin-Cyclophosphamide, followed by 2 cycles of Paclitaxel alone.

Regimen: **Dose Dense Epirubicin-Cyclophosphamide.** *Cycle*: 14 days for 6 cycles

Epirubicin 120 mg/m² IV, day 1
Cyclophosphamide 830 mg/m² IV, day 1
Filgrastim 5 mcg/kg/day subcutaneously, days 2 through 13
Epoetin alfa 40,000 units subcutaneously, weekly, days 1 and 8

followed by

Paclitaxel alone. *Cycle*: 21 days for 4 cycles

Paclitaxel 175 mg/m² IV (infusion duration not specified), day 1
Filgrastim 5 mcg/kg/day subcutaneously, days 2 through 13
Epoetin alfa 40,000 units subcutaneously, weekly, days 1, 8, and 15

Epirubicin-Paclitaxel

Use: Breast cancer.

Cycle: 21 days for 6 cycles

Regimen: Epirubicin 75 mg/m² IV, day 1
Paclitaxel 200 mg/m² IV over 3 hours, day 1

Epirubicin-Paclitaxel-Cyclophosphamide, Sequential, Dose Dense

Use: Breast cancer.

Cycle: 14 days. Give 3 cycles of Treatment A followed by 3 cycles of Treatment B followed by 3 cycles of Treatment C.

Regimen: **Treatment A** (cycles 1 through 3)

Epirubicin 150 mg/m^2 IV, day 1 for 3 cycles
Filgrastim 5 mcg/kg/day subcutaneously, days 3 through 10

Treatment B (cycles 4 through 6)

Paclitaxel 225 mg/m^2 IV (infusion duration not specified), day 1 for 3 cycles
Filgrastim 5 mcg/kg/day subcutaneously, days 3 through 10

Treatment C (cycles 7 through 9)

Cyclophosphamide 2,500 mg/m^2 IV, day 1 for 3 cycles
Filgrastim 5 mcg/kg/day subcutaneously, days 3 through 10
may be given with
Mesna 20% of cyclophosphamide dose IV before, then every 3 hours after cyclophosphamide infusion for a total of 3 to 6 doses, day 1*

*Note: Mesna dose not specified in original abstract; the dose given here is derived from the *Cancer Chemotherapy Manual* and the *Pediatric Drug Information Handbook*, both tertiary resources.

EPOCH

Use: Lymphoma (non-Hodgkin).

Cycle: 21 days for at least 6 cycles

Regimen:
Etoposide 50 mg/m^2/day continuous IV infusion, days 1 through 4
Prednisone 60 mg/m^2/day PO, days 1 through 6
Vincristine* 0.4 mg/m^2/day continuous IV infusion, days 1 through 4†
Doxorubicin 10 mg/m^2/day continuous IV infusion, days 1 through 4†
Cyclophosphamide 750 mg/m^2 IV, day 5
Cotrimoxazole double-strength (160/800) 1 tablet PO twice daily, given for 3 consecutive days each week

*Note: The vincristine dose is not capped in this protocol. Consult the prescriber if there is any question about the intended vincristine dose.

†Note: Vincristine and doxorubicin may be mixed and administered in the same infusion bag, if diluted with 0.9% Sodium Chloride Injection. Etoposide is usually infused in a separate line.

EPOCH, Dose-Adjusted

Use: Lymphoma (non-Hodgkin) associated with HIV infection.

Cycle: 21 days for up to 6 cycles

Regimen:
Etoposide 50 mg/m^2/day continuous IV infusion, days 1 through 4
Prednisone 60 mg/m^2/day PO, days 1 through 5
Vincristine* 0.4 mg/m^2/day continuous IV infusion, days 1 through 4†
Doxorubicin 10 mg/m^2/day continuous IV infusion, days 1 through 4†
with
Cyclophosphamide dose based on cell counts for first and subsequent cycles:

- Patients with baseline CD4+ cell counts at least 100 cells/mm^3: Cyclophosphamide 375 mg/m^2 IV, day 5 for the first cycle; adjust dose for subsequent cycles based on nadir
- Patients with baseline CD4+ cell counts less than 100 cells/mm^3: Cyclophosphamide 187 mg/m^2 IV, day 5 for the first cycle; adjust dose for subsequent cycles based on nadir
- Nadir absolute neutrophil count (ANC) above 500 cells/mm^3 after first cycle: May increase dose in increments of 187 mg/m^2 (up to 750 mg/m^2 maximum) for subsequent cycles
- Nadir ANC less than 500 cells/mm^3 or platelet nadir less than 25,000 cells/mm^3 after first cycle: Decrease dose in increments of 187 mg/m^2 for subsequent cycles

plus
Filgrastim 5 mcg/kg/day subcutaneously, from day 6 until ANC is at least 5,000 cells/mm^3
used in conjunction with antimicrobial prophylaxis‡

Cotrimoxazole (either 80/400 or 160/800 strength) 1 tablet PO daily, throughout entire course
plus
Azithromycin 1,200 mg PO once weekly, throughout entire course
or
Clarithromycin 500 mg PO twice weekly, throughout entire course

*Note: The vincristine dose is not capped in this protocol. Consult the prescriber if there is any question about the intended vincristine dose.

†Note: Vincristine and doxorubicin may be mixed and administered in the same infusion bag, if diluted with 0.9% Sodium Chloride Injection. Etoposide is usually infused in a separate line.

‡Note: Antimicrobial prophylaxis drugs and doses not specified in original articles; the doses given here are derived from *Infectious Diseases Handbook*, 6th ed., a tertiary resource.

(continued on next page)

EPOCH, Dose-Adjusted (cont.)

Use: Lymphoma (B-cell).
Cycle: 21 days for 6 to 8 cycles

Regimen: Prednisone 60 mg/m²/day PO, days 1 through 5
Vincristine* 0.4 mg/m²/day continuous IV infusion, days 1 through 4†
Etoposide 50 mg/m²/day continuous IV infusion, days 1 through 4, of first cycle only
Etoposide continuous IV infusion, day 1 through 4, except for first cycle, dose based on twice-weekly cell counts after previous cycle:
Nadir absolute neutrophil count (ANC) above 500 cells/mm³: May increase dose by 10 mg/m²/day from previous cycle
Nadir ANC less than 500 cells/mm³ on no more than 2 measurements: Give same dose as previous cycle
Nadir ANC less than 500 cells/mm³ on at least 3 measurements, or platelet nadir less than 25,000 cells/mm³ on at least 1 measurement: Decrease dose by 10 mg/m²/day from previous cycle (down to 50 mg/m²/day minimum)
Doxorubicin 10 mg/m²/day continuous IV infusion, days 1 through 4,† of first cycle only
Doxorubicin continuous IV infusion, days 1 through 4,† except for first cycle, dose based on twice-weekly cell counts after previous cycle:
Nadir absolute neutrophil count (ANC) above 500 cells/mm³: May increase dose by 2 mg/m²/day from previous cycle
Nadir ANC less than 500 cells/mm³ on no more than 2 measurements: Give same dose as previous cycle
Nadir ANC less than 500 cells/mm³ on at least 3 measurements, or platelet nadir less than 25,000 cells/mm³ on at least 1 measurement: Decrease dose by 2 mg/m²/day from previous cycle (down to 10 mg/m²/day minimum)
Cyclophosphamide 750 mg/m² IV, day 5, of first cycle only
Cyclophosphamide IV, day 5, except for first cycle, dose based on twice-weekly cell counts after previous cycle:
Nadir absolute neutrophil count (ANC) above 500 cells/mm³: May increase dose by 187 mg/m² from previous cycle
Nadir ANC less than 500 cells/mm³ on no more than 2 measurements: Give same dose as previous cycle
Nadir ANC less than 500 cells/mm³ on at least 3 measurements, or platelet nadir less than 25,000 cells/mm³ on at least 1 measurement: Decrease dose by 187 mg/m² from previous cycle
plus
Filgrastim 5 mcg/kg/day subcutaneously, from day 6 until the ANC is at least 5,000 cells/mm³
used in conjunction with antimicrobial prophylaxis
Cotrimoxazole (either 80/400 or 160/800 strength) 1 tablet PO twice daily, given 3 times weekly (eg, Monday, Wednesday, Friday), throughout entire course
*Note: The vincristine dose is not capped in this protocol. Consult the prescriber if there is any question about the intended vincristine dose.
†Note: Vincristine and doxorubicin may be mixed and administered in the same infusion bag, if diluted with 0.9% Sodium Chloride Injection. Etoposide is usually infused in a separate line.

EPOCH-R

Use: Lymphoma (B-cell, mantle cell).
Cycle: 21 days for at least 6 cycles, delay subsequent cycles until hematologic recovery

Regimen: Rituximab 375 mg/m² IV, day 1
Etoposide 50 mg/m²/day continuous IV infusion, days 1 through 4
Vincristine* 0.4 mg/m²/day continuous IV infusion, days 1 through 4†
Doxorubicin 10 mg/m²/day continuous IV infusion, days 1 through 4†
Prednisone 60 mg/m²/dose (120 mg/m²/day) PO twice daily, days 1 through 5
Cyclophosphamide 750 mg/m² IV, day 5
Filgrastim 5 mcg/kg/day subcutaneously, starting on day 6 and continued until granulocyte count exceeds 5,000 cells/mm³
Cotrimoxazole double-strength (160/800) 1 tablet PO twice daily, given on Monday, Wednesday, and Friday of each week
*Note: The vincristine dose is not capped in this protocol. Consult the prescriber if there is any question about the intended vincristine dose.
†Note: Vincristine and doxorubicin may be mixed and administered in the same infusion bag, if diluted with 0.9% Sodium Chloride Injection. Etoposide is usually infused in a separate line.

Erlotinib-Bevacizumab

Use: Lung cancer (non-small cell).
Cycle: 21 days for up to 52 weeks, or until disease progression or intolerable toxicity

Regimen: Erlotinib 150 mg/day PO, throughout entire course
Bevacizumab 15 mg/kg IV, day 1

ESHAP

Use: Lymphoma (non-Hodgkin).
Cycle: 21 to 28 days for up to 6 to 8 cycles

Regimen: Etoposide 40 to 60 mg/m²/day IV, days 1 through 4
Methylprednisolone 250 to 500 mg/day IV, days 1 through 4 or days 1 through 5
Cisplatin 25 mg/m²/day continuous IV infusion, days 1 through 4
Cytarabine 2,000 mg/m² IV, day 5 (give after etoposide and cisplatin are completed)

Estramustine-Cyclophosphamide

Use: Prostate cancer.
Cycle: 28 days, continue until disease progression or intolerable toxicity

Regimen: Estramustine 10 mg/kg/day PO given in 2 to 3 divided doses, days 1 through 14
Cyclophosphamide 2 mg/kg/day PO given in 2 to 3 divided doses, days 1 through 14

Estramustine-Etoposide

Use: Prostate cancer.
Cycle: 28 days, continue until disease progression or intolerable toxicity

Regimen: Estramustine 3.75 mg/kg/dose (15 mg/kg/day) PO 4 times daily, days 1 through 21
Etoposide 25 mg/m^2/dose (50 mg/m^2/day) PO twice daily, days 1 through 21

Estramustine/Vinblastine (EM-V)

Use: Prostate cancer.
Cycle: 8 weeks, continue until disease progression or intolerable toxicity

Regimen: Vinblastine 4 mg/m^2 IV weekly, weeks 1 through 6
with
Estramustine 3.33 mg/kg/dose (10 mg/kg/day) PO 3 times daily, days 1 through 42
or
Estramustine 600 mg/m^2/day PO given in 2 to 3 divided doses, days 1 through 42

EVA

Use: Lymphoma (Hodgkin).
Cycle: 28 days for up to 6 cycles

Regimen: Etoposide 100 mg/m^2/day IV, days 1 through 3
Vinblastine 6 mg/m^2 IV, day 1
Doxorubicin 50 mg/m^2 IV, day 1

F-CL (FU/LV)

Use: Pancreatic cancer.
Cycle: 4 weeks for 6 cycles

Regimen: Leucovorin 20 mg/m^2/day IV, days 1 through 5
Fluorouracil 425 mg/m^2/day IV, days 1 through 5 (give after leucovorin)

Use: Ovarian cancer.
Cycle: 4 weeks for cycles 1 and 2, then 5 weeks for subsequent cycles, continue until disease progression or intolerable toxicity

Regimen: Leucovorin 200 mg/m^2/day IV, days 1 through 5
Fluorouracil 370 mg/m^2/day IV, days 1 through 5 (give after leucovorin)

Use: Hepatocellular cancer.
Cycle: 28 days, continue until disease progression or intolerable toxicity

Regimen: Leucovorin 200 mg/m^2/day IV, days 1 through 5
Fluorouracil 370 mg/m^2/day IV, days 1 through 5 (give after leucovorin)

F-CL (FU/LV), Biweekly Regimen (de Gramont)

Use: Colorectal cancer.
Cycle: 14 days, continue until disease progression or intolerable toxicity

Regimen: Leucovorin 200 mg/m^2/day IV, days 1 and 2
Fluorouracil 400 mg/m^2/day IV bolus, days 1 and 2 (give after starting leucovorin)
then
Fluorouracil 600 mg/m^2/dose continuous IV infusion for 22 hours, days 1 and 2

F-CL (FU/LV), Mayo Clinic Regimen

Use: Colorectal cancer.
Cycle: 4 to 5 weeks

Regimen 1: Low-dose leucovorin:
Leucovorin 20 mg/m^2/day IV, days 1 through 5
Fluorouracil 370 to 425 mg/m^2/day IV, days 1 through 5 (give after starting leucovorin)

Regimen 2: High-dose leucovorin:
Leucovorin 200 mg/m^2/day IV, days 1 through 5
Fluorouracil 370 to 400 mg/m^2/day IV, days 1 through 5 (give after starting leucovorin)

F-CL (FU/LV), Post-Gastrectomy

Use: Gastric cancer.
Cycle: Give a single cycle after gastrectomy

Regimen: Fluorouracil 425 mg/m^2/day IV, days 1 through 5
Leucovorin 20 mg/m^2/day IV, days 1 through 5
followed by
Radiation therapy, 5 days per week for 5 weeks, days 29 through 33, days 36 through 40, days 43 though 47, days 50 through 54, and days 57 through 61
Fluorouracil 400 mg/m^2/day IV, days 29 through 32 and days 59 through 61
Leucovorin 20 mg/m^2/day IV, days 29 through 32 and days 59 through 61
followed 1 month later by
Fluorouracil 425 mg/m^2/day IV, days 85 through 89 and days 113 through 117
Leucovorin 20 mg/m^2/day IV, days 85 through 89 and days 113 through 117

F-CL (FU/LV), Roswell Park Regimen

Use: Colorectal cancer.
Cycle: 8 weeks

Regimen: Leucovorin 500 mg/m^2 IV, weekly for 6 weeks, then 2 weeks of rest
Fluorouracil 600 mg/m^2 IV, weekly for 6 weeks (give after starting leucovorin), then 2 weeks of rest

Use: Colorectal cancer.
Cycle: 8 weeks

Regimen: Leucovorin 500 mg/m^2 IV, weekly for 6 weeks, then 2 weeks of rest
Fluorouracil 500 mg/m^2 IV, weekly for 6 weeks (give after starting leucovorin), then 2 weeks of rest

F-CL (FU/LV), Weekly Regimen (Douillard Schedule)

Use: Colorectal cancer.
Cycle: 7 days, continue until disease progression

Regimen: Leucovorin 500 mg/m^2 IV, day 1
Fluorouracil 2,600 mg/m^2/day continuous IV infusion, day 1 (start after leucovorin)

F-CL (FU/LV), Weekly Regimen (German Schedule)

Use: Colorectal cancer.
Cycle: Ongoing, continue until disease progression

Regimen: Leucovorin 20 mg/m^2 IV, weekly
Fluorouracil 500 mg/m^2 IV, weekly (give after starting leucovorin)

F-CL (FU/LV) + Radiation ➡ Surgery ➡ F-CL

Use: Rectal cancer.
Cycle: See below, cycle length varies throughout protocol. Give a single cycle of F-CL + Radiation prior to surgical resection, followed by 4 cycles of F-CL after surgical resection.

Regimen: **F-CL + Radiation.** *Cycle*: 33 days. Give a single cycle.
Leucovorin 20 mg/m^2/day IV, days 1 through 5 and days 29 through 33
Fluorouracil 350 mg/m^2/day IV, days 1 through 5 and days 29 through 33 (give after leucovorin)
used in conjunction with
Radiation therapy
followed after 3 to 10 weeks by
Surgical resection
followed after 3 to 10 weeks by
F-CL. *Cycle*: 21 to 28 days for 4 cycles
Leucovorin 20 mg/m^2/day IV, days 1 through 5
Fluorouracil 350 mg/m^2/day IV, days 1 through 5 (give after leucovorin)

FAC

Use: Breast cancer.
Cycle: 21 to 28 days, for up to 8 cycles

Regimen: Fluorouracil 500 mg/m^2 IV, days 1 and 4 or days 1 and 8
Cyclophosphamide 500 mg/m^2 IV, day 1
with
Doxorubicin 50 mg/m^2 IV, day 1
or
Doxorubicin 16.7 mg/m^2/day continuous IV infusion, days 1 through 3

FAM

Use: Adenocarcinoma, gastric cancer, pancreatic cancer.
Cycle: 8 weeks, continue until disease progression or intolerable toxicity

Regimen: Fluorouracil 600 mg/m^2 IV, days 1, 8, 29, and 36
Doxorubicin 30 mg/m^2 IV, days 1 and 29
Mitomycin 10 mg/m^2 IV, day 1

FAMTX

Use: Gastric cancer.
Cycle: 28 days

Regimen: Methotrexate 1,500 mg/m^2 IV, day 1
Fluorouracil 1,500 mg/m^2 IV, day 1 (give after methotrexate)
Leucovorin 15 mg/m^2/dose PO every 6 hours for 8 doses (start 24 hours after methotrexate); increase dose to 30 mg/m^2/dose PO every 6 hours for 16 doses if 24-hour methotrexate level is 2.5 mol/L or higher
Doxorubicin 30 mg/m^2 IV, day 15

FAP

Use: Gastric cancer.
Cycle: 5 weeks, continue until disease progression or intolerable toxicity

Regimen: Fluorouracil 300 mg/m^2/day IV, days 1 through 5
Doxorubicin 40 mg/m^2 IV, day 1
Cisplatin 60 mg/m^2 IV, day 1

FAS

Use: Islet cell carcinoma.
Cycle: 28 days, continue until disease progression or intolerable toxicity

Regimen: Fluorouracil 400 mg/m^2/day IV, days 1 through 5
Doxorubicin 40 mg/m^2 IV, day 1
Streptozocin 400 mg/m^2/day IV, days 1 through 5

FBEC

Use: Head and neck cancer (nasopharyngeal).
Cycle: 21 days for 6 cycles

Regimen: Fluorouracil 700 mg/m^2/day continuous IV infusion, days 1 through 4
Bleomycin 10 mg IV, day 1 of cycles 1 through 3
Bleomycin 12 mg/m^2/day continuous IV infusion, days 1 through 4 of cycles 1 through 3 (start after bleomycin bolus on day 1)
Epirubicin 70 mg/m^2 IV, day 1
Cisplatin 100 mg/m^2 IV, day 5

FC (also see Fludarabine-Cyclophosphamide)

Use: Lymphoma (non-Hodgkin).
Cycle: 28 days for up to 8 cycles

Regimen: Fludarabine 20 mg/m^2/day IV, days 1 through 5
Cyclophosphamide 1,000 mg/m^2 IV, day 1
*used in conjunction with antimicrobial prophylaxis**
Cotrimoxazole double-strength (160/800) 1 tablet PO daily, throughout entire course
plus
Acyclovir 200 mg PO 3 times daily, throughout entire course
or
Acyclovir 400 mg PO twice daily, throughout entire course
*Note: Antimicrobial prophylaxis doses not specified in original article; the doses given here are derived from the *Infectious Diseases Handbook,* 6th ed., and *AHFS 2008 Drug Information,* both tertiary resources.

FCM + Rituximab (FCM-R, R-FCM)

Use: Lymphoma (non-Hodgkin).
Cycle: 28 days for 4 cycles

Regimen: Rituximab 375 mg/m^2 IV, day 1
Fludarabine 25 mg/m^2/day IV, days 2 through 4
Cyclophosphamide 200 mg/m^2 IV, days 2 through 4
Mitoxantrone 8 mg/m^2 IV, day 2

Use: Chronic lymphocytic leukemia (CLL).
Cycle: 28 to 42 days for 6 cycles, delay subsequent cycles until hematologic recovery

Regimen: Fludarabine 25 mg/m^2/day IV, days 1 through 3, except for day 1 of first cycle
Fludarabine 25 mg/m^2/day IV, day 4 of first cycle only
Cyclophosphamide 250 mg/m^2 IV, days 1 through 3, except for day 1 of first cycle
Cyclophosphamide 250 mg/m^2 IV, day 4 of first cycle only
Mitoxantrone 6 mg/m^2 IV, day 1, except for first cycle
Mitoxantrone 6 mg/m^2 IV, day 2 of first cycle only
Rituximab 375 mg/m^2 IV, day 1 of first cycle only
Rituximab 500 mg/m^2 IV, day 1, except for first cycle
Pegfilgrastim 6 mg subcutaneously, day 4 or 5 (give at least 24 hours after completion of chemotherapy infusions)*
*used in conjunction with antimicrobial prophylaxis**
Cotrimoxazole (either 80/400 or 160/800 strength) 1 tablet PO daily, throughout entire course
or
Pentamidine 300 mg inhaled once monthly, throughout entire course
plus
Valacyclovir 500 mg/day PO, throughout entire course
or
Acyclovir 200 mg PO 3 times daily, throughout entire course
or
Acyclovir 400 mg PO twice daily, throughout entire course
*Note: Pegfilgrastim and antimicrobial prophylaxis doses not specified in original article; the doses given here are derived from the *Infectious Diseases Handbook,* 6th ed., and *AHFS 2009 Drug Information,* both tertiary resources.

FCR

Use: Chronic lymphocytic leukemia (CLL).

Cycle: 28 days for up to 6 cycles. Delay each subsequent cycle until absolute neutrophil count (ANC) is greater than 1,000 cells/mm^3 and platelet count is at least 80,000 cells/mm^3.

Regimen:
Fludarabine 25 mg/m^2/day IV, days 1 through 3, except for day 1 of first cycle
Fludarabine 25 mg/m^2 IV, day 4 of first cycle only
Cyclophosphamide 250 mg/m^2/day IV, days 1 through 3, except for day 1 of first cycle
Cyclophosphamide 250 mg/m^2 IV, day 4 of first cycle only
Rituximab 375 mg/m^2 IV, day 1 of first cycle only
Rituximab 500 mg/m^2 IV, day 1 except for first cycle
used in conjunction with antimicrobial prophylaxis
Valacyclovir 500 mg/day PO, throughout entire course
plus
Cotrimoxazole (either 80/400 or 160/800 strength) 1 tablet PO daily, throughout entire course*
or
Pentamidine 300 mg inhaled once monthly, throughout entire course*
*Note: Pneumocystis prophylaxis doses not specified in original articles; the dose given here is derived from the *Infectious Diseases Handbook*, 6th ed., a tertiary resource.

Use: Lymphoma (non-Hodgkin).

Cycle: 21 days for 4 cycles

Regimen:
Fludarabine 25 mg/m^2/day IV, days 1 through 3
Cyclophosphamide 300 mg/m^2/day IV, days 1 through 3
Rituximab 375 mg/m^2 IV, day 1, except for first cycle
Rituximab 375 mg/m^2 IV, day 14 of first cycle only

FEC (also see CEF)

Use: Breast cancer.

Cycle: 21 days for 4 to 6 cycles

Regimen:
Fluorouracil 500 mg/m^2 IV, day 1
Epirubicin 100 mg/m^2 IV, day 1
Cyclophosphamide 500 mg/m^2 IV, day 1

FEC/Docetaxel, Sequential (FEC ➡ T)

Use: Breast cancer.

Cycle: 21 days

Regimen:
Give 3 cycles of FEC regimen for breast cancer
followed by
Docetaxel 100 mg/m^2 IV, day 1 for 3 cycles

FED

Use: Lung cancer (non-small cell).

Cycle: 21 days for up to 3 cycles

Regimen:
Cisplatin 100 mg/m^2 IV, day 1
Fluorouracil 960 mg/m^2/day continuous IV infusion, days 2 through 4
Etoposide 80 mg/m^2/day IV, days 2 through 4

FL

Use: Prostate cancer.

Cycle: Ongoing

Regimen:
Flutamide 250 mg/dose PO every 8 hours
with
Leuprolide acetate 1 mg subcutaneously daily
or
Leuprolide depot 7.5 mg/dose IM, every 28 days
or
Leuprolide depot 22.5 mg/dose IM, every 3 months

FLAG

Use: Acute myelocytic leukemia (AML; remission induction).

Cycle: Give a single cycle. May be given a second time based on individual response. Time between cycles not specified.

Regimen:
Filgrastim 300 mcg/day subcutaneously, from day 1 until neutropenia resolves
Fludarabine 30 mg/m^2/day IV, days 2 through 6
Cytarabine 2,000 mg/m^2/day IV, days 2 through 6 (begin 4 hours after starting fludarabine)

FLAG-Ida

Use: Acute myelocytic leukemia (AML; remission induction).
Cycle: Give a single cycle. May be given a second time based on individual response. Time between cycles not specified.

Regimen:
Filgrastim 300 mcg/day subcutaneously, from day 1 until neutropenia resolves
Fludarabine 30 mg/m^2/day IV, days 2 through 6
Cytarabine 2,000 mg/m^2/day IV, days 2 through 6 (begin 4 hours after starting fludarabine)
Idarubicin 8 mg/m^2/day IV, days 2 through 4

Fle

Use: Colorectal cancer.
Cycle: 1 year

Regimen:
Fluorouracil 450 mg/m^2/day IV, days 1 through 5
Fluorouracil 450 mg/m^2/week IV, weeks 5 through 52
Levamisole 50 mg/dose PO every 8 hours, days 1 through 3 of every other week for 1 year*
*Note: Levamisole is no longer available in the United States. The manufacturer discontinued this product in October 2000 for commercial reasons, not for safety or efficacy reasons.

FLO

Use: Gastric cancer, esophageal cancer.
Cycle: 14 days, continue until disease progression or intolerable toxicity

Regimen:
Oxaliplatin 85 mg/m^2 IV, day 1
Leucovorin 200 mg/m^2 IV, day 1
Fluorouracil 2,600 mg/m^2/day continuous IV infusion, day 1 (given after leucovorin and oxaliplatin)

FLOX

Use: Colorectal cancer.
Cycle: 8 weeks for 3 cycles

Regimen:
Leucovorin 500 mg/m^2 IV, weekly for 6 weeks, days 1, 8, 15, 22, 29, and 36
Fluorouracil 500 mg/m^2 IV, weekly for 6 weeks, days 1, 8, 15, 22, 29, and 36 (give after starting leucovorin)
Oxaliplatin 85 mg/m^2 IV, days 1, 15, and 29

Floxuridine-Leucovorin-Dexamethasone-Heparin Hepatic Artery Infusion

Use: Colorectal cancer (liver metastases).
Cycle: 28 days

Regimen:
Floxuridine 0.21 mg/kg/day continuous hepatic artery infusion, days 1 through 14*
Leucovorin 10.5 mg/m^2/day continuous hepatic artery infusion, days 1 through 14*
Dexamethasone 14 mg/day continuous hepatic artery infusion, days 1 through 14*
Heparin 35,000 units/day continuous hepatic artery infusion, days 1 through 14*
*Note: Floxuridine, leucovorin, dexamethasone, and heparin may be mixed and administered in the same infusion bag. The infusion pump used in the protocol delivered 70% of the dose provided in the infusion bag, which was floxuridine 0.3 mg/kg/day, leucovorin 15 mg/m^2/day, dexamethasone 20 mg/day, and heparin 50,000 units/day.

Fludarabine-Cyclophosphamide (also see FC)

Use: Chronic lymphocytic leukemia (CLL).
Cycle: 4 to 6 weeks based on recovery of myelosuppression. Give up to 6 cycles.

Regimen:
Fludarabine 30 mg/m^2/day IV, days 1 through 3
Cyclophosphamide 300 mg/m^2/day IV, days 1 through 3

Use: Chronic lymphocytic leukemia (CLL).
Cycle: 28 days for up to 6 cycles

Regimen:
Fludarabine 20 mg/m^2/day IV, days 1 through 5
Cyclophosphamide 600 mg/m^2 IV, day 1
Filgrastim 5 mcg/kg/day subcutaneously, from day 8 until hematologic recovery
*used in conjunction with antimicrobial prophylaxis**
Cotrimoxazole (either 80/400 or 160/800 strength) 1 tablet PO daily, throughout entire course, starting 1 day prior to first chemotherapy dose
or
Pentamidine 300 mg inhaled once monthly, throughout entire course, starting 1 day prior to first chemotherapy dose
plus
Acyclovir 200 mg PO 3 times daily, throughout entire course, starting on day 8 of first chemotherapy cycle
or
Acyclovir 400 mg PO twice daily, throughout entire course, starting on day 8 of first chemotherapy cycle
*Note: Antimicrobial prophylaxis doses not specified in original article; the doses given here are derived from the *Infectious Diseases Handbook,* 6th ed., and *AHFS 2008 Drug Information,* both tertiary resources.

Fluorouracil-Gemcitabine

Use: Renal cell carcinoma.
Cycle: 28 days for at least 2 cycles

Regimen:
Fluorouracil 150 mg/m^2/day continuous IV infusion, days 1 through 21
Gemcitabine 600 mg/m^2 IV, days 1, 8, and 15

Fluorouracil-Interferon

Use:	Hepatocellular cancer. *Cycle:* 28 days for at least 2 cycles
Regimen:	Fluorouracil 200 mg/m²/day continuous IV infusion, days 1 through 21 Interferon alfa-2b 4 million units/m²/dose subcutaneously 3 times weekly, weeks 1, 2, and 3 (during fluorouracil therapy)
Use:	Hepatocellular cancer. *Cycle:* 28 days for at least 3 cycles
Regimen:	Fluorouracil 300 mg/m²/day continuous intraarterial infusion, days 1 through 5 and days 8 through 12 Interferon alfa-2b 5 million units/dose subcutaneously 3 times weekly, throughout entire course* *Note: Interferon dose is in units not units/m².

Fluorouracil-Mitomycin

Use:	Head and neck cancer. *Cycle:* 49 days. Give a single cycle.
Regimen:	Fluorouracil 600 mg/m²/day continuous IV infusion, days 1 through 5 Mitomycin 10 mg/m² IV, days 5 and 36 *used in conjunction with* Radiation therapy
Use:	Anal cancer. *Cycle:* 32 days. Give a single cycle prior to surgery.
Regimen:	Fluorouracil 1,000 mg/m²/day continuous IV infusion, days 1 through 4 and days 29 through 32 Mitomycin 15 mg/m² IV, day 1 *used in conjunction with* Radiation therapy
Use:	Anal cancer. *Cycle:* 35 days. Give a single cycle prior to surgery.
Regimen:	Fluorouracil 750 mg/m²/day continuous IV infusion, days 1 through 5 and days 29 through 33 Mitomycin 15 mg/m² IV, day 1 *used in conjunction with* Radiation therapy
Use:	Anal cancer. *Cycle:* 28 days for 2 cycles
Regimen:	Fluorouracil 1,000 mg/m²/day (2,000 mg/day maximum dose) continuous IV infusion, days 1 through 4 Mitomycin 10 mg/m² (20 mg maximum dose) IV, day 1 *used in conjunction with* Radiation therapy
Use:	Anal cancer. *Cycle:* 59 days. Give a single cycle.
Regimen:	Fluorouracil 200 mg/m²/day continuous IV infusion, days 1 through 26 and days 43 through 59 Mitomycin 10 mg/m²/day IV, days 1 and 43 *used in conjunction with* Radiation therapy

Fluorouracil-Oxaliplatin-Radiation

Use:	Rectal cancer. *Cycle:* 36 days. Give a single cycle prior to surgery.
Regimen:	Fluorouracil 200 mg/m²/day continuous IV infusion, throughout entire course Oxaliplatin 60 mg/m² IV, weekly, days 1, 8, 15, 22, 29, and 36 *used in conjunction with* Radiation therapy *followed after 4 to 6 weeks by* Surgical resection

Fluorouracil-Streptozocin

Use:	Islet cell carcinoma. *Cycle:* 42 days, continue until disease progression or intolerable toxicity
Regimen:	Fluorouracil 400 mg/m²/day IV, days 1 through 5 Streptozocin 500 mg/m²/day IV, days 1 through 5

FM (FN)

Use:	Lymphoma (non-Hodgkin). *Cycle:* 21 days for up to 6 cycles, or until disease progression
Regimen:	Fludarabine 25 mg/m²/day IV, days 1 through 3 Mitoxantrone 10 mg/m² IV, day 1

FMD—see FND

FNC—see CNF

FND (FMD)

Use: Lymphoma (non-Hodgkin).
Cycle: 28 days for up to 8 cycles

Regimen: Fludarabine 25 mg/m^2/day IV, days 1 through 3
Mitoxantrone 10 mg/m^2 IV, day 1
Dexamethasone 20 mg/day IV or PO, days 1 through 5
Cotrimoxazole double-strength (160/800) 2 tablets PO daily for 2 consecutive days each week (usually given every Saturday and Sunday)

FND-R—see FND + Rituximab, Concurrent

FND + Rituximab, Concurrent (FND-R)

Use: Lymphoma (non-Hodgkin).
Cycle: 28 days for up to 8 cycles

Regimen: Rituximab 375 mg/m^2 IV, days 1 and 8 of first cycle only; then rituximab 375 mg/m^2 IV, day 1 for cycles 2 through 5
Fludarabine 25 mg/m^2/day IV, days 2 through 4
Mitoxantrone 10 mg/m^2 IV, day 2
Dexamethasone 20 mg/day IV or PO, days 2 through 4
Cotrimoxazole double-strength (160/800) 1 tablet PO twice daily for 2 consecutive days each week (usually given every Saturday and Sunday)

FOLFIRI

Use: Colorectal cancer.
Cycle: 14 days, continue until disease progression or intolerable toxicity

Regimen: Leucovorin 400 mg/m^2 IV, day 1
or
Levoleucovorin 200 mg/m^2 IV, day 1
with
Irinotecan 180 mg/m^2 IV, day 1 (begin with leucovorin or levoleucovorin)
then
Fluorouracil 400 mg/m^2 IV bolus, day 1
then
Fluorouracil 2,400 mg/m^2/dose continuous IV infusion over 46 hours for 2 cycles, starting on day 1. Increase to 3,000 mg/m^2/dose for remaining cycles if tolerated.

FOLFIRI + Bevacizumab

Use: Colorectal cancer.
Cycle: 14 days, continue until disease progression or intolerable toxicity

Regimen: Bevacizumab 5 mg/kg IV, day 1
Leucovorin 400 mg/m^2 IV, day 1
Irinotecan 180 mg/m^2 IV, day 1 (begin with leucovorin)
then
Fluorouracil 400 mg/m^2 IV bolus, day 1
then
Fluorouracil 2,400 mg/m^2/dose continuous IV infusion over 46 hours, starting day 1

FOLFIRI + Cetuximab

Use: Colorectal cancer.
Cycle: 14 days, continue until disease progression or intolerable toxicity

Regimen: Cetuximab 400 mg/m^2 IV, day 1 of first cycle only (loading dose)
Cetuximab 250 mg/m^2 IV weekly, days 1 and 8, except for day 1 of first cycle
Leucovorin 400 mg/m^2 IV, day 1
Irinotecan 180 mg/m^2 IV, day 1 (begin with leucovorin)
then
Fluorouracil 400 mg/m^2 IV bolus, day 1
then
Fluorouracil 2,400 mg/m^2/dose continuous IV infusion over 46 hours, starting on day 1

FOLFOX-2

Use: Colorectal cancer.
Cycle: 14 days, continue until disease progression or intolerable toxicity

Regimen: Oxaliplatin 100 mg/m^2 IV, day 1 (begin with leucovorin)
Leucovorin 500 mg/m^2/day IV, days 1 and 2
then
Fluorouracil 1,500 mg/m^2/dose continuous IV infusion over 22 hours, days 1 and 2, for 2 cycles. Increase to 2,000 mg/m^2/dose for remaining cycles if toxicity was below WHO grade 2 during first 2 cycles.

FOLFOX-3

Use: Colorectal cancer.
Cycle: 14 days, continue until disease progression or intolerable toxicity

Regimen: Oxaliplatin 85 mg/m^2 IV, day 1 (begin with leucovorin)
Leucovorin 500 mg/m^2/day IV, days 1 and 2
then
Fluorouracil 1,500 mg/m^2/dose continuous IV infusion over 22 hours, days 1 and 2, for 2 cycles. Increase to 2,000 mg/m^2/dose for remaining cycles if toxicity was below WHO grade 2 during first 2 cycles.

FOLFOX-4

Use: Colorectal cancer.
Cycle: 14 days, continue until disease progression or intolerable toxicity

Regimen: Oxaliplatin 85 mg/m^2 IV, day 1 (begin with leucovorin)
Leucovorin 200 mg/m^2/day IV, days 1 and 2
then
Fluorouracil 400 mg/m^2/day IV bolus, days 1 and 2
then
Fluorouracil 600 mg/m^2/dose continuous IV infusion over 22 hours, days 1 and 2

FOLFOX-4 + Bevacizumab

Use: Colorectal cancer.
Cycle: 14 days for up to 48 weeks, or until disease progression or intolerable toxicity

Regimen: Bevacizumab 5 or 10 mg/kg IV, day 1
Oxaliplatin 85 mg/m^2 IV, day 1 (begin with leucovorin)
Leucovorin 200 mg/m^2/day IV, days 1 and 2
then
Fluorouracil 400 mg/m^2/day IV bolus, days 1 and 2
then
Fluorouracil 600 mg/m^2/dose continuous IV infusion over 22 hours, days 1 and 2

FOLFOX-4 + Cetuximab

Use: Colorectal cancer.
Cycle: 14 days, continue until disease progression or intolerable toxicity

Regimen: Cetuximab 400 mg/m^2 IV, day 1 of first cycle only (loading dose)
Cetuximab 250 mg/m^2 IV weekly, days 1 and 8, except for day 1 of first cycle
Oxaliplatin 85 mg/m^2 IV, day 1 (begin with leucovorin)
Leucovorin 200 mg/m^2/day IV, days 1 and 2
then
Fluorouracil 400 mg/m^2/day IV bolus, days 1 and 2
then
Fluorouracil 600 mg/m^2/dose continuous IV infusion over 22 hours, days 1 and 2

FOLFOX-6

Use: Colorectal cancer.
Cycle: 14 days, continue until disease progression or intolerable toxicity

Regimen: Oxaliplatin 100 mg/m^2 IV, day 1 (begin with leucovorin)
Leucovorin 400 mg/m^2 IV, day 1
then
Fluorouracil 400 mg/m^2 IV bolus, day 1
then
Fluorouracil 2,400 mg/m^2/dose continuous IV infusion over 46 hours for 2 cycles, starting on day 1. Increase to 3,000 mg/m^2/dose for remaining cycles if tolerated.

FOLFOX-6, Modified (mFOLFOX-6)

Use: Colorectal cancer.
Cycle: 14 days, continue until disease progression or intolerable toxicity

Regimen: Leucovorin 350 mg/m^2 IV, day 1
or
Levoleucovorin 175 mg/m^2 IV, day 1
with
Oxaliplatin 85 mg/m^2 IV, day 1 (begin with leucovorin)
then
Fluorouracil 400 mg/m^2 IV bolus, day 1
then
Fluorouracil 2,400 mg/m^2/dose continuous IV infusion over 46 hours, starting day 1

FOLFOX-6, Modified + Bevacizumab (mFOLFOX-6 + Bevacizumab)

Use: Colorectal cancer.
Cycle: 14 days, continue until disease progression or intolerable toxicity

Regimen: Bevacizumab 5 mg/kg IV, day 1 (before chemotherapy)
with
Leucovorin 350 mg/m^2 IV, day 1
or
Levoleucovorin 175 mg/m^2 IV, day 1
with
Oxaliplatin 85 mg/m^2 IV, day 1 (begin with leucovorin)
then
Fluorouracil 400 mg/m^2 IV bolus, day 1
then
Fluorouracil 2,400 mg/m^2/dose continuous IV infusion over 46 hours, starting day 1

FOLFOX-6, Modified + Cetuximab (mFOLFOX-6 + Cetuximab)

Use: Colorectal cancer.
Cycle: 14 days

Regimen: Cetuximab 400 mg/m^2 IV, day 1 of first cycle only (loading dose)
Cetuximab 250 mg/m^2 IV weekly, days 1 and 8, except for day 1 of first cycle
Oxaliplatin 85 mg/m^2 IV, day 1 (begin with leucovorin)
Leucovorin 400 mg/m^2 IV, day 1
then
Fluorouracil 400 mg/m^2 IV bolus, day 1
then
Fluorouracil 2,400 mg/m^2/dose continuous IV infusion over 46 hours, starting on day 1

FOLFOX-7

Use: Colorectal cancer.
Cycle: 14 days for up to 8 cycles

Regimen: Leucovorin 400 mg/m^2 IV, day 1
or
Levoleucovorin 200 mg/m^2 IV, day 1
with
Oxaliplatin 130 mg/m^2 IV, day 1 (begin with leucovorin or levoleucovorin)
then
Fluorouracil 400 mg/m^2 IV bolus, day 1
then
Fluorouracil 2,400 mg/m^2/dose continuous IV infusion over 46 hours, starting on day 1

FOLFOX-7, Modified (mFOLFOX-7)

Use: Colorectal cancer.
Cycle: 14 days for up to 6 cycles

Regimen: Leucovorin 400 mg/m^2 IV, day 1
Oxaliplatin 100 mg/m^2 IV, day 1 (begin with leucovorin)
then
Fluorouracil 3,000 mg/m^2/dose continuous IV infusion over 46 hours, starting on day 1

FOLFOX-7, Modified + Bevacizumab (mFOLFOX-7 + Bevacizumab)

Use: Colorectal cancer.
Cycle: 14 days

Regimen: Leucovorin 400 mg/m^2 IV, day 1
Oxaliplatin 130 mg/m^2 IV, day 1 (begin with leucovorin)
then
Fluorouracil 2,400 mg/m^2/dose continuous IV infusion over 46 hours, starting on day 1
Bevacizumab 5 mg/kg IV, day 3

FOLFOXIRI

Use: Colorectal cancer.
Cycle: 14 days for up to 12 cycles

Regimen: Irinotecan 165 mg/m^2 IV, day 1
Oxaliplatin 85 mg/m^2 IV, day 1
Levoleucovorin 200 mg/m^2 IV, day 1
Fluorouracil 1,600 mg/m^2/day continuous IV infusion, days 1 and 2 (for 48 hours total)

FP

Use: Chronic lymphocytic leukemia (CLL).
Cycle: 28 days for up to 6 cycles

Regimen: Fludarabine 30 mg/m^2/day IV, days 1 through 5
Prednisone 30 mg/m^2/day PO, days 1 through 5

FR

Use: Chronic lymphocytic leukemia (CLL).
Cycle: 28 days for 6 cycles

Regimen:
Fludarabine 25 mg/m^2/day IV, days 1 through 5
Rituximab 375 mg/m^2 IV, day 1
Rituximab 375 mg/m^2 IV, day 4 of first cycle only (loading dose)
or
Fludarabine 25 mg/m^2/day IV, days 1 through 5
Rituximab 50 mg/m^2 IV, day 1 of first cycle only (incremental loading dose)
Rituximab 325 mg/m^2 IV, day 3 of first cycle only (incremental loading dose)
Rituximab 375 mg/m^2 IV, day 5 of first cycle only (loading dose)
Rituximab 375 mg/m^2 IV, day 1, except for first cycle

FU/LV—see F-CL

FU/LV/Bevacizumab

Use: Colorectal cancer.
Cycle: 8 weeks

Regimen:
Fluorouracil 600 mg/m^2 IV, weekly for 6 weeks, followed by 2 weeks of rest; administer on days 1, 8, 15, 22, 29, and 35
Leucovorin 500 mg/m^2 IV, weekly for 6 weeks, followed by 2 weeks of rest; administer on days 1, 8, 15, 22, 29, and 35
Bevacizumab 5 mg/kg IV, days 1, 15, 29, and 43

FU/LV/CPT-11 (IFL Douillard Regimen)

Use: Colorectal cancer.
Cycle: 14 days, continue until disease progression or intolerable toxicity

Regimen:
Fluorouracil 400 mg/m^2 IV bolus, day 1
then
Fluorouracil 600 mg/m^2/dose continuous IV infusion over 22 hours, day 1
Leucovorin 200 mg/m^2/day IV, days 1 and 2
Irinotecan 180 mg/m^2 IV, day 1
or
Fluorouracil 2,300 mg/m^2/day continuous IV infusion, weekly on days 1 and 8
Leucovorin 500 mg/m^2 IV, weekly, on days 1 and 8
Irinotecan 80 mg/m^2 IV, weekly, on days 1 and 8

FU/LV/CPT-11 (IFL Saltz Regimen)

Use: Colorectal cancer.*
Cycle: 42 days, continue until disease progression or intolerable toxicity

Regimen:
Fluorouracil 500 mg/m^2 IV, weekly for 4 weeks, on days 1, 8, 15, and 22
Leucovorin 20 mg/m^2 IV, weekly for 4 weeks, on days 1, 8, 15, and 22
Irinotecan 125 mg/m^2 IV, weekly for 4 weeks, on days 1, 8, 15, and 22
*Note: A study analysis found an increased risk of early deaths (within 60 days of initiating treatment) with use of this regimen. Specific risk factors that may have contributed to death were not identified. Intensive patient monitoring and dosage modification are recommended to reduce the risk of severe adverse effects.

FU/LV/CPT-11, Modified (Modified IFL Saltz Regimen)

Use: Colorectal cancer.
Cycle: 21 days, continue until disease progression or intolerable toxicity

Regimen:
Fluorouracil 500 mg/m^2 IV, days 1 and 8
Leucovorin 20 mg/m^2 IV, days 1 and 8
Irinotecan 125 mg/m^2 IV, days 1 and 8

FUFOX

Use: Colorectal cancer.
Cycle: 35 days, continue until disease progression or intolerable toxicity

Regimen:
Oxaliplatin 50 mg/m^2 IV, weekly for 4 weeks, on days 1, 8, 15, and 22 of cycles 1 through 4
Oxaliplatin 50 mg/m^2 IV, days 1 and 15 of subsequent cycles (ie, from cycle 5 until end of therapy)
then
Leucovorin 500 mg/m^2 IV, weekly for 4 weeks, on days 1, 8, 15, and 22
Fluorouracil 2,000 mg/m^2/dose continuous IV infusion over 22 hours, weekly for 4 weeks, on days 1, 8, 15, and 22

FUFOX + Cetuximab

Use: Gastric cancer.
Cycle: 35 days

Regimen:
Oxaliplatin 50 mg/m^2 IV, weekly for 4 weeks, on days 1, 8, 15, and 22
then
Leucovorin 200 mg/m^2 IV, weekly for 4 weeks, on days 1, 8, 15, and 22
Fluorouracil 2,000 mg/m^2/dose continuous IV infusion over 22 hours, weekly for 4 weeks, on days 1, 8, 15, and 22
Cetuximab 400 mg/m^2 IV, day 1 of first cycle only (loading dose)
Cetuximab 250 mg/m^2 IV weekly, except for day 1 of first cycle

FUOX

Use: Colorectal cancer.
Cycle: 14 days for up to 18 cycles

Regimen: Fluorouracil 1,125 mg/m^2/day continuous IV infusion, days 1 and 2 (for 48 hours total), and days 8 and 9 (for 48 hours total)
Oxaliplatin 85 mg/m^2 IV, day 1

FUP (also see CF; also see Cisplatin-Fluorouracil)

Use: Gastric cancer, biliary tract cancer.
Cycle: 28 days, continue until disease progression or intolerable toxicity

Regimen: Fluorouracil 1,000 mg/m^2/day continuous IV infusion, days 1 through 5
Cisplatin 100 mg/m^2 IV, day 2

FZ

Use: Prostate cancer.
Cycle: Ongoing

Regimen: Flutamide 250 mg/dose PO every 8 hours
with
Goserelin acetate 3.6 mg/dose implant subcutaneously every 28 days
or
Goserelin acetate 10.8 mg/dose implant subcutaneously every 12 weeks

FZ + Radiation

Use: Prostate cancer.
Cycle: 4 months. Give a single cycle.

Regimen: Flutamide 250 mg/dose PO every 8 hours, days 1 through 112
Goserelin acetate 3.6 mg/dose implant subcutaneously every 28 days, days 1 through 112
used in conjunction with
Radiation therapy, days 57 through 112

FZ + Radiation ➡ Z

Use: Prostate cancer.
Cycle: See below, cycle length varies throughout protocol. Give a single cycle of FZ + Radiation, followed by 2 years of Hormone therapy.

Regimen: **FZ + Radiation.** *Cycle:* 4 months. Give a single cycle.
Flutamide 250 mg/dose PO every 8 hours, days 1 through 112
Goserelin acetate 3.6 mg/dose implant subcutaneously every 28 days, days 1 through 112
used in conjunction with
Radiation therapy, days 57 through 112
followed by
Hormone therapy. *Cycle:* 2 years. Give a single cycle.
Goserelin acetate 3.6 mg/dose implant subcutaneously every 28 days

G + V (also see Gemcitabine-Vinorelbine)

Use: Lung cancer (non-small cell).
Cycle: 21 days for up to 6 cycles

Regimen: Gemcitabine 1,000 to 1,200 mg/m^2 IV, days 1 and 8
Vinorelbine 25 to 30 mg/m^2 IV, days 1 and 8

GCP (also see PCG)

Use: Adenocarcinoma (unknown primary).
Cycle: See below, cycle length varies throughout protocol. Give 4 cycles of GCP, followed by 3 cycles of Paclitaxel alone.

Regimen: **GCP.** *Cycle:* 21 days for 4 cycles
Gemcitabine 1,000 mg/m^2 IV, days 1 and 8
Carboplatin IV dose by Calvert equation to AUC 5 mg/mL/min, day 1 (sequence of administration not specified)
Paclitaxel 200 mg/m^2 IV over 1 hour, day 1
followed by
Paclitaxel alone. *Cycle:* 56 days for 3 cycles
Paclitaxel 70 mg/m^2 IV (infusion duration not specified), weekly for 6 weeks then 2 weeks of rest; administer on days 1, 8, 15, 22, 29, and 36

Gemcitabine-Bevacizumab

Use: Pancreatic cancer.
Cycle: 28 days, continue until disease progression or intolerable toxicity

Regimen: Gemcitabine 1,000 mg/m^2 IV, days 1, 8, and 15
Bevacizumab 10 mg/kg IV, days 1 and 15 (give after gemcitabine)

Gemcitabine-Capecitabine (Gem-Cap)

Use: Pancreatic cancer, biliary tract cancer.
Cycle: 21 days for up to 8 cycles, or until disease progression or intolerable toxicity
Regimen: Gemcitabine 1,000 mg/m^2 IV, days 1 and 8
Capecitabine 650 mg/m^2/dose PO twice daily, days 1 through 14

Use: Pancreatic cancer.
Cycle: 28 days, continue until disease progression or intolerable toxicity
Regimen: Gemcitabine 1,000 mg/m^2 IV, days 1, 8, and 15
Capecitabine 880 mg/m^2/dose PO twice daily, days 1 through 21

Gemcitabine-Carboplatin

Use: Lung cancer (non-small cell).
Cycle: 28 days for up to 6 cycles
Regimen: Gemcitabine 1,000 or 1,100 mg/m^2 IV, days 1 and 8
Carboplatin IV dose by Calvert equation to AUC 5 mg/mL/min, day 8

Use: Lung cancer (non-small cell).
Cycle: 21 days for up to 6 cycles
Regimen: Gemcitabine 1,250 mg/m^2 IV, days 1 and 8
Carboplatin IV dose by Calvert equation to AUC 5 mg/mL/min, day 1 (give after gemcitabine)

Use: Mesothelioma.
Cycle: 28 days for up to 6 cycles
Regimen: Gemcitabine 1,000 mg/m^2 IV, days 1, 8, and 15
Carboplatin IV dose by Calvert equation to AUC 5 mg/mL/min, day 1

Use: Ovarian cancer, bladder cancer.
Cycle: 21 days for up to 6 cycles
Regimen: Gemcitabine 1,000 mg/m^2 IV, days 1 and 8
Carboplatin IV dose by Calvert equation to AUC 4 mg/mL/min, day 1 (give after gemcitabine)

Gemcitabine-Cis (also see Gemcitabine-Cisplatin)

Use: Lung cancer (non-small cell).
Cycle: 28 days for up to 6 cycles
Regimen: Gemcitabine 1,000 to 1,200 mg/m^2 IV, days 1, 8, and 15
Cisplatin 100 mg/m^2 IV, day 15*
*Note: Some references state that a single dose of cisplatin may be given on day 1, 2, or 15 of each cycle. However, the best results are seen when cisplatin is given on day 15.

Use: Lung cancer (non-small cell).
Cycle: 21 days for up to 6 cycles
Regimen: Cisplatin 100 mg/m^2 IV, day 1 (give before gemcitabine)
Gemcitabine 1,250 mg/m^2 IV, days 1 and 8

Use: Mesothelioma.
Cycle: 28 days for up to 6 cycles
Regimen: Cisplatin 100 mg/m^2 IV, day 1 (give before gemcitabine)
Gemcitabine 1,000 mg/m^2 IV, days 1, 8, and 15

Gemcitabine-Cisplatin (also see Gemcitabine-Cis)

Use: Bladder cancer.
Cycle: 28 days for up to 6 cycles
Regimen: Gemcitabine 1,000 mg/m^2 IV, days 1, 8, and 15
Cisplatin 70 mg/m^2 IV, day 2

Use: Bladder cancer.
Cycle: 28 days for up to 6 cycles, or until disease progression or intolerable toxicity
Regimen: Gemcitabine 1,000 mg/m^2 IV, days 1, 8, and 15
Cisplatin 75 mg/m^2 IV, day 1 (give after gemcitabine)

Use: Biliary tract cancer.
Cycle: 21 days, continue until disease progression or intolerable toxicity
Regimen: Gemcitabine 1,250 mg/m^2 IV, days 1 and 8
Cisplatin 75 mg/m^2 IV, day 1

Use: Cervical cancer.
Cycle: 21 days for up to 6 cycles
Regimen: Gemcitabine 1,000 to 1,250 mg/m^2 IV, days 1 and 8
Cisplatin 50 mg/m^2 IV, day 1 (give after gemcitabine)

Gemcitabine-Cisplatin (also see Gemcitabine-Cis) (cont.)

Use:	Ovarian cancer. *Cycle:* 21 days
Regimen 1:	Patients treated with less than 2 prior chemotherapy regimens: Cisplatin 30 mg/m^2 IV, days 1 and 8 Gemcitabine 750 mg/m^2 IV, days 1 and 8 (give after cisplatin)
Regimen 2:	Patients treated with 2 or more prior chemotherapy regimens: Cisplatin 30 mg/m^2 IV, days 1 and 8 Gemcitabine 600 mg/m^2 IV, days 1 and 8 (give after cisplatin)
Use:	Pancreatic cancer. *Cycle:* 28 days, continue until disease progression or intolerable toxicity
Regimen:	Gemcitabine 1,000 mg/m^2 IV, days 1, 8, and 15 Cisplatin 50 mg/m^2 IV, days 1 and 15 (give after gemcitabine)
Use:	Pancreatic cancer. *Cycle:* 28 days
Regimen:	Gemcitabine 1,000 mg/m^2 IV, days 1 and 15 Cisplatin 50 mg/m^2 IV, days 1 and 15 (give after gemcitabine)
Use:	Head and neck cancer (nasopharyngeal). *Cycle:* 28 days for at least 6 cycles
Regimen:	Gemcitabine 1,000 mg/m^2 IV, days 1, 8, and 15 Cisplatin 50 mg/m^2 IV, days 1 and 8 *may be used in conjunction with* Radiation therapy

Gemcitabine-Cisplatin-Bevacizumab

Use:	Lung cancer (non-small cell). *Cycle:* 21 days for 6 cycles
Regimen:	Gemcitabine 1,250 mg/m^2 IV, days 1 and 8 Cisplatin 80 mg/m^2 IV, day 1 Bevacizumab 7.5 or 15 mg/kg IV, day 1 *followed by* Bevacizumab 7.5 or 15 mg/kg IV, every 3 weeks until disease progression or intolerable toxicity

Gemcitabine-Docetaxel

Use:	Lung cancer (non-small cell). *Cycle:* 21 days for up to 6 cycles or until disease progression or intolerable toxicity
Regimen:	Gemcitabine 1,100 mg/m^2 IV, days 1 and 8 Docetaxel 100 mg/m^2 IV, day 8 (give after gemcitabine) Filgrastim 150 mcg/m^2/day subcutaneously, days 9 through 15
Use:	Sarcoma (uterine). *Cycle:* 21 days for up to 6 cycles
Regimen 1:	Patients with no prior radiation therapy: Gemcitabine 900 mg/m^2 IV, days 1 and 8 Docetaxel 100 mg/m^2 IV, day 8 (give after gemcitabine on day 8) Filgrastim 150 mcg/m^2/day subcutaneously (rounded to 300 or 480 mcg), days 9 through 15
Regimen 2:	Patients with prior radiation therapy: Gemcitabine 675 mg/m^2 IV, days 1 and 8 Docetaxel 75 mg/m^2 IV, day 8 (give after gemcitabine on day 8) Filgrastim 150 mcg/m^2/day subcutaneously (rounded to 300 or 480 mcg), days 9 through 15

Gemcitabine-Erlotinib

Use:	Pancreatic cancer. *Cycle:* 56 days, continue until disease progression or intolerable toxicity
Regimen:	Gemcitabine 1,000 mg/m^2 IV, weekly for 7 weeks for first cycle; for subsequent cycles, give weekly for 3 weeks followed by 1 week of rest; administer on days 1, 8, 15, 29, 36, and 43 Erlotinib 100 mg/day PO, throughout entire course

Gemcitabine-Irinotecan

Use:	Pancreatic cancer. *Cycle:* 21 days for at least 6 cycles
Regimen:	Gemcitabine 1,000 mg/m^2 IV, days 1 and 8 Irinotecan 100 mg/m^2 IV, days 1 and 8 (give after gemcitabine)

Gemcitabine-Liposomal Doxorubicin

Use: Ovarian cancer.
Cycle: 21 days

Regimen: Gemcitabine 1,000 mg/m^2 IV, days 1 and 8
Liposomal doxorubicin 30 mg/m^2 IV, day 1

Gemcitabine-Liposomal Doxorubicin/CP

Use: Ovarian cancer.
Cycle: 21 days for 8 cycles. Give Treatment A, then follow with Treatment B; repeat alternating treatments for a total of 8 cycles (ie, 4 cycles of Treatment A and 4 cycles of Treatment B).

Regimen: **Treatment A** (cycles 1, 3, 5, and 7)
Gemcitabine 800 mg/m^2 IV, days 1 and 8
Liposomal doxorubicin 30 mg/m^2 IV, day 1
Treatment B (cycles 2, 4, 6, and 8)
Cyclophosphamide 600 mg/m^2 IV, day 1
Cisplatin 60 mg/m^2 IV, day 1

Gemcitabine-Vinorelbine (also see G + V)

Use: Lung cancer (non-small cell).
Cycle: 28 days for up to 6 cycles

Regimen: Gemcitabine 800 or 1,000 mg/m^2 IV, days 1, 8, and 15
Vinorelbine 20 mg/m^2 IV, days 1, 8, and 15

Use: Mesothelioma.
Cycle: 21 days for up to 6 cycles, or until disease progression or intolerable toxicity

Regimen: Gemcitabine 1,000 mg/m^2 IV, days 1 and 8
Vinorelbine 25 mg/m^2 IV, days 1 and 8 (give after gemcitabine)

Use: Sarcoma (soft-tissue).
Cycle: 21 days, continue until disease progression or intolerable toxicity

Regimen: Vinorelbine 25 mg/m^2 IV, days 1 and 8
Gemcitabine 800 mg/m^2 IV, days 1 and 8 (give after vinorelbine)

GEMOX

Use: Biliary tract adenocarcinoma, pancreatic cancer, hepatocellular cancer.
Cycle: 14 days for up to 6 cycles or until disease progression or intolerable toxicity

Regimen: Gemcitabine 1,000 mg/m^2 IV, day 1
Oxaliplatin 100 mg/m^2 IV, day 2

Use: Pancreatic cancer.
Cycle: 14 days, continue until disease progression or intolerable toxicity

Regimen: Gemcitabine 1,000 mg/m^2 IV, day 1
Oxaliplatin 100 mg/m^2 IV, day 1 (give after gemcitabine)

GEMOX-B—see GEMOX + Bevacizumab

GEMOX + Bevacizumab (GEMOX-B)

Use: Hepatocellular cancer.
Cycle: See below, cycle length varies throughout protocol. Give a single cycle of Treatment A, followed by Treatment B.

Regimen: **Treatment A (cycle 1).** *Cycle:* 14 days. Give a single cycle.
Bevacizumab 10 mg/kg IV, day 1
followed immediately by
Treatment B (all subsequent cycles). *Cycle:* 28 days, continued until disease progression or intolerable toxicity
Bevacizumab 10 mg/kg IV, days 1 and 15
Gemcitabine 1,000 mg/m^2 IV, days 2 and 16
Oxaliplatin 85 mg/m^2 IV, days 2 and 16

GEMOX + Rituximab (R-GEMOX)

Use: Lymphoma (B-cell).
Cycle: 14 days for up to 8 cycles

Regimen: Rituximab 375 mg/m^2 IV, day 1
Gemcitabine 1,000 mg/m^2 IV, day 2
Oxaliplatin 100 mg/m^2 IV, day 2 (give after gemcitabine)

Use: Lymphoma (mantle cell).
Cycle: 14 to 21 days for up to 8 cycles

Regimen: Rituximab 375 mg/m^2 IV, day 1
Gemcitabine 1,000 mg/m^2 IV, day 1
Oxaliplatin 100 mg/m^2 IV, day 1

GOLF

Use: Pancreatic cancer.
Cycle: 14 days

Regimen: Gemcitabine 1,000 mg/m^2 IV, day 1
Oxaliplatin 85 mg/m^2 IV, day 2
Levoleucovorin 100 mg/m^2/day IV, days 1 and 2
with
Fluorouracil 400 mg/m^2/day IV bolus, days 1 and 2
then
Fluorouracil 800 mg/m^2/day continuous IV infusion, days 1 and 2 (for 48 hours total)

GT

Use: Breast cancer.
Cycle: 21 days, continue until disease progression or intolerable toxicity

Regimen: Paclitaxel 175 mg/m^2 IV over 3 hours, day 1 (give before gemcitabine)
Gemcitabine 1,250 mg/m^2 IV, days 1 and 8

Use: Lung cancer (non-small cell).
Cycle: 21 days for up to 6 cycles

Regimen: Paclitaxel 200 mg/m^2 IV over 3 hours, day 1 (before gemcitabine)
Gemcitabine 1,000 mg/m^2 IV, days 1 and 8

Use: Bladder cancer.
Cycle: 21 days for up to 6 cycles

Regimen: Gemcitabine 1,000 mg/m^2 IV weekly, on days 1, 8, and 15
Paclitaxel 200 mg/m^2 IV over 1 hour, day 1 (sequence of administration not specified)

Use: Bladder cancer.
Cycle: 14 days for up to 12 cycles

Regimen: Paclitaxel 150 mg/m^2 IV over 3 hours, day 1 (give before gemcitabine)
Gemcitabine 2,500 mg/m^2 IV, day 1

GTX

Use: Pancreatic cancer.
Cycle: 21 days

Regimen: Capecitabine 750 mg/m^2/dose PO twice daily, days 1 through 14
Gemcitabine 750 mg/m^2 IV, days 4 and 11
Docetaxel 30 mg/m^2 IV, days 4 and 11 (give after gemcitabine)

GVD

Use: Lymphoma (Hodgkin).
Cycle: 21 days for up to 6 cycles, or until disease progression or intolerable toxicity

Regimen 1: Patients who have not undergone hematopoietic stem cell transplantation (HSCT):
Vinorelbine 20 mg/m^2 IV, days 1 and 8
Gemcitabine 1,000 mg/m^2 IV, days 1 and 8 (give after vinorelbine)
Liposomal doxorubicin 15 mg/m^2 IV, days 1 and 8 (give after gemcitabine)

Regimen 2: Patients who have undergone HSCT:
Vinorelbine 15 mg/m^2 IV, days 1 and 8
Gemcitabine 800 mg/m^2 IV, days 1 and 8 (give after vinorelbine)
Liposomal doxorubicin 10 mg/m^2 IV, days 1 and 8 (give after gemcitabine)

HDCA (High-Dose Cytarabine)—see professional monograph for Cytarabine

HDMTX

Use: Sarcoma (bone).
Cycle: 1 to 4 weeks

Regimen: Methotrexate 8,000 to 12,000 mg/m^2 (20,000 mg maximum dose) IV, day 1
Leucovorin 15 mg/m^2/dose IV or PO every 6 hours for 10 doses, beginning 20 to 30 hours after beginning of methotrexate infusion

HEC (also see Epirubicin-Cyclophosphamide)

Use: Breast cancer.
Cycle: 21 days for up to 8 cycles

Regimen: Epirubicin 100 mg/m^2 IV, day 1
Cyclophosphamide 830 mg/m^2 IV, day 1

Hexa-CAF

Use: Ovarian cancer.
Cycle: 28 days for at least 6 cycles

Regimen: Altretamine 150 $mg/m^2/day$ PO, days 1 through 14
Cyclophosphamide 100 to 150 $mg/m^2/day$ PO, days 1 through 14
Methotrexate 40 mg/m^2 IV, days 1 and 8
Fluorouracil 600 mg/m^2 IV, days 1 and 8

Hi-C DAZE

Use: Acute myelocytic leukemia (AML; induction—pediatrics).
Cycle: Give a single cycle

Regimen: Cytarabine 3,000 $mg/m^2/dose$ IV every 12 hours for 8 doses, days 1 through 4
Daunorubicin 30 $mg/m^2/day$ IV, days 1 through 3
Etoposide 200 $mg/m^2/day$ IV, days 1 through 3 and days 6 through 8
Azacitidine 150 $mg/m^2/day$ IV, days 3 through 5 and days 8 through 10

HIDAC (High-Dose Cytarabine)—see professional monograph for Cytarabine

Hyper-CVAD/HD MTX Ara-C*

Use: Lymphoma (mantle cell).
Cycle: 21 days, delay subsequent cycles until hematologic recovery. Give up to 4 cycles.

Regimen: **Hyper-CVAD** (cycles 1 and 3)
Cyclophosphamide 300 $mg/m^2/dose$ IV every 12 hours for 6 doses, days 1 through 3
Dexamethasone 40 mg/day IV or PO, days 1 through 4 and days 11 through 14
Vincristine 2 mg (dose is not in mg/m^2) IV, day 4 (given 12 hours after last cyclophosphamide dose) and day 11
Doxorubicin 25 $mg/m^2/day$ continuous IV infusion, days 4 and 5
Filgrastim 5 mcg/kg/day subcutaneously, starting on day 6 and continued until granulocyte count exceeds 4,500 $cells/mm^3$

HD MTX Ara-C (cycles 2 and 4)
Methotrexate 200 mg/m^2 IV bolus, day 1
then
Methotrexate 800 $mg/m^2/day$ continuous IV infusion, day 1
Cytarabine dose based on age and renal function:
Patients aged 60 years and younger, or patients with serum creatinine no more than 1.5 mg/dL: Cytarabine 3,000 $mg/m^2/dose$ IV every 12 hours for 4 doses, days 2 and 3
Patients older than 60 years of age, or patients with serum creatinine greater than 1.5 mg/dL: Cytarabine 1,000 $mg/m^2/dose$ IV every 12 hours for 4 doses, days 2 and 3 Leucovorin 50 mg PO, day 3, given 24 hours after methotrexate infusion is completed
Leucovorin 15 mg/dose PO every 6 hours for 8 doses, days 3 through 5, starting 30 hours after methotrexate infusion is completed
Filgrastim 5 mcg/kg/day subcutaneously, starting on day 6 and continued until granulocyte count exceeds 4,500 $cells/mm^3$

used in conjunction with
Autologous stem cell transplantation
*Note: These 2 regimens are normally used in combination with each other and are rarely given alone.

Use: Acute lymphocytic leukemia (ALL; induction—adults).
Cycle: 21 days, delay subsequent cycles until hematologic recovery. Give 8 cycles.

Regimen: **Hyper-CVAD** (cycles 1, 3, 5, and 7)
Cyclophosphamide 300 $mg/m^2/dose$ IV every 12 hours for 6 doses, days 1 through 3
Mesna 600 $mg/m^2/day$ continuous IV infusion, days 1 through 3 (begin with cyclophosphamide)
Dexamethasone 40 mg/day IV or PO, days 1 through 4 and days 11 through 14
Doxorubicin 50 mg/m^2 IV, day 4
Vincristine 2 mg (dose is not in mg/m^2) IV, days 4 and 11
Filgrastim 10 mcg/kg/day subcutaneously, starting on day 5 and continued until granulocyte count exceeds 3,000 $cells/mm^3$

HD MTX Ara-C (cycles 2, 4, 6, and 8)
Methotrexate 200 mg/m^2 IV bolus, day 1
then
Methotrexate 800 $mg/m^2/day$ continuous IV infusion, day 1
Cytarabine dose based on age and renal function:
Patients 60 years of age and younger, or patients with serum creatinine no more than 1.5 mg/dL: Cytarabine 3,000 $mg/m^2/dose$ IV every 12 hours for 4 doses, days 2 and 3
Patients older than 60 years of age, or patients with serum creatinine greater than 1.5 mg/dL: Cytarabine 1,000 $mg/m^2/dose$ IV every 12 hours for 4 doses, days 2 and 3 Leucovorin 15 mg/dose IV or PO every 6 hours for 8 doses, beginning on day 3, starting 24 hours after methotrexate infusion is completed and continued until methotrexate concentration is less than 0.1 microMol/L; increase dose to 50 mg/dose IV or PO every 6 hours if the methotrexate concentration is greater than 20 microMol/L at the end of the infusion or greater than 1 microMol/L 24 hours after the end of the infusion, or greater than 0.1 microMol/L 48 hours after the end of the infusion.
Methylprednisolone 50 mg/dose IV twice daily, days 1 through 3
Filgrastim 10 mcg/kg/day subcutaneously, starting on day 4 and continued until granulocyte count exceeds 3,000 $cells/mm^3$

used in conjunction with
(continued on next page)

Hyper-CVAD/HD MTX Ara-C* (cont.)

CNS prophylaxis. Give for cycles 1 and 2 for low-risk patients, cycles 1 through 4 for unknown risk, and all 8 cycles for high-risk patients.
Methotrexate 12 mg intrathecal, day 2
Cytarabine 100 mg intrathecal, day 8
used in conjunction with antimicrobial prophylaxis
Fluconazole 200 mg/day PO, throughout entire course
plus
Ciprofloxacin 500 mg PO twice daily, throughout entire course
or
Levofloxacin 500 mg/day PO, throughout entire course
plus
Acyclovir 200 mg PO twice daily, throughout entire course
or
Valacyclovir 500 mg/day PO, throughout entire course
*Note: These 2 regimens are normally used in combination with each other and are rarely given alone.

Hyper-CVAD/HD MTX Ara-C + Rituximab*

Use: Lymphoma (mantle cell).
Cycle: 21 days, delay subsequent cycles until hematologic recovery. Give up to 8 cycles.

Regimen: **R-Hyper-CVAD** (cycles 1, 3, 5, and 7)
Rituximab 375 mg/m^2 IV, day 1
Mesna 600 mg/m^2/day continuous IV infusion, days 2 through 5 (start 1 hour before cyclophosphamide and continue for 12 hours after last cyclophosphamide dose)
Cyclophosphamide 300 mg/m^2/dose IV every 12 hours for 6 doses, days 2 through 4
Dexamethasone 40 mg/day IV or PO, days 2 through 5 and days 12 through 15
Vincristine 1.4 mg/m^2 (2 mg maximum dose) IV, day 5 (given 12 hours after last cyclophosphamide dose) and day 12
Doxorubicin 16.7 mg/m^2/day continuous IV infusion, days 5 through 7 (start 12 hours after last cyclophosphamide dose)
Filgrastim 5 mcg/kg/day subcutaneously, starting on day 8 and continued until white blood cell count (WBC) is at least 3,000 cells/mm^3

R-HD MTX Ara-C (cycles 2, 4, 6, and 8)
Rituximab 375 mg/m^2 IV, day 1
Methotrexate 200 mg/m^2 IV bolus, day 2
then
Methotrexate 800 mg/m^2 continuous IV infusion over 22 hours, day 2
Cytarabine dose based on age and renal function
Patients 60 years of age and younger, or patients with serum creatinine no more than 1.5 mg/dL: Cytarabine 3,000 mg/m^2/dose IV every 12 hours for 4 doses, days 3 and 4
Patients older than 60 years of age, or patients with serum creatinine greater than 1.5 mg/dL: Cytarabine 1,000 mg/m^2/dose IV every 12 hours for 4 doses, days 3 and 4 Leucovorin 50 mg PO, day 3, given 24 hours after methotrexate infusion is completed
Leucovorin 15 mg/dose PO every 6 hours for 8 doses, days 4 through 6, starting 30 hours after methotrexate infusion is completed
Filgrastim 5 mcg/kg/day subcutaneously, starting on day 6 and continued until WBC is at least 3,000 cells/mm^3
used in conjunction with antimicrobial prophylaxis
Fluconazole 100 mg/day PO, days 8 through 17
Valacyclovir 500 mg/day PO, days 8 through 17
plus
Ciprofloxacin 500 mg PO twice daily, days 8 through 17
or
Levofloxacin 500 mg/day PO, days 8 through 17
*Note: These 2 regimens are normally used in combination with each other and are rarely given alone.

ICE—see MICE

ICE + Autologous Stem Cell Transplantation

Use: Lymphoma (non-Hodgkin—adults).
Cycle: 14 days for 3 cycles

Regimen: Etoposide 100 mg/m^2/day IV, days 1 through 3
Ifosfamide 5,000 mg/m^2/day continuous IV infusion, day 2*
Mesna 5,000 mg/m^2/day continuous IV infusion, day 2*
Carboplatin IV dose by Calvert equation to AUC 5 mg/mL/min (800 mg maximum dose), day 2
Filgrastim 5 mcg/kg/day subcutaneously, days 5 through 12; increased in third cycle to 10 mcg/kg/day subcutaneously, from day 5 until leukapheresis
used in conjunction with
Autologous stem cell transplantation
*Note: Ifosfamide and mesna may be mixed and administered in the same infusion bag.

ICE Protocol—see Idarubicin, Cytarabine, Etoposide

ICE + Rituximab (R-MICE, RICE)

Use: Lymphoma (non-Hodgkin—adults).
Cycle: 14 days for 3 cycles

Regimen:
Rituximab 375 mg/m^2 IV, day −1 of first cycle only (loading dose, given 2 days before starting other agents)
Rituximab 375 mg/m^2 IV, day 1
Etoposide 100 mg/m^2/day IV, days 3 through 5
Ifosfamide 5,000 mg/m^2/day continuous IV infusion, day 4*
Mesna 5,000 mg/m^2/day continuous IV infusion, day 4*
Carboplatin IV dose by Calvert equation to AUC 5 mg/mL/min (800 mg maximum dose), day 4
Filgrastim 5 mcg/kg/day subcutaneously, days 7 through 14 for first 2 cycles; increased in third cycle to 10 mcg/kg/day subcutaneously, from day 7 until leukapheresis
used in conjunction with
Autologous stem cell transplantation
*Note: Ifosfamide and mesna may be mixed and administered in the same infusion bag.

ICE-T

Use: Breast cancer, sarcoma, lung cancer (non-small cell).
Cycle: 28 days

Regimen:
Ifosfamide 1,250 mg/m^2/day IV, days 1 through 3
Carboplatin 300 mg/m^2 IV, day 1
Etoposide 80 mg/m^2/day IV, days 1 through 3
Paclitaxel 175 mg/m^2 IV over 3 hours, day 4
with
Mesna 20% of ifosfamide dose IV before ifosfamide, then mesna 40% of ifosfamide dose PO 4 and 8 hours after ifosfamide, days 1 through 3
or
Mesna 1,250 mg/m^2/day IV, days 1 through 3

ICE-V

Use: Lung cancer (small cell).
Cycle: 28 days for up to 6 cycles

Regimen:
Carboplatin 300 mg/m^2 IV, day 1
Ifosfamide 5,000 mg/m^2/day continuous IV infusion, day 1*
Mesna 5,000 mg/m^2/day continuous IV infusion, day 1*
Mesna 3,000 mg/m^2/dose continuous IV infusion over 12 hours, day 2 (start at end of ifosfamide infusion)
Etoposide 120 mg/m^2/day IV, days 1 and 2
Etoposide 240 mg/m^2 PO, day 3
Vincristine 1 mg/m^2 IV, day 14
*Note: Ifosfamide and mesna may be mixed and administered in the same infusion bag.

IDA-Based BF12—see Idarubicin, Cytarabine, Etoposide

Idarubicin, Cytarabine, Etoposide (ICE Protocol)

Use: Acute myelocytic leukemia (AML; induction—adults).
Cycle: Give a single cycle

Regimen:
Idarubicin 6 mg/m^2/day IV, days 1 through 5
Cytarabine 600 mg/m^2/day IV, days 1 through 5
Etoposide 150 mg/m^2/day IV, days 1 through 3

Idarubicin, Cytarabine, Etoposide (IDA-Based BF12)

Use: Acute myelocytic leukemia (AML; induction—adults).
Cycle: Usually 1 cycle is given. A second cycle may be considered for patients with partial response. Time between cycles not specified.

Regimen:
Idarubicin 5 mg/m^2/day IV, days 1 through 5
Cytarabine 2,000 mg/m^2/dose IV every 12 hours for 10 doses, days 1 through 5
Etoposide 100 mg/m^2/day IV, days 1 through 5

IDMTX

Use: Acute lymphocytic leukemia (ALL; intensification—pediatrics).
Cycle: 14 days, for 12 cycles

Regimen:
Methotrexate 1,000 mg/m^2/day continuous IV infusion, day 1 (24-hour infusion)
Mercaptopurine 1,000 mg/m^2 IV over 6 hours following methotrexate, day 2
Leucovorin 5 mg/m^2/dose IV every 6 hours for at least 5 doses, days 3 and 4, starting 48 hours after the start of the methotrexate infusion and continued until methotrexate concentration is less than 0.1 microMol/L
Methotrexate 20 mg/m^2 IM, day 8
Mercaptopurine 50 mg/m^2/day PO, days 8 through 14

IDMTX/6-MP

Use: Acute lymphocytic leukemia (ALL; consolidation—pediatrics).
Cycle: 2 weeks for up to 12 cycles

Regimen: **Week 1:** Methotrexate 200 mg/m^2 IV bolus, day 1
Mercaptopurine 200 mg/m^2 IV bolus, day 1
then
Methotrexate 800 mg/m^2/day continuous IV infusion, day 1
Mercaptopurine 800 mg/m^2 IV over 8 hours, day 1
Leucovorin 5 mg/m^2/dose IV or PO every 6 hours for 5 to 13 doses, beginning 24 hours after methotrexate infusion is completed
Week 2: Methotrexate 20 mg/m^2 IM, day 8
Mercaptopurine 50 mg/m^2/day PO, days 8 through 14

IDO

Use: Gastric cancer.
Cycle: 21 days for up to 8 cycles, or until disease progression or intolerable toxicity

Regimen: Irinotecan 150 mg/m^2 IV, day 1
Docetaxel 60 mg/m^2 IV, day 1
Oxaliplatin 85 mg/m^2 IV, day 2

IE (also see IfoVP)

Use: Sarcoma (soft tissue).
Cycle: 21 days for up to 6 cycles

Regimen: Ifosfamide 1,800 mg/m^2/day IV, days 1 through 5
Etoposide 100 mg/m^2/day IV, days 1 through 5
with
Mesna 1,800 mg/m^2/day IV, days 1 through 5
or
Mesna 20% of ifosfamide dose IV before, then 4 and 8 hours after each ifosfamide infusion, days 1 through 5

IFL—see FU/LV/CPT-11

IFL + Bevacizumab

Use: Colorectal cancer.
Cycle: 42 days, continue until disease progression or intolerable toxicity

Regimen: Irinotecan 125 mg/m^2 IV, weekly for 4 weeks, followed by 2 weeks of rest; administer on days 1, 8, 15, and 22
Fluorouracil 500 mg/m^2 IV, weekly for 4 weeks, followed by 2 weeks of rest; administer on days 1, 8, 15, and 22
Leucovorin 20 mg/m^2 IV, weekly for 4 weeks, followed by 2 weeks of rest; administer on days 1, 8, 15, and 22
Bevacizumab 5 mg/kg IV, days 1, 15, and 29

IFN + DTIC

Use: Malignant melanoma.
Cycle: 28 days for at least 2 to 3 cycles, or until disease progression or intolerable toxicity

Regimen: Interferon alfa-2b 15 million units/m^2/day IV, days 1 through 5, days 8 through 12, and days 15 through 19 of first cycle only
Interferon alfa-2b 10 million units/m^2/dose subcutaneous 3 times weekly throughout entire course, except for first cycle
Dacarbazine 200 mg/m^2/day IV, days 22 through 26

Ifosfamide-Paclitaxel

Use: Endometrial cancer.
Cycle: 21 days for up to 8 cycles

Regimen: Ifosfamide dose based on history of radiation therapy:
Patients without prior radiation therapy: Ifosfamide 1,600 mg/m^2/day IV, days 1 through 3
Patients with prior radiation therapy: Ifosfamide 1,200 mg/m^2/day IV, days 1 through 3
Paclitaxel 135 mg/m^2/day IV over 3 hours, day 1
with
Mesna 2,000 mg/dose continuous IV infusion over 12 hours, days 1 through 3 (start 15 minutes before ifosfamide each day)
or
Mesna 1,330 mg/dose PO, given 1 hour before, then 4 and 8 hours after each ifosfamide infusion, days 1 through 3 (for 3 doses total each day)
with
Filgrastim 5 mcg/kg/day subcutaneously, from day 4 until granulocyte count is at least 2,000 cells/mm^3

IfoVP (also see IE)

Use: Sarcoma (osteosarcoma—pediatrics).
Cycle: 21 days for up to 6 cycles

Regimen: Ifosfamide 1,800 mg/m^2/day IV, days 1 through 5
Etoposide 100 mg/m^2/day IV, days 1 through 5
Mesna 1,800 mg/m^2/day IV, days 1 through 5

IGeV

Use: Lymphoma (Hodgkin).
Cycle: 21 days for up to 4 cycles

Regimen:
Ifosfamide 2,000 mg/m²/day IV, days 1 through 4
Mesna 2,600 mg/m²/day continuous IV infusion, days 1 through 4
Gemcitabine 800 mg/m² IV, days 1 and 4
Vinorelbine 20 mg/m² IV, day 1
Prednisone 100 mg/day PO, days 1 through 4*
Filgrastim 300 mcg/day subcutaneously, days 7 through 13
used in conjunction with
Autologous stem cell transplantation
*Note: Prednisolone is recommended in the European literature. In the United States, prednisone is the preferred corticosteroid. The doses of these 2 corticosteroids are equivalent (ie, prednisone 40 mg PO = prednisolone 40 mg PO).

ILF (also see FU/LV/CPT-11)

Use: Gastric cancer.
Cycle: 14 days for at least 4 cycles, or until disease progression or intolerable toxicity

Regimen:
Fluorouracil 400 mg/m²/day IV bolus, days 1 and 2
then
Fluorouracil 600 mg/m²/dose continuous IV infusion over 22 hours, days 1 and 2
Leucovorin 200 mg/m²/day IV, days 1 and 2
Irinotecan 180 mg/m² IV, day 1

Use: Gastric cancer.
Cycle: 7 weeks, continue until disease progression or intolerable toxicity

Regimen:
Irinotecan 80 mg/m² IV, day 1, weekly for 6 weeks, then 1 week of rest
Leucovorin 500 mg/m²/day IV, weekly for 6 weeks, then 1 week of rest
then
Fluorouracil 2,000 mg/m²/dose continuous IV infusion over 22 hours, weekly for 6 weeks, then 1 week of rest

Interferon-Cytarabine-Hydroxyurea

Use: Chronic myelocytic leukemia (CML).
Cycle: 28 days for at least 6 cycles

Regimen:
Interferon alfa-2b 5 million units/day subcutaneously, throughout entire course; adjust dose to white blood cell count (WBC)
Hydroxyurea 50 mg/kg/day PO, throughout entire course; adjust dose to WBC
Cytarabine 20 mg/m²/day subcutaneously, days 15 through 24 (therapy modified based on WBC and therapeutic response)

Interleukin 2-Interferon alfa 2

Use: Renal cell carcinoma.
Cycle: 56 days, continue until disease progression or intolerable toxicity

Regimen:
Aldesleukin 20 million units/m²/dose subcutaneously 3 times weekly, weeks 1 and 4
Aldesleukin 5 million units/m²/dose subcutaneously 3 times weekly, weeks 2, 3, 5, and 6
Interferon alfa 6 million units/m²/dose subcutaneously once weekly, weeks 1 and 4
Interferon alfa 6 million units/m²/dose subcutaneously 3 times weekly, weeks 2, 3, 5, and 6

Use: Renal cell carcinoma.
Cycle: 42 days for up to 6 cycles

Regimen:
Aldesleukin 5 million units/m²/dose subcutaneously 3 times weekly, weeks 1 through 4
Interferon alfa-2b 5 million units/m²/dose subcutaneously every 8 hours for 3 doses, day 1 of week 1
Interferon alfa-2b 5 million units/m²/dose subcutaneously, days 2 through 5 of weeks 2 through 4
Interferon alfa-2b 5 million units/m²/dose subcutaneously 5 times weekly (eg, Sunday through Thursday), weeks 2 through 4

Use: Renal cell carcinoma

Regimen:
Remission induction. *Cycle*: 11 days for 2 cycles
Aldesleukin 18 million units/m²/day continuous IV infusion, days 1 through 5
Interferon alfa-2a* 6 million units/dose subcutaneously, days 1, 3, and 5
Maintenance. *Cycle*: 26 days for 4 cycles
Aldesleukin 18 million units/m²/day continuous IV infusion, days 1 through 5
Interferon alfa-2a* 6 million units/dose subcutaneously, days 1, 3, and 5
*Note: Interferon alfa-2a is no longer available in the United States. The manufacturer discontinued this product in October 2007 for commercial reasons, not for safety or efficacy reasons.

Interleukin 2-Interferon alfa 2-Fluorouracil

Use: Renal cell carcinoma.

Cycle: 8 weeks for up to 2 cycles

Regimen:
Aldesleukin 20 million units/m²/dose subcutaneously 3 times weekly, weeks 1 and 4
Aldesleukin 5 million units/m²/dose subcutaneously 3 times weekly, weeks 2 and 3
Interferon alfa-2a* 6 million units/m²/dose subcutaneously once weekly, weeks 1 and 4
Interferon alfa-2a* 6 million units/m²/dose subcutaneously 3 times weekly, weeks 2 and 3
Interferon alfa-2a* 9 million units/m²/dose subcutaneously 3 times weekly, weeks 5 through 8
Fluorouracil 750 mg/m²/dose IV bolus once weekly, weeks 5 through 8
*Note: Interferon alfa-2a is no longer available in the United States. The manufacturer discontinued this product in October 2007 for commercial reasons, not for safety or efficacy reasons.

Use: Renal cell carcinoma.

Cycle: 8 weeks for up to 3 cycles

Regimen:
Aldesleukin 10 million units/m²/dose subcutaneously twice daily, days 3 through 5, of weeks 1 and 4
Aldesleukin 5 million units/m² subcutaneously once daily, days 1, 3, and 5, of weeks 2 and 3
Interferon alfa-2a* 5 million units/m²/dose subcutaneously, day 1, of weeks 1 and 4
Interferon alfa-2a* 5 million units/m² subcutaneously once daily, days 1, 3, and 5, of weeks 2 and 3
Interferon alfa-2a* 10 million units/m² subcutaneously once daily, days 1, 3, and 5, of weeks 5 through 8
Fluorouracil 1,000 mg/m²/dose IV, day 1, of weeks 5 through 8
*Note: Interferon alfa-2a is no longer available in the United States. The manufacturer discontinued this product in October 2007 for commercial reasons, not for safety or efficacy reasons.

IPA

Use: Hepatoblastoma (pediatrics).

Cycle: 21 days for up to 4 cycles

Regimen:
Ifosfamide 500 mg/m² IV bolus, day 1
Ifosfamide 1,000 mg/m²/day continuous IV infusion, days 1 through 3
Cisplatin 20 mg/m²/day IV, days 4 through 8
Doxorubicin 30 mg/m²/day continuous IV infusion, days 9 and 10

IPB (Cisplatin-Irinotecan-Bevacizumab)

Use: Gastric cancer.

Cycle: 21 days

Regimen:
Cisplatin 30 mg/m² IV, days 1 and 8
Irinotecan 65 mg/m² IV, days 1 and 8
Bevacizumab 15 mg/kg IV, day 1

IROX

Use: Colorectal cancer.

Cycle: 21 days, continue until disease progression or intolerable toxicity

Regimen:
Irinotecan 200 mg/m² IV, day 1
Oxaliplatin 85 mg/m² IV, day 1

ITP

Use: Bladder cancer.

Cycle: 21 to 28 days for up to 6 cycles

Regimen:
Paclitaxel 200 mg/m² IV over 3 hours, day 1
Cisplatin 70 mg/m² IV, day 1 (give after paclitaxel)
Ifosfamide 1,500 mg/m²/day IV, days 1 through 3 (give after cisplatin and paclitaxel)
Mesna 20% of ifosfamide dose IV, given 30 minutes before, then 4 and 8 hours after each ifosfamide infusion, days 1 through 3 (for 3 doses total each day)
Filgrastim 5 mcg/kg/day subcutaneously, days 6 through 17, or until white blood cell count (WBC) exceeds 10,000 cells/mm³ for 2 days (whichever occurs earlier)

Ixabepilone-Capecitabine (XI)

Use: Breast cancer.

Cycle: 21 days, continue until disease progression or intolerable toxicity

Regimen:
Ixabepilone 40 mg/m² IV, day 1
Capecitabine 1,000 mg/m²/dose PO twice daily, days 1 through 14

Ketoconazole-Hydrocortisone

Use: Prostate cancer.

Cycle: Ongoing, continue until disease progression or intolerable toxicity

Regimen:
Ketoconazole 400 mg PO 3 times daily, throughout entire course
Hydrocortisone 30 mg PO every morning, throughout entire course
Hydrocortisone 10 mg PO every evening, throughout entire course

Lapatinib-Capecitabine

Use: Breast cancer.
Cycle: 21 days, continue until disease progression or intolerable toxicity

Regimen: Lapatinib 1,250 mg PO daily, throughout entire course
Capecitabine 1,000 mg/m^2/dose PO twice daily, days 1 through 14

Lapatinib-Paclitaxel

Use: Breast cancer.
Cycle: 21 days for up to 6 cycles

Regimen: Lapatinib 1,500 mg PO daily, throughout entire course
Paclitaxel 175 mg/m^2 IV over 3 hours, day 1
followed by
Lapatinib 1,500 mg PO daily, continued until disease progression or intolerable toxicity

Lapatinib-Trastuzumab (L + T)

Use: Breast cancer.
Cycle: Ongoing, continue until disease progression or intolerable toxicity

Regimen: Lapatinib 1,000 mg PO daily, throughout entire course
Trastuzumab 4 mg/kg IV, day 1 (loading dose)
Trastuzumab 2 mg/kg IV, weekly except for day 1

Larson Regimen (CAL-G, CALGB 8811)

Use: Acute lymphocytic leukemia (ALL—adults)

Regimen: **Remission induction.** *Cycle*: 28 days. Give a single cycle.

Patients 60 years of age and younger:
Cyclophosphamide 1,200 mg/m^2 IV, day 1
Daunorubicin 45 mg/m^2/day IV, days 1 through 3
Vincristine 2 mg (dose is not in mg/m^2) IV weekly, on days 1, 8, 15, and 22
Prednisone 60 mg/m^2/day IV or PO, days 1 through 21
Asparaginase 6,000 units/m^2/dose subcutaneously for 6 doses, on days 5, 8, 11, 15, 18, and 22

Patients older than 60 years of age:
Cyclophosphamide 800 mg/m^2 IV, day 1
Daunorubicin 30 mg/m^2/day IV, days 1 through 3
Vincristine 2 mg (dose is not in mg/m^2) IV weekly, on days 1, 8, 15, and 22
Prednisone 60 mg/m^2/day IV or PO, days 1 through 7
Asparaginase 6,000 units/m^2/dose subcutaneously for 6 doses, on days 5, 8, 11, 15, 18, and 22

Early intensification. *Cycle*: 28 days. Give 2 cycles.
Methotrexate 15 mg intrathecally, day 1
Cyclophosphamide 1,000 mg/m^2 IV, day 1
Mercaptopurine 60 mg/m^2/day PO, days 1 through 14
Cytarabine 75 mg/m^2/day subcutaneously, days 1 through 4 and days 8 through 11
Vincristine 2 mg (dose is not in mg/m^2) IV, days 15 and 22
Asparaginase 6,000 units/m^2/dose subcutaneously for 4 doses, days 15, 18, 22, and 25

CNS prophylaxis and interim maintenance. *Cycle*: 84 days. Give a single cycle.
Methotrexate 15 mg intrathecally, weekly for 5 weeks, on days 1, 8, 15, 22, and 29
Methotrexate 20 mg/m^2/dose PO, days 36, 43, 50, 57, and 64
Mercaptopurine 60 mg/m^2/day PO, days 1 through 70
used in conjunction with
Cranial irradiation
*used in conjunction with antimicrobial prophylaxis**
Cotrimoxazole (either 80/400 or 160/800 strength) 1 tablet PO daily, throughout entire course
or
Pentamidine 300 mg inhaled once monthly, throughout entire course

Late intensification. *Cycle*: 56 days. Give a single cycle.
Doxorubicin 30 mg/m^2/dose IV, days 1, 8, and 15
Vincristine 2 mg (dose is not in mg/m^2) IV, days 1, 8, and 15
Dexamethasone 10 mg/m^2/day PO, days 1 through 14
Cyclophosphamide 1,000 mg/m^2 IV, day 29
Thioguanine 60 mg/m^2/day PO, days 29 through 42
Cytarabine 75 mg/m^2/dose subcutaneously, days 29 through 32 and days 36 through 39
*used in conjunction with antimicrobial prophylaxis**
Cotrimoxazole (either 80/400 or 160/800 strength) 1 tablet PO daily, throughout entire course
or
Pentamidine 300 mg inhaled once monthly, throughout entire course

Prolonged maintenance. *Cycle*: 28 days, continue until 24 months after diagnosis
Vincristine 2 mg (dose is not in mg/m^2) IV, day 1
Prednisone 60 mg/m^2/day PO, days 1 through 5
Methotrexate 20 mg/m^2/dose PO weekly, on days 1, 8, 15, and 22, of first cycle only
Mercaptopurine 60 mg/m^2/day PO, days 1 through 28, of first cycle only
*used in conjunction with antimicrobial prophylaxis**
Cotrimoxazole (either 80/400 or 160/800 strength) 1 tablet PO daily, throughout entire course
or
Pentamidine 300 mg inhaled once monthly, throughout entire course

*Note: Antimicrobial prophylaxis doses not specified in original articles; the dose given here is derived from the *Infectious Diseases Handbook,* 6th ed., a tertiary resource.

Larson Regimen (CAL-G, CALGB 9111)

Use: Acute lymphocytic leukemia (ALL—adults)

Regimen: **Remission induction.** *Cycle:* 28 days. Give a single cycle.

Patients 60 years of age and younger:
Cyclophosphamide 1,200 mg/m^2 IV, day 1
Daunorubicin 45 mg/m^2/day IV, days 1 through 3
Vincristine 2 mg (dose is not in mg/m^2) IV weekly, on days 1, 8, 15, and 22
Prednisone 60 mg/m^2/day IV or PO, days 1 through 21
Asparaginase 6,000 units/m^2/dose subcutaneously for 6 doses, days 5, 8, 11, 15, 18, and 22
Filgrastim 5 mcg/kg/day subcutaneously, from day 4 until the absolute neutrophil count (ANC) is greater than 1,000 cells/mm^3 for 2 consecutive days

Patients older than 60 years of age:
Cyclophosphamide 800 mg/m^2 IV, day 1
Daunorubicin 30 mg/m^2/day IV, days 1 through 3
Vincristine 2 mg (dose is not in mg/m^2) IV weekly, on days 1, 8, 15, and 22
Prednisone 60 mg/m^2/day PO, days 1 through 7
Asparaginase 6,000 units/m^2/dose subcutaneously for 6 doses, days 5, 8, 11, 15, 18, and 22
Filgrastim 5 mcg/kg/day subcutaneously, from day 4, continued for at least 7 days and until the ANC is greater than 1,000 cells/mm^3 for 2 consecutive days

Early intensification. *Cycle:* 28 days. Give 2 cycles.
Methotrexate 15 mg intrathecally, day 1
Cyclophosphamide 1,000 mg/m^2 IV, day 1
Mercaptopurine 60 mg/m^2/day PO, days 1 through 14
Cytarabine 75 mg/m^2/day subcutaneously, days 1 through 4 and days 8 through 11
Vincristine 2 mg (dose is not in mg/m^2) IV, days 15 and 22
Asparaginase 6,000 units/m^2/dose subcutaneously for 4 doses, days 15, 18, 22, and 25
Filgrastim 5 mcg/kg/day subcutaneously, from day 2, continued for at least 14 days and until the ANC is at least 5,000 cells/mm^3 for 2 consecutive days

CNS prophylaxis and interim maintenance. *Cycle:* 84 days. Give a single cycle.
Methotrexate 15 mg intrathecally, weekly for 5 weeks, on days 1, 8, 15, 22, and 29
Methotrexate 20 mg/m^2/dose PO, days 36, 43, 50, 57, and 64
Mercaptopurine 60 mg/m^2/day PO, days 1 through 70
used in conjunction with
Cranial irradiation
*used in conjunction with antimicrobial prophylaxis**
Cotrimoxazole (either 80/400 or 160/800 strength) 1 tablet PO daily, throughout entire course
or
Pentamidine 300 mg inhaled once monthly, throughout entire course

Late intensification. *Cycle:* 56 days. Give a single cycle.
Doxorubicin 30 mg/m^2/dose IV, days 1, 8, and 15
Vincristine 2 mg (dose is not in mg/m^2) IV, days 1, 8, and 15
Dexamethasone 10 mg/m^2/day PO, days 1 through 14
Cyclophosphamide 1,000 mg/m^2 IV, day 29
Thioguanine 60 mg/m^2/day PO, days 29 through 42
Cytarabine 75 mg/m^2/dose subcutaneously, days 29 through 32 and days 36 through 39
*used in conjunction with antimicrobial prophylaxis**
Cotrimoxazole (either 80/400 or 160/800 strength) 1 tablet PO daily, throughout entire course
or
Pentamidine 300 mg inhaled once monthly, throughout entire course

Prolonged maintenance. *Cycle:* 28 days, continue until 24 months after diagnosis.
Vincristine 2 mg (dose is not in mg/m^2) IV, day 1
Prednisone 60 mg/m^2/day PO, days 1 through 5
Methotrexate 20 mg/m^2/dose PO weekly, on days 1, 8, 15, and 22, of first cycle only
Mercaptopurine 60 mg/m^2/day PO, days 1 through 28, of first cycle only
*used in conjunction with antimicrobial prophylaxis**
Cotrimoxazole (either 80/400 or 160/800 strength) 1 tablet PO daily, throughout entire course
or
Pentamidine 300 mg inhaled once monthly, throughout entire course

*Note: Antimicrobial prophylaxis doses not specified in original articles; the dose given here is derived from the *Infectious Diseases Handbook,* 6th ed., a tertiary resource.

Lenalidomide-Dexamethasone

Use: Multiple myeloma.
Cycle: 28 days, continue until disease progression or intolerable toxicity

Regimen 1: Low-dose dexamethasone:
Lenalidomide 25 mg/day PO, days 1 through 21
Dexamethasone 40 mg/dose PO, weekly, on days 1, 8, 15, and 22
used in conjunction with antithrombotic prophylaxis
Aspirin 80 or 325 mg PO once daily, throughout entire course

Regimen 2: High-dose dexamethasone:
Lenalidomide 25 mg/day PO, days 1 through 21
Dexamethasone 40 mg/day PO, days 1 through 4 of all cycles
Dexamethasone 40 mg/day PO, days 9 through 12 and days 17 through 20 of cycles 1 through 4
used in conjunction with antithrombotic prophylaxis
Aspirin 80 or 325 mg PO once daily, throughout entire course

Linker Protocol

Use: Acute lymphocytic leukemia (ALL; induction and consolidation)

Regimen: **Remission induction.** *Cycle*: Give 1 cycle only

Daunorubicin 50 mg/m^2/day IV, days 1 through 3
Vincristine 2 mg (dose is not in mg/m^2) IV, weekly, on days 1, 8, 15, and 22
Prednisone 60 mg/m^2/day PO, days 1 through 28
Asparaginase 6,000 units/m^2/day IM, days 17 through 28
If residual leukemia in marrow on day 14:
Daunorubicin 50 mg/m^2 IV, day 15
If residual leukemia in marrow on day 28:
Daunorubicin 50 mg/m^2/day IV, days 29 and 30
Vincristine 2 mg (dose is not in mg/m^2) IV, days 29 and 36
Prednisone 60 mg/m^2/day PO, days 29 through 42
Asparaginase 6,000 units/m^2/day IM, days 29 through 35

Consolidation therapy. *Cycle*: 28 days

Treatment A (cycles 1, 3, 5, and 7)
Daunorubicin 50 mg/m^2/day IV, days 1 and 2
Vincristine 2 mg (dose is not in mg/m^2) IV, days 1 and 8
Prednisone 60 mg/m^2/day PO, days 1 through 14
Asparaginase 12,000 units/m^2/dose IM 3 times weekly for 6 doses, days 2, 4, 7, 9, 11, and 14
Treatment B (cycles 2, 4, 6, and 8)
Teniposide 165 mg/m^2 IV, days 1, 4, 8, and 11
Cytarabine 300 mg/m^2 IV, days 1, 4, 8, and 11
Treatment C (cycle 9)
Methotrexate 690 mg/m^2 IV over 42 hours, starting on day 1
Leucovorin 15 mg/m^2/dose IV every 6 hours for 12 doses (start at end of methotrexate infusion), days 2 through 5

M-2

Use: Multiple myeloma.
Cycle: 5 weeks, continue until disease progression or intolerable toxicity

Regimen: Vincristine 0.03 mg/kg (2 mg maximum dose) IV, day 1
Carmustine 0.5 mg/kg IV, day 1
Cyclophosphamide 10 mg/kg IV, day 1
Prednisone 1 mg/kg/day PO, days 1 through 7, tapered over next 14 days
with
Melphalan 0.25 mg/kg/day PO, days 1 through 4
or
Melphalan 0.1 mg/kg/day PO, days 1 through 7 or days 1 through 10

m-BACOD (also see M-BACOD)*

Use: Lymphoma (non-Hodgkin).
Cycle: 21 days for at least 4 cycles

Regimen: Bleomycin 4 units/m^2 IV, day 1
Doxorubicin 45 mg/m^2 IV, day 1
Cyclophosphamide 600 mg/m^2 IV, day 1
Vincristine 1 mg/m^2 (2 mg maximum dose) IV, day 1
Dexamethasone 6 mg/m^2/day PO, days 1 through 5
Methotrexate 200 mg/m^2 IV, days 8 and 15
Leucovorin 10 mg/m^2/dose PO every 6 hours for 8 doses, begin 24 hours after each methotrexate dose, days 9 through 10 and days 16 through 17
Sargramostim 5 mcg/kg/day subcutaneously, days 4 through 13
used in conjunction with
Intrathecal chemotherapy
*Note: m-BACOD and M-BACOD differ in the dose and timing of the methotrexate dose. Leucovorin dose not specified in original articles; the dose given here is derived from *The Chemotherapy Source Book,* 3rd ed., a tertiary resource.

m-BACOD (Reduced Dose)*

Use: Lymphoma (non-Hodgkin) associated with HIV infection.
Cycle: 21 days for at least 4 cycles

Regimen: Bleomycin 4 units/m^2 IV, day 1
Doxorubicin 25 mg/m^2 IV, day 1
Cyclophosphamide 300 mg/m^2 IV, day 1
Vincristine 1.4 mg/m^2 (2 mg maximum dose) IV, day 1
Dexamethasone 3 mg/m^2/day PO, days 1 through 5
Methotrexate 200 mg/m^2 IV, day 15
Sargramostim 5 mcg/kg/day subcutaneously, days 4 through 13 (added during subsequent cycles), for granulocyte count less than 500 cells/mm^3 at any time during the cycle or less than 1,000 cells/mm^3 on day 22 of any chemotherapy cycle
used in conjunction with
Intrathecal chemotherapy
*Note: m-BACOD (reduced dose) has decreased doses of cyclophosphamide and dexamethasone, and decreased number of methotrexate doses compared with m-BACOD.

M-BACOD (also see m-BACOD)*

Use:	Lymphoma (non-Hodgkin). *Cycle:* 21 days
Regimen:	Bleomycin 4 units/m^2 IV, day 1 Doxorubicin 45 mg/m^2 IV, day 1 Cyclophosphamide 600 mg/m^2 IV, day 1 Vincristine 1 mg/m^2 (2 mg maximum dose) IV, day 1 Dexamethasone 6 mg/m^2/day PO, days 1 through 5 Methotrexate 3,000 mg/m^2 IV, day 15 Leucovorin 10 mg/m^2/dose PO every 6 hours for 8 doses, begin 24 hours after each methotrexate dose, days 16 and 17 Sargramostim 5 mcg/kg/day subcutaneously, days 4 through 13 *Note: m-BACOD and M-BACOD differ in the dose and timing of the methotrexate dose. Leucovorin dose not specified in original articles; the dose given here is derived from *The Chemotherapy Source Book*, 3rd ed., a tertiary resource.

M-VAC

Use:	Bladder cancer. *Cycle:* 28 days
Regimen:	Methotrexate 30 mg/m^2 IV, days 1, 15, and 22 Vinblastine 3 mg/m^2 IV, days 2, 15, and 22 Doxorubicin 30 mg/m^2 IV, day 2 Cisplatin 70 mg/m^2 IV, day 2

MAC III

Use:	Gestational trophoblastic neoplasm (high-risk). *Cycle:* 21 days
Regimen:	Methotrexate 1 mg/kg IM, days 1, 3, 5, and 7 Leucovorin 0.1 mg/kg IM, days 2, 4, 6, and 8 (give 24 hours after each methotrexate dose) Dactinomycin 0.012 mg/kg/day IV, days 1 through 5 Cyclophosphamide 3 mg/kg/day IV, days 1 through 5

MACC

Use:	Lung cancer (non-small cell). *Cycle:* 21 days
Regimen:	Methotrexate 30 to 40 mg/m^2 IV, day 1 Doxorubicin 30 to 40 mg/m^2 IV, day 1 (total cumulative dose 550 mg/m^2) Cyclophosphamide 400 mg/m^2 IV, day 1 Lomustine 30 mg/m^2/day PO, day 1

MACOP-B

Use:	Lymphoma (non-Hodgkin). *Cycle:* Give only a single cycle
Regimen:	Methotrexate 400 mg/m^2 IV weekly, weeks 2, 6, and 10 Leucovorin 15 mg/dose PO every 6 hours for 6 doses, begin 24 hours after each methotrexate dose, during weeks 2, 6, and 10 Doxorubicin 50 mg/m^2 IV weekly, weeks 1, 3, 5, 7, 9, and 11 Cyclophosphamide 350 mg/m^2 IV weekly, weeks 1, 3, 5, 7, 9, and 11 Vincristine 1.4 mg/m^2 (2 mg maximum dose) IV weekly, weeks 2, 4, 6, 8, 10, and 12 Prednisone 75 mg/day PO for 12 weeks, tapered over last 2 weeks Bleomycin 10 units/m^2 IV weekly, weeks 4, 8, and 12 *used in conjunction with* Intrathecal chemotherapy *used in conjunction with antimicrobial prophylaxis* Ketoconazole 200 mg/day PO, throughout entire course Cotrimoxazole double-strength (160/800) 2 tablets PO twice daily, throughout entire course

MAID

Use:	Sarcoma (bone, soft tissue). *Cycle:* 21 days, continue until disease progression or intolerable toxicity
Regimen:	Mesna 2,000 mg/m^2/day continuous IV infusion, days 1 through 4* Doxorubicin 15 mg/m^2/day continuous IV infusion, days 1 through 4 Ifosfamide 2,000 mg/m^2/day continuous IV infusion, days 1 through 3* Dacarbazine 250 mg/m^2/day continuous IV infusion, days 1 through 4 *Note: Ifosfamide and mesna may be mixed and administered in the same infusion bag.

MBC

Use:	Head and neck cancer. *Cycle:* 21 days for up to 2 cycles
Regimen:	Methotrexate 40 mg/m^2 IV, days 1 and 14 Bleomycin 10 units/m^2 IM or IV, days 1, 7, and 14 Cisplatin 50 mg/m^2 IV, day 4

MC

Use: Acute myelocytic leukemia (AML; induction—adults).
Cycle: Give a single cycle

Regimen: Mitoxantrone 12 mg/m^2/day IV, days 1 through 3
Cytarabine 100 to 200 mg/m^2/day continuous IV infusion or IV, days 1 through 7

MCF

Use: Gastric cancer.
Cycle: 42 days for up to 4 cycles

Regimen: Mitomycin 7 mg/m^2 (14 mg maximum dose) IV, day 1
Cisplatin 60 mg/m^2 IV, days 1 and 22
Fluorouracil 300 mg/m^2/day continuous IV infusion, days 1 through 180

MCP + Rituximab (R-MCP)

Use: Lymphoma (non-Hodgkin).
Cycle: 28 days for 8 cycles

Regimen: Rituximab 375 mg/m^2 IV, day 1
Mitoxantrone 8 mg/m^2 IV, days 3 through 4
Chlorambucil 3 mg/m^2/dose (9 mg/m^2/day) PO 3 times daily, days 3 through 7
Prednisone 25 mg/m^2/day PO, days 3 through 7*
*Note: Prednisolone is recommended in the European literature. In the United States, prednisone is the preferred corticosteroid. The doses of these 2 corticosteroids are equivalent (ie, prednisone 40 mg PO = prednisolone 40 mg PO).

MF

Use: Breast cancer.
Cycle: 28 days for up to 12 cycles

Regimen: Methotrexate 100 mg/m^2 IV, days 1 and 8
Fluorouracil 600 mg/m^2 IV, days 1 and 8, given 1 hour after methotrexate
Leucovorin 10 mg/m^2/dose IV or PO every 6 hours for 6 doses, starting 24 hours after each methotrexate dose, days 2 through 3 and days 9 through 10

MICE (ICE)

Use: Sarcoma (adults), osteosarcoma (pediatrics), lung cancer.
Cycle: 21 to 28 days

Regimen: Ifosfamide 1,250 to 1,500 mg/m^2/day IV, days 1 through 3
Carboplatin 300 to 635 mg/m^2 IV, once on day 1 or 3
Etoposide 80 to 100 mg/m^2/day IV, days 1 through 3
with
Mesna 1,250 mg/m^2/day IV, days 1 through 3
or
Mesna 20% of ifosfamide dose IV before, then 4 and 8 hours after each ifosfamide infusion, days 1 through 3

MidAC

Use: Acute myelocytic leukemia (AML; consolidation—pediatrics).
Cycle: Give a single cycle

Regimen: Mitoxantrone 10 mg/m^2/day IV, days 1 through 5
Cytarabine 1,000 mg/m^2/dose IV every 12 hours for 6 doses, days 1 through 3
used in conjunction with
Autologous stem cell transplantation

MINE

Use: Lymphoma (non-Hodgkin).
Cycle: 21 days for up to 6 cycles

Regimen: Ifosfamide 1,330 mg/m^2/day IV, days 1 through 3
Mesna 1,330 mg/m^2/day IV, days 1 through 3, given with ifosfamide
Mesna 500 mg/dose PO, 4 hours after ifosfamide, days 1 through 3
Mitoxantrone 8 mg/m^2 IV, day 1
Etoposide 65 mg/m^2/day IV, days 1 through 3

MINE-ESHAP

Use: Lymphoma (non-Hodgkin).
Cycle: 21 days

Regimen: Give MINE for 6 cycles, then give ESHAP for 3 to 6 cycles

mini-BEAM

Use: Lymphoma (Hodgkin).
Cycle: 4 to 6 weeks

Regimen:
Carmustine 60 mg/m^2 IV, day 1
Etoposide 75 mg/m^2/day IV, days 2 through 5
Cytarabine 100 mg/m^2/dose IV every 12 hours for 8 doses, days 2 through 5
Melphalan 30 mg/m^2 IV, day 6

Mitoxantrone-Etoposide-Cytarabine

Use: Acute myelocytic leukemia (AML; consolidation).
Cycle: Give a single cycle.

Regimen:
Cytarabine 75 mg/m^2/dose IV every 12 hours for 10 doses, days 1 through 5
Mitoxantrone 8 mg/m^2/day IV, days 1 through 5
Etoposide 75 mg/m^2/day IV, days 1 through 5

MOBP

Use: Cervical cancer.
Cycle: 6 weeks for up to 2 cycles

Regimen:
Bleomycin 30 units/day continuous IV infusion, days 1 through 4
Vincristine* 0.5 mg/m^2 IV, days 1 and 4
Cisplatin 50 mg/m^2 IV, days 1 and 22
Mitomycin 10 mg/m^2 IV, day 2
*Note: The vincristine dose is not capped in this protocol. Consult the prescriber if there is any question about the intended vincristine dose.

MOP

Use: Brain tumors (pediatrics).
Cycle: 28 days, continue until patient is 2 years of age

Regimen:
Mechlorethamine 6 mg/m^2 IV, days 1 and 8
Vincristine 1.5 mg/m^2 (2 mg maximum dose) IV, days 1 and 8
Procarbazine 100 mg/m^2/day PO, days 1 through 14

MOPP

Use: Lymphoma (Hodgkin—adults).
Cycle: 28 days for up to 6 cycles

Regimen:
Mechlorethamine 6 mg/m^2 IV, days 1 and 8
Vincristine 1.4 mg/m^2 (2 mg maximum dose) IV, days 1 and 8
Procarbazine 100 mg/m^2/day PO, days 1 through 14
Prednisone 40 mg/m^2/day PO, cycles 1 and 4,* days 1 through 14
*Note: Some clinicians give prednisone with every cycle of MOPP. The original clinical trials gave prednisone only with the first and fourth cycles.

Use: Lymphoma (Hodgkin—pediatrics).
Cycle: 28 days for up to 6 cycles

Regimen:
Mechlorethamine 6 mg/m^2 IV, days 1 and 8
Vincristine 1.4 mg/m^2 (2 mg maximum dose) IV, days 1 and 8
Procarbazine 50 mg PO, day 1
Procarbazine 100 mg/m^2/day PO, days 2 through 14
Prednisone 40 mg/m^2/day PO, cycles 1 and 4,* days 1 through 14
*Note: Some clinicians give prednisone with every cycle of MOPP. The original clinical trials gave prednisone only with the first and fourth cycles.

Use: Brain cancer (medulloblastoma).
Cycle: 28 days for up to 12 cycles

Regimen:
Mechlorethamine 3 mg/m^2 IV, days 1 and 8
Vincristine 1.4 mg/m^2 (2 mg maximum dose) IV, days 1 and 8
Prednisone 40 mg/m^2/day PO, days 1 through 10
Procarbazine 50 mg PO, day 1
Procarbazine 100 mg PO, day 2
Procarbazine 100 mg/m^2/day PO, days 3 through 10

MOPP/ABV

Use: Lymphoma (Hodgkin).
Cycle: 28 days for up to 10 cycles

Regimen:
Mechlorethamine 6 mg/m^2 IV, day 1
Vincristine 1.4 mg/m^2 (2 mg maximum dose) IV, day 1
Procarbazine 100 mg/m^2/day PO, days 1 through 7
Prednisone 40 mg/m^2/day PO, days 1 through 14
Doxorubicin 35 mg/m^2 IV, day 8
Bleomycin 10 units/m^2 IV, day 8
Vinblastine 6 mg/m^2 IV, day 8

MOPP/ABVD

Use:	Lymphoma (Hodgkin). *Cycle:* 28 days for up to 12 cycles (6 MOPP cycles and 6 ABVD cycles)
Regimen:	Alternate MOPP and ABVD regimens every month

MP

Use:	Multiple myeloma. *Cycle:* 21 to 28 days, continue for 6 to 12 months
Regimen:	Melphalan 8 mg/m^2/day PO, days 1 through 4 Prednisone 60 mg/m^2/day PO, days 1 through 4
Use:	Multiple myeloma. *Cycle:* 42 days
Regimen:	Melphalan 9 to 10 mg/m^2/day PO, days 1 through 4 Prednisone 60 mg/m^2/day PO, days 1 through 4
Use:	Multiple myeloma. *Cycle:* 42 days for 12 cycles
Regimen:	Melphalan 0.25 mg/kg/day PO, days 1 through 4 Prednisone 2 mg/kg/day PO, days 1 through 4
Use:	Prostate cancer. *Cycle:* 21 days, for up to 10 cycles
Regimen:	Mitoxantrone 12 mg/m^2 IV, day 1 Prednisone 5 mg/dose PO twice daily, throughout entire course

MPL

Use:	Multiple myeloma.
Regimen:	**Induction.** *Cycle:* 28 days for 9 cycles Melphalan 0.18 mg/kg/day PO, days 1 through 4 Prednisone 2 mg/kg/day PO, days 1 through 4 Lenalidomide 10 mg/day PO, days 1 through 21 *used in conjunction with antithrombotic prophylaxis* Aspirin 100 mg/day PO, throughout entire course *used in conjunction with antimicrobial prophylaxis** Ciprofloxacin 500 mg PO twice daily, throughout entire course **Maintenance.** *Cycle:* 28 days, continue until disease progression Lenalidomide 10 mg/day PO, days 1 through 21 *used in conjunction with antithrombotic prophylaxis* Aspirin 100 mg/day PO, throughout entire course *used in conjunction with antimicrobial prophylaxis** Ciprofloxacin 500 mg PO twice daily, throughout entire course *Note: Antimicrobial prophylaxis doses not specified in original article; the dose given here is derived from *AHFS 2009 Drug Information,* a tertiary resource.

MPT

Use:	Multiple myeloma.
Regimen:	**Induction.** *Cycle:* 28 days for 6 cycles Melphalan 4 mg/m^2/day PO, days 1 through 7 Prednisone 40 mg/m^2/day PO, days 1 through 7 Thalidomide 100 mg/day PO, throughout entire course *used in conjunction with antithrombotic prophylaxis* Enoxaparin 40 mg/day subcutaneously, days 1 through 28, cycles 1 through 4 **Maintenance.** *Cycle:* Ongoing, continue until disease progression Thalidomide 100 mg/day PO, throughout entire course
Use:	Multiple myeloma. *Cycle:* 42 days for 12 cycles
Regimen:	Melphalan 0.25 mg/kg/day PO, days 1 through 4 Prednisone 2 mg/kg/day PO, days 1 through 4 Thalidomide 100 to 400 mg/day PO, throughout entire course

MPV + RT + Ara-C

Use: Lymphoma (central nervous system).

Regimen: **Induction.** *Cycle:* 14 days for 5 cycles

Methotrexate 3,500 mg/m^2 IV, day 1
Leucovorin 10 mg IV or PO every 6 hours for 12 doses, starting 24 hours after IV methotrexate dose, days 2 through 4
Vincristine 1.4 mg/m^2 (2.8 mg maximum dose) IV, day 1
Procarbazine 100 mg/m^2/day PO once daily, days 1 through 7, of odd-numbered cycles only (ie, cycles 1, 3, and 5)
Dexamethasone 16 mg/day PO, throughout entire course, then taper off during radiation therapy
Methotrexate 12 mg intrathecal via Ommaya reservoir, day 8
Leucovorin 10 mg IV or PO every 12 hours for 8 doses, starting 24 hours after each intrathecal methotrexate dose, days 9 through 12

followed by 3 to 5 weeks of rest then
Radiation therapy
followed by 3 weeks of rest then
Consolidation. *Cycle:* 28 days for 2 cycles
Cytarabine 3,000 mg/m^2/day IV, days 1 and 2

MPV + RT + Ara-C + Rituximab (R-MPV + RT + Ara-C)

Use: Lymphoma (central nervous system).

Regimen: **Induction.** *Cycle:* 14 days for 5 to 7 cycles

Rituximab 500 mg/m^2 IV, day 1
Methotrexate 3,500 mg/m^2 IV, day 2
Leucovorin 20 to 25 mg IV or PO every 6 hours for at least 12 doses, starting 24 hours after IV methotrexate dose and continued until the methotrexate concentration is below 1×10^{-8} mg/dL (concentration is not in microMol/L); increase dose to 40 mg/dose IV or PO every 4 hours if the methotrexate concentration is greater than 1×10^{-5} mg/dL (concentration is not in microMol/L) 48 hours after the end of the infusion, or greater than 1×10^{-8} mg/dL (concentration is not in microMol/L) 72 hours after the end of the infusion.
Vincristine 1.4 mg/m^2 (2.8 mg maximum dose) IV, day 2
Procarbazine 100 mg/m^2/day PO once daily, days 1 through 7, of odd-numbered cycles only (ie, cycles 1, 3, and 5)
Filgrastim 5 mcg/kg/day subcutaneously for 3 to 5 days each cycle:
- Odd-numbered cycles: start at least 24 hours after last procarbazine dose
- Even-numbered cycles: start at least 96 hours after completion of methotrexate infusion or when methotrexate concentration is less than 1×10^{-8} mg/dL (concentration is not in microMol/L)

Patients with positive CNS cytology receive intrathecal methotrexate during each cycle:
- Methotrexate 12 mg intrathecal via Ommaya reservoir, given once between days 5 and 12

followed by 3 to 5 weeks of rest then
Radiation therapy
followed by 3 weeks of rest then
Consolidation. *Cycle:* 28 days for 2 cycles
Cytarabine 3,000 mg/m^2/day IV (6,000 mg/day maximum dose), days 1 and 2
Filgrastim 5 mcg/kg/day subcutaneously, days 4 through 13 (start at least 48 hours after completion of chemotherapy infusions)

MTX/6-MP

Use: Acute lymphocytic leukemia (ALL; continuation—pediatrics).
Cycle: Ongoing, weeks 25 through 130

Regimen:
Methotrexate 20 mg/m^2 IM weekly
Mercaptopurine 50 mg/m^2/day PO
used in conjunction with
Intrathecal therapy once every 12 weeks

MTX/6-MP/VP

Use: Acute lymphocytic leukemia (ALL; continuation—pediatrics).
Cycle: Ongoing, 2 to 3 years

Regimen:
Methotrexate 20 mg/m^2/dose PO weekly
Mercaptopurine 75 mg/m^2/day PO
Vincristine* 1.5 mg/m^2 IV, once monthly
Prednisone 40 mg/m^2/day PO for 5 days each month
*Note: The vincristine dose is not capped in this pediatric protocol. Consult the prescriber if there is any question about the intended vincristine dose.

MTX + Ara-C + Autologous Stem Cell Transplantation + Radiation Therapy

Use: Lymphoma (central nervous system).
Cycle: Give a single cycle.

Regimen:
Methotrexate 8,000 mg/m^2 IV, days 1, 10, and 20
Leucovorin 15 mg/m^2/dose IV or PO every 6 hours for at least 10 doses, starting 24 hours after each methotrexate infusion finished and continued until methotrexate concentration is less than 0.1 microMol/L
Cytarabine 3,000 mg/m^2/day IV, days 30 and 31
Thiotepa 40 mg/m^2 IV, day 31
Filgrastim 300 mcg/day (patients weighing less than 75 kg) to 480 mcg/day (patients weighing 75 kg or more) subcutaneously, days 35 through 40
Carmustine 400 mg/m^2 IV, day 50
Thiotepa 5 mg/kg IV, days 51 and 52
Autologous stem cell transplantation, day 56
Radiation therapy, starting on day 90

MTX-CDDPAdr

Use: Osteosarcoma (pediatrics).
Cycle: 28 days for 2 to 4 cycles

Regimen: Methotrexate 12,000 mg/m^2 IV, days 1 and 8
Leucovorin 20 mg/m^2/dose IV every 3 hours for 8 doses, then give PO every 6 hours for 8 doses (begin 16 hours after end of each methotrexate infusion), days 2 through 5 and days 9 through 12
Cisplatin 75 mg/m^2 IV, day 15 of cycles 1 through 7
Doxorubicin 25 mg/m^2/day IV, days 15 through 17 of cycles 1 through 7
Cisplatin 120 mg/m^2 IV, day 15 of cycles 8 through 10

MV

Use: Breast cancer.
Cycle: 6 to 8 weeks

Regimen: Mitomycin 20 mg/m^2 IV, day 1
Vinblastine 0.15 mg/kg IV, days 1 and 21

Use: Acute myelocytic leukemia (AML; induction).
Cycle: Give 1 cycle. Second cycle may be considered if complete response not achieved (eg, persistent blasts present on day 21).

Regimen: Mitoxantrone 10 mg/m^2/day IV, days 1 through 5
Etoposide 100 mg/m^2/day IV, days 1 through 5

MVP

Use: Lung cancer (non-small cell).
Cycle: 6 weeks for up to 6 cycles

Regimen: Mitomycin 8 mg/m^2 IV, day 1
Vinblastine 6 mg/m^2 IV, days 1 and 22
Cisplatin 50 mg/m^2 IV, days 1 and 22

MVPP

Use: Lymphoma (Hodgkin).
Cycle: 6 weeks for 6 to 8 cycles

Regimen: Mechlorethamine 6 mg/m^2 (10 mg maximum dose) IV, days 1 and 8
Vinblastine 4 to 6 mg/m^2 (10 mg maximum dose) IV, days 1 and 8
Procarbazine 100 mg/m^2/day (150 mg maximum dose) PO, days 1 through 14
Prednisone 40 mg/m^2/day (50 mg maximum dose) PO, cycles 1 and 4,* days 1 through 14
*Note: Some clinicians give prednisone with every cycle of MVPP. The original clinical trials gave prednisone only with the first and fourth cycles. Prednisolone is recommended in the British literature. In the United States, prednisone is the preferred corticosteroid. The doses of these 2 corticosteroids are equivalent (ie, prednisone 40 mg PO = prednisolone 40 mg PO).

NA—see Vinorelbine-Doxorubicin

NFL

Use: Breast cancer.
Cycle: 21 days for 6 to 8 cycles

Regimen: Mitoxantrone 12 mg/m^2 IV, day 1
Leucovorin 300 mg/day IV, days 1 through 3
Fluorouracil 350 mg/m^2/day IV, days 1 through 3 after leucovorin

Use: Breast cancer.
Cycle: 21 days for at least 2 cycles

Regimen: Mitoxantrone 10 mg/m^2 IV, day 1
Leucovorin 100 mg/m^2/day IV, days 1 through 3, give before fluorouracil on day 1
Fluorouracil 1,000 mg/m^2/day continuous IV infusion, days 1 through 3

NOVP

Use: Lymphoma (Hodgkin).
Cycle: 21 days for up to 3 cycles

Regimen: Mitoxantrone 10 mg/m^2 IV, day 1
Vinblastine 6 mg/m^2 IV, day 1
Prednisone 100 mg/day PO, days 1 through 5
Vincristine 1.4 mg/m^2 (2 mg maximum dose) IV, day 8

OFAR

Use: Chronic lymphocytic leukemia (CLL).
Cycle: 28 days for up to 6 cycles

Regimen:
Oxaliplatin 25 mg/m^2/day IV, days 1 through 4
Fludarabine 30 mg/m^2/day IV, days 2 and 3 (give after oxaliplatin)
Cytarabine 1,000 mg/m^2/day IV, days 2 and 3 (give after fludarabine)
Rituximab 375 mg/m^2 IV, day 1, except for first cycle
Rituximab 375 mg/m^2 IV, day 3 of first cycle only
Pegfilgrastim 6 mg subcutaneously, day 6
*used in conjunction with antimicrobial prophylaxis**
Cotrimoxazole (either 80/400 or 160/800 strength) 1 tablet PO daily, throughout entire course
or
Pentamidine 300 mg inhaled once monthly, throughout entire course
plus
Valacyclovir 500 mg/day PO, throughout entire course
or
Acyclovir 200 mg PO 3 times daily, throughout entire course
or
Acyclovir 400 mg PO twice daily, throughout entire course

*Note: Antimicrobial prophylaxis doses not specified in original article; the doses given here are derived from the *Infectious Diseases Handbook*, 6th ed., and the *AHFS 2009 Drug Information*, both tertiary resources.

OFF

Use: Pancreatic cancer.
Cycle: 42 days

Regimen:
Leucovorin 200 mg/m^2 IV, weekly for 4 weeks, followed by 2 weeks of rest; administer on days 1, 8, 15, and 22
Fluorouracil 2,000 mg/m^2/day continuous IV infusion, weekly for 4 weeks, followed by 2 weeks of rest; administer on days 1, 8, 15, and 22
Oxaliplatin 85 mg/m^2 IV, days 8 and 22

OPA

Use: Lymphoma (Hodgkin—pediatrics).
Cycle: 15 days for up to 2 cycles. Time between cycles not specified.

Regimen:
Vincristine 1.5 mg/m^2 (2 mg maximum dose) IV, days 1, 8, and 15
Prednisone 20 mg/m^2/dose PO 3 times daily, days 1 through 15
Doxorubicin 40 mg/m^2 IV, days 1 and 15

OPPA

Use: Lymphoma (Hodgkin—pediatrics).
Cycle: 15 days for up to 2 cycles. Time between cycles not specified.

Regimen: **Add to OPA:** Procarbazine 100 mg/m^2/day PO in 2 to 3 divided doses, days 1 through 15

P6

Use: Sarcoma (bone).
Cycle: Repeat for 7 cycles based on hematologic recovery, delay subsequent cycles until neutrophil count is greater than 500 cells/mm^3 post-nadir and platelet count is at least 100,000 cells/mm^3 after cycles 1 through 3 or platelet count is at least 75,000 cells/mm^3 after cycles 4 through 7.

Regimen:
Treatment A (cycles 1, 2, 3, and 6)
Patients younger than 10 years of age:
Cyclophosphamide 70 mg/kg/day IV, days 1 and 2
Mesna 70 mg/kg/day continuous IV infusion, days 1 and 2
Doxorubicin 25 mg/m^2/day continuous IV infusion, days 1 through 3*
Vincristine 0.67 mg/m^2/day (0.67 mg maximum/day, or 2 mg maximum/cycle) continuous IV infusion, days 1 through 3*
Filgrastim 5 mcg/kg/day subcutaneously, from day 5 until hematologic recovery (start at least 24 hours after completion of chemotherapy infusions)
Patients 10 years of age and older:
Cyclophosphamide 2,100 mg/m^2/day IV, days 1 and 2
Mesna 2,100 mg/m^2/day continuous IV infusion, days 1 and 2
Doxorubicin 25 mg/m^2/day continuous IV infusion, days 1 through 3*
Vincristine 0.67 mg/m^2/day (0.67 mg maximum/day, or 2 mg maximum/cycle) continuous IV infusion, days 1 through 3*
Filgrastim 5 mcg/kg/day subcutaneously, from day 5 until hematologic recovery (start at least 24 hours after completion of chemotherapy infusions)

(continued on next page)

P6 (cont.)

Treatment B (cycles 4, 5, and 7)
Ifosfamide 1,800 mg/m²/day IV, days 1 through 5†
Etoposide 100 mg/m²/day IV, days 1 through 5†
with
Mesna 1,800 mg/m²/day IV, days 1 through 5
or
Mesna 20% of ifosfamide dose IV before, then 4 and 8 hours after each ifosfamide infusion, days 1 through 5
plus
Filgrastim 5 mcg/kg/day subcutaneously, from day 6 until hematologic recovery (start at least 24 hours after completion of chemotherapy infusions)

used in conjunction with antimicrobial prophylaxis‡
Cotrimoxazole (either 80/400 or 160/800 strength) 1 tablet PO daily, throughout entire course
or
Pentamidine 300 mg inhaled once monthly, throughout entire course

*Note: Vincristine and doxorubicin may be mixed and administered in the same infusion bag, if diluted with 0.9% Sodium Chloride Injection.

†Note: Ifosfamide and mesna may be mixed and administered in the same infusion bag.

‡Note: Antimicrobial prophylaxis doses not specified in original articles; the dose given here is derived from the *Infectious Diseases Handbook,* 6th ed., a tertiary resource.

PA-CI

Use: Hepatoblastoma (pediatrics).
Cycle: 21 days for up to 4 cycles

Regimen: Cisplatin 90 mg/m² IV, day 1
Doxorubicin 20 mg/m²/day continuous IV infusion, days 2 through 5

PAC

Use: Ovarian cancer, endometrial cancer.
Cycle: 28 days for up to 6 cycles

Regimen: Cisplatin 50 mg/m² IV, day 1
Doxorubicin 50 mg/m² IV, day 1
Cyclophosphamide 500 mg/m² IV, day 1

Use: Thymoma.
Cycle: 21 days for up to 8 cycles

Regimen: Cisplatin 50 mg/m² IV, day 1
Doxorubicin 50 mg/m² IV, day 1
Cyclophosphamide 500 mg/m² IV, day 1

PAC-I (Indiana Protocol)

Use: Ovarian cancer.
Cycle: 21 days for up to 6 cycles

Regimen: Cisplatin 50 mg/m² IV, day 1 (total cumulative dose 300 mg/m²)
Doxorubicin 50 mg/m² IV, day 1
Cyclophosphamide 750 mg/m² IV, day 1

PACA

Use: Ovarian cancer.
Cycle: 28 days for up to 9 cycles

Regimen: Liposomal doxorubicin 30 mg/m² IV, day 1
Carboplatin IV dose by Calvert equation to AUC 5 mg/mL/min, day 1 (give after liposomal doxorubicin)

Use: Endometrial cancer.
Cycle: 28 days for up to 6 cycles

Regimen: Carboplatin IV dose by Calvert equation to AUC 5 mg/mL/min, day 1
Liposomal doxorubicin 40 mg/m² IV, day 1 (give after carboplatin)

Paclitaxel-Bevacizumab

Use: Breast cancer.
Cycle: 28 days, continue until disease progression or intolerable toxicity

Regimen: Paclitaxel 90 mg/m² IV (infusion duration not specified), days 1, 8, and 15
Bevacizumab 10 mg/kg IV, days 1 and 15

Paclitaxel-Carboplatin (also see Carbo-Tax; also see CaT; also see CT; also see PC)

Use: Endometrial cancer.
Cycle: 28 days for up to 6 cycles

Regimen: Paclitaxel 175 mg/m² IV over 3 hours, day 1
Carboplatin IV dose by Calvert equation to AUC 5 to 7 mg/mL/min, day 1 (give after paclitaxel)

(continued on next page)

Paclitaxel-Carboplatin (also see Carbo-Tax; also see CaT; also see CT; also see PC) (cont.)

Use: Head and neck cancer.
Cycle: 28 days

Regimen: Paclitaxel 200 mg/m^2 IV over 3 hours, day 1
Carboplatin IV dose by Calvert equation to AUC 7 mg/mL/min, day 1 (give after paclitaxel)
Filgrastim 5 mcg/kg/day subcutaneously, days 2 through 12

Paclitaxel-Carboplatin-Bevacizumab

Use: Lung cancer (non-small cell).
Cycle: 21 days for up to 6 cycles

Regimen: Paclitaxel 200 mg/m^2 IV over 3 hours, day 1
Carboplatin IV dose by Calvert equation to AUC 6 mg/mL/min, day 1 (give after paclitaxel)
Bevacizumab 15 mg/kg IV, day 1
followed by
Bevacizumab 15 mg/kg IV, every 3 weeks until disease progression or intolerable toxicity

Paclitaxel-Carboplatin-Etoposide

Use: Adenocarcinoma (unknown primary), lung cancer (small cell).
Cycle: 21 days for up to 4 cycles

Regimen: Paclitaxel 200 mg/m^2 IV over 1 hour, day 1
Carboplatin IV dose by Calvert equation to AUC 6 mg/mL/min, day 1 (give after paclitaxel)
Etoposide 50 mg/day PO alternated with 100 mg/day PO, days 1 through 10

Paclitaxel-Carboplatin-Fluorouracil

Use: Esophageal cancer.
Cycle: 21 days for 2 cycles prior to surgery

Regimen: Paclitaxel 200 mg/m^2 IV over 1 hour, day 1
Carboplatin IV dose by Calvert equation to AUC 6 mg/mL/min, day 1 (administration sequence not specified)
Fluorouracil 225 mg/m^2/day continuous IV infusion, days 1 through 21
used in conjunction with
Radiation therapy

Paclitaxel-Carboplatin + Sequential Radiation

Use: Lung cancer (non-small cell).
Cycle: 21 days for 2 cycles

Regimen: Paclitaxel 200 mg/m^2 IV over 3 hours, day 1
Carboplatin IV dose by Calvert equation to AUC 6 mg/mL/min, day 1 (give after paclitaxel)
followed by
Radiation therapy

Paclitaxel-Cetuximab

Use: Head and neck cancer.
Cycle: 21 days, continue until disease progression or intolerable toxicity

Regimen: Paclitaxel 80 mg/m^2 IV (infusion duration not specified), weekly, days 1, 8, and 15
Cetuximab 400 mg/m^2 IV, day 1 of first cycle only (loading dose)
Cetuximab 250 mg/m^2 IV weekly, days 1, 8, and 15, except for day 1 of first cycle

Paclitaxel-Gemcitabine

Use: Testicular cancer, germ cell tumors.
Cycle: 28 days for up to 6 cycles

Regimen: Paclitaxel 100 to 110 mg/m^2 IV over 1 hour, days 1, 8, and 15
Gemcitabine 1,000 mg/m^2 IV, days 1, 8, and 15 (give after paclitaxel)

Paclitaxel-Herceptin

Use: Breast cancer.
Cycle: 7 days, continue until death or intolerable toxicity

Regimen: Trastuzumab 4 mg/kg IV, day 1 of first cycle only (loading dose); then trastuzumab 2 mg/kg IV, day 1 of subsequent cycles
Paclitaxel 70 to 90 mg/m^2 IV over 1 hour, day 1 (give after trastuzumab)

Paclitaxel + Herceptin ➡ FEC + Herceptin, Sequential

Use: Breast cancer.

Cycle: 21 days. Give 4 cycles of Paclitaxel + Herceptin, followed by 4 cycles of FEC + Herceptin, for a total of 24 weeks of trastuzumab throughout the protocol.

Regimen: **Paclitaxel + Herceptin** (cycles 1 through 4)

Trastuzumab 4 mg/kg IV, day 1 of first cycle only (loading dose)
Trastuzumab 2 mg/kg IV weekly, on days 1, 8, 15, and 22, except for day 1 of first cycle
Paclitaxel 225 mg/m²/day continuous IV infusion over 24 hours, day 1, except for first cycle (give after trastuzumab)
Paclitaxel 225 mg/m²/day continuous IV infusion over 24 hours, day 2, of first cycle only (give after trastuzumab)

followed immediately by

FEC + Herceptin (cycles 5 through 8)

Trastuzumab 2 mg/kg IV weekly, on days 1, 8, 15, and 22
Fluorouracil 500 mg/m² IV, days 1 and 4
Epirubicin 75 mg/m² IV, day 1
Cyclophosphamide 500 mg/m² IV, day 1

Paclitaxel-Vinorelbine

Use: Breast cancer.

Cycle: 28 days, continue until disease progression or intolerable toxicity

Regimen: Vinorelbine 30 mg/m² IV, days 1 and 8
Paclitaxel 135 mg/m² IV over 3 hours, day 1 (give after vinorelbine infusion)

Use: Lung cancer (non-small cell).

Cycle: 14 days for 9 cycles

Regimen: Paclitaxel 135 mg/m² IV over 3 hours, day 1
Vinorelbine 25 mg/m² IV, day 1

PAD

Use: Multiple myeloma.

Cycle: 21 days for 4 cycles

Regimen: Bortezomib 1.3 mg/m² IV, days 1, 4, 8, and 11
Doxorubicin 4.5 or 9 mg/m²/day continuous IV infusion, days 1 through 4
Dexamethasone 40 mg/day PO, days 1 through 4 of all cycles
Dexamethasone 40 mg/day PO, days 8 through 11 and days 15 through 18 of first cycle only

used in conjunction with

Autologous stem cell transplantation

PBF

Use: Head and neck cancer (nasopharyngeal).

Cycle: 28 days for 3 cycles

Regimen: Cisplatin 100 mg/m² IV, day 1
Fluorouracil 650 mg/m²/day continuous IV infusion, days 1 through 5
Bleomycin 15 mg IV, day 1
Bleomycin 16 mg/m²/day continuous IV infusion, days 1 through 5 (start after bleomycin bolus on day 1)

PC (also see Carbo-Tax; also see CaT; also see CT; also see Paclitaxel-Carboplatin)

Use: Lung cancer (non-small cell).

Cycle: 21 days for 6 cycles

Regimen: Paclitaxel 135 mg/m²/day continuous IV infusion over 24 hours, day 1
Carboplatin IV dose by Calvert equation to AUC 7.5 mg/mL/min, day 2 (give after paclitaxel)
Filgrastim 5 mcg/kg/day subcutaneously (rounded to 300 or 480 mcg), days 3 through 17, of cycles 2 through 6

Use: Lung cancer (non-small cell).

Cycle: 21 days for 4 to 6 cycles

Regimen: Paclitaxel 175 mg/m² IV over 3 hours, day 1
Cisplatin 70 to 80 mg/m² IV, day 1 (give after paclitaxel)

Use: Head and neck cancer.

Cycle: 21 days for at least 6 cycles

Regimen: Paclitaxel 175 mg/m² IV over 3 hours, day 1
Cisplatin 75 mg/m² IV, day 1 (sequence of administration not specified)

Use: Endometrial cancer.

Cycle: 21 days for up to 6 cycles

Regimen: Paclitaxel 175 mg/m² IV over 3 hours, day 1
Cisplatin 75 mg/m² IV, day 1 (give after paclitaxel)
Filgrastim 5 mcg/kg/day subcutaneously (rounded to 300 or 480 mcg), from day 5 until the white blood cell count (WBC) exceeds 10,000 cells/mm³

(continued on next page)

PC (also see Carbo-Tax; also see CaT; also see CT; also see Paclitaxel-Carboplatin) (cont.)

Use: Bladder cancer, esophageal cancer.
Cycle: 21 days for up to 8 cycles, or until disease progression or intolerable toxicity

Regimen: Paclitaxel 200 or 225 mg/m^2 IV over 3 hours, day 1
Carboplatin IV dose by Calvert equation to AUC 5 to 6 mg/mL/min, day 1 (give after paclitaxel)

Use: Cervical cancer.
Cycle: 28 days for 6 to 9 cycles

Regimen 1: Patients without prior pelvic radiation therapy:
Paclitaxel 175 mg/m^2 IV over 3 hours, day 1
Carboplatin IV dose by Calvert equation to AUC 5 to 6 mg/mL/min, day 1 (give after paclitaxel)

Regimen 2: Patients with prior pelvic radiation therapy:
Paclitaxel 155 mg/m^2 IV over 3 hours, day 1
Carboplatin IV dose by Calvert equation to AUC 5 to 6 mg/mL/min, day 1 (give after paclitaxel)

PCG (also see GCP)

Use: Bladder cancer.
Cycle: 21 days

Regimen: Paclitaxel 200 mg/m^2 IV over 3 hours, day 1
Carboplatin IV dose by Calvert equation to AUC 5 mg/mL/min, day 1 (give after paclitaxel)
Gemcitabine 800 mg/m^2 IV, days 1 and 8 (give after carboplatin)

Use: Bladder cancer.
Cycle: 21 days for up to 6 cycles

Regimen: Paclitaxel 80 mg/m^2 IV over 1 hour, days 1 and 8
Cisplatin 70 mg/m^2 IV, day 1 (give after paclitaxel)
Gemcitabine 1,000 mg/m^2 IV, days 1 and 8 (give after cisplatin)

Use: Lung cancer (non-small cell).
Cycle: 21 days for at least 6 cycles

Regimen: Paclitaxel 200 mg/m^2/day IV over 3 hours, day 1
Carboplatin IV dose by Calvert equation to AUC 6 mg/mL/min, day 1 (give after paclitaxel)
Gemcitabine 1,000 mg/m^2 IV, days 1 and 8 (give after carboplatin)

PCR

Use: Chronic lymphocytic leukemia (CLL).
Cycle: 21 days for 6 cycles

Regimen: Pentostatin 2 mg/m^2 IV, day 1
Cyclophosphamide 600 mg/m^2 IV, day 1
Rituximab 100 mg/m^2 IV, day 1 of first cycle only
Rituximab 375 mg/m^2 IV, days 3 and 5 of first cycle only (loading dose)
Rituximab 375 mg/m^2 IV, day 1, except for first cycle
Filgrastim 5 mcg/kg/day subcutaneously, days 3 through 12 or until absolute neutrophil count (ANC) is greater than 1,000 cells/mm^3 for 2 consecutive days

*used in conjunction with antimicrobial prophylaxis**
Cotrimoxazole (either 80/400 or 160/800 strength) 1 tablet PO daily, days 1 through 365
plus
Acyclovir 200 mg PO 3 times daily, days 1 through 365
or
Acyclovir 400 mg PO twice daily, days 1 through 365

*Note: Antimicrobial prophylaxis doses not specified in original article; the doses given here are derived from *Infectious Diseases Handbook*, 6th ed., and *AHFS 2008 Drug Information*, both tertiary resources.

Use: Chronic lymphocytic leukemia (CLL).
Cycle: 21 days for 6 cycles

Regimen: Cyclophosphamide 600 mg/m^2 IV, day 1
Pentostatin 4 mg/m^2 IV, day 1 (give after cyclophosphamide)
Rituximab 375 mg/m^2 IV, day 1, except for first cycle (give after pentostatin)
Filgrastim 300 mcg/day (patients weighing less than 70 kg) to 480 mcg/day (patients weighing 70 kg or more) subcutaneously, starting on day 3 and continued until the absolute neutrophil count (ANC) is greater than 1,500 cells/mm^3 for 2 consecutive days or greater than 5,000 cells/mm^3

used in conjunction with antimicrobial prophylaxis
Cotrimoxazole double-strength (160/800) 1 tablet PO twice daily, given 3 times weekly (eg, Monday, Wednesday, Friday), throughout entire course
Acyclovir 800 mg PO twice daily, throughout entire course

PCV

Use: Brain tumor.
Cycle: 6 to 8 weeks, continue for 1 year or until disease progression

Regimen: Lomustine 110 mg/m^2 PO, day 1
Procarbazine 60 mg/m^2/day PO, days 8 through 21
Vincristine 1.4 mg/m^2 (2 mg maximum dose) IV, days 8 and 29

(continued on next page)

PCV (cont.)

Use: Brain tumor.
Cycle: 6 weeks for up to 12 cycles

Regimen: Procarbazine 100 mg/m^2/day PO, days 1 through 10
Lomustine 100 mg/m^2 PO, day 1
Vincristine 1.5 mg/m^2 (2 mg maximum dose) IV, day 1

Use: Advanced brain tumor.
Cycle: 8 weeks for up to 6 cycles

Regimen: Lomustine 130 mg/m^2 PO, day 1
Procarbazine 75 mg/m^2/day PO, days 8 through 21
Vincristine* 1.4 mg/m^2 IV, days 8 and 29
*Note: The vincristine is not capped in this protocol. Consult the prescriber if there is any question about the intended vincristine dose.

PE

Use: Prostate cancer.
Cycle: 21 days, continue until disease progression or intolerable toxicity

Regimen: Estramustine 600 mg/m^2/day PO given in 2 to 3 divided doses throughout entire course (start 24 hours before first paclitaxel infusion)
Paclitaxel 30 mg/m^2/day continuous IV infusion over 24 hours, days 1 through 4

Use: Prostate cancer.
Cycle: 28 days, continue until disease progression or intolerable toxicity. Delay each subsequent cycle until absolute neutrophil count (ANC) is at least 1,200 cells/mm^3 and platelet count is at least 75,000 cells/mm^3.

Regimen: Estramustine 140 mg/dose (420 mg/day) PO 3 times daily, days 1 through 3 (start 24 hours before first paclitaxel infusion); decrease to 140 mg/dose (280 mg/day) PO twice daily, days 1 through 3 for subsequent cycles if patient experiences significant nonhematologic toxicity
Paclitaxel 90 mg/m^2 IV over 1 hour, days 2, 9, and 16; decrease to paclitaxel 70 mg/m^2 IV, days 2, 9, and 16 for subsequent cycles if ANC is less than 1,800 cells/mm^3 or platelet count is less than 100,000 cells/mm^3 at start of cycle, or if patient experiences significant nonhematologic toxicity

PEB—see BEP

Pemetrexed-Bevacizumab

Use: Lung cancer (non-small cell).
Cycle: 21 days for up to 52 weeks, or until disease progression or intolerable toxicity

Regimen: Pemetrexed 500 mg/m^2 IV, day 1
Bevacizumab 15 mg/kg IV, day 1
used in conjunction with vitamin B supplementation
Folic acid 0.35 to 1 mg/day PO throughout entire course, starting at least 7 days before first chemotherapy dose and continued for 21 days after the last pemetrexed dose
Cyanocobalamin 1 mg/dose IM every 9 weeks throughout entire course, starting at least 7 days before first chemotherapy dose and continued throughout chemotherapy

Pemetrexed-Carboplatin

Use: Mesothelioma, lung cancer (non-small cell).
Cycle: 21 days for 4 or more cycles

Regimen: Pemetrexed 500 mg/m^2 IV, day 1
Carboplatin IV dose by Calvert equation to AUC 5 mg/mL/min, day 1 (give after pemetrexed)
used in conjunction with vitamin B supplementation
Folic acid 0.35 to 1 mg/day PO throughout entire course, starting 7 to 14 days before first chemotherapy dose and continued for 21 days after the last pemetrexed dose
Cyanocobalamin 1 mg/dose IM every 9 weeks throughout entire course, starting 7 to 14 days before first chemotherapy dose and continued throughout chemotherapy

Pemetrexed-Cisplatin

Use: Mesothelioma, lung cancer (non-small cell).
Cycle: 21 days

Regimen: Pemetrexed 500 mg/m^2 IV, day 1
Cisplatin 75 mg/m^2 IV, day 1 (give after pemetrexed)
used in conjunction with vitamin B supplementation
Folic acid 0.35 to 1 mg/day PO throughout entire course, starting 7 to 21 days before first chemotherapy dose and continued for 21 days after the last pemetrexed dose
Cyanocobalamin 1 mg/dose IM every 9 weeks, starting 7 to 21 days before first chemotherapy dose and continued throughout entire chemotherapy course

Pemetrexed-Gemcitabine

Use: Mesothelioma.
Cycle: 21 days for up to 6 cycles, or until disease progression

Regimen: Pemetrexed 500 mg/m^2 IV, day 8 (give before gemcitabine)
Gemcitabine 1,250 mg/m^2 IV, days 1 and 8
used in conjunction with vitamin B supplementation
Folic acid 0.35 to 1 mg/day PO throughout entire course, starting at least 7 days before first chemotherapy dose and continued for 21 days after the last pemetrexed dose
Cyanocobalamin 1 mg/dose IM every 9 weeks throughout entire course, starting at least 7 days before first chemotherapy dose and continued throughout chemotherapy

PFL

Use: Head and neck cancer, gastric cancer.
Cycle: 28 days for 2 to 3 cycles

Regimen: Cisplatin 25 mg/m^2/day continuous IV infusion, days 1 through 5
Leucovorin 500 mg/m^2/day continuous IV infusion, days 1 through 6
Fluorouracil 800 mg/m^2/day continuous IV infusion, days 2 through 6

Use: Head and neck cancer, gastric cancer.
Cycle: 21 days, continue until disease progression or intolerable toxicity

Regimen: Cisplatin 100 mg/m^2 IV, day 1
Fluorouracil 600 to 800 mg/m^2/day continuous IV infusion, days 1 through 5
Leucovorin 50 mg/m^2/dose PO every 4 to 6 hours, days 1 through 6

PIAF

Use: Hepatocellular cancer.
Cycle: 21 days for up to 6 cycles

Regimen: Cisplatin 20 mg/m^2/day IV, days 1 through 4
Interferon alfa-2b 5 million units/m^2/day subcutaneously, days 1 through 4
Doxorubicin 40 mg/m^2 IV, day 1
Fluorouracil 400 mg/m^2/day IV, days 1 through 4

PNET-3 Protocol

Use: Brain tumors (pediatrics).
Cycle: 21 days for 4 cycles

Regimen: Alternate cycles ABAB.
Cycle A: Vincristine* 1.5 mg/m^2 IV, days 1, 7, and 14
Etoposide 100 mg/m^2/day IV, days 1 through 3
Carboplatin 500 mg/m^2/day IV, days 1 and 2
Cycle B: Vincristine* 1.5 mg/m^2 IV, days 1, 7, and 14 of first Cycle B (ie, cycle 2), then day 1 of next Cycle B (ie, cycle 4)
Etoposide 100 mg/m^2/day IV, days 1 through 3
Cyclophosphamide 1,500 mg/m^2 IV, day 1
Mesna 750 mg/m^2/dose IV given 15 minutes before, and 4 and 8 hours after cyclophosphamide, day 1
*Note: The vincristine dose is not capped in this protocol. Consult the prescriber if there is any question about the intended vincristine dose.

POC

Use: Brain tumors (pediatrics).
Cycle: 6 weeks for up to 8 cycles

Regimen: Prednisone 40 mg/m^2/day PO, days 1 through 14
Vincristine 1.5 mg/m^2 IV (2 mg maximum dose), days 1, 8, and 15
Lomustine 100 mg/m^2 PO, day 1

ProMACE

Use: Lymphoma (non-Hodgkin).
Cycle: 28 days for up to 6 cycles

Regimen: Prednisone 60 mg/m^2/day PO, days 1 through 14
Doxorubicin 25 mg/m^2 IV, days 1 and 8
Cyclophosphamide 650 mg/m^2 IV, days 1 and 8
Etoposide 120 mg/m^2 IV, days 1 and 8
Methotrexate 750 mg/m^2 IV, day 14
Leucovorin 50 mg/m^2/dose IV every 6 hours for 5 doses, starting on day 15 (start 24 hours after methotrexate)

ProMACE/cytaBOM

Use: Lymphoma (non-Hodgkin).
Cycle: 21 days for at least 6 cycles

Regimen:
Prednisone 60 mg/m²/day PO, days 1 through 14
Doxorubicin 25 mg/m² IV, day 1
Cyclophosphamide 650 mg/m² IV, day 1
Etoposide 120 mg/m² IV, day 1
Cytarabine 300 mg/m² IV, day 8
Bleomycin 5 units/m² IV, day 8
Vincristine 1.4 mg/m² (2 mg maximum dose) IV, day 8
Methotrexate 120 mg/m² IV, day 8
Leucovorin 25 mg/m²/dose PO every 6 hours for 4 doses, starting on day 9 (start 24 hours after methotrexate dose)
Cotrimoxazole double-strength (160/800) 2 tablets PO twice daily, days 1 through 21

ProMACE/MOPP

Use: Lymphoma (non-Hodgkin).
Cycle: 28 days for at least 6 cycles

Regimen:
Prednisone 60 mg/m²/day PO, days 1 through 14
Doxorubicin 25 mg/m² IV, day 1
Cyclophosphamide 650 mg/m² IV, day 1
Etoposide 120 mg/m² IV, day 1
Mechlorethamine 6 mg/m² IV, day 8
Vincristine 1.4 mg/m² (2 mg maximum dose) IV, day 8
Procarbazine 100 mg/m²/day PO, days 8 through 14
Methotrexate 500 mg/m² IV, day 15
Leucovorin 50 mg/m²/dose PO every 6 hours for 4 doses, starting on day 16 (start 24 hours after methotrexate dose)

Pt/VM

Use: Neuroblastoma (pediatrics).
Cycle: 21 to 28 days for up to 5 cycles

Regimen:
Cisplatin 90 mg/m² IV, day 1
Teniposide 100 mg/m² IV, day 3

PVA

Use: Acute lymphocytic leukemia (ALL; induction—pediatrics).
Cycle: 28 days. Give a single cycle.

Regimen:
Prednisone 13.33 mg/m²/dose (40 mg/m²/day, or 60 mg/day maximum dose) PO 3 times daily, days 1 through 28
Vincristine 1.5 mg/m² (2 mg maximum dose) IV weekly, on days 1, 8, 15, and 22
with
Asparaginase 6,000 units/m²/dose IM, 3 times weekly for 6 doses total (eg, days 2, 5, 7, 9, 12, and 14)
or
Asparaginase 6,000 units/m²/dose IM twice weekly for 6 doses total, days 2, 5, 8, 12, 15, and 19
or
Asparaginase 5,000 units/m²/dose IM twice weekly for 6 doses total, days 2, 5, 8, 12, 15, and 18
used in conjunction with
Intrathecal therapy

PVB

Use: Testicular cancer, adenocarcinoma.
Cycle: 21 days for up to 4 cycles

Regimen:
Cisplatin 20 mg/m²/day IV, days 1 through 5
Vinblastine 0.15 mg/kg/day IV, days 1 and 2
Bleomycin 30 units IV, days 2, 9, and 16

PVDA

Use: Acute lymphocytic leukemia (ALL; induction—pediatrics).
Cycle: 28 days. Give a single cycle.

Regimen:
Prednisone 40 mg/m²/day PO, days 1 through 28
Vincristine 1.5 mg/m² (2 mg maximum dose) IV weekly, on days 1, 8, 15, and 22
Daunorubicin 25 mg/m² IV weekly, on days 1, 8, 15, and 22
Asparaginase 10,000 units/m²/dose IM, 3 times weekly for 12 doses, beginning on day 1
used in conjunction with
Intrathecal therapy
Cotrimoxazole 2.5 mg/kg/dose (as trimethoprim) PO twice daily, days 1 through 28

(continued on next page)

PVDA (cont.)

Use: Acute lymphocytic leukemia (ALL; induction—pediatrics).
Cycle: 28 days. Give a single cycle.

Regimen: Prednisone 40 mg/m^2/day PO, days 1 through 28
Vincristine 1.5 mg/m^2 (2 mg maximum dose) IV, days 2, 8, 15, and 22
Daunorubicin 25 mg/m^2 IV, days 2, 8, 15, and 22
Asparaginase 5,000 units/m^2/dose IM twice weekly for 6 doses, days 2, 5, 8, 12, 15, and 19
used in conjunction with
Intrathecal therapy

R-CHOP—see CHOP + Rituximab

R-CHOP-14—see CHOP-14 + Rituximab

R-CHOP + Maintenance Rituximab

Use: Lymphoma (B-cell).
Cycle: See below, cycle length varies throughout protocol. Give 6 cycles of R-CHOP, followed by up to 8 cycles (ie, 24 months) of maintenance rituximab.

Regimen: **R-CHOP.** *Cycle:* 21 days for 6 cycles
Add to CHOP: Rituximab 375 mg/m^2 IV, day 1

Maintenance Rituximab. *Cycle:* 3 months for up to 8 cycles, or until disease progression
Rituximab 375 mg/m^2 IV every 3 months

R-CVP—see CVP + Rituximab

R-FCM—see FCM + Rituximab

R-FCM + Maintenance Rituximab

Use: Lymphoma (non-Hodgkin).
Cycle: See below, cycle length varies throughout protocol. Give 4 cycles of R-FCM, followed by maintenance rituximab.

Regimen: **R-FCM.** *Cycle:* 28 days for 4 cycles
Rituximab 375 mg/m^2 IV, day 1
Fludarabine 25 mg/m^2/day IV, days 2 through 4
Cyclophosphamide 200 mg/m^2/day IV, days 2 through 4
Mitoxantrone 8 mg/m^2 IV, day 2
followed by 3 months of rest then
Maintenance Rituximab. *Cycle:* Give a single cycle.
Rituximab 375 mg/m^2 IV weekly for 4 weeks, followed by 5 months of rest, on days 1, 8, 15, and 22, and days 181, 188, 195, and 202

R-GEMOX—see GEMOX + Rituximab

R-MCP—see MCP + Rituximab

R-MICE—see ICE + Rituximab

RICE—see ICE + Rituximab

Rituximab ➡ R-CHOP

Use: Lymphoma (non-Hodgkin).
Cycle: See below, cycle length varies throughout protocol. Give a single cycle of rituximab, then 3 cycles of R-CHOP, then a single cycle of maintenance rituximab.

Regimen: **Rituximab.** *Cycle:* Give a single cycle (weeks 1 through 4)
Rituximab 375 mg/m^2 IV weekly for 4 weeks
R-CHOP. *Cycle:* 21 days for 3 cycles (weeks 5 through 13)
Add to CHOP: Rituximab 375 mg/m^2 IV, day 1
Maintenance Rituximab. *Cycle:* Give a single cycle (weeks 14 and 15)
Rituximab 375 mg/m^2 IV weekly for 2 weeks

Rituximab ➡ R-CVP

Use: Lymphoma (B-cell).
Cycle: See below, cycle length varies throughout protocol. Give a single cycle of rituximab, then 3 cycles of R-CVP, then a single cycle of maintenance rituximab.

Regimen: **Rituximab.** *Cycle:* Give a single cycle (weeks 1 through 4)
Rituximab 375 mg/m^2 IV weekly for 4 weeks
R-CVP. *Cycle:* 21 days for 3 cycles (weeks 5 through 13)
Cyclophosphamide 1,000 mg/m^2/day IV, day 1
Vincristine 1.4 mg/m^2 (2 mg maximum dose) IV, day 1
Prednisone 100 mg/day PO, days 1 through 5
Rituximab 375 mg/m^2 IV, day 1
Maintenance Rituximab. *Cycle:* Give a single cycle (weeks 14 and 15)
Rituximab 375 mg/m^2 IV weekly for 2 weeks

Rituximab-Bendamustine

Use: Lymphoma (B-cell, mantle cell).
Cycle: 28 days for 4 to 6 cycles

Regimen: Rituximab 375 mg/m^2 IV, day −7 of first cycle only (loading dose, given 7 days before starting other agents)
Rituximab 375 mg/m^2 IV, day 1
Rituximab 375 mg/m^2 IV, day 29 of last cycle only
Bendamustine 90 mg/m^2/day IV, days 2 and 3

Rituximab-Lenalidomide

Use: Lymphoma (mantle cell).
Cycle: 28 days

Regimen: Rituximab 375 mg/m^2 IV weekly, on days 1, 8, 15, and 22
Lenalidomide 20 mg/day PO, days 1 through 21

Use: Chronic lymphocytic leukemia (CLL).
Cycle: 28 days for 6 cycles

Regimen: Rituximab 375 mg/m^2 IV, days 1 and 15
Rituximab 375 mg/m^2 IV, day 8 of first cycle only (loading dose)
Lenalidomide 25 mg/day PO, days 1 through 21

Rituximab-Thalidomide

Use: Lymphoma (mantle cell).
Cycle: Ongoing, continue until disease progression

Regimen: Rituximab 375 mg/m^2 IV weekly for 4 weeks, on days 1, 8, 15, and 22
Thalidomide 200 mg/day PO, days 1 through 14
Thalidomide 400 mg/day PO, throughout entire course, except for days 1 through 14

RTOG 93-10

Use: Lymphoma (central nervous system).
Cycle: Give a single cycle

Regimen: Methotrexate 2,500 mg/m^2/dose IV, days 1, 15, 29, 43, and 57
Leucovorin 20 mg PO every 6 hours for 12 doses, starting 24 hours after each IV methotrexate dose, days 2 through 4, days 16 through 18, days 30 through 32, days 44 through 46, and days 58 through 60
Vincristine 1.4 mg/m^2 (2.8 mg maximum dose) IV, days 1, 15, 29, 43, and 57
Procarbazine 100 mg/m^2/day PO once daily, days 1 through 7, days 29 through 35, and days 57 through 63
Dexamethasone 16 mg/day PO, days 1 through 7; then dexamethasone 12 mg/day PO, days 8 through 14; then dexamethasone 8 mg/day PO, days 15 through 21; then dexamethasone 6 mg/day PO, days 22 through 28; then dexamethasone 4 mg/day PO, days 29 through 35; then dexamethasone 2 mg/day PO, days 36 through 42
Methotrexate 12 mg intrathecal via Ommaya reservoir, days 8, 22, 36, 50, and 64
Leucovorin 10 mg PO twice daily for 8 doses, beginning the evening after each intrathecal methotrexate dose, days 9 through 12, days 23 through 26, days 37 through 40, days 51 through 54, and days 65 through 68
followed by
Radiation therapy
followed by
Cytarabine 3,000 mg/m^2/day IV, days 106, 107, 127, and 128
*used in conjunction with antimicrobial prophylaxis**
Cotrimoxazole (either 80/400 or 160/800 strength) 1 tablet PO daily, throughout entire course
plus
Clotrimazole lozenge 10 mg PO 3 times daily, throughout entire course
*Note: Antimicrobial prophylaxis doses not specified in original article; the doses given here are derived from the *Infectious Diseases Handbook,* 6th ed., and *AHFS 2008 Drug Information,* both tertiary resources.

RTOG 97-04 Chemoradiation Regimen

Use: Pancreatic cancer.
Cycle: See below, cycle length varies throughout protocol. Give 3 cycles of Gemcitabine pre-chemoradiation, followed by concurrent chemoradiation, followed by 3 cycles of Gemcitabine post-chemoradiation.

Regimen: **Gemcitabine Pre-radiation.** *Cycle:* 7 days for 3 cycles
Gemcitabine 1,000 mg/m^2 IV, day 1
followed by 1 to 2 weeks of rest then
Concurrent Chemoradiation. *Cycle:* 6 weeks. Give a single cycle.
Fluorouracil 250 mg/m^2/day continuous IV infusion, throughout entire course until end of radiation therapy
used in conjunction with
Radiation therapy
followed by 3 to 5 weeks of rest then
Gemcitabine Post-radiation. *Cycle:* 28 days for 3 cycles
Gemcitabine 1,000 mg/m^2 IV, weekly for 3 weeks, on days 1, 8, and 15

Sequential AC/Paclitaxel—see AC/Paclitaxel, Sequential

Sequential Dox ➡ CMF—see Dox ➡ CMF, Sequential

SMF

Use: Pancreatic cancer.
Cycle: 8 weeks

Regimen: Streptozocin 1,000 mg/m^2 IV, days 1, 8, 29, and 36
Mitomycin 10 mg/m^2 IV, day 1
Fluorouracil 600 mg/m^2 IV, days 1, 8, 29, and 36

Stanford V

Use: Lymphoma (Hodgkin).
Cycle: 28 days for 3 cycles

Regimen 1: Patients younger than 50 years of age:
Mechlorethamine 6 mg/m^2 IV, day 1
Doxorubicin 25 mg/m^2 IV, days 1 and 15
Vinblastine 6 mg/m^2 IV, days 1 and 15
Prednisone 40 mg/m^2/dose PO, every other day continually for 10 weeks, then taper off by 10 mg every other day for next 14 days
Vincristine 1.4 mg/m^2 (2 mg maximum dose) IV, days 8 and 22
Bleomycin 5 units/m^2 IV, days 8 and 22
Etoposide 60 mg/m^2/day IV, days 15 and 16
used in conjunction with antimicrobial prophylaxis
Cotrimoxazole double-strength (160/800) 1 tablet PO twice daily, throughout entire course
Ketoconazole 200 mg/day PO, throughout entire course
Acyclovir 200 mg PO 3 times daily, throughout entire course

Regimen 2: Patients 50 years of age and older:
Mechlorethamine 6 mg/m^2 IV, day 1
Doxorubicin 25 mg/m^2 IV, days 1 and 15
Vinblastine 6 mg/m^2 IV, days 1 and 15 for cycles 1 and 2 only; then vinblastine 4 mg/m^2 IV, days 1 and 15 for cycle 3
Prednisone 40 mg/m^2/dose PO, every other day continually for 10 weeks, then taper off by 10 mg every other day for next 14 days
Vincristine 1.4 mg/m^2 (2 mg maximum dose) IV, days 8 and 22 for cycles 1 and 2 only; then vincristine 1 mg/m^2 (2 mg maximum dose) IV, days 1 and 15 for cycle 3
Bleomycin 5 units/m^2 IV, days 8 and 22
Etoposide 60 mg/m^2/day IV, days 15 and 16
used in conjunction with antimicrobial prophylaxis
Cotrimoxazole double-strength (160/800) 1 tablet PO twice daily, throughout entire course
Ketoconazole 200 mg/day PO, throughout entire course
Acyclovir 200 mg PO 3 times daily, throughout entire course

TAC

Use: Breast cancer.
Cycle: 21 days for up to 8 cycles

Regimen: Doxorubicin 50 mg/m^2 IV, day 1
Cyclophosphamide 500 mg/m^2 IV, day 1 (give after doxorubicin)
Docetaxel 75 mg/m^2 IV, day 1 (give after cyclophosphamide)
Ciprofloxacin 500 mg PO twice daily, days 5 through 15

TAD

Use: Acute myelocytic leukemia (AML; induction—adults).
Cycle: 21 days for 2 cycles

Regimen: Cytarabine 100 mg/m^2/day continuous IV infusion, days 1 and 2
Cytarabine 100 mg/m^2/dose IV every 12 hours for 12 doses, days 3 through 8
Daunorubicin 60 mg/m^2/day IV, days 3 through 5
Thioguanine 100 mg/m^2/dose PO every 12 hours for 14 doses, days 3 through 9

Tamoxifen-Epirubicin

Use: Breast cancer.
Cycle: 28 days for 6 cycles

Regimen: Tamoxifen 20 mg PO daily, continuously for 4 years
Epirubicin 50 mg/m^2 IV, on days 1 and 8

Tamoxifen-Exemestane

Use: Breast cancer.
Cycle: Ongoing for 5 years

Regimen: Tamoxifen 20 mg PO daily, continuously for 2 to 3 years
followed by
Exemestane 25 mg PO daily, continuously for remainder of 5 years

Tamoxifen-Goserelin

Use:	Breast cancer. *Cycle:* Ongoing for 3 years
Regimen:	Tamoxifen 20 mg PO daily, continuously Goserelin acetate 3.6 mg/dose implant subcutaneously, every 28 days

Tamoxifen-Goserelin-Zoledronic Acid

Use:	Breast cancer. *Cycle:* Ongoing for 3 years
Regimen:	Tamoxifen 20 mg PO daily, continuously Goserelin acetate 3.6 mg/dose implant subcutaneously, every 28 days Zoledronic acid 4 mg IV, every 6 months

Tamoxifen-Letrozole

Use:	Breast cancer. *Cycle:* Ongoing for 10 years
Regimen:	Tamoxifen 20 mg PO daily, continuously for 5 years* *followed by* Letrozole 2.5 mg PO daily, continuously for 5 years *Note: Tamoxifen dose not specified in original articles; the dose given here is derived from *AHFS 2009 Drug Information*, a tertiary resource.

TAP

Use:	Endometrial cancer. *Cycle:* 21 days for up to 7 cycles
Regimen:	Doxorubicin 45 mg/m^2 IV, day 1 Cisplatin 50 mg/m^2 IV, day 1 Paclitaxel 160 mg/m^2 IV over 3 hours, day 2 Filgrastim 5 mcg/kg/day subcutaneously, days 3 through 12

TC (also see Cisplatin-Docetaxel; also see Docetaxel-Cisplatin)

Use:	Gastric cancer. *Cycle:* 21 days for up to 9 cycles, or until disease progression or intolerable toxicity
Regimen:	Docetaxel 75 to 85 mg/m^2 IV, day 1 Cisplatin 75 mg/m^2 IV, day 1 (give after docetaxel)

TCF

Use:	Esophageal cancer. *Cycle:* 28 days
Regimen:	Paclitaxel 175 mg/m^2 IV over 3 hours, day 1 Cisplatin 20 mg/m^2/day IV, days 1 through 5 (give after paclitaxel) for first 3 cycles; decrease to cisplatin 15 mg/m^2/day IV, days 1 through 5 for subsequent cycles Fluorouracil 750 mg/m^2/day continuous IV infusion, days 1 through 5

TCH

Use:	Breast cancer. *Cycle:* 21 days for up to 6 cycles
Regimen:	Docetaxel 75 mg/m^2 IV, day 1 Carboplatin IV dose by Calvert equation to AUC 6 mg/mL/min, day 1 (sequence of administration not specified) Trastuzumab 4 mg/kg IV, day 1 of first cycle only (loading dose) Trastuzumab 2 mg/kg IV, weekly, on days 1, 8, and 15, except for day 1 of first cycle *followed by* Trastuzumab 6 mg/kg IV, every 3 weeks, on day 1 of weeks 19, 22, 25, 28, 31, 34, 37, 40, 43, 46, 49, and 52 (for a total of 52 weeks of trastuzumab throughout protocol)
Use:	Breast cancer. *Cycle:* 28 days, continued until disease progression or intolerable toxicity
Regimen:	Paclitaxel 80 mg/m^2 IV over 1 hour, days 1, 8, and 15 Carboplatin IV dose by Calvert equation to AUC 2 mg/mL/min, days 1, 8, and 15 Trastuzumab 4 mg/kg IV, day 1 of first cycle only (loading dose) Trastuzumab 2 mg/kg IV, weekly, on days 1, 8, 15, and 22, except for day 1 of first cycle

TEC

Use:	Prostate cancer. *Cycle:* 28 days for up to 10 cycles
Regimen:	Estramustine 3.33 mg/kg/dose (10 mg/kg/day or 840 mg/day maximum dose) PO 3 times daily, start 2 days before chemotherapy and continue for 2 days after chemotherapy, 5 days total (days −1 to +3 of each cycle) Paclitaxel 100 mg/m^2 IV over 1 hour weekly, on days 1, 8, 15, and 22 Carboplatin IV dose by Calvert equation to AUC 6 mg/mL/min (1,000 mg maximum dose), day 1

Temozolomide-IFN

Use: Malignant melanoma.
Cycle: 28 days, continued until disease progression or intolerable toxicity

Regimen:
Temozolomide 200 mg/m^2/day PO, days 1 through 5
Interferon alfa-2b 5 million units/m^2/dose subcutaneously 3 times weekly throughout entire course

Temozolomide-IL-2I + GM-CSF

Use: Malignant melanoma.
Cycle: 28 days for up to 8 cycles, or until disease progression or intolerable toxicity

Regimen 1: Patients who have not received prior chemotherapy:
Temozolomide 200 mg/m^2/day PO, days 1 through 5
Aldesleukin 4 million units/m^2/day subcutaneously, days 6 through 17
Interferon alfa-2b 5 million units/m^2/day subcutaneously, days 6 through 17
Sargramostim 125 mcg/m^2/day (250 mcg maximum dose) subcutaneously, days 6 through 17

Regimen 2: Patients who have received prior chemotherapy:
Temozolomide 150 mg/m^2/day PO, days 1 through 5
Aldesleukin 4 million units/m^2/day subcutaneously, days 6 through 17
Interferon alfa-2b 5 million units/m^2/day subcutaneously, days 6 through 17
Sargramostim 125 mcg/m^2/day (250 mcg maximum dose) subcutaneously, days 6 through 17

Temozolomide-Thalidomide

Use: Malignant melanoma.
Cycle: 56 days

Regimen 1: Patients younger than 70 years of age:
Temozolomide 75 mg/m^2/day PO, days 1 through 42
Thalidomide 200 mg/day PO, days 1 through 14 of first cycle only
Thalidomide 300 mg/day PO, days 15 through 27 of first cycle only
Thalidomide 400 mg/day PO, days 1 through 56, except for days 1 through 27 of first cycle

Regimen 2: Patients 70 years of age and older:
Temozolomide 75 mg/m^2/day PO, days 1 through 42
Thalidomide 100 mg/day PO, days 1 through 14 of first cycle only
Thalidomide 150 mg/day PO, days 15 through 27 of first cycle only
Thalidomide 200 mg/day PO, days 1 through 56, except for days 1 through 27 of first cycle

Thalidomide-Dexamethasone

Use: Multiple myeloma.
Cycle: 28 days for at least 4 cycles

Regimen:
Thalidomide 50 mg/day PO, days 1 through 14 of first cycle only
Thalidomide 100 mg/day PO, days 15 through 28 of first cycle only
Thalidomide 200 mg/day PO, days 1 through 28, except for first cycle
Dexamethasone 40 mg/day PO, days 1 through 4 of all cycles
Dexamethasone 40 mg/day PO, days 9 through 12 and days 17 through 20 of odd-numbered cycles only (eg, cycle 1, 3, 5)

TIC

Use: Head and neck cancer.
Cycle: 21 to 28 days

Regimen:
Paclitaxel 175 mg/m^2 IV over 3 hours, day 1
Ifosfamide 1,000 mg/m^2/day IV, days 1 through 3
Mesna 200 mg/m^2/day IV pre-ifosfamide, days 1 through 3
Mesna 400 mg/m^2/dose IV given 4 hours after ifosfamide, days 1 through 3
Carboplatin IV dose by Calvert equation to AUC 6 mg/mL/min, day 1

TIP

Use: Head and neck cancer, esophageal cancer.
Cycle: 21 to 28 days

Regimen:
Paclitaxel 175 mg/m^2 IV over 3 hours, day 1
Ifosfamide 1,000 mg/m^2/day IV, days 1 through 3
Mesna 400 mg/m^2/day IV pre-ifosfamide, days 1 through 3
Mesna 200 mg/m^2/dose IV given 4 hours after ifosfamide, days 1 through 3
Cisplatin 60 mg/m^2 IV, day 1 (give after paclitaxel infusion)

Use: Testicular cancer.
Cycle: 21 days for 4 cycles

Regimen:
Paclitaxel 175 to 250 mg/m^2/day continuous IV infusion over 24 hours, day 1
Ifosfamide 1,200 mg/m^2/day IV, days 2 through 6
Mesna 400 mg/m^2/dose IV before, then 4 and 8 hours after each ifosfamide infusion, days 2 through 6
Cisplatin 20 mg/m^2/day IV, days 2 through 6

(continued on next page)

TIP (cont.)

Use: Testicular cancer.
Cycle: 21 days for 4 cycles

Regimen: Paclitaxel 250 mg/m^2/day continuous IV infusion over 24 hours, day 1
Ifosfamide 1,500 mg/m^2/day IV, days 2 through 5
Mesna 500 mg/m^2/dose IV before, then 4 and 8 hours after each ifosfamide infusion, days 2 through 5
Cisplatin 25 mg/m^2/day IV, days 2 through 5
Filgrastim 5 mcg/kg/day subcutaneously, days 7 through 18

TIT

Use: Acute lymphocytic leukemia (ALL; CNS prophylaxis—pediatrics).

Regimen: Doses are based on patient's age. Give during weeks 1, 2, 3, 7, 13, 19, and 25 of intensification and every 12 weeks during maintenance.*

Age 1 to 2 years:
- Methotrexate 8 mg intrathecal
- Cytarabine 16 mg intrathecal
- Hydrocortisone 8 mg intrathecal

Age 2 to 3 years:
- Methotrexate 10 mg intrathecal
- Cytarabine 20 mg intrathecal
- Hydrocortisone 10 mg intrathecal

Age 3 to 9 years:
- Methotrexate 12 mg intrathecal
- Cytarabine 24 mg intrathecal
- Hydrocortisone 12 mg intrathecal

Age 9 years and older:
- Methotrexate 15 mg intrathecal
- Cytarabine 30 mg intrathecal
- Hydrocortisone 15 mg intrathecal

*Note: All 3 drugs may be mixed and administered in a single syringe, if diluted with preservative-free 0.9% Sodium Chloride Injection. Regimen is used in combination with an induction/maintenance regimen.

Use: Acute lymphocytic leukemia (ALL; CNS prophylaxis—pediatrics).

Regimen: Doses are based on patient's age. Give on day 1 of induction, during weeks 1, 2, 3, 6, 11, 16, 21, and 26 of intensification, during week 31, and every 12 weeks during maintenance.*

Age 1 year:
- Methotrexate 10 mg intrathecal
- Cytarabine 20 mg intrathecal
- Hydrocortisone 10 mg intrathecal

Age 2 years:
- Methotrexate 12.5 mg intrathecal
- Cytarabine 25 mg intrathecal
- Hydrocortisonee 12.5 mg intrathecal

Age greater than 3 years:
- Methotrexate 15 mg intrathecal
- Cytarabine 30 mg intrathecal
- Hydrocortisone 15 mg intrathecal

*Note: All 3 drugs may be mixed and administered in a single syringe, if diluted with preservative-free 0.9% Sodium Chloride Injection. Regimen is used in combination with an induction/maintenance regimen.

Use: Acute lymphocytic leukemia (ALL; CNS prophylaxis—adults).

Regimen: Give on days 1 and 5 of week 1, day 1 of week 4, days 1 and 5 of week 7, day 1 of week 10, days 1 and 5 of week 13, and day 1 of week 16.
Methotrexate 15 mg intrathecal
Cytarabine 40 mg intrathecal
Dexamethasone 4 mg intrathecal*

*Note: No preservative-free product is available; dexamethasone 4 mg/mL injection contains benzyl alcohol 10 mg/mL, a preservative that is unsuitable for intrathecal injection. Because other intrathecal regimens are available that do not include benzyl alcohol-containing products, this regimen should be reserved for use when no other options are available and the benefit to the patient clearly outweighs the risk of benzyl alcohol toxicity. Regimen is used in combination with an induction/maintenance regimen.

Topo/CTX (Cyclophosphamide-Topotecan)

Use: Sarcomas (bone and soft tissue—pediatrics).
Cycle: 21 days, continue until disease progression or intolerable toxicity

Regimen: Cyclophosphamide 250 mg/m^2/day IV, days 1 through 5
Mesna 150 mg/m^2/dose IV before and 3 hours after each cyclophosphamide infusion, days 1 through 5
Topotecan 0.75 mg/m^2/day IV, days 1 through 5 after cyclophosphamide
Filgrastim 5 mcg/kg/day subcutaneously, from day 6 until absolute neutrophil count (ANC) is at least 1,500 cells/mm^3

TPC

Use: Breast cancer.
Cycle: 21 days for 6 cycles

Regimen: Trastuzumab 4 mg/kg IV, day 1 of first cycle only (loading dose)
Trastuzumab 2 mg/kg IV weekly, on days 1, 8, and 15, except for day 1 of first cycle
Paclitaxel 175 mg/m^2/dose IV over 3 hours, day 2
Carboplatin IV dose by Calvert equation to AUC 6 mg/mL/min, day 2
followed after 6 cycles by
Trastuzumab 2 mg/kg IV, day 1 of each week until disease progression or intolerable toxicity

TPF (also see DCF)

Use: Head and neck cancer.
Cycle: 21 days for up to 4 cycles

Regimen: Docetaxel 75 mg/m^2 IV, day 1
Cisplatin 75 mg/m^2 IV, day 1 (give after docetaxel)
Fluorouracil 750 mg/m^2/day continuous IV infusion, days 1 through 5 (for 120 hours total)
used in conjunction with antimicrobial prophylaxis
Ciprofloxacin 500 mg PO twice daily, days 5 through 15

Use: Head and neck cancer.
Cycle: 21 days for up to 3 cycles

Regimen: Docetaxel 75 mg/m^2 IV, day 1
Cisplatin 75 or 100 mg/m^2 IV, day 1 (give after docetaxel)
Fluorouracil 1,000 mg/m^2/day continuous IV infusion, days 1 through 4 (for 96 hours total)
used in conjunction with antimicrobial prophylaxis
Ciprofloxacin 500 mg PO twice daily, days 5 through 15

TPF ➡ Carboplatin + Radiation, Sequential

Use: Head and neck cancer.
Cycle: See below, cycle length varies throughout protocol. Give 3 cycles of TPF, followed by 7 cycles of Carboplatin + Radiation.

Regimen: **TPF.** *Cycle:* 21 days for 3 cycles
Docetaxel 75 mg/m^2 IV, day 1
Cisplatin 100 mg/m^2 IV, day 1 (give after docetaxel)
Fluorouracil 1,000 mg/m^2/day continuous IV infusion, days 1 through 4 (for 96 hours total)
used in conjunction with antimicrobial prophylaxis
Ciprofloxacin 500 mg PO twice daily, days 5 through 14
followed after 3 to 8 weeks by
Carboplatin + Radiation. *Cycle:* 7 days for 7 cycles
Carboplatin IV dose by Calvert equation to AUC 1.5 mg/mL/min, day 1
used in conjunction with
Radiation therapy
may be followed after 6 to 12 weeks by
Surgical resection

TPF ➡ Radiation, Sequential

Use: Head and neck cancer.
Cycle: 21 days for 4 cycles

Regimen: Docetaxel 75 mg/m^2 IV, day 1
Cisplatin 75 mg/m^2 IV, day 1 (give after docetaxel)
Fluorouracil 750 mg/m^2/day continuous IV infusion, days 1 through 5 (for 120 hours total)
used in conjunction with antimicrobial prophylaxis
Ciprofloxacin 500 mg PO twice daily, days 5 through 15
followed after 4 to 7 weeks by
Radiation therapy

Trastuzumab-Anastrozole

Use: Breast cancer.
Cycle: Ongoing, continue until disease progression or intolerable toxicity

Regimen: Trastuzumab 4 mg/kg IV, day 1 (loading dose)
Trastuzumab 2 mg/kg IV weekly, except for day 1
Anastrozole 1 mg PO daily, throughout entire course

Trastuzumab-Docetaxel

Use: Breast cancer.
Cycle: 28 days, continue until disease progression or intolerable toxicity

Regimen: Trastuzumab 4 mg/kg IV, day 1 of first cycle only (loading dose)
Trastuzumab 2 mg/kg IV weekly, on days 1, 8 and 15, except for day 1 of first cycle
Docetaxel 35 mg/m^2 IV, days 1, 8, and 15

(continued on next page)

Trastuzumab-Docetaxel (cont.)

Use: Breast cancer.
Cycle: 21 days for 6 to 8 cycles

Regimen: Docetaxel 100 mg/m^2 IV, day 1
Trastuzumab 4 mg/kg IV, day 1 of first cycle only (loading dose)
Trastuzumab 2 mg/kg IV weekly, on days 1, 8, and 15, except for day 1 of first cycle
followed by
Trastuzumab 2 mg/kg IV weekly, continued until disease progression or intolerable toxicity

Trastuzumab-Gemcitabine

Use: Breast cancer.
Cycle: 21 days, continue until disease progression or intolerable toxicity

Regimen: Trastuzumab 8 mg/kg IV, day 1 of first cycle only (loading dose)
Trastuzumab 6 mg/kg IV, day 1, except for first cycle
Gemcitabine 1,250 mg/m^2 IV, days 1 and 8

Trastuzumab-Paclitaxel

Use: Breast cancer.
Cycle: 21 days for at least 6 cycles

Regimen: Trastuzumab 4 mg/kg IV, day 1 of first cycle only (loading dose)
Trastuzumab 2 mg/kg IV weekly, on days 1, 8, and 15, except for day 1 of first cycle
Paclitaxel 175 mg/m^2 IV over 3 hours, day 1

Use: Breast cancer.
Cycle: 21 days for 8 cycles

Regimen: Paclitaxel 175 mg/m^2 IV over 3 hours, day 1
Trastuzumab 8 mg/kg IV, day 2 of first cycle only (loading dose)
Trastuzumab 6 mg/kg IV, day 1, except for first cycle, continued until disease progression or intolerable toxicity

Trastuzumab-Vinorelbine

Use: Breast cancer.
Cycle: 7 days, continue until disease progression or intolerable toxicity

Regimen: Trastuzumab 4 mg/kg IV, day 1 of first cycle only (loading dose)
Trastuzumab 2 mg/kg IV, day 1, except for first cycle
Vinorelbine 25 mg/m^2 IV, day 1

V-TAD

Use: Acute myelocytic leukemia (AML; induction).
Cycle: 7 days. Give 1 cycle. Up to 3 cycles have been given, but time between cycles was not specified.

Regimen: Etoposide 50 mg/m^2/day IV, days 1 through 3
Thioguanine 75 mg/m^2/dose PO every 12 hours for 10 doses, days 1 through 5
Daunorubicin 20 mg/m^2/day IV, days 1 and 2
Cytarabine 75 mg/m^2/day continuous IV infusion, days 1 through 5

VAB-6

Use: Testicular cancer.
Cycle: 21 to 28 days for 3 to 12 cycles

Regimen: Cyclophosphamide 600 mg/m^2 IV, day 1
Dactinomycin 1 mg/m^2 IV, day 1
Vinblastine 4 mg/m^2 IV, day 1
Bleomycin 30 units IV push, day 1 (omit from cycle 3)
Bleomycin 20 units/m^2/day continuous IV infusion, days 1 through 3 (omit from cycle 3) (give after IV push dose)
Cisplatin 120 mg/m^2 IV, day 4

VAC for lung cancer—see CAV

VAC Pediatric

Use: Sarcoma (pediatrics).
Cycle: 21 days

Regimen: Vincristine 2 mg/m^2 IV (2 mg maximum dose), day 1
Dactinomycin 1 mg/m^2 IV, day 1
Cyclophosphamide 600 mg/m^2 IV, day 1

(continued on next page)

VAC Pediatric (cont.)

Use: Sarcoma (pediatrics).
Cycle: 21 days

Regimen: Vincristine 1.5 mg/m^2 IV (2 mg maximum dose) weekly, on days 1, 8, and 15
Dactinomycin 0.015 mg/kg/day (0.5 mg/day maximum dose) continuous IV infusion, days 1 through 5
Cyclophosphamide 2,200 mg/m^2 IV, day 1
Mesna 440 mg/m^2/dose IV given 15 minutes before, and 4 and 8 hours after cyclophosphamide, day 1
Filgrastim 5 mcg/kg/day subcutaneously, from day 6 until hematologic recovery (start at least 24 hours after completion of chemotherapy infusions)

VAC Pulse

Use: Sarcomas.
Cycle: Give a single cycle

Regimen: Vincristine 2 mg/m^2 (2 mg maximum dose) IV weekly, for 12 weeks
Dactinomycin 0.015 mg/kg/day (0.5 mg/day maximum dose) continuous IV infusion, days 1 through 5, every 3 months for 5 courses
Cyclophosphamide 10 mg/kg/day IV or PO, days 1 through 7, every 6 weeks

VAC Standard

Use: Sarcomas.
Cycle: Give a single cycle

Regimen: Vincristine 2 mg/m^2 (2 mg maximum dose) IV weekly, for 12 weeks
Dactinomycin 0.015 mg/kg/day (0.5 mg/day maximum dose) continuous IV infusion, days 1 through 5, every 3 months for 5 courses
Cyclophosphamide 2.5 mg/kg/day PO, daily for 2 years

VACAdr

Use: Sarcoma (bone and soft tissue—pediatrics).
Cycle: Give a single cycle

Regimen: Vincristine 1.5 mg/m^2 (2 mg maximum dose) IV, weekly for 6 weeks, on days 1, 8, 15, 22, 29, and 36
Cyclophosphamide 500 mg/m^2 IV, weekly for 6 weeks, on days 1, 8, 15, 22, 29, and 36
Doxorubicin 60 mg/m^2 IV, day 36
followed by 6-week rest period, then
Dactinomycin 0.015 mg/kg/day IV, days 1 through 5
Vincristine 1.5 mg/m^2 (2 mg maximum dose) IV, days 14, 21, 28, 35, and 42
Cyclophosphamide 500 mg/m^2 IV, days 14, 21, 28, 35, and 42
Doxorubicin 60 mg/m^2 IV, day 42 (give on day of final vincristine and cyclophosphamide doses)

VAD

Use: Multiple myeloma.
Cycle: 3 to 4 weeks, continue for 6 months or indefinitely

Regimen: Vincristine 0.4 mg/day (dose is not in mg/m^2) continuous IV infusion, days 1 through 4*
Doxorubicin 9 mg/m^2/day continuous IV infusion, days 1 through 4*
Dexamethasone 40 mg/day PO, days 1 through 4, days 9 through 12, and days 17 through 20†
*Note: Vincristine and doxorubicin may be mixed and administered in the same infusion bag, if diluted with 0.9% Sodium Chloride Injection.
†Note: After completing the first 2 cycles of VAD, some clinicians give dexamethasone only on days 1 through 4 of each cycle to reduce the risk of infection. Antibiotic prophylaxis with cotrimoxazole also has been used for this purpose.

Use: Acute lymphocytic leukemia (ALL).
Cycle: 24 to 28 days, may give a single cycle or repeat indefinitely

Regimen: Vincristine 0.4 mg/day (dose is not in mg/m^2) continuous IV infusion, days 1 through 4*
Doxorubicin 9 to 12 mg/m^2/day continuous IV infusion, days 1 through 4*
Dexamethasone 40 mg/day PO, days 1 through 4, days 9 through 12, and days 17 through 20
*Note: Vincristine and doxorubicin may be mixed and administered in the same infusion bag, if diluted with 0.9% Sodium Chloride Injection.

Use: Wilms tumor (pediatrics).
Cycle: 1 year for 1 cycle only

Regimen 1: Vincristine 1.5 mg/m^2 (2 mg maximum dose) IV, weekly for first 10 to 11 weeks then every 3 weeks for 15 more weeks
Dactinomycin 1.5 mg/m^2 IV every 6 weeks, starting week 1, for 9 doses
Doxorubicin 40 mg/m^2 IV every 6 weeks, starting week 4, for 9 doses

Regimen 2: Vincristine 1.5 mg/m^2 (2 mg maximum dose) IV, given every 6 weeks for 6 to 15 months
with
Dactinomycin 0.015 mg/kg/day IV for 5 doses, given every 6 weeks for 6 to 15 months
or
Dactinomycin 0.06 mg/kg IV, given every 6 weeks for 6 to 15 months
may or may not give with
Doxorubicin 20 mg/m^2 IV, given every 6 weeks for 6 to 15 months

VAD/CVAD

Use: Acute lymphocytic leukemia (ALL; induction—adults).
Cycle: Give 1 cycle only

Regimen:
Vincristine 0.4 mg/day (dose is not in mg/m^2) continuous IV infusion, days 1 through 4 and days 24 through 27*
Doxorubicin 12 mg/m^2/day continuous IV infusion, days 1 through 4 and days 24 through 27*
Dexamethasone 40 mg/day PO, days 1 through 4, days 9 through 12, days 17 through 20, days 24 through 27, days 32 through 35, and days 40 through 43
Cyclophosphamide 1,000 mg/m^2 IV, day 24
*Note: Vincristine and doxorubicin may be mixed and administered in the same infusion bag, if diluted with 0.9% Sodium Chloride Injection.

VAD-Liposomal (VLAD)

Use: Multiple myeloma.
Cycle: 28 days for up to 6 cycles

Regimen:
Vincristine 2 mg (dose is not in mg/m^2) IV, day 1
Liposomal doxorubicin 30 to 40 mg/m^2 IV, day 1
Dexamethasone 40 mg/day PO, days 1 through 4, days 9 through 12, and days 17 through 20

VAD, Rapid Infusion

Use: Multiple myeloma.
Cycle: 28 days for 3 to 4 cycles

Regimen:
Vincristine 0.4 mg/day (dose is not in mg/m^2) IV over 30 minutes, days 1 through 4*
Doxorubicin 9 mg/m^2/day IV over 30 minutes, days 1 through 4*
Dexamethasone 40 mg/day PO, days 1 through 4 of all cycles
Dexamethasone 40 mg/day PO, days 9 through 12 and days 17 through 20 of odd-numbered cycles only (eg, cycle 1, 3, 5)
used in conjunction with antimicrobial prophylaxis
Fluconazole 200 mg PO daily, throughout entire course
Cotrimoxazole double-strength (160/800) PO twice daily, throughout entire course
*Note: Vincristine and doxorubicin may be mixed and administered in the same infusion bag, if diluted with 0.9% Sodium Chloride Injection.

VATH

Use: Breast cancer.
Cycle: 21 days

Regimen:
Vinblastine 4.5 mg/m^2 IV, day 1
Doxorubicin 45 mg/m^2 IV, day 1
Thiotepa 12 mg/m^2 IV, day 1
Fluoxymesterone 10 mg/dose (30 mg/day) PO 3 times daily, throughout entire course

VBAP

Use: Multiple myeloma.
Cycle: 21 days for 6 to 12 months

Regimen:
Vincristine 1 mg/m^2 (1.5 mg maximum dose) IV, day 1
Carmustine 30 mg/m^2 IV, day 1
Doxorubicin 30 mg/m^2 IV, day 1
Prednisone 60 mg/m^2/day PO, days 1 through 4

VBCMP

Use: Multiple myeloma.
Cycle: 35 days for up to 10 cycles

Regimen:
Vincristine 1.2 mg/m^2 (2 mg maximum dose) IV, day 1
Carmustine 20 mg/m^2 IV, day 1
Cyclophosphamide 400 mg/m^2 IV, day 1
Melphalan 8 mg/m^2/day PO, days 1 through 4
Prednisone 40 mg/m^2/day PO, days 1 through 7 of all cycles
Prednisone 20 mg/m^2/day PO, days 8 through 14 of first 3 cycles only

VCAP

Use: Multiple myeloma.
Cycle: 21 days for 6 to 12 months

Regimen:
Vincristine 1 mg/m^2 (1.5 mg maximum dose) IV, day 1
Cyclophosphamide 125 mg/m^2/day PO, days 1 through 4
Doxorubicin 30 mg/m^2 IV, day 1
Prednisone 60 mg/m^2/day PO, days 1 through 4

VCMP—see VMCP

VD

Use: Breast cancer.
Cycle: 21 days

Regimen: Vinorelbine 25 mg/m² IV, days 1 and 8
Doxorubicin 50 mg/m² IV, day 1

VeIP

Use: Genitourinary cancer, testicular cancer.
Cycle: 21 days for up to 4 cycles

Regimen: Vinblastine 0.11 mg/kg/day IV, days 1 and 2
Ifosfamide 1,200 mg/m²/day IV, days 1 through 5
Mesna 1,200 mg/m²/day continuous IV infusion, days 1 through 5
Cisplatin 20 mg/m²/day IV, days 1 through 5

VIC—see CVI

Vinblastine-Interferon alfa

Use: Renal cell carcinoma.
Cycle: 21 days

Regimen: Vinblastine 0.1 mg/kg IV, day 1
Interferon alfa-2a* 3 million units/dose subcutaneously 3 times weekly, week 1 of first cycle only
Interferon alfa-2a* 18 million units/dose subcutaneously 3 times weekly, except for week 1 of first cycle; may decrease to interferon alfa-2a 9 million units/dose subcutaneously 3 times weekly if adverse effects are intolerable
*Note: Interferon alfa-2a is no longer available in the United States. The manufacturer discontinued this product in October 2007 for commercial reasons, not for safety or efficacy reasons.

Vinblastine-Methotrexate

Use: Desmoid tumor.
Cycle: 7 to 10 days for up to 12 months

Regimen: Vinblastine 6 mg/m² IV, day 1
Methotrexate 30 mg/m² IV, day 1

Vinorelbine-Carboplatin

Use: Lung cancer (non-small cell).
Cycle: 21 days for up to 6 cycles

Regimen: Vinorelbine 25 mg/m² IV, days 1 and 8
Carboplatin IV dose by Calvert equation to AUC 6 mg/mL/min, day 1

Use: Lung cancer (non-small cell).
Cycle: 21 days for up to 6 cycles

Regimen: Vinorelbine 30 mg/m² IV, days 1 and 8
Carboplatin IV dose by Calvert equation to AUC 5 mg/mL/min, day 1

Vinorelbine-Cisplatin (VC; also see Cisplatin-Vinorelbine)

Use: Lung cancer (non-small cell).
Cycle: 42 days, continue until disease progression or intolerable toxicity

Regimen: Vinorelbine 30 mg/m² IV, weekly, throughout entire course
Cisplatin 120 mg/m² IV, days 1 and 29 for first cycle; then day 1 of subsequent cycles

Use: Lung cancer (non-small cell).
Cycle: 28 days for up to 6 cycles, continue until disease progression or intolerable toxicity

Regimen: Vinorelbine 25 mg/m² IV weekly, on days 1, 8, 15, and 22
Cisplatin 100 mg/m² IV, day 1

Use: Cervical cancer.
Cycle: 21 days

Regimen: Vinorelbine 30 mg/m² IV, days 1 and 8
Cisplatin 50 mg/m² IV, day 1

Vinorelbine-Doxorubicin (NA)

Use: Breast cancer.
Cycle: 21 days for up to 11 cycles

Regimen: Vinorelbine 25 mg/m² IV, days 1 and 8
Doxorubicin 50 mg/m² IV, day 1

Vinorelbine-Gemcitabine

Use: Lung cancer (non-small cell).
Cycle: 28 days for up to 6 cycles

Regimen: Vinorelbine 20 mg/m² IV, days 1, 8, and 15
Gemcitabine 800 mg/m² IV, days 1, 8, and 15

VIP

Use: Genitourinary cancer, testicular cancer, sarcoma (bone).
Cycle: 21 days for up to 4 cycles

Regimen:
Etoposide 75 mg/m²/day IV, days 1 through 5
Ifosfamide 1,200 mg/m²/day IV, days 1 through 5
Mesna 1,200 mg/m²/day continuous IV infusion, days 1 through 5
Cisplatin 20 mg/m²/day IV, days 1 through 5

Use: Thymoma.
Cycle: 21 days for up to 4 cycles, or until disease progression or intolerable toxicity

Regimen:
Etoposide 75 mg/m²/day IV, days 1 through 4
Ifosfamide 1,200 mg/m²/day IV, days 1 through 4
Mesna 240 mg/m²/dose IV before, then 4 and 8 hours after each ifosfamide infusion, days 1 through 4
Cisplatin 20 mg/m²/day IV, days 1 through 4
Filgrastim 5 mcg/kg/day subcutaneously (rounded to 300 or 480 mcg), days 5 through 15, or until the white blood cell count (WBC) is at least 10,000 cells/mm³ post-nadir (whichever occurs earlier)

Use: Lung cancer (small cell).
Cycle: 21 to 28 days for up to 4 cycles

Regimen:
Ifosfamide 1,200 mg/m²/day IV, days 1 through 4
Mesna 120 to 300 mg/m² IV, day 1 (give before ifosfamide is started)
Mesna 1,200 mg/m²/day continuous IV infusion, days 1 through 4 (after mesna bolus is given)
Cisplatin 20 mg/m²/day IV, days 1 through 4
with
Etoposide 37.5 mg/m²/day PO, days 1 through 14
or
Etoposide 75 mg/m²/day IV, days 1 through 4

Use: Lung cancer (non-small cell).
Cycle: 28 days for up to 4 cycles

Regimen:
Ifosfamide 1,000 to 1,200 mg/m²/day IV, days 1 through 3
Cisplatin 100 mg/m² IV, days 1 and 8
Etoposide 60 to 75 mg/m²/day IV, days 1 through 3
with
Mesna 300 mg/m²/dose IV every 4 hours, days 1 through 4 (for 24 doses total)
or
Mesna 20% of ifosfamide dose IV before, then 4 and 8 hours after each ifosfamide infusion, days 1 through 4

VLAD—see VAD-Liposomal

VM

Use: Breast cancer.
Cycle: 6 to 8 weeks

Regimen:
Vinblastine 5 mg/m² IV, days 1, 14, 28, and 42 for 2 cycles, then days 1 and 21 only
Mitomycin 10 mg/m² IV, days 1 and 28 for 2 cycles, then day 1 only

VMCP (VCMP)

Use: Multiple myeloma.
Cycle: 21 days for 6 to 12 months

Regimen:
Vincristine 1 mg/m² (2 mg maximum dose) IV, day 1
Melphalan 6 mg/m²/day PO, days 1 through 4
Cyclophosphamide 125 mg/m²/day PO, days 1 through 4
Prednisone 60 mg/m²/day PO, days 1 through 4

VMP

Use: Multiple myeloma.

Regimen:
Induction. *Cycle:* 42 days. Give 4 cycles.
Bortezomib 1 or 1.3 mg/m² IV, days 1, 4, 8, 11, 22, 25, 29, and 32
Melphalan 9 mg/m²/day PO, days 1 through 4
Prednisone 60 mg/m²/day PO, days 1 through 4
Maintenance. *Cycle:* 35 to 42 days. Give 5 cycles.
Bortezomib 1 or 1.3 mg/m² IV, weekly for 4 weeks, on days 1, 8, 15, and 22
Melphalan 9 mg/m²/day PO, days 1 through 4
Prednisone 60 mg/m²/day PO, days 1 through 4

VMPT

Use: Multiple myeloma.
Cycle: 35 days for 6 cycles

Regimen:
Bortezomib 1 or 1.3 mg/m^2 IV, days 1, 4, 15, and 22
Melphalan 6 mg/m^2/day PO, days 1 through 5
Prednisone 60 mg/m^2/day PO, days 1 through 5
Thalidomide 50 mg/day PO, throughout entire course
*used in conjunction with antimicrobial prophylaxis**
Acyclovir 200 mg PO 3 times daily, throughout entire course
or
Acyclovir 400 mg PO twice daily, throughout entire course
*Note: Antimicrobial prophylaxis doses not specified in original article; the doses given here are derived from *AHFS 2009 Drug Information,* a tertiary resource.

VP

Use: Lung cancer (small cell).
Cycle: 21 days for up to 4 cycles

Regimen:
Etoposide 100 mg/m^2/day IV, days 1 through 4
Cisplatin 20 mg/m^2/day IV, days 1 through 4

X + T—see Capecitabine-Docetaxel

XELIRI (also see CAPIRI)

Use: Colorectal cancer.
Cycle: 21 days for up to 12 cycles

Regimen 1: Patients younger than 65 years of age, patients with creatinine clearance greater than 50 mL/min, or patients without prior pelvic radiation therapy:
Capecitabine 1,000 mg/m^2/dose PO twice daily, days 1 through 14
Irinotecan 250 mg/m^2 IV, day 1

Regimen 2: Patients 65 years of age and older, patients with creatinine clearance of 30 to 50 mL/min, or patients with prior pelvic radiation therapy:
Capecitabine 750 mg/m^2/dose PO twice daily, days 1 through 14
Irinotecan 200 mg/m^2 IV, day 1

XELIRI + Bevacizumab

Use: Colorectal cancer.
Cycle: 21 days, continue until disease progression or intolerable toxicity

Regimen:
Capecitabine 1,000 mg/m^2/dose PO twice daily, days 1 through 14
Irinotecan 200 mg/m^2 IV, day 1
Bevacizumab 7.5 mg/kg IV, day 1

XELOX (CAPOX)

Use: Colorectal cancer.
Cycle: 21 days for up to 11 cycles, or until disease progression or intolerable toxicity

Regimen 1: Patients who have not received prior chemotherapy:
Capecitabine 1,250 mg/m^2/dose PO twice daily, days 1 through 14
Oxaliplatin 130 mg/m^2 IV, day 1

Regimen 2: Patients who have received prior chemotherapy:
Capecitabine 1,000 mg/m^2/dose PO twice daily, days 1 through 14
Oxaliplatin 130 mg/m^2 IV, day 1

Use: Colorectal cancer.
Cycle: 21 days for up to 12 cycles

Regimen:
Capecitabine 1,000 mg/m^2/dose PO twice daily, days 1 through 14
Oxaliplatin 70 mg/m^2 IV, day 1 of all cycles
Oxaliplatin 70 mg/m^2 IV, day 8 of cycles 1 through 6

Use: Colorectal cancer.
Cycle: 14 days for up to 12 cycles

Regimen:
Capecitabine 1,750 mg/m^2/dose PO twice daily, days 1 through 7
Oxaliplatin 85 mg/m^2 IV, day 1

Use: Hepatocellular cancer.
Cycle: 21 days, continue until disease progression or intolerable toxicity

Regimen:
Capecitabine 1,000 mg/m^2/dose PO twice daily, days 1 through 14
Oxaliplatin 130 mg/m^2 IV, day 1

Use: Esophageal cancer, colorectal cancer.
Cycle: 21 days, continue for up to 8 to 12 cycles, or until disease progression or intolerable toxicity

Regimen:
Capecitabine 850 to 1,000 mg/m^2/dose PO twice daily, days 1 through 14
Oxaliplatin 130 mg/m^2 IV, day 1

XELOX + Bevacizumab (also see CapeOx-B, Modified)

Use: Colorectal cancer.
Cycle: 21 days, continue until disease progression or intolerable toxicity

Regimen: Capecitabine 850 to 1,000 mg/m^2/dose PO twice daily, days 1 through 14
Oxaliplatin 130 mg/m^2 IV, day 1
Bevacizumab 7.5 mg/kg IV, day 1

XELOX-RT

Use: Rectal cancer.
Cycle: 42 days. Give a single cycle prior to surgery.

Regimen: Capecitabine 825 mg/m^2/dose PO twice daily, days 1 through 14 and days 22 through 35
Oxaliplatin 50 mg/m^2 IV, days 1, 8, 22, and 29
used in conjunction with
Radiation therapy

XN

Use: Breast cancer.
Cycle: 21 days

Regimen: Capecitabine 1,000 mg/m^2/dose PO twice daily, days 1 through 14
Vinorelbine 25 mg/m^2 IV, days 1 and 8

XP

Use: Breast cancer.
Cycle: 21 days, continue until disease progression or intolerable toxicity

Regimen: Capecitabine 825 mg/m^2/dose PO twice daily, days 1 through 14
with
Paclitaxel 175 mg/m^2 IV over 3 hours, day 1
or
Paclitaxel 80 mg/m^2 IV (infusion duration not specified), days 1 and 8

ALKYLATING AGENTS

Nitrogen Mustards

CHLORAMBUCIL

Rx	**Leukeran** (GlaxoSmithKline)	**Tablets:** 2 mg	(GX EG3 L). Brown. Film coated. In 50s.

CHLORAMBUCIL — ORAL

WARNING

Chlorambucil can severely suppress bone marrow function. Chlorambucil is a carcinogen in humans. Chlorambucil is probably mutagenic and teratogenic in humans. Chlorambucil produces human infertility.

Indications

➤*Leukemia/Lymphomas:* For the treatment of chronic lymphatic (lymphocytic) leukemia, malignant lymphomas including lymphosarcoma, giant follicular lymphoma, and Hodgkin disease. It is not curative in any of these disorders but may produce clinically useful palliation.

➤*Off-label uses:* Chlorambucil has shown activity in other malignancies such as ovarian and testicular carcinoma, non-Hodgkin lymphoma, and Waldenström macroglobulinemia. Treatment of polycythemia vera.

Chlorambucil has been used safely and effectively in children for chronic lymphocytic leukemia, lymphomas, and nephrotic syndrome. (See Administration and Dosage.)

Administration and Dosage

➤*General dosing considerations:* Radiation and cytotoxic drugs render the bone marrow more vulnerable to damage, and chlorambucil should be used with particular caution within 4 weeks of a full course of radiation therapy or chemotherapy. However, small doses of palliative radiation over isolated foci remote from the bone marrow will not usually depress the neutrophil and platelet count. In these cases, chlorambucil may be given in the customary dosage.

➤*Adults:*

Chronic lymphocytic leukemia or lymphomas –

Usual dosage: 0.1 to 0.2 mg/kg daily for 3 to 6 weeks. This usually amounts to 4 to 10 mg/day for the average patient. The entire daily dose may be given at one time.

Patients with Hodgkin disease usually require 0.2 mg/kg/day, whereas patients with other lymphomas or chronic lymphocytic leukemia usually require only 0.1 mg/kg/day. When lymphocytic infiltration of the bone marrow is present, or when the bone marrow is hypoplastic, the daily dose should not exceed 0.1 mg/kg (about 6 mg for the average patient).

These dosages are for initiation of therapy or for short courses of treatment.

Maintenance dosage: Doses should not exceed 0.1 mg/kg/day and may be as low as 0.03 mg/kg/day. Doses of 2 to 4 mg/day or less are typical but depend on the status of the blood counts.

It is presently felt that short courses of treatment are safer than continuous maintenance therapy, although both methods have been effective. It must be recognized that continuous therapy may give the appearance of

Combinations of antineoplastic agents are frequently superior to single-drug therapy in the management of many diseases, leading to higher response-"maintenance" in patients who are actually in remission and have no immediate need for further drug. Therefore, it may be desirable to withdraw the drug after maximal control has been achieved, because intermittent therapy reinstituted at time of relapse may be as effective as continuous treatment.

Dosage adjustment: The dosage must be carefully adjusted according to the response of the patient and must be reduced as soon as there is an abrupt fall in the white blood cell count. (See also Dosage adjustment for toxicity.)

Pulse dosage: Initial single dose of 0.4 mg/kg. Doses are then given at biweekly or monthly intervals, increasing by 0.1 mg/kg increments until lymphocytosis is controlled or toxicity occurs. Subsequent doses are modified to produce mild hematologic toxicity.

Off-label dosing –

Macroglobulinemia: 2 to 10 mg/day has been used continuously for up to 9 years.

➤*Children:*

Off-label dosing –

Chronic lymphocytic leukemia:

• *Remission induction* – 0.1 to 0.2 mg/kg/day (4 to 10 mg/day) for 3 to 6 weeks. Alternatively, 4.5 mg/m^2/day may be given.

• *Maintenance dosage* – 0.03 to 0.1 mg/kg/day. Doses of 2 to 4 mg/day are typical.

• *Pulse dosage* – Initial single dose of 0.4 mg/kg. Doses are then given at biweekly or monthly intervals, increasing by 0.1 mg/kg increments until lymphocytosis is controlled or toxicity occurs. Subsequent doses are modified to produce mild hematologic toxicity.

Hodgkin disease: 0.2 mg/kg/day.

Non-Hodgkin lymphoma: 0.1 mg/kg/day.

Nephrotic syndrome: 0.1 to 0.2 mg/kg/day for 5 to 15 weeks, given in combination with prednisone.

CHLORAMBUCIL — ORAL

➤*Renal function impairment:* Dosage adjustment may be necessary in patients with more severe renal impairment, as shown in the following table.

Chlorambucil Dosage Adjustment Based on Renal Function	
Creatinine clearance	Percentage of usual dose
≥ 50 mL/min	100%
10 to 50 mL/min	75%
< 10 mL/min	50%
Hemodialysis	50%, no supplemental dosing needed.
Peritoneal dialysis	50%, no supplemental dosing needed.

➤*Dosage adjustment for toxicity:* Dosage reductions are required if the patient has received full-dose radiation or myelotoxic drugs within the last month or has a low leukocyte or platelet count. Do not exceed 0.1 mg/kg/day when lymphocytic infiltration of bone marrow is present or bone marrow is hypoplastic.

Monitor complete blood cell count (CBC) 1 to 2 times per week; reduce dose immediately if there is an abrupt fall in white blood cell count (WBC). WBC may continue to drop for up to 10 days after the last chlorambucil dose.

Discontinue chlorambucil immediately if skin reactions occur.

➤*Preparation for administration:* Chlorambucil is considered a cytotoxic agent. Follow safe handling procedures when preparing, administering, or dispensing chlorambucil.

➤*Administration:* To be administered orally either once daily or in divided doses given on an empty stomach (1 hour before or 2 hours after meals). Food reduces bioavailability by 10% to 20%.

➤*Storage/Stability:* Store in a refrigerator at 2° to 8°C (36° to 46°F).

Actions

➤*Pharmacokinetics:*

Absorption – Chlorambucil is rapidly and completely absorbed from the GI tract. After single oral doses of 0.6 to 1.2 mg/kg, peak plasma chlorambucil levels C_{max} are reached within 1 hour and the terminal half-life of the parent drug is estimated at 1.5 hours.

Distribution – Chlorambucil and its metabolites are extensively bound to plasma and tissue proteins. In vitro, chlorambucil is 99% bound to plasma proteins, specifically albumin. Cerebrospinal fluid levels of chlorambucil have not been determined. Evidence of human teratogenicity suggests that the drug crosses the placenta.

Metabolism – Chlorambucil is extensively metabolized in the liver primarily to phenylacetic acid mustard which has antineoplastic activity. Chlorambucil and its major metabolite spontaneously degrade in vivo forming monohydroxy and dihydroxy derivatives.

Excretion – After a single dose of radiolabeled chlorambucil (^{14}C), approximately 15% to 60% of the radioactivity appears in the urine after 24 hours. Again, less than 1% of the urinary radioactivity is in the form of chlorambucil or phenylacetic acid mustard. In summary, the pharmacokinetic data suggest that oral chlorambucil undergoes rapid GI absorption and plasma clearance and that it is almost completely metabolized, having extremely low urinary excretion.

Contraindications

Resistance to the agent; hypersensitivity to chlorambucil. There may be cross-hypersensitivity (skin rash) between chlorambucil and other alkylating agents.

Warnings/Precautions

➤*Bone marrow damage:* Many patients develop a slowly progressive lymphopenia during treatment. The lymphocyte count usually rapidly returns to normal levels upon completion of drug therapy. Most patients have some neutropenia after the third week of treatment and this may continue for up to 10 days after the last dose. Subsequently, the neutrophil count usually rapidly returns to normal. Severe neutropenia appears to be related to dosage and usually occurs only in patients who have received a total dosage of 6.5 mg/kg or more in one course of therapy with continuous dosing. About one-fourth of all patients receiving the continuous-dose schedule, and one-third of those receiving this dosage in 8 weeks or less may be expected to develop severe neutropenia.

While it is not necessary to discontinue chlorambucil at the first evidence of a fall in neutrophil count, it must be remembered that the fall may continue for 10 days after the last dose, and that as the total dose approaches 6.5 mg/kg, there is a risk of causing irreversible bone marrow damage. Decrease the dose of chlorambucil if leukocyte or platelet counts fall below normal values, and discontinue the dose for more severe depression.

Persistently low neutrophil and platelet counts or peripheral lymphocytosis suggest bone marrow infiltration. If confirmed by bone marrow examination, the daily dosage of chlorambucil should not exceed 0.1 mg/kg. Chlorambucil appears to be relatively free from GI side effects or other evidence of toxicity apart from the bone marrow-depressant action. In humans, single oral doses of 20 mg or more may produce nausea and vomiting.

➤*Radiation and chemotherapy:* Do not give chlorambucil at full dosages before 4 weeks after a full course of radiation therapy or chemotherapy because of the vulnerability of the bone marrow to damage under these conditions. If the pretherapy leukocyte or platelet counts are depressed from bone marrow disease process prior to institution of therapy, institute the treatment at a reduced dosage.

➤*Seizures:* Children with nephrotic syndrome and patients receiving high pulse doses of chlorambucil may have an increased risk of seizures. As with any potentially epileptogenic drug, exercise caution when administering chlorambucil to patients with a history of seizure disorder or head trauma, or to patients who are receiving other potentially epileptogenic drugs.

➤*Hypersensitivity reactions:* See Adverse Reactions for more information.

➤*Pregnancy: Category D.* Chlorambucil can cause fetal harm when administered to a pregnant woman. Unilateral renal agenesis has been observed in 2 offspring whose mothers received chlorambucil during the first trimester. Urogenital malformations, including absence of a kidney, were found in fetuses of rats given chlorambucil. There are no adequate and well-controlled studies in pregnant women. If this drug is used during pregnancy, or if the patient becomes pregnant while taking this drug, apprise the patient of the potential hazard to the fetus. Advise women of childbearing potential to avoid becoming pregnant.

Fertility impairment – A high incidence of sterility has been documented when chlorambucil is administered to prepubertal and pubertal males. Prolonged or permanent azoospermia has also been observed in adult males. While most reports of gonadal dysfunction secondary to chlorambucil have related to males, the induction of amenorrhea in females with alkylating agents is well documented and chlorambucil is capable of producing amenorrhea. Autopsy studies of the ovaries from women with malignant lymphoma treated with combination chemotherapy including chlorambucil have shown varying degrees of fibrosis, vasculitis, and depletion of primordial follicles.

➤*Lactation:* It is not known whether this drug is excreted in human milk. Because many drugs are excreted in human milk and because of the potential for serious adverse reactions in nursing infants from chlorambucil, decide whether to discontinue nursing or discontinue the drug, taking into account the importance of the drug to the mother.

➤*Children:* The safety and efficacy in pediatric patients have not been established.

➤*Monitoring:* Patients must be followed carefully to avoid life-endangering damage to the bone marrow during treatment. Perform weekly blood examinations to determine hemoglobin levels, total and differential leukocyte counts, and quantitative platelet counts. Also, during the first 3 to 6 weeks of therapy, it is recommended that white blood cell counts be made 3 or 4 days after each of the weekly complete blood counts. It has been suggested that in following patients it is helpful to plot the blood counts on a chart at the same time that body weight, temperature, and spleen size are recorded. It is considered dangerous to allow a patient to go greater than 2 weeks without hematological and clinical examination during treatment.

Drug Interactions

There are no known drug/drug interactions with chlorambucil.

Adverse Reactions

Chlorambucil is considered to have very low emetogenic potential (less than 10% incidence of emesis).

➤*CNS:* Tremors, muscular twitching, myoclonia, confusion, agitation, ataxia, flaccid paresis, and hallucinations have been reported as rare adverse reactions to chlorambucil that resolve upon discontinuation of drug. Rare, focal, or generalized seizures have been reported to occur in both children and adults at both therapeutic daily doses and pulse-dosing regimens, and in acute overdose.

➤*GI:* GI disturbances such as nausea and vomiting, diarrhea, and oral ulceration occur infrequently.

➤*Hematologic:* See Warnings/Precautions for more information.

➤*Hypersensitivity:* Allergic reactions such as urticaria and angioneurotic edema have been reported following initial or subsequent dosing. Skin hypersensitivity (including rare reports of skin rash progressing to erythema multiforme, toxic epidermal necrolysis, and Stevens-Johnson syndrome) has been reported.

➤*Miscellaneous:* Other reported adverse reactions include pulmonary fibrosis, hepatotoxicity and jaundice, drug fever, peripheral neuropathy, interstitial pneumonia, sterile cystitis, infertility, leukemia, and secondary malignancies.

Overdosage

➤*Symptoms:* Reversible pancytopenia was the main finding of inadvertent overdoses of chlorambucil. Neurological toxicity ranging from agitated behavior and ataxia to multiple grand mal seizures has also occurred.

➤*Treatment:* As there is no known antidote, closely monitor the blood picture and institute general supportive measures, together with appropriate blood transfusions, if necessary. Chlorambucil is not dialyzable.

Patient Information

Inform patients that the major toxicities of chlorambucil are related to hypersensitivity, drug fever, myelosuppression, hepatotoxicity, infertility, seizures, GI toxicity, and secondary malignancies. Patients should never be allowed to take the drug without medical supervision and should consult their doctor if they experience skin rash, bleeding, fever, jaundice, persistent cough, seizures, nausea, vomiting, amenorrhea, or unusual lumps/masses. Advise women of childbearing potential to avoid becoming pregnant.

CYCLOPHOSPHAMIDE

Rx	Cyclophosphamide (Roxane)	Tablets; oral: 25 mg	Lactose. (54 639). Lt. blue, round. In 100s.
		50 mg	Lactose. (54 980). Lt. blue, round. In 100s.
Rx	Cyclophosphamide (Baxter)	Injection, powder for solution: 500 mg	In single-dose vials.
		1 g	In single-dose vials.
		2 g	In single-dose vials.

CYCLOPHOSPHAMIDE — ORAL

Indications

➤*Malignant diseases:* Although effective alone in susceptible malignancies, cyclophosphamide is more frequently used concurrently or sequentially with other antineoplastic drugs. The following malignancies are often susceptible to cyclophosphamide treatment:

1.) Malignant lymphomas (stages III and IV of the Ann Arbor staging system), Hodgkin disease, lymphocytic lymphoma (nodular or diffuse), mixed-cell type lymphoma, histiocytic lymphoma, Burkitt lymphoma.
2.) Multiple myeloma.
3.) Leukemias: chronic lymphocytic leukemia, chronic granulocytic leukemia (it is usually ineffective in acute blastic crisis), acute myelogenous and monocytic leukemia, acute lymphoblastic (stem cell) leukemia in children (cyclophosphamide given during remission is effective in prolonging its duration).
4.) Mycosis fungoides (advanced disease).
5.) Neuroblastoma (disseminated disease).
6.) Adenocarcinoma of the ovary.
7.) Retinoblastoma.
8.) Carcinoma of the breast.

➤*Nephrotic syndrome in children:* Cyclophosphamide is useful in carefully selected cases of biopsy-proven "minimal change" nephrotic syndrome in children but should not be used as primary therapy. In children whose disease fails to respond adequately to appropriate adrenocorticosteroid therapy or in whom the adrenocorticosteroid therapy produces or threatens to produce intolerable adverse effects, cyclophosphamide may induce a remission. Cyclophosphamide is not indicated for nephrotic syndrome in adults or for any other renal disease.

➤*Off-label uses:*

Multiple sclerosis – [4] = Insufficient documentation. Cyclophosphamide has been studied for the treatment of multiple sclerosis (MS) for several decades in varying dosing regimens. Currently available data and consensus guidelines state that pulse cyclophosphamide therapy has no effect on altering the course of disease. Cyclophosphamide use is not without potentially significant safety concerns. Until additional data are available, use of cyclophosphamide in patients with MS is discouraged.

Rheumatoid arthritis – [3] = Safety concerns. Data evaluating the safety and efficacy of cyclophosphamide for the treatment of rheumatoid arthritis (RA) are dated and show inconsistent efficacy results. Because of concerns with safety and the availability of alternative agents, its use is not recommended for the treatment of RA.

Other possible off-label uses – Cyclophosphamide has been used for bronchogenic, small cell lung, endometrial, prostate, and testicular carcinomas; sarcomas; hematopoietic stem cell transplantation (see Administration and Dosage); systemic lupus erythematosus (see Administration and Dosage); vasculitis and other autoimmune diseases; and Wegener granulomatosis (see Administration and Dosage).

Administration and Dosage

➤*General dosing considerations:* Many other regimens of cyclophosphamide have been reported.

Cyclophosphamide is dosed in mg/kg for some indications, but may be dosed in mg/m^2 for other indications.

➤*Adults:*

Malignancies –

Usual dosage: 1 to 5 mg/kg/day for initial and maintenance dosing.

Dosage adjustment: Dosages must be adjusted in accordance with evidence of antitumor activity and/or leukopenia. The total leukocyte count is a good objective guide for regulating dosage. Transient decreases in the total white blood cell count to 2,000 cells/mm^3 (following short courses) or more persistent reduction to 3,000 cells/mm^3 (with continuing therapy) are tolerated without serious risk of infection if there is no marked granulocytopenia.

When used in combined cytotoxic regimens, it may be necessary to reduce the cyclophosphamide dose as well as that of the other drugs.

Off-label dosing –

Malignancies: Dosage regimens that include cyclophosphamide are too numerous to list. Refer to individual protocols. Usual oral dose ranges from 60 to 120 mg/m^2/day for initial and maintenance therapy.

Multiple sclerosis: [4] = Insufficient documentation. Dosing regimens and routes used in studies varied considerably; consult primary literature.

Rheumatoid arthritis: [3] = Safety concerns. 50 to 150 mg daily or 1 to 3.5 mg/kg daily for up to 1 year.

Systemic lupus erythematosus: One suggested dosage regimen is 1.5 to 3 mg/kg daily. Cyclophosphamide was used with glucocorticoids in the trials showing efficacy.

Wegener granulomatosis: Oral cyclophosphamide 2 mg/kg daily plus glucocorticoids has been shown to be an effective treatment. Monitor leukocyte count closely and adjust cyclophosphamide dosage in order to maintain leukocyte count above 3,000 cells/mm^3. After induction of complete remission, cyclophosphamide has been continued for 1 year and then gradually tapered and discontinued thereafter.

➤*Children:*

Malignant diseases – See Adults for dosing.

Nephrotic syndrome –

Usual dosage: 2.5 to 3 mg/kg/day.

Duration of therapy: 60 to 90 days. In men, the incidence of oligospermia and azoospermia increases if the duration of cyclophosphamide treatment exceeds 60 days. Treatment beyond 90 days increases the probability of sterility.

Concomitant therapy: Adrenocorticosteroid therapy may be tapered and discontinued during the course of cyclophosphamide therapy.

Off-label dosing –

Malignancies: See Adults for off-label dosing.

➤*Renal function impairment:* Dosage reduction to 75% of the usual dosage may be necessary in patients with severe renal failure (creatinine clearance, 0 to 10 mL/min).

Dialysis – Conventional hemodialysis is moderately effective (50% to 74%) in removing cyclophosphamide.

After hemodialysis, some health care providers recommend supplementing with 50% of the original dose.

➤*Hepatic function impairment:* Dosage adjustment is necessary in patients with hepatic dysfunction, as shown in the following table.

Cyclophosphamide Empiric Dosage Reductions for Hepatic Dysfunction	
Liver function tests	Percentage of dose
Bilirubin level 3.1 to 5 mg/dL or AST > 180 units/L	75%
Bilirubin level > 5 mg/dL	Do not give

➤*Concomitant therapy:* When cyclophosphamide is included in combined cytotoxic regimens, it may be necessary to reduce the dose of cyclophosphamide as well as that of the other drugs.

Concomitant treatment with mesna (a uroprotectant) may be required to prevent hemorrhagic cystitis in patients receiving higher doses of cyclophosphamide. Mesna prophylaxis should be considered when cyclophosphamide doses of more than 1,000 mg/m^2 are administered.

➤*Hydration:* Vigorous hydration and frequent urination reduces the risk of hemorrhagic cystitis. Patients may be hydrated with 1.5 to 2 L of fluids for 3 hours prior to cyclophosphamide to ensure adequate urine output. Patients should be encouraged to drink extra fluids (especially water) during the 24 hours following administration to maintain urine output.

➤*Preparation for administration:* Cyclophosphamide is considered a cytotoxic agent. Follow safe handling procedures when preparing, administering, or dispensing cyclophosphamide.

To minimize the risk of dermal exposure, always wear impervious gloves when handling bottles containing cyclophosphamide tablets. This includes all handling activities in clinical settings, pharmacies, storerooms, and home health care settings, including during unpacking and inspection, transportation within a facility, and dose preparation and administration.

➤*Administration:* Oral tablets should be taken on an empty stomach.

➤*Storage / Stability:* Store at or below 25°C (77°F); tablets will withstand brief exposure to temperatures of up to 30°C (86°F), but should be protected from temperatures higher than 30°C (86°F).

Actions

➤*Pharmacology:* Cyclophosphamide is a synthetic antineoplastic drug chemically related to the nitrogen mustards. Cyclophosphamide metabolites interfere with the growth of susceptible rapidly proliferating malignant cells. The mechanism of action is thought to involve cross-linking of tumor cell DNA.

➤*Pharmacokinetics:*

Absorption / Distribution – Cyclophosphamide is well absorbed after oral administration with a bioavailability greater than 75%. Plasma protein binding of unchanged drug is low but some metabolites are bound to an extent greater than 60%.

Metabolism / Excretion – Cyclophosphamide is biotransformed principally in the liver to active alkylating metabolites by a mixed function microsomal oxidase system. The unchanged drug has an elimination half-life of 3 to 12 hours. It is eliminated primarily in the form of metabolites, but from 5% to 25% of the dose is excreted in urine as unchanged drug. Several cytotoxic and noncytotoxic metabolites have been identified in urine and in plasma. Concentrations of metabolites reach a maximum in plasma 2 to

CYCLOPHOSPHAMIDE — ORAL

3 hours after an intravenous (IV) dose. It has not been demonstrated that any single metabolite is responsible for the therapeutic or toxic effects of cyclophosphamide.

Special populations –

Renal function impairment: Although elevated levels of metabolites of cyclophosphamide have been observed in patients with renal failure, increased clinical toxicity in such patients has not been demonstrated.

Contraindications

Continued use in severely depressed bone marrow function; hypersensitivity to cyclophosphamide.

Warnings/Precautions

➤*Urinary system:* Hemorrhagic cystitis may develop in patients treated with cyclophosphamide. Rarely, this condition can be severe and even fatal. Fibrosis of the urinary bladder, sometimes extensive, also may develop with or without accompanying cystitis. Atypical urinary bladder epithelial cells may appear in the urine. These adverse effects appear to depend on the dose of cyclophosphamide and the duration of therapy. Such bladder injury is thought to be because of cyclophosphamide metabolites excreted in the urine. Forced fluid intake helps to ensure an ample output of urine, necessitates frequent voiding, and reduces the time the drug remains in the bladder. This helps to prevent cystitis. Hematuria usually resolves in a few days after cyclophosphamide treatment is stopped, but it may persist. Medical and/or surgical supportive treatment may be required, rarely, to treat protracted cases of severe hemorrhagic cystitis. It is usually necessary to discontinue cyclophosphamide therapy in instances of severe hemorrhagic cystitis.

➤*Cardiac toxicity:* Although a few instances of cardiac dysfunction have been reported following the use of the recommended dose of cyclophosphamide, no causal relationship has been established. Acute cardiac toxicity has been reported with doses as low as 2.4 g/m^2 to as high as 26 g/m^2, usually as a portion of an intensive antineoplastic multidrug regimen or in conjunction with transplantation procedures. In a few instances with high doses of cyclophosphamide, severe, and sometimes fatal, congestive heart failure has occurred after the first cyclophosphamide dose. Histopathologic examination has primarily shown hemorrhagic myocarditis. Hemopericardium has occurred secondary to hemorrhagic myocarditis and myocardial necrosis. Pericarditis has been reported independent of any hemopericardium.

No residual cardiac abnormalities, as evidenced by electrocardiogram or echocardiogram, appear to be present in patients surviving episodes of apparent cardiac toxicity associated with high doses of cyclophosphamide.

➤*Immunosuppression:* Treatment with cyclophosphamide may cause significant suppression of immune response. Serious, sometimes fatal, infections may develop in severely immunosuppressed patients. Cyclophosphamide treatment may not be indicated, or should be interrupted, or the dose reduced, in patients who have or develop viral, bacterial, fungal, protozoan, or helminthic infections.

➤*Adrenalectomy:* Because cyclophosphamide has been reported to be more toxic in adrenalectomized dogs, adjustment of the doses of both replacement steroids and cyclophosphamide may be necessary for adrenalectomized patients.

➤*Wound healing:* Cyclophosphamide may interfere with normal wound healing.

➤*Reproductive and hormonal effects:* Amenorrhea associated with decreased estrogen and increased gonadotropin secretion develops in a significant proportion of women treated with cyclophosphamide. Affected patients generally resume regular menses within a few months after cessation of therapy. Girls treated with cyclophosphamide during prepubescence generally develop secondary sexual characteristics normally and have regular menses. Ovarian fibrosis with apparently complete loss of germ cells after prolonged cyclophosphamide treatment in late prepubescence has been reported. Girls treated with cyclophosphamide during prepubescence subsequently have conceived.

Men treated with cyclophosphamide may develop oligospermia or azoospermia associated with increased gonadotropin but normal testosterone secretion. Sexual potency and libido are unimpaired in these patients. Boys treated with cyclophosphamide during prepubescence develop secondary sexual characteristics normally, but may have oligospermia or azoospermia and increased gonadotropin secretion. Some degree of testicular atrophy may occur. Cyclophosphamide-induced azoospermia is reversible in some patients, though the reversibility may not occur for several years after cessation of therapy. Men temporarily rendered sterile by cyclophosphamide have subsequently fathered healthy children.

➤*Hypersensitivity reactions:* Anaphylactic reactions have been reported; death has also been reported in association with this event. Possible cross-sensitivity with other alkylating agents has been reported.

➤*Special risk:* Exercise special attention to the possible development of toxicity in patients being treated with cyclophosphamide if any of the following conditions are present: leukopenia, thrombocytopenia, tumor cell infiltration of bone marrow, previous radiation therapy, previous therapy with other cytotoxic agents, impaired hepatic function, or impaired renal function.

➤*Pregnancy: Category D.* Cyclophosphamide is contraindicated during the first trimester of pregnancy. Cyclophosphamide can cause fetal harm when administered to pregnant women, and such abnormalities have been reported following cyclophosphamide therapy in pregnant women. Abnormalities were found in 2 infants and a fetus 6 months of age born to women treated with cyclophosphamide. Ectrodactylia was found in 2 of the 3 cases. There have been other case reports in which newborns exposed in utero to cyclophosphamide or its metabolites have developed various abnormalities. In many instances, cyclophosphamide was given in combination with other agents of radiation. The authors of 1 study thought that cyclophosphamide is a human teratogen and that a distinct phenotype exists. Healthy infants have also been born to women treated with cyclophosphamide during pregnancy, including the first trimester. If this drug is used during pregnancy, or if the patient becomes pregnant while taking (receiving) this drug, apprise the patient of the potential hazard to the fetus. Advise women of childbearing potential to avoid becoming pregnant.

➤*Lactation:* Cyclophosphamide is excreted in breast milk and is contraindicated in breast-feeding. The American Academy of Pediatrics classified cyclophosphamide as a drug that may interfere with cellular metabolism of the breast-feeding infant. Because of the reported cases of neutropenia and thrombocytopenia and the potential for adverse effects relating to immune suppression, growth, and carcinogenesis, advise women receiving this drug not to breast-feed.

➤*Children:* The safety profile of cyclophosphamide in children is similar to that of the adult population.

➤*Elderly:* Subset analyses (younger than 65 years of age vs older than 65 years of age) from these trials, published reports of clinical trials of cyclophosphamide-containing regimens in breast cancer and non-Hodgkin lymphoma, and postmarketing experience suggest that elderly patients may be more susceptible to cyclophosphamide toxicities. In general, be cautious in dose selection for an elderly patient, usually starting at the low end of the dosing range and adjusting as necessary based on patient response.

➤*Monitoring:* During treatment, regularly monitor the patient's hematologic profile (particularly neutrophils and platelets) to determine the degree of hematopoietic suppression. Examine urine regularly for red cells, which may precede hemorrhagic cystitis.

Drug Interactions

Be alert for possible combined drug actions, desirable or undesirable, involving cyclophosphamide, even though cyclophosphamide has been used successfully concurrently with other drugs, including other cytotoxic drugs.

➤*General anesthesia:* If a patient has been treated with cyclophosphamide within 10 days of general anesthesia, alert the anesthesiologist.

➤*Adrenalectomy:* Adjustment of the doses of both replacement steroids and cyclophosphamide may be necessary for the adrenalectomized patient.

Cyclophosphamide Drug Interactions

Precipitant drug	Object drug[a]		Description
Allopurinol	Cyclophosphamide	⬆	The myelosuppressive effects of cyclophosphamide may be enhanced, possibly increasing the risk of bleeding or infection. Monitor hematologic function. If an interaction is suspected, it may be necessary to discontinue allopurinol.
Azole antifungal agents (eg, itraconazole)	Cyclophosphamide	⬆	Exposure to cyclophosphamide and its metabolites may be increased, increasing the risk of adverse reactions. Closely monitor for cyclophosphamide adverse reactions.
Carbamazepine	Cyclophosphamide	⬆	Cyclophosphamide plasma concentrations may be elevated, increasing the pharmacologic effects and risk of toxicity. Careful laboratory and clinical monitoring is indicated during coadministration of carbamazepine. Adjust the cyclophosphamide dose as needed to minimize toxicity. Alternatively, use of anticonvulsants that do not influence CYP-450[b] (eg, gabapentin, levetiracetam, valproic acid) may be acceptable alternatives to carbamazepine.
Chloramphenicol	Cyclophosphamide	⬇	Cyclophosphamide half-life may be increased and metabolite concentrations may be decreased. Use an alternative antibiotic if possible.

CYCLOPHOSPHAMIDE — ORAL

Cyclophosphamide Drug Interactions

Precipitant drug	Object drug[a]		Description
Hydantoins (eg, phenytoin)	Cyclophosphamide	↑	Exposure to the active metabolite of cyclophosphamide may be increased; the risk of toxicity may be increased. If administration of hydantoins cannot be avoided, consider reducing the initial dose of cyclophosphamide and monitoring the concentration of the 4-hydroxycyclophosphamide metabolite as a guide to cyclophosphamide dosing. Valproic acid derivatives or gabapentin may be alternatives to the use of hydantoins.
Pentostatin	Cyclophosphamide	↑	Additive or synergistic toxicity. Respiratory distress, hypotension, hypothermia, confusion, and death may occur after coadministration of pentostatin and cyclophosphamide. Avoid coadministration if possible.
Cyclophosphamide	Pentostatin		
Phenobarbital	Cyclophosphamide	↓	The rate of metabolism and the leukopenic activity of cyclophosphamide reportedly are increased by long-term administration of high doses of phenobarbital.
Thiazide diuretics	Cyclophosphamide[c]	↑	Antineoplastic-induced leukopenia may be prolonged. Monitor hematologic function. Use with caution.
TNF[b] blocking agents (eg, etanercept)	Cyclophosphamide	↑	The incidence of noncutaneous solid malignancies may be increased in patients receiving TNF blocking agents with cyclophosphamide. Coadministration is not recommended.
Cyclophosphamide	Anticoagulants (eg, warfarin)	↑	Anticoagulant effect is increased. Monitor coagulation parameters during and after cyclophosphamide therapy. Adjust the warfarin dose as needed.
Cyclophosphamide	Digoxin	↓	Digoxin serum levels may be reduced. Monitor digoxin serum concentrations and the clinical response of the patient. Adjust the digoxin dose as needed.
Cyclophosphamide	Doxorubicin	↑	Doxorubicin-induced cardiotoxicity is potentiated. Use with caution. Monitor for symptoms of cardiotoxicity.
Cyclophosphamide	Quinolones (eg, ciprofloxacin)	↓	The antimicrobial effects of quinolones may be decreased. Monitor the clinical response of the patient and adjust the quinolone dose as needed.
Cyclophosphamide	Succinylcholine	↑	Neuromuscular blockade may be prolonged because of inhibition of cholinesterase activity. Prolonged respiratory depression with extended periods of apnea may occur. Use with caution. If this combination is used, prior measurement of plasma cholinesterase activity with close monitoring of neuromuscular function and appropriate adjustment of succinylcholine dosage is recommended.
Cyclophosphamide	Trastuzumab	↑	The risk of trastuzumab-induced cardiac dysfunction may be increased by coadministration of cyclophosphamide. Close clinical monitoring for signs of cardiac dysfunction is indicated when trastuzumab and cyclophosphamide are coadministered.
Cyclophosphamide	Vaccines, live	↑	The risk of live vaccine–induced adverse reactions may be increased by coadministration of cyclophosphamide. Defer the use of live vaccines in patients receiving cyclophosphamide.

[a] ↑ = object drug increased; ↓ = object drug decreased.
[b] CYP-450 = cytochrome P450; TNF = tumor necrosis factor.
[c] Cyclophosphamide used in combination with other antineoplastics.

Adverse Reactions

The adverse reactions are listed in order of decreasing incidence.

➤*Emetogenic potential:* Cyclophosphamide IV in doses of at least 1,500 mg/m^2 is considered to have very high emetogenic potential (more than 90% incidence of emesis). Cyclophosphamide IV in doses of 750 to 1,500 mg/m^2 is considered to have moderately high emetogenic potential (60% to 90% incidence of emesis). Cyclophosphamide taken orally or in IV doses of 750 mg/m^2 or less is considered to have moderate emetogenic potential (30% to 60% incidence of emesis).

➤*Dermatologic:* Alopecia occurs commonly in patients treated with cyclophosphamide. The hair can be expected to grow back after treatment with the drug or even during continued drug treatment, though it may be different in texture or color. Skin rash occurs occasionally in patients receiving the drug. Pigmentation of the skin and changes in nails can occur. Very rare reports of Stevens-Johnson syndrome and toxic epidermal necrolysis have been received during postmarketing surveillance. Because of the nature of spontaneous adverse reaction reporting, a definitive causal relationship to cyclophosphamide has not been established.

➤*GI:* Nausea and vomiting commonly occur with cyclophosphamide therapy. Anorexia and, less frequently, abdominal discomfort or pain and diarrhea may occur. There are isolated reports of hemorrhagic colitis, oral mucosal ulceration, and jaundice occurring during therapy. These adverse drug effects generally remit when cyclophosphamide treatment is stopped.

➤*GU:* Hemorrhagic cystitis may develop in patients treated with cyclophosphamide. Rarely, this condition can be severe and even fatal. Fibrosis of the urinary bladder, sometimes extensive, also may develop with or without accompanying cystitis. Atypical urinary bladder epithelial cells may appear in the urine. These adverse effects appear to depend on the dose of cyclophosphamide and the duration of therapy. Such bladder injury is thought to be due to cyclophosphamide metabolites excreted in the urine. Forced fluid intake helps to ensure an ample output of urine, necessitates frequent voiding, and reduces the time the drug remains in the bladder. This helps to prevent cystitis. Hematuria usually resolves in a few days after cyclophosphamide treatment is stopped, but it may persist (see also Warnings/Precautions).

Hemorrhagic ureteritis and renal tubular necrosis have been reported to occur in patients treated with cyclophosphamide. Such lesions usually resolve following cessation of therapy.

Cyclophosphamide interferes with oogenesis and spermatogenesis. It may cause sterility in both sexes. Amenorrhea associated with decreased estrogen and increased gonadotropin secretion develops in a significant proportion of women treated with cyclophosphamide. Affected patients generally resume regular menses within a few months after cessation of therapy. Ovarian fibrosis with apparently complete loss of germ cells after prolonged cyclophosphamide treatment in late prepubescence has been reported. Men treated with cyclophosphamide may develop oligospermia or azoospermia associated with increased gonadotropin but normal testosterone secretion. Some degree of testicular atrophy may occur. Cyclophosphamide-induced azoospermia is reversible in some patients, though the reversibility may not occur for several years after cessation of therapy (see also Warnings/Precautions).

➤*Hematologic:* Leukopenia occurs in patients treated with cyclophosphamide and is related to the dose of drug and can be used as a dosage guide. Leukopenia of less than 2,000 cells/mm^3 develops commonly in patients treated with an initial loading dose of the drug and less frequently in patients maintained on smaller doses. The degree of neutropenia is particularly important because it correlates with a reduction in resistance to infections. Fever without documented infection has been reported in neutropenic patients.

Thrombocytopenia or anemia develop occasionally in patients treated with cyclophosphamide. These hematologic effects usually can be reversed by reducing the drug dose or by interrupting treatment. Recovery from leukopenia usually begins 7 to 10 days after cessation of therapy.

➤*Hypersensitivity:* Anaphylactic reactions have been reported; death has also been reported in association with this reaction. Possible cross-sensitivity with other alkylating agents has been reported.

➤*Respiratory:* Interstitial pneumonitis has been reported as part of the postmarketing experience. Interstitial pulmonary fibrosis has been reported in patients receiving high doses of cyclophosphamide over a prolonged period.

➤*Miscellaneous:* Syndrome of inappropriate antidiuretic hormone secretion has been reported with use of cyclophosphamide. Malaise and asthenia have been reported as part of the postmarketing experience.

CYCLOPHOSPHAMIDE — ORAL

Overdosage

➤*Treatment:* No specific antidote for cyclophosphamide overdosage is known. Manage overdosage with supportive measures, including appropriate treatment for any concurrent infection, myelosuppression, or cardiac toxicity if it occurs.

Patient Information

Inform patient that cyclophosphamide may cause irreversible sterility in both sexes.

Advise female patients that cyclophosphamide may cause fetal harm and is contraindicated during the first trimester. The use of birth control is recommended.

Advise women that cyclophosphamide is excreted in breast milk and is, therefore, contraindicated with breast-feeding.

Instruct patients to drink extra fluids and void frequently.

CYCLOPHOSPHAMIDE — INJECTION

Indications

➤*Malignant diseases:* Cyclophosphamide, although effective alone in susceptible malignancies, is more frequently used concurrently or sequentially with other antineoplastic drugs. The following malignancies are often susceptible to cyclophosphamide treatment:

1.) Malignant lymphomas (stages III and IV of the Ann Arbor staging system), Hodgkin disease, lymphocytic lymphoma (nodular or diffuse), mixed-cell type lymphoma, histiocytic lymphoma, Burkitt lymphoma.
2.) Multiple myeloma.
3.) Leukemias: chronic lymphocytic leukemia, chronic granulocytic leukemia (it is usually ineffective in acute blastic crisis), acute myelogenous and monocytic leukemia, acute lymphoblastic (stem cell) leukemia in children (cyclophosphamide given during remission is effective in prolonging its duration).
4.) Mycosis fungoides (advanced disease).
5.) Neuroblastoma (disseminated disease).
6.) Adenocarcinoma of the ovary.
7.) Retinoblastoma.
8.) Carcinoma of the breast.

➤*Nephrotic syndrome in children:* Cyclophosphamide is useful in carefully selected cases of biopsy-proven "minimal change" nephrotic syndrome in children, but should not be used as primary therapy. In children whose disease fails to respond to appropriate adrenocorticosteroid therapy or in whom the adrenocorticosteroid therapy produces or threatens to produce intolerable adverse effects, cyclophosphamide may induce a remission. Cyclophosphamide is not indicated for nephrotic syndrome in adults or for any other renal disease.

➤*Off-label uses:*

Juvenile idiopathic arthritis – [4] = Insufficient documentation. Data evaluating the safety and efficacy of IV cyclophosphamide for the treatment of juvenile idiopathic arthritis (JIA) are limited to a small open-label study and a few case reports in a limited number of patients. In all reports, IV cyclophosphamide was administered in combination with IV methylprednisolone as pulse therapy given every 1 to 3 months. While the reports show promise, there are concerns with potential long-term toxicity. For this reason, use should only be considered in patients who are refractory to other treatment options. Currently, there are no national guidelines for the management of JIA.

Other possible off-label uses – Cyclophosphamide has been used for bronchogenic, small cell lung, endometrial, prostate, and testicular carcinomas; sarcomas; hematopoietic stem cell transplantation (HSCT) (see Administration and Dosage); systemic lupus erythematosus (see Administration and Dosage), vasculitis, rheumatoid arthritis, and other autoimmune diseases; and Wegener granulomatosis (see Administration and Dosage).

Administration and Dosage

➤*General dosing considerations:* Many other regimens of cyclophosphamide have been reported.

Cyclophosphamide is dosed in mg/kg for some indications but may be dosed in mg/m^2 for other indications.

➤*Adults:*

Malignancies – For a list of malignancies, see Indications. See also Off-Label Dosing.

Initial dosage: 40 to 50 mg/kg intravenously (IV) in divided doses over a period of 2 to 5 days when given as the only oncolytic for patients with no hematologic deficiency.

In myelosuppressed patients, reduce initial dose by 33% to 50%.

Alternate dosage: 10 to 15 mg/kg IV 7 to 10 days or 3 to 5 mg/kg twice weekly.

Dosage adjustment: Dosages must be adjusted in accordance with evidence of antitumor activity and/or leukopenia. The total leukocyte count is a good objective guide for regulating dosage. Transient decreases in the total white blood cell count to 2,000 cells/mm^3 (following short courses) or more persistent reduction to 3,000 cells/mm^3 (with continuing therapy) are tolerated without serious risk of infection if there is no marked granulocytopenia.

When used in combined cytotoxic regimens, it may be necessary to reduce the cyclophosphamide dose as well as that of the other drugs.

Off-label dosing –

Hematopoietic stem cell transplantation: 120 to 200 mg/kg IV in divided doses (50 mg/kg/day for 4 doses or 60 mg/kg/day for 2 doses) in combination with other drugs has been used in HSCT conditioning. Doses as high as 7,200 mg/m^2 have been used.

For pretransplant conditioning ("priming") before autologous HSCT, cyclophosphamide 3,000 to 4,000 mg/m^2 IV as a single dose has been used alone or in combination with other drugs.

Malignancies: Dosage regimens that include cyclophosphamide are too numerous to list. Refer to individual protocols. Usual oral dose ranges from 500 to 1,500 mg/m^2/day per course of therapy.

Multiple sclerosis: [4] = Insufficient documentation. When used IV, cyclophosphamide has been given in induction regimens over a 2- to 3-week period. Examples of IV doses used include the following: 200 mg daily for 4 to 6 weeks, 100 to 300 mg daily for 16 to 33 days, 4 to 5 mg/kg/day for 10 days, and 400 to 800 mg/m^2 monthly. It has also been studied as pulse therapy, the most common way it used in clinical practice.

Systemic lupus erythematosus: One suggested dosage regimen is 7 to 25 mg/kg IV once monthly for 6 months. Consider concomitant therapy with mesna. Cyclophosphamide was used with glucocorticoids in the trials showing efficacy.

Wegener granulomatosis: The use of cyclophosphamide as an intermittent bolus injection (1 g/m^2 per month) has been used. However, some health care providers recommend the use of oral cyclophosphamide because of the increased rate of relapse that has been seen with bolus cyclophosphamide therapy.

➤*Children:*

Malignant diseases – See Adults for dosing.

Nephrotic syndrome – See the Cyclophosphamide Oral monograph for dosing.

Off-label dosing –

Juvenile idiopathic arthritis: [4] = Insufficient documentation. For children 2 to 17 years of age with refractory JIA, the most common pulse therapy dosages were cyclophosphamide 500 to 1,000 mg/kg IV in combination with methylprednisolone 30 mg/kg IV (maximum dose, 1,000 mg). Pulses ranged from once monthly to once every 3 months. Many patients also received methotrexate (oral or subcutaneous) weekly, and some also received oral prednisone and nonsteroidal anti-inflammatory drugs (NSAIDs). Therapy continued for up to 1 year in some reports.

Malignancies: See Adults for off-label dosing.

Neuroblastoma: 3,000 mg/m^2/day IV for 2 days or 2,000 mg/m^2/day for 3 consecutive days.

Hematopoietic stem cell transplantation: 150 to 200 mg/kg IV in divided doses (50 mg/kg/day for 3 to 4 doses) in combination with other drugs has been used in HSCT conditioning.

➤*Renal function impairment:* Dosage reduction to 75% of the usual dosage may be necessary in patients with severe renal failure (creatinine clearance, 0 to 10 mL/min).

Dialysis – Conventional hemodialysis is moderately effective (50% to 74%) in removing cyclophosphamide.

After hemodialysis, some health care providers recommend supplementing with 50% of the original dose.

➤*Hepatic function impairment:* Dosage adjustment is necessary in hepatic dysfunction, as shown in the following table.

Cyclophosphamide Empiric Dosage Reductions for Hepatic Dysfunction	
Liver function tests	Percentage of dose
Bilirubin level 3.1 to 5 mg/dL or AST > 180 units/L	75%
Bilirubin level > 5 mg/dL	Do not give

➤*Concomitant therapy:* When cyclophosphamide is included in combined cytotoxic regimens, it may be necessary to reduce the dose of cyclophosphamide as well as that of the other drugs.

Concomitant treatment with mesna (a uroprotectant) may be required to prevent hemorrhagic cystitis in patients receiving higher doses of cyclophosphamide. Mesna prophylaxis should be considered when cyclophosphamide doses of more than 1,000 mg/m^2 are administered.

➤*Hydration:* Vigorous hydration and frequent urination reduces the risk of hemorrhagic cystitis. Patients may be hydrated with 1.5 to 2 L of fluids for 3 hours prior to cyclophosphamide to ensure adequate urine output. Patients should be encouraged to drink extra fluids (especially water) during the 24 hours following administration to maintain urine output.

➤*Preparation for administration:* Cyclophosphamide is considered a cytotoxic agent. Follow safe handling procedures when preparing, administering, or dispensing cyclophosphamide.

The maximum concentration of cyclophosphamide for IV infusion is 20 mg/mL.

Cyclophosphamide should be prepared by adding sodium chloride 0.9% injection if injected directly.

Cyclophosphamide should be prepared by adding sterile water for injection if administered by infusion.

CYCLOPHOSPHAMIDE — INJECTION

Cyclophosphamide, reconstituted in water, is hypotonic and should not be injected directly.

Add the diluent to the vial and shake vigorously to dissolve. If the powder fails to dissolve immediately and completely, allow the vial to stand for a few minutes. Use the quantity of diluent shown in the following table to reconstitute the product to give a 20 mg/mL final concentration.

Reconstitution of Cyclophosphamide Injection

Vial size	Volume of diluent
500 mg	25 mL
1 g	50 mL
2 g	100 mL

Solutions reconstituted with sodium chloride 0.9% injection are isotonic (osmolarity 374 mOsm/L) and may be injected IV, intramuscularly (IM), intraperitoneally, or intrapleurally, or may be infused IV in the following: dextrose 5% injection, dextrose 5%/sodium chloride 0.9% injection, Ringer's/dextrose 5% injection, Ringer's lactate injection, sodium chloride 0.45% injection, or 1/6 Molar sodium lactate injection.

Solutions reconstituted with sterile water for injection are hypotonic (osmolarity 74 mOsm/L) and must be further diluted with dextrose 5% injection, dextrose 5%/sodium chloride 0.9% injection, Ringer's/dextrose 5% injection, Ringer's lactate injection, sodium chloride 0.45% injection, or 1/6 molar sodium lactate injection.

For use in HSCT regimens (off-label use), reconstitute powder with sterile water for injection. The reconstituted 20 mg/mL solution may be infused without further dilution.

➤*Administration:* Solutions of cyclophosphamide may be administered by IV injection, IV infusion (over 1 to 2 hours), IM, intraperitoneally, or intrapleurally. See Preparation for Administration for more information.

➤*Storage/Stability:* Store at or below 25°C (77°F). During transport or storage of cyclophosphamide vials, temperature influences can lead to melting of cyclophosphamide. Vials containing melted substance can be visually differentiated. Melted cyclophosphamide is a clear or yellowish viscous liquid usually found as a connected phase or in droplets in the affected vials. Do not use cyclophosphamide vials if there are signs of melting.

Solutions for injection are stable for 24 hours at room temperature or up to 6 days under refrigeration. However, reconstituted solutions are preservative free and should be used within 24 hours.

Discard vial within 6 hours of the initial needle puncture if opened within an ISO class 5 biological safety cabinet, or within 1 hour of the initial needle puncture if opened outside of such an environment, based on the USP < 797 > standards.

Actions

➤*Pharmacology:* Cyclophosphamide is a synthetic antineoplastic drug chemically related to the nitrogen mustards. Cyclophosphamide metabolites interfere with the growth of susceptible rapidly proliferating malignant cells. The mechanism of action is thought to involve cross-linking of tumor cell DNA.

➤*Pharmacokinetics:*

Distribution – Plasma protein binding of unchanged drug is low, but some metabolites are bound to an extent greater than 60%.

Metabolism/Excretion – Cyclophosphamide is biotransformed principally in the liver to active alkylating metabolites by a mixed-function microsomal oxidase system. The unchanged drug has an elimination half-life of 3 to 12 hours. It is eliminated primarily in the form of metabolites, but 5% to 25% of the dose is excreted in urine as unchanged drug. Several cytotoxic and noncytotoxic metabolites have been identified in urine and in plasma. Concentrations of metabolites reach a maximum in plasma 2 to 3 hours after an IV dose. It has not been demonstrated that any single metabolite is responsible for the therapeutic or toxic effects of cyclophosphamide.

Special populations –

Renal function impairment: Although elevated levels of metabolites of cyclophosphamide have been observed in patients with renal failure, increased clinical toxicity in such patients has not been demonstrated.

Contraindications

Continued use in severely depressed bone marrow function, hypersensitivity to cyclophosphamide.

Warnings/Precautions

➤*Urinary system:* Hemorrhagic cystitis may develop in patients treated with cyclophosphamide. Rarely, this condition can be severe and even fatal. Fibrosis of the urinary bladder, sometimes extensive, also may develop with or without accompanying cystitis. Atypical urinary bladder epithelial cells may appear in the urine. These adverse effects appear to depend on the dose of cyclophosphamide and the duration of therapy. Such bladder injury is thought to be because of cyclophosphamide metabolites excreted in the urine. Forced fluid intake helps to ensure an ample output of urine, necessitates frequent voiding, and reduces the time the drug remains in the bladder. This helps to prevent cystitis. Hematuria usually resolves in a few days after cyclophosphamide treatment is stopped, but it may persist. Medical and/or surgical supportive treatment may be required, rarely, to treat protracted cases of severe hemorrhagic cystitis. It is usually necessary to discontinue cyclophosphamide therapy in instances of severe hemorrhagic cystitis.

➤*Cardiac toxicity:* Although a few instances of cardiac dysfunction have been reported following use of the recommended dose of cyclophosphamide, no causal relationship has been established. Acute cardiac toxicity has been reported with doses as low as 2.4 g/m^2 to as high as 26 g/m^2, usually as a portion of an intensive antineoplastic multidrug regimen or in conjunction with transplantation procedures. In a few instances with high doses of cyclophosphamide, severe, and sometimes fatal, congestive heart failure has occurred after the first cyclophosphamide dose. Histopathologic examination has primarily shown hemorrhagic myocarditis. Hemopericardium has occurred secondary to hemorrhagic myocarditis and myocardial necrosis. Pericarditis has been reported independent of any hemopericardium.

No residual cardiac abnormalities, as evidenced by electrocardiogram or echocardiogram, appear to be present in patients surviving episodes of apparent cardiac toxicity associated with high doses of cyclophosphamide.

➤*Immunosuppression:* Treatment with cyclophosphamide may cause significant suppression of immune response. Serious, sometimes fatal, infections may develop in severely immunosuppressed patients. Cyclophosphamide treatment may not be indicated, or should be interrupted or the dose reduced, in patients who have or who develop viral, bacterial, fungal, protozoan, or helminthic infections.

➤*Adrenalectomy:* Because cyclophosphamide has been reported to be more toxic in adrenalectomized dogs, adjustment of the doses of both replacement steroids and cyclophosphamide may be necessary for adrenalectomized patients.

➤*Wound healing:* Cyclophosphamide may interfere with normal wound healing.

➤*Reproductive and hormonal effects:* Amenorrhea associated with decreased estrogen and increased gonadotropin secretion develops in a significant proportion of women treated with cyclophosphamide. Affected patients generally resume regular menses within a few months after cessation of therapy. Girls treated with cyclophosphamide during prepubescence generally develop secondary sexual characteristics normally and have regular menses. Ovarian fibrosis with apparently complete loss of germ cells after prolonged cyclophosphamide treatment in late prepubescence has been reported. Girls treated with cyclophosphamide during prepubescence subsequently have conceived.

Men treated with cyclophosphamide may develop oligospermia or azoospermia associated with increased gonadotropin but normal testosterone secretion. Sexual potency and libido are unimpaired in these patients. Boys treated with cyclophosphamide during prepubescence develop secondary sexual characteristics normally but may have oligospermia or azoospermia and increased gonadotropin secretion. Some degree of testicular atrophy may occur. Cyclophosphamide-induced azoospermia is reversible in some patients, though the reversibility may not occur for several years after cessation of therapy. Men temporarily rendered sterile by cyclophosphamide have subsequently fathered healthy children.

➤*Hypersensitivity reactions:* Anaphylactic reactions have been reported; death has also been reported in association with this event. Possible cross-sensitivity with other alkylating agents has been reported.

➤*Special risk:* Exercise special attention to the possible development of toxicity in patients being treated with cyclophosphamide if any of the following conditions are present: leukopenia, thrombocytopenia, tumor cell infiltration of bone marrow, previous radiation therapy, previous therapy with other cytotoxic agents, impaired hepatic function, or impaired renal function.

➤*Pregnancy: Category D.* Cyclophosphamide is contraindicated during the first trimester of pregnancy. Cyclophosphamide can cause fetal harm when administered to pregnant women, and such abnormalities have been reported following cyclophosphamide therapy in pregnant women. Abnormalities were found in 2 infants and a fetus 6 months of age born to women treated with cyclophosphamide. Ectrodactylia was found in 2 of the 3 cases. There have been other case reports in which newborns exposed in utero to cyclophosphamide or its metabolites have developed various abnormalities. In many instances, cyclophosphamide was given in combination with other agents of radiation. The authors of 1 study thought that cyclophosphamide is a human teratogen and that a distinct phenotype exists. Healthy infants have also been born to women treated with cyclophosphamide during pregnancy, including the first trimester. If this drug is used during pregnancy, or if the patient becomes pregnant while taking (receiving) this drug, apprise the patient of the potential hazard to the fetus. Advise women of childbearing potential to avoid becoming pregnant.

➤*Lactation:* Cyclophosphamide is excreted in breast milk and is contraindicated in breast-feeding. The American Academy of Pediatrics classified cyclophosphamide as a drug that may interfere with cellular metabolism of the breast-feeding infant. Because of the reported cases of neutropenia and thrombocytopenia and the potential for adverse effects relating to immune suppression, growth, and carcinogenesis, advise women receiving this drug not to breast-feed.

➤*Children:* The safety profile of cyclophosphamide in children is similar to that of the adult population.

➤*Elderly:* Subset analyses (younger than 65 years of age vs older than 65 years of age) from these trials, published reports of clinical trials of cyclophosphamide-containing regimens in breast cancer and non-Hodgkin lymphoma, and postmarketing experience suggest that elderly patients may be more susceptible to cyclophosphamide toxicities. In general, be cautious in dose selection for an elderly patient, usually starting at the low end of the dosing range and adjusting as necessary based on patient response.

CYCLOPHOSPHAMIDE — INJECTION

➤*Monitoring:* During treatment, regularly monitor the patient's hematologic profile (particularly neutrophils and platelets) to determine the degree of hematopoietic suppression. Examine urine regularly for red cells, which may precede hemorrhagic cystitis.

Drug Interactions

Be alert for possible combined drug actions, desirable or undesirable, involving cyclophosphamide, even though cyclophosphamide has been used successfully concurrently with other drugs, including other cytotoxic drugs.

➤*General anesthesia:* If a patient has been treated with cyclophosphamide within 10 days of general anesthesia, alert the anesthesiologist.

➤*Adrenalectomy:* Adjustment of the doses of replacement steroids and cyclophosphamide may be necessary for the adrenalectomized patient.

Cyclophosphamide Drug Interactions

Precipitant drug	Object drug[a]		Description
Allopurinol	Cyclophosphamide	⬆	The myelosuppressive effects of cyclophosphamide may be enhanced, possibly increasing the risk of bleeding or infection. Monitor hematologic function. If an interaction is suspected, it may be necessary to discontinue allopurinol.
Azole antifungal agents (eg, itraconazole)	Cyclophosphamide	⬆	Exposure to cyclophosphamide and its metabolites may be increased, increasing the risk of adverse reactions. Closely monitor for cyclophosphamide adverse reactions.
Carbamazepine	Cyclophosphamide	⬆	Cyclophosphamide plasma concentrations may be elevated, increasing the pharmacologic effects and risk of toxicity. Careful laboratory and clinical monitoring is indicated during coadministration of carbamazepine. Adjust the cyclophosphamide dose as needed to minimize toxicity. Alternatively, use of anticonvulsants that do not influence CYP-450[b] (eg, gabapentin, valproic acid, levetiracetam) may be acceptable alternatives to carbamazepine.
Chloramphenicol	Cyclophosphamide	⬇	Cyclophosphamide half-life may be increased and metabolite concentrations may be decreased. Use an alternative antibiotic if possible.
Hydantoins (eg, phenytoin)	Cyclophosphamide	⬆	Exposure to the active metabolite of cyclophosphamide may be increased; the risk of toxicity may be increased. If administration of hydantoins cannot be avoided, consider reducing the initial dose of cyclophosphamide and monitoring the concentration of the 4-hydroxycyclophosphamide metabolite as a guide to cyclophosphamide dosing. Valproic acid derivatives or gabapentin may be alternatives to the use of hydantoins.
Pentostatin	Cyclophosphamide	⬆	Additive or synergistic toxicity. Respiratory distress, hypotension, hypothermia, confusion, and death may occur after coadministration of pentostatin and cyclophosphamide. Avoid coadministration if possible.
Cyclophosphamide	Pentostatin		
Phenobarbital	Cyclophosphamide	⬇	The rate of metabolism and the leukopenic activity of cyclophosphamide reportedly are increased by chronic administration of high doses of phenobarbital.
Thiazide diuretics	Cyclophosphamide[c]	⬆	Antineoplastic-induced leukopenia may be prolonged. Monitor hematologic function. Use with caution.
TNF[d] blocking agents (eg, etanercept)	Cyclophosphamide	⬆	The incidence of noncutaneous solid malignancies may be increased in patients receiving TNF blocking agents with cyclophosphamide. Coadministration is not recommended.
Cyclophosphamide	Anticoagulants (eg, warfarin)	⬆	Anticoagulant effect is increased. Monitor coagulation parameters during and after cyclophosphamide therapy. Adjust the warfarin dose as needed.
Cyclophosphamide	Digoxin	⬇	Digoxin serum levels may be reduced. Monitor digoxin serum concentrations and the clinical response of the patient. Adjust the digoxin dose as needed.
Cyclophosphamide	Doxorubicin	⬆	Doxorubicin-induced cardiotoxicity is potentiated. Use with caution. Monitor for symptoms of cardiotoxicity.
Cyclophosphamide	Quinolones (eg, ciprofloxacin)	⬇	The antimicrobial effects of quinolones may be decreased. Monitor the clinical response of the patient and adjust the quinolone dose as needed.
Cyclophosphamide	Succinylcholine	⬆	Neuromuscular blockade may be prolonged because of inhibition of cholinesterase activity. Prolonged respiratory depression with extended periods of apnea may occur. Use with caution. If this combination is used, prior measurement of plasma cholinesterase activity with close monitoring of neuromuscular function and appropriate adjustment of succinylcholine dosage is recommended.
Cyclophosphamide	Trastuzumab	⬆	The risk of trastuzumab-induced cardiac dysfunction may be increased by coadministration of cyclophosphamide. Close clinical monitoring for signs of cardiac dysfunction is indicated when trastuzumab and cyclophosphamide are coadministered.
Cyclophosphamide	Vaccines, live	⬆	The risk of live vaccine–induced adverse reactions may be increased by coadministration of cyclophosphamide. Defer the use of live vaccines in patients receiving cyclophosphamide.

[a] ⬆ = object drug increased; ⬇ = object drug decreased.
[b] CYP-450 = cytochrome P450.
[c] Cyclophosphamide used in combination with other antineoplastics.
[d] TNF = tumor necrosis factor.

Adverse Reactions

The adverse reactions are listed in order of decreasing incidence.

➤*Emetogenic potential:* Cyclophosphamide IV in doses of at least 1,500 mg/m^2 is considered to have very high emetogenic potential (over 90% incidence of emesis). Cyclophosphamide IV in doses of 750 to 1,500 mg/m^2 is considered to have moderately high emetogenic potential (60% to 90% incidence of emesis). Cyclophosphamide taken orally or in IV doses of 750 mg/m^2 or less is considered to have moderate emetogenic potential (30% to 60% incidence of emesis).

➤*Dermatologic:* Alopecia commonly occurs in patients treated with cyclophosphamide. Hair can be expected to grow back after treatment with the drug or even during continued drug treatment, though it may be different in texture or color. Skin rash occurs occasionally in patients receiving the drug. Pigmentation of the skin and changes in nails can occur. Very rare reports of Stevens-Johnson syndrome and toxic epidermal necrolysis have been received during postmarketing surveillance; because of the nature of spontaneous adverse reaction reporting, a definitive causal relationship to cyclophosphamide has not been established.

➤*GI:* Nausea and vomiting commonly occur with cyclophosphamide therapy. Anorexia and, less frequently, abdominal discomfort or pain and diarrhea may occur. There are isolated reports of hemorrhagic colitis, oral mucosal ulceration, and jaundice occurring during therapy. These adverse drug effects generally remit when cyclophosphamide treatment is stopped.

CYCLOPHOSPHAMIDE — INJECTION

➤*GU:* Hemorrhagic cystitis may develop in patients treated with cyclophosphamide. Rarely, this condition can be severe and even fatal. Fibrosis of the urinary bladder, sometimes extensive, also may develop with or without accompanying cystitis. Atypical urinary bladder epithelial cells may appear in the urine. These adverse effects appear to depend on the dose of cyclophosphamide and the duration of therapy. Such bladder injury is thought to be due to cyclophosphamide metabolites excreted in the urine. Forced fluid intake helps to ensure an ample output of urine, necessitates frequent voiding, and reduces the time the drug remains in the bladder. This helps to prevent cystitis. Hematuria usually resolves in a few days after cyclophosphamide treatment is stopped, but it may persist (see also Warnings/Precautions).

Hemorrhagic ureteritis and renal tubular necrosis have been reported to occur in patients treated with cyclophosphamide. Such lesions usually resolve following cessation of therapy.

Cyclophosphamide interferes with oogenesis and spermatogenesis. It may cause sterility in both sexes. Amenorrhea associated with decreased estrogen and increased gonadotropin secretion develops in a significant proportion of women treated with cyclophosphamide. Affected patients generally resume regular menses within a few months after cessation of therapy. Ovarian fibrosis with apparently complete loss of germ cells after prolonged cyclophosphamide treatment in late prepubescence has been reported. Men treated with cyclophosphamide may develop oligospermia or azoospermia associated with increased gonadotropin but normal testosterone secretion. Some degree of testicular atrophy may occur. Cyclophosphamide-induced azoospermia is reversible in some patients, though the reversibility may not occur for several years after cessation of therapy (see also Warnings/Precautions).

➤*Hematologic:* Leukopenia occurs in patients treated with cyclophosphamide, is related to the dose of drug, and can be used as a dosage guide. Leukopenia of less than 2,000 cells/mm^3 develops commonly in patients treated with an initial loading dose of the drug and less frequently in patients maintained on smaller doses. The degree of neutropenia is particularly important because it correlates with a reduction in resistance to infections. Fever without documented infection has been reported in neutropenic patients.

Thrombocytopenia or anemia develop occasionally in patients treated with cyclophosphamide. These hematologic effects usually can be reversed by reducing the drug dose or by interrupting treatment. Recovery from leukopenia usually begins 7 to 10 days after cessation of therapy.

➤*Hypersensitivity:* Anaphylactic reactions have been reported; death has also been reported in association with this reaction. Possible cross-sensitivity with other alkylating agents has been reported.

➤*Respiratory:* Interstitial pneumonitis has been reported as part of the postmarketing experience. Interstitial pulmonary fibrosis has been reported in patients receiving high doses of cyclophosphamide over a prolonged period.

➤*Miscellaneous:* Syndrome of inappropriate antidiuretic hormone secretion has been reported with use of cyclophosphamide. Malaise and asthenia have been reported as part of the postmarketing experience.

Overdosage

➤*Treatment:* No specific antidote for cyclophosphamide overdosage is known. Manage overdosage with supportive measures, including appropriate treatment for any concurrent infection, myelosuppression, or cardiac toxicity if it occurs.

Patient Information

Inform patients that cyclophosphamide may cause irreversible sterility in both sexes.

Advise female patients that cyclophosphamide may cause fetal harm and is contraindicated during the first trimester. The use of birth control is recommended.

Advise women that cyclophosphamide is excreted in breast milk and is, therefore, contraindicated with breast-feeding.

Instruct patients to drink extra fluids and void frequently.

IFOSFAMIDE

Rx	**Ifosfamide** (American Pharmaceutical Partners)	**Powder for Injection:** 1 g	In single-dose vials.
Rx	**Ifex** (Baxter Medication Delivery)		In single-dose vials.
Rx	**Ifosfamide** (American Pharmaceutical Partners)	**Powder for Injection:** 3 g	In single-dose vials.
Rx	**Ifex** (Baxter Medication Delivery)		In single-dose vials.

IFOSFAMIDE — INJECTION

WARNING

Ifosfamide for injection should be administered under the supervision of a qualified physician experienced in the use of cancer chemotherapeutic agents. Urotoxic side effects, especially hemorrhagic cystitis, as well as CNS toxicities such as confusion and coma have been associated with the use of ifosfamide. When they occur, they may require cessation of ifosfamide therapy. Severe myelosuppression has been reported.

Indications

➤*Germ cell testicular cancer:* In combination with certain other approved antineoplastic agents for third-line chemotherapy of germ cell testicular cancer. It should ordinarily be used in combination with a prophylactic agent for hemorrhagic cystitis, such as mesna.

➤*Off-label uses:* Ifosfamide has shown activity in lung, breast, ovarian, pancreatic and gastric cancer, sarcomas, acute leukemias (except AML) and malignant lymphomas. Further studies are needed with ifosfamide alone and with other agents.

Treatment of soft-tissue, Ewing's and osteogenic sarcomas; non-Hodgkin's lymphomas; bladder and cervical carcinoma.

Ifosfamide has been used safely and effectively in children for the treatment of bone and soft-tissue sarcomas.

Administration and Dosage

➤*General dosing considerations:* Ifosfamide should be given with extensive hydration and mesna. (See Concomitant Therapy.)

➤*Adults:*

Germ cell testicular cancer –

Usual dosage: 1.2 g/m^2 daily by IV infusion for 5 consecutive days. Treatment is repeated every 3 weeks or after recovery from hematologic toxicity (platelets greater than or equal to 100,000 cells/mm^3, WBC greater than or equal to 4,000 cells/mm^3). (See also Off-Label Dosing.)

Dosage adjustment: Delay further courses until platelets are at least 100,000 cells/mm^3 and white blood cell (WBC) count is at least 4,000 cells/mm^3. Although no specific guidelines are available, consider dosage reduction if severe myelosuppression occurs.

Off-label dosing –

Germ cell testicular cancer: Other regimens use ifosfamide 2 g/m^2 daily by IV infusion on days 1 through 3 (MAID regimen, total dose is 6 g/m^2 over 72 hours), or doses as high as 5 g/m^2 daily by continuous IV infusion over 24 hours in combination with other antineoplastic agents.

➤*Children:*

Off-label dosing –

Bone and soft tissue sarcomas:

• *Usual dose* – 1.2 to 1.8 g/m^2 daily by IV infusion for 5 days, repeating this course every 3 to 4 weeks.

• *Dosage adjustment* – Delay further courses until platelets are at least 100,000 cells/mm^3 and WBC count is at least 4,000 cells/mm^3. Although no specific guidelines are available, consider dosage reduction if severe myelosuppression occurs.

• *Alternative dosage* – Other regimens use ifosfamide 3 g/m^2 daily by IV infusion on days 1 and 2, or doses as high as 5 g/m^2 daily by continuous IV infusion over 24 hours in combination with other antineoplastic agents.

➤*Renal function impairment:* Dosage reduction is necessary in renal insufficiency, as shown in the following table.

Ifosfamide Dosage Reduction in Renal Insufficiency

Glomerular filtration rate	Percent of usual dose
> 60 mL/min	100%
30 to 60 mL/min	75%
10 to 30 mL/min	50%
< 10 mL/min	0%

Dialysis – Conventional hemodialysis is effective (75% to 100%) in removing ifosfamide.

Some health care providers recommend a supplemental dose after hemodialysis, although specific recommendations are not available.

➤*Hepatic function impairment:* Dosage reduction may be necessary in hepatic dysfunction. Consider decreasing ifosfamide to 25% of usual dose if serum AST is greater than 300 units/L or if bilirubin is greater than 3 mg/dL.

➤*Concomitant therapy:* In order to prevent bladder toxicity, ifosfamide should be given with extensive hydration consisting of at least 2 L of oral or IV fluid per day. A protector, such as mesna, should also be used to prevent hemorrhagic cystitis.

➤*Preparation for administration:* Ifosfamide is considered a cytotoxic agent. Follow safe handling procedures when preparing, administering, or dispensing ifosfamide.

Skin reactions associated with accidental exposure to ifosfamide may occur. The use of gloves is recommended. If ifosfamide solution contacts the skin or mucosa, immediately wash the skin thoroughly with soap and water or rinse the mucosa with copious amounts of water.

Injections are prepared for parenteral use by adding Sterile Water for Injection or Sterile Bacteriostatic Water for Injection (benzyl alcohol or parabens

IFOSFAMIDE — INJECTION

preserved), to the vial and shaking to dissolve. Use the quantity of diluent shown in the information following to constitute the product:

Reconstitution of Ifosfamide		
Dosage strength	Quantity of diluent	Final concentration
1 g	20 mL	50 mg/mL
3 g	60 mL	50 mg/mL

Solutions of ifosfamide may be diluted further to achieve concentrations of 0.6 to 20 mg/mL in the following fluids: 5% Dextrose Injection, 0.9% Sodium Chloride Injection, Lactated Ringer's Injection, Sterile Water for Injection.

Because essentially identical stability results were obtained for Sterile Water admixtures as for the other admixtures (5% Dextrose Injection, 0.9% Sodium Chloride Injection, and Lactated Ringer's Injection), the use of large volume parenteral glass bottles, *Viaflex* bags or *PAB* bags that contain intermediate concentrations or mixtures of excipients (eg, 2.5% Dextrose Injection, 0.45% Sodium Chloride Injection, or 5% Dextrose and 0.9% Sodium Chloride Injection) is also acceptable.

➤*Administration:* Ifosfamide should be administered as a slow IV infusion lasting at least 30 minutes.

Ifosfamide has also been given as a continuous infusion (off-label) (see Adults).

➤*Extravasation:* Ifosfamide is considered an irritant and may cause phlebitis, but it is not known to cause tissue damage with extravasation. If signs or symptoms of extravasation occur, stop the infusion immediately. If possible, withdraw 3 to 5 mL of blood to remove some of the drug. Remove the infusion needle. Delineate the infiltrated area on the patient's skin with a felt tip marker. Elevate for 48 hours above heart level using a sling or stockinette dressing with an observation window cut in the dressing. Avoid pressure or friction. Do not rub the area. Observe for signs of increased erythema, pain, or skin necrosis. If increased symptoms occur, consult a plastic surgeon. After 48 hours, encourage the patient to use the extremity normally to promote full range of motion.

➤*Admixture compatibility:* Ifosfamide, at a concentration of 100 mg/mL, is incompatible with Bacteriostatic Water for Injection with benzyl alcohol. It is compatible with ifosfamide concentrations of up to 60 mg/mL.

➤*Storage/Stability:* Store at 20° to 25°C (68° to 77°F). Protect from temperatures above 30°C (86°F).

According to the manufacturer, constituted or constituted and further diluted solutions of ifosfamide should be refrigerated and used within 24 hours. Another reference states that solutions reconstituted with Bacteriostatic Water for Injection are stable for 1 week at room temperature or 3 weeks under refrigeration and that diluted solutions are chemically stable for up to 1 week at room temperature and for up to 6 weeks under refrigeration in glass containers or plastic bags. The possibility of microbial contamination of diluted solutions must be considered. Preservative-free solutions should be used within 24 hours.

Discard vial within 6 hours of the initial needle puncture if opened within an ISO Class 5 biological safety cabinet, or within 1 hour of the initial needle puncture if opened outside of such an environment, based on the USP Chapter <797> standards.

Actions

➤*Pharmacology:* Ifosfamide has been shown to require metabolic activation by microsomal liver enzymes to produce biologically active metabolites. Activation occurs by hydroxylation at the ring carbon atom 4 to form the unstable intermediate 4-hydroxyifosfamide. This metabolite rapidly degrades to the stable urinary metabolite 4-ketoifosfamide. Opening of the ring results in formation of the stable urinary metabolite, 4-carboxyifosfamide. These urinary metabolites have not been found to be cytotoxic. N, N-bis (2-chloroethyl)-phosphoric acid diamide (ifosphoramide) and acrolein are also found. Enzymatic oxidation of the chloroethyl side chains and subsequent dealkylation produces the major urinary metabolites, dechloroethyl ifosfamide and dechloroethyl cyclophosphamide. The alkylated metabolites of ifosfamide have been shown to interact with DNA.

➤*Pharmacokinetics:*

Absorption/Distribution – Ifosfamide exhibits dose-dependent pharmacokinetics in humans.

Metabolism/Excretion – At single doses of 3.8 to 5 g/m², the plasma concentrations decay biphasically and the mean terminal elimination half-life is about 15 hours. At doses of 1.6 to 2.4 g/m²/day, the plasma decay is monoexponential and the terminal elimination half-life is about 7 hours. Ifosfamide is extensively metabolized in humans, and the metabolic pathways appear to be saturated at high doses.

After administration of doses of 5 g/m² of ^{14}C-labeled ifosfamide, from 70% to 86% of the dosed radioactivity was recovered in the urine, with about 61% of the dose excreted as parent compound. At doses of 1.6 to 2.4 g/m² only 12% to 18% of the dose was excreted in the urine as unchanged drug within 72 hours.

Contraindications

Severely depressed bone marrow function; hypersensitivity to ifosfamide.

Warnings/Precautions

➤*Urotoxic side effects:* See Adverse Reactions for more information.

➤*Myelosuppression:* See Adverse Reactions for more information.

➤*CNS:* See Adverse Reactions for more information.

➤*Wound healing:* Ifosfamide may interfere with normal wound healing.

➤*Extravasation:* See Administration and Dosage for more information.

➤*Special risk:* Ifosfamide should be given cautiously to patients with impaired renal function as well as to those with compromised bone marrow reserve, as indicated by the following: Leukopenia, granulocytopenia, extensive bone marrow metastases, prior radiation therapy, or prior therapy with other cytotoxic agents.

➤*Pregnancy: Category D.* Animal studies indicate that the drug is capable of causing gene mutations and chromosomal damage in vivo. Embryotoxic and teratogenic effects have been observed in mice, rats and rabbits at doses 0.05 to 0.075 times the human dose. Ifosfamide can cause fetal damage when administered to a pregnant woman. If ifosfamide is used during pregnancy, or if the patient becomes pregnant while taking this drug, the patient should be apprised of the potential hazard to the fetus.

➤*Lactation:* Ifosfamide is excreted in breast milk. Because of the potential for serious adverse events and the tumorigenicity shown for ifosfamide in animal studies, a decision should be made whether to discontinue nursing or to discontinue the drug, taking into account the importance of the drug to the mother.

➤*Children:* Safety and effectiveness in pediatric patients have not been established.

➤*Monitoring:* During treatment, the patient's hematologic profile (particularly neutrophils and platelets) should be monitored regularly to determine the degree of hematopoietic suppression. Urine should also be examined regularly for red cells which may precede hemorrhagic cystitis.

Drug Interactions

The physician should be alert for possible combined drug actions, desirable or undesirable; involving ifosfamide even though ifosfamide has been used successfully concurrently with other drugs, including other cytotoxic drugs.

Adverse Reactions

Ifosfamide has moderate potential for nausea and vomiting.

Ifosfamide Adverse Reactions	
Adverse reaction	Incidence[a] (%)
Alopecia	83%
Nausea/vomiting	58%
Hematuria	46%
Gross hematuria	12%
CNS toxicity	12%
Infection	8%
Renal impairment	6%
Liver dysfunction	3%
Phlebitis	2%
Fever	1%
Allergic reaction	< 1%
Anorexia	< 1%
Cardiotoxicity	< 1%
Coagulopathy	< 1%
Constipation	< 1%
Dermatitis	< 1%
Diarrhea	< 1%
Fatigue	< 1%
Hypertension	< 1%
Hypotension	< 1%
Malaise	< 1%
Polyneuropathy	< 1%
Pulmonary symptoms	< 1%
Salivation	< 1%
Stomatitis	< 1%

[a] Based upon 2070 patients from the published literature in 30 single-agent studies.

➤*CNS:* CNS adverse effects were observed in 12% of patients treated with ifosfamide. Those most commonly seen were somnolence, confusion, depressive psychosis, and hallucinations. Other less frequent symptoms include dizziness, disorientation, and cranial nerve dysfunction. Seizures and coma with death were occasionally reported. The incidence of CNS toxicity may be higher in patients with altered renal function.

➤*GI:* Nausea and vomiting occurred in 58% of the patients who received ifosfamide. They were usually controlled by standard antiemetic therapy. Other GI side effects include anorexia, diarrhea, and in some cases, constipation.

➤*GU:* Urotoxicity consisted of hemorrhagic cystitis, dysuria, urinary frequency and other symptoms of bladder irritation. Hematuria occurred in 6% to 92% of patients treated with ifosfamide. The incidence and severity of hematuria can be significantly reduced by using vigorous hydration, a fractionated dose schedule and a protector such as mesna. At daily doses of

IFOSFAMIDE — INJECTION

1.2 g/m² for 5 consecutive days without a protector, microscopic hematuria is expected in about one-half of the patients and gross hematuria in about 8% of patients.

➤*Hematologic:* Myelosuppression was dose related and dose limiting. It consisted mainly of leukopenia and, to a lesser extent, thrombocytopenia. A WBC count less than 3000/mcL is expected in 50% of the patients treated with ifosfamide single agent at doses of 1.2 g/m²/day for 5 consecutive days. At this dose level, thrombocytopenia (platelets less than 100,000/ mcL) occurred in about 20% of the patients. At higher dosages, leukopenia was almost universal, and at total dosages of 10 to 12 g/m²/cycle, one-half of the patients had a WBC count less than 1000/mcL and 8% of patients had platelet counts less than 50,000/mcL. Myelosuppression was usually reversible and treatment can be given every 3 to 4 weeks. When ifosfamide is used in combination with other myelosuppressive agents, adjustments in dosing may be necessary. Patients who experience severe myelosuppression are potentially at increased risk for infection. Anemia has been reported as part of postmarketing surveillance.

➤*Renal:* Renal toxicity occurred in 6% of the patients treated with ifosfamide as a single agent. Clinical signs, such as elevation in BUN or serum creatinine or decrease in creatinine clearance, were usually transient. They were most likely to be related to tubular damage. One episode of renal tubular acidosis which progressed into chronic renal failure was reported. Proteinuria and acidosis also occurred in rare instances. Metabolic acidosis was reported in 31% of patients in 1 study when ifosfamide was administered at doses of 2 to 2.5 g/m²/day for 4 days. Renal tubular acidosis, Fanconi syndrome, renal rickets and acute renal failure have been reported. Close clinical monitoring of serum and urine chemistries including phosphorus, potassium, alkaline phosphatase and other appropriate laboratory studies is recommended. Appropriate replacement therapy should be administered as indicated.

➤*Miscellaneous:* Alopecia occurred in approximately 83% of the patients treated with ifosfamide as a single agent. In combination, this incidence may be as high as 100%, depending on the other agents included in the chemotherapy regimen. Increases in liver enzymes or bilirubin were noted in 3% of the patients. Other less frequent side effects included phlebitis, pulmonary symptoms, fever of unknown origin, allergic reactions, stomatitis, cardiotoxicity, and polyneuropathy.

Overdosage

➤*Treatment:* No specific antidote for ifosfamide is known. Management of overdosage would include general supportive measures to sustain the patient through any period of toxicity that might occur.

MECHLORETHAMINE HYDROCHLORIDE (Nitrogen Mustard; HN_2)

Rx	**Mustargen** (Merck)	**Powder for Injection:** 10 mg	In sets of 4 vials.

MECHLORETHAMINE HYDROCHLORIDE — INJECTION

WARNING

Administer mechlorethamine injection only under the supervision of a physician who is experienced in the use of cancer chemotherapeutic agents.

This drug is highly toxic, and both powder and solution must be handled and administered with care. Inhalation of dust or vapors and contact with skin or mucous membranes, especially those of the eyes, must be avoided. Avoid exposure during pregnancy. Due to the toxic properties of mechlorethamine (eg, corrosivity, carcinogenicity, mutagenicity, teratogenicity), review special handling procedures prior to handling and follow them diligently.

Extravasation of the drug into subcutaneous tissues results in a painful inflammation. The area usually becomes indurated and sloughing may occur. If leakage of drug is obvious, prompt infiltration of the area with sterile isotonic sodium thiosulfate (1/6 molar) and application of an ice compress for 6 to 12 hours may minimize the local reaction. For a 1/6 molar solution of sodium thiosulfate, use 4.14 g of sodium thiosulfate per 100 mL of sterile water for injection or 2.64 g of anhydrous sodium thiosulfate per 100 mL or dilute 4 mL of sodium thiosulfate injection (10%) with 6 mL of sterile water for injection.

Indications

➤*Leukemia/Lymphomas/Polycythemia vera/Mycosis fungoides/Bronchogenic carcinoma (intravenous only):* For the palliative treatment of Hodgkin disease (stages III and IV), lymphosarcoma, chronic myelocytic or chronic lymphocytic leukemia, polycythemia vera, mycosis fungoides, and bronchogenic carcinoma.

➤*Metastatic carcinoma:* Intrapleurally, intraperitoneally, or intrapericardially for the palliative treatment of metastatic carcinoma resulting in effusion.

➤*Off-label uses:* A topical mechlorethamine solution has been used to treat patients with mycosis fungoides. Also used for non-Hodgkin lymphoma.

Mechlorethamine has also been used safely and effectively in lymphoma and brain tumors.

Administration and Dosage

March 15, 1949.

➤*General dosing considerations:* The margin of safety in therapy with mechlorethamine is narrow, and considerable care must be exercised in the matter of dosage. Repeated examinations of blood are mandatory as a guide to subsequent therapy.

Base dosage on ideal dry body weight. The presence of edema or ascites must be considered so that dosage will be based on actual weight unaugmented by these conditions.

Within a few minutes after IV injection, mechlorethamine undergoes chemical transformation, combines with reactive compounds, and is no longer present in its active form in the bloodstream. Do not give subsequent courses until the patient has recovered hematologically from the previous course; this is best determined by repeated studies of the peripheral blood elements awaiting their return to normal levels. It is often possible to give repeated courses of mechlorethamine as early as 3 weeks after treatment.

➤*Adults:*

Leukemia/Lymphomas/Polycythemia vera/Mycosis fungoides/Bronchogenic carcinoma – For a list of uses, see Indications.

A total dose of 0.4 mg/kg IV for each course usually is given either as a single dose or in divided doses of 0.1 to 0.2 mg/kg/day. (See also Off-label dosing.)

Metastatic carcinoma – 0.4 mg/kg by intracavitary administration. A dose of 0.2 mg/kg (or 10 to 20 mg) has been used by the intrapericardial route. (See also Administration.)

Off-label dosing –

Advanced Hodgkin disease:

• *Usual dose* – When used in MOPP regimen, dose is 6 mg/m² body surface area IV on days 1 and 8 of a 28-day cycle.

• *Dosage adjustment* – When used in the MOPP regimen, adjust the dose based on hematologic parameters, as shown in the following table. Delay additional courses until the white blood cell count (WBC) is at least 1,000 cells/mm³ and platelets are at least 50,000 cells/mm³.

Mechlorethamine Dosage Adjustment in MOPP Regimen for Hematologic Effects

Nadir after prior dose (cells/mm³)		
Leukocytes	Platelets	Percentage of prior dose to be given
> 4,000	> 100,000	100
3,000 to 3,999	–	75
1,000 to 2,999	50,000 to 100,000	50
< 1,000	< 50,000	0

Mycosis fungoides: Apply compounded solutions or ointments to the entire body surface once daily for 6 to 12 months. If the lesions do not reappear, continue to apply every 2 to 7 days for a total of 3 years. (See also Preparation for Administration.)

➤*Children:*

Off-label dosing –

Advanced Hodgkin disease: When used in MOPP regimen, dose is 6 mg/m² body surface area IV on days 1 and 8 of a 28-day cycle.

Brain tumor: When used in MOPP regimen, dose is 6 mg/m² body surface area IV on days 1 and 8 of a 28-day cycle.

➤*Preparation for administration:*

Special handling – Mechlorethamine is considered a cytotoxic agent. Follow safe handling procedures when preparing, administering, or dispensing mechlorethamine.

This drug is highly toxic, and both powder and solution must be handled and administered with care. Because mechlorethamine is a powerful vesicant, it is intended primarily for IV use, and in most instances is given by this route. Inhalation of dust or vapors and contact with skin or mucous membranes, especially those of the eyes, must be avoided. Wear appropriate protective equipment when handling mechlorethamine.

Animal studies have shown mechlorethamine to be corrosive to skin and eyes, a powerful vesicant, irritating to the mucous membranes of the respiratory tract and highly toxic by the oral route. It has also been shown to be carcinogenic, mutagenic, and teratogenic. Due to the drug's toxic properties, appropriate precautions, including the use of appropriate safety equipment, are recommended for the preparation of mechlorethamine for parenteral administration. Avoid exposure during pregnancy. The National Institutes of Health presently recommends that the preparation of injectable antineoplastic drugs should be performed in a class II laminar flow biological safety cabinet. Personnel preparing drugs of this class should wear chemical-resistant, impervious gloves, safety goggles, outer garments, and shoe covers. Based upon the task being performed, use additional body garments (eg, sleevelets, apron, gauntlets, disposable suits) to avoid exposed skin surfaces and inhalation of vapors and dust. Use appropriate techniques to remove potentially contaminated clothing.

Accidental contact – If accidental eye contact occurs, institute copious irrigation for at least 15 minutes with water, normal saline, or a balanced salt, ophthalmic, irrigating solution immediately, followed by prompt ophthalmologic consultation. If accidental skin contact occurs, the affected part

MECHLORETHAMINE HYDROCHLORIDE — INJECTION

must be irrigated immediately with copious amounts of water, for at least 15 minutes, followed by 2% sodium thiosulfate solution. To prepare a 2% solution of sodium thiosulfate, dilute 2 mL of a 10% solution of sodium thiosulfate with 8 mL of sterile water or dilute 0.8 mL of a 25% solution of sodium thiosulfate with 9.2 mL of sterile water. Seek medical attention immediately. Destroy contaminated clothing.

Preparation of IV solution – Using a sterile 10 mL syringe, inject 10 mL of sterile water for injection or 10 mL sodium chloride injection into a vial of mechlorethamine. With the needle (syringe attached) still in the rubber stopper, shake the vial several times to dissolve the drug completely. The resultant solution contains mechlorethamine 1 mg/mL.

Preparation of intracavitary solution – For intracavitary use, mechlorethamine has been diluted in up to 100 mL 0.9% sodium chloride.

Extemporaneous compounding – Topical preparations must be prepared in a fume hood to prevent circulation of toxic vapors into room air.

Topical solution: Dissolve mechlorethamine 10 mg in 50 to 60 mL of water.

Topical ointment: Dissolve mechlorethamine in dehydrated alcohol, filter resulting solution, and add into a petrolatum or anhydrous ointment base.

➤*Administration:*

IV administration – Withdraw into the syringe the calculated volume of solution required for a single injection. Dispose of any remaining solution after neutralization. Although the drug may be injected directly into any suitable vein, it is injected preferably into the rubber or plastic tubing of a flowing IV infusion set. This reduces the possibility of severe local reactions due to extravasation or high concentration of the drug. Injecting the drug into the tubing rather than adding it to the entire volume of the infusion fluid minimizes a chemical reaction between the drug and the solution. The rate of injection apparently is not critical, provided it is completed within a few minutes.

Intracavitary administration – The technique and the dose used by any of these routes varies. Therefore, if mechlorethamine is given by the intracavitary route, consult the published articles concerning such use. Because of the inherent risks involved, the physician should be experienced in the appropriate injection techniques, and be thoroughly aware of the indications, dosages, hazards, and precautions as set forth in the published literature. When using mechlorethamine by the intracavitary route, keep in mind the general precautions concerning this agent.

Topical (off-label) – Use rubber gloves to apply. Product should be used only in well-ventilated areas with chemotherapy spill kits in close proximity.

Decontamination – To clean rubber gloves, tubing, and glassware after giving mechlorethamine, soak them in an aqueous solution containing equal volumes of sodium thiosulfate (5%) and sodium bicarbonate (5%) for 45 minutes. Excess reagents and reaction products are washed away easily with water. Neutralize any unused injection solution by mixing with an equal volume of sodium thiosulfate/sodium bicarbonate solution. Allow the mixture to stand for 45 minutes. Treat vials that have contained mechlorethamine the same way with thiosulfate/bicarbonate solution before disposal.

➤*Extravasation:* Mechlorethamine is considered a vesicant. Extravasation of the drug into subcutaneous tissue results in a painful inflammation. The area usually becomes indurated and sloughing may occur. If signs or symptoms of extravasation occur, stop the infusion immediately. If possible, withdraw 3 to 5 mL of blood to remove some of the drug. Administer sodium thiosulfate (1/6 molar) within the first few minutes to 1 hour after extravasation, if possible. To prepare a 1/6 molar solution, dilute 4 mL of 10% sodium thiosulfate with 6 mL sterile water for injection or dilute 1.6 mL of 25% sodium thiosulfate with 8.4 mL sterile water for injection. Cleanse the extravasation site with povidone iodine. Use 0.5 mL of sodium thiosulfate for each estimated mg of mechlorethamine extravasated. Administer sodium thiosulfate through the extravasated IV site if possible; it may be injected subcutaneously around the site of extravasation. Application of cold compresses for 15 minutes every 6 hours for 48 hours may be useful. Delineate the infiltrated area on the patient's skin with a felt-tip marker. Elevate for 48 hours above heart level using a sling or stockinette dressing with an observation window cut in the dressing. Avoid pressure or friction. Do not rub the area. Observe for signs of increased erythema, pain, or skin necrosis. If increased symptoms occur, consult a plastic surgeon. Ensure that no medication is given distally to extravasation site. After 48 hours, encourage the patient to use the extremity normally to promote full range of motion.

➤*Storage/Stability:* Store at 15° to 30°C (59° to 86°F). Protect from light and humidity. Solutions of mechlorethamine decompose on standing; therefore, prepare solutions of the drug immediately before use.

Actions

➤*Pharmacology:* Mechlorethamine, a biologic alkylating agent, has a cytotoxic action which inhibits rapidly proliferating cells.

➤*Pharmacokinetics:* In water or body fluids, mechlorethamine undergoes rapid chemical transformation and combines with water or reactive compounds of cells, so that the drug is no longer present in active form a few minutes after administration.

Contraindications

Infectious diseases; previous anaphylactic reactions to mechlorethamine.

Warnings/Precautions

➤*Amyloidosis:* As nitrogen mustard therapy may contribute to extensive and rapid development of amyloidosis, only use it if foci of acute and chronic suppurative inflammation are absent.

➤*Safe handling:* See Administration and Dosage for more information.

➤*Inoperable neoplasms/terminal stage:* Because of the toxicity of mechlorethamine, and the unpleasant side effects following its use, the potential risk and discomfort from the use of this drug in patients with inoperable neoplasms or in the terminal stage of the disease must be balanced against the limited gain obtainable. These gains will vary with the nature and the status of the disease under treatment. The routine use of mechlorethamine in all cases of widely disseminated neoplasms is to be discouraged.

➤*Tumors:* Tumors of bone and nervous tissue have responded poorly to therapy. Results are unpredictable in disseminated and malignant tumors of different types.

➤*Concomitant therapy:* Precautions must be observed with the use of mechlorethamine and x-ray therapy or other chemotherapy in alternating courses. Hematopoietic function is characteristically depressed by either form of therapy, and neither mechlorethamine following x-ray therapy nor x-ray therapy subsequent to the drug should be given until bone marrow function has recovered. In particular, irradiation of such areas as sternum, ribs, and vertebrae shortly after a course of nitrogen mustard may lead to hematologic complications.

➤*Immunosuppression:* Mechlorethamine has been reported to have immunosuppressive activity. Therefore, keep in mind that use of the drug may predispose the patient to bacterial, viral, or fungal infection.

➤*Hyperuricemia:* Hyperuricemia may develop during therapy with mechlorethamine. The problem of urate precipitation should be anticipated, particularly in the treatment of the lymphomas; institute adequate methods for control of hyperuricemia and direct careful attention toward adequate fluid intake before treatment.

➤*Hematologic:* The use of mechlorethamine in patients with leukopenia, thrombocytopenia, and anemia, due to invasion of the bone marrow by tumor carries a greater risk. In such patients, a good response to treatment, with disappearance of the tumor from the bone marrow, may be associated with improvement of bone marrow function. However, in the absence of a good response, or in patients who have been previously treated with chemotherapeutic agents, hematopoiesis may be further compromised, and leukopenia, thrombocytopenia, and anemia may become more severe and lead to the demise of the patient.

➤*Chronic lymphatic leukemia:* Because drug toxicity, especially sensitivity to bone marrow failure, seems to be more common in chronic lymphatic leukemia than in other conditions, give the drug with great caution in this condition, if at all.

➤*Extravasation:* See Administration and Dosage for more information.

➤*Pregnancy: Category D.* Mechlorethamine can cause fetal harm when administered to a pregnant woman. Mechlorethamine has been shown to produce fetal malformations in the rat and ferret when given as single subcutaneous injections of 1 mg/kg (2 to 3 times the maximum recommended human dose). There are no adequate and well-controlled studies in pregnant women. If this drug is used during pregnancy, or if the patient becomes pregnant while taking this drug, apprise the patient of the potential hazard to the fetus. Advise women of childbearing potential to avoid becoming pregnant.

➤*Lactation:* It is not known whether this drug is excreted in human milk. Because many drugs are excreted in human milk and because of the potential for serious adverse reactions in nursing infants from mechlorethamine, make a decision whether to discontinue nursing or to discontinue the drug, taking into account the importance of the drug to the mother.

➤*Children:* Safety and efficacy in pediatric patients have not been established by well-controlled studies. Use of mechlorethamine in pediatric patients has been quite limited. Mechlorethamine has been used in Hodgkin's disease, stages III and IV, in combination with other oncolytic agents (MOPP schedule). The MOPP chemotherapy combination includes mechlorethamine, vincristine, procarbazine, and prednisone or prednisolone.

➤*Monitoring:* Many abnormalities of renal, hepatic, and bone marrow function have been reported in patients with neoplastic disease and receiving mechlorethamine. It is advisable to check renal, hepatic, and bone marrow functions frequently.

Adverse Reactions

Mechlorethamine is considered to have very high emetogenic potential (over 90% incidence of emesis).

➤*Dermatologic:* Occasionally, a maculopapular skin eruption occurs, but this may be idiosyncratic and does not necessarily recur with subsequent courses of the drug. Erythema multiforme has been observed. Herpes zoster, a common complicating infection in patients with lymphomas, may first appear after therapy is instituted, and on occasion may be precipitated by treatment. Discontinue further treatment during the acute phase of this illness to avoid progression to generalized herpes zoster.

➤*GI:* Mechlorethamine is given preferably at night in case sedation for side effects is required. Nausea and vomiting usually occur 1 to 3 hours after use of the drug. Emesis may disappear in the first 8 hours, but nausea may persist for 24 hours. Nausea and vomiting may be so severe as to precipitate vascular accidents in patients with a hemorrhagic tendency. Premedication with antiemetics, in addition to sedatives, may help control severe nausea and vomiting. Anorexia, weakness, and diarrhea may also occur.

➤*GU:* Since the gonads are susceptible to mechlorethamine, treatment may be followed by delayed catamenia, oligomenorrhea, or temporary or permanent amenorrhea. Impaired spermatogenesis, azoospermia, and total ger-

MECHLORETHAMINE HYDROCHLORIDE — INJECTION

minal aplasia have been reported in male patients treated with alkylating agents, especially in combination with other drugs. In some instances, spermatogenesis may return in patients in remission, but this may occur only several years after intensive chemotherapy has been discontinued. Warn patients of the potential risk to their reproductive capacity.

➤*Hematologic:* The usual course of mechlorethamine (total dose of 0.4 mg/kg either given as a single IV dose or divided into 2 or 4 daily doses of 0.2 or 0.1 mg/kg, respectively) generally produces a lymphocytopenia within 24 hours after the first injection; significant granulocytopenia occurs within 6 to 8 days and lasts for 10 days to 3 weeks. Agranulocytosis appears to be relatively infrequent and recovery from leukopenia in most cases is complete within 2 weeks of the maximum reduction. Thrombocytopenia is variable, but the time course of the appearance and recovery from reduced platelet counts generally parallels the sequence of granulocyte levels. In some cases, severe thrombocytopenia may lead to bleeding from the gums and GI tract, petechiae, and small subcutaneous hemorrhages; these symptoms appear to be transient, and, in most cases, disappear with return to a normal platelet count. However, a severe and even uncontrollable depression of the hematopoietic system occasionally may follow the usual dose of mechlorethamine, particularly in patients with widespread disease and debility and in patients previously treated with other antineoplastic agents or x-ray. Persistent pancytopenia has been reported. In rare instances, hemorrhagic complications may be due to hyperheparinemia. Erythrocyte and hemoglobin levels may decline during the first 2 weeks after therapy but rarely significantly. Depression of the hematopoietic system may be found up to 50 days or more after starting therapy.

➤*Local:* Thrombosis and thrombophlebitis may result from direct contact of the drug with the intima of the injected vein. Avoid high concentration and prolonged contact with the drug, especially in cases of elevated pressure in the antebrachial vein (eg, in mediastinal tumor compression from severe vena cava syndrome).

➤*Miscellaneous:* Hypersensitivity reactions, including anaphylaxis, have been reported. Nausea, vomiting, and depression of formed elements in the circulating blood are dose-limiting side effects and usually occur with the use of full doses of mechlorethamine. Jaundice, alopecia, vertigo, tinnitus, and diminished hearing may occur infrequently. Rarely, hemolytic anemia associated with such diseases as the lymphomas and chronic lymphocytic leukemia may be precipitated by treatment with alkylating agents including mechlorethamine. Also, various chromosomal abnormalities have been reported in association with nitrogen mustard therapy.

Overdosage

➤*Symptoms:* With total doses exceeding 0.4 mg/kg of body weight for a single course, severe leukopenia, anemia, thrombocytopenia, and a hemorrhagic diathesis with subsequent delayed bleeding may develop. Death may follow.

➤*Treatment:* The only treatment in instances of excessive dosage appears to be repeated blood-product transfusions, antibiotic treatment of complicating infections, and general supportive measures.

MELPHALAN (Phenylalanine mustard, L-PAM; L-Phenylalanine Mustard; L-Sarcolysin)

Rx	**Alkeran** (GlaxoSmithKline)	**Tablets; oral:** 2 mg	(GX EH3 A). Film-coated. In amber glass bottles. In 50s.
Rx	**Melphalan** (Bioniche Pharma Group)	**Injection, lyophilized powder for solution:** 50 mg	As melphalan hydrochloride. In single-use vials[a] with 10 mL vial of sterile diluent.[b]
Rx	**Alkeran** (GlaxoSmithKline)		As melphalan hydrochloride. In single-use vials[a] with 10 mL vial of sterile diluent.[b]

[a] With povidone 20 mg.

[b] With sodium citrate 0.2 g, propylene glycol 6 mL, and ethanol (96%) 0.52 mL.

MELPHALAN — ORAL

WARNING

Administer melphalan under the supervision of a qualified health care provider experienced in the use of cancer chemotherapeutic agents. Severe bone marrow suppression with resulting infection or bleeding may occur. Melphalan is leukemogenic in humans.

Melphalan produces chromosomal aberrations in vitro and in vivo and, therefore, should be considered potentially mutagenic in humans.

Indications

➤*Epithelial ovarian cancer:* For the palliation of nonresectable epithelial carcinoma of the ovary.

➤*Multiple myeloma:* For the palliative treatment of multiple myeloma.

➤*Off-label uses:* Treatment of breast cancer, testicular cancer, and hematopoietic stem cell transplantation (HSCT).

Melphalan has been used safely and effectively in children for rhabdomyosarcoma, neuroblastoma, and acute hematologic malignancies.

Administration and Dosage

➤*General dosing considerations:* Because of the patient-to-patient variation in melphalan plasma levels following oral administration of the drug, several investigators have recommended that the dosage of melphalan be cautiously escalated until some myelosuppression is observed in order to ensure that potentially therapeutic levels of the drug have been reached.

➤*Adults:*

Epithelial ovarian cancer – 0.2 mg/kg/day for 5 days as a single course. Courses are repeated every 4 to 5 weeks depending upon hematologic tolerance.

Multiple myeloma –

Initial dosage: 6 mg (3 tablets) daily. The entire daily dose may be given at 1 time.

Maintenance dosage: 2 mg daily may be instituted when the white blood cell count (WBC) and platelet count are rising.

Dosage adjustment: The dose is adjusted, as required, on the basis of blood cell counts done at approximately weekly intervals. After 2 to 3 weeks of treatment, the drug should be discontinued for up to 4 weeks, during which time the blood cell count should be followed carefully.

All doses should be adjusted based on hematological parameters at nadir, as described in the following table.

Melphalan Dosage Adjustments Based on Nadirs

Nadir after prior dose (cells/mm³)		
White blood cell	Platelet	Percentage of prior dose to be given
≥ 4,000	≥ 100,000	100
3,000 to 3,999	75,000 to 99,999	75
2,000 to 2,999	50,000 to 74,999	50
< 2,000	≥ 50,000	0

Alternative dosage: Investigators in one study have used an initial course of 10 mg/day for 7 to 10 days. They report that maximal suppression of the leukocyte and platelet counts occurs within 3 to 5 weeks and recovery within 4 to 8 weeks. Continuous maintenance therapy with 2 mg/day is instituted when the WBC is more than 4,000 cells/mcL and the platelet count is more than 100,000 cells/mcL. Dosage is adjusted to between 1 and 3 mg/day, depending upon the hematological response. It is desirable to try to maintain a significant degree of bone marrow depression so as to keep the leukocyte count in the range of 3,000 to 3,500 cells/mcL.

One study reports starting treatment with 0.15 mg/kg/day for 7 days. This is followed by a rest period of at least 14 days, but it may be as long as 5 to 6 weeks. Maintenance therapy is started when the WBC and platelet count are rising. The maintenance dose is 0.05 mg/kg/day or less and is adjusted according to the blood cell count.

Another study has shown that the use of melphalan in combination with prednisone significantly improves the percentage of patients with multiple myeloma who achieve palliation. One regimen has been to administer courses of melphalan at 0.25 mg/kg/day for 4 consecutive days (or 0.2 mg/kg/day for 5 consecutive days) for a total dose of 1 mg/kg per course. These 4- to 5-day courses are then repeated every 4 to 6 weeks if the granulocyte count and platelet count have returned to normal levels.

It is to be emphasized that response may be very gradual over many months. It is important that repeated courses or continuous therapy be given because improvement may continue slowly over many months, and the maximum benefit may be missed if treatment is abandoned too soon.

➤*Children:*

Off-label dosing –

Various (consult protocols):

• *Usual dose* – 4 to 20 mg/m²/day orally for 1 to 21 days has been used in children.

• *Dosage adjustment* – All doses should be adjusted based on hematological parameters at nadir, as described in the following table.

Melphalan Dosage Adjustments Based on Nadirs

Nadir after prior dose (cells/mm³)		
White blood cell	Platelet	Percentage of prior dose to be given
≥ 4,000	≥ 100,000	100
3,000 to 3,999	75,000 to 99,999	75
2,000 to 2,999	50,000 to 74,999	50
< 2,000	≥ 50,000	0

➤*Preparation for administration:* Melphalan is considered a cytotoxic agent. Follow safe handling procedures when preparing, administering, or dispensing melphalan.

➤*Administration:* Give oral melphalan on an empty stomach. Food markedly reduces bioavailability.

➤*Storage / Stability:* Store in a refrigerator at 2° to 8°C (36° to 46°F). Protect from light.

MELPHALAN — ORAL

Actions

➤*Pharmacology:* Melphalan, also known as L-phenylalanine mustard, phenylalanine mustard, L-PAM, or L-sarcolysin, is a phenylalanine derivative of nitrogen mustard. Melphalan is an alkylating agent of the bischloroethylamine type. As a result, its cytotoxicity appears to be related to the extent of its interstrand cross-linking with DNA, probably by binding at the N^7 position of guanine. Like other bifunctional alkylating agents, it is active against both resting and rapidly dividing tumor cells.

➤*Pharmacokinetics:*

Absorption/Distribution – The pharmacokinetics of melphalan after oral administration have been extensively studied in adult patients. Plasma melphalan levels are highly variable after oral dosing, both with respect to the time of the first appearance of melphalan in plasma (range, approximately 0 to 6 hours) and to the peak plasma concentration (C_{max}) (range, 70 to 4,000 ng/mL, depending on the dose) achieved. These results may be due to incomplete intestinal absorption, a variable "first-pass" hepatic metabolism, or rapid hydrolysis. Five patients were studied after oral and intravenous (IV) dosing with 0.6 mg/kg as a single bolus dose by each route. The areas under the curve (AUCs) after oral administration averaged 61% ± 26% (± standard deviation [SD]) (range, 25% to 89%) of those following IV administration.

The steady-state volume of distribution of melphalan is 0.5 L/kg. Penetration into cerebrospinal fluid is low. The extent of melphalan binding to plasma proteins ranges from 60% to 90%. Serum albumin is the major binding protein, while alpha-1 acid glycoprotein appears to account for about 20% of the plasma protein binding. Approximately 30% of melphalan is (covalently) irreversibly bound to plasma proteins. Interactions with immunoglobulins have been found to be negligible.

Metabolism/Excretion – In 18 patients given a single oral dose of melphalan 0.6 mg/kg, the terminal plasma half-life ($t_{½}$) of parent drug was 1.5 ± 0.83 hours. The 24-hour urinary excretion of parent drug in these patients was 10% ± 4.5%, suggesting that renal clearance is not a major route of elimination of parent drug.

In a separate study in 18 patients given single oral doses of melphalan 0.2 to 0.25 mg/kg, C_{max} and AUC, when dose adjusted to a dose of 14 mg, were (mean ± SD) 212 ± 74 ng/mL and 498 ± 137 ng•h/mL, respectively. Elimination phase $t_{½}$ in these patients was approximately 1 hour and the median time to maximal concentration (T_{max}) was 1 hour.

Melphalan is eliminated from plasma primarily by chemical hydrolysis to monohydroxymelphalan and dihydroxymelphalan. Aside from these hydrolysis products, no other melphalan metabolites have been observed in humans. Although the contribution of renal elimination to melphalan clearance appears to be low, one pharmacokinetic study showed a significant positive correlation between the elimination rate constant for melphalan and renal function and a significant negative correlation between renal function and the area under the plasma melphalan concentration/time curve.

Contraindications

Prior resistance to this agent; hypersensitivity to melphalan.

Warnings/Precautions

➤*Bone marrow suppression:* As with other nitrogen mustard drugs, excessive dosage will produce marked bone marrow suppression. Bone marrow suppression is the most significant toxicity associated with melphalan in most patients. Therefore, perform the following tests at the start of therapy and prior to each subsequent course of melphalan: platelet count, hemoglobin, WBC, and differential. Thrombocytopenia and/or leukopenia are indications to withhold further therapy until the blood cell counts have sufficiently recovered. Frequent blood cell counts are essential to determine optimal dosage and to avoid toxicity. Consider dose adjustment on the basis of blood cell counts at the nadir and day of treatment.

➤*Prior irradiation or chemotherapy:* Use melphalan with extreme caution in patients whose bone marrow reserve may have been compromised by prior irradiation or chemotherapy, or whose marrow function is recovering from previous cytotoxic therapy. If the leukocyte count falls below 3,000 cells/mcL, or the platelet count below 100,000 cells/mcL, discontinue melphalan until the peripheral blood cell counts have recovered.

➤*Hypersensitivity reactions:* Hypersensitivity reactions, including anaphylaxis, have occurred rarely. These reactions have occurred after multiple courses of treatment and have recurred in patients who experienced a hypersensitivity reaction to IV melphalan. If a hypersensitivity reaction occurs, do not readminister oral or IV melphalan.

➤*Renal function impairment:* A recommendation as to whether dosage reduction should be made routinely in patients with renal function impairment cannot be made because 1) there is considerable inherent patient-to-patient variability in the systemic availability of melphalan in patients with healthy renal function, and 2) only a small amount of the administered dose appears as parent drug in the urine of patients with healthy renal function.

Closely observe patients with azotemia in order to make dosage reductions, if required, at the earliest possible time.

➤*Pregnancy: Category D.* Melphalan may cause fetal harm when administered to a pregnant woman. Melphalan was embryolethal and teratogenic in rats following oral (6 to 18 mg/m²/day for 10 days) and intraperitoneal (18 mg/m²) administration. Malformations resulting from melphalan included alterations of the brain (underdevelopment, deformation, meningocele, and encephalocele) and eye (anophthalmia and microphthalmos), reduction of the mandible and tail, as well as hepatocele (exomphaly).

There are no adequate and well-controlled studies in pregnant women. However, the molecular weight of melphalan is low enough; therefore, expect the transfer across the placenta to the fetus. Melphalan is contraindicated during the first trimester of pregnancy. If this drug is used during pregnancy, or if the patient becomes pregnant while taking this drug, apprise the patient of the potential hazard to the fetus. Advise women of childbearing potential to avoid becoming pregnant.

Fertility impairment – Melphalan causes suppression of ovarian function in premenopausal women, resulting in amenorrhea in a significant number of patients. Reversible and irreversible testicular suppression have also been reported.

➤*Lactation:* It is not known whether this drug is excreted in human milk. However, the molecular weight of melphalan is relatively low; expect excretion into breast milk. Do not give melphalan to breast-feeding mothers.

➤*Children:* The safety and efficacy of melphalan in children have not been established.

➤*Elderly:* Dose selection for an elderly patient should be cautious, usually starting at the low end of the dosing range, reflecting the greater frequency of decreased hepatic, renal, or cardiac function, and of concomitant disease or other drug therapy.

➤*Monitoring:* Perform periodic complete blood cell counts with differentials during the course of treatment with melphalan. Obtain at least 1 determination prior to each treatment course.

Closely observe patients for consequences of bone marrow suppression, which include severe infections, bleeding, and symptomatic anemia.

Drug Interactions

Melphalan Drug Interactions

Precipitant drug	Object drug[a]		Description
Cisplatin	Melphalan	↑	Cisplatin may affect melphalan kinetics by inducing renal function impairment and subsequently altering melphalan clearance.
Melphalan	Nalidixic acid	↑	Coadministration is contraindicated because of the risk of serious GI toxicity, such as hemorrhagic ulcerative colitis or intestinal necrosis.
Melphalan	Carmustine	↑	Carmustine lung toxicity threshold may be reduced.
Melphalan	Cyclosporine	↑	An increase in the toxicity of cyclosporine, particularly nephrotoxicity, has been observed following coadministration.
Melphalan	Vaccines, live	↓	Avoid administration of live vaccines to immunocompromised patients.

[a] ↑ = object drug increased; ↓ = object drug decreased.

Adverse Reactions

Melphalan has very low potential for nausea and vomiting with oral use.

➤*Cardiovascular:* Cardiac arrest (rare), vasculitis.

➤*Dermatologic:* Alopecia, maculopapular rashes, skin hypersensitivity.

➤*GI:* Diarrhea, nausea, oral ulceration, vomiting.

➤*Hematologic:* The most common adverse reaction is bone marrow suppression leading to leukopenia, thrombocytopenia, and anemia. Hemolytic anemia has also been reported. Although bone marrow suppression frequently occurs, it is usually reversible if melphalan is withdrawn early enough. However, irreversible bone marrow failure has been reported.

➤*Hepatic:* Hepatic disorders ranging from abnormal liver function tests to clinical manifestations, such as hepatitis and jaundice, have been reported.

➤*Hypersensitivity:* Allergic reactions, including urticaria, edema, skin rashes, and rare anaphylaxis, have occurred after multiple courses of treatment.

➤*Respiratory:* Interstitial pneumonitis, pulmonary fibrosis (including fatal outcomes).

Overdosage

➤*Symptoms:* Overdoses, including doses of up to 50 mg/day for 16 days, have been reported. Immediate effects are likely to be vomiting, ulceration of the mouth, diarrhea, and hemorrhage of the GI tract. The principal toxic effect is bone marrow suppression.

➤*Treatment:* Closely follow hematologic parameters for 3 to 6 weeks. An uncontrolled study suggests that administration of autologous bone marrow or hematopoietic growth factors (ie, sargramostim, filgrastim) may shorten the period of pancytopenia. Institute general supportive measures together with appropriate blood transfusions and antibiotics as deemed necessary. This drug is not removed from plasma to any significant degree by hemodialysis.

MELPHALAN — ORAL

Patient Information

Inform patients that the major toxicities of melphalan are related to bone marrow suppression, hypersensitivity reactions, GI toxicity, and pulmonary toxicity. The major long-term toxicities are related to infertility and secondary malignancies.

Never allow patients to take the drug without close medical supervision; advise them to consult their health care provider if they experience skin rash, vasculitis, bleeding, fever, persistent cough, nausea, vomiting, amenorrhea, weight loss, or unusual lumps/masses.

Advise women of childbearing potential to avoid becoming pregnant. Women taking melphalan should not breast-feed.

MELPHALAN HYDROCHLORIDE — INJECTION

WARNING

Administer melphalan under the supervision of a qualified health care provider experienced in the use of cancer chemotherapeutic agents. Severe bone marrow suppression with resulting infection or bleeding may occur. Controlled trials comparing intravenous (IV) to oral melphalan have shown more myelosuppression with the IV formulation. Hypersensitivity reactions, including anaphylaxis, have occurred in approximately 2% of patients who received the IV formulation. Melphalan is leukemogenic in humans. Melphalan produces chromosomal aberrations in vitro and in vivo and, therefore, should be considered potentially mutagenic in humans.

Indications

➤*Multiple myeloma:* For the palliative treatment of patients with multiple myeloma for whom oral therapy is not appropriate.

➤*Off-label uses:* Treatment of breast cancer, testicular cancer, and hematopoietic stem cell transplantation (HSCT).

Melphalan has been used safely and effectively in children for rhabdomyosarcoma, neuroblastoma, and acute hematologic malignancies.

Administration and Dosage

➤*General dosing considerations:* Hydrate patient prior to administration. (See Administration.)

Repeated courses should be given because improvement may continue slowly over many months, and the maximum benefit may be missed if treatment is abandoned prematurely.

➤*Adults:*

Multiple myeloma –

Usual dosage: 16 mg/m^2 given as a single IV infusion over 15 to 20 minutes. Administer at 2-week intervals for 4 doses, then, after adequate recovery from toxicity, at 4-week intervals.

Dosage adjustment: All doses should be adjusted based on hematological parameters at nadir, as described in the following table.

Melphalan Dosage Adjustments Based on Nadirs

Nadir after prior dose (cells/mm^3)		
White blood cell	Platelet	Percentage of prior dose to be given
≥ 4,000	≥ 100,000	100
3,000 to 3,999	75,000 to 99,999	75
2,000 to 2,999	50,000 to 74,999	50
< 2,000	≥ 50,000	0

Off-label dosing –

HSCT: Doses of melphalan, alone or in combination with other cytotoxic agents, have ranged from 40 to 200 mg/m^2.

➤*Children:*

Off-label dosing –

Rhabdomyosarcoma: 10 to 35 mg/m^2 IV every 21 to 28 days.

HSCT for neuroblastoma: 100 to 220 mg/m^2 IV given in 1 to 4 divided doses (70 to 100 mg/m^2/day for 2 doses, or 140 to 220 mg/m^2 as a single dose, or 50 mg/m^2/day for 4 doses, or 70 mg/m^2/day for 3 doses) has been used for HSCT conditioning.

HSCT for hematologic malignancies: 140 to 220 mg/m^2 IV given as a single dose prior to HSCT.

Dosage adjustments: All doses should be adjusted based on hematological parameters at nadir, as described in the following table.

Melphalan Dosage Adjustments Based on Nadirs

Nadir after prior dose (cells/mm^3)		
White blood cell	Platelet	Percentage of prior dose to be given
≥ 4,000	≥ 100,000	100
3,000 to 3,999	75,000 to 99,999	75
2,000 to 2,999	50,000 to 74,999	50
< 2,000	≥ 50,000	0

➤*Renal function impairment:* Dosage reduction of up to 50% should be considered in patients with renal function impairment (serum urea nitrogen [BUN] of 30 mg/dL or greater).

IV Melphalan Dosage Reduction for Renal Impairment

Creatinine clearance	BUN	Serum creatinine	Percentage of usual dose
> 60 mL/min	< 30 mg/dL	< 1.5 mg/dL	100
10 to 60 mL/min	—	—	75
< 10 mL/min	≥ 30 mg/dL	≥ 1.5 mg/dL	50

➤*Preparation for administration:* Melphalan is considered a cytotoxic agent. Follow safe handling procedures when preparing, administering, or dispensing melphalan.

Skin reactions associated with accidental exposure may occur. The use of gloves is recommended. If the solution of melphalan contacts the skin or mucosa, immediately wash the skin or mucosa thoroughly with soap and water.

Preparation of solution –

1.) Rapidly inject 10 mL of the supplied diluent directly into the vial of lyophilized powder using a sterile needle (20-gauge or larger needle diameter) and syringe.
2.) Immediately shake vial vigorously until a clear solution is obtained. This provides a 5 mg/mL solution of melphalan. Rapid addition of the diluent followed by immediate vigorous shaking is important for proper dissolution.
3.) Immediately dilute the dose to be administered in sodium chloride 0.9% injection to a concentration of not more than 0.45 mg/mL.

The time between reconstitution/dilution and administration of melphalan should be kept to a minimum because reconstituted and diluted solutions of melphalan are unstable. Over as short a time as 30 minutes, a citrate derivative of melphalan has been detected in reconstituted material from the reaction of melphalan with sterile diluent for melphalan. Upon further dilution with saline, nearly 1% label strength of melphalan hydrolyzes every 10 minutes.

Melphalan has also been given undiluted through a central venous catheter.

➤*Administration:* For patients receiving IV melphalan, hydrate with IV fluids beginning up to 12 hours before the dose and continuing up to 24 hours after the dose to reduce precipitation in the renal tubules. Furosemide may also be given to induce diuresis.

Administer the diluted product over a minimum of 15 minutes. Complete administration within 60 minutes of reconstitution. Administer by injecting slowly into a fast-running IV infusion via an injection port or central venous line. Do not administer by direct injection into a peripheral vein. Care should be taken to avoid possible extravasation of melphalan, and, in cases of poor peripheral venous access, consideration should be given to use of a central venous line.

Bolus doses of undiluted solution are also tolerated via a central venous catheter.

➤*Extravasation:* Melphalan is a considered vesicant. Melphalan for injection may cause local tissue damage if extravasation occurs; consequently, it should not be administered by direct injection into a peripheral vein. It is recommended that melphalan for injection be administered by injecting slowly into a fast-running IV infusion via an injection port or central venous line.

If signs or symptoms of extravasation occur, stop the infusion immediately. If possible, withdraw 3 to 5 mL of blood to remove some of the drug. Remove the infusion needle. Ice compresses may be applied to the site for 15 minutes every 6 hours for 48 hours. Delineate the infiltrated area on the patient's skin with a felt-tip marker. Elevate for 48 hours above heart level using a sling or stockinette dressing with an observation window cut in the dressing. Avoid pressure or friction. Do not rub the area. Observe for signs of increased erythema, pain, or skin necrosis. If increased symptoms occur, consult a plastic surgeon. Ensure that no medication is given distally to extravasation site. After 48 hours, encourage the patient to use the extremity normally to promote full range of motion.

➤*Storage/Stability:* Store the unreconstituted vials at 15° to 30°C (59° to 86°F) and protect from light.

A precipitate forms if the reconstituted solution is stored at 5°C (41°F). Do not refrigerate the reconstituted product.

Melphalan injection is rapidly hydrolyzed. The undiluted solution is stable for 90 minutes. With further dilution immediately after reconstitution, it is stable for 60 minutes.

Discard vial within 90 minutes of the initial needle puncture if opened within an ISO Class 5 biological safety cabinet, or within 60 minutes of the initial needle puncture if opened outside of such an environment, based on the USP Chapter <797> standards.

Actions

➤*Pharmacology:* Melphalan, also known as L-phenylalanine mustard, phenylalanine mustard, L-PAM, or L-sarcolysin, is a phenylalanine derivative of nitrogen mustard. Melphalan is an alkylating agent of the bischloroethylamine type. As a result, its cytotoxicity appears to be related to the extent of its interstrand cross-linking with DNA, probably by binding at the N^7 position of guanine. Like other bifunctional alkylating agents, it is active against both resting and rapidly dividing tumor cells.

➤*Pharmacokinetics:*

Absorption/Distribution – The pharmacokinetics of melphalan after IV administration have been extensively studied in adult patients. Following injection, drug plasma concentrations declined rapidly in a biexponential

MELPHALAN HYDROCHLORIDE — INJECTION

manner, with distribution phase and terminal elimination phase half-lives of approximately 10 and 75 minutes, respectively. Mean (± standard deviation [SD]) peak melphalan plasma concentrations in myeloma patients given IV melphalan at doses of 10 or 20 mg/m^2 were 1.2 ± 0.4 and 2.8 ± 1.9 mcg/mL, respectively.

The steady-state volume of distribution of melphalan is 0.5 L/kg. Penetration into cerebrospinal fluid is low. The extent of melphalan binding to plasma proteins ranges from 60% to 90%. Serum albumin is the major binding protein, while alpha-1 acid glycoprotein appears to account for approximately 20% of the plasma protein binding. Approximately 30% of the drug is (covalently) irreversibly bound to plasma proteins. Interactions with immunoglobulins have been found to be negligible.

Metabolism / Excretion – Melphalan is eliminated from plasma primarily by chemical hydrolysis to monohydroxymelphalan and dihydroxymelphalan. Aside from these hydrolysis products, no other melphalan metabolites have been observed in humans. Although the contribution of renal elimination to melphalan clearance appears to be low, one study noted an increase in the occurrence of severe leukopenia in patients with elevated BUN after 10 weeks of therapy.

Estimates of average total body clearance varied among studies, but typical values of approximately 7 to 9 mL/min/kg (250 to 325 mL/min/m^2) were observed. One study has reported that upon repeat dosing of 0.5 mg/kg every 6 weeks, the clearance of melphalan decreased from 8.1 mL/min/kg after the first course to 5.5 mL/min/kg after the third course but did not decrease appreciably after the third course.

Contraindications

Prior resistance to this agent; hypersensitivity to melphalan.

Warnings/Precautions

➤*Bone marrow suppression:* As with other nitrogen mustard drugs, excessive dosage will produce marked bone marrow suppression. Bone marrow suppression is the most significant toxicity associated with melphalan in most patients. Therefore, perform the following tests at the start of therapy and prior to each subsequent dose of melphalan: platelet count, hemoglobin, WBC, and differential. Thrombocytopenia and/or leukopenia are indications to withhold further therapy until the blood cell counts have sufficiently recovered. Frequent blood cell counts are essential to determine optimal dosage and avoid toxicity. Consider dose adjustment on the basis of blood cell counts at the nadir and day of treatment.

➤*Prior irradiation or chemotherapy:* Use melphalan with extreme caution in patients whose bone marrow reserve may have been compromised by prior irradiation or chemotherapy or whose marrow function is recovering from previous cytotoxic therapy.

➤*Extravasation:* See Administration and Dosage for more information.

➤*Hypersensitivity reactions:* Hypersensitivity reactions, including anaphylaxis, have occurred in approximately 2% of patients who received the IV formulation. These reactions usually occur after multiple courses of treatment. Treatment is symptomatic. The infusion should be terminated immediately, followed by the administration of volume expanders, pressor agents, corticosteroids, or antihistamines at the discretion of the health care provider. If a hypersensitivity reaction occurs, do not readminister IV or oral melphalan because hypersensitivity reactions have also been reported with oral melphalan.

➤*Renal function impairment:* Consider dose reduction in patients with renal function impairment receiving IV melphalan. In one trial, increased bone marrow suppression was observed in patients with BUN levels of 30 mg/dL or more. A 50% reduction in the IV melphalan dose decreased the incidence of severe bone marrow suppression in the latter portion of this study.

➤*Pregnancy: Category D.* Melphalan may cause fetal harm when administered to a pregnant woman. While adequate animal studies have not been conducted with IV melphalan, oral (6 to 18 mg/m^2/day for 10 days) and intraperitoneal (18 mg/m^2) administration in rats was embryolethal and teratogenic. Malformations resulting from melphalan included alterations of the brain (underdevelopment, deformation, meningocele, and encephalocele) and eye (anophthalmia and microphthalmos), reduction of the mandible and tail, as well as hepatocele (exomphaly).

There are no adequate and well-controlled studies in pregnant women. However, the molecular weight of melphalan is low enough; therefore, expect the transfer across the placenta to the fetus. Melphalan is contraindicated during the first trimester of pregnancy. If this drug is used during pregnancy, or if the patient becomes pregnant while taking this drug, apprise the patient of the potential hazard to the fetus. Advise women of childbearing potential to avoid becoming pregnant.

Fertility impairment – Melphalan causes suppression of ovarian function in premenopausal women, resulting in amenorrhea in a significant number of patients. Reversible and irreversible testicular suppression have also been reported.

➤*Lactation:* It is not known whether this drug is excreted in human milk. However, the molecular weight of melphalan is relatively low; expect excretion into breast milk. Do not give IV melphalan to breast-feeding mothers.

➤*Children:* Safety and efficacy in children have not been established.

➤*Elderly:* Dose selection for an elderly patient should be cautious, usually starting at the low end of the dosing range, reflecting the greater frequency of decreased hepatic, renal, or cardiac function, and of concomitant disease or other drug therapy.

➤*Monitoring:* Perform periodic complete blood cell counts with differentials during the course of treatment with melphalan. Obtain at least 1 determination prior to each dose.

Closely observe patients for consequences of bone marrow suppression, which include severe infections, bleeding, and symptomatic anemia.

Drug Interactions

Melphalan Drug Interactions

Precipitant drug	Object drug[a]		Description
Cisplatin	Melphalan	↑	Cisplatin may affect melphalan kinetics by inducing renal function impairment and subsequently altering melphalan clearance.
Melphalan	Nalidixic acid	↑	Coadministration is contraindicated because of the risk of serious GI toxicity, such as hemorrhagic ulcerative colitis or intestinal necrosis.
Melphalan	Carmustine	↑	Carmustine lung toxicity threshold may be reduced.
Melphalan	Cyclosporine	↑	An increase in the toxicity of cyclosporine, particularly nephrotoxicity, has been observed following coadministration.
Melphalan	Vaccines, live	↓	Avoid administration of live vaccines to immunocompromised patients.

[a] ↑ = object drug increased; ↓ = object drug decreased.

Adverse Reactions

Melphalan has very high potential for nausea and vomiting when used IV.

➤*Cardiovascular:* Cardiac arrest (rare), vasculitis.

➤*Dermatologic:* Alopecia, maculopapular rashes, skin hypersensitivity, skin necrosis rarely requiring skin grafting, skin ulceration at injection site.

➤*GI:* GI disturbances, such as nausea, vomiting, diarrhea, and oral ulceration, occur infrequently.

➤*Hematologic:* The most common adverse reaction is bone marrow suppression leading to leukopenia, thrombocytopenia, and anemia. Hemolytic anemia has also been reported. WBC and platelet count nadirs usually occur 2 to 3 weeks after treatment, with recovery in 4 to 5 weeks after treatment. Irreversible bone marrow failure has been reported.

➤*Hepatic:* Hepatic disorders ranging from abnormal liver function tests to clinical manifestations such as jaundice, hepatitis, and hepatic venoocclusive disease have been reported.

➤*Hypersensitivity:* Acute hypersensitivity reactions, including anaphylaxis, were reported in 2.4% of 425 patients receiving melphalan injection for myeloma. These reactions were characterized by urticaria, pruritus, edema, and, in some patients, tachycardia, bronchospasm, dyspnea, and hypotension. These patients appeared to respond to antihistamine and corticosteroid therapy. If a hypersensitivity reaction occurs, do not readminister IV or oral melphalan because hypersensitivity reactions have also been reported with oral melphalan.

➤*Respiratory:* Interstitial pneumonitis, pulmonary fibrosis (including fatal outcomes).

➤*Miscellaneous:* Other reported adverse reactions include allergic reactions. Temporary significant elevation of the blood urea has been seen in the early stages of therapy in patients with renal damage. Subjective and transient sensation of warmth and/or tingling.

Overdosage

➤*Symptoms:* Overdoses resulting in death have been reported. Overdoses, including doses of up to 290 mg/m^2, have produced the following symptoms: severe nausea and vomiting, decreased consciousness, convulsions, muscular paralysis, and cholinomimetic effects. Severe mucositis, stomatitis, colitis, diarrhea, and hemorrhage of the GI tract occur at high doses (more than 100 mg/m^2).

Elevations in liver enzymes and venoocclusive disease occur infrequently. Significant hyponatremia caused by an associated syndrome of inappropriate antidiuretic hormone secretion has been observed. Nephrotoxicity and adult respiratory distress syndrome have been reported rarely. The principal toxic effect is bone marrow suppression.

➤*Treatment:* Closely follow hematologic parameters for 3 to 6 weeks. An uncontrolled study suggests that administration of autologous bone marrow or hematopoietic growth factors (ie, sargramostim, filgrastim) may shorten the period of pancytopenia. Institute general supportive measures together with appropriate blood transfusions and antibiotics as deemed necessary. This drug is not removed from plasma to any significant degree by hemodialysis or hemoperfusion. A child survived a 254 mg/m^2 overdose treated with standard supportive care.

MELPHALAN HYDROCHLORIDE — INJECTION

Patient Information

Inform patients that the major acute toxicities of melphalan are related to bone marrow suppression, hypersensitivity reactions, GI toxicity, and pulmonary toxicity. The major long-term toxicities are related to infertility and secondary malignancies.

Never allow patients to take the drug without close medical supervision, and advise them to consult their health care provider if they experience skin rash, signs or symptoms of vasculitis, bleeding, fever, persistent cough, nausea, vomiting, amenorrhea, weight loss, or unusual lumps/masses.

Advise women of childbearing potential to avoid becoming pregnant. Women taking melphalan should not breast-feed.

ESTRAMUSTINE PHOSPHATE SODIUM

Rx	**Emcyt** (Pharmacia)	**Capsules:** 140 mg (as estramustine phosphate)	White. In 100s.

ESTRAMUSTINE PHOSPHATE SODIUM — ORAL

Indications

➤*Metastatic/Progressive prostate cancer:* Palliative treatment of metastatic and/or progressive carcinoma of the prostate.

➤*Off-label uses:* Treatment of metastatic renal cell carcinoma.

Administration and Dosage

➤*Adults:*

Metastatic/Progressive prostate cancer –

Usual dosage: 14 mg/kg/day (ie, one 140 mg capsule for each 10 kg or 22 lb) given in 3 or 4 divided doses (dosage range, 10 to 16 mg/kg/day).

Duration of therapy: Treat for 30 to 90 days before assessing the possible benefits of continued therapy. Continue therapy as long as response is favorable. Some patients have been maintained on therapy for more than 3 years at doses ranging from 10 to 16 mg/kg/day.

➤*Preparation for administration:* Estramustine is considered a cytotoxic agent. Follow safe handling procedures when preparing, administering, or dispensing estramustine.

➤*Administration:* Take with water at least 1 hour before or 2 hours after meals.

Milk, milk products, and calcium-rich foods or drugs (such as calcium-containing antacids) must not be taken simultaneously with estramustine.

➤*Storage/Stability:* Refrigerate at 2° to 8°C (36° to 46°F). Capsules may be left out of the refrigerator for 24 to 48 hours without affecting potency.

Actions

➤*Pharmacology:* Estramustine phosphate combines estradiol and nornitrogen mustard by a carbamate link. The molecule is phosphorylated to make it water soluble. The intent of the molecule design was for the estradiol portion to facilitate the uptake of the alkylating agent into the hormone-sensitive prostate cancer cells. However, it was determined that estramustine does not function in vivo as an alkylating agent and not all of its effects can be attributed to the estrogenic hormones. Estramustine has been shown to have weaker estrogenic effects than estradiol. It has been called an antimicrotubule agent because it covalently binds to microtubule-associated proteins, thereby inhibiting microtubule assembly and eventually causing their disassembly.

➤*Pharmacokinetics:*

Absorption/Distribution – After oral administration, estramustine is well absorbed with a bioavailability of at least 75%. Estramustine phosphate is readily dephosphorylated during absorption, and the major metabolites in plasma are estramustine, the estrone analog, estradiol, and estrone.

Prolonged treatment produces elevated total plasma concentrations of estradiol that are within ranges similar to the elevated estradiol levels found in prostatic cancer patients given conventional estradiol therapy. Estrogenic effects, as demonstrated by changes in circulating levels of steroids and pituitary hormones, are similar in patients treated with either estramustine phosphate or conventional estradiol.

Metabolism/Excretion – Estramustine is found in the body mainly as estromustine (17-keto analog).

The metabolic urinary patterns of estradiol and the estradiol moiety of estramustine phosphate are very similar, although the metabolites derived from estramustine phosphate are excreted at a slower rate. The nornitrogen mustard and estradiol metabolites are excreted independently into the bile, feces, and urine.

Contraindications

Hypersensitivity to estradiol or nitrogen mustard.

Active thrombophlebitis or thromboembolic disorders, except where the actual tumor mass is the cause of the thromboembolic phenomenon and the benefits of therapy outweigh the risks.

Warnings/Precautions

➤*Thrombosis:* The risk of thrombosis, including fatal and nonfatal myocardial infarction, increases in men receiving estrogens for prostatic cancer. Use with caution in patients with a history of thrombophlebitis, thrombosis or thromboembolic disorders, especially if they were associated with estrogen therapy. Use with caution in patients with cerebral vascular or coronary artery disease.

➤*Glucose tolerance:* Tolerance to glucose may be decreased; observe diabetic patients receiving this drug.

➤*Elevated blood pressure:* Blood pressure elevation may occur; monitor blood pressure periodically during therapy.

➤*Fluid retention:* Exacerbation of pre-existing or incipient peripheral edema or congestive heart disease may occur in some patients. Other conditions potentially influenced by fluid retention, such as epilepsy, migraine, or renal dysfunction, require careful observation.

➤*Calcium/Phosphorus metabolism:* Calcium/Phosphorus metabolism may be influenced by estramustine; use with caution in patients with metabolic bone diseases associated with hypercalcemia or in patients with renal insufficiency.

➤*Gynecomastia/Impotence:* Gynecomastia and impotence are known estrogenic effects.

➤*Hypersensitivity reactions:* Allergic reactions and angioedema at times involving the airway have been reported.

➤*Hepatic function impairment:* Estramustine may be poorly metabolized in patients with impaired liver function. Administer with caution.

➤*Pregnancy: Category X* (estradiol); *Category D* (nitrogen mustards). Because estradiol and nitrogen mustard are mutagenic, avoid use in pregnant women. Advise women of childbearing age to use effective contraception.

➤*Lactation:* It is unknown if this medication is excreted in breast milk. The American Academy of Pediatrics classifies estradiol as compatible with breast-feeding. Women taking nitrogen mustards should not breast-feed.

➤*Lab test abnormalities:* Certain endocrine and liver function tests may be affected by estrogen-containing drugs. Estramustine phosphate sodium may depress testosterone levels. Abnormalities of hepatic enzymes and of bilirubin have occurred. Perform such tests at appropriate intervals during therapy and repeat after the drug has been withdrawn for 2 months.

Drug Interactions

➤*Drug/Food interactions:* Milk, milk products, and calcium-rich foods or drugs may impair the absorption of estramustine phosphate sodium.

Adverse Reactions

Estramustine is considered to have low potential for nausea and vomiting.

Estramustine Phosphate Sodium Adverse Reactions

Adverse reactions	Estramustine phosphate sodium (11.5 to 15.9 mg/kg/day) (n = 93)	Diethylstilbestrol (3 mg/day) (n = 93)
Cardiovascular		
Cardiac arrest	0	2
Cerebrovascular accident	2	0
MI	3	1
Thrombophlebitis	3	7
Pulmonary emboli	2	5
CHF	3	2
CNS		
Lethargy alone	4	3
Depression	0	2
Emotional lability	2	0
Insomnia	3	0
Headache	1	1
Anxiety	1	0
Dermatologic		
Rash	1	4
Pruritus	2	2
Dry skin	2	0
Pigment changes	0	3
Easy bruising	3	0
Flushing	1	0
Night sweats	0	1
Fingertip (peeling skin)	1	0
Thinning hair	1	1

Estrogen/Nitrogen Mustard

ESTRAMUSTINE PHOSPHATE SODIUM — ORAL

Estramustine Phosphate Sodium Adverse Reactions		
Adverse reactions	Estramustine phosphate sodium (11.5 to 15.9 mg/kg/day) (n = 93)	Diethylstilbestrol (3 mg/day) (n = 93)
GI		
Nausea	15	8
Diarrhea	12	11
Minor GI upset	11	6
Anorexia	4	3
Flatulence	2	0
Vomiting	1	1
GI bleeding	1	0
Burning throat	1	0
Thirst	1	0
GU		
Breast tenderness	66	64
Breast enlargement		
Mild	60	54
Moderate	10	16
Marked	0	5
Respiratory		
Dyspnea	11	3
Upper respiratory discharge	1	1
Hoarseness	1	0
Special senses		
Pain in eyes	0	1
Tearing of eyes	1	1
Tinnitus	0	1

Estramustine Phosphate Sodium Adverse Reactions		
Adverse reactions	Estramustine phosphate sodium (11.5 to 15.9 mg/kg/day) (n = 93)	Diethylstilbestrol (3 mg/day) (n = 93)
Laboratory test abnormalities		
Hematologic		
Leukopenia	4	2
Thrombopenia	1	2
Hepatic		
Bilirubin alone	1	5
Bilirubin and LDH	0	1
Bilirubin and AST	2	1
Bilirubin, LDH, AST	2	0
LDH and/or AST	31	28
Miscellaneous		
Hypercalcemia (transient)	0	1
Leg cramps	8	11
Edema	19	17
Chest pain	1	1
Hot flashes	0	1

Overdosage

Although there has been no experience with overdosage, it may produce pronounced manifestations of the adverse reactions. In the event of overdosage, evacuate gastric contents by gastric lavage and initiate symptomatic therapy. Monitor hematologic and hepatic parameters for at least 6 weeks after overdosage.

Patient Information

Because of the possibility of mutagenic effects, use contraceptive measures.

Take with water at least 1 hour before or 2 hours after meals.

Milk, milk products, and calcium-rich foods or drugs (such as calcium-containing antacids) must not be taken simultaneously with estramustine phosphate sodium.

Nitrosoureas

CARMUSTINE (BCNU)

Rx	**BiCNU** (Bristol Labs Oncology)	**Powder for Injection, lyophilized:** 100 mg	Preservative-free. In single-dose vials with 3 mL sterile diluent.
Rx	**Gliadel** (Guilford Pharm.)	**Wafer:** 7.7 mg	Preservative-free. In single-dose treatment box with 8 individually pouched wafers.

CARMUSTINE — INJECTION

WARNING

Carmustine for injection should be administered under the supervision of a qualified physician experienced in the use of cancer chemotherapeutic agents.

Bone marrow suppression, notably thrombocytopenia and leukopenia, which may contribute to bleeding and overwhelming infections in an already compromised patient, is the most common and severe of the toxic effects of carmustine for injection (see Warnings and Adverse Reactions).

Since the major toxicity is delayed bone marrow suppression, blood counts should be monitored weekly for at least 6 weeks after a dose (see Adverse Reactions). At the recommended dosage, courses of carmustine for injection should not be given more frequently than every 6 weeks.

The bone marrow toxicity of carmustine for injection is cumulative and therefore dosage adjustment must be considered on the basis of nadir blood counts from prior dose (see Administration and Dosage).

Pulmonary toxicity from carmustine for injection appears to be dose related. Patients receiving greater than 1400 mg/m² cumulative dose are at significantly higher risk than those receiving less.

Delayed pulmonary toxicity can occur years after treatment, and can result in death, particularly in patients treated in childhood (see Adverse Reactions, and Warnings; Children).

Indications

➤*General information:* As palliative therapy as a single agent or in established combination therapy with other approved chemotherapeutic agents in the following:

➤*Brain tumors:* Brain tumors including glioblastoma, brainstem glioma, medulloblastoma, astrocytoma, ependymoma, and metastatic brain tumors.

➤*Multiple myeloma:* Multiple myeloma in combination with prednisone.

➤*Hodgkin's disease:* Hodgkin's disease as secondary therapy in combination with other approved drugs in patients who relapse while being treated with primary therapy, or who fail to respond to primary therapy.

➤*Non-Hodgkin's lymphomas:* Non-Hodgkin's lymphomas as secondary therapy in combination with other approved drugs for patients who relapse while being treated with primary therapy, or who fail to respond to primary therapy.

➤*Off-label uses:* Treatment of hematopoietic stem cell transplantation (HSCT), mycosis fungoides, colorectal carcinoma, malignant melanoma.

Administration and Dosage

➤*General dosing considerations:* Because the major toxicity is delayed bone marrow suppression, blood counts should be monitored weekly for at least 6 weeks after a dose (see Adverse Reactions). At the recommended dosage, courses of carmustine for injection should not be given more frequently than every 6 weeks.

The bone marrow toxicity of carmustine is cumulative; therefore, dosage adjustment must be considered on the basis of nadir blood counts from prior dose.

➤*Adults:*

Malignancies – For a list of malignancies, see Indications.

Usual dosage: 150 to 200 mg/m² intravenously (IV) every 6 weeks as a single agent in previously untreated patients. This may be given as a single dose or divided into daily injections such as 75 to 100 mg/m² on 2 successive days.

Dosage adjustment: Doses subsequent to the initial dose should be adjusted according to the hematologic response of the patient to the preceding dose. The following schedule is suggested as a guide to dosage adjustment:

Carmustine Injection Dosage Adjustment		
Nadir after prior dose		
Leukocytes/mm³	Platelets/mm³	Percentage of prior dose to be given
> 4,000	> 100,000	100%
3,000 to 3,999	75,000 to 99,999	100%
2,000 to 2,999	25,000 to 74,999	70%

CARMUSTINE — INJECTION

Carmustine Injection Dosage Adjustment		
Nadir after prior dose		
Leukocytes/mm^3	Platelets/mm^3	Percentage of prior dose to be given
< 2,000	< 25,000	50%

A repeat course of carmustine should not be given until circulating blood elements have returned to acceptable levels (platelets above 100,000/mm^3, leukocytes above 4,000/mm^3), and this is usually in 6 weeks. Adequate number of neutrophils should be present on a peripheral blood smear. Blood counts should be monitored weekly and repeat courses should not be given before 6 weeks because the hematologic toxicity is delayed and cumulative.

When carmustine is used in combination with other myelosuppressive drugs or in patients in whom bone marrow reserve is depleted, the doses should be adjusted accordingly.

Off-label dosing –

Bone marrow ablation:

• *Usual dose* – 300 to 600 mg/m^2 IV before HSCT, given in combination therapy.

• *Maximum dose* – Doses above 1,200 mg/m^2 are not tolerated because of pulmonary or hepatic toxicity.

➤*Children:*

Off-label dosing –

Malignancies:

• *Usual dose* – 200 to 250 mg/m^2 IV every 4 to 6 weeks as a single dose.

• *Dosage adjustment* – Compromised bone marrow function or therapy with other myelosuppressive drugs requires a reduction in dose. Do not administer repeat courses until acceptable leukocyte and platelet counts have recovered (usually 4,000 cells/mm^3 for leukocytes and 100,000 cells/mm^3 for platelet counts). Subsequent doses are determined by the clinical and hematologic tolerance of the previous dose (See table in Adults).

Follow dosage adjustment guidelines recommended for adults (See Adults).

➤*Premedication:* Premedication with an antiemetic may reduce nausea and vomiting after IV administration.

➤*Preparation for administration:* Carmustine is considered a cytotoxic agent. Follow safe handling procedures when preparing, administering, or dispensing carmustine.

Accidental contact of reconstituted carmustine for injection with the skin has caused transient hyperpigmentation of the affected areas. The use of gloves is recommended. If carmustine lyophilized material or solution contacts the skin or mucosa, immediately wash the skin or mucosa thoroughly with soap and water.

First, dissolve 1 vial of carmustine with 3 mL of the supplied sterile diluent (dehydrated alcohol injection). Second, aseptically add sterile water 27 mL for injection for a resulting solution of 3.3 mg/mL of carmustine in ethanol. 10%. This solution may be further diluted with dextrose 5% injection in glass containers only. Protect from light.

High doses – When preparing doses of carmustine over 900 mg/m^2, only 50% of the alcohol will be used to reconstitute carmustine powder. Reconstituted carmustine is further diluted with 500 mL of dextrose 5% injection and infused over 2 hours.

Important note – The lyophilized dosage formulation contains no preservatives and is not intended for use as a multiple dose vial.

➤*Administration:* The reconstituted solution is administered by IV drip over 1 to 2 hours. Shorter infusion times may produce intense pain and burning at the injection site.

When administered with polyvinyl chloride (PVC) tubing, longer infusion times may result in unacceptable drug loss. In static testing in PVC sets, 10% of carmustine was lost in the first 5 minutes and 65% was lost in 2 hours. With further testing at a simulated infusion rate of 530 mL/h, 4.6% of carmustine was lost in the first hour. At an infusion rate of 265 mL/h, 8.1% of carmustine was lost in the first hour. To avoid drug loss, polyethylene tubing, such as nitroglycerin tubing, can be utilized for infusions of carmustine.

➤*Extravasation:* Carmustine is considered an irritant and may cause phlebitis, but it is not known to cause tissue damage with extravasation. If signs or symptoms of extravasation occur, stop the infusion immediately. If possible, withdraw 3 to 5 mL of blood to remove some of the drug. Remove the infusion needle. Delineate the infiltrated area on the patient's skin with a felt tip marker. Elevate for 48 hours above heart level using a sling or stockinette dressing with an observation window cut in the dressing. Avoid pressure or friction. Do not rub the area. Observe for signs of increased erythema, pain, or skin necrosis. If increased symptoms occur, consult a plastic surgeon. Ensure that no medication is given distally to the extravasation site. After 48 hours, encourage the patient to use the extremity normally to promote full range of motion.

➤*Storage/Stability:* Glass containers were used for the stability data provided in this section. Only use glass containers for carmustine administration.

Before reconstitution – Store unopened vials in a refrigerator (2° to 8°C; 36° to 46°F). The recommended storage of unopened vials provides a stable product for 3 years.

After reconstitution – Carmustine is stable for 24 hours under refrigeration (2° to 8°; 36° to 46°F). Reconstituted vials should be examined for crystal formation prior to use. If crystals are observed, they may be redissolved by warming the vial to room temperature with agitation.

Discard vial within 6 hours of the initial needle puncture if opened within an ISO Class 5 biological safety cabinet, or within 1 hour of the initial needle puncture if opened outside of such an environment, based on the USP Chapter <797> standards.

After further dilution – Vials reconstituted as directed and further diluted to a concentration of 0.2 mg/mL in dextrose 5% injection, should be stored at room temperature, protected from light, and utilized within 8 hours.

Important note – Carmustine has a low melting point (30.5° to 32°C; 86.9° to 89.6°F). Exposure of the drug to this temperature or above will cause the drug to liquefy and appear as an oil film on the vials. This is a sign of decomposition and vials should be discarded. If there is a question of adequate refrigeration upon receipt of this product, immediately inspect the larger vial in each individual carton. Hold the vial to a bright light for inspection. The carmustine will appear as a very small amount of dry flakes or dry congealed mass. If this is evident, the carmustine is suitable for use and should be refrigerated immediately.

Actions

➤*Pharmacology:* Although it is generally agreed that carmustine alkylates DNA and RNA, it is not cross-resistant with other alkylators. As with other nitrosoureas, it may also inhibit several key enzymatic processes by carbamoylation of amino acids in proteins.

➤*Pharmacokinetics:* Intravenously administered carmustine is rapidly degraded, with no intact drug detectable after 15 minutes. However, in studies with C^{14}-labeled drug, prolonged levels of the isotope were detected in the plasma and tissue, probably representing radioactive fragments of the parent compound.

It is thought that the antineoplastic and toxic activities of carmustine may be due to metabolites. Approximately 60% to 70% of a total dose is excreted in the urine in 96 hours and about 10% as respiratory CO_2. The fate of the remainder is undetermined.

Because of the high lipid solubility and the relative lack of ionization at physiological pH, carmustine crosses the blood-brain barrier quite effectively. Levels of radioactivity in the CSF are ≥ 50% of those measured concurrently in plasma.

Contraindications

Hypersensitivity to carmustine.

Warnings/Precautions

➤*Bone marrow suppression:* See the Warning box for more information.

➤*Pulmonary toxicity:* See the Warning box for more information.

➤*Long-term use:* Long-term use of nitrosoureas has been reported to be associated with the development of secondary malignancies.

➤*Ocular:* Carmustine for injection has been administered through an intraarterial intracarotid route; this procedure is investigational and has been associated with ocular toxicity.

➤*Extravasation:* See Administration and Dosage for more information.

➤*Renal/Hepatic function impairment:* Liver and renal function tests should be monitored periodically (see Adverse Reactions).

➤*Pregnancy:* *Category D.* Carmustine for injection may cause fetal harm when administered to a pregnant woman. Carmustine for injection has been shown to be embryotoxic in rats and rabbits and teratogenic in rats when given in doses equivalent to the human dose. There are no adequate and well-controlled studies in pregnant women. If this drug is used during pregnancy, or if the patient becomes pregnant while taking (receiving) this drug, the patient should be apprised of the potential hazard to the fetus. Women of childbearing potential should be advised to avoid becoming pregnant.

➤*Lactation:* It is not known whether this drug is excreted in human milk. Because of the potential for serious adverse events in nursing infants, nursing should be discontinued while taking carmustine for injection.

➤*Children:* Safety and effectiveness in children have not been established. Delayed onset pulmonary fibrosis occurring up to 17 years after treatment, has been reported in a long-term study of patients who received carmustine for injection in childhood and early adolescence (1 to 16 years of age). Eight out of the 17 patients (47%) who survived childhood brain tumors, including all the 5 patients initially treated at younger than 5 years of age, died of pulmonary fibrosis. Therefore, the risks and benefits of carmustine for injection therapy must be carefully considered, due to the extremely high risk of pulmonary toxicity (see Adverse Reactions, Pulmonary toxicity).

➤*Monitoring:* In all instances where the use of carmustine for injection is considered for chemotherapy, the physician must evaluate the need and usefulness of the drug against the risks of toxic effects or adverse reactions. Most such adverse reactions are reversible if detected early. When such effects or reactions do occur, the drug should be reduced in dosage or discontinued and appropriate corrective measures should be taken according to the clinical judgment of the physician. Reinstitution of carmustine for injection therapy should be carried out with caution, and with adequate consideration of the further need for the drug and alertness as to possible recurrence of toxicity.

Due to delayed bone marrow suppression, blood counts should be monitored weekly for at least 6 weeks after a dose.

Baseline pulmonary function studies should be conducted along with frequent pulmonary function tests during treatment. Patients with a baseline

CARMUSTINE — INJECTION

below 70% of the predicted Forced Vital Capacity (FVC) or Carbon Monoxide Diffusing Capacity (DL_{CO}) are particularly at risk.

See Warnings/Precautions for more information.

Drug Interactions

Carmustine Drug Interactions

Precipitant drug	Object drug[a]		Description
Cimetidine	Carmustine	↑	Cimetidine may enhance the myelosuppressive effects of carmustine, possibly to the point of toxicity. Avoid if possible.
Carmustine	Digoxin	↓	Digoxin serum levels may be reduced, and its actions may be decreased by a combination chemotherapy regimen including carmustine.
Carmustine	Phenytoin	↓	Phenytoin serum concentrations may be decreased by a combination chemotherapy regimen including carmustine.

[a] ↑ = Object drug increased. ↓ = Object drug decreased.

Adverse Reactions

Carmustine in dosages of greater than 250 mg/m^2 is considered to have very high emetogenic potential (over 90% incidence of emesis). Carmustine in dosages of 250 mg/m^2 or less is considered to have high emetogenic potential (60% to 90% incidence of emesis).

➤*GI:* Nausea and vomiting after IV administration of carmustine for injection are noted frequently. This toxicity appears within 2 hours of dosing, usually lasting 4 to 6 hours, and is dose related. Prior administration of antiemetics is effective in diminishing and sometimes preventing this adverse effect.

➤*Hematologic:* A frequent and serious toxicity of carmustine for injection is delayed myelosuppression. It usually occurs 4 to 6 weeks after drug administration and is dose related. Thrombocytopenia occurs at about 4 weeks postadministration and persists for 1 to 2 weeks. Leukopenia occurs at 5 to 6 weeks after a dose of carmustine for injection and persists for 1 to 2 weeks. Thrombocytopenia is generally more severe than leukopenia. However, both may be dose-limiting toxicities.

Carmustine for injection may produce cumulative myelosuppression, manifested by more depressed indices or longer duration of suppression after repeated doses.

The occurrence of acute leukemia and bone marrow dysplasias have been reported in patients following long-term nitrosourea therapy.

Anemia also occurs, but is less frequent and less severe than thrombocytopenia or leukopenia.

➤*Hepatic:* A reversible type of hepatic toxicity, manifested by increased transaminase, alkaline phosphatase, and bilirubin levels, has been reported in a small percentage of patients receiving carmustine for injection.

➤*Pulmonary:* Pulmonary toxicity characterized by pulmonary infiltrates and/or fibrosis has been reported to occur from 9 days to 43 months after treatment with carmustine for injection and related nitrosoureas. Most of these patients were receiving prolonged therapy with total doses of carmustine for injection greater than 1400 mg/m^2. However, there have been reports of pulmonary fibrosis in patients receiving lower total doses. Other risk factors include past history of lung disease and duration of treatment. Cases of fatal pulmonary toxicity with carmustine for injection have been reported.

Additionally, delayed onset pulmonary fibrosis occurring up to 17 years after treatment has been reported in a long-term study with 17 patients who received carmustine for injection in childhood and early adolescence (1 to 16 years) in cumulative doses ranging from 770 to 1800 mg/m^2 combined with cranial radiotherapy for intracranial tumors. Chest x-rays demonstrated pulmonary hypoplasia with upper zone contraction. Gallium scans were normal in all cases. Thoracic CT scans have demonstrated an unusual pattern of upper zone fibrosis. There was some late reduction of pulmonary function in all long-term survivors. This form of lung fibrosis may be slowly progressive and has resulted in death in some cases. In this long-term study, 8 of 17 died of delayed pulmonary lung fibrosis, including all those initially treated (5 of 17) at younger than 5 years of age.

➤*Renal:* Renal abnormalities consisting of progressive azotemia, decrease in kidney size and renal failure have been reported in patients who received large cumulative doses after prolonged therapy with carmustine for injection and related nitrosoureas. Kidney damage has also been reported occasionally in patients receiving lower total doses.

➤*Miscellaneous:* Accidental contact of reconstituted carmustine for injection with skin has caused burning and hyperpigmentation of the affected areas.

Rapid IV infusion of carmustine for injection may produce intensive flushing of the skin and suffusion of the conjunctiva within 2 hours, lasting about 4 hours. It is also associated with burning at the site of injection although true thrombosis is rare.

Neuroretinitis, chest pain, headache, allergic reaction, hypotension and tachycardia have been reported as part of ongoing surveillance.

Overdosage

No proven antidotes have been established for carmustine for injection overdosage.

Patient Information

Contraceptive measures are recommended during therapy.

CARMUSTINE — IMPLANT

WARNING

Delayed pulmonary toxicity can occur years after treatment and can result in death, particularly in patients treated in childhood.

Indications

➤*Brain tumors:* As an adjunct to surgery and radiation in newly diagnosed high-grade malignant glioma patients; in recurrent glioblastoma multiforme patients as an adjunct to surgery.

➤*Off-label uses:* Topical carmustine has been shown to be effective in the treatment of primary cutaneous T-cell lymphoma (ie, mycosis fungoides and Sezary syndrome). Carmustine, alone or in combination therapy, has also shown some benefit in the management of malignant melanoma.

Administration and Dosage

➤*Adults:*

Malignant glioma and glioblastoma multiforme –

Usual dosage: Eight wafers should be placed in the resection cavity if the size and shape of cavity allow. Should the size and shape not accommodate 8 wafers, the maximum number of wafers allowed should be used to cover as much of the resection cavity as possible.

Maximum dose: No more than 8 wafers should be used per surgical procedure.

➤*Preparation for administration:* Carmustine is considered a cytotoxic agent. Follow safe handling procedures when preparing, administering, or dispensing carmustine wafers for implantation.

Use of double gloves is recommended because exposure to carmustine can cause severe burning and hyperpigmentation of the skin. Use surgical instruments dedicated to the handling of the wafers for implantation. Deliver the aluminum foil laminate pouches containing the wafer to the operating room and leave unopened until ready to implant the wafers.

➤*Administration:* Open the foil pouches containing the wafer in the operating room immediately prior to implantation. The inner foil pouch is sterile; the outside surface of the outer foil pouch is not.

Use a dedicated surgical instrument for handling the wafers during implantation.

Wafers may overlap slightly and should cover as much of the resection cavity as possible.

Wafers may be used if broken in half. Do not use if broken in more than 2 pieces; dispose of as hazardous chemical waste.

Oxidized regenerated cellulose may be placed on top of the wafers to secure them against the cavity surface.

After placement of the wafers, the resection cavity should be irrigated and the dura closed in a water-tight fashion.

Avoid communication between the resection cavity and the ventricular system to prevent wafers from migrating and causing obstructive hydrocephalus. Close any existing communication prior to wafer implantation.

➤*Storage/Stability:* Unopened foil pouches may be kept at ambient room temperature for a maximum of 6 hours at a time. Store at or below −20°C (−4°F).

Actions

➤*Pharmacology:* Carmustine alkylates deoxyribonucleic acid (DNA) and ribonucleic acid (RNA) and also inhibits several enzymes by carbamoylation of amino acids in proteins. Carmustine is not cross resistant with other alkylators. Antineoplastic and toxic activities may be caused by metabolites.

➤*Pharmacokinetics:* Wafers are biodegradable in the human brain when implanted into the cavity after tumor resection. The carmustine released from the wafer diffuses into the surrounding brain tissue. The rate of biodegradation is variable from patient to patient. A wafer remnant may be observed on brain imaging scans or at re-operation even though extensive degradation of all components has occurred. The absorption, distribution, metabolism, and excretion of the copolymer in humans is unknown.

Contraindications

Hypersensitivity to carmustine or to any components of the wafer formulation.

Warnings/Precautions

➤*Hematologic:* The most frequent and serious toxic effect of injectable carmustine is delayed myelosuppression, which usually occurs 4 to 6 weeks after administration and is dose related (see Warning Box). Thrombocytopenia occurs at about 4 weeks postadministration and persists for 1 to 2 weeks. Leukopenia occurs at 5 to 6 weeks after a dose and persists for 1 to

CARMUSTINE — IMPLANT

2 weeks Thrombocytopenia is generally more severe than leukopenia; however, both may have dose-limiting toxicities.

➤*Ocular:* Carmustine administration through an intra-arterial intracarotid route is investigational and has been associated with ocular toxicity.

➤*Brain herniation:* Cases of intracerebral mass effect unresponsive to corticosteroids have been described in patients treated with the wafer, including one case leading to brain herniation.

➤*Seizures:* In the initial surgery trial, the incidence of seizures was 33.3% in patients receiving carmustine wafer and 37.5% in patients receiving placebo. Grand mal seizures occurred in 5% of wafer-treated patients and 4.2% of placebo-treated patients. The incidence of seizures within the first 5 days after wafer implantation was 2.5% in the wafer group and 4.2% in the placebo group. The time from surgery to the onset of the first postoperative seizure did not differ between the wafer and placebo-treated patients.

In the surgery for recurrent disease trial, the incidence of postoperative seizures was the same for the wafer treatment group and placebo (19%). Of the 22 patients, 54% of wafer-treated patients and 9% of placebo patients experienced the first new or worsened seizure within the first 5 postoperative days; the median time to onset was 3.5 days and 61 days, respectively.

➤*Brain edema:* Brain edema was noted in 22.5% of patients treated with the wafer and in 19.2% of placebo patients. Development of brain edema with mass effect (caused by tumor recurrence, intracranial infection, or necrosis) may necessitate re-operation and, in some cases, removal of the wafer or its remnants.

➤*Intracranial infection:* In the initial surgery trial, the incidence of brain abscess or meningitis was 5% in patients treated with carmustine wafer and 6% in patients receiving placebo. In the recurrent setting, the incidence of brain abscess or meningitis was 4% in patients treated with the wafer and 1% in patients receiving placebo.

➤*Obstructive hydrocephalus:* Avoid communication between the surgical resection cavity and the ventricular system to prevent the wafers from migrating into the ventricular system and causing obstructive hydrocephalus. If a communication exists larger than the diameter of a wafer, close it prior to wafer implantation.

➤*Healing abnormalities:* The following healing abnormalities have been reported in clinical trials of carmustine wafer: Wound dehiscence, delayed wound healing, subdural, subgaleal, or wound effusions, and cerebrospinal fluid lead. In the initial surgery trial, healing abnormalities occurred in 15.8% of carmustine wafer-treated patients and in 11.7% of placebo recipients. Cerebrospinal fluid leaks occurred in 5% of carmustine wafer recipients and 0.8% of those given placebo. During surgery, obtain a water-tight dural closure to minimize the risk of cerebrospinal fluid leak.

In the surgery for recurrent disease trial, the incidence of healing abnormalities was 14% in carmustine-wafer treated patients and 5% in patients receiving placebo wafers.

➤*Pregnancy: Category D.* Carmustine is embryotoxic and teratogenic in rats and embryotoxic in rabbits at dose levels equivalent to the human dose. Carmustine may cause fetal harm when administered to a pregnant woman. There are no adequate and well-controlled studies in pregnant women. If this drug is used during pregnancy, or if the patient becomes pregnant while taking this drug, advise her of the potential hazard to the fetus. Advise women of childbearing potential to avoid becoming pregnant.

➤*Lactation:* It is not known whether this drug is excreted in breast milk. Because of the potential for serious adverse reactions in breastfeeding infants from carmustine, discontinue nursing.

➤*Children:* Safety and efficacy for use in children have not been established. Delayed-onset pulmonary fibrosis occurring up to 17 years after treatment, has been reported in a long-term study of patients who received carmustine injection in childhood and early adolescence (1 to 16 years of age). Eight out of the 17 patients (47%) who survived childhood brain tumors, including all of the 5 patients initially treated at less than 5 years of age, died of pulmonary fibrosis. Therefore, the risks and benefits of carmustine injection therapy must be carefully considered, because of the extremely high risk of pulmonary toxicity (see Adverse Reactions).

➤*Monitoring:* Monitor patients undergoing craniotomy for malignant glioma and implantation of the wafer closely for known complications of craniotomy, including seizures, intracranial infections, abnormal wound healing, and brain edema.

Computed tomography and magnetic resonance imaging of the head may demonstrate enhancement in the brain tissue surrounding the resection cavity after implantation of carmustine wafers. This enhancement may represent edema and inflammation caused by the wafer or tumor progression.

Drug Interactions

Carmustine Drug Interactions

Precipitant drug	Object drug[a]		Description
Cimetidine	Carmustine	↑	Cimetidine may enhance the myelosuppressive effects of carmustine, possibly to the point of toxicity. Avoid if possible.
Carmustine	Digoxin	↓	Digoxin serum levels may be reduced, and its actions may be decreased by a combination chemotherapy regimen including carmustine.
Carmustine	Phenytoin	↓	Phenytoin serum concentrations may be decreased by a combination chemotherapy regimen including carmustine.

[a] ↑ = Object drug increased. ↓ = Object drug decreased.

Adverse Reactions

Adverse Events Observed in Patients Receiving Carmustine Wafer at Initial Surgery (≥ 5%)

Adverse reaction	Carmustine wafer (N = 120)	Placebo (N = 120)
Cardiovascular		
Deep thrombophlebitis	10	9
Pulmonary embolus	8	8
Hemorrhage	7	6
CNS		
Headache	28	37
Hemiplegia	41	44
Convulsion	33	38
Confusion	23	21
Brain edema	23	19
Aphasia	18	18
Depression	16	10
Somnolence	11	15
Speech disorder	11	8
Amnesia	9	10
Intracranial hypertension	9	2
Personality disorder	8	8
Anxiety	7	4
Facial paralysis	7	4
Neuropathy	7	10
Ataxia	6	4
Hypesthesia	6	5
Paresthesia	6	8
Thinking abnormal	6	8
Abnormal gait	5	5
Dizziness	5	9
Grand mal convulsion	5	4
Hallucinations	5	3
Insomnia	5	6
Tremor	5	7
Coma	4	5
Incoordination	3	7
Hypokinesia	2	7
Endocrine system		
Diabetes mellitus	5	4
Cushing syndrome	3	5
Alopecia	10	12
GI		
Nausea	22	17
Vomiting	21	16
Constipation	19	12
Abdominal pain	8	2
Diarrhea	5	4
Liver function tests abnormal	1	5
GU		
Urinary tract infection	8	11
Urinary incontinence	8	8

CARMUSTINE — IMPLANT

Adverse Events Observed in Patients Receiving Carmustine Wafer at Initial Surgery (≥ 5%)

Adverse reaction	Carmustine wafer (N = 120)	Placebo (N = 120)
Metabolic/Nutritional disorders		
Healing abnormal	16	12
Peripheral edema	9	9
Respiratory		
Pneumonia	8	8
Dyspnea	3	7
Special senses		
Conjunctival edema	7	7
Abnormal vision	6	6
Visual field defect	5	7
Eye disorder	3	5
Diplopia	1	5
Miscellaneous		
Aggravation reaction[a]	82	79
Asthenia	22	15
Infection	18	20
Fever	18	18
Pain	13	15
Rash	12	11
Back pain	7	3
Face edema	6	5
Abscess	5	3
Accidental injury	5	7
Chest pain	5	0
Allergic reaction	2	5
Myasthenia	4	5

[a] Adverse events coded to "aggravation reaction" were usually events involving tumor/disease progression or general deterioration of condition (eg, condition/health/Karnofsky/neurological/physical deterioration).

Adverse Reactions: Carmustine Wafer vs Placebo for Recurrent Disease (≥ 4%)

Adverse reaction	Wafer with carmustine (n=110; %)	Wafer without carmustine (n=112; %)
CNS		
Convulsion	19	19
Hemiplegia	19	20
Headache	15	13
Somnolence	14	11
Confusion	10	8
Aphasia	9	11
Stupor	6	6
Brain edema	4	1
Intracranial hypertension	4	6
Meningitis or abscess	4	1
Miscellaneous		
Urinary tract infection	21	17
Healing abnormal	14	5
Fever	12	8
Nausea and vomiting	8	6
Pain	7	1
Rash	5	4

➤*Cardiovascular:* Hypertension (3%); hypotension (1%).

➤*CNS:* Seizures, brain edema (see Warnings); hydrocephalus, depression (3%); abnormal thinking, ataxia, dizziness, insomnia, monoplegia (2%); coma, amnesia, diplopia, paranoid reaction (1%); cerebral hemorrhage and cerebral infarct (less than 1%).

➤*GI:* Diarrhea, constipation (2%); dysphagia, GI hemorrhage, fecal incontinence (1%).

➤*Hematologic/Lymphatic:* Thrombocytopenia, leukocytosis (1%).

➤*Metabolic/Nutritional:* Hyponatremia, hyperglycemia (3%); hypokalemia (1%).

➤*Respiratory:* Infection (2%); aspiration pneumonia (1%).

➤*Special senses:* Visual field defect (2%); eye pain (1%).

➤*Miscellaneous:* Healing abnormalities, intracranial infection (see Warnings and Precautions); peripheral edema, neck pain, rash, urinary incontinence (2%); accidental injury, back pain, allergic reaction, asthenia, chest pain, sepsis (1%).

Overdosage

No proven antidotes have been established for carmustine overdosage.

Patient Information

Contraceptive measures are recommended during therapy.

LOMUSTINE (CCNU)

Rx	CeeNU (Bristol Labs Oncology)	**Capsules:** 10 mg	Mannitol. Two-tone white. In 20s.
		40 mg	Mannitol. White/green. In 20s.
		100 mg	Mannitol. Two-tone green. In 20s.

LOMUSTINE — ORAL

WARNING

Bone marrow suppression, notably thrombocytopenia and leukopenia, which may contribute to bleeding and overwhelming infections in an already compromised patient, is the most common and severe of the toxic effects of lomustine.

Because the major toxicity is delayed bone marrow suppression, monitor blood counts weekly for greater than or equal to 6 weeks after a dose. At the recommended dosage, do not give courses of lomustine more frequently than every 6 weeks.

Bone marrow toxicity is cumulative. Consider dosage adjustments on the basis of nadir blood counts from prior dosage (see Administration and Dosage and Warnings).

Indications

➤*Brain tumors:* Both primary and metastatic, in patients who have already received appropriate surgical and/or radiotherapeutic procedures.

➤*Hodgkin Disease:* Secondary therapy in combination with other approved drugs in patients who relapse while being treated with primary therapy, or who fail to respond to primary therapy.

➤*Off-label uses:* Non-Hodgkin lymphoma, melanoma, renal carcinoma, lung cancer, colon cancer, breast cancer, multiple myeloma.

Administration and Dosage

➤*General dosing considerations:* Round the dose to the nearest 10 mg. Patients should be told to wear gloves when handling lomustine capsules.

Directions to the pharmacist – The dose pack contains a total of 300 mg and will provide enough medication for titration of a single dose. The total dose prescribed by the physician can be obtained (to within 10 mg) by determining the appropriate combination of the enclosed capsule strengths.

The appropriate number of capsules of each size should be placed in a single vial to which the patient information label (gummed label provided) explaining the differences in the appearance of the capsules is affixed. Each color-coded capsule is imprinted with the dose in milligrams.

A patient information sticker, to be placed on dispensing container, is enclosed in the manufacturer's prescribing information.

➤*Adults:*

Brain tumors –

Usual dosage: 100 to 130 mg/m^2 as a single oral dose every 6 weeks as a single agent in previously untreated patients.

Dosage adjustment: In individuals with compromised bone marrow function, the dose should be reduced to 100 mg/m^2 every 6 weeks.

Doses subsequent to the initial dose should be adjusted according to the hematologic response of the patient to the preceding dose. Compared with the manufacturer's recommendations (see the following table), some clinicians advocate more conservative dosage adjustment guidelines.

LOMUSTINE — ORAL

Lomustine Dosage Adjustment		
Nadir after prior dose		Percentage of prior dose to be given
Leukocytes	Platelets	
> 4,000	> 100,000	100%
3,000 to 3,999	75,000 to 99,999	100%
2,000 to 2,999	25,000 to 74,999	70%
< 2,000	< 25,000	50%

A repeat course of lomustine should not be given until circulating blood elements have returned to acceptable levels (platelets above 100,000/mm^2, leukocytes above 4,000/mm^2) and this is usually in 6 weeks. Adequate number of neutrophils should be present on a peripheral blood smear. Blood counts should be monitored weekly and repeat courses should not be given before 6 weeks because the hematologic toxicity is delayed and cumulative.

Concomitant therapy: When lomustine is used in combination with other myelosuppressive drugs, the doses should be adjusted accordingly.

Hodgkin disease – See Brain tumors for dosing.

➤*Children:*

Brain tumors –

Usual dosage: 130 mg/m^2 as a single oral dose every 6 weeks as a single agent in previously untreated patients. See also Off-label dosing.

Dosage adjustment: In individuals with compromised bone marrow function, the dose should be reduced to 100 mg/m^2 every 6 weeks.

Doses subsequent to the initial dose should be adjusted according to the hematologic response of the patient to the preceding dose. Compared with the manufacturer's recommendations (see the following table), some clinicians advocate more conservative dosage adjustment guidelines.

Lomustine Dosage Adjustment		
Nadir after prior dose		Percentage of prior dose to be given
Leukocytes	Platelets	
> 4,000	> 100,000	100%
3,000 to 3,999	75,000 to 99,999	100%
2,000 to 2,999	25,000 to 74,999	70%
< 2,000	< 25,000	50%

A repeat course of lomustine should not be given until circulating blood elements have returned to acceptable levels (platelets above 100,000/mm^2, leukocytes above 4,000/mm^2) and this is usually in 6 weeks. Adequate number of neutrophils should be present on a peripheral blood smear. Blood counts should be monitored weekly and repeat courses should not be given before 6 weeks because the hematologic toxicity is delayed and cumulative.

Concomitant therapy: When lomustine is used in combination with other myelosuppressive drugs, the doses should be adjusted accordingly.

Hodgkin disease – See Brain tumors in Children for dosing. See also Off-label dosing.

Off-label dosing –

Brain tumors: 75 to 150 mg/m^2 administered as a single oral dose every 6 weeks.

Hodgkin disease: 75 to 150 mg/m^2 administered as a single oral dose every 6 weeks.

➤*Renal function impairment:* Dosage adjustment is required in renal dysfunction, as shown in the following table.

Lomustine Dosage Reduction for Renal Function Impairment	
Creatinine clearance	Percent of usual dose
> 50 mL/min	100
10 to 50 mL/min	75
< 10 mL/min	50

➤*Preparation for administration:* Lomustine is considered a cytotoxic agent. Follow safe handling procedures when preparing, administering, or dispensing lomustine.

Lomustine capsules should not be broken. Personnel should avoid exposure to broken capsules. If contact occurs, wash immediately and thoroughly.

➤*Administration:* Take lomustine on an empty stomach and avoid alcohol on that day.

➤*Storage/Stability:* Store in well closed containers at 25°C (77°F); excursions permitted to 15° to 30°C (59° to 86°F). Avoid excessive heat (over 40°C; 104°F).

Actions

➤*Pharmacology:* Although it is generally agreed that lomustine alkylates DNA and RNA, it is not cross resistant with other alkylators. As with other nitrosoureas, it may also inhibit several key enzymatic processes by carbamoylation of amino acids in proteins.

➤*Pharmacokinetics:*

Absorption/Distribution – Because of the high lipid solubility and the relative lack of ionization at physiological pH, lomustine crosses the blood-brain barrier quite effectively. Levels of radioactivity in the CSF are 50% or greater than those measured concurrently in plasma.

Metabolism/Excretion – Following oral administration of radioactive lomustine at doses ranging from 30 mg/m^2 to 100 mg/m^2, about half of the radioactivity given was excreted in the form of degradation products within 24 hours.

The serum half-life of the metabolites ranges from 16 hours to 2 days. Tissue levels are comparable to plasma levels at 15 minutes after intravenous administration.

Contraindications

Hypersensitivity to lomustine.

Warnings/Precautions

➤*Hematologic:* Since the major toxicity is delayed bone marrow suppression, blood counts should be monitored weekly for at least 6 weeks after a dose (see Adverse Reactions). At the recommended dosage, courses of lomustine should not be given more frequently than every 6 weeks.

See Administration and Dosage for more information.

➤*Pulmonary toxicity:* See Adverse Reactions for more information.

➤*Long-term use:* Long-term use of nitrosoureas has been reported to be possibly associated with the development of secondary malignancies.

➤*Pregnancy: Category D.* Lomustine can cause fetal harm when administered to a pregnant woman. Lomustine is embryotoxic and teratogenic in rats and embryotoxic in rabbits at dose levels equivalent to the human dose. There are no adequate and well controlled studies in pregnant women. If this drug is used during pregnancy, or if the patient becomes pregnant while taking (receiving) this drug, the patient should be apprised of the potential hazard to the fetus. Women of childbearing potential should be advised to avoid becoming pregnant.

➤*Lactation:* It is not known whether this drug is excreted in human milk. Because many drugs are excreted in human milk and because of the potential for serious adverse reactions in nursing infants from lomustine, a decision should be made whether to discontinue nursing or to discontinue the drug, taking into account the importance of the drug to the mother.

➤*Lab test abnormalities:* See Administration and Dosage for more information.

Baseline pulmonary function studies should be conducted along with frequent pulmonary function tests during treatment. Patients with a baseline below 70% of the predicted Forced Vital Capacity (FVC) or Carbon Monoxide Diffusing Capacity (DL_{co}) are particularly at risk.

➤*Monitoring:* Since lomustine may cause liver dysfunction, it is recommended that liver function tests be monitored periodically.

Renal function tests should also be monitored periodically.

Adverse Reactions

Lomustine in doses of greater than 60 mg/m^2 is considered to have very high emetogenic potential (over 90% incidence of emesis). Lomustine in doses of 60 mg/m^2 or less is considered to have moderately high emetogenic potential (60% to 90% incidence of emesis).

➤*CNS:* Neurological reactions such as disorientation, lethargy, ataxia, and dysarthria have been noted in some patients receiving lomustine. However, the relationship to medication in these patients is unclear.

➤*GI:* Nausea and vomiting may occur 3 to 6 hours after an oral dose and usually lasts less than 24 hours. Prior administration of antiemetics is effective in diminishing and sometimes preventing this side effect. Nausea and vomiting can also be reduced if lomustine capsules is administered to fasting patients.

➤*Hematologic:* The most frequent and most serious toxicity of lomustine is delayed myelosuppression. It usually occurs 4 to 6 weeks after drug administration and is dose related. Thrombocytopenia occurs at about 4 weeks postadministration and persists for 1 to 2 weeks. Leukopenia occurs at 5 to 6 weeks after a dose of lomustine and persists for 1 to 2 weeks. Approximately 65% of patients receiving 130 mg/m^2 develop white blood counts below 5000 wbc/mm^3. 36% develop white blood counts below 3000 wbc/mm^3. Thrombocytopenia is generally more severe than leukopenia. However, both may be dose-limiting toxicities.

Lomustine may produce cumulative myelosuppression, manifested by more depressed indices or longer duration of suppression after repeated doses.

The occurrence of acute leukemia and bone marrow dysplasias have been reported in patients following long term nitrosourea therapy.

Anemia also occurs, but is less frequent and less severe than thrombocytopenia or leukopenia.

➤*Hepatic:* A reversible type of hepatic toxicity, manifested by increased transaminase, alkaline phosphatase and bilirubin levels, has been reported in a small percentage of patients receiving lomustine.

➤*Pulmonary:* Pulmonary toxicity characterized by pulmonary infiltrates and/or fibrosis has been reported rarely with lomustine. Onset of toxicity has occurred after an interval of 6 months or longer from the start of therapy with cumulative doses of lomustine usually greater than 1100 mg/m^2. There is one report of pulmonary toxicity at a cumulative dose of only 600 mg.

Delayed onset pulmonary fibrosis occurring up to 17 years after treatment has been reported in patients who received related nitrosoureas in childhood and early adolescence (1 to 16 years) combined with cranial radiotherapy for intracranial tumors. There appeared to be some late reduction of pulmonary function of all long-term survivors. This form of lung fibrosis may be slowly progressive and has resulted in death in some cases. In this long-term study

LOMUSTINE — ORAL

of carmustine, all those initially treated at less than five years of age died of delayed pulmonary fibrosis.

➤*Renal:* Renal abnormalities consisting of progressive azotemia, decrease in kidney size and renal failure have been reported in patients who received large cumulative doses after prolonged therapy with lomustine. Kidney damage has also been reported occasionally in patients receiving lower total doses.

➤*Miscellaneous:* Stomatitis, alopecia, optic atrophy, and visual disturbances such as blindness have been reported infrequently.

Overdosage

No proven antidotes have been established for lomustine overdosage.

Patient Information

In order to provide the proper dose of lomustine, patients should be aware that there may be two or more different types and colors of capsules in the container dispensed by the pharmacist.

Patients should be told that lomustine is given as a single oral dose and will not be repeated for at least 6 weeks.

Patients should be told that nausea and vomiting usually last less than 24 hours, although loss of appetite may last for several days.

If any of the following reactions occur, notify the physician: fever, chills, sore throat, unusual bleeding or bruising, shortness of breath, dry cough, swelling of feet or lower legs, mental confusion, or yellowing of eyes and skin.

STREPTOZOCIN

Rx	**Zanosar** (Gensia Sicor)	**Powder for Injection:** 1 g (100 mg/ml)	In vials.

STREPTOZOCIN — INJECTION

WARNING

Streptozocin sterile powder should be administered under the supervision of a physician experienced in the use of cancer chemotherapeutic agents.

A patient need not be hospitalized but should have access to a facility with a laboratory and supportive resources sufficient to monitor drug tolerance and to protect and maintain a patient compromised by drug toxicity. Renal toxicity is dose-related and cumulative and may be severe or fatal. Other major toxicities are nausea and vomiting, which may be severe and at times treatment-limiting. In addition, liver dysfunction, diarrhea and hematological changes have been observed in some patients. Streptozocin is mutagenic. When administered parenterally, it has been found to be tumorigenic or carcinogenic in some rodents.

The physician must judge the possible benefit to the patient against the known toxic effects of this drug in considering the advisability of therapy with streptozocin. The physician should be familiar with the following text before making a judgment and beginning treatment.

Indications

➤*Metastatic islet cell carcinoma of the pancreas:* For the treatment of metastatic islet cell carcinoma of the pancreas. Responses have been obtained with both functional and nonfunctional carcinomas. Because of its inherent renal toxicity, therapy with this drug should be limited to patients with symptomatic or progressive metastatic disease.

➤*Off-label uses:* Treatment of Hodgkin disease, palliative treatment of metastatic carcinoid tumor, palliative treatment of colorectal cancer, pancreatic adenocarcinoma, metastatic pheochromocytoma.

Administration and Dosage

➤*Adults:*

Metastatic islet cell carcinoma of the pancreas –

Daily regimen:

• *Usual dosage* – 500 mg/m^2 body surface area IV for 5 consecutive days every 6 weeks until maximum benefit or until treatment-limiting toxicity is observed. Dose escalation on this schedule is not recommended.

Weekly regimen:

• *Initial dosage* – 1,000 mg/m^2 of body surface area administered IV at weekly intervals for the first 2 courses (weeks).

• *Dosage adjustment* – In subsequent courses, drug doses may be escalated in patients who have not achieved a therapeutic response and who have not experienced significant toxicity with the previous course of treatment. However, a single dose of 1,500 mg/m^2 body surface area should not be exceeded because a greater dose may cause azotemia. When administered on this schedule, the median time to onset of response is about 17 days, and the median time to maximum response is about 35 days. The median total dose to onset of response is about 2,000 mg/m^2 body surface area, and the median total dose to maximum response is about 4,000 mg/m^2 body surface area.

• *Response to therapy* – For patients with functional tumors, serial monitoring of fasting insulin levels allows a determination of biochemical response to therapy. For patients with either functional or nonfunctional tumors, response to therapy can be determined by measurable reductions of tumor size (reduction of organomegaly, masses, or lymph nodes).

➤*Renal function impairment:* Dosage adjustment is necessary in renal dysfunction, as shown in the following table. Reduce dose or discontinue therapy in patients who develop significant renal toxicity during streptozocin therapy.

Streptozocin Dosage Adjustment in Renal Dysfunction

Creatinine clearance	Percent of usual dose
> 50 mL/min	100%
10 to 50 mL/min	75%
< 10 mL/min	50%

➤*Preparation for administration:* Streptozocin is considered a cytotoxic agent. Follow safe handling procedures when preparing, administering, or dispensing streptozocin.

The use of gloves is recommended. If streptozocin contacts the skin or mucosae, immediately wash the affected area with soap and water.

Reconstitute streptozocin with 9.5 mL of dextrose injection, or sodium chloride 0.9% injection. The resulting pale-gold solution will contain streptozocin 100 mg/mL and citric acid 22 mg/mL. Where more dilute infusion solutions are desirable, further dilution in the above vehicles is recommended. The total storage time for streptozocin after it has been placed in solution should not exceed 12 hours. This product contains no preservatives and is not intended as a multiple-dose vial.

➤*Administration:* Administer by rapid IV injection, or IV infusion over 15 minutes to 6 hours. Bolus IV administration may cause intense venous pain.

Maintain adequate hydration to reduce the risk of nephrotoxicity.

Continuous infusions for 5 days may cause increased CNS toxicity.

Streptozocin is not active orally. Although it has been administered intra-arterially, this is not recommended pending further evaluation of the possibility that adverse renal effects may be evoked more rapidly by this route of administration.

➤*Extravasation:* Extravasation may cause severe tissue lesions and necrosis. If signs or symptoms of extravasation occur, stop the infusion immediately. If possible, withdraw 3 to 5 mL of blood to remove some of the drug. Remove the infusion needle. Delineate the infiltrated area on the patient's skin with a felt tip marker. Elevate for 48 hours above heart level using a sling or stockinette dressing with an observation window cut in the dressing. Avoid pressure or friction. Do not rub the area. Observe for signs of increased erythema, pain, or skin necrosis. If increased symptoms occur, consult a plastic surgeon. Ensure that no medication is given distally to the extravasation site. After 48 hours, encourage the patient to use the extremity normally to promote full range of motion.

➤*Storage/Stability:* Unopened vials of streptozocin should be stored at refrigeration temperatures (2° to 8°C; 35.6° to 46.4°F) and protected from light (preferably stored in carton).

Reconstituted solutions and diluted solutions prepared with dextrose 5% injection or sodium chloride 0.9% injection are stable for up to 48 hours at room temperature and for up to 96 hours under refrigeration. Streptozocin solutions should be used within 24 hours because they are preservative-free. The manufacturer recommends use within 12 hours of reconstitution. A color change from pale gold to dark brown indicates decomposition.

Discard vial within 6 hours of the initial needle puncture if opened within an ISO Class 5 biological safety cabinet, or within 1 hour of the initial needle puncture if opened outside of such an environment, based on the USP Chapter <797> standards.

Actions

➤*Pharmacology:* Streptozocin inhibits DNA synthesis in bacterial and mammalian cells. In bacterial cells, a specific interaction with cytosine moieties leads to degradation of DNA. The biochemical mechanism leading to mammalian cell death has not been definitely established; streptozocin inhibits cell proliferation at a considerably lower level than that needed to inhibit precursor incorporation into DNA or to inhibit several of the enzymes involved in DNA synthesis. Although streptozocin inhibits the progression of cells into mitosis, no specific phase of the cell cycle is particularly sensitive to its lethal effects.

Streptozocin is active in the L1210 leukemic mouse over a fairly wide range of parenteral dosage schedules. In experiments in many animal species, streptozocin induced a diabetes that resembles human hyperglycemic nonketotic diabetes mellitus. This phenomenon, which has been extensively studied, appears to be mediated through a lowering of beta cell nicotinamide adenine dinucleotide (NAD) and consequent histopathologic alteration of pancreatic islet beta cells.

➤*Pharmacokinetics:* The metabolism and the chemical dissociation of streptozocin that occurs under physiologic conditions has not been extensively studied. When administered intravenously to a variety of experimental animals, streptozocin disappears from the blood very rapidly. In all species tested, it was found to concentrate in the liver and kidney. As much as 20% of the drug (or metabolites containing an N-nitrosourea group) is metabolized or excreted by the kidney. Metabolic products have not yet been identified.

STREPTOZOCIN — INJECTION

Warnings/Precautions

➤*Usage:* Streptozocin sterile powder should be administered under the supervision of a physician experienced in the use of cancer chemotherapeutic agents.

The physician must judge the possible benefit to the patient against the known toxic effects of this drug in considering the advisability of therapy with streptozocin. The physician should be familiar with the following text before making a judgment and beginning treatment.

➤*Toxicities:* A patient need not be hospitalized but should have access to a facility with a laboratory and supportive resources sufficient to monitor drug tolerance and to protect and maintain a patient compromised by drug toxicity. Renal toxicity is dose-related and cumulative and may be severe or fatal. Other major toxicities are nausea and vomiting, which may be severe and at times treatment-limiting. In addition, liver dysfunction, diarrhea and hematological changes have been observed in some patients. Streptozocin is mutagenic. When administered parenterally, it has been found to be tumorigenic or carcinogenic in some rodents.

➤*Topical exposure:* When exposed dermally, some rats developed benign tumors at the site of application of streptozocin. Consequently, streptozocin may pose a carcinogenic hazard following topical exposure if not properly handled (see Administration and Dosage).

➤*Renal toxicity:* Many patients treated with streptozocin sterile powder have experienced renal toxicity, as evidenced by azotemia, anuria, hypophosphatemia, glycosuria and renal tubular acidosis. Such toxicity is dose-related and cumulative and may be severe or fatal. Renal function must be monitored before and after each course of therapy. Serial urinalysis, blood urea nitrogen, plasma creatinine, serum electrolytes and creatinine clearance should be obtained prior to, at least weekly during, and for 4 weeks after drug administration. Serial urinalysis is particularly important for the early detection of proteinuria and should be quantitated with a 24 hour collection when proteinuria is detected. Mild proteinuria is one of the first signs of renal toxicity and may herald further deterioration of renal function. Reduction of the dose of streptozocin or discontinuation of treatment is suggested in the presence of significant renal toxicity. Adequate hydration may help reduce the risk of nephrotoxicity to renal tubular epithelium by decreasing renal and urinary concentration of the drug and its metabolites.

Use of streptozocin in patients with preexisting renal disease requires a judgment by the physician of potential benefit as opposed to the known risk of serious renal damage.

This drug should not be used in combination with or concomitantly with other potential nephrotoxins.

➤*Extravasation:* See Administration and Dosage for more information.

➤*Pregnancy: Category D.* Reproduction studies revealed that streptozocin is teratogenic in the rat and has abortifacient effects in rabbits. When administered intravenously to pregnant monkeys, it appears rapidly in the fetal circulation. There are no studies in pregnant women. Streptozocin should be used during pregnancy only if the potential benefit justifies the potential risk to the fetus.

➤*Lactation:* It is not known whether streptozocin is excreted in human milk. Because many drugs are excreted in human milk and because of the potential for serious adverse reactions in nursing infants, nursing should be discontinued in patients receiving streptozocin.

➤*Monitoring:* Patients who are treated with streptozocin must be monitored closely, particularly for evidence of renal, hepatic, and hematopoietic toxicity. Renal function tests are described in the Warnings section. Patients should also be monitored closely for evidence of hematopoietic and hepatic toxicities. Complete blood counts and liver function tests should be done at least weekly. Dosage adjustments or discontinuance of the drug may be indicated, depending upon the degree of toxicity noted.

Drug Interactions

Streptozocin may demonstrate additive toxicity when used in combination with other cytotoxic drugs. Streptozocin has been reported to prolong the elimination half-life of doxorubicin and may lead to severe bone marrow suppression; a reduction of the doxorubicin dosage should be considered in patients receiving streptozocin concurrently. The concurrent use of streptozocin and phenytoin has been reported in one case to result in reduced streptozocin cytotoxicity.

Adverse Reactions

Streptozocin is considered to have very high emetogenic potential (over 90% incidence of emesis).

➤*GI:* Most patients treated with streptozocin sterile powder have experienced severe nausea and vomiting, occasionally requiring discontinuation of drug therapy. Some patients experienced diarrhea.

➤*Hepatic:* A number of patients have experienced hepatic toxicity, as characterized by elevated liver enzyme (AST and LDH) levels and hypoalbuminemia.

➤*Hematologic:* Hematological toxicity has been rare, most often involving mild decreases in hematocrit values. However, fatal hematological toxicity with substantial reductions in leukocyte and platelet count has been observed.

➤*Metabolic:* Mild to moderate abnormalities of glucose tolerance have been noted in some patients treated with streptozocin. These have generally been reversible, but insulin shock with hypoglycemia has been observed.

➤*Renal:* See Warnings. Two cases of nephrogenic diabetes insipidus following therapy with streptozocin have been reported. One had spontaneous recovery and the second responded to indomethacin.

➤*Postmarketing experience:* Spontaneous reports have been received of local inflammation (ie, edema, erythema, burning, tenderness) following extravasation of the product. In most cases, these events resolved the same day or within a few days.

Overdosage

No specific antidote for streptozocin is known.

Patient Information

Confusion, lethargy, and depression have been reported in a limited number of patients receiving continuous intravenous infusion of streptozocin for 5 days. Patients should be informed that there may be a potential risk in driving or using complex machinery.

Triazenes

DACARBAZINE (DTIC; Imidazole Carboxamide)

Rx	**Dacarbazine** (Various, eg, American Pharmaceutical Partners, Bedford, Mayne, Gensia Sicor)	**Powder for injection:** 100 mg	May contain mannitol. In vials.
Rx	**DTIC-Dome** (Bayer Pharmaceuticals)		May contain mannitol. In vials.
Rx	**Dacarbazine** (Various, eg, American Pharmaceutical Partners, Bedford, Mayne, Gensia Sicor)	**Powder for injection:** 200 mg	May contain mannitol. In vials.
Rx	**DTIC-Dome** (Bayer Pharmaceuticals)		May contain mannitol. In vials.

DACARBAZINE — INJECTION

WARNING

It is recommended that dacarbazine for injection be administered under the supervision of a qualified physician experienced in the use of cancer chemotherapeutic agents.

Hemopoietic depression is the most common toxicity with dacarbazine for injection.

Hepatic necrosis has been reported.

Studies have demonstrated this agent to have a carcinogenic and teratogenic effect when used in animals.

In treatment of each patient, the physician must weigh carefully the possibility of achieving therapeutic benefit against the risk of toxicity.

Indications

➤*Metastatic malignant melanoma/Hodgkin disease:* For the treatment of metastatic malignant melanoma. In addition, dacarbazine is also indicated for Hodgkin's disease as a secondary-line therapy when used in combination with other effective agents.

➤*Off-label uses:* In combination with cyclophosphamide and vincristine for malignant pheochromocytoma; in combination with other agents for the treatment of advanced metastatic soft tissue sarcoma; alone or in combination with other agents for the management of Kaposi sarcoma; treatment of soft-tissue sarcomas, neuroblastomas, fibrosarcomas, rhabdomyosarcoma, islet cell carcinomas,medullary carcinoma of the thyroid.

Dacarbazine has been used safely and effectively in children. (See Administration and Dosage).

Administration and Dosage

➤*General dosing considerations:* Dacarbazine is dosed in mg/kg for some indications, but may be dosed in mg/m^2 for other indications.

➤*Adults:*

Hodgkin disease –

Usual dosage: 150 mg/m^2 body surface area given daily IV for 5 days, in combination with other effective drugs. Treatment may be repeated every 4 weeks.

Alternative dosage: 375 mg/m^2 body surface area given daily IV on day 1, in combination with other effective drugs, to be repeated every 15 days.

Malignant melanoma –

Usual dosage: 2 to 4.5 mg/kg/day IV for 10 days. Treatment may be repeated at 4-week intervals.

Alternative dosage: 250 mg/m^2 body surface area given daily IV for 5 days. Treatment may be repeated every 3 weeks.

DACARBAZINE — INJECTION

Off-label dosing –

Sarcoma: 250 mg/m^2 body surface area given daily by continuous IV infusion on days 1 through 4 of MAID regimen (total dacarbazine dose is 1,000 mg/m^2 over 96 hours).

➤*Children:*

Off-label dosing –

Hodgkin lymphoma, combination therapy: 375 mg/m^2 body surface area given IV on day 1; repeated every 15 days.

Neuroblastoma, combination therapy: 800 to 900 mg/m^2 body surface area given IV as a single dose on day 1 of chemotherapy; may be repeated every 3 to 4 weeks.

Solid tumors: 200 to 470 mg/m^2 body surface area given daily IV for 5 days; may be repeated at 3 to 4 week intervals.

➤*Renal function impairment:* Dosage adjustment in renal insufficiency is warranted; however, there are no specific guidelines.

Dialysis – Conventional hemodialysis is moderately effective (50% to 74%) in removing dacarbazine.

➤*Hepatic function impairment:* Dosage adjustment in hepatic insufficiency is warranted; however, there are no specific guidelines.

➤*Preparation for administration:* Dacarbazine is considered a cytotoxic agent. Follow safe handling procedures when preparing, administering, or dispensing dacarbazine.

Dacarbazine for injection 100 mg/vial and 200 mg/vial are reconstituted with 9.9 mL and 19.7 mL, respectively, of sterile water for injection. The resulting solution contains dacarbazine 10 mg/mL, having a pH of 3 to 4. The calculated dose of the resulting solution is drawn into a syringe and administered only IV.

Reconstituted 10 mg/mL solution may be further diluted with up to 250 mL of dextrose 5% injection or sodium chloride 0.9% injection for IV infusion.

Solution should be pale yellow to ivory in color. Visually inspect reconstituted solution and discard if particulates or discoloration (ie, pink or red) are present.

➤*Administration:* Administer by IV injection, IV infusion, continuous IV infusion.

Administer reconstituted 10 mg/mL solution by IV push over 1 to 2 minutes in freely running IV solution.

Diluted solutions may be infused IV over 15 to 30 minutes or by continuous infusion over 24 hours.

Limit patient's food intake for 4 to 6 hours before administration to reduce risk of emesis.

➤*Extravasation:* Extravasation of the drug subcutaneously during IV administration may result in tissue damage and severe pain. Local pain, burning sensation, and irritation at the site of injection may be relieved by locally applied hot packs.

If signs or symptoms of extravasation occur, stop the infusion immediately. If possible, withdraw 3 to 5 mL of blood to remove some of the drug. Remove the infusion needle. Delineate the infiltrated area on the patient's skin with a felt tip marker. Elevate for 48 hours above heart level using a sling or stockinette dressing with an observation window cut in the dressing. Avoid pressure or friction. Do not rub the area. Observe for signs of increased erythema, pain, or skin necrosis. If increased symptoms occur, consult a plastic surgeon. Ensure that no medication is given distally to the extravasation site. After 48 hours, encourage the patient to use the extremity normally to promote full range of motion.

➤*Admixture compatibility:* For continuous infusion regimens, dacarbazine may be mixed in the same bag with doxorubicin.

➤*Storage/Stability:* Store in a refrigerator 2° to 8°C (36° to 46°F). Protect from light. Dacarbazine solutions must be protected from sunlight; protection from normal room lighting is unnecessary. Color change of solution to pink or red indicates decomposition.

After reconstitution and prior to use, the solution in the vial may be stored at 4°C (39.2°F) for up to 72 hours or at normal room conditions (temperature and light) for up to 8 hours. If the reconstituted solution is further diluted in dextrose 5% injection or sodium chloride injection the resulting solution may be stored at 4°C (39.2°F) for up to 24 hours or at normal room conditions for up to 8 hours.

Discard vial within 6 hours of the initial needle puncture if opened within an ISO Class 5 biological safety cabinet, or within 1 hour of the initial needle puncture if opened outside of such an environment, based on the USP Chapter <797> standards.

Actions

➤*Pharmacology:* Although the exact mechanism of action of dacarbazine for injection is not known, the following 3 hypotheses have been offered:

- Inhibition of DNA synthesis by acting as a purine analog.
- Action as an alkylating agent.
- Interaction with sulfhydryl (SH) groups.

➤*Pharmacokinetics:*

Absorption/Distribution – After IV administration of dacarbazine for injection, the volume of distribution exceeds total body water content, suggesting localization in some body tissue, probably the liver. At therapeutic concentrations, dacarbazine is not appreciably bound to human plasma protein.

Metabolism/Excretion – Its disappearance from the plasma is biphasic with initial half-life of 19 minutes and a terminal half-life of 5 hours. In a patient with renal and hepatic dysfunctions, the half-lives were lengthened to 55 minutes and 7.2 hours.

The average cumulative excretion of unchanged dacarbazine in the urine is 40% of the injected dose in 6 hours. Dacarbazine is subject to renal tubular secretion rather than glomerular filtration.

In man, dacarbazine is extensively degraded. Besides unchanged dacarbazine, 5-aminoimidazole-4 carboxamide (AIC) is a major metabolite of dacarbazine excreted in the urine. AIC is not derived endogenously but from the injected dacarbazine, because the administration of radioactive dacarbazine labeled with ^{14}C in the imidazole portion of the molecule (dacarbazine-2-^{14}C) gives rise to AIC-2-^{14}C.

Contraindications

Hypersensitivity to dacarbazine.

Warnings/Precautions

➤*Hemopoietic depression:* Hemopoietic depression is the most common toxicity with dacarbazine for injection, and involves primarily the leukocytes and platelets, although anemia may sometimes occur. Leukopenia and thrombocytopenia may be severe enough to cause death. The possible bone marrow depression requires careful monitoring of white blood cells, red blood cells, and platelet levels. Hemopoietic toxicity may warrant temporary suspension or cessation of therapy with dacarbazine for injection.

➤*Hepatotoxicity:* Hepatic toxicity accompanied by hepatic vein thrombosis and hepatocellular necrosis resulting in death, has been reported. The incidence of such reactions has been low; approximately 0.01% of patients treated. This toxicity has been observed mostly when dacarbazine for injection has been administered concomitantly with other antineoplastic drugs; however, it has also been reported in some patients treated with dacarbazine for injection alone.

➤*Usage:* Hospitalization is not always necessary, but adequate laboratory study capability must be available.

➤*Extravasation:* See Administration and Dosage for more information.

See Administration and Dosage for more information.

➤*Hypersensitivity reactions:* Anaphylaxis can occur following the administration of dacarbazine for injection.

➤*Pregnancy: Category C.*

Teratogenic – Dacarbazine for injection has been shown to be teratogenic in rats when given in doses 20 times the human daily dose on day 12 of gestation. Dacarbazine, when administered in 10 times the human daily dose to male rats (twice weekly for 9 weeks), did not affect the male libido; although, female rats mated to male rats had higher incidence of resorptions than controls. In rabbits, dacarbazine daily dose 7 times the human daily dose given on days 6 to 15 of gestation resulted in fetal skeletal anomalies. There are no adequate and well-controlled studies in pregnant women. Dacarbazine for injection should be used during pregnancy only if the potential benefit justifies the potential risk to the fetus.

➤*Lactation:* It is not known whether this drug is excreted in human milk. Because many drugs are excreted in human milk and because of the potential for tumorigenicity shown for dacarbazine for injection in animal studies, a decision should be made whether to discontinue nursing or to discontinue the drug, taking into account the importance of the drug to the mother.

Adverse Reactions

Dacarbazine is considered to have very high emetogenic potential (over 90% incidence of emesis).

➤*Dermatologic:* Alopecia has been noted, as has facial flushing and facial paresthesia.

Erythematous and urticarial rashes have been observed infrequently after administration of dacarbazine for injection. Rarely, photosensitivity reactions may occur.

➤*GI:* Symptoms of anorexia, nausea, and vomiting are the most frequently noted of all toxic reactions. Over 90% of patients are affected with the initial few doses. The vomiting lasts 1 to 12 hours, and is incompletely and unpredictably palliated with phenobarbital or prochlorperazine. Rarely, intractable nausea and vomiting have necessitated discontinuance of therapy with dacarbazine for injection. Rarely, dacarbazine for injection has caused diarrhea. Some helpful suggestions include restricting the patient's oral intake of food for 4 to 6 hours prior to treatment. The rapid toleration of these symptoms suggests that a CNS mechanism may be involved, and usually these symptoms subside after the first 1 or 2 days.

➤*Lab test abnormalities:* There have been few reports of significant liver or renal function test abnormalities in man. However, these abnormalities have been observed more frequently in animal studies.

➤*Miscellaneous:* There are a number of minor toxicities that are infrequently noted. Patients have experienced an influenza-like syndrome of fever up to 39°C (102.2°F), myalgias and malaise. These symptoms occur usually after large single doses, may last for several days, and they may occur with successive treatments.

Overdosage

➤*Treatment:* Give supportive treatment and monitor blood cell counts.

Triazenes

DACARBAZINE — INJECTION

Patient Information

Advise patients of common side effects, which include the following: increased risk of infection or bleeding for 21 to 25 days after therapy; nausea, vomiting, or loss of appetite for 1 to 2 days after each dose (restricting food intake for 4 to 6 hours before treatment may help); reversible hair loss.

Alkyl Sulfonates

BUSULFAN

Rx	**Myleran** (GlaxoSmithKline)	**Tablets; oral:** 2 mg	Lactose. (GX EF3 M). White. Film coated. In 25s.
Rx	**Busulfex** (Otsuka America)	**Injection; solution:** 6 mg/mL	PEG-400. In 10 mL single-use ampules with syringe filters.

BUSULFAN — ORAL

WARNING

Busulfan is a potent drug. Do not use it unless a diagnosis of chronic myelogenous leukemia (CML) has been adequately established and the responsible health care provider is knowledgeable in assessing response to chemotherapy.

Busulfan can induce severe bone marrow hypoplasia. Reduce or discontinue the dosage immediately at the first sign of any unusual depression of bone marrow function as reflected by an abnormal decrease in any of the formed elements of the blood. Perform a bone marrow examination if the bone marrow status is uncertain.

Malignant tumors and acute leukemias have been reported in patients who have received busulfan therapy, and this drug may be a human carcinogen. The World Health Organization (WHO) has concluded that there is a causal relationship between busulfan exposure and the development of secondary malignancies. Four cases of acute leukemia occurred among 243 patients treated with busulfan as adjuvant chemotherapy following surgical resection of bronchogenic carcinoma. All 4 cases were from a subgroup of 19 of these 243 patients who developed pancytopenia while taking busulfan 5 to 8 years before leukemia became clinically apparent. These findings suggest that busulfan is leukemogenic, although its mode of action is uncertain.

Indications

➤*CML:* Busulfan is indicated for the palliative treatment of chronic myelogenous (myeloid, myelocytic, granulocytic) leukemia.

➤*Off-label uses:* Other myeloproliferative disorders, including severe thrombocytosis and polycythemia vera, myelofibrosis; bone marrow transplantation (BMT).

Administration and Dosage

➤*General dosing considerations:* A decrease in the leukocyte (white blood cell [WBC]) count is not usually seen during the first 10 to 15 days of treatment. The WBC count may actually increase during this period; do not interpret it as resistance to the drug, and do not increase the dose. Because the WBC count may continue to fall for more than 1 month after discontinuing the drug, it is important that busulfan be discontinued prior to the WBC count falling into the normal range. When the WBC count has declined to approximately 15,000 cells/mm^3, withhold the drug.

With a constant dose of busulfan, the WBC count declines exponentially; a weekly plot of the WBC count on semilogarithmic graph paper aids in predicting the time when therapy should be discontinued. With the recommended dose of busulfan, a normal WBC count is usually achieved in 12 to 20 weeks.

Obesity has been reported to increase busulfan clearance. Consider dosing based on body surface area or adjusted ideal body weight (defined as an ideal body weight plus 25% of the difference between actual and ideal body weight) in obese patients.

➤*Adults:*

Chronic myelogenous leukemia –

Remission induction: 4 to 8 mg/day (60 mcg/kg or 1.8 mg/m^2 daily) for remission induction. Because the rate of fall of the WBC count is dose related, reserve daily doses exceeding 4 mg daily for patients with the most compelling symptoms; the greater the total daily dose, the greater the possibility of inducing bone marrow aplasia.

When the total WBC count has declined to approximately 15,000/mm^3, withhold the drug.

The patient is examined at monthly intervals and treatment resumed with the induction dosage when the WBC count reaches approximately 50,000 cells/mm^3.

Maintenance dosage: If remission lasts less than 3 months, maintenance therapy of 1 to 3 mg/day (range, 1 to 4 mg/day to 2 mg/week) may be advisable in order to keep the hematological status under control and prevent rapid relapse. Titrate dose to maintain WBC between 10,000 and 20,000 cells/mm^3.

Off-label dosing –

Bone marrow ablation prior to hematopoietic stem cell transplantation:

• *Usual dose* – 1 mg/kg every 6 hours for 16 doses (for a total dose of 16 mg/kg over 4 days) in combination with other agents.

Base dose on either ideal body weight or actual body weight, whichever is lower. For obese patients, dosage should be based on adjusted body weight.

• *Alternative dosage* – 0.4375 to 0.5 mg/kg every 6 hours for 16 doses (total dose of 7 to 8 mg/kg, respectively, over 4 days), alone or in combination with other chemotherapy agents.

Base dose on ideal body weight or actual body weight, whichever is lower. For obese patients, dosage should be based on adjusted body weight.

• *Concomitant therapy* – Administer antiemetics prior to the first dose of busulfan to reduce nausea and vomiting. Continue antiemetic therapy throughout the busulfan regimen.

Administer phenytoin concurrently to reduce the risk of seizures. Some health care providers administer a loading dose of phenytoin 15 to 18 mg/kg orally prior to starting busulfan, followed by a maintenance dose of phenytoin 300 mg/day orally until 24 to 48 hours after administering the final busulfan dose. Maintenance doses ranging from 4 to 8 mg/kg/day orally have also been given and are titrated to achieve therapeutic phenytoin serum levels (10 to 20 mcg/mL).

Administer ursodiol 9 to 12 mg/kg/day to reduce the risk of hepatotoxicity.

• *Risk of vomiting* – Some health care providers place patients on a clear liquid diet to decrease the risk of vomiting. Additional doses of busulfan may also be prescribed if tablets are visible in emesis. A full replacement dose may be given if vomiting occurs within 30 minutes of a dose and pill fragments are visible in the vomitus. If vomiting occurs more than 30 minutes after a dose, the replacement dose may be estimated based on the number of visible pill fragments; patients typically receive 50% of the usual dose. (See also Administration.)

Polycythemia vera: 2 to 6 mg/day.

Thrombocytosis: 4 to 6 mg/day.

➤*Children:*

Chronic myelogenous leukemia –

Remission induction: 60 to 120 mcg/kg or 1.8 to 4.6 mg/m^2 orally once daily for remission induction. Because the rate of fall of the leukocyte count is dose related, reserve daily doses exceeding 4 mg daily for patients with the most compelling symptoms; the greater the total daily dose, the greater the possibility of inducing bone marrow aplasia.

When total leukocyte count is less than 15,000 cells/mm^3, withhold drug.

During remission, treatment is resumed when WBC reaches 50,000 cells/mm^3.

Dosage adjustment: Reduce dose by 50% for WBC between 30,000 and 40,000 cells/mm^3. Discontinue therapy if WBC count falls to 20,000 cells/mm^3 or less.

Off-label dosing –

Bone marrow ablation prior to hematopoietic stem cell transplantation:

• *Usual dose* – 1 mg/kg orally every 6 hours for 16 doses (for a total dose of 16 mg/kg over 4 days) in combination with other agents.

• *Alternative dosage* – Alternatively, some health care providers have given busulfan 0.5 mg/kg every 6 hours orally for 16 doses (for a total dose of 8 mg/kg over 4 days) in combination with other chemotherapy agents. Calculate dose using ideal body weight.

• *Concomitant therapy* – Administer antiemetics prior to the first dose of busulfan to reduce nausea and vomiting. Continue antiemetic therapy throughout the busulfan regimen.

Administer phenytoin concurrently to reduce the risk of seizures. Some health care providers administer a loading dose of phenytoin 15 to 18 mg/kg orally prior to starting busulfan, followed by a maintenance dose of phenytoin 300 mg/day orally until 24 to 48 hours after administering the final busulfan dose. Maintenance doses ranging from 4 to 8 mg/kg/day orally have also been given and are titrated to achieve therapeutic phenytoin serum levels (10 to 20 mcg/mL).

Administer ursodiol 9 to 12 mg/kg/day to reduce the risk of hepatotoxicity.

• *Risk of vomiting* – Some health care providers place patients on a clear liquid diet to decrease the risk of vomiting. Additional doses of busulfan may also be prescribed if tablets are visible in emesis. A full replacement dose may be given if vomiting occurs within 30 minutes of a dose and pill fragments are visible in the vomitus. If vomiting occurs more than 30 minutes after a dose, the replacement dose may be estimated based on the number of visible pill fragments; patients typically receive 50% of the usual dose.

➤*Renal function impairment:*

Dialysis – Conventional hemodialysis is minimally effective (25% to 49%) in removing busulfan.

➤*Dosage adjustment/discontinuation:* Consider reducing the dose or temporarily discontinuing therapy if the leukocyte count decreases dramatically to prevent irreversible bone marrow depression. For uses other than HSCT, withhold drug when the WBC count is less than 15,000 cells/mm^3.

➤*Preparation for administration:* Busulfan is considered a cytotoxic agent. Follow safe handling procedures when preparing, administering, or dispensing busulfan.

BUSULFAN — ORAL

➤*Administration:* For patients unable to swallow tablets whole, place tablet in a half glass of noncarbonated water; do not crush tablet. Stir until dispersed; then have the patient drink the mixture immediately. To ensure that the entire dose is administered, rinse the inside of the container with another half glass of water and have the patient drink it immediately.

Tablets may be placed inside gelatin capsules to simplify oral administration of the high doses used for HSCT.

Shake suspension well before using.

➤*Storage/Stability:* Store at 25°C (77°F); excursions are permitted to 15° to 30°C (59° to 77°F).

Extemporaneous oral suspension is stable for up to 30 days refrigerated.

Actions

➤*Pharmacology:* In aqueous media, busulfan undergoes a wide range of nucleophilic substitution reactions. While this chemical reactivity is relatively nonspecific, alkylation of the deoxyribonucleic acid (DNA) is thought to be an important biological mechanism for its cytotoxic effect. Coliphage T7 exposed to busulfan had the DNA crosslinked by intrastrand crosslinkages, but no interstrand linkages were found.

The metabolic fate of busulfan has been studied in rats and humans using ^{14}C- and ^{35}S-labeled materials. In humans, as in the rat, almost all of the radioactivity in ^{35}S-labeled busulfan is excreted in the urine in the form of ^{35}S-methanesulfonic acid. No unchanged drug was found in human urine, although a small amount has been reported in rat urine. It was demonstrated that the formation of methanesulfonic acid in vivo in the rat was not caused by a simple hydrolysis of busulfan to 1, 4-butanediol because only about 4% of 2, 3-^{14}C-busulfan was excreted as carbon dioxide, whereas 2, 3-^{14}C-1, 4-butanediol was converted almost exclusively to carbon dioxide. The predominant reaction of busulfan in the rat is the alkylation of sulfhydryl groups (particularly cysteine and cysteine-containing compounds) to produce a cyclic sulfonium compound, which is the precursor of the major urinary metabolite of the 4-carbon portion of the molecule, 3-hydroxytetrahydrothiophene-1, 1-dioxide. This has been termed a "sulfur-stripping" action of busulfan, and it may modify the function of certain sulfur-containing amino acids, polypeptides, and proteins; whether this action makes an important contribution to the cytotoxicity of busulfan is unknown.

The biochemical basis for acquired resistance to busulfan is largely a matter of speculation. Although altered transport of busulfan into the cell is one possibility, increased intracellular inactivation of the drug before it reaches the DNA is also possible. Experiments with other alkylating agents have shown that resistance to this class of compounds may reflect an acquired ability of the resistant cell to repair alkylation damage more effectively.

➤*Pharmacokinetics:*

Absorption/Distribution – Busulfan is a small, highly lipophilic molecule that easily crosses the blood brain barrier. Following absorption, 32% and 47% of busulfan are bound to plasma proteins and red blood cells, respectively. Busulfan is reported to have a volume of distribution of 0.64 ± 0.12 L/kg in adults.

Busulfan absorption from the GI tract is essentially complete. This has been demonstrated in radioactive studies after both intravenous (IV) and oral administration of ^{35}S-busulfan, ^{14}C-busulfan and ^{3}H-busulfan. Following the IV administration of a single therapeutic dose of ^{35}S-busulfan, there was rapid disappearance of radioactivity from the blood, and 90% to 95% of the ^{35}S-label disappeared within 3 to 5 minutes after injection.

A study compared a single 2 mg IV bolus injection with a single oral dose of a 2 mg tablet of nonradioactive busulfan in 8 adult patients 13 to 60 years of age. The study demonstrated mean bioavailability of 80% in adults with large interpatient variability ranging from 47% to 103%. However, mean bioavailability for 8 children 18 months to 6 years of age was 68%, ranging from 22% to 120%.

In another study, busulfan 2, 4, and 6 mg given as a single oral dose on consecutive days (starting with the lowest dose) in 5 adult patients, the mean dose-normalized (to 2 mg dose) area under the plasma concentration time curve (AUC) was about 130 ng•h/mL, while the mean intrapatient and interpatient variability was approximately 16% and 21%, respectively. Busulfan was eliminated with a plasma terminal elimination half-life of approximately 2.6 hours, and demonstrated linear kinetics within the range of 2 to 6 mg for both the maximum plasma concentration (C_{max}) and AUC. The mean C_{max} for the 2, 4, and 6 mg doses (after dose normalization to 2 mg) was approximately 30 ng/mL. A recent study of 4 to 8 mg as single oral doses in 12 patients showed that the mean ± standard deviation (SD) C_{max} (after dose normalization to 4 mg) was 68.2 ± 24.4 ng/mL, occurring at approximately 0.9 hours, and the mean ± SD AUC (after dose normalization to 4 mg) was 269 ± 62 ng•h/mL. These results are consistent with previous results. In addition, the mean ± SD elimination half-life was 2.69 ± 0.49 hours.

Currently, there are no available data on the effect of food on busulfan bioavailability.

Metabolism/Excretion – After oral or IV administration of ^{35}S-busulfan to humans, 45% to 60% of the radioactivity was recovered in the urine in the 48 hours after administration; the majority of the total urinary excretion occurred in the first 24 hours. In humans, more than 95% of the urinary ^{35}S-label occurs as ^{35}S-methanesulfonic acid. Oral and IV administration of 1, 4-^{14}C-busulfan showed the same rapid initial disappearance of plasma radioactivity with a subsequent low-level plateau as observed following the administration of ^{35}S-labeled drug. Cumulative radioactivity in the urine after 48 hours was 25% to 30% of the administered dose (contrasting with 45% to 60% for ^{35}S-busulfan) and suggests a slower excretion of the alkylating portion of the molecule and its metabolites than for the sulfonoxymethyl moieties. Regardless of the route of administration, 1, 4-^{14}C-busulfan yielded a complex mixture of at least 12 radiolabeled metabolites in urine; the main metabolite being 3-hydroxytetrahydrothiophene-1, 1-dioxide. Pharmacokinetic studies employing ^{3}H-busulfan labeled on the tetramethylene chain confirmed a rapid initial clearance of the radioactivity from plasma, irrespective of whether the drug was given orally or IV.

Busulfan clearance in adult patients is 2.4 to 2.6 mL/min/kg. The elimination of busulfan appears to be independent of renal function. This probably reflects the extensive metabolism of the drug in the liver because less that 2% of the administered dose is excreted in the urine unchanged within 24 hours. Busulfan metabolism occurs in the liver and is mediated by gluthathione-S-transferase. The drug is metabolized by enzymatic activity to at least 12 metabolites, among which tetrahydrothiophene, tetrahydrothiophene 12-oxide, sulfolane, and 3-hydroxysulfolane were identified. These metabolites do not have cytotoxic activity.

There is no experience with the use of dialysis in an attempt to modify the clinical toxicity of busulfan. One technical difficulty would derive from the extremely poor water solubility of busulfan. Additionally, all studies of the metabolism of busulfan employing radiolabeled materials indicate rapid chemical reactivity of the parent compound with prolonged retention of some of the metabolites (particularly the metabolites arising from the "alkylating" portion of the molecule). The efficacy of dialysis at removing significant quantities of unreacted drug would be expected to be minimal in such a situation.

Special populations –

Renal function impairment: The impact of hemodialysis on the clearance of busulfan was determined in a patient with chronic renal failure undergoing autologous stem cell transplantation. The apparent oral clearance of busulfan during a 4-hour hemodialysis session was increased 65%, but the 24-hour oral clearance of busulfan was increased only 11%.

The incidence of venoocclusive disease was higher (33.3% vs 3%) in patients with busulfan $AUC_{0\text{-}6h}$ greater than 1,500 mcM•min (C_{ss} greater than 900 mcg/mL) compared with patients with busulfan $AUC_{0\text{-}6h}$ less than 1,500 mcM•min (C_{ss} less than 900 mcg/L).

Children: The bioavailability of oral busulfan shows large intrapatient variability ranging from 22% to 120% (mean 68%) in children. Plasma clearance is reported to be 2 to 4 times higher in children than adults when receiving 1 mg/kg every 6 hours for 4 days. Oral dosing children according to body surface yields AUC and C_{max} values and the colony-stimulating factor-:plasma ratio similar to those seen in adults. Busulfan is reported to have a volume of distribution of 1.15 + 0.52 L/kg in children.

Obese patients: Obesity has been reported to increase busulfan clearance. Consider dosing based on body surface area or adjusted ideal body weight (defined as an ideal body weight plus 25% of the difference between actual and ideal body weight) in obese patients.

Drug interactions: Itraconazole reduced busulfan clearance by up to 25% in patients receiving itraconazole compared with patients who did not receive itraconazole. Higher busulfan exposure caused by concomitant itraconazole or metronidazole could lead to toxic plasma levels in some patients. Fluconazole had no effect on the clearance of busulfan. Patients treated with concomitant cyclophosphamide and busulfan with phenytoin pretreatment have increased cyclophosphamide and busulfan clearance, which may lead to decreased concentrations of cyclophosphamide and busulfan. However, busulfan clearance may be reduced in the presence of cyclophosphamide alone, presumably because of competition for glutathione.

Diazepam had no effect on the clearance of busulfan.

No information is available regarding the penetration of busulfan into brain or cerebrospinal fluid.

Contraindications

Busulfan is contraindicated in patients in whom a definitive diagnosis of CML has not been firmly established.

Busulfan is contraindicated in patients who have previously suffered a hypersensitivity reaction to busulfan or any other component of the preparation.

Warnings/Precautions

➤*Hematologic effects:* The most frequent, serious side effect of treatment with busulfan is the induction of bone marrow failure (which may or may not be anatomically hypoplastic), resulting in severe pancytopenia. The pancytopenia caused by busulfan may be more prolonged than that induced with other alkylating agents. It is generally thought that the usual cause of busulfan-induced pancytopenia is the failure to stop administration of the drug soon enough; individual idiosyncrasy to the drug does not seem to be an important factor. Use busulfan with extreme caution and exceptional vigilance in patients whose bone marrow reserve may have been compromised by prior irradiation or chemotherapy, or whose marrow function is recovering from previous cytotoxic therapy. Although recovery from busulfan-induced pancytopenia may take from 1 month to 2 years, this complication is potentially reversible; vigorously support the patient through any period of severe pancytopenia.

The most consistent, dose-related toxicity is bone marrow suppression. This may be manifested by anemia, leukopenia, thrombocytopenia, or any combination of these. It is imperative that patients be instructed to promptly report the development of fever, sore throat, signs of local infection, bleeding from any site, or symptoms suggestive of anemia. Any one of these findings may indicate busulfan toxicity; however, they also may indicate transformation of the disease to acute blastic form. Because busulfan may have a delayed effect, it is important to withdraw the medication temporarily at the first sign of an abnormally large or exceptionally rapid fall in any of the formed elements of the blood. Never allow patients to take the drug without close medical supervision.

BUSULFAN — ORAL

➤*Pulmonary effects:* A rare, important complication of busulfan therapy is the development of bronchopulmonary dysplasia with pulmonary fibrosis. Symptoms have been reported to occur within 8 months to 10 years after initiation of therapy, the average duration of therapy being 4 years. The histologic findings associated with busulfan lung mimic those seen following pulmonary irradiation. Clinically, patients have reported the insidious onset of cough, dyspnea, and low-grade fever. In some cases, however, onset of symptoms may be acute. Pulmonary function studies have revealed diminished diffusion capacity and decreased pulmonary compliance. It is important to exclude more common conditions (such as opportunistic infections or leukemic infiltration of the lungs) with appropriate diagnostic techniques. If measures such as exfoliative cytology, sputum cultures, and virologic studies fail to establish an etiology for pulmonary infiltrates, lung biopsy may be necessary to establish the diagnosis. Treatment of established, busulfan-induced pulmonary fibrosis is unsatisfactory; in most cases, the patients have died within 6 months after the diagnosis was established. There is no specific therapy for this complication. Discontinue busulfan if this lung toxicity develops. The administration of corticosteroids has been suggested, but the results have not been impressive or uniformly successful.

Pulmonary toxicity consistent with idiopathic pneumonia syndrome commonly occurs following high-dose of busulfan, often in combination with cyclophosphamide, as part of a preparatory regimen for BMT. The syndrome usually manifests within 3 months of transplantation.

➤*Cardiac effects:* Cardiac tamponade has been reported in a small number of patients with thalassemia (2% in 1 series) who received busulfan and cyclophosphamide as the preparatory regimen for BMT. In this series, the cardiac tamponade often was fatal. Abdominal pain and vomiting preceded the tamponade in most patients.

➤*Hepatic effects:* Hepatic venoocclusive disease (HVOD), which may be life-threatening, has been reported in patients receiving busulfan, usually in combination with cyclophosphamide or other chemotherapeutic agents prior to BMT. Possible risk factors for the development of HVOD include the following: total busulfan dose exceeding 16 mg/kg based on ideal body weight; concurrent use of multiple, alkylating agents.

A clear cause-and-effect relationship with busulfan has not been demonstrated. Periodic measurement of serum transaminases, alkaline phosphatase, and bilirubin is indicated for early detection of hepatotoxicity. A reduced incidence of HVOD and other regimen-related toxicities have been observed in patients treated with high-dose busulfan and cyclophosphamide when the first dose of cyclophosphamide has been delayed for more than 24 hours after the last dose of busulfan.

➤*Cellular dysplasia:* Busulfan may cause cellular dysplasia in many organs in addition to the lung. Cytologic abnormalities characterized by giant, hyperchromatic nuclei have been reported in adrenal glands, bone marrow, lymph nodes, pancreas, and thyroid, liver. This cytologic dysplasia may be severe enough to cause difficulty in interpretation of exfoliative cytologic examinations from the bladder, breast, lung, and the uterine cervix.

➤*Bone marrow suspension:* The most consistent, dose-related toxicity is bone marrow suppression. This may be manifested by anemia, leukopenia, thrombocytopenia, or any combination of these. It is imperative to instruct patients to promptly report the development of fever, sore throat, signs of local infection, bleeding from any site, or symptoms suggestive of anemia. Any one of these findings may indicate busulfan toxicity; however, they also may indicate transformation of the disease to acute blastic form. Because busulfan may have a delayed effect, it is important to withdraw the medication temporarily at the first sign of an abnormally large or exceptionally rapid fall in any of the formed elements of the blood. Never allow patient to take the drug without close medical supervision.

➤*Seizures:* Seizures have been observed in patients receiving higher than recommended doses of busulfan. As with any potentially epileptogenic drug, exercise caution when administering busulfan to patients with a history of seizure disorder or head trauma, or to patients receiving other potentially epileptogenic drugs. Some investigators have used prophylactic anticonvulsant therapy in this setting.

➤*Vaccinations:* Avoid administration of live vaccines to immunocompromised patients.

➤*Pregnancy:* *Category D.* Busulfan may cause fetal harm when administered to a pregnant woman. Although there have been a number of cases reported where apparently healthy children have been born after busulfan treatment during pregnancy, 1 case has been cited in which a malformed baby was delivered by a mother treated with busulfan. During the pregnancy that resulted in the malformed infant, the mother received x-ray therapy early in the first trimester, mercaptopurine until the third month, then busulfan until delivery. In pregnant rats, busulfan produces sterility in male and female offspring because of the absence of germinal cells in testes and ovaries. Germinal cell aplasia or sterility in offspring of mothers receiving busulfan during pregnancy has not been reported in humans. There are no adequate and well-controlled studies in pregnant women. If this drug is used during pregnancy, or if the patient becomes pregnant while taking this drug, apprise the patient of the potential hazard to the fetus. Advise women of childbearing potential to avoid becoming pregnant.

Fertility impairment – Ovarian suppression and amenorrhea with menopausal symptoms commonly occur during busulfan therapy in premenopausal patients. Busulfan has been associated with ovarian failure, including failure to achieve puberty in women. Busulfan interferes with spermatogenesis in experimental animals, and there have been clinical reports of azoospermia, sterility, and testicular atrophy in men.

Nonteratogenic – There have been reports in the literature of small infants being born after the mothers received busulfan during pregnancy, in particular, during the third trimester. One case was reported in which an infant had mild anemia and neutropenia at birth after busulfan was administered to the mother from the eighth week of pregnancy to term.

➤*Lactation:* It is not known whether this drug is excreted in breast milk. Because of the potential for tumorigenicity shown for busulfan in animal and human studies, decide whether to discontinue breast-feeding or the drug, taking into account the importance of the drug to the mother.

➤*Children:* Dosing on a weight basis is the same for children and adults, approximately 60 mcg/kg of body weight or 1.8 mg/m^2 of body surface, daily. Because the rate of fall of the leukocyte count is dose related, reserve daily doses exceeding 4 mg for patients with the most compelling symptoms; the greater the total daily dose, the greater the possibility of inducing bone marrow aplasia.

➤*Elderly:* Clinical studies of busulfan did not include sufficient numbers of subjects 65 years of age and older to determine whether they respond differently from younger subjects. Other reported clinical experience has not identified differences in responses between the elderly and younger patients. In general, use caution in dose selection for an elderly patient, usually starting at the low end of the dosing range, reflecting the greater frequency of decreased cardiac, hepatic, or renal function and of concomitant disease or other drug therapy.

➤*Monitoring:* It is recommended that evaluation of the hemoglobin or hematocrit, total white blood cell count and differential count, and quantitative platelet count be obtained weekly while the patient is on busulfan therapy. In cases in which the cause of fluctuation in the formed elements of the peripheral blood is obscure, bone marrow examination may be useful for evaluation of marrow status. A decision to increase, decrease, continue, or discontinue a given dose of busulfan must be based not only on the absolute hematologic values, but also on the rapidity with which changes are occurring. The dosage of busulfan may need to be reduced if this agent is combined with other drugs whose primary toxicity is myelosuppression. Occasional patients may be unusually sensitive to busulfan administered at standard dosage and suffer neutropenia or thrombocytopenia after a relatively short exposure to the drug. Do not use busulfan where facilities for complete blood counts, including quantitative platelet counts, are not available at weekly (or more frequent) intervals.

Drug Interactions

Busulfan may cause additive myelosuppression when used with other myelosuppressive drugs.

Busulfan-induced pulmonary toxicity may be additive to the effects produced by other cytotoxic agents.

The concomitant systemic administration of itraconazole to patients receiving high-dose busulfan may result in reduced busulfan clearance. Monitor patients for signs of busulfan toxicity when itraconazole is used concomitantly with busulfan. The coadministration of metronidazole and high-dose busulfan may result in increased trough levels of busulfan, and, therefore, it is not recommended.

Busulfan Oral Drug Interactions

Precipitant drug	Object drug[a]		Description
Cyclophosphamide	Busulfan	↑	Coadministration may cause a decrease in busulfan clearance.
Itraconazole	Busulfan	↑	Itraconazole reduced busulfan clearance up to 25%. This may result in toxic busulfan levels. Monitor closely.
Metronidazole	Busulfan	↑	Metronidazole may increase busulfan trough concentrations, increasing the risk of serious toxicities. Coadministration is not recommended.
Phenytoin	Busulfan	↓	Patients treated with concomitant cyclophosphamide and busulfan with phenytoin pretreatment have increased cyclophosphamide and busulfan clearance.

[a] ↑ = Object drug increased. ↓ = Object drug decreased.

Adverse Reactions

Busulfan oral is considered to have very low potential for nausea and vomiting.

➤*Cardiovascular:* Cardiac tamponade has been reported in a small number of patients with thalassemia who received busulfan and cyclophosphamide as the preparatory regimen for BMT. In this series, the cardiac tamponade often was fatal. Abdominal pain and vomiting preceded the tamponade in most patients.

One case of endocardial fibrosis has been reported in a 79-year-old woman who received a total dose of busulfan 7,200 mg over a period of 9 years for the management of CML. At autopsy, she had endocardial fibrosis of the left ventricle in addition to interstitial pulmonary fibrosis.

➤*CNS:* Seizures have been observed in patients receiving higher than recommended doses of busulfan. As with any potentially epileptogenic drug, exercise caution when administering busulfan to patients with a history of seizure disorder or head trauma, or to patients receiving other potentially epileptogenic drugs. Some investigators have used prophylactic anticonvulsant therapy in this setting.

BUSULFAN — ORAL

➤*Dermatologic:* Hyperpigmentation is the most common adverse skin reaction and occurs in 5% to 10% of patients, particularly those with a dark complexion.

➤*Hematologic:* The most frequent, serious, toxic effect of busulfan is dose-related myelosuppression, resulting in leukopenia, thrombocytopenia, and anemia. Myelosuppression is most frequently the result of a failure to discontinue dosage in the face of an undetected decrease in leukocyte or platelet counts.

Aplastic anemia (sometimes irreversible) has been reported rarely, often following long-term conventional doses and high doses of busulfan.

➤*Hepatic:* HVOD, which may be life-threatening, has been reported in patients receiving busulfan, usually in combination with cyclophosphamide or other chemotherapeutic agents prior to BMT.

➤*Metabolic:* In a few cases, a clinical syndrome closely resembling adrenal insufficiency and characterized by anorexia, melanoderma, nausea, severe fatigue, vomiting, weakness, and weight loss has developed after prolonged busulfan therapy. The symptoms have sometimes been reversible when busulfan was withdrawn. Adrenal responsiveness to exogenously administered adrenocorticotropic hormone usually has been normal. However, pituitary function testing with metyrapone revealed a blunted urinary 17-hydroxycorticosteroid excretion in 2 patients. Following the discontinuation of busulfan (which was associated with clinical improvement), rechallenge with metyrapone revealed normal pituitary-adrenal function.

Hyperuricemia and/or hyperuricosuria are not uncommon in patients with CML. Additional rapid destruction of granulocytes may accompany the initiation of chemotherapy and increase the urate pool. Adverse reactions can be minimized by increased hydration, urine alkalinization, and the prophylactic administration of a xanthine oxidase inhibitor such as allopurinol.

➤*Ophthalmic:* Busulfan is capable of inducing cataracts in rats; there have been several reports indicating that this is a rare complication in humans.

➤*Pulmonary:* Interstitial pulmonary fibrosis has been reported rarely, but it is a clinically significant adverse reaction when observed and calls for immediate discontinuation of further administration of the drug. The role of corticosteroids in arresting or reversing the fibrosis has been reported to be beneficial in some cases and without effect in others.

➤*Miscellaneous:* Other reported adverse reactions include the following: alopecia, cheilosis, cholestatic jaundice, dryness of the oral mucous membranes, erythema multiforme, erythema nodosum, excessive dryness and fragility of the skin with anhidrosis, gynecomastia, myasthenia gravis, porphyria cutanea tarda, urticaria. Most of these are single case reports, and in many, a clear cause-and-effect relationship with busulfan has not been demonstrated.

➤*Adverse reactions observed during clinical practice:* The following reactions have been identified during postapproval use of busulfan. Because they are reported voluntarily from a population of unknown size, estimates of frequency cannot be made. These reactions have been chosen for inclusion because of a combination of their seriousness, frequency of reporting, or potential causal connection to busulfan.

Dermatologic – Rash; an increased local cutaneous reaction has been observed in patients receiving radiotherapy soon after busulfan.

Hematologic/Lymphatic – Aplastic anemia.

Hepatic – Centrilobular sinusoidal fibrosis, hepatocellular atrophy, hepatocellular necrosis, HVOD, hyperbilirubinemia.

Ophthalmic – Cataracts, corneal thinning, lens changes.

Respiratory – Pneumonia.

Miscellaneous – Infection, mucositis, sepsis.

Overdosage

➤*Symptoms:* GI toxicity with diarrhea, mucositis, nausea, and vomiting and has been observed when busulfan was used in association with BMT.

Oral median lethal doses (LD_{50}) in mice are singles doses of busulfan 120 mg/kg. Two distinct types of toxic response are seen at median lethal doses given intraperitoneally. Within a matter of hours, there are signs of stimulation of the CNS with convulsions and death on the first day. Mice are more sensitive to this effect than rats. With doses at the LD_{50} there is also delayed death because of damage to the bone marrow. At 3 times the LD_{50}, atrophy of the mucosa of the large intestine is found after a week, whereas that of the small intestine is little affected. After doses in the order of 10 times those used therapeutically were added to the diet of rats, irreversible cataracts were produced after several weeks. Small doses had no such effect.

➤*Treatment:* There is no known antidote to busulfan. The principal toxic effects are bone marrow depression and pancytopenia. Closely monitor the hematologic status and institute vigorous supportive measures if necessary. Gastric lavage followed by administration of charcoal would be indicated if ingestion were recent. Dialysis may be considered in the management of overdose as there is 1 report of successful dialysis of busulfan. The 1 report of the impact of hemodialysis on the oral clearance was in a patient with chronic renal failure undergoing autologous peripheral stem cell transplantation for non-Hodgkin lymphoma. A 4-hour hemodialysis session increased the apparent oral clearance of busulfan by about 65%. The factors that favor hemodialysis of busulfan include the following: low molecular weight, low plasma protein binding, and a blood-to-plasma partition ratio of close to 1. However, with a 4-hour hemodialysis, the mean daily (24 hours) oral clearance of busulfan was only increased about 10%.

Patient Information

Inform patients beginning therapy with busulfan of the importance of having periodic blood counts and of immediate reporting of any unusual fever or bleeding. Aside from the major toxicity of myelosuppression, instruct patients to report any difficulty in breathing, congestion, or persistent cough. Tell patients that diffuse pulmonary fibrosis is an infrequent, but serious and potentially life-threatening, complication of long-term busulfan therapy. Alert patients to report any signs of abrupt weakness, anorexia, melanoderma, nausea and vomiting, unusual fatigue, and weight loss that could be associated with a syndrome resembling adrenal insufficiency. Never allow patients to take the drug without medical supervision, and inform them that other encountered toxicities to busulfan include amenorrhea, drug hypersensitivity, dryness of the mucous membranes, infertility, skin hyperpigmentation, and, rarely, cataract formation. Advise women of child-bearing potential to avoid becoming pregnant. Explain the increased risk of a second malignancy to the patient.

BUSULFAN — INJECTION

WARNING

Busulfan injection is a potent cytotoxic drug that causes profound myelosuppression at the recommended dosage. It should be administered under the supervision of a qualified health care provider who is experienced in allogeneic hematopoietic stem-cell transplantation, the use of cancer chemotherapeutic drugs, and the management of patients with severe pancytopenia. Appropriate management of therapy and complications is only possible when adequate diagnostic and treatment facilities are readily available.

Indications

➤*Chronic myelogenous leukemia:* For use in combination with cyclophosphamide as a conditioning regimen prior to allogeneic hematopoietic progenitor cell transplantation for CML.

➤*Off-label uses:* Busulfan injection has been used safely and effectively in children 5 months to 16 years of age undergoing allogenic HSCT.

Administration and Dosage

➤*General dosing considerations:* Busulfan clearance is best predicted when the busulfan dose is administered based on adjusted ideal body weight (AIBW). Dosing busulfan based on actual body weight (ABW), ideal body weight (IBW), or other factors can produce significant differences in busulfan clearance among lean, healthy, and obese patients.

➤*Adults:*

Chronic myelogenous leukemia –

Usual dosage: 0.8 mg/kg of IBW or actual body weight (ABW), whichever is lower, administered intravenously (IV) via a central venous catheter as a 2-hour infusion every 6 hours for 4 consecutive days (a total of 16 doses).

Dosage adjustment:

• *Obese patients* – For obese or severely obese patients, busulfan should be administered based on AIBW. IBW should be calculated according to the following (height in cm and weight in kg):

$$\text{IBW (kg; men)} = 50 + 0.91 \times (\text{height in cm} - 152)$$

$$\text{IBW (kg; women)} = 45 + 0.91 \times (\text{height in cm} - 152)$$

AIBW should be calculated as follows:

$$\text{AIBW} = \text{IBW} + 0.25 \times (\text{actual weight} - \text{IBW})$$

• *Based on therapeutic drug monitoring* – Instructions for measuring the AUC of busulfan at dose 1 (see Blood Sample Collection for AUC Determination) and the formula for adjustment of subsequent doses to achieve the desired target AUC (1,125 mcM•min) as follows:

$$\text{Adjusted dose (mg)} = \frac{\text{actual dose (mg)} \times \text{target AUC (mcM•min)}}{\text{actual AUC (mcM•min).}}$$

For example, if a patient received a dose of busulfan 11 mg and if the corresponding AUC measured was 800 mcM•min, for a target AUC of 1,125 mcM•min, the target mg dose would be:

$$\text{Mg dose} = 11\text{ mg} \times 1{,}125\text{ mcM•min} / 800\text{ mcM•min} = 15.5\text{ mg.}$$

Busulfan dose adjustment may be made using this formula and the following instructions.

• *Blood sample collection for AUC determination* – Calculate the AUC (mcM•min) based on blood samples collected at the following time points:

For dose 1: Two hours (end of infusion), 4 and 6 hours (immediately prior to the next scheduled busulfan administration). Actual sampling times should be recorded.

For doses other than dose 1: Pre-infusion (baseline), 2 hours (end of infusion), 4 and 6 hours (immediately prior to the next scheduled busulfan administration).

BUSULFAN — INJECTION

AUC calculations based on fewer than the 3 specified samples may result in inaccurate AUC determinations.

For each scheduled blood sample, collect 1 to 3 mL of blood into heparinized (Na or Li heparin) *Vacutainer* tubes. The blood samples should be placed on wet ice immediately after collection and should be centrifuged (at 4°C [39.2°F]) within 1 hour. The plasma, harvested into appropriate cryovial storage tubes, should be frozen immediately at −20°C (−4°F). All plasma samples should be sent in a frozen state (on dry ice) to the assay laboratory for the determination of plasma busulfan concentrations.

Calculation of AUC: Busulfan AUC calculations may be made using the following instructions and appropriate standard pharmacokinetic formula:

Dose 1 AUC_∞ calculation:

$AUC_\infty = AUC_{0\text{-}6h} + AUC_{extrapolated}$, where $AUC_{0\text{-}6h}$ should be estimated using the linear trapezoidal rule, and AUC extrapolated can be computed by taking the ratio of the busulfan concentration at hour 6 and the terminal elimination rate constant, λ_z. The λ_z must be calculated from the terminal elimination phase of the busulfan concentration versus time curve. An "O" predose busulfan concentration should be assumed and used in the calculation of AUC.

If the AUC is assessed subsequent to dose 1, steady-state AUC_{ss} ($AUC_{0\text{-}6h}$) should be estimated from the trough, 2-, 4-, and 6-hour concentrations using the linear trapezoidal rule.

• *Toxicity* – Consider reducing the dose or temporarily discontinuing therapy if the leukocyte count decreases dramatically to prevent irreversible bone marrow depression.

Concomitant therapy: Cyclophosphamide is given on each of 2 days as a 1-hour infusion at a dose of 60 mg/kg beginning on bone marrow transplantation (BMT) day −3, no sooner than 6 hours following the 16th dose of busulfan.

Phenytoin should be given to all patients as premedication because busulfan is known to cross the blood-brain barrier and induce seizures. Some clinicians administer a loading dose of phenytoin 15 to 18 mg/kg orally prior to starting busulfan, followed by a maintenance dose of phenytoin 300 mg/day orally until 24 to 48 hours after administering the final busulfan dose. Maintenance doses ranging from 4 to 8 mg/kg/day orally have also been given and are titrated to achieve therapeutic phenytoin serum levels (10 to 20 mcg/mL). Phenytoin reduces busulfan plasma area under the curve (AUC) 15%. Use of other anticonvulsants may result in higher busulfan plasma AUCs and an increased risk of venoocclusive disease or seizures. In cases where other anticonvulsants must be used, plasma busulfan exposure should be monitored.

Antiemetics should be administered prior to the first dose of busulfan and continued on a fixed schedule through administration of busulfan.

Ursodiol 9 to 12 mg/kg/day should be administered to reduce the risk of hepatotoxicity.

➤*Children:*

Off-label dosing –

Bone marrow ablation prior to hematopoietic stem cell transplantation:

• *5 months to 16 years of age* –

Initial dosage: Based on patient's ABW, as shown in the following. Administer IV every 6 hours for 16 doses in combination with other agents.

Weight 12 kg or more: 1.1 mg/kg/dose (4.4 mg/kg/day, total dose of 17.6 mg/kg over 4 days).

Weight less than 12 kg: 0.8 mg/kg/dose (3.2 mg/kg/day, total dose of 12.8 mg/kg over 4 days).

Dosage adjustment: Pharmacokinetics of IV busulfan are variable in children. The desired target AUC for bone marrow ablation is 1,125 mcM•min. The manufacturer recommends calculating subsequent doses based on the AUC obtained after the initial dose using the following formula:

Adjusted dose (mg) = Actual dose (mg) × Target AUC/Actual AUC

Obtain blood samples after the first dose of IV busulfan, at 2 hours (end of the infusion), 4 hours, and 6 hours (prior to the second dose). Record the actual collection time to ensure accurate calculations. If measuring AUC after any other dose, also obtain a baseline blood sample prior to starting the infusion.

Place blood samples on wet ice immediately after collection and centrifuge at 4°C within 1 hour. Harvest and freeze plasma at −20°C immediately after centrifuging. Keep plasma samples frozen during transport to the laboratory. Send on dry ice.

➤*Renal function impairment:* Busulfan undergoes minimal renal elimination. Dosage adjustment is unlikely to be necessary in renal impairment. Vigorous hydration reduces the risk of renal toxicity.

Dialysis – Conventional hemodialysis is minimally effective (25% to 49%) in removing busulfan.

➤*Hepatic function impairment:* Busulfan is extensively metabolized in the liver. Dosage adjustment may be necessary in patients with hepatic dysfunction, although no specific guidelines are available. Monitor these patients closely and adjust the dose as needed for toxicity.

➤*Preparation for administration:* Busulfan is considered a cytotoxic agent. Follow safe handling procedures when preparing, administering, or dispensing busulfan.

Skin reactions may occur with accidental exposure. The use of gloves is recommended. If busulfan or diluted busulfan solution contacts the skin or mucosa, wash the skin or mucosa thoroughly with water.

Busulfan is a clear, colorless solution. Parenteral drug products should be visually inspected for particulate matter and discoloration prior to administration whenever the solution and container permit. If particulate matter is seen in the busulfan ampule, the drug should not be used.

Preparation for IV administration – Busulfan must be diluted prior to use with either 0.9% sodium chloride injection (normal saline) or 5% dextrose injection (D5W). The diluent quantity should be 10 times the volume of busulfan, ensuring that the final concentration of busulfan is approximately greater than or equal to 0.5 mg/mL. Calculation of the dose for a 70 kg patient, would be performed as follows.

$$\frac{(70\text{ kg patient}) \times (0.8\text{ mg/kg})}{(6\text{ mg/mL})} = \text{busulfan } 9.3\text{ mL } (56\text{ mg total dose})$$

To prepare the final solution for infusion, add busulfan 9.3 mL to 93 mL of diluent (normal saline or D5W) as calculated: (busulfan 9.3 mL) × (10) = 93 mL of either diluent plus busulfan 9.3 mL to yield a final concentration of busulfan 0.54 mg/mL (9.3 mL × 6 mg/mL ÷ 102.3 mL = 0.54 mg/mL).

All transfer procedures require strict adherence to aseptic techniques, preferably employing a vertical laminar flow safety hood while wearing gloves and protective clothing. In accordance with pharmacy practices, filter busulfan using the 5 micron syringe filter provided with each package, using 1 filter per ampule. If using the enclosed syringe filter in the forward flow direction, the calculated volume of busulfan should allow for approximately 0.16 mL of residual busulfan that will remain in the filter.

Do not put the busulfan into an IV bag or large-volume syringe that does not contain normal saline of D5W. Always add the busulfan to the diluent, not the diluent to the busulfan. Mix thoroughly by inverting several times. Use of syringe filters other than the specific type included in this package with each ampule is not recommended. Do not use polycarbonate syringes or polycarbonate filter needles with busulfan.

➤*Administration:* Busulfan should be administered IV via a central venous catheter as a 2-hour infusion every 6 hours for 4 consecutive days for a total of 16 doses.

An administration set with minimal residual hold-up volume (2 to 5 mL) should be used for product administration.

Infusion pumps should be used to administer the diluted busulfan solution. Set the flow rate of the pump to deliver the entire prescribed busulfan dose over 2 hours. Prior to and following each infusion, flush the catheter line with approximately 5 mL of 0.9% sodium chloride injection or 5% dextrose injection. Do not infuse concomitantly with another IV solution of unknown compatibility.

Rapid infusion of busulfan has not been tested and is not recommended.

Instructions for drug administration and blood sample collection for therapeutic drug monitoring – An administration set with minimal residual hold-up (priming) volume (1 to 3 mL) should be used for drug infusion to ensure accurate delivery of the entire prescribed dose and to ensure accurate collection of blood samples for therapeutic drug monitoring and dose adjustment.

Prime the administration set tubing with drug solution to allow accurate documentation of the start time of busulfan infusion. Collect the blood sample from a peripheral IV line to avoid contamination with infusing drug. If the blood sample is taken directly from the existing central venous catheter (CVC), do not collect the blood sample while the drug is infusing to ensure that the end of infusion sample is not contaminated with any residual drug. At the end of infusion (2 hours), disconnect the administration tubing and flush the CVC line with 5 mL of normal saline prior to the collection of the end of infusion sample from the CVC port. Collect the blood samples from a different port than that used for the busulfan infusion. When recording the busulfan infusion stop time, do not include the time required to flush the indwelling catheter line. Discard the administration tubing at the end of the 2-hour infusion.

➤*Extravasation:* Busulfan is considered an irritant and may cause phlebitis, but it is not known to cause tissue damage with extravasation. If signs or symptoms of extravasation occur, stop the infusion immediately. If possible, withdraw 3 to 5 mL of blood to remove some of the drug. Remove the infusion needle. Delineate the infiltrated area on the patient's skin with a felt tip marker. Elevate for 48 hours above heart level using a sling or stockinette dressing with an observation window cut in the dressing. Avoid pressure or friction. Do not rub the area. Observe for signs of increased erythema, pain, or skin necrosis. If increased symptoms occur, consult a plastic surgeon. Ensure that no medication is given distally to the extravasation site. After 48 hours, encourage the patient to use the extremity normally to promote full range of motion.

➤*Storage/Stability:* Unopened ampules of busulfan are stable until the date indicated on the package when stored under refrigeration at 2° to 8°C (36° to 46°F). Discard ampules after a single use.

Busulfan diluted in 0.9% sodium chloride injection or 5% dextrose injection is stable at 25°C (73°F) for up to 8 hours, but the infusion must be completed within that time. Busulfan diluted in 0.9% sodium chloride injection is stable at refrigerated conditions (2° to 8°C [6° to 46°F]) for up to 12 hours, but the infusion must be completed within that time.

Actions

➤*Pharmacology:*

Mechanism of action – Busulfan is a bifunctional alkylating agent in which 2 labile methanesulfonate groups are attached to opposite ends of a

BUSULFAN — INJECTION

4-carbon alkyl chain. In aqueous media, busulfan hydrolyzes to release the methanesulfonate groups. This produces reactive carbonium ions that can alkylate deoxyribonucleic acid (DNA). DNA damage is thought to be responsible for much of the cytotoxicity of busulfan.

➤*Pharmacokinetics:*

Distribution – Studies of distribution, metabolism, and elimination of busulfan have not been done; however, the literature on oral busulfan is relevant.

Busulfan achieves concentrations in the cerebrospinal fluid approximately equal to those in plasma. Irreversible binding to plasma elements, primarily albumin, has been estimated to be 32.4 ± 2.2%, which is consistent with the reactive electrophilic properties of busulfan.

Metabolism – Busulfan is predominantly metabolized by conjugation with glutathione, both spontaneously and by glutathione S-transferase catalysis. This conjugate undergoes further extensive oxidative metabolism in the liver.

Excretion – Following administration of ^{14}C-labeled busulfan to humans, approximately 30% of the radioactivity was excreted into the urine over 48 hours; negligible amounts were recovered in feces. The incomplete recovery of radioactivity may be caused by to the formation of long-lived metabolites or nonspecific alkylation of macromolecules.

The pharmacokinetics of busulfan were studied in 59 patients participating in a prospective trial of a busulfan-cyclophosphamide preparatory regimen prior to allogeneic hematopoietic progenitor stem-cell transplantation. Patients received busulfan 0.8 mg/kg every 6 hours for a total of 16 doses over 4 days. Fifty-five of 59 patients (93%) administered busulfan maintained AUC values below the target value (less than 1,500 mcM•min).

Steady-State Pharmacokinetic Parameters Following Busulfan Infusion (0.8 mg/kg; n = 59)

Parameters	Mean	CV (%)[a]	Range
C_{max} (ng/mL)[b]	1,222	18%	496 to 1,684
AUC (mcM•min)	1,167	20%	556 to 1,673
CL (mL/min/kg)[c]	2.52	25%	1.49 to 4.31

[a] CV = coefficient of variation.
[b] C_{max} = maximum plasma concentration.
[c] CL = clearance normalized to actual body weight for all patients.

Contraindications

History of hypersensitivity to any of its components.

Warnings/Precautions

➤*Hematologic:* The most frequent serious consequence of treatment with busulfan at the recommended dose and schedule is profound myelosuppression, occurring in all patients. Severe granulocytopenia, thrombocytopenia, anemia, or any combination thereof may develop. Monitor frequent complete blood counts, including white blood cell differentials and quantitative platelet counts, during treatment and until recovery is achieved. Absolute neutrophil counts (ANCs) dropped below 0.5 × 10^9/L at a median of 4 days posttransplant in 100% of patients treated in the busulfan clinical trial. The ANC recovered at a median of 13 days following allogeneic transplantation when prophylactic granulocyte colony-stimulating factor (G-CSF) was used in the majority of patients.

Thrombocytopenia (less than 25,000/mm^3 or requiring platelet transfusion) occurred at a median of 5 to 6 days in 98% of patients. Anemia (hemoglobin less than 8 g/dL) occurred in 69% of patients. Use antibiotic therapy and platelet and red blood cell support when medically indicated.

➤*Neurological:* Seizures have been reported in patients receiving high-dose oral busulfan at doses producing plasma drug levels similar to those achieved following the recommended dosage of busulfan. Despite prophylactic therapy with phenytoin, 1 seizure (1/42 patients) was reported during an autologous transplantation clinical trial of busulfan. This episode occurred during the cyclophosphamide portion of the conditioning regimen, 36 hours after the last busulfan dose. Initiate anticonvulsant prophylactic therapy prior to busulfan treatment. Exercise caution when administering the recommended dose of busulfan to patients with a history of a seizure disorder or head trauma, or who are receiving other potentially epileptogenic drugs.

➤*Hepatic:* Current literature suggests that high busulfan AUC values (greater than 1,500 mcM•min) may be associated with an increased risk of developing hepatic venoocclusive disease (HVOD). Patients who have received prior radiation therapy, at least 3 cycles of chemotherapy, or a prior progenitor cell transplant may be at increased risk of developing HVOD with the recommended busulfan dose and regimen. Based on clinical examination and laboratory findings, HVOD was diagnosed in 8% (5/61) of patients treated with busulfan in the setting of allogeneic transplantation, was fatal in 2/5 cases (40%), and yielded an overall mortality from HVOD in the entire study population of 2/61 (3%). Three of the 5 patients diagnosed with HVOD were retrospectively found to meet the Jones criteria. The incidence of HVOD reported in the literature from the randomized, controlled trials was 7.7% to 12%.

➤*Cardiac:* Cardiac tamponade has been reported in children with thalassemia (8/400 or 2% in 1 series) who received high doses of oral busulfan and cyclophosphamide as the preparatory regimen for hematopoietic progenitor cell transplantation. Six of the 8 children died, and 2 were saved by rapid pericardiocentesis. Abdominal pain and vomiting preceded the tamponade in most patients. No patients treated in the busulfan clinical trials experienced cardiac tamponade.

➤*Pulmonary:* Bronchopulmonary dysplasia with pulmonary fibrosis is a rare but serious complication following chronic busulfan therapy. The average onset of symptoms is 4 years after therapy (range, 4 months to 10 years).

➤*Hematologic:* See Warnings/Precautions for more information.

➤*Cytologic dysplasia:* Busulfan may cause cellular dysplasia in many organs. Cytologic abnormalities characterized by giant, hyperchromatic nuclei have been reported in lymph nodes, pancreas, thyroid, adrenal glands, liver, lungs, and bone marrow. This cytologic dysplasia may be severe enough to cause difficulty in interpretation of exfoliative cytologic examinations of the lungs, bladder, breast, and the uterine cervix.

➤*Extravasation:* See Administration and Dosage for more information.

➤*Pregnancy: Category D.* Busulfan may cause fetal harm when administered to a pregnant woman. Busulfan produced teratogenic changes in the offspring of mice, rats, and rabbits when given during gestation. Malformations and anomalies included significant alterations in the musculoskeletal system, body weight gain, and size. In pregnant rats, busulfan produced sterility in male and female offspring because of the absence of germinal cells in the testes and ovaries. The solvent DMA also may cause fetal harm when administered to a pregnant woman. In rats, DMA doses of 400 mg/kg/day (approximately 40% of the daily dose of DMA in the busulfan dose on a mg/m^2 basis) given during organogenesis caused significant developmental anomalies. The most striking abnormalities included anasarca, cleft palate, vertebral anomalies, rib anomalies, and serious anomalies of the vessels of the heart. There are no adequate and well-controlled studies of busulfan or DMA in pregnant women. If busulfan is used during pregnancy, or if the patient becomes pregnant while receiving busulfan, inform the patient of the potential hazard to the fetus. Advise women of childbearing potential to avoid becoming pregnant.

Fertility impairment – Ovarian suppression and amenorrhea commonly occur in premenopausal women undergoing chronic, low-dose busulfan therapy for CML. Busulfan depleted oocytes of female rats. Busulfan induced sterility in male rats and hamsters. Sterility, azoospermia, and testicular atrophy have been reported in men. The solvent dimethylacetamide (DMA) also may impair fertility.

➤*Lactation:* It is not known whether this drug is excreted in breast milk. Because many drugs are excreted in breast milk, and because of the potential for tumorigenicity shown for busulfan in human and animal studies, decide whether to discontinue breast-feeding or the drug, taking into account the importance of the drug to the mother.

➤*Children:* The efficacy of busulfan in the treatment of CML has not been specifically studied in children. An open-label, uncontrolled study evaluated the pharmacokinetics of busulfan in 24 children receiving busulfan as part of a conditioning regimen administered prior to hematopoietic progenitor cell transplantation for a variety of malignant hematologic (n = 15) or nonmalignant diseases (n = 9). Patients ranged in age from 5 months to 16 years of age (median, 3 years of age). Busulfan dosing was targeted to achieve an AUC of 900 to 1,350 mcM•min, with an initial dose of 0.8 or 1 mg/kg (based on ABW) if the patient was older than 4 years of age or 4 years of age and younger, respectively. The dose was adjusted based on plasma concentration after completion of dose 1.

Patients received busulfan doses every 6 hours as a 2-hour infusion over 4 days for a total of 16 doses, followed by cyclophosphamide 50 mg/kg once daily for 4 days. After 1 rest day, hematopoietic progenitor cells were infused. All patients received phenytoin as seizure prophylaxis. The target AUC (900 to 1,350 ± 5% mcM•min) for busulfan was achieved at dose 1 in 71% (17/24) of patients. Steady-state pharmacokinetic testing was performed at doses 9 and 13. Busulfan levels were within the target range for 21 of 23 evaluable patients.

All 24 patients experienced neutropenia (ANC less than 0.5 × 10^9/L) and thrombocytopenia (platelet transfusions or platelet count less than 20,000/mm^3). Seventy-nine percent (19/24) of patients experienced lymphopenia (absolute lymphocyte count less than 0.1 × 10^9). In 23 patients, the ANC recovered to more than 0.5 × 10^9/L (median time to recovery = BMT day +13; range = BMT day +9 to +22). One patient who died on day +20 had not recovered to an ANC greater than 0.5 × 10^9/L.

Four (17%) patients died during the study. Two patients died within 28 days of transplant; 1 with pneumonia and capillary leak syndrome, and the other with pneumonia and venoocclusive disease. Two patients died prior to day 100; 1 because of progressive disease and 1 because of multiorgan failure.

Adverse reactions were reported in all 24 patients during the study period (BMT day −10 through BMT day +28) or poststudy surveillance period (day +29 through +100). These included vomiting (100%), nausea (83%), stomatitis (79%), HVOD (21%), graft-versus-host disease (GVHD) (25%), and pneumonia (21%).

Based on the results of this 24-patient clinical trial, a suggested dosing regimen of busulfan in children is shown in the following dosing nomogram:

Busulfan Injection Dosing Nomogram

Patient's ABW	Busulfan dosage
≤ 12 kg	1.1 (mg/kg)
> 12 kg	0.8 (mg/kg)

Simulations based on a pediatric population pharmacokinetic model indicate that approximately 60% of children will achieve a target busulfan exposure (AUC) between 900 to 1,350 mcM•min with the first dose of busulfan using this dosing nomogram. Therapeutic drug monitoring and dose adjustment following the first dose of busulfan is recommended.

BUSULFAN — INJECTION

➤*Monitoring:* Monitor patients receiving busulfan daily with a complete blood count, including differential count and quantitative platelet count, until engraftment has been demonstrated.

To detect hepatotoxicity, which may herald the onset of HVOD, evaluate serum transaminases, alkaline phosphatase, and bilirubin daily through BMT day +28.

Drug Interactions

Busulfan Injection Drug Interactions

Precipitant drug	Object drug[a]		Description
Acetaminophen	Busulfan	↑	Because busulfan is eliminated from the body via conjugation with glutathione, use of acetaminophen prior to (< 72 hours) or concurrently with busulfan may result in reduced busulfan clearance based on the known property of acetaminophen to decrease glutathione levels in the blood and tissues.
Cyclophosphamide	Busulfan	↑	Cardiac tamponade, which was often fatal, has been reported in a small number of patients with thalassemia (2% in 1 series) who received high doses of busulfan and cyclophosphamide (see Warnings/Precautions).
Itraconazole	Busulfan	↓	Itraconazole decreases busulfan clearance up to 25% and may produce AUCs > 1,500 mcM•min in some patients.
Phenytoin	Busulfan	↑	Phenytoin increases the clearance of busulfan ≥ 15%, possibly caused by the induction of glutathione-S-transferase.
Thioguanine	Busulfan	↑	In 1 study, ≈ 3.6% of patients receiving continuous (6 to 45 months) concomitant therapy for treatment of CML had esophageal varices associated with abnormal liver function tests. Liver biopsies performed in 33% of these patients all showed evidence of nodular regenerative hyperplasia. Use with caution in long-term continuous therapy.

[a] ↑ = Object drug increased. ↓ = Object drug decreased.

Adverse Reactions

Busulfan injection is considered to have moderate to high potential for nausea and vomiting.

DMA, the solvent used in the busulfan formulation, was studied in 1962 as a potential cancer chemotherapy drug. In a phase 1 trial, the maximum tolerated dose (MTD) was 14.8 g/m²/day for 4 days. The daily recommended dose of busulfan contains DMA equivalent to 42% of the MTD on a mg/m² basis. The dose-limiting toxicities in the phase 1 study were hepatotoxicity as evidenced by increased AST levels and neurological symptoms as evidenced by hallucinations. The hallucinations had a pattern of onset at 1 day postcompletion of DMA administration and were associated with electroencephalogram changes. The lowest dose at which hallucinations were recognized was equivalent to 1.9 times that delivered in a conditioning regimen utilizing busulfan 0.8 mg/kg every 6 hours × 16 doses. Other neurological toxicities included confusion, lethargy, and somnolence. The relative contribution of DMA and/or other concomitant medications to neurologic and hepatic toxicities observed with busulfan is difficult to ascertain.

Treatment with busulfan at the recommended dose and schedule will result in profound myelosuppression in 100% of patients, including anemia, granulocytopenia, thrombocytopenia, or a combined loss of formed elements of the blood.

Summary of the Incidence (20%) of Nonhematologic Adverse Reactions Through BMT Day +28 in Patients Who Received Busulfan Injection Prior to Allogeneic Hematopoietic Progenitor Cell Transplantation

Nonhematological adverse reactions[a]	Incidence (%)
Cardiovascular	
Hypertension	36%
Tachycardia	44%
Thrombosis	33%
Vasodilation	25%
CNS	
Anxiety	72%
Depression	23%
Dizziness	30%
Insomnia	84%
Dermatologic	
Pruritus	28%
Rash	57%
GI	
Abdominal enlargement	23%
Abdominal pain	72%
Anorexia	85%
Constipation	38%
Diarrhea	84%
Dry mouth	26%
Dyspepsia	44%
Nausea	98%
Rectal disorder	25%
Stomatitis (mucositis)	97%
Vomiting	95%
Metabolic/Nutritional	
AST elevation	31%
Creatinine increased	21%
Edema	36%
Hyperbilirubinemia	49%
Hyperglycemia	66%
Hypocalcemia	49%
Hypokalemia	64%
Hypomagnesemia	77%
Respiratory	
Cough	28%
Dyspnea	25%
Epistaxis	25%
Lung disorder	34%
Rhinitis	44%
Miscellaneous	
Allergic reaction	26%
Asthenia	51%
Back pain	23%
Chest pain	26%
Chills	46%
Edema, general	28%
Fever	80%
Headache	69%
Inflammation at injection site	25%
Pain	44%

[a] Includes all reported adverse reactions regardless of severity (toxicity grades 1 to 4).

The following sections describe clinically significant reactions occurring in the busulfan clinical trials, regardless of drug attribution.

➤*Cardiovascular:* Mild or moderate tachycardia was reported in 44% of patients. In 7 patients (11%), it was first reported during busulfan administration. Other rhythm abnormalities, which were all mild or moderate, included arrhythmia (5%), atrial fibrillation (2%), ventricular extrasystoles (2%), and third-degree heart block (2%). Mild or moderate thrombosis occurred in 33% of patients, and all episodes were associated with the central venous catheter. Hypertension was reported in 36% of patients and was grade 3/4 in 7%. Hypotension occurred in 11% of patients and was grade 3/4 in 3%. Mild vasodilation (flushing and hot flashes) was reported in 25% of patients. Other cardiovascular events included cardiomegaly (5%), mild electrocardiogram abnormality (2%), grade 3/4 left-sided heart failure in 1 patient (2%), and moderate pericardial effusion (2%). These reactions were reported primarily in the postcyclophosphamide phase.

➤*CNS:* The most commonly reported adverse reactions of the CNS were insomnia (84%), anxiety (75%), dizziness (30%), and depression (23%). Severity was mild or moderate except for 1 patient (1%) who experienced severe insomnia. One patient (1%) developed a life-threatening cerebral

Alkyl Sulfonates

BUSULFAN — INJECTION

hemorrhage and a coma as a terminal event following multiorgan failure after HVOD. Other reactions considered severe included delirium (2%), agitation (2%), and encephalopathy (2%). The overall incidence of confusion was 11% and 5% of patients were reported to have experienced hallucinations. The patient who developed delirium and hallucination on the allogeneic study had onset of confusion at the completion of busulfan. The overall incidence of lethargy in the allogeneic busulfan clinical trial was 7%, and somnolence was reported in 2%. One patient (2%) treated in an autologous transplantation study experienced a seizure while receiving cyclophosphamide, despite prophylactic treatment with phenytoin.

➤*Dermatologic:* Rash (57%) and pruritus (28%) were reported; both conditions were predominantly mild. Alopecia was mild in 15% of patients; mild vesicular rash and vesiculobullous rash were reported in 10% of patients. Moderate maculopapular rash and skin discoloration was reported in 8% of patients. Acne was reported in 7% of patients. Exfoliative dermatitis was reported in 5% of patients. Erythema nodosum and moderate alopecia were reported in 2% of patients.

➤*GI:* GI toxicities were frequent and generally considered to be related to the drug. Few were categorized as serious. Mild or moderate nausea occurred in 92% of patients in the allogeneic clinical trial, and mild or moderate vomiting occurred in 95% through BMT day 28; nausea was severe in 7% of patients. The incidence of vomiting during busulfan administration (BMT day −7 to −4) was 43% in the allogeneic clinical trial. Grade 3 to 4 stomatitis developed in 26% of the participants, and grade 3 esophagitis developed in 2%. Grade 3 to 4 diarrhea was reported in 5% of the allogeneic study participants, while mild or moderate diarrhea occurred in 75%. Mild or moderate constipation occurred in 38% of patients; ileus developed in 8% of patients and was severe in 2% of patients. Forty-four percent of patients reported mild or moderate dyspepsia. Two percent of patients experienced mild hematemesis. Pancreatitis developed in 2% of patients. Mild or moderate rectal discomfort occurred in 24% of patients. Severe anorexia occurred in 21% of patients and was mild/moderate in 64% of patients.

➤*Hematologic:* At the indicated dose and schedule, busulfan produced profound myelosuppression in 100% of patients. Following hematopoietic progenitor cell infusion, recovery of neutrophil counts to greater than or equal to 500 cells/mm^3 occurred at median day 13 when prophylactic G-CSF was administered to the majority of participants on the study. The median number of platelet transfusions per patient on study was 6, and the median number of red blood cell transfusions on study was 4. Prolonged prothrombin time was reported in 1 patient (2%).

➤*Hepatic:* Hyperbilirubinemia occurred in 49% of patients in the allogeneic BMT trial. Grade 3/4 hyperbilirubinemia occurred in 30% of patients within 28 days of transplantation and was considered life-threatening in 5% of these patients. Hyperbilirubinemia was associated with GVHD in 6 patients and with HVOD in 5 patients. Grade 3/4 AST elevations occurred in 7% of patients. Alkaline phosphatase increases were mild or moderate in 15% of patients. Mild or moderate jaundice developed in 12% of patients, and mild or moderate hepatomegaly developed in 6% of patients.

HVOD – See Warnings/Precautions for more information.

➤*Metabolic/Nutritional:* Hyperglycemia was observed in 67% of patients and grade 3/4 hyperglycemia was reported in 15%. Hypomagnesemia was mild or moderate in 77% of patients; hypokalemia was mild or moderate in 62% and severe in 2% of patients; hypocalcemia was mild or moderate in 46% and severe in 3% of patients; hypophosphatemia was mild or moderate in 17% of patients; and hyponatremia was reported in 2% of patients.

➤*Renal:* Creatinine was mildly or moderately elevated in 21% of patients. BUN was increased in 3% of patients and to a grade 3/4 level in 2% of patients. Seven percent of patients experienced dysuria, 15% experienced oliguria, and 8% experienced hematuria. There were 4 (7%) grade 3/4 cases of hemorrhagic cystitis in the allogeneic clinical trial.

➤*Respiratory:* Mild or moderate dyspnea occurred in 25% of patients and was severe in 2% of patients. One patient (2%) experienced severe hyperventilation; and in 2 (3%) additional patients it was mild or moderate. Mild rhinitis and mild or moderate cough were reported in 44% and 28% of patients, respectively. Mild epistaxis events were reported in 25% of patients. Three patients (5%) on the allogeneic study developed documented alveolar hemorrhage. All required mechanical ventilatory support and all died. Nonspecific interstitial fibrosis was found on wedge biopsies performed with video-assisted thoracoscopy in 1 patient on the allogeneic study who subsequently died from respiratory failure on BMT day +98. Other pulmonary events, reported as mild or moderate, included pharyngitis (18%), hiccup (18%), asthma (8%), hemoptysis (3%), pleural effusion (3%), sinusitis (3%), atelectasis (2%), and hypoxia (2%).

➤*Miscellaneous:* Other reported reactions included headache (mild or moderate 64%, severe 5%), abdominal pain (mild or moderate 69%, severe 3%), asthenia (mild or moderate 49%, severe 2%), unspecified pain (mild or moderate 43%, severe 2%), allergic reaction (mild or moderate 24%, severe 2%), injection site inflammation (mild or moderate 25%), injection site pain (mild or moderate 15%), chest pain (mild or moderate 26%), back pain (mild or moderate 23%), myalgia (mild or moderate 16%), arthralgia (mild or moderate 13%), and ear disorder in 3%.

GVHD – GVHD developed in 18% of patients (11/61) receiving allogeneic transplants; it was severe in 3% and mild or moderate in 15% of patients. There were 3 deaths (5%) attributed to GVHD.

Edema – Patients receiving allogeneic transplant exhibited some form of edema (79%), hypervolemia, or documented weight increase (8%); all events were reported as mild or moderate.

Infection/Fever – Fifty-one percent of patients experienced at least 1 episode of infection. Pneumonia was fatal in 1 patient (2%) and life-threatening in 3% of patients. Fever was reported in 80% of patients; it was mild or moderate in 78% and severe in 3% of patients. Forty-six percent of patients experienced chills.

Deaths – There were 2 deaths through BMT day +28 in the allogeneic transplant setting. There were an additional 6 deaths BMT day +29 through BMT day +100 in the allogeneic transplant setting.

Overdosage

There is no known antidote to busulfan other than hematopoietic progenitor cell transplantation. In the absence of hematopoietic progenitor cell transplantation, the recommended dosage for busulfan would constitute an overdose of busulfan. The principal toxic effect is profound bone marrow hypoplasia/aplasia and pancytopenia but the CNS, liver, lungs, and GI tract may be affected. Closely monitor the hematologic status and institute vigorous supportive measures as medically indicated. Survival after a single dose of busulfan 140 mg tablets in an 18 kg, 4-year-old child has been reported. Inadvertent administration of a greater-than-normal dose of oral busulfan (2.1 mg/kg; total dose of 23.3 mg/kg) occurred in a 2-year-old child prior to a scheduled BMT without sequelae. An acute dose of 2.4 g was fatal in a 10-year-old boy. There is 1 report that busulfan is dialyzable, thus consider dialysis in the case of overdose. Busulfan is metabolized by conjugation with glutathione, thus administration of glutathione may be considered.

Patient Information

Explain the increased risk of a second malignancy to the patient.

Ethylenimines/Methylmelamines

ALTRETAMINE (Hexamethylmelamine)

Rx	**Hexalen** (Eisai)	**Capsules; oral:** 50 mg	Lactose. (USB001 Hexalen 50 mg). Clear. In 100s.

ALTRETAMINE (Hexamethylmelamine) — ORAL

WARNING

Administer only under the supervision of a physician experienced in the use of antineoplastic agents.

Monitor peripheral blood counts at least monthly, prior to the initiation of each course of altretamine therapy and as clinically indicated (see Adverse Reactions).

Because of the possibility of altretamine-related neurotoxicity, perform neurologic examination regularly during administration (see Adverse Reactions).

Indications

➤*Ovarian cancer:* For use as a single agent in the palliative treatment of patients with persistent or recurrent ovarian cancer following first-line therapy with a cisplatin- or alkylating agent-based combination.

Administration and Dosage

➤*Adults:*

Ovarian cancer –

Usual dosage: 260 mg/m^2/day for either 14 or 21 days in a 28-day cycle. Give the total daily dose in 3 to 4 divided doses (round dose to the nearest 50 mg) after meals and at bedtime. The usual dose is 400 mg/day.

Rechallenge: Temporarily discontinue altretamine (for 14 days or more) and subsequently restart at 200 mg/m^2/day for any of the following situations: GI intolerance unresponsive to symptomatic measures; WBC less than 2,000/mm^3 or granulocyte count less than 1,000/mm^3; platelet count less than 75,000/mm^3; progressive neurotoxicity.

If neurologic symptoms fail to stabilize on the reduced dose schedule, discontinue altretamine indefinitely.

➤*Preparation for administration:* Altretamine is considered a cytotoxic agent. Follow safe handling procedures when preparing, administering, or dispensing altretamine.

➤*Administration:* Take capsules after meals.

➤*Storage/Stability:* Store up to 25°C (77°F); excursions permitted to 15° to 30°C (59° to 86°F).

Actions

➤*Pharmacology:* Altretamine, formerly known as hexamethylmelamine, is a synthetic cytotoxic antineoplastic s-triazine derivative. The precise mechanism by which altretamine exerts its cytotoxic effect is unknown, although a number of theoretical possibilities have been studied. Structurally, altretamine resembles the alkylating agent triethylenemelamine, yet in vitro tests for alkylating activity of altretamine and its metabolites have been negative. Altretamine is efficacious for certain ovarian tumors resistant to classical alkylating agents. Metabolism of altretamine is a require-

ALTRETAMINE (Hexamethylmelamine) — ORAL

ment for cytotoxicity. Synthetic monohydroxymethylmelamines and products of altretamine metabolism in vitro and in vivo can form covalent adducts with tissue macromolecules including DNA, but the relevance of these reactions to antitumor activity is unknown.

➤*Pharmacokinetics:* Altretamine is well absorbed following oral administration, but undergoes rapid and extensive demethylation in the liver, producing variations in altretamine plasma levels. The principal metabolites are pentamethylmelamine and tetramethylmelamine. After oral administration to 11 patients with advanced ovarian cancer in doses of 120 to 300 mg/m^2, peak plasma levels were reached between 0.5 and 3 hours, varying from 0.2 to 20.8 mg/L. Half-life of the β-phase of elimination ranged from 4.7 to 10.2 hours. Altretamine and metabolites show binding to plasma proteins. The free fractions of altretamine, pentamethylmelamine and tetramethylmelamine are 6%, 25% and 50%, respectively.

Following oral administration of 4 mg/kg, urinary recovery was 61% at 24 hours and 90% at 72 hours. Human urinary metabolites were N-demethylated homologues of altretamine with less than 1% unmetabolized altretamine excreted at 24 hours. After intraperitoneal administration to mice, tissue distribution was rapid in all organs, reaching a maximum at 30 minutes. The excretory organs (liver and kidney) and the small intestine showed high concentrations, whereas relatively low concentrations were found in other organs, including the brain.

Contraindications

Hypersensitivity to altretamine.

Pre-existing severe bone marrow depression or severe neurologic toxicity; however, altretamine has been administered safely to patients heavily pretreated with cisplatin or alkylating agents including patients with pre-existing cisplatin neuropathies. Careful monitoring of neurologic function in these patients is essential.

Warnings/Precautions

➤*Neurotoxicity:* Altretamine causes mild to moderate neurotoxicity. Peripheral neuropathy and CNS symptoms (eg, mood disorders, disorders of consciousness, ataxia, dizziness, vertigo) have occurred. They are more likely to occur in patients receiving continuous high-dose daily altretamine than moderate-dose altretamine administered on an intermittent schedule. Neurologic toxicity appears to be reversible when therapy is discontinued. It has been suggested that the incidence and severity of neurotoxicity may be decreased by concomitant administration of pyridoxine, but this remains unproven. Perform a neurologic examination prior to the initiation of each course of therapy.

➤*Hematologic:* Altretamine causes mild to moderate dose-related myelosuppression. Leukopenia less than 3000 WBC/mm^3 occurred in less than 15% of patients on a variety of intermittent or continuous dose regimens; less than 1% had leukopenia less than 1000 WBC/mm^3. Thrombocytopenia less than 50,000 platelets/mm^3 was seen in less than 10% of patients. When given in doses of 8 to 12 mg/kg/day over a 21 day course, nadirs of leukocyte and platelet counts were reached by 3 to 4 weeks, and normal counts were regained by 6 weeks. With continuous administration at doses of 6 to 8 mg/kg/day, nadirs are reached in 6 to 8 weeks (median). Monitor peripheral blood counts prior to the initiation of each course of therapy, monthly, and as clinically indicated. Adjust the dose as necessary (see Administration and Dosage).

➤*Nausea and vomiting:* With continuous high-dose daily altretamine, nausea and vomiting of gradual onset occur frequently. In most instances, these symptoms are controllable with antiemetics; at times, however, the severity requires dose reduction or, rarely, discontinuation of therapy. In some instances, a tolerance of these symptoms develops after several weeks of therapy. The incidence and severity of nausea and vomiting are reduced with moderate-dose administration of altretamine. In two clinical studies of single-agent altretamine using a moderate, intermittent dose and schedule, only 1 patient (1%) discontinued altretamine due to severe nausea and vomiting.

➤*Pregnancy: Category D.* Altretamine is embryotoxic and teratogenic in rats and rabbits when given at doses 2 and 10 times the human dose, and it may cause fetal damage when administered to a pregnant woman. If altretamine is used during pregnancy, or if the patient becomes pregnant while taking the drug, apprise the patient of the potential hazard to the fetus. Advise women to avoid becoming pregnant.

➤*Lactation:* It is not known whether altretamine is excreted in breast milk. Because there is a possibility of toxicity in nursing infants secondary to altretamine treatment of the mother, it is recommended that breastfeeding be discontinued if the mother is treated with altretamine.

➤*Children:* Safety and efficacy in children have not been established.

Drug Interactions

Altretamine Drug Interactions

Precipitant drug	Object drug[a]		Description
Cimetidine	Altretamine	↑	Cimetidine, an inhibitor of microsomal drug metabolism, increased altretamine's half-life and toxicity in a rat model.
Altretamine	Monoamine oxidase inhibitors	↑	Monoamine oxidase inhibitors and concurrent altretamine may cause severe orthostatic hypotension. Four patients, all > 60 years of age, experienced symptomatic hypotension after 4 to 7 days of concomitant therapy.

[a] ↑ = Object drug increased.

Adverse Reactions

Altretamine is considered to have moderately low emetogenic potential (10% to 30% incidence of emesis).

The most common adverse reactions are: Nausea and vomiting (see Warnings/Precautions); peripheral neuropathy, CNS symptoms and myelosuppression (see Warnings/Precautions).

Altretamine Adverse Reactions in Previously Treated Ovarian Cancer Patients (n = 76)

Adverse reaction	Incidence (%)
GI	
Nausea and vomiting	
Mild to moderate	32
Severe	1
Increased alkaline phosphatase	9
Hematologic	
Leukopenia	
WBC 2000 to 2999/mm^3	4
WBC < 2000/mm^3	1
Thrombocytopenia	
Platelets 75,000 to 99,000/mm^3	6
Platelets < 75,000/mm^3	3
Anemia	
Mild	20
Moderate to severe	13
Neurologic	
Peripheral sensory neuropathy	
Mild	22
Moderate to severe	9
Anorexia and fatigue	1
Seizures	1
Renal	
Serum creatinine 1.6 to 3.75 mg/dL	7
BUN	
25-40 mg/dL	5
41-60 mg/dL	3
Greater than 60 mg/dL	1

THIOTEPA (Triethylenethiophosphoramide; TSPA; TESPA)

Rx	**Thioplex** (Amgen)	**Powder for injection, lyophilized:** 15 mg	In vials.
Rx	**Thiotepa** (Sicor)		In single-dose vials.
Rx	**Thiotepa** (Sicor)	**Powder for injection, lyophilized:** 30 mg	In single-dose vials.

THIOTEPA — INJECTION

Indications

➤*Neoplastic diseases:* Thiotepa has been tried with varying results in the palliation of a wide variety of neoplastic diseases. However, the most consistent results have been seen in the following tumors: adenocarcinoma of the breast; adenocarcinoma of the ovary; for controlling intracavitary effusions secondary to diffuse or localized neoplastic diseases of various serosal cavities; for the treatment of superficial papillary carcinoma of the urinary bladder.

While now largely superseded by other treatments, thiotepa has been effective against other lymphomas, such as lymphosarcoma and Hodgkin disease.

➤*Off-label uses:* Prevention of pterygium recurrence after postoperative β-irradiation, autologous bone marrow transplantation, intrathecal use for CNS leukemia, lymphoma, or metastases. Thiotepa has been used safely and effectively in children. (See Administration and Dosage.)

Administration and Dosage

➤*General dosing considerations:* Thiotepa is dosed in mg/kg for some indications, but may be dosed in mg/m^2 body surface area (BSA) for other indications.

Dosage must be carefully individualized. A slow response to thiotepa does not necessarily indicate a lack of effect. Therefore, increasing the frequency

THIOTEPA — INJECTION

of dosing may only increase toxicity. After maximum benefit is obtained by initial therapy, it is necessary to continue the patient on maintenance therapy (1- to 4-week intervals). In order to continue optimal effect, maintenance doses should not be administered more frequently than weekly in order to preserve correlation between dose and blood counts.

➤*Adults:*

Neoplastic diseases –

Initial dosage: Initially, the higher dose in the given range is commonly administered. (See the following dosage regimens.)

Maintenance dosage: The maintenance dose should be adjusted weekly on the basis of pretreatment control blood counts and subsequent blood counts.

IV administration: 0.3 to 0.4 mg/kg by rapid IV administration, every 1 to 4 weeks. (See also Off-Label Dosing.)

Intracavitary administration: 0.6 to 0.8 mg/kg instilled into the affected cavity every 1 to 4 weeks. (See also Off-Label Dosing.)

Intravesical administration: Patients with papillary carcinoma of the bladder are dehydrated for 8 to 12 hours prior to treatment. Then 30 to 60 mg (in 60 mL of sodium chloride 0.9% injection) is instilled intravesically once weekly for 4 weeks. Retain fluid in bladder for 2 hours. If patient cannot retain for 2 hours, dilute successive doses in 30 mL of sodium chloride 0.9% injection instead of 60 mL. It may be necessary to repeat the course of therapy or give maintenance therapy with 30 to 60 mg intravesically once monthly for up to 1 year. Second and third courses must be given with caution since bone marrow depression may be increased. Deaths have occurred after intravesical administration, caused by bone marrow depression from systemically absorbed drug.

After local resection or fulguration of bladder tumors, prophylaxis with thiotepa 30 to 60 mg has been used.

Off-label dosing –

IV administration: Alternative regimens are thiotepa 0.2 mg/kg/day IV for 4 to 5 days every 2 to 4 weeks; or 6 mg/m^2 BSA daily for 4 to 5 days every 2 to 4 weeks; or 30 to 60 mg/m^2 BSA once weekly.

Intracavitary administration: Alternatively, 15 to 30 mg has been administered pericardially.

Intrathecal use: 1 to 10 mg/m^2 intrathecally given once or twice weekly. Alternatively, thiotepa 15 mg has been used.

Hematopoietic stem cell transplantation: Doses of thiotepa have ranged from 500 mg/m^2 BSA in combination regimens to a maximum tolerated dose of 1,125 mg/m^2 BSA as a single agent.

Prophylaxis for pterygium recurrence: Thiotepa 0.05% solution instilled in affected eye every 3 hours while awake for 6 to 8 weeks postoperatively.

➤*Children:*

Off-label dosing –

Sarcomas: 25 to 65 mg/m^2 BSA IV every 3 to 4 weeks.

Hematopoietic stem cell transplantation: Doses of thiotepa 300 mg/m^2 BSA daily for 3 days (total dose of 900 mg/m^2) in combination with other antineoplastic agents have been used.

➤*Preparation for administration:* Thiotepa is considered a cytotoxic agent. Follow safe handling procedures when preparing, administering, or dispensing thiotepa.

Skin reactions associated with accidental exposure to thiotepa may occur. The use of gloves is recommended. If thiotepa solution contacts the skin, immediately wash the skin thoroughly with soap and water. If thiotepa contacts mucous membranes, the membranes should be flushed thoroughly with water.

Thiotepa should be reconstituted with 1.5 or 3 mL of sterile water for injection, resulting in a drug concentration of approximately 10 mg/mL.

Thiotepa Quantities and Concentration

Label claim (mg/vial)	Actual content (mg/vial)	Amount of diluent to be added (mL)	Approximate withdrawable volume (mL)	Approximate withdrawable amount (mg/vial)	Approximate reconstituted concentration (mg/mL)
15	15.6	1.5	1.4	14.7	10.4
30	31.2	3	2.8	29.4	10.4

The reconstituted solution is hypotonic and should be further diluted with sodium chloride 0.9% injection before use.

Intracavitary solutions – Dilute desired dose with 10 to 20 mL sodium chloride 0.9% injection or dextrose 5% injection prior to administration.

Intrathecal solutions – Dilute prior to administration to a final concentration between 1 and 5 mg/mL with preservative-free sodium chloride 0.9% injection or Ringer's lactate injection, or to 1 mg/mL if diluted with preservative-free sterile water for injection.

In order to eliminate haze, filter solutions through a 0.22 micron filter (polysulfone membrane [*Gelman's Sterile Acrodisc*, Single Use] or triton-free mixed ester of cellulose/PVC [*Millipore's MILLEX*-GS Filter Unit]) prior to administration. Filtering does not alter solution potency. Reconstituted solutions should be clear. Solutions that remain opaque or precipitate after filtration should not be used.

➤*Administration:* Thiotepa may be administered IV, by intravesical instillation, by intracavitary effusion, intrathecally (off-label), or by ophthalmic instillation (off-label).

Intravesical instillation – Prior to intravesical instillation, patients should not drink fluids for 8 to 12 hours. While thiotepa is instilled, patients may be repositioned every 15 minutes to maximize area of contact.

Intracavitary neoplastic effusions – Administer through the same catheter used to drain effusion fluid from affected cavity.

Intrathecal solutions – Administer intrathecal solutions within 1 hour of preparation.

➤*Extravasation:* Thiotepa is considered an irritant and may cause phlebitis, but it is not known to cause tissue damage with extravasation. If signs or symptoms of extravasation occur, stop the infusion immediately. If possible, withdraw 3 to 5 mL of blood to remove some of the drug. Remove the infusion needle. Delineate the infiltrated area on the patient's skin with a felt tip marker. Elevate for 48 hours above heart level using a sling or stockinette dressing with an observation window cut in the dressing. Avoid pressure or friction. Do not rub the area. Observe for signs of increased erythema, pain, or skin necrosis. If increased symptoms occur, consult a plastic surgeon. Ensure that no medication is given distally to the extravasation site. After 48 hours, encourage the patient to use the extremity normally to promote full range of motion.

➤*Storage/Stability:* Store at 2° to 8°C (36° to 46°F). Protect from light at all times.

Reconstituted solution is stable for at least 24 hours under refrigeration. However, thiotepa contains no preservative and the manufacturer recommends using the product within 8 hours.

Diluted 5 mg/mL solutions prepared with sodium chloride 0.9% injection are stable for up to 24 hours at room temperature or refrigerated. Solutions diluted to 1 to 3 mg/mL are stable for at least 24 hours refrigerated and for up to 24 hours at room temperature. Diluted 0.5 mg/mL solutions must be used within 8 hours.

Discard vial within 6 hours of the initial needle puncture if opened within an ISO Class 5 biological safety cabinet, or within 1 hour of the initial needle puncture if opened outside of such an environment, based on the USP Chapter < 797 > standards.

Intrathecal solutions – Administer intrathecal solutions within 1 hour of preparation.

Actions

➤*Pharmacology:* Thiotepa is a cytotoxic agent of the polyfunctional type, related chemically and pharmacologically to nitrogen mustard. The radiomimetic action of thiotepa is believed to occur through the release of ethylenimine radicals which, like irradiation, disrupt the bonds of DNA. One of the principal bond disruptions is initiated by alkylation of guanine at the N-7 position, which severs the linkage between the purine base and the sugar and liberates alkylated guanines.

➤*Pharmacokinetics:* TEPA, which possesses cytotoxic activity, appears to be the major metabolite of thiotepa found in human serum and urine. Urinary excretion of ^{14}C-labeled thiotepa and metabolites in a 34-year-old patient with metastatic carcinoma of the cecum who received a dose of 0.3 mg/kg IV was 63%. Thiotepa and TEPA in urine each accounts for less than 2% of the administered dose.

The pharmacokinetics of thiotepa and TEPA in 13 female patients (45 to 84 years) with advanced stage ovarian cancer receiving 60 mg and 80 mg thiotepa by IV infusion on subsequent courses given at 4-week intervals are presented in the following table:

Pharmacokinetics of Thiotepa and TEPA

Pharmacokinetic parameters	Thiotepa		TEPA	
	60 mg	80 mg	60 mg	80 mg
Peak serum concentration (ng/mL)	1331 ± 119	1828 ± 135	273 ± 46	353 ± 46
Elimination half-life (hr)	2.4 ± 0.3	2.3 ± 0.3	17.6 ± 3.6	15.7 ± 2.7
Area under the curve (ng•hr/mL)	2832 ± 412	4127 ± 668	4789 ± 1022	7452 ± 1667
Total body clearance (mL/min)	446 ± 63	419 ± 56		

Contraindications

Hypersensitivity (allergy) to this preparation.

Therapy is probably contraindicated in cases of existing hepatic, renal, or bone marrow damage. However, if the need outweighs the risk in such patients, thiotepa may be used in low dosage, and accompanied by hepatic, renal and hemopoietic function tests.

Warnings/Precautions

➤*Hematologic:* Death from septicemia and hemorrhage has occurred as a direct result of hematopoietic depression by thiotepa.

Thiotepa is highly toxic to the hematopoietic system. A rapidly falling white blood cell or platelet count indicates the necessity for discontinuing or reducing the dosage of thiotepa. Weekly blood and platelet counts are recommended during therapy and for at least 3 weeks after therapy has been discontinued.

➤*Bone marrow depression:* The serious complication of excessive thiotepa therapy, or sensitivity to the effects of thiotepa, is bone marrow depression. If proper precautions are not observed, thiotepa may cause leukopenia, thrombocytopenia, and anemia.

THIOTEPA — INJECTION

➤*Extravasation:* See Administration and Dosage for more information.

➤*Pregnancy: Category D.* Thiotepa can cause fetal harm when administered to a pregnant woman. Thiotepa given by the IP route was teratogenic in mice at doses greater than or equal to 1 mg/kg (3.2 mg/m^2), approximately 8-fold less than the maximum recommended human therapeutic dose based on body-surface area. Thiotepa given by the IP route was teratogenic in rats at doses greater than or equal to 3 mg/kg (21 mg/m^2), approximately equal to the maximum recommended human therapeutic dose based on body surface area. Thiotepa was lethal to rabbit fetuses at a dose of 3 mg/kg (41 mg/m^2), approximately 2 times the maximum recommended human therapeutic dose based on body surface area. Patients of childbearing potential should be advised to avoid pregnancy. There are no adequate and well-controlled studies in pregnant women. If thiotepa is used during pregnancy, or if pregnancy occurs during thiotepa therapy, the patient and partner should be apprised of the potential hazard to the fetus.

➤*Lactation:* It is not known whether thiotepa is excreted in human milk. Because many drugs are excreted in human milk and because of the potential for tumorigenicity shown for thiotepa in animal studies, a decision should be made whether to discontinue nursing or to discontinue the drug, taking into account the importance of the drug to the mother.

➤*Children:* Safety and efficacy in pediatric patients have not been established.

➤*Monitoring:* The most reliable guide to thiotepa toxicity is the white blood cell count. If this falls to 3000 or less, the dose should be discontinued. Another good index of thiotepa toxicity is the platelet count; if this falls to 150,000, therapy should be discontinued. Red blood cell count is a less accurate indicator of thiotepa toxicity. If the drug is used in patients with hepatic or renal damage (see Contraindications), regular assessment of hepatic and renal function tests are indicated.

Drug Interactions

It is not advisable to combine, simultaneously or sequentially, cancer chemotherapeutic agents or a cancer chemotherapeutic agent and a therapeutic modality having the same mechanism of action. Therefore, thiotepa combined with other alkylating agents such as nitrogen mustard or cyclophosphamide or thiotepa combined with irradiation would serve to intensify toxicity rather than to enhance therapeutic response. If these agents must follow each other, it is important that recovery from the first agent, as indicated by white blood cell count, be complete before therapy with the second agent is instituted.

Other drugs which are known to produce bone marrow depression should be avoided.

Adverse Reactions

Thiotepa is considered to have low potential for nausea and vomiting.

In addition to its effect on the blood-forming elements (see Warnings and Precautions), thiotepa may cause other adverse reactions.

➤*Allergic:* Rash, urticaria, laryngeal edema, asthma, anaphylactic shock, wheezing.

➤*CNS:* Dizziness, headache, blurred vision.

➤*Dermatologic:* Dermatitis, alopecia. Skin depigmentation has been reported following topical use.

➤*GI:* Nausea, vomiting, abdominal pain, anorexia.

➤*GU:* Amenorrhea, interference with spermatogenesis.

➤*Local:* Contact dermatitis, pain at the injection site.

➤*Renal:* Dysuria, urinary retention. There have been rare reports of chemical cystitis or hemorrhagic cystitis following intravesical, but not parenteral administration of thiotepa.

➤*Respiratory:* Prolonged apnea has been reported when succinylcholine was administered prior to surgery, following combined use of thiotepa and other anticancer agents. It was theorized that this was caused by decrease of pseudocholinesterase activity caused by the anticancer drugs.

➤*Special senses:* Conjunctivitis.

➤*Miscellaneous:* Fatigue, weakness. Febrile reaction and discharge from a subcutaneous lesion may occur as the result of breakdown of tumor tissue.

Overdosage

➤*Symptoms:* Hematopoietic toxicity can occur following overdose, manifested by a decrease in the white cell count or platelets. Red blood cell count is a less accurate indicator of thiotepa toxicity. Bleeding manifestations may develop. The patient may become more vulnerable to infection, and less able to combat such infection.

Dosages within and minimally above the recommended therapeutic doses have been associated with potentially life-threatening hematopoietic toxicity. Thiotepa has a toxic effect on the hematopoietic system that is dose related.

➤*Treatment:* Thiotepa is dialyzable.

There is no known antidote for overdosage with thiotepa. Transfusions of whole blood or platelets have proven beneficial to the patient in combating hematopoietic toxicity.

Patient Information

The patient should notify the physician in the case of any sign of bleeding (eg, epistaxis, easy bruising, change in color of urine, black stool) or infection (eg, fever, chills) or for possible pregnancy to patient or partner.

Effective contraception should be used during thiotepa therapy if either the patient or the partner is of childbearing potential.

MECHLORETHAMINE DERIVATIVE
BENDAMUSTINE HYDROCHLORIDE

Rx	**Treanda** (Cephalon)	**Injection, lyophilized powder for solution:** 25 mg	Mannitol 42.5 mg. Preservative free. In 8 mL single-use vials.
		100 mg	Mannitol 170 mg. Preservative free. In 20 mL single-use vials.

BENDAMUSTINE HYDROCHLORIDE — INJECTION

Indications

➤*Chronic lymphocytic leukemia:* For the treatment of patients with chronic lymphocytic leukemia (CLL).

➤*Non-Hodgkin lymphoma:* For the treatment of patients with indolent B-cell non-Hodgkin lymphoma (NHL) that has progressed during or within 6 months of treatment with rituximab or a rituximab-containing regimen.

Administration and Dosage

➤*General dosing considerations:* Reconstituted solution must be further diluted before administration. (See Preparation for Administration.)

Consider using allopurinol for the first few weeks of treatment to prevent tumor lysis syndrome in patients at high risk.

➤*Adults:*

Chronic lymphocytic leukemia –

Usual dosage: 100 mg/m^2 administered intravenously (IV) over 30 minutes on days 1 and 2 of a 28-day cycle for up to 6 cycles.

Dosage adjustment: Bendamustine administration should be delayed in the event of grade 4 hematologic toxicity or clinically significant grade 2 or higher nonhematologic toxicity. Once nonhematologic toxicity has recovered to grade 1 or lower and/or the blood cell counts have improved (absolute neutrophil count [ANC] 1 × 10^9/L or higher, platelets 75 × 10^9/L or higher), bendamustine can be reinitiated at the discretion of the treating health care provider. Dose reduction may be warranted.

• *Hematologic toxicity* – For grade 3 or greater toxicity, reduce the dose to 50 mg/m^2 on days 1 and 2 of each cycle; if grade 3 or greater toxicity recurs, reduce the dose to 25 mg/m^2 on days 1 and 2 of each cycle.

• *Nonhematologic toxicity* – For clinically significant grade 3 or greater toxicity, reduce the dose to 50 mg/m^2 on days 1 and 2 of each cycle.

Dose re-escalation in subsequent cycles may be considered at the discretion of the treating health care provider.

Non-Hodgkin lymphoma –

Usual dosage: 120 mg/m^2 administered IV over 60 minutes on days 1 and 2 of a 21-day cycle for up to 8 cycles.

Dosage adjustment: Bendamustine administration should be delayed in the event of grade 4 hematologic toxicity or clinically significant grade 2 or higher nonhematologic toxicity. Once nonhematologic toxicity has recovered to grade 1 or less and/or the blood cell counts have improved (ANC 1 × 10^9/L or higher, platelets 75 × 10^9/L or higher), bendamustine can be reinitiated at the discretion of the treating health care provider. Dose reduction may be warranted.

• *Hematologic toxicity* – For grade 4 toxicity, reduce the dose to 90 mg/m^2 on days 1 and 2 of each cycle; if grade 4 toxicity recurs, reduce the dose to 60 mg/m^2 on days 1 and 2 of each cycle.

• *Nonhematologic toxicity* – For grade 3 or greater toxicity, reduce the dose to 90 mg/m^2 on days 1 and 2 of each cycle; if grade 3 or greater toxicity recurs, reduce the dose to 60 mg/m^2 on days 1 and 2 of each cycle.

➤*Renal function impairment:* Use with caution in patients with mild or moderate renal impairment. Bendamustine should not be used in patients with creatinine clearance (CrCl) less than 40 mL/min.

➤*Hepatic function impairment:* Use with caution in patients with mild hepatic impairment. Bendamustine should not be used in patients with moderate (AST or ALT 2.5 to 10 × the upper limit of normal [ULN] and total bilirubin 1.5 to 3 × the ULN) or severe (total bilirubin more than 3 × the ULN) hepatic impairment.

➤*Infusion reactions:* Consider measures to prevent severe reactions, including antihistamines, antipyretics, and corticosteroids, in subsequent cycles in patients who have previously experienced grade 1 or 2 infusion reactions. Consider discontinuation in patients with grade 3 or 4 infusion reactions.

➤*Preparation for administration:* Aseptically reconstitute each bendamustine vial as follows: for the 25 mg vial, add 5 mL of only sterile water for injection; for the 100 mg vial, add 20 mL of only sterile water for injection.

BENDAMUSTINE HYDROCHLORIDE — INJECTION

Shake well to yield a clear, colorless to pale yellow solution with a bendamustine concentration of 5 mg/mL. The lyophilized powder should completely dissolve in 5 minutes.

Aseptically withdraw the volume needed for the required dose (based on the 5 mg/mL concentration) and immediately transfer to a 500 mL infusion bag of sodium chloride 0.9% injection (normal saline). As an alternative to sodium chloride 0.9% injection, a 500 mL infusion bag of dextrose 2.5%/sodium chloride 0.45% injection may be considered. The resulting final concentration of bendamustine in the infusion bag should be within 0.2 to 0.6 mg/mL. The reconstituted solution must be transferred to the infusion bag within 30 minutes of reconstitution. After transferring, thoroughly mix the contents of the infusion bag. The admixture should be a clear and colorless to slightly yellow solution.

Bendamustine contains no antimicrobial preservative. The admixture should be prepared as close as possible to the time of patient administration.

Safe handling and disposal – As with other potentially toxic anticancer agents, care should be exercised in the handling and preparation of solutions prepared from bendamustine. The use of gloves and safety glasses is recommended to avoid exposure in case of vial breakage or other accidental spillage. If bendamustine solution contacts the skin, immediately wash the skin thoroughly with soap and water. If bendamustine contacts the mucous membranes, flush thoroughly with water.

Procedures for the proper handling and disposal of anticancer drugs should be considered. Several guidelines on the subject have been published. There is no general agreement that all of the procedures recommended in the guidelines are necessary or appropriate.

Any unused solution should be discarded according to institutional procedures for antineoplastics.

➤*Administration:* Once diluted, the final admixture is stable for 24 hours under refrigeration, or 3 hours at room temperature and room light. Administration of bendamustine must be completed within this period.

Administer bendamustine via IV infusion over 60 minutes for NHL or over 30 minutes for CLL.

➤*Admixture compatibility:* Use sterile water for injection for reconstitution, and then either sodium chloride 0.9% injection or dextrose 2.5%/sodium chloride 0.45% injection for dilution. No other diluents have been shown to be compatible.

➤*Storage/Stability:* Vials may be stored at up to 25°C (77°F); excursions are permitted up to 30°C (86°F). Keep in the original package until time of use to protect from light. Once diluted with sodium chloride 0.9% injection or dextrose 2.5%/sodium chloride 0.45% injection, the final admixture is stable for 24 hours when refrigerated (2° to 8°C [36° to 47°F]), or for 3 hours when stored at room temperature (15° to 30°C [59° to 86°F]) and at room light.

Actions

➤*Pharmacology:* Bendamustine is a bifunctional mechlorethamine derivative containing a purine-like benzimidazole ring. Mechlorethamine and its derivatives form electrophilic alkyl groups. These groups form covalent bonds with electron-rich nucleophilic moieties, resulting in interstrand DNA crosslinks. The bifunctional covalent linkage can lead to cell death via several pathways. Bendamustine is active against both quiescent and dividing cells. The exact mechanism of action of bendamustine remains unknown.

➤*Pharmacokinetics:*

Absorption – Following a single IV dose of bendamustine, maximum drug concentration (C_{max}) typically occurred at the end of infusion. The dose proportionality of bendamustine has not been studied.

Distribution – In vitro, the binding of bendamustine to human serum plasma proteins ranged from 94% to 96% and was concentration independent from 1 to 50 mcg/mL. Data suggest that bendamustine is not likely to displace or to be displaced by highly protein-bound drugs. The blood to plasma concentration ratios in human blood ranged from 0.84 to 0.86 over a concentration range of 10 to 100 mcg/mL, indicating that bendamustine distributes freely in human red blood cells. In humans, the mean steady-state volume of distribution was approximately 25 L.

Metabolism – In vitro data indicate that bendamustine is primarily metabolized via hydrolysis to metabolites with low cytotoxic activity. In vitro, studies indicate that 2 active minor metabolites, M3 and M4, are primarily formed via CYP1A2. However, concentrations of these metabolites in plasma are 1/10 and 1/100 that of the parent compound, respectively, suggesting that the cytotoxic activity is primarily caused by bendamustine.

In vitro studies using human liver microsomes indicate that bendamustine does not inhibit CYP1A2, 2C9/10, 2D6, 2E1, or 3A4/5. Bendamustine did not induce metabolism of CYP1A2, 2A6, 2B6, 2C8, 2C9, 2C19, 2E1, or 3A4/5 enzymes in primary cultures of human hepatocytes.

Excretion – No mass balance study has been undertaken in humans. Preclinical radiolabeled bendamustine studies showed that approximately 90% of the administered drug was recovered in excreta, primarily in the feces.

Bendamustine clearance in humans is approximately 700 mL/min. After a single IV dose of bendamustine 120 mg/m^2 over 1 hour, the intermediate half-life of the parent compound is approximately 40 minutes. The mean apparent terminal elimination half-lives of M3 and M4 are approximately 3 hours and 30 minutes, respectively. Little or no accumulation in plasma is expected for bendamustine administered on days 1 and 2 of a 28-day cycle.

Special populations –

Renal function impairment: In a population pharmacokinetic analysis of bendamustine in patients receiving 120 mg/m^2, there was no meaningful effect of renal impairment (CrCl 40 to 80 mL/min; N = 31) on the pharmacokinetics of bendamustine. Bendamustine has not been studied in patients with CrCl less than 40 mL/min.

These results are limited; therefore, use bendamustine with caution in patients with mild or moderate renal impairment. Do not use bendamustine in patients with CrCl less than 40 mL/min.

Hepatic function impairment: In a population pharmacokinetic analysis of bendamustine in patients receiving 120 mg/m^2, there was no meaningful effect of mild (total bilirubin less than or equal to the ULN, AST more than or equal to the ULN to 2.5 × the ULN, and/or alkaline phosphatase more than or equal to the ULN to 5 × the ULN; N = 26) hepatic impairment on the pharmacokinetics of bendamustine. Bendamustine has not been studied in patients with moderate or severe hepatic impairment.

These results are limited; therefore, use bendamustine with caution in patients with mild hepatic impairment. Do not use bendamustine in patients with moderate (AST or ALT 2.5 to 10 × the ULN and total bilirubin 1.5 to 3 × the ULN) or severe (total bilirubin more than 3 × the ULN) hepatic impairment.

Race: The effect of race on the safety and/or efficacy of bendamustine has not been established. Based on a cross-study comparison, Japanese patients (n = 6), on average, had exposures that were 40% higher than non-Japanese patients receiving the same dose. The significance of this difference on the safety and efficacy of bendamustine in Japanese patients has not been established.

Contraindications

Known hypersensitivity (eg, anaphylactic and anaphylactoid reactions) to bendamustine or mannitol.

Warnings/Precautions

➤*Myelosuppression:* Patients treated with bendamustine are likely to experience myelosuppression. In the 2 NHL studies, 98% of patients had grade 3 to 4 myelosuppression. Three (2%) patients died from myelosuppression-related adverse reactions; one each from neutropenic sepsis, diffuse alveolar hemorrhage with grade 3 thrombocytopenia, and pneumonia from an opportunistic infection (eg, cytomegalovirus).

In the event of treatment-related myelosuppression, monitor leukocytes, platelets, hemoglobin, and neutrophils closely. In the clinical trials, blood cell counts were monitored every week initially. Hematologic nadirs were observed predominantly in the third week of therapy. Hematologic nadirs may require dose delays if recovery to the recommended values have not occurred by the first day of the next scheduled cycle. Prior to the initiation of the next cycle of therapy, ensure that the ANC is at least 1 × 10^9/L and the platelet count is at least 75 × 10^9/L.

➤*Infections:* Infection, including pneumonia and sepsis, has been reported in patients in clinical trials and in postmarketing reports. Infection has been associated with hospitalization, septic shock, and death. Patients with myelosuppression following treatment with bendamustine are more susceptible to infections.

➤*Infusion reactions and anaphylaxis:* Infusion reactions to bendamustine have occurred commonly in clinical trials. Symptoms include chills, fever, pruritus, and rash. In rare instances, severe anaphylactic and anaphylactoid reactions have occurred, particularly in the second and subsequent cycles of therapy. Clinically monitor and discontinue the drug if there are severe reactions. Ask patients about symptoms suggestive of infusion reactions after their first cycle of therapy. Patients who experienced grade 3 or worse allergic-type reactions were not typically rechallenged. Consider measures to prevent severe reactions, including antihistamines, antipyretics, and corticosteroids, in subsequent cycles in patients who have previously experienced grade 1 or 2 infusion reactions. Consider discontinuation in patients with grade 3 or 4 infusion reactions.

➤*Tumor lysis syndrome:* Tumor lysis syndrome associated with bendamustine treatment has been reported in patients in clinical trials and in postmarketing reports. The onset tends to be within the first treatment cycle of bendamustine and, without intervention, may lead to acute renal failure and death. Preventive measures include maintaining adequate volume status, and close monitoring of blood chemistry, particularly potassium and uric acid levels. Allopurinol has also been used during the beginning of bendamustine therapy. However, there may be an increased risk of severe skin toxicity when bendamustine and allopurinol are coadministered.

➤*Skin reactions:* A number of skin reactions have been reported in clinical trials and postmarketing safety reports. These reactions have included rash, toxic skin reactions, and bullous exanthema. Some reactions occurred when bendamustine was given in combination with other anticancer agents, so the precise relationship to bendamustine is uncertain.

In a study of bendamustine 90 mg/m^2 in combination with rituximab, one case of toxic epidermal necrolysis (TEN) occurred. TEN has been reported for rituximab. Cases of Stevens-Johnson syndrome and TEN, some fatal, have been reported when bendamustine was coadministered with allopurinol and other medications known to cause these syndromes. The relationship to bendamustine cannot be determined.

When skin reactions occur, they may be progressive and increase in severity with further treatment. Therefore, monitor patients with skin reactions closely. If skin reactions are severe or progressive, withhold or discontinue bendamustine.

➤*Other malignancies:* There are reports of premalignant and malignant diseases that have developed in patients who have been treated with bendamustine, including myelodysplastic syndrome, myeloproliferative disorders, acute myeloid leukemia, and bronchial carcinoma. The association with bendamustine therapy has not been determined.

BENDAMUSTINE HYDROCHLORIDE — INJECTION

➤*Renal function impairment:* No formal studies assessing the impact of renal impairment on the pharmacokinetics of bendamustine have been conducted. See Administration and Dosage for more information.

➤*Hepatic function impairment:* No formal studies assessing the impact of hepatic impairment on the pharmacokinetics of bendamustine have been conducted. See Administration and Dosage for more information.

➤*Pregnancy: Category D.* Bendamustine can cause fetal harm when administered to a pregnant woman. There are no adequate and well-controlled studies in pregnant women. If this drug is used during pregnancy or if the patient becomes pregnant while taking this drug, apprise the patient of the potential hazard to the fetus.

Single intraperitoneal doses of bendamustine 210 mg/m^2 (70 mg/kg) administered in mice during organogenesis caused an increase in resorptions, skeletal and visceral malformations (exencephaly, cleft palates, accessory rib, and spinal deformities), and decreased fetal body weights. This dose did not appear to be maternally toxic, and lower doses were not evaluated. Repeat intraperitoneal dosing in mice on gestation days 7 to 11 resulted in an increase in resorptions from 75 mg/m^2 (25 mg/kg) and an increase in abnormalities from 112.5 mg/m^2 (37.5 mg/kg) similar to those seen after a single intraperitoneal administration. Single intraperitoneal doses of bendamustine from 120 mg/m^2 (20 mg/kg) administered in rats on gestation days 4, 7, 9, 11, or 13 caused embryo and fetal lethality as indicated by increased resorptions and a decrease in live fetuses. A significant increase in external (effect on tail, head, and herniation of external organs [exomphalos]) and internal (hydronephrosis and hydrocephalus) malformations were seen in rats administered bendamustine.

Fertility impairment – Impaired spermatogenesis, azoospermia, and total germinal aplasia have been reported in men treated with alkylating agents, especially in combination with other drugs. In some instances, spermatogenesis may return in patients in remission, but this may occur only several years after intensive chemotherapy has been discontinued. Warn patients of the potential risk to their reproductive capacities.

➤*Lactation:* It is not known whether this drug is excreted in human milk. The molecular weight of the parent compound (about 359 for the free base) and the presence of two active metabolites suggest that excretion into breast milk will occur. Because many drugs are excreted in human milk and because of the potential for serious adverse reactions in breast-feeding infants and tumorigenicity shown for bendamustine in animal studies, decide whether to discontinue breast-feeding or the drug, taking into account the importance of the drug to the mother.

➤*Children:* The safety and effectiveness of bendamustine in children have not been established.

➤*Elderly:* In CLL and NHL studies, there were no clinically significant differences in the adverse reactions profile between elderly (65 years of age and older) and younger patients.

➤*Monitoring:* In the event of treatment-related myelosuppression, monitor leukocytes, platelets, hemoglobin, and neutrophils closely. Monitor hemoglobin and white blood cell differential counts every week initially, and monitor platelet counts each cycle.

Monitor for infusion reactions and anaphylaxis; discontinue drug for severe reactions.

Monitor blood chemistry, particularly potassium and uric acid levels, for the development of tumor lysis syndrome.

Closely monitor patients with skin reactions.

Drug Interactions

➤*Cytochrome P450 enzyme system:* Bendamustine's active metabolites, gamma-hydroxy bendamustine (M3) and N-desmethyl-bendamustine (M4), are formed via CYP1A2. Inhibitors of CYP1A2 have the potential to increase plasma concentrations of bendamustine and decrease plasma concentrations of active metabolites. Inducers of CYP1A2 (eg, smoking) have the potential to decrease plasma concentrations of bendamustine and increase plasma concentrations of its active metabolites. Use caution or consider alternative treatments if concomitant treatment with CYP1A2 inhibitors or inducers is needed.

Bendamustine Drug Interactions

Precipitant drug	Object drug[a]		Description
Ciprofloxacin	Bendamustine	↑↓	Inhibitors of CYP1A2, such as ciprofloxacin, have the potential to increase plasma concentrations of bendamustine and decrease plasma concentrations of its active metabolites. Coadminister with caution.
Fluvoxamine	Bendamustine	↑↓	Inhibitors of CYP1A2, such as fluvoxamine, have the potential to increase plasma concentrations of bendamustine and decrease plasma concentrations of its active metabolites. Coadminister with caution.
Omeprazole	Bendamustine	↑↓	Inducers of CYP1A2, such as omeprazole, have the potential to decrease plasma concentrations of bendamustine and increase plasma concentrations of its active metabolites. Coadminister with caution.
Smoking	Bendamustine	↑↓	Inducers of CYP1A2, such as smoking, have the potential to decrease plasma concentrations of bendamustine and increase plasma concentrations of its active metabolites. Use with caution in patients who start or stop smoking while receiving bendamustine.

[a] ↑↓ = object drug both increased and decreased.

Adverse Reactions

➤*Chronic lymphocytic leukemia:*

Most common adverse reactions – In the randomized CLL clinical study, nonhematologic adverse reactions (any grade) in the bendamustine group that occurred with a frequency of more than 15% were pyrexia (24%), nausea (20%), and vomiting (16%).

Discontinuation – The most frequent adverse reactions leading to study withdrawal for patients receiving bendamustine were hypersensitivity (2%) and pyrexia (1%).

Adverse reactions (5% or more) –

Bendamustine Adverse Reactions in Patients Treated for Chronic Lymphocytic Leukemia (≥ 5%)

Adverse reactions	Bendamustine (n = 153) All grades	Bendamustine (n = 153) Grade 3/4	Chlorambucil (n = 143) All grades	Chlorambucil (n = 143) Grade 3/4
Total number of patients with ≥ 1 adverse reaction	79%	34%	67%	17%
CNS				
Asthenia	8%	0%	4%	0%
Chills	6%	0%	< 1%	0%
Fatigue	9%	1%	6%	0%
Dermatologic				
Pruritus	5%	0%	1%	0%
Rash	8%	3%	5%	2%
GI				
Diarrhea	9%	1%	3%	0%
Nausea	20%	< 1%	15%	< 1%
Vomiting	16%	< 1%	6%	0%
Metabolic/Nutritional				
Hyperuricemia	7%	2%	1%	0%
Weight decreased	7%	0%	3%	0%
Respiratory				
Cough	4%	< 1%	5%	<1%
Nasopharyngitis	7%	0%	8%	0%
Miscellaneous				
Herpes simplex	3%	0%	5%	0%
Hypersensitivity	5%	1%	2%	0%
Infection	6%	2%	< 1%	< 1%
Pyrexia	24%	4%	6%	1%

Other adverse reactions – Other adverse reactions seen frequently in 1 or more studies included asthenia, fatigue, malaise, and weakness; constipation; cough; dry mouth; headache; mucosal inflammation and stomatitis; somnolence.

In the randomized CLL clinical study, worsening hypertension was reported in 4 patients treated with bendamustine and in no patients treated with chlorambucil. Three of these 4 adverse reactions were described as a hypertensive crisis and were managed with oral medications and resolved.

Lab test abnormalities – The grade 3 and 4 hematology laboratory test values confirm the myelosuppressive effects seen in patients treated with bendamustine. Red blood cell transfusions were administered to 20% of patients receiving bendamustine compared with 6% of patients receiving chlorambucil.

BENDAMUSTINE HYDROCHLORIDE — INJECTION

Bendamustine or Chlorambucil Hematology Laboratory Abnormalities in Patients Treated for Chronic Lymphocytic Leukemia

	Bendamustine (n = 150)		Chlorambucil (n = 141)	
Laboratory abnormality	All grades	Grade 3/4	All grades	Grade 3/4
Hemoglobin decreased	89%	13%	82%	9%
Leukocytes decreased	61%	28%	18%	3%
Lymphocytes decreased	68%	47%	19%	4%
Neutrophils decreased	75%	43%	61%	21%
Platelets decreased	77%	11%	78%	10%

In the randomized CLL clinical study, 34% of patients had bilirubin elevations, some without associated significant elevations in AST and ALT. Grade 3 or 4 increased bilirubin occurred in 3% of patients. Increases in AST and ALT of grade 3 or 4 were limited to 1% and 3% of patients, respectively. Patients treated with bendamustine may also have changes in creatinine levels. If abnormalities are detected, continue monitoring these parameters to ensure that significant deterioration does not occur.

➤*Non-Hodgkin lymphoma:*

Most common adverse reactions – The most common nonhematologic adverse reactions (at least 30%) were nausea (75%), fatigue (57%), vomiting (40%), diarrhea (37%), and pyrexia (34%). The most common nonhematologic grade 3 or 4 adverse reactions (at least 5%) were fatigue (11%), febrile neutropenia (6%), and pneumonia, hypokalemia, and dehydration, each reported in 5% of patients.

Serious adverse reactions – In both studies, serious adverse reactions, regardless of causality, were reported in 37% of patients receiving bendamustine. The most common serious adverse reactions occurring in at least 5% of patients were febrile neutropenia and pneumonia. Other important serious adverse reactions reported in clinical trials and/or postmarketing experience were acute renal failure, cardiac failure, hypersensitivity, myelodysplastic syndrome, pulmonary fibrosis, and skin reactions.

Serious drug-related adverse reactions reported in clinical trials included infections, infusion reactions, myelosuppression, pneumonia, and tumor lysis syndrome. Adverse reactions occurring less frequently but possibly related to bendamustine treatment were atypical pneumonia, dermatitis, dysgeusia/taste disorder, erythema, hemolysis, herpes zoster, sepsis, and skin necrosis.

Adverse reactions (5% or more) –

Bendamustine Nonhematologic Adverse Reactions in Patients Treated for Non-Hodgkin Lymphoma (≥ 5%)[a]

Adverse reactions	All grades	Grade 3/4
Total number of patients with ≥ 1 adverse reaction	100%	53%
Cardiovascular		
Hypotension	6%	1%
Tachycardia	7%	0%
CNS		
Anxiety	8%	< 1%
Asthenia	11%	2%
Chills	14%	0%
Depression	6%	0%
Dizziness	14%	0%
Dysgeusia	7%	0%
Fatigue	57%	11%
Headache	21%	0%
Insomnia	13%	0%
Dermatologic		
Dry skin	5%	0%
Hyperhidrosis	5%	0%
Night sweats	5%	0%
Pruritus	6%	0%
Rash	16%	< 1%
GI		
Abdominal distension	5%	0%
Abdominal pain	13%	1%
Abdominal pain, upper	5%	0%
Constipation	29%	< 1%
Diarrhea	37%	3%
Dry mouth	9%	< 1%
Dyspepsia	11%	0%
Gastroesophageal reflux disease	10%	0%
Nausea	75%	4%
Oral candidiasis	6%	1%
Stomatitis	15%	< 1%
Vomiting	40%	3%
Local		
Catheter-site pain	5%	0%
Infusion-site pain	6%	0%
Metabolic/Nutritional		
Anorexia	23%	2%
Decreased appetite	13%	< 1%
Dehydration	14%	5%
Edema peripheral	13%	< 1%
Hypokalemia	9%	5%
Weight decreased	18%	2%
Musculoskeletal		
Arthralgia	6%	0%
Back pain	14%	3%
Bone pain	5%	0%
Pain in extremity	5%	1%
Respiratory		
Cough	22%	< 1%
Dyspnea	16%	2%
Nasal congestion	5%	0%
Nasopharyngitis	6%	0%
Pharyngolaryngeal pain	8%	< 1%
Pneumonia	8%	5%
Sinusitis	9%	0%
Upper respiratory tract infection	10%	0%
Wheezing	5%	0%
Miscellaneous		
Chest pain	6%	< 1%
Febrile neutropenia	6%	6%
Herpes zoster	10%	3%
Pain	6%	0%
Pyrexia	34%	2%
Urinary tract infection	10%	2%

[a] Patients may have reported more than 1 adverse reaction. Patients counted only once in each preferred term category and once in each system organ class category.

Lab test abnormalities – Clinically important chemistry laboratory values that were new or worsened from baseline and occurred in more than 1% of patients at grade 3 or 4 in NHL patients treated in both single-arm studies combined were hyperglycemia (3%), elevated creatinine (2%), hypocalcemia (2%), and hyponatremia (2%).

Bendamustine Hematology Laboratory Abnormalities in Patients Treated for Non-Hodgkin Lymphoma

Laboratory abnormality	All grades	Grade 3/4
Hemoglobin decreased	88%	11%
Leukocytes decreased	94%	56%
Lymphocytes decreased	99%	94%
Neutrophils decreased	86%	60%
Platelets decreased	86%	25%

➤*Postmarketing:* The following adverse reactions have been identified during postapproval use of bendamustine. Because these reactions are reported voluntarily from a population of uncertain size, it is not always possible to reliably estimate their frequency or establish a causal relationship to drug exposure: anaphylaxis and injection- or infusion-site reactions, including pruritus, irritation, pain, and swelling.

Skin reactions, including Stephens-Johnson syndrome and TEN, have occurred when bendamustine was coadministered with allopurinol and other medications known to cause these syndromes.

Overdosage

➤*Symptoms:* Across all clinical experience, the reported maximum single dose received was 280 mg/m². Of 4 patients treated at this dose, 3 showed electrocardiogram (ECG) changes considered dose-limiting at 7 and 21 days after dosing. These changes included QT prolongation (1 patient), sinus tachycardia (1 patient), ST-segment and T-wave deviations (2 patients), and

Ethylenimines/Methylmelamines

BENDAMUSTINE HYDROCHLORIDE — INJECTION

left anterior fascicular block (1 patient). Cardiac enzymes and ejection fractions remained normal in all patients.

➤*Treatment:* No specific antidote for bendamustine overdose is known. Management of overdosage should include general supportive measures, including monitoring of hematologic parameters and ECGs.

Patient Information

Inform patients of the possibility of mild or serious allergic reactions, and advise them to immediately report rash, facial swelling, or difficulty breathing during or soon after infusion.

Inform patients of the likelihood that bendamustine will cause a decrease in white blood cells, platelets, and red blood cells. They will need frequent monitoring of these parameters. Instruct them to report shortness of breath, significant fatigue, bleeding, fever, or other signs of infection.

Advise patients with myelosuppression following bendamustine treatment to contact a health care provider if they have symptoms or signs of infection.

Bendamustine can cause fetal harm. Advise women to avoid becoming pregnant throughout treatment and for 3 months after bendamustine therapy has stopped. Advise men receiving bendamustine to use reliable contraception for the same time period. Advise patients to immediately report pregnancy. Advise patients to avoid breast-feeding while receiving bendamustine.

Advise patients that bendamustine may cause tiredness and to avoid driving any vehicle or operating any dangerous tools or machinery if they experience this adverse reaction.

Advise patients that bendamustine may cause nausea and/or vomiting. Instruct patients to report nausea and vomiting so that symptomatic treatment may be provided.

Advise patients that bendamustine may cause diarrhea. Instruct them to report diarrhea to their health care provider so that symptomatic treatment may be provided.

Advise patients that a mild rash or itching may occur during treatment with bendamustine. Advise patients to immediately report a severe or worsening rash or itching.

ANTIMETABOLITES

Folic Acid Antagonists

METHOTREXATE (Amethopterin; MTX)

Rx	**Methotrexate** (Various, eg, Major, Roxane, UDL)	**Tablets**: 2.5 mg	In 36s, 100s, and UD 20s.
Rx	**Rheumatrex Dose Pack** (STADA)		(LLM1). Yellow, scored. In 5, 7.5, 10, 12.5, and 15 mg/week dose packs.
Rx	**Trexall** (Barr)	**Tablets**: 5 mg	Lactose. (b 927 5). Green, oval, scored. Film-coated. In 30s, 60s, and 100s.
		7.5	Lactose (b 928 7½). Blue, oval, scored. Film-coated. In 30s, 60s, and 100s.
		10 mg	Lactose. (b 929 10). Pink, oval, scored. Film-coated. In 30s, 60s, and 100s.
		15 mg	Lactose. (b 945 15). Purple, oval, scored. Film-coated. In 30s, 60s, and 100s.
Rx	**Methotrexate Sodium** (Various, eg, American Pharmaceutical Partners[a], Bedford Labs)	**Injection**: 25 mg/mL (as base)	Preservative free. In 2, 4, 8, 10, 20, and 40 mL single-use vials.
Rx	**Methotrexate Sodium** (Various, eg, American Pharmaceutical Partners, Xanodyne)		In 2 and 10 mL vials.[b]
Rx	**Methotrexate LPF Sodium** (Xanodyne)		Preservative free. In 2, 4, and 10 mL single-use vials.[c]
Rx	**Methotrexate Sodium** (Various, eg, American Pharmaceutical Partners, Xanodyne)	**Powder for injection, lyophilized**: 1 g (as base)	Preservative free. In single-use vials.[d]

[a] The 2, 4, 8, 10, 20, and 40 mL solutions contain approximately 0.43, 0.86, 1.72, 2.15, 4.3, and 8.6 mEq sodium per vial, respectively.
[b] Contains 0.9% benzyl alcohol as a preservative; must not be used for intrathecal or high dose therapy.
[c] The 2, 4, and 10 mL vials contain approximately 0.43, 0.86, and 2.15 mEq sodium per vial, respectively.
[d] Approximately 0.14 mEq sodium in the 20 mg vial; 7 mEq sodium in the 1 g vial.

METHOTREXATE — ORAL

WARNING

The high-dose regimens recommended for osteosarcoma require meticulous care.

Deaths – Use methotrexate only in life-threatening neoplastic diseases, or in patients with psoriasis or rheumatoid arthritis (RA) with severe, recalcitrant, disabling disease that is not adequately responsive to other forms of therapy. Deaths have occurred with the use of methotrexate in malignancy, psoriasis, and RA. Closely monitor patients for bone marrow, liver, lung, and kidney toxicities.

Bone marrow depression: Marked bone marrow depression may occur with resultant anemia, leukopenia, or thrombocytopenia.

Unexpectedly severe (sometimes fatal) bone marrow suppression, aplastic anemia, and GI toxicity have occurred with coadministration of methotrexate (usually in high dosage) along with some NSAIDs (see Drug Interactions).

Monitoring – Periodic monitoring for toxicity, including CBC with differential and platelet counts, and liver and renal function testing is mandatory. Periodic liver biopsies may be indicated in some situations. Monitor patients at increased risk for impaired methotrexate elimination (eg, renal dysfunction, pleural effusions, ascites) more frequently.

WARNING (cont.)

Liver – Methotrexate causes hepatotoxicity, fibrosis, and cirrhosis, but generally only after prolonged use. Acutely, liver enzyme elevations are frequent, usually transient and asymptomatic, and also do not appear predictive of subsequent hepatic disease. Liver biopsy after sustained use often shows histologic changes, and fibrosis and cirrhosis have occurred; these latter lesions often are not preceded by symptoms or abnormal liver function tests. For this reason, periodic liver biopsies are usually recommended for psoriatic patients who are under long-term treatment. Persistent abnormalities in liver function tests may precede appearance of fibrosis or cirrhosis in the RA population.

Methotrexate-induced lung disease – Methotrexate-induced lung disease is a potentially dangerous lesion that may occur acutely at any time during therapy and has occurred at doses as low as 7.5 mg/week. It is not always fully reversible. Pulmonary symptoms (especially a dry, nonproductive cough) may require interruption of treatment and careful investigation.

Pregnancy – Fetal death and/or congenital anomalies have occurred; do not use in women of childbearing potential unless benefits outweigh possible risks. Pregnant women with psoriasis or RA should not receive methotrexate (see Contraindications).

Renal use – Use methotrexate in patients with impaired renal function with extreme caution, and at reduced dosages, because renal dysfunction will prolong elimination.

GI – Diarrhea and ulcerative stomatitis require interruption of therapy; hemorrhagic enteritis and death from intestinal perforation may occur.

Diluents – Do not use methotrexate formulations and diluents containing preservatives for intrathecal or experimental high dose MTX therapy.

METHOTREXATE — ORAL

WARNING (cont.)

Malignant lymphomas – Malignant lymphomas, which may regress following withdrawal of methotrexate, may occur in patients receiving low-dose methotrexate and, thus, may not require cytotoxic treatment. Discontinue methotrexate first and, if the lymphoma does not regress, appropriate treatment should be instituted.

Tumor lysis syndrome – Like other cytotoxic drugs, methotrexate may induce tumor lysis syndrome in patients with rapidly growing tumors.

Skin reactions – Severe, occasionally fatal skin reactions have been reported following single or multiple doses of methotrexate. Reactions have occurred within days of methotrexate administration. Recovery has been reported with discontinuation of therapy.

Potentially fatal opportunistic infections – Potentially fatal opportunistic infections, especially *Pneumocystis carinii* pneumonia, may occur with methotrexate therapy.

Radiotherapy – Methotrexate given concomitantly with radiotherapy may increase the risk of soft tissue necrosis and osteonecrosis.

Severe reactions – Because of the possibility of severe toxic reactions (which can be fatal), fully inform patients of the risks involved and assure constant supervision.

Indications

➤*Antineoplastic chemotherapy:* Treatment of gestational choriocarcinoma, chorioadenoma destruens, and hydatidiform mole.

Methotrexate alone or in combination with other anticancer agents for treatment of breast cancer, epidermoid cancers of the head and neck, advanced mycosis fungoides (cutaneous T-cell lymphoma) and lung cancer, particularly squamous cell and small cell types; in combination therapy in the treatment of advanced-stage non-Hodgkin lymphomas.

Methotrexate in high doses followed by leucovorin rescue in combination with other chemotherapeutic agents is effective in prolonging relapse-free survival in patients with nonmetastatic osteosarcoma who have undergone surgical resection or amputation for the primary tumor.

➤*Psoriasis:* Symptomatic control of severe, recalcitrant, disabling psoriasis that is not adequately responsive to other forms of therapy but only when the diagnosis has been established, as by biopsy and/or after dermatologic consultation. It is important to ensure that a psoriasis "flare" is not due to an undiagnosed concomitant disease affecting immune responses.

➤*RA:* Management of selected adults with severe, active RA (ACR criteria), or children with active polyarticular-course juvenile rheumatoid arthritis (JRA) who have had an insufficient therapeutic response to, or are intolerant of, an adequate trial of first-line therapy including full dose NSAIDs.

➤*Off-label uses:*

Multiple sclerosis – [4] = Insufficient documentation. Data evaluating efficacy of oral methotrexate monotherapy for the treatment of multiple sclerosis (MS) are limited. Methotrexate monotherapy has demonstrated modest efficacy. Methotrexate in combination with interferon beta-1a also showed only modest efficacy. While low-dose oral methotrexate appears to be safe, it may not offer sufficient benefits in efficacy to warrant therapy. Clinical practice guidelines for the use of disease-modifying therapies in MS state that methotrexate may favorably alter the disease course in patients with progressive MS (level C recommendation). Until additional data from larger, controlled trials are available, routine use of oral methotrexate for MS is not recommended.

Psoriasis (children/adolescents) – [3] = Safety concerns. American Academy of Dermatology guidelines state that although only a few reports describe the use of methotrexate for pediatric psoriasis, experience had been reported using methotrexate in children with several different dermatologic and rheumatologic conditions. It was concluded that low-dose weekly methotrexate was generally well tolerated and effective in children.

Other possible off-label uses – Used as maintenance regimen for Wegener granulomatosis; dermatomyositis; myositis; ulcerative colitis; refractory Crohn disease; uveitis; systemic lupus erythematosus; psoriatic arthritis.

In a study of 10 children (mean age 6.8 years) with localized scleroderma, methotrexate with early high doses of corticosteroids was shown to be both effective and well tolerated.

Administration and Dosage

➤*General dosing considerations:* Oral administration is often preferred when low doses are being administered.

Acute lymphatic (lymphoblastic) leukemia in children and young adolescents is most responsive. In young adults and older patients, clinical remission is more difficult to obtain, and early relapse is more common.

➤*Adults:*

Choriocarcinoma and similar trophoblastic diseases –

Usual dosage: 15 to 30 mg daily for a 5-day course. Repeat courses 3 to 5 times, as required, with rest periods of 1 or more weeks between courses, until any toxic symptoms subside. Evaluate the effectiveness of therapy by 24-hour quantitative analysis of urinary chorionic gonadotropin hormone (hCG), which should return to normal or less than 50 units per 24 hours, usually after the third or fourth course and is usually followed by a complete resolution of measurable lesions in 4 to 6 weeks. One to 2 courses of methotrexate after normalization of hCG is usually recommended. Careful clinical assessment is essential before each course. Cyclic combination therapy with other antitumor drugs may be useful.

Because hydatidiform mole may precede choriocarcinoma, prophylaxis chemotherapy with methotrexate has been recommended. Chorioadenoma destruens is an invasive form of hydatidiform mole. Administer methotrexate in doses similar to those for choriocarcinoma.

Leukemia –

Usual dosage: When used for induction, methotrexate in doses of 3.3 mg/m^2, in combination with prednisone 60 mg/m^2 given daily, produced remission in 50% of patients, usually within 4 to 6 weeks. Corticosteroid therapy, in combination with other antileukemic drugs or in cyclic combinations with methotrexate included, has appeared to produce rapid and effective remissions. Methotrexate in combination with other agents is the drug of choice for maintenance of remissions. When remission is achieved and supportive care has produced general clinical improvement, initiate maintenance therapy.

Maintenance dosage: Give methotrexate 2 times weekly in total weekly doses of 30 mg/m^2. If relapse occurs, repeat initial induction regimen.

Lymphomas (Burkitt tumor, stages I and II) – 10 to 25 mg/day for 4 to 8 days. In stage III, give methotrexate concomitantly with other antitumor agents. Treatment in all stages generally consists of several courses with 7 to 10 day rest periods. Lymphosarcomas in stage III may respond to combined drug therapy with methotrexate given in doses of 0.625 to 2.5 mg/kg/day.

Mycosis fungoides (cutaneous T-cell lymphoma) –

Usual dosage: 5 to 50 mg once weekly in early stages.

Dosage adjustment: Dose reduction or cessation is guided by patient response and hematologic monitoring. Methotrexate therapy produces clinical responses in 50% of cases.

Alternative dosage: Methotrexate has also been administered twice weekly in doses ranging from 15 to 37.5 mg in patients who have responded poorly to weekly therapy.

Concomitant therapy: Combination chemotherapy regimens that include IV methotrexate administered at higher doses with leucovorin rescue have been utilized in advanced stages of the disease.

Psoriasis –

Usual dosage: 10 to 25 mg once weekly until adequate response is achieved.

Maximum dose: 30 mg/week.

Dosage adjustment: Dosages may be gradually adjusted to achieve optimal clinical response. Once this occurs, reduce dosage to the lowest possible amount of drug and to the longest possible rest period. The use of methotrexate may permit the return to conventional topical therapy, which should be encouraged.

Alternative dosage: Divided oral doses of 2.5 mg at 12-hour intervals for 3 doses.

Rheumatoid arthritis –

Usual dosage: Weekly therapy may be instituted to provide doses over a range of 5 to 15 mg administered as a single weekly dose. All schedules should be continually tailored to the individual patient. An initial test dose may be given prior to the regular dosing schedule to detect any extreme sensitivity to adverse reactions. Maximal myelosuppression usually occurs in 7 to 10 days.

Maximum dose: 20 mg/week.

Initial dosage: 7.5 mg once weekly; or as divided doses of 2.5 mg at 12-hour intervals for 3 doses given as a course once weekly.

Dosage adjustment: Dosages may be adjusted gradually to achieve an optimal response. Limited experience shows a significant increase in the incidence and severity of serious toxic reactions, especially bone marrow suppression, at doses greater than 20 mg/week in adults.

Duration of therapy: Therapeutic response usually begins within 3 to 6 weeks, and the patient may continue to improve for another 12 weeks or more. The optimal duration of therapy is unknown. Limited data available from long-term studies in adults indicate that the initial clinical improvement is maintained for at least 2 years with continued therapy. When methotrexate is discontinued, the arthritis usually worsens within 3 to 6 weeks.

Off-label dosing –

Multiple sclerosis: [4] = Insufficient documentation. In published reports, oral methotrexate 7.5 or 20 mg was given once weekly, either alone or as add-on therapy to interferon beta-1a.

➤*Children:* Safety and efficacy in children have not been established, other than in cancer chemotherapy and in polyarticular-course JRA.

Leukemia – See Adults for dosing.

Polyarticular-course juvenile rheumatoid arthritis –

Usual dosage: The recommended starting dose is 10 mg/m^2 given once weekly. Dosages may be adjusted gradually to achieve an optimal response. Although there is experience with doses up to 30 mg/m^2/week in children, there are too few published data to assess how doses over 20 mg/m^2/week might affect the risk of serious toxicity in children. Experience does suggest, however, that children receiving 20 to 30 mg/m^2/week (0.65 to 1 mg/kg/week) may have better absorption and fewer GI adverse reactions if methotrexate is administered IM or subcutaneously.

Duration of therapy: Therapeutic response usually begins within 3 to 6 weeks, and the patient may continue to improve for another 12 weeks or more. The optimal duration of therapy is unknown. Limited data available from long-term studies in adults indicate that the initial clinical improvement is maintained for at least 2 years with continued therapy. When methotrexate is discontinued, the arthritis usually worsens within 3 to 6 weeks.

Off-label dosing –

Localized scleroderma: The dosage regimen used in a small study was methotrexate 0.3 to 0.6 mg/kg/week (mean duration of 22.3 months). Of 10

METHOTREXATE — ORAL

children, 9 were also treated with methylprednisone 30 mg/kg IV for 3 days each month for 3 months at the initiation of therapy.

Psoriasis (children/adolescents): [3] = Safety concerns. 0.2 to 0.4 mg/kg/wk (3.75 to 25 mg/wk) orally. Methotrexate has been studied at this dose in children for up to 46 weeks.

➤*Elderly:* Because of diminished hepatic and renal function and decreased folate stores in this population, consider relatively low doses. Closely monitor for early signs of toxicity.

➤*Renal function impairment:* Use methotrexate in patients with impaired renal function with extreme caution, and at reduced dosages, because renal dysfunction will prolong elimination.

➤*Preparation for administration:* Methotrexate is considered a cytotoxic agent. Follow safe handling procedures when preparing, administering, or dispensing methotrexate.

➤*Storage/Stability:* Store at 20° to 25°C (68° to 77°F); excursions permitted from 15° to 30°C (59° to 86°F). Protect from light.

Actions

➤*Pharmacology:* Methotrexate competitively inhibits dihydrofolic acid reductase. Dihydrofolates must be reduced to tetrahydrofolates by this enzyme before they can be utilized as carriers of one-carbon groups in the synthesis of purine nucleotides and thymidylate. Therefore, methotrexate interferes with DNA synthesis, repair, and cellular replication.

Actively proliferating tissues such as malignant cells, bone marrow, fetal cells, buccal and intestinal mucosa, and cells of the urinary bladder are generally more sensitive to this effect of methotrexate. Cellular proliferation in malignant tissue is greater than in most normal tissue; thus, methotrexate may impair malignant growth without irreversibly damaging normal tissues.

The original rationale for high-dose methotrexate therapy was based on the concept of selective rescue of normal tissues by leucovorin. More recent evidence suggests that high-dose methotrexate may also overcome methotrexate resistance caused by impaired active transport, decreased affinity of dihydrofolic acid reductase for methotrexate, increased levels of dihydrofolic acid reductase resulting from gene amplification, or decreased polyglutamation of methotrexate. The actual mechanism of action is unknown.

➤*Pharmacokinetics:*

Absorption/Distribution – In adults, oral absorption appears to be dose-dependent. After oral doses of 30 mg/m^2 or less, methotrexate is generally well absorbed with a mean bioavailability of about 60%. The absorption of doses greater than 80 mg/m^2 is significantly less, possibly due to a saturation effect. Peak serum levels are usually reached in 1 to 2 hours. In leukemic children, oral absorption reportedly varies widely (23% to 95%). A 20-fold difference between highest and lowest peak levels was reported. Significant interindividual variability was also noted in time to peak concentration and fraction of dose absorbed. Food delayed absorption and reduced peak concentration.

Following oral administration of methotrexate in doses of 6.4 to 11.2 mg/m^2/week in pediatric patients with JRA, mean serum concentrations were approximately 0.59 micromolar at 1 hour, 0.44 micromolar at 2 hours, and 0.29 micromolar at 3 hours. Methotrexate competes with reduced folates for active transport across cell membranes by means of a single carrier-mediated active transport process. At serum concentrations greater than 100 micromolar, passive diffusion becomes a major pathway by which effective intracellular concentrations can be achieved. Approximately 50% of the absorbed drug is bound to serum protein. Methotrexate does not penetrate the blood-cerebrospinal fluid barrier in therapeutic amounts. High CSF drug concentrations may be attained by direct intrathecal administration.

Metabolism/Excretion – After absorption, methotrexate undergoes hepatic and intracellular metabolism to polyglutamated forms which can be converted back to methotrexate by hydrolase enzymes. These polyglutamates act as inhibitors of dihydrofolate reductase and thymidylate synthetase. Small amounts of methotrexate polyglutamates may remain in tissues for extended periods. The retention and prolonged drug action of these active metabolite(s) vary among different cells, tissues, and tumors. A small amount of metabolism to 7-hydroxymethotrexate may occur at doses commonly prescribed. Accumulation of this metabolite may become significant at the high doses used in osteogenic sarcoma. The aqueous solubility of 7-hydroxymethotrexate is threefold to fivefold lower than the parent compound. Methotrexate is partially metabolized by intestinal flora after oral administration.

The terminal half-life is approximately 3 to 10 hours for patients receiving treatment for psoriasis, RA, or low-dose antineoplastic therapy (less than 30 mg/m^2). For patients on high doses, the terminal half-life is 8 to 15 hours. In pediatric patients receiving methotrexate for acute lymphocytic leukemia (6.3 to 30 mg/m^2), or for JRA (3.75 to 26.2 mg/m^2), the terminal half-life has been reported to range from 0.7 to 5.8 hours or 0.9 to 2.3 hours, respectively.

Renal excretion is the primary route of elimination and is dependent upon dosage and route of administration. With IV administration, 80% to 90% of the administered dose is excreted unchanged in the urine within 24 hours. There is limited biliary excretion of 10% or less. Enterohepatic recirculation of methotrexate has been proposed. Renal excretion occurs by glomerular filtration and active tubular secretion. Impaired renal function, as well as concurrent use of drugs such as weak organic acids that also undergo tubular secretion, can markedly increase serum levels. Excellent correlation has been reported between methotrexate clearance and endogenous creatinine clearance.

Clearance rates vary widely and are generally decreased at higher doses. Delayed drug clearance is one of the major factors responsible for toxicity because the toxicity for normal tissues appears more dependent upon the duration of exposure to the drug than the peak level achieved. When a patient has delayed drug elimination due to compromised renal function or other causes, methotrexate serum concentrations may remain elevated for prolonged periods.

The potential for toxicity from high-dose regimens or delayed excretion is reduced by leucovorin calcium during the final phase of methotrexate plasma elimination. Guidelines for monitoring serum methotrexate levels, and for adjustment of leucovorin dosing to reduce the risk of toxicity, are provided in Administration and Dosage.

Contraindications

Hypersensitivity to the drug.

Patients with psoriasis or RA with alcoholism, alcoholic liver disease, or other chronic liver disease should not receive methotrexate. Patients with psoriasis or RA who have overt or laboratory evidence of immunodeficiency syndromes should not receive methotrexate.

Patients with psoriasis or RA who have pre-existing blood dyscrasias (eg, bone marrow hypoplasia, leukopenia, thrombocytopenia, significant anemia) should not receive methotrexate.

➤*Pregnancy:* Methotrexate can cause fetal death or teratogenic effects when administered to a pregnant woman. Methotrexate is contraindicated in pregnant women with psoriasis or RA and should be used in the treatment of neoplastic diseases only when the potential benefit outweighs the risk to the fetus. Women of childbearing potential should not be started on methotrexate until pregnancy is excluded and should be fully counseled on the serious risk to the fetus should they become pregnant while undergoing treatment. Pregnancy should be avoided if either partner is receiving methotrexate; during and for a minimum of 3 months after therapy for male patients, and during and for at least 1 ovulatory cycle after therapy for female patients.

Lactation – Because of the potential for serious adverse reactions from methotrexate in breastfed infants, it is contraindicated in nursing mothers.

Warnings/Precautions

➤*Toxic effects:* Toxic effects, potentially serious, may be related in frequency and severity to dose or frequency of administration, but have been seen at all doses. These effects can occur at any time during therapy; follow patients closely. Most adverse reactions are reversible if detected early. When reactions occur, reduce dosage or discontinue drug and take appropriate corrective measures; this could include use of leucovorin calcium. Use caution if therapy is reinstituted. Consider further need for the drug and possibility of recurrence of toxicity.

➤*Organ system toxicity:*

GI – If vomiting, diarrhea, or stomatitis occur, which may result in dehydration, discontinue methotrexate until recovery occurs. Use with extreme caution in the presence of peptic ulcer disease or ulcerative colitis.

Hematologic – Methotrexate can suppress hematopoiesis and cause anemia, aplastic anemia, pancytopenia, leukopenia, neutropenia and/or thrombocytopenia. Use with caution, if at all, in patients with malignancy and preexisting hematopoietic impairment. In controlled clinical trials in RA (n = 128), leukopenia (WBC less than 3000/mm^3) was seen in 2 patients, thrombocytopenia (platelets less than 100,000/mm^3) in 6 patients, and pancytopenia in 2 patients.

In psoriasis and RA, methotrexate should be stopped immediately if there is a significant drop in blood counts. In the treatment of neoplastic diseases, continue methotrexate only if potential benefit warrants risk of severe myelosuppression. Evaluate those with profound granulocytopenia and fever immediately; they usually require parenteral broad-spectrum antibiotics.

Hepatic – See the Warning box for more information.
Psoriasis: See the Warning box for more information.
RA: See the Warning box for more information.

Infection or immunologic states – Use with extreme caution in the presence of active infection; usually contraindicated in patients with overt or laboratory evidence of immunodeficiency syndromes. Hypogammaglobulinemia occurs rarely.

See the Warning box for more information.

Neurologic – There have been reports of leukoencephalopathy following IV administration of methotrexate to patients who have had craniospinal irradiation. Serious neurotoxicity, frequently manifested as generalized or focal seizures, has been reported with unexpectedly increased frequency among pediatric patients with acute lymphoblastic leukemia who were treated with intermediate-dose IV methotrexate (1 g/m^2). Symptomatic patients were commonly noted to have leukoencephalopathy and/or microangiopathic calcifications on diagnostic imaging studies. Chronic leukoencephalopathy has also occurred in patients who received repeated doses of high-dose methotrexate with leucovorin rescue even without cranial irradiation. Discontinuation of methotrexate does not always result in complete recovery.

A transient acute neurologic syndrome has been observed in patients treated with high dosage regimens. Manifestations of this stroke-like encephalopathy may include confusion, hemiparesis, transient blindness, seizures, and coma. The exact cause is unknown.

Pulmonary – Pulmonary symptoms (especially a dry, nonproductive cough) or a nonspecific pneumonitis occurring during therapy indicate a potentially dangerous lesion and require interruption of treatment and care-

METHOTREXATE — ORAL

ful investigation. The typical patient presents with fever, cough, dyspnea, hypoxemia, and an infiltrate on chest x-ray; infection (including pneumonia) needs to be excluded. This lesion can occur at all dosages.

Renal – Methotrexate may cause renal damage that may lead to acute renal failure. High doses used in the treatment of osteosarcoma may cause renal damage leading to acute renal failure. Nephrotoxicity is due primarily to the precipitation of methotrexate and 7-hydroxymethotrexate in the renal tubules. Close attention to renal function including adequate hydration, urine alkalinization and measurement of serum methotrexate and creatinine levels are essential for safe administration.

Skin – See the Warning box for more information.

➤*Vaccines:* Immunization may be ineffective when given during methotrexate therapy. Immunization with live virus vaccines is generally not recommended. Disseminated vaccinia infections after smallpox immunization have occurred in patients receiving methotrexate.

➤*Debility:* Use with extreme caution in the presence of debility.

➤*Pleural effusions or ascites:* Methotrexate exits slowly from third space compartments (eg, pleural effusions or ascites). This results in a prolonged terminal plasma half-life and unexpected toxicity. In patients with significant third space accumulations, evacuate the fluid before treatment and monitor plasma methotrexate levels.

➤*Psoriasis lesions:* Lesions of psoriasis may be aggravated by concomitant exposure to ultraviolet radiation. Radiation dermatitis and sunburn may be "recalled" by the use of methotrexate.

➤*Folate deficiency:* Folate deficiency states may increase methotrexate toxicity.

➤*Renal function impairment:* Methotrexate is excreted principally by the kidneys. Its use in impaired renal function may result in accumulation of toxic amounts or additional renal damage. Determine the patient's renal status prior to and during therapy. Exercise caution should significant renal impairment occur. Reduce or discontinue drug dosage until renal function improves or is restored. The potential for toxicity from high dose regimens or delayed excretion is reduced by the administration of leucovorin calcium during the final phase of methotrexate plasma elimination.

➤*Pregnancy: Category X.* See Contraindications for more information.

Fertility impairment – Impairment of fertility, oligospermia, and menstrual dysfunction in humans has been reported during and for a short period after cessation of therapy.

➤*Lactation:* See Contraindications for more information.

➤*Children:* Safety and efficacy in children have not been established, other than in cancer chemotherapy and in polyarticular-course JRA.

➤*Elderly:* Clinical pharmacology has not been well studied in these patients. Due to diminished hepatic and renal function and decreased folate stores in this population, consider relatively low doses. Closely monitor for early signs of toxicity.

Since decline in renal function may be associated with increases in adverse events and serum creatinine measurements may overestimate renal function in the elderly, more accurate methods (ie, creatinine clearance) should be considered. Elderly patients should be closely monitored for early signs of hepatic, bone marrow, and renal toxicity. Postmarketing experience suggests that the occurrence of bone marrow suppression, thrombocytopenia, and pneumonitis may increase with age.

➤*Monitoring:* Baseline assessment should include complete blood count with differential and platelet counts; hepatic enzymes; renal function tests; and chest x-ray. During therapy of RA and psoriasis, monitoring of these parameters is recommended: Hematology at least monthly, renal function and liver function every 1 to 2 months. More frequent monitoring is usually indicated during antineoplastic therapy. During initial or changing doses, or during periods of increased risk of elevated methotrexate blood levels (eg, dehydration), more frequent monitoring may be indicated. Pulmonary function tests may be useful if methotrexate-induced lung disease is suspected, especially if baseline measurements are available. Appropriate steps should be taken to avoid conception during methotrexate therapy.

Hepatic – A relationship between abnormal liver function tests and fibrosis or cirrhosis of the liver has not been established. Transient liver function test abnormalities are observed frequently after methotrexate administration and are usually not cause for modification of methotrexate therapy. Persistent liver function test abnormalities or depression of serum albumin may indicate serious liver toxicity; they require evaluation.

RA: Liver function tests should be performed at baseline and at 4 to 8 week intervals in patients receiving methotrexate for RA. Pretreatment liver biopsy should be performed for patients with a history of excessive alcohol consumption, persistently abnormal baseline liver function test values, or chronic hepatitis B or C infection. During therapy, liver biopsy should be performed if there are persistent liver function test abnormalities or there is a decrease in serum albumin below the normal range (in the setting of well-controlled RA).

Drug Interactions

➤*NSAIDS / Salicylates:* Nonsteroidal anti-inflammatory drugs (NSAIDs) should not be administered prior to or concomitantly with the high doses of methotrexate used in the treatment of osteosarcoma. Concomitant administration of some NSAIDs with high-dose methotrexate therapy has been reported to elevate and prolong serum methotrexate levels, resulting in deaths from severe hematologic and GI toxicity.

Caution should be used when NSAIDs and salicylates are administered concomitantly with lower doses of methotrexate. These drugs have been reported to reduce the tubular secretion of methotrexate in an animal model and may enhance its toxicity.

➤*Salicylates, phenylbutazone, phenytoin, sulfonamides, probenecid:* Methotrexate is partially bound to serum albumin, and toxicity may be increased because of displacement by certain drugs, such as salicylates, phenylbutazone, phenytoin, and sulfonamides. Renal tubular transport is also diminished by probenecid; use of methotrexate with this drug should be carefully monitored.

➤*Cisplatin:* In the treatment of patients with osteosarcoma, caution must be exercised if high-dose methotrexate is administered in combination with a potentially nephrotoxic chemotherapeutic agent (eg, cisplatin).

➤*Mercaptopurine:* Methotrexate increases the plasma levels of mercaptopurine. The combination of methotrexate and mercaptopurine may therefore require dose adjustment.

➤*Oral antibiotics:* Oral antibiotics such as tetracycline, chloramphenicol, and nonabsorbable broad-spectrum antibiotics, may decrease intestinal absorption of methotrexate or interfere with the enterohepatic circulation by inhibiting bowel flora and suppressing metabolism of the drug by bacteria.

➤*Hepatotoxic agents:* The potential for increased hepatotoxicity when methotrexate is administered with other hepatotoxic agents has not been evaluated. However, hepatotoxicity has been reported in such cases. Therefore, patients receiving concomitant therapy with methotrexate and other potential hepatotoxins (eg, azathioprine, retinoids, sulfasalazine) should be monitored closely for possible increased risk of hepatotoxicity.

Methotrexate Oral Drug Interactions

Precipitant drug	Object drug[a]		Description
Aminoglycosides, oral	Methotrexate	⬇	The antitumorigenic actions of methotrexate may be decreased, but not predictably. Consider parenteral methotrexate if oral aminoglycosides are being coadministered.
Charcoal	Methotrexate	⬇	Charcoal can reduce absorption of methotrexate and remove it from systemic circulation. Depending on the clinical situation, this will reduce the effectiveness or toxicity of methotrexate.
Chloramphenicol	Methotrexate	⬇	Oral chloramphenicol may decrease intestinal absorption of methotrexate or interfere with the enterohepatic circulation by inhibiting bowel flora and suppressing metabolism of the drug by bacteria.
Folic acid	Methotrexate	⬇	Vitamin preparations containing folic acid or its derivatives may decrease responses to systemically administered methotrexate.
NSAIDs	Methotrexate	⬆	Concomitant administration of some NSAIDs with high dose methotrexate has been reported to elevate and prolong serum methotrexate levels, resulting in deaths from severe hematologic and GI toxicity. NSAIDs may reduce tubular secretion of methotrexate and enhance toxicity. Monitor renal impairment that could predispose to methotrexate toxicity, for signs of methotrexate toxicity, and methotrexate levels if indicated.
Penicillins	Methotrexate	⬆	Serum methotrexate concentrations may be elevated, increasing the risk of toxicity. Monitor for methotrexate toxicity and measure methotrexate concentrations twice a week for at least the first 2 weeks. If a broad-spectrum antibiotic is needed, ceftazidime may be less likely to interact.
Probenecid	Methotrexate	⬆	Methotrexate plasma levels, therapeutic effects, and toxicity may be enhanced. Monitor methotrexate concentrations and adjust dose accordingly.

METHOTREXATE — ORAL

Methotrexate Oral Drug Interactions

Precipitant drug	Object drug[a]		Description
Salicylates	Methotrexate	↑	Increased toxic effects of methotrexate may occur. Salicylates may reduce tubular secretion of methotrexate and enhance toxicity. Consider monitoring methotrexate levels.
Sulfonamides	Methotrexate	↑	Sulfonamides may increase the risk of methotrexate-induced bone marrow suppression. Methotrexate may predispose patients to trimethoprim-sulfamethoxazole (TMP-SMZ)-induced megaloblastic anemia. Closely monitor patients for signs of hematologic toxicity.
Methotrexate	Sulfonamides		
Tetracyclines	Methotrexate	↑	Methotrexate concentrations may be elevated, increasing the risk of toxicity (eg, bone marrow suppression). If tetracyclines cannot be avoided in patients receiving high-dose methotrexate, closely monitor methotrexate plasma concentrations and patients for signs and symptoms of toxicity.
Trimethoprim	Methotrexate	↑	Trimethoprim may increase the risk of methotrexate-induced bone marrow suppression and megaloblastic anemia. If this drug combination cannot be avoided, closely monitor for signs of hematologic toxicity.
Methotrexate	Digoxin	↓	Serum levels of digoxin may be reduced and actions may be decreased. Monitor patient for signs of reduction in pharmacologic effect of digoxin and increase digoxin dose if necessary. Serum level monitoring may facilitate tailoring dosage.
Methotrexate	Phenytoin	↓	Serum concentrations of phenytoin may be decreased, resulting in a loss of therapeutic effect. Monitor phenytoin serum levels and adjust the phenytoin dosage appropriately. IV phenytoin may be useful.
Methotrexate	Theophylline	↑	Methotrexate may decrease the clearance of theophylline. Theophylline levels should be monitored when used concomitantly with methotrexate.
Methotrexate	Thiopurines (eg, azathioprine)	↑	The actions of thiopurines may be enhanced. Reduced thiopurine dosage may be used during coadministration with methotrexate.

[a] ↑ = object drug increased; ↓ = object drug decreased.

➤*Drug/Food interactions:* Food may delay the absorption and reduce the peak concentration of methotrexate.

Adverse Reactions

The incidence and severity of acute side effects are generally related to dose and dosing frequency. See also Precautions section under "Organ System Toxicity."

The most common adverse reactions are: Ulcerative stomatitis; leukopenia; nausea; abdominal distress; malaise; fatigue; chills; fever; dizziness; decreased resistance to infection.

Methotrexate in doses of 250 mg/m^2 or more is considered to have moderate to high potential for nausea and vomiting. Methotrexate in doses of 100 to 250 mg/m^2 has moderate emetogenic potential. Methotrexate in lower doses has moderate to low emetogenic potential.

➤*Cardiovascular:* Pericarditis, pericardial effusion, hypotension, and thromboembolic events (including arterial thrombosis, cerebral thrombosis, deep vein thrombosis, retinal vein thrombosis, thrombophlebitis, and pulmonary embolus).

➤*CNS:* Headaches; drowsiness; blurred vision; aphasia; hemiparesis; paresis; convulsions; transient blindness; speech impairment, including dysarthria. Following low doses, there have been occasional reports of transient subtle cognitive dysfunction, mood alteration, unusual cranial sensations, leukoencephalopathy, or encephalopathy.

After intrathecal use, the CNS toxicity that may occur can be classified as follows:

1.) Acute chemical arachnoiditis (headache, back pain, nuchal rigidity, fever);
2.) subacute myelopathy (paraparesis/paraplegia with involvement of spinal nerve roots);
3.) chronic leukoencephalopathy (confusion, irritability, somnolence, ataxia, dementia, seizures, and coma).

➤*Dermatologic:* Erythematous rashes; pruritus; urticaria; photosensitivity; pigmentary changes; alopecia; ecchymosis; telangiectasia; acne; furunculosis; erythema multiforme; toxic epidermal necrolysis; Stevens-Johnson syndrome; skin necrosis; skin ulceration; exfoliative dermatitis; photosensitivity; "burning of skin lesions"; rash; plaque erosions (rare).

➤*GI:* Gingivitis; stomatitis; pharyngitis; anorexia; nausea; vomiting; diarrhea; hematemesis; melena; GI ulceration and bleeding; enteritis; pancreatitis.

➤*GU:* Renal failure; azotemia; cystitis; hematuria; severe nephropathy; defective oogenesis or spermatogenesis; transient oligospermia; menstrual dysfunction and vaginal discharge; infertility; abortion; fetal defects; gynecomastia; dysuria; vaginal discharge.

➤*Hematologic:* Bone marrow depression; leukopenia; thrombocytopenia; suppressed hematopoiesis causing anemia; aplastic anemia; pancytopenia; neutropenia; decreased hematocrit; lymphadenopathy and lymphoproliferative disorders (including reversible); hypogammaglobulinemia (rare).

➤*Hepatic:* Hepatotoxicity; acute hepatitis; chronic fibrosis; cirrhosis; decrease in serum albumin; liver enzyme elevations.

➤*Musculoskeletal:* Stress fracture, arthralgias, chest pain.

➤*Pulmonary:* Chronic interstitial obstructive pulmonary disease has occasionally occurred; deaths from respiratory fibrosis, respiratory failure, and interstitial pneumonitis have been reported. Upper respiratory infections, coughing, and epistaxis have occurred.

➤*Special senses:* Conjunctivitis; serious visual changes of unknown etiology; eye discomfort; tinnitus.

➤*Miscellaneous:* Rare reactions related to the use of methotrexate include arthralgia/myalgia, diabetes, osteoporosis and sudden death. Cases of anaphylactoid reactions have occurred; nodulosis; vasculitis, loss of libido/impotence; reversible lymphomas; tumor lysis syndrome; soft tissue necrosis; osteonecrosis; sweating.

Infection – The following also occurred. Infections, pneumonia, sepsis, nocardiosis, histoplasmosis, cryptococcosis, herpes zoster, herpes simplex hepatitis, and disseminated herpes simplex. There have been case reports of sometimes fatal opportunistic infections. *Pneumocystis carinii* pneumonia was the most common infection.

Overdosage

➤*Symptoms:* Reports of oral overdose often indicate accidental daily administration instead of weekly (single or divided doses). Symptoms commonly reported following oral overdose include those symptoms and signs reported at pharmacologic doses, particularly hematologic and GI reaction. For example, leukopenia, thrombocytopenia, anemia, pancytopenia, bone marrow suppression, mucositis, stomatitis, oral ulceration, nausea, vomiting, GI ulceration, and GI bleeding. In some cases, no symptoms were reported. There have been reports of death following overdose. In these cases, events such as sepsis or septic shock, renal failure, and aplastic anemia were also reported.

➤*Treatment:* Leucovorin (citrovorum factor) is used to diminish the toxicity and counteract the effect of inadvertent overdosage of methotrexate. Administer leucovorin as promptly as possible. As the time interval between administration and leucovorin rescue increases, leucovorin's effectiveness in counteracting toxicity diminishes. Monitoring of the serum methotrexate concentration is essential in determining the optimal dose and duration of leucovorin treatment.

In cases of massive overdosage, hydration and urinary alkalinization may be necessary to prevent the precipitation of methotrexate and its metabolites in the renal tubules. Neither hemodialysis nor peritoneal dialysis improves methotrexate elimination. Effective clearance of methotrexate has been reported with acute intermittent hemodialysis using a high-flux dialyzer.

Patient Information

Avoid alcohol, salicylates, and prolonged exposure to sunlight or sunlamps (particularly patients with psoriasis).

Use contraceptive measures during and for at least 3 months (males) or 1 ovulatory cycle (females) after cessation of therapy. The risk of effects on reproduction should be discussed with both males and females on methotrexate.

Notify physician if any of the following occurs: Diarrhea; abdominal pain; black stools; fever and chills; sore throat; sores in or around the mouth; cough; yellow discoloration of the skin or eyes; swelling of the feet or legs; joint pain. May cause nausea, vomiting, loss of appetite, hair loss, skin rash, fever, or dizziness. Notify the physician if these effects persist.

Inform patients of the early signs of toxicity, of the need to see their physician promptly if they occur, and the need for close follow-up, including laboratory tests to monitor toxicity.

METHOTREXATE SODIUM — INJECTION

WARNING

Methotrexate should be used only by physicians whose knowledge and experience include the use of antimetabolite therapy.

Because of the possibility of serious toxic reactions (which can be fatal):
Methotrexate should be used only in life-threatening neoplastic diseases, or in patients with psoriasis or rheumatoid arthritis (RA) with severe, recalcitrant, disabling disease which is not adequately responsive to other forms of therapy.
Deaths have been reported with the use of methotrexate in the treatment of malignancy, psoriasis, and RA.
Patients should be closely monitored for bone marrow, liver, lung and kidney toxicities.
Patients should be informed by their physicians of the risks involved and be under a physician's care throughout therapy.

The use of methotrexate high-dose regimens recommended for osteosarcoma requires meticulous care. High-dose regimens for other neoplastic diseases are investigational, and a therapeutic advantage has not been established.

Methotrexate formulations and diluents containing preservatives must not be used for intrathecal or high-dose methotrexate therapy.

1.) Methotrexate has been reported to cause fetal death or congenital anomalies. Therefore, it is not recommended for women of childbearing potential unless there is clear medical evidence that the benefits can be expected to outweigh the considered risks. Pregnant women with psoriasis or RA should not receive methotrexate.
2.) Methotrexate elimination is reduced in patients with impaired renal function, ascites, or pleural effusions. Such patients require especially careful monitoring for toxicity, and require dose reduction or, in some cases, discontinuation of methotrexate administration.
3.) Unexpectedly severe (sometimes fatal) bone marrow suppression and GI toxicity have been reported with concomitant administration of methotrexate (usually in high dosage) along with some nonsteroidal anti-inflammatory drugs (NSAIDs).
4.) Methotrexate causes hepatotoxicity, fibrosis and cirrhosis, but generally only after prolonged use. Acutely, liver enzyme elevations are frequently seen. These are usually transient and asymptomatic, and also do not appear predictive of subsequent hepatic disease. Liver biopsy after sustained use often shows histologic changes, and fibrosis and cirrhosis have been reported; these latter lesions may not be preceded by symptoms or abnormal liver function tests in the psoriasis population. For this reason, periodic liver biopsies are usually recommended for psoriatic patients who are under long-term treatment. Persistent abnormalities in liver function tests may precede appearance of fibrosis or cirrhosis in the RA population.
5.) Methotrexate-induced lung disease is a potentially dangerous lesion, which may occur acutely at any time during therapy and which has been reported at doses as low as 7.5 mg/week. It is not always fully reversible. Pulmonary symptoms (especially a dry, nonproductive cough) may require interruption of treatment and careful investigation.
6.) Diarrhea and ulcerative stomatitis require interruption of therapy; otherwise, hemorrhagic enteritis and death from intestinal perforation may occur.
7.) Malignant lymphomas, which may regress following withdrawal of methotrexate, may occur in patients receiving low-dose methotrexate and, thus, may not require cytotoxic treatment. Discontinue methotrexate first and, if the lymphoma does not regress, institute appropriate treatment.
8.) Like other cytotoxic drugs, methotrexate may induce "tumor lysis syndrome" in patients with rapidly growing tumors. Appropriate supportive and pharmacologic measures may prevent or alleviate this complication.
9.) Severe, occasionally fatal, skin reactions have been reported following single or multiple doses of methotrexate. Reactions have occurred within days of methotrexate administration. Recovery has been reported with discontinuation of therapy.
10.) Potentially fatal opportunistic infections, especially *Pneumocystis carinii* pneumonia, may occur with methotrexate therapy.
11.) Methotrexate given concomitantly with radiotherapy may increase the risk of soft tissue necrosis and osteonecrosis.

Indications

➤*Antineoplastic chemotherapy:* Treatment of gestational choriocarcinoma, chorioadenoma destruens and hydatidiform mole.

In acute lymphocytic leukemia, methotrexate is indicated in the prophylaxis of meningeal leukemia and is used in maintenance therapy in combination with other chemotherapeutic agents. Methotrexate is also indicated in the treatment of meningeal leukemia.

Methotrexate is used alone or in combination with other anticancer agents in the treatment of breast cancer, epidermoid cancers of the head and neck, advanced mycosis fungoides (cutaneous T cell lymphoma), and lung cancer, particularly squamous cell and small cell types. Methotrexate is also used in combination with other chemotherapeutic agents in the treatment of advanced stage non-Hodgkin's lymphomas.

Methotrexate in high doses followed by leucovorin rescue in combination with other chemotherapeutic agents is effective in prolonging relapse-free survival in patients with nonmetastatic osteosarcoma who have undergone surgical resection or amputation for the primary tumor.

➤*Psoriasis:* Methotrexate is indicated in the symptomatic control of severe, recalcitrant, disabling psoriasis that is not adequately responsive to other forms of therapy, but only when the diagnosis has been established, as by biopsy and/or after dermatologic consultation. It is important to ensure that a psoriasis "flare" is not due to an undiagnosed concomitant disease affecting immune responses.

➤*RA:* Methotrexate is indicated in the management of selected adults with severe, active, classical or definite RA (American Rheumatism Association [ARA] criteria), or children with active polyarticular-course juvenile RA, who have had an insufficient therapeutic response to, or are intolerant of, an adequate trial of first-line therapy, including full-dose NSAIDs.

➤*Off-label uses:*

Ectopic pregnancy – [1] = Good documentation. The use of methotrexate in the management of ectopic pregnancy in selected patients is recognized in national guidelines. The selection of appropriate candidates and patient monitoring during and after therapy are essential to optimize the safe use of this treatment.

Other possible off-label uses – Treatment of testicular carcinoma, bladder carcinoma, prevention of acute graft-versus-host disease (GVHD).

Administration and Dosage

➤*General dosing considerations:* Oral administration is often preferred when low doses are being administered because absorption is rapid, and effective serum levels are obtained. Methotrexate sodium injection and methotrexate for injection may be given by the IM, IV, intra-arterial, or intrathecal route. However, the preserved formulation contains benzyl alcohol and must not be used for intrathecal or high-dose therapy.

➤*Adults:*

Choriocarcinoma and similar trophoblastic diseases – 15 to 30 mg IM daily for a 5-day course. Such courses are usually repeated for 3 to 5 times as required, with rest periods of 1 or more weeks interposed between courses, until any manifesting toxic symptoms subside. The effectiveness of therapy is ordinarily evaluated by 24-hour quantitative analysis of urinary chorionic gonadotropin (hCG), which should return to normal or less than 50 units per 24 hours usually after the third or fourth course and usually be followed by a complete resolution of measurable lesions in 4 to 6 weeks. One to 2 courses of methotrexate after normalization of hCG is usually recommended. Before each course of the drug, careful clinical assessment is essential. Cyclic combination therapy of methotrexate with other antitumor drugs has been reported as being useful.

Because hydatidiform mole may precede choriocarcinoma, prophylactic chemotherapy with methotrexate has been recommended.

Chorioadenoma destruens is considered to be an invasive form of hydatidiform mole. Methotrexate is administered in these disease states in doses similar to those recommended for choriocarcinoma.

Leukemia –

Usual dosage: 3.3 mg/m^2 in combination with 60 mg/m^2 of prednisone, given daily, produced remissions in 50% of patients treated, usually within a period of 4 to 6 weeks. Methotrexate, alone or in combination with steroids, was used initially for induction of remission in acute lymphoblastic leukemias. More recently, corticosteroid therapy, in combination with other antileukemic drugs or in cyclic combinations with methotrexate included, has appeared to produce rapid and effective remissions. Methotrexate in combination with other agents appears to be the drug of choice for securing maintenance of drug-induced remissions. When remission is achieved and supportive care has produced general clinical improvement, maintenance therapy is initiated.

Maintenance dosage: Methotrexate is administered 2 times weekly IM in total weekly doses of 30 mg/m^2. It has also been given in doses of 2.5 mg/kg IV every 14 days. If and when relapse does occur, reinduction of remission can again usually be obtained by repeating the initial induction regimen.

Meningeal leukemia (intrathecal) – In the treatment or prophylaxis of meningeal leukemia, methotrexate must be administered intrathecally. Preservative-free methotrexate is diluted to a concentration of 1 mg/mL in an appropriate sterile, preservative-free medium such as 0.9% sodium chloride injection.

Usual dosage: The following intrathecal dosage regimen is based on age instead of body surface area.

Methotrexate Intrathecal Dosing According to Age for the Treatment of Meningeal Leukemia

Age (years)	Dose (mg)
< 1	6
1	8
2	10
3 or older	12

The cerebrospinal fluid (CSF) volume is dependent on age and not on body surface area. The CSF is at 40% of the adult volume at birth and reaches the adult volume in several years.

Intrathecal methotrexate administration at a dose of 12 mg/m^2 has been reported to result in low CSF methotrexate concentrations and reduced efficacy in children and high concentrations and neurotoxicity in adults.

Because the CSF volume and turnover may decrease with age, a dose reduction may be indicated in elderly patients.

For the treatment of meningeal leukemia, intrathecal methotrexate may be given at intervals of 2 to 5 days. However, administration at intervals of less than 1 week may result in increased subacute toxicity. Methotrexate is

METHOTREXATE SODIUM — INJECTION

administered until the cell count of the CSF returns to normal. At this point, one additional dose is advisable. For prophylaxis against meningeal leukemia, the dosage is the same as for treatment except for the intervals of administration. On this subject, it is advisable for the health care provider to consult the medical literature.

Untoward adverse reactions may occur with any given intrathecal injection and are commonly neurological in character. Large doses may cause convulsions. Methotrexate given by the intrathecal route appears significantly in the systemic circulation and may cause systemic methotrexate toxicity. Therefore, systemic antileukemic therapy with the drug should be appropriately adjusted, reduced, or discontinued. Focal leukemic involvement of the CNS may not respond to intrathecal chemotherapy and is best treated with radiotherapy.

Maximum dose: 15 mg.

Mycosis fungoides (cutaneous T-cell lymphoma) –

Usual dosage: Dosage in early stages is usually 5 to 50 mg once weekly.

Dosage adjustment: Dose reduction or cessation is guided by patient response and hematologic monitoring. Methotrexate therapy produces clinical responses in 50% of cases.

Alternative dosage: Methotrexate has also been administered twice weekly in doses ranging from 15 to 37.5 mg in patients who have responded poorly to weekly therapy.

Concomitant therapy: Combination chemotherapy regimens that include IV methotrexate administered at higher doses with leucovorin rescue have been utilized in advanced stages of the disease.

Osteosarcoma – An effective adjuvant chemotherapy regimen requires the administration of several cytotoxic chemotherapeutic agents. In addition to high-dose methotrexate with leucovorin rescue, these agents may include doxorubicin, cisplatin, and the combination of bleomycin, cyclophosphamide, and dactinomycin in the following doses and schedule.

Usual dosage: The starting dose for high-dose methotrexate treatment is 12 g/m^2. If this dose is not sufficient to produce a peak serum methotrexate concentration of 1,000 mcM (10^{-3} mol/L) at the end of the methotrexate infusion, the dose may be escalated to 15 g/m^2 in subsequent treatments. If the patient is vomiting or is unable to tolerate oral medication, leucovorin is given IV or IM at the same dose and schedule.

Osteosarcoma Chemotherapy Regimens: Dose and Schedules

Drug[a]	Dose[a]	Treatment week after surgery
Methotrexate	12 g/m^2 IV as 4-hour infusion (starting dose)	4, 5, 6, 7, 11, 12, 15, 16, 29, 30, 44, 45
Leucovorin	15 mg orally every 6 hours for 10 doses starting at 24 hours after start of methotrexate infusion	
Doxorubicin[b] as a single drug	30 mg/m^2/day IV × 3 days	8, 17
Doxorubicin[b]	50 mg/m^2 IV	20, 23, 33, 36
Cisplatin[b]	100 mg/m^2	20, 23, 33, 36
Bleomycin[b]	15 units/m^2 IV × 2 days	2, 13, 26, 39, 42
Cyclophosphamide[b]	600 mg/m^2 IV × 2 days	2, 13, 26, 39, 42
Dactinomycin[b]	0.6 mg/m^2 IV × 2 days	2, 13, 26, 39, 42

[a] Link MP, Goorin AM, Miser AW, et al: The effect of adjuvant chemotherapy on relapse-free survival in patients with osteosarcoma of the extremity. *N Engl J Med.* 1986;314(25):1600-1606.

[b] For the information following, please see respective monographs for each drug for full prescribing information. Dosage modifications may be necessary because of drug-induced toxicity.

When these higher doses of methotrexate are to be administered, the methotrexate safety with leucovorin rescue guidelines should be closely observed.

Guidelines for methotrexate therapy with leucovorin rescue – Administration of methotrexate should be delayed until recovery, if any, of the following occurs:

- The WBC count is less than 1,500/mcL.
- The neutrophil count is less than 200/mcL.
- The platelet count is less than 75,000/mcL.
- The serum bilirubin level is greater than 1.2 mg/dL.
- The ALT level is more than 450 units.
- Mucositis is present, until there is evidence of healing.
- Persistent pleural effusion is present; this should be drained dry prior to infusion.

Adequate renal function must be documented.

1.) Serum creatinine must be normal, and creatinine clearance must be greater than 60 mL/min, before initiation of therapy.
2.) Serum creatinine must be measured prior to each subsequent course of therapy. If serum creatinine has increased by 50% or more compared to a prior value, the creatinine clearance must be measured and documented to be greater than 60 mL/min (even if the serum creatinine is still within the normal range).

Patients must be well hydrated, and must be treated with sodium bicarbonate for urinary alkalinization.

1.) Administer 1,000 mL/m^2 of IV fluid over 6 hours prior to initiation of the methotrexate infusion. Continue hydration at 125 mL/m^2/h (3 L/m^2/day) during the methotrexate infusion and for 2 days after the infusion has been completed.
2.) Alkalinize urine to maintain pH above 7 during methotrexate infusion and leucovorin calcium therapy. This can be accomplished by the administration of sodium bicarbonate orally or by incorporation into a separate IV solution.

Repeat serum creatinine and serum methotrexate 24 hours after starting methotrexate and at least once daily until the methotrexate level is less than 5×10^{-8} mol/L (0.05 mcM).

Leucovorin Rescue Schedules Following Treatment with Higher Doses of Methotrexate

Clinical situation	Laboratory findings	Leucovorin dosage and duration
Normal methotrexate elimination	Serum methotrexate level approximately 10 mcM at 24 hours after administration, 1 mcM at 48 hours, and < 0.2 mcM at 72 hours	15 mg orally, IM, or IV every 6 hours for 60 hours (10 doses starting at 24 hours after start of methotrexate infusion)
Delayed late methotrexate elimination	Serum methotrexate level remaining above 0.2 mcM at 72 hours, and > 0.05 mcM at 96 hours after administration	Continue 15 mg orally, IM, or IV every 6 hours, until methotrexate level is < 0.05 mcM
Delayed early methotrexate elimination or evidence of acute renal injury	Serum methotrexate level of 50 mcM or more at 24 hours, or 5 mcM or more at 48 hours after administration, or a 100% or greater increase in serum creatinine level at 24 hours after methotrexate administration (eg, an increase from 0.5 mg/dL to a level of 1 mg/dL or more)	150 mg IV every 3 hours, until methotrexate level is < 1 mcM, then 15 mg IV every 3 hours until methotrexate level is < 0.05 mcM

Patients who experience delayed early methotrexate elimination are likely to develop nonreversible oliguric renal failure. In addition to appropriate leucovorin therapy, these patients require continuing hydration and urinary alkalization, and close monitoring of fluid and electrolyte status, until the serum methotrexate level has fallen to less than 0.05 mcM and the renal failure has resolved. If necessary, acute, intermittent hemodialysis with a high-flux dialyzer may also be beneficial in these patients.

Some patients will have abnormalities in methotrexate elimination or abnormalities in renal function following methotrexate administration, which are significant but less severe than the abnormalities described previously. These abnormalities may or may not be associated with significant clinical toxicity. If significant clinical toxicity is observed, leucovorin rescue should be extended for an additional 24 hours (total, 14 doses over 84 hours) in subsequent courses of therapy. The possibility that the patient is taking other medications that interact with methotrexate (eg, medications that may interfere with elimination or methotrexate binding to serum albumin) should always be reconsidered when laboratory abnormalities or clinical toxicities are observed.

Caution: Do not administer leucovorin intrathecally.

Rheumatoid arthritis – See Methotrexate Oral.

Psoriasis – See also Methotrexate Oral

Usual dosage: Weekly single IM or IV dose of 10 to 25 mg/week until adequate response is achieved.

Maximum dose: 30 mg/week.

Dosage adjustment: Dosages may be gradually adjusted to achieve optimal clinical response. Once optimal clinical response has been achieved, dosage should be reduced to the lowest possible amount of drug and to the longest possible rest period. The use of methotrexate may permit the return to conventional topical therapy, which should be encouraged.

Off-label dosing –

Ectopic pregnancy: [1] = Good documentation. Multiple- and single-dose treatment protocols have been recommended (see the following tables). Prior to the first dose of methotrexate, recommended laboratory testing includes complete blood cell count, liver function tests, serum creatinine, blood type, and Rh testing. A chest x-ray should be performed in women with a history of pulmonary disease because of an increased risk of interstitial pneumonitis in patients with underlying lung disease.

The multiple-dose regimen was adapted from early experience with treatment of ectopic pregnancy. "Single-dose" regimen is a misnomer as it includes the potential for multiple methotrexate injections when response is inadequate.

METHOTREXATE SODIUM — INJECTION

Single-Dose Methotrexate Regimen

Treatment day	Laboratory evaluation	Intervention
1	hCG	Methotrexate 50 mg/m^2 IM
4	hCG	None
7	hCG	•If hCG levels decrease < 15% between days 4 and 7, administer methotrexate 50 mg/m^2 IM. •If hCG levels decrease ≥ 15% between days 4 and 7, stop treatment and measure hCG weekly until reaching nonpregnant levels.
If during follow-up hCG levels plateau or increase, consider repeating methotrexate.		

Two-Dose Methotrexate Regimen

Treatment day	Laboratory evaluation	Intervention
0	hCG	Methotrexate 50 mg/m^2 IM
4	hCG	Methotrexate 50 mg/m^2 IM
7	hCG	•If hCG levels decrease < 15% between days 4 and 7, administer methotrexate 50 mg/m^2 IM. •If hCG levels decrease ≥ 15% between days 4 and 7, stop treatment and measure hCG weekly until reaching nonpregnant levels.
11	hCG	•If hCG levels decrease < 15% between days 7 and 11, consider administering methotrexate 50 mg/m^2 IM or surgical treatment. •If hCG levels decrease ≥ 15% between days 7 and 11, measure hCG weekly until reaching nonpregnant levels.

Multiple-Dose Methotrexate Regimen

Treatment day	Laboratory evaluation	Intervention[a]
1	hCG	Methotrexate 1 mg/kg IM
2		Leucovorin 0.1 mg/kg IM
3	hCG	•If hCG levels decrease < 15% between days 1 and 3, administer methotrexate 1 mg/kg IM. •If hCG levels decrease ≥ 15% between days 1 and 3, stop treatment and start surveillance.
4		Leucovorin 0.1 mg/kg IM
5	hCG	•If hCG levels decrease < 15% between days 3 and 5, administer methotrexate 1 mg/kg IM. •If hCG levels decrease ≥ 15% between days 3 and 5, stop treatment and start surveillance.
6		Leucovorin 0.1 mg/kg IM
7	hCG	•If hCG levels decrease < 15% between days 5 and 7, administer methotrexate 1 mg/kg IM. •If hCG levels decrease ≥ 15% between days 5 and 7, stop treatment and start surveillance.
8		Leucovorin 0.1 mg/kg IM

[a] Methotrexate is continued until hCG levels decrease by at least 15% from previous measurement. Approximately 50% of patients will not require full 8-day regimen.

➤*Children:*

Leukemia – See Adults for dosing.

Meningeal leukemia (intrathecal) – See Adults for dosing.

Osteosarcoma – See Adults for dosing.

Guidelines for methotrexate therapy with leucovorin rescue – See Adults for dosing.

Polyarticular-course juvenile rheumatoid arthritis –

Usual dosage: The recommended starting dose is 10 mg/m^2 given once weekly.

All schedules should be continually tailored to the individual patient. An initial test dose may be given prior to the regular dosing schedule to detect any extreme sensitivity to adverse effects. Maximal myelosuppression usually occurs in 7 to 10 days.

Dosage adjustment: Dosage may be adjusted gradually to achieve an optimal response. Although there is experience with doses up to 30 mg/m^2/week in children, there are too few published data to assess how doses over 20 mg/m^2/week might affect the risk of serious toxicity in children. Experience does suggest, however, that children receiving 20 to 30 mg/m^2/week (0.65 to 1 mg/kg/week) may have better absorption and fewer GI adverse reactions if methotrexate is administered IM or subcutaneously.

Duration of therapy: Therapeutic response usually begins within 3 to 6 weeks, and the patient may continue to improve for another 12 weeks or more. The optimal duration of therapy is unknown. Limited data available from long-term studies in adults indicate that the initial clinical improvement is maintained for at least 2 years with continued therapy. When methotrexate is discontinued, the arthritis usually worsens within 3 to 6 weeks.

➤*Elderly:* Because the CSF volume and turnover may decrease with age, a dose reduction may be indicated in intrathecal dosing for elderly patients.

➤*Preparation for administration:* Methotrexate is considered a cytotoxic agent. Follow safe handling procedures when preparing, administering, or dispensing methotrexate.

Reconstitution of lyophilized powders – Reconstitute immediately prior to use.

Methotrexate sodium for injection should be reconstituted with an appropriate sterile, preservative-free medium such as 5% dextrose solution or sodium chloride injection. Reconstitute the 20 mg vial to a concentration no greater than 25 mg/mL. The 1 g vial should be reconstituted with 19.4 mL to a concentration of 50 mg/mL. When high doses of methotrexate are administered by IV infusion, the total dose is diluted in 5% dextrose solution.

For intrathecal injection, reconstitute to a concentration of 1 mg/mL with an appropriate sterile, preservative-free medium such as sodium chloride injection.

Dilution instructions for liquid methotrexate sodium injection products –

Methotrexate sodium injection, isotonic liquid (contains preservative): If desired, the solution may be further diluted with a compatible medium such as sodium chloride injection. Storage for 24 hours at a temperature of 21° to 25°C (69° to 77°F) results in a product that is within 90% of label potency.

Methotrexate sodium injection, isotonic liquid (preservative-free, for single use only): If desired, the solution may be further diluted immediately prior to use with an appropriate sterile, preservative-free medium such as 5% dextrose solution or sodium chloride injection.

➤*Storage/Stability:* Store at 20° to 25°C (68° to 77°F); excursions are permitted to 15° to 30°C (59° to 86°F). Protect from light.

Actions

➤*Pharmacology:* Methotrexate inhibits dihydrofolic acid reductase. Dihydrofolates must be reduced to tetrahydrofolates by this enzyme before they can be utilized as carriers of 1-carbon groups in the synthesis of purine nucleotides and thymidylate. Therefore, methotrexate interferes with DNA synthesis, repair, and cellular replication. Actively proliferating tissues such as malignant cells, bone marrow, fetal cells, buccal and intestinal mucosa, and cells of the urinary bladder are in general more sensitive to this effect of methotrexate. When cellular proliferation in malignant tissues is greater than in most normal tissues, methotrexate may impair malignant growth without irreversible damage to healthy tissues.

Methotrexate in high doses, followed by leucovorin rescue, is used as a part of the treatment of patients with nonmetastatic osteosarcoma. The original rationale for high-dose methotrexate therapy was based on the concept of selective rescue of normal tissues by leucovorin. More recent evidence suggests that high-dose methotrexate may also overcome methotrexate resistance caused by impaired active transport, decreased affinity of dihydrofolic acid reductase for methotrexate, increased levels of dihydrofolic acid reductase resulting from gene amplification, or decreased polyglutamation of methotrexate. The actual mechanism of action is unknown.

➤*Pharmacokinetics:*

Absorption – Methotrexate is generally completely absorbed from parenteral routes of injection. After IM injection, peak serum concentrations occur in 30 to 60 minutes. As in leukemic pediatric patients, a wide interindividual variability in the plasma concentrations of methotrexate has been reported in pediatric patients with JRA.

Distribution – After IV administration, the initial volume of distribution is approximately 0.18 L/kg (18% of body weight) and steady-state volume of distribution is approximately 0.4 to 0.8 L/kg (40% to 80% of body weight). Methotrexate competes with reduced folates for active transport across cell membranes by means of a single carrier-mediated active transport process. At serum concentrations greater than 100 mcM, passive diffusion becomes a major pathway by which effective intracellular concentrations can be achieved. Methotrexate in serum is approximately 50% protein bound. Laboratory studies demonstrate that it may be displaced from plasma albumin by various compounds including sulfonamides, salicylates, tetracyclines, chloramphenicol, and phenytoin.

Methotrexate does not penetrate the blood-CSF barrier in therapeutic amounts when given orally or parenterally. High CSF concentrations of the drug may be attained by intrathecal administration.

Metabolism – After absorption, methotrexate undergoes hepatic and intracellular metabolism to polyglutamated forms which can be converted

METHOTREXATE SODIUM — INJECTION

back to methotrexate by hydrolase enzymes. These polyglutamates act as inhibitors of dihydrofolate reductase and thymidylate synthetase. Small amounts of methotrexate polyglutamates may remain in tissues for extended periods. The retention and prolonged drug action of these active metabolites vary among different cells, tissues and tumors. A small amount of metabolism to 7-hydroxymethotrexate may occur at doses commonly prescribed. Accumulation of this metabolite may become significant at the high doses used in osteogenic sarcoma. The aqueous solubility of 7-hydroxymethotrexate is 3- to 5-fold lower than the parent compound.

Excretion – Renal excretion is the primary route of elimination and is dependent upon dosage and route of administration. With IV administration, 80% to 90% of the administered dose is excreted unchanged in the urine within 24 hours. There is limited biliary excretion amounting to 10% or less of the administered dose. Enterohepatic recirculation of methotrexate has been proposed.

Renal excretion occurs by glomerular filtration and active tubular secretion. Nonlinear elimination due to saturation of renal tubular reabsorption has been observed in psoriatic patients at doses between 7.5 and 30 mg. Impaired renal function, as well as concurrent use of drugs such as weak organic acids that also undergo tubular secretion, can markedly increase methotrexate serum levels. Excellent correlation has been reported between methotrexate clearance and endogenous creatinine clearance.

Methotrexate clearance rates vary widely and are generally decreased at higher doses. Delayed drug clearance has been identified as 1 of the major factors responsible for methotrexate toxicity. It has been postulated that the toxicity of methotrexate for normal tissues is more dependent upon the duration of exposure to the drug rather than the peak level achieved. When a patient has delayed drug elimination due to compromised renal function, a third-space effusion, or other causes, methotrexate serum concentrations may remain elevated for prolonged periods. In pediatric patients receiving methotrexate for acute lymphocytic leukemia (6.3 to 30 mg/m^2), or for JRA (3.75 to 26.2 mg/m^2), the terminal half-life has been reported to range from 0.7 to 5.8 hours or 0.9 to 2.3 hours, respectively.

The terminal half-life reported for methotrexate is approximately 3 to 10 hours for patients receiving treatment for psoriasis, or RA or low-dose antineoplastic therapy (less than 30 mg/m^2). For patients receiving high doses of methotrexate, the terminal half-life is 8 to 15 hours.

The potential for toxicity from high-dose regimens or delayed excretion is reduced by the administration of leucovorin calcium during the final phase of methotrexate plasma elimination. Pharmacokinetic monitoring of methotrexate serum concentrations may help identify those patients at high risk for methotrexate toxicity and aid in proper adjustment of leucovorin dosing. Guidelines for monitoring serum methotrexate levels, and for adjustment of leucovorin dosing to reduce the risk of methotrexate toxicity, are available.

Contraindications

Methotrexate can cause fetal death or teratogenic effects when administered to a pregnant woman. Methotrexate is contraindicated in pregnant women with psoriasis or RA and should be used in the treatment of neoplastic diseases only when the potential benefit outweighs the risk to the fetus. Women of childbearing potential should not be started on methotrexate until pregnancy is excluded and should be fully counseled on the serious risk to the fetus should they become pregnant while undergoing treatment. Pregnancy should be avoided if either partner is receiving methotrexate; during and for a minimum of 3 months after therapy for male patients, and during and for at least 1 ovulatory cycle after therapy for female patients.

Because of the potential for serious adverse reactions from methotrexate in breastfed infants, it is contraindicated in nursing mothers.

Patients with psoriasis or RA with alcoholism, alcoholic liver disease or other chronic liver disease should not receive methotrexate.

Patients with psoriasis or RA who have overt or laboratory evidence of immunodeficiency syndromes should not receive methotrexate.

Patients with psoriasis or RA who have preexisting blood dyscrasias, such as bone marrow hypoplasia, leukopenia, thrombocytopenia or significant anemia, should not receive methotrexate.

Patients with a known hypersensitivity to methotrexate should not receive the drug.

Warnings/Precautions

➤*Intrathecal use/high dose:* Methotrexate formulations and diluents containing preservatives must not be used for intrathecal or high-dose methotrexate therapy.

➤*Renal effects:* High doses of methotrexate used in the treatment of osteosarcoma may cause renal damage leading to acute renal failure. Nephrotoxicity is due primarily to the precipitation of methotrexate and 7-hydroxymethotrexate in the renal tubules. Close attention to renal function including adequate hydration, urine alkalinization and measurement of serum methotrexate and creatinine levels are essential for safe administration.

➤*Hepatic effects:* Methotrexate has the potential for acute (elevated transaminases) and chronic (fibrosis and cirrhosis) hepatotoxicity. Chronic toxicity is potentially fatal; it generally has occurred after prolonged use (generally 2 years or more) and after a total dose of at least 1.5 g. In studies in psoriatic patients, hepatotoxicity appeared to be a function of total cumulative dose and appeared to be enhanced by alcoholism, obesity, diabetes and advanced age. An accurate incidence rate has not been determined; the rate of progression and reversibility of lesions is not known. Special caution is indicated in the presence of preexisting liver damage or impaired hepatic function.

In psoriasis, liver function tests, including serum albumin, should be performed periodically prior to dosing, but are often normal in the face of developing fibrosis or cirrhosis. These lesions may be detectable only by biopsy. The usual recommendation is to obtain a liver biopsy at pretherapy or shortly after initiation of therapy (2 to 4 months), at a total cumulative dose of 1.5 g, and after each additional 1 to 1.5 g. Moderate fibrosis or any cirrhosis normally leads to discontinuation of the drug; mild fibrosis normally suggests a repeat biopsy in 6 months. Milder histologic findings such as fatty change and low-grade portal inflammation are relatively common pretherapy. Although these mild changes are usually not a reason to avoid or discontinue methotrexate therapy, the drug should be used with caution.

In RA, age at first use of methotrexate and duration of therapy have been reported as risk factors for hepatotoxicity; other risk factors, similar to those observed in psoriasis, may be present in RA but have not been confirmed to date. Persistent abnormalities in liver function tests may precede appearance of fibrosis or cirrhosis in this population. There is a combined reported experience in 217 RA patients with liver biopsies both before and during treatment (after a cumulative dose of at least 1.5 g) and in 714 patients with a biopsy only during treatment. There are 64 (7%) cases of fibrosis and 1 (0.1%) case of cirrhosis. Of the 64 cases of fibrosis, 60 were deemed mild. The reticulin stain is more sensitive for early fibrosis, and its use may increase these figures. It is unknown whether even longer use will increase these risks.

Liver function tests should be performed at baseline and at 4- to 8-week intervals in patients receiving methotrexate for RA. Pretreatment liver biopsy should be performed for patients with a history of excessive alcohol consumption, persistently abnormal baseline liver function test values or chronic hepatitis B or C infection. During therapy, liver biopsy should be performed if there are persistent liver function test abnormalities or there is a decrease in serum albumin below the normal range (in the setting of well-controlled RA). If the results of a liver biopsy show mild changes (Roenigk grades I, II, IIIa), methotrexate may be continued and the patient monitored as per recommendations listed above. Methotrexate should be discontinued in any patient who displays persistently abnormal liver function tests and refuses liver biopsy or in any patient whose liver biopsy shows moderate-to-severe changes (Roenigk grade IIIb or IV).

➤*Neurologic:* There have been reports of leukoencephalopathy following IV administration of methotrexate to patients who have had craniospinal irradiation. Serious neurotoxicity, frequently manifested as generalized or focal seizures, has been reported with unexpectedly increased frequency among pediatric patients with acute lymphoblastic leukemia who were treated with intermediate-dose IV methotrexate (1 g/m^2). Symptomatic patients were commonly noted to have leukoencephalopathy or microangiopathic calcifications on diagnostic imaging studies. Chronic leukoencephalopathy has also been reported in patients who received repeated doses of high-dose methotrexate with leucovorin rescue even without cranial irradiation. Discontinuation of methotrexate does not always result in complete recovery.

A transient acute neurologic syndrome has been observed in patients treated with high-dosage regimens. Manifestations of this stroke-like encephalopathy may include confusion, hemiparesis, seizures and coma. The exact cause is unknown.

After the intrathecal use of methotrexate, the CNS toxicity which may occur can be classified as follows: Acute chemical arachnoiditis manifested by such symptoms as headache, back pain, nuchal rigidity, and fever; subacute myelopathy characterized by paraparesis/paraplegia associated with involvement with 1 or more spinal nerve roots; chronic leukoencephalopathy manifested by confusion, irritability, somnolence, ataxia, dementia, seizures and coma. This condition can be progressive and even fatal.

➤*Pulmonary:* Pulmonary symptoms (especially a dry, nonproductive cough) or a nonspecific pneumonitis occurring during methotrexate therapy may be indicative of a potentially dangerous lesion and require interruption of treatment and careful investigation. Although clinically variable, the typical patient with methotrexate-induced lung disease presents with fever, cough, dyspnea, hypoxemia, and an infiltrate on chest x-ray; infection needs to be excluded. This lesion can occur at all dosages.

➤*Skin:* Severe, occasionally fatal, dermatologic reactions, including toxic epidermal necrolysis, Stevens-Johnson syndrome, exfoliative dermatitis, skin necrosis, and erythema multiforme, have been reported in children and adults, within days of oral, IM, IV, or intrathecal methotrexate administration. Reactions were noted after single or multiple, low, intermediate or high doses of methotrexate in patients with neoplastic and nonneoplastic diseases.

➤*Pleural effusions or ascites:* Methotrexate exits slowly from third space compartments (eg, pleural effusions or ascites). This results in a prolonged terminal plasma half-life and unexpected toxicity. In patients with significant third-space accumulations, it is advisable to evacuate the fluid before treatment and to monitor plasma methotrexate levels.

➤*Psoriasis lesions:* Lesions of psoriasis may be aggravated by concomitant exposure to ultraviolet radiation. Radiation dermatitis and sunburn may be "recalled" by the use of methotrexate.

➤*Debility:* Methotrexate should be used with extreme caution in the presence of debility.

➤*Gastrointestinal:* If vomiting, diarrhea, or stomatitis occur, which may result in dehydration, methotrexate should be discontinued until recovery occurs. Methotrexate should be used with extreme caution in the presence of peptic ulcer disease or ulcerative colitis.

➤*Hematologic:* Methotrexate can suppress hematopoiesis and cause anemia, aplastic anemia, pancytopenia, leukopenia, neutropenia, or thrombocytopenia. In patients with malignancy and preexisting hematopoietic

METHOTREXATE SODIUM — INJECTION

impairment, the drug should be used with caution, if at all. In controlled clinical trials in RA (n = 128), leukopenia (WBC less than 3,000/mm^3) was seen in 2 patients, thrombocytopenia (platelets less than 100,000/mm^3) in 6 patients, and pancytopenia in 2 patients.

In psoriasis and RA, methotrexate should be stopped immediately if there is a significant drop in blood counts. In the treatment of neoplastic diseases, methotrexate should be continued only if the potential benefit warrants the risk of severe myelosuppression. Patients with profound granulocytopenia and fever should be evaluated immediately and usually require parenteral broad-spectrum antibiotic therapy.

➤*Infection or immunologic states:* Methotrexate should be used with extreme caution in the presence of active infection, and is usually contraindicated in patients with overt or laboratory evidence of immunodeficiency syndromes. Immunization may be ineffective when given during methotrexate therapy. Immunization with live virus vaccines is generally not recommended. There have been reports of disseminated vaccinia infections after smallpox immunization in patients receiving methotrexate therapy. Hypogammaglobulinemia has been reported rarely.

See Adverse Reactions for more information.

➤*Pregnancy: Category X.* Methotrexate causes embryotoxicity, abortion, and fetal defects in humans.

Methotrexate can cause fetal death or teratogenic effects when administered to a pregnant woman. Methotrexate is contraindicated in pregnant women with psoriasis or RA and should be used in the treatment of neoplastic diseases only when the potential benefit outweighs the risk to the fetus. Women of childbearing potential should not be started on methotrexate until pregnancy is excluded and should be fully counseled on the serious risk to the fetus should they become pregnant while undergoing treatment. Pregnancy should be avoided if either partner is receiving methotrexate; during and for a minimum of 3 months after therapy for male patients, and during and for at least 1 ovulatory cycle after therapy for female patients.

Fertility impairment – Impairment of fertility, oligospermia, and menstrual dysfunction in humans has been reported during and for a short period after cessation of therapy.

➤*Lactation:* Because of the potential for serious adverse reactions from methotrexate in breastfed infants, it is contraindicated in nursing mothers.

➤*Children:* Safety and efficacy in children have been established only in cancer chemotherapy and in polyarticular-course JRA.

Published clinical studies evaluating the use of methotrexate in children and adolescents (ie, patients 2 to 16 years of age) with JRA demonstrated safety comparable to that observed in adults with RA.

Methotrexate injectable formulations containing the preservative benzyl alcohol are not recommended for use in neonates. There have been reports of fatal "gasping syndrome" in neonates (children less than 1 month of age) following the administrations of IV solutions containing the preservative benzyl alcohol. Symptoms including a striking onset of gasping respiration, hypotension, bradycardia, and cardiovascular collapse.

➤*Elderly:* Clinical studies of methotrexate did not include sufficient numbers of subjects aged 65 years and older to determine whether they respond differently from younger subjects. In general, dose selection for an elderly patient should be cautious, reflecting the greater frequency of decreased hepatic and renal function, decreased folate stores, concomitant disease or other drug therapy (ie, that interfere with renal function, methotrexate or folate metabolism) in this population. Since decline in renal function may be associated with increases in adverse events and serum creatinine measurements may overestimate renal function in the elderly, more accurate methods (ie, creatinine clearance) should be considered. Serum methotrexate levels may also be helpful. Elderly patients should be closely monitored for early signs of hepatic, bone marrow, and renal toxicity. In chronic use situations, certain toxicities may be reduced by folate supplementation. Postmarketing experience suggests that the occurrence of bone marrow suppression, thrombocytopenia, and pneumonitis may increase with age.

➤*Lab test abnormalities:* Transient liver function test abnormalities are observed frequently after methotrexate administration and are usually not cause for modification of methotrexate therapy. Persistent liver function test abnormalities, or depression of serum albumin may be indicators of serious liver toxicity and require evaluation.

A relationship between abnormal liver function tests and fibrosis or cirrhosis of the liver has not been established for patients with psoriasis. Persistent abnormalities in liver function tests may precede appearance of fibrosis or cirrhosis in the RA population.

Pulmonary function tests may be useful if methotrexate-induced lung disease is suspected, especially if baseline measurements are available.

➤*Monitoring:* Patients undergoing methotrexate therapy should be closely monitored so that toxic effects are detected promptly. Baseline assessment should include a complete blood count with differential and platelet counts, hepatic enzymes, renal function tests, and a chest x-ray. During therapy of RA and psoriasis, monitoring of these parameters is recommended: Hematology at least monthly, renal function and liver function every 1 to 2 months. More frequent monitoring is usually indicated during antineoplastic therapy. During initial or changing doses, or during periods of increased risk of elevated methotrexate blood levels (eg, dehydration), more frequent monitoring may also be indicated.

Toxic effects – Methotrexate has the potential for serious toxicity. Toxic effects may be related in frequency and severity to dose or frequency of administration but have been seen at all doses. Because they can occur at any time during therapy, it is necessary to follow patients on methotrexate closely. Most adverse reactions are reversible if detected early. When such reactions do occur, the drug should be reduced in dosage or discontinued, and appropriate corrective measures should be taken. If necessary, this could include the use of leucovorin calcium or acute, intermittent hemodialysis with a high-flux dialyzer. If methotrexate therapy is reinstituted, it should be carried out with caution, with adequate consideration of further need for the drug and with increased alertness as to possible recurrence of toxicity.

Drug Interactions

➤*NSAIDS/Salicylates:* Nonsteroidal anti-inflammatory drugs (NSAIDs) should not be administered prior to or concomitantly with the high doses of methotrexate used in the treatment of osteosarcoma. Concomitant administration of some NSAIDs with high-dose methotrexate therapy has been reported to elevate and prolong serum methotrexate levels, resulting in deaths from severe hematologic and GI toxicity.

Caution should be used when NSAIDs and salicylates are administered concomitantly with lower doses of methotrexate. These drugs have been reported to reduce the tubular secretion of methotrexate in an animal model and may enhance its toxicity.

➤*Salicylates, phenylbutazone, phenytoin, sulfonamides, probenecid:* Methotrexate is partially bound to serum albumin, and toxicity may be increased because of displacement by certain drugs, such as salicylates, phenylbutazone, phenytoin, and sulfonamides. Renal tubular transport is also diminished by probenecid; use of methotrexate with this drug should be carefully monitored.

➤*Cisplatin:* In the treatment of patients with osteosarcoma, caution must be exercised if high-dose methotrexate is administered in combination with a potentially nephrotoxic chemotherapeutic agent (eg, cisplatin).

➤*Mercaptopurine:* Methotrexate increases the plasma levels of mercaptopurine. The combination of methotrexate and mercaptopurine may therefore require dose adjustment.

➤*Oral antibiotics:* Oral antibiotics such as tetracycline, chloramphenicol, and nonabsorbable broad-spectrum antibiotics, may decrease intestinal absorption of methotrexate or interfere with the enterohepatic circulation by inhibiting bowel flora and suppressing metabolism of the drug by bacteria.

➤*Hepatotoxic agents:* The potential for increased hepatotoxicity when methotrexate is administered with other hepatotoxic agents has not been evaluated. However, hepatotoxicity has been reported in such cases. Therefore, patients receiving concomitant therapy with methotrexate and other potential hepatotoxins (eg, azathioprine, retinoids, sulfasalazine) should be monitored closely for possible increased risk of hepatotoxicity.

Methotrexate Injection Drug Interactions

Precipitant drug	Object drug[a]		Description
Aminoglycosides, oral	Methotrexate	⬇	The antitumorigenic actions of methotrexate may be decreased, but not predictably. Consider parenteral methotrexate if oral aminoglycosides are being coadministered.
Chloramphenicol	Methotrexate	⬇	Oral chloramphenicol may decrease intestinal absorption of methotrexate or interfere with the enterohepatic circulation by inhibiting bowel flora and suppressing metabolism of the drug by bacteria.
Folic acid	Methotrexate	⬇	Vitamin preparations containing folic acid or its derivatives may decrease responses to systemically administered methotrexate.
NSAIDs	Methotrexate	⬆	Concomitant administration of some NSAIDs with high dose methotrexate has been reported to elevate and prolong serum methotrexate levels, resulting in deaths from severe hematologic and GI toxicity. NSAIDs may reduce tubular secretion of methotrexate and enhance toxicity. Monitor renal impairment that could predispose to methotrexate toxicity, for signs of methotrexate toxicity, and methotrexate levels if indicated.
Penicillins	Methotrexate	⬆	Serum methotrexate concentrations may be elevated, increasing the risk of toxicity. Monitor for methotrexate toxicity and measure methotrexate concentrations twice a week for at least the first 2 weeks. If a broad-spectrum antibiotic is needed, ceftazidime may be less likely to interact.

METHOTREXATE SODIUM — INJECTION

Methotrexate Injection Drug Interactions

Precipitant drug	Object drug[a]		Description
Probenecid	Methotrexate	↑	Methotrexate plasma levels, therapeutic effects, and toxicity may be enhanced. Monitor methotrexate concentrations and adjust dose accordingly.
Salicylates	Methotrexate	↑	Increased toxic effects of methotrexate may occur. Salicylates may reduce tubular secretion of methotrexate and enhance toxicity. Consider monitoring methotrexate levels.
Sulfonamides	Methotrexate	↑	Sulfonamides may increase the risk of methotrexate-induced bone marrow suppression. Methotrexate may predispose patients to trimethoprim-sulfamethoxazole (TMP-SMZ)-induced megaloblastic anemia. Closely monitor patients for signs of hematologic toxicity.
Methotrexate	Sulfonamides		
Tetracyclines	Methotrexate	↑	Methotrexate concentrations may be elevated, increasing the risk of toxicity (eg, bone marrow suppression). If tetracyclines cannot be avoided in patients receiving high-dose methotrexate, closely monitor methotrexate plasma concentrations and patients for signs and symptoms of toxicity.
Trimethoprim	Methotrexate	↑	Trimethoprim may increase the risk of methotrexate-induced bone marrow suppression and megaloblastic anemia. If this drug combination cannot be avoided, closely monitor for signs of hematologic toxicity.
Methotrexate	Digoxin	↓	Serum levels of digoxin may be reduced and actions may be decreased. Monitor patient for signs of reduction in pharmacologic effect of digoxin and increase digoxin dose if necessary. Serum level monitoring may facilitate tailoring dosage.
Methotrexate	Phenytoin	↓	Serum concentrations of phenytoin may be decreased, resulting in a loss of therapeutic effect. Monitor phenytoin serum levels and adjust the phenytoin dosage appropriately. IV phenytoin may be useful.
Methotrexate	Theophylline	↑	Methotrexate may decrease the clearance of theophylline. Theophylline levels should be monitored when used concomitantly with methotrexate.
Methotrexate	Thiopurines (eg, azathioprine)	↑	The actions of thiopurines may be enhanced. Reduced thiopurine dosage may be used during coadministration with methotrexate.

[a] ↑ = object drug increased; ↓ = object drug decreased.

Adverse Reactions

The most frequently reported adverse reactions include ulcerative stomatitis, leukopenia, nausea, and abdominal distress. Other frequently reported adverse effects are malaise, undue fatigue, chills and fever, dizziness and decreased resistance to infection.

Methotrexate in doses of 250 mg/m^2 or more is considered to have moderate to high potential for nausea and vomiting. Methotrexate in doses of 100 to 250 mg/m^2 has moderate emetogenic potential. Methotrexate in lower doses has moderate to low emetogenic potential.

➤*Adverse reactions in oncology setting:*

Cardiovascular – Pericarditis, pericardial effusion, hypotension, and thromboembolic events (including arterial thrombosis, cerebral thrombosis, deep vein thrombosis, retinal vein thrombosis, thrombophlebitis, and pulmonary embolus).

CNS – Headaches, drowsiness, blurred vision, transient blindness, speech impairment including dysarthria and aphasia, hemiparesis, paresis and convulsions have also occurred following administration of methotrexate. Following low doses, there have been occasional reports of transient subtle cognitive dysfunction, mood alteration, unusual cranial sensations, leukoencephalopathy, or encephalopathy.

Dermatologic – Erythematous rashes, pruritus, urticaria, photosensitivity, pigmentary changes, alopecia, ecchymosis, telangiectasia, acne, furunculosis, erythema multiforme, toxic epidermal necrolysis, Stevens-Johnson syndrome, skin necrosis, and exfoliative dermatitis.

GI – Gingivitis, pharyngitis, stomatitis, anorexia, nausea, vomiting, diarrhea, hematemesis, melena, GI ulceration and bleeding, enteritis, pancreatitis.

GU – Severe nephropathy or renal failure, azotemia, cystitis, hematuria, proteinuria; defective oogenesis or spermatogenesis, transient oligospermia, menstrual dysfunction, vaginal discharge and gynecomastia; infertility, abortion, fetal death, fetal defects.

Hepatic – Hepatotoxicity, acute hepatitis, chronic fibrosis and cirrhosis, hepatic failure, decrease in serum albumin, liver enzyme elevations.

Hematologic/Lymphatic – Suppressed hematopoiesis, anemia, aplastic anemia, pancytopenia, leukopenia, neutropenia, thrombocytopenia, agranulocytosis, eosinophilia, lymphadenopathy, and lymphoproliferative disorders (including reversible).

Hypogammaglobulinemia has been reported rarely.

Musculoskeletal – Stress fracture.

Ophthalmic – Conjunctivitis, serious visual changes of unknown etiology.

Pulmonary – Respiratory fibrosis, respiratory failure, alveolitis, interstitial pneumonitis deaths have been reported, and chronic interstitial obstructive pulmonary disease has occasionally occurred.

Miscellaneous –

Infection: There have been case reports of sometimes fatal opportunistic infections in patients receiving methotrexate therapy for neoplastic and non-neoplastic diseases. *Pneumocystis carinii* pneumonia was the most common opportunistic infection. There have also been reports of infections, pneumonia, cytomegalovirus infection, including cytomegaloviral pneumonia, sepsis, fatal sepsis, nocardiosis; histoplasmosis, cryptococcosis, *Herpes zoster*, *H. simplex* hepatitis, and disseminated *H. simplex*.

Other: Other rarer reactions related to or attributed to the use of methotrexate such as nodulosis; vasculitis; arthralgia/myalgia; loss of libido/impotence; diabetes; osteoporosis; sudden death; lymphoma, including reversible lymphomas; tumor lysis syndrome; soft tissue necrosis; and osteonecrosis. Anaphylactoid reactions have been reported.

➤*Adverse reactions in double-blind RA studies:*

Incidence greater than 10% – Elevated liver function tests 15%, nausea/vomiting 10%.

Incidence 3% to 10% – Stomatitis, thrombocytopenia (platelet count less than 100,000/mm^3).

Incidence 1% to 3% – Rash/pruritus/dermatitis, diarrhea, alopecia, leukopenia (WBC less than 3,000/mm^3), pancytopenia, dizziness.

Two other controlled trials of patients (n = 680) with RA on 7.5 mg to 15 mg/week oral doses showed an incidence of interstitial pneumonitis of 1%.

Other less common reactions included decreased hematocrit, headache, upper respiratory tract infection, anorexia, arthralgias, chest pain, coughing, dysuria, eye discomfort, epistaxis, fever, infection, sweating, tinnitus, and vaginal discharge.

➤*Adverse reactions in JRA studies:* The approximate incidences of adverse reactions reported in pediatric patients with JRA treated with oral, weekly doses of methotrexate (5 to 20 mg/m^2/week or 0.1 to 0.65 mg/kg/week) were as follows (virtually all patients were receiving concomitant nonsteroidal anti-inflammatory drugs, and some also were taking low-dose corticosteroids): Elevated liver function tests, 14%; GI reactions (eg, nausea, vomiting, diarrhea), 11%; stomatitis, 2%; leukopenia, 2%; headache, 1.2%; alopecia, 0.5%; dizziness, 0.2%; and rash, 0.2%. Although there is experience with dosing up to 30 mg/m^2/week in JRA, the published data for doses above 20 mg/m^2/week are too limited to provide reliable estimates of adverse reaction rates.

Overdosage

➤*Symptoms:* Symptoms of intrathecal overdosage are generally CNS symptoms, including headache, nausea and vomiting, seizure and convulsion, and acute toxic encephalopathy. In some cases, no symptoms were reported. There have been reports of death following intrathecal overdose. In these cases, cerebellar herniation associated with increased intracranial pressure, and acute toxic encephalopathy have also been reported.

➤*Treatment:* Leucovorin is indicated to diminish the toxicity and counteract the effect of inadvertently administered overdosages of methotrexate. Leucovorin administration should begin as promptly as possible. As the time interval between methotrexate administration and leucovorin initiation increases, the effectiveness of leucovorin in counteracting toxicity decreases. Monitoring of the serum methotrexate concentration is essential in determining the optimal dose and duration of treatment with leucovorin.

In cases of massive overdosage, hydration and urinary alkalinization may be necessary to prevent the precipitation of methotrexate or its metabolites in the renal tubules. Generally speaking, neither hemodialysis nor peritoneal dialysis have been shown to improve methotrexate elimination. However, effective clearance of methotrexate has been reported with acute intermittent hemodialysis using a high-flux dialyzer (Wall SM, et al. *Am J Kidney Dis.* 1996;28[6]:846-854.)

METHOTREXATE SODIUM — INJECTION

Accidental intrathecal overdosage may require intensive systemic support, high-dose systemic leucovorin, alkaline diuresis and rapid CSF drainage and ventriculolumbar perfusion.

There are published case reports of IV and intrathecal carboxypeptidase G2 treatment to hasten clearance of methotrexate in cases of overdose.

Patient Information

Patients should be informed of the early signs and symptoms of toxicity, of the need to see their physicians promptly if they occur, and the need for close follow-up, including periodic laboratory tests to monitor toxicity.

Both the physician and pharmacist should emphasize to the patient that the recommended dose is taken weekly in RA and psoriasis, and that mistaken daily use of the recommended dose has led to fatal toxicity. Patients should be encouraged to read the Patient Instructions sheet within the dose pack. Prescriptions should not be written or refilled on an as-needed basis.

Patients should be informed of the potential benefit and risk in the use of methotrexate. The risk of effects on reproduction should be discussed with both male and female patients taking methotrexate.

PEMETREXED

Rx	Alimta (Eli Lilly)	Injection, lyophilized powder for solution: 100 mg	As pemetrexed disodium. Preservative free. Mannitol 106 mg. In single-use vials.
		500 mg	As pemetrexed disodium. Preservative free. Mannitol 500 mg. In single-use vials.

PEMETREXED DISODIUM — INJECTION

Indications

➤*Malignant pleural mesothelioma:* In combination with cisplatin for the treatment of patients with malignant pleural mesothelioma whose disease is unresectable or who are otherwise not candidates for curative surgery.

➤*Nonsquamous non–small cell lung cancer:* As a single agent for the treatment of patients with locally advanced or metastatic nonsquamous non–small cell lung cancer after prior chemotherapy; in combination with cisplatin therapy for the initial treatment of patients with locally advanced or metastatic nonsquamous non–small cell lung cancer; for the maintenance treatment of patients with locally advanced or metastatic nonsquamous non–small cell lung cancer whose disease has not progressed after 4 cycles of platinum-based first-line chemotherapy.

Administration and Dosage

➤*Adults:*

Malignant pleural mesothelioma –

Usual dosage: 500 mg/m^2 administered as an intravenous (IV) infusion over 10 minutes on day 1 of each 21-day cycle.

Dosage adjustment: Dose adjustments at the start of a subsequent cycle should be based on nadir hematologic counts or maximum nonhematologic toxicity from the preceding cycle of therapy. Treatment may be delayed to allow sufficient time for recovery.

Patients should not begin a new cycle of treatment unless the absolute neutrophil count (ANC) is 1,500 cells/mm^3 or more, the platelet count is 100,000 cells/mm^3 or more, and creatine clearance (CrCl) is 45 mL/min or more. Upon recovery, re-treat patients. If patients develop nonhematologic toxicities (excluding neurotoxicity) of grade 3 or higher, withhold treatment until resolution to less than or equal to the patient's pretherapy value.

• *Hematologic toxicity –*

Dose Reduction for Pemetrexed (Single Agent or in Combination) and Cisplatin: Hematologic Toxicities	
Nadir ANC < 500/mm^3 and nadir platelets ≥ 50,000/mm^3	75% of previous dose (pemetrexed and cisplatin)
Nadir platelets < 50,000/mm^3 without bleeding regardless of nadir ANC	75% of previous dose (pemetrexed and cisplatin)
Nadir platelets < 50,000/mm^3 with bleeding[a] regardless of nadir ANC	50% of previous dose (pemetrexed and cisplatin)

[a] These criteria meet Common Toxicity Criteria (CTC) version 2.0 (National Cancer Institute [NCI] 1998) definition of ≥ CTC grade 2 bleeding.

• *Nonhematologic toxicity –*

Dose Reduction for Pemetrexed (Single Agent or in Combination) and Cisplatin: Nonhematologic Toxicities[a,b]	Dose of pemetrexed (mg/m^2)	Dose of cisplatin (mg/m^2)
Any grade 3 or 4 toxicities except mucositis	75% of previous dose	75% of previous dose
Any diarrhea requiring hospitalization (irrespective of grade) or grade 3 or 4 diarrhea	75% of previous dose	75% of previous dose
Grade 3 or 4 mucositis	50% of previous dose	100% of previous dose

[a] NCI CTC.
[b] Excluding neurotoxicity.

• *Neurotoxicity –*

CTC grade	Dose of pemetrexed (mg/m^2)	Dose of cisplatin (mg/m^2)
0 to 1	100% of previous dose	100% of previous dose
2	100% of previous dose	50% of previous dose

Table title: Dose Reduction for Pemetrexed (Single Agent or in Combination) and Cisplatin: Neurotoxicity

Concomitant therapy: Cisplatin 75 mg/m^2 infused over 2 hours beginning approximately 30 minutes after the end of pemetrexed administration. Give patients appropriate hydration prior to and/or after receiving cisplatin. Refer to the cisplatin monograph for more information.

Nonsquamous non–small cell lung cancer –

Usual dosage: 500 mg/m^2 administered as an IV infusion over 10 minutes on day 1 of each 21-day cycle when used as a single agent or in combination with cisplatin.

Dosage adjustment: See Malignant Pleural Mesothelioma.

Concomitant therapy: See Malignant Pleural Mesothelioma.

➤*Elderly:* Pemetrexed is known to be substantially excreted by the kidney, and the risk of adverse reactions to this drug may be greater in patients with impaired renal function. Because elderly patients are more likely to have decreased renal function, care should be taken in dose selection.

➤*Renal function impairment:* Exercise caution when coadministering pemetrexed with nonsteroidal anti-inflammatory drugs (NSAIDs) to patients whose CrCl is less than 80 mL/min.

Insufficient numbers of patients with CrCl less than 45 mL/min have been treated to make dosage recommendations for this group of patients. Therefore, pemetrexed should not be administered to patients whose CrCl is less than 45 mL/min using the standard Cockcroft and Gault formula or glomerular filtration rate measured by Tc99m-DPTA serum clearance method.

➤*Premedication:*

Corticosteroid – Pretreatment with dexamethasone (or equivalent) reduces the incidence and severity of cutaneous reaction. In clinical trials, dexamethasone 4 mg was given by mouth twice daily the day before, the day of, and the day after pemetrexed administration. Skin rash has been reported more frequently in patients not pretreated with a corticosteroid.

Vitamin supplementation – To reduce toxicity, instruct patients treated with pemetrexed to take a low-dose oral folic acid preparation or multivitamin with folic acid on a daily basis. At least 5 daily doses of folic acid must be taken during the 7-day period preceding the first dose of pemetrexed; dosing should continue during the full course of therapy and for 21 days after the last dose of pemetrexed. Patients must also receive 1 intramuscular (IM) injection of vitamin B_{12} during the week preceding the first dose of pemetrexed and every 3 cycles thereafter. Subsequent vitamin B_{12} injections may be given the same day as pemetrexed. In clinical trials, the dose of folic acid studied ranged from 350 to 1,000 mcg, and the dose of vitamin B_{12} was 1,000 mcg. The most commonly used dose of oral folic acid in clinical trials was 400 mcg.

➤*Discontinuation of therapy:* Discontinue pemetrexed therapy if a patient experiences any hematologic or nonhematologic grade 3 or 4 toxicity after 2 dose reductions, or immediately if grade 3 or 4 neurotoxicity is observed.

➤*Preparation for administration:* Reconstitute each 100 mg vial with 4.2 mL of sodium chloride 0.9% injection (preservative free). Reconstitute 500 mg vials with 20 mL of sodium chloride 0.9% injection (preservative free). Reconstitution of either size vial gives a solution containing pemetrexed 25 mg/mL. Gently swirl each vial until the powder is completely dissolved. Further dilution is required.

An appropriate quantity of the reconstituted pemetrexed solution must be further diluted into a solution of sodium chloride 0.9% injection (preservative free), so that the total volume of solution is 100 mL.

➤*Administration:* Pemetrexed is administered as an IV infusion over 10 minutes. Pemetrexed is compatible with standard polyvinyl chloride (PVC) administration sets and IV solution bags.

➤*Admixture compatibility:* Reconstitution and further dilution prior to IV infusion is only recommended with sodium chloride 0.9% injection (preservative free). Pemetrexed is physically incompatible with diluents containing calcium, including Ringer's lactate injection and Ringer's injection; therefore, these should not be used. Coadministration of pemetrexed with other drugs and diluents has not been studied and is therefore not recommended.

➤*Storage/Stability:* Store at 25°C (77°F); excursions are permitted between 15° and 30°C (59° and 86°F).

Chemical and physical stability of reconstituted and infusion solutions of pemetrexed were demonstrated for up to 24 hours following initial reconstitution when stored refrigerated between 2° and 8°C (36° and 46°F) or at 25°C (77°F); excursions are permitted to 15° to 30°C (59° to 86°F). When pre-

PEMETREXED DISODIUM — INJECTION

pared as directed, reconstituted and infusion solutions of pemetrexed contain no antimicrobial preservatives. Discard unused portion.

Actions

➤*Pharmacology:* Pemetrexed is a folate analog metabolic inhibitor that exerts its action by disrupting folate-dependent metabolic processes essential for cell replication. In vitro studies have shown that pemetrexed inhibits thymidylate synthase (TS), dihydrofolate reductase (DHFR), and glycinamide ribonucleotide formyltransferase (GARFT), all folate-dependent enzymes involved in the de novo biosynthesis of thymidine and purine nucleotides. Pemetrexed is transported into cells by both the reduced folate carrier and membrane folate binding protein transport systems. Once in the cell, pemetrexed is converted to polyglutamate forms by the enzyme folylpolyglutamate synthetase. The polyglutamate forms are retained in cells and are inhibitors of TS and GARFT. Polyglutamation is a time- and concentration-dependent process that occurs in tumor cells and, to a lesser extent, in normal tissues. Polyglutamated metabolites have an increased intracellular half-life, resulting in prolonged drug action in malignant cells.

➤*Pharmacokinetics:*

Absorption/Distribution – Pemetrexed total AUC and maximum plasma concentration (C_{max}) increase proportionally with dose. Pemetrexed has a steady-state volume of distribution of 16.1 L. In vitro studies indicate that pemetrexed is approximately 81% bound to plasma proteins. Binding is not affected by degree of renal impairment.

Metabolism/Excretion – Pemetrexed is not metabolized to an appreciable extent.

Pemetrexed is primarily eliminated in the urine, with 70% to 90% of the dose recovered unchanged within the first 24 hours following administration. The total systemic clearance of pemetrexed is 91.8 mL/min, and the elimination half-life of pemetrexed is 3.5 hours in patients with healthy renal function (CrCl of 90 mL/min). The clearance decreases and exposure (AUC) increases as renal function decreases.

Special populations –

Renal function impairment: Pharmacokinetic analyses of pemetrexed included 127 patients with reduced renal function. Plasma clearance of pemetrexed decreases as renal function decreases, with increase in systemic exposure. Patients with CrCl of 45, 50, and 80 mL/min had 65%, 54%, and 13% increases, respectively, in pemetrexed total AUC compared with patients with CrCl of 100 mL/min.

Contraindications

History of severe hypersensitivity reaction to pemetrexed or any other ingredient used in the formulation.

Warnings/Precautions

➤*Premedication:* Patients treated with pemetrexed must be instructed to take folic acid and vitamin B_{12} as a prophylactic measure to reduce treatment-related hematologic and GI toxicity. In clinical studies, less overall toxicity and reductions in grade 3 or 4 hematologic and nonhematologic toxicities, such as neutropenia, febrile neutropenia, and infection with grade 3 or 4 neutropenia, were reported when pretreatment with folic acid and vitamin B_{12} was administered. (See Administration and Dosage for more information.)

Skin rash has been reported more frequently in patients not pretreated with a corticosteroid in clinical trials. Pretreatment with dexamethasone (or equivalent) reduces the incidence and severity of cutaneous reaction.

➤*Bone marrow suppression:* Pemetrexed can suppress bone marrow function, manifested by neutropenia, thrombocytopenia, and anemia (or pancytopenia); myelosuppression is usually the dose-limiting toxicity. Dose reductions for subsequent cycles are based on nadir ANC, platelet count, and maximum nonhematologic toxicity seen in the previous cycle.

➤*Third space fluid:* The effect of third space fluid, such as pleural effusion and ascites, on pemetrexed is unknown. In patients with clinically significant third space fluid, consider draining the effusion prior to pemetrexed administration.

➤*Renal function impairment:* See Administration and Dosage for more information.

One patient with severe renal impairment (CrCl 19 mL/min) who did not receive folic acid and vitamin B_{12} died of drug-related toxicity following administration of pemetrexed alone.

➤*Pregnancy: Category D.* Based on its mechanism of action, pemetrexed can cause fetal harm when administered to a pregnant woman. There are no adequate and well controlled studies of pemetrexed in pregnant women. Pemetrexed administered intraperitoneally to mice during organogenesis was embryotoxic, fetotoxic, and teratogenic. In mice, repeated intraperitoneal doses of pemetrexed when given during organogenesis caused fetal malformations (incomplete ossification of talus and skull bone; about 1/833 the recommended IV human dose on a mg/m^2 basis), and cleft palate (1/33 the recommended IV human dose on a mg/m^2 basis). Embryotoxicity was characterized by increased embryo-fetal deaths and reduced litter sizes. If pemetrexed is used during pregnancy, or if the patient becomes pregnant while taking this drug, apprise the patient of the potential hazard to the fetus. Advise women to avoid becoming pregnant. Advise women to use effective contraceptive measures to prevent pregnancy during treatment with pemetrexed.

➤*Lactation:* It is not known whether pemetrexed or its metabolites are excreted in human milk. The molecular weight (about 471 for the nonhydrated form), moderate (81%) plasma protein binding, and the elimination half-life (3.5 hours) suggest that the drug will be excreted into breast milk. Because many drugs are excreted in human milk, and because of the potential for serious adverse reactions in breast-feeding infants from pemetrexed, it is recommended that breast-feeding be discontinued if the mother is treated with pemetrexed.

Holding breastfeeding for 18 to 24 hours while "pumping and dumping," would allow the drug to be nearly eliminated from the mother's circulation and lessen the risk to a nursing infant. However, breastfeeding is not recommended if the therapy includes cisplatin.

➤*Children:* The safety and effectiveness of pemetrexed in children have not been established.

➤*Elderly:* Pemetrexed is known to be substantially excreted by the kidney, and the risk of adverse reactions to this drug may be greater in patients with impaired renal function. Because elderly patients are more likely to have decreased renal function, care should be taken in dose selection. Renal function monitoring is recommended with administration of pemetrexed.

➤*Monitoring:* Perform complete blood cell counts, including platelet counts, on all patients receiving pemetrexed. Monitor patients for nadir and recovery (which were tested in the clinical study before each dose and on days 8 and 15 of each cycle). Patients should not begin a new cycle of treatment unless the ANC is 1,500 cells/mm^3 or more, the platelet count is 100,000 cells/mm^3 or more, and CrCl is 45 mL/min or higher. Perform periodic chemistry tests to evaluate renal and hepatic function.

Drug Interactions

Pemetrexed Drug Interactions

Precipitant drug	Object drug[a]		Description
Nephrotoxic agents	Pemetrexed	↑	Coadministration of nephrotoxic drugs could result in delayed clearance of pemetrexed. Coadministration of substances that also are tubularly secreted (eg, probenecid) could potentially result in delayed clearance of pemetrexed.
NSAIDs (eg, ibuprofen)	Pemetrexed	↑	Daily ibuprofen dosages of 400 mg 4 times per day reduce pemetrexed's clearance about 20% (and increase AUC 20%) in patients with healthy renal function. Use caution when coadministering ibuprofen with pemetrexed to patients with mild to moderate renal insufficiency (CrCl of 45 to 79 mL/min), and avoid giving NSAIDs with short elimination half-lives 2 days before, the day of, and 2 days following pemetrexed administration. Interrupt dosing in all patients taking NSAIDs with long elimination half-lives for at least 5 days before, the day of, and 2 days following pemetrexed administration. If coadministration of an NSAID is necessary, closely monitor patients for toxicity, especially myelosuppression, renal toxicity, and GI toxicity.

[a] ↑ = object drug increased.

Adverse Reactions

➤*Malignant pleural mesothelioma:*

Pemetrexed Adverse Reactions in Patients With Malignant Pleural Mesothelioma (> 5%)[a,b]

Adverse reaction[c]	Pemetrexed/Cisplatin (n = 168)		Cisplatin (n = 163)	
	All grades	Grade 3 to 4	All grades	Grade 3 to 4
CNS				
Fatigue	48%	10%	42%	9%
Neuropathy-sensory	10%	0%	10%	1%
Dermatologic				
Alopecia	11%	0%[d]	6%	0%[d]
Rash	16%	1%	5%	0%
GI				
Anorexia	20%	1%	14%	1%
Constipation	12%	1%	7%	1%
Diarrhea	17%	4%	8%	0%
Dyspepsia	5%	1%	1%	0%

PEMETREXED DISODIUM — INJECTION

Pemetrexed Adverse Reactions in Patients With Malignant Pleural Mesothelioma (> 5%)[a,b]				
Adverse reaction[c]	Pemetrexed/Cisplatin (n = 168)		Cisplatin (n = 163)	
Nausea	82%	12%	77%	6%
Stomatitis/ Pharyngitis	23%	3%	6%	0%
Taste disturbance	8%	0%[d]	6%	0%[d]
Vomiting	57%	11%	50%	4%
Hematologic				
Anemia	26%	4%	10%	0%
Leukopenia	53%	15%	17%	1%
Neutropenia	56%	23%	13%	3%
Thrombocytopenia	23%	5%	9%	0%
Renal				
CrCl decreased	16%	1%	18%	2%
Creatinine elevation	11%	1%	10%	1%
Miscellaneous				
Conjunctivitis	5%	0%	1%	0%
Dehydration	7%	4%	1%	1%

[a] For the purpose of this table, a cutoff of 5% was used for inclusion of all reactions in which the reporter considered a possible relationship to pemetrexed.
[b] In both treatment arms, these chemo-naive patients were fully supplemented with folic acid and vitamin B_{12}.
[c] Refer to NCI CTC version 2.0 for each grade of toxicity, except the term "creatinine clearance decreased," which is derived from the CTC term "renal/genitourinary-other."
[d] According to NCI CTC version 2.0, this adverse reaction term should only be reported as grade 1 or 2.

Additional adverse reactions –
Metabolic/Nutritional: Increased ALT, increased AST, increased gamma-glutamyl transferase (1% to 5%).
Miscellaneous: Chest pain, febrile neutropenia, infection, pyrexia, renal failure, urticaria (1% to 5%); arrhythmia, motor neuropathy (less than 1%).

➤*Non–small cell lung cancer, combination use with cisplatin:* All patients received study therapy as initial treatment for locally advanced or metastatic non–small cell lung cancer, and patients in both treatment groups were fully supplemented with folic acid and vitamin B_{12}.

Pemetrexed + Cisplatin Adverse Reactions in Fully Supplemented Patients With Non–Small Cell Lung Cancer (≥ 5%)[a]				
	Pemetrexed/Cisplatin (n = 839)		Gemcitabine/Cisplatin (n = 830)	
Adverse reaction[b]	All grades	Grade 3 to 4	All grades	Grade 3 to 4
All adverse reactions	90%	37%	91%	53%
CNS				
Fatigue	43%	7%	45%	5%
Neuropathy-sensory	9%	0%	12%	1%
Dermatologic				
Alopecia	12%	0%[c]	21%	1%[c]
Rash/Desquamation	7%	0%	8%	1%
GI				
Anorexia	27%	2%	24%	1%
Constipation	21%	1%	20%	0%
Diarrhea	12%	1%	13%	2%
Dyspepsia/Heartburn	5%	0%	6%	0%
Nausea	56%	7%	53%	4%
Stomatitis/Pharyngitis	14%	1%	12%	0%
Taste disturbance	8%	0%[c]	9%	0%[c]
Vomiting	40%	6%	36%	6%
Hematologic/Lymphatic				
Anemia	33%	6%	46%	10%
Leukopenia	18%	5%	21%	8%
Neutropenia	29%	15%	38%	27%
Thrombocytopenia	10%	4%	27%	13%
Miscellaneous				
Creatinine elevation	10%	1%	7%	1%

[a] For the purpose of this table, a cutoff of 5% was used for inclusion of all reactions in which the reporter considered a possible relationship to pemetrexed.
[b] Refer to NCI CTC version 2.0 for each grade of toxicity.
[c] According to NCI CTC version 2.0, this adverse reaction term should only be reported as grade 1 or 2.

Additional adverse reactions –
Metabolic/Nutritional: Increased ALT, increased AST (1% to 5%); increased gamma-glutamyl transferase (less than 1%).
Renal: CrCl decrease, renal failure (1% to 5%).
Miscellaneous: Conjunctivitis, dehydration, febrile neutropenia, infection, pyrexia (1% to 5%); arrhythmia, chest pain, motor neuropathy (less than 1%).

➤*Non–Small Cell Lung Cancer — maintenance:* All patients received study therapy immediately following 4 cycles of platinum-based treatment for locally advanced or metastatic non–small cell lung cancer. Patients in both study arms were fully supplemented with folic acid and vitamin B_{12}.

Pemetrexed Adverse Reactions in Non–Small Cell Lung Cancer[a]				
	Pemetrexed (n = 438)		Placebo (n = 218)	
Adverse reaction[b]	All grades	Grade 3 to 4	All grades	Grade 3 to 4
All adverse reactions	66%	16%	37%	4%
CNS				
Fatigue	25%	5%	11%	1%
Neuropathy-sensory	9%	1%	4%	0%
GI				
Anorexia	19%	2%	5%	0%
Diarrhea	5%	1%	3%	0%
Mucositis/Stomatitis	7%	1%	2%	0%
Nausea	19%	1%	6%	1%
Vomiting	9%	0%	1%	0%
Hematologic/Lymphatic				
Anemia	15%	3%	6%	1%
Leukopenia	6%	2%	1%	1%
Neutropenia	6%	3%	0%	0%
Hepatic				
Increased ALT	10%	0%	4%	0%
Increased AST	8%	0%	4%	0%
Miscellaneous				
Infection	5%	2%	2%	0%
Rash/Desquamation	10%	0%	3%	0%

[a] For the purpose of this table a cut off of 5% was used for inclusion of all reactions where the reporter considered a possible relationship to pemetrexed.
[b] Refer to NCI Common Terminology Criteria for Adverse Events version 3.0 for each grade of toxicity.

No clinically relevant differences in grade 3/4 adverse reactions were seen in patients based on age, gender, ethnic origin, or histology except a higher incidence of grade 3/4 fatigue for white patients compared with nonwhite patients (6.5% vs 0.6%).

Safety was assessed by exposure for patients who received at least 1 dose of pemetrexed (n = 438). The incidence of adverse reactions was evaluated for patients who received 6 cycles or less of pemetrexed, and compared with patients who received more than 6 cycles of pemetrexed. Increases in adverse reactions (all grades) were observed with longer exposure; however, no clinically relevant differences in grade 3/4 adverse reactions were seen.

Consistent with the higher incidence of anemia (all grades) on the pemetrexed arm, use of transfusions (mainly RBC) and erythropoiesis stimulating agents (ESAs) erythropoietin and darbepoetin) were higher in the pemetrexed arm compared with the placebo arm (transfusions 9.5% vs 3.2%, ESAs 5.9% vs 1.8%).

Additional adverse reactions –
Dermatologic: Alopecia, pruritus/itching (1% to 5%); erythema multiforme (less than 1%).
Hematologic: Thrombocytopenia (1% to 5%); febrile neutropenia (less than 1%).
Renal: Decreased CrCl, decreased glomerular filtration rate (1% to 5%), increased creatinine; renal failure (less than 1%).
Special senses: Increased lacrimation (1% to 5%), ocular surface disease (including conjunctivitis).

PEMETREXED DISODIUM — INJECTION

Miscellaneous: Constipation, edema, fever (in the absence of neutropenia) (1% to 5%); allergic reaction/hypersensitivity, motor neuropathy, supraventricular arrhythmia (less than 1%).

➤*Non–small cell lung cancer, after prior chemotherapy:*

Pemetrexed Adverse Reactions in Fully Supplemented Patients With Non-Small Cell Lung Cancer Who Had Received Prior Chemotherapy (> 5%)[a,b]

Adverse reaction	Pemetrexed (n = 265) All grades	Pemetrexed (n = 265) Grade 3 to 4	Docetaxel (n = 276) All grades	Docetaxel (n = 276) Grade 3 to 4
CNS				
Fatigue	34%	5%	36%	5%
Fever	8%	0%	8%	0%
Dermatologic				
Alopecia	6%	1%[c]	38%	2%[c]
Pruritus	7%	0%	2%	0%
Rash/Desquamation	14%	0%	6%	0%
GI				
Anorexia	22%	2%	24%	3%
Constipation	6%	0%	4%	0%
Diarrhea	13%	0%	24%	3%
Nausea	31%	3%	17%	2%
Stomatitis/Pharyngitis	15%	1%	17%	1%
Vomiting	16%	2%	12%	1%
Hematologic				
Anemia	19%	4%	22%	4%
Leukopenia	12%	4%	34%	27%
Neutropenia	11%	5%	45%	40%
Thrombocytopenia	8%	2%	1%	0%
Hepatic				
ALT elevation	8%	2%	1%	0%
AST elevation	7%	1%	1%	0%

[a] For the purpose of this table, a cutoff of 5% was used for inclusion of all reactions in which the reporter considered a possible relationship to pemetrexed.
[b] Refer to NCI CTC for lab values for each grade of toxicity (version 2.0).
[c] According to NCI CTC version 2.0, report this adverse reaction term as grade 1 or 2.

Additional adverse reactions –

Cardiovascular: Supraventricular arrhythmias (less than 1%).
CNS: Motor neuropathy, sensory neuropathy (1% to 5%).
Dermatologic: Erythema multiforme (1% to 5%).
GI: Abdominal pain (1% to 5%).
Renal: Increased creatinine (1% to 5%).
Miscellaneous: Allergic reaction/hypersensitivity, febrile neutropenia, infection (1% to 5%).

➤*Effects of vitamin supplementations:*

Selected Grade 3/4 Adverse Reactions Comparing Fully Supplemented[a] vs Never Supplemented Patients in the Pemetrexed + Cisplatin Arm

Adverse reaction[b]	Fully supplemented patients (n = 168)	Never supplemented patients (n = 32)
GI		
Diarrhea	4%	9%
Vomiting	11%	31%
Hematologic/Lymphatic		
Febrile neutropenia	1%	9%
Infection with grade 3/4 neutropenia	0%	6%
Neutropenia/Granulocytopenia	23%	38%
Thrombocytopenia	5%	9%

[a] Daily folic acid and vitamin B_{12} supplementation.
[b] Refer to NCI CTC for lab and nonlaboratory values for each grade of toxicity (version 2.0). The following adverse reactions were greater in the fully supplemented group compared with the never supplemented group: chest pain (8%, 6%), hypertension (11%, 3%), and thrombosis/embolism (6%, 3%).

➤*Postmarketing:* These reactions have occurred with pemetrexed when used as a single agent and in combination therapies.

GI – Colitis.

Respiratory – Interstitial pneumonitis.

Miscellaneous – Edema; radiation recall has been reported in patients who have previously received radiotherapy.

Overdosage

➤*Symptoms:* There have been few cases of pemetrexed overdose. Reported toxicities included neutropenia, anemia, thrombocytopenia, mucositis, and rash. Anticipated complications of overdose include bone marrow suppression as manifested by neutropenia, thrombocytopenia, and anemia. In addition, infection with or without fever, diarrhea, and mucositis may be seen.

➤*Treatment:* If an overdose occurs, institute general supportive measures as deemed necessary by the treating health care provider.

In clinical trials, leucovorin was permitted for CTC grade 4 leukopenia lasting 3 days or longer, CTC grade 4 neutropenia lasting 3 days or longer, and immediately for CTC grade 4 thrombocytopenia, bleeding associated with grade 3 thrombocytopenia, or grade 3 or 4 mucositis. The following IV dose and schedule of leucovorin was recommended for IV use: 100 mg/m^2 IV once, followed by 50 mg/m^2 IV every 6 hours for 8 days.

The ability of pemetrexed to be dialyzed is unknown.

Patient Information

Instruct patients treated with pemetrexed to take folic acid and vitamin B_{12} as a prophylactic measure to reduce treatment-related hematologic and GI toxicity.

Inform patients of the risk of low blood cell counts and instruct them to immediately contact their health care provider if any sign of infection develop, including fever. Instruct patients to contact their health care provider if bleeding or symptoms of anemia occur.

Instruct patients to contact their health care provider if persistent vomiting, diarrhea, or signs of dehydration appear.

Instruct patients to inform their health care provider if they are taking any concomitant prescription or nonprescription medications, including those for pain or inflammation, such as NSAIDs.

Advise women to use effective contraceptive measures to prevent pregnancy during treatment with pemetrexed.

PRALATREXATE

Rx	**Folotyn** (Allos Therapeutics Inc)	**Injection, solution:** 20 mg/mL	Preservative free. In 1 mL and 2 mL single-use vials.

PRALATREXATE — INJECTION

Indications

➤*Peripheral T-cell lymphoma:* For the treatment of patients with relapsed or refractory peripheral T-cell lymphoma.

Administration and Dosage

➤*General dosing considerations:* Dosage may need to be adjusted based on hematologic and nonhematologic toxicities. (See Dosage Adjustment.)

➤*Adults:*

Peripheral T-cell lymphoma –

Usual dosage: 30 mg/m^2 administered as an intravenous (IV) push over 3 to 5 minutes via the side port of a free flowing sodium chloride 0.9% injection IV line once weekly for 6 weeks in 7-week cycles until progressive disease or unacceptable toxicity.

Dosage adjustment: Prior to administering any dose of pralatrexate, mucositis should be grade 1 or less, platelet count should be 100,000/mcL or more for the first dose and 50,000/mcL for all subsequent doses, and absolute neutrophil count (ANC) should be 1,000/mcL or more.

Management of severe or intolerable adverse reactions may require dose omission, reduction, or interruption of pralatrexate therapy.

Doses may be omitted or reduced based on patient tolerance. Omitted doses will not be made up at the end of the cycle; once a dose reduction occurs for toxicity, do not re-escalate.

Pralatrexate Dose Modifications for Mucositis

Mucositis grade[a] on day of treatment	Action	Dose upon recovery to ≤ grade 1
Grade 2	Omit dose	Continue prior dose
Grade 2 recurrence	Omit dose	20 mg/m^2
Grade 3	Omit dose	20 mg/m^2
Grade 4	Stop therapy	

[a] Per the National Cancer Institute Common Terminology Criteria for Adverse Events (NCI CTCAE, version 3.0).

PRALATREXATE — INJECTION

Pralatrexate Dose Modifications for Hematologic Toxicities			
Blood cell count on day of treatment	Duration of toxicity	Action	Dose upon restart
Platelet < 50,000/mcL	1 week	Omit dose	Continue prior dose
	2 weeks	Omit dose	20 mg/m^2
	3 weeks	Stop therapy	
ANC 500 to 1,000/mcL and no fever	1 week	Omit dose	Continue prior dose
ANC 500 to 1,000/mcL with fever or ANC < 500/mcL	1 week	Omit dose, give G-CSF[a] or GM-CSF[a] support	Continue prior dose with G-CSF or GM-CSF support
	2 weeks or recurrence	Omit dose, give G-CSF or GM-CSF support	20 mg/m^2 with G-CSF or GM-CSF support
	3 weeks or second recurrence	Stop therapy	

[a] G-CSF = granulocyte colony-stimulating factor; GM-CSF = granulocyte-macrophage colony-stimulating factor.

Pralatrexate Dose Modifications for All Other Treatment-Related Toxicities		
Toxicity grade[a] on day of treatment	Action	Dose upon recovery to ≤ grade 2
Grade 3	Omit dose	20 mg/m^2
Grade 4	Stop therapy	

[a] Per NCI CTCAE, version 3.0.

Concomitant therapy:

• *Folic acid* – Patients should take low-dose (1 to 1.25 mg) oral folic acid on a daily basis. Folic acid should be initiated during the 10-day period preceding the first dose of pralatrexate, and dosing should continue during the full course of therapy and for 30 days after the last dose of pralatrexate.

• *Vitamin B_{12}* – Patients should also receive a vitamin B_{12} (1 mg) intramuscular injection no more than 10 weeks prior to the first dose of pralatrexate and every 8 to 10 weeks thereafter. Subsequent vitamin B_{12} injections may be given the same day as treatment with pralatrexate.

Monitoring: Complete blood cell counts and severity of mucositis should be monitored weekly. Serum chemistry tests, including renal and hepatic function, should be performed prior to the start of the first and fourth dose of a given cycle.

➤*Preparation for administration:* The calculated dose of pralatrexate should be aseptically withdrawn into a syringe for immediate use. Do not dilute pralatrexate.

Handling/Disposal – If pralatrexate comes in contact with the skin, immediately and thoroughly wash with soap and water. If pralatrexate comes in contact with mucous membranes, flush thoroughly with water.

➤*Administration:* Administer pralatrexate as an IV push over 3 to 5 minutes via the side port of a free flowing sodium chloride 0.9% injection IV line.

➤*Storage/Stability:* Vials must be stored refrigerated at 2° to 8°C (36° to 46°F) in original carton to protect from light.

Unopened vial(s) of pralatrexate are stable if stored in the original carton at room temperature for 72 hours. Any vials left at room temperature for more than 72 hours should be discarded.

Each vial of pralatrexate is intended for single use only. Any unused drug remaining after injection must be discarded.

Actions

➤*Pharmacology:* Pralatrexate is a folate analog metabolic inhibitor that competitively inhibits dihydrofolate reductase. It is also a competitive inhibitor for polyglutamylation by the enzyme folylpolyglutamyl synthetase. This inhibition results in the depletion of thymidine and other biological molecules, the synthesis of which depends on single carbon transfer.

➤*Pharmacokinetics:* The pharmacokinetics of pralatrexate administered as a single agent at a dose of 30 mg/m^2 administered as an IV push over 3 to 5 minutes once weekly for 6 weeks in 7-week cycles have been evaluated in 10 patients with peripheral T-cell lymphoma.

Absorption – Pralatrexate total systemic exposure (area under the curve [AUC]) and maximum plasma concentration (C_{max}) increased proportionally with dose (dose range, 30 to 325 mg/m^2, including pharmacokinetics data from high-dose solid tumor clinical studies). The pharmacokinetics of pralatrexate did not change significantly over multiple treatment cycles, and no accumulation of pralatrexate was observed.

Distribution – Pralatrexate diastereomers showed a steady-state volume of distribution of 105 L (S-diastereomer) and 37 L (R-diastereomer). In vitro studies indicate that pralatrexate is approximately 67% bound to plasma proteins. In in vitro studies using MDR1-MDCK and Caco-2 cell systems, pralatrexate was not a substrate for P-glycoprotein (Pgp)–mediated transport, nor did it inhibit Pgp-mediated transport.

Metabolism – In vitro studies using human hepatocytes, liver microsomes, and S9 fractions, and recombinant human cytochrome P450 (CYP-450) isozymes showed that pralatrexate is not significantly metabolized by the phase 1 hepatic CYP-450 isozymes or phase 2 hepatic glucuronidases. In vitro studies indicated that pralatrexate has low potential to induce or inhibit the activity of CYP-450 isozymes.

Excretion – The total systemic clearance of pralatrexate diastereomers was 417 mL/min (S-diastereomer) and 191 mL/min (R-diastereomer), and the terminal elimination half-life was 12 to 18 hours (coefficient of variance [CV], 62% to 120%). A mass balance study has not been performed. The mean fraction of unchanged pralatrexate diastereomers excreted in urine following a pralatrexate dose of 30 mg/m^2 administered as an IV push over 3 to 5 minutes was 31% (S-diastereomer) (CV, 47%) and 38% (R-diastereomer) (CV, 45%), respectively.

Special populations –

Renal function impairment: Approximately 34% of pralatrexate was excreted unchanged in the urine following a single dose of 30 mg/m^2 administered as an IV push over 3 to 5 minutes. In a population pharmacokinetic analysis, drug clearance decreased with decreasing creatinine clearance.

Elderly: Because of the contribution of renal excretion to overall clearance of pralatrexate, age-related decline in renal function may lead to a reduction in clearance and a commensurate increase in plasma exposure.

Contraindications

None known.

Warnings/Precautions

➤*Bone marrow suppression:* Pralatrexate can suppress bone marrow function, manifested by thrombocytopenia, neutropenia, and anemia. Dose modifications are based on ANC and platelet count prior to each dose. (See also Administration and Dosage for more information.)

➤*Mucositis:* Treatment with pralatrexate may cause mucositis. If grade 2 or higher mucositis is observed, modify the dose. (See also Administration and Dosage for more information.)

➤*Vitamin supplementation:* Instruct patients to take folic acid and receive vitamin B_{12} to potentially reduce treatment-related hematological toxicity and mucositis. (See also Administration and Dosage for more information.)

➤*Hepatic effects:* Liver function test abnormalities have been observed after pralatrexate administration. Persistent liver function test abnormalities may be indicators of liver toxicity and require dose modification. Monitor patients for liver function.

➤*Renal function impairment:* Although pralatrexate has not been formally tested in patients with renal impairment, caution is advised when administering pralatrexate to patients with moderate to severe impairment. Monitor patients for renal function and systemic toxicity caused by increased drug exposure.

➤*Hepatic function impairment:* Formal studies have not been performed with pralatrexate in patients with hepatic impairment. Patients with the following laboratory values were excluded from the pralatrexate lymphoma clinical trials: total bilirubin greater than 1.5 mg/dL; AST or ALT greater than 2.5 times the upper limit of normal (ULN); and AST or ALT greater than 5 times the ULN if documented hepatic involvement with lymphoma.

➤*Pregnancy: Category D.* Pralatrexate can cause fetal harm when administered to a pregnant woman. Pralatrexate was embryotoxic and fetotoxic in rats at IV dosages of 0.06 mg/kg/day (0.36 mg/m^2/day or approximately 1.2% of the clinical dose on a mg/m^2 basis) given on gestation days 7 through 20. Treatment with pralatrexate caused a dose-dependent decrease in fetal viability manifested as an increase in late, early, and total resorptions. There was also a dose-dependent increase in postimplantation loss. In rabbits, IV dosages of 0.03 mg/kg/day (0.36 mg/m^2/day) or greater given on gestation days 8 through 21 also caused abortion and fetal lethality. This toxicity manifested as early and total resorptions, postimplantation loss, and a decrease in the total number of live fetuses. If this drug is used during pregnancy, or if the patient becomes pregnant while taking this drug, apprise the patient of the potential hazard to the fetus.

➤*Lactation:* It is not known whether pralatrexate is excreted in human milk. The molecular weight (about 477) and the long terminal elimination half-life (12 to 18 hours) suggest that the drug will be excreted into breast milk. Because many drugs are excreted in human milk and because of the potential for serious adverse reactions in breast-feeding infants from this drug, decide whether to discontinue breast-feeding or the drug, taking into account the importance of pralatrexate to the mother.

➤*Children:* Children were not included in clinical studies with pralatrexate. The safety and effectiveness of pralatrexate in children have not been established.

➤*Elderly:* In the peripheral T-cell lymphoma efficacy study, 36% of patients (n = 40) were 65 years of age and older. No overall differences in efficacy and safety were observed in patients based on age (younger than 65 years of age compared with 65 years of age and older).

➤*Monitoring:* Monitor complete blood cell counts and severity of mucositis weekly. Perform serum chemistry tests, including renal and hepatic function, prior to the start of the first and fourth dose of a given cycle. Monitor patients for systemic toxicity caused by increased drug exposure.

PRALATREXATE — INJECTION

Drug Interactions

Pralatrexate Drug Interactions

Precipitant drug	Object drug[a]		Description
NSAIDs (eg, ibuprofen)	Pralatrexate	↑	NSAIDs may delay pralatrexate clearance, increasing drug exposure. Observe the clinical response of the patient and adjust the pralatrexate dose as needed.
Probenecid	Pralatrexate	↑	Probenecid may delay pralatrexate clearance, increasing drug exposure. Observe the clinical response of the patient and adjust the pralatrexate dose as needed.
Trimethoprim/Sulfamethoxazole	Pralatrexate	↑	Trimethoprim/sulfamethoxazole may delay pralatrexate clearance, increasing drug exposure. Observe the clinical response of the patient and adjust the pralatrexate dose as needed.

[a] ↑ = Object drug increased.

Adverse Reactions

The safety of pralatrexate was evaluated in 111 peripheral T-cell lymphoma patients in a single-arm clinical study in which patients received a starting dosage of 30 mg/m^2 once weekly for 6 weeks in 7-week cycles. The median duration of treatment was 70 days (range, 1 to 540 days).

➤*Most frequent adverse reactions:*

Pralatrexate Adverse Reactions in Peripheral T-Cell Lymphoma Patients (≥ 10%)

	(N = 111)		
Adverse reaction	Total	Grade 3	Grade 4
CNS			
Asthenia	10%	1%	0%
Fatigue	36%	5%	2%
Dermatological			
Pruritus	14%	2%	0%
Rash	15%	0%	0%
GI			
Abdominal pain	12%	4%	0%
Anorexia	15%	3%	0%
Constipation	33%	0%	0%
Diarrhea	21%	2%	0%
Nausea	40%	4%	0%
Vomiting	25%	2%	0%
Hematologic			
Anemia	34%	15%	2%
Leukopenia	11%	3%	4%
Neutropenia	24%	13%	7%
Thrombocytopenia[a]	41%	14%	19%[a]
Respiratory			
Cough	28%	1%	0%
Dyspnea	19%	7%	0%
Epistaxis	26%	0%	0%
Pharyngolaryngeal pain	14%	1%	0%
Upper respiratory tract infection	10%	1%	0%
Miscellaneous			
Back pain	11%	3%	0%
Edema	30%	1%	0%
Hypokalemia	15%	4%	1%
Liver function test abnormal[b]	13%	5%	0%
Mucositis[c]	70%	17%	4%
Night sweats	11%	0%	0%
Pain in extremity	12%	0%	0%
Pyrexia	32%	1%	1%
Tachycardia	10%	0%	0%

[a] Five patients with platelets < 10,000/mcL.
[b] ALT, AST, and transaminases increased.
[c] Stomatitis or mucosal inflammation of the GI and GU tracts.

➤*Serious adverse reactions:* Forty-four percent of patients experienced a serious adverse reaction while on study or within 30 days after their last dose of pralatrexate. The most common serious adverse reactions (more than 3%), regardless of causality, were dehydration, dyspnea, febrile neutropenia, mucositis, pyrexia, sepsis, and thrombocytopenia. One death from cardiopulmonary arrest in a patient with mucositis and febrile neutropenia was reported in this trial. Deaths from febrile neutropenia, mucositis, pancytopenia, and sepsis occurred in 1.2% of patients treated in all pralatrexate trials at doses ranging from 30 to 325 mg/m^2.

➤*Discontinuation:* Twenty-three percent of patients discontinued treatment with pralatrexate because of adverse reactions. The adverse reactions reported most frequently as the reason for discontinuation of treatment were mucositis (6%) and thrombocytopenia (5%).

➤*Dose modifications:* The target dosage of pralatrexate was 30 mg/m^2 once weekly for 6 weeks in 7-week cycles. The majority of patients (69%) remained at the target dose for the duration of treatment. Overall, 85% of scheduled doses were administered.

Overdosage

➤*Treatment:* No specific information is available on the treatment of overdosage of pralatrexate. If an overdose occurs, institute general supportive measures as deemed necessary by the treating health care provider. Based on pralatrexate's mechanism of action, consider the prompt administration of leucovorin.

Patient Information

Instruct patients to take folic acid and vitamin B_{12} as a prophylactic measure to potentially reduce possible adverse effects.

Inform patients of the signs and symptoms of mucositis. Instruct patients on ways to reduce the risk of its development and/or ways to maintain nutrition and control discomfort from mucositis if it occurs.

Inform patients of the risk of low blood cell counts and instruct them to immediately contact their health care provider should any signs of infection develop, including fever. Instruct patients to contact their health care provider if bleeding or symptoms of anemia occur.

Instruct patients to inform their health care provider if they are taking any concomitant medications, including prescription drugs (such as trimethoprim/sulfamethoxazole) and nonprescription drugs (such as NSAIDs).

Instruct patients to tell their health care provider if they are pregnant or plan to become pregnant because of the risk of fetal harm. Instruct patients to tell their health care provider if they are breast-feeding.

CAPECITABINE

Rx	**Xeloda** (Roche)	**Tablets:** 150 mg	Lactose. (Xeloda 150). Light peach, oblong. Film-coated. In 60s.
		500 mg	Lactose. (Xeloda 500). Peach, oblong. Film-coated. In 120s.

CAPECITABINE — ORAL

WARNING

Warfarin interaction – Frequently monitor the anticoagulant response (international normalized ratio [INR] or prothrombin time [PT]) of patients receiving concomitant capecitabine and oral coumarin-derivative anticoagulant therapy in order to adjust the anticoagulant dose accordingly. A clinically important capecitabine-warfarin drug interaction was demonstrated in a clinical pharmacology trial. Altered coagulation parameters and/or bleeding, including death, have been reported in patients taking capecitabine concomitantly with coumarin-derivative anticoagulants such as warfarin and phenprocoumon. Postmarketing reports have shown clinically significant increases in PT and INR in patients who were stabilized on anticoagulants at the time capecitabine was introduced. These events occurred within several days and up to several months after initiating capecitabine therapy and, in a few cases, within 1 month after stopping capecitabine. These events occurred in patients with and without liver metastases. Age older than 60 years and a diagnosis of cancer independently predispose patients to an increased risk of coagulopathy.

Indications

➤*Colorectal cancer:* Capecitabine is indicated as a single agent for adjuvant treatment in patients with Duke stage C colon cancer who have undergone complete resection of the primary tumor when treatment with fluoropyrimidine therapy alone is preferred. Capecitabine was noninferior to 5-fluorouracil and leucovorin for disease-free survival. Although neither capecitabine nor combination chemotherapy prolongs overall survival, combination chemotherapy has been demonstrated to improve disease-free survival compared with 5-fluorouracil/leucovorin. Consider these results when prescribing single-agent capecitabine in the adjuvant treatment of Duke stage C colon cancer.

Capecitabine is indicated as first-line treatment of patients with metastatic colorectal carcinoma when treatment with fluoropyrimidine therapy alone is preferred. Combination chemotherapy has shown a survival benefit compared with 5-fluorouracil/leucovorin alone. A survival benefit over 5-fluorouracil/leucovorin has not been demonstrated with capecitabine monotherapy. Use of capecitabine instead of 5-fluorouracil/leucovorin in combinations has not been adequately studied to ensure safety or preservation of the survival advantage.

➤*Breast cancer:* Capecitabine in combination with docetaxel is indicated for the treatment of patients with metastatic breast cancer after failure of prior anthracycline-containing chemotherapy.

Capecitabine monotherapy is indicated for the treatment of patients with metastatic breast cancer resistant to both paclitaxel and an anthracycline-containing chemotherapy regimen or resistant to paclitaxel and for whom further anthracycline therapy is not indicated (eg, patients who have received cumulative doses of 400 mg/m^2 of doxorubicin or doxorubicin equivalents). Resistance is defined as progressive disease while on treatment, with or without an initial response, or relapse within 6 months of completing treatment with an anthracycline-containing adjuvant regimen.

➤*Off-label uses:* As adjuvant treatment for pancreatic cancer. Treatment of advanced or metastatic breast cancer given in combination with lapatinib in women with HER2-overexpressing tumors who have been previously treated with an anthracycline, a taxane, and trastuzumab; treatment of advanced or metastatic breast cancer given in combination with ixabepilone in women who have been previously treated with an anthracycline and a taxane.

Administration and Dosage

➤*General dosing considerations:* Round to the nearest dose that gives a whole tablet rather than cutting tablets in half. (See Dosage Calculation.)

➤*Adults:*

Breast cancer –

Usual dosage: 1,250 mg/m^2 twice daily (morning and evening; equivalent to 2,500 mg/m^2 total daily dose) for 2 weeks. After a 1-week rest period, repeat this 3-week cycle.

Concomitant therapy: If given in combination with docetaxel, the docetaxel dosage is 75 mg/m^2 as a 1-hour intravenous (IV) infusion every 3 weeks. Premedication, according to the docetaxel labeling, should be started prior to docetaxel administration for patients receiving the capecitabine plus docetaxel combination.

Duke stage C colon cancer – 1,250 mg/m^2 twice daily for 2 weeks followed by a 1-week rest period, given as 3-week cycles for a total of 8 cycles (24 weeks).

Metastatic colorectal cancer – 1,250 mg/m^2 twice daily (morning and evening; equivalent to 2,500 mg/m^2 total daily dose) for 2 weeks followed by a 1-week rest period given as 3-week cycles.

Off-label dosing –

Advanced or metastatic breast cancer in combination with ixabepilone: Capecitabine 1,000 mg/m^2 twice daily (approximately 12 hours apart) for 2 weeks. After a 1-week rest period, repeat this 3-week cycle. Note: Ixabepilone is given once every 21 days.

Advanced or metastatic breast cancer in combination with lapatinib: Capecitabine 1,000 mg/m^2 twice daily (approximately 12 hours apart) for 2 weeks. After a 1-week rest period, repeat this 3-week cycle. Note: Lapatinib is given continuously (regimen given in Lapatinib monograph).

➤*Elderly:*

Breast cancer – To minimize toxicity, consider reducing the initial capecitabine dosage by 25% (ie, 1,900 mg/m^2/day in 2 divided doses) in patients 60 years of age and older when used in combination with docetaxel.

➤*Renal function impairment:*

Moderate renal impairment (CrCl 30 to 50 mL/min) – A dose reduction to 75% of the capecitabine starting dose (from 1,250 to 950 mg/m^2 twice daily) is recommended when used as monotherapy or in combination with docetaxel. Subsequent dose adjustment is recommended as outlined in the following tables if a patient develops a grade 2 to 4 adverse event. (See also Dose Modification Guidelines.)

Severe renal impairment (CrCl less than 30 mL/min) – Use is contraindicated.

Dialysis – Conventional hemodialysis is minimally effectively (25% to 49%) in removing capecitabine.

➤*Hepatic function impairment:* Avoid concomitant use of capecitabine and ixabepilone in patients with bilirubin levels greater than the upper limit of normal (ULN) or in patients with AST or ALT greater than 2.5 times the ULN. These patients may be at increased risk for toxicity. Neutropenia-related death was more common in patients with impaired hepatic function (29%) compared with those with normal or mildly impaired hepatic function (1.9%).

➤*Dosage Calculation:* Round to the nearest dose that gives a whole tablet rather than cutting tablets in half.

Capecitabine Dose Calculation According to Body Surface Area

Dosage level 1,250 mg/m^2 twice a day		Number of tablets per dose (morning and evening)	
Surface area (m^2)	Total daily[a] dose (mg)	150 mg	500 mg
≤ 1.25	3,000	0	3
1.26 to 1.37	3,300	1	3
1.38 to 1.51	3,600	2	3
1.52 to 1.65	4,000	0	4
1.66 to 1.77	4,300	1	4
1.78 to 1.91	4,600	2	4
1.92 to 2.05	5,000	0	5
2.06 to 2.17	5,300	1	5
≥ 2.18	5,600	2	5

[a] Total daily dose divided by 2 to allow equal morning and evening doses.

➤*Dose modification guidelines:* Capecitabine dosage may need to be individualized to optimize patient management. Patients should be carefully monitored for toxicity, and doses of capecitabine should be modified as necessary to accommodate individual patient tolerance to treatment. Toxicity due to capecitabine administration may be managed by symptomatic treatment, dose interruptions, and adjustment of capecitabine dose. Once the dose has been reduced it should not be increased at a later time.

CAPECITABINE — ORAL

Capecitabine combination therapy with docetaxel –

Capecitabine in Combination with Docetaxel Dose Reduction Schedule			
Toxicity NCIC grades[a]	Grade 2	Grade 3	Grade 4
1st appearance	Grade 2 occurring during the 14 days of capecitabine treatment: Interrupt capecitabine treatment until resolved to grade 0 to 1. Treatment may be resumed during the cycle at the same dose of capecitabine. Doses of capecitabine missed during a treatment cycle are not to be replaced. Prophylaxis for toxicities should be implemented where possible. Grade 2 persisting at the time the next capecitabine/docetaxel treatment is due: Delay treatment until resolved to grade 0 to 1, then continue at 100% of the original capecitabine and docetaxel dose. Prophylaxis for toxicities should be implemented where possible.	Grade 3 occurring during the 14 days of capecitabine treatment: Interrupt the capecitabine treatment until resolved to grade 0 to 1. Treatment may be resumed during the cycle at 75% of the capecitabine dose. Doses of capecitabine missed during a treatment cycle are not to be replaced. Prophylaxis for toxicities should be implemented where possible. Grade 3 persisting at the time the next capecitabine/docetaxel treatment is due: Delay treatment until resolved to grade 0 to 1. For patients developing grade 3 toxicity at any time during the treatment cycle, upon resolution to grade 0 to 1, subsequent treatment cycles should be continued at 75% of the original capecitabine dose and at 55 mg/m^2 of docetaxel. Implement prophylaxis for toxicities where possible.	Discontinue treatment unless the treating health care provider considers it to be in the best interest of the patient to continue with capecitabine at 50% of original dose.
2nd appearance of same toxicity	Grade 2 occurring during the 14 days of capecitabine treatment: Interrupt capecitabine treatment until resolved to grade 0 to 1. Treatment may be resumed during the cycle at 75% of original capecitabine dose. Doses of capecitabine missed during a treatment cycle are not to be replaced. Implement prophylaxis for toxicities where possible. Grade 2 persisting at the time the next capecitabine/docetaxel treatment is due: Delay treatment until resolved to grade 0 to 1. For patients developing 2nd occurrence of grade 2 toxicity at any time during the treatment cycle, upon resolution to grade 0 to 1, subsequent treatment cycles should be continued at 75% of the original capecitabine dose and at 55 mg/m^2 of docetaxel. Implement prophylaxis for toxicities where possible.	Grade 3 occurring during the 14 days of capecitabine treatment: Interrupt the capecitabine treatment until resolved to grade 0 to 1. Treatment may be resumed during the cycle at 50% of the capecitabine dose. Doses of capecitabine missed during a treatment cycle are not to be replaced. Implement prophylaxis for toxicities where possible. Grade 3 persisting at the time the next capecitabine/docetaxel treatment is due: Delay treatment until resolved to grade 0 to 1. For patients developing grade 3 toxicity at any time during the treatment cycle, upon resolution to grade 0 to 1, subsequent treatment cycles should be continued at 50% of the original capecitabine dose and the docetaxel discontinued. Implement prophylaxis for toxicities where possible.	Discontinue treatment.
3rd appearance of same toxicity	Grade 2 occurring during the 14 days of capecitabine treatment: Interrupt capecitabine treatment until resolved to grade 0 to 1. Treatment may be resumed during the cycle at 50% of the original capecitabine dose. Doses of capecitabine missed during a treatment cycle are not to be replaced. Prophylaxis for toxicities should be implemented where possible. Grade 2 persisting at the time the next capecitabine/docetaxel treatment is due: Delay treatment until resolved to grade 0 to 1. For patients developing 3rd occurrence of grade 2 toxicity at any time during the treatment cycle, upon resolution to grade 0 to 1, subsequent treatment cycles should be continued at 50% of the original capecitabine dose and the docetaxel discontinued. Implement prophylaxis for toxicities where possible.	Discontinue treatment.	
4th appearance of same toxicity	Discontinue treatment.		

[a] National Cancer Institute of Canada (NCIC) Common Toxicity Criteria were used except for hand-and-foot syndrome.

CAPECITABINE — ORAL

➤*Capecitabine monotherapy:*

Recommended Dose Modifications with Capecitabine Monotherapy		
Toxicity NCIC grades[a]	During a course of therapy	Dose adjustment for next treatment (% of starting dose)
Grade 1	Maintain dose level	Maintain dose level
Grade 2		
1st appearance	Interrupt until resolved to grade 0 to 1	100%
2nd appearance	Interrupt until resolved to grade 0 to 1	75%
3rd appearance	Interrupt until resolved to grade 0 to 1	50%
4th appearance	Discontinue treatment permanently	
Grade 3		
1st appearance	Interrupt until resolved to grade 0 to 1	75%
2nd appearance	Interrupt until resolved to grade 0 to 1	50%
3rd appearance	Discontinue treatment permanently	
Grade 4		
1st appearance	Discontinue permanently or if the health care provider deems it to be in the patient's best interest to continue, interrupt until resolved to grade 0 to 1	50%

[a] NCIC Common Toxicity Criteria were used except for the hand-and-foot syndrome.

Dosage modifications are not recommended for grade 1 events. Therapy with capecitabine should be interrupted upon the occurrence of a grade 2 or 3 adverse experience. Once the adverse event has resolved or decreased in intensity to grade 1, then capecitabine therapy may be restarted at full dose or as adjusted according to the previous tables. If a grade 4 experience occurs, therapy should be discontinued or interrupted until resolved or decreased to grade 1, and therapy should be restarted at 50% of the original dose. Doses of capecitabine omitted for toxicity are not replaced or restored; instead the patient should resume the planned treatment cycles.

➤*Concomitant therapy:* The dose of phenytoin and the dose of coumarin-derivative anticoagulants may need to be reduced when either drug is coadministered with capecitabine. (See Drug Interactions.)

➤*Preparation for administration:* Capecitabine is considered a cytotoxic agent. Follow safe handling procedures when preparing, administering, or dispensing capecitabine.

➤*Administration:* Capecitabine tablets should be swallowed with water within 30 minutes after a meal (breakfast and dinner).

For patients unable to swallow tablets whole, crush tablets and mix with 40 mL of water. Stir until dispersed, then have the patient drink the mixture immediately. The suspension may also be administered via an enteral feeding tube.

➤*Storage/Stability:* Store at 25°C (77°F); excursions are permitted to 15° to 30°C (59° to 86°F). Keep tightly closed.

Actions

➤*Pharmacology:* Capecitabine is relatively noncytotoxic in vitro. This drug is enzymatically converted to 5-fluorouracil in vivo.

Both normal and tumor cells metabolize 5-fluorouracil to 5-fluoro-2'-deoxyuridine monophosphate and 5-fluorouridine triphosphate. These metabolites cause cell injury by 2 different mechanisms. First, 5-fluoro-2'-deoxyuridine monophosphate and the folate cofactor, N^{5-10}-methylenetetrahydrofolate, bind to thymidylate synthase to form a covalently bound ternary complex. This binding inhibits the formation of thymidylate from 2'-deoxy-uridylate. Thymidylate is the necessary precursor of thymidine triphosphate, which is essential for the synthesis of deoxyribonucleic acid (DNA), so that a deficiency of this compound can inhibit cell division. Second, nuclear transcriptional enzymes can mistakenly incorporate 5-fluorouridine triphosphate in place of uridine triphosphate during the synthesis of ribonucleic acid (RNA). This metabolic error can interfere with RNA processing and protein synthesis.

➤*Pharmacokinetics:*

Absorption – Capecitabine is readily absorbed from the GI tract. Capecitabine reached peak blood levels in about 1.5 hours (T_{max}) with peak 5-fluorouracil levels occurring slightly later, at 2 hours. Food reduced both the rate and extent of absorption of capecitabine with mean maximum plasma concentration (C_{max}) and area under the curve ($AUC_{0-\infty}$) decreased by 60% and 35%, respectively. The C_{max} and $AUC_{0-\infty}$ of 5-fluorouracil were also reduced by food by 43% and 21%, respectively. Food delayed T_{max} of both parent and 5-fluorouracil by 1.5 hours.

The pharmacokinetics of capecitabine and its metabolites have been evaluated in about 200 cancer patients over a dosage range of 500 to 3,500 mg/m²/day. Over this range, the pharmacokinetics of capecitabine and its metabolite, 5'-deoxy-5-fluorocytidine were dose proportional and did not change over time. The increases in the AUCs of 5'-deoxy-5-fluorouridine and 5-fluorouracil, however, were greater than proportional to the increase in dose, and the AUC of 5-fluorouracil was 34% higher on day 14 than on day 1.

The interpatient variability in the C_{max} and AUC of 5-fluorouracil was greater than 85%.

Distribution – Plasma protein binding of capecitabine and its metabolites is less than 60% and is not concentration-dependent. Capecitabine was primarily bound to human albumin (approximately 35%).

Metabolism – Capecitabine is extensively metabolized enzymatically to 5-fluorouracil. The enzyme dihydropyrimidine dehydrogenase hydrogenates 5-fluorouracil, the product of capecitabine metabolism, to the much less toxic 5-fluoro-5,6-dihydro-fluorouracil. Dihydropyrimidinase cleaves the pyrimidine ring to yield 5-fluoro-ureido-propionic acid. Finally, beta-ureido-propionase cleaves 5-fluoro-ureido-propionic acid to alpha-fluoro-beta-alanine, which is cleared in the urine.

Excretion – Capecitabine and its metabolites are predominantly excreted in urine; 95.5% of administered capecitabine dose is recovered in urine. Fecal excretion is minimal (2.6%). The major metabolite excreted in urine is alpha-fluoro-beta-alanine, which represents 57% of the administered dose. About 3% of the administered dose is excreted in urine as unchanged drug.

The elimination half-life of both parent capecitabine and 5-fluorouracil was about three fourths of an hour.

Special populations –

Renal function impairment: Following oral administration of 1,250 mg/m² capecitabine twice a day to cancer patients with varying degrees of renal impairment, patients with moderate (creatinine clearance = 30 to 50 mL/min) and severe (creatinine clearance less than 30 mL/min) renal impairment showed 85% and 258% higher systemic exposure to alpha-fluoro-beta-alanine on day 1 compared with healthy renal function patients (creatinine clearance greater than 80 mL/min). Systemic exposure to 5'-deoxy-5-fluorouridine was 42% and 71% greater in moderately and severely renal impaired patients, respectively, than in healthy patients. Systemic exposure to capecitabine was about 25% greater in both moderately and severely renal impaired patients. Capecitabine is contraindicated in patients with severe renal impairment (creatinine clearance less than 30 mL/min [Cockroft and Gault]).

Hepatic function impairment: Capecitabine has been evaluated in 13 patients with mild to moderate hepatic dysfunction due to liver metastases defined by a composite score, including bilirubin, AST/ALT, and alkaline phosphatase following a single 1,255 mg/m² dose of capecitabine. Both $AUC_{0-\infty}$ and C_{max} of capecitabine increased by 60% in patients with hepatic dysfunction compared with patients with healthy hepatic function (n = 14). The $AUC_{0-\infty}$ and C_{max} of 5-fluorouracil were not affected. In patients with mild to moderate hepatic dysfunction due to liver metastases, exercise caution when capecitabine is administered. The effect of severe hepatic dysfunction on capecitabine is not known.

Contraindications

Capecitabine is contraindicated in patients who have a known hypersensitivity to capecitabine or to any of its components. Capecitabine is contraindicated in patients who have a known hypersensitivity to 5-fluorouracil. Capecitabine is contraindicated in patients with known dihydropyrimidine dehydrogenase (DPD) deficiency. Capecitabine is contraindicated in patients with severe renal impairment (creatinine clearance less than 30 mL/min [Cockroft and Gault]).

Warnings/Precautions

➤*Coagulopathy:* See Black Box Warning for more information.

➤*Diarrhea:* Capecitabine can induce diarrhea, sometimes severe. Carefully monitor patients with severe diarrhea and give fluid and electrolyte replacement if they become dehydrated. In 875 patients with either metastatic breast or colorectal cancer who received capecitabine monotherapy, the median time to first occurrence of grade 2 to 4 diarrhea was 34 days (range, 1 to 369 days). The median duration of grade 3 to 4 diarrhea was 5 days. NCIC grade 2 diarrhea is defined as an increase of 4 to 6 stools/day or nocturnal stools, grade 3 diarrhea as an increase of 7 to 9 stools/day or incontinence and malabsorption, and grade 4 diarrhea as an increase of greater than or equal to 10 stools/day or grossly bloody diarrhea or the need for parenteral support. If grade 2, 3, or 4 diarrhea occurs, immediately interrupt administration of capecitabine until the diarrhea resolves or decreases in intensity to grade 1. Following a reoccurrence of grade 2 diarrhea or occurrence of any grade 3 or 4 diarrhea, decrease subsequent doses of capecitabine. Standard antidiarrheal treatments (eg, loperamide) are recommended.

Necrotizing enterocolitis (typhlitis) has been reported.

➤*Hand-and-foot syndrome:* Hand-and-foot syndrome (palmar-plantar erythrodysesthesia or chemotherapy-induced acral erythema) is a cutaneous toxicity. Median time to onset was 79 days (range, 11 to 360 days) with a severity range of grades 1 to 3 for patients receiving capecitabine monotherapy in the metastatic setting. Grade 1 is characterized by any of the following: numbness, dysesthesia/paresthesia, tingling, painless swelling or erythema of the hands and/or feet, and/or discomfort that does not disrupt normal activities. Grade 2 hand-and-foot syndrome is defined as painful erythema and swelling of the hands and/or feet, and/or discomfort affecting the patient's activities of daily living. Grade 3 hand-and-foot syndrome is

CAPECITABINE — ORAL

defined as moist desquamation, ulceration, blistering or severe pain of the hands and/or feet, and/or severe discomfort that causes the patient to be unable to work or perform activities of daily living. If grade 2 or 3 hand-and-foot syndrome occurs, interrupt administration of capecitabine until the event resolves or decreases in intensity to grade 1. Following grade 3 hand-and-foot syndrome, decrease subsequent doses of capecitabine.

➤*Cardiotoxicity:* The cardiotoxicity observed with capecitabine includes myocardial infarction/ischemia, angina, dysrhythmias, cardiac arrest, cardiac failure, sudden death, electrocardiographic changes, and cardiomyopathy. These adverse reactions may be more common in patients with a history of coronary artery disease.

➤*DPD:* Rarely, unexpected, severe toxicity (eg, stomatitis, diarrhea, neutropenia and neurotoxicity) associated with 5-fluorouracil has been attributed to a deficiency of DPD activity. A link between decreased levels of DPD and increased, potentially fatal, toxic effects of 5-fluorouracil therefore cannot be excluded.

➤*Hyperbilirubinemia:* In 875 patients with either metastatic breast or colorectal cancer who received at least 1 dose of capecitabine 1,250 mg/m^2 twice daily as monotherapy for 2 weeks followed by a 1-week rest period, grade 3 (1.5 to 3 × ULN) hyperbilirubinemia occurred in 15.2% (n = 133) of patients and grade 4 (greater than 3 × ULN) hyperbilirubinemia occurred in 3.9% (n = 34) of patients. Of 566 patients who had hepatic metastases at baseline and 309 patients without hepatic metastases at baseline, grade 3 or 4 hyperbilirubinemia occurred in 22.8% and 12.3%, respectively. Of the 167 patients with grade 3 or 4 hyperbilirubinemia, 18.6% (n = 31) also had postbaseline elevations (grades 1 to 4, without elevations at baseline) in alkaline phosphatase and 27.5% (n = 46) had postbaseline elevations in transaminases at any time (not necessarily concurrent). The majority of these patients, 64.5% (n = 20) and 71.7% (n = 33), had liver metastases at baseline. In addition, 57.5% (n = 96) and 35.3% (n = 59) of the 167 patients had elevations (grades 1 to 4) at both prebaseline and postbaseline in alkaline phosphatase or transaminases, respectively. Only 7.8% (n = 13) and 3% (n = 5) had grade 3 or 4 elevations in alkaline phosphatase or transaminases.

In the 596 patients treated with capecitabine as first-line therapy for metastatic colorectal cancer, the incidence of grade 3 or 4 hyperbilirubinemia was similar to the overall clinical trial safety database of capecitabine monotherapy. The median time to onset for grade 3 or 4 hyperbilirubinemia in the colorectal cancer population was 64 days and median total bilirubin increased from 8 mcm/L at baseline to 13 mcm/L during treatment with capecitabine. Of the 136 colorectal cancer patients with grade 3 or 4 hyperbilirubinemia, 49 patients had grade 3 or 4 hyperbilirubinemia as their last measured value, of which 46 had liver metastases at baseline.

In 251 patients with metastatic breast cancer who received a combination of capecitabine and docetaxel, grade 3 (1.5 to 3 × ULN) hyperbilirubinemia occurred in 7% (n = 17) and grade 4 (greater than 3 × ULN) hyperbilirubinemia occurred in 2% (n = 5).

If drug-related grade 2 to 4 elevations in bilirubin occur, immediately interrupt administration of capecitabine until the hyperbilirubinemia resolves or decreases in intensity to grade 1. NCIC grade 2 hyperbilirubinemia is defined as 1.5 × normal, grade 3 hyperbilirubinemia as 1.5 to 3 × normal and grade 4 hyperbilirubinemia as greater than 3 × normal.

➤*Hematologic:* In 875 patients with either metastatic breast or colorectal cancer who received a dose of 1,250 mg/m^2 administered twice daily as monotherapy for 2 weeks followed by a 1-week rest period, 3.2%, 1.7%, and 2.4% of patients had grade 3 or 4 neutropenia, thrombocytopenia, or decreases in hemoglobin, respectively. In 251 patients with metastatic breast cancer who received a dose of capecitabine in combination with docetaxel, 68% had grade 3 or 4 neutropenia, 2.8% had grade 3 or 4 thrombocytopenia, and 9.6% had grade 3 or 4 anemia.

➤*Renal function impairment:* Patients with moderate renal impairment at baseline require dose reduction. Carefully monitor patients with mild and moderate renal impairment at baseline for adverse reactions. Prompt interruption of therapy with subsequent dose adjustments is recommended if a patient develops a grade 2 to 4 adverse reaction. Once the adverse reaction has resolved or decreased in intensity to grade 1, then capecitabine therapy may be restarted at full dose or reduced by 25% for each subsequent appearance of grade 2 toxicity. With the fourth appearance of grade 2 toxicity, discontinue treatment permanently. Interrupt therapy with capecitabine upon the occurrence of a grade 3 adverse experience. Once the adverse reaction has resolved or decreased in intensity to grade 1, then capecitabine therapy may be restarted at 75% of starting dose or reduced by 25% for the second appearance of a grade 3 adverse experience. Discontinue treatment permanently at the third appearance. If a grade 4 experience occurs, discontinue therapy permanently or interrupt until resolved or decreased to grade 1, and then restart at 50% of the original dose if it is in the patient's best interest to continue. Doses of capecitabine omitted for toxicity are not replaced or restored; instead the patient should resume the planned treatment cycles.

➤*Hepatic function impairment:* Carefully monitor patients with mild to moderate hepatic dysfunction due to liver metastases when capecitabine is administered. The effect of severe hepatic dysfunction on the disposition of capecitabine is not known.

➤*Pregnancy: Category D.* Advise women of childbearing potential to avoid becoming pregnant while receiving treatment with capecitabine.

Capecitabine may cause fetal harm when given to a pregnant woman. Capecitabine at dosages of 198 mg/kg/day during organogenesis caused teratogenic malformations and embryo death in mice. In separate pharmacokinetic studies, this dose in mice produced 5′-deoxy-5-fluorouridine AUC values about 0.2 times the corresponding values in patients administered the recommended daily dose. Teratogenic malformations in mice included cleft palate, anophthalmia, microphthalmia, oligodactyly, polydactyly, syndactyly, kinky tail, and dilation of cerebral ventricles. At dosages of 90 mg/kg/day, capecitabine given to pregnant monkeys during organogenesis caused fetal death. This dose produced 5′-deoxy-5-fluorouridine AUC values about 0.6 times the corresponding values in patients administered the recommended daily dose. There are no adequate and well-controlled studies in pregnant women using capecitabine. If the drug is used during pregnancy, or if the patient becomes pregnant while receiving this drug, apprise the patient of the potential hazard to the fetus. Advise women of childbearing potential to avoid becoming pregnant while receiving treatment with capecitabine.

➤*Lactation:* Lactating mice given a single oral dose of capecitabine excreted significant amounts of capecitabine metabolites into the milk. Because of the potential for serious adverse reactions in breast-feeding infants from capecitabine, it is recommended that breast-feeding be discontinued when receiving capecitabine therapy.

➤*Children:* The safety and efficacy of capecitabine in patients younger than 18 years of age have not been established.

➤*Elderly:* Patients 80 years of age or older may experience a greater incidence of grade 3 or 4 adverse reactions. In 875 patients with either metastatic breast of colorectal cancer who received capecitabine monotherapy, 62% of the 21 patients greater than or equal to 80 years of age treated with capecitabine experienced a treatment-related grade 3 or 4 adverse reaction: Diarrhea in 6 (28.6%), nausea in 3 (14.3%), hand-and-foot syndrome in 3 (14.3%), and vomiting in 2 (9.5%) patients. Among the 10 patients 70 years of age and older (no patients were older than 80 years of age) treated with capecitabine in combination with docetaxel, 30% (3 out of 10) of patients experienced grade 3 or 4 diarrhea and stomatitis, and 40% (4 out of 10) experienced grade 3 hand-and-foot syndrome.

Among the 67 patients 60 years of age and older receiving capecitabine in combination with docetaxel, the incidence of grade 3 or 4 treatment-related adverse reactions, treatment-related serious adverse reactions, withdrawals due to adverse reactions, treatment discontinuations due to adverse reactions, and treatment discontinuations within the first 2 treatment cycles was higher than in the less than 60 years of age patient group.

In 995 patients receiving capecitabine as adjuvant therapy for Duke stage C colon cancer after resection of the primary tumor, 41% of the 398 patients 65 years of age and older treated with capecitabine experienced a treatment-related grade 3 or 4 adverse reaction: hand-and-foot syndrome in 75 (18.8%), diarrhea in 52 (13.1%), stomatitis in 12 (3%), neutropenia/granulocytopenia in 11 (2.8%), vomiting in 6 (1.5%), and nausea in 5 (1.3%) patients. In patients 65 years of age and older (all randomized population; capecitabine 188 patients, 5-fluorouracil/leucovorin 208 patients) treated for Duke stage C colon cancer after resection of the primary tumor, the hazard ratios for disease-free survival and overall survival for capecitabine compared with 5-fluorouracil/leucovorin were 1.01 (95% CI, 0.8 to 1.27) and 1.04 (95% CI, 0.79 to 1.37), respectively.

Pay particular attention to monitoring the adverse effects of capecitabine in the elderly.

➤*Monitoring:* A health care provider experienced in the use of cancer chemotherapeutic agents should monitor patients receiving therapy with capecitabine. Most adverse reactions are reversible and do not need to result in discontinuation, although doses may need to be withheld or reduced.

Drug Interactions

Capecitabine Drug Interactions

Precipitant drug	Object drug[a]		Description
Antacids	Capecitabine	↑	When 20 mL of an aluminum hydroxide- and magnesium hydroxide–containing antacid was administered immediately after capecitabine, AUC and C_{max} increased by 16% and 35%, respectively, for capecitabine and by 18% and 22%, respectively, for 5′-deoxy-5-fluorocytidine.
Leucovorin	Capecitabine	↑	The concentration of 5-fluorouracil is increased and its toxicity may be enhanced by leucovorin. Deaths from severe enterocolitis, diarrhea, and dehydration have been reported in elderly patients receiving weekly leucovorin and fluorouracil.
Capecitabine	Phenytoin	↑	Carefully monitor phenytoin levels in patients taking capecitabine. The phenytoin dose may need to be reduced. The mechanism of interaction is presumed to be inhibition of the CYP2C9 isoenzyme by capecitabine or its metabolites.

CAPECITABINE — ORAL

Capecitabine Drug Interactions			
Precipitant drug	Object drug[a]		Description
Capecitabine	Warfarin	↑	Altered coagulation parameters and/or bleeding have been reported in patients taking capecitabine concomitantly with warfarin. Monitor patients regularly for PT or INR alterations and adjust anticoagulant dose as necessary.

[a] ↑ = Object drug increased.

➤*Drug/Food interactions:* In all clinical trials, patients were instructed to administer capecitabine within 30 minutes after a meal. Since current safety and efficacy data are based upon administration with food, it is recommended that capecitabine be administered with food. Capecitabine tablets should be swallowed with water within 30 minutes after a meal.

Adverse Reactions

Capecitabine is considered to have moderate potential for nausea and vomiting.

➤*Adjuvant colon cancer:* The following table shows the adverse reactions occurring in at least 5% of patients from one phase 3 trial in patients with Duke stage C colon cancer who received at least 1 dose of study medication and had at least 1 safety assessment. A total of 995 patients were treated with 1,250 mg/m^2 twice a day of capecitabine administered for 2 weeks followed by a 1-week rest period, and 974 patients were administered 5-fluorouracil and leucovorin (20 mg/m^2 leucovorin IV followed by 425 mg/m^2 IV bolus 5-fluorouracil, on days 1 to 5, every 28 days). The median duration of treatment was 164 days for capecitabine-treated patients and 145 days for 5-fluorouracil/leucovorin–treated patients. A total of 112 (11%) and 73 (7%) capecitabine and 5-fluorouracil/leucovorin–treated patients, respectively, discontinued treatment because of adverse reactions. A total of 18 deaths due to all causes occurred either on study or within 28 days of receiving study drug: 8 (0.8%) patients randomized to capecitabine and 10 (1%) randomized to 5-fluorouracil/leucovorin.

The second table that follows shows grade 3/4 laboratory abnormalities occurring in at least 1% of patients from 1 phase 3 trial in patients with Duke stage C colon cancer who received at least 1 dose of study medication and had at least 1 safety assessment.

Adverse Reactions in Patients Treated with Capecitabine or 5-Fluorouracil/Leucovorin for Colon Cancer in the Adjuvant Setting (≥ 5%)

	Adjuvant treatment for colon cancer (N = 1,969)			
	Capecitabine (n = 995)		5-Fluorouracil/Leucovorin (n = 974)	
Adverse reaction	All grades	Grade 3/4	All grades	Grade 3/4
CNS				
Asthenia	10%	< 1%	10%	1%
Dizziness	6%	< 1%	6%	—
Fatigue	16%	< 1%	16%	1%
Headache	5%	< 1%	6%	< 1%
Lethargy	10%	< 1%	9%	< 1%
Dermatologic				
Alopecia	6%	—	22%	< 1%
Erythema	6%	1%	5%	< 1%
Hand-and-foot syndrome	60%	17%	9%	< 1%
Rash	7%	—	8%	—
GI				
Abdominal pain	14%	3%	16%	2%
Anorexia	9%	< 1%	11%	< 1%
Constipation	9%	—	11%	< 1%
Diarrhea	47%	12%	65%	14%
Dysgeusia	6%	—	9%	—
Dyspepsia	6%	< 1%	5%	—
Nausea	34%	2%	47%	2%
Stomatitis	22%	2%	60%	14%
Upper abdominal pain	7%	< 1%	7%	< 1%
Vomiting	15%	2%	21%	2%
Hematologic				
Neutropenia	2%	< 1%	8%	5%
Respiratory				
Epistaxis	2%	—	5%	—
Special senses				
Conjunctivitis	5%	< 1%	6%	< 1%
Miscellaneous				
Pyrexia	7%	< 1%	9%	< 1%

Grade 3/4 Laboratory Abnormalities in Patients Receiving Capecitabine Monotherapy for Adjuvant Treatment of Colon Cancer (≥ 1%)

Adverse reaction	Capecitabine (n = 995) Grade 3/4	IV 5-Fluorouracil/Leucovorin (n = 974) Grade 3/4
Decreased calcium	2.3%	2.2%
Decreased hemoglobin	1%	1.2%
Decreased lymphocytes	13%	13%
Decreased neutrophils[a]	2.2%	26.2%
Decreased neutrophils/granulocytes	2.4%	26.4%
Decreased platelets	1%	0.7%
Increased ALT	1.6%	0.6%
Increased bilirubin[b]	20%	6.3%
Increased calcium	1.1%	0.7%

[a] The incidence of grade 3/4 white blood cells abnormalities was 1.3% in the capecitabine arm and 4.9% in the IV 5-fluorouracil/leucovorin.

[b] It should be noted that grading was according to NCIC CTC Version 1 (May, 1994). In the NCIC-CTC Version 1, hyperbilirubinemia grade 3 indicates a bilirubin value of 1.5 to 3 × ULN range, and grade 4 value of greater than 3 × ULN. The NCI CTC Version 2 and above define a grade 3 bilirubin value of greater than 3 to 10 × ULN, and grade 4 values greater than 10 × ULN.

➤*Metastatic colorectal cancer:* The following table shows the adverse reactions occurring in greater than or equal to 5% of patients from pooling the 2 phase 3 trials in first line metastatic colorectal cancer. A total of 596 patients with metastatic colorectal cancer were treated with 1,250 mg/m^2 twice a day of capecitabine administered for 2 weeks followed by a 1-week rest period, and 593 patients were administered 5-fluorouracil and leucovorin in the Mayo regimen (20 mg/m^2 leucovorin IV followed by 425 mg/m^2 IV bolus 5-fluorouracil, on days 1 to 5, every 28 days). In the pooled colorectal database the median duration of treatment was 139 days for capecitabine-treated patients and 140 days for 5-fluorouracil/leucovorin-treated patients. A total of 78 (13%) and 63 (11%) capecitabine and 5-fluorouracil/leucovorin-treated patients, respectively, discontinued treatment because of adverse reactions/intercurrent illness. A total of 82 deaths due to all causes occurred either on study or within 28 days of receiving study drug: 50 (8.4%) patients randomized to capecitabine and 32 (5.4%) randomized to 5-fluorouracil/leucovorin.

Phase 3 Colorectal Trials with Capecitabine vs 5-Fluorouracil/Leucovorin; Incidence Related or Unrelated to Treatment (≥ 5%)

	Capecitabine (n = 596)			5-Fluorouracil/Leucovorin (n = 593)		
	Total %	Grade 3 %	Grade 4 %	Total %	Grade 3 %	Grade 4 %
Number of patients with greater than 1 adverse reaction	96	52	9	94	45	9
CNS						
Depression	5%	—[a]	—[a]	4%	< 1%	—[a]
Dizziness[c]	8%	< 1%	—[a]	8%	< 1%	—[a]
Fatigue/Weakness	42%	4%	—[a]	46%	4%	—[a]
Headache	10%	1%	—[a]	7%	—[a]	—[a]
Insomnia	7%	—[a]	—[a]	7%	—[a]	—[a]
Mood alteration	5%	—[a]	—[a]	6%	< 1%	—[a]
Peripheral sensory neuropathy	10%	—[a]	—[a]	4%	—[a]	—[a]
Dermatologic						
Alopecia	6%	—[a]	—[a]	21%	< 1%	—[a]
Dermatitis	27%	1%	—[a]	26%	1%	—[a]
Hand-and-foot syndrome	54%	17%	NA[b]	6%	1%	NA
Skin discoloration	7%	< 1%	—[a]	5%	—[a]	—[a]
GI						
Abdominal pain	35%	9%	< 1%	31%	5%	—[a]
Constipation	14%	1%	< 1%	17%	1%	—[a]
Diarrhea	55%	13%	2%	61%	10%	2%
GI hemorrhage	6%	1%	< 1%	3%	1%	—[a]
GI motility disorder	10%	< 1%	—[a]	7%	< 1%	—[a]
Ileus	6%	4%	1%	5%	2%	1%
Nausea	43%	4%	—[a]	51%	3%	< 1%
Oral discomfort	10%	—[a]	—[a]	10%	—[a]	—[a]
Stomatitis	25%	2%	< 1%	62%	14%	1%
Taste disturbance	6%	1%	—[a]	11%	< 1%	1%

CAPECITABINE — ORAL

Phase 3 Colorectal Trials with Capecitabine vs 5-Fluorouracil/Leucovorin; Incidence Related or Unrelated to Treatment (≥ 5%)

	Capecitabine (n = 596)			5-Fluorouracil/Leucovorin (n = 593)		
	Total %	Grade 3 %	Grade 4 %	Total %	Grade 3 %	Grade 4 %
Upper GI inflammatory disorders	8%	< 1%	—[a]	10%	1%	—[a]
Vomiting	27%	4%	< 1%	30%	4%	< 1%
Hematologic/ Lymphatic						
Anemia	80%	2%	< 1%	79%	1%	< 1%
Neutropenia	13%	1%	2%	46%	8%	13%
Metabolic						
Appetite decreased	26%	3%	< 1%	31%	2%	< 1%
Dehydration	7%	2%	< 1%	8%	3%	1%
Edema	15%	1%	—[a]	9%	1%	—[a]
Musculoskeletal						
Arthralgia	8%	1%	—[a]	6%	1%	—[a]
Back pain	10%	2%	—[a]	9%	< 1%	—[a]
Respiratory						
Cough	7%	< 1%	1%	8%	—[a]	—[a]
Dyspnea	14%	1%	—[a]	10%	< 1%	1%
Epistaxis	3%	< 1%	—[a]	6%	—[a]	—[a]
Pharyngeal disorder	5%	—[a]	—[a]	5%	—[a]	—[a]
Sore throat	2%	—[a]	—[a]	6%	—[a]	—[a]
Special senses						
Eye irritation	13%	—[a]	—[a]	10%	< 1%	—[a]
Vision abnormal	5%	—[a]	—[a]	2%	—[a]	—[a]
Miscellaneous						
Chest pain	6%	1%	—[a]	6%	1%	< 1%
Hyperbilirubinemia	48%	18%	5%	17%	3%	3%
Pain	12%	1%	—[a]	10%	1%	—[a]
Pyrexia	18%	1%	—[a]	21%	2%	—[a]
Venous thrombosis	8%	3%	< 1%	6%	2%	—[a]
Viral infection	5%	< 1%	—[a]	5%	< 1%	—[a]

[a] Not observed.
[b] NA = Not applicable.
[c] Excluding vertigo.

➤*Breast cancer combination:* The following data are shown for the combination study with capecitabine and docetaxel in patients with metastatic breast cancer. In the capecitabine and docetaxel combination arm the treatment was capecitabine administered orally 1,250 mg/m² twice daily as intermittent therapy (2 weeks of treatment followed by 1 week without treatment) for at least 6 weeks and docetaxel administered as a 1-hour IV infusion at a dose of 75 mg/m² on the first day of each 3-week cycle for at least 6 weeks. In the monotherapy arm, docetaxel was administered as a 1-hour IV infusion at a dose of 100 mg/m² on the first day of each 3-week cycle for at least 6 weeks. The mean duration of treatment was 129 days in the combination arm and 98 days in the monotherapy arm. A total of 66 patients (26%) in the combination arm and 49 (19%) in the monotherapy arm withdrew from the study because of adverse reactions. The percentage of patients requiring dose reductions due to adverse reactions were 65% in the combination arm and 36% in the monotherapy arm. The percentage of patients requiring treatment interruptions due to adverse reactions in the combination arm was 79%. Treatment interruptions were part of the dose modification scheme for the combination therapy arm but not for the docetaxel monotherapy-treated patients.

Adverse Reactions Considered Related or Unrelated to Treatment in Capecitabine and Docetaxel Combination vs Docetaxel Monotherapy Study (≥ 5%)

	Capecitabine 1,250 mg/m² twice daily with docetaxel 75 mg/m²/3 weeks (n = 251)			Docetaxel 100 mg/m²/3 weeks (n = 255)		
Adverse reaction	Total %	Grade 3 %	Grade 4 %	Total %	Grade 3 %	Grade 4 %
Number of patients with at least 1 adverse reaction	99	76.5	29.1	97	57.6	31.8
CNS						
Asthenia	26%	4%	< 1%	25%	6%	—[a]
Depression	5%	—[a]	—[a]	5%	1%	—[a]
Dizziness	12%	—[a]	—[a]	8%	< 1%	—[a]
Fatigue	22%	4%	—[a]	27%	6%	—[a]
Headache	15%	3%	—[a]	15%	2%	—[a]
Hypoesthesia	4%	< 1%	—[a]	8%	< 1%	—[a]
Insomnia	8%	—[a]	—[a]	10%	< 1%	—[a]
Lethargy	7%	—[a]	—[a]	6%	2%	—[a]
Paresthesia	12%	< 1%	—[a]	16%	1%	—[a]
Peripheral neuropathy	6%	—[a]	—[a]	10%	1%	—[a]
Weakness	16%	2%	—[a]	11%	2%	—[a]
Dermatologic						
Alopecia	41%	6%	—[a]	42%	7%	—[a]
Dermatitis	8%	—[a]	—[a]	11%	1%	—[a]
Hand-and-foot syndrome	63%	24%	NA[b]	8%	1%	NA
Nail discoloration	6%	—[a]	—[a]	4%	< 1%	—[a]
Nail disorder	14%	2%	—[a]	15%	—[a]	—[a]
Onycholysis	5%	1%	—[a]	5%	1%	—[a]
Pruritus	4%	—[a]	—[a]	5%	—[a]	—[a]
Rash erythematous	9%	< 1%	—[a]	5%	—[a]	—[a]
GI						
Abdominal pain	30%	< 3%	< 1%	24%	2%	—[a]
Anorexia	13%	1%	—[a]	11%	< 1%	—[a]
Constipation	20%	2%	—[a]	18%	—[a]	—[a]
Diarrhea	67%	14%	< 1%	48%	5%	< 1%
Dry mouth	6%	< 1%	—[a]	5%	—[a]	—[a]
Dyspepsia	14%	—[a]	—[a]	8%	1%	—[a]
Nausea	45%	7%	—[a]	36%	2%	—[a]
Stomatitis	67%	17%	< 1%	43%	5%	—[a]
Taste disturbance	16%	< 1%	—[a]	14%	< 1%	—[a]
Vomiting	35%	4%	1%	24%	2%	—[a]
Infection						
Oral candidiasis	7%	< 1%	—[a]	8%	< 1%	—[a]
Upper respiratory tract	4%	—[a]	—[a]	5%	1%	—[a]
Urinary tract	6%	< 1%	—[a]	4%	—[a]	—[a]
Laboratory test abnormalities						
Anemia	80%	7%	3%	83%	5%	< 1%
Hyperbilirubinemia	20%	7%	2%	6%	2%	2%
Leukopenia	91%	37%	24%	88%	42%	33%
Lymphocytopenia	99%	48%	41%	98%	44%	40%
Neutropenia/ Granulocytopenia	86%	20%	49%	87%	10%	66%
Thrombocytopenia	41%	2%	1%	23%	1%	2%
Metabolic/ Nutritional						
Appetite decreased	10%	—[a]	—[a]	5%	—[a]	—[a]
Dehydration	10%	2%	—[a]	7%	< 1%	< 1%
Edema	33%	< 2%	—[a]	34%	< 3%	1%
Weight decreased	7%	—[a]	—[1]	5%	—[a]	—[a]
Musculoskeletal						
Arthralgia	15%	2%	—[a]	24%	3%	—[a]
Back pain	12%	< 1%	—[a]	11%	3%	—[a]
Bone pain	8%	< 1%	—[a]	10%	2%	—[a]
Myalgia	15%	2%	—[a]	25%	2%	—[a]
Respiratory						
Cough	13%	1%	—[a]	22%	< 1%	—[a]
Dyspnea	14%	2%	< 1%	16%	2%	—[a]
Epistaxis	7%	< 1%	—[a]	6%	—[a]	—[a]
Pleural effusion	2%	1%	—[a]	7%	4%	—[a]
Rhinorrhea	5%	—[a]	—[a]	3%	—[a]	—[a]

CAPECITABINE — ORAL

Adverse Reactions Considered Related or Unrelated to Treatment in Capecitabine and Docetaxel Combination vs Docetaxel Monotherapy Study (≥ 5%)

	Capecitabine 1,250 mg/m^2 twice daily with docetaxel 75 mg/m^2/3 weeks (n = 251)			Docetaxel 100 mg/m^2/3 weeks (n = 255)		
Adverse reaction	Total %	Grade 3 %	Grade 4 %	Total %	Grade 3 %	Grade 4 %
Sore throat	12%	2%	—[a]	11%	< 1%	—[a]
Special senses						
Conjunctivitis	5%	—[a]	—[a]	4%	—[a]	—[a]
Eye irritation	5%	—[a]	—[a]	1%	—[a]	—[a]
Lacrimation increased	12%	—[a]	—[a]	7%	< 1%	—[a]
Miscellaneous						
Chest pain (noncardiac)	4%	< 1%	—[a]	6%	2%	—[a]
Flushing	5%	—[a]	—[a]	5%	—[a]	—[a]
Influenza-like illness	5%	—[a]	—[a]	5%	—[a]	—[a]
Lymphedema	3%	< 1%	—[a]	5%	1%	—[a]
Neutropenic fever	16%	3%	13%	21%	5%	16%
Pain	7%	< 1%	—[a]	5%	1%	—[a]
Pain in limb	13%	< 1%	—[a]	13%	2%	—[a]
Pyrexia	28%	2%	—[a]	34%	2%	—[a]

[a] Not observed.
[b] NA = Not applicable.

➤*Breast cancer capecitabine monotherapy:* The following data are shown for the study in stage IV breast cancer patients who received a dose of 1,250 mg/m^2 administered twice daily for 2 weeks followed by a 1-week rest period. The mean duration of treatment was 114 days. A total of 13 out of 162 patients (8%) discontinued treatment because of adverse reactions/intercurrent illness.

Adverse Reactions Considered Remotely, Possibly, or Probably Related to Capecitabine Treatment in the Single Arm Trial in Stage IV Breast Cancer

	Phase 2 trial in stage IV breast cancer (n = 162)		
Adverse reaction	Total	Grade 3	Grade 4
CNS			
Dizziness	8%	—[a]	—[a]
Fatigue	41%	8%	—[a]
Headache	9%	1%	—[a]
Insomnia	8%	—[a]	—[a]
Paresthesia	21%	1%	—[a]
Dermatologic			
Dermatitis	37%	1%	—[a]
Hand-and-foot syndrome	57%	11%	NA[b]
Nail disorder	7%	—[a]	—[a]
GI			
Abdominal pain	20%	4%	—[a]
Anorexia	23%	3%	—[a]
Constipation	15%	1%	—[a]
Diarrhea	57%	12%	3%
Dyspepsia	8%	—[1]	—[a]
Nausea	53%	4%	—[a]
Stomatitis	24%	7%	—[a]
Vomiting	37%	4%	—[a]
Hematologic			
Anemia	72%	3%	1%
Lymphopenia	94%	44%	15%
Neutropenia	26%	2%	2%
Thrombocytopenia	24%	3%	1%
Metabolic			
Dehydration	7%	4%	1%
Edema	9%	1%	—[a]
Musculoskeletal			
Myalgia	9%	—[a]	—[a]
Miscellaneous			
Eye irritation	15%	—[a]	—[a]
Hyperbilirubinemia	22%	9%	2%
Pain in limb	6%	1%	—[a]
Pyrexia	12%	1%	—[a]

[a] Not observed.
[b] NA = Not applicable.

➤*Capecitabine and docetaxel in combination:* Shown by body system are the clinically relevant adverse reactions in less than 5% of patients in the overall clinical trial safety database of 251 patients (study details) reported as related to the administration of capecitabine in combination with docetaxel and that were clinically at least remotely relevant. In parentheses is the incidence of grade 3 and 4 occurrences of each adverse reaction. It is anticipated that the same types of adverse reactions observed in the capecitabine monotherapy studies may be observed in patients treated with the combination of capecitabine plus docetaxel.

Cardiovascular – Hypotension (1.2%), postural hypotension (0.8%), supraventricular tachycardia (0.39%), syncope (1.2%), venous phlebitis and thrombophlebitis (0.39%).

CNS – Ataxia (0.39%), polyneuropathy (0.39%), migraine (0.39%).

GI – Ileus (0.39%), necrotizing enterocolitis (0.39%), esophageal ulcer (0.39%), hemorrhagic diarrhea (0.8%), taste loss (0.8%).

Hematologic/Lymphatic – Agranulocytosis (0.39%), prothrombin decreased (0.39%).

Hepatic – Abnormal liver function tests, hepatic coma, hepatic failure, hepatotoxicity, jaundice (0.39%).

Miscellaneous – Bronchopneumonia (0.39%), hypersensitivity (1.2%), neutropenic sepsis (2.39%), renal failure (0.39%), sepsis (0.39%).

➤*Capecitabine monotherapy metastatic breast and colorectal cancer:* Shown by body system are the clinically relevant adverse reactions in less than 5% of patients in the overall clinical trial safety database of 875 patients (phase 3 colorectal studies [596 patients], phase 2 colorectal study [34 patients], phase 2 breast cancer studies [245 patients]) reported as related to the administration of capecitabine and that were clinically at least remotely relevant. In parentheses is the incidence of grade 3 or 4 occurrences of each adverse reaction.

Cardiovascular – Atrial fibrillation, bradycardia, cerebrovascular accident, extrasystoles, hypertension, myocarditis, tachycardia, ventricular extrasystoles (0.1%), hypotension, pulmonary embolism (0.2%), pericardial effusion.

CNS – Ataxia, insomnia (0.5%), confusion, depression, difficulty walking, dysphasia, encephalopathy, irritability, tremor (0.1%), abnormal coordination, dysarthria, loss of consciousness (0.2%), impaired balance, sedation, vertigo.

Dermatologic – Nail disorder, photosensitivity reaction, sweating increased (0.1%), pruritus, radiation recall syndrome, skin ulceration (0.2%).

GI – Abdominal distension, ascites, dysphagia, gastric ulcer, gastroenteritis, proctalgia, toxic dilation of intestine (0.1%), ileus (0.3%).

Hematologic/Lymphatic – Leukopenia (0.2%), bone marrow depression, coagulation disorder, lymphoedema, pancytopenia (0.1%), idiopathic thrombocytopenia purpura (1%).

Hepatic – Cholestatic hepatitis, hepatic fibrosis, hepatitis (0.1%), abnormal liver function tests.

Metabolic/Nutritional – Cachexia, increased weight (0.4%), hypertriglyceridemia (0.1%), edema, hypokalemia, hypomagnesemia.

Musculoskeletal – Arthritis, bone pain, myalgia (0.1%), muscle weakness.

Respiratory – Cough, epistaxis, hemoptysis, respiratory distress (0.1%), asthma, bronchitis, bronchopneumonia, pneumonia (0.2%), dyspnea.

Miscellaneous – Laryngitis (1%), chest pain, fungal infections (including candidiasis) (0.2%), chest mass, collapse, drug hypersensitivity, fibrosis, hoarseness, hot flushes, influenza-like illness, pain, thirst (0.1%), renal impairment (0.6%), keratoconjunctivitis, sepsis (0.3%), conjunctivitis, hemorrhage.

Postmarketing: Hepatic failure, lacrimal duct stenosis.

Overdosage

➤*Symptoms:* The manifestations of acute overdose would include nausea, vomiting, diarrhea, GI irritation and bleeding, and bone marrow depression.

➤*Treatment:* Medical management of overdose should include customary supportive medical interventions aimed at correcting the presenting clinical manifestations. Although no clinical experience using dialysis as a treatment for capecitabine overdose has been reported, dialysis may be of benefit in reducing circulating concentrations of 5′-deoxy-5-fluorouridine, a low-molecular weight metabolite of the parent compound.

Patient Information

Inform patients and patients' caregivers of the expected adverse effects of capecitabine, particularly nausea, vomiting, diarrhea, and hand-and-foot syndrome, and make them aware that patient specific dose adaptations during therapy are expected and necessary. Encourage patients to recognize the common grade 2 toxicities associated with capecitabine treatment.

➤*Diarrhea:* Instruct patients experiencing grade 2 or greater diarrhea (an increase of 4 to 6 stools/day or nocturnal stools) to stop taking capecitabine immediately. Standard antidiarrheal treatments (eg, loperamide) are recommended.

➤*Nausea:* Instruct patients experiencing grade 2 or greater nausea (food intake significantly decreased but able to eat intermittently) to stop taking capecitabine immediately. Initiation of symptomatic treatment is recommended.

CAPECITABINE — ORAL

➤*Vomiting:* Instruct patients experiencing grade 2 or greater vomiting (2 to 5 episodes in a 24-hour period) to stop taking capecitabine immediately. Initiation of symptomatic treatment is recommended.

➤*Hand-and-foot syndrome:* Instruct patients experiencing grade 2 or greater hand-and-foot syndrome (painful erythema and swelling of the hands and/or feet and/or discomfort affecting the patients' activities of daily living) to stop taking capecitabine immediately.

➤*Stomatitis:* Instruct patients experiencing grade 2 or greater stomatitis (painful erythema, edema or ulcers of the mouth or tongue, but able to eat) to stop taking capecitabine immediately. Initiation of symptomatic treatment is recommended.

➤*Fever and neutropenia:* Instruct patients who develop a fever of 38°C (100.5°F) or greater or other evidence of potential infection to call their health care provider.

CYTARABINE

Rx	**Cytarabine** (Mayne)	**Injection:** 20 mg/mL	In 5 mL single- and multi-[a] dose vials and preservative free 50 mL flip-top vial (pharmacy bulk package).
Rx	**Tarabine PFS** (Adria)		Preservative free. In 5 mL single vials and 50 mL bulk package vials.
Rx	**Cytarabine** (Abraxis)	**Injection:** 100 mg/mL	In 20 mL single-dose vials.
Rx	**Cytarabine** (Various, eg, Bedford)	**Powder for Injection:** 100 mg	In vials.
		500 mg	In vials.
		1 g	In vials.
		2 g	In vials.
Rx	**DepoCyt** (Enzon)	**Injection:** 10 mg/mL (liposomal)[b]	Preservative free. In 5 mLvials.

[a] With 0.9% benzyl alcohol.

[b] In Sodium Chloride 0.9% w/v in Water for Injection.

CYTARABINE — INJECTION

WARNING

Conventional cytarabine – Only physicians experienced in cancer chemotherapy should use cytarabine for injection and cytarabine sterile powder for injection.

For induction therapy, patients should be treated in a facility with laboratory and supportive resources sufficient to monitor drug tolerance and protect and maintain a patient compromised by drug toxicity. The main toxic effect of cytarabine for injection is bone marrow suppression with leukopenia, thrombocytopenia, and anemia. Less serious toxicity includes nausea, vomiting, diarrhea and abdominal pain, oral ulceration, and hepatic dysfunction.

The physician must judge possible benefit to the patient against known toxic effects of this drug in considering the advisability of therapy with cytarabine for injection. Before making this judgment or beginning treatment, the physician should be familiar with the following text.

Liposome injection – Intrathecal cytarabine liposome injection should be administered only under the supervision of a qualified physician experienced in the use of intrathecal cancer chemotherapeutic agents. Appropriate management of complications is possible only when adequate diagnostic and treatment facilities are readily available. In all clinical studies, chemical arachnoiditis, a syndrome manifested primarily by nausea, vomiting, headache, and fever was a common adverse event. If left untreated, chemical arachnoiditis may be fatal. The incidence and severity of chemical arachnoiditis can be reduced by coadministration of dexamethasone. Patients receiving intrathecal cytarabine should be treated concurrently with dexamethasone to mitigate the symptoms of chemical arachnoiditis.

Indications

➤*Conventional cytarabine:* Cytarabine solution for injection and cytarabine powder for injection, in combination with other approved anticancer drugs, is indicated for remission induction in acute nonlymphocytic leukemia of adults and pediatric patients. It has also been found useful in the treatment of acute lymphocytic leukemia and the blast phase of chronic myelocytic leukemia. Intrathecal administration of cytarabine injection (preservative-free preparations only) is indicated in the prophylaxis and treatment of meningeal leukemia.

➤*Liposome injection:* For the intrathecal treatment of lymphomatous meningitis. This indication is based on demonstration of increased complete response rate compared to unencapsulated cytarabine. There are no controlled trials that demonstrate a clinical benefit resulting from this treatment, such as improvement in disease-related symptoms, or increased time to disease progression, or increased survival.

➤*Off-label uses:* Treatment of Hodgkin disease; bone marrow transplantation.

Administration and Dosage

➤*General dosing considerations:* Thrombophlebitis has occurred at the site of drug injection or infusion in some patients, and rarely patients have noted pain and inflammation at subcutaneous injection sites. In most instances, however, the drug has been well tolerated.

Patients can tolerate higher total doses when they receive the conventional cytarabine by rapid IV injection as compared with slow infusion. This phenomenon is related to the drug's rapid inactivation and brief exposure of susceptible normal and neoplastic cells to significant levels after rapid injection. Normal and neoplastic cells seem to respond in somewhat parallel fashion to these different modes of administration, and no clear-cut clinical advantage has been demonstrated for either.

Intrathecal use – Cytarabine solution for injection and sterile powder for injection given intrathecally may cause systemic toxicity, and careful monitoring of the hemopoietic system is indicated. Modification of other antileukemic therapy may be necessary. Major toxicity is rare. The most frequently reported reactions after intrathecal administration were nausea, vomiting, and fever; these reactions are mild and self-limiting. Paraplegia has been reported. Necrotizing leukoencephalopathy occurred in 5 children; these patients had also been treated with intrathecal methotrexate and hydrocortisone, as well as by CNS radiation. Isolated neurotoxicity has been reported. Blindness occurred in 2 patients in remission whose treatment had consisted of combination systemic chemotherapy, prophylactic CNS radiation and intrathecal cytarabine.

When cytarabine is administered both intrathecally and IV within a few days, there is an increased risk of spinal cord toxicity; however, in serious life-threatening disease, concurrent use of IV and intrathecal cytarabine is left to the discretion of the treating physician.

Focal leukemic involvement of the CNS may not respond to intrathecal cytarabine and may better be treated with radiotherapy.

➤*Adults:*

Conventional cytarabine –

Acute nonlymphocytic leukemia: As induction therapy, 100 mg/m²/day by continuous IV infusion (days 1 to 7) or 100 mg/m² IV every 12 hours (days 1 to 7). Given in combination with other anticancer drugs. (See also Off-Label Dosing.)

Meningeal leukemia: Dosages have ranged from 5 mg/m² to 75 mg/m² of body surface area intrathecally once a day for 4 days to once every 4 days. The most frequently used dose was 30 mg/m² every 4 days until cerebrospinal fluid findings were normal, followed by 1 additional treatment. The dosage schedule is usually governed by the type and severity of CNS manifestations and the response to previous therapy.

Liposome injection –

Lymphomatous meningitis:

- *Induction therapy* – 50 mg administered intrathecally (intraventricular or lumbar puncture) every 14 days for 2 doses (weeks 1 and 3).
- *Consolidation therapy* – 50 mg administered intrathecally (intraventricular or lumbar puncture) every 14 days for 3 doses (weeks 5, 7, and 9), followed by 1 additional dose at week 13.
- *Maintenance therapy* – 50 mg administered intrathecally (intraventricular or lumbar puncture) every 28 days for 4 doses (weeks 17, 21, 25, and 29).
- *Dosage adjustment* – If drug-related neurotoxicity develops, the dose should be reduced to 25 mg. If it persists, treatment with intrathecal cytarabine should be discontinued.
- *Pretreatment* – Dexamethasone 4 mg twice daily either orally or IV for 5 days beginning on the day of intrathecal cytarabine injection to reduce the incidence of chemical arachnoiditis.

Off-label dosing –

Conventional cytarabine:

- *Acute leukemia* –
  - *Induction therapy:* 100 to 200 mg/m²/day or 2 to 6 mg/kg/day as a continuous IV infusion over 24 hours or in divided doses by rapid injection for 5 to 10 days, with the courses repeated approximately every 2weeks.
  - *Maintenance therapy:* 1 to 1.5 mg/kg/dose subcutaneously or IM every 1 to 4 weeks.
- *Acute nonlymphocytic leukemia* – 10 mg/m² subcutaneously twice daily for 7 to 14 days in combination with other chemotherapeutic drugs.
- *Hematopoietic stem cell transplantation* – Cytarabine 3,000 mg/m² IV every 12 hours for 3 days has been used.
- *Refractory acute leukemia or lymphomas* – 2,000 to 3,000 mg/m² IV every 12 hours for 2 to 6 days. Suspend or modify the dose of cytarabine if absolute neutrophil count (ANC) is below 1,000 cells/mm³ or the platelet count is below 50,000 cells/mm³.

CYTARABINE — INJECTION

➤*Children:*

Conventional cytarabine –

Acute nonlymphocytic leukemia: As induction therapy, 100 mg/m^2/day by continuous IV infusion (days 1 to 7) or 100 mg/m^2 IV every 12 hours (days 1 to 7). Given in combination with other anticancer drugs. (See also Off-Label Dosing.)

Meningeal leukemia: Dosages have ranged from 5 mg/m^2 to 75 mg/m^2 of body surface area intrathecally once a day for 4 days to once every 4 days. The most frequently used dose was 30 mg/m^2 every 4 days until cerebrospinal fluid findings were normal, followed by 1 additional treatment. The dosage schedule is usually governed by the type and severity of CNS manifestations and the response to previous therapy. (See also Off-Label Dosing.)

Off-label dosing –

Conventional cytarabine:

• *Acute leukemia –*

Induction therapy: 100 to 200 mg/m^2/day as a continuous IV infusion over 24 hours or in divided doses by rapid injection for 5 to 10 days, with the courses repeated approximately every 2weeks.

Maintenance therapy: 1 to 1.5 mg/kg/dose subcutaneously or IM every 1 to 4 weeks. Alternatively, 70 to 200 mg/m^2/day IV for 2 to 5 days repeated every month.

• *Meningeal leukemia –* Many clinicians recommend dosing intrathecal cytarabine by the child's age, as shown in the following table. Because the volume of the intrathecal space is related to age and not body surface area (BSA), dosing based on BSA may result in inadequate cerebrospinal fluid (CSF) concentrations in children and high, potentially neurotoxic concentrations in adults.

Intrathecal Cytarabine Dosing in Children According to Age

Patient age	Intrathecal cytarabine dose
< 1 year	20 mg
1 to 2 years	30 mg
2 to 3 years	50 mg
> 3 years	70 to 75 mg

• *Refractory acute leukemia or lymphomas –* 1,000 to 3,000 mg/m^2 IV every 12 hours for 2 to 6 days. Suspend or modify the dose of cytarabine if ANC is below 1,000 cells/mm^3 or the platelet count is below 50,000 cells/mm^3.

➤*Renal function impairment:*

Conventional cytarabine –

Dialysis: Supplemental dosing may be necessary after high-permeability hemodialysis.

➤*Conjunctivitis/Keratitis:* Prophylactic use of corticosteroid eye drops decreases the risk of conjunctivitis or keratitis with cytarabine. Begin prophylactic therapy prior to chemotherapy and continue for 2 to 7 days after the last dose of cytarabine. Effective regimens include prednisolone 1% eye drops (2 drops in both eyes every 4 hours) or dexamethasone 0.1% eye drops (1 to 2 drops in both eyes every 4 to 6 hours).

➤*Preparation for administration:* Cytarabine is considered a cytotoxic agent. Follow safe handling procedures when preparing, administering, or dispensing cytarabine.

Powder for injection –

Warning: Do not use bacteriostatic water for injection with benzyl alcohol as a diluent for intrathecal use.

IV: Reconstitute cytarabine lyophilized powder with bacteriostatic water for injection (with benzyl alcohol 0.9%) for IV use. Cytarabine may be further diluted with more than 50 mL of sodium chloride 0.9% injection for IV infusion.

Intrathecal: For intrathecal use, reconstitute lyophilized cytarabine with an isotonic buffered diluent without preservative, such as Ringer's lactate injection or sodium chloride 0.9% injection. Do not use a diluent containing benzyl alcohol.

High dose: For high doses, dilute cytarabine with preservative-free sodium chloride 0.9% injection.

Reconstitution of Cytarabine

Vial size	Volume of diluent: IV use[a]	Volume of diluent: Intrathecal use[b]	Resulting concentration
100 mg	5 mL	5 mL	20 mg/mL
500 mg	10 mL	10 mL	50 mg/mL
1,000 mg	10 mL	Not used	100 mg/mL
2,000 mg	20 mL	Not used	100 mg/mL

[a] Reconstitute with bacteriostatic water for injection (with benzyl alcohol 0.9%).
[b] Reconstitute with an isotonic buffered diluent without preservative, such as Ringer's lactate injection or sodium chloride 0.9% injection. Do not use a diluent containing benzyl alcohol.

Subcutaneous: Smaller volumes of diluent (1 to 2 mL) can be used to prepare a 100 mg/mL solution for subcutaneous injection.

Liposome injection – Vials of intrathecal cytarabine should be allowed to warm to room temperature and gently agitated or inverted to re-suspend the particles immediately prior to withdrawal from the vial. Avoid aggressive agitation. No further reconstitution or dilution is required. Further dilution is not recommended.

The use of gloves is recommended. If intrathecal cytarabine suspension contacts the skin, wash immediately with soap and water. If it contacts mucous membranes, flush thoroughly with water.

Intrathecal cytarabine particles are more dense than the diluent and have a tendency to settle with time.

➤*Administration:*

Conventional cytarabine – Cytarabine solution for injection and sterile powder for injection are not active orally. The schedule and method of administration varies with the program of therapy to be used. Cytarabine may be given by IV infusion or injection, subcutaneously, intrathecally (preservative-free preparation only), or IM.

Rotate injection sites for subcutaneous or IM administration.

When large IV doses are given quickly, patients are frequently nauseated and may vomit for several hours postinjection. This problem tends to be less severe when the drug is infused.

IV: Give by bolus injection over 1 to 3 minutes through a running IV line; infuse IV over 15 minutes in more than 50 mL of sodium chloride 0.9% injection; or give as a continuous IV infusion over 5 days. Cytarabine doses often are infused over 30 minutes.

High-dose therapy: Give IV infusion over 1 to 3 hours. Faster infusions of high doses may increase the risk of CNS adverse effects.

Liposome injection – Intrathecal cytarabine liposome injection should be withdrawn from the vial immediately before administration. Unused portions of each vial should be discarded properly. Do not save any unused portions for later administration. Do not mix intrathecal cytarabine with any other medications.

In-line filters must not be used when administering intrathecal cytarabine liposome injection. Intrathecal cytarabine is administered directly into the cerebral spinal fluid (CSF) via an intraventricular reservoir or by direct injection into the lumbar sac. Intrathecal cytarabine should be injected slowly over a period of 1 to 5 minutes. Following drug administration by lumbar puncture, the patient should be instructed to lie flat for 1 hour. Patients should be observed by the physician for immediate toxic reactions.

Intrathecal cytarabine liposome injection must only be administered by the intrathecal route.

➤*Extravasation:* Cytarabine is considered an irritant and may cause phlebitis, but it is not known to cause tissue damage with extravasation. If signs or symptoms of extravasation occur, stop the infusion immediately. If possible, withdraw 3 to 5 mL of blood to remove some of the drug. Remove the infusion needle. Delineate the infiltrated area on the patient's skin with a felt tip marker. Elevate for 48 hours above heart level using a sling or stockinette dressing with an observation window cut in the dressing. Avoid pressure or friction. Do not rub the area. Observe for signs of increased erythema, pain, or skin necrosis. If increased symptoms occur, consult a plastic surgeon. Ensure that no medication is given distally to the extravasation site. After 48 hours, encourage the patient to use the extremity normally to promote full range of motion.

➤*Storage/Stability:* Discard single-dose vials within 6 hours of the initial needle puncture if opened within an ISO Class 5 biological safety cabinet, or within 1 hour of the initial needle puncture if opened outside of such an environment, based on the USP Chapter < 797 > standards.

Multiple-dose vials may be used for up to 28 days after the initial needle puncture, based on the USP Chapter <797> standards.

Solution for injection – Store vials at 15° to 30°C (59° to 86°F). Protect from light. Retain in carton until time of use.

Chemical stability studies were performed by ultraviolet assay on cytarabine injection in infusion solutions. These studies showed that when reconstituted cytarabine or cytarabine solution for injection was added to sterile water for injection, dextrose 5% injection or sodium chloride injection, 94% to 96% of the cytarabine was present after 192 hours of storage at room temperature.

Discard pharmacy bulk package vials within 4 hours of the initial needle puncture.

Powder for injection – Store vials at 25°C (77°F); excursions are permitted to 15° to 30°C (59° to 86°F).

The pH of the reconstituted cytarabine for injection solutions is about 5. Solutions reconstituted with bacteriostatic water for injection with benzyl alcohol 0.945% w/v may be stored at 20° to 25°C (68° to 77°F) for 48 hours. Discard any solutions in which a slight haze develops. The manufacturer recommends that solutions reconstituted without a preservative be used immediately. However, preservative-free cytarabine solutions should be used within 24 hours of reconstitution.

Liposome injection – Refrigerate vials at 2° to 8°C (36° to 46°F). Protect from freezing and avoid aggressive agitation.

Unopened vials are stable at room temperature for up to 72 hours. Accelerated degradation occurs at temperatures above 37°C (98°F).

Liposomal cytarabine is preservative free. The manufacturer recommends using the suspension within 4 hours after removing it from the vial. Discard preservative-free liposomal cytarabine within 24 hours of preparation.

Actions

➤*Pharmacology:* Cytarabine is cytotoxic to a wide variety of proliferating mammalian cells in culture. It exhibits cell phase specificity, primarily killing cells undergoing DNA synthesis (S-phase) and under certain conditions blocking the progression of cells from the G_1 phase to the S-phase. Although the mechanism of action is not completely understood, it appears that cytarabine acts through the inhibition of DNA polymerase. A limited, but

CYTARABINE — INJECTION

significant, incorporation of cytarabine into both DNA and RNA has also been reported. Extensive chromosomal damage, including chromatoid breaks, have been produced by cytarabine and malignant transformation of rodent cells in culture has been reported. Deoxycytidine prevents or delays (but does not reverse) the cytotoxic activity.

Cytarabine is metabolized by deoxycytidine kinase and other nucleotide kinases to the nucleotide triphosphate, an effective inhibitor of DNA polymerase; it is inactivated by a pyrimidine nucleoside deaminase, which converts it to the nontoxic uracil derivative. It appears that the balance of kinase and deaminase levels may be an important factor in determining sensitivity or resistance of the cell to cytarabine.

Cytarabine is capable of obliterating immune responses in man during administration with little or no accompanying toxicity. Suppression of antibody responses to *E. coli*-VI antigen and tetanus toxoid have been demonstrated. This suppression was obtained during both primary and secondary antibody responses.

Cytarabine also suppressed the development of cell-mediated immune responses such as delayed hypersensitivity skin reaction to dinitrochlorobenzene. However, it had no effect on already established delayed hypersensitivity reactions.

Following 5-day courses of intensive therapy with cytarabine solution for injection or sterile powder for injection, the immune response was suppressed, as indicated by the following parameters: Macrophage ingress into skin windows; circulating antibody response following primary antigenic stimulation; lymphocyte blastogenesis with phytohemagglutinin. A few days after termination of therapy there was a rapid return to normal.

Liposome injection –

Mechanism of action: Intrathecal cytarabine liposome injection is a sustained-release formulation of the active ingredient cytarabine designed for direct administration into the CSF. Cytarabine is a cell cycle phase-specific antineoplastic agent, affecting cells only during the S-phase of cell division. Intracellularly, cytarabine is converted into cytarabine-5'-triphosphate (ara-CTP), which is the active metabolite. The mechanism of action is not completely understood, but it appears that ara-CTP acts primarily through inhibition of DNA polymerase. Incorporation into DNA and RNA may also contribute to cytarabine cytotoxicity. Cytarabine is cytotoxic to a wide variety of proliferating mammalian cells in culture.

➤*Pharmacokinetics:*

Absorption / Distribution –

Solution for injection and sterile powder for injection: Cytarabine is rapidly metabolized and is not effective orally; less than 20% of the orally administered dose is absorbed from the GI tract.

Relatively constant plasma levels can be achieved by continuous IV infusion.

After SC or IM administration of cytarabine labeled with tritium, peak plasma levels of radioactivity are achieved about 20 to 60 minutes after injection and are considerably lower than those after IV administration.

Cerebrospinal fluid levels of cytarabine are low in comparison to plasma levels after single IV injection. However, in 1 patient in whom cerebrospinal levels were examined after 2 hours of constant IV infusion, levels approached 40% of the steady state plasma level. With intrathecal administration, levels of cytarabine in the cerebrospinal fluid declined with a first order half-life of about 2 hours. Because cerebrospinal fluid levels of deaminase are low, little conversion to 1-β-D-arabinofuranosyluracil (ara-U) was observed.

Liposome injection: The pharmacokinetics of liposomal cytarabine administered intrathecally to patients at a 50 mg dose every 2 weeks is currently under investigation. However, preliminary analysis of the pharmacokinetic data show that following intrathecal cytarabine administration in patients, in either the lumbar sac or by intraventricular reservoir, peak levels of free cytarabine were observed within 5 hours in both the ventricle and lumbar sac. These peak levels were followed by a biphasic elimination profile with a terminal phase half-life of 100 to 263 hours over a dose range of 12.5 mg to 75 mg. In contrast, intrathecal administration of 30 mg of free cytarabine showed a biphasic CSF concentration profile with a terminal phase half-life of 3.4 hours. Since the transfer rate of cytarabine from the CSF to plasma is slow and the conversion of cytarabine to ara-U in the plasma is fast, systemic exposure to cytarabine was negligible following intrathecal administration of intrathecal cytarabine, 50 mg or 75 mg.

Metabolism / Excretion –

Solution for injection and powder for injection: Following rapid IV injection of cytarabine labeled with tritium, the disappearance from plasma is biphasic. There is an initial distributive phase with a half-life of about 10 minutes, followed by a second elimination phase with a half-life of about 1 to 3 hours. After the distributive phase, more than 80% of plasma radioactivity can be accounted for by the inactive metabolite ara-U. Within 24 hours about 80% of the administered radioactivity can be recovered in the urine, approximately 90% of which is excreted as ara-U.

Liposome injection: The primary route of elimination of intrathecal cytarabine liposome injection is metabolism to the inactive compound ara-U (1-β-D-arabinofuranosyluracil or uracilarabinoside), followed by urinary excretion of ara-U. In contrast to systemically administered cytarabine, which is rapidly metabolized to ara-U, conversion to ara-U in the CSF is negligible after intrathecal administration because of the significantly lower cytidine deaminase activity in the CNS tissues and CSF. The CSF clearance rate of cytarabine is similar to the CSF bulk flow rate of 0.24 mL/min.

Contraindications

Hypersensitivity to cytarabine or any component of the formulation; active meningeal infection (liposomal cytarabine only).

Warnings/Precautions

➤*Hematologic:* Cytarabine is a potent bone-marrow suppressant. Therapy should be started cautiously in patients with preexisting drug-induced bone marrow suppression. Patients receiving this drug must be under close medical supervision and, during induction therapy, should have leukocyte and platelet counts performed daily. Bone marrow examinations should be performed frequently after blasts have disappeared from the peripheral blood. Facilities should be available for management of complications, possibly fatal, of bone marrow suppression (infection resulting from granulocytopenia and other impaired body defenses, and hemorrhage secondary to thrombocytopenia). One case of anaphylaxis that resulted in acute cardiopulmonary arrest and required resuscitation has been reported. This occurred immediately after the IV administration of cytarabine solution for injection or powder for injection.

➤*Experimental doses:* Severe and at times fatal CNS, GI, and pulmonary toxicity (different from that seen with conventional therapy regimens of cytarabine) has been reported following some experimental dose schedules for cytarabine solution for injection and sterile powder for injection. These reactions include reversible corneal toxicity, and hemorrhagic conjunctivitis, which may be prevented or diminished by prophylaxis with a local corticosteroid eye drop; cerebral and cerebellar dysfunction, including personality changes, somnolence and coma, usually reversible; severe gastrointestinal ulceration, including pneumatosis cystoides intestinalis leading to peritonitis; sepsis and liver abscess; pulmonary edema, liver damage with increased hyperbilirubinemia; bowel necrosis; and necrotizing colitis. Rarely, severe skin rash, leading to desquamation has been reported. Complete alopecia is more commonly seen with experimental high dose therapy than with standard treatment programs using cytarabine solution for injection or powder for injection. If experimental high-dose therapy is used, do not use a preparation or diluent containing benzyl alcohol.

Cases of cardiomyopathy with subsequent death have been reported following experimental high dose therapy with cytarabine in combination with cyclophosphamide when used for bone marrow transplant preparation.

A syndrome of sudden respiratory distress, rapidly progressing to pulmonary edema and radiographically pronounced cardiomegaly has been reported following experimental high dose therapy with cytarabine used for the treatment of relapsed leukemia from 1 institution in 16 of 72 patients. The outcome of this syndrome can be fatal.

➤*Benzyl alcohol:* Benzyl alcohol is contained in the diluent for this product. Benzyl alcohol has been reported to be associated with a fatal "gasping syndrome" in premature infants.

➤*Delayed progressive ascending paralysis:* Two patients with childhood acute myelogenous leukemia who received intrathecal and IV cytarabine solution for injection or sterile powder for injection at conventional doses (in addition to a number of other concomitantly administered drugs) developed delayed progressive ascending paralysis resulting in death in 1 of the 2 patients.

➤*Liposome injection:* See the Warning box for more information.

Death – During the clinical studies, 2 deaths related to intrathecal liposomal cytarabine were reported. One patient died after developing encephalopathy 36 hours after an intraventricular dose of intrathecal cytarabine, 125 mg. This patient was receiving concurrent whole-brain irradiation and had previously received systemic chemotherapy with cyclophosphamide, doxorubicin, and fluorouracil, as well as intraventricular methotrexate. The other patient received intrathecal cytarabine 50 mg by the intraventricular route and developed focal seizures progressing to status epilepticus. This patient died approximately 8 weeks after the last dose of study medication. The death of 1 additional patient was considered "possibly" related to intrathecal cytarabine. He was a 63-year-old with extensive lymphoma involving the nasopharynx, brain, and meninges with multiple neurologic deficits who died of apparent disease progression 4 days after his second dose of intrathecal cytarabine.

Intrathecal use – After intrathecal administration of free cytarabine, the most frequently reported reactions are nausea, vomiting and fever. Intrathecal administration of free cytarabine may cause myelopathy and other neurologic toxicity and can rarely lead to a permanent neurologic deficit. Administration of intrathecal cytarabine in combination with other chemotherapeutic agents or with cranial/spinal irradiation may increase this risk of neurotoxicity.

Blockage to CSF flow may result in increased free cytarabine concentrations in the CSF and an increased risk of neurotoxicity.

➤*Rapid administration:* When large IV doses are given quickly, patients are frequently nauseated and may vomit for several hours postinjection. This problem tends to be less severe when the drug is infused.

➤*Acute pancreatitis:* Acute pancreatitis has been reported to occur in a patient receiving cytarabine for injection by continuous infusion and in patients being treated with cytarabine for injection who have had prior treatment with L-asparaginase.

➤*Neoplastic meningitis:* Some patients with neoplastic meningitis receiving treatment with intrathecal cytarabine may require concurrent radiation or systemic therapy with other chemotherapeutic agents; this may increase the rate of adverse events.

➤*CSF elevations:* Transient elevations in CSF protein and white blood cells have been observed in patients following intrathecal cytarabine administration and have also been noted after intrathecal treatment with methotrexate or cytarabine.

➤*Extravasation:* See Administration and Dosage for more information.

CYTARABINE — INJECTION

➤*Hypersensitivity reactions:* One case of anaphylaxis that resulted in acute cardiopulmonary arrest and required resuscitation has been reported. This occurred immediately after the IV administration of cytarabine for injection.

Liposome injection – Anaphylactic reactions following IV administration of free cytarabine have been reported.

➤*Renal/Hepatic function impairment:* The human liver apparently detoxifies a substantial fraction of an administered dose. In particular, patients with renal or hepatic function impairment may have a higher likelihood of CNS toxicity after high-dose cytarabine solution for injection or sterile powder for injection treatment. Use the drug with caution and possibly at reduced dose in patients whose liver or kidney function is poor.

➤*Pregnancy:*

Cytarabine solution for injection and sterile powder for injection – Category D. Cytarabine can cause fetal harm when administered to a pregnant woman. Cytarabine causes abnormal cerebellar development in the neonatal hamster and is teratogenic to the rat fetus. There are no adequate and well-controlled studies in pregnant women. Women of childbearing potential should be advised to avoid becoming pregnant.

A review of the literature has shown 32 reported cases where cytarabine solution for injection or sterile powder for injection was given during pregnancy, either alone or in combination with other cytotoxic agents:

Eighteen healthy infants were delivered. Four of these had first trimester exposure. Five infants were premature or of low birth weight. Twelve of the 18 healthy infants were followed up at ages ranging from 6 weeks to 7 years, and showed no abnormalities. One apparently healthy infant died at 90 days of gastroenteritis.

Two cases of congenital abnormalities have been reported, one with upper and lower distal limb defects, and the other with extremity and ear deformities. Both of these cases had first trimester exposure.

There were 7 infants with various problems in the neonatal period, including pancytopenia; transient depression of WBC, hematocrit or platelets; electrolyte abnormalities; transient eosinophilia; and 1 case of increased IgM levels and hyperpyrexia possibly due to sepsis. Six of the 7 infants were also premature. The child with pancytopenia died at 21 days of sepsis.

Therapeutic abortions were done in 5 cases. Four fetuses were grossly healthy, but one had an enlarged spleen and another showed Trisomy C chromosome abnormality in the chorionic tissue.

Because of the potential for abnormalities with cytotoxic therapy, particularly during the first trimester, a patient who is or who may become pregnant while on cytarabine solution for injection or sterile powder for injection should be apprised of the potential risk to the fetus and the advisability of pregnancy continuation. There is a definite, but considerably reduced risk if therapy is initiated during the second or third trimester. Although healthy infants have been delivered to patients treated in all 3 trimesters of pregnancy, follow-up of such infants would be advisable.

➤*Lactation:*

Solution for injection and sterile powder for injection – It is not known whether this drug is excreted in human milk. Because many drugs are excreted in human milk, and because of the potential for serious adverse reactions in nursing infants from cytarabine, a decision should be made whether to discontinue nursing or to discontinue the drug, taking into account the importance of the drug to the mother.

Liposome injection – It is not known whether cytarabine is excreted in human milk following intrathecal cytarabine liposome injection administration. The systemic exposure to free cytarabine following intrathecal treatment with intrathecal cytarabine was negligible. Despite the low apparent risk, because many drugs are excreted in human milk and because of the potential for serious adverse reactions in nursing infants, the use of intrathecal cytarabine is not recommended in nursing women.

➤*Children:*

Solution for injection and sterile powder for injection – Cytarabine solution for injection and sterile powder for injection, in combination with other approved anticancer drugs, is indicated for remission induction in acute nonlymphocytic leukemia of pediatric patients.

Liposome injection – The safety and efficacy of intrathecal cytarabine liposome injection in pediatric patients has not been established.

➤*Monitoring:*

Solution for injection and sterile powder for injection – Patients receiving cytarabine must be monitored closely. Frequent platelet and leukocyte counts and bone marrow examinations are mandatory. Consider suspending or modifying therapy when drug-induced marrow depression has resulted in a platelet count under 50,000 or a polymorphonuclear granulocyte count under 1000/mm^3. Counts of formed elements in the peripheral blood may continue to fall after the drug is stopped and reach lowest values after drug-free intervals of 12 to 24 days. When indicated, restart therapy when definite signs of marrow recovery appear (on successive bone marrow studies). Patients whose drug is withheld until "normal" peripheral blood values are attained may escape from control.

Periodic checks of bone marrow, liver and kidney functions should be performed in patients receiving cytarabine.

Like other cytotoxic drugs, cytarabine may induce hyperuricemia secondary to rapid lysis of neoplastic cells. The clinician should monitor the patient's blood uric acid level and be prepared to use such supportive and pharmacologic measures as might be necessary to control this problem.

Liposome injection – Intrathecal cytarabine liposome injection has the potential of producing serious toxicity. All patients receiving intrathecal cytarabine should be treated concurrently with dexamethasone to mitigate the symptoms of chemical arachnoiditis. Toxic effects may be related to a single dose or to cumulative administration. Because toxic effects can occur at any time during therapy (although they are most likely within 5 days of drug administration), patients receiving intrathecal therapy with intrathecal cytarabine liposome injection should be monitored continuously for the development of neurotoxicity. If patients develop neurotoxicity, subsequent doses of intrathecal cytarabine should be reduced, and intrathecal cytarabine should be discontinued if toxicity persists.

Although significant systemic exposure to free cytarabine following intrathecal treatment is not expected, some effect on bone marrow function cannot be excluded. Systemic toxicity due to IV administration of cytarabine consists primarily of bone marrow suppression with leukopenia, thrombocytopenia, and anemia. Accordingly, careful monitoring of the hematopoietic system is advised.

Drug Interactions

Cytarabine Drug Interactions

Precipitant drug	Object drug[a]		Description
Cytarabine	Digoxin	⬇	Combination chemotherapy (including cytarabine) may decrease digoxin absorption even several days after stopping chemotherapy. Digoxin capsules and digitoxin do not appear to be affected.
Cytarabine	Gentamicin	⬇	An in vitro interaction between gentamicin and cytarabine showed a cytarabine-related antagonism for the susceptibility of *K. pneumoniae* strains. This study suggests that in patients on cytarabine being treated with gentamicin for a *K. pneumoniae* infection, the lack of a prompt therapeutic response may indicate the need for reevaluation of antibacterial therapy.

[a] ⬇ = Object drug decreased.

➤*Digoxin:* Reversible decreases in steady-state plasma digoxin concentrations and renal glycoside excretion were observed in patients receiving beta-acetyldigoxin and chemotherapy regimens containing cyclophosphamide, vincristine and prednisone with or without cytarabine solution for injection or sterile powder for injection or procarbazine. Steady-state plasma digitoxin concentrations did not appear to change. Therefore, monitoring of plasma digoxin levels may be indicated in patients receiving similar combination chemotherapy regimens. The utilization of digitoxin for such patients may be considered as an alternative.

➤*Gentamicin:* An in vitro interaction study between gentamicin and cytarabine showed a cytarabine-related antagonism for the susceptibility of *K. pneumoniae* strains. This study suggests that in patients on cytarabine being treated with gentamicin for a *K. pneumoniae* infection, the lack of a prompt therapeutic response may indicate the need for reevaluation of antibacterial therapy.

➤*Fluorocytosine:* Clinical evidence in 1 patient showed possible inhibition of fluorocytosine efficacy during therapy with cytarabine solution for injection or sterile powder for injection. This may be due to potential competitive inhibition of its uptake.

➤*Drug/Lab test interactions:*

Liposome injection – See Warnings/Precautions for more information.

Adverse Reactions

Conventional cytarabine has very high potential for nausea and vomiting with doses above 1,000 mg/m^2 or rapid administration, moderate to high emetogenic potential with doses of 250 to 1,000 mg/m^2, and moderate emetogenic potential with lower doses. Liposomal cytarabine is considered to have low potential for nausea and vomiting.,

➤*Conventional cytarabine:*

Hematologic – Because cytarabine is a bone-marrow suppressant, anemia, leukopenia, thrombocytopenia, megaloblastosis and reduced reticulocytes can be expected as a result of administration with cytarabine. The severity of these reactions are dose and schedule dependent. Cellular changes in the morphology of bone marrow and peripheral smears can be expected. Following 5-day constant infusions or acute injections of 50 mg/m^2 to 600 mg/m^2, white cell depression follows a biphasic course. Regardless of initial count, dosage level, or schedule, there is an initial fall starting the first 24 hours with a nadir at days 7 to 9. This is followed by a brief rise which peaks around the twelfth day. A second and deeper fall reaches nadir at days 15 to 24. Then there is rapid rise to above baseline in the next 10 days. Platelet depression is noticeable at 5 days with a peak depression occurring between days 12 to 15. Thereupon, a rapid rise to above baseline occurs in the next 10 days.

Infection (solution for injection and sterile powder for injection) – Viral, bacterial, fungal, parasitic, or saprophytic infections, in any location in the body may be associated with the use of cytarabine for injection or ster-

CYTARABINE — INJECTION

ile powder for injection alone or in combination with other immunosuppressive agents following immunosuppressant doses that affect cellular or humoral immunity. These infections may be mild, but can be severe and at times fatal.

Cytarabine (Ara-C) syndrome – A cytarabine syndrome has been described. It is characterized by fever, myalgia, bone pain, occasionally chest pain, maculopapular rash, conjunctivitis and malaise. It usually occurs 6 to 12 hours following drug administration. Corticosteroids have been shown to be beneficial in treating or preventing this syndrome. If the symptoms of the syndrome are deemed treatable, corticosteroids should be contemplated as well as continuation of therapy with cytarabine solution for injection or sterile powder for injection.

Most frequent adverse reactions – Anorexia; oral and anal inflammation or ulceration; rash; nausea; thrombophlebitis; vomiting; hepatic dysfunction; bleeding (all sites); diarrhea; fever. Nausea and vomiting are most frequent following rapid IV injection.

Less frequent adverse reactions – Sepsis; esophageal ulceration; conjunctivitis (may occur with rash); esophagitis; pneumonia; dizziness; cellulitis at injection site; chest pain; alopecia; skin ulceration; pericarditis; anaphylaxis (see Warnings); urinary retention; bowel necrosis; allergic edema; renal dysfunction; abdominal pain; pruritus; neuritis; pancreatitis; shortness of breath; neural toxicity; freckling; urticaria; sore throat; jaundice; headache.

➤*Experimental doses:*

Miscellaneous – See Warnings/Precautions for more information.

Two patients with adult acute nonlymphocytic leukemia developed peripheral motor and sensory neuropathies after consolidation with high-dose cytarabine solution for injection or sterile powder for injection, daunorubicin, and asparaginase. Patients treated with high-dose cytarabine solution for injection or sterile powder for injection should be observed for neuropathy since dose schedule alterations may be needed to avoid irreversible neurologic disorders.

Ten patients treated with experimental intermediate doses of cytarabine solution for injection or sterile powder for injection (1 g/m^2) with and without other chemotherapeutic agents (meta-AMSA, daunorubicin, etoposide) at various dose regimens developed a diffuse interstitial pneumonitis without clear cause that may have been related to the cytarabine.

Two cases of pancreatitis have been reported following experimental doses of cytarabine and numerous other drugs. Cytarabine could have been the causative agent.

➤*Liposome injection:* Arachnoiditis is an expected and well-documented side effect of both neoplastic meningitis and of intrathecal chemotherapy. For clinical studies of intrathecal cytarabine, chemical arachnoiditis was defined as the occurrence of any one of the symptoms of neck rigidity, neck pain, meningism, or any 2 of the symptoms of nausea, vomiting, headache, fever, back pain, or CSF pleocytosis; the grade assigned to an episode of chemical arachnoiditis was the highest severity grade of its component symptoms. Since most of the adverse events reported in the trials were transient episodes associated with drug exposure, the incidence of these events is best expressed by drug cycle. A cycle of treatment for all treatment groups was defined as the 14-day period between intrathecal cytarabine doses. The duration of reported symptoms was from 1 to 5 days. Although it was sometimes difficult to distinguish between drug-related chemical arachnoiditis, infectious meningitis, or disease progression, greater than 90% of the chemical arachnoiditis cases reported occurred within 48 hours of the administration of intrathecal drug, indicating a drug etiology.

In the early study, chemical arachnoiditis was observed in 100% of cycles without dexamethasone prophylaxis; with concurrent administration of dexamethasone, chemical arachnoiditis was observed in 33% of cycles. Patients receiving intrathecal liposome injection should be treated concurrently with dexamethasone to mitigate the symptoms of chemical arachnoiditis.

Comparison of adverse events occurring in greater than or equal to 10% of patients, by cycle –

Patients with Lymphomatous Meningitis Receiving Intrathecal Cytarabine Liposome Injection or Cytarabine (Ara-C) in the Randomized Study				
	All adverse reactions %		Grade 3 or 4 adverse reactions %	
Body system/ adverse reaction	Intrathecal cytarabine liposome injection (n = 74)	Cytarabine (n = 45)	Intrathecal cytarabine liposome injection (n = 74)	Cytarabine (n = 45)
CNS	45%	53%	18%	18%
Confusion	14%	7%	4%	2%
Somnolence	12%	11%	4%	2%
Abnormal gait	4%	11%	1%	2%
GI	27%	44%	7%	9%
Nausea[a]	11%	16%	0%	4%
Vomiting[a]	12%	18%	3%	2%
Constipation	7%	11%	0%	0%
Hematologic	19%	22%	11%	13%
Neutropenia	9%	11%	8%	11%
Thrombocytopenia	8%	16%	5%	11%
Anemia	1%	13%	1%	4%
Metabolic/nutritional	16%	24%	0%	0%
Peripheral edema	7%	11%	0%	0%
GU	11%	20%	3%	2%
Urinary incontinence	3%	11%	0%	0%
Special senses	16%	18%	1%	2%
Miscellaneous	53%	60%	18%	22%
Headache	28%	9%	5%	2%
Asthenia	19%	33%	5%	9%
Fever[a]	11%	24%	4%	0%
Back pain[a]	7%	11%	0%	2%
Pain	11%	20%	3%	0%

[a] Components of chemical arachnoiditis.

Overdosage

➤*Conventional cytarabine:* There is no antidote for overdosage of cytarabine solution for injection or sterile powder for injection. Doses of 4.5 g/m^2 by IV infusion over 1 hour every 12 hours for 12 doses has caused an unacceptable increase in irreversible CNS toxicity and death. Single doses as high as 3 g/m^2 have been administered by rapid IV infusion without apparent toxicity.

➤*Liposome injection:* No overdosages with intrathecal cytarabine have been reported. An overdose with intrathecal cytarabine may be associated with severe chemical arachnoiditis including encephalopathy.

In an early uncontrolled study without dexamethasone prophylaxis, single doses up to 125 mg were administered. One patient at the 125 mg dose level died of encephalopathy 36 hours after receiving an intraventricular dose of intrathecal cytarabine. This patient, however, was also receiving concomitant whole brain irradiation and had previously received intraventricular methotrexate.

There is no antidote for overdose of intrathecal cytarabine or unencapsulated cytarabine released from intrathecal cytarabine. Exchange of CSF with isotonic saline has been carried out in a case of intrathecal overdose of free cytarabine, and such a procedure may be considered in the case of intrathecal cytarabine overdose. Management of overdose should be directed at maintaining vital functions.

Patient Information

Patients should be informed about the expected adverse events of headache, nausea, vomiting, and fever, and about the early signs and symptoms of neurotoxicity. The importance of concurrent dexamethasone administration should be emphasized at the initiation of each cycle of intrathecal cytarabine treatment. Patients should be instructed to seek medical attention if signs or symptoms of neurotoxicity develop, or if oral dexamethasone is not well tolerated.

FLUOROURACIL (5-Fluorouracil; 5-FU)

Rx	**Fluorouracil** (Various, eg, American Pharmaceutical Partners)	**Injection:** 50 mg/mL	In 10, 20, and 100 mL vials and 10 mL amps.
Rx	**Adrucil** (Gensia Sicor)		In 10, 50, and 100 mL vials.

FLUOROURACIL — INJECTION

WARNING

It is recommended that fluorouracil injection be given only by or under the supervision of a qualified physician who is experienced in cancer chemotherapy and who is well versed in the use of potent antimetabolites. Because of the possibility of severe toxic reactions, it is recommended that patients be hospitalized at least during the initial course of therapy. These instructions should be thoroughly reviewed before administration of fluorouracil.

Indications

➤*Cancer:* For the palliative management of carcinoma of the colon, rectum, breast, stomach, and pancreas.

➤*Off-label uses:* Treatment of ovarian, cervical, bladder, hepatic, prostate, endometrial, esophageal, and head and neck carcinoma.

Administration and Dosage

➤*General dosing considerations:* It is recommended that patients be hospitalized during their first course of treatment.

All dosages are based on the patient's actual weight. However, the estimated lean body mass (dry weight) is used if the patient is obese or if there has been a spurious weight gain due to edema, ascites, or other forms of abnormal fluid retention.

It is recommended that prior to treatment each patient be carefully evaluated in order to estimate as accurately as possible the optimum initial dosage of fluorouracil. Fluorouracil should be used with extreme caution in poor risk patients with a history of high-dose pelvic irradiation or previous use of alkylating agents, those who have a widespread involvement of bone marrow by metastatic tumors or those with impaired hepatic or renal function.

Rarely, unexpected, severe toxicity (eg, stomatitis, diarrhea, neutropenia, neurotoxicity) associated with 5-fluorouracil has been attributed to deficiency of dipyrimidine dehydrogenase activity. A few patients have been rechallenged with 5-fluorouracil and despite 5-fluorouracil dose lowering, toxicity recurred and progressed with worse morbidity. Absence of this catabolic enzyme appears to result in prolonged clearance of 5-fluorouracil.

➤*Adults:*

Carcinoma of the colon, rectum, breast, stomach, and pancreas –

Initial dosage: 12 mg/kg once daily by IV bolus for 4 successive days. The daily dose should not exceed 800 mg. If no toxicity is observed, 6 mg/kg should be given on days 6, 8, 10, and 12 unless toxicity occurs. No therapy is given on days 5, 7, 9, and 11. Therapy is to be discontinued at the end of day 12, even if no toxicity has become apparent.

Maintenance dosage: In instances where toxicity has not been a problem, it is recommended that therapy be continued using either of the following schedules:

1.) Repeat dosage of first course every 30 days after the last day of the previous course of treatment.
2.) When toxic signs resulting from the initial course of therapy have subsided, administer a maintenance dosage of 10 to 15 mg/kg/week as a single dose. Do not exceed 1 g/week.

The patient's reaction to the previous course of therapy should be taken into account in determining the amount of the drug to be used, and the dosage should be adjusted accordingly.

Duration of therapy: Some patients have received from 9 to 45 courses of treatment during periods that ranged from 12 to 60 months.

In poor-risk patients and those with inadequate nutritional status: 6 mg/kg/day IV for 3 days. If no toxicity is observed, 3 mg/kg may be given on days 5, 7, and 9 unless toxicity occurs. No therapy is given on days 4, 6, or 8. The daily dose should not exceed 400 mg. Poor-risk patients may require a reduced maintenance dose.

Off-label dosing –

Carcinoma of the colon, rectum, breast, stomach, and pancreas:

• *Continuous IV infusion* – 750 to 1,000 mg/m^2/day by continuous IV infusion for 4 to 5 days, in combination with other chemotherapy agents. Repeat every 21 to 28 days.

➤*Children:*

Off-label dosing – Follow dosage adjustment guidelines recommended for adults (see Adults).

IV bolus:

• *Initial dosage* – 12 mg/kg/day IV for 4 successive days. Then, give 6 mg/kg on days 6, 8, 10, and 12. The manufacturer does not recommend giving daily doses greater than 800 mg. Repeat every 4 weeks.

• *Alternative dosage* – 15 mg/kg/dose IV once a week. Adjust maintenance dose for toxicity. Usual range is 5 to 15 mg/kg/dose IV once a week. Weekly maintenance dosage should not exceed 1,000 mg.

Continuous IV infusion: 800 to 1,200 mg/m^2/day by continuous IV infusion for 1 to 5 days, in combination with other chemotherapy agents. Repeat every 21 to 28 days.

➤*Renal function impairment:* Use with extreme caution in patients with renal function impairment. Dosage adjustment may be necessary in renal dysfunction, although no specific guidelines are available. Monitor these patients closely.

Dialysis – Conventional hemodialysis and peritoneal dialysis are ineffective (0% to 24%) in removing fluorouracil. High permeability dialysis is minimally effective (25% to 49%) in removing fluorouracil.

After hemodialysis, some clinicians recommend supplementing with 50% of the original dose.

➤*Hepatic function impairment:* Use with extreme caution in patients with hepatic function impairment. Dosage adjustment may be necessary in hepatic dysfunction, although no specific guidelines are available. Monitor these patients closely. Some clinicians recommend not giving fluorouracil to patients with a bilirubin greater than 5 mg/dL.

➤*Discontinuation of therapy:* Therapy is to be discontinued promptly whenever 1 of the following signs of toxicity appears:

- Stomatitis or esophagopharyngitis, at the first visible sign.
- Leukopenia (white blood cells less than 3500), or a rapidly falling white blood count.
- Vomiting, intractable.
- Diarrhea, frequent bowel movements or watery stools.
- GI ulceration and bleeding.
- Thrombocytopenia, (platelets less than 100,000).
- Hemorrhage from any site.

➤*Preparation for administration:* Fluorouracil is considered a cytotoxic agent. Follow safe handling procedures when preparing, administering, or dispensing fluorouracil.

Fluorouracil solution for injection may be given undiluted or mixed with dextrose 5% injection or sodium chloride 0.9% injection prior to IV administration.

If a precipitate occurs due to exposure to low temperatures, resolubilize by heating to 60°C (140°F) and shake vigorously; allow to cool to body temperature before using.

➤*Administration:* Fluorouracil injection should be administered by IV push as undiluted product or infuse over 2 to 24 hours to decrease toxicity, using care to avoid extravasation.

Pharmacy bulk package – Not for direct infusion.

➤*Extravasation:* Fluorouracil is considered an irritant and may cause phlebitis, but it is not known to cause tissue damage with extravasation. If signs or symptoms of extravasation occur, stop the infusion immediately. If possible, withdraw 3 to 5 mL of blood to remove some of the drug. Remove the infusion needle. Delineate the infiltrated area on the patient's skin with a felt tip marker. Elevate for 48 hours above heart level using a sling or stockinette dressing with an observation window cut in the dressing. Avoid pressure or friction. Do not rub the area. Observe for signs of increased erythema, pain, or skin necrosis. If increased symptoms occur, consult a plastic surgeon. Ensure that no medication is given distally to the extravasation site. After 48 hours, encourage the patient to use the extremity normally to promote full range of motion.

➤*Storage/Stability:* Store at 15° to 30°C (59° to 86°F). Do not freeze. Protect from light. Retain in carton until time of use. Discard any unused portion. Although the fluorouracil solution may discolor slightly during storage, the potency and safety are not adversely affected.

Discard single-dose vials within 6 hours of the initial needle puncture if opened within an ISO Class 5 biological safety cabinet, or within 1 hour of the initial needle puncture if opened outside of such an environment, based on USP Chapter <797> standards.

Fluorouracil solutions diluted in dextrose 5% injection or sodium chloride 0.9% injection are chemically stable for up to 5 days at room temperature, unprotected from light. However, because fluorouracil injection is preservative-free, use solutions within 24 hours of preparation.

Actions

➤*Pharmacology:* There is evidence that the metabolism of fluorouracil in the anabolic pathway blocks the methylation reaction of deoxyuridylic acid to thymidylic acid. In this manner fluorouracil interferes with the synthesis of deoxyribonucleic acid (DNA) and to a lesser extent inhibits the formation of ribonucleic acid (RNA). Since DNA and RNA are essential for cell division and growth, the effect of fluorouracil may be to create a thymine deficiency which provokes unbalanced growth and death of the cell. The effects of DNA and RNA deprivation are most marked in those cells which grow more rapidly and which take up fluorouracil at a more rapid rate.

➤*Pharmacokinetics:*

Absorption/Distribution – Following IV injection, fluorouracil distributes into tumors, intestinal mucosa, bone marrow, liver and other tissues throughout the body. In spite of its limited lipid solubility, fluorouracil diffuses readily across the blood-brain barrier and distributes into cerebrospinal fluid and brain tissue.

Metabolism – The catabolic metabolism of fluorouracil results in degradation products (eg, CO_2 urea and α-fluoro-β-alanine) which are inactive.

Excretion – 7% to 20% of the parent drug is excreted unchanged in the urine in 6 hours; of this over 90% is excreted in the first hour. The remaining percentage of the administered dose is metabolized, primarily in the liver. The inactive metabolites are excreted in the urine over the next 3 to 4 hours.

FLUOROURACIL — INJECTION

When fluorouracil is labeled in the 6 carbon position, thus preventing the ^{14}C metabolism to CO_2, approximately 90% of the total radioactivity is excreted in the urine. When fluorouracil is labeled in the 2 carbon position approximately 90% of the total radioactivity is excreted in expired CO_2. Ninety percent (90%) of the dose is accounted for during the first 24 hours following IV administration.

Following IV administration of fluorouracil, the mean half-life of elimination from plasma is approximately 16 minutes, with a range of 8 to 20 minutes, and is dose dependent. No intact drug can be detected in the plasma 3 hours after an IV injection.

Contraindications

Poor nutritional state; depressed bone marrow function; potentially serious infections; hypersensitivity to fluorouracil.

Warnings/Precautions

➤*Toxic reactions:* Rarely, unexpected, severe toxicity (eg, stomatitis, diarrhea, neutropenia, neurotoxicity) associated with 5-fluorouracil has been attributed to deficiency of dipyrimidine dehydrogenase activity. A few patients have been rechallenged with 5-fluorouracil and despite 5-fluorouracil dose lowering, toxicity recurred and progressed with worse morbidity. Absence of this catabolic enzyme appears to result in prolonged clearance of 5-fluorouracil.

➤*Combination therapy:* Any form of therapy which adds to the stress of the patient, interferes with nutrition or depresses bone marrow function will increase the toxicity of fluorouracil.

➤*Severe toxicity:* Fluorouracil is a highly toxic drug with a narrow margin of safety. Therefore, patients should be carefully supervised, since therapeutic response is unlikely to occur without some evidence of toxicity. Severe hematological toxicity, gastrointestinal hemorrhage and even death may result from the use of fluorouracil despite meticulous selection of patients and careful adjustment of dosage. Although severe toxicity is more likely in poor risk patients, fatalities may be encountered occasionally even in patients in relatively good condition.

➤*Discontinuation:* Therapy is to be discontinued promptly whenever 1 of the following signs of toxicity appears:

- Stomatitis or esophagopharyngitis, at the first visible sign.
- Leukopenia (white blood cells less than 3,500), or a rapidly falling white blood count.
- Vomiting, intractable.
- Diarrhea, frequent bowel movements or watery stools.
- Gastrointestinal ulceration and bleeding.
- Thrombocytopenia (platelets less than 100,000).
- Hemorrhage from any site.

➤*Hand/Foot syndrome:* The administration of 5-fluorouracil has been associated with the occurrence of palmar-plantar erythrodysesthesia syndrome, also known as hand-foot syndrome. This syndrome has been characterized as a tingling sensation of hands and feet which may progress over the next few days to pain when holding objects or walking. The palms and soles become symmetrically swollen and erythematous with tenderness of the distal phalanges, possibly accompanied by desquamation. Interruption of therapy is followed by gradual resolution over 5 to 7 days. Although pyridoxine has been reported to ameliorate the palmar-plantar erythrodysesthesia syndrome, its safety and effectiveness have not been established.

➤*Extravasation:* See Administration and Dosage for more information.

➤*Special risk:* Use with extreme caution in poor risk patients with a history of high-dose pelvic irradiation or previous use of alkylating agents, those who have a widespread involvement of bone marrow by metastatic tumors or those with impaired hepatic or renal function.

➤*Pregnancy: Category D.*

Teratogenic – Fluorouracil may cause fetal harm when administered to a pregnant woman. Fluorouracil has been shown to be teratogenic in laboratory animals. Fluorouracil exhibited maximum teratogenicity when given to mice as single intraperitoneal injections of 10 to 40 mg/kg on day 10 or 12 of gestation. Similarly, intraperitoneal doses of 12 to 37 mg/kg given to rats between days 9 and 12 of gestation and IM doses of 3 to 9 mg given to hamsters between days 8 and 11 of gestation were teratogenic. Malformations included cleft palates, skeletal defects, and deformed appendages, paws, and tails. The dosages which were teratogenic in animals are 1 to 3 times the maximum recommended human therapeutic dose. In monkeys, divided doses of 40 mg/kg given between days 20 and 24 of gestation were not teratogenic.

There are no adequate and well-controlled studies with fluorouracil in pregnant women. While there is no evidence of teratogenicity in humans due to fluorouracil, it should be kept in mind that other drugs which inhibit DNA synthesis (eg, methotrexate, aminopterin) have been reported to be teratogenic in humans. Women of childbearing potential should be advised to avoid becoming pregnant. If the drug is used during pregnancy, or if the patient becomes pregnant while taking the drug, the patient should be told of the potential hazard to the fetus. Fluorouracil should be used during pregnancy only if the potential benefit justifies the potential risk to the fetus.

Nonteratogenic – Fluorouracil has not been studied in animals for its effects on peri- and postnatal development. However, fluorouracil has been shown to cross the placenta and enter into fetal circulation in the rat. Administration of fluorouracil has resulted in increased resorption and embryolethality in rats. In monkeys, maternal doses higher than 40 mg/kg resulted in abortion of all embryos exposed to fluorouracil. Compounds which inhibit DNA, RNA and protein synthesis might be expected to have adverse effects on peri- and postnatal development.

➤*Lactation:* It is not known whether fluorouracil is excreted in human milk. Because fluorouracil inhibits DNA, RNA and protein synthesis, mothers should not nurse while receiving this drug.

➤*Children:* Safety and efficacy in pediatric patients have not been established.

➤*Monitoring:* White blood counts with differential are recommended before each dose.

Drug Interactions

➤*Leucovorin calcium:* Leucovorin calcium may enhance the toxicity of fluorouracil.

Adverse Reactions

Fluorouracil in doses of 1,000 mg/m^2 or greater is considered to have moderate emetogenic potential (30% to 60% incidence of emesis). Fluorouracil in doses of less than 1,000 mg/m^2 is considered to have moderately low emetogenic potential (10% to 30% incidence of emesis).

➤*GI:* Stomatitis and esophagopharyngitis (which may lead to sloughing and ulceration), diarrhea, anorexia, nausea, and emesis are commonly seen during therapy.

➤*Hematologic:* Leukopenia usually follows every course of adequate therapy with fluorouracil. The lowest white blood cell counts are commonly observed between the ninth and fourteenth days after the first course of treatment, although uncommonly the maximal depression may be delayed for as long as 20 days. By the thirtieth day the count has usually returned to the normal range.

➤*Dermatologic:* Alopecia and dermatitis may be seen in a substantial number of cases. The dermatitis most often seen is a pruritic maculopapular rash usually appearing on the extremities and less frequently on the trunk. It is generally reversible and usually responsive to symptomatic treatment.

➤*Other adverse reactions:*

Allergic – Anaphylaxis and generalized allergic reactions.

Cardiovascular – Myocardial ischemia, angina.

CNS – Acute cerebellar syndrome (which may persist following discontinuance of treatment), nystagmus, headache.

Dermatologic – Dry skin, fissuring, photosensitivity, as manifested by erythema or increased pigmentation of the skin; vein pigmentation; palmar-plantar erythrodysesthesia syndrome, as manifested by tingling of the hands and feet following by pain, erythema, and swelling.

GI – Gastrointestinal ulceration and bleeding.

Hematologic – Pancytopenia, thrombocytopenia, agranulocytosis, anemia.

Ophthalmic – Lacrimal duct stenosis, visual changes, lacrimation, photophobia.

Psychiatric – Disorientation, confusion, euphoria.

Miscellaneous – Thrombophlebitis, epistaxis, nail changes (including loss of nails).

Overdosage

The possibility of overdosage with fluorouracil is unlikely in view of the mode of administration. Nevertheless, the anticipated manifestations would be nausea, vomiting, diarrhea, gastrointestinal ulceration and bleeding, bone marrow depression (including thrombocytopenia, leukopenia and agranulocytosis). No specific antidotal therapy exists. Patients who have been exposed to an overdose of fluorouracil should be monitored hematologically for at least 4 weeks. Should abnormalities appear, appropriate therapy should be utilized.

Patient Information

Patients should be informed of expected toxic effects, particularly oral manifestations. Patients should be alerted to the possibility of alopecia as a result of therapy and should be informed that it is usually a transient effect.

FLOXURIDINE

Rx	**Floxuridine** (Various, eg, Abraxis, Bedford)	**Injection, lyophilized powder for solution:** 500 mg	In 5 mL vials.
Rx	**FUDR** (Hospira)		In 5 mL vials.

FLOXURIDINE — INJECTION

WARNING

It is recommended that floxuridine be given only by or under the supervision of a qualified health care provider who is experienced in cancer chemotherapy and intraarterial drug therapy, and is well versed in the use of potent antimetabolites.

Because of the possibility of severe toxic reactions, hospitalize all patients for initiation of the first course of therapy.

Indications

➤*GI adenocarcinoma metastatic to the liver:* For the palliative management of GI adenocarcinoma metastatic to the liver when given by continuous regional intraarterial infusion in carefully selected patients who are considered incurable by surgery or other means. Patients with known disease extending beyond an area capable of infusion via a single artery should, except in unusual circumstances, be considered for systemic therapy with other chemotherapeutic agents.

➤*Off-label uses:* Treatment of tumors of the liver, ovaries, or kidneys.

Administration and Dosage

➤*Adults:*

GI adenocarcinoma metastatic to the liver –

Usual dosage: 0.1 to 0.6 mg/kg/day administered by continuous regional arterial infusion (using an implantable pump). The higher dose ranges (0.4 to 0.6 mg) are usually employed for hepatic artery infusion because the liver metabolizes the drug, thus reducing the potential for systemic toxicity.

Duration of therapy: According to the manufacturer, therapy can be given until adverse reactions appear. When these adverse reactions have subsided, therapy may be resumed. The patient should be maintained on therapy as long as response to floxuridine continues.

An alternative suggestion is to continue for 1 to 6 weeks, followed by a 14-day rest period between courses. Repeat cycles as long as response continues.

Discontinuation of therapy: Therapy is to be discontinued promptly whenever one of the following signs of toxicity appears:

- myocardial ischemia
- stomatitis or esophagopharyngitis, at the first visible sign
- leukopenia (white blood cell [WBC] count under 3,500) or a rapidly falling WBC count
- vomiting, intractable
- diarrhea, frequent bowel movements, or watery stools
- GI ulceration and bleeding
- thrombocytopenia (platelet count under 100,000)
- hemorrhage from any site

Off-label dosing –

Solid tumors: 0.5 to 1 mg/kg/day by IV infusion for 6 to 15 days or until toxicity occurs.

➤*Preparation for administration:* Floxuridine is considered a cytotoxic agent. Follow safe handling procedures when preparing, administering, or dispensing floxuridine.

Each vial must be reconstituted with 5 mL of sterile water for injection to yield a solution containing approximately 100 mg/mL of floxuridine. The calculated daily dose(s) of the drug is then diluted with dextrose 5% or sodium chloride 0.9% injection to a volume appropriate for the infusion apparatus to be used.

➤*Administration:* The administration of floxuridine is best achieved with the use of an appropriate pump to overcome pressure in large arteries and to ensure a uniform rate of infusion.

➤*Admixture compatibility:* Heparin and floxuridine are compatible in the same infusion. Heparin may be added to floxuridine infusions to prevent thrombotic complications.

➤*Storage/Stability:* The sterile powder should be stored at 15° to 30°C (59° to 86°F). Reconstituted vials should be stored under refrigeration (2° to 8°C; 36° to 46°F) for no more than 2 weeks.

Discard single-dose vials within 6 hours of the initial needle puncture if opened within an ISO Class 5 biological safety cabinet, or within 1 hour of the initial needle puncture if opened outside of such an environment, based on the USP Chapter < 797 > standards.

Actions

➤*Pharmacology:* Floxuridine, an antineoplastic antimetabolite, when given by rapid intraarterial injection, is apparently rapidly catabolized to 5-fluorouracil. Thus, rapid injection of floxuridine produces the same toxic and antimetabolic effects as does 5-fluorouracil. The primary effect is to interfere with the synthesis of DNA and, to a lesser extent, inhibit the formation of RNA. However, when floxuridine is given by continuous intraarterial infusion, its direct anabolism to floxuridine-monophosphate is enhanced, thus increasing the inhibition of DNA.

➤*Pharmacokinetics:*

Metabolism – Floxuridine is metabolized in the liver.

Excretion – The drug is excreted intact and as urea, fluorouracil, alpha-fluoro-beta-ureidopropionic acid, dihydrofluorouracil, alpha-fluoro-beta-guanidopropionic acid, and alpha-fluoro-beta-alanine in the urine; it is also expired as respiratory carbon dioxide.

Contraindications

Poor nutritional state; depressed bone marrow function; potentially serious infections.

Warnings/Precautions

➤*First course of therapy:* Because of the possibility of severe toxic reactions, hospitalize all patients for the first course of therapy.

➤*Combination therapy:* Any form of therapy that adds to the stress of the patient, interferes with nutrition, or depresses bone marrow function will increase the toxicity of floxuridine.

➤*Renal/Hepatic function impairment:* Use floxuridine with extreme caution in poor-risk patients with impaired hepatic or renal function.

➤*Special risk:* Use floxuridine with extreme caution in poor risk patients with a history of high-dose pelvic irradiation or previous use of alkylating agents. The drug is not intended as an adjuvant to surgery.

Toxicity – Floxuridine is a highly toxic drug with a narrow margin of safety; therefore, carefully supervise patients since therapeutic response is unlikely to occur without some evidence of toxicity. Severe hematological toxicity, GI hemorrhage, and even death may result from the use of floxuridine despite meticulous selection of patients and careful adjustment of dosage. Although severe toxicity is more likely in poor risk patients, fatalities may be encountered occasionally, even in patients in relatively good condition.

Discontinuation of therapy: Therapy is to be discontinued promptly whenever one of the following signs of toxicity appears:

- myocardial ischemia
- stomatitis or esophagopharyngitis, at the first visible sign
- leukopenia (white blood cell [WBC] count under 3,500) or a rapidly falling WBC count
- vomiting, intractable
- diarrhea, frequent bowel movements, or watery stools
- GI ulceration and bleeding
- thrombocytopenia (platelet count under 100,000)
- hemorrhage from any site

➤*Pregnancy: Category D.* There are no adequate and well-controlled studies with floxuridine in pregnant women. If this drug is used during pregnancy or if the patient becomes pregnant while taking it, apprise the patient of the potential hazard to the fetus. Advise women of childbearing potential to avoid becoming pregnant.

Teratogenic – While there is no evidence of teratogenicity in humans because of floxuridine, keep in mind that other drugs that inhibit DNA synthesis (eg, methotrexate, aminopterin) have been reported to be teratogenic in humans. Use floxuridine during pregnancy only if the potential benefit justifies the potential risk to the fetus.

Floxuridine may cause fetal harm when administered to a pregnant woman. It has been shown to be teratogenic in the chick embryo, mouse (at doses of 2.5 to 100 mg/kg), and rat (at doses of 75 to 150 mg/kg). Malformations included cleft palates, skeletal defects, and deformed appendages, paws, and tails. The doses that were teratogenic in animals are 4.2 to 125 times the recommended human therapeutic dose.

Nonteratogenic – Floxuridine has not been studied in animals for its effects on peri- and postnatal development. However, compounds that inhibit DNA, RNA, and protein synthesis might be expected to have adverse effects on peri- and postnatal development.

➤*Lactation:* It is not known whether floxuridine is excreted in human milk. Because floxuridine inhibits DNA and RNA synthesis, advise mothers not to breast-feed while receiving this drug.

➤*Children:* Safety and effectiveness in children have not been established.

➤*Monitoring:* Careful monitoring of the WBC count and platelet count is recommended.

Adverse Reactions

Adverse reactions to the arterial infusion of floxuridine are generally related to the procedural complications of regional arterial infusion.

The more common adverse reactions to the drug are diarrhea, enteritis, localized erythema, nausea, stomatitis, and vomiting. The more common laboratory abnormalities are anemia, leukopenia, thrombocytopenia and elevations of alkaline phosphatase, serum transaminase, serum bilirubin, and lactic dehydrogenase.

Floxuridine is considered to have low potential for nausea and vomiting.

➤*Cardiovascular:* Myocardial ischemia.

FLOXURIDINE — INJECTION

➤*CNS:* Lethargy, malaise, weakness.

➤*Dermatologic:* Alopecia, dermatitis, nonspecific skin toxicity, rash.

➤*GI:* Abdominal pain, acalculus cholecystitis, anorexia, bleeding, cramps, duodenal ulcer, duodenitis, gastritis, gastroenteritis, glossitis, pharyngitis, and possible intra- and extrahepatic biliary sclerosis.

➤*Lab test abnormalities:* Bromsulphthalein, prothrombin, sedimentation rate, thrombopenia, total proteins.

➤*Local:* Abscesses; arterial aneurysm; arterial ischemia; arterial thrombosis; bleeding at catheter site; catheter blocked, displaced, or leaking; embolism; fever; fibromyositis; hepatic necrosis; infection at catheter site; thrombophlebitis.

Overdosage

➤*Symptoms:* The possibility of overdosage with floxuridine is unlikely in view of the mode of administration. Nevertheless, the anticipated manifestations would be bone marrow depression (including, agranulocytosis, leucopenia, and thrombocytopenia), diarrhea, GI ulceration and bleeding, nausea, and vomiting.

➤*Treatment:* No specific antidotal therapy exists. Hematologically monitor patients who have been exposed to an overdosage of floxuridine for at least 4 weeks. Should abnormalities appear, utilize appropriate therapy.

Patient Information

Inform patients of expected toxic effects, particularly oral manifestations. Alert patients to the possibility of alopecia as a result of therapy and inform patients that it is usually a transient effect.

GEMCITABINE

Rx	**Gemcitabine** (Sandoz)	**Injection, lyophilized powder for solution:** 200 mg	As gemcitabine hydrochloride. Mannitol. In 10 mL single-use vials.
Rx	**Gemzar** (Eli Lilly)		As gemcitabine hydrochloride. Mannitol. In 10 mL single-use vials.
Rx	**Gemcitabine** (Sandoz)	**Injection, lyophilized powder for solution:** 1 g	As gemcitabine hydrochloride. Mannitol. In 50 mL single-use vials.
Rx	**Gemzar** (Eli Lilly)		As gemcitabine hydrochloride. Mannitol. In 50 mL single-use vials.
Rx	**Gemcitabine** (APP Pharmaceuticals)	**Injection, lyophilized powder for solution:** 2 g	As gemcitabine hydrochloride. Mannitol. In 100 mL single-use vials.

GEMCITABINE HYDROCHLORIDE — INJECTION

Indications

➤*Breast cancer:* In combination with paclitaxel as first-line treatment of patients with metastatic breast cancer after failure of prior anthracycline-containing adjuvant chemotherapy, unless anthracyclines were clinically contraindicated.

➤*Non-small cell lung cancer (NSCLC):* In combination with cisplatin as first-line treatment of patients with inoperable, locally advanced (stage IIIA or IIIB), or metastatic (stage IV) NSCLC.

➤*Ovarian cancer:* In combination with carboplatin for treatment of patients with advanced ovarian cancer that has relapsed at least 6 months after completion of platinum-based therapy.

➤*Pancreatic cancer:* As first-line treatment for patients with locally advanced (nonresectable stage II or stage III) or metastatic (stage IV) adenocarcinoma of the pancreas. Gemcitabine is indicated for patients previously treated with 5-fluorouracil (5-FU).

➤*Off-label uses:* Treatment of biliary cancer, bladder cancer, relapsed or refractory testicular cancer, squamous cell carcinoma of the head and neck.

Administration and Dosage

➤*Adults:*

Breast cancer –

Usual dosage: 1,250 mg/m^2 IV over 30 minutes on days 1 and 8 of each 21-day cycle.

Dosage adjustment: Gemcitabine dosage adjustments for hematologic toxicity are based on the granulocyte and platelet counts taken on day 8 of therapy. If marrow suppression is detected, modify gemcitabine dosage according to the following guidelines.

Day 8 Dosage Reduction Guidelines for Gemcitabine in Combination with Paclitaxel

AGC (× 10^6/L)		Platelet count (× 10^6/L)	% of full dose
≥ 1,200	and	> 75,000	100%
1,000 to 1,199	or	50,000 to 75,000	75%
700 to 999	and	≥ 50,000	50%
< 700	or	< 50,000	Hold

In general, for severe (grade 3 and 4) nonhematological toxicity, except alopecia and nausea/vomiting, therapy with gemcitabine should be held or decreased 50%, depending on the judgment of the treating health care provider. For paclitaxel dosage adjustment, see the paclitaxel monograph.

Concomitant therapy: Paclitaxel 175 mg/m^2 on day 1 as a 3-hour IV infusion before gemcitabine administration.

Monitoring: Patients should be monitored prior to each dose with a complete blood cell count (CBC), including differential counts. Patients should have an absolute granulocyte count (AGC) at least 1,500 × 10^6/L and a platelet count at least 100,000 × 10^6/L prior to each cycle.

Non–small cell lung cancer –

Usual dosage: Two schedules have been investigated, and the optimum schedule has not been determined.

• *4-week schedule* – 1,000 mg/m^2 IV over 30 minutes on days 1, 8, and 15 of each 28-day cycle.

• *3-week schedule* – 1,250 mg/m^2 IV over 30 minutes on days 1 and 8 of each 21-day cycle.

Dosage adjustment: Dosage adjustments for hematologic toxicity may be required for gemcitabine and cisplatin. Gemcitabine dosage adjustment for hematological toxicity is based on the granulocyte and platelet counts taken on the day of therapy. If marrow suppression is detected, modify or suspend therapy according to the following table.

Gemcitabine Dosage Reduction Guidelines

AGC (× 10^6/L)		Platelet count (× 10^6/L)	% of full dose
≥ 1,000	and	≥ 100,000	100%
500 to 999	or	50,000 to 99,000	75%
< 500	or	< 50,000	Hold

In general, for severe (grade 3 and 4) nonhematological toxicity, except alopecia and nausea/vomiting, therapy with gemcitabine plus cisplatin should be held or decreased 50%, depending on the judgment of the treating health care provider.

Concomitant therapy: Cisplatin 100 mg/m^2 IV on day 1 after the infusion of gemcitabine.

Monitoring: Patients receiving gemcitabine should be monitored prior to each dose with a CBC, including differential and platelet counts. During combination therapy with cisplatin, serum creatinine, serum potassium, serum calcium, and serum magnesium should be carefully monitored (grade 3 and 4 serum creatinine toxicity for gemcitabine plus cisplatin was 5% vs 2% for cisplatin alone).

Ovarian cancer –

Usual dosage: 1,000 mg/m^2 IV over 30 minutes on days 1 and 8 of each 21-day cycle.

Dosage adjustment: Gemcitabine dosage adjustments for hematological toxicity within a cycle of treatment are based on the granulocyte and platelet counts taken on day 8 of therapy. If marrow suppression is detected, gemcitabine dosage should be modified according to the guidelines in the following table.

Day 8 Dosage Reduction Guidelines for Gemcitabine in Combination With Carboplatin

AUC (× 10^6/L)		Platelet count (× 10^6/L)	% of full dose
≥ 1,500	and	≥ 100,000	100%
1,000 to 1,499	and/or	75,000 to 99,999	50%
< 1,000	and/or	< 75,000	Hold

In general, for severe (grade 3 and 4) nonhematological toxicity, except nausea/vomiting, therapy with gemcitabine should be held or decreased by 50%, depending on the judgment of the treating health care provider.

Dose adjustment for gemcitabine in combination with carboplatin for subsequent cycles is based on observed toxicity. The dose of gemcitabine in subsequent cycles should be reduced to 800 mg/m^2 on days 1 and 8 in case of any of the following hematologic toxicities: AGC less than 500 × 10^6/L for more than 5 days; AGC less than 100 × 10^6/L for more than 3 days; febrile neutropenia; platelets less than 25,000 × 10^6/L; cycle delay of more than 1 week because of toxicity.

If any of the previous toxicities recur after the initial dose reduction, gemcitabine should be given on day 1 only at 800 mg/m^2 for the subsequent cycle.

Concomitant therapy: Carboplatin area under the curve (AUC) 4 should be administered IV on day 1 after gemcitabine administration.

GEMCITABINE HYDROCHLORIDE — INJECTION

Monitoring: Patients should be monitored prior to each dose with a CBC, including differential counts. Patients should have an AGC of 1,500 × 10^6/L or greater and a platelet count of 100,000 × 10^6/L or greater prior to each cycle.

Pancreatic cancer –

Usual dosage: 1,000 mg/m^2 IV over 30 minutes once weekly for up to 7 weeks (or until toxicity necessitates reducing or holding a dose), followed by 1 week of rest from treatment. Subsequent cycles should consist of infusions once weekly for 3 consecutive weeks out of every 4 weeks.

Dosage adjustment: Dosage adjustment is based on the degree of hematologic toxicity experienced by the patient. Clearance in women and elderly patients is reduced, and women are somewhat less able to progress to subsequent cycles.

Patients receiving gemcitabine should be monitored prior to each dose with a CBC, including differential and platelet counts. If marrow suppression is detected, modify or suspend therapy according to the guidelines in the following table.

Gemcitabine Dosage Reduction Guidelines			
AGC (10^6/L)		Platelet count (10^6/L)	% of full dose
≥ 1,000	and	≥ 100,000	100%
500 to 999	or	50,000 to 99,000	75%
< 500	or	< 50,000	Hold

Patients treated with gemcitabine who complete an entire cycle of therapy may have the dose for subsequent cycles increased by 25%, provided that the AGC and platelet nadirs exceed 1,500 × 10^6/L and 100,000 × 10^6/L, respectively, and if nonhematologic toxicity has not been greater than World Health Organization (WHO) grade 1. If patients tolerate the subsequent course of gemcitabine at the increased dose, the dose for the next cycle can be further increased by 20%, provided again that the AGC and platelet nadirs exceed 1,500 × 10^6/L and 100,000 × 10^6/L, respectively, and that nonhematologic toxicity has not been greater than WHO grade 1.

Monitoring: Patients receiving gemcitabine should be monitored prior to each dose with a CBC, including differential and platelet counts. Laboratory evaluation of renal and hepatic function, including transaminases and serum creatinine, should be performed prior to initiation of therapy and periodically thereafter.

➤*Renal function impairment:*

Dialysis – Conventional hemodialysis is minimally effective (25% to 49%) in removing gemcitabine. Peritoneal dialysis is ineffective (0% to 24%) in removing gemcitabine.

Some health care providers recommend supplemental dosing after hemodialysis.

➤*Preparation for administration:* Gemcitabine is considered a cytotoxic agent. Follow safe handling procedures when preparing, administering, or dispensing gemcitabine.

The use of gloves is recommended. If gemcitabine solution comes in contact with the skin or mucosa, immediately wash the skin thoroughly with soap and water or rinse the mucosa with copious amounts of water. Although acute dermal irritation has not been observed in animal studies, 2 of 3 rabbits exhibited drug-related systemic toxicities (eg, death, hypoactivity, nasal discharge, shallow breathing) caused by dermal absorption.

To reconstitute, add 5 mL of sodium chloride 0.9% injection to the 200 mg vial or 25 mL of sodium chloride 0.9% injection to the 1 g vial. Shake to dissolve. These dilutions each yield a gemcitabine concentration of 38 mg/mL, which includes accounting for the displacement volume of the lyophilized powder (0.26 mL for the 200 mg vial or 1.3 mL for the 1 g vial). The total volume upon reconstitution will be 5.26 or 26.3 mL, respectively. Complete withdrawal of the vial contents will provide gemcitabine 200 mg or 1 g, respectively. The appropriate amount of drug may be administered as prepared or further diluted with sodium chloride 0.9% injection or dextrose 5% injection to concentrations as low as 0.1 mg/mL.

➤*Administration:* Gemcitabine is for IV use only. Gemcitabine may be administered on an outpatient basis.

Give by IV infusion over 30 minutes. Prolonging infusions past 60 minutes increases the risk of toxicity.

➤*Extravasation:* Gemcitabine is considered an irritant and may cause phlebitis, but it is not known to cause tissue damage with extravasation. If signs or symptoms of extravasation occur, stop the infusion immediately. If possible, withdraw 3 to 5 mL of blood to remove some of the drug. Remove the infusion needle. Delineate the infiltrated area on the patient's skin with a felt tip marker. Elevate for 48 hours above heart level using a sling or stockinette dressing with an observation window cut in the dressing. Avoid pressure or friction. Do not rub the area. Observe for signs of increased erythema, pain, or skin necrosis. If increased symptoms occur, consult a plastic surgeon. Ensure that no medication is given distally to the extravasation site. After 48 hours, encourage the patient to use the extremity normally to promote full range of motion.

➤*Storage/Stability:* Store unopened vials at 20° to 25°C (68° to 77°F).

Reconstituted gemcitabine solutions are chemically stable for up to 35 days at room temperature. However, reconstituted solutions are preservative-free and should be discarded after 24 hours. Do not refrigerate reconstituted product because crystals may form in the bag or bottle. Discard unused portion.

Gemcitabine 0.1 and 10 mg/mL solutions diluted with sodium chloride 0.9% injection or dextrose 5% injection are chemically stable for up to 35 days at room temperature or under refrigeration when stored in polyvinyl chloride bags. Because these solutions contain no preservative, they should be used within 24 hours of preparation.

Discard vial within 6 hours of the initial needle puncture if opened within an ISO Class 5 biological safety cabinet, or within 1 hour of the initial needle puncture if opened outside of such an environment, based on the USP Chapter <797> standards.

Actions

➤*Pharmacology:* Gemcitabine exhibits cell phase specificity, primarily killing cells undergoing DNA synthesis (S-phase) and also blocking the progression of cells through the G1/S-phase boundary. Gemcitabine is metabolized intracellularly by nucleoside kinases to the active diphosphate (dFdCDP) and triphosphate (dFdCTP) nucleosides. The cytotoxic effect of gemcitabine is attributed to a combination of 2 actions of the diphosphate and the triphosphate nucleosides, which leads to inhibition of DNA synthesis. First, gemcitabine diphosphate inhibits ribonucleotide reductase, which is responsible for catalyzing the reactions that generate the deoxynucleoside triphosphates for DNA synthesis. Inhibition of this enzyme by the diphosphate nucleoside causes a reduction in the concentrations of deoxynucleotides, including deoxycytidine triphosphate (dCTP). Second, gemcitabine triphosphate competes with dCTP for incorporation into DNA. The reduction in the intracellular concentration of dCTP (by the action of the diphosphate) enhances the incorporation of gemcitabine triphosphate into DNA (self-potentiation). After the gemcitabine nucleoside is incorporated into DNA, only 1 additional nucleoside is added to the growing DNA strands. After this addition, there is inhibition of further DNA synthesis. DNA polymerase epsilon is unable to remove the gemcitabine nucleotide and repair the growing DNA strands (masked chain termination). In CEM T lymphoblastoid cells, gemcitabine induces internucleosomal DNA fragmentation, one of the characteristics of programmed cell death.

Gemcitabine demonstrated dose-dependent synergistic activity with cisplatin in vitro. No effect of cisplatin on gemcitabine triphosphate accumulation or DNA double-strand breaks was observed. In vivo, gemcitabine showed activity in combination with cisplatin against the LX-1 and CALU-6 human lung xenografts, but minimal activity was seen with the NCI-H460 or NCI-H520 xenografts. Gemcitabine was synergistic with cisplatin in the Lewis lung murine xenograft. Sequential exposure to gemcitabine 4 hours before cisplatin produced the greatest interaction.

➤*Pharmacokinetics:*

Absorption/Distribution – Gemcitabine pharmacokinetics are linear and described by a 2-compartment model. Population pharmacokinetic analyses of combined single- and multiple-dose studies showed that the volume of distribution (Vd) of gemcitabine was significantly influenced by duration of infusion and gender.

Vd was increased with infusion length. Vd of gemcitabine was 50 L/m^2 following infusions lasting less than 70 minutes, indicating that gemcitabine, after short infusions, is not extensively distributed into tissues. For long infusions, the Vd rose to 370 L/m^2, reflecting slow equilibration of gemcitabine within the tissue compartment.

Gemcitabine plasma protein binding is negligible.

Metabolism/Excretion – Gemcitabine disposition was studied in 5 patients who received a single 1,000 mg/m^2 per 30-minute infusion of radiolabeled drug. Within 1 week, 92% to 98% of the dose was recovered, almost entirely in the urine. Gemcitabine (less than 10%) and the inactive uracil metabolite, 2′-deoxy-2′,2′-difluorouridine (dFdU), accounted for 99% of the excreted dose; the metabolite dFdU is also found in plasma.

Clearance was affected by age and gender. Differences in either clearance or Vd (based on patient characteristics or the duration of infusion) result in changes in half-life and plasma concentrations.

The following table shows plasma clearance and half-life of gemcitabine following short infusions for typical patients by age and gender.

Gemcitabine Clearance and Half-Life for the "Typical" Patient				
Age (years)	Clearance men (L/h/m^2)	Clearance women (L/h/m^2)	Half-life[a] men (min)	Half-life[a] women (min)
29	92.2	69.4	42	49
45	75.7	57	48	57
65	55.1	41.5	61	73
79	40.7	30.7	79	94

[a] Half-life for patients receiving a short infusion (less than 70 minutes).

Gemcitabine half-life for short infusions ranged from 42 to 94 minutes, and the value for long infusions varied from 245 to 638 minutes (depending on age and gender), reflecting a greatly increased Vd with longer infusions.

The maximum plasma concentrations of dFdU (inactive metabolite) were achieved up to 30 minutes after discontinuation of the infusions and the metabolite was excreted in urine without undergoing further biotransformation. The metabolite did not accumulate with weekly dosing, but its elimination is dependent on renal excretion and could accumulate with decreased renal function.

The active metabolite, gemcitabine triphosphate, can be extracted from peripheral blood mononuclear cells. The half-life of the terminal phase for gemcitabine triphosphate from mononuclear cells ranges from 1.7 to 19.4 hours.

GEMCITABINE HYDROCHLORIDE — INJECTION

Special populations –

Elderly/Women: The lower clearance in women and elderly patients results in higher concentrations of gemcitabine for any given dose.

Contraindications

Hypersensitivity to the drug.

Warnings/Precautions

➤*Infusion time/frequency:* Prolongation of the infusion time beyond 60 minutes and more frequently than weekly dosing has been shown to increase toxicity.

➤*Hematologic effects:* Gemcitabine can suppress bone marrow function as manifested by leukopenia, thrombocytopenia, or anemia, and myelosuppression is usually the dose-limiting toxicity. Monitor patients for myelosuppression during therapy. Dosage adjustment is based on the degree of hematologic toxicity the patient experiences.

➤*Pulmonary effects:* Pulmonary toxicity has been reported with the use of gemcitabine. In cases of severe lung toxicity, discontinue gemcitabine therapy immediately and institute appropriate supportive care measures.

➤*Gender:* Gemcitabine clearance is affected by gender. However, in the single-agent safety database (n = 979 patients), there is no evidence that unusual dose adjustments (other than those recommended) are necessary in women. In general, in single-agent studies of gemcitabine, adverse reaction rates were similar in men and women, but women, especially older women, were more likely not to proceed to a subsequent cycle and to experience grade 3 and 4 neutropenia and thrombocytopenia.

➤*Extravasation:* See Administration and Dosage for more information.

➤*Renal function impairment:* Use gemcitabine with caution in patients with preexisting renal function impairment. There is insufficient information from clinical studies to allow clear dose recommendations for these patient populations.

Hemolytic uremic syndrome (HUS) and/or renal failure have been reported following 1 or more doses of gemcitabine. Renal failure leading to death or requiring dialysis, despite discontinuation of therapy, has rarely been reported. The majority of the cases of renal failure leading to death were caused by HUS.

➤*Hepatic function impairment:* Use gemcitabine with caution in patients with preexisting hepatic function impairment, as there is insufficient information from clinical studies to allow clear dose recommendation for these patient populations. Administration of gemcitabine in patients with concurrent liver metastases or a preexisting medical history of alcoholism, hepatitis, or liver cirrhosis may lead to exacerbation of the underlying hepatic function impairment.

Serious hepatotoxicity, including liver failure and death, has been reported very rarely in patients receiving gemcitabine alone or in combination with other potentially hepatotoxic drugs.

➤*Pregnancy: Category D.* Gemcitabine can cause fetal harm when administered to a pregnant woman. Gemcitabine is embryotoxic, causing fetal malformations (eg, cleft palate, incomplete ossification) at doses of 1.5 mg/kg/day in mice (about 1/200 the recommended human dose on an mg/m² basis). Gemcitabine is fetotoxic, causing fetal malformations (eg, absence of gallbladder, fused pulmonary artery) at doses of 0.1 mg/kg/day in rabbits (about 1/600 the recommended human dose on an mg/m² basis). Embryotoxicity was characterized by decreased fetal viability, developmental delays, and reduced live litter sizes. There are no studies of gemcitabine in pregnant women. If gemcitabine is used during pregnancy or if the patient becomes pregnant while taking gemcitabine, inform the patient of the potential hazard to the fetus.

➤*Lactation:* It is not known whether gemcitabine or its metabolites are excreted in human milk. The molecular weight (about 264 for the free base) and negligible plasma protein binding suggest that the drug will be excreted into milk, but the very short elimination half-life (49 to 57 minutes) should mitigate the amount entering milk. Because many drugs are excreted in human milk and because of the potential for serious adverse reactions in breast-feeding infants from gemcitabine, warn the mother and decide whether to discontinue breast-feeding or the drug, taking into account the importance of the drug to the mother and the potential risk to the infant.

➤*Children:* Gemcitabine has not been studied in children. Safety and efficacy in children have not been established. Gemcitabine was evaluated in a phase 1 trial in children with refractory leukemia. It was determined that the maximum tolerated dose was 10 mg/m²/min for 360 minutes 3 times weekly followed by a 1-week rest period. Gemcitabine also was evaluated in a phase 2 trial in patients with relapsed acute lymphoblastic leukemia (22 patients) and acute myelogenous leukemia (10 patients) using 10 mg/m²/min for 360 minutes 3 times weekly followed by a 1-week rest period. Toxicities observed included bone marrow suppression, elevation of serum transaminases, febrile neutropenia, nausea, and rash/desquamation, which were similar to those reported in adults. No meaningful clinical activity was observed in this phase 2 trial.

➤*Elderly:* See Actions for more information.

In the randomized clinical trial of gemcitabine in combination with carboplatin for recurrent ovarian cancer, 125 women treated with gemcitabine plus carboplatin were younger than 65 years of age and 50 women were 65 years of age and older. Similar efficacy was observed between older and younger women. There was significantly higher grade 3 and 4 neutropenia in women 65 years of age and older. Overall, there were no substantial differences in the toxicity profile of gemcitabine plus carboplatin based on age.

➤*Monitoring:* Patients receiving gemcitabine therapy should be monitored closely by a health care provider experienced in the use of cancer chemotherapeutic agents. Most adverse reactions are reversible and do not require discontinuation, although doses may need to be withheld or reduced. There was a greater tendency in women, especially older women, not to proceed to the next cycle.

Perform laboratory evaluation of renal and hepatic function prior to initiation of therapy and periodically thereafter.

Monitor patients for myelosuppression during therapy.

See Administration and Dosage for more information.

Adverse Reactions

Gemcitabine is considered to have moderately low emetogenic potential (10% to 30% incidence of emesis).

➤*Single-agent use:* Myelosuppression is the principal dose-limiting toxicity with gemcitabine therapy. Dosage adjustments for hematologic toxicity are frequently needed.

Adverse Reactions in Patients Receiving Single-Agent Gemcitabine (≥ 10%)[a]

Adverse reactions	All patients[b]			Patients with pancreatic cancer[c]			Discontinuations[d]
	All grades	Grade 3	Grade 4	All grades	Grade 3	Grade 4	All patients
Laboratory[e]							
Hematologic							
Anemia	68%	7%	1%	73%	8%	2%	< 1%
Leukopenia	62%	9%	< 1%	64%	8%	1%	< 1%
Neutropenia	63%	19%	6%	61%	17%	7%	—
Thrombocytopenia	24%	4%	1%	36%	7%	< 1%	< 1%
Hepatic							< 1%
Alkaline phosphatase	55%	7%	2%	77%	16%	4%	
ALT	68%	8%	2%	72%	10%	1%	
AST	67%	6%	2%	78%	12%	5%	
Bilirubin	13%	2%	< 1%	26%	6%	2%	
Renal							< 1%
BUN[f]	16%	0%	0%	15%	0%	0%	
Creatinine	8%	< 1%	0%	6%	0%	0%	
Hematuria	35%	< 1%	0%	23%	0%	0%	
Proteinuria	45%	< 1%	0%	32%	< 1%	0%	
Nonlaboratory[g]							
CNS							
Paresthesias	10%	< 1%	0%	10%	< 1%	0%	0%
Somnolence	11%	< 1%	< 1%	11%	2%	< 1%	< 1%

GEMCITABINE HYDROCHLORIDE — INJECTION

Adverse Reactions in Patients Receiving Single-Agent Gemcitabine (≥ 10%)[a]

Adverse reactions	All patients[b]			Patients with pancreatic cancer[c]			Discontinuations[d]
	All grades	Grade 3	Grade 4	All grades	Grade 3	Grade 4	All patients
Dermatologic							
Alopecia	15%	< 1%	0%	16%	0%	0%	0%
Rash	30%	< 1%	0%	28%	< 1%	0%	< 1%
GI							
Constipation	23%	1%	< 1%	31%	3%	< 1%	0%
Diarrhea	19%	1%	0%	30%	3%	0%	0%
Nausea and vomiting	69%	13%	1%	71%	10%	2%	< 1%
Stomatitis	11%	< 1%	0%	10%	< 1%	0%	< 1%
Hematologic							
Hemorrhage	17%	< 1%	< 1%	4%	2%	< 1%	< 1%
Respiratory							
Dyspnea	23%	3%	< 1%	10%	0%	< 1%	< 1%
Miscellaneous							
Fever	41%	2%	0%	38%	2%	0%	< 1%
Infection	16%	1%	< 1%	10%	2%	< 1%	< 1%
Pain	48%	9%	< 1%	42%	6%	< 1%	< 1%

[a] Grade based on criteria from the WHO.
[b] N = 699 to 974; all patients with laboratory or nonlaboratory data.
[c] N = 161 to 241; all pancreatic cancer patients with laboratory or nonlaboratory data.
[d] N = 979.
[e] Regardless of causality.
[f] BUN = serum urea nitrogen.
[g] Table includes nonlaboratory data with incidence for all patients at least 10%. For approximately 60% of the patients, nonlaboratory reactions were graded only if assessed to be possibly drug-related.

Adverse Reactions of Gemcitabine and 5-Fluorouracil in Patients With Pancreatic Cancer[a]

Adverse reaction	Gemcitabine[b]			5-fluorouracil[c]		
	All grades	Grade 3	Grade 4	All grades	Grade 3	Grade 4
Laboratory[d]						
Hematologic						
Anemia	65%	7%	3%	45%	0%	0%
Leukopenia	71%	10%	0%	15%	2%	0%
Neutropenia	62%	19%	7%	18%	2%	3%
Thrombocytopenia	47%	10%	0%	15%	2%	0%
Hepatic						
Alkaline phosphatase	71%	16%	0%	64%	10%	3%
ALT	72%	8%	2%	38%	0%	0%
AST	72%	10%	2%	52%	2%	0%
Bilirubin	16%	2%	2%	25%	6%	3%
Renal						
BUN	8%	0%	0%	10%	0%	0%
Creatinine	2%	0%	0%	0%	0%	0%
Hematuria	13%	0%	0%	0%	0%	0%
Proteinuria	10%	0%	0%	2%	0%	0%
Nonlaboratory[e]						
CNS						
Paresthesias	2%	0%	0%	2%	0%	0%
Somnolence	5%	2%	0%	7%	2%	0%
Dermatologic						
Alopecia	18%	0%	0%	16%	0%	0%
Rash	24%	0%	0%	13%	0%	0%
GI						
Constipation	10%	3%	0%	11%	2%	0%
Diarrhea	24%	2%	0%	31%	5%	0%
Nausea and vomiting	64%	10%	3%	58%	5%	0%
Stomatitis	14%	0%	0%	15%	0%	0%
Hematologic						
Hemorrhage	0%	0%	0%	2%	0%	0%
Respiratory						
Dyspnea	6%	0%	0%	3%	0%	0%
Miscellaneous						
Fever	30%	0%	0%	16%	0%	0%
Infection	8%	0%	0%	3%	2%	0%
Pain	10%	2%	0%	7%	0%	0%

[a] Grade based on criteria from the WHO.
[b] N = 58 to 63; all gemcitabine patients with laboratory or nonlaboratory data.
[c] N = 61 to 63; all 5-fluorouracil patients with laboratory or nonlaboratory data.
[d] Regardless of causality.
[e] Nonlaboratory reactions were graded only if assessed to be possibly drug-related.

Allergic – Bronchospasm was reported for less than 2% of patients. Anaphylactoid reaction has been reported rarely. Do not administer gemcitabine to patients with a known hypersensitivity to this drug.

Cardiovascular – During clinical trials, 2% of patients discontinued therapy with gemcitabine because of cardiovascular reactions, such as arrhythmia, cerebrovascular accident, hypertension, and myocardial infarction. Many of these patients had a history of cardiovascular disease.

CNS – There was a 10% incidence of mild paresthesias and a less than 1% rate of severe paresthesias.

Dermatologic – Rash was reported in 30% of patients. The rash was typically a macular or finely granular maculopapular pruritic eruption of mild to moderate severity involving the trunk and extremities. Pruritus was reported in 13% of patients. Alopecia, usually minimal, was reported in 15% of patients.

GI – Nausea and vomiting were commonly reported (69%) but were usually of mild to moderate severity. Severe nausea and vomiting (WHO grade 3 and 4) occurred in less than 15% of patients. Diarrhea was reported by 19% of patients, and stomatitis by 11% of patients.

Hematologic – In studies in pancreatic cancer, myelosuppression is the dose-limiting toxicity with gemcitabine, but less than 1% of patients discontinued therapy for either anemia, leukopenia, or thrombocytopenia. Red blood cell (RBC) transfusions were required by 19% of patients. The incidence of sepsis was less than 1%. Petechiae or mild blood loss (hemorrhage), from any cause, was reported in 16% of patients; less than 1% of patients required platelet transfusions. Monitor patients for myelosuppression during gemcitabine therapy and modify or suspend dosage according to the degree of hematologic toxicity.

Hepatic – In clinical trials, gemcitabine was associated with transient elevations of 1 or both serum transaminases in approximately 70% of patients, but there was no evidence of increasing hepatic toxicity with longer duration of exposure to gemcitabine or with greater total cumulative dose. Serious hepatotoxicity, including liver failure and death, has been reported very rarely in patients receiving gemcitabine alone or in combination with other potentially hepatotoxic drugs.

GEMCITABINE HYDROCHLORIDE — INJECTION

Local – Injection-site related reactions were reported for 4% of patients. There were no reports of injection-site necrosis. Gemcitabine is not a vesicant.

Metabolic – Edema (13%), generalized edema (less than 1%), and peripheral edema (20%) were reported. Less than 1% of patients discontinued because of edema.

Renal – In clinical trials, mild proteinuria and hematuria were commonly reported. Clinical findings consistent with HUS were reported in 6 of 2,429 (0.25%) patients receiving gemcitabine in clinical trials. Four patients developed HUS on gemcitabine therapy, 2 immediately post-therapy. Consider the diagnosis of HUS if the patient develops anemia with evidence of microangiopathic hemolysis, as indicated by elevation of bilirubin or lactate dehydrogenase, evidence of renal failure (elevation of serum creatinine or BUN), reticulocytosis, and/or severe thrombocytopenia. Discontinue gemcitabine therapy immediately. Renal failure may not be reversible even with discontinuation of therapy, and dialysis may be required.

Respiratory – In clinical trials, dyspnea, unrelated to underlying disease, has been reported in association with gemcitabine therapy. Dyspnea was occasionally accompanied by bronchospasm. Pulmonary toxicity has been reported with the use of gemcitabine. The etiology of these effects is unknown. If such effects develop, discontinue gemcitabine. Early use of supportive care measures may help ameliorate these conditions.

Miscellaneous – The overall incidence of fever was 41%. This is in contrast to the incidence of infection (16%) and indicates that gemcitabine may cause fever in the absence of clinical infection. Fever was frequently associated with other flu-like symptoms and was usually mild and clinically manageable.

"Flu syndrome" was reported for 19% of patients. Individual symptoms of fever, asthenia, anorexia, headache, cough, chills, and myalgia were commonly reported. Fever and asthenia were also reported frequently as isolated symptoms. Insomnia, rhinitis, sweating, and malaise were reported infrequently. Less than 1% of patients discontinued because of flu-like symptoms.

Infections were reported for 16% of patients. Sepsis was rarely reported (less than 1%).

➤*Combination use in NSCLC:*

Adverse Reactions of Gemcitabine Plus Cisplatin Versus Single-Agent Cisplatin in NSCLC[a]

	Gemcitabine plus cisplatin[b]			Cisplatin[c]		
Adverse reactions	All grades	Grade 3	Grade 4	All grades	Grade 3	Grade 4
Laboratory[d]						
Hematologic						
Anemia	89%	22%	3%	67%	6%	1%
Leukopenia	82%	35%	11%	25%	2%	1%
Lymphocytes	75%	25%	18%	51%	12%	5%
Neutropenia	79%	22%	35%	20%	3%	1%
Platelet transfusions[e]	21%			< 1%		
RBC transfusion[e]	39%			13%		
Thrombocytopenia	85%	25%	25%	13%	3%	1%
Hepatic						
Alkaline phosphatase	19%	1%	0%	13%	0%	0%
Transaminase	22%	2%	1%	10%	1%	0%
Renal						
Creatinine	38%	4%	< 1%	31%	2%	< 1%
Hematuria	15%	0%	0%	13%	0%	0%
Proteinuria	23%	0%	0%	18%	0%	0%
Other laboratory						
Hyperglycemia	30%	4%	0%	23%	3%	0%
Hypocalcemia	18%	2%	0%	7%	0%	< 1%
Hypomagnesemia	30%	4%	3%	17%	2%	0%
Nonlaboratory[f]						
Cardiovascular						
Hypotension	12%	1%	0%	7%	1%	0%
CNS						
Neuro cortical	16%	3%	1%	9%	1%	0%
Neuro headache	14%	0%	0%	7%	0%	0%
Neuro hearing	25%	6%	0%	21%	6%	0%
Neuro mood	16%	1%	0%	10%	1%	0%
Neuro motor	35%	12%	0%	15%	3%	0%
Neuro sensory	23%	1%	0%	18%	1%	0%
Dermatologic						
Alopecia	53%	1%	0%	33%	0%	0%
Rash	11%	0%	0%	3%	0%	0%
GI						
Constipation	28%	3%	0%	21%	0%	0%
Diarrhea	24%	2%	2%	13%	0%	0%
Nausea	93%	25%	2%	87%	20%	< 1%
Stomatitis	14%	1%	0%	5%	0%	0%
Vomiting	78%	11%	12%	71%	10%	9%
Hematologic						
Hemorrhage	14%	1%	0%	4%	0%	0%
Respiratory						
Dyspnea	12%	4%	3%	11%	3%	2%
Miscellaneous						
Fever	16%	0%	0%	5%	0%	0%
Infection	18%	3%	2%	12%	1%	0%
Local	15%	0%	0%	6%	0%	0%

[a] Grade based on CTC. Table includes data for adverse reactions with incidence at least 10% in either arm.
[b] N = 217 to 253; all gemcitabine plus cisplatin patients with laboratory or nonlaboratory data. Gemcitabine at 1,000 mg/m^2 on days 1, 8, and 15, and cisplatin at 100 mg/m^2 on day 1 every 28 days.
[c] N = 213 to 248; all cisplatin patients with laboratory or nonlaboratory data. Cisplatin at 100 mg/m^2 on day 1 every 28 days.
[d] Regardless of causality.
[e] Percent of patients receiving transfusions. Percent transfusions are not CTC-graded reactions.
[f] Nonlaboratory reactions were graded only if assessed to be possibly drug-related.

Adverse Reactions of Gemcitabine Plus Cisplatin Versus Etoposide Plus Cisplatin in NSCLC[a]

	Gemcitabine plus cisplatin[b]			Etoposide plus cisplatin[c]		
Adverse reactions	All grades	Grade 3	Grade 4	All grades	Grade 3	Grade 4
Laboratory[d]						
Hematologic						
Anemia	88%	22%	0%	77%	13%	2%
Leukopenia	86%	26%	3%	87%	36%	7%
Neutropenia	88%	36%	28%	87%	20%	56%
Platelet transfusions[e]	3%			8%		
RBC transfusions[e]	29%			21%		
Thrombocytopenia	81%	39%	16%	45%	8%	5%
Hepatic						
Alkaline phosphatase	16%	0%	0%	11%	0%	0%
ALT	6%	0%	0%	12%	0%	0%
AST	3%	0%	0%	11%	0%	0%
Bilirubin	0%	0%	0%	0%	0%	0%
Renal						
BUN	6%	0%	0%	4%	0%	0%
Creatinine	2%	0%	0%	2%	0%	0%
Hematuria	22%	0%	0%	10%	0%	0%
Proteinuria	12%	0%	0%	5%	0%	0%
Nonlaboratory[f,g]						
CNS						
Paresthesias	38%	0%	0%	16%	2%	0%
Somnolence	3%	0%	0%	3%	2%	0%
Dermatologic						
Alopecia	77%	13%	0%	92%	51%	0%
Rash	10%	0%	0%	3%	0%	0%
GI						
Constipation	17%	0%	0%	15%	0%	0%
Diarrhea	14%	1%	1%	13%	0%	2%
Nausea and vomiting	96%	35%	4%	86%	19%	7%
Stomatitis	20%	4%	0%	18%	2%	0%
Hematologic						
Hemorrhage	9%	0%	3%	3%	0%	3%

GEMCITABINE HYDROCHLORIDE — INJECTION

Adverse Reactions of Gemcitabine Plus Cisplatin Versus Etoposide Plus Cisplatin in NSCLC[a]

Adverse reactions	Gemcitabine plus cisplatin[b]			Etoposide plus cisplatin[c]		
	All grades	Grade 3	Grade 4	All grades	Grade 3	Grade 4
Respiratory						
Dyspnea	1%	0%	1%	3%	0%	0%
Miscellaneous						
Fever	6%	0%	0%	3%	0%	0%
Infection	28%	3%	1%	21%	8%	0%

[a] Grade based on criteria from the WHO.
[b] N = 67 to 69; all gemcitabine plus cisplatin patients with laboratory or nonlaboratory data. Gemcitabine at 1,250 mg/m² on days 1 and 8 and cisplatin at 100 mg/m² on day 1 every 21 days.
[c] N = 57 to 63; all cisplatin plus etoposide patients with laboratory or nonlaboratory data. Cisplatin at 100 mg/m² on day 1 and etoposide IV at 100 mg/m² on days 1, 2, and 3 every 21 days.
[d] Regardless of causality.
[e] Percent of patients receiving transfusions. Percent transfusions are not WHO-graded reactions.
[f] Nonlaboratory reactions were graded only if assessed to be possibly drug-related.
[g] Pain data were not collected.

➤*Combination use in breast cancer:*

Adverse Reactions of Gemcitabine Plus Paclitaxel Versus Single-Agent Paclitaxel in Breast Cancer[a] (≥ 10%)

Adverse reactions	Gemcitabine plus paclitaxel (n = 262)			Paclitaxel (n = 259)		
	All grades	Grade 3	Grade 4	All grades	Grade 3	Grade 4
Laboratory[b]						
Hematologic						
Anemia	69%	6%	1%	51%	3%	< 1%
Leukopenia	21%	10%	1%	12%	2%	0%
Neutropenia	69%	31%	17%	31%	4%	7%
Thrombocytopenia	26%	5%	< 1%	7%	< 1%	< 1%
Hepatobiliary						
ALT	18%	5%	< 1%	6%	< 1%	0%
AST	16%	2%	0%	5%	< 1%	0%
Nonlaboratory[c]						
CNS						
Fatigue	40%	6%	< 1%	28%	1%	< 1%
Myalgia	33%	4%	0%	33%	3%	< 1%
Neuropathy, motor	15%	2%	< 1%	10%	< 1%	0%
Neuropathy, sensory	64%	5%	< 1%	58%	3%	0%
Dermatologic						
Alopecia	90%	14%	4%	92%	19%	3%
Rash/Desquamation	11%	< 1%	< 1%	5%	0%	0%
GI						
Anorexia	17%	0%	0%	12%	< 1%	0%
Constipation	11%	< 1%	0%	12%	0%	0%
Diarrhea	20%	3%	0%	13%	2%	0%
Nausea	50%	1%	0%	31%	2%	0%
Stomatitis/Pharyngitis	13%	1%	< 1%	8%	< 1%	0%
Vomiting	29%	2%	0%	15%	2%	0%
Miscellaneous						
Arthralgia	24%	3%	0%	22%	2%	< 1%
Bone pain	11%	2%	0%	10%	< 1%	0%
Fever	13%	< 1%	0%	3%	0%	0%
Pain, other	11%	< 1%	0%	8%	< 1%	0%

[a] Grade based on CTC Version 2.0 (all grades at least 10%).
[b] Regardless of causality.
[c] Nonlaboratory reactions were graded only if assessed to be possibly drug-related.

The following are the clinically relevant adverse reactions that occurred in more than 1% and less than 10% (all grades) of patients on either arm. In parentheses are the incidences of grade 3 and 4 adverse reactions (gemcitabine plus paclitaxel vs paclitaxel): febrile neutropenia (5% vs 1.2%), infection (0.8% vs 0.8%), dyspnea (1.9% vs 0%), and allergic reaction/hypersensitivity (0% vs 0.8%).

➤*Combination use in ovarian cancer:*

Adverse Reactions of Gemcitabine Plus Carboplatin Versus Single-Agent Carboplatin in Ovarian Cancer[a] (≥ 10%)

Adverse reactions	Gemcitabine plus carboplatin (n = 175)			Carboplatin (n = 174)		
	All grades	Grade 3	Grade 4	All grades	Grade 3	Grade 4
Laboratory[b]						
Hematologic						
Anemia	86%	22%	6%	75%	9%	2%
Leukopenia	86%	48%	5%	70%	6%	< 1%
Neutropenia	90%	42%	29%	58%	11%	1%
Platelet transfusion[c]	9%			3%		
RBC transfusions[c]	38%			15%		
Thrombocytopenia	78%	30%	5%	57%	10%	1%
Nonlaboratory[b]						
CNS						
Fatigue	40%	3%	< 1%	32%	5%	0%
Neuropathy-sensory	29%	1%	0%	27%	2%	0%
Dermatologic						
Alopecia	49%	0%	0%	17%	0%	0%
GI						
Anorexia	16%	1%	0%	13%	0%	0%
Constipation	42%	6%	1%	37%	3%	0%
Diarrhea	25%	3%	0%	14%	< 1%	0%
Nausea	69%	6%	0%	61%	3%	0%
Stomatitis/Pharyngitis	22%	< 1%	0%	13%	0%	0%
Vomiting	46%	6%	0%	36%	2%	< 1%

[a] Grade based on CTC Version 2.0 (all grades at least 10%).
[b] Regardless of causality.
[c] Percent of patients receiving transfusions. Transfusions are not CTC-graded reactions. Blood transfusions included both packed red blood cells and whole blood.

In addition to blood product transfusions as listed in the previous table, myelosuppression also was managed with hematopoetic agents. These agents were administered more frequently with combination therapy than with monotherapy (granulocyte growth factors: 23.6% and 10.1%, respectively; erythropoetic agents: 7.3% and 3.9%, respectively).

The following are the clinically relevant adverse reactions, regardless of causality, that occurred in more than 1% and less than 10% (all grades) of patients on either arm. In parentheses are the incidences of grade 3 and 4 adverse reactions (gemcitabine plus carboplatin vs carboplatin): AST or ALT elevation (0% vs 1.2%), dyspnea (3.4% vs 2.9%), febrile neutropenia (1.1% vs 0%), hemorrhagic reaction (2.3% vs 1.1%), hypersensitivity reaction (2.3% vs 2.9%), motor neuropathy (1.1% vs 0.6%), and rash/desquamation (0.6% vs 0%).

➤*Postmarketing:*

Cardiovascular – Congestive heart failure and myocardial infarction have been reported very rarely with the use of gemcitabine. Arrhythmias, predominantly supraventricular in nature, have been reported very rarely.

Dermatologic – Cellulitis and nonserious injection site reactions in the absence of extravasation have been rarely reported. Severe skin reactions, including bullous skin eruptions and desquamation, have been reported very rarely.

Hepatic – Increased liver function tests, including elevations in AST, ALT, alkaline phosphatase, bilirubin levels, and gamma-glutamyl transferase, have been reported rarely. Serious hepatotoxicity, including liver failure and death, has been reported very rarely in patients receiving gemcitabine alone or in combination with other potentially hepatotoxic drugs.

Renal – HUS and/or renal failure have been reported following 1 or more doses of gemcitabine. Renal failure leading to death or requiring dialysis, despite discontinuation of therapy, has been rarely reported. The majority of the cases of renal failure leading to death were caused by HUS.

Respiratory – Parenchymal toxicity, including adult respiratory distress syndrome, interstitial pneumonitis, pulmonary edema, and pulmonary fibrosis, has been rarely reported following 1 or more doses of gemcitabine administered to patients with various malignancies. Some patients experienced the onset of pulmonary symptoms up to 2 weeks after the last gemcitabine dose. Respiratory failure and death occurred very rarely in some patients despite discontinuation of therapy.

Miscellaneous – Clinical signs of gangrene and vasculitis have been reported very rarely.

Radiation recall reactions have been reported.

GEMCITABINE HYDROCHLORIDE — INJECTION

Overdosage

➤*Symptoms:* Myelosuppression, paresthesias, and severe rash were the principal toxicities seen when a single dose as high as 5,700 mg/m^2 was administered by IV infusion over 30 minutes every 2 weeks to several patients in a phase 1 study.

➤*Treatment:* There is no known antidote for overdoses of gemcitabine. In the event of suspected overdose, monitor the patient with appropriate blood counts and give supportive therapy as necessary.

Patient Information

Advise patients that this medication may reduce the number of clot-forming cells (platelets) in their blood. To prevent bleeding, patients should avoid situations in which bruising or injury may occur.

Advise patients that this medicine may lower the body's ability to fight infection and to notify a health care provider of any signs of infection, including chills, fever, rashes, or sore throat.

Instruct patients to avoid vaccinations with live virus vaccines (eg, measles, mumps, oral polio) while taking this medication. Vaccinations may be less effective.

CLADRIBINE (2-chlorodeoxyadenosine; CdA)

Rx	**Cladribine** (Bedford)	**Solution for Injection:** 1 mg/mL	9 mg NaCl/ml. In 10 mL fill in a 20 mL single-use vial.
Rx	**Leustatin** (Ortho Biotech)		Preservative free. In 10 mL or 10 mL fill in 20 mL single-use vials.

CLADRIBINE — INJECTION

WARNING

Cladribine should be administered under the supervision of a qualified physician experienced in the use of antineoplastic therapy. Suppression of bone marrow function should be anticipated. This is usually reversible and appears to be dose dependent. Serious neurological toxicity (including irreversible paraparesis and quadraparesis) has been reported in patients who received cladribine by continuous infusion at high doses (4 to 9 times the recommended dose for hairy cell leukemia). Neurologic toxicity appears to demonstrate a dose relationship; however, severe neurological toxicity has been reported rarely following treatment with standard cladribine dosing regimens.

Acute nephrotoxicity has been observed with high doses of cladribine (4 to 9 times the recommended dose for hairy cell leukemia), especially when given concomitantly with other nephrotoxic agents/therapies.

Indications

➤*Hairy cell leukemia:* For the treatment of active hairy cell leukemia as defined by clinically significant anemia, neutropenia, thrombocytopenia, or disease-related symptoms.

➤*Off-label uses:*

Multiple sclerosis – [4] = Insufficient documentation. Cladribine has been studied in patients with MS most commonly as a subcutaneous regimen given over 5 days, with cycles repeated monthly. The data showing the effect of cladribine on reducing enhancing lesions are consistently favorable. However, therapy has not been shown to prevent disease progression. Additional data are needed to determine the optimal dosing regimen and the patient population that would most benefit from therapy. (See Administration and Dosage.)

Other possible off-label uses – Treatment of chronic lymphocytic leukemia; non-Hodgkin lymphoma; acute myeloid leukemia; Waldenström macroglobulinemia. (See also Administration and Dosage.)

Cladribine has also been used safely and effectively in patients 1 to 21 years of age with acute leukemia. (See also Administration and Dosage.)

Administration and Dosage

➤*General dosing considerations:* Cladribine is dosed in mg/kg for hairy cell leukemia, but may be dosed in mg/m^2 for other indications. A dose of 0.9 mg/kg/day is approximately equal to 4 mg/m^2/day.

Specific risk factors predisposing to increased toxicity from cladribine have not been defined. In view of the known toxicities of agents of this class, it would be prudent to proceed carefully in patients with known or suspected renal insufficiency or severe bone marrow impairment of any etiology. Patients should be monitored closely for hematologic and non-hematologic toxicity.

➤*Adults:*

Hairy cell leukemia – 0.09 to 0.1 mg/kg/day as a single course given by continuous infusion for 7 consecutive days. (See also Off-label Dosing). According to the manufacturer, deviations from this dosage regimen are not advised. If the patient does not respond to the initial course of cladribine for hairy cell leukemia, it is unlikely that they will benefit from additional courses. However, some clinicians support repeating the course every 4 to 5 weeks.

Physicians should consider delaying or discontinuing the drug if neurotoxicity or renal toxicity occurs.

Off-label dosing –

Chronic lymphocytic leukemia: 0.1 mg/kg/day continuous intravenous (IV) infusion for 7 days. An alternate regimen is 0.028 to 0.14 mg/kg/day by IV infusion over 2 hours for 5 days.

Chronic myelogenous leukemia: 15 mg/m^2 body surface area given daily by IV infusion over 1 hour for 5 days. If no response to first course of therapy, may increase dose to 20 mg/m^2/day and give a second course after hematologic recovery.

Hairy cell leukemia: 3.4 mg/m^2 body surface area given daily subcutaneously for 7 days.

Multiple sclerosis: [4] = Insufficient documentation. Cladribine has been studied in various doses. The dose in the only published phase 3 trial was 0.07 mg/kg/day administered as a 5-day course every month for 4 to 6 months (cumulative dose, 2.1 mg/kg). Higher doses are not recommended because they have been shown to produce increased rates of myelosuppression and infection. Subcutaneous administration produced an equivalent therapeutic effect to IV administration.

➤*Children:*

Off-label dosing –

Acute leukemias:

• *1 year of age and older* – 6.2 to 7.5 mg/m^2 body surface area given daily by continuous IV infusion for 5 days.

➤*Preparation for administration:* Cladribine is considered a cytotoxic agent. Follow safe handling procedures when preparing, administering, or dispensing cladribine.

The use of disposable gloves and protective garments is recommended. If cladribine contacts the skin or mucous membranes, wash the involved surface immediately with copious amounts of water.

Cladribine must be diluted with the designated diluent prior to administration. Because the drug product does not contain any antimicrobial preservative or bacteriostatic agent, aseptic technique and proper environmental precautions must be observed in preparation of cladribine solutions.

To prepare a single daily dose – Add the calculated dose (0.09 mg/kg or 0.09 mL/kg) of cladribine to an infusion bag containing 500 mL of 0.9% sodium chloride injection. The use of 5% dextrose as a diluent is not recommended because of increased degradation of cladribine. Admixtures of cladribine are chemically and physically stable for at least 24 hours at room temperature under normal room fluorescent light in PVC infusion containers.

Cladribine 1-Day Infusion

	Dose of cladribine injection	Recommended diluent	Quantity of diluent
24-hour-infusion method	1 (day) × 0.09 mg/kg	0.9% sodium chloride injection	500 mL

To prepare a 7-day infusion – The 7-day infusion solution should only be prepared with bacteriostatic 0.9% sodium chloride injection (0.9% benzyl alcohol preserved). In order to minimize the risk of microbial contamination, both cladribine and the diluent should be passed through a sterile 0.22 micron disposable hydrophilic syringe filter as each solution is being introduced into the infusion reservoir. First add the calculated dose of cladribine (7 days times 0.09 mg/kg or mL/kg) to the infusion reservoir through the sterile filter. Then add a calculated amount of bacteriostatic 0.9% sodium chloride injection (0.9% benzyl alcohol preserved) also through the filter to bring the total volume of the solution to 100 mL. After completing solution preparation, clamp off the line, disconnect and discard the filter. Aseptically aspirate air bubbles from the reservoir as necessary using the syringe and a dry second sterile filter or a sterile vent filter assembly. Reclamp the line and discard the syringe and filter assembly. Infuse continuously over 7 days.

Solutions prepared with bacteriostatic sodium chloride injection for individuals weighing more than 85 kg may have reduced preservative effectiveness due to greater dilution of the benzyl alcohol preservative.

Admixtures for the 7-day infusion have demonstrated acceptable chemical and physical stability for at least 7 days in the *SIMS Deltec Medication Cassette Reservoir*.

Cladribine 7-Day Infusion

	Dose of cladribine injection	Recommended diluent	Quantity of diluent
7-day infusion method (use sterile 0.22 micron filter when preparing infusion solution)	7 (days) × 0.09 mg/kg	Bacteriostatic 0.9% sodium chloride injection (0.9% benzyl alcohol)	Quantity required up to 100 mL

➤*Administration:* Infuse continuously over 24 hours or continuously for 5 to 7 days. Cladribine has also been given subcutaneously (see Off-Label Dosing).

➤*Extravasation:* Cladribine is considered an irritant and may cause phlebitis, but it is not known to cause tissue damage with extravasation. If signs

CLADRIBINE — INJECTION

or symptoms of extravasation occur, stop the infusion immediately. If possible, withdraw 3 to 5 mL of blood to remove some of the drug. Remove the infusion needle. Delineate the infiltrated area on the patient's skin with a felt tip marker. Elevate for 48 hours above heart level using a sling or stockinette dressing with an observation window cut in the dressing. Avoid pressure or friction. Do not rub the area. Observe for signs of increased erythema, pain, or skin necrosis. If increased symptoms occur, consult a plastic surgeon. Ensure that no medication is given distally to the extravasation site. After 48 hours, encourage the patient to use the extremity normally to promote full range of motion.

➤*Admixture compatibility:* The use of 5% dextrose as a diluent is not recommended because of increased degradation of cladribine.

Because limited compatibility data are available, adherence to the recommended diluents and infusion systems is advised. Solutions containing cladribine should not be mixed with other IV drugs or additives or infused simultaneously via a common IV line because compatibility testing has not been performed.

➤*Storage/Stability:* Store vials in refrigerated conditions between 2° to 8°C (36° to 46°F) and protect from light.

Once diluted, solutions of cladribine should be administered promptly or stored in the refrigerator at 2° to 8°C (36° to 46°F) for no more than 8 hours prior to start of administration. Vials of cladribine are for single use only. Any unused portion should be discarded in an appropriate manner.

Admixtures of cladribine are chemically and physically stable for at least 24 hours at room temperature under normal room fluorescent light in PVC infusion containers. Admixtures for the 7-day infusion have demonstrated acceptable chemical and physical stability for at least 7 days in the *SIMS Deltec Medication Cassette Reservoir*.

A precipitate may occur during the exposure of cladribine to low temperatures; it may be resolubilized by allowing the solution to warm naturally to room temperature and by shaking vigorously. Do not heat or microwave. Freezing does not adversely affect the solution. Once thawed, the vial of cladribine is stable until expiry if refrigerated. Do not refreeze.

Actions

➤*Pharmacology:* The selective toxicity of 2-chloro-2′-deoxy-β-D-adenosine towards certain normal and malignant lymphocyte and monocyte populations is based on the relative activities of deoxycytidine kinase and deoxynucleotidase. Cladribine passively crosses the cell membrane. In cells with a high ratio of deoxycytidine kinase to deoxynucleotidase, it is phosphorylated by deoxycytidine kinase to 2-chloro-2′-deoxy-β-D-adenosine monophosphate (2-CdAMP). Since 2-chloro-2′-deoxy-β-D-adenosine is resistant to deamination by adenosine deaminase and there is little deoxynucleotide deaminase in lymphocytes and monocytes, 2-CdAMP accumulates intracellularly and is subsequently converted into the active triphosphate deoxynucleotide, 2-chloro-2′-deoxy-β-D-adenosine triphosphate (2-CdATP). It is postulated that cells with high deoxycytidine kinase and low deoxynucleotidase activities will be selectively killed by 2-chloro-2′-deoxy-β-D-adenosine as toxic deoxynucleotides accumulate intracellularly.

Cells containing high concentrations of deoxynucleotides are unable to properly repair single-strand DNA breaks. The broken ends of DNA activate the enzyme poly (ADP-ribose) polymerase resulting in NAD and ATP depletion and disruption of cellular metabolism. There is evidence, also, that 2-CdATP is incorporated into the DNA of dividing cells, resulting in impairment of DNA synthesis. Thus, 2-chloro-2′-deoxy-β-D-adenosine can be distinguished from other chemotherapeutic agents affecting purine metabolism in that it is cytotoxic to both actively dividing and quiescent lymphocytes and monocytes, inhibiting both DNA synthesis and repair.

➤*Pharmacokinetics:* In a clinical investigation, 17 patients with hairy cell leukemia and normal renal function were treated for 7 days with the recommended treatment regimen of cladribine injection (0.09 mg/kg/day) by continuous intravenous infusion. The mean steady-state serum concentration was estimated to be 5.7 ng/mL with an estimated systemic clearance of 663.5 mL/hr/kg when cladribine was given by continuous infusion over 7 days. In hairy cell leukemia patients, there does not appear to be a relationship between serum concentrations and ultimate clinical outcome.

In another study, 8 patients with hematologic malignancies received a 2-hour infusion of cladribine injection (0.12 mg/kg). The mean end-of-infusion plasma cladribine concentration was 48 ± 19 ng/mL. For 5 of these patients, the disappearance of cladribine could be described by either a biphasic or triphasic decline. For these patients with normal renal function, the mean terminal half-life was 5.4 hours. Mean values for clearance and steady-state volume of distribution were 978 ± 422 mL/hr/kg and 4.5 ± 2.8 L/kg, respectively.

Plasma concentrations are reported to decline multiexponentially after intravenous infusions with terminal half-lives ranging from approximately 3 to 22 hours. In general, the apparent volume of distribution of cladribine is very large (mean approximately 9 L/kg), indicating an extensive distribution of cladribine in body tissues. The mean half-life of cladribine in leukemic cells has been reported to be 23 hours.

Cladribine penetrates into cerebrospinal fluid. One report indicates that concentrations are approximately 25% of those in plasma.

Cladribine is bound approximately 20% to plasma proteins.

Except for some understanding of the mechanism of cellular toxicity, no other information is available on the metabolism of cladribine in humans. An average of 18% of the administered dose has been reported to be excreted in urine of patients with solid tumors during a 5-day continuous intravenous infusion of 3.5 to 8.1 mg/m²/day of cladribine. The effect of renal and hepatic impairment on the elimination of cladribine has not been investigated in humans.

Contraindications

Hypersensitivity to this drug or any of its components.

Warnings/Precautions

➤*Bone marrow suppression:* Severe bone marrow suppression, including neutropenia, anemia and thrombocytopenia, has been commonly observed in patients treated with cladribine, especially at high doses. At initiation of treatment, most patients in the clinical studies had hematologic impairment as a manifestation of active hairy cell leukemia. Following treatment with cladribine, further hematologic impairment occurred before recovery of peripheral blood counts began. During the first 2 weeks after treatment initiation, mean platelet count, ANC, and hemoglobin concentration declined and subsequently increased with normalization of mean counts by day 12, week 5 and week 8, respectively. The myelosuppressive effects of cladribine were most notable during the first month following treatment. Forty-four percent (44%) of patients received transfusions with RBCs and 14% received transfusions with platelets during month 1. Careful hematologic monitoring, especially during the first 4 to 8 weeks after treatment with cladribine, is recommended (see Precautions).

➤*Fever:* Fever (greater than or equal to 100°F) was associated with the use of cladribine in approximately two-thirds of patients (131/196) in the first month of therapy. Virtually all of these patients were treated empirically with parenteral antibiotics. Overall, 47% (93/196) of all patients had fever in the setting of neutropenia (ANC less than or equal to 1000), including 62 patients (32%) with severe neutropenia (ie, ANC less than or equal to 500).

Fever was a frequently observed side effect during the first month of study. Since the majority of fevers occurred in neutropenic patients, patients should be closely monitored during the first month of treatment and empiric antibiotics should be initiated as clinically indicated. Although 69% of patients developed fevers, less than ⅓ of febrile events were associated with documented infection. Given the known myelosuppressive effects of cladribine, practitioners should carefully evaluate the risks and benefits of administering this drug to patients with active infections.

➤*Nephrotoxicity/Neurotoxicity:* In a Phase I investigational study using cladribine in high doses (4 to 9 times the recommended dose for hairy cell leukemia) as part of a bone marrow transplant conditioning regimen, which also included high dose cyclophosphamide and total body irradiation, acute nephrotoxicity and delayed onset neurotoxicity were observed. Thirty-one (31) poor-risk patients with drug-resistant acute leukemia in relapse (29 cases) or non-Hodgkins lymphoma (2 cases) received cladribine for 7 to 14 days prior to bone marrow transplantation. During infusion, 8 patients experienced GI symptoms. While the bone marrow was initially cleared of all hematopoietic elements, including tumor cells, leukemia eventually recurred in all treated patients. Within 7 to 13 days after starting treatment with cladribine, 6 patients (19%) developed manifestations of renal dysfunction (eg, acidosis, anuria, elevated serum creatinine) and 5 required dialysis. Several of these patients were also being treated with other medications having known nephrotoxic potential. Renal dysfunction was reversible in 2 of these patients. In the 4 patients whose renal function had not recovered at the time of death, autopsies were performed; in 2 of these, evidence of tubular damage was noted. Eleven (11) patients (35%) experienced delayed onset neurologic toxicity. In the majority, this was characterized by progressive irreversible motor weakness (paraparesis/quadriparesis), of the upper or lower extremities, first noted 35 to 84 days after starting high-dose therapy with cladribine. Noninvasive testing (electromyography and nerve conduction studies) was consistent with demyelinating disease. Severe neurologic toxicity has also been noted with high doses of another drug in this class.

Axonal peripheral polyneuropathy was observed in a dose escalation study at the highest dose levels (approximately 4 times the recommended dose for hairy cell leukemia) in patients not receiving cyclophosphamide or total body irradiation. Severe neurological toxicity has been reported rarely following treatment with standard cladribine dosing regimens.

In patients with hairy cell leukemia treated with the recommended treatment regimen (0.09 mg/kg/day for 7 consecutive days), there have been no reports of nephrologic toxicities.

➤*Death:* Of the 196 hairy cell leukemia patients entered in the 2 trials, there were 8 deaths following treatment. Of these, 6 were of infectious etiology, including 3 pneumonias, and 2 occurred in the first month following cladribine therapy. Of the 8 deaths, 6 occurred in previously treated patients who were refractory to α-interferon.

➤*Tymor lysis syndrome:* Rare cases of tumor lysis syndrome have been reported in patients treated with cladribine with other hematologic malignancies having a high tumor burden.

➤*Extravasation:* See Administration and Dosage for more information.

➤*Special risk:* See Administration and Dosage for more information.

➤*Pregnancy: Category D.* Cladribine should not be given during pregnancy.

Cladribine is teratogenic in mice and rabbits and consequently has the potential to cause fetal harm when administered to a pregnant woman. A significant increase in fetal variations was observed in mice receiving 1.5 mg/kg/day (4.5 mg/m²) and increased resorptions, reduced litter size and increased fetal malformations were observed when mice received 3 mg/kg/day (9 mg/m²). Fetal death and malformations were observed in rabbits that

CLADRIBINE — INJECTION

received 3 mg/kg/day (33 mg/m^2). No fetal effects were seen in mice at 0.5 mg/kg/day (1.5 mg/m^2) or in rabbits at 1 mg/kg/day (11 mg/m^2).

Although there is no evidence of teratogenicity in humans due to cladribine, other drugs which inhibit DNA synthesis (eg, methotrexate and aminopterin) have been reported to be teratogenic in humans. Cladribine has been shown to be embryotoxic in mice when given at doses equivalent to the recommended dose.

There are no adequate and well-controlled studies in pregnant women. If cladribine is used during pregnancy, or if the patient becomes pregnant while taking this drug, the patient should be apprised of the potential hazard to the fetus. Women of child-bearing age should be advised to avoid becoming pregnant.

➤*Lactation:* It is not known whether this drug is excreted in human milk. The molecular weight (about 286), low plasma protein binding (about 20%), terminal half-life (5.4 hours), and long infusion time (7 consecutive days) suggest that the drug will be excreted into breast milk. Because many drugs are excreted in human milk and because of the potential for serious adverse reactions in nursing infants from cladribine, a decision should be made whether to discontinue nursing or discontinue the drug, taking into account the importance of the drug for the mother.

➤*Children:* Safety and effectiveness in pediatric patients have not been established. In a Phase I study involving patients 1 to 21 years old with relapsed acute leukemia, cladribine was given by continuous intravenous infusion in doses ranging from 3 to 10.7 mg/m^2/day for 5 days (one-half to twice the dose recommended in hairy cell leukemia). In this study, the dose-limiting toxicity was severe myelosuppression with profound neutropenia and thrombocytopenia. At the highest dose (10.7 mg/m^2/day), 3 of 7 patients developed irreversible myelosuppression and fatal systemic bacterial or fungal infections. No unique toxicities were noted in this study.

See Administration and Dosage for more information.

➤*Monitoring:* Cladribine is a potent antineoplastic agent with potentially significant toxic side effects. It should be administered only under the supervision of a physician experienced with the use of cancer chemotherapeutic agents. Patients undergoing therapy should be closely observed for signs of hematologic and non-hematologic toxicity. Periodic assessment of peripheral blood counts, particularly during the first 4 to 8 weeks post-treatment, is recommended to detect the development of anemia, neutropenia and thrombocytopenia and for early detection of any potential sequelae (eg, infection or bleeding). As with other potent chemotherapeutic agents, monitoring of renal and hepatic function is also recommended, especially in patients with underlying kidney or liver dysfunction.

Drug Interactions

There are no known drug interactions with cladribine. Caution should be exercised if cladribine is administered before, after, or in conjunction with other drugs known to cause immunosuppression or myelosuppression.

Adverse Reactions

Cladribine is considered to have very low emetogenic potential (less than 10% incidence of emesis).

➤*Most frequent adverse reactions:* Safety data are based on 196 patients with hairy cell leukemia: The original cohort of 124 patients plus an additional 72 patients enrolled at the same 2 centers after the original enrollment cutoff. In month 1 of the hairy cell leukemia clinical trials, severe neutropenia was noted in 70% of patients, fever in 69%, and infection was documented in 28%. Other adverse experiences reported frequently during the first 14 days after initiating treatment included fatigue (45%), nausea (28%), rash (27%), headache (22%) and injection site reactions (19%). Most nonhematologic adverse experiences were mild to moderate in severity.

➤*Myelosuppression:* Myelosuppression was frequently observed during the first month after starting treatment. Neutropenia (ANC less than 500 times 10^6/L) was noted in 70% of patients, compared with 26% in whom it was present initially. Severe anemia (hemoglobin less than 8.5 g/dL) developed in 37% of patients, compared with 10% initially and thrombocytopenia (platelets less than 20 times 10^9/L) developed in 12% of patients, compared to 4% in whom it was noted initially.

➤*Infection/Fever:* During the first month, 54 of 196 patients (28%) exhibited documented evidence of infection. Serious infections (eg, septicemia, pneumonia) were reported in 6% of all patients; the remainder were mild or moderate. Several deaths were attributable to infection and/or complications related to the underlying disease. During the second month, the overall rate of documented infection was 6%; these infections were mild to moderate and no severe systemic infections were seen. After the third month, the monthly incidence of infection was either less than or equal to that of the months immediately preceding cladribine therapy.

During the first month, 11% of patients experienced severe fever (ie, greater than or equal to 104°F). Documented infections were noted in fewer than one-third of febrile episodes. Of the 196 patients studied, 19 were noted to have a documented infection in the month prior to treatment. In the month following treatment, there were 54 episodes of documented infection: 23 (42%) were bacterial, 11 (20%) were viral and 11 (20%) were fungal. Seven (7) of 8 documented episodes of herpes zoster occurred during the month following treatment. Fourteen (14) of 16 episodes of documented fungal infections occurred in the first 2 months following treatment. Virtually all of these patients were treated empirically with antibiotics.

➤*Prolonged depressed CD4 counts:* Analysis of lymphocyte subsets indicates that treatment with cladribine is associated with prolonged depression of the CD4 counts. Prior to treatment, the mean CD4 count was 766/mcL. The mean CD4 count nadir, which occurred 4 to 6 months following treatment, was 272/mcL. Fifteen (15) months after treatment, mean CD4 counts remained below 500/mcL. CD8 counts behaved similarly, though increasing counts were observed after 9 months. The clinical significance of the prolonged CD4 lymphopenia is unclear.

➤*Prolonged bone marrow hypocellularity:* Another event of unknown clinical significance includes the observation of prolonged bone marrow hypocellularity. Bone marrow cellularity of less than 35% was noted after 4 months in 42 of 124 patients (34%) treated in the 2 pivotal trials. This hypocellularity was noted as late as day 1010. It is not known whether the hypocellularity is the result of disease related marrow fibrosis or if it is the result of cladribine toxicity. There was no apparent clinical effect on the peripheral blood counts.

➤*Dermatologic:* The vast majority of rashes were mild and occurred in patients who were receiving or had recently been treated with other medications (eg, allopurinol or antibiotics) known to cause rash.

➤*GI:* Most episodes of nausea were mild, not accompanied by vomiting, and did not require treatment with antiemetics. In patients requiring antiemetics, nausea was easily controlled, most frequently with chlorpromazine.

➤*Adverse reactions in greater than 5% of patients:* Adverse reactions reported during the first 2 weeks following treatment initiation (regardless of relationship to drug) by greater than 5% of patients included:

Cardiovascular – Edema (6%), tachycardia (6%)

CNS – Headache (22%), dizziness (9%), insomnia (7%).

Dermatologic – Rash (27%), injection site reactions (19%), pruritus (6%), pain (6%), erythema (6%).

GI – Nausea (28%), decreased appetite (17%), vomiting (13%), diarrhea (10%), constipation (9%), abdominal pain (6%).

Hematologic/Lymphatic – Purpura (10%), petechiae (8%), epistaxis (5%).

Musculoskeletal – Myalgia (7%), arthralgia (5%).

Respiratory – Abnormal breath sounds (11%), cough (10%), abnormal chest sounds (9%), shortness of breath (7%).

Miscellaneous – Fever (69%), fatigue (45%), chills (9%), asthenia (9%), diaphoresis (9%), malaise (7%), trunk pain (6%).

➤*Miscellaneous:* Adverse experiences related to intravenous administration included injection site reactions (9%) (ie, redness, swelling, pain), thrombosis (2%), phlebitis (2%) and a broken catheter (1%). These appear to be related to the infusion procedure and/or indwelling catheter, rather than the medication or the vehicle.

From day 15 to the last follow-up visit, the only events reported by greater than or equal to 5% of patients were fatigue (11%), rash (10%), headache (7%), cough (7%), and malaise (5%).

➤*Postmarketing reports:*

CNS – Neurological toxicity; however, severe neurotoxicity has been reported rarely following treatment with standard cladribine dosing regimens.

Dermatologic – Urticaria, hypereosinophilia. In isolated cases Stevens-Johnson and toxic epidermal necrolysis have been reported in patients who were receiving or had recently been treated with other medications (eg, allopurinol or antibiotics) known to cause these syndromes.

Hematologic – Bone marrow suppression with prolonged pancytopenia, including some reports of aplastic anemia; hemolytic anemia, which was reported in patients with lymphoid malignancies, occurring within the first few weeks following treatment.

Hepatic – Reversible, generally mild increases in bilirubin and transaminases.

Immunologic – Opportunistic infections have occurred in the acute phase of treatment due to the immunosuppression mediated by cladribine.

Respiratory – Pulmonary interstitial infiltrates; in most cases, an infectious etiology was identified.

Overdosage

High doses of cladribine have been associated with: irreversible neurologic toxicity (paraparesis/quadriparesis), acute nephrotoxicity, and severe bone marrow suppression resulting in neutropenia, anemia and thrombocytopenia. There is no known specific antidote to overdosage. Treatment of overdosage consists of discontinuation of cladribine, careful observation and appropriate supportive measures. It is not known whether the drug can be removed from the circulation by dialysis or hemofiltration.

FLUDARABINE PHOSPHATE

Rx	**Oforta** (Sanofi-Aventis)	**Tablets; oral:** 10 mg	Lactose. (LN). Salmon-pink, capsule shape. Film-coated. In UD 15s and UD 20s.
Rx	**Fludarabine Phosphate** (Various, eg, APP, Teva)	**Injection, solution:** 25 mg/mL	May contain mannitol. Preservative free. In 2 mL single-dose vials.
Rx	**Fludarabine Phosphate** (Various, eg, APP, Teva)	**Injection, lyophilized cake for solution:** 50 mg	May contain mannitol. Preservative free. In single-dose vials.
Rx	**Fludara** (Genzyme Corporation)		Mannitol 50 mg. Preservative free. In single-dose vials.

FLUDARABINE PHOSPHATE — ORAL

WARNING

Severe neurologic effects, including blindness, coma, and death, were observed in dose-ranging studies in patients with acute leukemia when fludarabine was administered at high doses. This severe CNS toxicity occurred in 36% of patients treated with doses approximately 4 times greater (96 mg/m^2/day for 5 to 7 days) than the recommended intravenous (IV) dose (25 mg/m^2/day). Similar severe CNS toxicity has been rarely (0.2% or less) reported in patients treated at doses in the range of the dose recommended for chronic lymphocytic leukemia (CLL). Periodic neurological assessments are recommended.

Instances of life-threatening and sometimes fatal autoimmune hemolytic anemia have been reported after 1 or more cycles of treatment with fludarabine. Patients undergoing treatment with fludarabine should be evaluated and closely monitored for hemolysis.

High incidence of fatal pulmonary toxicity was observed in a clinical investigation using fludarabine in combination with pentostatin (deoxycoformycin) for the treatment of refractory CLL. Therefore, the use of fludarabine in combination with pentostatin is not recommended.

Indications

➤*B-cell chronic lymphocytic leukemia:* As a single agent for the treatment of adult patients with B-cell CLL whose disease has not responded to or has progressed during or after treatment with at least 1 standard alkylating agent–containing regimen.

Administration and Dosage

➤*General dosing considerations:* The oral dose of fludarabine is different than the IV fludarabine dose.

A number of clinical settings may predispose to increased toxicity from fludarabine. These include advanced age, renal insufficiency, and bone marrow impairment. Such patients should be monitored closely for excessive toxicity, and the dose modified accordingly.

➤*Adults:*

B-cell chronic lymphocytic leukemia –

Usual dosage: 40 mg/m^2 daily for 5 consecutive days. Each 5-day course of treatment should commence every 28 days.

Dosage adjustment: Dosage may be decreased or delayed based on evidence of hematologic or nonhematologic toxicity. Health care providers should consider delaying or discontinuing the drug if neurotoxicity occurs.

Bone marrow impairment may predispose to increased toxicity from fludarabine. Patients with bone marrow impairment should be monitored closely for excessive toxicity and the dose modified accordingly.

Duration of therapy: The optimal duration of treatment has not been clearly established. It is recommended that 3 additional cycles of fludarabine be administered following the achievement of a maximal response and then the drug should be discontinued.

➤*Elderly:* Advanced age may predispose patients to increased toxicity from fludarabine. Monitor patients closely for excessive toxicity and modify the dose accordingly.

➤*Renal function impairment:* Reduce dose by 20% in patients with mild to moderate renal impairment (creatinine clearance [CrCl] 30 to 70 mL/min per 1.73 m^2). Reduce dose by 50% in patients with severe renal impairment (CrCl less than 30 mL/min per 1.73 m^2).

➤*Administration:* Fludarabine can be taken either on an empty stomach or with food. The tablets have to be swallowed whole with water; they should not be chewed or broken.

Handling/Disposal – Procedures for proper handling and disposal should be considered. Consideration should be given to handling and disposal according to guidelines issued for cytotoxic drugs. Several guidelines on this subject have been published. Caution should be exercised in the handling of fludarabine. Push tablets through foil to open. Do not remove tablets from individual blisters until immediately prior to taking or administering each scheduled dose. Do not crush tablets. Avoid exposure by direct contact of the skin or mucous membranes or by inhalation. If contact occurs, wash thoroughly with soap and water or wash the eyes immediately with gently flowing water for at least 15 minutes. Consult health care provider in case of a skin reaction or if the drug gets in the eyes.

➤*Storage/Stability:* Store at 25°C (77°F); excursions are permitted between 15° and 30°C (59° and 86°F).

Actions

➤*Pharmacology:* Fludarabine phosphate (2F-ara-AMP) is a synthetic purine nucleotide antimetabolite agent. Upon administration, 2F-ara-AMP is rapidly dephosphorylated in the plasma to 2F-ara-A, which then enters into the cell. Intracellularly, 2F-ara-A is converted to the 5'-triphosphate, 2-fluoro-ara-ATP (2F-ara-ATP). 2F-ara-ATP competes with deoxyadenosine triphosphate for incorporation into DNA. Once incorporated into DNA, 2F-ara-ATP functions as a DNA chain terminator; inhibits DNA polymerase alpha, gamma, and delta; and inhibits ribonucleoside diphosphate reductase. 2F-ara-A also inhibits DNA primase and DNA ligase I. The mechanism of action of this antimetabolite is not completely characterized and may be multifaceted.

➤*Pharmacokinetics:*

Absorption – 2F-ara-A exhibits dose proportional increases in area under the curve (AUC) and maximum plasma concentration (C_{max}) after single oral doses of 50, 70, or 90 mg of 2F-ara-AMP. C_{max} of 2F-ara-A occurs 1 to 2 hours after single or multiple oral doses and is approximately 20% to 30% of the maximum plasma concentrations produced at the end of a 30-minute IV infusion of the same dose. The absolute oral bioavailability of 2F-ara- A is 50% to 65% following single and repeated doses of fludarabine. Similar systemic exposure (AUC) was observed after a single 40 mg/m^2 fludarabine oral dose and a single 25 mg/m^2 fludarabine IV dose.

After 5 daily 30-minute IV infusions of 25 mg 2F-ara-AMP/m^2 to cancer patients, trough concentrations of 2F-ara-A increased by a factor of approximately 2.

A correlation was noted between the degree of absolute granulocyte count nadir and increased AUC.

Food effect: The C_{max}, AUC, and terminal half-life of 2F-ara-A are unaffected when administered with a high-fat meal, although time to reach maximum concentration is slightly delayed from 1.3 to 2.2 hours.

Distribution – Plasma protein binding of 2F-ara-A was approximately 19% to 29%.

Metabolism – Studies with the IV product have demonstrated that fludarabine is converted to the active metabolite, 2F-ara-A. Following administration of the IV product, systemic plasma clearance of 2F-ara-A is approximately 117 to 145 mL/min.

Excretion – The terminal half-life of 2F-ara-A was similar to that following IV administration (approximately 20 hours).

Following IV administration, renal clearance of 2F-ara-A represents approximately 40% of the total body clearance of fludarabine, and total body clearance is inversely correlated with serum creatinine and CrCl. The mean total body clearance was 172 mL/min for patients with healthy renal function.

Special populations –

Renal function impairment: In 2 patients with median CrCl of 22 mL/min per 1.73 m^2, 2F-ara-A clearance was reduced by 56%. Dosage adjustment based on CrCl is recommended. The mean total body clearance was 124 mL/min for patients with mildly to moderately impaired rental function and 71 mL/min for 2 patients with severe renal impairment.

See Administration and Dosage for more information.

Contraindications

None well documented.

Warnings/Precautions

➤*Neurotoxicity:* Dose-dependent neurotoxicity has been observed with fludarabine. Dose levels approximately 4 times greater (96 mg/m^2/day for 5 to 7 days) than the recommended IV dose (25 mg/m^2/day for 5 days) were associated with a syndrome characterized by delayed blindness, coma, and death. Symptoms appeared from 21 to 60 days following the last dose. Of patients who received fludarabine IV at high doses (at least 96 mg/m^2/day for 5 to 7 days per course), 36.1% developed severe neurotoxicity, while only 0.2% of patients who received the drug IV at low doses (40 mg/m^2/day or less for 5 days per course) developed toxicity. In the pivotal clinical study conducted with fludarabine tablets administered at 40 mg/m^2, severe impairment of consciousness was reported in 1 patient. The effect of long-term administration of fludarabine on the CNS is unknown; however, patients have received the recommended dose for up to 15 courses of therapy. Consider delaying or discontinuing the drug if neurotoxicity occurs.

➤*Hematologic effects:*

Bone marrow suppression – Severe bone marrow suppression, notably anemia, thrombocytopenia, and neutropenia, has been reported in patients treated with fludarabine. In a study in adults with solid tumors, the median time to nadir counts was 13 days (range, 3 to 25 days) for granulocytes and 16 days (range, 2 to 32 days) for platelets. Most patients had hematologic impairment at baseline either as a result of disease or as a result of prior myelosuppressive therapy. Cumulative myelosuppression may be seen. While chemotherapy-induced myelosuppression is often reversible, administration of fludarabine requires careful hematologic monitoring.

FLUDARABINE PHOSPHATE — ORAL

Bone marrow hypoplasia or aplasia – Several instances of trilineage bone marrow hypoplasia or aplasia resulting in pancytopenia, sometimes resulting in death, have been reported in adult patients. The duration of clinically significant cytopenia in the reported cases has ranged from approximately 2 months to approximately 1 year. These episodes have occurred both in previously treated or untreated patients. One case of pancytopenia was reported in the pivotal clinical study conducted with fludarabine tablets.

Autoimmune hemolytic anemia – Instances of life-threatening, and sometimes fatal, autoimmune hemolytic anemia have been reported to occur after 1 or more cycles of treatment with fludarabine in patients with or without a history of autoimmune hemolytic anemia or a positive Coombs test and who may or may not be in remission from their disease. Steroids may or may not be effective in controlling these hemolytic episodes. The majority of patients rechallenged with fludarabine developed a recurrence in the hemolytic process. The mechanism(s) that predispose patients to the development of this complication has not been identified. Evaluate and closely monitor for hemolysis in patients undergoing treatment with fludarabine.

➤*Fatalities:* Of 133 adult patients with CLL who received IV fludarabine in 2 clinical trials, there were 29 fatalities during study. Approximately 50% of the fatalities were due to infection and 25% due to progressive disease. Of 183 adult patients with CLL who received fludarabine tablets in 2 clinical trials, there were 13 deaths. Approximately 50% of the deaths were due to progressive disease, while 2 (15%) patient deaths were attributed to infection. Monitor for signs and symptoms of infection.

➤*Tumor lysis syndrome:* Tumor lysis syndrome associated with fludarabine treatment has been reported in patients with CLL with large tumor burdens. Since fludarabine can induce a response as early as the first week of treatment, take precautions in those patients at risk of developing this complication.

➤*Transfusion-associated graft-versus-host disease:* Transfusion-associated graft-versus-host disease (GVHD) has been observed rarely after transfusion of nonirradiated blood in fludarabine-treated patients. Therefore, consider the use of irradiated blood products in those patients requiring transfusions while undergoing treatment with fludarabine.

➤*Vaccination:* During and after treatment with fludarabine, avoid vaccination with live vaccines.

➤*Renal function impairment:* Fludarabine must be administered cautiously in patients with renal impairment. Following dosing of the IV product, the total body clearance of 2-fluoroara-A has been shown to be directly correlated with CrCl, indicating the importance of the renal excretion pathway for the elimination of the drug. See Administration and Dosage for more information. In patients with severe impairment of renal function (CrCl less than 30 mL/min per 1.73 m^2), reduce the fludarabine dose by 50% and monitor closely.

➤*Pregnancy: Category D.* Based on its mechanism of action, fludarabine can cause fetal harm when administered to a pregnant woman. There are no adequate and well-controlled studies of fludarabine in pregnant women. If fludarabine is used during pregnancy, or if the patient becomes pregnant while taking this drug, apprise the patient of the potential hazard to the fetus. Advise women of childbearing potential to avoid becoming pregnant. Women of childbearing potential and fertile males must take contraceptive measures during and for at least 6 months after the cessation of therapy.

Fludarabine was embryolethal and teratogenic in both rats and rabbits. In rats, repeated IV doses of fludarabine at 1.5 times and 4.5 times the recommended human oral dose (40 mg/m^2) administered during organogenesis caused an increase in resorptions, skeletal and visceral malformations (cleft palate, exencephaly, and fetal vertebrae deformities), and decreased fetal body weights. Maternal toxicity was not apparent at 1.5 times the human oral dose, and was limited to slight body weight decreases at 4.5 times the human oral dose. In rabbits, repeated IV doses of fludarabine at 2.4 times the human oral dose administered during organogenesis increased embryo and fetal lethality as indicated by increased resorptions and a decrease in live fetuses. A significant increase in malformations, including cleft palate, hydrocephaly, adactyly, brachydactyly, fusions of the digits, diaphragmatic hernia, heart/great vessel defects, and vertebrae/rib anomalies, were seen in all dose levels (0.3 times the human oral dose or greater).

➤*Lactation:* It is not known whether fludarabine phosphate is excreted in human milk. Because many drugs are excreted in human milk and because of the potential for serious adverse reactions, including tumorigenicity, in breast-feeding infants, decide whether to discontinue breast-feeding or the drug, taking into account the importance of the drug to the mother.

➤*Children:* Safety and effectiveness in children have not been established.

➤*Elderly:* See Administration and Dosage for more information.

➤*Monitoring:* Fludarabine is an antineoplastic agent with potentially significant toxic adverse effects. Closely observe patients undergoing therapy for signs of hematologic and nonhematologic toxicity. Periodic assessment of peripheral blood cell counts is recommended to detect the development of anemia, neutropenia, and thrombocytopenia.

During treatment, regularly monitor the patient's hematologic profile (particularly neutrophils and platelets) to determine the degree of hematopoietic suppression.

Monitor for signs and symptoms of infection. Monitor patients with advanced age, renal impairment, and bone marrow impairment closely for excessive toxicity and modify the dose accordingly.

Drug Interactions

➤*Vaccination:* See Warnings/Precautions for more information.

Fludarabine Oral Drug Interactions[a]

Precipitant drug	Object drug		Description
Fludarabine	Digoxin	⬇	Pharmacologic effects of digoxin may be decreased because of decreased GI absorption caused by fludarabine. Monitor serum digoxin concentrations and the patient for evidence of clinical deterioration and adjust dosage accordingly.
Fludarabine	Pentostatin	⬆	The use of fludarabine in combination with pentostatin is not recommended because of the risk of severe pulmonary toxicity.
Pentostatin	Fludarabine		

[a] ⬆ = object drug increased; ⬇ = object drug decreased.

Adverse Reactions

➤*Common adverse reactions:* Based on experience with the IV and oral use of fludarabine, the most common adverse reactions include myelosuppression (neutropenia, thrombocytopenia, and anemia), fever and chills, infection, and nausea and vomiting. Other commonly reported reactions include malaise, fatigue, anorexia, and weakness. Serious opportunistic infections have occurred in patients with CLL treated with fludarabine.

➤*Frequent adverse reactions:*

Cardiovascular – Edema has been frequently reported. One patient developed a pericardial effusion possibly related to treatment with fludarabine tablets.

CNS – Objective weakness, agitation, confusion, visual disturbances, and coma have occurred in patients with CLL treated with fludarabine at the recommended dose. Peripheral neuropathy and 1 case of wrist-drop have been observed with IV administration of fludarabine. In study 1 for fludarabine tablets, there was 1 report of severe impairment of consciousness that presented concurrent with hemolytic anemia. This patient had enrolled in the study with preexisting peripheral neurotoxicity.

Dermatologic – Skin toxicity, consisting primarily of skin rashes, has been reported.

GI – GI disturbances such as nausea and vomiting, anorexia, diarrhea, stomatitis, and GI bleeding have been reported in patients treated with fludarabine. Nausea and vomiting occurred in up to 38% of patients following treatment with fludarabine tablets in the clinical trials.

GU – Hemorrhagic cystitis has been reported in patients treated IV with fludarabine.

Hematologic – Hematologic events (neutropenia, thrombocytopenia, and/or anemia) were reported in the majority of patients with CLL treated with fludarabine. During IV fludarabine treatment of 133 patients with CLL, the absolute neutrophil count decreased to less than 500/mm^3 in 59% of patients, hemoglobin decreased from pretreatment values by at least 2 grams percent in 60%, and platelet count decreased from pretreatment values by at least 50% in 55%. Among 78 patients with B-CLL who were treated with fludarabine, the absolute neutrophil count decreased to less than 500/mm^3 in 37% of patients, hemoglobin decreased from pretreatment values by at least 2 grams percent in 14%, and platelet count decreased from pretreatment values by at least 50% in 17% of patients. Myelosuppression may be severe, cumulative, and may affect multiple cell lines. Bone marrow fibrosis occurred in 1 patient with CLL treated with fludarabine IV. In the pivotal oral fludarabine study (study 1), there was 1 report of a nonfatal case of pancytopenia. Similarly, there was 1 case of nonfatal pancytopenia reported among the 133 patients with CLL treated with IV fludarabine.

See Warnings/Precautions for more information.

Metabolic – Tumor lysis syndrome has been reported in patients with CLL treated with IV fludarabine. This complication may include hyperuricemia, hyperphosphatemia, hypocalcemia, metabolic acidosis, hyperkalemia, hematuria, urate crystalluria, and renal failure. The onset of this syndrome may be heralded by flank pain and hematuria.

Respiratory – Pneumonia, a frequent manifestation of infection in patients with CLL, was observed in 2 clinical trials conducted with IV fludarabine (16% and 22%) and in 2 clinical trials with fludarabine tablets (8% and 3%). Pulmonary hypersensitivity reactions to fludarabine characterized by dyspnea, cough, and interstitial pulmonary infiltrate have been observed. In study 1 conducted with fludarabine tablets, severe pulmonary toxicity was reported in 5 of 78 patients, often in conjunction with respiratory or pulmonary infections and hence not regarded as isolated drug-related pulmonary toxicity.

FLUDARABINE PHOSPHATE — ORAL

➤*Other adverse reactions:*

Fludarabine Nonhematologic Adverse Reactions in Patients With Chronic Lymphocytic Leukemia (≥ 5%)		
Adverse reactions	Study 1 (n = 78)	Study 2 (n = 81)
Any adverse reaction	82%	89%
CV, NOS[a]	14%	17%
Chest pain	0%	5%
CNS, NOS	19%	41%
Headache	9%	9%
Weakness/Fatigue (asthenia)	13%	31%
Dermatologic, NOS	22%	25%
Herpes simplex	8%	7%
Rash	5%	4%
Skin disorder	0%	6%
Sweating increased	0%	14%
GI, NOS	41%	28%
Abdominal pain	8%	10%
Anorexia	19%	0%
Diarrhea	6%	5%
Nausea	5%	1%
GU, NOS	8%	14%
Urinary tract infection	4%	5%
Metabolic and nutritional, NOS	3%	31%
Lactic dehydrogenase increased	0%	6%
Peripheral edema	0%	7%
Weight decreased	1%	6%
Musculoskeletal, NOS	10%	19%
Back pain	4%	9%
Respiratory, NOS	37%	53%
Bronchitis	6%	9%
Cough	21%	0%
Cough increased	0%	6%
Dyspnea	1%	5%
Pneumonia	8%	3%
Rhinitis	3%	11%
Sinusitis	1%	5%
Upper respiratory infection	9%	14%
Miscellaneous	59%	77%
Diaphoresis	8%	0%
Fever	26%	11%
Flu syndrome	8%	5%
Infection	12%	17%
Pain	5%	19%

[a] NOS = not otherwise specified.

➤*Postmarketing:*

CNS – Cases of progressive multifocal leukoencephalopathy have been reported. Most cases had a fatal outcome. Many of these cases were confounded by prior and/or concurrent chemotherapy. The median time to onset was approximately 1 year.

Hematologic – Several instances of trilineage bone marrow hypoplasia or aplasia resulting in pancytopenia, sometimes resulting in death, have been reported. The duration of clinically significant cytopenia in the reported cases has ranged from approximately 2 months to approximately 1 year. These episodes have occurred both in previously treated or untreated patients.

Respiratory – Cases of severe pulmonary toxicity have been observed with fludarabine use, which resulted in acute respiratory distress syndrome, respiratory distress, pulmonary hemorrhage, pulmonary fibrosis, and respiratory failure. After exclusion of an infectious origin, some patients experienced symptom improvement with corticosteroids.

Overdosage

➤*Symptoms:* High doses of fludarabine have been associated with an irreversible CNS toxicity characterized by delayed blindness, coma, and death. High doses are also associated with severe thrombocytopenia and neutropenia caused by bone marrow suppression. In study 2, two patients ingested an overdose of 20% to 33% of oral fludarabine phosphate. No serious side effects were reported.

➤*Treatment:* There is no known specific antidote for fludarabine overdosage. Treatment consists of drug discontinuation and supportive therapy.

Patient Information

Inform patients that fludarabine decreases blood cell count such as white blood cells, platelets, and red blood cells. Thus, it is important that periodic assessment of their blood count be performed to detect the development of neutropenia, thrombocytopenia, and anemia.

Advise patient to immediately report any of the following to health care provider: bleeding or unusual bruising; dark urine; difficulty breathing; fever, chills, or other signs of infection; hives; pain, redness, or swelling at the injection site; rash; sores in the mouth; yellowing of the skin or eyes.

Advise patients that fludarabine may reduce the ability to drive or use machinery.

Caution women of childbearing potential to avoid becoming pregnant.

Advise women of childbearing potential and fertile males to take contraceptive measures during and at least 6 months after stopping therapy with fludarabine.

Instruct patients that caution should be exercised in the handling of fludarabine. Do not crush tablets. Avoid exposure by direct contact of the skin or mucous membranes or by inhalation. If contact occurs, wash thoroughly with soap and water or wash the eyes immediately with gently flowing water for at least 15 minutes. Consult health care provider in case of a skin reaction or if the drug gets in the eyes. Ask your health care prover or pharmacist for directions about how to safely dispose of fludarabine.

FLUDARABINE PHOSPHATE — INJECTION

WARNING

Ensure that fludarabine is administered under the supervision of a qualified health care provider experienced in the use of antineoplastic therapy. Fludarabine can severely suppress bone marrow function. When used at high doses in dose-ranging studies in patients with acute leukemia, fludarabine was associated with severe neurologic effects, including blindness, coma, and death. This severe CNS toxicity occurred in 36% of patients treated with dosages approximately 4 times more (96 mg/m²/day for 5 to 7 days) than the recommended dosage. Similar severe CNS toxicity, including agitation, coma, confusion, and seizures, has been reported in patients treated at doses in the range of the dose recommended for chronic lymphocytic leukemia (CLL).

Instances of life-threatening and sometimes fatal autoimmune phenomena, such as acquired hemophilia, autoimmune thrombocytopenia/thrombocytopenic purpura (ITP), Evan syndrome, and hemolytic anemia, have been reported to occur after 1 or more cycles of treatment with fludarabine. Evaluate and closely monitor patients undergoing treatment with fludarabine for hemolysis.

In a clinical investigation using fludarabine in combination with pentostatin (deoxycoformycin) for the treatment of refractory CLL, there was an unacceptably high incidence of fatal pulmonary toxicity. Therefore, the use of fludarabine in combination with pentostatin is not recommended.

Indications

➤*B-cell chronic lymphocytic leukemia:* For the treatment of adult patients with B-cell CLL who have not responded to or whose disease has progressed during treatment with at least 1 standard alkylating agent–containing regimen.

➤*Off-label uses:* Treatment of non-Hodgkin lymphoma; may be used in combination therapy for the treatment of primary resistant or relapsing acute myelogenous leukemia (AML), acute lymphoblastic leukemia (ALL), and secondary AML.

Administration and Dosage

➤*General dosing considerations:* A number of clinical settings may predispose to increased toxicity from fludarabine. These include advanced age, renal insufficiency, and bone marrow impairment. Such patients should be monitored closely for excessive toxicity, and the dose modified accordingly.

➤*Adults:*

B-cell chronic lymphocytic leukemia –

Usual dosage: 25 mg/m² intravenously (IV) over a period of approximately 30 minutes daily for 5 consecutive days. Each 5-day course of treatment should commence every 28 days.

Dosage adjustment: Dosage may be decreased or delayed based on evidence of hematologic or nonhematologic toxicity. Health care providers should consider delaying or discontinuing the drug if neurotoxicity occurs.

FLUDARABINE PHOSPHATE — INJECTION

Duration of therapy: The optimal duration of treatment has not been clearly established. It is recommended that 3 additional cycles of fludarabine be administered following the achievement of a maximal response, and then the drug should be discontinued.

➤*Children:*

Off-label dosing –

Acute myelogenous leukemia: 10 mg/m² IV over 15 minutes as a single dose, followed by a continuous IV infusion of 30.5 mg/m²/day for 5 consecutive days.

In combination with other antineoplastics, 30 mg/m²/day IV for 5 days.

Solid tumors: 9 mg/m² IV bolus as a single dose, followed by a continuous IV infusion of 27 mg/m²/day for 5 days.

➤*Elderly:* Advanced age may predispose patients to increased toxicity from fludarabine. Monitor patients closely for excessive toxicity and modify the dose accordingly.

➤*Renal function impairment:*

Fludarabine Initial Dosage Recommendations in Renal Impairment	
CrCl[a]	Initial dosage
≥ 80 mL/min	25 mg/m² (full dose)
50 to 79 mL/min	20 mg/m²
30 to 49 mL/min	15 mg/m²
< 30 mL/min	Do not administer

[a] CrCl = creatinine clearance.

➤*Preparation for administration:*

Handling/Disposal – Fludarabine is considered a cytotoxic agent. Follow safe handling procedures when preparing, administering, or dispensing fludarabine.

Caution should be exercised in the handling and preparation of fludarabine. The use of latex gloves and safety glasses is recommended to avoid exposure in case of breakage of the vial or other accidental spillage. If the solution contacts the skin or mucous membranes, wash thoroughly with soap and water; rinse eyes thoroughly with plain water. Avoid exposure by inhalation or by direct contact of the skin or mucous membranes.

Lyophilized cake – Fludarabine should be prepared for parenteral use by aseptically adding sterile water for injection. When reconstituted with 2 mL of sterile water for injection, the solid cake should fully dissolve in 15 seconds or less; each milliliter of the resulting solution will contain fludarabine 25 mg.

Solution – In clinical studies, the product has been diluted in 100 or 125 mL of dextrose 5% injection or sodium chloride 0.9%.

➤*Administration:* Administer IV over a period of approximately 30 minutes.

➤*Admixture compatibility:* Fludarabine should not be mixed with other drugs.

➤*Storage/Stability:* Store between 2° and 8°C (36° and 46°F). Reconstituted fludarabine should be used within 8 hours of reconstitution.

Actions

➤*Pharmacology:* Fludarabine is a fluorinated nucleotide antimetabolite. Fludarabine phosphate is rapidly dephosphorylated to 2-fluoro-ara-A and then phosphorylated intracellularly by deoxycytidine kinase to the active triphosphate, 2-fluoro-ara-ATP. This metabolite appears to act by inhibiting DNA polymerase alpha, ribonucleotide reductase, and DNA primase, thus inhibiting DNA synthesis. The mechanism of action of this antimetabolite is not completely characterized and may be multifaceted.

➤*Pharmacokinetics:*

Absorption/Distribution – After the 5 daily doses of 25 mg of 2-fluoro-ara-AMP/m² to cancer patients infused over 30 minutes, 2-fluoro-ara-A concentrations show a moderate accumulation. During a 5-day treatment schedule, 2-fluoro-ara-A plasma trough levels increased by a factor of approximately 2. In vitro, plasma protein binding of fludarabine ranged between 19% and 29%.

A correlation was noted between the degree of absolute granulocyte count nadir and increased area under the curve (AUC).

Metabolism/Excretion – Fludarabine is rapidly dephosphorylated to 2-fluoro-ara and then phosphorylated intracellularly by deoxycytidine kinase to the active triphosphate, 2-fluoro-ara-ATP. The terminal half-life of 2-fluoro-ara-A was estimated as approximately 20 hours. Renal clearance represents approximately 40% of the total body clearance. Total body clearance was 172 mL/min for healthy patients.

Special populations –

Renal function impairment: The total body clearance of the principal metabolite, 2-fluoro-ara-A, correlated with the CrCl, indicating the importance of the renal excretion pathway for the elimination of the drug.

The mean total body clearance was 124 mL/min for patients with moderately impaired renal function.

Contraindications

Hypersensitivity to this drug or its components.

Warnings/Precautions

➤*Neurotoxicity:* There are clear dose-dependent toxic effects seen with fludarabine. Dose levels approximately 4 times more (96 mg/m²/day for 5 to 7 days) than that recommended for CLL (25 mg/m²/day for 5 days) were associated with a syndrome characterized by delayed blindness, coma, and death. Symptoms appeared from 21 to 60 days following the last dose. Thirty-six percent of patients who received fludarabine at high doses (96 mg/m²/day for 5 to 7 days) developed this severe neurotoxicity. Similar severe CNS toxicity, including agitation, coma, confusion, and seizures, has been rarely reported in patients treated at doses in the range of the dose recommended for CLL (25 mg/m²/day for 5 days every 28 days). This syndrome has been reported rarely in patients treated with doses in the range of the recommended CLL dose of 25 mg/m²/day for 5 days every 28 days. The effect of long-term administration of fludarabine on the CNS is unknown; however, patients have received the recommended dose for up to 15 courses of therapy.

➤*Hematologic effects:*

Bone marrow suppression – Severe bone marrow suppression, notably anemia, thrombocytopenia, and neutropenia, has been reported in patients treated with fludarabine. In a phase 1 study in adult solid tumor patients, the median time to nadir counts was 13 days (range, 3 to 25 days) for granulocytes and 16 days (range, 2 to 32) for platelets. Most patients had hematologic impairment at baseline as a result of disease or as a result of prior myelosuppressive therapy. Cumulative myelosuppression may be seen. While chemotherapy-induced myelosuppression is often reversible, administration of fludarabine requires careful hematologic monitoring.

Bone marrow hypoplasia or aplasia – Several instances of trilineage bone marrow hypoplasia or aplasia resulting in pancytopenia, sometimes resulting in death, have been reported in adult patients. The duration of clinically significant cytopenia in the reported cases has ranged from approximately 2 months to approximately 1 year. These episodes have occurred in previously treated or untreated patients.

Autoimmune phenomena – Instances of life-threatening and sometimes fatal autoimmune phenomena (eg, acquired hemophilia, autoimmune thrombocytopenia/thrombocytopenic purpura, Evan syndrome, hemolytic anemia) have been reported to occur after 1 or more cycles of treatment with fludarabine in patients with or without a history of autoimmune hemolytic anemia or a positive Coombs test and who may or may not be in remission from their disease. Steroids may or may not be effective in controlling these hemolytic episodes. The majority of patients rechallenged with fludarabine developed a recurrence in the hemolytic process. The mechanism(s) that predispose patients to the development of this complication has not been identified. Evaluate and closely monitor patients undergoing treatment with fludarabine for hemolysis. Discontinuation of therapy with fludarabine is recommended in cases of hemolysis.

➤*Transfusion-associated graft-versus-host disease:* Transfusion-associated graft-versus-host disease (GVHD) has been observed rarely after transfusion of nonirradiated blood in fludarabine-treated patients. Fatal outcome as a consequence of this disease has been reported. Therefore, to minimize the risk of transfusion-associated GVHD, ensure that patients who require blood transfusion and who are undergoing, or who have received, treatment with fludarabine receive irradiated blood only.

➤*Fatalities:* Of the 133 patients with CLL in the 2 trials, there were 29 fatalities during study. Approximately 50% of the fatalities were caused by infection, and 25% caused by progressive disease.

➤*Tumor lysis syndrome:* Tumor lysis syndrome associated with fludarabine treatment has been reported in patients with CLL with large tumor burdens. Since fludarabine can induce a response as early as the first week of treatment, take precautions in those patients at risk of developing this complication.

➤*Vaccination:* During and after treatment with fludarabine, advise patients to avoid vaccination with live vaccines.

➤*Disease progression:* Disease progression and transformation (eg, Richter syndrome) have been reported in patients with CLL.

➤*Renal function impairment:* There are inadequate data on dosing of patients with renal insufficiency. Fludarabine must be administered cautiously in patients with renal insufficiency. The total body clearance of 2-fluoro-ara-A was directly correlated with the CrCl.

See Administration and Dosage for more information.

➤*Special risk:* In patients with an impaired state of health, give fludarabine with caution and after careful risk/benefit consideration. This applies especially for patients with severe impairment of bone marrow function (thrombocytopenia, anemia, and/or granulocytopenia), immunodeficiency, or a history of opportunistic infection. Consider prophylactic treatment in patients at increased risk of developing opportunistic infections.

➤*Hazardous tasks:* Fludarabine may reduce the ability to drive or use machines because agitation, confusion, fatigue, seizures, visual disturbances, and weakness have been observed.

➤*Pregnancy:* *Category D.* Based on its mechanism of action, fludarabine can cause fetal harm when administered to a pregnant woman. There are no adequate and well-controlled studies of fludarabine in pregnant women. If fludarabine is used during pregnancy, or if the patient becomes pregnant while taking this drug, apprise the patient of the potential hazard to the fetus. Advise women of childbearing potential to avoid becoming pregnant.

FLUDARABINE PHOSPHATE — INJECTION

Women of childbearing potential and fertile men must take contraceptive measures during and at least for 6 months after cessation of treatment with fludarabine.

Fludarabine was embryolethal and teratogenic in rats and rabbits. Fludarabine was administered at dosages of 0, 1, 10, or 30 mg/kg/day (0.24, 2.4, and 7.2 times the recommended human dose on a mg/m^2 basis, respectively) to pregnant rats on days 6 to 15 of gestation. At 10 and 30 mg/kg/day administered during organogenesis, there was a dose-related increase in various skeletal variations and a decrease in mean fetal body weights. Maternal toxicity was not apparent at 10 mg/kg/day, and was limited to slight body weight decreases at 30 mg/kg/day. In a dose-finding study, malformations, such as limb and tail defects, were induced at 40 mg/kg/day (9.6 times the recommended human dose on a mg/m^2 basis). In a reproduction toxicity study on rabbits, fludarabine was administered IV at dosages of 0, 1, 5, or 8 mg/kg/day (approximately 0.5, 2.4, and 3.8 times the recommended human dose on a mg/m^2 basis) on days 6 to 18 of gestation. A dosage of 8 mg/kg/day administered during organogenesis increased embryo and fetal lethality, as indicated by a higher number of resorptions and a decrease in live fetuses. Compound-related teratogenic effects manifested by external deformities and skeletal malformations were observed at 5 and 8 mg/kg/day. The most frequent external malformations observed in rabbits were cleft palate, adactyly, brachydactyly, and syndactyly, along with skeletal malformations such as fused metatarsals, phalanges, sternebrae, and limb bones, and some soft tissue malformations (diaphragmatic herniae). Fetal body weights were decreased in rabbits given 8 mg/kg/day. Drug-related toxic effects on maternal weights were not observed.

➤*Lactation:* It is not known whether fludarabine is excreted in human milk. Because many drugs are excreted in human milk and because of the potential for serious adverse reactions, including tumorigenicity, in breast-feeding infants, decide whether to discontinue breast-feeding or the drug, taking into account the importance of the drug to the mother.

➤*Children:* Data submitted to the Food and Drug Administration were insufficient to establish efficacy in any childhood malignancy.

➤*Elderly:* See Administration and Dosage for more information.

➤*Monitoring:* Fludarabine is a potent antineoplastic agent with potentially significant toxic adverse reactions. Closely observe patients undergoing therapy for signs of hematologic and nonhematologic toxicity. Periodic assessment of peripheral blood cell counts is recommended to detect the development of anemia, neutropenia, and thrombocytopenia.

During treatment, monitor the patient's hematologic profile (particularly neutrophils and platelets) regularly to determine the degree of hematopoietic suppression.

Monitor for signs and symptoms of infection. Monitor patients with advanced age, renal impairment, and bone marrow impairment closely for excessive toxicity and modify the dose accordingly.

Drug Interactions

Fludarabine Injection Drug Interactions

Precipitant drug	Object drug[a]		Description
Fludarabine	Digoxin	⬇	Pharmacologic effects of digoxin may be decreased because of decreased GI absorption caused by fludarabine. Monitor serum digoxin concentrations and the patient for evidence of clinical deterioration and adjust the dose accordingly.
Fludarabine	Pentostatin	⬆	The use of fludarabine in combination with pentostatin is not recommended because of the risk of severe pulmonary toxicity.
Pentostatin	Fludarabine		

[a] ⬆ = object drug increased; ⬇ = object drug decreased.

➤*Vaccination:* See Warnings/Precautions for more information.

Adverse Reactions

➤*Common adverse reactions:* The most common adverse reactions include myelosuppression (anemia, neutropenia, and thrombocytopenia), fever and chills, infection, and nausea and vomiting. Other commonly reported reactions include anorexia, fatigue, malaise, and weakness. Serious opportunistic infections have occurred in patients with CLL treated with fludarabine.

➤*Frequent adverse reactions:* The most frequently reported adverse reactions and those reactions that are more clearly related to the drug are arranged according to body system.

Cardiovascular – Edema has been frequently reported. One patient developed a pericardial effusion possibly related to treatment with fludarabine.

CNS – Agitation, blindness, coma, confusion, objective weakness, optic neuritis, optic neuropathy, seizures, and visual disturbances have occurred in patients with CLL treated with fludarabine. Peripheral neuropathy has been observed and 1 case of wrist-drop was reported.

Dermatologic – Skin toxicity, consisting primarily of skin rashes, has been reported. Erythema multiforme, pemphigus, Stevens-Johnson syndrome, and toxic epidermal necrolysis have been reported, with fatal outcomes in some cases.

Worsening or flare-up of preexisting skin cancer lesions, as well as new onset of skin cancer, has been reported in patients during or after treatment.

GI – GI disturbances such as anorexia, diarrhea, GI bleeding, nausea and vomiting, and stomatitis have been reported.

GU – Rare cases of hemorrhagic cystitis have been reported.

Hematologic – Hematologic reactions (neutropenia, thrombocytopenia, and/or anemia) were reported in the majority of patients with CLL treated with fludarabine. During fludarabine treatment of 133 patients with CLL, the absolute neutrophil count decreased to less than 500/mm^3 in 59% of patients, hemoglobin decreased from pretreatment values by at least 2 grams percent in 60%, and platelet count decreased from pretreatment values by at least 50% in 55%. Myelosuppression may be severe and cumulative and may affect multiple cell lines. Bone marrow fibrosis occurred in 1 patient with CLL treated with fludarabine.

See Warnings/Precautions for more information.

Metabolic – Tumor lysis syndrome has been reported in CLL patients treated with fludarabine. This complication may include hematuria, hyperkalemia, hyperphosphatemia, hyperuricemia, hypocalcemia, metabolic acidosis, renal failure, and urate crystalluria. The onset of this syndrome may be heralded by flank pain and hematuria.

Respiratory – Pneumonia, a frequent manifestation of infection in CLL patients, occurred in 16% and 22% of those treated with fludarabine in the MD Anderson Cancer Center (MDAH) and Southwest Oncology Group (SWOG) studies, respectively. Pulmonary hypersensitivity reactions to fludarabine characterized by cough, dyspnea, and interstitial pulmonary infiltrate have been observed.

Miscellaneous – Serious, and sometimes fatal, infections, including opportunistic infections and reactivations of latent viral infections such as herpes zoster, Epstein-Barr virus, and John Cunningham virus (progressive multifocal leukoencephalopathy), have been reported.

Rare cases of Epstein-Barr virus–associated lymphoproliferative disorders have been reported.

➤*Other adverse reactions:*

Fludarabine Nonhematologic Adverse Reactions in Patients With Chronic Lymphocytic Leukemia

Adverse reactions	MDAH (n = 101)	SWOG (n = 32)
Any adverse reaction	88%	91%
Cardiovascular, NOS[a]	12%	38%
Aneurysm	1%	0%
Angina	0%	6%
Arrhythmia	0%	3%
Cerebrovascular accident	0%	3%
Congestive heart failure	0%	3%
Deep venous thrombosis	1%	3%
Myocardial infarction	0%	3%
Phlebitis	1%	3%
Supraventricular tachycardia	0%	3%
Transient ischemic attack	1%	0%
CNS, NOS	21%	69%
Cerebellar syndrome	1%	0%
Depression	1%	0%
Fatigue	10%	38%
Headache	3%	0%
Impaired mentation	1%	0%
Malaise	8%	6%
Paresthesia	4%	12%
Sleep disorder	1%	3%
Weakness	9%	65%
Dermatologic, NOS	17%	18%
Alopecia	0%	3%
Pruritus	1%	3%
Rash	15%	15%
Seborrhea	1%	0%
GI, NOS	46%	63%
Anorexia	7%	34%
Constipation	1%	3%
Diarrhea	15%	13%
Dysphagia	1%	0%
Esophagitis	3%	0%
GI bleeding	3%	13%

FLUDARABINE PHOSPHATE — INJECTION

Fludarabine Nonhematologic Adverse Reactions in Patients With Chronic Lymphocytic Leukemia		
Adverse reactions	MDAH (n = 101)	SWOG (n = 32)
Mucositis	2%	0%
Nausea/Vomiting	36%	31%
Stomatitis	9%	0%
GU, NOS	12%	22%
Abnormal renal function test	1%	0%
Dysuria	4%	3%
Hematuria	2%	3%
Hesitancy	0%	3%
Proteinuria	1%	0%
Renal failure	1%	0%
Urinary infection	2%	15%
Hepatic		
Abnormal liver function test	1%	3%
Cholelithiasis	0%	3%
Liver failure	1%	0%
Musculoskeletal, NOS	7%	16%
Arthralgia	1%	0%
Myalgia	4%	16%
Osteoporosis	2%	0%
Respiratory, NOS	35%	69%
Allergic pneumonitis	0%	6%
Bronchitis	1%	0%
Cough	10%	44%
Dyspnea	9%	22%
Epistaxis	1%	0%
Hemoptysis	1%	6%
Hypoxia	1%	0%
Pharyngitis	0%	9%
Pneumonia	16%	22%
Sinusitis	5%	0%
Upper respiratory tract infection	2%	16%
Special senses		
Hearing loss	2%	6%
Visual disturbance	3%	15%
Miscellaneous	72%	84%
Anaphylaxis	1%	0%
Chills	11%	19%
Dehydration	1%	0%
Diaphoresis	1%	13%
Edema	8%	19%
Fever	60%	69%
Hemorrhage	1%	0%
Hyperglycemia	1%	6%
Infection	33%	44%
Pain	20%	22%
Tumor lysis syndrome	1%	0%

[a] NOS = not otherwise specified.

➤*Postmarketing:*

CNS – Cases of progressive multifocal leukoencephalopathy have been reported. Most cases had a fatal outcome. Many of these cases were confounded by prior and/or concurrent chemotherapy. The time to onset has ranged from a few weeks to approximately 1 year after initiating treatment.

Hematologic – Several instances of trilineage bone marrow hypoplasia or aplasia resulting in pancytopenia, sometimes resulting in death, have been reported. The duration of clinically significant cytopenia in the reported cases has ranged from approximately 2 months to approximately 1 year. These episodes have occurred in previously treated or untreated patients.

Cases of myelodysplastic syndrome and acute myeloid leukemia, mainly associated with prior, concomitant, or subsequent treatment with alkylating agents, topoisomerase inhibitors, or irradiation, have been reported.

Respiratory – Cases of severe pulmonary toxicity have been observed that resulted in acute respiratory distress syndrome, respiratory distress, pulmonary hemorrhage, pulmonary fibrosis, and respiratory failure. After exclusion of an infectious origin, some patients experienced symptom improvement with corticosteroids.

Overdosage

➤*Symptoms:* High doses of fludarabine have been associated with an irreversible CNS toxicity characterized by delayed blindness, coma, and death. High doses are also associated with severe thrombocytopenia and neutropenia due to bone marrow suppression.

➤*Treatment:* There is no known specific antidote for fludarabine overdosage. Treatment consists of drug discontinuation and supportive therapy.

Patient Information

Advise patient that medication will be prepared and administered by health care provider.

Advise patients to immediately report any of the following to the health care provider: bleeding or unusual bruising; dark urine; difficulty breathing; fever, chills, or other signs of infection; hives; pain, redness, or swelling at the injection site; rash; sores in the mouth; yellowing of the skin or eyes.

Advise patients that fludarabine may reduce the ability to drive or use machinery.

Caution women of childbearing potential to avoid becoming pregnant.

Advise women of childbearing potential and fertile males to take contraceptive measures during and at least 6 months after stopping therapy with fludarabine.

MERCAPTOPURINE (6-Mercaptopurine; 6-MP)

Rx	**Mercaptopurine** (Par)	**Tablets:** 50 mg	Lactose. (P02). Lt. yellow to off-white, diamond shape, scored. In 60s.
Rx	**Purinethol** (Gate Pharmaceuticals)		(Purinethol O4A). Off-white, scored. In 25s and 250s.

MERCAPTOPURINE — ORAL

WARNING

Mercaptopurine is a potent drug. It should not be used unless a diagnosis of acute lymphatic leukemia has been adequately established, and the responsible physician is knowledgeable in assessing response to chemotherapy.

Indications

➤*Acute lymphatic leukemia:* For remission induction and maintenance therapy of acute lymphatic leukemia. The response to this agent depends upon the particular subclassification of acute lymphatic leukemia and the age of the patient (pediatric patient or adult).

Given as a single agent for remission induction, mercaptopurine induces complete remission in approximately 25% of pediatric patients and approximately 10% of adults. However, reliance upon mercaptopurine alone is not justified for initial remission induction of acute lymphatic leukemiabecause combination chemotherapy with vincristine, prednisone, and L-asparaginase results in more frequent complete remission induction than with mercaptopurine alone or in combination. The duration of complete remission induced in acute lymphatic leukemia is so brief without the use of maintenance therapy that some form of drug therapy is considered essential. Mercaptopurine, as a single agent, is capable of significantly prolonging complete remission duration; however, combination therapy has produced remission duration longer than that achieved with mercaptopurine alone.

➤*Acute myelogenous (and acute myelomonocytic) leukemia:* As a single agent, mercaptopurine will induce complete remission in approximately 10% of pediatric patients and adults with acute myelogenous leukemia or its subclassifications. These results are inferior to those achieved with combination chemotherapy employing optimum treatment schedules.

➤*Off-label uses:*

Other possible off-label uses – Non-Hodgkin lymphoma (see Administration and Dosage), Crohn disease, ulcerative colitis.

Administration and Dosage

➤*General dosing considerations:* Frequency and duration of remission is greater when given with other antineoplastic agents. As such, mercaptopurine is rarely used as a single agent.

The dosage which will be tolerated and effective varies from patient to patient, and, therefore, careful titration is necessary to obtain the optimum therapeutic effect without incurring excessive, unintended toxicity.

MERCAPTOPURINE — ORAL

➤*Adults:*

Acute lymphatic leukemia –

Initial dosage: For remission induction, the dosage is 2.5 mg/kg/day, calculated to the nearest multiple of 25 mg (100 to 200 mg in the average adult). The total daily dosage may be given at 1 time.

A dosage of 2.5 mg/kg/day may result in a rapid fall in leukocyte count within 1 to 2 weeks in some adults with acute lymphatic leukemia and high total leukocyte counts.

Dosage titration: If, after 4 weeks at the initial dosage, there is no clinical improvement and no definite evidence of leukocyte or platelet depression, the dosage may be increased up to 5 mg/kg daily.

Maintenance dosage: 1.5 to 2.5 mg/kg/day as a single dose. Once a complete hematologic remission is obtained, maintenance therapy is considered essential. Maintenance doses will vary from patient to patient. Mercaptopurine should rarely be relied upon as a single agent for the maintenance of remissions induced in acute leukemia.

Alternative dosage: Initiate therapy with 80 to 100 mg/m²/day, rounded to the nearest 25 mg.

Concomitant therapy: The dosage of mercaptopurine should be reduced to one-third to one-fourth of the usual dose if allopurinol is given concurrently.

Discontinuation of therapy: Because the drug may have a delayed action, it should be discontinued at the first sign of an abnormally large or rapid fall in the leukocyte or platelet count. If subsequently the leukocyte count or platelet count remains constant for 2 or 3 days, or rises, treatment may be resumed.

➤*Children:*

Acute lymphatic leukemia –

Initial dosage: Initial dosage: For remission induction, the dosage is 2.5 mg/kg/day, calculated to the nearest multiple of 25 mg (50 mg in an average child 5 years of age). The total daily dosage may be given at 1 time.

Dosage titration: If, after 4 weeks at the initial dosage, there is no clinical improvement and no definite evidence of leukocyte or platelet depression, the dosage may be increased up to 5 mg/kg daily.

Maintenance dosage: 1.5 to 2.5 mg/kg/day as a single dose. Once a complete hematologic remission is obtained, maintenance therapy is considered essential. Maintenance doses will vary from patient to patient. It is to be emphasized that in pediatric patients with acute lymphatic leukemia in remission, superior results have been obtained when mercaptopurine has been combined with other agents (most frequently with methotrexate) for remission maintenance. Mercaptopurine should rarely be relied on as a single agent for the maintenance of remissions induced in acute leukemia.

Alternative dosage:

- *Induction* – Initiate therapy with 70 to 100 mg/m²/day, rounded to the nearest 25 mg.
- *Maintenance* – 75 mg/m²/day, rounded to the nearest 25 mg.

Concomitant therapy: The dosage of mercaptopurine should be reduced to one-third to one-fourth of the usual dose if allopurinol is given concurrently.

Discontinuation of therapy: Because the drug may have a delayed action, it should be discontinued at the first sign of an abnormally large or rapid fall in the leukocyte or platelet count. If subsequently the leukocyte count or platelet count remains constant for 2 or 3 days, or rises, treatment may be resumed.

Off-label dosing –

Non-Hodgkin lymphoma:

- *Induction* – 60 mg/m²/day in combination with other antineoplastic agents. Refer to specific protocols for recommended treatment intervals.
- *Consolidation* – 25 mg/m²/day in combination with other antineoplastic agents. Refer to specific protocols for recommended treatment intervals.
- *Maintenance dosage* – 50 mg/m²/day in combination with other antineoplastic agents. Refer to specific protocols for recommended treatment intervals.

➤*Renal function impairment:* Dosage reduction may be needed in renal dysfunction, as shown in the following table.

Mercaptopurine Dosage Adjustment for Renal Function	
Renal function	Recommended dosage interval
Creatinine clearance (CrCl) ≥ 50 mL/min	Every 24 hours (ie, once daily)
CrCl < 50 mL/min	Every 48 hours
Hemodialysis, continuous ambulatory peritoneal dialysis, or continuous renal replacement therapy	Every 48 hours

Dialysis – Conventional hemodialysis is minimally effective (25% to 49%) in removing mercaptopurine.

➤*Preparation for administration:* Mercaptopurine is considered a cytotoxic agent. Follow safe handling procedures when preparing, administering, or dispensing mercaptopurine.

➤*Administration:* Give on an empty stomach because food may reduce bioavailability.

Shake suspension well before using.

Risk of relapse is lower with evening administration than with morning administration.

➤*Storage/Stability:* Store at 15° to 25°C (59° to 77°F) in a dry place.

Actions

➤*Pharmacology:* Mercaptopurine competes with hypoxanthine and guanine for the enzyme hypoxanthine-guanine phosphoribosyltransferase (HGPRTase) and is itself converted to thioinosinic acid (TIMP). This intracellular nucleotide inhibits several reactions involving inosinic acid (IMP), including the conversion of IMP to xanthylic acid (XMP) and the conversion of IMP to adenylic acid (AMP) via adenylosuccinate (SAMP). In addition, 6-methylthioinosinate (MTIMP) is formed by the methylation of TIMP. Both TIMP and MTIMP have been reported to inhibit glutamine-5-phosphoribosylpyrophosphate amidotransferase, the first enzyme unique to the de novo pathway for purine ribonucleotide synthesis.

Experiments indicate that radiolabeled mercaptopurine may be recovered from the DNA in the form of deoxythioguanosine. Some mercaptopurine is converted to nucleotide derivatives of 6-thioguanine (6-TG) by the sequential actions of inosinate (IMP) dehydrogenase and xanthylate (XMP) aminase, converting TIMP to thioguanylic acid (TGMP).

Animal tumors that are resistant to mercaptopurine often have lost the ability to convert mercaptopurine to TIMP. However, it is clear that resistance to mercaptopurine may be acquired by other means as well, particularly in human leukemias.

➤*Pharmacokinetics:* Monitoring of plasma levels of mercaptopurine during therapy is of questionable value. There is technical difficulty in determining plasma concentrations which are seldom greater than 1 to 2 mcg/mL after a therapeutic oral dose. More significantly, mercaptopurine enters rapidly into the anabolic and catabolic pathways for purines, and the active intracellular metabolites have appreciably longer half-lives than the parent drug. The biochemical effects of a single dose of mercaptopurine are evident long after the parent drug has disappeared from plasma. Because of this rapid metabolism of mercaptopurine to active intracellular derivatives, hemodialysis would not be expected to appreciably reduce toxicity of the drug. There is no known pharmacologic antagonist to the biochemical actions of mercaptopurine in vivo.

Absorption – Clinical studies have shown that the absorption of an oral dose of mercaptopurine in humans is incomplete and variable, averaging ≈ 50% of the administered dose. The factors influencing absorption are unknown.

Distribution – IV administration of an investigational preparation of mercaptopurine revealed a plasma half-disappearance time of 21 minutes in pediatric patients and 47 minutes in adults. The volume of distribution usually exceeded that of the total body water.

There is negligible entry of mercaptopurine into cerebrospinal fluid.

Plasma protein binding averages 19% over the concentration range 10 to 50 mcg/mL (a concentration only achieved by IV administration of mercaptopurine at doses exceeding 5 to 10 mg/kg).

Metabolism/Excretion – Following the oral administration of ³⁵S-6-mercaptopurine in 1 subject, a total of 46% of the dose could be accounted for in the urine (as parent drug and metabolites) in the first 24 hours. Metabolites of mercaptopurine were found in urine within the first 2 hours after administration. Radioactivity (in the form of sulfate) could be found in the urine for weeks afterwards.

Contraindications

Mercaptopurine should not be used unless a diagnosis of acute lymphatic leukemia has been adequately established and the responsible physician is knowledgeable in assessing response to chemotherapy.

Mercaptopurine should not be used in patients whose disease has demonstrated prior resistance to this drug. In animals and humans, there is usually complete cross-resistance between mercaptopurine and thioguanine.

Warnings/Precautions

➤*Mercaptopurine/Azathioprine:* Mercaptopurine is a metabolite of azathioprine; therefore, avoid coadministration due to the risk of severe myelosuppression.

➤*Bone marrow toxicity:* The most consistent, dose-related toxicity is bone marrow suppression. This may be manifest by anemia, leukopenia, thrombocytopenia, or any combination of these. Any of these findings may also reflect progression of the underlying disease. Since mercaptopurine may have a delayed effect, it is important to withdraw the medication temporarily at the first sign of an abnormally large fall in any of the formed elements of the blood.

There are rare individuals with an inherited deficiency of the enzyme thiopurine methyltransferase (TPMT) who may be unusually sensitive to the myelosuppressive effects of mercaptopurine and prone to developing rapid bone marrow suppression following the initiation of treatment. Substantial dosage reductions may be required to avoid the development of life-threatening bone marrow suppression in these patients. This toxicity may be more profound in patients treated with concomitant allopurinol (see Drug Interactions).

➤*Immunosuppression:* Mercaptopurine recipients may manifest decreased cellular hypersensitivities and impaired allograft rejection. Induction of immunity to infectious agents or vaccines will be subnormal in these patients; the degree of immunosuppression will depend on antigen dose and temporal relationship to drug. This immunosuppressive effect should be carefully considered with regard to intercurrent infections and risk of subsequent neoplasia.

➤*Hematologic:* The most frequent, serious, toxic effect of mercaptopurine is myelosuppression, resulting in leukopenia, thrombocytopenia, and anemia. These toxic effects are often unavoidable during the induction phase of adult acute leukemia if remission induction is to be successful. Whether or not these manifestations demand modification or cessation of dosage depends both upon the response of the underlying disease and a careful consideration of supportive facilities (granulocyte and platelet transfusions) which may be available. Life-threatening infections and bleeding have been

MERCAPTOPURINE — ORAL

observed as a consequence of mercaptopurine-induced granulocytopenia and thrombocytopenia. Severe hematologic toxicity may require supportive therapy with platelet transfusions for bleeding, and antibiotics and granulocyte transfusions if sepsis is documented.

If it is not the intent to deliberately induce bone marrow hypoplasia, it is important to discontinue the drug temporarily at the first evidence of an abnormally large fall in white blood cell count, platelet count, or hemoglobin concentration. In many patients with severe depression of the formed elements of the blood due to mercaptopurine, the bone marrow appears hypoplastic on aspiration or biopsy, whereas in other cases it may appear normocellular. The qualitative changes in the erythroid elements toward the megaloblastic series, characteristically seen with the folic acid antagonists and some other antimetabolites, are not seen with this drug.

➤*Renal function impairment:* It is probably advisable to start with smaller dosages in patients with impaired renal function, since the latter might result in slower elimination of the drug and metabolites and a greater cumulative effect.

➤*Hepatic function impairment:* Mercaptopurine is heptotoxic in animals and humans. A small number of deaths have been reported which may have been attributed to hepatic necrosis due to administration of mercaptopurine. Hepatic injury can occur with any dosage, but seems to occur with more frequency when doses of 2.5 mg/kg/day are exceeded. The histologic pattern of mercaptopurine hepatotoxicity includes features of both intrahepatic cholestasis and parenchymal cell necrosis, either of which may predominate. It is not clear how much of the hepatic damage is due to direct toxicity from the drug and how much may be due to a hypersensitivity reaction. In some patients jaundice has cleared following withdrawal of mercaptopurine and reappeared with its reintroduction.

Monitoring of serum transaminase levels, alkaline phosphatase, and bilirubin levels may allow early detection of hepatotoxicity. It is advisable to monitor these liver function tests at weekly intervals when first beginning therapy and at monthly intervals thereafter. Liver function tests may be advisable more frequently in patients who are receiving mercaptopurine with other hepatotoxic drugs or with known preexisting liver disease.

The concomitant administration of mercaptopurine with other hepatotoxic agents requires especially careful clinical and biochemical monitoring of hepatic function. Combination therapy involving mercaptopurine with other drugs not felt to be hepatotoxic should nevertheless be approached with caution. The combination of mercaptopurine with doxorubicin was reported to be hepatotoxic in 19 of 20 patients undergoing remission-induction therapy for leukemia resistant to previous therapy.

The hepatotoxicity has been associated in some cases with anorexia, diarrhea, jaundice, and ascites. Hepatic encephalopathy has occurred.

The onset of clinical jaundice, hepatomegaly, or anorexia with tenderness in the right hypochondrium are immediate indications for withholding mercaptopurine until the exact etiology can be identified. Likewise, any evidence of deterioration in liver function studies, toxic hepatitis, or biliary stasis should prompt discontinuation of the drug and a search for an etiology of the hepatotoxicity.

➤*Pregnancy: Category D.* Mercaptopurine can cause fetal harm when administered to a pregnant woman. Women receiving mercaptopurine in the first trimester of pregnancy have an increased incidence of abortion; the risk of malformation in offspring surviving first trimester exposure is not accurately known. In a series of 28 women receiving mercaptopurine after the first trimester of pregnancy, 3 mothers died undelivered, 1 delivered a stillborn child, and 1 aborted; there were no cases of macroscopically abnormal fetuses. Since such experience cannot exclude the possibility of fetal damage, mercaptopurine should be used during pregnancy only if the benefit clearly justifies the possible risk to the fetus, and particular caution should be given to the use of mercaptopurine in the first trimester of pregnancy.

There are no adequate and well-controlled studies in pregnant women. If this drug is used during pregnancy or if the patient becomes pregnant while taking the drug, the patient should be apprised of the potential hazard to the fetus. Women of childbearing potential should be advised to avoid becoming pregnant.

➤*Lactation:* It is not known whether this drug is excreted in human milk. Because many drugs are excreted in human milk, and because of the potential for serious adverse reactions in nursing infants from mercaptopurine, a decision should be made whether to discontinue nursing or to discontinue the drug, taking into account the importance of the drug to the mother.

➤*Children:* See Administration and Dosage.

➤*Monitoring:* It is recommended that evaluation of the hemoglobin or hematocrit, total white blood cell count and differential count, and quantitative platelet count be obtained weekly while the patient is on therapy with mercaptopurine. In cases where the cause of fluctuations in the formed elements in the peripheral blood is obscure, bone marrow examination may be useful for the evaluation of marrow status. The decision to increase, decrease, continue, or discontinue a given dosage of mercaptopurine must be based not only on the absolute hematologic values, but also upon the rapidity with which changes are occurring. In many instances, particularly during the induction phase of acute leukemia, complete blood counts will need to be done more frequently than once weekly in order to evaluate the effect of the therapy.

Drug Interactions

➤*Thioguanine:* There is usually complete cross-resistance between mercaptopurine and thioguanine.

Mercaptopurine Drug Interactions

Precipitant drug	Object drug[a]		Description
Allopurinol	Mercaptopurine	↑	When administered concomitantly with mercaptopurine, reduce mercaptopurine to ⅓ to ¼ the usual dose. Failure to observe this dosage reduction will delay catabolism of mercaptopurine and increase likelihood of severe toxicity.
Trimethroprim-sulfamethoxazole	Mercaptopurine	↑	When coadministered with mercaptopurine, enhanced marrow suppression has occurred.

[a] ↑ = Object drug increased.

Adverse Reactions

Mercaptopurine is considered to have very low emetogenic potential (less than 10% incidence of emesis).

➤*Dermatologic:* Dermatologic reactions can occur as a consequence of disease. The administration of mercaptopurine has been associated with skin rashes and hyperpigmentation.

➤*GI:* Intestinal ulceration has been reported. Nausea, vomiting, and anorexia are uncommon during initial administration. Mild diarrhea and sprue-like symptoms have been noted occasionally, but it is difficult at present to attribute these to the medication. Oral lesions are rarely seen, and when they occur they resemble thrush rather than antifolic ulcerations.

An increased risk of pancreatitis may be associated with the investigational use of mercaptopurine in inflammatory bowel disease.

➤*Hematologic:* See Warnings/Precautions for more information.

➤*Renal:* Hyperuricemia may occur in patients receiving mercaptopurine as a consequence of rapid cell lysis accompanying the antineoplastic effect. Adverse effects can be minimized by increased hydration, urine alkalinization, and the prophylactic administration of a xanthine oxidase inhibitor such as allopurinol. The dosage of mercaptopurine should be reduced to one third to one quarter of the usual dose if allopurinol is given concurrently.

➤*Miscellaneous:* Drug fever has been very rarely reported with mercaptopurine. Before attributing fever to mercaptopurine, every attempt should be made to exclude more common causes of pyrexia, such as sepsis, in patients with acute leukemia.

Overdosage

➤*Symptoms:* Signs and symptoms of overdosage may be immediate (eg, anorexia, nausea, vomiting, diarrhea); or delayed (eg, myelosuppression, liver dysfunction, gastroenteritis). The oral LD_{50} of mercaptopurine was determined to be 480 mg/kg in the mouse and 425 mg/kg in the rat.

➤*Treatment:* There is no known pharmacologic antagonist of mercaptopurine. The drug should be discontinued immediately if unintended toxicity occurs during treatment. If a patient is seen immediately following an accidental overdosage of the drug, it may be useful to induce emesis.

Dialysis cannot be expected to clear mercaptopurine. Hemodialysis is thought to be of marginal use due to the rapid intracellular incorporation of mercaptopurine into active metabolites with long persistence.

Patient Information

Patients should be informed that the major toxicities of mercaptopurine are related to myelosuppression, hepatotoxicity, and GI toxicity. Patients should never be allowed to take the drug without medical supervision and should be advised to consult their physician if they experience fever, sore throat, jaundice, nausea, vomiting, signs of local infection, bleeding from any site, or symptoms suggestive of anemia. Women of childbearing potential should be advised to avoid becoming pregnant.

PENTOSTATIN (2′-deoxycoformycin; DCF)

Rx	Pentostatin (Bedford Laboratories)	Injection, lyophilized powder for solution: 10 mg per vial	50 mg mannitol per vial. In single dose vials.
Rx	Nipent (Hospira)		50 mg mannitol per vial. In single-dose vials.

PENTOSTATIN — INJECTION

WARNING

Pentostatin should be administered under the supervision of a physician qualified and experienced in the use of cancer chemotherapeutic agents. The use of higher doses than those specified (see Administration and Dosage) is not recommended. Dose-limiting severe renal, liver, pulmonary, and CNS toxicities occurred in Phase 1 studies that used pentostatin at higher doses (20 to 50 mg/m² in divided doses over 5 days) than recommended.

In a clinical investigation in patients with refractory chronic lymphocytic leukemia using pentostatin at the recommended dose in combination with fludarabine phosphate, 4 of 6 patients entered in the study had severe or fatal pulmonary toxicity. The use of pentostatin in combination with fludarabine phosphate is not recommended.

Indications

➤*Hairy-cell leukemia:* Single-agent treatment for both untreated and alpha-interferon-refractory hairy-cell leukemia patients with active disease as defined by clinically significant anemia, neutropenia, thrombocytopenia, or disease-related symptoms.

➤*Off-label uses:* Treatment of prolymphocytic leukemia or cutaneous T-cell lymphoma; palliative therapy of chronic lymphocytic leukemia, refractory acute lymphocytic leukemia, mycosis fungoides.

There has been limited experience with use of pentostatin in children for Langerhans cell histiocytosis and chronic graft versus host disease (GVHD). (See Administration and Dosage).

Administration and Dosage

➤*Maximum dose:* 4 mg/m² every other week according to the prescribing information.

➤*Adults:*

Hairy-cell leukemia –

Usual dosage: 4 mg/m² IV every other week until complete response is achieved, then give 2 additional doses. Higher doses are not recommended.

Dosage adjustment: Delay further therapy in patients whose absolute neutrophil count (ANC) falls below 200 cells/mm³ from a baseline value above 500 cells/mm³ and in patients with active infections, severe rash, or nervous system toxicity. Therapy may be resumed when these conditions resolve.

Duration of therapy: The optimal duration of treatment has not been determined. In the absence of major toxicity and with observed continuing improvement, the patient should be treated until a complete response has been achieved. Although not established as required, the administration of two additional doses has been recommended following the achievement of a complete response.

All patients receiving pentostatin at 6 months should be assessed for response to treatment. If the patient has not achieved a complete or partial response, treatment with pentostatin should be discontinued.

If the patient has achieved a partial response, pentostatin treatment should be continued in an effort to achieve a complete response. At any time thereafter that a complete response is achieved, 2 additional doses of pentostatin are recommended. Pentostatin treatment should then be stopped. If the best response to treatment at the end of 12 months is a partial response, it is recommended that treatment with pentostatin be stopped.

➤*Children:*

Off-label dosing –

Chronic graft versus host disease: 4 mg/m² IV every other week for 24 weeks.

Langerhans cell histiocytosis: 4 mg/m² IV every week for 8 weeks, then 4 mg/m² IV every other week for 16 weeks, or until disease progression.

➤*Renal function impairment:* Patients with impaired renal function should be treated only when the potential benefit justifies the potential risk. Dosage reduction may be required in patients with impaired renal function (CrCl less than 60 mL/min). Two patients with impaired renal function (creatinine clearances 50 to 60 mL/min) achieved complete response without unusual adverse events when treated with 2 mg/m² every other week.

Dialysis – Conventional hemodialysis is moderately effective (50% to 74%) in removing pentostatin.

➤*Preparation for administration:* Pentostatin is considered a cytotoxic agent. Follow safe handling procedures when preparing, administering, or dispensing pentostatin.

Preparation of IV solution –

1.) Procedures for proper handling and disposal of anticancer drugs should be followed. There is no general agreement that all of the procedures recommended in the guidelines are necessary or appropriate. Spills and wastes should be treated with a 5% sodium hypochlorite solution prior to disposal.
2.) Protective clothing including polyethylene gloves must be worn.
3.) Transfer 5 mL of sterile water for injection to the vial containing pentostatin and mix thoroughly to obtain complete dissolution of a solution yielding 2 mg/mL. Parenteral drug products should be inspected visually for particulate matter and discoloration prior to administration.
4.) Pentostatin may be given IV by bolus injection or diluted in a larger volume (25 to 50 mL) with dextrose 5% injection or sodium chloride 0.9% injection. Dilution of the entire contents of a reconstituted vial with 25 mL or 50 mL provides a pentostatin concentration of 0.33 mg/mL or 0.18 mg/mL, respectively, for the diluted solutions.
5.) Pentostatin solution when diluted for infusion with dextrose 5% injection or sodium chloride 0.9% injection does not interact with PVC infusion containers or administration sets at concentrations of 0.18 mg/mL to 0.33 mg/mL

➤*Administration:* Pentostatin may be administered by IV bolus injection over 5 minutes or diluted in a larger volume and given over 20 to 30 minutes. (See Preparation for administration).

It is recommended that patients receive hydration with 500 to 1,000 mL of dextrose 5% injection with sodium chloride 0.45% injection (or the equivalent) before pentostatin administration. An additional 500 mL of dextrose 5% injection or equivalent should be administered after pentostatin is given.

➤*Storage/Stability:* Store unopened vials in the refrigerator (2° to 8°C [36° to 46°F]).

Pentostatin solutions contain no preservative and should be used within 24 hours. Reconstituted solutions of pentostatin 2 mg/mL are stable for up to 72 hours at room temperature, although the possibility of microbial contamination must be considered. After further dilution, pentostatin solutions are stable at room temperature for 24 hours. The manufacturer recommends use of pentostatin solutions within 8 hours of reconstitution.

Discard vial within 6 hours of the initial needle puncture if opened within an ISO Class 5 biological safety cabinet, or within 1 hour of the initial needle puncture if opened outside of such an environment, based on the USP Chapter <797> standards.

Actions

➤*Pharmacology:* Pentostatin is a potent transition state inhibitor of the enzyme adenosine deaminase (ADA). The greatest activity of ADA is found in cells of the lymphoid system with T-cells having higher activity than B-cells and T-cell malignancies higher ADA activity than B-cell malignancies. Pentostatin inhibition of ADA, particularly in the presence of adenosine or deoxyadenosine, leads to cytoxicity, and this is believed to be due to elevated intracellular levels of dATP which can block DNA synthesis through inhibition of ribonucleotide reductase. Pentostatin can also inhibit RNA synthesis as well as cause increased DNA damage. In addition to elevated dATP, these mechanisms may also contribute to the overall cytotoxic effect of pentostatin. The precise mechanism of pentostatin's antitumor effect, however, in hairy-cell leukemia is not known.

➤*Pharmacokinetics:*

Excretion – The mean terminal half-life was 5.7 hours, the mean plasma clearance was 68 mL/min/m², and approximately 90% of the dose was excreted in the urine as unchanged pentostatin and/or metabolites as measured by adenosine deaminase inhibitory activity.

Special populations –

Renal function impairment: A positive correlation was observed between pentostatin clearance and creatinine clearance (CrCl) in patients with creatinine clearance values ranging from 60 mL/min to 130 mL/min. Pentostatin half-life in patients with renal impairment (CrCl less than 50 mL/min, n = 2) was 18 hours, which was much longer than that observed in patients with normal renal function (CrCl greater than 60 mL/min, n = 14), about 6 hours.

Contraindications

Hypersensitivity to pentostatin.

Warnings/Precautions

➤*Myelosuppression:* Patients with hairy-cell leukemia may experience myelosuppression primarily during the first few courses of treatment. Patients with infections prior to pentostatin treatment have in some cases developed worsening of their condition leading to death, whereas others have achieved complete response. Patients with infection should be treated only when the potential benefit of treatment justifies the potential risk to the patient. Efforts should be made to control the infection before treatment is initiated or resumed.

In patients with progressive hairy-cell leukemia, the initial courses of pentostatin treatment were associated with worsening of neutropenia. Therefore, frequent monitoring of complete blood counts during this time is necessary. If severe neutropenia continues beyond the initial cycles, patients should be evaluated for disease status, including a bone marrow examination.

➤*Rashes:* Rashes, occasionally severe, were commonly reported and may worsen with continued treatment. Withholding of treatment may be required. (See Administration and Dosage.)

PENTOSTATIN — INJECTION

➤*Combination therapy:* Acute pulmonary edema and hypotension, leading to death, have been reported in the literature in patients treated with pentostatin in combination with carmustine, etoposide and high dose cyclophosphamide as part of the ablative regimen for bone marrow transplant.

➤*Renal function impairment:*

Toxicity – Renal toxicity was observed at higher doses in early studies; however, in patients treated at the recommended dose, elevations in serum creatinine were usually minor and reversible. There were some patients who began treatment with normal renal function who had evidence of mild to moderate toxicity at a final assessment. (See Administration and Dosage.)

➤*Pregnancy: Category D.* Pentostatin can cause fetal harm when administered to a pregnant woman. Pentostatin was administered intravenously at doses of 0, 0.01, 0.1, or 0.75 mg/kg/day (0, 0.06, 0.6, and 4.5 mg/m^2) to pregnant rats on days 6 through 15 of gestation. Drug-related maternal toxicity occurred at doses of 0.1 and 0.75 mg/kg/day (0.6 and 4.5 mg/m^2). Teratogenic effects were observed at 0.75 mg/kg/day (4.5 mg/m^2) manifested by increased incidence of various skeletal malformations. In a dose range-finding study, pentostatin was administered intravenously to rats at doses of 0, 0.05, 0.1, 0.5, 0.75, or 1 mg/kg/day (0, 0.3, 0.6, 3, 4.5, 6 mg/m^2), on days 6 through 15 of gestation. Fetal malformations that were observed were an omphalocele at 0.05 mg/kg (0.3 mg/m^2), gastroschisis at 0.75 mg/kg and 1 mg/kg (4.5 and 6 mg/m^2), and a flexure defect of the hind limbs at 0.75 mg/kg (4.5 mg/m^2). Pentostatin was also shown to be teratogenic in mice when administered as a single 2 mg/kg (6 mg/m^2) intraperitoneal injection on day 7 of gestation. Pentostatin was not teratogenic in rabbits when administered intravenously on days 6 through 18 of gestation at doses of 0, 0.005, 0.01, or 0.02 mg/kg/day (0, 0.015, 0.03, or 0.06 mg/m^2); however maternal toxicity, abortions, early deliveries, and deaths occurred in all drug-treated groups. There are no adequate and well-controlled studies in pregnant women. If pentostatin is used during pregnancy, or if the patient becomes pregnant while taking (receiving) this drug, the patient should be apprised of the potential hazard to the fetus. Women of childbearing potential receiving pentostatin should be advised to avoid becoming pregnant.

➤*Lactation:* It is not known whether pentostatin is excreted in human milk. Because many drugs are excreted in human milk, and because of the potential for serious adverse reactions in nursing infants from pentostatin, a decision should be made whether to discontinue nursing or discontinue the drug, taking into account the importance of pentostatin to the mother.

➤*Children:* Safety and effectiveness in children or adolescents have not been established.

➤*Lab test abnormalities:* Elevations in liver function tests occurred during treatment with pentostatin and were generally reversible.

➤*Monitoring:* Therapy with pentostatin requires regular patient observation and monitoring of hematologic parameters and blood chemistry values. If severe adverse reactions occur, the drug should be withheld (see Administration and Dosage), and appropriate corrective measures should be taken according to the clinical judgment of the physician.

Prior to initiating therapy with pentostatin, renal function should be assessed with a serum creatinine and/or a creatinine clearance assay (see Pharmacology and Administration and Dosage). Complete blood counts and serum creatinine should be performed before each dose of pentostatin and at other appropriate periods during therapy (see Administration and Dosage). Severe neutropenia has been observed following the early courses of treatment with pentostatin and therefore frequent monitoring of complete blood counts is recommended during this time. If hematologic parameters do not improve with subsequent courses, patients should be evaluated for disease status, including a bone marrow examination. Periodic monitoring of the peripheral blood for hairy cells should be performed to assess the response to treatment.

In addition, bone marrow aspirates and biopsies may be required at 2 to 3 month intervals to assess the response to treatment.

Drug Interactions

➤*Allopurinol:* Allopurinol and pentostatin are both associated with skin rashes. Based on clinical studies in 25 refractory patients who received both pentostatin and allopurinol, the combined use of pentostatin and allopurinol did not appear to produce a higher incidence of skin rashes than observed with pentostatin alone. There has been a report of one patient who received both drugs and experienced a hypersensitivity vasculitis that resulted in death. It was unclear whether this adverse event and subsequent death resulted from the drug combination.

➤*Vidarabine:* Biochemical studies have demonstrated that pentostatin enhances the effects of vidarabine, a purine nucleoside with antiviral activity. The combined use of vidarabine and pentostatin may result in an increase in adverse reactions associated with each drug. The therapeutic benefit of the drug combination has not been established.

➤*Fludarabine:* See the Warning box for more information.

➤*Carmustine / Etoposide / Cyclophosphamide:* See Warnings/Precautions for more information.

Adverse Reactions

Pentostatin is considered to have moderate potential for nausea and vomiting.

Adverse Reactions for Pentostatin When Used as Front-Line and IFN-Refractory Therapy (%)

All adverse reactions[b]	Frontline, treated with pentostatin (n = 180)	Frontline, treated with IFN (n = 176)	IFN-refractory, treated with pentostatin (n = 197)
Nausea/vomiting	63%	22%	53%[c]
Fever	46%	59%	42%
Rash	43%	30%	26%
Fatigue	42%	55%	29%
Leukopenia	22%	15%	60%
Pruritus	21%	6%	10%
Coughing/increased cough	20%	15%	17%
Myalgia	19%	36%	11%
Chills	19%	34%	11%
Headache	17%	29%	13%
Diarrhea	17%	17%	15%
Abdominal pain	16%	15%	4%
Anorexia	13%	10%	16%
Upper respiratory tract infection	13%	8%	16%
Asthenia	12%	13%	10%
Stomatitis	12%	7%	5%
Rhinitis	11%	15%	10%
Dyspnea	11%	13%	8%
Anemia	8%	5%	35%
Pain	8%	19%	20%
Pharyngitis	8%	11%	10%
Sweating/increased sweating	8%	21%	10%
Viral infection	8%	17%	NR[a]
Infection	7%[d]	2%[d]	36%
Arthralgia	6%	14%	3%
Thrombocytopenia	6%	6%	32%
Skin disorder	4%	5%	17%
Allergic reaction	2%	1%	11%
Hepatic disorder/elevated liver function tests[e]	2%	2%	19%
Neurologic disorder, CNS/CNS toxicity	1%	NR[a]	11%
Lung disorder/disease	NR[a]	1%	12%
Nausea	NR[a]	NR[a]	22%
Genitourinary disorder	NR[a]	NR[a]	15%

[a] Not reported.
[b] Occurring in > 10% of patients, in any group, regardless of drug association.
[c] Includes only nausea with vomiting.
[d] These figures represent only unspecified infections. Refer to infection table.
[e] Elevated liver enzymes and liver disorder for SWOG.

Pentostatin Adverse Reactions in the SWOG study (%)

Type of infection	Frontline, treated with pentostatin (n = 180)	Frontline, treated with IFN (n = 176)
Upper respiratory tract infection	13%	8%
Rhinitis	11%	15%
Herpes zoster	8%	1%
Pharyngitis	8%	11%
Viral infection	8%	17%
Infection (unspecified)	7%	2%
Sinusitis	6%	4%
Cellulitis	6%	3%
Bacterial infection	5%	4%
Pneumonia	5%	7%
Conjunctivitis	4%	2%
Furunculosis	4%	< 1%
Herpes simplex	4%	1%
Bronchitis	3%	2%
Sepsis	3%	2%
Urinary tract infection	3%	3%
Abscess, skin	2%	4%
Moniliasis, oral	2%	< 1%

PENTOSTATIN — INJECTION

Pentostatin Adverse Reactions in the SWOG study (%)		
Type of infection	Frontline, treated with pentostatin (n = 180)	Frontline, treated with IFN (n = 176)
Mycotic infection, skin	< 1%	3%
Osteomyelitis	1%	0%

➤*The drug relatedness of the adverse events listed below cannot be excluded. The following adverse events occurred in 3% to 10% of pentostatin-treated patients in the initial phase of the SWOG study:*

Cardiovascular – Hemorrhage, hypotension.

CNS – Confusion, dizziness, insomnia, paresthesia, somnolence.

Dermatologic – Skin dry, urticaria.

GI – Dental abnormalities, dyspepsia, flatulence, gingivitis.

Hematologic/Lymphatic – Agranulocytosis.

Lab test abnormalities – Elevated creatinine.

Musculoskeletal – Arthralgia.

Psychiatric – Anxiety, depression, nervousness.

Respiratory – Asthma.

Miscellaneous – Chest pain, death, face edema, peripheral edema.

➤*The remaining adverse events which occurred in less than 3% of pentostatin-treated patients during the initial phase of the SWOG study:*

Cardiovascular – Angina pectoris, arrhythmia, A-V block, bradycardia, extrasystoles ventricular, heart arrest, heart failure, hypertension, pericardial effusion, phlebitis, pulmonary embolus, sinus arrest, tachycardia, thrombophlebitis (deep), vasculitis.

CNS – Amnesia, ataxia, convulsions, dreaming abnormal, dysarthria, encephalitis, hyperkinesia, meningism, neuralgia, neuritis, neuropathy, paralysis, syncope, twitching, vertigo.

Dermatologic – Acne, alopecia, eczema, petechial rash, photosensitivity reaction.

GI – Constipation, dysphagia, glossitis, ileus.

GU – Amenorrhea, breast lump, impotence, kidney function abnormal, nephropathy, renal failure, renal insufficiency, renal stone.

Hematologic/Lymphatic – Acute leukemia, hemolytic anemia, aplastic anemia.

Lab test abnormalities – Hypercalcemia, hyponatremia.

Musculoskeletal – Arthritis, gout.

Psychiatric – Decrease/loss of libido, emotional lability, hallucination, hostility, neurosis, thinking abnormal.

Respiratory – Bronchospasm, larynx edema.

Special senses – Amblyopia, deafness, earache, eyes dry, labyrinthitis, lacrimation disorder, nonreactive eye, photophobia, retinopathy, tinnitus, unusual taste, vision abnormal, watery eyes.

Miscellaneous – Flu-like symptoms, hangover effect, neoplasm. One patient with hairy-cell leukemia treated with pentostatin during another clinical study developed unilateral uveitis with vision loss.

Nineteen (5%) patients withdrew from the Phase 3 SWOG 8691 study because of adverse events; 9 during initial pentostatin treatment, 4 during pentostatin crossover, 5 during initial IFN treatment, and 1 during both initial IFN treatment and pentostatin crossover. In the Phase 2 studies in IFN-refractory hairy-cell leukemia, 11% of patients withdrew from treatment with pentostatin due to an adverse event.

Overdosage

No specific antidote for pentostatin overdose is known. Pentostatin administered at higher doses (20 to 50 mg/m² in divided doses over 5 days) than recommended was associated with deaths due to severe renal, hepatic, pulmonary, and CNS toxicity. In case of overdose, management would include general supportive measures through any period of toxicity that occurs.

Patient Information

Patients should be advised of the signs and symptoms of adverse events associated with pentostatin therapy (see Adverse Reactions).

THIOGUANINE (TG; 6-Thioguanine)

Rx	**Tabloid** (GlaxoSmithKline)	**Tablets:** 40 mg	Lactose. (Wellcome U3B). Greenish yellow, scored. In 25s.

THIOGUANINE — ORAL

Indications

➤*Acute nonlymphocytic leukemias:* For remission induction and remission consolidation treatment of acute nonlymphocytic leukemias. However, it is not recommended for use during maintenance therapy or similar long-term continuous treatments because of the high risk of liver toxicity.

The response to this agent depends upon the age of the patient (younger patients faring better than older) and whether thioguanine is used in previously treated or previously untreated patients. Reliance upon thioguanine alone is seldom justified for initial remission induction of acute nonlymphocytic leukemias because combination chemotherapy including thioguanine results in more frequent remission induction and longer duration of remission than thioguanine alone.

➤*Other neoplasms:* Thioguanine is not effective in chronic lymphocytic leukemia, Hodgkin lymphoma, multiple myeloma, or solid tumors. Although thioguanine is one of several agents with activity in the treatment of the chronic phase of chronic myelogenous leukemia, more objective responses are observed with busulfan, and therefore busulfan is usually regarded as the preferred drug.

➤*Off-label uses:*

Crohn disease – [3] = Safety concerns. Thioguanine may offer an alternative therapy for patients with Crohn disease who are unable to tolerate azathioprine or mercaptopurine. Thioguanine is not a benign drug, and clinically significant, therapy-limiting adverse effects have been observed.

Psoriasis – [2] = Fair documentation. The American Academy of Dermatology guidelines recommend methotrexate, cyclosporine, and acitretin as first-line systemic agents for psoriasis, but thioguanine may be an appropriate alternative for patients with treatment-resistant disease or multiple intolerant adverse effects with first-tier agents.

Other possible off-label uses – Chronic myelogenous leukemia; second-line treatment for ulcerative colitis.

Administration and Dosage

➤*General dosing considerations:* Round dose to the nearest 20 mg.

Thioguanine may be dosed in mg/kg or mg/m² body surface area.

Thiopurine methyltransferase deficiency – See Warnings/Precautions for more information.

➤*Adults:*

Acute nonlymphocytic leukemias –

Initial dosage: 2 mg/kg/day when used as a single agent. See Off-Label Dosing for combination therapy dosing.

Dosage adjustment: If after 4 weeks on the initial dosage there is no clinical improvement and no leukocyte or platelet depression, the dosage may be cautiously increased to 3 mg/kg/day. The total daily dose may be given at 1 time.

Consider temporarily discontinuing thioguanine if severe or rapid myelosuppression occurs (ie, large or rapid fall in leukocytes, platelets, or hemoglobin). Resume therapy at lower dose once blood counts stabilize for 2 to 3 days or increase.

Dosage reduction may be necessary in patients who develop stomatitis or severe diarrhea. However, no specific recommendations are currently available.

Discontinuation of therapy: Discontinue thioguanine in patients who experience liver toxicity.

Off-label dosing –

Crohn disease: [3] = Safety concerns. 20 mg (one-half tablet) to 40 mg once daily. Dosages of up to 120 mg/day have been used in selected patients based on individual response and tolerance. A dosage of 20 mg 3 times per week was used in 2 cases in pregnant women. Ongoing therapy is required to maintain remission.

Psoriasis: [2] = Fair documentation. The recommended starting dosage is 80 mg orally 2 times per week, increased in 20 mg increments every 2 to 4 weeks up to a maximum of 160 mg 3 times per week. Pulsed dosing 2 or 3 times per week is preferable to daily dosing to limit the incidence of myelotoxicity. Therapy may be continued for as long as needed because there are no known cumulative toxicities; safe use has been demonstrated for up to 145 months.

Acute nonlymphocytic leukemias: When used in combination therapy, the dosage is 75 to 200 mg/m² body surface area daily, in 1 or 2 divided doses for 5 to 7 days in each course of therapy until remission occurs.

➤*Children:*

Acute nonlymphocytic leukemias – See Adults for dosing.

Off-label dosing –

Acute nonlymphocytic leukemias:

- *3 years of age and older* – When used in combination therapy, the dosage is 75 to 200 mg/m² body surface area, in 1 or 2 divided doses for 5 to 7 days in each course of therapy until remission occurs.
- *Younger than 3 years of age* – When used in combination therapy, the dosage is 3.3 mg/kg/day in 2 divided doses for 4 days in each course of therapy until remission occurs.

➤*Preparation for administration:* Thioguanine is considered a cytotoxic agent. Follow safe handling procedures when preparing, administering, or dispensing thioguanine.

➤*Administration:* Give on an empty stomach to facilitate absorption.

➤*Storage/Stability:* Store at 15° to 25°C (59° to 77°F) in a dry place.

THIOGUANINE — ORAL

The extemporaneous suspension is stable for 84 days stored at room temperature in amber glass bottles. Shake the extemporaneous suspensions well before using.

Actions

➤*Pharmacology:* Thioguanine is one of a large series of purine analogues that interferes with nucleic acid biosynthesis, and has been found active against selected human neoplastic diseases.

Thioguanine competes with hypoxanthine and guanine for the enzyme hypoxanthine-guanine phosphoribosyltransferase (HGPRTase) and is itself converted to 6-thioguanylic acid (TGMP). This nucleotide reaches high intracellular concentrations at therapeutic doses. TGMP interferes at several points with the synthesis of guanine nucleotides. It inhibits de novo purine biosynthesis by pseudo-feedback inhibition of glutamine-5-phosphoribosylpyrophosphate aminotransferase, the first enzyme unique to the de novo pathway for purine ribonucleotide synthesis. TGMP also inhibits the conversion of inosinic acid (IMP) to xanthylic acid (XMP) by competition for the enzyme IMP dehydrogenase. At one time, TGMP was felt to be a significant inhibitor of ATP:GMP phosphotransferase (guanylate kinase), but recent results have shown this not to be so.

Thioguanylic acid is further converted to the di- and triphosphates, thioguanosine diphosphate (TGDP) and thioguanosine triphosphate (TGTP) (as well as their 2′-deoxyribosyl analogues), by the same enzymes that metabolize guanine nucleotides. Thioguanine nucleotides are incorporated into the RNA and the DNA by phosphodiester linkages, and it has been argued that incorporation of such fraudulent bases contributes to the cytotoxicity of thioguanine.

Thus, thioguanine has multiple metabolic effects and at present it is not possible to designate 1 major site of action. Its tumor inhibitory properties may be caused by 1 or more of its effects on feedback inhibition of de novo purine synthesis, inhibition of purine nucleotide interconversions, or incorporation into the DNA and the RNA. The net consequence of its actions is a sequential blockade of the synthesis and utilization of the purine nucleotides.

In some animal tumors, resistance to the effect of thioguanine correlates with the loss of HGPRTase activity and the resulting inability to convert thioguanine to thioguanylic acid. However, other resistance mechanisms, such as increased catabolism of TGMP by a nonspecific phosphatase, may be operative. Although not invariable, it is usual to find cross-resistance between thioguanine and its close analogue, mercaptopurine.

➤*Pharmacokinetics:*

Absorption – Clinical studies have shown that the absorption of an oral dose of thioguanine in humans is incomplete and variable, averaging approximately 30% of the administered dose (range, 14% to 46%). Following oral administration of ^{35}S-6-thioguanine, total plasma radioactivity reached a maximum at 8 hours and declined slowly thereafter. Parent drug represented only a very small fraction of the total plasma radioactivity at any time, being virtually undetectable throughout the period of measurements.

Distribution – Intravenous administration of ^{35}S-6-thioguanine disclosed a median plasma half-disappearance time of 80 minutes (range, 25 to 240 minutes) when the compound was given in single doses of 65 to 300 mg/m^2. Although initial plasma levels of thioguanine did correlate with the dose level, there was no correlation between the plasma half-disappearance time and the dose.

Thioguanine is incorporated into the DNA and the RNA of human bone marrow cells. Studies with IV ^{35}S-6-thioguanine have shown that the amount of thioguanine incorporated into nucleic acids is more than 100 times higher after 5 daily doses than after a single dose. With the 5-dose schedule, from one half to virtually all of the guanine in the residual DNA was replaced by thioguanine. Tissue distribution studies of ^{35}S-6-thioguanine in mice showed only traces of radioactivity in brain after oral administration. No measurements have been made of thioguanine concentrations in human cerebrospinal fluid (CSF), but observations on tissue distribution in animals, together with the lack of CNS penetration by the closely related compound, mercaptopurine, suggest that thioguanine does not reach therapeutic concentrations in the CSF.

Metabolism – Monitoring of plasma levels of thioguanine during therapy is of questionable value. There is technical difficulty in determining plasma concentrations, which are seldom greater than 1 to 2 mcg/mL after a therapeutic oral dose. More significantly, thioguanine enters rapidly into the anabolic and catabolic pathways for purines, and the active intracellular metabolites have appreciably longer half-lives than the parent drug. The biochemical effects of a single dose of thioguanine are evident long after the parent drug has disappeared from plasma. Because of this rapid metabolism of thioguanine to active intracellular derivatives, hemodialysis would not be expected to appreciably reduce toxicity of the drug.

The catabolism of thioguanine and its metabolites is complex and shows significant differences between humans and mice. In both humans and mice, after oral administration of ^{35}S-6-thioguanine, urine contains virtually no detectable intact thioguanine. While deamination and subsequent oxidation to thiouric acid occurs only to a small extent in humans, it is the main pathway in mice. The product of deamination by guanase, 6-thioxanthine is inactive, having negligible antitumor activity. This pathway of thioguanine inactivation is not dependent on the action of xanthine oxidase, and an inhibitor of that enzyme (eg, allopurinol) will not block the detoxification of thioguanine even though the inactive 6-thioxanthine is normally further oxidized by xanthine oxidase to thiouric acid before it is eliminated. In humans, methylation of thioguanine is much more extensive than in the mouse. The product of methylation, 2-amino-6-methylthiopurine, is also substantially less active and less toxic than thioguanine, and its formation is likewise unaffected by the presence of allopurinol. Appreciable amounts of inorganic sulfate are also found in both murine and human urine, presumably arising from further metabolism of the methylated derivatives.

Excretion – The oral administration of radiolabeled thioguanine revealed only trace quantities of parent drug in the urine. However, a methylated metabolite, 2-amino-6-methylthiopurine (MTG), appeared very early, rose to a maximum 6 to 8 hours after drug administration, and was still being excreted after 12 to 22 hours. Radiolabeled sulfate appeared somewhat later than MTG but was the principal metabolite after 8 hours. Thiouric acid and some unidentified products were found in the urine in small amounts.

Contraindications

Prior resistance to this drug. In animals and humans, there is usually complete cross-resistance between mercaptopurine and thioguanine.

Warnings/Precautions

➤*Hepatic toxicity:* Thioguanine is not recommended for maintenance therapy or similar long-term continuous treatments because of the high risk of liver toxicity associated with vascular endothelial damage. This liver toxicity has been observed in a high proportion of children receiving thioguanine as part of maintenance therapy for acute lymphoblastic leukemia and in other conditions associated with continuous use of thioguanine. This liver toxicity is particularly prevalent in men. Liver toxicity usually presents as the clinical syndrome of hepatic veno-occlusive disease (hyperbilirubinemia, tender hepatomegaly, weight gain caused by fluid retention, and ascites) or with signs of portal hypertension (splenomegaly, thrombocytopenia, esophageal varices). Histopathological features associated with this toxicity include hepatoportal sclerosis, nodular regenerative hyperplasia, peliosis hepatitis, and periportal fibrosis.

Discontinue thioguanine therapy in patients with evidence of liver toxicity because reversal of signs and symptoms of liver toxicity have been reported upon withdrawal.

A few cases of jaundice have been reported in patients with leukemia receiving thioguanine. Among these were 2 adult men and 4 children with acute myelogenous leukemia and a man with acute lymphocytic leukemia who developed hepatic veno-occlusive disease while receiving chemotherapy for their leukemia. Six patients had received cytarabine prior to treatment with thioguanine, and some were receiving other chemotherapy in addition to thioguanine when they became symptomatic. While hepatic veno-occlusive disease has not been reported in patients treated with thioguanine alone, it is recommended that thioguanine be withheld if there is evidence of toxic hepatitis or biliary stasis, and that appropriate clinical and laboratory investigations be initiated to establish the etiology of the hepatic dysfunction. Deterioration in liver function studies during thioguanine therapy should prompt discontinuation of treatment and a search for an explanation of the hepatotoxicity.

Carefully monitor patients. Early indications of liver toxicity are signs associated with portal hypertension, such as thrombocytopenia out of proportion with neutropenia and splenomegaly. Elevations of liver enzymes have also been reported in association with liver toxicity but do not always occur.

➤*Bone marrow suppression:* The most consistent, dose-related toxicity is bone marrow suppression. This may be manifested by anemia, leukopenia, thrombocytopenia, or any combination of these. Any one of these findings also may reflect progression of the underlying disease. Because thioguanine may have a delayed effect, it is important to withdraw the medication temporarily at the first sign of an abnormally large fall in any of the formed elements of the blood.

There are individuals with an inherited deficiency of the TPMT who may be unusually sensitive to the myelosuppressive effects of thioguanine and prone to developing rapid bone marrow suppression following initiation of treatment. Substantial dose reductions may be required to avoid the development of life-threatening bone marrow suppression in these patients. Be aware that some laboratories offer testing for TPMT deficiency. Because bone marrow suppression may be associated with factors other than TPMT deficiency, TPMT testing may not identify all patients at risk for severe toxicity. Therefore, close monitoring of clinical and hematologic parameters is important. Bone marrow suppression could be exacerbated by coadministration with drugs that inhibit TPMT, such as olsalazine, mesalazine, and sulfasalazine.

Myelosuppression is often unavoidable during the induction phase of adult acute nonlymphocytic leukemias if remission induction is to be successful. Whether or not this demands modification or cessation of dosage depends upon the response of the underlying disease and a careful consideration of supportive facilities (granulocyte and platelet transfusions) that may be available. Life-threatening infections and bleeding have been observed as consequences of thioguanine-induced granulocytopenia and thrombocytopenia.

See Warnings/Precautions for more information.

➤*Immunization:* Avoid administration of live vaccines to immunocompromised patients.

➤*Other toxicities:* Although the primary toxicity of thioguanine is myelosuppression, other toxicities have occasionally been observed, particularly when thioguanine is used in combination with other cancer chemotherapeutic agents.

➤*Pregnancy: Category D.* Drugs such as thioguanine are potential mutagens and teratogens. Thioguanine may cause fetal harm when administered to a pregnant woman. Thioguanine has been shown to be teratogenic in rats when given in doses 5 times the human dose. When given to the rat on the fourth and fifth days of gestation, 13% of surviving placentas did not contain fetuses, and 19% of offspring were malformed or stunted. The malformations noted included generalized edema, cranial defects, and general skeletal hypoplasia, hydrocephalus, ventral hernia, situs inversus, and incomplete

THIOGUANINE — ORAL

development of the limbs. There are no adequate and well-controlled studies in pregnant women. If this drug is used during pregnancy, or if the patient becomes pregnant while taking the drug, apprise the patient of the potential hazard to the fetus. Advise women of childbearing potential to avoid becoming pregnant.

➤*Lactation:* It is not known whether this drug is excreted in human milk. Because of the potential for tumorigenicity shown for thioguanine, decide whether to discontinue breast-feeding or to discontinue the drug, taking into account the importance of the drug to the mother.

➤*Children:* Ninety-six (59%) of 163 pediatric patients with previously untreated acute nonlymphocytic leukemia obtained complete remission with a multiple-drug protocol including thioguanine, prednisone, cytarabine, cyclophosphamide, and vincristine. Remission was maintained with daily thioguanine, 4-day pulses of cytarabine and cyclophosphamide, and a single dose of vincristine every 28 days. The median duration of remission was 11.5 months.

➤*Elderly:* Clinical studies of thioguanine did not include sufficient numbers of subjects 65 years of age and older to determine whether they respond differently from younger subjects. Other reported clinical experience has not identified differences in responses between the elderly and younger patients. In general, dose selection for an elderly patient should be cautious, usually starting at the low end of the dosing range, reflecting the greater frequency of decreased hepatic, renal, or cardiac function, and of concomitant disease or other drug therapy.

➤*Monitoring:* See Warnings/Precautions for more information.

It is advisable to monitor liver function tests (serum transaminases, alkaline phosphatase, bilirubin) at weekly intervals when first beginning therapy and at monthly intervals thereafter. It may be advisable to perform liver function tests more frequently in patients with known preexisting liver disease or in patients who are receiving thioguanine and other hepatotoxic drugs. Instruct patients to discontinue thioguanine immediately if clinical jaundice is detected.

It is recommended that evaluation of the hemoglobin concentration or hematocrit, total WBC count and differential count, and quantitative platelet count be obtained frequently while the patient is on thioguanine therapy. In cases where the cause of fluctuations in the formed elements in the peripheral blood is obscure, bone marrow examination may be useful for the evaluation of marrow status. Base the decision to increase, decrease, continue, or discontinue a given dosage of thioguanine not only on the absolute hematologic values, but also upon the rapidity with which changes are occurring. In many instances, particularly during the induction phase of acute leukemia, complete blood counts will need to be done more frequently in order to evaluate the effect of the therapy. The dosage of thioguanine may need to be reduced when this agent is combined with other drugs whose primary toxicity is myelosuppression.

Drug Interactions

➤*Aminosalicylate derivatives:* Because there is in vitro evidence that aminosalicylate derivatives (eg, olsalazine, mesalazine, sulfasalazine) inhibit the TPMT enzyme, administer them with caution to patients receiving concurrent thioguanine therapy.

➤*Mercaptopurine:* There is usually complete cross-resistance between mercaptopurine and thioguanine.

Adverse Reactions

Thioguanine is considered to have very low emetogenic potential (less than 10% incidence of emesis).

➤*GI:* Less frequent adverse reactions include nausea, vomiting, anorexia, and stomatitis. Intestinal necrosis and perforation have been reported in patients who received multiple-drug chemotherapy including thioguanine.

➤*Hematologic:* The most frequent adverse reaction to thioguanine is myelosuppression. The induction of complete remission of acute myelogenous leukemia usually requires combination chemotherapy in dosages that produce marrow hypoplasia. Because consolidation and maintenance of remission are also affected by multiple-drug regimens whose component agents cause myelosuppression, pancytopenia is observed in nearly all patients. Adjust dosages and schedules to prevent life-threatening cytopenias whenever these adverse reactions are observed.

➤*Hepatic:* See Warnings/Precautions for more information.

Liver toxicity during short-term cyclical therapy presents as veno-occlusive disease. Reversal of signs and symptoms of this liver toxicity has been reported upon withdrawal of short-term or long-term continuous therapy.

Centrilobular hepatic necrosis has been reported in a few cases; however, the reports are confounded by the use of high doses of thioguanine, other chemotherapeutic agents, and oral contraceptives and chronic alcohol abuse.

➤*Metabolic:* Hyperuricemia frequently occurs in patients receiving thioguanine as a consequence of rapid cell lysis accompanying the antineoplastic effect. Adverse reactions can be minimized by increased hydration, urine alkalinization, and the prophylactic administration of a xanthine oxidase inhibitor such as allopurinol. Unlike mercaptopurine and azathioprine, thioguanine may be continued in the usual dosage when allopurinol is used conjointly to inhibit uric acid formation.

Overdosage

➤*Symptoms:* Signs and symptoms of overdosage may be immediate, such as nausea, vomiting, malaise, hypotension, and diaphoresis; or delayed, such as myelosuppression and azotemia. The oral LD_{50} of thioguanine was determined to be 823 mg/kg ± 50.73 mg/kg and 740 mg/kg ± 45.24 mg/kg for male and female rats, respectively. Symptoms of overdosage may occur after a single dose of as little as thioguanine 2 to 3 mg/kg. As much as 35 mg/kg has been given in a single oral dose with reversible myelosuppression observed.

➤*Treatment:* There is no known pharmacologic antagonist of thioguanine. Immediately discontinue the drug if unintended toxicity occurs during treatment. Severe hematologic toxicity may require supportive therapy with platelet transfusions for bleeding, and granulocyte transfusions and antibiotics if sepsis is documented. It is not known whether thioguanine is dialyzable. Hemodialysis is thought to be of marginal use because of the rapid intracellular incorporation of thioguanine into active metabolites with long persistence.

Patient Information

Inform patients that the major toxicities of thioguanine are related to myelosuppression, hepatotoxicity, and GI toxicity. Never allow patients to take the drug without medical supervision and advise them to consult their physicians if they experience fever, sore throat, jaundice, nausea, vomiting, signs of local infection, bleeding from any site, or symptoms suggestive of anemia. Advise women of childbearing potential to avoid becoming pregnant.

ALLOPURINOL

Rx	**Allopurinol** (Various, eg, Boots, Geneva, Major, Mylan, Parmed, Vangard)	**Tablets:** 100 mg	In 100s, 500s, 1000s, and UD 100s.
Rx	**Zyloprim** (GlaxoWellcome)		Lactose. (Zyloprim 100). White, scored. In 100s.
Rx	**Allopurinol** (Various, eg, Boots, Geneva, Major, Mylan, Parmed, Vangard)	**Tablets:** 300 mg	In 100s, 500s, 1000s, and UD 100s.
Rx	**Zyloprim** (GlaxoWellcome)		Lactose. (Zyloprim 300). Peach, scored. In 100s and 500s.
Rx	**Allopurinol Sodium** (Bedford Labs)	**Power for injection, lyophilized:** 500 mg	Preservative free. In 30 mL vials with rubber stoppers.
Rx	**Aloprim** (Nabi)		Preservative free. In 30 mL vials with rubber stoppers.

ALLOPURINOL — INJECTION

For more complete prescribing information on tablets, see the Allopurinol monograph in the Agents for Gout section.

Indications

➤*Elevated uric acid levels:* For the management of patients with leukemia, lymphoma, and solid tumor malignancies who are receiving cancer therapy that causes elevations of serum and urinary uric acid levels and who cannot tolerate oral therapy.

Administration and Dosage

➤*General dosing considerations:* A fluid intake sufficient to yield a daily urinary output of 2 L or more in adults and the maintenance of a neutral or, preferably, slightly alkaline urine is desirable.

The dosage of allopurinol to lower serum uric acid to normal or near-normal varies according to disease severity.

The amount and frequency of dosage for maintaining the serum uric acid just within the normal range is best determined by using the serum uric acid level as an index.

➤*Adults:*

Elevated uric acid levels –
Usual dosage: 200 to 400 mg/m^2/day.
Maximum dose: 600 mg/day.

➤*Children:*

Elevated uric acid levels –
Initial dosage: 200 mg/m^2/day.

➤*Renal function impairment:* Reduce the dose of allopurinol in patients with impaired renal function to avoid accumulation of allopurinol and its metabolites.

ALLOPURINOL — INJECTION

Dosage adjustment – According to the manufacturer's prescribing information, the dose of allopurinol in patients with renal function impairment should be adjusted based on the following recommendations.

Creatinine clearance (CrCl) 10 to 20 mL/min: 200 mg/day.
CrCl 3 to 10 mL/min: 100 mg.
CrCl less than 3 mL/min: 100 mg/day at extended intervals.

Alternative dosage adjustment – An alternative dosing regimen is:
CrCl greater than 50 mL/min: 75% of usual daily dose.
CrCl 10 to 50 mL/min: 50% of usual daily dose.
CrCl less than 10 mL/min: 25% of usual daily dose.

Hemodialysis – Administer 50% supplemental dose after dialysis.
Continuous renal replacement therapy: Dose as CrCl 10 to 50 mL/min.

➤*Preparation for administration:* Allopurinol for injection must be reconstituted and diluted. Dissolve the contents of each 30 mL vial with 25 mL of sterile water for injection. Reconstitution yields a clear, almost colorless solution with no more than a slight opalescence. This concentration solution has a pH of 11.1 to 11.8. Dilute it to the desired concentration with sodium chloride 0.9% injection or dextrose 5% for injection. Do not use sodium bicarbonate-containing solutions. A final concentration of 6 mg/mL or less is recommended. Begin administration within 10 hours of reconstitution.

➤*Administration:* In adults and children, the daily dose can be given as a single infusion or in equally divided infusions at 6-, 8-, or 12-hour intervals at the recommended final concentration of 6 mg/mL or less. The rate of infusion depends on the volume of infusate. Whenever possible, initiate therapy with allopurinol 24 to 48 hours before the start of chemotherapy known to cause tumor lysis (including adrenocorticosteroids). Do not mix allopurinol with or administer through the same IV port with agents that are incompatible in solution with allopurinol. (see Admixture Compatibilities)

➤*Admixture compatibility:* Drugs that are physically incompatible in a solution with allopurinol include the following: amikacin sulfate, amphotericin B, carmustine, cefotaxime sodium, chlorpromazine hydrochloride, cimetidine hydrochloride, clindamycin phosphate, cytarabine, dacarbazine, daunorubicin HCl, diphenhydramine hydrochloride, doxorubicin hydrochloride, doxycycline hyclate, droperidol, floxuridine, gentamicin sulfate, haloperidol lactate, hydroxyzine hydrochloride, idarubicin hydrochloride, imipenem-cilastatin sodium, mechlorethamine hydrochloride, meperidine hydrochloride, metoclopramide hydrochloride, methylprednisolone sodium succinate, minocycline hydrochloride, nalbuphine hydrochloride, netilmicin sulfate, ondansetron hydrochloride, prochlorperazine edisylate, promethazine hydrochloride, sodium bicarbonate, streptozocin, tobramycin sulfate, and vinorelbine tartrate.

➤*Storage/Stability:* Store unreconstituted powder at 25°C (77°F). Excursions permitted to 15° to 30°C (59° to 86°F). Store the reconstituted solution at 20° to 25°C (68° to 77°F). Do not refrigerate the reconstituted and/or diluted product. Begin administration within 10 hours of reconstitution.

Actions

➤*Pharmacology:* Allopurinol acts on purine catabolism without disrupting the biosynthesis of purines. It reduces the production of uric acid by inhibiting the biochemical reactions immediately preceding its formation. The degree of this decrease is dose-dependent.

Allopurinol is a structural analog of the natural purine base, hypoxanthine. It is an inhibitor of xanthine oxidase, the enzyme responsible for the conversion of hypoxanthine to xanthine and of xanthine to uric acid, the end product of purine metabolism in humans. Allopurinol is metabolized to the corresponding xanthine analog, oxypurinol (alloxanthine), which also is an inhibitor of xanthine oxidase.

Reutilization of both hypoxanthine and xanthine for nucleotide and nucleic acid synthesis is markedly enhanced when their oxidations are inhibited by allopurinol and oxypurinol. However, this reutilization does not disrupt normal nucleic acid anabolism because feedback inhibition is an integral part of purine biosynthesis. As a result of xanthine oxidase inhibition, the serum concentration of hypoxanthine plus xanthine in patients receiving allopurinol for treatment of hyperuricemia is usually in the range of 0.3 to 0.4 mg/dl compared with a normal level of approximately 0.15 mg/dl. A maximum of 0.9 mg/dl of these oxypurines has been reported when the serum urate was lowered to less than 2 mg/dl by high doses of allopurinol. These values are far below the saturation levels, at which point their precipitation would be expected to occur (greater than 7 mg/dl).

The renal clearance of hypoxanthine and xanthine is 10 or more times greater than that of uric acid. The increased xanthine and hypoxanthine in the urine have not been accompanied by problems of nephrolithiasis. There are isolated case reports of xanthine crystalluria in patients who were treated with oral allopurinol. The action of oral allopurinol differs from that of uricosuric agents, which lower the serum uric acid level by increasing urinary excretion of uric acid. Allopurinol reduces both the serum and urinary uric acid levels by inhibiting the formation of uric acid. The use of allopurinol to block the formation of urates avoids the hazard of increased renal excretion of uric acid posed by uricosuric drugs.

➤*Pharmacokinetics:* Following IV administration in 6 healthy male and female subjects, allopurinol was rapidly eliminated from the systemic circulation primarily via oxidative metabolism to oxypurinol, with no detectable plasma concentration of allopurinol after 5 hours post-dosing. Approximately 12% of the allopurinol IV dose was excreted unchanged, 76% excreted as oxypurinol, and the remaining dose excreted as riboside conjugates in the urine. The rapid conversion of allopurinol to oxypurinol was not significantly different after repeated allopurinol dosing. Oxypurinol was present in systemic circulation in much higher concentrations and for a much longer period than allopurinol; thus, it is generally believed the pharmacological action of allopurinol is mediated via oxypurinol. Oxypurinol was primarily eliminated unchanged in urine by glomerular filtration and tubular reabsorption, with a net renal clearance of approximately 30 mL/min.

To compare the pharmacokinetics of allopurinol and oxypurinol between IV and oral administration of allopurinol sodium for injection, a well-controlled, 4-way crossover study was conducted in 16 healthy male volunteers. Allopurinol sodium for injection was administered via an IV infusion over 30 minutes. Pharmacokinetic parameter estimates of allopurinol (mean ± S.D.) following single IV and oral administration of allopurinol sodium for injection are summarized as follows:

Administration of Allopurinol Injection				
Allopurinol parameters	100 mg IV	300 mg IV	100 mg PO (n = 7)	300 mg PO
C_{max} (mcg/ml)	1.58	5.12	0.53	1.35
T_{max} (hr)	0.5	0.5	1	1.67
$T_{1/2}$ (hr)	1	1.21	0.98	1.32
$AUC_{0-\infty}$ (hr•mcg/ml)	1.99	7.1	1.03	3.69
CL (ml/min/kg)	12.2	9.94		
V_{ss} (L/kg)	0.84	0.87		
$F_{absolute}$ (%)[a]			48.8	52.7

[a] Absolute bioavailability.

Oxypurinol was measurable in the plasma within 10 to 15 minutes following the administration of allopurinol sodium for injection. Pharmacokinetic parameter estimates of oxypurinol following IV and oral administration of allopurinol sodium for injection are shown below:

Administration of Allopurinol Injection				
Oxypurinol parameters	100 mg IV	300 mg IV	100 mg PO	300 mg PO
C_{max} (mcg/ml)	2.2	6.18	2.36	6.36
T_{max} (hr)	3.89	4.16	3.1	4.13
$T_{1/2}$ (hr)	24.1	23.5	24.9	23.7
$AUC_{0-\infty}$ (hr•mcg/ml)	80	231	83	245
$F_{relative}$ (%)[a]			107	108

[a] Relative bioavailability.

In general, the ratio of the area under the plasma concentration vs time curve ($AUC_{0-\infty}$) between oxypurinol and allopurinol was in the magnitude of 30 to 40. The C_{max} and $AUC_{0-\infty}$ for both allopurinol and oxypurinol following IV administration of allopurinol sodium for injection were dose-proportional in the dose range of 100 to 300 mg. The half-life of allopurinol and oxypurinol was not influenced by the route of allopurinol sodium for injection administration. Oral and IV administration of allopurinol sodium for injection at equal doses produced nearly superimposable oxypurinol plasma concentration vs time profiles, and the relative bioavailability of oxypurinol, ($F_{relative}$) was approximately 100%. Thus, the pharmacokinetics and plasma profiles of oxypurinol, the major pharmacological components derived from allopurinol, are similar after IV and oral administration of allopurinol sodium for injection.

Contraindications

Patients who previously have developed a severe reaction to allopurinol.

Warnings/Precautions

➤*Hepatotoxicity:* A few cases of reversible clinical hepatotoxicity have been noted in patients taking oral allopurinol, and in some patients asymptomatic rises in serum alkaline phosphatase or serum transaminase have been observed. If anorexia, weight loss, or pruritus develop in patients on allopurinol, include an evaluation of liver function as part of their diagnostic workup. In patients with preexisting liver disease, periodic liver function tests are recommended during the early stages of therapy.

➤*Fluid intake:* See Administration and Dosage for more information.

➤*Bone marrow suppression:* Bone marrow suppression has been reported in patients receiving allopurinol; however, most of these patients were receiving concomitant medications with the known potential to cause such an effect. The suppression has occurred from as early as 6 weeks to as long as 6 years after the initiation of allopurinol therapy.

➤*Hypersensitivity reactions:* Discontinue allopurinol at the first appearance of skin rash or other signs that may indicate an allergic reaction. In some instances with oral allopurinol, a skin rash may be followed by more severe hypersensitivity reactions such as exfoliative, urticarial, and purpuric lesions as well as Stevens-Johnson syndrome (erythema multiforme exudativum), and/or generalized vasculitis, irreversible hepatotoxicity and, on rare occasions, death.

➤*Renal function impairment:* The occurrence of hypersensitivity reactions to allopurinol may be increased in patients with decreased renal function receiving thiazides and allopurinol concurrently. Administer such combinations with caution in patients with decreased renal function.

A few patients with preexisting renal disease or poor urate clearance have shown a rise in BUN during allopurinol administration, although a decrease in BUN has also been observed. In patients with hyperuricemia due to malignancy, the vast majority of changes in renal function are attributable to the underlying malignancy rather than to therapy with allopurinol. Concurrent conditions such as multiple myeloma and congestive myocardial disease were present among those patients whose renal function deteriorated

ALLOPURINOL — INJECTION

after allopurinol was begun. Renal failure is rarely associated with hypersensitivity reactions to allopurinol.

See Administration and Dosage for more information.

➤*Hazardous tasks:* Because of the occasional occurrence of drowsiness, alert patients to the need for caution when engaging in activities where alertness is mandatory.

➤*Pregnancy: Category C.* There is a published report in pregnant mice that single intraperitoneal doses of 50 or 100 mg/kg (≈ ⅓ or ¾ the human dose on a mg/m^2 basis) of allopurinol on gestation days 10 or 13 produced significant increases in fetal deaths and teratogenic effects (cleft palate, harelip, and digital defects). It is uncertain whether these findings represented a fetal effect or an effect secondary to maternal toxicity. There are, however, no adequate or well-controlled studies in pregnant women. Because animal reproduction studies are not always predictive of human response, use this drug during pregnancy only if the potential benefit justifies the potential risk to the fetus. Experience with allopurinol during human pregnancy has been limited partly because women of reproductive age rarely require treatment with allopurinol. Two unpublished reports and one published paper describe women giving birth to normal offspring after receiving oral allopurinol during pregnancy. There have been no pregnancies reported in patients receiving allopurinol sodium for injection, but it is assumed that the same risks would apply.

➤*Lactation:* Allopurinol and oxypurinol have been found in the milk of a mother who was receiving allopurinol. Because the effect of allopurinol on the nursing infant is unknown, exercise caution when allopurinol is administered to a nursing woman.

➤*Children:* Clinical data are available on approximately 200 children treated with allopurinol sodium for injection. The efficacy and safety profile observed in this patient population were similar to that observed in adults (see Indications and Administration and Dosage).

➤*Elderly:* Clinical studies of allopurinol sodium for injection did not include sufficient numbers of patients greater than or equal to 65 years of age to determine whether they respond differently than younger patients. Other reported clinical experience has not identified differences in responses between the elderly and younger patients. In general, start at the low end of the dosing range when selecting a dose for the elderly.

➤*Monitoring:* The correct dosage and schedule for maintaining the serum uric acid within the normal range is best determined by using the serum uric acid as an index. In patients with pre-existing liver disease, periodic liver function tests are recommended during the early stages of therapy (see Warnings). Allopurinol and its primary active metabolite, oxypurinol, are eliminated by the kidneys; therefore, changes in renal function have a profound effect on dosage. In patients with decreased renal function, or who have concurrent illnesses that can affect renal function such as hypertension and diabetes mellitus, periodic laboratory parameters of renal function, particularly BUN and serum creatinine or creatinine clearance, should be performed and the patient's allopurinol dosage reassessed. Assess prothrombin time periodically in patients receiving dicumarol who are given allopurinol.

Drug Interactions

Allopurinol Injection Drug Interactions

Precipitant drug	Object drug[a]		Description
Uricosuric agents	Allopurinol	↑	Because the excretion of oxypurinol is similar to that of urate, uricosuric agents, which increase the excretion of urate, are also likely to increase the excretion of oxypurinol. As a result, the concomitant administration of uricosuric agents decreases the inhibition of xanthine oxidase by oxypurinol and increases the urinary excretion of uric acid.
Allopurinol	Ampicillin/ Amoxicillin	↑	An increase in the frequency of skin rash has been reported among patients receiving ampicillin or amoxicillin concurrently with allopurinol compared with patients who are not receiving both drugs. The cause of this reaction has not been established.
Allopurinol	Chlorpropamide	↑	The half-life of chlorpropamide in the plasma may be prolonged by allopurinol, because allopurinol and chlorpropamide may compete for excretion in the renal tubule. The risk of hypoglycemia secondary to this mechanism may be increased if allopurinol and chlorpropamide are given concomitantly in the presence of renal insufficiency.
Allopurinol	Cyclosporine	↑	Reports indicate that cyclosporine levels may be increased during concomitant treatment with allopurinol sodium for injection. Monitor cyclosporine levels, and adjust cyclosporine dosage when these drugs are co-administered.
Allopurinol	Cytotoxic agents	↑	Enhanced bone marrow suppression by cyclophosphamide and other cytotoxic agents has been reported among patients with neoplastic disease, except leukemia, in the presence of allopurinol. However, in a well-controlled study of patients with lymphoma on combination therapy, allopurinol did not increase the marrow toxicity of patients treated with cyclophosphamide, doxorubicin, bleomycin, procarbazine, or mechlorethamine.
Allopurinol	Dicumarol	↑	It has been reported that allopurinol prolongs the half-life of the anticoagulant, dicumarol. Consequently, reassess prothrombin time periodically in patients receiving both drugs. The clinical basis of this drug interaction has not been established.
Allopurinol	Mercaptopurine/ Azathioprine	↑	Allopurinol inhibits the enzymatic oxidation of mercaptopurine and azathioprine to 6-thiouric acid (inactive). This results in increased levels of the active drug. Therefore, the concomitant administration of 300 to 600 mg of oral allopurinol per day will require a reduction in dose to approximately one-third to one-fourth of the usual dose of mercaptopurine or azathioprine. Make subsequent adjustment of doses of mercaptopurine or azathioprine on the basis of therapeutic response and the appearance of toxic effects.

[a] ↑ = Object drug increased.

Adverse Reactions

In an uncontrolled, compassionate plea protocol, 125 of 1378 patients reported a total of 301 adverse reactions while receiving allopurinol sodium for injection. Most of the patients had advanced malignancies or serious underlying diseases and were taking multiple concomitant medications. Side effects directly attributable to allopurinol sodium for injection were reported in 19 patients. Fifteen of these adverse experiences were allergic in nature (rash, eosinophilia, local injection site reaction). One adverse experience of severe diarrhea and one incidence of nausea were also reported as being possibly attributable to allopurinol sodium for injection. Two patients had serious adverse experiences (decreased renal function and generalized seizure) reported as being possibly attributable to allopurinol sodium for injection.

A listing of the adverse reactions regardless of causality reported from clinical trials follows:

➤*Cardiovascular:* Bradycardia, cardiorespiratory arrest, cardiovascular disorder, decreased venous pressure, ECG abnormality, flushing, headache, heart failure, hemorrhage, hypertension, hypotension, pulmonary embolus, septic shock, stroke, thrombophlebitis, ventricular fibrillation (less than 1%).

➤*CNS:* Agitation, cerebral infarction, coma, dystonia, mental status changes, myoclonus, paralysis, seizure, status epilepticus, tremor, twitching (less than 1%).

➤*Dermatologic:* Rash (1.5%); local injection site reaction, pruritus, urticaria (less than 1%).

➤*GI:* Nausea (1.3%); vomiting (1.2%); diarrhea, GI bleeding, splenomegaly, hepatomegaly, intestinal obstruction, flatulence, constipation, proctitis (less than 1%).

➤*GU:* Renal failure/insufficiency (1.2%); hematuria, increased creatinine, kidney function abnormality, oliguria, urinary tract infection (less than 1%).

➤*Hematologic:* Anemia, bone marrow suppression, disseminated intravascular coagulation, ecchymosis, eosinophilia, leukopenia, marrow aplasia, neutropenia, pancytopenia, thrombocytopenia (less than 1%).

ALLOPURINOL — INJECTION

➤*Hepatic:* Hepatomegaly, hyperbilirubinemia, liver failure, jaundice (less than 1%).

➤*Hypersensitivity:* See Warnings/Precautions for more information.

➤*Metabolic:* Edema, electrolyte abnormality, glycosuria, hypercalcemia, hyperglycemia, hyperkalemia, hypernatremia, hyperphosphatemia, hyperuricemia, hypocalcemia, hypokalemia, hypomagnesemia, hyponatremia, lactic acidosis, metabolic acidosis, water intoxication (less than 1%).

➤*Respiratory:* Apnea, ARDS, respiratory failure/insufficiency, increased respiration rate (less than 1%).

➤*Miscellaneous:* Alopecia, blast crisis, cellulitis, chills, diaphoresis, enlarged abdomen, fever, hypervolemia, hypotonia, infection, mucositis/pharyngitis, pain, sepsis, tumor lysis syndrome, arthralgia (less than 1%).

Overdosage

Massive overdosing or acute poisoning by allopurinol sodium for injection has not been reported. In mice, the minimal lethal dose is 45 mg/kg given IV or 500 mg/kg orally (approximately ⅓ or 4 times the usual human dose on a mg/m^2 basis). Hypoactivity was observed with these doses. In rats, the minimum lethal dose is 100 mg/kg IV and 5000 mg/kg orally (approximately 1.5 and 75 times the usual human dose on a mg/m^2 basis). In the management of overdosage, there is no specific antidote for allopurinol sodium for injection. There has been no clinical experience in the management of a patient who has taken massive amounts of allopurinol. Both allopurinol and oxypurinol are dialyzable; however, the usefulness of hemodialysis or peritoneal dialysis in the management of an overdose of allopurinol sodium for injection is unknown.

RASBURICASE

Rx	**Elitek** (Sanofi-Aventis)	**Injection, lyophilized powder for solution:** 1.5 mg	Mannitol 10.6 mg. In cartons with single-use vials and diluent.
		7.5 mg	Mannitol 53 mg. In cartons with single-use vials and diluent.

RASBURICASE — INJECTION

WARNING

Anaphylaxis – Rasburicase may cause severe hypersensitivity reactions, including anaphylaxis. Immediately and permanently discontinue rasburicase in any patient developing clinical evidence of a serious hypersensitivity reaction.

Hemolysis – Do not administer rasburicase to patients with glucose-6-phosphate dehydrogenase (G6PD) deficiency. Immediately and permanently discontinue rasburicase in patients developing hemolysis. It is recommended that patients at higher risk for G6PD deficiency (eg, patients of African or Mediterranean ancestry) be screened prior to starting rasburicase therapy.

Methemoglobinemia – Rasburicase can result in methemoglobinemia in some patients. Immediately and permanently discontinue rasburicase in patients developing methemoglobinemia.

Interference with uric acid measurements – Rasburicase enzymatically degrades uric acid in blood samples left at room temperature. Collect blood samples in prechilled tubes containing heparin and immediately immerse and maintain sample in an ice water bath. Assay plasma samples within 4 hours of collection.

Indications

➤*Hyperuricemia:* For the initial management of plasma uric acid levels in children and adults with leukemia, lymphoma, and solid tumor malignancies who are receiving anticancer therapy expected to result in tumor lysis and subsequent elevation of plasma uric acid.

➤*Off-label uses:*

Gout – [4] = Insufficient documentation. Initial data from limited case reports suggest that rasburicase may be useful in nonmalignancy-related gout that is refractory to conventional therapy. However, this drug has some safety risks, including a black box warning, and is significantly more expensive than conventional therapy. More controlled data are needed. (See Administration and Dosage.)

Administration and Dosage

➤*Adults:*

Hyperuricemia –

Usual dosage: 0.2 mg/kg as a 30-minute intravenous (IV) infusion daily for up to 5 days.

Duration of therapy: Dosing beyond 5 days or administration of more than 1 course is not recommended.

Off-label dosing –

Gout: [4] = Insufficient documentation. 0.15 to 0.2 mg/kg infusion, administered in various dosage regimens. One patient received 10 infusions over a 16-month period (exact schedule was not reported). Other regimens have included an infusion every other week for approximately 6 months, followed by monthly infusions for up to 3 years or daily infusions for 4 days, followed by weekly infusions.

➤*Children:*

Hyperuricemia – See Adults for dosing.

➤*Preparation for administration:* Rasburicase must be reconstituted with the diluent provided in the carton. Reconstitute the 1.5 mg vial of rasburicase with 1 mL of diluent. Reconstitute the 7.5 mg vial of rasburicase with 5 mL of diluent. Mix by swirling gently. Do not shake or vortex. Inject the calculated dose of reconstituted rasburicase solution into an infusion bag containing the appropriate volume of sterile sodium chloride 0.9%, to achieve a final total volume of 50 mL. Do not use filters during reconstitution or infusion of rasburicase.

➤*Administration:* Administer by IV infusion. Do not administer as a bolus injection. Infuse over 30 minutes through a separate line or flush line with at least 15 mL of normal saline prior to and after rasburicase infusion.

Begin rasburicase therapy 4 to 24 hours prior to giving cytotoxic chemotherapy.

Administer rasburicase through a separate IV line from other medications. If separate IV line is not available, flush the IV line with at least 15 mL of sodium chloride 0.9% injection before and after rasburicase administration.

Observe the patient closely for at least the first 5 minutes of the rasburicase infusion.

Adequately hydrate patients during rasburicase therapy. Urine should be neutral or slightly alkaline.

➤*Storage/Stability:* Store at 2° to 8°C (36° to 46°F). Do not freeze. Protect from light. Store reconstituted or diluted solution at 2° to 8°C (36° to 46°F). Discard unused product solution 24 hours following reconstitution.

Actions

➤*Pharmacology:* Rasburicase is a recombinant urate-oxidase. In humans, uric acid is the final step in the catabolic pathway of purines. Rasburicase catalyzes enzymatic oxidation of poorly soluble uric acid into an inactive and more soluble metabolite (allantoin).

Pharmacodynamics – The measurement of plasma uric acid was used to evaluate the effectiveness of rasburicase in clinical studies. Following administration of either 0.15 or 0.2 mg/kg of rasburicase daily for up to 5 days, plasma uric acid levels decreased within 4 hours and were maintained below 7.5 mg/dL in 98% of adult and 90% of pediatric patients for at least 7 days. There was no evidence of a dose-response effect on uric acid control for doses between 0.15 and 0.2 mg/kg of rasburicase.

➤*Pharmacokinetics:*

Absorption/Distribution – Rasburicase exposure, as measured by area under the curve ($AUC_{0\text{-}24h}$) and maximal drug concentration, tended to increase with a dose range from 0.15 to 0.2 mg/kg. The mean volume of distribution of rasburicase ranged from 110 to 127 mL/kg in children and from 75.8 to 138 mL/kg in adults, respectively. Minimal accumulation of rasburicase (less than 1.3-fold) was observed between days 1 and 5 of dosing.

Excretion – The mean terminal half-life was similar between children and adults and ranged from 15.7 to 22.5 hours.

Special populations –

Race: A cross-study comparison revealed that after administration of rasburicase at 0.15 or 0.2 mg/kg, the geometric mean values of body weight normalized clearance were approximately 40% lower in Japanese (n = 20) than in white patients (n = 22).

Contraindications

Deficiency in G6PD; history of anaphylaxis or hypersensitivity reactions, hemolytic reactions, or methemoglobinemia reactions to rasburicase or any of the excipients.

Warnings/Precautions

➤*Hemolysis:* Rasburicase is contraindicated in patients with G6PD deficiency because hydrogen peroxide is one of the major by-products of the conversion of uric acid to allantoin. In clinical studies, hemolysis occurs in less than 1% of patients receiving rasburicase; severe hemolytic reactions occurred within 2 to 4 days of the start of rasburicase. Immediately and permanently discontinue rasburicase administration in any patient developing hemolysis. Institute appropriate patient monitoring and support measures (eg, transfusion support). Screen patients at higher risk for G6PD deficiency (eg, patients of African or Mediterranean ancestry) prior to starting rasburicase.

➤*Methemoglobinemia:* In clinical studies, methemoglobinemia occurred in less than 1% of patients receiving rasburicase. These included cases of serious hypoxemia requiring intervention with medical support measures. It is not known whether patients with deficiency of cytochrome b_5 reductase (formerly known as methemoglobin reductase) or of other enzymes with antioxidant activity are at increased risk for methemoglobinemia or hemolytic anemia. Immediately and permanently discontinue rasburicase administration in any patient identified as having developed methemoglobinemia. Institute appropriate monitoring and support measures (eg, transfusion support, methylene blue administration).

RASBURICASE — INJECTION

➤*Immunogenicity:* As with all therapeutic proteins, there is potential for immunogenicity. Rasburicase can elicit antiproduct antibodies that bind to rasburicase and in some instances inhibit the activity of rasburicase in vitro.

In clinical trials of pediatric patients with hematologic malignancies, 11% of patients tested developed antibodies by day 28 following rasburicase administration, as assessed by qualitative enzyme-linked immunosorbent assay (ELISA).

Using quasi-quantitative immunoassays in rasburicase-naive adult patients with hematological malignancies, 18% of patients were positive for anti-rasburicase immunoglobulin G (IgG), 8% of patients were positive for anti-rasburicase neutralizing IgG, and 6% of patients were positive for anti-rasburicase IgE from day 14 to 24 months after 5 daily doses of rasburicase.

➤*Hypersensitivity reactions:* Rasburicase can cause severe allergic reactions, including anaphylaxis. In clinical studies, anaphylaxis was reported in less than 1% of patients receiving rasburicase. This can occur at any time during treatment, including the first dose. Signs and symptoms of these reactions include bronchospasm, chest pain and tightness, dyspnea, hypoxia, hypotension, shock, and urticaria. Immediately and permanently discontinue rasburicase administration in any patient developing clinical evidence of a serious hypersensitivity reaction.

➤*Pregnancy: Category C.* There are no studies of rasburicase in pregnant women. Reproductive toxicity studies in rabbits treated during organogenesis (gestation day 6 to 19) with approximately 10 to 100 times the recommended human dose of rasburicase resulted in teratogenicity, including weight loss and mortality, decreases in uterine weights and viable fetuses, increased fetal resorptions, postimplantation losses and abortions, and heart and great vessel malformations at all dose levels. Multiple heart and great vessel malformations were also observed in offspring of pregnant rats treated with approximately 250 times the recommended human dose of rasburicase.

Other adverse effects were observed in rasburicase-treated pregnant rabbits at all dose levels tested and included pre- and postimplantation losses, abortions, and decreased uterine weights.

It is unknown whether rasburicase can cross the placental barrier in humans and result in fetal harm. Because of the observed teratogenic effects of rasburicase in animal reproductive studies, use rasburicase during pregnancy only if the potential benefit to the mother justifies the potential risk to the fetus.

➤*Lactation:* It is not known whether this drug is excreted in human milk. Because many drugs are excreted in human milk and because of the potential for serious adverse reactions in breast-feeding infants, decide whether to discontinue breast-feeding or rasburicase, taking into account the importance of the drug to the mother.

➤*Monitoring:* Monitor all patients for allergic reactions (eg, bronchospasm, chest pain and tightness, dyspnea, hypoxia, hypotension, shock, urticaria), hemolysis, and methemoglobinemia.

Drug Interactions

➤*Drug/Lab test interactions:* At room temperature, rasburicase causes enzymatic degradation of the uric acid in blood/plasma/serum samples, potentially resulting in spuriously low plasma uric acid assay readings. The following special sample handling procedure must be followed to avoid ex vivo uric acid degradation.

Uric acid must be analyzed in plasma. Blood must be collected into prechilled tubes containing heparin anticoagulant. Samples must be immediately immersed in an ice water bath. Plasma samples must be prepared by centrifugation in a precooled centrifuge (4°C). Finally, the plasma must be maintained in an ice water bath and analyzed for uric acid within 4 hours of collection.

Adverse Reactions

➤*Hypersensitivity:* Hypersensitivity reactions occurred in 4.3% of rasburicase-treated patients and 1.1% of rasburicase/allopurinol-treated patients in study 4. Clinical manifestations of hypersensitivity included arthralgia, injection-site irritation, peripheral edema, and rash.

➤*Anaphylaxis/Hemolysis/Methemoglobinemia:* The incidence of anaphylaxis, hemolysis, and methemoglobinemia was less than 1% of the 887 rasburicase-treated patients entered in these clinical trials.

Overdosage

➤*Treatment:* Monitor patients who receive an overdose and initiate supportive measures if required.

Patient Information

Instruct patients to notify their health care provider immediately if any of the following occur: allergic reaction, bronchospasm, chest pain or tightness, dyspnea, hypoxia, hypotension, shock, or urticaria.

CLOFARABINE

Rx	**Clolar** (Genzyme Corporation)	**Injection, solution, concentrate:** 1 mg/mL	Preservative free. In 20 mL single-use vials.

CLOFARABINE — INJECTION

Indications

➤*Acute lymphoblastic leukemias:* For the treatment of patients 1 to 21 years of age with relapsed or refractory acute lymphoblastic leukemia (ALL) after at least 2 prior regimens.

➤*Off-label uses:* Treatment of other relapsed or refractory leukemias including acute myelocytic leukemia (AML), myelodysplastic syndrome, and chronic myeloid leukemia in blast phase.

Administration and Dosage

➤*General dosing considerations:* The dosage is based on the patient's body surface area (BSA), calculated using the actual height and weight before the start of each cycle.

Consider avoiding drugs with known renal toxicity during the 5 days of clofarabine administration and use of medications known to induce hepatic toxicity.

Monitor cardiac, renal, and hepatic function during the 5 days of administration.

➤*Adults:*

Acute lymphoblastic leukemia – Limited experience with use in adults older than 21 years of age.

21 years of age and younger: See Children for dosing.

Off-label dosing –

Acute lymphoblastic leukemia: 40 mg/m²/day intravenous (IV) for 5 days, with the courses repeated every 28 days.

➤*Children:*

Acute lymphoblastic leukemia –

1 year of age and older:

• *Usual dosage* – 52 mg/m² administered by IV infusion over 2 hours daily for 5 consecutive days. Treatment cycles are repeated following recovery or return to baseline organ function, approximately every 2 to 6 weeks.

• *Dosage adjustment* –

Hematologic toxicity: Administer subsequent cycles no sooner than 14 days from the starting day of the previous cycle, provided the patient's absolute neutrophil count (ANC) is 0.75×10^9/L or more. If a patient experiences a grade 4 neutropenia (ANC of less than 0.5×10^9/L) lasting 4 weeks or more, reduce dose by 25% for the next cycle.

Nonhematologic toxicity: Withhold clofarabine if a patient develops a clinically significant infection until the infection is clinically controlled and then restart at the full dose. Withhold clofarabine if a grade 3 noninfectious nonhematologic toxicity (excluding transient elevations in serum transaminases and/or serum bilirubin and/or nausea/vomiting that were controlled by antiemetic therapy) occurs. Reinstitute clofarabine administration at a 25% dose reduction when resolution or return to baseline occurs.

➤*Concomitant therapy:* Provide supportive care, such as IV fluids and allopurinol, and alkalinize urine throughout the 5 days of clofarabine administration to reduce the effects of tumor lysis and other adverse events. Consider the use of prophylactic steroids (ie, hydrocortisone 100 mg/m² on days 1 through 3) to prevent signs or symptoms of systemic inflammatory response syndrome, or capillary leak syndrome (eg, hypotension, pulmonary edema, tachycardia, tachypnea).

If hyperuricemia is anticipated (tumor lysis), prophylactically administer allopurinol.

Consider prophylactic antiemetic medications because clofarabine is moderately emetogenic.

➤*Discontinuation of therapy:* Discontinue clofarabine if hypotension develops during the 5 days of administration.

Discontinue administration if a grade 4 noninfectious nonhematologic toxicity occurs or if a patient shows early signs or symptoms of systemic inflammatory response syndrome or capillary leak syndrome (eg, hypotension, pulmonary edema, tachycardia, tachypnea) and provide appropriate supportive measures.

Discontinue clofarabine administration if grade 3 or higher increases in creatinine or bilirubin are noted. Reinstitute clofarabine when the patient is stable and organ function has returned to baseline, generally with a 25% dose reduction.

➤*Preparation for administration:* Filter clofarabine through a sterile 0.2 micron syringe filter and then further dilute with dextrose 5% injection or sodium chloride 0.9% injection prior to IV infusion to a final concentration between 0.15 and 0.4 mg/mL.

➤*Administration:* Administer by IV infusion over 2 hours. Some clinical trials used 1-hour infusions.

➤*Admixture compatibility:* Do not administer any other medications through the same IV line.

➤*Storage/Stability:* Store vials containing undiluted clofarabine solution at 25°C (77°F); excursions are permitted between 15° and 30°C (59° and 86°F). After dilution, store at 15° to 30°C (59° to 86°F) and use within 24 hours of preparation.

Actions

➤*Pharmacology:* Clofarabine is a purine nucleoside metabolic inhibitor and is sequentially metabolized intracellularly to the 5′-monophosphate metabolite by deoxycytidine kinase and mono- and di-phosphokinases to the active 5′-triphosphate metabolite. Clofarabine has high affinity for the acti-

CLOFARABINE — INJECTION

vating phosphorylating enzyme, deoxycytidine kinase, equal to or greater than that of the natural substrate, deoxycytidine. Clofarabine inhibits DNA synthesis by decreasing cellular deoxynucleotide triphosphate pools through an inhibitory action on ribonucleotide reductase and by terminating DNA chain elongation and inhibiting repair through incorporation into the DNA chain by competitive inhibition of DNA polymerases. The affinity of clofarabine triphosphate for these enzymes is similar to or greater than that of deoxyadenosine triphosphate. In preclinical models, clofarabine has demonstrated the ability to inhibit DNA repair by incorporation into the DNA chain during the repair process. Clofarabine 5′-triphosphate also disrupts the integrity of the mitochondrial membrane, leading to the release of the proapoptotic mitochondrial proteins, cytochrome C and apoptosis-inducing factor, leading to programmed cell death.

Clofarabine is cytotoxic to rapidly proliferating and quiescent cancer cell types in vitro.

➤*Pharmacokinetics:*

Absorption / Distribution – The population pharmacokinetics of clofarabine were studied in 40 children 2 to 19 years of age (21 boys/19 girls) with relapsed or refractory ALL or AML. At the given 52 mg/m^2 dose, similar concentrations were obtained over a wide range of BSAs. Clofarabine was 47% bound to plasma proteins, predominantly to albumin. Based on noncompartmental analysis, volume of distribution at steady state was 172 L/m^2.

Metabolism / Excretion – Based on noncompartmental analysis, systemic clearance was estimated to be 28.8 L/h/m^2. The terminal half-life was estimated to be 5.2 hours.

Based on 24-hour urine collections in the pediatric studies, 49% to 60% of the dose is excreted in the urine unchanged. In vitro studies using isolated human hepatocytes indicate very limited metabolism (0.2%). The pathways of nonhepatic elimination remain unknown.

Contraindications

None well documented.

Warnings/Precautions

➤*Hematologic toxicity:* Monitor complete blood cell counts and platelet counts during clofarabine therapy.

Anticipate suppression of bone marrow function. This is usually reversible and appears to be dose dependent.

Severe bone marrow suppression, including neutropenia, anemia, and thrombocytopenia, has been observed in patients treated with clofarabine. At initiation of treatment, most patients in the clinical studies had hematological impairment as a manifestation of leukemia. Because of the preexisting immunocompromised condition of these patients and prolonged neutropenia that can result from treatment with clofarabine, patients are at increased risk for severe opportunistic infections.

➤*Infections:* The use of clofarabine is likely to increase the risk of infection, including severe sepsis, as a result of bone marrow suppression. Monitor patients for signs and symptoms of infection and treat promptly.

➤*Hyperuricemia (tumor lysis):* Administration of clofarabine may result in a rapid reduction in peripheral leukemia cells. Evaluate and monitor patients undergoing treatment for signs and symptoms of tumor lysis syndrome. Provide IV infusion fluids throughout the 5 days of clofarabine administration to reduce the effects of tumor lysis and other adverse reactions. Administer allopurinol if hyperuricemia is expected.

➤*Systemic inflammatory response syndrome and capillary leak syndrome:* Evaluate and monitor patients undergoing treatment with clofarabine for signs and symptoms of cytokine release (eg, hypotension, pulmonary edema, tachycardia, tachypnea) that could develop into systemic inflammatory response syndrome, capillary leak syndrome, and organ dysfunction. Discontinue clofarabine immediately in the event of clinically significant signs or symptoms of systemic inflammatory response syndrome or capillary leak syndrome, either of which can be fatal, and consider use of steroids, diuretics, and albumin. Reinstitute clofarabine when the patient is stable, generally with a 25% dose reduction. The use of prophylactic steroids may be of benefit in preventing signs and symptoms of cytokine release.

➤*Hepatic effects:* Hepatobiliary enzyme elevations were frequently observed in children during treatment with clofarabine. Some patients discontinued treatment because of hepatic enzyme abnormalities.

Patients who have previously received a hematopoietic stem cell transplant (HSCT) may be at higher risk for hepatotoxicity, suggestive of venoocclusive disease following treatment in children (40 mg/m^2) when used in combination with etoposide (100 mg/m^2) and cyclophosphamide (440 mg/m^2). Severe hepatotoxic events have been reported in an ongoing phase 1/2 combination study of clofarabine in children with relapsed or refractory acute leukemia.

➤*Adults with hematologic malignancies:* Safety and effectiveness have not been established in adults.

In a phase 1 study of adults with refractory and/or relapsed hematologic malignancies, the recommended pediatric dosage of 52 mg/m^2/day was not tolerated.

➤*Renal / Hepatic function impairment:* Clofarabine has not been studied in patients with hepatic or renal dysfunction. Undertake its use in such patients only with the greatest caution.

➤*Pregnancy: Category D.* Clofarabine may cause fetal harm when administered to a pregnant woman.

It is not known if clofarabine crosses the human placenta. The molecular weight (about 304), plasma protein binding, and elimination half-life suggest that exposure of the embryo and fetus will occur.

Clofarabine was teratogenic in rats and rabbits. Developmental toxicity (reduced fetal body weight and increased postimplantation loss) and increased incidences of malformations and variations (gross external, soft tissue, skeletal, and retarded ossification) were observed in rats receiving 54 mg/m^2/day (approximately equivalent to the recommended clinical dosage on a mg/m^2 basis), and in rabbits receiving 12 mg/m^2/day (approximately 23% of the recommended clinical dosage on a mg/m^2 basis).

There are no adequate and well-controlled studies in pregnant women using clofarabine. If this drug is used during pregnancy, or if the patient becomes pregnant while taking this drug, apprise the patient of the potential hazard to the fetus.

Advise women of childbearing potential to avoid becoming pregnant while receiving treatment with clofarabine. Advise all patients to use effective contraceptive measures to prevent pregnancy.

➤*Lactation:* It is not known whether clofarabine or its metabolites are excreted in human milk. The molecular weight (about 304), plasma protein binding (47%), and elimination half-life (5.2 hours) suggest that the drug will be excreted into breast milk. The effects of this exposure on a breast-feeding infant are unknown, but severe toxicity potentially involving multiple systems throughout the body is a concern. Because of the potential for tumorigenicity shown for clofarabine in animal studies and the potential for serious adverse reactions, instruct women treated with clofarabine not to breast-feed.

➤*Children:* Safety and effectiveness have been established in patients 1 to 21 years of age with relapsed or refractory ALL.

➤*Elderly:* Safety and effectiveness of clofarabine have not been established in elderly patients 65 years of age and older.

➤*Monitoring:* Obtain complete blood cell counts and platelet counts at regular intervals during clofarabine therapy and more frequently in patients who develop cytopenias. In addition, frequently monitor liver and kidney function during the 5 days of clofarabine administration.

Monitor patients taking medications known to affect blood pressure.

Monitor patients for signs and symptoms of infection and treat promptly. Monitor patients undergoing treatment with clofarabine for signs and symptoms of cytokine release (eg, hypotension, pulmonary edema, tachycardia, tachypnea) that could develop into capillary leak syndrome, organ dysfunction, and systemic inflammatory response syndrome.

Adverse Reactions

➤*Most common adverse reactions:* The most common adverse reactions with clofarabine are anxiety, diarrhea, fatigue, febrile neutropenia, flushing, headache, mucosal inflammation, nausea, palmar-plantar erythrodysesthesia syndrome, pruritus, pyrexia, rash, and vomiting.

➤*Adverse reactions (5% or more):*

Clofarabine Adverse Reactions (≥ 5%)

Adverse reactions[a]	ALL/AML (n = 115)	Worst NCI common ALL/AML terminology criteria grade[a,b]		
	%	3	4	5
Cardiovascular				
Flushing	19.1%			
Hypertension	13%	5.2%		
Hypotension	28.7%	11.3%	7.8%	
Pericardial effusion	7.8%		0.9%	
Tachycardia	34.8%	5.2%		

CLOFARABINE — INJECTION

Clofarabine Adverse Reactions (≥ 5%)				
	ALL/AML (n = 115)	Worst NCI common ALL/AML terminology criteria grade[a,b]		
Adverse reactions[a]	%	3	4	5
CNS				
Agitation	5.2%	0.9%		
Anxiety	20.9%	1.7%		
Asthenia	10.4%	0.9%	0.9%	
Chills	33.9%	2.6%		
Fatigue	33.9%	2.6%	1.7%	
Headache	42.6%	5.2%		
Irritability	9.6%	0.9%		
Lethargy	10.4%	0.9%		
Somnolence	9.6%	0.9%		
Dermatologic				
Cellulitis	7.8%	6.1%		
Erythema	11.3%			
Palmar-plantar erythrodysesthesia syndrome	15.7%	7%		
Petechiae	26.1%	6.1%		
Pruritic rash	7.8%			
Pruritus	42.6%	0.9%		
Rash	38.3%	7%		
GI				
Abdominal pain	34.8%	7%		
Abdominal pain, upper	7.8%	0.9%		
Clostridium colitis	7%	5.2%		
Diarrhea	55.7%	12.2%		
Gingival bleeding	13.9%	6.1%	0.9%	
Mouth hemorrhage	5.2%	1.7%		
Nausea	73%	13.9%	0.9%	
Oral candidiasis	11.3%	1.7%		
Oral mucosal petechiae	5.2%	3.5%		
Proctalgia	7.8%	1.7%		
Stomatitis	7%	0.9%		
Vomiting	78.3%	7.8%	0.9%	
Hematologic				
Febrile neutropenia	54.8%	51.3%	2.6%	
Neutropenia	9.6%	2.6%	7%	
Metabolic/Nutritional				
Anorexia	29.6%	5.2%	7%	
Edema	12.2%	1.7%		
Musculoskeletal				
Arthralgia	8.7%	2.6%		
Back pain	10.4%	2.6%		
Bone pain	9.6%	2.6%		
Myalgia	13.9%			
Pain in extremity	29.6%	5.2%		
Respiratory				
Dyspnea	13%	5.2%	1.7%	
Epistaxis	27%	13%		
Pleural effusion	12.2%	3.5%	1.7%	
Pneumonia	9.6%	5.2%	0.9%	0.9%
Respiratory distress	10.4%	4.4%	3.5%	0.9%
Tachypnea	8.7%	3.5%	0.9%	
Upper respiratory tract infection	5.2%	0.9%		
Miscellaneous				
Bacteremia	8.7%	8.7%		
Candidiasis	7%	0.9%		
Catheter-related infection	12.2%	11.3%		
Hematuria	13%	1.7%		
Herpes simplex	9.6%	5.2%		
Herpes zoster	7%	5.2%		

CLOFARABINE — INJECTION

Clofarabine Adverse Reactions (≥ 5%)				
	ALL/AML (n = 115)	Worst NCI common ALL/AML terminology criteria grade[a,b]		
Adverse reactions[a]	%	3	4	5
Jaundice	7.8%	1.7%		
Mucosal inflammation	15.7%	1.7%		
Pain	14.8%	6.1%	0.9%	
Pyrexia	39.1%	13.9%		
Sepsis	9.6%	4.4%	1.7%	3.5%
Septic shock	7%	0.9%	1.7%	4.4%
Staphylococcal bacteremia	6.1%	4.4%	0.9%	
Staphylococcal sepsis	5.2%	4.4%	0.9%	
Tumor lysis syndrome	6.1%	6.1%		

[a] Patients with > 1 preferred term within a system organ class are counted only once in the system organ class totals. Patients with > 1 occurrence of the same preferred term are counted only once within that term and at the highest severity grade.

[b] NCI = National Cancer Institute.

➤*Other adverse reactions (1% to 4%):*

GI – Cecitis, gastroenteritis adenovirus, pancreatitis.

Respiratory – Pneumonia fungal, pneumonia primary atypical, pulmonary edema, respiratory syncytial virus infection, sinusitis.

Miscellaneous – Bacterial infection, *Enterococcal* bacteremia, *Escherichia* bacteremia, *Escherichia* sepsis, fungal infection, fungal sepsis, infection, influenza, *Parainfluenzae* virus infection, staphylococcal infection. Blood creatinine increased, hyperbilirubinemia, hypersensitivity, mental status change.

➤*Hematologic:* The most frequently reported hematologic adverse reactions in children included febrile neutropenia (55%) and nonfebrile neutropenia (10%).

➤*Hepatic:* Hepatobiliary toxicities were frequently observed in children during treatment with clofarabine. Grade 3 or 4 elevated AST occurred in 36% of patients and grade 3 or 4 elevated ALT occurred in 44% of patients. Grade 3 or 4 elevated bilirubin occurred in 13% of patients, with 2 events reported as grade 4 hyperbilirubinemia (2%), one of which resulted in treatment discontinuation, 1 patient had multiorgan failure and died. Two reports (2%) of venoocclusive disease were considered related to study drug.

For patients with follow-up data, elevations in AST and ALT were transient and typically were 15 days duration or fewer. The majority of AST and ALT elevations occurred within 10 days of clofarabine administration and returned to grade 2 or less within 15 days. Where follow-up data are available, the majority of bilirubin elevations returned to grade 2 or less within 10 days. Eight patients had grade 3 or 4 elevations in serum bilirubin at the last time point measured; these patients died due to sepsis and/or multiorgan failure.

➤*Renal:* The most prevalent renal toxicity in children was elevated creatinine. Grade 3 or 4 elevated creatinine occurred in 8% of patients. Acute renal failure was reported in 3% of patients with grade 3 and 2% of patients with grade 4. Nephrotoxic medications, tumor lysis, and tumor lysis with hyperuricemia may contribute to renal toxicity. Hematuria was observed in 13% of patients overall.

➤*Miscellaneous:*

Infection – At baseline, 48% of children had 1 or more concurrent infections. A total of 83% of patients experienced at least 1 infection after clofarabine treatment, including fungal, viral, and bacterial infections.

Systemic inflammatory response syndrome – Adverse reactions of systemic inflammatory response syndrome were reported in 2% of patients (see Warnings/Precautions for more information).

➤*Capillary leak syndrome:* Adverse reactions of capillary leak syndrome were reported in 4% of patients. Symptoms included rapid onset of respiratory distress, hypotension, pleural and pericardial effusion, and multiorgan failure.

Close monitoring for this syndrome and early intervention are recommended. The use of prophylactic steroids (eg, hydrocortisone 100 mg/m^2 on days 1 through 3) may be of benefit in preventing signs or symptoms of systemic inflammatory response syndrome or capillary leak syndrome. Be alert to early indications of these syndromes and immediately discontinue clofarabine administration if they occur and provide appropriate supportive measures. After the patient is stabilized and organ function has returned to baseline, retreatment with clofarabine can be considered with a 25% dose reduction.

➤*Lab test abnormalities:*

Clofarabine Laboratory Abnormalities		
Laboratory parameters	Any grade	Grade 3 or higher
Hematologic		
Anemia (n = 114)	83.3%	75.4%
Leukopenia (n = 114)	87.7%	87.7%
Lymphopenia (n =113)	82.3%	82.3%
Neutropenia (n = 113)	63.7%	63.7%
Thrombocytopenia (n = 114)	80.7%	79.8%
Hepatic		
Elevated total bilirubin (n = 114)	44.7%	13.2%
Elevated ALT (n = 113)	80.5%	43.4%
Elevated AST (n = 100)	74%	36%
Miscellaneous		
Elevated creatinine (n = 115)	49.5%	7.8%

➤*Postmarketing:*

Dermatologic – Occurrences of Stevens-Johnson syndrome and toxic epidermal necrolysis have been reported in patients who were receiving or had recently been treated with clofarabine and other medications (eg, allopurinol, antibiotics) known to cause these syndromes.

Hematologic – Bone marrow failure.

Hepatic – Serious hepatotoxic adverse reactions of venoocclusive disease have been reported in adult patients following HSCT. These patients received conditioning regimens that included busulfan, melphalan, and/or the combination of cyclophosphamide and total body irradiation.

Overdosage

There were no known overdoses of clofarabine. The highest daily dosage administered to a human to date (on a mg/m^2 basis) has been 70 mg/m^2/day for 5 days (2 children with ALL). The toxicities reported in these 2 patients included grade 4 hyperbilirubinemia, grade 2 and 3 vomiting, and grade 3 maculopapular rash.

Patient Information

Advise patients to have regular blood count testing and to report any symptoms associated with hematologic toxicity (eg, easy bruising, fatigue, fever, pallor, petechiae, purpura, shortness of breath, weakness) to their health care provider.

Advise patients of the signs or symptoms of infection (eg, fever) and to notify their health care provider immediately if any occur.

Advise patients to avoid medications including over-the-counter and herbal medications, which may be hepatotoxic or nephrotoxic, during the 5 days of clofarabine administration.

Advise patients of the signs or symptoms of systemic inflammatory response syndrome, such as fever, tachycardia, tachypnea, dyspnea, and symptoms suggestive of hypotension.

Advise men and women with reproductive potential to use effective contraceptive measures to prevent pregnancy. Advise women to avoid breastfeeding during clofarabine treatment.

VINBLASTINE SULFATE (VLB)

Rx	**Vinblastine Sulfate** (Various)	**Powder for injection:** 10 mg	In vials.
Rx	**Velban** (Lilly)		In vials.
Rx	**Vinblastine Sulfate** (Various)	**Injection:** 1 mg/ml	In 10 and 25 ml vials.[a]

[a] With 0.9% benzyl alcohol.

VINBLASTINE SULFATE (VLB) — INJECTION

WARNING

It is extremely important the needle be properly positioned in the vein before this product is injected. If leakage into surrounding tissue should occur during IV administration of vinblastine sulfate, it may cause considerable irritation. Immediately discontinue the injection, and introduce any remaining portion of the dose into another vein. Local injection of hyaluronidase and the application of moderate heat to the area of leakage will help disperse the drug and may minimize the discomfort and the possibility of cellulitis.

Fatal if given intrathecally. For IV use only.

Indications

➤*General information:* Palliative treatment of the following:

➤*Frequently responsive malignancies:* Generalized Hodgkin's disease (stages III and IV, Ann Arbor modification of Rye staging system), lymphocytic lymphoma (nodular and diffuse, poorly and well differentiated); histiocytic lymphoma; mycosis fungoides (advanced stages); advanced testicular carcinoma; Kaposi's sarcoma and Letterer-Siwe disease (histiocytosis X).

➤*Less frequently responsive malignancies:* Choriocarcinoma resistant to other chemotherapy; breast cancer unresponsive to endocrine surgery and hormonal therapy.

➤*Multiple drug protocols:* Vinblastine, effective as a single agent, is usually administered with other antineoplastics. Combination therapy enhances therapeutic effect without additive toxicity when agents with different dose-limiting toxicities and mechanisms of action are selected.

➤*Hodgkin's disease:* Vinblastine used as a single agent; advanced Hodgkin's disease also has been successfully treated with multiple-drug regimens that included vinblastine.

➤*Advanced testicular germinal-cell cancers (embryonal carcinoma, teratocarcinoma, and choriocarcinoma):* Advanced testicular germinal-cell cancers are sensitive to vinblastine alone, but better clinical results are achieved with combination therapy. Vinblastine enhances the effect of bleomycin if given 6 to 8 hours prior to bleomycin administration; this schedule permits more cells to be arrested during metaphase, the stage in which bleomycin is active.

➤*Off-label uses:* Treatment of non-small cell lung carcinoma; bladder cancer; refractory idiopathic thrombocytopenic purpura.

Administration and Dosage

➤*General dosing considerations:* Fatal if given intrathecally. For IV use only. (See Administration).

Leukopenic responses vary following therapy. For this reason, do not administer drug more than once weekly.

➤*Adults:*

Malignancies – For a list of malignancies, see Indications.

Usual dosage: 5.5 to 7.4 mg/m^2 weekly.

Initial dosage: 3.7 mg/m^2 as a single IV dose. Thereafter, measure WBC counts to determine patient's sensitivity to vinblastine.

Dosage titration: A simplified and conservative incremental approach to dosage at weekly intervals for adults may be as follows:

Incremental Vinblastine Dosage (Weekly Intervals)

	Adult dose (mg/m^2)
First dose	3.7
Second dose	5.5
Third dose	7.4
Fourth dose	9.25
Fifth dose	11.1

Use the same increments until a maximum dose not exceeding 18.5 mg/m^2 is reached. Do not increase dose after WBC count is reduced to approximately 3,000 cells/mm^3. For most adults, the weekly dosage range is 5.5 to 7.4 mg/m^2.

Maintenance dosage: When the dose produces the above degree of leukopenia, administer a dose one increment smaller every 7 to 14 days.

Even though 7 days have elapsed, do not give the next dose until the WBC count has returned to at least 4,000 cells/mm^3. In some cases, oncolytic activity may be encountered before leukopenic effect but do not increase the size of subsequent doses.

Duration of therapy: For an adequate trial, vinblastine must be continued for at least 4 to 6 weeks. Duration of maintenance therapy varies according to the disease and the combination of antineoplastics used. Prolonged chemotherapy for maintaining remission involves several risks: life-threatening infections, sterility, secondary cancers through suppression of immune surveillance. In some disorders, survival following complete remission may not be as prolonged as that achieved with shorter periods of maintenance therapy. Conversely, failure to provide maintenance therapy may lead to unnecessary relapse; complete remission in patients with testicular cancer, unless maintained for at least 2 years, often results in early relapse.

➤*Children:*

Malignancies – For a list of malignancies, see Indications. See also Off-label dosing.

Initial dosage:

- *Hodgkin disease* – 6 mg/m^2 IV when used in combination with other chemotherapeutic agents.
- *Letterer-Siwe disease (histiocytosis X)* – 6.5 mg/m^2 IV as a single agent.
- *Testicular germ cell carcinomas* – 3 mg/m^2 IV when used in combination with other chemotherapeutic agents.

Dosage adjustment: Dose modifications should be guided by hematologic tolerance.

Duration of therapy: For an adequate trial, vinblastine must be continued for at least 4 to 6 weeks.

Off-label dosing –

Germ cell tumors: 3 mg/m^2/day continuous IV infusion, days 1 through 5 of each cycle. Given in combination with other antineoplastics.

Hodgkin lymphoma: Various regimens have been reported (see the following). Given in combination with other antineoplastics.

- 6 mg/m^2/dose IV given every 14 days.
- 5 mg/m^2/dose IV given every 28 days.
- 4 to 6 mg/m^2/dose (10 mg/dose maximum) IV given on days 1 and 8 of each 28-day cycle.
- 6 mg/m^2/dose or 10 mg/dose IV given every 28 days.
- 6 mg/m^2/dose IV given every 21 days.

Testicular cancer: 0.11 to 0.15 mg/kg/day IV, days 1 and 2 of each 21-day cycle. An alternative regimen is vinblastine 4 mg/m^2/dose IV given every 21 to 28 days. Given in combination with other antineoplastics.

➤*Hepatic function impairment:* Vinblastine undergoes extensive hepatic metabolism. The package labeling states that a 50% dose reduction is recommended for patients having a direct serum bilirubin value greater than 3 mg/dL.

Alternative recommendations are to reduce the dose for patients with hepatic dysfunction, as shown in the following table.

Vinblastine Dosage Adjustment Based on Hepatic Function

Serum bilirubin	AST	Percent of usual dose
< 1.5 mg/dL	< 60 units/L	100%
1.5 to 3 mg/dL	60 to 180 units/L	50%
3 to 5 mg/dL	—	25%
> 5 mg/dL	> 180 units/L	Do not administer

➤*Preparation for administration:* Vinblastine is considered a cytotoxic agent. Follow safe handling procedures when preparing, administering, or dispensing vinblastine.

Reconstitute lyophilized powder by adding 10 mL of bacteriostatic sodium chloride injection (preserved with phenol or benzyl alcohol) to the vial for a concentration of 1 mg/mL. Powder may also be reconstituted with 10 mL preservative-free sodium chloride 0.9% injection. The drug dissolves instantly to give a clear solution. A preservative-containing solvent is unnecessary if unused portions are discarded immediately.

Do not dilute the dose in large volumes of diluent (ie, 100 to 250 mL) or give IV for prolonged periods (30 min or longer), because this often results in vein irritation and increases the chance of extravasation.

➤*Administration:* Fatal if given intrathecally. For IV use only. Inject into either the tubing of a running IV infusion or directly into a vein over 1 minute. To prevent cellulitis or phlebitis, secure the needle within the vein so that no solution extravasates. To further minimize extravasation, rinse syringe and needle with venous blood before withdrawal of needle.

Do not dilute the dose in large volumes of diluent (ie, 100 to 250 mL) or give IV for prolonged periods (30 min or longer), because this often results in vein irritation and increases the chance of extravasation.

Because of the enhanced possibility of thrombosis, do not inject solution into an extremity in which circulation is impaired or potentially impaired by conditions such as compressing or invading neoplasm, phlebitis, or varicosity.

➤*Extravasation:* Vinblastine is considered a vesicant. If signs or symptoms of extravasation occur, stop the infusion immediately. If possible, withdraw 3 to 5 mL of blood to remove some of the drug. Remove the infusion needle. Administer hyaluronidase 150 units/mL solution within the first few minutes to 1 hour after extravasation. Cleanse the area with povidone-iodine. Reconstitute 1 mL vial of hyaluronidase. (Note: Some products do not

VINBLASTINE SULFATE (VLB) — INJECTION

require dilution.) Inject locally, subcutaneously or intradermally, using a 25-gauge needle or smaller. The dose is 150 units (1 mL) given as 5 injections (0.2 mL each). Application of warm compresses to the area for 15 minutes every 6 hours for 48 hours may be useful. Delineate the infiltrated area on the patient's skin with a felt-tip marker. Elevate for 48 hours above heart level using a sling or stockinette dressing with an observation window cut in the dressing. Avoid pressure or friction. Do not rub the area. Observe for signs of increased erythema, pain, or skin necrosis. If increased symptoms occur, consult a plastic surgeon. Ensure that no medication is given distally to extravasation site. After 48 hours, encourage the patient to use the extremity normally to promote full range of motion.

➤*Admixture compatibility:* Do not dilute with solvents that raise or lower the pH of the resulting solution from between 3.5 and 5. Make solutions with either normal saline or sodium chloride 0.9% injection (each with or without preservative) and do not combine in the same container with any other chemical.

➤*Storage/Stability:* Refrigerate unopened vials at 2° to 8°C (36° to 46°F). Unopened vials are stable at room temperature for 2 weeks, but this is not recommended for storage.

Solutions reconstituted with bacteriostatic sodium chloride injection are stable for 28 days in the refrigerator. Solutions reconstituted with preservative-free sodium chloride 0.9% injection should be used within 24 hours.

Multiple-dose vials may be used for up to 28 days after the initial needle puncture, based on the USP Chapter <797> standards.

Discard single-dose vials within 6 hours of the initial needle puncture if opened within an ISO Class 5 biological safety cabinet, or within 1 hour of the initial needle puncture if opened outside of such an environment, based on the USP Chapter <797> standards.

Actions

➤*Pharmacology:* Vinblastine sulfate, an alkaloid extracted from Vinca rosea Linn, interferes with metabolic pathways of amino acids leading from glutamic acid to the citric acid cycle and urea. Studies have demonstrated a stathmokinetic effect and various atypical mitotic figures. However, therapeutic responses are not fully explained by the cytologic changes, because these changes are sometimes observed clinically and experimentally in the absence of any oncolytic effects.

Vinblastine has an effect on cell energy production required for mitosis and interferes with nucleic acid synthesis. In vitro, the drug arrests growing cells in metaphase.

Reversal of the antitumor effect by glutamic acid or tryptophan has occurred.

➤*Pharmacokinetics:*

Absorption/Distribution – Similar to vincristine, vinblastine undergoes rapid distribution and extensive tissue binding following IV injection. Vinblastine also localizes in platelets and leukocyte fractions of whole blood.

Metabolism/Excretion – Vinblastine is partially metabolized to deacetyl vinblastine, which is more active than the parent drug. Plasma decline follows a triphasic pattern. The initial, middle, and terminal half-lives are 3.7 minutes, 1.6 hours and 24.8 hours, respectively. Toxicity may be increased if liver disease is present.

Vinblastine is metabolized by the hepatic P450 3A cytochromes, and the major route of excretion may be through the biliary system.

Contraindications

Leukopenia; presence of bacterial infection (infections must be under control prior to initiating therapy); significant granulocytopenia unless it is a result of the disease being treated.

Warnings/Precautions

➤*For IV use only:* The intrathecal administration of vinblastine has resulted in death. Label syringes containing this product "Vinblastine Sulfate for Intravenous Use Only."

Extemporaneously prepared syringes containing this product must be packaged in an overwrap that is labeled "Do Not Remove Covering Until Moment of Injection. Fatal if Given Intrathecally. For Intravenous Use Only."

➤*Hematologic effects:* Leukopenia is expected; leukocyte count is an important guide to therapy. In general, the larger the dose, the more profound and longer lasting the leukopenia will be. If the WBC count returns to normal after drug-induced leukopenia, the white cell-producing mechanism is not permanently depressed. Usually, WBC count has completely returned to normal after virtual disappearance of white cells from peripheral blood. The nadir in WBC count occurs 5 to 10 days after the last dose of drug is given. Recovery of the WBC count is fairly rapid and usually complete within 7 to 14 days. With smaller doses employed for maintenance therapy, leukopenia may not occur.

Although the thrombocyte count ordinarily is not significantly lowered by therapy, recently impaired bone marrow by prior therapy with radiation or with other oncolytic drugs may show thrombocytopenia (less than 200,000 platelets/mm^3). When other chemotherapy or radiation has not been previously employed, thrombocytopenia is rare, even when vinblastine may be causing significant leukopenia. Rapid recovery (within a few days) from thrombocytopenia is the rule.

The effect on red blood cell count and hemoglobin is usually insignificant in the absence of other therapy; however, patients with malignant disease may exhibit anemia in the absence of any therapy.

If leukopenia (less than 2000 WBC/mm^3) occurs following a dose of this drug, carefully watch the patient for evidence of infection until a safe WBC count has returned.

When cachexia or ulcerated skin surface occurs, a more profound leukopenic response may occur; avoid use in older persons suffering from these conditions.

In patients with malignant cell infiltration of bone marrow, leukocyte and platelet counts have sometimes fallen precipitously after moderate doses, making further use of the drug inadvisable.

Leukopenia (granulocytopenia) may reach dangerously low levels following use of the higher recommended doses. Follow recommended dosage technique. Stomatitis and neurologic toxicity, although not common or permanent, can be disabling.

➤*Long-term use:* Using small amounts of drug daily for long periods is not advised, even though the resulting total weekly dose may be similar to that recommended. Strict adherence to the recommended dosage schedule is very important. When amounts equal to several times the recommended weekly dosage were given in 7 daily installments for long periods, convulsions, severe and permanent CNS damage and death occurred.

➤*Avoid eye contamination:* Severe irritation or corneal ulceration (if the drug was delivered under pressure) may result. Thoroughly wash the eye with water immediately.

➤*Pulmonary reactions:* Acute shortness of breath and severe bronchospasm have occurred following use of vinca alkaloids. These reactions occur most frequently when the vinca alkaloid is used with mitomycin. Onset may be within minutes or several hours after the vinca is injected and may occur up to 2 weeks after the dose of mitomycin. (See Drug Interactions.)

➤*Benzyl alcohol:* Benzyl alcohol, contained in some of these products as a preservative, has been associated with a fatal "gasping syndrome" in premature infants.

➤*Extravasation:* See Administration and Dosage for more information.

➤*Hepatic function impairment:* See Administration and Dosage for more information.

➤*Pregnancy: Category D.* Information is very limited. Animal studies suggest teratogenicity may occur. Animals given the drug early in pregnancy suffered resorption of the conceptus; surviving fetuses demonstrated gross deformities. There are no adequate and well controlled studies in pregnant women, but the drug can cause fetal harm. If the drug is used during pregnancy, or if the patient becomes pregnant while receiving this drug, apprise her of the potential hazard to the fetus. Advise women of childbearing potential to avoid becoming pregnant.

Fertility impairment – Aspermia has been reported. Amenorrhea has occurred in some patients treated with a combination of an alkylating agent, procarbazine, prednisone and vinblastine. Its occurrence was related to the total dose of these agents. Recovery of menses was frequent. The same combination of drugs given to male patients produced azoospermia; if spermatogenesis did return, it was not likely to do so with less than 2 years of unmaintained remission.

➤*Lactation:* It is not known whether this drug is excreted in breast milk. Because of the potential for serious adverse reactions in nursing infants, decide whether to discontinue nursing or to discontinue the drug, taking into account the importance of the drug to the mother.

Drug Interactions

Vinblastine Drug Interactions

Precipitant drug	Object drug[a]		Description
Vinblastine	Mitomycin	⬆	Acute shortness of breath and severe bronchospasm have occurred following use of vinca alkaloids in patients who had previously or simultaneously received mitomycin. Onset may be within minutes or several hours after the vinca alkaloid is injected and may occur up to 2 weeks after the dose of mitomycin.
Vinblastine	Phenytoin	⬇	Combination chemotherapy (including vinblastine) may reduce phenytoin plasma levels and increase seizure activity. Adjust the dosage based on serial blood level monitoring.
Erythromycin	Vinblastine	⬆	May cause toxicity of vinblastine. Severe myalgia, neutropenia and constipation have been reported.
Agents that inhibit the cytochrome P450 pathway	Vinblastine	⬆	Vinblastine is metabolized by the P450 3A enzyme. Use caution when coadministering drugs that inhibit P450 enzymes.

[a] ⬆ = Object drug increased. ⬇ = Object drug decreased.

VINBLASTINE SULFATE (VLB) — INJECTION

Adverse Reactions

Incidence of adverse reactions is dose-related. Except for epilation, leukopenia and neurologic side effects, adverse reactions have not usually persisted for longer than 24 hours. Neurologic side effects are not common; when they occur, they often last for more than 24 hours. Leukopenia, the most common adverse reaction, is usually the dose-limiting factor.

Vinblastine is considered to have very low emetogenic potential (less than 10% incidence of emesis).

➤*Cardiovascular:* Hypertension. Cases of unexpected myocardial infarction and cerebrovascular accidents have occurred in patients undergoing combination chemotherapy with vinblastine, bleomycin and cisplatin.

➤*CNS:* Numbness of digits; paresthesias; peripheral neuritis; mental depression; loss of deep tendon reflexes; headache; convulsions.

➤*Dermatologic:* Alopecia is common. Total epilation infrequently develops. In some cases, hair regrows during maintenance therapy. A single case of light sensitivity has been associated with this drug.

➤*GI:* Nausea and vomiting (may be controlled by antiemetics); pharyngitis; vesiculation of the mouth; ileus; diarrhea; constipation; anorexia; abdominal pain; rectal bleeding; hemorrhagic enterocolitis; bleeding from an old peptic ulcer.

➤*Hematologic:* Leukopenia (granulocytopenia), anemia, thrombocytopenia (myelosuppression). See Warnings.

➤*Miscellaneous:* Malaise; weakness; dizziness; pain in tumor site; bone and jaw pain. The syndrome of inappropriate secretion of antidiuretic hormone has occurred with higher than recommended doses.

Extravasation during IV injection may lead to cellulitis and phlebitis; sloughing may occur (see Administration and Dosage).

There are isolated reports of Raynaud's phenomenon occurring in patients with testicular carcinoma treated with bleomycin, cisplatin and vinblastine sulfate. It is unknown whether the cause was the disease, the drugs or a combination of these.

Overdosage

➤*Symptoms:* Side effects are dose-related. After an overdose, expected exaggerated effects. In addition, neurotoxicity similar to that with vincristine may occur.

➤*Treatment:* Supportive care should include prevention of side effects that result from the syndrome of inappropriate secretion of antidiuretic hormone (ie, restriction of the volume of daily fluid intake to that of the urine output plus insensible loss and perhaps use of a diuretic affecting the function of the loop of Henle and the distal tubule); administration of an anticonvulsant; prevention of ileus; monitoring the cardiovascular system; and determining daily blood counts for guidance in transfusion requirements and assessing the risk of infection. The major effect of excessive doses will be myelosuppression, which may be life-threatening. There is no information regarding the effectiveness of dialysis nor of cholestyramine for the treatment of overdosage.

In the dry state, the drug is irregularly and unpredictably absorbed from the GI tract following oral administration. Absorption of the solution has not been studied. If vinblastine is swallowed, oral activated charcoal in a water slurry may be given along with a cathartic. The use of cholestyramine in this situation has not been reported.

Patient Information

Immediately report sore throat, fever, chills or sore mouth to the physician.

The following may occur: Alopecia, jaw pain, pain in the organs containing tumor tissue, nausea and vomiting. Scalp hair will regrow to its pretreatment extent, even with continued treatment. Report any other serious medical event to the physician.

Avoid constipation.

VINCRISTINE SULFATE (VCR; LCR)

Rx	**Vincristine Sulfate** (Various)	**Injection:** 1 mg/ml	In 1, 2 and 5 ml vials.
Rx	**Vincasar PFS** (Sicor)		In 1, 2, 5 ml flip-top vials.[a]

[a] With 100 mg mannitol. Refrigerate.

VINCRISTINE SULFATE (VCR; LCR) — INTRAVENOUS

WARNING

It is extremely important that the IV needle or catheter be properly positioned before injection. Leakage into surrounding tissue may cause considerable irritation.

This preparation is for IV use only. Intrathecal use usually results in death.

Indications

➤*Acute leukemia:* For acute leukemia.

➤*Combination therapy:* Combination therapy in Hodgkin's disease, non-Hodgkin's malignant lymphomas (lymphocytic, mixed-cell, histiocytic, undifferentiated, nodular and diffuse types), rhabdomyosarcoma, neuroblastoma and Wilms' tumor.

➤*Off-label uses:*

Postherpetic neuralgia (iontophoretic) – [5] = Poor documentation.
Use of vincristine ionophoresis for the treatment of postherpetic neuralgia (PHN) has been studied in 2 trials that showed conflicting results. American Academy of Neurology clinical practice guidelines state that the efficacy of vincristine iontophoresis is not better than that of placebo in patients with PHN.

Other possible off-label uses – Vincristine has been used in the treatment of idiopathic thrombocytopenic purpura, Kaposi's sarcoma, breast cancer, bladder cancer, small cell lung carcinoma, brain tumors, multiple myeloma, chronic lymphocytic and myelocytic leukemias, and autoimmune hemolytic anemia.

Administration and Dosage

➤*General dosing considerations:* Cautiously calculate and administer dose; overdosage may be serious or fatal.

For IV use only. Intrathecal use usually results in death.

➤*Adults:*

Malignancies – For a list of malignancies, see Indications.
Usual dosage: 1.4 mg/m² IV once weekly (typical dose 2 mg). (See also Off-label dosing.)

Off-label dosing –
Malignancies: 0.4 to 0.5 mg/day as a continuous IV infusion for 4 days, repeated every 4 weeks.

➤*Children:*

Malignancies – For a list of malignancies, see Indications.
Usual dosage:
• *Body weight more than 10 kg or body surface area of 1 m² or more* – 1 to 2 mg/m² IV once weekly.
• *Body weight less than or equal to 10 kg or BSA less than 1 m²* – 0.05 mg/kg IV once weekly initially. Titrate dose as tolerated, up to 2 mg/dose.
Duration of therapy: 3 to 6 weeks.

Off-label dosing –
Neuroblastoma: For children weighing more than 10 kg (or BSA 1 m² or more), the dosage is 1 mg/m²/day by continuous IV infusion over 24 hours for 3 days (total dose of 3 mg/m² over a 3-day period). Vincristine is part of a combination therapy.

➤*Hepatic function impairment:* Vincristine undergoes extensive hepatic metabolism. The package labeling states that a 50% dose reduction is recommended for patients having a direct serum bilirubin value greater than 3mg/dL.

Alternative recommendations are to reduce the dosage for patients with hepatic dysfunction, as shown in the following table.

Vincristine Dosage Adjustment Based on Hepatic Function

Serum bilirubin	AST	Percent of usual dose
< 1.5 mg/dL	< 60 units/L	100%
1.5 to 3 mg/dL	60 to 180 units/L	50%
3 to 5 mg/dL	—	25%
> 5 mg/dL	> 180 units/L	Do not administer

➤*Preparation for administration:* Vincristine is considered a cytotoxic agent. Follow safe handling procedures when preparing, administering, or dispensing vincristine.

Vincristine should not be diluted for routine IV use. For continuous IV infusion, vincristine may be diluted with sodium chloride 0.9% injection or dextrose 5% injection.

➤*Administration:* Administer IV only; intrathecal administration is uniformly fatal.

Do not filter.

Inject solution either directly into a vein or into the tubing of a running IV infusion. Injection may be completed in about 1 minute.

Continuous infusions of vincristine can only be administered through a central venous catheter resting in the vena cava. A peripherally inserted central catheter, or PICC line, may also be appropriate.

VINCRISTINE SULFATE (VCR; LCR) — INTRAVENOUS

➤*Extravasation:* Vincristine is considered a vesicant. If signs or symptoms of extravasation occur, stop the infusion immediately. If possible, withdraw 3 to 5 mL of blood to remove some of the drug. Remove the infusion needle. Administer hyaluronidase 150 units/mL solution within the first few minutes to 1 hour after extravasation. Cleanse the area with povidone-iodine. Reconstitute 1 mL vial of hyaluronidase. (Note: Some products do not require dilution.) Inject locally, subcutaneously or intradermally, using a 25-gauge needle or smaller. The dose is 150 units (1 mL) given as 5 injections (0.2 mL each). Application of warm compresses to the area for 15 minutes every 6 hours for 48 hours may be useful. Delineate the infiltrated area on the patient's skin with a felt-tip marker. Elevate for 48 hours above heart level using a sling or stockinette dressing with an observation window cut in the dressing. Avoid pressure or friction. Do not rub the area. Observe for signs of increased erythema, pain, or skin necrosis. If increased symptoms occur, consult a plastic surgeon. Ensure that no medication is given distally to extravasation site. After 48 hours, encourage the patient to use the extremity normally to promote full range of motion.

➤*Admixture compatibility:* Do not dilute in solutions that raise or lower the pH outside the range of 3.5 to 5.5. Do not mix with anything other than normal saline or glucose in water.

➤*Storage/Stability:* Store refrigerated (2° to 8°C; 36° to 46°F). Protect from light.

Discard vial within 6 hours of the initial needle puncture if opened within an ISO Class 5 biological safety cabinet, or within 1 hour of the initial needle puncture if opened outside of such an environment, based on the USP Chapter <797> standards.

Actions

➤*Pharmacology:* Vincristine sulfate is an alkaloid obtained from the periwinkle (*Vinca rosea* Linn). Mode of action is unknown. In vitro, it arrests mitotic division at metaphase. Antineoplastic effects are related to interference with intracellular tubulin function. It reversibly binds to microtubule and spindle proteins in the S phase.

Combination cancer chemotherapy involves simultaneous use of several agents. Generally, each agent has a unique toxicity and mechanism so that therapeutic enhancement occurs without additive toxicity. It is rarely possible to achieve equally good results with single agent treatment. Vincristine is often chosen as part of polychemotherapy because of lack of significant bone marrow suppression (at recommended doses) and of unique clinical toxicity (neuropathy). See Administration and Dosage for possible increased toxicity when used in combination therapy.

➤*Pharmacokinetics:*

Absorption/Distribution – Within 15 to 30 minutes following IV administration, greater than 90% of the drug is distributed from blood into tissue where it remains tightly, but not irreversibly, bound. Penetration across the blood-brain barrier is poor.

Metabolism/Excretion – Studies in cancer patients show a triphasic serum decay pattern following rapid IV injection. Initial, middle and terminal half-lives are 5 min, 2.3 hrs and 85 hrs, respectively; the range of the terminal half-life is 19 to 155 hrs. The liver is the major excretory organ; ≈ 80% of a dose appears in feces and 10% to 20% in urine. Hepatic dysfunction may alter elimination kinetics and augment toxicity.

Contraindications

Do not give to patients with demyelinating form of Charcot-Marie-Tooth syndrome.

Warnings/Precautions

➤*Administer IV only:* See the Warning box for more information.

➤*Acute uric acid nephropathy:* Acute uric acid nephropathy has occurred.

➤*CNS leukemia:* CNS leukemia has occurred in patients undergoing otherwise successful therapy with vincristine. If CNS leukemia is diagnosed, additional agents may be required, since this drug does not adequately cross the blood-brain barrier.

➤*Leukopenia or complicating infection:* In the presence of these conditions, administration of the next dose warrants careful consideration.

➤*Neuromuscular disease:* Pay particular attention to dosage and neurological side effects if administered to patients with preexisting neuromuscular disease or when other neurotoxic drugs are used.

➤*Eye contamination:* Eye contamination should be avoided with concentrations used clinically. If accidental contamination occurs, severe irritation (or, if drug was delivered under pressure, even corneal ulceration) may result. Wash eyes immediately and thoroughly.

➤*Pulmonary reactions:* Acute shortness of breath and severe bronchospasm have followed administration of vinca alkaloids, most frequently when the drug was used with mitomycin-C. The onset may be within minutes or several hours after the vinca is injected and may occur up to 2 weeks following the dose of mitomycin.

➤*Concomitant radiation therapy:* Do not give to patients receiving radiation therapy through ports that include the liver.

➤*Extravasation:* See Administration and Dosage for more information.

➤*Hypersensitivity reactions:* Hypersensitivity temporally related to vincristine therapy, has occurred. Refer to Management of Acute Hypersensitivity Reactions. See Adverse Reactions.

➤*Pregnancy: Category D.* Vincristine can cause fetal harm when administered to a pregnant woman. In several animal species, it induces teratogenic effects and embryolethality with doses that are nontoxic to the mother. There are no adequate and well controlled studies in pregnant women. If this drug is used during pregnancy or if the patient becomes pregnant while receiving it, apprise her of the potential hazard to the fetus. Advise women of childbearing potential to avoid becoming pregnant.

Fertility impairment – Reports of both males and females who received multiple agent chemotherapy that included vincristine indicate azoospermia and amenorrhea can occur in postpubertal patients. Recovery occurred many months after chemotherapy completion in some. It is much less likely to cause permanent azoospermia and amenorrhea in prepubertal patients.

➤*Lactation:* It is not known whether this drug is excreted in breast milk. Because of the potential for serious adverse reactions in nursing infants, decide whether to discontinue nursing or the drug, taking into account importance of the drug to the mother.

➤*Monitoring:* Dose-limiting clinical toxicity is manifested as neurotoxicity; clinical evaluation (history, physical examination) is necessary to detect need for dosage modification. Following vincristine, some patients may have a fall in WBC or platelet counts, particularly when previous therapy or the disease has reduced bone marrow function. Perform complete blood count before each dose. Acute serum uric acid elevation may occur during induction of remission in acute leukemia; thus determine such levels frequently during the first 3 to 4 treatment weeks or take appropriate measures to prevent uric acid nephropathy.

Drug Interactions

Vincristine Drug Interactions

Precipitant drug	Object drug[a]		Description
Vincristine	Digoxin	⬇	Combination chemotherapy (including vincristine) may decrease digoxin plasma levels and renal excretion.
L-asparaginase	Vincristine	⬆	Administering L-asparaginase first may reduce hepatic clearance of vincristine. Give vincristine 12 to 24 hrs before L-asparaginase to minimize toxicity.
Mitomycin	Vincristine	⬆	Acute pulmonary reactions may occur (see Precautions).
Vincristine	Phenytoin	⬇	Combination chemotherapy (including vincristine) may reduce phenytoin plasma levels, requiring increased dosage to maintain therapeutic plasma levels.

[a] ⬆ = object drug increased; ⬇ = object drug decreased.

Adverse Reactions

Adverse reactions are generally reversible and dose-related. With single weekly doses, leukopenia, neuritic pain, and constipation may occur and are usually of short duration (ie, less than 7 days). When dosage is reduced, reactions may lessen or disappear. They seem to increase when the drug is given in divided doses. Other adverse reactions, such as hair loss, sensory loss, paresthesia, difficulty in walking, slapping gait, loss of deep tendon reflexes, and muscle wasting may persist for at least as long as therapy is continued. Generalized sensorimotor dysfunction may become progressively more severe with continued treatment. Neuromuscular difficulties usually disappear by the sixth week after treatment is discontinued, but they may persist for prolonged periods in some patients. Hair regrowth may occur while maintenance therapy continues.

Vincristine is considered to have very low emetogenic potential (less than 10% incidence of emesis).

SIADH – The syndrome of inappropriate antidiuretic hormone secretion (SIADH), including high urinary sodium excretion in the presence of hyponatremia, occurs rarely. Renal or adrenal disease, hypotension, dehydration, azotemia, and clinical edema are absent. With fluid deprivation, hyponatremia and renal sodium loss improve.

➤*CNS:* Loss of deep-tendon reflexes, ataxia, footdrop, and paralysis have been seen with continued use. Cranial nerve manifestations, including isolated paresis or paralysis of muscles may occur; extraocular and laryngeal muscles are most commonly involved. Severe pain may occur in the jaw, pharynx, parotid gland, bones, back, and limbs. Myalgias have occurred. Reduced intestinal motility results in constipation. Convulsions, often with hypertension, have occurred in a few patients. Convulsions followed by coma have been seen in children. Frequently, there is a sequence in the development of neuropathy: Initially, sensory impairment and paresthesias, then neuritic pain may appear and later, motor difficulties. Neurotoxicity is dose-related and cumulative to where therapy must be stopped after a cumulative dose of 30 to 50 mg. It is reversible upon discontinuation, but recovery may take several months.

In one study, the administration of glutamic acid (500 mg 3 times daily) decreased the neurotoxicity induced by vincristine.

➤*GI:* Oral ulceration; abdominal cramps; nausea; vomiting; diarrhea; anorexia; intestinal necrosis or perforation.

Constipation – Constipation may take the form of upper colon impaction, and, on examination, the rectum may be empty. Colicky abdominal pain may

VINCRISTINE SULFATE (VCR; LCR) — INTRAVENOUS

accompany an empty rectum. A flat film of the abdomen demonstrates this condition. Cases respond to high enemas and laxatives. Use routine prophylaxis for constipation.

Paralytic ileus – Paralytic ileus that mimics the "surgical abdomen" may occur, particularly in young children. The ileus will reverse itself upon temporary discontinuation of vincristine and with symptomatic care.

➤*GU:* Polyuria; dysuria; urinary retention due to bladder atony. Discontinue other drugs known to cause urinary retention (particularly in the elderly), if possible, for the first few days following administration.

➤*Hematologic:* Serious bone marrow depression (usually not dose-limiting); anemia; leukopenia; thrombocytopenia. Thrombocytopenia, if present when therapy is begun, may improve before the appearance of marrow remission.

➤*Hypersensitivity:* Rare cases of allergic type reactions, such as anaphylaxis, rash and edema, that are temporally related to vincristine therapy have occurred in patients receiving vincristine as a part of multi-drug chemotherapy regimens (see Warnings).

➤*Ophthalmic:* Optic atrophy with blindness; transient cortical blindness; ptosis; diplopia; photophobia.

➤*Pulmonary:* See Warnings/Precautions for more information.

➤*Miscellaneous:* Hyper- or hypotension; weight loss; fever; alopecia; rash; headache.

Overdosage

➤*Symptoms:* Side effects are dose-related. After an overdose, expect exaggerated side effects. In children less than 13 years of age, death has occurred after doses 10 times those recommended; severe symptoms may occur with 3 to 4 mg/m². Adults may experience severe symptoms after single doses greater than or equal to 3 mg/m².

➤*Treatment:* Supportive care should include prevention of side effects resulting from SIADH (eg, fluid intake restriction; perhaps a diuretic affecting function of Henle's loop and distal tubule); phenobarbital (anticonvulsant); enemas or cathartics to prevent ileus (in some instances, GI tract decompression may be necessary); monitor cardiovascular system; determine daily blood counts to guide transfusion requirements.

Folinic acid, 100 mg IV every 3 hours for 24 hours, then every 6 hours for at least 48 hours, may help treat overdose. Folinic acid does not eliminate the need for supportive measures.

Most of an IV dose is excreted into the bile after rapid tissue binding. Hemodialysis is not likely to be helpful. Patients with liver disease sufficient to decrease biliary excretion may experience increased severity of side effects.

VINORELBINE TARTRATE

Rx	**Vinorelbine Tartrate** (GensiaSicor)	**Injection:** 10 mg/ml	In 1 and 5 mL vials.
Rx	**Navelbine** (Pierre Fabre Pharmaceuticals)		Preservative free. In 1 and 5 mL single-use vials.

VINORELBINE TARTRATE — INJECTION

WARNING

Vinorelbine tartrate injection should be administered under the supervision of a physician experienced in the use of cancer chemotherapeutic agents. This product is for intravenous (IV) use only. Intrathecal administration of other vinca alkaloids has resulted in death. Syringes containing this product should be labeled "Warning — for IV use only. Fatal if given intrathecally."

Severe granulocytopenia resulting in increased susceptibility to infection may occur. Granulocyte counts should be greater than or equal to 1000 cells/mm³ prior to the administration of vinorelbine tartrate. The dosage should be adjusted according to complete blood counts with differentials obtained on the day of treatment.

Caution – It is extremely important that the IV's needle or catheter be properly positioned before vinorelbine tartrate is injected. Administration of vinorelbine tartrate may result in extravasation causing local tissue necrosis or thrombophlebitis.

Indications

➤*Non-small cell lung cancer:* As a single agent or in combination with cisplatin for the first-line treatment of ambulatory patients with unresectable, advanced non-small cell lung cancer (NSCLC). In patients with stage IV NSCLC, vinorelbine tartrate is indicated as a single agent or in combination with cisplatin. In stage III NSCLC, vinorelbine tartrate is indicated in combination with cisplatin.

➤*Off-label uses:* Metastatic breast cancer; carcinoma of the uterine cervix; desmoid tumors and fibromatosis; advanced Kaposi sarcoma; ovarian cancer; cervical cancer; Hodgkin lymphoma; non-Hodgkin lymphoma.

Administration and Dosage

➤*Adults:*

Non-small cell lung cancer –

Single-agent therapy: 30 mg/m² administered IV over 6 to 10 minutes once weekly. In controlled trials, single-agent vinorelbine was given weekly until progression or dose-limiting toxicity.

Combination therapy with cisplatin:

• *Usual dosage* – 25 mg/m² administered IV once weekly in combination with cisplatin 100 mg/m² every 4 weeks.

• *Dosage adjustment* – Blood counts should be checked weekly to determine whether dose reductions of vinorelbine or cisplatin are necessary. In the Southwest Oncology Group (SWOG) study, most patients required a 50% dose reduction of vinorelbine at day 15 of each cycle and a 50% dose reduction of cisplatin by cycle 3.

• *Alternative dosage* – 30 mg/m² administered IV once weekly in combination with cisplatin 120 mg/m², given on days 1 and 29, then every 6 weeks.

Dosage adjustment: The dosage should be adjusted according to hematologic toxicity or hepatic insufficiency, whichever results in the lower dose for the corresponding starting dose of vinorelbine. (See Hepatic Function Impairment and Hematologic Toxicity.)

Discontinuation of therapy: If grade greater than or equal to 2 neurotoxicity develops, vinorelbine should be discontinued.

➤*Hepatic function impairment:* Vinorelbine should be administered with caution to patients with hepatic insufficiency. In patients who develop hyperbilirubinemia during treatment with vinorelbine, the dose should be adjusted for total bilirubin according to the following table:

Vinorelbine Dose Modification Based on Total Bilirubin

Total bilirubin (mg/dL)	Percentage of starting dose
≤ 2	100%
2.1 to 3	50%
> 3	25%

➤*Hematologic toxicity:* Granulocyte counts should be greater than or equal to 1,000 cells/mm³ prior to the administration of vinorelbine. Adjustments in the dosage of vinorelbine should be based on granulocyte counts obtained on the day of treatment according to the following table:

Vinorelbine Dose Adjustments Based on Granulocyte Counts

Granulocytes on day of treatment (cells/mm³)	Percentage of starting dose of vinorelbine injection
≥ 1,500	100%
1,000 to 1,499	50%
< 1,000	Do not administer. Repeat granulocyte count in 1 week. If 3 consecutive weekly doses are held because granulocyte count is < 1,000 cells/mm³, discontinue vinorelbine.
Note: For patients who, during treatment with vinorelbine, experienced fever or sepsis while granulocytopenic or had 2 consecutive weekly doses held due to granulocytopenia, subsequent doses of vinorelbine should be:	
≥ 1,500	75%
1,000 to 1,499	37.5%
< 1,000	See above

➤*Concurrent hematologic toxicity and hepatic function impairment:* In patients with both hematologic toxicity and hepatic function impairment, the lower of the doses based on the corresponding starting dose of vinorelbine determined from the previous information should be administered.

➤*Preparation for administration:* Vinorelbine is considered a cytotoxic agent. Follow safe handling procedures when preparing, administering, or dispensing vinorelbine.

Skin reactions may occur with accidental exposure. The use of gloves is recommended. If the solution of vinorelbine contacts the skin or mucosa, immediately wash the skin or mucosa thoroughly with soap and water. Severe irritation of the eye has been reported with accidental contamination of the eye with another vinca alkaloid. If this happens with vinorelbine, the eye should be flushed with water immediately and thoroughly.

Vinorelbine injection must be diluted in either a syringe or IV bag using 1 of the recommended solutions.

Syringe – The calculated dose of vinorelbine should be diluted to a concentration between 1.5 and 3 mg/mL. The following solutions may be used for dilution: dextrose 5% injection or sodium chloride 0.9% injection.

IV bag – The calculated dose of vinorelbine should be diluted to a concentration between 0.5 and 2 mg/mL. The following solutions may be used for dilution: dextrose 5% injection, sodium chloride 0.9% injection, sodium chloride 0.45% injection, dextrose 5% and sodium chloride 0.45% injection, Ringer's injection, Ringer's lactate injection.

➤*Administration:* Diluted vinorelbine must be administered IV over 6 to 10 minutes into the side port of a free-flowing IV closest to the IV bag fol-

VINORELBINE TARTRATE — INJECTION

lowed by flushing with at least 75 to 125 mL of dextrose 5% injection or sodium chloride 0.9% injection.

It is extremely important that the IV needle or catheter be properly positioned before any vinorelbine is injected. Leakage into surrounding tissue during IV administration may cause considerable irritation, local tissue necrosis, or thrombophlebitis. If extravasation occurs, the injection should be discontinued immediately and any remaining portion of the dose should then be introduced into another vein. Because there are no established guidelines for the treatment of extravasation injuries with vinorelbine, institutional guidelines may be used.

➤*Extravasation:* Administration of vinorelbine tartrate may result in extravasation causing local tissue necrosis or thrombophlebitis. If signs or symptoms of extravasation occur, stop the infusion immediately. If possible, withdraw 3 to 5 mL of blood to remove some of the drug. Remove the infusion needle. Administer hyaluronidase 150 units/mL solution within the first few minutes to 1 hour after extravasation. Cleanse the area with povidone-iodine. Reconstitute 1 mL vial of hyaluronidase. (Note: Some products do not require dilution.) Inject locally, subcutaneously or intradermally, using a 25-gauge needle or smaller. The dose is 150 units (1 mL) given as 5 injections (0.2 mL each). Application of warm compresses to the area for 15 minutes every 6 hours for 48 hours may be useful. Delineate the infiltrated area on the patient's skin with a felt-tip marker. Elevate for 48 hours above heart level using a sling or stockinette dressing with an observation window cut in the dressing. Avoid pressure or friction. Do not rub the area. Observe for signs of increased erythema, pain, or skin necrosis. If increased symptoms occur, consult a plastic surgeon. Ensure that no medication is given distally to extravasation site. After 48 hours, encourage the patient to use the extremity normally to promote full range of motion.

➤*Storage / Stability:* Store unopened vials under refrigeration at 2° to 8°C (36° to 46°F) in the carton. Protect from light. Do not freeze. Unopened vials are stable at temperatures up to 25°C (77°F) for up to 72 hours. Product should not be frozen.

Diluted vinorelbine may be used for up to 24 hours under normal room light when stored in polypropylene syringes or polyvinyl chloride bags at 5° to 30°C (41° to 86°F).

Discard vial within 6 hours of the initial needle puncture if opened within an ISO Class 5 biological safety cabinet, or within 1 hour of the initial needle puncture if opened outside of such an environment, based on the USP Chapter <797> standards.

Actions

➤*Pharmacology:* Vinorelbine is a vinca alkaloid that interferes with microtubule assembly. The vinca alkaloids are structurally similar compounds comprised of 2 multiringed units, vindoline and catharanthine. Unlike other vinca alkaloids, the catharanthine unit is the site of structural modification for vinorelbine. The antitumor activity of vinorelbine is thought to be due primarily to inhibition of mitosis at metaphase through its interaction with tubulin. Like other vinca alkaloids, vinorelbine may also interfere with: 1) amino acid, cyclic AMP, and glutathione metabolism, 2) calmodulin-dependent Ca^{++}-transport ATPase activity, 3) cellular respiration, and 4) nucleic acid and lipid biosynthesis. In intact tectal plates from mouse embryos, vinorelbine, vincristine, and vinblastine inhibited mitotic microtubule formation at the same concentration (2 mcM), inducing a blockade of cells at metaphase. Vincristine produced depolymerization of axonal microtubules at 5 mcM, but vinblastine and vinorelbine did not have this effect until concentrations of 30 mcM and 40 mcM, respectively. These data suggest relative selectivity of vinorelbine for mitotic microtubules.

➤*Pharmacokinetics:* The pharmacokinetics of vinorelbine were studied in 49 patients who received doses of 30 mg/m^2 in 4 clinical trials. Doses were administered by 15- to 20-minute constant-rate infusions. Following intravenous administration, vinorelbine concentration in plasma decays in a triphasic manner. The initial rapid decline primarily represents distribution of drug to peripheral compartments followed by metabolism and excretion of the drug during subsequent phases. The prolonged terminal phase is due to relatively slow efflux of vinorelbine from peripheral compartments. The terminal phase half-life averages 27.7 to 43.6 hours and the mean plasma clearance ranges from 0.97 to 1.26 L/hr per kg. Steady-state volume of distribution (V_{ss}) values range from 25.4 to 40.1 L/kg.

Vinorelbine demonstrated high binding to human platelets and lymphocytes. The free fraction was approximately 0.11 in pooled human plasma over a concentration range of 234 to 1169 ng/mL. The binding to plasma constituents in cancer patients ranged from 79.6% to 91.2%. Vinorelbine binding was not altered in the presence of cisplatin, 5-fluorouracil, or doxorubicin.

Vinorelbine undergoes substantial hepatic elimination in humans, with large amounts recovered in feces after intravenous administration to humans. Two metabolites of vinorelbine have been identified in human blood, plasma, and urine; vinorelbine N-oxide and deacetylvinorelbine. Deacetylvinorelbine has been demonstrated to be the primary metabolite of vinorelbine in humans, and has been shown to possess antitumor activity similar to vinorelbine. Therapeutic doses of vinorelbine (30 mg/m^2) yield very small, if any, quantifiable levels of either metabolite in blood or urine. The metabolism of vinca alkaloids has been shown to be mediated by hepatic cytochrome P450 isoenzymes in the CYP3A subfamily. This metabolic pathway may be impaired in patients with hepatic dysfunction or who are taking concomitant potent inhibitors of these isoenzymes. The effects of renal or hepatic dysfunction on the disposition of vinorelbine have not been assessed, but based on experience with other anticancer vinca alkaloids, dose adjustments are recommended for patients with impaired hepatic function.

The disposition of radiolabeled vinorelbine given intravenously was studied in a limited number of patients. Approximately 18% of the administered dose was recovered in the urine and 46% in the feces. Incomplete recovery in humans is consistent with results in animals where recovery is incomplete, even after prolonged sampling times. A separate study of the urinary excretion of vinorelbine using specific chromatographic analytical methodology showed that 10.9% ± 0.7% of a 30 mg/m^2 intravenous dose was excreted unchanged in the urine. Although the pharmacokinetics of vinorelbine are not influenced by the concurrent administration of cisplatin, the incidence of granulocytopenia with vinorelbine tartrate used in combination with cisplatin is significantly higher than with single-agent vinorelbine tartrate.

Contraindications

Pretreatment granulocyte counts less than 1000 cells/mm^3.

Warnings/Precautions

➤*Myelosuppression:* Patients treated with vinorelbine tartrate should be frequently monitored for myelosuppression both during and after therapy. Granulocytopenia is dose-limiting. Granulocyte nadirs occur between 7 and 10 days after dosing with granulocyte count recovery usually within the following 7 to 14 days. Complete blood counts with differentials should be performed and results reviewed prior to administering each dose of vinorelbine tartrate. Vinorelbine tartrate should not be administered to patients with granulocyte counts less than 1000 cells/mm^3. Patients developing severe granulocytopenia should be monitored carefully for evidence of infection or fever. Patients with a granulocyte count of greater than or equal to 1500 cells/mm^3 on treatment days should receive 100% starting dose of vinorelbine. Patients with a granulocyte count of 1000 to 1499 cells/mm^3 on treatment days should receive 50% starting dose of vinorelbine. Patients with a granulocyte count less than 1000 cells/mm^3 on treatment days should not receive vinorelbine; repeat the granulocyte count in 1 week and if 3 consecutive weekly doses are held because of the granulocyte less than 1000 cells/mm^3, discontinue vinorelbine.

➤*Pulmonary toxicity:* Reported cases of interstitial pulmonary changes and acute respiratory distress syndrome (ARDS), most of which were fatal, occurred in patients treated with single-agent vinorelbine tartrate. The mean time to onset of these symptoms after vinorelbine administration was 1 week (range 3 to 8 days). Patients with alterations in their baseline pulmonary symptoms or with new onset of dyspnea, cough, hypoxia, or other symptoms should be evaluated promptly.

➤*Discontinuation:* Most drug-related adverse events of vinorelbine tartrate are reversible. If severe adverse events occur, vinorelbine tartrate should be reduced in dosage or discontinued and appropriate corrective measures taken. Reinstitution of therapy with vinorelbine tartrate should be carried out with caution and alertness as to possible recurrence of toxicity.

➤*Bone marrow:* Vinorelbine tartrate should be used with extreme caution in patients whose bone marrow reserve may have been compromised by prior irradiation or chemotherapy, or whose marrow function is recovering from the effects of previous chemotherapy.

➤*Prior radiation therapy:* Administration to patients with prior radiation therapy may result in radiation recall reactions.

➤*Bronchospasm:* Acute shortness of breath and severe bronchospasm have been reported infrequently, following the administration of vinorelbine tartrate and other vinca alkaloids, most commonly when the vinca alkaloid was used in combination with mitomycin. These adverse events may require treatment with supplemental oxygen, bronchodilators, or corticosteroids, particularly when there is preexisting pulmonary dysfunction.

➤*Pulmonary toxicity:* See Warnings/Precautions for more information.

➤*GI:* Vinorelbine tartrate has been reported to cause severe constipation (eg, grade 3 to 4), paralytic ileus, intestinal obstruction, necrosis, or perforation. Some events have been fatal.

➤*Eye contact:* Care must be taken to avoid contamination of the eye with concentrations of vinorelbine tartrate used clinically. Severe irritation of the eye has been reported with accidental exposure to another vinca alkaloid. If exposure occurs, the eye should immediately be thoroughly flushed with water.

➤*Extravasation:* See Administration and Dosage for more information.

➤*Hepatic function impairment:* See Administration and Dosage for more information.

➤*Pregnancy: Category D.* Vinorelbine tartrate may cause fetal harm if administered to a pregnant woman. A single dose of vinorelbine has been shown to be embryo- or fetotoxic in mice and rabbits at doses of 9 mg/m^2 and 5.5 mg/m^2, respectively (one third and one sixth the human dose). At nonmaternotoxic doses, fetal weight was reduced and ossification was delayed. There are no studies in pregnant women. If vinorelbine tartrate is used during pregnancy, or if the patient becomes pregnant while receiving this drug, the patient should be apprised of the potential hazard to the fetus. Women of childbearing potential should be advised to avoid becoming pregnant during therapy with vinorelbine tartrate.

➤*Lactation:* It is not known whether the drug is excreted in human milk. Because many drugs are excreted in human milk and because of the potential for serious adverse reactions in nursing infants from vinorelbine tartrate, it is recommended that nursing be discontinued in women who are receiving therapy with vinorelbine tartrate.

➤*Children:* Safety and effectiveness in pediatric patients have not been established. Data from a single-arm study in 46 patients with recurrent solid malignant tumors, including rhabdomyosarcoma/undifferentiated sar-

VINORELBINE TARTRATE — INJECTION

coma, neuroblastoma, and CNS tumors, at doses similar to those used in adults, showed no meaningful clinical activity. Toxicities were similar to those reported in adults.

➤*Elderly:* Of the total number of patients in North American clinical studies of IV vinorelbine tartrate, approximately one third were 65 years of age or greater. No overall differences in effectiveness or safety were observed between these patients and younger patients. Other reported clinical experience has not identified differences in responses between the elderly and younger patients, but greater sensitivity of some older individuals cannot be ruled out.

➤*Lab test abnormalities:* Since dose-limiting clinical toxicity is the result of depression of the white blood cell count, it is imperative that complete blood counts with differentials be obtained and reviewed on the day of treatment prior to each dose of vinorelbine tartrate.

➤*Monitoring:* Patients with a history or preexisting neuropathy, regardless of etiology, should be monitored for new or worsening signs and symptoms of neuropathy while receiving vinorelbine tartrate.

Drug Interactions

➤*P-450 enzymes:* Caution should be exercised in patients concurrently taking drugs known to inhibit drug metabolism by hepatic cytochrome P450 isoenzymes in the CYP3A subfamily, or in patients with hepatic dysfunction. Concurrent administration of vinorelbine tartrate with an inhibitor of this metabolic pathway may cause an earlier onset or an increased severity of side effects.

Vinorelbine Drug Interactions

Precipitant drug	Object drug[a]		Description
Cisplatin	Vinorelbine	↑	Although the pharmacokinetics of vinorelbine are not influenced by the concurrent administration of cisplatin, the incidence of granulocytopenia with vinorelbine used in combination with cisplatin is significantly higher than with single-agent vinorelbine.
Mitomycin	Vinorelbine	↑	Acute pulmonary reactions have been reported with vinorelbine and other anticancer vinca alkaloids used in conjunction with mitomycin.
Paclitaxel	Vinorelbine	↑	Monitor for signs and symptoms of neuropathy for patients who receive vinorelbine and paclitaxel, either concomitantly or sequentially.

[a] ↑ = Object drug increased.

Adverse Reactions

Vinorelbine is considered to have very low emetogenic potential (less than 10% incidence of emesis).

Summary of Adverse Reactions in 365 Patients Receiving Single-Agent Vinorelbine Tartrate[a,b]

Adverse reaction	All patients (n = 365)	NSCLC (n = 143)
Bone marrow		
Granulocytopenia < 2000 cells/mm³	90%	80%
Granulocytopenia < 500 cells/mm³	36%	29%
Leukopenia < 4000 cells/mm³	92%	81%
Leukopenia < 1000 cells/mm³	15%	12%
Thrombocytopenia < 100,000 cells/mm³	5%	4%
Thrombocytopenia < 50,000 cells/mm³	1%	1%
Anemia < 11 g/dL	83%	77%
Anemia < 8 g/dL	9%	1%
Hospitalizations due to granulocytopenic complications	9%	8%

[a] None of the reported toxicities were influenced by age. Grade based on modified criteria from the National Cancer Institute.
[b] Patients with NSCLC had not received prior chemotherapy. The majority of the remaining patients had received prior chemotherapy.

Vinorelbine Adverse Reactions (%)

Adverse reaction	All grades		Grade 3		Grade 4	
	All patients	NSCLC	All patients	NSCLC	All patients	NSCLC
Clinical chemistry elevations						
Total bilirubin (n = 351)	13%	9%	4%	3%	3%	2%
AST (n = 346)	67%	54%	5%	2%	1%	1%
GI						
Nausea	44%	34%	2%	1%	0%	0%
Vomiting	20%	15%	2%	1%	0%	0%
Constipation	35%	29%	3%	2%	0%	0%
Diarrhea	17%	13%	1%	1%	0%	0%
Peripheral neuropathy[a]	25%	20%	1%	1%	< 1%	0%
Dyspnea	7%	3%	2%	2%	1%	0%
Alopecia	12%	12%	≤ 1%	1%	0%	0%
Miscellaneous						
Asthenia	36%	27%	7%	5%	0%	0%
Injection site reactions	28%	38%	2%	5%	0%	0%
Injection site pain	16%	13%	2%	1%	0%	0%
Phlebitis	7%	10%	< 1%	1%	0%	0%

[a] Incidence of paresthesia plus hypesthesia.

➤*Cardiovascular:* Chest pain was reported in 5% of patients. Most reports of chest pain were in patients who had either a history of cardiovascular disease or tumor within the chest. There have been rare reports of myocardial infarction.

➤*CNS:* Loss of deep tendon reflexes occurred in less than 5% of patients. The development of severe peripheral neuropathy was infrequent (1%) and generally reversible.

➤*Dermatologic:* Like other anticancer vinca alkaloids, vinorelbine tartrate is a moderate vesicant. Injection site reactions, including erythema, pain at injection site, and vein discoloration occurred in approximately one third of patients; 5% were severe. Chemical phlebitis along the vein proximal to the site of injection was reported in 10% of patients.

➤*GI:* Prophylactic administration of antiemetics was not routine in patients treated with single-agent vinorelbine tartrate. Due to the low incidence of severe nausea and vomiting with single-agent vinorelbine tartrate, the use of serotonin antagonists is generally not required.

➤*Hematologic:* Granulocytopenia was the major dose-limiting toxicity with vinorelbine tartrate. Dose adjustments are required for hematologic toxicity and hepatic insufficiency. Granulocytopenia was generally reversible and not cumulative over time. Granulocyte nadirs occurred 7 to 10 days after the dose, with granulocyte recovery usually within the following 7 to 14 days. Granulocytopenia resulted in hospitalizations for fever and/or sepsis in 8% of patients. Septic deaths occurred in approximately 1% of patients. Prophylactic hematologic growth factors have not been routinely used with vinorelbine tartrate. If medically necessary, growth factors may be administered at recommended doses no earlier than 24 hours after the administration of cytotoxic chemotherapy. Growth factors should not be administered in the period 24 hours before the administration of chemotherapy.

Whole blood or packed red blood cells were administered to 18% of patients who received vinorelbine tartrate.

➤*Hepatic:* Transient elevations of liver enzymes were reported without clinical symptoms.

➤*Pulmonary:* Shortness of breath was reported in 3% of patients; it was severe in 2%. Interstitial pulmonary changes were documented.

➤*Miscellaneous:* Fatigue occurred in 27% of patients. It was usually mild or moderate but tended to increase with cumulative dosing. Other toxicities that have been reported in less than 5% of patients include jaw pain, myalgia, arthralgia, and rash. Hemorrhagic cystitis and the syndrome of inappropriate ADH secretion were each reported in less than 1% of patients.

➤*Postmarketing:*

Cardiovascular – Hypertension, hypotension, vasodilation, tachycardia, and pulmonary edema have been reported.

CNS – Peripheral neurotoxicities such as, but not limited to, muscle weakness and disturbance of gait, have been observed in patients with and without prior symptoms. There may be increased potential for neurotoxicity in patients with preexisting neuropathy, regardless of etiology, who receive vinorelbine tartrate. Vestibular and auditory deficits have been observed with vinorelbine tartrate, usually when used in combination with cisplatin.

Dermatologic – Injection site reactions, including localized rash and urticaria, blister formation, and skin sloughing have been observed in clinical practice. Some of these reactions may be delayed in appearance.

GI – Dysphagia, mucositis, and pancreatitis have been reported.

Hematologic – Thromboembolic events including pulmonary embolus and deep venous thrombosis have been reported primarily in seriously ill and debilitated patients with known predisposing risk factors for these events.

VINORELBINE TARTRATE — INJECTION

Hypersensitivity – Systemic allergic reactions reported as anaphylaxis, pruritus, urticaria, and angioedema; flushing; and radiation recall events such as dermatitis and esophagitis have been reported.

Musculoskeletal – Headache has been reported, with and without other musculoskeletal aches and pains.

Pulmonary – Pneumonia has been reported.

Miscellaneous – Pain in tumor-containing tissue, back pain, and abdominal pain have been reported. Electrolyte abnormalities, including hyponatremia with or without the syndrome of inappropriate ADH secretion, have been reported in seriously ill and debilitated patients.

Overdosage

There is no known antidote for overdoses of vinorelbine tartrate. Overdoses involving quantities up to 10 times the recommended dose (30 mg/m^2) have been reported. The toxicities described were consistent with the adverse reactions, including paralytic ileus, stomatitis, and esophagitis. Bone marrow aplasia, sepsis, and paresis have also been reported. Fatalities have occurred following overdose of vinorelbine tartrate. If overdosage occurs, general supportive measures together with appropriate blood transfusions, growth factors, and antibiotics should be instituted as deemed necessary by the physician.

Patient Information

Patients should be informed that the major acute toxicities of vinorelbine tartrate are related to bone marrow toxicity, specifically granulocytopenia with increased susceptibility to infection. They should be advised to report fever or chills immediately. Women of childbearing potential should be advised to avoid becoming pregnant during treatment.

Patients should be advised to contact their physician if they experience increased shortness of breath, cough, or other new pulmonary symptoms, or if they experience symptoms of abdominal pain or constipation.

PACLITAXEL

Rx	**Paclitaxel** (SuperGen)	**Injection:** 6 mg/mL	In 5 and 16.7 mL multi-dose vials.[a]
Rx	**Onxol** (Zenith Goldline Pharmaceuticals)		In 5, 25, and 50 mL multi-dose vials.[b]
Rx	**Abraxane** (Abraxis Oncology)	**Powder for injection, lyophilized (albumin-bound):** 100 mg	In single-use vials.[c]

[a] With 527 mg/mL polyoxyethylated castor oil (*Cremophor EL*) and 49.7% dehydrated alcohol.
[b] With 527 mg/mL polyoxyl 35 castor oil and 49.7% dehydrated alcohol.
[c] With 900 mg human albumin.

PACLITAXEL — INJECTION

WARNING

Administer paclitaxel under the supervision of a health care provider experienced in the use of cancer chemotherapeutic agents. Appropriate management of complications is possible only when adequate diagnostic and treatment facilities are readily available.

Paclitaxel injection – Do not give paclitaxel therapy to patients with solid tumors who have baseline neutrophil counts of less than 1,500 cells/mm^3, and do not give to patients with AIDS-related Kaposi sarcoma if the baseline neutrophil count is less than 1,000 cells/mm^3. In order to monitor the occurrence of bone marrow suppression, primarily neutropenia, which may be severe and result in infection, perform frequent peripheral blood cell counts on all patients receiving paclitaxel.

Anaphylaxis and severe hypersensitivity reactions characterized by dyspnea and hypotension requiring treatment, angioedema, and generalized urticaria have occurred in 2% to 4% of patients receiving paclitaxel in clinical trials. Fatal reactions have occurred in patients despite premedication. Pretreat all patients with corticosteroids, diphenhydramine, and H_2 antagonists. Do not rechallenge patients who experience severe hypersensitivity reactions to paclitaxel with the drug.

Abraxane – Do not give paclitaxel therapy to patients with metastatic breast cancer who have baseline neutrophil counts of less than 1,500 cells/mm^3. In order to monitor the occurrence of bone marrow suppression, primarily neutropenia, which may be severe and result in infection, perform frequent peripheral blood cell counts on all patients receiving paclitaxel.

An albumin form of paclitaxel may substantially affect a drug's functional properties relative to those of drug in solution. Do not substitute for or with other paclitaxel formulations.

Indications

➤*Taxol*:

Ovarian cancer – As first-line and subsequent therapy for the treatment of advanced carcinoma of the ovary. As first-line therapy, paclitaxel is indicated in combination with cisplatin.

Breast cancer – Adjuvant treatment of node-positive breast cancer administered sequentially to standard doxorubicin-containing combination chemotherapy. In the clinical trial, there was an overall favorable effect on disease-free and overall survival in the total population of patients with receptor-positive and receptor-negative tumors, but the benefit has been specifically demonstrated by available data (median follow-up, 30 months) only in the patients with estrogen and progesterone receptor-negative tumors.

Indicated for the treatment of breast cancer after failure of combination chemotherapy for metastatic disease or relapse within 6 months of adjuvant chemotherapy. Previous therapy should have included an anthracycline unless clinically contraindicated.

Non-small cell lung cancer (NSCLC) – In combination with cisplatin, for the first-line treatment of NSCLC in patients who are not candidates for potentially curative surgery or radiation therapy.

AIDS-related Kaposi sarcoma – For the second-line treatment of AIDS-related Kaposi sarcoma.

➤*Onxol*:

Ovarian cancer – As subsequent therapy for the treatment of advanced carcinoma of the ovary.

Breast cancer – For the treatment of breast cancer after failure of combination chemotherapy for metastatic disease or relapse within 6 months of adjuvant chemotherapy. Previous therapy should have included an anthracycline unless clinically contraindicated.

➤*Abraxane*:

Breast cancer – For the treatment of breast cancer after failure of combination chemotherapy for metastatic disease or relapse within 6 months of adjuvant chemotherapy. Previous therapy should have included an anthracycline unless clinically contraindicated.

➤*Off-label uses:* Squamous cell head and neck cancer, small-cell lung cancer, bladder cancer, endometrial cancer, esophageal cancer, prostate cancer, gastric cancer, testicular cancer, and germ cell tumors. Paclitaxel has also been used for refractory leukemia and recurrent Wilms tumor in children. (See Administration and Dosage.)

Albumin-bound paclitaxel has been used for non–small cell lung cancer; metastatic melanoma; squamous cell cancer of the tongue, head and neck, or anal canal. (See Administration and Dosage).

Administration and Dosage

➤*General dosing considerations:* The dose of paclitaxel protein-bound particles is different from the dose of conventional paclitaxel.

The dose of paclitaxel protein-bound particles is calculated based on the paclitaxel content of the formulation (ie, paclitaxel 5 mg/mL).

➤*Adults:*

Abraxane –

Breast cancer:

• *Usual dosage* – 260 mg/m^2 administered IV over 30 minutes every 3 weeks. Indicated after failure of combination chemotherapy for metastatic breast cancer or relapse within 6 months of adjuvant chemotherapy. (See also Off-Label Dosing.)

• *Dosage adjustment* – According to the prescribing information, in patients who experience severe neutropenia (neutrophil counts less than 500 cells/mm^3 for 1 week or longer) or severe sensory neuropathy during paclitaxel protein-bound particles therapy, reduce the dosage to 220 mg/m^2 for subsequent courses of paclitaxel protein-bound particles. For recurrence of severe neutropenia or severe sensory neuropathy, make an additional dose reduction to 180 mg/m^2. For grade 3 sensory neuropathy, hold treatment until resolution to grade 1 or 2, followed by a dose reduction for all subsequent courses of paclitaxel protein-bound particles.

The following are additional recommendations from an additional reference. Delay subsequent courses of therapy until the absolute neutrophil count (ANC) is at least 1,500 cells/mm^3 and platelet count is at least 100,000 cells/mm^3. Monitor blood counts at least weekly during therapy. If severe neutropenia occurs (ANC below 500 cells/mm^3 for 1 week or more), reduce dose for subsequent cycles, as shown in the following table.

Adverse Effects Requiring Paclitaxel Protein-Bound Particles Dosage Modification

Adverse effect and grade of severity[a]	Dosage adjustment[b]
Hematologic toxicity:[a]	
NCI Toxicity grade 2 (ANC 1,000 to 1,500 cells/mm^3, or platelets 50,000 to 100,000 cells/mm^3)	Withhold therapy. When ANC at least 1,500 cells/mm^3 and platelets at least 100,000 cells/mm^3, resume therapy at usual dose.
NCI Toxicity grade 3 (ANC 500 to 1,000 cells/mm^3, or platelets 25,000 to 50,000 cells/mm^3)	Withhold therapy. When ANC at least 1,500 cells/mm^3 and platelets at least 100,000 cells/mm^3, resume therapy at usual dose.

PACLITAXEL — INJECTION

Adverse Effects Requiring Paclitaxel Protein-Bound Particles Dosage Modification	
Adverse effect and grade of severity[a]	Dosage adjustment[b]
NCI Toxicity grade 4 (ANC less than 500 cells/mm³, or platelets less than 25,000 cells/mm³)	•ANC remains below 500 cells/mm³ for less than 1 week: Withhold therapy. When ANC at least 1,500 cells/mm³ and platelets at least 100,000 cells/mm³, resume therapy at usual dose. •ANC remains below 500 cells/mm³ for 1 week or more, first occurrence: Withhold therapy. When ANC at least 1,500 cells/mm³ and platelets at least 100,000 cells/mm³, decrease dose to 220 mg/m²/course for all subsequent courses and resume therapy. •ANC remains below 500 cells/mm³ for 1 week or more, second occurrence: Withhold therapy. When ANC at least 1,500 cells/mm³ and platelets at least 100,000 cells/mm³, decrease dose to 180 mg/m²/course for all subsequent courses and resume therapy.
Sensory neuropathy:[a]	
NCI Toxicity grade 3 (sensory alteration or paresthesia; interferes with activities of daily living)	•First occurrence: Withhold therapy. When toxicity resolves to grade 1 to 2, decrease dose to 220 mg/m²/course for all subsequent courses and resume therapy. •Second occurrence: Withhold therapy. When toxicity resolves to grade 1 to 2, decrease dose to 180 mg/m²/course for all subsequent courses and resume therapy.
NCI Toxicity grade 4 (disabling sensory alteration or paresthesia)	Permanently discontinue therapy.

[a] Refer to Common Toxicity Criteria for additional information on toxicity grading.
[b] All dosage adjustments are based on the labeled initial dose of 260 mg/m²/cycle.

Onxol –

Breast cancer:

• *Usual dosage* – After failure of initial chemotherapy for metastatic disease or relapse within 6 months of adjuvant chemotherapy, paclitaxel 175 mg/m² administered IV over 3 hours every 3 weeks has been shown to be effective.

• *Repeat courses* – Do not repeat courses of paclitaxel until the neutrophil count is at least 1,500 cells/mm³ and the platelet count is at least 100,000 cells/mm³.

• *Dose reduction* – In patients who experience severe neutropenia (neutrophil counts less than 500 cells/mm³ for 1 week or longer) or severe peripheral neuropathy during paclitaxel, reduce the dosage 20% for subsequent courses of paclitaxel. The incidence of neurotoxicity and the severity of neutropenia increase with dose.

Ovarian cancer:

• *Usual dosage* – In patients previously treated with chemotherapy for carcinoma of the ovary, paclitaxel has been used at several doses and schedules; however, the optimal regimen is not yet clear. One regimen is paclitaxel 135 or 175 mg/m² administered IV over 3 hours every 3 weeks.

• *Repeat courses* – Do not repeat courses of paclitaxel until the neutrophil count is at least 1,500 cells/mm³ and the platelet count is at least 100,000 cells/mm³.

• *Dose reduction* – In patients who experience severe neutropenia (neutrophil counts less than 500 cells/mm³ for 1 week or longer) or severe peripheral neuropathy during paclitaxel, reduce the dosage 20% for subsequent courses of paclitaxel. The incidence of neurotoxicity and the severity of neutropenia increase with dose.

Taxol –

AIDS-related Kaposi sarcoma: Do not give to patients with AIDS-related Kaposi sarcoma if the baseline or subsequent neutrophil count is less than 1,000 cells/mm³.

• *Usual dosage* – 135 mg/m² given IV over 3 hours once every 3 weeks or at a dose of 100 mg/m² given IV over 3 hours once every 2 weeks is recommended (dose intensity 45 to 50 mg/m²/wk). In the 2 clinical trials evaluating these schedules, the former schedule (135 mg/m² every 3 weeks) was more toxic than the latter. In addition, all patients with low performance status were treated with the latter schedule (100 mg/m² every 2 weeks).

• *Dosage adjustment* – Based upon the immunosuppression in patients with advanced HIV disease, the following modifications are recommended in these patients:

1.) Reduce the dose of dexamethasone (as 1 of the 3 premedication drugs) to 10 mg orally (instead of 20 mg orally).
2.) Initiate or repeat treatment with paclitaxel only if the neutrophil count is at least 1,000 cells/mm³.
3.) Reduce the dose of subsequent courses of paclitaxel 20% for patients who experience severe neutropenia (neutrophil less than 500 cells/mm³ for a week or longer).
4.) Initiate concomitant hematopoietic growth factor (G-CSF) as clinically indicated.

In patients who experience severe neutropenia (neutrophil counts less than 500 cells/mm³ for 1 week or longer) or severe peripheral neuropathy during paclitaxel, reduce the dosage 20% for subsequent courses of paclitaxel. The incidence of neurotoxicity and the severity of neutropenia increase with dose.

Breast cancer:

• *Adjuvant treatment* – For the adjuvant treatment of node-positive breast cancer, paclitaxel 175 mg/m² IV over 3 hours once every 3 weeks for 4 courses administered sequentially to doxorubicin-containing combination chemotherapy. The clinical trial used 4 courses of doxorubicin and cyclophosphamide.

• *After treatment failure or relapse* – After failure of initial chemotherapy for metastatic disease or relapse within 6 months of adjuvant chemotherapy, paclitaxel 175 mg/m² administered IV over 3 hours once every 3 weeks has been shown to be effective.

• *Repeated course* – Do not repeat courses until neutrophil count is at least 1,500 cells/mm³ and the platelet count is at least 100,000 cells/mm³.

• *Dose reduction* – In patients who experience severe neutropenia (neutrophil counts less than 500 cells/mm³ for 1 week or longer) or severe peripheral neuropathy during paclitaxel, reduce the dosage 20% for subsequent courses of paclitaxel. The incidence of neurotoxicity and the severity of neutropenia increase with dose.

Non–small cell lung cancer:

• *Usual dosage* – Given every 3 weeks, paclitaxel 135 mg/m² is administered IV over 24 hours followed by cisplatin 75 mg/m².

• *Repeated course* – Do not repeat courses until neutrophil count is at least 1,500 cells/mm³ and the platelet count is at least 100,000 cells/mm³.

• *Dose reduction* – In patients who experience severe neutropenia (neutrophil counts less than 500 cells/mm³ for 1 week or longer) or severe peripheral neuropathy during paclitaxel, reduce the dosage 20% for subsequent courses of paclitaxel. The incidence of neurotoxicity and the severity of neutropenia increase with dose.

Ovarian cancer:

• *Previously untreated* – For previously untreated patients, 1 of the following recommended regimens may be given every 3 weeks. In selecting the appropriate regimen, consider differences in toxicities.

1.) Paclitaxel 175 mg/m² administered IV over 3 hours followed by cisplatin 75 mg/m².
2.) Paclitaxel 135 mg/m² administered IV over 24 hours followed by cisplatin 75 mg/m².

• *Previously treated* – In patients previously treated with chemotherapy, paclitaxel has been used at several doses and schedules; however, the optimal regimen is not yet clear. One regimen is paclitaxel 135 or 175 mg/m² administered IV over 3 hours once every 3 weeks.

• *Repeated course* – Do not repeat courses until neutrophil count is at least 1,500 cells/mm³ and the platelet count is at least 100,000 cells/mm³.

• *Dose reduction* – In patients who experience severe neutropenia (neutrophil counts less than 500 cells/mm³ for 1 week or longer) or severe peripheral neuropathy during paclitaxel, reduce the dosage 20% for subsequent courses of paclitaxel. The incidence of neurotoxicity and the severity of neutropenia increase with dose.

Off-label dosing –

Abraxane:

• *Breast cancer* – An alternative dosage regimen is 100 to 150 mg/m² IV once weekly for 3 weeks of a 4-week cycle.

• *Metastatic melanoma –*

Previously treated patients: 100 mg/m² IV once weekly for 3 weeks of a 4-week cycle, given alone or combined with other antineoplastic agents.

Treatment-naive patients: 100 to 150 mg/m² IV once weekly for 3 weeks of a 4-week cycle, given alone or combined with other antineoplastic agents.

• *Non–small cell lung cancer –*

Single agent: 260 mg/m² IV on day 1 every 3 weeks.

Alternative dosage: 125 mg/m² IV once weekly for 3 weeks of a 4-week cycle.

• *Squamous cell tongue cancer* – 150 mg/m² intraarterially on day 1 every 3 weeks. Given as a single agent.

➤*Children:*

Off-label dosing –

Onxol/Taxol:

• *Refractory leukemia* – 250 to 360 mg/m² by IV infusion over 24 hours once every 2 weeks. Follow dosage adjustment guidelines recommended for adults.

• *Wilms tumor* – 250 to 350 mg/m² by IV infusion over 24 hours once every 3 weeks. Follow dosage adjustment guidelines recommended for adults.

➤*Hepatic function impairment:*

Abraxane – Dosage reduction is necessary in patients with hepatic impairment (eg, serum bilirubin greater than 1.25 times the upper limit of normal [ULN]), as shown in the following table.

PACLITAXEL — INJECTION

Albumin-Bound Paclitaxel Dosage Adjustment in Hepatic Dysfunction	
Hepatic function	Recommended dose[a]
Moderate: serum bilirubin 1.26 to 2 times the ULN, and AST 1 to 10 times the ULN	200 mg/m²/dose
Severe: serum bilirubin 2.01 to 5 times the ULN, and AST 1 to 10 times the ULN	130 mg/m²/dose initially; may increase to 200 mg/m²/dose as tolerated
Very severe: serum bilirubin > 5 times the ULN, or AST > 10 times the ULN	Do not administer

[a] All dosage adjustments are based on the labeled initial dose of 260 mg/m²/cycle.

Onxol – There is evidence that the toxicity of paclitaxel is enhanced in patients with elevated liver enzymes. Exercise caution when administering paclitaxel to patients with moderate to severe hepatic impairment and consider dose adjustments.

Taxol – Patients with hepatic impairment may be at increased risk of toxicity, particularly grade 3 to 4 myelosuppression. Recommendations for dosage adjustment for the first course of therapy are shown in the following table for 3- and 24-hour infusions. Base further dose reduction in subsequent courses on individual tolerance. Monitor patients closely for the development of profound myelosuppression.

Paclitaxel Dosing Recommendations in Patients With Hepatic Impairment[a]			
Transaminase levels		Bilirubin levels[b]	Recommended paclitaxel dose[c]
24-hour infusion			
< 2 × ULN	and	≤ 1.5 mg/dL	135 mg/m²
2 to < 10 × ULN	and	≤ 1.5 mg/dL	100 mg/m²
< 10 × ULN	and	1.6 to 7.5 mg/dL	50 mg/m²
≥ 10 × ULN	or	> 7.5 mg/dL	Not recommended
3-hour infusion			
< 10 × ULN	and	≤ 1.25 × ULN	175 mg/m²
< 10 × ULN	and	1.26 to 2 × ULN	135 mg/m²
< 10 × ULN	and	2.01 to 5 × ULN	90 mg/m²
≥ 10 × ULN	or	> 5 × ULN	Not recommended

[a] These recommendations are based on doses for patients without hepatic impairment of 135 mg/m² over 24 hours or 175 mg/m² over 3 hours; data are not available to make dose adjustment recommendations for other regimens (eg, for AIDS-related Kaposi sarcoma).

[b] Differences in criteria for bilirubin levels between the 3- and 24-hour infusion are caused by differences in clinical trial design.

[c] Dose recommendations are for the first course of therapy; base further dose reduction in subsequent courses on individual tolerance.

➤*Premedication:*

Onxol/Taxol – Premedicate all patients prior to paclitaxel administration to prevent severe hypersensitivity reactions.

- Dexamethasone 20 mg orally or IV 12 hours and 6 hours before paclitaxel administration. Reduce each dexamethasone dose to 10 mg in AIDS patients. Some clinicians give a third dexamethasone dose immediately prior to paclitaxel. An alternative regimen is to give a single IV dose 30 minutes prior to the paclitaxel dose.
- Diphenhydramine 50 mg IV 30 to 60 minutes before paclitaxel.
- Cimetidine 300 mg, ranitidine 50 mg, or famotidine 20 mg IV 30 to 60 minutes before paclitaxel administration.

➤*Preparation for administration:* Paclitaxel is considered a cytotoxic agent. Follow safe handling procedures when preparing, administering, or dispensing paclitaxel.

Use gloves. If paclitaxel solution contacts the skin, wash the skin immediately and thoroughly with soap and water. After topical exposure, adverse reactions have included burning, redness, and tingling. If paclitaxel contacts mucous membranes, thoroughly flush the membranes with water. Upon inhalation, burning eyes, chest pain, dyspnea, nausea, and sore throat have been reported.

Onxol/Taxol – Prior to infusion, dilute paclitaxel concentrate in sodium chloride 0.9% injection; dextrose 5% injection; dextrose 5% and sodium chloride 0.9% injection; or dextrose 5% in Ringer's injection to a final concentration of 0.3 to 1.2 mg/mL. The solutions are physically and chemically stable for up to 27 hours at ambient temperature (approximately 25°C [77°F]) and room lighting conditions.

Upon preparation, solutions may show haziness, which is attributed to the formulation vehicle. No significant losses in potency have been noted following simulated delivery of the solution through IV tubing containing an in-line (0.22 micron) filter.

Abraxane – Paclitaxel protein-bound particles are supplied as a sterile lyophilized powder for reconstitution before use. To avoid errors, read entire preparation instructions prior to reconstitution.

Reconstitute each vial by slowly (over a minimum of 1 minute) injecting 20 mL of sodium chloride 0.9% injection, using the sterile syringe to direct the solution flow onto the inside wall of the vial. Do not inject the sodium chloride 0.9% injection directly onto the lyophilized cake, as this will result in foaming. Allow the vial to sit for a minimum of 5 minutes to ensure proper wetting of the lyophilized cake/powder. Gently swirl and/or invert the vial slowly for at least 2 minutes until complete dissolution of any cake/powder occurs. Avoid generation of foam. If foaming or clumping occurs, let solution sit for at least 15 minutes until foam subsides.

The reconstituted sample should be milky and homogenous without visible particulates. If particulates or settling are visible, gently invert the vial again to ensure complete resuspension prior to use.

The use of an in-line (0.22 micron) filter is not recommended with *Abraxane*.

➤*Administration:* Given the possibility of extravasation, it is advisable to closely monitor the infusion site for possible infiltration during drug administration. (See Extravasation).

Onxol/Taxol – Premedication is required. (See Premedication.)

Give by IV infusion over 1 to 24 hours via non–polyvinyl chloride (PVC)-containing administration sets (eg, low-adsorption tubing, polyethylene-lined tubing).

Administer paclitaxel through an in-line filter with a microporous membrane not more than 0.22 microns. Use of filter devices, such as *IVEX-2* filters that incorporate short inlet and outlet PVC-coated tubing, has not resulted in significant leaching of di-(2-ethylhexyl)phthalate (DEHP).

Do not use the *Chemo Dispensing Pin* device or similar devices with spikes with vials of paclitaxel because they can cause the stopper to collapse, resulting in loss of sterile integrity of the paclitaxel solution.

PVC equipment: Contact of the undiluted paclitaxel concentrate with plasticized PVC equipment or devices used to prepare solutions for infusion is not recommended. Data collected for the presence of the extractable plasticizer DEHP show that levels increase with time and concentration when dilutions are prepared in PVC containers. In order to minimize patient exposure to the plasticizer DEHP, which may be leached from PVC infusion bags or sets, store diluted paclitaxel solutions in bottles (glass, polypropylene) or plastic bags (polypropylene, polyolefin) and administer through polyethylene-lined administration sets.

Abraxane – Each milliliter of the reconstituted formulation will contain paclitaxel 5 mg/mL.

Calculate the exact total dosing volume of 5 mg/mL suspension required for the patient:

$$\text{Dosing volume (mL)} = \frac{\text{total dose (mg)}}{5 \text{ (mg/mL)}}$$

For IV or intraarterial infusion over 30 minutes. Do not filter.

PVC equipment: Inject the appropriate amount of reconstituted paclitaxel into an empty, sterile, PVC-type IV bag. Albumin-bound paclitaxel does not contain *Cremophor EL* and is not expected to leach DEHP from PVC infusion sets or bags. Unlike with conventional paclitaxel, it is not necessary to use glass, polypropylene, or polyolefin containers and polyethylene-lined administration sets for preparation, storage, and administration of albumin-bound paclitaxel. The use of an in-line filter is not recommended.

➤*Extravasation:* It is unknown whether albumin-bound paclitaxel is a vesicant or an irritant; mild injection-site reactions have been reported.

Paclitaxel is considered a vesicant. If signs or symptoms of extravasation occur, stop the infusion immediately. If possible, withdraw 3 to 5 mL of blood to remove some of the drug. Remove the infusion needle. Ice compresses may be applied to the site for 15 minutes every 6 hours for 24 hours. Delineate the infiltrated area on the patient's skin with a felt tip marker. Elevate for 48 hours above heart level using a sling or stockinette dressing with an observation window cut in the dressing. Avoid pressure or friction. Do not rub the area. Observe for signs of increased erythema, pain, or skin necrosis. If increased symptoms occur, consult a plastic surgeon. After 48 hours, encourage the patient to use the extremity normally to promote full range of motion.

➤*Admixture compatibility:* One study indicates compatibility in dextrose 5% injection or normal saline at 0.1 and 1 mg/mL concentrations, at 4°, 22°, or 32°C (39.2°, 71.6°, or 89.6°F) for 3 days. Small, needle-like crystals form after 3 days.

Another study showed admixtures of paclitaxel 0.3 and 1.2 mg/mL with carboplatin 2 mg/mL in normal saline injection or dextrose 5% injection were stable for at least 24 hours at 4°, 23°, and 32°C (39.2°, 71.6°, or 89.6°F). Paclitaxel 0.2 mg/mL mixed with cisplatin 0.2 mg/mL in normal saline injection showed unacceptable cisplatin loss in 24 hours. Utility time of paclitaxel mixed with carboplatin or cisplatin is limited due to paclitaxel microcrystalline precipitation and decomposition of carboplatin and cisplatin.

Paclitaxel 0.3 or 1.2 mg/mL combined with doxorubicin 200 mcg/mL in normal saline injection or dextrose 5% injection was found to be stable for at least 24 hours at temperatures of 4°, 23°, and 32°C (39.2°, 71.6°, or 89.6°F). Microcrystalline precipitation of paclitaxel developed within 3 days.

➤*Storage/Stability:*

Onxol/Taxol – Store between 20° and 25°C (68° and 77°F) in the original package. Upon refrigeration, components in the paclitaxel vial may precipitate, but will redissolve upon reaching room temperature with little or no agitation. There is no impact on product quality under these circumstances. If the solution remains cloudy or if an insoluble precipitate is noted, discard the vial. Solutions for infusion prepared as recommended are stable at ambient temperature (approximately 25°C [77°F]) and lighting conditions for up to 27 hours.

Multiple-dose vials may be used for up to 28 days after the initial needle puncture, based on the USP Chapter <797> standards.

Abraxane: Store between 20° and 25°C (68° and 77°F) in the original package. Use reconstituted paclitaxel protein-bound particles immediately; may

PACLITAXEL — INJECTION

be refrigerated at 2° to 8°C (36° to 46°F) for a maximum of 8 hours if necessary. If not used immediately, place each vial of reconstituted suspension in the original carton to protect it from bright light. Discard any unused portion. Neither freezing nor refrigeration adversely affects the stability of the product. Some settling of the reconstituted suspension may occur. Ensure complete resuspension by mild agitation before use. Discard the reconstituted suspension if precipitates are observed. The suspension for infusion prepared as recommended in an infusion bag is stable at ambient temperature (approximately 25°C [77°F]) and lighting conditions for up to 8 hours.

Actions

➤*Pharmacology:* Paclitaxel is a novel antimicrotubule agent that promotes the assembly of microtubules from tubulin dimers and stabilizes microtubules by preventing depolymerization. This stability results in the inhibition of the normal dynamic reorganization of the microtubule network that is essential for vital interphase and mitotic cellular functions. Paclitaxel induces abnormal arrays or "bundles" of microtubules throughout the cell cycle and multiple asters of microtubules during mitosis.

➤*Pharmacokinetics:* The pharmacokinetics of paclitaxel also were evaluated in adult cancer patients who received single doses of 15 to 135 mg/m² given by 1-hour infusions (n = 15), 30 to 275 mg/m² given by 6-hour infusions (n = 36), and 200 to 275 mg/m² given by 24-hour infusions (n = 54) in phase 1 and 2 studies. Values for total body clearance (CL_T) and volume of distribution were consistent with the findings in the phase 3 study. The pharmacokinetics of paclitaxel in patients with AIDS-related Kaposi sarcoma have not been studied.

Summary of Paclitaxel Pharmacokinetic Parameters (Mean Values)[a]

Dose (mg/m²)	Infusion duration (h)	Patients (n)	C_{max} (ng/mL)	$AUC_{(0-\infty)}$ (ng•h/mL)	t½ (h)	CL_T (L/h/m²)
135	24	2	195	6,300	52.7	21.7
175	24	4	365	7,993	15.7	23.8
135	3	7	2,170	7,952	13.1	17.7
175	3	5	3,650	15,007	20.2	12.2

[a] C_{max}, $AUC_{(0-\infty)}$, and CL_T.

Absorption/Distribution – Following IV administration of paclitaxel, paclitaxel plasma concentrations declined in a biphasic manner. The initial rapid decline represents distribution to the peripheral compartment and elimination of the drug. The later phase is due, in part, to a relatively slow efflux of paclitaxel from the peripheral compartment.

It appeared that with the 24-hour infusion of paclitaxel, a 30% increase in dose (135 mg/m² versus 175 mg/m²) increased the maximum plasma concentration (C_{max}) by 87%, whereas the area under the plasma concentration-time curve [$AUC_{(0-\infty)}$] remained proportional. However, with a 3-hour infusion for a 30% increase in dose, the C_{max} and $AUC_{(0-\infty)}$ were increased by 68% and 89%, respectively. The mean apparent volume of distribution at steady state with the 24-hour infusion of paclitaxel ranged from 227 to 688 L/m², indicating extensive extravascular distribution or tissue binding of paclitaxel.

In vitro studies of binding to human serum proteins using paclitaxel concentrations ranging from 0.1 to 50 mcg/mL indicate that between 89% to 98% of drug is bound; the presence of cimetidine, ranitidine, dexamethasone, or diphenhydramine did not affect protein binding of paclitaxel.

Metabolism – In vitro studies with human liver microsomes and tissue slices showed that paclitaxel was metabolized primarily to 6α-hydroxypaclitaxel by the cytochrome P-450 isozyme CYP2C8; and to 2 minor metabolites, 3′-p-hydroxypaclitaxel and 6α, 3′-p-dihydroxypaclitaxel, by CYP3A4. In vitro, the metabolism of paclitaxel to 6α-hydroxypaclitaxel was inhibited by a number of agents (eg, ketoconazole, verapamil, diazepam, quinidine, dexamethasone, cyclosporine, teniposide, etoposide, and vincristine), but the concentrations used exceeded those found in vivo following normal therapeutic doses. Testosterone, 17α-ethinyl estradiol, retinoic acid, and quercetin, a specific inhibitor of CYP2C8, also inhibited the formation of 6α-hydroxypaclitaxel in vitro. The pharmacokinetics of paclitaxel may also be altered in vivo as a result of interactions with compounds that are substrates, inducers, or inhibitors of CYP2C8 or CYP3A4.

Excretion – After IV administration of 15 to 275 mg/m² doses of paclitaxel as 1-, 6-, or 24-hour infusions, mean values for cumulative urinary recovery of unchanged drug ranged from 1.3% to 12.6% of the dose, indicating extensive nonrenal clearance. In 5 patients administered a 225 or 250 mg/m² dose of radiolabeled paclitaxel as a 3-hour infusion, a mean of 71% of the radioactivity was excreted in the feces in 120 hours, and 14% was recovered in the urine. Total recovery of radioactivity ranged from 56% to 101% of the dose. Paclitaxel represented a mean of 5% of the administered radioactivity recovered in the feces, while metabolites, primarily 6α-hydroxypaclitaxel, accounted for the balance.

Special populations –

Hepatic function impairment: The disposition and toxicity of a paclitaxel 3-hour infusion were evaluated in 35 patients with varying degrees of hepatic function. Relative to patients with normal bilirubin, plasma paclitaxel exposure in patients with abnormal serum bilirubin less than or equal to 2 times ULN administered 175 mg/m² was increased, but with no apparent increase in the frequency or severity of toxicity. In 5 patients with serum total bilirubin greater than 2 times ULN, there was a statistically nonsignificant higher incidence of severe myelosuppression, even at a reduced dose (110 mg/m²), but no observed increase in plasma exposure.

Abraxane – The pharmacokinetics of total paclitaxel following 30- and 180-minute infusions of paclitaxel protein-bound particles at dose levels of 80 to 375 mg/m² were determined in clinical studies. Following IV administration of paclitaxel protein-bound particles, paclitaxel plasma concentrations declined in a biphasic manner, the initial rapid decline representing distribution to the peripheral compartment and the slower second phase representing drug elimination.

Absorption/Distribution: The terminal half-life was approximately 27 hours.

The drug exposure (AUCs) was dose proportional over 80 to 375 mg/m² and the pharmacokinetics of paclitaxel for paclitaxel protein-bound particles were independent of the duration of administration. At the recommended paclitaxel protein-bound particles clinical dose, 260 mg/m², the mean maximum concentration of paclitaxel, which occurred at the end of the infusion, was 18,741 ng/mL. The mean total clearance was 15 L/h/m². The mean volume of distribution was 632 L/m²; the large volume of distribution indicates extensive extravascular distribution and/or tissue binding of paclitaxel.

In vitro studies of binding to human serum proteins using paclitaxel concentrations ranging from 0.1 to 50 mcg/mL indicate that between 89% to 98% of drug is bound; the presence of cimetidine, ranitidine, dexamethasone, or diphenhydramine did not affect protein binding of paclitaxel.

The pharmacokinetic data of paclitaxel protein-bound particles 260 mg/m² administered over 30 minutes was compared with the pharmacokinetics of paclitaxel 175 mg/m² injection over 3 hours. The clearance of paclitaxel protein-bound particles was larger (43%) than the clearance of paclitaxel injection, and the volume of distribution of paclitaxel protein-bound particles was also higher (53%). Differences in C_{max} and C_{max} corrected for dose reflected differences in total dose and rate of infusion. There were no differences in terminal half-lives.

Metabolism: In vitro studies with human liver microsomes and tissue slices showed that paclitaxel was metabolized primarily to 6α-hydroxypaclitaxel by the cytochrome P-450 isozyme CYP2C8; and to 2 minor metabolites, 3′-p-hydroxypaclitaxel and 6α, 3′-p-dihydroxypaclitaxel, by CYP3A4. In vitro, the metabolism of paclitaxel to 6α-hydroxypaclitaxel was inhibited by a number of agents (eg, ketoconazole, verapamil, diazepam, quinidine, dexamethasone, cyclosporine, teniposide, etoposide, vincristine), but the concentrations used exceeded those found in vivo following normal therapeutic doses. Testosterone, 17α-ethinyl estradiol, retinoic acid, and quercetin, a specific inhibitor of CYP2C8, also inhibited the formation of 6α-hydroxypaclitaxel in vitro. The pharmacokinetics of paclitaxel also may be altered in vivo as a result of interactions with compounds that are substrates, inducers, or inhibitors of CYP2C8 or CYP3A4. The effect of renal or hepatic dysfunction on the disposition of paclitaxel protein-bound particles have not been investigated.

Excretion: After a 30-minute infusion of 260 mg/m² doses of paclitaxel protein-bound particles, the mean values for cumulative urinary recovery of unchanged drug (4%) indicated extensive nonrenal clearance. Less than 1% of the total administered dose was excreted in urine as the metabolites 6α-hydroxypaclitaxel and 3′-*p*-hydroxypaclitaxel. Fecal excretion was approximately 20% of the total dose administered.

Contraindications

➤*Taxol/Onxol*: Paclitaxel is contraindicated in patients who have a history of hypersensitivity reactions with paclitaxel or other drugs formulated in polyoxyethylated castor oil (*Cremophor EL*).

See the Warning box for more information.

➤*Abraxane*: See the Warning box for more information.

Warnings/Precautions

➤*Bone marrow suppression:* Bone marrow suppression (primarily neutropenia) is dose dependent and is a dose-limiting toxicity. Neutrophil nadirs occurred at a median of 11 days. Do not administer paclitaxel to patients with baseline neutrophil counts of less than 1,500 cells/mm³ (less than 1,000 cells/mm³ for patients with Kaposi's sarcoma). Institute frequent monitoring of blood counts during paclitaxel treatment. Do not retreat patients with subsequent cycles of paclitaxel until neutrophils recover to a level greater than 1,500 cells/mm³ (greater than 1,000 cells/mm³ for patients with Kaposi sarcoma) and platelets recover to a level greater than 100,000 cells/mm³.

➤*Cardiac effects:*

Taxol/Onxol – Severe conduction abnormalities have been documented in less than 1% of patients during paclitaxel therapy and in some cases requiring pacemaker placement. If patients develop significant conduction abnormalities during paclitaxel infusion, administer appropriate therapy and perform continuous cardiac monitoring during subsequent therapy with paclitaxel.

Hypotension, bradycardia, and hypertension have been observed during administration of paclitaxel, but generally do not require treatment. Occasionally paclitaxel infusions must be interrupted or discontinued because of initial or recurrent hypertension. Frequent vital sign monitoring, particularly during the first hour of paclitaxel infusion, is recommended. Continuous cardiac monitoring is not required except for patients with serious conduction abnormalities.

➤*Albumin (human):*

Abraxane – Paclitaxel protein-bound particles contains albumin (human), a derivative of human blood. Based on effective donor screening and product manufacturing processes, it carries an extremely remote risk for transmission of viral disease. A theoretical risk for transmission of Creutzfeldt-Jakob disease also is considered extremely remote. No cases of transmission of viral diseases or Creutzfeldt-Jakob disease have ever been identified for albumin.

PACLITAXEL — INJECTION

➤*Use in men:* Advise men not to father a child while receiving treatment with paclitaxel.

➤*PVC equipment/devices:*

Taxol/Onxol – See Administration and Dosage for more information.

➤*CNS:*

Taxol/Onxol – Although the occurrence of peripheral neuropathy is frequent, the development of severe symptomatology is unusual and requires a dose reduction of 20% for all subsequent courses of paclitaxel.

Paclitaxel contains dehydrated alcohol 396 mg/mL; consider possible CNS and other effects of alcohol. There have been reports of CNS toxicity (rarely associated with death) in a clinical trial in pediatric patients in which paclitaxel was infused IV over 3 hours at doses ranging from 350 to 420 mg/m^2. The toxicity is most likely attributable to the high dose of the ethanol component of the paclitaxel vehicle given over a short infusion time. The use of concomitant antihistamines may intensify this effect. Although a direct effect of the paclitaxel itself cannot be discounted, consider the high doses used in this study (over twice the recommended adult dose) in assessing the safety of paclitaxel for use in this population.

Abraxane – Sensory neuropathy occurs frequently with paclitaxel protein-bound particles. The occurrence of grade 1 or 2 sensory neuropathy generally does not require dose modification. If grade 3 sensory neuropathy develops, withhold treatment until resolution to grade 1 or 2 followed by a dose reduction for all subsequent courses of paclitaxel protein-bound particles.

➤*Injection-site reactions:*

Taxol/Onxol – Injection site reactions, including reactions secondary to extravasation, were usually mild and consisted of erythema, tenderness, skin discoloration, or swelling at the injection site. These reactions have been observed more frequently with the 24-hour infusion than with the 3-hour infusion. Recurrence of skin reactions at a site of previous extravasation following administration of paclitaxel at a different site ("recall") has been reported rarely.

Rare reports of more severe events, such as phlebitis, cellulitis, induration, skin exfoliation, necrosis, and fibrosis, have been received as part of the continuing surveillance of paclitaxel safety. In some cases, the onset of the injection site reaction occurred during a prolonged infusion or was delayed by a week to 10 days.

Closely monitor the infusion site for possible infiltration during drug administration.

Abraxane – Injection-site reactions occur infrequently with paclitaxel protein-bound particles and were mild in the randomized clinical trial. Given the possibility of extravasation, closely monitor the infusion site for possible infiltration during drug administration.

➤*Extravasation:* See Administration and Dosage for more information.

➤*Hypersensitivity reactions:*

Taxol/Onxol – See the Warning box for more information.

Do not treat patients with a history of severe hypersensitivity reactions to products containing polyoxyethylated castor oil (eg, cyclosporin for injection concentrate and teniposide for injection concentrate) with paclitaxel. Minor symptoms, such as flushing, skin reactions, dyspnea, hypotension, or tachycardia, do not require interruption of therapy. However, severe reactions, such as hypotension requiring treatment, dyspnea requiring bronchodilators, angioedema, or generalized urticaria, require immediate discontinuation of paclitaxel and aggressive symptomatic therapy. Do not rechallenge patients who have developed severe hypersensitivity reactions with paclitaxel.

Abraxane – See Administration and Dosage for more information.

➤*Hepatic function impairment:*

Taxol – See Actions for more information.

Onxol – There is evidence that the toxicity of paclitaxel is enhanced in patients with elevated liver enzymes. Exercise caution when administering paclitaxel to patients with moderate to severe hepatic impairment and consider dose adjustments.

➤*Pregnancy:* *Category D.*

Taxol/Onxol – Paclitaxel can cause fetal harm when administered to a pregnant woman. Administration of paclitaxel during the period of organogenesis to rabbits at dosages of 3 mg/kg/day (about 0.2 times the daily maximum recommended human dosage on a mg/m^2 basis) caused embryo- and fetotoxicity, as indicated by intrauterine mortality, increased resorptions, and increased fetal deaths. Maternal toxicity also was observed at this dosage. No teratogenic effects were observed at 1 mg/kg/day (about 1/15 the daily maximum recommended human dosage on a mg/m^2 basis); teratogenic potential could not be assessed at higher doses because of extensive fetal mortality.

Abraxane – Paclitaxel protein-bound particles can cause fetal harm when administered to a pregnant woman. Administration of paclitaxel protein-bound particles to rats on gestation days 7 to 17 at dose of 6 mg/m^2 (approximately 2% of the daily maximum recommended human dose on a mg/m^2 basis) caused embryo- and fetotoxicity, as indicated by intrauterine mortality, increased resorptions (up to 5-fold), reduced numbers of litters and live fetuses, reduction in fetal body weight, and increase in fetal anomalies. Fetal anomalies included soft tissue and skeletal malformations, such as eye bulge, folded retina, microphthalmia, and dilation of brain ventricles. A lower incidence of soft tissue and skeletal malformations also was exhibited at 3 mg/m^2 (approximately 1% of the daily maximum recommended human dose on a mg/m^2 basis).

There are no adequate and well-controlled studies in pregnant women. If paclitaxel is used during pregnancy, or if the patient becomes pregnant while receiving this drug, apprise the patient of the potential hazard to the fetus. Advise women of childbearing potential to avoid becoming pregnant while receiving paclitaxel treatment.

➤*Lactation:* It is not known whether paclitaxel is excreted in human milk. Following IV administration of C^{14}-labeled paclitaxel to rats on days 9 to 10 postpartum, concentrations of radioactivity in milk were higher than in plasma and declined in parallel with the plasma concentrations. Because many drugs are excreted in human milk and because of the potential for serious adverse reactions in nursing infants, it is recommended that breast-feeding be discontinued when receiving paclitaxel therapy.

➤*Children:* The safety and efficacy of paclitaxel in pediatric patients have not been established.

Taxol/Onxol – There have been reports of CNS toxicity (rarely associated with death) in a clinical trial in pediatric patients in which paclitaxel was infused IV over 3 hours at doses ranging from 350 to 420 mg/m^2. The toxicity is most likely attributable to the high dose of the ethanol component of the paclitaxel vehicle given over a short infusion time. The use of concomitant antihistamines may intensify this effect. Although a direct effect of the paclitaxel itself cannot be discounted, consider the high doses used in this study (over twice the recommended adult dosage) in assessing the safety of paclitaxel for use in this population.

➤*Elderly:*

Taxol – Of 2,228 patients who received paclitaxel in 8 clinical studies evaluating its safety and effectiveness in the treatment of advanced ovarian cancer, breast carcinoma, or NSCLC, and 1,570 patients who were randomized to receive paclitaxel in the adjuvant breast cancer study, 649 patients (17%) were 65 years of age or older and 49 patients (1%) were 75 years of age or older. In most studies, severe myelosuppression was more frequent in elderly patients; in some studies, severe neuropathy was more common in elderly patients. In 2 clinical studies in NSCLC, the elderly patients treated with paclitaxel had a higher incidence of cardiovascular events. Estimates of efficacy appeared similar in elderly patients and in younger patients; however, comparative efficacy cannot be determined with confidence because of the small number of elderly patients studied. In a study of first-line treatment with ovarian cancer, elderly patients had a lower median survival than younger patients, but no other efficacy parameters favored the younger group. The table below presents the incidences of grade IV neutropenia and severe neuropathy in clinical studies according to age.

Selected Adverse Reactions in Elderly Patients Receiving Paclitaxel Injection in Clinical Studies

Indication (study/regimen)	Patients [n/total (%)] Neutropenia (grade 4) Age (years) ≥ 65	< 65	Peripheral neuropathy (grades 3/4) Age (years) ≥ 65	< 65
Ovarian cancer				
Intergroup first-line/ T175/3 c75[a]	34/83 (41%)	78/252 (31%)	24/84 (29%)[b,c]	46/255 (18%)[c]
GOG-111 first-line/ T135/24 c75[a]	48/61 (79%)	106/129 (82%)	3/62 (5%)	2/134 (1%)
Phase 3 second-line/ T175/3[d]	5/19 (26%)	21/76 (28%)	1/19 (5%)	0/76 (0%)
Phase 3 second-line/ T175/24[d]	21/25 (84%)	57/79 (72%)	0/25 (0%)	2/80 (3%)
Phase 3 second-line/ T135/3[d]	4/16 (25%)	10/81 (12%)	0/17 (0%)	0/81 (0%)
Phase 3 second-line/ T135/24[d]	17/22 (77%)	53/83 (64%)	0/22 (0%)	0/83 (0%)
Phase 3 second-line pooled	47/82 (57%)[b]	141/319 (44%)	1/83 (1%)	2/320 (1%)
Adjuvant breast cancer				
Intergroup/ AC followed by T[e]	56/102 (55%)	734/1468 (50%)	5/102 (5%)[f]	46/1468 (3%)[f]
Phase 3/T175/3[d]	7/24 (29%)	56/200 (28%)	3/25 (12%)	12/204 (6%)
Phase 3/T135/3[d]	7/20 (35%)	37/207 (18%)	0/20 (0%)	6/209 (3%)

PACLITAXEL — INJECTION

Selected Adverse Reactions in Elderly Patients Receiving Paclitaxel Injection in Clinical Studies				
	Patients [n/total (%)]			
	Neutropenia (grade 4) Age (years)		Peripheral neuropathy (grades 3/4) Age (years)	
Indication (study/regimen)	≥ 65	< 65	≥ 65	< 65
NSCLC				
ECOG/T135/ 24 c75[a]	58/71 (82%)	86/124 (69%)	9/71 (13%)[g]	16/124 (13%)[g]
Phase 3/T175/ 3 c80[a]	37/89 (42%)[b]	56/267 (21%)	11/91 (12%)[b]	11/271 (4%)

[a] Paclitaxel dose in mg/m²/infusion duration in hours; cisplatin doses in mg/m².
[b] $P < 0.05$.
[c] Peripheral neuropathy was included within the neurotoxicity category in the Intergroup First-Line Ovarian Cancer study.
[d] Paclitaxel dose in mg/m²/infusion duration in hours.
[e] Paclitaxel (T) following 4 courses of doxorubicin and cyclophosphamide (AC) at a dose of 175 mg/m² every 3 hours every 3 weeks for 4 courses.
[f] Peripheral neuropathy reported as neurosensory toxicity in the Intergroup Adjuvant Breast Cancer study.
[g] Peripheral neuropathy reported as neurosensory toxicity in the ECOG NSCLC study.

➤*Monitoring:* Do not administer paclitaxel therapy to patients with baseline neutrophil counts of less than 1,500 cells/mm³. In order to monitor the occurrence of myelotoxicity, it is recommended that frequent peripheral blood cell counts be performed on all patients receiving paclitaxel. Do not retreat patients with subsequent cycles of paclitaxel until neutrophils recover to a level greater than 1,500 cells/mm³ and platelets recover to a level greater than 100,000 cells/mm³. In the case of severe neutropenia (less than 500 cells/mm³ for 7 days or more) during a course of paclitaxel therapy (*Taxol* or *Onxol*), a 20% reduction in dose for subsequent courses of therapy is recommended. For patients with advanced HIV disease and poor-risk AIDS-related Kaposi sarcoma, paclitaxel (*Taxol*), at the recommended dose for this disease, can be initiated and repeated if the neutrophil count is at least 1,000 cells/mm³.

In patients who experience severe neutropenia (neutrophil counts less than 500 cells/mm³ for a week or longer) or severe sensory neuropathy during *Abraxane* therapy, reduce the dose to 220 mg/m² for subsequent courses of *Abraxane*. For recurrence of severe neutropenia or severe sensory neuropathy, additionally reduce the dose to 180 mg/m². For grade 3 sensory neuropathy, hold treatment until resolution to grade 1 or 2, followed by a dose reduction for all subsequent courses of *Abraxane*.

Drug Interactions

Paclitaxel Drug Interactions			
Precipitant drug	Object drug[a]		Description
Cisplatin	Paclitaxel	⬆	In a phase 1 trial using escalating doses of paclitaxel (110 to 200 mg/m²) and cisplatin (50 or 75 mg/m²) given as sequential infusions, myelosuppression was more profound when paclitaxel was given after cisplatin than with paclitaxel before cisplatin. Data demonstrated a decrease in paclitaxel clearance of approximately 33% when paclitaxel was administered following cisplatin.
CYP2C8 inhibitors (eg, 17α-ethinylestradiol, diazepam, doxorubicin, felodipine, ketoconazole, midazolam, retinoic acid)	Paclitaxel	⬆	Metabolism of paclitaxel may be decreased through the inhibition of CYP2C8 by any of these drugs.
CYP3A4 inducers (eg, carbamazepine, phenobarbital)	Paclitaxel	⬇	Coadministration of either of these drugs may induce the metabolism of paclitaxel through the cytochrome CYP3A4 isoenzyme.
CYP3A4 inhibitors (eg, cyclosporin, doxorubicin, felodipine, ketoconazole)	Paclitaxel	⬆	Metabolism of paclitaxel may be decreased through the inhibition of CYP3A4 by any of these drugs.
Paclitaxel	Doxorubicin	⬆	Doxorubicin and its active metabolite doxorubicinol may be increased when coadministered with paclitaxel.

[a] ⬆ = Object drug increased. ⬇ = Object drug decreased.

Adverse Reactions

Paclitaxel is considered to have moderately low emetogenic potential (10% to 30% incidence of emesis).

➤*Pooled analysis of adverse reactions from single-agent studies: Taxol/Onxol* – Data in the following table are based on the experience of 812 patients (493 with ovarian cancer and 319 with breast cancer) enrolled in 10 studies who received single-agent paclitaxel. Two hundred seventy-five patients were treated in 8 phase 2 studies with paclitaxel doses ranging from 135 to 300 mg/m² administered over 24 hours (in 4 of these studies, G-CSF was administered as hematopoietic support). Three hundred one patients were treated in the randomized phase 3 ovarian cancer study that compared 2 doses (135 or 175 mg/m²) and 2 schedules (3 or 24 hours) of paclitaxel. Two hundred and thirty-six patients with breast carcinoma received paclitaxel (135 or 175 mg/m²) administered over 3 hours in a controlled study.

Summary[a] of Adverse Reactions in Patients with Solid Tumors Receiving Single-Agent Paclitaxel (%)	
Adverse reactions	Patients (N = 812)
Cardiovascular	
Abnormal electrocardiogram (ECG)	
All patients	23%
Patients with normal baseline (n = 559)	14%
Vital sign changes[b]	
Bradycardia (n = 537)	3%
Hypotension (n = 532)	12%
Significant cardiovascular events	1%
CNS	
Peripheral neuropathy	
Any symptoms	60%
Severe symptoms[c]	3%
Dermatologic	
Alopecia	87%
GI	
Diarrhea	38%
Mucositis	31%
Nausea/Vomiting	52%
Hematologic	
Anemia hemoglobin < 11 g/dL	78%
Anemia hemoglobin < 8 g/dL	16%
Bleeding	14%
Leukopenia [3]	90%
Leukopenia [3]	17%
Neutropenia [3]	90%
Neutropenia [3]	52%
Platelet transfusions	2%
Red cell transfusions	25%
Thrombocytopenia [3]	20%
Thrombocytopenia [3]	7%
Hepatic[d]	
Alkaline phosphatase elevations (n = 575)	22%
AST elevations (n = 591)	19%
Bilirubin elevations (n = 765)	7%
Hypersensitivity[e]	
All	41%
Severe[c]	2%
Musculoskeletal	
Myalgia/arthralgia	
Any symptoms	60%
Severe symptoms[c]	8%

PACLITAXEL — INJECTION

Summary[a] of Adverse Reactions in Patients with Solid Tumors Receiving Single-Agent Paclitaxel (%)	
Adverse reactions	Patients (N = 812)
Miscellaneous	
Infections	30%
Injection site reaction	13%

[a] Based on worst course analysis.
[b] During the first 3 hours of infusion.
[c] Severe reactions are defined as at least grade 3 toxicity.
[d] Patients with normal baseline and on study data
[e] All patients received premedication.

Paclitaxel Frequency[a] of Important Adverse Reactions in the Phase 3 First-Line Ovarian Cancer Studies (%)				
	Intergroup		GOG-111	
Adverse reactions	Paclitaxel 175 mg/m² over 3 hours followed by cisplatin 75 mg/m² (n = 339)	Cyclophosphamide 750 mg/m² followed by cisplatin 75 mg/m² (n = 336)	Paclitaxel 135 mg/m² over 24 hours followed by cisplatin 75 mg/m² (n = 196)	Cyclophosphamide 750 mg/m² followed by cisplatin 75 mg/m² (n = 213)
CNS				
Neurotoxicity[b]				
Any symptoms	87%[c]	52%[c]	25%	20%
Severe symptoms[d]	21%[c]	2%[c]	3%[c]	0%[c]
Dermatologic				
Alopecia				
Any symptoms	96%[c]	89%[c]	55%[c]	37%[c]
Severe symptoms	51%[c]	21%[c]	6%	8%
GI				
Diarrhea				
Any symptoms	37%[c]	29%[c]	16%[c]	8%[c]
Severe symptoms[d]	2%	3%	4%	1%
Nausea/Vomiting				
Any symptoms	88%	93%	65%	69%
Severe symptoms[d]	18%	24%	10%	11%
Hematologic				
Anemia hemoglobin < 11 g/dL[e]	96%	97%	88%	86%
Anemia hemoglobin < 8 g/dL	3%[c]	8%[c]	13%	9%
Febrile neutropenia	4%	7%	15%[c]	4%[c]
Neutropenia < 2,000/mm³	91%[c]	95%[c]	96%	92%
Neutropenia < 500/mm³	33%[c]	43%[c]	81%[c]	58%[c]
Thrombocytopenia < 100,000/mm³[f]	21%[c]	33%[c]	26%	30%
Thrombocytopenia < 50,000/mm³	3%[c]	7%[c]	10%	9%
All	11%[c]	6%[c]	8%[c,f]	1%[c,g]
Severe[d]	1%	1%	3%[c,f]	[c,g]
Musculoskeletal				
Myalgia/Arthralgia				
Any symptoms	60%[c]	27%[c]	9%[c]	2%[c]
Severe symptoms[d]	6%[c]	1%[c]	1%	0%
Miscellaneous				
Asthenia				
Any symptoms	NC[h]	NC	17%[c]	10%[c]
Severe symptoms[d]	NC	NC	1%	1%
Infections	25%	27%	21%	15%

[a] Based on worst course analysis.
[b] In the GOG-111 study, neurotoxicity was collected as peripheral neuropathy and in the Intergroup study, neurotoxicity was collected as either neuromotor or neurosensory symptoms.
[c] $P < 0.05$ by Fisher exact test.
[d] Severe reactions are defined as at least grade 3 toxicity.
[e] Less hemoglobin than 12 g/dL in the Intergroup study.
[f] Less than 130,000/mm³ in the Intergroup study.
[g] All patients received premedication.
[h] NC = not collected.

➤*Disease-specific adverse reactions: first-line ovary cancer in combination:*

Taxol – For the 1,084 patients who were evaluable for safety in the phase 3 first-line ovary combination therapy studies, the following table shows the incidence of important adverse reactions. For both studies, the analysis of safety was based on all courses of therapy (6 courses for the GOG-111 study and up to 9 courses for the Intergroup study.

➤*Second-line ovarian cancer:*

Taxol/Onxol – For the 403 patients who received single-agent paclitaxel in the phase 3 second-line ovarian cancer study, the following table shows the incidence of important adverse reactions.

Paclitaxel Frequency[a] of Important Adverse Reactions in the Phase 3 Second-Line Ovarian Cancer Study (%)				
Adverse reactions	Paclitaxel 175 mg/m² over 3 hours (n = 95)	Paclitaxel 175 mg/m² over 24 hours (n = 105)	Paclitaxel 135 mg/m² over 3 hours (n = 98)	Paclitaxel 135 mg/m² over 24 hours (n = 105)
CNS				
Peripheral neuropathy				
Any symptoms	63%	60%	55%	42%

PACLITAXEL — INJECTION

Paclitaxel Frequency[a] of Important Adverse Reactions in the Phase 3 Second-Line Ovarian Cancer Study (%)

Adverse reactions	Paclitaxel 175 mg/m² over 3 hours (n = 95)	Paclitaxel 175 mg/m² over 24 hours (n = 105)	Paclitaxel 135 mg/m² over 3 hours (n = 98)	Paclitaxel 135 mg/m² over 24 hours (n = 105)
Severe symptoms[b]	1%	2%	0%	0%
GI				
Mucositis				
Any symptoms	17%	35%	21%	25%
Severe symptoms[b]	0%	3%	0%	2%
Hematologic				
Anemia hemoglobin < 11 g/dL	84%	90%	68%	88%
Anemia hemoglobin < 8 g/dL	11%	12%	6%	10%
Neutropenia < 2,000/mm³	78%	98%	78%	98%
Neutropenia < 500/mm³	27%	75%	14%	67%
Thrombocytopenia < 100,000/mm³	4%	18%	8%	6%

Paclitaxel Frequency[a] of Important Adverse Reactions in the Phase 3 Second-Line Ovarian Cancer Study (%)

Adverse reactions	Paclitaxel 175 mg/m² over 3 hours (n = 95)	Paclitaxel 175 mg/m² over 24 hours (n = 105)	Paclitaxel 135 mg/m² over 3 hours (n = 98)	Paclitaxel 135 mg/m² over 24 hours (n = 105)
Thrombocytopenia < 50,000/mm³	1%	7%	2%	1%
Hypersensitivity[c]				
All	41%	45%	38%	45%
Severe[b]	2%	0%	2%	1%
Miscellaneous				
Infections	26%	29%	20%	18%

[a] Based on worst course analysis.
[b] Severe reactions are defined as at least grade 3 toxicity.
[c] All patients received premedication.

Myelosuppression was dose and schedule related, with the schedule effect being more prominent. The development of severe hypersensitivity reactions was rare, 1% of the patients and 0.2% of the courses overall. There was no apparent dose or schedule effect seen for the hypersensitivity reactions. Peripheral neuropathy was clearly dose-related, but schedule did not appear to affect the incidence.

➤*Adjuvant breast cancer:*

Taxol – For the phase 3 adjuvant breast cancer study, the following table shows the incidence of important severe adverse reactions for the 3,121 patients (total population) who were evaluable for safety as well as for a group of 325 patients (early population) who, per the study protocol, were monitored more intensively than other patients.

Paclitaxel Frequency[a] of Important Severe[b] Adverse Reactions in the Phase 3 Adjuvant Breast Cancer Study (%)

Adverse reactions	Early population: Cyclophosphamide plus doxorubicin[c] (n = 166)	Early population: Cyclophosphamide plus doxorubicin[c] followed by paclitaxel[d] (n = 159)	Total population: Cyclophosphamide plus doxorubicin[c] (n = 1,551)	Total population: Cyclophosphamide plus doxorubicin[c] followed by paclitaxel[d] (n = 1,570)
CNS				
Neuromotor toxicity	1%	1%	< 1%	1%
Neurosensory toxicity	-	3%	< 1%	3%
GI				
Mucositis	13%	4%	6%	5%
Nausea/Vomiting	13%	18%	8%	9%
Hematologic[e]				
Anemia hemoglobin < 8 g/dL	17%	21%	8%	8%
Cardiovascular	1%	2%	1%	2%
Fever without infection	-	3%	< 1%	1%
Hypersensitivity[f]	1%	4%	1%	2%
Neutropenia < 500/mm³	79%	76%	48%	50%
Thrombocytopenia < 50,000/mm³	27%	25%	11%	11%
Musculoskeletal				
Myalgia/Arthralgia	-	2%	< 1%	2%
Miscellaneous				
Infections	6%	14%	5%	6%

[a] Based on worst course analysis.
[b] Severe reactions are defined as at least grade 3 toxicity.
[c] Patients received 600 mg/m² cyclophosphamide and doxorubicin (AC) at doses of either 60 mg/m², 75 mg/m², or 90 mg/m² (with prophylactic G-CSF support and ciprofloxacin), every 3 weeks for 4 courses.
[d] Paclitaxel (T) following 4 courses of AC at a dose of 175 mg/m² over 3 hours every 3 weeks for 4 courses.
[e] The incidence of febrile neutropenia was not reported in this study.
[f] All patients were to receive premedication.

The incidence of an adverse reaction for the total population likely represents an underestimation of the actual incidence given that safety data were collected differently based on enrollment cohort. However, because safety data were collected consistently across regimens, the safety of the sequential addition of paclitaxel injection following AC therapy may be compared with AC therapy alone. Compared with patients who received AC alone, patients who received AC followed by paclitaxel experienced grade 3/4 neurosensory toxicity, grade 3/4 myalgia/arthralgia, grade 3/4 neurologic pain (5% vs 1%), grade 3/4 flu-like symptoms (5% vs 3%), and grade 3/4 hyperglycemia (3% vs 1%). During the additional 4 courses of treatment with paclitaxel, 2 deaths (0.1%) were attributed to treatment. During paclitaxel treatment, grade 4 neutropenia was reported in 15% of patients, grade 2/3 neurosensory toxicity in 15%, grade 2/3 myalgias in 23%, and alopecia in 46%.

The incidences of severe hematologic toxicities, infections, mucositis, and cardiovascular reactions increased with higher doses of doxorubicin.

➤*Breast cancer after failure of initial chemotherapy:*

Taxol/Onxol – For the 458 patients who received single-agent paclitaxel in the phase 3 breast cancer study, the following table shows the incidence of important adverse reactions by treatment arm (each arm was administered by a 3-hour infusion).

Paclitaxel Frequency[a] of Important Adverse Reactions in the Phase 3 Study of Breast Cancer After Failure of Initial Chemotherapy or Within 6 Months of Adjuvant Chemotherapy (%)

Adverse reactions	Paclitaxel 175 mg/m² over 3 hours (n = 229)	Paclitaxel 135 mg/m² over 3 hours (n = 229)
CNS		
Peripheral neuropathy		
Any symptoms	70%	46%
Severe symptoms[b]	7%	3%
GI		
Mucositis		
Any symptoms	23%	17%
Severe symptoms[b]	3%	< 1%

PACLITAXEL — INJECTION

Paclitaxel Frequency[a] of Important Adverse Reactions in the Phase 3 Study of Breast Cancer After Failure of Initial Chemotherapy or Within 6 Months of Adjuvant Chemotherapy (%)

Adverse reactions	Paclitaxel 175 mg/m² over 3 hours (n = 229)	Paclitaxel 135 mg/m² over 3 hours (n = 229)
Hematologic		
Anemia hemoglobin < 11 g/dL	55%	47%
Anemia hemoglobin < 8 g/dL	4%	2%
Febrile neutropenia	2%	2%
Neutropenia < 2,000/mm³	90%	81%
Neutropenia < 500/mm³	28%	19%
Thrombocytopenia < 100,000/mm³	11%	7%
Thrombocytopenia < 50,000/ mm³	3%	2%
Hypersensitivity[c]		
All	36%	31%
Severe[b]	0%	< 1%
Miscellaneous		
Infections	23%	15%

[a] Based on worst course analysis.
[b] Severe reactions are defined as at least grade 3 toxicity.
[c] All patients received premedication.

Myelosuppression and peripheral neuropathy were dose related. There was 1 severe hypersensitivity reaction observed at the dose of 135 mg/m².

➤*First-line NSCLC in combination:*

Taxol – In the ECOG study, patients were randomized to either paclitaxel (T) 135 mg/m² as a 24-hour infusion in combination with cisplatin (c) 75 mg/m², paclitaxel (T) 250 mg/m² as a 24-hour infusion in combination with cisplatin (c) 75 mg/m² with G-CSF support, or cisplatin (c) 75 mg/m² on day 1, followed by etoposide (VP) 100 mg/m² on days 1, 2, and 3 (control).

Paclitaxel Frequency[a] of Important Adverse Reactions in the Phase 3 Study for First-Line NSCLC (%)

Adverse reactions	Paclitaxel 135 mg/m² over 24 hours with cisplatin 75 mg/m² (n = 195)	Paclitaxel 250 mg/m² over 24 hours with cisplatin 75 mg/m² with G-CSF support (n = 197)	Cisplatin 75 mg/m² on day 1 followed by etoposide 100 mg/m² on days 1, 2, 3[b] (n = 196)
Cardiovascular			
Any symptoms	33%	39%	24%
Severe symptoms[c]	13%	12%	8%
CNS			
Neuromotor toxicity			
Any symptoms	37%	47%	44%
Severe symptoms[c]	6%	12%	7%
Neurosensory toxicity			
Any symptoms	48%	61%	25%
Severe symptoms[c]	13%	28%[d]	8%
GI			
Mucositis			
Any symptoms	18%	28%	16%
Severe symptoms[c]	1%	4%	2%
Nausea/Vomiting			
Any symptoms	85%	87%	81%
Severe symptoms[c]	27%	29%	22%
Hematologic			
Anemia hemoglobin < normal	94%	96%	95%
Anemia hemoglobin < 8 g/dL	22%	19%	28%
Neutropenia < 2000/mm³	89%	86%	84%
Neutropenia < 500/mm³	74%[d]	65%	55%
Thrombocytopenia < normal	48%	68%	62%
Thrombocytopenia < 50,000/mm³	6%	12%	16%
Hypersensitivity[e]			
All	16%	27%	13%
Severe[c]	1%	4%[d]	1%
Musculoskeletal			
Arthralgia/Myalgia			
Any symptoms	21%[d]	42%[d]	9%
Severe symptoms[c]	3%	11%	1%
Miscellaneous			
Infections	38%	31%	35%

[a] Based on worst course analysis.
[b] Etoposide (VP) dose in mg/m² was administered IV on days 1, 2, and 3; cisplatin dose in mg/m².
[c] Severe reactions are defined as at least grade 3 toxicity.
[d] $P < 0.05$.
[e] All patients received premedication.

Toxicity was generally more severe in the high-dose paclitaxel treatment arm (paclitaxel 250 mg/cisplatin 75 mg) than in the low-dose paclitaxel arm (paclitaxel 135 mg/cisplatin 75 mg). Compared with the cisplatin/etoposide arm, patients in the low-dose paclitaxel arm experienced more arthralgia/myalgia of any grade and more severe neutropenia. The incidence of febrile neutropenia was not reported in this study.

Kaposi sarcoma –

Taxol: The following table shows the frequency of important adverse reactions in the 85 patients with Kaposi sarcoma treated with 2 different single-agent paclitaxel regimens.

Paclitaxel Frequency[a] of Important Adverse Reactions in the AIDS-Related Kaposi Sarcoma Studies (%)

Adverse reactions	Study CA139-174 Paclitaxel 135 mg/m² over 3 hours every 3 weeks (n = 29)	Study CA139-281 Paclitaxel 100 mg/m² over 3 hours every 2 weeks (n = 56)
Cardiovascular		
Bradycardia	3%	-
Hypotension	17%	9%
CNS		
Peripheral neuropathy		
Any	79%	46%
Severe[b]	10%	2%
GI		
Diarrhea	90%	73%
Mucositis	45%	20%
Nausea/Vomiting	69%	70%
Hematologic		
Anemia hemoglobin < 11 g/dL	86%	73%
Anemia hemoglobin < 8 g/dL	34%	25%
Febrile neutropenia	55%	9%
Neutropenia < 2,000/mm³	100%	95%
Neutropenia < 500/mm³	76%	35%
Thrombocytopenia < 100,000/mm³	52%	27%
Thrombocytopenia < 50,000/mm³	17%	5%
Hypersensitivity[c]		
All	14%	9%
Musculoskeletal		
Myalgia/Arthralgia		
Any	93%	48%
Severe[b]	14%	16%

PACLITAXEL — INJECTION

Paclitaxel Frequency[a] of Important Adverse Reactions in the AIDS-Related Kaposi Sarcoma Studies (%)

Adverse reactions	Study CA139-174 Paclitaxel 135 mg/m^2 over 3 hours every 3 weeks (n = 29)	Study CA139-281 Paclitaxel 100 mg/m^2 over 3 hours every 2 weeks (n = 56)
Opportunistic infection		
Any	76%	54%
Candidiasis, esophageal	7%	9%
Cryptosporidiosis	7%	7%
Cryptococcal meningitis	3%	2%
Cytomegalovirus	45%	27%
Herpes simplex	38%	11%
Leukoencephalopathy		2%
Mycobacterium avium intracellulare	24%	4%
Pneumocystis carinii	14%	21%
Renal (creatinine elevation)		
Any	34%	18%
Severe[b]	7%	5%
Discontinuation for drug toxicity	7%	16%

[a] Based on worst course analysis.
[b] Severe reactions are defined as at least grade 3 toxicity.
[c] All patients received premedication. As demonstrated previously, toxicity was more pronounced in the study utilizing paclitaxel at a dose of 135 mg/m^2 every 3 weeks than in the study utilizing paclitaxel at a dose of 100 mg/m^2 every 2 weeks. Notably, severe neutropenia (76% vs 35%), febrile neutropenia (55% vs 9%), and opportunistic infections (76% vs 54%) were more common with the former dose and schedule. Take into account the differences between the 2 studies with respect to dose escalation and use of hematopoietic growth factors, as described previously. Note also that only 26% of the 85 patients in these studies received concomitant treatment with protease inhibitors, whose effect on paclitaxel metabolism has not yet been studied.

➤*Abraxane*: The following table shows the frequency of important adverse reactions in the randomized comparative trial for the patients who received either single-agent *Abraxane* or paclitaxel injection for the treatment of metastatic breast cancer.

Paclitaxel Frequency[a] of Important Treatment Emergent Adverse Reactions in the Randomized Study on an Every-3-Weeks Schedule (%)

Adverse reactions	Paclitaxel protein-bound particles 260 mg/m^2 over 30 minutes (n = 229)	Paclitaxel injection 175 mg/m^2 over 3 hours[b] (n = 225)
Cardiovascular		
Abnormal ECG		
All patients	60%	52%
Patients with normal baseline	35%	30%
Vital sign changes[c]		
Bradycardia	< 1%	< 1%
Hypotension	5%	5%
Severe cardiovascular events[d]	3%	4%
CNS		
Sensory neuropathy		
Any symptoms	71%	56%
Severe symptoms[d]	10%	2%
Dermatologic		
Alopecia	90%	94%
GI		
Diarrhea		
Any symptoms	26%	15%
Severe symptoms[d]	< 1%	1%
Mucositis		
Any symptoms	7%	7%
Severe symptoms[d]	< 1%	0%
Nausea		
Any symptoms	30%	21%
Severe symptoms[d]	3%	< 1%
Vomiting		
Any symptoms	18%	9%
Severe symptoms[d]	4%	1%
Hematologic		
Anemia		
Bleeding	2%	2%
Febrile neutropenia	2%	1%
Hemoglobin		
< 11 g/L	33%	25%
< 8 g/L	1%	< 1%
Neutropenia		
< 2,000/mm^3	80%	82%
^{3}	9%	22%
Thrombocytopenia		
< 100,000/mm^3	2%	3%
^{3}	< 1%	1%
Hepatic (patients with normal baseline)		
Alkaline phosphatase elevations	36%	31%
AST elevations	39%	32%
Bilirubin elevations	7%	7%
Hypersensitivity[e]		
All	4%	12%
Severe[d]	0%	2%
Musculoskeletal		
Myalgia/arthralgia		
Any symptoms	44%	49%
Severe symptoms[d]	8%	4%
Respiratory		
Cough	6%	6%
Dyspnea	12%	9%
Miscellaneous		
Asthenia		
Any symptoms	47%	38%
Severe symptoms[d]	8%	3%
Fluid retention/Edema		
Any symptoms	10%	8%
Severe symptoms[d]	0%	< 1%
Infections	24%	20%
Injection site reaction	1%	1%

[a] Based on worst grade.
[b] Paclitaxel injection patients received premedication.
[c] During study drug dosing.
[d] Severe events are defined as at least grade 3 toxicity.
[e] Includes treatment-related events related to hypersensitivity (eg, flushing, dyspnea, chest pain, hypotension) that began on a day of dosing.

Miscellaneous – Myelosuppression and sensory neuropathy were dose related.

➤*Adverse reactions by body system:*

Cardiovascular –

Taxol/Onxol: Hypotension during the first 3 hours of infusion occurred in 12% of all patients and 3% of all courses administered. Bradycardia during the first 3 hours of infusion occurred in 3% of all patients and 1% of all courses. In the phase 3 second-line ovarian study, neither dose nor schedule had an effect on the frequency of hypotension and bradycardia. These vital sign changes most often caused no symptoms and required neither specific therapy nor treatment discontinuation. The frequency of hypotension and bradycardia were not influenced by prior anthracycline therapy.

Significant cardiovascular reactions, possibly related to single-agent paclitaxel, occurred in approximately 1% of all patients. These reactions included syncope, rhythm abnormalities, hypertension, and venous thrombosis. One of the patients with syncope treated with paclitaxel at 175 mg/m^2 over 24 hours had progressive hypotension and died. The arrhythmias included

PACLITAXEL — INJECTION

asymptomatic ventricular tachycardia, bigeminy, and complete atrioventricular block requiring pacemaker placement.

ECG abnormalities were common among patients at baseline. ECG abnormalities on study did not usually result in symptoms, were not dose-limiting, and required no intervention. ECG abnormalities were noted in 23% of all patients. Among patients with a normal ECG prior to study entry, 14% of all patients developed an abnormal tracing while on study. The most frequently reported ECG modifications were nonspecific repolarization abnormalities, sinus bradycardia, sinus tachycardia, and premature beats. Among patients with normal ECGs at baseline, prior therapy with anthracyclines did not influence the frequency of ECG abnormalities.

Cases of myocardial infarction have been reported rarely. Congestive heart failure has been reported typically in patients who have received other chemotherapy, notably anthracyclines.

Rare reports of atrial fibrillation and supraventricular tachycardia have been received as part of the continuing surveillance of paclitaxel safety.

Taxol: Among patients with NSCLC treated with paclitaxel in combination with cisplatin in the phase 3 study, significant cardiovascular reactions occurred in 12% to 13%. This apparent increase in cardiovascular reactions is possibly caused by an increase in cardiovascular risk factors in patients with lung cancer.

Abraxane: Hypotension during the 30-minute infusion occurred in 5% of patients in the randomized metastatic breast cancer trial. Bradycardia, during the 30-minute infusion, occurred in less than 1% of patients. These vital sign changes most often caused no symptoms and required neither specific therapy nor treatment discontinuation.

Severe cardiovascular events, possibly related to single-agent paclitaxel protein-bound particles, occurred in approximately 3% of patients in the randomized trial. These events included chest pain, cardiac arrest, supraventricular tachycardia, edema, thrombosis, pulmonary thromboembolism, pulmonary emboli, and hypertension. Cases of cerebrovascular attacks (strokes) and transient ischemic attacks have been reported rarely.

ECG abnormalities were common among patients at baseline. ECG abnormalities on study did not usually result in symptoms, were not dose-limiting, and required no intervention. ECG abnormalities were noted in 60% of all patients in the metastatic breast cancer randomized trial. Among patients with a normal ECG prior to study entry, 35% of all patients developed an abnormal tracing while on study. The most frequently reported ECG modifications were nonspecific repolarization abnormalities, sinus bradycardia, and sinus tachycardia.

CNS –

Taxol/Onxol: The frequency and severity of neurologic manifestations were dose-dependent but were not influenced by infusion duration. Peripheral neuropathy was observed in 60% of all patients (3% severe) and in 52% (2% severe) of the patients without preexisting neuropathy.

The frequency of peripheral neuropathy increased with cumulative dose. Neurologic symptoms were observed in 27% of the patients after the first course of treatment and in 34% to 51% from course 2 to 10.

Peripheral neuropathy was the cause of paclitaxel discontinuation in 1% of all patients. Sensory symptoms have usually improved or resolved within several months of paclitaxel discontinuation. The incidence of neurologic symptoms did not increase in the subset of patients previously treated with cisplatin. Preexisting neuropathies resulting from prior therapies are not a contraindication for paclitaxel therapy.

Other than peripheral neuropathy, serious neurologic reactions following paclitaxel administration have been rare (less than 1%) and have included grand mal seizures, syncope, ataxia, and neuroencephalopathy.

Rare reports of autonomic neuropathy, resulting in paralytic ileus, have been received as part of the continuing surveillance of paclitaxel safety. Optic nerve or visual disturbances (scintillating scotomata) have also been reported, particularly in patients who have received higher doses than those recommended. These effects generally have been reversible. However, rare reports of abnormal visual in the literature evoked potentials in patients have suggested persistent optic nerve damage.

Taxol: The assessment of neurologic toxicity was conducted differently among the studies as evident from the data reported in each individual study (see previous tables). Moreover, the frequency and severity of neurologic manifestations were influenced by prior and/or concomitant therapy with neurotoxic agents.

In the Intergroup first-line ovarian cancer study, neurotoxicity included reports of neuromotor and neurosensory events. The regimen with *Taxol* 175 mg/m^2 given by 3-hour infusion plus cisplatin 75 mg/m^2 resulted in a greater incidence and severity of neurotoxicity than the regimen containing cyclophosphamide and cisplatin, 87% (21% severe) versus 52% (2% severe), respectively. The duration of grade 3 or 4 neurotoxicity cannot be determined with precision for the Intergroup study because the resolution dates of adverse reactions were not collected in the case report forms for this trial and complete follow-up documentation was available only in a minority of these patients. In the GOG first-line ovarian cancer study, neurotoxicity was reported as peripheral neuropathy. The regimen with *Taxol* 135 mg/m^2 injection given by 24-hour infusion plus cisplatin 75 mg/m^2 resulted in an incidence of neurotoxicity that was similar to the regimen containing cyclophosphamide plus cisplatin, 25% (3% severe) versus 20% (0% severe), respectively. Cross-study comparison of neurotoxicity in the Intergroup and GOG trials suggests that when *Taxol* is given in combination with cisplatin 75 mg/m^2, the incidence of severe neurotoxicity is more common at a *Taxol* dose of 175 mg/m^2 given by 3-hour infusion (21%) than at a dose of 135 mg/m^2 given by 24-hour infusion (3%).

In patients with NSCLC, administration of paclitaxel followed by cisplatin resulted in greater incidence of severe neurotoxicity compared with the incidence in patients with ovarian or breast cancer treated with single-agent paclitaxel. Severe neurosensory symptoms were noted in 13% of NSCLC patients receiving paclitaxel 135 mg/m^2 by 24-hour infusion followed by cisplatin 75 mg/m^2 and 8% of NSCLC patients receiving cisplatin/etoposide.

Abraxane: The frequency and severity of neurologic manifestations were influenced by prior and/or concomitant therapy with neurotoxic agents.

In general, the frequency and severity of neurologic manifestation were dose-dependent in patients receiving single-agent paclitaxel protein-bound particles. In the randomized trial, sensory neuropathy was observed in 71% of patients (10% severe) in the paclitaxel protein-bound particles arm and in 56% of patients (2% severe) in the paclitaxel injection arm. The frequency of sensory neuropathy increased with cumulative dose. Sensory neuropathy was the cause of paclitaxel protein-bound particles discontinuation in 7/229 (3%) patients in the randomized trial. In the randomized comparative study, 24 patients (10%) treated with paclitaxel protein-bound particles developed grade 3 peripheral neuropathy; of these patients, 14 had documented improvement after a median of 22 days; 10 patients resumed treatment at a reduced dose of paclitaxel protein-bound particles and 2 discontinued because of peripheral neuropathy. Of the 10 patients without documented improvement, 4 discontinued the study because of peripheral neuropathy.

No incidences of grade 4 sensory neuropathies were reported in the clinical trial. Only 1 incident of motor neuropathy (grade 1) was observed in either arm of the controlled trial.

Reports of autonomic neuropathy, resulting in paralytic ileus, have been received as part of the continuing surveillance of paclitaxel injection safety.

Dermatologic –

Taxol/Onxol: Alopecia was observed in almost all (87%) of the patients. Transient skin changes caused by paclitaxel-related hypersensitivity reactions have been observed, but no other skin toxicities were significantly associated with paclitaxel administration. Nail changes (changes in pigmentation or discoloration of nail bed) were uncommon (2%). Edema was reported in 21% of all patients (17% of those without baseline edema); only 1% had severe edema and none of these patients required treatment discontinuation. Edema was most commonly focal and disease-related. Edema was observed in 5% of all courses for patients with normal baseline and did not increase with time on study.

Rare reports of skin abnormalities related to radiation recall as well as reports of maculopapular rash and pruritus have been received as part of the continuing surveillance of paclitaxel safety.

Abraxane: Alopecia was observed in almost all of the patients. Nail changes (changes in pigmentation or discoloration of nail bed) were uncommon. Edema (fluid retention) was infrequent (10% of randomized trial patients); no patients had severe edema.

GI –

Taxol/Onxol: Nausea/Vomiting, diarrhea, and mucositis were reported by 52%, 38%, and 31% of all patients, respectively. These manifestations were usually mild to moderate. Mucositis was schedule dependent and occurred more frequently with the 24-hour than with the 3-hour infusion.

Rare reports of intestinal obstruction, intestinal perforation, pancreatitis, ischemic colitis, and dehydration have been received as part of the continuing surveillance of paclitaxel safety. Rare reports of neutropenic enterocolitis (typhlitis), despite the coadministration of G-CSF, were observed in patients treated with paclitaxel alone and in combination with other chemotherapeutic agents.

Taxol: In patients with poor-risk AIDS-related Kaposi sarcoma, nausea/vomiting, diarrhea, and mucositis were reported by 69%, 79%, and 28% of patients, respectively. One third of patients with Kaposi sarcoma complained of diarrhea prior to study start.

In the first-line, phase 3 ovarian cancer studies, the incidence of nausea and vomiting when paclitaxel injection was administered in combination with cisplatin appeared to be greater compared with the database for single-agent paclitaxel in ovarian and breast cancer. In addition, diarrhea of any grade was reported more frequently compared with the control arm, but there was no difference for severe diarrhea in these studies.

Abraxane: Nausea/Vomiting, diarrhea, and mucositis were reported by 33%, 27%, and 7% of paclitaxel protein-bound particles treated patients in the randomized trial.

Rare reports of intestinal obstruction, intestinal perforation, pancreatitis, and ischemic colitis have been received as part of the continuing surveillance of paclitaxel injection safety and may occur following paclitaxel protein-bound particles treatment. Rare reports of neutropenic enterocolitis (typhlitis), despite the coadministration of G-CSF, were observed in patients treated with paclitaxel injection alone and in combination with other chemotherapeutic agents.

Hematologic –

Taxol/Onxol: Bone marrow suppression was the major dose-limiting toxicity of paclitaxel. Neutropenia, the most important hematologic toxicity, was dose-dependent, schedule-dependent, and generally rapidly reversible. Among patients treated in the phase 3 second-line ovarian study with a 3-hour infusion, neutrophil counts declined below 500 cells/mm^3 in 14% of the patients treated with a dose of 135 mg/m^2 compared with 27% at a dose of 175 mg/m^2 ($P = 0.05$). In the same study, severe neutropenia (less than 500 cells/mm^3) was more frequent with the 24-hour than with the 3-hour infusion; infusion duration had a greater impact on myelosuppression than dose. Neutropenia did not appear to increase with cumulative exposure and did not appear to be more frequent nor more severe for patients previously treated with radiation therapy.

Fever was frequent (12% of all treatment courses). Infectious episodes occurred in 30% of all patients and 9% of all courses; these episodes were

PACLITAXEL — INJECTION

fatal in 1% of all patients, and included sepsis, pneumonia, and peritonitis. In the phase 3, second-line ovarian study, infectious episodes were reported in 20% and 26% of the patients treated with a dose of 135 or 175 mg/m^2 given as 3-hour infusions, respectively. Urinary tract infections and upper respiratory tract infections were the most frequently reported infectious complications.

Thrombocytopenia was uncommon and almost never severe (less than 50,000 cells/mm^3). Twenty percent of the patients experienced a drop in their platelet count below 100,000 cells/mm^3 at least once while on treatment; 7% had a platelet count less than 50,000 cells/mm^3 at the time of their worst nadir. Bleeding episodes were reported in 4% of all courses and by 14% of all patients. Most of the hemorrhagic episodes were localized, and the frequency of these reactions was unrelated to the paclitaxel injection dose and schedule. In the phase 3, second-line ovarian study, bleeding episodes were reported in 10% of the patients; no patients treated with the 3-hour infusion received platelet transfusions.

Anemia (hemoglobin less than 11 g/dL) was observed in 78% of all patients and was severe (hemoglobin less than 8 g/dL) in 16% of the cases. No consistent relationship between dose or schedule and the frequency of anemia was observed. Among all patients with normal baseline hemoglobin, 69% became anemic on study but only 7% had severe anemia. Red cell transfusions were required in 25% of all patients and in 12% of those with normal baseline hemoglobin levels.

Taxol: In the study where paclitaxel was administered to patients with ovarian cancer at a dose of 135 mg/m^2 over 24 hours in combination with cisplatin versus the control arm of cyclophosphamide plus cisplatin, the incidences of grade 4 neutropenia and of febrile neutropenia were significantly greater in the paclitaxel plus cisplatin arm than in the control arm. Grade 4 neutropenia occurred in 81% on the paclitaxel plus cisplatin arm versus 58% on the cyclophosphamide plus cisplatin arm, and febrile neutropenia occurred in 15% and 4% respectively. On the paclitaxel/cisplatin arm, there were 35 out of 1,074 (3%) courses with fever in which grade 4 neutropenia was reported at some time during the course. When paclitaxel followed by cisplatin was administered to patients with advanced NSCLC in the ECOG study, the incidences of grade 4 neutropenia were 74% (paclitaxel 135 mg/m^2 over 24 hours followed by cisplatin) and 65% (paclitaxel 250 mg/m^2 over 24 hours followed by cisplatin and G-CSF) compared with 55% in patients who received cisplatin/etoposide.

In the immunosuppressed patient population with advanced HIV disease and poor-risk AIDS-related Kaposi sarcoma, 61% of the patients reported at least 1 opportunistic infection. The use of supportive therapy, including G-CSF, is recommended for patients who have experienced severe neutropenia.

In the adjuvant breast cancer trial, the incidence of severe thrombocytopenia and platelet transfusions increased with higher doses of doxorubicin.

Abraxane: Neutropenia, the most important hematologic toxicity, was dose dependent and reversible. Among patients with metastatic breast cancer in the randomized trial, neutrophil counts declined below 500 cells/mm^3 (grade 4) in 9% of the patients treated with a dose of 260 mg/m^2 compared with 22% in patients receiving paclitaxel injection at a dose of 175 mg/m^2.

In the randomized, metastatic breast cancer study, infectious episodes were reported in 24% of the patients treated with a dose of 260 mg/m^2 given as a 30-minute infusion. Oral candidiasis, respiratory tract infections, and pneumonia were the most frequently reported infectious complications. Febrile neutropenia was reported in 2% of patients in the paclitaxel protein-bound particles arm and 1% of patients in the paclitaxel injection arm.

Thrombocytopenia was uncommon. In the randomized, metastatic breast cancer study, bleeding episodes were reported in 2% of the patients in each treatment arm.

Anemia (hemoglobin less than 11 g/dL) was observed in 33% in the randomized trial and was severe (hemoglobin less than 8 g/dL) in 1% of the cases. Among all patients with normal baseline hemoglobin, 31% became anemic on study and 1% had severe anemia.

Hepatic – Rare reports of hepatic necrosis and hepatic encephalopathy leading to death have been received as part of the continuing surveillance of paclitaxel injection safety and may occur following paclitaxel protein-bound particles treatment.

Taxol/Onxol: No relationship was observed between liver function abnormalities and either dose or schedule of paclitaxel administration. Among patients with normal baseline liver function 7%, 22%, and 19% had elevations in bilirubin, alkaline phosphatase, and AST, respectively. Prolonged exposure to paclitaxel was not associated with cumulative hepatic toxicity.

Abraxane: Among patients with normal baseline liver function 7%, 36%, and 39% had elevations in bilirubin, alkaline phosphatase, and AST, respectively. Grade 3 or 4 elevations in gamma-glutamyltransferase (GGT) were reported for 14% of patients treated with paclitaxel protein-bound particles and 10% of patients treated with paclitaxel injection in the randomized trial.

Hypersensitivity –

Taxol/Onxol: All patients received premedication prior to paclitaxel. The frequency and severity of hypersensitivity reactions were not affected by the dose or schedule of paclitaxel administration. Premedicate all patients prior to paclitaxel administration in order to prevent severe hypersensitivity reactions. Such premedication may consist of dexamethasone 20 mg orally administered approximately 12 and 6 hours before paclitaxel, diphenhydramine (or its equivalent) 50 mg IV 30 to 60 minutes prior to paclitaxel, and cimetidine 300 mg or ranitidine 50 mg IV 30 to 60 minutes before paclitaxel. In the phase 3 second-line ovarian study, the 3-hour infusion was not associated with a greater increase in hypersensitivity reactions when compared with the 24-hour infusion. Hypersensitivity reactions were observed in 20% of all courses and in 41% of all patients. These reactions were severe in less than 2% of the patients and 1% of the courses. No severe reactions were observed after course 3 and severe symptoms occurred generally within the first hour of paclitaxel infusion. The most frequent symptoms observed during these severe reactions were dyspnea, flushing, chest pain, and tachycardia.

The minor hypersensitivity reactions consisted mostly of flushing (28%), rash (12%), hypotension (4%), dyspnea (2%), tachycardia (2%), and hypertension (1%). The frequency of hypersensitivity reactions remained relatively stable during the entire treatment period. Rare reports of chills and reports of back pain in association with hypersensitivity reactions have been received as part of the continuing surveillance of paclitaxel safety.

Local – Injection site reactions, including reactions secondary to extravasation, were usually mild and consisted of erythema, tenderness, skin discoloration, or swelling at the injection site. These reactions have been observed more frequently with the 24-hour infusion than with the 3-hour infusion. Recurrence of skin reactions at a site of previous extravasation following administration of paclitaxel at a different site ("recall") has been reported rarely.

Rare reports of more severe reactions, such as phlebitis, cellulitis, induration, skin exfoliation, necrosis, and fibrosis, have been received as part of the continuing surveillance of paclitaxel safety. In some cases the onset of the injection site reaction either occurred during a prolonged infusion or was delayed by a week to 10 days.

A specific treatment for extravasation reactions is unknown at this time. Given the possibility of extravasation, it is advisable to closely monitor the infusion site for possible infiltration during drug administration.

Musculoskeletal –

Taxol/Onxol: There was no consistent relationship between dose or schedule of paclitaxel and the frequency or severity of arthralgia/myalgia. Sixty percent of all patients treated experienced arthralgia/myalgia; 8% experienced severe symptoms. The symptoms were usually transient, occurred 2 or 3 days after paclitaxel administration, and resolved within a few days. The frequency and severity of musculoskeletal symptoms remained unchanged throughout the treatment period.

Abraxane: Forty-four percent of patients treated in the randomized trial experienced arthralgia/myalgia; 8% experienced severe symptoms. The symptoms were usually transient, occurred 2 or 3 days after paclitaxel protein-bound particles administration, and resolved within a few days.

Ophthalmic –

Abraxane: Ocular/Visual disturbances occurred in 13% of all patients (n = 366) treated with paclitaxel protein-bound particles in single arm and randomized trials and 1% were severe. The severe cases (keratitis and blurred vision) were reported in patients in a single arm study who received higher doses than those recommended (300 or 375 mg/m^2). These effects generally have been reversible. However, rare reports in the literature of abnormal visual evoked potentials in patients treated with paclitaxel injection have suggested persistent optic nerve damage.

Renal –

Taxol: Among the patients treated for Kaposi sarcoma with paclitaxel, 5 patients had renal toxicity of grade 3 or 4 severity. One patient with suspected HIV nephropathy of grade 4 severity had to discontinue therapy. The other 4 patients had renal insufficiency with reversible elevations of serum creatinine.

Abraxane: Overall 11% of patients experienced creatinine elevation; 1% was severe. No discontinuations, dose reductions, or dose delays were caused by renal toxicities.

Respiratory –

Taxol/Onxol: Rare reports of interstitial pneumonia, lung fibrosis, and pulmonary embolism have been received as part of the continuing surveillance of paclitaxel safety. Rare reports of radiation pneumonitis have been received in patients receiving concurrent radiotherapy.

Abraxane: Reports of dyspnea (12%) and cough (6%) were reported after treatment with paclitaxel protein-bound particles in the randomized trial. Rare reports (less than 1%) of pneumothorax were reported after treatment with paclitaxel protein-bound particles. There is no experience with the use of paclitaxel protein-bound particles with concurrent radiotherapy.

Miscellaneous –

Taxol: Reports of asthenia and malaise have been received as part of the continuing surveillance of paclitaxel safety. In the phase 3 trial of paclitaxel 135 mg/m^2 over 24 hours in combination with cisplatin as first-line therapy of ovarian cancer, asthenia was reported in 17% of the patients, significantly greater than the 10% incidence observed in the control arm of cyclophosphamide/cisplatin.

Abraxane: Asthenia was reported in 47% of patients (8% severe) treated with paclitaxel protein-bound particles in the randomized trial. Asthenia included reports of asthenia, fatigue, weakness, lethargy, and malaise.

Rare cases of cardiac ischemia/infarction and thrombosis/embolism, possibly related to paclitaxel protein-bound particles treatment, have been reported.

The following rare adverse reactions have been reported as part of the continuing surveillance of paclitaxel injection safety and may occur following paclitaxel protein-bound particles treatment: skin abnormalities related to radiation recall, as well as reports of maculopapular rash, Stevens-Johnson syndrome, toxic epidermal necrolysis, conjunctivitis, and increased lacrimation.

Postmarketing:

• *Taxol* – Postmarketing reports of ototoxicity (hearing loss and tinnitus) have been received.

Rare reports of conjunctivitis and increased lacrimation have been received as part of the continuing surveillance of paclitaxel injection safety.

Accidental exposure: No reports of accidental exposure to paclitaxel protein-bound particles have been received. However, upon inhalation of paclitaxel injection, dyspnea, chest pain, burning eyes, sore throat, and nau-

PACLITAXEL — INJECTION

sea have been reported. Following topical exposure, reactions have included tingling, burning, and redness.

Overdosage

➤*Symptoms:* The primary anticipated complications of overdosage would consist of bone marrow suppression, sensory neurotoxicity, and mucositis. Overdoses in pediatric patients may be associated with acute ethanol toxicity. There have been reports of CNS toxicity (rarely associated with death) in a clinical trial in pediatric patients in which paclitaxel was infused IV over 3 hours at doses ranging from 350 to 420 mg/m². The toxicity is most likely attributable to the high dose of the ethanol component of the paclitaxel vehicle given over a short infusion time. The use of concomitant antihistamines may intensify this effect. Although a direct effect of the paclitaxel itself cannot be discounted, the high doses used in this study (over twice the recommended adult dosage) must be considered in assessing the safety of paclitaxel for use in this population.

➤*Treatment:* There is no known antidote for paclitaxel overdosage.

DOCETAXEL

Rx	Taxotere (Aventis)	Injection: 20 mg per 0.5 mL	Polysorbate 80.[a] In single-dose vials with 1.5 mL diluent.[b]
		80 mg per 2 mL	Polysorbate 80.[a] In single-dose vials with 6 mL diluent.[b]

[a] 1,040 mg/mL polysorbate 80.

[b] Contains 13% ethanol (w/w) in water for injection.

DOCETAXEL — INJECTION

WARNING

Docetaxel should be administered under the supervision of a qualified health care provider experienced in the use of antineoplastic agents. Appropriate management of complications is possible only when adequate diagnostic and treatment facilities are readily available.

The incidence of treatment-related mortality associated with docetaxel therapy is increased in patients with abnormal liver function, patients receiving higher doses, and patients with non-small cell lung cancer (NSCLC) and a history of treatment with platinum-based chemotherapy who receive docetaxel as a single agent at a dose of 100 mg/m².

Hepatic function impairment – In general, do not give docetaxel to patients with bilirubin more than the upper limit of normal (ULN) or patients with AST and/or ALT more than 1.5 times ULN concomitant with alkaline phosphatase more than 2.5 times the ULN. Patients with elevations of bilirubin or abnormalities of transaminase concurrent with alkaline phosphatase are at increased risk for the development of grade 4 neutropenia, febrile neutropenia, infections, severe thrombocytopenia, severe stomatitis, severe skin toxicity, and toxic death. Patients with isolated elevations of transaminase more than 1.5 times the ULN also had a higher rate of febrile grade 4 neutropenia but did not have an increased incidence of toxic death. Obtain and review bilirubin, AST or ALT, and alkaline phosphatase values prior to each cycle of docetaxel therapy.

Neutropenia – Do not give docetaxel therapy to patients with neutrophil counts of less than 1,500 cells/mm³. In order to monitor the occurrence of neutropenia, which may be severe and result in infection, perform frequent blood cell counts on all patients receiving docetaxel.

Hypersensitivity – Severe hypersensitivity reactions, characterized by general rash/erythema, hypotension and/or bronchospasm, or, very rarely, fatal anaphylaxis, have been reported in patients who received the recommended 3-day dexamethasone premedication. Hypersensitivity reactions require immediate discontinuation of the docetaxel infusion and administration of appropriate therapy. Do not give docetaxel to patients who have a history of severe hypersensitivity reactions to docetaxel or to other drugs formulated with polysorbate 80.

Fluid retention – Severe fluid retention occurred in 6.5% (6/92) of patients despite the use of a 3-day dexamethasone premedication regimen. It was characterized by 1 or more of the following reactions: poorly tolerated peripheral edema, generalized edema, pleural effusion requiring urgent drainage, dyspnea at rest, cardiac tamponade, or pronounced abdominal distention (due to ascites).

Indications

➤*Breast cancer:* For the treatment of patients with locally advanced or metastatic breast cancer after failure of prior chemotherapy.

In combination with doxorubicin and cyclophosphamide for the adjuvant treatment of patients with operable node-positive breast cancer.

➤*Gastric adenocarcinoma:* In combination with cisplatin and fluorouracil for the treatment of patients with advanced gastric adenocarcinoma, including adenocarcinoma of the gastroesophageal junction, who have not received prior chemotherapy for advanced disease.

➤*Head and neck cancer:* In combination with cisplatin and fluorouracil for the induction treatment of patients with inoperable locally advanced squamous cell carcinoma of the head and neck (SCCHN).

➤*NSCLC:* As a single agent for the treatment of patients with locally advanced or metastatic NSCLC after failure of prior platinum-based chemotherapy.

In combination with cisplatin for the treatment of patients with unresectable, locally advanced, or metastatic NSCLC who have not previously received chemotherapy for this condition.

➤*Prostate cancer:* In combination with prednisone for the treatment of patients with androgen-independent (hormone-refractory) metastatic prostate cancer.

➤*Off-label uses:* Ovarian cancer, urothelial cancer, small-cell lung cancer, esophageal cancer.

Administration and Dosage

➤*General dosing considerations:* All patients should be premedicated with oral corticosteroids. (See Premedication.)

➤*Adults:*

Breast cancer –

Monotherapy:

• *Usual dosage* – 60 to 100 mg/m² administered intravenously (IV) over 1 hour every 3 weeks.

• *Dosage adjustment* – Patients who are dosed initially at 100 mg/m² and who experience febrile neutropenia, neutrophils less than 500 cells/mm³ for more than 1 week, or severe or cumulative cutaneous reactions during docetaxel therapy should have the dose adjusted from 100 to 75 mg/m². If the patient continues to experience these reactions, the dose should either be decreased from 75 to 55 mg/m² or treatment should be discontinued. Conversely, patients who are dosed initially at 60 mg/m² and do not experience febrile neutropenia, neutrophils less than 500 cells/mm³ for more than 1 week, severe or cumulative cutaneous reactions, or severe peripheral neuropathy during docetaxel therapy may tolerate higher doses. Patients who develop peripheral neuropathy grade 3 or higher should have docetaxel treatment discontinued entirely.

Combination therapy:

• *Usual dosage* – 75 mg/m² administered IV 1 hour after doxorubicin 50 mg/m² and cyclophosphamide 500 mg/m². Administer regimen every 3 weeks for 6 courses. Prophylactic granulocyte colony-stimulating factor (G-CSF) may be used to mitigate the risk of hematological toxicities.

• *Dosage adjustment* – Docetaxel in combination with doxorubicin and cyclophosphamide should be administered when the neutrophil count is 1,500 cells/mm³ or more. Patients who experience febrile neutropenia should receive G-CSF in all subsequent cycles. Patients who continue to experience this reaction should remain on G-CSF and have their docetaxel dose reduced to 60 mg/m². Patients who experience grade 3 or 4 stomatitis should have their docetaxel dose decreased to 60 mg/m². Patients who experience severe or cumulative cutaneous reactions or moderate neurosensory signs and/or symptoms during docetaxel therapy should have their dose of docetaxel reduced from 75 to 60 mg/m². If the patient continues to experience these reactions at 60 mg/m², treatment should be discontinued.

• *Concomitant therapy* – Doxorubicin 50 mg/m² and cyclophosphamide 500 mg/m² every 3 weeks for 6 courses. Prophylactic G-CSF may be used to mitigate the risk of hematological toxicities.

Gastric adenocarcinoma –

Usual dosage: 75 mg/m² as 1-hour IV infusion, followed by cisplatin 75 mg/m², as a 1- to 3-hour IV infusion (both on day 1 only), followed by fluorouracil 750 mg/m²/day given as a 24-hour continuous IV infusion for 5 days, starting at the end of the cisplatin infusion. Treatment is repeated every 3 weeks. Patients must receive premedication with antiemetics and appropriate hydration for cisplatin administration.

Dosage adjustment:

• *Hematologic abnormalities* – In both studies, G-CSF was recommended during the second and/or subsequent cycles in case of febrile neutropenia, documented infection with neutropenia, or neutropenia lasting longer than 7 days. If an episode of febrile neutropenia, prolonged neutropenia, or neutropenic infection occurs despite G-CSF use, the docetaxel dose should be reduced from 75 to 60 mg/m². If subsequent episodes of complicated neutropenia occur, the docetaxel dose should be reduced from 60 to 45 mg/m². In case of grade 4 thrombocytopenia, the docetaxel dose should be reduced from 75 to 60 mg/m². Patients should not be retreated with subsequent cycles of docetaxel until neutrophils recover to a level of more than 1,500 cells/mm³ and platelets recover to a level of more than 100,000 cells/mm³. Discontinue treatment if these toxicities persist.

• *GI toxicities* – Recommended dose modifications for GI toxicities in patients treated with docetaxel in combination with cisplatin and fluorouracil are shown in the following table.

DOCETAXEL — INJECTION

Recommended Dose Modifications for GI Toxicities in Patients Treated With Docetaxel in Combination With Cisplatin and Fluorouracil	
Toxicity	Dosage adjustment
Diarrhea grade 3	First episode: Reduce fluorouracil dose by 20%. Second episode: Reduce docetaxel dose by 20%.
Diarrhea grade 4	First episode: Reduce docetaxel and fluorouracil doses by 20%. Second episode: Discontinue treatment.
Stomatitis/mucositis grade 3	First episode: Reduce fluorouracil dose by 20%. Second episode: Discontinue fluorouracil only, at all subsequent cycles. Third episode: Reduce docetaxel dose by 20%.
Stomatitis/mucositis grade 4	First episode: Discontinue fluorouracil only, at all subsequent cycles. Second episode: Reduce docetaxel dose by 20%.

• *Hepatic toxicities* – In case of AST/ALT more than 2.5 to 5 times the ULN and alkaline phosphatase 2.5 times the ULN or less, or AST/ALT more than 1.5 to 5 times the ULN and alkaline phosphatase more than 2.5 to 5 times the ULN, docetaxel should be reduced by 20%. In case of AST/ALT more than 5 times the ULN and/or alkaline phosphatase more than 5 times the ULN, docetaxel should be stopped.

Head and neck cancer –

Usual dosage:

• *Induction chemotherapy followed by radiotherapy (TAX 323)* – 75 mg/m^2 as a 1-hour IV infusion followed by cisplatin 75 mg/m^2 IV over 1 hour, on day 1, followed by fluorouracil as a continuous IV infusion at 750 mg/m^2 per day for 5 days. Administer regimen every 3 weeks for 4 cycles. Following chemotherapy, patients should receive radiotherapy.

• *Induction chemotherapy followed by chemoradiotherapy (TAX 324)* – 75 mg/m^2 as a 1-hour IV infusion on day 1, followed by cisplatin 100 mg/m^2 administered as a 30-minute to 3-hour infusion, followed by fluorouracil 1,000 mg/m^2/day as a continuous infusion from day 1 to day 4. Administer regimen every 3 weeks for 3 cycles. Following chemotherapy, patients should receive chemoradiotherapy.

Dosage adjustment: See information in the Gastric adenocarcinoma section.

Premedication: Patients must receive premedication with antiemetics and appropriate hydration (prior to and after cisplatin administration). All patients on the docetaxel-containing arm of the TAX 323 and TAX 324 studies received prophylactic antibiotics.

Non-small cell lung cancer –

Monotherapy after failure of prior platinum-based chemotherapy:

• *Usual dosage* – 75 mg/m^2 administered IV over 1 hour every 3 weeks.

• *Dosage adjustment* – Patients who are dosed initially at 75 mg/m^2 and experience febrile neutropenia, neutrophils less than 500 cells/mm^3 for more than 1 week, severe or cumulative cutaneous reactions, or other grade 3/4 nonhematologic toxicities during docetaxel monotherapy should have treatment withheld until resolution of toxicity and then resumed at 55 mg/m^2. Patients who develop peripheral neuropathy that is grade 3 or higher should have docetaxel treatment discontinued entirely.

Combination therapy in chemotherapy-naive patients:

• *Usual dosage* – 75 mg/m^2 administered IV over 1 hour, immediately followed by cisplatin 75 mg/m^2 over 30 to 60 minutes every 3 weeks.

• *Dosage adjustment* – For patients who are dosed initially at 75 mg/m^2 in combination with cisplatin and whose nadir of platelet count during the previous course of therapy is less than 25,000 cells/mm^3, patients who experience febrile neutropenia, and patients with serious nonhematologic toxicities, the docetaxel dose should be reduced in subsequent cycles to 65 mg/m^2. In patients who require a further dose reduction, a dose of 50 mg/m^2 is recommended. For cisplatin dosage adjustments, see the Cisplatin monograph.

Prostate cancer –

Usual dosage: 75 mg/m^2 every 3 weeks as a 1-hour infusion.

Dosage adjustment: Docetaxel should be administered when the neutrophil count is 1,500 cells/mm^3 or more. Patients who experience febrile neutropenia, neutrophils less than 500 cells/mm^3 for more than 1 week, severe or cumulative cutaneous reactions, or moderate neurosensory signs and/or symptoms during docetaxel therapy should have the dose of docetaxel reduced from 75 to 60 mg/m^2. If the patient continues to experience these reactions at 60 mg/m^2, treatment should be discontinued.

Concomitant therapy: Prednisone 5 mg orally twice daily is administered continuously.

Off-label dosing –

Esophageal cancer: 75 mg/m^2 IV every 3 weeks, in combination with fluorouracil and cisplatin.

➤*Hepatic function impairment:* According to the manufacturer, in general, do not give docetaxel to patients with bilirubin more than the ULN or with AST and/or ALT more than 1.5 times the ULN concomitant with alkaline phosphatase more than 2.5 times the ULN (See also Black Box Warning). In case of AST/ALT more than 2.5 to 5 times the ULN and alkaline phosphatase 2.5 times the ULN or less, or AST/ALT more than 1.5 to 5 times the ULN and alkaline phosphatase more than 2.5 to 5 times the ULN, docetaxel should be reduced by 20%.

In case of AST/ALT more than 5 times the ULN and/or alkaline phosphatase more than 5 times the ULN, docetaxel should be stopped.

Another reference suggests the following:

Docetaxel Dosage Adjustment for Hepatic Function	
Liver function	Percent of usual dose
AST or ALT ≤ 1.5 times the ULN	100%
AST or ALT 1.6 to 6 times the ULN and alkaline phosphatase	75%
AST or ALT > 6 times the ULN and alkaline phosphatase	Use clinical judgement.
AST or ALT > 1.5 times the ULN and alkaline phosphatase ≥ 2.5 times the ULN	Do not administer

➤*Premedication:* All patients should be premedicated with oral corticosteroids, such as dexamethasone 16 mg/day (eg, 8 mg twice a day), for 3 days starting 1 day prior to docetaxel administration in order to reduce the incidence and severity of fluid retention as well as the severity of hypersensitivity reactions.

Prostate cancer – For hormone-refractory metastatic prostate cancer, given the concurrent use of prednisone, the recommended premedication regimen is dexamethasone 8 mg orally at 12, 3, and 1 hour(s) before the docetaxel infusion.

➤*Preparation for administration:* Docetaxel is considered a cytotoxic agent. Follow safe handling procedures when preparing, administering, or dispensing docetaxel.

The use of gloves is recommended. If docetaxel should come into contact with the skin, wash immediately and thoroughly with soap and water. If docetaxel comes into contact with mucosa, wash immediately and thoroughly with water.

Preparation of solution –

Polyvinyl chloride equipment: Contact of the docetaxel concentrate with plasticized polyvinyl chloride (PVC) equipment or devices used to prepare solutions for infusion is not recommended. In order to minimize patient exposure to the plasticizer diethylhexyl phthalate (DEHP), which may be leached from PVC infusion bags or sets, store diluted docetaxel solution in bottles (glass, polypropylene) or plastic bags (polypropylene, polyolefin) and administer through polyethylene-lined administration sets.

Preparation of the initial diluted solution:

1.) If the vials are refrigerated, allow the appropriate number of vials of docetaxel and diluent (ethanol 13% in water for injection) to stand at room temperature for approximately 5 minutes.
2.) Aseptically withdraw the entire contents of the appropriate diluent vial (approximately 1.8 mL for docetaxel 20 mg and approximately 7.1 mL for docetaxel 80 mg) into a syringe by partially inverting the vial and transfer it to the vial of docetaxel for injection concentrate. If the procedure is followed as described, an initial diluted solution of docetaxel 10 mg/mL will result.
3.) Mix the initial diluted solution vial by repeated inversions for at least 45 seconds to ensure full mixture of the concentrate and diluent. Do not shake.
4.) The initial diluted docetaxel solution (docetaxel 10 mg/mL) should be clear; however, there may be some foam on top of the solution because of the polysorbate 80. Allow the solution to stand for a few minutes to allow any foam to dissipate. It is not required that all foam dissipate prior to continuing the preparation process. The initial diluted solution may be used immediately or stored either in the refrigerator or at room temperature for a maximum of 8 hours.

Preparation of the final dilution for infusion:

1.) Aseptically withdraw the required amount of initial diluted docetaxel solution (docetaxel 10 mg/mL) with a calibrated syringe and inject into a 250 mL infusion bag or bottle of either sodium chloride 0.9% solution or dextrose 5% solution to produce a final concentration of 0.3 to 0.74 mg/mL. If a dose of more than docetaxel 200 mg is required, use a larger volume of the infusion vehicle so that a concentration of docetaxel 0.74 mg/mL is not exceeded.
2.) Thoroughly mix the infusion by manual rotation.
3.) If the docetaxel initial diluted solution or final dilution for infusion is not clear or appears to have precipitation, discard the dilution. Solutions should be clear and yellow to yellow-brown in color, although some foam may be present.

➤*Administration:* Administer the final docetaxel solution as a 1-hour IV infusion under ambient room temperature and lighting conditions.

➤*Extravasation:* Docetaxel is considered an irritant and may cause phlebitis, but it is not known to cause tissue damage with extravasation. If signs or symptoms of extravasation occur, stop the infusion immediately. If possible, withdraw 3 to 5 mL of blood to remove some of the drug. Remove the infusion needle. Delineate the infiltrated area on the patient's skin with a felt tip marker. Elevate for 48 hours above heart level using a sling or stockinette dressing with an observation window cut in the dressing. Avoid pressure or friction. Do not rub the area. Observe for signs of increased erythema, pain, or skin necrosis. If increased symptoms occur, consult a plastic surgeon. After 48 hours, encourage the patient to use the extremity normally to promote full range of motion.

➤*Storage/Stability:* Store undiluted between 2° and 25°C (36° and 77°F). Retain in the original package to protect from bright light. Freezing does not adversely affect the product.

DOCETAXEL — INJECTION

According to the manufacturer, the initial diluted solution (10 mg/mL) may be used immediately or stored either in the refrigerator or at room temperature for a maximum of 8 hours. However, in stability studies, the 10 mg/mL solution was stable for 28 days at room temperature or when stored in the refrigerator.

According to the manufacturer, fully prepared infusion solution (in either sodium chloride 0.9% solution or dextrose 5% solution) should be used within 4 hours (including the 1 hour IV administration). However, solutions diluted with sodium chloride 0.9% injection are stable for up to 28 days at room temperature when stored in glass or polyethylene containers. Solutions diluted with dextrose 5% injection are stable for up to 28 days at room temperature when stored in glass or polypropylene containers.

Docetaxel solutions contain no preservative and should be used within 24 hours of reconstitution to reduce the risk of microbial contamination.

Discard vials within 6 hours of the initial needle puncture if opened within an ISO Class 5 biological safety cabinet, or within 1 hour of the initial needle puncture if opened outside of such an environment, based on the USP Chapter <797> standards.

Actions

➤*Pharmacology:* Docetaxel is an antineoplastic agent that disrupts the microtubular network in cells, which is essential for mitotic and interphase cellular functions. Docetaxel binds to free tubulin and promotes the assembly of tubulin into stable microtubules while simultaneously inhibiting their disassembly. This leads to the production of microtubule bundles without healthy function and to the stabilization of microtubules, which results in the inhibition of mitosis in cells. Docetaxel's binding to microtubules does not alter the number of protofilaments in the bound microtubules, a feature that differs from most spindle poisons currently in clinical use.

➤*Pharmacokinetics:*

Absorption –

The area under the curve (AUC) was dose proportional following doses of 70 to 115 mg/m², with infusion times of 1 to 2 hours.

Distribution – Mean value for steady-state volume of distribution was 113 L.

In vitro studies showed that docetaxel is about 94% protein bound, mainly to alpha 1-acid glycoprotein, albumin, and lipoproteins. In 3 cancer patients, the in vitro binding to plasma proteins was found to be approximately 97%.

Metabolism – In vitro drug interaction studies revealed that docetaxel is metabolized by the CYP3A4 isoenzyme.

Excretion – A study of ^{14}C-docetaxel was conducted in 3 cancer patients. Docetaxel was eliminated in the urine and feces following oxidative metabolism of the tert-butyl ester group, but fecal excretion was the main elimination route. Within 7 days, urinary and fecal excretion accounted for approximately 6% and 75% of the administered radioactivity, respectively. About 80% of the radioactivity recovered in feces is excreted during the first 48 hours as 1 major and 3 minor metabolites with very small amounts (less than 8%) of unchanged drug.

Docetaxel's pharmacokinetic profile is consistent with a 3-compartment pharmacokinetic model, with half-lives for the α, β, and γ phases of 4 minutes, 36 minutes, and 11.1 hours, respectively. The initial rapid decline represents distribution to the peripheral compartments, and the late (terminal) phase is due, in part, to a relatively slow efflux of docetaxel from the peripheral compartment. Mean value for total body clearance was 21 L/h/m².

Special populations –

Hepatic function impairment: In patients with clinical chemistry data suggestive of mild to moderate liver function impairment (AST and/or ALT more than 1.5 times the ULN concomitant with alkaline phosphatase more than 2.5 times the ULN), total body clearance was lowered by an average of 27%, resulting in a 38% increase in systemic exposure (AUC). This average, however, includes a substantial range, and presently there is no measurement that would allow recommendation for dosage adjustment in such patients. In general, do not treat patients with combined abnormalities of transaminase and alkaline phosphatase with docetaxel.

Contraindications

History of severe hypersensitivity reactions to docetaxel or to other drugs formulated with polysorbate 80; See the Warning box for more information.

Warnings/Precautions

➤*Acute myeloid leukemia (AML):* Treatment-related AML has occurred in patients given anthracyclines and/or cyclophosphamide, including use in adjuvant therapy for breast cancer. In the adjuvant breast cancer trial (TAX 316), AML occurred in 3 of 744 patients who received docetaxel, doxorubicin, and cyclophosphamide and in 1 of 736 patients who received fluorouracil, doxorubicin, and cyclophosphamide.

➤*Fluid retention:* See the Warning box for more information.

Severe fluid retention has been reported following docetaxel therapy. Premedicate patients with oral corticosteroids prior to each docetaxel administration to reduce the incidence and severity of fluid retention. Closely monitor patients with preexisting effusions from the first dose for the possible exacerbation of the effusions.

When fluid retention occurs, peripheral edema usually starts in the lower extremities and may become generalized with a median weight gain of 2 kg.

➤*Hematologic effects:* Neutropenia (less than 2,000 neutrophils/mm³) occurs in virtually all patients given 60 to 100 mg/m² of docetaxel, and grade 4 neutropenia (less than 500 cells/mm³) occurs in 85% of patients given 100 mg/m² and 75% of patients given 60 mg/m². Frequent monitoring of blood cell counts is, therefore, essential so that the dose can be adjusted. Do not administer docetaxel to patients with neutrophils less than 1,500 cells/mm³.

Febrile neutropenia occurred in about 12% of patients given 100 mg/m² but was very uncommon in patients given 60 mg/m². Hematologic responses, febrile reactions and infections, and rates of septic death for different regimens are dose related.

Three breast cancer patients with severe liver function impairment (bilirubin more than 1.7 times the ULN) developed fatal GI bleeding associated with severe drug-induced thrombocytopenia.

In gastric cancer patients treated with docetaxel in combination with cisplatin and fluorouracil, febrile neutropenia and/or neutropenic infection occurred in 12% of patients receiving G-CSF compared with 28% who did not. Closely monitor patients receiving docetaxel plus cisplatin plus fluorouracil during the first and subsequent cycles for febrile neutropenia and neutropenic infection.

➤*Premedication regimen:* See Administration and Dosage for more information.

➤*Toxic deaths:*

Breast cancer – Docetaxel administered at 100 mg/m² was associated with deaths considered possibly or probably related to treatment in 2% (19/965) of metastatic breast cancer patients, both previously treated and untreated, with normal baseline liver function and in 11.5% (7/61) of patients with various tumor types who had abnormal baseline liver function (AST and/or ALT more than 1.5 times the ULN together with alkaline phosphatase more than 2.5 times the ULN). Among patients dosed at 60 mg/m², mortality related to treatment occurred in 0.6% (3/481) of patients with healthy liver function and in 3 of 7 patients with abnormal liver function. Approximately half of these deaths occurred during the first cycle. Sepsis accounted for the majority of the deaths.

NSCLC – Docetaxel administered at a dose 100 mg/m² in patients with locally advanced or metastatic NSCLC who had a history of platinum-based chemotherapy was associated with increased treatment-related mortality (14% and 5% in 2 randomized, controlled studies). There were 2.8% treatment-related deaths among the 176 patients treated at the 75 mg/m² dose in the randomized trials. Among patients who experienced treatment-related mortality at the 75 mg/m² dose level, 3 of 5 patients had a performance status of 2 at study entry.

➤*Asthenia:* Severe asthenia has been reported in 14.9% (144/965) of metastatic breast cancer patients but has led to treatment discontinuation in only 1.8%. Symptoms of fatigue and weakness may last a few days up to several weeks and may be associated with deterioration of performance status in patients with progressive disease.

➤*Dermatologic:* See Adverse Reactions for more information.

➤*Neurologic:* Severe neurosensory symptoms (paresthesia, dysesthesia, pain) were observed in 5.5% (53/965) of metastatic breast cancer patients and resulted in treatment discontinuation in 6.1% of patients. When these symptoms occur, adjust dosage. If symptoms persist, discontinue treatment. Patients who experienced neurotoxicity in clinical trials and for whom follow-up information on the complete resolution of the reaction was available had spontaneous reversal of symptoms with a median of 9 weeks from onset (range, 0 to 106 weeks). Severe peripheral motor neuropathy mainly manifested as distal extremity weakness occurred in 4.4% (42/965) of patients.

➤*Treatment response:* Responding patients may not experience an improvement in performance status on therapy and may experience worsening. The relationship between changes in performance status, response to therapy, and treatment-related adverse reactions has not been established.

➤*Extravasation:* See Administration and Dosage for more information.

➤*Hypersensitivity reactions:* See the Warning box for more information.

Hypersensitivity reactions may occur within a few minutes following initiation of a docetaxel infusion. If minor reactions, such as flushing or localized skin reactions, occur, interruption of therapy is not required. More severe reactions, however, require the immediate discontinuation of docetaxel and aggressive therapy. Premedicate all patients with an oral corticosteroid prior to the initiation of the infusion of docetaxel.

➤*Hepatic function impairment:* See the Warning box for more information.

➤*Pregnancy: Category D.* Docetaxel can cause fetal harm when administered to pregnant women. Studies in rats and rabbits at doses of 0.3 or more and 0.03 mg/kg/day, respectively (about 1/50 and 1/300 the daily maximum recommended human dose on a mg/m² basis, respectively), administered during the period of organogenesis, have shown that docetaxel is embryotoxic and fetotoxic (characterized by intrauterine mortality, increased resorption, reduced fetal weight, and fetal ossification delay). These dosages also caused maternal toxicity.

There are no adequate and well-controlled studies in pregnant women using docetaxel. If docetaxel is used during pregnancy or if the patient becomes pregnant while receiving this drug, apprise the patient of the potential hazard to the fetus or potential risk for loss of the pregnancy. Advise women of childbearing potential to avoid becoming pregnant during therapy with docetaxel.

➤*Lactation:* It is not known whether docetaxel is excreted in human milk. Because many drugs are excreted in human milk and because of the potential for serious adverse reactions in breast-feeding infants from docetaxel, advise mothers to discontinue breast-feeding prior to taking the drug.

DOCETAXEL — INJECTION

➤*Children:* The safety and efficacy of docetaxel in children have not been established.

➤*Elderly:* In patients 65 years of age or older treated with docetaxel plus cisplatin, diarrhea (55%), peripheral edema (39%), and stomatitis (28%) were observed more frequently than in the vinorelbine plus cisplatin group (diarrhea 24%, peripheral edema 20%, stomatitis 20%). Patients treated with docetaxel plus cisplatin who were 65 years of age and older were more likely to experience diarrhea (55%), infections (42%), peripheral edema (39%), and stomatitis (28%) compared with patients younger than 65 years of age administered the same treatment (43%, 31%, 31%, and 21%, respectively).

When docetaxel was combined with carboplatin for the treatment of chemotherapy-naïve advanced NSCLC, patients 65 years of age and older (28%) experienced a higher frequency of infection compared with similar patients treated with docetaxel plus cisplatin, and a higher frequency of diarrhea, infection, and peripheral edema than elderly patients treated with vinorelbine plus cisplatin.

Of the 333 patients treated with docetaxel every 3 weeks plus prednisone in the prostate cancer study (TAX 327), 209 patients were 65 years of age and older, and 68 patients were older than 75 years of age. In patients treated with docetaxel every 3 weeks, the following treatment-emergent adverse reactions occurred at rates of at least 10% and higher in patients 65 years of age and older, compared with younger patients: anemia (71% vs 59%), infection (37% vs 24%), nail changes (34% vs 23%), anorexia (21% vs 10%), and weight loss (15% vs 5%), respectively.

Among the 221 patients treated with docetaxel in combination with cisplatin and fluorouracil in the gastric cancer study, 54 were 65 years of age and older, and 2 patients were older than 75 years. In this study, the number of patients who were 65 years of age and older was insufficient to determine whether they respond differently from younger patients. However, the incidence of serious adverse reactions was higher in the elderly patients compared with younger patients. The incidence of the following adverse reactions (all grades): diarrhea, dizziness, edema, febrile neutropenia/neutropenic infection, lethargy, and stomatitis occurred at rates of 10% or more in patients who were 65 years of age and older, compared with younger patients. Closely monitor elderly patients treated with docetaxel plus cisplatin plus fluorouracil.

➤*Monitoring:* Perform frequent peripheral blood cell counts on all patients receiving docetaxel. Do not retreat patients with subsequent cycles of docetaxel until neutrophils recover to a level greater than 1,500 cells/mm^3 and platelets recover to a level greater than 100,000 cells/mm^3.

A 25% reduction in the dose of docetaxel is recommended during subsequent cycles following severe neutropenia (less than 500 cells/mm^3) lasting 7 days or more, febrile neutropenia, or a grade 4 infection in a docetaxel cycle.

Obtain bilirubin, AST or ALT, and alkaline phosphatase values prior to each cycle of docetaxel therapy.

Closely monitor patients with preexisting effusions from the first dose for the possible exacerbation of the effusions.

Drug Interactions

Docetaxel Drug Interactions

Precipitant drug	Object drug[a]		Description
Azole antifungals (eg, itraconazole, ketoconazole)	Docetaxel	↑	Docetaxel plasma concentrations may be elevated, increasing the pharmacologic effects and risk of toxicity (eg, neutropenia). Coadminister with caution and reduce dose as needed.
CYP-450 3A4 inhibitors (eg, clarithromycin, nefazodone, nelfinavir)	Docetaxel	↑	It is likely that CYP3A4 inhibitors may lead to substantial increases in docetaxel blood concentrations.

[a] ↑ = object drug increased.

Adverse Reactions

Docetaxel is considered to have moderately low emetogenic potential (10% to 30% incidence of emesis).

➤*Monotherapy with docetaxel for locally advanced or metastatic breast cancer after failure of prior chemotherapy:*

Docetaxel Adverse Reactions in Patients With Breast Cancer

Adverse reaction	All tumor types normal liver function tests[a] (n = 2,045)	All tumor types elevated liver function tests[b] (n = 61)	Breast cancer normal liver function tests[a] (n = 965)
CNS			
Asthenia (any)	61.8%	52.5%	66.3%
Asthenia (severe)	12.8%	24.6%	14.9%
Neurosensory (any)	49.3%	34.4%	58.3%
Neurosensory (severe)	4.3%	0%	5.5%
Dermatologic			
Alopecia	75.8%	62.3%	74.2%
Cutaneous (any)	47.6%	54.1%	47%
Cutaneous (severe)	4.8%	9.8%	5.2%
Nail changes (any)	30.6%	23%	40.5%
Nail changes (severe)	2.5%	4.9%	3.7%
GI			
Diarrhea	38.7%	32.8%	42.6%
Diarrhea (severe)	4.7%	4.9%	5.5%
Nausea	38.8%	37.7%	42.1%
Stomatitis (any)	41.7%	49.2%	51.7%
Stomatitis (severe)	5.5%	13%	7.4%
Vomiting	22.3%	23%	23.4%
Hematologic			
Anemia < 8 g/dL	8.8%	31.1%	7.7%
Anemia < 11 g/dL	90.4%	91.8%	93.6%
Febrile neutropenia[c]	11%	26.2%	12.3%
Leukopenia < 1,000 cells/mm^3	31.6%	46.6%	43.7%
Leukopenia < 4,000 cells/mm^3	95.6%	98.3%	98.6%
Neutropenia < 500 cells/mm^3	75.4%	87.5%	85.9%
Neutropenia < 2,000 cells/mm^3	95.5%	96.4%	98.5%
Thrombocytopenia < 100,000 cells/mm^3	8%	24.6%	9.2%
Hypersensitivity			
Regardless of premedication (any)	21%	19.7%	17.6%
Regardless of premedication (severe)	4.2%	9.8%	2.6%
With 3-day premedication	(n = 92)	(n = 3)	(n = 92)
Any	15.2%	33.3%	15.2%
Severe	2.2%	0%	2.2%
Metabolic			
Fluid retention			
Regardless of premedication (any)	47%	39.3%	59.7%
Regardless of premedication (severe)	6.9%	8.2%	8.9%
With 3-day premedication	(n = 92)	(n = 3)	(n = 92)
Any	64.1%	66.7%	64.1%
Severe	6.5%	33.3%	6.5%
Musculoskeletal			
Arthralgia	9.2%	6.6%	8.2%
Myalgia (any)	18.9%	16.4%	21.1%
Myalgia (severe)	1.5%	1.6%	1.8%
Miscellaneous			
Fever in absence of infection (any)	31.2%	41%	35.1%
Fever in absence of infection (severe)	2.1%	8.2%	2.2%
Infection (any)	21.6%	32.8%	22.2%
Infection (severe)	6.1%	16.4%	6.4%
Infusion-site reactions	4.4%	3.3%	4%

DOCETAXEL — INJECTION

Docetaxel Adverse Reactions in Patients With Breast Cancer			
Adverse reaction	All tumor types normal liver function tests[a] (n = 2,045)	All tumor types elevated liver function tests[b] (n = 61)	Breast cancer normal liver function tests[a] (n = 965)
Nonseptic death	0.6%	6.6%	0.6%
Septic death	1.6%	4.9%	1.4%

[a] Normal baseline liver function tests: transaminases ≤ 1.5 times the ULN or alkaline phosphatase ≤ 2.5 times the ULN or isolated elevations of transaminases or alkaline phosphatase ≤ 5 times the ULN.
[b] Elevated baseline liver function tests: AST and/or ALT > 1.5 times the ULN concurrent with alkaline phosphatase > 2.5 times the ULN.
[c] Febrile neutropenia: absolute neutrophil count (ANC) grade 4 with fever > 38°C (100.4°F) with IV antibiotics and/or hospitalization.

Cardiovascular – Hypotension occurred in 2.8% of patients with solid tumors; 1.2% required treatment. Clinically meaningful reactions, such as atrial flutter, dysrhythmia, heart failure, hypertension, pulmonary edema, sinus tachycardia, and unstable angina, occurred rarely. Seven of 86 (8.1%) metastatic breast cancer patients receiving docetaxel 100 mg/m^2 in a randomized trial and who had serial left ventricular ejection fraction (LVEF) assessed developed deterioration of LVEF by at least 10% that was associated with a drop below the institutional lower limit of normal.

CNS – See Warnings/Precautions for more information.

Dermatologic – Localized erythema of the extremities with edema followed by desquamation has been observed. In case of severe skin toxicity, a dosage adjustment is recommended. The discontinuation rate due to skin toxicity was 1.6% (15/965) for metastatic breast cancer patients. Among 92 breast cancer patients premedicated with 3-day corticosteroids, there were no cases of severe skin toxicity reported, and no patient discontinued docetaxel because of skin toxicity.

Reversible cutaneous reactions characterized by a rash, including localized eruptions, mainly on the feet and/or hands but also on the arms, face, or thorax, usually associated with pruritus, have been observed. Eruptions generally occurred within 1 week after docetaxel infusion, recovered before the next infusion, and were not disabling.

Severe nail disorders were characterized by hypo- or hyperpigmentation and occasionally by onycholysis (in 0.8% of patients with solid tumors) and pain.

GI – GI reactions (diarrhea, nausea, and/or vomiting) were generally mild to moderate. Severe reactions occurred in 3% to 5% of patients with solid tumors and, to a similar extent, among metastatic breast cancer patients. The incidence of severe reactions was 1% or less for the 92 breast cancer patients premedicated with 3-day corticosteroids.

Severe stomatitis occurred in 5.5% of patients with solid tumors, in 7.4% of patients with metastatic breast cancer, and in 1.1% of the 92 breast cancer patients premedicated with 3-day corticosteroids.

Hematologic – Reversible marrow suppression was the major dose-limiting toxicity of docetaxel. The median time to nadir was 7 days, while the median duration of severe neutropenia (less than 500 cells/mm^3) was 7 days. Among 2,045 patients with solid tumors and normal baseline liver function tests, severe neutropenia occurred in 75.4% of patients and lasted for more than 7 days in 2.9% of cycles.

Febrile neutropenia (less than 500 cells/mm^3 with fever higher than 38°C [100.4°F] with IV antibiotics and/or hospitalization) occurred in 11% of patients with solid tumors, 12.3% of patients with metastatic breast cancer, and 9.8% of 92 breast cancer patients premedicated with 3-day corticosteroids.

Severe infectious episodes occurred in 6.1% of patients with solid tumors, 6.4% of patients with metastatic breast cancer, and 5.4% of 92 breast cancer patients premedicated with 3-day corticosteroids.

Thrombocytopenia (less than 100,000 cells/mm^3) associated with fatal GI hemorrhage has been reported.

Hepatic – In patients with normal liver function tests at baseline, bilirubin values greater than the ULN occurred in 8.9% of patients. Increases in AST or ALT more than 1.5 times the ULN or alkaline phosphatase more than 2.5 times ULN, were observed in 18.9% and 7.3% of patients, respectively. While on docetaxel, increases in AST and/or ALT more than 1.5 times ULN concomitant with alkaline phosphatase more than 2.5 times ULN occurred in 4.3% of patients with normal liver function tests at baseline (whether these changes were related to the drug or underlying disease has not been established).

Hypersensitivity – See the Warning box for more information.

Minor reactions, including back pain, chest tightness, chills, drug fever, dyspnea, flushing, or rash with or without pruritus, have been reported and resolved after discontinuing the infusion and appropriate therapy.

Local – Infusion-site reactions were generally mild and consisted of extravasation, hyperpigmentation, inflammation, phlebitis, redness or dryness of the skin, or swelling of the vein.

Metabolic –

Fluid retention: See the Warning box for more information.

➤*Hematologic and other toxicity: relation to dose and baseline liver chemistry abnormalities:*

Docetaxel Adverse Reactions in Breast Cancer Patients By Liver Function Abnormalities			
	Docetaxel 100 mg/m^2		Docetaxel 60 mg/m^2
Adverse reaction	Normal liver function tests[a] (n = 730)	Elevated liver function tests[b] (n = 18)	Normal liver function tests[a] (n = 174)
CNS			
Asthenia (any)	65.2%	44.4%	65.5%
Asthenia (severe)	16.6%	22.2%	0%
Neurosensory (any)	56.8%	50%	19.5%
Neurosensory (severe)	5.8%	0%	0%
Dermatologic			
Cutaneous (any)	44.8%	61.1%	30.5%
Cutaneous (severe)	4.8%	16.7%	0%
GI			
Diarrhea (any)	42.2%	27.8%	NA[c]
Diarrhea (severe)	6.3%	11.1%	NA
Stomatitis (any)	53.3%	66.7%	19%
Stomatitis (severe)	7.8%	38.9%	0.6%
Hematologic			
Anemia < 11 g/dL	94.6%	94.4%	64.9%
Febrile neutropenia[d] (by course)	2.4%	8.6%	0%
Febrile neutropenia[d] (by patient)	11.8%	33.3%	0%
Neutropenia (any < 2,000 cells/mm^3)	98.4%	100%	95.4%
Neutropenia (grade 4 < 500 cells/mm^3)	84.4%	93.8%	74.9%
Thrombocytopenia (any < 100,000 cells/mm^3)	10.8%	44.4%	14.4%
Thrombocytopenia (grade 4 < 20,000 cells/mm^3)	0.6%	16.7%	1.1%
Miscellaneous			
Acute hypersensitivity reaction regardless of premedication (any)	13%	5.6%	0.6%
Acute hypersensitivity reaction regardless of premedication (severe)	1.2%	0%	0%
Fluid retention[e] regardless of premedication (any)	56.2%	61.1%	12.6%
Fluid retention[e] regardless of premedication (severe)	7.9%	16.7%	0%
Infection[f] (any)	22.5%	38.9%	1.1%
Infection[f] (grades 3 and 4)	7.1%	33.3%	0%
Myalgia	22.7%	33.3%	3.4%
Nonseptic death	1.1%	11.1%	0%
Septic death	1.5%	5.6%	1.1%

[a] Normal baseline liver function tests: transaminases ≤ 1.5 times the ULN or alkaline phosphatase ≤ 2.5 times the ULN or isolated elevations of transaminases or alkaline phosphatase ≤ 5 times the ULN.
[b] Elevated baseline liver function: AST and/or ALT > 1.5 times the ULN concurrent with alkaline phosphatase> 2.5 times the ULN.
[c] NA = not available.
[d] Febrile neutropenia: for 100 mg/m^2, ANC grade 4 and fever > 38°C with IV antibiotics and/or hospitalization; for 60 mg/m^2, ANC grade 3 or 4 and fever > 38.1°C.
[e] Fluid retention includes the following (by COSTART): edema (generalized, localized, lymphedema, peripheral, pulmonary edema, and edema otherwise not specified) and effusion (ascites, pericardial, and pleural); no premedication given with the 60 mg/m^2 dose.
[f] Incidence of infection requiring hospitalization and/or IV antibiotics was 8.5% (n = 62) among the 730 patients with normal liver function tests at baseline; 7 patients had concurrent grade 3 neutropenia, and 46 patients had grade 4 neutropenia.

In the 3-arm monotherapy trial, TAX 313, which compared docetaxel 60, 75, and 100 mg/m^2 in advanced breast cancer, the overall safety profile was consistent with the safety profile observed in previous docetaxel trials. Grade 3 or 4 or severe adverse reactions occurred in 49% of patients treated with docetaxel 60 mg/m^2 compared with 55.3% and 65.9% treated with 75 and

DOCETAXEL — INJECTION

100 mg/m², respectively. Discontinuation due to adverse reactions was reported in 5.3% of patients treated with 60 mg/m² versus 6.9% and 16.5% for patients treated at 75 and 100 mg/m², respectively. Deaths within 30 days of last treatment occurred in 4% of patients treated with 60 mg/m² compared with 5.3% and 1.6% for patients treated at 75 and 100 mg/m², respectively.

The following adverse reactions were associated with increasing docetaxel doses: anemia (87%, 94%, and 97%, respectively) febrile neutropenia (5%, 7%, and 14% respectively), fluid retention (26%, 38%, and 46% at 60, 75, and 100 mg/m², respectively), neutropenia (92%, 94%, and 97% respectively), thrombocytopenia (7%, 11%, and 12% respectively), and treatment-related grade 3 or 4 infection (2%, 3%, and 7% respectively).

➤*Adjuvant treatment of breast cancer:*

Docetaxel Adverse Reactions in Adjuvant Treatment of Breast Cancer

Adverse reaction	Docetaxel 75 mg/m² + doxorubicin 50 mg/m² + cyclophosphamide 500 mg/m² (TAC) (n = 744)		Fluorouracil 500 mg/m² + doxorubicin 50 mg/m² + cyclophosphamide 500 mg/m² (FAC) (n = 736)	
	Any	Grade 3 or 4	Any	Grade 3 or 4
Cardiovascular				
Cardiac dysrhythmias	7.9%	0.3%	6%	0.3%
Hypotension	2.6%	0%	1.1%	0.1%
Phlebitis	1.2%	0%	0.8%	0%
Syncope	1.6%	0.5%	1.2%	0.3%
Vasodilation	27%	1.1%	21.2%	0.5%
CNS				
Asthenia	80.8%	11.2%	71.2%	5.6%
Neurocerebellar	2.4%	0.1%	2%	0%
Neurocortical	5.1%	0.5%	6.4%	0.7%
Neuropathy, motor	3.8%	0.1%	2.2%	0%
Neuropathy, sensory	25.5%	0%	10.2%	0%
Dermatologic				
Alopecia	97.8%	NA	97.1%	NA
Nail disorders	18.5%	0.4%	14.4%	0.1%
Skin toxicity	26.5%	0.8%	17.7%	0.4%
GI				
Abdominal pain	10.9%	0.7%	5.3%	0%
Anorexia	21.6%	2.2%	17.7%	1.2%
Constipation	33.9%	1.1%	31.8%	1.4%
Diarrhea	35.2%	3.8%	27.9%	1.8%
Nausea	80.5%	5.1%	88%	9.5%
Stomatitis	69.4%	7.1%	52.9%	2%
Taste perversion	27.8%	0.7%	15.1%	0%
Vomiting	44.5%	4.3%	59.2%	7.3%
Hematologic				
Anemia	91.5%	4.3%	71.7%	1.6%
Febrile neutropenia	24.7%	NA	2.5%	NA
Neutropenia	71.4%	65.5%	82%	49.3%
Neutropenic infection	12.1%	NA	6.3%	NA
Thrombocytopenia	39.4%	2%	27.7%	1.2%
Metabolic				
Fluid retention[a]	35.1%	0.9%	14.7%	0.1%
Lymphedema	4.4%	0%	1.2%	0%
Peripheral edema	26.9%	0.4%	7.3%	0%
Weight gain	12.9%	0.3%	8.6%	0.3%
Musculoskeletal				
Arthralgia	19.4%	0.5%	9%	0.3%
Myalgia	26.7%	0.8%	9.9%	0%
Special senses				
Conjunctivitis	5.1%	0.3%	6.9%	0.1%
Lacrimation disorder	11.3%	0.1%	7.1%	0%
Miscellaneous				
Amenorrhea	61.7%	NA	52.4%	NA
Cough	13.7%	0%	9.8%	0.1%
Fever in absence of infection	46.5%	1.3%	17.1%	0%
Hypersensitivity reactions	13.4%	1.3%	3.7%	0.1%
Infection	39.4%	3.9%	36.3%	2.2%

[a] COSTART term and grading system for reactions related to treatment.

Of the 744 patients treated with TAC, 36.3% experienced severe treatment-emergent adverse reactions compared with 26.6% of the 736 patients treated with FAC. Dose reductions due to hematologic toxicity occurred in 1% of cycles in the TAC arm versus 0.1% of cycles in the FAC arm. Six percent of patients treated with TAC discontinued treatment because of adverse reactions compared with 1.1% treated with FAC; allergy and fever in the absence of infection were the most common reasons for withdrawal among TAC-treated patients. Two patients died in each arm within 30 days of their last study treatment; 1 death per arm was attributed to study drugs.

Cardiovascular – More cardiovascular reactions were reported in the TAC arm versus the FAC arm: congestive heart failure (1.6% vs 0.5%); dysrhythmias, all grades (7.9% vs 6%); and hypotension, all grades (2.6% vs 1.1%). One patient in each arm died because of heart failure.

GI – In addition to GI reactions reflected in the preceding table, 7 patients in the TAC arm were reported to have colitis/enteritis/large intestine perforation versus 1 patient in the FAC arm. Five of the 7 TAC-treated patients required treatment discontinuation; no deaths due to these reactions occurred.

Miscellaneous –

Fever and infection: Fever in the absence of infection was seen in 46.5% of TAC-treated patients and in 17.1% of FAC-treated patients. Grade 3/4 fever in the absence of infection was seen in 1.3% and 0% of TAC- and FAC-treated patients, respectively. Infection was seen in 39.4% of TAC-treated patients compared with 36.3% of FAC-treated patients. Grade 3/4 infection was seen in 3.9% and 2.2% of TAC-treated and FAC-treated patients, respectively. There were no septic deaths in either treatment arm.

AML: See Warnings/Precautions for more information.

Gastric adenocarcinoma –

Docetaxel Adverse Reactions in Gastric Cancer[a]

Adverse reaction	Docetaxel + cisplatin + fluorouracil (n = 221)		Cisplatin + fluorouracil (n = 224)	
	Any	Grade 3 or 4	Any	Grade 3 or 4
Cardiovascular				
Cardiac dysrhythmias	4.5%	2.3%	2.2%	0.9%
Myocardial ischemia	0.9%	0%	2.7%	2.2%
CNS				
Dizziness	15.8%	4.5%	8%	1.8%
Lethargy	62.9%	21.3%	58%	17.9%
Neuromotor	8.6%	3.2%	7.6%	2.7%
Neurosensory	38%	7.7%	24.6%	3.1%
Dermatologic				
Alopecia	66.5%	5%	41.1%	1.3%
Nail changes	8.1%	0%	0%	0%
Rash/Itch	11.8%	0.9%	8.5%	0%
Skin desquamation	1.8%	0%	0.4%	0%
GI				
Anorexia	50.7%	13.1%	54%	11.6%
Constipation	25.3%	1.8%	33.9%	3.1%
Diarrhea	77.8%	20.4%	49.6%	8%
Esophagitis/ Dysphagia/ Odynophagia	16.3%	1.8%	13.8%	4.9%
GI pain/cramping	11.3%	1.8%	7.1%	2.7%
Nausea	73.3%	15.8%	76.3%	18.8%
Stomatitis	59.3%	20.8%	61.2%	27.2%

DOCETAXEL — INJECTION

Docetaxel Adverse Reactions in Gastric Cancer[a]				
	Docetaxel + cisplatin + fluorouracil (n = 221)		Cisplatin + fluorouracil (n = 224)	
Adverse reaction	Any	Grade 3 or 4	Any	Grade 3 or 4
Vomiting	66.5%	14.9%	73.2%	18.8%
Hematologic				
Anemia	96.8%	18.2%	93.3%	25.6%
Febrile neutropenia	16.4%	NA	4.5%	NA
Neutropenia	95.5%	82.3%	83.3%	56.8%
Neutropenic infection	15.9%	NA	10.4%	NA
Thrombocytopenia	25.5%	7.7%	39%	13.5%
Special senses				
Altered hearing	6.3%	0%	12.5%	1.8%
Tearing	8.1%	0%	2.2%	0.4%
Miscellaneous				
Allergic reactions	10.4%	1.8%	5.8%	0%
Edema[b]	13.1%	0%	3.1%	0.4%
Fever in the absence of infection	35.7%	1.8%	22.8%	1.3%
Fluid retention[b]	14.9%	0%	4%	0.4%
Infection	29.4%	16.3%	22.8%	10.3%

[a] Clinically important treatment-emergent adverse reactions were determined based upon frequency, severity, and clinical impact of the adverse reaction.
[b] Related to treatment.

➤*Head and neck cancer:*

Docetaxel Adverse Reactions in SCCHN				
	Docetaxel 75 mg/m² + cisplatin 75 mg/m² + fluorouracil 750 mg/m² (n = 174)		Cisplatin 100 mg/m² + fluorouracil 1,000 mg/m² (n = 181)	
Adverse reaction	Any	Grade 3 or 4	Any	Grade 3 or 4
Cardiovascular				
Cardiac dysrhythmia	1.7%	1.7%	1.7%	0.6%
Myocardial ischemia	1.7%	1.7%	0.6%	0%
Venous	3.4%	2.3%	5.5%	1.7%
CNS				
Dizziness	2.3%	0%	5%	0.6%
Lethargy	40.8%	3.4%	38.1%	3.3%
Neurosensory	17.8%	0.6%	10.5%	0.6%
Dermatologic				
Alopecia	81%	10.9%	43.1%	0%
Desquamation	4%	0.6%	5.5%	0%
Dry skin	5.7%	0%	1.7%	0%
Rash/Itch	11.5%	0%	6.1%	0%

Docetaxel Adverse Reactions in SCCHN				
	Docetaxel 75 mg/m² + cisplatin 75 mg/m² + fluorouracil 750 mg/m² (n = 174)		Cisplatin 100 mg/m² + fluorouracil 1,000 mg/m² (n = 181)	
Adverse reaction	Any	Grade 3 or 4	Any	Grade 3 or 4
GI				
Anorexia	16.1%	0.6%	24.9%	3.3%
Constipation	16.7%	0.6%	16%	1.1%
Diarrhea	32.8%	2.9%	23.8%	4.4%
Esophagitis/Dysphagia/Odynophagia	12.6%	1.1%	18.2%	2.8%
GI bleeding	4%	1.7%	0%	0%
GI pain/cramping	7.5%	0.6%	8.8%	0.6%
Heartburn	6.3%	0%	6.1%	0%
Nausea	47.1%	0.6%	51.4%	7.2%
Stomatitis	42.5%	4%	47%	11%
Vomiting	26.4%	0.6%	38.7%	5%
Hematologic				
Anemia	89.1%	9.2%	87.8%	13.8%
Febrile neutropenia[a]	5.2%	NA	2.2%	NA
Neutropenia	93.1%	76.3%	86.7%	52.8%
Neutropenic infection	13.9%	NA	8.3%	NA
Thrombocytopenia	23.6%	5.2%	47%	18.2%
Metabolic/Nutritional				
Fluid retention	20.1%	0%	14.4%	0.6%
Edema only	12.6%	0%	6.6%	0%
Weight gain only	5.7%	0%	6.1%	0%
Weight loss	20.7%	6.6%	26.5%	0.6%
Special senses				
Altered hearing	5.7%	0%	9.9%	2.8%
Conjunctivitis	1.1%	0%	1.1%	0%
Taste, sense of smell altered	10.3%	0%	5%	0%
Tearing	1.7%	0%	0.6%	0%
Miscellaneous				
Allergy	6.3%	0%	2.8%	0%
Cancer pain	20.7%	4.6%	16%	3.3%
Fever in the absence of infection	31.6%	0.6%	36.5%	0%
Infection	27%	8.6%	26%	7.7%
Myalgia	9.8%	1.1%	7.2%	0%

[a] Febrile neutropenia: grade ≥ 2 fever concomitant with grade 4 neutropenia requiring IV antibiotics and/or hospitalization.

➤*Treatment of NSCLC:*

Docetaxel Adverse Reactions in NSCLC Patients					
	Previously treated with platinum-based chemotherapy[a]			Chemotherapy-naïve	
Adverse reaction	Docetaxel 75 mg/m² (n = 176)	Best supportive care (n = 49)	Vinorelbine/ifosfamide (n = 119)	Docetaxel 75 mg/m² + cisplatin 75 mg/m² (n = 406)	Vinorelbine 25 mg/m² + cisplatin 100 mg/m² (n = 396)
CNS					
Asthenia (any)[b]	52.8%	57.1%	53.8%	74%	75%
Asthenia (severe or life-threatening)[b]	18.2%	38.8%	22.7%	12%	14%
Neuromotor (any)	15.9%	8.2%	10.1%	19%	17%
Neuromotor (grade 3 and 4)	4.5%	6.1%	3.4%	3%	6%
Neurosensory (any)	23.3%	14.3%	28.6%	47%	42%
Neurosensory (grade 3 and 4)	1.7%	6.1%	5%	4%	4%
Dermatologic					
Alopecia (any)	56.3%	34.7%	49.6%	75%	42%

DOCETAXEL — INJECTION

Docetaxel Adverse Reactions in NSCLC Patients

Adverse reaction	Previously treated with platinum-based chemotherapy[a]			Chemotherapy-naïve	
	Docetaxel 75 mg/m² (n = 176)	Best supportive care (n = 49)	Vinorelbine/ifosfamide (n = 119)	Docetaxel 75 mg/m² + cisplatin 75 mg/m² (n = 406)	Vinorelbine 25 mg/m² + cisplatin 100 mg/m² (n = 396)
Alopecia (grade 3)	—	—	—	< 1%	0%
Dermatologic (any)	19.9%	6.1%	16.8%	16%	14%
Dermatologic (grade 3 and 4)	0.6%	2%	0.8%	< 1%	1%
Nail disorder (any)[b]	11.4%	0%	1.7%	14%	< 1%
Nail disorder (severe)[b]	1.1%	0%	0%	< 1%	0%
GI					
Anorexia (any)[b]	—	—	—	42%	40%
Anorexia (severe or life-threatening)[b]	—	—	—	5%	5%
Diarrhea (any)	22.7%	6.1%	11.8%	47%	25%
Diarrhea (grade 3 and 4)	2.8%	0%	4.2%	7%	3%
Nausea (any)	33.5%	30.6%	31.1%	72%	76%
Nausea (grade 3 and 4)	5.1%	4.1%	7.6%	10%	17%
Stomatitis (any)	26.1%	6.1%	7.6%	24%	21%
Stomatitis (grade 3 and 4)	1.7%	0%	0.8%	2%	1%
Taste perversion (any)	5.7%	0%	0%	—	—
Taste perversion (severe)[b]	0.6%	0%	0%	—	—
Vomiting (any)	21.6%	26.5%	21.8%	55%	61%
Vomiting (grade 3 and 4)	2.8%	2%	5.9%	8%	16%
Hematologic					
Anemia (any)	91%	55.1%	90.8%	89%	94%
Anemia (grade 3 and 4)	9.1%	12.2%	14.3%	7%	25%
Febrile neutropenia[c]	6.3%	NA	0.8%	5%	5%
Leukopenia (any)	83.5%	6.1%	89.1%	—	—
Leukopenia (grade 3 and 4)	49.4%	0%	42.9%	—	—
Neutropenia (any)	84.1%	14.3%	83.2%	91%	90%
Neutropenia (grade 3 and 4)	65.3%	12.2%	57.1%	74%	78%
Thrombocytopenia (any)	8%	0%	7.6%	15%	15%
Thrombocytopenia (grade 3 and 4)	2.8%	0%	1.7%	3%	4%
Hypersensitivity					
Hypersensitivity reactions (any)[d]	5.7%	0%	0.8%	12%	4%
Hypersensitivity reactions (grade 3 and 4)[d]	2.8%	0%	0%	3%	< 1%
Metabolic/Nutritional					
Fluid retention (any)[b]	33.5%	ND[e]	22.7%	54%	42%
Fluid retention (severe or life-threatening)[b]	2.8%	ND	3.4%	2%	2%
Peripheral edema (any)	—	—	—	34%	18%
Peripheral edema (severe or life-threatening)	—	—	—	< 1%	< 1%
Weight gain (any)			—	15%	9%
Weight gain (severe or life-threatening)			—	< 1%	< 1%
Musculoskeletal					
Arthralgia (any)	3.4%	2%	1.7%	—	—
Arthralgia (severe)[b]	0%	0%	0.8%	—	—
Myalgia (any)[b]	6.3%	0%	2.5%	18%	12%
Myalgia (severe)[b]	0%	0%	0%	< 1%	< 1%
Respiratory					
Pleural effusion (any)	—	—	—	23%	22%
Pleural effusion (severe or life-threatening)	—	—	—	2%	2%
Pulmonary (any)	40.9%	49%	45.4%	—	—
Pulmonary (grade 3 and 4)	21%	28.6%	18.5%	—	—
Miscellaneous					
Fever in absence of infection (any)	—	—	—	33%	29%
Fever in absence of infection (grade 3 and 4)	—	—	—	< 1%	1%
Infection (any)	33.5%	28.6%	30.3%	35%	37%
Infection (grade 3 and 4)	10.2%	6.1%	9.2%	8%	8%

DOCETAXEL — INJECTION

Docetaxel Adverse Reactions in NSCLC Patients					
	Previously treated with platinum-based chemotherapy[a]			Chemotherapy-naïve	
Adverse reaction	Docetaxel 75 mg/m² (n = 176)	Best supportive care (n = 49)	Vinorelbine/ifosfamide (n = 119)	Docetaxel 75 mg/m² + cisplatin 75 mg/m² (n = 406)	Vinorelbine 25 mg/m² + cisplatin 100 mg/m² (n = 396)
Treatment-related mortality	2.8%	NA	3.4%	—	—

[a] Normal baseline liver function tests: transaminases ≤ to 1.5 times ULN, alkaline phosphatase ≤ 2.5 times ULN, or isolated elevations of transaminases or alkaline phosphatase ≤ 5 times ULN.
[b] COSTART term and grading system.
[c] Febrile neutropenia: ANC grade 4 with fever > 38°C (100.4°F) with IV antibiotics and/or hospitalization.
[d] Replaces NCI term "allergy."
[e] ND = not done.

Deaths within 30 days of last study treatment occurred in 31 patients (7.6%) in the docetaxel plus cisplatin arm and 37 patients (9.3%) in the vinorelbine plus cisplatin arm. Deaths within 30 days of last study treatment attributed to study drug occurred in 9 patients (2.2%) in the docetaxel plus cisplatin arm and 8 patients (2%) in the vinorelbine plus cisplatin arm.

The second comparison in the study, vinorelbine plus cisplatin versus docetaxel plus carboplatin (which did not demonstrate a superior survival associated with docetaxel) demonstrated a higher incidence of alopecia, diarrhea, fluid retention, hypersensitivity reactions, nail changes, skin toxicity, and thrombocytopenia on the docetaxel plus carboplatin arm, while a higher incidence of anemia, anorexia, asthenia, nausea, neurosensory toxicity, and vomiting was observed on the vinorelbine plus cisplatin arm.

➤*Prostate cancer:*

Docetaxel Adverse Reactions in Prostate Cancer Patients				
	Docetaxel 75 mg/m² every 3 weeks + prednisone 5 mg twice daily (n = 332)		Mitoxantrone 12 mg/m² every 3 weeks + prednisone 5 mg twice daily (n = 335)	
Adverse reaction	Any	Grade 3 or 4	Any	Grade 3 or 4
CNS				
Fatigue	53.3%	4.5%	34.6%	5.1%
Neuropathy, motor	7.2%	1.5%	3%	0.9%
Neuropathy, sensory	30.4%	1.8%	7.2%	0.3%
Dermatologic				
Alopecia	65.1%	NA	12.8%	NA
Nail changes	29.5%	0%	7.5%	0%
Rash/ Desquamation	6%	0.3%	3.3%	0.6%
GI				
Anorexia	16.6%	1.2%	14.3%	0.3%
Diarrhea	31.6%	2.1%	9.6%	1.2%
Nausea	41%	2.7%	35.5%	1.5%
Stomatitis/ Pharyngitis	19.6%	0.9%	8.4%	0%
Taste disturbance	18.4%	0%	6.6%	0%
Vomiting	16.9%	1.5%	14%	1.5%
Hematologic				
Anemia	66.5%	4.9%	57.8%	1.8%
Febrile neutropenia	2.7%	NA	1.8%	NA
Neutropenia	40.9%	32%	48.2%	21.7%
Thrombocytopenia	3.4%	0.6%	7.8%	1.2%
Metabolic/Nutritional				
Fluid retention[a]	24.4%	0.6%	4.5%	0.3%
Peripheral edema[a]	18.1%	0.3%	1.5%	0%
Weight gain[a]	7.5%	0.3%	3%	0%
Musculoskeletal				
Arthralgia	8.1%	0.6%	5.1%	1.2%
Myalgia	14.5%	0.3%	12.8%	0.9%
Respiratory				
Cough	12.3%	0%	7.8%	0%
Dyspnea	15.1%	2.7%	8.7%	0.9%
Epistaxis	5.7%	0.3%	1.8%	0%
Miscellaneous				
Allergic reactions	8.4%	0.6%	0.6%	0%
Cardiac left ventricular function	9.6%	0.3%	22.1%	1.2%
Infection	32.2%	5.7%	20.3%	4.2%
Tearing	9.9%	0.6%	1.5%	0%

[a] Related to treatment.

➤*Postmarketing:*

Cardiovascular – Atrial fibrillation, deep vein thrombosis, electrocardiogram (ECG) abnormalities, myocardial infarction, pulmonary embolism, syncope, tachycardia, thrombophlebitis.

CNS – Confusion, rare cases of seizures or transient loss of consciousness have been observed, sometimes appearing during the infusion of the drug.

Dermatologic – Very rare cases of cutaneous lupus erythematous and rare cases of bullous eruption, such as erythema multiforme, Stevens-Johnson syndrome, and toxic epidermal necrolysis. In some cases, multiple factors may have contributed to the development of these reactions. Severe hand and foot syndrome has been reported.

GI – Abdominal pain, anorexia, colitis, constipation, dehydration as a consequence of GI reactions, duodenal ulcer, esophagitis, GI hemorrhage, GI perforation, ileus, intestinal obstruction, and ischemic colitis and neutropenic enterocolitis have been reported.

Hepatic – Rare cases of hepatitis (sometimes fatal), primarily in patients with preexisting liver disorder, have been reported.

Hypersensitivity – Rare cases of anaphylactic shock have been reported. Very rarely these cases resulted in a fatal outcome in patients who received premedication.

Respiratory – Acute pulmonary edema, acute respiratory distress syndrome, dyspnea, interstitial pneumonia. Pulmonary fibrosis has been rarely reported. Rare cases of radiation pneumonitis have been reported in patients receiving concomitant radiotherapy.

Special senses – Conjunctivitis, lacrimation, or lacrimation with or without conjunctivitis. Excessive tearing that may be attributable to lacrimal duct obstruction has been reported.

Rare cases of transient visual disturbances (flashes, flashing lights, scotomata) typically occurring during drug infusion and in association with hypersensitivity reactions have been reported. These were reversible upon discontinuation of the infusion. Rare cases of ototoxicity, hearing disorders, and/or hearing loss have been reported, including cases associated with other ototoxic drugs.

Miscellaneous – Bleeding episodes, chest pain, diffuse pain, radiation recall phenomenon, renal function impairment.

Overdosage

➤*Symptoms:* There were 2 reports of overdose. One patient received 150 mg/m², and the other received 200 mg/m² as 1-hour infusions. Both patients experienced severe neutropenia, mild asthenia, cutaneous reactions, and mild paresthesia and recovered without incident. Anticipated complications of overdosage include bone marrow suppression, peripheral neurotoxicity, and mucositis.

➤*Treatment:* There is no known antidote for docetaxel overdosage. In case of overdosage, keep the patient in a specialized unit where vital functions can be monitored closely. Give patients therapeutic G-CSF as soon as possible after discovery of overdose. Take other appropriate symptomatic measures as needed.

DOCETAXEL — INJECTION

Patient Information

Inform patients that adverse reactions associated with docetaxel may include low white blood cell count, hair loss, fatigue, fluid retention, numbness, mouth irritation, cutaneous changes, nausea, and diarrhea.

Inform patients that their health care provider may prescribe other medications, including a corticosteroid such as dexamethasone, that help to avoid or lessen some of the adverse reactions of treatment.

Inform patients that if they have a fever of more than 100°F, to call their health care provider immediately. Other symptoms of infection, such as sore throat, cough, or burning sensation while urinating, also should be reported.

Advise patients to tell their health care provider immediately if they feel a warm sensation, tightness in the chest, difficulty breathing, or itching during or shortly after treatment.

Inform patients to alert their health care provider if there are any signs of fluid retention (ie, increased weight, swelling of the feet or hands).

Advise patients to tell their health care provider if they feel prolonged fatigue during the course of treatment.

Patients receiving docetaxel may develop a red, blotchy rash. This usually occurs on the feet and hands but may also appear on the arms, face, or body. If it occurs, the rash generally appears within the week after docetaxel treatment and usually disappears after a week or two. Advise patients to inform their health care provider if this occurs.

Some patients receiving docetaxel experience numbness, tingling, or burning sensations in their fingers and/or toes.

Advise patients that changes in the color of the nails may occur. Occasionally, nails become soft and tender. In rare cases, nails may fall off.

CABAZITAXEL

Rx	**Jevtana** (Sanofi-Aventis)	**Injection, solution, concentrate:** 40 mg/mL	Polysorbate 80. In single-use vials with diluent.

CABAZITAXEL — INJECTION

WARNING

Neutropenia – Neutropenic deaths have been reported. In order to monitor the occurrence of neutropenia, frequent blood cell counts should be performed on all patients receiving cabazitaxel. Cabazitaxel should not be given to patients with neutrophil counts of 1,500 cells/mm^3 or less.

Hypersensitivity – Severe hypersensitivity reactions can occur and may include generalized rash/erythema, hypotension, and bronchospasm. Severe hypersensitivity reactions require immediate discontinuation of the cabazitaxel infusion and administration of appropriate therapy. Patients should receive premedication. Cabazitaxel must not be given to patients who have a history of severe hypersensitivity reactions to cabazitaxel or to other drugs formulated with polysorbate 80.

Indications

➤*Prostate cancer:* In combination with prednisone for the treatment of patients with hormone-refractory metastatic prostate cancer previously treated with a docetaxel-containing treatment regimen.

Administration and Dosage

➤*General dosing considerations:* Premedication is recommended prior to treatment (see Premedication).

Dilution is required twice prior to administration. (See Preparation for Administration.)

➤*Adults:*

Prostate cancer –

Usual dosage: 25 mg/m^2 administered as a 1-hour intravenous (IV) infusion every 3 weeks in combination with oral prednisone 10 mg administered daily throughout cabazitaxel treatment.

Dose modifications –

Cabazitaxel Dosage Modifications

Toxicity	Dosage modification
Prolonged grade ≥ 3 neutropenia (> 1 week) despite appropriate medication including G-CSF[a]	Delay treatment until neutrophil count is > 1,500 cells/mm^3, then reduce dosage of cabazitaxel to 20 mg/m^2. Use G-CSF for secondary prophylaxis. Discontinue cabazitaxel treatment if a patient continues to experience any of these reactions at 20 mg/m^2.
Febrile neutropenia	Delay treatment until improvement or resolution, and until neutrophil count is > 1,500 cells/mm^3, then reduce dosage of cabazitaxel to 20 mg/m^2. Use G-CSF for secondary prophylaxis. Discontinue cabazitaxel treatment if a patient continues to experience any of these reactions at 20 mg/m^2.
≥ Grade 3 diarrhea or persisting diarrhea despite appropriate medication, fluid, and electrolyte replacement	Delay treatment until improvement or resolution, then reduce dosage of cabazitaxel to 20 mg/m^2. Discontinue cabazitaxel treatment if a patient continues to experience any of these reactions at 20 mg/m^2.

[a] G-CSF = granulocyte colony-stimulating factor.

Premedication – Premedicate at least 30 minutes prior to each dose of cabazitaxel with the following IV medications to reduce the risk and/or severity of hypersensitivity: antihistamine (dexchlorpheniramine 5 mg, or diphenhydramine 25 mg or equivalent antihistamine), corticosteroid (dexamethasone 8 mg or equivalent steroid), and H_2 antagonist (ranitidine 50 mg or equivalent H_2 antagonist).

Antiemetic prophylaxis is recommended and can be given orally or IV as needed.

➤*Hepatic function impairment:* Cabazitaxel should not be given to patients with hepatic impairment (total bilirubin at greater than or equal to the upper limits of normal [ULN], or AST and/or ALT at least 1.5 × ULN).

➤*Preparation for administration:* Cabazitaxel is a cytotoxic anticancer drug and caution should be exercised when handling and preparing cabazitaxel solutions, taking into account the use of containment devices, personal protective equipment (eg, gloves), and preparation procedures. If cabazitaxel should come into contact with the skin, immediately and thoroughly wash with soap and water. If cabazitaxel should come into contact with mucosa, immediately and thoroughly wash with water.

Do not use polyvinyl chloride (PVC) infusion containers or polyurethane infusions sets for preparation and administration of cabazitaxel infusion solution. Cabazitaxel requires 2 dilutions prior to administration. Both the cabazitaxel injection and the diluent vials contain an overfill to compensate for liquid loss during preparation. This overfill ensures that after dilution with the entire contents of the accompanying diluent, there is an initial diluted solution containing 10 mg/mL cabazitaxel.

Initial dilution – Each vial of cabazitaxel 60 mg per 1.5 mL must first be mixed with the entire contents of supplied diluent. Once reconstituted, the resultant solution contains cabazitaxel 10 mg/mL.

When transferring the diluent, direct the needle onto the inside wall of cabazitaxel vial and inject slowly to limit foaming. Remove the syringe and needle and gently mix the initial diluted solution by repeated inversions for at least 45 seconds to assure full mixing of the drug and diluent. Do not shake. Let the solution stand for a few minutes to allow any foam to dissipate, and check that the solution is homogeneous and contains no visible particulate matter. It is not required that all foam dissipate prior to continuing the preparation process.

The resulting initial diluted cabazitaxel solution (cabazitaxel 10 mg/mL) requires further dilution before administration. The final dilution should be done immediately (within 30 minutes).

Final dilution – Withdraw the recommended dose from the cabazitaxel solution containing 10 mg/mL as prepared using a calibrated syringe and further dilute into a sterile 250 mL PVC-free container of sodium chloride 0.9% solution or dextrose 5% solution for infusion. If a dose greater than cabazitaxel 65 mg is required, use a larger volume of the infusion vehicle so that a concentration of cabazitaxel 0.26 mg/mL is not exceeded. The concentration of the cabazitaxel final infusion solution should be between 0.1 and 0.26 mg/mL.

Remove the syringe and thoroughly mix the final infusion solution by gently inverting the bag or bottle. Cabazitaxel final infusion solution (in sodium chloride 0.9% solution or dextrose 5% solution) should be used immediately or within 8 hours at ambient temperature (including the 1-hour infusion) or within a total of 24 hours if refrigerated (including the 1-hour infusion).

Because the final infusion solution is supersaturated, it may crystallize over time. Do not use and discard if this occurs.

➤*Administration:* Administer IV as a 1-hour infusion at room temperature using an in-line filter of 0.22 micrometer nominal pore size.

➤*Admixture compatibility:* Cabazitaxel should not be mixed with any other drugs.

➤*Storage/Stability:* Store at 25°C (77°F); excursions permitted between 15° and 30°C (59° and 86°F). Do not refrigerate. Use initial diluted cabazitaxel solution immediately (within 30 minutes). Discard any unused portion. Fully prepared cabazitaxel infusion solution (in sodium chloride 0.9% solution or dextrose 5% solution) should be used within 8 hours at ambient temperature (including the 1-hour infusion), or for a total of 24 hours (including the 1-hour infusion) under the refrigerated conditions. Discard the unused portion.

Actions

➤*Pharmacology:* Cabazitaxel, a microtubule inhibitor, is an antineoplastic agent belonging to the taxane class. Cabazitaxel binds to tubulin and promotes its assembly into microtubules while simultaneously inhibiting disassembly. This leads to the stabilization of microtubules, which results in the inhibition of mitotic and interphase cellular functions.

➤*Pharmacokinetics:*

Absorption – Based on the population pharmacokinetic analysis, after an IV dose of cabazitaxel 25 mg/m^2 every 3 weeks, the mean maximal drug concentration (C_{max}) in patients with metastatic prostate cancer was 226 ng/mL (coefficient of variation [CV], 107%) and was reached at the end of the 1-hour infusion (time of maximal concentration). The mean area under the curve in patients with metastatic prostate cancer was 991 ng•h/mL (CV, 34%). No

CABAZITAXEL — INJECTION

major deviation from the dose proportionality was observed from 10 to 30 mg/m^2 in patients with advanced solid tumors.

Distribution – The volume of distribution at steady state was 4,864 L (2,643 L/m^2 for a patient with a median body surface area (BSA) of 1.84 m^2).

In vitro, the binding of cabazitaxel to human serum proteins was 89% to 92% and was not saturable up to 50,000 ng/mL, which covers the maximum concentration observed in clinical trials. Cabazitaxel is mainly bound to human serum albumin (82%) and lipoproteins (88% for high-density lipoprotein, 70% for low-density lipoprotein, and 56% for very low density lipoprotein). The in vitro blood-to-plasma concentration ratio in human blood ranged from 0.9 to 0.99, indicating that cabazitaxel was equally distributed between blood and plasma.

Metabolism – Cabazitaxel is extensively metabolized in the liver (more than 95%), mainly by the cytochrome P450 (CYP-450) 3A4/5 isoenzyme (80% to 90%), and to a lesser extent by CYP2C8. Cabazitaxel is the main circulating moiety in human plasma. Seven metabolites were detected in plasma (including the 3 active metabolites issued from O-demethylation), with the main one accounting for 5% of cabazitaxel exposure. Around 20 metabolites of cabazitaxel are excreted into human urine and feces.

Excretion – After a 1-hour IV infusion of [^{14}C]-cabazitaxel 25 mg/m^2, approximately 80% of the administered dose was eliminated within 2 weeks. Cabazitaxel is mainly excreted in the feces as numerous metabolites (76% of the dose); while renal excretion of cabazitaxel and metabolites account for 3.7% of the dose (2.3% as unchanged drug in urine).

Based on the population pharmacokinetic analysis, cabazitaxel has a plasma clearance of 48.5 L/h (CV, 39%; 26.4 L/h/m for a patient with a median BSA of 1.84 m^2) in patients with metastatic prostate cancer. Following a 1-hour IV infusion, plasma concentrations of cabazitaxel can be described by a 3-compartment pharmacokinetic model with alpha, beta, and gamma half-lives of 4 minutes, 2 hours, and 95 hours, respectively.

Special populations –

Renal function impairment: Cabazitaxel is minimally excreted via the kidney. No formal pharmacokinetic trials have been conducted with cabazitaxel in patients with renal impairment. The population pharmacokinetic analysis carried out in 170 patients including 14 patients with moderate renal impairment (creatinine clearance [CrCl] at least 30 mL/min to less than 50 mL/min) and 59 patients with mild renal impairment (CrCl at least 50 mL/min to less than 80 mL/min) showed that mild to moderate renal impairment did not have meaningful effects on the pharmacokinetics of cabazitaxel. No data are available for patients with severe renal impairment or ESRD.

Hepatic function impairment: No formal trials in patients with hepatic impairment have been conducted. Because cabazitaxel is extensively metabolized in the liver, hepatic impairment is likely to increase the cabazitaxel concentrations.

Elderly: Based on a population pharmacokinetic analysis, no significant difference was observed in the pharmacokinetics of cabazitaxel between patients younger than 65 years of age (n = 100) and those older than 65 years of age (n = 70).

Contraindications

Neutrophil count of 1,500/mm^3 or less; history of severe hypersensitivity reactions to cabazitaxel or to other drugs formulated with polysorbate 80.

Warnings/Precautions

➤*Neutropenia:* Five patients experienced fatal infectious adverse reactions (sepsis or septic shock). All had grade 4 neutropenia and 1 had febrile neutropenia. One additional patient's death was attributed to neutropenia without a documented infection.

G-CSF may be administered to reduce the risks of neutropenia complications associated with cabazitaxel use. Consider primary prophylaxis with G-CSF in patients with high-risk clinical features (older than 65 years of age, poor performance status, previous episodes of febrile neutropenia, extensive prior radiation ports, poor nutritional status, or other serious comorbidities) that predispose them to increased complications from prolonged neutropenia. Consider therapeutic use of G-CSF and secondary prophylaxis in all patients considered to be at increased risk of neutropenia complications.

Monitoring of complete blood counts is essential on a weekly basis during cycle 1 and before each treatment cycle thereafter so that the dose can be adjusted, if needed.

Do not administer cabazitaxel to patients with neutrophils 1,500/mm^3 or less.

If a patient experiences febrile neutropenia or prolonged neutropenia (longer than 1 week) despite appropriate medication (eg, G-CSF), reduce the dose of cabazitaxel. Patients can restart treatment with cabazitaxel only when neutrophil counts recover to a level greater than 1,500/mm^3.

➤*GI effects:* Nausea, vomiting, and severe diarrhea, at times, may occur. Death related to diarrhea and electrolyte imbalance occurred in the randomized clinical trial. Intensive measures may be required for severe diarrhea and electrolyte imbalance. Treat patients with rehydration, antidiarrheal, or antiemetic medications as needed. Treatment delay or dosage reduction may be necessary if patients experience grade 3 or greater diarrhea.

➤*Renal effects:* Renal failure, including 4 cases with fatal outcome, was reported in the randomized clinical trial. Most cases occurred in association with sepsis, dehydration, or obstructive uropathy. Some deaths because of renal failure did not have a clear cause. Take appropriate measures to identify causes of renal failure and treat aggressively.

➤*Hypersensitivity reactions:* Premedicate all patients prior to the initiation of the infusion of cabazitaxel. Observe patients closely for hypersensitivity reactions, especially during the first and second infusions. Hypersensitivity reactions may occur within a few minutes following the initiation of the infusion of cabazitaxel, thus ensure that facilities and equipment for the treatment of hypotension and bronchospasm are available. Severe hypersensitivity reactions can occur and may include generalized rash/erythema, hypotension and bronchospasm. Severe hypersensitivity reactions require immediate discontinuation of the cabazitaxel infusion and appropriate therapy. Do not rechallenge patients with a history of severe hypersensitivity reactions with cabazitaxel.

➤*Renal function impairment:* Use caution in patients with severe renal impairment (CrCl less than 30 mL/min) and patients with ESRD.

➤*Hepatic function impairment:* See Actions for more information.

Hepatic impairment increases the risk of severe and life-threatening complications in patients receiving other drugs belonging to the same class as cabazitaxel. Do not give cabazitaxel to patients with hepatic impairment (total bilirubin at or greater than ULN, or AST and/or ALT 1.5 × ULN or greater).

➤*Pregnancy: Category D.* Cabazitaxel can cause fetal harm when administered to a pregnant woman. There are no adequate and well-controlled studies in pregnant women using cabazitaxel. If this drug is used during pregnancy or if the patient becomes pregnant while taking this drug, apprise the patient of the potential hazard to the fetus. Advise women of childbearing potential to avoid becoming pregnant during treatment with cabazitaxel.

In non-clinical studies in rats and rabbits, cabazitaxel was embryotoxic, fetotoxic, and abortifacient at exposures significantly lower than those expected at the recommended human dose level. Cabazitaxel was shown to cross the placenta barrier within 24 hours of a single IV administration of a 0.08 mg/kg dose (approximately 0.02 times the maximum recommended human dose [MRHD]) to pregnant rats at gestational day 17.

Cabazitaxel administered once daily to female rats during organogenesis at a dosage of 0.16 mg/kg/day (approximately 0.02 to 0.06 times the C_{max} in patients with cancer at the recommended human dose) caused maternal and embryofetal toxicity consisting of increased postimplantation loss, embryolethality, and fetal deaths. Decreased mean fetal birth weight associated with delays in skeletal ossification were observed at doses of at least 0.08 mg/kg (approximately 0.02 times the C_{max} at the MRHD). In utero exposure to cabazitaxel did not result in fetal abnormalities in rats or rabbits at exposure levels significantly lower than the expected human exposures.

➤*Lactation:* Cabazitaxel or cabazitaxel metabolites are excreted in maternal milk of lactating rats. It is not known whether this drug is excreted in human milk. Within 2 hours of a single IV administration of cabazitaxel to lactating rats at a dose of 0.08 mg/kg (approximately 0.02 times the MRHD), radioactivity related to cabazitaxel was detected in the stomachs of nursing pups. This was detectable for up to 24 hours post-dose. Approximately 1.5% of the dose delivered to the mother was calculated to be delivered in the maternal milk. Because many drugs are excreted in human milk and because of the potential for serious adverse reactions in breast-feeding infants from cabazitaxel, decide whether to discontinue breast-feeding or to discontinue the drug, taking into account the importance of the drug to the mother.

➤*Children:* The safety and effectiveness of cabazitaxel in children have not been established.

➤*Elderly:* In the randomized clinical trial, 2% of patients younger than 65 years of age and 6% of patients 65 years of age and older died of causes other than disease progression within 30 days of the last cabazitaxel dose. Patients 65 years of age or older are more likely to experience certain adverse reactions, including neutropenia and febrile neutropenia.

See Adverse Reactions for more information.

➤*Monitoring:* Monitoring of complete blood counts is essential on a weekly basis during cycle 1 and before each treatment cycle thereafter, so that the dose can be adjusted if needed. Patients should be observed closely for hypersensitivity reactions, especially during the first and second infusions.

Drug Interactions

Cabazitaxel Drug Interactions

Precipitant drug	Object drug[a]		Description
CYP3A inducers (eg, carbamazepine, phenobarbital, phenytoin, rifabutin, rifampin, rifapentine, St. John's wort)	Cabazitaxel	⬇	Coadministration of strong CYP3A inducers is expected to decrease cabazitaxel concentrations. Avoid coadministration.

CABAZITAXEL — INJECTION

Cabazitaxel Drug Interactions

Precipitant drug	Object drug[a]		Description
CYP3A inhibitors (eg, atazanavir, clarithromycin, indinavir, itraconazole, ketoconazole, nefazodone, nelfinavir, ritonavir, saquinavir, telithromycin, voriconazole)	Cabazitaxel	↑	Coadministration of strong CYP3A inhibitors is expected to increase concentrations of cabazitaxel. Avoid coadministration with strong CYP3A inhibitors. Coadminister moderate CYP3A inhibitors with caution.

[a] ↑ = object drug increased; ↓ = object drug decreased.

Adverse Reactions

➤*Mortality:* Deaths due to causes other than disease progression within 30 days of the last study drug dose were reported in 5% of cabazitaxel-treated patients and less than 1% of mitoxantrone-treated patients. The most common fatal adverse reactions in cabazitaxel-treated patients were infections (n = 5) and renal failure (n = 4). The majority (4 of 5 patients) of fatal infection-related adverse reactions occurred after a single dose of cabazitaxel. Other fatal adverse reactions in cabazitaxel-treated patients included ventricular fibrillation, cerebral hemorrhage, and dyspnea.

➤*Most common adverse reactions:* The most common (10% or greater) grade 1 to 4 adverse reactions were abdominal pain, alopecia, anemia, anorexia, arthralgia, asthenia, back pain, constipation, cough, diarrhea, dysgeusia, dyspnea, fatigue, hematuria, leukopenia, nausea, neutropenia, peripheral neuropathy, pyrexia, thrombocytopenia, and vomiting.

The most common (5% or greater) grade 3 to 4 adverse reactions in patients who received cabazitaxel were anemia, asthenia, diarrhea, fatigue, febrile neutropenia, leukopenia, and neutropenia.

➤*Discontinuations / Dose modifications:* Treatment discontinuations because of adverse drug reactions occurred in 18% of patients who received cabazitaxel and 8% of patients who received mitoxantrone. The most common adverse reactions leading to treatment discontinuation in the cabazitaxel group were neutropenia and renal failure. Dose reductions were reported in 12% of cabazitaxel-treated patients and 4% of mitoxantrone-treated patients. Dose delays were reported in 28% of cabazitaxel-treated patients and 15% of mitoxantrone-treated patients.

Cabazitaxel in Combination With Prednisone Adverse Reactions (≥ 5%)

	Cabazitaxel 25 mg/m² every 3 weeks with prednisone 10 mg daily (n = 371)		Mitoxantrone 12 mg/m² every 3 weeks with prednisone 10 mg daily (n = 371)	
	Grade 1 to 4	Grade 3 to 4	Grade 1 to 4	Grade 3 to 4
Median duration of treatment	6 cycles		4 cycles	
Adverse reactions				
Cardiovascular				
Arrhythmia[a]	5%	1%	2%	< 1%
Hypotension	5%	< 1%	2%	< 1%
CNS				
Asthenia	20%	5%	12%	2%
Dizziness	8%	0%	6%	< 1%
Dysgeusia	11%	0%	4%	0%
Fatigue	37%	5%	27%	3%
Headache	8%	0%	5%	0%
Peripheral neuropathy[b]	13%	< 1%	3.2%	< 1%
GI				
Abdominal pain[c]	17%	2%	6%	0%
Constipation	20%	1%	15%	< 1%
Diarrhea	47%	6%	11%	< 1%
Dyspepsia[d]	10%	0%	2%	0%
Nausea	34%	2%	23%	< 1%
Vomiting	22%	2%	10%	0%
Hematologic				
Anemia[e]	98%	11%	82%	5%
Febrile neutropenia	7%	7%	1%	1%
Leukopenia[e]	96%	69%	93%	42%
Neutropenia[e]	94%	82%	87%	58%
Thrombocytopenia[e]	48%	4%	43%	2%

Cabazitaxel in Combination With Prednisone Adverse Reactions (≥ 5%)

	Cabazitaxel 25 mg/m² every 3 weeks with prednisone 10 mg daily (n = 371)		Mitoxantrone 12 mg/m² every 3 weeks with prednisone 10 mg daily (n = 371)	
	Grade 1 to 4	Grade 3 to 4	Grade 1 to 4	Grade 3 to 4
Median duration of treatment	6 cycles		4 cycles	
Adverse reactions				
Metabolic/Nutritional				
Anorexia	16%	< 1%	11%	< 1%
Dehydration	5%	2%	3%	< 1%
Weight decreased	9%	0%	8%	< 1%
Musculoskeletal				
Arthralgia	11%	1%	8%	1%
Back pain	16%	4%	12%	3%
Muscle spasms	7%	0%	3%	0%
GU				
Dysuria	7%	0%	1%	0%
Hematuria	17%	2%	4%	< 1%
Urinary tract infections[f]	8%	2%	3%	1%
Respiratory				
Cough	11%	0%	6%	0%
Dyspnea	12%	1%	4%	< 1%
Miscellaneous				
Alopecia	10%	0%	5%	0%
Mucosal inflammation	6%	< 1%	3%	< 1%
Pain	5%	1%	5%	2%
Peripheral edema	9%	< 1%	9%	< 1%
Pyrexia	12%	1%	6%	< 1%

[a] Includes atrial fibrillation, atrial flutter, atrial tachycardia, atrioventricular block complete, bradycardia, palpitations, supraventricular tachycardia, tachyarrhythmia, and tachycardia.
[b] Includes peripheral motor neuropathy and peripheral sensory neuropathy.
[c] Includes abdominal discomfort, abdominal pain lower, abdominal pain upper, abdominal tenderness, and GI pain.
[d] Includes gastroesophageal reflux disease and reflux gastritis.
[e] Based on laboratory values, cabazitaxel, n = 369; mitoxantrone, n = 370.
[f] Includes urinary tract infection enterococcal and urinary tract infection fungal.

➤*Neutropenia and associated reactions:* See Warnings/Precautions for more information. Six percent of patients discontinued cabazitaxel treatment because of neutropenia, febrile neutropenia, infection, or sepsis. The most common adverse reaction leading to treatment discontinuation in the cabazitaxel group was neutropenia (2%).

➤*Hematuria:* Adverse reactions of hematuria, including those requiring medical intervention, were more common in cabazitaxel-treated patients. The incidence of grade 2 or greater hematuria was 6% in cabazitaxel-treated patients and 2% in mitoxantrone-treated patients. Other factors associated with hematuria were well-balanced between arms and do not account for the increased rate of hematuria on the cabazitaxel arm.

➤*Lab test abnormalities:* The incidences of grade 3 to 4 increased AST, increased ALT, and increased bilirubin were each 1% or less.

➤*Elderly:* The following grade 1 to 4 adverse reactions were reported at rates at least 5% higher in patients 65 years of age and older compared with younger patients: fatigue (40% vs 30%), neutropenia (97% vs 89%), asthenia (24% vs 15%), pyrexia (15% vs 8%), dizziness (10% vs 5%), urinary tract infection (10% vs 3%) and dehydration (7% vs 2%), respectively.

The incidence of the following grade 3 to 4 adverse reactions were higher in patients 65 years of age and older compared with younger patients; neutropenia (87% vs 74%), and febrile neutropenia (8% vs 6%).

Overdosage

➤*Symptoms:* Anticipated complications of overdose include exacerbation of adverse reactions, such as bone marrow suppression and GI disorders.

➤*Treatment:* There is no known antidote for cabazitaxel overdose. In case of overdose, keep the patient in a specialized unit where vital signs, chemistry, and particular functions can be closely monitored. Ensure that patients receive therapeutic G-CSF as soon as possible after discovery of overdose. Take other appropriate symptomatic measures as needed.

Patient Information

Inform patients about the risk of potential hypersensitivity associated with cabazitaxel. Confirm that patients do not have a history of severe hypersensitivity reactions to cabazitaxel or to other drugs formulated with polysorbate 80. Instruct patients to immediately report signs of a hypersensitivity reaction.

Taxoids

CABAZITAXEL — INJECTION

Explain the importance of routine blood cell counts. Instruct patients to monitor their temperature frequently and immediately report any occurrence of fever to the treating health care provider.

Inform patients that it is important to take the oral prednisone as prescribed. Instruct patients to report if they were not compliant with oral corticosteroid regimen.

Advise patients that severe and fatal infections, dehydration, and renal failure have been associated with cabazitaxel exposure. Instruct patients to immediately report fever, significant vomiting or diarrhea, decreased urinary output, and hematuria to the treating health care provider.

Advise patients about the risk of drug interactions and the importance of providing a list of prescription and nonprescription drugs to the treating health care provider.

Advise elderly patients that certain adverse reactions may be more frequent or severe.

Epothilones

IXABEPILONE

Rx	**Ixempra** (Bristol-Myers Squibb)	**Injection, lyophilized, powder for solution, concentrate:** 15 mg	In single-use kits. Kit contains 1 vial of ixabepilone and 1 vial of diluent.[a]
		45 mg	In single-use kits. Kit contains 1 vial of ixabepilone and 1 vial of diluent.[a]

[a] Diluent contains 52.8% purified polyoxyethylated castor oil and 39.8% dehydrated alcohol.

IXABEPILONE — INJECTION

WARNING

Toxicity in hepatic function impairment – Ixabepilone in combination with capecitabine is contraindicated in patients with AST or ALT greater than 2.5 times the upper limit of normal (ULN) or bilirubin greater than 1 times ULN because of an increased risk of toxicity and neutropenia-related death.

Indications

➤*Breast cancer:* In combination with capecitabine for the treatment of patients with metastatic or locally advanced breast cancer resistant to treatment with an anthracycline and a taxane, or in patients whose cancer is taxane-resistant and for whom further anthracycline therapy is contraindicated; as monotherapy for the treatment of metastatic or locally advanced breast cancer in patients whose tumors are resistant or refractory to anthracyclines, taxanes, and capecitabine.

Administration and Dosage

➤*General dosing considerations:* To minimize the chance of occurrence of a hypersensitivity reaction, all patients must be premedicated. (See Premedication.)

Consider discontinuing ixabepilone if cardiac ischemia or dysfunction occur.

➤*Adults:*

Breast cancer –

Usual dosage: 40 mg/m^2 administered intravenously (IV) over 3 hours every 3 weeks. Doses for patients with body surface area greater than 2.2 m^2 should be calculated based on 2.2 m^2.

Dosage adjustment:

• *During treatment* – Patients should be evaluated during treatment by periodic clinical observation and laboratory tests, including complete blood cell counts. If toxicities are present, treatment should be delayed to allow recovery. Dosing adjustment guidelines for monotherapy and combination therapy are shown in the following tables. If toxicities recur, an additional 20% dose reduction should be made.

Ixabepilone Dose Adjustment Guidelines[a]

Ixabepilone monotherapy or combination therapy	Ixabepilone dose modification
Nonhematologic	
Grade 2 neuropathy (moderate) lasting ≥ 7 days	Decrease the dose by 20%
Grade 3 neuropathy (severe) lasting < 7 days	Decrease the dose by 20%
Grade 3 neuropathy (severe) lasting ≥ 7 days or disabling neuropathy	Discontinue treatment
Any grade 3 toxicity (severe) other than neuropathy	Decrease the dose by 20%
Transient grade 3 arthralgia/myalgia or fatigue	No change in the dose of ixabepilone
Grade 3 hand-foot syndrome (palmar-plantar erythrodysesthesia)	
Any grade 4 toxicity (disabling)	Discontinue treatment
Hematologic	
Neutrophil < 500 cells/mm^3 for ≥ 7 days	Decrease the dose by 20%
Febrile neutropenia	Decrease the dose by 20%
Platelets < 25,000/mm^3 or platelets ^{3} with bleeding	Decrease the dose by 20%

[a] Toxicities graded in accordance with National Cancer Institute Common Toxicity Criteria for Adverse Events (NCI-CTCAE), version 3.0.

Capecitabine Dose Adjustment Guidelines When Used in Combination With Ixabepilone[a]

Capecitabine dose adjustment (in combination with ixabepilone)	Capecitabine dose modification
Nonhematologic	Follow capecitabine label
Hematologic	
Platelets < 25,000/mm^3 or < 50,000/mm^3 with bleeding	Hold for concurrent diarrhea or stomatitis until platelet count > 50,000/mm^3, then continue at same dose
Neutrophils < 500 cells/mm^3 for ≥ 7 days or febrile neutropenia	Hold for concurrent diarrhea or stomatitis until neutrophil count > 1,000 cells/mm^3, then continue at same dose

[a] Toxicities graded in accordance with NCI-CTCAE, version 3.0.

• *Re-treatment criteria* – Dose adjustments at the start of a cycle should be based on nonhematologic toxicity or blood cell counts from the preceding cycle and should follow the guidelines in the previous tables. Patients should not begin a new cycle of treatment unless the neutrophil count is at least 1,500 cells/mm^3, the platelet count is at least 100,000 cells/mm^3, and nonhematologic toxicities have improved to grade 1 (mild) or resolved.

Duration of therapy: Continue ixabepilone as long as response is favorable and drug is tolerated. Assess therapeutic response after every 2 cycles of therapy.

➤*Hepatic function impairment:*

Combination therapy – Ixabepilone in combination with capecitabine is contraindicated in patients with AST or ALT more than 2.5 times ULN or bilirubin more than 1 times ULN because of an increased risk of toxicity and neutropenia-related death. Patients receiving combination treatment who have AST and ALT less than or equal to 2.5 times ULN and bilirubin less than or equal to 1 times ULN may receive the standard dose of ixabepilone (40 mg/m^2).

Monotherapy – Patients with hepatic function impairment should be dosed with ixabepilone based on the guidelines in the following table. Patients with moderate hepatic function impairment should be started at 20 mg/m^2; the dosage in subsequent cycles may be escalated up to, but not exceeding, 30 mg/m^2 if tolerated. Use in patients with AST or ALT more than 10 times ULN or bilirubin more than 3 times ULN is not recommended. Limited data are available for patients with baseline AST or ALT more than 5 times ULN. Caution should be used when treating these patients.

Ixabepilone Dose Adjustments as Monotherapy in Patients With Hepatic Function Impairment

	Transaminase levels		Bilirubin levels[a]	Ixabepilone[b] (mg/m^2)
Mild	AST and ALT ≤ 2.5 times ULN	and	≤ 1 times ULN	40
	AST and ALT ≤ 10 times ULN	and	≤ 1.5 times ULN	32
Moderate	AST and ALT ≤ 10 times ULN	and	> 1.5 times ULN to ≤ 3 times ULN	20 to 30

[a] Excluding patients whose total bilirubin is elevated because of Gilbert disease.
[b] Dosage recommendations are for first course of therapy; further decreases in subsequent courses should be based on individual tolerance.

➤*Concomitant therapy:* The use of concomitant strong CYP3A4 inhibitors should be avoided (eg, ketoconazole, itraconazole, clarithromycin, atazanavir, nefazodone, saquinavir, telithromycin, ritonavir, amprenavir, indinavir, nelfinavir, delavirdine, voriconazole). Grapefruit juice may also increase plasma concentrations of ixabepilone and should be avoided. Based on pharmacokinetic studies, if a strong CYP3A4 inhibitor must be coadministered, a dose reduction of 20 mg/m^2 is predicted to adjust the ixabepilone area under the curve (AUC) to the range observed without inhibitors and should be considered. If the strong inhibitor is discontinued, a washout

IXABEPILONE — INJECTION

period of approximately 1 week should be allowed before the ixabepilone dose is adjusted upward to the indicated dose.

➤*Premedication:* To minimize the chance of occurrence of a hypersensitivity reaction, all patients must be premedicated approximately 1 hour before the infusion of ixabepilone with an H_1 antagonist (eg, diphenhydramine 50 mg orally or equivalent) and an H_2 antagonist (eg, ranitidine 150 to 300 mg orally, famotidine 20 to 40 mg, or nizatidine 150 to 300 mg orally or equivalent).

Patients who experienced a hypersensitivity reaction to ixabepilone required premedication with corticosteroids (eg, dexamethasone 20 mg IV 30 minutes before infusion or orally 60 minutes before infusion) in addition to pretreatment with H_1 and H_2 antagonists.

➤*Preparation for administration:* Ixabepilone is considered a cytotoxic agent. Follow safe handling procedures when preparing, administering, or dispensing ixabepilone.

To minimize the risk of dermal exposure, impervious gloves should be worn when handling vials containing ixabepilone, regardless of the setting, including unpacking and inspection, transport within a facility, and dose preparation and administration.

The ixabepilone kit contains 2 vials, a vial labeled ixabepilone for injection that contains ixabepilone powder and a vial containing diluent for ixabepilone. Only supplied diluent must be used for reconstituting ixabepilone for injection. Prior to reconstituting ixabepilone for injection, the kit should be removed from the refrigerator and allowed to stand at room temperature for approximately 30 minutes. When the vials are first removed from the refrigerator, a white precipitate may be observed in the diluent vial. This precipitate will dissolve to form a clear solution once the diluent warms to room temperature. To allow for withdrawal losses, the vial labeled ixabepilone 15 mg for injection contains ixabepilone 16 mg and the vial labeled ixabepilone 45 mg for injection contains ixabepilone 47 mg.

Reconstitution – With a suitable syringe, aseptically withdraw the diluent and slowly inject it into the ixabepilone for injection vial. The ixabepilone 15 mg kit is supplied with a vial providing 8 mL of the diluent, and the ixabepilone 45 mg kit is supplied with a vial providing 23.5 mL of the diluent. Gently swirl and invert the vial until the powder in ixabepilone is completely dissolved. After reconstituting with the diluent, the concentration of ixabepilone is 2 mg/mL.

Dilution – Before administration, the reconstituted solution must be further diluted only with Ringer's lactate injection, supplied in di-(2-ethylhexyl)phthalate (DEHP)–free bags. For most doses, a 250 mL bag of Ringer's lactate injection is sufficient. However, it is necessary to check the final infusion concentration of each dose based on the volume of Ringer's lactate injection to be used. The final concentration for infusion must be between 0.2 and 0.6 mg/mL. To calculate the final infusion concentration, use the following formulas:

Total infusion volume = mL of reconstituted solution + mL of Ringer's Lactate injection

Final infusion concentration = dose of ixabepilone (mg)/total infusion volume (mL).

Aseptically, withdraw the appropriate volume of reconstituted solution containing ixabepilone 2 mg/mL. Aseptically, transfer to an IV bag containing an appropriate volume of Ringer's lactate injection to achieve the final desired concentration of ixabepilone. Thoroughly mix the infusion bag by manual rotation.

➤*Administration:* Administer IV over 3 hours. The infusion solution must be administered through an appropriate inline filter with a microporous membrane of 0.2 to 1.2 microns. DEHP-free infusion containers and administration sets must be used. Any remaining solution should be discarded according to institutional procedures for antineoplastics.

➤*Extravasation:* Ixabepilone is considered an irritant and may cause phlebitis, but it is not known to cause tissue damage with extravasation. If signs or symptoms of extravasation occur, stop the infusion immediately. If possible, withdraw 3 to 5 mL of blood to remove some of the drug. Remove the infusion needle. Delineate the infiltrated area on the patient's skin with a felt-tip marker. Elevate for 48 hours above heart level using a sling or stockinette dressing with an observation window cut in the dressing. Avoid pressure or friction. Do not rub the area. Observe for signs of increased erythema, pain, or skin necrosis. If increased symptoms occur, consult a plastic surgeon. Ensure that no medication is given distally to extravasation site. After 48 hours, encourage the patient to use the extremity normally to promote full range of motion.

➤*Storage/Stability:* The ixabepilone kit must be stored in a refrigerator at 36° to 46°F (2° to 8°C) in the original package to protect from light. After reconstituting ixabepilone, the reconstituted solution should be further diluted with Ringer's lactate injection as soon as possible, but may be stored in the vial (not the syringe) for a maximum of 1 hour at room temperature and room light. Once diluted with Ringer's lactate injection, the solution is stable at room temperature and room light for a maximum of 6 hours. Ringer's lactate injection is specified because it has a pH range of 6 to 7.5, which is required to maintain ixabepilone stability.

Actions

➤*Pharmacology:* Ixabepilone is a semisynthetic analog of epothilone B. Ixabepilone binds directly to β-tubulin subunits on microtubules, leading to suppression of microtubule dynamics. Ixabepilone suppresses the dynamic instability of αβ-II and αβ-III microtubules. Ixabepilone possesses low in vitro susceptibility to multiple tumor resistance mechanisms, including efflux transporters, such as MRP-1 and P-glycoprotein (P-gp). Ixabepilone blocks cells in the mitotic phase of the cell division cycle, leading to cell death.

Pharmacodynamics – In cancer patients, ixabepilone has a plasma concentration–dependent effect on tubulin dynamics in peripheral blood mononuclear cells that is observed as the formation of microtubule bundles. Ixabepilone has antitumor activity in vivo against multiple human tumor xenografts, including drug-resistant types that overexpress P-gp, MRP-1, and β-III tubulin isoforms, or harbor tubulin mutations. Ixabepilone is active in xenografts that are resistant to multiple agents, including taxanes, anthracyclines, and vinca alkaloids. Ixabepilone demonstrated synergistic antitumor activity in combination with capecitabine in vivo. In addition to direct antitumor activity, ixabepilone has antiangiogenic activity.

➤*Pharmacokinetics:*

Absorption – Following administration of a single 40 mg/m² dose of ixabepilone in patients with cancer, the mean maximum plasma concentration (C_{max}) was 252 ng/mL (coefficient of variation [CV], 56%) and the mean area under the curve (AUC) was 2,143 ng•h/mL (CV, 48%). Typically, C_{max} occurred at the end of the 3-hour infusion. In cancer patients, the pharmacokinetics of ixabepilone were linear at doses of 15 to 57 mg/m².

Distribution – The mean volume of distribution of ixabepilone 40 mg/m² at steady state was in excess of 1,000 L. In vitro, the binding of ixabepilone to human serum proteins ranged from 67% to 77%, and the blood-to-plasma concentration ratios in human blood ranged from 0.65 to 0.85 over a concentration range of 50 to 5,000 ng/mL.

Metabolism – Ixabepilone is extensively metabolized in the liver. In vitro studies indicated that the main route of oxidative metabolism of ixabepilone is via CYP3A4. More than 30 metabolites of ixabepilone are excreted into human urine and feces. No single metabolite accounted for more than 6% of the administered dose. The biotransformation products generated from ixabepilone by human liver microsomes were not active when tested for in vitro cytotoxicity against a human tumor cell line.

In vitro studies using human liver microsomes indicate that clinically relevant concentrations of ixabepilone do not inhibit CYP3A4, CYP1A2, CYP2A6, CYP2B6, CYP2C8, CYP2C9, CYP2C19, or CYP2D6. At clinically relevant concentrations, ixabepilone does not induce the activity or the corresponding mRNA levels of CYP1A2, CYP2B6, CYP2C9, or CYP3A4 in cultured human hepatocytes. Therefore, it is unlikely that ixabepilone will affect the plasma levels of drugs that are substrates of CYP enzymes.

Excretion – Ixabepilone is eliminated primarily as metabolized drug. After an IV ^{14}[C]-ixabepilone dose, approximately 86% of the dose was eliminated within 7 days in feces (65% of the dose) and in urine (21% of the dose). Unchanged ixabepilone accounted for approximately 1.6% and 5.6% of the dose in feces and urine, respectively. Ixabepilone has a terminal elimination half-life of approximately 52 hours. No accumulation in plasma is expected for ixabepilone administered every 3 weeks.

Contraindications

Patients with a history of a severe (CTC grade 3/4) hypersensitivity reaction to agents containing polyoxyethylated castor oil; patients who have neutrophil count less than 1,500 cells/mm³ or a platelet count less than 100,000 cells/mm³; ixabepilone in combination with capecitabine is contraindicated in patients with AST or ALT greater than 2.5 times ULN or bilirubin greater than 1 times ULN.

Warnings/Precautions

➤*Peripheral neuropathy:* Peripheral neuropathy was common (see the following table). Monitor patients treated with ixabepilone for symptoms of neuropathy, such as burning sensation, hyperesthesia, hypoesthesia, paresthesia, discomfort, or neuropathic pain. Neuropathy occurred early during treatment; approximately 75% of new-onset or worsening neuropathy occurred during the first 3 cycles. Patients experiencing new or worsening symptoms may require a reduction or delay in the dose of ixabepilone. In clinical studies, peripheral neuropathy was managed through dose reductions, dose delays, and treatment discontinuation. Neuropathy was the most frequent cause of treatment discontinuation because of drug toxicity. In studies 046 and 081, 80% and 87%, respectively, of patients with peripheral neuropathy who received ixabepilone had improvement or no worsening of their neuropathy following dose reduction. For patients with grade 3/4 neuropathy in studies 046 and 081, 76% and 79%, respectively, had documented improvement to baseline or grade 1, twelve weeks after onset.

Ixabepilone Treatment-Related Peripheral Neuropathy

	Ixabepilone with capecitabine (study 046)	Ixabepilone as monotherapy (study 081)
Peripheral neuropathy (all grades)[a,b]	67%	63%
Peripheral neuropathy (grades 3/4)[a,b]	23%	14%
Discontinuation because of neuropathy	21%	6%
Median number of cycles to onset of grade 3/4 neuropathy	4	4
Median time to improvement of grade 3/4 neuropathy to baseline or to grade 1	6	4.6

[a] Sensory and motor neuropathy combined.
[b] Twenty-four percent and 27% of patients in 046 and 081, respectively, had preexisting neuropathy (grade 1).

IXABEPILONE — INJECTION

A pooled analysis of 945 cancer patients treated with ixabepilone indicated that patients with diabetes mellitus may be at increased risk of severe neuropathy. The presence of grade 1 neuropathy and prior therapy with neurotoxic chemotherapy agents did not predict the development or worsening of neuropathy. Patients with moderate to severe neuropathy (grade 2 or greater) were excluded from studies with ixabepilone. Use caution when treating patients with diabetes mellitus or existing moderate to severe neuropathy.

➤*Myelosuppression:* Myelosuppression is dose-dependent and primarily manifested as neutropenia. In clinical studies, grade 4 neutropenia (less than 500 cells/mm^3) occurred in 36% of patients treated with ixabepilone in combination with capecitabine and 23% of patients treated with ixabepilone monotherapy. Febrile neutropenia and infection with neutropenia were reported in 5% and 6% of patients treated with ixabepilone in combination with capecitabine, respectively, and in 3% and 5% of patients treated with ixabepilone as monotherapy, respectively. Neutropenia-related death occurred in 1.9% of 414 patients with healthy hepatic function or mild hepatic function impairment who were treated with ixabepilone in combination with capecitabine. The rate of neutropenia-related deaths was higher (29%, 5/17) in patients with AST or ALT greater than 2.5 times ULN or bilirubin greater than 1.5 times ULN. Neutropenia-related death occurred in 0.4% of 240 patients treated with ixabepilone as monotherapy. No neutropenia-related deaths were reported in 24 patients with AST or ALT greater than 2.5 times ULN or bilirubin greater than 1.5 times ULN who were treated with ixabepilone monotherapy. Ixabepilone must not be administered to patients with a neutrophil count less than 1,500 cells/mm^3. To monitor for myelosuppression, frequent peripheral blood cell counts are recommended for all patients receiving ixabepilone. Patients who experience severe neutropenia or thrombocytopenia should have their dose reduced.

➤*Cardiac effects:* The frequency of cardiac adverse reactions (myocardial ischemia and ventricular dysfunction) was higher in ixabepilone in combination with capecitabine (1.9%) than in the capecitabine alone (0.3%) treatment group. Supraventricular arrhythmias were observed in the combination arm (0.5%) but not in the capecitabine alone arm. Exercise caution in patients with a history of cardiac disease. Consider discontinuation of ixabepilone in patients who develop cardiac ischemia or impaired cardiac function.

➤*Cognitive impairment from excipients:* Because ixabepilone contains dehydrated alcohol, consider the possibility of CNS and other effects of alcohol.

➤*Extravasation:* See Administration and Dosage for more information.

➤*Hypersensitivity reactions:* Do not treat patients with a history of a severe hypersensitivity reaction to agents containing polyoxyethylated castor oil with ixabepilone. Premedicate all patients with an H_1 and an H_2 antagonist approximately 1 hour before ixabepilone infusion and observe them for hypersensitivity reactions (eg, flushing, rash, dyspnea, bronchospasm). In case of severe hypersensitivity reactions, stop infusion of ixabepilone and start aggressive supportive treatment (eg, epinephrine, corticosteroids). Of the 1,323 patients treated with ixabepilone in clinical studies, 9 (1%) patients experienced severe hypersensitivity reactions, including anaphylaxis. Three of the 9 patients were able to be re-treated. Patients who experience a hypersensitivity reaction in 1 cycle of ixabepilone must be premedicated in subsequent cycles with a corticosteroid in addition to the H_1 and H_2 antagonists, and consider extension of the infusion time.

➤*Renal function impairment:* Ixabepilone is minimally excreted via the kidney. No controlled pharmacokinetic studies were conducted with ixabepilone in patients with renal function impairment. Ixabepilone in combination with capecitabine has not been evaluated in patients with calculated creatinine clearance (CrCl) of less than 50 mL/min. Ixabepilone as monotherapy has not been evaluated in patients with creatinine greater than 1.5 times ULN. In a population pharmacokinetic analysis of ixabepilone as monotherapy, there was no meaningful effect of mild and moderate renal function impairment (CrCl greater than 30 mL/min) on the pharmacokinetics of ixabepilone.

➤*Hepatic function impairment:* Patients with baseline AST or ALT greater than 2.5 times ULN or bilirubin greater than 1.5 times ULN experienced greater toxicity than patients with baseline AST or ALT less than or equal to 2.5 times ULN or bilirubin less than or equal to 1.5 times ULN when treated with ixabepilone at 40 mg/m^2 in combination with capecitabine or as monotherapy in breast cancer studies. In combination with capecitabine, the overall frequency of grade 3/4 adverse reactions, febrile neutropenia, serious adverse reactions, and toxicity-related deaths was greater. With monotherapy, grade 4 neutropenia, febrile neutropenia, and serious adverse reactions were more frequent. The safety and pharmacokinetics of ixabepilone as monotherapy were evaluated in a dose escalation study in 56 patients with varying degrees of hepatic function impairment. Exposure was increased in patients with elevated AST or bilirubin.

Ixabepilone in combination with capecitabine is contraindicated in patients with AST or ALT greater than 2.5 times ULN or bilirubin greater than 1 times ULN because of increased risk of toxicity and neutropenia-related death. Patients who are treated with ixabepilone as monotherapy should receive a reduced dose depending on the degree of hepatic function impairment. Use in patients with AST or ALT greater than 10 times ULN or bilirubin greater than 3 times ULN is not recommended. Limited data are available for patients with AST or ALT greater than 5 times ULN. Use caution when treating these patients.

Ixabepilone was evaluated in 56 patients with mild to severe hepatic function impairment, defined by bilirubin levels and AST levels. Compared with patients with healthy hepatic function (n = 17), the $AUC_{0\text{-infinity}}$ of ixabepilone increased by 22% in patients with a) bilirubin greater than 1 to 1.5 times ULN or b) AST greater than ULN but bilirubin less than 1.5 times ULN; 30% in patients with bilirubin greater than 1.5 to 3 times ULN and any AST level; and 81% in patients with bilirubin greater than 3 times ULN and any AST level.

Doses of 10 and 20 mg/m^2 as monotherapy were tolerated in 17 patients with severe hepatic function impairment (bilirubin greater than 3 times ULN).

Ixabepilone in combination with capecitabine must not be given to patients with AST or ALT greater than 2.5 times ULN or bilirubin greater than 1 times ULN. Dose reduction is recommended when administering ixabepilone as monotherapy to patients with hepatic function impairment. Because there is a need for dosage adjustment based upon hepatic function, assessment of hepatic function is recommended before initiation of ixabepilone and periodically thereafter.

➤*Pregnancy: Category D.* Ixabepilone may cause fetal harm when administered to pregnant women. There are no adequate and well-controlled studies with ixabepilone in pregnant women. Advise women not to become pregnant when taking ixabepilone. If this drug is used during pregnancy or if the patient becomes pregnant while taking this drug, apprise the patient of the potential hazard to the fetus.

Ixabepilone was studied for effects on embryo-fetal development in pregnant rats and rabbits given IV doses of 0.02, 0.08, and 0.3 mg/kg/day, and 0.01, 0.03, 0.11 and 0.3 mg/kg/day, respectively. There were no teratogenic effects. In rats, an increase in resorptions and postimplantation loss and a decrease in the number of live fetuses and fetal weight was observed at the maternally toxic dose of 0.3 mg/kg/day (approximately one-tenth the human clinical exposure based on AUC). Abnormalities included a reduced ossification of caudal vertebrae, sternebrae, and metacarpals. In rabbits, ixabepilone caused maternal toxicity (death) and embryo-fetal toxicity (resorptions) at 0.3 mg/kg/day (approximately one-tenth the human clinical dose based on body surface area). No fetuses were available at this dose for evaluation.

➤*Lactation:* It is not known whether ixabepilone is excreted into human milk. Following IV administration of radiolabeled ixabepilone to rats on days 7 to 9 postpartum, concentrations of radioactivity in milk were comparable with those in plasma and declined in parallel with the plasma concentrations. Because many drugs are excreted in human milk and because of the potential for serious adverse reactions in breast-feeding infants from ixabepilone, a decision must be made whether to discontinue breast-feeding or ixabepilone, taking into account the importance of the drug to the mother.

➤*Children:* The safety and effectiveness of ixabepilone in children have not been established.

➤*Elderly:* Forty-five of 431 patients treated with ixabepilone in combination with capecitabine were 65 years of age and older and 3 patients were 75 years of age and older. Overall, the incidence of grade 3/4 adverse reactions was higher in patients 65 years of age and older versus those younger than 65 years of age (82% vs 68%), including grade 3/4 stomatitis (9% vs 1%), diarrhea (9% vs 6%), palmar-plantar erythrodysesthesia syndrome (27% vs 20%), peripheral neuropathy (24% vs 22%), febrile neutropenia (9% vs 3%), fatigue (16% vs 12%), and asthenia (11% vs 6%). Toxicity-related deaths occurred in 2 of 43 (4.7%) patients 65 years of age and older with normal baseline hepatic function or mild impairment.

➤*Monitoring:* Monitor patients treated with ixabepilone for symptoms of neuropathy, such as burning sensation, hyperesthesia, hypoesthesia, paresthesia, discomfort, or neuropathic pain. To monitor for myelosuppression, frequent peripheral blood cell counts are recommended for all patients receiving ixabepilone. Because there is a need for dosage adjustment based upon hepatic function, assessment of hepatic function is recommended before initiation of ixabepilone and periodically thereafter. Closely monitor patients receiving CYP3A4 inhibitors (eg, azole antifungals, protease inhibitors, macrolide antibiotics) during treatment with ixabepilone for acute toxicities (eg, frequent monitoring of peripheral blood cell counts between cycles).

Drug Interactions

➤*Cytochrome P450 system:* Because ixabepilone is metabolized mainly by the CYP3A enzyme systems, substances known to inhibit these enzymes may decrease metabolism or increase bioavailability of ixabepilone as indicated by increased whole blood or plasma concentrations. Drugs known to induce these enzyme systems may result in an increased metabolism of ixabepilone or decreased bioavailability, as indicated by decreased whole blood or plasma concentrations. Monitoring of blood concentrations and appropriate dosage adjustments are essential when such drugs are used concomitantly.

IXABEPILONE — INJECTION

Ixabepilone Drug Interactions

Precipitant drug	Object drug[a]		Description
Azole antifungals (eg, fluconazole, itraconazole, ketoconazole, voriconazole)	Ixabepilone	↑	Coadministration of ixabepilone with ketoconazole, a potent CYP3A4 inhibitor, increased ixabepilone AUC by 79%. If alternative treatment cannot be administered, consider a dose adjustment (see Administration and Dosage). The effect of fluconazole, a moderate CYP3A4 inhibitor, has not been studied. Therefore, use mild or moderate CYP3A4 inhibitors with caution and consider alternative therapy. Monitor closely for acute toxicities (eg, frequent peripheral blood counts between ixabepilone cycles).
Capecitabine	Ixabepilone	↔	In patients who received ixabepilone in combination with capecitabine, ixabepilone C_{max} decreased by 19%, capecitabine C_{max} decreased by 27%, and 5-fluorouracil AUC increased by 14%, compared with ixabepilone or capecitabine administered separately. This interaction is not considered clinically significant, given that the combination treatment is supported by efficacy data. However, coadministration of ixabepilone and capecitabine is contraindicated in patients with AST or ALT > 2.5 times the ULN or bilirubin > 1 times the ULN due to an increased risk of toxicity and neutropenia-related death.
Ixabepilone	Capecitabine		
Carbamazepine	Ixabepilone	↓	Carbamazepine, a strong CYP3A4 inducer, may decrease ixabepilone concentrations, leading to subtherapeutic levels. If coadministration cannot be avoided, a gradual ixabepilone dose adjustment may be considered.
Delavirdine	Ixabepilone	↑	Delavirdine, a strong CYP3A4 inhibitor, may increase ixabepilone concentrations (see Administration and Dosage). Avoid coadministration. If coadministration cannot be avoided, monitor closely for acute toxicities (eg, frequent peripheral blood counts between ixabepilone cycles).
Dexamethasone	Ixabepilone	↓	Dexamethasone, a strong CYP3A4 inducer, may decrease ixabepilone concentrations, leading to subtherapeutic levels. If coadministration cannot be avoided, a gradual ixabepilone dose adjustment may be considered.
Macrolide antibiotics (eg, clarithromycin, erythromycin)	Ixabepilone	↑	Macrolide antibiotics, CYP3A4 inhibitors, may increase ixabepilone plasma concentrations (see Administration and Dosage). Avoid coadministration. If coadministration cannot be avoided, monitor closely for acute toxicities (eg, frequent peripheral blood counts between ixabepilone cycles).
Nefazodone	Ixabepilone	↑	Nefazodone, a strong CYP3A4 inhibitor, may increase ixabepilone concentrations (see Administration and Dosage). Avoid coadministration. If coadministration cannot be avoided, monitor closely for acute toxicities (eg, frequent peripheral blood counts between ixabepilone cycles).
Phenobarbital	Ixabepilone	↓	Phenobarbital, a strong CYP3A4 inducer, may decrease ixabepilone concentrations, leading to subtherapeutic levels. If coadministration cannot be avoided, a gradual ixabepilone dose adjustment may be considered.
Phenytoin	Ixabepilone	↓	Phenytoin, a strong CYP3A4 inducer, may decrease ixabepilone concentrations, leading to subtherapeutic levels. If coadministration cannot be avoided, a gradual ixabepilone dose adjustment may be considered.
Protease inhibitors (eg, amprenavir, atazanavir, indinavir, nelfinavir, ritonavir, saquinavir)	Ixabepilone	↑	Coadministration of strong CYP3A4 inhibitors such as protease inhibitors may increase ixabepilone concentrations. If alternative treatment cannot be administered, consider an ixabepilone dose adjustment (see Administration and Dosage).
Rifamycins (eg, rifabutin, rifampin)	Ixabepilone	↓	Rifamycins, strong CYP3A4 inducers, may decrease ixabepilone concentrations, leading to subtherapeutic levels. If coadministration cannot be avoided, a gradual ixabepilone dose adjustment may be considered.
St. John's wort	Ixabepilone	↓	St. John's wort may decrease ixabepilone plasma concentrations unpredictably and should be avoided.
Telithromycin	Ixabepilone	↑	Coadministration of a strong CYP3A4 inhibitor such as telithromycin may increase ixabepilone concentrations and should be avoided (see Administration and Dosage). If coadministration cannot be avoided, monitor closely for acute toxicities (eg, frequent peripheral blood counts between ixabepilone cycles).
Verapamil	Ixabepilone	↑	Verapamil, a CYP3A4 inhibitor, may increase ixabepilone plasma concentrations. Use with caution and monitor closely for acute toxicities.
Ixabepilone	Disulfiram, metronidazole	↑	Ixabepilone diluent contains alcohol. Therefore, administration of ixabepilone to patients receiving disulfiram or metronidazole may produce acute alcohol intolerance. The effects of this interaction are dose-dependent. Avoid use of alcohol-containing products in patients taking disulfiram or metronidazole.
Ixabepilone	Vaccines, live	↑	Severe complications have occurred following the use of live attenuated vaccines in immunocompromised patients. The risk of live vaccine-induced adverse reactions may be increased by coadministration of ixabepilone. Defer the use of live vaccines in patients receiving ixabepilone.

[a] ↑ = object drug increased; ↓ = object drug decreased; ↔ = undetermined clinical effect.

➤*Drug/Food interactions:* Grapefruit juice may increase ixabepilone plasma concentrations and should be avoided.

Adverse Reactions

Unless otherwise specified, assessment of adverse reactions is based on 1 randomized study (study 046) and 1 single-arm study (study 081). In study 046, 369 patients with metastatic breast cancer were treated with ixabepilone 40 mg/m^2 administered IV over 3 hours every 21 days, combined with capecitabine 1,000 mg/m^2 twice daily for 2 weeks followed by a 1-week rest period. Patients treated with capecitabine as monotherapy (n = 368) in this study received 1,250 mg/m^2 twice daily for 2 weeks every 21 days. In study

IXABEPILONE — INJECTION

081, 126 patients with metastatic or locally advanced breast cancer were treated with ixabepilone 40 mg/m^2 administered IV over 3 hours every 3 weeks.

The most common adverse reactions (at least 20%) reported by patients receiving ixabepilone were alopecia, diarrhea, fatigue/asthenia, musculoskeletal pain, myalgia/arthralgia, peripheral sensory neuropathy, stomatitis/mucositis, nausea, and vomiting. The following additional reactions occurred in at least 20% in combination treatment: palmar-plantar erythrodysesthesia (hand-foot) syndrome, anorexia, abdominal pain, nail disorder, and constipation. The most common hematologic abnormalities (more than 40%) included anemia, leukopenia, neutropenia, and thrombocytopenia.

The following table presents nonhematologic adverse reactions reported in 5% or more of patients. Hematologic abnormalities are presented in the second following table.

Ixabepilone Nonhematologic Adverse Reactions (≥ 5%)

Adverse reaction[a]	Study 046				Study 081	
	Ixabepilone with capecitabine (n = 369)		Capecitabine (n = 368)		Ixabepilone monotherapy (n = 126)	
	Total	Grade 3/4	Total	Grade 3/4	Total	Grade 3/4
Cardiovascular						
Hot flush[b]	5%	0%	2%	0%	6%	0%
CNS						
Dizziness	8%	1%[c]	5%	1%[c]	7%	0%
Headache	8%	< 1%[c]	3%	0%	11%	0%
Fatigue/asthenia[b]	60%	16%	29%	4%	56%	13%
Insomnia[b]	9%	< 1%[c]	2%	0%	5%	0%
Motor neuropathy[b]	16%	5%[c]	< 1%	0%	10%	1%[c]
Sensory neuropathy[b,d]	65%	21%	16%	0%	62%	14%
Dermatologic						
Alopecia[b]	31%	0%	3%	0%	48%	0%
Nail disorder[b]	24%	2%[c]	10%	< 1%[c]	9%	0%
Palmar-plantar erythrodysesthesia syndrome[b,e]	64%	18%[c]	63%	17%[c]	8%	2%[c]
Pruritus	5%	0%	2%	0%	6%	1%[c]
Skin exfoliation[b]	5%	< 1%[c]	3%	0%	2%	0%
Skin hyperpigmentation[b]	11%	0%	14%	0%	2%	0%
GI						
Abdominal pain[b]	24%	2%[c]	14%	1%[c]	13%	2%[c]
Anorexia[b]	34%	3%[c]	15%	1%[c]	19%	2%[c]
Constipation	22%	0%	6%	< 1%[c]	16%	2%[c]
Diarrhea[b]	44%	6%[c]	39%	9%	22%	1%[c]
Gastroesophageal reflux disease[b]	7%	1%[c]	8%	0%	6%	0%
Nausea	53%	3%[c]	40%	2%[c]	42%	2%[c]
Stomatitis/mucositis[b]	31%	4%	20%	3%[c]	29%	6%
Taste disorder[b]	12%	0%	4%	0%	6%	0%
Vomiting[b]	39%	4%[c]	24%	2%	29%	1%[c]
Hematologic/Lymphatic						
Febrile neutropenia	5%	4%[f]	1%	1%[c]	3%	3%[c]
Metabolic/Nutritional						
Dehydration[b]	5%	2%	2%	< 1%[c]	2%	1%[c]
Weight decreased	11%	0%	3%	0%	6%	0%
Musculoskeletal						
Musculoskeletal pain[b]	23%	2%[c]	5%	0%	20%	3%[c]
Myalgia/arthralgia[b]	39%	8%[c]	5%	< 1%[c]	49%	8%[c]
Respiratory						
Cough[b]	6%	0%	2%	0%	2%	0%
Dyspnea[b]	7%	1%	4%	1%	9%	1%[c]
Upper respiratory tract infection[b]	4%	0%	3%	0%	6%	0%
Special senses						
Lacrimation increased	5%	0%	4%	< 1%[c]	4%	0%
Miscellaneous						
Chest pain[b]	4%	1%[c]	< 1%	0%	5%	1%[c]
Edema[b]	8%	0%	5%	< 1%[c]	9%	1%[c]
Hypersensitivity[b]	2%	1%[c]	0%	0%	5%	1%[c]
Pain[b]	9%	1%[c]	2%	0%	8%	3%[c]
Pyrexia	10%	1%[c]	4%	0%	8%	1%[c]

[a] System organ class presented as outlined in Guidelines for Preparing Core Clinical Safety Information on Drugs by the Council for International Organizations of Medical Sciences.
[b] A composite of multiple Medical Dictionary for Regulatory Activities Preferred Terms.
[c] No grade 4 reports.
[d] Peripheral sensory neuropathy (graded with the NCI-CTC scale) was defined as the occurrence of any of the following: areflexia, burning sensation, dysesthesia, hyperesthesia, hypoesthesia, hyporeflexia, neuralgia, neuritis, neuropathy, neuropathy peripheral, neurotoxicity, painful response to normal stimuli, paresthesia, pallanesthesia, peripheral sensory neuropathy, polyneuropathy, polyneuropathy toxic and sensorimotor disorder. Peripheral motor neuropathy was defined as the occurrence of any of the following: multifocal motor neuropathy, neuromuscular toxicity, peripheral motor neuropathy, and peripheral sensorimotor neuropathy.
[e] Palmar-plantar erythrodysesthesia (hand-foot syndrome) was graded on a 1 to 3 severity scale in study 046.
[f] NCI-CTC grading for febrile neutropenia ranges from grade 3 to 5. Three (1%) patients experienced grade 5 (fatal) febrile neutropenia. Other neutropenia-related deaths (9) occurred in the absence of reported febrile neutropenia.

Ixabepilone Hematologic Abnormalities (≥ 2%)

Hematology parameter	Study 046				Study 081	
	Ixabepilone with capecitabine (n = 369)		Capecitabine (n = 368)		Ixabepilone monotherapy (n = 126)	
	Grade 3	Grade 4	Grade 3	Grade 4	Grade 3	Grade 4
Anemia (Hgb[a])	8%	2%	4%	1%	6%	2%
Leukopenia (WBC[b])	41%	16%	5%	1%	36%	13%
Neutropenia[c]	32%	36%	9%	2%	31%	23%
Thrombocytopenia	5%	3%	2%	2%	5%	2%

[a] Hgb = hemoglobin.
[b] WBC = white blood cell count.
[c] Granulocyte colony-stimulating factor or granulocyte-macrophage colony-stimulating factor was used in 20% and 17% of patients who received ixabepilone in studies 046 and 081, respectively

➤*Other adverse reactions:* The following serious adverse reactions were also reported in 1,323 patients treated with ixabepilone as monotherapy or in combination with other therapies in phase 2 and 3 studies.

Cardiovascular – Angina pectoris, atrial flutter, cardiomyopathy, embolism, hemorrhage, hypotension, hypovolemic shock, left ventricular dysfunction, myocardial infarction, myocardial ischemia, supraventricular arrhythmia, thrombosis, vasculitis.

CNS – Abnormal coordination, cerebral hemorrhage, cognitive disorder, lethargy, syncope.

Dermatologic – Erythema multiforme.

GI – Colitis, dysphagia, enterocolitis, esophagitis, gastritis, GI hemorrhage, ileus, impaired gastric emptying.

GU – Urinary tract infection.

Hematologic/Lymphatic – Coagulopathy, increased blood alkaline phosphatase, lymphopenia, neutropenic infection.

Hepatic – Acute hepatic failure, increased gamma-glutamyltransferase, increased transaminases, jaundice.

Metabolic/Nutritional – Hypokalemia, hyponatremia, hypovolemia, metabolic acidosis.

Musculoskeletal – Muscle spasms, muscular weakness, trismus.

Renal – Nephrolithiasis, renal failure.

Respiratory – Acute pulmonary edema, dysphonia, hypoxia, laryngitis, lower respiratory tract infection, pharyngolaryngeal pain, pneumonia, pneumonitis, respiratory failure.

Miscellaneous – Bacterial infection, chills, infection, sepsis.

Epothilones

IXABEPILONE — INJECTION

Overdosage

➤*Symptoms:* One case of overdose of ixabepilone has been reported. The patient mistakenly received 100 mg/m^2 (total dose, 185 mg) and was admitted to the hospital for observation. The patient experienced myalgia (grade 1) and fatigue (grade 1) one day after infusion and was treated with a centrally acting analgesic. The patient recovered and was discharged without incident.

➤*Treatment:* There is no known antidote for overdosage of ixabepilone. In case of overdosage, monitor the patient closely, and administer supportive treatment. Management of overdose should include supportive medical interventions to treat the presenting clinical manifestations.

Patient Information

Advise patients to report to their health care provider any numbness and tingling of the hands or feet.

Instruct patients to call their health care provider if a fever of 100.5°F or greater or other evidence of potential infection such as chills, cough, or burning or pain on urination develops.

Advise patients to call their health care provider if they experience urticaria, pruritus, rash, flushing, swelling, dyspnea, chest tightness, or other hypersensitivity-related symptoms following an infusion of ixabepilone.

Advise patients to use effective contraceptive measures to prevent pregnancy and to avoid breast-feeding during treatment with ixabepilone.

Advise patients to report to their health care provider chest pain, difficulty breathing, palpitations, or unusual weight gain.

Halichondrin B Analog

ERIBULIN MESYLATE

Rx	**Halaven** (Eisai)	**Injection, solution:** 0.5 mg/mL	Ethanol. In 2 mL single-use vial.

ERIBULIN MESYLATE — INJECTION

Indications

➤*Metastatic breast cancer:* For the treatment of patients with metastatic breast cancer who have previously received at least 2 chemotherapeutic regimens for the treatment of metastatic disease. Prior therapy should have included an anthracycline and a taxane in either the adjuvant or metastatic setting.

Administration and Dosage

➤*Adults:*

Metastatic breast cancer –

Usual dosage: 1.4 mg/m^2 intravenously (IV) over 2 to 5 minutes on days 1 and 8 of a 21-day cycle.

Dosage adjustment: Assess for peripheral neuropathy and obtain complete blood cell counts prior to each dose.

• *Dose delays –* Do not administer eribulin on day 1 or day 8 for any of the following: absolute neutrophil count (ANC) less than 1,000/mm^3, platelets less than 75,000/mm^3, grade 3 or 4 nonhematological toxicities.

The day 8 dose may be delayed for a maximum of 1 week. If toxicities do not resolve or improve to grade 2 severity or less by day 15, omit the dose. If toxicities resolve or improve to grade 2 severity or less by day 15, administer eribulin at a reduced dose and initiate the next cycle no sooner than 2 weeks later.

• *Dose reductions –* If a dose has been delayed for toxicity and toxicities have recovered to grade 2 severity or less, resume eribulin at a reduced dose. Do not re-escalate eribulin dose after it has been reduced.

Eribulin Recommended Dose Reductions[a]

Event description	Eribulin recommended dose
ANC < 500/mm^3 for > 7 days	Permanently reduce the dose to 1.1 mg/m^2
ANC < 1,000 /mm^3 with fever or infection	
Platelets < 25,000/mm^3	
Platelets < 50,000/mm^3 requiring transfusion	
Nonhematologic grade 3 or 4 toxicities	
Omission or delay of day 8 eribulin dose in previous cycle for toxicity	
Occurrence of any event requiring permanent dose reduction while receiving eribulin 1.1 mg/m^2	Permanently reduce the dose to 0.7 mg/m^2
Occurrence of any event requiring permanent dose reduction while receiving eribulin 0.7 mg/m^2	Discontinue eribulin

[a] Toxicities graded in accordance with National Cancer Institute (NCI) Common Terminology Criteria for Adverse Events (CTCAE) version 3.0.

➤*Renal function impairment:*

Mild renal impairment – No dosage adjustment is necessary in patients with creatinine clearance (CrCl) of 50 to 80 mL/min.

Moderate renal impairment – 1.1 mg/m^2 over 2 to 5 minutes on days 1 and 8 of a 21-day cycle in patients with CrCl of 30 to 50 mL/min.

➤*Hepatic function impairment:*

Mild hepatic impairment (Child-Pugh class A) – 1.1 mg/m^2 IV over 2 to 5 minutes on days 1 and 8 of a 21-day cycle.

Moderate hepatic impairment (Child-Pugh class B) – 0.7 mg/m^2 IV over 2 to 5 minutes on days 1 and 8 of a 21-day cycle.

➤*Preparation for administration:* Aseptically withdraw the required amount of eribulin from the single-use vial and administer undiluted or diluted in 100 mL of sodium chloride 0.9% injection.

➤*Administration:* Administer IV over 2 to 5 minutes on days 1 and 8 of a 21-day cycle.

➤*Admixture compatibility:* Do not dilute in or administer through an IV line containing solutions with dextrose. Do not administer in the same IV line concurrent with the other medicinal products.

➤*Storage/Stability:* Store the vials in their original cartons at 25°C (77°F); excursions are permitted between 15° and 30°C (59° and 86°F). Do not freeze. Store undiluted eribulin in the syringe for up to 4 hours at room temperature or for up to 24 hours under refrigeration (4°C [40°F]). Store diluted solutions of eribulin for up to 4 hours at room temperature or up to 24 hours under refrigeration. Discard unused portions of the vial.

Actions

➤*Pharmacology:* Eribulin is a nontaxane microtubule dynamics inhibitor that inhibits the growth phase of microtubules without affecting the shortening phase, and sequesters tubulin into nonproductive aggregates. Eribulin exerts its effects via a tubulin-based antimitotic mechanism leading to G_2/M cell-cycle block, disruption of mitotic spindles, and, ultimately, apoptotic cell death after prolonged mitotic blockage.

➤*Pharmacokinetics:*

Absorption/Distribution – Eribulin has a mean volume of distribution of 43 to 114 L/m^2 over the dosage range of 0.25 to 4 mg/m^2. The human plasma protein binding of eribulin at concentrations of 100 to 1,000 ng/mL ranges from 49% to 65%.

Metabolism – Unchanged eribulin was the major circulating species in plasma following administration of ^{14}C-eribulin to patients. Metabolite concentrations represented less than 0.6% of parent compound, confirming that there are no major human metabolites of eribulin.

Cytochrome P450 3A4 (CYP3A4) negligibly metabolizes eribulin in vitro. Eribulin inhibits CYP3A4 activity in human liver microsomes, but it is unlikely that eribulin will substantially increase the plasma levels of CYP3A4 substrates.

Excretion – Eribulin has a mean elimination half-life of approximately 40 hours and a mean clearance of 1.16 to 2.42 L/h/m^2 over the dose range of 0.25 to 4 mg/m^2.

Eribulin is eliminated primarily in feces unchanged. After administration of ^{14}C-eribulin to patients, approximately 82% of the dose was eliminated in feces and 9% in urine. Unchanged eribulin accounted for approximately 88% and 91% of the dose in feces and urine, respectively.

Special populations –

Renal function impairment: For patients with moderate renal impairment (CrCl 30 to 50 mL/min), the geometric mean dose-normalized systemic exposure increased 2-fold compared with patients with normal renal function. The safety of eribulin was not studied in patients with severe renal impairment (CrCl less than 30 mL/min).

Hepatic function impairment: Compared with patients with normal hepatic function, eribulin exposure increased 1.8- and 2.5-fold in patients with mild and moderate hepatic impairment, respectively. Administration of eribulin at a dose of 1.1 mg/m^2 to patients with mild hepatic impairment and 0.7 mg/m^2 to patients with moderate hepatic impairment resulted in similar exposure to eribulin as a dose of 1.4 mg/m^2 to patients with normal hepatic function. Eribulin was not studied in patients with severe hepatic impairment (Child-Pugh class C).

Contraindications

None well documented.

Warnings/Precautions

➤*Neutropenia:* Severe neutropenia (ANC less than 500/mm^3) lasting more than 1 week occurred in 12% of patients in study 1, leading to discontinuation in less than 1% of patients. Patients with ALT or AST greater than 3 × upper limit of normal (ULN) experienced a higher incidence of grade 4 neutropenia and febrile neutropenia than patients with normal aminotransferase levels. Patients with bilirubin greater than 1.5 × ULN also had a higher incidence of grade 4 neutropenia and febrile neutropenia.

Monitor complete blood cell counts prior to each dose; increase the frequency of monitoring in patients who develop grade 3 or 4 cytopenias. Delay administration of eribulin and reduce subsequent doses in patients who experience

ERIBULIN MESYLATE — INJECTION

febrile neutropenia or grade 4 neutropenia lasting longer than 7 days. Clinical studies of eribulin did not include patients with baseline neutrophil counts below 1,500/mm^3.

➤*Peripheral neuropathy:* Grade 3 peripheral neuropathy occurred in 8% of patients, and grade 4 in 0.4% of patients in study 1. Peripheral neuropathy was the most common toxicity leading to discontinuation of eribulin (5% of patients). Neuropathy lasting more than 1 year occurred in 5% of patients. A total of 22% of patients developed a new or worsening neuropathy that had not recovered within a median follow-up duration of 269 days (range, 25 to 662 days). Monitor patients closely for signs of peripheral motor and sensory neuropathy. Withhold eribulin in patients who experience grade 3 or 4 peripheral neuropathy until resolution to grade 2 or less.

➤*QT prolongation:* In an uncontrolled open-label electrocardiogram (ECG) study in 26 patients, QT prolongation was observed on day 8, independent of eribulin concentration, with no QT prolongation observed on day 1. ECG monitoring is recommended if therapy is initiated in patients with congestive heart failure, bradyarrhythmias, drugs known to prolong the QT interval (including class Ia and III antiarrhythmics), and electrolyte abnormalities. Correct hypokalemia or hypomagnesemia prior to initiating eribulin and monitor these electrolytes periodically during therapy. Avoid eribulin in patients with congenital long QT syndrome.

➤*Renal function impairment:* See Administration and Dosage for more information.

➤*Hepatic function impairment:* See Administration and Dosage for more information.

➤*Pregnancy: Category D.* There are no adequate and well-controlled studies with eribulin in pregnant women. Eribulin is a microtubule inhibitor; therefore, it is expected to cause fetal harm when administered to a pregnant woman. Embryofetal toxicity and teratogenicity occurred in rats that received eribulin at approximately half of the recommended human dose based on body surface area (BSA). If this drug is used during pregnancy, or if the patient becomes pregnant while taking this drug, apprise the patient of the potential hazard to the fetus.

In a developmental toxicity study, pregnant rats received IV infusion of eribulin during organogenesis (gestation days 8, 10, and 12) at doses approximately 0.04, 0.13, 0.43 and 0.64 times the recommended human dose, based on BSA (mg/m^2). Increased abortion and severe external or soft tissue malformations were observed in offspring at doses 0.64 times the recommended human dose based on BSA (mg/m^2), including the absence of a lower jaw, tongue, stomach and spleen. Increased embryofetal death/resorption, reduced fetal weights, and minor skeletal anomalies consistent with developmental delay were also reported at or above doses of 0.43 times the recommended human dose.

Maternal toxicity of eribulin was reported in rats at or above doses of 0.43 times the recommended human dose (mg/m^2), and included enlarged spleen, reduced maternal weight gain and decreased food consumption.

➤*Lactation:* It is not known whether eribulin is excreted into human milk. No studies in humans or animals were conducted to determine if eribulin is excreted into milk. Because many drugs are excreted into human milk and because of the potential for serious adverse reactions in breast-fed infants from eribulin, decide whether to discontinue breast-feeding or to discontinue eribulin, taking into account the importance of the drug to the mother.

➤*Children:* The safety and effectiveness in children younger than 18 years of age have not been established.

➤*Monitoring:* Assess for peripheral neuropathy and obtain complete blood cell counts prior to each dose. Increase the frequency of monitoring in patients who develop grade 3 or 4 cytopenias. Monitor patients closely for signs and symptoms of peripheral motor and sensory neuropathy. ECG monitoring is recommended if therapy is initiated in patients with congestive heart failure, bradyarrhythmias, drugs known to prolong the QT interval, including class Ia and III antiarrhythmics, and electrolyte abnormalities. Monitor for hypokalemia and hypomagnesia prior to therapy and periodically throughout therapy.

Drug Interactions

➤*QT prolongation:* An additive effect of eribulin with other drugs that prolong the QT interval cannot be excluded. The following drugs may prolong the QT interval and increase the risk of life-threatening cardiac arrhythmias, including torsade de pointes: antiarrhythmic agents (eg, amiodarone, bretylium, disopyramide, dofetilide, procainamide, quinidine, sotalol), arsenic trioxide, chlorpromazine, cisapride, dolasetron, droperidol, gatifloxacin, halofantrine, levomethadyl, mefloquine, mesoridazine, moxifloxacin, pentamidine, pimozide, probucol, sparfloxacin, thioridazine, ziprasidone. (See Drug-Induced Prolongation of the QT Interval and Torsades De Pointes.)

Adverse Reactions

➤*Most common adverse reactions:* The most common adverse reactions (25% or more) reported in patients receiving eribulin were neutropenia, anemia, asthenia/fatigue, alopecia, peripheral neuropathy, nausea, and constipation. The most common serious adverse reactions reported in patients receiving eribulin were febrile neutropenia (4%) and neutropenia (2%).

➤*Discontinuation:* The most common adverse reaction resulting in discontinuation of eribulin was peripheral neuropathy (5%).

➤*Adverse reactions (10% or more):*

Eribulin Adverse Reactions (≥ 10%)

Adverse reactions	Eribulin (n = 503)		Control group (n = 247)	
	All grades	≥ Grade 3	All grades	≥ Grade 3
CNS				
Asthenia/Fatigue	54%	10%	40%	11%
Headache	19%	< 1%	12%	< 1%
Peripheral neuropathy[b]	35%	8%	16%	2%
GI				
Anorexia	20%	1%	13%	1%
Constipation	25%	1%	21%	1%
Diarrhea	18%	0%	18%	0%
Nausea	35%	1%	28%	3%
Vomiting	18%	1%	18%	1%
Weight decreased	21%	1%	14%	< 1%
Hematologic[a]				
Anemia	58%	2%	55%	4%
Neutropenia	82%	57%	53%	23%
Musculoskeletal				
Arthralgia/Myalgia	22%	< 1%	12%	1%
Back pain	16%	1%	7%	2%
Bone pain	12%	2%	9%	2%
Pain in extremity	11%	1%	10%	1%
Respiratory				
Cough	14%	0%	9%	0%
Dyspnea	16%	4%	13%	4%
Miscellaneous				
Alopecia	45%	NA[c]	10%	NA
Mucosal inflammation	9%	1%	10%	2%
Pyrexia	21%	< 1%	13%	< 1%
Urinary Tract Infection	10%	1%	5%	0%

[a] Based on laboratory data.
[b] Includes neuropathy peripheral, neuropathy, peripheral motor neuropathy, polyneuropathy, peripheral sensory neuropathy, and paresthesia.
[c] NA = not applicable (grading system does not specify greater than grade 2 for alopecia).

➤*Hematologic:* Grade 3 neutropenia occurred in 28% of patients who received eribulin in study 1, and 29% of patients experienced grade 4 neutropenia. Febrile neutropenia occurred in 5% of patients; 2 patients died from complications of febrile neutropenia. Dose reduction because of neutropenia was required in 12% of patients and discontinuation was required in less than 1% of patients. The mean time to nadir was 13 days and the mean time to recovery from severe neutropenia (less than 500/mm^3) was 8 days. Grade 3 or greater thrombocytopenia occurred in 1% of patients. Granulocyte colony-stimulating factor or granulocyte-macrophage colony-stimulating factor was used in 19% of patients who received eribulin.

➤*Peripheral neuropathy:* In study 1, 17% of enrolled patients had grade 1 peripheral neuropathy and 3% of patients had grade 2 peripheral neuropathy at baseline. Dose reduction because of peripheral neuropathy was required by 3% of patients who received eribulin. A total of 4% of patients experienced peripheral motor neuropathy of any grade and 2% of patients developed grade 3 peripheral motor neuropathy.

➤*Other adverse reactions (5% to less than 10%):*

CNS – Depression, dizziness, insomnia.

GI – Abdominal pain, dry mouth, dyspepsia, stomatitis.

Musculoskeletal – Muscle spasms, muscular weakness.

Special senses – Dysgeusia, increased lacrimation.

Miscellaneous – Hypokalemia, peripheral edema, rash, upper respiratory tract infection.

➤*Lab test abnormalities:* Among patients with grade 0 or 1 ALT levels at baseline, 18% of eribulin-treated patients experienced grade 2 or greater ALT elevation. One eribulin-treated patient without documented liver metastases had concomitant grade 2 elevations in bilirubin and ALT; these abnormalities resolved and did not recur with re-exposure to eribulin.

Halichondrin B Analog

ERIBULIN MESYLATE — INJECTION

Overdosage

➤*Symptoms:* Overdosage of eribulin has been reported at approximately 4 times the recommended dose, which resulted in grade 3 neutropenia lasting 7 days and a grade 3 hypersensitivity reaction lasting 1 day.

Patient Information

Advise patients to contact their health care provider if they experience a fever of 38°C (100.5°F) or greater or other signs or symptoms of infection, such as chills, cough, or burning or pain on urination.

Advise women of childbearing potential to avoid pregnancy and to use effective contraception during treatment.

EPIPODOPHYLLOTOXINS

Podophyllotoxin Derivatives

WARNING

Etoposide and teniposide are cytotoxic drugs that should be administered under the supervision of a qualified health care provider experienced in the use of cancer chemotherapeutic agents. Appropriate management of therapy and complications is possible only when adequate treatment facilities are readily available.

Severe myelosuppression – Severe myelosuppression with resulting infection or bleeding may occur.

Hypersensitivity reactions – Hypersensitivity reactions, including anaphylaxis-like symptoms, may occur with initial dosing or at repeated exposure. Epinephrine, with or without corticosteroids and antihistamines, has been employed to alleviate hypersensitivity reaction symptoms.

Indications

➤*Acute lymphoblastic leukemia:* Teniposide is indicated for use in combination with other approved anticancer agents for induction therapy in patients with refractory childhood acute lymphoblastic leukemia (ALL).

➤*Refractory testicular tumors:* Etoposide and etoposide phosphate injection are indicated in combination with other chemotherapeutic agents for refractory testicular tumors in patients who have received surgery, chemotherapy, and radiotherapy. Adequate data on the use of oral etoposide are not available.

➤*Small cell lung cancer:* Etoposide, oral and injection, and etoposide phosphate injection are indicated for small cell lung cancer in combination with other agents as first-line treatment.

➤*Off-label uses:* Etoposide has been used alone or in combination in acute non-lymphocytic leukemias (monocytic), Hodgkin disease, non-Hodgkin lymphomas, Kaposi sarcoma, neuroblastoma, bladder carcinoma, Ewing sarcoma, brain tumors, gestational trophoblastic tumors, ovarian germ cell tumors, Wilms tumor, and bone marrow transplantation. Other tumors with a response rate of 5% to 20% to etoposide as a single agent include choriocarcinoma; rhabdomyosarcoma; hepatocellular carcinoma; epithelial ovarian, small and non-small cell lung, testicular, gastric, and endometrial and breast cancers; acute lymphocytic leukemia; and soft tissue sarcoma.

Teniposide has been used in the treatment of adult acute lymphocytic leukemia and non-Hodgkin lymphoma.

Actions

➤*Pharmacology:* Etoposide and teniposide are semisynthetic derivatives of podophyllotoxin.

The main effect of etoposide appears to be at the G_2 portion of the cell cycle. Two different dose-dependent responses are seen. At high concentrations (10 mcg/mL or more), lysis of cells entering mitosis is observed. At low concentrations (0.3 to 10 mcg/mL), cells are inhibited from entering prophase. Etoposide does not interfere with microtubular assembly. The predominant macromolecular effect of etoposide appears to be the induction of DNA strand breaks by an interaction with DNA-topoisomerase II or the formation of free radicals.

Teniposide, also commonly known as VM-26, is a phase-specific cytotoxic drug, acting in the late S or early G_2 phase of the cell cycle, thus preventing cells from entering mitosis. Teniposide causes dose-dependent single- and double-stranded breaks in DNA and DNA-protein crosslinks. The mechanism of action appears to be related to the inhibition of type II topoisomerase activity because teniposide does not intercalate into DNA or bind strongly to DNA. The cytotoxic effects of teniposide are related to the relative number of double-stranded DNA breaks produced in cells, which are a reflection of the stabilization of a topoisomerase II–DNA intermediate.

Teniposide has a broad spectrum of in vivo antitumor activity against murine tumors, including hematologic malignancies and various solid tumors. Notably, teniposide is active against sublines of certain murine leukemias with acquired resistance to cisplatin, doxorubicin, amsacrine, daunorubicin, mitoxantrone, or vincristine.

➤*Pharmacokinetics:*

Summary of Podophyllotoxin Derivative Pharmacokinetics

Pharmacokinetic parameter	Etoposide	Teniposide
Total body clearance	16 to 36 mL/min/m² (33 to 48 mL/min)	10.3 mL/min/m² (children)
Terminal half-life	4 to 11 h	5 h (children)
Volume of distribution	7 to 17 L/m² (18 to 29 L)	3 to 11 L/m² (children) 8 to 44 L/m² (adults)
Protein binding	97%	> 99%
Elimination	Renal (56%) and fecal (44%)	Renal (44%) and fecal (≤ 10%)
Excreted unchanged in urine	< 50%	4% to 12%

Absorption/Distribution – Following intravenous (IV) administration of etoposide phosphate, the drug is rapidly and completely converted to etoposide in plasma. Upon IV administration, the disposition of etoposide is a biphasic process with a distribution half-life of approximately 1.5 hours. The areas under the curve (AUCs) and maximum plasma concentration (C_{max}) values increase linearly with dose. Etoposide does not accumulate in the plasma following daily administration of 100 mg/m² for 4 to 5 days. After either IV infusion or oral administration, C_{max} and AUC values exhibit marked intra- and intersubject variability. This results in variability in the estimates of the absolute oral bioavailability of etoposide oral capsules. The overall mean oral bioavailability for etoposide capsules is approximately 50% (range, 25% to 75%).

Etoposide enters the cerebrospinal fluid (CSF) poorly. Although detectable in CSF and intracerebral tumors, the concentrations are lower than in extracerebral tumors and plasma. Concentrations are higher in healthy lung than in lung metastases and are similar in primary tumors and healthy tissues of the myometrium.

An inverse relationship between plasma albumin levels and renal clearance is found in children. Etoposide binding ratio correlates directly with serum albumin. The unbound fraction significantly correlated with bilirubin in patients with cancer. Data have suggested a significant inverse correlation between serum albumin concentration and free fraction of etoposide.

C_{max} and AUC values for orally administered etoposide capsules consistently fall in the same range as the C_{max} and AUC values for an IV dose of one-half the size of the oral dose. The overall mean value of oral capsule bioavailability is approximately 50% (range, 25% to 75%). The bioavailability of etoposide capsules appears to be linear up to a dose of at least 250 mg/m².

Teniposide plasma drug levels declined biexponentially following IV infusion in children with newly diagnosed ALL. In adults, plasma levels increased linearly with dose. Drug accumulation did not occur after daily administration for 3 days. In children, C_{max} after infusions of 137 to 203 mg/m² over a period of 1 to 2 hours exceeded 40 mcg/mL; by 20 to 24 hours after infusion, plasma levels were generally less than 2 mcg/mL.

The pharmacokinetic characteristics of teniposide differ from those of etoposide. Teniposide is more extensively bound to plasma proteins, and its cellular uptake is greater. Steady-state volume of distribution of teniposide increases with a decrease in plasma albumin levels. The blood-brain barrier appears to limit diffusion of teniposide into the brain, although in a study in patients with brain tumors, CSF levels were higher than in patients without brain tumors.

Metabolism/Excretion – Biliary excretion of unchanged drug and/or metabolites is an important route of etoposide elimination, as fecal recovery of radioactivity is 44% of the IV dose. The hydroxy acid metabolite [4′-demethylepipodophyllic acid-9-(4, 6-0-(R)-ethylidene-β-D-glucopyranoside)], formed by opening of the lactone ring, is found in the urine of adults and children. It is also present in human plasma, presumably as the trans isomer. Glucuronide and/or sulfate conjugates of etoposide are also excreted in human urine. Only 8% or less of an IV dose is excreted in the urine as radiolabeled metabolites of ^{14}C-etoposide. In addition, O-demethylation of the dimethoxyphenol ring occurs through the CYP3A4 isoenzyme pathway to produce the corresponding catechol.

After IV administration of ^{14}C-etoposide (100 to 124 mg/m²), mean recovery of radioactivity in the urine was 56% of the dose at 120 hours, 45% of which was excreted as etoposide; fecal recovery of radioactivity was 44% of the dose at 120 hours.

In children, approximately 55% of the dose is excreted in the urine as etoposide in 24 hours. The mean renal clearance of etoposide is 7 to 10 mL/min/m² or approximately 35% of the total body clearance over a dose range of 80 to 600 mg/m^2. Therefore, etoposide is cleared by both renal and nonrenal processes (ie, metabolism and biliary excretion). The effect of renal disease on plasma etoposide clearance is not known.

Renal clearance of parent teniposide accounts for approximately 10% of total body clearance. In adults, after IV administration of 10 mg/kg or 67 mg/m^2 of tritium-labeled teniposide, 44% of the radiolabel was recovered in urine (parent drug and metabolites) within 120 hours after dosing.

Special populations –

Renal function impairment: Patients with renal function impairment receiving etoposide have exhibited reduced total body clearance, increased AUC, and a lower volume of distribution at steady state.

Hepatic function impairment: There appears to be some association between an increase in serum alkaline phosphatase or gamma-glutamyl transpeptidase and a decrease in plasma clearance of teniposide. Therefore, exercise caution if teniposide is to be administered to patients with hepatic function impairment.

Children: In children, elevated serum ALT levels are associated with reduced etoposide total body clearance.

Contraindications

Hypersensitivity to etoposide, teniposide, and/or any other component of the products, such as polyoxyethylated castor oil, which is contained in teniposide injection solution.

Warnings/Precautions

➤*Myelosuppression:* Patients being treated with etoposide or teniposide must be frequently observed for myelosuppression during and after therapy. Dose-limiting bone marrow suppression is the most significant toxicity associated with therapy. Therefore, obtain the following laboratory tests at the start of therapy and prior to each subsequent cycle: platelet count, hemoglobin, white blood cell count (WBC), and differential. The occurrence of a platelet count below 50,000/mm^3 or an absolute neutrophil count (ANC) below 500/mm^3 is an indication to withhold further etoposide therapy until the blood cell counts have sufficiently recovered. If necessary, repeat bone marrow examination prior to the decision to continue teniposide therapy in the setting of severe myelosuppression.

Myelosuppression resulting in death has been reported following etoposide administration.

➤*Toxicity:* In all instances in which the use of etoposide or teniposide is considered for chemotherapy, evaluate the need and usefulness of the drug against the risk of adverse reactions. Most such adverse reactions are reversible if detected early. If severe reactions occur, reduce the drug dosage or discontinue and institute appropriate corrective measures. Carry out reinstitution of therapy with caution, with adequate consideration of the further need for the drug and alertness as to possible recurrence of toxicity.

The toxicity of rapidly infused etoposide phosphate in patients with renal or hepatic function impairment has not been adequately evaluated. The toxicity profile of etoposide phosphate, when infused at doses greater than 175 mg/m^2, has not been delineated.

➤*Cardiovascular effects:* One episode of sudden death, attributed to probable arrhythmia and intractable hypotension, has been reported in an elderly patient receiving teniposide combination therapy for a nonleukemic malignancy. Continuously observe patients receiving teniposide treatment for at least the first 60 minutes following the start of the infusion and at frequent intervals thereafter.

Give etoposide and teniposide only by slow IV infusion (usually over at least a 30- to 60-minute period) because hypotension has been reported as a possible adverse reaction of rapid IV injection. With teniposide, it may also be due to a direct effect of the polyoxyethylated castor oil component. If clinically significant hypotension develops, discontinue the teniposide infusion. The blood pressure usually normalizes within hours in response to cessation of the infusion and administration of fluids or other supportive therapy as appropriate. If the infusion is restarted, use a lower administration rate and monitor the patient carefully.

➤*Administration/Extravasation:* Teniposide must be administered as an IV infusion. Hypotension has been reported following rapid IV administration; it is recommended that the teniposide solution be administered over at least a 30- to 60-minute period. Do not give teniposide by rapid IV injection. Take care to ensure that the IV catheter or needle is in the proper position and is functional prior to infusion. Improper administration may result in extravasation causing local tissue necrosis and/or thrombophlebitis. In some instances, occlusion of central venous access devices has occurred during 24-hour infusion of teniposide at a concentration of 0.1 to 0.2 mg/mL. Frequent observation during these infusions is necessary to minimize risk.

➤*Benzyl alcohol:* Teniposide injection solution and some etoposide solution formulations contain benzyl alcohol as a preservative, which has been associated with a fatal "gasping syndrome" in premature infants.

➤*CNS depression:* Acute CNS depression and hypotension have occurred in patients receiving investigational infusions of high-dose teniposide who were pretreated with antiemetic drugs. The depressant effects of the antiemetic agents and the alcohol content of the teniposide formulation may place patients receiving higher than recommended doses at risk for CNS depression.

➤*Hypersensitivity reactions:* Anaphylactic reactions, characterized by chills, fever, tachycardia, bronchospasm, dyspnea, and/or hypotension, have been reported in patients receiving etoposide or teniposide. These reactions have usually responded promptly to the cessation of the infusion and administration of pressor agents, corticosteroids, antihistamines, or volume expanders as appropriate; however, these reactions can be fatal. Hypertension and/or flushing have also been reported. Blood pressure usually normalizes within a few hours after cessation of the infusion. This reaction may occur during the first dose or initial infusion.

Facial/tongue swelling, coughing, diaphoresis, cyanosis, tightness in throat, laryngospasm, back pain, and/or loss of consciousness have sometimes occurred with the previous reactions. In addition, an apparent hypersensitivity-associated apnea has been reported rarely with etoposide. Rash, urticaria, and/or pruritus have infrequently been reported at recommended doses. At investigational doses of etoposide, a generalized erythematous maculopapular rash, consistent with perivasculitis, has been reported.

Higher rates of anaphylactic-like reactions have been reported in children who received infusions of etoposide at concentrations higher than those recommended. The role that concentration of infusion (or rate of infusion) and/or the polyoxyethylated castor oil component of the vehicle of teniposide play in the development of anaphylactic-like reactions is uncertain. Patients who have experienced prior hypersensitivity reactions are at risk for recurrence of symptoms and should only be treated if the benefit clearly outweighs the risk. When a decision is made to re-treat in spite of an earlier hypersensitivity reaction, pretreat the patient with corticosteroids and antihistamines and perform careful clinical observations during and after the infusion.

If symptoms or signs of anaphylaxis occur, stop the infusion immediately and follow with the administration of epinephrine, corticosteroids, antihistamines, pressor agents, or volume expanders. Make available an aqueous solution of epinephrine 1:1,000 and a source of oxygen at the bedside.

➤*Renal function impairment:* In patients with renal function impairment, consider etoposide dose modifications based on measured creatinine clearance. See etoposide individual monographs for more information. Teniposide dose adjustments may be necessary for patients with significant renal function impairment.

➤*Hepatic function impairment:* There appears to be some association between an increase in serum alkaline phosphatase or gamma-glutamyl transpeptidase and a decrease in plasma clearance of teniposide. Therefore, exercise caution if teniposide is administered to patients with hepatic function impairment. In children, elevated serum ALT levels are associated with reduced drug total body clearance of etoposide.

➤*Special risk:* Patients with low serum albumin may be at an increased risk for etoposide-associated toxicities.

Patients with Down syndrome – Patients with both Down syndrome and leukemia may be especially sensitive to myelosuppressive chemotherapy; therefore, reduce initial dosing with teniposide in these patients. It is suggested that the first course be given at half the usual dose. Subsequent courses may be administered at higher dosages depending on the degree of myelosuppression and mucositis encountered in earlier courses in an individual patient.

➤*Pregnancy: Category D.* Etoposide and teniposide can cause fetal harm when administered to a pregnant woman. Etoposide and teniposide have both been shown to be teratogenic in mice and rats.

There are no adequate and well-controlled studies of podophyllotoxin derivative use in pregnant women. Advise women of childbearing potential to avoid becoming pregnant. If etoposide and/or teniposide are used during pregnancy, or if the patient becomes pregnant while receiving these drugs, warn the patient of the potential hazard to the fetus.

Etoposide is teratogenic and embryocidal in rats and mice at doses of 1% to 3% of the recommended clinical dose based on body surface area. In rats, an IV etoposide dosage of 0.4 mg/kg/day (approximately one-twentieth of the human dose on a mg/m^2 basis) during organogenesis caused maternal toxicity, embryotoxicity, and teratogenicity (skeletal abnormalities, exencephaly, encephalocele, and anophthalmia); higher dosages of 1.2 and 3.6 mg/kg/day (approximately one-seventh and one-half of the human dose on a mg/m^2 basis) resulted in 90% and 100% embryonic resorptions. In mice, a single 1 mg/kg (one-sixteenth of the human dose on a mg/m^2 basis) dose of etoposide administered intraperitoneally on days 6, 7, and 8 of gestation caused embryotoxicity, cranial abnormalities, and major skeletal malformations. An intraperitoneal dose of 1.5 mg/kg (about one-tenth of the human dose on a mg/m^2 basis) on day 7 of gestation caused an increase in the incidence of intrauterine death and fetal malformations and a significant decrease in the average fetal body weight.

In pregnant rats, IV administration of teniposide 0.1 to 3 mg/kg (0.6 to 18 mg/m^2) every second day from day 6 to day 16 postcoitum caused dose-related embryotoxicity and teratogenicity. Major anomalies included spinal and rib defects, deformed extremities, anophthalmia, and celosomia.

➤*Lactation:* Etoposide is excreted into breast milk and is contraindicated. It is recommended to stop breast-feeding for at least 55 hours after the last dose of etoposide. Severe toxicities in a breast-fed infant may include myelosuppression, alopecia, and carcinogenicity. It is not known whether teniposide is excreted in breast milk. Decide whether to discontinue breast-feeding or the drug, taking into account the importance of the drug to the mother.

➤*Children:* Safety and effectiveness of the use of etoposide in children have not been established. Higher rates of anaphylactic-like reactions have been reported in children who received infusions of etoposide at concentrations higher than those recommended. Teniposide is indicated for use in children.

Polysorbate 80 – Etoposide injection contains polysorbate 80. In premature infants, a life-threatening syndrome consisting of liver and renal failure, pulmonary deterioration, thrombocytopenia, and ascites has been associated with an injectable vitamin E product containing polysorbate 80.

Benzyl alcohol – Teniposide and some etoposide solution formulations contain benzyl alcohol, which has been associated with a fatal "gasping syndrome" in premature infants.

➤*Elderly:* World Health Organization grade 3 or 4 leukopenia, granulocytopenia, and asthenia were more frequent among elderly patients treated with etoposide phosphate injection. In one study, elderly patients also had more anorexia, mucositis, dehydration, somnolence, and elevated serum urea nitrogen levels than younger patients. Postmarketing experience also suggests that elderly patients may be more sensitive to some of the known adverse effects of etoposide, including myelosuppression, GI reactions, infectious complications, and alopecia.

Etoposide and its metabolites are known to be substantially excreted by the kidney, and the risk of adverse reactions may be greater in patients with renal function impairment. Because elderly patients are more likely to have decreased renal function, take care in dose selection, and it may be useful to monitor renal function.

One episode of sudden death, attributed to probable arrhythmia and intractable hypotension, has been reported in an elderly patient receiving teniposide combination therapy for nonleukemic malignancy.

➤*Monitoring:* Monitor patients receiving teniposide infusions for at least the first 60 minutes following the start of infusion and at frequent intervals thereafter.

Frequently observe patients being treated with etoposide and teniposide for myelosuppression, both during and after therapy. Therefore, obtain a complete blood cell count, including hemoglobin, WBC and differential, and platelet count during the course of etoposide and teniposide therapy (prior to each cycle of therapy and at appropriate intervals during and after therapy). Perform these tests prior to therapy and at clinically appropriate intervals during and after therapy. There should be at least 1 determination of hematologic status prior to therapy.

Monitor renal and hepatic function at baseline and periodically during etoposide and teniposide therapy.

Drug Interactions

Podophyllotoxin Derivatives Drug Interactions

Precipitant drug	Object drug[a]		Description
Cyclosporine	Podophyllotoxin derivatives Etoposide	↑	Serum etoposide concentrations may be elevated, resulting in increased toxicity. Monitor complete blood cell count and adjust the dose of etoposide as needed.
Levamisole[b]	Podophyllotoxin derivatives Etoposide phosphate	↑	Exercise caution when administering etoposide phosphate with drugs that are known to inhibit phosphatase activities, such as levamisole.
Salicylates Sulfonamides Tolbutamide	Podophyllotoxin derivatives Teniposide	↑	Teniposide was displaced from protein-binding sites by these agents to a small but significant extent. Because of the extremely high binding of teniposide to plasma proteins, these small decreases in binding could cause substantial increases in free drug levels, resulting in potentiation of toxicity.
Podophyllotoxin derivatives Teniposide	Methotrexate	↑↓	Plasma clearance of methotrexate may be slightly increased. However, increased intracellular levels were observed in vitro.
Podophyllotoxin derivatives Etoposide	Warfarin	↑	The anticoagulant effect of warfarin may be increased. Carefully monitor coagulation parameters during and after chemotherapy.

[a] ↑ = object drug increased; ↑↓ = object drug both increased and decreased.
[b] No longer marketed in the United States.

Adverse Reactions

Podophyllotoxin Derivatives Adverse Reactions[a]

Adverse reaction	Etoposide (oral and injection)	Teniposide[b]
Cardiovascular		
Hypertension	✓	—
Hypotension	1% to 2%	2%
CNS		
Asthenia/Malaise	39%[d]	—
Dizziness	5%[e]	—
Peripheral neurotoxicity	1% to 2%	< 1%
Dermatologic		
Alopecia (reversible)[f]	8% to 66%	9%
Pigmentation	✓[c]	—
Rash	✓[c]	3%
Stevens-Johnson syndrome	✓[c]	—
Toxic epidermal necrolysis	✓[c]	—
GI		
Abdominal pain	≤ 7%	—
Aftertaste	✓[c]	—
Anorexia	10% to 16%	—
Constipation	≤ 8%	—
Diarrhea	1% to 13%	33%
Dysphagia	✓	—
Hepatic dysfunction/toxicity	≤ 3%[e]	< 1%
Mucositis	11%[d]	76%
Nausea/Vomiting	31% to 43%	29%
Stomatitis	1% to 6%	—
Taste alteration	6%[d]	—
Hematologic		
Anemia	≤ 33%	88%
Anemia < 11 g/dL	72%[d]	—
Anemia < 8 g/dL	19%[d]	—
Bleeding	—	5%
Leukopenia (WBC/mm^3)		
< 4,000	60% to 91%	—
< 3,000	—	89%
< 1,000	3% to 17%	—
Myelosuppression, nonspecified	✓[c]	75%
Neutropenia (ANC/mm^3)		
< 2,000	88%[d]	95%
< 500	37%[d]	—
Thrombocytopenia (platelets/mm^3)		
< 100,000	22% to 41%	85%
< 50,000	1% to 20%	—
Miscellaneous		
Chills and/or fever	24%[d]	—
Extravasation/Phlebitis	5%[d]	—
Fever	—	3%
Hypersensitivity/Anaphylactic reactions[g]	1% to 3%[g,h]	5%[h]
Infection	—	12%
Metabolic abnormalities	✓[c,e]	< 1%
Renal dysfunction	—	< 1%

[a] Data are pooled from different studies and are not necessarily comparable.
[b] Adverse reactions reported in children.
[c] ✓ = adverse reaction observed, incidence not reported.
[d] Etoposide phosphate injection.
[e] Generally reported in patients receiving higher doses of the drug than recommended.
[f] Sometimes progressing to total baldness.
[g] See Warnings and Precautions for more information.
[h] Characterized by blood pressure changes (hypertension or hypotension), bronchospasm, chills, dyspnea, fever, flushing, and tachycardia.

➤*Other etoposide (oral and injection) adverse reactions:*

CNS – Fatigue, seizures (occasionally associated with allergic reactions), somnolence.

Dermatologic – Pruritus, rash, and/or urticaria have infrequently been reported at recommended doses. At investigational doses, a generalized pruritic erythematous maculopapular rash, consistent with perivasculitis, has been reported. A single report of radiation recall dermatitis has been reported.

GI – Mild to severe mucositis/esophagitis may occur. GI toxicities are slightly more frequent after oral administration than after IV infusion.

Hematologic – Myelosuppression is dose related and dose limiting, with granulocyte nadirs occurring 7 to 14 days after etoposide administration and 12 to 19 days after etoposide phosphate administration, and platelet nadirs occurring 9 to 16 days after etoposide administration and 10 to 15 days after etoposide phosphate administration. Leukocyte nadirs occurred from day 15 to day 22 after initiation of etoposide phosphate. Bone marrow recovery is usually complete by day 20, and no cumulative toxicity has been reported. Fever and infection have also been reported in patients with neutropenia. Death associated with myelosuppression has been reported.

Hypersensitivity – See Warnings and Precautions for more information.

Local – Extravasation has been reported with necrosis and venous induration rarely.

Miscellaneous – Interstitial pneumonitis/pulmonary fibrosis, optic neuritis, transient cortical blindness.

Overdosage

➤*Symptoms:* The anticipated complications of overdosage are secondary to bone marrow suppression.

➤*Treatment:* There is no known antidote for etoposide or teniposide overdosage. Treatment should consist of supportive care, including blood products and antibiotics, as indicated.

Patient Information

Inform patients that etoposide capsules may be taken with or without food and to store the capsules in a refrigerator, away from heat and moisture.

Advise women of childbearing potential to avoid becoming pregnant during treatment. Etoposide and teniposide have the potential to cause serious adverse effects to a fetus.

Inform patients to report any signs or symptoms of severe skin reactions.

Advise patients that podophyllotoxin derivatives may cause loss of hair, a sore or tender mouth, fever, nausea, vomiting, and diarrhea.

Advise patients to immediately report any swelling, pain, burning, or redness at the infusion site.

Advise patients to report to their health care provider any signs of an infection, such as fever, chills, cough, or flu-like symptoms. Podophyllotoxin derivatives may decrease the body's ability to fight infections.

ETOPOSIDE (VP-16, VP-16-213)

Rx	**Etoposide** (Various, eg, Mylan, UDL)	**Capsules; oral:** 50 mg	May be liquid filled. PEG. Dark pink. (E50). In blister pack 10s.
Rx	**Etoposide** (Various, eg, Abraxis, Bedford)	**Injection, solution, concentrate:** 20 mg/mL	In 5, 12.5, 25, and 50 mL multiple-dose vials.[a]
Rx	**Toposar** (Teva)		In 5, 25, and 50 mL multiple-dose vials.[b]
Rx	**Etopophos** (Bristol-Myers Squibb)	**Injection, lyophilized powder for solution:** 100 mg	As etoposide phosphate. In single-dose vials.

[a] May contain alcohol, benzyl alcohol, citric acid, polyethylene glycol, or polysorbate 80.

[b] With dehydrated alcohol 33.2%, 650 mg of polyethylene glycol 300, and 80 mg of polysorbate 80.

ETOPOSIDE — ORAL

For complete and comparative prescribing information, refer to the Podophyllotoxin Derivatives group monograph.

WARNING

Administer etoposide under the supervision of a qualified health care provider who is experienced in the use of cancer chemotherapeutic agents. Severe myelosuppression, with resulting infection or bleeding, may occur.

Indications

➤*Small cell lung cancer:* In combination with other approved chemotherapeutic agents, as first-line treatment in patients with small cell lung cancer.

➤*Off-label uses:*

Other possible off-label uses – Treatment of bladder carcinoma, bone marrow transplantation, brain tumors, Ewing sarcoma, gestational trophoblastic tumors, Kaposi sarcoma, leukemias, lymphomas, ovarian germ cell tumors, rhabdomyosarcomas, Wilms tumor.

Administration and Dosage

➤*Adults:*

Small cell lung cancer –

Usual dosage: 2 times the intravenous (IV) dose rounded to the nearest 50 mg (ie, 2 times 35 mg/m²/day for 4 days to 50 mg/m²/day for 5 days). See also Off-label dosing.

Dosage adjustment: The dosage should be modified to take into account the myelosuppressive effects of other drugs in the combination or the effects of prior x-ray therapy or chemotherapy that may have compromised bone marrow reserve.

Off-label dosing –

Small cell lung cancer: Alternatively, 50 mg/m²/day for 21 days has been given. Repeat regimen after a 1- to 2-week rest period.

➤*Renal function impairment:* The following initial dose modification should be considered based on measured creatinine clearance (CrCl). Subsequent etoposide dosing should be based on patient tolerance and clinical effect.

Etoposide Dosage Adjustment Based on Renal Function

CrCl	Alternative dosage recommendation	Manufacturer package insert
> 50 mL/min	100%	100%
15 to 50 mL/min	75%	75%
10 to 15 mL/min	75%	Consider further dose reduction
< 10 mL/min	50%	Consider further dose reduction
Hemodialysis	50%, no supplemental dosing needed	No recommendation
Peritoneal dialysis	50%, no supplemental dosing needed	No recommendation
Continuous renal replacement therapy	75%, no supplemental dosing needed	No recommendation

➤*Hepatic function impairment:* In patients with a bilirubin level greater than 1 mg/dL there may be a reduced amount of albumin for binding. A dosage adjustment may be necessary, see the following table.

Etoposide Dosage Adjustment Based on Hepatic Function

Serum bilirubin	AST	Percentage of usual dose
< 1.5 mg/dL	< 60 units/L	100%
1.5 to 3 mg/dL	60 to 180 units/L	50%
3 to 5 mg/dL	> 180 units/L	25%
> 5 mg/dL	—	Do not administer

➤*Preparation for administration:* Etoposide is considered a cytotoxic agent. Follow safe handling procedures when preparing, administering, or dispensing etoposide.

➤*Administration:* Take capsules with or without food. Administer as a single daily dose for doses of 400 mg/day or less. For doses greater than 400 mg/day, give 2 to 4 divided doses.

➤*Storage/Stability:* Refrigerate capsules at 2° to 8°C (36° to 46°F). Do not freeze. The capsules are stable for 24 months under such refrigeration conditions.

ETOPOSIDE — INJECTION

For complete and comparative prescribing information, refer to the Podophyllotoxin Derivatives group monograph.

WARNING

Administer etoposide under the supervision of a qualified health care provider experienced in the use of cancer chemotherapeutic agents. Severe myelosuppression with resulting infection or bleeding may occur.

Indications

➤*Refractory testicular tumors:* In combination therapy with other approved chemotherapeutic agents in patients with refractory testicular tumors who have already received appropriate surgical, chemotherapeutic, and radiotherapeutic therapy.

➤*Small cell lung cancer:* In combination with other approved chemotherapeutic agents as first-line treatment in patients with small cell lung cancer.

➤*Off-label uses:*

Other possible off-label uses – Treatment of bladder carcinoma, lymphomas, leukemias, Ewing sarcoma, Kaposi sarcoma, brain tumors, gestational trophoblastic tumors, ovarian germ cell tumors, rhabdomyosarcomas, Wilms tumor, bone marrow transplantation.

Administration and Dosage

➤*General dosing considerations:* Cyclophosphamide is dosed in mg/m^2 for most indications, but may be dosed in mg/kg for other indications.

Etoposide solution (20 mg/mL) must be further diluted prior to administration.

➤*Adults:*

Small cell lung cancer –

Usual dosage: Ranges from 35 mg/m^2/day IV for 4 days each cycle to 50 mg/m^2/day for 5 days each cycle. Repeat cycles every 3 to 4 weeks. Give in combination with other approved chemotherapeutic drugs.

Dosage adjustment: The dosage should be modified to take into account the myelosuppressive effects of other drugs in the combination or the effects of prior x-ray therapy or chemotherapy that may have compromised bone marrow reserve.

Hold etoposide if the platelet count is lower than 50,000 cells/mm^3 or the absolute neutrophil count (ANC) is lower than 500 cells/mm^3. Resume therapy when counts recover.

Testicular tumors (refractory) –

Usual dosage: 50 to 100 mg/m^2/day IV on days 1 through 5 of each cycle, or 100 mg/m^2/day IV on days 1, 3, and 5 of each cycle. Repeat cycles every 3 to 4 weeks. Give in combination with other approved chemotherapeutic agents.

Dosage adjustment: The dosage should be modified to take into account the myelosuppressive effects of other drugs in the combination or the effects of prior x-ray therapy or chemotherapy that may have compromised bone marrow reserve.

Hold etoposide if the platelet count is lower than 50,000 cells/mm^3 or the absolute neutrophil count (ANC) is lower than 500 cells/mm^3. Resume therapy when counts recover.

Off-label dosing –

AIDS-related Kaposi sarcoma: 150 mg/m^2/day IV for 3 days every 4 weeks.

Hematopoietic stem cell transplantation: 60 mg/kg body weight IV as a single dose has been used in combination with other agents.

Dosages used for pretransplant conditioning ("priming") have ranged from 900 to 2,000 mg/m^2 IV. Etoposide has been used alone or in combination with colony-stimulating factors.

➤*Children:* Some etoposide for injection products contain benzyl alcohol 3%. Avoid use in infants because toxicity may occur.

Etoposide for injection may contain polysorbate 80. Avoid use in premature infants because toxicity may occur.

Off-label dosing –

Acute nonlymphocytic leukemia:

- *Induction* – 150 mg/m^2/day IV for 2 to 3 days for 2 to 3 courses.
- *Consolidation or intensification* – 250 mg/m^2/day IV for 3 consecutive days on courses 2 to 5 of chemotherapy.

Brain tumor: 150 mg/m^2/day IV on days 2 and 3 of each treatment course.

Neuroblastoma: 100 mg/m^2/day IV on days 1 to 5 of each 28-day cycle.

Hematopoietic stem cell transplantation: 60 mg/kg body weight IV as a single dose has been used in combination with other agents.

➤*Renal function impairment:* The following dose modification should be considered based on measured creatinine clearance (CrCl). Subsequent etoposide dosing should be based on patient tolerance and clinical effect.

Etoposide Dosage Adjustment Based on Renal Function

CrCl	Alternative dosage recommendation	Manufacturer package insert
> 50 mL/min	100%	100%
15 to 50 mL/min	75%	75%
10 to 15 mL/min	75%	Consider further dose reduction
< 10 mL/min	50%	Consider further dose reduction
Hemodialysis	50%, no supplemental dosing needed	No recommendation
Peritoneal dialysis	50%, no supplemental dosing needed	No recommendation
Continuous renal replacement therapy	75%, no supplemental dosing needed	No recommendation

➤*Hepatic function impairment:* In patients with a bilirubin level greater than 1 mg/dL there may be a reduced amount of albumin for binding. A dosage adjustment may be necessary, see the following table.

Etoposide Dosage Adjustment Based on Hepatic Function

Serum bilirubin	AST	Percentage of usual dose
< 1.5 mg/dL	< 60 units/L	100%
1.5 to 3 mg/dL	60 to 180 units/L	50%
3 to 5 mg/dL	> 180 units/L	25%

➤*Preparation for administration:* Etoposide is considered a cytotoxic agent. Follow safe handling procedures when preparing, administering, or dispensing etoposide.

Skin reactions associated with accidental exposure to etoposide may occur. The use of gloves is recommended. If etoposide solution contacts the skin or mucosa, immediately and thoroughly wash the skin with soap and water and flush the mucosa with water.

Dilution – Etoposide must be diluted prior to use with dextrose 5% injection or sodium chloride 0.9% injection to give a final concentration of 0.2 to 0.4 mg/mL. If solutions are prepared at concentrations above 0.4 mg/mL, precipitation may occur.

➤*Administration:* Infuse over at least 30 to 60 minutes. Do not give by rapid IV injection due to the risk of hypotension. Monitor blood pressure before and after infusion. A longer duration of administration may be used if the volume of fluid to be infused is a concern.

For high-dose HSCT regimens (off-label use), infuse over 4 hours directly into a central venous line. If undiluted etoposide is used, solutions should be prepared in sterile glass containers and administered through non-ABS tubing (eg, nitroglycerin tubing) to avoid cracking of plastic. A special infusion-pump device may be required. For example, an *IVAC* infusion pump and *IVAC* tubing may be used.

➤*Admixture compatibility:* Plastic devices made of acrylic or a polymer composed of acrylonitrile, butadiene, and styrene (ABS) have been reported to crack and leak when used with undiluted etoposide injection.

➤*Storage/Stability:* Store at 15° to 30°C (59° to 86°F). Do not freeze. Unopened vials of etoposide are stable for 24 months at room temperature, 25°C (77°F). Vials diluted as recommended to a concentration of 0.2 or 0.4 mg/mL are stable for 96 and 24 hours, respectively, at room temperature, 25°C (77°F), under normal room fluorescent lights in both glass and plastic containers.

ETOPOSIDE PHOSPHATE — INJECTION

For complete and comparative prescribing information, refer to the Podophyllotoxin Derivatives group monograph.

WARNING

Etoposide should be administered under the supervision of a qualified health care provider experienced in the use of cancer chemotherapeutic agents. Severe myelosuppression with resulting infection or bleeding may occur.

Indications

➤*Refractory testicular tumors:* In combination therapy with other approved chemotherapeutic agents in patients with refractory testicular tumors who have already received appropriate surgical, chemotherapeutic, and radiotherapeutic therapy.

➤*Small cell lung cancer:* In combination with other approved chemotherapeutic agents as first-line treatment in patients with small cell lung cancer.

➤*Off-label uses:*

Other possible off-label uses – Treatment of bladder carcinoma, lymphomas, leukemias, Ewing sarcoma, Kaposi sarcoma, brain tumors, gestational trophoblastic tumors, ovarian germ cell tumors, rhabdomyosarcomas, Wilms tumor, bone marrow transplantation.

Administration and Dosage

➤*General dosing considerations:* The dose of etoposide phosphate should always be expressed as the desired etoposide dose, rather than as the etoposide phosphate dose. One appropriate way to write orders is "Etoposide phosphate equivalent to ___ mg etoposide". Etoposide phosphate may be substituted for etoposide in any regimen, although its use is usually limited to high-dose regimens. All doses are given as etoposide equivalents.

ETOPOSIDE PHOSPHATE — INJECTION

Cyclophosphamide is dosed in mg/m^2 for most indications, but may be dosed in mg/kg for other indications.

➤*Adults:*

Small cell lung cancer –

Usual dosage: Ranges from 35 mg/m^2/day IV for 4 days to 50 mg/m^2/day for 5 days each cycle. Repeat cycles every 3 to 4 weeks. Give in combination with other approved chemotherapeutic drugs. Equivalent doses of etoposide base injection (eg, *Toposar*) should be used.

Dosage adjustment: The dosage should be modified to take into account the myelosuppressive effect of other drugs in the combination or the effects of prior x-ray therapy or chemotherapy that may have compromised bone marrow reserve.

Hold etoposide if the platelet count is lower than 50,000 cells/mm^3 or the absolute neutrophil count (ANC) is lower than 500 cells/mm^3. Resume therapy when counts recover.

Testicular tumors (refractory) –

Usual dosage: 50 to 100 mg/m^2/day IV on days 1 through 5 of each cycle, or 100 mg/m^2/day IV on days 1, 3, and 5 of each cycle. Repeat cycles every 3 to 4 weeks. Give in combination with other approved chemotherapeutic agents. Equivalent doses of etoposide (eg, *Toposar*) should be used.

Dosage adjustment: The dosage should be modified to take into account the myelosuppressive effect of other drugs in the combination or the effects of prior x-ray therapy or chemotherapy that may have compromised bone marrow reserve. Hold etoposide if the platelet count is lower than 50,000 cells/mm^3 or the absolute neutrophil count (ANC) is lower than 500 cells/mm^3. Resume therapy when counts recover.

Off-label dosing –

AIDS-related Kaposi sarcoma: 150 mg/m^2/day IV for 3 days every 4 weeks.

Hematopoietic stem cell transplantation: 60 mg/kg body weight IV as a single dose has been used in combination with other agents.

Dosages used for pretransplant conditioning ("priming") have ranged from 900 to 2,000 mg/m^2 IV. Etoposide has been used alone or in combination with colony-stimulating factors.

➤*Children:*

Off-label dosing –

Acute nonlymphocytic leukemia:

- *Induction* – 150 mg/m^2/day IV for 2 to 3 days for 2 to 3 courses.
- *Consolidation or intensification* – 250 mg/m^2/day IV for 3 consecutive days on courses 2 to 5 of chemotherapy.

Brain tumor: 150 mg/m^2/day IV on days 2 and 3 of each treatment course.

Neuroblastoma: 100 mg/m^2/day IV on days 1 to 5 of each 28-day cycle.

Hematopoietic stem cell transplantation: 60 mg/kg body weight IV as a single dose has been used in combination with other agents.

➤*Elderly:* Because elderly patients are more likely to have decreased renal function, take care in dose selection. It may also be useful to monitor renal function.

➤*Renal function impairment:* The following dose modification should be considered based on measured creatinine clearance (CrCl). Subsequent etoposide dosing should be based on patient tolerance and clinical effect.

Etoposide Dosage Adjustment Based on Renal Function

CrCl	Alternative dosage recommendation	Manufacturer package insert
> 50 mL/min	100%	100%
15 to 50 mL/min	75%	75%
10 to 15 mL/min	75%	Consider further dose reduction
< 10 mL/min	50%	Consider further dose reduction
Hemodialysis	50%, no supplemental dosing needed	No recommendation
Peritoneal dialysis	50%, no supplemental dosing needed	No recommendation
Continuous renal replacement therapy	75%, no supplemental dosing needed	No recommendation

➤*Hepatic function impairment:* In patients with a bilirubin level greater than 1 mg/dl there may be a reduced amount of albumin for binding. A dosage adjustment may be necessary, see the following table.

Etoposide Dosage Adjustment Based on Hepatic Function

Serum bilirubin	AST	Percentage of usual dose
< 1.5 mg/dL	< 60 units/L	100%
1.5 to 3 mg/dL	60 to 180 units/L	50%
3 to 5 mg/dL	> 180 units/L	25%

➤*Preparation for administration:* Etoposide is considered a cytotoxic agent. Follow safe handling procedures when preparing, administering, or dispensing etoposide.

Skin reactions associated with accidental exposure to etoposide may occur. The use of gloves is recommended. If etoposide solution contacts the skin or mucosa, immediately and thoroughly wash the skin with soap and water and flush the mucosa with water.

Reconstitution – Prior to use, the content of each vial must be reconstituted with sterile water for injection, dextrose 5% injection, sodium chloride 0.9% injection, bacteriostatic water for injection with benzyl alcohol, or bacteriostatic sodium chloride for injection with benzyl alcohol to a concentration equivalent to etoposide 20 mg/mL or 10 mg/mL (etoposide phosphate 22.7 or 11.4 mg/mL, respectively). Use the quantity of diluent shown in the following table to reconstitute the product.

Volume of Diluent for Etoposide Phosphate Administration

Vial strength	Volume of diluent	Final concentration
100 mg	5 mL	20 mg/mL
	10 mL	10 mg/mL

Dilution – Following reconstitution, etoposide can be further diluted to concentrations as low as etoposide 0.1 mg/mL with dextrose 5% injection or sodium chloride 0.9% injection.

➤*Administration:* Etoposide solutions may be administered at infusion rates from 5 to 210 minutes. The toxicity profile of etoposide when infused at doses greater than 175 mg/m^2 has not been delineated. Do not give by rapid IV injection due to the risk of hypotension. Monitor blood pressure before and after infusion.

For high-dose HSCT regimens (off-label use), infuse over 4 hours directly into a central venous line. If undiluted etoposide is used, solutions should be prepared in sterile glass containers and administered through non-ABS tubing (eg, nitroglycerin tubing) to avoid cracking of plastic. A special infusion-pump device may be required. For example, an *IVAC* infusion pump and *IVAC* tubing may be used.

➤*Storage / Stability:* Store the unopened vials under refrigeration between 2° and 8°C (36° and 46°F). Retain in original package to protect from light.

When reconstituted as directed, etoposide phosphate solutions can be stored in glass or plastic containers under refrigeration between 2° and 8°C (36° and 46°F) for 7 days; at controlled room temperature between 20° and 25°C (68° and 77°F) for 24 hours following reconstitution with sterile water for injection, dextrose 5% injection, or sodium chloride 0.9% injection; or at controlled room temperature between 20° and 25°C (68° and 77°F) for 48 hours following reconstitution with bacteriostatic water for injection with benzyl alcohol or bacteriostatic sodium chloride for injection with benzyl alcohol. Etoposide solutions further diluted as directed can be stored under refrigeration between 2° and 8°C (36° and 46°F) or at controlled room temperature between 20° and 25°C (68° and 77°F) for 24 hours.

Discard single-dose vial within 6 hours of the initial needle puncture if opened within an ISO Class 5 biological safety cabinet, or within 1 hour of the initial needle puncture if opened outside of such an environment, based on the USP Chapter <797> standards.

Podophyllotoxin Derivatives

TENIPOSIDE (VM-26)

Rx	Vumon (Bristol-Myers Squibb)	**Injection, solution, concentrate:** 10 mg/mL (50 mg per 5 mL)	Benzyl alcohol 30 mg, *Cremophor EL* (polyoxyethylated castor oil) 500 mg, and dehydrated alcohol 42.7%. In 5 mL amps.

TENIPOSIDE — INJECTION

For complete and comparative prescribing information, refer to the Podophyllotoxin Derivatives group monograph.

WARNING

Teniposide is a cytotoxic drug. Administer under the supervision of a qualified health care provider experienced in the use of cancer chemotherapeutic agents. Appropriate management of therapy and complications is possible only when adequate treatment facilities are readily available.

Severe myelosuppression with resulting infection or bleeding may occur. Hypersensitivity reactions, including anaphylaxis-like symptoms, may occur with initial dosing or with repeated exposure to teniposide. Epinephrine, with or without corticosteroids and antihistamines, has been employed to alleviate hypersensitivity reaction symptoms.

Indications

➤*Acute lymphoblastic leukemia:* In combination with other approved anticancer agents for induction therapy in patients with refractory childhood acute lymphoblastic leukemia (ALL).

➤*Off-label uses:* Treatment of adult acute lymphocytic leukemia; non-Hodgkin lymphoma.

Administration and Dosage

➤*General dosing considerations:* Dosing adjustment suggested for patients with both Down syndrome and leukemia. (See Patients with Down syndrome.)

➤*Adults:*

Off-label dosing –

Acute lymphoblastic leukemia: 165 mg/m^2 by IV infusion on days 1, 4, 8, and 11 during consolidation on the "Linker" regimen.

Non-Hodgkin lymphoma: 30 mg/m^2/day for 10 days; or 50 to 100 mg/m^2 once a week as a single agent or 60 to 70 mg/m^2/day once a week in combination with other chemotherapeutic drugs.

➤*Children:*

Acute lymphoblastic leukemia –

Patients refractory to cytarabine-containing regimens: 165 mg/m^2 (in combination with cytarabine 300 mg/m^2) by IV infusion, twice weekly for 8 to 9 doses.

Patients refractory to vincristine/prednisone-containing regimens: 250 mg/m^2 (in combination with vincristine 1.5 mg/m^2) by IV infusion, weekly for 4 to 8 weeks, and prednisone 40 mg/m^2 orally for 28 days.

➤*Renal function impairment:*

Dialysis – Conventional hemodialysis and peritoneal dialysis are ineffective (0% to 24%) in removing teniposide.

Supplemental doses are not required after hemodialysis.

➤*Patients with Down syndrome:* For patients with both Down syndrome and leukemia, the initial dosing with teniposide should be reduced. It is suggested that the first course of teniposide should be given at half the usual dose. Subsequent courses may be administered at higher dosages, depending on the degree of myelosuppression and mucositis encountered in earlier courses in an individual patient.

➤*Preparation for administration:* Teniposide is considered a cytotoxic agent. Follow safe handling procedures when preparing, administering, or dispensing teniposide.

Skin reactions associated with accidental exposure to teniposide may occur. The use of gloves is recommended. If teniposide solution contacts the skin, immediately wash the skin thoroughly with soap and water. If teniposide contacts mucous membranes, the membranes should be flushed thoroughly with water.

Aseptically withdraw the desired dose from the ampule using a filter needle to withdraw the dose; then remove the filter needle and use a new needle to add teniposide to the diluent.

Teniposide must be diluted with either dextrose 5% injection or sodium chloride 0.9% injection to give final teniposide concentrations of 0.1, 0.2, 0.4, or 1 mg/mL.

Although solutions are chemically stable under the conditions indicated, precipitation of teniposide may occur at the recommended concentrations, especially if the diluted solution is subjected to more agitation than is recommended to prepare the drug solution for parenteral administration. In addition, storage time prior to administration should be minimized and care should be taken to avoid contact of the diluted solution with other drugs or fluids.

➤*Administration:* Hypotension has been reported following rapid IV administration; it is recommended that the teniposide solution be administered over at least a 30- to 60-minute period. Teniposide should not be given by rapid IV injection.

Observe patients during and after the infusion for signs of hypersensitivity.

Precipitation has been reported during 24-hour infusions of teniposide diluted to teniposide concentrations of 0.1 to 0.2 mg/mL, resulting in occlusion of central venous access catheters in several patients. Heparin solution can cause precipitation of teniposide; therefore, the administration apparatus should be flushed thoroughly with dextrose 5% injection or sodium chloride 0.9% injection before and after administration of teniposide.

The use of nondiethylhexyl phthalate (DEHP) IV administration sets is recommended. The use of polyvinyl chloride (PVC) containers is not recommended.

Similarly, the use of non-DEHP IV administration sets is recommended. Lipid administration sets or low DEHP-containing nitroglycerin sets will keep patients' exposure to DEHP at low levels and are suitable for use. The diluted solutions are chemically and physically compatible with the recommended IV administration sets and large-volume parenteral (LVP) containers for up to 24 hours at ambient room temperature and lighting conditions. A polyethylene administration set is also suitable for use. Undiluted teniposide may cause cracking of plastic devices made of acrylic or acrylonitrite butadiene styrene (ABS).

Although not recommended by the manufacturer, PVC tubing may be used for administration of teniposide; however, the drug must then be administered faster, at a rate of 250 mL/h.

➤*Extravasation:* Improper administration of teniposide may result in extravasation, causing local tissue necrosis and/or thrombophlebitis. In some instances, occlusion of central venous access devices has occurred during 24-hour infusion of teniposide at a concentration of 0.1 to 0.2 mg/mL. Frequent observation during these infusions is necessary to minimize this risk.

If signs or symptoms of extravasation occur, stop the infusion immediately. If possible, withdraw 3 to 5 mL of blood to remove some of the drug. Remove the infusion needle. Delineate the infiltrated area on the patient's skin with a felt tip marker. Elevate for 48 hours above heart level using a sling or stockinette dressing with an observation window cut in the dressing. Avoid pressure or friction. Do not rub the area. Observe for signs of increased erythema, pain, or skin necrosis. If increased symptoms occur, consult a plastic surgeon. Ensure that no medication is given distally to the extravasation site. After 48 hours, encourage the patient to use the extremity normally to promote full range of motion.

➤*Admixture compatibility:* Because of the potential for precipitation, compatibility with other drugs, infusion materials, or IV pumps cannot be ensured.

Heparin solution can cause precipitation of teniposide. Contact of undiluted teniposide with plastic equipment or devices used to prepare solutions for infusion may result in softening or cracking and possible drug product leakage. This effect has not been reported with diluted solutions of teniposide.

In order to prevent extraction of the plasticizer DEHP, solutions of teniposide should be prepared in non–DEHP-containing LVP containers, such as glass or polyolefin plastic bags or containers.

➤*Storage/Stability:* Store the unopened ampules under refrigeration, 2° to 8°C (36° to 46°F). Retain in original package to protect from light. Unopened vials of teniposide are stable until the date indicated on the package when stored under refrigeration in the original package. Freezing does not adversely affect the product.

Solutions prepared in dextrose 5% injection or sodium chloride 0.9% injection at teniposide concentrations of 0.1, 0.2, or 0.4 mg/mL are stable at room temperature for up to 24 hours after preparation. Teniposide solutions prepared at a final teniposide concentration of 1 mg/mL should be administered within 4 hours of preparation to reduce the potential for precipitation. Refrigeration of teniposide solutions is not recommended. Stability and use times are identical in glass and plastic parenteral solution containers.

DAUNORUBICIN HYDROCHLORIDE

Rx	**Daunorubicin HCl for Injection** (Various, eg, Abbott, Bedford)	**Injection**: 5 mg/ml (equivalent to 5.34 mg daunorubicin HCl)[a]	Preservative-free. In 4 and 10 ml single-use vials.
Rx	**Daunorubicin HCl** (Various, eg, Abbott, Gensia Sicor)	**Powder for Injection, lyophilized**: 21.4 mg (equivalent to 20 mg daunorubicin)	100 mg mannitol. In 10 ml single-dose vials.
Rx	**Cerubidine** (Bedford)		100 mg mannitol. In single-dose vials.
Rx	**Daunorubicin HCl** (Various, eg, Abbott, Gensia Sicor)	**Powder for Injection, lyophilized**: 53.5 mg (equivalent to 50 mg daunorubicin)	250 mg mannitol. In 20 ml single-dose vials.

[a] 9 mg NaCl.

DAUNORUBICIN HYDROCHLORIDE — INJECTION

WARNING

Give daunorubicin into a rapidly flowing IV infusion. Do not administer IM or SC. Severe local tissue necrosis will result if extravasation occurs.

Myocardial toxicity, in its most severe form, as potentially fatal congestive heart failure, may occur when total cumulative dosage exceeds 400 to 550 mg/m^2 in adults, 300 mg/m^2 in children older than 2 years of age, or 10 mg/kg in children younger than 2 years of age. This may occur during therapy or several months to years after therapy.

It is recommended that daunorubicin be administered only by physicians who are experienced in leukemia chemotherapy and in facilities with laboratory and supportive resources adequate to monitor drug tolerance and protect and maintain a patient compromised by drug toxicity.

The physician and institution must be capable of responding rapidly and completely to severe hemorrhagic conditions or overwhelming infection.

Severe myelosuppression occurs when used in therapeutic doses; this may lead to infection or hemorrhage.

Reduce dosage in patients with impaired hepatic or renal function.

Indications

➤*Acute nonlymphocytic/lymphocytic leukemia:* In combination with other approved anticancer drugs, for remission induction in acute nonlymphocytic leukemia (myelogenous, monocytic, erythroid) of adults and for remission induction in acute lymphocytic leukemia of children and adults.

➤*Off-label uses:* Treatment of chronic myelogenous leukemia. Daunorubicin has been used safely and effectively in children for the treatment of acute myelocytic leukemia and anaplastic large cell lymphoma. (See Administration and Dosage.)

Administration and Dosage

➤*General dosing considerations:* To eradicate the leukemic cells and induce a complete remission, a profound suppression of bone marrow is usually required. Evaluation of both the peripheral blood and bone marrow are mandatory in the formulation of treatment plans.

Risk of cardiotoxicity increases with the cumulative daunorubicin dose. (See Maximum dose and Warnings/Precautions.)

➤*Adults:*

Acute lymphocytic leukemia (remission induction) – The following combination regimen is according to the manufacturer; however, other combinations have been used.

Usual dosage: Daunorubicin 45 mg/m^2/day IV on days 1, 2, and 3.

Concomitant therapy: Vincristine 2 mg IV on days 1, 8, and 15; prednisone 40 mg/m^2/day orally on days 1 through 22, then tapered between days 22 to 29; L-asparaginase 500 units/kg/day for 10 days IV on days 22 through 32.

Acute nonlymphocytic leukemia – The following combination regimen is according to the manufacturer; however, other combinations have been used.

Usual dosage: Daunorubicin 45 mg/m^2/day IV on days 1, 2, and 3 of the first course and on days 1 and 2 of subsequent courses.

Duration of therapy: Attaining a normal appearing bone marrow may require up to 3 courses of induction therapy. Evaluate bone marrow following recovery from the previous induction course to determine the need for a further course of induction treatment.

Concomitant therapy: Cytosine arabinoside 100 mg/m^2/day IV infusion for 7days for the first course and for 5 days for subsequent courses.

Off-label dosing –

Chronic myelogenous leukemia (accelerated phase or blast crisis): Daunorubicin 30 to 45 mg/m^2/day IV on days 1 to 3, using induction regimens similar to those for acute lymphocytic leukemia or acute myelocytic leukemia, depending on disease histology and patient age.

➤*Children:* For children younger than 2 years of age or with less than 0.5 m^2 body surface area, calculate dosage on the basis of weight (mg/kg) instead of body surface area. Some clinicians recommend giving daunorubicin 1 mg/kg/dose IV for 1 to 3 days. Administration frequency is specific to each combination chemotherapy regimen.

Acute lymphocytic leukemia (remission induction) – The following combination regimen is according to the manufacturer; however, other combinations have been used.

Usual dosage: Daunorubicin 25 mg/m^2 IV on day 1 every week. (See also Off-label doses).

Duration of therapy: Generally, complete remission will be obtained with 4 courses of therapy; however, if after 4 courses the patient is in partial remission, an additional 1 or, if necessary, 2 courses may be given in an effort to obtain a complete remission.

Concomitant therapy: Vincristine 1.5 mg/m^2 IV on day 1 every week with oral prednisone 40 mg/m^2/day.

Off-label dosing –

Acute lymphocytic leukemia (remission induction): Alternatively, daunorubicin 25 to 45 mg/m^2/day IV has been given on days 1 and 8 of each cycle. Other protocols have used daunorubicin 30 to 45 mg/m^2/day IV on days 1 to 3 of each cycle. Schedule is specific to each combination chemotherapy regimen.

Acute myelocytic leukemia (remission induction): Daunorubicin 30 to 60 mg/m^2/day by continuous IV infusion over 24 hours on days 1 to 3 of each cycle. Alternatively, daunorubicin 20 mg/m^2/day by continuous infusion over 24 hours on days 1 to 4 of each 14-day cycle. Given in combination with other antineoplastics.

Anaplastic large cell lymphoma, induction: Daunorubicin 60 mg/m^2/day IV on days 9 and 10 of the 29-day induction phase.

➤*Elderly:* Cardiotoxicity may be more frequent in the elderly. Use caution in patients who have inadequate bone marrow reserves due to age. In addition, elderly patients are more likely to have age-related renal function impairment, which may require reduction of dosage in patients receiving daunorubicin.

Acute nonlymphocytic leukemia –

60 years of age and older: The following combination regimen is according to the manufacturer; however, other combinations have been used.

- *Usual dose* – Daunorubicin 30 mg/m^2/day IV on days 1, 2, and 3 of the first course and on days 1 and 2 of subsequent courses.
- *Duration of therapy* – Attaining a normal appearing bone marrow may require up to 3 courses of induction therapy. Evaluate bone marrow following recovery from the previous induction course to determine the need for a further course of induction treatment.
- *Concomitant therapy* – Cytosine arabinoside 100 mg/m^2/day IV infusion for 7 days for the first course and for 5 days for subsequent courses.

➤*Renal function impairment:* If serum creatinine is greater than 3 mg/dL, administer 50% of the usual dose.

➤*Hepatic function impairment:* If the serum bilirubin is 1.2 to 3 mg/dL, administer 75% of the usual dose. If the serum bilirubin is greater than 3 mg/dL, administer 50% of the usual dose.

➤*Preparation for administration:* Daunorubicin is considered a cytotoxic agent. Follow safe handling procedures when preparing, administering, or dispensing daunorubicin.

Powder for solution (20 mg/vial) – Reconstitute vial contents with 4 mL sterile water for injection to prepare a solution of daunorubicin 5 mg/mL. Shake vial gently to dissolve contents. Solution will be red. Withdraw the desired dose into a syringe containing 10 to 15 mL of sodium chloride 0.9% injection; inject into the tubing or sidearm of a rapidly flowing IV infusion of dextrose 5% injection or sodium chloride 0.9% injection.

Solution (5 mg/mL) – Withdraw the desired dose into a syringe containing 10 to 15 mL of sodium chloride 0.9% injection; inject into the tubing or sidearm of a rapidly flowing IV infusion of dextrose 5% injection or sodium chloride 0.9% injection.

Solution for IV infusion – Daunorubicin solution has also been diluted in 100 mL of dextrose 5% injection or sodium chloride 0.9% injection for infusion via a central venous catheter.

➤*Administration:* For IV use only (IV push or IV infusion). Do not administer IM or subcutaneously. Severe local tissue necrosis will result if extravasation occurs.

Diluted 5 mg/mL solution with 10 to 15 mL of sodium chloride 0.9% injection should be given by direct IV injection or by IV sidearm through a running IV line.

Daunorubicin solution diluted in 100 mL of dextrose 5% injection or sodium chloride 0.9% injection may be infused IV over 30 to 45 minutes. However, many clinicians consider the risk of extravasation unacceptable unless infused through a central venous catheter.

➤*Extravasation:* Severe local tissue necrosis will result if extravasation occurs. If signs or symptoms of extravasation occur, stop the infusion immediately. If possible, withdraw 3 to 5 mL of blood to remove some of the drug. Remove the infusion needle.

There are currently 2 treatments for extravasation resulting from anthracycline IV therapy: topical dimethyl sulfoxide and dexrazoxane IV. Both treatments are effective for treating anthracycline extravasation injury, although no comparative trials have been conducted.

- Apply dimethyl sulfoxide (DMSO) 99% by saturating a gauze pad and painting on an area twice the size of the extravasation. Allow the site to air dry and repeat the application every 6 hours for 14 days. Do not cover the area with dressing.

DAUNORUBICIN HYDROCHLORIDE — INJECTION

- Dexrazoxane (*Totect*) is FDA-approved for the treatment of extravasation resulting from anthracycline IV therapy. The first infusion of dexrazoxane should be administered as soon as possible and within the first 6 hours following the extravasation. Topical cooling, such as ice packs, should be removed for at least 15 minutes prior to and during dexrazoxane administration. Concurrent extravasation treatment, such as topical dimethyl sulfoxide application should not be used in conjunction with dexrazoxane, and if administered, may worsen extravasation-induced tissue injury. The recommended dose of dexrazoxane for day 1 is 1,000 mg/m^2 (up to 2,000 mg), the dose for day 2 is 1,000 mg/m^2 (up to 2,000 mg), and the dose for day 3 is 500 mg/m^2 (up to 1,000 mg). Dexrazoxane is administered as an IV infusion over 1 to 2 hours.

Application of ice compresses to the area for 15 minutes every 6 hours for 48 hours may be useful. Delineate the infiltrated area on the patient's skin with a felt-tip marker. Elevate for 48 hours above heart level using a sling or stockinette dressing with an observation window cut in the dressing. Avoid pressure or friction. Do not rub the area. Observe for signs of increased erythema, pain, or skin necrosis. If increased symptoms occur, consult a plastic surgeon. Ensure that no medication is given distally to extravasation site. After 48 hours, encourage the patient to use the extremity normally to promote full range of motion.

➤*Admixture compatibility:* Do not mix with other drugs or heparin.

➤*Storage/Stability:* Store unopened vials of solution at 2° to 8°C (36° to 46°F). Store unreconstituted powder at 15° to 30°C (59° to 86°F). Store prepared solution for infusion at room temperature, 15° to 30°C (59° to 86°F) for up to 24 hours. However, the reconstituted solution is chemically stable under refrigeration for up to 48 hours. Contains no preservative. Color change of solution from red to blue-purple indicates decomposition. Discard unused portion. Protect from light.

Discard vial within 6 hours of the initial needle puncture if opened within an ISO Class 5 biological safety cabinet, or within 1 hour of the initial needle puncture if opened outside of such an environment, based on the USP Chapter < 797 > standards.

Actions

➤*Pharmacology:* Daunorubicin has antimitotic and cytotoxic activity through a number of proposed mechanisms of action. It forms complexes with DNA by intercalation between base pairs. It inhibits topoisomerase II activity by stabilizing the DNA-topoisomerase II complex, preventing the religation portion of the ligation-religation reaction that topoisomerase II catalyzes. Single-strand and double-strand DNA breaks result. Daunorubicin may also inhibit polymerase activity, affect regulation of gene expression, and produce free radical damage to DNA.

➤*Pharmacokinetics:*

Absorption/Distribution – Following IV injection, daunorubicin undergoes rapid tissue uptake and concentration. It does not cross the blood-brain barrier. Plasma and tissue protein binding is rapid and extensive; highest concentrations occur in the spleen, kidneys, liver, lungs, and heart.

Metabolism/Excretion – Daunorubicin is extensively metabolized in the liver and other tissues, mainly by cytoplasmic aldo-keto reductases, producing daunorubicinol, the major metabolite, which has antineoplastic activity. Approximately 40% of the drug in the plasma is present as daunorubicinol within 30 minutes and 60% in 4 hours after a dose of daunorubicin. Further metabolism via reduction cleavage of the glycosidic bond, 4-O demethylation and conjugation with both sulfate and glucuronide have been demonstrated. Terminal half-lives for daunorubicin and daunorubicinol are 18.5 and 26.7 hours, respectively. About 25% is eliminated in active form by urinary excretion and 40% by biliary excretion.

Contraindications

Hypersensitivity to daunorubicin or any component of the product.

Warnings/Precautions

➤*Previous cumulative dose:* Do not use in patients who have previously received the recommended maximum cumulative dose of either doxorubicin or daunorubicin.

➤*Bone marrow suppression:* Bone marrow suppression will occur in all patients given a therapeutic dose of this drug. Do not start therapy in patients with preexisting drug-induced bone marrow suppression unless the benefit from such treatment warrants the risk. Persistent, severe myelosuppression may result in superinfection or hemorrhage.

➤*Cardiotoxicity:* Preexisting heart disease or previous doxorubicin therapy are cofactors of increased risk of cardiotoxicity; weigh benefit-to-risk ratio before starting therapy. Give attention to the drug's potential cardiac toxicity, particularly in infants and children.

In adults, at total cumulative doses less than 550 mg/m^2, acute CHF is seldom encountered. However, rare instances of pericarditis-myocarditis, not dose-related, have occurred. At cumulative doses more than 550 mg/m^2, there is an increased incidence of CHF. This limit appears lower (400 mg/m^2) in patients receiving radiation therapy that encompassed the heart. In infants and children, there is a greater susceptibility to anthracycline-induced cardiotoxicity compared with adults, which is more clearly dose-related. However, there is little risk for children older than 2 years of age below a cumulative dose of 300 mg/m^2 or in children younger than 2 years of age (or less than 0.5 m^2 body surface area) below a cumulative dose of 10 mg/kg. Furthermore, the total dose given to children and adults should take into account any previous or concomitant therapy with other potentially cardiotoxic agents or related compounds such as doxorubicin.

There is no reliable method for predicting patients who will develop acute CHF; certain ECG changes and a decrease in the systolic injection fraction from pretreatment baseline may aid in recognizing those patients at greatest risk. A decrease of at least 30% in limb lead QRS voltage has been associated with significant risk of drug-induced cardiomyopathy. Perform an ECG or determine systolic ejection fraction before each course. If one or the other of these predictive parameters occurs, weigh the benefit of continued therapy against the risk of producing cardiac damage.

➤*Secondary leukemias:* There have been reports of secondary leukemias in patients exposed to topoisomerase II inhibitors when used in combination with other antineoplastic agents or radiation therapy.

➤*Urine discoloration:* Urine discoloration (red) may occur transiently; advise patient appropriately.

➤*Infections:* Control any systemic infection before beginning therapy.

➤*Hyperuricemia:* Hyperuricemia may be induced secondary to rapid lysis of leukemic cells. As a precaution, administer allopurinol prior to initiating antileukemic therapy. Monitor serum uric acid levels; initiate therapy if hyperuricemia develops.

➤*Extravasation:* See Administration and Dosage for more information.

➤*Renal/Hepatic function impairment:* Hepatic and renal function impairment can enhance toxicity; assess hepatic and renal function prior to therapy.

➤*Pregnancy: Category D.* Due to its teratogenic potential, daunorubicin can cause fetal harm if administered to a pregnant woman. An increased incidence of fetal abnormalities (parieto-occipital cranioschisis, umbilical hernias, or rachischisis) and abortions occurred in rabbits at doses of 0.05 mg/kg/day or approximately 1/100 of the highest recommended human dose on a body-surface-area basis. Decreases in fetal birth weight and post-delivery growth rate were observed in mice. There are no adequate and well-controlled studies in pregnant women. Advise women of childbearing potential to avoid becoming pregnant.

➤*Lactation:* It is not known whether this drug is excreted in breast milk. Due to the potential for serious adverse reactions in nursing infants from daunorubicin, advise mothers to discontinue nursing during daunorubicin therapy.

➤*Monitoring:* Observe patient closely and monitor chemical and laboratory tests extensively. Evaluate cardiac, renal, and hepatic function prior to each course of treatment.

Drug Interactions

Daunorubicin HCl Drug Interactions

Precipitant drug	Object drug[a]		Description
Cyclophosphamide	Daunorubicin	↑	Cyclophosphamide used concurrently with daunorubicin may result in increased cardiotoxicity.
Myelosuppressive agents	Daunorubicin	↑	Dosage reduction of daunorubicin may be required when used concurrently with other myelosuppressive agents.
Hepatotoxic medications (eg, methotrexate)	Daunorubicin	↑	Hepatotoxic medications, such as high-dose methotrexate, may impair liver function and increase the risk of toxicity.

[a] ↑ = Object drug increased.

Adverse Reactions

Daunorubicin is considered to have moderate potential for nausea and vomiting.

Dose-limiting toxicity includes myelosuppression and cardiotoxicity (see Warnings).

➤*Dermatologic:* Reversible alopecia; rash; contact dermatitis; urticaria.

➤*GI:* Acute nausea and vomiting (usually mild). Antiemetic therapy may help. Mucositis may occur 3 to 7 days after administration. Diarrhea and abdominal pain occur occasionally.

➤*Local:* If extravasation occurs, tissue necrolysis, severe cellulitis, thrombophlebitis, or painful induration can result at the site.

➤*Miscellaneous:* Rarely, anaphylactoid reactions, fever, and chills can occur. Hyperuricemia may occur, especially in patients with leukemia; monitor serum uric levels.

DAUNORUBICIN CITRATE LIPOSOMAL

Rx	DaunoXome (Gilead Sciences)	Injection: 2 mg/mL (equivalent to 50 mg daunorubicin base)	In single-use vials and single-unit packs.

DAUNORUBICIN CITRATE LIPOSOMAL — INJECTION

WARNING

Monitor cardiac function regularly in patients receiving liposomal daunorubicin because of the potential risk for cardiac toxicity and congestive heart failure (CHF). Cardiac monitoring is especially advised in those patients who have received prior anthracyclines, have had preexisting cardiac disease, or who have had prior radiotherapy encompassing the heart. Severe myelosuppression may occur.

Administer liposomal daunorubicin only under the supervision of a physician who is experienced in the use of cancer chemotherapeutic agents.

Reduce dosage in patients with impaired hepatic function (see Administration and Dosage).

A triad of back pain, flushing, and chest tightness has been reported in 13.8% of the patients (16/116) treated with liposomal daunorubicin in the phase 3 clinical trial, and in 2.7% of treatment cycles (27/994). This triad generally occurs during the first 5 minutes of the infusion, subsides with interruption of the infusion, and generally does not recur if the infusion is then resumed at a slower rate.

Indications

➤*Advanced HIV-associated Kaposi sarcoma:* As first-line cytotoxic therapy for advanced HIV-associated Kaposi sarcoma.

Administration and Dosage

➤*Adults:*

Advanced HIV-associated Kaposi sarcoma –

Usual dosage: 40 mg/m^2 administered IV over 60 minutes. Repeat every 2 weeks. Repeat blood counts prior to each dose and withhold therapy if the absolute granulocyte count is less than 750 cells/mm^3.

Duration of therapy: Continue treatment until there is evidence of progressive disease (eg, based on best response achieved, new visceral sites of involvement or progression of visceral disease, development of 10 or more new cutaneous lesions or a 25% increase in the number of lesions compared with baseline, a change in the character of at least 25% of all previously counted flat lesions to raised, increase in surface area of the indicator lesions) or until other intercurrent complications of HIV disease preclude continuation of therapy.

➤*Renal function impairment:* If serum creatinine is more than 3 mg/dL, administer 50% of the usual dose.

➤*Hepatic function impairment:* If the serum bilirubin is 1.2 to 3 mg/dL, administer 75% of the usual dose. If the serum bilirubin is more than 3 mg/dL, administer 50% of the usual dose.

➤*Infusion reactions:* Daunorubicin liposomal is associated with infusion reactions that may occur within the first 5 minutes of starting the infusion and manifest as back pain, flushing, and chest tightness. The reaction may be controlled by temporarily stopping the infusion and re-initiating it at a slower rate.

➤*Preparation for administration:* Daunorubicin is considered a cytotoxic agent. Follow safe handling procedures when preparing, administering, or dispensing daunorubicin citrate liposomal.

Dilute liposomal daunorubicin 1:1 with dextrose 5% injection before administration. The recommended concentration after dilution is daunorubicin 1 mg/mL of solution.

➤*Administration:* IV infusion over 60 minutes. Do not filter.

➤*Extravasation:* Conventional daunorubicin has been associated with local tissue necrosis at the site of drug extravasation. Although grade 3 to 4 injection-site inflammation was reported in 2 patients treated with liposomal daunorubicin, no instances of local tissue necrosis were observed with extravasation. Take care to ensure there is no extravasation of the drug when liposomal daunorubicin is administered.

Liposomal daunorubicin is considered an irritant and may cause phlebitis, but it is not known to cause tissue damage with extravasation. If signs or symptoms of extravasation occur, stop the infusion immediately. If possible, withdraw 3 to 5 mL of blood to remove some of the drug. Remove the infusion needle. Delineate the infiltrated area on the patient's skin with a felt tip marker. Elevate for 48 hours above heart level using a sling or stockinette dressing with an observation window cut in the dressing. Avoid pressure or friction. Do not rub the area. Observe for signs of increased erythema, pain, or skin necrosis. If increased symptoms occur, consult a plastic surgeon. Ensure that no medication is given distally to the extravasation site. After 48 hours, encourage the patient to use the extremity normally to promote full range of motion.

➤*Admixture compatibility:* Do not mix liposomal daunorubicin with other drugs.

➤*Storage/Stability:* Refrigerate between 2° and 8°C (36° and 46°F). If not used immediately, store reconstituted solution for a maximum of 6 hours under refrigeration. Do not freeze. Protect from light.

Discard vial within 6 hours of the initial needle puncture if opened within an ISO Class 5 biological safety cabinet, or within 1 hour of the initial needle puncture if opened outside of such an environment, based on the USP Chapter < 797 > standards of practice.

Actions

➤*Pharmacology:* Liposomal daunorubicin contains an aqueous solution of the citrate salt of daunorubicin encapsulated within lipid vesicles (liposomes) composed of a lipid bilayer of distearoylphosphatidylcholine and cholesterol (2:1 molar ratio). Daunorubicin is an anthracycline antibiotic with antineoplastic activity originally obtained from *Streptomyces peucetius*. It may also be isolated from *Streptomyces coeruleorubidus*. Daunorubicin has a 4-ring anthracycline moiety linked by a glycosidic bond to daunosamine, an amino sugar.

Liposomal daunorubicin is a liposomal preparation of daunorubicin formulated to maximize the selectivity of daunorubicin for solid tumors in situ. In the circulation, the liposomal daunorubicin formulation helps to protect the entrapped daunorubicin from chemical and enzymatic degradation, minimizes protein binding, and generally decreases uptake by normal (nonreticuloendothelial system) tissues. The specific mechanism by which liposomal daunorubicin is able to deliver daunorubicin to solid tumors in situ is not known. However, it is believed to be a function of increased permeability of the tumor neovasculature to some particles in the size range of liposomal daunorubicin. Once within the tumor environment, daunorubicin is released over time, enabling it to exert its antineoplastic activity.

➤*Pharmacokinetics:*

Absorption/Distribution –

Liposomal Daunorubicin Pharmacokinetic Parameters

Parameters (units)	Daunorubicin citrate liposomal (n = 30)	Conventional daunorubicin (n = 4)
Plasma clearance (mL/min)	17.3 ± 6.1	236 ± 181[a]
Volume of distribution (L)	6.4 ± 1.5	1006 ± 622
Distribution half-life (h)	4.41 ± 2.33	0.77 ± 0.3
Elimination half-life (h)	4.4 (apparent)	55.4 ± 13.7

[a] Calculated.

The plasma pharmacokinetics of liposomal daunorubicin differ significantly from conventional daunorubicin HCl. The differences in the volume of distribution and clearance result in a higher daunorubicin exposure (in terms of AUC) from liposomal daunorubicin than with conventional daunorubicin HCl. The apparent elimination half-life of liposomal daunorubicin is far shorter than that of daunorubicin HCl, and probably represents a distribution half-life. Preclinical biodistribution data in animals suggest that liposomal daunorubicin crosses the normal blood-brain barrier, however, it is unknown if this occurs in humans.

Metabolism – Daunorubicinol, the major active metabolite of daunorubicin, was detected at low levels in the plasma.

Contraindications

Hypersensitivity reaction to previous doses of liposomal daunorubicin or to any of its constituents.

Warnings/Precautions

➤*Myelosuppression:* The primary toxicity of liposomal daunorubicin is myelosuppression, especially of the granulocytic series, which may be severe and associated with fever and may result in infection. Effects on the platelets and erythroid series are much less marked. Careful hematologic monitoring is required. Because patients with HIV infection are immunocompromised, carefully observe patients for evidence of intercurrent or opportunistic infections.

➤*Potential cardiac toxicity:* Give special attention to the potential cardiac toxicity of liposomal daunorubicin. Although there is no reliable means of predicting CHF, cardiomyopathy induced by anthracyclines is usually associated with a decrease of the left ventricular ejection fraction (LVEF). Evaluate cardiac function in each patient by means of a history and physical examination before each course of liposomal daunorubicin, and perform determination of LVEF at total cumulative doses of liposomal daunorubicin 320 mg/m^2 and every 160 mg/m^2 thereafter.

Patients who have received prior therapy with anthracyclines (doxorubicin greater than 300 mg/m^2 or equivalent), have preexisting cardiac disease, or have received previous radiotherapy encompassing the heart may be less "cardiac" tolerant to treatment with liposomal daunorubicin. Therefore, monitor LVEF at cumulative liposomal daunorubicin doses prior to therapy and every 160 mg/m^2 of liposomal daunorubicin.

In patients with Kaposi sarcoma, CHF has been reported in 1 patient at a cumulative dose of 340 mg/m^2 of liposomal daunorubicin. In 8 Kaposi sarcoma patients, LVEF decreases were reported at cumulative doses ranging from 200 to 2100 mg/m^2 (median dose 320 mg/m^2) of liposomal daunorubicin. In clinical studies in malignancies other than Kaposi sarcoma treated with doses of liposomal daunorubicin greater than the recommended dose of 40 mg/m^2, CHF has been reported at a cumulative dose as low as 200 mg/m^2 of liposomal daunorubicin; 7 patients have been reported with LVEF decreases. The proportion of patients at risk for cardiotoxicity is unknown

DAUNORUBICIN CITRATE LIPOSOMAL — INJECTION

because the denominator is uncertain since there were several instances of missing repeat cardiac evaluations.

➤*Back pain, flushing, and chest tightness:* See the Warning box for more information.

➤*Extravasation:* See Administration and Dosage for more information.

See Administration and Dosage for more information.

➤*Hepatic function impairment:* See Administration and Dosage for more information.

➤*Pregnancy: Category D.* Liposomal daunorubicin can cause fetal harm when administered to a pregnant woman. If liposomal daunorubicin is used during pregnancy or if the patient becomes pregnant while taking liposomal daunorubicin, warn the patient of the potential hazard to the fetus.

➤*Children:* Safety and efficacy in children have not been established.

Adverse Reactions

Daunorubicin (liposomal) is considered to have moderate potential for nausea and vomiting.

Adverse Reactions of Liposomal Daunorubicin Compared with ABV (%)

Adverse reaction	Liposomal daunorubicin (n = 116)		ABV (n = 111)	
	Mild/ Moderate	Severe	Mild/ Moderate	Severe
CNS				
Depression	7	3	6	-
Dizziness	8	-	9	-
Fatigue	43	6	44	7
Headache	22	3	23	2
Insomnia	6	-	14	-
Malaise	9	1	11	1
Neuropathy	12	1	38	3
Dermatologic				
Alopecia	8	-	36	-
Pruritus	7	-	14	-
GI				
Abdominal pain	20	3	23	4
Anorexia	21	2	26	2
Constipation	7	-	18	-
Diarrhea	34	4	29	6
Nausea	51	3	45	5
Stomatitis	9	1	8	-
Vomiting	20	3	26	2
Musculoskeletal				
Arthralgia	7	-	6	-
Back pain	16	-	8	-
Myalgia	7	-	12	-
Rigors	19	-	23	-
Respiratory				
Cough	26	2	19	-
Dyspnea	23	3	17	3
Rhinitis	12	-	6	-
Sinusitis	8	-	5	1
Miscellaneous				
Abnormal vision	3	2	3	-
Allergic reaction	21	3	19	2
Chest pain	9	1	7	-
Edema	9	2	8	1
Fever	42	5	49	5
Influenza-like symptoms	5	-	5	-
Sweating increased	12	2	12	-
Tenesmus	4	1	1	-

Summary of Important Safety Data (Liposomal Daunorubicin vs ABV)

Adverse reaction	Daunorubicin citrate liposomal (n = 116)	ABV (n = 111)
Neutropenia (less than 1000 cells/mm³) Neutropenia (less than 500 cells/mm³)	36% 15%	35% 5%
Opportunistic infections/illnesses	40%	27%
Median time to first opportunistic infections/illnesses	214 days	412 days[b]
Number of cases with absolute reduction in ejection fraction of 20% to 25%	3	1
Number of cases removed from therapy because of cardiac causes[a]	2	0
Alopecia (all grades)	8%	36%[c]
Neuropathy (all grades)	13%	41%[c]

[a] The denominator is uncertain because there were several instances of missing repeat cardiac evaluations.
[b] $P = 0.21$.
[c] $P < 0.001$.

➤*Cardiovascular:* Angina pectoris; atrial fibrillation; cardiac arrest; hot flushes; hypertension; myocardial infarction; palpitation; pericardial effusion; pericardial tamponade; pulmonary hypertension; sinus tachycardia; supraventricular tachycardia; syncope; tachycardia; ventricular extrasystoles (5% or less).

➤*CNS:* Abnormal gait; abnormal thinking; amnesia; anxiety; ataxia; confusion; convulsions; emotional lability; hallucinations; hyperkinesia; hypertonia; meningitis; somnolence; tremors (5% or less).

➤*Dermatologic:* Dry skin; folliculitis; seborrhea (5% or less).

➤*GI:* Dry mouth; dysphagia; gastritis; GI hemorrhage; gingival bleeding; hemorrhoids; hepatomegaly; melena; tooth caries (5% or less).

➤*GU:* Dysuria; nocturia; polyuria (5% or less).

➤*Respiratory:* Hemoptysis; hiccups; increased sputum; pulmonary infiltration (5% or less).

➤*Special senses:* Conjunctivitis; deafness; earache; eye pain; taste perversion; tinnitus (5% or less).

➤*Miscellaneous:* Dehydration; increased appetite; injection-site inflammation; lymphadenopathy; splenomegaly; thirst (5% or less).

Overdosage

Symptoms of acute overdosage are increased severities of the observed dose-limiting toxicities of therapeutic doses, myelosuppression (especially granulocytopenia), fatigue, nausea, and vomiting.

Patient Information

Advise patients that this medicine will be prepared and administered by a health care provider in a medical setting.

Advise patients that lab tests will be required to monitor therapy. Instruct patients to be sure to keep appointments.

Advise patients not to take any otc or prescription medications or dietary supplements without talking with their health care provider.

Advise patients to avoid becoming pregnant during therapy.

DOXORUBICIN HYDROCHLORIDE CONVENTIONAL

Rx	**Doxorubicin Hydrochloride** (Bedford Labs)	**Injection, lyophilized powder for solution:** 10 mg	50 mg lactose. In single-dose flip-top vials.
Rx	**Adriamycin RDF** (Pharmacia & Upjohn)		In single-dose vials.[b] *Rapid dissolution formula.*
Rx	**Doxorubicin Hydrochloride** (Bedford Labs)	**Powder for Injection (lyophilized):** 20 mg	100 mg lactose. In single-dose flip-top vials.
Rx	**Adriamycin RDF** (Pharmacia & Upjohn)		In single-dose vials.[b] *Rapid dissolution formula.*
Rx	**Doxorubicin Hydrochloride** (Bedford Labs)	**Injection, lyophilized powder for solution:** 50 mg	250 mg lactose. In single-dose flip-top vials.
Rx	**Adriamycin RDF** (Pharmacia & Upjohn)		In single-dose vials.[b] *Rapid dissolution formula.*
Rx	**Adriamycin RDF** (Pharmacia & Upjohn)	**Injection, lyophilized powder for solution:** 150 mg[a]	In single-dose vials.[b] *Rapid dissolution formula.*
Rx	**Doxorubicin Hydrochloride** (Bedford Labs)	**Injection:** 2 mg/mL	0.9% NaCl, hydrochloric acid. In 5, 10, 25, and 100 mL vials.
Rx	**Adriamycin PFS** (Pharmacia & Upjohn)	**Injection:** 2 mg/mL	Preservative-free. In 5, 10, 25, and 37.5 mL single-dose vials and 100 ml multidose vials.

[a] Multiple-dose vial.
[b] With methylparaben and 50, 100, 250, and 750 mg lactose, respectively.

DOXORUBICIN HYDROCHLORIDE CONVENTIONAL — INJECTION

Note: The following monograph pertains to the conventional form of doxorubicin only. For complete prescribing information for the liposomal form of doxorubicin, refer to the Doxorubicin, Liposomal monograph.

WARNING

Severe local tissue necrosis will occur if there is extravasation during administration. On IV administration of doxorubicin, extravasation may occur, with or without an accompanying burning or stinging sensation, even if blood returns well on aspiration of the infusion needle. If any signs or symptoms of extravasation have occurred, the injection or infusion should be immediately terminated and restarted in another vein. If extravasation is suspected, intermittent application of ice to the site for 15 minutes 4 times daily for 3 days may be useful. The benefit of local administration of drugs has not been clearly established. Because of the progressive nature of extravasation reactions, close observation and plastic surgery consultation is recommended. Blistering, ulceration or persistent pain are indications for wide excision surgery, followed by split-thickness skin grafting.

Doxorubicin must not be given by the IM or SC route.

Myocardial toxicity manifested in its most severe form by potentially fatal congestive heart failure may occur either during therapy or months to years after termination of therapy. The probability of developing impaired myocardial function based on a combined index of signs, symptoms, and decline in left ventricular ejection fraction (LVEF) is estimated to be 1% to 2% at a total cumulative dose of 300 mg/m^2 of doxorubicin, 3% to 5% at a dose of 400 mg/m^2, 5% to 8% at 450 mg/m^2, and 6% to 20% at 500 mg/m^2. The risk of developing CHF increases rapidly with increasing total cumulative doses of doxorubicin in excess of 450 mg/m^2. This toxicity may occur at lower cumulative doses in patients with prior mediastinal irradiation or on concurrent cyclophosphamide therapy or with preexisting heart disease. Pediatric patients are at increased risk for developing delayed cardiotoxicity.

Dosage should be reduced in patients with impaired hepatic function.

Severe myelosuppression may occur.

Doxorubicin should be administered only under the supervision of a physician who is experienced in the use of cancer chemotherapeutic agents.

Indications

➤*Disseminated neoplastic conditions:* Doxorubicin HCl has been used successfully to produce regression in disseminated neoplastic conditions such as acute lymphoblastic leukemia, acute myeloblastic leukemia, Wilms' tumor, neuroblastoma, soft tissue and bone sarcomas, breast carcinoma, ovarian carcinoma, transitional cell bladder carcinoma, thyroid carcinoma, gastric carcinoma, Hodgkin disease, malignant lymphoma and bronchogenic carcinoma in which the small cell histologic type is the most responsive compared to other cell types.

➤*Off-label uses:* Treatment of refractory multiple myeloma; endometrial, islet cell, and lung cancers; AIDS-related Kaposi sarcoma.

Administration and Dosage

➤*General dosing considerations:* The lower dosage should be given to patients with inadequate marrow reserves due to old age, or prior therapy, or neoplastic marrow infiltration.

Risk of cardiotoxicity increases with the cumulative doxorubicin dose. (See also Black Box Warning and Warnings/Precautions.)

Caregivers of children receiving doxorubicin should be counseled to take precautions (such as wearing latex gloves) to prevent contact with the patient's urine and other body fluids for at least 5 days after each treatment.

➤*Adults:*

Disseminated neoplastic conditions –

Single-agent therapy: 60 to 75 mg/m^2 as a single IV injection administered at 21-day intervals. (See also Off-Label Dosing).

Combination therapy: 40 to 60 mg/m^2 given as a single IV injection every 21 to 28 days. Given with other chemotherapeutic agents.

Off-label dosing –

Disseminated neoplastic conditions: 30 mg/m^2/day IV for 3 successive days every 4 weeks or 20 mg/m^2 IV once weekly.

Intravesical: Instill 50 mg in the bladder every 3 to 4 weeks, retaining the solution in the bladder for 30 to 120 minutes.

➤*Children:*

Disseminated neoplastic conditions –

Single-agent therapy: 60 to 75 mg/m^2 as a single IV injection administered at 21-day intervals. (See also Off-Label Dosing).

Combination therapy: 40 to 60 mg/m^2 given as a single IV injection every 21 to 28 days. Given with other chemotherapeutic agents.

Evidence is available that in some types of neoplastic disease combination chemotherapy is superior to single agents. The benefits and risks of such therapy continue to be elucidated.

Off-label dosing –

Disseminated neoplastic conditions: 35 to 75 mg/m^2 IV, as a single dose every 21 days. Alternative doses are 20 to 30 mg/m^2 IV once weekly for 3 weeks, 20 mg/m^2/day IV for 3 successive days every 3 to 4 weeks, or 15 to 20 mg/m^2/day as a continuous infusion for 4 days every 3 to 4 weeks.

➤*Renal function impairment:* For creatinine clearance of less than 10 mL/min, consider reducing the dosage to 75% of the usual dosage.

➤*Hepatic function impairment:* Doxorubicin dosage must be reduced in case of hyperbilirubinemia as follows:

Doxorubicin Dosage Adjustment According to Bilirubin Concentration

Plasma bilirubin concentration	Dosage reduction
1.2 to 3 mg/dL	50%
3.1 to 5 mg/dL	75%

Some clinicians do not recommend administering doxorubicin to patients with a bilirubin greater than 5 mg/dL.

➤*Preparation for administration:* Doxorubicin is considered a cytotoxic agent. Follow safe handling procedures when preparing, administering, or dispensing doxorubicin.

Skin reactions associated with doxorubicin have been reported. Skin accidentally exposed to doxorubicin should be rinsed copiously with soap and warm water, and if the eyes are involved, standard irrigation techniques should be used immediately. The use of goggles, gloves, and protective gowns is recommended during preparation and administration of the drug.

Powder for solution – Doxorubicin powder 10 mg, 20 mg, 50 mg, and 150 mg vials should be reconstituted with 5 mL, 10 mL, 25 mL, and 75 mL, respectively, of sodium chloride 0.9% injection to give a final concentration of 2 mg/mL of doxorubicin. An appropriate volume of air should be withdrawn from the vial during reconstitution to avoid excessive pressure buildup. Bacteriostatic diluents are not recommended. After adding the diluent, the vial should be shaken and the contents allowed to dissolve. Solution will be red. Further dilution is not recommended for IV administration.

For intravesical instillation in the bladder, doxorubicin may be diluted in 50 to 150 mL of sterile water or sodium chloride 0.9%.,

➤*Administration:* May be given as an IV injection or IV continuous infusion. Doxorubicin must not be given by the IM or subcutaneous route.

Continuous infusion of doxorubicin should only be given through a central venous catheter resting in the vena cava.

It is recommended that doxorubicin be slowly administered into the tubing of a freely running IV infusion of sodium chloride injection, or dextrose 5% injection. The tubing should be attached to a *Butterfly* needle and inserted, preferably into a large vein. If possible, avoid veins over joints or in extremities with compromised venous or lymphatic drainage.

The rate of administration is dependent on the size of the vein and the dosage. However, the dose should be administered in not less than 3 to 5 minutes. Local erythematous streaking along the vein as well as facial flushing may be indicative of too rapid an administration. A burning or stinging sensation may be indicative of perivenous infiltration, and the infusion should be immediately terminated and restarted in another vein. Perivenous infiltration may occur painlessly.

➤*Extravasation:* Severe local tissue necrosis will occur if there is extravasation during administration. Care in the administration of doxorubicin hydrochloride will reduce the chance of perivenous infiltration. It may also decrease the chance of local reactions such as urticaria and erythematous streaking. On IV administration of doxorubicin, extravasation may occur with or without an accompanying burning or stinging sensation, even if blood returns well on aspiration of the infusion needle.

If signs or symptoms of extravasation occur, stop the infusion immediately. If possible, withdraw 3 to 5 mL of blood to remove some of the drug. Remove the infusion needle.

There are currently 2 treatments for extravasation resulting from anthracycline IV therapy: topical dimethyl sulfoxide and dexrazoxane IV. Both treatments are effective for treating anthracycline extravasation injury, although no comparative trials have been conducted.

- Apply dimethyl sulfoxide (DMSO) 99% by saturating a gauze pad and painting on an area twice the size of the extravasation. Allow the site to air dry and repeat the application every 6 hours for 14 days. Do not cover the area with dressing.
- Dexrazoxane (*Totect*) is FDA-approved for the treatment of extravasation resulting from anthracycline IV therapy. The first infusion of dexrazoxane should be administered as soon as possible and within the first 6 hours following the extravasation. Topical cooling, such as ice packs, should be removed for at least 15 minutes prior to and during dexrazoxane administration. Concurrent extravasation treatment, such as topical dimethyl sulfoxide application should not be used in conjunction with dexrazoxane, and if administered, may worsen extravasation-induced tissue injury. The recommended dose of dexrazoxane for day 1 is 1,000 mg/m^2 (up to 2,000 mg), the dose for day 2 is 1,000 mg/m^2 (up to 2,000 mg), and the dose for day 3 is 500 mg/m^2 (up to 1,000 mg). Dexrazoxane is administered as an IV infusion over 1 to 2 hours.

Application of ice compresses to the area for 15 minutes every 6 hours for 48 hours may be useful. Delineate the infiltrated area on the patient's skin with a felt-tip marker. Elevate for 48 hours above heart level using a sling or stockinette dressing with an observation window cut in the dressing. Avoid pressure or friction. Do not rub the area. Observe for signs of increased erythema, pain, or skin necrosis. If increased symptoms occur, consult a plastic surgeon. Ensure that no medication is given distally to extravasation site. After 48 hours, encourage the patient to use the extremity normally to promote full range of motion.

➤*Admixture compatibility:* Doxorubicin should not be mixed with heparin or fluorouracil, since it has been reported that these drugs are incompat-

DOXORUBICIN HYDROCHLORIDE CONVENTIONAL — INJECTION

ible to the extent that a precipitate may form. Until specific compatibility data are available, it is not recommended that doxorubicin be mixed with other drugs.

➤*Storage/Stability:*

Powder for solution – Store powder at 15° to 30°C (59° to 86°F). Protect from light. Retain in carton until time of use. Discard unused portion from single-dose vials. Reconstituted doxorubicin does not contain a preservative and should be used within 24 hours. However, doxorubicin is chemically stable for a longer period of time.

Solution – Store refrigerated at 2° to 8°C (36° to 46°F). Protect from light. Retain in carton until time of use. Discard unused portion.

Discard single-dose vials within 6 hours of the initial needle puncture if opened within an ISO Class 5 biological safety cabinet, or within 1 hour of the initial needle puncture if opened outside of such an environment, based on the USP Chapter <797> standards.

Actions

➤*Pharmacology:* The cytotoxic effect of doxorubicin on malignant cells and its toxic effects on various organs are thought to be related to nucleotide base intercalation and cell membrane lipid-binding activities of doxorubicin. Intercalation inhibits nucleotide replication and action of DNA and RNA polymerases. The interaction of doxorubicin with topoisomerase II to form DNA-cleavable complexes appears to be an important mechanism of doxorubicin cytocidal activity. Doxorubicin cellular membrane-binding may effect a variety of cellular functions. Enzymatic electron reduction of doxorubicin by a variety of oxidases, reductases and dehydrogenases generate highly reactive species including the hydroxyl-free radical OH•. Free radical formation has been implicated in doxorubicin cardiotoxicity by means of Cu (II) and Fe (III) reduction at the cellular level. Cells treated with doxorubicin have been shown to manifest the characteristic morphologic changes associated with apoptosis or programmed cell death. Doxorubicin-induced apoptosis may be an integral component of the cellular mechanism of action relating to therapeutic effects, toxicities, or both.

Animal studies have shown activity in a spectrum of experimental tumors, immunosuppression, carcinogenic properties in rodents, induction of a variety of toxic effects, including delayed and progressive cardiac toxicity, myelosuppression in all species and atrophy to testes in rats and dogs.

➤*Pharmacokinetics:*

Absorption/Distribution – Pharmacokinetic studies, determined in patients with various types of tumors undergoing either single or multiagent therapy have shown that doxorubicin follows a multiphasic disposition after IV injection.

The initial distributive half-life of approximately 5 minutes suggests rapid tissue uptake of doxorubicin, while its slow elimination from tissues is reflected by a terminal half-life of 20 to 48 hours. Steady-state distribution volumes exceed 20 to 30 L/kg and are indicative of extensive drug uptake into tissues.

Metabolism/Excretion – Plasma clearance is in the range of 8 to 20 mL/min/kg and is predominately by metabolism and biliary excretion. Approximately 40% of the dose appears in the bile in 5 days, while only 5% to 12% of the drug and its metabolites appear in the urine during the same time period. Binding of doxorubicin and its major metabolite, doxorubicinol to plasma proteins is about 74% to 76% and is independent of plasma concentration of doxorubicin up to 2 mcM. Enzymatic reduction at the 7 position and cleavage of the daunosamine sugar yields aglycones which are accompanied by free radical formation, the local production of which may contribute to the cardiotoxic activity of doxorubicin. Disposition of doxorubicinol (DOX-OL) in patients is formation rate limited. The terminal half-life of DOX-OL is similar to doxorubicin. The relative exposure of DOX-OL, compared to doxorubicin ranges between 0.4 to 0.6. In urine, less than 3% of the dose was recovered as DOX-OL over 7 days.

Contraindications

Doxorubicin therapy should not be started in patients who have marked myelosuppression induced by previous treatment with other antitumor agents or by radiotherapy. Doxorubicin treatment is contraindicated in patients who received previous treatment with complete cumulative doses of doxorubicin, daunorubicin, idarubicin, or other anthracyclines and anthracenes.

This medication is contraindicated in patients with a history of hypersensitivity reactions to conventional or liposomal doxorubicin or their components.

Warnings/Precautions

➤*Cardiac toxicity:* Special attention must be given to the cardiotoxicity induced by doxorubicin. Irreversible myocardial toxicity, manifested in its most severe form by life-threatening or fatal congestive heart failure, may occur either during therapy or months to years after termination of therapy. The probability of developing impaired myocardial function, based on a combined index of signs, symptoms and decline in left ventricular ejection fraction (LVEF) is estimated to be 1% to 2% at a total cumulative dose of 300 mg/m^2 of doxorubicin, 3% to 5% at a dose of 400 mg/m^2, 5% to 8% at a dose of 450 mg/m^2 and 6% to 20% at a dose of 500 mg/m^2 given in a schedule of a bolus injection once every 3 weeks. In a retrospective review by Von Hoff et al, the probability of developing congestive heart failure (CHF) was reported to be 5/168 (3%) at a cumulative dose of 430 mg/m^2 of doxorubicin, 8/110 (7%) at 575 mg/m^2 and 3/14 (21%) at 728 mg/m^2. The cumulative incidence of CHF was 2.2%. In a prospective study of doxorubicin in combination with cyclophosphamide, fluorouracil or vincristine in patients with breast cancer or small cell lung cancer, the cumulative incidence of CHF was 5% to 6%. The probability of CHF at various cumulative doses of doxorubicin was 1.5% at 300 mg/m^2, 4.9% at 400 mg/m^2, 7.7% at 450 mg/m^2 and 20.5% at 500 mg/m^2.

Cardiotoxicity may occur at lower doses in patients with prior mediastinal irradiation, concurrent cyclophosphamide therapy exposure at an early age and advanced age. Data also suggest that preexisting heart disease is a cofactor for increased risk of doxorubicin cardiotoxicity. In such cases, cardiac toxicity may occur at doses lower than the respective recommended cumulative dose of doxorubicin. Studies have suggested that concomitant administration of doxorubicin and calcium channel entry blockers may increase the risk of doxorubicin cardiotoxicity. The total dose of doxorubicin administered to the individual patient should also take into account previous or concomitant therapy with related compounds such as daunorubicin, idarubicin and mitoxantrone. Cardiomyopathy or congestive heart failure may be encountered several months or years after discontinuation of doxorubicin therapy.

Treatment of doxorubicin-induced CHF includes the use of digitalis, diuretics, after load reducers such as angiotensin I-converting enzyme (ACE) inhibitors, low salt diet, and bed rest. Such intervention may relieve symptoms and improve the functional status of the patient.

➤*Monitoring of cardiac function:* See Warnings/Precautions for more information.

➤*Hematologic monitoring:* See Warnings/Precautions for more information.

➤*Concurrent chemotherapy:* See Drug Interactions for more information.

➤*Necrotizing colitis:* Necrotizing colitis manifested by typhlitis (cecal inflammation), bloody stools and severe and sometimes fatal infections have been associated with a combination of doxorubicin given by IV push daily for 3 days and cytarabine given by continuous infusion daily for 7 or more days.

➤*Extravasation:* See Administration and Dosage for more information.

➤*Hepatic function impairment:* Since metabolism and excretion of doxorubicin occurs predominantly by the hepatobiliary route, toxicity to recommended doses of doxorubicin can be enhanced by hepatic impairment; therefore, prior to the individual dosing, evaluation of hepatic function is recommended using conventional laboratory tests such as AST, ALT, alkaline phosphatase and bilirubin.

➤*Pregnancy: Category D.* Safe use of doxorubicin in pregnancy has not been established. Doxorubicin is embryotoxic and teratogenic in rats and embryotoxic and abortifacient in rabbits. There are no adequate and well-controlled studies in pregnant women. If doxorubicin is to be used during pregnancy, or if the patient becomes pregnant during therapy, the patient should be apprised of the potential hazard to the fetus. Women of childbearing age should be advised to avoid becoming pregnant.

➤*Lactation:* Because of the potential for serious adverse reactions in nursing infants from doxorubicin, mothers should be advised to discontinue nursing during doxorubicin therapy.

➤*Children:* Pediatric patients are at increased risk for developing delayed cardiotoxicity. Follow-up cardiac evaluations are recommended periodically to monitor for this delayed cardiotoxicity. Doxorubicin, as a component of intensive chemotherapy regimens administered to pediatric patients, may contribute to prepubertal growth failure. It may also contribute to gonadal impairment, which is usually temporary.

The risk of congestive heart failure and other acute manifestations of doxorubicin cardiotoxicity in pediatric patients may be as much or lower than in adults. Pediatric patients appear to be at particular risk for developing delayed cardiac toxicity in that doxorubicin induced cardiomyopathy impairs myocardial growth as pediatric patients mature, subsequently leading to possible development of congestive heart failure during early adulthood. As many as 40% of pediatric patients may have subclinical cardiac dysfunction and 5% to 10% of pediatric patients may develop congestive heart failure on long-term follow-up. This late cardiac toxicity may be related to the dose of doxorubicin. The longer the length of follow-up the greater the increase in the detection rate.

➤*Monitoring:* Initial treatment with doxorubicin requires observation of the patient and periodic monitoring of complete blood counts, hepatic function tests, and radionuclide left ventricular ejection fraction. Like other cytotoxic drugs, doxorubicin may induce "tumor lysis syndrome" and hyperuricemia in patients with rapidly growing tumors. Appropriate supportive and pharmacologic measures may prevent or alleviate this complication.

Monitoring of cardiac function – In adult patients severe cardiac toxicity may occur precipitously without antecedent ECG changes. Cardiomyopathy induced by anthracyclines is usually associated with very characteristic histopathologic changes on an endomyocardial biopsy (EM biopsy), and a decrease of LVEF, as measured by multigated radionuclide angiography (MUGA scans) or echocardiogram (ECHO), from pretreatment baseline values. However, it has not been demonstrated that monitoring of the ejection fraction will predict when individual patients are approaching their maximally tolerated cumulative dose of doxorubicin. Cardiac function should be carefully monitored during treatment to minimize the risk of cardiac toxicity. A baseline cardiac evaluation with an ECG, LVEF, or an echocardiogram (ECHO) is recommended especially in patients with risk factors for increased cardiac toxicity (preexisting heart disease, mediastinal irradiation, or concurrent cyclophosphamide therapy). Subsequent evaluations should be obtained at a cumulative dose of doxorubicin of at least 400 mg/m^2 and periodically thereafter during the course of therapy. Pediatric patients

DOXORUBICIN HYDROCHLORIDE CONVENTIONAL — INJECTION

are at increased risk for developing delayed cardiotoxicity following doxorubicin administration and therefore a follow-up cardiac evaluation is recommended periodically to monitor for this delayed cardiotoxicity.

In adults, a 10% decline in LVEF to below the lower limit of normal or an absolute LVEF of 45%, or a 20% decline in LVEF at any level is indicative of deterioration in cardiac function. In pediatric patients, deterioration in cardiac function during or after the completion of therapy with doxorubicin is indicated by a drop in fractional shortening (FS) by an absolute value of greater than or equal to 10 percentile units or below 29%, and a decline in LVEF of 10 percentile units or an LVEF below 55%. In general, if test results indicate deterioration in cardiac function associated with doxorubicin, the benefit of continued therapy should be carefully evaluated against the risk of producing irreversible cardiac damage.

Acute life-threatening arrhythmias have been reported to occur during or within a few hours after doxorubicin administration.

Hematologic monitoring – There is a high incidence of bone-marrow depression, primarily of leukocytes, requiring careful hematologic monitoring. With the recommended dose schedule, leukopenia is usually transient, reaching its nadir 10 to 14 days after treatment with recovery usually occurring by the 21st day. White blood counts as low as 1000/mm^3 are to be expected during treatment with appropriate doses of doxorubicin. Red blood cell and platelet levels should also be monitored since they may also be depressed. Hematologic toxicity may require dose reduction or suspension or delay of doxorubicin therapy. Persistent severe myelosuppression may result in superinfection or hemorrhage.

Drug Interactions

➤*QT prolongation:* An additive effect of doxorubicin with other drugs that prolong the QT interval cannot be excluded. The following drugs may prolong the QT interval and increase the risk of life-threatening cardiac arrhythmias, including torsades de pointes: Antiarrhythmic agents (eg, amiodarone, bretylium, disopyramide, dofetilide, procainamide, quinidine, and sotalol), arsenic trioxide, chlorpromazine, cisapride, dolasetron, droperidol, mefloquine, mesoridazine, moxifloxacin, pentamidine, pimozide, tacrolimus, thioridazine, and ziprasidone. For a more complete list of drugs that may prolong the QT interval, see the appendix, Drug-Induced Prolongation of the QT Interval and Torsades de Pointes.

➤*Concurrent chemotherapy:* Doxorubicin may potentiate the toxicity of other anticancer therapies. Exacerbation of cyclophosphamide-induced hemorrhagic cystitis and enhancement of the hepatotoxicity of 6-mercaptopurine have been reported. Radiation-induced toxicity to the myocardium, mucosae, skin and liver have been reported to be increased by the administration of doxorubicin. Pediatric patients receiving concomitant doxorubicin and actinomycin-D have manifested acute "recall" pneumonitis at variable times after local radiation therapy.

Literature reports have also described the following drug interactions: Phenobarbital increases the elimination of doxorubicin, phenytoin levels may be decreased by doxorubicin, streptozocin may inhibit hepatic metabolism of doxorubicin, and administration of live vaccines to immunosuppressed patients including those undergoing cytotoxic chemotherapy may be hazardous.

Doxorubicin Drug Interactions

Precipitant drug	Object drug[a]		Description
Cyclosporine	Doxorubicin	⬆	The addition of cyclosporine to doxorubicin may result in increases in AUC for doxorubicin and doxorubicinol possibly because of a decrease in clearance of parent drug and a decrease in metabolism of doxorubicinol. Literature reports suggest that adding cyclosporine to doxorubicin results in more profound and prolonged hematologic toxicity than doxorubicin alone. Coma or seizures have also been described.
Paclitaxel	Doxorubicin	⬆	Two published studies report that initial administration of paclitaxel infused over 24 hours followed by doxorubicin administered over 48 hours resulted in a significant decrease in doxorubicin clearance with more profound neutropenic and stomatitis episodes than the reverse sequence of administration.
Phenobarbital	Doxorubicin	⬇	Phenobarbital increases doxorubicin elimination.
Progesterone	Doxorubicin	⬆	In a published study, progesterone was given IV to patients with advanced malignancies (ECOG PS < 2) at high doses (up to 10 g over 24 hours) concomitantly with a fixed doxorubicin dose (60 mg/m^2) via bolus. Enhanced doxorubicin-induced neutropenia and thrombocytopenia were observed.
Streptozocin	Doxorubicin	⬆	Streptozocin may inhibit hepatic metabolism of doxorubicin.
Verapamil	Doxorubicin	⬆	A study of the effects of verapamil on the acute toxicity of doxorubicin in mice revealed higher initial peak concentrations of doxorubicin in the heart with a higher incidence and severity of degenerative changes in cardiac tissue resulting in shorter survival.
Doxorubicin	Actinomycin-D	⬆	Pediatric patients receiving concomitant doxorubicin and actinomycin-D have manifested acute "recall" pneumonitis at variable times after local radiation therapy.
Doxorubicin	Cyclophosphamide Mercaptopurine	⬆	Exacerbation of cyclophosphamide-induced hemorrhagic cystitis and enhancement of 6-mercaptopurine have occurred.
Doxorubicin	Digoxin	⬇	Serum levels may be decreased by combination chemotherapy (including doxorubicin). Digitoxin and digoxin capsules do not appear to be affected.
Doxorubicin	Phenytoin	⬇	Phenytoin levels may be decreased by doxorubicin.
Doxorubicin	Radiation	⬆	Radiation-induced toxicity to the myocardium, mucosa, skin, and liver have been increased by doxorubicin administration.

[a] ⬆ = Object drug increased. ⬇ = Object drug decreased.

Adverse Reactions

Doxorubicin in doses greater than 60 mg/m^2 is considered to have moderate to high emetogenic potential. Doxorubicin in doses of 20 to 60 mg/m^2 is considered to have moderate emetogenic potential.

➤*CNS:*

Neurological – Peripheral neurotoxicity in the form of local-regional sensory or motor disturbances have been reported in patients treated intra-arterially with doxorubicin, mostly in combination with cisplatin. Animal studies have demonstrated seizures and coma in rodents and dogs treated with intracarotid doxorubicin. Seizures and coma have been reported in patients treated with doxorubicin in combination with cisplatin or vincristine.

➤*Dermatologic:* Reversible complete alopecia occurs in most cases. Hyperpigmentation of nail beds and dermal crease, primarily in pediatric patients, and onycholysis have been reported in a few cases. Recall of skin reaction due to prior radiotherapy has occurred with doxorubicin administration.

➤*GI:* Acute nausea and vomiting occurs frequently and may be severe. This may be alleviated by antiemetic therapy. Mucositis (stomatitis and esophagitis) may occur 5 to 10 days after administration. The effect may be severe leading to ulceration and represents a site of origin for severe infections. The dosage regimen consisting of administration of doxorubicin on 3 successive days results in greater incidence and severity of mucositis. Ulceration and necrosis of the colon, especially the cecum, may occur leading to bleeding or severe infections which can be fatal. This reaction has been reported in patients with acute nonlymphocytic leukemia treated with a 3-day course of doxorubicin combined with cytarabine. Anorexia and diarrhea have been occasionally reported.

➤*Hematologic:* The occurrence of secondary acute myeloid leukemia with or without a preleukemic phase has been reported rarely in patients concurrently treated with doxorubicin in association with DNA-damaging antineoplastic agents. Such cases could have a short (1 to 3 years) latency period. Pediatric patients are also at risk of developing secondary acute myeloid leukemia.

➤*Hypersensitivity:* Fever, chills and urticaria have been reported occasionally. Anaphylaxis may occur. A case of apparent cross-sensitivity to lincomycin has been reported.

DOXORUBICIN HYDROCHLORIDE CONVENTIONAL — INJECTION

➤*Local:* Severe cellulitis, vesication and tissue necrosis will occur if extravasation of doxorubicin occurs during administration. Erythematous streaking along the vein proximal to the site of injection had been reported. A burning or stinging sensation may be indicative of perivenous infiltration, and the infusion should be immediately terminated and restarted in another vein. Perivenous infiltration may occur painlessly.

Phlebosclerosis has been reported especially when small veins are used or a single vein is used for repeated administration. Facial flushing may occur if the injection is given too rapidly.

➤*Miscellaneous:* Conjunctivitis and lacrimation occur rarely.

Overdosage

Acute overdosage with doxorubicin enhances the toxic effect of mucositis, leukopenia and thrombocytopenia. Treatment of acute overdosage consists of treatment of the severely myelosuppressed patient with hospitalization, antimicrobials, platelet transfusions and symptomatic treatment of mucositis. Use of hemopoietic growth factor (G-CSF, GM-CSF) may be considered.

The 150 mg doxorubicin HCl powder and the 75 mL and 100 mL (2 mg/mL) doxorubicin HCl solution vials are packaged as multiple-dose vials and caution should be exercised to prevent inadvertent overdosage.

Cumulative dosage with doxorubicin increases the risk of cardiomyopathy and resultant congestive heart failure. Treatment consists of vigorous management of congestive heart failure with digitalis preparations, diuretics, and afterload reducers such as ACE inhibitors.

Patient Information

Doxorubicin HCl imparts a red coloration to the urine for 1 to 2 days after administration, and patients should be advised to expect this during active therapy.

DOXORUBICIN HYDROCHLORIDE, LIPOSOMAL (Pegylated Liposomal Doxorubicin)

Rx	**Doxil** (Ortho Biotech)	**Injection, suspension, liposomal concentrate:** 2 mg/mL	Sucrose. Preservative free. In 10 and 30 mL single-use vials.

DOXORUBICIN HYDROCHLORIDE, LIPOSOMAL — INJECTION

Note: The following monograph pertains to the liposomal form of doxorubicin only. For conventional prescribing information, refer to the Doxorubicin, Conventional monograph.

WARNING

Cardiotoxicity – The use of liposomal doxorubicin may lead to cardiac toxicity. Myocardial damage may lead to congestive heart failure (CHF) and may occur as the total cumulative dose of doxorubicin (conventional or liposomal) approaches 550 mg/m². Cardiac toxicity also may occur at lower cumulative doses in patients with prior mediastinal irradiation or who are receiving concurrent cyclophosphamide therapy.

Infusion reactions – Acute infusion-related reactions, sometimes reversible upon terminating or slowing infusions, have occurred in up to 10% of patients. Serious and sometimes life-threatening or fatal allergic/anaphylactoid-like infusion reactions have been reported. Make medications to treat such reactions, as well as emergency equipment, available for immediate use. Administer liposomal doxorubicin at an initial rate of 1 mg/min to minimize the risk of infusion reactions.

Myelosuppression – Severe myelosuppression may occur.

Hepatic function impairment – Reduce dosage in patients with hepatic function impairment.

Accidental substitution – Accidental substitution of liposomal doxorubicin for conventional doxorubicin has resulted in severe adverse reactions. Do not substitute liposomal doxorubicin for conventional doxorubicin on a milligram per milligram basis.

Indications

➤*AIDS-related Kaposi sarcoma (KS):* For the treatment of AIDS-related KS in patients with disease that has progressed on prior combination chemotherapy or in patients who are intolerant to such therapy.

➤*Multiple myeloma:* In combination with bortezomib for the treatment of patients with multiple myeloma who have not previously received bortezomib and have received at least 1 prior therapy.

➤*Ovarian cancer:* For the treatment of patients with ovarian cancer whose disease has progressed or recurred after platinum-based chemotherapy.

➤*Off-label uses:* Refractory metastatic breast cancer.

Administration and Dosage

➤*General dosing considerations:* The dose of liposomal doxorubicin is different from the dose of conventional doxorubicin. Do not substitute liposomal doxorubicin for conventional doxorubicin on a mg per mg basis.

Risk of cardiotoxicity increases with the cumulative doxorubicin dose. (See also Warning Box and Warnings/Precautions.)

➤*Adults:*

AIDS-related Kaposi sarcoma –

Usual dosage: 20 mg/m² (doxorubicin hydrochloride equivalent) intravenously (IV) at an initial rate of 1 mg/min to minimize the risk of infusion-related reactions. If no infusion-related adverse reactions are observed, the infusion rate should be increased to complete the administration of the drug over 1 hour. Repeat once every 3 weeks.

Duration of therapy: For as long as the patient responds satisfactorily and tolerates treatment.

Multiple myeloma –

Usual dosage: 30 mg/m² IV on day 4 following bortezomib (which is administered at 1.3 mg/m² bolus on days 1, 4, 8, and 11) every 3 weeks. With the first liposomal doxorubicin dose, an initial rate of 1 mg/min should be used to minimize the risk of infusion-related reactions. If no infusion-related adverse reactions are observed, the infusion rate should be increased to complete the administration of the drug over 1 hour.

Dosage adjustment: For patients who experience hand-foot syndrome or stomatitis, the liposomal doxorubicin dose should be modified. (See Dosage Modification.) For additional bortezomib dosing and dosage adjustments, see the Bortezomib monograph.

Dosage Adjustments for Liposomal Doxorubicin and Bortezomib Combination Therapy

Patient status	Liposomal doxorubicin	Bortezomib
Fever ≥ 38°C (100.4°F) and ANC [3]	Do not dose this cycle if before day 4; if after day 4, reduce next dose by 25%.	Reduce the next dose by 25%.
On any day of drug administration after day 1 of each cycle: platelet count < 25,000/mm³, hemoglobin < 8 g/dL, ANC < 500/mm³	Do not dose this cycle if before day 4; if after day 4, reduce next dose by 25% in the following cycles if bortezomib is reduced for hematologic toxicity.	Do not dose; if 2 or more doses are not given in a cycle, reduce dose by 25% in following cycles.
Grade 3 or 4 nonhematologic drug-related toxicity	Do not dose until recovered to grade < 2; reduce dose by 25% for all subsequent doses.	Do not dose until recovered to grade < 2; reduce dose by 25% for all subsequent doses.
Neuropathic pain or peripheral neuropathy	No dosage adjustments.	See Bortezomib monograph for dosage adjustments in patients with neuropathic pain.

Duration of therapy: Patient may be treated for up to 8 cycles, until disease progression or the occurrence of unacceptable toxicity.

Ovarian cancer –

Usual dosage: 50 mg/m² (doxorubicin hydrochloride equivalent) IV at an initial rate of 1 mg/min to minimize the risk of infusion reactions. If no infusion-related adverse reactions are observed, the rate of infusion can be increased to complete administration of the drug over 1 hour. Administer once every 4 weeks.

Dosage adjustment: To manage adverse reactions, such as hand-foot syndrome, hematologic toxicity, or stomatitis, the doses may be delayed or reduced. Pretreatment with or concomitant use of antiemetics should be considered. (See Dosage Modification.)

Duration of therapy: A minimum of 4 courses is recommended because the median time to response in clinical trials was 4 months. Administer for as long as the patient does not progress, shows no evidence of cardiotoxicity, and continues to tolerate treatment.

Off-label dosing –

Refractory metastatic breast cancer: 30 to 50 mg/m² IV over 1 hour every 2 to 4 weeks.

➤*Renal function impairment:*

Dialysis – Conventional hemodialysis is minimally effective (25% to 49%) in removing liposomal doxorubicin.

➤*Hepatic function impairment:*

Liposomal Doxorubicin Dosage Adjustment According to Bilirubin Concentration

Plasma bilirubin concentration (mg/dL)	Dosage reduction (%)
1.2 to 3	50
> 3	75

➤*Dosage modification:* Liposomal doxorubicin exhibits nonlinear pharmacokinetics at 50 mg/m²; therefore, dose adjustments may result in a nonproportional greater change in plasma concentration and exposure to the drug.

Patients should be carefully monitored for toxicity. Adverse reactions, such as hand-foot syndrome, hematologic toxicities, and stomatitis, may be managed by dose delays and adjustments. Following the first appearance of a grade 2 or higher adverse reaction, the dosing should be adjusted or delayed, as described in the following tables. Once the dose has been reduced, it should not be increased at a later time.

DOXORUBICIN HYDROCHLORIDE, LIPOSOMAL — INJECTION

➤*Hand-foot syndrome:*

Liposomal Doxorubicin Dose Modification for Hand-Foot Syndrome		
Toxicity grade	Symptoms	Dose adjustment
1	Mild erythema, swelling, or desquamation not interfering with daily activities	Redose unless patient has experienced previous grade 3 or 4 HFS. If so, delay up to 2 weeks and decrease dose by 25%. Return to original dosing interval.
2	Erythema, desquamation, or swelling interfering with, but not precluding, normal physical activities; small blisters or ulcerations less than 2 cm in diameter	Delay dosing up to 2 weeks or until resolved to grade 0 to 1. If after 2 weeks there is no resolution, liposomal doxorubicin should be discontinued. If resolved to grade 0 to 1 within 2 weeks, and if there was no prior grade 3 to 4 HFS, continue treatment at previous dose and return to original dosing interval. If patient experienced previous grade 3 or 4 toxicity, continue treatment with a 25% dose reduction and return to original dosing interval.
3	Blistering, ulceration, or swelling interfering with walking or normal daily activities; cannot wear regular clothing	Delay dosing up to 2 weeks or until resolved to grade 0 to 1. Decrease dose by 25% and return to original dosing interval. If after 2 weeks there is no resolution, liposomal doxorubicin should be discontinued.
4	Diffuse or local process causing infectious complications, or a bedridden state or hospitalization	Delay dosing up to 2 weeks or until resolved to grade 0 to 1. Decrease dose by 25% and return to original dosing interval. If after 2 weeks there is no resolution, liposomal doxorubicin should be discontinued.

➤*Hematologic toxicity:* The following dose modifications apply to liposomal doxorubicin monotherapy. See the Multiple Myeloma Dose Modification table for recommendations when liposomal doxorubicin is combined with bortezomib.

Liposomal Doxorubicin Dose Modification for Hematological Toxicity			
Grade	ANC[a]	Platelets	Modification
1	1,500 to 1,900	75,000 to 150,000	Resume treatment with no dose reduction.
2	1,000 to < 1,500	50,000 to < 75,000	Wait until ANC ≥ 1,500 and platelets ≥ 75,000; redose with no dose reduction.
3	500 to 999	25,000 to < 50,000	Wait until ANC ≥ 1,500 and platelets ≥ 75,000; redose with no dose reduction.
4	< 500	< 25,000	Wait until ANC ≥ 1,500 and platelets ≥ 75,000; redose at 25% dose reduction or continue full dose with cytokine support.

[a] ANC = absolute neutrophil count.

➤*Stomatitis:*

Liposomal Doxorubicin Dose Modification for Stomatitis		
Toxicity grade	Symptoms	Dose adjustment
1	Painless ulcers, erythema, or mild soreness	Redose unless patient has experienced previous grade 3 or 4 toxicity. If so, delay up to 2 weeks and decrease dose by 25%. Return to original dosing interval.
2	Painful erythema, edema, or ulcers, but can eat	Delay dosing up to 2 weeks or until resolved to grade 0 to 1. If after 2 weeks there is no resolution, liposomal doxorubicin should be discontinued. If resolved to grade 0 to 1 within 2 weeks and there was no prior grade 3 or 4 stomatitis, continue treatment at previous dose and return to original dosing interval. If patient experienced previous grade 3 or 4 toxicity, continue treatment with a 25% dose reduction and return to original dosing interval.
3	Painful erythema, edema, or ulcers, and cannot eat	Delay dosing up to 2 weeks or until resolved to grade 0 to 1. Decrease dose by 25% and return to original dosing interval. If after 2 weeks there is no resolution, liposomal doxorubicin should be discontinued.
4	Requires parenteral or enteral support	Delay dosing up to 2 weeks or until resolved to grade 0 to 1. Decrease dose by 25% and return to liposomal doxorubicin original dosing interval. If after 2 weeks there is no resolution, liposomal doxorubicin should be discontinued.

➤*Drug substitution:* Liposomal encapsulation can substantially affect a drug's functional properties relative to those of the unencapsulated drug. In addition, different liposomal drug products may vary in chemical composition and physical form of the liposomes. Such differences can substantially affect the functional properties of liposomal drug products. Do not substitute.

➤*Preparation for administration:* Doxorubicin is considered a cytotoxic agent. Follow safe handling procedures when preparing, administering, or dispensing liposomal doxorubicin.

The use of gloves is required. If liposomal doxorubicin comes into contact with skin or mucosa, immediately wash thoroughly with soap and water.

Liposomal doxorubicin doses of up to 90 mg must be diluted in 250 mL of dextrose 5% injection prior to administration. Doses exceeding 90 mg should be diluted in 500 mL of dextrose 5% injection prior to administration. Aseptic technique must be strictly observed because no preservative or bacteriostatic agent is present in liposomal doxorubicin.

➤*Administration:* Do not administer as a bolus injection or an undiluted solution. Rapid infusion may increase the risk of infusion-related reactions. (See Warnings/Precautions.) Administer at an initial rate of 1 mg/min to minimize the risk of infusion-related reactions. If no infusion-related adverse reactions are observed, the infusion rate should be increased to complete the administration of the drug over 1 hour.

Liposomal doxorubicin must not be given by the intramuscular (IM) or subcutaneous route.

Do not use an in-line filter or administer via small peripheral veins.

Rapid flushing of the infusion line should be avoided.

➤*Extravasation:* Liposomal doxorubicin is considered an irritant, and precautions should be taken to avoid extravasation. With IV administration of liposomal doxorubicin, extravasation may occur with or without an accompanying stinging or burning sensation, even if blood returns well on aspiration of the infusion needle.

If signs or symptoms of extravasation occur, stop the infusion immediately. If possible, withdraw 3 to 5 mL of blood to remove some of the drug. Remove the infusion needle. Delineate the infiltrated area on the patient's skin with a felt tip marker. Elevate for 48 hours above heart level using a sling or stockinette dressing with an observation window cut in the dressing. Avoid pressure or friction. Do not rub the area. Observe for signs of increased erythema, pain, or skin necrosis. If increased symptoms occur, consult a plastic surgeon. After 48 hours, encourage the patient to use the extremity normally to promote full range of motion.

➤*Admixture compatibility:* Do not mix with other drugs. Do not use with any diluent other than dextrose 5% injection. Do not use any bacteriostatic agent, such as benzyl alcohol.

➤*Storage/Stability:* Refrigerate unopened vials at 2° to 8°C (36° to 46°F). Diluted liposomal doxorubicin should be refrigerated at 2° to 8°C (36° to 46°F) and administered within 24 hours. Avoid freezing. Prolonged freezing may adversely affect liposomal drug products; however, short-term freezing (less than 1 month) does not appear to have a deleterious effect on liposomal doxorubicin.

Discard vial within 6 hours of the initial needle puncture if opened within an ISO Class 5 biological safety cabinet, or within 1 hour of the initial needle puncture if opened outside of such an environment, based on the USP Chapter <797> standards.

Actions

➤*Pharmacology:* The active ingredient of liposomal doxorubicin is doxorubicin hydrochloride. The mechanism of action of doxorubicin hydrochloride is thought to be related to its ability to bind DNA and inhibit nucleic acid synthesis. Cell structure studies have demonstrated rapid cell penetration and perinuclear chromatin binding, rapid inhibition of mitotic activity and nucleic acid synthesis, and induction of mutagenesis and chromosomal aberrations.

Liposomal doxorubicin is doxorubicin hydrochloride encapsulated in long-circulating *STEALTH* liposomes. Liposomes are microscopic vesicles composed of a phospholipid bilayer that are capable of encapsulating active drugs. The *STEALTH* liposomes of liposomal doxorubicin are formulated with surface-bound methoxypolyethylene glycol, a process often referred to as pegylation, to protect liposomes from detection by the mononuclear phagocyte system and increase blood circulation time.

STEALTH liposomes have a half-life of approximately 55 hours in humans. They are stable in blood, and direct measurement of liposomal doxorubicin shows that at least 90% of the drug (the assay used cannot quantify less than 5% to 10% of free doxorubicin) remains liposome-encapsulated during circulation.

It is hypothesized that because of their small size (approximately 100 nm) and persistence in the circulation, the pegylated liposomal doxorubicin liposomes are able to penetrate the altered and often compromised vasculature of tumors. This hypothesis is supported by studies using colloidal gold-containing *STEALTH* liposomes, which can be visualized microscopically. Evidence of penetration of *STEALTH* liposomes from blood vessels and their entry and accumulation in tumors has been seen in mice with C-26 colon carcinoma tumors and in transgenic mice with KS-like lesions. Once the *STEALTH* liposomes distribute to the tissue compartment, the encapsulated doxorubicin becomes available. The exact mechanism of release is not understood.

DOXORUBICIN HYDROCHLORIDE, LIPOSOMAL — INJECTION

➤*Pharmacokinetics:*

Pharmacokinetic Parameters of Liposomal Doxorubicin in Patients With AIDS-Related KS[a]		
	Dose	
Parameter (units)	10 mg/m²	20 mg/m²
Peak plasma concentration (mcg/mL)	4.12 ± 0.215	8.34 ± 0.49
Plasma clearance (L/h/m²)	0.056 ± 0.01	0.041 ± 0.004
Steady-state volume of distribution (L/m²)	2.83 ± 0.145	2.72 ± 0.12
AUC[b] (mcg•h/mL)	277 ± 32.9	590 ± 58.7
First phase (λ_1) half-life (h)	4.7 ± 1.1	5.2 ± 1.4
Second phase (λ_1) half-life (h)	52.3 ± 5.6	55 ± 4.8

[a] N = 23.
[b] AUC = area under the curve.

Absorption – The plasma pharmacokinetics of liposomal doxorubicin were evaluated in 42 patients with AIDS-related KS who received single doses of 10 or 20 mg/m² administered by a 30-minute infusion. Twenty-three of these patients received single doses of both 10 and 20 mg/m², with a 3-week washout period between doses. The pharmacokinetic parameter values of liposomal doxorubicin, given for total doxorubicin (mostly liposomally bound), are presented in the following table.

Liposomal doxorubicin displayed linear pharmacokinetics over the range of 10 to 20 mg/m². Disposition occurred in 2 phases after liposomal doxorubicin administration, with a relatively short first phase (approximately 5 hours) and a prolonged second phase (approximately 55 hours) that accounted for the majority of the AUC.

The pharmacokinetics of liposomal doxorubicin at a 50 mg/m² dose is reported to be nonlinear. At this dose, the elimination half-life of liposomal doxorubicin is expected to be longer and the clearance lower compared with a 20 mg/m² dose. The exposure (AUC) is thus expected to be more than proportional at a 50 mg/m² dose compared with lower doses.

Distribution – In contrast to the pharmacokinetics of doxorubicin, which display a large volume of distribution ranging from 700 to 1,100 L/m², the small steady-state volume of distribution of liposomal doxorubicin shows that liposomal doxorubicin is confined mostly to the vascular fluid volume. The plasma protein binding of liposomal doxorubicin has not been determined; the plasma protein binding of doxorubicin is approximately 70%.

Metabolism – Doxorubicinol, the major metabolite of doxorubicin, was detected at very low levels (range, 0.8 to 26.2 ng/mL) in the plasma of patients who received liposomal doxorubicin 10 or 20 mg/m².

Excretion – The plasma clearance of liposomal doxorubicin was slow, with a mean clearance value of 0.041 L/h/m² at a dose of 20 mg/m². This is in contrast to doxorubicin, which displays a plasma clearance value ranging from 24 to 35 L/h/m².

Because of its slower clearance, the AUC of liposomal doxorubicin, primarily representing the circulation of liposome-encapsulated doxorubicin, is approximately 2 to 3 orders of magnitude larger than the AUC for a similar dose of conventional doxorubicin, as reported in the literature.

Contraindications

Hypersensitivity to a conventional formulation of doxorubicin or the components of liposomal doxorubicin; breast-feeding mothers.

Warnings/Precautions

➤*Cardiac toxicity:* Give special attention to the risk of myocardial damage from cumulative doses of doxorubicin. Include prior use of other anthracyclines or anthracenodiones in calculations of total cumulative dosage. Acute left ventricular failure may occur with doxorubicin, particularly in patients who have received a total cumulative dosage of doxorubicin exceeding the currently recommended limit of 550 mg/m². Lower (400 mg/m²) doses appear to cause heart failure in patients who have received radiotherapy to the mediastinal area or concomitant therapy with other potentially cardiotoxic agents, such as cyclophosphamide.

CHF or cardiomyopathy may be encountered after discontinuation of anthracycline therapy. Administer liposomal doxorubicin to patients with a history of cardiovascular disease only when the potential benefit of treatment outweighs the risk.

Carefully monitor cardiac function in patients treated with liposomal doxorubicin. The most definitive test for anthracycline myocardial injury is endomyocardial biopsy. Other methods, such as echocardiography or multigated radionuclide scans, have been used to monitor cardiac function during anthracycline therapy. Employ any of these methods to monitor potential cardiac toxicity in patients treated with liposomal doxorubicin. If these test results indicate possible cardiac injury associated with liposomal doxorubicin therapy, carefully weigh the benefit of continued therapy against the risk of myocardial injury.

➤*Infusion reactions:* Acute infusion-related reactions were reported in 7.1% of patients treated with liposomal doxorubicin in a randomized ovarian cancer study. These reactions were characterized by 1 or more of the following symptoms: apnea, asthma, back pain, bronchospasm, chest pain, chills, cyanosis, facial swelling, fever, flushing, headache, hypotension, pruritus, rash, shortness of breath, syncope, tachycardia, and tightness in the chest and throat. In most patients, these reactions resolve over the course of several hours to a day once the infusion is terminated. In some patients, the reaction resolved when the rate of infusion was slowed. In this study, 2 (0.8%) patients treated with liposomal doxorubicin discontinued because of infusion-related reactions. In clinical studies, 6 (0.9%) patients with AIDS-related KS and 13 (1.7%) patients with solid tumors discontinued liposomal doxorubicin therapy because of infusion-related reactions.

Serious and sometimes life-threatening or fatal allergic/anaphylactoid-like infusion reactions have been reported. Have medications to treat such reactions, as well as emergency equipment, available for immediate use.

The majority of infusion-related reactions occurred during the first infusion. Similar reactions have not been reported with conventional doxorubicin; they presumably represent a reaction to the liposomal doxorubicin liposomes or one of its surface components.

The initial rate of infusion should be 1 mg/min to help minimize the risk of infusion reactions.

➤*Myelosuppression:* Because of the potential for bone marrow suppression, careful hematologic monitoring is required during use of liposomal doxorubicin, including white blood cell count (WBC), neutrophil, platelet counts, and hemoglobin/hematocrit. With the recommended dosage schedule, leukopenia is usually transient. Hematologic toxicity may require dose reduction or delay or suspension of liposomal doxorubicin therapy. Persistent severe myelosuppression may result in hemorrhage, neutropenic fever, or superinfection. Development of sepsis in the setting of neutropenia has resulted in discontinuation of treatment and, in rare cases, death.

Liposomal doxorubicin may potentiate the toxicity of other anticancer therapies. In particular, hematologic toxicity may be more severe when liposomal doxorubicin is administered in combination with other agents that cause bone marrow suppression.

For patients with AIDS-related KS who often present with baseline myelosuppression because of such factors as their HIV disease or concomitant medications, myelosuppression appears to be the dose-limiting adverse reaction at the recommended dose of 20 mg/m². Leukopenia is the most common adverse reaction experienced in this population; anemia and thrombocytopenia also can be expected. Sepsis occurred in 5% of patients; for 0.7% of patients, the reaction was considered possibly or probably related to liposomal doxorubicin. Eleven (1.6%) patients discontinued the study because of bone marrow suppression or neutropenia.

➤*HFS:* HFS was generally observed after 2 or 3 cycles of treatment but may occur earlier. In most patients, the reaction is mild and resolves in 1 to 2 weeks so that prolonged delay of therapy need not occur. However, dose modification may be required to manage HFS. The reaction can be severe and debilitating in some patients and may require discontinuation of treatment.

➤*Radiation recall therapy:* Recall reaction has occurred with liposomal doxorubicin administration after radiotherapy.

➤*Toxicity potentiation:* Liposomal doxorubicin may potentiate the toxicity of other anticancer therapies. Exacerbation of cyclophosphamide-induced hemorrhagic cystitis and enhancement of the hepatotoxicity of 6-mercaptopurine have been reported with the conventional formulation of doxorubicin. Radiation-induced toxicity to the liver, mucosae, myocardium, and skin has been reported to be increased by the administration of doxorubicin.

➤*Extravasation:* See Administration and Dosage for more information.

See Administration and Dosage for more information.

➤*Hepatic function impairment:* See Administration and Dosage for more information.

➤*Pregnancy: Category D.* Liposomal doxorubicin can cause fetal harm when administered to a pregnant woman. Liposomal doxorubicin is embryotoxic at doses of 1 mg/kg/day in rats and is embryotoxic and abortifacient at 0.5 mg/kg/day in rabbits (both doses are about one-eighth of the 50 mg/m² human dose on a mg/m² basis). Embryotoxicity was characterized by increased embryofetal deaths and reduced live litter sizes.

There are no adequate and well-controlled studies in pregnant women. If liposomal doxorubicin is to be used during pregnancy or the patient becomes pregnant during therapy, apprise the patient of the potential hazard to the fetus. If pregnancy occurs in the first few months following treatment with liposomal doxorubicin, consider the prolonged half-life of the drug. Advise women of childbearing potential to avoid pregnancy during treatment with liposomal doxorubicin.

➤*Lactation:* It is not known whether this drug is excreted in human milk. Because many drugs, including anthracyclines, are excreted in human milk and because of the potential for serious adverse reactions in breast-feeding infants from liposomal doxorubicin, instruct mothers to discontinue breast-feeding prior to taking this drug.

➤*Children:* The safety and effectiveness of liposomal doxorubicin in children have not been established.

➤*Monitoring:* Patients receiving therapy with liposomal doxorubicin should be monitored by a health care provider experienced in the use of cancer chemotherapeutic agents. Most adverse reactions are manageable with dose reductions or delays.

Obtain complete blood cell counts, including platelet counts, frequently and, at a minimum, prior to each dose of liposomal doxorubicin.

Prior to liposomal doxorubicin administration, evaluation of hepatic function, using conventional clinical laboratory tests such as alkaline phosphatase, ALT, AST, and bilirubin, is recommended.

DOXORUBICIN HYDROCHLORIDE, LIPOSOMAL — INJECTION

Drug Interactions

No formal drug interaction studies have been conducted with liposomal doxorubicin. Until specific compatibility data are available, it is not recommended that liposomal doxorubicin be mixed with other drugs. Liposomal doxorubicin may interact with drugs known to interact with the conventional formulation of doxorubicin.

Drug-drug interactions between liposomal doxorubicin and other drugs, including antiviral agents, have not been adequately evaluated in patients with AIDS-related KS, multiple myeloma, or ovarian cancer.

➤*QT prolongation:* An additive effect of doxorubicin with other drugs that prolong the QT interval cannot be excluded. The following drugs may prolong the QT interval and increase the risk of life-threatening cardiac arrhythmias, including torsades de pointes: Antiarrhythmic agents (eg, amiodarone, bretylium, disopyramide, dofetilide, procainamide, quinidine, and sotalol), arsenic trioxide, chlorpromazine, cisapride, dolasetron, droperidol, mefloquine, mesoridazine, moxifloxacin, pentamidine, pimozide, tacrolimus, thioridazine, and ziprasidone. For a more complete list of drugs that may prolong the QT interval, see the appendix, Drug-Induced Prolongation of the QT Interval and Torsades de Pointes.

Conventional Doxorubicin Drug Interactions

Precipitant drug	Object drug[a]		Description
Barbiturates (eg, phenobarbital)	Doxorubicin	↓	Phenobarbital may increase doxorubicin metabolism, decreasing its therapeutic effect.
Cyclophosphamide	Doxorubicin	↑	Concurrent use may potentiate cardiotoxicity of both agents.
Doxorubicin	Cyclophosphamide		Doxorubicin may enhance hemorrhagic cystitis caused by cyclophosphamide.
Cyclosporine	Doxorubicin	↑	Cyclosporine may increase serum doxorubicin levels, causing more profound hematologic toxicity.
Paclitaxel	Doxorubicin	↑	Paclitaxel may cause increased plasma concentrations of doxorubicin and its active metabolite, doxorubicinol, which may increase adverse reactions.
Progesterone	Doxorubicin	↑	Progesterone may enhance neutropenia and thrombocytopenia associated with doxorubicin.
Streptozocin	Doxorubicin	↑	Streptozocin may enhance neutropenia and thrombocytopenia associated with doxorubicin.
Verapamil	Doxorubicin	↑	Verapamil may inhibit doxorubicin metabolism, potentially leading to toxicity.
Doxorubicin	Digoxin	↓	Oral absorption of digoxin may be decreased. Digitoxin and digoxin capsules do not appear to be affected.
Doxorubicin	Mercaptopurine	↑	Doxorubicin may enhance hepatotoxicity caused by mercaptopurine.
Doxorubicin	Phenytoin	↓	Doxorubicin may decrease serum phenytoin levels. Monitor phenytoin levels during concomitant therapy and adjust the dose as needed.
Doxorubicin	Quinolone antibiotics (eg, ciprofloxacin, levofloxacin)	↓	Doxorubicin may decrease oral absorption of quinolone antibiotics.
Doxorubicin	Zidovudine	↓	Doxorubicin may decrease the antiviral activity of zidovudine.

[a] ↑ = object drug increased; ↓ = object drug decreased.

Adverse Reactions

Doxorubicin (liposomal) is considered to have moderate to low potential for nausea and vomiting.

The most common adverse reactions observed with liposomal doxorubicin are anemia, anorexia, asthenia, constipation, diarrhea, fatigue, fever, HFS, nausea, rash and neutropenia, stomatitis, thrombocytopenia, and vomiting.

The following safety data reflect exposure to liposomal doxorubicin in 1,310 patients, including 239 patients with ovarian cancer, 753 patients with AIDS-related KS, and 318 patients with multiple myeloma.

➤*Ovarian cancer:*

Liposomal Doxorubicin Hematology Data in Patients With Ovarian Cancer

	Liposomal doxorubicin (n = 239)	Topotecan (n = 235)
Neutropenia		
500 to < 1,000/mm³	19 (7.9%)	33 (14%)
< 500/mm³	10 (4.2%)	146 (62.1%)
Anemia		
6.5 to < 8 g/dL	13 (5.4%)	59 (25.1%)
< 6.5 g/dL	1 (0.4%)	10 (4.3%)
Thrombocytopenia		
10,000 to < 50,000/mm³	3 (1.3%)	40 (17%)
< 10,000/mm³	0 (0%)	40 (17%)

Ovarian Cancer Nonhematologic Adverse Reactions With Liposomal Doxorubicin (≥ 10%)

	Liposomal doxorubicin (n = 239)		Topotecan (n = 235)	
Adverse reaction	All grades	Grades 3 to 4	All grades	Grades 3 to 4
CNS				
Asthenia	40.2%	7.1%	51.5%	8.1%
Dizziness	4.2%	0%	10.2%	0%
Headache	10.5%	0.8%	14.9%	0%
Dermatologic				
Alopecia	19.2%	NA[a]	52.3%	NA
HFS	50.6%	23.8%	0.9%	0%
Rash	28.5%	4.2%	12.3%	0.4%
GI				
Anorexia	20.1%	2.5%	21.7%	1.3%
Diarrhea	20.9%	2.5%	34.9%	4.2%
Dyspepsia	12.1%	0.8%	14%	0%
Nausea	46%	5.4%	63%	8.1%
Stomatitis	41.4%	8.3%	15.3%	0.4%
Vomiting	32.6%	7.9%	43.8%	9.8%
Respiratory				
Cough increased	9.6%	0%	11.5%	0%
Dyspnea	15.1%	4.1%	23.4%	4.3%
Pharyngitis	15.9%	0%	17.9%	0.4%
Miscellaneous				
Back pain	11.7%	1.7%	10.2%	0.9%
Fever	21.3%	0.8%	30.6%	5.5%
Infection	11.7%	2.1%	6.4%	0.9%
Mucous membrane disorder	14.2%	3.8%	3.4%	0%

[a] NA = not applicable.

The following additional adverse reactions (not included in the table) were observed in patients with ovarian cancer with doses administered every 4 weeks. The incidence was 1% to 10% for these reactions.

Cardiovascular – Cardiac arrest, deep thrombophlebitis, hypotension, tachycardia, vasodilation.

CNS – Depression, dizziness, somnolence.

Dermatologic – Acne, dry skin, exfoliative dermatitis, fungal dermatitis, furunculosis, herpes simplex, herpes zoster, maculopapular rash, pruritus, skin discoloration, vesiculobullous rash.

GI – Dysphagia, esophagitis, ileus, mouth ulceration, oral moniliasis, rectal bleeding.

GU – Hematuria, urinary tract infection, vaginal moniliasis.

Hematologic/Lymphatic – Ecchymosis.

Metabolic/Nutritional – Dehydration, hyperbilirubinemia, hypercalcemia, hypokalemia, hyponatremia, weight loss.

Respiratory – Epistaxis, pneumonia, rhinitis, sinusitis.

Special senses – Conjunctivitis, dry eyes, taste perversion.

DOXORUBICIN HYDROCHLORIDE, LIPOSOMAL — INJECTION

➤*AIDS-related KS:*

Liposomal Doxorubicin Hematology Data in Patients With AIDS-Related KS

	Patients with refractory or intolerant AIDS-related KS (n = 74)	Total patients with AIDS-related KS (N = 720)
Neutropenia		
< 1,000/mm^3	34 (45.9%)	352 (48.9%)
< 500/mm^3	8 (10.8%)	96 (13.3%)
Anemia		
< 10 g/dL	43 (58.1%)	399 (55.4%)
< 8 g/dL	12 (16.2%)	131 (18.2%)
Thrombocytopenia		
< 150,000/mm^3	45 (60.8%)	439 (60.9%)
< 25,000/mm^3	1 (1.4%)	30 (4.2%)

Liposomal Doxorubicin Nonhematologic Adverse Reactions in Patients With AIDS-Related KS (≥ 5%)

Adverse reaction	Patients with refractory or intolerant AIDS-related KS (n = 77)	Total patients with AIDS-related KS (N = 705)
GI		
Diarrhea	4 (5.2%)	55 (7.8%)
Nausea	14 (18.2%)	119 (16.9%)
Stomatitis	4 (5.2%)	48 (6.8%)
Vomiting	6 (7.8%)	55 (7.8%)
Miscellaneous		
Alkaline phosphatase increase	1 (1.3%)	55 (7.8%)
Alopecia	7 (9.1%)	63 (8.9%)
Asthenia	5 (6.5%)	70 (9.9%)
Fever	6 (7.8%)	64 (9.1%)
Oral moniliasis	1 (1.3%)	39 (5.5%)

The following additional adverse reactions (not included in the previous table) were observed in patients with AIDS-related KS.

Cardiovascular – Chest pain, hypotension, tachycardia (1% to 5%); bundle branch block, cardiomyopathy, CHF, heart arrest, palpitation, thrombophlebitis, thrombosis, ventricular arrhythmia (less than 1%).

CNS – Chills, dizziness, headache, somnolence (1% to 5%).

Dermatologic – Herpes simplex, itching, rash (1% to 5%); herpes zoster, maculopapular rash (less than 1%).

GI – Anorexia, dysphagia, mouth ulceration (1% to 5%).

Hepatic – Hepatitis (less than 1%).

Metabolic/Nutritional – ALT increase, hyperbilirubinemia, weight loss (1% to 5%); dehydration (less than 1%).

Respiratory – Dyspnea, pneumonia (1% to 5%); cough increase, pharyngitis (less than 1%).

Special senses – Conjunctivitis, taste perversion (less than 1%).

Miscellaneous – Allergic reaction, back pain, infection (1% to 5%); cryptococcosis, moniliasis, sepsis (less than 1%).

➤*Multiple myeloma:*

Multiple Myeloma Adverse Reactions With Liposomal Doxorubicin Plus Bortezomib (≥ 10%)

	Liposomal doxorubicin + bortezomib (N = 318)			Bortezomib (N = 318)		
Adverse reaction	Any	Grade 3	Grade 4	Any	Grade 3	Grade 4
CNS						
Neuralgia	17%	3%	0%	20%	4%	1%
Paresthesia/ dysesthesia	13%	< 1%	0%	10%	0%	0%
Peripheral neuropathy[a]	42%	7%	< 1%	45%	10%	1%
Dermatologic						
HFS	19%	6%	0%	< 1%	0%	0%
Rash[b]	22%	1%	0%	18%	1%	0%
GI						
Abdominal pain	11%	1%	0%	8%	1%	0%
Anorexia	19%	2%	0%	14%	< 1%	0%
Constipation	31%	1%	0%	31%	1%	0%
Diarrhea	46%	7%	0%	39%	5%	0%
Mucositis/ Stomatitis	20%	2%	0%	5%	< 1%	0%
Nausea	48%	3%	0%	40%	1%	0%
Vomiting	32%	4%	0%	22%	1%	0%
Hematologic						
Anemia	25%	7%	2%	21%	8%	2%
Neutropenia	36%	22%	10%	22%	11%	5%
Thrombocytopenia	33%	11%	13%	28%	9%	8%
Respiratory						
Cough	18%	0%	0%	12%	0%	0%
Miscellaneous						
Asthenia	22%	6%	0%	18%	4%	0%
Fatigue	36%	6%	1%	28%	3%	0%
Herpes simplex	10%	0%	0%	6%	1%	0%
Herpes zoster	11%	2%	0%	9%	2%	0%
Pyrexia	31%	1%	0%	22%	1%	0%
Weight decreased	12%	0%	0%	4%	0%	0%

[a] Peripheral neuropathy includes the following adverse reactions: peripheral motor neuropathy, peripheral neuropathy, peripheral sensory neuropathy, polyneuropathy, and neuropathy not otherwise specified.
[b] Rash includes the following adverse reactions: exfoliative rash, rash, rash erythematous, rash generalized, rash macular, rash maculopapular, and rash pruritic.

➤*Postmarketing:* The following additional adverse reactions have been identified during postapproval use of liposomal doxorubicin. Because these reactions are reported voluntarily from a population of uncertain size, it is not always possible to reliably estimate their frequency or establish a causal relationship to drug exposure.

Musculoskeletal – Rare cases of muscle spasms.

Respiratory – Rare cases of pulmonary embolism (in some cases fatal).

Hematologic – Secondary acute myelogenous leukemia, with and without fatal outcomes, has been reported in patients whose treatment included liposomal doxorubicin.

Overdosage

➤*Symptoms:* Acute overdosage with doxorubicin causes increases in leukopenia, mucositis, and thrombocytopenia.

➤*Treatment:* Treatment of acute overdosage consists of treatment of the severely myelosuppressed patient with hospitalization, antibiotics, platelet and granulocyte transfusions, and symptomatic treatment of mucositis.

Patient Information

Inform patients and patients' caregivers of the expected adverse reactions of liposomal doxorubicin, particularly HFS, neutropenia, and stomatitis, and related complications of infection, neutropenic fever, and sepsis.

Instruct patients who experience tingling or burning, redness, flaking, bothersome swelling, small blisters, or small sores on the palms of their hands or soles of their feet (symptoms of HFS) to notify their health care provider.

Instruct patients who experience painful redness, swelling, or sores in the mouth (symptoms of stomatitis) to notify their health care provider.

Instruct patients who develop neutropenia and a fever of 38°C (100.5°F) or higher to notify their health care provider.

Instruct patients who develop mild hair loss, nausea, rash, tiredness, vomiting, or weakness to notify their health care provider.

Following its administration, liposomal doxorubicin may impart a reddish-orange color to the urine and other body fluids. This nontoxic reaction is caused by the color of the product and will dissipate as the drug is eliminated from the body.

EPIRUBICIN HYDROCHLORIDE

Rx	**Epirubicin Hydrochloride** (Mayne)	**Injection, lyophilized powder for solution:** 50 mg	Lactose. In single-use vials.
		200 mg	Lactose. In single-use vials.
Rx	**Epirubicin Hydrochloride** (Bedford)	**Injection, solution:** 2 mg/mL	Preservative-free. In 25 and 100 mL single-use vials.
Rx	**Ellence** (Pharmacia & Upjohn)		

EPIRUBICIN HYDROCHLORIDE — INJECTION

WARNING

Severe local tissue necrosis will occur if there is extravasation during administration. It is recommended that epirubicin HCl be slowly administered into the tubing of a freely running intravenous infusion usually between 3 and 20 minutes depending upon dosage and volume of the infusion solution. If possible, veins over joints or in extremities with compromised venous or lymphatic drainage should be avoided. A burning or stinging sensation may be indicative of perivenous infiltration, and the infusion should be immediately terminated and restarted in another vein. Perivenous infiltration may occur without causing pain. Epirubicin must not be given by the intramuscular or subcutaneous route.

Myocardial toxicity, manifested in its most severe form by potentially fatal congestive heart failure (CHF), may occur either during therapy with epirubicin or months to years after termination of therapy. The probability of developing clinically evident CHF is estimated as approximately 0.9% at a cumulative dose of 550 mg/m², 1.6% at 700 mg/m², and 3.3% at 900 mg/m². In the adjuvant treatment of breast cancer, the maximum cumulative dose used in clinical trials was 720 mg/m². The risk of developing CHF increases rapidly with increasing total cumulative doses of epirubicin in excess of 900 mg/m²; this cumulative dose should only be exceeded with extreme caution. Active or dormant cardiovascular disease, prior or concomitant radiotherapy to the mediastinal/pericardial area, previous therapy with other anthracyclines or anthracenediones, or concomitant use of other cardiotoxic drugs may increase the risk of cardiac toxicity. Cardiac toxicity with epirubicin may occur at lower cumulative doses whether or not cardiac risk factors are present.

Secondary acute myelogenous leukemia (AML) has been reported in patients with breast cancer treated with anthracyclines, including epirubicin. The occurrence of refractory secondary leukemia is more common when such drugs are given in combination with DNA-damaging antineoplastic agents, when patients have been heavily pretreated with cytotoxic drugs, or when doses of anthracyclines have been escalated. The cumulative risk of developing treatment-related AML, in 3844 patients with breast cancer who received adjuvant treatment with epirubicin-containing regimens, was estimated as 0.2% at 3 years and 0.8% at 5 years.

Dosage should be reduced in patients with impaired hepatic function. Definitive recommendation regarding use of epirubicin HCl in patients with hepatic dysfunction are not available because patients with hepatic abnormalities were excluded from participation in adjuvant trials of FEC-100/CEF-120 therapy. In patients with elevated serum AST or serum total bilirubin concentrations, the following dose reductions were recommended in clinical trials, although few patients experienced hepatic impairment:

- Bilirubin 1.2 to 3 mg/dL or AST 2 to 4 times upper limit of normal: ½ of recommended starting dose.
- Bilirubin greater than 3 mg/dL or AST greater than 4 times upper limit of normal: ¼ of recommended starting dose.

Severe myelosuppression may occur.

Epirubicin should be administered only under the supervision of a physician who is experienced in the use of cancer chemotherapeutic agents.

Indications

➤*Breast cancer:* Epirubicin HCl injection is indicated as a component of adjuvant therapy in patients with evidence of axillary node tumor involvement following resection of primary breast cancer.

➤*Off-label uses:* For the treatment of small cell lung cancer, non–small cell lung cancer, esophageal cancer, ovarian cancer, gastric cancer, soft tissue sarcoma, Hodgkin lymphoma, and non-Hodgkin lymphoma. (See Administration and Dosage.)

Administration and Dosage

➤*Maximum dose:*

Adults – The recommended lifetime maximum dose is 900 mg/m² (or 650 mg/m² in adults who have received mediastinal radiation or treatment with other anthracyclines) according to the prescribing information. (See also Maximum lifetime cumulative dose.)

➤*General dosing considerations:* Epirubicin is given in repeated 3- to 4-week cycles. The total dose of epirubicin may be given on day 1 of each cycle or divided equally and given on days 1 and 8 of each cycle.

In patients receiving 120 mg/m²/cycle, administer prophylactic antimicrobials for the duration of chemotherapy to reduce the risk of serious infections. (See Concomitant therapy.)

➤*Adults:*

Breast cancer –

Initial dosage: 100 to 120 mg/m² by intravenous (IV) infusion once every 3- to 4-week cycle. The total dose of epirubicin may be given on day 1 of each cycle or divided equally and given on days 1 and 8 of each cycle. (See also Off-Label Dosing.) The following regimens were used in the trials supporting use of epirubicin as a component of adjuvant therapy in patients with axillary-node positive breast cancer:

Epirubicin Regimens in Adjuvant Therapy		
CEF-120	Cyclophosphamide	75 mg/m² orally days 1 to 14
	Epirubicin	60 mg/m² IV days 1, 8
	5-flourouracil	500 mg/m² IV days 1, 8
	Repeated every 28 days for 6 cycles	
FEC-100	5-fluorouracil	500 mg/m²
	Epirubicin	100 mg/m²
	Cyclophosphamide	500 mg/m²
	All drugs were administered IV on day 1 and repeated every 21 days for 6 cycles.	

Dosage adjustment: Dosage adjustments after the first treatment cycle should be made based on hematologic and nonhematologic toxicities. Patients experiencing nadir platelet counts less than 50,000/mm³, absolute neutrophil counts (ANC) less than 250/mm³, neutropenic fever, or grades 3/4 nonhematologic toxicity during treatment cycle should have the day 1 dose in subsequent cycles reduced to 75% of the day 1 dose given in the current cycle. Day 1 chemotherapy in subsequent courses of treatment should be delayed until platelet counts are at least 100,000/mm³, ANC are at least 1,500/mm³, and nonhematologic toxicities have recovered to grade 1 or less.

For patients receiving a divided dose of epirubicin (day 1 and day 8), the day 8 dose should be 75% of day 1 if platelet counts are 75,000 to 100,000/mm³ and ANC is 1,000 to 1,499/mm³. If day 8 platelet counts are less than 75,000/mm³, ANC are less than 1,000/mm³, or grade 3/4 nonhematologic toxicity has occurred, the day 8 dose should be omitted.

Off-label dosing –

Breast cancer: 100 mg/m² IV on day 1 of each 21-day cycle. An alternative regimen is 60 mg/m² IV on day 1 and day 8 of a 28-day cycle (for a total dose of 120 mg/m² during each cycle). Give a total of 6 cycles.

Esophageal cancer:

- *Combination therapy* – 50 mg/m² IV on day 1 of each 21-day cycle.
- *Alternative dosage* – 50 to 60 mg/m² IV on day 1 of each 28-day cycle, or 20 mg/m² IV on days 1 to 3 of each 28-day cycle.

Gastric cancer:

- *Combination therapy* – 80 mg/m² IV on day 1 of each 21-day cycle.
- *Single-agent therapy* – 75 to 100 mg/m² IV on day 1 of each 21-day cycle.

Hodgkin lymphoma:

- *Combination therapy* – 35 mg/m²/day IV on day 1 of each 14-day cycle.
- *Alternative dosage* – 70 mg/m²/day IV on day 1 of each cycle, repeated every 3 to 4 weeks.

Non–Hodgkin lymphoma:

- *Combination therapy* – 60 to 75 mg/m² IV on day 1 of each cycle, repeated every 21 to 28 days.
- *Single-agent therapy* – 75 to 90 mg/m² IV on day 1 of each 21-day cycle.

Non–small cell lung cancer:

- *Combination therapy* – 90 to 120 mg/m² IV on day 1 of each cycle, repeated every 3 to 4 weeks.
- *Single-agent therapy* – 120 to 150 mg/m² IV on day 1 of each cycle, repeated every 3 to 4 weeks.

Ovarian cancer: 50 to 90 mg/m² IV on day 1 of each cycle, repeated every 3 to 4 weeks, given in combination or as a single dose.

Small cell lung cancer:

- *Combination therapy* – 50 to 90 mg/m² IV on day 1 of each 21-day cycle.
- *Single-agent therapy* – 90 to 120 mg/m²/day IV on day 1 of each 21-day cycle.

➤*Renal function impairment:* While no specific dose recommendation can be made based on the limited available data in patients with renal impairment, consider reducing the dose by 50% in patients with severe renal impairment (serum creatinine greater than 5 mg/dL).

➤*Hepatic function impairment:* Definitive recommendations regarding use of epirubicin in patients with hepatic function impairment are not available because patients with hepatic abnormalities were excluded from participation in adjuvant trials of FEC-100/CEF-120 therapy. In patients with

EPIRUBICIN HYDROCHLORIDE — INJECTION

elevated serum AST or serum total bilirubin concentrations, the following dose reductions were recommended in clinical trials, although few patients experienced hepatic impairment:

- Bilirubin 1.2 to 3 mg/dL or AST 2 to 4 times the upper limit of normal (ULN): give 50% of recommended starting dose.
- Bilirubin greater than 3 mg/dL or AST greater than 4 times the ULN: give 25% of recommended starting dose.

➤*Bone marrow dysfunction:* Consideration should be given to administration of lower starting doses (75 to 90 mg/m^2) for heavily pretreated patients, patients with preexisting bone marrow depression, or in the presence of neoplastic bone marrow infiltration.

➤*Concomitant therapy:* In patients receiving 120 mg/m^2/cycle, administer prophylactic antimicrobials for the duration of chemotherapy to reduce the risk of serious infections. Although the manufacturer recommends co-trimoxazole or a fluoroquinolone, other agents with similar spectrums of activity may be used. Clinical trials have used any of the following regimens:

- Co-trimoxazole 800 mg/160 mg orally twice daily,
- Norfloxacin 400 mg orally twice daily, or
- Ciprofloxacin 500 mg orally twice daily.

➤*Maximum lifetime cumulative dose:* Risk of cardiotoxicity increases with cumulative epirubicin dose. (See also Warnings/Precautions.) The recommended lifetime maximum dose differs in various patient groups, as shown in the following table.

Lifetime Cumulative Doses of Epirubicin Above Which Frequency of Cardiotoxicity Increases

Demographics/Risk factor	Lifetime cumulative dose
Adults	≤ 900 mg/m^2
Adults who have received mediastinal radiation or treatment with other anthracyclines	≤ 650 mg/m^2

➤*Preparation for administration:* Epirubicin is considered a cytotoxic agent. Follow safe handling procedures when preparing, administering, or dispensing epirubicin.

The solution should be red to red-orange in color; slight pinkish discoloration is acceptable. Do not use the solution if precipitation or significant discoloration is present.

➤*Administration:* Epirubicin should be administered into the tubing of a freely flowing IV infusion (0.9% sodium chloride or 5% glucose solution). The usual infusion time ranges between 3 and 20 minutes, depending on dosage and volume of the infusion solution. This technique is intended to minimize the risk of thrombosis or perivenous extravasation, which could lead to severe cellulitis, vesication, or tissue necrosis. A direct push injection is not recommended because of the risk of extravasation, which may occur even in the presence of adequate blood return on needle aspiration. Venous sclerosis may result from injection into small vessels or repeated injections into the same vein.

Flush well with a heparin-free solution before and after epirubicin administration.

➤*Extravasation:* Extravasation of epirubicin during the infusion may cause local pain, severe tissue lesions (vesication, severe cellulitis), and necrosis. If signs or symptoms of extravasation occur, stop the infusion immediately. If possible, withdraw 3 to 5 mL of blood to remove some of the drug. Remove the infusion needle.

There are currently 2 treatments for extravasation resulting from anthracycline IV therapy: topical dimethyl sulfoxide and dexrazoxane IV. Both treatments are effective for treating anthracycline extravasation injury, although no comparative trials have been conducted.

- Apply dimethyl sulfoxide (DMSO) 99% by saturating a gauze pad and painting on an area twice the size of the extravasation. Allow the site to air dry and repeat the application every 6 hours for 14 days. Do not cover the area with dressing.
- Dexrazoxane (*Totect*) is FDA-approved for the treatment of extravasation resulting from anthracycline IV therapy. The first infusion of dexrazoxane should be administered as soon as possible and within the first 6 hours following the extravasation. Topical cooling, such as ice packs, should be removed for at least 15 minutes prior to and during dexrazoxane administration. Concurrent extravasation treatment, such as topical dimethyl sulfoxide application should not be used in conjunction with dexrazoxane, and if administered, may worsen extravasation-induced tissue injury. The recommended dose of dexrazoxane for day 1 is 1,000 mg/m^2 (up to 2,000 mg), the dose for day 2 is 1,000 mg/m^2 (up to 2,000 mg), and the dose for day 3 is 500 mg/m^2 (up to 1,000 mg). Dexrazoxane is administered as an IV infusion over 1 to 2 hours.

Application of ice compresses to the area for 15 minutes every 6 hours for 48 hours may be useful. Delineate the infiltrated area on the patient's skin with a felt-tip marker. Elevate for 48 hours above heart level using a sling or stockinette dressing with an observation window cut in the dressing. Avoid pressure or friction. Do not rub the area. Observe for signs of increased erythema, pain, or skin necrosis. If increased symptoms occur, consult a plastic surgeon. Ensure that no medication is given distally to extravasation site. After 48 hours, encourage the patient to use the extremity normally to promote full range of motion.

➤*Admixture compatibility:* Epirubicin can be used in combination with other antitumor agents, but it is not recommended that it be mixed with other drugs in the same syringe.

Prolonged contact with any solution of an alkaline pH should be avoided as it will result in hydrolysis of the drug. Epirubicin should not be mixed with heparin or fluorouracil due to chemical incompatibility that may lead to precipitation.

➤*Storage/Stability:* Store vials of injection solution in a refrigerator between 2° and 8°C (36° and 46°F). Do not freeze. Store vials of powder for solution at 25°C (77°F); excursions are permitted to 15°C to 30°C (59°F to 86°F). Protect from light. Discard unused portion. Store upright.

Reconstituted solutions are stable for 24 hours when stored at 2° to 8°C (36° to 46°F) and protected from light, or 25°C (77°F) in normal lighting conditions.

Epirubicin solution is preservative-free and should be used within 24 hours of the first penetration of the rubber stopper.

Discard the vial within 6 hours of the initial needle puncture if opened within an ISO Class 5 biological safety cabinet, or within 1 hour of the initial needle puncture if opened outside of such an environment, based on the USP Chapter <797> standards.

Actions

➤*Pharmacology:* Epirubicin is an anthracycline cytotoxic agent. Although it is known that anthracyclines can interfere with a number of biochemical and biological functions within eukaryotic cells, the precise mechanisms of epirubicin's cytotoxic and/or antiproliferative properties have not been completely elucidated.

Epirubicin forms a complex with DNA by intercalation of its planar rings between nucleotide base pairs, with consequent inhibition of nucleic acid (DNA and RNA) and protein synthesis. Such intercalation triggers DNA cleavage by topoisomerase II, resulting in cytocidal activity. Epirubicin also inhibits DNA helicase activity, preventing the enzymatic separation of double-stranded DNA and interfering with replication and transcription. Epirubicin is also involved in oxidation/reduction reactions by generating cytotoxic free radicals. The antiproliferative and cytotoxic activity of epirubicin is thought to result from these or other possible mechanisms.

Epirubicin is cytotoxic in vitro to a variety of established murine and human cell lines and primary cultures of human tumors. It is also active in vivo against a variety of murine tumors and human xenografts in athymic mice, including breast tumors.

➤*Pharmacokinetics:*

Summary of Mean Pharmacokinetic Parameters in Patients[a] with Solid Tumors Receiving IV Epirubicin 60 to 150 mg/m^2

Dose[b] (mg/m^2)	C_{max}[c] (mcg/mL)	AUC[d] (mcg•hr/mL)	$t_{1/2}$[e] (hours)	CL[f] (L/hour)	V_{ss}[g] (L/kg)
60	5.7 ± 1.6	1.6 ± 0.2	35.3 ± 9	65 ± 8	21 ± 2
75	5.3 ± 1.5	1.7 ± 0.3	32.1 ± 5	83 ± 14	27 ± 11
120	9 ± 3.5	3.4 ± 0.7	33.7 ± 4	65 ± 13	23 ± 7
150	9.3 ± 2.9	4.2 ± 0.8	31.1 ± 6	69 ± 13	21 ± 7

[a] Advanced solid tumor cancers, primarily of the lung.
[b] N = 6 patients per dose level.
[c] Plasma concentration at the end of 6- to 10-minute infusion.
[d] Area under the plasma concentration curve.
[e] Half-life of terminal phase.
[f] Plasma clearance.
[g] Steady-state volume of distribution.

Absorption – Epirubicin pharmacokinetics are linear over the dose range of 60 to 150 mg/m^2 and plasma clearance is not affected by the duration of infusion or administration schedule. Pharmacokinetic parameters for epirubicin following 6- to 10-minute, single-dose intravenous infusions of epirubicin at doses of 60 to 150 mg/m^2 in patients with solid tumors are shown in the table below. The plasma concentration declined in a triphasic manner with mean half-lives for the alpha, beta, and gamma phases of about 3 minutes, 2.5 hours, and 33 hours, respectively.

Distribution – Following intravenous administration, epirubicin is rapidly and widely distributed into the tissues. Binding of epirubicin to plasma proteins, predominantly albumin, is about 77% and is not affected by drug concentration. Epirubicin also appears to concentrate in red blood cells; whole blood concentrations are approximately twice those of plasma.

Metabolism – Epirubicin is extensively and rapidly metabolized by the liver and is also metabolized by other organs and cells, including red blood cells. Four main metabolic routes have been identified:

1.) Reduction of the C-13 keto-group with the formation of the 13(S)-dihydro derivative, epirubicinol.
2.) Conjugation of both the unchanged drug and epirubicinol with glucuronic acid.
3.) Loss of the amino sugar moiety through a hydrolytic process with the formation of the doxorubicin and doxorubicinol aglycones.
4.) Loss of the amino sugar moiety through a redox process with the formation of the 7-deoxy-doxorubicin aglycone and 7-deoxy-doxorubicinol aglycone. Epirubicinol has in vitro cytotoxic activity one-tenth that of epirubicin. As plasma levels of epirubicinol are lower than those of the unchanged drug, they are unlikely to reach in vivo concentrations sufficient for cytotoxicity. No significant activity or toxicity has been reported for the other metabolites.

EPIRUBICIN HYDROCHLORIDE — INJECTION

Excretion – Epirubicin and its major metabolites are eliminated through biliary excretion and, to a lesser extent, by urinary excretion. Mass-balance data from one patient found about 60% of the total radioactive dose in feces (34%) and urine (27%). These data are consistent with those from 3 patients with extrahepatic obstruction and percutaneous drainage, in whom approximately 35% and 20% of the administered dose were recovered as epirubicin or its major metabolites in bile and urine, respectively, in the 4 days after treatment.

Special populations –

Renal function impairment: No significant alterations in the pharmacokinetics of epirubicin or its major metabolite, epirubicinol, have been observed in patients with serum creatinine less than 5 mg/dL. A 50% reduction in plasma clearance was reported in 4 patients with serum creatinine greater than or equal to 5 mg/dL. Patients on dialysis have not been studied.

Hepatic function impairment: Epirubicin is eliminated by both hepatic metabolism and biliary excretion and clearance is reduced in patients with hepatic dysfunction. In a study of the effect of hepatic dysfunction, patients with solid tumors were classified into 3 groups. Patients in group 1 (n = 22) had serum AST levels above the upper limit of normal (median, 93 IU/L) and normal serum bilirubin levels (median, 0.5 mg/dL) and were given epirubicin doses of 12.5 to 90 mg/m^2. Patients in group 2 had alterations in both serum AST (median, 175 IU/L) and bilirubin levels (median, 2.7 mg/dL) and were treated with an epirubicin dose of 25 mg/m^2 (n = 8). Their pharmacokinetics were compared to those of patients with normal serum AST and bilirubin values, who received epirubicin doses of 12.5 to 120 mg/m^2. The median plasma clearance of epirubicin was decreased compared to patients with normal hepatic function by about 30% in patients in group 1 and by 50% in patients in group 2. Patients with more severe hepatic impairment have not been evaluated. Definitive recommendation regarding use of epirubicin HCl in patients with hepatic dysfunction are not available because patients with hepatic abnormalities were excluded from participation in adjuvant trials of FEC-100/CEF-120 therapy. In patients with elevated serum AST or serum total bilirubin concentrations, the following dose reductions were recommended in clinical trials, although few patients experienced hepatic impairment:

- Bilirubin 1.2 to 3 mg/dL or AST 2 to 4 times upper limit of normal: ½ of recommended starting dose.
- Bilirubin greater than 3 mg/dL or AST greater than 4 times upper limit of normal: ¼ of recommended starting dose.

Elderly: A population analysis of plasma data from 36 cancer patients (13 males and 23 females, 20 to 73 years) showed that age affects plasma clearance of epirubicin in female patients. The predicted plasma clearance for a female patient of 70 years of age was about 35% lower than that for a female patient of 25 years of age. An insufficient number of males greater than 50 years of age were included in the study to draw conclusions about age-related alterations in clearance in males. Although a lower epirubicin starting dose does not appear necessary in elderly female patients, and was not used in clinical trials, particular care should be taken in monitoring toxicity when epirubicin is administered to female patients greater than 70 years of age.

Contraindications

Baseline neutrophil count less than 1500 cells/mm^3; severe myocardial insufficiency, recent myocardial infarction, severe arrhythmias; previous treatment with anthracyclines up to the maximum cumulative dose; hypersensitivity to epirubicin, other anthracyclines, or anthracenediones; or severe hepatic dysfunction.

Warnings/Precautions

➤*Administration:* Epirubicin HCl injection should be administered only under the supervision of qualified physicians experienced in the use of cytotoxic therapy. Before beginning treatment with epirubicin, patients should recover from acute toxicities (eg, stomatitis, neutropenia, thrombocytopenia, and generalized infections) of prior cytotoxic treatment. Also, initial treatment with epirubicin HCl should be preceded by a careful baseline assessment of blood counts; serum levels of total bilirubin, AST, and creatinine; and cardiac function as measured by left ventricular ejection function (LVEF). Patients should be carefully monitored during treatment for possible clinical complications due to myelosuppression. Supportive care may be necessary for the treatment of severe neutropenia and severe infectious complications. Monitoring for potential cardiotoxicity is also important, especially with greater cumulative exposure to epirubicin.

➤*Hematologic toxicity:* A dose-dependent, reversible leukopenia and/or neutropenia is the predominant manifestation of hematologic toxicity associated with epirubicin and represents the most common acute dose-limiting toxicity of this drug. In most cases, the white blood cell (WBC) nadir is reached 10 to 14 days from drug administration. Leukopenia/neutropenia is usually transient, with WBC and neutrophil counts generally returning to normal values by day 21 after drug administration. As with other cytotoxic agents, epirubicin HCl at the recommended dose in combination with cyclophosphamide and fluorouracil can produce severe leukopenia and neutropenia. Severe thrombocytopenia and anemia may also occur. Clinical consequences of severe myelosuppression include fever, infection, septicemia, septic shock, hemorrhage, tissue hypoxia, symptomatic anemia, or death. If myelosuppressive complications occur, appropriate supportive measures (eg, intravenous antibiotics, colony-stimulating factors, transfusions) may be required. Myelosuppression requires careful monitoring. Total and differential WBC, red blood cell (RBC), and platelet counts should be assessed before and during each cycle of therapy with epirubicin HCl.

➤*Cardiac function:* Cardiotoxicity is a known risk of anthracycline treatment. Anthracycline-induced cardiac toxicity may be manifested by early (or acute) or late (delayed) events. Early cardiac toxicity of epirubicin consists mainly of sinus tachycardia or ECG abnormalities such as non-specific ST-T wave changes, but tachyarrhythmias, including premature ventricular contractions and ventricular tachycardia, bradycardia, as well as atrioventricular and bundle-branch block have also been reported. These effects do not usually predict subsequent development of delayed cardiotoxicity, are rarely of clinical importance, and are generally not considered an indication for the suspension of epirubicin treatment. Delayed cardiac toxicity results from a characteristic cardiomyopathy that is manifested by reduced LVEF and/or signs and symptoms of congestive heart failure (CHF) (eg, tachycardia, dyspnea, pulmonary edema, dependent edema, hepatomegaly, ascites, pleural effusion, gallop rhythm). Life-threatening CHF is the most severe form of anthracycline-induced cardiomyopathy. This toxicity appears to be dependent on the cumulative dose of epirubicin HCl and represents the cumulative dose-limiting toxicity of the drug. If it occurs, delayed cardiotoxicity usually develops late in the course of therapy with epirubicin HCl or within 2 to 3 months after completion of treatment, but later events (several months to years after treatment termination) have been reported.

Given the risk of cardiomyopathy, a cumulative dose of 900 mg/m^2 epirubicin HCl should be exceeded only with extreme caution. Risk factors (active or dormant cardiovascular disease, prior or concomitant radiotherapy to the mediastinal/pericardial area, previous therapy with other anthracyclines or anthracenediones, concomitant use of other drugs with the ability to suppress cardiac contractility) may increase the risk of cardiac toxicity. Although not formally tested, it is probable that the toxicity of epirubicin and other anthracyclines or anthracenediones is additive. Cardiac toxicity with epirubicin HCl may occur at lower cumulative doses whether or not cardiac risk factors are present.

Although endomyocardial biopsy is recognized as the most sensitive diagnostic tool to detect anthracycline-induced cardiomyopathy, this invasive examination is not practically performed on a routine basis. Electrocardiogram (ECG) changes such as dysrhythmias, a reduction of the QRS voltage, or a prolongation beyond normal limits of the systolic time interval may be indicative of anthracycline-induced cardiomyopathy, but ECG is not a sensitive or specific method for following anthracycline-related cardiotoxicity. The risk of serious cardiac impairment may be decreased through regular monitoring of LVEF during the course of treatment with prompt discontinuation of epirubicin HCl at the first sign of impaired function. The preferred method for repeated assessment of cardiac function is evaluation of LVEF measured by multi-gated radionuclide angiography (MUGA) or echocardiography (ECHO). A baseline cardiac evaluation with an ECG and a MUGA scan or an ECHO is recommended, especially in patients with risk factors for increased cardiac toxicity. Repeated MUGA or ECHO determinations of LVEF should be performed, particularly with higher, cumulative anthracycline doses. The technique used for assessment should be consistent through follow-up. In patients with risk factors, particularly prior anthracycline or anthracenedione use, the monitoring of cardiac function must be particularly strict and the risk-benefit of continuing treatment with epirubicin HCl in patients with impaired cardiac function must be carefully evaluated.

➤*Secondary leukemia:* The occurrence of secondary acute myelogenous leukemia, with or without a preleukemic phase, has been reported in patients treated with anthracyclines. Secondary leukemia is more common when such drugs are given in combination with DNA-damaging antineoplastic agents, when patients have been heavily pretreated with cytotoxic drugs, or when doses of the anthracyclines have been escalated. These leukemias can have a short 1- to 3-year latency period. An analysis of 3844 patients who received adjuvant treatment with epirubicin in controlled clinical trials, showed a cumulative risk of secondary acute myelogenous leukemia of about 0.2% (approximately 95% CI: 0.05 to 0.4) at 3 years and approximately 0.8% (approximately 95% CI: 0.3 to 1.2) at 5 years. Epirubicin HCl is mutagenic, clastogenic, and carcinogenic in animals.

➤*Tumor lysis syndrome:* As with other cytotoxic agents, epirubicin HCl may induce hyperuricemia as a consequence of the extensive purine catabolism that accompanies drug-induced rapid lysis of highly chemosensitive neoplastic cells (tumor lysis syndrome). Other metabolic abnormalities may also occur. While not generally a problem in patients with breast cancer, physicians should consider the potential for tumor lysis syndrome in potentially susceptible patients and should consider monitoring serum uric acid, potassium, calcium phosphate, and creatinine immediately after initial chemotherapy administration. Hydration, urine alkalinization, and prophylaxis with allopurinol to prevent hyperuricemia may minimize potential complications of tumor lysis syndrome.

➤*Injection-site reactions:* Epirubicin HCl injection is administered by intravenous infusion. Venous sclerosis may result from an injection into a small vessel or from repeated injections into the same vein. Extravasation of epirubicin during the infusion may cause local pain, severe tissue lesions (vesication, severe cellulitis) and necrosis. It is recommended that epirubicin HCl be slowly administered into the tubing of a freely running intravenous infusion usually between 3 and 20 minutes depending upon dosage and volume of the infusion solution. If possible, veins over joints or in extremities with compromised venous or lymphatic drainage should be avoided. A burning or stinging sensation may be indicative of perivenous infiltration, and the infusion should be immediately terminated and restarted in another vein. Perivenous infiltration may occur without causing pain.

Facial flushing, as well as local erythematous streaking along the vein, may be indicative of excessively rapid administration. It may precede local phlebitis or thrombophlebitis.

➤*Prophylactic antibiotics:* Patients administered the 120 mg/m^2 regimen of epirubicin HCl as a component of combination chemotherapy should also receive prophylactic antibiotic therapy with trimethoprim-sulfamethoxazole or a fluoroquinolone.

➤*Antiemetics:* Epirubicin is emetigenic. Antiemetics may reduce nausea and vomiting; prophylactic use of antiemetics should be considered before

EPIRUBICIN HYDROCHLORIDE — INJECTION

administration of epirubicin HCl, particularly when given in conjunction with other emetigenic drugs.

➤*Inflammatory recall reactions:* As with other anthracyclines, administration of epirubicin HCl after previous radiation therapy may induce an inflammatory recall reaction at the site of the irradiation.

➤*Thrombophlebitis/Thromboembolism:* As with other cytotoxic agents, thrombophlebitis and thromboembolic phenomena, including pulmonary embolism (in some cases fatal) have been coincidentally reported with the use of epirubicin.

➤*Extravasation:* See Administration and Dosage for more information.

➤*Renal function impairment:* See Administration and Dosage for more information.

➤*Hepatic function impairment:* See the Warning box for more information.

➤*Pregnancy: Category D.* Epirubicin HCl may cause fetal harm when administered to a pregnant woman. Administration of 0.8 mg/kg/day intravenously of epirubicin to rats (about 0.04 times the maximum recommended single human dose on a body surface area basis) during days 5 to 15 of gestation was embryotoxic (increased resorptions and postimplantation loss) and caused fetal growth retardation (decreased body weight), but was not teratogenic up to this dose. Administration of 2 mg/kg/day intravenously of epirubicin to rats (approximately 0.1 times the maximum recommended single human dose on a body surface area basis) on days 9 and 10 of gestation was embryotoxic (increased late resorptions, postimplantation losses, and dead fetuses; and decreased live fetuses), retarded fetal growth (decreased body weight), and caused decreased placental weight. This dose was also teratogenic, causing numerous external (anal atresia, misshapen tail, abnormal genital tubercle), visceral (primarily gastrointestinal, urinary, and cardiovascular systems), and skeletal (deformed long bones and girdles, rib abnormalities, irregular spinal ossification) malformations. Administration of intravenous epirubicin to rabbits at doses up to 0.2 mg/kg/day (approximately 0.02 times the maximum recommended single human dose on a body surface area basis) during days 6 to 18 of gestation was not embryotoxic or teratogenic, but a maternally toxic dose of 0.32 mg/kg/day increased abortions and delayed ossification. Administration of a maternally toxic intravenous dose of 1 mg/kg/day epirubicin to rabbits (approximately 0.1 times the maximum recommended single human dose on a body surface area basis) on days 10 to 12 of gestation induced abortion, but no other signs of embryofetal toxicity or teratogenicity were observed. When doses up to 0.5 mg/kg/day epirubicin were administered to rat dams from day 17 of gestation to day 21 after delivery (approximately 0.025 times the maximum recommended single human dose on a body surface area basis), no permanent changes were observed in the development, functional activity, behavior, or reproductive performance of the offspring.

There are no adequate and well-controlled studies in pregnant women. Two pregnancies have been reported in women taking epirubicin. A 34-year-old woman, 28 weeks pregnant at her diagnosis of breast cancer, was treated with cyclophosphamide and epirubicin every 3 weeks for 3 cycles. She received the last dose at 34 weeks of pregnancy and delivered a healthy baby at 35 weeks. A second 34-year-old woman with breast cancer metastatic to the liver was randomized to FEC-50 but was removed from study because of pregnancy. She experienced a spontaneous abortion. If epirubicin is used during pregnancy, or if the patient becomes pregnant while taking this drug, the patient should be apprised of the potential hazard to the fetus. Women of childbearing potential should be advised to avoid becoming pregnant.

Fertility impairment – Although experimental data are not available, epirubicin HCl could induce chromosomal damage in human spermatozoa due to its genotoxic potential. Men undergoing treatment with epirubicin HCl should use effective contraceptive methods. Epirubicin HCl may cause irreversible amenorrhea (premature menopause) in premenopausal women.

➤*Lactation:* Epirubicin was excreted into the milk of rats treated with 0.5 mg/kg/day of epirubicin during peri- and postnatal periods. It is not known whether epirubicin is excreted in human milk. Because many drugs, including other anthracyclines, are excreted in human milk and because of the potential for serious adverse reactions in nursing infants from epirubicin, mothers should discontinue nursing prior to taking this drug.

➤*Children:* The safety and effectiveness of epirubicin in pediatric patients have not been established in adequate and well-controlled clinical trials. Pediatric patients may be at greater risk for anthracycline-induced acute manifestations of cardiotoxicity and for chronic CHF.

➤*Elderly:* Although a lower starting dose of epirubicin HCl was not used in trials in elderly female patients, particular care should be taken in monitoring toxicity when epirubicin HCl is administered to female patients greater than or equal to 70 years of age.

➤*Monitoring:* Blood counts, including absolute neutrophil counts and liver function should be assessed before and during each cycle of therapy with epirubicin. Repeated evaluations of LVEF should be performed during therapy.

Drug Interactions

➤*Cytotoxic drugs:* Epirubicin HCl when used in combination with other cytotoxic drugs may show on-treatment additive toxicity, especially hematologic and gastrointestinal effects.

➤*Cardioactive compounds:* Concomitant use of epirubicin HCl with other cardioactive compounds that could cause heart failure (eg, calcium channel blockers) requires close monitoring of cardiac function throughout treatment.

➤*Radiation therapy:* There are few data regarding the coadministration of radiation therapy and epirubicin. In adjuvant trials of epirubicin-containing CEF-120 or FEC-100 chemotherapies, breast irradiation was delayed until after chemotherapy was completed. This practice resulted in no apparent increase in local breast cancer recurrence relative to published accounts in the literature. A small number of patients received epirubicin-based chemotherapy concomitantly with radiation therapy but had chemotherapy interrupted in order to avoid potential overlapping toxicities. It is likely that use of epirubicin with radiotherapy may sensitize tissues to the cytotoxic actions of irradiation. Administration of epirubicin HCl after previous radiation therapy may induce an inflammatory recall reaction at the site of the irradiation.

➤*Cimetidine:* Cimetidine increased the AUC of epirubicin by 50%. Cimetidine treatment should be stopped during treatment with epirubicin.

Adverse Reactions

Epirubicin has moderate to high potential for nausea and vomiting.

➤*Delayed reactions:* The table below describes the incidence of delayed adverse reactions in patients participating in the MA-5 and GFEA-05 trials.

Epirubicin Long-Term Adverse Reactions in Patients with Early Breast Cancer (%)

Adverse reaction	FEC-100/CEF-120 (n = 620)	FEC-50 (n = 280)	CMF (n = 360)
Cardiac toxicity			
Asymptomatic drops in LVEF	1.8%	1.4%	0.8%
CHF	1.5%	0.4%	0.3%
Leukemia			
AML	0.8%	0%	0.3%

Two cases of acute lymphoid leukemia (ALL) were also observed in patients receiving epirubicin. However, an association between anthracyclines such as epirubicin and ALL has not been clearly established.

➤*Overview of acute and delayed toxicities:*

Cardiovascular – See Warnings/Precautions for more information.

Dermatologic – Alopecia occurs frequently, but is usually reversible, with hair regrowth occurring within 2 to 3 months from the termination of therapy. Flushes, skin and nail hyperpigmentation, photosensitivity, and hypersensitivity to irradiated skin (radiation-recall reaction) have been observed. Urticaria and anaphylaxis have been reported in patients treated with epirubicin; signs and symptoms of these reactions may vary from skin rash and pruritus to fever, chills, and shock.

GI – A dose-dependent mucositis (mainly oral stomatitis, less often esophagitis) may occur in patients treated with epirubicin. Clinical manifestations of mucositis may include a pain or burning sensation, erythema, erosions, ulcerations, bleeding, or infections. Mucositis generally appears early after drug administration and, if severe, may progress over a few days to mucosal ulcerations; most patients recover from this adverse event by the third week of therapy. Hyperpigmentation of the oral mucosa may also occur.

Nausea, vomiting, and occasionally diarrhea and abdominal pain can also occur. Severe vomiting and diarrhea may produce dehydration. Antiemetics may reduce nausea and vomiting; prophylactic use of antiemetics should be considered before therapy, particularly if epirubicin is given in conjunction with other emetigenic drugs.

Hematologic – See Warnings/Precautions for more information.

Local – Venous sclerosis may result from an injection into a small vessel or from repeated injections into the same vein. Extravasation of epirubicin during the infusion may cause local pain, severe tissue lesions (vesication, severe cellulitis) and necrosis.

Secondary leukemia – See Warnings/Precautions for more information.

Overdosage

➤*Symptoms:* A 36-year-old man with non-Hodgkin's lymphoma received a daily 95 mg/m^2 dose of epirubicin HCl injection for 5 consecutive days. Five days later, he developed bone marrow aplasia, grade 4 mucositis, and gastrointestinal bleeding. No signs of acute cardiac toxicity were observed. He was treated with antibiotics, colony-stimulating factors, and antifungal agents, and recovered completely. A 63-year-old women with breast cancer and liver metastasis received a single 320 mg/m^2 dose of epirubicin HCl. She was hospitalized with hyperthermia and developed multiple organ failure (respiratory and renal), with lactic acidosis, increased lactate dehydrogenase, and anuria. Death occurred within 24 hours after administration of epirubicin HCl. Additional instances of administration of doses higher than recommended have been reported at doses ranging from 150 to 250 mg/m^2. The observed adverse reactions in these patients were qualitatively similar to known toxicities of epirubicin. Most of the patients recovered with appropriate supportive care.

➤*Treatment:* If an overdose occurs, supportive treatment (including antibiotic therapy, blood and platelet transfusions, colony-stimulating factors, and intensive care as needed) should be provided until the recovery of toxicities. Delayed CHF has been observed months after anthracycline administration. Patients must be observed carefully over time for signs of CHF and provided with appropriate supportive therapy.

EPIRUBICIN HYDROCHLORIDE — INJECTION

Patient Information

Patients should be informed of the expected adverse effects of epirubicin, including gastrointestinal symptoms (nausea, vomiting, diarrhea, and stomatitis) and potential neutropenic complications.

Patients should consult their physicians if vomiting, dehydration, fever, evidence of infection, symptoms of CHF, or injection-site pain occurs following therapy with epirubicin HCl. Patients should be informed that they will almost certainly develop alopecia.

Patients should be advised that their urine may appear red for 1 to 2 days after administration of epirubicin HCl and that they should not be alarmed.

Patients should understand that there is a risk of irreversible myocardial damage associated with treatment with epirubicin HCl, as well as a risk of treatment-related leukemia.

Because epirubicin may induce chromosomal damage in sperm, men undergoing treatment with epirubicin HCl should use effective contraceptive methods.

Women treated with epirubicin HCl may develop irreversible amenorrhea, or premature menopause.

IDARUBICIN HYDROCHLORIDE

Rx	**Idarubicin Hydrochloride** (GensiaSicor)	**Injection:** 1 mg/mL	Preservative-free. In 5, 10, and 20 mL single-use vials.
Rx	**Idamycin PFS** (Pfizer)		Preservative-free. In 5, 10, and 20 mL single-use vials.

IDARUBICIN HYDROCHLORIDE — INJECTION

WARNING

Idarubicin HCl should be given slowly into a freely flowing IV infusion; it must never be given IM or subcutaneously. Severe local tissue necrosis can occur if there is extravasation during administration.

As is the case with other anthracyclines, the use of idarubicin HCl can cause myocardial toxicity leading to congestive heart failure. Cardiac toxicity is more common in patients who have received prior anthracyclines or who have preexisting cardiac disease.

As is usual with antileukemic agents, severe myelosuppression occurs when idarubicin HCl is used at effective therapeutic doses.

It is recommended that idarubicin HCl be administered only under the supervision of a physician who is experienced in leukemia chemotherapy and in facilities with laboratory and supportive resources adequate to monitor drug tolerance and protect and maintain a patient compromised by drug toxicity. The physician and institution must be capable of responding rapidly and completely to severe hemorrhagic conditions or overwhelming infection.

Dosage should be reduced in patients with impaired hepatic or renal function. In patients with hepatic or renal impairment, a dose reduction of idarubicin hydrochloride should be considered. Idarubicin hydrochloride should not be administered if the bilirubin level exceeds 5 mg/dL.

Indications

➤*Acute myeloid leukemia:* In combination with other approved antileukemic drugs for the treatment of acute myeloid leukemia (AML) in adults. This includes French-American-British (FAB) classifications M1 through M7.

➤*Off-label uses:* Acute lymphocytic leukemia, chronic myelogenous leukemia, breast cancer, and autologous hematopoietic stem cell transplantation (HSCT). In children, idarubicin has been used safely and effectively for acute lymphocytic and nonlymphocytic leukemia and solid tumors. (See Administration and Dosage.)

Administration and Dosage

➤*Maximum dose:*

Adults – There is no well-established maximum dose for the approved indication according to the prescribing information. However, a maximum lifetime cumulative dosage has been suggested off-label. (See Off-label dosing.)

➤*Adults:*

Acute myeloid leukemia –

Induction therapy:

• *Initial dosage* – 12 mg/m² daily for 3 days by slow (10 to 15 minute) IV injection.

• *Concomitant therapy* – Give in combination with cytarabine. Cytarabine may be given as 100 mg/m² daily by continuous infusion for 7 days or as cytarabine 25 mg/m² IV bolus followed by cytarabine 200 mg/m² daily for 5 days continuous infusion.

• *Second course of therapy* – In patients with unequivocal evidence of leukemia after the first induction course, a second course may be administered. Administration of the second course should be delayed in patients who experience severe mucositis, until recovery from this toxicity has occurred, and a dose reduction of 25% is recommended.

Off-label dosing –

Acute myeloid leukemia:

• *Consolidation therapy* – 10 to 12 mg/m²/day IV for 2 days.

Autologous hematopoietic stem cell transplantation (combination therapy): 20 mg/m²/day continuous IV infusion for 3 days. An alternate regimen is 21 mg/m²/day continuous IV infusion for 2 days.

➤*Children:*

Off-label dosing –

Acute lymphocytic leukemia: As induction therapy in combination with other chemotherapeutic drugs, the dosage is idarubicin 10 to 12 mg/m²/day IV for 3 days during each treatment course; may repeat courses every 3 weeks. Delay therapy until recovery from mucositis occurs.

Acute nonlymphocytic leukemia: As induction therapy in combination with other chemotherapeutic drugs, the dosage is idarubicin 10 to 12 mg/m²/day IV for 3 days during each treatment course; may repeat courses every 3 weeks. Delay therapy until recovery from mucositis occurs.

Solid tumors: 5 mg/m²/day IV for 3 days during each treatment course; may repeat courses every 3 weeks.

➤*Renal function impairment:* For patients with renal function impairment, a dosage reduction of idarubicin should be considered if the creatinine levels are above the normal range. For patients with serum creatinine greater than 2 mg/dL, give 75% of usual dose.

Dialysis – Conventional hemodialysis and peritoneal dialysis are ineffective (0% to 24%) in removing idarubicin.

➤*Hepatic function impairment:* For patients with hepatic function impairment, a dosage reduction of idarubicin should be considered. Idarubicin should not be administered if the bilirubin level exceeds 5 mg/dL. If serum bilirubin is 2.6 to 5 mg/dL, then give 50% of usual dose. If AST is between 60 and 180 units/L, give 50% of usual dose.

➤*Maximum lifetime cumulative dose:* Risk of cardiotoxicity increases with the cumulative idarubicin dose. No maximum cumulative lifetime dose for cardiotoxicity has yet been determined. However, some clinicians recommend not exceeding a lifetime maximum dose of idarubicin 150 mg/m².

➤*Preparation for administration:* Idarubicin is considered a cytotoxic agent. Follow safe handling procedures when preparing, administering, or dispensing idarubicin.

Caution in handling of the solution must be exercised as skin reactions associated with idarubicin may occur. Skin accidently exposed to idarubicin should be washed thoroughly with soap and water and if the eyes are involved, standard irrigation techniques should be used immediately. The use of goggles, gloves, and protective gowns is recommended during preparation and administration of the drug.

Further dilution is not necessary. Solution is a red-orange color.

➤*Administration:* Idarubicin should be administered slowly (over 10 to 15 minutes) by IV push injection or IV sidearm into the tubing of a freely running IV infusion of sodium chloride 0.9% injection or dextrose 5% injection. The tubing should be attached to a butterfly needle or other suitable device and inserted preferably into a large vein.

Idarubicin should not be given IM or subcutaneously.

➤*Extravasation:* Severe local tissue necrosis can occur if there is extravasation during administration. Care in the administration of idarubicin will reduce the chance of perivenous infiltration. It may also decrease the chance of local reactions such as urticaria and erythematous streaking. During IV administration of idarubicin, extravasation may occur with or without an accompanying stinging or burning sensation even if blood returns well on aspiration of the infusion needle.

If signs or symptoms of extravasation occur, stop the infusion immediately. If possible, withdraw 3 to 5 mL of blood to remove some of the drug. Remove the infusion needle. Ice compresses may be applied to the site for 15 minutes every 6 hours for 48 hours. Dexrazoxane (*Totect*) is FDA-approved for the treatment of extravasation resulting from anthracycline IV therapy. The first infusion of dexrazoxane should be administered as soon as possible and within the first 6 hours following the extravasation. Topical cooling, such as ice packs, should be removed for at least 15 minutes prior to and during dexrazoxane administration. Concurrent extravasation treatment, such as topical dimethyl sulfoxide (DMSO) application, should not be used in conjunction with dexrazoxane, and if administered, may worsen the extravasation-induced tissue injury. The recommended dose of dexrazoxane for day 1 is 1,000 mg/m² (up to 2,000 mg), the dose for day 2 is 1,000 mg/m² (up to 2,000 mg), and the dose for day 3 is 500 mg/m² (up to 1,000 mg). Dexrazoxane is administered as an IV infusion over 1 to 2 hours.

Delineate the infiltrated area on the patient's skin with a felt-tip marker. Elevate for 48 hours above heart level using a sling or stockinette dressing with an observation window cut in the dressing. Avoid pressure or friction. Do not rub the area. Observe for signs of increased erythema, pain, or skin necrosis. If increased symptoms occur, consult a plastic surgeon. Ensure that no medication is given distally to extravasation site. After 48 hours, encourage the patient to use the extremity normally to promote full range of motion.

IDARUBICIN HYDROCHLORIDE — INJECTION

➤*Admixture compatibility:* Unless specific compatibility data are available, idarubicin should not be mixed with other drugs. Precipitation occurs with heparin. Flush well with a heparin-free solution before and after idarubicin administration. Prolonged contact with any solution of an alkaline pH will result in degradation of the drug.

➤*Storage/Stability:* Store under refrigeration 2° to 8°C (36° to 46°F), and protect from light. Retain in carton until the time of use. Preservative-free; use solution within 24 hours of opening the vial.

Discard vial within 6 hours of the initial needle puncture if opened within an ISO Class 5 biological safety cabinet, or within 1 hour of the initial needle puncture if opened outside of such an environment, based on the USP Chapter <797> standards.

Actions

➤*Pharmacology:* Idarubicin hydrochloride is a DNA-intercalating analog of daunorubicin which has an inhibitory effect on nucleic acid synthesis and interacts with the enzyme topoisomerase II. The absence of a methoxy group at position 4 of the anthracycline structure gives the compound a high lipophilicity which results in an increased rate of cellular uptake compared with other anthracyclines.

➤*Pharmacokinetics:*

Absorption – Pharmacokinetic studies have been performed in adult leukemia patients with normal renal and hepatic function following IV administration of 10 to 12 mg/m^2 of idarubicin daily for 3 to 4 days as a single agent or combined with cytarabine. The plasma concentrations of idarubicin are best described by a 2 or 3 compartment open model.

Distribution – The disposition profile shows a rapid distributive phase with a very high volume of distribution presumably reflecting extensive tissue binding. Studies of cellular (nucleated blood and bone marrow cells) drug concentrations in leukemia patients have shown that peak cellular idarubicin concentrations are reached a few minutes after injection. Concentrations of idarubicin and idarubicinol in nucleated blood and bone marrow cells are greater than 100 times the plasma concentrations. Idarubicin disappearance rates in plasma and cells were comparable with a terminal half-life of about 15 hours. The terminal half-life of idarubicinol in cells was about 72 hours. The extent of drug and metabolic accumulation predicted in leukemia patients for days 2 and 3 of dosing, based on the mean plasma levels and half-life obtained after the first dose, is 1.7- and 2.3-fold, respectively, and suggests no change in kinetics following a daily × 3 regimen. The percentages of idarubicin and idarubicinol bound to human plasma proteins averaged 97% and 94%, respectively, at concentrations similar to maximum plasma levels obtained in the pharmacokinetic studies. The binding is concentration independent. The plasma clearance is twice the expected hepatic plasma flow indicating extensive extrahepatic metabolism.

Metabolism – The primary active metabolite formed is idarubicinol. As idarubicinol has cytotoxic activity, it presumably contributes to the effects of idarubicin.

Excretion – The elimination rate of idarubicin from plasma is slow with an estimated mean terminal half-life of 22 hours (range, 4 to 48 hours) when used as a single agent and 20 hours (range, 7 to 38 hours) when used in combination with cytarabine. The elimination of the primary active metabolite, idarubicin, is considerably slower than that of the parent drug with an estimated mean terminal half-life that exceeds 45 hours; hence, its plasma levels are sustained for a period greater than 8 days. The drug is eliminated predominately by biliary and to a lesser extent by renal excretion, mostly in the form of idarubicinol.

Special populations –

Renal function impairment: See Warnings/Precautions for more information.

Hepatic function impairment: See Warnings/Precautions for more information.

Warnings/Precautions

➤*Bone marrow suppression:* Idarubicin HCl is a potent bone marrow suppressant. Idarubicin HCl should not be given to patients with preexisting bone marrow suppression induced by previous drug therapy or radiotherapy unless the benefit warrants the risk.

➤*Severe myelosuppression:* Severe myelosuppression will occur in all patients given a therapeutic dose of this agent for induction, consolidation or maintenance. Careful hematologic monitoring is required. Deaths due to infection or bleeding have been reported during the period of severe myelosuppression. Facilities with laboratory and supportive resources adequate to monitor drug tolerability and protect and maintain a patient compromised by drug toxicity should be available. It must be possible to treat rapidly and completely a severe hemorrhagic condition or a severe infection.

➤*Cardiotoxicity:* Preexisting heart disease and previous therapy with anthracyclines at high cumulative doses or other potentially cardiotoxic agents are cofactors for increased risk of idarubicin-induced cardiac toxicity and the benefit to risk ratio of idarubicin therapy in such patients should be weighed before starting treatment with idarubicin HCl.

Myocardial toxicity as manifested by potentially fatal congestive heart failure, acute life-threatening arrhythmias or other cardiomyopathies may occur following therapy with idarubicin HCl. Appropriate therapeutic measures for the management of congestive heart failure or arrhythmias are indicated.

Cardiac function should be carefully monitored during treatment in order to minimize the risk of cardiac toxicity of the type described for other anthracycline compounds. The risk of such myocardial toxicity may be higher following concomitant or previous radiation to the mediastinal-pericardial area or in patients with anemia, bone marrow depression, infections, leukemic pericarditis or myocarditis. While there are no reliable means for predicting congestive heart failure, cardiomyopathy induced by anthracyclines is usually associated with a decrease of the left ventricular ejection fraction (LVEF) from pretreatment baseline values.

➤*Extravasation:* See Administration and Dosage for more information.

➤*Renal/Hepatic function impairment:* Since hepatic or renal function impairment can affect the disposition of idarubicin HCl, liver and kidney function should be evaluated with conventional clinical laboratory tests (using serum bilirubin and serum creatinine as indicators) prior to and during treatment. In a number of phase III clinical trials, treatment was not given if bilirubin or creatinine serum levels exceeded 2 mg/dL. However, in 1 phase III trial, patients with bilirubin levels between 2.6 mg/dL and 5 mg/dL received the anthracycline with a 50% reduction in dose. Dose reduction of idarubicin HCl should be considered if the bilirubin or creatinine levels are above the normal range (greater than 5 mg/dL).

➤*Pregnancy: Category D.* Idarubicin was embryotoxic and teratogenic in the rat at a dose of 1.2 mg/m^2/day or one-tenth the human dose, which was nontoxic to dams, idarubicin was embryotoxic but not teratogenic in the rabbit even at a dose of 2.4 mg/m^2/day or two-tenths the human dose, which was toxic to dams.

There is no conclusive information about idarubicin adversely affecting human fertility or causing teratogenesis. There has been 1 report of a fetal fatality after maternal exposure to idarubicin during the second trimester.

There are no adequate and well-controlled studies in pregnant women. If idarubicin HCl is to be used during pregnancy, or if the patient becomes pregnant during therapy, the patient should be apprised of the potential hazard to the fetus. Women of childbearing potential should be advised to avoid pregnancy.

➤*Lactation:* It is not known whether this drug is excreted in human milk. Because many drugs are excreted in human milk and because of the potential for serious adverse reactions in nursing infants from idarubicin, mothers should discontinue nursing prior to taking this drug.

➤*Children:* Safety and effectiveness in children have not been established.

➤*Elderly:* Patients over 60 years of age who were undergoing induction therapy experienced congestive heart failure, serious arrhythmias, chest pain, MI, and asymptomatic declines in LVEF more frequently than younger patients.

➤*Monitoring:* Frequent complete blood counts and monitoring of hepatic and renal function tests are recommended.

Therapy with idarubicin HCl requires close observation of the patient and careful laboratory monitoring. Hyperuricemia secondary to rapid lysis of leukemic cells may be induced. Appropriate measures must be taken to prevent hyperuricemia and to control any systemic infection before beginning therapy.

Adverse Reactions

Idarubicin is considered to have moderate emetogenic potential (30% to 60% incidence of emesis).

Idarubicin Induction Phase Adverse Reactions (%)

Adverse reactions	IDR (n = 110)	DNR (n = 118)
Infection	95%	97%
Nausea/vomiting	82%	80%
Hair loss	77%	72%
Abdominal cramps/diarrhea	73%	68%
Hemorrhage	63%	65%
Mucositis	50%	55%
Dermatologic	46%	40%
Mental status	41%	34%
Pulmonary (clinical)	39%	39%
Fever (not elsewhere classified)	26%	28%
Headache	20%	24%
Cardiac (clinical)	16%	24%
Neurologic (peripheral nerves)	7%	9%
Pulmonary allergy	2%	4%
Seizure	4%	5%
Cerebellar	4%	4%

The duration of aplasia and incidence of mucositis were greater on the IDR arm than the DNR arm, especially during consolidation in some US controlled trials.

➤*Cardiovascular:* Congestive heart failure (frequently attributed to fluid overload), serious arrhythmias including atrial fibrillation, chest pain, MI and asymptomatic declines in LVEF have been reported in patients undergoing induction therapy for AML. Myocardial insufficiency and arrhythmias were usually reversible and occurred in the setting of sepsis, anemia and aggressive IV fluid administration. The events were reported more frequently in patients greater than 60 years of age and in those with preexisting cardiac disease.

IDARUBICIN HYDROCHLORIDE — INJECTION

➤*Dermatologic:* Alopecia was reported frequently and dermatologic reactions including generalized rash, urticaria and a bullous erythrodermatous rash of the palms and soles have occurred. The dermatologic reactions were usually attributed to concomitant antibiotic therapy. Recall of skin reaction due to prior radiotherapy has occurred with idarubicin HCl injection administration.

➤*GI:* Nausea or vomiting, mucositis, abdominal pain and diarrhea were reported frequently, but were severe (equivalent to WHO grade 4) in less than 5% of patients. Severe enterocolitis with perforation has been reported rarely. The risk of perforation may be increased by instrumental intervention. The possibility of perforation should be considered in patients who develop severe abdominal pain and appropriate steps for diagnosis and management should be taken.

➤*Hepatic:* Changes in hepatic function tests have been observed. These changes were usually transient and occurred in the setting of sepsis and while patients were receiving potentially hepatotoxic antibiotics and antifungal agents. Severe changes in hepatic function (equivalent to WHO grade 4) occurred in less than 5% of patients.

➤*Immunologic:* Severe myelosuppression is the major toxicity associated with idarubicin HCl therapy, but this effect of the drug is required in order to eradicate the leukemic clone. During the period of myelosuppression, patients are at risk of developing infection and bleeding which may be life-threatening or fatal.

➤*Local:* Local reactions including hives at the injection site have been reported.

➤*Renal:* Changes in renal function tests have been observed. These changes were usually transient and occurred in the setting of sepsis and while patients were receiving potentially nephrotoxic antibiotics and antifungal agents. Severe changes in renal function (equivalent to WHO grade 4) occurred in no more than 1% of patients.

Overdosage

➤*Symptoms:* Two cases of fatal overdosage in patients receiving therapy for AML have been reported. The doses were 135 mg/m^2 over 3 days and 45 mg/m^2 of idarubicin and 90 mg/m^2 of daunorubicin over a 3-day period.

It is anticipated that overdosage with idarubicin will result in severe and prolonged myelosuppression and possibly in increased severity of GI toxicity. Adequate supportive care including platelet transfusions, antibiotics and symptomatic treatment of mucositis is required. The effect of acute overdose on cardiac function is not fully known, but severe arrhythmia occurred in 1 of the 2 patients exposed. It is anticipated that very high doses of idarubicin may cause acute cardiac toxicity and may be associated with a higher incidence of delayed cardiac failure.

➤*Treatment:* There is no known antidote to idarubicin HCl injection.

Disposition studies with idarubicin in patients undergoing dialysis have not been carried out. The profound multicompartment behavior, extensive extravascular distribution and tissue binding, coupled with the low unbound fraction available in the plasma pool make it unlikely that therapeutic efficacy or toxicity would be altered by conventional peritoneal or hemodialysis.

VALRUBICIN

Rx	**Valstar** (Indevus)	**Injection, solution, concentrate**: 40 mg/mL[a]	Preservative free. In single-use vials.

[a] In 50% polyoxyl castor oil/50% dehydrated alcohol.

VALRUBICIN — INTRAVESICAL

Indications

➤*Bacillus Calmette-Guérin-refractory carcinoma in situ:* For intravesical therapy of Bacillus Calmette-Guérin (BCG)-refractory carcinoma in situ (CIS) of the urinary bladder in patients for whom immediate cystectomy would be associated with unacceptable morbidity or mortality.

Administration and Dosage

➤*Adults:*

Bacillus Calmette-Guérin-refractory carcinoma in situ – 800 mg administered intravesically once a week for 6 weeks. Administration should be delayed at least 2 weeks after transurethral resection and/or fulguration.

➤*Preparation for administration:* Valrubicin is considered a cytotoxic agent. Follow safe handling procedures when preparing, administering, or dispensing valrubicin.

Allow solution to warm slowly to room temperature. Do not heat or microwave.

For each instillation, four 5 mL vials (valrubicin 200 mg per 5 mL vial) should be allowed to warm slowly to room temperature but should not be heated. 20 mL of valrubicin should then be withdrawn from the 4 vials and diluted with 55 mL of sodium chloride 0.9% injection, providing 75 mL of a diluted valrubicin solution.

Valrubicin for intravesical instillation is a clear red solution. It should be visually inspected for particulate matter and discoloration prior to administration. At temperatures below 4°C (39°F), polyoxyl castor oil may begin to form a waxy precipitate. If this happens, the vial should be warmed in the hand until the solution is clear. If particulate matter is still seen, valrubicin should not be administered.

Contact toxicity, common and severe with other anthracyclines, is not typical with valrubicin and, when observed, has been mild. Skin reactions may occur with accidental exposure, and the use of gloves during dose preparation and administration is recommended. Irritation of the eye has also been reported with accidental exposure. If this happens, the eye should be flushed with water immediately and thoroughly.

Valrubicin sterile solution contains polyoxyl castor oil, which has been known to cause leaching of di(2-ethylhexyl)phthalate (DEHP), a hepatotoxic plasticizer, from polyvinyl chloride (PVC) bags and intravenous tubing. Valrubicin solutions should be prepared and stored in glass, polypropylene, or polyolefin containers and tubing. It is recommended that non-DEHP–containing administration sets, such as those that are polyethylene-lined, be used.

Spills should be cleaned up with undiluted chlorine bleach.

➤*Administration:* Valrubicin for intravesical instillation is intended for intravesical administration in the urinary bladder. To ensure that the patient can retain the solution for the necessary 2-hour period, patients should not drink fluids for several hours before administration. They should void before instillation of valrubicin into the bladder. A urethral catheter should be inserted into the patient's bladder under aseptic conditions, the bladder drained, and the diluted valrubicin 75 mL solution instilled slowly via gravity flow over a period of several minutes. The catheter should then be withdrawn. The patient should retain the drug for 2 hours before voiding. At the end of 2 hours, all patients should void. Some patients will be unable to retain the drug for the full 2 hours. Patients should be instructed to maintain adequate hydration following treatment.

Patients receiving valrubicin for refractory CIS must be monitored closely for disease recurrence or progression. Recommended evaluations include cystoscopy, biopsy, and urine cytology every 3 months.

Valrubicin may cause red discoloration of urine for up to 24 hours after administration; patients should be counseled to expect this effect.

➤*Extravasation:* Valrubicin is considered an irritant and may cause phlebitis, but it is not known to cause tissue damage with extravasation. If signs or symptoms of extravasation occur, stop the infusion immediately. If possible, withdraw 3 to 5 mL of blood to remove some of the drug. Remove the infusion needle. Delineate the infiltrated area on the patient's skin with a felt tip marker. Elevate for 48 hours above heart level using a sling or stockinette dressing with an observation window cut in the dressing. Avoid pressure or friction. Do not rub the area. Observe for signs of increased erythema, pain, or skin necrosis. If increased symptoms occur, consult a plastic surgeon. Ensure that no medication is given distally to extravasation site. After 48 hours, encourage the patient to use the extremity normally to promote full range of motion.

➤*Storage/Stability:* Store vials under refrigeration at 2° to 8°C (36° to 46°F) in the carton. Do not freeze. Vials should not be heated. Valrubicin diluted in sodium chloride 0.9% injection for administration is stable for 12 hours at temperatures up to 25°C (77°F).

Discard vial within 6 hours of the initial needle puncture if opened within an ISO Class 5 biological safety cabinet, or within 1 hour of the initial needle puncture if opened outside of such an environment, based on the USP Chapter <797> standards.

Valrubicin solutions can leach phthalates from PVC containers. To avoid this, prepare valrubicin in glass, polypropylene, or polyolefin containers.

For intravesical administration, phthalate leaching may be minimized by placing the solution in a non-PVC container (eg, glass, polypropylene, polyolefin) and using a non–PVC-containing, polyethylene-lined administration set. Nitroglycerin tubing may be used to administer intravesical valrubicin.

Actions

➤*Pharmacology:* Valrubicin is an anthracycline that affects a variety of interrelated biological functions, most of which involve nucleic acid metabolism. It readily penetrates into cells, where it inhibits the incorporation of nucleosides into nucleic acids, causes extensive chromosomal damage, and arrests cell cycle in G2. Although valrubicin does not bind strongly to DNA, a principal mechanism of its action, mediated by valrubicin metabolites, is interference with the normal DNA breaking-resealing action of DNA topoisomerase II.

➤*Pharmacokinetics:*

Absorption – When valrubicin 800 mg was administered intravesically to patients with CIS, valrubicin penetrated into the bladder wall. The mean total anthracycline concentration measured in bladder tissue exceeded the levels, causing 90% cytotoxicity to human bladder cells cultured in vitro. During the 2-hour dose-retention period, only nanogram quantities of valrubicin were absorbed into the plasma.

Total systemic exposure to anthracyclines during and after intravesical administration of valrubicin is dependent upon the condition of the bladder wall. The mean $AUC_{0\text{-}6\ h}$ (total anthracyclines exposure) for an intravesical dose of valrubicin 900 mg administered 2 weeks after transurethral resection of bladder tumors (n = 6) was 78 nmol/L•h. In patients receiving valrubicin 800 mg 5 to 51 minutes after typical (n = 8) and extensive (n = 5) transurethral resection of bladder tumors (TURBs), the mean $AUC_{0\text{-}6\ h}$ values for total anthracyclines were 409 and 788 nmol/L•h, respectively. The

VALRUBICIN — INTRAVESICAL

$AUC_{0\text{-}6\ h}$ total exposure to anthracyclines was 18,382 nmol/L•h in 1 patient who experienced a perforated bladder following a transurethral resection that occurred 5 minutes before administration of an intravesical dose of valrubicin 800 mg. Administration of a comparable intravenous dose of valrubicin (600 mg/m^2; n = 2) as a 24-hour infusion resulted in an $AUC_{0\text{-}6\ h}$ for total anthracyclines of 11,975 nmol/L•h.

The patient with a perforated bladder who received valrubicin 800 mg intravesically developed severe leukopenia and neutropenia approximately 2 weeks after drug administration. Systemic hematologic toxicity from valrubicin was not seen after an intravesical dose of valrubicin 800 mg unless perforation of the urinary bladder occurred.

Metabolism / Excretion – During the 2-hour dose-retention period, the metabolism of valrubicin to its major metabolites, N-trifluoroacetyladriamycin and N-trifluoroacetyladriamycinol, was negligible. After retention, the drug was almost completely excreted by voiding the instillate. Mean percent recovery of valrubicin, N-trifluoroacetyladriamycin, and total anthracyclines in 14 urine samples from 6 patients was 98.6%, 0.4%, and 99% of the total administered drug, respectively. Valrubicin metabolites N-trifluoroacetyladriamycin and N-trifluoroacetyladriamycinol were measured in blood.

Contraindications

Known hypersensitivity to anthracyclines or polyoxyl castor oil; concurrent urinary tract infection; patients with a small bladder capacity (unable to tolerate a 75 mL instillation).

Warnings/Precautions

➤*Limited patient response:* Inform patients that valrubicin has been shown to induce complete response in only about 1 in 5 patients with BCG-refractory CIS, and that delaying cystectomy could lead to development of metastatic bladder cancer, which is lethal. The exact risk of developing metastatic bladder cancer from such a delay may be difficult to assess but increases the longer cystectomy is delayed in the presence of persisting CIS. If there is not a complete response of CIS to treatment after 3 months or if CIS recurs, cystectomy must be reconsidered.

➤*Compromised bladder:* In order to avoid possible dangerous systemic exposure to valrubicin for the patients undergoing transurethral resection of the bladder, evaluate the status of the bladder before the intravesical instillation of drug. In case of bladder perforation, delay the administration of valrubicin until bladder integrity has been restored.

Do not administer valrubicin to patients with a perforated bladder or to those in whom the integrity of the bladder mucosa has been compromised.

➤*Chemotherapy-experienced health care provider:* Administer valrubicin under the supervision of a health care provider experienced in the use of intravesical cancer chemotherapeutic agents.

➤*Aseptic techniques:* Aseptic techniques must be used during administration of intravesical valrubicin to avoid introducing contaminants into the urinary tract or unduly traumatizing the urinary mucosa.

➤*Irritable bladder symptoms:* Use valrubicin with caution in patients with severe irritable bladder symptoms. Bladder spasm and spontaneous discharge of the intravesical instillate may occur; clamping of the urinary catheter is not advised, and, if performed, should be executed under medical supervision and with caution.

➤*Extravasation:* See Administration and Dosage for more information.

➤*Pregnancy: Category C.* Valrubicin can cause fetal harm if a pregnant woman is exposed to the drug systemically. Such exposure could occur after perforation of the urinary bladder during valrubicin therapy.

There are no preclinical studies of the effects of intravesical valrubicin on fetal development and no adequate and well-controlled studies of valrubicin in pregnant women. If valrubicin is used during pregnancy, or if the patient becomes pregnant while receiving this drug, apprise the patient of the potential hazard to the fetus. Use during pregnancy only if the potential benefit justifies the potential risk to the fetus. Advise women who might become pregnant to avoid doing so during therapy with valrubicin.

➤*Lactation:* It is not known whether valrubicin is excreted in human milk. Nevertheless, the drug is highly lipophilic, and any exposure of infants to valrubicin could pose serious health risks. Women should discontinue breast-feeding before the initiation of valrubicin therapy.

➤*Children:* Safety and effectiveness in pediatric patients have not been established.

Drug Interactions

Because systemic exposure to valrubicin is negligible following intravesical administration, the potential for drug interactions is low. No drug interaction studies were conducted.

Adverse Reactions

Approximately 84% of patients who received intravesical valrubicin in clinical studies experienced local adverse reactions, but approximately 50% of the patients reported irritable bladder symptoms prior to treatment. The local adverse reactions associated with valrubicin usually occur during or shortly after instillation and resolve within 1 to 7 days after the instillate is removed from the bladder.

Local Adverse Reactions Before and During Treatment With Intravesical Valrubicin (% of Patients)

Adverse reactions	Patients who received multiple-cycle treatment regimen at 800 mg/dose (N = 170)	
	Before treatment	During 6-wk course of treatment
Any local bladder symptom	45%	88%
Bladder pain	6%	28%
Bladder spasm	3%	31%
Cystitis	4%	15%
Dysuria	11%	56%
Hematuria	11%	29%
Hematuria (gross)	0%	1%
Local burning symptoms, procedure related	0%	5%
Nocturia	2%	7%
Pelvic pain	1%	1%
Urethral pain	0%	3%
Urinary frequency	30%	61%
Urinary incontinence	7%	22%
Urinary urgency	27%	57%

Most systemic adverse reactions associated with use of valrubicin have been mild in nature and self-limited, resolving within 24 hours after drug administration. The following table displays the adverse reactions other than local bladder symptoms that occurred in 1% or more of the 230 patients who received at least one dose of valrubicin (200 to 900 mg) in a clinical trial. It cannot be determined whether these reactions are drug-related.

Most Commonly Reported Systemic Adverse Reactions Following Intravesical Administration of Valrubicin (% of Patients)

Adverse reactions	All patients receiving valrubicin (N = 230)
CNS	
Asthenia	4%
Dizziness	3%
Headache	4%
GI	
Abdominal pain	5%
Diarrhea	3%
Flatulence	1%
Nausea	5%
Vomiting	2%
GU	
Hematuria (microscopic)	3%
Urinary retention	4%
Urinary tract infection	15%
Metabolic/Nutritional	
Hyperglycemia	1%
Peripheral edema	1%
Miscellaneous	
Anemia	2%
Back pain	3%
Chest pain	3%
Fever	2%
Malaise	4%
Myalgia	1%
Pneumonia	1%
Rash	3%
Vasodilation	2%

The following are adverse reactions other than local reactions that occurred in less than 1% of the patients who received valrubicin intravesically in clinical trials. This list includes only adverse reactions that were suspected of being related to treatment.

➤*Dermatologic:* Local skin irritation, pruritus. Inadvertent paravenous extravasation of valrubicin was not associated with skin ulceration or necrosis.

➤*GI:* Tenesmus.

VALRUBICIN — INTRAVESICAL

➤*GU:* Poor urine flow, urethritis.

➤*Metabolic/Nutritional:* Nonprotein nitrogen increased.

➤*Special senses:* Taste loss.

Overdosage

➤*Symptoms:* Myelosuppression is possible if valrubicin is inadvertently administered systemically or if significant systemic exposure occurs following intravesical administration (eg, in patients with bladder rupture/perforation). The maximum tolerated dose in humans by either intraperitoneal or intravenous administration is 600 mg/m^2. Dose limiting toxicities are leukopenia and neutropenia, beginning within 1 week of dose administration, with nadirs by the second week, and recovery generally by the third week.

➤*Treatment:* There is no known antidote for overdoses of valrubicin. The primary anticipated complications of overdosage associated with intravesical administration would be consistent with irritable bladder symptoms. If valrubicin is administered when bladder rupture or perforation is suspected, weekly monitoring of complete blood cell counts should be performed for 3 weeks.

Patient Information

Inform patients that valrubicin has been shown to induce complete responses in only about 1 in 5 patients, and that delaying cystectomy could lead to development of metastatic bladder cancer, which is lethal. Discuss with patients the relative risk of cystectomy versus the risk of metastatic bladder cancer and make patients aware that the risk increases the longer cystectomy is delayed in the presence of persisting CIS.

Inform patients that the major acute toxicities from valrubicin are related to irritable bladder symptoms that may occur during instillation and retention of valrubicin and for a limited period following voiding. For the first 24 hours following administration, red-tinged urine is typical. Instruct patients to report prolonged irritable bladder symptoms or prolonged passage of red-colored urine immediately to their health care provider.

Advise women of child-bearing potential not to become pregnant during treatment. Advise men to refrain from engaging in procreative activities while receiving therapy with valrubicin. Advise all patients of reproductive age to use an effective contraception method during the treatment period.

BLEOMYCIN

Rx	**Bleomycin** (Various, eg, APP Pharmaceuticals, Bedford Laboratories, Teva)	**Injection, lyophilized powder for solution:** 15 units[a]	As bleomycin sulfate. In vials.
		30 units[a]	As bleomycin sulfate. In vials.

[a] A unit of bleomycin is equal to the formerly used milligram activity.

BLEOMYCIN SULFATE — INJECTION

WARNING

It is recommended that bleomycin be administered under the supervision of a qualified physician experienced in the use of cancer chemotherapeutic agents. Appropriate management of therapy and complications is possible only when adequate diagnostic and treatment facilities are readily available.

Pulmonary fibrosis is the most severe toxicity associated with bleomycin. The most frequent presentation is pneumonitis occasionally progressing to pulmonary fibrosis. Its occurrence is higher in elderly patients and in those receiving more than 400 units total dose, but pulmonary toxicity has been observed in young patients and those treated with low doses.

A severe idiosyncratic reaction consisting of hypotension, mental confusion, fever, chills, and wheezing has been reported in approximately 1% of lymphoma patients treated with bleomycin.

Indications

➤*Lymphomas:* As palliative treatment for Hodgkin disease and non-Hodgkin lymphoma, either as a single agent or in proven combinations with other approved chemotherapeutic agents.

➤*Malignant pleural effusion:* As a sclerosing agent for the treatment of malignant pleural effusion and prevention of recurrent pleural effusions.

➤*Squamous cell carcinoma:* As palliative treatment for head and neck (including mouth, tongue, tonsil, nasopharynx, oropharynx, sinus, palate, lip, buccal mucosa, gingiva, epiglottis, skin, larynx), penis, cervix, and vulva neoplasms as a single agent or in proven combinations with other approved chemotherapeutic agents.

➤*Testicular carcinoma:* As palliative treatment for embryonal cell, choriocarcinoma, and teratocarcinoma neoplasms as a single agent or in proven combinations with other approved chemotherapeutic agents.

➤*Off-label uses:*

Malignant pericardial effusion – [1] = Good documentation. Intrapericardial bleomycin, following pericardiocentesis, appears to be an effective agent in the treatment of malignant pericardial effusion and has an excellent safety profile. Further studies comparing bleomycin with other sclerosing agents are needed to determine the preferred agent.

Malignant peritoneal effusion – [2] = Fair documentation. Intraperitoneal bleomycin appears to be an effective strategy in the management of malignant peritoneal effusion or malignant ascites; however, based on the limited available evidence, further studies are needed to determine its place in therapy.

Warts (intralesional) – [1] = Good documentation. Intralesional bleomycin appears to be an effective therapy for the treatment of previously untreated or recalcitrant warts on the hands and feet. Although pain and discomfort following injection are common, the good clearance rate and ease of administration make intralesional bleomycin a good therapeutic option.

Other possible off-label uses – Treatment of mycosis fungoides; osteosarcoma; AIDS-related Kaposi sarcoma. Bleomycin has been used in children for palliative treatment of lymphomas; testicular carcinoma; germ cell tumors; sclerosis of pleural effusions.

Administration and Dosage

➤*General dosing considerations:* Pulmonary toxicity of bleomycin appears to be dose related, with a striking increase when the total dose is more than 400 units. Total doses of more than 400 units should be given with great caution.

When bleomycin is used in combination with other antineoplastic agents, pulmonary toxicities may occur at lower doses.

Improvement of Hodgkin disease and testicular tumors is prompt and noted within 2 weeks. If no improvement is seen by this time, improvement is unlikely. Squamous cell cancers respond more slowly, sometimes requiring as long as 3 weeks before any improvement is noted.

➤*Adults:*

Lymphoma –

Hodgkin disease:

• *Initial dosage* – Treat with 2 units or less for the first 2 doses because of the possibility of an anaphylactoid reaction. If no acute reaction occurs, then the regular dosage schedule may be followed.

• *Maintenance dosage* – 0.25 to 0.5 units/kg (10 to 20 units/m^2) given intravenously (IV), intramuscularly (IM), or subcutaneously weekly or twice weekly. After a 50% response, a maintenance dose of 1 unit daily or 5 units weekly IV or IM should be given.

Non-Hodgkin lymphoma:

• *Initial dosage* – Treat with 2 units or less for the first 2 doses because of the possibility of an anaphylactoid reaction. If no acute reaction occurs, then the regular dosage schedule may be followed.

• *Maintenance dosage* – 0.25 to 0.5 units/kg (10 to 20 units/m^2) given IV, IM, or subcutaneously weekly or twice weekly.

Malignant pleural effusion – 60 units as a single-dose bolus intrapleural injection.

Squamous cell carcinoma – 0.25 to 0.5 units/kg (10 to 20 units/m^2) given IV, IM, or subcutaneously weekly or twice weekly.

Testicular carcinoma – 0.25 to 0.5 units/kg (10 to 20 units/m^2) given IV, IM, or subcutaneously weekly or twice weekly.

Off-label dosing –

Malignant pericardial effusion: [1] = Good documentation. Dissolve bleomycin 5 to 20 mg in 10 to 20 mL of normal saline and instill via catheter into the pericardial space following pericardiocentesis. Clamp the catheter for up to 6 hours. Continue drainage of effusions until the volume of fluid is less than 20 to 30 mL/day. Repeat intrapericardial infusion, if needed, to reach the desired level of drainage.

Malignant peritoneal effusion: [2] = Fair documentation. Bleomycin 30 to 60 mg in 100 mL of normal saline administered via intraperitoneal infusion. The duration of therapy is unknown; however, bleomycin was dosed every 1 to 2 weeks for a total cumulative dose of 720 mg in 1 case report.

Warts (intralesional): [1] = Good documentation. Bleomycin must be reconstituted, and the most common method involves using normal saline to reach a concentration of 0.5 to 1 unit/mL. The dose ranges from 0.1 to 2 units, depending on lesion size. The injection technique typically involves inserting a large gauge needle at the base of the wart until blanching occurs. Other methods of injecting bleomycin include using multiple puncture sites following topically applied bleomycin dermatography (method of tattooing), dermajet, or using a pulsed dye lased prior to injection.

One study used a higher dose of bleomycin that was reconstituted with bupivacaine 0.5% and epinephrine 1:200,000 to reach a concentration of 1.5 units/mL. The dose injected ranged from 0.25 to 3 mL, depending on the size of the lesion.

BLEOMYCIN SULFATE — INJECTION

➤*Renal function impairment:*

Bleomycin Dosage in Renal Impairment	
CrCl[a] (mL/min)	Bleomycin dose
≥ 50 mL/min	100%
40 to 50 mL/min	70%
30 to 40 mL/min	60%
20 to 30 mL/min	55%
10 to 20 mL/min	45%
5 to 10 mL/min	40%

[a] CrCl = creatinine clearance.

➤*Preparation for administration:* Bleomycin is considered a cytotoxic agent. Follow safe handling procedures when preparing, administering, or dispensing bleomycin.

IM or subcutaneous – The 15 unit vial should be reconstituted with 1 to 5 mL of sterile water for injection, sodium chloride 0.9% injection, or sterile bacteriostatic water for injection. The 30 unit vial should be reconstituted with 2 to 10 mL of the previously listed diluents.

IV – The contents of the 15 or 30 unit vial should be dissolved in 5 or 10 mL, respectively, of sodium chloride 0.9% injection and administered slowly over a period of 10 minutes.

Intrapleural – 60 units of bleomycin are dissolved in 50 to 100 mL of sodium chloride 0.9% injection and administered through a thoracostomy tube following drainage of excess pleural fluid and confirmation of complete lung expansion.

The thoracostomy tube is clamped after bleomycin instillation. The patient is moved from the supine to the left and right lateral positions several times during the next 4 hours. The clamp is then removed and suction reestablished. The amount of time the chest tube remains in place following sclerosis is dictated by the clinical situation.

➤*Administration:* Administer IV, IM, subcutaneously, or intrapleurally.

➤*Extravasation:* Bleomycin is considered an irritant and may cause phlebitis, but it is not known to cause tissue damage with extravasation. If signs or symptoms of extravasation occur, stop the infusion immediately. If possible, withdraw 3 to 5 mL of blood to remove some of the drug. Remove the infusion needle. Delineate the infiltrated area on the patient's skin with a felt tip marker. Elevate for 48 hours above heart level using a sling or stockinette dressing with an observation window cut in the dressing. Avoid pressure or friction. Do not rub the area. Observe for signs of increased erythema, pain, or skin necrosis. If increased symptoms occur, consult a plastic surgeon. Ensure that no medication is given distally to the extravasation site. After 48 hours, encourage the patient to use the extremity normally to promote full range of motion.

➤*Admixture compatibility:* Bleomycin should not be reconstituted or diluted with dextrose 5% in water or other dextrose-containing diluents.

➤*Storage/Stability:* The sterile powder is stable at 2° to 8°C (36° to 46°F).

Bleomycin is stable for 24 hours at room temperature in sodium chloride injection.

Actions

➤*Pharmacology:* Although the exact mechanism of action of bleomycin, a cytotoxic glycopeptide antibiotic, is unknown, available evidence would seem to indicate that the main mode of action is the inhibition of DNA synthesis with some evidence of lesser inhibition of RNA and protein synthesis.

Bleomycin is known to cause single- and, to a lesser extent, double-stranded breaks in DNA. In in vitro and in vivo experiments, bleomycin has been shown to cause cell cycle arrest in G2 and in mitosis.

When administered into the pleural cavity in the treatment of malignant pleural effusions, bleomycin acts as a sclerosing agent.

➤*Pharmacokinetics:*

Absorption – Bleomycin is rapidly absorbed following IM, subcutaneous, intraperitoneal, or intrapleural administration, reaching peak plasma concentrations in 30 to 60 minutes. Systemic bioavailability of bleomycin is 100% and 70% following IM and subcutaneous administrations, respectively, and 45% following both intraperitoneal and intrapleural administrations, compared with IV bolus administration.

Following IM doses of 1 to 10 units/m^2, both peak plasma concentration and area under the curve (AUC) increased in proportion with the increase of dose.

Following IV bolus administration of 30 units of bleomycin to 1 patient with a primary germ cell tumor of the brain, a peak cerebrospinal fluid (CSF) level was 40% of the simultaneously obtained plasma level and was attained in 2 hours after drug administration. The area under the bleomycin CSF concentration × time curve was 25% of the area of the bleomycin plasma concentration × time curve.

Distribution – Bleomycin is widely distributed throughout the body, with a mean volume of distribution of 17.5 L/m^2 in patients following a 15 unit/m^2 IV bolus dose.

Metabolism – Bleomycin is inactivated by a cytosolic cysteine proteinase enzyme, bleomycin hydrolase. The enzyme is widely distributed in normal tissues, with the exception of the skin and lungs, both targets of bleomycin toxicity. Systemic elimination of the drug by enzymatic degradation is probably only important in patients with severely compromised renal function.

Excretion – The primary route of elimination is via the kidneys. Approximately 65% of the administered IV dose is excreted in urine within 24 hours. In patients with healthy renal function, plasma concentrations of bleomycin decline biexponentially, with a mean terminal half-life of 2 hours following IV bolus administration. Total body clearance and renal clearance averaged 51 and 23 mL/min/m^2, respectively.

Following intrapleural administration to patients with healthy renal function, a lower percentage of drug (40%) is recovered in the urine, compared with that found in the urine after IV administration.

Special populations –

Renal function impairment: Renal insufficiency markedly alters bleomycin elimination. In patients with a CrCl of more than 35 mg/min, the serum or plasma terminal elimination half-life of bleomycin is approximately 115 minutes. In patients with a CrCl of less than 35 mL/min, the plasma or serum terminal elimination half-life increases exponentially as the CrCl decreases. It was reported that patients with moderately severe renal failure excreted less than 20% of the dose in the urine. This result would suggest that severe renal impairment could lead to accumulation of the drug in blood.

See Administration and Dosage for more information.

Children: Children younger than 3 years of age have higher total body clearance than adults (71 mL/min/m^2 vs 51 mL/min/m^2, respectively) following IV bolus administration.

Contraindications

Hypersensitivity or an idiosyncratic reaction to bleomycin.

Warnings/Precautions

➤*Pulmonary effects:* Pulmonary toxicities occur in 10% of treated patients. In approximately 1%, the nonspecific pneumonitis induced by bleomycin progresses to pulmonary fibrosis and death. Although this is age and dose related, the toxicity is unpredictable. Frequent roentgenograms are recommended. Use bleomycin with extreme caution in patients with compromised pulmonary function.

➤*Renal/Hepatic effects:* Renal or hepatic toxicity, beginning as a deterioration in renal or liver function tests, have been reported infrequently. These toxicities may occur, however, at any time after initiation of therapy.

➤*Extravasation:* See Administration and Dosage for more information.

➤*Hypersensitivity reactions:* See the Warning box for more information.

➤*Renal function impairment:* Treat patients with CrCl values of less than 50 mL/min with caution and carefully monitor renal function during the administration of bleomycin. Lower doses of bleomycin may be required in these patients than in those with healthy renal function.

Bleomycin should be used with extreme caution in patients with significant impairment of renal function.

➤*Pregnancy: Category D.* Bleomycin can cause fetal harm when administered to a pregnant woman. It has been shown to be teratogenic in rats. Administration of intraperitoneal dosages of 1.5 mg/kg/day to rats (approximately 1.6 times the recommended human dose on a unit/m^2 basis) on days 6 to 15 of gestation caused skeletal malformations, shortened innominate artery, and hydroureter. Bleomycin is abortifacient but not teratogenic in rabbits at IV dosages of 1.2 mg/kg/day (approximately 2.4 times the recommended human dose on a unit/m^2 basis) given on gestation days 6 to 18.

There have been no studies in pregnant women. Chromosomal aberrations in human marrow cells have been reported, but the significance to the fetus is unknown. If bleomycin is used during pregnancy, or if the patient becomes pregnant while receiving this drug, apprise the patient of the potential hazard to the fetus. Advise women of childbearing potential to avoid becoming pregnant during therapy with bleomycin.

➤*Lactation:* It is not known whether the drug is excreted in human milk. Because many drugs are excreted in human milk and because of the potential for serious adverse reactions in breast-feeding infants, it is recommended that breast-feeding be discontinued by women receiving bleomycin therapy.

➤*Children:* Safety and effectiveness of bleomycin in children have not been established.

➤*Elderly:* In clinical trials, pulmonary toxicity was more common in patients older than 70 years of age than in younger patients. Other reported clinical experience has not identified other differences in responses between elderly and younger patients, but greater sensitivity of some older individuals cannot be ruled out.

Bleomycin is known to be substantially excreted by the kidney, and the risk of toxic reactions to this drug may be greater in patients with impaired renal function. Because elderly patients are more likely to have decreased renal function, take care in dose selection; it may be useful to monitor renal function.

➤*Monitoring:* Monitor patients carefully and frequently for pulmonary toxicity and hypersensitivity reactions during and after therapy.

Monitor renal function during administration in patients with CrCl less than 50 mL/min. Monitor patient for extravasation during therapy.

To monitor the onset of pulmonary toxicity, take roentgenograms of the chest every 1 to 2 weeks. If pulmonary changes are noted, discontinue treatment until it can be determined if they are drug related. Recent studies have suggested that sequential measurement of the pulmonary diffusion capacity for carbon monoxide (DL_{CO}) during treatment with bleomycin may be an indicator of subclinical pulmonary toxicity. It is recommended that the DL_{CO} be monitored monthly if it is to be employed to detect pulmonary toxicities, and thus the drug should be discontinued when the DL_{CO} falls below 30% to 35% of the pretreatment value.

BLEOMYCIN SULFATE — INJECTION

Drug Interactions

Bleomycin Drug Interactions

Precipitant drug	Object drug[a]		Description
Cisplatin	Bleomycin	⬆	Elimination of bleomycin may be decreased secondary to cisplatin-induced renal dysfunction, increasing the risk of bleomycin toxicity. Use with caution. Monitor renal function and adjust the bleomycin dose as needed.
Oxygen	Bleomycin	⬆	Risk for pulmonary toxicity is increased (see Warnings/Precautions).
Bleomycin	Oxygen		
Bleomycin	Digoxin	⬇	Digoxin serum levels may be decreased by combination chemotherapy (including bleomycin). Digoxin capsules do not appear to be affected. Monitor patients for signs of reduction in pharmacologic effect (eg, deteriorating heart failure). Increase digoxin dose if necessary; serum level monitoring may facilitate tailoring dosage.
Bleomycin	Hydantoins (eg, phenytoin)	⬇	Phenytoin serum concentrations may be decreased by combination chemotherapy. Monitor serum phenytoin levels and adjust the phenytoin dosage appropriately. IV phenytoin may be useful.

[a] ⬆ = object drug increased; ⬇ = object drug decreased.

Adverse Reactions

➤*Hypersensitivity:* See the Warning box for more information.

➤*Cardiovascular:* Vascular toxicities coincident with the use of bleomycin in combination with other antineoplastic agents have been reported rarely. The reactions are clinically heterogeneous and may include cerebral arteritis, cerebrovascular accident, myocardial infarction, or thrombotic microangiopathy (hemolytic uremic syndrome). Various mechanisms have been proposed for these vascular complications. There are also reports of Raynaud phenomenon occurring in patients treated with bleomycin in combination with vinblastine with or without cisplatin or, in a few cases, with bleomycin as a single agent. It is currently unknown if the cause of Raynaud phenomenon in these cases is the disease, underlying vascular compromise, bleomycin, vinblastine, hypomagnesemia, or a combination of any of these factors. Hypotension possibly requiring symptomatic treatment has been reported infrequently with intrapleural administration.

➤*Dermatologic:* The most frequent adverse reactions, reported in approximately 50% of treated patients, included erythema, hyperpigmentation, rash, striae, vesiculation, and tenderness of the skin. Alopecia, hyperkeratosis, nail changes, pruritus, and stomatitis have also been reported. It was necessary to discontinue bleomycin therapy in 2% of treated patients because of these toxicities.

Skin toxicity is a relatively late manifestation, usually developing in the second and third week of treatment after 150 to 200 units of bleomycin have been administered, and appears to be related to the cumulative dose.

Intrapleural administration of bleomycin has occasionally been associated with local pain.

➤*Pulmonary:* This is potentially the most serious adverse effect, occurring in approximately 10% of patients treated with bleomycin. The most frequent presentation is pneumonitis occasionally progressing to pulmonary fibrosis. Approximately 1% of patients treated have died of pulmonary fibrosis. Pulmonary toxicity is both dose and age related, being more common in patients older than 70 years of age and in those receiving more than 400 units total dose. This toxicity, however, is unpredictable and has been seen occasionally in young patients receiving low doses.

Because of lack of specificity of the clinical syndrome, the identification of patients with pulmonary toxicity caused by bleomycin has been extremely difficult. The earliest symptom associated with bleomycin pulmonary toxicity is dyspnea. The earliest sign is fine rales.

Radiographically, bleomycin-induced pneumonitis produces nonspecific patchy opacities, usually of the lower lung fields. The most common changes in pulmonary function tests are a decrease in total lung volume and a decrease in vital capacity. However, these changes are not predictive of the development of pulmonary fibrosis.

The microscopic tissue changes caused by bleomycin toxicity include atypical alveolar epithelial cells, bronchiolar squamous metaplasia, fibrinous edema, interstitial fibrosis, and reactive macrophages. The acute stage may involve capillary changes and subsequent fibrinous exudation into alveoli, producing a change similar to hyaline membrane formation and progressing to a diffuse interstitial fibrosis resembling the Hamman-Rich syndrome. These microscopic findings are nonspecific (eg, similar changes are seen in radiation pneumonitis and pneumocystic pneumonitis).

Because of bleomycin's sensitization of lung tissue, patients who have received bleomycin are at greater risk of developing pulmonary toxicity when oxygen is administered in surgery. While long exposure to very high oxygen concentrations is a known cause of lung damage, after bleomycin administration, lung damage can occur at lower concentrations that are usually considered safe. Suggestive preventive measures are to maintain fraction of inspired oxygen (FiO_2) at concentrations approximating that of room air (25%) during surgery and the postoperative period and to carefully monitor fluid replacement, focusing more on colloid administration rather than crystalloid.

Sudden onset of an acute chest pain syndrome suggestive of pleuropericarditis has been rarely reported during bleomycin infusions. Although each patient must be individually evaluated, further courses of bleomycin do not appear to be contraindicated.

➤*Miscellaneous:* Fever, chills, and vomiting were frequently reported adverse reactions. Anorexia and weight loss are common and may persist long after termination of this medication. Pain at tumor site, phlebitis, and other local reactions were reported infrequently.

Death has been very rarely reported in association with bleomycin pleurodesis in these very seriously ill patients.

➤*Postmarketing:*

Miscellaneous – Malaise, scleroderma-like skin changes.

Patient Information

Inform patients that antibacterial drugs, including bleomycin, should only be used to treat bacterial infections. They do not treat viral infections (eg, the common cold).

Advise patients to immediately report any of the following to their health care provider: rash; hives, difficulty breathing or unexplained shortness of breath; chest pain, fever, chills, or other signs of infection; sores in mouth; pain, redness, or swelling at the injection site; and skin changes.

Advise women of childbearing potential to avoid becoming pregnant during therapy.

Advise breast-feeding women not to breast-feed during therapy.

DACTINOMYCIN (Actinomycin D; ACT)

Rx	**Dactinomycin** (Bedford Labs)	**Injection, powder for solution, lyophilized:** 500 mcg	In single-dose vials.[a]
Rx	**Cosmegen** (Merck)		In vials.[a]

[a] With mannitol 20 mg.

DACTINOMYCIN — INJECTION

WARNING

Dactinomycin should be administered only under the supervision of a physician who is experienced in the use of cancer chemotherapeutic agents.

This drug is highly toxic and both powder and solution must be handled and administered with care. Inhalation of dust or vapors and contact with skin or mucous membranes, especially those of the eyes, must be avoided. Avoid exposure during pregnancy. Due to the toxic properties of dactinomycin (eg, corrosivity, carcinogenicity, mutagenicity, teratogenicity), special handling procedures should be reviewed prior to handling and followed diligently.

Dactinomycin is extremely corrosive to soft tissue. If extravasation occurs during IV use, severe damage to soft tissues will occur. In at least one instance, this has led to contracture of the arms.

Indications

➤*Wilms' tumor, rhabdomyosarcoma, Ewing's sarcoma, nonseminomatous testicular cancer:* As part of a combination chemotherapy and/or multi-modality treatment regimen for the treatment of Wilms' tumor, childhood rhabdomyosarcoma, Ewing's sarcoma and metastatic, nonseminomatous testicular cancer.

➤*Gestational trophoblastic neoplasia:* As a single agent or as part of a combination chemotherapy regimen for the treatment of gestational trophoblastic neoplasia.

➤*Solid malignancies:* As a component of regional perfusion for the palliative and/or adjunctive treatment of locally recurrent or locoregional solid malignancies.

➤*Off-label uses:* Treatment of osteosarcoma; malignant melanoma; Paget disease of the bone.

DACTINOMYCIN — INJECTION

Administration and Dosage

➤*General dosing considerations:* Dactinomycin is dosed in mcg/kg for some indications, but may be dosed in mcg/m^2 for other indications.

The dosage of dactinomycin varies depending on the tolerance of the patient, the size, and location of the neoplasm, and the use of other forms of therapy. It may be necessary to decrease the usual dosages when other chemotherapy or radiation therapy is used concomitantly or has been used previously.

Toxic reactions due to dactinomycin are frequent and may be severe, thus limiting in many instances the amount that may be administered. However, the severity of toxicity varies markedly and is only partly dependent on the dose employed.

It may be advisable to use lower doses in obese patients, or when previous chemotherapy or radiation therapy has been employed.

Calculation of the dosage for obese or edematous patients should be performed on the basis of surface area in an effort to more closely relate dosage to lean body mass.

➤*Adults:*

Ewing's sarcoma –

Usual dosage: 15 mcg/kg/day IV for 5 days administered in various combinations and schedules with other chemotherapeutic agents. Repeat in 3 weeks if necessary.

Maximum dose: 15 mcg/kg/day or 400 to 600 mcg/m^2/day IV for 5 days.

Gestational trophoblastic neoplasia –

Single agent: 12 mcg/kg/day IV for 5 days.

Combination regimen: 500 mcg IV on days 1 and 2 with etoposide, methotrexate, leucovorin (folinic acid), vincristine, cyclophosphamide, and cisplatin.

Metastatic nonseminomatous testicular cancer – 1,000 mcg/m^2 body surface area IV on day 1 as part of a combination regimen with cyclophosphamide, bleomycin, vinblastine, and cisplatin.

Rhabdomyosarcoma –

Usual dosage: 15 mcg/kg/day IV for 5 days administered in various combinations and schedules with other chemotherapeutic agents. Repeat in 3 to 6 weeks if necessary.

Maximum dose: 15 mcg/kg/day or 400 to 600 mcg/m^2/day IV for 5 days.

Solid malignancies – The dosage schedules and the technique itself vary from one investigator to another; the published literature, therefore, should be consulted for details. In general, the following doses are suggested:

Lower extremity or pelvis: 50 mcg/kg IV.

Upper extremity: 35 mcg/kg IV.

Wilms' tumor –

Usual dosage: 15 mcg/kg/day IV for 5 days administered in various combinations and schedules with other chemotherapeutic agents. Repeat in 3 weeks if necessary.

Maximum dose: 15 mcg/kg/day or 400 to 600 mcg/m^2/day IV for 5 days.

➤*Children:*

Childhood rhabdomyosarcoma –

Older than 6 months of age:

- *Usual dosage* – 15 mcg/kg/day IV for 5 days administered in various combinations and schedules with other chemotherapeutic agents. Repeat in 3 to 6 weeks if necessary. (See also Off-label dosing.)
- *Maximum dose* – 15 mcg/kg/day or 400 to 600 mcg/m^2/day IV for 5 days.

Ewing's sarcoma – See Childhood rhabdomyosarcoma for dosing.

Metastatic nonseminomatous testicular cancer –

Older than 6 months of age: 1,000 mcg/m^2 body surface area IV on day 1 as part of a combination regimen with cyclophosphamide, bleomycin, vinblastine, and cisplatin.

Solid malignancies –

Older than 6 months of age: The dosage schedules and the technique itself vary from one investigator to another; the published literature, therefore, should be consulted for details. In general, the following doses are suggested:

- *Lower extremity or pelvis* – 50 mcg/kg IV.
- *Upper extremity* – 35 mcg/kg IV.

Wilms' tumor – See Childhood rhabdomyosarcoma for dosing.

Off-label dosing –

Alternative schedule: 0.357 mg/m^2/day by continuous infusion over 24 hours for 7 days (total dose is 2.5 mg/m^2 over 1 week).

➤*Preparation for administration:*

Special handling – This drug is highly toxic and powder and solution must be handled and administered with care. Dactinomycin is considered a carcinogen, mutagen, and teratogen. Follow safe handling procedures when preparing, administering, or dispensing dactinomycin.

Inhalation of dust or vapors and contact with skin or mucous membranes, especially those of the eyes, must be avoided. Appropriate protective equipment should be worn when handling dactinomycin.

Accidental contact measures – Should accidental eye contact occur, copious irrigation for at least 15 minutes with water, normal saline, or a balanced salt ophthalmic irrigating solution should be instituted immediately, followed by prompt ophthalmologic consultation. Should accidental skin contact occur, the affected part must be irrigated immediately with copious amounts of water for at least 15 minutes while removing contaminated clothing and shoes. Medical attention should be sought immediately. Contaminated clothing should be destroyed and shoes cleaned thoroughly before reuse.

Preparation of solution – Reconstitute dactinomycin by adding 1.1 mL of sterile water for injection (without preservative) using aseptic precautions. The resulting solution of dactinomycin will contain approximately 500 mcg (0.5 mg) per mL.

Once reconstituted, the solution of dactinomycin can be added to infusion solutions of dextrose injection 5% or sodium chloride injection either directly or to the tubing of a running IV infusion.

➤*Administration:* Not for oral administration. Administer by IV push injection or by IV sidearm.

If the drug is given directly into the vein without the use of an infusion, the two-needle technique should be used. Reconstitute and withdraw the calculated dose from the vial with one sterile needle. Use another sterile needle for direct injection into the vein.

Once reconstituted, the solution of dactinomycin can be added to infusion solutions of dextrose injection 5% or sodium chloride injection either directly or to the tubing of a running IV infusion.

Partial removal of dactinomycin from IV solutions by cellulose ester membrane filters used in some IV in-line filters has been reported.

➤*Extravasation:* Dactinomycin is extremely corrosive to soft tissue. If extravasation occurs during IV use, severe damage to soft tissue will occur. In at least one instance, this has led to contracture of the arms. Care in the administration of dactinomycin will reduce the chance of perivenous infiltration. It may also decrease the chance of local reactions, such as urticaria and erythematous streaking. On IV administration of dactinomycin, extravasation may occur with or without an accompanying burning or stinging sensation, even if blood returns well on aspiration of the infusion needle.

If signs or symptoms of extravasation occur, stop the infusion immediately. If possible, withdraw 3 to 5 mL of blood to remove some of the drug. Remove the infusion needle. May apply ice compresses to the site for 15 minutes every 6 hours for 48 hours. Delineate the infiltrated area on the patient's skin with a felt-tip marker. Elevate for 48 hours above heart level using a sling or stockinette dressing with an observation window cut in the dressing. Avoid pressure or friction. Do not rub the area. Observe for signs of increased erythema, pain, or skin necrosis. If increased symptoms occur, consult a plastic surgeon. Ensure that no medication is given distally to extravasation site. After 48 hours, encourage the patient to use the extremity normally to promote full range of motion.

➤*Admixture compatibility:* Use of water containing preservatives (benzyl alcohol or parabens) to reconstitute dactinomycin, results in the formation of a precipitate.

➤*Storage/Stability:* Store at 25°C (77°F); excursions are permitted to 15° to 30°C (59° to 86°F). Protect from light and humidity.

Discard vial within 6 hours of the initial needle puncture if opened within an ISO Class 5 biological safety cabinet, or within 1 hour of the initial needle puncture if opened outside of such an environment, based on the USP Chapter < 797 > standards.

Because the reconstituted solution does not contain preservatives, discard within 24 hours.

Actions

➤*Pharmacology:* Generally, the actinomycins exert an inhibitory effect on gram-positive and gram-negative bacteria and on some fungi. However, the toxic properties of the actinomycins (including dactinomycin) in relation to antibacterial activity are such as to preclude their use as antibiotics in the treatment of infectious diseases.

Because the actinomycins are cytotoxic, they have an antineoplastic effect that has been demonstrated in experimental animals with various types of tumor implant. This cytotoxic action is the basis for their use in the palliative treatment of certain types of cancer. Dactinomycin is believed to produce its cytotoxic effects by binding DNA and inhibiting RNA synthesis.

Dactinomycin anchors into a purine-pyrimidine (DNA) base pair by intercalation, inhibiting messenger RNA synthesis. Although maximal cell-kill is noted in G^1 phase, the cytotoxic action is primarily cell cycle nonspecific. Activity proliferating cells are more sensitive.

➤*Pharmacokinetics:* Very little active drug can be detected in circulating blood 2 minutes after IV injection.Results of a study in patients with malignant melanoma indicate that dactinomycin (^{3}H actinomycin D) is minimally metabolized, is concentrated in nucleated cells, and does not penetrate the blood-brain barrier. Approximately 30% of the dose was recovered in urine and feces in 1 week. The terminal plasma half-life for radioactivity was approximately 36 hours.

Contraindications

Dactinomycin should not be given at or about the time of infection with chickenpox or herpes zoster because of the risk of severe generalized disease which may result in death.

Warnings/Precautions

➤*Highly toxic:* This drug is highly toxic and both powder and solution must be handled and administered with care. Since dactinomycin is extremely corrosive to soft tissues, it is intended for intravenous use.

Inhalation of dust or vapors and contact with skin or mucous membranes, especially those of the eyes, must be avoided. Appropriate protective equipment should be worn when handling dactinomycin. Should accidental eye contact occur, copious irrigation for at least 15 minutes with water, normal saline or a balanced salt ophthalmic irrigating solution should be instituted immediately, followed by prompt ophthalmologic consultation. Should accidental skin contact occur, the affected part must be irrigated immediately with copious amounts of water for at least 15 minutes, while removing con-

DACTINOMYCIN — INJECTION

taminated clothing and shoes. Medical attention should be sought immediately. Contaminated clothing should be destroyed and shoes cleaned thoroughly before reuse.

➤*Toxicities:* As with all antineoplastic agents, dactinomycin is a toxic drug and very careful and frequent observation of the patient for adverse reactions is necessary. These reactions may involve any tissue of the body, most commonly the hematopoietic system resulting in myelosuppression. The possibility of an anaphylactoid reaction should be borne in mind.

It is extremely important to observe the patient daily for toxic side effects when combination chemotherapy is employed, since a full course of therapy occasionally is not tolerated. If stomatitis, diarrhea, or severe hematopoietic depression appear during therapy, these drugs should be discontinued until the patient has recovered.

➤*Radiation therapy:* An increased incidence of gastrointestinal toxicity and marrow suppression has been reported with combined therapy incorporating dactinomycin and radiation. Moreover, the normal skin, as well as the buccal and pharyngeal mucosa, may show early erythema. A smaller than usual radiation dose administered in combination with dactinomycin causes erythema and vesiculation, which progress more rapidly through the stages of tanning and desquamation. Healing may occur in 4 to 6 weeks rather than 2 to 3 months. Erythema from previous radiation therapy may be reactivated by dactinomycin alone, even when radiotherapy was administered many months earlier, and especially when the interval between the 2 forms of therapy is brief. This potentiation of radiation effect represents a special problem when the radiotherapy involves the mucous membrane. When irradiation is directed toward the nasopharynx, the combination may produce severe oropharyngeal mucositis. Severe reactions may ensue if high doses of both dactinomycin and radiation therapy are used or if the patient is particularly sensitive to such combined therapy.

Particular caution is necessary when administering dactinomycin within 2 months of irradiation for the treatment of right-sided Wilms' tumor, since hepatomegaly and elevated AST levels have been noted. In general, dactinomycin should not be concomitantly administered with radiotherapy in the treatment of Wilms' tumor unless the benefit outweighs the risk.

➤*Regional perfusion therapy:* Complications of the perfusion technique are related mainly to the amount of drug that escapes into the systemic circulation and may consist of hematopoietic depression, absorption of toxic products from massive destruction of neoplastic tissue, increased susceptibility to infection, impaired wound healing, and superficial ulceration of the gastric mucosa. Other side effects may include edema of the extremity involved, damage to soft tissues of the perfused area, and (potentially) venous thrombosis.

➤*Extravasation:* See Administration and Dosage for more information.

See Administration and Dosage for more information.

➤*Pregnancy: Category D* per manufacturer's prescribing information. *Category C* per Briggs' *Drugs in Pregnancy and Lactation*. Dactinomycin may cause fetal harm when administered to a pregnant woman. Dactinomycin has been shown to cause malformations and embryotoxicity in rat, rabbit, and hamster when given in doses of 50 to 100 mcg/kg (approximately 0.5 to 2 times the maximum recommended daily human dose on a body surface area basis). If this drug is used during pregnancy, or if the patient becomes pregnant while receiving this drug, the patient should be apprised of the potential hazard to the fetus. Women of childbearing potential must be warned to avoid becoming pregnant.

➤*Lactation:* It is not known whether this drug is excreted in human milk. Because many drugs are excreted in human milk and because of the potential for serious adverse reactions in nursing infants from dactinomycin, a decision should be made whether to discontinue nursing or to discontinue the drug, taking into account the importance of the drug to the mother.

➤*Children:* The greater frequency of toxic effects of dactinomycin in infants suggests that this drug should be given to infants only over the age of 6 to 12 months.

➤*Elderly:* Clinical studies of dactinomycin did not include sufficient numbers of subjects aged 65 and over to determine whether they respond differently from younger subjects. Other reported clinical experience has not identified differences in responses between the elderly and younger patients. However, a published meta-analysis of all studies performed by the Eastern Cooperative Oncology Group (ECOG) over a 13-year period suggests that administration of dactinomycin to elderly patients may be associated with an increased risk of myelosuppression compared to younger patients. In general, dose selection for an elderly patient should be cautious, usually starting at the low end of the dosing range, reflecting the greater frequency of decreased hepatic, renal, or cardiac function, and of concomitant disease or other drug therapy.

➤*Monitoring:* Many abnormalities of renal, hepatic, and bone marrow function have been reported in patients with neoplastic diseases receiving dactinomycin. Renal, hepatic, and bone marrow functions should be assessed frequently.

Drug Interactions

➤*Drug/Lab test interactions:* Dactinomycin may interfere with bioassay procedures for the determination of antibacterial drug levels.

Adverse Reactions

Dactinomycin is considered to have moderate to high potential for nausea and vomiting.

Toxic effects (except nausea and vomiting) usually do not become apparent until 2 to 4 days after a course of therapy is stopped, and may not be maximal before 1 to 2 weeks have elapsed. Deaths have been reported. However, adverse reactions are usually reversible on discontinuance of therapy. They include the following:

➤*Dermatologic:* Alopecia; skin eruptions; acne; flare-up of erythema or increased pigmentation of previously irradiated skin. Dactinomycin is extremely corrosive. If extravasation occurs during IV use, severe damage to soft tissues will occur. In at least one instance, this has led to contracture of the arms. Epidermolysis, erythema, and edema, at times severe, have been reported with regional limb perfusion.

➤*GI:* Anorexia; nausea; vomiting; abdominal pain; diarrhea; gastrointestinal ulceration; liver toxicity including ascites; hepatomegaly; hepatic veno-occlusive disease; hepatitis; and liver function test abnormalities. Nausea and vomiting, which occur early during the first few hours after administration, may be alleviated by giving antiemetics. Cheilitis; dysphagia; esophagitis; ulcerative stomatitis; pharyngitis.

➤*Hematologic:* Anemia, even to the point of aplastic anemia; agranulocytosis; leukopenia; thrombopenia; pancytopenia; reticulopenia. Platelet and white cell counts should be performed frequently daily to detect severe hemopoietic depression. If either count markedly decreases, the drug should be withheld to allow marrow recovery. This often takes up to 3 weeks.

➤*Pulmonary:* Pneumonitis.

➤*Miscellaneous:* Malaise; fatigue; lethargy; fever; myalgia; proctitis; hypocalcemia, growth retardation, infection.

Overdosage

Dactinomycin was lethal to mice and rats at intravenous doses of 700 and 500 mcg/kg, respectively (approximately 3.8 and 5.4 times the maximum recommended daily human dose on a body surface area basis, respectively). The oral LD_{50} of dactinomycin is 7.8 mg/kg and 7.2 mg/kg in the mouse and rat, respectively.

MITOMYCIN (Mitomycin-C; MTC)

Rx	**Mitomycin** (Various, eg, American Pharmaceutical Partners, Bedford)	**Powder for Injection:** 5 mg	10 mg mannitol. In vials.
	Mitomycin (Various, eg, Bedford)	**Powder for Injection:** 20 mg	40 mg mannitol. In vials.
	Mitomycin (Various, eg, American Pharmaceutical Partners, Bedford)	**Powder for Injection:** 40 mg	80 mg mannitol. In vials.

MITOMYCIN — INJECTION

WARNING

Mitomycin should be administered under the supervision of a qualified physician experienced in the use of cancer chemotherapeutic agents. Appropriate management of therapy and complications is possible only when adequate diagnostic and treatment facilities are readily available.

Bone marrow suppression, notably thrombocytopenia and leukopenia, which may contribute to overwhelming infections in an already compromised patient, is the most common and severe of the toxic effects of mitomycin.

Hemolytic uremic syndrome (HUS), a serious complication of chemotherapy, consisting primarily of microangiopathic hemolytic anemia, thrombocytopenia, and irreversible renal failure has been reported in patients receiving systemic mitomycin. The syndrome may occur at any time during systemic therapy with mitomycin as a single agent or in combination with other cytotoxic drugs; however, most cases occur at doses greater than or equal to 60 mg of mitomycin. Blood product transfusion may exacerbate the symptoms associated with this syndrome.

The incidence of the syndrome has not been defined.

Indications

➤*Disseminated adenocarcinoma of the stomach or pancreas:* Mitomycin for injection is not recommended as single-agent, primary therapy. It has been shown to be useful in the therapy of disseminated adenocarcinoma of the stomach or pancreas in proven combinations with other approved chemotherapeutic agents and as palliative treatment when other modalities have failed. Mitomycin is not recommended to replace appropriate surgery or radiotherapy.

➤*Off-label uses:* Mitomycin has been given by the intravesical route for the management of superficial bladder cancer. Mitomycin as an ophthalmic solution appears beneficial as an adjunct to surgical excision in primary or recurrent pterygia.

Treatment of anal cancer, colorectal cancer, breast cancer, squamous cell carcinoma of head and neck, lungs or cervix; hepatocellular cancer (intraarterial use); topically for otolaryngologic procedures; and to treat tracheal stenosis.

Miomycin has been used safely and effectively in children; has been used topically for otolaryngologic procedures and to treat tracheal stenosis.

MITOMYCIN — INJECTION

Administration and Dosage

➤*General dosing considerations:* Patients receiving mitomycin should be observed for evidence of renal toxicity.

➤*Adults:*

Disseminated adenocarcinoma of the stomach or pancreas –

Usual dosage: 10 to 20 mg/m^2/dose IV, may repeat this course every 6 to 8 weeks. Reevaluate patient fully after each course of mitomycin therapy (see Dosage adjustment.)

According to the manufacturer, repeat doses of mitomycin have only been evaluated at a dose of 15 mg/m^2 at 6- to 8-week intervals after full hematological recovery (see the following Dosage adjustment table.)

Dosage adjustment: Because of cumulative myelosuppression, patients should be fully reevaluated after each course of mitomycin, and the dose reduced if the patient has experienced any toxicities. Doses greater than 20 mg/m^2 have not been shown to be more effective and are more toxic than lower doses. The following schedule is suggested as a guide to dosage adjustment.

Mitomycin Dose Adjustments		
Nadir After Prior Mitomycin Dose		
Leukocytes/mm^3	Platelets/mm^3	Percentage of prior dose to be given
> 3,000	> 75,000	100%
2,000 to 2,999	25,000 to 74,999	70%
< 2,000	< 25,000	50%

No repeat dosage should be given until leukocyte count has returned to 4,000/mm^3 and platelet count to 100,000/mm^3.

Discontinuation of therapy: Discontinue therapy if disease progression continues after 2 courses of therapy.

Off-label dosing –

Bladder cancer (intravesicular use): 20 to 40 mg instilled into the bladder up to 3 times weekly, repeated up to 20 times per course.

Hepatocellular cancer (intraarterial use): 10 mg/dose given intraarterially, as a single dose or repeated every 4 to 8 weeks. Given in combination with other antineoplastic agents.

➤*Children:*

Off-label dosing – Mitomycin has been used safely and effectively in children. See Adults for dosing.

➤*Renal function impairment:* According to the manufacturer, mitomycin should not be used in patients with severe renal dysfunction (creatinine clearance [CrCl] less than 30 mL/min). The manufacturer also recommends avoiding mitomycin use in patients with serum creatinine above 1.7 mg/dL.

Dosage adjustment is recommended in renal dysfunction, as shown in the following table.

Mitomycin Dosage Adjustment Based on Renal Function		
	Chemotherapy Source Book	Alternative reference
CrCl	Percent of Usual Dose	Percent of Usual Dose
> 60 mL/minute	100	100
30 to 60 mL/minute	75	100
10 to 29 mL/minute	50	100
< 10 mL/minute	0	75
Continuous ambulatory peritoneal dialysis	No recommendation	75

Dialysis – Conventional hemodialysis is minimally effectively (25% to 49%) in removing mitomycin.

➤*Concomitant therapy:* When mitomycin is used in combination with other myelosuppressive agents, the doses should be adjusted accordingly.

➤*Discontinuation of therapy:* If the disease continues to progress after 2 courses of mitomycin, the drug should be stopped since chances of response are minimal.

➤*Preparation for administration:* Mitomycin is considered a cytotoxic agent. Follow safe handling procedures when preparing, administering, or dispensing mitomycin.

Dilute with volume of sterile water for injection specified in the following table. Shake the vial to enhance dissolution; allow to stand at room temperature for complete dissolution. The solution should be clear to pale blue. Maximum concentration is 0.5 mg/mL; more concentrated solutions crystallize easily. Protect from light.

Reconstitution of Mannitol Formulation of Mitomycin		
Vial size	Sterile Water for Injection	Concentration
5 mg	10 mL	0.5 mg/mL
20 mg	40 mL	0.5 mg/mL
40 mg	80 mL	0.5 mg/mL

Mitomycin 0.2 mg/mL (0.02%) eye drops for pterygium (off-label use) – Reconstitute 5 mg vial of mitomycin with 10 mL sterile water for injection for a concentration of 0.5 mg/mL. Transfer 6 mL (3 mg) to a sterile 15 mL eye dropper bottle. Add 9 mL of sterile water for injection for a final concentration of 0.2 mg/mL (0.02% solution).

Mitomycin 0.2 mg/mL ophthalmic solution for intraoperative use (off-label use) – Reconstitute 5 mg vial of mitomycin with 10 mL sterile water for injection. Transfer the contents of the vial to a 30 mL sterile vial. Add 15 mL of sterile water for injection for a final volume of 25 mL (0.2 mg/mL).

Intravesical administration (off-label use) – Reconstitute 20 mg vial of mitomycin with 20 mL of sterile water for injection, to give a final concentration of 1 mg/mL.

Intraarterial administration (off-label use) – Mix mitomycin 10 mg with cisplatin 50 to 100 mg, doxorubicin 50 mg, and radiopaque contrast media in a quantity sufficient to give a total volume of 10 to 20 mL. This mixture may be given alone or mixed with *Gelfoam* powder 25 to 30 mg/mL or polyvinyl alcohol immediately prior to administration.

➤*Administration:* Mitomycin should be given IV, using care to avoid extravasation. Administer by IV push injection or IV sidearm into a running infusion.

When administered by the intravesical route (off-label use), instill into bladder and retain solution for up to 3 hours.

For intraarterial administration (off-label use), infuse with an appropriate pump to overcome pressure in large arteries.

➤*Extravasation:* If extravasation occurs, cellulitis, ulceration, and slough may result. Extravasation may occur with or without an accompanying stinging or burning sensation and even if there is adequate blood return when the injection needle is aspirated. There have been reports of delayed erythema or ulceration occurring either at or distant from the injection site, weeks to months after mitomycin, even when no obvious evidence of extravasation was observed during administration. Skin grafting has been required in some cases.

If signs or symptoms of extravasation occur, stop the infusion immediately. If possible, withdraw 3 to 5 mL of blood to remove some of the drug. Remove the infusion needle. Apply dimethyl sulfoxide (DMSO) 99% by saturating a gauze pad and painting on an area twice the size of the extravasation. Allow the site to air dry and repeat the application every 6 hours for 14 days. Do not cover the area with dressing. Application of ice compresses to the area for 15 minutes every 6 hours for 48 hours may be useful. Delineate the infiltrated area on the patient's skin with a felt-tip marker. Elevate for 48 hours above heart level using a sling or stockinette dressing with an observation window cut in the dressing. Avoid pressure or friction. Do not rub the area. Observe for signs of increased erythema, pain, or skin necrosis. If increased symptoms occur, consult a plastic surgeon. Ensure that no medication is given distally to extravasation site. After 48 hours, encourage the patient to use the extremity normally to promote full range of motion.

➤*Admixture compatibility:* The combination of mitomycin (5 to 15 mg) and heparin (1,000 to 10,000 units) in 30 mL of sodium chloride 0.9% injection is stable for 48 hours at room temperature.

Mitomycin 1 mg/mL mixed with cisplatin 10 mg/mL, and doxorubicin 5 mg/mL in sodium chloride 0.9% injection is stable for up to 12 hours refrigerated.

Mitomycin 1 mg/mL mixed with cisplatin 10 mg/mL, and doxorubicin 5 mg/mL in a 1:1 mixture of sodium chloride 0.9% injection and Ioversal 68% is stable for up to 72 hours refrigerated or for up to 24 hours at room temperature.

➤*Storage/Stability:*

Prior to reconstitution – Store dry powder at 15° to 30°C (59° to 86°F) and protect from light. Avoid excessive heat over 40°C (104°F). Dry powder is stable for the lot life indicated on the package.

Discard single-dose vials within 6 hours of the initial needle puncture if opened within an ISO Class 5 biological safety cabinet, or within 1 hour of the initial needle puncture if opened outside of such an environment, based on the USP Chapter <797> standards.

After reconstitution – Reconstituted mitomycin solutions contain no preservative and should be used within 24 hours; solutions are stable for 14 days refrigerated or 7 days at room temperature if protected from light.

After dilution – According to the manufacturer, mitomycin diluted in various IV fluids to a concentration of 20 to 40 mcg/mL is stable at room temperature for the time periods stated in the following table.

Mitomycin Dilution Stability	
IV fluid	Stability
Dextrose 5% injection	No more than 3 hours
Sodium chloride 0.9% injection	No more than 12 hours
Sodium lactate injection	No more than 24 hours

Mitomycin 0.02% eye drops for pterygium (mannitol formulation) – The 0.2 mg/mL (0.02%) solution is stable for 1 week at room temperature and 2 weeks refrigerated.

Mitomycin 0.2 mg/mL ophthalmic solution for intraoperative use (mannitol formulation) – The 0.2 mg/mL solution is stable for 52 weeks frozen, 2 weeks under refrigeration, and 24 hours at room temperature.

MITOMYCIN — INJECTION

Intravesical administration – The 1 mg/mL intravesical solution is stable for up to 24 hours at room temperature, protected from light or under fluorescent lighting.

Actions

➤*Pharmacology:* Mitomycin selectively inhibits the synthesis of deoxyribonucleic acid (DNA). The guanine and cytosine content correlates with the degree of mitomycin-induced cross-linking. At high concentrations of the drug, cellular RNA and protein synthesis are also suppressed.

➤*Pharmacokinetics:*

Absorption / Distribution – *Mitozytrex* was found bioequivalent to mitomycin in an open-label randomized crossover study in cancer patients who received single doses (15 mg/m² by a 30-minute infusion) of each formulation. In another open-label study, sequential cycles of mitomycin showed similar pharmacokinetics to mitomycin when administered every 6 weeks (15 mg/m² by a 30-minute infusion). The maximal serum concentration of mitomycin ranged from 0.38 to 1.89 mcg/mL after a 30-minute infusion of 15 mg/m² mitomycin. The disposition of mitomycin is biphasic with a mean terminal half life of 46 minutes.

Metabolism – In humans, mitomycin is rapidly cleared from the serum after intravenous administration. Time required to reduce the serum concentration by 50% after a 30 mg bolus injection is 17 minutes. After injection of 30 mg, 20 mg, or 10 mg IV, the maximal serum concentrations were 2.4 mcg/mL, 1.7 mcg/mL, and 0.52 mcg/mL, respectively. Clearance is effected primarily by metabolism in the liver, but metabolism occurs in other tissues as well. The rate of clearance is inversely proportional to the maximal serum concentration because, it is thought, of saturation of the degradative pathways.

Excretion – Approximately 10% of a dose of mitomycin is excreted unchanged in the urine. Since metabolic pathways are saturated at relatively low doses, the percentage of a dose excreted in urine increases with increasing dose. In children, excretion of intravenously administered mitomycin is similar.

Approximately 80% to 90% of HPβCD, the solubilizing agent in mitomycin, is eliminated through the kidneys, and greater than 93% is excreted unchanged in the urine within 12 hours after dosing.

Special populations –

Renal function impairment: See Warnings/Precautions for more information.

Contraindications

Hypersensitivity or idiosyncratic reaction to mitomycin; thrombocytopenia, coagulation disorder, or an increase in bleeding tendency due to other causes.

Warnings/Precautions

➤*Bone marrow suppression:* The use of mitomycin results in a high incidence of bone marrow suppression, particularly thrombocytopenia and leukopenia. Therefore, the following studies should be obtained repeatedly during therapy and for at least 8 weeks following therapy: Platelet count, white blood cell count, differential, and hemoglobin. The occurrence of a platelet count below 100,000/mm³ or a WBC below 4000/mm³ or a progressive decline in either is an indication to withhold further therapy until blood counts have recovered above these levels.

Patients should be advised of the potential toxicity of this drug, particularly bone marrow suppression. Deaths have been reported due to septicemia as a result of leukopenia due to the drug.

➤*Pulmonary toxicity:* This has occurred infrequently but can be severe and may be life threatening. Dyspnea with a nonproductive cough and radiographic evidence of pulmonary infiltrates may be indicative of mitomycin-induced pulmonary toxicity. If other etiologies are eliminated, mitomycin therapy should be discontinued. Steroids have been employed as treatment of this toxicity, but the therapeutic value has not been determined.

Acute shortness of breath and severe bronchospasm have been reported following the administration of vinca alkaloids in patients who had previously or simultaneously received mitomycin. The onset of this acute respiratory distress occurred within minutes to hours after the vinca alkaloid injection. The total number of doses for each drug has varied considerably. Bronchodilators, steroids or oxygen have produced symptomatic relief.

A few cases of adult respiratory distress syndrome have been reported in patients receiving mitomycin in combination with other chemotherapy and maintained at FIO_2 concentrations greater than 50% perioperatively. Therefore, caution should be exercised using only enough oxygen to provide adequate arterial saturation since oxygen itself is toxic to the lungs. Careful attention should be paid to fluid balance and overhydration should be avoided.

➤*Hemolytic uremic syndrome (HUS):* This serious complication of chemotherapy, consisting primarily of microangiopathic hemolytic anemia (hematocrit less than or equal to 25%), thrombocytopenia (less than or equal to 100,000/mm³, and irreversible renal failure (serum creatinine greater than or equal to 1.6 mg/dL) has been reported in patients receiving systemic mitomycin. Microangiopathic hemolysis with fragmented red blood cells on peripheral blood smears has occurred in 98% of patients with the syndrome. Other less frequent complications of the syndrome may include pulmonary edema (65%), neurologic abnormalities (16%), and hypertension. Exacerbation of the symptoms associated with HUS has been reported in some patients receiving blood product transfusions. A high mortality rate (52%) has been associated with this syndrome.

The syndrome may occur at any time during systemic therapy with mitomycin as a single agent or in combination with other cytotoxic drugs. Less frequently, HUS has also been reported in patients receiving combinations of cytotoxic drugs not including mitomycin. Of 83 patients studied, 72 developed the syndrome at total doses exceeding 60 mg of mitomycin. Consequently, patients receiving greater than or equal to 60 mg of mitomycin should be monitored closely for unexplained anemia with fragmented cells on peripheral blood smear, thrombocytopenia, and decreased renal function.

➤*Cardiac toxicity:* Congestive heart failure, often treated effectively with diuretics and cardiac glycosides, has rarely been reported. Almost all patients who experienced this side effect had received prior doxorubicin therapy.

➤*Bladder toxicity:* Bladder fibrosis/contraction has been reported with intravesical administration of mitomycin (not an approved route of administration), which in rare cases has required cystectomy. The safety of intravesical administration of mitomycin and its HPβCD excipient has not been studied. Evidence of bladder toxicities have been observed following parenteral administration of the HPβCD excipient of mitomycin as single and repeat doses equal to or greater than 0.15 g/m² and 0.5 g/m² in rodents and dogs, respectively (about 1/60 and 1/20 the amount of HPβCD administered per recommended human intravenous dose of mitomycin on a mg/m² basis). Findings included edema, inflammation, cellular inclusions and bladder stones associated with metaplasia; findings persisted at least 3 months following dosing.

➤*Bladder toxicity:* See Warnings/Precautions for more information.

➤*Extravasation:* See Administration and Dosage for more information.

➤*Renal function impairment:* Patients receiving mitomycin should be observed for evidence of renal toxicity. Mitomycin should not be given to patients with a serum creatinine greater than 1.7 mg/dL.

Renal toxicity – Two percent (2%) of 1281 patients demonstrated a statistically significant rise in creatinine. There appeared to be no correlation between total dose administered or duration of therapy and the degree of renal impairment. In a study where a single intravenous dose of 200 mg of HPβCD was given to subjects with severe renal impairment (creatinine clearance less than or equal to 19 mL/min), clearance of HPβCD was reduced 6-fold compared to subjects with normal renal function.

➤*Pregnancy: Category D.* Mitomycin can cause fetal harm when administered to a pregnant woman. If mitomycin is used during pregnancy, or if the patient becomes pregnant while receiving this drug, the patient should be apprised of the potential hazard to the fetus or potential risk for loss of the pregnancy.

Studies in both mice and rats at mitomycin doses equal to or greater than 0.5 mg/kg/day (about 1/10 and 1/5, respectively, of the recommended human dose on a mg/m² basis), administered intraperitoneally during the period of organogenesis showed a significant decrease in number of live fetuses; mitomycin was lethal to dams at 2 mg/kg/day (about 4/10's the recommended human dose on a mg/m² basis) in mice. Evidence of fetotoxicity, including delayed fetal development (eg, depressed fetal body weights, incomplete ossification), fetal external anomalies (eg, exencephaly, club foot, cleft palate, maldirection of digits, kinked tail), and neonatal anomalies (hydronephrosis, retarded development of reproductive organs) was observed in mice and rats administered doses equal to or greater than 0.05 mg/kg/day (about 1/100 and 1/50, respectively, of the recommended human dose on a mg/m² basis). In a separate study, mitomycin was administered to pregnant female mice; offspring exhibited significantly retarded reproductive tract development.

In 2 separate studies, HPβCD, the excipient for mitomycin, was fetotoxic (decreased number of live fetuses, depressed fetal body weight, incomplete ossification) in rats dosed by gavage and intravenously at doses equal to or greater than 50 and 250mg/kg/day, respectively (about 1/30 and 1/6 the amount of HPβCD administered per recommended human dose of mitomycin on a mg/m² basis).

➤*Lactation:* It is not known if mitomycin is excreted in human milk. Because many drugs are excreted in human milk and because of the potential for serious adverse reactions in nursing infants from mitomycin, it is recommended that nursing be discontinued when receiving mitomycin therapy.

➤*Children:* Safety and effectiveness in pediatric patients have not been established.

➤*Elderly:* Clinical studies of mitomycin did not include sufficient numbers of subjects aged 65 and over to determine whether they tolerate the drug differently than younger subjects. In general, elderly patients should be treated with caution due to the greater frequency of decreased hepatic, renal, or cardiac function, and concomitant disease or other drug therapy.

➤*Monitoring:* Patients being treated with mitomycin must be observed carefully and frequently during and after therapy.

Patients receiving mitomycin should be observed for evidence of renal toxicity. Mitomycin should not be given to patients with a serum creatinine greater than 1.7 mg/dL.

Nephrotoxicity, including irreversible renal necrosis, was observed in rodents and non-rodents following parenteral administration of HPβCD, the excipient contained in mitomycin. This nephrotoxicity appeared to be the result of the accumulation and recrystallization of HPβCD in the proximal tubules of the kidney.

As severe renal impairment prolongs the elimination rate of HPβCD, mitomycin should not be used in patients with severe renal dysfunction (creatinine clearance less than 30 mL/min).

Adverse Reactions

Mitomycin is considered to have moderate to low potential for nausea and vomiting.

MITOMYCIN — INJECTION

➤*Bone marrow toxicity:* This was the most common and most serious toxicity, occurring in 605 of 937 patients (64.4%) treated with mitomycin. Thrombocytopenia or leukopenia may occur anytime within 8 weeks after onset of therapy with an average time of 4 weeks. Recovery after cessation of therapy was within 10 weeks. About 25% of the leukopenic or thrombocytopenic episodes did not recover. Mitomycin produces cumulative myelosuppression.

➤*Integument and mucous membrane toxicity:* This has occurred in approximately 4% of patients treated with mitomycin. Cellulitis at the injection site has been reported and is occasionally severe. Stomatitis and alopecia also occur frequently. Rashes are rarely reported. The most important dermatological problem with this drug, however, is the necrosis and consequent sloughing of tissue which results if the drug is extravasated during injection. Extravasation may occur with or without an accompanying stinging or burning sensation and even if there is adequate blood return when the injection needle is aspirated. There have been reports of delayed erythema or ulceration occurring either at or distant from the injection site, weeks to months after mitomycin, even when no obvious evidence of extravasation was observed during administration. Skin grafting has been required in some of the cases.

➤*Renal toxicity:* See Warnings/Precautions for more information.

➤*Pulmonary toxicity:* See Warnings/Precautions for more information.

➤*Hemolytic uremic syndrome (HUS):* See Warnings/Precautions for more information.

➤*Cardiac toxicity:* See Warnings/Precautions for more information.

➤*Acute side effects due to mitomycin:* Fever, anorexia, nausea, and vomiting. They occurred in about 14% of 1281 patients.

➤*Other:* Headache, blurring of vision, confusion, drowsiness, syncope, fatigue, edema, thrombophlebitis, hematemesis, diarrhea, and pain. These did not appear to be dose related and were not unequivocally drug related. They may have been due to the primary or metastatic disease processes. Malaise and asthenia have been reported as part of postmarketing surveillance. Bladder fibrosis/contraction has been reported with intravesical administration (not an approved route of administration). The safety of intravesical administration of mitomycin and its HPβCD excipient has not been studied.

HORMONES

Antiandrogens

BICALUTAMIDE

Rx	**Bicalutamide** (Various, eg, Accord, Teva)	**Tablets; oral:** 50 mg	May contain lactose, PEG. In 30s, 100s, 500s, 1,000s, and UD 30s.
Rx	**Casodex** (AstraZeneca)		Lactose, PEG. (CDX50 Casodex). White. Film-coated. In 30s, 100s, and UD 30s.

BICALUTAMIDE — ORAL

Indications

➤*Prostate cancer:* For the treatment of stage D2 metastatic carcinoma of the prostate in combination therapy with a luteinizing hormone–releasing hormone (LHRH) analog.

Administration and Dosage

➤*Adults:*

Prostate cancer –

Usual dosage: One 50 mg tablet once daily (morning or evening).

Concomitant therapy: Take in combination with an LHRH analog. Treatment with bicalutamide should be started at the same time as treatment with an LHRH analog.

➤*Hepatic function impairment:* Bicalutamide should be used with caution in patients with moderate to severe hepatic impairment.

➤*Administration:* May take with or without food. It is recommended that bicalutamide be taken at the same time each day.

➤*Storage/Stability:* Store at 20° to 25°C (68° to 77°F).

Actions

➤*Pharmacology:* Bicalutamide is a nonsteroidal androgen receptor inhibitor. It competitively inhibits the action of androgens by binding to cytosol androgen receptors in the target tissue. Prostatic carcinoma is known to be androgen sensitive and responds to treatment that counteracts the effect of androgen and/or removes the source of androgen.

➤*Pharmacokinetics:*

Bicalutamide Pharmacokinetic Parameters

Parameter	Mean	Standard deviation
Healthy men (n = 30)		
Apparent oral clearance (L/h)	0.32	0.103
Single-dose peak concentration (mcg/mL)	0.768	0.178
Single-dose time to peak concentration (h)	31.3	14.6
Half-life (days)	5.8	2.29
Patients with prostate cancer (n = 40)		
C_{ss}[a] (mcg/mL)	8.939	3.504

[a] C_{ss} = mean steady-state concentration.

Absorption – Bicalutamide is well absorbed following oral administration, although the absolute bioavailability is unknown.

Distribution – Bicalutamide is highly protein-bound (96%).

Metabolism/Excretion – Bicalutamide undergoes stereospecific metabolism. The S (inactive) isomer is metabolized primarily by glucuronidation. The R (active) isomer also undergoes glucuronidation but is predominantly oxidized to an inactive metabolite followed by glucuronidation. Both the parent and metabolite glucuronides are eliminated in the urine and feces. The S-enantiomer is rapidly cleared relative to the R-enantiomer, with the R-enantiomer accounting for about 99% of total steady-state plasma levels.

Contraindications

Women; pregnancy; hypersensitivity reaction to the drug or any of the tablet's components.

Warnings/Precautions

➤*Hepatitis:* Rare cases of death or hospitalization because of severe liver injury have been reported during postmarketing in association with the use of bicalutamide. Hepatotoxicity in these reports generally occurred within the first 3 to 4 months of treatment. Hepatitis or marked increases in liver enzymes leading to drug discontinuation occurred in approximately 1% of bicalutamide patients in controlled clinical trials.

Measure serum transaminase levels prior to starting treatment with bicalutamide, at regular intervals for the first 4 months of treatment, and periodically thereafter. If clinical symptoms or signs suggestive of liver dysfunction occur (eg, nausea, vomiting, abdominal pain, fatigue, anorexia, flu-like symptoms, dark urine, jaundice, or right upper quadrant tenderness), measure the serum transaminases, in particular the serum ALT, immediately. If at any time a patients has jaundice or their ALT rises above 2 times the upper limit of normal (ULN), immediately discontinue bicalutamide, with close follow-up of liver function.

➤*Gynecomastia and breast pain:* In clinical trials with bicalutamide 150 mg as a single agent for prostate cancer, gynecomastia and breast pain have been reported in up to 38% and 39% of patients, respectively.

➤*Glucose tolerance:* A reduction in glucose tolerance has been observed in men receiving LHRH agonists. This may manifest as diabetes or loss of glycemic control in those with preexisting diabetes. Therefore, give careful consideration to monitoring blood glucose in patients receiving bicalutamide in combination with LHRH agonists.

➤*Hypersensitivity reactions:* Hypersensitivity reactions, including angioneurotic edema and urticaria, have been reported.

➤*Hepatic function impairment:* Use bicalutamide with caution in patients with moderate to severe hepatic impairment. Bicalutamide is extensively metabolized by the liver. Limited data in subjects with severe hepatic impairment suggest that excretion of bicalutamide may be delayed and could lead to further accumulation. Consider periodic liver function tests for hepatically impaired patients on long-term therapy.

➤*Pregnancy: Category X.* Bicalutamide may cause fetal harm when administered to a pregnant woman. Bicalutamide is contraindicated in women, including those who are or may become pregnant. There are no studies in pregnant women using bicalutamide. If this drug is used during pregnancy or if the patient becomes pregnant while taking this drug, apprise the patient of the potential hazard to the fetus.

While there are no human data on the use of bicalutamide in pregnancy and bicalutamide is not for use in women, it is important to know that maternal use of an androgen receptor inhibitor could affect development of the fetus.

In animal reproduction studies, male offspring of rats receiving dosages of at least 10 mg/kg/day (approximately two-thirds of clinical exposure at the recommended dose) had reduced anogenital distance and hypospadias. These pharmacological effects have been observed with other antiandrogens.

Fertility impairment – Administration of bicalutamide may lead to inhibition of spermatogenesis. The long-term effects of bicalutamide on male fertility have not been studied.

➤*Lactation:* Bicalutamide is not indicated for use in women, and its use in women is contraindicated.

BICALUTAMIDE — ORAL

➤*Children:* Safety and effectiveness of bicalutamide in children have not been established.

➤*Monitoring:* Measure serum transaminase levels prior to starting treatment with bicalutamide, at regular intervals for the first 4 months of treatment, and periodically thereafter. If clinical symptoms or signs suggestive of liver dysfunction occur (eg, nausea, vomiting, abdominal pain, fatigue, anorexia, flu-like symptoms, dark urine, jaundice, right upper quadrant tenderness), measure the serum transaminases, in particular the serum ALT, immediately. If at any time a patient has jaundice, or their ALT rises above 2 times the upper limit of normal, discontinue bicalutamide immediately, with close follow-up of liver function.

Regular assessments of serum prostate-specific antigen (PSA) may be helpful in monitoring the patient's response. If PSA levels rise during bicalutamide therapy, evaluate the patient for clinical progression. For patients who have objective progression of disease together with an elevated PSA, a treatment-free period of antiandrogen, while continuing the LHRH analog, may be considered.

Monitor blood glucose.

Drug Interactions

➤*Anticoagulants:* In vitro studies have shown bicalutamide can displace coumarin anticoagulants, such as warfarin, from their protein-binding sites. It is recommended that if bicalutamide is started in patients already receiving coumarin anticoagulants, closely monitor prothrombin times and adjust the anticoagulant dose if necessary.

➤*Cytochrome P-450 system:* R-bicalutamide is an inhibitor of CYP3A4. Coadministration with midazolam has shown mean midazolam levels increased 1.5-fold (for maximum plasma concentration) and 1.9-fold (for area under the curve). Exercise caution when bicalutamide is coadministered with CYP3A4 substrates.

Adverse Reactions

➤*Most frequent adverse reaction:* In patients with advanced prostate cancer treated with bicalutamide in combination with an LHRH analog, the most frequent adverse reaction was hot flashes (53%).

➤*Clinical trial:*

Bicalutamide Adverse Reactions (≥ 5%)		
Adverse reaction	Bicalutamide + LHRH analog (n = 401)	Flutamide + LHRH analog (n = 407)
Cardiovascular		
Hot flashes	53%	53%
Hypertension	8%	7%
CNS		
Anxiety	5%	2%
Asthenia	22%	21%
Depression	4%	8%
Dizziness	10%	9%
Headache	7%	7%
Insomnia	7%	10%
Paresthesia	8%	10%
Dermatologic		
Rash	9%	7%
Sweating	6%	5%
GI		
Abdominal pain	11%	11%
Anorexia	6%	7%
Constipation	22%	17%
Diarrhea	12%	26%
Dyspepsia	7%	6%
Flatulence	6%	5%
Liver enzyme test increased	7%	11%
Nausea	15%	14%
Vomiting	6%	8%
GU		
Breast pain	6%	4%
Gynecomastia	9%	7%
Hematuria	12%	6%
Impaired urination	5%	4%
Impotence	7%	9%
Nocturia	12%	14%
Urinary frequency	6%	7%
Urinary incontinence	4%	8%
Urinary retention	5%	3%
Urinary tract infection	9%	9%
Metabolic/Nutritional		
Hyperglycemia	6%	7%
Increased alkaline phosphatase	5%	6%
Peripheral edema	13%	10%
Weight gain	5%	4%
Weight loss	7%	10%
Musculoskeletal		
Arthritis	5%	7%
Back pain	25%	26%
Bone pain	9%	11%
Myasthenia	7%	5%
Pathological fracture	4%	8%
Respiratory		
Bronchitis	6%	3%
Cough increased	8%	6%
Dyspnea	13%	8%
Pharyngitis	8%	6%
Pneumonia	4%	5%
Rhinitis	4%	5%
Miscellaneous		
Anemia	11%	13%
Chest pain	8%	8%
Flu syndrome	7%	7%
General pain	35%	31%
Infection	18%	14%
Pelvic pain	21%	17%

➤*Other adverse reactions:*

Cardiovascular – Angina pectoris, congestive heart failure, coronary artery disorder, heart arrest, myocardial infarct, syncope (at least 2% but less than 5%).

CNS – Confusion, hypertonia, libido decreased, nervousness, neuropathy, somnolence (at least 2% but less than 5%).

Dermatologic – Alopecia, dry skin, herpes zoster, pruritus, skin carcinoma, skin disorder (at least 2% but less than 5%).

GI – Dry mouth, dysphagia, GI carcinoma, GI disorder, melena, periodontal abscess, rectal hemorrhage (at least 2% but less than 5%).

GU – Dysuria, hydronephrosis, urinary tract disorder, urinary urgency (at least 2% but less than 5%).

Lab test abnormalities – Elevated AST, ALT, bilirubin, serum urea nitrogen (BUN), and creatinine; decreased hemoglobin and white blood cell count.

Metabolic/Nutritional – BUN increased, creatinine increased, dehydration, edema, gout, hypercholesteremia (at least 2% but less than 5%).

Musculoskeletal – Leg cramps, myalgia (at least 2% but less than 5%).

Respiratory – Asthma, epistaxis, lung disorder, sinusitis (at least 2% but less than 5%).

Miscellaneous – Cataract specified, chills, cyst, fever, hernia, neck pain, neoplasm, sepsis (at least 2% but less than 5%).

➤*Postmarketing:*

Endocrine – Reduction in glucose tolerance, manifesting as diabetes or a loss of glycemic control in those with preexisting diabetes, has been reported during treatment with LHRH agonists.

Hypersensitivity – Uncommon cases of hypersensitivity reactions, including angioneurotic edema and urticaria.

Respiratory – Uncommon cases of interstitial lung disease, including interstitial pneumonitis and pulmonary fibrosis.

Overdosage

➤*Treatment:* There is no specific antidote; treatment of an overdose should be symptomatic.

In this patient population, multiple drugs may have been taken. Dialysis is not likely to be helpful since bicalutamide is highly protein bound and is extensively metabolized. General supportive care, including frequent monitoring of vital signs and close observation of the patient, is indicated.

BICALUTAMIDE — ORAL

Patient Information

Inform patients that therapy with bicalutamide and the LHRH analog should be initiated concomitantly, and that they should not interrupt or stop taking these medications without consulting their health care provider.

During treatment with bicalutamide, somnolence has been reported. Advise those patients who experience this symptom to observe caution when driving or operating machines.

Inform patients that diabetes or loss of glycemic control in patients with preexisting diabetes has been reported during treatment with LHRH agonists. Therefore, consider monitoring blood glucose in patients receiving bicalutamide in combination with LHRH agonists.

FLUTAMIDE

Rx	**Flutamide** (Various, eg, Eon, Ivax, Zenith Goldline)	**Capsules:** 125 mg	May contain lactose. In 100s, 180s, 500s, and UD 100s.

FLUTAMIDE — ORAL

WARNING

Hepatic injury – There have been postmarketing reports of hospitalization and rarely death due to liver failure in patients taking flutamide. Evidence of hepatic injury included elevated serum transaminase levels, jaundice, hepatic encephalopathy and death related to acute hepatic failure. The hepatic injury was reversible after discontinuation of therapy in some patients. Approximately half of the reported cases occurred within the initial 3 months of treatment with flutamide.

Serum transaminase levels should be measured prior to starting treatment with flutamide. Flutamide is not recommended in patients whose ALT values exceed twice the upper limit of normal. Serum transaminase levels should then be measured monthly for the first 4 months of therapy, and periodically thereafter. Liver function tests also should be obtained at the first signs and symptoms suggestive of liver dysfunction (eg, nausea, vomiting, abdominal pain, fatigue, anorexia, "flu-like" symptoms, hyperbilirubinuria, jaundice, right upper quadrant tenderness). If at any time, a patient has jaundice, or their ALT rises above 2 times the upper limit of normal, flutamide should be immediately discontinued with close follow-up of liver function tests until resolution.

Indications

➤*Prostatic carcinoma:* For use in combination with LHRH-agonists for the management of locally confined Stage B_2-C and Stage D_2 metastatic carcinoma of the prostate.

Stage B_2-C prostatic carcinoma – Treatment with flutamide capsules and the goserelin acetate implant should start 8 weeks prior to initiating radiation therapy and continue during radiation therapy.

Stage D_2 metastatic carcinoma – To achieve benefit from treatment, flutamide capsules should be initiated with the LHRH-agonist and continued until progression.

➤*Off-label uses:*

Hirsutism in women – [1] = Good documentation. Guidelines primarily based on expert consensus recommend the use of an antiandrogen such as flutamide in combination with an oral contraceptive for treatment of polycystic ovary syndrome hirsutism. Trials performed to date, which have been small and not well designed, have demonstrated benefit in patients with PCOS and idiopathic hirsutism. (See Administration and Dosage.)

Administration and Dosage

➤*Adults:*

Prostatic carcinoma –

Usual dosage: 250 mg (2 capsules) every 8 hours (total daily dose 750 mg).

Alternative dosage: 500 to 1,500 mg once daily has been used.

Off-label dosing –

Hirsutism in women: [1] = Good documentation. Used as monotherapy or in combination therapy at doses ranging from 125 to 500 mg daily in 1 to 2 divided doses.

➤*Renal function impairment:*

Dialysis – Conventional and peritoneal hemodialysis are ineffective (0% to 24%) in removing flutamide.

Supplemental doses are not required after hemodialysis.

➤*Preparation for administration:* Flutamide is a hormonal agent and is considered a potential teratogen. Follow safe handling procedures when preparing, administering, or dispensing flutamide.

➤*Administration:* May be taken without regard to food.

For patients unable to swallow capsules, open the capsule and mix the contents with applesauce, pudding, or other semisolid food. Administer immediately. Do not mix with beverages.

Initiate therapy simultaneously with or 24 hours prior to LHRH analog therapy.

➤*Storage/Stability:* Store at 25°C (77°F); excursions permitted to 15° to 30°C (59° to 86°F). Dispense with a child-resistant closure in a tight, light-resistant container.

Actions

➤*Pharmacology:* In animal studies, flutamide demonstrates potent antiandrogenic effects. It exerts its antiandrogenic action by inhibiting androgen uptake or by inhibiting nuclear binding of androgen in target tissues or both. Prostatic carcinoma is known to be androgen sensitive and responds to treatment that counteracts the effect of androgen or removes the source of androgen, (eg, castration). Elevations of plasma testosterone and estradiol levels have been noted following flutamide administration.

➤*Pharmacokinetics:*

Absorption – Analysis of plasma, urine, and feces following a single oral 200 mg dose of tritium-labeled flutamide to human volunteers showed that the drug is rapidly and completely absorbed. Following a single 250 mg oral dose to healthy adult volunteers, the biologically active alpha-hydroxylated metabolite reaches maximum plasma concentrations in about 2 hours, indicating that it is rapidly formed from flutamide. Food has no effect on the bioavailability of flutamide.

Distribution – In male rats administered an oral 5 mg/kg dose of ^{14}C-flutamide, neither flutamide nor any of its metabolites is preferentially accumulated in any tissue except the prostate. Total drug levels were highest 6 hours after drug administration in all tissues. Levels declined at roughly similar rates to low levels at 18 hours. Flutamide, in vivo, at steady-state plasma concentrations of 24 to 78 ng/mL, is 94% to 96% bound to plasma proteins. The active metabolite of flutamide, in vivo, at steady-state plasma concentrations of 1556 to 2284 ng/mL, is 92% to 94% bound to plasma proteins.

The major metabolite was present at higher concentrations than flutamide in all tissues studied. Following a single 250 mg oral dose to healthy adult volunteers, low plasma concentrations of flutamide were detected. The plasma half-life for the alpha-hydroxylated metabolite of flutamide is approximately 6 hours.

Metabolism – The composition of plasma radioactivity, following a single 200 mg oral dose of tritium-labeled flutamide to healthy adult volunteers, showed that flutamide is rapidly and extensively metabolized, with flutamide comprising only 2.5% of plasma radioactivity 1 hour after administration. At least 6 metabolites have been identified in plasma. The major plasma metabolite is a biologically active alpha-hydroxylated derivative which accounts for 23% of the plasma tritium 1 hour after drug administration. The major urinary metabolite is 2-amino-5-nitro-4-(trifluoromethyl)phenol.

Excretion – Flutamide and its metabolites are excreted mainly in the urine with only 4.2% of a single dose excreted in the feces over 72 hours.

Contraindications

Hypersensitivity to flutamide or any component of this preparation; severe hepatic impairment (baseline hepatic enzymes should be evaluated prior to treatment).

Warnings/Precautions

➤*Use in women:* Flutamide capsules are for use only in men. This product has no indication for women, and should not be used in this population, particularly for non-serious or non-life-threatening conditions.

➤*Fetal toxicity:* Flutamide may cause fetal harm when administered to a pregnant woman (see Pregnancy).

➤*Aniline toxicity:* One metabolite of flutamide is 4-nitro-3-fluoromethylaniline. Several toxicities consistent with aniline exposure, including methemoglobinemia, hemolytic anemia and cholestatic jaundice have been observed in both animals and humans after flutamide administration. In patients susceptible to aniline toxicity (eg, persons with glucose-6-phosphate dehydrogenase deficiency, hemoglobin M disease and smokers), monitoring of methemoglobin levels should be considered.

➤*Hepatic function impairment:* See Warning Box.

➤*Pregnancy: Category D.* There was decreased 24-hour survival in the offspring of pregnant rats treated with flutamide at doses of 30, 100 or 200 mg/kg/day (approximately 3, 9 and 19 times the human dose). A slight increase in minor variations in the development of the sternebrae and vertebrae was seen in fetuses of rats treated with 2 higher doses. Feminization of the male rats also occurred at the 2 higher dose levels. There was a decreased survival rate in the offspring of rabbits receiving the highest dose (15 mg/kg/day, equal 1.4 times the human dose).

➤*Lactation:* Flutamide is not recommended for use in women and should not be used by this population, particularly for nonserious or non–life-threatening conditions.

➤*Monitoring:* Regular assessment of serum prostate specific antigen (PSA) may be helpful in monitoring the patient's response. If PSA levels rise significantly and consistently during flutamide therapy, the patient should be evaluated for clinical progression. For patients who have objective pro-

FLUTAMIDE — ORAL

gression of disease together with an elevated PSA, a treatment period free of antiandrogen while continuing the LHRH analog may be considered.

Drug Interactions

➤*Anticoagulants:* Increases in prothrombin time have been noted in patients receiving long-term warfarin therapy after flutamide was initiated. Therefore close monitoring of prothrombin time is recommended, and adjustment of the anticoagulant dose may be necessary when flutamide capsules are administered concomitantly with warfarin.

Adverse Reactions

Gynecomastia – In clinical trials, gynecomastia occurred in 9% of patients receiving flutamide together with medical castration.

➤*Stage B_2-C prostatic carcinoma:*

Flutamide Adverse Reactions During Acute Radiation Therapy (%)

Adverse reactions	Goserelin acetate implant and flutamide and radiation (n = 231)	Radiation only (n = 235)
Rectum/large bowel	80%	76%
Bladder	58%	60%
Skin	37%	37%

Flutamide Adverse Reactions During Late Radiation Phase (%)

Adverse reactions	Goserelin acetate implant and flutamide and radiation (n = 231)	Radiation only (n = 235)
Diarrhea	36%	40%
Cystitis	16%	16%
Rectal bleeding	14%	20%
Proctitis	8%	8%
Hematuria	7%	12%

Additional adverse event data were collected for the combination therapy with radiation group over both the hormonal treatment and hormonal treatment plus radiation phases of the study. Adverse experiences occurring in more than 5% of patients in this group, over both parts of the study, were hot flashes (46%), diarrhea (40%), nausea (9%), and skin rash (8%).

➤*Stage D_2 metastatic carcinoma:* The following adverse experiences were reported during a multicenter clinical trial comparing flutamide and LHRH agonist vs placebo and LHRH agonist.

Flutamide Adverse Reactions (%)

Adverse reactions	Flutamide and LHRH agonist (n = 294)	Placebo and LHRH agonist (n = 285)
Hot flashes	61%	57%
Loss of libido	36%	31%
Impotence	33%	29%
Diarrhea	12%	4%
Nausea/vomiting	11%	10%
Gynecomastia	9%	11%
Other	7%	9%
Other GI	6%	4%

As shown in the table, for both treatment groups, the most frequently occurring adverse experiences (hot flashes, impotence, loss of libido) were those known to be associated with low serum androgen levels and known to occur with LHRH agonists alone.

The only notable difference was the higher incidence of diarrhea in the flutamide and LHRH agonist group (12%), which was severe in 5% as opposed to the placebo and LHRH agonist (4%), which was severe in less than 1%.

➤*Additional adverse reactions:*

Cardiovascular – Hypertension in 1% of patients.

CNS – Drowsiness, confusion, depression, anxiety, or nervousness occurred in 1% of patients.

GI – Anorexia 4%, and other GI disorders occurred in 6% of patients.

Hematologic – Anemia occurred in 6%, leukopenia in 3%, and thrombocytopenia in 1% of patients.

Hepatic – Hepatitis and jaundice in less than 1% of patients.

Lab test abnormalities – Laboratory abnormalities including elevated AST, ALT, bilirubin values, SGGT, blood urea nitrogen (BUN), and serum creatinine have been reported.

Local – Irritation at the injection site and rash occurred in 3% of patients.

Miscellaneous – Edema occurred in 4%, GU and neuromuscular symptoms in 2%, and pulmonary symptoms in less than 1% of patients. Malignant breast neoplasms have occurred rarely in male patients being treated with flutamide.

Postmarketing: In addition, the following spontaneous adverse experiences have been reported during the marketing of flutamide: Hemolytic anemia, macrocytic anemia, methemoglobinemia, sulfhemoglobinemia, photosensitivity reactions (including erythema, ulceration, bullous eruptions, and epidermal necrolysis), and urine discoloration. The urine was noted to change to an amber or yellow-green appearance which can be attributed to the flutamide or its metabolites. Also reported were cholestatic jaundice, hepatic encephalopathy, and hepatic necrosis. The hepatic conditions were often reversible after discontinuing therapy; however, there have been reports of death following severe hepatic injury associated with use of flutamide.

Overdosage

➤*Symptoms:* In animal studies with flutamide alone, signs of overdose included hypoactivity, piloerection, slow respiration, ataxia, or lacrimation, anorexia, tranquilization, emesis, and methemoglobinemia.

Clinical trials have been conducted with flutamide in doses up to 1500 mg/day for periods up to 36 weeks with no serious adverse effects reported. Those adverse reactions reported included gynecomastia, breast tenderness, and some increases in AST. The single dose of flutamide ordinarily associated with symptoms of overdose or considered to be life-threatening has not been established.

➤*Treatment:* Flutamide is highly protein bound and is not cleared by hemodialysis. As in the management of overdosage with any drug, it should be borne in mind that multiple agents may have been taken. If vomiting does not occur spontaneously, it should be induced if the patient is alert. General supportive care, including frequent monitoring of the vital signs and close observation of the patient, is indicated.

Patient Information

Patients should be informed that flutamide capsules and the drug used for medical castration should be administered concomitantly, and that they should not interrupt their dosing or stop taking these medications without consulting their physician.

NILUTAMIDE

Rx	Nilandron (Sanofi-Aventis)	Tablets; oral: 150 mg	Lactose. (168D). White, cylindrical. In UD 30s.

NILUTAMIDE — ORAL

WARNING

Interstitial pneumonitis – Interstitial pneumonitis has been reported in 2% of patients in controlled clinical trials in patients exposed to nilutamide. A small study in Japanese patients showed that 17% of patients developed interstitial pneumonitis. Reports of interstitial changes, including pulmonary fibrosis that led to hospitalization and death, have been reported rarely in postmarketing. Symptoms included exertional dyspnea, cough, chest pain, and fever. X-rays showed interstitial or alveolo-interstitial changes, and pulmonary function tests revealed a restrictive pattern with decreased diffusing capacity of lungs for carbon monoxide. Most cases occurred within the first 3 months of treatment with nilutamide, and most reversed with discontinuation of therapy. Perform a routine chest x-ray prior to initiating treatment with nilutamide. Consider baseline pulmonary function tests. Instruct patients to report any new or worsening shortness of breath that they experience while on nilutamide. If symptoms occur, immediately discontinue nilutamide until it can be determined if the symptoms are drug related.

Indications

➤*Metastatic prostate cancer:* For use in combination with surgical castration for the treatment of metastatic prostate cancer (stage D2).

➤*Off-label uses:* Treatment of metastatic prostate cancer alone or in combination with luteinizing hormone-releasing hormone agonists.

Administration and Dosage

➤*Adults:*

Metastatic prostate cancer –

Initial dosage: 300 mg once a day for 30 days.

Maintenance dosage: 150 mg once a day.

➤*Preparation for administration:* Nilutamide is a hormonal agent and is considered a potential teratogen. Follow safe handling procedures when preparing, administering, or dispensing nilutamide.

➤*Administration:* Nilutamide can be taken with or without food. Nilutamide should be started on the day of or on the day after surgical castration.

NILUTAMIDE — ORAL

➤*Storage/Stability:* Store at 25°C (77°F); excursions are permitted between 15° and 30°C (59° to 86°F). Protect from light.

Actions

➤*Pharmacology:* Prostate cancer is known to be androgen-sensitive and responds to androgen ablation. In animal studies, nilutamide has demonstrated antiandrogenic activity without other hormonal (ie, estrogen, progesterone, mineralocorticoid, glucocorticoid) effects. In vitro, nilutamide blocks the effects of testosterone at the androgen receptor level. In vivo, nilutamide interacts with the androgen receptor and prevents the normal androgenic response.

➤*Pharmacokinetics:*

Absorption – Analysis of blood, urine, and feces samples following a single oral 150 mg dose of (^{14}C)-nilutamide in patients with metastatic prostate cancer showed that the drug is rapidly and completely absorbed and that it yields high and persistent plasma concentrations.

During multiple dosing of nilutamide 150 mg (given as 3 times 50 mg) twice a day, steady state was reached within 2 to 4 weeks for most patients, and mean steady-state area under the curve $(AUC)_{0-12}$ was 110% higher than the $AUC_{0-\infty}$ obtained from the first 150 mg dose. These data and in vitro metabolism data suggest that, upon multiple dosing, metabolic enzyme inhibition may occur for this drug.

Distribution – After absorption of the drug, there is a detectable distribution phase. There is moderate binding of the drug to plasma proteins and low binding to erythrocytes. The binding is nonsaturable, except in the case of alpha-1-glycoprotein, which makes a minor contribution to the total concentration of proteins in the plasma. The results of binding studies do not indicate any effects that would cause nonlinear pharmacokinetics.

Metabolism – The results of a human metabolism study using ^{14}C-radiolabeled tablets show that nilutamide is extensively metabolized and less than 2% of the drug is excreted unchanged in urine after 5 days. Five metabolites have been isolated from human urine. Two metabolites display an asymmetric center caused by oxidation of a methyl group, resulting in the formation of D- and L-isomers. In vitro, 1 of the metabolites was shown to possess 25% to 50% of the pharmacological activity of the parent drug, and the D-isomer of the active metabolite showed equal or greater potency compared with the L-isomer. However, the pharmacokinetics and the pharmacodynamics of the metabolites have not been fully investigated.

Excretion – The majority (62%) of orally administered (^{14}C)-nilutamide is eliminated in the urine during the first 120 hours after a single 150 mg dose. Fecal elimination is negligible, ranging from 1.4% to 7% of the dose after 4 to 5 days. Excretion of radioactivity in urine likely continues beyond 5 days. The mean elimination half-life of nilutamide determined in studies in which subjects received a single dose of 100 to 300 mg ranged from 38 to 59.1 hours, with most values between 41 and 49 hours. The elimination of at least 1 metabolite is generally longer than that of unchanged nilutamide (59 to 126 hours).

Contraindications

Severe hepatic impairment; severe respiratory insufficiency; hypersensitivity to nilutamide or any component of this preparation.

Warnings/Precautions

➤*Interstitial pneumonitis:* See the Warning box for more information.

➤*Hepatic effects:* Rare cases of death or hospitalization because of severe liver injury have been reported during postmarketing in association with the use of nilutamide. Hepatotoxicity in these reports generally occurred within the first 3 to 4 months of treatment. Hepatitis or marked increases in liver enzymes leading to drug discontinuation occurred in 1% of nilutamide patients in controlled clinical trials.

Measure serum transaminase levels prior to starting treatment with nilutamide, at regular intervals for the first 4 months of treatment, and periodically thereafter. Obtain liver function tests at the first sign or symptom suggestive of liver dysfunction (eg, abdominal pain, anorexia, dark urine, fatigue, flu-like symptoms, jaundice, nausea, right upper quadrant tenderness, vomiting). If at any time a patient has jaundice or their ALT rises above 2 times the upper limit of normal, immediately discontinue nilutamide, with close follow-up of liver function tests until resolution.

➤*Use in women:* Nilutamide has no indication for women; do not use in this population, particularly for nonserious or non–life-threatening conditions.

➤*Aplastic anemia:* Foreign postmarketing surveillance has revealed isolated cases of aplastic anemia in which a causal relationship with nilutamide could not be ascertained.

➤*Antiandrogen withdrawal syndrome:* Patients whose disease progresses while being treated with an antiandrogen may experience clinical improvement with discontinuation of the antiandrogen.

➤*Pregnancy: Category C.* Animal reproduction studies have not been conducted with nilutamide. It is also not known whether nilutamide can cause fetal harm when administered to a pregnant woman or if it affects reproductive capacity. Administer nilutamide to a pregnant woman only if clearly needed. Nilutamide is not indicated for use in women.

➤*Lactation:* Nilutamide is not indicated for use in women.

➤*Children:* Safety and efficacy in children have not been determined.

➤*Monitoring:* Perform a routine chest x-ray prior to initiating treatment with nilutamide and consider baseline pulmonary function tests. Measure serum transaminase levels prior to starting treatment with nilutamide, at regular intervals for the first 4 months of treatment, and periodically thereafter. Obtain liver function tests at the first sign or symptom suggestive of liver dysfunction (eg, abdominal pain, anorexia, dark urine, fatigue, flu-like symptoms, jaundice, nausea, right upper quadrant tenderness, vomiting).

Drug Interactions

➤*Cytochrome P450:* In vitro, nilutamide has been shown to inhibit the activity of liver cytochrome P450 (CYP-450) isoenzymes and, therefore, may reduce the metabolism of compounds requiring these systems.

➤*Low therapeutic margin:* Drugs with a low therapeutic margin, such as vitamin K antagonists, phenytoin, and theophylline, could have a delayed elimination and increases in their serum half-life, leading to a toxic level. The dosage of these drugs or others with a similar metabolism may need to be modified if they are coadministered with nilutamide. For example, when vitamin K antagonists are coadministered with nilutamide, carefully monitor prothrombin time and, if necessary, reduce the dosage of vitamin K antagonists.

Adverse Reactions

➤*Nilutamide plus surgical castration:* Some frequently occurring adverse reactions (eg, decreased libido, hot flushes, impotence) are known to be associated with low serum androgen levels and occur with medical or surgical castration alone. Of note was the higher incidence of visual disturbances (variously described as abnormal vision, colored vision, and impaired adaptation to darkness), which led to treatment discontinuation in 1% to 2% of patients.

Nilutamide Plus Surgical Castration Adverse Reactions (> 5%)

Adverse reactions	Nilutamide + surgical castration (n = 225)	Placebo + surgical castration (n = 232)
GI		
Constipation	7.1%	3.9%
Nausea	9.8%	6%
Hepatic		
Increased ALT	7.6%	4.3%
Increased AST	8%	3.9%
Special senses		
Abnormal vision	6.7%	1.7%
Impaired adaptation to dark	12.9%	1.3%
Miscellaneous		
Dizziness	7.1%	3.4%
Dyspnea	6.2%	7.3%
Hot flushes	28.4%	22.4%
Hypertension	5.3%	2.6%
Urinary tract infection	8%	9.1%

➤*Nilutamide plus leuprolide:*

Nilutamide Plus Leuprolide Adverse Reactions (> 5%)

Adverse reactions	Nilutamide + leuprolide (n = 209)	Placebo + leuprolide (n = 202)
CNS		
Asthenia	19.1%	20.8%
Depression	8.6%	7.4%
Dizziness	10%	11.4%
Headache	13.9%	10.4%
Hypesthesia	5.3%	2%
Insomnia	16.3%	15.8%
Dermatologic		
Body hair loss	5.7%	0.5%
Dry skin	5.3%	2.5%
Rash	5.3%	4%
Sweating	6.2%	3%
GI		
Abdominal pain	10%	5.4%
Anorexia	11%	6.4%
Constipation	19.6%	16.8%
Dyspepsia	6.7%	4.5%
Nausea	23.9%	8.4%
Vomiting	5.7%	4%

Antiandrogens

NILUTAMIDE — ORAL

Nilutamide Plus Leuprolide Adverse Reactions (> 5%)		
Adverse reactions	Nilutamide + leuprolide (n = 209)	Placebo + leuprolide (n = 202)
GU		
Gynecomastia	10.5%	11.9%
Hematuria	8.1%	7.9%
Impotence	11%	12.9%
Libido decreased	11%	4.5%
Nocturia	6.7%	6.4%
Testicular atrophy	16.3%	12.4%
Urinary tract disorder	7.2%	10.4%
Urinary tract infection	8.6%	21.3%
Hepatic		
Increased ALT	9.1%	8.9%
Increased AST	12.9%	13.9%
Musculoskeletal		
Back pain	11.5%	16.8%
Bone pain	6.2%	5%
Respiratory		
Dyspnea	10.5%	7.4%
Pneumonia	5.3%	3.5%
Upper respiratory tract infection	8.1%	10.9%
Special senses		
Abnormal vision	6.2%	4.5%
Chromatopsia	8.6%	0%
Impaired adaptation to dark	56.9%	5.4%
Impaired adaptation to light	7.7%	1%
Miscellaneous		
Anemia	7.2%	6.4%
Chest pain	7.2%	4.5%
Fever	5.3%	6.4%
Flu syndrome	7.2%	3%
Hot flushes	66.5%	59.4%
Hypertension	9.1%	9.9%
Pain	26.8%	27.7%
Peripheral edema	12.4%	17.3%

➤*Interstitial pneumonitis:* See the Warning box for more information.

➤*Other adverse reactions:*

Cardiovascular – Heart failure (3%); angina, syncope (2%).

CNS – Paresthesia (3%); malaise, nervousness (2%).

GI – Diarrhea, dry mouth, GI disorder, GI hemorrhage, melena (2%).

Lab test abnormalities – Hyperglycemia (4%); alkaline phosphatase increased, leukopenia (3%); creatinine increased, increased blood urea nitrogen, increased haptoglobin (2%).

Metabolic/Nutritional – Alcohol intolerance (5%); edema, weight loss (2%).

Respiratory – Lung disorder (4%); increased cough, interstitial lung disease (2%).

Special senses – Cataract, photophobia, rhinitis (2%).

Miscellaneous – Arthritis, pruritus (2%).

Overdosage

➤*Symptoms:* One case of massive overdosage has been published. A man 79 years of age attempted suicide by ingesting nilutamide 13 g (ie, 43 times the maximum recommended dose). Despite immediate gastric lavage and oral administration of activated charcoal, plasma nilutamide levels peaked at 6 times the normal range 2 hours after ingestion. There were no clinical signs or symptoms or changes in parameters, such as transaminases or chest x-ray. Maintenance treatment (150 mg/day) was resumed 30 days later.

In repeated-dose tolerance studies, dosages of 600 and 900 mg/day were administered to 9 and 4 patients, respectively. The ingestion of these doses was associated with GI disorders, including nausea and vomiting, malaise, headache, and dizziness. In addition, a transient elevation in hepatic enzyme levels was noted in 1 patient.

➤*Treatment:* Because nilutamide is protein bound, dialysis may not be useful as treatment for overdose. As in the management of overdosage with any drug, multiple agents may have been taken. General supportive care, including frequent monitoring of the vital signs and close observation of the patient, is indicated.

Patient Information

Inform patients that nilutamide should be started on the day of or on the day after surgical castration. Advise patients not to interrupt their dosing of nilutamide or stop taking this medication without consulting their health care providers.

Because of the possibility of interstitial pneumonitis, inform patients to immediately report any dyspnea or aggravation of preexisting dyspnea.

Because of the possibility of hepatitis, tell patients to consult with their health care provider if nausea, vomiting, abdominal pain, or jaundice occur.

Because of the possibility of an intolerance to alcohol (eg, facial flushes, hypotension, malaise) following ingestion of nilutamide, advise patients who experience this reaction to avoid the intake of alcoholic beverages.

In clinical trials, patients receiving nilutamide reported a delay in adaptation to dark, ranging from seconds to a few minutes, when passing from a lighted area to a dark area. This effect sometimes does not abate as drug treatment is continued. Caution patients who experience this effect about driving at night or through tunnels. This effect can be alleviated by the wearing of tinted glasses.

Progestins

MEGESTROL ACETATE

For complete prescribing information, refer to the Megestrol monograph in the Endocrine chapter.

MEDROXYPROGESTERONE ACETATE

For complete prescribing information refer to the Medroxyprogesterone Acetate monograph in the Contraceptive Hormones section of the Endocrine chapter.

Antiestrogens

TAMOXIFEN CITRATE

Rx	**Tamoxifen Citrate** (Various, eg, Barr, Ivax, Mylan, Teva)	**Tablets:** 10 mg (as base)	In 60s, 180s, 500s, 1,000s, and UD 100s.
Rx	**Tamoxifen Citrate** (Various, eg, Barr, Ivax, Mylan, Teva)	**Tablets:** 20 mg (as base)	In 30s, 90s, 100s, 500s, 1,000s, and UD 100s.

TAMOXIFEN CITRATE — ORAL

WARNING

For women with ductal carcinoma in situ (DCIS) and women at high risk for breast cancer – Serious and life-threatening events associated with tamoxifen in the risk-reduction setting (women at high risk for cancer and women with DCIS) include uterine malignancies, stroke, and pulmonary embolism (PE). Incidence rates for these events were estimated from the National Surgical Adjuvant Breast and Bowel Project (NSABP) P-1 trial. Uterine malignancies consist of both endometrial adenocarcinoma (incidence rate per 1,000 women years of 2.2 for tamoxifen versus 0.71 for placebo) and uterine sarcoma (incidence rate per 1,000 women years of 0.17 for tamoxifen versus 0.4 for placebo). (Updated long-term follow-up data [median length of follow-up is 6.9 years] from NSABP P-1 study.)

For stroke, the incidence rate per 1,000 women years was 1.43 for tamoxifen versus 1 for placebo. For PE, the incidence rate per 1,000 women years was 0.75 for tamoxifen versus 0.25 for placebo.

Some of the strokes, PE, and uterine malignancies were fatal.

Discuss the potential benefits versus the potential risks of these serious events with women at high risk of breast cancer and with women with DCIS considering tamoxifen to reduce their risks of developing breast cancer.

The benefits of tamoxifen outweigh its risks in women already diagnosed with breast cancer.

Indications

➤*Adjuvant treatment of breast cancer:* For the treatment of node-positive breast cancer in postmenopausal women following total mastectomy or segmental mastectomy, axillary dissection, and breast irradiation. In some tamoxifen adjuvant studies, most of the benefit to date has been in the subgroup with 4 or more positive axillary nodes.

For the treatment of axillary node-negative breast cancer in women following total mastectomy or segmental mastectomy, axillary dissection, and breast irradiation.

The ER- and progesterone-receptor values may help to predict whether adjuvant tamoxifen therapy is likely to be beneficial.

Tamoxifen reduces the occurrence of contralateral breast cancer in patients receiving adjuvant tamoxifen therapy for breast cancer.

➤*DCIS:* In women with DCIS, following breast surgery and radiation, tamoxifen is indicated to reduce the risk of invasive breast cancer. Base the decisions regarding therapy with tamoxifen for the reduction in breast cancer incidence upon an individual assessment of the benefits and risks of tamoxifen therapy.

Current data from clinical trials support 5 years of adjuvant tamoxifen therapy for patients with breast cancer.

➤*Metastatic breast cancer:* Effective in the treatment of metastatic breast cancer in women and men. In premenopausal women with metastatic breast cancer, tamoxifen is an alternative to oophorectomy or ovarian irradiation. Available evidence indicates that patients whose tumors are estrogen receptor (ER) positive are more likely to benefit from tamoxifen therapy.

➤*Reduction of breast cancer incidence in high-risk women:* To reduce the incidence of breast cancer in women at high risk for breast cancer. This effect was shown in a study of 5 years planned duration, with a median follow-up of 4.2 years. Twenty-five percent of the participants received the drug for 5 years. The longer-term effects are not known. In this study, there was no impact of tamoxifen on overall or breast cancer–related mortality.

Tamoxifen is indicated only for high-risk women. "High risk" is defined as women at least 35 years of age with a 5-year predicted risk of breast cancer greater than or equal to 1.67%, as calculated by the Gail model.

Examples of combinations of factors predicting a 5-year risk greater than or equal to 1.67% are the following –

35 years of age or older and any of the following combination of factors:

- one first-degree relative with a history of breast cancer, 2 or more benign biopsies, and a history of a breast biopsy showing atypical hyperplasia
- at least 2 first-degree relatives with a history of breast cancer and a personal history of at least 1 breast biopsy
- lobular cancer in situ (LCIS)

40 years of age or older and any of the following combination of factors:

- one first-degree relative with a history of breast cancer, 2 or more benign biopsies, age at first live birth 25 years or older, and age at menarche 11 years or younger
- at least 2 first-degree relatives with a history of breast cancer and age at first live birth 19 years or younger
- one first-degree relative with a history of breast cancer and a personal history of a breast biopsy showing atypical hyperplasia

45 years of age or older and any of the following combination of factors:

- at least 2 first-degree relatives with a history of breast cancer and age at first live birth 24 years or younger
- one first-degree relative with a history of breast cancer with a history of a benign breast biopsy, age at menarche 11 years or younger, and age at first live birth 20 years or older

50 years of age or older and any of the following combination of factors:

- at least 2 first-degree relatives with a history of breast cancer
- history of 1 breast biopsy showing atypical hyperplasia, age at first live birth 30 years or older, and age at menarche 11 years or younger
- history of at least 2 breast biopsies with a history of atypical hyperplasia, and age at first live birth 30 years or older

55 years of age or older and any of the following combination of factors:

- one first-degree relative with a history of breast cancer with a personal history of a benign breast biopsy and age at menarche 11 years or younger
- history of at least 2 breast biopsies with a history of atypical hyperplasia and age at first live birth 20 years or older

60 years of age or older and the following:

- five-year predicted risk of breast cancer greater than or equal to 1.67%, as calculated by the Gail model For women whose risk factors are not described in the preceding examples, the Gail model is necessary to estimate absolute breast cancer risk. Health care providers can obtain a Gail model risk assessment tool by calling 1-800-544-2007.

There are no data available regarding the effect of tamoxifen on breast cancer incidence in women with inherited mutations (BRCA1, BRCA2) to be able to make specific recommendations on the efficacy of tamoxifen in these patients.

After an assessment of the risk of developing breast cancer, base the decision regarding therapy with tamoxifen for the reduction in breast cancer incidence upon an individual assessment of the benefits and risks. In the NSABP P-1 trial, tamoxifen treatment lowered the risk of developing breast cancer during the follow-up period of the trial but did not eliminate breast cancer risk.

➤*Off-label uses:*

Gynecomastia – [1] = Good documentation. Tamoxifen has been demonstrated to have a significant role in the treatment of primary or secondary gynecomastia.

Mastalgia – [3] = Safety concerns. The use of tamoxifen for the treatment of mastalgia is supported by a meta-analysis of controlled trials that showed a consistent improvement in breast pain in the studies. Tamoxifen was recommended as the drug of first choice because of its favorable safety profile compared with other evidence-based therapies for mastalgia. However, tamoxifen has a black box warning for women at high risk of breast cancer, which should be considered when weighing the risks and benefits for each patient.

McCune-Albright syndrome in girls – [3] = Safety concerns. Tamoxifen may be effective in slowing the rate of bone maturation in girls with McCune-Albright syndrome, but study data are limited and long-term data on tamoxifen's effects on final adult height are lacking. Tamoxifen may reverse precocious puberty and reduce vaginal bleeding. Periodic pelvic ultrasounds have been recommended to assess uterine size during tamoxifen treatment of McCune-Albright syndrome. Tamoxifen has a black box warning for women at high risk of breast cancer, which should be considered as part of the risk-benefit analysis.

Menstrual migraine – [4] = Insufficient documentation. Tamoxifen appears to be a potentially effective preventative therapy for migraine headaches associated with menstruation, but published clinical experience to date is extremely limited. The optimal dosage has not been established, and serious safety risks have been identified in women taking tamoxifen for other indications. National guidelines for the prevention of migraine associated with menstruation recommend standard prophylactic migraine therapies. When these are ineffective, the guidelines state that hormonal therapy may be considered, but the therapy of choice is supplemental estrogen in the form of estradiol.

Oligospermia – [2] = Fair documentation. In the most successful study, in which improved pregnancy rates were observed, the mean sperm count at baseline in tamoxifen plus testosterone–treated men exceeded 29 million/mL, the typical threshold below which men are considered to be oligospermic. Other trials of combination tamoxifen and testosterone have demonstrated improvements in seminal parameters. In contrast, several small studies with tamoxifen alone found minimal or no benefits on seminal parameters, hormonal parameters, or pregnancy rates. Thus, any improvements observed with tamoxifen therapy may be dependent on or the direct result of concurrent use with testosterone. The potential for tamoxifen to improve pregnancy rates remains to be proven in men with severe oligospermia, who are least likely to achieve conception without intervention.

Ovulation disorders – [3] = Safety concerns. Tamoxifen is recommended by the United Kingdom's National Institute for Clinical Excellence as a reasonable first-line treatment alternative to clomiphene for inducing ovulation in anovulatory women. Evidence from meta-analyses of comparative studies does not support a significant benefit of tamoxifen over clomiphene and confirms that they are equally efficacious. Tamoxifen has a black box warning for women with high risk for breast cancer, which should be considered during patient assessment. Guidelines recommend that women taking either clomiphene or tamoxifen for ovulation induction be warned about the risk of multiple pregnancy.

Other possible off-label uses – Malignant carcinoid tumor and carcinoid syndrome; migraine associated with menstruation; metastatic melanoma; desmoid tumors.

There is limited experience in children with brain tumors and precocious puberty secondary to McCune-Albright syndrome.

Administration and Dosage

➤*General dosing considerations:* Initiate therapy during menstruation in sexually active premenopausal women. In women with menstrual irregularity, initiate therapy immediately after a negative pregnancy test result (ie, beta-hCG in urine).

TAMOXIFEN CITRATE — ORAL

➤*Adults:*

Breast cancer –

Usual dosage: 20 to 40 mg/day. Dosages greater than 20 mg/day should be given in divided doses (morning and evening).

Ductal carcinoma in situ – 20 mg/day for 5 years.

Reduction of breast cancer incidence in high-risk women – 20 mg/day for 5 years; there are no data to support the use of tamoxifen for other than for 5 years.

Off-label dosing –

Gynecomastia: [1] = Good documentation. 20 mg/day for 1 to 12 months.

Mastalgia: [3] = Safety concerns. 10 to 20 mg/day for 3 to 6 months.

McCune-Albright syndrome in girls: [3] = Safety concerns. 10 to 40 mg/day given once daily or divided for twice-daily administration. In a case report, tamoxifen was administered continuously for 3 years.

Menstrual migraine: [4] = Insufficient documentation. 10 to 20 mg/day for 7 to 14 days before menses, followed by 5 to 10 mg/day during menses, repeated with each cycle.

Oligospermia: [2] = Fair documentation. 10 mg twice daily is the most commonly reported dosage, although total dosages of 10 to 40 mg/day have been used. Increasing the dosage from 10 mg twice daily after 6 months to 20 mg twice daily did not increase sperm count. Tamoxifen has been administered for oligospermia for up to 18 months. Tamoxifen has been shown to be most effective when used in combination with testosterone.

Ovulation disorders: [3] = Safety concerns. 20 to 80 mg/day, adjusted based on response, for days 2 through 6, days 3 through 7, or days 5 through 9 of each cycle. Therapy may be administered for up to 12 months in women who respond to therapy with ovulation. In one study, tamoxifen was administered for up to 133 cycles.

Metastatic melanoma: 20 mg/day, used in combination with antineoplastic agents.

➤*Children:*

Off-label dosing –

Malignant brain tumors: Limited information available. Sixty to 200 mg/m^2/day in 2 divided doses has been used in some case series.

➤*Preparation for administration:* Tamoxifen is a hormonal agent and a potential teratogen. Follow safe handling procedures when preparing, administering, or dispensing tamoxifen.

➤*Administration:* Dosages greater than 20 mg/day should be given in divided doses (morning and evening). May be taken with or without food. Swallow tablets whole.

➤*Storage/Stability:* Store at 20° to 25°C (68° to 77°F). Keep in a well-closed, light-resistant container. Keep out of the reach of children.

Actions

➤*Pharmacology:* Tamoxifen is a nonsteroidal agent that has demonstrated potent antiestrogenic properties in animal test systems. The antiestrogenic effects may be related to its ability to compete with estrogen for binding sites in target tissues such as breast. Tamoxifen inhibits the induction of rat mammary carcinoma induced by dimethylbenzanthracene (DMBA) and causes the regression of already established DMBA-induced tumors. In this rat model, tamoxifen appears to exert its antitumor effects by binding the estrogen receptors.

In cytosols derived from human breast adenocarcinomas, tamoxifen competes with estradiol for ER protein.

➤*Pharmacokinetics:*

Absorption/Distribution –

Tablets: Following a single, oral dose of tamoxifen 20 mg, an average peak plasma concentration (C_{max}) of 40 ng/mL (range, 35 to 45 ng/mL) occurred approximately 5 hours after dosing. The decline in plasma concentrations of tamoxifen is biphasic, with a terminal elimination half-life of about 5 to 7 days. The average C_{max} of N-desmethyl tamoxifen is 15 ng/mL (range, 10 to 20 ng/mL). Chronic administration of tamoxifen 10 mg given twice daily for 3 months to patients results in average steady-state plasma concentrations of 120 ng/mL (range, 67 to 183 ng/mL) for tamoxifen and 336 ng/mL (range, 148 to 654 ng/mL) for N-desmethyl tamoxifen. The average steady-state plasma concentrations (C_{ss}) of tamoxifen and N-desmethyl tamoxifen after administration of tamoxifen 20 mg once daily for 3 months are 122 ng/mL (range, 71 to 183 ng/mL) and 353 ng/mL (range, 152 to 706 ng/mL), respectively. After initiation of therapy, C_{ss} for tamoxifen are achieved in about 4 weeks, and C_{ss} for N-desmethyl tamoxifen are achieved in about 8 weeks, suggesting a half-life of approximately 14 days for this metabolite. In a steady-state, crossover study of tamoxifen 10 mg tablets given twice a day versus a tamoxifen 20 mg tablet given once daily, the tamoxifen 20 mg tablet was bioequivalent to the tamoxifen 10 mg tablets.

Metabolism – Tamoxifen is extensively metabolized after oral administration. N-desmethyl tamoxifen is the major metabolite found in patients' plasma. The biological activity of N-desmethyl tamoxifen appears to be similar to that of tamoxifen. Four-hydroxytamoxifen and a side chain primary alcohol derivative of tamoxifen have been identified as minor metabolites in plasma. Tamoxifen is a substrate of cytochrome P-450 3A, 2C9, and 2D6, and an inhibitor of P-glycoprotein.

Excretion – Studies in women receiving 20 mg of ^{14}C (radiolabeled) tamoxifen have shown that approximately 65% of the administered dose was excreted from the body over a period of 2 weeks, with fecal excretion as the primary route of elimination. The drug is excreted mainly as polar conjugates, with unchanged drug and unconjugated metabolites accounting for less than 30% of the total fecal radioactivity.

Special populations –

Children: In pediatric patients, an average $C_{ss,\ max}$ and AUC were of 187 ng/mL and 4,110 ng h/mL, respectively, and $C_{ss,\ max}$ occurred approximately 8 hours after dosing. Clearance (CL/F) as body weight adjusted in female pediatric patients was approximately 2.3-fold higher than in female breast cancer patients. In the youngest cohort of female pediatric patients (2 to 6 years of age), CL/F was 2.6-fold higher; in the oldest cohort (7 to 10.9 years of age), CL/F was approximately 1.9-fold higher. Exposure to N-desmethyl tamoxifen was comparable between the pediatric and adult patients. The safety and efficacy of tamoxifen for girls 2 to 10 years of age with McCune-Albright syndrome and precocious puberty have not been studied beyond 1 year of treatment. The long-term effects of tamoxifen therapy in girls have not been established. In adults treated with tamoxifen, an increase in incidence of uterine malignancies, stroke, and PE has been noted.

Contraindications

Known hypersensitivity to the drug or any of its ingredients.

➤*Reduction of breast cancer incidence in high-risk women:* In women who require concomitant coumarin-type anticoagulant therapy or in women with a history of deep vein thrombosis (DVT) or PE.

Warnings/Precautions

➤*Hypercalcemia:* As with other additive hormonal therapy (estrogens and androgens), hypercalcemia has been reported in some breast cancer patients with bone metastases within a few weeks of starting treatment with tamoxifen. If hypercalcemia does occur, take appropriate measures and, if severe, discontinue tamoxifen.

➤*Uterus (endometrial cancer) and uterine sarcoma effects:* An increased incidence of uterine malignancies has been reported in association with tamoxifen treatment. The underlying mechanism is unknown, but may be related to the estrogen-like effect of tamoxifen. Most uterine malignancies seen in association with tamoxifen are classified as adenocarcinoma of the endometrium. However, rare uterine sarcomas, including malignant mixed mullerian tumors, have also been reported. Uterine sarcoma is generally associated with a higher International Federation of Gynecology and Obstetrics (FIGO) stage (III/IV) at diagnosis, poorer prognosis, and shorter survival. Uterine sarcoma has been reported to occur more frequently among long-term users (greater than or equal to 2 years) of tamoxifen than nonusers. Some of the uterine malignancies (endometrial carcinoma or uterine sarcoma) have been fatal.

In the NSABP P-1 trial, among participants randomized to tamoxifen, there was a statistically significant increase in the incidence of endometrial cancer: 33 cases of invasive endometrial cancer compared with 14 cases among participants randomized to placebo (relative risk [RR], 2.48; 95% confidence interval [CI], 1.27 to 4.92). The 33 cases in participants receiving tamoxifen were FIGO stage I, including 20 IA, 12 IB, and 1 IC endometrial adenocarcinomas. In participants randomized to placebo, 13 were FIGO stage 1 (8 IA and 5 IB) and 1 was FIGO stage IV. Five women on tamoxifen and 1 on placebo received postoperative radiation therapy in addition to surgery. This increase was observed primarily among women at least 50 years of age at the time of randomization (26 cases of invasive endometrial cancer, compared with 6 cases among participants randomized to placebo (RR, 4.5; 95% CI, 1.78 to 13.16). Among women 49 years of age or younger at the time of randomization, there were 7 cases of invasive endometrial cancer, compared with 8 cases among participants randomized to placebo (RR, 0.94; 95% CI, 0.28 to 2.89). If age at the time of diagnosis is considered, there were 4 cases of endometrial cancer among participants 49 years of age or younger randomized to tamoxifen compared with 2 among participants randomized to placebo (RR, 2.21; 95% CI, 0.4 to 12). For women 50 years of age or older at the time of diagnosis, there were 29 cases among participants randomized to tamoxifen compared with 12 among women on placebo (RR, 2.5; 95% CI, 1.3 to 4.9). The risk ratios were similar in the 2 groups, although fewer events occurred in younger women. Most (29 of 33 cases in the tamoxifen group) endometrial cancers were diagnosed in symptomatic women, although 5 of 33 cases in the tamoxifen group occurred in asymptomatic women. Among women receiving tamoxifen, the events appeared between 1 and 61 months (average, 32 months) from the start of treatment.

In an updated review of long-term data (median length of total follow-up is 6.9 years, including blind follow-up) on 8,306 women with an intact uterus at randomization in the NSABP P-1 risk reduction trial, the incidence of both adenocarcinomas and rare uterine sarcomas was increased in women taking tamoxifen. During blinded follow-up, there were 36 cases of FIGO stage I endometrial adenocarcinoma (22 were FIGO stage IA, 13 IB, and 1 IC) in women receiving tamoxifen and 15 cases in women receiving placebo (14 were FIGO stage I [9 IA and 5 IB], and 1 case was FIGO stage IV). Of the patients receiving tamoxifen who developed endometrial cancer, 1 with stage IA and 4 with stage IB cancers received radiation therapy. In the placebo group, 1 patient with FIGO stage 1B cancer received radiation therapy and the patient with FIGO stage IVB cancer received chemotherapy and hormonal therapy. During total follow-up, endometrial adenocarcinoma was reported in 53 women randomized to tamoxifen (30 cases of FIGO stage IA, 20 were stage IB, 1 was stage IC, and 2 were stage IIIC) and 17 women randomized to placebo (9 cases were FIGO stage IA, 6 were stage IB, 1 was stage IIIC, and 1 was stage IVB) (incidence per 1,000 women-years of 2.2 and 0.71, respectively). Some patients received postoperative radiation therapy in addition to surgery. Uterine sarcomas were reported in 4 women randomized to tamoxifen (1 was FIGO IA, 1 was FIGO IB, 1 was FIGO IIA, and 1 was FIGO IIIC) and 1 patient randomized to placebo (FIGO 1A) (incidence per 1,000 women-years of 0.17 and 0.04, respectively). Of the patients randomized to tamoxifen, the FIGO IA and IB cases were a malignant mixed

TAMOXIFEN CITRATE — ORAL

mullerian tumor (MMMT) and sarcoma, respectively; the FIGO II was an MMMT; and the FIGO III was a sarcoma; and the 1 patient randomized to placebo had an MMMT. A similar increased incidence in endometrial adenocarcinoma and uterine sarcoma was observed among women receiving tamoxifen in 5 other NSABP clinical trials.

Promptly evaluate any patient receiving or who has previously received tamoxifen who reports abnormal vaginal bleeding. Perform annual gynecological exams on patients receiving or who have previously received tamoxifen, and they should be advised to promptly inform their health care provider if they experience any abnormal gynecological symptoms (eg, menstrual irregularities, abnormal vaginal bleeding, changes in vaginal discharge, pelvic pain or pressure).

In the P-1 trial, endometrial sampling did not alter the endometrial cancer detection rate compared with women who did not undergo endometrial sampling (0.6% with sampling, 0.5% without sampling) for women with an intact uterus. There are no data to suggest that routine endometrial sampling in asymptomatic women taking tamoxifen to reduce the incidence of breast cancer would be beneficial.

Nonmalignant effects on the uterus – An increased incidence of endometrial changes including hyperplasia and polyps have been reported in association with tamoxifen treatment. The incidence and pattern of this increase suggest that the underlying mechanism is related to the estrogenic properties of tamoxifen.

There have been a few reports of endometriosis and uterine fibroids in women receiving tamoxifen. The underlying mechanism may be due to the partial estrogenic effect of tamoxifen. Ovarian cysts have also been observed in a small number of premenopausal patients with advanced breast cancer who have been treated with tamoxifen.

Tamoxifen has been reported to cause menstrual irregularity or amenorrhea.

➤*Thromboembolic effects:* There is evidence of an increased incidence of thromboembolic events, including DVT and PE, during tamoxifen therapy. When tamoxifen is coadministered with chemotherapy, there may be a further increase in the incidence of thromboembolic effects. For treatment of breast cancer, carefully consider the risks and benefits of tamoxifen in women with a history of thromboembolic events.

Data from the NSABP P-1 trial show that participants receiving tamoxifen without a history of PE had a statistically significant increase in PE (18, tamoxifen; 6, placebo; RR, 3.01; 95% CI, 1.15 to 9.27). Three of the PE, all in the tamoxifen arm, were fatal. Eighty-seven percent of the cases of PE occurred in women at least 50 years of age at randomization. Among women receiving tamoxifen, the events appeared between 2 and 60 months (average, 27 months) from start of treatment.

In this same population, a nonstatistically significant increase in DVT was seen in the tamoxifen group (30, tamoxifen; 19, placebo; RR, 1.59; 95% CI, 0.86 to 2.98). The same increase in RR was seen in women 49 years of age or younger and in women 50 years of age or older, although fewer events occurred in younger women. Women with thromboembolic events were at risk for a second related event (7 out of 25 women on placebo, 5 out of 48 women on tamoxifen) and were at risk for complications of the event and its treatment (0 out of 25 on placebo, 4 out of 48 on tamoxifen). Among women receiving tamoxifen, DVT events occurred between 2 and 57 months (average, 19 months) from the start of treatment.

There was a nonstatistically significant increase in stroke among patients randomized to tamoxifen (24, placebo; 34, tamoxifen; RR, 1.42; 95% CI, 0.82 to 2.51). Six of the 24 strokes in the placebo group were considered hemorrhagic in origin, and 10 of the 34 strokes in the tamoxifen group were categorized as hemorrhagic. Seventeen of the 34 strokes in the tamoxifen group were considered occlusive, and 7 were considered to be of unknown etiology. Fourteen of the 24 strokes on the placebo arm were reported to be occlusive and 4 of unknown etiology. Among these strokes, 3 strokes in the placebo group and 4 strokes in the tamoxifen group were fatal. Eighty-eight percent of the strokes occurred in women 50 years of age or older at the time of randomization. Among women receiving tamoxifen, the events occurred between 1 and 63 months (average, 30 months) from the start of treatment.

➤*Ophthalmic effects:* Ocular disturbances, including corneal changes, decrement in color perception, retinal vein thrombosis, and retinopathy have been reported in patients receiving tamoxifen. An increased incidence of cataracts and the need for cataract surgery have been reported in patients receiving tamoxifen.

In the NSABP P-1 trial, an increased risk of borderline significance of developing cataracts among those women without cataracts at baseline (540, tamoxifen; 483, placebo; RR, 1.13; 95% CI, 1 to 1.28) was observed. Among these same women, tamoxifen was associated with an increased risk of having cataract surgery (101, tamoxifen; 63, placebo; RR, 1.62; 95% CI, 1.18 to 2.22). Among all women on the trial (with or without cataracts at baseline), tamoxifen was associated with an increased risk of having cataract surgery (201, tamoxifen; 129, placebo; RR, 1.58; 95% CI, 1.26 to 1.97). Eye examinations were not required during the study. No other conclusions regarding noncataract ophthalmic events can be made.

➤*Hepatic effects:*

Liver cancer – In the Swedish trial using adjuvant tamoxifen 40 mg/day for 2 to 5 years, 3 cases of liver cancer have been reported in the tamoxifen-treated group versus 1 case in the observation group. In other clinical trials evaluating tamoxifen, no cases of liver cancer have been reported to date.

One case of liver cancer was reported in NSABP P-1 in a participant randomized to tamoxifen.

Nonmalignant effects – Tamoxifen has been associated with changes in liver enzyme levels, and on rare occasions, a spectrum of more severe liver abnormalities including fatty liver, cholestasis, hepatitis, and hepatic necrosis. A few of these serious cases included fatalities. In most reported cases, the relationship to tamoxifen is uncertain. However, some positive rechallenges and dechallenges have been reported.

In the NSABP P-1 trial, few grade 3 to 4 changes in liver function (AST, ALT, bilirubin, alkaline phosphatase) were observed (10 on placebo, 6 on tamoxifen). Serum lipids were not systematically collected.

➤*Reduction of invasive breast cancer and DCIS in women with DCIS:* Women with DCIS treated with lumpectomy and radiation therapy who are considering tamoxifen to reduce the incidence of a second breast cancer event should assess the risks and benefits of therapy, since treatment with tamoxifen decreased the incidence of invasive breast cancer but has not been shown to affect survival.

➤*Reduction of breast cancer incidence in high-risk women:* Women who are at high risk for breast cancer can consider taking tamoxifen therapy to reduce the incidence of breast cancer. Whether the benefits of treatment are considered to outweigh the risks depends on a woman's personal health history and how she weighs the benefits and risks. Tamoxifen therapy to reduce the incidence of breast cancer may therefore not be appropriate for all women at high risk for breast cancer. Women who are considering tamoxifen therapy should consult their health care provider for an assessment of the potential benefits and risks prior to starting therapy for reduction in breast cancer incidence. Women should understand that tamoxifen reduces the incidence of breast cancer but may not eliminate risk. Tamoxifen decreased the incidence of small ER-positive tumors but did not alter the incidence of ER-negative tumors or larger tumors. In women with breast cancer who are at high risk of developing a second breast cancer, treatment with about 5 years of tamoxifen reduced the annual incidence rate of a second breast cancer by approximately 50%.

➤*Pregnancy: Category D.* Tamoxifen may cause fetal harm when administered to a pregnant woman. Advise women not to become pregnant while taking tamoxifen or within 2 months of discontinuing tamoxifen and to use barrier or nonhormonal contraceptive measures if sexually active. Tamoxifen does not cause infertility, even in the presence of menstrual irregularity. Effects on reproductive functions are expected from the antiestrogenic properties of the drug. In reproductive studies in rats at dose levels equal to or below the human dose, nonteratogenic developmental skeletal changes were seen and were found reversible. In addition, in fertility studies in rats and in teratology studies in rabbits using doses at or below those used in humans, a lower incidence of embryo implantation and a higher incidence of fetal death or retarded in utero growth were observed, with slower learning behavior in some rat pups when compared with historical controls. Several pregnant marmosets were dosed with 10 mg/kg/day (about 2-fold the daily MRHD on a mg/m^2 basis) during organogenesis or in the last half of pregnancy. No deformations were seen and, although the dose was high enough to terminate pregnancy in some animals, those that did maintain pregnancy showed no evidence of teratogenic malformations.

In rodent models of fetal reproductive tract development, tamoxifen (at dosages 0.002- to 2.4-fold the MRHD on a mg/m^2 basis) caused changes in both sexes that are similar to those caused by estradiol, ethinylestradiol, and diethylstilbestrol. Although the clinical relevance of these changes is unknown, some of these changes, especially vaginal adenosis, are similar to those seen in young women who were exposed to diethylstilbestrol in utero and who have a 1 in 1,000 risk of developing clear cell adenocarcinoma of the vagina or cervix. To date, in utero exposure to tamoxifen has not been shown to cause vaginal adenosis or clear cell adenocarcinoma of the vagina or cervix in young women. However, only a small number of young women have been exposed to tamoxifen in utero, and a smaller number have been followed long enough (to 15 to 20 years of age) to determine whether vaginal or cervical neoplasia could occur as a result of this exposure.

There are no adequate and well-controlled trials of tamoxifen in pregnant women. There have been a small number of reports of vaginal bleeding, spontaneous abortions, birth defects, and fetal deaths in pregnant women. If this drug is used during pregnancy, or the patient becomes pregnant while taking this drug, or within approximately 2 months after discontinuing therapy, inform the patient of the potential risks to the fetus, including the potential long-term risk of a diethylstilbestrol-like syndrome.

Reduction of breast cancer incidence in high-risk women – For sexually active women of childbearing potential, initiate tamoxifen therapy during menstruation. In women with menstrual irregularity, a negative chorionic gonadotropin immediately prior to the initiation of therapy is sufficient.

Women who are pregnant or who plan to become pregnant should not take tamoxifen to reduce their risk of breast cancer. Effective nonhormonal contraception must be used by all premenopausal women taking tamoxifen if they are sexually active. Tamoxifen does not cause infertility, even in the presence of menstrual irregularity. For sexually active women of childbearing potential, initiate tamoxifen therapy during menstruation. In women with menstrual irregularity, a negative chorionic gonadotropin immediately prior to the initiation of therapy is sufficient.

➤*Lactation:* It is not known whether this drug is excreted in human milk. Because many drugs are excreted in human milk and because of the potential for serious adverse reactions in breast-feeding infants from tamoxifen, decide whether to discontinue breast-feeding or the drug, taking into account the importance of the drug to the mother.

Tamoxifen has been reported to inhibit lactation. Two placebo-controlled studies in over 150 women have shown that tamoxifen significantly inhibits early postpartum milk production. In both studies tamoxifen was adminis-

TAMOXIFEN CITRATE — ORAL

tered within 24 hours of delivery for between 5 and 18 days. The effect of tamoxifen on established milk production is not known.

There are no data that address whether tamoxifen is excreted into human milk. If excreted, there are no data regarding the effects of tamoxifen in breast milk on the breast-fed infant or breast-fed animals. However, direct neonatal exposure of tamoxifen to mice and rats (not via breast milk) produced (1) reproduction tract lesions in female rodents (similar to those seen in humans after intrauterine exposure to diethylstilbestrol) and (2) functional defects of the reproductive tract in male rodents such as testicular atrophy and arrest of spermatogenesis.

Because of the potential for serious adverse reactions in breast-feeding infants from tamoxifen, women taking tamoxifen should not breast-feed.

➤*Children:* The safety and efficacy of tamoxifen for girls 2 to 10 years of age with McCune-Albright syndrome and precocious puberty have not been studied beyond 1 year of treatment. The long-term effects of tamoxifen therapy for girls have not been established. In adults treated with tamoxifen, an increase in incidence of uterine malignancies, stroke, and PE has been noted.

➤*Lab test abnormalities:* Decreases in platelet counts, usually to 50,000 to 100,000/mm^3, infrequently lower, have been occasionally reported in patients taking tamoxifen for breast cancer. In patients with significant thrombocytopenia, rare hemorrhagic episodes have occurred, but it is uncertain if these episodes are due to tamoxifen therapy. Leukopenia has been observed, sometimes in association with anemia or thrombocytopenia. There have been rare reports of neutropenia and pancytopenia in patients receiving tamoxifen; this can sometimes be severe.

In the NSABP P-1 trial, 6 women on tamoxifen and 2 on placebo experienced grade 3 to 4 drops in platelet counts (less than or equal to 50,000/mm^3).

➤*Monitoring:* Perform periodic complete blood cell counts, including platelet counts and periodic liver function tests.

Instruct women who are taking or having previously taken tamoxifen to seek prompt medical attention for new breast lumps, vaginal bleeding, gynecologic symptoms (eg, menstrual irregularities, changes in vaginal discharge, pelvic pain or pressure), symptoms of leg swelling or tenderness, unexplained shortness of breath, or changes in vision. Women should inform all health care providers, regardless of the reason for evaluation, that they take tamoxifen.

Women taking tamoxifen to reduce the incidence of breast cancer should have a breast examination, a mammogram, and a gynecologic examination prior to the initiation of therapy. These studies should be repeated at regular intervals while on therapy, in keeping with good medical practice. Women taking tamoxifen as adjuvant breast cancer therapy should follow the same monitoring procedures as women taking tamoxifen for the reduction in the incidence of breast cancer. Women taking tamoxifen as treatment for metastatic breast cancer should review this monitoring plan with their health care provider and select the appropriate modalities and schedule of evaluation.

Drug Interactions

➤*QT prolongation:* An additive effect of tamoxifen with other drugs that prolong the QT interval cannot be excluded. The following drugs may prolong the QT interval and increase the risk of life-threatening cardiac arrhythmias, including torsades de pointes: Antiarrhythmic agents (eg, amiodarone, bretylium, disopyramide, dofetilide, procainamide, quinidine, and sotalol), arsenic trioxide, chlorpromazine, cisapride, dolasetron, droperidol, mefloquine, mesoridazine, moxifloxacin, pentamidine, pimozide, tacrolimus, thioridazine, and ziprasidone. For a more complete list of drugs that may prolong the QT interval, see the appendix, Drug-Induced Prolongation of the QT Interval and Torsades de Pointes.

➤*Rifampin/aminoglute thimide:* Tamoxifen and N-desmethyl tamoxifen plasma concentrations have been shown to be reduced when coadministered with rifampin or aminoglutethimide. Induction of CYP3A4-mediated metabolism is considered to be the mechanism by which these reductions occur; other CYP3A4-inducing agents have not been studied to confirm this effect.

Rifampin induced the metabolism of tamoxifen and significantly reduced the plasma concentrations of tamoxifen in 10 patients. Aminoglutethimide reduces tamoxifen and N-desmethyl tamoxifen plasma concentrations.

➤*Medroxyprogesterone:* Medroxyprogesterone reduces plasma concentrations of N-desmethyl, but not tamoxifen.

➤*Bromocriptine:*

Tamoxifen Drug Interactions

Precipitant drug	Object drug[a]		Description
Aminoglutethimide	Tamoxifen	⬇	Aminoglutethimide reduces tamoxifen and N-desmethyl tamoxifen plasma concentrations.
Bromocriptine	Tamoxifen	⬆	Bromocriptine may elevate serum tamoxifen and N-desmethyl tamoxifen levels.
Cytotoxic agents	Tamoxifen	⬆	The risk of thromboembolic events increases with coadministration.
Medroxyprogesterone	Tamoxifen	⬇	Medroxyprogesterone reduces plasma concentrations of N-desmethyl tamoxifen (metabolite) but not tamoxifen.
Phenobarbital	Tamoxifen	⬇	One patient receiving tamoxifen with concomitant phenobarbital exhibited a steady-state serum level of tamoxifen lower than that observed for other patients (ie, 26 ng/mL vs mean value of 122 ng/mL). The clinical significance of this is unknown.
Rifamycins	Tamoxifen	⬇	Plasma concentrations of tamoxifen may be reduced. Rifampin reduced tamoxifen AUC and C_{max} by 86% and 55%, respectively. It may be necessary to increase the tamoxifen dose during coadministration.
Tamoxifen	Anticoagulants	⬆	The hypoprothrombinemic effect may be increased by concurrent tamoxifen. Carefully monitor prothrombin time.
Tamoxifen	Letrozole	⬇	Tamoxifen reduced plasma letrozole concentrations by 37% when these drugs were coadministered.

[a] ⬆ = object drug increased; ⬇ = object drug decreased.

➤*Drug/Lab test interactions:* During postmarketing surveillance, thyroxine elevations were reported for a few postmenopausal patients, which may be explained by increases in thyroid-binding globulin. These elevations were not accompanied by clinical hyperthyroidism.

Variations in the karyopyknotic index on vaginal smears and various degrees of estrogen effect on Pap smears have been infrequently seen in postmenopausal patients given tamoxifen.

In the postmarketing experience with tamoxifen, infrequent cases of hyperlipidemias have been reported. Periodic monitoring of plasma triglycerides and cholesterol may be indicated in patients with preexisting hyperlipidemias.

Adverse Reactions

Adverse reactions to tamoxifen are relatively mild and rarely severe enough to require discontinuation of treatment in breast cancer patients.

Continued clinical studies have resulted in further information that better indicates the incidence of adverse reactions with tamoxifen as compared with placebo.

➤*Metastatic breast cancer:* Increased bone and tumor pain and local disease flare have occurred, which are sometimes associated with a good tumor response. Patients with increased bone pain may require additional analgesics. Patients with soft tissue disease may have sudden increases in the size of preexisting lesions, sometimes associated with marked erythema within and surrounding the lesions or the development of new lesions. When they occur, the bone pain or disease flare are seen shortly after starting tamoxifen and generally subside rapidly.

In patients treated with tamoxifen for metastatic breast cancer, the most frequent adverse reaction to tamoxifen is hot flashes.

Other adverse reactions which are seen infrequently are hypercalcemia, peripheral edema, distaste for food, pruritus vulvae, depression, dizziness, light-headedness, headache, hair thinning or partial hair loss, and vaginal dryness.

➤*Premenopausal women:* The following table summarizes the incidence of adverse reactions reported at a frequency of greater than or equal to 2% from clinical trials (Ingle, Pritchard, Buchanan) that compared tamoxifen therapy with ovarian ablation in premenopausal patients with metastatic breast cancer.

Tamoxifen Adverse Reactions vs Ovarian Ablation (≥ 2%)

Adverse reaction[a]	Tamoxifen (all effects) (n = 104)	Ovarian ablation (all effects) (n = 100)
CNS		
Depression	2%	2%
Fatigue	4%	1%
Dermatologic		
Flush	33%	46%
GI		
Abdominal cramps	1%	2%
Anorexia	1%	2%
Nausea	5%	4%

TAMOXIFEN CITRATE — ORAL

Tamoxifen Adverse Reactions vs Ovarian Ablation (≥ 2%)		
Adverse reaction[a]	Tamoxifen (all effects) (n = 104)	Ovarian ablation (all effects) (n = 100)
GU		
Altered menses	13%	5%
Amenorrhea	16%	69%
Menstrual disorder	6%	4%
Oligomenorrhea	9%	1%
Ovarian cyst(s)	3%	2%
Musculoskeletal		
Bone pain	6%	6%
Musculoskeletal pain	3%	0%
Respiratory		
Cough/coughing	4%	1%
Miscellaneous		
Edema	4%	1%
Pain	3%	4%

[a] Some women had more than 1 adverse reaction.

➤*Male breast cancer:* Tamoxifen is well tolerated in men with breast cancer. Reports from the literature and case reports suggest that the safety profile of tamoxifen in men is similar to that seen in women. Loss of libido and impotence have resulted in discontinuation of tamoxifen therapy in male patients. Also, in oligospermic men treated with tamoxifen, luteinizing hormone, follicle-stimulating hormone, testosterone, and estrogen levels were elevated. No significant clinical changes were reported.

➤*Adjuvant breast cancer:* In the NSABP B-14 study, women with axillary node–negative breast cancer were randomized to 5 years of tamoxifen 20 mg/day or placebo following primary surgery. The reported adverse reactions are given in the following table (mean follow-up of approximately 6.8 years), showing adverse reactions more common on tamoxifen than on placebo. The incidence of hot flashes (64% vs 48%), vaginal discharge (30% vs 15%), and irregular menses (25% vs 19%) were higher with tamoxifen compared with placebo. All other adverse reactions occurred with similar frequency in the 2 treatment groups, with the exception of thrombotic events, a higher incidence was seen in tamoxifen-treated patients (through 5 years, 1.7% vs 0.4%). Two of the patients treated with tamoxifen who had thrombotic events died.

Tamoxifen Adverse Reaction in NSABP B-14 Study		
Adverse reaction	Tamoxifen (n = 1,422)	Placebo (n = 1,437)
Cardiovascular		
DVT	0.8%	0.2%
Dermatologic		
Skin changes	19%	15%
GI		
Nausea	26%	24%
GU		
Irregular menses	25%	19%
Vaginal discharge	30%	15%
Hematologic		
Thrombocytopenia[a]	2%	1%
Hepatic		
Increased AST	5%	3%
Increased bilirubin	2%	1%
Renal		
Increased creatinine	2%	1%
Respiratory		
PE	0.5%	0.2%
Miscellaneous		
Fluid retention	32%	30%
Hot flashes	64%	48%
Superficial phlebitis	0.4%	0%
Weight loss (> 5%)	23%	18%

[a] Defined as a platelet count of less than 100,000/mm^3.

In the ECOG adjuvant breast cancer trial, tamoxifen or placebo was administered for 2 years to women following mastectomy. When compared with placebo, tamoxifen showed a significantly higher incidence of hot flashes (19% vs 8% for placebo). The incidence of all other adverse reactions was similar in the 2 treatment groups with the exception of thrombocytopenia where the incidence for tamoxifen was 10% versus 3% for placebo, an observation of borderline statistical significance.

In other adjuvant studies, Toronto and NATO, women received either tamoxifen or no therapy. In the Toronto study, hot flashes were observed in 29% of patients for tamoxifen versus 1% in the untreated group. In the NATO trial, hot flashes and vaginal bleeding were reported in 2.8%, and 2% of women, respectively, for tamoxifen versus 0.2% for each in the untreated group.

➤*DCIS:* The type and frequency of adverse reactions in the NSABP B-24 trial were consistent with those observed in the other adjuvant trials conducted with tamoxifen.

➤*Reduction in breast cancer incidence in high-risk women:*

NSABP-1 trial – In the NSABP P-1 trial, there was an increase in 5 serious adverse reactions in the tamoxifen group: endometrial cancer (33 cases in the tamoxifen group vs 14 in the placebo group), PE (18 cases in the tamoxifen group vs 6 in the placebo group), DVT (30 cases in the tamoxifen group vs 19 in the placebo group), stroke (34 cases in the tamoxifen group vs 24 in the placebo group), cataract formation (540 cases in the tamoxifen group vs 483 in the placebo group), and cataract surgery (101 cases in the tamoxifen group vs 63 in the placebo group).

The following table presents the adverse reactions observed in NSABP P-1 by treatment arm. Only adverse reactions more common on tamoxifen than on placebo are shown.

Tamoxifen Adverse Reactions in NSABP P-1 Trial		
Adverse reactions	Tamoxifen (n = 6,681)	Placebo (n = 6,707)
Self-reported symptoms	n = 6,441 [a]	n = 6,469 [a]
Hot flashes	80%	68%
Vaginal bleeding	23%	22%
Vaginal discharges	55%	35%
Laboratory test abnormalities	n = 6,520 [b]	n = 6,535 [b]
Platelets decreased	0.7%	0.3%

[a] Number with quality of life questionnaires.
[b] Number with treatment follow-up questionnaires.

Tamoxifen Adverse Reactions in NSABP P-1 Trial		
Adverse reaction	n = 6,492 [a]	n = 6,484 [a]
CNS		
Mood	11.6%	10.8%
Dermatologic		
Alopecia	5.2%	4.4%
Skin	5.6%	4.7%
GI		
Constipation	4.4%	3.2%
Miscellaneous		
Allergy	2.5%	2.1%
Infection/sepsis	6%	5.1%

[a] Number with adverse drug reaction forms.

In the NSABP P-1 trial, 15% and 9.7% of participants receiving tamoxifen and placebo therapy, respectively, withdrew from the trial for medical reasons. The medical reasons for withdrawal from tamoxifen and placebo therapy, respectively, were hot flashes (3.1% vs 1.5%) and vaginal discharge (0.5% vs 0.1%).

In the NSABP P-1 trial, 8.7% and 9.6% of participants receiving tamoxifen and placebo therapy, respectively, withdrew for nonmedical reasons.

On the NSABP P-1 trial, hot flashes of any severity occurred in 68% of women on placebo and in 80% of women on tamoxifen. Severe hot flashes occurred in 28% of women on placebo and 45% of women on tamoxifen. Vaginal discharge occurred in 35% and 55% of women on placebo and tamoxifen, respectively, and was severe in 4.5% and 12.3%, respectively. There was no difference in the incidence of vaginal bleeding between treatment arms.

➤*Pediatric patients:*

McCune-Albright syndrome – Mean uterine volume increased after 6 months of treatment and doubled at the end of the 1-year study. A causal relationship has not been established; however, as an increase in the incidence of endometrial adenocarcinoma and uterine sarcoma has been noted in adults treated with tamoxifen, continued monitoring of McCune-Albright patients treated with tamoxifen for long-term effects is recommended. The safety and efficacy of tamoxifen for girls 2 to 10 years of age with McCune-Albright syndrome and precocious puberty have not been studied beyond 1 year of treatment. The long-term effects of tamoxifen therapy in girls have not been established.

➤*Postmarketing:*

Miscellaneous – Less frequently reported adverse reactions are vaginal bleeding, vaginal discharge, menstrual irregularities, skin rash, and headaches. Usually these have not been of sufficient severity to require dosage reduction or discontinuation of treatment. Very rare reports of erythema multiforme, Stevens-Johnson syndrome, bullous pemphigoid, interstitial pneumonitis, and rare reports of hypersensitivity reactions including angioedema have been reported with tamoxifen therapy. In some of these cases, the time to onset was more than 1 year. Rarely, elevation of serum triglyceride levels, in some cases with pancreatitis, may be associated with the use of tamoxifen.

Overdosage

➤*Symptoms:* Signs observed at the highest doses following studies to determine the median lethal dose in animals were respiratory difficulties and convulsions.

Acute overdosage in humans has not been reported. In a study of advanced metastatic cancer patients that specifically determined the maximum tolerated dose of tamoxifen in evaluating the use of very high doses to reverse multidrug resistance, acute neurotoxicity manifested by tremor, hyper-

TAMOXIFEN CITRATE — ORAL

reflexia, unsteady gait, and dizziness were noted. These symptoms occurred within 3 to 5 days of beginning tamoxifen and cleared within 2 to 5 days after stopping therapy. No permanent neurologic toxicity was noted. One patient experienced a seizure several days after tamoxifen was discontinued and neurotoxic symptoms had resolved. The causal relationship of the seizure to tamoxifen therapy is unknown. Doses given in these patients were all greater than 400 mg/m^2 loading dose, followed by maintenance doses of 150 mg/m^2 of tamoxifen given twice a day.

In the same study, prolongation of the QT interval on the electrocardiogram was noted when patients were given doses greater than 250 mg/m^2 loading dose, followed by maintenance doses of 80 mg/m^2 of tamoxifen given twice a day. For a woman with a body surface area of 1.5 m^2, the minimal loading dose and maintenance doses given at which neurological symptoms and QT changes occurred were at least 6-fold higher in respect to the maximum recommended dose.

➤*Treatment:* No specific treatment for overdosage is known; treatment must be symptomatic.

Patient Information

Advise patients that tamoxifen reduces the incidence of breast cancer but may not eliminate risk. Instruct patients on the benefits of tamoxifen versus the risk.

Women with DCIS treated with lupectomy and radiation therapy who are considering tamoxifen to reduce the incidence of a second breast cancer event should assess the risks and benefits of therapy because treatment with tamoxifen decreased the incidence of invasive breast cancer but has not been shown to affect survival.

Advise women who are receiving or who have previously received tamoxifen to have regular gynecologic examinations and promptly inform their health care provider of menstrual irregularities, abnormal vaginal bleeding, change in vaginal discharge, or pelvic pain or pressure.

Women who are pregnant or who plan to become pregnant should not take tamoxifen to reduce the risk of breast cancer. Effective nonhormonal contraception must be used by all premenopausal women taking tamoxifen and for approximately 2 months after discontinuing therapy if they are sexually active. Tamoxifen does not cause infertility, even in the presence of menstrual irregularity. For sexually active women of childbearing potential, initiate tamoxifen therapy during menstruation. In women with menstrual irregularity, a negative chorionic gonadotropin immediately prior to the initiation of therapy is sufficient.

Advise patients to notify their health care provider of pain/swelling/tenderness of legs, unexplained shortness of breath, changes in vision, new breast lumps, vaginal bleeding, or gynecologic symptoms (eg, menstrual irregularities, changes in vaginal discharge, pelvic pain or pressure).

TOREMIFENE

Rx	**Fareston** (GTx)	**Tablets; oral:** 60 mg	Equiv. to toremifene citrate 88.5 mg. Lactose. (TO 60). White, round. In 30s.

TOREMIFENE CITRATE — ORAL

WARNING

QT prolongation – Toremifene has been shown to prolong the QTc interval in a dose- and concentration-related manner. Prolongation of the QT interval can result in a type of ventricular tachycardia called torsades de pointes, which may result in syncope, seizure, and/or death. Toremifene should not be prescribed to patients with congenital/acquired QT prolongation, uncorrected hypokalemia, or uncorrected hypomagnesemia. Drugs known to prolong the QT interval and strong CYP3A4 inhibitors should be avoided.

Indications

➤*Breast cancer:* For the treatment of metastatic breast cancer in postmenopausal women with estrogen receptor–positive or unknown tumors.

➤*Off-label uses:* Desmoid tumors.

Administration and Dosage

➤*Adults:*

Breast cancer –

Usual dosage: 60 mg once a day.

Duration of therapy: Treatment is generally continued until disease progression is observed.

➤*Preparation for administration:* Toremifene is a hormonal agent and is considered a potential teratogen. Follow safe handling procedures when preparing, administering, or dispensing toremifene.

➤*Administration:* May be taken without regard to food.

➤*Storage/Stability:* Store at 25°C (77°F); excursions are permitted between 15° and 30°C (59° and 86°F). Protect from heat and light.

Actions

➤*Pharmacology:* Toremifene is a nonsteroidal triphenylethylene derivative. Toremifene binds to estrogen receptors and may exert estrogenic, antiestrogenic, or both activities, depending upon the duration of treatment, animal species, gender, target organ, or endpoint selected. In general, however, nonsteroidal triphenylethylene derivatives are predominantly antiestrogenic in rats and humans and estrogenic in mice. In rats, toremifene causes regression of established dimethylbenzanthracene (DMBA)-induced mammary tumors. The antitumor effect of toremifene in breast cancer is believed to be mainly due to its antiestrogenic effects (ie, its ability to compete with estrogen for binding sites in the cancer, blocking the growth-stimulating effects of estrogen in the tumor).

Toremifene causes a decrease in the estradiol-induced vaginal cornification index in some postmenopausal women, indicative of its antiestrogenic activity. Toremifene also has estrogenic activity as shown by decreases in serum gonadotropin concentration (follicle-stimulating hormone and luteinizing hormone).

➤*Pharmacokinetics:*

Absorption/Distribution – Toremifene is well absorbed after oral administration and absorption is not influenced by food. Peak plasma concentrations are obtained within 3 hours. Toremifene displays linear pharmacokinetics after single oral doses of 10 to 680 mg. After multiple dosing, dose proportionality was observed for doses of 10 to 400 mg. Steady-state concentrations were reached in about 4 to 6 weeks. Toremifene has an apparent volume of distribution of 580 L and binds extensively (greater than 99.5%) to serum proteins, mainly to albumin.

The plasma concentration time profile of toremifene declines biexponentially after absorption with a mean distribution half-life of about 4 hours and an elimination half-life of about 5 days.

Metabolism/Excretion – Elimination half-lives of major metabolites, N-demethyltoremifene and (deaminohydroxy) toremifene were 6 and 4 days, respectively. Mean total clearance of toremifene was approximately 5 L/hr.

Toremifene is extensively metabolized, principally by CYP3A4 to N-demethyltoremifene, which is also antiestrogenic but with weak in vivo antitumor potency. Serum concentrations of N-demethyltoremifene are 2 to 4 times higher than toremifene at steady state. Toremifene is eliminated as metabolites predominantly in the feces, with about 10% excreted in the urine during a 1-week period. Elimination of toremifene is slow, in part because of enterohepatic circulation.

Special populations –

Hepatic function impairment: The mean elimination half-life of toremifene was increased by less than 2-fold in 10 patients with hepatic impairment (cirrhosis or fibrosis) compared to subjects with healthy hepatic function. The pharmacokinetics of N-demethyltoremifene were unchanged in these patients. Ten patients on anticonvulsants (phenobarbital, clonazepam, phenytoin, and carbamazepine) showed a 2-fold increase in clearance and a decrease in the elimination half-life of toremifene.

Elderly: The pharmacokinetics of toremifene were studied in 10 healthy young males and 10 elderly females following a single 120 mg dose under testing conditions. Increases in the elimination half-life (4.2 vs 7.2 days) and the volume of distribution (457 vs 627 L) of toremifene were seen in the elderly females without any change in clearance or AUC.

Contraindications

Hypersensitivity to the drug; congenital/acquired QT prolongation (long QT syndrome), uncorrected hypokalemia, or uncorrected hypomagnesemia.

Warnings/Precautions

➤*Hypercalcemia and tumor flare:* As with other antiestrogens, hypercalcemia and tumor flare have been reported in some breast cancer patients with bone metastases during the first weeks of treatment with toremifene citrate. Tumor flare is a syndrome of diffuse musculoskeletal pain and erythema with increased size of tumor lesions that later regress. It is often accompanied by hypercalcemia. Tumor flare does not imply failure of treatment or represent tumor progression. If hypercalcemia occurs, appropriate measures should be instituted and if hypercalcemia is severe, discontinue toremifene citrate treatment.

➤*Tumorigenicity:* Since most toremifene trials have been conducted in patients with metastatic disease, adequate data on the potential endometrial tumorigenicity of long-term treatment with toremifene citrate are not available. Endometrial hyperplasia has been reported. Some patients treated with toremifene citrate have developed endometrial cancer, but circumstances (short duration of treatment or prior antiestrogen treatment of premalignant conditions) make it difficult to establish the role of toremifene citrate.

➤*Thromboembolic disease/pre-existing endometrial hyperplasia:* Patients with a history of thromboembolic diseases should generally not be treated with toremifene citrate. In general, patients with preexisting endometrial hyperplasia should not be given long-term toremifene citrate treatment.

➤*Pregnancy: Category D.* Toremifene citrate may cause fetal harm when administered to pregnant women. Studies in rats at doses greater than or equal to 1 mg/kg/day (about ¼ the daily maximum recommended human dose on a mg/m^2 basis) administered during the period of organogenesis, have shown that toremifene is embryotoxic and fetotoxic, as indicated by intrauterine mortality, increased resorption, reduced fetal weight, and fetal anomalies, including malformation of limbs, incomplete ossification, misshapen bones, ribs/spine anomalies, hydroureter, hydronephrosis, testicular displacement, and subcutaneous edema. Fetal anomalies may have been a

TOREMIFENE CITRATE — ORAL

consequence of maternal toxicity. Toremifene has been shown to cross the placenta and accumulate in the rodent fetus.

Embryotoxicity and fetotoxicity were observed in rabbits at doses greater than or equal to 1.25 mg/kg/day and 2.5 mg/kg/day, respectively (about ⅓ and ⅔ the daily maximum recommended human dose on a mg/m^2 basis); fetal anomalies included incomplete ossification and anencephaly.

There are no studies in pregnant women. If toremifene citrate is used during pregnancy, or if the patient becomes pregnant while receiving this drug, apprise the patient of the potential hazard to the fetus or potential risk for loss of the pregnancy.

➤*Lactation:* Toremifene has been shown to be excreted in the milk of lactating rats. It is not known if this drug is excreted in human milk.

➤*Children:* There is no indication for use of toremifene in children.

➤*Monitoring:* Periodic complete blood counts, calcium levels, and liver function tests should be obtained.

Patients with bone metastases should be monitored closely for hypercalcemia during the first weeks of treatment. Leukopenia and thrombocytopenia have been reported rarely; leukocyte and platelet counts should be monitored when using toremifene citrate in patients with leukopenia and thrombocytopenia.

Drug Interactions

➤*Thiazide diuretics:* Drugs that decrease renal calcium excretion (eg, thiazide diuretics) may increase the risk of hypercalcemia in patients receiving toremifene citrate.

➤*Anticoagulants:* There is a known interaction between antiestrogenic compounds of the triphenylethylene derivative class and coumarin-type anticoagulants (eg, warfarin), leading to an increased prothrombin time. When concomitant use of anticoagulants with toremifene citrate is necessary, careful monitoring of the prothrombin time is recommended.

➤*CYP450 isoenzymes:* Cytochrome P450 3A4 enzyme inducers, such as phenobarbital, phenytoin, and carbamazepine, increase the rate of toremifene metabolism, lowering the steady-state concentration in serum. Metabolism of toremifene may be inhibited by drugs known to inhibit the CYP3A4-6 enzymes. Examples of such drugs are ketoconazole and similar antimycotics as well as erythromycin and similar macrolides. This interaction has not been studied and its clinical relevance is uncertain.

Adverse Reactions

Adverse drug reactions are principally due to the antiestrogenic hormonal actions of toremifene citrate and typically occur at the beginning of treatment.

Toremifene Citrate Adverse Reactions in the North American Study (%)

Adverse reactions	FAR60 (n = 221)	TAM20 (n = 215)
Dizziness	9%	7%
Edema	5%	5%
Hot flashes	35%	30%
Nausea	14%	15%
Sweating	20%	17%
Vaginal bleeding	2%	4%
Vaginal discharge	13%	16%
Vomiting	4%	2%

Approximately 1% of patients receiving toremifene citrate (n = 592) in the 3 controlled studies discontinued treatment as a result of adverse events (nausea and vomiting, fatigue, thrombophlebitis, depression, lethargy, anorexia, ischemic attack, arthritis, pulmonary embolism, and myocardial infarction).

Toremifene Citrate Adverse Events in 3 Controlled Studies (%)

Adverse events	North American				Eastern European				Nordic			
	FAR60 (n = 221)		TAM20 (n = 215)		FAR60 (n = 157)		TAM40 (n = 149)		FAR60 (n = 214)		TAM40 (n = 201)	
Cardiovascular												
Angina pectoris	a		—		1	(< 1)	a		1	(< 1)	2	(1)
Arrhythmia	a		—		—		a		3	(1.5)	1	(< 1)
Cardiac failure	2	(1)	1	(< 1)	—		1	(< 1)	2	(1)	3	(1.5)
Myocardial infarction	2	(1)	3	(1.5)	1	(< 1)	2	(1)	—		1	(< 1)
Elevated liver tests[b]												
Alkaline phosphatase	41	(19)	24	(11)	16	(10)	13	(9)	18	(8)	31	(15)
AST	11	(5)	4	(2)	30	(19)	22	(15)	32	(15)	35	(17)
Bilirubin	3	(1.5)	4	(2)	2	(1)	1	(< 1)	2	(1)	3	(1.5)
Hypercalcemia	6	(3)	6	(3)	1	(< 1)	—		—		—	
Ocular[a]												
Abnormal vision/diplopia	a		—		—		a		3	(1.5)	—	
Abnormal visual fields	8	(4)	10	(5)	a		a		—		1	(< 1)
Cataracts	22	(10)	16	(7.5)	—		a				5	(3)
Corneal keratopathy	4	(2)	2	(1)	—		a		—		—	
Dry eyes	20	(9)	16	(7.5)	—		—		—		a	
Glaucoma	3	(1.5)	2	(1)	1	(< 1)					1	(< 1)
Thromboembolic												
CVA/TIA	1	(< 1)	—		—		1	(< 1)	4	(2)	4	(2)
Pulmonary embolism	4	(2)	2	(1)	1	(< 1)	—		a		1	(< 1)
Thrombophlebitis	—		2	(1)	1	(< 1)	1	(< 1)	4	(2)	3	(1.5)
Thrombosis	—		1	(< 1)	1	(< 1)	—		3	(1.5)	4	(2)

[a] Most of the ocular abnormalities were observed in the North American study in which on-study and biannual ophthalmic examinations were performed. No cases of retinopathy were observed in any arm.

[b] Elevated defined as follows: North American study; AST greater than 100 Units/L; alkaline phosphatase greater than 200 Units/L; bilirubin greater than 2 mg/dL. Eastern European and Nordic studies; AST, alkaline phosphatase, and bilirubin - WHO Grade 1 (1.25 times the upper limit of normal).

Other adverse events of unclear causal relationship to toremifene citrate included leukopenia and thrombocytopenia, skin discoloration or dermatitis, constipation, dyspnea, paresis, tremor, vertigo, pruritus, anorexia, reversible corneal opacity (corneal verticulata), asthenia, alopecia, depression, jaundice, and rigors.

In the 200 and 240 mg toremifene citrate-dose arms, the incidence of AST elevation and nausea was higher. Approximately 4% of patients were withdrawn for toxicity from the high-dose toremifene citrate-treatment arms. Reasons for withdrawal included hypercalcemia, abnormal liver function tests, and 1 case each of toxic hepatitis, depression, dizziness, incoordination, ataxia, blurry vision, diffuse dermatitis, and a constellation of symptoms consisting of nausea, sweating, and tremor.

Overdosage

Lethality was observed in rats following single oral doses that were greater than or equal to 1,000 mg/kg (about 150 times the recommended human dose on a mg/m^2 basis) and was associated with gastric atony/dilatation leading to interference with digestion and adrenal enlargement.

➤*Symptoms:* Vertigo, headache, and dizziness were observed in healthy volunteer studies at a daily dose of 680 mg for 5 days. The symptoms occurred in 2 of the 5 subjects during the third day of the treatment and disappeared within 2 days of discontinuation of the drug. No immediate concomitant changes in any measured clinical chemistry parameters were found. In a study in postmenopausal breast cancer patients, toremifene 400 mg/m^2/day caused dose-limiting nausea, vomiting, and dizziness, as well as reversible hallucinations and ataxia in one patient.

Theoretically, overdose may be manifested as an increase of antiestrogenic effects, such as hot flashes; estrogenic effects, such as vaginal bleeding; or nervous system disorders, such as vertigo, dizziness, ataxia, and nausea.

➤*Treatment:* There is no specific antidote and the treatment is symptomatic.

TOREMIFENE CITRATE — ORAL

Patient Information

Vaginal bleeding has been reported in patients using toremifene citrate. Inform patients about this and instruct them to contact their physicians if such bleeding occurs.

Inform patients with bone metastases about the typical signs and symptoms of hypercalcemia and instruct them to contact their physicians for further assessment if such signs or symptoms occur.

FULVESTRANT

Rx	**Faslodex** (AstraZeneca)	**Injection, solution:** 50 mg/mL	Alcohol, benzyl alcohol, castor oil. In 5 mL prefilled syringes.

FULVESTRANT — INJECTION

Indications

➤*Breast cancer:* For the treatment of hormone receptor–positive metastatic breast cancer in postmenopausal women with disease progression following antiestrogen therapy.

Administration and Dosage

➤*Adults:*

Breast cancer – 500 mg intramuscularly (IM) on days 1, 15, 29, and once monthly thereafter.

➤*Renal function impairment:* No dosage adjustment required.

Dialysis – Conventional and peritoneal hemodialysis are ineffective (0% to 24%) in removing fulvestrant.

Fulvestrant is approximately 99% protein bound. The volume of distribution is 3 to 5 L/kg. Fulvestrant is metabolized extensively in the liver. It is primarily eliminated in the feces as metabolites (90%); less than 1% is excreted renally.

➤*Hepatic function impairment:* 250 mg IM for patients with moderate hepatic impairment (Child-Pugh class B) on days 1, 15, 29, and once monthly thereafter.

➤*Preparation for administration:* Fulvestrant is considered a potential teratogen. Follow safe handling procedures when preparing, administering, or dispensing fulvestrant.

The injection may be warmed before use to maximize patient comfort. Suitable warming methods include storing the injection at room temperature for 1 hour or rolling the injection gently in the hands.

➤*Administration:* Administered by slow IM injection (1 to 2 minutes per injection) into the buttocks as two 5 mL injections, one in each buttock.

➤*Storage/Stability:* Refrigerate, 2° to 8°C (36° to 46°F). Store in the original package to protect from light.

Actions

➤*Pharmacology:* Many breast cancers have estrogen receptors, and the growth of these tumors can be stimulated by estrogen. Fulvestrant is an estrogen receptor antagonist that binds to the estrogen receptor in a competitive manner with affinity comparable to that of estradiol. Fulvestrant downregulates the estrogen receptor protein in human breast cancer cells.

In vitro studies demonstrated that fulvestrant is a reversible inhibitor of the growth of tamoxifen-resistant, as well as estrogen-sensitive human breast cancer (MCF-7) cell lines. In in vivo tumor studies, fulvestrant delayed the establishment of tumors from xenografts of human breast cancer MCF-7 cells in nude mice. Fulvestrant inhibited the growth of established MCF-7 xenografts and of tamoxifen-resistant breast tumor xenografts.

Pharmacodynamics – In a clinical study in postmenopausal women with primary breast cancer treated with single doses of fulvestrant 15 to 22 days prior to surgery, there was evidence of increasing down regulation of estrogen receptor with increasing dose. This was associated with a dose-related decrease in the expression of the progesterone receptor, an estrogen-regulated protein. These effects on the estrogen receptor pathway were also associated with a decrease in Ki67 labeling index, a marker of cell proliferation.

➤*Pharmacokinetics:*

Absorption –

Fulvestrant Pharmacokinetic Parameters After Intramuscular Administration of the 500 mg + Additional Dose Dosing Regimen[a]

		C_{max} (ng/mL)	C_{min} (ng/mL)	AUC (ng•h/mL)
500 mg + additional dose[b]	Single dose	25.1 (35.3)	16.3 (25.9)	11,400 (33.4)
	Multidose steady state[c]	28 (27.9)	12.2 (21.7)	13,100 (23.4)

[a] C_{max} = maximum plasma concentration; C_{min} = minimum plasma concentration; AUC = area under the curve.
[b] Additional 500 mg dose given on day 15.
[c] Month 3.

The additional dose of fulvestrant given 2 weeks after the initial dose allows for steady-state concentrations to be reached within the first month of dosing.

Distribution – The apparent volume of distribution at steady state was approximately 3 to 5 L/kg. This suggests that distribution is largely extravascular. Fulvestrant was highly (99%) bound to plasma proteins; very low density lipoprotein, low density lipoprotein, and high density lipoprotein fractions appear to be the major binding components. The role of sex hormone-binding globulin, if any, could not be determined.

Metabolism – Fulvestrant is metabolized primarily in the liver. Biotransformation and disposition of fulvestrant in humans have been determined following IM and intravenous (IV) administration of ^{14}C-labeled fulvestrant. Metabolism of fulvestrant appears to involve combinations of a number of possible biotransformation pathways analogous to those of endogenous steroids, including oxidation, aromatic hydroxylation, conjugation with glucuronic acid and/or sulphate at the 2, 3, and 17 positions of the steroid nucleus, and oxidation of the side chain sulphoxide. Identified metabolites are either less active or exhibit similar activity to fulvestrant in antiestrogen models. Studies using human liver preparations and recombinant human enzymes indicate that cytochrome P450 3A4 (CYP3A4) is the only P450 isoenzyme involved in the oxidation of fulvestrant; however, the relative contribution of P450 and non-P450 routes in vivo is unknown.

Excretion – Fulvestrant was rapidly cleared by the hepatobiliary route, with excretion primarily via the feces (approximately 90%). Renal elimination was negligible (less than 1%). After an IM injection of 250 mg, the clearance (mean ± standard deviation) was 690 ± 226 mL/min, with an apparent half-life of approximately 40 days.

Special populations –

Hepatic function impairment: In subjects with moderate hepatic impairment (Child-Pugh class B), the average AUC of fulvestrant increased by 70% compared with patients with normal hepatic function. AUC was positively correlated with total bilirubin concentration ($P = 0.012$).

Contraindications

Hypersensitivity to the drug or any of its components.

Warnings/Precautions

➤*Bleeding tendencies:* Because fulvestrant is administered IM, use with caution in patients with bleeding diatheses, thrombocytopenia, or patients taking anticoagulants.

➤*Hepatic function impairment:* See Administration and Dosage for more information.

➤*Pregnancy: Category D.* Fulvestrant can cause fetal harm when administered to a pregnant woman. Fulvestrant caused fetal loss or abnormalities in animals when administered during the period of organogenesis at doses significantly smaller than the maximum recommended human dose based on the body surface area. Advise women of childbearing potential not to become pregnant while receiving fulvestrant. There are no adequate and well-controlled studies in pregnant women using fulvestrant. If fulvestrant is used during pregnancy or if the patient becomes pregnant while receiving this drug, apprise the patient of the potential hazard to the fetus.

➤*Lactation:* Fulvestrant is found in rat milk at levels significantly higher (approximately 12-fold) than plasma after administration of 2 mg/kg. Drug exposure in rodent pups from fulvestrant-treated lactating dams was estimated as 10% of the administered dose. It is not known if fulvestrant is excreted in human milk. Because many drugs are excreted in milk, and because of the potential for serious adverse reactions from fulvestrant in breast-feeding infants, decide whether to discontinue breast-feeding or the drug, taking into account the importance of the drug to the mother.

➤*Children:* Safety and efficacy have not been established.

Drug Interactions

➤*Disulfiram, metronidazole:* Because fulvestrant injection contains alcohol, patients receiving disulfiram or metronidazole may experience an acute alcohol intolerance reaction if fulvestrant is administered concurrently. Avoid fulvestrant administration to patients receiving disulfiram or metronidazole.

Adverse Reactions

➤*Comparison of fulvestrant 500 and 250 mg:*

Most frequent – The most frequently reported adverse reactions in the fulvestrant 500 mg group were injection-site pain (11.6%), nausea (9.7%), and bone pain (9.4%); the most frequently reported adverse reactions in the fulvestrant 250 mg group were nausea (13.6%), back pain (10.7%), and injection-site pain (9.1%).

FULVESTRANT — INJECTION

Adverse reactions (5% or more) –

Fulvestrant Adverse Reactions (Study 1) (≥ 5%)		
Adverse reactions	Fulvestrant 500 mg (n = 361)	Fulvestrant 250 mg (n = 374)
CNS		
Asthenia	5.8%	6.1%
Fatigue	7.5%	6.4%
Headache	7.8%	6.7%
GI		
Anorexia	6.1%	3.7%
Constipation	5%	3.5%
Nausea	9.7%	13.6%
Vomiting	6.1%	5.6%
Musculoskeletal		
Arthralgia	8%	7.8%
Back pain	7.5%	10.7%
Bone pain	9.4%	7.5%
Musculoskeletal pain	5.5%	3.2%
Respiratory		
Cough	5.3%	5.3%
Dyspnea	4.4%	5.1%
Miscellaneous		
Hot flash	6.6%	5.9%
Injection-site pain	11.6%	9.1%
Pain in extremity	6.9%	7%

Hepatic – In the pooled safety population (N = 1,127) from clinical trials comparing fulvestrant 500 mg with fulvestrant 250 mg, post-baseline increases of at least 1 common toxicity criteria grade in either AST, ALT, or alkaline phosphatase were observed in more than 15% of patients receiving fulvestrant. Grade 3 to 4 increases were observed in 1% to 2% of patients. The incidence and severity of increased hepatic enzymes (ALT, AST, alkaline phosphatase) did not differ between the 250 and 500 mg fulvestrant arms.

➤*Comparison of fulvestrant 250 mg and anastrozole:*

Most common – The most commonly reported adverse reactions in the fulvestrant and anastrozole treatment groups, regardless of the investigator's assessment of causality, were GI symptoms (including nausea, vomiting, constipation, diarrhea, and abdominal pain), headache, back pain, vasodilatation (hot flashes), and pharyngitis.

Adverse reactions (5% or more) –

Fulvestrant vs Anastrozole: Adverse Reactions (≥ 5%)		
Adverse reactions[a]	Fulvestrant 250 mg/month (n = 423)	Anastrozole 1 mg/day (n = 423)
Cardiovascular, NOS[b]	30.3%	27.9%
Vasodilation	17.7%	17.3%
CNS, NOS	34.3%	33.8%
Anxiety	5%	3.8%
Asthenia	22.7%	27%
Depression	5.7%	6.9%
Dizziness	6.9%	6.6%
Headache	15.4%	16.8%
Insomnia	6.9%	8.5%
Paresthesia	6.4%	7.6%
Dermatologic, NOS	22.2%	23.4%
Rash	7.3%	8%
Sweating	5%	5.2%
GI, NOS	51.5%	48%
Abdominal pain	11.8%	11.6%
Anorexia	9%	10.9%
Constipation	12.5%	10.6%
Diarrhea	12.3%	12.8%
Nausea	26%	25.3%
Vomiting	13%	11.8%
GU, NOS	18.2%	14.9%
Urinary tract infection	6.1%	3.5%
Hematologic/Lymphatic, NOS	13.7%	13.5%
Anemia	4.5%	5%
Metabolic/Nutritional, NOS	18.2%	17.7%
Peripheral edema	9%	10.2%
Musculoskeletal, NOS	25.5%	27.9%
Arthritis	2.8%	6.1%
Back pain	14.4%	13.2%
Bone pain	15.8%	13.7%
Respiratory, NOS	38.5%	33.6%
Cough increased	10.4%	10.4%
Dyspnea	14.9%	12.3%
Pharyngitis	16.1%	11.6%
Miscellaneous, NOS	68.3%	67.6%
Accidental injury	4.5%	5.7%
Chest pain	7.1%	5%
Fever	6.4%	6.4%
Flu syndrome	7.1%	6.4%
Injection-site pain[c]	10.9%	6.6%
Pain	18.9%	20.3%
Pelvic pain	9.9%	9%

[a] A patient may have more than one adverse reaction.
[b] NOS = not otherwise specified.
[c] All patients on fulvestrant received injections, but only those anastrozole patients who were in the North American study (study 2) received placebo injections.

Local – Injection-site reactions with mild transient pain and inflammation were seen with fulvestrant and occurred in 7% of patients (1% of treatments) given the single 5 mL injection (European trial; study 3) and in 27% of patients (4.6% of treatments) given the 2 × 2.5 mL injections (North American trial; study 2).

➤*Postmarketing:*

GU – Vaginal bleeding has been reported infrequently (less than 1%), mainly in patients during the first 6 weeks after changing from existing hormonal therapy to treatment with fulvestrant. If bleeding persists, consider further evaluation.

Miscellaneous – For fulvestrant 250 mg, other adverse reactions reported as drug-related and seen infrequently (less than 1%) include leukopenia, myalgia, thromboembolic phenomena, vertigo, and hypersensitivity reactions including angioedema and urticaria.

Overdosage

➤*Symptoms:* There is no clinical experience with overdosage in humans. No adverse reactions were seen in healthy male and female volunteers who received IV fulvestrant, which resulted in peak plasma concentrations at the end of the infusion that were approximately 10 to 15 times those seen after IM injection.

Patient Information

Advise women of childbearing potential not to become pregnant while receiving fulvestrant. Fulvestrant can cause fetal harm when administered to a pregnant woman.

Inform patients that because fulvestrant is administered IM, it should be used with caution in patients with bleeding disorders, decreased platelet count, or in patients receiving anticoagulants (eg, warfarin).

HISTRELIN ACETATE

Rx	Supprelin LA (Indevus)	Implant; subcutaneous: 50 mg	In carton with implantation kit.
Rx	Vantas (Endo Pharmaceuticals)		In carton with implantation kit.

HISTRELIN ACETATE — SUBCUTANEOUS

Indications

➤*Advanced prostate cancer (Vantas only)*: For the palliative treatment of advanced prostate cancer.

➤*Central precocious puberty (Supprelin LA only)*: For the treatment of children with central precocious puberty.

Prior to initiation of treatment, a clinical diagnosis of central precocious puberty should be confirmed by measurement of blood concentrations of total sex steroids, luteinizing hormone (LH) and follicle-stimulating hormone (FSH) following stimulation with a gonadotropin-releasing hormone (GnRH) analog, and assessment of bone age versus chronological age. Baseline evaluations should include height and weight measurements, diagnostic imaging of the brain (to rule out intracranial tumor), pelvic/testicular/adrenal ultrasound (to rule out steroid secreting tumors), human chorionic gonadotropin levels (to rule out chorionic gonadotropin secreting tumor), and adrenal steroids to exclude congenital adrenal hyperplasia.

Administration and Dosage

➤*Adults:*

Advanced prostate cancer (Vantas only) –

Usual dosage: 1 implant inserted subcutaneously every 12 months.

Duration of therapy: Continue therapy until disease progression. In clinical trials, patients have been treated continuously for more than 4 years.

➤*Children:*

Central precocious puberty (Supprelin LA only) –

2 years of age and older:

- *Usual dosage* – 1 implant inserted subcutaneously every 12 months.
- *Discontinuation of therapy* – Discontinuation of *Supprelin LA* should be considered at the discretion of the health care provider and at the appropriate time point for the onset of puberty (approximately 11 years of age for females and 12 years of age for males).

➤*Renal function impairment:* No dosing adjustment required.

Dialysis – Conventional and peritoneal dialysis are minimally effective (25% to 49%) in removing histrelin.

➤*Administration:* The implant is inserted subcutaneously in the inner aspect of the upper arm and provides continuous release of histrelin (65 mcg/day for *Supprelin LA* and 50 to 60 mcg/day for *Vantas*) for 12 months of hormonal therapy.

Histrelin implant must be removed after 12 months of therapy (the implant has been designed to allow for a few additional weeks of histrelin release in order to allow for flexibility of medical appointments). At the time an implant is removed, another implant may be inserted to continue therapy.

➤*Storage/Stability:* Upon receipt, refrigerate the small carton containing the amber plastic pouch and glass vial (with the implant inside) until the day of insertion. Store the implant refrigerated, 2° to 8°C (36° to 46°F), in the unopened glass vial with the sterile sodium chloride 1.8% solution, overwrapped in the amber plastic pouch and carton. Protect from light. Do not freeze. The kit itself does not require refrigeration.

Actions

➤*Pharmacology:* Histrelin, an LH-releasing hormone (LH-RH) agonist, acts as a potent inhibitor of gonadotropin secretion when given continuously in therapeutic doses. Both animal and human studies indicate that following an initial stimulatory phase, chronic, subcutaneous administration of histrelin desensitizes responsiveness of the pituitary gonadotropin, which, in turn, causes a reduction in ovarian (*Supprelin LA* only) and testicular steroidogenesis (*Supprelin LA* and *Vantas*).

In humans, administration of histrelin acetate results in an initial increase in circulating levels of LH and FSH, leading to a transient increase in concentration of gonadal steroids (testosterone and dihydrotestosterone in males, and estrone and estradiol in premenopausal females). However, continuous administration of histrelin causes a reversible down-regulation of the GnRH receptors in the pituitary gland and desensitization of the pituitary gonadotropes. These inhibitory effects result in decreased levels of LH and FSH. In males, testosterone is reduced to castrate levels. These decreases occur within 2 to 4 weeks after initiation of treatment.

The histrelin implant is designed to provide continuous subcutaneous release of histrelin at a nominal rate of 50 to 60 mcg/day (*Vantas*) or approximately histrelin 65 mcg per day (*Supprelin LA*) over 12 months.

Pharmacodynamics –

Supprelin LA: Long-term treatment with histrelin suppresses the LH response to GnRH, causing LH levels to decrease to prepubertal levels within 1 month of treatment. As a result, serum concentrations of sex steroids (estrogen or testosterone) also decrease. Consequently, secondary sexual development ceases to progress in most patients. Additionally, linear growth velocity is slowed, which improves the chance of attaining predicted adult height.

➤*Pharmacokinetics:*

Absorption –

Supprelin LA: Pharmacokinetics of histrelin after implantation were evaluated in a total of 47 children with central precocious puberty (11 subjects in study 1 and 36 subjects in study 2). Patients were examined at 4 weeks after implant insertion and a few times throughout the treatment period. Median serum histrelin concentrations remained above the limit of quantification for the treatment period. Histrelin levels were sustained throughout the study period for most subjects. The median of maximum serum histrelin concentrations over the study period was 0.43 ng/mL, which is expected to maintain gonadotropins at prepubertal levels. There was no apparent pharmacokinetic difference between naive subjects to a LH-RH agonist treatment and subjects who had previous treatment with a LH-RH agonist.

Vantas: Following subcutaneous insertion of one histrelin 50 mg implant in advanced prostate cancer patients (n = 17), peak serum concentrations of 1.1 ± 0.375 ng/mL (mean ± standard deviation [SD]) occurred at a median of 12 hours. Continuous subcutaneous release was evident, as serum levels were sustained throughout the 52-week dosing period. The mean serum histrelin concentration at the end of the 52-week treatment duration was 0.13 ± 0.065 ng/mL. When histrelin serum concentrations were measured following a second implant inserted after 52 weeks, the observed serum concentrations over 8 weeks following the second implant were comparable with the same period following the first implant. The average rate of subcutaneous drug release from 41 implants assayed for residual drug content was 56.7 ± 7.71 mcg/day over the 52-week dosing period. The relative bioavailability for the histrelin implant in prostate cancer patients with healthy renal and hepatic function compared with a subcutaneous bolus dose in healthy male volunteers was 92%. Serum histrelin concentrations were proportional to dose after one, two, or four histrelin 50 mg implants (50, 100, or 200 mg of histrelin) in 42 prostate cancer patients.

Distribution –

Vantas: The apparent volume of distribution of histrelin following a subcutaneous bolus dose (500 mcg) in healthy volunteers was 58.4 ± 7.86 L. The fraction of drug unbound in plasma measured in vitro was 29.5% ± 8.9% (mean ± SD).

Metabolism –

Vantas: An in vitro drug metabolism study using human hepatocytes identified a single histrelin metabolite resulting from C-terminal dealkylation. Peptide fragments resulting from hydrolysis also are likely metabolites. Following a subcutaneous bolus dose in healthy volunteers, the apparent clearance of histrelin was 179 ± 37.8 mL/min (mean ± SD), and the terminal half-life was 3.92 ± 1.01 hours (mean ± SD). The apparent clearance following a histrelin 50 mg implant in 17 prostate cancer patients was 174 ± 56.5 mL/min (mean ± SD).

Contraindications

Hypersensitivity to GnRH or GnRH agonist analogs or any components in the histrelin implant; females who are or may become pregnant while receiving the drug (*Supprelin LA* only); use in women and children (*Vantas* only).

Anaphylactic reactions to synthetic LH-RH or LH-RH agonist analogs have been reported in the literature.

Warnings/Precautions

➤*Worsening of signs and symptoms:*

Supprelin LA – Histrelin, like other GnRH agonists, initially causes a transient increase in serum concentrations of estradiol in females and testosterone in both sexes during the first week of treatment. Patients may experience worsening of symptoms or onset of new symptoms during this period. However, within 4 weeks of histrelin therapy, suppression of gonadal steroids occurs and manifestations of puberty decrease.

Vantas – Histrelin, like other LH-RH agonists, causes a transient increase in serum concentrations of testosterone during the first week of treatment. Patients may experience worsening of symptoms or onset of new symptoms, including bone pain, neuropathy, hematuria, or ureteral or bladder outlet obstruction. Cases of ureteral obstruction and spinal cord compression, which may contribute to paralysis with or without fatal complications, have been reported with LH-RH agonists. If spinal cord compression or renal function impairment develops, institute standard treatment of these complications.

➤*Implant insertion and removal:* Implant insertion is a surgical procedure and it is important that the insertion instructions are followed to avoid potential complications. The insertion and removal of the implant should be done aseptically. Proper surgical technique is critical in minimizing adverse reactions related to the insertion and the removal of the histrelin implant. On occasion, localizing and/or removal of implant products have been difficult and imaging techniques were used, including ultrasound, computerized tomography (CT), or magnetic resonance imaging (MRI) (note: the histrelin implant is not radiopaque). Rare events of spontaneous extrusion of the implant have been observed in clinical trials. Detailed instructions on the insertion and removal procedures of the implant are provided in previous sections. In addition, instruct patients to refrain from wetting the arm for 24 hours and from heavy lifting or strenuous exertion of the inserted arm for 7 days after implant insertion.

In all clinical trials combined, an implant was not recovered in 8 patients. For 2 of these, serum testosterone rose above castrate level and the implant was neither palpable nor visualized with ultrasound. These 2 implants were believed to have been extruded without appreciation by the patients. In the

HISTRELIN ACETATE — SUBCUTANEOUS

other 6, serum testosterone remained below the castrate level, but the implant was not palpable. No further diagnostic tests were conducted. One of these patients underwent in-clinic surgical exploration that did not locate the implant. Based upon these findings, it is important to know that histrelin implant is not radiopaque and, therefore, will not be visible through x-ray. However, if the implant is difficult to locate by palpation, ultrasound and CT scan may be used.

➤*Pregnancy: Category X.* Histrelin is contraindicated in females who are or may become pregnant while receiving the drug. Histrelin can cause fetal harm when administered to a pregnant patient. The possibility exists that spontaneous abortion may occur.

Major fetal abnormalities were observed in rabbits at 3 times human therapeutic exposure but not in rats after administration of histrelin throughout gestation.

➤*Lactation:* Vantas is contraindicated in women.

➤*Children:*

Supprelin LA – Safety and efficacy in children younger than 2 years of age have not been established. The use of histrelin in children younger than 2 years of age is not recommended.

Vantas – Histrelin is contraindicated in children and was not studied in children.

➤*Monitoring:*

Supprelin LA – During treatment, patients should be evaluated for evidence of clinical and biochemical suppression of central precocious puberty manifestations. LH, FSH, and estradiol or testosterone should be monitored at 1 month postimplantation then every 6 months thereafter. Additionally, height (for calculation of height velocity) and bone age should be assessed every 6 to 12 months.

Vantas – Monitor response to histrelin by measuring serum concentrations of testosterone and PSA periodically, especially if the anticipated clinical or biochemical response to treatment has not been achieved.

Closely observe patients with metastatic vertebral lesions and/or urinary tract obstruction during the first few weeks of therapy.

Drug Interactions

➤*Drug/Lab test interactions:* Therapy with histrelin results in suppression of the pituitary-gonadal system. Results of diagnostic tests of pituitary-gonadotropic and gonadal functions conducted during and after histrelin therapy may be affected.

Supprelin LA decreased mean serum insulin-like growth factor-1 levels by approximately 11% in study 1. *Supprelin LA* increased the serum concentration of dehydroepiandrosterone in 8 of 36 patients in study 2.

Adverse Reactions

➤*Supprelin LA:* The most common adverse reactions with histrelin involved the implant site. Local reactions after implant insertion include bruising, pain, soreness, erythema, and swelling.

During the early phase of therapy, gonadotropins and sex steroids rise above baseline because of the natural stimulatory effect of the drug. Therefore, an increase in clinical signs and symptoms may be observed.

The safety of histrelin in children with central precocious puberty was evaluated in 2 single-arm clinical trials conducted in a total of 47 patients (44 females and 3 males) over a period of time ranging from 9 to 18 months. The most commonly reported adverse reaction was implant-site reaction, which was reported by 24 of 47 (51.1%) patients. Implant-site reaction includes discomfort, bruising, soreness, pain, tingling, itching, and implant-area protrusion and swelling. Two subjects experienced a serious adverse reaction: one subject who coincidentally had Stargardt disease experienced amblyopia, and one subject had a benign pituitary tumor (pituitary adenoma). One subject discontinued the study because of an adverse reaction of infection at the implant site. There were no clinically meaningful findings in standard clinical hematology and chemistry tests and/or in vital signs. The incidence of implantation adverse reactions reported by more than 2 patients are summarized in the following table.

Supprelin LA Adverse Reactions in Children with Central Precocious Puberty (≥ 2%)

Adverse reactions	(n = 47)
Local	
Application-site pain	4.3%
Implant-site reaction	51.1%
Keloid scar	6.4%
Postprocedural pain	4.3%
Scar	6.4%
Suture-related complication	6.4%

The following adverse reactions were reported as possibly related or related in one patient each: breast tenderness, disease progression, dysmenorrhea, epistaxis, erythema, feeling cold, gynecomastia, headache, influenza-like illness, menorrhagia, migraine, mood swings, pituitary tumor benign, pruritus, weight increased, and wound infection. The adverse reaction metrorrhagia was reported as possibly related or related in 2 patients.

➤*Vantas:* Histrelin, like other LH-RH analogs, caused a transient increase in serum testosterone concentrations during the first week of treatment. Therefore, potential exacerbations of signs and symptoms of the disease during the first few weeks of treatment are of concern in patients with vertebral metastases and/or urinary obstruction or hematuria. If these conditions are aggravated, it may lead to neurological problems such as weakness and/or paresthesia of the lower limbs or worsening of urinary symptoms.

Local – In the first 12 months after initial insertion of the implant, an implant extruded through the incision site in 8 of 171 patients in the clinical trials.

In the pivotal study (study 301), a detailed evaluation for implant-site reactions was conducted. Of the 138 patients in the study, 19 (13.8%) patients experienced local or insertion-site reactions. All local site reactions were reported as mild in severity. The majority were associated with initial insertion or removal and insertion of a new implant, and began and resolved within the first 2 weeks following implant insertion. Reactions persisted in 4 (2.8%) patients. An additional 4 (2.8%) patients developed application-site reactions after the first 2 weeks following insertion.

Local reactions after implant insertion included bruising (7.2%) and pain/soreness/tenderness (3.6%). Other, less frequently reported reactions included erythema (2.8%) and swelling (0.7%). In this study, 2 patients had events described as local infections/inflammations, one that resolved after treatment with oral antibiotics and the other without treatment.

Local reactions following insertion of a subsequent implant were comparable with those seen after initial insertion.

Systemic – The following possibly or probably related systemic adverse reactions occurred during clinical trials of up to 24 months of treatment with histrelin and were reported in 2% or more of patients (see the following table).

Vantas Adverse Reactions (≥ 2%)

Adverse reaction	%
CV	
Hot flashes[a]	65.5%
CNS	
Fatigue	9.9%
Headache	2.9%
Insomnia	2.9%
Libido decreased[a]	2.3%
Dermatologic	
Implant-site reaction	5.8%
GI	
Constipation	3.5%
GU	
Erectile dysfunction[a]	3.5%
Gynecomastia[a]	4.1%
Renal function impairment[b]	4.7%
Testicular atrophy[a]	5.3%
Miscellaneous	
Weight increased	2.3%

[a] Expected pharmacological consequences of testosterone suppression.
[b] Five of the 8 patients had a single occurrence of mild renal function impairment (defined as creatinine clearance [CrCl] 30 mL/min to less than 60 mL/min), which returned to a healthy range by the next visit.

Hot flashes were the most common adverse reaction reported (65.5%). In terms of severity, 2.3% of patients reported severe hot flashes, 25.4% reported moderate hot flashes, and 37.7% reported mild hot flashes. In addition, the following possibly or probably related systemic adverse reactions were reported by less than 2% of patients using histrelin implant in clinical studies.

Cardiovascular – Flushing, hematoma, palpitations, ventricular extrasystoles.

CNS – Depression, dizziness, irritability, lethargy, malaise, tremor, weakness.

Dermatologic – Contusion, hypotrichosis, night sweats, pruritus, sweating increased.

GI – Abdominal discomfort, nausea.

GU – Breast pain, breast tenderness, calculus renal, dysuria, genital pruritus male, gynecomastia aggravated, hematuria aggravated, renal failure aggravated, sexual dysfunction, urinary frequency, urinary frequency aggravated, urinary retention.

Hematologic – Anemia.

Hepatic – Hepatic disorder.

Lab test abnormalities – AST increased, blood glucose increased, blood lactate dehydrogenase increased, blood testosterone increased, CrCl decreased, prostatic acid phosphatase increased.

Metabolic/Nutritional – Appetite increased, fluid retention, food craving, hypercalcemia, hypercholesterolemia, peripheral edema, weight decreased.

Musculoskeletal – Arthralgia, back pain, back pain aggravated, bone pain, muscle twitching, myalgia, neck pain, pain in limb.

HISTRELIN ACETATE — SUBCUTANEOUS

Respiratory – Dyspnea exertional.

Miscellaneous – Feeling cold, pain, pain exacerbated, stent occlusion.

Bone density – In men who have had orchiectomy or have been treated with an LH-RH agonist analog, decreased bone density has been reported in the medical literature. It can be anticipated that long periods of medical castration in men will have effects on bone density.

Overdosage

There have been no reports of overdose in *Supprelin LA* clinical trials. High doses of histrelin injection in animal studies were generally associated only with effects attributed to the expected pharmacology. The method of drug delivery makes accidental or intentional overdosage unlikely.

Vantas injection of up to 200 mcg/kg (rats, rabbits) or 2,000 mcg/kg (mice) resulted in no systemic toxicity. This represents 20 to 200 times the maximal recommended human dose of 10 mcg/kg/day. Adverse reaction profiles were similar in patients receiving 1, 2, or 4 *Vantas* implants.

Patient Information

Advise patients that a transient worsening of symptoms of puberty or onset of new symptoms may occur initially with *Supprelin LA*. However, within 4 weeks of *Supprelin LA* therapy, complete suppression of gonadal steroids occurs and manifestations of puberty decrease.

Instruct patients to refrain from getting the inserted arm wet for 24 hours and from strenuous exertion of the inserted arm for 7 days after implant insertion to allow the incision to fully close. The adhesive elastic bandage can be removed at that time. Instruct the patient not to remove the surgical strips; rather, the strips should be allowed to fall off on their own after several days.

Advise patients to report to their health care provider any severe pain, redness, or swelling in and around the implant site. Infrequently, histrelin implant may be expelled from the body through the original incision site, rarely without the patient noticing. Instruct the patient to monitor the incision site until it is healed. Instruct the patient to return for routine checks of their condition and to ensure that histrelin implant is present and functioning in his/her body.

LEUPROLIDE ACETATE

Rx	**Leuprolide Acetate Injection** (Various, eg, Bedford Laboratories)	**Injection:** 5 mg/mL	In 2.8 mL multiple-dose vials.[a]
Rx	**Lupron for Pediatric Use** (Abbott)		In 2.8 mL multiple-dose vials.[a]
Rx	**Eligard** (Sanofi-Synthelabo)	**Powder for Injection, lyophilized:** 7.5 mg	In single-use kits with a 2-syringe mixing system and 20-gauge, ½-inch needle.
Rx	**Eligard** (Sanofi-Synthelabo)	**Injection:** 22.5 mg (3-month depot)	In single-use kits with a 2-syringe mixing system and 20-gauge, ½-inch needle.
		30 mg (4-month depot)	In single-use kit with 2-syringe mixing system and syringe containing *Atrigel*.
		45 mg (6-month depot)	In single-use kit with 2-syringe mixing system and syringe containing *Atrigel*.
Rx	**Lupron Depot** (Abbott)	**Microspheres for Injection, lyophilized:**[b] 3.75 mg	Mannitol. Preservative free. In single kits, multi-packs, and prefilled dual-chamber syringe.
		7.5 mg	Mannitol. Preservative free. In single kits, multi-packs, and prefilled dual-chamber syringe.
Rx	**Lupron Depot-Ped** (Abbott)	**Microspheres for Injection, lyophilized:**[b] 7.5 mg	Mannitol. Preservative free. In single-dose kit and pre-filled dual-chamber syringe.
		11.25 mg	Mannitol. Preservative free. In single-dose kit and pre-filled dual-chamber syringe.
		15 mg	Mannitol. Preservative free. In single-dose kit and pre-filled dual-chamber syringe.
Rx	**Lupron Depot - 3 Month** (Abbott)	**Microspheres for Injection, lyophilized:**[b] 11.25 mg	Mannitol. Preservative free. In single-use kit containing 11.25 mg vial leuprolide with 1.5 mL diluent and in pre-filled dual-chamber syringes.
		22.5 mg	Mannitol. Preservative free. In single-use kit containing 22.5 mg vial leuprolide with 1.5 mL diluent and in pre-filled dual-chamber syringes.
Rx	**Lupron Depot - 4 Month** (Abbott)	**Microspheres for Injection, lyophilized:**[b] 30 mg	Mannitol. Preservative free. In single-use kit containing 30 mg vial leuprolide with 1.5 mL diluent and in pre-filled dual-chamber syringes.

[a] With 9 mg/mL benzyl alcohol as preservative and sodium chloride.

[b] Listed as total dose; vials are combined to provide proper strength.

LEUPROLIDE ACETATE — INJECTION

Indications

➤*Advanced prostatic cancer (injection, implant, or depot 7.5, 22.5, 30, and 45 mg):* Palliative treatment of advanced prostatic cancer that offers an alternative when orchiectomy or estrogen administration are not indicated or are unacceptable to the patient.

➤*Endometriosis (depot 3.75 and 11.25 mg):* Management of endometriosis, including pain relief and reduction of endometriotic lesions. Experience is limited to women greater than or equal to 18 years of age treated for less than or equal to 6 months.

➤*Uterine leiomyomata (fibroids) (depot 3.75 and 11.25 mg):* Concomitantly with iron therapy for the preoperative hematologic improvement of patients with anemia caused by uterine leiomyomata. Experience with leuprolide depot in females has been limited to women greater than or equal to 18 years of age and treated for less than or equal to 6 months.

➤*Central precocious puberty (CPP) (pediatric injection or Depot-Ped):* Treatment of children with CPP.

➤*Off-label uses:* Treatment of breast cancer, ovarian carcinoma.

Administration and Dosage

➤*General dosing considerations:* Because of different release characteristics, a fractional dose of the 3-, 4-, or 6-month depot formulation is not equivalent to the same dose of the monthly formulation and should not be given.

➤*Adults:*

Advanced prostate cancer –

Depot: 7.5 mg monthly, 22.5 mg every 3 months (84 days), 30 mg every 4 months (16 weeks), or 45 mg every 6 months. *Lupron* should be administered IM, and *Eligard* should be administered subcutaneously.

Injection: 1 mg daily subcutaneously.

Endometriosis –

Depot:

• *Usual dosage* – 3.75 mg IM monthly or 11.25 mg IM every 3 months.

• *Duration of therapy* – 6 months.

• *Re-treatment* – Re-treatment cannot be recommended because safety data are not available. If the symptoms of endometriosis recur after a course of therapy and further treatment is contemplated, it is recommended that bone density be assessed before re-treatment begins to ensure that values are within normal limits.

Uterine leiomyomata –

Depot: The health care provider may wish to consider a 1-month trial period of iron alone because some patients may respond to iron alone.

• *Usual dosage* – 3.75 mg IM monthly or one 11.25 mg IM injection with concomitant iron therapy. 11.25 mg is indicated only for women for whom 3 months of hormonal suppression is deemed necessary.

• *Duration of therapy* – 3 months or less.

• *Re-treatment* – The symptoms associated with uterine leiomyomata will recur following discontinuation of therapy. If additional treatment is contemplated, assess bone density prior to initiation of therapy to ensure that values are within normal limits.

LEUPROLIDE ACETATE — INJECTION

➤*Children:*

Central precocious puberty – Individualize dosage based on mg/kg ratio of drug to body weight. Younger children require higher doses on mg/kg ratio.

Initial dosage:

• *Depot-Ped* (7.5, 11.25, and 15 mg) – 0.3 mg/kg once every 4 weeks (minimum, 7.5 mg) as a single IM injection. Determine the starting dose as follows:

Leuprolide Depot Starting Dose for CPP	
Weight (kg)	Intramuscular dose (mg)
> 37.5	15
> 25 to 37.5	11.25
≤ 25	7.5

• *Injection* – 50 mcg/kg/day as a single subcutaneous injection.

Dosage titration: Titrate the dose upwards until no progression of the condition is noted, either clinically or by lab parameters. The first dose to result in adequate downregulation can probably be maintained for the duration of therapy in most children. However, there are insufficient data to guide dosage adjustment as patients move into higher weight categories. Verify adequate downregulation in patients whose weight has increased significantly while on therapy.

• *Depot-Ped* (7.5, 11.25, and 15 mg) – If total downregulation is not achieved, titrate upward in 3.75 mg increments every 4 weeks.

• *Injection* – If total downregulation is not achieved, titrate upward by 10 mcg/kg/day.

Discontinuation of therapy: Consider discontinuation of therapy in females before they reach 11 years of age and in males before they reach 12 years of age.

Monitoring: After 1 to 2 months of initiating therapy or changing doses, monitor with a GnRH stimulation test, sex steroids, and Tanner staging to confirm downregulation. Monitor measurements of bone age for advancement every 6 to 12 months.

➤*Preparation for administration:*

Depot –

Single-use kit: Reconstitute the lyophilized microspheres with diluent provided. Using a 22-gauge needle, withdraw appropriate amount of diluent from ampule (1 or 1.5 mL); inject into vial. Shake well to obtain uniform suspension. It will appear milky. Withdraw entire contents of vial into syringe and inject immediately.

Prefilled dual-chamber syringe: See prescribing information. The suspension will appear milky. If the microspheres (particles) adhere to the stopper, tap the syringe against your finger. The suspension settles very quickly following reconstitution; therefore, it is preferable to mix and use immediately. Reshake suspension if settling occurs.

➤*Administration:*

Adults –

Depot:

• *Single-use kit* – For a single IM injection.

• *Prefilled dual-chamber syringe* – Remove the needle guard and advance the plunger to expel air from the syringe. Inject the entire contents of the syringe IM (*Lupron*) or subcutaneously (*Eligard*) as you would for a normal injection.

Injection: Vary the injection site periodically. Use the syringes provided in the kit; if alternate syringes are needed, use insulin syringes.

Children – Vary the injection site periodically.

Depot-Ped: Must be administered under physician supervision as a single IM injection.

Injection: May be administered by a patient/parent or health care provider as a single subcutaneous injection.

➤*Storage/Stability:*

Injection – Store below room temperature (25°C [77°F]). Avoid freezing. Protect from light; store vial in carton until use.

Depot –

Lupron: Store at 25°C (77°F); excursions are permitted to 15° to 30°C (59° to 86°F). The product does not contain a preservative; therefore, discard if not used immediately.

Eligard: Store at 2° to 3°C (35.6° to 46.4°F). Once mixed, the product must be administered within 30 minutes.

Actions

➤*Pharmacology:* Leuprolide, an LH-RH and GnRH agonist, acts as a potent inhibitor of gonadotropin secretion when given continuously in therapeutic doses. Animal and human studies indicate that following an initial stimulation, chronic administration of leuprolide results in suppression of ovarian and testicular steroidogenesis. This effect is reversible upon discontinuation of drug therapy. Administration of leuprolide has resulted in inhibition of the growth of certain hormone-dependent tumors (prostatic tumors in Noble and Dunning male rats and DMBA-induced mammary tumors in female rats) as well as atrophy of the reproductive organs.

In humans, administration of leuprolide results in an initial increase in circulating levels of luteinizing hormone (LH) and follicle-stimulating hormone (FSH), leading to a transient increase in levels of the gonadal steroids (testosterone and dihydrotestosterone in males, and estrone and estradiol in premenopausal females). However, continuous administration of leuprolide results in decreased levels of LH and FSH in all patients; in males, testosterone is reduced to castrate levels or to below the castrate threshold (less than or equal to 50 ng/dL). These decreases occur within 2 to 4 weeks after initiation of treatment.

➤*Pharmacokinetics:*

Absorption – In adults, bioavailability by subcutaneous administration is comparable to that by IV administration.

Daily injection: Leuprolide is not active when given orally. Leuprolide acetate has a plasma half-life of approximately 3 hours. The metabolism, distribution, and excretion of leuprolide in humans have not been determined. A pharmacokinetic study of leuprolide in children has not been performed.

7.5 mg (monthly) injection: The pharmacokinetics/pharmacodynamics was observed during 3 once-monthly injections (7.5 mg) in 20 patients with advanced carcinoma of the prostate.Mean serum leuprolide concentrations following the initial injection rose to 25.3 ng/mL (C_{max}) at approximately 5 hours after injection. After the initial increase following each injection, serum concentrations remained relatively constant (0.28 to 2 ng/mL). There was no evidence of significant accumulation during repeated dosing. Nondetectable leuprolide plasma concentrations have been observed during chronic leuprolide 7.5 mg administration, but testosterone levels were maintained at castrate levels.

22.5 mg (3-month) injection: The pharmacokinetics/pharmacodynamics was observed during 2 injections every 3 months (leuprolide 22.5 mg) in 22 patients with advanced carcinoma of the prostate. Mean serum leuprolide concentrations rose to 127 ng/mL and 107 ng/mL at approximately 5 hours following the initial and second injections, respectively. After the initial increase following each injection, serum leuprolide concentrations remained relatively constant (0.2 to 2 ng/mL). There was no evidence of significant accumulation during repeated dosing. Nondetectable leuprolide plasma concentrations have been observed during chronic leuprolide 22.5 mg administration, but testosterone levels were maintained at castrate levels.

30 mg (4-month) injection: The pharmacokinetics/pharmacodynamics was observed during injections administered initially and at 4 months (leuprolide 30 mg) in 24 patients with advanced carcinoma of the prostate. Mean serum leuprolide concentrations following the initial injection rose rapidly to 150 ng/mL (C_{max}) at approximately 3.3 hours after injection. After the initial increase following each injection, mean serum concentrations remained relatively constant (0.1 to 1 ng/mL). There was no evidence of significant accumulation during repeated dosing. Nondetectable leuprolide plasma concentrations have been occasionally observed during leuprolide 30 mg administration, but testosterone levels were maintained at castrate levels.

3.75 mg (monthly) depot suspension: A single dose of leuprolide 3.75 mg depot suspension was administered by IM injection to healthy female volunteers. The absorption of leuprolide was characterized by an initial increase in plasma concentration, with peak concentration ranging from 4.6 to 10.2 ng/mL at 4 hours postdosing. However, intact leuprolide and an inactive metabolite could not be distinguished by the assay used in the study. Following the initial rise, leuprolide concentrations started to plateau within 2 days after dosing and remained relatively stable for about 4 to 5 weeks with plasma concentrations of about 0.3 ng/mL.

7.5 mg (monthly) depot suspension and pediatric formulations: Following a single leuprolide 7.5 mg depot suspension injection to adult patients, mean peak leuprolide plasma concentration was almost 20 ng/mL at 4 hours and then declined to 0.36 ng/mL at 4 weeks. However, intact leuprolide and an inactive major metabolite could not be distinguished by the assay which was employed in the study. Nondetectable leuprolide plasma concentrations have been observed during chronic leuprolide 7.5 mg depot suspension administration, but testosterone levels appear to be maintained at castrate levels.

11.25 mg (3-month) depot suspension: Following a single injection of the 3-month formulation of leuprolide for 11.25 mg (3-month) depot suspension in female subjects, a mean plasma leuprolide concentration of 36.3 ng/mL was observed at 4 hours. Leuprolide appeared to be released at a constant rate following the onset of steady-state levels during the third week after dosing, and mean levels then declined gradually to near the lower limit of detection by 12 weeks. The mean (± standard deviation) leuprolide concentration from 3 to 12 weeks was 0.23 ± 0.09 ng/mL. However, intact leuprolide and an inactive major metabolite could not be distinguished by the assay which was employed in the study. The initial burst, followed by the rapid decline to a steady-state level, was similar to the release pattern seen with the monthly formulation.

22.5 mg (3-month) depot suspension: Following a single injection of the 3-month formulation of leuprolide 22.5 mg (3-month) depot suspension in patients, mean peak plasma leuprolide concentration of 48.9 ng/mL was observed at 4 hours and then declined to 0.67 ng/mL at 12 weeks. Leuprolide appeared to be released at a constant rate following the onset of steady-state levels during the third week after dosing, providing steady plasma concentrations through the 12-week dosing interval. However, intact leuprolide and an inactive major metabolite could not be distinguished by the assay which was employed in the study. Detectable levels of leuprolide were present at all measurement points in all patients. The initial burst, followed by the rapid decline to a steady-state level, was similar to the release pattern seen with the monthly formulation.

30 mg (4-month) depot suspension: Following a single injection of leuprolide 30 mg (4-month) depot suspension in 16 orchiectomized prostate cancer patients, mean plasma leuprolide concentration of 59.3 ng/mL was observed at 4 hours, and the mean concentration then declined to 0.3 ng/mL at 16 weeks. The mean plasma concentration of leuprolide from weeks 3.5 to 16 was 0.44 ± 0.2 ng/mL (range 0.2 to 1.06). Leuprolide appeared to be released at a constant rate following the onset of steady-state levels during the fourth week after dosing, providing steady plasma concentrations throughout the 16-week dosing interval. However, intact leuprolide and an inactive major metabolite could not be distinguished by the assay which was employed in the study. The initial burst, followed by the rapid decline to a steady-state level, was similar to the release pattern seen with the other depot formulations.

LEUPROLIDE ACETATE — INJECTION

Distribution – The mean steady-state volume of distribution of leuprolide following IV bolus administration to healthy male volunteers was 27 L. In vitro binding to human plasma proteins ranged from 43% to 49%.

Metabolism –

7.5 mg (monthly) injection, 22.5 mg (3-month), 30 mg (4-month): In healthy male volunteers, a 1 mg bolus of leuprolide administered IV revealed that the mean systemic clearance was 8.34 L/hr, with a terminal elimination half-life of approximately 3 hours based on a 2-compartment model.

No drug metabolism study was conducted with leuprolide 7.5 mg, 22.5 mg (3-month), or 30 mg (4-month) injections. Upon administration with different leuprolide formulations, the major metabolite of leuprolide is a pentapeptide (M-1) metabolite.

Daily pediatric injection and pediatric depot suspensions, 3.75 (monthly) depot suspension, 7.5 mg (monthly) depot suspension, 11.25 mg (3-month) depot suspension, 22.5 mg (3-month) depot suspension, 30 mg (4-month) depot suspension: In healthy male volunteers, a 1 mg bolus of leuprolide administered IV revealed that the mean systemic clearance was 7.6 L/hr, with a terminal elimination half-life of approximately 3 hours based on a 2-compartment model.

In a pharmacokinetic/pharmacodynamic study of endometriosis patients, IM 3.75 mg (monthly) leuprolide depot suspension (n = 15) every 4 weeks or IM 11.25 mg (3-month) depot suspension (n = 19) every 12 weeks was administered for 24 weeks. There was no statistically significant difference in changes of serum estradiol concentration from baseline between the 2 treatment groups.

M-I plasma concentrations measured in 5 prostate cancer patients reached maximum concentration 2 to 6 hours after dosing and were approximately 6% of the peak parent drug concentration. One week after dosing, mean plasma M-I concentrations were approximately 20% of mean leuprolide concentrations.

Excretion – Following administration of leuprolide for depot suspension 3.75 mg to 3 patients, less than 5% of the dose was recovered as parent and M-I metabolite in the urine.

7.5 mg (monthly), 22.5 mg (3–month), 30 mg (4-month) injections: No drug excretion study was conducted with leuprolide 7.5 mg (monthly), 22.5 mg (3-month), or 30 mg (4-month) injections.

Contraindications

Hypersensitivity to GnRH, GnRH agonist analogs, or any of the components in the various formulations of leuprolide for injection. Reports of anaphylactic reactions to synthetic GnRH or GnRH agonist analogs have been reported in the medical literature.

Leuprolide is contraindicated in women with undiagnosed abnormal vaginal bleeding.

All doses of leuprolide injections and depot suspensions are contraindicated in women who are or may become pregnant while receiving the drug. Leuprolide may cause fetal harm when administered to a pregnant woman. Major fetal abnormalities were observed in rabbits but not in rats after administration of leuprolide throughout gestation. There was increased fetal mortality and decreased fetal weights in rats and rabbits. The effects on fetal mortality are expected consequences of the alterations in hormonal levels brought about by this drug. Therefore, the possibility exists that spontaneous abortion may occur if the drug is administered during pregnancy. If this drug is used during pregnancy, or if the patient becomes pregnant while taking this drug, apprise the patient of the potential hazard to the fetus.

Leuprolide is contraindicated in women who are breastfeeding.

➤*7.5 mg (monthly), 22.5 mg (3-month), 30 mg (4-month) injections:* Leuprolide 7.5 mg (monthly), 22.5 mg (3-month), and 30 mg (4-month) injections are contraindicated in women and in pediatric patients and were not studied in women or children.

Warnings/Precautions

➤*Worsening of symptoms:*

Central precocious puberty – During the early phase of therapy, gonadotropins and sex steroids rise above baseline because of the natural stimulatory effect of the drug. Therefore, an increase in clinical signs and symptoms may be observed.

Noncompliance with drug regimen or inadequate dosing may result in inadequate control of the pubertal process. The consequences of poor control include the return of pubertal signs such as menses, breast development, and testicular growth. The long-term consequences of inadequate control of gonadal steroid secretion are unknown, but may include a further compromise of adult stature.

Advanced prostatic cancer – Initially, leuprolide, like other LH-RH agonists, causes transient increases in serum levels of testosterone to approximately 50% above baseline during the first week of treatment. Isolated cases of worsening of signs and symptoms during the first weeks of treatment have been reported with LH-RH analogs. Transient worsening of symptoms, or the occurrence of additional signs and symptoms of prostate cancer, may occasionally develop during the first few weeks of leuprolide treatment, including bone pain, neuropathy, hematuria, or bladder outlet obstruction. As with other LH-RH agonists, isolated cases of ureteral obstruction and spinal cord compression have been observed, which may contribute to paralysis, with or without fatal complications.

For patients at risk, the physician may consider initiating therapy with daily leuprolide injection for the first 2 weeks to facilitate withdrawal of treatment if that is considered necessary.

If spinal cord compression or renal impairment develops, institute standard treatment of these complications.

Endometriosis and uterine leiomyomata – Safe use of leuprolide in pregnancy has not been established clinically. Before starting treatment with leuprolide depot suspensions, pregnancy must be excluded.

When used at the recommended dose and dosing interval, leuprolide 3.75 mg (monthly) depot suspension and 11.25 mg (3-month) depot suspension usually inhibit ovulation and stop menstruation. Contraception is not ensured, however, by taking leuprolide. Therefore, patients should use nonhormonal methods of contraception. Advise patients to see their physicians if they believe they may be pregnant. If a patient becomes pregnant during treatment, the drug must be discontinued, and the patient must be apprised of the potential risk to the fetus.

During the early phase of therapy, sex steroids temporarily rise above baseline because of the physiologic effect of the drug. Therefore, an increase in clinical signs and symptoms may be observed during the initial days of therapy, but these will dissipate with continued therapy.

➤*Hypersensitivity reactions:* Patients with known allergies to benzyl alcohol, an ingredient of the vehicle of leuprolide daily injection and daily pediatric injection, may present symptoms of hypersensitivity, usually local, in the form of erythema and induration at the injection site.

Symptoms consistent with an anaphylactoid or asthmatic process have been rarely reported postmarketing.

➤*Renal function impairment:* If renal impairment develops, institute standard treatment of this complication.

➤*Pregnancy: Category X.* See Contraindications for more information.

➤*Lactation:* It is not known whether leuprolide is excreted in human milk. Because many drugs are excreted in human milk, and because the effects of leuprolide on lactation or the breastfed child have not been determined, leuprolide should not be used by nursing mothers.

➤*Children:* The safety and effectiveness of leuprolide, apart from the pediatric formulations for the treatment of central precocious puberty, have not been established in pediatric patients. See the labeling for the pediatric formulations for their safety and effectiveness in children with central precocious puberty.

3.75 (monthly) and 11.25 mg (3-month) depot suspension – Experience with leuprolide 3.75 monthly depot suspension for the treatment of endometriosis has been limited to women 18 years of age and older.

7.5 mg (monthly), 22.5 mg (3-month), and 30 mg (4-month) injections – Leuprolide 7.5 mg (monthly), 22.5 mg (3-month), and 30 mg (4-month) injections are contraindicated in pediatric patients and were not studied in children.

➤*Monitoring:*

Central precocious puberty –

Pediatric formulations: Monitor response to leuprolide pediatric formulations 1 to 2 months after the start of therapy with a GnRH stimulation test and sex steroid levels. Perform measurement of bone age for advancement every 6 to 12 months.

Sex steroids may increase or rise above prepubertal levels if the dose is inadequate. Once a therapeutic dose has been established, gonadotropin and sex steroid levels will decline to prepubertal levels.

Advanced prostatic cancer – Closely observe patients with metastatic vertebral lesions or with urinary tract obstruction during the first few weeks of therapy.

Monitor response to leuprolide by measuring serum levels of testosterone, as well as prostate-specific antigen and prostatic acid phosphatase.

7.5 mg (monthly) injection and depot suspension and 22.5 mg (3-month) injection and depot suspension, 30 mg (4-month) injection and depot suspension – Transient increases in prostatic acid phosphatase levels may occur sometime early in treatment. However, by the fourth week, the elevated levels can be expected to decrease to values at or near baseline.

Results of testosterone determinations are dependent on assay methodology. It is advisable to be aware of the type and precision of the assay methodology to make appropriate clinical and therapeutic decisions.

3.75 mg (monthly) depot suspension –

Endometriosis: During early clinical trials with leuprolide 3.75 mg monthly depot suspension for endometriosis, regular laboratory monitoring revealed that AST levels were more than twice the upper limit of normal in only 1 patient. There was no clinical or other laboratory evidence of abnormal liver function.

In 2 other clinical trials, 6 of 191 patients receiving leuprolide 3.75 mg monthly depot suspension plus norethindrone acetate 5 mg daily for up to 12 months developed an elevated (at least twice the upper limit of normal) ALT or gamma-glutamyl-transferase (GGT). Five of the 6 increases were observed beyond 6 months of treatment. None was associated with elevated bilirubin concentration.

Triglycerides were increased above the upper limit of normal in 12% of the endometriosis patients who received leuprolide 3.75 mg monthly depot suspension.

Uterine leiomyomata (fibroids): In clinical trials with leuprolide 3.75 mg monthly depot suspension for uterine leiomyomata, five (3%) patients had a post-treatment transaminase value that was at least twice the baseline value and above the upper limit of the normal range. None of the laboratory increases was associated with clinical symptoms.

LEUPROLIDE ACETATE — INJECTION

Lipids: Of those endometriosis and uterine fibroid patients whose pretreatment cholesterol values were in the normal range, mean change following therapy was +16 mg/dL to +17 mg/dL in endometriosis patients and +11 mg/dL to +29 mg/dL in uterine fibroid patients. In the endometriosis-treated patients, increases from the pretreatment values were statistically significant (P less than 0.03).

Chemistry: Slight to moderate mean increases were noted for glucose, uric acid, blood urea nitrogen, creatinine, total protein, albumin, bilirubin, alkaline phosphatase, LDH, calcium, and phosphorus. None of these increases was clinically significant.

Drug Interactions

➤*Drug/Lab test interactions:* Administration of leuprolide in therapeutic doses results in suppression of the pituitary-gonadal system. Normal function is usually restored within 4 to 12 weeks after treatment is discontinued. Therefore, diagnostic tests of pituitary gonadotropic and gonadal functions conducted during treatment and for up to 3 months after discontinuation of leuprolide or leuprolide depot suspensions may be misleading.

Adverse Reactions

➤*Central precocious puberty (CPP):* Potential exacerbation of signs and symptoms during the first few weeks of treatment is a concern in patients with rapidly advancing central precocious puberty.

Leuprolide Adverse Reactions in Children With CPP (≥ 2%)

Adverse reaction	Patients (n = 395)	(%)
Dermatologic		
Acne/seborrhea	7	2%
Injection site reactions, including abscess	21	5%
Rash, including erythema multiforme	8	2%
GU		
Vaginitis/bleeding/discharge	7	2%
Miscellaneous		
General pain	7	2%

In those same studies, the following adverse reactions were reported in less than 2% of the patients.

Cardiovascular – Syncope, vasodilation.

CNS – Emotional lability, nervousness, personality disorder, somnolence.

Dermatologic – Alopecia, skin striae.

Endocrine – Accelerated sexual maturity.

GI – Dysphagia, gingivitis, nausea/vomiting.

GU – Cervix disorder, gynecomastia/breast disorders, urinary incontinence.

Metabolic/Nutritional – Peripheral edema, weight gain.

Respiratory – Epistaxis.

Miscellaneous – Body odor, fever, headache, infection.

➤*CPP (postmarketing):* Symptoms consistent with an anaphylactoid or asthmatic process have been rarely (incidence rate of about 0.002%) reported. Rash, urticaria, and photosensitivity reactions have also been reported.

Cardiovascular – Hypotension, pulmonary embolism.

CNS – Peripheral neuropathy, spinal fracture/paralysis.

Dermatologic – Hair growth.

GU – Prostate pain.

Hematologic/Lymphatic – Decreased white blood cells.

Hepatic – Hepatic dysfunction.

Local – Localized reactions, including induration and abscess, have been reported at the site of injection.

Musculoskeletal – Tenosynovitis-like symptoms.

Respiratory – Respiratory disorders.

Special senses – Hearing disorder.

Miscellaneous – Hard nodule in throat, weight gain, increased uric acid. Symptoms consistent with fibromyalgia (eg, joint and muscle pain, headaches, sleep disorders, GI distress, shortness of breath) have been reported individually and collectively.

Changes in bone density – Decreased bone density has been reported in the medical literature in men who have had orchiectomy or who have been treated with an LH-RH agonist analog. In a clinical trial, 25 men with prostate cancer, 12 of whom had been treated previously with leuprolide for at least 6 months, underwent bone density studies as a result of pain. The leuprolide-treated group had lower bone density scores than the nontreated control group. The effects on bone density in children are unknown.

➤*Advanced prostate cancer (daily injection):* In the majority of patients, testosterone levels increased above baseline during the first week, declining thereafter to baseline levels or below by the end of the second week of treatment. This transient increase was occasionally associated with a temporary worsening of signs and symptoms, usually manifested by an increase in bone pain. In a few cases, a temporary worsening of existing hematuria and urinary tract obstruction occurred during the first week. Temporary weakness and paresthesia of the lower limbs have been reported in a few cases.

Potential exacerbations of signs and symptoms during the first few weeks of treatment is a concern in patients with vertebral metastases or urinary obstruction which, if aggravated, may lead to neurological problems or increase the obstruction.

Leuprolide Adverse Reactions (≥ 5%) in Advanced Prostate Cancer

Adverse reaction	Leuprolide (n = 98)	DES (n = 101)
Cardiovascular		
Congestive heart failure	1	5
ECG changes/ischemia	19	22
High blood pressure	8	5
Murmur	3	8
Peripheral edema	12	30
Phlebitis/thrombosis	2	10
CNS/peripheral nervous system		
Dizziness/lightheadedness	5	7
General pain	13	13
Headache	7	4
Insomnia/sleep disorders	7	5
Dermatologic		
Dermatitis	5	8
Endocrine		
Decreased testicular size[a]	7	11
Gynecomastia/breast tenderness or pain[a]	7	63
Hot flashes[a]	55	12
Impotence[a]	4	12
GI		
Anorexia	6	5
Constipation	7	9
Nausea/vomiting	5	17
GU		
Frequency/urgency	6	8
Hematuria	6	4
Urinary tract infection	3	7
Hematologic-lymphatic		
Anemia	5	5
Musculoskeletal		
Bone pain	5	2
Myalgia	3	9
Respiratory		
Dyspnea	2	8
Sinus congestion	5	6
Miscellaneous		
Asthenia	10	10

[a] Physiologic effect of decreased testosterone.

In this same study, the following adverse reactions were reported in less than 5% of the patients on leuprolide:

Cardiovascular – Angina, cardiac arrhythmias, myocardial infarction, pulmonary emboli.

CNS – Anxiety, blurred vision, lethargy, memory disorder, mood swings, nervousness, numbness, paresthesia, peripheral neuropathy, syncope/blackouts.

Dermatologic – Carcinoma of skin/ear, dry skin, ecchymosis, hair loss, itching, local skin reactions, pigmentation, skin lesions.

Endocrine – Decreased libido, thyroid enlargement.

GI – Diarrhea, dysphagia, gastrointestinal bleeding, gastrointestinal disturbance, peptic ulcer, rectal polyps.

GU – Bladder spasms, dysuria, incontinence, testicular pain, urinary obstruction.

Musculoskeletal – Joint pain.

Ophthalmic – Swelling (temporal bone).

Respiratory – Cough, pleural rub, pneumonia, pulmonary fibrosis.

Special senses – Taste disorders.

Miscellaneous – Depression, diabetes, fatigue, fever/chills. hypoglycemia, increased BUN, increased calcium, increased creatinine, infection/inflammation.

LEUPROLIDE ACETATE — INJECTION

➤*Advanced prostate cancer (additional adverse reactions reported with leuprolide daily injection during other clinical trials or during postmarketing surveillance):*

Cardiovascular – Hypotension, transient ischemic attack/stroke.

CNS – Hearing disorder, peripheral neuropathy, spinal fracture/paralysis.

Dermatologic – Hair growth.

Endocrine – Increased libido.

GU – Penile swelling, prostate pain.

Hepatic – Hepatic dysfunction.

Hematologic/Lymphatic – Decreased WBC, hemoptysis.

Musculoskeletal – Ankylosing spondylosis, pelvic fibrosis.

Respiratory – Pulmonary infiltrate, respiratory disorders.

Miscellaneous – Hypoproteinemia, hard nodule in throat, increased uric acid, weight gain.

➤*Advanced prostate cancer (7.5 mg [monthly] injection):* See Warnings/Precautions for more information.

In Study AGL9904, 120 patients were dosed with leuprolide 7.5 mg for up to 6 months, and injection sites were closely monitored. In all, 716 injections of leuprolide 7.5 mg (monthly) injection were administered. Transient burning/stinging was reported following 248 (34.6%) injections, with the majority (84%) of these events reported as mild. Pain was reported following 4.3% of study injections (18.3% of patients) and was generally reported as brief in duration and mild in intensity.

Erythema was reported following 2.6% of injections (12.5% of patients). These events were all reported as mild and generally resolved within a few days postinjection. Mild bruising was reported following 2.5% of injections (11.7% of patients). Pruritus, induration, and ulceration was reported following 1.4% (11 patients), 0.4% (3 patients), and 0.1% (1 patient) of study injections, respectively.

Adverse Reactions with Leuprolide 7.5 mg for ≤ 6 months in Study AGL9904 (≥ 2%)

Body system	Adverse event	Patients (n = 120)
Cardiovascular	Hot flashes/sweats[a]	68 (56.7%)
GI	Gastroenteritis/colitis	3 (2.5%)
GU	Atrophy of testes[a]	6 (5%)
Miscellaneous	Malaise and fatigue	21 (17.5%)
	Dizziness	4 (3.3%)

[a] Expected pharmacological consequences of testosterone suppression. In the patient populations studied, a total of 86 hot flashes/sweats adverse events were reported in 70 patients. Of these, 71 events (83%) were mild; 14 (16%) were moderate; 1 (1%) were severe.

Adverse Reactions Reported by Surgically Castrated Patients Treated with a Single-Dose of Leuprolide 7.5 mg in Study AGL9802 (≥ 2%)

Body system	Adverse event	Number (n = 8)
Cardiovascular	Hot flashes/sweats[a]	2 (25%)

[a] Expected pharmacological consequences of testosterone suppression. In the patient populations studied, a total of 86 hot flashes/sweats adverse events were reported in 70 patients. Of these, 71 events (83%) were mild; 14 (16%) were moderate; 1 (1%) were severe.

In addition, the following possibly or probably related systemic adverse events were reported by less than 2% of the patients using leuprolide 7.5 mg (monthly) injection in clinical studies.

CNS – Depression, disturbance of smell and taste, vertigo.

Dermatologic – Alopecia.

GI – Constipation, flatulence.

GU – Breast soreness, decreased libido, testicular soreness; gynecomastia, impotence (expected pharmacological consequences of testosterone suppression. In the patient populations studied, a total of 86 hot flashes/sweats adverse events were reported in 70 patients. Of these, 71 events (83%) were mild; 14 (16%) were moderate; 1 (1%) were severe).

Hematologic – Decreased red blood cell count, hematocrit and hemoglobin.

Metabolic – Weight gain.

Musculoskeletal – Backache, joint pain, tremor.

Miscellaneous – Insomnia, sweating, syncope.

Changes in bone density (7.5 mg [monthly] injection) – Decreased bone density has been reported in the medical literature in men who have had orchiectomy or who have been treated with an LH-RH agonist analog. It can be anticipated that long periods of medical castration in men will have effects on bone density.

➤*Advanced prostate cancer (22.5 mg [3-month] injection):* See Warnings/Precautions for more information.

In Study AGL9909, 117 patients were dosed with leuprolide 22.5 mg (3-month) injection every 3 months for up to 6 months, and injection sites were closely monitored. In all, 230 injections of leuprolide 22.5 mg (3-month) injection were administered. Transient burning/stinging was reported following 50 injections (21.7%), with the majority (86%) of these events reported as mild. Pain was reported following 3.5% of study injections (6% of patients) and was generally reported as brief in duration and mild in intensity.

Erythema was reported following 2 injections (0.9% of study injections, 1.7% of patients). One of the reports characterized the erythema as mild and resolved within 7 days. The other was moderate and resolved within 15 days. Neither patient experienced erythema at multiple injections. Mild bruising was reported following 4 injections (1.7% of study injections, 3.4% of patients). Mild pruritus was reported following 1 injection (0.4% of study injections, 0.9% of patients).

Adverse Events Reported by Patients Treated with Leuprolide 22.5 mg (3-Month) Injection for ≤ 6 months; Study AGL9909 (≥ 2%)

Body system	Adverse event	Number (n = 117)
Cardiovascular		
Vascular disorders	Hot flashes/sweats[a]	66 (56.4%)
Dermatologic	Pruritus	3 (2.6%)
GI	Nausea	4 (3.4%)
GU	Urinary frequency	3 (2.6%)
Musculoskeletal	Arthralgia	4 (3.4%)
Miscellaneous	Fatigue	7 (6%)

[a] Expected pharmacological consequence of testosterone suppression. In the patient population studied, a total of 84 hot flashes/sweats events were reported in 66 patients. Of these, 73 events (87%) were described as mild; 11 (13%) as moderate; none were severe.

In addition, the following possibly or probably related systemic adverse events were reported by less than 2% of the patients using leuprolide 22.5 mg (3-month) injection in the clinical study.

Cardiovascular –
Vascular: Hypertension, hypotension.

Dermatologic – Clamminess; increased sweating, night sweats (expected pharmacological consequences of testosterone suppression. In the patient populations studied, a total of 86 hot flashes/sweats adverse events were reported in 70 patients. Of these, 71 events (83%) were mild; 14 (16%) were moderate; 1 (1%) were severe).

GI – Dyspepsia.

GU – Testicular pain; breast tenderness, gynecomastia, impotence, testicular atrophy (expected pharmacological consequences of testosterone suppression. In the patient populations studied, a total of 86 hot flashes/sweats adverse events were reported in 70 patients. Of these, 71 events (83%) were mild; 14 (16%) were moderate; 1 (1%) were severe).

Renal – Bladder spasm, blood in urine, difficulties with urination, pain on urination, scanty urination, and urinary retention.

Miscellaneous – Lethargy, rigors, weakness.

Changes in bone density (22.5 mg [3-month] injection) – Decreased bone density has been reported in the medical literature in men who have had orchiectomy or who have been treated with an LH-RH agonist analog. It can be anticipated that long periods of medical castration in men will have effects on bone density.

➤*Advanced prostate cancer (30 mg [4-month] injection):* See Warnings/Precautions for more information.

In Study AGL0001, 90 patients were dosed with leuprolide 30 mg (4-month) every 4 months for up to 8 months, and injection sites were closely monitored. In all, 175 injections of leuprolide 30 mg (4-month) injection were administered. Transient burning/stinging was reported at the injection site following 35 (20%) injections, with all (100%) of these events reported as mild. Pain was reported following 2.3% of study injections (3.3% of patients) and was generally reported as mild in intensity. A single event reported as moderate pain resolved within 2 minutes, and all 3 mild pain events resolved within several days. Erythema was reported following 1.1% of injections (2.2% of patients). These events were all reported as mild and generally resolved within a few days postinjection.

Adverse Events Reported by Patients Treated with Leuprolide 30 mg (4-Month) Injection for up to 8 Months in Study AGL0001 (≥ 2%)

Body system	Adverse event	Number (N = 90)
Cardiovascular	Hot flashes[a]	66 (73.3%)
CNS	Dizziness	4 (4.4%)
Dermatologic	Alopecia	2 (2.2%)
	Clamminess[a]	
	Night sweats[a]	3 (3.3%)
GI	Nausea	2 (2.2%)
GU	Gynecomastia[a]	2 (2.2%)
	Testicular atrophy*	4 (4.4%)
	Testicular pain	2 (2.2%)
Musculoskeletal	Myalgia	2 (2.2%)

LEUPROLIDE ACETATE — INJECTION

Adverse Events Reported by Patients Treated with Leuprolide 30 mg (4-Month) Injection for up to 8 Months in Study AGL0001 (≥ 2%)		
Body system	Adverse event	Number (N = 90)
Renal/Urinary	Nocturia	2 (2.2%)
	Urinary frequency	2 (2.2%)
Miscellaneous	Fatigue	12 (13.3%)

[a] Expected pharmacological consequences of testosterone suppression. In the patient population studied, a total of 75 hot flash adverse events were reported in 66 patients. Of these, 57 events (76%) were mild; 16 (21%) were moderate; 2 (3%) were severe.

In addition, the following possibly or probably related systemic adverse events were reported by 1.1% of patients using leuprolide 30 mg (4-month) injection in the clinical study.

GU – Reduced penis size; breast enlargement, erectile dysfunction (expected pharmacological consequences of testosterone suppression. In the patient population studied, a total of 75 hot flash adverse events were reported in 66 patients. Of these, 57 events (76%) were mild; 16 (21%) were moderate; 2 (3%) were severe).

Musculoskeletal – Limb pain, muscle atrophy.

Psychiatric – Depression, insomnia.

Renal – Incontinence, urinary urgency.

Miscellaneous – Lethargy.

Changes in bone density (30 mg [4-month] injection) – Decreased bone density has been reported in the medical literature in men who have had orchiectomy or who have been treated with an LH-RH agonist analog. It can be anticipated that long periods of medical castration in men will have effects on bone density.

➤*Advanced prostate cancer (7.5 mg [monthly] depot formulation):* See Warnings/Precautions for more information.

Leuprolide 7.5 mg (Monthly) Depot Suspension Adverse Reactions in Advanced Prostate Cancer		
Adverse reaction	(n = 56)	(%)
Cardiovascular		
Hot flashes/sweats[a]	32	(57.1%)
CNS		
Decreased libido[a]	3	(5.4%)
GI		
GI disorders	8	(14.3%)
GU		
Impotence[a]	3	(5.4%)
Testicular atrophy[a]	3	(5.4%)
Urinary disorder	7	(12.5%)
Metabolic/nutritional		
Edema	8	(14.3%)
Respiratory		
Respiratory disorder	6	(10.7%)
Miscellaneous		
General pain	13	(23.2%)
Infection	3	(5.4%)

[a] Due to the expected physiologic effect of decreased testosterone levels.

In the same study, the following adverse reactions were reported in less than 5% of the patients on leuprolide 7.5 mg (monthly) depot suspension.

Cardiovascular – Angina, congestive heart failure.

CNS – Agitation, insomnia/sleep disorders, neuromuscular disorders.

Dermatologic – Hair disorder, skin reaction.

GI – Anorexia, dysphagia, eructation, peptic ulcer.

GU – Balanitis, breast enlargement, urinary tract infection.

Hematologic/Lymphatic – Ecchymosis.

Lab test abnormalities – Abnormalities of certain parameters were observed, but their relationship to drug treatment are difficult to assess in this population. The following were recorded in greater than or equal to 5% of patients at final visit: Decreased albumin, decreased hemoglobin/hematocrit, decreased prostatic acid phosphatase, decreased total protein, decreased urine-specific gravity, hyperglycemia, hyperuricemia, increased BUN, increased creatinine, increased liver function tests (AST, LDH), increased phosphorus, increased platelets, increased prostatic acid phosphatase, increased total cholesterol, increased urine-specific gravity, leukopenia.

Musculoskeletal – Myalgia.

Respiratory – Emphysema, hemoptysis, increased sputum, lung edema.

Miscellaneous – Asthenia, cellulitis, fever, headache, injection-site reaction, neoplasm.

➤*Advanced prostate cancer (postmarketing, 7.5 mg [monthly] depot suspension):* Symptoms consistent with an anaphylactoid or asthmatic process have been rarely (incidence rate of about 0.002%) reported. Rash, urticaria, and photosensitivity reactions have also been reported.

Localized reactions, including induration and abscess have been reported at the site of injection.

Symptoms consistent with a fibromyalgia (eg, joint and muscle pain, headaches, sleep disorders, GI distress, and shortness of breath) have been reported individually and collectively.

Cardiovascular – Hypotension, pulmonary embolism.

CNS – Peripheral neuropathy, spinal fracture/paralysis.

GU – Prostate pain.

Hematologic/Lymphatic – Decreased white blood cells.

Musculoskeletal – Tenosynovitis-like symptoms.

Changes in bone density (7.5 mg [monthly] depot suspension) – Decreased bone density has been reported in the medical literature in men who have had orchiectomy or who have been treated with an LH-RH agonist analog. In a clinical trial, 25 men with prostate cancer, 12 of whom had been treated previously with leuprolide for at least 6 months, underwent bone density scans as a result of pain. The leuprolide-treated group had lower bone density scores than the nontreated control group. It can be anticipated that long periods of medical castration in men will have effects on bone density.

➤*Advanced prostate cancer (22.5 mg [3-month] depot suspension):* See Warnings/Precautions for more information.

Leuprolide 22.5 mg (3-Month) Depot Suspension Adverse Reactions in Advanced Prostate Cancer		
Adverse reaction	n = 94	(%)
Cardiovascular		
Hot flashes/sweats[a]	55	(58.5%)
CNS		
Dizziness/vertigo	6	(6.4%)
Insomnia/sleep disorders	8	(8.5%)
Neuromuscular disorders	9	(9.6%)
Dermatologic		
Skin reaction	8	(8.5%)
GI		
GI disorders	15	(16%)
GU		
Testicular atrophy[a]	19	(20.2%)
Urinary disorders	14	(14.9%)
Musculoskeletal		
Joint disorders	11	(11.7%)
Respiratory		
Respiratory disorders	6	(6.4%)
Miscellaneous		
Asthenia	7	(7.4%)
General pain	25	(26.6%)
Headache	6	(6.4%)
Injection site reaction	13	(13.8%)

[a] Physiologic effect of decreased testosterone.

In these same studies, the following adverse reactions were reported in less than 5% of the patients on leuprolide for depot suspension 22.5 mg (3-month).

Cardiovascular – Arrhythmia, bradycardia, heart failure, hypertension, hypotension, varicose vein.

CNS – Anxiety, delusions, depression, hypesthesia, decreased libido (physiologic effect of decreased testosterone), nervousness, paresthesia.

GI – Anorexia, duodenal ulcer, increased appetite, thirst/dry mouth.

GU – Gynecomastia, impotence (physiologic effect of decreased testosterone), penis disorders, testis disorders.

Hematologic/Lymphatic – Anemia, lymphedema.

Lab test abnormalities – Abnormalities of certain parameters were observed, but are difficult to assess in this population. The following were recorded in greater than or equal to 5% of patients: Increased BUN, hyperglycemia, hyperlipidemia (total cholesterol, LDL cholesterol, triglycerides), hyperphosphatemia, abnormal liver function tests, increased PT, increased PTT. Additional laboratory abnormalities reported were decreased platelets, decreased potassium, and increased WBC.

Metabolic/Nutritional – Dehydration, edema.

Respiratory – Epistaxis, pharyngitis, pleural effusion, pneumonia.

Special senses – Abnormal vision, amblyopia, dry eyes, tinnitus.

Miscellaneous – Enlarged abdomen, fever.

LEUPROLIDE ACETATE — INJECTION

➤*Advanced prostate cancer (postmarketing, 22.5 [3-month] depot suspension):* Symptoms consistent with an anaphylactoid or asthmatic process have been reported rarely (incidence rate of about 0.002%). Rash, urticaria, and photosensitivity reactions have also been reported.

Localized reactions, including induration and abscess, have been reported at the site of injection.

Symptoms consistent with fibromyalgia (eg, joint and muscle pain, headaches, sleep disorders, GI distress, and shortness of breath) have been reported individually and collectively.

Cardiovascular – Hypotension, pulmonary embolism.

CNS – Peripheral neuropathy, spinal fracture/paralysis.

GU – Prostate pain.

Hematologic/Lymphatic – Decreased white blood cells.

Musculoskeletal – Tenosynovitis-like symptoms.

➤*Advanced prostate cancer (30 mg, [4-month] depot suspension):* See Warnings/Precautions for more information.

Adverse Reactions Reported in Patients Regardless of Causality (Leuprolide for Depot Suspension 30 mg [4-month]) in Advanced Prostate Cancer (≥ 5%)				
	Nonorchiectomized (n = 49) Study 013		Orchiectomized (n = 24) Study 012	
Adverse reactions	n	(%)	n	(%)
Cardiovascular				
Hot flashes/sweats[a]	23	(46.9%)	2	(8.3%)
CNS				
Dizziness/vertigo	3	(6.1%)	2	(8.3%)
Neuromuscular disorders	3	(6.1%)	1	(4.2%)
Paresthesia	4	(8.2%)	1	(4.2%)
Dermatologic				
Skin reaction	6	(12.2%)	0	(0%)
GI				
GI disorders	5	(10.2%)	3	(12.5%)
GU				
Urinary disorders	5	(10.2%)	4	(16.7%)
Metabolic/Nutritional				
Dehydration	4	(8.2%)	0	(0%)
Edema	4	(8.2%)	5	(20.8%)
Musculoskeletal				
Joint disorder	8	(16.3%)	1	(4.2%)
Myalgia	4	(8.2%)	0	(0%)
Respiratory				
Respiratory disorder	4	(8.2%)	1	(4.2%)
Miscellaneous				
Asthenia	6	(12.2%)	1	(4.2%)
Flu syndrome	6	(12.2%)	0	(0%)
General pain	16	(32.7%)	1	(4.2%)
Headache	5	(10.2%)	1	(4.2%)
Injection-site reaction	4	(8.2%)	9	(37.5%)

[a] Due to the expected physiologic effects of decreased testosterone levels.

In these same studies, the following adverse reactions were reported in less than 5% of the patients on leuprolide 30 mg (4–month) depot suspension.

Cardiovascular – Atrial fibrillation, deep thrombophlebitis, hypertension.

CNS – Abnormal thinking, amnesia, confusion, convulsion, dementia, depression, insomnia/sleep disorders, libido decreased (due to the expected physiologic effects of decreased testosterone levels), neuropathy, paralysis.

Dermatologic – Herpes zoster, melanosis.

GI – Anorexia, eructation, gastrointestinal hemorrhage, gingivitis, gum hemorrhage, hepatomegaly, increased appetite, intestinal obstruction, periodontal abscess.

GU – Bladder carcinoma, epididymitis, impotence (due to the expected physiologic effects of decreased testosterone levels), prostate disorder, testicular atrophy (due to the expected physiologic effects of decreased testosterone levels), urinary incontinence, urinary tract infection.

Hematologic/Lymphatic – Lymphadenopathy.

Lab test abnormalities – Abnormalities of certain parameters were observed, but their relationship to drug treatment are difficult to assess in this population. The following were recorded in greater than or equal to 5% of patients: Decreased bicarbonate, decreased hemoglobin/hematocrit/RBC, hyperlipidemia (total cholesterol, LDL cholesterol, triglycerides), decreased HDL cholesterol, eosinophilia, increased glucose, increased liver function tests (ALT, AST, GGTP, LDH), increased phosphorus. Additional laboratory abnormalities were reported: Increased BUN and PT, leukopenia, thrombocytopenia, uricaciduria.

Metabolic/Nutritional – Abnormal healing, hypoxia, weight loss.

Musculoskeletal – Leg cramps, pathological fracture, ptosis.

Respiratory – Asthma, bronchitis, hiccup, lung disorder, sinusitis, voice alteration.

Miscellaneous – Abscess, accidental injury, allergic reaction, cyst, fever, generalized edema, hernia, neck pain, neoplasm.

➤*Postmarketing advanced prostate cancer (30 mg [4-month] depot suspension):* Symptoms consistent with an anaphylactoid or asthmatic process have been rarely (incidence rate of about 0.002%) reported. Rash, urticaria, and photosensitivity reactions have also been reported.

Localized reactions, including induration and abscess, have been reported at the site of injection.

Symptoms consistent with fibromyalgia (eg, joint and muscle pain, headaches, sleep disorders, GI distress, and shortness of breath) have been reported individually and collectively.

Cardiovascular – Hypotension, pulmonary embolism.

CNS – Peripheral neuropathy, spinal fracture/paralysis.

GU – Prostate pain.

Hematologic/Lymphatic – Decreased white blood cells.

Musculoskeletal – Tenosynovitis-like symptoms.

Changes in bone density (22.5 mg [3-month] and 30 mg [4-month] depot suspensions) – Decreased bone density has been reported in the medical literature in men who have had orchiectomies or who have been treated with LH-RH agonist analogs. In a clinical trial, 25 men with prostate cancer, 12 of whom had been treated previously with leuprolide for at least 6 months, underwent bone density studies as a result of pain. The leuprolide-treated group had lower bone density scores than the nontreated control group. It can be anticipated that long periods of medical castration in men will have effects on bone density.

➤*Endometriosis (3.75 mg [monthly] depot suspension):* Estradiol levels may increase during the first weeks following the initial injection, but then decline to menopausal levels. This transient increase in estradiol can be associated with a temporary worsening of signs and symptoms.

As would be expected with a drug that lowers serum estradiol levels, the most frequently reported adverse reactions were those related to hypoestrogenism.

In controlled studies for endometriosis comparing leuprolide for depot suspension 3.75 mg monthly and danazol (800 mg/day) or placebo, adverse reactions included the following:

Cardiovascular – Palpitations, syncope, tachycardia.

CNS – Anxiety (possible effect of decreased estrogen), delusions, memory disorder, personality disorder.

Dermatologic – Alopecia, ecchymosis, hair disorder.

GI – Appetite changes, dry mouth, thirst.

GU – Dysuria (possible effect of decreased estrogen), lactation.

Miscellaneous – Lymphadenopathy, ophthalmologic disorders (possible effect of decreased estrogen).

Potentially drug-related adverse events observed in at least 5% of patients in any treatment group during the first 6 months of treatment in the add-back clinical studies (3.75 mg [monthly] depot suspension) – The following table lists the potentially drug-related adverse events observed in at least 5% of patients in any treatment group during the first 6 months of treatment in the add–back clinical studies.

Leuprolide Treatment-Related Adverse Events (≥ 5%) in the Add-Back Clinical Studies (3.75 mg [Monthly] Depot Suspension)						
	Controlled study				Open-label study	
	LD-only[a] (n = 51)		LD/N[b] (n = 55)		LD/N[b] (n = 136)	
Adverse events	n	(%)	n	(%)	n	(%)
Any adverse event	50	(98%)	53	(96%)	126	(93%)
Cardiovascular						
Hot flashes/sweats	50	(98%)	48	(87%)	78	(57%)
CNS						
Anxiety	3	(6%)	0	(0%)	11	(8%)
Depression/emotional lability	16	(31%)	15	(27%)	46	(34%)
Dizziness/vertigo	8	(16%)	6	(11%)	10	(7%)
Insomnia/sleep disorder	16	(31%)	7	(13%)	20	(15%)
Libido changes	5	(10%)	2	(4%)	10	(7%)
Memory disorder	3	(6%)	1	(2%)	6	(4%)
Nervousness	4	(8%)	2	(4%)	15	(11%)

LEUPROLIDE ACETATE — INJECTION

Leuprolide Treatment-Related Adverse Events (≥ 5%) in the Add-Back Clinical Studies (3.75 mg [Monthly] Depot Suspension)

	Controlled study				Open-label study	
	LD-only[a] (n = 51)		LD/N[b] (n = 55)		LD/N[b] (n = 136)	
Adverse events	n	(%)	n	(%)	n	(%)
Neuromuscular disorder	1	(2%)	5	(9%)	4	(3%)
Dermatologic						
Alopecia	0	(0%)	5	(9%)	4	(3%)
Androgen-like effects	2	(4%)	3	(5%)	24	(18%)
Skin/mucous membrane reaction	2	(4%)	5	(9%)	15	(11%)
GI						
Altered bowel function	7	(14%)	8	(15%)	14	(10%)
Changes in appetite	2	(4%)	0	(0%)	8	(6%)
GI disturbance	2	(4%)	4	(7%)	6	(4%)
Nausea/vomiting	13	(25%)	16	(29%)	17	(13%)
GU						
Breast changes/pain/tenderness	3	(6%)	7	(13%)	11	(8%)
Menstrual disorders	1	(2%)	0	(0%)	7	(5%)
Vaginitis	10	(20%)	8	(15%)	11	(8%)
Metabolic/Nutritional						
Edema	0	(0%)	5	(9%)	9	(7%)
Weight changes	6	(12%)	7	(13%)	6	(4%)
Miscellaneous						
Asthenia	9	(18%)	10	(18%)	15	(11%)
Headache/migraine	33	(65%)	28	(51%)	63	(46%)
Injection site reaction	1	(2%)	5	(9%)	4	(3%)
Pain	12	(24%)	16	(29%)	29	(21%)

[a] LD-only = leuprolide 3.75 mg (monthly) depot suspension.
[b] LD/N = leuprolide 3.75 mg plus norethindrone acetate 5 mg.

In the controlled clinical trial, 50 of 51 (98%) patients in the LD group and 48 of 55 (87%) patients in the LD/N group reported experiencing hot flashes on 1 or more occasions during treatment. During month 6 of treatment, 32 of 37 (86%) patients in the LD group and 22 of 38 (58%) patients in the LD/N group reported having experienced hot flashes. The mean number of days on which hot flashes were reported during this month of treatment was 19 and 7 in the LD and LD/N treatment groups, respectively. The mean maximum number of hot flashes in a day during this month of treatment was 5.8 and 1.9 in the LD and LD/N treatment groups, respectively.

➤*Uterine leiomyomata (fibroids) (3.75 mg [monthly] depot suspension):*

Leuprolide Adverse Reactions Observed in Patients and Thought to be Potentially Related to Drug (> 5%) in Uterine Leiomyomata

	Leuprolide 3.75 mg monthly depot suspension		Placebo	
Adverse reactions	(n = 166)	(%)	(n = 163)	(%)
Cardiovascular				
Hot flashes/sweats[a]	121	(72.9%)	29	(17.8%)
CNS				
Depression/emotional lability[a]	18	(10.8%)	7	(4.3%)
GU				
Vaginitis[a]	19	(11.4%)	3	(1.8%)
Metabolic/Nutritional				
Edema	9	(5.4%)	2	(1.2%)
Musculoskeletal				
Joint disorder[a]	13	(7.8%)	5	(3.1%)
Miscellaneous				
Asthenia	14	(8.4%)	8	(4.9%)
General pain	14	(8.4%)	10	(6.1%)
Headache[a]	43	(25.9%)	29	(17.8%)

[a] Possible effect of decreased estrogen.

Symptoms reported in less than 5% of patients included:

Cardiovascular – Tachycardia.

CNS – Anxiety, decreased libido (possible effect of decreased estrogen), dizziness, insomnia, nervousness (possible effect of decreased estrogen), neuromuscular disorders (possible effect of decreased estrogen), paresthesias.

Dermatologic – Androgen-like effects, nail disorder, skin reactions.

GI – Appetite changes, dry mouth, GI disturbances, nausea/vomiting.

GU – Breast changes (possible effect of decreased estrogen), menstrual disorders.

Metabolic/Nutritional – Weight changes.

Musculoskeletal – Myalgia.

Respiratory – Rhinitis.

Special senses – Conjunctivitis, taste perversion.

Miscellaneous – Body odor, flu syndrome, injection-site reactions.

In 1 controlled clinical trial, patients received a higher dose (7.5 mg) of leuprolide for depot suspension. Events seen with this dose that were thought to be potentially related to drug and were not seen at the lower dose included palpitations, syncope, glossitis, ecchymosis, hypesthesia, confusion, lactation, pyelonephritis, and urinary disorders. Generally, a higher incidence of hypoestrogenic effects was observed at the higher dose.

Changes in bone density (3.75 mg [monthly] and 11.25 mg [3-month] depot suspensions) – In controlled clinical studies, patients with endometriosis (6 months of therapy) or uterine fibroids (3 months of therapy) were treated with leuprolide 3.75 mg monthly depot suspension. In endometriosis patients, vertebral bone density as measured by dual energy x-ray absorptiometry (DEXA) decreased by an average of 3.2% at 6 months compared with the pretreatment value. Clinical studies demonstrate that concurrent hormonal therapy (norethindrone acetate 5 mg daily) and calcium supplementation is effective in significantly reducing the loss of bone mineral density that occurs with leuprolide treatment, without compromising the efficacy of leuprolide in relieving symptoms of endometriosis.

Leuprolide 3.75 mg (monthly) depot suspension plus norethindrone acetate 5 mg daily was evaluated in 2 clinical trials. The results from this regimen were similar in both studies. Leuprolide 3.75 mg (monthly) depot suspension was used as a control group in 1 study. The bone mineral density data of the lumbar spine from these 2 studies are presented in the following table:

Leuprolide Mean Percent Change from Baseline in Bone Mineral Density of Lumbar Spine

	Leuprolide 3.75 mg monthly depot suspension		Leuprolide 3.75 mg monthly depot suspension plus norethindrone acetate 5 mg daily			
	Controlled study		Controlled study		Open-label study	
	n	Change	n	Change	n	Change
Week 24[a]	41	−3.2%	42	−0.3%	115	−0.2%
Week 52[b]	29	−6.3%	32	−1%	84	−1.1%

[a] Includes on-treatment measurements that fell within 2 to 252 days after the first day of treatment.
[b] Includes on-treatment measurements greater than 252 days after the first days of treatment.

In the phase IV 6-month pharmacokinetic/pharmacodynamic study in endometriosis patients who were treated with leuprolide 3.75 mg (monthly) depot suspension or leuprolide 11.25 mg (3-month) depot suspension, vertebral bone density measured by DEXA decreased compared with baseline by an average of 3% and 2.8% at 6 months for the 2 groups, respectively.

When leuprolide 3.75 mg (monthly) depot suspension was administered for 3 months in uterine fibroid patients, vertebral trabecular bone mineral density as assessed by quantitative digital radiography (QDR) revealed a mean decrease of 2.7% compared with baseline. Six months after discontinuation of therapy, a trend toward recovery was observed. Use of leuprolide 3.75 mg (monthly) depot suspension for longer than 3 months (uterine fibroids) or 6 months (endometriosis) or in the presence of other known risk factors for decreased bone mineral content may cause additional bone loss and is not recommended.

➤*Endometriosis and uterine leiomyomata, fibroids (changes in laboratory values during treatment, 3.75 mg [monthly] depot suspension):*

Plasma enzymes –

Endometriosis: During early clinical trials with leuprolide 3.75 mg monthly depot suspension for endometriosis, regular laboratory monitoring revealed that AST levels were more than twice the upper limit of normal in only 1 patient. There was no clinical or other laboratory evidence of abnormal liver function.

In 2 other clinical trials, 6 of 191 patients receiving leuprolide 3.75 mg (monthly) depot suspension plus norethindrone acetate 5 mg daily for up to 12 months developed an elevated (at least twice the upper limit of normal) ALT or gamma-glutamyl-transferase (GGT). Five of the 6 increases were observed beyond 6 months of treatment. None was associated with elevated bilirubin concentration.

Uterine leiomyomata (fibroids): In clinical trials with leuprolide 3.75 mg (monthly) depot suspension for uterine leiomyomata, five (3%) patients had a post-treatment transaminase value that was at least twice the baseline value and above the upper limit of the normal range. None of the laboratory increases was associated with clinical symptoms.

LEUPROLIDE ACETATE — INJECTION

➤*Endometriosis and uterine leiomyomata, fibroids (3.75 mg [monthly] depot suspension):*

Lipids –

Endometriosis: Triglycerides were increased above the upper limit of normal in 12% of the endometriosis patients who received leuprolide 3.75 mg (monthly) depot suspension and in 32% of the subjects receiving leuprolide 11.25 mg (3-month) depot suspension.

Of those endometriosis and uterine fibroid patients whose pretreatment cholesterol values were in the normal range, mean change following therapy was +16 mg/dL to +17 mg/dL in endometriosis patients and +11 mg/dL to +29 mg/dL in uterine fibroid patients. In the endometriosis-treated patients, increases from the pretreatment values were statistically significant (P less than 0.03). There was essentially no increase in the LDL/HDL ratio in patients from either population receiving leuprolide 3.75 mg (monthly) depot suspension.

In 2 other clinical trials, leuprolide 3.75 mg (monthly) depot suspension plus norethindrone acetate 5 mg daily were evaluated for 12 months of treatment. Leuprolide 3.75 mg (monthly) depot suspension was used as a control group in 1 study. Percent changes from baseline for serum lipids and percentages of patients with serum lipid values outside of the normal range in the 2 studies are summarized in the following tables:

Serum Lipids: Leuprolide Mean Percent Changes from Baseline Values at Treatment Week 24

Lipids	Leuprolide		Leuprolide plus norethindrone acetate 5 mg daily			
	Baseline value[a]	Week 24 (% change)	Baseline value[a]	Week 24 (% change)	Baseline value[a]	Week 24 (% change)
Total cholesterol	170.5	9.2%	179.3	0.2%	181.2	2.8%
HDL cholesterol	52.4	7.4%	51.8	−18.8%	51	−14.6%
LDL cholesterol	96.6	10.9%	101.5	14.1%	109.1	13.1%
LDL/HDL ratio	2[b]	5%	2.1[b]	43.4%	2.3[b]	39.4%
Triglycerides	107.8	17.5%	130.2	9.5%	105.4	13.8%

[a] mg/dL.
[b] ratio.

Changes from baseline tended to be greater at week 52. After treatment, mean serum lipid levels from patients with follow-up data returned to pretreatment values.

Percentage of Leuprolide-Treated Patients with Serum Lipid Values Outside of the Normal Range

Lipids	Leuprolide Controlled study (n = 39) Week 0	Week 24[a]	Leuprolide plus norethindrone acetate 5 mg daily Controlled study (n = 41) Week 0	Week 24[a]	Open-label study (n = 117) Week 0	Week 24[a]
Total cholesterol (> 240 mg/dL)	15%	23%	15%	20%	6%	7%
HDL cholesterol (< 40 mg/dL)	15%	10%	15%	44%	15%	41%
LDL cholesterol (> 160 mg/dL)	0%	8%	5%	7%	9%	11%
LDL/HDL ratio (> 4)	0%	3%	2%	15%	7%	21%
Triglycerides (> 200 mg/dL)	13%	13%	12%	10%	5%	9%

[a] Includes all patients regardless of baseline value.

Low HDL cholesterol (less than 40 mg/dL) and elevated LDL cholesterol (greater than 160 mg/dL) are recognized risk factors for cardiovascular disease. The long-term significance of the observed treatment-related changes in serum lipids in women with endometriosis is unknown. Therefore, consider assessment of cardiovascular risk factors prior to initiation of concurrent treatment with leuprolide 3.75 mg (monthly) depot suspension and norethindrone acetate.

• *Chemistry* – Slight-to-moderate mean increases were noted for glucose, uric acid, blood urea nitrogen, creatinine, total protein, albumin, bilirubin, alkaline phosphatase, LDH, calcium, and phosphorus. None of these increases were clinically significant. In the hormonal add-back studies, leuprolide 11.25 mg (3-month) depot suspension in combination with norethindrone acetate was associated with elevations of GGT and ALT in 6% to 7% of patients.

Uterine leiomyomata (fibroids): In patients receiving leuprolide 3.75 mg monthly depot suspension, mean changes in cholesterol (+11 mg/dL to +29 mg/dL), LDL cholesterol (+8 mg/dL to +22 mg/dL), HDL cholesterol (0 to +6 mg/dL), and the LDL/HDL ratio (−0.1 to +0.5) were observed across studies. In the 1 study in which triglycerides were determined, the mean increase from baseline was 32 mg/dL.

➤*Endometriosis and uterine leiomyomata (fibroids) (3.75 mg [monthly] depot suspension):*

Other changes –

Endometriosis: The following changes were seen in approximately 5% to 8% of patients. In the earlier comparative studies, leuprolide 3.75 mg (monthly) depot suspension was associated with elevations of LDH and phosphorus, and decreases in WBC counts. Danazol therapy was associated with increases in hematocrit, platelet count, and LDH. In the hormonal add-back studies leuprolide 3.75 mg (monthly) depot suspension in combination with norethindrone acetate was associated with elevations of GGT and ALT.

Uterine leiomyomata (fibroids):

• *Hematology* – In leuprolide 3.75 mg (monthly) depot suspension-treated patients, although there were statistically significant mean decreases in platelet counts from baseline to final visit, the last mean platelet counts were within the normal range. Decreases in total WBC count and neutrophils were observed, but were not clinically significant.

• *Chemistry* – Slight to moderate mean increases were noted for glucose, uric acid, blood urea nitrogen, creatinine, total protein, albumin, bilirubin,alkaline phosphatase, LDH, calcium, and phosphorus. None of these increases were clinically significant.

➤*Endometriosis and uterine leiomyomata (postmarketing, 3.75 mg [monthly] and 11.25 mg [3-month] depot suspensions):* During postmarketing surveillance, the following adverse events were reported. Like other drugs in this class, mood swings, including depression, have been reported as a physiologic effect of decreased sex steroids. There have been rare reports of suicidal ideation and attempt. Many, but not all, of these patients had histories of depression or other psychiatric illness. Counsel patients on the possibility of development or worsening of depression during treatment with leuprolide.

Symptoms consistent with an anaphylactoid or asthmatic process have been rarely reported. Rash, urticaria, and photosensitivity reactions have also been reported.

Localized reactions, including induration and abscess, have been reported at the site of injection.

Symptoms consistent with fibromyalgia (eg, joint and muscle pain, headaches, sleep disorder, GI distress, and shortness of breath) have been reported individually and collectively. Other events reported are as follows:

Cardiovascular – Hypotension, pulmonary embolism.

CNS – Peripheral neuropathy, spinal fracture/paralysis.

GU – Prostate pain.

Hematologic/Lymphatic – Decreased white blood cells.

Musculoskeletal – Tenosynovitis-like symptoms.

➤*Endometriosis and uterine fibroids (11.25 mg [3-month] depot suspension):* The monthly formulation of leuprolide 3.75 mg depot suspension was utilized in controlled clinical trials that studied the drug in 166 endometriosis and 166 uterine fibroids patients. Adverse events reported in greater than or equal to 5% of patients in either of these populations and thought to be potentially related to the drug are noted in the following table.

Leuprolide Adverse Reactions Reported to be Causally Related to Drug (≥ 5%) inEndometriosis and Uterine Fibroids

	Endometriosis (2 studies)						Uterine fibroids (4 studies)			
	Leuprolide 3.75 mg depot suspension (n = 166)		Danazol (n = 136)		Placebo (n = 31)		Leuprolide 3.75 mg depot suspension (n = 166)		Placebo (n = 163)	
Adverse reaction	n	(%)	n	(%)	n	(%)	n	(%)	n	(%)
Cardiovascular										
Hot flashes/sweats[a]	139	(84%)	77	(57%)	9	(29%)	121	(72.9%)	29	(17.8%)

LEUPROLIDE ACETATE — INJECTION

Leuprolide Adverse Reactions Reported to be Causally Related to Drug (≥ 5%) in Endometriosis and Uterine Fibroids

	Endometriosis (2 studies)						Uterine fibroids (4 studies)			
	Leuprolide 3.75 mg depot suspension (n = 166)		Danazol (n = 136)		Placebo (n = 31)		Leuprolide 3.75 mg depot suspension (n = 166)		Placebo (n = 163)	
Adverse reaction	n	(%)	n	(%)	n	(%)	n	(%)	n	(%)
CNS										
Decreased libido[a]	19	(11%)	6	(4%)	0	(0%)	3	(1.8%)	0	(0%)
Depression/emotional lability[a]	36	(22%)	27	(20%)	1	(3%)	18	(10.8%)	7	(4.3%)
Dizziness	19	(11%)	4	(3%)	0	(0%)	3	(1.8%)	6	(3.7%)
Nervousness[a]	8	(5%)	11	(8%)	0	(0%)	8	(4.8%)	1	(0.6%)
Neuromuscular disorders[a]	11	(7%)	17	(13%)	0	(0%)	3	(1.8%)	0	(0%)
Paresthesias	12	(7%)	11	(8%)	0	(0%)	2	(1.2%)	1	(0.6%)
Dermatologic										
Skin reactions	17	(10%)	20	(15%)	1	(3%)	5	(3%)	2	(1.2%)
Endocrine										
Acne	17	(10%)	27	(20%)	0	(0%)	0	(0%)	0	(0%)
Hirsutism	2	(1%)	9	(7%)	1	(3%)	1	(0.6%)	0	(0%)
GI										
Nausea/vomiting	21	(13%)	17	(13%)	1	(3%)	8	(4.8%)	6	(3.7%)
GI disturbances[a]	11	(7%)	8	(6%)	1	(3%)	5	(3%)	2	(1.2%)
GU										
Breast changes/tenderness/pain[a]	10	(6%)	12	(9%)	0	(0%)	3	(1.8%)	7	(4.3%)
Vaginitis[a]	46	(28%)	23	(17%)	0	(0%)	19	(11.4%)	3	(1.8%)
Metabolic/Nutritional										
Edema	12	(7%)	17	(13%)	1	(3%)	9	(5.4%)	2	(1.2%)
Weight gain/loss	22	(13%)	36	(26%)	0	(0%)	5	(3%)	2	(1.2%)
Musculoskeletal										
Joint disorder[a]	14	(8%)	11	(8%)	0	(0%)	13	(7.8%)	5	(3.1%)
Myalgia[a]	1	(1%)	7	(5%)	0	(0%)	1	(0.6%)	0	(0%)
Miscellaneous										
Asthenia	5	(3%)	9	(7%)	0	(0%)	14	(8.4%)	8	(4.9%)
General pain	31	(19%)	22	(16%)	1	(3%)	14	(8.4%)	10	(6.1%)
Headache[a]	53	(32%)	30	(22%)	2	(6%)	43	(25.9%)	29	(17.8%)

[a] Physiologic effect of the drug.

In these same studies, symptoms reported in less than 5% of patients included:

Cardiovascular – Palpitations, syncope, tachycardia.

CNS – Anxiety (physiologic effect of the drug), delusions, insomnia/sleep disorders (physiologic effect of the drug), memory disorder, personality disorder.

Dermatologic – Alopecia, hair disorder, nail disorder.

Endocrine – Androgen-like effects.

GI – Appetite changes, dry mouth, thirst.

GU – Dysuria (physiologic effect of the drug), lactation, menstrual disorders.

Hematologic / Lymphatic – Ecchymosis, lymphadenopathy.

Respiratory – Rhinitis.

Special senses – Conjunctivitis, ophthalmologic disorders (physiologic effect of the drug), taste perversion.

Miscellaneous – Body odor, flu syndrome, injection site reactions. In 1 controlled clinical trial utilizing the monthly formulation of leuprolide for depot suspension, patients diagnosed with uterine fibroids received a higher dose (7.5 mg) of leuprolide for depot suspension. Events seen with this dose that were thought to be potentially related to drug and were not seen at the lower dose included glossitis, hypesthesia, lactation, pyelonephritis, and urinary disorders. Generally, a higher incidence of hypoestrogenic effects was observed at the higher dose.

In a pharmacokinetic trial involving 20 healthy female subjects receiving leuprolide 11.25 mg (3-month) depot suspension a few adverse events were reported with this formulation that were not reported previously. These included face edema, agitation, laryngitis, and ear pain.

The following table lists the potentially drug-related adverse events observed in at least 5% of patients in any treatment group, during the first 6 months of treatment in the add-back clinical studies, in which patients were treated with monthly leuprolide 3.75 mg (monthly) depot suspension with or without norethindrone acetate cotreatment.

Leuprolide Treatment-Related Adverse Events (≥ 5%) in the Add-Back Clinical Studies (3.75 mg [Monthly] Depot Suspension)

	Controlled study		Open-label study
Adverse events	Leuprolide 3.75 mg monthly depot suspension[a] (n = 51)	Leuprolide 3.75 mg monthly depot suspension/ norethindrone acetate[b] (n = 55)	Leuprolide 3.75 mg monthly depot suspension[b]/ norethindrone acetate (n = 136)
Any adverse event	50 (98%)	53 (96%)	126 (93%)
Cardiovascular			
Hot flashes/sweats	50 (98%)	48 (87%)	78 (57%)
CNS			
Anxiety	3 (6%)	0 (0%)	11 (8%)
Depression/emotional lability	16 (31%)	15 (27%)	46 (34%)
Dizziness/vertigo	8 (16%)	6 (11%)	10 (7%)
Insomnia/sleep disorder	16 (31%)	7 (13%)	20 (15%)
Libido changes	5 (10%)	2 (4%)	10 (7%)
Memory disorder	3 (6%)	1 (2%)	6 (4%)
Nervousness	4 (8%)	2 (4%)	15 (11%)
Neuromuscular disorder	1 (2%)	5 (9%)	4 (3%)
Dermatologic			
Alopecia	0 (0%)	5 (9%)	4 (3%)

LEUPROLIDE ACETATE — INJECTION

Leuprolide Treatment-Related Adverse Events (≥ 5%) in the Add-Back Clinical Studies (3.75 mg [Monthly] Depot Suspension)			
	Controlled study		Open-label study
Adverse events	Leuprolide 3.75 mg monthly depot suspension[a] (n = 51)	Leuprolide 3.75 mg monthly depot suspension/ norethindrone acetate[b] (n = 55)	Leuprolide 3.75 mg monthly depot suspension[b]/ norethindrone acetate (n = 136)
Androgen-like effects	2 (4%)	3 (5%)	24 (18%)
Skin/mucous membrane reaction	2 (4%)	5 (9%)	15 (11%)
GI			
Altered bowel function	7 (14%)	8 (15%)	14 (10%)
Changes in appetite	2 (4%)	0 (0%)	8 (6%)
GI disturbance	2 (4%)	4 (7%)	6 (4%)
Nausea/vomiting	13 (25%)	16 (29%)	17 (13%)
GU			
Breast changes/ pain/tenderness	3 (6%)	7 (13%)	11 (8%)
Menstrual disorders	1 (2%)	0 (0%)	7 (5%)
Vaginitis	10 (20%)	8 (15%)	11 (8%)
Metabolic/Nutritional			
Edema	0 (0%)	5 (9%)	9 (7%)
Weight changes	6 (12%)	7 (13%)	6 (4%)
Miscellaneous			
Asthenia	9 (18%)	10 (18%)	15 (11%)
Headache/migraine	33 (65%)	28 (51%)	63 (46%)
Injection-site reaction	1 (2%)	5 (9%)	4 (3%)
Pain	12 (24%)	16 (29%)	29 (21%)

[a] Leuprolide acetate 3.75 mg (monthly) depot suspension.
[b] Leuprolide acetate/norethindrone acetate 3.75 mg (monthly) depot suspension plus norethindrone acetate 5 mg.

In the controlled clinical trial, 50 of 51 (98%) patients in the leuprolide 3.75 mg monthly depot suspension and 48 of 55 (87%) patients in the leuprolide 3.75 mg (monthly) depot suspension plus norethindrone acetate 5 mg daily reported experiencing hot flashes on 1 or more occasions during treatment. During month 6 of treatment, 32 of 37 (86%) patients in the leuprolide depot suspension group and 22 of 38 (58%) patients in the leuprolide 3.75 mg (monthly) depot suspension plus norethindrone acetate group reported having experienced hot flashes. The mean number of days on which hot flashes were reported during this month of treatment was 19 and 7 in the leuprolide depot suspension group and the leuprolide depot suspension plus norethindrone acetate treatment groups, respectively. The mean maximum number of hot flashes in a day during this month of treatment was 5.8 and 1.9 in the leuprolide depot suspension group and the leuprolide depot suspension plus norethindrone acetate treatment groups, respectively.

➤*Endometriosis and uterine leiomyomata (changes in laboratory values during treatment, 11.25 mg [3-month] depot suspension):*

Liver enzymes – Three percent of uterine fibroid patients treated with 3.75 mg monthly depot suspension manifested posttreatment transaminase values that were at least twice the baseline value and above the upper limit of normal range. None of the laboratory increases was associated with clinical symptoms.

Lipids – Triglycerides were increased above the upper limit of normal in 12% of the endometriosis patients who received leuprolide 3.75 mg (monthly) depot suspension and in 32% of the subjects receiving leuprolide 11.25 mg (3-month) depot suspension.

Of those endometriosis and uterine fibroid patients whose pretreatment cholesterol values were in the normal range, mean change following therapy was + 16 mg/dL to + 17 mg/dL in endometriosis patients and +11 mg/dL to +29 mg/dL in uterine fibroid patients. In the endometriosis-treated patients, increases from the pretreatment values were statistically significant (*P* less than 0.03). There was essentially no increase in the LDL/HDL ratio in patients from either population receiving leuprolide 3.75 mg (monthly) suspension.

Overdosage

In rats, subcutaneous administration of 125 to 500 times the recommended human pediatric dose, expressed on a per body weight basis, resulted in dyspnea, decreased activity, and local irritation at the injection site. There is no evidence at present that there is a clinical counterpart of this phenomenon.

In early clinical trials using daily subcutaneous leuprolide in adult patients, doses as high as 20 mg/day for up to 2 years caused no adverse effects differing from those observed with the 1 mg/day dose.

GOSERELIN ACETATE

Rx	**Zoladex** (AstraZeneca)	**Implant:** 3.6 mg	In preloaded syringes (16-gauge needle).
		10.8 mg	In preloaded syringes (14-gauge needle).

GOSERELIN ACETATE — SUBCUTANEOUS

Indications

➤*Advanced breast cancer (3.6 mg only):* For use in the palliative treatment of advanced breast cancer in pre- and postmenopausal women.

The estrogen and progesterone receptor values may help to predict whether goserelin therapy is likely to be beneficial.

➤*Endometrial thinning (3.6 mg only):* For use as an endometrial-thinning agent prior to endometrial ablation for dysfunctional uterine bleeding.

➤*Endometriosis (3.6 mg only):* For the management of endometriosis, including pain relief and reduction of endometriotic lesions for the duration of therapy. Experience with goserelin for the management of endometriosis has been limited to women 18 years of age and older treated for 6 months.

➤*Prostatic carcinoma:* In the palliative treatment of advanced carcinoma of the prostate.

➤*Stage B2 to C prostatic carcinoma:* For use in combination with flutamide for the management of locally confined stage T2b to T4 (stage B2-C) carcinoma of the prostate. Treatment with goserelin and flutamide should start 8 weeks prior to initiating radiation therapy and continue during radiation therapy.

Administration and Dosage

➤*General dosing considerations:* The 10.8 mg goserelin implant is not indicated in women because the data are insufficient to support reliable suppression of serum estradiol. For women requiring treatment with goserelin, refer to the use of the goserelin 3.6 mg implant in the following information.

➤*Adults:*

Advanced breast cancer –

Usual dosage: 3.6 mg administered subcutaneously every 28 days. While the delay of a few days is permissible, make every effort to adhere to the 28-day schedule.

Duration of therapy: For long-term administration unless clinically inappropriate.

Endometrial thinning – 1 or 2 depot injections of goserelin 3.6 mg administered subcutaneously. If 2 depot injections are to be given, administer them 4 weeks apart. For use prior to endometrial ablation. When 1 depot is administered, perform surgery at 4 weeks. When 2 depots are administered, perform surgery within 2 to 4 weeks following administration of the second depot.

Endometriosis –

Usual dosage: 3.6 mg administered subcutaneously every 28 days. While the delay of a few days is permissible, make every effort to adhere to the 28-day schedule.

Duration of therapy: 6 months.

Re-treatment: Re-treatment cannot be recommended for the management of endometriosis because safety data for re-treatment are not available. If the symptoms of endometriosis recur after a course of therapy and further treatment with goserelin is contemplated, consider monitoring bone mineral density. Clinical studies suggest the addition of hormone replacement therapy (estrogens and/or progestins) to goserelin is effective in reducing the bone mineral loss that occurs with goserelin alone without compromising the efficacy of goserelin in relieving the symptoms of endometriosis. The addition of hormone replacement therapy also may reduce the occurrence of vasomotor symptoms and vaginal dryness associated with hypoestrogenism. The optimal drugs, dose, and duration of treatment have not been established.

Prostatic carcinoma –

Usual dosage: 3.6 mg administered subcutaneously every 28 days or one 10.8 mg implant administered subcutaneously every 12 weeks.

Duration of therapy: For long-term administration, unless clinically inappropriate.

Stage B2 to C prostatic carcinoma: When goserelin is given in combination with radiotherapy and flutamide for patients with stage T2b to T4 (stage B2 to C) prostatic carcinoma, start treatment 8 weeks prior to initiating radio-

GOSERELIN ACETATE — SUBCUTANEOUS

therapy and continue during radiation therapy. Administer a treatment regimen using one goserelin 3.6 mg depot 8 weeks before radiotherapy, followed in 28 days by one goserelin 10.8 mg depot. Alternatively, 4 injections of 3.6 mg depot can be administered at 28-day intervals (2 depots preceding and 2 during radiotherapy).

➤*Renal function impairment:*

Dialysis – Conventional hemodialysis is moderately effective (50% to 74%) in removing goserelin.

➤*Administration:*

Monthly (3.6 mg) implant – Administer goserelin 3.6 mg implant subcutaneously every 28 days into the anterior abdominal wall below the navel line using an aseptic technique. While the delay of a few days is permissible, make every effort to adhere to the 28-day schedule.

3-Month (10.8 mg) implant – Administer goserelin 10.8 mg implant subcutaneously every 12 weeks into the upper abdominal wall using an aseptic technique. While a delay of a few days is permissible, make every effort to adhere to the 12-week schedule.

Removal of implant – In the unlikely event of the need to surgically remove goserelin, it may be localized by ultrasound.

➤*Storage/Stability:* The unit is sterile and comes in a sealed, light- and moisture-proof, aluminum foil laminate pouch containing a desiccant capsule. Store at room temperature (do not exceed 25°C; 77°F).

Actions

➤*Pharmacology:* Goserelin is a synthetic decapeptide analogue of LHRH. Goserelin acts as a potent inhibitor of pituitary gonadotropin secretion when administered in the biodegradable formulation.

Following initial administration in males, goserelin causes an initial increase in serum-luteinizing hormone (LH) and follicle-stimulating hormone (FSH) levels with subsequent increases in serum levels of testosterone. Chronic administration of goserelin leads to sustained suppression of pituitary gonadotropins, and serum levels of testosterone consequently fall into the range normally seen in surgically castrated men approximately 2 to 4 weeks after initiation of therapy. This leads to accessory sex organ regression.

In animal and in vitro studies, administration of goserelin resulted in the regression or inhibition of growth of the hormonally sensitive dimethylbenzanthracene (DMBA)-induced rat mammary tumor and Dunning R3327 prostate tumor.

In clinical trials using 3.6 mg goserelin with follow-up of more than 2 years, suppression of serum testosterone to castrate levels has been maintained for the duration of therapy.

In women, a similar down-regulation of the pituitary gland by chronic exposure to goserelin leads to suppression of gonadotropin secretion, a decrease in serum estradiol to levels consistent with the postmenopausal state, and would be expected to lead to a reduction of ovarian size and function, reduction in the size of the uterus and mammary gland, as well as a regression of sex hormone-responsive tumors, if present. Serum estradiol is suppressed to levels similar to those observed in postmenopausal women within 3 weeks following initial administration; however, after suppression was attained, isolated elevations of estradiol were seen in 10% of the patients enrolled in clinical trials. Serum LH and FSH are suppressed to follicular phase levels within 4 weeks after initial administration of drug and are usually maintained at that range with continued use of goserelin. In 5% or less of women treated with goserelin, FSH and LH levels may not be suppressed to follicular phase levels on day 28 post treatment with use of a single 3.6 mg depot injection. In certain individuals, suppression of any of these hormones to such levels may not be achieved with goserelin. Estradiol, LH, and FSH levels return to pretreatment values within 12 weeks following the last implant administration in all but rare cases.

➤*Pharmacokinetics:*

Absorption –

3.6 mg: The absorption of radiolabeled drug was rapid, and the peak blood radioactivity levels occurred between 0.5 and 1 hour after dosing. The mean (± standard deviation) pharmacokinetic parameter estimates of goserelin after administration of 3.6 mg depot for 2 months in males (n = 7) and females (n = 7) are presented in the following table.

Goserelin Pharmacokinetic Parameters for the 3.6 mg Depot

Parameters (units)	Men (n = 7)	Women (n = 7)
Peak plasma concentration (ng/mL)	2.84 ± 1.81	1.46 ± 0.82
Time to peak concentration (days)	12 to 15	8 to 22
AUC (0 to 28 days) (ng•hr/mL)	27.8 ± 15.3	18.5 ± 10.3
Systemic clearance (mL/min)	110.5 ± 47.5	163.9 ± 71
Apparent volume of distribution (L)[a]	44.1 ± 13.6	20.3 ± 4.1
Elimination half-life (h)[a]	4.2 ± 1.1	2.3 ± 0.6

[a] The apparent volume of distribution and the elimination half-life were determined after subcutaneous administration of 250 mcg aqueous solution of goserelin.

Goserelin is released from the depot at a much slower rate initially for the first 8 days, and then there is more rapid and continuous release for the remainder of the 28-day dosing period. Despite the change in the releasing rate of goserelin, administration of goserelin every 28 days resulted in testosterone levels that were suppressed to and maintained in the range normally seen in surgically castrated men.

10.8 mg: The pharmacokinetics of goserelin have been determined in healthy male volunteers and patients. In healthy males, radiolabeled goserelin was administered as a single 250 mcg (aqueous solution) dose by the subcutaneous route. The absorption of radiolabeled drug was rapid, and the peak blood radioactivity levels occurred between 0.5 and 1 hour after dosing.

The overall pharmacokinetic profile of goserelin following administration of a 10.8 mg goserelin depot to patients with prostate cancer was determined. The initial release of goserelin from the depot was relatively rapid resulting in a peak concentration at 2 hours after dosing. From day 4 until the end of the 12-week dosing interval, the sustained release of goserelin from the depot produced reasonably stable systemic exposure. Mean (standard deviation) pharmacokinetic data are presented below. There is no clinically significant accumulation of goserelin following administration of 4 depots administered at 12-week intervals. Pharmacokinetic data were obtained using an RIA method, which has been shown to be specific for goserelin in the presence of its metabolites.

Goserelin Pharmacokinetic Parameters for the 10.8 mg Depot

Parameter	n	Mean	(SD)[b]	95% CI[c] Lower	95% CI[c] Upper
Systemic clearance (mL/min)	41	121	(42.4)	108	134
C_{max} (ng/mL)	41	8.85	(2.83)	7.96	9.74
T_{max} (hr)	41	1.8	(0.34)	1.7	1.92
C_{min} (ng/mL)	44	0.37	(0.21)	0.3	0.43
Elimination half-life (hr)[a]	7	4.16	(1.12)	3.12	5.2

[a] Determined after subcutaneous administration of 250 mcg aqueous solution of goserelin.
[b] Standard deviation.
[c] 95% confidence interval.

Serum goserelin concentrations in prostate cancer patients administered three 3.6 mg depots followed by one 10.8 mg depot are displayed below. The profiles for both formulations are primarily dependent upon the rate of drug release from the depots. For the 3.6 mg depot, mean concentrations gradually rise to reach a peak of about 3 ng/mL at around 15 days after administration and then decline to approximately 0.5 ng/mL by the end of the treatment period. For the 10.8 mg depot, mean concentrations increase to reach a peak of about 8 ng/mL within the first 24 hours and then decline rapidly up to day 4. Thereafter, mean concentrations remain relatively stable in the range of about 0.3 to 1 ng/mL up to the end of the treatment period.

Administration of four 10.8 mg goserelin depots to patients with prostate cancer resulted in testosterone levels that were suppressed to and maintained within the range normally observed in surgically castrated men (0 to 1.73 nmol/L or 0 to 50 ng/dL), over the dosing interval in approximately 91% (145 out of 160) of patients studied. In 6 of 15 patients that escaped from castrate range, serum testosterone levels were maintained below 2 nmol/L (58 ng/dL), and in only 1 of the 15 patients did the depot completely fail to maintain serum testosterone levels to within the castrate range over a 336-day period (4 depot injections). In the 8 additional patients, a transient escape was followed 14 days later by a level within the castrate range.

Distribution –

3.6 mg: The apparent volumes of distribution determined after subcutaneous administration of 250 mcg aqueous solution of goserelin were 44.1 and 20.3 L for males and females, respectively. The plasma protein binding of goserelin obtained from one sample was found to be 27.3%.

10.8 mg: The apparent volume of distribution determined after subcutaneous administration of 250 mcg aqueous solution of goserelin was 44.1 ± 13.6 L for healthy males. The plasma protein binding of goserelin was found to be 27%.

Metabolism – Metabolism of goserelin, by hydrolysis of the C-terminal amino acids, is the major clearance mechanism. The major circulating component in serum appeared to be 1 to 7 fragment, and the major component present in urine of 1 healthy male volunteer was 5 to 10 fragment. The metabolism of goserelin in humans yields a similar but narrow profile of metabolites to that found in other species. All metabolites found in humans also have been found in toxicology species.

Excretion – Clearance of goserelin following subcutaneous administration of a radiolabeled solution of goserelin was very rapid and occurred via a combination of hepatic and urinary excretion. More than 90% of a subcutaneous radiolabeled solution formulation dose of goserelin was excreted in urine. Approximately 20% of the dose recovered in urine was accounted for by unchanged goserelin.

Special populations –

Weight: A decline of approximately 1% to 2.5% in the AUC after administration of a 10.8 mg depot was observed with a kg increase in body weight. In obese patients who have not responded clinically, closely monitor testosterone levels.

GOSERELIN ACETATE — SUBCUTANEOUS

Contraindications

Hypersensitivity to LHRH, LHRH agonist analogues, or any of the components in goserelin; women who are breastfeeding; women being treated for endometriosis or endometrial thinning who are or may become pregnant while receiving the drug. Goserelin can cause fetal harm when administered to a pregnant woman. Effects on reproductive function, as a result of antigonadotrophic properties of the drug, are expected to occur on chronic administration.

Effective nonhormonal contraception must be used by all premenopausal women during goserelin therapy and for 12 weeks following discontinuation of therapy. There are no adequate and well-controlled studies in pregnant women using goserelin. If this drug is used during pregnancy, or if the patient being treated for endometriosis or endometrial thinning becomes pregnant while taking this drug, apprise the patient of the potential hazard to the fetus or potential risk for loss of the pregnancy. Advise women of childbearing potential to avoid becoming pregnant.

The 10.8 mg goserelin implant is not indicated in women as the data are insufficient to support reliable suppression of serum estradiol.

Goserelin is contraindicated in women who are or may become pregnant while receiving the drug. In studies in rats and rabbits, goserelin increased preimplantation loss, resorptions, and abortions. In rats and dogs, goserelin suppressed ovarian function, decreased ovarian weight and size, and led to atrophic changes in secondary sex organs. Further evidence suggests that fertility was reduced in female rats that became pregnant after goserelin was stopped. These effects are an expected consequence of the hormonal alterations produced by goserelin in humans. If a patient becomes pregnant during treatment, the drug must be discontinued and the patient must be apprised of the potential risk for loss of the pregnancy because of possible hormonal imbalance as a result of the expected pharmacologic action of goserelin treatment. In animal studies, there was no evidence that goserelin possessed the potential to cause teratogenicity in rabbits; however, in rats the incidence of umbilical hernia was significantly increased with treatment.

Warnings/Precautions

➤*Prostate and breast cancer:* Initially, goserelin, like other LHRH agonists, causes transient increases in serum levels of testosterone in men with prostate cancer, and estrogen in women with breast cancer. Transient worsening of symptoms or the occurrence of additional signs and symptoms of prostate or breast cancer, may occasionally develop during the first few weeks of goserelin treatment. A small number of patients may experience a temporary increase in bone pain, which can be managed symptomatically. As with other LHRH agonists, isolated cases of ureteral obstruction and spinal cord compression have been observed. If spinal cord compression or renal impairment develops, institute standard treatment of these complications. For extreme cases in prostate cancer patients, consider an immediate orchiectomy.

As with other LHRH agonists or hormonal therapies (eg, antiestrogens, estrogens), hypercalcemia has been reported in some prostate and breast cancer patients with bone metastases after starting treatment with goserelin. If hypercalcemia does occur, initiate appropriate treatment measures.

➤*Antibody formation:* Of 115 women worldwide treated with 3.6 mg goserelin and tested for development of binding to goserelin following treatment with goserelin, 1 patient showed low-titer binding to goserelin. On further testing of this patient's plasma obtained following treatment, her goserelin binding component was found not to be precipitated with rabbit antihuman immunoglobulin polyvalent sera. These findings suggest the possibility of antibody formation.

➤*Endometrial ablation:* The pharmacologic action of goserelin on the uterus and cervix may cause an increase in cervical resistance. Therefore, exercise caution when dilating the cervix for endometrial ablation.

➤*Hypersensitivity reactions:* Hypersensitivity, antibody formation and acute anaphylactic reactions have been reported with LHRH agonist analogues.

➤*Pregnancy: Category D* (breast cancer 3.6 mg strength); *Category X* (endometriosis, endometrial thinning 3.6 mg strength; prostatic cancer 10.8 mg strength).

See Contraindications for more information.

There are no adequate and well-controlled studies in pregnant women using goserelin. Advise women of childbearing potential to avoid becoming pregnant.

➤*Lactation:* Goserelin has been shown to be excreted in the milk of lactating rats. It is not known if this drug is excreted in human milk. Because many drugs are excreted in human milk and there is a potential for serious adverse reactions in nursing infants of mothers receiving goserelin, mothers should discontinue nursing prior to taking the drug.

See Contraindications for more information.

➤*Children:* Safety and efficacy have not been established.

Drug Interactions

➤*Drug/Lab test interactions:* Administration of goserelin in therapeutic doses results in suppression of the pituitary-gonadal system. Because of this suppression, diagnostic tests of pituitary-gonadotropic and gonadal functions conducted during treatment and until resumption of menses may show results which are misleading. Normal function is usually restored within 12 weeks after treatment is discontinued.

Adverse Reactions

➤*Hypersensitivity:* Rarely, hypersensitivity reactions (including urticaria and anaphylaxis) have been reported in patients receiving goserelin.

➤*Hypocalcemia:* As with other endocrine therapies, hypercalcemia (increased calcium) has rarely been reported in cancer patients with bone metastases following initiation of treatment with goserelin or other LHRH agonists.

➤*Hypotension/Hypertension:* Changes in blood pressure, manifested as hypotension or hypertension, have been occasionally observed in patients administered goserelin. The changes are usually transient, resolving either during continued therapy or after cessation of therapy with goserelin. Rarely, such changes have been sufficient to require medical intervention including withdrawal of treatment from goserelin.

➤*Pituitary apoplexy:* As with other agents in this class, very rare cases of pituitary apoplexy have been reported following initial administration.

➤*Postmarketing:* There have been postmarketing reports of osteoporosis, decreased bone mineral density, and bony fracture in men treated with goserelin for prostate cancer.

➤*Men - Prostatic carcinoma:* Goserelin has been found to be generally well tolerated in clinical trials. Adverse reactions reported in these trials were rarely severe enough to result in the patients' withdrawal from goserelin treatment. As seen with other hormonal therapies, the most commonly observed adverse reactions during goserelin therapy were caused by the expected physiological effects from decreased testosterone levels. These included hot flashes, sexual dysfunction, and decreased erections.

Initially, goserelin, like other LHRH agonists, causes transient increases in serum levels of testosterone. A small percentage of patients experienced a temporary worsening of signs and symptoms, usually manifested by an increase in cancer-related pain which was managed symptomatically. Isolated cases of exacerbation of disease symptoms, either ureteral obstruction or spinal cord compression, occurred at similar rates in controlled clinical trials with both goserelin and orchiectomy. The relationship of these reactions to therapy is uncertain.

Two controlled clinical trials using 10.8 mg goserelin vs 3.6 mg goserelin were conducted. During a comparative phase, patients were randomized to receive either a single 10.8 mg implant or 3 consecutive 3.6 mg implants every 4 weeks over weeks 0 to 12. During this phase, the only adverse reaction reported in greater than 5% of patients was hot flashes, with an incidence of 47% in the 10.8 mg goserelin group and 48% in the 3.6 mg goserelin group.

From weeks 12 to 48, all patients were treated with a 10.8 mg implant every 12 weeks. During this noncomparative phase, the following adverse reactions were reported in greater than 5% of patients:

Goserelin 10.8 mg Adverse Reactions in Patients with Prostatic Carcinoma (%)

Adverse reaction	Goserelin 10.8 mg (n = 157)
Asthenia	5%
Bone pain	6%
Gynecomastia	8%
Hot flashes	64%
Pain (general)	14%
Pelvic pain	6%

➤*Goserelin vs orchiectomy:*

Adverse Reactions of Goserelin 3.6 mg versus Orchiectomy (%)

Adverse reaction	Goserelin (n = 242)	Orchiectomy (n = 254)
Anorexia	5%	2%
Chronic obstructive pulmonary disease	5%	3%
Complications of surgery	0%	18%[a]
CHF	5%	1%
Decreased erections	18%	16%
Dizziness	5%	4%
Edema	7%	8%
Hot flashes	62%	53%
Insomnia	5%	1%
Lethargy	8%	4%
Lower urinary tract symptoms	13%	8%
Nausea	5%	2%
Pain (worsened in the first 30 days)	8%	3%
Rash	6%	1%
Sexual dysfunction	21%	15%
Sweating	6%	4%
Upper respiratory tract infection	7%	2%

[a] Complications related to surgery were reported in 18% of the orchiectomy patients, while only 3% of goserelin patients reported adverse reactions at the injection site. The surgical complications included scrotal infections (5.9%), groin pain (4.7%), wound seepage (3.1%), scrotal hematoma (2.8%), incisional discomfort (1.6%), and skin necrosis (1.2%).

GOSERELIN ACETATE — SUBCUTANEOUS

➤*The following adverse reactions were reported in greater than 1%, but less than 5% of patients treated with 10.8 mg goserelin implant every 12 weeks. Some of these are commonly reported in elderly patients:*

Cardiovascular – Angina pectoris, cerebral ischemia, cerebrovascular accident, heart failure, pulmonary embolus, varicose veins.

CNS – Dizziness, headache, paresthesia.

Dermatologic – Herpes simplex, pruritus.

Endocrine – Diabetes mellitus.

GI – Abdominal pain, diarrhea, hematemesis.

GU – Bladder neoplasm, breast pain, hematuria, impotence, urinary frequency, urinary incontinence, urinary tract disorder, urinary tract infection, urination impaired, urinary retention.

Hematologic – Anemia.

Metabolic – Peripheral edema.

Respiratory – Cough increased, dyspnea, pneumonia.

Miscellaneous – Back pain, flu syndrome, sepsis, aggravation reaction.

➤*Men - Stage B2 to C prostatic carcinoma:* Treatment with goserelin and flutamide did not add substantially to the toxicity of radiation treatment alone. The following adverse reactions were reported during a multicenter clinical trial comparing goserelin + flutamide + radiation vs radiation alone. The most frequently reported (greater than 5%) adverse reactions are listed below.

Adverse Reactions During Acute Radiation Therapy (%)

Adverse reaction	Flutamide + goserelin + radiation (n = 231)	Radiation only (n = 235)
Bladder	58%	60%
Rectum/large bowel	80%	76%
Skin	37%	37%

Adverse Reactions During Late Radiation Therapy (%)

Adverse reaction	Flutamide + goserelin + radiation (n = 231)	Radiation only (n = 235)
Cystitis	16%	16%
Diarrhea	36%	40%
Hematuria	7%	12%
Proctitis	8%	8%
Rectal bleeding	14%	20%

Additional adverse reaction data were collected for the combination therapy with radiation group over both the hormonal treatment and hormonal treatment plus radiation phases of the study. Adverse reactions occurring in more than 5% of patients in this group, over both parts of the study, were hot flashes (46%), diarrhea (40%), nausea (9%), and skin rash (8%).

Lab test abnormalities –

Plasma enzymes: Elevation of liver enzymes (ALT, AST) have been reported in female patients exposed to 3.6 mg goserelin (representing less than 1% of all patients). There was no other evidence of abnormal liver function. Causality between these changes and goserelin have not been established.

Lipids: In a controlled trial in females, 3.6 mg goserelin therapy resulted in a minor, but statistically significant effect on serum lipids. In patients treated for endometriosis at 6 months following initiation of therapy, danazol treatment resulted in a mean increase in LDL cholesterol of 33.3 mg/dL and a decrease in HDL cholesterol of 21.3 mg/dL compared with increases of 21.3 and 2.7 mg/dL in LDL cholesterol and HDL cholesterol, respectively, for goserelin-treated patients. Triglycerides increased by 8 mg/dL in goserelin-treated patients compared with a decrease of 8.9 mg/dL in danazol-treated patients.

In patients treated for endometriosis, goserelin increased total cholesterol and LDL cholesterol during 6 months of treatment. However, goserelin therapy resulted in HDL cholesterol levels which were significantly higher relative to danazol therapy. At the end of 6 months of treatment, HDL cholesterol fractions (HDL_2 and HDL_3) were decreased by 13.5 and 7.7 mg/dL, respectively, for danazol-treated patients compared with treatment increases of 1.9 and 0.8 mg/dL, respectively, for goserelin-treated patients.

➤*Women:* As would be expected with a drug that results in hypoestrogenism, the most frequently reported adverse reactions were those related to this effect.

As with other LHRH agonists, there have been reports of ovarian cyst formation and, when 3.6 mg goserelin is used in combination with gonadotropins, of ovarian hyperstimulation syndrome (OHSS).

Endometriosis –

Goserelin Adverse Reactions (%)

Adverse reaction	Goserelin (n = 411)	Danazol (n = 207)
Abdominal pain	7%	7%
Acne	42%	55%
Application site reaction	6%	0%
Asthenia	11%	13%
Back pain	7%	13%
Breast atrophy	33%	42%
Breast enlargement	18%	15%
Breast pain	7%	4%
Decreased libido	61%	44%
Depression	54%	48%
Dizziness	6%	4%
Dyspareunia	14%	5%
Emotional lability	60%	56%
Flu syndrome	5%	5%
Hair disorders	4%	11%
Headache	75%	63%
Hirsutism	7%	15%
Hot flashes	96%	67%
Hypertonia	1%	10%
Increased appetite	2%	5%
Increased libido	12%	19%
Infection	13%	11%
Insomnia	11%	4%
Leg cramps	2%	6%
Myalgia	3%	11%
Nausea	8%	14%
Nervousness	3%	5%
Pain	17%	16%
Pelvic symptoms	18%	23%
Peripheral edema	21%	34%
Pharyngitis	5%	2%
Pruritus	2%	6%
Seborrhea	26%	52%
Sweating	45%	30%
Vaginitis	75%	43%
Voice alterations	3%	8%
Weight gain	3%	23%

➤*The following adverse reactions not already listed above were reported at a frequency of 1% or greater, regardless of causality, in goserelin-treated women from all clinical trials:*

Cardiovascular – Hemorrhage, hypertension, migraine, palpitations, tachycardia.

CNS – Anxiety, paresthesia, somnolence, abnormal thinking.

Dermatologic – Alopecia, dry skin, rash, skin discoloration.

GI – Constipation, diarrhea, dry mouth, dyspepsia, flatulence.

GU – Dysmenorrhea, urinary frequency, urinary tract infection, vaginal hemorrhage.

Hematologic – Ecchymosis.

Metabolic/Nutritional – Edema.

Musculoskeletal – Arthralgia, joint disorder.

Respiratory – Bronchitis, increased cough, epistaxis, rhinitis, sinusitis.

Special senses – Amblyopia, dry eyes.

Miscellaneous – Allergic reaction, chest pain, fever, malaise, anorexia.

➤*Hormone replacement therapy:* Clinical studies suggest the addition of hormone replacement therapy (estrogens and/or progestins) to goserelin may decrease the occurrence of vasomotor symptoms and vaginal dryness associated with hypoestrogenism without compromising the efficacy of goserelin in relieving pelvic symptoms. The optimal drugs, dose, and duration of treatment have not been established.

➤*Changes in bone mineral density:* After 6 months of goserelin treatment, 109 female patients treated with goserelin showed an average 4.3% decrease of vertebral trabecular bone mineral density (BMD) as compared with pretreatment values. BMD was measured by dual-photon absorptiometry or dual energy x-ray absorptiometry. Sixty-six of these patients were assessed for BMD loss 6 months after the completion (posttherapy) of the

GOSERELIN ACETATE — SUBCUTANEOUS

6-month therapy period. Data from these patients showed an average 2.4% BMD loss compared with pretreatment values. Twenty-eight of the 109 patients were assessed for BMD at 12 months posttherapy. Data from these patients showed an average decrease of 2.5% in BMD compared with pretreatment values. These data suggest a possibility of partial reversibility. Clinical studies suggest the addition of hormone replacement therapy (estrogens and/or progestins) to goserelin is effective in reducing the bone mineral loss which occurs with goserelin alone without compromising the efficacy of goserelin in relieving the symptoms of endometriosis. The optimal drugs, dose, and duration of treatment have not been established.

➤*Breast cancer:* The adverse reaction profile for women with advanced breast cancer treated with goserelin is consistent with the profile described above for women treated with goserelin for endometriosis. In a controlled clinical trial (SWOG-8692) comparing goserelin with oophorectomy in premenopausal and perimenopausal women with advanced breast cancer, the following reactions were reported at a frequency of 5% or greater in either treatment group regardless of causality.

Goserelin Adverse Reactions (%)		
Adverse reaction	Goserelin (n = 57)	Oophorectomy (n = 55)
Edema	5%	0%
Hot flashes	70%	47%
Malaise/fatigue/lethargy	5%	2%
Nausea	11%	7%
Tumor flare	23%	4%
Vomiting	4%	7%

In the phase 2 clinical trial program in 333 pre- and perimenopausal women with advanced breast cancer, hot flashes were reported in 75.9% of patients and decreased libido was noted in 47.7% of patients. These 2 adverse reactions reflect the pharmacological actions of goserelin.

Injection site reactions were reported in less than 1% of patients.

➤*Endometrial thinning:* The following adverse reactions were reported at a frequency of 5% or greater in premenopausal women presenting with dysfunctional uterine bleeding in Trial 0022 for endometrial thinning. These results indicate that headache, hot flushes, and sweating were more common in the goserelin group than in the placebo group.

Goserelin Adverse Reactions (≥ 5%)		
Adverse reaction	Goserelin 3.6 mg (n = 180)	Placebo (n = 177)
Cardiovascular		
Hypertension	6%	2%
Migraine	7%	4%
Vasodilation	57%	18%
CNS		
Depression	3%	7%
Headache	32%	22%
Nervousness	5%	3%
Dermatologic		
Sweating	16%	5%
GI		
Abdominal pain	11%	10%
Nausea	5%	6%
GU		
Dysmenorrhea	7%	9%
Menorrhagia	4%	5%
Uterine hemorrhage	6%	4%
Vaginitis	1%	6%
Vulvovaginitis	5%	1%
Respiratory		
Pharyngitis	6%	9%
Sinusitis	3%	6%
Miscellaneous		
Back pain	4%	7%
Pelvic pain	9%	6%

Overdosage

The pharmacologic properties of goserelin and its mode of administration make accidental or intentional overdosage unlikely. There is no experience of overdosage from clinical trials. Animal studies indicate that no increased pharmacologic effect occurred at higher doses or more frequent administration. Subcutaneous doses of the drug as high as 1 mg/kg/day in rats and dogs did not produce any nonendocrine related sequelae; this dose is greater than 400 times that proposed for human use. If overdosage occurs, it should be managed symptomatically.

Patient Information

➤*Men:* Carefully consider the use of goserelin in patients at particular risk of developing ureteral obstruction or spinal cord compression and closely monitor the patients during the first month of therapy. Patients with ureteral obstruction or spinal cord compression should have appropriate treatment prior to initiation of goserelin therapy.

➤*Women:* Since menstruation should stop with effective doses of goserelin, the patient should notify her physician if regular menstruation persists. Patients missing 1 or more successive doses of goserelin may experience breakthrough menstrual bleeding.

Do not prescribe goserelin if the patient is pregnant, breastfeeding, lactating, has nondiagnosed abnormal vaginal bleeding, or is allergic to any of the components of goserelin.

Use of goserelin in pregnancy is contraindicated in women being treated for endometriosis or endometrial thinning. Therefore, a nonhormonal method of contraception should be used during treatment. Advise patients that if they miss 1 or more successive doses of goserelin, breakthrough menstrual bleeding or ovulation may occur with the potential for conception. If a patient becomes pregnant during treatment for endometriosis or endometrial thinning, discontinue goserelin treatment and advise the patient on the possible risks to the pregnancy and fetus. In studies in rats and rabbits, 10.8 mg goserelin increased preimplantation loss, resorptions, and abortions. In rats and dogs, 10.8 mg goserelin suppressed ovarian function, decreased ovarian weight and size, and led to atrophic changes in secondary sex organs. Further evidence suggests that fertility was reduced in female rats that became pregnant after goserelin was stopped. These effects are an expected consequence of the hormonal alterations produced by goserelin in humans. In animal studies, there was no evidence that goserelin possessed the potential to cause teratogenicity in rabbits; however, in rats, the incidence of umbilical hernia was significantly increased with treatment.

Those adverse reactions occurring most frequently in clinical studies with goserelin are associated with hypoestrogenism; of these, the most frequently reported are hot flashes (flushes), headaches, vaginal dryness, emotional lability, change in libido, depression, sweating and change in breast size. Clinical studies in endometriosis suggest the addition of hormone replacement therapy (estrogens and/or progestins) to goserelin may decrease the occurrence of vasomotor symptoms and vaginal dryness associated with hypoestrogenism without compromising the efficacy of goserelin in relieving pelvic symptoms. The optimal drugs, dose, and duration of treatment have not been established.

As with other LHRH agonist analogues, treatment with goserelin induces a hypoestrogenic state which results in a loss of bone mineral density (BMD) over the course of treatment, some of which may not be reversible. In patients with a history of prior treatment that may have resulted in bone mineral density loss or in patients with major risk factors for decreased bone mineral density, such as chronic alcohol abuse or tobacco abuse, significant family history of osteoporosis, or chronic use of drugs that can reduce bone density such as anticonvulsants and corticosteroids, goserelin therapy may pose an additional risk. In these patients, the risks and benefits must be weighed carefully before therapy with goserelin is instituted. Clinical studies suggest the addition of hormone replacement therapy (estrogens and/or progestins) to goserelin is effective in reducing the bone mineral loss which occurs with goserelin alone. The optimal drugs, dose, and duration of treatment have not been established.

Currently, there are no clinical data on the effects of retreatment or treatment of benign gynecological conditions with goserelin for periods in excess of 6 months.

As with other hormonal interventions that disrupt the pituitary-gonadal axis, some patients may have delayed return to menses. The rare patient, however, may experience persistent amenorrhea.

TRIPTORELIN PAMOATE

Rx	**Trelstar** (Watson)	**Injection, lyophilized microgranules for suspension:** 3.75 mg	Mannitol, polysorbate 80. In single-dose vials and in single-dose *Mixject* delivery system with 2 mL of diluent.
		11.25 mg	Mannitol, polysorbate 80. In single-dose vials and in single-dose *Mixject* delivery system with 2 mL of diluent.
		22.5 mg	Mannitol, polysorbate 80. In single-dose vials and in single-dose *Mixject* delivery system with 2 mL of diluent.

TRIPTORELIN PAMOATE — INJECTION

Indications

➤*Advanced prostate cancer:* For palliative treatment of advanced prostate cancer.

➤*Off-label uses:* Treatment of ovarian cancer, pancreatic carcinoma, endometriosis, hyperandrogenism, growth hormone deficiency, in vitro fertilization, uterine leiomyomata.

Triptorelin has been used safely and effectively in children for central precocious puberty.

Administration and Dosage

➤*Adults:*

Advanced prostate cancer – Recommended dosage is 3.75 mg intramuscularly (IM) once every 4 weeks, 11.25 mg IM once every 12 weeks, or 22.5 mg IM once every 24 weeks.

➤*Children:*

Off-label dosing –

Central precocious puberty: 3.75 mg IM monthly. Calcium supplementation should be considered.

➤*Preparation for administration:*

Vials – Wash your hands with soap and hot water and put on gloves immediately prior to preparing the injection. Place the vial in a standing upright position on a clean, flat surface that is covered with a sterile pad or cloth. Remove *Flip-Off* button from the top of the vial, revealing the rubber stopper. Disinfect the rubber stopper with an alcohol wipe. Discard the alcohol wipe and allow the stopper to dry. Using a syringe fitted with a sterile 21-gauge needle, withdraw 2 mL of sterile water for injection and inject into the vial. Shake well to thoroughly disperse particles to obtain a uniform suspension. The suspension will appear milky. Slowly withdraw the entire contents of the reconstituted suspension into the syringe. Administer immediately after reconstitution.

Mixject system – Wash your hands with soap and hot water and put on gloves immediately prior to preparing the injection. Place the sealed tray on a clean, flat surface that is covered with a sterile pad or cloth. Peel the cover away from the tray and remove the *Mixject* components and the vial. Remove the *Flip-Off* button from the top of the vial, revealing the rubber stopper. Place the vial in a standing upright position on the prepared surface. Disinfect the rubber stopper with the alcohol wipe. Discard the alcohol wipe and allow the stopper to dry.

Peel the cover away from the blister pack containing the vial adapter. Do not remove the vial adapter from the blister pack. Place the blister pack containing the vial adapter firmly on the vial top, piercing the vial. Push down gently until you feel it snap in place. Remove the blister pack from the vial adapter.

Screw the plunger rod into the barrel end of the syringe. Remove the cap from the syringe barrel.

Connect the syringe to the vial adapter by screwing it clockwise into the opening on the side of the vial adapter. Be sure to gently twist the syringe until it stops turning to ensure a tight connection.

While holding the vial, place your thumb on the plunger rod and push the plunger rod in all the way to transfer the diluent from the pre-filled syringe into the vial. Do not release the plunger rod.

Keeping the plunger rod depressed, gently swirl the vial so that the diluent rinses the sides of the vial. This will ensure complete mixing of triptorelin and the sterile water diluent. The suspension will now have a milky appearance. In order to avoid separation of the suspension, proceed to the next steps without delay.

Invert the *Mixject* system so that the vial is at the top. Grasp the *Mixject* system firmly by the syringe and pull back the plunger rod slowly to draw the reconstituted triptorelin into the syringe.

Return the vial to its upright position and disconnect the vial adapter and vial from the *Mixject* syringe assembly by turning the plastic cap of the vial adapter clockwise. Grasp only the plastic cap when removing.

Lift up the safety cover and remove the clear plastic needle shield by pulling it from the assembly. The safety cover should be perpendicular to the needle, with the needle facing away from you. The syringe containing triptorelin suspension is now ready for administration. Administer immediately after reconstitution.

➤*Administration:* Triptorelin should only be administered IM immediately after reconstitution. Inject suspension into either buttock. Rotate injection sites.

Mixject system – After administering the injection, immediately activate the safety mechanism by centering your thumb or forefinger on the textured finger pad area of the safety cover and pushing it forward over the needle until you hear or feel it lock. Use the one-handed technique and activate the mechanism away from yourself and others. Activation of the safety cover causes virtually no splatter. Immediately discard the syringe assembly after a single use into a suitable sharps container.

Vials – Administer triptorelin with a 21-gauge needle.

➤*Admixture compatibility:* Reconstitute in sterile water. Do not use any other diluent.

➤*Storage/Stability:* Store between 20° and 25°C (68° and 77°F). Do not freeze.

Actions

➤*Pharmacology:* Triptorelin is a synthetic decapeptide agonist analog of gonadotropin-releasing hormone (GnRH).

Pharmacodynamics – Following the first administration, there is a transient surge in circulating levels of luteinizing hormone (LH), follicle-stimulating hormone (FSH), testosterone, and estradiol. After long-term and continuous administration (usually 2 to 4 weeks after initiation of therapy), a sustained decrease in LH and FSH secretion and marked reduction of testicular steroidogenesis are observed. A reduction of serum testosterone concentration to a level typically seen in surgically castrated men is obtained. Consequently, tissues and functions that depend on these hormones for maintenance become quiescent. These effects are usually reversible after cessation of therapy.

➤*Pharmacokinetics:*

Triptorelin Pharmacokinetic Parameters[a]

Group	C_{max} (ng/mL)	AUC_{inf} (h•ng/mL)	Cl_p (mL/min)	Cl_{renal} (mL/min)	t½ (h)	CrCl (mL/min)
6 healthy men	48.2 ± 11.8	36.1 ± 5.8	211.9 ± 31.6	90.6 ± 35.3	2.81 ± 1.21	149.9 ± 7.3
6 men with moderate renal impairment	45.6 ± 20.5	69.9 ± 24.6	120 ± 45	23.3 ± 17.6	6.56 ± 1.25	39.7 ± 22.5
6 men with severe renal impairment	46.5 ± 14	88 ± 18.4	88.6 ± 19.7	4.3 ± 2.9	7.65 ± 1.25	8.9 ± 6
6 men with liver disease	54.1 ± 5.3	131.9 ± 18.1	57.8 ± 8	35.9 ± 5	7.58 ± 1.17	89.9 ± 15.1

[a] C_{max} = maximum plasma concentration; AUC = area under the curve; Cl_p = plasma clearance; Cl_{renal} = renal clearance; t½ = half-life; CrCl = creatinine clearance.

Absorption – Following a single IM injection of triptorelin to patients with prostate cancer, mean peak serum concentrations of 28.4, 38.5, and 44.1 ng/mL occurred 1 to 3 hours after the 3.75, 11.25, and 22.5 mg formulations, respectively.

Triptorelin 3.75 mg: Following a single IM injection of triptorelin 3.75 mg to healthy male volunteers, serum testosterone levels first increased, peaking on day 4, and thereafter declined to low levels by week 4.

Triptorelin 11.25 mg: Following a single IM injection of triptorelin 11.25 mg to men with advanced prostate cancer, serum testosterone levels first increased, peaking on days 2 to 3, and thereafter declined to low levels by weeks 3 to 4.

Triptorelin 22.5 mg: Following a single IM injection of triptorelin 22.5 mg to men with advanced prostate cancer, serum testosterone levels first increased, peaking on day 3, and declined thereafter to low levels by weeks 3 to 4.

Distribution – The volume of distribution following a single intravenous (IV) bolus dose of triptorelin peptide 0.5 mg was 30 to 33 L in healthy male volunteers. There is no evidence that triptorelin, at clinically relevant concentrations, binds to plasma proteins.

Results of pharmacokinetic investigations conducted in healthy men indicate that after IV bolus administration, triptorelin is distributed and eliminated according to a 3-compartment model, and corresponding half-lives are approximately 6 minutes, 45 minutes, and 3 hours.

Metabolism – Thus far, no metabolites of triptorelin have been identified. Pharmacokinetic data suggest that C-terminal fragments produced by tissue degradation are completely degraded in the tissues, rapidly degraded in plasma, or cleared by the kidneys.

Excretion – Triptorelin is eliminated by the liver and the kidneys. Following IV administration of triptorelin peptide 0.5 mg to 6 healthy male volunteers with a CrCl of 149.9 mL/min, 41.7% of the dose was excreted in urine as intact peptide with a total triptorelin clearance of 211.9 mL/min. This percentage increased to 62.3% in patients with liver disease who have a lower CrCl (89.9 mL/min). It has also been observed that the nonrenal clearance of triptorelin (patient anuric, CrCl = 0) was 76.2 mL/min, thus indicating that the nonrenal elimination of triptorelin is mainly dependent on the liver.

Special populations –

Renal function impairment: Renal impairment led to a decrease in total triptorelin clearance proportional to the decrease in CrCl, as well as an increase in volume of distribution and, consequently, an increase in elimination half-life. Patients with renal impairment had 2- to 4-fold higher exposure (AUC) values than younger healthy males.

TRIPTORELIN PAMOATE — INJECTION

Pharmacokinetic data obtained in young, healthy men 20 to 22 years of age with an elevated CrCl (approximately 150 mL/min) indicate that triptorelin was eliminated twice as fast in this young population compared with patients with moderate renal impairment.

Hepatic function impairment: In patients with hepatic insufficiency, a decrease in triptorelin clearance was more pronounced than that observed with renal insufficiency. Because of minimal increases in the volume of distribution, the elimination half-life in subjects with hepatic insufficiency was similar to subjects with renal insufficiency. Patients with hepatic impairment had 2- to 4-fold higher exposure (AUC) values than younger, healthy men.

Elderly: Triptorelin clearance is partly correlated to total CrCl, which is well known to decrease with age.

Contraindications

Hypersensitivity to triptorelin or any other component of the product, other GnRH agonists, or GnRH; women who are or may become pregnant.

Warnings/Precautions

➤*Worsening of signs and symptoms:* Initially, triptorelin, like other GnRH agonists, causes a transient increase in serum testosterone levels. As a result, isolated cases of worsening of signs and symptoms of prostate cancer during the first weeks of treatment have been reported with GnRH agonists. Patients may experience worsening of symptoms or onset of new symptoms, including bone pain, neuropathy, hematuria, or urethral or bladder outlet obstruction. Cases of spinal cord compression, which may contribute to weakness or paralysis with or without fatal complications, have been reported with the use of GnRH agonists.

If spinal cord compression or renal impairment develops, institute standard treatment of these complications, and, in extreme cases, consider an immediate orchiectomy.

➤*Hypersensitivity reactions:* Anaphylactic shock, hypersensitivity, and angioedema related to triptorelin administration have been reported. In the event of a hypersensitivity reaction, immediately discontinue therapy and administer the appropriate supportive and symptomatic care.

➤*Pregnancy: Category X.* Triptorelin is contraindicated in women who are or may become pregnant while receiving the drug. Triptorelin injections may cause fetal harm when administered to pregnant women. Expected hormonal changes that occur with triptorelin treatment increase the risk for pregnancy loss. If this drug is used during pregnancy or if the patient becomes pregnant while taking this drug, apprise the patient of the potential hazard to the fetus.

Studies in pregnant rats administered triptorelin at dosages of 2, 10, and 100 mcg/kg/day (approximately equivalent to 0.2, 0.8, and 8 times the estimated human daily dose based on body surface area) during the period of organogenesis demonstrated maternal toxicity and embryofetal toxicities. Embryofetal toxicities consisted of preimplantation loss, increased resorption, and reduced mean number of viable fetuses at the high dose.

➤*Lactation:* Triptorelin is not indicated for use in women. It is not known whether triptorelin is excreted in human milk. Because many drugs are excreted in human milk and because of the potential for serious adverse reactions in breast-feeding infants, make a decision to discontinue breast-feeding or the drug, taking into account the importance of the drug to the mother.

➤*Children:* Safety and effectiveness in children have not been established.

➤*Monitoring:* Monitor response to triptorelin by measuring serum levels of testosterone periodically or as indicated.

Closely observe patients with metastatic vertebral lesions and/or upper or lower urinary tract obstruction during the first few weeks of therapy.

Drug Interactions

➤*Hyperprolactinemic drugs:* No drug-drug interaction studies involving triptorelin have been conducted. In the absence of relevant data and as a precaution, do not prescribe hyperprolactinemic drugs concomitantly with triptorelin because hyperprolactinemia reduces the number of pituitary GnRH receptors.

➤*Drug/Lab test interactions:* Long-term or continuous administration of triptorelin in therapeutic doses results in suppression of the pituitary-gonadal axis. Diagnostic tests of the pituitary-gonadal function conducted during treatment and after cessation of therapy may, therefore, be misleading.

Adverse Reactions

The safety of the 3 triptorelin formulations was evaluated in clinical trials involving patients with advanced prostate cancer. Mean testosterone levels increased above baseline during the first week following the initial injection, declining thereafter to baseline levels or below by the end of the second week of treatment. The transient increase in testosterone levels may be associated with temporary worsening of disease signs and symptoms, including bone pain, hematuria, neuropathy, and urethral or bladder outlet obstruction. Isolated cases of spinal cord compression with weakness or paralysis of the lower extremities have occurred.

The majority of adverse reactions related to triptorelin are a result of its pharmacological action (ie, the induced variation in serum testosterone levels, either an increase in testosterone at the initiation of treatment, or a decrease in testosterone once castration is achieved). Local reactions at the injection site or allergic reactions may occur.

Triptorelin 3.75 mg –

Triptorelin 3.75 mg Adverse Reactions (≥ 1%)	
Adverse reaction	(n = 140)
CNS	
Dizziness	1.4%
Emotional lability	1.4%
Fatigue	2.1%
Headache	5%
Insomnia	2.1%
GI	
Diarrhea	1.4%
Vomiting	2.1%
GU	
Impotence	7.1%
Urinary retention	1.4%
Urinary tract infection	1.4%
Musculoskeletal	
Leg pain	2.1%
Skeletal pain	12.1%
Miscellaneous	
Anemia	1.4%
Hot flushes	58.6%
Hypertension	3.6%
Injection-site pain	3.6%
Pain	2.1%
Pruritus	1.4%

Triptorelin 11.25 mg –

Triptorelin 11.25 mg Adverse Reactions (≥ 1%)	
Adverse reaction	(n = 174)
CNS	
Asthenia	1.1%
Dizziness	2.9%
Fatigue	2.3%
Headache	6.9%
Insomnia	1.7%
GI	
Abdominal pain	1.1%
Anorexia	1.7%
Constipation	1.7%
Diarrhea	1.1%
Dyspepsia	1.7%
Nausea	2.9%
GU	
Breast pain	2.3%
Decreased libido	2.3%
Dysuria	4.6%
Gynecomastia	1.7%
Impotence	2.3%
Urinary retention	1.1%
Metabolic/Nutritional	
Dependent edema	2.3%
Edema in legs	6.3%
Increased alkaline phosphatase	1.7%
Peripheral edema	1.1%
Musculoskeletal	
Arthralgia	2.3%
Back pain	2.9%
Injection-site pain	4%
Leg cramps	1.7%
Leg pain	5.2%
Myalgia	1.1%
Skeletal pain	13.2%
Respiratory	
Coughing	1.7%

TRIPTORELIN PAMOATE — INJECTION

Triptorelin 11.25 mg Adverse Reactions (≥ 1%)	
Adverse reaction	(n = 174)
Dyspnea	1.1%
Pharyngitis	1.1%
Special senses	
Conjunctivitis	1.1%
Eye pain	1.1%
Miscellaneous	
Abnormal hepatic function	1.1%
Chest pain	1.7%
Hot flushes	73%
Hypertension	4%
Pain	3.4%
Rash	1.7%

Triptorelin 22.5 mg –

Triptorelin 22.5 mg Adverse Reactions (≥ 5%) (n = 120)		
Adverse reaction	Treatment-emergent	Treatment-related
CNS		
Headache	7.5%	1.7%
Insomnia	5%	0.8%
GU		
Erectile dysfunction	10%	10%
Testicular atrophy	7.5%	7.5%
Urinary retention	5%	0%
Urinary tract infection	11.6%	0%
Musculoskeletal		
Arthralgia	7.5%	0.8%
Back pain	10.8%	0.8%
Pain in extremity	7.5%	0.8%
Miscellaneous		
Bronchitis	5%	0%
Diabetes mellitus/ hyperglycemia	5%	0%
Edema peripheral	5%	0%
Hot flush	72.5%	71.7%
Hypertension	14.2%	0.8%
Influenza	15.8%	0%

➤*Lab test abnormalities (10% or more):*

Triptorelin 11.25 mg – Decreased hemoglobin and red blood cell count and increased glucose, serum urea nitrogen, AST, ALT, and alkaline phosphatase at the day 253 visit.

Triptorelin 22.5 mg – Decreased hemoglobin and increased glucose and hepatic transaminases were detected during the study. The majority of the changes were mild to moderate.

➤*Postmarketing:* During postmarketing surveillance, rare cases of pituitary apoplexy (a clinical syndrome secondary to infarction of the pituitary gland) have been reported after the administration of GnRH agonists. In a majority of these cases, a pituitary adenoma was diagnosed with a majority of pituitary apoplexy cases occurring within 2 weeks of the first dose, and some within the first hour. In these cases, pituitary apoplexy has presented as sudden headache, vomiting, visual changes, ophthalmoplegia, altered mental status, and sometimes cardiovascular collapse. Immediate medical attention has been required.

Overdosage

➤*Treatment:* There is no experience of overdosage in clinical trials. If overdosage occurs, discontinue therapy immediately and administer the appropriate supportive and symptomatic treatment.

Patient Information

Instruct patients that they will likely experience an increase in serum testosterone levels following their initial injection. This may cause a worsening of their symptoms of prostate cancer during the first weeks of treatment. These symptoms may include bone pain, spinal cord injury, hematuria, and urethral or bladder outlet obstruction. This increase in serum testosterone levels and associated symptoms should decline 3 to 4 weeks following their injection. Discuss the use of drugs appropriate for alleviating the risk associated with the increase with patients prior to administration of the products.

Advise patients that allergic reactions, including serious allergic reactions, could occur and that serious reactions require immediate treatment. Advise patients to report any previous hypersensitivity reactions to triptorelin, other GnRH agonists, or GnRH.

ANASTROZOLE

Rx	**Anastrozole** (Various, eg, APP Pharmaceutical, Cypress Pharmaceutical, Dr. Reddy's Labs, Mylan, Roxane, Sandoz, Teva)	**Tablets; oral:** 1 mg	May contain lactose, PEG, polydextrose. In 30s, 90s, and 500s.
Rx	**Arimidex** (AstraZeneca)		Lactose, PEG. (A/Adx 1). White. Film-coated. In 30s.

ANASTROZOLE — ORAL

Indications

➤*Breast cancer:* For adjuvant treatment of postmenopausal women with hormone receptor–positive early breast cancer.

For the first-line treatment of postmenopausal women with hormone receptor–positive or hormone receptor–unknown locally advanced or metastatic breast cancer.

For the treatment of advanced breast cancer in postmenopausal women with disease progression following tamoxifen therapy.

Patients with estrogen receptor–negative disease and patients who did not respond to previous tamoxifen therapy rarely responded to anastrozole.

➤*Off-label uses:*

Breast cancer prevention – [4] = Insufficient documentation. Although results were considered too preliminary for the American Society of Clinical Oncology to recommend the routine use of anastrozole for breast cancer chemoprevention, the available information on aromatase inhibitors and inactivators is encouraging. Anastrozole may have the potential to offer improved efficacy in preventing breast cancer, coupled with a more favorable safety profile, relative to tamoxifen.

Male infertility – [4] = Insufficient documentation. In noncontrolled trials, mean testosterone levels increased and mean estradiol levels decreased significantly in men treated with anastrozole for infertility and hypogonadotropic hypogonadism with premature ejaculation. The rate of paternity or pregnancy after treatment with anastrozole was not measured in the studies. Further studies are required to establish the role of anastrozole in the treatment of male infertility.

Administration and Dosage

➤*Adults:*

Breast cancer – 1 mg once a day.

Off-label dosing –

Breast cancer prevention: [4] = Insufficient documentation. 1 mg/day for 5 years.

Male infertility: [4] = Insufficient documentation. 1 mg orally once daily for a mean duration of 4.7 months (range, 1 to 24 months).

➤*Hepatic function impairment:* No changes in dose are recommended for patients with mild to moderate hepatic impairment. Anastrozole has not been studied in patients with severe hepatic impairment.

➤*Duration of therapy:* For patients with advanced breast cancer, anastrozole should be continued until tumor progression.

For adjuvant treatment of early breast cancer in postmenopausal women, the optimal duration of therapy is unknown. In the ATAC trial anastrozole was administered for 5 years.

➤*Administration:* Anastrozole can be taken with or without food.

➤*Storage/Stability:* Store at 20° to 25°C (68° to 77°F).

Actions

➤*Pharmacology:* The growth of many cancers of the breast is stimulated or maintained by estrogens. In postmenopausal women, estrogens are mainly derived from the action of the aromatase enzyme, which converts adrenal androgens (primarily androstenedione and testosterone) to estrone and estradiol. The suppression of estrogen biosynthesis in peripheral tissues

ANASTROZOLE — ORAL

and in the cancer tissue itself can, therefore, be achieved by specifically inhibiting the aromatase enzyme.

Anastrozole is a potent and selective nonsteroidal aromatase inhibitor. It significantly lowers serum estradiol concentrations and has no detectable effect on formation of adrenal corticosteroids or aldosterone.

➤*Pharmacokinetics:*

Absorption – Inhibition of aromatase activity is primarily due to anastrozole, the parent drug. Absorption of anastrozole is rapid and maximum plasma concentrations typically occur within 2 hours of dosing under fasted conditions. Studies with radiolabeled drug have demonstrated that orally administered anastrozole is well absorbed into the systemic circulation. The pharmacokinetics of anastrozole are linear over the dose range of 1 to 20 mg, and do not change with repeated dosing. The pharmacokinetics of anastrozole were similar in patients and healthy volunteers.

Effect of food: Food reduces the rate but not the overall extent of anastrozole absorption. The mean maximum plasma concentration (C_{max}) of anastrozole decreased by 16% and the median time to C_{max} (T_{max}) was delayed from 2 to 5 hours when anastrozole was administered 30 minutes after food.

Distribution – Steady-state plasma levels are approximately 3- to 4-fold higher than levels observed after a single dose of anastrozole. Plasma concentrations approach steady-state levels at about 7 days of once daily dosing. Anastrozole is 40% bound to plasma proteins in the therapeutic range.

Metabolism – Metabolism of anastrozole occurs by N-dealkylation, hydroxylation, glucuronidation. Three metabolites of anastrozole (triazole, a glucuronide conjugate of hydroxy-anastrozole, and a glucuronide conjugate of anastrozole itself) have been identified in human plasma and urine. The major circulating metabolite of anastrozole, triazole, lacks pharmacologic activity.

Anastrozole inhibited reactions catalyzed by cytochrome P450 1A2, 2C8/9, and 3A4 in vitro with Ki values which were approximately 30 times higher than the mean steady-state C_{max} values observed following a 1 mg daily dose. Anastrozole had no inhibitory effect on reactions catalyzed by CYP450 2A6 or 2D6 in vitro. Administration of a single 30 mg/kg or multiple 10 mg/kg doses of anastrozole to healthy subjects had no effect on the clearance of antipyrine or urinary recovery of antipyrine metabolites.

Special populations –

Renal function impairment: Anastrozole pharmacokinetics have been investigated in subjects with renal impairment. Anastrozole renal clearance decreased proportionally with creatinine clearance (CrCl) and was approximately 50% lower in volunteers with severe renal impairment (CrCl less than 30 mL/min/1.73 m^2) compared with controls. Total clearance was only reduced 10%. No dosage adjustment is needed for renal impairment.

Hepatic function impairment: Anastrozole pharmacokinetics have been investigated in subjects with hepatic cirrhosis related to alcohol abuse. The apparent oral clearance (CL/F) of anastrozole was approximately 30% lower in subjects with stable hepatic cirrhosis than in control subjects with healthy liver function. However, these plasma concentrations were still within the range of concentrations seen in healthy subjects. The effect of severe hepatic impairment was not studied. No dose adjustment is necessary for stable hepatic cirrhosis.

Children: Following 1 mg once daily multiple administration in children, the mean T_{max} was 1 hour. The mean (range) disposition parameters of anastrozole in children were described by a CL/F of 1.54 L/h (0.77 to 4.53 L/h) and apparent volume of distribution (V/F) of 98.4 L (50.7 to 330 L). The terminal elimination half-life was 46.8 hours, which was similar to that observed in postmenopausal women treated with anastrozole for breast cancer. Based on a population pharmacokinetic analysis, the pharmacokinetics of anastrozole were similar in boys with pubertal gynecomastia and girls with McCune-Albright syndrome.

Contraindications

Anastrozole is contraindicated in women who are or may become pregnant and in any patient who has shown a hypersensitivity reaction to the drug or to any of the excipients. Observed reactions include anaphylaxis, angioedema, and urticaria.

Warnings/Precautions

➤*Usage:* Anastrozole should be administered under the supervision of a qualified physician experienced in the use of anticancer agents.

➤*Ischemic cardiovascular events:* In women with preexisting ischemic heart disease, an increased incidence of ischemic cardiovascular events was observed with anastrozole in the ATAC trial (17% of patients on anastrozole and 10% of patients on tamoxifen). Consider the risks and benefits of anastrozole therapy in patients with preexisting ischemic heart disease.

➤*Bone effects:* Results from the ATAC trial bone substudy at 12 and 24 months demonstrated that patients receiving anastrozole had a mean decrease in both lumbar spine and total hip bone mineral density (BMD) compared with baseline. Patients receiving tamoxifen had a mean increase in both lumbar spine and total hip BMD compared with baseline.

➤*Cholesterol:* During the ATAC trial, more patients receiving anastrozole were reported to have elevated serum cholesterol compared with patients receiving tamoxifen (9% vs 3.5%, respectively).

➤*Renal function impairment:* Since only about 10% of anastrozole is excreted unchanged in the urine, renal impairment does not influence the total body clearance. Dosage adjustment in patients with renal impairment is not necessary.

➤*Hepatic function impairment:* The plasma anastrozole concentrations in subjects with hepatic cirrhosis were within the range of concentrations seen in healthy subjects across all clinical trials. Therefore, dosage adjustment is also not necessary in patients with stable hepatic cirrhosis. Anastrozole has not been studied in patients with severe hepatic impairment.

➤*Pregnancy: Category X.* Anastrozole can cause fetal harm when administered to a pregnant woman and offers no clinical benefit to premenopausal women with breast cancer. Anastrozole is contraindicated in women who are or may become pregnant. There are no studies of anastrozole use in pregnant women. If anastrozole is used during pregnancy, or if the patient becomes pregnant while receiving this drug, apprise the patient of the potential hazard to the fetus and potential risk for pregnancy loss.

In animal studies, anastrozole caused pregnancy failure, increased pregnancy loss, and signs of delayed fetal development. In animal reproduction studies, pregnant rats and rabbits received anastrozole during organogenesis at doses at least 1 (rats) and one-third (rabbits) the recommended human dose on a mg/m^2 basis. In both species, anastrozole crossed the placenta, and there was increased pregnancy loss (increased pre- and/or post-implantation loss, increased resorption, and decreased numbers of live fetuses). In rats, these effects were dose related, and placental weights were significantly increased. Fetotoxicity, including delayed fetal development (ie, incomplete ossification and depressed fetal body weights), occurred in rats at anastrozole doses that produced peak plasma levels 19 times higher than serum levels in humans at the therapeutic dose (AUC_{0-24h} 9 times higher). In rabbits, anastrozole caused pregnancy failure at doses of 16 times or more the recommended human dose on a mg/m^2 basis.

➤*Lactation:* It is not known if anastrozole is excreted in human milk. Because many drugs are excreted in human milk and because of tumorigenicity shown for anastrozole in animal studies, or the potential for serious adverse reactions in breast-feeding infants, decide whether to discontinue breast-feeding or the drug, taking into account the importance of the drug to the mother.

➤*Children:* Clinical studies in children included a placebo-controlled trial in pubertal boys of adolescent age with gynecomastia and a single-arm trial in girls with McCune-Albright syndrome and progressive precocious puberty. The efficacy of anastrozole in the treatment of pubertal gynecomastia in adolescent boys and in the treatment of precocious puberty in girls with McCune Albright syndrome has not been demonstrated.

➤*Monitoring:* Consider periodic monitoring of BMD. Monitor cholesterol levels periodically.

Drug Interactions

Anastrozole Drug Interactions

Precipitant drug	Object drug[a]		Description
Estrogen	Anastrozole	⬇	Estrogen may diminish the pharmacologic action of anastrozole. Coadministration not recommended.
Tamoxifen	Anastrozole	⬇	Coadministration of anastrozole and tamoxifen reduced anastrozole plasma concentration by 27%. The combination of anastrozole and tamoxifen did not demonstrate any efficacy benefit. Based on clinical and pharmacokinetic results from the ATAC trial, tamoxifen should not be administered with anastrozole.

[a] ⬇ = object drug decreased.

Adverse Reactions

For more information on ischemic cardiovascular events, bone effects, and cholesterol, refer to Warnings/Precautions.

➤*Serious adverse reactions:* Serious adverse reactions with anastrozole occurring in less than 1 in 10,000 patients are skin reactions, such as lesions, ulcers, or blisters; allergic reactions with swelling of the face, lips, tongue, and/or throat that may cause difficulty in swallowing and/or breathing; and changes in blood tests of liver function, including inflammation of the liver with symptoms that may include a general feeling of not being well, with or without jaundice, liver pain, or liver swelling.

➤*Common adverse reactions:* Common adverse reactions (occurring with an incidence of more than 10%) in women taking anastrozole include: hot flashes, asthenia, arthritis, pain, arthralgia, pharyngitis, hypertension, depression, nausea and vomiting, rash, osteoporosis, fractures, back pain, insomnia, headache, bone pain, peripheral edema, increased cough, dyspnea, pharyngitis, and lymphedema.

➤*Discontinuation of therapy:* In the ATAC trial, the most common reported adverse reaction (more than 0.1%) leading to discontinuation of therapy for both treatment groups was hot flashes, although there were fewer patients who discontinued therapy as a result of hot flashes in the anastrozole group.

ANASTROZOLE — ORAL

➤*Adjuvant therapy:*

Anastrozole Adverse Reactions (≥ 5%) in the ATAC Trial[a]		
Adverse reactions[a]	Anastrozole 1 mg (n = 3,092)	Tamoxifen 20 mg (n = 3,094)
Cardiovascular		
Hypertension	13%	11%
Vasodilatation	36%	41%
CNS		
Anxiety	6%	6%
Asthenia	19%	18%
Depression	13%	12%
Dizziness	8%	8%
Headache	10%	8%
Insomnia	10%	9%
Paresthesia	7%	5%
Dermatologic		
Rash	11%	13%
Sweating	5%	6%
GI		
Abdominal pain	9%	9%
Constipation	8%	8%
Diarrhea	9%	7%
Dyspepsia	7%	6%
GI disorder	7%	5%
Nausea	11%	11%
GU		
Breast neoplasm	5%	5%
Breast pain	8%	6%
Leukorrhea	3%	9%
Urinary tract infection	8%	10%
Vaginal hemorrhage[b]	4%	6%
Vaginitis	4%	5%
Vulvovaginitis	6%	5%
Hematologic/Lymphatic		
Anemia	4%	5%
Lymphoedema	10%	11%
Metabolic		
Hypercholesteremia	9%	3.5%
Peripheral edema	10%	11%
Weight gain	9%	9%
Musculoskeletal		
Arthralgia	15%	11%
Arthritis	17%	14%
Arthrosis	7%	5%
Back pain	10%	10%
Bone pain	7%	6%
Fracture	10%	7%
Joint disorder	6%	5%
Myalgia	6%	5%
Osteoporosis	11%	7%
Respiratory		
Bronchitis	5%	5%
Dyspnea	8%	8%
Increased cough	8%	9%
Pharyngitis	14%	14%
Sinusitis	6%	5%
Miscellaneous		
Accidental injury	10%	10%
Cataract specified	6%	7%
Chest pain	7%	5%
Cyst	5%	5%
Flu syndrome	6%	6%
Infection	9%	9%
Neoplasm	5%	5%
Pain	17%	16%

[a] The combination arm was discontinued due to lack of efficacy benefit at 33 month follow-up. A patient may have had > 1 adverse reaction, including > 1 adverse reaction in the same body system. n = number of patients receiving treatment.
[b] Vaginal hemorrhage without further diagnosis.

Certain adverse reactions and combinations of adverse reactions were prospectively specified for analysis, based on the known pharmacologic properties and side effect profiles of the 2 drugs (see the following table).

Anastrozole Patients with Prespecified Adverse Reaction in ATAC Trial (%)[a]				
Adverse reactions	Anastrozole (n = 3,092) (%)	Tamoxifen (n = 3,094) (%)	Odds ratio	95% Confidence interval
Cardiovascular				
Deep venous thromboembolic events	2%	2%	0.64	0.45 to 0.93
Ischemic cardiovascular disease	4%	3%	1.23	0.95 to 1.6
Ischemic cerebrovascular event	2%	3%	0.7	0.5 to 0.97
Venous thromboembolic events	3%	5%	0.61	0.47 to 0.8
CNS				
Fatigue/Asthenia	19%	18%	1.07	0.94 to 1.22
Mood disturbances	19%	18%	1.1	0.97 to 1.25
GU				
Endometrial cancer[b]	0.2%	0.6%	0.31	0.10 to 0.94
Vaginal bleeding	5%	10%	0.5	0.41 to 0.61
Vaginal discharge	4%	13%	0.24	0.19 to 0.3
Musculoskeletal				
All fractures	10%	7%	1.57	1.3 to 1.88
Fractures of spine, hip, wrist	4%	3%	1.48	1.13 to 1.95
Hip	1%	1%		
Spine	1%	1%		
Wrists/Colles	2%	2%		
Musculoskeletal events[c]	36%	29%	1.32	1.19 to 1.47
Miscellaneous				
Cataracts	6%	7%	0.85	0.69 to 1.04
Hot flashes	36%	41%	0.8	0.73 to 0.89
Nausea and vomiting	13%	12%	1.03	0.88 to 1.19

[a] Patients with multiple events in the same category are counted only once in that category.
[b] Percentages calculated based upon the numbers of patients with an intact uterus at baseline.
[c] Refers to joint symptoms, including arthritis, arthrosis, arthralgia, and joint disorders.

Ischemic cardiovascular events – Between treatment arms in the overall populations of 6,186 patients, there was no statistical difference in ischemic cardiovascular events (4% anastrozole vs 3% tamoxifen).

In the overall population, angina pectoris was reported in 71 of 3,092 (2.3%) patients in the anastrozole arm and 51 of 3,094 (1.6%) patients in the tamoxifen arm; myocardial infarction (MI) was reported in 37 of 3,092 (1.2%) patients in the anastrozole arm and 34 of 3,094 (1.1%) patients in the tamoxifen arm.

In women with preexisting ischemic heart disease 465 of 6,186 (7.5%), the incidence of ischemic cardiovascular events was 17% in patients on anastrozole and 10% in patients on tamoxifen. In this patient population, angina pectoris was reported in 25 of 216 (11.6%) patients receiving anastrozole and 13 of 249 (5.2%) patients receiving tamoxifen; MI was reported in 2 of 216 (0.9%) patients receiving anastrozole and 8 of 249 (3.2%) patients receiving tamoxifen.

Bone mineral density findings – See Warnings/Precautions for more information.

Cholesterol – See Warnings/Precautions for more information.

ANASTROZOLE — ORAL

Other adverse reactions – Patients receiving anastrozole had an increase in joint disorders (including arthritis, arthrosis, and arthralgia) compared with patients receiving tamoxifen.

Patients receiving anastrozole had a higher incidence of carpal tunnel syndrome (78 [2.5%]) compared with patients receiving tamoxifen (22 [0.7%]).

➤*First-line therapy:*

Anastrozole Adverse Reactions (≥ 5%) in Trials 0030 and 0027[a]

Adverse reactions	Anastrozole (n = 506)	Tamoxifen (n = 511)
Cardiovascular		
Hypertension	5%	7%
Vasodilation	25%	21%
CNS		
Asthenia	16%	16%
Depression	5%	6%
Dizziness	6%	4%
Headache	9%	8%
Hypertonia	3%	5%
Insomnia	6%	7%
GI		
Abdominal pain	8%	7%
Anorexia	5%	9%
Constipation	9%	13%
Diarrhea	8%	6%
Nausea	19%	21%
Vomiting	8%	7%
Musculoskeletal		
Back pain	12%	13%
Bone pain	11%	10%
Respiratory		
Cough increased	11%	10%
Dyspnea	10%	9%
Pharyngitis	10%	13%
Miscellaneous		
Chest pain	7%	7%
Flu syndrome	7%	6%
Leukorrhea	2%	6%
Pain	14%	14%
Pelvic pain	5%	6%
Peripheral edema	10%	8%
Rash	8%	8%

[a] A patient may have had > 1 adverse reaction.

Anastrozole Patients With Prespecified Adverse Reactions in Trial 0030 and 0027[a]

Adverse reactions	Anastrozole 1 mg (n = 506)	Tamoxifen 20 mg (n = 511)
Cardiovascular		
Coronary and cerebral thromboembolic disease[b]	3%	4%
Thromboembolic disease	4%	6%
Venous thromboembolic disease[c]	1%	3%
CNS		
Depression	5%	6%
Lethargy	1%	3%
GU		
Vaginal bleeding	1%	2%
Vaginal dryness	2%	1%
Miscellaneous		
GI disturbance	34%	38%
Hot flushes	26%	23%
Tumor flare	3%	4%
Weight gain	2%	2%

[a] A patient may have had > 1 adverse reaction.
[b] Includes MI, myocardial ischemia, angina pectoris, cerebrovascular accident, cerebral ischemia, and cerebral infarct.
[c] Includes pulmonary embolus, thrombophlebitis, and retinal vein thrombosis.

➤*Second-line therapy:*

Anastrozole Adverse Reactions (≥ 5%) in Trials 0004 and 0005[a]

Adverse reactions	Anastrozole 1 mg (n = 262)	Anastrozole 10 mg (n = 246)	Megestrol acetate 160 mg (n = 253)
CNS			
Asthenia	16%	13%	19%
Depression	5%	2%	2%
Dizziness	6%	5%	6%
Headache	13%	18%	9%
Paresthesia	5%	6%	4%
Dermatologic			
Rash	6%	6%	8%
Sweating	2%	1%	6%
GI			
Abdominal pain	7%	6%	7%
Anorexia	7%	8%	4%
Appetite increased	0%	0%	5%
Constipation	7%	7%	8%
Diarrhea	8%	7%	3%
Dry mouth	6%	4%	5%
Nausea	16%	20%	11%
Vomiting	9%	11%	6%
Metabolic			
Peripheral edema	5%	9%	11%
Weight gain	2%	4%	12%
Musculoskeletal			
Back pain	11%	11%	8%
Bone pain	6%	12%	8%
Respiratory			
Cough increased	8%	7%	8%
Dyspnea	9%	11%	21%
Pharyngitis	6%	9%	6%
Miscellaneous			
Chest pain	5%	7%	5%
Hot flashes	12%	11%	8%
Pain	11%	15%	11%
Pelvic pain	5%	7%	5%
Vaginal hemorrhage	2%	2%	5%

[a] A patient may have > 1 adverse reaction.

➤*Other less frequent (2% to 5%) adverse reactions:* Other less frequent (2% to 5%) adverse reactions reported in patients receiving anastrozole 1 mg in trial 0004 or trial 0005 are listed in the following.

Cardiovascular – Hypertension; thrombophlebitis.

CNS – Anxiety; confusion; insomnia; nervousness; somnolence.

Dermatologic – Hair thinning; pruritus.

GU – Breast pain; urinary tract infection.

Hematologic – Anemia; leukopenia.

Hepatic – ALT increased; AST increased; gamma-glutamyl transferase increased.

Metabolic/Nutritional – Alkaline phosphatase increased; weight loss.

Mean serum total cholesterol levels increased by 0.5 mmol/L among patients receiving anastrozole. Increases in low-density lipoprotein cholesterol have been shown to contribute to these changes.

Musculoskeletal – Arthralgia; myalgia; neck pain; pathological fracture.

Respiratory – Bronchitis; rhinitis; sinusitis.

Miscellaneous – Accidental injury; fever; flu syndrome; infection; malaise.

➤*Adverse reactions related to 1 or both of the therapies:* The incidences of the following adverse reaction groups potentially causally related to 1 or both of the therapies because of their pharmacology, were statistically analyzed: weight gain, edema, thromboembolic disease, GI disturbance, hot flushes, and vaginal dryness. These 6 groups, and the adverse reactions captured in the groups, were prospectively defined.

ANASTROZOLE — ORAL

Anastrozole Adverse Reactions Prespecified in Trials 0004 and 0005			
Adverse reaction	Anastrozole 1 mg (n = 262)	Anastrozole 10 mg (n = 246)	Megestrol acetate 160 mg (n = 253)
Metabolic			
Edema	7%	11%	14%
Weight gain	2%	4%	12%
Miscellaneous			
GI disturbance	29%	33%	21%
Hot flushes	13%	12%	14%
Thromboembolic disease	3%	2%	5%
Vaginal dryness	2%	1%	1%

➤*Postmarketing:* Hepatobiliary events, including increases in alkaline phosphatase, alanine aminotransferase, and aspartate aminotransferase have been reported commonly (more than 1% and less than 10%) and gamma-GT, bilirubin, and hepatitis have been reported uncommonly (more than 0.1% and less than 1%) in patients receiving anastrozole.

Anastrozole may also be associated with rash, including cases of mucocutaneous disorders, such as erythema multiforme and Stevens-Johnson syndrome.

Cases of allergic reactions, including angioedema, urticaria, and anaphylaxis, have been reported in patients receiving anastrozole.

Overdosage

➤*Animal toxicology:* Anastrozole can cause fetal harm when administered to a pregnant woman. Anastrozole has been found to cross the placenta following oral administration of 0.1 mg/kg in rats and rabbits (about 1 and 1.9 times the recommended human dose, respectively, on a mg/m^2 basis). Studies in both rats and rabbits at dosages greater than or equal to 0.1 and 0.02 mg/kg/day, respectively (about 1 and ⅓, respectively, the recommended human dose on a mg/m^2 basis), administered during the period of organogenesis showed that anastrozole increased pregnancy loss (increased pre- or postimplantation loss, increased resorption, and decreased numbers of live fetuses); effects were dose related in rats. Placental weights were significantly increased in rats at dosages of 0.1 mg/kg/day or more.

Evidence of fetotoxicity, including delayed fetal development (ie, incomplete ossification and depressed fetal body weights), was observed in rats administered dosages of 1 mg/kg/day (which produced plasma anastrozole $C_{ss\ max}$ and AUC_{0-24h} that were 19 times and 9 times higher than the respective values found in healthy postmenopausal humans at the recommended dose). There was no evidence of teratogenicity in rats administered dosages up to 1 mg/kg/day. In rabbits, anastrozole caused pregnancy failure at dosages equal to or greater than 1 mg/kg/day (about 16 times the recommended human dose on a mg/m^2 basis); there was no evidence of teratogenicity in rabbits administered 0.2 mg/kg/day (about 3 times the recommended human dose on a mg/m^2 basis).

Clinical trials have been conducted with anastrozole, up to 60 mg in a single dose given to healthy male volunteers and up to 10 mg daily given to postmenopausal women with advanced breast cancer; these dosages were well tolerated. A single dose of anastrozole that results in life-threatening symptoms has not been established.

➤*Treatment:* There is no specific antidote to overdosage and treatment must be symptomatic. In the management of an overdose, consider that multiple agents may have been taken. Dialysis may be helpful because anastrozole is not highly protein bound. General supportive care, including frequent monitoring of vital signs and close observation of the patient, is indicated.

Patient Information

Advise patients that anastrozole may cause fetal harm. Also advise them that anastrozole is not for use in premenopausal women; therefore, if they become pregnant, they should stop taking anastrozole and immediately contact their doctor.

Inform patients of the possibility of serious allergic reactions with swelling of the face, lips, tongue, and/or throat (angioedema), which may cause difficulty in swallowing and/or breathing and to immediately report this to their health care provider.

Inform patients with preexisting ischemic heart disease that an increased incidence of cardiovascular events has been observed with anastrozole use compared with tamoxifen use.

Inform patients that anastrozole lowers the level of estrogen. This may lead to a loss of the mineral content of bones, which might decrease bone strength. A possible consequence of decreased mineral content of bones is an increase in the risk of fractures.

Inform patients that an increased level of cholesterol might be seen while receiving anastrozole.

Advise patients not to take anastrozole with tamoxifen.

LETROZOLE

Rx	**Femara** (Novartis)	**Tablets; oral:** 2.5 mg	Lactose, PEG. (FV CG). Dark yellow, round. Film-coated. In 30s.

LETROZOLE — ORAL

Indications

➤*Breast cancer:* For the adjuvant treatment of postmenopausal women with hormone receptor–positive early breast cancer; for first-line treatment of postmenopausal women with hormone receptor–positive or hormone receptor–unknown locally advanced or metastatic breast cancer; for the treatment of advanced breast cancer in postmenopausal women with disease progression following antiestrogen therapy; for the extended adjuvant treatment of early breast cancer in postmenopausal women who have received 5 years of adjuvant tamoxifen therapy.

➤*Off-label uses:*

Delayed puberty in adolescent males – [4] = Insufficient documentation. The use of letrozole in delayed puberty has been studied by 1 group and results have been published in 3 different journals. Although growth benefits associated with estrogen inhibition may be valid, these results need to be confirmed in larger, long-term, controlled trials before routine use can be recommended in boys with delayed puberty. (See Administration and Dosage.)

Other possible off-label uses – For ovulation stimulation to improve the chances of pregnancy.

Administration and Dosage

➤*General dosing considerations:* Letrozole may reduce bone mineral density (BMD), increasing the risk of osteoporosis in postmenopausal women. Monitor BMD by dual energy x-ray absorptiometry (DEXA) bone scan at baseline and annually during therapy. Administer a bisphosphonate in patients with osteoporosis and monitor BMD closely in patients with osteopenia. Counsel all patients on osteoporosis prevention, including calcium and vitamin D supplements and weight-bearing exercise.

➤*Adults:*

Breast cancer –

Usual dosage: 2.5 mg once daily.

Duration of therapy: In patients with advanced disease, continue treatment with letrozole until tumor progression is evident.

In the extended adjuvant setting, the optimal treatment duration with letrozole is not known. The planned duration of treatment in the study was 5 years. In the final updated analysis conducted at a median follow-up of 62 months, the median treatment duration was 60 months. Seventy-one percent of patients were treated for at least 3 years and 58% of patients completed at least 4.5 years of extended adjuvant treatment.

Discontinuation of therapy: Treatment should be discontinued at tumor relapse.

➤*Children:*

Off-label dosing –

Delayed puberty in adolescent males: [4] = Insufficient documentation. 2.5 mg once daily for 1 year coadministered with 6 doses of testosterone enanthate (intramuscularly) given every 4 weeks.

➤*Hepatic function impairment:*

Severe hepatic impairment/cirrhosis – 2.5 mg administered every other day.

➤*Administration:* Take without regard to meals.

➤*Storage/Stability:* Store at 25°C (77°F); excursions are permitted between 15° and 30°C (59° and 86°F).

Actions

➤*Pharmacology:* Letrozole is a nonsteroidal competitive inhibitor of the aromatase enzyme system; it inhibits the conversion of androgens to estrogens. In adult nontumor- and tumor-bearing female animals, letrozole is as effective as an ovariectomy in reducing uterine weight, elevating serum luteinizing hormone, and causing the regression of estrogen-dependent tumors. In contrast to an ovariectomy, treatment with letrozole does not lead to an increase in serum follicle-stimulating hormone. Letrozole selectively inhibits gonadal steroidogenesis but has no significant effect on adrenal mineralocorticoid or glucocorticoid synthesis.

Letrozole inhibits the aromatase enzyme by competitively binding to the heme of the cytochrome P450 (CYP-450) subunit of the enzyme, resulting in a reduction of estrogen biosynthesis in all tissues. Treatment of women with letrozole significantly lowers serum estrone, estradiol, and estrone sulfate, and has not been shown to significantly affect adrenal corticosteroid synthesis, aldosterone synthesis, or synthesis of thyroid hormones.

➤*Pharmacokinetics:*

Absorption/Distribution – Letrozole is rapidly and completely absorbed from the GI tract. Steady-state plasma concentrations after daily 2.5 mg dosing is reached in 2 to 6 weeks. Plasma concentrations at steady state are 1.5 to 2 times higher than predicted from the concentrations measured after a single dose, indicating a slight nonlinearity in the pharmacokinetics upon daily administration of letrozole 2.5 mg. However, these steady-state levels are maintained over extended periods and continuous

LETROZOLE — ORAL

accumulation of letrozole does not occur. Letrozole is weakly protein bound and has a large volume of distribution (approximately 1.9 L/kg).

Metabolism/Excretion – The major pathway of letrozole clearance is metabolism to a pharmacologically inactive carbinol metabolite (4,4′-methanol-bisbenzonitrile) and renal excretion of the glucuronide conjugate of this metabolite. About 90% of radiolabeled letrozole is recovered in urine. Of the radiolabel drug recovered in urine, at least 75% was the glucuronide of the carbinol metabolite, approximately 9% was 2 unidentified metabolites, and 6% was unchanged letrozole. Letrozole's terminal elimination half-life is about 2 days.

In human microsomes with specific CYP isozyme activity, CYP3A4 metabolized letrozole to the carbinol metabolite, while CYP2A6 formed this metabolite and its ketone analog. In human liver microsomes, letrozole strongly inhibited CYP2A6 and moderately inhibited CYP2C19.

Special populations –

Hepatic function impairment: In a study of subjects with mild to moderate nonmetastatic hepatic dysfunction (eg, cirrhosis, Child-Pugh class A and B), the mean area under the curve (AUC) values of the volunteers with moderate hepatic impairment were 37% higher than in healthy subjects, but still within the range seen in subjects without impaired function. In a pharmacokinetics study, subjects with liver cirrhosis and severe hepatic impairment (Child-Pugh class C, which included bilirubins about 2 to 11 times the upper limit of normal [ULN] with minimal to severe ascites) had 2-fold increases in exposure (AUC) and a 47% reduction in systemic clearance. Breast cancer patients with severe hepatic impairment are thus expected to be exposed to higher levels of letrozole than patients with healthy liver function receiving similar doses of this drug.

Contraindications

Women who are or may become pregnant.

Warnings/Precautions

➤*Bone effects:* Use of letrozole may cause decreases in BMD. Results of a substudy to evaluate safety in the adjuvant setting comparing the effect on lumbar spine (L2-L4) BMD of adjuvant treatment of letrozole with that of tamoxifen showed at 24 months a median decrease in lumbar spine BMD of 4.1% in the letrozole arm compared with a median increase of 0.3% in the tamoxifen arm (difference of 4.4%) (*P*

In the adjuvant trial, the incidence of bone fractures at any time after randomization was 13.8% for letrozole and 10.5% for tamoxifen. The incidence of osteoporosis was 5.1% for letrozole and 2.7% for tamoxifen. In the extended adjuvant trial, the incidence of bone fractures at any time after randomization was 13.3% for letrozole and 7.8% for placebo. The incidence of new osteoporosis was 14.5% for letrozole and 7.8% for placebo.

➤*Cholesterol:* In the adjuvant trial, hypercholesterolemia was reported in 52.3% of letrozole patients and 28.6% of tamoxifen patients. Common Toxicity Criteria (CTC) grade 3 to 4 hypercholesterolemia was reported in 0.4% of letrozole patients and 0.1% of tamoxifen patients. Also in the adjuvant setting, an increase of at least 1.5 times the ULN in total cholesterol (generally nonfasting) was observed in patients on monotherapy who had baseline total serum cholesterol within the normal range (ie, less than 1.5 times the ULN) in 8.2% on letrozole versus 3.2%. Lipid-lowering medications were required for 25% of patients on letrozole and 16% on tamoxifen.

➤*Hepatic function impairment:* See Actions for more information.

➤*Hazardous tasks:* Because fatigue, dizziness, and somnolence have been reported with the use of letrozole, caution is advised when driving or using machinery until it is known how the patient reacts to letrozole use.

➤*Pregnancy: Category X.* Letrozole may cause fetal harm when administered to a pregnant woman and the clinical benefit to premenopausal women with breast cancer has not been demonstrated. Letrozole is contraindicated in women who are or may become pregnant. If this drug is used during pregnancy or if the patient becomes pregnant while taking this drug, apprise the patient of the potential hazard to a fetus.

Letrozole caused adverse pregnancy outcomes, including congenital malformations, in rats and rabbits at doses much smaller than the daily maximum recommended human dose (MRHD) on a mg/m^2 basis. Effects included increased postimplantation pregnancy loss and resorptions, fewer live fetuses, and fetal malformations affecting the renal and skeletal systems. Animal data and letrozole's mechanism of action raise concerns that letrozole could be a human teratogen as well.

Reproduction studies in rats showed embryo and fetal toxicity at letrozole doses during organogenesis equal to or greater than 1/100 the daily MRHD on a mg/m^2 basis. Adverse effects included intrauterine mortality; increased resorptions and postimplantation loss; decreased numbers of live fetuses; and fetal anomalies, including absence and shortening of renal papilla, dilation of ureter, edema, and incomplete ossification of frontal skull and metatarsals. Letrozole doses 1/10 the daily MRHD (mg/m^2 basis) caused fetal domed head and cervical/centrum vertebral fusion. In rabbits, letrozole caused embryo and fetal toxicity at doses about 1/100,000 and 1/10,000 the daily MRHD (mg/m^2 basis), respectively. Fetal anomalies included incomplete ossification of the skull, sternebrae, and fore- and hind legs.

Discuss the need for adequate contraception with women who are recently menopausal. Advise patients to use contraception until postmenopausal status is clinically well-established.

➤*Lactation:* It is not known if letrozole is excreted in human milk. Letrozole has a very long half-life, which is concerning in a breast-feeding infant and could lead to higher plasma levels over time. The transfer of small amounts of letrozole to an infant could seriously impair bone growth or sexual development.

Because many drugs are excreted in human milk and because of the potential for serious adverse reactions from letrozole in breast-feeding infants, make a decision whether to discontinue breast-feeding or the drug, taking into account the importance of the drug to the mother.

➤*Children:* Safety and efficacy in children have not been established.

➤*Elderly:* The median age of patients in all studies of first- and second-line treatment for metastatic breast cancer was 64 to 65 years of age. About one-third of the patients were 70 years of age and older. In the first-line study, patients 70 years of age and older experienced longer time to tumor progression and higher response rates than patients younger than 70 years of age.

➤*Lab test abnormalities:* No dose-related effect of letrozole on any hematologic or clinical chemistry parameter was evident. Moderate decreases in lymphocyte counts, of uncertain clinical significance, were observed in some patients receiving letrozole 2.5 mg. This depression was transient in about half of those affected. Two patients on letrozole developed thrombocytopenia; the relationship to the study drug was unclear. Whether related to study treatment or not, patient withdrawal because of laboratory abnormalities was infrequent.

➤*Monitoring:* Monitor BMD by DEXA bone scan at baseline and annually during therapy. Monitor BMD closely in patients with osteopenia. Monitor serum cholesterol. Closely monitor for clinical and laboratory signs of reduced letrozole antitumor effects in patients taking letrozole immediately after tamoxifen.

Drug Interactions

➤*Tamoxifen:* Coadministration of letrozole and tamoxifen 20 mg daily resulted in a reduction of letrozole plasma levels by 38% on average. Clinical experience in the second-line breast cancer pivotal trials indicates that the therapeutic effect of letrozole therapy is not impaired if letrozole is administered immediately after tamoxifen. Closely monitor for clinical and laboratory signs of reduced letrozole antitumor effects.

Adverse Reactions

➤*Adjuvant treatment of early breast cancer:*

Adverse reactions (grades 1 to 4) –

Letrozole Adverse Reactions in Adjuvant Treatment of Early Breast Cancer[a]

Adverse reactions	Grades 1 to 4		Grades 3 to 4	
	Letrozole (n = 2,448)	Tamoxifen (n = 2,447)	Letrozole (n = 2,448)	Tamoxifen (n = 2,447)
Any adverse reaction	94.4%	90.5%	25.9%	24.7%
Cardiovascular				
Angina[b]	1.1%	1%	–	–
Angina[c]	1.3%	1.3%	–	–
Cerebrovascular accident[b]	2.1%	1.9%	–	–
Cerebrovascular accident[c]	2.9%	2.6%	–	–
Hot flashes/flushes	33.5%	38%	0	0
Myocardial infarction[b]	1%	0.5%	–	–
Myocardial infarction[c]	1.5%	1%	–	–
Myocardial ischemia	0.2%	0.4%	–	–
Other cardiovascular[b]	0.6%	10.5%	–	–
Other cardiovascular[c]	12.7%	13.8%	–	–
Thromboembolic event[b]	2.1%	3.6%	–	–
Thromboembolic event[c]	2.9%	4.5%	–	–
CNS				
Depression	4.9%	4.7%	0.7%	0.6%
Dizziness/light-headedness	3.4%	3.4%	< 0.1%	0.2%
Fatigue (lethargy, malaise, asthenia)	9.6%	10.2%	0.2%	0.3%
Headache	4.3%	3.8%	0.4%	0.2%
GI				
Anorexia	0.8%	0.8%	< 0.1%	< 0.1%
Constipation	2%	2.9%	0.1%	< 0.1%
Nausea	11.6%	11.3%	0.2%	0.4%
Vomiting	3.3%	3.3%	0.1%	0.2%

LETROZOLE — ORAL

Letrozole Adverse Reactions in Adjuvant Treatment of Early Breast Cancer[a]				
	Grades 1 to 4		Grades 3 to 4	
Adverse reactions	Letrozole (n = 2,448)	Tamoxifen (n = 2,447)	Letrozole (n = 2,448)	Tamoxifen (n = 2,447)
GU				
Breast pain	1.5%	1.8%	< 1%	0
Endometrial hyperplasia/ cancer[c,d]	0.6%	3.6%	–	–
Endometrial hyperplasia/ cancer[b,d]	0.3%	2.9%	–	–
Endometrial proliferation disorders	0.3%	1.8%	0	0.6%
Other endometrial disorders	< 0.1%	0.1%	0	0
Vaginal bleeding	5.2%	13.1%	< 0.1%	0.3%
Vaginal irritation	4.5%	3.1%	< 0.1%	< 0.1%
Metabolic				
Edema	6.7%	6.5%	0.1%	< 0.1%
Weight decrease	5.7%	5.3%	0.3%	0.2%
Weight increase	12.9%	15.4%	1.1%	1.6%
Musculoskeletal				
Arthralgia/Arthritis	25.2%	20.4%	3.5%	2%
Back pain	5.1%	5.6%	0.3%	0.4%
Bone fractures[b]	10.1%	7.1%	–	–
Bone fractures[c]	13.8%	10.5%	–	–
Bone pain	5%	4.5%	0.2%	0.2%
Myalgia	8.9%	8.7%	0.7%	0.6%
Osteopenia	3.6%	3%	0	< 0.1%
Osteoporosis NOS[e]	5.1%	2.7%	0.4%	0.2%
Miscellaneous				
Alopecia	3.4%	3.4%	0	0
Cataract	2%	2.2%	0.7%	0.7%
Hypercholesterol-emia	52.3%	28.6%	0.4%	0.2%
Night sweats	14.6%	17.4%	0	0
Pain in extremity	4.2%	3.2%	0.2%	0.2%
Second malignancies[b]	2.2%	3.2%	–	–
Second malignancies[c]	4.2%	34.9%	–	–

[a] Cardiovascular (including cerebrovascular and thromboembolic), skeletal, and urogenital/endometrial reactions and second malignancies were collected lifelong. All of these reactions were assumed to be of CTC grade 3 through 5 and were not individually graded.
[b] During study treatment, based on safety monotherapy population.
[c] Any time after randomization, including post-treatment follow-up.
[d] Excluding women who had undergone hysterectomy before study entry.
[e] NOS = not otherwise specified.

Adverse reactions (all grades) – When considering all grades during study treatment, a higher incidence of reactions was seen for letrozole regarding fractures (10.1% vs 7.1%), myocardial infarctions (1% vs 0.5%), and arthralgia (25.2% vs 20.4%) (letrozole vs tamoxifen, respectively). A higher incidence was seen for tamoxifen regarding thromboembolic reactions (2.1% vs 3.6%), endometrial hyperplasia/cancer (0.3% vs 2.9%), and endometrial proliferative disorders (0.3% vs 1.8%) (letrozole vs tamoxifen, respectively).

At a median follow-up of 73 months, a higher incidence of reactions was seen for letrozole (13.8%) than for tamoxifen (10.5%) regarding fractures. A higher incidence was seen for tamoxifen compared with letrozole regarding thromboembolic reactions (4.5% vs 2.9%), and endometrial hyperplasia or cancer (2.9% vs 0.4%) (tamoxifen vs letrozole, respectively).

Musculoskeletal – Results of a phase 3 safety trial in 262 postmenopausal women with resected receptor-positive early breast cancer in the adjuvant setting comparing the effect on lumbar spine (L2-L4) BMD of adjuvant treatment with letrozole compared with tamoxifen showed at 24 months a median decrease in lumbar spine BMD of 4.1% in the letrozole arm compared with a median increase of 0.3% in the tamoxifen arm (difference of 4.4%) (*P*

Lipids – In a phase 3 safety trial in 262 postmenopausal women with resected receptor-positive early breast cancer at 24 months comparing the effects on lipid profiles of adjuvant letrozole with tamoxifen, 12% of patients on letrozole had at least 1 total cholesterol value of a higher CTC for Adverse Events grade than at baseline compared with 4% of patients on tamoxifen.

➤*Extended adjuvant treatment of early breast cancer:*

Letrozole Adverse Reactions (≥ 5%) in Extended Adjuvant Treatment of Early Breast Cancer				
	Grade 1 to 4		Grade 3 to 4	
Adverse reactions	Letrozole (n = 2,563)	Placebo (n = 2,573)	Letrozole (n = 2,563)	Placebo (n = 2,573)
CNS	33.7%	31.8%	2.5%	2.3%
Asthenia	33.6%	32.1%	0.6%	0.3%
Dizziness	14.2%	13.3%	0.4%	0.2%
Headache	20.1%	19.7%	0.7%	0.7%
Insomnia	5.8%	4.7%	< 0.1%	< 0.1%
Psychiatric disorders	12.5%	10.7%	0.8%	0.6%
Dermatologic	32.4%	30.6%	0.7%	0.6%
Increased sweating	24.2%	22.4%	< 0.1%	0
GI	28.3%	28.4%	1.7%	1.6%
Constipation	11.3%	11.8%	0.2%	< 0.1%
Diarrhea NOS	5%	5.6%	0.5%	0.3%
Nausea	8.6%	8.2%	0.1%	0.4%
GU	11.8%	13.9%	0.4%	0.3%
Vaginal hemorrhage	4.8%	6.6%	< 0.1%	0.2%
Vulvovaginal dryness	5.3%	4.9%	0	0
Musculoskeletal	38.2%	32.5%	2.8%	1.9%
Arthralgia	22%	18.1%	1%	0.8%
Arthritis NOS	6.7%	4.8%	0.4%	0.2%
Back pain	5%	4.4%	0.3%	0.3%
Myalgia	6.7%	4.7%	0.3%	0.2%
Metabolic/Nutritional	21.5%	20.9%	0.9%	1.2%
Edema NOS	18.4%	16.2%	0.2%	0.1%
Hypercholesterolemia	15.6%	15.5%	< 0.1%	0.2%
Respiratory	10.9%	10.1%	1.2%	1.1%
Dyspnea	5.5%	5.3%	0.8%	0.7%
Miscellaneous	45%	42.4%	1.2%	1.1%
Any adverse reaction	87.1%	84.5%	16.3%	15.1%
Flushing	49.7%	43.3%	0.1%	0
Infections and infestations	6.5%	6.3%	1.6%	1.3%
Investigations	7.2%	5.7%	0.5%	0.5%
Renal disorders	5.1%	3.9%	0.5%	0.2%
Vascular disorders	53.6%	47.8%	2.3%	2.9%

Musculoskeletal – Based on a median follow-up of patients for 28 months, the incidence of clinical fractures from the core randomized study in patients who received letrozole was 5.9% and 5.5% with placebo. The incidence of self-reported osteoporosis was higher in patients who received letrozole (6.9%) than in patients who received placebo (5.5%). Bisphosphonates were administered to 21.1% of the patients who received letrozole and 18.7% of the patients who received placebo.

Cardiovascular – The incidence of cardiovascular ischemic reactions from the core randomized study was comparable between patients who received letrozole (6.8%) and placebo (6.5%).

GU – A patient-reported measure that captures treatment impact on important symptoms associated with estrogen deficiency demonstrated a difference in favor of placebo for vasomotor and sexual symptom domains.

Updated analysis, extended adjuvant treatment of early breast cancer –

Musculoskeletal: During treatment or within 30 days of stopping treatment (median duration of treatment, 60 months), a higher rate of fractures was observed for letrozole (10.4%) compared with placebo (5.8%), and also a higher rate of osteoporosis (letrozole 12.2% vs placebo 6.4%).

Based on 62 months median duration of follow-up in the randomized letrozole arm in the safety population, the incidence of new fractures at any time after randomization was 13.3% for letrozole and 7.8% for placebo. The incidence of new osteoporosis was 14.5% for letrozole and 7.8% for placebo.

Cardiovascular: During treatment or within 30 days of stopping treatment (median duration of treatment, 60 months) the incidence of cardiovascular events was 9.8% for letrozole and 7% for placebo.

Based on 62 months median duration of follow-up in the randomized letrozole arm in the safety population, the incidence of cardiovascular disease at any time after randomization was 14.4% for letrozole and 9.8% for placebo.

➤*Advanced breast cancer:*

First-line treatment –

Most frequent adverse reactions: The most frequently reported adverse reactions were arthralgia, back pain, bone pain, dyspnea, hot flushes, and nausea.

LETROZOLE — ORAL

Discontinuation: Discontinuations for adverse reactions other than progression of tumor occurred in 2% of patients on letrozole and in 3% of patients on tamoxifen.

Adverse reactions (5% or more):

Letrozole Adverse Reactions (> 5%) as First-Line Treatment in Advanced Breast Cancer

Adverse reactions	Letrozole 2.5 mg (n = 455)	Tamoxifen 20 mg (n = 455)
Cardiovascular		
Hot flushes	19%	16%
Hypertension	8%	4%
CNS		
Fatigue	13%	13%
Headache NOS	8%	7%
Insomnia	7%	4%
Weakness	6%	4%
GI		
Anorexia	4%	6%
Constipation	10%	11%
Diarrhea	8%	4%
Nausea	17%	17%
Vomiting	7%	8%
GU		
Breast pain	7%	7%
Postmastectomy lymphedema	7%	7%
Urinary tract infection NOS	6%	3%
Metabolic		
Decreased weight	7%	5%
Peripheral edema	5%	6%
Musculoskeletal		
Arthralgia	16%	15%
Back pain	18%	19%
Bone pain	22%	21%
Limb pain	10%	8%
Respiratory		
Chest wall pain	6%	6%
Cough	13%	13%
Dyspnea	18%	17%
Miscellaneous		
Chest pain	8%	9%
Influenza	6%	4%
Pain NOS	5%	7%

Adverse reactions (less than 2%):

- *Cardiovascular* – Angina, coronary heart disease, myocardial infarction, myocardial ischemia, portal vein thrombosis, pulmonary embolism, thrombophlebitis, thrombotic or hemorrhagic strokes, transient ischemic attacks, venous thrombosis.
- *CNS* – Development of hemiparesis.

Second-line treatment – There were fewer thromboembolic reactions at both letrozole doses than on the megestrol acetate arm (0.6% vs 4.7%). There also was less vaginal bleeding (0.3% vs 3.2%) on letrozole than on megestrol.

Discontinuation: Study discontinuations in the megestrol comparison study for adverse reactions other than progression of tumor occurred in 2.7% of patients on letrozole 0.5 mg, in 2.3% of patients on letrozole 2.5 mg, and in 7.9% of patients on megestrol. In the aminoglutethimide comparison study, discontinuations for reasons other than progression occurred in 3.1% of patients on letrozole 0.5 mg, 3.8% of patients on letrozole 2.5 mg, and 3.9% of patients on aminoglutethimide.

Adverse reactions (5% or more):

Letrozole Adverse Reactions (5% or more) as Second-Line Treatment in Advanced Breast Cancer

Adverse reactions	Pooled letrozole 2.5 mg (n = 359)	Pooled letrozole 0.5 mg (n = 380)	Megestrol 160 mg (n = 189)	Aminoglutethimide 500 mg (n = 178)
Cardiovascular				
Hot flushes	6%	5%	4%	3%
Hypertension	5%	7%	5%	6%
CNS				
Asthenia	4%	5%	4%	5%
Dizziness	3%	5%	7%	3%
Fatigue	8%	6%	11%	3%
Headache	9%	12%	9%	7%
Somnolence	3%	2%	2%	9%
Dermatologic				
Pruritus	1%	2%	5%	3%
Rash[a]	5%	4%	3%	12%
GI				
Abdominal pain	6%	5%	9%	8%
Anorexia	5%	3%	5%	5%
Constipation	6%	7%	9%	7%
Diarrhea	6%	5%	3%	4%
Dyspepsia	3%	4%	6%	5%
Nausea	13%	15%	9%	14%
Vomiting	7%	7%	5%	9%
Metabolic				
Hypercholesterolemia	3%	3%	0%	6%
Peripheral edema[b]	5%	5%	8%	3%
Weight increase	2%	2%	9%	3%
Musculoskeletal				
Arthralgia	8%	8%	8%	3%
Musculoskeletal pain[c]	21%	22%	30%	14%
Respiratory				
Coughing	6%	5%	7%	5%
Dyspnea	7%	9%	16%	5%
Miscellaneous				
Chest pain	6%	3%	7%	3%
Viral infection	6%	5%	6%	3%

[a] Includes rash, erythematous rash, maculopapular rash, psoriaform rash, vesicular rash.
[b] Includes peripheral edema, leg edema, dependent edema, edema.
[c] Includes musculoskeletal pain, skeletal pain, back pain, arm pain, leg pain.

Adverse reactions (less than 5%):

- *CNS* – Anxiety, depression, vertigo.
- *Dermatologic* – Alopecia, increased sweating.
- *Miscellaneous* – Fracture, hypercalcemia, pleural effusion.

First- and second-line treatment –

CNS: Dysesthesia (including hypesthesia/paresthesia), irritability, memory impairment, nervousness.

Cardiovascular: Arterial thrombosis, cardiac failure, palpitations, tachycardia.

GU: Increased urinary frequency, vaginal discharge.

Special senses: Cataract, disturbances of taste and thirst, eye irritation.

Miscellaneous: Appetite increase, dryness of skin and mucosa (including dry mouth), leukopenia, pyrexia, stomatitis cancer pain, urticaria.

➤*Postmarketing:*

Dermatologic – Erythema multiforme, toxic epidermal necrolysis.

Hepatic – Hepatitis, increased hepatic enzymes.

Hypersensitivity – Anaphylactic reactions, angioedema.

Special senses – Blurred vision.

Overdosage

➤*Animal toxicology:* Lethality was observed in mice and rats following single oral doses of 2,000 mg/kg or more (approximately 4,000 to 8,000 times the daily MRHD on a mg/m^2 basis); death was associated with reduced motor activity, ataxia, and dyspnea. Lethality was observed in cats following single intravenous doses of 10 mg/kg or more (approximately 50 times the daily MRHD on a mg/m^2 basis); death was preceded by depressed blood pressure and arrhythmias.

➤*Treatment:* Because of the limited data available, no firm recommendations for treatment can be made. In general, supportive care and frequent monitoring of vital signs are appropriate.

Patient Information

Inform patients of the necessity of adequate contraception in women who have the potential to become pregnant, including women who are perimenopausal or who recently became postmenopausal, until their postmenopausal status is fully established.

Advise patients that fatigue and dizziness have been observed with the use of letrozole and somnolence was uncommonly reported; therefore, caution is advised when driving or using machinery.

Inform patients that they may require BMD monitoring.

EXEMESTANE

Rx	**Aromasin** (Pharmacia & Upjohn)	**Tablets:** 25 mg	Mannitol, methylparaben, polyvinyl alcohol. (7663). Off-white to gray. Biconvex. In 30s.

EXEMESTANE — ORAL

Indications

➤*Breast cancer:* For the treatment of advanced breast cancer in postmenopausal women whose disease has progressed following tamoxifen therapy.

➤*Off-label uses:*

Breast cancer prevention – [4] = Insufficient documentation. Although results were considered too preliminary for the American Society of Clinical Oncology to recommend the routine use of exemestane for breast cancer chemoprevention, the available information on aromatase inhibitors and inactivators is encouraging. Exemestane may have the potential to offer improved efficacy in preventing breast cancer, coupled with a more favorable safety profile, relative to tamoxifen. Ongoing studies are needed to establish the role of exemestane in breast cancer chemoprevention.

Other possible off-label uses – Prevention of prostate carcinogenesis.

Administration and Dosage

➤*Adults:*

Breast cancer –

Usual dosage: 25 mg once daily after a meal.

Duration of therapy: Treatment should continue until tumor progression is evident.

Off-label dosing –

Breast cancer prevention: [4] = Insufficient documentation. 25 mg/day orally for 5 years.

➤*Preparation for administration:* Exemestane is a hormonal agent and is considered a potential teratogen. Follow safe handling procedures when preparing, administering, or dispensing exemestane.

➤*Administration:* Take after a meal to increase absorption.

➤*Storage/Stability:* Store at 25°C (77°F); excursions permitted between 15° and 30°C (59° and 86°F).

Actions

➤*Pharmacology:* Breast cancer cell growth may be estrogen-dependent. Exemestane is the principal enzyme that converts androgens to estrogens both in pre- and postmenopausal women. While the main source of estrogen (primarily estradiol) is the ovary in premenopausal women, the principal source of circulating estrogens in postmenopausal women is from conversion of adrenal and ovarian androgens (androstenedione and testosterone) to estrogens (estrone and estradiol) by the aromatase enzyme in peripheral tissues. Estrogen deprivation through aromatase inhibition is an effective and selective treatment for some postmenopausal patients with hormone-dependent breast cancer.

Exemestane is an irreversible, steroidal aromatase inactivator, structurally related to the natural substrate androstenedione. It acts as a false substrate for the aromatase enzyme, and is processed to an intermediate that binds irreversibly to the active site of the enzyme causing its inactivation, an effect also known as "suicide inhibition." Exemestane significantly lowers circulating estrogen concentrations in postmenopausal women, but has no detectable effect on adrenal biosynthesis of corticosteroids or aldosterone. Exemestane has no effect on other enzymes involved in the steroidogenic pathway up to a concentration at least 600 times higher than that inhibiting the aromatase enzyme.

➤*Pharmacokinetics:*

Absorption – Following oral administration to healthy postmenopausal women, exemestane is rapidly absorbed. The pharmacokinetics of exemestane are dose proportional after single (10 to 200 mg) or repeated oral doses (0.5 to 50 mg). Following repeated daily doses of exemestane 25 mg, plasma concentrations of unchanged drug are similar to levels measured after a single dose.

Pharmacokinetic parameters in postmenopausal women with advanced breast cancer following single or repeated doses have been compared with those in healthy, postmenopausal women. Exemestane appeared to be more rapidly absorbed in the women with breast cancer than in the healthy women, with a mean T_{max} of 1.2 hours in the women with breast cancer and 2.9 hours in the healthy women. After repeated dosing, the average oral clearance in women with advanced breast cancer was 45% lower than the oral clearance in healthy postmenopausal women, with corresponding higher systemic exposure. Mean AUC values following repeated doses in women with breast cancer (75.4 ng•hr/mL) were about twice those in healthy women (41.4 ng•hr/mL).

Following oral administration of radiolabeled exemestane, at least 42% of radioactivity was absorbed from the gastrointestinal tract. Exemestane plasma levels increased by approximately 40% after a high-fat breakfast.

Distribution – Exemestane is extensively distributed and is cleared from the systemic circulation primarily by metabolism.

Exemestane is distributed extensively into tissues. Exemestane is 90% bound to plasma proteins and the fraction bound is independent of the total concentration. Albumin and α_1-acid glycoprotein both contribute to the binding. The distribution of exemestane and its metabolites into blood cells is negligible.

Metabolism/Excretion – After maximum plasma concentration is reached, levels decline polyexponentially with a mean terminal half-life of about 24 hours.

Following administration of radiolabeled exemestane to healthy postmenopausal women, the cumulative amounts of radioactivity excreted in urine and feces were similar (42 ± 3% in urine and 42 ± 6% in feces over a 1-week collection period). The amount of drug excreted unchanged in urine was less than 1% of the dose.

Exemestane is extensively metabolized, with levels of the unchanged drug in plasma accounting for less than 10% of the total radioactivity. The initial steps in the metabolism of exemestane are oxidation of the methylene group in position 6 and reduction of the 17-keto group with subsequent formation of many secondary metabolites. Each metabolite accounts only for a limited amount of drug-related material. The metabolites are inactive or inhibit aromatase with decreased potency compared with the parent drug. One metabolite may have androgenic activity. Studies using human liver preparations indicate that cytochrome P450 3A4 (CYP3A4) is the principal isoenzyme involved in the oxidation of exemestane.

Special populations –

Renal function impairment: See Warnings/Precautions for more information.

Hepatic function impairment: See Warnings/Precautions for more information.

Contraindications

Hypersensitivity to the drug or to any of the excipients.

Warnings/Precautions

➤*Premenopausal women:* Exemestane tablets should not be administered to premenopausal women. Exemestane should not be coadministered with estrogen-containing agents as these could interfere with its pharmacologic action.

➤*Renal function impairment:* The AUC of exemestane after a single 25 mg dose was approximately 3 times higher in subjects with moderate or severe renal insufficiency (creatinine clearance less than 35 mL/min/1.73 m^2) compared with the AUC in healthy volunteers. The safety of chronic dosing in patients with moderate or severe renal impairment has not been studied. Based on experience with exemestane at repeated doses up to 200 mg daily that demonstrated a moderate increase in non-life threatening adverse events, dosage adjustment does not appear to be necessary.

➤*Hepatic function impairment:* The pharmacokinetics of exemestane have been investigated in subjects with moderate or severe hepatic insufficiency (Childs-Pugh class B or C). Following a single 25 mg oral dose, the AUC of exemestane was approximately 3 times higher than that observed in healthy volunteers. The safety of chronic dosing in patients with moderate or severe hepatic impairment has not been studied. Based on experience with exemestane at repeated doses up to 200 mg daily that demonstrated a moderate increase in non-life threatening adverse events, dosage adjustment does not appear to be necessary.

➤*Pregnancy: Category D.* Exemestane tablets may cause fetal harm when administered to a pregnant woman. Radioactivity related to ^{14}C-exemestane crossed the placenta of rats following oral administration of 1 mg/kg exemestane. The concentration of exemestane and its metabolites was approximately equivalent in maternal and fetal blood. When rats were administered exemestane from 14 days prior to mating until either days 15 or 20 of gestation, and resuming for the 21 days of lactation, an increase in placental weight was seen at 4 mg/kg/day (approximately 1.5 times the recommended human daily dose on a mg/m^2 basis). Prolonged gestation and abnormal or difficult labor was observed at doses greater than or equal to 20 mg/kg/day. Increased resorption, reduced number of live fetuses, decreased fetal weight, and retarded ossification were also observed at these doses. No malformations were noted when exemestane was administered to pregnant rats during the organogenesis period at doses up to 810 mg/kg/day (approximately 320 times the recommended human dose on a mg/m^2 basis). Daily doses of exemestane, given to rabbits during organogenesis caused a decrease in placental weight at 90 mg/kg/day (approximately 70 times the recommended human daily dose on a mg/m^2 basis). Abortions, an increase in resorptions, and a reduction in fetal body weight were seen at 270 mg/kg/day. There was no increase in the incidence of malformations in rabbits at doses up to 270 mg/kg/day (approximately 210 times the recommended human dose on a mg/m^2 basis).

There are no studies in pregnant women using exemestane. Exemestane is indicated for postmenopausal women. If there is exposure to exemestane during pregnancy, the patient should be apprised of the potential hazard to the fetus and potential risk for loss of the pregnancy.

➤*Lactation:* Exemestane is only indicated in postmenopausal women. However, radioactivity related to exemestane appeared in rat milk within 15 minutes of oral administration of radiolabeled exemestane. Concentrations of exemestane and its metabolites were approximately equivalent in the milk and plasma of rats for 24 hours after a single oral dose of 1 mg/kg ^{14}C-exemestane. It is not known whether exemestane is excreted in human milk. Because many drugs are excreted in human milk, caution should be exercised if a nursing woman is inadvertently exposed to exemestane.

EXEMESTANE — ORAL

➤*Children:* The safety and effectiveness of exemestane in pediatric patients have not been established.

➤*Lab test abnormalities:* Approximately 20% of patients receiving exemestane in clinical studies experienced common toxicity criteria (CTC) grade 3 or 4 lymphocytopenia. Of these patients, 89% had a preexisting lower grade lymphopenia. Forty percent of patients either recovered or improved to a lesser severity while on treatment. Patients did not have a significant increase in viral infections, and no opportunistic infections were observed. Elevations of serum levels of AST, ALT, alkaline phosphatase, and gamma glutamyl transferase greater than 5 times the upper value of the healthy range (ie, greater than or equal to CTC grade 3) have been rarely reported but appear mostly attributable to the underlying presence of liver or bone metastases. In the comparative study, CTC grade 3 or 4 elevation of gamma glutamyl transferase without documented evidence of liver metastasis was reported in 2.7% of patients treated with exemestane and in 1.8% of patients treated with megestrol acetate.

Adverse Reactions

A total of 1058 patients were treated with exemestane 25 mg once daily in the clinical trials program. Exemestane was generally well tolerated, and adverse events were usually mild to moderate. Only 1 death was considered possibly related to treatment with exemestane; an 80-year-old woman with known coronary artery disease had a myocardial infarction with multiple organ failure after 9 weeks on study treatment. In the clinical trials program, only 3% of the patients discontinued treatment with exemestane because of adverse events, mainly within the first 10 weeks of treatment; late discontinuations because of adverse events were uncommon (0.3%).

In the comparative study, adverse reactions were assessed for 358 patients treated with exemestane and 400 patients treated with megestrol acetate. Fewer patients receiving exemestane discontinued treatment because of adverse events than those treated with megestrol acetate (2% vs 5%). Adverse events that were considered drug related or of indeterminate cause included hot flashes (13% vs 5%), nausea (9% vs 5%), fatigue (8% vs 10%), increased sweating (4% vs 8%), and increased appetite (3% vs 6%). The proportion of patients experiencing an excessive weight gain (greater than 10% of their baseline weight) was significantly higher with megestrol acetate than with exemestane (17% versus 8%). The data below shows the adverse events of all CTC grades, regardless of causality, reported in 5% or greater of patients in the study treated either with exemestane or megestrol acetate.

Exemestane Adverse Reactions (≥ 5%)		
Adverse reaction	Exemestane 25 mg once daily (n = 358)	Megestrol acetate 40 mg 4 times/day (n = 400)
Autonomic nervous system		
Increased sweating	6	9
Cardiovascular		
Hypertension	5	6
CNS		
Depression	13	9
Insomnia	11	9
Anxiety	10	11
Dizziness	8	6
Headache	8	7
GI		
Nausea	18	12
Vomiting	7	4
Abdominal pain	6	11
Anorexia	6	5
Constipation	5	8
Diarrhea	4	5
Increased appetite	3	6
Respiratory		
Dyspnea	10	15
Coughing	6	7
Miscellaneous		
Fatigue	22	29
Hot flashes	13	6
Pain	13	13
Influenza-like symptoms	6	5
Edema (includes edema, peripheral edema, leg edema)	7	6

[a] Graded according to Common Toxicity Criteria.

➤*Less frequent adverse events (from 2% to 5%):* Less frequent adverse events of any cause (from 2% to 5%) reported in the comparative study for patients receiving exemestane 25 mg once daily were fever, generalized weakness, paresthesia, pathological fracture; bronchitis, sinusitis, rash, itching, urinary tract infection, and lymphedema.

➤*Additional adverse events:* Additional adverse events of any cause observed in the overall clinical trials program (n = 1058) in 5% or greater of patients treated with exemestane 25 mg once daily but not in the comparative study included the following: Pain at tumor sites (8%), asthenia (6%), and fever (5%). Adverse events of any cause reported in 2% to 5% of all patients treated with exemestane 25 mg in the overall clinical trials program but not in the comparative study included the following: Chest pain, hypoesthesia, confusion, dyspepsia, arthralgia, back pain, skeletal pain, infection, upper respiratory tract infection, pharyngitis, rhinitis, and alopecia.

Overdosage

Clinical trials have been conducted with exemestane given as a single dose to healthy female volunteers at doses as high as 800 mg and daily for 12 weeks to postmenopausal women with advanced breast cancer at doses as high as 600 mg. These dosages were well tolerated. There is no specific antidote to overdosage and treatment must be symptomatic. General supportive care, including frequent monitoring of vital signs and close observation of the patient, is indicated.

A male child (age unknown) accidentally ingested a 25 mg tablet of exemestane. The initial physical examination was normal, but blood tests performed 1 hour after ingestion indicated leucocytosis (WBC 25,000/mm^3 with 90% neutrophils). Blood tests were repeated 4 days after the incident and were healthy. No treatment was given.

In mice, mortality was observed after a single oral dose of exemestane of 3200 mg/kg, the lowest dose tested (about 640 times the recommended human dose on a mg/m^2 basis). In rats and dogs, mortality was observed after single oral doses of exemestane of 5000 mg/kg (about 2000 times the recommended human dose on a mg/m^2 basis) and 3000 mg/kg (about 4000 times the recommended human dose on a mg/m^2 basis), respectively.

Convulsions were observed after single doses of exemestane of 400 mg/kg and 3000 mg/kg in mice and dogs (≈ 80 and 4000 times the recommended human dose on a mg/m^2 basis), respectively.

ENZYMES

ASPARAGINASE

Rx	Elspar (Lundbeck)	Injection, lyophilized, powder for solution: 10,000 units	Mannitol 80 mg. Preservative free. In single-dose vials.

ASPARAGINASE — INJECTION

Indications

➤*Acute lymphoblastic leukemia:* For the treatment of patients with acute lymphoblastic leukemia (ALL) as a component of a multiagent chemotherapeutic regimen.

Administration and Dosage

➤*Adults:*

Acute lymphoblastic leukemia – 6,000 units/m^2 intramuscularly (IM) or intravenously (IV) 3 times a week.

➤*Children:*

Acute lymphoblastic or acute undifferentiated leukemia –

Younger than 16 years of age: 6,000 units/m^2 IM 3 times a week for a total of 9 doses.

Off-label dosing –

Acute lymphocytic leukemia:

• *Combination therapy* –

Usual dosage:

IV: 1,000 units/kg daily for 10 days.

IM: 6,000 units/m^2 per dose every third day for 3 weeks.

Alternative dosage: A high dose of 25,000 units/m^2 IM has also been given once weekly for 9 weeks.

• *Monotherapy* – 200 units/kg daily for 28 days. Monotherapy is not recommended if the patient can tolerate combination therapy.

➤*Preparation for administration:*

IM – Reconstitute by adding 2 mL of sodium chloride injection to the vial. Withdraw volume of reconstituted asparaginase containing calculated dose into sterile syringe. The reconstituted solution contains 5,000 units/mL. Use within 8 hours.

IV – Reconstitute by adding 5 mL of sterile water for injection or sodium chloride injection to the vial. Withdraw volume of reconstituted asparaginase containing calculated dose into sterile syringe. The reconstituted solution contains 2,000 units/mL. Use within 8 hours.

ASPARAGINASE — INJECTION

Occasionally, a very small number of gelatinous fiber-like particles may develop on standing. Filtration through a 5 micron filter during administration will remove the particles with no resultant loss in potency.

➤*Administration:*

IM – The volume at a single injection site should be limited to 2 mL. If a volume greater than 2 mL is to be administered, 2 injection sites should be used.

IV – Give over a period of not less than 30 minutes through the sidearm of an infusion of sodium chloride injection or dextrose 5% injection.

➤*Storage/Stability:* Store unreconstituted vials at 2° to 8°C (36° to 46°F). Store unused, reconstituted solution at 2° to 8°C (36° to 46°F). Discard after 8 hours or sooner if it becomes cloudy. Discard unused portion.

Actions

➤*Pharmacology:* Asparaginase contains the enzyme L-asparagine amidohydrolase, type EC-2, derived from *Escherichia coli*. The mechanism of action of asparaginase is thought to be based on selective killing of leukemic cells caused by depletion of plasma asparagine. Some leukemic cells are unable to synthesize asparagine because of a lack of asparagine synthetase and are dependent on an exogenous source of asparagine for survival. Depletion of asparagine, which results from treatment with the enzyme L-asparaginase, kills the leukemic cells. However, normal cells are less affected by the depletion because of their ability to synthesize asparagine.

➤*Pharmacokinetics:*

Absorption/Distribution – In a study in patients with metastatic cancer and leukemia, daily IV administration of L-asparaginase resulted in a cumulative increase in plasma levels. Apparent volume of distribution was slightly greater than the plasma volume. Asparaginase levels in cerebrospinal fluid were less than 1% of concurrent plasma levels.

In a study in which patients with leukemia and metastatic cancer received IM L-asparaginase, peak plasma levels of asparaginase were reached 14 to 24 hours after dosing.

Excretion – Plasma half-life was 34 to 49 hours for IM administration and 8 to 30 hours for IV administration.

Contraindications

Serious allergic reactions to asparaginase or other *E. coli*–derived L-asparaginases; serious thrombosis with prior L-asparaginase therapy; pancreatitis with prior L-asparaginase therapy; serious hemorrhagic events with prior L-asparaginase therapy.

Warnings/Precautions

➤*Thrombosis:* Serious thrombotic events, including sagittal sinus thrombosis, can occur in patients receiving asparaginase. Discontinue asparaginase in patients with serious thrombotic events.

➤*Pancreatitis:* Pancreatitis, in some cases fulminant or fatal, can occur in patients receiving asparaginase. Evaluate patients with abdominal pain for evidence of pancreatitis. Discontinue asparaginase in patients with pancreatitis.

➤*Glucose intolerance:* Glucose intolerance can occur in patients receiving asparaginase. In some cases, glucose intolerance is irreversible. Monitor serum glucose.

➤*Coagulopathy:* Hypofibrinogenemia, increased partial thromboplastin time, and increased prothrombin time can occur in patients receiving asparaginase. CNS hemorrhages have been observed. Monitor coagulation parameters at baseline and periodically during and after treatment. Initiate treatment with fresh-frozen plasma to replace coagulation factors in patients with severe or symptomatic coagulopathy.

➤*Immunogenicity:* As with all therapeutic proteins, there is a potential for immunogenicity, defined as development of binding and/or neutralizing antibodies to the product.

➤*Hepatic effects:* Fulminant hepatic failure may occur. Hepatotoxicity and abnormal liver function, including elevations of AST, ALT, alkaline phosphatase, bilirubin (direct and indirect), and depression of serum albumin, and plasma fibrinogen can occur. Fatty changes in the liver have been documented on biopsy. Evaluate hepatic enzymes and bilirubin pretreatment and periodically during treatment.

➤*Vaccines:* See Drug Interactions for more information.

➤*Hypersensitivity reactions:* Serious allergic reactions can occur in patients receiving asparaginase. The risk of serious allergic reactions is higher in patients with prior exposure to asparaginase or other *E. coli*–derived L-asparaginases. Observe patients for 1 hour after administration of asparaginase in a setting with resuscitation equipment and other agents necessary to treat anaphylaxis (eg, antihistamines, epinephrine, IV steroids, oxygen). Discontinue asparaginase in patients with serious allergic reactions.

➤*Pregnancy: Category C.* There are no adequate and well-controlled studies in pregnant women. Give asparaginase to a pregnant woman only if clearly needed.

In mice and rats, asparaginase has been shown to retard the weight gain of mothers and fetuses when given in doses of more than 1,000 units/kg (approximately equivalent to the recommended human dose, when adjusted for total body surface area [BSA]). Gross abnormalities, resorptions, and skeletal abnormalities were observed. The IV administration of 50 or 100 units/kg (approximately equivalent to 10% to 20% of the recommended human dose, when adjusted for total BSA) to pregnant rabbits on day 8 and 9 of gestation resulted in dose-dependent embryotoxicity and gross abnormalities.

➤*Lactation:* It is not known whether asparaginase is excreted in human milk. Because many drugs are excreted in human milk and because of the potential for serious adverse reactions in breast-feeding infants from asparaginase, decide whether to discontinue breast-feeding or the drug, taking into account the importance of the drug to the mother.

➤*Monitoring:* Monitor coagulation parameters and serum glucose and evaluate hepatic enzymes and bilirubin at baseline and periodically during and after treatment.

Observe patients for 1 hour after administration of asparaginase in a setting with resuscitation equipment and other agents necessary to treat anaphylaxis (eg, antihistamines, epinephrine, IV steroids, oxygen).

Drug Interactions

➤*Vaccines:* The risk of live vaccine-induced adverse reactions may be increased by coadministration. Defer the use of live vaccines in patients receiving asparaginase.

Adverse Reactions

➤*Common adverse reactions:* Allergic reactions (including anaphylaxis); azotemia; CNS thrombosis; coagulopathy; elevated transaminases; hyperbilirubinemia; hyperglycemia; liver function abnormalities, including hyperbilirubinemia, and elevated transaminases; pancreatitis.

➤*Serious adverse reactions:*

Cardiovascular – Serious thrombosis, including sagittal sinus thrombosis.

CNS – CNS effects, including coma, hallucinations, and seizures.

Hematologic – Coagulopathy, including increased prothrombin time, increased partial thromboplastin time, and decreased fibrinogen, protein C, protein S, and antithrombin III; CNS hemorrhages.

Hepatic – Hepatotoxicity, in some cases fatal.

Hypersensitivity – Anaphylaxis and serious allergic reactions.

Miscellaneous – Pancreatitis, in some cases fulminant or fatal; glucose intolerance, in some cases irreversible.

➤*Other adverse reactions:* Hyperlipidemia, including hypertriglyceridemia and hypercholesterolemia.

Patient Information

Advise patient, family, or caregiver that medication will be used in combination with other agents to achieve maximum benefit possible.

Advise patient, family, or caregiver to contact a health care provider immediately to report any of the following: acute difficulty in breathing/shortness of breath; new-onset chest pain; severe abdominal pain; severe headache, seizures, change in mental status; swelling of the face, arms, or legs, with or without pain in the arm or leg.

Advise patients to inform their health care provider of excessive thirst or an increase in the volume or frequency of urination or pregnancy.

PEGASPARGASE (PEG-L-ASPARAGINASE)

Rx	**Oncaspar** (Enzon)	**Injection:** 750 units/mL	Preservative free. In single-use vials.

PEGASPARGASE (PEG-L-ASPARAGINASE) — INJECTION

Indications

➤*Acute lymphoblastic leukemia and hypersensitivity to asparaginase:* As a component of a multiagent chemotherapeutic regimen for the treatment of patients with acute lymphoblastic leukemia (ALL) and hypersensitivity to native forms of L-asparaginase.

➤*First-line acute lymphoblastic leukemia:* As a component of a multiagent chemotherapeutic regimen for the first-line treatment of patients with ALL.

➤*Off-label uses:* Chronic lymphocytic leukemia in blast crisis, non-Hodgkin lymphoma (salvage therapy).

Administration and Dosage

➤*General dosing considerations:* Pegaspargase is used as a single agent only in unusual circumstances, such as when the toxicity of combination therapy is unacceptable, other patient-specific factors preclude combination therapy, or the tumor is refractory to combination therapy.

➤*Adults:*

Acute lymphoblastic leukemia – 2,500 units/m^2 intramuscularly (IM) or intravenously (IV), administered no more frequently than every 14 days.

➤*Children:*

Acute lymphoblastic leukemia – 2,500 units/m^2 IM or IV, administered no more frequently than every 14 days. (See also Off-label dosing.)

PEGASPARGASE (PEG-L-ASPARAGINASE) — INJECTION

Off-label dosing –

Acute lymphoblastic leukemia:

• *Body surface area less than 0.6 m²* – 82.5 units/kg body weight administered IM or IV no more frequently than every 14 days; given in combination with other antineoplastics or as a single agent.

• *Body surface area 0.6 m² or more* – 2,500 units/m² administered IM or IV no more frequently than every 14 days; given in combination with other antineoplastics or as a single agent.

➤*Preparation for administration:* Pegaspargase is considered a cytotoxic agent. Follow safe handling procedures when preparing, administering, or dispensing pegaspargase.

➤*Administration:* IM administration is preferred. IV administration of pegaspargase is associated with a higher incidence of adverse effects (eg, hepatotoxicity, coagulopathy, renal effects, GI effects) than IM administration and is not recommended unless IM administration is contraindicated.

Intramuscular – When administering IM, the volume at a single injection site should be limited to 2 mL. If the volume to be administered is greater than 2 mL, multiple injection sites should be used.

Intravenous – When administering IV, pegaspargase should be given over a period of 1 to 2 hours in 100 mL of sodium chloride or dextrose 5% injection through an infusion that is already running. Do not filter.

➤*Storage/Stability:* Keep refrigerated at 2° to 8°C (36° to 46°F). Use only 1 dose per vial; do not reenter the vial. Discard unused portions. Do not save unused drug for later administration.

Do not administer pegaspargase if the drug has been frozen, stored at room temperature (15° to 25°C; 59° to 77°F) for more than 48 hours, or shaken or vigorously agitated; or if it is cloudy, discolored, or precipitate is present.

Because these preparations contain no preservatives, use them within 24 hours of preparation.

Actions

➤*Pharmacology:* The mechanism of action of pegaspargase is thought to be based on selective killing of leukemic cells due to depletion of the plasma asparagine. Some leukemic cells are unable to synthesize asparagine because of a lack of asparagine synthetase and are dependent on an exogenous source of asparagine for survival. Depletion of asparagine, which results from treatment with the enzyme L-asparaginase, kills the leukemic cells. Normal cells, however, are less affected by the depletion because of their ability to synthesize asparagine.

➤*Pharmacokinetics:* Pharmacokinetic assessments were based on an enzymatic assay measuring asparaginase activity. Serum pharmacokinetics were assessed in 34 newly diagnosed children with standard-risk ALL in study 1 following IM administration of 2,500 units/m². The elimination half-life of pegaspargase was approximately 5.8 days during the induction phase. Similar elimination half-lives were observed during delayed intensification 1 and 2. Concentrations greater than 0.1 units/mL were observed in more than 90% of the samples from patients treated with pegaspargase during induction, delayed intensification 1, and delayed intensification 2 for approximately 20 days.

In 3 pharmacokinetic studies, 37 patients with relapsed ALL received pegaspargase IM at 2,500 units/m² every 2 weeks. The plasma half-life of pegaspargase was 3.2 ± 1.8 days in 9 patients who were previously hypersensitive to native *Escherichia coli* L-asparaginase and 5.7 ± 3.2 days in 28 nonhypersensitive patients. The area under the plasma concentration-time curve was 9.5 ± 4 units/mL/day in the previously hypersensitive patients and 9.8 ± 6 units/mL/day in the nonhypersensitive patients.

Contraindications

History of serious allergic reactions to pegaspargase, serious thrombosis with prior L-asparaginase therapy, pancreatitis with prior L-asparaginase therapy, and/or serious hemorrhagic events with prior L-asparaginase therapy.

Warnings/Precautions

➤*Thrombosis:* Serious thrombotic events, including sagittal sinus thrombosis, can occur in patients receiving pegaspargase. Discontinue pegaspargase in patients with serious thrombotic events.

➤*Pancreatitis:* Pancreatitis can occur in patients receiving pegaspargase. Evaluate patients with abdominal pain for evidence of pancreatitis. Discontinue pegaspargase in patients with pancreatitis.

➤*Glucose intolerance:* Glucose intolerance can occur in patients receiving pegaspargase. In some cases, glucose intolerance is irreversible.

➤*Coagulopathy:* Increased prothrombin time, increased partial thromboplastin time, and hypofibrinogenemia can occur in patients receiving pegaspargase. Monitor coagulation parameters at baseline and periodically during and after treatment. Initiate treatment with fresh-frozen plasma to replace coagulation factors in patients with severe or symptomatic coagulopathy.

➤*Hypersensitivity reactions:* Serious allergic reactions can occur in patients receiving pegaspargase. The risk of serious allergic reactions is higher in patients with known hypersensitivity to other forms of L-asparaginase. Observe patients for 1 hour after administration of pegaspargase in a setting with resuscitation equipment and other agents necessary to treat anaphylaxis (eg, epinephrine, oxygen, IV steroids, antihistamines). Discontinue pegaspargase in patients with serious allergic reactions.

➤*Pregnancy: Category C.* Animal reproduction studies have not been conducted with pegaspargase. It is also not known whether pegaspargase can cause fetal harm when administered to a pregnant woman or can affect reproduction capacity. Give pegaspargase to a pregnant woman only if clearly needed.

➤*Lactation:* It is not known whether pegaspargase is excreted in human milk. Because many drugs are excreted in human milk and because of the potential for serious adverse reactions due to pegaspargase in breast-feeding infants, decide whether to discontinue breast-feeding or the drug, taking into account the importance of the drug to the mother.

➤*Children:* Safety and efficacy have been established in clinical trials in children 1 to 9 years of age.

➤*Elderly:* Clinical studies of pegaspargase did not include sufficient numbers of subjects 65 years of age and older to determine whether they respond differently than younger subjects.

➤*Monitoring:* Pegaspargase may affect a number of plasma proteins; therefore, monitoring of fibrinogen, prothrombin time, and partial thromboplastin time may be indicated.

Monitor serum amylase, glucose, and liver function tests at periodic intervals throughout therapy.

Drug Interactions

No formal drug interaction studies between pegaspargase and other drugs have been performed.

Adverse Reactions

The following serious adverse reactions can occur with pegaspargase treatment: anaphylaxis and serious allergic reactions, coagulopathy, glucose intolerance, pancreatitis, and serious thrombosis.

The most common adverse reactions with pegaspargase are allergic reactions (including anaphylaxis), CNS thrombosis, coagulopathy, elevated transaminases, hyperbilirubinemia, hyperglycemia, and pancreatitis.

Pegaspargase is considered to have low potential for nausea and vomiting.

First-line ALL –

Pegaspargase Grade 3 and 4 Adverse Reactions		
	Pegaspargase (n = 58)	Native *E. coli* L-asparaginase (n = 59)
Abnormal liver tests	3 (5%)	5 (8%)
Elevated transaminases[a]	2 (3%)	4 (7%)
Hyperbilirubinemia	1 (2%)	1 (2%)
Hyperglycemia	3 (5%)	2 (3%)
CNS thrombosis	2 (3%)	2 (3%)
Coagulopathy[b]	1 (2%)	3 (5%)
Pancreatitis	1 (2%)	1 (2%)
Clinical allergic reactions to asparaginase	1 (2%)	0 (0%)

[a] AST, ALT.

[b] Prolonged prothrombin time or partial thromboplastin time, or hypofibrinogenemia.

Safety data were collected in study 2 only for National Cancer Institute Common Toxicity Criteria version 2.0, grade 3 and 4 nonhematologic toxicities. In this study, the per-patient incidence for the following adverse reactions occurring during treatment courses in which patients received pegaspargase were: elevated transaminases, 11%; coagulopathy, 7%; hyperglycemia, 5%; CNS thrombosis/hemorrhage, 2%; pancreatitis, 2%; clinical allergic reaction, 1%; and hyperbilirubinemia, 1%. There were 3 deaths due to pancreatitis.

Previously treated ALL – The most common adverse reactions of pegaspargase were clinical allergic reactions, elevated transaminases, hyperbilirubinemia, and coagulopathies. The most common serious adverse reactions due to pegaspargase treatment were thrombosis (4%), hyperglycemia requiring insulin therapy (3%), and pancreatitis (1%).

➤*Hypersensitivity:* Clinical allergic reactions include the following: bronchospasm, hypotension, laryngeal edema, local erythema or swelling, systemic rash, and urticaria.

Previously treated ALL – Among 62 patients with relapsed ALL and prior hypersensitivity reactions to asparaginase, 35 (56%) patients had a history of clinical allergic reactions to native *E. coli* L-asparaginase, and 27 (44%) patients had a history of clinical allergic reactions to both native *E. coli* and native *Erwinia* L-asparaginase.

Pegaspargase Hypersensitivity Reactions					
	Toxicity grade, n (%)				
	1	2	3	4	Total
Previously hypersensitive patients (n = 62)	7 (11%)	8 (13%)	4 (6%)	1 (2%)	20 (32%)
Nonhypersensitive patients (n = 112)	5 (4%)	4 (4%)	1 (1%)	1 (1%)	11 (10%)
First line (n = 58)	1 (2%)	0 (0%)	1 (2%)	0 (0%)	2 (3%)

PEGASPARGASE (PEG-L-ASPARAGINASE) — INJECTION

➤*Immunogenicity:* As with all therapeutic proteins, there is a potential for immunogenicity, defined as the development of binding and/or neutralizing antibodies to the product.

In study 1, pegaspargase-treated patients were assessed for evidence of binding antibodies using an enzyme-linked immunosorbent assay method. The incidence of protocol-specified "high-titer" antibody formation was 2% in induction (n = 48), 10% in delayed intensification 1 (n = 50), and 11% in delayed intensification 2 (n = 44). There is insufficient information to determine whether the development of antibodies is associated with an increased risk of clinical allergic reactions, altered pharmacokinetics, or loss of antileukemic efficacy.

Overdosage

Three patients received pegaspargase 10,000 units/m² as an IV infusion. One patient experienced a slight increase in liver enzymes. A second patient developed a rash 10 minutes after the start of the infusion, which was controlled with the administration of an antihistamine and by slowing down the infusion rate. The third patient did not experience any adverse reactions.

Patient Information

Inform patients of the possibility of serious allergic reactions, including anaphylaxis, and tell them to immediately report any swelling or difficulty breathing.

Advise patients to immediately report any severe headache, arm or leg swelling, acute shortness of breath, or chest pain.

Advise patients to immediately report any severe abdominal pain.

Advise patients to report excessive thirst or any increase in the volume or frequency of urination.

RADIOPHARMACEUTICALS

SODIUM IODIDE I 131

Rx	**Sodium Iodide I 131** (Mallinckrodt)	**Capsules; oral:** Radioactivity ranging from 0.75 to 100 mCi per capsule.	Various strengths.
		Solution; oral: Radioactivity ranging from 3.5 to 150 mCi/vial.	0.1% sodium bisulfite and 0.2% EDTA. In vials.
Rx	**Hicon** (Draximage)	**Solution, concentrated; oral:** 1000 mci/mL	Disodium edetate dihydrate. In 0.25, 0.5, and 1 mL vial kit. Kit includes 10 small gelatin capsules containing approx 300 mg dibasic sodium phosphate and 10 empty large hard gelatin capsules.

SODIUM IODIDE I 131 — ORAL

Sodium Iodide I 131 is also used for treatment of hyperthyroidism. Refer to the Antithyroid Agents group monograph in the Endocrine/Metabolic chapter.

Indications

➤*Diagnostic capsules:* For use in performance of the radioactive iodide (RAI) uptake test to evaluate thyroid function. Diagnostic doses may also be employed in localizing metastases associated with thyroid malignancies.

➤*Therapeutic capsules and oral solution:* For the treatment of hyperthyroidism and selected cases of carcinoma of the thyroid. Palliative effects may be seen in patients with papillary or follicular carcinoma of the thyroid. Stimulation of radioiodide uptake may be achieved by the administration of thyrotropin. (Radioiodide will not be taken up by giant cell and spindle cell carcinoma of the thyroid nor by amyloid solid carcinomas.)

Administration and Dosage

➤*General dosing considerations:* The patient dose should be measured by a suitable radioactivity calibration system immediately prior to administration.

Patients should be adequately hydrated before and after administration of radioiodide to ensure rapid urinary elimination of the iodide that is not absorbed by the thyroid gland.

➤*Adults:*

Hyperthyroidism (therapeutic capsules and oral solution) –

Usual dosage: 148 to 370 megabecquerels (MBq) (4 to 10 millicuries [mCi]) administered orally. Toxic nodular goiter and other special situations will require the use of larger doses.

Antithyroid therapy of a severely hyperthyroid patient is usually discontinued 3 to 4 days before administration of radioiodide.

Sodium iodide I 131 is not usually used for treatment of hyperthyroidism in patients younger than 30 years of age unless circumstances preclude other methods of treatment.

Thyroid carcinoma –

Initial dosage: 1.1 to 3.7 gigabecquerels (GBq) (30 to 100 mCi) administered orally.

Subsequent dose: Subsequent ablation of metastases with 3.7 to 7.4 GBq (100 to 200 mCi) administered orally.

Thyroid function evaluation (diagnostic capsules) – The suggested oral dosage ranges employed in the average patient (70 kg) for diagnostic procedures for thyroid function are as follows:

Localization of extra-thyroidal metastases: 37 MBq (1,000 microcuries).
Scintiscanning: 1.85 to 3.7 MBq (50 to 100 microcuries).
Thyroid uptake: 0.185 to 0.555 MBq (5 to 15 microcuries).

➤*Preparation for administration:* Sodium iodide I 131 is a radioactive agent. Follow safe handling procedures when preparing, administering, or dispensing sodium iodide I 131. Waterproof gloves should be used during the entire handling and administration procedure.

Hicon must be diluted prior to administration. See the manufacturer's information for preparation details.

➤*Administration:* Administer sodium iodide I 131 orally.

➤*Storage/Stability:* Store at 20° to 25°C (68° to 77°F).

Actions

➤*Pharmacokinetics:*

Absorption/Distribution – Sodium iodide is readily absorbed from the GI tract. Following absorption, the iodide is distributed primarily within the extracellular fluid of the body.

Sodium iodide I 131 therapeutic capsules and oral solution: About 90% of local irradiation is the result of beta radiation and 10% is the result of gamma radiation.

Physical characteristics (diagnostic use and therapeutic use): Iodine I-131 decays by beta and associated gamma emissions with a physical half-life of 8.04 days. The principle beta emissions and gamma photons are listed in the following table:

Principal Radiation Emission Data Used for Iodine I 131

Radiation	Mean % per disintegration	Energy (keV)
Beta-1	2.12	69.4 Avg
Beta-3	7.36	96.6 Avg
Beta-4	89.3	191.6 Avg
Gamma-7	6.05	284.3
Gamma-14	81.2	364.5
Gamma-17	7.26	637

External radiation (diagnostic use and therapeutic use): The specific gamma ray constant for iodine I-131 is 2.27 R/hr-mCi at 1 cm. The first half-value thickness of lead (Pb) for iodine I-131 is 0.24 cm. A range of values for the relative attenuation of the radiation emitted by this radionuclide that results from interposition of various thicknesses of Pb is shown in the information below. For example, the use of 4.6 cm of Pb will decrease the external radiation exposure by a factor of about 1000.

Radiation (Emitted by Iodine I 131) Attenuation by Lead Shielding

Shield thickness (Pb), cm	Coefficient of attenuation
0.24	0.5
0.95	10^{-1}
2.6	10^{-2}
4.6	10^{-3}
6.5	10^{-4}

To correct for physical decay of this radionuclide, the fractions that remain at selected time intervals after the date of calibration are shown in the following table:

Physical Decay Chart, Iodine I 131, Half-life 8.04 days

Days	Fraction remaining	Days	Fraction remaining
0[a]	1	16	0.252
1	0.917	17	0.231
2	0.842	18	0.212
3	0.772	19	0.194

SODIUM IODIDE I 131 — ORAL

Physical Decay Chart, Iodine I 131, Half-life 8.04 days			
Days	Fraction remaining	Days	Fraction remaining
4	0.708	20	0.178
5	0.65	21	0.164
6	0.596	22	0.15
7	0.547	23	0.138
8	0.502	24	0.126
9	0.46	25	0.116
10	0.422	26	0.106
11	0.387	27	0.098
12	0.355	28	0.089
13	0.326	29	0.082
14	0.299	30	0.075
15	0.274		

[a] Calibration day.

Metabolism/Excretion – It is concentrated and organified by the thyroid, and trapped but not organified by the stomach and salivary glands. It is also promptly excreted by the kidneys.

Contraindications

Vomiting and diarrhea represent contraindications to the use of radioiodide.

Therapeutic doses of sodium iodide I 131 may cause fetal harm when administered to a pregnant woman. Therapeutic doses of sodium iodide I 131 are contraindicated in women who are or may become pregnant. If this drug is used during pregnancy, or if the patient becomes pregnant while taking this drug, the patient should be apprised of the potential hazards to the fetus.

Warnings/Precautions

➤*Radiographic contrast media:* The uptake of radioiodide will be affected by recent intake of stable iodine in any form, or by the use of thyroid, antithyroid and certain other drugs. Accordingly, the patient should be questioned carefully regarding previous medication and procedures involving radiographic contrast media.

➤*Expiration date:* The expiration date is not later than 1 month after the calibration date. The calibration date and the expiration date are stated on the container label.

➤*Sulfite sensitivity:*

Therapeutic oral solution – Some of these products may contain sodium bisulfite, a sulfite that may cause allergic-type reactions, including anaphylactic symptoms and life-threatening or less severe asthmatic episodes in certain susceptible people. The overall prevalence of sulfite sensitivity in the general population is unknown and probably low. Sulfite sensitivity is seen more frequently in asthmatic than in nonasthmatic people.

➤*Pregnancy: Category C* – diagnostic capsules (per manufacturer's prescribing information); *Category X* – therapeutic capsules and oral solution (per manufacturer's prescribing information). *Category X* – Per Briggs' *Drugs in Pregnancy and Lactation*.

Diagnostic capsules – Animal reproduction studies have not been conducted with sodium iodide I 131 diagnostic capsules. It is also not known whether sodium iodide I 131 diagnostic capsules can cause fetal harm when administered to a pregnant woman or can affect reproduction capacity. Sodium iodide I 131 diagnostic capsules should be given to a pregnant woman only if clearly needed.

Childbearing women – Ideally, examinations using radiopharmaceutical drug products (especially those elective in nature) of women of childbearing capability should be performed during the first 10 days following the onset of menses.

Therapeutic capsules and oral solution – See Contraindications for more information.

Radioiodide therapy in women of childbearing capability should only be performed when appropriate contraceptive measures have been taken or when pregnancy testing is negative.

➤*Lactation:* Radioiodine is excreted in human milk during lactation. Therefore, formula feedings should be substituted for breast milk.

➤*Children:*

Diagnostic capsules – Safety and efficacy in pediatric patients have not been established.

Therapeutic capsules and oral solution – Sodium iodide I 131 is not usually used for treatment of hyperthyroidism in patients under 30 years of age.

Adverse Reactions

Diagnostic capsules – Although rare, reactions associated with the administration of iodine-containing radiopharmaceuticals for diagnostic use include, in decreasing order of frequency, nausea, vomiting, chest pain, tachycardia, itching skin, rash and hives.

➤*Therapeutic capsules and oral solution:* Although rare, reactions have been reported following the administration of iodine-containing radiopharmaceuticals, including, in decreasing order of frequency, nausea, vomiting, chest pain, tachycardia, itching skin, rash, and hives. Depression of the hematopoietic system may occur when large doses are employed. Such potential side effects include radiation sickness, increase in clinical symptoms, bone marrow depression, acute leukemia, anemia, chromosomal abnormalities, acute thyroid crisis, blood dyscrasia, leukopenia, thrombocytopenia, and death.

STRONTIUM-89 CHLORIDE

Rx	**Metastron** (Medi-Physics/Amersham)	**Injection:** 148 MBq, 4 mCi (10.9 to 22.6 mg/mL)	Preservative free. In 10 ml vials with Water for Injection.

STRONTIUM-89 CHLORIDE — INJECTION

Indications

➤*Bone pain due to skeletal metastases:* For the relief of bone pain in patients with painful skeletal metastases.

Administration and Dosage

➤*General dosing considerations:* The patient dose should be measured by a suitable radioactivity calibration system immediately prior to administration.

➤*Adults:*

Bone pain caused by skeletal metastases –

Usual dosage: 148 megabecquerels (MBq) (4 mCi) administered by slow IV injection (1 to 2 minutes).

Alternative dosage: 1.5 to 2.2 MBq/kg (40 to 60 microCi/kg) may be used.

Repeat doses: Repeated administrations of strontium-89 chloride should be based on the individual patient's response to therapy, current symptoms, and hematologic status, and are generally not recommended at intervals of fewer than 90 days.

Radiation dosimetry: The estimated radiation dose that would be delivered over time by the IV injection of 37 MBq, 1 mCi of strontium-89 to a healthy adult is given in the information below. Data are taken from the *ICRP* publication "Radiation Dose to Patients from Radiopharmaceuticals"-*ICRP* #53, Vol. 18, No. 1 to 4; 171, Pergamon Press, 1988.

Strontium-89 Dosimetry		
Organ	mGy/MBq	rad/mCi
Bone surface	17	63
Red bone marrow	11	40.7
Lower bowel wall	4.7	17.4
Bladder wall	1.3	4.8
Testes	0.8	2.9
Ovaries	0.8	2.9
Uterine wall	0.8	2.9
Kidneys	0.8	2.9

When blastic osseous metastases are present, significantly enhanced localization of the radiopharmaceutical will occur with correspondingly higher doses to the metastases compared with normal bones and other organs.

➤*Preparation for administration:* Strontium-89 chloride is considered a cytotoxic agent and a radioactive agent. Follow safe handling procedures when preparing, administering, or dispensing strontium-89 chloride.

The radiation dose hazard in handling strontium-89 chloride injection during dose dispensing and administration is similar to that from phosphorus-32. The beta emission has a range in water of about 8 mm (max) and in glass of about 3 mm, but the bremsstrahlung radiation may augment the contact dose.

Measured values of the dose on the surface of the unshielded vial are about 65 mR/min/mCi.

It is recommended that the vial be kept inside its transportation shield whenever possible.

➤*Administration:* Administer by slow IV injection (1 to 2 minutes).

➤*Storage/Stability:* The vial and its contents should be stored inside its transportation container at 15° to 25°C (59° to 77°F).

The calibration date (for radioactivity content) and expiration date are quoted on the vial label. The expiration date will be 28 days after calibration. Stability studies have shown no change in any of the product characteristics monitored during routine product quality control over the period from manufacture to expiration.

STRONTIUM-89 CHLORIDE — INJECTION

Actions

➤*Pharmacology:* Following IV injection, soluble strontium compounds behave like their calcium analogs, clearing rapidly from the blood and selectively localizing in bone mineral. Uptake of strontium by bone occurs preferentially in sites of active osteogenesis; thus, primary bone tumors and areas of metastatic involvement (blastic lesions) can accumulate significantly greater concentrations of strontium than surrounding normal bone.

Strontium-89 chloride is retained in metastatic bone lesions much longer than in normal bone, where turnover is about 14 days. In patients with extensive skeletal metastases, well over half of the injected dose is retained in the bones.

Strontium-89 is a pure beta emitter, and strontium-89 chloride selectively irradiates sites of primary and metastatic bone involvement with minimal irradiation of soft tissues distant from the bone lesions. (The maximum range in tissue is 8 mm; maximum energy is 1.463 MeV).

➤*Pharmacokinetics:*

Absorption/Distribution –

Physical characteristics: Strontium-89 decays by beta emission, with a physical half-life of 50.5 days. The maximum beta energy is 1.463 MeV (100%). The maximum range of beta- from strontium-89 in tissue is approximately 8 mm.

Radioactive decay factors to be applied to the stated value for radioactive concentration at calibration, when calculating injection volumes at the time of administration, are given in the following table:

Decay of Strontium-89	
Day[a]	Factor
−24	1.39
−22	1.35
−20	1.32
−18	1.28
−16	1.25
−14	1.21
−12	1.18
−10	1.15
−8	1.12
−6	1.09
−4	1.06
−2	1.03
0 = calibration	1
+6	0.92
+8	0.9
+10	0.87
+12	0.85
+14	0.83
+16	0
+18	0.78
+20	0.76
+22	0.74
+24	0.72
+26	0.7
+28	0.68

[a] Days before (−) or after (+) the calibration date stated on the vial.

Excretion – Excretion pathways are two-thirds urinary and one-third fecal in patients with bone metastases. Urinary excretion is higher in people without bone lesions. Urinary excretion is greatest in the first 2 days following injection.

Contraindications

None known.

Warnings/Precautions

➤*Hematologic toxicity:* Use of strontium-89 chloride in patients with evidence of seriously compromised bone marrow from previous therapy or disease infiltration is not recommended unless the potential benefit of the treatment outweighs its risks. Bone marrow toxicity is to be expected following the administration of strontium-89 chloride, particularly white blood cells and platelets. The extent of toxicity is variable. It is recommended that the patient's peripheral blood cell counts be monitored at least once every other week. Typically, platelets will be depressed by about 30% compared to preadministration levels. The nadir of platelet depression in most patients is found between 12 and 16 weeks following administration of strontium-89 chloride. White blood cells are usually depressed to a varying extent compared to preadministration levels. Thereafter, recovery occurs slowly, typically reaching preadministration levels 6 months after treatment unless the patient's disease or additional therapy intervenes.

➤*Repeat administration:* In considering repeat administration of strontium-89 chloride, the patient's hematologic response to the initial dose, current platelet level and other evidence of marrow depletion should be carefully evaluated.

Verification of dose and patient identification is necessary prior to administration because strontium-89 chloride delivers a relatively high dose of radioactivity.

➤*Short-life expectancy:* In view of the delayed onset of pain relief, typically 7 to 20 days postinjection, administration of strontium-89 chloride to patients with very short life expectancy is not recommended.

➤*Rapid administration:* A calcium-like flushing sensation has been observed in patients following a rapid (less than 30 second injection) administration.

➤*Incontinence:* Special precautions, such as urinary catheterization, should be taken following administration to patients who are incontinent to minimize the risk of radioactive contamination of clothing, bed linen and the patient's environment.

➤*Renal function impairment:* Strontium-89 chloride is excreted primarily by the kidneys. In patients with renal dysfunction, the possible risks of administering strontium-89 chloride should be weighed against the possible benefits.

➤*Special risk:* Strontium-89 chloride is not indicated for use in patients with cancer not involving bone. Strontium-89 chloride should be used with caution in patients with platelet counts below 60,000 and white cell counts below 2400.

➤*Pregnancy: Category D.* Strontium-89 chloride may cause fetal harm when administered to a pregnant woman. There are no adequate and well-controlled studies in pregnant women. If this drug is used during pregnancy, or if the patient becomes pregnant while receiving this drug, the patient should be apprised of the potential hazard to the fetus. Women of childbearing potential should be advised to avoid becoming pregnant.

➤*Lactation:* Because strontium acts as a calcium analog, secretion of strontium-89 chloride into human milk is likely. It is recommended that nursing be discontinued by mothers about to receive IV strontium-89 chloride. It is not known whether this drug is excreted in human milk.

➤*Children:* Safety and efficacy in children below the age of 18 years have not been established.

Adverse Reactions

➤*Fatal septicemia:* A single case of fatal septicemia following leukopenia was reported during clinical trials. Most severe reactions of marrow toxicity can be managed by conventional means.

➤*Other adverse reactions:* A small number of patients have reported a transient increase in bone pain at 36 to 72 hours after injection. This is usually mild and self-limiting, and controllable with analgesics. A single patient reported chills and fever 12 hours after injection without long-term sequelae.

Patient Information

The patient may feel a slight increase in pain for 2 or 3 days beginning 2 or 3 days after injection. The physician may suggest a temporary increase in the dose of pain medication until the pain is under control. After about 1 or 2 weeks, the pain should begin to diminish.

The patient can eat and drink normally and there is no need to avoid alcohol or caffeine unless already advised to do so. The physician may want to carry out periodic, routine blood tests.

Advise patients to tell any health practitioner who is giving them medical treatment that they have received strontium-89.

During the first week after injection, strontium-89 will be present in the blood and urine. It is therefore important to consider the following common sense precautions for 1 week: where a normal toilet is available, use in preference to a urinal. Flush the toilet twice. Wipe up any spilled urine with a tissue and flush it away. Always wash hands after using the toilet. Immediately wash any linen or clothes that become stained with urine or blood. Wash them separately from other clothes and rinse thoroughly. If any urine collection device is used, follow instructions on its use. Wash away any spilled blood if a cut occurs.

In many people who receive strontium-89, the effect lasts for several months. If pain returns, consult the physician.

SAMARIUM SM 153 LEXIDRONAM

Rx	**Quadramet** (Du Pont Pharma)	**Injection:** 1850 MBq/mL (50 mCi/mL) at calibration	Frozen, single-dose 10 mL vials. In 2 mL fill (3700 MBq) and 3 mL fill (5550 MBq).

SAMARIUM SM 153 LEXIDRONAM — INJECTION

Indications

➤*Pain due to osteoblastic metastatic bone lesions:* For relief of pain in patients with confirmed osteoblastic metastatic bone lesions that enhance on radionuclide bone scan.

Administration and Dosage

➤*General dosing considerations:* The dose should be measured by a suitable radioactivity calibration system, such as a radioisotope dose calibrator, immediately before administration.

The dose of radioactivity to be administered and the patient should be verified before administering samarium SM 153 lexidronam. Patients should not be released until their radioactivity levels and exposure rates comply with federal and local regulations.

➤*Adults:*

Pain caused by osteoblastic metastatic bone lesions –

Usual dosage: 1 mCi/kg administered intravenously (IV) over 1 minute through a secure indwelling catheter and followed with a saline flush.

➤*Preparation for administration:* Samarium Sm 153 is a radioactive agent. Follow safe handling procedures when preparing, administering, or dispensing samarium Sm 153.

Thaw at room temperature before administration and use within 8 hours of thawing.

➤*Administration:* Administer IV over 1 minute.

The patient should ingest (or receive by IV administration) a minimum of 500 mL (2 cups) of fluids prior to injection and should void as often as possible after injection to minimize radiation exposure to the bladder.

➤*Admixture compatibility:* Samarium SM 153 lexidronam contains calcium and may be incompatible with solutions that contain molecules that can complex with and form calcium precipitates.

Samarium SM 153 lexidronam should not be diluted or mixed with other solutions.

➤*Storage/Stability:* Store frozen at −10° to −20°C (14° to −4°F) in a lead shielded container.

Actions

➤*Pharmacology:* Samarium (Samarium Sm-153 EDTMP) has an affinity for bone and concentrates in areas of bone turnover in association with hydroxyapatite. In clinical studies employing planar imaging techniques, more samarium accumulates in osteoblastic lesions than in normal bone with a lesion-to-normal bone ratio of approximately 5. The mechanism of action of samarium in relieving the pain of bone metastases is not known.

➤*Pharmacokinetics:*

Absorption – The greater the number of metastatic lesions, the more skeletal uptake of Sm-153 radioactivity. The relationship between skeletal uptake and the size of the metastatic lesions has not been studied. The total skeletal uptake of radioactivity was 65.5% ± 15.5% of the injected dose in 453 patients with metastatic lesions from a variety of primary malignancies. In a study of 22 patients with a wide range in the number of metastatic sites, the percentage of the injected dose (% ID) taken up by bone ranged from 56.3% in a patient with 5 metastatic lesions to 76.7% in a patient with 52 metastatic lesions. If the number of metastatic lesions is fixed, over the range 0.1 to 3 mCi/kg, the percent ID taken up by bone is the same regardless of the dose.

Distribution – Human protein binding has not been studied; however, in dog, rat and bovine studies, less than 0.5% of samarium-153 EDTMP is bound to protein. At physiologic pH, greater than 90% of the complex is present as ^{153}Sm]$^{-5}$, and less than 10% as ^{153}SmH]$^{-4}$. The octanol/water partition coefficient is less than 10^{-5}.

Metabolism – The complex formed by samarium and EDTMP is excreted as an intact, single species that consists of 1 atom of the Sm-153 and 1 molecule of the EDTMP, as shown by an analysis of urine samples from patients (n = 5) administered samarium Sm-153 EDTMP. Metabolic products of samarium Sm-153 EDTMP were not detected in humans.

Excretion – For samarium, calculations of the percent ID detected in the whole body, urine and blood were corrected for radionuclide decay. The clearance of activity through the urine is expressed as the cumulated activity excreted. The whole body retention is the simple reciprocal of the cumulated urine activity. (See Absorption).

Urine: Samarium Sm-153 EDTMP radioactivity was excreted in the urine after intravenous injection. During the first 6 hours, 34.5% (± 15.5%) was excreted. Overall, the greater the number of metastatic lesions, the less radioactivity was excreted.

Blood: Clearance of radioactivity from the blood demonstrated biexponential kinetics after intravenous injection in 19 patients (10 men, 9 women) with a variety of primary cancers that were metastatic to bone. Over the first 30 minutes, the radioactivity (mean ± SD) in the blood decreased to 15% (± 8%) of the injected dose with a t ½ of 5.5 min (±1.1 min). After 30 minutes, the radioactivity cleared from the blood more slowly with a t½ of 65.4 min (± 9.6 min). Less than 1% of the dose injected remained in the blood 5 hours after injection.

Contraindications

Hypersensitivity to EDTMP or similar phosphonate compounds.

Warnings/Precautions

➤*Bone marrow suppression:* Samarium causes bone marrow suppression. In clinical trials, white blood cell counts and platelet counts decreased to a nadir of approximately 40% to 50% of baseline in 123 (95%) of patients within 3 to 5 weeks after samarium, and tended to return to pretreatment levels by 8 weeks. The grade of marrow toxicity is as follows.

In the clinical trials of samarium (1 mCi/kg), the number of patients who experienced marrow toxicity was assessed using the toxicity grade based on the National Cancer Institute criteria. Normal levels according to this criteria is a hemoglobin count greater than 10 g/dL, leucocyte count greater than or equal to 4 x 103/mcL, and a platelet count greater than or equal to 150,000/mcL. For the hemoglobin count, the number (and percent) of patients, as assessed by toxicity grade, for the placebo group (n = 85) and samarium group (n = 185), respectively, is as follows: Toxicity grade 0 to 2: 78 (92%) vs 162 (88%); toxicity grade 3: 6 (7%) vs 20 (11%); and toxicity grade 4: 1 (1%) vs 3 (2%). For the leucocyte count, the number (and percent) of patients, as assessed by toxicity grade, for the placebo group (n = 85) and samarium group (n = 184), respectively, is as follows: Toxicity grade 0-2: 85 (100%) vs. 169 (92%); toxicity grade 3: 0 vs. 15 (8%); and toxicity grade 4: 0 vs. 0. For the platelet count, the number (and percent) of patients, as assessed by toxicity grade, for the placebo group (n = 85) and samarium group (n = 185), respectively, is as follows: Toxicity grade 0 to 2: 85 (100%) vs. 173 (94%); toxicity grade 3: 0 vs 10 (5%); and toxicity grade 4: 0 vs 2 (1%).

Before samarium is administered, consideration should be given to the patient's current clinical and hematologic status and bone marrow response history to treatment with myelotoxic agents. Metastatic prostate and other cancers can be associated with disseminated intravascular coagulation (DIC); caution should be exercised in treating cancer patients whose platelet counts are falling or who have other clinical or laboratory findings suggesting DIC. Because of the unknown potential for additive effects on bone marrow, samarium should not be given concurrently with chemotherapy or external beam radiation therapy unless the clinical benefits outweigh the risks. Use of samarium in patients with evidence of compromised bone marrow reserve from previous therapy or disease involvement is not recommended unless the potential benefits of the treatment outweigh the risks. Blood counts should be monitored weekly for at least 8 weeks, or until recovery of adequate bone marrow function.

➤*Hypocalcemia:* In a subset of 31 patients who had serum calcium monitored during the first 2 hours after samarium infusion, a clear pattern of calcium change was not identified. However, 10 (32%) patients had at least 1 serum calcium level that was below normal (7.16 to 8.28). The extent to which samarium-153 EDTMP is related to this hypocalcemia is not known. Caution should be exercised when administering samarium to patients at risk for developing hypocalcemia.

➤*Skeletal:* Spinal cord compression frequently occurs in patients with known metastases to the cervical, thoracic or lumbar spine. In clinical studies of samarium, spinal cord compression was reported in 7% of patients who received placebo and in 8.3% of patients who received 1 mCi/kg samarium. Samarium is not indicated for treatment of spinal cord compression. Samarium administration for pain relief of metastatic bone cancer does not prevent the development of spinal cord compression. When there is a clinical suspicion of spinal cord compression, appropriate diagnostic and therapeutic measures must be taken immediately to avoid permanent disability.

➤*ECG changes:* EDTMP is a chelating agent. Although the chelating effects have not been evaluated thoroughly in humans, dogs that received non-radioactive samarium EDTMP (6 times the human dose based on body weight, 3 times based on surface area) developed a variety of electrocardiographic (ECG) changes (with or without the presence of hypocalcemia). The causal relationship between the hypocalcemia and ECG changes has not been studied. Whether samarium causes electrocardiographic changes or arrhythmias in humans has not been studied. Caution and appropriate monitoring should be given when administering samarium to patients.

➤*Bone marrow suppression:* This drug should be used with caution in patients with compromised bone marrow reserves. Samarium causes bone marrow suppression. In clinical trials, white blood cell counts and platelet counts decreased to a nadir of approximately 40% to 50% of baseline in 123 (95%) of patients within 3 to 5 weeks after samarium, and tended to return to pretreatment levels by 8 weeks.

➤*Incontinence:* Special precautions, such as bladder catheterization, should be taken with incontinent patients to minimize the risk of radioactive contamination of clothing, bed linen, and the patient's environment. Urinary excretion of radioactivity occurs over about 12 hours (with 35% occurring during the first 6 hours). Studies have not been done on the use of samarium in patients with renal impairment.

➤*Pregnancy: Category D.* As with other radiopharmaceutical drugs, samarium can cause fetal harm when administered to a pregnant woman. Adequate and well controlled studies have not been conducted in animals or pregnant women. Women of childbearing age should have a negative pregnancy test before administration of samarium. If this drug is used during pregnancy, or if a patient becomes pregnant after taking this drug, the

SAMARIUM SM 153 LEXIDRONAM — INJECTION

patient should be apprised of the potential hazard to the fetus. Women of childbearing potential should be advised to avoid becoming pregnant soon after receiving samarium. Men and women patients should be advised to use an effective method of contraception after the administration of samarium.

➤*Lactation:* It is not known whether samarium is excreted in human milk. Because of the potential for serious adverse reactions in nursing infants from samarium, a decision should be made whether to continue nursing or to administer the drug. If samarium is administered, formula feedings should be substituted for breastfeedings.

➤*Children:* Safety and effectiveness in pediatric patients below the age of 16 years have not been established.

➤*Monitoring:* Because concomitant hydration is recommended to promote the urinary excretion of samarium, appropriate monitoring and consideration of additional supportive treatment should be used in patients with a history of congestive heart failure or renal insufficiency.

Because of the potential for bone marrow suppression, beginning 2 weeks after samarium administration, blood counts should be monitored weekly for at least 8 weeks, or until recovery of adequate bone marrow function.

Drug Interactions

➤*Chemotherapy/Radiation:* The potential for additive bone marrow toxicity of samarium with chemotherapy or external beam radiation has not been studied. Samarium should not be given concurrently with chemotherapy or external beam radiation therapy unless the benefit outweighs the risks. Samarium should not be given after either of these treatments until there has been time for adequate marrow recovery. Drug-drug interaction studies have not been made.

Adverse Reactions

Of these patients, 472 (83%) had at least 1 adverse reaction. In a subgroup of 399 patients who received samarium 1 mCi/kg, there were 23 deaths and 46 serious adverse reactions. The deaths occurred an average of 67 days (9 to 130) after samarium. Serious reactions occurred an average of 46 days (1 - 118) after samarium. Although most of the patient deaths and serious adverse reactions appear to be related to the underlying disease, the relationship of end stage disease, marrow invasion by cancer cells, previous myelotoxic treatment and samarium toxicity can not be easily distinguished. In clinical studies, 2 patients with rapidly progressive prostate cancer developed thrombocytopenia and died 4 weeks after receiving samarium. One (1) of the patients showed evidence of disseminated intravascular coagulation (DIC); the other patient experienced a fatal cerebrovascular accident, with a suspicion of DIC. The relationship of the DIC to the bone marrow suppressive effect of samarium is not known. Marrow toxicity occurred in 277 (47%) patients.

In controlled studies, 7% of patients receiving 1 mCi/kg samarium (as compared to 6% of patients receiving placebo) reported a transient increase in bone pain shortly after injection (flare reaction). This was usually mild, self-limiting, and responded to analgesics.

Samarium Adverse Reactions in Controlled Clinical Trials (≥ 1 %)

Adverse reactions	Placebo (n = 90)	Samarium 1 mCi/kg (n = 199)
Patients with any adverse reaction	72 (80%)	169 (85%)
Cardiovascular	19 (21%)	32 (16%)
Arrhythmias	2 (2.2%)	10 (5%)
Chest pain	4 (4.4%)	8 (4%)
Hypertension	0	6 (3%)
Hypotension	2 (2.2%)	4 (2%)
CNS	39 (43%)	59 (30%)
Dizziness	1 (1.1%)	8 (4%)
Paresthesia	7 (7.8%)	4 (2%)
Spinal cord compression	5 (5.5%)	13 (6.5%)
Cerebrovascular accident/stroke	0	2 (1%)
Dermatologic	17 (19%)	13 (7%)
Purpura	0	2 (1%)
Rash	2 (2.2%)	2 (1%)
GI	44 (49%)	82 (41%)
Abdominal pain	7 (7.8%)	12 (6%)
Diarrhea	3 (3.3%)	12 (6%)
Nausea and/or vomiting	37 (41.1%)	65 (32.7%)
Hematologic/Lymphatic	12 (13%)	54 (27%)
Coagulation disorder	0	3 (1.5%)
Hemoglobin decreased	21 (23.3%)	81 (40.7%)
Leukopenia	6 (6.7%)	118 (59.3%)
Lymphadenopathy	0	4 (2%)
Thrombocytopenia	8 (8.9%)	138 (69.3%)
Any bleeding manifestations[a]	8 (8.9%)	32 (16.1%)
Ecchymosis	1 (1.1%)	3 (3%)
Epistaxis	1 (1.1%)	4 (2%)
Hematuria	3 (3.3%)	10 (5%)
Infection	10 (11.1%)	34 (17.1%)
Fever and/or chills	10 (11.1%)	17 (8.5%)
Infection, not specified	4 (4.4%)	14 (7%)
Oral moniliasis	1 (1.1%)	4 (2%)
Musculoskeletal	28 (31%)	55 (27%)
Myasthenia	8 (8.9%)	13 (6.5%)
Pathologic fracture	2 (2.2%)	5 (2.5%)
Respiratory	24 (27%)	35 (18%)
Bronchitis/cough increased	2 (2.2%)	8 (4%)
Pneumonia	1 (1.1%)	3 (1.5%)
Special senses	11 (12%)	11 (6%)
Miscellaneous	56 (62%)	100 (50%)
Pain flare reaction	5 (5.6%)	14 (7%)

Samarium Adverse Reactions in Controlled Clinical Trials (≥ 1 %)

[a] Includes hemorrhage (gastrointestinal, ocular) reported in < 1%.

In an additional 200 patients who received samarium in uncontrolled clinical trials, adverse events that were reported at a rate of greater than or equal to 1% were similar except for 9 (4.5%) patients who had agranulocytosis. Other selected adverse events that were reported in less than 1% of the patients who received samarium 1 mCi/kg in any clinical trial include alopecia, angina, congestive heart failure, sinus bradycardia, and vasodilation.

Overdosage

Overdosage with samarium has not been reported. An antidote for samarium overdosage is not known. The anticipated complications of overdosage would likely be secondary to bone marrow suppression from the radioactivity of ^{153}Sm, or secondary to hypocalcemia and cardiac arrhythmias related to the EDTMP.

Patient Information

Patients who receive samarium should be advised that for several hours following administration, radioactivity will be present in excreted urine. To help protect themselves and others in their environment, precautions need to be taken for 12 hours following administration. Whenever possible, a toilet should be used, rather than a urinal, and the toilet should be flushed several times after each use. Spilled urine should be cleaned up completely and patients should wash their hands thoroughly. If blood or urine gets onto clothing, the clothing should be washed separately, or stored for 1 to 2 weeks to allow for decay of the ^{153}Sm.

Some patients have reported a transient increase in bone pain shortly after injection (flare reaction). This is usually mild and self-limiting and occurs within 72 hours of injection. Such reactions are usually responsive to analgesics.

Patients who respond to samarium might begin to notice the onset of pain relief 1 week after samarium. Maximal pain relief generally occurs at 3 to 4 weeks after injection of samarium. Patients who experience a reduction in pain may be encouraged to decrease their use of opioid analgesics.

CARBOPLATIN

Rx	**Carboplatin** (Various, eg, Bedford Labs, Hospira)	**Injection, solution:** 10 mg/mL	In 5, 15, and 45 mL single-use vials.
Rx	**Carboplatin** (Baxter)	**Injection, lyophilized powder for solution:** 50 mg	Mannitol. In single-dose vials.
Rx	**Paraplatin** (Bristol-Myers Squibb)		Mannitol. In single-dose vials.
Rx	**Carboplatin** (Baxter)	**Injection, lyophilized powder for solution:** 150 mg	Mannitol. In single-dose vials.
Rx	**Paraplatin** (Bristol-Myers Squibb)		Mannitol. In single-dose vials.
Rx	**Carboplatin** (Baxter)	**Injection, lyophilized powder for solution:** 450 mg	Mannitol. In single-dose vials.
Rx	**Paraplatin** (Bristol-Myers Squibb)		Mannitol. In single-dose vials.

CARBOPLATIN — INJECTION

WARNING

Carboplatin should be administered under the supervision of a qualified physician experienced in the use of cancer chemotherapeutic agents. Appropriate management of therapy and complications is possible only when adequate treatment facilities are readily available.

Bone marrow suppression is dose related and may be severe, resulting in infection or bleeding. Anemia may be cumulative and may require transfusion support. Vomiting is another frequent drug-related side effect.

Anaphylactic-like reactions to carboplatin have been reported and may occur within minutes of carboplatin administration. Epinephrine, corticosteroids, and antihistamines have been employed to alleviate symptoms.

Indications

➤*Advanced ovarian carcinoma:* For the initial treatment of advanced ovarian carcinoma in established combination with other approved chemotherapeutic agents.

Carboplatin is indicated for the palliative treatment of patients with ovarian carcinoma recurrent after prior chemotherapy, including patients who have been previously treated with cisplatin.

➤*Off-label uses:* As a single agent in previously treated and untreated patients with small cell lung cancer and non-small cell lung cancer, but is most effective when combined with other agents (eg, etoposide); alone or in combination (usually with fluorouracil) in the treatment of advanced or recurrent squamous cell carcinoma of the head and neck; advanced endometrial cancer, in relapsed and refractory acute leukemia and for seminoma of testicular cancer.

Administration and Dosage

➤*General dosing considerations:* Before initial therapy, determine baseline renal function by evaluating BUN, serum creatinine, and creatinine clearance. Monitor BUN and creatinine before each course.

➤*Adults:*

Advanced ovarian carcinoma –

Single-agent therapy: A dosage regimen of 360 mg/m^2 IV on day 1 every 4 weeks has been shown to be effective in patients with recurrent ovarian carcinoma (alternately, see Calvert Formula Dosing). In general, however, single intermittent courses of carboplatin should not be repeated until the neutrophil count is at least 2,000 and the platelet count is at least 100,000.

Combination therapy with cyclophosphamide: In the chemotherapy of advanced ovarian cancer, an effective combination for previously untreated patients consists of:

- Carboplatin 300 mg/m^2 IV on day 1 every 4 weeks for 6 cycles (alternately, see Calvert Formula Dosing).
- Cyclophosphamide 600 mg/m^2 IV on day 1 every 4 weeks for 6 cycles. For directions regarding the use and administration of cyclophosphamide, please refer to the cyclophosphamide monograph. Intermittent courses of carboplatin in combination with cyclophosphamide should not be repeated until the neutrophil count is at least 2,000 and the platelet count is at least 100,000.

Dose adjustment: Pretreatment platelet count and performance status are important prognostic factors for severity of myelosuppression in previously treated patients.

The suggested dose adjustments for single agent or combination therapy below are modified from controlled trials in previously treated and untreated patients with ovarian carcinoma. Blood counts were done weekly, and the recommendations are based on the lowest posttreatment platelet or neutrophil value.

Carboplatin Dose Adjustments for Single Agent or Combination Therapy

Platelets	Neutrophils	Adjusted dose[a] (from prior course)
> 100,000	> 2000	125%
50 to 100,000	500 to 2000	No adjustment
< 50,000	< 500	75%

[a] Percentages apply to carboplatin injection as a single agent or to both carboplatin and cyclophosphamide in combination. In the controlled studies, dosages were also adjusted at a lower level (50% to 60%) for severe myelosuppression. Escalations above 125% were not recommended for these studies.

Calvert formula dosing: Another approach for determining the initial dose of carboplatin is the use of mathematical formulae, which are based on a patient's preexisting renal function or renal function and desired platelet nadir. Renal excretion is the major route of elimination for carboplatin. The use of dosing formulae, as compared to empirical dose calculation based on body surface area, allows compensation for patient variations in pretreatment renal function that might otherwise result in either underdosing (in patients with above average renal function) or overdosing (in patients with impaired renal function).

A simple formula for calculating dosage, based upon a patient's glomerular filtration rate (GFR in mL/min) and carboplatin target area under the concentration vs time curve (AUC in mg/mL•min), has been proposed by Calvert. In these studies, GFR was measured by ^{51}Cr-EDTA clearance.

Calvert Formula for Carboplatin Dosing
Total dose (mg) = (target AUC) × (GFR + 25)
Note: With the Calvert formula, the total dose of carboplatin is calculated in mg, not mg/m^2

The target AUC of 4 to 6 mg/mL•min using single agent carboplatin appears to provide the most appropriate dose range in previously treated patients. This study also showed a trend between the AUC of single agent carboplatin administered to previously treated patients and the likelihood of developing toxicity.

Actual Toxicity in Patients Previously Treated with Carboplatin (%)

AUC (mg/mL•min)	Grade 3 or 4 thrombocytopenia	Grade 3 or 4 leukopenia
4 to 5	16%	13%
6 to 7	33%	34%

➤*Children:*

Off-label dosing –

3 years of age and older:

- *Brain tumors* – 175 mg/m^2 IV once weekly for 4 weeks, followed by a 2-week rest period.
- *Solid tumors* – 300 to 600 mg/m^2 IV every 4 weeks.
- *Modified Calvert formula* – Carboplatin may be dosed to achieve a target AUC based on the patient's GFR using a modified Calvert formula. The desired target AUC depends on the disease and the patient's treatment status. However, target AUCs between 5 and 7 mg/mL•min are typical in children. Consult specific protocols for more information.

The modified Calvert formula calculates the carboplatin dose in milligrams as follows: Total dose (mg) = target AUC (mg/mL•min) × [GFR (mL/min) + (0.36 × weight in kg)].

In trials evaluating the predictability of the Calvert formula in adults, GFR was determined by ^{51}Cr-EDTA clearance. Limited information is available regarding the accuracy of other methods to determine GFR (eg, Cockcroft-Gault equation, Jelliffe equation). Although some clinicians may use methods other than ^{51}Cr-EDTA clearance to determine GFR, it is unknown whether similar clinical outcomes are achieved.

➤*Elderly:* Because renal function is often decreased in elderly patients, formula dosing of carboplatin based on estimates of GFR should be used in elderly patients to provide predictable plasma carboplatin AUCs and thereby minimize the risk of toxicity.

➤*Renal function impairment:* Patients with creatinine clearance values below 60 mL/min are at increased risk of severe bone marrow suppression. In renally impaired patients who received single agent carboplatin therapy, the incidence of severe leukopenia, neutropenia, or thrombocytopenia has been about 25% when the dosage modifications below have been used.

Initial dose –

Carboplatin Dosage Modifications in Renal Function Impairment

Baseline creatinine clearance	Recommended dose on Day 1
41 to 59 mL/min	250 mg/m^2
16 to 40 mL/min	200 mg/m^2

The data available for patients with severely impaired kidney function (creatinine clearance below 15 mL/min) are too limited to permit a recommendation for treatment.

Subsequent dosages – These dosing recommendations apply to the initial course of treatment. Subsequent dosages should be adjusted according to the patient's tolerance based on the degree of bone marrow suppression.

Dialysis – Literature describing the effectiveness of conventional hemodialysis in removing carboplatin has varied. Some sources state that conventional hemodialysis is ineffective (0% to 24%) in removing carboplatin while others state that it is minimally effective (25% to 49%) or even moderately effective (50% to 74%) in removing carboplatin. High permeability dialysis has been shown to be minimally effective (25% to 49%) in removing carboplatin.

After hemodialysis, some clinicians recommend supplementing with 50% of the original dose.

CARBOPLATIN — INJECTION

➤*Preparation for administration:* Carboplatin is considered a cytotoxic agent. Follow safe handling procedures when preparing, administering, or dispensing carboplatin.

Aluminum reacts with carboplatin causing precipitate formation and loss of potency; therefore, needles or intravenous sets containing aluminum parts that may come in contact with the drug must not be used for the preparation or administration of carboplatin.

Powder for injection – Reconstitute lyophilized powder with sterile water for injection, sodium chloride 0.9% injection, or dextrose 5% injection with volumes of diluent specified below.

Dilution for Carboplatin[a]		
Vial size	Volume of diluent	Concentration
50 mg	5 mL	10 mg/mL
150 mg	15 mL	10 mg/mL
450 mg	45 mL	10 mg/mL

[a] Can be further diluted to 0.5 mg/mL with sodium chloride 0.9% injection or dextrose 5% injection.

Solution for injection – Carboplatin injection is a premixed aqueous solution of 10 mg/mL carboplatin. Carboplatin can be further diluted to concentrations as low as 0.5 mg/mL with dextrose 5% injection or sodium chloride 0.9% injection.

➤*Administration:* Infuse IV over at least 15 minutes. Carboplatin doses may also be infused over 30 to 60 minutes. No pre- or post-treatment hydration or forced diuresis is required.

➤*Extravasation:* Carboplatin (in concentrations of 10 mg/mL or greater) is usually considered an irritant. However, necrosis associated with extravasation has been reported. If signs or symptoms of extravasation occur, stop the infusion immediately. If possible, withdraw 3 to 5 mL of blood to remove some of the drug. Remove the infusion needle. Delineate the infiltrated area on the patient's skin with a felt tip marker. Elevate for 48 hours above heart level using a sling or stockinette dressing with an observation window cut in the dressing. Avoid pressure or friction. Do not rub the area. Observe for signs of increased erythema, pain, or skin necrosis. If increased symptoms occur, consult a plastic surgeon. Ensure that no medication is given distally to the extravasation site. After 48 hours, encourage the patient to use the extremity normally to promote full range of motion.

➤*Admixture compatibility:* Aluminum reacts with carboplatin causing precipitate formation and loss of potency; therefore, needles or intravenous sets containing aluminum parts that may come in contact with the drug must not be used for the preparation or administration of carboplatin.

➤*Storage/Stability:* Store at 25°C (77°F); excursions permitted from 15° to 30°C (59° to 86°F). Protect from light.

Although chemically stable for longer periods of time, carboplatin solutions do not contain a preservative and the manufacturer recommends use within 8 hours of reconstitution or preparation when stored at room temperature (25°C; 77°F). Use carboplatin within 24 hours of reconstitution or preparation to reduce the risk of microbial contamination.

When stored in the original multidose vial, the commercially available aqueous solution is stable for up to 14 days at room temperature even with multiple needle entries.

Discard single-dose vials within 6 hours of the initial needle puncture if opened within an ISO Class 5 biological safety cabinet, or within 1 hour of the initial needle puncture if opened outside of such an environment, based on the USP Chapter <797> standards.

Actions

➤*Pharmacology:* Carboplatin, like cisplatin, produces predominantly interstrand DNA cross-links rather than DNA-protein cross-links. This effect is apparently cell-cycle nonspecific. The aquation of carboplatin, which is thought to produce the active species, occurs at a slower rate than in the case of cisplatin. Despite this difference, it appears that both carboplatin and cisplatin induce equal numbers of drug-DNA cross-links, causing equivalent lesions and biological effects. The differences in potencies for carboplatin and cisplatin appear to be directly related to the difference in aquation rates.

➤*Pharmacokinetics:*

Absorption/Distribution – Carboplatin is not bound to plasma proteins. No significant quantities of protein-free, ultrafilterable platinum-containing species other than carboplatin are present in plasma. However, platinum from carboplatin becomes irreversibly bound to plasma proteins and is slowly eliminated with a minimum half-life of 5 days.

Metabolism/Excretion – The major route of elimination of carboplatin is renal excretion. Patients with creatinine clearances of approximately 60 mL/min or greater excrete 65% of the dose in the urine within 12 hours and 71% of the dose within 24 hours. All of the platinum in the 24-hour urine is present as carboplatin. Only 3% to 5% of the administered platinum is excreted in the urine between 24 and 96 hours. There are insufficient data to determine whether biliary excretion occurs.

Special populations –

Renal function impairment: In patients with creatinine clearances below 60 mL/min the total body and renal clearances of carboplatin decrease as the creatinine clearance decreases. Carboplatin dosages should therefore be reduced in these patients.

In patients with creatinine clearances of about 60 mL/min or greater, plasma levels of intact carboplatin decay in a biphasic manner after a 30-minute intravenous infusion of 300 to 500 mg/m^2 of carboplatin. The initial plasma half-life (alpha) was found to be 1.1 to 2 hours (n = 6), and the postdistribution plasma half-life (beta) was found to be 2.6 to 5.9 hours (n = 6). The total body clearance, apparent volume of distribution and mean residence time for carboplatin are 4.4 L/hour, 16 L and 3.5 hours, respectively. The C_{max} values and areas under the plasma concentration vs time curves from 0 to infinity (AUC inf) increase linearly with dose, although the increase was slightly more than dose proportional. Carboplatin, therefore, exhibits linear pharmacokinetics over the dosing range studied (300 to 500 mg/m^2).

The primary determinant of carboplatin clearance is glomerular filtration rate (GFR) and this parameter of renal function is often decreased in elderly patients. Dosing formulas incorporating estimates of GFR to provide predictable carboplatin plasma AUCs should be used in elderly patients to minimize the risk of toxicity.

Contraindications

Severe allergic reactions to cisplatin or other platinum-containing compounds, or mannitol; severe bone marrow depression or significant bleeding.

Warnings/Precautions

➤*Bone marrow suppression:* Bone marrow suppression (leukopenia, neutropenia, and thrombocytopenia) is dose-dependent and is also the dose-limiting toxicity. Peripheral blood counts should be frequently monitored during carboplatin treatment and, when appropriate, until recovery is achieved. Median nadir occurs at day 21 in patients receiving single-agent carboplatin.By day 28, 90% of patients have platelet counts greater than 100,000/mm^3; 74% have neutrophil counts greater than 2,000/mm^3; 67% have leukocyte counts greater than 4,000/mm^3. In general, single intermittent courses of carboplatin should not be repeated until leukocyte, neutrophil, and platelet counts have recovered.

Since anemia is cumulative, transfusions may be needed during treatment with carboplatin, particularly in patients receiving prolonged therapy.

Bone marrow suppression is increased in patients who have received prior therapy, especially regimens including cisplatin. Marrow suppression is also increased in patients with impaired kidney function. Initial carboplatin dosages in these patients should be appropriately reduced and blood counts should be carefully monitored between courses. The use of carboplatin in combination with other bone marrow suppressing therapies must be carefully managed with respect to dosage and timing in order to minimize additive effects.

➤*Toxicity:* Carboplatin has limited nephrotoxic potential, but concomitant treatment with aminoglycosides has resulted in increased renal or audiologic toxicity, and caution must be exercised when a patient receives both drugs. Clinically significant hearing loss has been reported to occur in pediatric patients when carboplatin was administered at higher than recommended doses in combination with other ototoxic agents.

➤*Emesis:* Carboplatin can induce emesis, which can be more severe in patients previously receiving emetogenic therapy. The incidence and intensity of emesis have been reduced by using premedication with antiemetics. Although no conclusive efficacy data exist with the following schedules of carboplatin, lengthening the duration of single intravenous administration to 24 hours or dividing the total dose over 5 consecutive daily pulse doses has resulted in reduced emesis.

➤*Peripheral neurotoxicity:* Although peripheral neurotoxicity is infrequent, its incidence is increased in patients greater than 65 years of age and in patients previously treated with cisplatin. Preexisting cisplatin-induced neurotoxicity does not worsen in about 70% of the patients receiving carboplatin as secondary treatment.

➤*Ophthalmic:* Loss of vision, which can be complete for light and colors, has been reported after the use of carboplatin for injection with doses higher than those recommended. Vision appears to recover totally or to a significant extent within weeks of stopping these high doses.

➤*Allergic reactions:* As in the case of other platinum coordination compounds, allergic reactions to carboplatin have been reported. These may occur within minutes of administration and should be managed with appropriate supportive therapy. There is increased risk of allergic reactions including anaphylaxis in patients previously exposed to platinum therapy. Carboplatin is contraindicated in patients with a history of severe allergic reactions to cisplatin or other platinum-containing compounds.

➤*Lab test abnormalities:* See Adverse Reactions for more information.

➤*Aluminum:* See Administration and Dosage for more information.

➤*Extravasation:* See Administration and Dosage for more information.

➤*Pregnancy: Category D.* Carboplatin may cause fetal harm when administered to a pregnant woman. Carboplatin has been shown to be embryotoxic and teratogenic in rats. There are no adequate and well-controlled studies in pregnant women. If this drug is used during pregnancy, or if the patient becomes pregnant while receiving this drug, the patient should be apprised of the potential hazard to the fetus. Women of childbearing potential should be advised to avoid becoming pregnant.

➤*Lactation:* It is not known whether carboplatin is excreted in human milk. Because there is a possibility of toxicity in nursing infants secondary to carboplatin treatment of the mother, it is recommended that breastfeeding be discontinued if the mother is treated with carboplatin.

➤*Children:* Safety and effectiveness in children have not been established.

➤*Elderly:* Of the 789 patients in initial treatment combination therapy studies (NCIC and SWOG), 395 patients were treated with carboplatin in combination with cyclophosphamide. Of these, 141 were over 65 years of age and 22 were 75 years of age or older. In these trials, age was not a prognostic factor for survival. In terms of safety, elderly patients treated with carbo-

CARBOPLATIN — INJECTION

platin were more likely to develop severe thrombocytopenia than younger patients. In a combined database of 1,942 patients (414 were greater than or equal to 65 years of age) that received single-agent carboplatin for different tumor types, a similar incidence of adverse events was seen in patients 65 years and older and in patients less than 65. Other reported clinical experience has not identified differences in responses between elderly and younger patients, but greater sensitivity of some older individuals cannot be ruled out. Because renal function is often decreased in the elderly, renal function should be considered in the selection of carboplatin dosage.

Drug Interactions

Carboplatin Drug Interactions

Precipitant drug	Object drug[a]		Description
Aminoglycosides	Carboplatin	↑	Coadministration has resulted in increased renal and/or audiologic toxicity. Use with caution.
Carboplatin	Aminoglycosides		
Carboplatin	Phenytoin	↓	Serum concentrations of phenytoin may be decreased, resulting in a loss of therapeutic effect. Monitor phenytoin levels and adjust dose appropriately.
Carboplatin	Warfarin	↑	The anticoagulant effect of warfarin may be increased. Monitor coagulation parameters and adjust warfarin as needed.

[a] ↑ = object drug increased; ↓ = object drug decreased.

Adverse Reactions

Carboplatin is considered to have moderately high emetogenic potential (60% to 90% incidence of emesis).

➤*Allergic:* Hypersensitivity to carboplatin has occurred in 2% of the patients and may occur within minutes of administration; manage with appropriate supportive therapy. These allergic reactions have been similar in nature and severity to those reported with other platinum-containing compounds, ie, rash, urticaria, erythema, pruritus, and rarely bronchospasm and hypotension. Anaphylactic reactions have been reported as part of postmarketing surveillance. These reactions have been successfully managed with standard epinephrine, corticosteroid, and antihistamine therapy.

➤*CNS:* Peripheral neuropathies have been observed in 4% of the patients receiving carboplatin (6% of pretreated ovarian cancer patients) with mild paresthesias occurring most frequently. Carboplatin therapy produces significantly fewer and less severe neurologic side effects than does therapy with cisplatin. However, patients greater than 65 years of age or previously treated with cisplatin appear to have an increased risk (10%) for peripheral neuropathies. In 70% of the patients with preexisting cisplatin-induced peripheral neurotoxicity, there was no worsening of symptoms during therapy with carboplatin. Clinical ototoxicity and other sensory abnormalities such as visual disturbances and change in taste have been reported in only 1% of the patients. Central nervous system symptoms have been reported in 5% of the patients and appear to be most often related to the use of antiemetics.

Although the overall incidence of peripheral neurologic side effects induced by carboplatin is low, prolonged treatment, particularly in cisplatin pretreated patients, may result in cumulative neurotoxicity.

➤*Electrolyte disturbance:* The incidences of abnormally decreased serum electrolyte values reported were as follows: Sodium, 29%; potassium, 20%; calcium, 22%; and magnesium, 29%; (47%, 28%, 31%, and 43%, respectively, in pretreated ovarian cancer patients). Electrolyte supplementation was not routinely administered concomitantly with carboplatin, and these electrolyte abnormalities were rarely associated with symptoms.

➤*GI:* Vomiting occurs in 65% of the patients (81% of previously treated ovarian cancer patients) and in about one-third of these patients it is severe. Carboplatin, as a single agent or in combination, is significantly less emetogenic than cisplatin; however, patients previously treated with emetogenic agents, especially cisplatin, appear to be more prone to vomiting. Nausea alone occurs in an additional 10% to 15% of patients. Both nausea and vomiting usually cease within 24 hours of treatment and are often responsive to antiemetic measures. Although no conclusive efficacy data exist with the following schedules, prolonged administration of carboplatin, either by continuous 24-hour infusion or by daily pulse doses given for 5 consecutive days, was associated with less severe vomiting than the single dose intermittent schedule. Emesis was increased when carboplatin was used in combination with other emetogenic compounds. Other gastrointestinal effects observed frequently were pain in 17% of the patients; diarrhea in 6%; and constipation also in 6%.

➤*Hematologic:* Bone marrow suppression is the dose-limiting toxicity of carboplatin. Thrombocytopenia with platelet counts below 50,000/mm^3 occurs in 25% of the patients (35% of pretreated ovarian cancer patients); neutropenia with granulocyte counts below 1,000/mm^3 occurs in 16% of the patients (21% of pretreated ovarian cancer patients); leukopenia with WBC counts below 2,000/mm^3 occurs in 15% of the patients (26% of pretreated ovarian cancer patients). The nadir usually occurs about day 21 in patients receiving single-agent therapy. By day 28, 90% of patients have platelet counts above 100,000/mm^3; 74% have neutrophil counts above 2,000/mm^3; 67% have leukocyte counts above 4,000/mm^3.

Marrow suppression is usually more severe in patients with impaired kidney function. Patients with poor performance status have also experienced a higher incidence of severe leukopenia and thrombocytopenia.

The hematologic effects, although usually reversible, have resulted in infectious or hemorrhagic complications in 5% of the patients treated with carboplatin for injection, with drug related death occurring in less than 1% of the patients. Fever has also been reported in patients with neutropenia.

Anemia with hemoglobin less than 11 g/dL has been observed in 71% of the patients who started therapy with a baseline above that value. The incidence of anemia increases with increasing exposure to carboplatin. Transfusions have been administered to 26% of the patients treated with carboplatin (44% of previously treated ovarian cancer patients).

Bone marrow depression may be more severe when carboplatin is combined with other bone marrow suppressing drugs or with radiotherapy.

➤*Hepatic:* The incidences of abnormal liver function tests in patients with normal baseline values were reported as follows: Total bilirubin, 5%; AST, 15%; and alkaline phosphatase, 24% (5%, 19%, and 37%, respectively, in pretreated ovarian cancer patients). These abnormalities have generally been mild and reversible in about one-half of the cases, although the role of metastatic tumor in the liver may complicate the assessment in many patients. In a limited series of patients receiving very high dosages of carboplatin and autologous bone marrow transplantation, severe abnormalities of liver function tests were reported.

➤*Local:* Injection site reactions, including redness, swelling, and pain have been reported during postmarketing surveillance. Necrosis associated with extravasation has also been reported.

➤*Lab test abnormalities:* High dosages of carboplatin (greater than 4 times the recommended dose) have resulted in severe abnormalities of liver function tests. Total bilirubin, AST, and alkaline phosphatase abnormalities have generally been mild and reversible in approximately 50% of the cases.

➤*Renal:* Renal toxicity is limited, but concomitant treatment with aminoglycosides has resulted in increased renal or audiologic toxicity. Exercise caution when a patient receives both drugs. Development of abnormal renal function test results is uncommon, despite the fact that carboplatin, unlike cisplatin, has usually been administered without high-volume fluid hydration or forced diuresis. The incidences of abnormal renal function tests reported are 6% for serum creatinine and 14% for blood urea nitrogen (10% and 22%, respectively, in pretreated ovarian cancer patients). Most of these reported abnormalities have been mild and about one-half of them were reversible.

Creatinine clearance has proven to be the most sensitive measure of kidney function in patients receiving carboplatin, and it appears to be the most useful test for correlating drug clearance and bone marrow suppression. Twenty-seven percent (27%) of the patients who had a baseline value of 60 mL/min or more demonstrated a reduction below this value during carboplatin therapy.

➤*Miscellaneous:* Pain and asthenia were the most frequently reported miscellaneous adverse effects; their relationship to the tumor and to anemia was likely. Alopecia was reported (3%). Cardiovascular, respiratory, genitourinary, and mucosal side effects have occurred in 6% or less of the patients. Cardiovascular events (cardiac failure, embolism, cerebrovascular accidents) were fatal in less than 1% of the patients and did not appear to be related to chemotherapy. Cancer-associated hemolytic uremic syndrome has been reported rarely.

Malaise, anorexia, and hypertension have been reported as part of postmarketing surveillance.

Carboplatin Adverse Reactions in Patients with Ovarian Cancer (%)

Adverse reactions	First line combination therapy[a]	Second line single agent therapy[b]
Bone marrow		
Thrombocytopenia		
< 100,000/mm^3	66%	62%
< 50,000/mm^3	33%	35%
Neutropenia		
< 2000 cells/mm^3	96%	67%
< 1000 cells/mm^3	82%	21%
Leukopenia		
< 4000 cells/mm^3	97%	85%
< 2000 cells/mm^3	71%	26%
Anemia		
< 11 g/dL	90%	90%
< 8 g/dL	14%	21%
Infections	16%	5%
Bleeding	8%	5%
Transfusions	35%	44%
CNS		
Peripheral neuropathies	15%	6%
Ototoxicity	12%	1%
Other sensory side effects	5%	1%

CARBOPLATIN — INJECTION

Carboplatin Adverse Reactions in Patients with Ovarian Cancer (%)		
Adverse reactions	First line combination therapy[a]	Second line single agent therapy[b]
Central neurotoxicity	26%	5%
Electrolytes loss		
Sodium	10%	47%
Potassium	16%	28%
Calcium	16%	31%
Magnesium	61%	43%
GI		
Nausea and vomiting	93%	92%
Vomiting	83%	81%
Other GI side effects	46%	21%
Hepatic		
Bilirubin elevations	5%	5%
AST elevations	20%	19%
Alkaline phosphatase elevations	29%	37%
Renal		
Serum creatinine elevations	6%	10%
Blood urea elevations	17%	22%
Miscellaneous		
Pain	44%	23%
Asthenia	41%	11%
Cardiovascular	19%	6%
Respiratory	10%	6%
Allergic	11%	2%
GU	10%	2%
Alopecia	49%	2%
Mucositis	8%	1%

[a] Use with cyclophosphamide for initial treatment of ovarian cancer: Data are based on the experience of 393 patients with ovarian cancer (regardless of baseline status) who received initial combination therapy with carboplatin and cyclophosphamide in 2 randomized controlled studies conducted by SWOG and NCIC.Combination with cyclophosphamide as well as duration of treatment may be responsible for the differences that can be noted in the adverse experiences table.

[b] Single agent use for the secondary treatment of ovarian cancer: Data are based on the experience of 553 patients with previously treated ovarian carcinoma (regardless of baseline status) who received single-agent carboplatin.

Overdosage

There is no known antidote for carboplatin overdosage. The anticipated complications of overdosage would be secondary to bone marrow suppression or hepatic toxicity.

CISPLATIN (CDDP)

Rx	**Cisplatin** (Various, eg, Abbott, American Pharmaceutical, Bedford Labs)	**Injection:** 1 mg/mL	In 50, 100, and 200 ml multi-dose vials.

CISPLATIN (CDDP) — INJECTION

WARNING

Cisplatin should be administered under the supervision of a qualified physician experienced in the use of cancer chemotherapeutic agents. Appropriate management of therapy and complications is possible only when adequate diagnostic and treatment facilities are readily available.

Cumulative renal toxicity – Cumulative renal toxicity associated with cisplatin is severe (see Warnings). Other major dose-related toxicities are myelosuppression, nausea, and vomiting.

Ototoxicity – Ototoxicity, which may be more pronounced in children, and is manifested by tinnitus or loss of high frequency hearing and, occasionally, deafness, is significant.

Anaphylactic-like reactions – Anaphylactic-like reactions have occurred (see Warnings). Facial edema, bronchoconstriction, tachycardia, and hypotension may occur within minutes of cisplatin administration. Epinephrine, corticosteroids, and antihistamines have been effectively employed to alleviate symptoms (see Warnings and Adverse Reactions).

Exercise caution to prevent inadvertent cisplatin overdose. Doses greater than 100 mg/m²/cycle once every 3 to 4 weeks are rarely used. Care must be taken to avoid inadvertent cisplatin overdose due to confusion with carboplatin or prescribing practices that fail to differentiate daily doses from total dose per cycle.

Indications

➤*Metastatic testicular tumors:* In combination therapy in patients who have received appropriate surgical or radiotherapeutic procedures.

➤*Metastatic ovarian tumors:* In combination therapy (eg, cyclophosphamide) in patients who have received appropriate surgical or radiotherapeutic procedures. Cisplatin, as a single agent, is indicated as secondary therapy in patients refractory to standard chemotherapy who have not previously received cisplatin.

➤*Advanced bladder cancer:* As a single agent for patients with transitional cell bladder cancer no longer amenable to local treatments (eg, surgery or radiotherapy).

➤*Off-label uses:* Treatment of squamous cell carcinoma of the head and neck, cervix; lung carcinomas; osteogenic sarcoma; brain tumors; advanced esophageal, adrenal cortex, breast, endometrial, and liver carcinoma; bone marrow transplantation. (See Administration and Dosage.)

Cisplatin has been used safely and effectively in children for the treatment of brain tumors, neuroblastoma, and osteosarcoma. (See Administration and Dosage).

Administration and Dosage

➤*General dosing considerations:* Perform pretreatment hydration prior to dose. (See Preparation for administration).

Note to pharmacist – Exercise caution to prevent inadvertent cisplatin overdosage. Please call prescriber if dose is greater than 100 mg/m² per cycle. Aluminum and flip-off seal of vial have been imprinted with the following statement: Call Dr. if dose greater than 100 mg/m²/cycle.

➤*Adults:*

Advanced bladder cancer – 50 to 70 mg/m² IV once every 3 to 4 weeks (single agent therapy), depending on prior radiation therapy or chemotherapy. For heavily pretreated patients, give an initial dose of 50 mg/m² IV once every 4 weeks.

Metastatic ovarian tumors –

Combination regimen:

- *Cisplatin* – 75 to 100 mg/m² IV once every 4 weeks.
- *Cyclophosphamide* – 600 mg/m² IV once every 4 weeks (day 1).

In combination therapy, administer cisplatin and cyclophosphamide sequentially.

Single agent dosing: 100 mg/m² IV once every 4 weeks.

Metastatic testicular tumors – 20 mg/m²/day IV for 5 days every 3 weeks for 3 courses (combination regimen). Single doses of cisplatin up to 120 mg/m² in combination with other antineoplastics have been used.

Off-label dosing –

Cervical cancer: Cisplatin doses range from 40 mg/m² IV once weekly to 75 mg/m² IV once every 3 weeks. Given in combination with radiation therapy.

Hepatocellular cancer (chemoembolization): Cisplatin 40 to 100 mg/m² administered intraarterially with or without ethiodized oil and embolizing agents such as *Gelfoam*.

Intraperitoneal administration: Cisplatin 90 to 270 mg/m² instilled peritoneally every 3 to 4 weeks.

Other cancers: Single doses of up to 100 to 120 mg/m² IV have been used for multiple indications including osteogenic sarcoma and cancer of the lungs, bladder, and head and neck.

➤*Children:*

Off-label dosing –

Recurrent brain tumors: 60 mg/m²/day IV for 2 consecutive days every 3 to 4 weeks.

Other cancers: Single doses of 30 to 100 mg/m² IV have been used for multiple indications, including osteogenic sarcoma and neuroblastoma. Doses similar to those found in adult regimens may be used, calculated based on body surface area (BSA).

➤*Renal function impairment:* The manufacturer does not recommend the use of cisplatin in patients with renal function impairment. Some clinicians recommend not giving cisplatin to patients with a CrCl below 30 mL/min.

Dosage adjustment is recommended in renal impairment as shown in the following table.

Cisplatin Dosage Adjustment Based on Renal Function	
Baseline CrCl	Percentage of dose
30 to 50 mL/min	50%
10 to 29 mL/min	50%, consider avoiding use
0 to 9 mL/min	Do not give.

Dialysis – Conventional hemodialysis is ineffective (0% to 24%) in removing cisplatin. High permeability is minimally effective (25% to 49%) in removing cisplatin.

CISPLATIN (CDDP) — INJECTION

➤*Repeat courses:* Do not give a repeat course until the serum creatinine is less than 1.5 mg/dL or the BUN is less than 25 mg/dL or until circulating blood elements are at an acceptable level (platelets greater than or equal to 100,000/mm^3, WBC greater than or equal to 4,000/mm^3). Do not give subsequent doses until an audiometric analysis indicates that auditory acuity is within normal limits.

➤*Concomitant therapy:* Delayed emesis typically occurs 24 to 72 hours after cisplatin administration. Severity may be reduced by administration of a prophylactic regimen of dexamethasone in combination with metoclopramide or prochlorperazine. Begin prophylactic therapy 16 to 24 hours after cisplatin administration and continue for a total of 4 days. Add additional antiemetics if breakthrough nausea and vomiting occur.

Amifostine may decrease the risk of cumulative renal toxicity with repeated courses in ovarian cancer patients.

➤*Preparation for administration:* Cisplatin is considered a cytotoxic agent. Skin reactions associated with accidental exposure may occur. Use gloves. If solution contacts skin or mucosa, wash immediately and thoroughly with soap and water and flush mucosa with water. Follow safe handling procedures when preparing, administering, or dispensing cisplatin.

Note – Do not use needles or IV sets containing aluminum parts for preparation or administration. Aluminum reacts with cisplatin, causing black precipitation and a loss of potency.

Hydration – Adequately hydrate patients before and for 24 hours after administration of cisplatin to increase urine output and minimize nephrotoxicity. The manufacturer recommends hydrating patients with 1 to 2 L of fluid infused for 8 to 12 hours before cisplatin administration. Patients may be given 1 L of 0.9% sodium chloride (with or without potassium chloride) over 2 to 4 hours prior to cisplatin administration to establish good urine output.

Then dilute the drug in 2 L of 5% dextrose in one-half or one-third normal saline containing mannitol 37.5 g and infuse over 6 to 8 hours. If diluted solution is not to be used within 6 hours, protect from light. Do not dilute cisplatin in just 5% dextrose injection. Maintain adequate hydration and urinary output during the following 24 hours. More concentrated solutions, up to a maximum concentration of 0.7 mg/mL, have been used. In some hospitals, cisplatin (up to 200 mg) may also be diluted in 500 mL of 0.9% sodium chloride with mannitol 12.5 to 25 g.

Chemoembolization solution – The 1 mg/mL solution may be used without further dilution. If desired, a cisplatin/oil emulsion may be used. Mix the desired dose of cisplatin with ethiodized oil 10 to 20 mL. Emulsify using 2 syringes and a 3-way stopcock.Safe handling techniques may be difficult to maintain when preparing this emulsion.

Intraperitoneal solution – Dilute with 2 L of 0.9% sodium chloride. Allow solution to warm before instillation.

➤*Administration:*

IV – Infuse cisplatin over 6 to 8 hours. More rapid administration rates (30 minutes to 2 hours) are commonly used.

Chemoembolization (off-label) – Chemoembolization procedures are performed using arteriography. The chemoembolization solution is injected intra-arterially and may be followed by gelatin-sponge (*Gelfoam*) particles. Angiography is typically performed after the procedure to evaluate the degree of vascular occlusion.

Intraperitoneal administration (off-label) – Drain peritoneal cavity prior to administration. Instill cisplatin into peritoneal cavity by gravity flow over 10 minutes through a percutaneously inserted peritoneal dialysis catheter. Allow to dwell for 4 hours, then drain peritoneal cavity.

➤*Extravasation:* Cisplatin in volumes of more than 20 mL and in concentrations of 0.5 mg/mL or more is considered a vesicant. If signs or symptoms of extravasation occur, stop the infusion immediately. If possible, withdraw 3 to 5 mL of blood to remove some of the drug. If possible, administer sodium thiosulfate (⅙ molar) within the first few minutes to 1 hour after extravasation. To prepare a ⅙ molar solution, dilute 4 mL of 10% sodium thiosulfate with 6 mL of sterile water for injection or dilute 1.6 mL of 25% sodium thiosulfate with 8.4 mL of sterile water for injection. Cleanse the extravasation site with povidone-iodine. Use 2 mL of sodium thiosulfate for each estimated mg of cisplatin extravasated. If possible, administer sodium thiosulfate through the extravasated IV site and inject subcutaneously around the site of extravasation. Application of cold compresses for 15 minutes every 6 hours for 48 hours may be useful. Delineate the infiltrated area on the patient's skin with a felt tip marker. Elevate for 48 hours above heart level using a sling or stockinette dressing with an observation window cut in the dressing. Avoid pressure or friction. Do not rub the area. Observe for signs of increased erythema, pain, or skin necrosis. If increased symptoms occur, consult a plastic surgeon. Ensure that no medication is given distally to extravasation site. After 48 hours, encourage the patient to use the extremity normally to promote full range of motion.

Cisplatin in volumes of less than 20 mL and in concentrations less than 0.5 mg/mL is considered an irritant. It may cause phlebitis, but it is not known to cause tissue damage with extravasation. If signs or symptoms of extravasation occur, stop the infusion immediately. If possible, withdraw 3 to 5 mL of blood to remove some of the drug. Remove the infusion needle. Delineate the infiltrated area on the patient's skin with a felt tip marker. Elevate for 48 hours above heart level using a sling or stockinette dressing with an observation window cut in the dressing. Avoid pressure or friction. Do not rub the area. Observe for signs of increased erythema, pain, or skin necrosis. If increased symptoms occur, consult a plastic surgeon. Ensure that no medication is given distally to extravasation site. After 48 hours, encourage the patient to use the extremity normally to promote full range of motion.

➤*Admixture compatibility:* Cisplatin and fluorouracil admixtures are stable in 0.9% normal saline for 1 hour.

➤*Storage/Stability:* Store vials at 15° to 25°C. Protect unopened container from light. Do not refrigerate. Commercially available cisplatin solution is preservative free. Although chemically stable for longer periods of time, use diluted solutions within 24 hours of preparation.

Vials of commercially available cisplatin solution for injection that have been entered are stable at room temperature for 7 days under fluorescent light and for 28 days if protected from light.

Chemoembolization solution – No stability information is available for cisplatin/oil emulsion. Prepare chemoembolization emulsions just prior to injection. Discard any unused product.

Actions

➤*Pharmacology:* Cisplatin is an inorganic heavy metal coordination complex containing a central atom of platinum surrounded by 2 chloride atoms and 2 ammonia molecules in the cis position. The antitumor effect of cisplatin has been correlated with binding to DNA, production of intrastrand crosslinks and formation of DNA adducts.

➤*Pharmacokinetics:*

Absorption/Distribution – Plasma concentrations of the parent compound, cisplatin, have a half-life of approximately 20 to 30 minutes; the total body clearance and volume of distribution at steady-state are approximately 15 L/hr/m^2 and approximately 11 L/m^2, respectively. The ratios of cisplatin to total free platinum in the plasma vary considerably between patients and range from 0.5 to 1.1. Cisplatin does not undergo binding to plasma proteins; however, platinum is 90% bound to several plasma proteins including albumin, transferrin, and gamma globulin. The albumin-platinum complexes do not dissociate significantly and are slowly eliminated with a minimum half-life of greater than or equal to 5 days.

Maximum red blood cell concentrations of platinum are reached within 90 to 150 minutes and have a terminal half-life of 36 to 47 days. Concentrations of platinum are highest in liver, prostate, and kidney, somewhat lower in bladder, muscle, testicle, pancreas, and spleen, and lowest in bowel, adrenal, heart, lung, cerebrum, and cerebellum. Platinum is present in tissues for as long as 180 days after the last administration.

Metabolism/Excretion – 90% of the drug is removed by renal mechanisms whereas less than 10% is removed by biliary excretion. The parent compound, cisplatin, is excreted in the urine and accounts for 13% to 17% of the administered dose excreted within 1 hour of administration. The renal clearance of cisplatin and platinum exceed creatinine clearance, indicating active secretion by the kidney. The mean renal clearance of cisplatin is 50 to 62 ml/min/m^2; platinum clearance is non-linear, variable, and dependent on dose, urine flow rate, and individual variability of active secretion and possible tubular reabsorption. Approximately 10% to 40% of the administered platinum is excreted in the urine within 24 hours with a mean of 35% to 51% excreted in the urine over 5 days.

Contraindications

Preexisting renal impairment; myelosuppression; hearing impairment; history of allergic reactions to cisplatin or other platinum-containing compounds.

Warnings/Precautions

➤*Renal toxicity:* Dose-related and cumulative renal insufficiency is the major dose-limiting toxicity. Renal toxicity has been noted in 28% to 36% of patients treated with a single dose of 50 mg/m^2. First noted during the second week after a dose, it is manifested by elevations in BUN and creatinine, serum uric acid, or a decrease in creatinine clearance. Renal toxicity becomes more prolonged and severe with repeated courses of the drug. Renal function must return to normal before another dose can be given.

Amifostine can be used to reduce cumulative renal toxicity in patients with advanced ovarian cancer receiving repeated cisplatin administration.

Impairment of renal function is associated with renal tubular damage. The administration of cisplatin using a 6- to 8-hour infusion with IV hydration and mannitol has been used to reduce nephrotoxicity. However, renal toxicity can still occur (see Precautions).

➤*Ototoxicity:* Ototoxicity has occurred in less than or equal to 31% of patients given a single 50 mg/m^2 dose. It is manifested by tinnitus or hearing loss in the high frequency range (4000 to 8000 Hz); decreased ability to hear normal conversational tones occurs occasionally. Ototoxic effects may be more severe in children. Hearing loss can be unilateral or bilateral and is more frequent and severe with repeated doses. Ototoxicity may be enhanced with prior or simultaneous cranial irradiation. It is unclear whether ototoxicity is reversible. Ototoxic effects may be related to the peak plasma concentration of cisplatin. Because ototoxicity of cisplatin is cumulative, carefully perform audiometry before starting therapy and prior to subsequent doses. Vestibular toxicity has occurred. Deafness after the initial dose of cisplatin has been reported rarely.

Ototoxicity may become more severe in patients being treated with other drugs with nephrotoxic potential.

➤*Hematologic:* Myelosuppression occurs in 25% to 30% of patients treated with cisplatin. The nadirs in circulating platelets and leukocytes occur between days 18 and 23 (range, 7.5 to 45); most patients recover by day 39 (range, 13 to 62). Leukopenia and thrombocytopenia are more pronounced at doses greater than 50 mg/m^2. Anemia (decrease of 2 g hemoglobin/dL) occurs at the same frequency and with the same timing as leukopenia and thrombocytopenia. Fever and infection also have been reported in patients with neutropenia.

In addition to anemia secondary to myelosuppression, a Coombs' positive hemolytic anemia has been reported. In the presence of cisplatin hemolytic

CISPLATIN (CDDP) — INJECTION

anemia, a further course of treatment may be accompanied by increased hemolysis and this risk should be weighed by the treating physician.

The development of acute leukemia coincident with the use of cisplatin has rarely been reported in humans. In these reports, cisplatin was generally given in combination with other leukemogenic agents.

➤*Hepatotoxicity:* Transient elevations of liver enzymes, especially AST, as well as bilirubin, have been reported to be associated with cisplatin administration at the recommended doses.

➤*Vascular toxicities:* Vascular toxicities coincident with use of cisplatin in combination with other antineoplastic agents have occurred rarely. The events are clinically heterogeneous and may include MI, cerebrovascular accident, thrombotic microangiopathy, or cerebral arteritis. Various mechanisms have been proposed for these vascular complications. There are also reports of Raynaud's phenomenon occurring in patients treated with the combination of bleomycin and vinblastine with or without cisplatin. Hypomagnesemia developing coincident with use of cisplatin may be an added, although not essential, factor associated with this event. However, it is currently unknown if the cause of Raynaud's phenomenon in these cases is the disease, underlying vascular compromise, bleomycin, vinblastine, hypomagnesemia, or a combination of any of these factors.

➤*Hyperuricemia:* Hyperuricemia occurs at approximately the same frequency as increases in BUN and serum creatinine. It is more pronounced after doses greater than 50 mg/m^2, and peak uric acid levels generally occur 3 to 5 days after the dose. Allopurinol therapy is effective.

➤*Electrolyte disturbance:* Hypomagnesemia, hypocalcemia, hyponatremia, hypokalemia, and hypophosphatemia have occurred and are probably related to renal tubular damage. Tetany has occasionally occurred in those patients with hypocalcemia and hypomagnesemia. Generally, normal serum electrolyte levels are restored by administering supplemental electrolytes and discontinuing cisplatin.

Increased plasma iron levels and inappropriate antidiuretic hormone syndrome also have occurred.

➤*Ophthalmic effects:* Optic neuritis, papilledema, and cerebral blindness have occurred infrequently in patients receiving standard recommended cisplatin doses. Improvement or total recovery usually occurs after drug discontinuation. Steroids with or without mannitol have been used; however, efficacy has not been established.

Blurred vision and altered color perception have occurred after the use of regimens with higher doses or greater dose frequencies than those recommended. The altered color perception manifests as a loss of color discrimination, particularly in the blue-yellow axis. The only finding on funduscopic exam is irregular retinal pigmentation of the macular area.

➤*Neuropathies:* Neurotoxicity, usually characterized by peripheral neuropathy, has occurred. Severe neuropathies have occurred in patients receiving higher doses of cisplatin or greater dose frequencies than those recommended or after prolonged therapy (4 to 7 months); however, neurologic symptoms have been reported to occur after a single dose. Although symptoms and signs of cisplatin neuropathy usually develop during treatment, symptoms of neuropathy may begin 3 to 8 weeks after the last dose of cisplatin (rare). These neuropathies may be irreversible and are seen as paresthesias in a stocking-glove distribution, areflexia, and loss of proprioception and vibratory sensation. Loss of motor function also has occurred. Discontinue therapy when symptoms are first observed. Neuropathy may progress further even after stopping treatment. Preliminary evidence suggests peripheral neuropathy may be irreversible in some patients.

➤*High/Cumulative doses:* Muscle cramps, defined as localized, painful, involuntary skeletal muscle contractions of sudden onset and short duration, have occurred and were usually associated in patients receiving a relatively high cumulative dose of cisplatin and with a relatively advanced symptomatic stage of peripheral neuropathy.

➤*GI:* Marked nausea and vomiting occur in almost all patients and are occasionally so severe that the drug must be discontinued. Nausea and vomiting usually begin 1 to 4 hours after treatment and last up to 24 hours; nausea and anorexia may persist for up to 1 week after treatment. Metoclopramide in high doses has been used in the prophylaxis of vomiting associated with cisplatin therapy. Delayed nausea and vomiting (beginning or persisting greater than or equal to 24 hours after chemotherapy) has occurred in patients attaining complete emetic control on the day of therapy.

➤*Extravasation:* See Administration and Dosage for more information.

➤*Hypersensitivity reactions:* Anaphylactic-like reactions have occurred. Facial edema, wheezing, tachycardia, and hypotension may occur within minutes of use in patients with prior drug exposure. Symptoms are alleviated by use of epinephrine, corticosteroids, and antihistamines. Refer to Management of Acute Hypersensitivity Reactions.

➤*Pregnancy: Category D.* Of 7 reported pregnancy cases, 1 infant developed profound leukopenia with neutropenia, which resolved after 10 days. The mother had developed profound neutropenia just prior to delivery. By 12 weeks of age, the child was developing normally, except for moderate bilateral hearing loss. Advise patients to avoid becoming pregnant.

➤*Lactation:* Cisplatin has been reported to be found in breast milk; patients receiving cisplatin should not breastfeed.

➤*Children:* Safety and efficacy in children have not been established.

➤*Monitoring:* Monitor peripheral blood counts weekly and liver function periodically. Measure serum creatinine, BUN, creatinine clearance, magnesium, sodium, calcium, and potassium levels prior to initiating therapy and prior to each subsequent course. Do not give more frequently than once every 3 to 4 weeks at the recommended dosage. Perform neurologic and auditory examinations regularly. Carefully perform audiometry before starting therapy and prior to subsequent doses.

Drug Interactions

Cisplatin Drug Interactions

Precipitant drug	Object drug[a]		Description
Aminoglycosides	Cisplatin	↑	Cisplatin produces cumulative nephrotoxicity that is potentiated by aminoglycosides (see Warnings).
Loop diuretics	Cisplatin	↑	Concomitant use of loop diuretics and cisplatin may produce additive ototoxicity (see Warnings).
Cisplatin	Phenytoin	↓	Combination chemotherapy (including cisplatin) may reduce phenytoin plasma levels.

[a] ↑ = Object drug increased. ↓ = Object drug decreased.

Adverse Reactions

Cisplatin in dosages above 50 mg/m^2 is considered to have very high potential for nausea and vomiting. Cisplatin in lower dosages is considered to have moderate to high emetogenic potential.

➤*CNS:* Peripheral neuropathies; seizures; dorsal column myelopathy; malaise; Lhermitte's sign; autonomic neuropathy (see Warnings).

➤*Dermatologic:* Local soft tissue toxicity has rarely been reported following extravasation of cisplatin. Severity of the local tissue toxicity appears to be related to the concentration of the cisplatin solution. Infusion of solutions with a cisplatin concentration greater than 0.5 mg/mL may result in tissue cellulitis, fibrosis, and necrosis.

➤*Electrolyte disturbance:* Hypomagnesemia; hypocalcemia; hyponatremia; hypokalemia; hypophosphatemia; increased plasma iron levels; antidiuretic hormone syndrome (see Warnings).

➤*GI:* Nausea, vomiting, anorexia (see Precautions); diarrhea; loss of taste.

➤*Hematologic:* Myelosuppression (25% to 30%); leukopenia; thrombocytopenia; anemia (see Warnings).

➤*Ophthalmic:* Optic neuritis, papilledema, cerebral blindness (infrequent); blurred vision; altered color perception (see Warnings).

➤*Renal:* Renal insufficiency, renal tubular damage (see Warnings).

➤*Special senses:* Tinnitus, high frequency hearing loss, vestibular toxicity (see Warnings).

➤*Miscellaneous:* Vascular toxicities (rare); hyperuricemia, ototoxicity, anaphylactic-like reactions (see Warnings); elevated AST; alopecia; asthenia.

Infrequent – Cardiac abnormalities; hiccups; rash; elevated serum amylase.

Overdosage

➤*Symptoms:* Exercise caution to prevent inadvertent overdosage with cisplatin. Acute overdosage with this drug may result in kidney failure, liver failure, deafness, ocular toxicity (including detachment of the retina), significant myelosuppression, intractable nausea and vomiting, or neuritis. In addition, death can occur following overdosage.

➤*Treatment:* No proven antidotes have been established for cisplatin overdosage. Hemodialysis, even when initiated 4 hours after the overdosage, appears to have little effect on removing platinum from the body because of cisplatin's rapid and high degree of protein binding. Management of overdosage should include general supportive measures to sustain the patient through any period of toxicity that may occur. Refer to General Management of Acute Overdosage.

OXALIPLATIN

Rx	**Oxaliplatin** (Various, eg, Teva)	**Injection, solution, concentrate:** 5 mg/mL	Preservative free. In 10 and 20 mL single-use vials.
Rx	**Eloxatin** (Sanofi-Aventis)		Preservative free. In 10, 20, and 40 mL single-use vials.
Rx	**Oxaliplatin** (Various, eg, APP Pharmaceuticals)	**Injection, lyophilized powder for solution:** 50 mg	Preservative free. May contain lactose. In single-use vials.
Rx	**Oxaliplatin** (Various, eg, APP Pharmaceuticals)	**Injection, lyophilized powder for solution:** 100 mg	Preservative free. May contain lactose. In single-use vials.

OXALIPLATIN — INJECTION

WARNING

Anaphylactic reactions – Anaphylactic-like reactions to oxaliplatin have been reported and may occur within minutes of administration. Epinephrine, corticosteroids, and antihistamines have been employed to alleviate symptoms.

Indications

➤*Adjuvant treatment of stage III colon cancer:* In combination with infusional 5-fluorouracil/leucovorin for adjuvant treatment of stage III colon cancer patients who have undergone complete resection of the primary tumor.

➤*Advanced colorectal cancer:* In combination with infusional 5-fluorouracil/leucovorin for the treatment of advanced colorectal cancer.

➤*Off-label uses:* Treatment of relapsed or refractory non-Hodgkin lymphoma; treatment of advanced ovarian cancer.

Administration and Dosage

➤*General dosing considerations:* Prior to subsequent therapy cycles, patients should be evaluated for clinical toxicities and laboratory tests. Prolongation of infusion time for oxaliplatin from 2 to 6 hours may mitigate acute toxicities. The infusion times for infusional 5-fluorouracil and leucovorin do not need to be changed.

Premedication is recommended (see Premedication).

➤*Adults:*

Advanced colorectal cancer –

Usual dosage:

• *Day 1* – Oxaliplatin 85 mg/m^2 intravenous (IV) infusion in dextrose 5% in water (D5W) 250 to 500 mL and leucovorin 200 mg/m^2 IV infusion in D5W, both given over 120 minutes at the same time in separate bags using a Y-line, followed by 5-fluorouracil 400 mg/m^2 IV bolus given over 2 to 4 minutes, followed by 5-fluorouracil 600 mg/m^2 IV infusion in D5W 500 mL (recommended) as a 22-hour continuous infusion.

• *Day 2* – Leucovorin 200 mg/m^2 IV infusion over 120 minutes, followed by 5-fluorouracil 400 mg/m^2 IV bolus given over 2 to 4 minutes, followed by 5-fluorouracil 600 mg/m^2 IV infusion in D5W 500 mL (recommended) as a 22-hour continuous infusion. Repeat cycle every 2 weeks.

Dosage adjustment: For patients who experience persistent grade 2 neurosensory events that do not resolve, a dose reduction of oxaliplatin to 65 mg/m^2 should be considered. For patients with persistent grade 3 neurosensory events, discontinuing therapy should be considered. The 5-fluorouracil/leucovorin regimen need not be altered.

A dose reduction of oxaliplatin to 65 mg/m^2 and 5-fluorouracil by 20% (300 mg/m^2 bolus and 500 mg/m^2 22-hour infusion) is recommended for patients after recovery from grade 3/4 GI (despite prophylactic treatment), grade 4 neutropenia, or grade 3/4 thrombocytopenia. The next dose should be delayed until neutrophils are at least 1.5×10^9/L and platelets are at least 75×10^9/L.

Duration of therapy: Treatment is recommended until disease progression or unacceptable toxicity.

Stage III colon cancer –

Usual dosage:

• *Day 1* – Oxaliplatin 85 mg/m^2 IV infusion in D5W 250 to 500 mL and leucovorin 200 mg/m^2 IV infusion in D5W, both given over 120 minutes at the same time in separate bags using a Y-line, followed by 5-fluorouracil 400 mg/m^2 IV bolus given over 2 to 4 minutes, followed by 5-fluorouracil 600 mg/m^2 IV infusion in D5W 500 mL (recommended) as a 22-hour continuous infusion.

• *Day 2* – Leucovorin 200 mg/m^2 IV infusion over 120 minutes, followed by 5-fluorouracil 400 mg/m^2 IV bolus given over 2 to 4 minutes, followed by 5-fluorouracil 600 mg/m^2 IV infusion in D5W 500 mL (recommended) as a 22-hour continuous infusion. Repeat cycle every 2 weeks.

Dosage adjustment: For patients who experience persistent grade 2 neurosensory events that do not resolve, a dose reduction of oxaliplatin to 75 mg/m^2 should be considered. For patients with persistent grade 3 neurosensory events, discontinuing therapy should be considered. The infusional 5-fluorouracil/leucovorin regimen need not be altered.

A dose reduction of oxaliplatin to 75 mg/m^2 and infusional 5-fluorouracil to 300 mg/m^2 bolus and 500 mg/m^2 22-hour infusion is recommended for patients after recovery from grade 3/4 GI (despite prophylactic treatment), grade 4 neutropenia, or grade 3/4 thrombocytopenia. The next dose should be delayed until neutrophils are at least 1.5×10^9/L and platelets are at least 75×10^9/L.

Duration of therapy: Recommended for a total of 6 months (ie, 12 cycles, every 2 weeks).

➤*Premedication:* Premedication with antiemetics, including 5-HT$_3$ blockers with or without dexamethasone, is recommended. The administration of oxaliplatin does not require prehydration.

➤*Preparation for administration:* Oxaliplatin is considered a cytotoxic agent. Follow safe handling procedures when preparing, administering, or dispensing oxaliplatin.

The use of gloves is recommended. If a solution of oxaliplatin contacts the skin, wash the skin immediately and thoroughly with soap and water. If oxaliplatin contacts the mucous membranes, flush thoroughly with water.

Powder – Reconstitute by adding 10 mL (for the 50 mg vial) or 20 mL (for the 100 mg vial) of water for injection or dextrose 5% injection. Do not administer the reconstituted solution without further dilution. The reconstituted solution must be further diluted in an infusion solution of 250 to 500 mL of dextrose 5% injection. Reconstitution or final dilution must never be performed with a sodium chloride solution or other chloride-containing solution.

Solution – The solution must be further diluted in an infusion solution of 250 to 500 mL of dextrose 5% injection. A final dilution must never be performed with a sodium chloride solution or other chloride-containing solutions.

➤*Extravasation:* Extravasation may result in local pain and inflammation that may be severe and lead to complications, including necrosis. If signs or symptoms of extravasation occur, stop the infusion immediately. If possible, withdraw 3 to 5 mL of blood to remove some of the drug. Remove the infusion needle. May apply ice compresses to the site for 15 minutes every 6 hours for 48 hours. Delineate the infiltrated area on the patient's skin with a felt-tip marker. Elevate for 48 hours above heart level using a sling or stockinette dressing with an observation window cut in the dressing. Avoid pressure or friction. Do not rub the area. Observe for signs of increased erythema, pain, or skin necrosis. If increased symptoms occur, consult a plastic surgeon. Ensure that no medication is given distally to extravasation site. After 48 hours, encourage the patient to use the extremity normally to promote full range of motion.

➤*Admixture compatibility:* Oxaliplatin is incompatible in solution with alkaline medications or media (such as basic solutions of 5-fluorouracil) and must not be mixed with these or administered simultaneously through the same infusion line. The infusion line should be flushed with D5W prior to administration of any concomitant medications.

Needles or IV administration sets containing aluminum parts that may come in contact with oxaliplatin should not be used for the preparation or mixing of the drug. Aluminum has been reported to cause degradation of platinum compounds.

To screen for specific compatibilities, see *Trissel's IV-Chek*.

➤*Storage/Stability:*

Powder – Store at 25°C (77°F); excursions are permitted between 15° and 30°C (59° and 86°F). After reconstitution in the original vial, the solution may be stored for up to 24 hours at 2° to 8°C (36° to 46°F). After final dilution with 250 to 500 mL of dextrose 5% injection, the shelf life is 6 hours at 20° to 25°C (68° to 77°F) or up to 24 hours at 2° to 8°C (36° to 46°F). Oxaliplatin is not light sensitive.

Solution – Store at 25°C (77°F); excursions are permitted between 15° and 30°C (59° and 86°F). Do not freeze. Protect from light (keep in original outer carton). After dilution with 250 to 500 mL of dextrose 5% injection, the shelf life is 6 hours at 20° to 25°C (68° to 77°F) or up to 24 hours at 2° to 8°C (36° to 46°F). After final dilution, protection from light is not required.

Actions

➤*Pharmacology:* Oxaliplatin undergoes nonenzymatic conversion in physiologic solutions to active derivatives via displacement of the labile oxalate ligand. Several transient reactive species are formed, including monoaquo and diaquo 1,2-diaminocyclohexane (DACH) platinum, which covalently bind with macromolecules. Both interstrand and intrastrand Pt-DNA crosslinks are formed. Crosslinks are formed between the N7 positions of 2 adjacent guanines, adjacent adenine-guanines, and guanines separated by an intervening nucleotide. These crosslinks inhibit DNA replication and transcription. Cytotoxicity is cell-cycle nonspecific. In vivo studies have shown antitumor activity of oxaliplatin against colon carcinoma.

➤*Pharmacokinetics:*

Absorption/Distribution – Pharmacokinetic parameters obtained after a single 2-hour IV infusion of oxaliplatin at a dose of 85 mg/m^2 expressed as an ultrafilterable platinum were a maximum plasma concentration (C_{max}) of 0.814 mcg/mL and a volume of distribution of 440 L.

Interpatient and intrapatient variability in ultrafilterable platinum exposure (area under the curve [$AUC_{0\text{-}48h}$]) assessed over 3 cycles was moderate to low (23% and 6%, respectively).

At the end of a 2-hour infusion of oxaliplatin, approximately 15% of the administered platinum is present in the systemic circulation. The remaining 85% is rapidly distributed into tissues or eliminated in the urine. In patients, plasma protein binding of platinum is irreversible and is greater than 90%. The main binding proteins are albumin and gamma-globulins. Platinum also binds irreversibly and accumulates (approximately 2-fold) in erythrocytes, where it appears to have no relevant activity. No platinum accumulation was observed in plasma ultrafiltrate following 85 mg/m^2 every 2 weeks.

Metabolism – Oxaliplatin undergoes rapid and extensive nonenzymatic biotransformation. There is no evidence of cytochrome P450–mediated metabolism in vitro.

Up to 17 platinum-containing derivatives have been observed in plasma ultrafiltrate samples from patients, including several cytotoxic species (monochloro DACH platinum, dichloro DACH platinum, and monoaquo and diaquo DACH platinum) and a number of noncytotoxic, conjugated species.

Excretion – The major route of platinum elimination is renal excretion. At 5 days after a single 2-hour infusion of oxaliplatin, urinary elimination accounted for about 54% of the platinum eliminated, with fecal excretion accounting for only about 2%. Platinum was cleared from plasma at a rate (10 to 17 L/h) that was similar to or exceeded the average human glomerular filtration rate (GFR) (7.5 L/h). The renal clearance of ultrafilterable platinum is significantly correlated with GFR.

The reactive oxaliplatin derivatives are present as a fraction of the unbound platinum in plasma ultrafiltrate. The decline of ultrafilterable platinum levels following oxaliplatin administration is triphasic, characterized by 2 relatively short distribution phases (distribution half-life alpha, 0.43 hours;

OXALIPLATIN — INJECTION

distribution half-life beta, 16.8 hours) and a long terminal elimination phase (terminal elimination half-life gamma, 391 hours).

Special populations –

Renal function impairment: The AUC $_{0-48h}$ of platinum in the plasma ultrafiltrate increases as renal function decreases. The AUC $_{0-48h}$ of platinum in patients with mild (creatinine clearance [CrCl] 50 to 80 mL/min), moderate (CrCl 30 to less than 50 mL/min), and severe (CrCl less than 30 mL/min) renal function impairment is increased by approximately 60%, 140%, and 190%, respectively, compared with patients with healthy renal function (CrCl greater than 80 mL/min). Clearance of ultrafilterable platinum is decreased in patients with mild, moderate, and severe renal impairment.

Children: The pharmacokinetic parameters of ultrafiltrable platinum have been evaluated in 105 children during the first cycle. The mean clearance in children estimated by the population pharmacokinetic analysis was 4.7 L/h. The interpatient variability of platinum clearance in pediatric cancer patients was 41%. Mean platinum pharmacokinetic parameters in ultrafiltrate were C_{max} of 0.75 ± 0.24 mcg/mL, AUC_{0-48} of 7.52 ± 5.07 mcg•h/mL, and AUC_{inf} of 8.83 ± 1.57 mcg•h/mL at oxaliplatin 85 mg/m^2; and C_{max} of 1.1 ± 0.43 mcg/mL, AUC_{0-48} of 9.74 ± 2.52 mcg•h/mL, and AUC_{inf} of 17.3 ± 5.34 mcg•h/mL at oxaliplatin 130 mg/m^2.

Contraindications

History of known allergy to oxaliplatin or other platinum compounds.

Warnings/Precautions

➤*Neuropathy:* Oxaliplatin is associated with 2 types of neuropathy:

- An acute, reversible, primarily peripheral sensory neuropathy that is of early onset, occurring within hours or 1 to 2 days of dosing, that resolves within 14 days, and that frequently recurs with further dosing. The symptoms may be precipitated or exacerbated by exposure to cold temperature or cold objects, and they usually present as transient paresthesia, dysesthesia, and hypoesthesia in the hands, feet, perioral area, or throat. Jaw spasm, abnormal tongue sensation, dysarthria, eye pain, and a feeling of chest pressure also have been observed. The acute, reversible pattern of sensory neuropathy was observed in about 56% of study patients who received oxaliplatin with infusional 5-fluorouracil/leucovorin. In any individual cycle, acute neurotoxicity was observed in approximately 30% of patients. In adjuvant patients, the median cycle of onset for grade 3 peripheral sensory neuropathy was 9; in previously treated patients, the median number of cycles administered on the oxaliplatin plus 5-fluorouracil/leucovorin combination arm was 6.
- An acute syndrome of pharyngolaryngeal dysesthesia seen in 1% to 2% (grade 3/4) of patients previously untreated for advanced colorectal cancer and previously treated patients is characterized by subjective sensations of dysphagia or dyspnea, without any laryngospasm or bronchospasm (no stridor or wheezing). Avoid using ice (mucositis prophylaxis) during the infusion of oxaliplatin because cold temperature can exacerbate acute neurological symptoms.
- A persistent (longer than 14 days), primarily peripheral, sensory neuropathy that is usually characterized by paresthesias, dysesthesias, hypesthesias, but may also include deficits in proprioception that can interfere with daily activities (eg, writing, buttoning, swallowing, difficulty walking from impaired proprioception) has been observed. These forms of neuropathy occurred in 48% of the study patients receiving oxaliplatin with infusional 5-fluorouracil/leucovorin. Persistent neuropathy can occur without any prior acute neuropathy event. The majority (80%) of the patients who developed grade 3 persistent neuropathy progressed from prior grade 1 or 2 events. These symptoms may improve in some patients upon discontinuation of oxaliplatin.

Colon cancer – Peripheral sensory neuropathy was reported in adjuvant patients treated with the oxaliplatin combination with a frequency of 92% (all grades) and 13% (grade 3). At the 28-day follow-up after the last treatment cycle, 60% of all patients had any grade (grade 1 = 40%, grade 2 = 16%, grade 3 = 5%) peripheral sensory neuropathy decreasing to 39% at 6 months' follow-up (grade 1 = 31%, grade 2 = 7%, grade 3 = 1%) and 21% at 18 months' follow-up (grade 1 = 17%, grade 2 = 3%, grade 3 = 1%).

Advanced colorectal cancer – The grading scale for paresthesias/dysesthesias in advanced colorectal cancer patients was: grade 1, resolved and did not interfere with functioning; grade 2, interfered with function but not daily activities; grade 3, pain or functional impairment that interfered with daily activities; and grade 4, persistent impairment that is disabling or life-threatening.

Overall, neuropathy was reported in patients previously untreated for advanced colorectal cancer in 82% (all grades) and 19% (grade 3/4), and in the previously treated patients in 74% (all grades) and 7% (grade 3/4) events. Information regarding reversibility of neuropathy was not available from the trial for patients who had not been previously treated for colorectal cancer.

➤*Pulmonary toxicity:* Oxaliplatin has been associated with pulmonary fibrosis (less than 1% of study patients), which may be fatal. The combined incidence of cough and dyspnea was 7.4% (any grade) and less than 1% (grade 3), with no grade 4 events in the oxaliplatin plus infusional 5-fluorouracil/leucovorin arm compared with 4.5% (any grade) and no grade 3 and 0.1% grade 4 events in the infusional 5-fluorouracil/leucovorin alone arm in adjuvant colon cancer patients. In this study, 1 patient died from eosinophil pneumonia in the oxaliplatin combination arm. The combined incidence of cough, dyspnea, and hypoxia was 43% (any grade) and 7% (grade 3 and 4) in the oxaliplatin plus 5-fluorouracil/leucovorin arm compared with 32% (any grade) and 5% (grade 3 and 4) in the irinotecan plus 5-fluorouracil/leucovorin arm of unknown duration for patients with previously untreated colorectal cancer. In case of unexplained respiratory symptoms, such as nonproductive cough, dyspnea, crackles, or radiological pulmonary infiltrates, discontinue oxaliplatin until further pulmonary investigation excludes interstitial lung disease or pulmonary fibrosis.

➤*Hepatotoxicity:* Hepatotoxicity, as evidenced in the adjuvant study by an increase in transaminases (57% vs 34%) and alkaline phosphatase (42% vs 20%), was observed more commonly in the oxaliplatin combination arm. The incidence of increased bilirubin was similar on both arms. Changes noted on liver biopsies include peliosis, nodular regenerative hyperplasia or sinusoidal alterations, perisinusoidal fibrosis, and veno-occlusive lesions. Consider hepatic vascular disorders and, if appropriate, investigate in case of abnormal liver function test results or portal hypertension that cannot be explained by liver metastases.

➤*Extravasation:* See Administration and Dosage for more information.

➤*Hypersensitivity reactions:* Grade 3/4 hypersensitivity, including anaphylactic/anaphylactoid reactions, to oxaliplatin has been observed in 2% to 3% of colon cancer patients. These allergic reactions, which can be fatal, can occur within minutes of administration and at any cycle, and are similar in nature and severity to those reported with other platinum-containing compounds, such as rash, urticaria, erythema, pruritus, and, rarely, bronchospasm and hypotension. The symptoms associated with hypersensitivity reactions reported in the previously untreated patients were urticaria, pruritus, flushing of the face, diarrhea associated with oxaliplatin infusion, shortness of breath, bronchospasm, diaphoresis, chest pains, hypotension, disorientation, and syncope. These reactions are usually managed with standard epinephrine, corticosteroid, and antihistamine therapy and may require discontinuation of therapy. Drug-related deaths associated with platinum compounds from anaphylaxis have been reported.

➤*Renal function impairment:* The safety and efficacy of the combination of oxaliplatin and 5-fluorouracil/leucovorin in patients with renal impairment have not been evaluated. Use caution with the combination of oxaliplatin and 5-fluorouracil/leucovorin in patients with preexisting renal impairment because the primary route of platinum elimination is renal.

➤*Pregnancy: Category D.* Based on direct interaction with DNA, oxaliplatin may cause fetal harm when administered to a pregnant woman. There are no adequate and well-controlled studies of oxaliplatin in pregnant women. Reproductive toxicity studies in rats demonstrated adverse effects on fertility and embryo-fetal development at maternal doses that were below the recommended human dose based on body surface area. If this drug is used during pregnancy or if the patient becomes pregnant while taking this drug, apprise the patient of the potential hazard to the fetus. Advise women of childbearing potential to avoid becoming pregnant and use effective contraception while receiving treatment with oxaliplatin.

Pregnant rats were administered oxaliplatin at less than one-tenth the recommended human dose based on BSA during gestation days 1 to 5 (preimplantation), 6 to 10, or 11 to 16 (during organogenesis). Oxaliplatin caused developmental mortality (increased early resorptions) when administered on days 6 to 10 and 11 to 16, and adversely affected fetal growth (decreased fetal weight, delayed ossification) when administered on days 6 to 10. Administration of oxaliplatin to male and female rats prior to mating resulted in 97% postimplantation loss in animals that received approximately one-seventh the recommended human dose based on BSA.

➤*Lactation:* It is not known whether oxaliplatin or its derivatives are excreted in human milk. Because many drugs are excreted in human milk and because of the potential for serious adverse reactions in breast-feeding infants from oxaliplatin, decide whether to discontinue breast-feeding or delay the use of the drug, taking into account the importance of the drug to the mother.

➤*Children:* The effectiveness of oxaliplatin in children has not been established.

➤*Elderly:* See Adverse Reactions for more information.

Patients 65 years of age and older receiving oxaliplatin combination therapy experienced more grade 3 to 4 granulocytopenia than patients younger than 65 years of age (45% versus 39%).

➤*Monitoring:* Standard monitoring of the white blood cell count with differential, hemoglobin, platelet count, and blood chemistries (including ALT, AST, bilirubin, creatinine) is recommended before each oxaliplatin cycle. Patients receiving oxaliplatin plus 5-fluorouracil/leucovorin and requiring oral anticoagulants may require closer monitoring.

Drug Interactions

Oxaliplatin Drug Interactions

Precipitant Drug	Object Drug[a]		Description
Nephrotoxic drugs (eg, gentamicin)	Oxaliplatin	⬆	Because platinum-containing species are eliminated primarily through the kidney, clearance of these products may be decreased by coadministration of potentially nephrotoxic compounds; although, this has not been specifically studied.

OXALIPLATIN — INJECTION

Oxaliplatin Drug Interactions			
Precipitant Drug	Object Drug[a]		Description
Oxaliplatin	5-fluorouracil/ leucovorin	↑	No pharmacokinetic interaction between oxaliplatin 85 mg/m² and 5-fluorouracil/leucovorin has been observed in patients treated every 2 weeks. Increases of 5-fluorouracil/leucovorin plasma concentrations by approximately 20% have been observed with doses of 130 mg/m² oxaliplatin dosed every 3 weeks.
Oxaliplatin plus 5-fluorouracil	Anticoagulants (eg, warfarin)	↑	There have been reports while in study and from postmarketing surveillance of prolonged prothrombin time and international normalized ratio occasionally associated with hemorrhage in patients who received oxaliplatin plus 5-fluorouracil/leucovorin while taking anticoagulants. Monitor coagulation parameters and adjust the anticoagulant dose as needed.

[a] ↑ = Object drug increased.

Adverse Reactions

➤*Most common adverse reactions:* The most common adverse reactions in patients with stage II or III colon cancer receiving adjuvant therapy were anemia, diarrhea, emesis, fatigue, increase in transaminases and alkaline phosphatase, nausea, neutropenia, peripheral sensory neuropathy, stomatitis, and thrombocytopenia. The most common adverse reactions in previously untreated and treated patients were diarrhea, emesis, fatigue, nausea, neutropenia, and peripheral sensory neuropathies.

Both 5-fluorouracil/leucovorin and oxaliplatin are associated with GI or hematologic adverse reactions. When oxaliplatin is administered in combination with infusional 5-fluorouracil/leucovorin, the incidence of these reactions is increased.

➤*Colon cancer:*

Discontinuation – Discontinuation of treatment because of adverse reactions occurred in 15% of the patients receiving oxaliplatin and infusional 5-fluorouracil/leucovorin.

Mortality – The incidence of death within 28 days of the last treatment, regardless of causality, was 0.5% in the oxaliplatin combination and infusional 5-fluorouracil/leucovorin arms, respectively. Deaths within 60 days from initiation of therapy were 0.3% in the oxaliplatin combination and infusional 5-fluorouracil/leucovorin arms, respectively. In the oxaliplatin combination arm, 3 deaths were because of sepsis/neutropenic sepsis, 2 from intracerebral bleeding, and 1 from eosinophilic pneumonia. In the 5-fluorouracil/leucovorin arm, 1 death was because of suicide, 2 from Stevens-Johnson syndrome (1 patient also had sepsis), 1 unknown cause, 1 anoxic cerebral infarction, and 1 probable abdominal aorta rupture.

In addition, the number of cardiovascular deaths was 1.4% in the oxaliplatin combination arm compared with 0.7% in the infusional 5-fluorouracil/ leucovorin arm. Clinical significance of these findings is unknown.

Adverse reactions (5% or more) –

Oxaliplatin Adverse Reactions (≥ 5%) in Colon Cancer Patients				
	Oxaliplatin + 5-fluorouracil/leucovorin (n = 1,108)		5-fluorouracil/leucovorin (n = 1,111)	
Adverse reaction	All grades	Grade 3/4	All grades	Grades 3/4
Any reaction	100%	70%	99%	31%
CNS				
Fatigue	44%	4%	38%	1%
Headache	7%	< 1%	5%	< 1%
Overall peripheral sensory neuropathy	92%	12%	16%	< 1%
Sensory disturbance	8%	< 1%	1%	< 1%
Dermatologic				
Alopecia	30%	< 1%	28%	< 1%
Skin disorder	32%	2%	36%	2%
GI				
Abdominal pain	18%	1%	17%	2%
Anorexia	13%	1%	8%	< 1%
Constipation	22%	< 1%	19%	< 1%
Diarrhea	56%	11%	48%	7%
Dyspepsia	8%	< 1%	5%	< 1%
Nausea	74%	5%	61%	2%
Stomatitis	42%	3%	40%	2%
Taste perversion	12%	< 1%	8%	< 1%
Vomiting	47%	6%	24%	1%
Metabolic/Nutritional				
Phosphate alkaline increased	42%	< 1%	20%	< 1%
Weight increase	10%	< 1%	10%	< 1%
Respiratory				
Dyspnea	5%	< 1%	3%	< 1%
Epistaxis	16%	< 1%	12%	< 1%
Rhinitis	6%	< 1%	8%	< 1%
Special senses				
Conjunctivitis	9%	< 1%	15%	< 1%
Lacrimation abnormal	4%	< 1%	12%	< 1%
Miscellaneous				
Allergic reaction	10%	3%	2%	< 1%
Fever	27%	1%	12%	1%
Infection	25%	4%	25%	3%
Injection-site reaction[a]	11%	3%	10%	3%
Pain	5%	< 1%	5%	< 1%

[a] Includes thrombosis related to the catheter.

Elderly / Race / Gender – Although specific reactions can vary, the overall frequency of adverse reactions was similar in men and women and in patients younger than 65 years of age and 65 years of age and older. However, the following grade 3/4 reactions were more common in women: diarrhea, fatigue, granulocytopenia, nausea, and vomiting. In patients 65 years of age and older, the incidence of grade 3/4 diarrhea and granulocytopenia was higher than in younger patients. Insufficient subgroup sizes prevented analysis of safety by race.

Additional adverse reactions – The following additional adverse reactions were reported in at least 2% and less than 5% of the patients in the oxaliplatin and infusional 5-fluorouracil/leucovorin combination arm: coughing, leukopenia, pain, weight decrease.

Secondary malignancy – The number of patients who developed secondary malignancies was similar; 62 in the oxaliplatin combination arm and 68 in the infusional 5- fluorouracil/leucovorin arm. An exploratory analysis showed that the number of deaths due to secondary malignancies was 1.96% in the oxaliplatin combination arm and 0.98% in the infusional 5-fluorouracil/leucovorin arm.

➤*Previously untreated advanced colorectal cancer:*

Mortality – The incidence of death within 30 days of treatment in the previously untreated advanced colorectal cancer study, regardless of causality, was 3% with oxaliplatin and 5-fluorouracil/leucovorin combination, 5% with irinotecan plus 5-fluorouracil/leucovorin, and 3% with oxaliplatin plus irinotecan. Deaths within 60 days from initiation of therapy were 2.3% with the oxaliplatin and 5-fluorouracil/leucovorin combination, 5.1% with irinotecan plus 5-fluorouracil/leucovorin, and 3.1% with oxaliplatin plus irinotecan.

Adverse reactions (5% or more) –

Oxaliplatin Adverse Reactions (≥ 5%) in Patients With Previously Untreated Colorectal Cancer[a]						
	Oxaliplatin + 5-fluorouracil/ leucovorin (n = 259)		Irinotecan + 5-fluorouracil/ leucovorin (n = 256)		Oxaliplatin + irinotecan (n = 258)	
Adverse reaction	All grades	Grade 3/4	All grades	Grade 3/4	All grades	Grade 3/4
Any reaction	99%	82%	98%	70%	99%	76%
Cardiovascular						
Hypotension	5%	3%	6%	3%	4%	3%
Thrombosis	6%	5%	6%	6%	3%	3%
CNS						
Anxiety	5%	< 1%	2%	< 1%	6%	< 1%
Depression	9%	< 1%	5%	< 1%	7%	< 1%
Dizziness	8%	< 1%	6%	< 1%	10%	< 1%
Dysphasia	5%	< 1%	3%	< 1%	3%	< 1%
Fatigue	70%	7%	58%	11%	66%	16%

OXALIPLATIN — INJECTION

Oxaliplatin Adverse Reactions (≥ 5%) in Patients With Previously Untreated Colorectal Cancer[a]						
	Oxaliplatin + 5-fluorouracil/ leucovorin (n = 259)		Irinotecan + 5-fluorouracil/ leucovorin (n = 256)		Oxaliplatin + irinotecan (n = 258)	
Adverse reaction	All grades	Grade 3/4	All grades	Grade 3/4	All grades	Grade 3/4
Headache	13%	< 1%	6%	< 1%	9%	< 1%
Insomnia	13%	< 1%	9%	< 1%	11%	< 1%
Neuralgia	5%	0%	0%	0%	2%	1%
Neuro NOS	1%	0%	1%	0%	1%	0%
Neurosensory	12%	1%	2%	0%	9%	1%
Overall neuropathy	82%	19%	18%	2%	69%	7%
Paresthesias	77%	18%	16%	2%	62%	6%
Pharyngolaryngeal dysesthesias	38%	2%	1%	0%	28%	1%
Dermatologic						
Alopecia	38%	< 1%	44%	< 1%	67%	< 1%
Dry skin	6%	< 1%	2%	< 1%	5%	< 1%
Flushing	7%	< 1%	2%	< 1%	5%	< 1%
Pruritus	6%	< 1%	4%	< 1%	2%	< 1%
Rash	11%	< 1%	4%	< 1%	7%	< 1%
Skin reaction, hand/foot	7%	1%	2%	1%	1%	0%
Sweating	5%	1%	6%	< 1%	12%	< 1%
GI						
Abdominal pain	29%	8%	31%	7%	39%	10%
Anorexia	35%	2%	25%	4%	27%	5%
Constipation	32%	4%	27%	2%	21%	2%
Diarrhea	56%	12%	65%	29%	76%	25%
Diarrhea-colostomy	13%	2%	16%	7%	16%	3%
Dyspepsia	12%	< 1%	7%	< 1%	5%	< 1%
Flatulence	9%	< 1%	6%	< 1%	5%	< 1%
GI NOS	5%	2%	4%	2%	3%	2%
Mouth dryness	5%	< 1%	2%	< 1%	3%	< 1%
Nausea	71%	6%	67%	15%	83%	19%
Stomatitis	38%	0%	25%	1%	19%	1%
Taste perversion	14%	< 1%	6%	< 1%	8%	< 1%
Vomiting	41%	4%	43%	13%	64%	23%
Hematologic						
Febrile neutropenia	4%	4%	15%	14%	12%	11%
Lymphopenia	6%	2%	4%	1%	5%	2%
Metabolic/Nutritional						
Dehydration	9%	5%	16%	11%	14%	7%
Edema	15%	< 1%	13%	< 1%	10%	< 1%
Elevated creatinine	4%	< 1%	4%	< 1%	5%	< 1%
Hyperglycemia	14%	2%	11%	3%	12%	3%
Hypoalbuminemia	8%	0%	5%	2%	9%	1%
Hypocalcemia	7%	< 1%	5%	< 1%	4%	< 1%
Hypokalemia	11%	3%	7%	4%	6%	2%
Hyponatremia	8%	2%	7%	4%	4%	1%
Weight loss	11%	< 1%	9%	< 1%	11%	< 1%
Musculoskeletal						
Arthralgia	5%	< 1%	5%	< 1%	8%	< 1%
Myalgia	14%	2%	6%	0%	9%	2%
Rigors	8%	< 1%	2%	< 1%	7%	< 1%
Respiratory						
Cough	35%	1%	25%	2%	17%	1%
Dyspnea	18%	7%	14%	3%	11%	2%
Epistaxis	10%	< 1%	2%	< 1%	2%	< 1%
Rhinitis, allergic	10%	< 1%	6%	< 1%	6%	< 1%
Special senses						
Abnormal vision	5%	0%	2%	1%	6%	1%
Tearing	9%	< 1%	1%	< 1%	2%	< 1%
Miscellaneous						
Fever, normal ANC	16%	< 1%	9%	< 1%	9%	< 1%
Hiccups	5%	1%	2%	0%	3%	2%
Hypersensitivity	12%	2%	5%	0%	6%	1%
Infection, low ANC	8%	8%	12%	11%	9%	8%
Infection, normal ANC	10%	4%	5%	1%	7%	2%
Injection-site reaction	6%	0%	1%	0%	4%	1%
Pain	7%	1%	5%	1%	6%	1%
Urinary frequency	5%	1%	2%	1%	3%	1%

[a] NOS = not otherwise specified; ANC = absolute neutrophil count.

Elderly / Gender – Adverse reactions were similar in men and women and in patients younger than 65 years of age and 65 years of age and older, but older patients may have been more susceptible to dehydration, diarrhea, hypokalemia, leukopenia, fatigue, and syncope.

Additional adverse reactions –

CV: Hypertension, syncope.
Dermatologic: Nail changes, pigmentation changes, urticaria.
GI: Rectal bleeding, rectal pain.
Respiratory: Hypoxia, pneumonitis, pulmonary.
Miscellaneous: Bone pain, catheter infection, chest pain, dysuria, metabolic, prothrombin time, unknown infection, vertigo.

➤*Previously treated advanced colorectal cancer:*

Discontinuation – Thirteen percent of patients in the oxaliplatin and 5-fluorouracil/leucovorin combination arm and 18% in the 5-fluorouracil/leucovorin arm of the previously treated study had to discontinue treatment because of adverse reactions related to GI or hematologic adverse reactions or neuropathies.

Mortality – The incidence of death within 30 days of treatment in the previously treated study, regardless of causality, was 5% with the oxaliplatin and 5-fluorouracil/leucovorin combination, 8% with oxaliplatin alone, and 7% with 5-fluorouracil/leucovorin. Of the 7 deaths that occurred on the oxaliplatin and 5-fluorouracil/leucovorin combination arm within 30 days of stopping treatment, 3 may have been treatment related, associated with GI bleeding or dehydration.

Adverse reactions (5% or more) –

Oxaliplatin Adverse Reactions in Patients With Previously Treated Colorectal Cancer (≥ 5%)						
	Oxaliplatin + 5-fluorouracil/ leucovorin (n = 150)		5-fluorouracil/ leucovorin (n = 142)		Oxaliplatin (n = 153)	
Adverse reaction	All grades	Grade 3/4	All grades	Grade 3/4	All grades	Grade 3/4
Any reaction	99%	73%	98%	41%	100%	46%
CNS						
Acute neuropathy	56%	2%	10%	0%	65%	5%
Dizziness	13%	< 1%	8%	< 1%	7%	< 1%
Fatigue	68%	7%	52%	6%	61%	9%
Headache	17%	< 1%	8%	< 1%	13%	< 1%
Insomnia	9%	< 1%	4%	< 1%	11%	< 1%
Neuropathy	74%	7%	17%	0%	76%	7%
Persistent neuropathy	48%	6%	9%	0%	43%	3%
Dermatologic						
Alopecia	7%	< 1%	3%	< 1%	3%	< 1%
Flushing	10%	< 1%	2%	< 1%	3%	< 1%
Hand-foot syndrome	11%	< 1%	13%	< 1%	1%	< 1%
Rash	9%	< 1%	5%	< 1%	5%	< 1%

OXALIPLATIN — INJECTION

Oxaliplatin Adverse Reactions in Patients With Previously Treated Colorectal Cancer (≥ 5%)						
	Oxaliplatin + 5-fluorouracil/ leucovorin (n = 150)		5-fluorouracil/ leucovorin (n = 142)		Oxaliplatin (n = 153)	
Adverse reaction	All grades	Grade 3/4	All grades	Grade 3/4	All grades	Grade 3/4
GI						
Abdominal pain	33%	4%	31%	5%	31%	7%
Anorexia	29%	3%	20%	1%	20%	2%
Constipation	32%	< 1%	23%	< 1%	31%	< 1%
Diarrhea	67%	11%	44%	3%	46%	4%
Dyspepsia	14%	< 1%	10%	< 1%	7%	< 1%
Flatulence	5%	< 1%	6%	< 1%	3%	< 1%
Gastroesophageal reflux	5%	2%	3%	0%	1%	0%
Mucositis	7%	< 1%	10%	< 1%	2%	< 1%
Nausea	65%	11%	59%	4%	64%	4%
Stomatitis	37%	3%	32%	3%	14%	0%
Taste perversion	13%	< 1%	1%	< 1%	5%	< 1%
Vomiting	40%	9%	27%	4%	37%	4%
GU						
Dysuria	6%	< 1%	1%	< 1%	1%	< 1%
Hematuria	6%	< 1%	4%	< 1%	0%	< 1%
Metabolic/Nutritional						
Dehydration	8%	3%	6%	4%	5%	3%
Edema	15%	1%	13%	1%	10%	1%
Hypokalemia	9%	4%	3%	1%	3%	2%
Peripheral edema	10%	< 1%	11%	< 1%	5%	< 1%
Musculoskeletal						
Arthralgia	10%	< 1%	10%	< 1%	7%	< 1%
Back pain	19%	3%	16%	4%	11%	0%
Rigors	7%	< 1%	6%	< 1%	9%	< 1%
Respiratory						
Coughing	19%	1%	9%	0%	11%	0%
Dyspnea	20%	4%	11%	2%	13%	7%
Epistaxis	9%	< 1%	1%	< 1%	2%	< 1%
Hiccups	5%	< 1%	0%	< 1%	2%	< 1%
Pharyngitis	9%	< 1%	10%	< 1%	2%	< 1%
Rhinitis	15%	< 1%	4%	< 1%	6%	< 1%
Upper respiratory tract infection	10%	< 1%	4%	< 1%	7%	< 1%
Miscellaneous						
Abnormal lacrimation	7%	< 1%	6%	< 1%	1%	< 1%
Allergic reaction	10%	< 1%	1%	< 1%	3%	< 1%
Chest pain	8%	1%	4%	1%	5%	1%
Febrile neutropenia	6%	6%	1%	1%	0%	0%
Fever	29%	1%	23%	1%	25%	1%
Injection-site reaction	10%	3%	5%	1%	9%	0%
Pain	15%	2%	9%	3%	14%	3%
Thromboembolism	9%	8%	4%	2%	2%	1%

Elderly/Gender – Adverse reactions were similar in men and women and in patients younger than 65 years of age and 65 years of age and older, but older patients may have been more susceptible to dehydration, diarrhea, hypokalemia, and fatigue.

Additional adverse reactions –

CNS: Anxiety, ataxia, depression, involuntary muscle contractions, nervousness, somnolence.

Dermatologic: Dry skin, erythematous rash, hot flashes, increased sweating, pruritus, purpura.

GI: Ascites, dry mouth, enlarged abdomen, gingivitis, hemorrhoids, intestinal obstruction, melena, proctitis, rectal hemorrhage, tenesmus.

GU: Abnormal micturition frequency, urinary incontinence, vaginal hemorrhage, weight decrease.

Musculoskeletal: Muscle weakness, myalgia.

Respiratory: Hemoptysis, pneumonia.

Miscellaneous: Conjunctivitis, tachycardia.

➤*Cardiovascular:* The incidence of thromboembolic reactions in adjuvant patients with colon cancer was 6% (grade 3/4, 1.8%) in the infusional 5-fluorouracil/leucovorin arm and 6% (grade 3/4, 1.2%) in the oxaliplatin and infusional 5-fluorouracil/leucovorin combined arm, respectively. The incidence was 6% and 9% of the patients previously untreated for advanced colorectal cancer and previously treated patients in the oxaliplatin and infusional 5-fluorouracil/leucovorin combination arm, respectively.

➤*Dermatologic:* Oxaliplatin did not increase the incidence of alopecia compared with infusional 5-fluorouracil/leucovorin alone. No complete alopecia was reported. The incidence of grade 3/4 skin disorders was 2% in both the oxaliplatin plus infusional 5-fluorouracil/leucovorin and the infusional 5-fluorouracil/leucovorin alone arms in the adjuvant colon cancer patients. The incidence of hand-foot syndrome in patients previously untreated for advanced colorectal cancer was 2% in the irinotecan plus 5-fluorouracil/leucovorin arm and 7% in the oxaliplatin and 5-fluorouracil/leucovorin combination arm. The incidence of hand-foot syndrome in previously treated patients was 13% in the 5-fluorouracil/leucovorin arm and 11% in the oxaliplatin and 5-fluorouracil/leucovorin combination arm.

➤*GI:* In patients receiving the combination of oxaliplatin plus infusional 5-fluorouracil/leucovorin for adjuvant treatment for colon cancer, the incidence of grade 3/4 nausea and vomiting was greater than those receiving infusional 5-fluorouracil/leucovorin alone. In patients previously untreated for advanced colorectal cancer receiving the combination of oxaliplatin and 5-fluorouracil/leucovorin, the incidence of grade 3 and 4 vomiting and diarrhea was less compared with irinotecan plus 5-fluorouracil/leucovorin controls. In previously treated patients receiving the combination of oxaliplatin and 5-fluorouracil/leucovorin, the incidence of grade 3 and 4 nausea, vomiting, diarrhea, and mucositis/stomatitis increased compared with 5-fluorouracil/leucovorin controls.

The incidence of GI adverse reactions in the previously untreated and previously treated patients appears to be similar across cycles. Premedication with antiemetics, including 5-HT_3 blockers, is recommended. Diarrhea and mucositis may be exacerbated by the addition of oxaliplatin to 5-fluorouracil/leucovorin; manage with appropriate supportive care. Because cold temperature can exacerbate acute neurological symptoms, avoid using ice (mucositis prophylaxis) during the infusion of oxaliplatin.

➤*Hematologic:*

Oxaliplatin Adverse Hematologic Reactions in Colon Cancer (≥ 5%)				
	Oxaliplatin + 5-fluorouracil/leucovorin (n = 1,108)		5-fluorouracil/leucovorin (n = 1,111)	
Hematologic adverse reaction	All grades	Grade 3/4	All grades	Grade 3/4
Anemia	76%	1%	67%	< 1%
Neutropenia	79%	41%	40%	5%
Thrombocytopenia	77%	2%	19%	< 1%

Oxaliplatin Adverse Hematologic Reactions in Previously Untreated Colorectal Cancer (≥ 5%)						
	Oxaliplatin + 5-fluorouracil/ leucovorin (n = 259)		Irinotecan + 5-fluorouracil/ leucovorin (n = 256)		Oxaliplatin + irinotecan (n = 258)	
Hematologic adverse reaction	All grades	Grade 3/4	All grades	Grade 3/4	All grades	Grade 3/4
Anemia	27%	3%	28%	4%	25%	3%
Leukopenia	85%	20%	84%	23%	76%	24%
Neutropenia	81%	53%	77%	44%	71%	36%
Thrombocytopenia	71%	5%	26%	2%	44%	4%

Adverse Hematologic Reactions in Previously Treated Colorectal Cancer (≥ 5%)						
	Oxaliplatin + 5-fluorouracil/ leucovorin (n = 150)		5-fluorouracil/ leucovorin (n = 142)		Oxaliplatin (n = 153)	
Hematologic adverse reactions	All grades	Grade 3/4	All grades	Grade 3/4	All grades	Grade 3/4
Anemia	81%	2%	68%	2%	64%	1%
Leukopenia	76%	19%	34%	1%	13%	0%
Neutropenia	73%	44%	25%	5%	7%	0%
Thrombocytopenia	64%	4%	20%	0%	30%	3%

Thrombocytopenia – Thrombocytopenia was frequently reported with the combination of oxaliplatin and infusional 5-fluorouracil/leucovorin. The incidence of all hemorrhagic reactions in the adjuvant and previously treated patients was higher in the oxaliplatin combination arm compared with the infusional 5-fluorouracil/leucovorin arm. These reactions included GI bleeding, hematuria, and epistaxis. In the adjuvant trial, 2 patients died from intracerebral hemorrhages.

The incidence of grade 3/4 thrombocytopenia was 2% in adjuvant patients with colon cancer. In patients treated for advanced colorectal cancer, the incidence of grade 3/4 thrombocytopenia was 3% to 5%, and the incidence of these reactions was greater for the combination of oxaliplatin and

OXALIPLATIN — INJECTION

5-fluorouracil/leucovorin over the irinotecan plus 5-fluorouracil/leucovorin or 5-fluorouracil/leucovorin control groups. Grade 3/4 GI bleeding was reported in 0.2% of adjuvant patients receiving oxaliplatin and 5-fluorouracil/leucovorin. In the previously untreated patients, the incidence of epistaxis was 10% in the oxaliplatin and 5-fluorouracil/leucovorin arm, and 2% and 1%, respectively, in the irinotecan plus 5-fluorouracil/leucovorin or irinotecan plus oxaliplatin arms.

Neutropenia – Neutropenia was frequently observed with the combination of oxaliplatin and 5-fluorouracil/leucovorin, with grade 3 and 4 reactions reported in 29% and 12% of adjuvant patients with colon cancer, respectively. In the adjuvant trial, 3 patients died from sepsis/neutropenic sepsis. Grade 3 and 4 reactions were reported in 35% and 18% of the patients previously untreated for advanced colorectal cancer, respectively. Grade 3 and 4 reactions were reported in 27% and 17% of previously treated patients, respectively. In adjuvant patients, the incidence of either febrile neutropenia (0.7%) or documented infection with concomitant grade 3/4 neutropenia (1.1%) was 1.8% in the oxaliplatin and 5-fluorouracil/leucovorin arm. The incidence of febrile neutropenia in the patients previously untreated for advanced colorectal cancer was 15% (3% of cycles) in the irinotecan plus 5-fluorouracil/leucovorin arm and 4% (less than 1% of cycles) in the oxaliplatin and 5-fluorouracil/leucovorin combination arm. Additionally, in this same population, infection with grade 3 or 4 neutropenia was 12% in the irinotecan plus 5-fluorouracil/leucovorin arm and 8% in the oxaliplatin and 5-fluorouracil/leucovorin combination arm. The incidence of febrile neutropenia in the previously treated patients was 1% in the 5-fluorouracil/leucovorin arm and 6% (less than 1% of cycles) in the oxaliplatin and 5-fluorouracil/leucovorin combination arm.

➤*Hepatic:*

Oxaliplatin Adverse Hepatic Reactions in Patients With Colon Cancer (≥ 5%)

Hepatic adverse reaction	Oxaliplatin + 5-fluorouracil/ leucovorin (n = 1,108) All grades	Grade 3/4	5-fluorouracil/ leucovorin (n = 1,111) All grades	Grade 3/4
Alkaline phosphatase increased	42%	< 1%	20%	< 1%
Bilirubinemia	20%	4%	20%	5%
Increase in transaminases	57%	2%	34%	1%

Oxaliplatin Adverse Hepatic Reactions in Patients Previously Untreated for Advanced Colorectal Cancer (≥ 5%)

Hepatic adverse reaction	Oxaliplatin + 5-fluorouracil/ leucovorin (n = 259) All grades	Grade 3/4	Irinotecan + 5-fluorouracil/ leucovorin (n = 256) All grades	Grade 3/4	Oxaliplatin + irinotecan (n = 258) All grades	Grade 3/4
Alkaline phosphatase	16%	0%	8%	0%	14%	2%
ALT	6%	1%	2%	0%	5%	2%
AST	17%	1%	2%	1%	11%	1%
Total bilirubin	6%	1%	3%	1%	3%	2%

Oxaliplatin Adverse Hepatic Reactions in Patients Previously Treated for Advanced Colorectal Cancer (≥ 5%)

Hepatic adverse reaction	Oxaliplatin + 5-fluorouracil/ leucovorin (n = 150) All grades	Grade 3/4	5-fluorouracil/ leucovorin (n = 142) All grades	Grade 3/4	Oxaliplatin (n = 153) All grades	Grade 3/4
ALT	31%	0%	28%	3%	36%	1%
AST	47%	0%	39%	2%	54%	4%
Total bilirubin	13%	1%	22%	6%	13%	5%

➤*Local:* Extravasation may result in local pain and inflammation that may be severe and lead to complications, including necrosis. Injection-site reaction, including redness, swelling, and pain, have been reported.

➤*Renal:* About 5% to 10% of patients in all groups had some degree of elevation of serum creatinine. The incidence of grade 3/4 elevations in serum creatinine in the oxaliplatin and infusional 5-fluorouracil/leucovorin combination arm was 1% in previously treated patients. Serum creatinine measurements were not reported in the adjuvant trial.

➤*Postmarketing:*

CNS – Convulsion, cranial nerve palsies, dysarthria, fasciculations, Lhermitte sign, loss of deep tendon reflexes.

GI – Colitis (including *Clostridium difficile* diarrhea), ileus, intestinal obstruction, pancreatitis, severe diarrhea/vomiting resulting in hypokalemia.

GU – Acute tubular necrosis, acute interstitial nephritis, acute renal failure.

Hematologic – Hemolytic uremic syndrome, immuno-allergic hemolytic anemia, immuno-allergic thrombocytopenia, prolongation of prothrombin time and of international normalized ratio in patients receiving anticoagulants.

Hepatic – Perisinusoidal fibrosis (which, rarely, may progress), veno-occlusive disease of liver (also known as sinusoidal obstruction syndrome).

Respiratory – Pulmonary fibrosis, other interstitial lung diseases (sometimes fatal).

Special senses – Deafness, decrease of visual acuity, optic neuritis, transient vision loss (reversible following therapy discontinuation), visual field disturbance.

Miscellaneous – Anaphylactic shock, angioedema, metabolic acidosis.

Overdosage

➤*Symptoms:* Several cases of overdoses have been reported with oxaliplatin. Adverse reactions observed were grade 4 thrombocytopenia (less than 25,000/mm^3) without any bleeding; anemia; sensory neuropathy, such as paresthesia, dysesthesia, laryngospasm and facial muscle spasms; GI disorders, such as nausea, vomiting, stomatitis, flatulence, abdomen enlarged, and grade 4 intestinal obstruction; grade 4 dehydration; dyspnea; wheezing; chest pain; respiratory failure; severe bradycardia; and death.

In addition to thrombocytopenia, the anticipated complications of an oxaliplatin overdose include hypersensitivity reaction, myelosuppression, nausea, vomiting, diarrhea, and neurotoxicity.

The maximum dose of oxaliplatin that has been administered in a single infusion is 825 mg.

➤*Treatment:* There is no known antidote for oxaliplatin overdose. Monitor patients suspected of receiving an overdose and administer supportive treatment.

Patient Information

Inform patients and patient caregivers of the expected side effects of oxaliplatin, particularly its neurologic effects, both the acute, reversible effects and the persistent neurosensory toxicity. Inform patients that the acute neurosensory toxicity may be precipitated or exacerbated by exposure to cold or cold objects.

Instruct patients to avoid cold drinks and the use of ice, and to cover exposed skin prior to exposure to cold temperature or cold objects.

Adequately inform patients of the risk of low blood cell counts and instruct them to contact their health care provider immediately if fever, particularly if associated with persistent diarrhea, or evidence of infection develop.

Instruct patients to contact their health care provider if persistent vomiting, diarrhea, signs of dehydration, coughing, breathing difficulties, or signs of allergic reaction occur.

Caution women of childbearing potential to avoid becoming pregnant during therapy.

Inform patients that oxaliplatin treatment resulting in an increased risk of dizziness, nausea and vomiting, and other neurologic symptoms that affect gait and balance may lead to a minor or moderate influence on the ability to drive and use machines.

Inform patients that vision abnormalities, in particular transient vision loss (reversible following therapy discontinuation), may affect patients' ability to drive and use machines. Warn patients of the potential effect of these events on the ability to drive or use machines.

ANTHRACENEDIONE

MITOXANTRONE

Rx	Mitoxantrone Hydrochloride (Various, eg, APP, Dabur)	Injection, solution, concentrate: 2 mg/mL	As mitoxantrone hydrochloride. In 10, 12.5, and 15 mL multidose vials.
Rx	Novantrone (Serono Laboratories, Inc)		As mitoxantrone hydrochloride. Preservative free. In 10 mL multidose vial.[a]

[a] With sodium chloride 0.8%, sodium acetate 0.005%, and acetic acid 0.046%.

MITOXANTRONE HYDROCHLORIDE — INJECTION

WARNING

Mitoxantrone should be administered under the supervision of a health care provider experienced in the use of cytotoxic chemotherapy agents.

Mitoxantrone should be given slowly into a freely flowing intravenous (IV) infusion. It must never be given subcutaneously, intramuscularly (IM), or intra-arterially. Severe local tissue damage may occur if there is extravasation during administration.

Not for intrathecal use. Severe injury with permanent sequelae can result from intrathecal administration.

Except for the treatment of acute nonlymphocytic leukemia, mitoxantrone therapy generally should not be given to patients with baseline neutrophil counts of less than 1,500 cells/mm^3. In order to monitor the occurrence of bone marrow suppression (primarily neutropenia, which may be severe and result in infection), it is recommended that frequent peripheral blood cell counts be performed on all patients receiving mitoxantrone.

Cardiotoxicity – Congestive heart failure (CHF), potentially fatal, may occur during therapy with mitoxantrone or months to years after termination of therapy. Cardiotoxicity risk increases with cumulative mitoxantrone dose and may occur whether or not cardiac risk factors are present. Presence or history of cardiovascular disease, radiotherapy to the mediastinal/pericardial area, previous therapy with other anthracyclines or anthracenediones, or use of other cardiotoxic drugs may increase this risk. In patients with cancer, the risk of symptomatic CHF was estimated to be 2.6% for patients receiving up to a cumulative dose of 140 mg/m^2. To mitigate the cardiotoxicity risk with mitoxantrone, consider the following:

- All patients should be assessed for cardiac signs and symptoms by history, physical examination, and electrocardiogram (ECG) prior to start of mitoxantrone therapy.
- All patients should have baseline quantitative evaluation of left ventricular ejection fraction (LVEF) using appropriate methodology (eg, echocardiogram, multigated radionuclide angiogram [MUGA], magnetic resonance imaging [MRI]).
- Patients with multiple sclerosis (MS) with a baseline LVEF below the lower limit of normal should not be treated with mitoxantrone.
- Patients with MS should be assessed for cardiac signs and symptoms by history, physical examination, and ECG prior to each dose.
- Patients with MS should undergo quantitative reevaluation of LVEF prior to each dose using the same methodology that was used to assess baseline LVEF. Additional doses of mitoxantrone should not be administered to MS patients who have experienced a drop in LVEF to below the lower limit of normal or a clinically significant reduction in LVEF during mitoxantrone therapy.
- Patients with MS should not receive a cumulative mitoxantrone dose higher than 140 mg/m^2.
- Patients with MS should undergo yearly quantitative LVEF evaluation after stopping mitoxantrone to monitor for late-occurring cardiotoxicity.

Secondary leukemia – Mitoxantrone therapy in MS patients and in patients with cancer increases the risk of developing secondary acute myeloid leukemia (AML).

Indications

➤*Acute nonlymphocytic leukemia:* In the initial therapy of acute nonlymphocytic leukemia in adults in combination with other approved drug(s). This category includes myelogenous, promyelocytic, monocytic, and erythroid acute leukemias.

➤*Multiple sclerosis:* For reducing neurologic disability and/or the frequency of clinical relapses in patients with secondary (long-term) progressive, progressive relapsing, or worsening relapsing remitting MS (ie, patients whose neurologic status is significantly abnormal between relapses).

➤*Prostate cancer:* As initial chemotherapy for the treatment of patients with pain related to advanced hormone-refractory prostate cancer in combination with corticosteroids.

➤*Off-label uses:* Treatment of breast cancer, non-Hodgkin lymphoma, autologous bone marrow transplantation; treatment of acute nonlymphocytic leukemia or solid tumors in children.

Administration and Dosage

➤*General dosing considerations:* In patients with MS, complete blood cell counts, including platelets, should be monitored prior to each course of mitoxantrone and in the event that signs or symptoms of infection develop. Liver function tests should also be monitored prior to each course in MS patients. Mitoxantrone therapy in MS patients with abnormal liver function tests is not recommended because mitoxantrone clearance is reduced by hepatic impairment and no laboratory measurement can predict drug clearance and dose adjustments.

In patients with MS, LVEF should be evaluated by echocardiogram or MUGA prior to administration of the initial dose of mitoxantrone and all subsequent doses. In addition, LVEF evaluations are recommended if signs or symptoms of CHF develop at any time during treatment with mitoxantrone. Mitoxantrone should not be administered to MS patients with an LVEF less than 50% or with a clinically significant reduction in LVEF. Mitoxantrone generally should not be administered to MS patients with neutrophil counts less than 1,500 cells/mm^3.

Mitoxantrone must be diluted prior to administration (see Preparation for Administration).

➤*Adults:*

Acute nonlymphocytic leukemia –

Induction therapy: 12 mg/m^2 daily on days 1 through 3 given as an IV infusion, and 100 mg/m^2 of cytarabine for 7 days given as a continuous 24-hour infusion on days 1 through 7. Most complete remissions will occur following the initial course of induction therapy. In the event of an incomplete antileukemic response, a second induction course may be given. Mitoxantrone should be given for 2 days and cytarabine for 5 days using the same daily dosage levels.

If severe or life-threatening nonhematologic toxicity is observed during the first induction course, the second induction course should be withheld until toxicity resolves.

Consolidation therapy: 12 mg/m^2 IV infusion daily on days 1 and 2 and cytarabine 100 mg/m^2 for 5 days given as a continuous 24-hour infusion on days 1 through 5. The first course was given approximately 6 weeks after the final induction course; the second was generally administered 4 weeks after the first. Severe myelosuppression occurred.

Multiple sclerosis – 12 mg/m^2 given as a short (approximately 5 to 15 minutes) IV infusion every 3 months. Mitoxantrone should not be administered to patients who have received a cumulative lifetime dose of 140 mg/m^2 or more.

Prostate cancer – 12 to 14 mg/m^2 given as a short IV infusion every 21 days.

➤*Children:*

Off-label dosing –

Acute nonlymphocytic leukemia:

- *Older than 2 years of age* – 12 mg/m^2/day IV on days 1 through 3 of each course. In patients with relapse, 8 to 12 mg/m^2/day IV on day 1 through 5 of each course may be given.
- *2 years of age and younger* – 0.4 mg/kg/day IV for 3 to 5 days.

Solid tumors: 18 to 20 mg/m^2 IV every 3 to 4 weeks, or 5 to 8 mg/m^2 IV once weekly.

➤*Hepatic function impairment:* Ordinarily, do not treat MS patients who have hepatic impairment with mitoxantrone. Administer mitoxantrone with caution to other patients with hepatic impairment; dosage adjustment may be required. In patients with severe hepatic impairment, the area under the curve (AUC) is more than 3 times higher than the value observed in patients with healthy hepatic function.

➤*Preparation for administration:*

Safe handling – Mitoxantrone is considered a cytotoxic agent. Follow safe handling procedures when preparing, administering, or dispensing mitoxantrone.

Avoid contact of mitoxantrone with the skin, mucous membranes, or eyes. Skin accidentally exposed to mitoxantrone should be rinsed copiously with warm water and, if the eyes are involved, standard irrigation techniques should be used immediately. The use of goggles, gloves, and protective gowns is recommended during preparation and administration of the drug.

Dilution – Mitoxantrone concentrate must be diluted prior to use. The dose of mitoxantrone should be diluted to at least 50 mL with either sodium chloride 0.9% injection or dextrose 5% injection. Mitoxantrone may be further diluted in dextrose 5% in water, normal saline, or dextrose 5% with normal saline and used immediately. Do not freeze.

➤*Administration:* The diluted solution should be introduced slowly into the tubing as a freely running IV infusion of sodium chloride 0.9% injection or dextrose 5% injection over a period of not less than 3 minutes. The tubing should be attached to a butterfly needle or other suitable device and inserted preferably into a large vein. If possible, avoid veins over joints or in extremities with compromised venous or lymphatic drainage. Mitoxantrone should not be administered subcutaneously.

➤*Extravasation:* Mitoxantrone may rarely act as a vesicant; injury is more likely to occur if a large amount of concentrated solution is extravasated. Care in the administration of mitoxantrone will reduce the chance of extravasation. If any signs or symptoms of extravasation have occurred, including burning, pain, pruritus, erythema, swelling, blue discoloration, or ulceration, the injection or infusion should be immediately terminated and restarted in another vein. During IV administration of mitoxantrone, extravasation may occur with or without an accompanying stinging or burning sensation, even if blood returns well on aspiration of the infusion needle. If it is known or suspected that subcutaneous extravasation has occurred, the manufacturers recommend that intermittent ice packs be placed over the area of extravasation and that the affected extremity be elevated. Because of the progressive nature of extravasation reactions, the area of injection should be frequently examined and surgery consultation obtained early if there is any sign of a local reaction. Alternatively, if possible, withdraw 3 to 5 mL of blood to remove some of the drug. Remove the infusion needle. Delineate the infiltrated area on the patient's skin with a felt tip marker. Elevate for 48 hours above heart level using a sling or stockinette dressing with an observation window cut in the dressing. Avoid pressure or friction. Do not rub the area. Observe for signs of increased erythema, pain, or skin necrosis. If increased symptoms occur, consult a plastic surgeon. Ensure that no medication is given distally to extravasation site. After 48 hours, encourage the patient to use the extremity normally to promote full range of motion.

➤*Admixture compatibility:* Mitoxantrone should not be mixed in the same infusion as heparin because a precipitate may form. Because specific compatibility data are not available, it is recommended that mitoxantrone not be mixed in the same infusion with other drugs.

MITOXANTRONE HYDROCHLORIDE — INJECTION

➤*Storage/Stability:* Store between 15° and 25°C (59° and 77°F). Do not freeze. Unused infusion solutions should be discarded immediately in an appropriate fashion. In the case of multidose use, after penetration of the stopper, the remaining portion of the undiluted mitoxantrone concentrate should be stored no longer than 7 days between 15° and 25°C (59° and 77°F) or 14 days under refrigeration. Do not freeze.

Actions

➤*Pharmacology:* Mitoxantrone, a DNA-reactive agent that intercalates into DNA through hydrogen bonding, causes crosslinks and strand breaks. Mitoxantrone also interferes with RNA and is a potent inhibitor of topoisomerase II, an enzyme responsible for uncoiling and repairing damaged DNA. It has a cytocidal effect on proliferating and nonproliferating cultured human cells, suggesting lack of cell-cycle phase specificity.

Mitoxantrone has been shown in vitro to inhibit B cell, T cell, and macrophage proliferation, and impair antigen presentation, as well as the secretion of interferon gamma, tumor necrosis factor alpha, and interleukin-2.

➤*Pharmacokinetics:*

Absorption/Distribution – In patients administered 15 to 90 mg/m^2 of mitoxantrone IV, there is a linear relationship between dose and AUC.

Mitoxantrone is 78% bound to plasma proteins in the observed concentration range of 26 to 455 ng/mL. This binding is independent of concentration. Distribution to tissues is extensive; steady-state volume of distribution exceeds 1,000 L/m^2. Tissue concentrations of mitoxantrone appear to exceed those in the blood during the terminal elimination phase. In healthy monkeys, distribution to the brain, spinal cord, eye, and spinal fluid is low.

Metabolism/Excretion – Mitoxantrone is excreted in urine and feces as unchanged or as inactive metabolites. In human studies, 11% and 25% was recovered in urine and feces, respectively, as parent drug or metabolite during the 5-day period following drug administration. Of the material recovered in the urine, 65% is unchanged drug. The remaining 35% is comprised primarily of a monocarboxylic and dicarboxylic acid derivatives and their glucuronide conjugates. The pathways leading to metabolism of mitoxantrone have not been elucidated.

Pharmacokinetics of mitoxantrone in patients following a single IV administration of mitoxantrone can be characterized by a 3-compartment model. The mean alpha half-life of mitoxantrone is 6 to 12 minutes, the mean beta half-life is 1.1 to 3.1 hours, and the mean gamma (terminal or elimination) half-life is 23 to 215 hours (median, approximately 75 hours).

Special populations –

Hepatic function impairment: Mitoxantrone clearance is reduced by hepatic impairment. Patients with severe hepatic dysfunction (bilirubin more than 3.4 mg/dL) have an AUC more than 3 times greater than that of patients with healthy hepatic function receiving the same dose.

Patients with MS who have hepatic impairment should not ordinarily be treated with mitoxantrone. Treat other patients with hepatic impairment with caution; dosage adjustment may be required.

Elderly: In elderly patients with breast cancer, the systemic mitoxantrone clearance was 21.3 L/h/m^2, compared with 28.3 L/h/m^2 and 16.2 L/h/m^2 for nonelderly patients with nasopharyngeal carcinoma and malignant lymphoma, respectively.

Contraindications

Hypersensitivity to mitoxantrone.

Warnings/Precautions

➤*Myelosuppression:* When mitoxantrone is used in high doses (more than 14 mg/m^2/day × 3 days), such as indicated for the treatment of leukemia, severe myelosuppression will occur. Therefore, it is recommended that mitoxantrone be administered only by health care providers experienced in the chemotherapy of this disease. Laboratory and supportive services must be available for hematologic and chemistry monitoring and adjunctive therapies, including antibiotics. Blood and blood products must be available to support patients during the expected period of medullary hypoplasia and severe myelosuppression. Give particular care to ensuring full hematologic recovery before undertaking consolidation therapy (if this treatment is used) and monitor patients closely during this phase. Mitoxantrone administered at any dose can cause myelosuppression.

Patients with preexisting myelosuppression as the result of prior drug therapy should not receive mitoxantrone unless it is felt that the possible benefit from such treatment warrants the risk of further medullary suppression.

Topoisomerase II inhibitors, including mitoxantrone, have been associated with the development of secondary AML and myelosuppression.

➤*Administration:* Safety for use by routes other than IV administration has not been established. Mitoxantrone is not indicated for subcutaneous, IM, or intra-arterial injection. There have been reports of local/regional neuropathy, some irreversible, following intra-arterial injection.

Mitoxantrone must not be given by intrathecal injection. There have been reports of central and peripheral neuropathy and neurotoxicity following intrathecal injection. These reports have included seizures leading to coma and severe neurologic sequelae, and paralysis with bowel and bladder dysfunction.

➤*Cardiac effects:* Because of the possible danger of cardiac effects in patients previously treated with daunorubicin or doxorubicin, determine the benefit-to-risk ratio of mitoxantrone therapy in such patients before starting therapy.

Functional cardiac changes, including decreases in LVEF and irreversible CHF, can occur with mitoxantrone. Cardiac toxicity may be more common in patients with prior treatment with anthracyclines, prior mediastinal radiotherapy, or with preexisting cardiovascular disease. Such patients should have regular cardiac monitoring of LVEF from the initiation of therapy.

Patients who have cancer who received cumulative doses of 140 mg/m^2 alone or in combination with other chemotherapeutic agents had a cumulative 2.6% probability of clinical CHF. In comparative oncology trials, the overall cumulative probability rate of moderate or severe decreases in LVEF at this dose was 13%.

Multiple sclerosis – Changes in cardiac function may occur in patients with MS treated with mitoxantrone. In one controlled trial (study 1), 2% of patients receiving mitoxantrone had LVEF values that decreased to below 50%: one received a 5 mg/m^2 dose and the other received a 12 mg/m^2 dose. An additional patient receiving 12 mg/m^2 who did not have LVEF measured had a decrease in another echocardiographic measurement of ventricular function (fractional shortening) that led to discontinuation from the trial. There were no reports of CHF in either controlled trial.

Assess MS patients for cardiac signs and symptoms by history, physical examination, ECG, and quantitative LVEF evaluation using appropriate methodology (eg, echocardiogram, MRI, MUGA) prior to the start of mitoxantrone therapy. Do not treat MS patients with a baseline LVEF below the lower limit of normal with mitoxantrone. Subsequent LVEF and ECG evaluations are recommended if signs or symptoms of CHF develop and prior to every dose administered to MS patients. Do not administer mitoxantrone to MS patients who experience a reduction in LVEF to below the lower limit of normal, to those who experience a clinically significant reduction in LVEF, or to those who have received a cumulative lifetime dose of more than 140 mg/m^2. Patients with MS should have yearly quantitative LVEF evaluation after stopping mitoxantrone to monitor for late-occurring cardiotoxicity.

Acute nonlymphocytic leukemia: Acute CHF may occasionally occur in patients treated with mitoxantrone for acute nonlymphocytic leukemia. In first-line comparative trials of mitoxantrone and cytarabine versus daunorubicin and cytarabine in adult patients with previously untreated acute nonlymphocytic leukemia, therapy was associated with CHF in 6.5% of patients in each arm. A causal relationship between drug therapy and cardiac effects is difficult to establish in this setting because myocardial function is frequently depressed by anemia, fever and infection, and hemorrhage that often accompany the underlying disease.

Prostate cancer: Functional cardiac changes, such as decreases in LVEF and CHF, may occur in patients with hormone-refractory prostate cancer treated with mitoxantrone. In a randomized comparative trial of mitoxantrone plus low-dose prednisone versus low-dose prednisone, 5.5% of patients treated with mitoxantrone had a cardiac event, defined as any decrease in LVEF below the normal range, CHF (n = 3), or myocardial ischemia. Two patients had a history of cardiac disease. The total mitoxantrone dose administered to patients with cardiac effects ranged from more than 48 to 212 mg/m^2.

Among 112 patients evaluable for safety on the mitoxantrone and hydrocortisone arm of the CALGB trial, 19% of patients had a reduction in cardiac function, 5% of patients had cardiac ischemia, and 2% of patients experienced pulmonary edema. The range of total mitoxantrone doses administered to these patients is not available.

➤*Secondary leukemia:* Mitoxantrone therapy increases the risk of developing secondary leukemia in patients with cancer and in MS patients.

In a study of patients with prostate cancer, AML occurred in 1% of mitoxantrone-treated patients versus no cases in the control group not receiving mitoxantrone at 4.7 years follow-up.

In a prospective, open-label tolerability and safety monitoring study of MS patients treated with mitoxantrone followed for up to 5 years (median of 2.8 years), leukemia occurred in 0.6% of patients. Publications describe leukemia risks of 0.25% to 2.8% in cohorts of MS patients treated with mitoxantrone and followed for varying periods of time. This leukemia risk exceeds the risk of leukemia in the general population. The most commonly reported types were acute promyelocytic leukemia and acute myelocytic leukemia.

In 1,774 patients with breast cancer who received mitoxantrone concomitantly with other cytotoxic agents and radiotherapy, the cumulative risk of developing treatment-related AML was estimated as 1.1% and 1.6% at 5 and 10 years, respectively. The second largest report involved 449 patients with breast cancer treated with mitoxantrone, usually in combination with radiotherapy and/or other cytotoxic agents. In this study, the cumulative probability of developing secondary leukemia was estimated to be 2.2% at 4 years.

Secondary AML has also been reported in patients with cancer treated with anthracyclines. Mitoxantrone is an anthracenedione, a related drug. The occurrence of refractory secondary leukemia is more common when anthracyclines are given in combination with DNA-damaging antineoplastic agents, when patients have been heavily pretreated with cytotoxic drugs, or when doses of anthracyclines have been escalated. Symptoms of acute leukemia may include excessive bruising, bleeding, and recurrent infections.

➤*Systemic infections:* Treat systemic infections concomitantly with or just prior to commencing therapy with mitoxantrone.

➤*Extravasation:* See Administration and Dosage for more information.

➤*Hepatic function impairment:* The safety of mitoxantrone in patients with hepatic insufficiency is not established.

Do not ordinarily treat MS patients who have hepatic impairment with mitoxantrone. Administer mitoxantrone with caution to other patients with hepatic impairment. In patients with severe hepatic impairment, the AUC is more than 3 times greater than the value observed in patients with healthy hepatic function.

➤*Pregnancy: Category D.* Mitoxantrone may cause fetal harm when administered to a pregnant woman. Advise women of childbearing potential to avoid becoming pregnant. Mitoxantrone is considered a potential human

MITOXANTRONE HYDROCHLORIDE — INJECTION

teratogen because of its mechanism of action and the developmental effects demonstrated by related agents. Treatment of pregnant rats during the organogenesis period of gestation was associated with fetal growth retardation at dosages of at least 0.1 mg/kg/day (0.01 times the recommended human dose on a mg/m² basis). When pregnant rabbits were treated during organogenesis, an increased incidence of premature delivery was observed at dosages of at least 0.1 mg/kg/day (0.01 times the recommended human dose on a mg/m² basis). No teratogenic effects were observed in these studies, but the maximum doses tested were well below the recommended human dose (0.02 and 0.05 times in rats and rabbits, respectively, on a mg/m² basis). There are no adequate and well-controlled studies in pregnant women. Women with MS who are biologically capable of becoming pregnant should have a pregnancy test prior to each dose, and the results should be known prior to administration of the drug. If this drug is used during pregnancy or if the patient becomes pregnant while taking this drug, apprise the patient of the potential risk to the fetus.

➤*Lactation:* Mitoxantrone is excreted in human milk; significant concentrations (18 ng/mL) have been reported for 28 days after the last administration. Mitoxantrone accumulates in the plasma and tissue after multiple doses and is slowly eliminated from the body. The long-term consequences of such exposure are unknown. Because of the potential for serious adverse reactions in infants from mitoxantrone, discontinue breast-feeding before starting treatment.

➤*Children:* Safety and efficacy in children have not been established.

➤*Monitoring:* Accompany therapy with mitoxantrone by close and frequent monitoring of hematologic and chemical laboratory parameters, as well as frequent patient observation.

In leukemia treatment, hyperuricemia may occur as a result of rapid lysis of tumor cells by mitoxantrone. Monitor serum uric acid levels and institute hypouricemic therapy prior to the initiation of antileukemic therapy.

Obtain a complete blood cell count, including platelets, prior to each course of mitoxantrone and in the event that signs and symptoms of infection develop. Generally, do not administer mitoxantrone to MS patients with neutrophil counts less than 1,500 cells/mm³.

Perform liver function tests prior to each course of therapy. Mitoxantrone therapy in MS patients with abnormal liver function tests is not recommended because mitoxantrone clearance is reduced by hepatic impairment and no laboratory measurement can predict drug clearance and dose adjustments.

Advise MS patients to have yearly quantitative LVEF evaluation after stopping mitoxantrone to monitor for late-occurring cardiotoxicity.

Carefully assess all patients for cardiac signs and symptoms by history and physical examination prior to start of therapy. Perform baseline evaluation of LVEF by echocardiogram or MUGA. Assess cardiac signs and symptoms by history, physical examination, and ECG. Reevaluate LVEF prior to each dose administered to MS patients.

Women with MS who are biologically capable of becoming pregnant, even if they are using birth control, should have a pregnancy test and the results should be obtained before receiving each dose of mitoxantrone.

Drug Interactions

Mitoxantrone Drug Interactions

Precipitant drug	Object drug[a]		Description
Cyclosporine	Mitoxantrone	↑	Therapeutic and toxic effects of mitoxantrone may be increased by cyclosporine. Close clinical and laboratory monitoring are indicated.
Palifermin	Mitoxantrone	↑	Coadministration of palifermin and mitoxantrone within the same 24-hour time period may increase the severity and duration of mitoxantrone-induced oral mucositis. Do not administer palifermin within 24 hours before, during, or after administration of mitoxantrone.
Mitoxantrone	Digoxin	↓	Digoxin plasma concentrations may be reduced, decreasing the pharmacologic effects. Monitor digoxin concentrations and the patient for signs of clinical deterioration (eg, CHF). Adjust the digoxin dose as needed.
Mitoxantrone	Hydantoins (eg, phenytoin)	↓	Plasma concentrations and therapeutic effectiveness of hydantoins may be reduced by mitoxantrone, increasing the risk of seizures. Monitor plasma hydantoin concentrations and seizure frequency when starting or stopping mitoxantrone. Adjust the hydantoin dose as needed.
Mitoxantrone	Live vaccines	↑	The risk of live vaccine–induced adverse reactions may be increased by coadministration of mitoxantrone. If possible, defer the use of live vaccines in patients receiving mitoxantrone.
Mitoxantrone	Trastuzumab	↑	The risk of trastuzumab-induced cardiac dysfunction may be increased by coadministration of mitoxantrone. Closely monitor for signs of cardiac dysfunction.

[a] ↑ = object drug increased; ↓ = object drug decreased.

Adverse Reactions

Mitoxantrone in doses less than 15 mg/m² has moderate potential for nausea and vomiting. Mitoxantrone at higher doses may be more emetogenic.

➤*Multiple sclerosis:*

Study 1 –

Discontinuation: In study 1, the proportion of patients who discontinued treatment because of adverse reaction was 9.7% (n = 6) in the mitoxantrone 12 mg/m² arm (bone pain and emesis, decreased left ventricular function, depression, leukopenia, renal failure, and 1 discontinuation to prevent future complications from repeated urinary tract infections) compared with 3.1% (n = 2) in the placebo arm (hepatitis and myocardial infarction).

Adverse reactions (5% or more):

Mitoxantrone Adverse Reactions in Multiple Sclerosis Patients (≥ 5%): Study 1

Adverse reactions	Mitoxantrone 5 mg/m² (n = 65)	Mitoxantrone 12 mg/m² (n = 62)	Placebo (n = 64)
Cardiovascular			
Arrhythmia	6%	18%	8%
ECG abnormal	5%	11%	3%
GI			
Constipation	14%	10%	6%
Diarrhea	25%	16%	11%
Nausea	55%	76%	20%
Stomatitis	15%	19%	8%
GU			
Amenorrhea[a]	28%	43%	3%
Menstrual disorder[a]	51%	61%	26%
Urinary tract infection	29%	32%	13%
Urine abnormal	5%	11%	6%
Respiratory			
Sinusitis	3%	6%	2%
Upper respiratory tract infection	51%	53%	52%
Miscellaneous			
Alopecia	38%	61%	31%
Back pain	6%	8%	5%
Headache	6%	6%	5%

[a] Percentage of female patients.

Cardiovascular: Two of the 127 patients treated with mitoxantrone in study 1 had decreased LVEF to below 50% at some point during the 2 years of treatment. An additional patient receiving 12 mg/m² did not have LVEF measured, but had another echocardiographic measure of ventricular function (fractional shortening) that led to discontinuation from the study.

Infection: The proportion of patients experiencing any infection during study 1 was 67% for the placebo group, 85% for the 5 mg/m² group, and 81% for the 12 mg/m² group. However, few of these infections required hospitalization: one placebo patient (tonsillitis), three 5 mg/m² patients (enteritis, urinary tract infection, viral infection), and four 12 mg/m² patients (tonsillitis, urinary tract infection [two], endometritis).

• *Laboratory abnormalities –*

Mitoxantrone Lab Test Abnormalities in Multiple Sclerosis Patients[a] (≥ 5%): Study 1

Reactions	Mitoxantrone 5 mg/m² (n = 65)	Mitoxantrone 12 mg/m² (n = 62)	Placebo (n = 64)
ALT increased	6%	5%	3%
Anemia	9%	6%	2%
AST increased	9%	8%	8%
Gamma-glutamyltransferase increased	3%	15%	3%
Granulocytopenia[b]	6%	6%	2%

MITOXANTRONE HYDROCHLORIDE — INJECTION

Mitoxantrone Lab Test Abnormalities in Multiple Sclerosis Patients[a] (≥ 5%): Study 1			
Reactions	Mitoxantrone 5 mg/m² (n = 65)	Mitoxantrone 12 mg/m² (n = 62)	Placebo (n = 64)
Leukopenia[c]	9%	19%	0%

[a] Assessed using World Health Organization toxicity criteria.
[b] Less than 2,000 cells/mm³.
[c] Less than 4,000 cells/mm³.

Study 2 –

Mitoxantrone Adverse Reactions in Multiple Sclerosis Patients (≥ 5%): Study 2[a]		
Adverse reactions	Mitoxantrone + methylprednisolone (n = 21)	Methylprednisolone (n = 21)
Dermatologic		
Alopecia	33%	0%
Cutaneous mycosis	10%	0%
GI		
Aphthosis	10%	0%
Gastralgia/Stomach burn/ Epigastric pain	14%	5%
Nausea	29%	0%
GU		
Amenorrhea[b]	53%	0%
Menorrhagia[b]	7%	0%
Respiratory		
Pharyngitis/Throat infection	19%	5%
Rhinitis	10%	0%
Miscellaneous		
Asthenia	24%	0%

[a] Assessed using National Cancer Institute (NCI) common toxicity criteria.
[b] Percentage of female patients.

Mitoxantrone Lab Test Abnormalities in Multiple Sclerosis Patients (≥ 5%): Study 2[a]		
Adverse reactions	Mitoxantrone + methylprednisolone (n = 21)	Methylprednisolone (n = 21)
WBC low[b]	100%	14%
ANC low[c]	100%	10%
Lymphocytes low	95%	43%
Hemoglobin low	43%	48%
Platelets low[d]	33%	0%
AST high	15%	5%
ALT high	15%	10%
Glucose high	10%	5%
Potassium low	10%	0%

[a] Assessed using NCI common toxicity criteria.
[b] WBC = white blood cell count. Less than 4,000 cells/mm³.
[c] ANC = absolute neutrophil count. Less than 1,500 cells/mm³.
[d] Less than 100,000 cells/mm³.

Leukopenia and neutropenia were reported in the mitoxantrone plus methylprednisolone group. Neutropenia occurred within 3 weeks after mitoxantrone administration and was always reversible. Only mild to moderate intensity infections were reported in 9 of 21 patients in the mitoxantrone plus methylprednisolone group and in 3 of 21 patients in the methylprednisolone group; none of these required hospitalization.

➤Acute nonlymphocytic leukemia:

Mitoxantrone Adverse Reactions in Acute Nonlymphocytic Leukemia Patients				
	Induction		Consolidation	
	% patients entering induction		% patients entering induction	
Adverse reactions	Mitoxantrone (n = 102)	Daunorubicin (n = 102)	Mitoxantrone (n = 55)	Daunorubicin (n = 49)
Cardiovascular	26%	28%	11%	24%
Arrhythmias	3%	3%	4%	4%
CHF	5%	6%	0%	0%
CNS	30%	30%	34%	35%
Headache	10%	9%	13%	8%
Seizures	4%	4%	2%	8%
GI	88%	85%	58%	51%
Abdominal pain	15%	9%	9%	4%
Diarrhea	47%	47%	18%	8%
GI bleeding	16%	12%	2%	2%
Mucositis/ Stomatitis	29%	33%	18%	8%
Nausea/Vomiting	72%	67%	31%	31%
Hepatic	10%	11%	14%	2%
Jaundice	3%	8%	7%	0%
Respiratory	43%	43%	24%	14%
Cough	13%	9%	9%	2%
Dyspnea	18%	20%	6%	0%
Pneumonia	9%	7%	9%	0%
Special senses				
Conjunctivitis	5%	1%	0%	0%
Eye adverse reactions	7%	6%	2%	4%
Miscellaneous				
Alopecia	37%	40%	22%	16%
Bleeding	37%	41%	20%	6%
Fever	78%	71%	24%	18%
Fungal infections	15%	13%	9%	6%
Infections	66%	73%	60%	43%
Petechiae/ Ecchymoses	7%	9%	11%	2%
Renal failure	8%	6%	0%	2%
Sepsis	34%	36%	31%	18%
Urinary tract infection	7%	2%	7%	2%

➤Prostate cancer:

Trial CCI-NOV22 –

Mitoxantrone Adverse Reactions in Prostate Cancer Patients (≥ 5%): Trial CCI-NOV22		
Adverse reactions	Mitoxantrone + prednisone (n = 80)	Prednisone (n = 81)
CNS		
Anxiety/Depression	5%	3%
Fatigue	39%	14%
Dermatologic		
Alopecia	29%	0%
Skin infection	5%	3%
GI		
Anorexia	25%	6%
Constipation	16%	14%
Dyspepsia	5%	6%
Emesis	9%	5%
Mucositis	10%	0%
Nausea	61%	35%
Respiratory		
Cough	5%	0%
Dyspnea	11%	5%
Miscellaneous		
Anemia	5%	3%
Blurred vision	3%	5%
Decreased LVEF	5%	0%
Edema	10%	4%
Fever	6%	3%

MITOXANTRONE HYDROCHLORIDE — INJECTION

Mitoxantrone Adverse Reactions in Prostate Cancer Patients (≥ 5%): Trial CCI-NOV22		
Adverse reactions	Mitoxantrone + prednisone (n = 80)	Prednisone (n = 81)
Hemorrhage/Bruise	6%	1%
Nail bed changes	11%	0%
Pain	8%	9%
Systemic infection	10%	7%
Urinary tract infection	9%	4%

Trial CALCB 9182 –

Mitoxantrone Adverse Reactions in Prostate Cancer Patients (≥ 5%): Trial CALGB 9182		
Adverse reactions	Mitoxantrone + hydrocortisone (n = 112)	Hydrocortisone (n = 113)
Cardiovascular		
Abnormal cardiac function	18%	0%
Cardiac dysrhythmia	7%	3%
Cardiac ischemia	5%	1%
Hypertension	4%	5%
CNS		
Malaise/Fatigue	34%	14%
Neurologic/Mood disorder	6%	2%
Neurologic/Motor disorder	7%	3%
Other neurologic problems	11%	5%
Dermatologic		
Alopecia	20%	1%
Skin disorder	6%	4%
Sweats	9%	2%
GI		
Anorexia	22%	14%
Diarrhea	14%	4%
Nausea	26%	8%
Neurologic/Constipation	7%	2%
Other GI problems	14%	11%
Stomatitis	8%	1%
Vomiting	11%	5%
Weight gain	14%	15%
Weight loss	17%	12%
GU		
Abnormal blood urea nitrogen	22%	20%
Abnormal creatinine	13%	10%
Hematuria	11%	6%
Impotence/Libido	7%	3%
Other kidney or bladder problems	5%	3%
Proteinuria	6%	3%
Sterility	5%	3%
Hematologic		
Abnormal granulocytes/bands	79%	3%
Abnormal lymphocyte count	72%	25%
Abnormal platelet count	39%	7%
Decreased hemoglobin	75%	39%
Decreased WBC	87%	4%
Hemorrhage	5%	3%
Hepatic		
Abnormal alkaline phosphatase	37%	38%
Abnormal transaminase	20%	14%
Other liver problems	8%	8%
Metabolic		
Edema	30%	14%
Hyperglycemia	31%	30%
Hypocalcemia	10%	5%
Hypokalemia	7%	4%
Hyponatremia	9%	3%
Other endocrine problems	6%	4%
Respiratory		
Dyspnea	15%	8%
Other pulmonary problems	5%	3%
Miscellaneous		
Chills	5%	0%
Fever in absence of infection	14%	6%
Infection	17%	4%
Myalgias/Arthralgias	5%	3%
Pain	41%	39%

➤*Other adverse reactions:*

Cardiovascular – CHF, tachycardia, ECG changes including arrhythmias, chest pain, and asymptomatic decreases in LVEF have occurred.

GI – Nausea and vomiting occurred acutely in most patients and may have contributed to reports of dehydration, but were generally mild to moderate and could be controlled through the use of antiemetics. Stomatitis/mucositis occurred within 1 week of therapy.

Hematologic – Topoisomerase II inhibitors, including mitoxantrone, in combination with other antineoplastic agents have been associated with the development of acute leukemia.

Acute nonlymphocytic leukemia: Myelosuppression is rapid in onset and is consistent with the requirement to produce significant marrow hypoplasia to achieve a response in acute leukemia. The incidences of infection and bleeding seen in the United States trial are consistent with those reported for other standard induction regimens.

Prostate cancer: In a randomized study where dose escalation was required for nadir neutrophil counts greater than 1,000/mm^3, grade 4 neutropenia (ANC less than 500/mm^3) was observed in 54% of patients treated with mitoxantrone plus low-dose prednisone. In a separate randomized trial in which patients were treated with 14 mg/m^2, grade 4 neutropenia in 23% of patients treated with mitoxantrone plus hydrocortisone was observed. Neutropenic fever/infection occurred in 11% and 10% of patients receiving mitoxantrone plus corticosteroids, respectively, on the 2 trials. Platelets less than 50,000/mm^3 were noted in 4% and 3% of patients receiving mitoxantrone plus corticosteroids on these trials, and there was 1 patient death on mitoxantrone plus hydrocortisone caused by intracranial hemorrhage after a fall.

Hypersensitivity – Dyspnea, hypotension, rashes, and urticaria have been reported occasionally. Anaphylaxis/anaphylactoid reactions have been reported rarely.

Pulmonary – Interstitial pneumonitis has been reported in cancer patients receiving combination chemotherapy that included mitoxantrone.

Miscellaneous – Extravasation at the infusion site has been reported, which may result in erythema, swelling, pain, burning, and/or blue discoloration of the skin. Extravasation can result in tissue necrosis with resultant need for debridement and skin grafting. Phlebitis has also been reported at the site of infusion.

Overdosage

➤*Symptoms:* Accidental overdoses have been reported. Four patients receiving 140 to 180 mg/m^2 as a single bolus injection died as a result of severe leukopenia with infection.

➤*Treatment:* There is no known specific antidote for mitoxantrone. Hematologic support and antimicrobial therapy may be required during prolonged periods of severe myelosuppression.

Although patients with severe renal failure have not been studied, mitoxantrone is extensively tissue bound, and it is unlikely that the therapeutic effect or toxicity would be mitigated by peritoneal dialysis or hemodialysis.

Patient Information

Mitoxantrone may impart a blue-green color to the urine for 24 hours after administration; advise patients to expect this during therapy. Bluish discoloration of the sclera may also occur.

Advise patients of the signs and symptoms of myelosuppression.

Provide MS patients with the patient information leaflet at the time the decision is made to treat with mitoxantrone and prior to and in close temporal proximity to each treatment. In addition, discuss the issues addressed in the patient information leaflet with the patient.

HYDROXYUREA

Rx	**Droxia** (Bristol-Myers Squibb Oncology)	**Capsules:** 200 mg	Lactose. (Droxia 6335). Blue-green. In 60s.
		300 mg	Lactose. (Droxia 6336). Purple. In 60s.
		400 mg	Lactose. (Droxia 6337). Reddish-orange. In 60s.
Rx	**Hydroxyurea** (Various, eg, Barr, Major, Par, Roxane)	**Capsules:** 500 mg	In 100s and UD 100s.
Rx	**Hydrea** (Bristol-Myers Squibb)		Lactose. (Hydrea 830). Green and pink. In 100s.

HYDROXYUREA — ORAL

Indications

➤*Droxia*: To reduce the frequency of painful crises and to reduce the need for blood transfusions in adult patients with sickle cell anemia with recurrent moderate to severe painful crises (generally at least 3 during the preceding 12 months).

➤*Hydrea*: Significant tumor response to *Hydrea* (**hydroxyurea** capsules, USP) has been demonstrated in melanoma, resistant chronic myelocytic leukemia, and recurrent, metastatic, or inoperable carcinoma of the ovary.

Hydroxyurea used concomitantly with irradiation therapy is intended for use in the local control of primary squamous cell (epidermoid) carcinomas of the head and neck, excluding the lip.

➤*Off-label uses:*

Refractory psoriasis – [4] = Insufficient documentation. Initial research suggests that hydroxyurea may be effective in treating refractory psoriasis in adults; however, sample sizes have been small and data are equivocal. Hydroxyurea may be most useful in patients who have failed other therapies. Long-term effects of therapy are unknown, and the risk of severe and potentially life-threatening secondary malignancies must be weighed against potential benefits of treatment.

Thrombocythemia – [1] = Good documentation. Hydroxyurea is effective at controlling platelet counts in patients with thrombocythemia. When compared with anagrelide, hydroxyurea treatment resulted in a lower incidence of thrombosis, hemorrhage, and death. However, venous thrombosis was more common in patients receiving hydroxyurea than in patients receiving anagrelide. Hydroxyurea use has been associated with secondary malignancies, especially in patients who received prior treatment with busulfan. Larger, long-term studies are needed to further assess the risk of secondary malignancies with hydroxyurea treatment.

Other possible off-label uses – Treatment of cervical carcinoma, polycythemia vera, essential thrombocytosis. In combination with radiation therapy, used as a radiation sensitizer in brain tumors, cervical cancer, and head and neck cancer.

HIV: Potential antiviral activity of hydroxyurea may be enhanced by didanosine.

Administration and Dosage

➤*General dosing considerations:* Dosage should be based on the patient's actual or ideal weight, whichever is less.

Concurrent use of *Hydrea* with other myelosuppressive agents may require adjustment of dosages.

An increase in fluid intake is recommended while taking hydroxyurea.

➤*Adults:*

Carcinoma of the head and neck (with radiation) (Hydrea, generics only) – 80 mg/kg as a single dose every third day, beginning at least 7 days before radiation and continued during and after irradiation.

Resistant chronic myelocytic leukemia (Hydrea, generics only) –

Usual dosage: 20 to 30 mg/kg as a single daily dose daily. (See also Off-label dosing).

An adequate trial period for determining the antineoplastic effectiveness of hydroxyurea is 6 weeks of therapy. When there is regression in tumor size or arrest in tumor growth, therapy should be continued indefinitely.

Dosage adjustment: Therapy should be interrupted if the white blood cell count drops below 2,500/mm^3 or if the platelet count is below 100,000/mm^3. In these cases, the counts should be reevaluated after 3 days, and therapy resumed when the counts return to acceptable levels. Because the hematopoietic rebound is prompt, it is usually necessary to omit only a few doses. If prompt rebound has not occurred during combined *Hydrea* and irradiation therapy, irradiation may also be interrupted. However, the need for postponement of irradiation has been rare; radiotherapy has usually been continued using the recommended dosage and technique.

Concomitant therapy: Because hematopoiesis may be compromised by extensive irradiation or by other antineoplastic agents, it is recommended that hydroxyurea be administered cautiously to patients who have recently received extensive radiation therapy or chemotherapy with other cytotoxic drugs.

Anemia: Severe anemia, if it occurs, should be corrected without interrupting hydroxyurea therapy.

Mucositis: Pain or discomfort from inflammation of the mucous membranes at the irradiated site (mucositis) is usually controlled by measures such as topical anesthetics and orally administered analgesics. If the reaction is severe, hydroxyurea therapy may be temporarily interrupted; if it is extremely severe, irradiation dosage may, in addition, be temporarily postponed. However, it has rarely been necessary to terminate these therapies.

Gastric effects: Severe gastric distress (eg, nausea, vomiting, and anorexia) resulting from combined therapy may usually be controlled by temporary interruption of hydroxyurea administration.

Sickle cell anemia (Droxia only) –

Maximum dose: 35 mg/kg/day.

Initial dosage: 15 mg/kg as a single daily dose.

Dosage adjustment: The patient's blood count must be monitored every 2 weeks (see Warnings/Precautions). If blood counts are in an acceptable range, the dose may be increased by 5 mg/kg/day every 12 weeks until a maximum tolerated dose (the highest dose that does not produce toxic blood counts over 24 consecutive weeks), or 35 mg/kg/day, is reached.

If blood counts are between the acceptable range and toxic (see parameters for acceptable and toxic below) the dose is not increased.

If blood counts are considered toxic, *Droxia* should be discontinued until hematologic recovery. Treatment may then be resumed after reducing the dose by 2.5 mg/kg/day from the dose associated with hematologic toxicity. *Droxia* may then be titrated up or down, every 12 weeks in 2.5 mg/kg/day increments, until the patient is at a stable dose that does not result in hematologic toxicity for 24 weeks. Any dosage on which a patient develops hematologic toxicity twice should not be tried again.

• *Acceptable ranges* – Neutrophils at least 2,500 cells/mm^3, platelets at least 95,000/mm^3, hemoglobin more than 5.3 g/dL, and reticulocytes at least 95,000/mm^3 if the hemoglobin concentration is less than 9 g/dL.

• *Toxic* – Neutrophils less than 2,000 cells/mm^3, platelets less than 80,000/mm^3, hemoglobin less than 4.5 g/dL, and reticulocytes less than 80,000/mm^3 if the hemoglobin concentration is less than 9 g/dL.

Solid tumors (Hydrea, generics only) –

Intermittent therapy: 80 mg/kg (2,000 to 3,000 mg/m^2) as a single dose every third day. Hold therapy for white blood cell count (WBC) below 2,500 cells/mm^3 or platelet count below 100,000 cells/mm^3.

Continuous therapy: 20 to 30 mg/kg as a single daily dose.

Off-label dosing –

Refractory psoriasis: [4] = Insufficient documentation. 0.5 to 1.5 g orally daily in 2 or 3 divided doses.

Thrombocythemia: [1] = Good documentation. 15 to 20 mg/kg/day initially, titrated to maintain platelet levels of 400 × 10^9/L or less and an absolute neutrophil count (ANC) greater than 1,000 cells/mm^3.

Resistant chronic myelocytic leukemia: Initial doses of 20 to 50 mg/kg may be used to control hyperleukocytosis.

➤*Children:*

Off-label dosing –

Astrocytoma, medulloblastoma, neuroectodermal tumors, combination therapy: 1,500 to 3,000 mg/m^2 body surface area as a single dose repeated every 4 to 6 weeks.

Resistant chronic myelocytic leukemia: 10 to 20 mg/kg as a single daily dose. Adjust dose according to hematologic response.

Sickle cell disease:

• *Maximum dose* – 35 mg/kg/day.

• *Initial dosage* – 15 mg/kg as a single daily dose initially.

• *Dosage adjustment* – May increase by 5 mg/kg/day at intervals of 12 weeks if WBC is at least 2,500 cells/mm^3, platelet count is at least 95,000 cells/mm^3, hemoglobin is below 9 g/dL with reticulocyte count at least 95,000 cells/mm^3, or hemoglobin is at least 5.3 g/dL. Do not exceed 35 mg/kg/day.

Hold therapy for WBC below 2,000 cells/mm^3, platelet count below 80,000 cells/mm^3, hemoglobin below 9 g/dL with reticulocyte count below 80,000 cells/mm^3, or hemoglobin below 4.5 g/dL. When counts recover, reduce dose by 2.5 mg/kg/day and resume therapy. Avoid further increases if hematologic toxicity occurs twice on the same dose level.

➤*Renal function impairment:*

Hydroxyurea Dosage Adjustment Based on Renal Function

Creatinine clearance	Percentage of usual dose to be given: Drug prescribing in renal failure	Manufacturer package insert
≥ 60 mL/min	100%	100%
51 to 59 mL/min	100%	50%
10 to 50 mL/min	50%	50%
< 10 mL/min	20%	50%
Hemodialysis	20%, given after dialysis on dialysis days	50%, given after dialysis on dialysis days
Continuous renal replacement therapy	50%	No recommendation

Dialysis – Conventional hemodialysis is moderately effective (50% to 74%) in removing hydroxyurea. Peritoneal dialysis is ineffective (0% to 24%) in removing hydroxyurea.

Supplemental doses are not required after hemodialysis.

➤*Administration:* Administer orally. May administer with food to minimize GI adverse effects.

For patients unable to swallow capsules, empty capsule contents into a glass of water and administer immediately. Inert materials may float on the surface of the water. Capsule contents may also be mixed with juice or sprinkled on food immediately before administration.

HYDROXYUREA — ORAL

➤*Storage/Stability:* Store at 25°C (77°F); excursions permitted to 15° to 30°C (59° to 86°F). Keep tightly closed.

Actions

➤*Pharmacology:* Various studies support the hypothesis that hydroxyurea causes an immediate inhibition of DNA synthesis by acting as a ribonucleotide reductase inhibitor, without interfering with the synthesis of ribonucleic acid or of protein.

Droxia – The precise mechanism by which hydroxyurea produces its cytotoxic and cytoreductive effects is not known. The mechanisms by which *Droxia* produces its beneficial effects in patients with sickle cell anemia (SCA) are uncertain. Known pharmacologic effects of *Droxia* that may contribute to its beneficial effects include increasing hemoglobin F levels in RBCs, decreasing neutrophils, increasing the water content of RBCs, increasing deformability of sickled cells, and altering the adhesion of RBCs to endothelium.

Hydrea – The precise mechanism by which *Hydrea* produces its antineoplastic effects cannot, at present, be described. Three mechanisms of action have been postulated for the increased effectiveness of concomitant use of hydroxyurea therapy with irradiation on squamous cell (epidermoid) carcinomas of the head and neck. In vitro studies utilizing Chinese hamster cells suggest the following: *Hydrea* is lethal to normally radioresistant S-stage cells; *Hydrea* holds other cells of the cell cycle in the G1 or pre-DNA synthesis stage where they are most susceptible to the effects of irradiation; the third mechanism of action has been theorized on the basis of in vitro studies of HeLa cells: it appears that hydroxyurea, by inhibition of DNA synthesis, hinders the normal repair process of cells damaged but not killed by irradiation, thereby decreasing their survival rate; RNA and protein syntheses have shown no alteration.

➤*Pharmacokinetics:*

Absorption – Hydroxyurea is readily absorbed after oral administration. Peak plasma levels are reached in 1 to 4 hours after an oral dose. With increasing doses, disproportionately greater mean peak plasma concentrations and AUCs are observed.

Distribution – Hydroxyurea distributes rapidly and widely in the body with an estimated volume of distribution approximating total body water.

Plasma to ascites fluid ratios range from 2:1 to 7.5:1. Hydroxyurea concentrates in leukocytes and erythrocytes.

Metabolism – Up to 50% of an oral dose undergoes conversion through metabolic pathways that are not fully characterized. In 1 minor pathway, hydroxyurea may be degraded by urease found in intestinal bacteria. Acetohydroxamic acid was found in the serum of 3 leukemic patients receiving hydroxyurea and may be formed from hydroxylamine resulting from action of urease on hydroxyurea.

Excretion – Excretion of hydroxyurea in humans is a nonlinear process occurring through 2 pathways. One is saturable, probably hepatic metabolism; the other is first-order renal excretion. In adults with SCA, mean cumulative urinary hydroxyurea excretion was 62% of the administered dose at 8 hours.

Special populations –

Renal function impairment: See Administration and Dosage for more information.

Contraindications

Hypersensitivity to hydroxyurea or any other component of its formulation.

➤*Hydrea*: *Hydrea* is contraindicated in patients with marked bone marrow depression (ie, leukopenia [less than 2500 WBC] or thrombocytopenia [less than 100,000]) or severe anemia.

Warnings/Precautions

➤*Bone marrow suppression:*

Droxia – *Droxia* is a cytotoxic and myelosuppressive agent. *Droxia* should not be given if bone marrow function is markedly depressed, as indicated by neutrophils less than 2,000 cells/mm^3; a platelet count less than 80,000/mm^3; a hemoglobin level less than 4.5 g/dL; or reticulocytes less than 80,000/mm^3 when the hemoglobin concentration is less than 9 g/dL. Neutropenia is generally the first and most common manifestation of hematologic suppression (see Administration and Dosage, *Droxia*). Thrombocytopenia and anemia occur less often, and are seldom seen without a preceding leukopenia. Recovery from myelosuppression is usually rapid when therapy is interrupted. *Droxia* causes macrocytosis, which may mask the incidental development of folic acid deficiency. Prophylactic administration of folic acid is recommended.

Hydrea – Treatment with hydroxyurea should not be initiated if bone marrow function is markedly depressed (see Contraindications). Bone marrow suppression may occur, and leukopenia is generally its first and most common manifestation. Thrombocytopenia and anemia occur less often, and are seldom seen without a preceding leukopenia. However, the recovery from myelosuppression is rapid when therapy is interrupted. It should be borne in mind that bone marrow depression is more likely in patients who have previously received radiotherapy or cytotoxic cancer chemotherapeutic agents; hydroxyurea should be used cautiously in such patients.

Patients who have received irradiation therapy in the past may have an exacerbation of postirradiation erythema.

Severe anemia must be corrected before initiating therapy with hydroxyurea.

Erythrocytic abnormalities: Megaloblastic erythropoiesis, which is self-limiting, is often seen early in the course of *Hydrea* therapy. The morphologic change resembles pernicious anemia, but is not related to vitamin B_{12} or folic acid deficiency. Hydroxyurea may also delay plasma iron clearance and reduce the rate of iron utilization by erythrocytes, but it does not appear to alter the red blood cell survival time.

In patients receiving long-term hydroxyurea for myeloproliferative disorders, such as polycythemia vera and thrombocythemia, secondary leukemia has been reported. It is unknown whether this leukemogenic effect is secondary to hydroxyurea or associated with the patients' underlying disease.

➤*Fatal and nonfatal pancreatitis in HIV-infected patients:* Fatal and nonfatal pancreatitis have occurred in HIV-infected patients during therapy with hydroxyurea and didanosine, with or without stavudine. Hepatotoxicity and hepatic failure resulting in death have been reported during postmarketing surveillance in HIV-infected patients treated with hydroxyurea and other antiretroviral agents. Fatal hepatic events were reported most often in patients treated with the combination of hydroxyurea, didanosine, and stavudine. Peripheral neuropathy, which was severe in some cases, has been reported in HIV-infected patients receiving hydroxyurea in combination with antiretroviral agents, including didanosine, with or without stavudine.

➤*Droxia*: Some patients treated at the recommended initial dose of 15 mg/kg/day have experienced severe or life-threatening myelosuppression, requiring interruption of treatment and dose reduction. The hematologic status of the patient as well as kidney and liver function should be determined prior to, and repeatedly during, treatment. Treatment should be interrupted if neutrophil levels fall to less than 2000/mm^3; platelets fall to less than 80,000/mm^3; hemoglobin declines to less than 4.5 g/dL; or if reticulocytes fall less than 80,000/mm^3 when the hemoglobin concentration is less than 9 g/dL. Following recovery, treatment may be resumed at lower doses (see Administration and Dosage).

Patients must be able to follow directions regarding drug administration and their monitoring and care.

➤*Hydrea*: The complete status of the blood, including bone marrow examination, if indicated, as well as kidney function and liver function should be determined prior to, and repeatedly during, treatment. The determination of the hemoglobin level, total leukocyte counts, and platelet counts should be performed at least once a week throughout the course of hydroxyurea therapy. If the white blood cell count decreases to less than 2500/mm^3, or the platelet count to less than 100,000/mm^3, therapy should be interrupted until the values rise significantly toward normal levels. Severe anemia, if it occurs, should be managed without interrupting hydroxyurea therapy.

➤*HIV-infected patients:* Hydroxyurea is not indicated for the treatment of HIV infection; however, if HIV-infected patients are treated with hydroxyurea, and in particular, in combination with didanosine or stavudine, close monitoring for signs and symptoms of pancreatitis and hepatotoxicity is recommended. Patients who develop signs and symptoms of pancreatitis or hepatotoxicity should permanently discontinue therapy with hydroxyurea (see Warnings and Adverse Reactions).

➤*Renal function impairment:* Hydroxyurea should be used with caution in patients with renal dysfunction (see Administration and Dosage).

➤*Pregnancy: Category D.* Drugs that affect DNA synthesis, such as hydroxyurea, may be potential mutagenic agents. The physician should carefully consider this possibility before administering this drug to male or female patients who may contemplate conception.

Hydroxyurea can cause fetal harm when administered to a pregnant woman. Hydroxyurea has been demonstrated to be a potent teratogen in a wide variety of animal models, including mice, hamsters, cats, miniature swine, dogs and monkeys at doses within 1-fold of the human dose given on a mg/m^2 basis. Hydroxyurea is embryotoxic and causes fetal malformations (partially ossified cranial bones, absence of eye sockets, hydrocephaly, bipartite sternebrae, missing lumbar vertebrae) at 180 mg/kg/day (approximately 0.8 times the maximum recommended human daily dose on a mg/m^2 basis) in rats and at 30 mg/kg/day (approximately 0.3 times the maximum recommended human daily dose on a mg/m^2 basis) in rabbits. Embryotoxicity was characterized by decreased fetal viability, reduced live litter sizes, and developmental delays. Hydroxyurea crosses the placenta. Single doses of 375 mg/kg or more (approximately 1.7 times the maximum recommended human daily dose on a mg/m^2 basis) to rats caused growth retardation and impaired learning ability. There are no adequate and well-controlled studies in pregnant women. If this drug is used during pregnancy or if the patient becomes pregnant while taking this drug, the patient should be apprised of the potential harm to the fetus. Women of childbearing potential should be advised to avoid becoming pregnant.

➤*Lactation:* Hydroxyurea is excreted in human milk. Because of the potential for serious adverse reactions with hydroxyurea, a decision should be made either to discontinue nursing or to discontinue the drug, taking into account the importance of the drug to the mother.

➤*Children:* Safety and effectiveness in pediatric patients have not been established.

➤*Elderly:*

Hydrea – Elderly patients may be more sensitive to the effects of hydroxyurea, and may require a lower dose regimen.

➤*Monitoring:* Therapy with hydroxyurea requires close supervision.

Drug Interactions

➤*Hydrea*: Concurrent use of *Hydrea* and other myelosuppressive agents or radiation therapy may increase the likelihood of bone marrow depression or other adverse events (see Warnings and Adverse Reactions).

Uricosuric agents – Because hydroxyurea may raise the serum uric acid level, dosage adjustment of uricosuric medication may be necessary.

HYDROXYUREA — ORAL

Adverse Reactions

Hydroxyurea is considered to have low potential for nausea and vomiting.

➤*Adverse reactions:* Adverse reactions associated with the use of hydroxyurea, in the treatment of neoplastic diseases, in addition to hematologic effects include the following:

CNS – Neurological disturbances have occurred extremely rarely and were limited to headache, dizziness, disorientation, hallucinations, and convulsions.

Large doses may produce moderate drowsiness.

Dermatologic – Maculopapular rash, skin ulceration, dermatomyositis-like skin changes, peripheral erythema and facial erythema. Hyperpigmentation, atrophy of skin and nails, scaling, and violet papules have been observed in some patients after several years of long-term daily maintenance therapy with hydroxyurea. Skin cancer has been reported.

GI – Stomatitis, anorexia, nausea, vomiting, diarrhea, and constipation.

GU – Dysuria and alopecia occur very rarely.

Hematologic –

Hydrea: Adverse reactions have been primarily bone marrow depression (leukopenia, anemia, and occasionally thrombocytopenia).

Lab test abnormalities – Abnormal BSP retention has been reported.

Elevation of hepatic enzymes have also been reported.

Renal – Hydroxyurea occasionally may cause temporary impairment of renal tubular function accompanied by elevations in serum uric acid, BUN, and creatinine levels.

Miscellaneous – Fever, chills, malaise, edema, asthenia.

➤*Acute pulmonary reactions:*

Respiratory – The association of hydroxyurea with the development of acute pulmonary reactions consisting of diffuse pulmonary infiltrates, fever and dyspnea has been rarely reported. Pulmonary fibrosis also has been reported rarely.

➤*Fatal and nonfatal pancreatitis and hepatotoxicity:* Fatal and nonfatal pancreatitis and hepatotoxicity, and severe peripheral neuropathy have been reported in HIV-infected patients who received hydroxyurea in combination with antiretroviral agents, in particular, didanosine plus stavudine. Patients treated with hydroxyurea in combination with didanosine, stavudine, and indinavir in study ACTG 5025 showed a median decline in CD4 cells of approximately 100/mm^3 (see Warnings and Precautions).

➤*Droxia:*

Sickle cell anemia – In patients treated for sickle cell anemia in the Multicenter Study of Hydroxyurea in Sickle Cell Anemia, the most common adverse reactions were hematologic, with neutropenia, and low reticulocyte and platelet levels necessitating temporary cessation in almost all patients. Hematologic recovery usually occurred in two weeks.

Nonhematologic events that possibly were associated with treatment include hair loss, skin rash, fever, gastrointestinal disturbances, weight gain, bleeding, and parvovirus B-19 infection; however, these nonhematologic events occurred with similar frequencies in the hydroxyurea and placebo treatment groups. Melanonychia has also been reported in patients receiving *Droxia* for SCA.

➤*Hydrea*:

Irradiation therapy – Adverse reactions observed with combined *Hydrea* and irradiation therapy are similar to those reported with the use of hydroxyurea or radiation treatment alone. These effects primarily include bone marrow depression (anemia and leukopenia), gastric irritation, and mucositis. Almost all patients receiving an adequate course of combined hydroxyurea and irradiation therapy will demonstrate concurrent leukopenia. Platelet depression (less than 100,000 cells/mm^3) has occurred rarely and only in the presence of marked leukopenia. *Hydrea* may potentiate some adverse reactions usually seen with irradiation alone, such as gastric distress and mucositis.

Overdosage

➤*Animal pharmacology and toxicology with Hydrea*: The oral LD_{50} of hydroxyurea is 7330 mg/kg in mice and 5780 mg/kg in rats, given as a single dose.

In subacute and chronic toxicity studies in the rat, the most consistent pathological findings were an apparent dose-related mild to moderate bone marrow hypoplasia as well as pulmonary congestion and mottling of the lungs. At the highest dosage levels (1260 mg/kg/day for 37 days then 2520 mg/kg/day for 40 days), testicular atrophy with absence of spermatogenesis occurred; in several animals, hepatic cell damage with fatty metamorphosis was noted. In the dog, mild to marked bone marrow depression was a consistent finding except at the lower dosage levels. Additionally, at the higher dose levels (140 to 420 mg or 140 to 1260 mg/kg/week given 3 or 7 days weekly for 12 weeks), growth retardation, slightly increased blood glucose values, and hemosiderosis of the liver or spleen were found; reversible spermatogenic arrest was noted. In the monkey, bone marrow depression, lymphoid atrophy of the spleen, and degenerative changes in the epithelium of the small and large intestines were found. At the higher, often lethal, doses (400 to 800 mg/kg/day for 7 to 15 days), hemorrhage and congestion were found in the lungs, brain, and urinary tract. Cardiovascular effects (changes in heart rate, blood pressure, orthostatic hypotension, EKG changes) and hematological changes (slight hemolysis, slight methemoglobinemia) were observed in some species of laboratory animals at doses exceeding clinical levels.

➤*Symptoms:* Acute mucocutaneous toxicity has been reported in patients receiving hydroxyurea at dosages several times the therapeutic dose. Soreness, violet erythema, edema on palms and soles followed by scaling of hands and feet, severe generalized hyperpigmentation of the skin, and stomatitis have been observed.

METHYLHYDRAZINE DERIVATIVES

PROCARBAZINE HYDROCHLORIDE (N-Methylhydrazine; MIH)

Rx	**Matulane** (Sigma-Tau)	**Capsules:** 50 mg	Talc, mannitol, parabens. (Matulane Sigma-Tau). Ivory. In 100s.

PROCARBAZINE HYDROCHLORIDE — ORAL

WARNING

It is recommended that procarbazine hydrochloride be given only by or under the supervision of a physician experienced in the use of potent antineoplastic drugs. Adequate clinical and laboratory facilities should be available to patients for proper monitoring of treatment.

Indications

➤*Hodgkin's disease:* Procarbazine hydrochloride is indicated for use in combination with other anticancer drugs for the treatment of Stage III and IV Hodgkin's disease. Procarbazine hydrochloride is used as part of the MOPP (nitrogen mustard, vincristine, procarbazine, prednisone) regimen.

➤*Off-label uses:* Treatment of non-Hodgkin lymphoma, brain tumors, small cell lung cancer, melanoma, mycosis fungoides, and multiple myeloma.

Administration and Dosage

➤*General dosing considerations:* All dosages are based on the patient's actual weight. However, the estimated lean body mass (dry weight) is used if the patient is obese or if there has been a spurious weight gain due to edema, ascites or other forms of abnormal fluid retention.

Round dosage to the nearest 50 mg.

Procarbazine is dosed in mg/kg for some indications, but may be dosed in mg/m^2 for other indications.

Continuous dosage regimens may increase the risk of secondary malignancy and should be avoided.

➤*Adults:*

Hodgkin disease –

Single agent therapy:

• *Initial dosage* – 2 to 4 mg/kg/day (in single or divided doses) for the 7 days to minimize the nausea and vomiting experienced by a high percentage of patients beginning procarbazine therapy.

• *Dosage titration* – After the initial dosage, increase dose to 4 to 6 mg/kg/day until maximum response is obtained or until the white blood count falls below 4,000 cells/mm^3 or the platelets fall below 100,000 cells/mm^3.

• *Maintenance dosage* – Reduce dosage to 1 to 2 mg/kg/day after maximum response is obtained.

• *Rechallenge* – After toxic side effects have subsided, therapy may then be resumed at the discretion of the physician, based on clinical evaluation and appropriate laboratory studies, at a dosage of 1 to 2 mg/kg/day.

• *Discontinuation of therapy* – Upon evidence of hematologic or other toxicity, the drug should be discontinued until there has been satisfactory recovery. (See the following Discontinuation of therapy.)

MOPP combination regimen: 100 mg/m^2 body surface area per day, on days 1 through 14 of 28-day cycle; treat with a minimum of 6 cycles of MOPP, plus 2 to 3 cycles of consolidation chemotherapy.

Off-label dosing –

Non-Hodgkin lymphoma, combination regimen: 100 mg/m^2 body surface area per day for 7 to 14 days of each 28-day cycle.

Non–small cell lung cancer, combination regimen: 100 mg/m^2 body surface area per day, on days 1 through 10 of 28-day cycle.

➤*Children:* Very close clinical monitoring is mandatory. Undue toxicity, evidenced by tremors, coma and convulsions, has occurred in a few cases. Dosage, therefore, should be individualized. The following dosage schedule is provided as a guideline only.

Hodgkin disease – See also Off-label dosing.

Single agent therapy:

• *Initial dosage* – 50 mg/m^2 body surface area per day for the first 7 days.

• *Dosage titration* – After the initial dosage, increase dosage to 100 mg/m^2 body surface area per day until maximum response is obtained or until leukopenia or thrombocytopenia occurs.

• *Maintenance dosage* – Reduce dosage to 50 mg/m^2 body surface area per day after maximum response is obtained.

• *Rechallenge* – After toxic side effects have subsided, therapy may then be resumed.

PROCARBAZINE HYDROCHLORIDE — ORAL

• *Discontinuation of therapy* – Upon evidence of hematologic or other toxicity, the drug should be discontinued until there has been satisfactory recovery, based on clinical evaluation and appropriate laboratory tests. (See the following Discontinuation of therapy.)

Off-label dosing –

Brain tumor: 75 mg/m² body surface area per day at hour 1 on day 1 of each cycle, repeat cycles every 2 to 4 weeks.

Alternatively, 100 mg/m² body surface area per day for 14 days of each 28-day cycle.

Hodgkin lymphoma (MOPP combination therapy): 50 mg on day 1 followed by 100 mg/m² body surface area on days 2 through 14. Treat with a minimum of 6 cycles of MOPP plus 2 to 3 cycles of consolidation chemotherapy.

➤*Hepatic function impairment:*

Procarbazine Dosage Adjustment Based on Hepatic Function

Serum bilirubin	AST or ALT	Percent of usual dose
≤ 5 mg/dL	< 1.6 times the ULN[a]	100%
	1.6 to 6 times the ULN	75%
	> 6 times the ULN	Use clinical judgment.
> 5 mg/dL		Do not administer.

[a] ULN = upper limit of normal.

➤*Discontinuation of therapy:* Prompt cessation of therapy is recommended if any one of the following occurs:

- CNS signs or symptoms such as paresthesias, neuropathies or confusion.
- Leukopenia (white blood count less than 4,000 cells/mm³).
- Thrombocytopenia (platelet count less than 100,000 cells/mm³).
- Hypersensitivity reaction.
- Stomatitis (the first small ulceration or persistent spot soreness around the oral cavity is a signal for cessation of therapy).
- Diarrhea (frequent bowel movements or watery stools).
- Hemorrhage or bleeding tendencies.

In adults, therapy may be resumed after toxic side effects have subsided at the discretion of the physician, based on clinical evaluation and appropriate laboratory studies, at a dosage of 1 to 2 mg/kg/day.

➤*Preparation for administration:* Procarbazine is considered a cytotoxic agent. Follow safe handling procedures when preparing, administering, or dispensing procarbazine.

➤*Administration:* Give with or after meals. May give once daily or in 2 to 3 divided doses.

➤*Storage/Stability:* Store capsules in light-resistant containers at room temperature.

Actions

➤*Pharmacology:* The precise mode of cytotoxic action of procarbazine has not been clearly defined. There is evidence that the drug may act by inhibition of protein, RNA and DNA synthesis. Studies have suggested that procarbazine may inhibit transmethylation of methyl groups of methionine into t-RNA. The absence of functional t-RNA could cause the cessation of protein synthesis and consequently DNA and RNA synthesis. In addition, procarbazine may directly damage DNA. Hydrogen peroxide, formed during the autooxidation of the drug, may attack protein sulfhydryl groups contained in residual protein which is tightly bound to DNA.

➤*Pharmacokinetics:*

Absorption – Procarbazine is rapidly and completely absorbed. Following oral administration of 30 mg of ^{14}C-labeled procarbazine, maximum peak plasma radioactive concentrations were reached within 60 minutes.

Distribution – Procarbazine crosses the blood-brain barrier and rapidly equilibrates between plasma and cerebrospinal fluid after oral administration.

Metabolism – Procarbazine is metabolized primarily in the liver and kidneys. The drug appears to be auto-oxidized to the azo derivative with the release of hydrogen peroxide. The azo derivative isomerizes to the hydrazone, and following hydrolysis splits into a benzylaldehyde derivative and methylhydrazine. The methylhydrazine is further degraded to CO_2 and CH_4 and possibly hydrazine, whereas the aldehyde is oxidized to N-isopropylterephthalamic acid, which is excreted in the urine.

Excretion – After intravenous injection, the plasma half-life of procarbazine is approximately 10 minutes. Approximately 70% of the radioactivity is excreted in the urine as N-isopropylterephthalamic acid within 24 hours following both oral and intravenous administration of ^{14}C-labeled procarbazine.

Contraindications

Procarbazine hydrochloride is contraindicated in patients with known hypersensitivity to the drug or inadequate marrow reserve as demonstrated by bone marrow aspiration. Due consideration of this possible state should be given to each patient who has leukopenia, thrombocytopenia or anemia.

Warnings/Precautions

➤*Drug/Food warnings:* To minimize CNS depression and possible potentiation, barbiturates, antihistamines, narcotics, hypotensive agents or phenothiazines should be used with caution. Ethyl alcohol should not be used since there may be a disulfiram-like reaction. Because procarbazine hydrochloride exhibits some monoamine oxidase inhibitory activity, sympathomimetic drugs, tricyclic antidepressant drugs (eg, amitriptyline HCl, imipramine HCl) and other drugs and foods with known high tyramine content, such as wine, yogurt, ripe cheese and bananas, should be avoided. A further phenomenon of toxicity common to many hydrazine derivatives is hemolysis and the appearance of Heinz-Ehrlich inclusion bodies in erythrocytes.

➤*Prior radiation/chemotherapy:* If radiation or a chemotherapeutic agent known to have marrow-depressant activity has been used, an interval of 1 month or longer without such therapy is recommended before starting treatment with procarbazine hydrochloride. The length of this interval may also be determined by evidence of bone marrow recovery based on successive bone marrow studies.

➤*Discontinuation:* Prompt cessation of therapy is recommended if any one of the following occurs: CNS signs or symptoms such as paresthesias, neuropathies, or confusion; leukopenia (white blood count under 4,000); thrombocytopenia (platelets under 100,000); hypersensitivity reaction; stomatitis (the first small ulceration or persistent spot soreness around the oral cavity is a signal for cessation of therapy); diarrhea (frequent bowel movements or watery stools); hemorrhage or bleeding tendencies.

➤*Bone marrow depression:* Bone marrow depression often occurs 2 to 8 weeks after the start of treatment. If leukopenia occurs, hospitalization of the patient may be needed for appropriate treatment to prevent systemic infection.

➤*Renal/Hepatic function impairment:* Undue toxicity may occur if procarbazine hydrochloride is used in patients with impairment of renal and/or hepatic function. When appropriate, hospitalization for the initial course of treatment should be considered.

➤*Pregnancy: Category D.*

Fertility impairment – Azoospermia and antifertility effects associated with procarbazine hydrochloride administration in combination with other chemotherapeutic agents for treating Hodgkin's disease have been reported in human clinical studies. Since these patients received multicombination therapy, it is difficult to determine to what extent procarbazine hydrochloride alone was involved in the male germ-cell damage. The usual Segment I fertility/reproduction studies in laboratory animals have not been carried out with procarbazine hydrochloride. However, compounds that inhibit DNA, RNA and/or protein synthesis might be expected to have adverse effects on gametogenesis. Unscheduled DNA synthesis in the testis of rabbits and decreased fertility in male mice treated with procarbazine hydrochloride have been reported.

Teratogenic – Procarbazine hydrochloride can cause fetal harm when administered to a pregnant woman. While there are no adequate and well-controlled studies with procarbazine hydrochloride in pregnant women, there are case reports of malformations in the offspring of women who were exposed to procarbazine hydrochloride in combination with other antineoplastic agents during pregnancy. Procarbazine hydrochloride should be used during pregnancy only if the potential benefit justifies the potential risk to the fetus. If this drug is used during pregnancy, or if the patient becomes pregnant while taking this drug, the patient should be apprised of the potential hazard to the fetus. Women of childbearing potential should be advised to avoid becoming pregnant. Procarbazine hydrochloride is teratogenic in the rat when given at doses approximately 4 to 13 times the maximum recommended human therapeutic dose of 6 mg/kg/day.

Nonteratogenic – Procarbazine hydrochloride has not been adequately studied in animals for its effects on peri- and postnatal development. However, neurogenic tumors were noted in the offspring of rats given intravenous injections of 125 mg/kg of procarbazine hydrochloride on day 22 of gestation. Compounds which inhibit DNA, RNA and protein synthesis might be expected to have adverse effects on peri- and postnatal development.

➤*Lactation:* It is not known whether procarbazine hydrochloride is excreted in human milk. Because of the potential for tumorigenicity shown for procarbazine hydrochloride in animal studies, mothers should not nurse while receiving this drug.

➤*Children:* Undue toxicity, evidenced by tremors, coma and convulsions, has occurred in a few cases. Dosage, therefore, should be individualized. All dosages are based on the patient's actual weight. However, the estimated lean body mass (dry weight) is used if the patient is obese or if there has been a spurious weight gain due to edema, ascites or other forms of abnormal fluid retention. Very close clinical monitoring is mandatory.

➤*Monitoring:* Baseline laboratory data should be obtained prior to initiation of therapy. The hematologic status as indicated by hemoglobin, hematocrit, white blood count (WBC), differential, reticulocytes and platelets should be monitored closely, at least every 3 or 4 days.

Hepatic and renal evaluation are indicated prior to beginning therapy. Urinalysis, transaminase, alkaline phosphatase and blood urea nitrogen tests should be repeated at least weekly.

Drug Interactions

Procarbazine Drug Interactions

Precipitant drug	Object drug[a]		Description
Procarbazine	CNS depressants (ie, narcotics, hypotensive agents, phenothiazines, antihistamines, barbiturates, sedatives)	⬆	Concomitant use may result in depressant effects on the CNS (ie, respiratory depression).

PROCARBAZINE HYDROCHLORIDE — ORAL

Procarbazine Drug Interactions			
Precipitant drug	Object drug[a]		Description
Procarbazine	Ethanol	↑	Concomitant ingestion has resulted in a disulfiram-like reaction (ie, flushing of the face).
Procarbazine	Methotrexate	↑	The nephrotoxicity of methotrexate may be increased; consider an interval of ≥ 72 hours between administration of the final dose of procarbazine and the initiation of a high-dose methotrexate infusion.
Procarbazine	Sympathomimetics (eg, ephedrine, epinephrine)	↑	May cause an abrupt increase in blood pressure, resulting in a potentially fatal hypertensive crisis.
Procarbazine	Tricyclic antidepressants (eg, amitriptyline, imipramine)	↑	Severe toxic and fatal reactions including excitability, fluctuations in blood pressure, convulsions, and coma may occur. However, some studies report uneventful concurrent use with MAOIs.
Procarbazine	Radiation or other chemotherapy	↑	If radiation or other chemotherapy known to have marrow depressant activity has been used, wait ≥ 1 month before starting procarbazine. Interval length may also be determined by evidence of bone marrow recovery based on successive bone marrow studies.

[a] ↑ = Object drug increased. ↓ = Object drug decreased.

Adverse Reactions

Leukopenia, anemia and thrombopenia occur frequently. Nausea and vomiting are the most commonly reported side effects.

Procarbazine is considered to have moderately high emetogenic potential (60% to 90% incidence of emesis).

➤*Other adverse reactions:*

Allergic – Generalized allergic reactions.

Cardiovascular – Hypotension, tachycardia, syncope.

CNS – Coma, convulsions, neuropathy, ataxia, paresthesia, nystagmus, diminished reflexes, falling, foot drop, headache, dizziness, unsteadiness.

Dermatologic – Herpes, dermatitis, pruritus, alopecia, hyperpigmentation, rash, urticaria, flushing.

Endocrine – Gynecomastia in prepubertal and early pubertal boys.

GI – Hepatic dysfunction, jaundice, stomatitis, hematemesis, melena, diarrhea, dysphagia, anorexia, abdominal pain, constipation, dry mouth.

GU – Hematuria, urinary frequency, nocturia.

Hematologic – Pancytopenia, eosinophilia, hemolytic anemia, bleeding tendencies such as petechiae, purpura, epistaxis and hemoptysis.

Musculoskeletal – Pain, including myalgia and arthralgia; tremors.

Ophthalmic – Retinal hemorrhage, papilledema, photophobia, diplopia, inability to focus.

Psychiatric – Hallucinations, depression, apprehension, nervousness, confusion, nightmares.

Respiratory – Pneumonitis, pleural effusion, cough.

Miscellaneous – Intercurrent infections, hearing loss, pyrexia, diaphoresis, lethargy, weakness, fatigue, edema, chills, insomnia, slurred speech, hoarseness, drowsiness.

Second nonlymphoid malignancies (including lung cancer, acute myelocytic leukemia and malignant myelosclerosis) and azoospermia have been reported in patients with Hodgkin's disease treated with procarbazine in combination with other chemotherapy and/or radiation. The risks of secondary lung cancer from treatment appear to be multiplied by tobacco use.

Overdosage

The major manifestations of overdosage with procarbazine hydrochloride would be anticipated to be nausea, vomiting, enteritis, diarrhea, hypotension, tremors, convulsions and coma. Treatment should consist of either the administration of an emetic or gastric lavage. General supportive measures such as intravenous fluids are advised. Since the major toxicity of procarbazine hydrochloride is hematologic and hepatic, patients should have frequent complete blood counts and liver function tests throughout their period of recovery and for a minimum of 2 weeks thereafter. Should abnormalities appear in any of these determinations, appropriate measures for correction and stabilization should be immediately undertaken.

The estimated mean lethal dose of procarbazine hydrochloride in laboratory animals varied from approximately 150 mg/kg in rabbits to 1300 mg/kg in mice.

Patient Information

Patients should be warned not to drink alcoholic beverages while on procarbazine hydrochloride therapy since there may be an disulfiram-like reaction. They should also be cautioned to avoid foods with known high tyramine content such as wine, yogurt, ripe cheese and bananas. Over-the-counter drug preparations which contain antihistamines or sympathomimetic drugs should also be avoided. Patients taking procarbazine hydrochloride should also be warned against the use of prescription drugs without the knowledge and consent of their physician. Patients should be advised to discontinue tobacco use.

IMIDAZOTETRAZINE DERIVATIVES

TEMOZOLOMIDE

Rx	Temodar (Schering-Plough Corp)	Capsules; oral: 5 mg	Opaque. White/Green. (5 mg Temodar). Lactose. In 5s and 14s.
		20 mg	Opaque. White/Yellow. (20 mg Temodar). Lactose. In 5s and 14s.
		100 mg	Opaque. White/Pink. (100 mg Temodar). Lactose. In 5s and 14s.
		140 mg	Opaque. White/Blue. (140 mg Temodar). Lactose. In 5s and 14s.
		180 mg	Opaque. White/Orange. (180 mg Temodar). Lactose. In 5s and 14s.
		250 mg	Opaque. White/White. (200 mg Temodar). Lactose. In 5s.
		Injection, lyophilized powder for solution: 100 mg	In single-use vials.

TEMOZOLOMIDE — ORAL

Indications

➤*Anaplastic astrocytoma:* For the treatment of adult patients with refractory anaplastic astrocytoma (ie, patients who have experienced disease progression on a drug regimen containing a nitrosourea and procarbazine).

➤*Glioblastoma multiforme:* For the treatment of adults with newly diagnosed glioblastoma multiforme concomitantly with radiotherapy and then as maintenance treatment.

➤*Off-label uses:* Metastatic melanoma.

Administration and Dosage

➤*General dosing considerations:* The dosage of temozolomide must be adjusted according to nadir neutrophil and platelet counts in the previous cycle and the neutrophil and platelet counts at the time of initiating the next cycle.

During treatment, a complete blood cell count (CBC) should be obtained weekly.

To reduce nausea and vomiting, temozolomide should be taken on an empty stomach.

Antiemetic therapy may be administered prior to and/or following administration of temozolomide.

Capsules should not be opened or chewed.

➤*Adults:*

Anaplastic astrocytoma –

Initial dosage: 150 mg/m^2 orally once daily for 5 consecutive days per 28-day treatment cycle.

Dosage adjustment: During treatment, a CBC should be obtained on day 22 (21 days after the first dose) or within 48 hours of that day, and weekly until the absolute neutrophil count (ANC) is above 1.5×10^9/L (1,500/mcL) and the platelet count exceeds 100×10^9/L (100,000 mcL). The next cycle of temozolomide should not be started until the ANC and platelet count exceed these levels. If the ANC falls to less than 1×10^9/L (1,000/mcL) or the platelet count is less than 50×10^9/L (50,000/mcL) during any cycle, the next cycle should be reduced by 50 mg/m^2, but not below 100 mg/m^2, the lowest recommended dose.

If both the nadir and day of dosing (day 29, day 1 of next cycle) ANC are 1.5×10^9/L (1,500/mcL) or more and both the nadir and day 29, day 1 of next cycle platelet counts are 100×10^9/L (100,000/mcL) or more, the temozolomide dose may be increased to 200 mg/m^2/day for 5 consecutive days per 28-day treatment cycle.

Duration of therapy: Temozolomide therapy can be continued until disease progression. In the clinical trial, treatment could be continued for a maximum of 2 years, but the optimal duration of therapy is not known.

TEMOZOLOMIDE — ORAL

Glioblastoma multiforme –

Concomitant phase:

• *Initial dosage* – 75 mg/m^2 daily for 42 days concomitant with focal radiotherapy (60 Gy administered in 30 fractions) followed by maintenance temozolomide for 6 cycles.

• *Dosage adjustment* – No dose reductions are recommended during the concomitant phase; however, dose interruptions or discontinuation may occur based on toxicity.

• *Duration of therapy* – The temozolomide dose should be continued throughout the 42-day concomitant period up to 49 days if all of the following conditions are met: ANC 1.5 × 10^9/L or more, platelet count 100 × 10^9/L or more, Common Toxicity Criteria (CTC) nonhematological toxicity grade 1 or less (except for alopecia, nausea, and vomiting).

• *Concomitant therapy* – *Pneumocystis carinii* pneumonia (PCP) prophylaxis is required during the coadministration of temozolomide and radiotherapy and should be continued in patients who develop lymphocytopenia until recovery from lymphocytopenia (CTC grade 1 or less).

• *Discontinuation of therapy* – Temozolomide dosing should be interrupted or discontinued during the concomitant phase according to the hematological and nonhematological toxicity criteria.

Temozolomide Dosing Interruption or Discontinuation During Concomitant Radiotherapy

Toxicity	Temozolomide interruption[a]	Temozolomide discontinuation
ANC	≥ 0.5 and < 1.5 × 10^9/L	< 0.5 × 10^9/L
Platelet count	≥ 10 and < 100 × 10^9/L	< 10 × 10^9/L
CTC nonhematological toxicity (except for alopecia, nausea, and vomiting)	CTC grade 2	CTC grade 3 or 4

[a] Treatment with concomitant temozolomide could be continued when all of the following conditions are met: ANC ≥ 1.5 × 10^9/L, platelet count ≥ 100 × 10^9/L, and CTC nonhematological toxicity grade ≤ 1 (except for alopecia, nausea, and vomiting).

Maintenance phase: Four weeks after completing the temozolomide plus radiotherapy phase, temozolomide is administered for an additional 6 cycles of maintenance treatment.

Cycle 1: Dosage in cycle 1 (maintenance) is 150 mg/m^2 once daily for 5 days, followed by 23 days without treatment.

Cycle 2 to 6: At the start of cycle 2, the dose is escalated to 200 mg/m^2 if CTC nonhematologic toxicity for cycle 1 is grade 2 or less (except for alopecia, nausea, and vomiting), ANC is 1.5 × 10^9/L or more, and the platelet count is 100 × 10^9/L or more. The dosage remains at 200 mg/m^2/day for the first 5 days of each subsequent cycle, unless toxicity occurs. If the dose is not escalated at cycle 2, escalation should not be done in subsequent cycles.

Temozolomide Dose Levels for Maintenance Treatment

Dose level	Dosage (mg/m^2/day)	Remarks
−1	100	Reduction for prior toxicity
0	150	Dose during cycle 1
1	200	Dose during cycles 2 to 6 in absence of toxicity

• *Dose reduction or discontinuation during maintenance* – During treatment, a CBC should be obtained on day 22 (21 days after the first dose of temozolomide) or within 48 hours of that day and weekly until the ANC is above 1.5 × 10^9/L (1,500/mcL) and the platelet count exceeds 100 × 10^9/L (100,000/mcL). The next cycle of temozolomide should not be started until the ANC and platelet count exceed these levels. Dose reductions during the next cycle should be based on the lowest blood counts and worst nonhematologic toxicity during the previous cycle. Dose reductions or discontinuations during the maintenance phase should be applied.

Temozolomide Dose Reduction or Discontinuation During Maintenance Treatment

Toxicity	Reduce temozolomide by 1 dose level[a]	Discontinue temozolomide
ANC	< 1 × 10^9/L	[b]
Platelet count	< 50 × 10^9/L	[b]
CTC nonhematological toxicity (except for alopecia, nausea, and vomiting)	CTC grade 3	CTC grade 4[b]

[a] Temozolomide dose levels are listed in the previous table.

[b] Temozolomide is to be discontinued if dose reduction to < 100 mg/m^2 is required or if the same grade 3 nonhematological toxicity (except for alopecia, nausea, and vomiting) recurs after dose reduction.

➤*Children:*

Off-label dosing –

Anaplastic astrocytoma and glioblastoma multiforme: Temozolomide has been used safely and effectively in children 3 years of age and older.

Doses are similar to those used in adult regimens, with calculation based on body surface area (BSA). Usual dosages range from 150 mg/m^2/day to 200 mg/m^2/day for 5 days during each 28-day course of therapy.

Follow dosage adjustment guidelines recommended for adults (see Adults for dosage).

➤*Elderly:* Dose selection for an elderly patient should be cautious, reflecting the greater frequency of decreased hepatic, renal, or cardiac function, and of concomitant disease or other drug therapy.

➤*Renal function impairment:* Exercise caution when temozolomide is administered to patients with severe renal function impairment.

➤*Hepatic function impairment:* Exercise caution when temozolomide is administered to patients with severe hepatic impairment.

➤*Preparation for administration:* Temozolomide is considered a cytotoxic agent. Follow safe handling procedures when preparing, administering, or dispensing temozolomide.

Capsules should not be opened. If capsules are accidentally opened or damaged, rigorous precautions should be taken with the capsule contents to avoid inhalation or contact with the skin or mucous membranes. The use of gloves and safety glasses is recommended to avoid exposure in case of breakage of the vial or capsules.

➤*Administration:* In clinical trials, temozolomide was administered under fasting and nonfasting conditions; however, absorption is affected by food and consistency of administration with respect to food is recommended. There are no dietary restrictions with temozolomide. To reduce nausea and vomiting, temozolomide should be taken on an empty stomach. Bedtime administration may be advised. Antiemetic therapy may be administered prior to and/or following administration of temozolomide.

Advise patients not to open or chew temozolomide capsules. Patients should swallow them whole with a glass of water. If capsules are accidentally opened or damaged, avoid inhalation or contact with the skin or mucous membranes.

➤*Storage/Stability:* Store at 25°C (77°F); excursions are permitted to 15° to 30°C (59° to 86°F).

Actions

➤*Pharmacology:* Temozolomide, an imidazotetrazine derivative, is not directly active but undergoes rapid nonenzymatic conversion at physiologic pH to the reactive compound 5-(3-methyltriazen-1-yl),imidazole-4-carboxamide (MTIC). The cytotoxicity of MTIC is thought to be caused primarily by alkylation of DNA. Alkylation (methylation) occurs mainly at the O^6 and N^7 positions of guanine.

➤*Pharmacokinetics:*

Absorption – Temozolomide is absorbed rapidly and completely after oral administration; peak plasma concentration (C_{max}) occurs in a median time to C_{max} (T_{max}) of 1 hour.

Effect of food: Food reduces the rate and extent of temozolomide absorption. Mean C_{max} and area under the curve (AUC) decreased 32% and 9%, respectively, and mean T_{max} increased 2-fold (1.1 to 2.25 hours) when temozolomide was administered after a modified high-fat breakfast.

Distribution – Temozolomide has a mean apparent volume of distribution of 0.4 L/kg (% coefficient of variation = 13%). It is weakly bound to human plasma proteins; the mean percent bound of drug-related total radioactivity is 15%.

Metabolism – Temozolomide is hydrolyzed spontaneously at physiologic pH to the active species, MTIC, and to temozolomide acid metabolite. MTIC is further hydrolyzed to 5-amino-imidazole-4-carboxamide (AIC), which is known to be an intermediate in purine and nucleic acid biosynthesis and to methylhydrazine, which is believed to be the active alkylating species. Cytochrome P450 (CYP-450) enzymes play only a minor role in the metabolism of temozolomide and MTIC. Relative to the AUC of temozolomide, the exposure to MTIC and AIC is 2.4% and 23%, respectively.

Excretion – Temozolomide is eliminated rapidly, with a mean elimination half-life of 1.8 hours, and exhibits linear kinetics over the therapeutic dosing range of 75 to 250 mg/m^2/day. About 38% of the administered temozolomide total radioactive dose is recovered over 7 days; 37.7% in urine and 0.8% in feces. The majority of the recovery of radioactivity in urine is as unchanged temozolomide (5.6%), AIC (12%), temozolomide acid metabolite (2.3%), and unidentified polar metabolite(s) (17%). Overall clearance of temozolomide is approximately 5.5 L/h/m^2.

Special populations –

Gender: Population pharmacokinetic analysis indicates that women have an approximate 5% lower clearance (adjusted for BSA) for temozolomide than men.

Contraindications

History of hypersensitivity reaction to temozolomide or any of its components; history of hypersensitivity to dacarbazine because both temozolomide and dacarbazine are metabolized to MTIC.

Warnings/Precautions

➤*Myelosuppression:* Patients treated with temozolomide may experience myelosuppression, including prolonged pancytopenia, which may result in aplastic anemia, which in some cases has resulted in a fatal outcome. In some cases, exposure to concomitant medications associated with aplastic anemia including carbamazepine, phenytoin, and sulfamethoxazole/trimethoprim complicates assessment. Prior to dosing, patients must have an ANC 1.5 × 10^9/L or more and a platelet count 100 × 10^9/L or more. Obtain a CBC on day 22 (21 days after the first dose) or within 48 hours of that day, and weekly until the ANC is above 1.5 × 10^9/L and platelet count exceeds 100 × 10^9/L. Elderly patients and women have been shown in clinical trials to have a higher risk of developing myelosuppression.

➤*Myelodysplastic syndrome/secondary malignancies:* Cases of myelodysplastic syndrome and secondary malignancies, including myeloid leukemia, have also been observed.

TEMOZOLOMIDE — ORAL

➤*Pneumocystis carinii pneumonia:* For the treatment of newly diagnosed glioblastoma multiforme, prophylaxis against PCP is required for all patients receiving concomitant temozolomide and radiotherapy for the 42-day regimen.

There may be a higher occurrence of PCP when temozolomide is administered during a longer dosing regimen. However, closely observe all patients receiving temozolomide, particularly patients receiving steroids, for the development of PCP regardless of the regimen.

➤*Renal/Hepatic function impairment:* Exercise caution when temozolomide is administered to patients with severe hepatic or severe renal impairment.

➤*Pregnancy: Category D.* Temozolomide can cause fetal harm when administered to a pregnant woman. Five consecutive days of oral administration of 75 mg/m^2/day in rats and 150 mg/m^2/day in rabbits during the period of organogenesis (0.38 and 0.75 the maximum recommended human dose [MRHD], respectively) caused numerous malformations of the external organs, soft tissues, and skeleton in both species. Dosages of 150 mg/m^2/day in rats and rabbits also caused embryolethality, as indicated by increased resorptions. There are no adequate and well-controlled studies in pregnant women. The molecular weight of the parent compound (about 194) and the minimal plasma protein binding suggest that the drug will cross to the embryo and fetus. However, after absorption, temozolomide undergoes rapid hydrolysis to MTIC, and this compound may also cross the placenta. If this drug is used during pregnancy, or if the patient becomes pregnant while taking this drug, inform the patient of the potential hazard to the fetus. Advise women of childbearing potential to avoid becoming pregnant during therapy with temozolomide.

➤*Lactation:* It is not known whether this drug is excreted in human milk. The molecular weight of the parent compound (about 194) and the minimal plasma protein binding (about 15%) suggest that the drug will be excreted into breast milk. Because many drugs are excreted in human milk and because of the potential for serious adverse reactions in breast-feeding infants and tumorigenicity shown for temozolomide in animal studies, decide whether to discontinue breast-feeding or to discontinue the drug, taking into account the importance of the drug to the mother.

➤*Children:* Safety and effectiveness in children have not been established.

➤*Elderly:* See Administration and Dosage for more information.

In the anaplastic astrocytoma study population, patients 70 years of age and older had a higher incidence of grade 4 neutropenia and grade 4 thrombocytopenia (2/8; 25%, $P = 0.31$ and 2/10; 20%, $P = 0.09$, respectively) in the first cycle of therapy than patients younger than 70 years of age.

➤*Monitoring:* For the concomitant treatment phase with radiotherapy, obtain a CBC prior to treatment and weekly during treatment.

For the 28-day treatment cycles, obtain a CBC prior to initiation of treatment on day 1 and on day 22 (21 days after the first dose) of each cycle or within 48 hours of that day. Perform blood counts weekly until recovery if the ANC falls below 1.5×10^9/L and the platelet count falls below 100×10^9/L.

Closely monitor all patients receiving temozolomide, particularly patients receiving steroids, for the development of PCP, regardless of the regimen.

Drug Interactions

➤*Valproic acid:* Administration of valproic acid decreases oral clearance of temozolomide about 5%. The clinical implication of this effect is not known.

➤*Drug/Food interactions:* See Actions for more information.

Adverse Reactions

Temozolomide is considered to have moderate potential for nausea and vomiting.

➤*Glioblastoma multiforme:*

Severe or life-threatening reactions – Forty-nine percent of patients treated with temozolomide reported one or more severe or life-threatening reactions, most commonly fatigue (13%), convulsions (6%), headache (5%), and thrombocytopenia (5%).

Temozolomide Adverse Reactions in Patients With Glioblastoma Multiforme ($\ge$ 5%)[a]

Adverse reactions	Concomitant phase: Radiotherapy alone (n = 285)		Concomitant phase: Radiotherapy + temozolomide (n = 288)[b]		Maintenance phase: Temozolomide (n = 224)	
	All reactions	Grade $\ge$ 3	All reactions	Grade $\ge$ 3	All reactions	Grade $\ge$ 3
Any adverse reaction	91%	26%	92%	28%	92%	37%
CNS						
Confusion	4%	2%	4%	1%	5%	2%
Convulsions	7%	3%	6%	3%	11%	3%
Dizziness	4%	0%	4%	1%	5%	0%
Fatigue	49%	5%	54%	7%	61%	9%
Headache	17%	4%	19%	2%	23%	4%
Insomnia	3%	< 1%	5%	0%	4%	0%
Memory impairment	4%	< 1%	3%	< 1%	7%	1%
Weakness	3%	1%	3%	2%	7%	2%
Dermatologic						
Alopecia	63%	0%	69%	0%	55%	0%
Dry skin	2%	0%	2%	0%	5%	< 1%
Erythema	5%	0%	5%	0%	1%	0%
Pruritus	1%	0%	4%	0%	5%	0%
Rash	15%	0%	19%	1%	13%	1%
GI						
Abdominal pain	1%	0%	2%	< 1%	5%	< 1%
Anorexia	9%	< 1%	19%	1%	27%	1%
Constipation	6%	0%	18%	1%	22%	0%
Diarrhea	3%	0%	6%	0%	10%	1%
Nausea	16%	< 1%	36%	1%	49%	1%
Stomatitis	5%	< 1%	7%	0%	9%	1%
Vomiting	6%	< 1%	20%	< 1%	29%	2%
Respiratory						
Coughing	1%	0%	5%	1%	8%	< 1%
Dyspnea	3%	1%	4%	2%	5%	< 1%
Special senses						
Blurred vision	9%	1%	9%	1%	8%	0%
Taste perversion	2%	0%	6%	0%	5%	0%
Miscellaneous						
Allergic reaction	2%	< 1%	5%	0%	3%	0%
Arthralgia	1%	0%	2%	< 1%	6%	0%

TEMOZOLOMIDE — ORAL

Temozolomide Adverse Reactions in Patients With Glioblastoma Multiforme (≥ 5%)[a]						
	Concomitant phase		Concomitant phase		Maintenance phase	
	Radiotherapy alone (n = 285)		Radiotherapy + temozolomide (n = 288)[b]		Temozolomide (n = 224)	
Adverse reactions	All reactions	Grade ≥ 3	All reactions	Grade ≥ 3	All reactions	Grade ≥ 3
Radiation injury NOS[c]	4%	< 1%	7%	0%	2%	0%
Thrombocytopenia	1%	0%	4%	3%	8%	4%

[a] Grade 5 (fatal) adverse reactions are included in the grade ≥ 3 column.
[b] One patient who was randomized to the radiotherapy-only arm received radiotherapy plus temozolomide.
[c] NOS = not otherwise specified.

Myelosuppression – Neutropenia and thrombocytopenia, which are known dose-limiting toxicities for most cytotoxic agents, including temozolomide, were observed. When laboratory abnormalities and adverse reactions were combined, grade 3 or 4 neutrophil abnormalities, including neutropenic reactions, were observed in 8% of the patients, and grade 3 or 4 platelet abnormalities, including thrombocytopenic reactions, were observed in 14% of the patients treated with temozolomide.

➤*Anaplastic astrocytoma:*

Myelosuppression – Myelosuppression occurred late in the treatment cycle and returned to normal, on average, within 14 days of nadir counts. The median nadirs occurred at 26 days for platelets (range, 21 to 40 days) and 28 days for neutrophils (range, 1 to 44 days). Only 14% (22/158) of patients had a neutrophil nadir, and 20% (32/158) of patients had a platelet nadir that may have delayed the start of the next cycle. Less than 10% of patients required hospitalization, blood transfusion, or discontinuation of therapy because of myelosuppression.

In clinical trial experience with 110 to 111 women and 169 to 174 men (depending on measurements), there were higher rates of grade 4 neutropenia (ANC less than 500 cells/mcL) and thrombocytopenia (less than 20,000 cells/mcL) in women than men in the first cycle of therapy (12% vs 5% and 9% vs 3%, respectively).

In the entire safety database for which hematologic data exist (N = 932), 7% (4/61) and 9.5% (6/63) of patients older than 70 years of age experienced grade 4 neutropenia or thrombocytopenia in the first cycle, respectively. For patients 70 years of age and younger, 7% (62/871) and 5.5% (48/879) experienced grade 4 neutropenia or thrombocytopenia in the first cycle, respectively. Pancytopenia, leukopenia, and anemia also have been reported.

Temozolomide Adverse Reactions in Patients With Anaplastic Astrocytoma (> 5%)		
Adverse reactions	All reactions (n = 158)	Grade 3/4 (n = 158)
Any adverse reaction	97%	50%
CNS		
Abnormal coordination	11%	1%
Abnormal gait	6%	1%
Amnesia	10%	4%
Anxiety	7%	1%
Asthenia	13%	6%
Ataxia	8%	2%
Confusion	5%	0%
Convulsions	23%	5%
Depression	6%	0%
Dizziness	12%	1%
Fatigue	34%	4%
Headache	41%	6%
Hemiparesis	18%	6%
Insomnia	10%	0%
Local convulsions	6%	0%
Paresis	8%	3%
Paresthesia	9%	1%
Somnolence	9%	3%
Dermatologic		
Pruritus	8%	1%
Rash	8%	0%
GI		
Abdominal pain	9%	1%
Anorexia	9%	1%
Constipation	33%	1%
Diarrhea	16%	2%
Dysphasia	7%	1%
Nausea	53%	10%
Vomiting	42%	6%
GU		
Breast pain, female	6%	
Micturition increased frequency	6%	0%
Urinary incontinence	8%	2%
Urinary tract infection	8%	0%
Ophthalmic		
Abnormal vision[a]	5%	
Diplopia	5%	0%
Respiratory		
Coughing	5%	0%
Pharyngitis	8%	0%
Sinusitis	6%	0%
Upper respiratory tract infection	8%	0%
Miscellaneous		
Adrenal hypercorticism	8%	0%
Back pain	8%	3%
Fever	13%	2%
Myalgia	5%	
Peripheral edema	11%	1%
Viral infection	11%	0%
Weight increase	5%	0%

[a] Blurred vision, visual deficit, vision changes, vision troubles.

Temozolomide Hematologic Adverse Reactions in Patients With Anaplastic Astrocytoma (Grade 3 to 4)	
Hematologic adverse reactions	Temozolomide[a]
Hemoglobin	4%
Lymphopenia	55%
Neutrophils	14%
Platelets	19%
WBC[b]	11%

[a] Change from grade 0 to 2 at baseline to grade 3 or 4 during treatment.
[b] WBC = white blood cell count.

➤*Children:* The following table shows the adverse reactions in 122 children in the COG phase 2 study.

Temozolomide Adverse Reactions in Children (≥ 10%)		
Adverse reactions	All reactions (n = 122)[a]	Grade 3 or 4 (n = 122)[a]
Subjects reporting adverse reaction	88%	57%
CNS		
Central cerebral CNS cortex	18%	11%
GI		
Nausea	46%	4%
Vomiting	51%	3%

TEMOZOLOMIDE — ORAL

Temozolomide Adverse Reactions in Children (≥ 10%)		
Adverse reactions	All reactions (n = 122)[a]	Grade 3 or 4 (n = 122)[a]
Hematologic/Lymphatic		
Decreased hemoglobin	51%	6%
Decreased WBC	58%	17%
Lymphopenia	60%	39%
Neutropenia	51%	20%
Thrombocytopenia	58%	25%

[a] These various tumors included the following: alveolar soft part sarcoma, brain stem tumor, ependymoma, Ewing sarcoma, glioblastoma, low-grade astrocytoma, mixed glioma, neuroblastoma, neurofibrosarcoma, oligodendroglioma, optic glioma, osteosarcoma, pineoblastoma, and PNET-medulloblastoma.

➤*Postmarketing:* Allergic reactions, including anaphylaxis have been reported. Erythema multiforme has been reported which resolved after discontinuation of temozolomide and, in some cases, recurred upon rechallenge. Cases of toxic epidermal necrolysis and Stevens-Johnson syndrome have been reported. Opportunistic infections including PCP have also been reported. Prolonged pancytopenia, which may result in aplastic anemia, has been reported, and in some cases has resulted in a fatal outcome.

Overdosage

➤*Symptoms:* Doses of 500, 750, 1,000, and 1,250 mg/m^2 (total dose per cycle over 5 days) have been evaluated clinically in patients. Dose-limiting toxicity was hematologic and was reported with any dose but is expected to be more severe at higher doses. An overdose of 2,000 mg/day for 5 days was taken by 1 patient, and the adverse reactions reported were multiorgan failure, pancytopenia, pyrexia, and death. There are reports of patients who have taken more than 5 days of treatment (up to 64 days) with adverse reactions reported, including bone marrow suppression, which in some cases was severe and prolonged, and infections, and resulted in death.

➤*Treatment:* In the event of an overdose, hematologic evaluation is needed. Provide supportive measures as necessary.

Patient Information

Advise patients to take temozolomide on an empty stomach to ease nausea. Nausea and vomiting are the most frequently occurring adverse reactions. These were usually either self-limiting or readily controlled with standard antiemetic therapy.

Instruct patients to swallow capsules whole with a full glass of water. Advise patients not to open or chew capsules. If capsules are accidentally opened or damaged, advise patients to take rigorous precautions with the capsule contents to avoid inhalation or contact with the skin or mucous membranes. Advise patients to keep this medication away from children and pets.

Advise women of childbearing potential to avoid becoming pregnant during therapy with temozolomide.

TEMOZOLOMIDE — INJECTION

Indications

➤*Anaplastic astrocytoma:* For the treatment of adults with refractory anaplastic astrocytoma (ie, patients who have experienced disease progression on a drug regimen containing a nitrosourea and procarbazine).

➤*Glioblastoma multiforme:* For the treatment of adult patients with newly diagnosed glioblastoma multiforme concomitantly with radiotherapy and then as maintenance treatment.

➤*Off-label uses:* Metastatic melanoma.

Administration and Dosage

➤*General dosing considerations:* The dosage of temozolomide must be adjusted according to nadir neutrophil and platelet counts in the previous cycle and the neutrophil and platelet counts at the time of initiating the next cycle.

During treatment, a complete blood cell count (CBC) should be obtained weekly.

Antiemetic therapy may be administered prior to and/or following administration of temozolomide.

➤*Adults:*

Anaplastic astrocytoma –

Initial dosage: 150 mg/m^2 intravenously (IV) once daily for 5 consecutive days per 28-day treatment cycle.

Dosage adjustment: During treatment, a CBC should be obtained on day 22 (21 days after the first dose) or within 48 hours of that day, and weekly until the absolute neutrophil count (ANC) is above 1.5 × 10^9/L (1,500/mcL) and the platelet count exceeds 100 × 10^9/L (100,000 mcL). The next cycle of temozolomide should not be started until the ANC and platelet count exceed these levels. If the ANC falls to less than 1 × 10^9/L (1,000/mcL) or the platelet count is less than 50 × 10^9/L (50,000/mcL) during any cycle, the next cycle should be reduced by 50 mg/m^2, but not below 100 mg/m^2, the lowest recommended dose.

If both the nadir and day of dosing (day 29, day 1 of next cycle) ANC are 1.5 × 10^9/L (1,500/mcL) or more and both the nadir and day 29, day 1 of next cycle platelet counts are 100 × 10^9/L (100,000/mcL) or more, the temozolomide dose may be increased to 200 mg/m^2/day for 5 consecutive days per 28-day treatment cycle.

Duration of therapy: Temozolomide therapy can be continued until disease progression. In the clinical trial, treatment could be continued for a maximum of 2 years, but the optimum duration of therapy is not known.

Glioblastoma multiforme –

Concomitant phase:

• *Initial dosage* – 75 mg/m^2 IV daily for 42 days concomitant with focal radiotherapy (60 Gy administered in 30 fractions), followed by maintenance temozolomide for 6 cycles.

• *Dosage adjustment* – No dose reductions are recommended during the concomitant phase; however, dose interruptions or discontinuation may occur based on toxicity.

• *Duration of therapy* – The temozolomide dose should be continued throughout the 42-day concomitant period up to 49 days if all of the following conditions are met: ANC 1.5 × 10^9/L or more, platelet count 100 × 10^9/L or more, Common Toxicity Criteria (CTC) nonhematological toxicity grade 1 or less (except for alopecia, nausea, and vomiting).

• *Concomitant therapy* – *Pneumocystis carinii* pneumonia (PCP) prophylaxis is required during the coadministration of temozolomide and radiotherapy and should be continued in patients who develop lymphocytopenia until recovery from lymphocytopenia (CTC grade 1 or less).

• *Discontinuation of therapy* – Temozolomide dosing should be interrupted or discontinued during the concomitant phase according to the hematological and nonhematological toxicity criteria.

Temozolomide Dosing Interruption or Discontinuation During Concomitant Radiotherapy		
Toxicity	Temozolomide interruption[a]	Temozolomide discontinuation
ANC	≥ 0.5 and < 1.5 × 10^9/L	< 0.5 × 10^9/L
Platelet count	≥ 10 and < 100 × 10^9/L	< 10 × 10^9/L
CTC nonhematological toxicity (except for alopecia, nausea, and vomiting)	CTC grade 2	CTC grade 3 or 4

[a] Treatment with concomitant temozolomide could be continued when all of the following conditions are met: ANC ≥ 1.5 × 10^9/L, platelet count ≥ 100 × 10^9/L, and CTC nonhematological toxicity grade ≤ 1 (except for alopecia, nausea, and vomiting).

Maintenance phase: Four weeks after completing the temozolomide plus radiotherapy phase, temozolomide is administered for an additional 6 cycles of maintenance treatment.

Cycle 1: Dosage in cycle 1 (maintenance) is 150 mg/m^2 once daily for 5 days followed by 23 days without treatment.

Cycle 2 to 6: At the start of cycle 2, the dose is escalated to 200 mg/m^2 if CTC nonhematologic toxicity for cycle 1 is grade 2 or less (except for alopecia, nausea, and vomiting), ANC is 1.5 × 10^9/L or more, and the platelet count is 100 × 10^9/L or more. The dosage remains at 200 mg/m^2/day for the first 5 days of each subsequent cycle, unless toxicity occurs. If the dose is not escalated at cycle 2, escalation should not be done in subsequent cycles.

Temozolomide Dose Levels for Maintenance Treatment		
Dose level	Dosage (mg/m^2/day)	Remarks
–1	100	Reduction for prior toxicity
0	150	Dose during cycle 1
1	200	Dose during cycles 2 to 6 in absence of toxicity

• *Dose reduction or discontinuation during maintenance* – During treatment, a CBC should be obtained on day 22 (21 days after the first dose of temozolomide) or within 48 hours of that day, and weekly until the ANC is above 1.5 × 10^9/L (1,500/mcL) and the platelet count exceeds 100 × 10^9/L (100,000/mcL). The next cycle of temozolomide should not be started until the ANC and platelet count exceed these levels. Dose reductions during the next cycle should be based on the lowest blood counts and worst nonhematologic toxicity during the previous cycle. Dose reductions or discontinuations during the maintenance phase should be applied.

Temozolomide Dose Reduction or Discontinuation During Maintenance Treatment		
Toxicity	Reduce temozolomide by 1 dose level[a]	Discontinue temozolomide
ANC	< 1 × 10^9/L	[b]
Platelet count	< 50 × 10^9/L	[b]
CTC nonhematological toxicity (except for alopecia, nausea, and vomiting)	CTC grade 3	CTC grade 4[b]

[a] Temozolomide dose levels are listed in the previous table.

[b] Temozolomide is to be discontinued if dose reduction to < 100 mg/m^2 is required or if the same grade 3 nonhematological toxicity (except for alopecia, nausea, and vomiting) recurs after dose reduction.

TEMOZOLOMIDE — INJECTION

➤*Children:*

Off-label dosing –

Anaplastic astrocytoma and glioblastoma multiforme: Temozolomide has been used safely and effectively in children 3 years of age and older.

Doses are similar to those used in adult regimens, with calculation based on body surface area (BSA). Usual dosages range from 150 mg/m^2/day to 200 mg/m^2/day for 5 days during each 28-day course of therapy.

Follow dosage adjustment guidelines recommended for adults (see Adults for dosage).

➤*Elderly:* Dose selection for an elderly patients should be cautious, reflecting the greater frequency of decreased hepatic, renal, or cardia function, and of concomitant disease or other drug therapy.

➤*Renal function impairment:* Exercise caution when temozolomide is administered to patients with severe renal function impairment.

➤*Hepatic function impairment:* Exercise caution when temozolomide is administered to patients with severe hepatic impairment.

➤*Preparation for administration:* Temozolomide is considered a cytotoxic agent. Follow safe handling procedures when preparing, administering, or dispensing temozolomide.

Vials should not be opened. If vials are accidentally opened or damaged, rigorous precautions should be taken with the contents to avoid inhalation or contact with the skin or mucous membranes. The use of gloves and safety glasses is recommended to avoid exposure in case of breakage of the vial.

Each vial of temozolomide contains sterile and pyrogen-free temozolomide lyophilized powder. When reconstituted with 41 mL of sterile water for injection, the resulting solution will contain temozolomide 2.5 mg/mL. Bring the vial to room temperature prior to reconstitution with sterile water for injection. The vials should be gently swirled and not shaken. Do not further dilute the reconstituted solution.

Using aseptic technique, withdraw up to 40 mL from each vial to make up the total dose based on calculations by BSA and transfer into an empty 250 mL polyvinyl chloride (PVC) infusion bag.

➤*Administration:* Temozolomide should be infused IV using a pump over a period of 90 minutes. Temozolomide for injection should be administered only by IV infusion. Flush the lines before and after each temozolomide infusion.

➤*Admixture compatibility:* Because no data are available on the compatibility of temozolomide with other IV substances or additives, other medications should not be infused simultaneously through the same IV line.

➤*Storage / Stability:* Store refrigerated at 2° to 8°C (36° to 46°F). After reconstitution, store at 25°C (77°F). Reconstituted product must be used within 14 hours, including infusion time.

Actions

➤*Pharmacology:* Temozolomide, an imidazotetrazine derivative, is not directly active but undergoes rapid nonenzymatic conversion at physiologic pH to the reactive compound 5-(3-methyltriazen-1-yl)imidazole-4-carboxamide (MTIC). The cytotoxicity of MTIC is thought to be caused primarily by alkylation of DNA. Alkylation (methylation) occurs mainly at the O^6 and N^7 positions of guanine.

➤*Pharmacokinetics:*

Absorption – Following a single 90-minute IV infusion of 150 mg/m^2, the geometric mean peak plasma concentration (C_{max}) values for temozolomide and MTIC were 7.3 mcg/mL and 276 ng/mL, respectively.

Following a single 90-minute IV infusion of 150 mg/m^2, the geometric mean area under the curve (AUC) values for temozolomide and MTIC were 24.6 mcg•h/mL and 891 ng•h/mL, respectively.

Distribution – Temozolomide has a mean apparent volume of distribution of 0.4 L/kg (% coefficient of variation = 13%). It is weakly bound to human plasma proteins; the mean percent bound of drug-related total radioactivity is 15%.

Metabolism – Temozolomide is hydrolyzed spontaneously at physiologic pH to the active species, MTIC, and to temozolomide acid metabolite. MTIC is further hydrolyzed to 5-amino-imidazole-4-carboxamide (AIC), which is known to be an intermediate in purine and nucleic acid biosynthesis and to methylhydrazine, which is believed to be the active alkylating species. Cytochrome P450 (CYP-450) enzymes play only a minor role in the metabolism of temozolomide and MTIC. Relative to the AUC of temozolomide, the exposure to MTIC and AIC is 2.4% and 23%, respectively.

Excretion – Temozolomide is eliminated rapidly, with a mean elimination half-life of 1.8 hours, and exhibits linear kinetics over the therapeutic dosing range of 75 to 250 mg/m^2/day. About 38% of the administered temozolomide total radioactive dose is recovered over 7 days; 37.7% in urine and 0.8% in feces. The majority of the recovery of radioactivity in urine is as unchanged temozolomide (5.6%), AIC (12%), temozolomide acid metabolite (2.3%), and unidentified polar metabolite(s) (17%). Overall clearance of temozolomide is approximately 5.5 L/h/m^2.

Special populations –

Gender: Population pharmacokinetic analysis indicates that women have an approximate 5% lower clearance (adjusted for BSA) for temozolomide than men.

Contraindications

History of hypersensitivity reaction to temozolomide or any of its components; history of hypersensitivity to dacarbazine because both temozolomide and dacarbazine are metabolized to MTIC.

Warnings/Precautions

➤*Myelosuppression:* Patients treated with temozolomide may experience myelosuppression, including prolonged pancytopenia, which may result in aplastic anemia, which in some cases has resulted in a fatal outcome. In some cases, exposure to concomitant medications associated with aplastic anemia including carbamazepine, phenytoin, and sulfamethoxazole/trimethoprim complicates assessment. Prior to dosing, patients must have an ANC 1.5 × 10^9/L or more and a platelet count 100 × 10^9/L or more. Obtain a CBC on day 22 (21 days after the first dose) or within 48 hours of that day and weekly until the ANC is above 1.5 × 10^9/L and platelet count exceeds 100 × 10^9/L. Elderly patients and women have been shown in clinical trials to have a higher risk of developing myelosuppression.

➤*Myelodysplastic syndrome / secondary malignancies:* Cases of myelodysplastic syndrome and secondary malignancies, including myeloid leukemia, have also been observed.

➤*Pneumocystis carinii pneumonia:* For the treatment of newly diagnosed glioblastoma multiforme, prophylaxis against PCP is required for all patients receiving concomitant temozolomide and radiotherapy for the 42-day regimen.

There may be a higher occurrence of PCP when temozolomide is administered during a longer dosing regimen. However, closely observe all patients receiving temozolomide, particularly patients receiving steroids, for the development of PCP regardless of the regimen.

➤*Infusion time:* As bioequivalence has been established only when temozolomide was given over 90 minutes, infusion over a shorter or longer period of time may result in suboptimal dosing. Additionally, the possibility of an increase in infusion related adverse reactions cannot be ruled out.

➤*Renal / Hepatic function impairment:* Exercise caution when temozolomide is administered to patients with severe hepatic or severe renal impairment.

➤*Pregnancy:* Category D. Temozolomide can cause fetal harm when administered to a pregnant woman. Five consecutive days of oral administration of 75 mg/m^2/day in rats and 150 mg/m^2/day in rabbits during the period of organogenesis (0.38 and 0.75 the maximum recommended human dose [MRHD], respectively) caused numerous malformations of the external organs, soft tissues, and skeleton in both species. Dosages of 150 mg/m^2/day in rats and rabbits also caused embryolethality, as indicated by increased resorptions. There are no adequate and well-controlled studies in pregnant women. The molecular weight of the parent compound (about 194) and the minimal plasma protein binding suggest that the drug will cross to the embryo and fetus. However, after absorption, temozolomide undergoes rapid hydrolysis to MTIC, and this compound may also cross the placenta. If this drug is used during pregnancy, or if the patient becomes pregnant while taking this drug, inform the patient of the potential hazard to the fetus. Advise women of childbearing potential to avoid becoming pregnant during therapy with temozolomide.

➤*Lactation:* It is not known whether this drug is excreted in human milk. The molecular weight of the parent compound (about 194) and the minimal plasma protein binding (about 15%) suggest that the drug will be excreted into breast milk. Because many drugs are excreted in human milk and because of the potential for serious adverse reactions in breast-feeding infants and tumorigenicity shown for temozolomide in animal studies, decide whether to discontinue breast-feeding or to discontinue the drug, taking into account the importance of the drug to the mother.

➤*Children:* Safety and effectiveness in children have not been established.

➤*Elderly:* See Administration and Dosage for more information.

In the anaplastic astrocytoma study population, patients 70 years of age and older had a higher incidence of grade 4 neutropenia and grade 4 thrombocytopenia (2/8; 25%, P = 0.31 and 2/10; 20%, P = 0.09, respectively) in the first cycle of therapy than patients younger than 70 years of age.

➤*Monitoring:* For the concomitant treatment phase with radiotherapy, obtain a CBC prior to initiation of treatment and weekly during treatment.

For the 28-day treatment cycles, obtain a CBC prior to treatment on day 1 and on day 22 (21 days after the first dose) of each cycle or within 48 hours of that day. Perform blood counts weekly until recovery if the ANC falls below 1.5 × 10^9/L and the platelet count falls below 100 × 10^9/L.

Closely monitor all patients receiving temozolomide, particularly patients receiving steroids, for the development of PCP, regardless of the regimen.

Drug Interactions

➤*Valproic acid:* Administration of valproic acid decreases oral clearance of temozolomide about 5%. The clinical implication of this effect is not known.

Adverse Reactions

Temozolomide is considered to have moderate potential for nausea and vomiting.

➤*Glioblastoma multiforme:*

Severe or life-threatening reactions – Forty-nine percent of patients treated with temozolomide reported 1 or more severe or life-threatening reactions, most commonly fatigue (13%), convulsions (6%), headache (5%), and thrombocytopenia (5%).

TEMOZOLOMIDE — INJECTION

Temozolomide Adverse Reactions in Patients With Glioblastoma Multiforme (≥ 5%)[a]

Adverse reactions	Concomitant phase: Radiotherapy alone (n = 285)		Concomitant phase: Radiotherapy + temozolomide (n = 288)[b]		Maintenance phase: Temozolomide (n = 224)	
	All reactions	Grade ≥ 3	All reactions	Grade ≥ 3	All reactions	Grade ≥ 3
Any adverse reaction	91%	26%	92%	28%	92%	37%
CNS						
Confusion	4%	2%	4%	1%	5%	2%
Convulsions	7%	3%	6%	3%	11%	3%
Dizziness	4%	0%	4%	1%	5%	0%
Fatigue	49%	5%	54%	7%	61%	9%
Headache	17%	4%	19%	2%	23%	4%
Insomnia	3%	< 1%	5%	0%	4%	0%
Memory impairment	4%	< 1%	3%	< 1%	7%	1%
Weakness	3%	1%	3%	2%	7%	2%
Dermatologic						
Alopecia	63%	0%	69%	0%	55%	0%
Dry skin	2%	0%	2%	0%	5%	< 1%
Erythema	5%	0%	5%	0%	1%	0%
Pruritus	1%	0%	4%	0%	5%	0%
Rash	15%	0%	19%	1%	13%	1%
GI						
Abdominal pain	1%	0%	2%	< 1%	5%	< 1%
Anorexia	9%	< 1%	19%	1%	27%	1%
Constipation	6%	0%	18%	1%	22%	0%
Diarrhea	3%	0%	6%	0%	10%	1%
Nausea	16%	< 1%	36%	1%	49%	1%
Stomatitis	5%	< 1%	7%	0%	9%	1%
Vomiting	6%	< 1%	20%	< 1%	29%	2%
Respiratory						
Coughing	1%	0%	5%	1%	8%	< 1%
Dyspnea	3%	1%	4%	2%	5%	< 1%
Special senses						
Blurred vision	9%	1%	9%	1%	8%	0%
Taste perversion	2%	0%	6%	0%	5%	0%
Miscellaneous						
Allergic reaction	2%	< 1%	5%	0%	3%	0%
Arthralgia	1%	0%	2%	< 1%	6%	0%
Radiation injury NOS[c]	4%	< 1%	7%	0%	2%	0%
Thrombocytopenia	1%	0%	4%	3%	8%	4%

[a] Grade 5 (fatal) adverse reactions are included in the grade ≥ 3 column.
[b] One patient who was randomized to the radiotherapy-only arm received radiotherapy plus temozolomide.
[c] NOS = not otherwise specified.

Myelosuppression – Neutropenia and thrombocytopenia, which are known dose-limiting toxicities for most cytotoxic agents, including temozolomide, were observed. When laboratory abnormalities and adverse reactions were combined, grade 3 or 4 neutrophil abnormalities, including neutropenic reactions, were observed in 8% of the patients, and grade 3 or 4 platelet abnormalities, including thrombocytopenic reactions, were observed in 14% of the patients treated with temozolomide.

➤*Anaplastic astrocytoma:*

Myelosuppression – Myelosuppression occurred late in the treatment cycle and returned to normal, on average, within 14 days of nadir counts. The median nadirs occurred at 26 days for platelets (range, 21 to 40 days) and 28 days for neutrophils (range, 1 to 44 days). Only 14% (22/158) of patients had a neutrophil nadir, and 20% (32/158) of patients had a platelet nadir that may have delayed the start of the next cycle. Less than 10% of patients required hospitalization, blood transfusion, or discontinuation of therapy because of myelosuppression.

In clinical trial experience with 110 to 111 women and 169 to 174 men (depending on measurements), there were higher rates of grade 4 neutropenia (ANC less than 500 cells/mcL) and thrombocytopenia (less than 20,000 cells/mcL) in women than men in the first cycle of therapy (12% vs 5% and 9% vs 3%, respectively).

In the entire safety database for which hematologic data exist (N = 932), 7% (4/61) and 9.5% (6/63) of patients older than 70 years of age experienced grade 4 neutropenia or thrombocytopenia in the first cycle, respectively. For patients 70 years of age and younger, 7% (62/871) and 5.5% (48/879) experienced grade 4 neutropenia or thrombocytopenia in the first cycle, respectively. Pancytopenia, leukopenia, and anemia also have been reported.

Temozolomide Adverse Reactions in Patients With Anaplastic Astrocytoma (> 5%)

Adverse reactions	All reactions (n = 158)	Grade 3/4 (n = 158)
Any adverse reaction	97%	50%
CNS		
Abnormal coordination	11%	1%
Abnormal gait	6%	1%
Amnesia	10%	4%
Anxiety	7%	1%
Asthenia	13%	6%
Ataxia	8%	2%
Confusion	5%	0%
Convulsions	23%	5%
Depression	6%	0%
Dizziness	12%	1%
Fatigue	34%	4%
Headache	41%	6%
Hemiparesis	18%	6%
Insomnia	10%	0%

TEMOZOLOMIDE — INJECTION

Temozolomide Adverse Reactions in Patients With Anaplastic Astrocytoma (> 5%)		
Adverse reactions	All reactions (n = 158)	Grade 3/4 (n = 158)
Local convulsions	6%	0%
Paresis	8%	3%
Paresthesia	9%	1%
Somnolence	9%	3%
Dermatologic		
Pruritus	8%	1%
Rash	8%	0%
GI		
Abdominal pain	9%	1%
Anorexia	9%	1%
Constipation	33%	1%
Diarrhea	16%	2%
Dysphasia	7%	1%
Nausea	53%	10%
Vomiting	42%	6%
GU		
Breast pain, female	6%	
Micturition increased frequency	6%	0%
Urinary incontinence	8%	2%
Urinary tract infection	8%	0%
Ophthalmic		
Abnormal vision[a]	5%	
Diplopia	5%	0%
Respiratory		
Coughing	5%	0%
Pharyngitis	8%	0%
Sinusitis	6%	0%
Upper respiratory tract infection	8%	0%
Miscellaneous		
Adrenal hypercorticism	8%	0%
Back pain	8%	3%
Fever	13%	2%
Myalgia	5%	
Peripheral edema	11%	1%
Viral infection	11%	0%
Weight increase	5%	0%

[a] Blurred vision, visual deficit, vision changes, vision troubles.

Temozolomide Hematologic Adverse Reactions in Patients With Anaplastic Astrocytoma (Grade 3 to 4)	
Hematologic adverse reactions	Temozolomide[a]
Hemoglobin	4%
Lymphopenia	55%
Neutrophils	14%
Platelets	19%
WBC[b]	11%

[a] Change from grade 0 to 2 at baseline to grade 3 or 4 during treatment.
[b] WBC = white blood cell count.

Local adverse reactions – Temozolomide delivers equivalent temozolomide dose and exposure to both temozolomide and MTIC as the corresponding temozolomide capsules. Adverse reactions probably related to treatment that were reported from the 2 studies with the IV formulation (n = 35) that were not reported in studies using the temozolomide capsules were pain, irritation, pruritus, warmth, swelling, and erythema at infusion site as well as petechiae and hematoma.

➤*Postmarketing:* Allergic reactions, including anaphylaxis, have been reported. Erythema multiforme has been reported which resolved after discontinuation of temozolomide and, in some cases, recurred upon rechallenge. Cases of toxic epidermal necrolysis and Stevens-Johnson syndrome have been reported. Opportunistic infections including PCP have also been reported. Prolonged pancytopenia, which may result in aplastic anemia, has been reported, and in some cases has resulted in a fatal outcome.

Overdosage

➤*Symptoms:* Doses of 500, 750, 1,000, and 1,250 mg/m^2 (total dose per cycle over 5 days) have been evaluated clinically in patients. Dose-limiting toxicity was hematologic and was reported with any dose, but it is expected to be more severe at higher doses. An overdose of 2,000 mg/day for 5 days was taken by 1 patient, and the adverse reactions reported were multiorgan failure, pancytopenia, pyrexia, and death. There are reports of patients who have taken more than 5 days of treatment (up to 64 days) with adverse reactions reported, including bone marrow suppression, which in some cases was severe and prolonged, and infections, and resulted in death.

➤*Treatment:* In the event of an overdose, hematologic evaluation is needed. Provide supportive measures as necessary.

Patient Information

Nausea and vomiting are the most frequently occurring adverse reactions. Advise patients that these were usually either self-limiting or readily controlled with standard antiemetic therapy.

If vials are accidentally opened or damaged, advise patients to take rigorous precautions with the vial contents to avoid inhalation or contact with the skin or mucous membranes. Advise patients to keep this medication away from children and pets.

Advise women of childbearing potential to avoid becoming pregnant during therapy with temozolomide.

CYTOPROTECTIVE AGENTS

AMIFOSTINE

Rx	**Amifostine** (Various, eg, Bedford Laboratories, Caraco Pharmaceutical)	**Injection, lyophilized powder for solution:** 500 mg	In 10 mL single-use vials.
Rx	**Ethyol** (MedImmune Pharma)		In 10 mL single-use vials.

AMIFOSTINE — INJECTION

Indications

➤*Renal toxicity:* Reduction of cumulative renal toxicity associated with repeated administration of cisplatin in patients with advanced ovarian cancer.

➤*Xerostomia:* Reduction of the incidence of moderate to severe xerostomia in patients undergoing postoperative radiation treatment for head and neck cancer, where the radiation port includes a substantial portion of the parotid glands.

➤*Off-label uses:*

Prevention of antineoplastic-induced bone marrow toxicity – [1] = Good documentation. Guidelines developed from clinical trials support the use of amifostine as prophylaxis for bone marrow toxicity. A limited number of randomized, controlled trials show no adverse impact of amifostine on tumor response, but this should not always be assumed. Use of amifostine with nonplatinum, nonalkylating cytotoxic agents is not recommended at this time. Further research is needed.

Radiation and/or chemotherapy-induced mucositis – [2] = Fair documentation. Guidelines support the use of amifostine to prevent mucositis in 2 specific situations. When assessing whether amifostine is an appropriate therapeutic option, the adverse reactions of nausea, vomiting, and hypotension must be weighed against its ability to reduce mucositis. More research is needed to delineate a broader role for amifostine in the management of mucositis.

Other possible off-label uses – To prevent or reduce cisplatin-induced neurotoxicity and cyclophosphamide-induced granulocytopenia; prevent or reduce toxicity of radiation therapy to other areas; reduce toxicity of paclitaxel.

Administration and Dosage

➤*General dosing considerations:* Adequately hydrate patients prior to amifostine infusion.

Monitor blood pressure during the infusion (see Administration). It is recommended that antiemetic medication be administered prior to and in conjunction with amifostine. (See Premedication).

➤*Adults:*

Renal toxicity –

Initial dosage: 910 mg/m^2 once daily as a 15-minute intravenous (IV) infusion, starting 30 minutes prior to chemotherapy.

Dosage adjustment: Interrupt the infusion if the systolic blood pressure decreases significantly from the baseline.

AMIFOSTINE — INJECTION

Guidelines for Interrupting Amifostine Infusion Because of Decrease in Systolic Blood Pressure

	Baseline systolic blood pressure (mm Hg)				
	< 100	100 to 119	120 to 139	140 to 179	≥ 180
Decrease in systolic blood pressure during infusion of amifostine	20	25	30	40	50

If the blood pressure returns to normal within 5 minutes and the patient is asymptomatic, the infusion may be restarted so that the full dose may be administered. If the full dose cannot be administered, the dose for subsequent cycles should be 740 mg/m^2.

Xerostomia –

Usual dosage: 200 mg/m^2 once daily as a 3-minute IV infusion 15 to 30 minutes prior to standard fraction radiation therapy (1.8 to 2 Gy).

Off-label dosing –

Prevention of antineoplastic-induced bone marrow toxicity: [2] = Fair documentation. 910 mg/m^2 IV infusion. Some studies suggest that 740 mg/m^2 IV may offer the same degree of protection with fewer adverse effects.

Radiation- and/or chemotherapy-induced mucositis: [1] = Good documentation. Dose for prevention of radiation proctitis in patients receiving standard-dose radiotherapy for rectal cancer is 340 mg/m^2 or more. Dose for prevention of esophagitis induced by concomitant chemotherapy and radiotherapy in patients with non–small cell lung cancer is 500 mg IV twice weekly before chemoradiation.

➤*Premedication:*

Renal toxicity – It is recommended that antiemetic medication, including dexamethasone 20 mg IV and a serotonin 5HT$_3$ receptor antagonist, be administered prior to and in conjunction with amifostine. Additional antiemetic agents may be required based on the chemotherapy drugs coadministered.

Xerostomia – Administer antiemetic medication prior to and in conjunction with amifostine. Oral 5HT$_3$ receptor antagonists, alone or in combination with other antiemetics, have been used effectively in the radiotherapy setting.

➤*Discontinuation of therapy:* Permanently discontinue amifostine for serious or severe cutaneous reactions or for cutaneous reactions associated with fever or other constitutional symptoms not known to be due to another etiology.

➤*Preparation for administration:* Reconstitute with 9.7 mL of sodium chloride 0.9% injection. Prior to infusion, dilute in sodium chloride to a final concentration of 5 to 40 mg/mL.

➤*Administration:* For IV infusion. Keep patients in a supine position during the infusion.

When used prior to chemotherapy, monitor blood pressure every 5 minutes during the infusion and thereafter as clinically indicated. When used prior to radiation therapy, monitor blood pressure at least before and immediately after the infusion and thereafter as clinically indicated.

➤*Admixture compatibility:* The compatibility of amifostine with solutions other than sodium chloride 0.9% for injection or sodium chloride solutions with other additives has not been studied and is not recommended. The use of other solutions is not recommended.

➤*Storage/Stability:* Store the powder between 20° and 25°C (68° and 77°F). The reconstituted solution is chemically stable for up to 5 hours at approximately 25°C (77°F) or up to 24 hours under refrigeration at 2° to 8°C (36° to 46°F). Amifostine prepared in polyvinylchloride (PVC) bags at concentrations ranging from 5 to 40 mg/mL is chemically stable for up to 5 hours when stored at approximately 25°C (77°F) or up to 24 hours when stored under refrigeration at 2° to 8°C (36° to 46°F).

Actions

➤*Pharmacology:* Amifostine is an organic thiophosphate cytoprotective agent. This prodrug is dephosphorylated by alkaline phosphatase in tissues to a pharmacologically active free thiol metabolite. This metabolite is believed to be responsible for the reduction of the cumulative renal toxicity of cisplatin and for the reduction of the toxic effects of radiation on healthy oral tissues. The ability to differentially protect healthy tissues is attributed to the higher capillary alkaline phosphatase activity, higher pH, and better vascularity of healthy tissues relative to tumor tissue. The result is a more rapid generation of the active thiol metabolite as well as a higher rate constant for uptake into cells. The higher concentration of the thiol metabolite in healthy tissues is, thus, available to bind to, and thereby detoxify, reactive metabolites of cisplatin. The thiol metabolites also scavenge reactive oxygen species generated by exposure to cisplatin or radiation.

➤*Pharmacokinetics:*

Distribution – Amifostine is rapidly cleared from the plasma with a distribution half-life of less than 1 minute. Less than 10% of amifostine remains in the plasma 6 minutes after drug administration.

Metabolism/Excretion – Amifostine has an elimination half-life of approximately 8 minutes. Amifostine is rapidly metabolized to an active free thiol metabolite. A disulfide metabolite is produced subsequently and is less active than the free thiol. After a 10-second bolus dose of amifostine 150 mg/m^2, renal excretion of the parent drug and its 2 metabolites was low during the hour following drug administration, averaging 0.69%, 2.64%, and 2.22% of the administered dose for the parent, thiol, and disulfide, respectively. Measurable levels of the free thiol metabolite have been found in bone marrow cells 5 to 8 minutes after IV infusion of amifostine.

Contraindications

Sensitivity to aminothiol compounds.

Warnings/Precautions

➤*Effectiveness of chemotherapy:* Limited data are available on the preservation of antitumor efficacy when amifostine is administered prior to cisplatin therapy in settings other than advanced ovarian cancer or non–small cell lung cancer. Although some animal data suggest interference is possible, in most tumor models, the antitumor effects of chemotherapy are not altered by amifostine. Therefore, do not use amifostine in patients receiving chemotherapy for malignancies in which chemotherapy can produce a significant survival benefit or cure (eg, certain malignancies of germ cell origin), except in the context of a clinical study.

➤*Effectiveness of radiotherapy:* Do not administer amifostine in patients receiving definitive radiotherapy, except during a clinical trial, because of insufficient data to exclude a tumor-protective effect in this setting. Amifostine was studied only with standard fractionated radiotherapy and when at least 75% of both parotid glands were exposed to radiation. Amifostine's effects on the incidence of xerostomia, on toxicity in the setting of combined chemotherapy and radiotherapy, and in the setting of accelerated and hyperfractionated therapy have not been systematically studied.

➤*Hypotension:* Do not administer amifostine in patients who are hypotensive or in a state of dehydration. Interrupt patients receiving amifostine as doses recommended for chemotherapy should have antihypertensive therapy 24 hours preceding administration of amifostine. Do not administer amifostine to patients receiving amifostine at doses recommended for chemotherapy who are taking antihypertensive therapy that cannot be stopped for 24 hours preceding amifostine treatment.

Prior to amifostine infusion, adequately hydrate patients. During amifostine infusion, keep patients in a supine position. Monitor blood pressure every 5 minutes during the infusion, and thereafter as clinically indicated. It is important that the duration of the 910 mg/m^2 infusion not exceed 15 minutes because administration of amifostine as a longer infusion is associated with a higher incidence of adverse effects. For infusion durations less than 5 minutes, monitor blood pressure at least before and immediately after the infusion, and thereafter as clinically indicated. If hypotension occurs, place patients in the Trendelenburg position and give an infusion of normal saline using a separate IV line. During and after amifostine infusion, take care to monitor the blood pressure of patients whose antihypertensive medication has been interrupted because hypertension may be exacerbated by discontinuation of antihypertensive medication and other causes such as IV hydration (see Administration and Dosage).

Hypotension may occur during or shortly after amifostine infusion, despite adequate hydration and positioning of the patient. Hypotension has been reported to be associated with dyspnea, apnea, hypoxia, and, in rare cases, seizures, unconsciousness, respiratory arrest, and respiratory failure.

➤*Cutaneous reactions:* Serious cutaneous reactions have been associated with amifostine administration. Serious cutaneous reactions have included erythema multiforme, Stevens-Johnson syndrome, toxic epidermal necrolysis, toxoderma, and exfoliative dermatitis, which have been reported more frequently when amifostine is used as a radioprotectant. Some of these reactions have been fatal or have required hospitalization and/or discontinuance of therapy. Carefully monitor patients prior to, during, and after amifostine administration. Serious cutaneous reactions may develop weeks after initiation of amifostine administration.

Cutaneous reactions may require permanent discontinuation of amifostine or urgent dermatological consultation and biopsy. Perform cutaneous evaluation of the patient prior to each amifostine administration. Pay particular attention to the development of the following: any rash involving the lips or involving mucosa not known to be due to another etiology (eg, herpes simplex, radiation mucositis); cutaneous reactions with associated fever or other constitutional symptoms; erythematous, edematous, or bullous lesions on the palms of the hands or soles of the feet; and/or other cutaneous reactions on the trunk (front, back, abdomen).

Permanently discontinue amifostine for serious or severe cutaneous reactions or for cutaneous reactions associated with fever or other constitutional symptoms not known to be because of another cause. Withhold amifostine and dermatological consultation and consider biopsy for cutaneous reactions or mucosal lesions of unknown etiology appearing outside of the injection site or radiation port and for erythematous, edematous, or bullous lesions on the palms of the hand or soles of the feet. Reinitiation of amifostine should be at the health care provider's discretion based on medical judgment and appropriate dermatological evaluation.

➤*Nausea and vomiting:* Administer antiemetic medication prior to and in conjunction with amifostine. When amifostine is administered with highly emetogenic chemotherapy, carefully monitor the fluid balance of the patient.

➤*Hypocalcemia:* Monitor serum calcium levels in patients at risk of hypocalcemia, such as those with nephrotic syndrome or patients receiving multiple doses. If necessary, administer calcium supplements.

➤*Hypersensitivity reactions:* Allergic manifestations, including anaphylaxis and severe cutaneous reactions, have been associated rarely with amifostine administration.

In case of severe acute allergic reactions, immediately and permanently discontinue amifostine. Have epinephrine and other appropriate measures available for treatment of serious allergic events, such as anaphylaxis.

➤*Special risk:* Safety has not been established in patients with preexisting cardiovascular or cerebrovascular conditions such as ischemic heart dis-

AMIFOSTINE — INJECTION

ease, arrhythmias, or congestive heart failure, or a history of stroke or transient ischemic attacks. Use amifostine with particular care in these and other patients in whom the common amifostine adverse reactions of nausea/vomiting and hypotension may be more likely to have serious consequences.

➤*Pregnancy: Category C.* Amifostine is embryotoxic in rabbits at doses of 50 mg/kg, approximately 60% of the recommended dose in humans on a body surface area basis. There are no adequate and well-controlled studies in pregnant women. It is not known if amifostine crosses the human placenta. The molecular weight of the prodrug (approximately 214) suggests that it will distribute to the embryo and/or fetus, but the very short plasma elimination half-life should limit the amount available for transfer.

Do not use during pregnancy unless the potential benefit justifies the potential risk to the fetus.

➤*Lactation:* No information is available on the excretion of amifostine or its metabolites into breast milk.

The molecular weight of the prodrug (approximately 214) suggests that it will be excreted into breast milk, but the very short plasma elimination half-life (approximately 8 minutes) should limit the amount. The effects of this potential exposure on a breast-feeding infant are unknown. However, because the drug is given as a short IV infusion immediately before chemotherapy or radiation and breast-feeding would be unlikely at this time, the risk of exposing an infant to amifostine when breast-feeding is later resumed appears to be nil.

Discontinue breast-feeding if the mother is treated with amifostine.

➤*Children:* Safety and efficacy have not been established.

➤*Elderly:* In general, use caution in dose selection and consider the greater frequency of decreased hepatic, renal, or cardiac function and of concomitant disease or other drug therapy in elderly patients.

➤*Monitoring:* Monitor serum calcium levels in patients at risk of hypocalcemia, such as those with nephrotic syndrome or patients receiving multiple doses of amifostine. When used prior to chemotherapy, monitor blood pressure every 5 minutes during the infusion and thereafter as clinically indicated. When used prior to radiation therapy, monitor blood pressure at least before and immediately after the infusion and thereafter as clinically indicated. Carefully monitor patients prior to, during, and after amifostine administration for cutaneous reactions.

When amifostine is administered with highly emetogenic chemotherapy, carefully monitor the fluid balance of the patient.

Drug Interactions

➤*Antihypertensives:* Give special consideration to amifostine administration in patients receiving antihypertensive medications or other drugs that could cause or potentiate hypotension. Interrupt patients receiving amifostine at chemotherapy doses 24 hours before amifostine administration. Do not administer amifostine if antihypertensive therapy cannot be stopped for 24 hours preceding amifostine treatment.

Adverse Reactions

➤*Hypotension:* In a randomized study of patients with ovarian cancer given 910 mg/m^2 amifostine prior to chemotherapy, transient hypotension occurred in 62% of patients treated. Mean time of onset was 14 minutes into the infusion; mean duration was 6 minutes. In some cases, the infusion had to be prematurely terminated because of a more pronounced drop in systolic pressure. In general, blood pressure returns to normal within 5 to 15 minutes. Fewer than 3% of patients discontinued amifostine because of blood pressure reductions. In the randomized study of patients with head and neck cancer given amifostine at a dose of 200 mg/m^2 prior to radiotherapy, hypotension was observed in 15% of patients treated.

Treat hypotension that requires interruption of the amifostine infusion with fluid infusion and postural management of the patient (supine or Trendelenburg position). If the blood pressure returns to normal within 5 minutes and the patient is asymptomatic, the infusion may be restarted, so that the full dose of amifostine can be administered. Short-term, reversible loss of consciousness has been reported rarely.

➤*Common adverse reactions:*

Amifostine Common Adverse Reactions

Adverse reactions	Ovarian cancer trial (WR-1) 910 mg/m^2		Head and neck cancer trial (WR-38) 200 mg/m^2	
	Per patient	Per infusion	Per patient	Per infusion
Nausea/Vomiting				
≥ Grade 3	30%	9%	8%	< 1%
All grades	96%	88%	53%	5%

Amifostine Common Adverse Reactions

Adverse reactions	Ovarian cancer trial (WR-1) 910 mg/m^2		Head and neck cancer trial (WR-38) 200 mg/m^2	
	Per patient	Per infusion	Per patient	Per infusion
Hypotension				
≥ Grade 3[a]	8%	27%	3%	1%
All grades	61%		15%	

[a] According to protocol-defined criteria, WR-1: requiring interruption of infusion; WR-38: drop of > 20 mm Hg.

➤*Discontinuation:* In the randomized study of patients with head and neck cancer, 17% discontinued amifostine because of adverse reactions. All but 1 of these patients continued to receive radiation treatment until completion.

➤*Cardiovascular:* Hypotension, usually brief systolic and diastolic, has been associated with 1 or more of the following adverse reactions: apnea, bradycardia, chest pain, convulsion, dyspnea, extrasystoles, hypoxia, myocardial ischemia, tachycardia. Rare cases of myocardial infarction and cardiac arrest have been observed during or after hypotension.

Rare cases of arrhythmias such as atrial fibrillation/flutter, cardiac arrest, and supraventricular tachycardia have been reported. These are sometimes associated with hypotension or allergic reactions.

Transient hypertension and exacerbations of preexisting hypertension have been observed rarely after amifostine administration.

➤*CNS:* Seizures and syncope have been reported rarely.

➤*Dermatologic:* Cutaneous eruptions have been commonly reported during clinical trials and were generally nonserious. Serious, sometimes fatal skin reactions, including erythema multiforme and, in rare cases, exfoliative dermatitis, Stevens-Johnson syndrome, and toxic epidermal necrolysis, have also occurred. The reported incidence of serious skin reactions associated with amifostine is higher in patients receiving amifostine as a radioprotectant than in patients receiving amifostine as a chemoprotectant.

➤*GI:* Nausea and/or vomiting occur frequently after amifostine infusion and may be severe. In the ovarian cancer randomized study, the incidence of severe nausea/vomiting on day 1 of cyclophosphamide-cisplatin chemotherapy was 10% in patients who did not receive amifostine and 19% in patients who did receive amifostine. In the randomized study of patients with head and neck cancer, the incidence of severe nausea/vomiting was 8% in patients who received amifostine and 1% in patients who did not receive amifostine.

➤*Hypersensitivity:* Allergic reactions characterized by one or more of the following manifestations have been observed during or after amifostine administration: chest tightness, chills/rigors, cutaneous eruptions, dyspnea, fever, hypotension, hypoxia, laryngeal edema, pruritus, urticaria. There have been rare reports of anaphylactoid reactions.

➤*Metabolic:* Decrease in serum calcium concentrations is a known pharmacological effect of amifostine. At the recommended doses, clinically significant hypocalcemia was reported in 1% of patients in the randomized head and neck cancer study.

➤*Miscellaneous:* Rare cases of renal failure and respiratory arrests have been observed during or after hypotension. Other effects, which have been described during or following administration of amifostine infusion are chills/feeling of coldness, dizziness, fever, flushing/feeling of warmth, hiccups, malaise, rash, sneezing, and somnolence. These effects have not generally precluded the completion of therapy.

Overdosage

➤*Symptoms:* In clinical trials, the maximum single dose of amifostine was 1,300 mg/m^2. Children have received single doses of up to 2,700 mg/m^2. At the higher doses, anxiety and reversible urinary retention occurred. Administration of amifostine at 2 and 4 hours after the initial dose has not led to increased nausea and vomiting or hypotension. The most likely symptom of overdosage is hypotension.

➤*Treatment:* Manage by infusion of normal saline and other supportive measures as clinically indicated.

Patient Information

Advise patients that medication will be prepared and administered by a health care provider in a health care setting just before chemotherapy or radiation therapy.

Advise patients to remain supine for 15 minutes after completion of infusion and to use caution when standing up.

Instruct patients to inform a health care provider if they note any of the following during the administration of the drug: anxiety, itching, rapid heartbeat, rash, shortness of breath or difficulty breathing, sweating, swelling of the throat.

DEXRAZOXANE

Rx	**Dexrazoxane** (Bedford)	**Injection, lyophilized, powder for solution:** 250 mg	As dexrazoxane hydrochloride. In single-use vials with 25 mL vial of sodium lactate injection.
Rx	**Zinecard** (Pfizer)		As dexrazoxane hydrochloride. In single-use vials with 25 mL vial of sodium lactate injection.
Rx	**Dexrazoxane** (Bedford)	**Injection, lyophilized, powder for solution:** 500 mg	As dexrazoxane hydrochloride. In single-use vials with 50 mL vial of sodium lactate injection.
Rx	**Totect** (Topo Target[a])		Equiv to dexrazoxane hydrochloride 589 mg. Preservative-free. In single-use vials with 50 mL vial of sodium lactate injection.
Rx	**Zinecard** (Pfizer)		As dexrazoxane hydrochloride. In single-use vials with 50 mL vial of sodium lactate injection.

[a] Topo Target USA Inc, 100 Enterprise Drive, NJ 07866.

DEXRAZOXANE — INJECTION

Indications

➤*Cardiomyopathy associated with doxorubicin use (except Totect):* For reducing the incidence and severity of cardiomyopathy associated with doxorubicin administration in women with metastatic breast cancer who have received a cumulative doxorubicin dose of 300 mg/m^2 and who will continue to receive doxorubicin therapy to maintain tumor control. It is not recommended for use with the initiation of doxorubicin therapy.

➤*Extravasation resulting from intravenous (IV) anthracycline chemotherapy (Totect only):* For the treatment of extravasation resulting from IV anthracycline chemotherapy.

➤*Off-label uses:* Cardioprotectant for other anthracyclines (epirubicin).

Administration and Dosage

➤*Maximum dose:*

Adults – 2,000 mg (days 1 and 2) or 1,000 mg (day 3) for the treatment of extravasation resulting from IV anthracycline chemotherapy (*Totect* only) according to the prescribing information. There is no well-established maximum dose for the other approved indication according to the prescribing information.

➤*Adults:*

Cardiomyopathy associated with doxorubicin use (Zinecard, generic products) – The recommended IV dose ratio of dexrazoxane:doxorubicin is 10:1 (eg, dexrazoxane 500 mg/m^2:doxorubicin 50 mg/m^2). Doxorubicin must be administered within 30 minutes of starting the dexrazoxane infusion.

Extravasation resulting from IV anthracycline chemotherapy (Totect) –

Usual dosage: 1,000 mg/m^2 (up to 2,000 mg/dose) IV once daily for 2 days, then 500 mg/m^2 (up to 1,000 mg) IV for 1 day. Start first dose within 6 hours of anthracycline extravasation, then give subsequent doses at approximately 24-hour intervals (range, 21 to 27 hours).

Maximum dose: 2,000 mg (days 1 and 2); 1,000 mg (day 3).

➤*Children:*

Off-label dosing –

Cardiomyopathy associated with doxorubicin use:

• *Zinecard*, generic products – The recommended IV dosage ratio of dexrazoxane:doxorubicin is 10:1 (eg, dexrazoxane 500 mg/m^2:doxorubicin 50 mg/m^2). Doxorubicin must be administered within 30 minutes of starting the dexrazoxane infusion.

➤*Renal function impairment:* The total dexrazoxane dose should be reduced by 50% in patients with CrCl values less than 40 mL/min.

➤*Preparation for administration:* Dexrazoxane is considered a mutagen and potential teratogen. Follow safe handling procedures when preparing, administering, or dispensing dexrazoxane.

The use of gloves is recommended. If dexrazoxane powder or solution contacts the skin or mucosae, immediately wash thoroughly with soap and water.

Cardiomyopathy associated with dexrazoxane (Zinecard, generic products) – Dexrazoxane must be reconstituted with 0.167 mol/L (M/6) of sodium lactate injection to give a concentration of dexrazoxane 10 mg/mL.

The reconstituted solution may be injected without further dilution. If desired, the reconstituted solution may be diluted with either sodium chloride 0.9% injection or dextrose 5% injection to a concentration range of 1.3 to 5 mg/mL in IV infusion bags.

Extravasation resulting for IV anthracycline chemotherapy (Totect only) – The individual dosage is based on calculation of the body surface area (BSA) up to a maximum dose of 2,000 mg (each on day 1 and 2) and 1,000 mg (day 3), corresponding to a BSA of 2 m^2.

1.) Each vial of dexrazoxane (500 mg) must be mixed with 50 mL of supplied diluent (sodium lactate) to give a concentration of dexrazoxane 10 mg/mL. The solution should be used immediately (within 2 hours) after preparation. It contains no antibacterial preservative.
2.) Inject the mixed volume into the infusion bag with 1,000 mL of sodium chloride 0.9%. Dexrazoxane must not be mixed with any other drugs.
3.) Repeat steps 1 and 2 in order to obtain the required dose, and inject all the required mixed solutions into the same sodium chloride 0.9% 1,000 mL bag. The infusion bag should be used immediately after preparation. The product is stable for 4 hours from the time of preparation when stored below 25°C (77°F).
4.) Dexrazoxane should be infused over 1 to 2 hours at room temperature and normal light conditions.

The solution of dexrazoxane is slightly yellow.

➤*Administration:*

Cardiomyopathy associated with dexrazoxane (Zinecard, generic products) – The reconstituted solution should be given by slow IV push or rapid-drip IV infusion from a bag. After completing the dexrazoxane infusion and prior to a total elapsed time of 30 minutes (from the beginning of the dexrazoxane infusion), the IV injection of doxorubicin should be given.

Extravasation resulting for IV anthracycline chemotherapy (Totect only) – Administer as an IV infusion over 1 to 2 hours in a large caliber vein in an extremity/area other than the one affected by the extravasation. Cooling procedures such as ice packs, if used, should be removed from the area at least 15 minutes before dexrazoxane administration to allow sufficient blood flow to the area of extravasation. Treatment on day 2 and day 3 should start at the same hour (± 3 hours) as on the first day.

➤*Admixture compatibility:* Dexrazoxane should not be mixed or administered with other drugs.

➤*Storage / Stability:*

Zinecard, generic products – Store at 25°C (77°F); excursions are permitted to 15° to 30°C (59° to 86°F). Reconstituted solutions of dexrazoxane are stable for 6 hours at 15° to 30°C (59° to 86°F), or under refrigeration at 2° to 8°C (36° to 46°F). Discard unused solutions.

Totect only – Store unreconstituted vials at 25°C (77°F); excursions are permitted between 15° and 30°C (59° and 86°F). Protect from light. Keep vials in carton until ready for use. The reconstituted product should be used immediately (within 2 hours) after mixing as it contains no antibacterial preservative. After further dilution, the product is stable for 4 hours when stored below 25°C (77°F). Discard vial within 6 hours of the initial needle puncture if opened within an ISO Class 5 biological safety cabinet, or within 1 hour of the initial needle puncture if opened outside of such an environment, based on the USP Chapter <797> standards.

Actions

➤*Pharmacology:*

Cardiomyopathy associated with doxorubicin use (except Totect) – Dexrazoxane, a potent intracellular chelating agent, is a cardioprotective agent for use in conjunction with doxorubicin. The mechanism by which dexrazoxane exerts its cardioprotective activity is not fully understood. Dexrazoxane is a cyclic derivative of ethylenediaminetetraacetic acid that readily penetrates cell membranes. Results of laboratory studies suggest that dexrazoxane is converted intracellularly to a ring-opened chelating agent that interferes with iron-mediated free radical generation thought to be responsible, in part, for anthracycline-induced cardiomyopathy.

Extravasation resulting from IV anthracycline chemotherapy (Totect only) – The mechanism by which dexrazoxane diminishes tissue damage resulting from the extravasation of anthracycline drugs is unknown. Some evidence suggests that dexrazoxane inhibits topoisomerase II reversibly.

➤*Pharmacokinetics:*

Dexrazoxane Pharmacokinetic Parameters (% CV[a]) at a 10:1 Dosage Ratio of Dexrazoxane:Doxorubicin

Dose doxorubicin (mg/m^2)	Dose dexrazoxane (mg/m^2)	Number of subjects	$t_{1/2}$[b] (h)	Plasma Cl[c] (L/h/m^2)	Renal Cl (L/h/m^2)	Steady-state Vd[d] (L/m^2)
50	500	10	2.5 (16)	7.88 (18)	3.35 (36)	22.4 (22)
60	600	5	2.1 (29)	6.25 (31)		22 (55)

[a] CV = coefficient of variation.
[b] $t_{1/2}$ = elimination half-life.
[c] Cl = clearance.
[d] Vd = volume of distribution.

Absorption – Generally, the pharmacokinetics of dexrazoxane can be adequately described by a 2-compartment open model with first-order elimination. Dexrazoxane has been administered as a 15-minute infusion over a dose range of 60 to 900 mg/m^2 with doxorubicin 60 mg/m^2, and at a fixed dose of 500 mg/m^2 with doxorubicin 50 mg/m^2.

The disposition kinetics of dexrazoxane are dose-independent, as shown by a linear relationship between the area under plasma concentration-time curves (AUCs) and administered doses ranging from 60 to 900 mg/m^2. The mean peak plasma concentration of dexrazoxane was 36.5 mcg/mL at the

DEXRAZOXANE — INJECTION

end of the 15-minute infusion of dexrazoxane 500 mg/m^2 administered 15 to 30 minutes prior to doxorubicin 50 mg/m^2.

Distribution – Following a rapid distributive phase (approximately 0.2 to 0.3 hours), dexrazoxane reaches postdistributive equilibrium within 2 to 4 hours. The estimated steady-state volume of distribution of dexrazoxane suggests its distribution is primarily in the total body water (25 L/m^2). In vitro studies have shown that dexrazoxane is not bound to plasma proteins.

Metabolism – Qualitative metabolism studies with dexrazoxane have confirmed the presence of unchanged drug, a diacid-diamide cleavage product, and 2 monoacid-monoamide ring products in the urine of animals and humans. The metabolite levels were not measured in the pharmacokinetic studies.

Excretion – Urinary excretion plays an important role in the elimination of dexrazoxane. Forty-two percent of the dose of dexrazoxane 500 mg/m^2 was excreted in the urine.

Special populations –

Renal function impairment: The pharmacokinetics of dexrazoxane were assessed following a single 15-minute IV infusion of dexrazoxane 150 mg/m^2 in men and women with varying degrees of renal function impairment as determined by CrCl based on a 24-hour urinary creatinine collection. Dexrazoxane clearance was reduced in subjects with renal function impairment. Compared with controls, the mean $AUC_{0-\infty}$ value was 2-fold greater in patients with moderate (CrCl 30 to 50 mL/min) to severe (CrCl less than 30 mL/min) renal function impairment. Modeling demonstrated that equivalent exposure ($AUC_{0-\infty}$) could be achieved if dosing were reduced by 50% in patients with CrCl values less than 40 mL/min compared with control subjects (CrCl greater than 80 mL/min).

Hepatic function impairment: The pharmacokinetics of dexrazoxane have not been evaluated in patients with hepatic function impairment. The dexrazoxane dose is dependent upon the dose of doxorubicin. Because a doxorubicin dose reduction is recommended in the presence of hyperbilirubinemia, the dexrazoxane dosage is proportionately reduced in patients with hepatic function impairment.

Race: The mean systemic clearance and steady-state volume of distribution of dexrazoxane in 2 Asian women at dexrazoxane 500 mg/m^2 along with doxorubicin 50 mg/m^2 were 15.15 L/h/m^2 and 36.27 L/m^2, respectively; however, their elimination half-life and renal clearance of dexrazoxane were similar to those of the 10 white patients from the same study.

Contraindications

Chemotherapy regimens that do not contain an anthracycline.

Warnings/Precautions

➤*Myelosuppression:* Dexrazoxane is a cytotoxic drug. Dexrazoxane may add to the myelosuppression caused by chemotherapeutic agents. While the myelosuppressive effects of dexrazoxane at the recommended dose are mild, additive effects upon the myelosuppressive activity of chemotherapeutic agents may occur. Because dexrazoxane may add to the myelosuppressive effects of cytotoxic drugs and because treatment with dexrazoxane is associated with leukopenia, neutropenia, and thrombocytopenia, frequent complete blood cell counts are recommended.

➤*Antitumor interference:* There is some evidence that the use of dexrazoxane concurrently with the initiation of fluorouracil, doxorubicin, and cyclophosphamide therapy interferes with the antitumor efficacy of the regimen; this use is not recommended. In the largest of 3 breast cancer trials, patients who received dexrazoxane starting with their first cycle of fluorouracil, doxorubicin, and cyclophosphamide therapy had a lower response rate (48% vs 63%; $P = 0.007$) and shorter time to progression than patients who did not receive dexrazoxane. Therefore, only use dexrazoxane in patients who have received a cumulative dose of doxorubicin 300 mg/m^2 and are continuing with doxorubicin therapy.

➤*Anthracycline-induced cardiac toxicity:* Although clinical studies have shown that patients receiving fluorouracil, doxorubicin, and cyclophosphamide with dexrazoxane may receive a higher cumulative dose of doxorubicin before experiencing cardiac toxicity than patients receiving fluorouracil, doxorubicin, and cyclophosphamide without dexrazoxane, the use of dexrazoxane in patients who have already received a cumulative dose of doxorubicin 300 mg/m^2 without dexrazoxane does not eliminate the potential for anthracycline-induced cardiac toxicity. Therefore, carefully monitor cardiac function.

➤*Hepatic effects:* Reversible elevations of liver enzymes may occur with dexrazoxane.

➤*Secondary malignancies:* Secondary malignancies (primarily acute myeloid leukemia) have been reported in patients treated chronically with oral razoxane. Razoxane is the racemic mixture, of which dexrazoxane is the S(+)-enantiomer. In these patients, the total cumulative dose of razoxane ranged from 26 to 480 g and the duration of treatment was from 42 to 319 weeks. One case of T-cell lymphoma, a case of B-cell lymphoma, and 6 to 8 cases of cutaneous basal cell or squamous cell carcinoma also have been reported in patients treated with razoxane.

➤*Dimethylsulfoxide:* Do not use dimethylsulfoxide in patients who are receiving dexrazoxane to treat anthracycline-induced extravasation.

➤*Renal function impairment:* See Administration and Dosage for more information.

➤*Pregnancy:* Category C (except *Totect*); Category D (*Totect* only). Dexrazoxane was maternotoxic at doses of 2 mg/kg (one-fortieth the human dose on a mg/m^2 basis; one-eightieth the human dose on a mg/m^2 basis [*Totect*]), and embryotoxic and teratogenic at 8 mg/kg (approximately one-tenth the human dose on a mg/m^2 basis; approximately one-twentieth the human dose on a mg/m^2 basis [*Totect*]) when given daily to pregnant rats during the period of organogenesis. Teratogenic effects in the rat included imperforate anus, microphthalmia, and anophthalmia. In offspring allowed to develop to maturity, fertility was impaired in the male and female rats treated in utero during organogenesis at 8 mg/kg. In rabbits, doses of 5 mg/kg (approximately one-tenth the human dose on a mg/m^2 basis; approximately one-sixteenth the human dose on a mg/m^2 basis [*Totect*]) daily during the period of organogenesis were maternotoxic and doses of 20 mg/kg (one-half the human dose on a mg/m^2 basis; one-fourth the human dose on a mg/m^2 basis [*Totect*]) were embryotoxic and teratogenic. Teratogenic effects in the rabbit included several skeletal malformations such as short tail, rib and thoracic malformations, and soft tissue variations, including subcutaneous, eye, and cardiac hemorrhagic areas, as well as agenesis of the gallbladder and intermediate lobe of the lung.

There is no adequate information about the use of dexrazoxane in pregnant women. If this drug is used during pregnancy, or if the patient becomes pregnant while taking this drug, apprise the patient of the potential hazard to the fetus.

➤*Lactation:* It is not known whether dexrazoxane or its metabolites are excreted in human milk. Because many drugs are excreted in human milk and because of the potential for serious adverse reactions in breast-feeding infants exposed to dexrazoxane, decide whether to discontinue breast-feeding or the drug, taking into account the importance of the drug to the mother.

➤*Children:* Safety and efficacy of dexrazoxane in children have not been established.

➤*Elderly:* This drug is known to be substantially excreted by the kidney, and the risk of toxic reactions to this drug may be greater in patient with renal function impairment. Because elderly patients are more likely to have decreased renal function, take care in dose selection and monitor renal function. In general, treat elderly patients with caution because of the greater frequency of decreased hepatic, renal, or cardiac function, and of concomitant disease or other drug therapy.

➤*Monitoring:* Because dexrazoxane will always be used with cytotoxic drugs, and because it may add to the myelosuppressive effects of cytotoxic drugs, frequent blood cell counts are recommended; carefully monitor cardiac function and liver enzymes.

Drug Interactions

None known.

Adverse Reactions

Dexrazoxane Adverse Reactions				
	Fluorouracil, doxorubicin, and cyclophosphamide + dexrazoxane		Fluorouracil, doxorubicin, and cyclophosphamide + placebo	
Adverse reaction	Courses 1 through 6 (n = 413)	Courses ≥ 7 (n = 102)	Courses 1 through 6 (n = 458)	Courses ≥ 7 (n = 99)
CNS				
Fatigue/Malaise	61%	48%	58%	55%
Neurotoxicity	17%	10%	13%	5%
Dermatological				
Alopecia	94%	100%	97%	98%
Recall skin reaction	1%	1%	2%	0%
Streaking/ Erythema	5%	4%	4%	2%
Urticaria	2%	2%	2%	0%
GI				
Anorexia	42%	27%	47%	38%
Diarrhea	21%	14%	24%	7%
Dysphagia	8%	0%	10%	5%
Esophagitis	6%	3%	7%	4%
Nausea	77%	51%	84%	60%
Stomatitis	34%	26%	41%	28%
Vomiting	59%	42%	72%	49%
Local				
Extravasation	1%	3%	1%	2%
Pain on injection	12%	13%	3%	0%
Phlebitis	6%	3%	3%	5%
Miscellaneous				
Fever	34%	22%	29%	18%
Hemorrhage	2%	3%	2%	1%
Infection	23%	19%	18%	21%
Sepsis	17%	12%	14%	9%

➤*Hematologic:* Patients receiving fluorouracil, doxorubicin, and cyclophosphamide with dexrazoxane experienced more severe leukopenia, granulocytopenia, and thrombocytopenia at nadir than patients receiving fluorouracil, doxorubicin, and cyclophosphamide without dexrazoxane, but recovery counts were similar for the 2 groups of patients.

➤*Lab test abnormalities:* Some patients receiving fluorouracil, doxorubicin, and cyclophosphamide plus dexrazoxane or fluorouracil, doxorubicin, and cyclophosphamide plus placebo experienced marked abnormalities in hepatic or renal function tests, but the frequency and severity of abnormalities in bilirubin, alkaline phosphatase, serum urea nitrogen, and creatinine

DEXRAZOXANE — INJECTION

were similar for patients receiving fluorouracil, doxorubicin, and cyclophosphamide with or without dexrazoxane.

➤*Totect only:*

Dexrazoxane Adverse Reactions (≥ 5%)[a]	
Adverse reaction	Study 1 and 2 combined (all causalities) (N = 80)
Cardiovascular	
Cardiac disorders	5%
Vascular disorders	15%
CNS	
Depression	8%
Dizziness	11%
Fatigue	13%
Headache	6%
Insomnia	5%
Nervous system disorders	24%
Psychiatric disorders	14%
Dermatological	
Alopecia	14%
Skin and subcutaneous disorders	18%
GI	
Abdominal pain	6%
Anorexia	5%
Constipation	6%
Diarrhea	11%
GI disorders	55%
Nausea	43%
Vomiting	19%
Hematologic	
Anemia	6%
Blood and lymphatic system disorders	14%
Local	
General disorders and administration-site conditions	58%
Injection-site pain	16%
Injection-site phlebitis	6%
Respiratory	
Cough	5%
Dyspnea	8%
Pneumonia	6%
Respiratory, thoracic, and mediastinal disorders	16%
Miscellaneous	
Edema peripheral	10%
Infections and infestations	30%
Metabolism and nutrition disorders	10%
Musculoskeletal and connective tissue disorders	13%
Postoperative infection	16%
Pyrexia	21%

[a] Eighty-five percent of patients experienced at least 1 reaction.

Neutropenia and febrile neutropenia each occurred in 2.5% of patients.

Lab test abnormalities –

Dexrazoxane Laboratory Test Abnormalities			
Laboratory parameters	CTC[a] grade 3	CTC grade 4	CTC grade 2 to 4
Hematologic			
Decreased hemoglobin	3%	0%	43%
Decreased neutrophils	22%	24%	61%
Decreased platelets	21%	0%	26%
Decreased white blood cells	25%	20%	73%
Hepatic			
Increased alkaline phosphatase	0%	0%	4%
Increased ALT	1%	5%	22%
Increased AST	1%	1%	28%
Increased bilirubin	2%	0%	11%
Increased LDH[b]	0%	0%	5%
Metabolic			
Increased calcium total	2%	2%	7%
Increased creatinine	2%	2%	14%
Decreased sodium	5%	1%	6%

[a] CTC = Common Toxicity Criteria.
[b] LDH = lactate dehydrogenase.

Overdosage

➤*Treatment:* Disposition studies with dexrazoxane have not been conducted in cancer patients undergoing dialysis, but retention of a significant dose fraction (greater than 0.4) of the unchanged drug in the plasma pool, minimal tissue partitioning or binding, and availability of greater than 90% of the systemic drug levels in the unbound form suggest that it could be removed using conventional peritoneal or hemodialysis.

There is no known antidote for dexrazoxane overdose. Manage instances of suspected overdose with good supportive care until resolution of myelosuppression and related conditions is complete. Management of overdose should include treatment of infections, fluid regulation, and maintenance of nutritional requirements.

Patient Information

Dexrazoxane is always used together with doxorubicin. Advise patients to tell their health care provider or pharmacist if any of the following occur: appetite loss, chills, diarrhea, difficulty swallowing, fever, general body discomfort, hair loss, hives, nausea, numbness or tingling, pain at injection site, sore throat, stomach pain, streaking or redness of the skin, tiredness, unusual bleeding, or vomiting.

Advise women who have the potential to become pregnant that dexrazoxane might cause fetal harm.

MESNA

Rx	**Mesna** (Baxter)	**Tablets:** 400 mg	Lactose. (M4). White, oblong, scored. Film coated. In 10 blisters.
Rx	**Mesnex** (Bristol-Myers Squibb)		Lactose, simethicone. (M4). White, oblong, scored. Film coated. In 10 blisters.
Rx	**Mesna** (Various, eg, American Pharmaceutical Partners, Baxter)	**Injection:** 100 mg/mL	With 0.25 mg/mL EDTA. In 10 mL multidose vials.[a]
Rx	**Mesnex** (Bristol-Myers Squibb)		With 0.25 mg/mL EDTA. In 10 mL multidose vials.[a]

[a] With 10.4 mg benzyl alcohol as a preservative.

MESNA — ORAL

Indications

➤*Ifosfamide-induced hemorrhagic cystitis:* As a prophylactic agent in reducing the incidence of ifosfamide-induced hemorrhagic cystitis.

➤*Off-label uses:* Prevention of cyclophosphamide-induced hemorrhagic cystitis. Mesna has been used safely and effectively in children. (See Administration and Dosage).

Administration and Dosage

➤*General dosing considerations:* Mesna may be given on a fractionated dosing schedule of 3 bolus IV injections or a single bolus injection followed by 2 oral administrations of mesna tablets as outlined in the following sections.

The efficacy and safety of the following ratio of IV and oral mesna has not been established as being effective for daily doses of ifosfamide higher than 2 g/m^2.

➤*Adults:*

Prevention of ifosfamide-induced hemorrhagic cystitis –

Usual dosage: Following the initial IV mesna dose (20% of ifosfamide dose), the oral mesna dose is 40% of the ifosfamide dose (w/w) administered 2 and 6 hours after each ifosfamide dose. The total daily dose of mesna is 100% of the ifosfamide dose.

The dosing schedule should be repeated on each day that ifosfamide is administered.

MESNA — ORAL

Recommended Mesna Dosing Schedule (IV and Oral Dosing Regimen)			
	0 hours	2 hours	6 hours
Ifosamide	1.2 g/m^2		
Mesna injection	240 mg/m^2		
Mesna tablets		480 mg/m^2	480 mg/m^2

Dosage adjustment: When the dosage of ifosfamide is adjusted (either increased or decreased), the ratio of mesna to ifosfamide should be maintained.

Alternative dosage: An alternative regimen for oral mesna is 40% of the ifosfamide dose given 4 and 8 hours after each ifosfamide dose.

Off-label dosing –

Prevention of cyclophosphamide-induced hemorrhagic cystitis: Following the initial IV mesna dose (20% of the cyclophosphamide dose), the oral mesna dose is 40% of the cyclophosphamide dose administered 4 and 8 hours after each cyclophosphamide dose.

➤*Children:*

Off-label dosing – The appropriate dose of mesna is determined by the dose of the antineoplastic agent. The mesna dose is calculated on a weight-per-weight basis.

Prevention of ifosfamide-induced hemorrhagic cystitis: Following the initial IV mesna dose (20% of the ifosfamide dose), the oral mesna dose is 40% of the ifosfamide dose administered 4 and 8 hours after each ifosfamide dose.

Prevention of cyclophosphamide-induced hemorrhagic cystitis: Following the initial IV mesna dose (20% of cyclophosphamide dose), the oral mesna dose is 40% of the cyclophosphamide dose administered 4 and 8 hours after each cyclophosphamide dose.

➤*Administration:* It is important for the patient to drink at least a quart (4 cups) of liquid a day whenever taking mesna.

Give an additional mesna dose (IV or orally) if the patient vomits within 2 hours of an oral mesna dose.

If mesna is given orally for the initial dose, it should be administered 1 hour before chemotherapy is given to allow for absorption.

➤*Storage/Stability:* Store at 20° to 25°C (68° to 77°F).

Actions

➤*Pharmacology:* Mesna was developed as a prophylactic agent to reduce the risk of hemorrhagic cystitis induced by ifosfamide.

Analogous to the physiological cysteine-cystine system, mesna is rapidly oxidized to its major metabolite, mesna disulfide (dimesna). Mesna disulfide remains in the intravascular compartment and is rapidly eliminated by the kidneys.

In the kidney, the mesna disulfide is reduced to the free thiol compound, mesna, which reacts chemically with the urotoxic ifosfamide metabolites (acrolein and 4-hydroxy-ifosfamide) resulting in their detoxification. The first step in the detoxification process is the binding of mesna to 4-hydroxy-ifosfamide forming a nonurotoxic 4-sulfoethylthioifosfamide. Mesna also binds to the double bonds of acrolein and to other urotoxic metabolites.

In multiple human xenograft or rodent tumor model studies of limited scope, using IV or intraperitoneal (IP) routes of administration, mesna, in combination with ifosfamide (at dose ratios of up to 20-fold as single or multiple courses), failed to demonstrate interference with antitumor efficacy.

➤*Pharmacokinetics:*

Absorption/Distribution –

IV-oral-oral regimen: The half-life of mesna ranged from 1.2 to 8.3 hours after administration of IV plus oral doses of mesna, as recommended in Administration and Dosage. The urinary bioavailability of oral mesna ranged from 45% to 79% of IV mesna. Food does not affect the urinary availability of orally administered mesna. Approximately 18% to 26% of the combined IV and oral mesna dose appears as free mesna in the urine. When compared to IV mesna, the IV plus oral dosing regimen increases systemic exposures (150%) and provides more sustained excretion of mesna in the urine over a 24-hour period. Approximately 5% of the mesna dose is excreted during the 12- to 24-hour interval, as compared to negligible amounts in patients given the IV regimen. The fraction of the administered dose of mesna excreted in the urine is independent of dose. Protein binding of mesna is in a moderate range (69% to 75%).

Metabolism/Excretion – At doses of 2 to 4 g/m^2, the terminal elimination half-life of ifosfamide is about 4 to 8 hours. As a result, in order to maintain adequate levels of mesna in the urinary bladder during the course of elimination of the urotoxic ifosfamide metabolites, repeated doses of mesna are required.

Contraindications

Hypersensitivity to mesna or other thiol compounds.

Warnings/Precautions

➤*Usage:* Mesna has been developed as an agent to reduce the risk of ifosfamide-induced hemorrhagic cystitis. It will not prevent or alleviate any of the other adverse reactions or toxicities associated with ifosfamide therapy.

➤*Hematuria:* Mesna does not prevent hemorrhagic cystitis in all patients. Up to 6% of patients treated with mesna have developed hematuria (greater than 50 RBC/hpf or World Health Organization [WHO] grade 2 and above). As a result, a morning specimen of urine should be examined for the presence of hematuria (microscopic evidence of red blood cells) each day prior to ifosfamide therapy. If hematuria develops when mesna is given with ifosfamide according to the recommended dosage schedule, depending on the severity of the hematuria, dosage reductions or discontinuation of ifosfamide therapy may be initiated.

In order to reduce the risk of hematuria, mesna must be administered with each dose of ifosfamide as outlined in Administration and Dosage. Mesna is not effective in reducing the risk of hematuria due to other pathological conditions such as thrombocytopenia.

➤*Hypersensitivity reactions:* Allergic reactions to mesna ranging from mild hypersensitivity to systemic anaphylactic reactions have been reported. Patients with autoimmune disorders who were treated with cyclophosphamide and mesna appeared to have a higher incidence of allergic reactions. The majority of these patients received mesna orally.

➤*Pregnancy: Category B.* There are no adequate and well-controlled studies in pregnant women. Because animal reproductive studies are not always predictive of human response, this drug should be used during pregnancy only if clearly needed.

➤*Lactation:* It is not known whether mesna or dimesna is excreted in human milk. Because many drugs are excreted in human milk and because of the potential for adverse reactions in nursing infants from mesna, a decision should be made whether to discontinue nursing or discontinue the drug, taking into account the importance of the drug to the mother.

➤*Children:* Safety and efficacy of mesna tablets in pediatric patients have not been established.

➤*Elderly:* In general, dose selection for an elderly patient should be cautious, reflecting the greater frequency of decreased hepatic, renal, or cardiac function, and of concomitant disease or other drug therapy. However, the ratio of ifosfamide to mesna should remain unchanged.

Drug Interactions

➤*Drug/Lab test interactions:* A false-positive test for urinary ketones may arise in patients treated with mesna. In this test, a red-violet color develops which, with the addition of glacial acetic acid, will return to violet.

Adverse Reactions

The most frequently reported side effects (observed in 2 or more patients) for patients receiving single doses of mesna IV were headache, injection-site reactions, flushing, dizziness, nausea, vomiting, somnolence, diarrhea, anorexia, fever, pharyngitis, hyperaesthesia, influenza-like symptoms, and coughing. Among patients who received a single 1200 mg dose as an oral solution, rigors, back pain, rash, conjunctivitis, and arthralgia were also reported. In 2 phase 1 multiple-dose studies where patients received mesna tablets alone or IV mesna followed by repeated doses of mesna tablets, flatulence and rhinitis were reported. In addition, constipation was reported by patients who had received repeated doses of IV mesna.

Incidence of Adverse Reactions and Incidence of Most Frequently Reported Adverse Reactions in Controlled Studies (%)		
Mesna regimen	IV-IV-IV (N = 119)	IV-oral-oral (N = 119)
Incidence of adverse reactions	101 (84.9%)	106 (89.1%)
Nausea	65 (54.6%)	64 (53.8%)
Vomiting	35 (29.4%)	45 (37.8%)
Constipation	28 (23.5%)	21 (17.6%)
Leukopenia	25 (21%)	21 (17.6%)
Fatigue	24 (20.2%)	24 (20.2%)
Fever	24 (20.2%)	18 (15.1%)
Anorexia	21 (17.6%)	19 (16%)
Thrombocytopenia	21 (17.6%)	16 (13.4%)
Anemia	20 (16.8%)	21 (17.6%)
Granulocytopenia	16 (13.4%)	15 (12.6%)
Asthenia	15 (12.6%)	21 (17.6%)
Abdominal pain	14 (11.8%)	18 (15.1%)
Alopecia	12 (10.1%)	13 (10.9%)
Dyspnea	11 (9.2%)	11 (9.2%)
Chest pain	10 (8.4%)	9 (7.6%)
Hypokalemia	10 (8.4%)	11 (9.2%)
Diarrhea	9 (7.6%)	17 (14.3%)
Dizziness	9 (7.6%)	5 (4.2%)
Headache	9 (7.6%)	13 (10.9%)
Pain	9 (7.6%)	10 (8.4%)
Increased sweating	9 (7.6%)	2 (1.7%)
Back pain	8 (6.7%)	6 (5%)
Hematuria[a]	8 (6.7%)	7 (5.9%)
Injection-site reaction	8 (6.7%)	10 (8.4%)
Edema	8 (6.7%)	9 (7.6%)
Peripheral edema	8 (6.7%)	8 (6.7%)
Somnolence	8 (6.7%)	12 (10.1%)
Anxiety	7 (5.9%)	4 (3.4%)

MESNA — ORAL

Incidence of Adverse Reactions and Incidence of Most Frequently Reported Adverse Reactions in Controlled Studies (%)		
Mesna regimen	IV-IV-IV (N = 119)	IV-oral-oral (N = 119)
Confusion	7 (5.9%)	6 (5%)
Face edema	6 (5%)	5 (4.2%)
Insomnia	6 (5%)	11 (9.2%)
Coughing	5 (4.2%)	10 (8.4%)
Dyspepsia	4 (3.4%)	6 (5%)
Hypotension	4 (3.4%)	6 (5%)
Pallor	4 (3.4%)	6 (5%)
Dehydration	3 (2.5%)	7 (5.9%)
Pneumonia	2 (1.7%)	8 (6.7%)
Tachycardia	1 (0.8%)	7 (5.9%)
Flushing	1 (0.8%)	6 (5.0%)

[a] All grades.

➤*Postmarketing surveillance:* Allergic reactions, decreased platelet counts associated with allergic reactions, hypertension, hypotension, increased heart rate, increased liver enzymes, injection site reactions (including pain and erythema), limb pain, malaise, myalgia, ST-segment elevation, tachycardia, and tachypnea have been reported as part of postmarketing surveillance.

Overdosage

➤*Symptoms:* Oral doses of 6.1 and 4.3 g/kg were lethal to mice and rats, respectively. These doses are approximately 15 and 22 times the maximum recommended human dose on a body surface area basis. Death was preceded by diarrhea, tremor, convulsions, dyspnea, and cyanosis.

➤*Treatment:* There is no known antidote for mesna.

Patient Information

It is important for the patient to drink at least a quart (4 cups) of liquid a day whenever taking mesna.

A small number of patients who take mesna get blood in their urine (hematuria). Therefore, laboratory testing of the urine will be performed by the health care provider each day of mesna therapy. The laboratory test can find low levels of blood in the urine that undetectable by viewing.

If the patient's urine has turned a pink or red color, contact the health care provider as soon as possible. Certain prescription medicines and foods, such as red beets, may also cause urine to change color. A laboratory test of urine will show if the source of the color is due to one of these causes or hematuria.

Mesna tablets should be taken at the exact times advised by the health care provider. If a dose is missed, it should be taken as soon as possible and the health care provider should be contacted for more instructions. The dose should not be doubled to make up for the missed dose.

Mesna should not be taken if the patient has had an allergic reaction to mesna or other medicines that contain sulfur.

Before beginning treatment with mesna, the patient should check with the health care provider regarding the following:

- Pregnancy. The patient and health care provider should discuss if mesna is the right therapy.
- Breast-feeding. The health care provider may advise the patient to stop breast-feeding or not to use mesna.
- Autoimmune disorders (eg, rheumatoid arthritis, systemic lupus erythematosis [SLE], or nephritis [a type of kidney problem]). The patient may be more likely to get an allergic reaction from mesna.

Mesna should be taken at the exact times in the exact amounts instructed by the health care provider. If the first dose is IV and the other doses are oral, the patient will get the IV dose at the same time as the ifosfamide. Tablets should be taken 2 and 6 hours after the ifosfamide.

The dose of mesna depends on the amount of the ifosfamide dose. Advise patients to pay careful attention to the number of tablets the health care provider instructs them to take. Half tablets for the dose may be required. Each tablet has a groove in the middle that makes it easy to break the tablets in half.

The most common side effects reported for mesna tablets are headache; digestive symptoms such as nausea, vomiting, diarrhea, stomach pain, and low or no appetite; flu-like symptoms including dizziness, flushing, and fever; sensitive skin; sleepiness; coughing; sore throat; cold-like symptoms; injection site reactions. Some patients may get allergic reactions, rash, constipation, paleness, fluid retention, and decreased blood pressure. These are not all the possible side effects of mesna. For a complete list, consult the health care provider.

If there is suspicion that someone may have taken more than the prescribed dose of mesna, contact the local poison control center or emergency room right away.

Store mesna tablets in a cool, dry place protected from excess moisture and heat. If possible, it should not be stored in the kitchen or bathroom. Any unused portion should be thrown away after the expiration date.

MESNA — INJECTION

Indications

➤*Ifosfamide-induced hemorrhagic cystitis:* Mesna has been shown to be effective as a prophylactic agent in reducing the incidence of ifosfamide-induced hemorrhagic cystitis.

➤*Off-label uses:* Mesna may be useful in reducing the incidence of cyclophosphamide-induced hemorrhagic cystitis. Mesna has been used safely and effectively in children. (See Administration and Dosage.)

Administration and Dosage

➤*General dosing considerations:* The appropriate dose of mesna is determined by the dose of the antineoplastic agent. The mesna dose is calculated on a weight-per-weight basis.

Mesna may be given on a fractionated dosing schedule of 3 bolus intravenous (IV) injections or a single bolus injection followed by 2 oral administrations of mesna tablets. See the Mesna Oral monograph for additional information.

➤*Adults:*

Prevention of ifosfamide-induced hemorrhagic cystitis –

IV only regimen: Mesna is given as IV bolus injections in a dosage equal to 20% of the ifosfamide dosage (w/w) at the time of ifosfamide administration and 4 and 8 hours after each dose of ifosfamide. The total daily dose of mesna is 60% of the ifosfamide dose. (See also Off-label dosing).

In order to maintain adequate protection, this dosing schedule should be repeated on each day that ifosfamide is administered.

Recommended Mesna Dosing Schedule (IV Only Regimen)			
	0 hours	4 hours	8 hours
Ifosfamide	1.2 g/m²	-	-
Mesna	240 mg/m²	240 mg/m²	240 mg/m²

IV and Oral Dosing Regimen: Mesna injection is given as IV bolus injections in a dosage equal to 20% of the ifosfamide dosage (w/w) at the time of ifosfamide administration. Mesna tablets are given orally in a dosage equal to 40% of the ifosfamide dose 2 and 6 hours after each dose of ifosfamide. The total daily dose of mesna is 100% of the ifosfamide dose.

Recommended Mesna Dosing Schedule (IV and Oral Dosing)			
	0 hours	2 hours	6 hours
Ifosfamide	1.2 g/m²	-	-
Mesna injection	240 mg/m²	-	-
Mesna tablets	-	480 mg/m²	480 mg/m²

Dosage adjustment: When the dosage of ifosfamide is adjusted (either increased or decreased), the ratio of mesna to ifosfamide should be maintained.

Off-label dosing –

Prevention of ifosfamide-induced hemorrhagic cystitis: Some regimens utilize a mesna dose equal to the ifosfamide dose given as a continuous infusion. Because the half-life of mesna is shorter than that of ifosfamide, some clinicians recommend giving additional mesna at the same infusion rate for 8 to 24 hours after the end of the ifosfamide infusion.

Prevention of cyclophosphamide-induced hemorrhagic cystitis: Mesna dose is 20% of cyclophosphamide dose at the time of, 4 hours after, and 8 hours after each cyclophosphamide dose.

Some clinicians recommend a mesna dose equal to the cyclophosphamide dose given as a continuous infusion. Because the half-life of mesna is shorter than that of cyclophosphamide, some clinicians recommend giving additional mesna at the same infusion rate for at least 24 hours after the end of the cyclophosphamide infusion.

➤*Children:*

Off-label dosing –

Prevention of ifosfamide-induced hemorrhagic cystitis: Mesna dose is 20% of ifosfamide dose at the time of, 4 hours after, and 8 hours after each ifosfamide. An alternative regimen is 20% of the ifosfamide dose given at the time of and every 3 hours after each ifosfamide dose for a total of 3 to 6 doses.

Some regimens utilize a mesna dose equal to the ifosfamide dose given as a continuous infusion. Because the half-life of mesna is shorter than that of ifosfamide, some clinicians recommend giving additional mesna at the same infusion rate for 8 to 24 hours after the end of the ifosfamide infusion.

Prevention of cyclophosphamide-induced hemorrhagic cystitis: Mesna dose is 20% of cyclophosphamide dose at the time of, 4 hours after, and 8hours after each cyclophosphamide dose. An alternative regimen is 20% of the cyclophosphamide dose given at the time of and every 3 hours after each cyclophosphamide dose for a total of 3 to 6 doses.

Some clinicians recommend a mesna dose equal to the cyclophosphamide dose given as a continuous infusion. Because the half-life of mesna is shorter than that of cyclophosphamide, some clinicians recommend giving additional mesna at the same infusion rate for at least 24 hours after the end of the cyclophosphamide infusion.

➤*Preparation for administration:* For IV administration, the drug can be diluted by adding the contents of a mesna injection ampule to any of the following fluids obtaining final concentrations of mesna 20 mg/mL fluid: dextrose 5% injection; dextrose 5% and sodium chloride 0.2% injection; dextrose 5% and sodium chloride 0.33% injection; dextrose 5% and sodium chloride 0.45% injection; sodium chloride injection 0.92%; or lactated Ringer's injection.

MESNA — INJECTION

➤*Administration:* Administer as an IV bolus, IV infusion over 15 to 30 minutes (off-label), or continuous IV infusion (off-label).

It is important for the patient to drink at least a quart (4 cups) of liquid a day whenever taking mesna.

Give an additional mesna dose (IV or orally) if the patient vomits within 2 hours of an oral mesna dose.

➤*Admixture compatibility:* Mesna is not compatible with cisplatin or carboplatin.

➤*Storage/Stability:* Store vials between 20° and 25°C (68° and 77°F). According to the manufacturer, the mesna multidose vials may be stored and used for up to 8 days. However, multiple-dose vials may be used for up to 28 days after the initial needle puncture, based on the USP Chapter < 797> standards.

Diluted solutions are chemically and physically stable for 24 hours at 25°C (77°F).

Actions

➤*Pharmacology:* Mesna was developed as a prophylactic agent to prevent the hemorrhagic cystitis induced by ifosfamide. Analogous to the physiological cysteine-cystine system, following IV administration, mesna is rapidly oxidized to its only metabolite, mesna disulfide (dimesna). Mesna disulfide remains in the intravascular compartment and is rapidly eliminated by the kidneys.

In the kidney, the mesna disulfide is reduced to the free thiol compound, mesna, which reacts chemically with the urotoxic ifosfamide metabolites (acrolein and 4-hydroxy-ifosfamide) resulting in their detoxification. The first step in the detoxification process is the binding of mesna to 4-hydroxy-ifosfamide forming a nonurotoxic 4-sulfoethylthioifosfamide. Mesna also binds to the double bonds of acrolein and other urotoxic metabolites.

In multiple human xenograft or rodent tumor model studies of limited scope, using IV or intraperitoneal (IP) routes of administration, mesna in combination with ifosfamide (at dose ratios of up to 20-fold as single or multiple courses) failed to demonstrate interference with antitumor efficacy.

➤*Pharmacokinetics:*

Absorption –

IV-oral-oral regimen: The urinary bioavailability of oral mesna ranged from 45% to 79% of IV mesna. Food does not affect the urinary availability of orally administered mesna.

Distribution –

IV-oral-oral regimen: Protein binding of mesna is in a moderate range (69% to 75%).

IV-IV-IV regimen: Mesna has a volume of distribution of 0.652 L/kg and a plasma clearance of 1.23 L/kg/h.

Excretion – At doses of 2 to 4 g/m^2, the terminal elimination half-life of ifosfamide is about 4 to 8 hours. As a result, in order to maintain adequate levels of mesna in the urinary bladder during the course of elimination of the urotoxic ifosfamide metabolites, repeated doses of mesna are required.

IV-oral-oral regimen: The half-life of mesna ranged from 1.2 to 8.3 hours after administration of IV plus oral doses of mesna, as recommended in Administration and Dosage. Approximately 18% to 26% of the combined IV and oral mesna dose appears as free mesna in the urine. When compared to IV mesna, the IV plus oral dosing regimen increases systemic exposures (150%) and provides more sustained excretion of mesna in the urine over a 24-hour period. Approximately 5% of the mesna dose is excreted during the 12- to 24-hour interval, as compared to negligible amounts in patients given the IV regimen. The fraction of the administered dose of mesna excreted in the urine is independent of dose.

IV-IV-IV regimen: After IV administration of an 800 mg dose the half-lives of mesna and dimesna in the blood are 0.36 hours and 1.17 hours, respectively. Approximately 32% and 33% of the administered dose was eliminated in the urine in 24 hours as mesna and dimesna, respectively. The majority of the dose recovered was eliminated within 4 hours.

Contraindications

Hypersensitivity to mesna or other thiol compounds.

Warnings/Precautions

➤*Usage:* Mesna has been developed as an agent to prevent ifosfamide-induced hemorrhagic cystitis. It will not prevent or alleviate any of the other adverse reactions or toxicities associated with ifosfamide therapy.

➤*Hematuria:* Mesna does not prevent hemorrhagic cystitis in all patients. Up to 6% of patients treated with mesna have developed hematuria (greater than 50 red blood cells/high powered field or WHO grade 2 and above). As a result, a morning specimen of urine should be examined for the presence of hematuria (red blood cells) each day prior to ifosfamide therapy. If hematuria develops when mesna is given with ifosfamide according to the recommended dosage schedule, depending on the severity of the hematuria, dosage reductions or discontinuation of ifosfamide therapy may be initiated.

➤*Administration with ifosfamide:* In order to reduce the risk of hematuria, mesna must be administered with each dose of ifosfamide as outlined: Mesna injection is given as IV bolus injections in a dosage equal to 20% of the ifosfamide dosage (w/w) at the time of ifosfamide administration. Mesna tablets are given orally in a dosage equal to 40% of the ifosfamide dose 2 and 6 hours after each dose of ifosfamide. The total daily dose of mesna is 100% of the ifosfamide dose. Mesna is not effective in reducing the risk of hematuria due to other pathological conditions such as thrombocytopenia.

➤*Hypersensitivity reactions:* Allergic reactions to mesna ranging from mild hypersensitivity to systemic anaphylactic reactions have been reported. Patients with autoimmune disorders who were treated with cyclophosphamide and mesna appeared to have a higher incidence of allergic reactions. The majority of these patients received mesna orally.

➤*Pregnancy: Category B.* There are no adequate and well-controlled studies in pregnant women. Because animal reproductive studies are not always predictive of human response, this drug should be used during pregnancy only if clearly needed.

➤*Lactation:* It is not known whether mesna or dimesna is excreted in human milk. Because many drugs are excreted in human milk and because of the potential for adverse reactions in nursing infants, from mesna, a decision should be made whether to discontinue nursing or discontinue the drug, taking into account the importance of the drug to the mother.

➤*Children:* Because of the benzyl alcohol content, the multidose vial should not be used in neonates or infants and should be used with caution in older pediatric patients.

➤*Elderly:* Clinical studies of mesna did not include sufficient numbers of subjects aged 65 and over to determine whether they respond differently from younger subjects. In general, dose selection for an elderly patient should be cautious, reflecting the greater frequency of decreased hepatic, renal, or cardiac function, and of concomitant disease or other drug therapy. However, the ratio of ifosfamide to mesna should remain unchanged.

➤*Lab test abnormalities:* A false-positive test for urinary ketones may arise in patients treated with mesna injection. In this test, a red-violet color develops which, with the addition of glacial acetic acid, will return to violet.

➤*Monitoring:* Health care providers should advise patients taking mesna to drink at least a quart of liquid a day. Patients should be informed to report if their urine has turned a pink or red color, if they vomit within 2 hours of taking oral mesna, or if they miss a dose of oral mesna.

Adverse Reactions

The most frequently reported side effects (observed in 2 or more patients) for patients receiving single doses of mesna IV were headache, injection site reactions, flushing, dizziness, nausea, vomiting, somnolence, diarrhea, anorexia, fever, pharyngitis, hyperaesthesia, influenza-like symptoms, and coughing. Among patients who received a single 1200 mg dose as an oral solution, rigors, back pain, rash, conjunctivitis, and arthralgia were also reported. In 2 phase I multiple-dose studies where patients received mesna tablets alone or IV mesna followed by repeated doses of mesna tablets, flatulence and rhinitis were reported. In addition, constipation was reported by patients who had received repeated doses of IV mesna.

In phase I studies in which IV bolus doses of 0.8 to 1.6 g/m^2 mesna were administered as single or 3 repeated doses to a total of 10 patients, a bad taste in the mouth (100%) and soft stools (70%) were reported. At IV and oral bolus doses of 2.4 g/m^2 which are approximately 10 times the recommended clinical doses (0.24 g/m^2) headache (50%), fatigue (33%), nausea (33%), diarrhea (83%), limb pain (50%), hypotension (17%) and allergy (17%) have also been reported in the 6 patients who participated in this study.

In controlled clinical studies, adverse reactions which can be reasonably associated with mesna were vomiting, diarrhea and nausea.

Incidence of Adverse Reactions and Incidence of Most Frequently Reported Adverse Reactions in Controlled Studies (%)

Mesna regimen	IV-IV-IV (N = 119)	IV-oral-oral (N = 119)
Incidence of AEs	101 (84.9%)	106 (89.1%)
Nausea	65 (54.6%)	64 (53.8%)
Vomiting	35 (29.4%)	45 (37.8%)
Constipation	28 (23.5%)	21 (17.6%)
Leukopenia	25 (21%)	21 (17.6%)
Fatigue	24 (20.2%)	24 (20.2%)
Fever	24 (20.2%)	18 (15.1%)
Anorexia	21 (17.6%)	19 (16%)
Thrombocytopenia	21 (17.6%)	16 (13.4%)
Anemia	20 (16.8%)	21 (17.6%)
Granulocytopenia	16 (13.4%)	15 (12.6%)
Asthenia	15 (12.6%)	21 (17.6%)
Abdominal pain	14 (11.8%)	18 (15.1%)
Alopecia	12 (10.1%)	13 (10.9%)
Dyspnea	11 (9.2%)	11 (9.2%)
Chest pain	10 (8.4%)	9 (7.6%)
Hypokalemia	10 (8.4%)	11 (9.2%)
Diarrhea	9 (7.6%)	17 (14.3%)
Dizziness	9 (7.6%)	5 (4.2%)
Headache	9 (7.6%)	13 (10.9%)
Pain	9 (7.6%)	10 (8.4%)
Sweating increased	9 (7.6%)	2 (1.7%)
Back pain	8 (6.7%)	6 (5%)
Hematuria[a]	8 (6.7%)	7 (5.9%)
Injection site reaction	8 (6.7%)	10 (8.4%)
Edema	8 (6.7%)	9 (7.6%)

MESNA — INJECTION

Incidence of Adverse Reactions and Incidence of Most Frequently Reported Adverse Reactions in Controlled Studies (%)		
Mesna regimen	IV-IV-IV (N = 119)	IV-oral-oral (N = 119)
Peripheral edema	8 (6.7%)	8 (6.7%)
Somnolence	8 (6.7%)	12 (10.1%)
Anxiety	7 (5.9%)	4 (3.4%)
Confusion	7 (5.9%)	6 (5%)
Face edema	6 (5%)	5 (4.2%)
Insomnia	6 (5%)	11 (9.2%)
Coughing	5 (4.2%)	10 (8.4%)
Dyspepsia	4 (3.4%)	6 (5%)
Hypotension	4 (3.4%)	6 (5%)
Pallor	4 (3.4%)	6 (5%)
Dehydration	3 (2.5%)	7 (5.9%)
Pneumonia	2 (1.7%)	8 (6.7%)
Tachycardia	1 (0.8%)	7 (5.9%)
Flushing	1 (0.8%)	6 (5%)

[a] All grades.

➤*Postmarketing surveillance:* Allergic reactions, decreased platelet counts associated with allergic reactions, hypertension, hypotension, increased heart rate, increased liver enzymes, injection site reactions (including pain and erythema), limb pain, malaise, myalgia, ST-segment elevation, tachycardia, and tachypnea have been reported as part of postmarketing surveillance.

Overdosage

There is no known antidote for mesna.

Oral doses of 6.1 and 4.3 g/kg were lethal to mice and rats, respectively. These doses are approximately 15 and 22 times the maximum recommended human dose on a body surface area basis. Death was preceded by diarrhea, tremor, convulsions, dyspnea, and cyanosis.

Patient Information

It is important for the patient to drink at least a quart (4 cups) of liquid a day whenever taking mesna.

A small number of patients taking mesna get blood in their urine (hematuria). Therefore, laboratory testing of the urine will be performed by the health care provider each day of mesna therapy. The laboratory test can find low levels of blood in the urine undetectable by viewing.

If the patient's urine has turned a pink or red color, contact the health care provider as soon as possible. Certain prescription medicines and foods, such as red beets, may also cause the urine to change color. A laboratory test of your urine will show if the source of the color is due to one of these causes or hematuria.

Mesna injection should be stored in a cool, dry place protected from excess moisture and heat. If possible, it should not be stored in the kitchen or bathroom. Any unused portion should be thrown away after the expiration date.

LEUCOVORIN CALCIUM (Folinic Acid; Citrovorum Factor)

Rx	**Leucovorin Calcium** (Various, eg, Barr)	**Tablets; oral:** 5 mg	In 30s, 100s and UD 50s.
Rx	**Leucovorin Calcium** (Lederle)	**Tablets; oral:** 15 mg	Lactose. (LL 15 C 35). Yellowish white, scored. Oval, convex. In 12s, 24s and UD 50s.
Rx	**Leucovorin Calcium** (Barr)	**Tablets; oral:** 25 mg	(485). Light green. In 25s.
Rx	**Leucovorin Calcium** (Various, eg, American Regent, Bedford)	**Injection, solution:** 10 mg/mL	In 5 mg single-dose vials (25s).
Rx	**Leucovorin Calcium** (Various, eg, Bedford, Lederle)	**Injection, solution, lyophilized:** 50 mg/vial	Preservative free. In vials.
Rx	**Leucovorin Calcium** (Various, eg, Bedford, Lederle)	**Injection, solution, lyophilized:** 100 mg/vial	Preservative free. In vials.
Rx	**Leucovorin Calcium** (Various, eg, APP Pharmaceutical, Bedford)	**Injection, solution, lyophilized:** 200 mg/vial	Preservative free. In vials.
		500 mg/vial	In vials.
Rx	**Leucovorin Calcium** (Various, eg, Bedford, Mayne)	**Injection, solution, lyophilized:** 350 mg/vial	Preservative free. In vials.

LEUCOVORIN CALCIUM — ORAL

Indications

➤*Methotrexate toxicity:* After high-dose methotrexate therapy in osteosarcoma. Leucovorin is also indicated to diminish the toxicity and counteract the effects of impaired methotrexate elimination and of inadvertent overdosages of folic acid antagonists.

➤*Off-label uses:* Treatment of non-Hodgkin lymphoma.

Administration and Dosage

➤*Adults:*

Leucovorin rescue after high-dose methotrexate therapy – The recommendations for leucovorin rescue are based on a methotrexate dose of 12 to 15 g/m^2 administered by IV infusion over 4 hours.

Some patients will have abnormalities in methotrexate elimination or renal function following methotrexate administration, which are significant but less severe than the abnormalities described. Those abnormalities may or may not be associated with significant clinical toxicity. If significant clinical toxicity is observed, leucovorin rescue should be extended for an additional 24 hours (total of 14 doses over 84 hours) in subsequent courses of therapy. The possibility that the patient is taking other medications that interact with methotrexate (eg, medications that may interfere with methotrexate elimination or binding to serum albumin) should always be reconsidered when laboratory abnormalities or clinical toxicities are observed.

Usual dosage: 15 mg (approximately 10 mg/m^2) every 6 hours for 10 doses starting 24 hours after the beginning of the methotrexate infusion. In the presence of GI toxicity, nausea, or vomiting, leucovorin should be administered parenterally.

Maximum dose: 25 mg/dose because absorption is saturable.

Dosage adjustment: Serum creatinine and methotrexate levels should be determined at least once daily. Adjust the dosage or duration of therapy according to the following table.

Leucovorin for Methotrexate Toxicity: Dosage Adjustment Guidelines[a]		
Clinical situation	Laboratory findings	Leucovorin dosage and duration
Normal methotrexate elimination	Methotrexate concentration after methotrexate dose: •24 hours after dose: 10 micromolar, •48 hours after dose: 1 micromolar, or •72 hours after dose: < 0.2 micromolar	15 mg orally, IM, or IV every 6 hours for 60 hours (10 doses), with the first dose given 24 hours after beginning methotrexate therapy.
Delayed late methotrexate elimination	Methotrexate concentration after methotrexate dose: •72 hours after dose: > 0.2 micromolar, or •96 hours after dose: > 0.05 micromolar	Continue 15 mg orally, IM, or IV every 6 hours until methotrexate level is < 0.05 micromolar.
Delayed early methotrexate elimination and/or evidence of acute renal injury	Methotrexate concentration after methotrexate dose: •24 hours after dose: ≥ 50 micromolar, or •48 hours after dose: ≥ 5 micromolar, or	Increase dose to 150 mg IV every 3 hours until methotrexate level is < 1 micromolar; then 15 mg IV every 3 hours until methotrexate level is < 0.05 micromolar.
	Serum creatinine after methotrexate dose: •24 hours after dose: increased ≥ 100% from baseline	

[a] IM = intramuscular; IV = intravenous.

Duration of therapy: Leucovorin, hydration, and urinary alkalinization (pH of 7 or higher) should be continued until the methotrexate level is below 5×10^{-8} M (0.05 micromolar).

Patients who experience delayed early methotrexate elimination are likely to develop reversible renal failure. In addition to appropriate leucovorin therapy, these patients require continuing hydration and urinary alkalinization and close monitoring of fluid and electrolyte status until the serum methotrexate level has fallen to below 0.05 micromolar and the renal failure has resolved.

LEUCOVORIN CALCIUM — ORAL

Concomitant therapy: Hydration and urinary alkalinization (pH of 7 or higher).

Impaired methotrexate elimination or inadvertent overdosage – The same dosage and administration guidelines may be used. However, leucovorin administration should begin as soon as possible after an inadvertent overdosage is recognized.

➤*Children:* See Adults for dosing.

➤*Elderly:* Care should be taken in dose selection. The risk of toxic reactions to the drug may be greater in patients with impaired renal function.

➤*Renal function impairment:* The risk of toxic reactions to the drug may be greater in patients with impaired renal function (See Warnings/Precautions).

➤*Storage/Stability:* Store between 15° to 30°C (59° to 86°F). Protect from light.

Actions

➤*Pharmacology:* Leucovorin is a mixture of the diastereoisomers of the 5-formyl derivative of tetrahydrofolic acid. The biologically active component of the mixture is the (−)-L-isomer, known as Citrovorum factor, or (−)-folinic acid. Leucovorin does not require reduction by the enzyme dihydrofolate reductase in order to participate in reactions utilizing folates as a source of "1-carbon" moieties. Following oral administration, leucovorin is rapidly absorbed and enters the general body pool of reduced folates.

The increase in plasma and serum reduced folate activity (determined microbiologically with *Lactobacillus casei*) seen after oral administration of leucovorin is predominantly due to 5-methyltetrahydrofolate.

Following a 20 mg dose of leucovorin calcium, the mean maximum serum total reduced folate concentrations were the following:

Tablet – Three hundred sixty-four ± 12.1 ng/mL at 2 ± 0.07 hours.

➤*Pharmacokinetics:*

Absorption – Oral tablets produced equivalent bioavailability (8% difference) when compared to the parenteral administration. The parenteral solution also provided equal bioavailability to the tablets when administered orally (2% difference). Oral absorption of leucovorin is saturable at doses above 25 mg. The apparent bioavailability of leucovorin was 97% for 25 mg, 75% for 50 mg and 37% for 100 mg.

Following oral administration, leucovorin is rapidly absorbed and expands the serum pool of reduced folates. After oral administration of leucovorin reconstituted with aromatic elixir, the mean peak concentration of serum total reduced folates was 393 ng/mL (range 160 to 550). At a dose of 25 mg, almost 100% of the l-isomer but only 20% of the d-isomer is absorbed. Oral absorption of leucovorin is saturable at doses above 25 mg. The apparent bioavailability of leucovorin was 97% for 25 mg, 75% for 50 mg, and 37% for 100 mg.

The mean time to peak was 2.3 hours and the terminal half-life was 5.7 hours. The mean peak of 5-methyl-THF was 367 ng/mL at 2.4 hours.

Metabolism – The major component was the metabolite 5-methyltetrahydrofolate to which leucovorin is primarily converted in the intestinal mucosa. The peak level of the parent compound was 51 ng/mL at 1.2 hours. The AUC of total reduced folates after oral administration of the 25 mg dose was 92% of the AUC after IV administration.

Excretion – The half-life of plasma 5-formyltetrahydrofolate was 1.5 ± 0.08 hours and that of the 5-methyltetrahydrofolate was 3 ± 0.09 hours. The terminal half-life was 5.7 hours.

Contraindications

Pernicious anemia and other megaloblastic anemias secondary to the lack of vitamin B_{12}.

Warnings/Precautions

➤*Folic acid antagonists overdosage:* In the treatment of accidental overdosages of folic acid antagonists, leucovorin should be administered as promptly as possible. As the time interval between antifolate administration (eg, methotrexate) and leucovorin rescue increases, leucovorin's effectiveness in counteracting toxicity diminishes.

➤*Methotrexate concentrations:* Monitoring of serum methotrexate concentration is essential in determining the optimal dose and duration of treatment with leucovorin.

Delayed methotrexate excretion may be caused by a third-space fluid accumulation (ie, ascites, pleural effusion), renal insufficiency, or inadequate hydration. Under such circumstances, higher doses of leucovorin or prolonged administration may be indicated. Doses higher than those recommended for oral use must be given IV.

➤*5-fluorouracil toxicity:* Leucovorin may enhance the toxicity of fluorouracil. Deaths from severe enterocolitis, diarrhea, and dehydration have been reported in elderly patients receiving weekly leucovorin and fluorouracil. Concomitant granulocytopenia and fever were present in some but not all of the patients.

➤*Seizures:* Seizures or syncope have been reported rarely in cancer patients receiving leucovorin, usually in association with fluoropyrimidine administration, and most commonly in those with CNS metastases or other predisposing factors; however, a causal relationship has not been established.

➤*Anemias:* Leucovorin is improper therapy for pernicious anemia and other megaloblastic anemias secondary to the lack of vitamin B_{12}. A hematologic remission may occur while neurologic manifestations remain progressive.

➤*Methotrexate toxicities:* Leucovorin has no effect on other established toxicities of methotrexate such as the nephrotoxicity resulting from drug or metabolite precipitation in the kidney.

➤*Parenteral administration:* Parenteral administration is preferable to oral dosing if there is a possibility that the patient may vomit or not absorb the leucovorin.

➤*Pregnancy: Category C.* Animal reproduction studies have not been conducted with leucovorin. It is also not known whether leucovorin can cause fetal harm when administered to a pregnant woman or can affect reproduction capacity. Leucovorin should be given to a pregnant woman only if clearly needed.

➤*Lactation:* It is not known whether this drug is excreted in human milk. Because many drugs are excreted in human milk, caution should be exercised when leucovorin is administered to a nursing mother.

➤*Children:* Folic acid in large amounts may counteract the antiepileptic effect of phenobarbital, phenytoin and primidone, and increase the frequency of seizures in susceptible children.

Drug Interactions

Leucovorin Drug Interactions

Precipitant drug	Object drug[a]		Description
Leucovorin	Anticonvulsants	⬇	Folic acid in large amounts may counteract the antiepileptic effect of phenobarbital, phenytoin and primidone, and increase the frequency of seizures in susceptible children. Although this interaction has not been reported with leucovorin, consider the possibility when using these drugs concomitantly.
Leucovorin	5-Fluorouracil	⬆	Leucovorin may enhance the toxicity of 5-FU (see Warnings).
Leucovorin	Methotrexate	⬇	Small quantities of systemically administered leucovorin enter the CSF primarily as 5-methyltetrahydrofolate and remain 1 to 3 orders of magnitude lower than the usual MTX concentrations following intrathecal administration. However, high doses of leucovorin may reduce the efficacy of intrathecally administered MTX.

[a] ⬆ = object drug increased; ⬇ = object drug decreased.

Adverse Reactions

Allergic sensitization, including anaphylactoid reactions and urticaria, has been reported following the administration of both oral and parenteral leucovorin.

Overdosage

Excessive amounts of leucovorin may nullify the chemotherapeutic effect of folic acid antagonists.

LEUCOVORIN CALCIUM — INJECTION

Indications

➤*Methotrexate toxicity:* After high-dose methotrexate therapy in osteosarcoma. Leucovorin calcium is also indicated to diminish the toxicity and counteract the effects of impaired methotrexate elimination and of inadvertent overdosage of folic acid antagonists.

➤*Megaloblastic anemia:* Treatment of megaloblastic anemias due to folic acid deficiency when oral therapy is not feasible.

➤*Advanced colorectal cancer:* For use in combination with 5-fluorouracil to prolong survival in the palliative treatment of patients with advanced colorectal cancer.

➤*Off-label uses:* Treatment of non-Hodgkin lymphoma.

Administration and Dosage

➤*General dosing considerations:* Leucovorin may be harmful or fatal if given intrathecally.

➤*Adults:*

Advanced colorectal cancer –

Usual dosage: Either of the 2 regimens is recommended:

- 200 mg/m^2 by slow intravenous (IV) injection over a minimum of 3 minutes, followed by 5-fluorouracil at 370 mg/m^2 by IV injection
- 20 mg/m^2 by IV injection followed by 5-fluorouracil at 425 mg/m^2 by IV injection.

5-flurouracil and leucovorin should be administered separately to avoid the formation of a precipitate.

LEUCOVORIN CALCIUM — INJECTION

Treatment is repeated daily for 5 days. This 5-day treatment course may be repeated at 4-week (28-day) intervals for 2 courses, and then repeated at 4- to 5-week (28- to 35-day) intervals, provided that the patient has completely recovered from the toxic effects of the prior treatment course.

Dosage adjustment: In subsequent treatment courses, the dosage of 5-fluorouracil should be adjusted based on patient tolerance of the prior treatment course. The daily dosage of 5-fluorouracil should be reduced by 20% for patients who experienced moderate hematologic or GI toxicity in the prior treatment course, and by 30% for patients who experienced severe toxicity. For patients who experienced no toxicity in the prior treatment course, 5-fluorouracil dosage may be increased by 10%. Leucovorin dosages are not adjusted for toxicity.

Leucovorin rescue after high-dose methotrexate therapy – The recommendations for leucovorin rescue are based on a methotrexate dose of 12 to 15 g/m^2 administered by IV infusion over 4 hours.

Some patients will have abnormalities in methotrexate elimination or renal function following methotrexate administration, which are significant but less severe than the abnormalities described below. Those abnormalities may or may not be associated with significant clinical toxicity. If significant clinical toxicity is observed, leucovorin rescue should be extended for an additional 24 hours (total of 14 doses over 84 hours) in subsequent courses of therapy. The possibility that the patient is taking other medications that interact with methotrexate (eg, medications that may interfere with methotrexate elimination or binding to serum albumin) should always be reconsidered when laboratory abnormalities or clinical toxicities are observed.

Usual dosage: 15 mg (approximately 10 mg/m^2) every 6 hours for 10 doses starting 24 hours after the beginning of the methotrexate infusion. In the presence of GI toxicity, nausea, or vomiting, leucovorin should be administered parenterally.

Dosage adjustment: Serum creatinine and methotrexate levels should be determined at least once daily. Adjust the dosage or duration of therapy according to the following table.

Leucovorin for Methotrexate Toxicity: Dosage Adjustment Guidelines

Clinical situation	Laboratory findings	Leucovorin dosage and duration
Normal methotrexate elimination	Methotrexate concentration after methotrexate dose: •24 hours after dose: 10 micromolar, •48 hours after dose: 1 micromolar, or •72 hours after dose: < 0.2 micromolar	15 mg orally, IM[a], or IV every 6 hours for 60 hours (10 doses), with the first dose given 24 hours after beginning methotrexate therapy.
Delayed late methotrexate elimination	Methotrexate concentration after methotrexate dose: •72 hours after dose: > 0.2 micromolar, or •96 hours after dose: > 0.05 micromolar	Continue 15 mg orally, IM, or IV every 6 hours, until methotrexate level is < 0.05 micromolar.
Delayed early methotrexate elimination and/or evidence of acute renal injury	Methotrexate concentration after methotrexate dose: •24 hours after dose: ≥ 50 micromolar, or •48 hours after dose: ≥ 5 micromolar, or Serum creatinine after methotrexate dose: •24 hours after dose: increased ≥ 100% from baseline	Increase dose to 150 mg IV every 3 hours until methotrexate level is < 1 micromolar; then 15 mg IV every 3 hours until methotrexate level is < 0.05 micromolar.

[a] IM = intramuscular.

Duration of therapy: Leucovorin, hydration, and urinary alkalinization (pH of 7 or higher) should be continued until the methotrexate level is below 5×10^{-8} M (0.05 micromolar).

Patients who experience delayed early methotrexate elimination are likely to develop reversible renal failure. In addition to appropriate leucovorin therapy, these patients require continuing hydration and urinary alkalinization, and close monitoring of fluid and electrolyte status, until the serum methotrexate level has fallen to below 0.05 micromolar and the renal failure has resolved.

Concomitant therapy: Hydration and urinary alkalinization (pH of 7 or higher).

Impaired methotrexate elimination or inadvertent overdosage – Leucovorin rescue should begin as soon as possible after an inadvertent overdosage and within 24 hours of methotrexate administration when there is delayed excretion. Delayed methotrexate excretion may be caused by a third-space fluid accumulation (ie, ascites, pleural effusion), renal insufficiency, or inadequate hydration. Under such circumstances, higher doses of leucovorin or prolonged administration may be indicated. Doses higher than those recommended for oral use must be given IV.

Usual dosage: 10 mg/m^2 administered IV, IM, or orally every 6 hours until the serum methotrexate level is less than 0.01 micromolar (1×10^{-8} M). In the presence of GI toxicity, nausea, or vomiting, leucovorin should be administered parenterally.

Dosage adjustment: Serum creatinine and methotrexate levels should be determined at 24-hour intervals. If the 24-hour serum creatinine has increased 50% over baseline or if the 24-hour methotrexate level is more than 5 micromolar (5×10^{-6} M) or the 48-hour level is more than 0.9 micromolar (9×10^{-7} M), the dose of leucovorin should be increased to 100 mg/m^2 IV every 3 hours until the methotrexate level is less than 0.01 micromolar.

Concomitant therapy: Hydration (3 L/day) and urinary alkalinization with sodium bicarbonate solution should be employed concomitantly. The bicarbonate dose should be adjusted to maintain the urine pH at 7 or higher.

Megaloblastic anemia due to folic acid deficiency – Up to 1 mg daily. There is no evidence that doses greater than 1 mg/day have greater efficacy than those of 1 mg; additionally, loss of folate in urine becomes roughly logarithmic as the amount administered exceeds 1 mg.

➤*Children:* See Adults for dosing.

➤*Elderly:* Care should be taken in dose selection. The risk of toxic reactions to the drug may be greater in patients with impaired renal function.

➤*Renal function impairment:* The risk of toxic reactions to the drug may be greater in patients with impaired renal function. (See Warnings/Precautions.)

➤*Preparation for administration:* Each leucovorin 350 mg vial when reconstituted with 17 mL of sterile diluent yields a leucovorin concentration of leucovorin 20 mg /mL. Leucovorin calcium for injection contains no preservative. Reconstitute with bacteriostatic water for injection, which contains benzyl alcohol, or with sterile water for injection. When reconstituted with bacteriostatic water for injection, the resulting solution must be used within 7 days. If the product is reconstituted with sterile water for injection, it must be used immediately.

When doses greater than 10 mg/m^2 are administered, leucovorin should be reconstituted with sterile water for injection and used immediately because of the benzyl alcohol contained in bacteriostatic water for injection.

➤*Administration:* Do not administer intrathecally. Leucovorin may be harmful or fatal if given intrathecally.

May be administered IV or IM. Because of the calcium content of the leucovorin solution, no more than 160 mg of leucovorin should be injected IV per minute (16 mL of a 10 mg/mL or 8 mL of a 20 mg/mL solution per minute).

➤*Admixture compatibility:* Leucovorin should not be mixed in the same infusion as 5-fluorouracil, because this may lead to the formation of a precipitate.

➤*Storage/Stability:*

10 mg/mL injection solution – Store in the refrigerator between 2° and 8°C (36° and 46°F). Protect from light.

Powders for solution – Store at 25°C (77°F): Excursions permitted between 15° and 30°C (59° and 86°F). Protect from light. When reconstituted with bacteriostatic water for injection, the resulting solution must be used within 7 days. If the product is reconstituted with sterile water for injection, it must be used immediately.

Actions

➤*Pharmacology:* Leucovorin is a mixture of the diastereoisomers of the 5-formyl derivative of tetrahydrofolic acid (THF). The biologically active compound of the mixture is the (−)-l-isomer, known as citrovorum factor or (−)-folinic acid. Leucovorin does not require reduction by the enzyme dihydrofolate reductase in order to participate in reactions utilizing folates as a source of "1-carbon" moieties. l-Leucovorin (l-5-formyltetrahydrofolate) is rapidly metabolized (via, 5,10-methenyltetrahydrofolate then 5,10-methylenetetrahydrofolate) to l-5-methyltetrahydrofolate. l – 5-Methyltetrahydrofolate can in turn be metabolized via other pathways back to 5,10-methylenetetrahydrofolate, which is converted to 5-methyltetrahydrofolate by an irreversible, enzyme catalyzed reduction using the cofactors $FADH_2$ and NADPH.

Administration of leucovorin can counteract the therapeutic and toxic effects of folic acid antagonists such as methotrexate, which act by inhibiting dihydrofolate reductase.

In contrast, leucovorin can enhance the therapeutic and toxic effects of fluoropyrimidines used in cancer therapy, such as 5-fluorouracil. Concurrent administration of leucovorin does not appear to alter the plasma pharmacokinetics of 5-fluorouracil. 5-fluorouracil is metabolized to fluorodeoxyuridylic acid, which binds to and inhibits the enzyme thymidylate synthase (an enzyme important in DNA repair and replication).

Leucovorin is readily converted to another reduced folate, 5, 10-methylenetetrahydrofolate, which acts to stabilize the binding of fluorodeoxyuridylic acid to thymidylate synthase and thereby enhances the inhibition of this enzyme.

➤*Pharmacokinetics:*

Absorption –

IV: The pharmacokinetics after IV, IM, and oral administration of a 25 mg dose of leucovorin were studied in male volunteers. After IV administration, serum total reduced folates (as measured by *Lactobacillus casei* assay) reached a mean peak of 1259 ng/mL (range 897 to 1625). The mean time to peak was 10 minutes. This initial rise in total reduced folates was primarily due to the parent compound 5-formyl-THF (measured by *Streptococcus faecalis* assay) which rose to 1206 ng/mL at 10 minutes. A sharp drop in parent compound followed and coincided with the appearance of the active metabolite 5-methyl-THF which became the predominant circulating form of the drug.

The mean peak of 5-methyl-THF was 258 ng/mL and occurred at 1.3 hours.

IM: After IM injection, the mean peak of serum total reduced folates was 436 mg/mL (range 240 to 725) and occurred at 52 minutes. Similar to IV administration, the initial sharp rise was due to the parent compound.

The mean peak of 5-formyl-THF was 360 ng/mL and occurred at 28 minutes. The level of the metabolite 5-methyl-THF increased subsequently over time until at 1.5 hours it represented 50% of the circulating total folates. The mean peak of 5-methyl-THF was 226 ng/mL at 2.8 hours.

LEUCOVORIN CALCIUM — INJECTION

Metabolism / Excretion –

IV: The terminal half-life for total reduced folates was 6.2 hours. The area under the concentration versus time curves (AUCs) for l-leucovorin, d-leucovorin and 5-methyltetrahydrofolate were 28.4 ± 3.5, 956 ± 97 and 129 ± 12 (mg.min/L ± S.E.). When a higher dose of d,l-leucovorin (200 mg/m^2) was used, similar results were obtained. The d-isomer persisted in plasma at concentrations greatly exceeding those of the l-isomer.

IM: The terminal half-life of total reduced folates was 6.2 hours. There was no difference of statistical significance between IM and IV administration in the AUC for total reduced folates. 5-formyl-THF, or 5-methyl-THF.

Contraindications

Pernicious anemia and other megaloblastic anemias secondary to the lack of vitamin B_{12}.

Warnings/Precautions

➤*Folic acid antagonists overdosage:* In the treatment of accidental overdosage of folic acid antagonists, IV leucovorin should be administered as promptly as possible. As the time interval between antifolate administration (eg, methotrexate) and leucovorin rescue increases, leucovorin's effectiveness in counteracting toxicity decreases. In the treatment of accidental overdosages of intrathecally administered folic acid antagonists, do not administer leucovorin intrathecally. Leucovorin may be harmful or fatal if given intrathecally.

➤*Methotrexate concentrations:* Monitoring of the serum methotrexate concentration is essential in determining the optimal dose and duration of treatment with leucovorin.

Delayed methotrexate excretion may be caused by a third-space fluid accumulation (ie, ascites, pleural effusion), renal insufficiency, or inadequate hydration. Under such circumstances, higher doses of leucovorin or prolonged administration may be indicated. Doses higher than those recommended for oral use must be given IV.

➤*Benzyl alcohol:* Because of the benzyl alcohol contained in certain diluents used for leucovorin calcium for injection, when doses greater than 10 mg/m^2 are administered, leucovorin calcium for injection should be reconstituted with Sterile Water for Injection, USP, and used immediately.

➤*Calcium content:* See Administration and Dosage for more information.

➤*5-fluorouracil dosage / toxicity:* Leucovorin enhances the toxicity of 5-fluorouracil. When those drugs are administered concurrently in the palliative therapy of advanced colorectal cancer, the dosage of 5-fluorouracil must be lower than usually administered. Although the toxicities observed in patients treated with the combination of leucovorin plus 5-fluorouracil are qualitatively similar to those observed in patients treated with 5-fluorouracil alone, GI toxicities (particularly stomatitis and diarrhea) are observed more commonly and may be more severe and of prolonged duration in patients treated with the combination.

In the first Mayo/NCCTG controlled trial, toxicity, primarily gastrointestinal, resulted in 7% of patients requiring hospitalization when treated with 5-fluorouracil alone or 5-fluorouracil in combination with 200 mg/m^2 of leucovorin and 20% when treated with 5-fluorouracil in combination with 20 mg/m^2 of leucovorin. In the second Mayo/NCCTG trial, hospitalizations related to treatment toxicity also appeared to occur more often in patients treated with the low-dose leucovorin/5-fluorouracil combination than in patients treated with the high-dose combination: 11% vs 3%. Therapy with leucovorin/5-fluorouracil must not be initiated or continued in patients who have symptoms of GI toxicity of any severity, until those symptoms have completely resolved. Patients with diarrhea must be monitored with particular care until the diarrhea has resolved, as rapid clinical deterioration leading to death can occur. In an additional study utilizing higher weekly doses of 5-FU and leucovorin, elderly or debilitated patients were found to be at greater risk for severe GI toxicity.

Since leucovorin enhances the toxicity of fluorouracil, leucovorin/5-fluorouracil combination therapy for advanced colorectal cancer should be administered under the supervision of a physician experienced in the use of antimetabolite cancer chemotherapy. Particular care should be taken in the treatment of elderly or debilitated colorectal cancer patients, as these patients may be at increased risk of severe toxicity.

➤*Seizures:* Seizures or syncope have been reported rarely in cancer patients receiving leucovorin, usually in association with fluoropyrimidine administration, and most commonly in those with CNS metastases or other predisposing factors; however, a causal relationship has not been established.

➤*Pneumocystis carinii pneumonia patients:* The concomitant use of leucovorin with trimethoprim-sulfamethoxazole for the acute treatment of *Pneumocystis carinii* pneumonia in patients with HIV infection was associated with increased rates of treatment failure and morbidity in a placebo-controlled study.

➤*Anemias:* Leucovorin is improper therapy for pernicious anemia and other megaloblastic anemias secondary to the lack of vitamin B_{12}. A hematologic remission may occur while neurologic manifestations continue to progress.

➤*Parenteral administration:* Parenteral administration is preferable to oral dosing if there is a possibility that the patient may vomit or not absorb the leucovorin. Leucovorin has no effect on nonhematologic toxicities of methotrexate such as the nephrotoxicity resulting from drug or metabolite precipitation in the kidney.

➤*Renal function impairment:* This drug is known to be excreted by the kidney, and the risk of toxic reactions to the drug may be greater in patients with impaired renal function.

➤*Pregnancy: Category C.* Adequate animal reproduction studies have not been conducted with leucovorin. It is also not known whether leucovorin can cause fetal harm when administered to a pregnant woman or can affect reproduction capacity. Leucovorin should be given to a pregnant woman only if clearly needed.

➤*Lactation:* It is not known whether this drug is excreted in human milk. Because many drugs are excreted in human milk, caution should be exercised when leucovorin is administered to a nursing mother.

➤*Children:* See Drug Interactions for more information.

➤*Elderly:* Clinical studies of leucovorin calcium did not show differences in safety or efficacy between subjects over age 65 and younger subjects. Other clinical experience has not identified differences in responses between the elderly and younger patients, but greater sensitivity of some older patients cannot be ruled out. This drug is known to be excreted by the kidney, and the risk of toxic reactions to the drug may be greater in patients with impaired renal function. Because elderly patients are more likely to have decreased renal function, care should be taken in dose selection in this patient population.

➤*Monitoring:* Patients being treated with the leucovorin/5-fluorouracil combination should have a CBC with differential and platelets prior to each treatment. During the first 2 courses, a CBC with differential and platelets has to be repeated weekly and thereafter once each cycle at the time of anticipated WBC nadir. Electrolytes and liver function tests should be performed prior to each treatment for the first 3 cycles then prior to every other cycle. Dosage modifications of fluorouracil should be instituted as follows, based on the most severe toxicities:

For moderate diarrhea or stomatitis, WBC nadir 1000 to 1900 mm^3, or platelet nadir 25 to 75,000 mm^3, decrease 5-FU dosage by 20%. For severe diarrhea or stomatitis, WBC nadir less than 1000 mm^3, or platelet nadir less than 25,000 mm^3, decrease 5-FU dosage by 30%.

If no toxicity occurs, the 5-fluorouracil dose may increase 10%. Treatment should be deferred until WBCs are 4000/mm^3 and platelets 130,000/mm^3. If blood counts do not reach these levels within 2 weeks, treatment should be discontinued. Patients should be followed up with physical examination prior to each treatment course and appropriate radiological examination as needed. Treatment should be discontinued when there is clear evidence of tumor progression.

Drug Interactions

Leucovorin Drug Interactions

Precipitant drug	Object drug[a]		Description
Leucovorin	Anticonvulsants	⬇	Folic acid in large amounts may counteract the antiepileptic effect of phenobarbital, phenytoin and primidone, and increase the frequency of seizures in susceptible children. Although this interaction has not been reported with leucovorin, consider the possibility when using these drugs concomitantly.
Leucovorin	5-Fluorouracil	⬆	Leucovorin may enhance the toxicity of 5-FU (see Warnings).
Leucovorin	Methotrexate	⬇	Small quantities of systemically administered leucovorin enter the CSF primarily as 5-methyltetrahydrofolate and remain 1 to 3 orders of magnitude lower than the usual MTX concentrations following intrathecal administration. However, high doses of leucovorin may reduce the efficacy of intrathecally administered MTX.

[a] ⬆ = object drug increased; ⬇ = object drug decreased.

Adverse Reactions

Allergic sensitization, including anaphylactoid reactions and urticaria, has been reported following administration of both oral and parenteral leucovorin. No other adverse reactions have been attributed to the use of leucovorin per se.

LEUCOVORIN CALCIUM — INJECTION

Percentage of Patients Treated With Leucovorin/Fluorouracil for Advanced Colorectal Carcinoma Reporting Adverse Reactions or Hospitalized for Toxicity

Adverse reaction	(High LV)[a]/5-FU (n = 155) Any[c] (%)	Grade 3+[d] (%)	(Low LV)[b]/5-FU (n = 161) Any[c] (%)	Grade 3+[d] (%)	5-FU alone (n = 70) Any[c] (%)	Grade 3+[d] (%)
Leukopenia	69%	14%	83%	23%	93%	48%
Thrombocytopenia	8%	2%	8%	1%	18%	3%
Infection	8%	1%	3%	1%	7%	2%
Nausea	74%	10%	80%	9%	60%	6%
Vomiting	46%	8%	44%	9%	40%	7%
Diarrhea	66%	18%	67%	14%	43%	11%
Stomatitis	75%	27%	84%	29%	59%	16%
Constipation	3%	0%	4%	0%	1%	
Lethargy/malaise/fatigue	13%	3%	12%	2%	6%	3%
Alopecia	42%	5%	43%	6%	37%	7%
Dermatitis	21%	2%	25%	1%	13%	
Anorexia	14%	1%	22%	4%	14%	
Hospitalization for toxicity	5%		15%		7%	

[a] High LV = leucovorin 200 mg/m².
[b] Low LV = leucovorin 20 mg/m².
[c] Any = percentage of patients reporting toxicity of any severity.
[d] Grade 3+ = percentage of patients reporting toxicity of grade 3 or higher.

Overdosage

Excessive amounts of leucovorin may nullify the chemotherapeutic effect of folic acid antagonists.

LEVOLEUCOVORIN

Rx	**Fusilev** (Spectrum Pharmaceuticals)	**Injection, lyophilized, powder for solution:** 50 mg	Equivalent to levoleucovorin calcium 64 mg. Contains mannitol 50 mg. In single-use vials.

LEVOLEUCOVORIN CALCIUM — INJECTION

Indications

➤*Rescue after high-dose methotrexate therapy:* Levoleucovorin rescue is indicated after high-dose methotrexate therapy in osteosarcoma.

➤*Impaired methotrexate elimination or inadvertent overdosage:* Levoleucovorin is also indicated to diminish the toxicity and counteract the effects of impaired methotrexate elimination and of inadvertent overdosage of folic acid antagonists.

Administration and Dosage

➤*General dosing considerations:* Levoleucovorin is dosed at one-half the usual dose of the racemic form.

Although levoleucovorin may ameliorate the hematologic toxicity associated with high-dose methotrexate, levoleucovorin has no effect on other established toxicities of methotrexate, such as the nephrotoxicity resulting from drug and/or metabolite precipitation in the kidney.

➤*Adults:*

Rescue after high-dose methotrexate therapy – The recommendations for levoleucovorin rescue are based on a methotrexate dose of 12 g/m² administered by intravenous (IV) infusion over 4 hours.

Usual dosage: 7.5 mg (approximately 5 mg/m²) IV every 6 hours for 10 doses starting 24 hours after the beginning of the methotrexate infusion.

Serum creatinine and methotrexate levels should be determined at least once daily. Levoleucovorin administration, hydration, and urinary alkalinization (pH of 7 or greater) should be continued until the methotrexate level is below 5×10^{-8} M (0.05 micromolar).

Dosage adjustment: The levoleucovorin dose should be adjusted or rescue extended based on the following guidelines.

Guidelines for Levoleucovorin Dosage and Administration

Clinical situation	Laboratory findings	Levoleucovorin dosage and duration
Normal methotrexate elimination	Serum methotrexate level approximately 10 micromolar at 24 h after administration, 1 micromolar at 48 h, and at 72 h	7.5 mg IV every 6 h for 60 h (10 doses starting at 24 h after start of methotrexate infusion).
Delayed late methotrexate elimination	Serum methotrexate level remaining above 0.2 micromolar at 72 h, and > 0.05 micromolar at 96 h after administration.	Continue 7.5 mg IV every 6 hours, until methotrexate level is < 0.05 micromolar.
Delayed early methotrexate elimination and/or evidence of acute renal injury	Serum methotrexate level of ≥ 50 micromolar at 24 h, or ≥ 5 micromolar at 48 h after administration, or a 100% or greater increase in serum creatinine level at 24 hours after methotrexate administration (eg, an increase from 0.5 mg/dL to a level of 1 mg/dL or more).	75 mg IV every 3 h until methotrexate level is 7.5 mg IV every 3 h until methotrexate level is < 0.05 micromolar.

Some patients will have abnormalities in methotrexate elimination or renal function following methotrexate administration, which are significant but less severe than the abnormalities described in the previous table. These abnormalities may or may not be associated with significant clinical toxicity. If significant clinical toxicity is observed, levoleucovorin rescue should be extended for an additional 24 hours (total of 14 doses over 84 hours) in subsequent courses of therapy. The possibility that the patient is taking other medications that interact with methotrexate (eg, medications that may interfere with methotrexate elimination or binding to serum albumin) should always be reconsidered when laboratory abnormalities or clinical toxicities are observed.

Delayed methotrexate excretion may be caused by accumulation in a third space fluid collection (ie, ascites, pleural effusion), renal function impairment, or inadequate hydration. Under such circumstances, higher doses of levoleucovorin or prolonged administration may be indicated.

Concomitant therapy: Patients who experience delayed early methotrexate elimination are likely to develop reversible renal failure. In addition to appropriate levoleucovorin therapy, these patients require continuing hydration and urinary alkalinization and close monitoring of fluid and electrolyte status until the serum methotrexate level has fallen to below 0.05 micromolar and the renal failure has resolved.

Impaired methotrexate elimination or inadvertent overdosage – Levoleucovorin rescue should begin as soon as possible after an inadvertent overdosage and within 24 hours of methotrexate administration when there is delayed excretion. As the time interval between antifolate administration (eg, methotrexate) and levoleucovorin rescue increases, levoleucovorin's effectiveness in counteracting toxicity may decrease.

Usual dosage: 7.5 mg (approximately 5 mg/m²) IV every 6 hours until the serum methotrexate level is less than 10^{-8} M.

Dosage adjustment: Serum creatinine and methotrexate levels should be determined at 24-hour intervals. If the 24-hour serum creatinine has increased 50% over baseline or if the 24-hour methotrexate level is more than 5×10^{-6} M or the 48-hour level is more than 9×10^{-7} M, the dose of levoleucovorin should be increased to 50 mg/m² IV every 3 hours until the methotrexate level is less than 10^{-8} M.

Concomitant therapy: Hydration (3 L/day) and urinary alkalinization with sodium bicarbonate should be employed concomitantly. The bicarbonate dose should be adjusted to maintain the urine pH at 7 or greater.

➤*Children:* The safety and efficacy of levoleucovorin rescue following high-dose methotrexate were evaluated in 16 patients 6 to 21 years of age who received 58 courses of therapy for osteogenic sarcoma. High-dose methotrexate was one component of several different combination chemotherapy regimens evaluated across several trials. Methotrexate 12 g/m² IV over 4 hours was administered to 13 patients who received levoleucovorin 7.5 mg every 6 hours for 60 hours or longer beginning 24 hours after completion of methotrexate. Three patients received methotrexate 12.5 g/m² IV over 6 hours, followed by levoleucovorin 7.5 mg every 3 hours for 18 doses beginning 12 hours after completion of methotrexate. The mean number of levoleucovorin doses per course was 18.2 and the mean total dose per course was 350 mg. The efficacy of levoleucovorin rescue following high-dose methotrexate was based on the adverse reaction profile.

➤*Preparation for administration:* Prior to IV injection, the 50 mg vial of levoleucovorin for injection is reconstituted with 5.3 mL of sodium chloride 0.9% injection to yield a levoleucovorin concentration of 10 mg/mL. Reconstitution with sodium chloride solutions with preservatives (eg, benzyl alco-

LEVOLEUCOVORIN CALCIUM — INJECTION

hol) has not been studied. The use of solutions other than sodium chloride 0.9% injection is not recommended.

The reconstituted levoleucovorin 10 mg/mL contains no preservative. Observe strict aseptic technique during reconstitution of the drug product.

Saline reconstituted levoleucovorin solutions may be further diluted, immediately, to concentrations of 0.5 to 5 mg/mL in sodium chloride 0.9% injection or dextrose 5% injection. Initial reconstitution or further dilution using sodium chloride 0.9% injection may be held at room temperature for not more than a total of 12 hours. Dilutions in dextrose 5% injection may be held at room temperature for not more than 4 hours.

➤*Administration:* Levoleucovorin is indicated for IV administration only. Do not administer intrathecally.

No more than 16 mL of reconstituted solutions (levoleucovorin 160 mg) should be injected IV per minute, because of the calcium content of the levoleucovorin solution.

➤*Admixture compatibility:* Because of the risk of precipitation, do not coadminister levoleucovorin with other agents in the same admixture.

➤*Storage/Stability:* Store at 25°C (77°F) in carton until contents are used. Excursions are permitted between 15° and 30°C (59° and 86°F). Protect from light.

Actions

➤*Pharmacology:* Levoleucovorin is a folate analog. Levoleucovorin is the pharmacologically active isomer of 5-formyl tetrahydrofolic acid. Levoleucovorin does not require reduction by the enzyme dihydrofolate reductase in order to participate in reactions utilizing folates as a source of one-carbon moieties. Administration of levoleucovorin can counteract the therapeutic and toxic effects of folic acid antagonists such as methotrexate, which act by inhibiting dihydrofolate reductase.

Pharmacodynamics – Levoleucovorin is actively and passively transported across cell membranes. In vivo, levoleucovorin is converted to 5-methyltetrahydrofolic acid (5-methyl-THF), the primary circulating form of active reduced folate. Levoleucovorin and 5-methyl-THF are polyglutamated intracellularly by the enzyme folylpolyglutamate synthetase. Folylpolyglutamates are active and participate in biochemical pathways that require reduced folate.

➤*Pharmacokinetics:*

Absorption – The pharmacokinetics of levoleucovorin after IV administration of a 15 mg dose were studied in healthy male volunteers. After rapid IV administration, serum total tetrahydrofolate (total-THF) concentrations reached a mean peak of 1,722 ng/mL. Serum (6S)-5-methyl-5,6,7,8-tetrahydrofolate concentrations reached a mean peak of 275 ng/mL, and the mean time to peak was 0.9 hours.

Excretion – The mean terminal half-life for total-THF and (6S)-5-methyl-5,6,7,8- tetrahydrofolate was 5.1 and 6.8 hours, respectively.

Contraindications

Previous allergic reactions attributed to folic acid or folinic acid.

Warnings/Precautions

➤*Rate of administration:* Because of the Ca^{++} content of the levoleucovorin solution, inject no more than 16 mL (levoleucovorin 160 mg) IV per minute.

➤*Pregnancy: Category C.* It is not known whether levoleucovorin can cause fetal harm when administered to a pregnant woman or if it can affect reproduction capacity. Animal reproduction studies have not been conducted with levoleucovorin. Give levoleucovorin to a pregnant woman only if clearly needed.

➤*Lactation:* It is not known whether this drug is excreted in human milk. Because many drugs are excreted in human milk, exercise caution when levoleucovorin is administered to a breast-feeding mother.

➤*Children:* The safety and efficacy of levoleucovorin rescue following high-dose methotrexate were evaluated in 16 patients 6 to 21 years of age who received 58 courses of therapy for osteogenic sarcoma. High-dose methotrexate was one component of several different combination chemotherapy regimens evaluated across several trials. Methotrexate 12 g/m² IV over 4 hours was administered to 13 patients who received levoleucovorin 7.5 mg every 6 hours for 60 hours or longer beginning 24 hours after completion of methotrexate. Three patients received methotrexate 12.5 g/m² IV over 6 hours, followed by levoleucovorin 7.5 mg every 3 hours for 18 doses beginning 12 hours after completion of methotrexate. The mean number of levoleucovorin doses per course was 18.2 and the mean total dose per course was 350 mg. The efficacy of levoleucovorin rescue following high-dose methotrexate was based on the adverse reaction profile.

➤*Elderly:* Deaths from severe enterocolitis, diarrhea, and dehydration have been reported in elderly patients receiving weekly d,l-leucovorin and 5-fluorouracil.

Drug Interactions

Levoleucovorin Drug Interactions			
Precipitant drug	Object drug[a]		Description
Levoleucovorin	Anticonvulsants	⬇	Folic acid in large amounts may counteract the antiepileptic effect of phenobarbital, phenytoin, and primidone, and increase the frequency of seizures in susceptible children. Although this interaction has not been reported with leucovorin, consider the possibility when using these drugs concomitantly.
Levoleucovorin	5-Fluorouracil	⬆	Leucovorin may enhance the toxicity of the 5-fluorouracil. Deaths from severe enterocolitis, diarrhea, and dehydration have been reported in elderly patients receiving weekly d,l-leucovorin and 5-fluorouracil.
Levoleucovorin	Methotrexate	⬇	Small quantities of systemically administered leucovorin enter the cerebrospinal fluid primarily as 5-methyltetra-hydrofolate and remain 1 to 3 order of magnitude lower than the usual methotrexate concentrations following intrathecal administration. However, high doses of leucovorin may reduce the efficacy of intrathecally administered methotrexate.
Levoleucovorin	Trimethoprim-Sulfamethoxazole	⬇	Concomitant use of d,l-leucovorin with trimethoprim-sulfamethoxazole for the acute treatment of *Pneumocystis carinii* pneumonia in patients with HIV infection was associated with increased rates of treatment failure and morbidity in a placebo-controlled study.

[a] ⬆ = object drug increased; ⬇ = object drug decreased.

Adverse Reactions

Because clinical trials are conducted under widely varying conditions, adverse reaction rates observed in the clinical trials of a drug cannot be directly compared with rates in the clinical trials of another drug and may not reflect the rates observed in practice. The following table presents the frequency of adverse reactions that occurred during the administration of 58 courses of high-dose methotrexate 12 g/m² followed by levoleucovorin rescue for osteosarcoma in 16 patients 6 to 21 years of age. Most patients received levoleucovorin 7.5 mg every 6 hours for 60 hours or longer beginning 24 hours after completion of methotrexate.

Levoleucovorin Adverse Reactions				
Adverse reactions	Number (%) of patients with adverse reactions (N = 16)		Number (%) of courses with adverse reactions (N = 58)	
	All	Grade 3+	All	Grade 3+
CNS				
Confusion	6.3%	0%	1.7%	0%
Neuropathy	6.3%	0%	1.7%	0%
GI				
Diarrhea	6.3%	0%	1.7%	0%
Dyspepsia	6.3%	0%	1.7%	0%
Nausea	18.8%	0%	5.2%	0%
Stomatitis	37.5%	6.3%	17.2%	1.7%
Taste perversion	6.3%	0%	1.7%	0%
Typhlitis	6.3%	6.3%	1.7%	1.7%
Vomiting	37.5%	0%	24.1%	0%
Dermatologic				
Dermatitis	6.3%	0%	1.7%	0%
Respiratory				
Dyspnea	6.3%	0%	1.7%	0%
Miscellaneous				
Renal function abnormal	6.3%	0%	5.2%	0%

LEVOLEUCOVORIN CALCIUM — INJECTION

The incidence of adverse reactions may be underestimated because not all patients were fully evaluable for toxicity for all cycles in the clinical trials. Leukopenia and thrombocytopenia were observed, but could not be attributed to high-dose methotrexate with levoleucovorin rescue because patients were receiving other myelosuppressive chemotherapy.

➤*Postmarketing:* Spontaneously reported adverse reactions collected by the World Health Organization Collaborating Center for International Drug Monitoring in Uppsala, Sweden have yielded 7 cases in which levoleucovorin was administered with a regimen of methotrexate. The events were dyspnea, pruritus, rash, temperature change, and rigors. For 217 adverse reactions (108 reports) for which levoleucovorin was a suspected or interacting medication, there were 40 occurrences of possible allergic reaction.

Overdosage

➤*Animal toxicology:* The acute IV median lethal dose (LD_{50}) values in adult mice and rats were 575 mg/kg (1,725 mg/m^2) and 378 mg/kg (2,268 mg/m^2), respectively. Signs of sedation, tremors, reduced motor activity, prostration, labored breathing, and/or convulsion were observed in these studies. Anticipated human dose for each administration is approximately 5 mg/m^2, which represents a 3-log safety margin.

DNA DEMETHYLATION AGENTS

AZACITIDINE

Rx	**Vidaza** (Celgene)	**Injection, lyophilized powder**[a]: 100 mg	Preservative free. In single-use vials.

[a] Reconstituted as a suspension for subcutaneous injection or as a solution with further dilution for intravenous (IV) infusion.

AZACITIDINE — INJECTION

Indications

➤*Myelodysplastic syndrome:* For the treatment of patients with the following French-American-British (FAB) myelodysplastic syndrome (MDS) subtypes: refractory anemia or refractory anemia with ringed sideroblasts (RARS) (if accompanied by neutropenia or thrombocytopenia or requiring transfusions), refractory anemia with excess blasts (RAEB), refractory anemia with excess blasts in transformation (RAEB-T), and chronic myelomonocytic leukemia (CMMoL).

➤*Off-label uses:* Refractory acute lymphocytic leukemia; refractory acute myelogenous leukemia.

Administration and Dosage

➤*General dosing considerations:* Patients should be premedicated for nausea and vomiting.

Patients should be monitored for hematologic response and renal toxicities.

Reduced doses may be needed in patients with renal impairment (see Renal Function Impairment).

➤*Adults:*

Myelodysplastic syndrome –

Initial dosage: 75 mg/m^2 subcutaneously or IV daily for 7 days.

Maintenance dosage: Cycles should be repeated every 4 weeks. It is recommended that patients be treated for a minimum 4 to 6 cycles; however, complete or partial response may require additional treatment cycles.

Dosage adjustment: The dose may be increased to 100 mg/m^2 if no beneficial effect is seen after 2 treatment cycles and if no toxicity other than nausea and vomiting has occurred.

For patients with baseline white blood cell count (WBC) of 3 × 10^9/L or more, absolute neutrophil count (ANC) of 1.5 × 10^9/L or more, and platelets of 75 × 10^9/L or more, adjust the dosage based on nadir counts for any given cycle.

Azacitidine Dosage Adjustment Based on Hematology Values

Nadir counts		% dose in the next course
ANC (× 10^9/L)	Platelets (× 10^9/L)	
< 0.5	< 25	50%
0.5 to 1.5	25 to 50	67%
> 1.5	> 50	100%

For patients whose baseline counts are WBC less than 3 × 10^9/L, ANC less than 1.5 × 10^9/L or platelets less than 75 × 10^9/L, dose adjustments should be based on nadir counts and bone marrow biopsy cellularity at the time of the nadir, unless there is clear improvement in differentiation (percentage of mature granulocytes is higher than ANC at onset of that course) at the time of the next cycle, in which case the dose of the current treatment should be continued.

Azacitidine Dose Adjustments Based on Nadir Counts and Bone Marrow Biopsy Cellularity

WBC or platelet nadir % decrease in counts from baseline	Bone marrow biopsy cellularity at time of nadir		
	30% to 60%	15% to 30%	< 15%
	% dose in the next course		
50% to 75%	100%	50%	33%
> 75%	75%	50%	33%

If a nadir, as defined in the previous table, has occurred, the next course of treatment should be given 28 days after the start of the preceding course, providing that both the WBC and the platelet counts are greater than 25% above the nadir and rising. If a greater than 25% increase above nadir is not seen by day 28, counts should be reassessed every 7 days. If a 25% increase is not seen by day 42, then the patient should be treated with 50% of the scheduled dose.

Duration of therapy: Treatment may be continued as long as the patient continues to benefit.

➤*Elderly:* Care should be taken in dose selection. It may be useful to monitor renal function.

➤*Renal function impairment:* Closely monitor patients with renal impairment for toxicity because azacitidine and its metabolites are primarily excreted by the kidneys. If unexplained elevations of serum urea nitrogen (BUN) or serum creatinine occur, the next cycle should be delayed until values return to normal or baseline, and the dose should be reduced by 50% on the next treatment course.

➤*Electrolytes:* If unexplained reduction in serum bicarbonate levels to less than 20 mEq/L occurs, the dosage should be reduced 50% on the next course.

➤*Preparation for administration:*

Subcutaneous administration – Reconstitute aseptically with 4 mL of sterile water for injection. The diluent should be injected slowly into the vial. Vigorously shake or roll the vial until a uniform suspension is achieved. The suspension will be cloudy. The resulting suspension will contain azacitidine 25 mg/mL.

For immediate subcutaneous administration, the product may be held at room temperature for up to 1 hour, but must be administered within 1 hour after reconstitution.

For delayed subcutaneous administration, the reconstituted product may be kept in the vial or drawn into a syringe. The product must be refrigerated immediately, and may be held under refrigerated conditions (2° to 8°C; 36° to 46°F) for up to 8 hours. After removal from refrigerated conditions, the suspension may be allowed to equilibrate to room temperature for up to 30 minutes prior to administration.

IV administration – Reconstitute the appropriate number of azacitidine vials to achieve the desired dose. Reconstitute each vial with 10 mL of sterile water for injection. Vigorously shake or roll the vial until all solids are dissolved. The resulting solution will contain azacitidine 10 mg/mL. The solution should be clear. Withdraw the required amount of azacitidine solution to deliver the desired dose and inject into a 50 to 100 mL infusion bag of sodium chloride 0.9% injection or Ringer's lactate injection.

➤*Administration:* Doses for more than 4 mL should be divided equally into 2 syringes.

Subcutaneous administration – To provide a homogeneous suspension, the contents of the syringe must be resuspended immediately prior to administration. To resuspend, vigorously roll the syringe between the palms until a uniform, cloudy suspension is achieved.

Azacitidine suspension is administered subcutaneously. Rotate sites for each injection (thigh, abdomen, or upper arm). New injections should be given at least 1 inch from an old site, and never into areas where the site is tender, bruised, red, or hard.

IV administration – Azacitidine solution is administered IV. Administer the total dose over a period of 10 to 40 minutes. The administration must be completed within 1 hour of reconstitution of the azacitidine vial.

➤*Admixture compatibility:* Azacitidine IV solution is incompatible with dextrose 5% solutions, *HESpan* (hetastarch 6% in sodium chloride 0.9% injection), or solutions that contain bicarbonate. These solutions have the potential to increase the rate of degradation of azacitidine and should therefore be avoided.

➤*Storage / Stability:* Store unreconstituted vials at 25°C (77°F); excursions are permitted to 15° to 30°C (59° to 86°F). Unused portions of each vial should be discarded properly. Do not save any unused portions for later administration.

Suspension – Store for up to 1 hour at 25°C (77°F) or for up to 8 hours between 2° and 8°C (36° and 46°F).

Solution – Store at 25°C (77°F), but administration must be completed within 1 hour of reconstitution.

Actions

➤*Pharmacology:* Azacitidine is a pyrimidine nucleoside analog of cytidine. Azacitidine is believed to exert its antineoplastic effects by causing hypomethylation of DNA and direct cytotoxicity on abnormal hematopoietic cells in the bone marrow. The concentration of azacitidine required for maximum inhibition of DNA methylation in vitro does not cause major suppression of DNA synthesis. Hypomethylation may restore normal function to genes that are critical for differentiation and proliferation. The cytotoxic effects of azacitidine cause the death of rapidly dividing cells, including cancer cells that are no longer responsive to normal growth control mechanisms. Nonproliferating cells are relatively insensitive to azacitidine.

AZACITIDINE — INJECTION

➤*Pharmacokinetics:*

Absorption / Distribution – Azacitidine is rapidly absorbed after subcutaneous administration; the peak plasma azacitidine concentration of 750 ± 403 ng/mL occurred in 0.5 hours. The bioavailability of subcutaneous azacitidine relative to IV azacitidine is approximately 89%, based on area under the curve (AUC). Mean volume of distribution following IV dosing is 76 ± 26 L.

Metabolism / Excretion – Mean apparent subcutaneous clearance is 167 ± 49 L/h, and mean half-life after subcutaneous administration is 41 ± 8 minutes. An in vitro study of azacitidine incubation in human liver fractions indicated that azacitidine may be metabolized by the liver.

Published studies indicate that urinary excretion is the primary route of elimination of azacitidine and its metabolites. Following IV administration of radioactive azacitidine to 5 patients with cancer, the cumulative urinary excretion was 85% of the radioactive dose. Fecal excretion accounted for less than 1% of administered radioactivity over 3 days. Mean excretion of radioactivity in urine following subcutaneous administration of ^{14}C-azacitidine was 50%. The mean elimination half-lives of total radioactivity (azacitidine and its metabolites) were similar after IV and subcutaneous administrations, about 4 hours.

Contraindications

Advanced malignant hepatic tumors; known hypersensitivities to azacitidine or mannitol.

Warnings/Precautions

➤*Hematologic effects:* Treatment with azacitidine is associated with anemia, neutropenia, and thrombocytopenia. Perform complete blood cell counts (CBCs) as needed to monitor response and toxicity, but at minimum, prior to each dosing cycle. After administration of the recommended dosage for the first cycle, reduce or delay dosage for subsequent cycles based on nadir counts and hematologic response.

➤*Use in men:* Advise men not to father a child while receiving treatment with azacitidine. In animal studies, preconception treatment of male mice and rats resulted in increased embryofetal loss in mated females.

➤*Renal function impairment:* Safety and effectiveness of azacitidine in patients with MDS and renal impairment have not been studied, because these patients were excluded from the clinical trials.

Closely monitor patients with renal impairment for toxicity because azacitidine and its metabolites are primarily excreted by the kidneys.

Renal abnormalities ranging from elevated serum creatinine to renal failure and death have been reported rarely in patients treated with azacitidine IV in combination with other chemotherapeutic agents for non-MDS conditions. In addition, renal tubular acidosis, defined as a fall in serum bicarbonate to less than 20 mEq/L in association with an alkaline urine and hypokalemia (serum potassium less than 3 mEq/L) developed in 5 patients with CML treated with azacitidine and etoposide. If unexplained reductions in serum bicarbonate of less than 20 mEq/L or elevations of serum urea nitrogen (BUN) or serum creatinine occur, reduce the dosage or hold as described previously.

➤*Hepatic function impairment:* Safety and effectiveness of azacitidine in patients with MDS and hepatic impairment have not been studied because these patients were excluded from the clinical trials.

Because azacitidine is potentially hepatotoxic in patients with severe preexisting hepatic impairment, caution is needed in patients with liver disease. Patients with extensive tumor burden caused by metastatic disease have been rarely reported to experience progressive hepatic coma and death during azacitidine treatment, especially in such patients with baseline albumin less than 30 g/L. Azacitidine is contraindicated in patients with advanced malignant hepatic tumors.

➤*Pregnancy: Category D.* There are no adequate and well-controlled studies in pregnant women using azacitidine. It is not known if azacitidine crosses the human placenta. The molecular weight (244) and elimination half-life suggest that the drug will cross to the embryo and/or fetus. Do not give pregnant women this drug, especially in the first trimester. If this drug is used during pregnancy, or if the patient becomes pregnant while taking this drug, apprise the patient of the potential hazard to the fetus.

Advise women of childbearing potential to avoid becoming pregnant while receiving treatment with azacitidine. Advise female partners of men receiving azacitidine not to become pregnant.

Teratogenic – Azacitidine may cause fetal harm when administered to a pregnant woman. Azacitidine caused congenital malformations in animals. Early embryotoxicity studies in mice revealed a 44% frequency of intrauterine embryonal death (increased resorption) after a single intraperitoneal injection of 6 mg/m^2 (approximately 8% of the recommended human daily dose on a mg/m^2 basis) azacitidine on gestation day 10. Developmental abnormalities in the brain have been detected in mice given azacitidine on or before gestation day 15 at doses of approximately 3 to 12 mg/m^2 (approximately 4% to 16% the recommended human daily dose on a mg/m^2 basis).

In rats, azacitidine was clearly embryotoxic when given intraperitoneally on gestation days 4 to 8 (postimplantation) at a dose of 6 mg/m^2 (approximately 8% of the recommended human daily dose on a mg/m^2 basis), although treatment in the preimplantation period (on gestation days 1 to 3) had no adverse effect on the embryos. Azacitidine caused multiple fetal abnormalities in rats after a single intraperitoneal dose of 3 to 12 mg/m^2 (approximately 8% the recommended human daily dose on a mg/m^2 basis) given on gestation day 9, 10, 11, or 12. In this study, azacitidine caused fetal death when administered at 3 to 12 mg/m^2 on gestation days 9 and 10; average live animals per litter was reduced to 9% of control at the highest dose on gestation day 9. Fetal anomalies included CNS anomalies (exencephaly/encephalocele), limb anomalies (micromelia, club foot, syndactyly, and oligodactyly), and others (micrognathia, gastroschisis, edema, and rib abnormalities).

➤*Lactation:* It is not known whether azacitidine or its metabolites are excreted in human milk. The molecular weight (244) and the elimination half-life (about 4 hours) suggest that the drug will be excreted into breast milk. The potential effects of this exposure on a breast-feeding infant are unknown, but the effects may be severe. Because of the potential for tumorigenicity shown for azacitidine in animal studies and the potential for serious adverse reactions in breast-feeding infants, decide whether to discontinue breast-feeding or the drug, taking into consideration the importance of the drug to the mother.

➤*Children:* Safety and effectiveness in children have not been established.

➤*Elderly:* Azacitidine and its metabolites are known to be substantially excreted by the kidney, and the risk of adverse reactions to this drug may be greater in patients with impaired renal function. Because elderly patients are more likely to have decreased renal function, take care in dose selection, and it may be useful to monitor renal function.

➤*Monitoring:* Obtain liver chemistries and serum creatinine prior to initiation of therapy.

Perform CBCs as needed to monitor response and toxicity, but at a minimum, prior to each dosing cycle. After administration of the recommended dosage for the first cycle, reduce or delay dosage for subsequent cycles based on nadir counts and hematologic response.

Closely monitor patients with renal impairment for toxicity because azacitidine and its metabolites are primarily excreted by the kidneys.

Drug Interactions

None known.

Adverse Reactions

For more information on anemia, elevated serum creatinine, hepatic coma, hypokalemia, neutropenia, renal failure, renal tubular acidosis, and/or thrombocytopenia, refer to Warnings/Precautions.

➤*Most common adverse reactions:* Anemia, constipation, diarrhea, ecchymosis, injection-site erythema, leukopenia, nausea, neutropenia, pyrexia, thrombocytopenia, vomiting. The most common adverse reactions by IV route also included hypokalemia, petechiae, rigors, and weakness.

➤*Discontinuation because of adverse reactions:* Leukopenia, neutropenia, thrombocytopenia (more than 2%).

➤*Dose held because of adverse reactions:* Febrile neutropenia, leukopenia, neutropenia, pneumonia, pyrexia, thrombocytopenia (more than 2%).

➤*Dose reduced because of adverse reactions:* Leukopenia, neutropenia, thrombocytopenia (more than 2%).

➤*Adverse reactions in clinical trials:*

Studies 1 and 2 (subcutaneous) –

Azacitidine Most Frequent Adverse Reactions (≥ 5%) (Studies 1 and 2)[a]		
Adverse reactions[a]	Azacitidine (n = 220)[b]	Observation (n = 92)[c]
Cardiovascular		
Hematoma	8.6%	0%
Hypotension	6.8%	2.2%
Petechiae	23.6%	8.7%
CNS		
Anxiety	13.2%	3.3%
Dizziness	18.6%	5.4%
Headache	21.8%	10.9%
Insomnia	10.9%	4.3%
Lethargy	7.7%	2.2%
Malaise	10.9%	1.1%
Dermatologic		
Dry skin	5%	1.1%
Ecchymosis	30.5%	15.2%
Erythema	16.8%	4.3%
Injection-site bruising	14.1%	0%
Injection-site erythema	35%	0%
Injection-site granuloma	5%	0%
Injection-site pain	22.7%	0%
Injection-site pigmentation changes	5%	0%
Injection-site pruritus	6.8%	0%
Injection-site reaction	13.6%	0%
Injection-site swelling	5%	0%
Rash	14.1%	9.8%
Skin nodule	5%	1.1%
Urticaria	5.9%	1.1%

AZACITIDINE — INJECTION

Azacitidine Most Frequent Adverse Reactions (≥ 5%) (Studies 1 and 2)[a]		
Adverse reactions[a]	Azacitidine (n = 220)[b]	Observation (n = 92)[c]
GI		
Abdominal tenderness	11.8%	1.1%
Anorexia	20.5%	6.5%
Constipation	33.6%	6.5%
Diarrhea	36.4%	14.1%
Gingival bleeding	9.5%	4.3%
Loose stools	5.5%	0%
Mouth hemorrhage	5%	1.1%
Nausea	70.5%	17.4%
Stomatitis	7.7%	0%
Vomiting	54.1%	5.4%
Hematologic/Lymphatic		
Aggravated anemia	5.5%	5.4%
Anemia	69.5%	64.1%
Febrile neutropenia	16.4%	4.3%
Leukopenia	48.2%	29.3%
Neutropenia	32.3%	10.9%
Thrombocytopenia	65.5%	45.7%
Respiratory		
Dyspnea	29.1%	12%
Nasopharyngitis	14.5%	3.3%
Pneumonia	10.9%	5.4%
Upper respiratory tract infection	12.7%	4.3%
Miscellaneous		
Arthralgia	22.3%	3.3%
Chest pain	16.4%	5.4%
Chest wall pain	5%	0%
Myalgia	15.9%	2.2%
Postprocedural hemorrhage	5.9%	1.1%
Pyrexia	51.8%	30.4%

[a] Multiple reports of the same preferred terms for a patient are only counted once within each treatment group.
[b] Includes reactions from all patients exposed to azacitidine, including patients after crossing over from observation.
[c] Includes reactions from observation period only; excludes any events after crossover to azacitidine.

Study 4 (subcutaneous) – Similar to studies 1 and 2 , duration of exposure to treatment with azacitidine was longer (mean, 12.2 months) compared with best supportive care (mean, 7.5 months).

Azacitidine Most Frequent Adverse Reactions (≥ 5%) (Study 4)[a]				
	Any grade		Grade 3/4	
Adverse reactions	Azacitidine (n = 175)	Best supportive care only (n = 102)	Azacitidine (n = 175)	Best supportive care only (n = 102)
CNS				
Anxiety	5.1%	1%	0%	0%
Fatigue	24%	11.8%	3.4%	2%
Insomnia	8.6%	2.9%	0%	0%
Lethargy	7.4%	2%	0%	1%
Dermatologic				
Erythema	7.4%	2.9%	0%	0%
Injection-site bruising	5.1%	0%	0%	0%
Injection-site erythema	42.9%	0%	0%	0%
Injection-site hematoma	6.3%	0%	0%	0%
Injection-site induration	5.1%	0%	0%	0%
Injection-site pain	18.9%	0%	0%	0%
Injection-site rash	5.7%	0%	0%	0%
Petechiae	11.4%	3.9%	1.1%	0%
Pruritus	12%	2%	0%	0%
Rash	10.3%	1%	0%	0%
GI				
Abdominal pain	12.6%	6.9%	4%	0%
Constipation	50.3%	7.8%	1.1%	0%
Dyspepsia	5.7%	2%	0%	0%
Nausea	48%	11.8%	1.7%	0%
Vomiting	26.9%	6.9%	0%	0%
GU				
Hematuria	6.3%	2%	2.3%	1%
Urinary tract infection	8.6%	2.9%	1.7%	0%
Hematologic				
Anemia	51.4%	44.1%	13.7%	8.8%
Febrile neutropenia	13.7%	9.8%	12.6%	6.9%
Leukopenia	18.3%	2%	14.9%	1%
Neutropenia	65.7%	28.4%	61.1%	21.6%
Thrombocytopenia	69.7%	34.3%	58.3%	28.4%
Respiratory				
Dyspnea	14.9%	4.9%	3.4%	2%
Dyspnea exertional	5.1%	1%	0%	0%
Pharyngolaryngeal pain	6.3%	2.9%	0%	0%
Rhinitis	5.7%	1%	0%	0%
Upper respiratory tract infection	9.1%	3.9%	1.7%	0%
Miscellaneous				
Hypertension	8.6%	3.9%	1.1%	2%
Hypokalemia	6.3%	2.9%	1.7%	2.9%
Injection-site reaction	29.1%	0%	0.6%	0%
Pyrexia	30.3%	17.6%	4.6%	1%
Weight decreased	8%	0%	0.6%	0%

[a] Multiple reports or the same preferred term from a patient were only counted once within each treatment.

In studies 1, 2, and 4 with subcutaneous administration of azacitidine, adverse reactions of neutropenia, thrombocytopenia, anemia, nausea, vomiting, diarrhea, constipation and injection-site erythema/reaction tended to increase in incidence with increasing doses of azacitidine. Adverse reactions that tended to be more pronounced during the first 1 to 2 cycles of subcutaneous treatment compared with later cycles included thrombocytopenia, neutropenia, anemia, nausea, vomiting, injection-site erythema/pain/bruising/reactions, constipation, petechiae, dizziness, anxiety, hypokalemia, and insomnia. There did not appear to be any adverse reactions that increased in frequency over the course of treatment.

➤*IV administration:* Overall, adverse reactions were qualitatively similar between the IV and subcutaneous studies. Adverse reactions that appeared to be specifically associated with the IV route of administration included infusion-site reactions (eg, erythema, pain) and catheter-site reactions (eg, infection, erythema, hemorrhage).

➤*Other adverse reactions (less than 5%):*

Cardiovascular – Atrial fibrillation, cardiac failure, cardiac failure congestive, cardiorespiratory arrest, congestive cardiomyopathy, orthostatic hypotension.

CNS – Cerebral hemorrhage, convulsions, intracranial hemorrhage.

Dermatologic – Cellulitis, pruritic rash, pyoderma gangrenosum, skin induration.

GI – Diverticulitis, GI hemorrhage, melena, perirectal abscess.

GU – Loin pain, renal failure.

Hematologic/Lymphatic – Agranulocytosis, bone marrow failure, pancytopenia, splenomegaly.

Hypersensitivity – Anaphylactic shock, hypersensitivity.

Musculoskeletal – Aggravated bone pain, muscle weakness, neck pain.

Respiratory – Hemoptysis, lung infiltration, pneumonitis, respiratory distress.

Miscellaneous – Bacterial infection, blastomycosis, catheter-site hemorrhage, cholecystectomy, cholecystitis, dehydration, eye hemorrhage, general physical health deterioration, injection-site infection, *Klebsiella* sepsis, leukemia cutis, limb abscess, neutropenic sepsis, pharyngitis streptococcal, pneumonia *Klebsiella*, sepsis, septic shock, staphylococcal bacteremia, staphylococcal infection, systemic inflammatory response syndrome, toxoplasmosis.

Overdosage

➤*Symptoms:* One case of overdose with azacitidine was reported during clinical trials. A patient experienced diarrhea, nausea, and vomiting after receiving a single IV dose of approximately 290 mg/m², almost 4 times the recommended starting dose. The events resolved without sequelae, and the correct dose was resumed the following day.

AZACITIDINE — INJECTION

➤*Treatment:* In the event of overdosage, monitor the patient with appropriate blood counts and receive supportive treatment, as necessary. There is no known specific antidote for azacitidine overdosage.

Patient Information

Advise patients to inform their health care provider about any underlying liver or renal disease.

Advise women of childbearing potential to avoid becoming pregnant while receiving treatment with azacitidine. For breast-feeding mothers, decide whether to discontinue breast-feeding or the drug, taking into consideration the importance of the drug to the mother.

Advise men not to father children while receiving treatment with azacitidine.

NELARABINE

Rx	**Arranon** (GlaxoSmithKline)	**Injection, solution:** 5 mg/mL	Sodium chloride 4.5 mg/mL. In vials.

NELARABINE — INJECTION

WARNING

Neurologic adverse reactions – Severe neurologic reactions have been reported with the use of nelarabine. These reactions have included the following: altered mental states, including severe somnolence; CNS effects, including convulsions; and peripheral neuropathy, ranging from numbness and paresthesias to motor weakness and paralysis. There have also been reports of reactions associated with demyelination and ascending peripheral neuropathies similar in appearance to Guillain-Barré syndrome.

Full recovery from these reactions has not always occurred with cessation of therapy with nelarabine. Close monitoring for neurologic reactions is strongly recommended; discontinue nelarabine for neurologic reactions of National Cancer Institute (NCI) Common Toxicity Criteria grade 2 or greater.

Indications

➤*Leukemia/Lymphoma:* Nelarabine is indicated for the treatment of patients with T-cell acute lymphoblastic leukemia and T-cell lymphoblastic lymphoma whose disease has not responded to or has relapsed following treatment with at least 2 chemotherapy regimens. This use is based on the induction of complete responses. Randomized trials demonstrating increased survival or other clinical benefit have not been conducted.

➤*Off-label uses:* Relapsed or refractory B-cell acute lymphocytic leukemia, prolymphocytic leukemia, chronic lymphocytic leukemia, chronic myeloid leukemia in blast phase, non-Hodgkin lymphoma.

Administration and Dosage

➤*Adults:*

Leukemia/Lymphoma – 1,500 mg/m^2 administered intravenously (IV) over 2 hours on days 1, 3, and 5, repeated every 21 days.

Off-label dosing –

Combination therapy (ie, fludarabine): 1,200 mg/m^2 administered IV over 1 hour for 3 doses each cycle, given on alternate days (days 1, 3, and 5). Repeat courses every 21 to 28 days.

➤*Children:*

Leukemia/Lymphoma – 650 mg/m^2 administered IV over 1 hour daily for 5 consecutive days, repeated every 21 days.

➤*Discontinuation of therapy:* Nelarabine should be discontinued for neurologic events of NCI Common Toxicity Criteria grade 2 or greater. Dosage may be delayed for other toxicities, including hematologic toxicity.

➤*Preparation for administration:* Nelarabine is considered a cytotoxic agent. Follow safe handling procedures when preparing, administering, or dispensing nelarabine.

Use of gloves and other protective clothing to prevent skin contact is recommended.

Nelarabine is not diluted prior to administration. The appropriate dose of nelarabine is transferred into polyvinyl chloride (PVC) infusion bags or glass containers and then administered.

➤*Administration:* Nelarabine is administered undiluted as a 2-hour infusion in adult patients and as a 1-hour infusion in pediatric patients.

Appropriate measures (eg, hydration, urine alkalinization, prophylaxis with allopurinol) must be taken to prevent hyperuricemia of tumor lysis syndrome.

➤*Storage/Stability:* Store at 25°C (77°F); excursions are permitted between 15° and 30°C (59° and 86°F). Nelarabine is stable in PVC infusion bags and glass containers for up to 8 hours at up to 30°C (86°F).

Discard vial within 6 hours of the initial needle puncture if opened within an ISO Class 5 biological safety cabinet, or within 1 hour of the initial needle puncture if opened outside of such an environment, based on the USP Chapter <797> standards.

Actions

➤*Pharmacology:* Nelarabine is a prodrug of the deoxyguanosine analog 9-β-D-arabinofuranosylguanine (ara-G). Nelarabine is demethylated by adenosine deaminase to ara-G, mono-phosphorylated by deoxyguanosine kinase and deoxycytidine kinase, and subsequently converted to the active 5′-triphosphate, ara-GTP. Accumulation of ara-GTP in leukemic blasts allows for incorporation into DNA, leading to inhibition of DNA synthesis and cell death. Other mechanisms may contribute to the cytotoxic and systemic toxicity of nelarabine.

➤*Pharmacokinetics:*

Absorption – Following IV administration of nelarabine to adult patients with refractory leukemia or lymphoma, plasma ara-G maximum plasma concentration (C_{max}) values generally occurred at the end of the nelarabine infusion and were generally higher than nelarabine C_{max} values, suggesting rapid and extensive conversion of nelarabine to ara-G. Mean plasma nelarabine and ara-G C_{max} values were 5 ± 3 mcg/mL and 31.4 ± 5.6 mcg/mL, respectively, after a nelarabine 1,500 mg/m^2 dose infused over 2 hours in adult patients. The area under the curve (AUC) of ara-G is 37 times higher than that for nelarabine on day 1 after nelarabine IV infusion of 1,500 mg/m^2 dose (162 ± 49 mcg•h/mL vs 4.4 ± 2.2 mcg•h/mL, respectively). Comparable C_{max} and AUC were obtained for nelarabine between days 1 and 5 at the nelarabine adult dose of 1,500 mg/m^2, indicating that nelarabine does not accumulate after multiple dosing. There are not enough data for ara-G to make a comparison between day 1 and day 5. After a nelarabine adult dose of 1,500 mg/m^2, intracellular C_{max} for ara-GTP appeared within 3 to 25 hours on day 1. Exposure (AUC) to intracellular ara-GTP was 532 times higher than that for nelarabine and 14 times higher than that for ara-G (2,339 ± 2,628 mcg•h/mL vs 4.4 ± 2.2 mcg•h/mL and 162 ± 49 mcg•h/mL, respectively).

Distribution – Nelarabine and ara-G are extensively distributed throughout the body. For nelarabine, apparent volume of distribution at steady state (V_{ss}) values were 197 ± 216 L/m^2 in adult patients. For ara-G, apparent volume of distribution at steady state after non-IV administration (V_{ss}/F) values were 50 ± 24 L/m^2 in adult patients.

Nelarabine and ara-G are not substantially bound to human plasma proteins (less than 25%) in vitro, and binding is independent of nelarabine or ara-G concentrations up to 600 mcM.

Metabolism – The principal route of metabolism for nelarabine is O-demethylation by adenosine deaminase to form ara-G, which undergoes hydrolysis to form guanine. In addition, some nelarabine is hydrolyzed to form methylguanine, which is O-demethylated to form guanine. Guanine is N-deaminated to form xanthine, which is further oxidized to yield uric acid.

Excretion – Nelarabine and ara-G are rapidly eliminated from plasma with a mean half-life of 18 minutes and 3.2 hours, respectively, in adult patients.

Combined phase 1 pharmacokinetic data at nelarabine doses of 199 to 2,900 mg/m^2 (n = 66 adult patients) indicate that the mean clearance of nelarabine is 197 ± 189 L/h/m^2 on day 1. The apparent clearance of ara-G (clearance/F) is 10.5 ± 4.5 L/h/m^2 on day 1.

Nelarabine and ara-G are partially eliminated by the kidneys. Mean urinary excretion of nelarabine and ara-G was 6.6% ± 4.7% and 27% ±15% of the administered dose, respectively, in 28 adult patients over the 24 hours after nelarabine infusion on day 1. Renal clearance averaged 24 ± 23 L/h for nelarabine and 6.2 ± 5 L/h for ara-G in 21 adult patients.

Special populations –

Children: Combined phase 1 pharmacokinetic data at doses of nelarabine 104 to 2,900 mg/m^2 indicate that the mean clearance of nelarabine is about 30% higher in children than in adult patients (259 ± 409 L/h/m^2 vs 197 ±189 L/h/m^2, respectively; n = 66 adults, n = 22 children) on day 1. The apparent clearance of ara-G (clearance/F) is comparable between the 2 groups (10.5 ± 4.5 L/h/m^2 in adult patients and 11.3 ± 4.2 L/h/m^2 in children) on day 1.

Nelarabine and ara-G are extensively distributed throughout the body. For nelarabine, V_{ss} values were 213 ± 358 L/m^2 in children. For ara-G, V_{ss}/F values were 33 ± 9.3 L/m^2 in children, respectively. Nelarabine and ara-G are rapidly eliminated from plasma in children, with a half-life of 13 minutes and 2 hours, respectively.

Contraindications

None well documented.

Warnings/Precautions

➤*Neurologic effects:* Neurotoxicity is the dose-limiting toxicity of nelarabine. Closely observe patients undergoing therapy with nelarabine for signs and symptoms of neurologic toxicity.

Common signs and symptoms of nelarabine-related neurotoxicity include somnolence, confusion, convulsions, ataxia, paresthesias, and hypesthesia. Severe neurologic toxicity can manifest as coma, status epilepticus, craniospinal demyelination, or ascending neuropathy similar in presentation to Guillain-Barré syndrome.

Patients treated previously or concurrently with intrathecal chemotherapy or previously with craniospinal irradiation may be at increased risk for neurologic adverse reactions.

NELARABINE — INJECTION

➤*Hematologic effects:* Leukopenia, thrombocytopenia, anemia, and neutropenia (including febrile neutropenia) have been associated with nelarabine therapy. Regularly monitor complete blood cell counts, including platelets.

➤*Hyperuricemia:* Patients receiving nelarabine should receive IV hydration according to standard medical practice for the management of hyperuricemia in patients at risk for tumor lysis syndrome. Consider the use of allopurinol in patients at risk of hyperuricemia.

➤*Vaccines:* Avoid administration of live vaccines to immunocompromised patients.

➤*Renal function impairment:* Because the risk of adverse reactions to this drug may be greater in patients with moderate (creatinine clearance [CrCl] = 30 to 50 mL/min) or severe (CrCl less than 30 mL/min) renal impairment, closely monitor these patients for toxicities when treated with nelarabine.

➤*Hepatic function impairment:* Because the risk of adverse reactions to this drug may be greater in patients with severe hepatic impairment (total bilirubin more than 3 times the upper limit of normal), closely monitor these patients for toxicities when treated with nelarabine.

➤*Hazardous tasks:* Because patients receiving nelarabine therapy may experience somnolence, caution them about operating hazardous machinery, including automobiles.

➤*Pregnancy: Category D.* Nelarabine may cause fetal harm when administered to a pregnant woman. There are no studies of nelarabine in pregnant women. It is not known if nelarabine or ara-G can cross the human placenta. The molecular weight (about 297) of nelarabine and the lack of protein binding suggest that these agents will reach the embryo and fetus. The short plasma half-lives should decrease the exposure. If this drug is used during pregnancy, or if the patient becomes pregnant while taking this drug, apprise the patient of the potential hazard to the fetus. Advise women of childbearing potential to avoid becoming pregnant while receiving treatment with nelarabine.

Nelarabine administration during the period of organogenesis caused increased incidences of fetal malformations, anomalies, and variations in rabbits at dosages 360 mg/m^2/day or more (8-hour IV infusion; approximately one-fourth the adult dosage compared on a mg/m^2 basis), which was the lowest dosage tested. Cleft palate was seen in rabbits given 3,600 mg/m^2/day (approximately 2-fold the adult dosage) and absent pollices (digits) was seen in rabbits given 1,200 mg/m^2/day or more (approximately three-fourths the adult dosage), while absent gallbladder, absent accessory lung lobes, fused or extra sternebrae, and delayed ossification was seen at all dosages. Maternal body weight gain and fetal body weights were reduced in rabbits given 3,600 mg/m^2/day (approximately 2-fold the adult dosage), but could not account for the increased incidence of malformations seen at this or lower administered dosages.

➤*Lactation:* It is not known whether nelarabine or ara-G are excreted in human milk. The molecular weight (about 297) and lack of protein binding suggest that nelarabine and ara-G will be excreted into breast milk. The short plasma half-lives of 30 minutes and 3 hours, respectively, should decrease the exposure, but the terminal elimination half-life of the intracellular active metabolite ara-GTP has not been determined. Because many drugs are excreted in human milk and because of the potential for serious adverse reactions in breast-feeding infants from nelarabine, decide whether to discontinue breast-feeding or the drug, taking into account the importance of the drug to the mother.

➤*Children:* The safety and effectiveness of nelarabine have been established in children.

➤*Elderly:* Because elderly patients are more likely to have decreased renal function, take care in dose selection; it may be useful to monitor renal function.

➤*Monitoring:* Regularly monitor complete blood cell counts, including platelets. Close monitoring for neurologic reactions is strongly recommended. Closely monitor patients with moderate (CrCl = 30 to 50 mL/min) or severe (CrCl less than 30 mL/min) renal impairment or severe hepatic impairment for toxicity.

Drug Interactions

➤*Vaccines:* See Warnings/Precautions for more information.

➤*Pentostatin:* Coadministration of nelarabine and pentostatin is not recommended. Administration of pentostatin, a strong inhibitor of adenosine deaminase, may result in a reduction in the conversion of the prodrug nelarabine to its active metabolite, reducing the efficacy of nelarabine and changing the adverse reaction profile of either drug.

Adverse Reactions

➤*Adults:*

Common adverse reactions –

Nelarabine Adverse Reactions in Adult Patients (≥ 5%)

Adverse reactions	Toxicity grade (N = 103)		
	Grade 3	Grade 4 and 5[a]	All grades
Cardiovascular			
Hypotension	1%	1%	8%
Sinus tachycardia	1%	0%	8%
CNS			
Abnormal gait	0%	0%	6%
Asthenia	0%	1%	17%
Confusional state	2%	0%	8%
Depression	1%	0%	6%
Fatigue	10%	2%	50%
Insomnia	0%	0%	7%
Rigors	0%	0%	8%
GI			
Abdominal distension	0%	0%	6%
Abdominal pain	1%	0%	9%
Anorexia	0%	0%	9%
Constipation	1%	0%	21%
Diarrhea	1%	0%	22%
Nausea	0%	0%	41%
Stomatitis	1%	0%	8%
Vomiting	1%	0%	22%
Hematologic/Lymphatic			
Anemia	20%	14%	99%
Febrile neutropenia	9%	1%	12%
Neutropenia	14%	49%	81%
Thrombocytopenia	37%	22%	86%
Metabolic/Nutritional			
Dehydration	3%	1%	7%
Edema	0%	0%	11%
Edema, peripheral	0%	0%	15%
Hyperglycemia	1%	0%	6%
Musculoskeletal			
Arthralgia	1%	0%	9%
Back pain	0%	0%	8%
Muscular weakness	5%	0%	8%
Myalgia	1%	0%	13%
Pain in extremity	1%	0%	7%
Respiratory			
Cough	0%	0%	25%
Dyspnea	4%	2%	20%
Dyspnea, exertional	0%	0%	7%
Epistaxis	0%	0%	8%
Pleural effusion	5%	1%	10%
Pneumonia	4%	1%	8%
Sinusitis	1%	0%	7%
Wheezing	0%	0%	5%
Miscellaneous			
AST increased	1%	1%	6%
Chest pain	0%	0%	5%
Chest pain, noncardiac	0%	1%	5%
Infection	2%	1%	9%
Pain	3%	0%	11%
Petechiae	2%	0%	12%
Pyrexia	5%	0%	23%

[a] Five patients had a fatal adverse reaction. Fatal reactions included hypotension (n = 1), respiratory arrest (n = 1), pleural effusion/pneumothorax (n = 1), pneumonia (n = 1), and cerebral hemorrhage/coma/leukoencephalopathy (n = 1).

Other adverse reactions – Blurred vision was also reported in 4% of adult patients.

There was a single report of biopsy-confirmed progressive multifocal leukoencephalopathy in the adult patient population.

CNS: Nervous system reactions, regardless of drug relationship, were reported for 76% of patients across the phase 1 and 2 studies.

NELARABINE — INJECTION

Nelarabine Neurologic Adverse Reactions (≥ 2%) in Adult Patients					
	(N = 103)				
Adverse reactions	Grade 1	Grade 2	Grade 3	Grade 4	All grades
Amnesia	2%	1%	0%	0%	3%
Ataxia	1%	6%	2%	0%	9%
Balance disorder	1%	1%	0%	0%	2%
Depressed level of consciousness	4%	1%	0%	1%	6%
Dizziness	14%	8%	0%	0%	21%
Dysgeusia	2%	1%	0%	0%	3%
Headache	11%	3%	1%	0%	15%
Hypesthesia	5%	10%	2%	0%	17%
Paresthesia	11%	4%	0%	0%	15%
Peripheral neurologic disorders, any reaction	8%	12%	2%	0%	21%
Neuropathy	0%	4%	0%	0%	4%
Peripheral motor neuropathy	3%	3%	1%	0%	7%
Peripheral neuropathy	2%	2%	1%	0%	5%
Peripheral sensory neuropathy	7%	6%	0%	0%	13%
Sensory loss	0%	2%	0%	0%	2%
Somnolence	20%	3%	0%	0%	23%
Tremor	2%	3%	0%	0%	5%

One patient had a fatal neurologic reaction, cerebral hemorrhage/coma/leukoencephalopathy.

• *Other neurologic adverse reactions* – Most nervous system reactions in the adult patients were evaluated as grade 1 or 2. The additional grade 3 reactions in adult patients, regardless of causality, were aphasia, convulsion, hemiparesis, and loss of consciousness, each reported in 1 (1%) patient. The additional grade 4 reactions, regardless of causality, were cerebral hemorrhage, coma, intracranial hemorrhage, leukoencephalopathy, and metabolic encephalopathy, each reported in 1 (1%) patient.

The other neurologic adverse reactions, regardless of causality, reported as grade 1, 2, or unknown in adult patients were abnormal coordination, burning sensation, disturbance in attention, dysarthria, hyporeflexia, neuropathic pain, nystagmus, peroneal nerve palsy, sciatica, sensory disturbance, sinus headache, and speech disorder, each reported in 1 (1%) patient.

➤*Children:*

Common adverse reactions –

Nelarabine Adverse Reactions in Children (≥ 5%)			
	(N = 84)		
	Toxicity grade		
Adverse reactions	Grade 3	Grade 4 and 5[a]	All grades
Hematologic/Lymphatic			
Anemia	45%	10%	95%
Leukopenia	14%	7%	38%
Neutropenia	17%	62%	94%
Thrombocytopenia	27%	32%	88%
Hepatic			
Blood albumin decreased	5%	1%	10%
Blood bilirubin increased	7%	2%	10%
Transaminases increased	4%	0%	12%
Lab test abnormalities			
Blood calcium decreased	1%	1%	8%
Blood creatinine increased	0%	0%	6%
Blood glucose decreased	4%	0%	6%
Blood magnesium decreased	2%	0%	6%
Blood potassium decreased	4%	2%	11%
Miscellaneous			
Asthenia	1%	0%	6%
Infection	2%	1%	5%
Vomiting	0%	0%	10%

[a] Three patients had a fatal adverse reaction. Fatal adverse reactions included neutropenia and pyrexia (n = 1), status epilepticus/seizure (n = 1), and fungal pneumonia (n = 1).

CNS – Nervous system adverse reactions, regardless of drug relationship, were reported for 42% of children across the phase 1 and 2 studies.

Nelarabine Neurologic Adverse Reactions in Children (≥ 2%)					
	(N = 84)				
Adverse reactions	Grade 1	Grade 2	Grade 3	Grade 4 and 5[a]	All grades
Ataxia	1%	0%	1%	0%	2%
CNS disorder	1%	2%	0%	0%	4%
Headache	8%	2%	4%	2%	17%
Hypesthesia	1%	1%	4%	0%	6%
Motor dysfunction	1%	1%	1%	0%	4%
Paresthesia	0%	2%	1%	0%	4%
Peripheral neurologic disorders, any reaction	1%	4%	7%	0%	12%
Peripheral motor neuropathy	1%	0%	2%	0%	4%
Peripheral neuropathy	0%	4%	2%	0%	6%
Peripheral sensory neuropathy	0%	0%	6%	0%	6%
Somnolence	1%	4%	1%	1%	7%
Seizures	0%	0%	0%	6%	6%
Convulsions	0%	0%	0%	3%	4%
Generalized tonic-clonic convulsions	0%	0%	0%	1%	1%
Status epilepticus	0%	0%	0%	1%	1%
Tremor	1%	2%	0%	0%	4%

[a] One patient had a fatal neurologic reaction, status epilepticus.

Other neurologic reactions: The other grade 3 reaction in children, regardless of causality, was hypertonia reported in 1 patient. The additional grade 4 reactions, regardless of causality, were third nerve paralysis, and sixth nerve paralysis, each reported in 1 patient. The other neurologic adverse reactions, regardless of causality, reported as grade 1, 2, or unknown in children were dysarthria, encephalopathy, hydrocephalus, hyporeflexia, lethargy, mental impairment, paralysis, and sensory loss, each reported in 1 patient.

➤*Postmarketing:*

CNS – Demyelination and ascending peripheral neuropathies similar in appearance to Guillain-Barré syndrome.

Miscellaneous – Fatal opportunistic infections, tumor lysis syndrome.

Overdosage

➤*Symptoms:* It is anticipated that overdosage would result in severe neurotoxicity (possibly including paralysis, coma), myelosuppression, and potentially death.

Nelarabine has been administered in clinical trials up to a dose of 2,900 mg/m^2 on days 1, 3, and 5 to 2 adult patients. At a dose of 2,200 mg/m^2 given on days 1, 3, and 5 every 21 days, 2 patients developed a significant grade 3 ascending sensory neuropathy. Magnetic resonance imaging evaluations of the 2 patients demonstrated findings consistent with a demyelinating process in the cervical spine.

➤*Treatment:* There is no known antidote for overdoses of nelarabine. In the event of overdose, provide supportive care consistent with good clinical practice.

Patient Information

Because patients receiving nelarabine therapy may experience somnolence, caution them about operating hazardous machinery, including automobiles.

Instruct patients to contact their health care provider if they experience new or worsening symptoms of peripheral neuropathy. These signs and symptoms include the following: tingling or numbness in fingers, hands, toes, or feet; difficulty with the fine motor coordination tasks, such as buttoning clothing; unsteadiness while walking; weakness arising from a low chair; weakness in climbing stairs; and increased tripping while walking over uneven surfaces.

Instruct patients that seizures have been known to occur in patients who receive nelarabine. If a seizure occurs, promptly inform the health care provider administering nelarabine.

Advise patients who develop fever or signs of infection while on therapy to notify their health care provider promptly.

Advise patients to use effective contraceptive measures to prevent pregnancy and to avoid breast-feeding during treatment with nelarabine.

DECITABINE

Rx	**Dacogen** (Eisai)	**Injection, lyophilized powder for solution:** 50 mg	In single-dose vials.

DECITABINE — INJECTION

Indications

➤*Myelodysplastic syndromes:* For treatment of patients with myelodysplastic syndromes, including previously treated and untreated, de novo and secondary myelodysplastic syndromes of all French-American-British (FAB) subtypes (refractory anemia, refractory anemia with ringed sideroblasts, refractory anemia with excess blasts, refractory anemia with excess blasts in transformation, and chronic myelomonocytic leukemia) and intermediate-1, intermediate-2, and high-risk International Prognostic Scoring System (IPSS) groups.

➤*Off-label uses:* Acute myelogenous leukemia, chronic myelogenous leukemia. (See Administration and Dosage.)

Administration and Dosage

➤*General dosing considerations:* Patients may be premedicated with standard antiemetic therapy.

➤*Adults:*

Myelodysplastic syndromes –

Usual dosage: 15 mg/m^2 administered by continuous intravenous (IV) infusion over 3 hours, repeated every 8 hours for 3 days. Repeat cycle every 6 weeks.

Dosage adjustment:

• *Hematological toxicities* – If hematologic recovery (absolute neutrophil count [ANC] at least 1,000/mcL and platelets at least 50,000/mcL) from a previous decitabine treatment cycle requires more than 6 weeks, then the next cycle of decitabine therapy should be delayed and dosing temporarily reduced by following this algorithm:

- For recovery requiring more than 6 but less than 8 weeks, decitabine dosing should be delayed for up to 2 weeks and the dose temporarily reduced to 11 mg/m^2 every 8 hours (33 mg/m^2/day, 99 mg/m^2/cycle) upon restarting therapy.
- For recovery requiring more than 8 but less than 10 weeks, the patient should be assessed for disease progression (by bone marrow aspirates); in the absence of progression, the decitabine dose should be delayed up to 2 more weeks and the dose reduced to 11 mg/m^2 every 8 hours (33 mg/m^2/day, 99 mg/m^2/cycle) upon restarting therapy, then maintained or increased in subsequent cycles as clinically indicated.

• *Nonhematological toxicities* – If any of the following nonhematologic toxicities are present, decitabine treatment should not be restarted until the toxicity is resolved: serum creatinine at least 2 mg/dL; ALT, total bilirubin at least 2 times the upper limit of normal (ULN); and active or uncontrolled infection.

Alternative dosage:

• *Usual dosage* – 20 mg/m^2 by continuous IV infusion over 1 hour repeated daily for 5 days. This cycle should be repeated every 4 weeks.

• *Dosage adjustment –*

Hematologic toxicities: If myelosuppression is present, subsequent treatment cycles of decitabine should be delayed until there is hematologic recovery (ANC at least 1,000/mcL and platelets at least 50,000/mcL).

Nonhematological toxicities: If any of the following nonhematologic toxicities are present, decitabine treatment should not be restarted until the toxicity is resolved: serum creatinine at least 2 mg/dL; ALT, total bilirubin at least 2 times the ULN; and active or uncontrolled infection.

Duration of therapy: For both treatment regimens, it is recommended that patients be treated for a minimum of 4 cycles; however, a complete or partial response may take longer than 4 cycles.

Off-label dosing –

Acute myelogenous leukemia: 15 mg/m^2 IV once daily on days 1 to 5 and 8 to 12 of each cycle; repeat cycles every 6 weeks. Infuse each dose over 1 hour.

Chronic myelogenous leukemia, chronic phase: 10 mg/m^2 IV once daily on days 1 to 5 and 8 to 12 of each cycle; repeat cycles every 6 weeks. Infuse each dose over 1 hour.

Chronic myelogenous leukemia, acute phase or blast phase: 15 mg/m^2 IV once daily on days 1 to 5 and 8 to 12 of each cycle; repeat cycles every 6 weeks. Infuse each dose over 1 hour.

➤*Renal function impairment:* Use decitabine with caution in patients with renal impairment. In patients with serum creatinine 2 mg/dL or more, do not administer decitabine until the toxicity has resolved.

➤*Hepatic function impairment:* Use decitabine with caution in patients with hepatic impairment. In patients with ALT or total bilirubin 2 times the ULN or more, do not administer decitabine until the toxicity has resolved.

➤*Preparation for administration:* Decitabine is considered a cytotoxic agent. Follow safe handling procedures when preparing, administering, or dispensing decitabine.

Decitabine should be aseptically reconstituted with 10 mL of sterile water for injection; upon reconstitution, each mL contains approximately 5 mg of decitabine at pH 6.7 to 7.3. Immediately after reconstitution, the solution should be further diluted with sodium chloride 0.9% injection, dextrose 5% injection, or Ringer's lactate injection to a final drug concentration of 0.1 to 1 mg/mL. Unless used within 15 minutes of reconstitution, the diluted solution must be prepared using cold (2° to 8°C) infusion fluids and stored at 2° to 8°C (36° to 46°F) for up to a maximum of 7 hours until administration.

➤*Administration:* For the treatment of myelodysplastic syndromes, administer by IV infusion over 3 hours (15 mg/m^2 dose) or over 1 hour (20 mg/m^2 dose). For the treatment of acute or chronic myelogenous leukemia (off-label uses), administer by IV infusion over 1 hour.

➤*Storage/Stability:* Store vials at 25°C (77°F); excursions are permitted to 15° to 30°C (59° to 86°F). Unless used within 15 minutes of reconstitution, the diluted solution must be prepared using cold (2° to 8°C) infusion fluids and stored at 2° to 8°C (36° to 46°F) for up to a maximum of 7 hours until administration.

Actions

➤*Pharmacology:* Decitabine is believed to exert its antineoplastic effects after phosphorylation and direct incorporation into DNA and inhibition of DNA methyltransferase, causing hypomethylation of DNA and cellular differentiation or apoptosis. Decitabine inhibits DNA methylation in vitro, which is achieved at concentrations that do not cause major suppression of DNA synthesis. Decitabine-induced hypomethylation in neoplastic cells may restore normal function to genes that are critical for the control of cellular differentiation and proliferation. In rapidly dividing cells, the cytotoxicity of decitabine also may be attributed to the formation of covalent adducts between DNA methyltransferase and decitabine incorporated into DNA. Nonproliferating cells are relatively insensitive to decitabine.

➤*Pharmacokinetics:*

Decitabine Pharmacokinetic Parameters[a]

Dose	C_{max} (ng/ mL)	$AUC_{0-\infty}$ (ng•h/mL)	t½ (h)	Clearance (L/h/m^2)	$AUC_{Cumulative}$[b] (ng•h/mL)
15 mg/m^2 3-hour infusion every 8 hours for 3 days (option 1) (n = 14)	73.8 (66)	163 (62)	0.62 (49)	125 (53)	1,332 (1,010 to 1,730)
20 mg/m^2 1-hour infusion daily for 5 days (option 2) (n = 11)	147 (49)	115 (43)	0.54 (43)	210 (47)	570 (470 to 700)

[a] C_{max} = maximum plasma concentration; t½ = half-life; AUC = area under the curve.
[b] N = 35 cumulative AUC per cycle.

Absorption/Distribution – Pharmacokinetic parameters were evaluated in patients. Eleven patients received 20 mg/m^2 infused over 1 hour IV (treatment option 2), Fourteen patients received 15 mg/m^2 infused over 3 hours (treatment option 1). Plasma concentration-time profiles after discontinuation of infusion showed a biexponential decline. Upon repeat doses there was no systemic accumulation of decitabine or any changes in pharmacokinetic parameters. Population pharmacokinetic analysis (N = 35) showed that the cumulative AUC per cycle for treatment option 2 was 2.3-fold lower than the cumulative AUC per cycle following treatment option 1.

Metabolism/Excretion – The clearance of decitabine was higher following treatment with a 20 mg/m^2 1 hour infusion daily for 5 days.

The exact route of elimination and metabolic fate of decitabine is not known in humans. One of the pathways of elimination of decitabine appears to be deamination by cytidine deaminase found principally in the liver, but also in granulocytes, intestinal epithelium, and whole blood.

Contraindications

None well documented.

Warnings/Precautions

➤*Hematologic effects:* Treatment with decitabine is associated with neutropenia and thrombocytopenia. Perform complete blood cell and platelet counts as needed to monitor response and toxicity, but at a minimum, prior to each dosing cycle. After administration of the recommended dosage for the first cycle, adjust dosage for subsequent cycles as described in Administration and Dosage. Consider the need for early institution of growth factors and/or antimicrobial agents for the prevention or treatment of infections in patients with myelodysplastic syndromes. Myelosuppression and worsening neutropenia may occur more frequently in the first or second treatment cycles, and may not necessarily indicate progression of underlying myelodysplastic syndromes.

➤*Use in men:* Advise men not to father a child while receiving treatment with decitabine and for 2 months afterwards. Men with female partners of childbearing potential should use effective contraception during this time. Based on its mechanism of action, decitabine alters DNA synthesis and can cause fetal harm.

➤*Renal/Hepatic function impairment:* There are no data on the use of decitabine in patients with renal or hepatic dysfunction; therefore, use decitabine with caution in these patients.

➤*Pregnancy: Category D.* Decitabine can cause fetal harm when administered to a pregnant woman. It is not known if decitabine crosses the human placenta. The molecular weight (approximately 228) and lack of plasma protein binding suggest that the drug will cross, but the very short terminal

DECITABINE — INJECTION

phase half-life will limit the amount of drug at the maternal-fetal interface. Based on its mechanism of action, decitabine is expected to result in adverse reproductive effects. In preclinical studies in mice and rats, decitabine was teratogenic, fetotoxic, and embryotoxic.

There are no adequate and well-controlled studies of decitabine in pregnant women. If this drug is used during pregnancy or if the patient becomes pregnant while receiving this drug, apprise the patient of the potential hazard to the fetus. Advise women of childbearing potential to avoid becoming pregnant while receiving decitabine and for 1 month following completion of treatment. Counsel women of childbearing potential to use effective contraception during this time.

Teratogenic – The developmental toxicity of decitabine was examined in mice exposed to single intraperitoneal injections (0, 0.9, and 3 mg/m^2, approximately 2% and 7% of the recommended daily clinical dose, respectively) over gestation days 8, 9, 10, or 11. No maternal toxicity was observed, but reduced fetal survival was observed after treatment at 3 mg/m^2 and decreased fetal weight was observed at both dose levels. The 3 mg/m^2 dose elicited characteristic fetal defects for each treatment day, including supernumerary ribs (both dose levels), fused vertebrae and ribs, cleft palate, vertebral defects, hind-limb defects, and digital defects of fore limbs and hind limbs. In rats given a single intraperitoneal injection of 2.4, 3.6, or 6 mg/m^2 (approximately 5%, 8%, or 13% the daily recommended clinical dose, respectively) on gestation days 9 to 12, no maternal toxicity was observed. No live fetuses were seen at any dose when decitabine was injected on gestation day 9. A significant decrease in fetal survival and reduced fetal weight at doses greater than 3.6 mg/m^2 were seen when decitabine was given on gestation day 10. Increased incidences of vertebral and rib anomalies were seen at all dose levels, and induction of exophthalmia, exencephaly, and cleft palate were observed at 6 mg/m^2. Increased incidence of foredigit defects was seen in fetuses at doses greater than 3.6 mg/m^2. Reduced size and ossification of long bones of the fore limb and hind limb were noted at 6 mg/m^2.

➤*Lactation:* It is not known whether decitabine or its metabolites are excreted in human milk. However, the molecular weight (about 228) and lack of plasma protein binding suggest that the drug will be excreted into breast milk, but the very short terminal phase half-life will limit the amount excreted. The effects of this exposure on a breast-feeding infant are unknown, but the potential effects may be severe. Because many drugs are excreted in human milk, and because of the potential for serious adverse reactions from decitabine in breast-feeding infants, decide whether to discontinue the drug, taking into account the importance of the drug to the mother.

➤*Children:* The safety and effectiveness in children have not been established.

➤*Monitoring:* Perform complete blood cell counts and platelet counts as needed to monitor response and toxicity, but at a minimum, prior to each cycle. Obtain liver chemistries and serum creatinine prior to initiation of treatment.

Adverse Reactions

For more information on hematologic toxicity, refer to Warnings/Precautions.

➤*Most common adverse reactions:* Anemia, constipation, cough, diarrhea, fatigue, hyperglycemia, nausea, neutropenia, petechiae, pyrexia, and thrombocytopenia.

➤*Most frequent adverse reactions (at least 1%) resulting in clinical intervention:*

Discontinuation – Abnormal liver function tests, cardiorespiratory arrest, increased blood bilirubin, intracranial hemorrhage, *Mycobacterium avium* complex infection, neutropenia, pneumonia, thrombocytopenia.

Dose delayed – Atrial fibrillation, central-line infection, febrile neutropenia, neutropenia, pulmonary edema.

Dose reduced – Anemia, depression, edema, lethargy, neutropenia, pharyngitis, tachycardia, thrombocytopenia.

➤*Adverse reactions (5% or more):*

Decitabine (15 mg/m^2 IV Every 8 hours for 3 days Every 6 Weeks) Adverse Reactions (≥ 5%)

Adverse reaction	Decitabine (n = 83)	Supportive care (n = 81)
Cardiovascular		
Cardiac murmur NOS[a]	16%	11%
Hypotension NOS	6%	5%
CNS		
Anxiety	11%	10%
Confusional state	12%	4%
Dizziness	18%	12%
Fall	8%	4%
Headache	28%	14%
Hypesthesia	11%	1%
Insomnia	28%	14%
Lethargy	12%	4%
Malaise	5%	1%

Decitabine (15 mg/m^2 IV Every 8 hours for 3 days Every 6 Weeks) Adverse Reactions (≥ 5%)

Adverse reaction	Decitabine (n = 83)	Supportive care (n = 81)
Dermatologic		
Alopecia	8%	1%
Cellulitis	12%	7%
Ecchymosis	22%	15%
Erythema	14%	6%
Pallor	23%	12%
Petechiae	39%	16%
Pruritus	11%	2%
Rash NOS	19%	9%
Skin lesion NOS	11%	4%
Swelling face	6%	0%
Urticaria NOS	6%	1%
GI		
Abdominal distension	5%	1%
Abdominal pain NOS	14%	6%
Anorexia	16%	10%
Appetite decreased NOS	16%	15%
Ascites	10%	2%
Constipation	35%	14%
Diarrhea NOS	34%	16%
Dyspepsia	12%	1%
Dysphagia	6%	2%
Gastroesophageal reflux disease	5%	0%
Gingival bleeding	8%	6%
Glossodynia	5%	0%
Hemorrhoids	8%	4%
Lip ulceration	5%	4%
Loose stools	7%	4%
Nausea	42%	16%
Oral mucosal petechiae	13%	5%
Oral soft tissue disorder NOS	6%	1%
Stomatitis	12%	6%
Tongue ulceration	7%	2%
Upper abdominal pain	5%	1%
Vomiting NOS	25%	9%
GU		
Dysuria	6%	4%
Urinary frequency	5%	1%
Urinary tract infection NOS	7%	1%
Hematologic/Lymphatic		
Anemia NOS	82%	74%
Febrile neutropenia	29%	6%
Hematoma NOS	5%	4%
Leukopenia NOS	28%	14%
Lymphadenopathy	12%	7%
Neutropenia	90%	72%
Thrombocythemia	5%	1%
Thrombocytopenia	89%	79%
Lab test abnormalities		
AST increased	10%	9%
Blood albumin decreased	7%	0%
Blood alkaline phosphatase NOS increased	11%	9%
Blood bicarbonate decreased	5%	1%
Blood bicarbonate increased	6%	1%
Blood bilirubin decreased	5%	1%
Blood chloride decreased	6%	1%
Blood lactate dehydrogenase increased	8%	6%
Blood urea increased	10%	1%
Protein total decreased	5%	4%

DECITABINE — INJECTION

Decitabine (15 mg/m² IV Every 8 hours for 3 days Every 6 Weeks) Adverse Reactions (≥ 5%)		
Adverse reaction	Decitabine (n = 83)	Supportive care (n = 81)
Local		
Catheter-related infection	8%	0%
Catheter-site erythema	5%	1%
Catheter-site pain	5%	0%
Injection-site swelling	5%	0%
Metabolic/Nutritional		
Dehydration	6%	5%
Edema NOS	18%	6%
Edema peripheral	25%	16%
Hyperbilirubinemia	14%	5%
Hyperglycemia NOS	33%	20%
Hyperkalemia	13%	4%
Hypoalbuminemia	24%	17%
Hypokalemia	22%	12%
Hypomagnesemia	24%	7%
Hyponatremia	19%	16%
Musculoskeletal		
Arthralgia	20%	10%
Back pain	17%	6%
Chest wall pain	7%	1%
Musculoskeletal discomfort	6%	0%
Myalgia	5%	1%
Pain in limb	19%	10%
Rigors	22%	17%
Respiratory		
Cough	40%	31%
Decreased breath sounds	10%	9%
Hypoxia	10%	5%
Lung crackles	14%	1%
Pharyngitis	16%	7%
Pneumonia NOS	22%	14%
Postnasal drip	5%	2%
Pulmonary edema NOS	6%	0%
Rales	8%	2%
Sinusitis NOS	5%	2%
Miscellaneous		
Abrasion NOS	5%	1%
Bacteremia	5%	0%
Candidal infection NOS	10%	1%
Chest discomfort	7%	4%
Crepitations NOS	5%	1%
Intermittent pyrexia	6%	4%
Oral candidiasis	6%	2%
Pain NOS	13%	6%
Pyrexia	53%	28%
Tenderness NOS	11%	0%
Transfusion reaction	7%	4%
Staphylococcal infection	7%	0%
Vision blurred	6%	0%

[a] NOS = not otherwise specified.

In the controlled trial using decitabine dosed at 15 mg/m², administered by continuous IV infusion over 3 hours repeated every 8 hours for 3 days, the highest incidence of grade 3 or 4 adverse reactions in the decitabine arm were neutropenia (87%), thrombocytopenia (85%), febrile neutropenia (23%), and leukopenia (22%). Bone marrow suppression was the most frequent cause of dose reduction, delay, and discontinuation. Six patients had fatal reactions associated with their underlying disease and myelosuppression (anemia, neutropenia, and thrombocytopenia) that were considered at least possibly related to drug treatment. Of the 83 decitabine-treated patients, 8 permanently discontinued therapy for adverse reactions; compared with 1 of 81 patients in the supportive care arm.

In a single-arm study (N = 99) decitabine was dosed at 20 mg/m² IV, infused over 1 hour daily for 5 consecutive days of a 4 week cycle.

Decitabine (20 mg/m² IV, Infused over 1 Hour Daily For 5 Consecutive Days of a 4 Week Cycle) Adverse Reactions (≥ 5%)[a]	
Adverse reaction	Decitabine (N = 99)
Cardiovascular	
Congestive cardiac failure	5%
Hypertension	6%
Hypotension	11%
Tachycardia	8%
CNS	
Anxiety	9%
Asthenia	15%
Chills	16%
Confusional state	8%
Depression	9%
Dizziness	21%
Fatigue	46%
Headache	23%
Insomnia	14%
Dermatologic	
Cellulitis	9%
Contusion	9%
Dry skin	8%
Ecchymosis	9%
Erythema	5%
Night sweats	5%
Petechiae	12%
Pruritus	9%
Rash	11%
Skin lesion	5%
GI	
Abdominal pain	14%
Constipation	30%
Diarrhea	28%
Dyspepsia	10%
Dysphagia	5%
Gastroesophageal reflux disease	5%
Nausea	40%
Oral pain	5%
Stomatitis	11%
Tooth abscess	5%
Toothache	6%
Upper abdominal pain	6%
Vomiting	16%
Hematologic	
Anemia	31%
Febrile neutropenia	20%
Leukopenia	6%
Neutropenia	38%
Pancytopenia	5%
Thrombocythemia	5%
Thrombocytopenia	27%
Metabolic/Nutritional	
Anorexia	23%
Decreased appetite	8%
Dehydration	8%
Edema	5%
Hyperglycemia	6%
Hypokalemia	12%
Hypomagnesemia	5%
Peripheral edema	27%
Weight decreased	9%
Musculoskeletal	
Arthralgia	17%
Back pain	18%
Bone pain	6%

DECITABINE — INJECTION

Decitabine (20 mg/m² IV, Infused over 1 Hour Daily For 5 Consecutive Days of a 4 Week Cycle) Adverse Reactions (≥ 5%)[a]	
Adverse reaction	Decitabine (N = 99)
Muscle spasms	7%
Muscular weakness	5%
Musculoskeletal pain	5%
Myalgia	9%
Pain in extremity	18%
Respiratory	
Abnormal breath sounds	5%
Cough	27%
Dyspnea	29%
Epistaxis	13%
Pharyngolaryngeal pain	8%
Pleural effusion	5%
Pneumonia	20%
Sinus congestion	5%
Sinusitis	6%
Upper respiratory tract infection	10%
Miscellaneous	
Chest pain	6%
Ear pain	6%
Increased blood bilirubin	6%
Mucosal inflammation	9%
Oral candidiasis	6%
Pain	5%
Pyrexia	36%
Staphylococcal bacteremia	8%
Urinary tract infection	7%

[a] In this single-arm study, investigators reported adverse reactions based on clinical signs and symptoms rather than predefined laboratory abnormalities. Thus, not all laboratory abnormalities were recorded as adverse events.

In the single-arm study (N = 99) when decitabine was dosed at 20 mg/m² IV, infused over 1 hour daily for 5 consecutive days, the highest incidence of grade 3 or grade 4 adverse reactions were neutropenia (37%), thrombocytopenia (24%), and anemia (22%). Seventy-eight percent of patients had dose delays, the median duration of this delay was 7 days, and the largest percentage of delays were due to hematologic toxicities. Hematologic toxicities and infections were the most frequent causes of dose delays and discontinuation. Eight patients had fatal events due to infection and/or bleeding (7 of which occurred in the clinical setting of myelosuppression) that were considered at least possibly related to drug treatment. Nineteen of 99 patients permanently discontinued therapy because of adverse events.

➤*Other serious adverse reactions:*

Cardiovascular – Atrial fibrillation, cardiomyopathy, cardiorespiratory arrest, myocardial infarction, supraventricular tachycardia.

CNS – Intracranial hemorrhage, mental status changes.

GI – Gingival pain, upper GI hemorrhage.

GU – Renal failure, urethral hemorrhage.

Hematologic/Lymphatic – Myelosuppression, splenomegaly.

Hypersensitivity – Hypersensitivity (anaphylactic reaction) to decitabine has been reported in a phase 2 trial.

Respiratory – Bronchopulmonary aspergillosis, hemoptysis, lung infiltration, pseudomonal lung infection, pulmonary mass, pulmonary embolism, respiratory arrest, respiratory tract infection.

Miscellaneous – Catheter site hemorrhage, chest pain, cholecystitis, fungal infection, *Mycobacterium avium* complex infection, peridiverticular abscess, postprocedural hemorrhage, postprocedural pain, sepsis.

➤*Postmarketing:* Cases of Sweet syndrome (acute febrile neutrophilic dermatosis) have been reported.

Overdosage

➤*Symptoms:* Higher doses are associated with increased myelosuppression, including prolonged neutropenia and thrombocytopenia.

➤*Treatment:* There is no known antidote for overdosage with decitabine. Take standard supportive measures in the event of an overdose.

Patient Information

Advise patients to monitor and report any symptoms of neutropenia, thrombocytopenia, or fever to their health care provider as soon as possible.

Advise women of childbearing potential to avoid becoming pregnant while receiving treatment with decitabine and for 1 month afterwards, and to use effective contraception during this time.

Advise men not to father a child while receiving treatment with decitabine, and for 2 months afterwards. During these times, advise men with female partners of childbearing potential to use effective contraception.

Advise women to consult a health care provider before breast-feeding.

DNA TOPOISOMERASE INHIBITORS

IRINOTECAN HYDROCHLORIDE

Rx	**Irinotecan Hydrochloride** (Various, eg, Abraxis, Dabur Pharma, Greenstone, Sandoz, Teva)	**Injection, solution:** 20 mg/mL	May contain sorbitol 45 mg/mL. In 2, 5, and 25 mL vials.
Rx	**Camptosar** (Pharmacia)		Sorbitol 45 mg. In 2 and 5 mL single-dose vials.

IRINOTECAN HYDROCHLORIDE — INJECTION

WARNING

Irinotecan should be administered only under the supervision of a health care provider who is experienced in the use of cancer chemotherapeutic agents. Appropriate management of complications is possible only when adequate diagnostic and treatment facilities are readily available. Irinotecan can induce both early and late forms of diarrhea that appear to be mediated by different mechanisms. Both forms of diarrhea may be severe. Early diarrhea (occurring during or shortly after infusion of irinotecan) may be accompanied by cholinergic symptoms of rhinitis, increased salivation, miosis, lacrimation, diaphoresis, flushing, and intestinal hyperperistalsis, which can cause abdominal cramping. Early diarrhea and other cholinergic symptoms may be prevented or ameliorated by atropine. Late diarrhea (generally occurring more than 24 hours after administration of irinotecan) can be life-threatening because it may be prolonged and lead to dehydration, electrolyte imbalance, or sepsis. Late diarrhea should be treated promptly with loperamide. Carefully monitor patients with diarrhea and give fluid and electrolyte replacement if they become dehydrated, or antibiotic therapy if they develop fever, ileus, or severe neutropenia. Administration of irinotecan should be interrupted and subsequent doses reduced if severe diarrhea occurs.

Severe myelosuppression may occur.

Indications

➤*Metastatic carcinoma of the colon or rectum:* As first-line therapy in combination with 5-fluorouracil and leucovorin for patients with metastatic carcinoma of the colon or rectum; for patients with metastatic carcinoma of the colon or rectum whose disease has recurred or progressed following initial fluorouracil-based therapy.

➤*Off-label uses:* Cervical cancer, lung cancer (small cell or non–small cell), gastric cancer, and tumors of the CNS.

Administration and Dosage

➤*General dosing considerations:* Irinotecan is emetogenic. It is recommended that patients receive premedication with antiemetic agents. (See Premedication.)

Irinotecan must be diluted prior to infusion. (See Preparation for Administration.)

➤*Adults:*

Metastatic carcinoma of the colon or rectum –

Combination therapy:

• *Usual dosage* – For all regimens, the dose of leucovorin should be administered immediately after irinotecan, with the administration of 5-fluorouracil to occur immediately after receipt of leucovorin.

Irinotecan/5-Fluorouracil/Leucovorin: Dosage Regimens and Dose Modifications[a,b]				
Regimen 1: 6-wk cycle with bolus 5-fluorouracil/leucovorin (next cycle begins on day 43)	Irinotecan	125 mg/m² IV[c] over 90 min, days 1, 8, 15, 22		
	Leucovorin	20 mg/m² IV bolus, days 1, 8, 15, 22		
	5-fluorouracil	500 mg/m² IV bolus, days 1, 8, 15, 22		
		Starting dose and modified dose levels (mg/m²)		
		Starting dose	Dose level −1	Dose level −2
	Irinotecan	125	100	75
	Leucovorin	20	20	20
	5-fluorouracil	500	400	300

IRINOTECAN HYDROCHLORIDE — INJECTION

Irinotecan/5-Fluorouracil/Leucovorin: Dosage Regimens and Dose Modifications[a,b]

Regimen 2: 6-wk cycle with infusional 5-fluorouracil/ leucovorin (next cycle begins on day 43)	Irinotecan	180 mg/m^2 IV over 90 min, days 1, 15, 29		
	Leucovorin	200 mg/m^2 IV over 2 h, days 1, 2, 15, 16, 29, 30		
	5-fluorouracil (bolus)	400 mg/m^2 IV bolus, days 1, 2, 15, 16, 29, 30		
	5-fluorouracil (infusion[d])	600 mg/m^2 IV over 22 h, days 1, 2, 15, 16, 29, 30		
		Starting dose and modified dose levels (mg/m^2)		
		Starting dose	Dose level −1	Dose level −2
	Irinotecan	180	150	120
	Leucovorin	200	200	200
	5-fluorouracil (bolus)	400	320	240
	5-fluorouracil (infusion[d])	600	480	360

[a] Dose reductions beyond dose level −2 by decrements of approximately 20% may be warranted for patients continuing to experience toxicity. Provided intolerable toxicity does not develop, treatment with additional cycles may be continued indefinitely as long as patients continue to experience clinical benefit.
[b] Dosing for patients with bilirubin greater than 2 mg/dL cannot be recommended because there is insufficient information to recommend a dose in these patients.
[c] IV = intravenous.
[d] Infusion follows bolus administration.

It is recommended that patients receive premedication with antiemetic agents. Prophylactic or therapeutic administration of atropine should be considered in patients experiencing cholinergic symptoms.

• *Dosage adjustment* – Patients should be carefully monitored for toxicity and assessed prior to each treatment. Doses of irinotecan and 5-fluorouracil should be modified as necessary to accommodate individual patient tolerance to treatment. Based on the recommended dose levels described in the previous table, subsequent doses should be adjusted as suggested in the following table. All dose modifications should be based on the worst preceding toxicity. After the first treatment, patients with active diarrhea should return to pretreatment bowel function without requiring antidiarrheal medications for at least 24 hours before the next chemotherapy administration.

A new cycle of therapy should not begin until the toxicity has recovered to National Cancer Institute (NCI) grade 1 or less. Treatment may be delayed 1 to 2 weeks to allow for recovery from treatment-related toxicity. If the patient has not recovered, consideration should be given to discontinuing therapy. Provided intolerable toxicity does not develop, treatment with additional cycles of irinotecan/5-fluorouracil/leucovorin may be continued indefinitely, as long as patients continue to experience clinical benefit.

Irinotecan/5-Fluorouracil/Leucovorin: Dose Modification According to Toxicity

Patients should return to pretreatment bowel function without requiring antidiarrheal medications for at least 24 h before the next chemotherapy administration. A new cycle of therapy should not begin until the granulocyte count has recovered to ≥ 1,500/mm^3, the platelet count has recovered to ≥ 100,000 mm^3, and treatment-related diarrhea is fully resolved. Treatment should be delayed 1 to 2 wk to allow for recovery from treatment-related toxicities. If the patient has not recovered after a 2-wk delay, consider discontinuing therapy.

Toxicity NCI-CTC [a]grade (value)	During a cycle of therapy	At the start of subsequent cycles of therapy[b]
No toxicity	Maintain dose level	Maintain dose level
Neutropenia		
1 (1,500 to 1,999/mm^3)	Maintain dose level	Maintain dose level
2 (1,000 to 1,499/mm^3)	↓ 1 dose level	Maintain dose level
3 (500 to 999/mm^3)	Omit dose until resolved to ≤ grade 2, then ↓ 1 dose level	↓ 1 dose level
4 (< 500/mm^3)	Omit dose until resolved to ≤ grade 2, then ↓ 2 dose levels	↓ 2 dose levels
Neutropenic fever	Omit dose until resolved, then ↓ 2 dose levels	
Other hematologic toxicities	Dose modifications for leukopenia or thrombocytopenia during a cycle of therapy and at the start of subsequent cycles of therapy are also based on NCI-CTC and are the same as previously recommended for neutropenia.	

Irinotecan/5-Fluorouracil/Leucovorin: Dose Modification According to Toxicity

Patients should return to pretreatment bowel function without requiring antidiarrheal medications for at least 24 h before the next chemotherapy administration. A new cycle of therapy should not begin until the granulocyte count has recovered to ≥ 1,500/mm^3, the platelet count has recovered to ≥ 100,000 mm^3, and treatment-related diarrhea is fully resolved. Treatment should be delayed 1 to 2 wk to allow for recovery from treatment-related toxicities. If the patient has not recovered after a 2-wk delay, consider discontinuing therapy.

Toxicity NCI-CTC [a]grade (value)	During a cycle of therapy	At the start of subsequent cycles of therapy[b]
Diarrhea		
1 (2 to 3 stools/day > pretreatment)	Delay dose until resolved to baseline, then give same dose	Maintain dose level
2 (4 to 6 stools/day > pretreatment)	Omit dose until resolved to baseline, then ↓ 1 dose level	Maintain dose level
3 (7 to 9 stools/day > pretreatment)	Omit dose until resolved to baseline, then ↓ 1 dose level	↓ 1 dose level
4 (≥ 10 stools/day > pretreatment)	Omit dose until resolved to baseline, then ↓ 2 dose level	↓ 2 dose levels
Other nonhematologic toxicities[c]		
1	Maintain dose level	Maintain dose level
2	Omit dose until resolved to ≤ grade 1, then ↓ 1 dose level	Maintain dose level
3	Omit dose until resolved to ≤ grade 2, then ↓ 1 dose level	↓ 1 dose level
4	Omit dose until resolved to ≤ grade 2, then ↓ 2 dose levels	↓ 2 dose levels
	For mucositis/stomatitis, decrease only 5-fluorouracil, not irinotecan	For mucositis/ stomatitis, decrease only 5-fluorouracil, not irinotecan

[a] NCI Common Toxicity Criteria (version 1.0).
[b] Relative to the starting dose used in the previous cycle.
[c] Excludes alopecia, anorexia, and asthenia.

Single-agent therapy:

• *Usual dosage* –

Irinotecan (Single Agent): Dosage Regimen and Dose Modifications

Weekly regimen[a]	125 mg/m^2 IV over 90 min, days 1, 8, 15, 22, then 2-wk rest		
	Starting dose and modified dose levels[b] (mg/m^2)		
	Starting dose	Dose level −1	Dose level −2
	125	100	75
Once-every-3-wk regimen[c]	350 mg/m^2 IV over 90 min, once every 3 wk[b]		
	Starting dose and modified dose levels (mg/m^2)		
	Starting dose	Dose level −1	Dose level −2
	350	300	250

[a] Subsequent doses may be adjusted as high as 150 mg/m^2 or as low as 50 mg/m^2 in 25 to 50 mg/m^2 decrements, depending on individual patient tolerance.
[b] Provided intolerable toxicity does not develop, treatment with additional cycles may be continued indefinitely, as long as patients continue to experience clinical benefit.
[c] Subsequent doses may be adjusted as low as 200 mg/m^2 in 50 mg/m^2 decrements, depending on individual patient tolerance.

• *Dosage adjustment* – A reduction in the starting dose by 1 dose level of irinotecan may be considered for patients with any of the following conditions: prior pelvic/abdominal radiotherapy, performance status of 2, or increased bilirubin levels. Dosing for patients with bilirubin greater than 2 mg/dL cannot be recommended because there is insufficient information to recommend a dose in these patients.

Patients should be carefully monitored for toxicity, and doses of irinotecan should be modified as necessary to accommodate individual patient tolerance to treatment. Based on recommended dose levels previously described, subsequent doses should be adjusted as suggested in the following table. All dose modifications should be based on the worst preceding toxicity.

IRINOTECAN HYDROCHLORIDE — INJECTION

A new cycle of therapy should not begin until the toxicity has recovered to NCI grade 1 or less. Treatment may be delayed 1 to 2 weeks to allow for recovery from treatment-related toxicity. If the patient has not recovered, consideration should be given to discontinuing this combination therapy. Provided intolerable toxicity does not develop, treatment with additional cycles of irinotecan may be continued indefinitely, as long as patients continue to experience clinical benefit.

Irinotecan (Single Agent): Dose Modification According to Toxicity[a]

A new cycle of therapy should not begin until the granulocyte count has recovered to ≥ 1,500/mm³, the platelet count has recovered to ≥ 100,000/mm³, and treatment-related diarrhea is fully resolved. Treatment should be delayed 1 to 2 wk to allow for recovery from treatment-related toxicities. If the patient has not recovered after a 2-wk delay, consider discontinuing irinotecan.

Worst toxicity NCI grade[b] (value)	During a cycle of therapy	At the start of the next cycle of therapy (after adequate recovery) compared with the starting dose in the previous cycle[a]	
	Weekly	Weekly	Once every 3 wk
No toxicity	Maintain dose level	↑ 25 mg/m² up to a maximum dose of 150 mg/m²	Maintain dose level
Neutropenia			
1 (1,500 to 1,999/mm³)	Maintain dose level	Maintain dose level	Maintain dose level
2 (1,000 to 1,499/mm³)	↓ 25 mg/m²	Maintain dose level	Maintain dose level
3 (500 to 999/mm³)	Omit dose until resolved to ≤ grade 2, then ↓ 25 mg/m²	↓ 25 mg/m²	↓ 50 mg/m²
4 (< 500/mm³)	Omit dose until resolved to ≤ grade 2, then ↓ 50 mg/m²	↓ 50 mg/m²	↓ 50 mg/m²
Neutropenic fever	Omit dose until resolved, then ↓ 50 mg/m² when resolved	↓ 50 mg/m²	↓ 50 mg/m²
Other hematologic toxicities	Dose modifications for leukopenia, thrombocytopenia, and anemia during a cycle of therapy and at the start of subsequent cycles of therapy are also based on NCI-CTC and are the same as previously recommended for neutropenia.		
Diarrhea			
1 (2 to 3 stools/day > pretreatment)	Maintain dose level	Maintain dose level	Maintain dose level
2 (4 to 6 stools/day > pretreatment)	↓ 25 mg/m²	Maintain dose level	Maintain dose level
3 (7 to 9 stools/day > pretreatment)	Omit dose until resolved to ≤ grade 2, then ↓ 25 mg/m²	↓ 25 mg/m²	↓ 50 mg/m²
4 (≥ 10 stools/day > pretreatment)	Omit dose until resolved to ≤ grade 2, then ↓ 50 mg/m²	↓ 50 mg/m²	↓ 50 mg/m²
Other nonhematologic[c] toxicities			
1	Maintain dose level	Maintain dose level	Maintain dose level
2	↓ 25 mg/m²	↓ 25 mg/m²	↓ 50 mg/m²
3	Omit dose until resolved to ≤ grade 2, then ↓ 25 mg/m²	↓ 25 mg/m²	↓ 50 mg/m²
4	Omit dose until resolved to ≤ grade 2, then ↓ 50 mg/m²	↓ 50 mg/m²	↓ 50 mg/m²

[a] All dose modifications should be based on the worst preceding toxicity.
[b] NCI-CTC (version 1.0).
[c] Excludes alopecia, anorexia, and asthenia.

Off-label dosing –
Malignant glioma:

- *Usual dose* – 300 mg/m² IV once every 21 days for 2 cycles, then increased to 350 mg/m² IV every 21 days. Do not increase the dose above 350 mg/m². Based on adverse effects, the dose may be decreased in 50 mg/m² increments.
- *Alternative dosage* – Irinotecan 125 mg/m² IV once weekly for 4 weeks, followed by 2 weeks of rest. For subsequent cycles, give irinotecan once weekly for 4 weeks, followed by 2 weeks of rest. Based on response and adverse effects, the dose may be adjusted in 25 to 50 mg/m² increments. The weekly dose may be increased in 25 mg/m² increments to a maximum of 150 mg/m² per dose.

➤*Elderly:*

70 years of age and older –
Initial dosage: 300 mg/m² for the once-every-3-week dosage schedule.

➤*Hepatic function impairment:* Irinotecan is not recommended in patients with a serum bilirubin above 2 mg/dL. Risk of profound neutropenia is increased in patients with increased bilirubin levels and a history of pelvic or abdominal irradiation. Consider dosage reduction, as shown in the following table.

Irinotecan Dosage Adjustment for Patients With Hepatic Dysfunction and Previous Abdominal or Pelvic Irradiation

Serum bilirubin	Recommended initial dose, monotherapy: Once-weekly regimen	Recommended initial dose, monotherapy: Every-21-days regimen
< 1 mg/dL	125 mg/m²	350 mg/m²
1 to 2 mg/dL	100 mg/m²	300 mg/m²
> 2 mg/dL	Not recommended	Not recommended

➤*Premedication:* It is recommended that patients receive premedication with antiemetic agents. In clinical studies of the weekly dosage schedule, the majority of patients received dexamethasone 10 mg given in conjunction with another type of antiemetic agent, such as a 5-HT_3 blocker (eg, granisetron, ondansetron). Antiemetic agents should be given on the day of treatment starting at least 30 minutes before administration of irinotecan. Also consider providing patients with an antiemetic regimen (eg, prochlorperazine) for subsequent use as needed. Prophylactic or therapeutic administration of IV or subcutaneous atropine 0.25 to 1 mg should be considered (unless clinically contraindicated) in patients experiencing abdominal cramping, diaphoresis, diarrhea (occurring during or shortly after infusion of irinotecan), flushing, increased salivation, lacrimation, miosis, or rhinitis. These symptoms are expected to occur more frequently with higher irinotecan doses.

➤*Previous abdominal or pelvic irradiation:* Risk of profound neutropenia is increased in patients with a history of pelvic or abdominal irradiation. Consider dosage reduction, as shown in the previous table. (See Hepatic Function Impairment.)

➤*Genetic polymorphism:* Risk of neutropenia is higher in patients who are homozygous for genetic polymorphism on allele 28 of UDP-glucuronosyl transferase 1A1 (UGT1A1*28), the primary enzyme responsible for inactivation of irinotecan's active metabolite (SN-38). When administered in combination with other agents or as a single agent, a reduction in the starting dose by at least 1 level of irinotecan should be considered for patients known to be homozygous for the UGT1A1*28 allele. However, the precise dose reduction in this patient population is not known and subsequent dose modifications should be considered based on individual patient tolerance to treatment.

Consider reducing the initial dose at least 1 level in these patients, as shown in the following table.

Irinotecan Dosage Adjustment in UGT1A1*28 Homozygous Patients

Dosage frequency	Irinotecan monotherapy	Combination regimens
Once weekly	Decrease initial dose by at least 25 mg/m²	Decrease initial dose by at least 25 mg/m²
Every 14 days	—	Decrease initial dose by at least 30 mg/m²
Every 21 days	Decrease initial dose by at least 50 mg/m²	—

➤*Preparation for administration:* Irinotecan is considered a cytotoxic agent. Follow safe handling procedures when preparing, administering, or dispensing irinotecan.

The use of gloves is recommended. If a solution of irinotecan contacts the skin, wash the skin immediately and thoroughly with soap and water. If irinotecan contacts the mucous membranes, flush thoroughly with water.

Irinotecan must be diluted prior to infusion. Irinotecan should be diluted in dextrose 5% injection (preferred) or sodium chloride 0.9% injection to a final concentration range of 0.12 to 2.8 mg/mL. In most clinical trials, irinotecan was administered in 250 to 500 mL of dextrose 5% injection.

➤*Administration:* Administer as an IV infusion over 90 minutes. Shorter infusions (30 minutes) are associated with a higher incidence of some adverse effects, including myelosuppression and cholinergic symptoms.

➤*Extravasation:* Take care to avoid extravasation and monitor the infusion site for signs of inflammation. If extravasation occurs, the manufacturers recommend flushing the site with sterile water and applying ice.

Irinotecan is considered an irritant and may cause phlebitis, but it is not known to cause tissue damage with extravasation. If signs or symptoms of

IRINOTECAN HYDROCHLORIDE — INJECTION

extravasation occur, stop the infusion immediately. If possible, withdraw 3 to 5 mL of blood to remove some of the drug. Remove the infusion needle. Delineate the infiltrated area on the patient's skin with a felt-tip marker. Elevate for 48 hours above heart level using a sling or stockinette dressing with an observation window cut in the dressing. Avoid pressure or friction. Do not rub the area. Observe for signs of increased erythema, pain, or skin necrosis. If increased symptoms occur, consult a plastic surgeon. Ensure that no medication is given distally to extravasation site. After 48 hours, encourage the patient to use the extremity normally to promote full range of motion.

➤*Admixture compatibility:* Other drugs should not be added to the infusion solution.

➤*Storage / Stability:* Store vials at 15° to 30°C (59° to 86°F). Protect from light. It is recommended that the vials remain in the carton until the time of use.

The diluted solution is physically and chemically stable for up to 24 hours at room temperature (approximately 25°C [77°F]) and in ambient fluorescent lighting. In the case of admixtures prepared with dextrose 5% injection or sodium chloride injection, the manufacturer recommends that the solutions be used within 6 hours if kept at room temperature (15° to 30°C [59° to 86°F]). Solutions diluted in dextrose 5% injection and stored at refrigerated temperatures (approximately 2° to 8°C [36° to 46°F]) and protected from light are physically and chemically stable for 48 hours. However, it is advisable to use the admixture prepared with dextrose 5% injection within 24 hours if refrigerated (2° to 8°C [36° to 46°F]) because of possible microbial contamination during dilution. Refrigeration of admixtures using sodium chloride 0.9% injection is not recommended because of a low and sporadic incidence of visible particulates. Freezing irinotecan and admixtures of irinotecan may result in precipitation of the drug and should be avoided.

Discard vial within 6 hours of the initial needle puncture if opened within an ISO Class 5 biological safety cabinet, or within 1 hour of the initial needle puncture if opened outside of such an environment, based on the USP Chapter <797> standards.

Actions

➤*Pharmacology:* Irinotecan, an antineoplastic agent of the topoisomerase inhibitor class, is a derivative of camptothecin. Camptothecins interact specifically with the enzyme topoisomerase I, which relieves torsional strain in DNA by inducing reversible single-strand breaks. Irinotecan and its active metabolite SN-38 bind to the topoisomerase I-DNA complex and prevent relegation of these single-strand breaks. Current research suggests that the cytotoxicity of irinotecan is due to double-strand DNA damage produced during DNA synthesis when replication enzymes interact with the ternary complex formed by topoisomerase I, DNA, and either irinotecan or SN-38. Mammalian cells cannot efficiently repair these double-strand breaks. Administration of irinotecan has resulted in antitumor activity in mice bearing cancers of rodent origin and in human carcinoma xenografts of various histological types.

➤*Pharmacokinetics:*

Irinotecan and SN-38 Mean (± SD) Pharmacokinetic Parameters in Patients With Solid Tumors[a]

	Irinotecan					SN-38		
Dose (mg/m²)	C_{max} (ng/mL)	AUC_{0-24} (ng•h/mL)	t½ (h)	V_z (L/m²)	CL (L/h/m²)	C_{max} (ng/mL)	AUC_{0-24} (ng•h/mL)	t½ (h)
125 (n = 64)	1,660 ± 797	10,200 ± 3,270	5.8[b] ± 0.7	110 ± 48.5	13.3 ± 6.01	26.3 ± 11.9	229 ± 108	10.4[b] ± 3.1
340 (n = 6)	3,392 ± 874	20,604 ± 6,027	11.7[c] ± 1	234 ± 69.6	13.9 ± 4	56 ± 28.2	474 ± 245	21[c] ± 4.3

[a] SD = standard deviation; C_{max} = maximum plasma concentration; AUC_{0-24} = area under the curve from 0 to 24 hours after the end of the 90-minute infusion; t½ = terminal elimination half-life; V_z = volume of distribution of terminal elimination phase; CL = total systemic clearance.
[b] Plasma specimens collected for 24 hours following the end of the 90-minute infusion.
[c] Plasma specimens were collected for 48 hours following the end of the 90-minute infusion. Because of the longer collection period, these values provide a more accurate reflection of the terminal elimination half-lives of irinotecan and SN-38.

Absorption / Distribution – Over the dose range of 50 to 350 mg/m², the AUC of irinotecan increases linearly with dose; the AUC of SN-38 increases less than proportionally with dose. The plasma AUC values for SN-38 are 2% to 8% of irinotecan. Maximum concentrations of the active metabolite SN-38 are generally seen within 1 hour following the end of a 90-minute infusion of irinotecan.

Irinotecan exhibits moderate plasma protein binding (30% to 68% bound). SN-38 is highly bound to human plasma proteins (approximately 95% bound). The plasma protein that irinotecan and SN-38 predominantly bind to is albumin.

Metabolism / Excretion – Irinotecan serves as a water-soluble precursor of the lipophilic metabolite SN-38. The metabolic conversion of irinotecan to the active metabolite SN-38 is mediated by carboxylesterase enzymes and primarily occurs in the liver. SN-38 is formed from irinotecan by carboxylesterase-mediated cleavage of the carbamate bond between the camptothecin moiety and the dipiperidino side chain. SN-38 is approximately 1,000 times as potent as irinotecan as an inhibitor of topoisomerase I purified from human and rodent tumor cell lines. In vitro cytotoxicity assays show that the potency of SN-38 relative to irinotecan varies from 2- to 2,000-fold. Therefore, the precise contribution of SN-38 to the activity of irinotecan is unknown. Both irinotecan and SN-38 exist in an active lactone form and an inactive hydroxy acid anion form. A pH-dependent equilibrium exists between the 2 forms such that an acid pH promotes the formation of the lactone, while a more basic pH favors the hydroxy acid anion form. SN-38 is subsequently conjugated predominantly by the enzyme UGT1A1 to form a glucuronide metabolite. UGT1A1 activity is reduced in individuals with genetic polymorphisms that lead to reduced enzyme activity, such as the UGT1A1*28 polymorphism. Approximately 10% of the North American population is homozygous for the UGT1A1*28 allele (also referred to as UGT1A1 7/7 genotype). SN-38 glucuronide had 1/50 to 1/100 the activity of SN-38 in cytotoxicity assays using 2 cell lines in vitro. The disposition of irinotecan has not been fully elucidated in humans.

After IV infusion of irinotecan in humans, irinotecan plasma concentrations decline in a multiexponential manner, with a mean terminal elimination half-life of approximately 6 to 12 hours. The mean terminal elimination half-life of the active metabolite SN-38 is approximately 10 to 20 hours. The half-lives of the lactone (active) forms of irinotecan and SN-38 are similar to those of total irinotecan and SN-38, as the lactone and hydroxy acid forms are in equilibrium. The urinary excretion of irinotecan is 11% to 20%; SN-38, less than 1%; and SN-38 glucuronide, 3%. The cumulative biliary and urinary excretion of irinotecan and its metabolites (SN-38 and SN-38 glucuronide) over a period of 48 hours following administration of irinotecan in 2 patients ranged from approximately 25% (100 mg/m²) to 50% (300 mg/m²).

Special populations –

Hepatic function impairment: Irinotecan clearance is diminished in patients with hepatic impairment, while exposure to the active metabolite SN-38 is increased relative to that in patients with healthy hepatic function. The magnitude of these effects is proportional to the degree of liver impairment as measured by elevations in total bilirubin and transaminase concentrations. However, the tolerability of irinotecan in patients with hepatic impairment (bilirubin greater than 2 mg/dL) has not been assessed sufficiently, and no recommendations for dosing can be made.

Elderly: In a study of 162 patients that was not prospectively designed to investigate the effect of age, small (less than 18%) but statistically significant differences in dose-normalized irinotecan pharmacokinetic parameters in patients younger than 65 years of age compared with patients at least 65 years of age were observed.

In studies using the weekly schedule, the terminal half-life of irinotecan was 6 hours in patients who were 65 years of age and older and 5.5 hours in patients younger than 65 years of age.

See Administration and Dosage for more information.

Children: Pharmacokinetic parameters for irinotecan and SN-38 were determined in 2 pediatric solid-tumor trials at dose levels of 50 mg/m² (60-minute infusion, n = 48) and 125 mg/m² (90-minute infusion, n = 6). Irinotecan clearance (mean ± standard deviation) was 17.3 ± 6.7 L/h/m² for the 50 mg/m² dose and 16.2 ± 4.6 L/h/m² for the 125 mg/m² dose, which is comparable with that in adults. Dose-normalized SN-38 AUC values were comparable between adults and children. Minimal accumulation of irinotecan and SN-38 was observed in children on daily dosing regimens (daily × 5 every 3 weeks or [daily × 5] × 2 weeks every 3 weeks).

UGT1A1 genotype – In a prospective study in which irinotecan was administered as a single agent (350 mg/m²) on a once-every-3-week schedule, patients who were homozygous for UGT1A1 7/7 genotype had a higher exposure to SN-38 than patients with the wild-type UGT1A1 allele (UGT1A1 6/6 genotype).

Contraindications

Known hypersensitivity to the drug or its excipients.

Warnings/Precautions

➤*Toxicities:* Outside of a well-designed clinical study, do not use irinotecan in combination with the "Mayo Clinic" regimen of 5-fluorouracil/leucovorin (administration for 4 to 5 consecutive days every 4 weeks) because of reports of increased toxicity, including toxic deaths. Use irinotecan as recommended.

➤*Diarrhea:* Irinotecan can induce both early and late forms of diarrhea that appear to be mediated by different mechanisms. Early diarrhea (occurring during or shortly after infusion of irinotecan) is cholinergic in nature. It is usually transient and only infrequently is severe. It may be accompanied by symptoms of diaphoresis, flushing, increased salvation, intestinal hyperperistalsis (which can cause abdominal cramping), lacrimation, miosis, and rhinitis. Early diarrhea and other cholinergic symptoms may be prevented or ameliorated by administration of atropine. Consider prophylactic or therapeutic administration of IV or subcutaneous atropine 0.25 to 1 mg (unless clinically contraindicated) in patients experiencing abdominal cramping, diaphoresis, diarrhea (occurring during or shortly after infusion of irinotecan), flushing, increased salivation, lacrimation, miosis, or rhinitis. These symptoms are expected to occur more frequently with higher irinotecan doses.

Late diarrhea (occurring more than 24 hours after administration of irinotecan) can be life-threatening because it may be prolonged and may lead to dehydration, electrolyte imbalance, or sepsis. Promptly treat late diarrhea with loperamide. Instruct each patient to have loperamide readily available and to begin treatment for late diarrhea (occurring more than 24 hours after administration of irinotecan) at the first episode of poorly formed or loose stools or at the earliest onset of bowel movements more frequent than normally expected for the patient. One dosage regimen for loperamide used in clinical trials consisted of the following (this dosage regimen exceeds the usual dosage recommendations for loperamide): 4 mg at the first onset of late diarrhea and then 2 mg every 2 hours until the patient is diarrhea-free for at least 12 hours. Loperamide is not recommended to be used for more than 48 consecutive hours at these doses because of the risk of paralytic ileus. During the night, the patient may take loperamide 4 mg every 4 hours. Premedication with loperamide is not recommended. Carefully monitor patients with diarrhea, give fluid and electrolyte replacement if

IRINOTECAN HYDROCHLORIDE — INJECTION

they become dehydrated, and give antibiotic support if they develop fever, ileus, or severe neutropenia. After the first treatment, delay subsequent weekly chemotherapy treatments in patients until return of pretreatment bowel function for at least 24 hours without need for antidiarrheal medication. If grade 2, 3, or 4 late diarrhea occurs, decrease subsequent doses of irinotecan within the current cycle.

➤*Neutropenia:* Deaths due to sepsis following severe neutropenia have been reported in patients treated with irinotecan. Promptly manage neutropenic complications with antibiotic support. Omit therapy with irinotecan temporarily during a cycle of therapy if neutropenic fever occurs or if the absolute neutrophil count (ANC) drops to less than 1,000/mm^3. After the patient recovers to an ANC of 1,000/mm^3 or more, reduce subsequent doses of irinotecan depending upon the level of neutropenia observed.

Routine administration of a colony-stimulating factor (CSF) is not necessary, but health care providers may wish to consider CSF use in individual patients experiencing significant neutropenia.

Reduced UGT1A1 activity – Individuals who are homozygous for the UGT1A1*28 allele (UGT1A1 7/7 genotype) are at an increased risk for neutropenia following initiation of irinotecan treatment. Consider a reduced initial dose for patients known to be homozygous for the UGT1A1*28 allele. Heterozygous patients (carriers of 1 variant allele and 1 wild-type allele, which results in intermediate UGT1A1*28 activity) may be at an increased risk for neutropenia; however, clinical results have been variable and such patients have been shown to tolerate normal starting doses.

When administered in combination with other agents or as a single-agent, consider a reduction in the starting dose by at least 1 level of irinotecan for patients known to be homozygous for the UGT1A1*28 allele. However, the precise dose reduction in this patient population is not known; consider subsequent dose modifications based on individual patient tolerance to treatment.

➤*Colitis/Ileus:* Cases of colitis complicated by bleeding, ileus, infection, and ulceration have been observed. Administer prompt antibiotic support to patients experiencing ileus.

➤*Renal effects:* Rare cases of renal impairment and acute renal failure have been identified, usually in patients who became volume-depleted from severe vomiting and/or diarrhea.

➤*Thromboembolism:* Thromboembolic reactions have been observed in patients receiving irinotecan-containing regimens; the specific cause of these reactions has not been determined.

➤*Pulmonary toxicity:* Interstitial pulmonary disease–like events, including fatalities, have been reported in patients receiving irinotecan (in combination and as monotherapy) for treatment of colorectal cancer and other advanced solid tumors. In the event of an acute onset of new or progressive, unexplained pulmonary symptoms, such as dyspnea, cough, and fever, interrupt irinotecan and other coprescribed chemotherapeutic agents pending diagnostic evaluation. If interstitial pulmonary disease is diagnosed, discontinue irinotecan and other chemotherapy and institute appropriate treatment as needed.

➤*Premedication with antiemetics:* See Administration and Dosage for more information.

➤*Vaccines:* Administration of live or live-attenuated vaccines in patients immunocompromised by chemotherapeutic agents, including irinotecan, may result in serious or fatal infections. Avoid vaccination with a live vaccine in patients receiving irinotecan. Killed or inactivated vaccines may be administered; however, the response to such vaccines may be diminished.

➤*Irradiation:* Patients who have previously received pelvic/abdominal irradiation are at an increased risk of severe myelosuppression following the administration of irinotecan. The coadministration of irinotecan with irradiation has not been adequately studied and is not recommended.

➤*Extravasation:* See Administration and Dosage for more information.

➤*Hypersensitivity reactions:* Hypersensitivity reactions, including severe anaphylactic or anaphylactoid reactions, have been observed.

➤*Renal function impairment:* Exercise caution in patients with renal impairment. Irinotecan is not recommended for use in patients on dialysis.

➤*Hepatic function impairment:* In clinical trials of the weekly dosage schedule, patients with modestly elevated baseline serum total bilirubin levels (1 to 2 mg/dL) had a significantly greater likelihood of experiencing first-cycle grade 3 or 4 neutropenia than those with bilirubin levels that were less than 1 mg/dL (50% vs 18%; $P < 0.001$). Patients with deficient glucuronidation of bilirubin, such as those with Gilbert syndrome, may be at greater risk of myelosuppression when receiving therapy with irinotecan. See Actions for more information.

➤*Special risk:* In patients receiving irinotecan/5-fluorouracil/leucovorin or 5-fluorouracil/leucovorin in clinical trials, higher rates of hospitalization, neutropenic fever, thromboembolism, first-cycle treatment discontinuation, and early deaths were observed in patients with a baseline performance status of 2 than in patients with a baseline performance status of 0 or 1.

Irinotecan commonly causes anemia, leucopenia, and neutropenia, any of which may be severe; therefore, do not use in patients with severe bone marrow failure. Patients must not be treated with irinotecan until resolution of the bowel obstruction. Do not give irinotecan in patients with hereditary fructose intolerance, because this product contains sorbitol.

➤*Pregnancy: Category D.* Irinotecan may cause fetal harm when administered to a pregnant woman. There are no adequate and well-controlled studies of irinotecan in pregnant women. If the drug is used during pregnancy or if the patient becomes pregnant while receiving this drug, apprise the patient of the potential hazard to the fetus. Advise women of childbearing potential to avoid becoming pregnant while receiving treatment with irinotecan.

Radioactivity related to ^{14}C-irinotecan crosses the placenta in rats following IV administration of 10 mg/kg (which in separate studies produced an irinotecan C_{max} and AUC approximately 3 and 0.5 times, respectively, the corresponding values in patients administered 125 mg/m^2). Administration of irinotecan 6 mg/kg/day IV to rats (which in separate studies produced an irinotecan C_{max} and AUC approximately 2 and 0.2 times, respectively, the corresponding values in patients administered 125 mg/m^2) and rabbits (approximately 50% the recommended human dose on a mg/m^2 basis) during the period of organogenesis is embryotoxic, as characterized by increased postimplantation loss and decreased numbers of live fetuses. Irinotecan was teratogenic in rats at dosages greater than 1.2 mg/kg/day (which in separate studies produced an irinotecan C_{max} and AUC approximately two-thirds and one-fortieth, respectively, of the corresponding values in patients administered 125 mg/m^2) and in rabbits at 6 mg/kg/day (approximately 50% the recommended weekly human dose on a mg/m^2 basis). Teratogenic effects included a variety of external, visceral, and skeletal abnormalities. Irinotecan administered to rat dams for the period following organogenesis through weaning at dosages of 6 mg/kg/day caused decreased learning ability and decreased female body weights in the offspring.

➤*Lactation:* Radioactivity appeared in rat's milk within 5 minutes of IV administration of radiolabeled irinotecan and was concentrated up to 65-fold at 4 hours after administration relative to plasma concentrations. The molecular weight of irinotecan (about 587 for the nonhydrated free base), moderate plasma protein binding, and long elimination half-life suggest that the drug will be excreted into breast milk. Because many drugs are excreted in human milk and because of the potential for serious adverse reactions in breast-feeding infants, it is recommended that breast-feeding be discontinued during therapy with irinotecan.

➤*Children:* The efficacy of irinotecan in children has not been established.

➤*Elderly:* Closely monitor patients older than 65 years because of a greater risk of late diarrhea in this population.

See Administration and Dosage for more information..

➤*Monitoring:* Carefully monitor patients with diarrhea and give fluid and electrolyte replacement if they become dehydrated, or antibiotic therapy if they develop fever, ileus, or severe neutropenia. It is recommended that the white blood cell count with differential, hemoglobin, and platelet count be carefully monitored before each dose of irinotecan. Closely monitor patients who have previously received pelvic/abdominal radiation and elderly patients with comorbid conditions. Closely monitor patients with risk factors for respiratory symptoms before and during irinotecan therapy.

Drug Interactions

➤*Vaccines:* The risk of live vaccine–induced adverse reactions may be increased by coadministration of irinotecan. The use of live vaccines in patients receiving irinotecan is not recommended under most circumstances and should be deferred.

Irinotecan Drug Interactions

Precipitant drug	Object drug[a]		Description
Antineoplastics	Irinotecan	⬆	The adverse reactions of irinotecan, such as myelosuppression and diarrhea, would be expected to be exacerbated by other antineoplastic agents having similar adverse reactions. Closely monitor for irinotecan adverse reactions.
CYP3A4 inducers (eg, carbamazepine, phenobarbital, phenytoin, rifabutin, rifampin, St. John's wort)	Irinotecan	⬇	Exposure to irinotecan and its active metabolite (SN-38) is substantially reduced when given concomitantly to patients receiving CYP3A4 enzyme–inducing anticonvulsants. For patients requiring anticonvulsant treatment, consider substituting a nonenzyme-inducing anticonvulsant at least 2 weeks prior to initiation of irinotecan therapy. Coadministration with St. John's wort is contraindicated. Discontinue St. John's wort at least 2 weeks prior to the first cycle of irinotecan.
CYP3A4 inhibitors (eg, atazanavir, ketoconazole)	Irinotecan	⬆	Coadministration may increase irinotecan and its active metabolite (SN-38). Coadministration with ketoconazole is contraindicated. Instruct patients to discontinue ketoconazole at least 1 week prior to initiating irinotecan therapy. Avoid concomitant use with atazanavir. Close clinical and laboratory monitoring is warranted when administering ritonavir-boosted lopinavir with IV irinotecan.

IRINOTECAN HYDROCHLORIDE — INJECTION

Irinotecan Drug Interactions			
Precipitant drug	Object drug[a]		Description
Dexamethasone	Irinotecan	↑	Lymphocytopenia has been reported in patients receiving irinotecan, and it is possible that the administration of dexamethasone as antiemetic prophylaxis may have enhanced the likelihood of this effect. Hyperglycemia has also been reported. It is probable that dexamethasone given as emetic prophylaxis contributed to hyperglycemia in some patients.
Laxatives	Irinotecan	↑	It would be expected that laxative use during therapy with irinotecan would worsen the incidence or severity of diarrhea, but this has not been studied.
Palifermin	Irinotecan	↑	Coadministration of palifermin and irinotecan within the same 24-hour time period may increase the severity and duration of oral mucositis. Do not administer palifermin within 24 hours before, during, or 24 hours after administration of irinotecan.
Prochlorperazine	Irinotecan	↑	The incidence of akathisia in clinical trials was greater (8.5%) when prochlorperazine was administered on the same day as irinotecan than when these drugs were given on separate days (1.3%). However, the 8.5% incidence of akathisia is within the range reported for use of prochlorperazine when given as a premedication for other chemotherapeutics.
Irinotecan	Depolarizing neuromuscular blocking agents (eg, succinylcholine)	↑	Irinotecan has anticholinesterase activity, which may prolong the neuromuscular blocking effects of succinylcholine.
Irinotecan	Diuretics (eg, furosemide)	↑	In view of the potential risk of dehydration secondary to vomiting and/or diarrhea induced by irinotecan, the health care provider may wish to withhold diuretics during dosing with irinotecan and during periods of active vomiting or diarrhea.
Irinotecan	Nondepolarizing neuromuscular blocking agents (eg, vecuronium)	↓	Irinotecan may antagonize the neuromuscular blockage of nondepolarizing neuromuscular blocking agents.

[a] ↑ = object drug increased; ↓ = object drug decreased.

Adverse Reactions

➤*Emetogenic potential:* Irinotecan is considered to have moderately high emetogenic potential (60% to 90% incidence of emesis).

➤*First-line combination therapy:*

Study 1: Deaths and discontinuations of therapy – In study 1, 7.3% of patients died within 30 days of last study treatment: 9.3% of patients received irinotecan in combination with 5-fluorouracil/leucovorin, 6.8% received 5-fluorouracil/leucovorin alone, and 5.8% received irinotecan alone. Deaths potentially related to treatment occurred in 2 (0.9%) patients who received irinotecan in combination with 5-fluorouracil/leucovorin (2 neutropenic fever/sepsis), 1.4% of patients who received 5-fluorouracil/leucovorin alone (1 neutropenic fever/sepsis, 1 CNS bleeding during thrombocytopenia, 1 unknown), and 0.9% of patients who received irinotecan alone (2 neutropenic fever). Deaths from any cause within 60 days of first study treatment were reported for 6.7% of patients who received irinotecan in combination with 5-fluorouracil/leucovorin, 7.3% of patients who received 5-fluorouracil/leucovorin alone, and 6.7% of patients who received irinotecan alone. Discontinuations due to adverse reactions were reported for 7.6% of patients who received irinotecan in combination with 5-fluorouracil/leucovorin, 6.4% of patients who received 5-fluorouracil/leucovorin alone, and 11.7% of patients who received irinotecan alone.

Study 2: Deaths and discontinuations of therapy – In study 2, 3.5% of patients died within 30 days of last study treatment: 4.1% received irinotecan in combination with 5-fluorouracil/leucovorin and 2.8% received 5-fluorouracil/leucovorin alone. There was 1 potentially treatment-related death that occurred in a patient who received irinotecan in combination with 5-fluorouracil/leucovorin (0.7%, neutropenic sepsis). Deaths from any cause within 60 days of first study treatment were reported for 2.1% of patients who received irinotecan in combination with 5-fluorouracil/leucovorin and 1.4% of patients who received 5-fluorouracil/leucovorin alone. Discontinuations due to adverse reactions were reported for 6.2% of patients who received irinotecan in combination with 5-fluorouracil/leucovorin and 0.7% of patients who received 5-fluorouracil/leucovorin alone.

Most significant adverse reactions – The most clinically significant adverse reactions for patients receiving irinotecan-based therapy were alopecia, diarrhea, nausea, neutropenia, and vomiting. The most clinically significant adverse reactions for patients receiving 5-fluorouracil/leucovorin therapy were diarrhea, mucositis, neutropenia, and neutropenic fever. In study 1, grade 4 neutropenia, neutropenic fever (defined as grade 2 fever and grade 4 neutropenia), and mucositis were observed less often with weekly irinotecan/5-fluorouracil/leucovorin than with monthly administration of 5-fluorouracil/leucovorin.

Study 1 adverse reactions –

Irinotecan Study 1: Adverse Reactions in Combination Therapies[a]						
	Irinotecan + bolus 5-fluorouracil/ leucovorin weekly × 4 every 6 wk (n = 225)		Bolus 5-fluorouracil/ leucovorin daily × 5 every 4 wk (n = 219)		Irinotecan weekly × 4 every 6 wk (n = 223)	
Adverse reaction	Grade 1 to 4	Grade 3 and 4	Grade 1 to 4	Grade 3 and 4	Grade 1 to 4	Grade 3 and 4
Total adverse reactions	100%	53.3%	100%	45.7%	99.6%	45.7%
Cardiovascular						
Hypotension	5.8%	1.3%	2.3%	0.5%	5.8%	1.7%
Thromboembolic reactions[b]	9.3%	—	11.4%	—	5.4%	—
Vasodilation	9.3%	0.9%	5%	0%	9%	0%
CNS						
Confusion	7.1%	1.8%	4.1%	0%	2.7%	0%
Dizziness	23.1%	1.3%	16.4%	0%	21.1%	1.8%
Somnolence	12.4%	1.8%	4.6%	1.8%	9.4%	1.3%
Dermatologic						
Alopecia[c]	43.1%	—	26.5%	—	46.1%	—
Exfoliative dermatitis	0.9%	0%	3.2%	0.5%	0%	0%
Rash	19.1%	0%	26.5%	0.9%	14.3%	0.4%
GI						
Abdominal pain	63.1%	14.6%	50.2%	11.5%	67.7%	13%
Anorexia	34.2%	5.8%	42%	3.7%	43.9%	7.2%
Constipation	41.3%	3.1%	31.5%	1.8%	32.3%	0.4%
Diarrhea (early)	45.8%	4.9%	31.5%	1.4%	43%	6.7%
Diarrhea (late)	84.9%	22.7%	69.4%	13.2%	83%	31%
Grade 3	—	15.1%	—	5.9%	—	18.4%
Grade 4	—	7.6%	—	7.3%	—	12.6%
Mucositis	32.4%	2.2%	76.3%	16.9%	29.6%	2.2%
Nausea	79.1%	15.6%	67.6%	8.2%	81.6%	16.1%
Vomiting	60.4%	9.7%	46.1%	4.1%	62.8%	12.1%
Hematologic						
Anemia	96.9%	8.4%	98.6%	5.5%	96.9%	4.5%
Leukopenia	96.9%	37.8%	98.6%	23.3%	96.4%	21.5%
Neutropenia	96.9%	53.8%	98.6%	66.7%	96.4%	31.4%
Grade 3	—	29.8%	—	23.7%	—	19.3%
Grade 4	—	24%	—	42.5%	—	12.1%
Neutropenic fever	—	7.1%	—	14.6%	—	5.8%
Neutropenic infection	—	1.8%	—	0%	—	2.2%
Thrombocytopenia	96%	2.6%	98.6%	2.7%	96%	1.7%
Respiratory						
Cough	26.7%	1.3%	18.3%	0%	20.2%	0.4%
Dyspnea	27.6%	6.3%	16%	0.5%	22%	2.2%
Pneumonia	6.2%	2.7%	1.4%	1%	3.6%	1.3%
Miscellaneous						
Asthenia	70.2%	19.5%	64.4%	11.9%	69.1%	13.9%
Fever	42.2%	1.7%	32.4%	3.6%	43.5%	0.4%
Increased bilirubin	87.6%	7.1%	92.2%	8.2%	83.9%	7.2%

IRINOTECAN HYDROCHLORIDE — INJECTION

Irinotecan Study 1: Adverse Reactions in Combination Therapies[a]						
	Irinotecan + bolus 5-fluorouracil/ leucovorin weekly × 4 every 6 wk (n = 225)		Bolus 5-fluorouracil/ leucovorin daily × 5 every 4 wk (n = 219)		Irinotecan weekly × 4 every 6 wk (n = 223)	
Adverse reaction	Grade 1 to 4	Grade 3 and 4	Grade 1 to 4	Grade 3 and 4	Grade 1 to 4	Grade 3 and 4
Infection	22.2%	0%	16%	1.4%	13.9%	0.4%
Pain	30.7%	3.1%	26.9%	3.6%	22.9%	2.2%

[a] Severity of adverse reactions based on NCI-CTC (version 1.0).
[b] Includes angina pectoris, arterial thrombosis, cerebral infarction, cerebrovascular accident, deep thrombophlebitis, embolus lower extremity, heart arrest, myocardial infarction, myocardial ischemia, peripheral vascular disorder, pulmonary embolus, sudden death, thrombophlebitis, thrombosis, vascular disorder.
[c] Complete hair loss = grade 2.

Study 2 adverse reactions –

Irinotecan Study 2: Adverse Reactions in Combination Therapies[a]				
	Irinotecan + 5-fluorouracil/ leucovorin by infusion on days 1 and 2 every 2 wk (n = 145)		5-fluorouracil/ leucovorin by infusion on days 1 and 2 every 2 wk (n = 143)	
Adverse reaction	Grade 1 to 4	Grade 3 and 4	Grade 1 to 4	Grade 3 and 4
Total adverse reactions	100%	72.4%	100%	39.2%
Cardiovascular				
Hypotension	3.4%	1.4%	0.7%	0%
Thromboembolic reactions[b]	11.7%	—	5.6%	—
Dermatologic				
Alopecia[c]	56.6%	—	16.8%	—
Cutaneous signs	17.2%	0.7%	20.3%	0%
Hand and foot syndrome	10.3%	0.7%	12.6%	0.7%
GI				
Abdominal pain	17.2%	2.1%	16.8%	0.7%
Anorexia	35.2%	2.1%	18.9%	0.7%
Cholinergic syndrome[d]	28.3%	1.4%	0.7%	0%
Constipation	30.3%	0.7%	25.2%	1.4%
Diarrhea (late)	72.4%	14.4%	44.8%	6.3%
Grade 3	—	10.3%	—	4.2%
Grade 4	—	4.1%	—	2.1%
Mucositis	40%	4.1%	28.7%	2.8%
Nausea	66.9%	2.1%	55.2%	3.5%
Vomiting	44.8%	3.5%	32.2%	2.8%
Hematologic				
Anemia	97.2%	2.1%	90.9%	2.1%
Leukopenia	81.3%	17.4%	42%	3.5%
Neutropenia	82.5%	46.2%	47.9%	13.4%
Grade 3	—	36.4%	—	12.7%
Grade 4	—	9.8%	—	0.7%
Neutropenic fever	—	3.4%	—	0.7%
Neutropenic infection	—	2.1%	—	0%
Thrombocytopenia	32.6%	0%	32.2%	0%
Miscellaneous				
Asthenia	57.9%	9%	48.3%	4.2%
Dyspnea	9.7%	1.4%	4.9%	0%
Fever	22.1%	0.7%	25.9%	0.7%
Increased bilirubin	19.1%	3.5%	35.9%	10.6%
Infection	35.9%	7.6%	33.6%	3.5%
Pain	64.1%	9.7%	61.5%	8.4%

[a] Severity of adverse reactions based on NCI-CTC (version 1.0).
[b] Includes angina pectoris, arterial thrombosis, cerebral infarction, cerebrovascular accident, deep thrombophlebitis, embolus lower extremity, heart arrest, myocardial infarction, myocardial ischemia, peripheral vascular disorder, pulmonary embolus, sudden death, thrombophlebitis, thrombosis, vascular disorder.
[c] Complete hair loss = grade 2.
[d] Includes abdominal cramping, diaphoresis, diarrhea (occurring during or shortly after infusion of irinotecan), flushing, increased salivation, lacrimation, miosis, or rhinitis.

➤*Second-line single-agent therapy:*

Weekly dosage schedule –

Death: Seventeen of the patients died within 30 days of administration of irinotecan; in 1.6% of cases, the deaths were potentially drug-related. These 5 patients experienced a constellation of medical reactions that included known effects of irinotecan. One of these patients died of neutropenic sepsis without fever. Neutropenic fever occurred in 3% of other patients; these patients recovered with supportive care.

Hospitalization: Of the 304 patients, 39.1% were hospitalized a total of 156 times because of adverse reactions; 26.6% of patients were hospitalized for reactions judged to be related to administration of irinotecan. The primary reasons for drug-related hospitalization were diarrhea, with or without nausea and/or vomiting (18.4%); neutropenia/leukopenia, with or without diarrhea and/or fever (8.2%); and nausea and/or vomiting (4.9%).

Dosage adjustments: Adjustments in the dose of irinotecan were made during the cycle of treatment and for subsequent cycles based on individual patient tolerance. The first dose of at least 1 cycle of irinotecan was reduced for 67% of patients who began the studies at the 125 mg/m^2 starting dose. Within-cycle dose reductions were required for 32% of the cycles initiated at the 125 mg/m^2 starting dose. The most common reasons for dose reduction were late diarrhea, leukopenia, and neutropenia. A total of 4.3% of patients discontinued treatment with irinotecan because of adverse reactions.

Adverse reactions (more than 10%):

Irinotecan Weekly Dosage Schedule Adverse Reactions in Previously Treated Patients (> 10%; N = 304)[a]		
Adverse reaction	NCI grades 1 to 4	NCI grades 3 and 4
CNS		
Dizziness	15%	0%
Headache	17%	1%
Insomnia	19%	0%
Dermatologic		
Alopecia	60%	NA[b]
Rash	13%	1%
Sweating	16%	0%
GI		
Abdominal cramping/pain	57%	16%
Abdominal enlargement	10%	0%
Anorexia	55%	6%
Constipation	30%	2%
Diarrhea (early)[c]	51%	8%
Diarrhea (late)[d]	88%	31%
7 to 9 stools/day (grade 3)	—	16%
≥ 10 stools/day (grade 4)	—	14%
Dyspepsia	10%	0%
Flatulence	12%	0%
Nausea	86%	17%
Stomatitis	12%	1%
Vomiting	67%	12%
Hematologic		
Anemia	60%	7%
Leukopenia	63%	28%
Neutropenia	54%	26%
500 to < 1,000/mm^3 (grade 3)		15%
< 500/mm^3 (grade 4)		12%

IRINOTECAN HYDROCHLORIDE — INJECTION

Irinotecan Weekly Dosage Schedule Adverse Reactions in Previously Treated Patients (> 10%; N = 304)[a]		
Adverse reaction	NCI grades 1 to 4	NCI grades 3 and 4
Metabolic/Nutritional		
Alkaline phosphatase increased	13%	4%
AST increased	10%	1%
Body weight decreased	30%	1%
Dehydration	15%	4%
Respiratory		
Coughing increased	17%	0%
Dyspnea	22%	4%
Rhinitis	16%	0%
Miscellaneous		
Asthenia	76%	12%
Back pain	14%	2%
Chills	14%	0%
Edema	10%	1%
Fever	45%	1%
Minor infection[e]	14%	0%
Pain	24%	2%
Vasodilation (flushing)	11%	0%

[a] Severity of adverse reactions based on NCI-CTC (version 1.0).
[b] Not applicable; complete hair loss = NCI grade 2.
[c] Occurring 24 hours or less after administration of irinotecan.
[d] Occurring 24 hours or more after administration of irinotecan.
[e] Primarily upper respiratory tract infections.

Once-every-3-week dosage schedule –

Death: A total of 3.5% of patients treated with irinotecan died within 30 days of treatment. In three (1%) of cases, the deaths were potentially related to irinotecan treatment and were attributed to neutropenic infection, grade 4 diarrhea, and asthenia, respectively. One (0.8%) patient treated with 5-fluorouracil died within 30 days of treatment; this death was attributed to grade 4 diarrhea.

Hospitalization: Hospitalizations due to serious adverse reactions (whether or not related to study treatment) occurred at least once in 60% of patients who received irinotecan, 63% who received best supportive care, and 39% who received 5-fluorouracil–based therapy. Eight percent of patients treated with irinotecan and 7% treated with 5-fluorouracil–based therapy discontinued treatment because of adverse reactions.

Significant adverse reactions: Of the 316 patients treated with irinotecan, the most clinically significant adverse reactions (all grades, 1 to 4) were diarrhea (84%), alopecia (72%), nausea (70%), vomiting (62%), cholinergic symptoms (47%), and neutropenia (30%).

Adverse reactions:

Irinotecan Once-Every-3-Week Therapy Grades 3 and 4 Adverse Reactions[a]				
	Study 1		Study 2	
Adverse reaction	Irinotecan (n = 189)	BSC[b] (n = 90)	Irinotecan (n = 127)	5-fluorouracil (n = 129)
Total grades 3 and 4 adverse reactions	79%	67%	69%	54%
Dermatologic				
Cutaneous signs[c]	2%	0%	1%	3%
Hand and foot syndrome	0%	0%	0%	5%
GI				
Abdominal pain	14%	16%	9%	8%
Anorexia	5%	7%	6%	4%
Constipation	10%	8%	8%	6%
Diarrhea	22%	6%	22%	11%
Mucositis	2%	1%	2%	5%
Nausea	14%	3%	11%	4%
Vomiting	14%	8%	14%	5%
Hematologic				
Anemia	7%	6%	6%	3%
Fever (with grade 3/4 neutropenia)	2%	0%	4%	2%
Fever (without grade 3/4 neutropenia)	2%	1%	2%	0%
Hemorrhage	5%	3%	1%	3%
Infection (with grade 3/4 neutropenia)	1%	0%	2%	0%
Infection (without grade 3/4 neutropenia)	8%	3%	1%	4%
Leukopenia/Neutropenia	22%	0%	14%	2%
Thrombocytopenia	1%	0%	4%	2%
Miscellaneous				
Asthenia	15%	19%	13%	12%
Cardiovascular[d]	9%	3%	4%	2%
CNS[e]	12%	13%	9%	4%
Hepatic[f]	9%	7%	9%	6%
Other[g]	32%	28%	12%	14%
Pain	19%	22%	17%	13%
Respiratory[h]	10%	8%	5%	7%

[a] Severity of adverse reactions based on NCI-CTC (version 1.0).
[b] BSC = best supportive care.
[c] Cutaneous signs include reactions such as rash.
[d] Cardiovascular includes reactions such as dysrhythmias, ischemia, and mechanical cardiac dysfunction.
[e] Neurologic includes reactions such as somnolence.
[f] Hepatic includes reactions such as ascites and jaundice.
[g] Other includes reactions such as accidental injury, hepatomegaly, syncope, vertigo, and weight loss.
[h] Respiratory includes reactions such as dyspnea and cough.

➤*Other adverse reactions:*

Cardiovascular – Bradycardia, thromboembolic reactions, vasodilation (flushing).

CNS – Dizziness, insomnia.

Dermatologic – Alopecia, rashes.

GI – Diarrhea, nausea, and vomiting are common adverse reactions following treatment with irinotecan and can be severe. When observed, nausea and vomiting usually occur during or shortly after infusion of irinotecan. An increased incidence of late diarrhea was observed in 2 studies, one using a 3-week schedule and the other using a weekly schedule. In the clinical studies testing the every-3-week dosage schedule, the median time to the onset of late diarrhea was 5 days after irinotecan infusion. In the clinical studies evaluating the weekly dosage schedule, the median time to onset of late diarrhea was 11 days following administration of irinotecan. For patients starting treatment at the 125 mg/m² weekly dose, the median duration of any grade of late diarrhea was 3 days. Among those patients treated at the 125 mg/m² weekly dose who experienced grade 3 or 4 late diarrhea, the median duration of the entire episode of diarrhea was 7 days. The frequency of grade 3 or 4 late diarrhea was somewhat greater in patients starting treatment at 125 mg/m² than in patients given a 100 mg/m² weekly starting dose (34% vs 23%; $P = 0.08$). The frequency of grade 3 and 4 late diarrhea by age was significantly greater in patients 65 years of age and older than in patients younger than 65 years of age (40% vs 23%; $P = 0.002$). In another study of 183 patients treated on the weekly schedule, the frequency of grade 3 or 4 late diarrhea in patients at least 65 years of age was 28.6% and in patients less than 65 years of age was 23.9%. In one study of the weekly dosage treatment, the frequency of grade 3 and 4 late diarrhea was significantly greater in men than in women (43% vs 16%; $P = 0.01$), but there were no gender differences in the frequency of grade 3 and 4 late diarrhea in the other 2 studies of the weekly dosage treatment schedule. Colonic ulceration, sometimes with GI bleeding, has been observed in association with administration of irinotecan.

Hematologic – Irinotecan commonly causes anemia, leukopenia (including lymphocytopenia), and neutropenia. Serious thrombocytopenia is uncommon. When evaluated in the trials of weekly administration, the frequency of grade 3 and 4 neutropenia was significantly higher in patients who received previous pelvic/abdominal irradiation than in those who had not received such irradiation (48% vs 24%; $P = 0.04$). In these same studies, patients with baseline serum total bilirubin levels of 1 mg/dL or more also had a significantly greater likelihood of experiencing first-cycle grade 3 or 4 neutropenia than those with bilirubin levels that were less than 1 mg/dL (50% vs 18%; P

Hepatic – In the clinical studies evaluating the weekly dosage schedule, NCI grade 3 or 4 liver enzyme abnormalities were observed in fewer than 10% of patients. These reactions typically occur in patients with known hepatic metastases.

Respiratory – Severe pulmonary reactions are infrequent. In the clinical studies evaluating the weekly dosage schedule, NCI grade 3 or 4 dyspnea was reported in 4% of patients. Over half the patients with dyspnea had lung metastases; the extent to which malignant pulmonary involvement or other preexisting lung disease may have contributed to dyspnea in these patients is unknown.

Interstitial pulmonary disease presenting as pulmonary infiltrates is uncommon during irinotecan therapy. Interstitial pulmonary disease can be fatal. Risk factors possibly associated with the development of interstitial pulmonary disease include preexisting lung disease, use of pneumotoxic drugs, radiation therapy, and CSFs.

IRINOTECAN HYDROCHLORIDE — INJECTION

Miscellaneous – Abdominal pain, asthenia, and fever.

Patients may have cholinergic symptoms of diaphoresis, flushing, increased salivation, intestinal hyperperistalsis (which can cause abdominal cramping and early diarrhea), lacrimation, miosis, and rhinitis. If these symptoms occur, they manifest during or shortly after drug infusion. They are thought to be related to the anticholinesterase activity of the irinotecan parent compound and are expected to occur more frequently with higher irinotecan doses.

➤*Postmarketing:*

GI – Infrequent cases of ulcerative and ischemic colitis have been observed. This can be complicated by bleeding, ileus, infection (including typhlitis), obstruction, and ulceration. Cases of intestinal perforation, symptomatic pancreatitis, asymptomatic elevated pancreatic enzymes, and megacolon have been reported.

Hypersensitivity – Hypersensitivity reactions, including severe anaphylactic or anaphylactoid reactions.

Metabolic/Nutritional – Cases of hyponatremia mostly related to diarrhea and vomiting;increases in serum levels of transaminases (ie, AST and ALT) in the absence of progressive liver metastasis; transient increase of amylase and occasionally transient increase of lipase.

Renal – Infrequent cases of renal impairment, including acute renal failure, hypotension, or circulatory failure, have been observed in patients who experienced episodes of dehydration associated with diarrhea and/or vomiting, or sepsis.

Miscellaneous – Myocardial ischemic events; transient dysarthria; muscular contraction or cramps and paresthesia; hiccups.

Overdosage

➤*Symptoms:* There have been reports of overdosage at doses up to approximately twice the recommended therapeutic dose, which may be fatal. The most significant adverse reactions reported were severe neutropenia and severe diarrhea.

➤*Treatment:* There is no known antidote for overdosage of irinotecan. Institute maximum supportive care to prevent dehydration due to diarrhea and to treat any infectious complications.

Patient Information

Inform patients and their caregivers of the expected toxic effects of irinotecan, particularly of its GI complications, such as abdominal cramping, diarrhea, infection, nausea, and vomiting. Instruct each patient to have loperamide readily available and to begin treatment for late diarrhea (occurring more than 24 hours after administration of irinotecan) at the first episode of poorly formed or loose stools or at the earliest onset of bowel movements more frequent than normally expected for the patient. Avoid the use of drugs with laxative properties because of the potential for exacerbation of diarrhea. Advise patients to contact their health care provider to discuss any laxative use.

Instruct patients to contact their health care provider if any of the following occur: diarrhea for the first time during treatment; black or bloody stools; symptoms of dehydration, such as dizziness, faintness, or light-headedness; inability to take fluids by mouth because of nausea or vomiting; inability to get diarrhea under control within 24 hours; fever or evidence of infection.

Warn patients about the potential for dizziness or visual disturbances, which may occur within 24 hours following the administration of irinotecan. Advise patients not to drive or operate machinery if these symptoms occur.

Alert patients to the possibility of alopecia.

TOPOTECAN

Rx	**Hycamtin** (GlaxoSmithKline)	**Capsules; oral:** 0.25 mg	As topotecan hydrochloride. Hydrogenated vegetable oil. (HYCAMTIN 0.25 mg). Opaque white to yellowish-white. In 10s.
		1 mg	As topotecan hydrochloride. Hydrogenated vegetable oil. (HYCAMTIN 1 mg). Opaque pink. In 10s.
Rx	**Topotecan** (Various, eg, Sagent Pharmaceutical, Three Rivers)	**Injection, lyophilized powder for solution:** 4 mg	As topotecan hydrochloride. Preservative free. May contain mannitol. In single-dose vials.
Rx	**Hycamtin** (GlaxoSmithKline)		As topotecan hydrochloride. Preservative free. In single-dose vials.

TOPOTECAN HYDROCHLORIDE — ORAL

WARNING

Bone marrow suppression – Administer topotecan only to patients with baseline neutrophil counts of 1,500 cells/mm^3 or more and a platelet count of 100,000 cells/mm^3 or more. In order to assess the occurrence of bone marrow suppression, monitor blood cell counts.

Indications

➤*Relapsed small cell lung cancer:* For the treatment of relapsed small cell lung cancer (SCLC) in patients with a prior complete or partial response who are at least 45 days from the end of first-line chemotherapy.

➤*Off-label uses:* Nonsmall cell lung cancer, relapsed or refractory ovarian cancer. (See Administration and Dosage.)

Administration and Dosage

➤*Adults:*

Relapsed small cell lung cancer –

Usual dosage: 2.3 mg/m^2 once daily for 5 consecutive days repeated every 21 days. Round the calculated oral daily dose to the nearest 0.25 mg, and prescribe the minimum number of 1 and 0.25 mg capsules. The same number of capsules should be prescribed for each of the 5 dosing days.

Dosage adjustment: Patients should not be treated with subsequent courses of topotecan until neutrophils recover to greater than 1,000 cells/mm^3, platelets recover to greater than 100,000 cells/mm^3, and hemoglobin levels recover to 9 g/dL or more (with transfusion if necessary).

For patients who experience severe neutropenia (neutrophils less than 500 cells/mm^3 associated with fever or infection or lasting for 7 days or more) or neutropenia (neutrophils 500 to 1,000 cells/mm^3 lasting beyond day 21 of the treatment course), the topotecan dose should be reduced by 0.4 mg/m^2/day for subsequent courses. Doses should be similarly reduced if the platelet count falls below 25,000 cells/mm^3.

For patients who experience grade 3 or 4 diarrhea, the topotecan dose should be reduced by 0.4 mg/m^2/day for subsequent courses. Patients with grade 2 diarrhea may need to follow the same dose modification guidelines.

Off-label dosing –

Nonsmall cell lung cancer: 2.3 mg/m^2 once daily for 5 consecutive days starting on day 1 of a 21-day cycle. Round the calculated dose to the nearest 0.25 mg using the smallest number of capsules.

Relapsed or refractory ovarian cancer: 2.3 mg/m^2 once daily for 5 consecutive days starting on day 1 of a 21-day cycle. Round the calculated dose to the nearest 0.25 mg using the smallest number of capsules.

➤*Renal function impairment:* A dose adjustment of topotecan to 1.8 mg/m^2/day is predicted to adjust the area under the curve (AUC) to normal range for patients with moderate renal function impairment (creatinine clearance [CrCl] = 30 to 49 mL/min). Insufficient data are available in patients with severe renal function impairment to provide a dosage recommendation for topotecan.

Topotecan Oral Dosage Adjustment for Adults Based on Renal Function

Baseline creatinine clearance	Percent of usual dose to be given: Manufacturer package insert	Alternative dosage recommendation
> 80 mL/min	100%	100%
50 to 80 mL/min	100%	75%
30 to 49 mL/min	78% (reduce initial dose to 1.8 mg/m^2/day)	50%
10 to 29 mL/min	Dose reduction necessary; no data available to determine dose.	50%
< 10 mL/min	Dose reduction necessary; no data available to determine dose.	25%
Hemodialysis	Do not administer.	Do not administer.
Peritoneal dialysis	Do not administer.	Do not administer.
Continuous renal replacement therapy	Do not administer.	50%

Dialysis – In one patient, conventional hemodialysis was shown to be ineffective (0% to 24%) in removing topotecan; however, conventional hemodialysis was shown to be moderately effective (50% to 74%) in removing topotecan in another patient.

Some clinicians recommend a supplemental dose after hemodialysis.

➤*Hepatic function impairment:* Monitor these patients and adjust dose as needed if toxicity occurs.

➤*Preparation for administration:* Topotecan is considered a cytotoxic agent. Follow safe handling procedures when preparing, administering, or dispensing topotecan.

Direct contact of the capsule contents with the skin or mucous membranes should be avoided. If such contact occurs, wash thoroughly with soap and water or wash the eyes immediately with gently flowing water for at least 15 minutes. Advise patients to consult the health care provider in case of a skin reaction or if the drug gets in the eyes.

➤*Administration:* Topotecan may be taken with or without food. The capsules must be swallowed whole and must not be chewed, crushed, or divided. For patients unable to swallow capsules whole, see Preparation for Administration.

If the patient vomits after taking the dose of topotecan, the patient should not take a replacement dose.

TOPOTECAN HYDROCHLORIDE — ORAL

➤*Storage/Stability:* Store refrigerated 2° to 8°C (36° to 46°F). Store bottles protected from light in the original outer cartons.

Actions

➤*Pharmacology:* Topoisomerase I relieves torsional strain in DNA by inducing reversible single strand breaks. Topotecan binds to the topoisomerase I–DNA complex and prevents relegation of these single strand breaks. The cytotoxicity of topotecan is thought to be due to double-strand DNA damage produced during DNA synthesis, when replication enzymes interact with the ternary complex formed by topotecan, topoisomerase I, and DNA. Mammalian cells cannot efficiently repair these double-strand breaks.

Pharmacodynamics – The dose-limiting toxicity of topotecan is leukopenia. White blood cell count decreases with increasing topotecan dose or topotecan AUC. There is a correlation between topotecan lactone AUC on day 1 and percent decrease of leukocytes.

➤*Pharmacokinetics:*

Absorption – Topotecan exhibits biexponential pharmacokinetics. Total exposure (AUC) increases approximately proportionally with dose.

Topotecan is rapidly absorbed, with peak plasma concentrations occurring between 1 to 2 hours following oral administration. The oral bioavailability of topotecan is about 40%.

Effect of food: Following a high-fat meal, the extent of exposure was similar in the fed and fasted states, while time to reach maximum plasma concentration was delayed from 1.5 to 3 hours (topotecan lactone) and from 3 to 4 hours (total topotecan), respectively. Topotecan capsules can be given without regard to food.

Distribution – Plasma protein binding of topotecan is about 35%.

Metabolism/Excretion – Topotecan undergoes a reversible pH-dependent hydrolysis of its lactone moiety; it is the lactone form that is pharmacologically active. At a pH of 4 or less, the lactone is exclusively present, whereas the ring-opened hydroxy-acid form predominates at physiologic pH. The mean metabolite:parent AUC ratio was less than 10% for total topotecan and topotecan lactone.

In a mass-balance study in 4 patients with advanced solid tumors, the overall recovery of drug-related material following 5 daily doses of topotecan was 57% of the administered oral dose. In the urine, 20% of the oral administered dose was excreted as total topotecan and 2% was excreted as N-desmethyl topotecan. Fecal elimination of total topotecan accounted for 33%, while fecal elimination of N-desmethyl topotecan was 1.5%. Overall, the N-desmethyl metabolite contributed a mean of less than 6% (range, 4% to 8%) of the total drug-related material accounted for in the urine and feces. O-glucuronides of both topotecan and N-desmethyl topotecan have been identified in the urine. Mean terminal half-life of topotecan is 3 to 6 hours.

Special populations –

Elderly: A cross-study analysis in 217 patients with advanced solid tumors indicated that age does not significantly affect the pharmacokinetics of oral topotecan.

Gender: A cross-study analysis in 217 patients with advanced solid tumors indicated that gender does not significantly affect the pharmacokinetics of oral topotecan.

Race: There are insufficient data to determine an effect of race on pharmacokinetics of oral topotecan.

Contraindications

History of severe hypersensitivity reactions (eg, anaphylactoid reactions) to topotecan or to any of its ingredients; pregnancy; breast-feeding; severe bone marrow depression.

Warnings/Precautions

➤*Bone marrow suppression:* Bone marrow suppression (primarily neutropenia) is a dose-limiting toxicity of topotecan. Neutropenia is not cumulative over time. The following data on myelosuppression are based on an integrated safety database from 4 thoracic malignancy studies (N = 682) using topotecan at 2.3 mg/m^2/day for 5 consecutive days. The median day for neutrophil, red blood cell, and platelet nadirs occurred on day 15.

See the Warning box for more information.

Neutropenia – Grade 4 neutropenia (less than 500 cells/mm^3) occurred in 32% of patients with a median duration of 7 days and was most common during course 1 of treatment (20% of patients). Infection, sepsis, and febrile neutropenia occurred in 17%, 2%, and 4% of patients, respectively. Death due to sepsis occurred in 1% of patients. Pancytopenia has been reported.

Topotecan-induced neutropenia can lead to neutropenic colitis. Fatalities due to neutropenic colitis have been reported. Consider the possibility of neutropenic colitis in patients presenting with fever, neutropenia, and a compatible pattern of abdominal pain.

Thrombocytopenia – Grade 4 thrombocytopenia (less than 10,000 cells/mm^3) occurred in 6% of patients, with a median duration of 3 days.

Anemia – Grade 3 or 4 anemia (less than 8 g/dL) occurred in 25% of patients.

➤*Diarrhea:* Diarrhea, including severe diarrhea requiring hospitalization, has been reported during treatment with topotecan. Diarrhea related to topotecan can occur at the same time as drug-related neutropenia and its sequelae. Communication with patients prior to drug administration regarding these adverse reactions and proactive management of early and all signs and symptoms of diarrhea is important. Treatment-related diarrhea is associated with significant morbidity and may be life-threatening. Should diarrhea occur during treatment with topotecan, health care providers are advised to aggressively manage diarrhea. Clinical guidelines describing the aggressive management of diarrhea include specific recommendations on patient communication and awareness, recognition of early warning signs, use of antidiarrheals and antibiotics, changes in fluid intake and diet, and need for hospitalization.

Of the 682 patients who received topotecan in the 4 thoracic cancer studies, the overall incidence of drug-related diarrhea was 22%, including 4% with grade 3 and 0.4% with grade 4. Drug-related diarrhea was more frequent in patients 65 years of age and older (28%) compared with those younger than 65 years of age (19%).

➤*Renal function impairment:* A cross-study analysis of data collected from 217 patients with advanced solid tumors indicated that exposure ($AUC_{0-\infty}$) to topotecan lactone, the pharmacologically active moiety, was 10% and 20% higher in patients with mild (CrCl = 50 to 80 mL/min) and moderate (CrCl = 30 to 49 mL/min) renal function impairment, respectively, than in patients with healthy renal function (CrCl greater than 80 mL/min).

➤*Hepatic function impairment:* In a population pharmacokinetic analysis involving oral topotecan administered at doses of 0.15 to 2.7 mg/m^2/day to 118 cancer patients, the pharmacokinetics of total topotecan did not differ significantly based on patient serum bilirubin, ALT, or AST. No dosage adjustment appeared to be required for patients with hepatic function impairment (serum bilirubin greater than 1.5 mg/dL).

➤*Hazardous tasks:* As with other chemotherapeutic agents, topotecan may cause asthenia or fatigue. Advise patients to use caution when driving or operating machinery if these symptoms occur.

➤*Pregnancy: Category D.* Topotecan may cause fetal harm when administered to a pregnant woman. The effects of topotecan on pregnant women have not been studied. Warn women to avoid becoming pregnant. In rabbits, an IV dose of 0.10 mg/kg/day (about equal to the clinical IV dose on a mg/m^2 basis) given on days 6 through 20 of gestation caused maternal toxicity, embryolethality, and reduced fetal body weight. In the rat, an IV dose of 0.23 mg/kg/day (about equal to the clinical IV dose on a mg/m^2 basis) given for 14 days before mating through gestation day 6 caused fetal resorption, microphthalmia, preimplant loss, and mild maternal toxicity. An IV dose of 0.10 mg/kg/day (about half the clinical IV dose on a mg/m^2 basis) given to rats on days 6 through 17 of gestation caused an increase in postimplantation mortality. This dose also caused an increase in total fetal malformations. The most frequent malformations were of the eye (microphthalmia, anophthalmia, rosette formation of the retina, coloboma of the retina, ectopic orbit), brain (dilated lateral and third ventricles), skull, and vertebrae. If this drug is used during pregnancy, or if a patient becomes pregnant while taking this drug, apprise the patient of the potential hazard to the fetus.

Fertility impairment – Topotecan may impair fertility in women and men.

➤*Lactation:* Topotecan is contraindicated during breast-feeding.

Rats excrete high concentrations of topotecan into milk. Lactating female rats given 4.72 mg/m^2 IV (about twice the clinical dose on a mg/m^2 basis) excreted topotecan into milk at concentrations up to 48-fold higher than those in plasma. It is not known whether the drug is excreted in human milk. Women receiving topotecan should discontinue breast-feeding.

➤*Children:* Safety and effectiveness in children have not been established.

➤*Elderly:* Treatment-related diarrhea was more frequent in patients 65 years of age and older (28%) compared with those younger than 65 years of age (19%). Among patients 65 years of age and older, those receiving topotecan plus best supportive care (BSC) showed a survival benefit compared with those receiving BSC alone.

There were no apparent differences in the pharmacokinetics of topotecan in elderly patients with CrCl of 60 mL/min or more.

This drug is known to be excreted by the kidney, and the risk of toxic reactions to this drug may be greater in patients with renal function impairment.

➤*Monitoring:* Institute frequent monitoring of peripheral blood cell counts during treatment with topotecan.

Drug Interactions

Topotecan Oral Drug Interactions

Precipitant drug	Object drug[a]		Description
Cytotoxic agents (eg, cisplatin)	Topotecan	↑	Greater myelosuppression is likely to be seen when topotecan is given in combination with other cytotoxic agents.
P-glycoprotein inhibitors (eg, cyclosporine A, elacridar, ketoconazole, ritonavir, saquinavir)	Topotecan	↑	Avoid coadministration. P-glycoprotein inhibitors can cause a significant increase in topotecan exposure.

[a] ↑ = object drug increased.

➤*Drug/Food interactions:* Following a high-fat meal, the time to reach maximum plasma concentration was delayed from 1.5 to 3 hours (topotecan lactone) and from 3 to 4 hours (total topotecan), respectively.

Adverse Reactions

Topotecan is considered to have moderately low emetogenic potential (10% to 30% incidence of emesis).

The following table describes the hematologic and nonhematologic adverse reactions in recurrent SCLC patients treated with topotecan capsules plus BSC and in the overall thoracic cancer patient population.

TOPOTECAN HYDROCHLORIDE — ORAL

Topotecan Capsules Adverse Reactions (≥ 5%)[a]						
	Topotecan + BSC (n[b] = 70)			Topotecan thoracic cancer population (N[b] = 682)		
Adverse reaction	All grades	Grade 3	Grade 4	All grades	Grade 3	Grade 4
CNS						
Asthenia	3%	0%	0%	7%	2%	0%
Fatigue	11%	0%	0%	19%	4%	0.1%
GI						
Anorexia	7%	0%	0%	14%	2%	0%
Diarrhea	14%	4%	1%	22%	4%	0.4%
Nausea	27%	1%	0%	33%	3%	0%
Vomiting	19%	1%	0%	21%	3%	0.4%
Hematologic						
Anemia	94%	15%	10%	98%	18%	7%
Leukopenia	90%	25%	16%	86%	29%	15%
Neutropenia	91%	28%	33%	83%	24%	32%
Thrombocytopenia	81%	30%	7%	81%	29%	6%
Miscellaneous						
Alopecia	10%	0%	0%	20%	0.1%	0%
Pyrexia	7%	1%	0%	5%	1%	1%

[a] Adverse reactions were graded using National Cancer Institute-Common Toxicity Criteria.
[b] n/N = total number of patients treated.

➤*Diarrhea adverse reactions:* Of the 70 patients who received topotecan capsules plus BSC, the incidence of drug-related diarrhea was 14%, with 4% grade 3 and 1% grade 4.

In the 682 patients who received topotecan capsules in the 4 thoracic cancer studies, the incidence of drug-related diarrhea was 22%, with 4% grade 3 and 0.4% grade 4. The overall incidence of drug-related diarrhea was more frequent in patients 65 years of age and older (28%, n = 225), with 10% grade 1, 9% grade 2, 7% grade 3, and 1% grade 4, compared with those younger than 65 years of age (19%, n = 457), with 7% grade 1, 9% grade 2, 3% grade 3, and 0% grade 4. The incidence of grade 3 or 4 diarrhea proximate (within 5 days) to grade 3 or 4 neutropenia events in the topotecan capsules treatment group was 5%. The median time to onset of grade 2 or worse diarrhea was 9 days in the topotecan capsules group.

➤*Death:* In the 682 patients who received topotecan capsules in the 4 thoracic cancer studies, 39 deaths occurred within 30 days after the last dose of study medication for a reason other than progressive disease; 13 of these deaths were attributed to hematologic toxicity, 5 were attributed to nonhematologic toxicity, and 21 were attributed to other causes. One patient death (68 years of age) was attributed to treatment-related diarrhea and 1 death (68 years of age) attributed diarrhea as a contributory event; both patients received topotecan capsules.

➤*Adverse reactions reported with topotecan injection:* In addition to the adverse reactions listed previously, the following adverse reactions have been reported with topotecan injection

CNS – Malaise (1% to 10%).

GI – Abdominal pain, constipation, stomatitis (greater than 10%).

Hematologic – Febrile neutropenia (greater than 10%); hyperbilirubinemia, sepsis (1% to 10%).

Hypersensitivity – Hypersensitivity reactions, including rash (1% to 10%).

➤*Postmarketing:* There is no postmarketing experience with topotecan capsules. The following adverse reactions have been identified during postapproval use of topotecan injection. Because these reactions are reported voluntarily from a population of uncertain size, it is not always possible to reliably estimate their frequency or establish a causal relationship to drug exposure.

Dermatologic – Angioedema, severe dermatitis, severe pruritus.

GI – Abdominal pain potentially associated with neutropenic colitis.

Hematologic / Lymphatic – Severe bleeding (in association with thrombocytopenia).

Hypersensitivity – Allergic manifestations, anaphylactoid reactions.

Overdosage

➤*Symptoms:* There is no known antidote for overdosage with topotecan capsules. The primary anticipated complication of overdosage would consist of hematological toxicity.

➤*Treatment:* Observe the patient closely for bone marrow suppression, and consider supportive measures (such as the prophylactic use of granulocyte colony–stimulating factor and/or antibiotic therapy).

Patient Information

Inform patients that topotecan decreases blood cell counts such as white blood cells, platelets, and red blood cells. Patients who develop fever or other signs of infection, including chills, cough, or burning pain on urination, while on therapy should promptly notify their health care provider. Inform patients that frequent blood tests will be performed to monitor for the occurrence of bone marrow suppression while taking topotecan.

Advise patients to use effective contraceptive measures to prevent pregnancy and to avoid breast-feeding during treatment with topotecan.

Inform patients that topotecan causes diarrhea, which may be severe in some cases. Tell patients how to manage and/or prevent diarrhea and to inform their health care provider if severe diarrhea occurs during treatment with topotecan.

TOPOTECAN HYDROCHLORIDE — INJECTION

WARNING

Administer topotecan under the supervision of a health care provider experienced in the use of cancer chemotherapeutic agents. Appropriate management of complications is possible only when adequate diagnostic and treatment facilities are readily available.

Do not give topotecan therapy to patients with baseline neutrophil counts of less than 1,500 cells/mm^3. In order to monitor the occurrence of bone marrow suppression, primarily neutropenia, which may be severe and result in infection and death, perform frequent peripheral blood cell counts on all patients receiving topotecan.

Indications

➤*Cervical cancer (in combination with cisplatin):* For the treatment of stage IVB, recurrent, or persistent carcinoma of the cervix that is not amenable to curative treatment with surgery and/or radiation therapy.

➤*Ovarian cancer:* For the treatment of metastatic carcinoma of the ovary after failure of initial or subsequent chemotherapy.

➤*Small cell lung cancer:* For the treatment of small cell lung cancer (SCLC)-sensitive disease after failure of first-line chemotherapy. In clinical studies submitted to support approval, sensitive disease was defined as disease responding to chemotherapy but subsequently progressing at least 60 days (in the phase 3 study) or at least 90 days (in the phase 2 studies) after chemotherapy.

➤*Off-label uses:* In combination with paclitaxel for the treatment of advanced non-small cell lung cancer (NSCLC); intrathecal use for neoplastic meningitis (see Administration and Dosage); limited experience with use in children for sarcoma, neuroblastoma, or refractory solid tumors (see Administration and Dosage).

Administration and Dosage

➤*General dosing considerations:* Prior to administration of the first course of topotecan, patients must have a baseline neutrophil count of more than 1,500 cells/mm^3 and a platelet count of more than 100,000 cells/mm^3.

➤*Adults:*

Cervical cancer –

Usual dosage: 0.75 mg/m^2 by intravenous (IV) infusion over 30 minutes on days 1, 2, and 3, followed by cisplatin 50 mg/m^2 by IV infusion on day 1, repeated every 21 days (21-day course).

Dosage adjustment: Dosage adjustments for subsequent courses of topotecan in combination with cisplatin are specific for each drug.

Delay additional doses until neutrophil count is above 1,500 cells/mm^3, platelet count is above 100,000 cells/mm^3, and hemoglobin is at least 9 g/dL.

In the event of severe febrile neutropenia (defined as ANC less than 1,000 cells/mm^3 with temperature of 38°C [100.4°F]), the dose of topotecan should be reduced by 20% to 0.6 mg/m^2 for subsequent courses. Alternatively, granulocyte colony-stimulating factor (G-CSF) may be administered following the subsequent course (before resorting to dose reduction) starting from day 4 of the course (24 hours after completion of topotecan administration). If febrile neutropenia occurs despite the use of G-CSF, the dose of topotecan should be reduced by another 20% to 0.45 mg/m^2 for subsequent courses.

Doses of topotecan should be similarly reduced (by 20% to 0.6 mg/m^2) if the platelet count falls below 10,000 cells/mm^3.

See the cisplatin monograph for cisplatin administration and hydration guidelines and cisplatin dosage adjustment in the event of hematologic toxicity.

Ovarian cancer –

Usual dosage: 1.5 mg/m^2 daily by IV infusion over 30 minutes for 5 consecutive days, starting on day 1 of a 21-day course. In the absence of tumor progression, a minimum of 4 courses is recommended because tumor response may be delayed. The median time to response in 3 ovarian cancer clinical trials was 9 to 12 weeks.

Dosage adjustment: Delay additional doses until neutrophil count is above 1,500 cells/mm^3, platelet count is above 100,000 cells/mm^3, and hemoglobin is at least 9 g/dL.

In the event of severe neutropenia during any course, the dose should be reduced by 0.25 mg/m^2 (to 1.25 mg/m^2) for subsequent courses. Alternatively, G-CSF may be administered following the subsequent course (before resorting to dose reduction) starting from day 6 of the course (24 hours after completion of topotecan administration).

Doses should be similarly reduced if the platelet count falls below 25,000 cells/mm^3.

TOPOTECAN HYDROCHLORIDE — INJECTION

Alternative dosage: 0.3 to 0.7 mg/m^2 daily by continuous IV infusion for 14 to 21 days of a 28-day cycle.

Small cell lung cancer –

Usual dosage: 1.5 mg/m^2 daily by IV infusion over 30 minutes for 5 consecutive days, starting on day 1 of a 21-day course. In the absence of tumor progression, a minimum of 4 courses is recommended because tumor response may be delayed. The median time to response in 4 SCLC trials was 5 to 7 weeks.

Dosage adjustment: Delay additional doses until neutrophil count is above 1,500 cells/mm^3, platelet count is above 100,000 cells/mm^3, and hemoglobin is at least 9 g/dL.

In the event of severe neutropenia during any course, the dose should be reduced by 0.25 mg/m^2 (to 1.25 mg/m^2) for subsequent courses. Alternatively, G-CSF may be administered following the subsequent course (before resorting to dose reduction) starting from day 6 of the course (24 hours after completion of topotecan administration).

Doses should be similarly reduced if the platelet count falls below 25,000 cells/mm^3.

Off-label dosing –

Neoplastic meningitis:

- *Initial dosage* – 0.4 mg intrathecally twice weekly for 4 weeks, then evaluate response before giving consolidation and maintenance regimens.
- *In patients with complete response after 4 weeks* – Give 0.4 mg intrathecally weekly for 4 weeks, then every 2 weeks for 4 months, then once monthly for up to 8 months.
- *In patients with partial response or stable disease after 4 weeks* – Give 0.4 mg intrathecally twice weekly for an additional 2 weeks. Then give 0.4 mg weekly for 4 weeks, then every 2 weeks for 4 months, then once monthly for up to 8 months.

➤*Children:*

Off-label dosing –

Solid tumors, single-agent therapy:

- *Usual dose* – 2.4 mg/m^2/day IV for 5 consecutive days starting on day 1 of a 21-day cycle. See Adults for dosage adjustment guidelines.
- *Alternative dosage* – 0.75 to 2 mg/m^2/day (usual dose, 1 mg/m^2/day) by continuous IV infusion for 3 days, repeated every 21 days.

Solid tumors, combination therapy: 0.75 mg/m^2/day IV for 5 consecutive days starting on day 1 of a 21-day cycle. See Adults for dosage adjustment guidelines.

➤*Renal function impairment:* Dosage adjustment of topotecan to 0.75 mg/m^2 is recommended for patients with moderate renal function impairment (creatinine clearance [CrCl] 20 to 39 mL/min.). Insufficient data are available in patients with severe renal function impairment to provide a dosage recommendation.

Topotecan in combination with cisplatin for the treatment of cervical cancer should only be initiated in patients with a serum creatinine of 1.5 mg/dL or less. In clinical trials, cisplatin was discontinued for a serum creatinine of more than 1.5 mg/dL. Insufficient data are available regarding continuing monotherapy with topotecan after cisplatin discontinuation in patients with cervical cancer.

Topotecan Injection Dosage Adjustment for Adults Based on Renal Function

Baseline creatinine clearance	Percent of usual dose to be given	
	Manufacturer package insert	Alternative dosage recommendation
> 80 mL/min	100%	100%
51 to 80 mL/min	100%	75%
40 to 50 mL/min	100%	50%
20 to 39 mL/min	50%	50%
10 to 19 mL/min	Dose reduction necessary; no data available to determine dose.	50%
< 10 mL/min	Dose reduction necessary; no data available to determine dose.	25%
Hemodialysis	Do not administer.	Do not administer.
Peritoneal dialysis	Do not administer.	Do not administer.
Continuous renal replacement therapy	Do not administer.	50%

Dialysis – In one patient, conventional hemodialysis was shown to be ineffective (0% to 24%) in removing topotecan; however, conventional hemodialysis was shown to be moderately effective (50% to 74%) in removing topotecan in another patient.

Some clinicians recommend a supplemental dose after hemodialysis.

➤*Hepatic function impairment:* Monitor these patients and adjust dose as needed if toxicity occurs.

➤*Preparation for administration:* Topotecan is considered a cytotoxic agent. Follow safe handling procedures when preparing, administering, or dispensing topotecan.

As with other potentially toxic compounds, topotecan should be prepared under a vertical laminar flow hood while wearing gloves and protective clothing. If topotecan solution contacts the skin, immediately wash the skin thoroughly with soap and water. If topotecan contacts mucous membranes, flush thoroughly with water.

Solutions should be clear and yellow or yellowish-green in color. Discard solutions that appear cloudy or contain particles.

IV infusion – Each topotecan 4 mg vial is reconstituted with 4 mL of sterile water for injection for a final concentration of 1 mg/mL. Then the appropriate volume of the reconstituted solution is diluted in sodium chloride 0.9% IV infusion or dextrose 5% IV infusion prior to administration. According to the manufacturer, because the lyophilized dosage form contains no antibacterial preservative, the reconstituted product should be used immediately. (See also Storage and Stability for additional information.)

Intrathecal (off-label): Dilute with preservative-free sodium chloride 0.9% injection to a final volume of 4 to 10 mL for intrathecal administration.

➤*Administration:* Give by IV infusion over 30 minutes, continuous IV infusion (off-label), or intrathecal (off-label).

➤*Extravasation:* Inadvertent extravasation with topotecan has been associated with mild local reactions, such as erythema and bruising. Topotecan is considered an irritant and may cause phlebitis, but it is not known to cause tissue damage with extravasation. If signs or symptoms of extravasation occur, stop the infusion immediately. If possible, withdraw 3 to 5 mL of blood to remove some of the drug. Remove the infusion needle. Delineate the infiltrated area on the patient's skin with a felt tip marker. Elevate for 48 hours above heart level using a sling or stockinette dressing with an observation window cut in the dressing. Avoid pressure or friction. Do not rub the area. Observe for signs of increased erythema, pain, or skin necrosis. If increased symptoms occur, consult a plastic surgeon. Ensure that no medication is given distally to extravasation site. After 48 hours, encourage the patient to use the extremity normally to promote full range of motion.

➤*Storage / Stability:* Unopened vials of topotecan are stable until the date indicated on the package when stored between 20° and 25°C (68° and 77°F) and protected from light in the original package.

The lyophilized powder contains no preservative and should be used within 6 hours of the initial needle puncture if opened within an ISO Class 5 biological safety cabinet, or within 1 hour of the initial needle puncture if opened outside of such an environment. Preservative-free topotecan solutions should be discarded within a similar timeframe, based on the USP Chapter <797> standards.

According to the manufacturer, reconstituted vials of topotecan diluted for infusion are stable at approximately 20° to 25°C (68° to 77°F) and in ambient lighting conditions when stored for 24 hours. Others have reported that diluted solutions are chemically stable for up to 4 days at room temperature or for up to 7 days under refrigeration.

Actions

➤*Pharmacology:* Topoisomerase I relieves torsional strain in DNA by inducing reversible single-strand breaks. Topotecan binds to the topoisomerase I-DNA complex and prevents religation of these single-strand breaks. The cytotoxicity of topotecan is thought to be due to double-strand DNA damage produced during DNA synthesis when replication enzymes interact with the ternary complex formed by topotecan, topoisomerase I, and DNA. Mammalian cells cannot efficiently repair these double-strand breaks.

Pharmacodynamics – The dose-limiting toxicity of topotecan is leukopenia. White blood cell count (WBC) decreases with increasing topotecan dose or topotecan area under the curve (AUC). When topotecan is administered at a dose of 1.5 mg/m^2/day for 5 days, an 80% to 90% decrease in WBC at nadir is typically observed after the first cycle of therapy.

➤*Pharmacokinetics:*

Absorption / Distribution – Total exposure (AUC) of topotecan is approximately dose proportional. Binding of topotecan to plasma proteins is approximately 35%.

Metabolism / Excretion – Topotecan exhibits multiexponential pharmacokinetics with a terminal half-life of 2 to 3 hours. Topotecan undergoes a reversible, pH-dependent hydrolysis of its lactone moiety; it is the lactone form that is pharmacologically active. At a pH of 4 or less, the lactone is exclusively present, whereas the ring-opened hydroxy-acid form predominates at physiologic pH. In vitro studies in human liver microsomes indicate that topotecan is metabolized to an N-desmethylated metabolite. The mean metabolite:parent AUC ratio was about 3% for total topotecan and topotecan lactone following IV administration.

Renal clearance is an important determinant of topotecan elimination. In a mass balance/excretion study in 4 patients with solid tumors, the overall recovery of total topotecan and its N-desmethyl metabolite in urine and feces over 9 days averaged 73.4% ± 2.3% of the administered IV dose. Mean values of 50.8% ± 2.9% as total topotecan and 3.1% ± 1% as N-desmethyl topotecan were excreted in the urine following IV administration. Fecal elimination of total topotecan accounted for 17.9% ± 3.6%, while fecal elimination of N-desmethyl topotecan was 1.7% ± 0.6%. An O-glucuronidation metabolite of topotecan and N-desmethyl topotecan has been identified in the urine. These metabolites, topotecan-O-glucuronide and N-desmethyl topotecan-O-glucuronide, were less than 2% of the administered dose.

Special populations –

Renal function impairment: In patients with mild renal function impairment (CrCl 40 to 60 mL/min), topotecan plasma clearance was decreased to approximately 67% of the value in patients with healthy renal function. In patients with moderate renal function impairment (CrCl 20 to 39 mL/min), topotecan plasma clearance was reduced to approximately 34% of the value in control patients, with an increase in half-life. Mean half-life, estimated in 3 patients with renal function impairment, was about 5 hours. Dosage adjustment is recommended for these patients.

Hepatic function impairment: Plasma clearance in patients with hepatic function impairment (serum bilirubin levels between 1.7 and 15 mg/dL) was decreased to approximately 67% of the value in patients without hepatic function impairment. Topotecan half-life increased slightly, from 2 to 2.5 hours, but these patients with hepatic function impairment tolerated the usual recommended topotecan dosage regimen.

TOPOTECAN HYDROCHLORIDE — INJECTION

Elderly: Decreased renal clearance, common in elderly patients, is a more important determinant of topotecan clearance than age as an individual factor.

Gender: The overall mean topotecan plasma clearance in men was approximately 24% higher than in women, largely reflecting difference in body size.

Contraindications

History of hypersensitivity reactions to topotecan or any other ingredient in the product; pregnancy; breast-feeding; severe bone marrow depression.

Warnings/Precautions

➤*Bone marrow suppression:* Bone marrow suppression (primarily neutropenia) is the dose-limiting toxicity of topotecan. Neutropenia is not cumulative over time.

➤*Neutropenia:*

Cervical cancer – Grades 3 and 4 neutropenia affected 264% and 48% of patients, respectively.

Ovarian cancer and SCLC – Grade 4 neutropenia (less than 500 cells/mm^3) was most common during course 1 of treatment (60% of patients) and occurred in 39% of all courses, with a median duration of 7 days. The nadir neutrophil count occurred at a median of 12 days. Therapy-related sepsis or febrile neutropenia occurred in 23% of patients, and sepsis was fatal in 1%. Pancytopenia has been reported.

Neutropenic colitis – Topotecan-induced neutropenia can lead to neutropenic colitis. Fatalities caused by neutropenic colitis have been reported in clinical trials with topotecan. In patients presenting with fever, neutropenia, and a compatible pattern of abdominal pain, consider the possibility of neutropenic colitis.

➤*Thrombocytopenia:*

Cervical cancer – Grades 3 and 4 thrombocytopenia affected 26% and 7% of patients, respectively.

Ovarian cancer and SCLC – Grade 4 thrombocytopenia (less than 25,000/mm^3) occurred in 27% of patients and 9% of courses, with a median duration of 5 days and platelet nadir at a median of 15 days. Platelet transfusions were given to 15% of patients in 4% of courses.

➤*Anemia:*

Cervical cancer – Grades 3 and 4 anemia affected 34% and 6% of patients, respectively.

Ovarian cancer and SCLC experience – Grades 3 and 4 anemia (less than 8 g/dL) occurred in 37% of patients and 14% of courses. Median nadir was at day 15. Transfusions were needed in 52% of patients in 22% of courses.

➤*Treatment-related death:* In ovarian cancer, the overall treatment-related death rate was 1%. However, in the comparative study in SCLC, the treatment-related death rates were 5% for topotecan and 4% for cyclophosphamide-doxorubicin-vincristine.

➤*Hepatic function impairment:* See Administration and Dosage for more information.

➤*Hazardous tasks:* As with other chemotherapeutic agents, topotecan may cause asthenia or fatigue; if these symptoms occur, patients should observe caution when driving or operating machinery.

➤*Pregnancy: Category D.* Topotecan may cause fetal harm when administered to a pregnant woman. The effects of topotecan on pregnant women have not been studied. If topotecan is used during a patient's pregnancy or if a patient becomes pregnant while taking topotecan, warn her of the potential hazard to the fetus. Warn women of child-bearing potential to avoid becoming pregnant.

In rabbits, a dose of 0.1 mg/kg/day (approximately equal to the clinical dose on a mg/m^2 basis) given on days 6 through 20 of gestation caused maternal toxicity, embryolethality, and reduced fetal body weight. In rats, a dose of 0.23 mg/kg/day (approximately equal to the clinical dose on a mg/m^2 basis) given for 14 days before mating through gestation day 6 caused fetal resorption, microphthalmia, preimplant loss, and mild maternal toxicity. A dose of 0.1 mg/kg/day (approximately half the clinical dose on a mg/m^2 basis) given to rats on days 6 through 17 of gestation caused an increase in postimplantation mortality. This dose also caused an increase in total fetal malformations. The most frequent malformations were of the eye (microphthalmia, anophthalmia, rosette formation of the retina, coloboma of the retina, ectopic orbit), brain (dilated lateral and third ventricles), skull, and vertebrae.

➤*Lactation:* Topotecan is contraindicated in breast-feeding women.

➤*Children:* The safety and efficacy of topotecan in children have not been established.

➤*Elderly:* No overall differences in efficacy or safety were observed between these patients and younger adult patients. Other reported clinical experience has not identified differences in responses between elderly and younger adult patients, but greater sensitivity of some older individuals cannot be ruled out.

This drug is known to be substantially excreted by the kidney, and the risk of toxic reactions to this drug may be greater in patients with renal function impairment. Because elderly patients are more likely to have decreased renal function, take care in dose selection; it may be useful to monitor renal function.

➤*Monitoring:* Only administer topotecan to patients with adequate bone marrow reserves, including a baseline neutrophil count of at least 1,500 cells/mm^3 and a platelet count of at least 100,000/mm^3. Institute frequent monitoring of peripheral blood cell counts during treatment with topotecan. Do not treat patients with subsequent courses of topotecan until neutrophils recover to more than 1,000 cells/mm^3, platelets recover to more than 100,000 cells/mm^3, and hemoglobin levels recover to 9 g/dL (with transfusion if necessary).

Drug Interactions

Topotecan Injection Drug Interactions

Precipitant drug	Object drug[a]		Description
Cytotoxic agents (eg, cisplatin)	Topotecan	↑	Myelosuppression is more severe when topotecan is given in combination with cisplatin. There are no adequate data to define a safe and effective regimen for topotecan and cisplatin in combination. Coadministration of a platinum agent on day 1 of topotecan dosing required lower doses of each agent compared with coadministration on day 5 of the topotecan dosing schedule. Greater myelosuppression is likely to be seen when topotecan is used in combination with other cytotoxic agents, thereby necessitating a dose reduction.
Filgrastim (G-CSF)	Topotecan	↑	Coadministration can prolong the duration of neutropenia. If G-CSF is used, do not initiate it until 24 hours after completion of topotecan treatment (day 4 of the course of therapy for cervical cancer or day 6 of the course of therapy for ovarian cancer or SCLC).

[a] ↑ = object drug increased.

Adverse Reactions

Topotecan is considered to have moderately low emetogenic potential (10% to 30% incidence of emesis).

➤*Cervical cancer:*

Topotecan Hematologic Adverse Reactions in Cervical Cancer Patients[a]

Adverse reaction	Topotecan + cisplatin (n = 140)	Cisplatin (n = 144)
Hematologic		
Anemia		
All grades (hemoglobin < 12 g/dL)	94%	90%
Grade 3 (hemoglobin 6.5 to 8 g/dL	34%	19%
Grade 4 (hemoglobin < 6.5 g/dL)	6%	3%
Leukopenia		
All grades (< 3,800 cells/mm^3)	91%	30%
Grade 3 (1,000 to 2,000 cells/mm^3)	41%	1%
Grade 4 (< 1,000 cells/mm^3)	25%	0%
Neutropenia		
All grades (< 2,000 cells/mm^3)	89%	19%
Grade 3 (< 1,000 to 500 cells/mm^3)	26%	1%
Grade 4 (< 500 cells/mm^3)	48%	1%
Thrombocytopenia		
All grades (< 130,000 cells/mm^3)	74%	15%
Grade 3 (< 50,000 to 10,000 cells/mm^3)	26%	3%
Grade 4 (< 10,000 cells/mm^3)	7%	0%

[a] Includes patients who were eligible and treated.

Nonhematologic adverse reactions –

Topotecan Nonhematologic Adverse Reactions in Cervical Cancer Patients[a] (≥ 5%)

Adverse reaction	Topotecan + cisplatin (n = 140) All grades[b]	Topotecan + cisplatin (n = 140) Grade 3	Topotecan + cisplatin (n = 140) Grade 4	Cisplatin (n = 144) All grades[b]	Cisplatin (n = 144) Grade 3	Cisplatin (n = 144) Grade 4
Cardiovascular						
Cardiovascular, NOS[c]	25%	5%	4%	15%	6%	2%

TOPOTECAN HYDROCHLORIDE — INJECTION

Topotecan Nonhematologic Adverse Reactions in Cervical Cancer Patients[a] (≥ 5%)						
	Topotecan + cisplatin (n = 140)			Cisplatin (n = 144)		
Adverse reaction	All grades[b]	Grade 3	Grade 4	All grades[b]	Grade 3	Grade 4
CNS						
Neuropathy	3%	< 1%	0%	2%	< 1%	0%
Other	35%	2%	< 1%	30%	5%	1%
Dermatologic						
Dermatologic, NOS	48%	< 1%	0%	20%	0%	0%
Endocrine						
Endocrine, NOS	6%	0%	0%	3%	1%	0%
GI						
Nausea	55%	13%	1%	55%	9%	0%
Stomatitis-pharyngitis	6%	< 1%	0%	0%	0%	0%
Vomiting	40%	14%	1%	37%	9%	0%
Other	63%	11%	3%	56%	8%	2%
GU						
GU, NOS	36%	6%	6%	34%	5%	5%
Sexual reproduction function	5%	0%	0%	7%	< 1%	0%
Hematologic						
Coagulation	6%	3%	2%	7%	5%	0%
Febrile neutropenia	28%	15%	4%	18%	18%	0%
Hemorrhage	15%	6%	< 1%	14%	2%	< 1%
Hepatic						
Hepatic, NOS	24%	4%	1%	16%	1%	0%
Metabolic						
Metabolic, NOS	39%	9%	5%	31%	10%	< 1%
Musculoskeletal						
Musculoskeletal, NOS	14%	2%	0%	5%	< 1%	< 1%
Respiratory						
Pulmonary, NOS	17%	3%	0%	16%	3%	2%
Special senses						
Ocular (visual)	5%	0%	0%	5%	< 1%	0%
Miscellaneous						
Allergy-immunology	6%	1%	< 1%	3%	0%	< 1%
Constitutional[d]	69%	8%	0%	62%	12%	0%
Pain[e]	59%	20%	2%	50%	13%	3%

[a] Includes patients who were eligible and treated.
[b] Grades 1 through 4 only. There were 3 patients who experienced grade 5 deaths with investigator-designated attribution. One was a grade 5 hemorrhage in which the drug-related thrombocytopenia aggravated the reaction. A second patient experienced bowel obstruction, cardiac arrest, pleural effusion, and respiratory failure, which were not treatment related but probably aggravated by treatment. A third patient experienced a pulmonary embolism and adult respiratory distress syndrome; the latter was indirectly treatment related.
[c] NOS = not otherwise specified.
[d] Includes chills, fatigue (lethargy, malaise, asthenia), fever (in the absence of neutropenia), rigors, sweating, and weight gain or loss.
[e] Pain includes abdominal pain or cramping, arthralgia, bone pain, chest pain (noncardiac and nonpleuritic), dysmenorrhea, dyspareunia, earache, headache, hepatic pain, myalgia, neuropathic pain, pain caused by radiation, pelvic pain, pleuritic pain, rectal or perirectal pain, and tumor pain.

➤*Ovarian cancer and SCLC:*

Topotecan Hematologic Adverse Reactions (≥ 15%)		
Hematologic adverse reactions	Patients (n = 879)	Courses (n = 4,124)
Neutropenia		
< 1,500 cells/mm³	97%	81%
< 500 cells/mm ³	78%	39%
Leukopenia		
< 3,000 cells/mm³	97%	80%
< 1,000 cells/mm³	32%	11%
Thrombocytopenia		
< 75,000/mm³	69%	42%
< 25,000/mm³	27%	9%
Anemia		
< 10 g/dL	89%	71%
< 8 g/dL	37%	14%
Platelet transfusions	15%	4%
RBC[a] transfusions	52%	22%

[a] RBC = red blood cell.

Nonhematologic adverse reactions –

Topotecan Nonhematologic Adverse Reactions (≥ 15%)[a]						
	All grades		Grade 3		Grade 4	
Nonhematologic adverse reactions	Patients (n = 879)	Courses (n = 4,124)	Patients (n = 879)	Courses (n = 4,124)	Patients (n = 879)	Courses (n = 4,124)
CNS						
Asthenia	25%	13%	4%	1%	2%	< 1%
Fatigue	29%	22%	5%	2%	0%	0%
Headache	18%	7%	1%	< 1%	< 1%	0%
Dermatologic						
Alopecia	49%	54%	NA	NA	NA	NA
Rash[b]	16%	6%	1%	< 1%	0%	0%
GI						
Abdominal pain	22%	10%	2%	1%	2%	< 1%
Anorexia	19%	9%	2%	1%	< 1%	< 1%
Constipation	29%	15%	2%	1%	1%	< 1%
Diarrhea	32%	14%	3%	1%	1%	< 1%
Nausea	64%	42%	7%	2%	1%	< 1%
Stomatitis	18%	8%	1%	< 1%	< 1%	< 1%
Vomiting	45%	22%	4%	1%	1%	< 1%
Respiratory						
Coughing	15%	7%	1%	< 1%	0%	0%
Dyspnea	22%	11%	5%	2%	3%	1%

TOPOTECAN HYDROCHLORIDE — INJECTION

Topotecan Nonhematologic Adverse Reactions (≥ 15%)[a]						
	All grades		Grade 3		Grade 4	
Nonhematologic adverse reactions	Patients (n = 879)	Courses (n = 4,124)	Patients (n = 879)	Courses (n = 4,124)	Patients (n = 879)	Courses (n = 4,124)
Miscellaneous						
Pain[c]	23%	11%	2%	1%	1%	< 1%
Pyrexia	28%	11%	1%	< 1%	< 1%	< 1%
Sepsis or pyrexia/infection with neutropenia[d]	43%	15%	NR	NR	23%	7%

[a] NA = not applicable; NR = not reported separately.
[b] Rash also includes bullous eruption, dermatitis, erythematous rash, maculopapular rash, pruritus, and urticaria.
[c] Pain includes back, body, and skeletal pain.
[d] Does not include grade 1 sepsis or pyrexia.

➤*Other adverse reactions:*

CNS – Headache (18% of patients) was the most frequently reported neurologic toxicity. Paresthesia occurred in 7% of patients but was generally grade 1.

Dermatologic – Total alopecia (grade 2) occurred in 31% of patients.

GI – The incidence of nausea was 64% (8% grade 3 and 4), and vomiting occurred in 45% (6% grade 3 and 4) of patients (see the preceding table). The prophylactic use of antiemetics was not routine in patients treated with topotecan. Thirty-two percent of patients had diarrhea (4% grade 3 and 4), 29% had constipation (2% grade 3 and 4), and 22% had abdominal pain (4% grade 3 and 4). Grade 3 and 4 abdominal pain occurred in 6% of ovarian cancer patients and 2% of SCLC patients.

Hematologic – See Warnings/Precautions.

Hepatic – Grade 1 transient elevations in hepatic enzymes occurred in 8% of patients. Greater elevations, grades 3 and 4, occurred in 4%. Grades 3 and 4 elevated bilirubin occurred in less than 2% of patients.

Respiratory – The incidence of grades 3 and 4 dyspnea was 4% in ovarian cancer patients and 12% in SCLC patients.

➤*Topotecan/paclitaxel comparator trial in ovarian cancer:*

Topotecan Adverse Reactions in Ovarian Cancer Patients				
	Topotecan		Paclitaxel	
Adverse reaction	Patients (n = 112)	Courses (n = 597)	Patients (n = 114)	Courses (n = 589)
CNS				
Asthenia	5%	2%	3%	1%
Fatigue	7%	2%	6%	2%
Headache	1%	< 1%	2%	1%
Malaise	2%	< 1%	2%	< 1%
Dermatologic				
Rash[a]	0%	0%	1%	< 1%
GI				
Abdominal pain	5%	1%	4%	1%
Anorexia	4%	1%	0%	0%
Constipation	5%	1%	0%	0%
Diarrhea	6%	2%	1%	< 1%
Intestinal obstruction	5%	1%	4%	1%
Nausea	10%	3%	2%	< 1%
Stomatitis	1%	< 1%	1%	< 1%
Vomiting	10%	2%	3%	< 1%
Hematologic grades 3 and 4				
Grades 3 and 4 anemia (hemoglobin < 8 g/dL)	41%	16%	6%	2%
Grade 4 neutropenia (< 500 cells/mm³)	80%	36%	21%	9%
Grade 4 thrombocytopenia (< 25,000 platelets/mm³)	27%	10%	3%	< 1%
Pyrexia/grade 4 neutropenia	23%	6%	4%	1%
Hepatic				
Increased hepatic enzymes[b]	1%	< 1%	1%	< 1%
Musculoskeletal				
Arthralgia	1%	< 1%	3%	< 1%
Myalgia	0%	0%	3%	2%
Pain[c]	5%	1%	7%	2%
Miscellaneous				
Chest pain	2%	< 1%	1%	< 1%
Death related to sepsis	2%	NA	0%	NA
Documented sepsis	5%	1%	2%	< 1%
Dyspnea	6%	2%	5%	1%

[a] Rash also includes bullous eruption, dermatitis, erythematous rash, maculopapular rash, pruritus, and urticaria.
[b] Increased hepatic enzymes include increased ALT, increased AST, and increased hepatic enzymes.
[c] Pain includes back, body, and skeletal pain.

➤*Topotecan/cyclophosphamide-doxorubicin-vincristine comparator trial in SCLC:*

Topotecan Adverse Reactions in SCLC Patients				
	Topotecan		Cyclophosphamide-doxorubicin-vincristine	
Adverse reaction	Patients (n = 107)	Courses (n = 446)	Patients (n = 104)	Courses (n = 359)
CNS				
Asthenia	9%	4%	7%	2%
Fatigue	6%	4%	10%	3%
Headache	0%	0%	2%	< 1%
Dermatologic				
Rash[a]	1%	< 1%	1%	< 1%
GI				
Abdominal pain	6%	1%	4%	2%
Anorexia	3%	1%	4%	2%
Constipation	1%	< 1	0%	0%
Diarrhea	1%	< 1	0%	0%
Nausea	8%	2%	6%	2%
Stomatitis	2%	< 1%	1%	< 1%
Vomiting	3%	< 1%	3%	1%
Hematologic grades 3 and 4				
Grades 3 and 4 anemia (hemoglobin < 8 g/dL)	42%	18%	20%	7%
Grade 4 neutropenia (< 500 cells/mm³)	70%	38%	72%	51%
Grade 4 thrombocytopenia (< 25,000 platelets/mm³)	29%	10%	5%	1%
Pyrexia/grade 4 neutropenia	28%	9%	26%	13%
Hepatic				
Increased hepatic enzymes[b]	1%	< 1%	0%	0%
Respiratory				
Coughing	2%	1%	0%	0%
Dyspnea	9%	5%	14%	7%
Pneumonia	8%	2%	6%	2%
Miscellaneous				
Death related to sepsis	3%	NA	1%	NA
Documented sepsis	5%	1%	5%	1%
Pain[c]	5%	2%	7%	4%

[a] Rash also includes bullous eruption, dermatitis, erythematous rash, maculopapular rash, pruritus, and urticaria.
[b] Increased hepatic enzymes includes increased ALT, increased AST, and increased hepatic enzymes.
[c] Pain includes back, body, and skeletal pain.

TOPOTECAN HYDROCHLORIDE — INJECTION

➤*Postmarketing:* Reports of adverse reactions in patients taking topotecan received after market introduction, which are not listed previously, include the following:

Dermatologic – Severe dermatitis, severe pruritus (rare).

GI – Abdominal pain potentially associated with neutropenic colitis.

Hematologic – Severe bleeding in association with thrombocytopenia (rare).

Hypersensitivity – Allergic manifestations (infrequent); angioedema, anaphylactoid reactions (rare).

Overdosage

➤*Symptoms:* The primary anticipated complication of overdose would consist of bone marrow suppression.

One patient on a single-dose regimen of 17.5 mg/m^2, given on day 1 of a 21-day cycle, had received a single dose of 35 mg/m^2. This patient experienced severe neutropenia (nadir of 320/mm^3) 14 days later but recovered without incident.

➤*Treatment:* There is no known antidote for topotecan overdosage.

Patient Information

As with other chemotherapeutic agents, topotecan may cause asthenia or fatigue; advise patients that if these symptoms occur, they should observe caution when driving or operating machinery.

Advise patients to contact their health care provider if they have symptoms of an infection (eg, chills, fever, painful urination, persistent sore throat), unusual bruising or bleeding, or unusual fatigue.

Advise patients to avoid contact with people who have colds or infection, as this medicine may lower their ability to fight infection.

BIOLOGICAL RESPONSE MODIFIERS

ALDESLEUKIN (Interleukin-2; IL-2)

Rx	**Proleukin** (Prometheus)	**Injection, lyophilized powder for solution:** 22 x 10^6 units/vial (18 million units [1.1 mg] per mL when reconstituted)	Preservative free. In single-use vials.[a]

[a] With 50 mg mannitol, 0.18 mg sodium dodecyl sulfate, and 0.17 mg monobasic and 0.89 mg dibasic sodium phosphate.

ALDESLEUKIN — INJECTION

WARNING

Restrict therapy with aldesleukin for injection to patients with normal cardiac and pulmonary functions as defined by thallium stress testing and formal pulmonary function testing. Use extreme caution in patients with a normal thallium stress test and a normal pulmonary function test who have a history of cardiac or pulmonary disease.

Administer aldesleukin in a hospital setting under the supervision of a qualified physician experienced in the use of anticancer agents. An intensive care facility and specialists skilled in cardiopulmonary or intensive care medicine must be available.

Aldesleukin administration has been associated with capillary leak syndrome (CLS) which is characterized by a loss of vascular tone and extravasation of plasma proteins and fluid into the extravascular space. CLS results in hypotension and reduced organ perfusion which may be severe and can result in death. CLS may be associated with cardiac arrhythmias (supraventricular and ventricular), angina, myocardial infarction, respiratory insufficiency requiring intubation, gastrointestinal bleeding or infarction, renal insufficiency, edema, and mental status changes.

Aldesleukin treatment is associated with impaired neutrophil function (reduced chemotaxis) and with an increased risk of disseminated infection, including sepsis and bacterial endocarditis. Consequently, preexisting bacterial infections should be adequately treated prior to initiation of aldesleukin therapy. Patients with indwelling central lines are particularly at risk for infection with gram-positive microorganisms. Antibiotic prophylaxis with oxacillin, nafcillin, ciprofloxacin, or vancomycin has been associated with a reduced incidence of staphylococcal infections.

Withhold aldesleukin administration in patients developing moderate to severe lethargy or somnolence; continued administration may result in coma.

Indications

➤*Metastatic renal cell carcinoma:* For the treatment of adults with metastatic renal cell carcinoma (metastatic RCC).

➤*Metastatic melanoma:* For the treatment of adults with metastatic melanoma.

➤*Patient selection:* Careful patient selection is mandatory prior to the administration of aldesleukin.

Evaluation of clinical studies to date reveals that patients with more favorable ECOG performance status (ECOG PS 0) at treatment initiation respond better to aldesleukin, with a higher response rate and lower toxicity. Therefore, selection of patients for treatment should include assessment of performance status.

Experience in patients with ECOG PS greater than 1 is extremely limited.

➤*Off-label uses:* May be beneficial when used in combination with highly active antiretroviral therapy (HAART) in the treatment of HIV patients; in combination for treatment of cutaneous T-cell lymphoma; treatment of colorectal cancer, non-Hodgkin lymphoma, acute myelogenous leukemia (AML), after hematopoietic stem cell transplantation (HSCT). (See Administration and Dosage).

Aldesleukin has been used safely and effectively in children with AML. (See Administration and Dosage).

Administration and Dosage

➤*General dosing considerations:* Before initiating treatment, carefully review the entire monograph, particularly regarding patient selection, possible serious adverse events, patient monitoring, and withholding dosage.

Each course of treatment consists of two 5-day treatment cycles separated by a rest period.

➤*Adults:*

Metastatic melanoma –

Dosage adjustment: If toxicity occurs, hold or interrupt doses rather than decreasing them. See Dose modifications for more information.

First course of therapy: 600,000 units/kg (0.037 mg/kg) administered every 8 hours by a 15-minute IV infusion for a maximum of 14 doses. Following 9 days of rest, the schedule is repeated for another 14 doses, for a maximum of 28 doses per course, as tolerated. Metastatic melanoma patients received a median of 18 doses during the first course of therapy.

Retreatment: Evaluate tumor response 4 weeks after therapy and again immediately prior to the scheduled start of the next treatment course. If tumor shrinkage is evident and further treatment is not contraindicated, another course of aldesleukin may be given using the same regimen. Allow at least 7 weeks between treatment courses (from date of hospital discharge).

Metastatic renal cell carcinoma –

Dosage adjustment: If toxicity occurs, hold or interrupt doses rather than decreasing them. See Dose modifications for more information.

First course of therapy: 600,000 units/kg (0.037 mg/kg) dose administered every 8 hours by a 15-minute IV infusion for a maximum of 14 doses. Following 9 days of rest, the schedule is repeated for another 14 doses, for a maximum of 28 doses per course, as tolerated. Metastatic RCC patients treated with this schedule received a median of 20 of the 28 doses during the first course of therapy.

Retreatment: Evaluate tumor response 4 weeks after therapy and again immediately prior to the scheduled start of the next treatment course. If tumor shrinkage is evident and further treatment is not contraindicated, another course of aldesleukin may be given using the same regimen. Allow at least 7 weeks between treatment courses (from date of hospital discharge).

Off-label dosing –

Acute myelogenous leukemia after autologous HSCT: An induction regimen is 3 million to 9 million units/m^2/day by continuous IV infusion for 4 to 5 days. After a 4- to 7-day rest period, begin maintenance therapy with aldesleukin 0.3 to 1.6 million units/m^2/day by continuous IV infusion for 10 days.

Breast cancer after autologous HSCT: Doses ranging from 0.6 million to 1.8 million units/m^2/day for 7 to 28 days have been given by subcutaneous injection or continuous IV infusion.

➤*Children:*

Off-label dosing –

Acute myelogenous leukemia: 9 million units/day for 4 days by continuous IV infusion, followed by a 4-day rest, then 1.6 million units/day for 10 days by continuous IV infusion.

➤*Renal function impairment:* Renal function is impaired during aldesleukin treatment. Use of concomitant nephrotoxic medications may further increase toxicity to the kidney. Serum creatinine should be 1.5 mg/dL or less prior to initiation of treatment. Dosage adjustment may be necessary in patients with renal impairment, although no specific guidelines are available.

Dialysis – Conventional hemodialysis and peritoneal dialysis are ineffective (0% to 24%) in removing aldesleukin.

➤*Hepatic function impairment:* Hepatic function is impaired during aldesleukin treatment. Use of concomitant hepatotoxic medications may further increase toxicity to the liver. If hepatic failure occurs, discontinue treatment for that course. Further courses may be given at least 7 weeks after resolution of hepatic failure or hospital discharge, whichever is most recent.

➤*Dose modifications:* Accomplish dose modification for toxicity by withholding or interrupting a dose rather than reducing the dose to be given. Decisions to stop, hold, or restart aldesleukin therapy must be made after a global assessment of the patient. With this in mind, use the following guidelines.

ALDESLEUKIN — INJECTION

Aldesleukin Dose Modification Based on Toxicity

Organ system	Permanently discontinue therapy	Delay subsequent doses	Continue with subsequent doses
Cardiovascular	Sustained ventricular tachycardia (≥ 5 beats)	Atrial fibrillation, supraventricular tachycardia, or bradycardia that requires therapy, recurs, or persists	Asymptomatic with full recovery to normal sinus rhythm
	Uncontrollable or unresponsive arrhythmias	Systolic blood pressure < 90 mm Hg with increasing pressor requirements	Systolic blood pressure ≥ 90 mm Hg with stable or improving pressor requirements
	Recurrent chest pain with ECG changes, documented angina, or myocardial infarction (MI)	ECG changes consistent with MI, myocarditis, or ischemia with or without chest pain; suspected ischemia	MI and myocarditis ruled out, angina not suspected, and patient asymptomatic; no ventricular hypokinesia present
	Pericardial tamponade		
CNS	Coma or toxic psychosis lasting > 48 hours	Mental status changes (eg, moderate confusion, agitation)	Complete resolution of mental status changes
	Repetitive or refractory seizures		
Dermatologic	—	Bullous dermatitis or marked worsening of preexisting skin condition (avoid topical steroids)	Complete resolution of bullous dermatitis.
GI	Bowel ischemia, perforation, or bleeding requiring surgery	Stool guaiac > 3 to 4+ repeatedly.	Negative stool guaiac
Hepatic	—	Signs of hepatic failure (eg, encephalopathy, increased ascites, liver pain, hypoglycemia), discontinue current course of therapy.	Resolution of hepatic failure; may consider starting another course of therapy at least 7 weeks after symptom resolution and hospital discharge
Renal	Dysfunction requiring dialysis for > 72 hours	Serum creatinine > 4.5 mg/dL or a serum creatinine ≥ 4 mg/dL with severe volume overload, acidosis, or hyperkalemia.	Serum creatinine < 4 mg/dL with stable fluid and electrolytes
	—	Persistent oliguria or urine output < 10 mL/h for 16 to 24 hours with increased serum creatinine.	Urine output > 10 mL/h with normalization or decrease (> 1.5 mg/dL) in creatinine.
Respiratory	Intubation required for > 72 hours	Oxygen saturation < 90%	Oxygen saturation ≥ 90%
Systemic	—	Sepsis syndrome, patient clinically unstable.	Resolution of sepsis syndrome, patient clinically stable, and infection being treated.

➤*Pretreatment:* Pretreatment with a nonsteroidal anti-inflammatory drug (NSAID) or acetaminophen may minimize the risk of developing fever or reduce its severity. Initiate premedication immediately before giving aldesleukin and continue for 12 hours after the final aldesleukin dose.

➤*Preparation for administration:* Reconstitution and dilution procedures other than those recommended may alter the delivery or pharmacology of aldesleukin, and thus should be avoided.

1.) Each vial contains 22 million units (1.3 mg) of aldesleukin and should be reconstituted aseptically with 1.2 mL of sterile water for injection. When reconstituted as directed, each mL contains 18 million units (1.1 mg) of aldesleukin. The resulting solution should be a clear, colorless to slightly yellow liquid. The vial is for single use only. Discard any unused portion.
2.) During reconstitution, direct the sterile water for injection at the side of the vial and gently swirl the contents to avoid excess foaming. Do not shake.
3.) Dilute the desired dose of aldesleukin in 50 mL of dextrose 5% injection to achieve a final aldesleukin concentration of 30 to 70 mcg/mL. The volume of dextrose 5% injection may be adjusted to keep the aldesleukin concentration within this range. Alternatively, the dose may be prepared with human serum albumin 0.1% (final concentration) for aldesleukin concentrations of less than 30 mcg/mL. Concentrations of aldesleukin below 30 mcg/mL and above 70 mcg/mL have shown increased variability in drug delivery. Avoid dilution and delivery of aldesleukin outside of this concentration range.
4.) Glass bottles and plastic (polyvinyl chloride) bags have been used in clinical trials with comparable results. It is recommended that plastic bags be used as the dilution container since experimental studies suggest that use of plastic containers results in more consistent drug delivery. Do not use in-line filters when administering aldesleukin.
5.) Before and after reconstitution and dilution, store in a refrigerator at 2° to 8°C (36° to 46°F). Do not freeze. Administer aldesleukin within 48 hours of reconstitution. Bring the solution to room temperature prior to infusion in the patient.

Pharmacia Deltec CADD infusion cassette – Dilute the desired dose of aldesleukin with dextrose 5% injection to achieve a final aldesleukin concentration of 100 to 500 mcg/mL. For aldesleukin concentrations between 5 and 60 mcg/mL, add human serum albumin to achieve a final albumin concentration of 0.1%.

➤*Administration:* To be given as an IV infusion (over 15 minutes), continuous IV infusion, or subcutaneous injection. Do not filter.

Continuous infusion – Infuse solution with the *Pharmacia Deltec CADD* infusion pump device. Contents of each cassette infuse over up to 6 days.

➤*Admixture compatibility:* Avoid reconstitution or dilution with bacteriostatic water for injection or sodium chloride 0.9% injection because of increased aggregation.

Do not coadminister aldesleukin with other drugs in the same container.

➤*Storage/Stability:* Store vials in a refrigerator at 2° to 8°C (36° to 46°F). Protect from light. Store in carton until time of use.

Reconstituted or diluted aldesleukin is stable for up to 48 hours at refrigerated and room temperatures, 2° to 25°C (36° to 77°F). However, since this product contains no preservative, store the reconstituted and diluted solutions in the refrigerator and use within 24 hours of reconstitution.

Diluted solutions containing dextrose 5% injection and human serum albumin 2% are stable for up to 6 days at room temperature. Because these preparations contain no preservatives, use them within 24 hours of preparation.

Discard vial within 6 hours of the initial needle puncture if opened within an ISO Class 5 biological safety cabinet, or within 1 hour of the initial needle puncture if opened outside of such an environment, based on the USP Chapter <797> standards.

Pharmacia Deltec CADD infusion cassette – Diluted solutions containing dextrose 5% injection and aldesleukin 100 to 500 mcg/mL are stable for up to 6 days at room temperature. Diluted solutions containing dextrose 5% injection, aldesleukin 5 to 60 mcg/mL, and human serum albumin 0.1% are also stable for up to 6 days at room temperature.

Actions

➤*Pharmacology:* Aldesleukin has been shown to possess the biological activities of human native interleukin-2. In vitro studies performed on human cell lines demonstrate the immunoregulatory properties of aldesleukin, including:

1.) Enhancement of lymphocyte mitogenesis and stimulation of long-term growth of human interleukin-2 dependent cell lines.
2.) Enhancement of lymphocyte cytotoxicity.
3.) Induction of killer cell (lymphokine-activated [LAK] and natural [NK]) activity.
4.) Induction of interferon-gamma production.

The in vivo administration of aldesleukin in animals and humans produces multiple immunological effects in a dose-dependent manner. These effects include activation of cellular immunity with profound lymphocytosis, eosinophilia, and thrombocytopenia, and the production of cytokines including tumor necrosis factor, IL-1, and gamma interferon. In vivo experiments in murine tumor models have shown inhibition of tumor growth. The exact mechanism by which aldesleukin mediates its antitumor activity in animals and humans is unknown.

➤*Pharmacokinetics:*

Absorption/Distribution – Aldesleukin exists as biologically active, noncovalently bound microaggregates with an average size of 27 recombinant interleukin-2 molecules. The solubilizing agent, sodium dodecyl sulfate, may have an effect on the kinetic properties of this product.

ALDESLEUKIN — INJECTION

The pharmacokinetic profile of aldesleukin is characterized by high plasma concentrations following a short IV infusion, rapid distribution into the extravascular space and elimination from the body by metabolism in the kidneys with little or no bioactive protein excreted in the urine. Studies of IV aldesleukin in sheep and humans indicate that upon completion of infusion, approximately 30% of the administered dose is detectable in plasma. This finding is consistent with studies in rats using radiolabeled aldesleukin, which demonstrate a rapid (less than 1 minute) uptake of the majority of the label into the lungs, liver, kidney, and spleen.

The serum half-life ($t_{1/2}$) curves of aldesleukin remaining in the plasma are derived from studies done in 52 cancer patients following a 5-minute IV infusion. These patients were shown to have a distribution and elimination $t_{1/2}$ of 13 and 85 minutes, respectively.

Metabolism/Excretion – Following the initial rapid organ distribution, the primary route of clearance of circulating aldesleukin is the kidney. In humans and animals, aldesleukin is cleared from the circulation by both glomerular filtration and peritubular extraction in the kidney. This dual mechanism for delivery of aldesleukin to the proximal tubule may account for the preservation of clearance in patients with rising serum creatinine values. Greater than 80% of the amount of aldesleukin distributed to plasma, cleared from the circulation and presented to the kidney is metabolized to amino acids in the cells lining the proximal convoluted tubules. In humans, the mean clearance rate in cancer patients is 268 mL/min.

The relatively rapid clearance of aldesleukin has led to dosage schedules characterized by frequent, short infusions. Observed serum levels are proportional to the dose of aldesleukin.

Contraindications

History of hypersensitivity to interleukin-2 or any component of the aldesleukin formulation; abnormal thallium stress test or abnormal pulmonary function tests; organ allografts. Retreatment with aldesleukin is contraindicated in patients who have experienced the following drug-related toxicities while receiving an earlier course of therapy: sustained ventricular tachycardia (greater than or equal to 5 beats); cardiac arrhythmias not controlled or unresponsive to management; chest pain with ECG changes, consistent with angina or myocardial infarction; cardiac tamponade; intubation for greater than 72 hours; renal failure requiring dialysis greater than 72 hours; coma or toxic psychosis lasting greater than 48 hours; repetitive or difficult to control seizures; bowel ischemia/perforation; GI bleeding requiring surgery.

Warnings/Precautions

➤*Severe adverse events:* Because of the severe adverse events which generally accompany aldesleukin therapy at the recommended dosages, perform thorough clinical evaluation to identify patients with significant cardiac, pulmonary, renal, hepatic, or CNS impairment in whom aldesleukin is contraindicated. Patients with normal cardiovascular, pulmonary, hepatic, and CNS function may experience serious, life-threatening, or fatal adverse events. Adverse events are frequent, often serious, and sometimes fatal.

Should adverse events, which require dose modification occur, withhold dosage rather than reduce it.

➤*Exacerbation of pre-existing diseases:* Aldesleukin has been associated with exacerbation of preexisting or initial presentation of autoimmune disease and inflammatory disorders. Exacerbation of Crohn's disease, scleroderma, thyroiditis, inflammatory arthritis, diabetes mellitus, oculobulbar myasthenia gravis, crescentic IgA glomerulonephritis, cholecystitis, cerebral vasculitis, Stevens-Johnson syndrome, and bullous pemphigoid has been reported following treatment with IL-2.

All patients should have thorough evaluation and treatment of CNS metastases and have a negative scan prior to receiving aldesleukin therapy. New neurologic signs, symptoms, and anatomic lesions following aldesleukin therapy have been reported in patients without evidence of CNS metastases. Clinical manifestations included changes in mental status, speech difficulties, cortical blindness, limb or gait ataxia, hallucinations, agitation, obtundation, and coma. Radiological findings included multiple and, less commonly, single cortical lesions on MRI and evidence of demyelination. Neurologic signs and symptoms associated with aldesleukin therapy usually improve after discontinuation of aldesleukin therapy; however, there are reports of permanent neurologic defects. One case of possible cerebral vasculitis, responsive to dexamethasone, has been reported. In patients with known seizure disorders, exercise extreme caution as aldesleukin may cause seizures.

➤*Immunogenicity:* 57 of 77 (74%) metastatic renal cell carcinoma patients treated with an every 8-hour aldesleukin regimen and 33 of 50 (66%) metastatic melanoma patients treated with a variety of IV regimens developed low titers of nonneutralizing antialdesleukin antibodies. Neutralizing antibodies were not detected in this group of patients, but have been detected in 1 of 106 (less than 1%) patients treated with IV aldesleukin using a wide variety of schedules and doses. The clinical significance of antialdesleukin antibodies is unknown.

➤*Capillary leak syndrome (CLS):* Patients should have normal cardiac, pulmonary, hepatic, and CNS function at the start of therapy. CLS begins immediately after aldesleukin treatment starts and is marked by increased capillary permeability to protein and fluids and reduced vascular tone. In most patients, this results in a concomitant drop in mean arterial blood pressure within 2 to 12 hours after the start of treatment. With continued therapy, clinically significant hypotension (defined as systolic blood pressure below 90 mm Hg or a 20 mm Hg drop from baseline systolic pressure) and hypoperfusion will occur. In addition, extravasation of protein and fluids into the extravascular space will lead to the formation of edema and creation of new effusions.

Medical management of CLS begins with careful monitoring of the patient's fluid and organ perfusion status. This is achieved by frequent determination of blood pressure and pulse, and by monitoring organ function, which includes assessment of mental status and urine output. Hypovolemia is assessed by catheterization and central pressure monitoring.

Fluid status – Flexibility in fluid and pressor management is essential for maintaining organ perfusion and blood pressure. Consequently, use extreme caution in treating patients with fixed requirements for large volumes of fluid (eg, patients with hypercalcemia). Administration of IV fluids, either colloids or crystalloids is recommended for treatment of hypovolemia. Correction of hypovolemia may require large volumes of IV fluids but caution is required because unrestrained fluid administration may exacerbate problems associated with edema formation or effusions. With extravascular fluid accumulation, edema is common and ascites, pleural or pericardial effusions may develop. Management of these events depends on a careful balancing of the effects of fluid shifts so that neither the consequences of hypovolemia (eg, impaired organ perfusion) nor the consequences of fluid accumulations (eg, pulmonary edema) exceed the patient's tolerance.

Dopamine – Clinical experience has shown that early administration of dopamine (1 to 5 mcg/kg/min) to patients manifesting capillary leak syndrome, before the onset of hypotension, can help to maintain organ perfusion particularly to the kidney and thus preserve urine output. Carefully monitor weight and urine output. If organ perfusion and blood pressure are not sustained by dopamine therapy, clinical investigators have increased the dose of dopamine to 6 to 10 mcg/kg/min or have added phenylephrine hydrochloride (1 to 5 mcg/kg/min) to low-dose dopamine. Prolonged use of pressors, either in combination or as individual agents, at relatively high doses, may be associated with cardiac rhythm disturbances. If there has been excessive weight gain or edema formation, particularly if associated with shortness of breath from pulmonary congestion, use of diuretics, once blood pressure has normalized, has been shown to hasten recovery. Note: Prior to the use of any product mentioned, the physician should refer to the package insert for the respective product.

Withhold aldesleukin treatment for failure to maintain organ perfusion as demonstrated by altered mental status, reduced urine output, a fall in the systolic blood pressure below 90 mm Hg, or onset of cardiac arrhythmias. Recovery from CLS begins soon after cessation of aldesleukin therapy. Usually, within a few hours, the blood pressure rises, organ perfusion is restored and reabsorption of extravasated fluid and protein begins.

CNS toxicity – Mental status changes including irritability, confusion, or depression which occur while receiving aldesleukin may be indicators of bacteremia or early bacterial sepsis, hypoperfusion, occult CNS malignancy, or direct aldesleukin-induced CNS toxicity. Alterations in mental status due solely to aldesleukin therapy may progress for several days before recovery begins. Rarely, patients have sustained permanent neurologic deficits.

Exacerbation of pre-existing diseases – Exacerbation of preexisting autoimmune disease or initial presentation of autoimmune and inflammatory disorders has been reported following aldesleukin alone or in combination with interferon. Hypothyroidism, sometimes preceded by hyperthyroidism, has been reported following aldesleukin treatment. Some of these patients required thyroid replacement therapy. Changes in thyroid function may be a manifestation of autoimmunity. Onset of symptomatic hyperglycemia or diabetes mellitus has been reported during aldesleukin therapy.

Transplant patients – Aldesleukin enhancement of cellular immune function may increase the risk of allograft rejection in transplant patients.

Pulmonary – All patients should have baseline pulmonary function tests with arterial blood gases. Document adequate pulmonary function (FEV_1 greater than 2 L or greater than or equal to 75% of predicted for height and age) prior to initiating therapy.

During treatment, monitor pulmonary function on a regular basis by clinical examination, assessment of vital signs, and pulse oximetry. Further assess patients with dyspnea or clinical signs of respiratory impairment (tachypnea or rales) with arterial blood gas determination. Repeat these tests as often as clinically indicated.

Stress thallium study – Screen all patients with a stress thallium study. Document normal ejection fraction and unimpaired wall motion. If a thallium stress test suggests minor wall motion abnormalities, further testing is suggested to exclude significant coronary artery disease.

Cardiac – Assess cardiac function daily by clinical examination and assessment of vital signs. Further assess patients with signs or symptoms of chest pain, murmurs, gallops, irregular rhythm or palpitations with an ECG examination and cardiac enzyme evaluation. Evidence of myocardial injury, including findings compatible with myocardial infarction or myocarditis, has been reported. Ventricular hypokinesia due to myocarditis may be persistent for several months. If there is evidence of cardiac ischemia or congestive heart failure, hold aldesleukin therapy, and perform a repeat thallium study.

➤*Hypersensitivity reactions:* Hypersensitivity reactions have been reported in patients receiving combination regimens containing sequential high-dose aldesleukin and antineoplastic agents, specifically, dacarbazine, cis-platinum, tamoxifen, and interferon-alfa. These reactions consisted of erythema, pruritus, and hypotension and occurred within hours of administration of chemotherapy. These events required medical intervention in some patients.

➤*Renal/Hepatic function impairment:* Kidney and liver function are impaired during aldesleukin treatment. Use of concomitant nephrotoxic or hepatotoxic medications may further increase toxicity to the kidney or liver. Serum creatinine should be less than or equal to 1.5 mg/dL prior to initiation of aldesleukin treatment.

➤*Pregnancy: Category C.* Aldesleukin has been shown to have embryolethal effects in rats when given in doses at 27 to 36 times the human dose (scaled by body weight). Significant maternal toxicities were observed in pregnant rats administered aldesleukin by IV injection at doses 2.1 to

ALDESLEUKIN — INJECTION

36 times higher than the human dose during critical period of organogenesis. No evidence of teratogenicity was observed other than that attributed to maternal toxicity. There are no adequate well-controlled studies of aldesleukin in pregnant women. Use aldesleukin during pregnancy only if the potential benefit justifies the potential risk to the fetus.

Fertility impairment – There have been no studies conducted assessing the effect of aldesleukin on fertility. It is recommended that this drug not be administered to fertile persons of either gender not practicing effective contraception.

➤*Lactation:* It is not known whether this drug is excreted in human milk. Because many drugs are excreted in human milk and because of the potential for serious adverse reactions in nursing infants from aldesleukin, a decision should be made whether to discontinue nursing or to discontinue the drug, taking into account the importance of the drug to the mother.

➤*Children:* Safety and effectiveness in children younger than 18 years of age have not been established.

➤*Elderly:* Aldesleukin is known to be substantially excreted by the kidney, and the risk of toxic reactions to this drug may be greater in patients with impaired renal function. The pattern of organ system toxicity and the proportion of patients with severe toxicities by organ system were generally similar in patients 65 and older and younger patients. There was a trend, however, towards an increased incidence of severe urogenital toxicities and dyspnea in the older patients.

➤*Monitoring:* Daily monitoring during therapy with aldesleukin should include vital signs (temperature, pulse, blood pressure, and respiration rate), weight, and fluid intake and output. In a patient with a decreased systolic blood pressure, especially less than 90 mm Hg, conduct constant cardiac rhythm monitoring. If an abnormal complex or rhythm is seen, perform an ECG. Take vital signs in these hypotensive patients hourly.

The following clinical evaluations are recommended for all patients, prior to beginning treatment and then daily during drug administration: standard hematologic tests, including CBC, differential and platelet counts; blood chemistries, including electrolytes, renal and hepatic function tests; chest x-rays.

Drug Interactions

➤*Current chemotherapy:* Hypersensitivity reactions have been reported in patients receiving combination regimens containing sequential high-dose aldesleukin and antineoplastic agents, specifically, dacarbazine, cisplatinum, tamoxifen and interferon-alfa. These reactions consisted of erythema, pruritus, and hypotension and occurred within hours of administration of chemotherapy. These events required medical intervention in some patients.

➤*Interferon-alfa:* Myocardial injury, including myocardial infarction, myocarditis, ventricular hypokinesia, and severe rhabdomyolysis appear to be increased in patients receiving aldesleukin and interferon-alfa concurrently.

Exacerbation or the initial presentation of a number of autoimmune and inflammatory disorders has been observed following concurrent use of interferon-alfa and aldesleukin, including crescentic IgA glomerulonephritis, oculo-bulbar myasthenia gravis, inflammatory arthritis, thyroiditis, bullous pemphigoid, and Stevens-Johnson syndrome.

➤*Iodinated contrast media:* A review of the literature revealed that 12.6% (range 11% to 28%) of 501 patients treated with various interleukin-2 containing regimens who were subsequently administered radiographic iodinated contrast media experienced acute, atypical adverse reactions. The onset of symptoms usually occurred within hours (most commonly 1 to 4 hours) following the administration of contrast media. These reactions include fever, chills, nausea, vomiting, pruritus, rash, diarrhea, hypotension, edema, and oliguria. Some clinicians have noted that these reactions resemble the immediate side effects caused by interleukin-2 administration; however, the cause of contrast reactions after interleukin-2 therapy is unknown. Most events were reported to occur when contrast media was given within 4 weeks after the last dose of interleukin-2. These events were also reported to occur when contrast media was given several months after interleukin-2 treatment.

Aldesleukin Drug Interactions

Precipitant drug	Object drug[a]		Description
Antihypertensives	Aldesleukin	↑	Antihypertensives may potentiate the hypotension seen with aldesleukin.
Corticosteroids	Aldesleukin	↓	Although glucocorticoids reduce the side effects of aldesleukin, coadministration may reduce the antitumor effectiveness of aldesleukin; avoid concurrent use.

Aldesleukin Drug Interactions

Precipitant drug	Object drug[a]		Description
Cardiotoxic agents (eg, doxorubicin)	Aldesleukin	↑	Increased toxicity in these organ systems may occur during coadministration.
Hepatotoxic agents (eg, methotrexate, asparaginase)			
Myelotoxic agents (eg, cytotoxic chemotherapy)			
Nephrotoxic agents (eg, aminoglycosides, indomethacin)			
Aldesleukin	Protease inhibitors (eg, indinavir)	↑	Protease concentrations may be elevated, increasing risk of toxicity. May need to adjust the dose of indinavir when aldesleukin is initiated or stopped.
Aldesleukin	Psychotropic agents (eg, narcotics, analgesics, sedatives, antiemetics, tranquilizers)	↔	Aldesleukin may affect CNS function. Therefore, interactions could occur following coadministration of these agents.

[a] ↑ = Object drug increased. ↓ = Object drug decreased. ↔ = Undetermined clinical effect.

Adverse Reactions

The rate of drug-related deaths in the 255 metastatic RCC patients who received single-agent aldesleukin was 4% (11 of 255); the rate of drug-related deaths in the 270 metastatic melanoma patients who received single-agent aldesleukin was 2% (6 of 270).

Aldesleukin Adverse Events (≥ 10%)

Adverse reactions	Patients (n = 525)
Cardiovascular	
Arrhythmia	10%
Cardiovascular disorder[a]	11%
Hypotension	71%
Supraventricular tachycardia	12%
Tachycardia	23%
Vasodilation	13%
CNS	
Anxiety	12%
Confusion	34%
Dizziness	11%
Somnolence	22%
Dermatologic	
Exfoliative dermatitis	18%
Pruritus	24%
Rash	42%
GI	
Anorexia	20%
Diarrhea	67%
Nausea	35%
Nausea and vomiting	19%
Stomatitis	22%
Vomiting	50%
GU	
Oliguria	63%
Hemic/Lymphatic	
Anemia	29%
Leukopenia	16%
Thrombocytopenia	37%
Metabolic/Nutritional	
Acidosis	12%
Alkaline phosphatase increase	10%

ALDESLEUKIN — INJECTION

Aldesleukin Adverse Events (≥ 10%)

Adverse reactions	Patients (n = 525)
AST increase	23%
Bilirubinemia	40%
Creatinine increase	33%
Edema	15%
Hypoglycemia	11%
Hypomagnesemia	12%
Peripheral edema	28%
Weight gain	16%
Respiratory	
Cough increase	11%
Dyspnea	43%
Lung disorder[b]	24%
Respiratory tract disorder[c]	11%
Rhinitis	10%
Miscellaneous	
Abdominal pain	11%
Asthenia	23%
Chills	52%
Enlarged abdomen	10%
Fever	29%
Infection	13%
Malaise	27%
Pain	12%

[a] Cardiovascular disorder: Fluctuations in blood pressure, asymptomatic ECG changes, CHF.
[b] Lung disorder: Physical findings associated with pulmonary congestion, rales, rhonchi.
[c] Respiratory disorder: ARDS, CXR infiltrates, unspecified pulmonary changes.

Life-Threatening (Grade 4) Aldesleukin Adverse Events (%)

Adverse reaction	Patients (n = 525)
Cardiovascular	
Cardiovascular disorder[a]	7 (1%)
Heart arrest	4 (1%)
Hypotension	15 (3%)
Myocardial infarction	7 (1%)
Supraventricular tachycardia	3 (1%)
Ventricular tachycardia	5 (1%)
CNS	
Coma	8 (2%)
Confusion	5 (1%)
Psychosis	7 (1%)
Stupor	3 (1%)
GI	
Diarrhea	10 (2%)
Vomiting	7 (1%)
GU	
Acute kidney failure	3 (1%)
Anuria	25 (5%)
Oliguria	33 (6%)
Hemic/Lymphatic	
Coagulation disorder[b]	4 (1%)
Thrombocytopenia	5 (1%)
Metabolic/Nutritional	
Acidosis	4 (1%)
AST increase	3 (1%)
Bilirubinemia	13 (2%)
Creatinine increase	5 (1%)
Respiratory	
Apnea	5 (1%)
Dyspnea	5 (1%)
Respiratory tract disorder[c]	14 (3%)
Miscellaneous	
Fever	5 (1%)
Infection	7 (1%)
Sepsis	6 (1%)

[a] Cardiovascular disorder: Fluctuations in blood pressure.
[b] Coagulation disorder: Intravascular coagulopathy.
[c] Respiratory disorder: ARDS, respiratory failure, intubation.

The following life-threatening (grade 4) events were reported by less than 1% of the 525 patients: Hypothermia; shock; bradycardia; ventricular extrasystoles; myocardial ischemia; syncope; hemorrhage; atrial arrhythmia; phlebitis; AV block second degree; endocarditis; pericardial effusion; peripheral gangrene; thrombosis; coronary artery disorder; stomatitis; nausea and vomiting; liver function tests abnormal; gastrointestinal hemorrhage; hematemesis; bloody diarrhea; gastrointestinal disorder; intestinal perforation; pancreatitis; anemia; leukopenia; leukocytosis; hypocalcemia; alkaline phosphatase increase; BUN increase; hyperuricemia; NPN increase; respiratory acidosis; somnolence; agitation; neuropathy; paranoid reaction; convulsion; grand mal convulsion; delirium; asthma; lung edema; hyperventilation; hypoxia; hemoptysis; hypoventilation; pneumothorax; mydriasis; pupillary disorder; kidney function abnormal; kidney failure; acute tubular necrosis.

➤*Serious adverse reactions:* In an additional population of greater than 1,800 patients treated with aldesleukin-based regimens using a variety of doses and schedules (eg, subcutaneous, continuous infusion, administration with LAK cells) the following serious adverse events were reported: Duodenal ulceration; bowel necrosis; myocarditis; supraventricular tachycardia; permanent or transient blindness secondary to optic neuritis; transient ischemic attacks; meningitis; cerebral edema; pericarditis; allergic interstitial nephritis; tracheoesophageal fistula.

➤*Fatal adverse reactions:* In the same clinical population, the following fatal events each occurred with a frequency of less than 1%: Malignant hyperthermia; cardiac arrest; myocardial infarction; pulmonary emboli; stroke; intestinal perforation; liver or renal failure; severe depression leading to suicide; pulmonary edema; respiratory arrest; respiratory failure. In patients with both metastatic RCC and metastatic melanoma, those with ECOG PS of 1 or higher had a higher treatment-related mortality and serious adverse events.

➤*Permanent sequelae:* Most adverse reactions are self-limiting and, usually, but not invariably, reverse or improve within 2 or 3 days of discontinuation of therapy. Examples of adverse reactions with permanent sequelae include myocardial infarction, bowel perforation/infarction, and gangrene.

➤*Postmarketing:* In postmarketing experience, the following serious adverse events have been reported in a variety of treatment regimens that include interleukin-2: Anaphylaxis; cellulitis; injection-site necrosis; retroperitoneal hemorrhage; cardiomyopathy; cerebral hemorrhage; fatal endocarditis; hypertension; cholecystitis; colitis; gastritis; hepatitis; hepatosplenomegaly; intestinal obstruction; hyperthyroidism; neutropenia; myopathy; myositis; rhabdomyolysis; cerebral lesions; encephalopathy; extrapyramidal syndrome; insomnia; neuralgia; neuritis; neuropathy (demyelination); urticaria; pneumonia (bacterial, fungal, viral).

➤*Exacerbation of pre-exisitng diseases:* Exacerbation or initial presentation of a number of autoimmune and inflammatory disorders have been reported. Persistent but nonprogressive vitiligo has been observed in malignant melanoma patients treated with interleukin-2. Synergistic, additive and novel toxicities have been reported with aldesleukin used in combination with other drugs. Novel toxicities include delayed adverse reactions to iodinated contrast media and hypersensitivity reactions to antineoplastic agents.

➤*Concurrent therapy:* Experience has shown the following concomitant medications to be useful in the management of patients on aldesleukin therapy:

1.) Standard antipyretic therapy, including nonsteroidal anti-inflammatories (NSAIDs), started immediately prior to aldesleukin to reduce fever. Monitor renal function, as some NSAIDs may cause synergistic nephrotoxicity.
2.) Meperidine used to control the rigors associated with fever.
3.) H_2 antagonists given for prophylaxis of gastrointestinal irritation and bleeding.
4.) Antiemetics and antidiarrheals used as needed to treat other gastrointestinal side effects. Generally these medications were discontinued 12 hours after the last dose of aldesleukin.

➤*Other:* Patients with indwelling central lines have a higher risk of infection with gram-positive organisms. A reduced incidence of staphylococcal infections in aldesleukin studies has been associated with the use of antibiotic prophylaxis which includes the use of oxacillin, nafcillin, ciprofloxacin, or vancomycin. Hydroxyzine or diphenhydramine has been used to control symptoms from pruritic rashes and continued until resolution of pruritus. Apply topical creams and ointments as needed for skin manifestations. Avoid preparations containing a steroid (eg, hydrocortisone). Note: Prior to the use of any product mentioned, the physician should refer to drug monograph for the respective product.

Overdosage

➤*Symptoms:* Side effects following the use of aldesleukin appear to be dose related. Exceeding the recommended dose has been associated with a more rapid onset of expected dose-limiting toxicities.

ALDESLEUKIN — INJECTION

➤*Treatment:* Monitor symptoms that persist after cessation of aldesleukin, and treat supportively. Life-threatening toxicities may be ameliorated by the IV administration of dexamethasone, which may also result in loss of the therapeutic effects of aldesleukin.

BCG LIVE

Rx	**Tice BCG** (Organon)	**Injection, lyophilized, powder for suspension**[a]: 1 to 8×10^8 CFU (equivalent to ≈ 50 mg wet weight)	Preservative free. In ≈ 50 mg vial.
Rx	**TheraCys** (Sanofi Pasteur)	**Injection, lyophilized, powder for suspension**[a]: 10.5 ± 8.7×10^8 CFU when resuspended (equivalent to ≈ 81 mg dry weight)	Monosodium glutamate. Preservative free. In 81 mg vial with 3 mL diluent vial.

[a] For intravesical administration.

BCG LIVE — INTRAVESICAL

The BCG vaccine for tuberculosis prevention is discussed in the Biologic and Immunological agents chapter.

WARNING

BCG live contains live, attenuated mycobacteria. Because of the potential risk for transmission, it should be prepared, handled, and disposed of as a biohazardous material.

BCG infections have been reported in health care workers, primarily from exposures resulting from accidental needle sticks or skin lacerations during the preparation of BCG live for administration. Nosocomial infections have been reported in patients, including immunosuppressed patients, receiving parenteral drugs that were prepared in areas in which BCG live was reconstituted. BCG live is capable of dissemination when administered by the intravesical route. Serious infections, including fatal infections, have been reported in patients receiving intravesical BCG live.

Indications

➤*Carcinoma in situ (CIS) of the urinary bladder:* For the treatment and prophylaxis of CIS of the urinary bladder.

➤*Stage Ta and/or T1 papillary tumors:* For the prophylaxis of primary or recurrent stage Ta and/or T1 papillary tumors following transurethral resection (TUR). BCG live is not recommended for stage TaG1 papillary tumors, unless they are judged to be at high risk of tumor recurrence.

BCG live is not indicated for papillary tumors of stages higher than T1 nor as an immunizing agent for the prevention of tuberculosis (TB).

➤*Off-label uses:* Local control of accessible tumor.

Administration and Dosage

➤*General dosing considerations: TheraCys* and *TICE BCG* are not bioequivalent and may not be used interchangeably. Do not switch patients between products without careful medical supervision.

➤*Adults:*

Carcinoma in situ (CIS) of the urinary bladder –

TheraCys:

• *Initial dosage* – After reconstitution, instill the contents of 1 vial (BCG 81 mg [dry weight]) into the bladder once weekly for 6 consecutive weeks, starting 7to 14 days after biopsy or transurethral resection.

• *Maintenance dosage* – After reconstitution, instill the contents of 1 vial (BCG 81 mg [dry weight]) into the bladder given 3, 6, 12, 18, and 24 months following the initial dose.

TICE BCG:

• *Initial dosage* – After reconstitution, instill the contents of 1 vial into the bladder once weekly for 6 consecutive weeks, starting 7 to 14 days after bladder biopsy.

This schedule may be repeated once if tumor remission has not been achieved and if the clinical circumstances warrant.

• *Maintenance dosage* – After reconstitution, instill the contents of 1 vial into the bladder at approximately monthly intervals for at least 6 to 12 months.

• *Duration of therapy* – At least 6 to 12 months.

Stage Ta and/or T1 papillary tumors – See Carcinoma in situ (CIS) of the Urinary Bladder for dosing.

➤*Instructions for disposal:* After use, unused product, packaging, and all equipment and materials used for instillation of the product (eg, syringes, catheters) should be placed immediately in a container for biohazardous materials and disposed of according to local requirements applicable to biohazardous materials.

Urine voided during the 6-hour period following BCG live instillation should be disinfected with an equal volume of hypochlorite 5% solution (undiluted household bleach) and allowed to stand for 15 minutes before flushing.

➤*Preparation for administration:* The preparation of BCG live should be done using aseptic technique. To avoid cross-contamination, parenteral drugs should not be prepared in areas where BCG live has been prepared. A separate area for the preparation of BCG live is recommended. Prepare in a vertical laminar flow hood. All equipment, supplies, and receptacles in contact with BCG live should be handled and disposed of as biohazardous. The pharmacist or individual responsible for mixing the agent should wear gloves and eye protection and take precautions to avoid contact of BCG live with broken skin. If the preparation cannot be performed in a biocontainment hood, then a mask and gown may be worn to avoid inhalation of BCG live organisms and inadvertent exposure to broken skin.

Suspension will appear cloudy. Discard if any clumping or flocculation is present.

TheraCys – *TheraCys* should not be handled by persons with an immunologic deficiency.

Do not remove the rubber stopper from the vial.

Apply a sterile piece of cotton moistened with a suitable antiseptic to the surface of the rubber stoppers of the vial of diluent and vial of *TheraCys*.

Reconstitute the freeze-dried material with the total 3 mL volume of the provided diluent. Shake the vial gently until a fine, even suspension results. Avoid foaming because this will prevent withdrawal of the proper dose. Withdraw the entire contents (approximately 3 mL) of the reconstituted material into the syringe.

The reconstituted material from the vial (1 dose) is further diluted in an additional 50 mL of sterile, preservative-free saline to a final volume of 53 mL for intravesical instillation.

TheraCys should be used immediately after reconstitution. However, if there is an unavoidable delay between reconstitution and administration, this delay must not exceed 2 hours. Any reconstituted product that exhibits flocculation or clumping that cannot be dispersed with gentle shaking should not be used.

Tice BCG – Draw 1 mL of sterile, preservative-free saline (sodium chloride 0.9% injection) at 4° to 25°C (39.2° to 77°F) into a small syringe (eg, 3 mL) and add to 1 vial of *Tice BCG* to resuspend. Gently swirl the vial until a homogenous suspension is obtained. Avoid forceful agitation that may cause clumping of the mycobacteria.

Dispense the cloudy *Tice BCG* suspension into the top end of a catheter-tip syringe that contains 49 mL of saline diluent, bringing the total volume to 50 mL. To mix, gently rotate the syringe.

Note: Do not filter the contents of the *Tice BCG* vial. Precautions should be taken to avoid exposing the *Tice BCG* cake to direct sunlight. Bacteriostatic solutions must be avoided. In addition, use only sterile, preservative-free saline, sodium chloride 0.9% injection, as diluent.

➤*Administration:* Give by intravesical instillation only. Do not inject subcutaneously or intravenously.

Wear gloves, a gown, and a mask while administering BCG live.

TheraCys – A urethral catheter is inserted into the bladder under aseptic conditions, the bladder is drained, and then 53 mL suspension of *TheraCys* is instilled slowly by gravity, following which, the catheter is withdrawn.

The patient retains the suspension for as long as possible for a total of up to 2 hours. During the first 15 minutes following instillation, the patient should lie prone. Thereafter, the patient is allowed to be up. At the end of 2 hours, all patients should void in a seated position for safety reasons. Patients should be instructed to increase fluid intake in order to flush the bladder in the hours following BCG treatment.

Tice BCG – Patients should not drink fluids for 4 hours before treatment and should empty their bladder prior to *Tice BCG* administration. The reconstituted *Tice BCG* is instilled into the bladder by gravity flow via the catheter. Do not depress plunger and force the flow of the *Tice BCG*. The *Tice BCG* is retained in the bladder 2 hours and then voided. Patients unable to retain the suspension for 2 hours should be allowed to void sooner, if necessary.

While the *Tice BCG* is retained in the bladder, the patient should ideally be repositioned from left side to right side and also should lie upon the back and the abdomen, changing these positions every 15 minutes to maximize bladder surface exposure to the agent.

➤*Storage/Stability:* Store vials (and the *TheraCys* diluent) in a refrigerator between 2° and 8°C (36° and 46°F). Do not expose to sunlight, direct or indirect. Exposure to artificial light should be kept to a minimum. Use immediately after reconstitution; maximum stability is 2 hours.

Actions

➤*Pharmacology:* When administered intravesically as a cancer therapy, BCG live promotes a local acute inflammatory and subacute granulomatous reaction with macrophage and lymphocyte infiltration in the urothelium, and lamina propria of the urinary bladder. The exact mechanism of action is unknown, but the antitumor effect appears to be T-lymphocyte–dependent.

Contraindications

Immunosuppressed patients or persons with congenital or acquired immune deficiencies, whether caused by concurrent disease (eg, AIDS, leukemia, lymphoma), cancer therapy (eg, cytotoxic drugs, radiation), or immunosuppressive therapy (eg, corticosteroids).

Postpone treatment until resolution of a concurrent febrile illness, urinary tract infection, or gross hematuria. Allow 7 to 14 days before BCG live is administered following biopsy, TUR, or traumatic catheterization.

BCG LIVE — INTRAVESICAL

Do not administer BCG live to persons with active TB. Rule out active TB in individuals who are purified protein derivative (PPD)-positive before starting treatment with BCG live. Perform test for detecting *Mycobacterium Tuberculosis* infection if PPD of tuberculin status is unknown.

A positive Mantoux test by itself is not a contraindication to using *TheraCys*, but an assessment must be made regarding whether the patient has signs, symptoms, and/or a chest x-ray consistent with active or latent TB that requires treatment with antimycobacterial drugs.

TheraCys is contraindicated for patients with current symptoms or a previous history of systemic BCG reaction.

Warnings/Precautions

➤*Systemic BCG reaction:* A systemic BCG reaction is a systemic granulomatous illness that may occur subsequent to exposure to BCG live.

Based on past clinical experience with intravesical BCG live, "systemic BCG reaction" may be defined as the presence of any of the following signs, if no other etiologies for such signs are detectable: fever at least 39.5°C (103.1°F) for at least 12 hours; fever at least 38.5°C (101.3°F) for at least 48 hours; pneumonitis; hepatitis; other organ dysfunction outside of the GU tract with granulomatous inflammation on biopsy; or the classical signs of sepsis, including circulatory collapse, acute respiratory distress, and disseminated intravascular coagulation.

If *TheraCys* is administered within 1 week of either biopsy, TUR, or traumatic bladder catheterization (association with hematuria), a systemic BCG reaction is much more likely to occur. Death has been reported with the use of *TheraCys* in association with systemic BCG reaction in postmarketing experience.

If a patient develops persistent fever or experiences an acute febrile illness consistent with BCG infection, permanently discontinue BCG instillations, evaluate and treat the patient immediately for BCG infection, and seek an infectious disease consultation.

➤*Management of serious BCG complications:* Acute, localized, irritative toxicities of BCG live may be accompanied by systemic manifestations consistent with a "flu-like" syndrome. Systemic adverse reactions such as malaise, fever, and chills of 1 to 2 days' duration often reflect hypersensitivity reactions. However, symptoms such as fever of at least 38.5°C (101.3°F), or acute localized inflammation such as epididymitis, prostatitis, or orchitis persisting longer than 2 to 3 days suggest active infection; consider evaluation for serious infectious complications.

In patients who develop persistent fever or experience an acute febrile illness consistent with BCG infection, administer 2 or more antimycobacterial agents while diagnostic evaluation, including cultures, is conducted. Discontinue BCG treatment. Negative cultures do not necessarily rule out infection.

See Warnings/Precautions for more information.

BCG live is sensitive to the most commonly used anti-TB agents (eg, isoniazid, rifampin, ethambutol). *Tice BCG* and *TheraCys* are not sensitive to pyrazinamide.

➤*Not for use as a vaccine:* *Tice BCG* and *TheraCys* are not vaccines for the prevention of cancer. Use BCG vaccine, not *Tice BCG*, for the prevention of TB. For vaccination use, refer to the BCG vaccine monograph.

➤*Infectious complications:* BCG live is an infectious agent. Be familiar with the literature on the prevention and treatment of BCG-related complications and be prepared in such emergencies to contact an infectious disease specialist with experience in treating the infectious complications of intravesical BCG live. The treatment of the infectious complications of BCG requires long-term, multiple-drug antibiotic therapy. Special culture media are required for mycobacteria, and health care providers administering intravesical BCG or those caring for these patients should have these media readily available.

➤*Administration/Handling precautions:* BCG live contains live mycobacteria; prepare and handle using aseptic technique. BCG infections have been reported in health care workers preparing BCG live for administration. Avoid needle-stick injuries during the handling and mixing of BCG live. Nosocomial infections have been reported in patients and immunosuppressed patients receiving parenteral drugs that were prepared in areas where BCG live was prepared.

BCG is capable of dissemination when administered by intravesical route. Serious reactions, including fatal infections, have been reported in patients receiving intravesical BCG. Take care not to traumatize the urinary tract or to introduce contaminants into the urinary system. Allow 7 to 14 days to elapse before BCG live is administered following TUR, biopsy, or traumatic catheterization.

➤*HIV:* Administer BCG live with extreme caution to persons at high risk for HIV infection only after careful evaluation of risk/benefit.

➤*Falsely positive tuberculin test:* See Drug Interactions for more information.

➤*Concurrent infections:* Postpone intravesical instillations of BCG live during treatment with antibiotics because antimicrobial therapy may interfere with the efficacy of BCG live. Do not use BCG live in individuals with concurrent infections.

➤*Bacterial urinary tract infection (UTI):* If a bacterial UTI occurs during the course of *TheraCys* treatment, withhold *TheraCys* instillation until complete resolution of the bacterial UTI because the combination of a UTI and BCG-induced cystitis may lead to more severe adverse reactions on the GU tract, and BCG bacilli are sensitive to a wide variety of antibiotics; therefore, antimicrobial administration may diminish the efficacy of *TheraCys*.

➤*Bleeding mucosa:* Instillation of BCG live into a patient with an actively bleeding mucosa may promote systemic BCG infection. Postpone treatment for at least 1 week following transurethral resection, biopsy, traumatic catheterization, or gross hematuria.

➤*Small bladder:* Small bladder capacity has been associated with increased risk of severe local reactions; consider this risk when deciding to use BCG live therapy. In patients with small bladder capacity, consider increased risk of bladder contracture in decisions to treat with *TheraCys*.

➤*Immunosuppression:* For patients with a condition that may, in the future, require mandatory immunosuppression (eg, awaiting an organ transplant, myasthenia gravis), carefully consider the decision to treat with *TheraCys*.

➤*Aneurysms/Prosthetic devices:* BCG infection of aneurysms and prosthetic devices (including arterial grafts, cardiac devices, and artificial joints) has been reported following intravesical administration of BCG live. The risk of these ectopic BCG infections has not been determined. The benefits of BCG live therapy must be carefully weighed against the possibility of an ectopic BCG infection in patients with preexisting arterial aneurysms or prosthetic devices of any kind.

➤*Latex:* The stopper of the vial for *TheraCys* contains natural rubber latex, which may cause allergic reactions.

➤*Pregnancy: Category C.*

Teratogenic – Animal reproduction studies have not been conducted with BCG live. It is also not known whether BCG live can cause fetal harm when administered to a pregnant woman or can affect reproduction capacity. Give BCG live to a pregnant woman only if clearly needed. Advise women not to become pregnant while on therapy.

➤*Lactation:* It is not known whether BCG live is excreted in human milk. Because many drugs are excreted in human milk and because of the potential for serious adverse reactions in breast-feeding infants from BCG live, it is advisable to discontinue breast-feeding or the drug, taking into account the importance of the drug to the mother.

➤*Children:* Safety and efficacy of BCG live for the treatment of superficial bladder cancer in children have not been established. Do not use *TheraCys* in children.

➤*Elderly:* Of the total number of subjects in clinical studies of *Tice BCG*, the average age was 66 years. No overall difference in safety or efficacy was observed between older and younger subjects.

➤*Lab test abnormalities:* The use of BCG live may cause tuberculin sensitivity. It is advisable to determine the tuberculin reactivity of patients receiving BCG live by PPD skin testing before treatment is initiated.

➤*Monitoring:* Deaths have been reported as a result of systemic BCG infection and sepsis. Monitor patients for the presence of symptoms and signs of toxicity after each intravesical treatment. Febrile episodes with flu-like symptoms lasting more than 72 hours, fever of at least 39.4°C (103°F), systemic manifestations increasing in intensity with repeated instillations, or persistent abnormalities of liver function tests suggest systemic BCG infection and may require anti-TB therapy. Local symptoms (eg, prostatitis, epididymitis, orchitis) lasting more than 2 to 3 days may also suggest active infection.

Drug Interactions

➤*Immunosuppressants/bone marrow depressants/radiation/antibiotics/anti-TB drugs:* Drug combinations containing immunosuppressants, bone marrow depressants, and/or radiation interfere with the development of the immune response; do not use in combination with BCG live.

Antimicrobial therapy for other infections may interfere with the efficacy of BCG live. There are no data to suggest that the acute, local urinary tract toxicity common with BCG live is because of mycobacterial infection; do not use anti-TB drugs (eg, isoniazid) to prevent or treat the local, irritative toxicities of BCG live.

See Warnings/Precautions for more information.

➤*Drug/Lab test interactions:*

Falsely positive tuberculin test – The use of BCG live may cause a falsely positive tuberculin reaction sensitivity. Therefore, it may be advisable to determine the true tuberculin reactivity before treatment.

Adverse Reactions

➤*Bladder irritability:* Administration of BCG live causes an inflammatory response in the bladder and has been frequently associated with transient fever, hematuria, urinary frequency, and dysuria; careful patient monitoring is required. Symptoms of bladder irritability related to the inflammatory response induced are reported in approximately 50% and 60% of patients receiving *TheraCys* and *Tice BCG*, respectively. The symptoms typically begin 4 to 6 hours after instillation and last 24 to 72 hours. The irritative adverse reactions are usually seen following the third instillation, and tend to increase in severity after each administration.

The irritative bladder adverse reactions can usually be managed symptomatically with products such as pyridium, propantheline bromide, oxybutynin chloride, and acetaminophen. The mechanism of action of the irritative adverse reactions has not been firmly established, but is most consistent with an immunological mechanism. There is no evidence that dose reduction or anti-TB drug therapy can prevent or lessen the irritative toxicity of BCG live.

BCG LIVE — INTRAVESICAL

Adverse reactions to BCG live tend to be progressive in frequency and severity with subsequent instillation. Delay or postponement of subsequent treatment may or may not reduce the severity of a reaction during subsequent instillation.

➤*Hypersensitivity:* Flu-like symptoms (eg, malaise, fever, chills), which may accompany the localized, irritative toxicities, often reflect hypersensitivity reactions, which can be treated symptomatically. Antihistamines also have been used.

➤*Serious infections:* Although uncommon, serious infectious complications of intravesical BCG live have been reported. The most serious infectious complication of BCG live is disseminated sepsis with associated mortality. In addition, BCG infections have been reported in eye, lung, liver, bone, bone marrow, kidney, regional lymph nodes, peritoneum, and prostate in patients who have received intravesical BCG live. Some male GU tract infections (orchitis/epididymitis) have been resistant to multiple-drug anti-TB therapy and required orchiectomy.

If a patient develops persistent fever or experiences an acute febrile illness consistent with BCG infection, discontinue BCG treatment and immediately evaluate and treat the patient for systemic infection.

➤*Tice BCG*: The local and systemic adverse reactions reported in a review of 674 patients with superficial bladder cancer, including 153 patients with CIS, are summarized in the following table.

Tice BCG Adverse Reactions in Patients With Superficial Bladder Cancer (%)		
Adverse reaction	Number of patients	Overall (grade ≥ 3)
GI		
Abdominal pain	10	2% (1%)
Anorexia/weight loss	15	2% (< 1%)
Nausea/vomiting	20	3% (< 1%)
GU		
Cystitis	40	6% (2%)
Dysuria	401	60% (11%)
Genital inflammation/abscess	12	2% (< 1%)
Hematuria	175	26% (7%)
Nocturia	30	5% (1%)
Urgency	39	6% (1%)
Urinary debris	15	2% (< 1%)
Urinary frequency	272	40% (7%)
Urinary incontinence	16	2% (0%)
UTI	10	2% (1%)
Miscellaneous		
Allergy	14	2% (< 1%)
Arthritis/myalgia	18	3% (< 1%)
Cardiac (unclassified)	13	2% (1%)
Cramps/pain	27	4% (1%)
Fever	134	20% (8%)
Flu-like syndrome	224	33% (9%)
Headache/dizziness	16	2% (0%)
Malaise/fatigue	50	7% (0%)
Respiratory (unclassified)	11	2% (< 1%)
Rigors	22	3% (1%)

Other adverse reactions (1% or less) – The following adverse reactions were reported in 1% or less of patients: anemia, BCG sepsis, coagulopathy, contracted bladder, diarrhea, epididymitis/prostatitis, hepatic granuloma, hepatitis, leukopenia, neurologic (unclassified), orchitis, pneumonitis, pyuria, rash, thrombocytopenia, urethritis, and urinary obstruction. In SWOG study 8795, toxicity evaluations were available on a total of 222 *Tice BCG*–treated patients and 220 mitomycin C–treated patients. Direct bladder toxicity (eg, cramps, dysuria, frequency, urgency, hematuria, hemorrhagic cystitis, incontinence) was seen more often with *Tice BCG*, with 356 events compared with 234 events for mitomycin C. Grade 2 or less toxicity was seen significantly more frequently following *Tice BCG* treatment ($P = 0.003$). No life-threatening toxicity was seen in either arm. Systemic toxicity with *Tice BCG* was markedly increased compared with that of mitomycin C, with 181 events for *Tice BCG* compared with 80 for mitomycin C. The frequency of toxicity was increased in all grades, particularly for grades 2 and 3. The most common complaints were malaise, fatigue and lethargy, fever, and abdominal pain. Thirty-two *Tice BCG* patients were reported to have been treated with isoniazid. Five *Tice BCG* patients had liver enzyme elevation, including 2 with grade 3 elevations. Eighteen (8.1%) of the 222*Tice BCG* patients failed to complete the prescribed protocol compared with 6.2% in the mitomycin C group.

Tice BCG Most Common Adverse Reactions in SWOG Study 8795[a]				
Adverse reaction	*Tice BCG* (n = 222)		Mitomycin C (n = 220)	
	All grades	Grade ≥ 3	All grades	Grade ≥ 3
Dermatologic				
Diaphoresis	3%	0%	< 1%	0%
Rash	3%	< 1%	7%	1%
GU				
Bladder cramps	8%	0%	4%	0%
Dysuria	52%	3%	35%	2%
Hematuria	38%	3%	25%	2%
Hemorrhagic cystitis	9%	1%	5%	0%
Urgency/frequency	50%	2%	29%	3%
Miscellaneous				
Chills	9%	0%	1%	1%
Fever	17%	< 1%	3%	0%
Flu-like symptoms	24%	< 1%	13%	0%
Incontinence	4%	0%	1%	0%
Myalgia/arthralgia	3%	0%	0%	0%
Nausea	7%	0%	5%	0%
Pain (not specified)	17%	2%	10%	< 1%

[a] The adverse reaction profile of *Tice BCG* was similar in the Nijmegen study.

➤*TheraCys*:

TheraCys Adverse Reactions (%)	
Adverse reaction	Percent of patients overall (grade ≥ 3)
GI	
Anorexia	11% (0%)
Diarrhea	6% (0%)
Nausea/vomiting	16% (0%)
GU	
Contracted bladder	5% (0%)
Cystitis	29% (0%)
Dysuria	52% (4%)
Genital pain	10% (0%)
Hematuria	39% (7%)
Renal toxicity (NOS[a])	10% (2%)
Urgency	18% (0%)
Urinary frequency	40% (2%)
Urinary incontinence	6% (0%)
UTI	18% (1%)
Miscellaneous	
Anemia	21% (0%)
Arthralgia/myalgia	7% (1%)
Chills	34% (3%)
Cramps/pain	6% (0%)
Fever (> 38°C; 100.4°F)	38% (3%)
Leukopenia	5% (0%)
Malaise	40% (2%)

[a] NOS = not otherwise specified.

The following adverse reactions were reported in less than 5% of patients: abdominal pain, cardiac (unclassified), coagulopathy, constipation, dizziness, fatigue, flank pain, headache, liver involvement, local infection, pulmonary infection, skin rash, systemic infection, thrombocytopenia, tissue in urine, and ureteral obstruction. In a US clinical trial, 112 patients received *TheraCys*. The incidence of adverse reactions associated with intravesical *TheraCys* is given in the following paragraph.

The following adverse reactions were reported in 1% or less of patients: constipation, dizziness, fatigue, flank pain, local infection, thrombocytopenia, and tissue in urine.

In this study, local irritative symptoms were more common with *TheraCys* than with doxorubicin; however, grade 3 or higher irritative toxicity was similar, occurring in approximately 2% to 7% of patients. Systemic symptoms (eg, fever, chills, malaise) were also more common with *TheraCys*. Overall, grade 3 or higher toxicities were seen in 26 patients (23%) treated with *TheraCys* and 25 patients (21%) treated with doxorubicin. "Systemic infection" was reported to occur in 3 patients treated with *TheraCys* (one grade 2 and two grade 3) and 1 patient treated with doxorubicin (grade 2). In 4 patients, treatment was discontinued because of toxicity (2 with irritative symptoms, 1 with severe hematuria, and 1 with possible BCG infection). In addition, 6 patients refused further treatment because of severe local toxic-

BCG LIVE — INTRAVESICAL

ity and/or chills. Six of these 10 patients received *TheraCys*. The following table compares the common adverse reactions reported in this study.

Comparative toxicity for TheraCys:

***TheraCys* Compared With Doxorubicin — Adverse Reactions (%)**				
	TheraCys (n = 112)		Doxorubicin (n = 119)	
Adverse reaction	All grades	Grade ≥ 3	All grades	Grade ≥ 3
GI				
Nausea/vomiting	16%	0%	8%	< 1%
GU				
Bladder cramps/pain	6%	0%	5%	1%
Cystitis	29%	0%	19%	< 1%
Dysuria	52%	4%	40%	6%
Frequency	40%	2%	29%	4%
Hematuria	39%	7%	28%	7%
Urgency	18%	< 1%	12%	2%
Miscellaneous				
Chills	34%	3%	6%	0%
Fever (> 38°C; 100.4°F)	38%	3%	9%	0%
Malaise	40%	2%	14%	0%

➤*Postmarketing:* The following reactions were reported voluntarily from a population of uncertain size. It is not possible to reliably calculate their frequencies.

Symptomatic granulomatous prostatitis, epididymoorchitis, and renal abscess associated with administration of intravesical BCG live have been reported.

Ocular symptoms (including uveitis, conjunctivitis, iritis, keratitis, and granulomatous choreoretinitis) alone or in combination with joint symptoms (arthritis or arthralgia), urinary symptoms, and/or skin rash have been reported following administration of intravesical BCG live. The risk appears to be elevated among patients who are positive for human leukocyte antigen B27 (HLA-B27).

Skin rash, arthralgia, and migratory arthritis may be allergic reactions.

Overdosage

Overdosage occurs if more than 1 vial of BCG live is administered per instillation. Closely monitor the patient for signs of active local or systemic infection. For acute local or systemic reactions suggesting active infection, consult an infectious disease specialist experienced in BCG complications.

Patient Information

BCG live is retained in the bladder for as long as possible, up to 2 hours, and then voided. To avoid transmission of BCG to others, instruct patients to void while seated in order to avoid splashing of urine. For the 6 hours after treatment, disinfect urine voided for 15 minutes with an equal volume of household bleach before flushing. Unless medically contraindicated, instruct patients to increase fluid intake in order to flush the bladder in the hours following BCG live treatment. Patients may experience burning with the first void after treatment.

Because BCG live contains live mycobacteria, excreted urine may also contain live bacteria. Advise patients on appropriate infection control procedures to protect family and close contacts from infection.

Advise patients to be attentive to adverse reactions such as fever, chills, malaise, flu-like symptoms, or increased fatigue. If the patient experiences severe urinary adverse reactions such as burning or pain on urination, urgency, frequency of urination, blood in urine, or other symptoms such as joint pain, eye complaints (eg, pain, irritation, redness), jaundice or vomiting, cough, or skin rash, instruct the patient to notify their health care provider.

DENILEUKIN DIFTITOX

Rx	Ontak (EISAI)	Injection, solution, concentrate: 150 mcg/mL	EDTA. In single-use vials.

DENILEUKIN DIFTITOX — INJECTION

WARNING

Serious infusion reactions, capillary leak syndrome, and loss of visual acuity – The following adverse reactions have been reported:

- Serious and fatal infusion reactions. Administer denileukin diftitox in a facility equipped and staffed for cardiopulmonary resuscitation. Immediately stop and permanently discontinue denileukin diftitox for serious infusion reactions.
- Capillary leak syndrome resulting in death. Monitor weight, edema, blood pressure, and serum albumin levels prior to and during denileukin diftitox treatment.
- Loss of visual acuity and color vision.

Indications

➤*Cutaneous T-cell lymphoma:* For the treatment of persistent or recurrent cutaneous T-cell lymphoma (CTCL) whose malignant cells express the CD25 component of the interleukin-2 (IL-2) receptor.

➤*Off-label uses:* Treatment of chronic lymphocytic leukemia refractory to fludarabine; non-Hodgkin lymphoma.

Administration and Dosage

➤*General dosing considerations:* Withhold administration of denileukin diftitox if serum albumin levels are less than 3 g/dL.

Discontinue for adverse infusion reactions.

Do not administer as a bolus injection or through an inline filter.

➤*Adults:*

Premedication – Premedicate with an antihistamine and acetaminophen prior to each denileukin diftitox infusion.

Usual dosage – 9 or 18 mcg/kg/day by intravenous (IV) infusion over 30 to 60 minutes for 5 consecutive days every 21 days for 8 cycles.

➤*Preparation for administration:* Denileukin diftitox is considered a biohazard. Follow safe handling procedures when preparing, administering, or dispensing denileukin diftitox.

Bring denileukin diftitox to room temperature before preparing the dose. Mix the solution in the vial by gentle swirling; do not shake.

Prepare and hold diluted denileukin diftitox in plastic syringes or soft plastic IV bags. Do not use glass containers.

Maintain concentration of denileukin diftitox at 15 mcg/mL or higher during all steps in the preparation of the solution for IV infusion.

Withdraw the calculated dose from the vial(s) and inject it into an empty IV infusion bag. Do not add more than 9 mL of sterile saline without preservative to the IV bag for each 1 mL of denileukin diftitox.

➤*Administration:* Do not administer denileukin diftitox as a bolus injection or through an inline filter.

Administer prepared solutions of denileukin diftitox within 6 hours, using a syringe pump or IV infusion bag.

➤*Admixture compatibility:* Do not mix denileukin diftitox with other drugs.

➤*Storage/Stability:* Store frozen, at or below −10°C (14°F). Thaw vials in the refrigerator at 2° to 8°C (36° to 46°F) for not more than 24 hours or at room temperature for 1 to 2 hours. Do not refreeze denileukin diftitox after thawing. Discard unused portions of denileukin diftitox immediately.

Actions

➤*Pharmacology:* Denileukin diftitox is a recombinant, DNA-derived, cytotoxic protein composed of the amino acid sequences for diphtheria toxin fragments A and B (Met_1-Thr_{387})-His and the sequences for human IL-2 (Ala_1-Thr_{133}). Denileukin diftitox is a fusion protein designed to direct the cytocidal action of diphtheria toxin to cells that express the IL-2 receptor. Ex vivo studies report that after binding to the IL-2 receptor on the cell surface, denileukin diftitox is internalized by receptor-medicated endocytosis. The fusion protein is subsequently cleaved, releasing diphtheria toxin enzymatic and translocation domains from the IL-2 fragment, resulting in the inhibition of protein synthesis and, ultimately, cell death.

➤*Pharmacokinetics:* Pharmacokinetic parameters associated with denileukin diftitox were determined over a range of dosages (3 to 31 mcg/kg/day) in patients with lymphoma. Denileukin diftitox was administered as an IV infusion following the schedule used in the clinical trials.

Distribution – Mean volume of distribution was similar to that of circulating blood (0.06 to 0.09 L/kg).

Following the first dose, denileukin diftitox displayed 2-compartment behavior with a distribution phase (half-life, approximately 2 to 5 minutes) and a terminal phase (half-life, approximately 70 to 80 minutes). Systemic exposure was variable but proportional to dose.

Excretion – Mean clearance was approximately 0.6 to 2 mL/min/kg. The mean clearance increased approximately 2- to 8-fold from course 1 to course 3, corresponding to a decrease in exposure of approximately 75%. No accumulation was evident between the first and fifth doses.

Contraindications

None known.

Warnings/Precautions

➤*Infusion reactions:* Infusion reactions, defined as symptoms occurring within 24 hours of infusion and resolving within 48 hours of the last infusion in that course, were reported in 70.5% (165/234) of denileukin diftitox–treated patients across 3 clinical studies utilizing the approved doses and schedule. Serious infusion reactions were reported in 8.1% (19/234) of denileukin diftitox–treated patients. There have been postmarketing reports of infusion reactions resulting in death.

For patients completing at least 4 courses of denileukin diftitox treatment in study 1, the incidence of infusion reactions was lower in the third and fourth cycles compared with the first and second cycles of denileukin diftitox.

Resuscitative equipment should be available during denileukin diftitox administration. Immediately stop and permanently discontinue denileukin diftitox for serious infusion reactions.

DENILEUKIN DIFTITOX — INJECTION

➤*Capillary leak syndrome:* Capillary leak syndrome was defined as the occurrence of at least 2 of the following 3 symptoms (hypotension, edema, serum albumin less than 3 g/dL) at any time during denileukin diftitox therapy. These symptoms were not required to occur simultaneously to be characterized as capillary leak syndrome. As defined, capillary leak syndrome was reported in 32.5% (76/234) of denileukin diftitox–treated patients. Among these 76 patients with capillary leak syndrome, one-third required hospitalization or medical intervention to prevent hospitalization. There have been postmarketing reports of capillary leak syndrome resulting in death.

The onset of symptoms in patients with capillary leak syndrome may be delayed, occurring up to 2 weeks following infusion. Symptoms may persist or worsen after the cessation of denileukin diftitox.

Regularly assess patients for weight gain, new onset or worsening edema, and hypotension (including orthostatic changes), and monitor serum albumin levels prior to the initiation of each course of therapy and more often as clinically indicated. Withhold denileukin diftitox for serum albumin levels of less than 3 g/dL.

➤*Visual loss:* Loss of visual acuity, usually with loss of color vision, with or without retinal pigment mottling, has been reported following administration of denileukin diftitox. Recovery was reported in some of the affected patients; however, most patients reported persistent visual impairment.

➤*CD25 tumor expression and evaluation:* Confirm that the patient's malignant cells express CD25 prior to administration of denileukin diftitox. A testing service for the assay of CD25 expression in tumor biopsy samples is available. For information on this service, call 1-877-873-4724.

➤*Immunogenicity:* An immune response to denileukin diftitox was assessed using 2 enzyme-linked immunoassays (ELISA). The first assay measured reactivity directed against intact denileukin diftitox calibrated against antidiphtheria toxin, and the second assay measured reactivity against the IL-2 portion of the protein. An additional in vitro cell-based assay that measured the ability of antibodies in serum to protect a human IL-2R–expressing cell line from toxicity by denileukin diftitox was used to detect the presence of neutralizing antibodies that inhibited functional activity. The immunogenicity data reflect the percentage of patients whose test results were considered positive for antibodies to the intact fusion protein denileukin diftitox. These results are highly dependent on the sensitivity and the specificity of the assays. Additionally, the observed incidence of the antibody positivity may be influenced by several factors, including sample handling, concomitant medication, and underlying disease. For these reasons, the comparison of the incidence of antibodies to denileukin diftitox with the incidence of antibodies to other products may be misleading.

In study 1, of 95 patients treated with denileukin diftitox, 66% tested positive for antibodies at baseline, probably because of a prior exposure to diphtheria toxin or its vaccine. After 1, 2, and 3 courses of treatment, 94%, 99%, and 100% of patients tested positive, respectively. Mean titers of anti–denileukin diftitox antibodies were similarly increased in the 9 and 18 mcg/kg/day dosage groups after 2 courses of treatment. Meanwhile, pharmacokinetic parameters decreased substantially (maximum plasma concentration approximately 57%, area under the curve approximately 80%), and clearance increased 2- to 8-fold.

In study 2, 131 patients were assessed for binding antibodies. Of these, 51 patients (39%) had antibodies at baseline. Seventy-six percent of patients tested positive after 1 course of treatment and 97% after 3 courses of treatment. Neutralizing antibodies were assessed in 60 patients; 45%, 73%, and 97% had evidence of inhibited functional activity in the cellular assay at baseline and after 1 and 3 courses of treatment, respectively.

➤*Pregnancy: Category C.* Animal reproduction studies have not been conducted with denileukin diftitox. The molecular weight of the protein, approximately 58,000, suggests that it does not cross the human placenta. It is also not known whether denileukin diftitox can cause fetal harm when administered to a pregnant woman or affect reproductive capacity. Give denileukin diftitox to a pregnant woman only if clearly needed.

➤*Lactation:* It is not known whether denileukin diftitox is excreted in human milk. The molecular weight of the protein, approximately 58,000, suggests that it will not be excreted into breast milk. Because many drugs are excreted in human milk, and because of the potential for serious adverse reactions in breast-feeding infants from denileukin diftitox, decide whether to discontinue breast-feeding or the drug, taking into account the importance of the drug to the mother. Waiting approximately 4 hours after a dose to breast-feed should limit the potential exposure of the infant.

➤*Children:* Safety and effectiveness in children have not been established.

➤*Monitoring:* Prior to administration of this product, test the patient's malignant cells for CD25 expression.

Carefully monitor weight, edema, and blood pressure prior to and during treatment.

Monitor serum albumin levels prior to the initiation of each treatment course. Delay administration of denileukin diftitox until serum albumin levels are at least 3 g/dL.

Adverse Reactions

The following adverse reactions are discussed in greater detail in other sections: capillary leak syndrome, infusion reactions, and visual loss. (See Warnings/Precautions section.)

Denileukin diftitox is considered to have moderate emetogenic potential (30% to 60% incidence of emesis).

➤*Most common adverse reactions:* Across all 3 studies, the most common adverse reactions in denileukin diftitox–treated patients (20% or greater) were cough, diarrhea, dyspnea, fatigue, headache, nausea, peripheral edema, pruritus, pyrexia, rigors, and vomiting. The most common serious adverse reactions were capillary leak syndrome (11.1%), infusion reactions (8.1%), and visual changes, including loss of visual acuity (4%). Denileukin diftitox was discontinued in 28.2% (66/234) of patients because of adverse reactions.

➤*Adverse reactions (more than 10%):*

Denileukin Diftitox Adverse Reactions (≥ 10%)			
Adverse reactions	Placebo (n = 44)	Denileukin diftitox 9 mcg/kg (n = 45)	Denileukin diftitox 18 mcg/kg (n = 55)
CNS			
Asthenia	4.5%	17.8%	18.2%
Dizziness	11.4%	11.1%	12.7%
Fatigue	31.8%	46.7%	43.6%
Headache	18.2%	28.9%	25.5%
Dermatologic			
Pruritus	9.1%	15.6%	18.2%
Rash	4.5%	24.4%	20%
GI			
Anorexia	4.5%	8.9%	20%
Diarrhea	9.1%	22.2%	21.8%
Dysgeusia	2.3%	0%	10.9%
Nausea	22.7%	46.7%	60%
Vomiting	6.8%	13.3%	34.5%
Musculoskeletal			
Arthralgia	11.4%	15.6%	12.7%
Back pain	2.3%	15.6%	18.2%
Myalgia	4.5%	17.8%	20%
Rigors	20.5%	42.2%	47.3%
Respiratory			
Cough	6.8%	20%	18.2%
Dyspnea	4.5%	13.3%	10.9%
Upper respiratory tract infection	11.4%	13.3%	12.7%
Miscellaneous			
Chest pain	2.3%	4.4%	12.7%
Edema, peripheral	22.7%	20%	25.5%
Hypotension	2.3%	6.7%	16.4%
Pain	6.8%	11.1%	12.7%
Pyrexia	15.9%	48.9%	63.6%

➤*Hepatic:* Increase in serum ALT or AST from baseline occurred in 84% of subjects treated with denileukin diftitox (197/234). In the majority of subjects, these enzyme elevations occurred during either the first or second cycle; enzyme elevation resolved without medical intervention and did not require discontinuation of denileukin diftitox.

Overdosage

➤*Symptoms:* Dosages of approximately twice the recommended dosage (31 mcg/kg/day) resulted in moderate to severe nausea, vomiting, fever, chills, and/or persistent asthenia.

Patient Information

Advise patients to report the following:

- fever, chills, breathing problems, chest pain, tachycardia, and urticaria following infusion.
- rapid weight gain, edema, and orthostatic hypotension following infusion. Instruct patients to weigh themselves daily.
- visual loss, including loss of color vision.

TRETINOIN (ALL-TRANS-RETINOIC ACID)

Rx	**Tretinoin** (Barr)	**Capsules; oral:** 10 mg	EDTA. (barr 808). Brown/Dk. yellow. In 100s.

TRETINOIN (all-trans retinoic acid) — ORAL

WARNING

Experienced health care provider and institution – Patients with acute promyelocytic leukemia (APL) are at high risk in general and can have severe adverse reactions to tretinoin. Therefore, administer tretinoin only to patients with APL under the strict supervision of a health care provider who is experienced in the management of patients with acute leukemia, and in a facility with laboratory and supportive services sufficient to monitor drug tolerance and protect and maintain a patient compromised by drug toxicity, including respiratory compromise. Use of tretinoin requires that the health care provider conclude the possible benefit to the patient outweighs the following known adverse reactions in therapy.

Retinoic acid-APL syndrome – Approximately 25% of patients with APL treated with tretinoin have experienced the retinoic acid-APL (RA-APL) syndrome, characterized by fever, dyspnea, acute respiratory distress, weight gain, radiographic pulmonary infiltrates, pleural and pericardial effusions, edema, and hepatic, renal, and multiorgan failure. This syndrome occasionally has been accompanied by impaired myocardial contractility and episodic hypotension. It has been observed with or without concomitant leukocytosis. Endotracheal intubation and mechanical ventilation have been required in some cases due to progressive hypoxemia, and several patients have expired with multiorgan failure. The syndrome generally occurs during the first month of treatment, with some cases reported following the first dose of tretinoin.

The management of the syndrome has not been defined rigorously, but high-dose steroids given at the first suspicion of the RA-APL syndrome appear to reduce morbidity and mortality. At the first signs suggestive of the syndrome (eg, unexplained fever, dyspnea and/or weight gain, abnormal chest auscultatory findings, radiographic abnormalities), initiate high-dose steroids (dexamethasone 10 mg intravenous [IV] administered every 12 hours for 3 days or until the resolution of symptoms) immediately, irrespective of the leukocyte count. The majority of patients do not require termination of tretinoin therapy during treatment of the RA-APL syndrome. However, in cases of moderate and severe RA-APL syndrome, consider temporary interruption of tretinoin therapy.

Leukocytosis – During tretinoin treatment, approximately 40% of patients will develop rapidly evolving leukocytosis. Patients who present with high white blood cell (WBC) at diagnosis (more than 5×10^9/L) have an increased risk of a further rapid increase in WBC counts. Rapidly evolving leukocytosis is associated with a higher risk of life-threatening complications.

If signs and symptoms of the RA-APL syndrome are present together with leukocytosis, immediately initiate treatment with high-dose steroids. Some investigators routinely add chemotherapy to tretinoin treatment in the case of patients presenting with a WBC count of more than 5×10^9/L or in the case of a rapid increase in WBC count for patients leukopenic at start of treatment, and have reported a lower incidence of the RA-APL syndrome. Consider adding full-dose chemotherapy (including an anthracycline if not contraindicated) to tretinoin therapy on day 1 or 2 for patients presenting with a WBC count of more than 5×10^9/L; immediately add for patients presenting with a WBC count of less than 5×10^9/L, if the WBC count reaches greater than or equal to 6×10^9/L by day 5, greater than or equal to 10×10^9/L by day 10, or greater than or equal to 15×10^9/L by day 28.

Teratogenic effects –

Pregnancy (Category D): There is a high risk that a severely deformed infant will result if tretinoin is administered during pregnancy. If, nonetheless, it is determined that tretinoin represents the best available treatment for a pregnant woman or a woman of childbearing potential, it must be assured that the patient has received full information and warnings of the risk to the fetus if she were to be pregnant and of the risk of possible contraception failure. Instruct the patient to use 2 reliable forms of contraception simultaneously during therapy and for 1 month following discontinuation of therapy, and emphasize the need for using dual contraception, unless abstinence is the chosen method.

Within 1 week prior to the institution of tretinoin therapy, collect blood or urine from the patient for a serum or urine pregnancy test with a sensitivity of at least 50 milliunits/mL. When possible, delay tretinoin therapy until a negative result from this test is obtained. When a delay is not possible, place the patient on 2 reliable forms of contraception. Repeat pregnancy testing and contraception counseling monthly throughout the period of tretinoin treatment.

Indications

➤*Induction of remission:* Tretinoin capsules are indicated for the induction of remission in patients with APL, French-American-British (FAB) classification M3 (including the M3 variant), characterized by the presence of the t(15;17) translocation and/or the presence of the PML/RARα gene, who are refractory to, or who have relapsed from, anthracycline chemotherapy, or for whom anthracycline-based chemotherapy is contraindicated. Tretinoin is for the induction of remission only. The optimal consolidation or maintenance regimens have not been defined, but all patients should receive an accepted form of remission consolidation and/or maintenance therapy for APL after completion of induction therapy with tretinoin.

➤*Off-label uses:*

Emphysema – [5] = Poor documentation. Preliminary data from a single, very small controlled trial did not demonstrate any benefit associated with the use of tretinoin (all-trans-retinoic acid) therapy in the management of emphysema. Before use of this drug can be recommended, additional studies are required to determine if higher doses or longer duration of treatment is needed for efficacy.

Other possible off-label uses – Maintain remission of acute promyelocytic leukemia.

Administration and Dosage

➤*General dosing considerations:* Tretinoin is for the induction of remission only. Optimal consolidation or maintenance regimens have not been determined. Therefore, all patients should receive a standard consolidation and/or maintenance chemotherapy regimen for APL after induction therapy with tretinoin, unless otherwise contraindicated.

If, after initiation of treatment of tretinoin, the presence of the t(15;17) translocation is not confirmed by cytogenetics and/or by polymerase chain reaction studies, and the patient has not responded to tretinoin, consider alternative therapy appropriate for acute myelogenous leukemia.

➤*Adults:*

Acute promyelocytic leukemia (induction of remission) –

Usual dosage: 45 mg/m^2/day administered as 2 or 3 evenly divided doses.

Duration of therapy: Discontinue therapy 30 days after achievement of complete remission or after 90 days of treatment, whichever occurs first.

Off-label dosing –

Acute promyelocytic leukemia (maintenance of remission): 45 to 200 mg/m^2/day in 2 to 3 divided doses. Continue therapy for up to 12 months. Because optimal regimens have not been determined, tretinoin is not considered first-line maintenance therapy.

➤*Children:*

Acute promyelocytic leukemia (induction of remission) – See Adults for dosing for children 1 to 16 years of age.

Off-label dosing –

Acute promyelocytic leukemia (maintenance of remission): See Adults for dosing for children 1 to 16 years of age.

➤*Preparation for administration:* Oral tretinoin is considered a teratogen. Follow safe handling procedures when preparing, administering, or dispensing tretinoin.

➤*Administration:* Take with food. Administration with a fatty meal may enhance absorption. Do not open, crush, or chew capsules.

For patients unable to swallow capsules, aspirate capsule contents into a 19-gauge syringe and immediately administer sublingually or via an enteral feeding tube. To allow aspiration of a greater portion of the capsule contents, prime the syringe with soybean oil 1 mL and flush the capsule with additional soybean oil.

➤*Storage/Stability:* Store at 15° to 30°C (59° to 86°F). Protect from light.

Actions

➤*Pharmacology:* Tretinoin is not a cytolytic agent, but, instead, it induces cytodifferentiation and decreased proliferation of APL cells in culture and in vivo. In APL patients, tretinoin treatment produces an initial maturation of the primitive promyelocytes derived from the leukemic clone, followed by a repopulation of the bone marrow and peripheral blood by normal, polyclonal hematopoietic cells in patients achieving complete remission (CR). The exact mechanism of action of tretinoin in APL is unknown.

➤*Pharmacokinetics:*

Absorption – Tretinoin activity primarily is caused by the parent drug. In human pharmacokinetics studies, an orally administered drug was well absorbed into the systemic circulation. A single 45 mg/m^2 (approximately 80 mg) oral dose to APL patients resulted in a mean ± SD peak tretinoin concentration of 347 ± 266 ng/mL. Time to reach peak concentration was between 1 and 2 hours.

Plasma tretinoin concentrations decrease on average to one third of their day 1 values during 1 week of continuous therapy. Mean ± SD peak tretinoin concentrations decreased from 394 ± 89 to 138 ± 139 ng/mL, while area under the curve (AUC) values decreased from 537 ± 191 ng•h/mL to 249 ± 185 ng•h/mL during 45 mg/m^2 daily dosing in 7 APL patients. Increasing the dose to "correct" for this change has not increased response.

Distribution – The apparent volume of distribution of tretinoin has not been determined. Tretinoin is more than 95% bound in plasma, predominately to albumin. Plasma protein binding remains constant over the concentration range of 10 to 500 ng/mL.

Metabolism – Tretinoin metabolites have been identified in plasma and urine. Cytochrome P-450 enzymes have been implicated in the oxidative metabolism of tretinoin. Metabolites include 13-cis retinoic acid, 4-oxo trans retinoic acid, 4-oxo cis retinoic acid, and 4-oxo trans retinoic acid glucuronide. In APL patients, daily administration of a 45 mg/m^2 dose of tretinoin resulted in an approximately 10-fold increase in the urinary excretion of 4-oxo trans retinoic acid glucuronide after 2 to 6 weeks of continuous dosing, when compared with baseline values. There is evidence that tretinoin induces its own metabolism.

TRETINOIN (all-trans retinoic acid) — ORAL

Excretion – Approximately two thirds of the administered radiolabeled dose was recovered in the urine. The terminal elimination half-life of tretinoin following initial dosing is 0.5 to 2 hours in patients with APL. Studies with radiolabeled drug have demonstrated that after the oral administration of 2.75 and 50 mg doses of tretinoin, more than 90% of the radioactivity was recovered in the urine and feces. Based upon data from 3 subjects, approximately 63% of radioactivity was recovered in the urine within 72 hours, and 31% appeared in the feces within 6 days.

Contraindications

Hypersensitivity to tretinoin, any of its components, or other retinoids. Do not give tretinoin to patients who are sensitive to parabens, which are used as preservatives in the gelatin capsule.

Warnings/Precautions

➤*Patients without the t(15;17) translocation:* Initiation of therapy with tretinoin may be based on the morphological diagnosis of APL. Seek confirmation of the diagnosis of APL by detection of the t(15;17) genetic marker by cytogenetic studies. If these are negative, seek PML/RARα fusion using molecular diagnostic techniques. The response rate of other AML subtypes to tretinoin has not been demonstrated; therefore, consider alternative treatment for patients who lack the genetic marker.

➤*RA-APL syndrome:* In up to 25% of patients with APL treated with tretinoin, RA-APL syndrome occurs, which can be fatal.

See the Warning box for more information.

➤*Leukocytosis:* See the Warning box for more information.

➤*Pseudotumor cerebri:* Retinoids, including tretinoin, have been associated with pseudotumor cerebri (benign intracranial hypertension), especially in children. The concomitant use of other agents known to cause pseudotumor cerebri/intracranial hypertension, such as tetracyclines, might increase the risk of this condition. Early signs and symptoms of pseudotumor cerebri include papilledema, headache, nausea, vomiting, and visual disturbances. Evaluate patients with these symptoms for pseudotumor cerebri, and, if present, institute appropriate care in concert with neurological assessment.

➤*Lipids:* Up to 60% of patients experienced hypercholesterolemia and/or hypertriglyceridemia, which was reversible upon completion of treatment. The clinical consequences of temporary elevation of triglycerides and cholesterol are unknown, but venous thrombosis and myocardial infarction (MI) have been reported in patients who ordinarily are at low risk for such complications.

➤*Thrombosis:* There is a risk of thrombosis (venous and arterial) that may involve any organ system during the first month of treatment. Therefore, exercise caution when treating patients with the combination of tretinoin and antifibrinolytic agents, such as tranexamic acid, aminocaproic acid, or aprotinin.

➤*Toxic adverse reactions:* Tretinoin has potentially significant toxic adverse reactions in APL patients. Closely observe patients undergoing therapy for signs of respiratory compromise and/or leukocytosis. Maintain supportive care appropriate for APL patients (eg, prophylaxis for bleeding, prompt therapy for infection) during therapy with tretinoin.

➤*Hazardous tasks:* The ability to drive or operate machinery might be impaired in patients treated with tretinoin, particularly if they are experiencing dizziness or severe headache.

➤*Pregnancy: Category D.* Tretinoin has teratogenic and embryotoxic effects in mice, rats, hamsters, rabbits, and pigtail monkeys, and may be expected to cause fetal harm when administered to a pregnant woman. Tretinoin causes fetal resorptions and a decrease in live fetuses in all animals studied. Gross external, soft tissue, and skeletal alterations occurred at dosages greater than 0.7 mg/kg/day in mice, 2 mg/kg/day in rats, 7 mg/kg/day in hamsters, and at a dosage of 10 mg/kg/day (the only dosage tested) in pigtail monkeys (about 1/20, 1/4, and 1/2, and 4 times the human dosage, respectively, on a mg/m^2 basis).

There are no adequate and well-controlled studies in pregnant women. Although experience with humans administered tretinoin is extremely limited, increased spontaneous abortions and major human fetal abnormalities related to the use of other retinoids have been documented in humans. Reported defects include abnormalities of the CNS, musculoskeletal system, external ear, eye, thymus, and great vessels; facial dysmorphia; cleft palate; and parathyroid hormone deficiency. Some of these abnormalities were fatal. Cases of intelligence quotient scores less than 85, with or without obvious CNS abnormalities, also have been reported. All fetuses exposed during pregnancy can be affected and, at the present time, there is no antepartum means of determining which fetuses are and are not affected.

Effective contraception must be used by all women during tretinoin therapy and for 1 month following discontinuation of therapy. Microdosed progesterone preparations (ie, minipill) may be an inadequate method of contraception during treatment with tretinoin. Contraception must be used even when there is a history of infertility or menopause, unless a hysterectomy has been performed. Whenever contraception is required, it is recommended that 2 reliable forms of contraception be used simultaneously, unless abstinence is the chosen method. If pregnancy does occur during treatment, the health care provider and patient should discuss the desirability of continuing or terminating the pregnancy.

➤*Lactation:* It is not known whether this drug is excreted in human milk. Because many drugs are excreted in human milk, and because of the potential for serious adverse reactions from tretinoin in breast-feeding infants, advise mothers to discontinue breastfeeding prior to taking this drug.

➤*Children:* There are limited clinical data on the pediatric use of tretinoin. Of 15 children (range, 1 to 16 years of age) treated with tretinoin, the incidence of complete remission was 67%. Safety and efficacy in children younger than 1 year of age have not been established. Some children experienced severe headache and pseudotumor cerebri, requiring analgesic treatment and lumbar puncture for relief. Increased caution is recommended in the treatment of children. Consider dose reduction for children experiencing serious and/or intolerable toxicity; however, the efficacy and safety of tretinoin at dosages less than 45 mg/m^2/day have not been evaluated in the pediatric population.

➤*Elderly:* Of the total number of subjects in clinical studies of tretinoin, 21.4% were 60 years of age and older. No overall differences in safety or efficacy were observed between these subjects and younger subjects, and other reported clinical experience has not identified differences in responses between the elderly and younger patients, but greater sensitivity of some older individuals cannot be ruled out.

➤*Lab test abnormalities:* Elevated liver function test results occur in 50% to 60% of patients during treatment. Carefully monitor liver function test results during treatment and give consideration to a temporary withdrawal of tretinoin if test results reach greater than 5 times the upper limit of normal values. However, the majority of these abnormalities resolve without interruption of tretinoin or after completion of treatment.

➤*Monitoring:* Frequently monitor the patient's hematologic profile, coagulation profile, liver function test results, and triglyceride and cholesterol levels.

Drug Interactions

➤*CYP-450 system:* As tretinoin is metabolized by the hepatic P-450 system, there is a potential for alteration of pharmacokinetic parameters in patients coadministered medications that also are inducers or inhibitors of this system. Medications that generally induce hepatic P-450 enzymes include rifampin, glucocorticoids, phenobarbital, and pentobarbital. Medications that generally inhibit hepatic P-450 enzymes include ketoconazole, cimetidine, erythromycin, verapamil, diltiazem, and cyclosporine. To date there are no data to suggest that coadministration with these medications increases or decreases either efficacy or toxicity of tretinoin.

In 13 patients who received daily doses of tretinoin for 4 consecutive weeks, administration of ketoconazole (400 to 1,200 mg oral dose) 1 hour prior to the administration of the tretinoin dose on day 29 led to a 72% increase (218 ± 224 vs 375 ± 285 ng•h/mL) in tretinoin mean plasma AUC. The precise cytochrome P-450 enzymes involved in these interactions have not been specified; CYP 3A4, 2C8, and 2E have been implicated in various preliminary reports.

Tretinoin Oral Drug Interactions

Precipitant drug	Object drug[a]		Description
Ketoconazole	Tretinoin	↑	In 13 patients given ketoconazole 400 to 1,200 mg 1 hour prior to tretinoin, a 72% increase in tretinoin mean plasma AUC occurred.
Tretinoin	Tetracyclines	↑	Coadministration of tretinoin and agents known to cause pseudotumor cerebri/intracranial hypertension, such as tetracyclines, may increase the risk of this condition.
Tetracyclines	Tretinoin		
Tretinoin	Vitamin A	↑	As with other retinoids, tretinoin must not be administered in combination with vitamin A because symptoms of hypervitaminosis A could be aggravated.
Antifibrinolytic agents (eg, tranexamic acid, aminocaproic acid, aprotinin)	Tretinoin	↑	Cases of fatal thrombotic complications have been reported rarely in patients coadministered tretinoin and antifibrinolytic agents. Use with caution.

[a] ↑ = object drug increased

➤*Agents known to cause pseudotumor cerebri/intracranial hypertension (such as tetracyclines):* Tretinoin may cause pseudotumor cerebri/intracranial hypertension. Coadministration of tretinoin and agents also known to cause pseudotumor cerebri/intracranial hypertension might increase the risk of this condition.

➤*Vitamin A:* As with other retinoids, do not administer tretinoin in combination with vitamin A because symptoms of hypervitaminosis A could be aggravated.

➤*Antifibrinolytic agents:* Cases of fatal thrombotic complications have been reported rarely in patients concomitantly treated with tretinoin and antifibrinolytic agents (eg, tranexamic acid, aminocaproic acid, aprotinin). Therefore, exercise caution when administering tretinoin concomitantly with these agents.

➤*Drug/Food interactions:* No data on the effect of food on the absorption of tretinoin are available. The absorption of retinoids as a class is enhanced when taken concurrently with food.

Adverse Reactions

Tretinoin is considered to have moderate to low potential for nausea and vomiting.

TRETINOIN (all-trans retinoic acid) — ORAL

Virtually all patients experience some drug-related toxicity, especially headache, fever, weakness, and fatigue. These adverse reactions seldom are permanent or irreversible, nor do they usually require interruption of therapy. Some of the adverse reactions are common in patients with APL, including hemorrhage, infections, GI hemorrhage, disseminated intravascular coagulation, pneumonia, septicemia, and cerebral hemorrhage. Respiratory system disorders were reported commonly in APL patients administered tretinoin. The majority of these reactions are symptoms of the RA-APL syndrome. The following describes the adverse reactions that were observed in patients treated with tretinoin, regardless of drug relationship.

➤*Cardiovascular:* Arrhythmias and flushing (23%); hypotension (14%); hypertension and phlebitis (11%); cardiac failure (6%); cardiac arrest, enlarged heart, heart murmur, ischemia, MI, myocarditis, pericarditis, pulmonary hypertension, secondary cardiomyopathy, and stroke (3%); thrombosis (venous and arterial) involving various sites (eg, cerebrovascular accident, MI, renal infarct) (rare).

➤*CNS:* Dizziness (20%); anxiety, paresthesia (17%); depression, insomnia, (14%); confusion (11%); agitation, cerebral hemorrhage, intracranial hypertension (9%); hallucination (6%); abnormal gait, agnosia, aphasia, asterixis, cerebellar disorders, cerebellar edema, CNS depression, coma, convulsions, dementia, dysarthria, encephalopathy, facial paralysis, forgetfulness, hemiplegia, hyporeflexia, hypotaxia, leg weakness, neurologic reaction, no light reflex, slow speech, somnolence, spinal cord disorder, tremor, unconsciousness (3%).

➤*Dermatologic:* Cellulitis (8%); pallor (6%); genital ulceration; vasculitis (predominantly involving the skin) (rare).

➤*GI:* GI hemorrhage (34%); abdominal pain (31%); other GI disorders (26%); diarrhea (23%); constipation, anorexia (17%); dyspepsia (14%); abdominal distention (11%); hepatosplenomegaly (9%); hepatitis, ulcer, unspecified liver disorder (3%).

➤*GU:* Renal impairment (11%); dysuria (9%); acute renal failure, enlarged prostate, micturition frequency, renal tubular necrosis (3%).

➤*Hematologic/Lymphatic:* Hemorrhage (60%); disseminated intravascular coagulation (26%); lymph disorders (6%); thrombocytosis (rare).

➤*Metabolic:* Peripheral edema (52%); edema (29%); weight increase (23%); weight decrease (17%); face edema, fluid imbalance (6%).

➤*Respiratory:* Upper respiratory tract disorders (63%); dyspnea (60%); respiratory insufficiency (26%); pleural effusion (20%); expiratory wheezing, pneumonia, rales (14%), lower respiratory tract disorders (9%); pulmonary infiltration (6%); bronchial asthma, larynx edema, pulmonary edema, unspecified pulmonary disease (3%).

➤*Special senses:* Earache or feeling of fullness in the ears (23%); hearing loss and other unspecified auricular disorders (6%); irreversible hearing loss (less than 1%).

➤*Miscellaneous:* Malaise (66%); shivering (63%); infections (58%); pain (37%); chest discomfort (32%); injection-site reactions (17%); myalgia (14%); flank pain (9%); acidosis, ascites, hypothermia (3%).

Isolated cases of basophilia, erythema nodosum, hypercalcemia, hyperhistaminemia, myositis, organomegaly, pancreatitis, and Sweet syndrome have been reported.

RA-APL syndrome – See the Warning box for more information.

Typical retinoid toxicity – The most frequently reported adverse reactions were similar to those described in patients taking high doses of vitamin A and included the following: headache (86%); fever (83%); skin/mucous membrane dryness, bone pain (77%); nausea/vomiting (57%); rash (54%); mucositis (26%); pruritus, increased sweating (20%); visual disturbances, ocular disorders (17%); alopecia and skin changes (14%); changed visual acuity (6%); bone inflammation and visual field defects (3%).

Overdosage

➤*Symptoms:* There has been no experience with acute overdosage in humans. The maximal tolerated dosage in patients with myelodysplastic syndrome or solid tumors was 195 mg/m²/day. The maximal tolerated dosage in children was lower at 60 mg/m²/day. Overdosage with other retinoids has been associated with transient headache, facial flushing, cheilosis, abdominal pain, dizziness, and ataxia. These symptoms quickly have resolved without apparent residual effects.

➤*Treatment:* There is no specific treatment in the case of an overdose; however, it is important the patient be treated in a special hematological unit.

REXINOIDS

BEXAROTENE

Rx	**Targretin** (Eisai Inc.)	**Capsules, softgel; oral:** 75 mg	(Targretin). Sorbitol. Off-white, oblong. In 100s.

BEXAROTENE — ORAL

WARNING

Bexarotene capsules are a member of the retinoid class of drugs that is associated with birth defects in humans. Bexarotene capsules also caused birth defects when administered orally to pregnant rats. Bexarotene capsules must not be administered to a pregnant woman.

Indications

➤*Cutaneous T-cell lymphoma (CTCL):* Bexarotene capsules are indicated for the treatment of cutaneous manifestations of CTCL in patients who are refractory to at least 1 prior systemic therapy.

Administration and Dosage

➤*General dosing considerations:* Women of childbearing potential should be advised to avoid becoming pregnant when bexarotene is used. (See also Warnings/Precautions).

➤*Adults:*

Cutaneous T-cell lymphoma –

Initial dosage: 300 mg/m²/day (see the following table), as a single oral daily dose with a meal.

An initial dose of 150 to 225 mg has also been used.

Bexarotene Capsule Initial Dose Calculation According to Body Surface Area		
Initial dose level (300 mg/m²/day)		
Body surface area (m²)	Total daily dose (mg/day)	Number of 75 mg bexarotene capsules
0.88 to 1.12	300	4
1.13 to 1.37	375	5
1.38 to 1.62	450	6
1.63 to 1.87	525	7
1.88 to 2.12	600	8
2.13 to 2.37	675	9
2.38 to 2.62	750	10

Maintenance dosage: Increase to 400 mg/m²/day if no tumor response after 8 weeks. A target maintenance dose of 450 to 525 mg has also been used.

Dosage adjustment: Adverse reactions requiring dosage adjustment include:

- AST, ALT, or bilirubin greater than 3 times the upper limit of normal,
- Leukopenia or neutropenia, or
- Hypertriglyceridemia unresponsive to therapy.

Reduce dose to 200 mg/m²/day. If reaction does not resolve, decrease to 100 mg/m²/day or temporarily discontinue. When toxicity is controlled, doses may be carefully readjusted upward.

Duration of therapy: In clinical trials in CTCL, bexarotene capsules were administered for up to 97 weeks. Bexarotene capsules should be continued as long as the patient is deriving benefit.

➤*Administration:* Take with food.

For patients unable to swallow capsules whole, cut capsule open and rinse the inside of the capsule with water to suspend contents in water, then administer immediately. Avoid contact between the gel inside the capsule and skin or mucous membranes.

In women of childbearing potential, initiate therapy on the second or third day of a normal menstrual period.

➤*Storage/Stability:* Store at 2° to 2°5C (36° to 77°F). Avoid exposing to high temperatures and humidity after the bottle is opened. Protect from light.

Actions

➤*Pharmacology:* Bexarotene selectively binds and activates retinoid X receptor subtypes (RXRα, RXRβ, RXRγ). RXRs can form heterodimers with various receptor partners such as RARs, vitamin D receptor, thyroid receptor, and peroxisome proliferator activator receptors (PPARs). Once activated, these receptors function as transcription factors that regulate the expression of genes that control cellular differentiation and proliferation. Bexarotene inhibits the growth in vitro of some tumor cell lines of hematopoietic and squamous cell origin. It also induces tumor regression in vivo in some animal models. The exact mechanism of action of bexarotene in the treatment of CTCL is unknown.

➤*Pharmacokinetics:*

Absorption/Distribution – After oral administration of bexarotene capsules, bexarotene is absorbed with a t_{max} of about 2 hours. Terminal half-life of bexarotene is about 7 hours. Studies in patients with advanced malignancies show approximate single dose linearity within the therapeutic range and low accumulation with multiple doses. Plasma bexarotene AUC and C_{max} values resulting from a 75 to 300 mg dose were 35% and 48% higher, respectively, after a fat-containing meal than after a glucose solution. Bexarotene is highly bound (greater than 99%) to plasma proteins. The plasma proteins to which bexarotene binds have not been elucidated, and the ability of bexarotene to displace drugs bound to plasma proteins and the ability of drugs to displace bexarotene binding have not been studied. The uptake of bexarotene by organs or tissues has not been evaluated.

Metabolism – Four bexarotene metabolites have been identified in plasma: 6- and 7-hydroxy-bexarotene and 6- and 7-oxo-bexarotene. In vitro studies suggest that cytochrome P450 3A4 is the major cytochrome P450

BEXAROTENE — ORAL

responsible for formation of the oxidative metabolites and that the oxidative metabolites may be glucuronidated. The oxidative metabolites are active in in vitro assays of retinoid receptor activation, but the relative contribution of the parent and any metabolites to the efficacy and safety of bexarotene capsules is unknown.

Excretion – The renal elimination of bexarotene and its metabolites was examined in patients with type 2 diabetes mellitus. Neither bexarotene nor its metabolites were excreted in urine in appreciable amounts. Bexarotene is thought to be eliminated primarily through the hepatobiliary system.

Special populations –

Renal function impairment: See Warnings/Precautions for more information.

Hepatic function impairment: See Warnings/Precautions for more information.

Contraindications

Bexarotene capsules are contraindicated in patients with a known hypersensitivity to bexarotene or other components of the product.

➤*Pregnancy:* Bexarotene capsules may cause fetal harm when administered to a pregnant woman. Bexarotene capsules must not be given to a pregnant woman or a woman who intends to become pregnant. If a woman becomes pregnant while taking bexarotene capsules, the capsules must be stopped immediately and the woman given appropriate counseling.

Bexarotene caused malformations when administered orally to pregnant rats during days 7 to 17 of gestation. Developmental abnormalities included incomplete ossification at 4 mg/kg/day and cleft palate, depressed eye bulge/microphthalmia, and small ears at 16 mg/kg/day. The plasma AUC of bexarotene in rats at 4 mg/kg/day is approximately one third the AUC in humans at the recommended daily dose. At doses greater than 10 mg/kg/day, bexarotene caused developmental mortality. The no effect dose for fetal effects in rats was 1 mg/kg/day (producing an AUC approximately one sixth of the AUC at the recommended human daily dose).

Women of childbearing potential should be advised to avoid becoming pregnant when bexarotene capsules are used. The possibility that a woman of childbearing potential is pregnant at the time therapy is instituted should be considered. A negative pregnancy test (eg, serum beta-human chorionic gonadotropin [beta-HCG]) with a sensitivity of at least 50 mIU/L should be obtained within 1 week prior to bexarotene capsules therapy, and the pregnancy test must be repeated at monthly intervals while the patient remains on bexarotene capsules. Effective contraception must be used for 1 month prior to the initiation of therapy, during therapy and for at least 1 month following discontinuation of therapy; it is recommended that 2 reliable forms of contraception be used simultaneously unless abstinence is the chosen method. Bexarotene can potentially induce metabolic enzymes and thereby theoretically reduce the plasma concentrations of hormonal contraceptives. Thus, if treatment with bexarotene capsules is intended in a woman with childbearing potential, it is strongly recommended that 1 of the 2 reliable forms of contraception should be nonhormonal. Male patients with sexual partners who are pregnant, possibly pregnant, or who could become pregnant must use condoms during sexual intercourse while taking bexarotene capsules and for at least 1 month after the last dose of drug. Bexarotene capsules therapy should be initiated on the second or third day of a normal menstrual period. No more than a 1 month supply of bexarotene capsules should be given to the patient so that the results of pregnancy testing can be assessed and counseling regarding avoidance of pregnancy and birth defects can be reinforced.

Warnings/Precautions

➤*Lipid abnormalities:* Bexarotene capsules induce major lipid abnormalities in most patients. These must be monitored and treated during long-term therapy. About 70% of patients with CTCL who received an initial dose of greater than or equal to 300 mg/m²/day of bexarotene capsules had fasting triglyceride levels greater than 2.5 times the upper limit of normal. About 55% had values over 800 mg/dL with a median of about 1200 mg/dL in those patients. Cholesterol elevations above 300 mg/dL occurred in approximately 60% and 75% of patients with CTCL who received an initial dose of 300 mg/m²/day or greater than 300 mg/m²/day, respectively. Decreases in high density lipoprotein (HDL) cholesterol to less than 25 mg/dL were seen in about 55% and 90% of patients receiving an initial dose of 300 mg/m²/day or greater than 300 mg/m²/day, respectively, of bexarotene capsules. The effects on triglycerides, HDL cholesterol, and total cholesterol were reversible with cessation of therapy, and could generally be mitigated by dose reduction or concomitant antilipemic therapy.

Fasting blood lipid determinations should be performed before bexarotene capsules therapy is initiated and weekly until the lipid response to bexarotene capsules is established, which usually occurs within 2 to 4 weeks, and at 8 week intervals thereafter. Fasting triglycerides should be normal or normalized with appropriate intervention prior to initiating bexarotene capsules therapy. Attempts should be made to maintain triglyceride levels below 400 mg/dL to reduce the risk of clinical sequelae. If fasting triglycerides are elevated or become elevated during treatment, antilipemic therapy should be instituted, and if necessary, the dose of bexarotene capsules reduced or suspended. In the 300 mg/m²/day initial dose group, 60% of patients were given lipid lowering drugs. Atorvastatin was used in 48% ($^{73}/_{152}$) of patients with CTCL. Because of a potential drug-drug interaction, gemfibrozil is not recommended for use with bexarotene capsules.

➤*Pancreatitis:* Acute pancreatitis has been reported in 4 patients with CTCL and in 6 patients with non-CTCL cancers treated with bexarotene capsules; the cases were associated with marked elevations of fasting serum triglycerides, the lowest being 770 mg/dL in 1 patient. One patient with advanced non-CTCL cancer died of pancreatitis. Patients with CTCL who have risk factors for pancreatitis (eg, prior pancreatitis, uncontrolled hyperlipidemia, excessive alcohol consumption, uncontrolled diabetes mellitus, biliary tract disease, and medications known to increase triglyceride levels or to be associated with pancreatic toxicity) should generally not be treated with bexarotene capsules.

➤*Liver function test abnormalities:* For patients with CTCL receiving an initial dose of 300 mg/m²/day of bexarotene capsules, elevations in liver function tests (LFTs) have been observed in 5% (AST), 2% (ALT), and 0% (bilirubin). In contrast, with an initial dose greater than 300 mg/m²/day of bexarotene capsules, the incidence of LFT elevations was higher at 7% (AST), 9% (ALT), and 6% (bilirubin). Two patients developed cholestasis, including 1 patient who died of liver failure. In clinical trials, elevation of LFTs resolved within 1 month in 80% of patients following a decrease in dose or discontinuation of therapy. Baseline LFTs should be obtained, and LFTs should be carefully monitored after 1, 2, and 4 weeks of treatment initiation, and if stable, at least every 8 weeks thereafter during treatment. Consideration should be given to a suspension or discontinuation of bexarotene capsules if test results reach greater than 3 times the upper limit of normal values for AST, ALT, or bilirubin.

➤*Thyroid axis alterations:* Bexarotene capsules induce biochemical evidence of or clinical hypothyroidism in about half of all patients treated, causing a reversible reduction in thyroid hormone (total thyroxine [total T_4]) and thyroid-stimulating hormone (TSH) levels. The incidence of decreases in TSH and total T_4 were about 60% and 45%, respectively, in patients with CTCL receiving an initial dose of 300 mg/m²/day. Hypothyroidism was reported as an adverse event in 29% of patients. Treatment with thyroid hormone supplements should be considered in patients with laboratory evidence of hypothyroidism. In the 300 mg/m²/day initial dose group, 37% of patients were treated with thyroid hormone replacement. Baseline thyroid function tests should be obtained and patients monitored during treatment.

➤*Leukopenia:* A total of 18% of patients with CTCL receiving an initial dose of 300 mg/m²/day of bexarotene capsules had reversible leukopenia in the range of 1000 to less than 3000 WBC/mm³. Patients receiving an initial dose greater than 300 mg/m²/day of bexarotene capsules had an incidence of leukopenia of 43%. No patient with CTCL treated with bexarotene capsules developed leukopenia of less than 1000 WBC/mm³. The time to onset of leukopenia was generally 4 to 8 weeks. The leukopenia observed in most patients was explained by neutropenia. In the 300 mg/m²/day initial dose group, the incidence of NCI grade 3 and grade 4 neutropenia, respectively, was 12% and 4%. The leukopenia and neutropenia experienced during bexarotene capsules therapy resolved after dose reduction or discontinuation of treatment, on average within 30 days in 93% of the patients with CTCL and 82% of patients with non-CTCL cancers. Leukopenia and neutropenia were rarely associated with severe sequelae or serious adverse events. Determination of WBC with differential should be obtained at baseline and periodically during treatment.

➤*Cataracts:* Posterior subcapsular cataracts were observed in preclinical toxicity studies in rats and dogs administered bexarotene daily for 6 months. In 15 of 79 patients who had serial slit lamp examinations, new cataracts or worsening of previous cataracts were found. Because of the high prevalence and rate of cataract formation in older patient populations, the relationship of bexarotene capsules and cataracts cannot be determined in the absence of an appropriate control group. Patients treated with bexarotene capsules who experience visual difficulties should have an appropriate ophthalmologic evaluation.

➤*Vitamin A supplementation:* In clinical studies, patients were advised to limit vitamin A intake to less than or equal to 15,000 IU/day. Because of the relationship of bexarotene to vitamin A, patients should be advised to limit vitamin A supplements to avoid potential additive toxic effects.

➤*Hypersensitivity reactions:* Bexarotene capsules should be used with caution in patients with a known hypersensitivity to retinoids. Clinical instances of cross-reactivity have not been noted.

➤*Renal function impairment:* No formal studies have been conducted with bexarotene capsules in patients with renal insufficiency. Urinary elimination of bexarotene and its known metabolites is a minor excretory pathway for bexarotene (less than 1% of administered dose), but because renal insufficiency can result in significant protein binding changes, and bexarotene is greater than 99% protein bound, pharmacokinetics may be altered in patients with renal insufficiency.

➤*Hepatic function impairment:* No specific studies have been conducted with bexarotene capsules in patients with hepatic insufficiency. Because less than 1% of the dose is excreted in the urine unchanged and there is in vitro evidence of extensive hepatic contribution to bexarotene elimination, hepatic impairment would be expected to lead to greatly decreased clearance. Bexarotene capsules should be used only with great caution in this population.

➤*Special risk:*

Diabetes mellitus – Caution should be used when administering bexarotene capsules in patients using insulin, agents enhancing insulin secretion (eg, sulfonylureas), or insulin-sensitizers (eg, troglitazone). Based on the mechanism of action, bexarotene capsules could enhance the action of these agents, resulting in hypoglycemia. Hypoglycemia has not been associated with the use of bexarotene capsules as monotherapy.

➤*Photosensitivity:* Retinoids as a class have been associated with photosensitivity. In vitro assays indicate that bexarotene is a potential photosensitizing agent. Mild phototoxicity manifested as sunburn and skin sensitivity to sunlight was observed in patients who were exposed to direct sunlight while receiving bexarotene capsules. Patients should be advised to minimize exposure to sunlight and artificial ultraviolet light while receiving bexarotene capsules.

➤*Pregnancy: Category X.* See Contraindications for more information.

➤*Lactation:* It is not known whether bexarotene is excreted in human milk. Because many drugs are excreted in human milk and because of the potential for serious adverse reactions in nursing infants from bexarotene, a

BEXAROTENE — ORAL

decision should be made whether to discontinue nursing or to discontinue the drug, taking into account the importance of the drug to the mother.

➤*Children:* Safety and effectiveness in pediatric patients have not been established.

➤*Elderly:* Of the total patients with CTCL in clinical studies of bexarotene capsules, 64% were 60 years or older, while 33% were 70 years or older. No overall differences in safety were observed between patients 70 years or older and younger patients, but greater sensitivity of some older individuals to bexarotene capsules cannot be ruled out. Responses to bexarotene capsules were observed across all age group decades, without preference for any individual age group decade.

➤*Monitoring:* Blood lipid determinations should be performed before bexarotene capsules are given. Fasting triglycerides should be normal or normalized with appropriate intervention prior to therapy. Hyperlipidemia usually occurs within the initial 2 to 4 weeks. Therefore, weekly lipid determinations are recommended during this interval. Subsequently, in patients not hyperlipidemic, determinations can be performed less frequently.

A white blood cell count with differential should be obtained at baseline and periodically during treatment. Baseline liver function tests should be obtained and should be carefully monitored after 1, 2, and 4 weeks of treatment initiation, and if stable, periodically thereafter during treatment. Baseline thyroid function tests should be obtained and then monitored during treatment as indicated.

Drug Interactions

Bexarotene Drug Interactions

Precipitant drug	Object drug[a]		Description
CYP450 inducers (eg, rifampin, phenytoin, phenobarbital)	Bexarotene	⬇	On the basis of bexarotene metabolism, cytochrome P450 3A4 inducers may reduce plasma bexarotene concentrations.
CYP450 inhibitors (eg, ketoconazole, itraconazole, erythromycin, grapefruit juice)	Bexarotene	⬆	On the basis of bexarotene metabolism, cytochrome P450 3A4 inhibitors may increase plasma bexarotene concentrations.
Gemfibrozil	Bexarotene	⬆	Coadministration of bexarotene and gemfibrozil resulted in substantial increases in plasma concentrations of bexarotene. Concomitant administration of gemfibrozil with bexarotene is not recommended.
Vitamin A	Bexarotene	⬆	Bexarotene is a member of the retinoids. Limit vitamin A supplements to avoid potential additive toxic effects (≤ 15,000 IU/day; see Precautions).
Bexarotene	Vitamin A		
Bexarotene	Antidiabetic agents	⬆	Bexarotene may enhance antidiabetic agents, resulting in hypoglycemia (see Precautions).
Bexarotene	Tamoxifen	⬇	Coadministration of bexarotene capsules and tamoxifen in women with breast cancer who were progressing on tamoxifen resulted in a modest decrease in plasma tamoxifen concentrations, possibly through an induction of cytochrome P450 3A4.
Bexarotene	Oral contraceptives	⬇	Bexarotene can potentially induce metabolic enzymes and thereby theoretically reduce plasma concentrations of hormonal contraceptives. It is strongly recommended that 2 reliable forms of contraception be used concurrently, 1 of which should be nonhormonal.

[a] ⬆ = Object drug increased. ⬇ = Object drug decreased.

➤*Drug/Lab test interactions:* CA125 assay values in patients with ovarian cancer may be increased by bexarotene capsule therapy.

➤*Drug/Food interactions:* In all clinical trials, patients were instructed to take bexarotene capsules with or immediately following a meal. In one clinical study, plasma bexarotene AUC and C_{max} values were substantially higher following a fat-containing meal versus those following the administration of a glucose solution. Because safety and efficacy data are based upon administration with food, it is recommended that bexarotene capsules be administered with food.

Adverse Reactions

The safety of bexarotene capsules has been evaluated in clinical studies of 152 patients with CTCL who received bexarotene capsules for up to 97 weeks and in 352 patients in other studies. The mean duration of therapy for the 152 patients with CTCL was 166 days. The most common adverse events reported with an incidence of at least 10% in patients with CTCL treated at an initial dose of 300 mg/m²/day of bexarotene capsules are shown below. The events at least possibly related to treatment are lipid abnormalities (elevated triglycerides, elevated total and LDL cholesterol and decreased HDL cholesterol), hypothyroidism, headache, asthenia, rash, leukopenia, anemia, nausea, infection, peripheral edema, abdominal pain, and dry skin. Most adverse events occurred at a higher incidence in patients treated at starting doses of greater than 300 mg/m²/day (see table).

Adverse events leading to dose reduction or study drug discontinuation in at least 2 patients were hyperlipemia, neutropenia/leukopenia, diarrhea, fatigue/lethargy, hypothyroidism, headache, liver function test abnormalities, rash, pancreatitis, nausea, anemia, allergic reaction, muscle spasm, pneumonia, and confusion.

The moderately severe (NCI grade 3) and severe (NCI grade 4) adverse events reported in 2 or more patients with CTCL treated at an initial dose of 300 mg/m²/day of bexarotene capsules were hypertriglyceridemia, pruritus, headache, peripheral edema, leukopenia, rash, and hypercholesterolemia. Most of these moderately severe or severe adverse events occurred at a higher rate in patients treated at starting doses of greater than 300 mg/m²/day than in patients treated at a starting dose of 300 mg/m²/day.

In patients with CTCL receiving an initial dose of 300 mg/m²/day, the incidence of NCI grade 3 or 4 elevations in triglycerides and total cholesterol was 28% and 25%, respectively. In contrast, in patients with CTCL receiving greater than 300 mg/m²/day, the incidence of NCI Grade 3 or 4 elevated triglycerides and total cholesterol was 45% and 45%, respectively. Other grade 3 and 4 laboratory abnormalities are shown below.

In addition to the 152 patients enrolled in the 2 CTCL studies, 352 patients received bexarotene capsules as monotherapy for various advanced malignancies at doses from 5 mg/m²/day to 1000 mg/m²/day. The common adverse events (incidence greater than 10%) were similar to those seen in patients with CTCL.

In the 504 patients (CTCL and non-CTCL) who received bexarotene capsules as monotherapy, drug-related serious adverse events that were fatal, in 1 patient each, were acute pancreatitis, subdural hematoma, and liver failure.

In the patients with CTCL receiving an initial dose of 300 mg/m²/day of bexarotene capsules, adverse events reported at an incidence of less than 10% and not included in other sections or discussed in other parts of labeling and possibly related to treatment were as follows:

➤*Cardiovascular:* Hemorrhage, hypertension, angina pectoris, right heart failure, syncope, and tachycardia.

➤*CNS:* Depression, agitation, ataxia, cerebrovascular accident, confusion, dizziness, hyperesthesia, hypesthesia, and neuropathy.

➤*Dermatologic:* Skin ulcer, acne, alopecia, skin nodule, maculopapular rash, pustular rash, serous drainage, and vesicular bullous rash.

➤*GI:* Constipation, dry mouth, flatulence, colitis, dyspepsia, cheilitis, gastroenteritis, and melena.

➤*GU:* Albuminuria, hematuria, urinary incontinence, urinary tract infection, urinary urgency, dysuria, kidney function abnormal, and breast pain.

➤*Hematologic/Lymphatic:* Eosinophilia, thrombocythemia, coagulation time increased, lymphocytosis, and thrombocytopenia.

➤*Metabolic/Nutritional:* LDH increased, creatinine increased, hypoproteinemia, hyperglycemia, weight decreased, weight increased, and amylase increased.

➤*Musculoskeletal:* Arthralgia, myalgia, bone pain, myasthenia, and arthrosis.

➤*Respiratory:* Pharyngitis, rhinitis, dyspnea, pleural effusion, bronchitis, cough increased, lung edema, hemoptysis, and hypoxia.

➤*Special senses:* Dry eyes, conjunctivitis, ear pain, blepharitis, corneal lesion, keratitis, otitis externa, and visual field defect.

➤*Miscellaneous:* Chills, cellulitis, chest pain, sepsis, gingivitis, liver failure, and monilia.

➤*Adverse reactions with incidence greater than or equal to 10% in CTCL trials:*

Bexarotene Adverse Reactions in CTCL Trials (≥ 10%)

Adverse reaction[a,b]	Initial assigned dose group 300 mg/m²/day (n = 84)	Initial assigned dose group > 300 mg/m²/day (n = 53)
Cardiovascular		
Peripheral edema	11 (13.1%)	6 (11.3%)
CNS		
Insomnia	4 (4.8%)	6 (11.3%)
Infection, bacterial	1 (1.2%)	7 (13.2%)
Dermatologic		
Rash	14 (16.7%)	12 (22.6%)
Dry skin	9 (10.7%)	5 (9.4%)
Exfoliative dermatitis	8 (9.5%)	15 (28.3%)
Alopecia	3 (3.6%)	6 (11.3%)

BEXAROTENE — ORAL

Bexarotene Adverse Reactions in CTCL Trials (≥ 10%)		
	Initial assigned dose group	
Adverse reaction[a,b]	300 mg/m²/day (n = 84)	> 300 mg/m²/day (n = 53)
Endocrine		
Hypothyroidism	24 (28.6%)	28 (52.8%)
GI		
Nausea	13 (15.5%)	4 (7.5%)
Diarrhea	6 (7.1%)	22 (41.5%)
Vomiting	3 (3.6%)	7 (13.2%)
Anorexia	2 (2.4%)	12 (22.6%)
Hematologic/Lymphatic		
Leukopenia	14 (16.7%)	25 (47.2%)
Anemia	5 (6%)	13 (24.5%)
Hypochromic anemia	3 (3.6%)	7 (13.2%)
Metabolic/Nutritional		
Hyperlipidemia	66 (78.6%)	42 (79.2%)
Hypercholesteremia	27 (32.1%)	33 (62.3%)
Lactic dehydrogenase increased	6 (7.1%)	7 (13.2%)
Miscellaneous		
Headache	25 (29.8%)	22 (41.5%)
Asthenia	17 (20.2%)	24 (45.3%)
Infection	11 (13.1%)	12 (22.6%)
Abdominal pain	9 (10.7%)	2 (3.8%)
Chills	8 (9.5%)	7 (13.2%)
Fever	4 (4.8%)	9 (17%)
Flu syndrome	3 (3.6%)	7 (13.2%)
Back pain	2 (2.4%)	6 (11.3%)

[a] Preferred English term coded according to Ligand-modified COSTART 5 Dictionary.
[b] Patients are counted at most once in each adverse reaction category.

➤*Incidence of moderately severe and severe adverse reactions reported in at least 2 patients (CTCL trials):*

Incidence of Moderately Severe and Severe Bexarotene Adverse Reactions Reported in ≥ 2 Patients (CTCL Trials) (%)				
	Initial assigned dose group			
	300 mg/m²/day (n = 84)		> 300 mg/m²/day (n = 53)	
Adverse reaction[a,b]	Moderate/ Severe	Severe	Moderate/ Severe	Severe
Cardiovascular				
Peripheral edema	2 (2.4%)	1 (1.2%)	0	0
Dermatologic				
Exfoliative dermatitis	0	1 (1.2%)	3 (5.7%)	1 (1.9%)
Rash	1 (1.2%)	2 (2.4%)	1 (1.9%)	0
Endocrine				
Hypothyroidism	1 (1.2%)	1 (1.2%)	2 (3.8%)	0
GI				
Anorexia	0	0	3 (5.7%)	0
Diarrhea	1 (1.2%)	1 (1.2%)	2 (3.8%)	1 (1.9%)
Pancreatitis	1 (1.2%)	0	3 (5.7%)	0
Vomiting	0	0	2 (3.8%)	0
Hematologic/Lymphatic				
Leukopenia	3 (3.6%)	0	6 (11.3%)	1 (1.9%)
Metabolic/Nutritional				
Bilirubinemia	0	1 (1.2%)	2 (3.8%)	0
Hypercholesteremia	2 (2.4%)	0	5 (9.4%)	0
Hyperlipemia	16 (19%)	6 (7.1%)	17 (32.1%)	5 (9.4%)
AST increased	0	0	2 (3.8%)	0
ALT increased	0	0	2 (3.8%)	0
Respiratory				
Pneumonia	0	0	2 (3.8%)	2 (3.8%)

Incidence of Moderately Severe and Severe Bexarotene Adverse Reactions Reported in ≥ 2 Patients (CTCL Trials) (%)				
	Initial assigned dose group			
	300 mg/m²/day (n = 84)		> 300 mg/m²/day (n = 53)	
Adverse reaction[a,b]	Moderate/ Severe	Severe	Moderate/ Severe	Severe
Miscellaneous				
Asthenia	1 (1.2%)	0	11 (20.8%)	0
Headache	3 (3.6%)	0	5 (9.4%)	1 (1.9%)
Infection, bacterial	1 (1.2%)	0	0	2 (3.8%)

[a] Preferred English term coded according to Ligand-modified COSTART 5 Dictionary.
[b] Patients are counted at most once in each adverse reaction category. Patients are classified by the highest severity within each row.

➤*Treatment-emergent abnormal laboratory values in CTCL trials:*

Treatment-Emergent Abnormal Laboratory Values in CTCL Trials (%)				
	Initial assigned dose			
	300 mg/m²/day (n = 83)[a]		> 300 mg/m²/day (n = 53)[a]	
Analyte	Grade 3[b]	Grade 4[b]	Grade 3	Grade 4
Triglycerides[c]	21.3%	6.7%	31.8%	13.6%
Total cholesterol[c]	18.7%	6.7%	15.9%	29.5%
Alkaline phosphatase	1.2%	0	0	1.9%
Hyperglycemia	1.2%	0	5.7%	0
Hypocalcemia	1.2%	0	0	0
Hyponatremia	1.2%	0	9.4%	0
ALT	1.2%	0	1.9%	1.9%
Hyperkalemia	0	0	1.9%	0
Hypernatremia	0	1.2%	0	0
AST	0	0	1.9%	1.9%
Total bilirubin	0	0	0	1.9%
ANC	12%	3.6%	18.9%	7.5%
ALC	7.2%	0	15.1%	0
WBC	3.6%	0	11.3%	0
Hemoglobin	0	0	1.9%	0

[a] Number of patients with at least 1 analyte value post-baseline.
[b] Adapted from NCI Common Toxicity Criteria, grade 3 and 4, Version 2.0. Patients are considered to have had a grade 3 or 4 value if either of the following occurred: Value becomes grade 3 or 4 during the study or value is abnormal at baseline and worsens to grade 3 or 4 on study, including all values beyond study drug discontinuation, as defined in data handling conventions.
[c] The denominator used to calculate the incidence rates for fasting total cholesterol and triglycerides were n = 75 for the 300 mg/m²/day initial dose group and n = 44 for the greater than 300 mg/m²/day initial dose group.

Overdosage

Doses up to 1000 mg/m²/day of bexarotene capsules have been administered in short-term studies in patients with advanced cancer without acute toxic effects. Single doses of 1500 mg/kg and 720 mg/kg were tolerated without significant toxicity in rats and dogs, respectively. These doses are approximately 30 and 50 times, respectively, the recommended human dose on a mg/m² basis.

No clinical experience with an overdose of bexarotene capsules has been reported. Any overdose with bexarotene capsules should be treated with supportive care for the signs and symptoms exhibited by the patient.

Patient Information

Bexarotene capsules can cause major damage to a fetus. Pregnancy must be avoided in patients receiving bexarotene capsules. The health care provider should be contacted immediately if pregnancy is suspected while taking bexarotene capsules and until 1 month after discontinuing bexarotene capsules. For women of childbearing potential, pregnancy tests are required within 1 week before starting bexarotene capsule therapy and monthly while taking bexarotene capsules, confirming absence of pregnancy. Effective contraception (birth control) is required continuously starting 1 month before beginning treatment with bexarotene capsules until 1 month after discontinuing bexarotene capsules. It is strongly recommended that 2 reliable forms of contraception be used together. At least 1 of these 2 forms of contraception should include condoms, diaphragms, cervical caps, IUDs, or spermicides. If the patient is a man and has a partner who is pregnant or capable of becoming pregnant, he should discuss with the partner the precautions that should be taken.

The most common side effect is an increase in blood lipids (fats in the blood). Periodic blood tests will be needed to determine blood levels of lipids, including triglycerides and cholesterol. Medication may be needed to control high fat levels in the blood.

Another common side effect is underactive thyroid. The symptoms of underactive thyroid may be difficult to detect because they may develop very gradually and may be very mild. For example, a patient may begin to always feel tired, low on energy, or unusually cold all the time. A thyroid hormone

BEXAROTENE — ORAL

medication is readily available to fully control these temporary symptoms, so the health care provider should be contacted early if the patient begins to experience any of these symptoms. Periodic blood tests will be needed to detect this.

The patient should not take bexarotene capsules if allergic to the medicine.

The patient should discuss the following conditions with the health care provider (if applicable) before starting to take this medicine: pregnancy or possibility of pregnancy, pancreatitis, breast-feeding, taking gemfibrozil (a medication to reduce high triglyceride and cholesterol levels in the blood), taking tamoxifen.

Because vitamin A in large doses may cause some side effects that are similar to those seen in patients taking bexarotene capsules, advise the patient not take more than the recommended daily dietary allowance of vitamin A (4,000 to 5,000 IU). If taking vitamins, instruct patient to check the label to see how much vitamin A they contain. If unsure, advise patient to ask the health care provider or pharmacist.

Skin may become more sensitive to sunlight while taking this medicine. Advise patient to minimize exposure to sunlight and to not use a sunlamp.

Advise patient to always take bexarotene capsules as instructed (ie, taking prescribed number of capsules each day; taking the daily dose of bexarotene capsules all at once; taking the dose once each day with or immediately following a meal. For example, a patient may take the daily amount of bexarotene capsules with the evening meal).

Capsules should be swallowed whole; not chewed or dissolved in liquid or in the mouth. Depending on the health and condition of the patient, the health care provider may change the daily dose (the number of capsules taken) during treatment.

If a dose is missed, advise the patient to take it as soon as possible with food. However, if it is nearing time for the next dose, instruct patient to skip the missed dose and continue the dose schedule as before and not double the dose.

If too many bexarotene capsules are taken or someone else accidentally takes the medicine, instruct patients to contact their health care provider, emergency room, or the nearest hospital immediately.

Although some patients see improvement within the first several weeks of bexarotene capsule treatment, most patients require several months or more of treatment to improve CTCL. The health care provider should determine how long to take bexarotene capsules and when treatment may be stopped.

As an infrequent side effect of bexarotene capsule treatment, pancreatitis (inflamed pancreas) may occur. Symptoms of pancreatitis include persistent nausea, vomiting, and abdominal or back pain. If the patient develops any of these symptoms while taking bexarotene capsules, contact the health care provider immediately.

Store capsules in a dry place in a closed container, away from light and heat, at room temperature. The capsules should not be used after the expiration date printed on the bottle. Keep this medicine out of the reach and sight of children. If bexarotene capsules are broken or leaking, advise patients not to touch the capsules or the contents and notify the pharmacist immediately. Should the contents of a broken capsule get on the skin, instruct patient to immediately wash the area with soap and water and notify the health care provider.

MONOCLONAL ANTIBODIES

RITUXIMAB

Rx	Rituxan (Genentech)	Injection, solution, concentrate: 10 mg/mL	Preservative free. Polysorbate 80, sodium chloride 9 mg/mL. In 10 and 50 mL single-use vials.

RITUXIMAB — INJECTION

WARNING

Fatal infusion reactions – Rituximab administration can result in serious, including fatal, infusion reactions. Deaths within 24 hours of rituximab infusion have been reported. Approximately 80% of fatal infusion reactions occurred in association with the first infusion.

Carefully monitor patients during infusions. Discontinue rituximab infusion and administer medical treatment in patients who develop severe (grade 3 or 4) infusion reactions.

Tumor lysis syndrome – Acute renal failure requiring dialysis, with instances of fatal outcome, has been reported in the setting of tumor lysis syndrome following rituximab monotherapy treatment in patients with non-Hodgkin lymphoma (NHL).

Severe mucocutaneous reactions – Severe, including fatal, mucocutaneous reactions can occur in patients receiving rituximab treatment.

Progressive multifocal leukoencephalopathy – JC virus infection resulting in progressive multifocal leukoencephalopathy (PML) and death can occur in patients treated with rituximab.

Indications

➤*Chronic lymphocytic leukemia:* In combination with fludarabine and cyclophosphamide for the treatment of patients with previously untreated and previously treated CD20-positive chronic lymphocytic leukemia (CLL).

➤*Non-Hodgkin lymphoma:* As a single agent for the treatment of patients with relapsed or refractory, low-grade or follicular, CD20-positive, B-cell NHL; for previously untreated follicular, CD20-positive, B-cell NHL in combination with first-line chemotherapy and, in patients achieving a complete or partial response to rituximab in combination with chemotherapy, as single-agent maintenance chemotherapy; for nonprogressing (including stable disease), low-grade, CD20-positive, B-cell NHL as a single agent following first-line treatment with cyclophosphamide, vincristine, and prednisone chemotherapy; for previously untreated diffuse large B-cell, CD20-positive NHL in combination with cyclophosphamide, doxorubicin, vincristine, and prednisone or other anthracycline-based chemotherapy regimens.

➤*Rheumatoid arthritis:* In combination with methotrexate for the treatment of adults with moderately to severely active rheumatoid arthritis (RA) who have had an inadequate response to 1 or more tumor necrosis factor (TNF) antagonist therapies.

➤*Off-label uses:*

Idiopathic thrombocytopenic purpura – [2] = Fair documentation. Rituximab in the management of refractory or relapsed idiopathic thrombocytopenic purpura has been primarily evaluated in noncontrolled settings, demonstrating benefit in the majority of patients either as complete or partial response. In consensus guidelines, rituximab is recommended as second-line therapy, although the optimal dose is not known and requires further study.

Juvenile idiopathic arthritis – [3] = Safety concerns. Data evaluating the safety and efficacy of rituximab for the treatment of juvenile idiopathic arthritis are limited to case reports in 5 patients, all of which only recently appeared in the published literature. While these reports are promising, additional studies are needed to define the optimal dose and patient population that would most benefit from therapy. Until additional data are available, routine use of rituximab for juvenile idiopathic arthritis is not recommended because safety concerns exist. Currently, there are no national guidelines for the management of juvenile idiopathic arthritis.

Neuropathy/Polyneuropathy – [4] = Insufficient documentation. Very preliminary data suggest that rituximab may have some benefit in the treatment of polyneuropathies related to immunoglobulin M (IgM) antibodies.

Peripheral ulcerative keratitis – [3] = Safety concerns. Beneficial results from case report data indicate that rituximab may be useful in the treatment of refractory peripheral ulcerative keratitis. However, larger, controlled trials are needed, particularly because of serious potential adverse events associated with other indications.

Waldenström macroglobulinemia – [1] = Good documentation. The role of rituximab in the treatment of Waldenström macroglobulinemia has been established in US, international, and British guidelines. Evidence suggests that the response to rituximab is inferior in patients with baseline serum monoclonal protein levels higher than 40 g/L or total IgM levels higher than 6 g/dL. In addition, serum IgM levels can increase abruptly after administration of rituximab. For these reasons, rituximab monotherapy is not recommended in patients with symptomatic hyperviscosity. In addition, rituximab-induced flares in IgM levels may precipitate clinically significant hyperviscosity requiring plasma exchange, which can result in loss of the rituximab antibody. Flares in IgM levels appear to be associated primarily with rituximab monotherapy and not combination therapy. One small study suggested that administering fludarabine daily for 4 days prior to rituximab could prevent rituximab-mediated increases in IgM levels.

Other possible off-label uses – Thrombocytopenic purpura.

Administration and Dosage

➤*Adults:*

Chronic lymphocytic leukemia –

Usual dosage: 375 mg/m^2 intravenous (IV) infusion the day prior to the initiation of fludarabine and cyclophosphamide chemotherapy, then 500 mg/m^2 on day 1 of cycles 2 to 6 (every 28 days).

Concomitant therapy: Pneumocystis jiroveci pneumonia and antiherpetic viral prophylaxis is recommended for patients with CLL during treatment and for up to 12 months following treatment as appropriate.

Non-Hodgkin lymphoma –

Relapsed or refractory, low-grade or follicular, CD20-positive, B-cell non-Hodgkin lymphoma:

- *Usual dosage* – 375 mg/m^2 IV infusion once weekly for 4 or 8 doses.
- *Re-treatment* – 375 mg/m^2 IV infusion given once weekly for 4 doses.

Previously untreated follicular, CD20-positive, B-cell non-Hodgkin lymphoma: 375 mg/m^2 IV infusion given on day 1 of each cycle of chemotherapy for up to 8 doses. In patients with complete or partial response, initiate rituximab maintenance 8 weeks following completion of rituximab in combination with chemotherapy as a single-agent every 8 weeks for 12 doses.

Nonprogressing, low-grade, CD20-positive, B-cell non-Hodgkin lymphoma: 375 mg/m^2 IV infusion once weekly for 4 doses every 6 months to a maximum of 16 doses following completion of 6 to 8 cycles of cyclophosphamide, vincristine, and prednisone chemotherapy.

Diffuse large B-cell non-Hodgkin lymphoma: 375 mg/m^2 IV infusion on day 1 of each cycle of chemotherapy for up to 8 infusions.

RITUXIMAB — INJECTION

Rheumatoid arthritis –

Usual dosage: Two 1,000 mg IV infusions separated by 2 weeks in combination with methotrexate.

Subsequent doses: Administer subsequent doses every 24 weeks or based on clinical evaluation, but not sooner than every 16 weeks.

Off-label dosing –

Idiopathic thrombocytopenic purpura: [2] = Fair documentation. 375 mg/m² IV once weekly for 4 doses. Lower weekly doses (100 mg) have been documented as effective with a longer time of response. Premedicants, including antihistamines, acetaminophen, and/or hydrocortisone, administered prior to rituximab infusion have been documented in some trials.

Juvenile idiopathic arthritis: [3] = Safety concerns. Given as a 2-dose regimen, with 1 g on days 1 and 15. A dose of 500 mg was used in a patient weighing only 40 kg. Treatment was repeated 6 to 12 months later in some patients.

Neuropathy/Polyneuropathy: [4] = Insufficient documentation. 375 mg/m² IV infusion once weekly for 4 weeks. All patients received acetaminophen, diphenhydramine, and granisetron to reduce the frequency of adverse effects.

Peripheral ulcerative keratitis: [3] = Safety concerns. 1,000 mg/wk IV infusion for 2 doses.

Waldenström macroglobulinemia: [1] = Good documentation. 375 mg/m² IV infusion once weekly for 4 doses. An extended-dose regimen of 375 mg/m² twice weekly for 4 weeks (weeks 1 through 4), and repeated at week 12 (weeks 12 through 15), has also been used. Maintenance use of rituximab has also been reported.

➤*Children:*

Off-label dosing –

Autoimmune hemolytic anemia: 375 mg/m² IV infusion once weekly for 3 to 6 doses.

B-cell acute lymphocytic leukemia: 375 mg/m² IV infusion to conventional salvage therapy.

Non-Hodgkin lymphoma:

- *CD-20 positive, B-cell non-Hodgkin lymphoma* –
  - *Initial dosage:* 375 mg/m² IV infusion once weekly for 4 to 8 doses as monotherapy or in combination with cyclophosphamide, doxorubicin, vincristine, and prednisone.
  - *Re-treatment therapy:* 375 mg/m² IV infusion once weekly for 4 doses or once weekly for 4 doses every 6 months for up to 2 years.
  - *Refractory therapy:* 375 mg/m² IV infusion on days 1 and 3 given in combination with ifosfamide, mesna, carboplatin, and etoposide.
- *Relapsed or refractory, low-grade, follicular, or transformed B-cell non-Hodgkin lymphoma* – 250 mg/m² IV infusion 4 hours prior to indium-111 (In-111) ibritumomabtiuxetan; 7 to 9 days later, administer rituximab 250 mg/m² within 4 hours of yttrium-90 (Y-90) ibritumomab tiuxetan.

Posttransplant lymphoproliferative disorder: 375 mg/m² IV infusion once weekly for 3 to 4 doses.

➤*Concomitant therapy with ibritumomab tiuxetan:* 250 mg/m² IV infusion within 4 hours prior to the administration of In-111 ibritumomab tiuxetan and within 4 hours prior to the administration of Y-90 ibritumomab tiuxetan. Administer rituximab and In-111 ibritumomab tiuxetan 7 to 9 days prior to rituximab and Y-90 ibritumomab tiuxetan.

➤*Premedication:* Premedicate before each infusion with acetaminophen and an antihistamine. For RA patients, methylprednisolone 100 mg IV or its equivalent is recommended 30 minutes prior to each infusion.

➤*Preparation for administration:* Withdraw the necessary amount of rituximab and dilute to a final concentration of 1 to 4 mg/mL into an infusion bag containing sodium chloride 0.9% or dextrose 5% in water. Gently invert the bag to mix the solution. Do not shake.

➤*Administration:* Do not administer as an IV push or bolus; administer only as an IV infusion.

First infusion – Initiate infusion at a rate of 50 mg/h. In the absence of infusion toxicity, increase infusion rate by 50 mg/h increments every 30 minutes to a maximum of 400 mg/h.

Subsequent infusions – Initiate infusion at a rate of 100 mg/h. In the absence of infusion toxicity, increase rate by 100 mg/h increments at 30-minute intervals to a maximum of 400 mg/h.

Infusion reactions – Interrupt the infusion or slow the infusion rate for infusion reactions. Continue the infusion at half the previous rate upon improvement of symptoms.

➤*Admixture compatibility:* Rituximab should not be mixed or diluted with other drugs.

➤*Storage/Stability:* Store vials between 2° and 8°C (36° and 46°F). Protect from direct sunlight; do not freeze. Discard any unused potion left in the vial. Diluted infusions may be stored between 2° and 8°C (36° and 46°F) for 24 hours and are stable for an additional 24 hours at room temperature.

Actions

➤*Pharmacology:* Rituximab is a genetically engineered, chimeric murine/human monoclonal immunoglobulin G1 (IgG1) kappa antibody directed against the CD20 antigen. Rituximab binds specifically to the antigen CD20 (human B-lymphocyte-restricted differentiation antigen, Bp35), a hydrophobic transmembrane protein with a molecular weight of approximately 35 kD located on pre-B and mature B lymphocytes. The antigen is expressed on more than 90% of B-cell NHLs but is not found on hematopoietic stem cells, pro-B cells, normal plasma cells, or other normal tissues. CD20 regulates an early step(s) in the activation process for cell cycle initiation and differentiation, and possibly functions as a calcium ion channel. CD20 is not shed from the cell surface and does not internalize upon antibody binding. Free CD20 antigen is not found in the circulation.

B cells are believed to play a role in the pathogenesis of RA and associated chronic synovitis. In this setting, B cells may be acting at multiple sites in the autoimmune/inflammatory process, including through production of rheumatoid factor (RF) and other autoantibodies, antigen presentation, T-cell activation, and/or proinflammatory cytokine production.

The Fab domain of rituximab binds to the CD20 antigen on B lymphocytes, and the Fc domain recruits immune effector functions to mediate B-cell lysis in vitro. Possible mechanisms of cell lysis include complement-dependent cytotoxicity and antibody-dependent, cell-mediated cytotoxicity. The antibody has been shown to induce apoptosis in the DHL-4 human B-cell lymphoma line.

➤*Pharmacokinetics:*

Absorption/Distribution –

Non-Hodgkin lymphoma: Rituximab 375 mg/m² IV infusion was administered at weekly intervals for 4 doses to 203 patients with NHL. Rituximab was detectable in the serum of patients 3 to 6 months after completion of treatment.

Rheumatoid arthritis: Following the administration of 2 doses of rituximab in patients with RA, the mean (± standard deviation, percent coefficient of variation) concentrations after the first infusion ($C_{max\ first}$) and second infusion ($C_{max\ second}$) were 157 (± 46; 29%) and 183 (± 55; 30%) mcg/mL, and 318 (± 86; 27%) and 381 (± 98; 26%) mcg/mL for the 2 × 500 mg and 2 × 1,000 mg doses, respectively. For RA patients, the volume of distribution was 3.1 L.

Excretion – The estimated median terminal elimination half-life was 22 days (range, 6.1 to 52 days) for NHL patients. Patients with higher CD19-positive cell counts or larger measurable tumor lesions at pretreatment had a higher clearance. However, dose adjustment for pretreatment CD19 count or size of tumor lesion is not necessary.

The estimated median terminal half-life of rituximab in patients with CLL was 32 days (range, 14 to 62 days).

The estimated clearance of rituximab in RA patients was 0.335 L/day and mean terminal elimination half-life was 18 days (range, 5.17 to 77.5 days).

Contraindications

None well documented.

Warnings/Precautions

➤*Severe infusion reactions:* Rituximab can cause severe, including fatal, infusion reactions. Severe reactions typically occurred during the first infusion, with time to onset of 30 to 120 minutes. Rituximab-induced infusion reactions and sequelae included acute respiratory distress syndrome, anaphylactic events, angioedema, bronchospasm, cardiogenic shock, hypotension, hypoxia, myocardial infarction (MI), pulmonary infiltrates, urticaria, ventricular fibrillation, or death.

Management of severe infusion reactions – Premedicate patients with an antihistamine and acetaminophen prior to dosing. For RA patients, methylprednisolone 100 mg IV or its equivalent is recommended 30 minutes prior to each infusion. Institute medical management (eg, glucocorticoids, epinephrine, bronchodilators, oxygen) for infusion reactions as needed. Depending on the severity of the infusion reaction and the required interventions, temporarily or permanently discontinue rituximab. Resume infusion at a minimum 50% reduction in rate after symptoms have resolved. Closely monitor those with preexisting cardiac or pulmonary conditions, those who experienced prior cardiopulmonary adverse reactions, and those with high numbers of circulating malignant cells (at least 25,000/mm³).

➤*Tumor lysis syndrome:* Acute renal failure, hyperkalemia, hypocalcemia, hyperuricemia, or hyperphosphatemia from tumor lysis, some fatal, can occur within 12 to 24 hours after the first infusion of rituximab in patients with NHL. A high number of circulating malignant cells (at least 25,000/mm³) or high tumor burden confers a greater risk of tumor lysis syndrome. Administer aggressive IV hydration and antihyperuricemic therapy in patients at high risk for tumor lysis syndrome. Correct electrolyte abnormalities, monitor renal function and fluid balance, and administer supportive care, including dialysis, as indicated.

➤*Severe mucocutaneous reactions:* Mucocutaneous reactions, some with fatal outcome, can occur in patients treated with rituximab. These reactions include lichenoid dermatitis, paraneoplastic pemphigus, Stevens-Johnson syndrome, toxic epidermal necrolysis, and vesiculobullous dermatitis. The onset of these reactions has varied from 1 to 13 weeks following rituximab exposure. Discontinue rituximab in patients who experience a severe mucocutaneous reaction. The safety of readministration of rituximab to patients with severe mucocutaneous reactions has not been determined.

➤*Progressive multifocal leukoencephalopathy:* JC virus infection, resulting in PML and death, can occur in rituximab-treated patients with hematologic malignancies or with autoimmune diseases. The majority of patients with hematologic malignancies diagnosed with PML received rituximab in combination with chemotherapy or as part of a hematopoietic stem cell transplant. The patients with autoimmune diseases had prior or concurrent immunosuppressive therapy. Most cases of PML were diagnosed within 12 months of their last infusion of rituximab.

Consider the diagnosis of PML in any patient presenting with new-onset neurologic manifestations. Evaluation of PML includes, but is not limited to, consultation with a neurologist, brain magnetic resonance imaging, and lumbar puncture. Discontinue rituximab and consider reducing or discontinuing any concomitant chemotherapy or immunosuppressive therapy in patients who develop PML.

RITUXIMAB — INJECTION

➤*Hepatitis B virus reactivation:* Hepatitis B virus (HBV) reactivation, with fulminant hepatitis, hepatic failure, and death, can occur in patients treated with rituximab. The median time to the diagnosis of hepatitis among patients with hematologic malignancies was approximately 4 months after the initiation of rituximab and approximately 1 month after the last dose.

Screen patients at high risk of HBV infection before initiating rituximab. Closely monitor carriers of HBV for clinical and laboratory signs of active HBV infection for several months following rituximab therapy. In patients who develop viral hepatitis, discontinue rituximab and any concomitant chemotherapy and initiate appropriate treatment, including antiviral therapy. There are insufficient data regarding the safety of resuming rituximab therapy in patients who develop hepatitis subsequent to HBV reactivation.

➤*Infections:* Serious, including fatal, bacterial, fungal, and new or reactivated viral infections can occur during and up to 1 year following the completion of rituximab-based therapy. New or reactivated viral infections included cytomegalovirus, herpes simplex virus, parvovirus B19, varicella zoster virus, West Nile virus, and hepatitis B and C. Discontinue rituximab for serious infections and institute appropriate anti-infective therapy.

➤*Cardiovascular effects:* Discontinue infusions in the event of serious or life-threatening cardiac arrhythmias. Perform cardiac monitoring for patients who develop clinically significant arrhythmias during and after subsequent infusions of rituximab or who have a history of arrhythmia or angina.

➤*Renal toxicity:* Severe, including fatal, renal toxicity can occur in patients with NHL after rituximab administration. Renal toxicity has occurred in patients who experience tumor lysis syndrome and in NHL patients coadministered cisplatin therapy during clinical trials. The combination of cisplatin and rituximab is not an approved treatment regimen. Monitor patients closely for signs of renal failure, and discontinue rituximab for those with rising serum creatinine or oliguria.

➤*GI effects:* Abdominal pain, bowel obstruction, and perforation, in some cases leading to death, can occur in patients receiving rituximab in combination with chemotherapy. In postmarketing reports, the mean time to documented GI perforation was 6 days (range, 1 to 77 days) in patients with NHL. Perform a thorough diagnostic evaluation and institute appropriate treatment for complaints of abdominal pain.

➤*Vaccines:* The safety of immunization with live viral vaccines following rituximab therapy has not been studied, and vaccination with live virus vaccines is not recommended.

For patients with RA, follow current immunization guidelines and administer non-live vaccines at least 4 weeks prior to a course of rituximab.

➤*Immunogenicity:* As with all therapeutic proteins, there is a potential for immunogenicity. The observed incidence of antibody (including neutralizing antibody) positivity in an assay is highly dependent on several factors, including assay sensitivity and specificity, assay methodology, sample handling, timing of sample collection, concomitant medications, and underlying disease. For these reasons, comparison of the incidence of antibodies to rituximab with the incidence of antibodies to other products may be misleading.

Using an enzyme-linked immunosorbent assay, anti–human antichimeric antibody (HACA) was detected in 1.1% of patients with low-grade or follicular NHL receiving single-agent rituximab. Three of the 4 patients had an objective clinical response.

A total of 11% of patients with RA tested positive for HACA at any time after receiving rituximab. HACA positivity was not associated with increased infusion reactions or other adverse reactions. Upon further treatment, the proportions of patients with infusion reactions were similar between HACA-positive and HACA-negative patients, and most reactions were mild to moderate. Four HACA-positive patients had serious infusion reactions, and the temporal relationship between HACA positivity and infusion reaction was variable. The clinical relevance of HACA formation in rituximab-treated patients is unclear.

➤*Pregnancy: Category C.* There are no adequate and well-controlled studies of rituximab in pregnant women. Rituximab crosses the human placenta at least near term. Very high levels of the antibody have been measured in the cord blood and the young infant. NHL and moderate to severe RA are serious conditions that require treatment. Use rituximab during pregnancy only if the potential benefit to the mother justifies the potential risk to the fetus. Reproduction studies in cynomolgus monkeys at maternal exposures similar to human therapeutic exposures showed no evidence of teratogenic effects. However, B-cell lymphoid tissue was reduced in the offspring of treated dams. The B-cell counts returned to normal levels, and immunologic function was restored within 6 months of birth. Patients of childbearing potential should use effective contraceptive methods during treatment and for up to 12 months following rituximab therapy.

Postmarketing data indicate that B-cell lymphocytopenia generally lasting less than 6 months can occur in infants exposed to rituximab in utero. Rituximab was detected postnatally in the serum of infants exposed in utero.

➤*Lactation:* It is not known whether rituximab is secreted into human milk. Rituximab is secreted in the milk of lactating cynomolgus monkeys, and IgG is excreted in human milk; therefore, rituximab also may be excreted. The effects of this potential exposure on a breast-feeding infant are unknown, but immunosuppression and other severe adverse reactions are potential complications. Published data suggest that antibodies in breast milk do not enter the neonatal and infant circulations in substantial amounts. Weigh the unknown risks to the infant from oral ingestion of rituximab against the known benefits of breast-feeding.

➤*Children:* The safety and efficacy of rituximab in children have not been established.

➤*Elderly:*

Diffuse large B-cell non-Hodgkin lymphoma and rheumatoid arthritis – No overall differences in efficacy were observed between these patients and younger patients.

Elderly patients were more likely to experience cardiac adverse reactions, mostly supraventricular arrhythmias, serious infections, and malignancies. Serious pulmonary adverse reactions, including pneumonia and pneumonitis, were also more common among elderly patients.

Chronic lymphocytic leukemia – The incidence of grade 3 and 4 adverse reactions was higher among patients receiving rituximab, fludarabine, and cyclophosphamide who were 70 years and older compared with younger patients for neutropenia (44% vs 31% [study 10]; 56% vs 39% [study 11]), febrile neutropenia (16% vs 6% [study 10]), anemia (5% vs 2% [study 10]; 21% vs 10% [study 11]), thrombocytopenia (19% vs 8% [study 11]), pancytopenia (7% vs 2% [study 10]; 7% vs 2% [study 11]), and infections (30% vs 14% [study 11]).

➤*Monitoring:* During treatment with rituximab monotherapy in patients with lymphoid malignancies, obtain complete blood cell counts (CBC) and platelet counts prior to each rituximab course. During treatment with rituximab and chemotherapy, obtain CBC and platelet counts at weekly to monthly intervals and more frequently in patients who develop cytopenias. In patients with RA, obtain CBC and platelet counts at 2- to 4-month intervals during rituximab therapy. The duration of cytopenias caused by rituximab can extend months beyond the treatment period.

Closely observe patients for signs of infection, particularly PML, especially if they are receiving rituximab in combination with chemotherapy or as part of a hematopoietic stem cell transplant or if biologic agents and/or disease-modifying antirheumatic drugs (DMARDs) are used concomitantly.

Because patients with RA are at an increased risk for cardiovascular events compared with the general population, monitor patients with RA throughout the infusion and discontinue rituximab in the event of a serious or life-threatening cardiac event. Perform cardiac monitoring during and after all infusions in patients who develop clinically significant arrhythmias or have a history of arrhythmia angina.

Monitor patients closely for infusion reactions. Monitor renal function and fluid balance.

Closely monitor carriers of hepatitis B for clinical and laboratory signs of active HBV infection for up to several months following rituximab therapy.

Closely monitor patients with preexisting cardiac or pulmonary conditions, those who experienced prior cardiopulmonary adverse reactions, and those with high numbers of circulating malignant cells (at least 25,000/mm^3).

Drug Interactions

➤*Vaccines:* See Warnings/Precautions for more information.

Rituximab Drug Interactions

Precipitant drug	Object drug[a]		Description
Biological agents or DMARDs	Rituximab	↑	Limited data are available on the safety of the use of biologic agents or DMARDs other than methotrexate in patients exhibiting peripheral B-cell depletion following treatment with rituximab. Risk for infection may be increased. Closely observe patients for signs of infection if biologic agents and/or DMARDs are coadministered with rituximab.
Cisplatin	Rituximab	↑	Renal toxicity has occurred in patients receiving rituximab and cisplatin concomitantly in clinical trials. Coadministration of these agents is not an approved treatment regimen.
Tocilizumab	Rituximab	↑	Coadministration of rituximab and tocilizumab may increase the risk of serious infection. Avoid coadministration.
Rituximab	Tocilizumab		

[a] ↑ = object drug increased.

Adverse Reactions

➤*Most common adverse reactions:* The most common adverse reactions of rituximab (incidence 25% or more) observed in patients with NHL are asthenia, chills, fever, infection, infusion reactions, and lymphopenia.

The most common adverse reactions of rituximab (incidence 25% or more) observed in clinical trials of patients with CLL were infusion reactions and neutropenia.

➤*Lymphoid malignancies:*

Infusion reactions – In the majority of patients with NHL, infusion reactions consisting of angioedema, bronchospasm, chills/rigors, dizziness, fever, headache, hypertension, hypotension, myalgia, nausea, pruritus, rash, urticaria, or vomiting occurred during the first rituximab infusion. Infusion reactions generally occurred within 30 to 120 minutes of beginning the first infusion and resolved with slowing or interruption of the rituximab infusion and with supportive care (diphenhydramine, acetaminophen, IV saline). The incidence of infusion reactions was highest during the first infusion (77%) and decreased with each subsequent infusion.

RITUXIMAB — INJECTION

Infections – Serious infections (National Cancer Institute Common Terminology Criteria for Adverse Events grade 3 or 4), including sepsis, occurred in less than 5% of patients with NHL in the single-arm studies. The overall incidence of infections was 31% (bacterial, 19%; viral, 10%; unknown, 6%; and fungal, 1%).

In randomized, controlled studies in which rituximab was administered following chemotherapy for the treatment of follicular or low-grade NHL, the rate of infection was higher among patients who received rituximab. In diffuse large B-cell lymphoma patients, viral infections occurred more frequently in those who received rituximab.

Hematologic – In patients with NHL receiving rituximab monotherapy, NCI-CTC grade 3 and 4 cytopenias were reported in 48% of patients. These included lymphopenia (40%), neutropenia (6%), leukopenia (4%), anemia (3%), and thrombocytopenia (2%). The median duration of lymphopenia was 14 days (range, 1 to 588 days) and of neutropenia was 13 days (range, 2 to 116 days). A single occurrence of transient aplastic anemia (pure red cell aplasia) and 2 occurrences of hemolytic anemia following rituximab therapy occurred during the single-arm studies. In studies of monotherapy, rituximab induced B-cell depletion in 70% to 80% of patients with NHL. Decreased IgM and IgG serum levels occurred in 14% of these patients.

Relapsed or refractory, low-grade or follicular, CD20-positive, B-cell non-Hodgkin lymphoma –

Rituximab Adverse Reactions in Relapsed or Refractory, Low Grade or Follicular, CD-20 Positive, B-cell Non-Hodgkin Lymphoma Patients (≥ 5%) (n = 356)[a,b]

Adverse reactions	All grades	Grade 3 and 4
Any adverse reaction	99%	57%
Cardiovascular	25%	3%
Hypertension	6%	1%
Hypotension	10%	1%
CNS	32%	1%
Anxiety	5%	1%
Asthenia	26%	1%
Dizziness	10%	1%
Headache	19%	1%
Dermatologic	44%	2%
Flushing	5%	0%
Night sweats	15%	1%
Pruritus	14%	1%
Rash	15%	1%
Urticaria	8%	1%
GI	37%	2%
Abdominal pain	14%	1%
Diarrhea	10%	1%
Nausea	23%	1%
Throat irritation	9%	0%
Vomiting	10%	1%
Hematologic/Lymphatic	67%	48%
Anemia	8%	3%
Leukopenia	14%	4%
Lymphopenia	48%	40%
Neutropenia	14%	6%
Thrombocytopenia	12%	2%
Metabolic/Nutritional	38%	3%
Hyperglycemia	9%	1%
LDH[c] increase	7%	0%
Peripheral edema	8%	0%
Musculoskeletal	26%	3%
Arthralgia	10%	1%
Back pain	10%	1%
Myalgia	10%	1%
Respiratory	38%	4%
Bronchospasm	8%	1%
Dyspnea	7%	1%
Increased cough	13%	1%
Rhinitis	12%	1%
Sinusitis	6%	0%
Miscellaneous		
Angioedema	11%	1%
Chills	33%	3%
Fever	53%	1%
Infection	31%	4%
Pain	12%	1%

[a] Most patients received single-agent rituximab 375 mg/m² weekly for 4 doses.
[b] N = 356; adverse reactions observed up to 12 months following rituximab therapy; graded for severity by NCI-CTC criteria.
[c] LDH = lactate dehydrogenase.

In these single-arm rituximab studies, bronchiolitis obliterans occurred during and up to 6 months after rituximab infusion.

Previously untreated, low-grade or follicular non-Hodgkin lymphoma – In study 4, patients in the rituximab, cyclophosphamide, vincristine, and prednisone arm had higher incidences of infusional toxicity and neutropenia compared with those in the cyclophosphamide, vincristine, and prednisone arm. The following adverse reactions occurred more frequently (at least 5%) in patients receiving rituximab, cyclophosphamide, vincristine, and prednisone, compared with cyclophosphamide, vincristine, and prednisone alone: rash (17% vs 5%), cough (15% vs 6%), flushing (14% vs 3%), rigors (10% vs 2%), pruritus (10% vs 1%), neutropenia (8% vs 3%), and chest tightness (7% vs 1%).

In study 5, detailed safety data collection was limited to serious adverse reactions, grade 2 or greater infections, and grade 3 or greater adverse reactions. In patients receiving rituximab as single-agent maintenance therapy following rituximab plus chemotherapy, infections were reported more frequently compared with the observation arm (37% vs 22%). Grade 3 to 4 adverse reactions occurring at a higher incidence (more than 2%) in the rituximab-only group were infections (4% vs 1%) and neutropenia (4% vs less than 1%).

In study 6, the following adverse reactions were reported more frequently (at least 5%) in patients receiving rituximab following cyclophosphamide, vincristine, and prednisone, compared with those who received no further therapy: fatigue (39% vs 14%), anemia (35% vs 20%), peripheral sensory neuropathy (30% vs 18%), infections (19% vs 9%), pulmonary toxicity (18% vs 10%), hepatobiliary toxicity (17% vs 7%), rash and/or pruritus (17% vs 5%), arthralgia (12% vs 3%), and weight gain (11% vs 4%). Neutropenia was the only grade 3 or 4 adverse reaction that occurred more frequently (at least 2%) in the rituximab arm, compared with those who received no further therapy (4% vs 1%).

Diffuse large B-cell lymphoma – In studies 7 and 8, the following adverse reactions, regardless of severity, were reported more frequently (5% or more) in patients 60 years and older receiving rituximab, cyclophosphamide, doxorubicin, vincristine, and prednisone, as compared with cyclophosphamide, doxorubicin, vincristine, and prednisone alone: pyrexia (56% vs 46%), lung disorder (31% vs 24%), cardiac disorder (29% vs 21%), and chills (13% vs 4%). Detailed safety data collection in these studies was primarily limited to grade 3 and 4 adverse reactions and serious adverse reactions.

In study 8, a review of cardiac toxicity revealed that supraventricular arrhythmias or tachycardia accounted for most of the difference in cardiac disorders, with incidences of 4.5% for rituximab, cyclophosphamide, doxorubicin, vincristine, and prednisone versus 1% for cyclophosphamide, doxorubicin, vincristine, and prednisone.

The following grade 3 or 4 adverse reactions were reported more frequently among patients in the rituximab, cyclophosphamide, doxorubicin, vincristine, and prednisone arm, compared with those in the cyclophosphamide, doxorubicin, vincristine, and prednisone arm: thrombocytopenia (9% vs 7%) and lung disorder (6% vs 3%). Other grade 3 or 4 adverse reactions occurring more frequently among patients receiving rituximab, cyclophosphamide, doxorubicin, vincristine, and prednisone were viral infection (study 8), neutropenia (studies 8 and 9), and anemia (study 9).

Chronic lymphocytic leukemia – In study 10, the following grade 3 and 4 adverse reactions occurred more frequently in patients receiving rituximab, fludarabine, and cyclophosphamide compared with patients receiving fludarabine and cyclophosphamide: infusion reactions (9% in the rituximab, fludarabine, and cyclophosphamide arm), neutropenia (30% vs 19%), febrile neutropenia (9% vs 6%), leukopenia (23% vs 12%), and pancytopenia (3% vs 1%).

In study 11, the following grade 3 or 4 adverse reactions occurred more frequently in patients receiving rituximab, fludarabine, and cyclophosphamide compared with patients receiving fludarabine and cyclophosphamide: infusion reactions (7% in the rituximab, fludarabine, and cyclophosphamide arm), neutropenia (49% vs 44%), febrile neutropenia (15% vs 12%), thrombocytopenia (11% vs 9%), hypotension (2% vs 0%), and hepatitis B (2% vs less than 1%). Fifty-nine percent of patients receiving rituximab, fludarabine, and cyclophosphamide experienced an infusion reaction of any severity.

RITUXIMAB — INJECTION

➤*Rheumatoid arthritis:*

Adverse reactions (5% or more) –

Respiratory: Bronchitis, nasopharyngitis, upper respiratory tract infection (greater than 10%); upper respiratory tract infection (greater than 5%).

Miscellaneous: Infusion-related reactions, urinary tract infection (greater than 10%); arthralgia, hypertension, nausea, pruritus, pyrexia (greater than 5%).

Adverse reactions (2% or more) –

Rituximab Adverse Reactions[a] in Patients With Rheumatoid Arthritis (≥ 2%)		
Adverse reactions	Rituximab + methotrexate (n = 540)	Placebo + methotrexate (n = 398)
CNS		
Anxiety	2%	1%
Asthenia	2%	< 1%
Migraine	2%	< 1%
Paresthesia	2%	< 1%
Dermatologic		
Pruritus	5%	1%
Urticaria	2%	< 1%
GI		
Dyspepsia	3%	< 1%
Nausea	8%	5%
Throat irritation	2%	0%
Upper abdominal pain	2%	1%
Respiratory		
Rhinitis	3%	2%
Upper respiratory tract infection	7%	6%
Miscellaneous		
Arthralgia	6%	4%
Chills	3%	2%
Hypertension	8%	5%
Pyrexia	5%	2%

[a] These data are based on 938 patients treated in phase 2 and 3 studies of rituximab (2 × 1,000 mg) or placebo administered in combination with methotrexate.

Infusion reactions – In rituximab RA placebo-controlled studies, 32% of rituximab-treated patients experienced an adverse reaction during or within 24 hours following their first infusion, compared with 23% of placebo-treated patients receiving their first infusion. The incidence of adverse reactions during the 24-hour period following the second infusion of rituximab or placebo decreased to 11% and 13%, respectively. Acute infusion reactions (manifested by angioedema, bronchospasm with or without associated hypotension or hypertension, chills, cough, fever, pruritus, rigors, sneezing, throat irritation, and/or urticaria/rash) were experienced by 27% of rituximab-treated patients following their first infusion, compared with 19% of placebo-treated patients receiving their first infusion. The incidence of these acute infusion reactions following the second infusion of rituximab or placebo decreased to 9% and 11%, respectively. Serious acute infusion reactions were experienced by less than 1% of patients in either treatment group. Acute infusion reactions required dose modification (stopping, slowing, or interrupting the infusion) after the first course in 10% and 2% of patients receiving rituximab or placebo, respectively. The proportion of patients experiencing acute infusion reactions decreased with subsequent courses of rituximab. The administration of IV glucocorticoids prior to rituximab infusions reduced the incidence and severity of such reactions; however, there was no clear benefit from the administration of oral glucocorticoids for the prevention of acute infusion reactions. Patients in clinical studies also received antihistamines and acetaminophen prior to rituximab infusions.

Infections – In the pooled, placebo-controlled studies, 39% of patients in the rituximab group experienced an infection of any type, compared with 34% of patients in the placebo group. The most common infections were bronchitis, nasopharyngitis, sinusitis, upper respiratory tract infections, and urinary tract infections.

The incidence of serious infections was 2% in the rituximab-treated patients and 1% in the placebo group.

In the experience with rituximab in 2,578 patients with RA, the rate of serious infection was 4.31 per 100 patient-years. The most common serious infections (0.5% or more) were cellulitis, pneumonia or lower respiratory tract infections, and urinary tract infections. Fatal serious infections included colitis, pneumonia, and sepsis. Rates of serious infection remain stable in patients receiving subsequent courses. In 185 rituximab-treated patients with RA with active disease, subsequent treatment with a biologic DMARD, the majority of which were TNF antagonists, did not appear to increase the rate of serious infection. Thirteen serious infections were observed in 186.1 patient-years (6.99 per 100 patient-years) prior to exposure and 10 were observed in 182.3 patient-years (5.49 per 100 patient-years) after exposure.

Cardiovascular – The proportion of patients with serious cardiovascular reactions in the pooled, placebo-controlled studies was 1.7% and 1.3% in rituximab and placebo treatment groups, respectively. Three cardiovascular deaths occurred during the double-blind period of the RA studies, including all rituximab regimens (0.4%) compared with none in the placebo treatment group.

In the experience with rituximab in 2,578 patients with RA, the rate of serious cardiac reactions was 1.93 per 100 patient-years. The rate of MI was 0.56 per 100 patient-years (28 events in 26 patients), which is consistent with MI rates in the general RA population. These rates did not increase over 3 courses of rituximab.

Hypophosphatemia and hyperuricemia – In the pooled, placebo-controlled studies, newly occurring hypophosphatemia (less than 2 mg/dL) was observed in 12% of patients on rituximab versus 10% of patients on placebo. Hypophosphatemia was more common in patients who received corticosteroids. Newly occurring hyperuricemia (more than 10 mg/dL) was observed in 1.5% of patients on rituximab versus 0.3% of patients on placebo.

In the experience with rituximab in RA patients, newly occurring hypophosphatemia was observed in 21% of patients and newly occurring hyperuricemia was observed in 2% of patients. The majority of the observed hypophosphatemia occurred at the time of the infusions and was transient.

➤*Postmarketing:*

Cardiovascular – Fatal cardiac failure, systemic vasculitis.

Dermatologic – Severe mucocutaneous reactions, vasculitis with rash.

GI – Bowel obstruction and perforation.

Hematologic – Hyperviscosity syndrome in Waldenström macroglobulinemia, late-onset neutropenia, marrow hypoplasia, prolonged pancytopenia.

Respiratory – Fatal bronchiolitis obliterans, fatal interstitial lung disease, pleuritis.

Special senses – Optic neuritis, uveitis.

Miscellaneous – Disease progression of Kaposi sarcoma, a reported increased incidence of grade 3 and 4 infections in patients with previously treated lymphoma without known HIV infection, increase in fatal infections in HIV-associated lymphoma, lupus-like syndrome, polyarticular arthritis, posterior reversible encephalopathy syndrome/reversible posterior leukoencephalopathy syndrome, serum sickness, viral infections, including PML.

Patient Information

Advise patients of childbearing potential to use effective contraceptive methods during treatment and for up to 12 months following rituximab therapy.

Inform patients that rituximab may lower the ability of the immune system to fight infections. Instruct patients of the importance of contacting their health care provider if they develop any symptoms of infection, including new-onset neurologic symptoms that may be suggestive of PML, including new or worsening medical problems, such as new or sudden change in thinking, walking, strength, or vision, or other problems that have lasted over several days.

Advise patients of the potential for serious, including fatal, infusion reactions and ask them to report promptly any symptoms suggestive of infusion reactions, including blurred vision, cough, dizziness, drowsiness, headache, hives, swelling, trouble breathing, or wheezing, while receiving or after receiving rituximab.

Counsel patients with NHL about the possible risk of tumor lysis syndrome while receiving rituximab.

Advise patients to report promptly any symptoms suggestive of severe mucocutaneous reactions, such as painful sores on skin or in mouth, ulcers, blisters, or peeling skin, while receiving or after receiving rituximab.

IBRITUMOMAB TIUXETAN

Rx	**Zevalin** (Cell Therapeutics)	**Injection, solution:** 3.2 mg	Preservative free. In 2 mL single-use vials. In In-111 ibritumomab tiuxetan and Y-90 ibritumomab tiuxetan kits with sodium acetate 50 mM vial, formulation buffer vial,[a] reaction vial, and identification labels.[b]

[a] Formulation buffer vial contains albumin (human) 750 mg, sodium chloride 76 mg, sodium phosphate dibasic dodecahydrate 28 mg, pentetic acid 4 mg, potassium phosphate monobasic 2 mg, and potassium chloride 2 mg in water for injection 10 mL.

[b] The indium-111 (In-111) chloride sterile solution must be ordered separately from GE Healthcare or Mallinckrodt/Covidien at the time the In-111 ibritumomab tiuxetan kit is ordered. The yttrium-90 (Y-90) chloride sterile solution will be shipped directly from MDS Nordion upon placement of an order for the Y-90 ibritumomab tiuxetan kit.

IBRITUMOMAB TIUXETAN — INJECTION

Because the ibritumomab tiuxetan therapeutic regimen includes the use of rituximab, see the Rituximab monograph.

WARNING

Serious infusion reactions – Deaths have occurred within 24 hours of rituximab infusion, an essential component of the ibritumomab tiuxetan therapeutic regimen. These fatalities were associated with acute respiratory distress syndrome, cardiogenic shock, hypoxia, myocardial infarction (MI), pulmonary infiltrates, or ventricular fibrillation. Approximately 80% of fatal infusion reactions occurred with the first rituximab infusion. Discontinue rituximab, In-111 ibritumomab tiuxetan, and Y-90 ibritumomab tiuxetan infusions in patients who develop severe infusion reactions.

Prolonged and severe cytopenias – Y-90 ibritumomab tiuxetan administration results in severe and prolonged cytopenias in most patients. Do not administer the ibritumomab tiuxetan therapeutic regimen to patients with at least 25% lymphoma marrow involvement and/or impaired bone marrow reserve.

Severe cutaneous and mucocutaneous reactions – Severe cutaneous and mucocutaneous reactions, some with fatal outcome, have been reported with the ibritumomab tiuxetan therapeutic regimen. Discontinue rituximab, In-111 ibritumomab tiuxetan, and Y-90 ibritumomab tiuxetan infusions in patients experiencing severe cutaneous or mucocutaneous reactions.

Dosing – The dose of Y-90 ibritumomab tiuxetan should not exceed 32 mCi (1,184 MBq). Do not administer Y-90 ibritumomab tiuxetan to patients with altered biodistribution as determined by imaging with In-111 ibritumomab tiuxetan.

Indications

➤*Non-Hodgkin lymphoma:* For the treatment of relapsed or refractory, low-grade or follicular B-cell non-Hodgkin lymphoma (NHL); for the treatment of previously untreated follicular NHL in patients who achieve a partial or complete response to first-line chemotherapy.

Administration and Dosage

➤*General dosing considerations:* Rituximab infusion is an essential component of the ibritumomab tiuxetan therapeutic regimen (see the Rituximab monograph for more information).

Initiate the ibritumomab tiuxetan therapeutic regimen following recovery of platelet counts to 150,000/mm^3 or higher at least 6 weeks, but no more than 12 weeks, following the last dose of first-line chemotherapy.

Monitor patients closely for evidence of extravasation during the injection of Y-90 ibritumomab tiuxetan. Immediately stop infusion and restart in another limb if any signs or symptoms of extravasation occur.

Premedication required. (See Premedication.)

➤*Adults:*

Non-Hodgkin lymphoma –

Day 1:

- *Rituximab* –
  - *Maximum dose:* 400 mg/h.
  - *Initial dosage:* 250 mg/m^2 intravenously (IV) at an initial rate of 50 mg/h.
  - *Dosage titration:* In the absence of infusion reactions, escalate the infusion rate in 50 mg/h increments every 30 minutes to a maximum of 400 mg/h.
  - *Dosage adjustment:* Immediately stop the rituximab infusion for serious infusion reactions and discontinue the ibritumomab tiuxetan therapeutic regimen. Temporarily slow or interrupt the rituximab infusion for less severe infusion reactions. If symptoms improve, continue the infusion at one-half the previous rate.
- *Ibritumomab tiuxetan* – 5 mCi of In-111 ibritumomab tiuxetan over 10 minutes as an IV injection within 4 hours following completion of the rituximab infusion.

Day 7, 8, or 9: Verify that expected biodistribution is present 48 to 72 hours after In-111 ibritumomab tiuxetan administration; do not proceed if biodistribution is not acceptable (see Image acquisition and interpretation of biodistribution.)

- *Rituximab* –
  - *Maximum dose:* 400 mg/h.
  - *Initial dosage:* 250 mg/m^2 IV at an initial rate of 100 mg/h.
  - *Dosage titration:* Increase rate by 100 mg/h increments at 30-minute intervals, to a maximum of 400 mg/h, as tolerated.
  - *Dosage adjustment:* If infusion reactions occurred during rituximab infusion on day 1 of treatment, administer rituximab at an initial rate of 50 mg/h and escalate the infusion rate in 50 mg/h increments every 30 minutes to a maximum of 400 mg/h.
- *Ibritumomab tiuxetan* –
  - *Maximum dose:* Do not administer more than 32 mCi (1,184 MBq) of Y-90 ibritumomab tiuxetan dose regardless of the patient's body weight.
  - *Platelet count 150,000/mm^3 or higher:* Y-90 ibritumomab tiuxetan over 10 minutes as an IV injection at a dose of Y-90 0.4 mCi/kg (14.8 MBq/kg) actual body weight.
  - *Platelet count 100,000 to 149,000/mm^3 in relapsed or refractory patients:* Y-90 ibritumomab tiuxetan over 10 minutes as an IV injection at a dose of Y-90 0.3 mCi/kg (11.1 MBq/kg) actual body weight.
  - *Platelets less than 100,000/mm^3:* Do not administer.

➤*Image acquisition and interpretation of biodistribution:* Assess the biodistribution of In-111 ibritumomab tiuxetan by a visual evaluation of whole body planar view anterior and posterior gamma images obtained at 48 to 72 hours after injection. Images at additional time points may be necessary to resolve ambiguities. Acquire whole body anterior/posterior planar images using a large field-of-view gamma camera and medium energy collimators. Suggested gamma camera settings are as follows: 256 × 1,024 matrix; dual energy photopeaks set at 172 and 247 keV; 15% symmetric window; scan speed of 10 cm/min for the 48- to 72-hour scan, and 7 to 10 cm/min for subsequent scans.

Expected biodistribution – Activity in the blood pool areas (heart, abdomen, neck, and extremities) may be faintly visible; moderately high to high uptake in healthy liver and spleen; moderately low or very low uptake in healthy kidneys, urinary bladder, and healthy (uninvolved) bowel; nonfixed areas within the bowel lumen that change position with time; delayed imaging, as described previously, may be necessary to confirm GI clearance; focal fixed areas of uptake in the bowel wall (localization to lymphoid aggregates in bowel wall).

Tumor uptake may be visualized; however, tumor visualization on the In-111 ibritumomab tiuxetan scan is not required for Y-90 ibritumomab tiuxetan therapy.

Altered biodistribution – The criteria for altered biodistribution are met if any of the following are detected on visual inspection of the required gamma images: intense localization of radiotracer in the liver and spleen and bone marrow indicative of reticuloendothelial system uptake; increased uptake in healthy organs (not involved by tumor) such as diffuse uptake in healthy lungs more intense than the liver, kidneys have greater intensity than the liver on the posterior view, fixed areas (unchanged with time) of uptake in the healthy bowel are greater than uptake in the liver. In less than 0.5% of patients receiving In-111 ibritumomab tiuxetan, prominent bone marrow uptake was observed, characterized by clear visualization of the long bones and ribs.

Consider bone marrow involvement by lymphoma, increased marrow activity caused by recent hematopoietic growth factor administration, and increased reticuloendothelial uptake in patients with human antimouse antibody (HAMA) and human antichimeric antibody (HACA) as possible causes of prominent bone marrow uptake. Reassess biodistribution after correction of underlying factors.

➤*Premedication:* Premedicate with acetaminophen 650 mg orally and diphenhydramine 50 mg orally prior to each rituximab infusion.

➤*Preparation for administration:* Two separate and distinctly labeled kits are required for preparation of In-111 ibritumomab tiuxetan and Y-90 ibritumomab tiuxetan. The procedures are different for the preparation of In-111 ibritumomab tiuxetan and of Y-90 ibritumomab tiuxetan.

Required materials not supplied in the kits – Indium-111 chloride sterile solution (In-111 chloride) from GE Healthcare or Mallinckrodt/Covidien, or Y-90 chloride sterile solution from MDS Nordion; 3 sterile 1 mL plastic syringes; 1 sterile 3 mL plastic syringe; 2 sterile 10 mL plastic syringes with 18- to 20-gauge needles; instant thin-layer chromatographic silica gel (ITLC-SG) strips; sodium chloride 0.9% aqueous solution for the chromatography solvent; developing chamber for chromatography; suitable radioactivity counting apparatus; filter, 0.22 micrometer, low-protein-binding; and appropriate lead shielding for reaction vial and syringe for In-111 or appropriate acrylic shielding for reaction vial and syringe for Y-90.

In-111 ibritumomab tiuxetan – Allow contents of the refrigerated In-111 ibritumomab tiuxetan kit (ibritumomab tiuxetan vial, sodium acetate 50 mM vial, formulation buffer vial, and empty reaction vial) to reach room temperature. Place the empty reaction vial in an appropriate lead shield. Determine the amount of each component needed as follows: a) calculate volume of In-111 chloride equivalent to 5.5 mCi based on the activity concentration of the In-111 chloride stock; b) the volume of sodium 50 mM acetate solution needed is 1.2 times the volume of In-111 chloride solution determined in the previous step; c) calculate volume of formulation buffer needed to bring the reaction vial contents to a final volume of 10 mL. Transfer the calculated volume of 50 mM of sodium acetate to the empty reaction vial. Coat the entire inner surface of the reaction vial by gentle inversion or rolling. Transfer 5.5 mCi of In-111 chloride to the reaction vial using a lead

IBRITUMOMAB TIUXETAN — INJECTION

shielded syringe. Mix the 2 solutions by gentle inversion or rolling. Transfer 1 mL of ibritumomab tiuxetan to the reaction vial. Do not shake or agitate the vial contents.

Allow the labeling reaction to proceed at room temperature for 30 minutes. A shorter or longer reaction time may adversely alter the final labeled product. Immediately after the 30-minute incubation period, transfer the calculated volume of formulation buffer determined previously to the reaction vial. Gently add the formulation buffer down the side of the reaction vial. If necessary, withdraw an equal volume of air to normalize pressure. Measure the final product for total activity using a radioactivity calibration system suitable for the measurement of In-111. Using supplied labels, record the date and time of preparation, total activity and volume, and date and time of expiration; affix these labels to the shielded reaction vial container.

Patient dose: Calculate the volume required for an In-111 ibritumomab tiuxetan dose of 5 mCi. Withdraw the required volume from the reaction vial into a sterile syringe. Assay the syringe in a dose calibrator suitable for the measurement of In-111. Using the supplied labels, record patient identifier, total activity and volume, and the date and time of expiration; affix these labels to the syringe and shielded unit dose container. Determine radiochemical purity. Immediately prior to administration, assay the syringe and contents using an appropriate radioactivity calibration system.

Y-90 ibritumomab tiuxetan – Allow contents of the refrigerated Y-90 ibritumomab tiuxetan kit (ibritumomab tiuxetan vial, sodium acetate 50 mM vial, and formulation buffer vial) to reach room temperature. Place the empty reaction vial in an appropriate acrylic shield. Determine the amount of each component needed as follows: a) calculate volume of Y-90 chloride equivalent to 40 mCi based on the activity concentration of the Y-90 chloride stock; b) the volume of sodium acetate 50 mM solution needed is 1.2 times the volume of Y-90 chloride solution determined previously; c) calculate the volume of formulation buffer needed to bring the reaction vial contents to a final volume of 10 mL. Transfer the calculated volume of 50 mM of sodium acetate to the empty reaction vial.

Coat the entire inner surface of the reaction vial by gentle inversion or rolling. Transfer 40 mCi of Y-90 chloride to the reaction vial using an acrylic shielded syringe. Mix the 2 solutions by gentle inversion or rolling. Transfer 1.3 mL of ibritumomab tiuxetan to the reaction vial. Do not shake or agitate the vial contents.

Allow the labeling reaction to proceed at room temperature for 5 minutes. A shorter or longer reaction time may adversely alter the final labeled product. Immediately after the 5-minute incubation period, transfer the calculated volume of formulation buffer determined previously to the reaction vial. Gently add the formulation buffer down the side of the reaction vial. If necessary, withdraw an equal volume of air to normalize pressure. Measure the final product for total activity using a radioactivity calibration system suitable for the measurement of Y-90. Using the supplied labels, record the date and time of preparation, the total activity and volume, and the date and time of expiration; affix these labels to the shielded reaction vial container.

Patient dose: Calculate the volume required for a Y-90 ibritumomab tiuxetan dose. Withdraw the required volume from the reaction vial. Assay the syringe in the dose calibrator suitable for the measurement of Y-90. The measured dose must be within 10% of the prescribed dose of Y-90 ibritumomab tiuxetan and must not exceed 32 mCi (1,184 MBq). Using the supplied labels, record the patient identifier, total activity and volume, and the date and time of expiration; affix these labels to the syringe and shielded unit dose container. Determine radiochemical purity. Immediately prior to administration, assay the syringe and contents using a radioactivity calibration system suitable for the measurement of Y-90.

Determining radiochemical purity – Place a small drop of either In-111 or Y-90 ibritumomab tiuxetan at the origin of an ITLC-SG strip. Place the ITLC-SG strip into a chromatography chamber with the origin at the bottom and the solvent front at the top. Allow the solvent (sodium chloride 0.9%) to migrate at least 5 cm from the bottom of the strip. Remove the strip from the chamber and cut the strip in half. Count each half of the ITLC-SG strip for 1 minute (count per minute [CPM]) with a suitable counting apparatus. Calculate the percent radiochemical purity as follows: percent radiochemical purity = (CPM bottom half divided by CPM bottom half + CPM top half) × 100. Repeat the ITLC procedure if the radiochemical purity is less than 95%. If repeat testing confirms that radiochemical purity is less than 95%, do not administer the In-111 or Y-90 ibritumomab tiuxetan dose.

➤*Administration:*

Ibritumomab tiuxetan – Use a 0.22 micron low-protein-binding in-line filter between the syringe and the infusion port. After injection, flush the line with at least 10 mL of normal saline.

Administer Y-90 ibritumomab tiuxetan through a free flowing IV line within 4 hours following completion of rituximab infusion.

➤*Admixture compatibility:* Do not mix or dilute rituximab with other drugs.

➤*Storage/Stability:* Store kits at 2° to 8°C (36° to 46°F). Do not freeze. Administer In-111 ibritumomab tiuxetan within 12 hours of radiolabeling. Administer Y-90 ibritumomab tiuxetan within 8 hours of radiolabeling.

Actions

➤*Pharmacology:* Ibritumomab tiuxetan is a monoclonal antibody that binds specifically to the CD20 antigen (human B-lymphocyte–restricted differentiation antigen, Bp35). The apparent affinity (K_D) of ibritumomab tiuxetan for the CD20 antigen ranges between approximately 14 and 18 nanomolar. The CD20 antigen is expressed on pre-B and mature B lymphocytes and on greater than 90% of B-cell NHL. The CD20 antigen is not shed from the cell surface and does not internalize upon antibody binding.

The chelate tiuxetan, which tightly binds In-111 or Y-90, is covalently linked to ibritumomab. The beta emission from Y-90 induces cellular damage by the formation of free radicals in the target and neighboring cells.

Ibritumomab tiuxetan binding was observed in vitro on lymphoid cells of the bone marrow, lymph node, thymus, red and white pulp of the spleen, and lymphoid follicles of the tonsil, as well as lymphoid nodules of other organs such as the large and small intestines.

Pharmacodynamics – In clinical studies, administration of the ibritumomab tiuxetan therapeutic regimen resulted in sustained depletion of circulating B cells. At 4 weeks, the median number of circulating B cells was zero (range, 0 to 1,084 cells/mm^3). B-cell recovery began at approximately 12 weeks following treatment, and the median level of B cells was within the normal range (32 to 341 cells/mm^3) by 9 months after treatment. Median serum levels of immunoglobulin G (IgG) and IgA remained within the normal range throughout the period of B-cell depletion. Median immunoglobulin M serum levels dropped below normal (median, 49 mg/dL; range, 13 to 3,990 mg/dL) after treatment and recovered to normal values by 6 months posttherapy.

➤*Pharmacokinetics:*

Absorption – In pharmacokinetic studies of patients receiving the ibritumomab tiuxetan therapeutic regimen, the mean area under the fraction of injected activity versus time curve in blood was 39 hours.

Excretion – The mean effective half-life for Y-90 activity in blood was 30 hours. Over 7 days, a median of 7.2% of the injected activity was excreted in urine.

Contraindications

None well documented.

Warnings/Precautions

➤*Serious infusion reactions:* Rituximab, alone or as a component of the ibritumomab tiuxetan therapeutic regimen, can cause severe, including fatal, infusion reactions. These reactions typically occur during the first rituximab infusion, with time to onset of 30 to 120 minutes. Signs and symptoms of severe infusion reactions may include urticaria, hypotension, angioedema, hypoxia, bronchospasm, pulmonary infiltrates, acute respiratory distress syndrome, MI, ventricular fibrillation, and cardiogenic shock. Temporarily slow or interrupt the rituximab infusion for less severe infusion reactions. Immediately stop rituximab, In-111 ibritumomab tiuxetan, or Y-90 ibritumomab tiuxetan administration for severe infusion reactions. (See the Rituximab monograph for more information.)

➤*Prolonged and severe cytopenias:* Cytopenias with delayed onset and prolonged duration, some complicated by hemorrhage and severe infection, are the most common severe adverse reactions of the ibritumomab tiuxetan therapeutic regimen. When used according to recommended doses, the incidences of severe thrombocytopenia and neutropenia are greater in patients with mild baseline thrombocytopenia (100,000 to 149,000 /mm^3) compared with those with normal pretreatment platelet counts. Severe cytopenias persisting more than 12 weeks following administration can occur.

Do not administer the ibritumomab tiuxetan therapeutic regimen to patients with at least 25% lymphoma marrow involvement and/or impaired bone marrow reserve. Monitor patients for cytopenias and their complications (eg, febrile neutropenia, hemorrhage) for up to 3 months after use of the ibritumomab tiuxetan therapeutic regimen. Avoid using drugs that interfere with platelet function or coagulation following the ibritumomab tiuxetan therapeutic regimen.

➤*Severe cutaneous and mucocutaneous reactions:* Erythema multiforme, Stevens-Johnson syndrome, toxic epidermal necrolysis, bullous dermatitis, and exfoliative dermatitis, some fatal, were reported in postmarketing experience. The time to onset of these reactions was variable, ranging from a few days to 4 months after administration of the ibritumomab tiuxetan therapeutic regimen. Discontinue the ibritumomab tiuxetan therapeutic regimen in patients experiencing a severe cutaneous or mucocutaneous reaction.

➤*Altered biodistribution:* Do not administer Y-90 ibritumomab tiuxetan to patients with altered biodistribution of In-111 ibritumomab tiuxetan. In a postmarketing registry designed to collect biodistribution images and other information in reported cases of altered biodistribution, 1.3% of patients reported to have altered biodistribution among 953 patients registered.

➤*Secondary malignancies:* Myelodysplastic syndrome and/or acute myelogenous leukemia (AML) were reported in 5.2% of patients with relapsed or refractory NHL enrolled in clinical studies and 1.5% of patients

IBRITUMOMAB TIUXETAN — INJECTION

included in the expanded-access trial, with median follow-up of 6.5 and 4.4 years, respectively. Among the 19 reported cases, the median time to the diagnosis of myelodysplastic syndrome or AML was 1.9 years following treatment with the ibritumomab tiuxetan therapeutic regimen; however, the cumulative incidence continues to increase.

Among 204 patients receiving Y-90 ibritumomab tiuxetan following first-line chemotherapy, 1% of patients were diagnosed with AML within 3 years of receiving ibritumomab tiuxetan.

➤*Extravasation:* Monitor patients closely for evidence of extravasation during ibritumomab tiuxetan infusion. Immediately terminate the infusion if signs or symptoms of extravasation occur and restart in another limb.

➤*Vaccines:* See Drug Interactions for more information.

➤*Radiation exposure:* During and after radiolabeling ibritumomab tiuxetan with In-111 or Y-90, minimize radiation exposure to patients and to medical personnel, consistent with institutional good radiation safety practices and patient management procedures.

➤*Viral disease:* The ibritumomab tiuxetan therapeutic regimen contains albumin, a derivative of human blood. Based on effective donor screening and product manufacturing processes, ibritumomab tiuxetan carries an extremely remote risk for transmission of viral diseases. A theoretical risk for transmission of Creutzfeldt-Jakob disease also is considered extremely remote. No cases of transmission of viral diseases or Creutzfeldt-Jakob disease have ever been identified for albumin.

➤*Immunogenicity:* As with all therapeutic proteins, there is a potential for immunogenicity. The incidence of antibody formation is highly dependent on the sensitivity and specificity of the assay. Additionally, the observed incidence of antibody (including neutralizing antibody) positivity in an assay may be influenced by several factors, including assay methodology, sample handling, timing of sample collection, concomitant medications, and underlying disease. For these reasons, comparisons of the incidence of HAMA/HACA to the ibritumomab tiuxetan therapeutic regimen with the incidence of antibodies to other products may be misleading.

HAMA and HACA response data on 446 patients from 8 clinical studies conducted over a 10-year time period are available. Overall, 2.5% had evidence of either HAMA formation (n = 8) or HACA formation (n = 4). Six of these patients developed HAMA/HACA after treatment with ibritumomab tiuxetan and 5 were HAMA/HACA positive at baseline. Of the 6 who were HAMA/HACA positive, only 1 was positive for both. Furthermore, in 6 of the 11 patients, the HAMA/HACA reverted to negative within 2 weeks to 3 months. No patients had increasing levels of HAMA/HACA at the end of the studies.

Only 1.3% of patients developed evidence of antibody formation after treatment with ibritumomab tiuxetan, and of these, many either reverted to negative or decreased over time. These data demonstrate that HAMA/HACA develop infrequently, are typically transient, and do not increase with time.

➤*Pregnancy: Category D.* Based on its radioactivity, Y-90 ibritumomab tiuxetan may cause fetal harm when administered to a pregnant woman. It is not known if ibritumomab tiuxetan or the components of the therapeutic regimen cross the human placenta. High molecular weight (approximately 148,000) of ibritumomab tiuxetan suggests that it will not cross the placenta. Immunoglobulins are known to cross the placenta and, therefore, ibritumomab tiuxetan with the tightly bound radioactive components may also cross. There are no adequate and well-controlled studies in pregnant women. Animal reproductive toxicology studies of ibritumomab tiuxetan have not been conducted.

Ibritumomab tiuxetan should not be used in pregnancy. Advise women of childbearing potential to use adequate contraception. Inform women who become pregnant while receiving ibritumomab tiuxetan of the potential fetal risks.

➤*Lactation:* The high molecular weight (approximately 148,000) of ibritumomab tiuxetan suggests that it will not be excreted into breast milk. However, because human IgG is excreted in human milk, it is expected that ibritumomab tiuxetan would be present in human milk. Because of the potential for adverse reactions in breast-feeding infants from ibritumomab tiuxetan, decide whether to discontinue breast-feeding or not administer the ibritumomab tiuxetan therapeutic regimen, taking into account the importance of the drug to the mother.

➤*Children:* The safety and efficacy of the ibritumomab tiuxetan therapeutic regimen in children have not been established.

➤*Elderly:* No overall differences in safety or efficacy were observed between these subjects and younger subjects, but greater sensitivity of some older patients cannot be ruled out.

➤*Monitoring:* Obtain complete blood cell counts (CBC) and platelet counts weekly following the ibritumomab tiuxetan therapeutic regimen, and continue until levels recover. Monitor CBC and platelet counts more frequently in patients who develop severe cytopenia, patients who are receiving medications that interfere with platelet function or coagulation, or as clinically indicated.

Drug Interactions

➤*Vaccines:* A reduced immune response may occur following administration of live vaccines. Avoid immunization with a live vaccine for 12 months following ibritumomab tiuxetan therapy.

Ibritumomab Tiuxetan Drug Interactions

Precipitant drug	Object drug[a]		Description
Anticoagulant agents (eg, enoxaparin, heparin, warfarin) or antiplatelet agents (eg, aspirin, clopidogrel, dipyridamole)	Ibritumomab	↑	Risk of bleeding or hemorrhage as well as cytopenias may be increased by concomitant therapy. Avoid coadministration. If coadministered, monitor anticoagulant function and frequently monitor for thrombocytopenia.
Ibritumomab	Anticoagulant agents (eg, enoxaparin, heparin, warfarin) or antiplatelet agents (eg, aspirin, clopidogrel, dipyridamole)		
Hematopoietic growth factors (eg, darbepoetin alfa, epoetin alfa, filgrastim, pegfilgrastim)	Ibritumomab	↑	May alter the biodistribution pattern by increasing bone marrow uptake of ibritumomab tiuxetan. Reassess biodistribution after correction of underlying factors.

[a] ↑ = object drug increased.

Adverse Reactions

➤*Common adverse reactions:* The most common adverse reactions of ibritumomab tiuxetan are abdominal pain, asthenia, cough, cytopenias, diarrhea, fatigue, nasopharyngitis, nausea, and pyrexia.

➤*Severe adverse reactions:* The most serious adverse reactions of ibritumomab tiuxetan are prolonged and severe cytopenias (anemia, lymphopenia, neutropenia, thrombocytopenia) and secondary malignancies.

➤*Non-Hodgkin lymphoma:*

Ibritumomab Tiuxetan Adverse Reactions (≥ 5%)[a]

Adverse reaction	Ibritumomab tiuxetan (n = 206) All grades[b]	Ibritumomab tiuxetan (n = 206) Grade[b] 3 to 4	Observation (n = 203) All grades[b]	Observation (n = 203) Grade[b] 3 to 4
CNS				
Asthenia	15%	1%	8%	< 1%
Dizziness	7%	0%	2%	0%
Fatigue	33%	1%	9%	0%
Dermatological				
Night sweats	8%	0%	2%	0%
Petechiae	8%	2%	0%	0%
Pruritus	7%	0%	1%	0%
Rash	7%	0%	< 1%	0%
GI				
Abdominal pain	17%	2%	13%	< 1%
Anorexia	8%	0%	2%	0%
Diarrhea	11%	0%	3%	0%
Nausea	18%	0%	2%	0%
Hematologic				
Anemia	22%	5%	4%	0%
Leukopenia	43%	36%	4%	1%
Lymphopenia	26%	18%	9%	5%
Neutropenia	45%	41%	3%	2%
Thrombocytopenia	62%	51%	1%	0%
Respiratory				
Bronchitis	8%	0%	3%	0%
Cough	11%	< 1%	5%	0%
Epistaxis	5%	2%	< 1%	0%
Nasopharyngitis	19%	0%	10%	0%
Pharyngolaryngeal pain	7%	0%	2%	0%

IBRITUMOMAB TIUXETAN — INJECTION

Ibritumomab Tiuxetan Adverse Reactions (≥ 5%)[a]

Adverse reaction	Ibritumomab tiuxetan (n = 206)		Observation (n = 203)	
	All grades[b]	Grade[b] 3 to 4	All grades[b]	Grade[b] 3 to 4
Special senses				
Rhinitis	8%	0%	2%	0%
Sinusitis	7%	< 1%	< 1%	0%
Miscellaneous				
Hypertension	7%	3%	2%	< 1%
Influenza-like illness	8%	0%	3%	0%
Myalgia	9%	0%	3%	0%
Pyrexia	10%	3%	4%	0%
Urinary tract infection	7%	< 1%	3%	0%

[a] Between-group difference of ≥ 5%.
[b] National Cancer Institute Common Terminology Criteria for Adverse Events version 2.0.

➤*Hematologic adverse reactions:* Grade 2 to 4 hematologic toxicity occurred in 86% of ibritumomab tiuxetan–treated patients.

Ibritumomab Tiuxetan Hematologic Adverse Reactions[a] (N = 349)

Hematologic adverse reactions	All grades	Grades 3 to 4
Anemia	61%	17%
Ecchymosis	7%	< 1%
Neutropenia	77%	60%
Thrombocytopenia	95%	63%

[a] Occurring within the 12 weeks following the first rituximab infusion of the ibritumomab tiuxetan therapeutic regimen.

Prolonged and severe cytopenias – Patients in clinical studies were not permitted to receive hematopoietic growth factors beginning 2 weeks prior to administration of the ibritumomab tiuxetan therapeutic regimen.

Ibritumomab Tiuxetan Severe Hematologic Toxicity

	Group 1 (n = 270)	Group 2 (n = 65) 100,000 to	Study 4 (n = 204)
Baseline platelet count	≥ 150,000/mm^3	149,000/mm^3	≥ 150,000/mm^3
Y-90 ibritumomab tiuxetan dose	0.4 mCi/kg (14.8 MBq/kg)	0.3 mCi/kg (11.1 MBq/kg)	0.4 mCi/kg (14.8 MBq/kg)
ANC			
Median nadir (cells/mm^3)	800	600	721
Per patient incidence ANC ^{3}	57%	74%	65%
Per patient incidence ANC ^{3}	30%	35%	26%
Median duration (days)[a] ANC < 1,000 cells/mm^3	22	29	29
Median time to recovery[b]	12	13	15
Platelets			
Median nadir (cells/mm^3)	41,000	24,000	42,000
Per patient incidence platelets < 50,000 cells/mm^3	61%	78%	61%
Per patient incidence platelets < 10,000 cells/mm^3	10%	14%	4%
Median duration (days)[c] platelets < 50,000 cells/mm^3	24	35	26
Median time to recovery[b]	13	14	14

[a] Day from last absolute neutrophil count (ANC) ≥ 1,000 cells/mm^3 to first ANC ≥ 1,000/mm^3 following nadir, censored at next treatment or death.
[b] Day from nadir to first count at level of grade 1 toxicity or baseline.
[c] Day from last platelet count ≥ 50,000 cells/mm^3 to day of first platelet count ≥ 50,000 cells/mm^3 following nadir, censored at next treatment or death.

Cytopenias were more severe and more prolonged among 5% of patients who received ibritumomab tiuxetan after first-line fludarabine or a fludarabine-containing chemotherapy regimen, compared with patients receiving nonfludarabine-containing regimens. Among these patients, the median platelet nadir was 13,000/mm^3, with a median duration of platelets below 50,000/mm^3 of 56 days, and the median time for platelet recovery from nadir to grade 1 toxicity or baseline was 35 days. The median ANC was 355/mm^3, with a median duration of ANC below 1,000/mm^3 of 37 days, and the median time for ANC recovery from nadir to grade 1 toxicity or baseline was 20 days.

The median time to cytopenia was similar across patients with relapsed/refractory NHL and those completing first-line chemotherapy, with median ANC nadir at 61 to 62 days, platelet nadir at 49 to 53 days, and hemoglobin nadir at 68 to 69 days after Y-90-ibritumomab tiuxetan administration.

Information on hematopoietic growth factor use and platelet transfusions is based on 211 patients with relapsed/refractory NHL and 206 patients following first-line chemotherapy. Filgrastim was given to 13% of patients and erythropoietin to 8% with relapsed or refractory disease; 14% of patients receiving ibritumomab tiuxetan following first-line chemotherapy received granulocyte colony-stimulating factors and 5% received erythopoiesis-stimulating agents. Platelet transfusions were given to approximately 22% of all ibritumomab tiuxetan–treated patients. Red blood cell transfusions were given to 20% of patients with relapsed or refractory NHL and 2% of patients receiving ibritumomab tiuxetan following first-line chemotherapy.

Leukemia and myelodysplastic syndrome – Among 746 patients with relapsed/refractory NHL, 2.6% of patients developed myelodysplastic syndrome/AML with a median follow-up of 4.4 years. The overall incidence of myelodysplastic syndrome/AML among the 211 patients included in the clinical studies was 5.2%, with a median follow-up of 6.5 years and median time to development of myelodysplastic syndrome/AML of 2.9 years. The cumulative Kaplan-Meier estimated incidence of myelodysplastic syndrome/secondary leukemia in this patient population was 2.2% at 2 years and 5.9% at 5 years. The incidence of myelodysplastic syndrome/AML among the 535 patients in the expanded access programs was 1.5%, with a median follow-up of 4.4 years and median time to development of myelodysplastic syndrome/AML of 1.5 years. Multiple cytogenetic abnormalities were described, most commonly involving chromosomes 5 and/or 7. The risk of myelodysplastic syndrome/AML was not associated with the number of prior treatments (0 to 1 vs 2 to 10).

Among 204 patients receiving Y-90 ibritumomab tiuxetan following first-line treatment, two (1%) developed AML at approximately 2 and 3.3 years after ibritumomab tiuxetan administration, respectively.

➤*Infections:* In relapsed or refractory NHL patients, infections occurred in 29% of patients during the first 3 months after initiating the ibritumomab tiuxetan therapeutic regimen, and 3% developed serious infections (cellulitis, colitis, diarrhea, febrile neutropenia, osteomyelitis, sepsis, pneumonia, urinary tract infection, and upper respiratory tract infection). Life-threatening infections were reported in 2% (biliary stent-associated cholangitis, empyema, febrile neutropenia, fever, pneumonia, and sepsis). From 3 months to 4 years after ibritumomab tiuxetan treatment, 6% of patients developed infections; 2% were serious (bacterial or viral pneumonia, febrile neutropenia, IV drug-associated viral hepatitis, pericarditis, perihilar infiltrate, and urinary tract infection) and 1% were life-threatening infections (bacterial pneumonia, respiratory disease, and sepsis).

When administered following first-line chemotherapy, grade 3 to 4 infections occurred in 8% of ibritumomab tiuxetan–treated patients and in 2% of controls and included neutropenic sepsis (1%), bronchitis, catheter sepsis, diverticulitis, herpes zoster, influenza, lower respiratory tract infection, sinusitis, and upper respiratory tract infection.

➤*Postmarketing:*

Dermatologic – Cutaneous and mucocutaneous reactions: bullous dermatitis, erythema multiforme, exfoliative dermatitis, Stevens-Johnson syndrome, and toxic epidermal necrolysis.

Local – Infusion-site erythema and ulceration following extravasation.

Miscellaneous – Radiation injury in tissues near areas of lymphomatous involvement within a month of ibritumomab tiuxetan administration.

Overdosage

➤*Animal toxicology:* Animal reproductive toxicology studies of the ibritumomab tiuxetan therapeutic regimen have not been conducted. Because the ibritumomab tiuxetan therapeutic regimen includes the use of rituximab, also see the monograph for rituximab.

➤*Symptoms:* Severe cytopenias that may require stem cell support have occurred at doses higher than the recommended maximum total dose of 32 mCi (1,184 MBq).

Patient Information

Advise patients to contact a health care provider for severe signs and symptoms of infusion reactions.

Advise patients to take premedications as prescribed.

Advise patients to report any signs or symptoms of cytopenias (bleeding, easy bruising, petechiae or purpura, pallor, weakness, or fatigue).

Advise patients to avoid medications that interfere with platelet function, except as directed by a health care provider.

Advise patients to seek prompt medical evaluation for diffuse rash, bullae, or desquamation of the skin or oral mucosa.

Advise patients to immediately report symptoms of infection (eg, pyrexia).

Advise patients that immunization with live viral vaccines is not recommended for 12 months following the ibritumomab tiuxetan therapeutic regimen.

Advise patients to discontinue breast-feeding during and after ibritumomab tiuxetan treatment.

Advise women of childbearing potential to avoid becoming pregnant, and to use effective contraceptive methods during treatment and for up to 12 months following the ibritumomab tiuxetan therapeutic regimen.

IPILIMUMAB

Rx	**Yervoy** (Bristol-Myers Squibb)	**Injection, solution, concentrate:** 5 mg/mL	Preservative free. Mannitol, polysorbate 80. In 10 and 40 mL single-use vials.

IPILIMUMAB — INJECTION

WARNING

Immune-mediated adverse reactions – Ipilimumab can result in severe and fatal immune-mediated adverse reactions due to T-cell activation and proliferation. These immune-mediated reactions may involve any organ system; however, the most common severe immune-mediated adverse reactions are enterocolitis, hepatitis, dermatitis (including toxic epidermal necrolysis), neuropathy, and endocrinopathy. The majority of these immune-mediated reactions initially manifested during treatment; however, a minority occurred weeks to months after discontinuation of ipilimumab.

Permanently discontinue ipilimumab and initiate systemic high-dose corticosteroid therapy for severe immune-mediated reactions.

Assess patients for signs and symptoms of enterocolitis, dermatitis, neuropathy, and endocrinopathy, and evaluate clinical chemistries, including liver function tests and thyroid function tests, at baseline and before each dose.

Indications

➤*Melanoma:* For the treatment of unresectable or metastatic melanoma.

Administration and Dosage

➤*Adults:*

Melanoma –

Usual dosage: 3 mg/kg intravenously (IV) over 90 minutes every 3 weeks for a total of 4 doses.

Dosage adjustment: Withhold scheduled dose of ipilimumab for any moderate immune-mediated adverse reactions or for symptomatic endocrinopathy. For patients with complete or partial resolution of adverse reactions (grade 0 to 1), and who are receiving less than 7.5 mg of prednisone or equivalent per day, resume ipilimumab at a dosage of 3 mg/kg every 3 weeks until administration of all 4 planned doses or 16 weeks from first dose, whichever occurs earlier.

Discontinuation of therapy: Permanently discontinue ipilimumab for any of the following: persistent moderate adverse reactions or inability to reduce corticosteroid dose to 7.5 mg of prednisone or equivalent per day; failure to complete full treatment course within 16 weeks from administration of first dose; severe or life-threatening adverse reactions, including any of the following: colitis with abdominal pain, fever, ileus, or peritoneal signs; increase in stool frequency (7 or more over baseline); stool incontinence; need for IV hydration for more than 24 hours; GI hemorrhage; GI perforation; AST or ALT more than 5 times the upper limit of normal (ULN), or total bilirubin more than 3 times the ULN; Stevens-Johnson syndrome; toxic epidermal necrolysis; rash complicated by full-thickness dermal ulceration, or necrotic, bullous, or hemorrhagic manifestations; severe motor or sensory neuropathy; Guillain-Barré syndrome; myasthenia gravis; severe immune-mediated reactions involving any organ system (eg, nephritis, pneumonitis, pancreatitis, noninfectious myocarditis); or immune-mediated ocular disease that is unresponsive to topical immunosuppressive therapy.

➤*Preparation for administration:* Do not shake. Allow the vials to stand at room temperature for approximately 5 minutes prior to preparation of infusion. Withdraw the required volume of ipilimumab and transfer into an IV bag. Dilute with sodium chloride 0.9% injection or dextrose 5% injection to prepare a diluted solution with a final concentration ranging from 1 to 2 mg/mL. Mix diluted solution by gentle inversion.

➤*Administration:* Administer diluted solution over 90 minutes through an IV line containing a sterile, non-pyrogenic, low-protein-binding in-line filter. Flush the IV line with sodium chloride 0.9% injection or dextrose 5% injection after each dose.

➤*Admixture compatibility:* Do not mix ipilimumab with, or administer as an infusion with, other medicinal products.

➤*Storage/Stability:* Store under refrigeration between 2° and 8°C (36° and 46° F). Do not freeze. Protect from light. Store the diluted solution for no more than 24 hours under refrigeration (2° to 8°C [36° to 46°F]) or at room temperature (20° to 25°C [68° to 77°F]). Discard partially used vials or empty vials of ipilimumab.

Actions

➤*Pharmacology:* Ipilimumab is a recombinant, human monoclonal antibody that binds to the cytotoxic T-lymphocyte–associated antigen 4 (CTLA-4). CTLA-4 is a negative regulator of T-cell activation. Ipilimumab binds to CTLA-4 and blocks the interaction of CTLA-4 with its ligands, CD80/CD86. Blockade of CTLA-4 has been shown to augment T-cell activation and proliferation. The mechanism of action of ipilimumab's effect in patients with melanoma is indirect, possibly through T-cell mediated antitumor immune responses.

➤*Pharmacokinetics:*

Absorption – Peak concentration, trough concentration (C_{min}), and area under the curve (AUC) of ipilimumab were found to be dose proportional within the dose range examined. The mean (± standard deviation [SD]) ipilimumab C_{min} achieved at steady state with the 3 mg/kg regimen was 21.8 mcg/mL (± 11.2). Ipilimumab steady-state concentration was reached by the third dose.

Distribution – Ipilimumab has a volume of distribution at steady state of 7.21 L (10.5%).

Excretion – Upon repeated dosing of ipilimumab administered every 3 weeks, ipilimumab clearance was found to be time-invariant, and minimal systemic accumulation was observed as evident by an accumulation index of 1.5-fold or less. The following mean (percent coefficient of variation) parameters were generated through population pharmacokinetic analysis: terminal half-life of 14.7 days (30.1%); systemic clearance of 15.3 mL/h (38.5%).

Special populations –

Weight: Ipilimumab clearance increased with increasing body weight; however, no dose adjustment of ipilimumab is required for body weight after administration on a mg/kg basis.

Contraindications

None well documented.

Warnings/Precautions

➤*Immune-mediated enterocolitis:* See the Warning box for more information.

In study 1, severe, life-threatening, or fatal (diarrhea of 7 or more stools above baseline, fever, ileus, peritoneal signs; grade 3 to 5) immune-mediated enterocolitis occurred in 7% of ipilimumab-treated patients, and moderate (diarrhea with up to 6 stools above baseline, abdominal pain, mucus or blood in stool; grade 2) enterocolitis occurred in 5% of ipilimumab-treated patients. Across all ipilimumab-treated patients (n = 511), 1% of patients developed intestinal perforation, 0.8% of patients died as a result of complications, and 5% of patients were hospitalized for severe enterocolitis.

The median time to onset was 7.4 weeks (range, 1.6 to 13.4) and 6.3 weeks (range, 0.3 to 18.9) after the initiation of ipilimumab for patients with grade 3 to 5 enterocolitis and with grade 2 enterocolitis, respectively.

Of the patients with grade 3 to 5 enterocolitis, 74% experienced complete resolution, 3% experienced improvement to grade 2 severity, and 24% did not improve. Among the patients with grade 2 enterocolitis, 79% experienced complete resolution, 11% improved, and 11% did not improve.

Permanently discontinue ipilimumab in patients with severe enterocolitis and initiate systemic corticosteroids at a dosage of prednisone 1 to 2 mg/kg/day or equivalent. Upon improvement to grade 1 or less, initiate corticosteroid taper and continue to taper over at least 1 month. In clinical trials, rapid corticosteroid tapering resulted in recurrence or worsening symptoms of enterocolitis in some patients.

Withhold ipilimumab dosing for moderate enterocolitis; administer antidiarrheal treatment and, if persistent for more than 1 week, initiate systemic corticosteroids at a dosage of prednisone 0.5 mg/kg/day or equivalent.

➤*Immune-mediated hepatitis:* In study 1, severe, life-threatening, or fatal hepatotoxicity (AST or ALT elevations of more than 5 times the ULN or total bilirubin elevations more than 3 times the ULN; grade 3 to 5) occurred in 2% of ipilimumab-treated patients, with fatal hepatic failure in 0.2% and hospitalization in 0.4% of ipilimumab-treated patients. An additional 2.5% of patients experienced moderate hepatotoxicity manifested by liver function test abnormalities (AST or ALT elevations of more than 2.5 times but not more than 5 times the ULN or total bilirubin elevation of more than 1.5 times but not more than 3 times the ULN; grade 2). The underlying pathology was not ascertained in all patients but in some instances included immune-mediated hepatitis. There were insufficient numbers of patients with biopsy-proven hepatitis to characterize the clinical course of this event.

Permanently discontinue ipilimumab in patients with grade 3 to 5 hepatotoxicity and administer systemic corticosteroids at a dosage of prednisone 1 to 2 mg/kg/day or equivalent. When liver function tests show sustained improvement or return to baseline, initiate corticosteroid tapering and continue to taper over 1 month. Across the clinical development program for ipilimumab, mycophenolate treatment has been administered in patients who have persistent severe hepatitis despite high-dose corticosteroids. Withhold ipilimumab in patients with grade 2 hepatotoxicity (see Monitoring).

➤*Immune-mediated dermatitis:* In study 1, severe, life-threatening, or fatal immune-mediated dermatitis (eg, Stevens-Johnson syndrome, toxic epidermal necrolysis, or rash complicated by full-thickness dermal ulceration, or necrotic, bullous, or hemorrhagic manifestations; grade 3 to 5) occurred in 2.5% of ipilimumab-treated patients. One (0.2%) patient died as a result of toxic epidermal necrolysis and 1 additional patient required hospitalization for severe dermatitis. Twelve percent of patients had moderate (grade 2) dermatitis.

IPILIMUMAB — INJECTION

The median time to onset of moderate, severe, or life-threatening immune-mediated dermatitis was 3.1 weeks and ranged up to 17.3 weeks from the initiation of ipilimumab.

Permanently discontinue ipilimumab in patients with Stevens-Johnson syndrome, toxic epidermal necrolysis, or rash complicated by full-thickness dermal ulceration, or necrotic, bullous, or hemorrhagic manifestations. Administer systemic corticosteroids at a dosage of prednisone 1 to 2 mg/kg/day or equivalent. When dermatitis is controlled, corticosteroid tapering should occur over a period of at least 1 month. Withhold ipilimumab dosing in patients with moderate to severe signs and symptoms (see Monitoring).

➤*Immune-mediated neuropathies:* In study 1, one case of fatal Guillain-Barré syndrome and one case of severe (grade 3) peripheral motor neuropathy were reported. Across the clinical development program of ipilimumab, myasthenia gravis and additional cases of Guillain-Barré syndrome have been reported (see Monitoring).

Permanently discontinue ipilimumab in patients with severe neuropathy (interfering with daily activities), such as Guillain-Barré–like syndromes. Institute medical intervention as appropriate for management of severe neuropathy. Consider initiation of systemic corticosteroids at a dosage of prednisone 1 to 2 mg/kg/day or equivalent for severe neuropathies. Withhold ipilimumab dosing in patients with moderate neuropathy (not interfering with daily activities).

➤*Immune-mediated endocrinopathies:* In study 1, severe to life-threatening immune-mediated endocrinopathies (requiring hospitalization, urgent medical intervention, or interfering with activities of daily living; grade 3 to 4) occurred in 1.8% of ipilimumab-treated patients. All patients had hypopituitarism and some had additional concomitant endocrinopathies, such as adrenal insufficiency, hypogonadism, and hypothyroidism. Of these patients, 61.7% were hospitalized for severe endocrinopathies. Moderate endocrinopathy (requiring hormone replacement or medical intervention; grade 2) occurred in 2.3% of patients and consisted of hypothyroidism, adrenal insufficiency, hypopituitarism, and 1 case each of hyperthyroidism and Cushing syndrome. The median time to onset of moderate to severe immune-mediated endocrinopathy was 11 weeks and ranged up to 19.3 weeks after the initiation of ipilimumab.

Withhold ipilimumab dosing in symptomatic patients. Initiate systemic corticosteroids at a dosage of prednisone 1 to 2 mg/kg/day or equivalent, and initiate appropriate hormone replacement therapy (see Monitoring).

➤*Other immune-mediated adverse reactions, including ocular manifestations:* The following clinically significant immune-mediated adverse reactions were seen in less than 1% of ipilimumab-treated patients in study 1: nephritis, pneumonitis, meningitis, pericarditis, uveitis, iritis, and hemolytic anemia.

Across the clinical development program for ipilimumab, the following likely immune-mediated adverse reactions were also reported with less than 1% incidence: myocarditis, angiopathy, temporal arteritis, vasculitis, polymyalgia rheumatica, conjunctivitis, blepharitis, episcleritis, scleritis, leukocytoclastic vasculitis, erythema multiforme, psoriasis, pancreatitis, arthritis, and autoimmune thyroiditis.

Permanently discontinue ipilimumab for clinically significant or severe immune-mediated adverse reactions. Initiate systemic corticosteroids at a dosage of prednisone 1 to 2 mg/kg/day or equivalent for severe immune-mediated adverse reactions.

Administer corticosteroid eye drops to patients who develop uveitis, iritis, or episcleritis. Permanently discontinue ipilimumab for immune-mediated ocular disease that is unresponsive to local immunosuppressive therapy.

➤*Immunogenicity:* In clinical studies, 1.1% of evaluable patients tested positive for binding antibodies against ipilimumab in an electrochemiluminescent (ECL)–based assay.

Because trough levels of ipilimumab interfere with the ECL assay results, a subset analysis was performed in the dose cohort with the lowest trough levels. In this analysis, 6.9% of evaluable patients treated with 0.3 mg/kg dose tested positive for binding antibodies against ipilimumab.

➤*Pregnancy: Category C.* There are no adequate and well-controlled studies of ipilimumab in pregnant women. Human IgG1 is known to cross the placental barrier and ipilimumab is an immunoglobulin G1 (IgG1); therefore, ipilimumab has the potential to be transmitted from the mother to the developing fetus. Use ipilimumab during pregnancy only if the potential benefit justifies the potential risk to the fetus.

The effects of ipilimumab on prenatal and postnatal development in monkeys have not been fully investigated. Preliminary results are available from an ongoing study in cynomolgus monkeys. Pregnant monkeys received ipilimumab every 21 days from the onset of organogenesis in the first trimester through delivery, at dose levels 2.6 or 7.2 times higher than the clinical dose of ipilimumab 3 mg/kg (by AUC). No treatment-related adverse effects on reproduction were detected during the first 2 trimesters of pregnancy. Beginning in the third trimester, the ipilimumab groups experienced higher incidences of abortion, stillbirth, premature delivery (with corresponding lower birth weight), and higher incidences of infant mortality in a dose-related manner compared with controls.

➤*Lactation:* It is not known whether ipilimumab is secreted in human milk. Because many drugs are secreted in human milk and because of the potential for serious adverse reactions in breast-feeding infants from ipilimumab, decide whether to discontinue breast-feeding or ipilimumab, taking into account the importance of ipilimumab to the woman.

➤*Children:* Safety and effectiveness of ipilimumab have not been established in children.

➤*Monitoring:* Monitor patients for signs and symptoms of enterocolitis (eg, diarrhea, abdominal pain, mucus or blood in stool, with or without fever) and of bowel perforation (eg, peritoneal signs, ileus). In symptomatic patients, rule out infectious etiologies and consider endoscopic evaluation for persistent or severe symptoms.

Monitor liver function tests (hepatic transaminase and bilirubin levels) and assess patients for signs and symptoms of hepatotoxicity before each dose of ipilimumab. In patients with hepatotoxicity, rule out infectious or malignant causes and increase frequency of liver function test monitoring until resolution.

Monitor patients for signs and symptoms of dermatitis, such as rash and pruritus. Unless an alternate etiology has been identified, consider signs or symptoms of dermatitis to be immune-mediated.

Monitor for symptoms of motor or sensory neuropathy, such as unilateral or bilateral weakness, sensory alterations, or paresthesia.

Monitor patients for clinical signs and symptoms of hypophysitis, adrenal insufficiency (including adrenal crisis), and hyper- or hypothyroidism. Patients may present with fatigue, headache, mental status changes, abdominal pain, unusual bowel habits, and hypotension, or nonspecific symptoms that may resemble other causes, such as brain metastasis or underlying disease. Unless an alternate etiology has been identified, consider signs or symptoms of endocrinopathies to be immune-mediated.

Monitor thyroid function tests and clinical chemistries at the start of treatment, before each dose, and as clinically indicated based on symptoms. In a limited number of patients, hypophysitis was diagnosed by imaging studies through enlargement of the pituitary gland.

Drug Interactions

None well documented.

Adverse Reactions

For more information on immune-mediated adverse reactions, including enterocolitis, hepatitis, dermatitis, neuropathies, endocrinopathies, and others, refer to Warnings/Precautions.

➤*Discontinuation:* Ipilimumab was discontinued for adverse reactions in 10% of patients.

➤*Adverse reactions (5% or more):*

Ipilimumab Adverse Reactions (5% or more)[a]

Adverse reactions	Ipilimumab 3 mg/kg (n = 131) Any grade	Grade 3 to 5	Ipilimumab 3 mg/kg+gp100 (n = 380) Any grade	Grade 3 to 5	gp100 (n = 132) Any grade	Grade 3 to 5
CNS						
Fatigue	41%	7%	34%	5%	31%	3%
Dermatologic						
Pruritus	31%	0%	21%	< 1%	11%	0%
Rash	29%	2%	25%	2%	8%	0%
GI						
Diarrhea	32%	5%	37%	4%	20%	1%
Colitis	8%	5%	5%	3%	2%	0%

[a] Incidences presented in this table are based on reports of adverse events regardless of causality.

➤*Severe to fatal immune-mediated adverse reactions:*

Ipilimumab Severe to Fatal Immune-Mediated Adverse Reactions

	Ipilimumab 3 mg/kg (n = 131)	Ipilimumab 3 mg/kg+gp100 (n = 380)
Any immune-mediated adverse reaction	15%	12%
Adrenal insufficiency	0%	1%
Dermatitis[a]	2%	3%
Enterocolitis[a,b]	7%	7%
Endocrinopathy	4%	1%
Hepatotoxicity[a]	1%	2%
Hypopituitarism	4%	1%
Neuropathy[a]	1%	< 1%

IPILIMUMAB — INJECTION

Ipilimumab Severe to Fatal Immune-Mediated Adverse Reactions		
	Ipilimumab 3 mg/kg (n = 131)	Ipilimumab 3 mg/kg+gp100 (n = 380)
Other		
Eosinophilia[c]	1%	0%
Meningitis	0%	< 1%
Nephritis	1%	0%
Pericarditis[a,c]	0%	< 1%
Pneumonitis	0%	< 1%

[a] Including fatal outcome.
[b] Including intestinal perforation.
[c] Underlying etiology not established.

➤*Other adverse reactions:* Urticaria (2%); large intestinal ulcer, esophagitis, acute respiratory distress syndrome, renal failure, and infusion reaction (less than 1%).

Patient Information

Inform patients of the potential risk of immune-mediated adverse reactions.

Advise patients to read the Medication Guide before each ipilimumab infusion.

Advise women that ipilimumab may cause fetal harm.

Advise breast-feeding women not to breast-feed while taking ipilimumab.

CETUXIMAB

Rx	**Erbitux** (Bristol-Myers Squibb)	**Injection, solution:** 2 mg/mL	Preservative free. In single-use 50 and 100 mL vials.[a]

[a] With sodium chloride 8.48 mg/mL, sodium phosphate dibasic heptahydrate 1.88 mg/mL, and sodium phosphate monobasic monohydrate 0.41 mg/mL.

CETUXIMAB — INJECTION

WARNING

Infusion reactions – Serious infusion reactions occurred with the administration of cetuximab in approximately 3% of patients in clinical trials, with fatal outcomes reported in less than 1 in 1,000. Immediately interrupt and permanently discontinue cetuximab infusion for serious infusion reactions.

Cardiopulmonary arrest – Cardiopulmonary arrest and/or sudden death occurred in 2% of 208 patients with squamous cell carcinoma of the head and neck treated with radiation therapy and cetuximab. Closely monitor serum electrolytes, including serum magnesium, potassium, and calcium, during and after cetuximab administration.

Indications

➤*Colorectal cancer:* Cetuximab, as a single agent, is indicated for the treatment of epidermal growth factor receptor (EGFR)-expressing metastatic colorectal cancer after failure of both irinotecan- and oxaliplatin-based regimens. Cetuximab, as a single agent, is also indicated for the treatment of EGFR-expressing metastatic colorectal cancer in patients who are intolerant to irinotecan-based regimens.

Cetuximab, in combination with irinotecan, is indicated for the treatment of EGFR-expressing metastatic colorectal carcinoma in patients who are refractory to irinotecan-based chemotherapy. The effectiveness of cetuximab in combination with irinotecan is based on objective response rates. Currently, no data are available that demonstrate an improvement in disease-related symptoms or increased survival with cetuximab in combination with irinotecan for the treatment of EGFR-expressing, metastatic colorectal carcinoma.

➤*Squamous cell carcinoma of the head and neck (SCCHN):* In combination with radiation therapy for the initial treatment of locally or regionally advanced SCCHN.

Cetuximab, as a single agent, is indicated for the treatment of patients with recurrent or metastatic SCCHN for whom prior platinum-based therapy has failed.

Administration and Dosage

➤*General dosing considerations:* Reduce incidence of infusion reactions with premedication. (See Premedication).

➤*Adults:*

Colorectal cancer –

Initial dosage: 400 mg/m^2 administered as a 120-minute intravenous (IV) infusion (maximum infusion rate, 10 mg/min), either as monotherapy or in combination with irinotecan.

Maintenance dosage: 250 mg/m^2 infused IV over 60 minutes (maximum infusion rate, 10 mg/min) once weekly, either as monotherapy or in combination with irinotecan.

Duration of therapy: Until disease progression or unacceptable toxicity occurs.

Squamous cell carcinoma of the head and neck (SCCHN) –

Combination with radiation therapy:

• *Initial dosage* – 400 mg/m^2 administered as a 120-minute IV infusion (maximum infusion rate, 10 mg/min) 1 week prior to initiation of radiation therapy.

• *Maintenance dosage* – 250 mg/m^2 infused over 60 minutes (maximum infusion rate, 10 mg/min) once weekly. Complete cetuximab administration 1 hour prior to radiation therapy.

• *Duration of therapy* – Continue for the duration of radiation therapy (6 to 7 weeks).

Monotherapy:

• *Initial dosage* – 400 mg/m^2 administered as a 120-minute IV infusion (maximum infusion rate, 10 mg/min).

• *Maintenance dosage* – 250 mg/m^2 infused over 60 minutes (maximum infusion rate, 10 mg/min) once weekly.

• *Duration of therapy* – Until disease progression or unacceptable toxicity occurs.

➤*Premedication:* Premedicate with an H_1 antagonist (eg, diphenhydramine 50 mg) IV 30 to 60 minutes prior to the first dose; premedication should be administered for subsequent cetuximab doses based on clinical judgment and presence and/or severity of prior infusion reactions.

Monitor patients for 1 hour following cetuximab infusions in a setting with resuscitation equipment and other agents necessary to treat anaphylaxis (eg, epinephrine, corticosteroids, IV antihistamines, bronchodilators, and oxygen). Monitor longer to confirm resolution of the event in patients requiring treatment for infusion reactions.

➤*Dosage adjustments:*

Infusion reactions – Reduce the infusion rate by 50% (maximum rate, 2.5 mL/min) for National Cancer Institute Common Toxicity Criteria (NCI-CTC) grade 1 or 2 and nonserious NCI-CTC grade 3 to 4 infusion reactions. Immediately and permanently discontinue cetuximab for serious infusion reactions requiring medical intervention and/or hospitalization.

Dermatologic toxicity – Recommended dose modifications for severe (NCI-CTC grade 3 or 4) acneform rash are specified in the following table.

Cetuximab Dose Modification Guidelines for Severe (NCI-CTC Grade 3 or 4) Acneform Rash			
Severe acneform rash	Cetuximab	Outcome	Cetuximab dose modification
First occurrence	Delay infusion 1 to 2 weeks	Improvement[a]	Continue at 250 mg/m^2
		No improvement	Discontinue cetuximab
Second occurrence	Delay infusion 1 to 2 weeks	Improvement[a]	Reduce dose to 200 mg/m^2
		No improvement	Discontinue cetuximab
Third occurrence	Delay infusion 1 to 2 weeks	Improvement[a]	Reduce dose to 150 mg/m^2
		No improvement	Discontinue cetuximab
Fourth occurrence	Discontinue cetuximab		

[a] Improvement to grade 0 to 2.

➤*Preparation for administration:* Cetuximab is considered a cytotoxic agent and a potential teratogen. Follow safe handling procedures when preparing, administering, or dispensing cetuximab.

Do not dilute cetuximab prior to administration. Avoid shaking cetuximab solution.

Using aseptic technique, withdraw the entire contents of the vial. If administering via an infusion pump, place entire calculated dose of solution in a sterile evacuated container or bag. If using a syringe pump, place contents of 1 vial in a sterile syringe and infuse 1 vial at a time; infuse remainder of dose using another syringe.

The solution should be clear and colorless and may contain a small amount of easily visible, white, amorphous, cetuximab particulates.

CETUXIMAB — INJECTION

➤*Administration:* Do not administer cetuximab as an IV push or bolus. Administer cetuximab via infusion pump or syringe pump. Administer initial dose over 120 minutes, then administer subsequent doses over 60 minutes. The maximum infusion rate is 5 mL/min (10 mg/min).

Administer cetuximab through a low protein-binding 0.22 micrometer in-line filter. Observe patient for 1 hour after administration.

Flush lines with sodium chloride 0.9% injection after IV injection.

➤*Storage/Stability:* Store vials under refrigeration at 2° to 8°C (36° to 46°F). Do not freeze. Increased particulate formation may occur at temperatures at or below 0°C (32°F). This product contains no preservatives. Preparations of cetuximab in infusion containers are chemically and physically stable for up to 12 hours at 2° to 8°C (36° to 46°F) and up to 8 hours at controlled room temperature (20° to 25°C; 68° to 77°F). Discard any remaining solution in the infusion container after 8 hours at controlled room temperature or after 12 hours at 2° to 8°C (36° to 46°F). Discard any unused portion of the vial.

Discard vial within 6 hours of the initial needle puncture if opened within an ISO Class 5 biological safety cabinet, or within 1 hour of the initial needle puncture if opened outside of such an environment, based on the USP Chapter <797> standards.

Actions

➤*Pharmacology:* The EGFR, human epidermal growth receptor 1 (HER-1), c-ErbB-1 is a transmembrane glycoprotein that is a member of a subfamily of type I receptor tyrosine kinases including EGFR, HER-2, HER-3, and HER-4. The EGFR is constitutively expressed in many normal epithelial tissues, including the skin and hair follicle. Expression of EGFR is also detected in many human cancers including those of the head and neck, colon, and rectum.

Cetuximab binds specifically to the EGFR on both normal and tumor cells, and competitively inhibits the binding of epidermal growth factor (EGF) and other ligands, such as transforming growth factor-alpha. In vitro assays and in vivo animal studies have shown that binding of cetuximab to the EGFR blocks phosphorylation and activation of receptor-associated kinases, resulting in inhibition of cell growth, induction of apoptosis, and decreased matrix metalloproteinase and vascular endothelial growth factor production. In vitro, cetuximab can mediate antibody-dependent cellular cytotoxicity against certain human tumor types.

In vitro assays and in vivo animal studies have shown that cetuximab inhibits the growth and survival of tumor cells that express the EGFR. No antitumor effects of cetuximab were observed in human tumor xenografts lacking EGFR expression. The addition of cetuximab to radiation therapy or irinotecan in human tumor xenograft models in mice resulted in an increase in antitumor effects compared with radiation therapy or chemotherapy alone.

➤*Pharmacokinetics:*

Absorption/Distribution – The pharmacokinetics of cetuximab were similar in patients with SCCHN and those with colorectal cancer. Cetuximab, administered as monotherapy or in combination with concomitant chemotherapy or radiation therapy, exhibits nonlinear pharmacokinetics. The area under the curve (AUC) increased in a greater than dose proportional manner, while clearance of cetuximab decreased from 0.08 to 0.02 L/h/m^2 as the dose increased from 20 to 200 mg/m^2, and at doses greater than 200 mg/m^2, it appeared to plateau. The volume of the distribution for cetuximab appeared to be independent of dose and approximated the vascular space of 2 to 3 L/m^2.

Metabolism/Excretion – Following the recommended dose regimen (400 mg/m^2 initial dose; 250 mg/m^2 weekly dose), concentrations of cetuximab reached steady-state levels by the third weekly infusion, with mean peak and trough concentrations across studies ranging from 168 to 235 and 41 to 85 mcg/mL, respectively. The mean half-life of cetuximab was approximately 112 hours (range, 63 to 230 hours).

Warnings/Precautions

➤*Infusion reactions:* Serious infusion reactions requiring medical intervention and immediate, permanent discontinuation of cetuximab included rapid onset of airway obstruction (bronchospasm, stridor, hoarseness), hypotension, and/or cardiac arrest. Severe (NCI-CTC Grade 3 and 4) infusion reactions occurred in 2% to 5% of 1,373 patients in clinical trials, with fatal outcome in 1 patient.

Approximately 90% of severe infusion reactions occurred with the first infusion, despite premedication with antihistamines.

Monitor patients for 1 hour following cetuximab infusions in a setting with resuscitation equipment and other agents necessary to treat anaphylaxis (eg, epinephrine, corticosteroids, IV antihistamines, bronchodilators, and oxygen). Monitor longer to confirm resolution of the event in patients requiring treatment for infusion reactions.

Immediately and permanently discontinue cetuximab in patients with serious infusion reactions.

➤*Cardiopulmonary arrest:* Cardiopulmonary arrest and/or sudden death occurred in 4 (2%) of 208 patients treated with radiation therapy and cetuximab compared with none of 212 patients treated with radiation therapy alone in a randomized, controlled trial in patients with SCCHN. Three patients with a history of coronary artery disease died at home, with myocardial infarction as the presumed cause of death. One of these patients had arrhythmia and one had congestive heart failure. Death occurred 27, 32, and 43 days after the last dose of cetuximab. One patient with no prior history of coronary artery disease died one day after the last dose of cetuximab. Carefully consider use of cetuximab in combination with radiation therapy in head and neck cancer patients with a history of coronary artery disease, congestive heart failure, or arrhythmias in light of these risks. Closely monitor serum electrolytes, including serum magnesium, potassium, and calcium, during and after cetuximab.

➤*Pulmonary toxicity:* Interstitial lung disease (ILD), including 1 fatality, occurred in 4 of 1,570 (less than 0.5%) patients receiving cetuximab in clinical trials. Interrupt cetuximab for acute onset or worsening of pulmonary symptoms. Permanently discontinue cetuximab for confirmed ILD.

➤*Dermatologic toxicity:* Dermatologic toxicities, including acneform rash, skin drying and fissuring, paronychial inflammation, and infectious sequelae (for example *Staphylococcus aureus* sepsis, abscess formation, cellulitis, blepharitis, cheilitis) occurred in patients receiving cetuximab therapy. Acneform rash occurred in 76% to 88% of 1,373 patients receiving cetuximab in clinical trials. Severe acneform rash occurred in 1% to 17% of patients.

Acneform rash usually developed within the first 2 weeks of therapy and resolved in a majority of the patients after cessation of treatment, although in nearly half, the event continued beyond 28 days. Monitor patients receiving cetuximab for dermatologic toxicities and infectious sequelae. Instruct patients to limit sun exposure during cetuximab.

➤*Combination with radiation and cisplatin:* The safety of cetuximab in combination with radiation therapy and cisplatin has not been established. Death and serious cardiotoxicity were observed in a single-arm trial with cetuximab, radiation therapy, and cisplatin (100 mg/m^2) in patients with locally advanced SCCHN. Two of 21 patients died, one as a result of pneumonia and one of an unknown cause. Four patients discontinued treatment because of adverse reactions. Two of these discontinuations were due to cardiac events.

➤*Electrolyte abnormalities:* In patients evaluated during clinical trials, hypomagnesemia occurred in 55% of patients (199/365) receiving cetuximab and was severe (NCI-CTC grade 3 and 4) in 6% to 17%. The onset of hypomagnesemia and accompanying electrolyte abnormalities occurred days to months after initiation of cetuximab. Periodically monitor patients for hypomagnesemia, hypocalcemia, and hypokalemia, during and for at least 8 weeks following the completion of cetuximab. Replete electrolytes as necessary.

➤*EGFR expression and response:*

Colorectal cancer – Patients enrolled in the colorectal cancer clinical studies were required to have immunohistochemical evidence of EGFR tumor expression. Primary tumor or tumor from a metastatic site was tested with the *DakoCytomation EGFR pharmDx* test kit. Specimens were scored based on the percentage of cells expressing EGFR and intensity (barely/faint, weak to moderate, and strong). The response rate did not correlate with the percentage of positive cells or the intensity of EGFR expression.

SCCHN – Because expression of EGFR has been detected in nearly all SCCHN tumor specimens, patients enrolled in the head and neck cancer clinical studies were not required to have immunohistochemical evidence of EGFR tumor expression prior to study entry.

➤*Immunogenicity:* As with all therapeutic proteins, there is potential for immunogenicity. Immunogenic responses to cetuximab were assessed using either a double antigen radiometric assay or an enzyme-linked immunosorbent assay. Because of limitations in assay performance and sampling timing, the incidence of antibody development in patients receiving cetuximab has not been adequately determined. Nonneutralizing anticetuximab antibodies were detected in 5% (49/1,001) of evaluable patients without apparent effect on the safety or antitumor activity of cetuximab.

The incidence of antibody formation is highly dependent on the sensitivity and specificity of the assay. Additionally, the observed incidence of antibody (including neutralizing antibody) positivity in an assay may be influenced by several factors, including assay methodology, sample handling, timing of sample collection, concomitant medications, and underlying disease. For these reasons, comparison of the incidence of antibodies to cetuximab with the incidence of antibodies to other products may be misleading.

➤*Photosensitivity:* Patients should wear sunscreen and hats and limit sun exposure while receiving cetuximab because sunlight can exacerbate any skin reactions that may occur.

CETUXIMAB — INJECTION

➤*Pregnancy: Category C.* Animal reproduction studies have not been conducted with cetuximab. However, the EGFR has been implicated in the control of prenatal development and may be essential for normal organogenesis, proliferation, and differentiation in the developing embryo. In addition, human immunoglobulin G1 (IgG1) is known to cross the placental barrier; therefore, cetuximab has the potential to be transmitted from the mother to the developing fetus. It is not known whether cetuximab can cause fetal harm when administered to a pregnant woman or whether cetuximab can affect reproductive capacity. There are no adequate and well-controlled studies of cetuximab in pregnant women. Give to a pregnant woman, or any woman not employing adequate contraception, only if the potential benefit justifies the potential risk to the fetus. Counsel all patients regarding the potential risk of cetuximab treatment to the developing fetus prior to initiation of therapy. If the patient becomes pregnant while receiving this drug, apprise her of the potential hazard to the fetus and/or the potential risk of loss of the pregnancy.

➤*Lactation:* It is not known whether cetuximab is secreted in human milk. IgG antibodies, such as cetuximab, can be excreted in human milk. Because many drugs are excreted in human milk and because of the potential for serious adverse reactions in breast-feeding infants from cetuximab, decide whether to discontinue breast-feeding or the drug, taking into account the importance of the drug to the mother. If breast-feeding is interrupted, based on the mean half-life of cetuximab, do not resume breast-feeding earlier than 60 days following the last dose of cetuximab.

➤*Children:* The safety and effectiveness of cetuximab in children have not been established. The pharmacokinetics of cetuximab have not been studied in children.

➤*Monitoring:* Monitor patients for 1 hour following cetuximab infusion. Longer observation periods may be required in those who experience infusion reactions.

Monitor patients for dermatologic toxicities and infectious sequelae while receiving cetuximab, and initiate appropriate treatment.

Periodically monitor patients for hypomagnesemia, hypocalcemia, and hypokalemia during and for at least 8 weeks following the completion of cetuximab therapy.

Adverse Reactions

Cetuximab is considered to have moderately low emetogenic potential (10% to 30% incidence of emesis).

The most common adverse reactions with cetuximab (incidence of 25% or more) are cutaneous adverse reactions (including rash, pruritus, and nail changes), headache, diarrhea, and infection.

The most serious adverse reactions with cetuximab are infusion reactions, cardiopulmonary arrest, dermatologic toxicity and radiation dermatitis, sepsis, renal failure, interstitial lung disease, and pulmonary embolus.

Across all studies, cetuximab was discontinued in 3% to 10% of patients because of adverse reactions.

➤*SCCHN:* The following table contains selected adverse reactions in 420 patients receiving radiation therapy either alone or with cetuximab for locally or regionally advanced SCCHN in study 1. Cetuximab was administered at the recommended dose and schedule (400 mg/m^2 initial dose, followed by 250 mg/m^2 weekly). Patients received a median of 8 infusions (range, 1 to 11).

Cetuximab Adverse Reactions (≥ 10%) in Patients With Locoregionally Advanced SCCHN

Adverse reaction	Cetuximab plus radiation (n = 208) Grades 1 to 4	Cetuximab plus radiation (n = 208) Grades 3 and 4	Radiation therapy alone (n = 212) Grades 1 to 4	Radiation therapy alone (n = 212) Grades 3 and 4
CNS				
Asthenia	56%	4%	49%	5%
Headache	19%	< 1%	8%	< 1%
Dermatologic				
Acneform rash[a]	87%	17%	10%	1%
Application-site reaction	18%	0%	12%	1%
Pruritus	16%	0%	4%	0%
Radiation dermatitis	86%	23%	90%	18%
GI				
Diarrhea	19%	2%	13%	1%
Dyspepsia	14%	0%	9%	1%
Emesis	29%	2%	23%	4%
Nausea	49%	2%	37%	2%
Metabolic/Nutritional				
Dehydration	25%	6%	19%	8%
Weight loss	84%	11%	72%	7%
Respiratory				
Pharyngitis	26%	3%	19%	4%
Miscellaneous				
Chills[b]	16%	0%	5%	0%
Fever[b]	29%	1%	13%	1%
Infection	13%	1%	9%	1%
Infusion reaction[c]	15%	3%	2%	0%

[a] Acneform rash is defined as any event described as acne, rash, maculopapular rash, pustular rash, dry skin, or exfoliative dermatitis.
[b] Includes cases also reported as infusion reaction.
[c] Infusion reaction is defined as any event described at any time during the clinical study as allergic reaction or anaphylactoid reaction, or any event occurring on the first day of dosing described as allergic reaction, anaphylactoid reaction, fever, chills, chills and fever, or dyspnea.

The incidence and severity of mucositis, stomatitis, and xerostomia were similar in both arms of the study.

➤*Late radiation toxicity:* The overall incidence of late radiation toxicities (any grade) was higher in cetuximab in combination with radiation therapy compared with radiation therapy alone. The following sites were affected: salivary glands (65% vs 56%), larynx (52% vs 36%), subcutaneous tissue (49% vs 45%), mucous membrane (48% vs 39%), esophagus (44% vs 35%), and skin (42% vs 33%). The incidence of grade 3 or 4 late radiation toxicities was similar between the radiation therapy alone and the cetuximab plus radiation treatment groups.

➤*Colorectal cancer:* Cetuximab was administered at the recommended dose and schedule (400 mg/m^2 initial dose, followed by 250 mg/m^2 weekly).

Cetuximab Monotherapy Adverse Reactions Occurring in Patients With Advanced Colorectal Carcinoma (≥ 10%)[a]

Adverse reaction	Cetuximab plus best supportive care (n = 288) Any grades[b]	Cetuximab plus best supportive care (n = 288) Grades 3 and 4	Best supportive care alone (n = 274) Any grades	Best supportive care alone (n = 274) Grades 3 and 4
CNS				
Anxiety	14%	2%	8%	1%
Confusion	15%	6%	9%	2%
Depression	13%	1%	6%	< 1%
Fatigue	89%	33%	76%	26%
Headache	33%	4%	11%	0%
Insomnia	30%	1%	15%	1%
Dermatologic				
Dry skin	49%	0%	11%	0%
Nail changes	21%	0%	4%	0%
Other (dermatology)	27%	1%	6%	1%
Pruritus	40%	2%	8%	0%
Rash/Desquamation	89%	12%	16%	< 1%
GI				
Abdominal pain	59%	14%	52%	16%
Constipation	46%	4%	38%	5%
Diarrhea	39%	2%	20%	2%
Mouth dryness	11%	0%	4%	0%
Other (GI)	23%	10%	18%	8%
Stomatitis	25%	1%	10%	< 1%
Vomiting	37%	6%	29%	6%
Musculoskeletal				
Bone pain	15%	3%	7%	2%
Pain, other	51%	16%	34%	7%
Pulmonary				
Cough	29%	2%	19%	1%
Dyspnea	48%	16%	43%	12%

CETUXIMAB — INJECTION

Cetuximab Monotherapy Adverse Reactions Occurring in Patients With Advanced Colorectal Carcinoma (≥ 10%)[a]

Adverse reaction	Cetuximab plus best supportive care (n = 288)		Best supportive care alone (n = 274)	
	Any grades[b]	Grades 3 and 4	Any grades	Grades 3 and 4
Miscellaneous				
Infection without neutropenia	35%	13%	17%	6%
Infusion reactions[c]	20%	5%		
Fever	30%	1%	18%	< 1%
Rigors, chills	13%	< 1%	4%	0%

[a] Adverse reactions occurring more frequently in cetuximab-treated patients than in controls.
[b] Adverse reactions were graded using the NCI-CTC, version 2.
[c] Infusion reaction is defined as any reaction (chills, rigors, dyspnea, tachycardia, bronchospasm, chest tightness, swelling, urticaria, hypotension, flushing, rash, hypertension, nausea, angioedema, pain, pruritus, sweating, tremors, shaking, cough, visual disturbances, or other) recorded by the investigator as infusion related.

The most frequently reported adverse reactions in 354 patients treated with cetuximab plus irinotecan in clinical trials were acneform rash (88%), asthenia/malaise (73%), diarrhea (72%), and nausea (55%). The most common grade 3/4 adverse reactions included diarrhea (22%), leukopenia (17%), asthenia/malaise (16%), and acneform rash (14%).

➤*Infusion reactions:* Infusion reactions, which included pyrexia, chills, rigors, dyspnea, bronchospasm, angioedema, urticaria, hypertension, and hypotension occurred in 15% to 21% of patients across studies. Grades 3 and 4 infusion reactions occurred in 2% to 5% of patients; infusion reactions were fatal in 1 patient.

➤*Infections:* The incidence of infection was variable across studies, ranging from 13% to 35%. Sepsis occurred in 1% to 4% of patients.

➤*Renal:* Renal failure occurred in 1% of patients with colorectal cancer.

Overdosage

The maximum single dose of cetuximab administered is 1,000 mg/m^2 in 1 patient. No adverse reactions were reported for this patient.

Patient Information

Advise patients to report signs and symptoms of infusion reactions such as fever, chills, or breathing problems.

Advise patients of the potential risks of using cetuximab during pregnancy or breast-feeding and of the need to use adequate contraception in both men and women during and for 6 months following the last dose of cetuximab therapy.

Inform patients that breast-feeding is not recommended during, and for 2 months following, the last dose of cetuximab therapy.

Advise patients to limit sun exposure (use sunscreen, wear hats) while receiving, and for 2 months following, the last dose of cetuximab.

BEVACIZUMAB

Rx	**Avastin** (Genentech)	**Injection, solution, concentrate:** 25 mg/mL	Preservative free. In single-use 4[a] and 16 mL[b] vials.

[a] With alpha,alpha-trehalose dihydrate 240 mg, sodium phosphate (monobasic, monohydrate) 23.2 mg, sodium phosphate (dibasic, anhydrous) 4.8 mg, 1.6 mg of polysorbate 20.

[b] With alpha,alpha-trehalose dihydrate 960 mg, sodium phosphate (monobasic, monohydrate) 92.8 mg, sodium phosphate (dibasic, anhydrous) 19.2 mg, 6.4 mg polysorbate 20.

BEVACIZUMAB — INJECTION

WARNING

GI perforations – The incidence of GI perforations, some fatal, in bevacizumab-treated patients ranges from 0.3% to 2.4%. Discontinue bevacizumab in patients with GI perforation.

Surgery and wound healing complications – The incidence of wound healing and surgical complications, including serious and fatal complications, is increased in bevacizumab-treated patients. Discontinue bevacizumab in patients with wound dehiscence. The appropriate interval between termination of bevacizumab and subsequent elective surgery required to reduce the risks of impaired wound healing/wound dehiscence has not been determined. Discontinue at least 28 days prior to elective surgery. Do not initiate bevacizumab for at least 28 days after surgery and until the surgical wound is fully healed.

Hemorrhage – Severe or fatal hemorrhage, including hemoptysis, GI bleeding, CNS hemorrhage, epistaxis, and vaginal bleeding, occurred up to 5-fold more frequently in patients receiving bevacizumab. Do not administer bevacizumab to patients with serious hemorrhage or recent hemoptysis.

Indications

➤*Glioblastoma:* As single agent therapy for the treatment of glioblastoma with progressive disease following prior therapy.

➤*Metastatic breast cancer:* In combination with paclitaxel for the treatment of patients who have not received chemotherapy for metastatic human epidermal growth factor receptor 2 (HER2)–negative breast cancer.

➤*Metastatic colorectal cancer:* In combination with intravenous (IV) 5-fluorouracil–based chemotherapy for first- or second-line treatment of patients with metastatic carcinoma of the colon or rectum.

➤*Metastatic renal cell carcinoma:* In combination with interferon alfa for the treatment of patients with metastatic renal cell carcinoma.

➤*Nonsquamous non–small cell lung cancer:* In combination with carboplatin and paclitaxel for the first-line treatment of patients with unresectable, locally advanced, recurrent or metastatic nonsquamous non–small cell lung cancer.

➤*Off-label uses:*

Age-related macular degeneration – [1] = Good documentation. The American Academy of Ophthalmology Preferred Practice Pattern guidelines recommend the use of intravitreal bevacizumab in the treatment of neovascular age-related macular degeneration.

Other possible off-label uses – In combination with erlotinib to treat metastatic renal cell carcinoma.

Administration and Dosage

➤*General dosing considerations:* Do not initiate bevacizumab therapy until at least 28 days following major surgery. (See Surgery.)

Patients should continue treatment until disease progression or unacceptable toxicity.

➤*Adults:*

Glioblastoma – 10 mg/kg as an IV infusion every 2 weeks.

Metastatic breast cancer – 10 mg/kg as an IV infusion every 14 days in combination with paclitaxel.

Metastatic colorectal cancer – 5 to 10 mg/kg as an IV infusion every 14 days in combination with IV 5-fluorouracil–based chemotherapy.

When used in combination with bolus irinotecan/5-fluorouracil/leucovorin, the dose of bevacizumab is 5 mg/kg.

When used in combination with 5-fluorouracil/leucovorin/oxaliplatin, the dose of bevacizumab is 10 mg/kg.

Metastatic renal cell carcinoma – 10 mg/kg as an IV injection every 14 days in combination with interferon alfa.

Nonsquamous non–small cell lung cancer – 15 mg/kg as an IV infusion every 3 weeks in combination with carboplatin and paclitaxel.

Off-label dosing –

Age-related macular degeneration: [1] = Good documentation. Intravitreal bevacizumab 1.25 to 2.5 mg monthly.

➤*Dosage adjustment:* There are no recommended dose reductions for the use of bevacizumab. If needed, discontinue or temporarily suspend bevacizumab therapy.

Discontinuation – Discontinue bevacizumab therapy in patients who develop GI perforation (GI perforation, fistula formation in the GI tract, intra-abdominal abscess), fistula formation involving an internal organ, wound dehiscence and wound-healing complications requiring medical intervention, serious hemorrhage (ie, requiring medical interventions), a severe arterial thromboembolic event, nephrotic syndrome, hypertensive crisis, reversible posterior leukoencephalopathy syndrome, or hypertensive encephalopathy.

Temporary suspension – Temporary suspension of bevacizumab therapy is recommended in patients with evidence of moderate to severe proteinuria pending further evaluation, with severe infusion reactions, and with severe hypertension that is not controlled with medical management.

Surgery – Suspend bevacizumab therapy at least 4 weeks prior to elective surgery and do not resume until the surgical incision is fully healed.

BEVACIZUMAB — INJECTION

➤*Preparation for administration:* Withdraw the necessary amount of bevacizumab and dilute in a total volume of 100 mL of sodium chloride 0.9% injection. Discard any unused portion left in the vial because the product contains no preservatives.

➤*Administration:* Do not administer as an IV push or bolus. Administer only as an IV infusion. Deliver the initial bevacizumab dose over 90 minutes as an IV infusion following chemotherapy. If the first infusion is well tolerated, the second infusion may be administered over 60 minutes. If the 60-minute infusion is well tolerated, all subsequent infusions may be administered over 30 minutes.

➤*Admixture compatibility:* Do not administer or mix bevacizumab infusions with dextrose solutions.

➤*Storage/Stability:* Bevacizumab vials are stable at 2° to 8°C (36° to 46°F). Protect vials from light. Store in the original carton until time of use. Do not freeze or shake. Diluted bevacizumab solutions for infusion may be stored at 2° to 8°C (36° to 46°F) for up to 8 hours.

Actions

➤*Pharmacology:* Bevacizumab binds vascular endothelial growth factor (VEGF) and prevents the interaction of VEGF to its receptors (Flt-1 and KDR) on the surface of endothelial cells. The interaction of VEGF with its receptors leads to endothelial cell proliferation and new blood vessel formation in in vitro models of angiogenesis. Administration of bevacizumab to xenotransplant models of colon cancer in nude (athymic) mice caused a reduction of microvascular growth and inhibition of metastatic disease progression.

➤*Pharmacokinetics:*

Absorption/Distribution – Based on a population pharmacokinetic analysis of 491 patients who received bevacizumab 1 to 20 mg/kg weekly, every 2 weeks, or every 3 weeks, the predicted time to reach steady state was 100 days. The accumulation ratio was 2.8 following a dose of bevacizumab 10 mg/kg every 2 weeks.

Metabolism/Excretion – The estimated half-life of bevacizumab was approximately 20 days (range, 11 to 50 days). The relationship between bevacizumab exposure and clinical outcomes has not been explored.

Special populations –

Gender: The clearance of bevacizumab varied by body weight and gender. After correcting for body weight, men had a higher bevacizumab clearance (0.262 vs 0.207 L/day) and a larger volume of distribution in the central compartment (3.25 vs 2.66 L) than women. In study 1, there was no evidence of lesser efficacy (hazard ratio [HR] for overall survival) in men treated with bevacizumab compared with women.

Tumor burden: The clearance of bevacizumab varied by tumor burden. Patients with higher tumor burden (at or above median value of tumor surface area) had a higher bevacizumab clearance (0.249 vs 0.199 L/day) than patients with tumor burdens below the median. In study 1, there was no evidence of lesser efficacy (HR for overall survival) in patients with higher tumor burden treated with bevacizumab compared with patients with low tumor burden.

Contraindications

None well documented.

Warnings/Precautions

➤*GI perforations:* See the Warning box for more information.

The typical presentation may include abdominal pain, nausea, emesis, constipation, and fever. Perforation can be complicated by intra-abdominal abscess and fistula formation. The majority of cases occurred within the first 50 days of initiation of bevacizumab.

➤*Surgery and wound healing complications:* Bevacizumab impairs wound healing in animal models. In clinical trials, administration of bevacizumab was not allowed until at least 28 days after surgery. In a controlled clinical trial, the incidence of wound healing complications, including serious and fatal complications, was 15% in patients with metastatic colorectal cancer who underwent surgery during the course of bevacizumab treatment, and was 4% in patients who did not receive bevacizumab.

See the Warning box for more information.

➤*Hemorrhage:* Bevacizumab can result in 2 distinct patterns of bleeding: minor hemorrhage (most commonly grade 1 epistaxis), and serious (in some cases fatal) hemorrhagic events.

Severe or fatal hemorrhage, including hemoptysis, GI bleeding, hematemesis, CNS hemorrhage, epistaxis, and vaginal bleeding, occurred up to 5-fold more frequently in patients receiving bevacizumab compared with patients receiving only chemotherapy. Across indications, the incidence of grade 3 or higher hemorrhagic events among patients receiving bevacizumab ranged from 1.2% to 4.6%.

Serious or fatal pulmonary hemorrhage occurred in 31% of patients with squamous cell histology and 4% of patients with nonsquamous non–small cell lung cancer receiving bevacizumab and chemotherapy compared with none of the patients receiving chemotherapy alone.

In clinical studies in non–small cell lung cancer where patients with CNS metastases who completed radiation and surgery more than 4 weeks prior to the start of bevacizumab were evaluated with serial CNS imaging, symptomatic grade 2 CNS hemorrhage was documented in 1 of 83 bevacizumab-treated patients (rate, 1.2%; 95% CI, 0.06% to 5.93%).

Intracranial hemorrhage occurred in 8 of 163 patients with previously treated glioblastoma; 2 patients had grade 3 to 4 hemorrhage.

Do not administer bevacizumab to patients with recent history of hemoptysis of one-half teaspoon or more of red blood. Discontinue bevacizumab therapy in patients with hemorrhage.

➤*Non-GI fistula formation:* Serious and sometimes fatal non-GI fistula formation involving tracheoesophageal, bronchopleural, biliary, vaginal, renal, and bladder sites occurred at a higher incidence in bevacizumab-treated patients compared with controls. The incidence of non-GI perforation was less than 0.3% in clinical studies. Most events occurred within the first 6 months of bevacizumab therapy.

Discontinue bevacizumab therapy in patients with fistula formation involving an internal organ.

➤*Arterial thromboembolic events:* Serious, sometimes fatal, arterial thromboembolic events, including cerebral infarction, transient ischemic attacks, myocardial infarction (MI), angina, and a variety of other arterial thromboembolic events, occurred at a higher incidence in patients receiving bevacizumab compared with those in the control arm.

Across indications, the incidence of grade 3 or higher arterial thromboembolic events in the bevacizumab-containing arms was 2.4% compared with 0.7% in the control arms. Among patients receiving bevacizumab in combination with chemotherapy, the risk of developing arterial thromboembolic events during therapy was increased in patients with a history of arterial thromboembolism, or age older than 65 years.

The safety of resumption of bevacizumab therapy after resolution of an arterial thromboembolic event has not been studied. Discontinue bevacizumab therapy in patients who experience a severe arterial thromboembolic event during treatment.

➤*Hypertension:* The incidence of severe hypertension was increased in patients receiving bevacizumab compared with controls. Across clinical studies, the incidence of grade 3 or 4 hypertension ranged from 5% to 18%.

Monitor blood pressure every 2 to 3 weeks during treatment with bevacizumab. Treat with appropriate antihypertensive therapy and monitor blood pressure regularly. Continue to monitor blood pressure at regular intervals in patients with bevacizumab-induced or bevacizumab-exacerbated hypertension after discontinuation of bevacizumab therapy.

Discontinue bevacizumab therapy in patients with hypertensive crisis or hypertensive encephalopathy. Temporarily suspend bevacizumab therapy in patients with severe hypertension not controlled with medical management.

➤*Reversible posterior leukoencephalopathy syndrome:* Reversible posterior leukoencephalopathy syndrome has been reported in clinical studies with an incidence of less than 0.1%. Reversible posterior leukoencephalopathy syndrome is a neurological disorder that can present with headache, seizure, lethargy, confusion, blindness, and other visual and neurologic disturbances. Mild to severe hypertension may be present. Magnetic resonance imaging is necessary to confirm the diagnosis of reversible posterior leukoencephalopathy syndrome. The onset of symptoms occurred from 16 hours to 1 year after initiation of bevacizumab therapy.

Discontinue bevacizumab therapy in patients who develop reversible posterior leukoencephalopathy syndrome. Symptoms usually resolve or improve within days, although some patients have experienced ongoing neurologic sequelae. The safety of reinitiating bevacizumab therapy in patients who have previously experienced reversible posterior leukoencephalopathy syndrome is not known.

➤*Proteinuria:* The incidence and severity of proteinuria are increased in patients receiving bevacizumab compared with control.

Nephrotic syndrome, in some cases with fatal outcome, occurred in less than 1% of patients receiving bevacizumab in the clinical trials. In a published case series, kidney biopsy of 6 patients with proteinuria showed findings consistent with thrombotic microangiopathy.

Monitor proteinuria by dipstick urine analysis for the development or worsening of proteinuria with serial urinalyses during bevacizumab therapy. Patients with a 2+ or greater urine dipstick reading should undergo further assessment (eg, a 24-hour urine collection).

Discontinue bevacizumab therapy in patients with nephrotic syndrome. Temporarily suspend bevacizumab therapy in patients with 2 g or more of proteinuria per 24 hours and resume when proteinuria is less than 2 g per 24 hours. Data from a postmarketing safety study showed poor correlation between urine protein/creatinine ratio (UPCR) and 24-hour urine protein (Pearson correlation, 0.39; 95% CI, 0.17% to 0.57%). The safety of continued bevacizumab treatment in patients with moderate to severe proteinuria has not been evaluated.

➤*Congestive heart failure:* The incidence of grade 3 or higher left ventricular dysfunction was 1% in patients receiving bevacizumab compared with 0.6% in the control arm across indications. In patients with metastatic breast cancer, the incidence of grade 3 to 4 congestive heart failure (CHF) was increased in patients in the bevacizumab plus paclitaxel arm (2.2%) compared with the control arm (0.3%). Among patients receiving prior anthracyclines for metastatic breast cancer, the rate of CHF was 3.8% for bevacizumab-treated patients and 0.6% for patients receiving paclitaxel alone.

The safety of continuation or resumption of bevacizumab in patients with cardiac dysfunction has not been studied.

BEVACIZUMAB — INJECTION

➤*Infusion reactions:* Infusion reactions reported in the clinical trials and postmarketing experience include hypertension, hypertensive crises associated with neurologic signs and symptoms, wheezing, oxygen desaturation, grade 3 hypersensitivity, chest pain, headaches, rigors, and diaphoresis. In clinical studies, infusion reactions with the first dose of bevacizumab were uncommon (less than 3%), and severe reactions occurred in 0.2% of patients. Stop infusion if a severe infusion reaction occurs and administer appropriate medical therapy.

➤*Immunogenicity:* As with all therapeutic proteins, there is a potential for immunogenicity. The incidence of antibody development in patients receiving bevacizumab has not been adequately determined because the assay sensitivity was inadequate to reliably detect lower titers. Enzyme-linked immunosorbent assays were performed on sera from approximately 500 patients treated with bevacizumab, primarily in combination with chemotherapy. High titer human antibevacizumab antibodies were not detected.

➤*Pregnancy: Category C.* There are no studies of bevacizumab in pregnant women. Reproduction studies in rabbits treated with approximately 1 to 12 times the recommended human dose of bevacizumab resulted in teratogenicity, including an increased incidence of specific gross and skeletal fetal alterations. Adverse fetal outcomes were observed at all doses tested. Other observed effects included decreases in maternal and fetal body weights and an increased number of fetal resorptions. Pregnant rabbits dosed with 1 to 12 times the human dose of bevacizumab every 3 days during the period of organogenesis (gestation days 6 to 18) exhibited teratogenic effects, decreases in maternal and fetal body weights, and increased number of fetal resorptions. Teratogenic effects included reduced or irregular ossification in the skull, jaw, spine, ribs, tibia, and bones of the paws; meningocele; fontanel, rib, and hind limb deformities; corneal opacity; and absent hind limb phalanges. There are no data available regarding the level of bevacizumab exposure in the offspring.

Human immunoglobulin G is known to cross the placental barrier; therefore, bevacizumab may be transmitted from the mother to the developing fetus, and has the potential to cause fetal harm when administered to pregnant women. Because of the observed teratogenic effects of known inhibitors of angiogenesis in humans, use bevacizumab during pregnancy only if the potential benefit justifies the potential risk to the fetus.

➤*Lactation:* It is not known whether bevacizumab is secreted in human milk, but human IgG is excreted in human milk. Therefore, expect the excretion into milk of the closely related bevacizumab. Published data suggest that breast milk antibodies do not enter the neonatal and infant circulation in substantial amounts. Because many drugs are secreted in human milk and because of the potential for serious adverse reactions in breast-feeding infants from bevacizumab, decide whether to discontinue breast-feeding or the drug, taking into account the half-life of the product (approximately 20 days [range, 11 to 50 days]), and the importance of the drug to the mother.

➤*Children:* The safety and effectiveness of bevacizumab therapy in children have not been established.

Juvenile cynomolgus monkeys with open growth plates exhibited physeal dysplasia following 4 to 26 weeks' exposure at 0.4 to 20 times the recommended human dose (based on mg/kg and exposure). The incidence and severity of physeal dysplasia were dose-related and were partially reversible upon cessation of treatment.

➤*Elderly:* In study 1, severe adverse reactions that occurred at a higher incidence (at least 2%) in patients 65 years of age and older compared with younger patients were anemia, anorexia, asthenia, CHF, constipation, dehydration, diarrhea, deep thrombophlebitis, hypertension, hypokalemia, hyponatremia, hypotension, leukopenia, MI, and sepsis. The effect of bevacizumab on overall survival was similar in elderly patients compared with younger patients.

In study 2, patients 65 years of age and older receiving bevacizumab plus 5-fluorouracil/leucovorin/oxaliplatin had a greater relative risk compared with younger patients for the following adverse reactions: emesis, fatigue, ileus, and nausea.

In study 4, patients 65 years of age and older receiving carboplatin, paclitaxel, and bevacizumab had a greater relative risk for proteinuria compared with younger patients.

Of the 742 patients enrolled in the manufacturer-sponsored clinical studies in which all adverse reactions were assessed, 29% were 65 years of age and older and 6% were 75 years of age and older. Adverse reactions of any severity that occurred at a higher incidence in elderly patients compared with younger patients, in addition to those previously described, were dyspepsia, edema, epistaxis, GI hemorrhage, increased cough, and voice alteration.

In an exploratory, pooled analysis of 1,745 patients treated in 5 randomized, controlled studies, there were 618 patients 65 years of age and older and 1,127 patients younger than 65 years of age. The overall incidence of arterial thromboembolic events was increased in all patients receiving bevacizumab with chemotherapy compared with those receiving chemotherapy alone, regardless of age. However, the increase in arterial thromboembolic events incidence was greater in patients 65 years of age and older (8.5% vs 2.9%) compared with those younger than 65 years of age (2.1% vs 1.4%).

➤*Monitoring:* Conduct blood pressure monitoring every 2 to 3 weeks during treatment with bevacizumab. Continue to monitor the blood pressure at regular intervals of patients with bevacizumab-induced or bevacizumab-exacerbated hypertension who discontinue bevacizumab therapy.

Monitor proteinuria by dipstick urine analysis and for worsening of proteinuria with serial urinalysis. Further assess (eg, a 24-hour urine collection) patients with a 2+ or greater urine dipstick reading.

Drug Interactions

A drug interaction study was performed in which irinotecan was administered as part of the leucovorin, fluorouracil, and irinotecan regimen with or without bevacizumab. The results demonstrated no significant effect of bevacizumab on the pharmacokinetics of irinotecan or its active metabolite SN38.

In a randomized study in 99 patients with nonsquamous non–small cell lung cancer, based on limited data, there did not appear to be a difference in the mean exposure of either carboplatin or paclitaxel when each was administered alone or in combination with bevacizumab. However, 3 of the 8 patients receiving bevacizumab plus paclitaxel/carboplatin had substantially lower paclitaxel exposure after 4 cycles of treatment (at day 63) than those at day 0, while patients receiving paclitaxel/carboplatin without bevacizumab had a greater paclitaxel exposure at day 63 than at day 0.

In study 9, there was no difference in the mean exposure of interferon alfa administered in combination with bevacizumab when compared with interferon alfa alone.

➤*Concomitant chemotherapy:* Bevacizumab plus paclitaxel/carboplatin resulted in substantially lower paclitaxel exposure after 4 cycles of treatment (at day 63) than those at day 0, and paclitaxel/carboplatin without bevacizumab resulted in a greater paclitaxel exposure at day 63 than at day 0.

Adverse Reactions

➤*Most common adverse reactions:* The most common adverse reactions observed in bevacizumab patients at a rate of greater than 10% and at least twice the control arm rate are back pain, dry skin, epistaxis, exfoliative dermatitis, headache, hypertension, lacrimation disorder, proteinuria, rectal hemorrhage, rhinitis, and taste alteration.

➤*Discontinuation:* Across all studies, bevacizumab was discontinued in 8.4% to 21% of patients because of adverse reactions.

➤*Metastatic colorectal cancer:*

Study 1 –

Bevacizumab Grade 3 to 4 Adverse Reactions in Patients With Metastatic Colorectal Cancer (≥ 2%)

Adverse reactions	Arm 1 irinotecan/ 5-fluorouracil/ leucovorin + placebo (n = 396)	Arm 2 irinotecan/ 5-fluorouracil/ leucovorin + bevacizumab (n = 392)
NCI-CTC[a] grade 3 to 4 reactions	74%	87%
Cardiovascular		
Deep vein thrombosis	5%	9%
Hypertension	2%	12%
Intra-abdominal thrombosis	1%	3%
Syncope	1%	3%
GI		
Abdominal pain	5%	8%
Constipation	2%	4%
Diarrhea	25%	34%
Hematologic/Lymphatic		
Leukopenia	31%	37%
Neutropenia[b]	14%	21%
Miscellaneous		
Asthenia	7%	10%
Pain	5%	8%

[a] NCI-CTC = National Cancer Institute Common Toxicity Criteria.
[b] Central laboratories were collected on days 1 and 21 of each cycle. Neutrophil counts are available in 303 patients in arm 1 and 276 in arm 2.

Bevacizumab NCI-CTC Grade 1 to 4 Adverse Reactions in Patients With Metastatic Colorectal Cancer (≥ 5%)

Adverse reactions	Arm 1 irinotecan/ 5-fluorouracil/ leucovorin + placebo (n = 98)	Arm 2 irinotecan/ 5-fluorouracil/ leucovorin + bevacizumab (n = 102)	Arm 3 5-fluorouracil/ leucovorin + bevacizumab (n = 109)
Cardiovascular			
Deep vein thrombosis	3%	9%	6%
Hypertension	14%	23%	34%
Hypotension	7%	15%	7%

BEVACIZUMAB — INJECTION

Bevacizumab NCI-CTC Grade 1 to 4 Adverse Reactions in Patients With Metastatic Colorectal Cancer (≥ 5%)			
Adverse reactions	Arm 1 irinotecan/ 5-fluorouracil/ leucovorin + placebo (n = 98)	Arm 2 irinotecan/ 5-fluorouracil/ leucovorin + bevacizumab (n = 102)	Arm 3 5-fluorouracil/ leucovorin + bevacizumab (n = 109)
CNS			
Dizziness	20%	26%	19%
Headache	19%	26%	26%
Dermatologic			
Alopecia	26%	32%	6%
Skin ulcer	1%	6%	6%
GI			
Abdominal pain	55%	61%	50%
Anorexia	30%	43%	35%
Colitis	1%	6%	1%
Constipation	29%	40%	29%
Dry mouth	2%	7%	4%
Dyspepsia	15%	24%	17%
GI hemorrhage	6%	24%	19%
Stomatitis	18%	32%	30%
Vomiting	47%	52%	47%
Respiratory			
Dyspnea	15%	26%	25%
Epistaxis	10%	35%	32%
Upper respiratory tract infection	39%	47%	40%
Special senses			
Taste disorder	9%	14%	21%
Voice alteration	2%	9%	6%
Miscellaneous			
Pain	55%	61%	62%
Proteinuria	24%	36%	36%
Thrombocytopenia	0%	5%	5%
Weight loss	10%	15%	16%

Study 2 – Only grade 3 to 5 nonhematologic and grade 4 to 5 hematologic adverse reactions related to treatment were collected in study 2. The most frequent adverse reactions (selected grade 3 to 5 nonhematologic and grade 4 to 5 hematologic adverse reactions) occurring at a higher incidence (2% or more) in 287 patients receiving 5-fluorouracil/leucovorin/oxaliplatin plus bevacizumab compared with 285 patients receiving 5-fluorouracil/leucovorin/oxaliplatin alone were fatigue (19% vs 13%), diarrhea (18% vs 13%), sensory neuropathy (17% vs 9%), nausea (12% vs 5%), vomiting (11% vs 4%), dehydration (10% vs 5%), hypertension (9% vs 2%), abdominal pain (8% vs 5%), hemorrhage (5% vs 1%), other neurological (5% vs 3%), ileus (4% vs 1%), and headache (3% vs 0%). These data are likely to underestimate the true adverse reaction rates because of the reporting mechanisms used in study 2.

➤*Unresectable nonsquamous non–small cell lung cancer:*

Study 4 – Only grade 3 to 5 nonhematologic and grade 4 to 5 hematologic adverse reactions were collected in study 4. Grade 3 to 5 nonhematologic and grade 4 to 5 hematologic adverse reactions occurring at a higher incidence (2% or more) in 427 patients receiving paclitaxel plus bevacizumab compared with 441 patients receiving paclitaxel alone were neutropenia (27% vs 17%), fatigue (16% vs 13%), hypertension (8% vs 0.7%), infection without neutropenia (7% vs 3%), venous thrombus/embolism (5% vs 3%), febrile neutropenia (5% vs 2%), pneumonitis/pulmonary infiltrates (5% vs 3%), infection with grade 3 or 4 neutropenia (4% vs 2%), hyponatremia (4% vs 1%), headache (3% vs 1%), and proteinuria (3% vs 0%).

➤*Metastatic breast cancer:*

Study 5 – Only grade 3 to 5 nonhematologic and grade 4 to 5 hematologic adverse reactions were collected in study 5. Grade 3 to 4 adverse reactions occurring at a higher incidence (2% or more) in 363 patients receiving paclitaxel plus bevacizumab compared with 348 patients receiving paclitaxel alone were sensory neuropathy (24% vs 18%), hypertension (16% vs 1%), fatigue (11% vs 5%), infection without neutropenia (9% vs 5%), neutrophils (6% vs 3%), vomiting (6% vs 2%), diarrhea (5% vs 1%), bone pain (4% vs 2%), headache (4% vs 1%), nausea (4% vs 1%), cerebrovascular ischemia (3% vs 0%), dehydration (3% vs 1%), infection with unknown absolute neutrophil count (3% vs 0.3%), rash/desquamation (3% vs 0.3%), and proteinuria (3% vs 0%).

Other adverse reactions: Fatigue, hypertension, and sensory neuropathy were reported at a 5% or more higher absolute incidence in the paclitaxel plus bevacizumab arm compared with the paclitaxel alone arm.

Fatal adverse reactions: Fatal adverse reactions occurred in 1.7% of patients who received paclitaxel plus bevacizumab. Causes of death were GI perforation (n = 2), MI (n = 2), and diarrhea/abdominal pain/weakness/hypotension (n = 2).

Study 6 – Bevacizumab is not approved for use in combination with capecitabine or for use in second- or third-line treatment of metastatic breast cancer. The following data are presented to provide information on the overall safety profile of bevacizumab in women with breast cancer because study 6 is the only randomized, controlled study in which all adverse reactions were collected for all patients. All patients in study 6 received prior anthracycline and taxane adjuvant therapy or for metastatic disease. Grade 1 to 4 events that occurred at a higher incidence (5% or more) in patients receiving capecitabine plus bevacizumab compared with the capecitabine alone arm are presented in the following table.

Bevacizumab NCI-CTC Grade 1 to 4 Adverse Reactions in Patients With Metastatic Breast Cancer (≥ 5%)		
Adverse reactions	Capecitabine + bevacizumab (n = 229)	Capecitabine (n = 215)
CNS		
Asthenia	57%	47%
Headache	33%	13%
Respiratory		
Dyspnea	27%	18%
Epistaxis	16%	1%
Miscellaneous		
Albuminuria	22%	7%
Exfoliative dermatitis	84%	75%
Hypertension	24%	2%
Myalgia	14%	8%
Pain	31%	25%
Stomatitis	25%	19%
Weight loss	9%	4%

➤*Glioblastoma:* In patients receiving bevacizumab alone (n = 84), the most frequently reported adverse reactions of any grade were infection (55%), fatigue (45%), headache (37%), hypertension (30%), epistaxis (19%), and diarrhea (21%). Of these, the incidence of grade 3 or higher adverse reactions was infection (10%), fatigue (4%), headache (4%), hypertension (8%), and diarrhea (1%). Two deaths during the study were possibly related to bevacizumab: 1 retroperitoneal hemorrhage and 1 neutropenic infection.

In patients receiving bevacizumab alone or bevacizumab plus irinotecan (n = 163), the incidence of bevacizumab-related adverse reactions (grade 1 to 4) were bleeding/hemorrhage (40%), hypertension (32%), epistaxis (26%), venous thromboembolic event (8%), arterial thromboembolic event, wound-healing complications (6%), CNS hemorrhage (5%), proteinuria (4%), GI perforation (2%), and reversible posterior leukoencephalopathy syndrome (1%). The incidence of grade 3 to 5 reactions in these 163 patients were venous thromboembolic event (7%), hypertension (5%), arterial thromboembolic event, wound-healing complications (3%), bleeding/hemorrhage, GI perforation (2%), and CNS hemorrhage, proteinuria (1%).

➤*Metastatic renal cell carcinoma:*

Study 9 – All grade adverse reactions were collected in study 9. Grade 3 to 5 adverse reactions occurring at a higher incidence (2% or more) in 337 patients receiving interferon alfa plus bevacizumab compared with 304 patients receiving interferon alfa plus placebo were fatigue (13% vs 8%), asthenia (10% vs 7%), proteinuria (7% vs 0%), hypertension (6% vs 1%; including hypertension and hypertensive crisis), and hemorrhage (3% vs 0.3%; including aneurysm ruptured, epistaxis, gastric ulcer hemorrhage, gingival bleeding, hemoptysis, hemorrhage intracranial, large intestinal hemorrhage, respiratory tract hemorrhage, small intestinal hemorrhage, and traumatic hematoma).

Grade 1 to 5 adverse reactions occurring at a higher incidence (5% or more) in patients receiving interferon alfa plus bevacizumab compared with the interferon alfa plus placebo arm are presented in the following table.

NCI-CTC Grades 1 to 5 Adverse Reactions (≥ 5%) in Interferon Alfa plus Bevacizumab vs Interferon Alfa plus Placebo		
Adverse reactions	Interferon alfa plus placebo (n = 304)	Interferon alfa plus bevacizumab (n = 337)
CNS		
Fatigue	27%	33%
Headache	16%	24%
GI		
Anorexia	31%	36%
Musculoskeletal		
Back pain	6%	12%
Myalgia	14%	19%

BEVACIZUMAB — INJECTION

NCI-CTC Grades 1 to 5 Adverse Reactions (≥ 5%) in Interferon Alfa plus Bevacizumab vs Interferon Alfa plus Placebo		
Adverse reactions	Interferon alfa plus placebo (n = 304)	Interferon alfa plus bevacizumab (n = 337)
Respiratory		
Dysphonia	0%	5%
Epistaxis	4%	27%
Miscellaneous		
Diarrhea	16%	21%
Hypertension	9%	28%
Proteinuria	3%	20%
Weight decreased	15%	20%

Other adverse reactions: The following adverse reactions were reported at a 5-fold greater incidence in the interferon alfa plus bevacizumab arm compared with interferon alfa alone and not represented in the previous table: gingival bleeding (13 patients vs 1 patient), rhinitis (9 vs 0), blurred vision (8 vs 0), gingivitis (8 vs 1), gastroesophageal reflux disease (8 vs 1), tinnitus (7 vs 1), tooth abscess (7 vs 0), mouth ulceration (6 vs 0), acne (5 vs 0), deafness (5 vs 0), gastritis (5 vs 0), gingival pain (5 vs 0), and pulmonary embolism (5 vs 1).

➤*Surgery and wound healing complications:* The incidence of postoperative wound healing and/or bleeding complications was increased in patients with metabolic colorectal cancer receiving bevacizumab compared with patients receiving only chemotherapy. Among patients requiring surgery on or within 60 days of receiving study treatment, wound healing and/or bleeding complications occurred in 15% of patients receiving bolus-irinotecan/5-fluorouracil/leucovorin plus bevacizumab compared with 4% of patients who received bolus-irinotecan/5-fluorouracil/leucovorin alone. In study 7, reactions of postoperative wound healing complications (craniotomy site wound dehiscence and cerebrospinal fluid leak) occurred in patients with previously treated glioblastoma: 3 of 84 patients in the bevacizumab-alone arm and 1 of 79 patients in the bevacizumab-plus-irinotecan arm.

➤*Hemorrhage:* The incidence of epistaxis was higher (35% vs 10%) in patients with metastatic colorectal cancer receiving bolus-irinotecan/5-fluorouracil/leucovorin plus bevacizumab compared with patients receiving bolus-irinotecan/5-fluorouracil/leucovorin plus placebo. All but 1 of these events were grade 1 in severity and resolved without medical intervention. Grade 1 or 2 hemorrhagic events were more frequent in patients receiving bolus-irinotecan/5-fluorouracil/leucovorin plus bevacizumab when compared with those receiving bolus-irinotecan/5-fluorouracil/leucovorin plus placebo and included GI hemorrhage (24% vs 6%), minor gum bleeding (2% vs 0%), and vaginal hemorrhage (4% vs 2%).

➤*Venous thromboembolic events:* The incidence of grade 3 to 4 venous thromboembolic events was higher in patients with metastatic colorectal cancer or non–small cell lung cancer receiving bevacizumab with chemotherapy compared with those receiving chemotherapy alone. In patients with metastatic colorectal cancer, the risk of developing a second subsequent thromboembolic event was increased in patients receiving bevacizumab and chemotherapy compared with patients receiving chemotherapy alone.

In study 1, 14% of patients on the bolus-irinotecan/5-fluorouracil/leucovorin plus bevacizumab arm and 8% of patients on the bolus-irinotecan/5-fluorouracil/leucovorin plus placebo arm received full-dose warfarin following a venous thromboembolic event. Among these patients, an additional thromboembolic event occurred in 21% of patients receiving bolus-irinotecan/5-fluorouracil/leucovorin plus bevacizumab and 3% of patients receiving bolus-irinotecan/5-fluorouracil/leucovorin alone.

The overall incidence of grade 3 to 4 venous thromboembolic events in study 1 was 15.1% in patients receiving bolus-irinotecan/5-fluorouracil/leucovorin plus bevacizumab and 13.6% in patients receiving bolus-irinotecan/5-fluorouracil/leucovorin plus placebo. In study 1, the incidence of the following grade 3 and 4 venous thromboembolic events was higher in patients receiving bolus-irinotecan/5-fluorouracil/leucovorin plus bevacizumab as compared with patients receiving bolus-irinotecan/5-fluorouracil/leucovorin plus placebo: deep venous thrombosis (34 vs 19 patients) and intra-abdominal venous thrombosis (10 vs 5 patients).

➤*Neutropenia and infection:* The incidences of neutropenia and febrile neutropenia are increased in patients receiving bevacizumab and chemotherapy compared with chemotherapy alone. In study 1, the incidence of grade 3 or 4 neutropenia was increased in patients with metastatic colorectal cancer receiving irinotecan/5-fluorouracil/leucovorin plus bevacizumab (21%) compared with patients receiving irinotecan/5-fluorouracil/leucovorin alone (14%). In study 4, the incidence of grade 4 neutropenia was increased in patients with non–small cell lung cancer receiving paclitaxel/carboplatin plus bevacizumab (26.2%) compared with patients receiving paclitaxel/carboplatin alone (17.2%). Febrile neutropenia was also increased (5.4% for paclitaxel/carboplatin plus bevacizumab vs 1.8% for paclitaxel/carboplatin alone). There were 4.5% infections with grade 3 or 4 neutropenia in the paclitaxel/carboplatin plus bevacizumab arm, 3 of which were fatal, compared with 2% neutropenic infections in patients receiving paclitaxel/carboplatin alone, none of which were fatal. During the first 6 cycles of treatment, the incidence of serious infections, including pneumonia, febrile neutropenia, catheter infections, and wound infections, was increased in the paclitaxel/carboplatin plus bevacizumab arm (13.6%) compared with the paclitaxel/carboplatin alone arm (6.6%).

In study 7, one fatal reaction of neutropenic infection occurred in a patient with previously treated glioblastoma receiving bevacizumab alone. The incidence of any grade of infection in patients receiving bevacizumab alone was 55%, and the incidence of grade 3 to 5 infection was 10%.

➤*Proteinuria:* Grade 3 to 4 proteinuria ranged from 0.7% to 7.4% in studies 1, 2, 4, and 9. The overall incidence of proteinuria (all grades) was only adequately assessed in study 9, in which the incidence was 20%. Median onset of proteinuria was 5.6 months (range, 15 days to 37 months) after initiation of bevacizumab. Median time to resolution was 6.1 months (95% CI, 2.8 to 11.3 months). Proteinuria did not resolve in 40% of patients after median follow-up of 11.2 months and required permanent discontinuation of bevacizumab in 30% of the patients who developed proteinuria (study 9).

➤*Congestive heart failure:* See Warnings/Precautions.

➤*Postmarketing:*

Cardiovascular – Pulmonary hypertension, reversible posterior leukoencephalopathy syndrome.

GI – Anastomotic ulceration, intestinal necrosis, mesenteric venous occlusion.

Renal – Renal thrombotic microangiopathy (manifested as severe proteinuria).

Respiratory – Dysphonia, nasal septum perforation.

Miscellaneous – Pancytopenia, polyserositis.

Overdosage

➤*Symptoms:* The highest dose tested in humans (bevacizumab 20 mg/kg IV) was associated with headache in 9 of 16 patients and with severe headache in 3 of 16 patients.

Patient Information

Advise patients to undergo routine blood pressure monitoring and to contact their health care provider if blood pressure is elevated.

Advise patients to immediately contact their health care provider for unusual bleeding, high fever, rigors, sudden onset of worsening neurological function, or persistent or severe abdominal pain, severe constipation, or vomiting.

Advise patients of increased risk of wound-healing complications during and following bevacizumab therapy.

Advise patients of increased risk of an arterial thromboembolic event.

Advise patients of the potential risk to the fetus during and following bevacizumab and the need to continue adequate contraception for at least 6 months following the last dose of bevacizumab.

PANITUMUMAB

Rx	**Vectibix** (Amgen)	**Injection, solution:** 20 mg/mL	Preservative free. Sodium acetate, sodium chloride. In 5, 10, and 20 mL single-use vials.

PANITUMUMAB — INJECTION

WARNING

Dermatologic toxicity – Dermatologic toxicities related to panitumumab blockade of epidermal growth factor (EGF)–binding and subsequent inhibition of epidermal growth factor receptor (EGFR)–mediated signaling pathways were reported in 89% of patients and were severe (National Cancer Institute Common Toxicity Criteria [NCI-CTC] grade 3 and higher) in 12% of patients receiving panitumumab monotherapy. The clinical manifestations included, but were not limited to, dermatitis acneiform, pruritus, erythema, rash, skin exfoliation, paronychia, dry skin, and skin fissures. Severe dermatologic toxicities were complicated by infections, including sepsis, septic death, and abscesses requiring incisions and drainage. Withhold or discontinue panitumumab and monitor for inflammatory or infectious sequelae in patients with severe dermatologic toxicities.

WARNING (cont.)

Infusion reactions – Severe infusion reactions occurred with the administration of panitumumab in approximately 1% of patients. Severe infusion reactions were identified by reports of anaphylactic reaction, bronchospasm, fever, chills, and hypotension. Although fatal infusion reactions have not been reported with panitumumab, fatalities have occurred with other monoclonal antibody products. Stop the infusion if a severe infusion reaction occurs. Depending on the severity and/or persistence of the reaction, permanently discontinue panitumumab.

Indications

➤*Colorectal carcinoma:* As a single agent for the treatment of EGFR-expressing, metastatic colorectal carcinoma with disease progression on or following fluoropyrimidine-, oxaliplatin-, and irinotecan-containing chemotherapy regimens.

PANITUMUMAB — INJECTION

Administration and Dosage

➤*General dosing considerations:* Appropriate medical resources for the treatment of severe infusion reactions should be available during panitumumab infusions. (See Infusion Reaction).

➤*Adults:*

Colorectal carcinoma – 6 mg/kg administered IV over 60 minutes once every 14 days. Administer through a peripheral line or indwelling catheter. Doses higher than 1,000 mg should be administered over 90 minutes.

➤*Infusion reaction:* Severe infusion reactions occurred with the administration of panitumumab in approximately 1% of patients. Severe infusion reactions were identified by reports of anaphylactic reaction, bronchospasm, fever, chills, and hypotension. Reduce the infusion rate 50% in patients experiencing a mild or moderate (grade 1 or 2) reaction for the duration of that infusion. Immediately and permanently discontinue panitumumab in patients experiencing severe (grade 3 or 4) infusion reactions. (See also Black Box Warning.)

➤*Dermatologic toxicity:* Withhold panitumumab for dermatologic toxicities that are grade 3 or higher or are considered intolerable. If toxicity does not improve to grade 2 or lower within 1 month, permanently discontinue panitumumab.

If dermatologic toxicity improves to grade 2 or lower and the patient is symptomatically improved after withholding up to 2 doses of panitumumab, treatment may be resumed at 50% of the original dose.

If toxicities do not recur, subsequent doses of panitumumab may be increased by increments of 25% of the original dose until the recommended dose of 6 mg/kg is reached. (See also Black Box Warning.)

➤*Discontinuation of therapy:* Discontinue panitumumab permanently if severe hypersensitivity reactions, interstitial lung disease, pneumonitis, or lung infiltration occur.

➤*Preparation for administration:* Panitumumab is considered a cytotoxic agent. Follow safe handling procedures when preparing, administering, or dispensing panitumumab.

Preparation of solution –

Although panitumumab should be colorless, the solution may contain a small amount of visible translucent to white, amorphous, proteinaceous panitumumab particulates (which will be removed by filtration). Panitumumab should not be administered if discoloration is observed.

Prepare the solution for infusion using aseptic technique as follows:

1.) Withdraw the necessary amount of panitumumab for a dose of 6 mg/kg.
2.) Dilute to a total volume of 100 mL with sodium chloride 0.9% injection. Doses higher than 1,000 mg should be diluted to 150 mL with sodium chloride 0.9% injection. Final concentration should not exceed 10 mg/mL.
3.) Mix diluted solution by gentle inversion. Do not shake.

Flush the line before and after panitumumab administration with sodium chloride 0.9% injection to avoid mixing with other drug products or IV solutions.

➤*Administration:* Infuse over 60 minutes through a peripheral line or indwelling catheter. Doses higher than 1,000 mg should be infused over 90 minutes. Do not administer as an IV push or bolus. Panitumumab must be administered by an IV infusion pump using a low-protein-binding 0.2 or 0.22 mcm in-line filter.

Flush the line before and after administration with sodium chloride 0.9% injection.

Routine premedication is not necessary to prevent infusion reactions with panitumumab. Observe patient during administration and for 1 hour afterward.

➤*Admixture compatibility:* Panitumumab should not be mixed with or administered as an infusion with other medicinal products. No other medications should be added to solutions containing panitumumab.

➤*Storage/Stability:* Store vials in the original cartons under refrigeration at 2° to 8°C (36° to 46°F) until the time of use. Protect the vials from direct sunlight. Do not freeze the vials. Because panitumumab does not contain preservatives, discard any unused portion remaining in the vial.

Use the diluted infusion solution of panitumumab within 6 hours of preparation if stored at room temperature or within 24 hours of dilution if stored at 2° to 8°C (36° to 46°F). Do not freeze the solution.

Actions

➤*Pharmacology:* Panitumumab is a recombinant human immunoglobulin G2 (IgG2) kappa monoclonal antibody that binds specifically to the human EGFR. The EGFR is a member of a subfamily of type I receptor tyrosine kinases, including EGFR (HER1, c-ErbB-1), and breast cancer genes HER2/neu, HER3, and HER4. EGFR is a transmembrane glycoprotein that is constitutively expressed in many normal epithelial tissues, including the skin and hair follicles. Overexpression of EGFR is also detected in many human cancers, including those of the colon and rectum. Interaction of EGFR with its normal ligands (eg, EGF, transforming growth factor-alpha) leads to phosphorylation and activation of a series of intracellular tyrosine kinases, which in turn regulate transcription of molecules involved with cellular growth and survival, motility, proliferation, and transformation.

Panitumumab binds specifically to EGFR on both normal and tumor cells and competitively inhibits the binding of ligands for EGFR. Nonclinical studies show that binding of panitumumab to the EGFR prevents ligand-induced receptor autophosphorylation and activation of receptor-associated kinases, resulting in inhibition of cell growth, induction of apoptosis, decreased proinflammatory cytokine and vascular growth factor production, and internalization of the EGFR. In vitro assays and in vivo animal studies demonstrate that panitumumab inhibits the growth and survival of selected human tumor cell lines expressing EGFR.

➤*Pharmacokinetics:*

Absorption/Distribution – Panitumumab administered as a single agent exhibits nonlinear pharmacokinetics.

Following a single-dose administration of panitumumab as a 1-hour infusion, the area under the curve (AUC) increased in a greater dose-proportional manner, and clearance of panitumumab decreased from 30.6 to 4.6 mL/kg/day as the dose increased from 0.75 to 9 mg/kg. However, at doses of more than 2 mg/kg, the AUC of panitumumab increases in an approximate dose-proportional manner.

Following the recommended dose regimen (6 mg/kg given once every 2 weeks as a 1-hour infusion), panitumumab concentrations reached steady-state levels by the third infusion, with mean (± standard deviation [SD]) peak and trough concentrations of 213 ± 59 mcg/mL and 39 ± 14 mcg/mL, respectively. The mean (± SD) $AUC_{0\text{-tau}}$ and clearance were 1,306 ± 374 mcg•day/mL and 4.9 ± 1.4 mL/kg/day, respectively.

Excretion – The elimination half-life was approximately 7.5 days (range, 3.6 to 10.9 days).

Contraindications

None known.

Warnings/Precautions

➤*Toxicities:* Weekly administration of panitumumab to cynomolgus monkeys for 4 to 26 weeks resulted in dermatologic findings, including dermatitis, pustule formation and exfoliative rash, and deaths secondary to bacterial infection and sepsis, at doses of 1.25- to 5-fold higher (on a mg/kg basis) than the recommended human dose.

In the randomized, controlled clinical trial of panitumumab, dermatologic toxicities related to panitumumab blockade of EGF binding and subsequent inhibition of EGFR-mediated signaling pathways were reported in 90% of patients and were severe (NCI-CTC grade 3 and higher) in 16% of patients with metastatic carcinoma of the colon or rectum and who were receiving panitumumab. The clinical manifestations included, but were not limited to, dermatitis acneiform, dry skin, erythema, paronychia, pruritus, rash, skin exfoliation, and skin fissures. Subsequent to the development of severe dermatologic toxicities, infectious complications, including abscesses requiring incisions and drainage, sepsis, and septic death, were reported. Toxicity involving GI mucosa, eye, and nail was also reported.

➤*Infusion reactions:* In the randomized, controlled clinical trial of panitumumab, 4% of patients experienced infusion reactions; in 1% of patients, reactions were graded as severe (NCI-CTC grade 3 to 4).

Across all clinical studies, severe infusion reactions occurred with the administration of panitumumab in approximately 1% of patients. Severe infusion reactions were identified from reports of anaphylactic reaction, bronchospasm, chills, fever, and hypotension. Although fatal infusion reactions have not been reported with panitumumab, fatalities have occurred with other monoclonal antibody products. Stop infusion if a severe infusion reaction occurs. Depending on the severity and/or persistence of the reaction, permanently discontinue panitumumab.

➤*Increased toxicity with combination chemotherapy:* Panitumumab is not indicated for use in combination with chemotherapy with or without bevacizumab. In an interim analysis of a randomized (1:1) clinical trial of patients with previously untreated metastatic colorectal cancer, the addition of panitumumab to the combination of bevacizumab and chemotherapy resulted in decreased PFS (n = 947) and increased incidence of NCI-CTC grade 3 to 5 (87% vs 72%) adverse reactions (n = 926). All patients received bevacizumab; 86% received an oxaliplatin–fluoroyrimidine-based regimen and 14% received an irinotecan–fluoropyrimidine-based regimen. NCI-CTC grade 3 to 4 adverse drug reactions occurring at a higher rate in panitumumab-treated patients included rash/dermatitis/acneiform (26% vs 1%), diarrhea (23% vs 12%), dehydration, primarily occurring in patients with diarrhea (16% vs 5%), hypokalemia (10% vs 4%), stomatitis/mucositis (4% vs less than 1%), and hypomagnesemia (4% vs 0%). NCI-CTC grade 3 to 5 pulmonary embolism occurred at a higher rate in panitumumab-treated patients (7% vs 4%) and included fatal events in 3 (less than 1%) panitumumab-treated patients.

As a result of the toxicities experienced, patients randomized to panitumumab, bevacizumab, and chemotherapy received a significantly lower mean relative dose intensity of each chemotherapeutic agent (oxaliplatin, irinotecan, bolus 5-fluorouracil, and/or infusional 5-fluorouracil) over the first 24 weeks on study, compared with those randomized to bevacizumab and chemotherapy.

In a single-arm study of 19 patients receiving panitumumab in combination with irinotecan plus bolus fluorouracil/leucovorin, the incidence of NCI-CTC grade 3 to 4 diarrhea was 58%; in addition, grade 5 diarrhea occurred in 1 patient. In a single-arm study of 24 patients receiving panitumumab plus irinotecan plus infusional fluorouracil/leucovorin, the incidence of NCI-CTC grade 3 diarrhea was 25%.

➤*Pulmonary fibrosis:* Pulmonary fibrosis occurred in less than 1% (2/1,467) of patients enrolled in clinical studies of panitumumab. Of these 2 cases, 1 case, occurring in a patient with underlying idiopathic pulmonary fibrosis and who received panitumumab in combination with chemotherapy, resulted in death from worsening pulmonary fibrosis after 4 doses of panitumumab. The second case was characterized by cough and wheezing 8 days following the initial dose, exertional dyspnea on the day of the seventh dose, and persistent symptoms and computerized tomography evidence of pulmonary fibrosis following the eleventh dose of panitumumab as monotherapy.

PANITUMUMAB — INJECTION

An additional patient died with bilateral pulmonary infiltrates of uncertain etiology with hypoxia after 23 doses of panitumumab in combination with chemotherapy. Following the initial fatality, patients with a history of interstitial pneumonitis or pulmonary fibrosis, or who exhibit evidence of interstitial pneumonitis or pulmonary fibrosis were excluded from clinical studies. Therefore, the estimated risk in a general population that may include such patients is uncertain. Permanently discontinue panitumumab therapy in patients developing interstitial lung disease, lung infiltrates, or pneumonitis.

➤*Electrolyte depletion:* In the randomized, controlled clinical trial of panitumumab, median magnesium levels decreased 0.1 mmol/L in the panitumumab arm; hypomagnesemia (NCI-CTC grade 3 or 4) requiring oral or IV electrolyte repletion occurred in 2% of patients. Hypomagnesemia occurred 6 weeks or longer after the initiation of panitumumab. In some patients, hypomagnesemia was associated with hypocalcemia. Periodically monitor patients' electrolytes during and for 8 weeks after the completion of panitumumab therapy.

➤*EGFR testing:* Detection of EGFR protein expression is necessary for selection of patients appropriate for panitumumab therapy because these are the only patients studied and the only patients who have benefited. Patients enrolled in the colorectal cancer clinical studies were required to have immunohistochemical evidence of EGFR expression using the *Dako EGFR pharmDx* test kit. Only laboratories with demonstrated proficiency in the specific technology being utilized should assess the EGFR expression. Improper assay performance, including use of suboptimally fixed tissue, failure to utilize specific reagents, deviation from specific assay instructions, and failure to include appropriate controls for assay validation can lead to unreliable results (refer to the package insert for the *Dako EGFR pharmDX* test kit or other test kits approved by the Food and Drug Administration (FDA) for identification of patients eligible for treatment with panitumumab and for full instructions on assay performance).

➤*Photosensitivity:* It is recommended that patients wear sunscreen and hats and limit sun exposure while receiving panitumumab because sunlight can exacerbate any skin reactions that may occur.

➤*Pregnancy: Category C.* There are no adequate and well-controlled studies in pregnant women. However, EGFR has been implicated in the control of prenatal development and may be essential for normal organogenesis, proliferation, and differentiation in the developing embryo. Panitumumab treatment was associated with significant increases in embryolethal or abortifacient effects in pregnant cynomolgus monkeys when administered weekly during the period of organogenesis (gestation days 20 to 50) at doses approximately 1.25- to 5-fold greater than the recommended human dose (based on body weight).

Human IgG is known to cross the placental barrier; therefore, panitumumab may be transmitted from the mother to the developing fetus. In women of childbearing potential, appropriate contraceptive measures must be used during treatment with panitumumab and for 6 months following the last dose of panitumumab. If panitumumab is used during pregnancy or if the patient becomes pregnant while receiving this drug, explain to her the potential risk for loss of the pregnancy and the potential hazard to the fetus.

Fertility impairment – Panitumumab may impair fertility in women of childbearing potential.

Teratogenic – There were no fetal malformations or other evidence of teratogenesis noted in the offspring of pregnant cynomolgus monkeys treated with panitumumab. While no panitumumab was detected in serum of neonates from panitumumab-treated dams, antipanitumumab antibody titers were present in 14 of 27 offspring delivered at gestation day 100. Therefore, while no teratogenic effects were observed in panitumumab-treated monkeys, panitumumab could potentially cause fetal harm when administered to pregnant women.

➤*Lactation:* Studies have not been conducted to assess the secretion of panitumumab in human milk. Because human IgG is secreted into human milk, panitumumab might also be secreted. The potential for absorption and harm to the infant after ingestion is unknown. Advise women to discontinue breast-feeding during treatment with panitumumab and for 2 months after the last dose of panitumumab.

➤*Children:* The safety and effectiveness of panitumumab have not been established in children.

➤*Monitoring:* Monitor vital signs (ie, heart rate, blood pressure, respiratory rate, temperature) every 15 to 30 minutes during infusion and for 1 hour afterward. Periodically monitor patients' electrolytes, including magnesium and calcium, during and for 8 weeks after the completion of panitumumab therapy. Institute appropriate treatment (eg, oral or IV electrolyte repletion) as needed. Monitor patients for inflammatory or infectious sequelae in patients with severe dermatologic toxicities. Monitor patients during administration for infusion reactions.

Drug Interactions

➤*Irinotecan:* The frequency and severity of diarrhea may increase when panitumumab is given concomitantly with irinotecan. To minimize the risk of severe diarrhea, avoid using panitumumab with irinotecan-containing regimens.

Adverse Reactions

➤*Common adverse reactions:* The most common adverse reactions observed in clinical studies of panitumumab (N = 1,467) were abdominal pain, diarrhea (including diarrhea resulting in dehydration), fatigue, hypomagnesemia, paronychia, nausea, and skin rash with variable presentations.

➤*Serious adverse reactions:* The most serious adverse reactions observed were abdominal pain, constipation, infusion reactions, hypomagnesemia, pulmonary fibrosis, nausea, severe dermatologic toxicity complicated by infectious sequelae and septic death, and vomiting. Adverse reactions requiring discontinuation of panitumumab were infusion reactions, paronychia, pulmonary fibrosis, and severe skin toxicity.

➤*Adverse reactions (5% or more):*

Panitumumab Adverse Reactions (≥ 5%)

	Panitumumab + best supportive care (n = 229)		Best supportive care alone (n = 234)	
	Grade[a]			
Adverse reaction	All grades	Grades 3 to 4	All grades	Grades 3 to 4
Dermatologic				
All skin/integument toxicity	90%	16%	9%	0%
Hair	9%	0%	1%	0%
Growth of eyelashes	6%	0%	0%	0%
Nail	29%	2%	0%	0%
Other nail disorders	9%	0%	0%	0%
Paronychia	25%	2%	0%	0%
Skin	90%	14%	6%	0%
Acne	13%	1%	0%	0%
Acneiform dermatitis	57%	7%	1%	0%
Dry skin	10%	0%	0%	0%
Erythema	65%	5%	1%	0%
Pruritus	57%	2%	2%	0%
Rash	22%	1%	1%	0%
Skin exfoliation	25%	2%	0%	0%
Skin fissures	20%	1%	< 1%	0%
GI				
Abdominal pain	25%	7%	17%	5%
Constipation	21%	3%	9%	1%
Diarrhea	21%	2%	11%	0%
Mucosal inflammation	6%	< 1%	1%	0%
Nausea	23%	1%	16%	< 1%
Stomatitis	7%	0%	1%	0%
Vomiting	19%	2%	12%	1%
Metabolic/Nutritional				
Hypomagnesemia (lab)	39%	4%	2%	0%
Peripheral edema	12%	1%	6%	< 1%
Respiratory				
Cough	14%	< 1%	7%	0%
Special senses				
Eye-related toxicities	15%	< 1%	2%	0%
Miscellaneous				
Fatigue	26%	4%	15%	3%
General deterioration	11%	8%	4%	3%

[a] Version 2 of the NCI-CTC was used for grading toxicities. Skin toxicity was coded based on a modification of the NCI-CTCAE, version 3.

➤*Infusion reactions:* Infusional toxicity was defined as any reaction described at any time during the clinical study as an allergic or anaphylactoid reaction, or any reaction occurring on the first day of dosing described as an allergic reaction, anaphylactoid reaction, chills, dyspnea, or fever. Vital signs and temperature were measured within 30 minutes prior to initiation and upon completion of the panitumumab infusion. The use of premedication was not standardized in the clinical trials. Thus, the utility of premedication in preventing the first or subsequent episodes of infusional toxicity is unknown. Of all panitumumab-treated patients, excluding those treated with panitumumab in combination with carboplatin and paclitaxel, 3% (43 of 1,336) experienced infusion reactions of which approximately 1% (6 of 1,136) were severe (NCI-CTC grades 3 to 4). In 1 patient, panitumumab was permanently discontinued for a serious infusion reaction.

➤*Dermatologic:* In the randomized, controlled clinical trial, skin-related toxicities were reported in 90% of patients receiving panitumumab. Skin toxicity was severe (NCI-CTC grade 3 and higher) in 16% of patients. The incidence of paronychia was 25% and was severe in 2% of patients. Other nail disorders were observed in 9% of patients.

Median time to the development of skin/eye-related toxicity was 14 days and the most severe skin/eye-related toxicity occurred 15 days after the first dose of panitumumab. The median time to resolution after the last dose of panitumumab was 84 days.

PANITUMUMAB — INJECTION

➤*GI:* Stomatitis (7%) and oral mucositis (6%) were reported. One patient experienced a NCI-CTC grade 3 mucosal inflammation reaction.

➤*Immunogenicity:* As with all therapeutic proteins, there is potential for immunogenicity. The immunogenicity of panitumumab has been evaluated using 2 different screening immunoassays for the detection of antipanitumumab antibodies: an acid dissociation bridging enzyme-linked immunosorbent assay (ELISA) that detects high-affinity antibodies and a *Biacore* biosensor immunoassay that detects both high- and low-affinity antibodies. The incidence of binding antibodies to panitumumab (excluding predose and transient-positive patients) was 2 of 612 (less than 1%), as detected by the acid dissociation ELISA, and 25 of 610 (4.1%), as detected by the *Biacore* assay.

For patients whose sera tested positive in screening immunoassays, an in vitro biological assay was performed to detect neutralizing antibodies. Excluding predose and transient-positive patients, 8 of the 604 patients (1.3%) with postdose samples and 1 of the 350 (less than 1%) patients with follow-up samples tested positive for neutralizing antibodies.

➤*Special senses:* Eye-related toxicities occurred in 15% of patients and included, but were not limited to, conjunctivitis (4%), ocular hyperemia (3%), increased lacrimation (2%), and eye/eyelid irritation (1%). Median time to the development of skin/eye-related toxicity was 14 days and the most severe skin/eye-related toxicity occurred 15 days after the first dose of panitumumab. The median time to resolution after the last dose of panitumumab was 84 days.

➤*Miscellaneous:* Infectious complications, including sepsis, septic death, and abscesses requiring incisions and drainage, were reported; secure toxicity necessitated dose interruption in 11% of panitumumab-treated patients.

Overdosage

The highest per-infusion dose administered in clinical studies was 9 mg/kg administered every 3 weeks. There is no experience with overdosage in human clinical trials.

Patient Information

Inform patients of the possible adverse reactions of panitumumab, including dermatologic toxicity, infusion reactions, pulmonary fibrosis, and potential embryofetal lethality. Instruct patients to report skin and ocular changes and dyspnea to their health care provider. Advise patients that periodic monitoring of electrolyte levels is required.

In women of childbearing potential, appropriate contraceptive measures must be used during treatment with panitumumab and for 6 months following the last dose of panitumumab.

Advise women to discontinue breast-feeding during treatment with panitumumab and for 2 months after the last dose of panitumumab.

It is recommended that patients wear sunscreen and hats and limit sun exposure while receiving panitumumab because sunlight can exacerbate any skin reactions that may occur.

TRASTUZUMAB

Rx	**Herceptin** (Genentech)	**Injection, lyophilized powder for solution:** 440 mg	In multiuse vials. With 20 mL diluent vials of bacteriostatic water for injection with benzyl alcohol 1.1%.

TRASTUZUMAB — INJECTION

WARNING

Cardiomyopathy – Trastuzumab can result in subclinical and clinical cardiac failure. The incidence and severity was highest in patients who received trastuzumab concurrently with anthracycline-containing chemotherapy regimens.

Evaluate left ventricular function in all patients prior to and during treatment with trastuzumab. Discontinue trastuzumab treatment in patients receiving adjuvant therapy, and withhold trastuzumab treatment in patients with metastatic disease for a clinically significant decrease in left ventricular function.

Infusion reactions and pulmonary toxicity – Trastuzumab administration can result in serious and fatal infusion reactions and pulmonary toxicity. Symptoms usually occur during or within 24 hours of administration of trastuzumab. Interrupt trastuzumab infusion for patients experiencing dyspnea or clinically significant hypotension. Monitor patients until signs and symptoms resolve completely. Discontinue trastuzumab for anaphylaxis, angioedema, interstitial pneumonitis, or acute respiratory distress syndrome.

Indications

➤*Breast cancer:*

Adjuvant breast cancer treatment – For adjuvant treatment of human epidermal growth receptor 2 (HER2)-overexpressing node positive or node negative (estrogen receptor/progesterone receptor negative or with one high risk feature) breast cancer as part of a treatment regimen consisting of doxorubicin, cyclophosphamide, and either paclitaxel or docetaxel; with docetaxel and carboplatin; or as a single agent following multimodality anthracycline-based therapy.

Metastatic breast cancer – In combination with paclitaxel for first-line treatment of HER2-overexpressing metastatic breast cancer; as a single agent for treatment of HER2-overexpressing breast cancer in patients who have received one or more chemotherapy regimens for metastatic disease.

➤*Metastatic gastric cancer:* In combination with cisplatin and capecitabine or 5-fluorouracil for the treatment of patients with HER2–overexpressing metastatic gastric or gastroesophageal junction adenocarcinoma who have not received prior treatment for metastatic disease.

Administration and Dosage

➤*General dosing considerations:* Assess left ventricular ejection fraction (LVEF) prior to initiation of trastuzumab and at regular intervals during treatment. Treatment regimen adjustments may be required. (See Cardiomyopathy.)

➤*Adults:*

Adjuvant breast cancer treatment –

During and following paclitaxel, docetaxel, or docetaxel/carboplatin:

• *Initial dosage* – 4 mg/kg as an intravenous (IV) infusion over 90 minutes, then 2 mg/kg as an IV infusion over 30 minutes weekly during chemotherapy for the first 12 weeks (paclitaxel or docetaxel) or 18 weeks (docetaxel/carboplatin).

• *Maintenance dosage* – One week following the last weekly dose of trastuzumab, administer trastuzumab 6 mg/kg as an IV infusion over 30 to 60 minutes every 3 weeks.

• *Duration of therapy* – A total of 52 weeks of trastuzumab therapy.

Following completion of multimodality anthracycline-based chemotherapy regimens:

• *Initial dosage* – 8 mg/kg as an IV infusion over 90 minutes within 3 weeks following completion of multimodality anthracycline-based chemotherapy.

• *Maintenance dosage* – 6 mg/kg as an IV infusion over 30 to 90 minutes every 3 weeks.

• *Duration of therapy* – A total of 52 weeks of trastuzumab therapy.

Metastatic breast cancer –

Initial dosage: 4 mg/kg as an IV infusion over 90 minutes, given alone or in combination with paclitaxel.

Maintenance dosage: 2 mg/kg as an IV infusion over 30 minutes, given once weekly until disease progression.

Metastatic gastric cancer –

Initial dosage: 8 mg/kg as an IV infusion over 90 minutes.

Maintenance dosage: 6 mg/kg as an IV infusion over 30 to 90 minutes every 3 weeks until disease progression.

➤*Renal function impairment:*

Dialysis – Conventional hemodialysis and peritoneal dialysis are ineffective (0% to 24%) in removing trastuzumab.

➤*Infusion reactions:* Decrease the rate of infusion for mild or moderate infusion reactions. Interrupt the infusion in patients with dyspnea or clinically significant hypotension. Discontinue trastuzumab for severe or life-threatening infusion reactions. Consider discontinuing therapy if the patient experiences a severe infusion reaction, such as anaphylaxis, angioedema, pneumonitis, or respiratory distress syndrome. Symptoms may be treated with diphenhydramine, acetaminophen, meperidine, epinephrine, corticosteroids, oxygen, bronchodilators, or IV fluids. Evaluate patients and monitor them carefully until complete resolution of signs and symptoms. Patients who react to the initial trastuzumab infusion may receive further doses. The infusion duration may be increased at the practitioner's discretion. In patients with more serious reactions, consider premedication with antihistamines or corticosteroids prior to subsequent courses.

➤*Cardiomyopathy:* Assess LVEF prior to initiation of trastuzumab and at regular intervals during treatment. Withhold trastuzumab dosing for at least 4 weeks if there is a 16% or more absolute decrease in LVEF from pretreatment values or if LVEF falls below institutional limits of normal and there is a 10% or more absolute decrease in LVEF from pretreatment values. Trastuzumab may be resumed if, within 4 to 8 weeks, the LVEF returns to normal limits and the absolute decrease from baseline is 15% or less. Permanently discontinue trastuzumab for a persistent (longer than 8 weeks) LVEF decline or for suspension of trastuzumab dosing on more than 3 occasions for cardiomyopathy.

➤*Preparation for administration:*

Reconstitution – Reconstitute each 440 mg vial of trastuzumab with 20 mL of bacteriostatic water for injection, containing benzyl alcohol 1.1% as a preservative, to yield a multidose solution containing trastuzumab 21 mg/mL. In patients with known hypersensitivity to benzyl alcohol, reconstitute with 20 mL of sterile water for injection without preservative (not supplied) to yield a single-use solution.

Using a sterile syringe, slowly inject 20 mL of the diluent into the vial containing the lyophilized cake of trastuzumab. The stream of diluent should be directed into the lyophilized cake. Swirl the vial gently to aid reconstitution. Do not shake. Slight foaming of the product may be present upon reconstitution. Allow the vial to stand undisturbed for approximately 5 minutes.

Dilution – Determine the dose (in milligrams) of trastuzumab. Calculate the volume of 21 mg/mL of reconstituted trastuzumab solution needed, withdraw this amount from the vial, and add it to an infusion bag containing

TRASTUZUMAB — INJECTION

250 mL of sodium chloride 0.9% injection. Do not use dextrose 5% solution. Gently invert the bag to mix the solution.

➤*Administration:* Give as an IV infusion. Do not administer as an IV push or bolus. Infuse the initial dose over 90 minutes. If the initial infusion is tolerated, subsequent doses may be administered over 30 minutes for weekly doses, or over 30 to 90 minutes if given every 3 weeks. Observe patients for infusion-related symptoms (eg, fever, chills). (See Infusion Reactions).

➤*Admixture compatibility:* Do not mix trastuzumab with other drugs. Do not reconstitute or dilute with dextrose 5% injection because aggregation may occur.

➤*Storage/Stability:* Vials are stable at 2° to 8°C (36° to 46°F) prior to reconstitution. A vial of trastuzumab reconstituted with bacteriostatic water for injection, as supplied, is stable for 28 days after reconstitution when refrigerated between 2° and 8°C (36° and 46°F). Discard any remaining multidose reconstituted solution after 28 days. A vial of trastuzumab reconstituted with unpreserved sterile water for injection (not supplied) should be used within 24 hours; however, the manufacturer states to use immediately. Any unused portion should be discarded.

The solution of trastuzumab for infusion diluted in polyvinylchloride or polyethylene bags containing sodium chloride 0.9% injection should be stored between 2° and 8°C (36° and 46°F) for no more than 24 hours prior to use.

Do not freeze reconstituted or diluted solutions.

Actions

➤*Pharmacology:* Trastuzumab is a humanized immunoglobulin G1 kappa monoclonal antibody that selectively binds with high affinity to the extracellular domain of the HER2 protein.

The HER2 (or c-erbB2) proto-oncogene encodes a transmembrane receptor protein of 185 kDa, which is structurally related to the epidermal growth factor receptor. Trastuzumab has been shown, in in vitro assays and in animals, to inhibit the proliferation of human tumor cells that overexpress HER2.

Trastuzumab is a mediator of antibody-dependent cellular cytotoxicity (ADCC). In vitro, trastuzumab-mediated ADCC has been shown to be preferentially exerted on HER2-overexpressing cancer cells compared with cancer cells that do not overexpress HER2.

➤*Pharmacokinetics:*

Absorption/Distribution –

Short duration IV infusion of trastuzumab 10 to 500 mg once weekly demonstrated dose-dependent pharmacokinetics. The volume of distribution of trastuzumab was approximately that of serum volume (44 mL/kg). At the highest weekly dose studied (500 mg), mean peak serum concentrations were 377 mcg/mL.

Between weeks 16 and 32, trastuzumab serum concentrations reached a steady state with mean trough and peak concentrations of approximately 79 and 123 mcg/mL, respectively.

Between weeks 6 and 37 in a study of women receiving adjuvant therapy for breast cancer, trastuzumab serum concentrations reached a steady-state with mean trough and peak concentrations of 63 and 216 mcg/mL, respectively.

In patients with metastatic gastric cancer (study 7), mean serum trastuzumab trough concentrations at steady state were 24% to 63% lower compared with the concentrations observed in patients with breast cancer receiving treatment for metastatic disease in combination with paclitaxel, as monotherapy for metastatic disease, or as adjuvant monotherapy.

Sixty-four percent of women with metastatic breast cancer had detectable circulating extracellular domain of the HER2 receptor (shed antigen), which ranged as high as 1,880 ng/mL (median, 11 ng/mL). Patients with higher baseline shed antigen levels were more likely to have lower serum trough concentrations.

Metabolism/Excretion – Mean half-life increased and clearance decreased with increasing dose level. The half-life averaged 2 and 12 days at the 10 and 500 mg dose levels, respectively. In studies using an initial dose of 4 mg/kg followed by a weekly dose of 2 mg/kg, a mean half-life of 6 days (range, 1 to 32 days) was observed. In a study of women receiving adjuvant therapy for breast cancer, a mean half-life of trastuzumab of 16 days (range, 11 to 23 days) was observed after an initial dose of 8 mg/kg followed by a dose of 6 mg/kg every 3 weeks.

Contraindications

None well documented.

Warnings/Precautions

➤*Cardiovascular effects:* Trastuzumab can cause left ventricular cardiac dysfunction, arrhythmias, hypertension, disabling cardiac failure, cardiomyopathy, and cardiac death. Trastuzumab can also cause asymptomatic decline in LVEF.

There is a 4- to 6-fold increase in the incidence of symptomatic myocardial dysfunction among patients receiving trastuzumab as a single agent or in combination therapy compared with those not receiving trastuzumab. The highest absolute incidence occurs when trastuzumab is administered with an anthracycline.

See Administration and Dosage for more information.

The safety of continuation or resumption of trastuzumab in patients with trastuzumab-induced left ventricular cardiac dysfunction has not been studied.

See Monitoring for information regarding the cardiac assessment of patients who are candidates for treatment with trastuzumab.

In study 1, 16% of patients discontinued trastuzumab due to clinical evidence of myocardial dysfunction or significant decline in LVEF. In study 3, the number of patients who discontinued trastuzumab due to cardiac toxicity was 2.6%. In study 4, a total of 2.9% of patients in the docetaxel and carboplatin plus trastuzumab arm (1.5% during the chemotherapy phase and 1.4% during the monotherapy phase) and 5.7% of patients in the doxorubicin and cyclophosphamide followed by docetaxel plus trastuzumab arm (1.5% during the chemotherapy phase and 4.2% during the monotherapy phase) discontinued trastuzumab due to cardiac toxicity.

Among 32 patients receiving adjuvant chemotherapy (studies 1 and 2) who developed CHF, 1 patient died of cardiomyopathy and all other patients were receiving cardiac medication at last follow-up. Approximately half of the surviving patients had recovery to a normal LVEF (defined as 50% or more) on continuing medical management at the time of last follow-up. The safety of continuation or resumption of trastuzumab in patients with trastuzumab-induced left ventricular cardiac dysfunction has not been studied.

In study 4, the incidence of National Cancer Institute-Common Toxicity Criteria (NCI-CTC) grade 3/4 cardiac ischemia/infarction was higher in the trastuzumab-containing regimens (doxorubicin and cyclophosphamide followed by docetaxel plus trastuzumab: 0.3% and docetaxel and carboplatin plus trastuzumab: 0.2%) compared with none in doxorubicin and cyclophosphamide followed by docetaxel.

➤*Infusion reactions:* Infusion reactions consisted of a symptom complex characterized by fever and chills and, on occasion, included nausea, vomiting, pain (in some cases at tumor sites), headache, dizziness, dyspnea, hypotension, rash, and asthenia.

In postmarketing reports, serious and fatal infusion reactions have been reported. Severe reactions, which include bronchospasm, anaphylaxis, angioedema, hypoxia, and severe hypotension, were usually reported during or immediately following the initial infusion. However, the onset and clinical course were variable, including progressive worsening, initial improvement followed by clinical deterioration, or delayed postinfusion events with rapid clinical deterioration. For fatal events, death occurred within hours to days following a serious infusion reaction.

Interrupt trastuzumab infusion in all patients experiencing dyspnea, clinically significant hypotension, and intervention with medical therapy, which may include epinephrine, corticosteroids, diphenhydramine, bronchodilators, and oxygen. Evaluate patients and monitor them carefully until complete resolution of signs and symptoms. Strongly consider permanent discontinuation in all patients with severe infusion reactions.

There are no data regarding the most appropriate method of identification of patients who may safely be re-treated with trastuzumab after experiencing a severe infusion reaction. Prior to resumption of trastuzumab infusion, the majority of patients who experienced a severe infusion reaction were premedicated with antihistamines and/or corticosteroids. While some patients tolerated trastuzumab infusions, others had recurrent severe infusion reactions despite premedications.

➤*Exacerbation of chemotherapy-induced neutropenia:* In randomized, controlled, clinical trials in women with metastatic breast cancer, the per patient incidences of NCI-CTC grade 3 to 4 neutropenia and of febrile neutropenia were higher in patients receiving trastuzumab in combination with myelosuppressive chemotherapy compared with those who received chemotherapy alone. The incidence of septic death was not significantly increased.

➤*Pulmonary toxicity:* Trastuzumab use can result in serious and fatal pulmonary toxicity. Pulmonary toxicity includes dyspnea, interstitial pneumonitis, pulmonary infiltrates, pleural effusions, noncardiogenic pulmonary edema, pulmonary insufficiency and hypoxia, acute respiratory distress syndrome, and pulmonary fibrosis. Such events may occur as sequelae of infusion reactions. Patients with symptomatic intrinsic lung disease or with extensive tumor involvement of the lungs, resulting in dyspnea at rest, appear to have more severe toxicity.

➤*HER2 testing:* Detection of HER2 protein overexpression is necessary for selection of patients appropriate for trastuzumab therapy because these are the only patients studied for whom benefit has been shown.

Limitations in assay precision make it inadvisable to rely on as a single method to rule out potential trastuzumab benefit.

Perform assessment of HER2 protein overexpression and HER2 gene amplification in metastatic gastric cancer using FDA-approved tests specifically for gastric cancers because of differences in gastric versus breast histopathology, including incomplete membrane staining and more frequent heterogeneous expression of HER2 seen in gastric cancers. Study 7 demonstrated that gene amplification and protein overexpression were not as well correlated as with breast cancer.

➤*Benzyl alcohol:* The trastuzumab diluent provided contains benzyl alcohol as a preservative. The administration of medications containing benzyl alcohol as a preservative to premature neonates has been associated with a fatal gasping syndrome.

➤*Immunogenicity:* As with all therapeutic proteins, there is potential for immunogenicity. Among 903 women with metastatic breast cancer, human antihuman antibody to trastuzumab was detected in 1 patient using an enzyme-linked immunosorbent assay. This patient did not experience an allergic reaction. Samples for assessment of human antihuman antibody were not collected in studies of adjuvant breast cancer.

➤*Pregnancy: Category D.* Trastuzumab can cause fetal harm when administered to a pregnant woman. Postmarketing case reports suggest that trastuzumab use during pregnancy increases the risk of oligohydramnios during the second and third trimester. If trastuzumab is used during pregnancy or

TRASTUZUMAB — INJECTION

if a woman becomes pregnant while taking trastuzumab, apprise her of the potential hazard to the fetus.

In the postmarketing setting, oligohydramnios was reported in women who received trastuzumab during pregnancy, either alone or in combination with chemotherapy. In half of these women, amniotic fluid index increased after trastuzumab was stopped. In 1 case, trastuzumab was resumed after the amniotic fluid index improved, and oligohydramnios recurred.

Monitor women using trastuzumab during pregnancy for oligohydramnios. If oligohydramnios occurs, perform fetal testing that is appropriate for gestational age and consistent with community standards of care. Additional IV hydration has been helpful when oligohydramnios has occurred following administration of other chemotherapy agents; however, the effects of additional IV hydration with trastuzumab treatment are not known.

Reproduction studies in cynomolgus monkeys at doses of up to 25 times the recommended weekly human dose of trastuzumab 2 mg/kg revealed no evidence of harm to the fetus. However, HER2 protein expression is high in many embryonic tissues, including cardiac and neural tissues; in mutant mice lacking HER2, embryos died in early gestation. Placental transfer of trastuzumab was detected at Caesarean section/delivery in offspring from monkeys dosed during the early (days 20 to 50 of gestation) and late (days 120 to 150 of gestation) fetal development periods at levels of 15% to 28% of the maternal blood levels.

Pregnancy registry – Pregnant women with breast cancer who are using trastuzumab are encouraged to enroll in MotHER- the *Herceptin* Pregnancy Registry by calling 1-800-690-6720.

➤*Lactation:* It is not known whether trastuzumab is excreted in human milk, but human immunoglobulin G is excreted in human milk. Published data suggest that breast milk antibodies do not enter the neonatal and infant circulation in substantial amounts.

Trastuzumab was present in the breast milk of lactating cynomolgus monkeys given 12.5 times the recommended weekly human dose of trastuzumab 2 mg/kg. Infant monkeys with detectable serum levels of trastuzumab did not have any adverse effects on growth or development from birth to 3 months of age; however, trastuzumab levels in animal breast milk may not accurately reflect human breast milk levels.

Because many drugs are secreted in human milk and because of the potential for serious adverse reactions in breast-feeding infants from trastuzumab, decide whether to discontinue breast-feeding or the drug, taking into account the elimination half-life of trastuzumab and the importance of the drug to the mother.

➤*Children:* The safety and effectiveness of trastuzumab in children have not been established.

➤*Elderly:* Trastuzumab has been administered to 386 patients who were 65 years of age and older (253 in the adjuvant treatment, 133 in metastatic breast cancer treatment settings). The risk of cardiac dysfunction was increased in elderly patients compared with younger patients in both those receiving treatment for metastatic disease or adjuvant therapy in studies 1 and 2.

➤*Monitoring:* Conduct thorough cardiac assessment, including history, physical examination, and determination of LVEF by echocardiogram or multiple gated acquisition scan. The following schedule is recommended: baseline LVEF measurement immediately prior to initiation of trastuzumab; LVEF measurements every 3 months during and upon completion of trastuzumab; repeat LVEF measurement at 4-week intervals if trastuzumab is withheld for significant left ventricular cardiac dysfunction; and LVEF measurements every 6 months for at least 2 years following completion of trastuzumab as a component of adjuvant therapy.

Monitor women using trastuzumab during pregnancy for oligohydramnios.

Drug Interactions

Trastuzumab Drug Interactions

Precipitant drug	Object drug[a]		Description
Antineoplastic agents (eg, anthracyclines, doxorubicin)	Trastuzumab	⬆	The risk of symptomatic cardiac dysfunction is increased in patients receiving trastuzumab in combination with chemotherapy agents. The incidence and severity is highest when trastuzumab is used with anthracycline-containing chemotherapy regiments. Close clinical monitoring for signs of cardiac dysfunction is warranted.
Paclitaxel	Trastuzumab	⬆	In clinical studies, administration of paclitaxel in combination with trastuzumab resulted in a 1.5-fold increase in trastuzumab serum levels. Close clinical monitoring for signs of cardiac dysfunction is warranted.

[a] ⬆ = object drug increased.

Adverse Reactions

➤*Emetogenic potential:* Trastuzumab is considered to have moderately low emetogenic potential (10% to 30% incidence of emesis).

➤*Common adverse reactions:* The most common adverse reactions in patients receiving trastuzumab in the adjuvant and metastatic breast cancer setting are anemia, diarrhea, dyspnea, fatigue, fever, headache, increased cough, infections, infusion reactions, myalgia, nausea, neutropenia, rash, and vomiting.

In the metastatic gastric cancer setting, the most common adverse reactions (10% or more) that were increased (at least 5% difference) in the trastuzumab arm compared with the chemotherapy-alone arm were anemia, diarrhea, dysgeusia, fatigue, fever, mucosal inflammation, nasopharyngitis, neutropenia, stomatitis, thrombocytopenia, upper respiratory tract infections, and weight loss.

➤*Discontinuation of therapy:* Adverse reactions requiring interruption or discontinuation of trastuzumab treatment in the adjuvant and metastatic breast cancer setting include congestive heart failure (CHF), pulmonary toxicity, severe infusion reactions, and significant decline in left ventricular cardiac function.

The most common adverse reactions in the metastatic gastric cancer setting that resulted in discontinuation of treatment on the trastuzumab-containing arm in the absence of disease progression were diarrhea, febrile neutropenia, and infection.

➤*Adjuvant breast cancer treatment:*

Trastuzumab Adjuvant Breast Cancer Treatment Adverse Reactions (Study 3) (%)[a]

Adverse reactions	Trastuzumab (1 year) (n = 1,678)	Observation (n = 1,708)
Cardiovascular		
Cardiac arrhythmias[b]	3%	1%
Cardiac disorder	0.3%	0%
Cardiac failure	0.5%	0.2%
CHF	2%	0.3%
Ejection fraction decreased	3.5%	0.6%
Hypertension	4%	2%
Palpitations	3%	0.7%
Ventricular dysfunction	0.2%	0%
CNS		
Asthenia	4.5%	2%
Chills	5%	0%
Dizziness	4%	2%
Headache	10%	3%
Paresthesia	2%	0.6%
Dermatologic		
Nail disorders	2%	0%
Pruritus	2%	0.6%
Rash	4%	0.6%
GI		
Constipation	2%	1%
Diarrhea	7%	1%
Dyspepsia	2%	0.5%
Nausea	6%	1%
Upper abdominal pain	2%	1%
Vomiting	3.5%	0.6%
Musculoskeletal		
Arthralgia	8%	6%
Back pain	5%	3%
Bone pain	3%	2%
Muscle spasm	3%	0.2%
Myalgia	4%	1%
Respiratory		
Cough	5%	2%
Dyspnea	3%	2%
Epistaxis	2%	0.06%
Influenza	4%	0.5%
Interstitial pneumonitis	0.2%	0%
Nasopharyngitis	8%	3%
Pharyngolaryngeal pain	2%	0.5%
Pulmonary hypertension	0.2%	0%
Rhinitis	2%	0.4%
Sinusitis	2%	0.3%
Upper respiratory tract infection	3%	1%

TRASTUZUMAB — INJECTION

Trastuzumab Adjuvant Breast Cancer Treatment Adverse Reactions (Study 3) (%)[a]

Adverse reactions	Trastuzumab (1 year) (n = 1,678)	Observation (n = 1,708)
Miscellaneous		
Autoimmune thyroiditis	0.3%	0%
Edema peripheral	5%	2%
Hypersensitivity	0.6%	0.06%
Influenza-like illness	2%	0.2%
Pyrexia	6%	0.4%
Sudden death	0.06%	0%
Urinary tract infection	3%	0.8%

[a] The incidence of grade 3/4 adverse reactions was < 1% in both arms for each listed term.
[b] Higher level grouping term.

In study 1, only grade 3 to 5 adverse reactions, treatment-related grade 2 events, and grade 2 to 5 dyspnea were collected during and for up to 3 months following protocol-specified treatment. The following noncardiac adverse reactions of grade 2 to 5 occurred at an incidence of at least 2% greater among patients randomized to trastuzumab plus chemotherapy compared with chemotherapy alone: arthralgia (31% vs 28%), fatigue (28% vs 22%), infection (22% vs 14%), hot flashes (17% vs 15%), anemia (13% vs 7%), dyspnea (12% vs 4%), rash/desquamation (11% vs 7%), neutropenia (7% vs 5%), headache (6% vs 4%), and insomnia (3.7% vs 1.5%). The majority of these events were grade 2 in severity.

In study 2, data collection was limited to the following investigator attributed treatment-related adverse reactions: National Cancer Institute-Common Toxicity Criteria (NCI-CTC) grade 4 and 5 hematologic toxicities, grade 3 through 5 nonhematologic toxicities, selected grade 2 through 5 toxicities associated with taxanes (arthralgias, motor neuropathy, myalgia, nail changes, sensory neuropathy), and grade 1 through 5 cardiac toxicities occurring during chemotherapy and/or trastuzumab treatment. The following noncardiac adverse reactions of grade 2 through 5 occurred at an incidence of at least 2% greater among patients randomized to trastuzumab plus chemotherapy compared with chemotherapy alone: arthralgia (11% vs 8.4%), myalgia (10% vs 8%), nail changes (9% vs 7%), and dyspnea (2.5% vs 0.1%). The majority of these reactions were grade 2 in severity.

In study 4, the toxicity profile was similar to that reported in studies 1, 2, and 3, with the exception of a low incidence of CHF in the docetaxel and carboplatin plus trastuzumab arm.

➤*Metastatic breast cancer:*

Trastuzumab Metastatic Breast Cancer Adverse Reactions (≥ 5%) (Studies 5 and 6)

Adverse reactions	Single agent trastuzumab[a] (n = 352)	Trastuzumab + paclitaxel (n = 91)	Paclitaxel alone (n = 95)	Trastuzumab + anthracycline (doxorubicin or epirubicin) and cyclophosphamide (n = 143)	Anthracycline (doxorubicin or epirubicin) and cyclophosphamide alone (n = 135)
Cardiovascular					
CHF	7%	11%	1%	28%	7%
Tachycardia	5%	12%	4%	10%	5%
CNS					
Asthenia	42%	62%	57%	54%	55%
Chills	32%	41%	4%	35%	11%
Depression	6%	12%	13%	20%	12%
Dizziness	13%	22%	24%	24%	18%
Headache	26%	36%	28%	44%	31%
Insomnia	14%	25%	13%	29%	15%
Neuropathy	1%	13%	5%	4%	4%
Paresthesia	9%	48%	39%	17%	11%
Peripheral neuritis	2%	23%	16%	2%	2%
Dermatologic					
Acne	2%	11%	3%	3%	< 1%
Herpes simplex	2%	12%	3%	7%	9%
Rash	18%	38%	18%	27%	17%
GI					
Abdominal pain	22%	34%	22%	23%	18%
Anorexia	14%	24%	16%	31%	26%
Diarrhea	25%	45%	29%	45%	26%
Nausea	33%	51%	9%	76%	77%
Nausea and vomiting	8%	14%	11%	18%	9%
Vomiting	23%	37%	28%	53%	49%
Hematologic					
Anemia	4%	14%	9%	36%	26%
Leukopenia	3%	24%	17%	52%	34%
Metabolic					
Edema	8%	10%	8%	11%	5%
Peripheral edema	10%	22%	20%	20%	17%
Musculoskeletal					
Arthralgia	6%	37%	21%	8%	9%
Back pain	22%	34%	30%	27%	15%
Bone pain	7%	24%	18%	7%	7%
Respiratory					
Cough increased	26%	41%	22%	43%	29%
Dyspnea	22%	27%	26%	42%	25%
Pharyngitis	12%	22%	14%	30%	18%
Rhinitis	14%	22%	5%	22%	16%
Sinusitis	9%	21%	7%	13%	6%
Miscellaneous					
Accidental injury	6%	13%	3%	9%	4%
Allergic reaction	3%	8%	2%	4%	2%
Fever	36%	49%	23%	56%	34%
Flu syndrome	10%	12%	5%	12%	6%
Infection	20%	47%	27%	47%	31%
Pain	47%	61%	62%	57%	42%
Urinary tract infection	5%	18%	14%	13%	7%

[a] Data for trastuzumab as a single agent were from 4 studies, including 213 patients from study 6.

➤*Metastatic gastric cancer:*

Trastuzumab Metastatic Gastric Cancer Adverse Reactions of All Grades (≥ 5%) or Grade 3 /4 (>1%) (Study 7)

Adverse reactions	Trastuzumab + Cisplatin + Capecitabine or 5-fluorouracil (n = 294)		Cisplatin + Capecitabine or 5-fluorouracil (n = 290)	
	All grades	Grades 3/4	All grades	Grades 3/4
CNS				
Chills	8%	≤ 1%	0%	0%
Dysgeusia	10%	0%	5%	0%
Fatigue	35%	4%	28%	2%
GI				
Diarrhea	37%	9%	28%	4%
Dysphagia	6%	2%	3%	≤1%
Stomatitis	24%	1%	15%	2%
Hematologic				
Anemia	28%	12%	21%	10%
Febrile Neutropenia		5%		3%
Neutropenia	78%	34%	73%	29%
Thrombocytopenia	16%	5%	11%	3%
Metabolic/Nutritional				
Hypokalemia	28%	10%	24%	6%
Weight decrease	23%	2%	14%	2%
Respiratory				
Nasopharyngitis	13%	0%	6%	0%
Upper respiratory tract infections	19%	0%	10%	0%
Miscellaneous				
Fever	18%	1%	12%	0%
Mucosal inflammation	13%	2%	6%	1%
Renal failure and impairment	18%	3%	15%	2%

➤*Cardiovascular:*

Thrombosis/Embolism – In 4 randomized, controlled clinical trials, the incidence of thrombotic adverse reactions was higher in patients receiving trastuzumab and chemotherapy compared with chemotherapy alone in 3 studies (3% vs 1.3% [study 1], 2.5% and 3.7% vs 2.2% [study 4], and 2.1% vs 0% [study 5]).

TRASTUZUMAB — INJECTION

Cardiomyopathy – Serial measurement of cardiac function (LVEF) was obtained in clinical trials in the adjuvant treatment of breast cancer. In studies 1 and 2, 6% of patients were not permitted to initiate trastuzumab following completion of doxorubicin and cyclophosphamide chemotherapy due to cardiac dysfunction (LVEF less than 50% or 15 point or more decline in LVEF from baseline to end of doxorubicin and cyclophosphamide). Following initiation of trastuzumab therapy, the incidence of new-onset, dose-limiting myocardial dysfunction was higher among patients receiving trastuzumab and paclitaxel compared with those receiving paclitaxel alone in studies 1 and 2, and in patients receiving trastuzumab monotherapy compared with observation in study 3.

Trastuzumab New-Onset Myocardial Dysfunction (by LVEF)[a]					
	LVEF < 50% and absolute decrease from baseline			Absolute LVEF decrease	
	LVEF < 50%	≥ 10% decrease	≥ 16% decrease	< 20% and ≥ 10%	≥ 20%
Studies 1 and 2					
Doxorubicin and cyclophosphamide followed by paclitaxel plus trastuzumab (n = 1,606)	22.8%	18.3%	11.7%	33.4%	9.2%
Doxorubicin and cyclophosphamide followed by paclitaxel (n = 1,488)	9.1%	5.4%	2.2%	18.3%	2.4%
Study 3					
Trastuzumab (n = 1,678)	8.6%	7%	3.8%	22.4%	3.5%
Observation (n = 1,708)	2.7%	2%	1.2%	11.9%	1.2%
Study 4					
Docetaxel and carboplatin plus trastuzumab (n = 1,056)	8.5%	5.9%	3.3%	34.5%	6.3%
Doxorubicin and cyclophosphamide followed by docetaxel plus trastuzumab (n = 1,068)	17%	13.3%	9.8%	44.3%	13.2%
Doxorubicin and cyclophosphamide followed by docetaxel (n = 1,050)	9.5%	6.6%	3.3%	34%	5.5%

[a] For studies 1, 2, and 3, events are counted from the beginning of trastuzumab treatment. For study 4, events are counted from the date of randomization.

The incidence of treatment-emergent CHF among patients in the metastatic breast cancer trials was classified for severity using the New York Heart Association (NYHA) classification system (I through IV, where IV is the most severe level of cardiac failure).

In the metastatic breast cancer trials, the probability of cardiac dysfunction was highest in patients who received trastuzumab concurrently with anthracyclines.

In study 7, 5% of patients in the trastuzumab plus chemotherapy arm compared with 1.1% of patients in the chemotherapy-alone arm had LVEF value below 50% with a 10% or more absolute decrease in LVEF from pretreatment values.

➤*GI:* Among women receiving adjuvant therapy for breast cancer, the incidence of NCI-CTC grade 2 to 5 diarrhea (6.2% vs 4.8% [study 1]), NCI-CTC grade 3 to 5 diarrhea (1.6% vs 0% [study 2]), and grade 1 to 4 diarrhea (7% vs 1% [study 3]) were higher in patients receiving trastuzumab compared with controls. In study 4, the incidence of grade 3 to 4 diarrhea was higher (5.7% doxorubicin and cyclophosphamide followed by docetaxel plus trastuzumab, 5.5% docetaxel and carboplatin plus trastuzumab vs 3% doxorubicin and cyclophosphamide followed by docetaxel) and of grade 1 to 4 was higher (51% doxorubicin and cyclophosphamide followed by docetaxel plus trastuzumab, 63% docetaxel and carboplatin plus trastuzumab vs 43% doxorubicin and cyclophosphamide followed by docetaxel) among women receiving trastuzumab. Of patients receiving trastuzumab as a single agent for the treatment of metastatic breast cancer, 25% experienced diarrhea. An increased incidence of diarrhea was observed in patients receiving trastuzumab in combination with chemotherapy for treatment of metastatic breast cancer.

➤*Hematologic:*

Anemia – In randomized, controlled clinical trials, the overall incidence of anemia (30% vs 21% [study 5]), of selected NCI-CTC grade 2 to 5 anemia (12.5% vs 6.6% [study 1]), and of anemia requiring transfusions (0.1% vs 0 patients [study 2]) was increased in patients receiving trastuzumab and chemotherapy compared with those receiving chemotherapy alone. Following the administration of trastuzumab as a single agent (study 6), the incidence of NCI-CTC grade 3 anemia was less than 1%. In study 7 (metastatic gastric cancer) on the trastuzumab-containing arm compared with the chemotherapy-alone arm, the overall incidence of anemia was 28% compared with 21% and of NCI-CTC grade 3/4 anemia was 12.2% compared with 10.3%.

Neutropenia – In randomized, controlled clinical trials in the adjuvant setting, the incidence of selected NCI-CTC grade 4 to 5 neutropenia (2% vs 0.7% [study 2]) and of selected grade 2 to 5 neutropenia (7.1% vs 4.5% [study 1]) was increased in patients receiving trastuzumab and chemotherapy compared with those receiving chemotherapy alone. In a randomized, controlled trial in patients with metastatic breast cancer, the incidences of NCI-CTC grade 3/4 neutropenia (32% vs 22%) and of febrile neutropenia (23% vs 17%) were also increased in patients randomized to trastuzumab in combination with myelosuppressive chemotherapy compared with chemotherapy alone. In study 7 (metastatic gastric cancer) on the trastuzumab-containing arm compared with the chemotherapy-alone arm, the incidence of NCI CTC grade 3/4 neutropenia was 36.8% compared with 28.9%; febrile neutropenia was 5.1% compared with 2.8%.

➤*Renal:* In study 7 (metastatic gastric cancer) on the trastuzumab-containing arm compared with the chemotherapy-alone arm, the incidence of renal impairment was 18% compared with 14.5%. Severe (grade 3/4) renal failure was 2.7% on the trastuzumab-containing arm compared with 1.7% on the chemotherapy-only arm. Treatment discontinuation for renal insufficiency/failure was 2% on the trastuzumab-containing arm and 0.3% on the chemotherapy-only arm.

In the postmarketing setting, rare cases of nephrotic syndrome with pathologic evidence of glomerulopathy have been reported. The time to onset ranged from 4 months to approximately 18 months from initiation of trastuzumab therapy. Pathologic findings included membranous glomerulonephritis, focal glomerulosclerosis, and fibrillary glomerulonephritis. Complications included volume overload and CHF.

➤*Respiratory:*

Adjuvant breast cancer treatment – Among women receiving adjuvant therapy for breast cancer, the incidence of selected NCI-CTC grade 2 to 5 pulmonary toxicity (14% vs 5% [study 1]), selected NCI-CTC grade 3 to 5 pulmonary toxicity, and spontaneously reported grade 2 dyspnea (3.4% vs 1% [study 2]) was higher in patients receiving trastuzumab and chemotherapy compared with chemotherapy alone. The most common pulmonary toxicity was dyspnea (NCI-CTC grade 2 to 5: 12% vs 4% [study 1]; NCI-CTC grade 2 to 5: 2.5% vs 0.1% [study 2]). Pneumonitis/pulmonary infiltrates occurred in 0.7% of patients receiving trastuzumab compared with 0.3% of those receiving chemotherapy alone. Fatal respiratory failure occurred in 3 patients receiving trastuzumab, one as a component of multi-organ system failure, compared with 1 patient receiving chemotherapy alone.

In study 3, there were 4 cases of interstitial pneumonitis in trastuzumab-treated patients compared with none in the control arm.

Metastatic breast cancer – Among women receiving trastuzumab for treatment of metastatic breast cancer, the incidence of pulmonary toxicity was also increased. Pulmonary adverse reactions have been reported in the postmarketing experience as part of the symptom complex of infusion reactions. Pulmonary reactions include acute respiratory distress syndrome, bronchospasm, dyspnea, hypoxia, noncardiogenic pulmonary edema, pleural effusions, and pulmonary infiltrates.

➤*Miscellaneous:*

Infection – The overall incidences of infection (46% vs 30% [study 5]), selected NCI-CTC grade 2 to 5 infection/febrile neutropenia (22% vs 14% [study 1]), and selected grade 3 to 5 infection/febrile neutropenia (3.3% vs 1.4% [study 2]) were higher in patients receiving trastuzumab and chemotherapy compared with those receiving chemotherapy alone. The most common site of infections in the adjuvant setting involved the upper respiratory tract, skin, and urinary tract.

In study 4, the overall incidence of infection was higher with the addition of trastuzumab to doxorubicin and cyclophosphamide followed by docetaxel but not to docetaxel and carboplatin plus trastuzumab (44% [doxorubicin and cyclophosphamide followed by docetaxel plus trastuzumab], 37% [docetaxel and carboplatin plus trastuzumab], 38% [doxorubicin and cyclophosphamide followed by docetaxel]). The incidences of NCI-CTC grade 3 to 4 infection were similar (25% [doxorubicin and cyclophosphamide followed by docetaxel plus trastuzumab], 21% [docetaxel and carboplatin plus trastuzumab], 23% [doxorubicin and cyclophosphamide followed by docetaxel]) across the 3 arms.

In a randomized, controlled trial in treatment of metastatic breast cancer, the reported incidence of febrile neutropenia was higher (23% vs 17%) in patients receiving trastuzumab in combination with myelosuppressive chemotherapy compared with chemotherapy alone.

Infusion reactions – During the first infusion with trastuzumab, the symptoms most commonly reported were chills and fever, occurring in approximately 40% of patients in clinical trials. Symptoms were treated with acetaminophen, diphenhydramine, and meperidine (with or without reduction in the rate of trastuzumab infusion); permanent discontinuation of trastuzumab for infusional toxicity was required in less than 1% of patients. Other signs and/or symptoms may include nausea, vomiting, pain (in some cases at tumor sites), rigors, headache, dizziness, dyspnea, hypotension, elevated blood pressure, rash, and asthenia. Infusional toxicity occurred in 21% and 35% of patients and was severe in 1.4% and 9% of patients on second or subsequent trastuzumab infusions administered as monotherapy or in combination with chemotherapy, respectively. In the postmarketing setting, severe infusion reactions, including hypersensitivity, anaphylaxis, and angioedema, have been reported.

➤*Postmarketing:* Glomerulopathy, infusion reaction, and oligohydramnios have been identified during postapproval use of trastuzumab.

TRASTUZUMAB — INJECTION

Overdosage

There is no experience with overdosage in human clinical trials. Single doses greater than 8 mg/kg have not been tested.

Patient Information

Advise patients to contact their health care provider immediately for any of the following: new onset or worsening shortness of breath, cough, swelling of the ankles/legs, swelling of the face, palpitations, weight gain of more than 5 pounds in 24 hours, dizziness, or loss of consciousness.

Advise pregnant women and women of childbearing potential that trastuzumab exposure can result in fetal harm.

Advise women with reproductive potential to use effective contraceptive methods during treatment and for a minimum of 6 months following trastuzumab.

Encourage pregnant women who are using trastuzumab to enroll in MotHER- the *Herceptin* Pregnancy Registry by calling 1-800-690-6720.

ALEMTUZUMAB

Rx	**Campath** (Bayer HealthCare)	**Injection, solution, concentrate:** 30 mg/mL	Sodium chloride 8 mg, dibasic sodium phosphate 1.44 mg, potassium chloride 0.2 mg, monobasic potassium phosphate 0.2 mg, 0.0187 mg EDTA. Preservative free. In single-use vials.

ALEMTUZUMAB — INJECTION

WARNING

Cytopenias – Serious, including fatal, pancytopenia/marrow hypoplasia, autoimmune idiopathic thrombocytopenia, and autoimmune hemolytic anemia have occurred in patients receiving alemtuzumab therapy. Single doses of alemtuzumab of more than 30 mg or cumulative doses of more than 90 mg per week increase the incidence of pancytopenia.

Infusion reactions – Alemtuzumab administration can result in serious, including fatal, infusion reactions. Carefully monitor patients during infusions and withhold alemtuzumab for grade 3 or 4 infusion reactions. Gradually escalate to the recommended dose at the initiation of therapy and after interruption of therapy for 7 days or more.

Infections – Serious, including fatal, bacterial, viral, fungal, and protozoan infections can occur in patients receiving alemtuzumab. Administer prophylaxis against *Pneumocystis jiroveci* pneumonia (PCP) and herpes virus infections.

Indications

➤*B-cell chronic lymphocytic leukemia (B-CLL):* As a single agent for the treatment of B-CLL.

➤*Off-label uses:*

Multiple sclerosis – [4] = Insufficient documentation. Data evaluating the efficacy of alemtuzumab for the treatment of multiple sclerosis (MS) are limited to open, noncontrolled trials in 2 patient cohorts and to interim results from a phase 2 trial. All published data currently available are from the same group of investigators. In patients with secondary progressive MS, alemtuzumab was found to reduce cerebral inflammation and the development of new lesions; however, disease progression continued. In patients with relapsing-remitting MS, there was a significant decrease in cerebral inflammation, reduced relapse rate, and improvement in disability. However, alemtuzumab use is not without potentially significant safety concerns. Alemtuzumab use in patients with MS is discouraged until additional data are available from randomized, controlled trials.

Rheumatoid arthritis – [5] = Poor documentation. The data evaluating the safety and efficacy of alemtuzumab for the treatment of rheumatoid arthritis (RA) are limited to open, noncontrolled, phase 1/2 trials. Overall, clinical response was rapid but short lived. Because published data suggest that the risks of therapy exceed the benefits, use in patients with RA is not recommended.

Administration and Dosage

➤*Maximum dose:*

Adults – 30 mg/day (single dose) or 90 mg/week (cumulative dose) according to the prescribing information.

➤*General dosing considerations:* Reduce incidence of infusion reactions with premedication. (See Infusion reactions.)

Gradually escalate to the recommended dose at the initiation of therapy and after interruption of therapy for 7 days or more.

➤*Adults:*

B-cell chronic lymphocytic leukemia (B-CLL) –

Initial dosage: 3 mg/day IV until infusion reactions are grade 2 or less.

Escalation is required at initiation of dosing or if dosing is withheld for at least 7 days during treatment.

Dosage titration: After the initial dose, administer 10 mg/day IV until infusion reactions are grade 2 or less. Gradually escalate to the maximum recommended single dose of 30 mg IV. Escalation to 30 mg ordinarily can be accomplished in 3 to 7 days.

Maintenance dosage: 30 mg/day IV 3 times per week on alternate days (eg, Monday, Wednesday, Friday).

Single doses of more than 30 mg or cumulative doses of more than 90 mg per week increase the incidence of pancytopenia.

Dosage adjustment: Withhold alemtuzumab therapy during serious infection, profound hematologic toxicity, or other serious adverse reactions until resolution.

Discontinue alemtuzumab therapy for autoimmune anemia or autoimmune thrombocytopenia.

There are no dose modifications recommended for lymphopenia.

Alemtuzumab Dosage Adjustment for Neutropenia or Thrombocytopenia

Hematologic values	Dose adjustment[a]
ANC[b] < 250/mcL and/or platelet count ≤ 25,000/mcL	
For first occurrence	Withhold alemtuzumab therapy. Resume alemtuzumab therapy at 30 mg when the ANC is ≥ 500/mcL and the platelet count is ≥ 50,000/mcL.
For second occurrence	Withhold alemtuzumab therapy. Resume alemtuzumab therapy at 10 mg when the ANC is ≥ 500/mcL and the platelet count is ≥ 50,000/mcL.
For third occurrence	Discontinue alemtuzumab therapy.
≥ 50% decrease from baseline in patients initiating therapy with a baseline ANC ≤ 250/mcL and/or a baseline platelet count ≤ 25,000/mcL	
For first occurrence	Withhold alemtuzumab therapy. Resume alemtuzumab therapy at 30 mg upon return to baseline value(s).
For second occurrence	Withhold alemtuzumab therapy. Resume alemtuzumab therapy at 10 mg upon return to baseline value(s).
For third occurrence	Discontinue alemtuzumab therapy.

[a] If the delay between dosing is ≥ 7 days, initiate therapy at alemtuzumab 3 mg and escalate to 10 mg and then to 30 mg as tolerated.
[b] ANC = absolute neutrophil count.

Duration of therapy: The total duration of therapy, including dose escalation, is 12 weeks.

Concomitant therapy: Premedicate with diphenhydramine 50 mg and acetaminophen 500 to 1,000 mg 30 minutes before the first dose, before dose escalation, and as needed.(See also Infusion reactions.)

In patients who experience severe infusion reactions, hydrocortisone sodium succinate 200 mg IV may be added to the pretreatment regimen prior to subsequent doses. (See also Infusion reactions.)

Administer trimethoprim/sulfamethoxazole double-strength twice daily 3 times per week (or equivalent) as PCP prophylaxis. Administer famciclovir 250 mg twice daily or equivalent as herpetic prophylaxis.

Continue PCP and herpes viral prophylaxis for a minimum of 2 months after completion of alemtuzumab therapy or until the CD4+ count is at least 200 cells/mcL, whichever occurs later.

Off-label dosing –

Multiple sclerosis: [4] = Insufficient documentation. 100 mg was given as 20 mg daily for 5 consecutive days by IV infusion over 4 hours. Most patients received only the single 100 mg dose. Repeat doses were given to a subset of patients to maintain or enhance improvement.

➤*Infusion reactions:* Premedicate with diphenhydramine 50 mg and acetaminophen 500 to 1,000 mg 30 minutes before the first dose, before dose escalation, and as needed.

Institute appropriate medical management (eg, epinephrine, meperidine, steroids) for infusion reactions as needed. If the patient experiences a reaction, the infusion may be continued at the same rate at the clinician's discretion. Temporarily interrupt the infusion or decrease the rate if severe reactions occur, including hypotension, hypertension, shortness of breath, or rash.

Symptoms may be treated with hydrocortisone sodium succinate 200 mg IV, diphenhydramine, acetaminophen, bronchodilators, oxygen, or IV fluids. Monitor the patient until symptoms resolve completely.

In patients who experience severe infusion reactions, hydrocortisone sodium succinate 200 mg IV may be added to the pretreatment regimen prior to subsequent doses. Patients who react to alemtuzumab infusions may receive additional doses.

➤*Preparation for administration:* Alemtuzumab is considered a cytotoxic agent. Follow safe handling procedures when preparing, administering, or dispensing alemtuzumab.

Do not shake vial.

ALEMTUZUMAB — INJECTION

Use aseptic technique during the preparation and administration of alemtuzumab. Withdraw the necessary amount of alemtuzumab from the vial into a syringe. Use within 8 hours after dilution.

- To prepare a 3 mg dose, withdraw 0.1 mL into a 1 mL syringe calibrated in increments of 0.01 mL.
- To prepare a 10 mg dose, withdraw 0.33 mL into a 1 mL syringe calibrated in increments of 0.01 mL.
- To prepare a 30 mg dose, withdraw 1 mL in either a 1 or 3 mL syringe calibrated in 0.1 mL increments.

Inject syringe contents into 100 mL of sterile sodium chloride 0.9% or dextrose 5% in water. Gently invert the bag to mix the solution. Discard the syringe. Discard the vial, including any unused portion, after withdrawal of the dose.

➤*Administration:* Administer as an IV infusion over 2 hours. Observe patients for infusion-related symptoms (eg, rigors, fever). (See also Infusion reactions.)

Do not administer as an IV push or bolus.

➤*Admixture compatibility:* Alemtuzumab is compatible with polyvinylchloride (PVC) bags and PVC or polyethylene-lined PVC administration sets. Do not add or simultaneously infuse other drug substances through the same IV line.

➤*Storage/Stability:* Store undiluted alemtuzumab at 2° to 8°C (36° to 46°F). Do not freeze. If accidentally frozen, thaw at 2° to 8°C (36° to 46°F) before administration. Protect from direct sunlight.

Store diluted alemtuzumab at room temperature, 15° to 30°C (59° to 86°F), or refrigerated, 2° to 8°C (36° to 46°F). Protect from light. Diluted solutions are preservative free and should be used within 24 hours to reduce the risk of microbial contamination. However, the manufacturer recommends use within 8 hours.

Discard any unused portion in vial after a single use. Discard vial within 6 hours of the initial needle puncture if opened within an ISO Class 5 biological safety cabinet, or within 1 hour of the initial needle puncture if opened outside of such an environment, based on the USP Chapter 797 standards.

Actions

➤*Pharmacology:* Alemtuzumab binds to CD52, a nonmodulating antigen present on the surface of B and T lymphocytes, a majority of monocytes, macrophages, and natural killer cells, and a subpopulation of granulocytes. A proportion of bone marrow cells, including some CD34+ cells, express variable levels of CD52. The proposed mechanism of action is antibody-dependent cellular-mediated lysis following cell surface binding of alemtuzumab to the leukemic cells.

➤*Pharmacokinetics:*

Absorption/Distribution – Alemtuzumab pharmacokinetics displayed nonlinear elimination kinetics. After the last 30 mg dose, the mean volume of distribution at steady state was 0.18 L/kg (range, 0.1 to 0.4 L/kg). Systemic clearance decreased with repeated administration because of decreased receptor-mediated clearance (ie, loss of CD52 receptors in the periphery). After 12 weeks of dosing, patients exhibited a 7-fold increase in mean area under the curve (AUC).

Excretion – Mean half-life was 11 hours (range, 2 to 32 hours) after the first 30 mg dose and was 6 days (range, 1 to 14 days) after the last 30 mg dose.

Warnings/Precautions

➤*Infusion reactions:* Adverse reactions occurring during or shortly after alemtuzumab infusion include bronchospasm, chills/rigors, dyspnea, emesis, hypotension, nausea, pyrexia, rash, and urticaria. In clinical trials, the frequency of infusion reactions was highest in the first week of treatment. Monitor for the signs and symptoms listed previously and withhold infusion for grade 3 or 4 infusion reactions. The following serious, including fatal, infusion reactions have been identified in postmarketing reports: acute cardiac insufficiency, acute respiratory distress syndrome, anaphylactoid shock, angioedema, cardiac arrest, cardiac arrhythmias, myocardial infarction, pulmonary infiltrates, respiratory arrest, and syncope. Initiate alemtuzumab according to the recommended dose-escalation scheme. Premedicate patients with an antihistamine and acetaminophen prior to dosing. Institute medical management (eg, epinephrine, glucocorticoids, meperidine) for infusion reactions as needed. If therapy is interrupted for 7 or more days, reinstitute alemtuzumab with gradual dose escalation.

➤*Immunosuppression/Infections:* Alemtuzumab treatment results in severe and prolonged lymphopenia with a concomitant increased incidence of opportunistic infections. Administer PCP and herpes viral prophylaxis during alemtuzumab therapy and for a minimum of 2 months following the last dose of alemtuzumab or until CD4+ counts are at least 200 cells/mcL, whichever occurs later. Prophylaxis does not eliminate these infections.

Routinely monitor patients for cytomegalovirus (CMV) infection during alemtuzumab treatment and for at least 2 months following completion of treatment. Withhold alemtuzumab for serious infections and during antiviral treatment for CMV infection or confirmed CMV viremia (defined as polymerase chain reaction-positive CMV in 2 or more consecutive samples obtained 1 week apart). Initiate therapeutic ganciclovir (or equivalent) for CMV infection or confirmed CMV viremia.

Administer only irradiated blood products to severely lymphopenic patients to avoid graft versus host disease, unless emergent circumstances dictate immediate transfusion.

In patients receiving alemtuzumab as initial therapy, recovery of CD4+ counts to at least 200 cells/mcL occurred by 6 months posttreatment; however at 2 months posttreatment, the median was 183 cells/mcL. In previously treated patients receiving alemtuzumab, the median time to recovery of CD4+ counts to at least 200 cells/mcL was 2 months; however, full recovery (to baseline) of CD4+ and CD8+ counts may take longer than 12 months.

➤*Cytopenias:* Severe, including fatal, autoimmune anemia and thrombocytopenia, and prolonged myelosuppression have been reported in patients receiving alemtuzumab.

In addition, bone marrow aplasia, hemolytic anemia, hypoplasia, and pure red cell aplasia have been reported after treatment with alemtuzumab at the recommended dose. Single doses of alemtuzumab of more than 30 mg or cumulative doses of more than 90 mg per week increase the incidence of pancytopenia.

Withhold alemtuzumab for severe cytopenias (except lymphopenia). Discontinue for autoimmune cytopenias or recurrent/persistent severe cytopenias (except lymphopenia). No data exist on the safety of alemtuzumab resumption in patients with autoimmune cytopenias or marrow aplasia.

➤*Immunization:* The safety of immunization with live viral vaccines following alemtuzumab therapy has not been studied. Do not administer live viral vaccines to patients who have recently received alemtuzumab. The ability to generate a primary or anamnestic humoral response to any vaccine following alemtuzumab therapy has not been studied.

➤*Immunogenicity:* As with all therapeutic proteins, there is potential for immunogenicity. Using an enzyme-linked immunoabsorbent assay, antihuman antibodies were detected in 11 of 133 (8.3%) previously untreated patients. In addition, 2 patients were weakly positive for neutralizing activity. Limited data suggest that anti-alemtuzumab antibodies did not adversely affect tumor response. Four of 211 (1.9%) previously treated patients were found to have antibodies to alemtuzumab following treatment.

The incidence of antibody formation is highly dependent on the sensitivity and specificity of the assay. Additionally, the observed incidence of antibody (including neutralizing antibody) positivity in an assay may be influenced by several factors, including assay methodology, sample handling, timing of sample collection, concomitant medications, and underlying disease. For these reasons, comparison of the incidence of antibodies to alemtuzumab with the incidence of antibodies to other products may be misleading.

➤*Pregnancy: Category C.* Animal reproduction studies have not been conducted with alemtuzumab. Immunoglobulin G (IgG) antibodies, such as alemtuzumab, can cross the placental barrier. It is not known whether alemtuzumab can cause fetal harm when administered to a pregnant woman or can affect reproduction capacity. Give alemtuzumab to a pregnant woman only if clearly needed.

➤*Lactation:* Excretion of alemtuzumab in human breast milk has not been studied. It is not known whether this drug is excreted in human milk. IgG antibodies, such as alemtuzumab, can be excreted in human milk. Because many drugs are excreted in human milk and because of the potential for serious adverse reactions in breast-feeding infants from alemtuzumab, decide whether to discontinue breast-feeding or the drug, taking into account the elimination half-life of alemtuzumab and the importance of the drug to the mother.

➤*Children:* The safety and efficacy of alemtuzumab in children have not been established.

➤*Monitoring:* Obtain complete blood cell counts at weekly intervals during alemtuzumab therapy and more frequently if worsening anemia, neutropenia, or thrombocytopenia occurs. Assess CD4+ counts after treatment until recovery to at least 200 cells/mcL. Monitor patient for signs and symptoms of an infusion reaction and CMV during treatment and for at least 2 months following completion of treatment.

Adverse Reactions

The following adverse reactions are discussed in greater detail in other sections of the monograph: cytopenias, immunosuppression/infections, and infusion reactions. The most common adverse reactions with alemtuzumab are cytopenias (eg, anemia, lymphopenia, neutropenia, thrombocytopenia), GI symptoms (eg, abdominal pain, emesis, nausea), infections (eg, CMV infection, CMV viremia, other infections), infusion reactions (eg, chills, dyspnea, hypotension, nausea, pyrexia, rash, tachycardia, urticaria), and neurological symptoms (eg, anxiety, insomnia). The most common serious adverse reactions are cytopenias, immunosuppression/infections, and infusion reactions.

Alemtuzumab is considered to have moderately low emetogenic potential (10% to 30% incidence of emesis).

➤*Previously treated/untreated patients:* The following data reflect exposure to alemtuzumab in 296 patients with CLL of whom 147 were previously untreated and 149 of whom received at least 2 prior chemotherapy regimens. The median duration of exposure was 11.7 weeks for previously untreated patients and 8 weeks for previously treated patients.

Infusion reactions – Infusion reactions, which included chills, dyspnea, hypotension, pyrexia, and urticaria, were common. Grade 3 and 4 pyrexia and/or chills occurred in approximately 10% of previously untreated patients and in approximately 35% of previously treated patients. The occurrence of infusion reactions was greatest during the initial week of treatment and decreased with subsequent doses of alemtuzumab. All patients were pretreated with antipyretics and antihistamines; additionally, 43% of previously untreated patients received glucocorticoid pretreatment.

Infections – In the study of previously untreated patients, patients were tested weekly for CMV using a polymerase chain reaction assay from initiation through completion of therapy, and every 2 weeks for the first 2 months following therapy. CMV infection occurred in 16% (23/147) of previously untreated patients; approximately one-third of these infections were serious or life threatening. In studies of previously treated patients in which routine

ALEMTUZUMAB — INJECTION

CMV surveillance was not required, CMV infection was documented in 6% (9/149) of patients; nearly all of these infections were serious or life-threatening.

Other infections were reported in approximately 50% of patients across all studies. Grade 3 to 5 sepsis ranged from 3% to 10% across studies and was higher in previously treated patients. Grade 3 to 4 febrile neutropenia ranged from 5% to 10% across studies and was higher in previously treated patients. Infection-related fatalities occurred in 2% of previously untreated patients and 16% of previously treated patients. There were 198 episodes of other infection in 109 previously untreated patients; 16% were bacterial, 7% were fungal, 4% were other viral, and in 73%, the organism was not identified.

Anemia – In previously untreated patients, the incidence of grade 3 or 4 anemia was 12% with a median time to onset of 31 days and a median duration of 8 days. In previously treated patients, the incidence of grade 3 or 4 anemia was 38%. Seventeen percent of previously untreated patients and 66% of previously treated patients received erythropoiesis-stimulating agents, transfusions, or both.

Neutropenia – In previously untreated patients, the incidence of grade 3 or 4 neutropenia was 42% with a median time to onset of 31 days and a median duration of 37 days. In previously treated patients, the incidence of grade 3 or 4 neutropenia was 64% with a median duration of 28 days. Ten percent of previously untreated patients and 17% of previously treated patients received granulocyte colony–stimulating factors.

Thrombocytopenia – In previously untreated patients, the incidence of grade 3 or 4 thrombocytopenia was 14% with a median time to onset of 9 days and a median duration of 14 days. In previously treated patients, the incidence of grade 3 or 4 thrombocytopenia was 52% with a median duration of 21 days. Autoimmune thrombocytopenia was reported in 2% of previously treated patients with 1 fatality.

Lymphopenia – Severe lymphopenia and a rapid and sustained decrease in lymphocyte subsets occurred in previously untreated and previously treated patients following administration of alemtuzumab. In previously untreated patients, the median CD4+ was 0 cells/mcL at 1 month after treatment and 238 cells/mcL (25% to 75% interquartile range, 115 to 418 cells/mcL at 6 months posttreatment).

Cardiac – Cardiac dysrhythmias occurred in approximately 14% of previously untreated patients. The majority were tachycardias and were temporally associated with infusion; dysrhythmias were grade 3 or 4 in 1% of patients.

➤*Previously untreated patients:* The following table contains selected adverse reactions observed in 294 patients randomized (1:1) to received alemtuzumab or chlorambucil as first line therapy for B-CLL. Alemtuzumab was administered at a dose of 30 mg IV, 3 times weekly for up to 12 weeks. The median duration of therapy was 11.7 weeks with a median weekly dose of 82 mg (25% to 75% interquartile range, 69 to 90 mg).

Alemtuzumab Adverse Reactions in Treatment Naive B-CLL Patients[a]

Adverse reaction	Alemtuzumab (n = 147)		Chlorambucil (n = 147)	
	All grades[b]	Grades 3 to 4	All grades	Grades 3 to 4
Cardiovascular				
Hypertension	14%	5%	2%	1%
Hypotension	16%	1%	0%	0%
Tachycardia	10%	0%	1%	0%
CNS				
Anxiety	8%	0%	1%	0%
Headache	14%	1%	8%	0%
Insomnia	10%	0%	3%	0%
Tremor	3%	0%	1%	0%
Dermatologic				
Erythema	4%	0%	1%	0%
Rash	13%	1%	4%	0%
Urticaria	16%	2%	1%	0%
Hematologic/Lymphatic				
Anemia	76%	13%	54%	18%
Lymphopenia	97%	97%	9%	1%
Neutropenia	77%	42%	51%	26%
Thrombocytopenia	71%	13%	70%	14%
Miscellaneous				
Chills	53%	3%	1%	0%
CMV infection	16%	5%	0%	0%
CMV viremia[c]	55%	4%	8%	0%
Diarrhea	10%	1%	4%	0%
Dyspnea	14%	4%	7%	3%
Other infections	74%	21%	65%	10%
Pyrexia	69%	10%	11%	1%

[a] Adverse reactions occurring at a higher relative frequency in the alemtuzumab arm.
[b] National Cancer Institute-Common Toxicity Criteria (NCI-CTC) version 2.0 for adverse reactions; NCI-Common Terminology Criteria for Adverse Events (CTCAE) version 3.0 for laboratory values.
[c] CMV viremia (without evidence of symptoms) included both cases of single polymerase reaction chain-positive test results and of confirmed CMV viremia (≥ 2 occasions in consecutive samples 1 week apart). For the latter, ganciclovir (or equivalent) was initiated per protocol.

➤*Previously treated patients:* Additional safety information was obtained from 3 single-arm studies of 149 previously treated patients with CLL administered alemtuzumab 30 mg IV, 3 times weekly for 4 to 12 weeks (median cumulative dose, 673 mg [range, 2 to 1,106 mg]; median duration of therapy, 8 weeks). Adverse reactions in these studies not listed in the previous table that occurred at an incidence rate of more than 5% were anorexia, bronchospasm, dysesthesia, emesis, fatigue, mucositis, musculoskeletal pain, and nausea.

➤*Postmarketing:* The following adverse reactions were identified during postapproval use of alemtuzumab. Because these reactions are reported voluntarily from a population of uncertain size, it is not always possible to reliably estimate their frequency or establish a causal relationship to alemtuzumab exposure. Decisions to include these reactions in labeling are typically based on 1 or more of the following factors: seriousness of the reaction, frequency of the reporting, or strength of causal connection to alemtuzumab.

Cardiovascular – Cardiomyopathy, decreased ejection fraction (in patients previously treated with cardiotoxic agents).

CNS – Chronic inflammatory demyelinating polyradiculoneuropathy, Guillain Barré syndrome, optic neuropathy.

Miscellaneous – Aplastic anemia, Epstein-Barr virus, fatal infusion reactions, Goodpasture syndrome, Grave disease, progressive multifocal leukoencephalopathy, serum sickness, tumor lysis syndrome.

Overdosage

➤*Symptoms:* Across all clinical experience, the reported maximum single dose received was 90 mg. Bone marrow aplasia, infections, or severe infusion reactions occurred in patients who received a dose higher than recommended.

➤*Treatment:* There is no known specific antidote for alemtuzumab overdosage. Treatment consists of drug discontinuation and supportive therapy.

Patient Information

Advise patients to report any signs or symptoms, such as bleeding, easy bruising, petechiae or purpura, pallor, weakness, or fatigue.

Advise patients of the signs and symptoms of infusion reactions and of the need to take premedications as prescribed.

Advise patients to immediately report symptoms of infection (eg, pyrexia) and to take prophylactic anti-infectives for PCP (trimethoprim/sulfamethoxazole double-strength or equivalent) and for herpes virus (famciclovir or equivalent) as prescribed.

Advise patients that irradiation of blood products is required until adequate lymphocyte recovery.

Advise patients that they should not be immunized with live viral vaccines if they have recently been treated with alemtuzumab.

Advise men and women with reproductive potential to use effective contraceptive methods during treatment and for a minimum of 6 months following alemtuzumab therapy.

OFATUMUMAB

Rx	**Arzerra** (GlaxoSmithKline)	**Injection, solution, concentrate:** 20 mg/mL	Preservative free. In 10 mL single-use vials.

OFATUMUMAB — INJECTION

Indications

➤*Chronic lymphocytic leukemia:* For the treatment of patients with chronic lymphocytic leukemia (CLL) refractory to fludarabine and alemtuzumab.

Administration and Dosage

➤*General dosing considerations:* Premedicate before each infusion.

➤*Adults:*

Chronic lymphocytic leukemia –

Usual dosage: 12 doses administered intravenously (IV) according to the following: 300 mg initial dose (dose 1), followed 1 week later by 2,000 mg weekly for 7 doses (doses 2 to 8), followed 4 weeks later by 2,000 mg every 4 weeks for 4 doses (doses 9 to 12).

Dosage adjustment: Interrupt infusion for infusion reactions of any severity. For grade 4 infusion reactions, do not resume the infusion.

OFATUMUMAB — INJECTION

For grade 1, 2, or 3 infusion reaction, if the infusion reaction resolves or remains grade 2 or less, resume infusion with the following modifications according to the initial grade of the infusion reaction. For grade 1 or 2, infuse at one-half of the previous infusion rate. For grade 3, infuse at a rate of 12 mL/h. After resuming the infusion, the infusion rate may be increased based on patient tolerance.

Premedication: Premedicate 30 minutes to 2 hours prior to each dose with oral acetaminophen 1,000 mg (or equivalent), oral or intravenous (IV) antihistamine (cetirizine 10 mg or equivalent), and IV corticosteroid (prednisolone 100 mg or equivalent).

Do not reduce corticosteroid dose for doses 1, 2, and 9. Corticosteroid dose may be reduced as follows for doses 3 to 8 and 10 to 12: for doses 3 through 8, gradually reduce corticosteroid dose with successive infusions if a grade 3 or greater infusion reaction did not occur with the preceding dose. For doses 10 through 12, administer prednisolone 50 to 100 mg or equivalent if a grade 3 or greater infusion reaction did not occur with dose 9.

➤*Preparation for administration:* Do not shake product.

Prepare all doses in 1,000 mL of sodium chloride 0.9% injection.

Preparation of solution –

300 mg dose: Withdraw and discard 15 mL from a 1,000 mL polyolefin bag of sodium chloride 0.9% injection. Withdraw 5 mL from each of 3 vials of ofatumumab and add to the bag. Mix diluted solution by gentle inversion.

2,000 mg dose: Withdraw and discard 100 mL from a 1,000 mL bag of sodium chloride 0.9% injection. Withdraw 5 mL from each of the 20 vials of ofatumumab and add to the bag. Mix diluted solution by gentle inversion.

➤*Administration:* Do not administer as an IV push or bolus.

Administer using an infusion pump, the in-line filter provided with the product, and polyvinyl chloride (PVC) administration sets.

Flush the IV line with sodium chloride 0.9% injection before and after each dose.

Start infusion within 12 hours of preparation.

Infusion rate –

Dose 1: Initiate infusion at a rate of 3.6 mg/h (12 mL/h).

Dose 2: Initiate infusion at a rate of 24 mg/h (12 mL/h).

Doses 3 through 12: Initiate infusion at a rate of 50 mg/h (25 mL/h). In the absence of infusion toxicity, the rate of infusion may be increased every 30 minutes. Do not exceed the infusion rates.

Ofatumumab Infusion Rates

Interval after start of infusion (min)	Dose 1[a] (mL/h)	Dose 2[b] (mL/h)	Doses 3 to 12[b] (mL/h)
0 to 30	12	12	25
31 to 60	25	25	50
61 to 90	50	50	100
91 to 120	100	100	200
> 120	200	200	400

[a] Dose 1 = 300 mg (0.3 mg/mL).
[b] Doses 2 and 3 to 12 = 2,000 mg (2 mg/mL).

➤*Admixture compatibility:* Do not mix ofatumumab with, or administer as an infusion with, other medicinal products.

➤*Storage/Stability:* Store refrigerated between 2° and 8°C (36° and 46°F). Do not freeze. Vials should be protected from light. Discard prepared solution after 24 hours.

Actions

➤*Pharmacology:* Ofatumumab binds specifically to the small and large extracellular loops of the CD20 molecule. The CD20 molecule is expressed on normal B lymphocytes (pre-B- to mature B-lymphocyte) and on B-cell CLL. The CD20 molecule is not shed from the cell surface and is not internalized following antibody binding. The Fab domain of ofatumumab binds to the CD20 molecule and the Fc domain mediates immune effector functions to result in B-cell lysis in vitro. Data suggest that possible mechanisms of cell lysis include complement-dependent cytotoxicity and antibody-dependent, cell-mediated cytotoxicity.

➤*Pharmacokinetics:*

Absorption – The maximum plasma concentration (C_{max}) and area under the curve ($AUC_{(0-\infty)}$) after the 8th infusion in study 1 were approximately 40% and 60% higher than after the 4th infusion in study 2.

Distribution – The mean volume of distribution (Vd) at steady-state values ranged from 1.7 to 5.1 L.

Excretion – Ofatumumab is eliminated through a target-independent route and a B cell-mediated route. Ofatumumab exhibited dose-dependent clearance in the dose range of 100 to 2,000 mg. Due to the depletion of B cells, the clearance of ofatumumab decreased substantially after subsequent infusions compared with the first infusion. The mean clearance between the 4th and 12th infusions was approximately 0.01 L/h and exhibited large intersubject variability with coefficient of variation (CV%) greater than 50%. The mean $t_{½}$ between the 4th and 12th infusions was approximately 14 days (range, 2.3 to 61.5 days).

Contraindications

None well documented.

Warnings/Precautions

➤*Infusion reactions:* Ofatumumab can cause serious infusion reactions manifesting as bronchospasm, dyspnea, laryngeal edema, pulmonary edema, flushing, hypertension, hypotension, syncope, cardiac ischemia/infarction, back pain, abdominal pain, pyrexia, rash, urticaria, and angioedema. Infusion reactions occur more frequently with the first 2 infusions.

Premedicate with acetaminophen, an antihistamine, and a corticosteroid. Interrupt infusion for infusion reactions of any severity. Institute medical management for severe infusion reactions including angina or other signs and symptoms of myocardial ischemia.

In a study of patients with moderate to severe chronic obstructive pulmonary disease, an indication for which ofatumumab is not approved, 2 of 5 patients developed grade 3 bronchospasm during infusion.

➤*Hematologic effects:* Prolonged (at least 1 week) severe neutropenia and thrombocytopenia can occur with ofatumumab. Monitor complete blood cell counts (CBC) and platelet counts at regular intervals during therapy, and increase the frequency of monitoring in patients who develop grade 3 or 4 cytopenias.

➤*Progressive multifocal leukoencephalopathy:* Progressive multifocal leukoencephalopathy (PML), including fatal PML, can occur with ofatumumab. Consider PML in any patient with new onset of or changes in preexisting neurological signs or symptoms. Discontinue ofatumumab if PML is suspected, and initiate evaluation for PML, including consultation with a neurologist, brain magnetic resonance imaging (MRI), and lumbar puncture.

➤*Hepatitis B reactivation:* Hepatitis B reactivation, including fulminant hepatitis and death, occurs with other monoclonal antibodies directed against CD20. Screen patients at high risk of hepatitis B virus (HBV) infection before initiation of ofatumumab. Closely monitor carriers of hepatitis B for clinical and laboratory signs of active HBV infection during treatment with ofatumumab and for 6 to 12 months following the last infusion of ofatumumab. Discontinue ofatumumab in patients who develop viral hepatitis or reactivation of viral hepatitis, and institute appropriate treatment.

Insufficient data exist regarding the safety of administration of ofatumumab in patients with active hepatitis.

➤*Intestinal obstruction:* Obstruction of the small intestine can occur in patients receiving ofatumumab. Perform a diagnostic evaluation if obstruction is suspected.

➤*Immunizations:* The safety of immunization with live viral vaccines during or following administration of ofatumumab has not been studied. Do not administer live viral vaccines to patients who have recently received ofatumumab. The ability to generate an immune response to any vaccine following administration of ofatumumab has not been studied.

➤*Pregnancy: Category C.* There are no adequate or well-controlled studies of ofatumumab in pregnant women. Ofatumumab should be used during pregnancy only if the potential benefit to the mother justifies the potential risk to the fetus. A reproductive study in pregnant cynomolgus monkeys that received ofatumumab at doses of up to 3.5 times the recommended human dose of ofatumumab did not demonstrate maternal toxicity or teratogenicity. Ofatumumab crossed the placental barrier, and fetuses exhibited depletion of peripheral B cells and decreased spleen and placental weights.

There are no human or animal data on the potential short-term and long-term effects of perinatal B-cell depletion in offspring following in-utero exposure to ofatumumab. Ofatumumab does not bind normal human tissues other than B lymphocytes. It is not known if binding occurs to unique embryonic or fetal tissue targets. In addition, the kinetics of B-lymphocyte recovery are unknown in offspring with B-cell depletion.

➤*Lactation:* It is not known whether ofatumumab is secreted in human milk; however, human immunoglobulin G is secreted in human milk. Published data suggest that neonatal and infant consumption of breast milk does not result in substantial absorption of these maternal antibodies into circulation. Because the effects of local gastrointestinal and limited systemic exposure to ofatumumab are unknown, exercise caution when ofatumumab is administered to a breast-feeding woman.

➤*Children:* Safety and effectiveness of ofatumumab have not been established in children.

➤*Monitoring:* Monitor CBC and platelet counts at regular intervals during therapy, and increase the frequency of monitoring in patients who develop grade 3 or 4 cytopenias. Closely monitor carriers of hepatitis B for clinical and laboratory signs of active HBV infection during treatment with ofatumumab and for 6 to 12 months following the last infusion of ofatumumab.

Drug Interactions

➤*Immunization:* See Warnings/Precautions.

Adverse Reactions

➤*Most common adverse reactions:* The most common adverse reactions (10% or greater) in study 1 were anemia, bronchitis, cough, diarrhea, dyspnea, fatigue, nausea, neutropenia, pneumonia, pyrexia, rash, and upper respiratory tract infections.

The most common serious adverse reactions in study 1 were infections (including pneumonia and sepsis), neutropenia, and pyrexia. Infections were the most common adverse reactions leading to drug discontinuation in study 1.

OFATUMUMAB — INJECTION

Clinical trials experience –

Ofatumumab Adverse Reactions (≥ 5%)				
	Total population (n = 154)		Fludarabine- and alemtuzumab-refractory (n = 59)	
Adverse reactions	All grades	Grade ≥ 3	All grades	Grade ≥ 3
Cardiovascular				
Edema peripheral	9%	< 1%	8%	2%
Hypertension	5%	0%	8%	0%
Hypotension	5%	0%	3%	0%
Tachycardia	5%	< 1%	7%	2%
CNS				
Chills	8%	0%	10%	0%
Fatigue	15%	0%	15%	0%
Headache	6%	0%	7%	0%
Insomnia	7%	0%	10%	0%
Dermatologic				
Hyperhidrosis	5%	0%	5%	0%
Rash[a]	14%	< 1%	17%	2%
Urticaria	8%	0%	5%	0%
GI				
Diarrhea	18%	0%	19%	0%
Nausea	11%	0%	12%	0%
Musculoskeletal				
Back pain	8%	1%	12%	2%
Muscle spasms	5%	0%	3%	0%
Respiratory				
Bronchitis	11%	< 1%	19%	2%
Cough	19%	0%	19%	0%
Dyspnea	14%	2%	19%	5%
Nasopharyngitis	8%	0%	8%	0%
Pneumonia[b]	23%	14%	25%	15%
Sinusitis	5%	2%	3%	2%
Upper respiratory tract infection	11%	0%	3%	0%
Miscellaneous				
Anemia	16%	5%	17%	8%
Herpes zoster	6%	1%	7%	2%
Pyrexia	20%	3%	25%	5%
Sepsis[c]	8%	8%	10%	10%

[a] Rash includes rash, rash macular, and rash vesicular.
[b] Pneumonia includes pneumonia, lung infection, lobar pneumonia, and bronchopneumonia.
[c] Sepsis includes sepsis, neutropenic sepsis, bacteremia, and septic shock.

➤*Other adverse reactions:*

Infusion reactions – Infusion reactions occurred in 44% of patients on the day of the first infusion (300 mg), 29% on the day of the second infusion (2,000 mg), and less frequently during subsequent infusions.

Infections – A total of 108 (70%) patients experienced bacterial, viral, or fungal infections. A total of 45 (29%) patients experienced at least grade 3 infections, of which 19 (12%) patients were fatal. The proportion of fatal infections in the fludarabine- and alemtuzumab-refractory group was 17%.

Neutropenia – Of 108 patients with normal neutrophil counts at baseline, 45 (42%) patients developed at least grade 3 neutropenia. Nineteen (18%) patients developed grade 4 neutropenia. Some patients experienced new-onset grade 4 neutropenia more than 2 weeks in duration.

➤*Immunogenicity:* There is a potential for immunogenicity with therapeutic proteins such as ofatumumab. Serum samples from patients with CLL in study 1 were tested by enzyme-linked immunosorbent assay for antiofatumumab antibodies during and after the 24-week treatment period. Results were negative in 46 patients after the 8th infusion and in 33 patients after the 12th infusion.

Immunogenicity assay results are highly dependent on several factors including assay sensitivity and specificity, assay methodology, sample handling, timing of sample collection, concomitant medications, and underlying disease. For these reasons, comparison of incidence of antibodies to ofatumumab with the incidence of antibodies to other products may be misleading.

Overdosage

None well documented.

Patient Information

Advise patients to contact a health care provider for any of the following: signs and symptoms of infusion reactions, including fever, chills, rash, or breathing problems within 24 hours of infusion; bleeding, easy bruising, petechiae, pallor, worsening weakness, or fatigue; signs of infections, including fever and cough; new neurological symptoms, such as confusion, dizziness or loss of balance, difficulty talking or walking, or vision problems; symptoms of hepatitis including worsening fatigue or yellow discoloration of skin or eyes; new or worsening abdominal pain or nausea; or if you are pregnant or breast-feeding.

Advise patients of the need for periodic monitoring for blood counts; avoiding vaccination with live viral vaccines.

TOSITUMOMAB AND IODINE ^{131}I-TOSITUMOMAB

Rx	**Bexxar Dosimetric Packaging**[a] (Corixa/GlaxoSmithKline)		A carton containing 2 single-use 225 mg vials and 1 single-use 35 mg vial of tositumomab. A package containing a single-use vial of ^{131}I-tositumomab.
Rx	**Tositumomab** (McKesson Biosciences)	**Injection:** 14 mg/mL	10% (w/v) maltose. Preservative free. In 35 and 225 mg single-use vials.
Rx	**Iodine ^{131}I-Tositumomab**[b] (MDS Nordion[c])	**Injection:** 0.1 mg/mL (0.61 mCi/mL at calibration)	Preservative free. Single-use vials.[d]
Rx	**Bexxar Therapeutic Packaging**[a] (GlaxoSmithKline)		A carton containing 2 single-use 225 mg vials and 1 single-use 35 mg vial of tositumomab. A package containing 1 or 2 single-use vials of ^{131}I-tositumomab.
Rx	**Tositumomab** (McKesson Biosciences)	**Injection:** 14 mg/mL	10% (w/v) maltose. Preservative free. In 35 and 225 mg single-use vials.
Rx	**Iodine ^{131}I-Tositumomab**[b] (MDS Nordion[c])	**Injection:** 1.1 mg/mL (5.6 mCi/mL at calibration)	Preservative free. Single-use vials.[e]

[a] The components are shipped from separate sites; when ordering, ensure that the components are scheduled to arrive on the same day. The components are shipped only to individuals who are participating in the certification program.
[b] Refer to the product specification sheet for the lot specific protein concentration, activity concentration, total activity, and expiration date.
[c] MDS Nordion, 447 March Road, Ottawa, ON K2K 1X8, Canada; (613) 592-2790, (800) 267-6211.
[d] Contains 5% to 6% povidone, 1 to 2 mg/mL maltose, 0.85 to 0.95 mg/mL sodium chloride, and 0.9 to 1.3 mg/mL ascorbic acid.
[e] Contains 5% to 6% povidone, 9 to 15 mg/mL maltose, 0.85 to 0.95 mg/mL sodium chloride, and 0.9 to 1.3 mg/mL ascorbic acid.

TOSITUMOMAB AND IODINE ^{131}I-TOSITUMOMAB — INJECTION

WARNING

Hypersensitivity reactions, including anaphylaxis – Serious hypersensitivity reactions, including some with fatal outcome, have been reported with therapy. Medications for the treatment of severe hypersensitivity reactions should be available for immediate use. Patients who develop severe hypersensitivity reactions should have infusions of the tositumomab therapeutic regimen discontinued and receive medical attention.

Prolonged and severe cytopenias – The majority of patients who received therapy experienced severe thrombocytopenia and neutropenia. Do not administer the therapeutic regimen to patients with more than 25% lymphoma marrow involvement and/or impaired bone marrow reserve.

Pregnancy – Category X. Tositumomab/^{131}I-tositumomab can cause fetal harm when administered to a pregnant woman.

Special requirements – Tositumomab/^{131}I-tositumomab contains a radioactive component and should be administered only by health care providers qualified by training in the safe use and handling of therapeutic radionuclides. The therapeutic regimen should be administered only by health care providers who are in the process of being or have been certified by the manufacturer in dose calculation and administration of the therapeutic regimen.

Indications

➤*Non-Hodgkin lymphoma (NHL):* For the treatment of patients with CD20 antigen-expressing, relapsed or refractory, low grade, follicular or transformed NHL, including patients with rituximab-refractory NHL. This regimen is not indicated for the initial treatment of patients with CD20 positive NHL.

Administration and Dosage

➤*General dosing considerations:* The therapeutic regimen consists of 4 components administered in 2 discrete steps: the dosimetric step, followed 7 to 14 days later by a therapeutic step. The safety of the therapeutic regimen was established only in the setting of patients receiving thyroid blocking agents and premedication to ameliorate/prevent infusion reactions.

The therapeutic regimen is intended as a single course of treatment. The safety of multiple courses of this drug regimen or combination of this regimen with other forms of irradiation or chemotherapy have not been evaluated.

Thyroid protective agents must be given with tositumomab/iodine ^{131}I-tositumomab to reduce damage to the thyroid gland.

➤*Adults:*

Non-Hodgkin lymphoma –

Dosimetric step:

• *Tositumomab* – Administer tositumomab 450 mg intravenously (IV) in 50 mL of sodium chloride 0.9% over 60 minutes. Reduce the rate of infusion by 50% for mild to moderate infusional toxicity; interrupt infusion for severe infusional toxicity. After complete resolution of severe infusional toxicity, infusion may be resumed with a 50% reduction in the rate of infusion.

• *Iodine ^{131}I-tositumomab* – Administer ^{131}I-tositumomab (containing ^{131}I 5 mCi and tositumomab 35 mg) IV in 30 mL of sodium chloride 0.9% over 20 minutes. Reduce the rate of infusion by 50% for mild to moderate infusional toxicity; interrupt infusion for severe infusional toxicity. After complete resolution of severe infusional toxicity, infusion may be resumed with a 50% reduction in the rate of infusion.

Therapeutic step: Therapeutic step is administered 7 to 14 days after the dosimetric step. Do not administer the therapeutic step if biodistribution is altered.

• *Tositumomab* – Administer tositumomab 450 mg IV in 50 mL of sodium chloride 0.9% over 60 minutes. Reduce the rate of infusion by 50% for mild to moderate infusional toxicity; interrupt infusion for severe infusional toxicity. After complete resolution of severe infusional toxicity, infusion may be resumed with a 50% reduction in the rate of infusion.

• *Iodine ^{131}I-tositumomab* – See the prescribing information for instructions on how to calculate the iodine^{131} activity for the therapeutic dose.

For ^{131}I-tositumomab, reduce the rate of infusion by 50% for mild to moderate infusional toxicity; interrupt infusion for severe infusional toxicity. After complete resolution of severe infusional toxicity, infusion may be resumed with a 50% reduction in the rate of infusion.

- In patients with 150,000 platelets/mm^3 or more, the recommended dose is the activity of ^{131}I calculated to deliver 75 cGy total body irradiation and tositumomab 35 mg, administered IV over 20 minutes.
- In patients with National Cancer Institute (NCI) grade 1 thrombocytopenia (platelet counts 100,000 to less than 150,000 platelets/mm^3), the recommended dose is the activity of ^{131}I calculated to deliver 65 cGy total body irradiation and tositumomab 35 mg, administered IV over 20 minutes.

Concomitant therapy:

• *Thyroid protective agents* – Saturated solution of potassium iodide 4 drops orally, 3 times daily; Lugol's solution 20 drops orally, 3 times daily; or potassium iodide 130 mg tablets orally, every day. Initiate thyroid protective agents at least 24 hours prior to administration of the ^{131}I-tositumomab dosimetric dose and continue until 2 weeks after administration of the ^{131}I-tositumomab therapeutic dose.

Do not administer the dosimetric dose of ^{131}I-tositumomab to patients if they have not yet received at least 3 doses of potassium iodide, 3 doses of Lugol's solution, or 1 dose of potassium iodide 130 mg tablets (at least 24 hours prior to the dosimetric dose).

• *Premedication* – Acetaminophen 650 mg orally and diphenhydramine 50 mg orally, 30 minutes prior to administration of tositumomab in the dosimetric and therapeutic steps.

➤*Dosimetry:* See prescribing information for dosimetry instructions.

➤*Calculation of ^{131}I activity for the therapeutic dose:* See prescribing information for calculation instructions.

➤*Preparation for administration:* ^{131}I-tositumomab is a radioactive regimen. Follow safe handling procedures when preparing, administering, or dispensing ^{131}I-tositumomab.

See prescribing information for specific preparation instructions.

➤*Administration:* To ensure that the correct dose is given, each dose must be measured by a radioactivity calibration system immediately before administration.

The therapeutic regimen is administered via an IV tubing set with an inline 0.22 micron filter. The same IV tubing set and filter must be used throughout the entire dosimetric or therapeutic step. A change in filter can result in loss of drug.

Nonradioactive tositumomab is administered by IV infusion over 60 minutes.

Radioactive iodine ^{131}I-tositumomab is administered by IV infusion over 20 minutes immediately following nonradioactive tositumomab.

See prescribing information for complete administration instructions.

➤*Storage / Stability:* Discard single-dose vials within 6 hours of the initial needle puncture if opened within an ISO Class 5 biological safety cabinet, or within 1 hour of the initial needle puncture if opened outside of such an environment, based on the USP Chapter <797> standards

Tositumomab – Refrigerate vials of tositumomab at 2° to 8°C (36° to 46°F) prior to dilution. Protect from strong light. Do not shake. Do not freeze. Discard any unused portions left in the vial.

Solutions of diluted tositumomab are stable for up to 24 hours when refrigerated at 2° to 8°C (36° to 46°F) and for up to 8 hours at room temperature (15° to 30°C [59° to 86°F]). It is recommended to refrigerate the diluted solution at 2° to 8°C (36° to 46°F) prior to administration because it does not contain preservatives. Any unused portion must be discarded. Do not freeze solutions of diluted tositumomab.

^{131}I-tositumomab – Store frozen in the original lead pots. Store in a freezer at a temperature of −20°C (−4°F) or below until it is removed for thawing prior to administration.

Thawed dosimetric and therapeutic doses of ^{131}I-tositumomab are stable for up to 8 hours at 2° to 8°C (36° to 46°F) or at room temperature (15° to 30°C; 59° to 86°F). Solutions of ^{131}I-tositumomab diluted for infusion contain no preservatives; store refrigerated at 2° to 8°C (36° to 46°F) prior to administration (do not freeze). Any unused portion must be discarded.

Actions

➤*Pharmacology:* The therapeutic regimen is an antineoplastic radioimmunotherapeutic monoclonal antibody-based regimen composed of the monoclonal antibody tositumomab, and the radiolabeled monoclonal antibody^{131}I-tositumomab.

Tositumomab is a murine Ig G_{2a} lambda monoclonal antibody that binds specifically to the CD20 (human B-lymphocyte–restricted differentiation antigen, Bp35 or B1) antigen. This antigen is a transmembrane phosphoprotein expressed on pre-B lymphocytes and at higher density on mature B lymphocytes. The antigen is also expressed on more than 90% of B-cell NHL. The recognition epitope for tositumomab is found within the extracellular domain of the CD20 antigen. CD20 does not shed from the cell surface and does not internalize following antibody binding.

Possible mechanisms of action include induction of apoptosis, complement-dependent cytotoxicity, and antibody-dependent cellular cytotoxicity mediated by the antibody. Additionally, cell death is associated with ionizing radiation from the radioisotope.

➤*Pharmacokinetics:* The principal beta emission has a mean energy of 191.6 keV and the principal gamma emission has an energy of 364.5 keV.

The phase 1 study of ^{131}I-tositumomab determined that a 475 mg predose of unlabeled antibody decreased splenic targeting and increased the terminal half-life of the radiolabeled antibody. The median blood clearance following administration of tositumomab 485 mg in 110 patients with NHL was 68.2 mg/h (range, 30.2 to 260.8 mg/h). Patients with high tumor burden, splenomegaly, or bone marrow involvement were noted to have a faster clearance, shorter terminal half-life, and larger volume of distribution. The total body clearance, as measured by total body gamma camera counts, was dependent on the same factors noted for blood clearance. Patient-specific dosing, based on total body clearance, provided a consistent radiation dose, despite variable pharmacokinetics, by allowing each patient's administered activity to be adjusted for individual patient variables. The median total body effective half-life, as measured by total gamma camera counts, in 980 patients with NHL was 67 hours (range, 28 to 115 hours).

^{131}I-tositumomab decays with beta and gamma emissions with a physical half-life of 8.04 days. Elimination of ^{131}I occurs by decay and excretion in the urine. Urine was collected for 49 dosimetric doses. After 5 days, the whole body clearance was 67% of the injected dose. Ninety-eight percent of the clearance was accounted for in the urine.

In clinical studies, administration of the therapeutic regimen resulted in sustained depletion of circulating CD20-positive cells. The impact of the therapeutic regimen on circulating CD20-positive cells was assessed in 2 clinical studies, 1 conducted in chemotherapy-naïve patients and 1 in heavily pretreated patients. The assessment of circulating lymphocytes did not distinguish normal from malignant cells. Consequently, assessment of recovery of normal B cell function was not directly assessed. At 7 weeks, the median number of circulating CD20-positive cells was 0 (range, 0 to 490 cells/mm^3). Lymphocyte recovery began at approximately 12 weeks fol-

TOSITUMOMAB AND IODINE ^{131}I-TOSITUMOMAB — INJECTION

lowing treatment. Among patients who had CD20-positive cell counts recorded at baseline and at 6 months, 14% (8 of 58) chemotherapy-naïve patients had CD20-positive cell counts below normal limits at 6 months, and 32% (6 of 19) of heavily pretreated patients had CD20-positive cell counts below normal limits at 6 months. There was no consistent effect of the therapeutic regimen on posttreatment serum IgG, IgA, or IgM levels.

Radiation dosimetry – Estimations of radiation-absorbed doses for ^{131}I-tositumomab were performed using sequential whole body images and the MIRDOSE 3 software program. Patients with apparent thyroid, stomach, or intestinal imaging were selected for organ dosimetry analyses. The estimated radiation-absorbed doses to organs and marrow from a course of the therapeutic regimen are in the following table.

Estimated Radiation-Absorbed Organ Doses from ^{131}I-tositumomab		
	^{131}I-tositumomab mGy/MBq median	^{131}I-tositumomab mGy/MBq range
From organ ROIs[a]		
Heart wall	1.25	0.5 to 1.8
Kidneys	1.96	1.5 to 2.5
Liver	0.82	0.6 to 1.3
LLI[b] wall	1.3	0.8 to 1.6
Lungs	0.79	0.5 to 1.1
Red marrow	0.65	0.5 to 1.1
Spleen	1.14	0.7 to 5.4
Stomach wall	0.4	0.2 to 0.8
Testes	0.83	0.3 to 1.3
Thyroid	2.71	1.4 to 6.2
ULI[c] wall	1.34	0.8 to 1.7
From whole body ROIs		
Adrenals	0.28	0.2 to 0.3
Bone surfaces	0.41	0.4 to 0.6
Brain	0.13	0.1 to 0.2
Breasts	0.16	0.1 to 0.2
Gallbladder wall	0.29	0.2 to 0.3
Muscle	0.18	0.1 to 0.2
Ovaries	0.25	0.2 to 0.3
Pancreas	0.31	0.2 to 0.4
Skin	0.13	0.1 to 0.2
Small intestine	0.23	0.2 to 0.3
Thymus	0.22	0.1 to 0.3
Total body	0.24	0.2 to 0.3
Urine bladder wall	0.64	0.6 to 0.9
Uterus	0.2	0.2 to 0.2

[a] ROI = region of interest.
[b] LLI = large lower intestine.
[c] ULI = upper large intestine.

Contraindications

Known hypersensitivity to murine proteins or any other component of the therapeutic regimen; pregnancy.

Warnings/Precautions

➤*Prolonged and severe cytopenias:* The most common adverse reactions associated with the therapeutic regimen were severe or life-threatening cytopenias (NCI common toxicity criteria grade 3 or 4), with 71% of the 230 patients enrolled in clinical studies experiencing grade 3 or 4 cytopenias. These consisted primarily of grade 3 or 4 thrombocytopenia (53%) and grade 3 or 4 neutropenia (63%). The time to nadir was 4 to 7 weeks, and the duration of cytopenias was approximately 30 days. Thrombocytopenia, neutropenia, and anemia persisted for more than 90 days following administration of the tositumomab-iodine drug complex in 7%, 7%, and 5% of the patients, respectively (this includes patients with transient recovery followed by current cytopenia). Because of the variable onset of cytopenias, obtain complete blood cell counts weekly for 10 to 12 weeks. The sequelae of severe cytopenias were commonly observed in clinical studies and included infections (45%), hemorrhage (12%), a requirement for growth factors (12% granulocyte- or granulocyte macrophage colony stimulating factor [CSF]; 7% epoetin alfa), and blood product support (15% platelet transfusions; 16% red blood cell transfusions). Prolonged cytopenias may also influence subsequent treatment decisions.

The safety of the therapeutic regimen has not been established in patients with more than 25% lymphoma marrow involvement, platelet count less than 100,000 cells/mm^3, or neutrophil count less than 1,500 cells/mm^3.

➤*Secondary malignancies:* Myelodysplastic syndrome (MDS) and/or acute leukemia were reported in 10% of patients enrolled in the clinical studies and 3% of patients included in expanded access programs with median follow-up of 39 and 27 months, respectively. Among the 44 reported cases, the median time to development of MDS/leukemia was 31 months following treatment; however, the cumulative rate continues to increase.

Additional nonhematological malignancies were also reported in 54 of the 995 patients enrolled in clinical studies or included in the expanded access program. Approximately half of these were nonmelanomatous skin cancers. The remainder, which occurred in 2 or more patients, included colorectal, head and neck, breast, lung, bladder, melanoma, and gastric cancer, in order of decreasing incidence. The relative risk of developing secondary malignancies in patients receiving the therapeutic regimen over the background rate cannot be determined because of the absence of controlled studies.

➤*Hypothyroidism:* Therapy may result in hypothyroidism. Initiate thyroid-blocking medications at least 24 hours before receiving the dosimetric dose, and continue until 14 days after the therapeutic dose. All patients must receive thyroid-blocking agents; do not administer this therapeutic regimen to any patient who is unable to tolerate thyroid-blocking agents. Evaluate patients for signs and symptoms of hypothyroidism and screen for biochemical evidence of hypothyroidism annually.

➤*Radionuclide:* ^{131}I-tositumomab is radioactive. To minimize exposure of medical personnel and other patients, exercise caution by staying consistent with the institutional radiation safety practices and applicable federal guidelines.

➤*Immunization:* The safety of immunization with live viral vaccines following administration of the therapeutic regimen has not been studied. The ability of patients who have received this therapeutic regimen to generate a primary or anamnestic humoral response to any vaccine has not been studied.

➤*Hypersensitivity reactions:* Serious hypersensitivity reactions, including some with fatal outcome, were reported during and following administration of the this therapeutic regimen. Make medications for the treatment of hypersensitivity reactions (eg, antihistamines, corticosteroids, epinephrine) available for immediate use in the event of an allergic reaction during administration of the therapeutic regimen. Screen patients who have received murine proteins for human antimouse antibodies (HAMA). Patients who are positive for HAMA may be at increased risk of anaphylaxis and serious hypersensitivity reactions during administration of the therapeutic regimen.

➤*Renal function impairment:* ^{131}I-tositumomab and ^{131}I are excreted primarily by the kidneys. Impaired renal function may decrease the rate of excretion of the radiolabeled iodine and increase patient exposure to the radioactive component of the therapeutic regimen. There are no data regarding the safety of administration of the therapeutic regimen in patients with impaired renal function.

➤*Pregnancy: Category X.* ^{131}I-tositumomab (a component of the therapeutic regimen) is contraindicated for use in women who are pregnant. ^{131}I may cause harm to the fetal thyroid gland when administered to pregnant women. Review of the literature has shown that transplacental passage of radioiodide may cause severe, and possibly irreversible, hypothyroidism in neonates. While there are no adequate and well-controlled studies of this drug complex in pregnant animals or humans, defer use of therapy in women of childbearing age until the possibility of pregnancy has been ruled out. If the patient becomes pregnant while being treated with the drug complex, apprise the patient of the potential hazard to the fetus. Advise patients to use effective contraceptive methods during treatment and for 12 months following administration.

Fertility impairment – Administration of this therapeutic regimen results in delivery of a significant radiation dose to the testes. There is a potential risk that the drug complex may cause toxic effects on the male and female gonads. Instruct patients to use effective contraceptive methods during treatment and for 12 months following administration of the therapeutic regimen.

➤*Lactation:* Radioiodine is excreted in breast milk and may reach concentrations equal to or greater than maternal plasma concentrations. Immunoglobulins are also known to be excreted in breast milk. The absorption potential and potential for adverse reactions of the monoclonal antibody component (tositumomab) in the infant are not known. Therefore, substitute formula feedings for breast-feedings before starting treatment. Advise women to discontinue breast-feeding.

➤*Children:* The safety and efficacy of the therapeutic regimen in children have not been established.

➤*Elderly:* Across all studies, the overall response rate was lower in patients 65 years of age and older (41% versus 61%), and the duration of responses was shorter (10 versus 16 months); however, these findings are primarily derived from 2 of the 5 studies. While the incidence of severe hematologic toxicity was lower, the duration of severe hematologic toxicity was longer in those 65 years of age and older as compared with patients younger than 65 years of age. Because of limited experience, greater sensitivity of some older individuals cannot be ruled out.

➤*Monitoring:* Obtain a complete blood cell count with differential and platelet count prior to and at least weekly following administration of the therapeutic regimen. Continue weekly monitoring of blood cell counts for a minimum of 10 weeks or, if persistent, until severe cytopenias have completely resolved. More frequent monitoring is indicated in patients with evidence of moderate or more severe cytopenias. Monitor thyroid-stimulating hormone (TSH) levels before treatment and annually thereafter. Measure serum creatinine levels immediately prior to administration of the therapeutic regimen.

Assess pregnancy status prior to administration in women of childbearing potential.

Drug Interactions

➤*Anticoagulants/Antiplatelet agents:* Because of the frequent occurrence of severe and prolonged thrombocytopenia, weigh the potential benefits of medications that interfere with platelet function and/or anticoagulation against the potential increased risk of bleeding and hemorrhage.

TOSITUMOMAB AND IODINE ^{131}I-TOSITUMOMAB — INJECTION

➤*Drug/Lab test interactions:* Administration of this therapeutic regimen may result in the development of HAMA. The presence of HAMA may affect the accuracy of the results of in vitro and in vivo diagnostic tests and may affect the toxicity profile and efficacy of therapeutic agents that rely on murine antibody technology. Patients who are HAMA positive may be at increased risk for serious allergic reactions and other adverse reactions if they undergo in vivo diagnostic testing or treatment with murine monoclonal antibodies.

Adverse Reactions

^{131}I-tositumomab is considered to have low potential for nausea and vomiting.

The most serious adverse reactions observed in the clinical trials were severe and prolonged cytopenias and the sequelae of cytopenias, which included infections (sepsis) and hemorrhage in thrombocytopenic patients, allergic reactions (bronchospasm and angioedema), secondary leukemia, and myelodysplasia.

The most common adverse reactions occurring in the clinical trials included neutropenia, thrombocytopenia, and anemia that are both prolonged and severe. Less common but severe adverse reactions included pneumonia, pleural effusion, and dehydration.

Nonhematologic Adverse Reactions in Patients Treated with Tositumomab/^{131}I-Tositumomab (N = 230) (≥ 5%)

Adverse reaction	All Grades (96%)	Grade 3/4 (48%)
Cardiovascular		
Hypotension	7%	1%
Vasodilation	5%	0%
CNS		
Dizziness	5%	0%
Headache	16%	0%
Somnolence	5%	0%
Dermatologic		
Rash	17%	< 1%
Pruritus	10%	0%
Sweating	8%	< 1%
GI		
Abdominal pain	15%	3%
Anorexia	14%	0%
Constipation	6%	1%
Diarrhea	12%	0%
Dyspepsia	6%	< 1%
Nausea	36%	3%
Vomiting	15%	1%
Metabolic		
Peripheral edema	9%	0%
Weight loss	6%	< 1%
Musculoskeletal		
Arthralgia	10%	1%
Myalgia	13%	< 1%
Respiratory		
Cough increased	21%	1%
Dyspnea	11%	3%
Pharyngitis	12%	0%
Pneumonia	6%	0%
Rhinitis	10%	0%
Miscellaneous		
Asthenia	46%	2%
Back pain	8%	1%
Chest pain	7%	0%
Chills	18%	1%
Fever	37%	2%
Hypothyroidism	7%	0%
Infection[a]	21%	< 1%
Neck pain	6%	1%
Pain	19%	1%

[a] Infection includes a subset of infections (eg, upper respiratory tract infection). Other terms are mapped to preferred terms (eg, pneumonia, sepsis).

Tositumomab/^{131}I-Tositumomab Hematologic Toxicity[a] (N = 230)

End point	Values
Platelets	
Median nadir (cells/mm^3)	43,000
Per patient incidence[a] platelets 3	53%
Median[b] duration of platelets < 50,000/mm^3 (days)	32
Grade 3/4 without recovery to grade 2	7%
Per patient incidence[c] platelets 3	21%
ANC[d]	
Median nadir (cells/mm^3)	690
Per patient incidence[a] ANC < 1,000 cells/mm^3	63%
Median[b] duration of ANC < 1,000 cells/mm^3 (days)	31
Grade 3/4 without recovery to grade 2	7%
Per patient incidence[c] ANC 3	25%
Hemoglobin	
Median nadir (g/dL)	10
Per patient incidence[a] < 8 g/dL	29%
Median[b] duration of hemoglobin < 8 g/dL (days)	23
Grade 3/4 without recovery to grade 2	5%
Per patient incidence[c] hemoglobin	5%

[a] Grade 3/4 toxicity was assumed if patient was missing 2 or more weeks of hematology data between weeks 5 and 9.
[b] Duration of Grade 3/4 of 1,000+ days (censored) was assumed for those patients with undocumented grade 3/4 and no hematologic data on or after week 9.
[c] Grade 4 toxicity was assumed if patient had documented grade 3 toxicity and was missing 2 or more weeks of hematology data between weeks 5 and 9.
[d] ANC = absolute neutrophil count.

➤*Hematologic:* Hematologic toxicity was the most frequently observed adverse reaction in clinical trials with the therapeutic regimen. Twenty-seven percent of the patients received 1 or more hematologic supportive care measures following the therapeutic dose. Twelve percent received granulocyte-CSF, 7% received epoetin alfa, 15% received platelet transfusions, and 16% received packed red blood cell transfusions. Twelve percent of patients experienced hemorrhagic events (the majority were mild to moderate).

➤*Infections:* Forty-five percent of patients experienced 1 or more adverse reactions possibly related to infection. The majority were viral (eg, herpes, flu symptoms, pharyngitis, rhinitis) or other minor infections. Nine percent of patients experienced infections that were considered serious because the patient was hospitalized to manage the infection. Documented infections included bacteremia, bronchitis, pneumonia, septicemia, and skin infections.

➤*Hypersensitivity:* Six percent experienced 1 or more of the following adverse reactions: allergic reaction, anaphylactic reaction, face edema, injection site hypersensitivity, laryngismus, and serum sickness.

➤*GI toxicity:* Thirty-eight percent of patients experienced 1 or more of the following GI adverse reactions: abdominal pain, diarrhea, emesis, nausea. These reactions were temporally related to the infusion of the antibody. Abdominal pain, nausea, and vomiting were often reported within days of infusion, whereas diarrhea was generally reported days to weeks after the infusion.

➤*Infusional toxicity:* Symptoms, including bronchospasm, chills, dyspnea, fever, hypotension, rigors, sweating, and nausea have been reported during or within 48 hours of infusion. Twenty-nine percent of patients reported fever, rigors/chills, or sweating within 14 days following the dosimetric dose. Although all patients in the clinical studies received pretreatment with acetaminophen and an antihistamine, the value of premedication in preventing infusion-related toxicity was not evaluated in any of the clinical studies. Infusional toxicities were managed by slowing and/or temporarily interrupting the infusion. Symptomatic management was required in more severe cases.

➤*Delayed adverse reactions:*

Secondary leukemia and MDS – There were 44 new cases of MDS/secondary leukemia reported among 4% of patients included in clinical studies and expanded access programs, with a median follow-up of 29 months.

Secondary malignancies – Of the 995 patients in clinical studies and the expanded access programs, there were 65 reports of second malignancies in 54 patients, excluding secondary leukemia. The most common included nonmelanomatous skin cancers, colorectal, head and neck, breast, lung and bladder cancers, melanoma, and gastric cancer. Some of these events included recurrence of an earlier diagnosis of cancer.

Hypothyroidism – With a median follow-up period of 46 months, the incidence of hypothyroidism based on elevated TSH or initiation of thyroid replacement therapy in the patients from the clinical studies was 18% with a median time to development of hypothyroidism of 16 months. The overall incidences of hypothyroidism at 2 and 5 years in these patients were 11% and 19%, respectively. New events have been observed up to 90 months' posttreatment.

With a median follow-up period of 33 months, the incidence of hypothyroidism based on elevated TSH or initiation of thyroid replacement therapy in these 455 patients from the expanded access programs was 13% with a median time to development of hypothyroidism of 15 months. The cumulative incidences of hypothyroidism at 2 and 5 years in these patients were 9% and 17%, respectively.

Immunogenicity – Of the 230 patients in the clinical studies, 220 patients were seronegative for HAMA prior to treatment, and 219 had at least 1 posttreatment HAMA value obtained. With a median observation period of 6 months, a total of 23 patients became seropositive for HAMA posttreatment. The median time of HAMA development was 6 months. The overall incidences of HAMA seropositivity at 6, 12, and 18 months were 6%, 17%, and 21%, respectively.

TOSITUMOMAB AND IODINE ^{131}I-TOSITUMOMAB — INJECTION

With a median observation period of 7 months, a total of 57 patients from the expanded access program became seropositive for HAMA posttreatment. The median time of HAMA development was 5 months. The overall incidences of HAMA seropositivity at 6, 12, and 18 months were 7%, 12%, and 13%, respectively.

In a study of 76 previously untreated patients with low-grade NHL who received the therapeutic regimen, the incidence of conversion to HAMA seropositivity was 70%, with a median time to development of HAMA of 27 days.

The data reflect the percentage of patients whose test results were considered positive for HAMA in an enzyme-linked immunoabsorbent assay that detects antibodies to the Fc portion of IgG_1 murine immunoglobulin and are highly dependent on the sensitivity and specificity of the assay. Additionally, the observed incidence of antibody positivity in an assay may be influenced by several factors including sample handling, concomitant medications, and underlying disease. For these reasons, comparison of the incidence of HAMA in patients treated with the therapeutic regimen with the incidence of HAMA in patients treated with other products may be misleading.

Postmarketing – Severe hypersensitivity reactions, including fatal anaphylaxis, have been reported.

Overdosage

➤*Symptoms:* The maximum dose of the tositumomab/^{131}I-tositumomab therapeutic regimen that was administered in clinical trials was 88 cGy. Three patients were treated with a total body dose of 85 cGy of iodine ^{131}I-tositumomab in a dose escalation study. Two of the 3 patients developed grade 4 toxicity of 5 weeks' duration with subsequent recovery. In addition, accidental overdose of the therapeutic regimen occurred in 1 patient at total body doses of 88 cGy. The patient developed grade 3 hematologic toxicity of 18 days' duration.

➤*Treatment:* Monitor patients who receive an accidental overdose of ^{131}I-tositumomab closely for cytopenias and radiation-related toxicity. The efficacy of hematopoietic stem cell transplantation as a supportive care measure for marrow injury has not been studied; however, the timing of such support should take into account the pharmacokinetics of the therapeutic regimen and decay rate of the ^{131}I in order to minimize the possibility of irradiation of infused hematopoietic stem cells.

Patient Information

Inform patients that they will have a radioactive material in their body for several days upon their release from the hospital or clinic.

After discharge, provide patients with oral and written instructions for minimizing exposure of family members, friends, and the general public. Give patients a copy of the written instructions for use as a reference for the recommended precautionary actions.

Assess the pregnancy status of women of childbearing potential, and advise these women of the potential risks to the fetus. Instruct women who are breast-feeding to discontinue breast-feeding. Apprise women of the resultant potential harmful effects to the infant if these instructions are not followed.

Advise patients of the potential risk of toxic effects on the male and female gonads following the therapeutic regimen, and instruct patients to use effective contraceptive methods during treatment and for 12 months following the administration of the therapeutic regimen.

Inform patients of the risks of hypothyroidism, and advise them of the importance of compliance with thyroid-blocking agents and the need for life long monitoring.

Inform patients of the risks of cytopenias and symptoms associated with cytopenia and the need for frequent monitoring for up to 12 weeks after treatment and the potential for persistent cytopenias beyond 12 weeks.

Inform patients that certain antineoplastic agents used in the treatment of malignancy, including this therapeutic regimen, have been associated with the development of MDS, secondary leukemia, and solid tumors.

Because of the lack of controlled clinical studies and high background incidence in the heavily pretreated patient population, the relative risk of development of MDS/acute leukemia and solid tumors caused by the therapeutic regimen cannot be determined.

Inform patients of the possibility of developing a HAMA immune response and that HAMA may affect the results of in vitro and in vivo diagnostic tests, as well as results of therapies that rely on murine antibody technology.

KINASE INHIBITORS

Tyrosine Kinase Inhibitors

DASATINIB

Rx	**Sprycel** (Bristol-Myers Squibb)	**Tablets; oral:** 20 mg	Lactose. (BMS 527). White to off-white, round. Film-coated. In 60s.
		50 mg	Lactose. (BMS 528). White to off-white, oval. Film-coated. In 60s.
		70 mg	Lactose. (BMS 524). White to off-white, round. Film-coated. In 60s.
		80 mg	Lactose. (BMS 80 855). White to off-white, triangular. Film-coated. In 30s.
		100 mg	Lactose. (BMS 100 852). White to off-white, oval. Film-coated. In 30s.
		140 mg	Lactose. (BMS 140 857). White to off-white, round. Film-coated. In 30s.

DASATINIB — ORAL

Indications

➤*Acute lymphoblastic leukemia:* For the treatment of adults with Philadelphia chromosome–positive (Ph+) acute lymphoblastic leukemia (ALL) with resistance or intolerance to prior therapy.

➤*Chronic myeloid leukemia:* For the treatment of adults with newly diagnosed Ph+ chronic myeloid leukemia (CML) in chronic phase; for the treatment of adults with chronic, accelerated, or myeloid or lymphoid blast phase Ph+ CML with resistance or intolerance to prior therapy, including imatinib.

Administration and Dosage

➤*Adults:*

Acute lymphoblastic leukemia –

Initial dosage: 140 mg once daily.

Dosage adjustment: May escalate dosage to 180 mg once daily in patients who do not achieve a hematologic or cytogenic response at the recommended dosage.

Chronic myeloid leukemia –

Accelerated phase, or myeloid or lymphoid blast phase: See Acute Lymphoblastic Leukemia for dosing.

Chronic phase:

- *Initial dosage* – 100 mg once daily.
- *Dosage adjustment* – May escalate dosage to 140 mg once daily in patients who do not achieve a hematologic or cytogenic response at the recommended dosage.

➤*Dose adjustment:*

Myelosuppression –

Dasatinib Dose Adjustments for Neutropenia and Thrombocytopenia

Indication and starting dosage	Laboratory parameters	Adjustment
Accelerated phase CML, blast phase CML, and Ph+ ALL (starting dosage 140 mg once daily)	ANC[a] $< 0.5 \times 10^9$/L or Platelets $< 10 \times 10^9$/L	1. Check if cytopenia is related to leukemia (marrow aspirate or biopsy). 2. If cytopenia is unrelated to leukemia, stop dasatinib until ANC $\geq 1 \times 10^9$/L and platelets $\geq 20 \times 10^9$/L and resume at the original starting dose. 3. If cytopenia recurs, repeat step 1 and resume dasatinib at a reduced dosage of 100 mg once daily (second episode) or 80 mg once daily (third episode). 4. If cytopenia is related to leukemia, consider dosage escalation to 180 mg once daily.

DASATINIB — ORAL

Dasatinib Dose Adjustments for Neutropenia and Thrombocytopenia

Indication and starting dosage	Laboratory parameters	Adjustment
Chronic phase CML (starting dosage 100 mg once daily)	ANC < 0.5 × 10^9/L or Platelets < 50 × 10^9/L	1. Stop dasatinib until ANC ≥ 1 × 10^9/L and platelets ≥ 50 × 10^9/L. 2. Resume treatment with dasatinib at the original starting dose if recovery occurs in ≤ 7 days. 3. If platelets ^{9}/L or recurrence of ANC ^{9}/L for > 7 days, repeat step 1 and resume dasatinib at a reduced dosage of 80 mg once daily (second episode). For the third episode, further reduce the dosage to 50 mg once daily (for newly diagnosed patients) or discontinue dasatinib (for patients resistant or intolerant to prior therapy, including imatinib.

[a] ANC = absolute neutrophil count.

Nonhematological adverse reactions – If a severe nonhematological adverse reaction develops with dasatinib use, treatment must be withheld until the event has resolved or improved. Thereafter, treatment can be resumed as appropriate at a reduced dose depending on the initial severity of the event.

➤*Concomitant therapy:*

Strong CYP3A4 inducers – The use of concomitant strong CYP3A4 inducers (eg, dexamethasone, phenytoin, carbamazepine, rifampin, rifabutin, phenobarbital) may decrease dasatinib plasma concentrations and should be avoided. St. John's wort may decrease dasatinib plasma concentrations unpredictably and should be avoided. If patients must be coadministered a strong CYP3A4 inducer, based on pharmacokinetic studies, an increased dasatinib dose should be considered. If the dose of dasatinib is increased, the patient should be monitored carefully for toxicity.

Strong CYP3A4 inhibitors – CYP3A4 inhibitors (eg, ketoconazole, itraconazole, clarithromycin, atazanavir, indinavir, nefazodone, nelfinavir, ritonavir, saquinavir, telithromycin, voriconazole) may increase dasatinib plasma concentrations. Grapefruit juice may also increase plasma concentrations of dasatinib and should be avoided.

The selection of an alternate concomitant medication with no or minimal enzyme inhibition potential is recommended. If dasatinib must be administered with a strong CYP3A4 inhibitor, a decreased dose should be considered. Based on pharmacokinetic studies, a dose decrease to 20 mg daily should be considered for patients taking dasatinib 100 mg daily. For patients taking dasatinib 140 mg daily, a decreased dose to 40 mg daily should be considered. These reduced doses of dasatinib are predicted to adjust the area under the curve (AUC) to the range observed without CYP3A4 inhibitors. However, there are no clinical data with these dose adjustments in patients receiving strong CYP3A4 inhibitors. If dasatinib is not tolerated after dose reduction, either the strong CYP3A4 inhibitor must be discontinued, or dasatinib should be stopped until treatment with the inhibitor has ceased. When the strong inhibitor is discontinued, a washout period of approximately 1 week should be allowed before the dasatinib dose is increased.

➤*Duration of therapy:* In clinical studies, treatment with dasatinib was continued until disease progression or until no longer tolerated by the patient. The effect of stopping treatment after the achievement of a complete cytogenetic response has not been investigated.

➤*Administration:* Tablets should not be crushed or cut. They should be swallowed whole and may be taken with or without a meal in the morning or in the evening.

Safe handling/disposal – Dasatinib is considered a cytotoxic agent. Follow safe handling procedures when preparing, administering, or dispensing dasatinib.

Dasatinib tablets consist of a core tablet (containing the active drug substance) surrounded by a film coating to prevent exposure of pharmacy and clinical personnel to the active drug substance. However, pharmacy and clinical personnel should wear disposable chemotherapy gloves in case tablets are inadvertently crushed or broken. Personnel who are pregnant should avoid exposure to crushed and/or broken tablets.

➤*Storage/Stability:* Store at 25°C (77°F); excursions are permitted between 15° and 30°C (59° and 86°F).

Actions

➤*Pharmacology:* Dasatinib, at nanomolar concentrations, inhibits the following kinases: BCR-ABL, SRC family (SRC, LCK, YES, FYN), c-KIT, EPHA2, and PDGFR-beta. Based on modeling studies, dasatinib is predicted to bind to multiple conformations of the ABL kinase.

In vitro, dasatinib was active in leukemic cell lines representing variants of imatinib mesylate sensitive and resistant disease. Dasatinib inhibited the growth of CML and ALL cell lines overexpressing BCR-ABL. Under the conditions of the assays, dasatinib was able to overcome imatinib resistance resulting from BCR-ABL kinase domain mutations, activation of alternate signaling pathways involving the SRC family kinases (LYN, HCK), and multidrug resistance gene overexpression.

➤*Pharmacokinetics:*

Absorption – Maximum plasma concentrations (C_{max}) of dasatinib are observed between 0.5 and 6 hours (time of maximum concentration [T_{max}]) following oral administration. Dasatinib exhibits dose proportional increases in AUC and linear elimination characteristics over the dose range of 15 to 240 mg/day.

Effect of food: Data from a study of 54 healthy subjects who were administered a single dose of dasatinib 100 mg 30 minutes following consumption of a high-fat meal resulted in a 14% increase in the mean AUC of dasatinib. The observed food effects were not clinically relevant.

Distribution – In patients, dasatinib has an apparent volume of distribution of 2,505 L, suggesting that the drug is extensively distributed in the extravascular space. Binding of dasatinib and its active metabolite to human plasma proteins in vitro was approximately 96% and 93%, respectively, with no concentration dependence over the range of 100 to 500 ng/mL.

Metabolism – Dasatinib is extensively metabolized in humans, primarily by the cytochrome P450 enzyme 3A4. CYP3A4 was the primary enzyme responsible for the formation of the active metabolite. Flavin-containing monooxygenase 3 and uridine diphosphate-glucuronosyltransferase enzymes are also involved in the formation of dasatinib metabolites.

The exposure of the active metabolite, which is equipotent to dasatinib, represents approximately 5% of the dasatinib AUC. This indicates that the active metabolite of dasatinib is unlikely to play a major role in the observed pharmacology of the drug. Dasatinib also had several other inactive oxidative metabolites.

Dasatinib is a weak time-dependent inhibitor of CYP3A4. At clinically relevant concentrations, dasatinib does not inhibit CYP1A2, 2A6, 2B6, 2C8, 2C9, 2C19, 2D6, or 2E1. Dastinib is not an inducer of human CYP enzymes.

Excretion – The overall mean terminal half-life of dasatinib is 3 to 5 hours. Elimination is primarily via the feces. Following a single oral dose of [^{14}C]-labeled dasatinib, approximately 4% and 85% of the administered radioactivity was recovered in the urine and feces, respectively, within 10 days. Unchanged dasatinib accounted for 0.1% and 19% of the administered dose in urine and feces, respectively, with the remainder of the dose being metabolites.

Special populations –

Hepatic function impairment: Dasatinib doses of 50 and 20 mg were evaluated in 8 patients with moderate (Child-Pugh class B) and 7 patients with severe (Child-Pugh class C) hepatic impairment, respectively. Matched controls with healthy hepatic function (n = 15) were also evaluated and received a dasatinib dose of 70 mg. Compared with subjects with healthy liver function, patients with moderate hepatic impairment had decreases in dose-normalized C_{max} and AUC by 47% and 8%, respectively. Patients with severe hepatic impairment had dose-normalized C_{max} decreased by 43% and AUC decreased by 28% compared with the healthy controls.

These differences in C_{max} and AUC are not clinically relevant. Dose adjustment is not necessary in patients with hepatic impairment.

Contraindications

None well documented.

Warnings/Precautions

➤*Myelosuppression:* Treatment with dasatinib is associated with severe (National Cancer Institute Common Toxicity Criteria [NCI-CTC] grade 3 or 4) thrombocytopenia, neutropenia, and anemia. The occurrence is more frequent in patients with advanced CML or Ph+ ALL than in chronic phase CML. Perform complete blood cell counts weekly for the first 2 months and then monthly thereafter, or as clinically indicated. Myelosuppression was generally reversible and usually managed by withholding dasatinib temporarily or by dose reduction. In a dose-optimization study in patients with resistance or intolerance to prior imatinib therapy and chronic phase CML, grade 3 or 4 myelosuppression was reported less frequently in patients treated with 100 mg once daily than in patients treated with other dosing regimens.

➤*Hemorrhage:* In addition to causing thrombocytopenia in human patients, dasatinib caused platelet dysfunction in vitro. In all clinical studies, severe CNS hemorrhages, including fatalities, occurred in 1% of patients receiving dasatinib. Severe GI hemorrhage, including fatalities, occurred in 4% of patients and generally required treatment interruptions and transfusions. Other cases of severe hemorrhage occurred in 2% of patients. Most bleeding reactions were associated with severe thrombocytopenia.

Patients were excluded from participation in dasatinib clinical studies if they took medications that inhibit platelet function or anticoagulants. In subsequent trials, the use of anticoagulants, aspirin, and nonsteroidal anti-inflammatory drugs (NSAIDs) was allowed concurrently with dasatinib if the platelet count was more than 50,000 to 75,000/mcL. Exercise caution if patients are required to take medications that inhibit platelet function or anticoagulants.

➤*Fluid retention:* Dasatinib is associated with fluid retention. In all clinical studies, severe fluid retention was reported in up to 10% of patients. Ascites and generalized edema were each reported in less than 1%. Severe pulmonary edema was reported in 1% of patients. Evaluate patients who

DASATINIB — ORAL

develop symptoms suggestive of pleural effusion, such as dyspnea or dry cough, by chest x-ray. Severe pleural effusion may require thoracentesis and oxygen therapy. Fluid retention reactions were typically managed by supportive care measures that included diuretics or short courses of steroids. In dose-optimization studies, fluid retention events were reported less frequently with once-daily dosing than with other dosing regimens.

➤*QT prolongation:* In vitro data suggest that dasatinib has the potential to prolong cardiac ventricular repolarization (QT interval). Of the 2,440 patients with CML treated with dasatinib in clinical studies, less than 1% of patients had QTc prolongation reported as an adverse reaction. One percent of patients experienced a QTcF more than 500 ms. In 865 patients with leukemia treated with dasatinib in five phase 2 single-arm studies, the maximum mean changes in QTcF (90% upper bound confidence interval [CI]) from baseline ranged from 7 to 13.4 ms.

Administer dasatinib with caution to patients who have or may develop prolongation of QTc. These include patients with hypokalemia or hypomagnesemia, patients with congenital long QT syndrome, patients taking antiarrhythmic medicines or other medicinal products that lead to QT prolongation, and cumulative high-dose anthracycline therapy. Correct hypokalemia or hypomagnesemia prior to dasatinib administration.

➤*Cardiovascular effects:* Cardiac adverse reactions were reported in 5.8% of 258 patients taking dasatinib, including 1.6% of patients with cardiomyopathy, congestive heart failure, diastolic dysfunction, fatal myocardial infarction, and left ventricular dysfunction. Monitor patients for signs or symptoms consistent with cardiac dysfunction and treat appropriately.

➤*Hepatic function impairment:* Caution is recommended when administering dasatinib to patients with hepatic impairment.

➤*Pregnancy: Category D.* Dasatinib may cause fetal harm when administered to a pregnant woman. There are no adequate and well-controlled studies of dasatinib in pregnant women. It is not known if dasatinib crosses the human placenta. The molecular weight (approximately 486 for the nonhydrated form) is low enough, but the short plasma elimination half-life and high plasma protein binding should limit the amount crossing to the embryo and fetus. However, the drug has a very high volume of distribution, suggesting that it is extensively distributed into extravasation space. Advise women of childbearing potential of the potential hazard to the fetus and to avoid becoming pregnant. If dasatinib is used during pregnancy, or if the patient becomes pregnant while taking dasatinib, apprise the patient of the potential hazard to the fetus.

In nonclinical studies, at plasma concentrations below those observed in humans receiving therapeutic doses of dasatinib, embryofetal toxicities were observed in rats and rabbits. Fetal death was observed in rats. In both rats and rabbits, the lowest dosages of dasatinib tested (rat, 2.5 mg/kg/day [15 mg/m²/day] and rabbit, 0.5 mg/kg/day [6 mg/m²/day]) resulted in embryofetal toxicities. These dosages produced maternal AUCs of 105 ng•h/mL (0.3-fold the human AUC in females at the recommended dosage of 70 mg twice daily) and 44 ng•h/mL (0.1-fold the human AUC) in rats and rabbits, respectively. Embryofetal toxicities included skeletal malformations at multiple sites (scapula, humerus, femur, radius, ribs, clavicle), reduced ossification (sternum; thoracic, lumbar, and sacral vertebrae; forepaw phalanges; pelvis; and hyoid body), edema, and microhepatia.

Fertility impairment – Results of repeat-dose toxicity studies in multiple species indicate the potential for dasatinib to impair reproductive function and fertility.

➤*Lactation:* It is unknown whether dasatinib is excreted in human milk. The molecular weight (about 486 for the nonhydrated form) of the parent compound is low enough, but the short plasma elimination half-lives of dasatinib and its active metabolite and the high plasma protein binding should limit the amounts excreted in breast milk. Because many drugs are excreted in human milk and because of the potential for serious adverse reactions in breast-feeding infants from dasatinib, a decision should be made whether to discontinue breast-feeding or the drug, taking into account the importance of the drug to the mother.

➤*Children:* The safety and efficacy of dasatinib in patients younger than 18 years of age have not been established.

➤*Elderly:* Compared with patients younger than 65 years of age, patients 65 years of age and older are more likely to experience toxicity.

➤*Monitoring:* Monitor patients for signs or symptoms consistent with cardiac dysfunction and treat appropriately. Perform complete blood cell counts weekly for the first 2 months and then monthly thereafter, or as clinically indicated. Evaluate patients who develop symptoms suggestive of pleural effusion, such as dyspnea or dry cough, by chest x-ray.

Drug Interactions

➤*QT prolongation:* An additive effect of dasatinib with other drugs that prolong the QT interval cannot be excluded. The following drugs may prolong the QT interval and increase the risk of life-threatening cardiac arrhythmias, including torsades de pointes: antiarrhythmic agents (eg, amiodarone, bretylium, disopyramide, dofetilide, procainamide, quinidine, sotalol), arsenic trioxide, chlorpromazine, cisapride, dolasetron, droperidol, gatifloxacin, halofantrine, levomethadyl, mefloquine, mesoridazine, moxifloxacin, pentamidine, pimozide, probucol, sparfloxacin, thioridazine, and ziprasidone. (See Drug-Induced Prolongation of the QT Interval and Torsades De Pointes.)

Dasatinib Drug Interactions

Precipitant drug	Object drug[a]		Description
Antacids (eg, aluminum hydroxide/ magnesium hydroxide, calcium carbonate)	Dasatinib	↑↓	Administration of aluminum hydroxide/magnesium hydroxide 2 hours prior to a single dose of dasatinib increased C_{max} by 26%, but when the doses were given concomitantly, AUC was decreased by 55% and C_{max} was reduced by 58%. Avoid simultaneous administration. Give antacids 2 hours before or after dasatinib.
CYP3A4 inducers (eg, carbamazepine, dexamethasone, rifabutin, rifampin, phenobarbital, phenytoin, St. John's wort)	Dasatinib	↓	CYP3A4 inducers may decrease dasatinib plasma concentrations. Coadministration of rifampin decreased dasatinib mean C_{max} and AUC by 81% and 82%, respectively. Avoid concurrent use. Selection of an alternate concomitant medication with no or minimal enzyme induction potential is recommended. If dasatinib must be administered with a strong CYP3A4 inducer, consider increasing the dose of dasatinib and carefully monitoring the patient for toxicity.
CYP3A4 inhibitors (eg, clarithromycin, itraconazole, ketoconazole, nefazodone, protease inhibitors [eg, atazanavir, indinavir, nelfinavir, ritonavir, saquinavir], telithromycin, voriconazole).	Dasatinib	↑	Dasatinib plasma concentrations may be elevated, increasing the pharmacologic effects and risk of adverse reactions. Ketoconazole coadministration increased dasatinib C_{max} and AUC 4- and 5- fold, respectively. Avoid strong inhibitors of CYP3A4. If dasatinib must be administered with a CYP3A4 inhibitor, closely monitor for toxicity, and consider reducing the dose of dasatinib to 20 mg daily in patients taking dasatinib 100 mg daily and 40 mg daily in patients taking dasatinib 140 mg daily. When the strong inhibitor is discontinued, allow a 1-week washout period before increasing the dasatinib dose. See Administration and Dosage for more information.
H_2 blockers (eg, famotidine), proton pump inhibitors (eg, omeprazole)	Dasatinib	↓	Long-term suppression of gastric acid secretion is likely to reduce dasatinib exposure. The concomitant use of H_2 blockers or proton pump inhibitors is not recommended. Single-dose administration of dasatinib 10 hours after famotidine reduced the AUC and C_{max} by 61% and 63%, respectively.
Dasatinib	CYP3A4 substrates (eg, alfentanil, cisapride,[b] cyclosporine, ergot derivatives [eg, dihydroergotamine, ergotamine], fentanyl, pimozide, quinidine, simvastatin, sirolimus, tacrolimus)	↑	The mean C_{max} and AUC of simvastatin were increased by 37% and 20%, respectively, with coadministration. Use with caution. Carefully monitor the patient and adjust the CYP3A4 substrate dose as needed.

[a] ↑ = object drug increased; ↓ = object drug decreased; ↑↓ = object drug both increased and decreased.
[b] Available from the manufacturer on a limited-access protocol.

➤*Drug/Food interactions:* Grapefruit juice may increase dasatinib plasma concentrations and should be avoided.

Adverse Reactions

➤*Chronic myeloid leukemia:*

Discontinuation of therapy – In the newly diagnosed chronic phase CML trial, drug was discontinued for adverse reactions in 6% of dasatinib-treated patients. Among patients with resistance or intolerance to prior imatinib therapy, the rates of discontinuation for adverse reactions were 15% of patients in chronic phase CML, 16% in accelerated phase CML, 15% in

DASATINIB — ORAL

myeloid blast phase CML, 8% in Ph± ALL, and 8% in lymphoid blast phase CML. In a dose-optimization study in patients with resistance or intolerance to prior imatinib therapy and chronic phase CML, the rate of discontinuation for adverse reactions was lower in patients treated with 100 mg once daily than in patients treated with other dosing regimens (10% and 16%, respectively).

Serious adverse reactions – The most frequently reported serious adverse reactions in patients with newly diagnosed chronic phase CML included pleural effusion (2%), hemorrhage (2%), congestive heart failure (1%), and pyrexia (1%).

The most frequently reported serious adverse reactions in patients with resistance or intolerance to prior imatinib therapy included pleural effusion (11%); febrile neutropenia, GI bleeding (4%); diarrhea, dyspnea, pneumonia, pyrexia (3%); congestive heart failure/cardiac dysfunction, infection (2%); CNS hemorrhage, pericardial effusion (1%).

Most common adverse reactions – The most frequently reported adverse reactions reported in at least 10% of patients in newly diagnosed chronic phase CML included myelosuppression, fluid retention events (pleural effusion, superficial localized edema, generalized edema), diarrhea, headache, musculoskeletal pain, and rash. Pleural effusions were reported in 31 patients.

The most frequently reported adverse reactions (20% or more of patients) with resistance or intolerance to prior imatinib therapy included diarrhea, dyspnea, fatigue, fluid retention events, headache, hemorrhage, myelosuppression, nausea, and skin rash.

Newly diagnosed chronic phase chronic myeloid leukemia –

Dasatinib Adverse Reactions in Newly Diagnosed Chronic Phase Chronic Myeloid Leukemia (≥ 10%)

Adverse reactions	All grades: Dasatinib (n = 258)	All grades: Imatinib (n = 258)	Grade 3/4: Dasatinib (n = 258)	Grade 3/4: Imatinib (n = 258)
Cardiovascular				
Congestive heart failure/cardiac dysfunction[a]	2%	1%	< 1%	< 1%
Pericardial effusion	2%	< 1%	< 1%	0%
CNS				
CNS bleeding	0%	< 1%	0%	< 1%
Fatigue	8%	11%	< 1%	0%
Headache	12%	10%	0%	0%
GI				
Diarrhea	18%	19%	< 1%	1%
GI bleeding	2%	< 1%	1%	0%
Nausea	9%	21%	0%	0%
Vomiting	5%	10%	0%	0%
Hematologic				
Hemorrhage[b]	6%	5%	1%	1%
Other bleeding[c]	5%	5%	0%	1%
Metabolic/Nutrition				
Fluid retention	23%	43%	1%	1%
Generalized edema	3%	7%	0%	0%
Superficial localized edema	10%	36%	0%	< 1%
Musculoskeletal				
Musculoskeletal pain	12%	16%	0%	< 1%
Muscle inflammation	4%	19%	0%	< 1%
Myalgia	6%	12%	0%	0%
Respiratory				
Pleural effusion	12%	0%	< 1%	0%
Pulmonary edema	< 1%	0%	0%	0%
Pulmonary hypertension	1%	0%	0%	0%
Miscellaneous				
Rash[d]	11%	17%	0%	1%

[a] Includes cardiac failure acute, cardiac failure congestive, cardiomyopathy, diastolic dysfunction, ejection fraction decreased, and left ventricular dysfunction.
[b] Adverse reaction of special interest with less than 10% frequency.
[c] Includes conjunctival hemorrhage, ear hemorrhage, ecchymosis, epistaxis, eye hemorrhage, gingival bleeding, hematoma, hematuria, hemoptysis, intra-abdominal hematoma, petechiae, scleral hemorrhage, uterine hemorrhage, and vaginal hemorrhage.
[d] Includes erythema, erythema multiforme, rash, rash generalized, rash macular, rash papular, rash pustular, skin exfoliation, and rash vesicular.

Chronic myeloid leukemia resistent or intolerant to prior imatinib therapy –

Dasatinib Adverse Reactions in Chronic Myeloid Leukemia Resistant or Intolerant to Prior Imatinib Therapy (≥ 10%)

	100 mg once daily		140 mg once daily					
	Chronic (n = 165)		Accelerated (n = 157)		Myeloid blast (n = 74)		Lymphoid blast (n = 33)	
Adverse reaction	All grades	Grade 3/4	All grades	Grade 3/4	All grades	Grade 3/4	All grades	Grade 3/4
Cardiovascular								
Congestive heart failure/cardiac dysfunction[a]	0%	0%	0%	0%	4%	0%	0%	0%
Pericardial effusion	2%	1%	3%	1%	0%	0%	0%	0%
CNS								
CNS bleeding	0%	0%	1%	1%	0%	0%	3%	3%
Fatigue	24%	2%	19%	2%	20%	1%	9%	3%
Headache	33%	1%	27%	1%	18%	1%	15%	3%
GI								
Abdominal pain	12%	1%	6%	0%	8%	3%	3%	0%
Diarrhea	27%	2%	31%	3%	20%	5%	18%	0%
GI bleeding	2%	1%	8%	6%	9%	7%	9%	3%
Nausea	18%	1%	19%	1%	23%	1%	21%	3%
Vomiting	7%	1%	11%	1%	12%	0%	15%	0%
Metabolic/Nutritional								
Fluid retention	34%	4%	35%	8%	34%	7%	21%	6%
Generalized edema	3%	0%	1%	0%	3%	0%	0%	0%
Superficial localized edema	18%	0%	18%	1%	14%	0%	3%	0%
Musculoskeletal								
Arthralgia	12%	1%	10%	0%	5%	1%	0%	0%
Musculoskeletal pain	19%	2%	11%	0%	8%	1%	0%	0%
Myalgia	13%	0%	7%	1%	7%	1%	3%	0%
Respiratory								
Dyspnea	20%	2%	20%	3%	15%	3%	3%	3%
Pleural effusion	18%	2%	21%	7%	20%	7%	21%	6%
Pulmonary edema	0%	0%	1%	0%	4%	3%	0%	0%
Miscellaneous								
Febrile neutropenia	1%	1%	4%	4%	12%	12%	12%	12%
Hemorrhage	11%	1%	26%	8%	19%	9%	24%	9%
Infection (including bacterial, viral, fungal, nonspecified)	12%	1%	10%	6%	14%	7%	9%	0%
Pyrexia	5%	1%	11%	2%	18%	3%	6%	0%
Skin rash[b]	17%	2%	15%	0%	16%	1%	21%	0%

[a] Includes cardiac failure, cardiac failure congestive, cardiomyopathy, congestive cardiomyopathy, diastolic dysfunction, ejection fraction decreased, ventricular failure, and ventricular dysfunction.
[b] Includes drug eruption, erythema, erythema multiforme, erythrosis, exfoliative rash, generalized erythema, genital rash, heat rash, milia, rash, rash erythematous, rash follicular, rash generalized, rash macular, rash maculopapular, rash papular, rash pruritic, rash pustular, skin exfoliation, skin irritation, urticaria vesiculosa, and rash vesicular.

➤*Acute lymphoblastic leukemia:*

Most frequent adverse reactions – The most frequently reported adverse reactions included fluid retention events (eg, pleural effusion [24%], superficial edema [19%]) and GI disorders (eg, diarrhea [31%], nausea [24%], vomiting [16%]). Hemorrhage (19%); pyrexia (17%); and rash and dyspnea (16%) were also frequently reported.

Serious adverse reactions – The most frequently reported serious adverse reactions included pleural effusion (11%); GI bleeding (7%); febrile neutropenia (6%); infection (5%); pyrexia (4%); pneumonia and diarrhea (3%); and nausea, vomiting, and colitis (2%).

➤*Other adverse reactions:*

Cardiovascular – Arrhythmia (including tachycardia), flushing, hypertension, palpitations (1% to less than 10%); angina pectoris, cardiomegaly, hypotension, pericarditis, syncope, thrombophlebitis, ventricular arrhythmia (including ventricular tachycardia) (0.1% to less than 1%); acute coronary syndrome, cerebrovascular accident, cor pulmonale, livedo reticularis, myocarditis, optic neuritis, transient ischemic attack (less than 0.1%).

DASATINIB — ORAL

CNS – Asthenia, depression, dizziness, dysgeusia, insomnia, neuropathy (including peripheral neuropathy), somnolence (1% to less than 10%); affect lability, amnesia, anxiety, confusional state, libido decreased, malaise, tremor, vertigo (0.1% to less than 1%); convulsion (less than 0.1%).

Dermatologic – Acne, alopecia, dermatitis (including eczema), dry skin, hyperhidrosis, pruritus, urticaria (1% to less than 10%); acute febrile neutrophilic dermatosis, bullous conditions, nail disorder, palmar-plantar erythrodysesthesia syndrome, panniculitis, photosensitivity, pigmentation disorder, skin ulcer (0.1% to less than 1%).

GI – Abdominal distension, colitis (including neutropenic colitis), constipation, dyspepsia, enterocolitis infection, gastritis, mucosal inflammation (including mucositis/stomatitis), oral soft tissue disorder (1% to less than 10%); anal fissure, ascites, cholecystitis, cholestasis, dysphagia, esophagitis, hepatitis, pancreatitis, upper GI ulcer (0.1% to less than 1%); protein losing gastroenteropathy (less than 0.1%).

GU – Gynecomastia, menstruation irregular, proteinuria, renal failure, urinary frequency (0.1% to less than 1%).

Hematologic/Lymphatic – Pancytopenia (1% to less than 10%); pure red cell aplasia (less than 0.1%).

Lab test abnormalities – Blood creatine phosphokinase increased (0.1% to less than 1%).

Metabolic/Nutritional – Anorexia, appetite disturbances, weight decreased, weight increased (1% to less than 10%); hyperuricemia, hypoalbuminemia (0.1% to less than 1%).

Musculoskeletal – Muscular weakness (1% to less than 10%); musculoskeletal stiffness, rhabdomyolysis (0.1% to less than 1%); tendonitis (less than 0.1%).

Respiratory – Cough, lung infiltration, pneumonia (including bacterial, viral, and fungal), pneumonitis, pulmonary hypertension, upper respiratory tract infection/inflammation (1% to less than 10%); asthma, bronchospasm (0.1% to less than 1%); acute respiratory distress syndrome (less than 0.1%).

Special senses – Dry eye, tinnitus, visual disorder (including visual disturbance, vision blurred, and visual acuity reduced) (1% to less than 10%); conjunctivitis (0.1% to less than 1%); optic neuritis (less than 0.1%).

Miscellaneous – Chest pain, chills, contusion, herpes virus infection, pain (1% to less than 10%); hypersensitivity (including erythema nodosum), sepsis (including fatal outcomes), temperature intolerance, tumor lysis syndrome (0.1% to less than 1%).

➤*Lab test abnormalities:*

Chronic myeloid leukemia – Myelosuppression was commonly reported in all patient populations. The frequency of grade 3 or 4 neutropenia, thrombocytopenia, and anemia was higher in patients with advanced phase CML than in chronic phase CML. Myelosuppression was reported in patients with normal baseline laboratory values as well as in patients with preexisting laboratory abnormalities.

In patients who experienced severe myelosuppression, recovery generally occurred following dose interruption or reduction; permanent discontinuation of treatment occurred in 2% of patients with newly diagnosed chronic phase CML and 5% of patients with resistance or intolerance to prior imatinib therapy.

Grade 3 or 4 elevations of transaminases or bilirubin and grade 3 or 4 hypocalcemia, hypokalemia, and hypophosphatemia were reported in patients with all phases of CML but were reported with an increased frequency in patients with myeloid or lymphoid blast phase CML. Elevations in transaminases or bilirubin were usually managed with dose reduction or interruption. Patients developing grade 3 or 4 hypocalcemia during the course of dasatinib therapy often had recovery with oral calcium supplementation.

Newly diagnosed chronic phase chronic myeloid leukemia –

Dasatinib CTC Grade 3/4 Laboratory Abnormalities in Newly Diagnosed Chronic Phase Chronic Myeloid Leukemia[a]

Laboratory parameters	Dasatinib (n = 258)	Imatinib (n = 258)
Anemia	11%	7%
Elevated bilirubin	1%	0%
Elevated creatinine	< 1%	1%
Elevated ALT	< 1%	1%
Elevated AST	< 1%	1%
Hypocalcemia	3%	2%
Hypokalemia	0%	2%
Hypophosphatemia	5%	24%
Neutropenia	22%	20%
Thrombocytopenia	19%	10%

[a] CTC grades: neutropenia (grade 3 ≥ 0.5 to less than 1 × 10^9/L, grade 4 < 0.5 × 10^9/L); thrombocytopenia (grade 3 ≥ 25 to < 50 × 10^9/L, grade 4 < 25 × 10^9/L); anemia (hemoglobin grade 3 ≥ 65 to < 80 g/L, grade 4 < 65 g/L); elevated creatinine (grade 3 > 3 to 6 × upper limit of normal [ULN], grade 4 > 6 × ULN), elevated bilirubin (grade 3 > 3 to 10 × ULN, grade 4 > 10 × ULN); elevated AST or ALT (grade 3 > 5 to 20 × ULN, grade 4 > 20 × ULN); hypocalcemia (grade 3 < 7 to 6 mg/dL, grade 4 < 6 mg/dL); hypophosphatemia (grade 3 < 2 to 1 mg/dL, grade 4 < 1 mg/dL; hypokalemia (grade 3 < 3 to 2.5 mmol/L, grade 4 2.5 mmol/L).

Chronic myeloid leukemia resistant or intolerant to prior imatinib therapy –

Dasatinib CTC Grades 3/4 Laboratory Abnormalities in Chronic Myeloid Leukemia Resistant or Intolerant to Prior Imatinib Therapy[a]

Laboratory parameters	Chronic phase CML	Advanced phase CML		
	100 mg once daily (n = 165)	Accelerated phase 140 mg once daily (n = 157)	Myeloid blast phase 140 mg once daily (n = 74)	Lymphoid blast phase 140 mg once daily (n = 33)
Anemia	13%	47%	74%	52%
Elevated ALT	0%	2%	5%	3%
Elevated AST	< 1%	0%	4%	3%
Elevated bilirubin	< 1%	1%	3%	6%
Elevated creatinine	0%	2%	8%	0%
Hypocalcemia	< 1%	4%	9%	12%
Hypokalemia	2%	7%	11%	15%
Hypophosphatemia	10%	13%	12%	18%
Neutropenia	36%	58%	77%	79%
Thrombocytopenia	23%	63%	78%	85%

[a] CTC grades: neutropenia (grade 3 ≥ 0.5 to less than 1 × 10^9/L, grade 4 < 0.5 × 10^9/L); thrombocytopenia (grade 3 ≥ 25 to < 50 × 10^9/L, grade 4 < 25 × 10^9/L); anemia (hemoglobin grade 3 ≥ 65 to < 80 g/L, grade 4 < 65 g/L); elevated creatinine (grade 3 > 3 to 6 × ULN, grade 4 > 6 × ULN); elevated bilirubin (grade 3 > 3 to 10 × ULN, grade 4 > 10 × ULN); elevated AST or ALT (grade 3 > 5 to 20 × ULN, grade 4 > 20 × ULN); hypocalcemia (grade 3 < 7 to 6 mg/dL, grade 4 < 6 mg/dL); hypophosphatemia (grade 3 < 2 to 1 mg/dL, grade 4 < 1 mg/dL); hypokalemia (grade 3 < 3 to 2.5 mmol/L, grade 4 < 2.5 mmol/L).

➤*Postmarketing:*

Cardiovascular – Atrial fibrillation/atrial flutter, thrombosis/embolism (including pulmonary embolism, deep vein thrombosis).

Respiratory – Interstitial lung disease.

Overdosage

➤*Symptoms:* Experience with overdose of dasatinib in clinical studies is limited to isolated cases. Overdosage of 280 mg/day for 1 week was reported in 2 patients and both developed severe myelosuppression and bleeding.

➤*Treatment:* Because dasatinib is associated with severe myelosuppression, closely monitor patients who ingested more than the recommended dosage for myelosuppression and give appropriate supportive treatment.

Patient Information

Advise patients not to crush or cut dasatinib tablets; they should be swallowed whole and may be taken with or without a meal.

Advise patients that dasatinib contains lactose 135 mg and 189 mg in a 100 mg and 140 mg daily dose, respectively.

Inform patients of the possibility of serious bleeding and advise them to immediately report any signs or symptoms suggestive of hemorrhage (unusual bleeding or easy bruising).

Inform patients of the possibility of developing low blood cell counts; instruct patients to immediately report development of fever, particularly in association with any suggestion of infection.

Advise patients of the possibility of developing fluid retention (swelling, weight gain, or shortness of breath) and to seek medical attention if those symptoms arise.

Instruct patients that dasatinib may cause fetal harm when administered to a pregnant woman. Advise women of the potential hazard to the fetus and to avoid becoming pregnant. If dasatinib is used during pregnancy, or if the patient becomes pregnant while taking dasatinib, apprise the patient of the potential hazard to the fetus.

Inform patients that they may experience nausea, vomiting, or diarrhea with dasatinib. If these symptoms are significant, they should seek medical attention.

Inform patients that they may experience headache or musculoskeletal pain with dasatinib. If these symptoms are significant, they should seek medical attention.

Inform patients that they may experience fatigue with dasatinib. If this symptom is significant, they should seek medical attention.

Patients should be informed that they may experience skin rash with dasatinib. If this symptom is significant, they should seek medical attention.

Inform patients that if they miss a dose of dasatinib to take the next scheduled dose at its regular time. The patient should not take 2 doses at the same time.

IMATINIB

Rx	**Gleevec** (Novartis)	**Tablets; oral:** 100 mg	As imatinib mesylate. (NVR SA). Very dark yellow to brownish-orange, round, scored. Film-coated. In 90s.
		400 mg	As imatinib mesylate. (SL 400). Very dark yellow to brownish-orange, ovaloid, scored. Film-coated. In 30s.

IMATINIB MESYLATE — ORAL

Indications

➤*Acute lymphoblastic leukemia:* Adults with relapsed or refractory Philadelphia chromosome–positive (Ph+) acute lymphoblastic leukemia (ALL).

➤*Aggressive systemic mastocytosis:* Adults with aggressive systemic mastocytosis without the D816V c-Kit mutation or with c-Kit mutational status unknown.

➤*Chronic myeloid leukemia:* Newly diagnosed adults and children with Ph+ chronic myeloid leukemia (CML) in chronic phase; adults with Ph+ CML in blast crisis, accelerated phase, or in chronic phase after failure of interferon alpha therapy; children with Ph+ chronic phase CML whose disease has recurred after stem cell transplant or who are resistant to interferon alpha therapy.

There are no controlled trials in children demonstrating a clinical benefit, such as improvement in disease-related symptoms or increased survival.

➤*Dermatofibrosarcoma protuberans:* Adults with unresectable, recurrent, and/or metastatic dermatofibrosarcoma protuberans.

➤*GI stromal tumors:* Patients with Kit (CD117)–positive unresectable and/or metastatic malignant GI stromal tumors (GIST); adjuvant treatment of patients following complete gross resection of Kit (CD117)–positive GIST.

➤*Hypereosinophilic syndrome and/or chronic eosinophilic leukemia:* Adults with hypereosinophilic syndrome and/or chronic eosinophilic leukemia who have the FIP1L1-platelet–derived growth factor receptor (PDGFR)α fusion kinase (mutational analysis or fluorescent in situ hybridization [FISH] demonstration of CHIC2 allele deletion) and for patients with hypereosinophilic syndrome and/or chronic eosinophilic leukemia who are FIP1L1-PDGFRα fusion kinase negative or unknown.

➤*Myelodysplastic/Myeloproliferative diseases:* Adults with myelodysplastic/myeloproliferative diseases associated with PDGFR gene rearrangements.

➤*Off-label uses:*

Rectal administration – [4] = Insufficient documentation. Based on a single case report, initial data suggest that rectal administration of twice the daily dose (administered as divided doses) of imatinib may offer similar area under the curve (AUC) parameters to oral dosing. However, additional trials are needed to establish this type of use. (See Administration and Dosage.)

Administration and Dosage

➤*General dosing considerations:* If a severe nonhematologic adverse reaction develops (such as severe hepatotoxicity or severe fluid retention), imatinib should be withheld until the reaction has resolved. Thereafter, treatment can be resumed as appropriate, depending on the initial severity of the event. (See Dosage Adjustment for more information.)

Dose reduction or treatment interruptions for severe neutropenia and thrombocytopenia are recommended. (See Dosage Adjustment for more information.)

➤*Adults:*

Acute lymphoblastic leukemia – 600 mg/day.

Aggressive systemic mastocytosis – 400 mg/day.

Aggressive systemic mastocytosis associated with eosinophilia –

Initial dosage: 100 mg/day.

Dosage adjustment: Dose increase from 100 to 400 mg may be considered in the absence of adverse drug reactions if assessments demonstrate an insufficient response to therapy.

Chronic eosinophilic leukemia – 400 mg/day.

Chronic eosinophilic leukemia with demonstrated FIP1L1-PDGFRα fusion kinase –

Initial dosage: 100 mg/day.

Dosage adjustment: Dose increase from 100 to 400 mg may be considered in the absence of adverse drug reactions if assessments demonstrate an insufficient response to therapy.

Chronic myeloid leukemia –

Accelerated phase or blast crisis:

• *Usual dosage* – 600 mg/day.

• *Dosage adjustment* – A dose increase from 600 to 800 mg (given as 400 mg twice daily) may be considered in the absence of severe adverse drug reaction and severe non–leukemia-related neutropenia or thrombocytopenia in the following circumstances: disease progression (at any time); failure to achieve a satisfactory hematologic response after at least 3 months of treatment; failure to achieve a cytogenetic response after 6 to 12 months of treatment; loss of a previously achieved hematologic or cytogenetic response.

Chronic phase:

• *Usual dosage* – 400 mg/day.

• *Dosage adjustment* – A dose increase from 400 to 600 mg may be considered in the absence of severe adverse drug reactions and severe non–leukemia-related neutropenia or thrombocytopenia in the following circumstances: disease progression (at any time); failure to achieve a satisfactory hematologic response after at least 3 months of treatment; failure to achieve a cytogenetic response after 6 to 12 months of treatment; loss of a previously achieved hematologic or cytogenetic response.

Dermatofibrosarcoma protuberans – 800 mg/day.

GI stromal tumors –

Adjuvant treatment of GI stromal tumors:

• *Initial dosage* – 400 mg/day.

• *Duration of therapy* – In the clinical study, imatinib was administered for 1 year. The optimal treatment duration with imatinib is not known.

Unresectable and/or metastatic, malignant GI stromal tumors:

• *Initial dosage* – 400 mg/day.

• *Dosage adjustment* – A dosage increase of up to 800 mg daily (given as 400 mg twice daily) may be considered, as clinically indicated, in patients showing clear signs or symptoms of disease progression at a lower dose and in the absence of severe adverse drug reactions.

Hypereosinophilic syndrome – 400 mg/day.

Hypereosinophilic syndrome with demonstrated FIP1L1-PDGFRα fusion kinase –

Initial dosage: 100 mg/day.

Dosage adjustment: Dose increase from 100 to 400 mg for these patients may be considered in the absence of adverse drug reactions if assessments demonstrate an insufficient response to therapy.

Myelodysplastic/Myeloproliferative diseases – 400 mg/day.

Off-label dosing –

Rectal administration: [4] = Insufficient documentation. Rectal administration of the oral tablets as 400 mg twice daily (prior oral dose was 400 mg daily).

➤*Children:*

Children 2 years of age and older –

Newly diagnosed chronic myeloid leukemia:

• *Usual dosage* – 340 mg/m²/day.

• *Maximum dose* – 600 mg/day.

Chronic phase chronic myeloid leukemia recurring after transplant or resistant to interferon: 260 mg/m²/day.

➤*Renal function impairment:* Patients with moderate renal impairment (creatinine clearance [CrCl], 20 to 39 mL/min) should receive a 50% decrease in the recommended starting dose and increase as tolerated. Doses more than 600 mg are not recommended in patients with mild renal impairment (CrCl, 40 to 59 mL/min). For patients with moderate renal impairment, doses of more than 400 mg are not recommended. Imatinib should be used with caution in patients with severe renal impairment. A dosage of 100 mg/day was tolerated in 2 patients with severe renal impairment.

➤*Hepatic function impairment:* Patients with mild and moderate hepatic impairment do not require a dose adjustment. A 25% decrease in the recommended dose should be used for patients with severe hepatic impairment.

➤*Concomitant therapy:* The use of concomitant strong CYP3A4 inducers should be avoided (eg, carbamazepine, dexamethasone, phenobarbital, phenytoin, rifampin, St. John's wort). If patients must be coadministered strong CYP3A4 inducers, based on pharmacokinetic studies, dosage of imatinib should be increased by at least 50%, and clinical response should be carefully monitored.

➤*Dosage adjustment:*

Hematologic dose reduction –

Adults:

Imatinib Dose Adjustments for Adults With Neutropenia and Thrombocytopenia

Aggressive systemic mastocytosis associated with eosinophilia (starting dose 100 mg)	ANC[a] 1 × 10⁹/L and/or platelets 50 × 10⁹/L	Stop imatinib until ANC ≥ 1.5 × 10⁹/L and platelets ≥ 75× 10⁹/L. Resume treatment with imatinib at the previous dose (ie, before severe adverse reaction).
Hypereosinophilic syndrome/chronic eosinophilic leukemia withFIP1L1-PDGFRα fusion kinase (starting dose 100 mg)	ANC 1 × 10⁹/L and/or platelets 50 × 10⁹/L	Stop imatinib until ANC ≥ 1.5 × 10⁹/L and platelets ≥ 75 × 10⁹/L. Resume treatment with imatinib at the previous dose (ie, before severe adverse reaction).

IMATINIB MESYLATE — ORAL

Imatinib Dose Adjustments for Adults With Neutropenia and Thrombocytopenia

Chronic phase chronic myeloid leukemia (starting dose 400 mg)	ANC 1×10^9/L and/or platelets 50×10^9/L	Stop imatinib until ANC $\geq 1.5 \times 10^9$/L and platelets $\geq 75 \times 10^9$/L. Resume treatment with imatinib at the original starting dose of 400 mg. If recurrence of ANC $< 1 \times 10^9$/L and/or platelets $< 50 \times 10^9$/L, repeat the previous step and resume imatinib at a reduced dose of 300 mg.
Myelodysplastic/Myeloproliferative diseases, aggressive systemic mastocytosis, and hypereosinophilic syndrome/chronic eosinophilic leukemia (starting dose 400 mg)		
GI stromal tumors (starting dose 400 mg)		
Ph+ chronic myeloid leukemia: accelerated phase and blast crisis (starting dose 600 mg)	ANC 0.5×10^9/L and/or platelets 10×10^9/L	Check if cytopenia is related to leukemia (marrow aspirate or biopsy). If cytopenia is unrelated to leukemia, reduce the dose of imatinib to 400 mg. If cytopenia persists 2 weeks, reduce further to 300 mg. If cytopenia persists 4 weeks and is still unrelated to leukemia, stop imatinib until ANC $\geq 1 \times 10^9$/L and platelets $\geq 20 \times 10^9$/L, and then resume treatment at 300 mg.
Ph+ acute lymphoblastic leukemia (starting dose 600 mg)		
Dermatofibrosarcoma protuberans (starting dose 800 mg)	ANC 1×10^9/L and/or platelets 50×10^9/L	Stop imatinib until ANC $\geq 1.5 \times 10^9$/L and platelets $\geq 75 \times 10^9$/L. Resume treatment with imatinib at 600 mg. In the event of recurrence of ANC $< 1 \times 10^9$/L and/or platelets ^{9}/L, repeat the previous step and resume imatinib at a reduced dose of 400 mg.

[a] ANC = absolute neutrophil count.

Children:

Imatinib Dose Adjustments for Children With Neutropenia and Thrombocytopenia

Children with newly diagnosed chronic phase CML (starting dose 340 mg/m^2)	ANC 1×10^9/L and/or platelets 50×10^9/L	Stop imatinib until ANC $\geq 1.5 \times 10^9$/L and platelets $\geq 75 \times 10^9$/L. Resume treatment with imatinib at previous dose (ie, before severe reaction). In the event of recurrence of ANC $< 1 \times 10^9$/L and/or platelets $< 50 \times 10^9$/L, repeat the previous step and resume imatinib at a reduced dose of 260 mg/m^2.
Children with chronic phase CML recurring after transplant or resistant to interferon (starting dose 260 mg/m^2)	ANC 1×10^9/L and/or platelets 50×10^9/L	Stop imatinib until ANC $\geq 1.5 \times 10^9$/L and platelets $\geq 75 \times 10^9$/L. Resume treatment with imatinib at previous dose (ie, before severe reaction). In the event of recurrence of ANC $< 1 \times 10^9$/L and/or platelets $< 50 \times 10^9$/L, repeat the previous step and resume imatinib at a reduced dose of 200 mg/m^2.

Hepatotoxicity –

Adults:

Imatinib Dose Adjustments for Adults With Hepatotoxicity

Toxicity	Recommendation	Dosage adjustment for next dose
Bilirubin $> 3 \times$ IULN[a]	Withhold imatinib until bilirubin levels have returned to $< 1.5 \times$ IULN	Treatment with imatinib may then be continued at a reduced daily dose (300 mg if previous dose was 400 mg, 400 mg if previous dose was 600 mg, or 600 mg if previous dose was 800 mg).
Liver transaminases $> 5 \times$ IULN	Withhold imatinib until transaminase levels have returned to $< 2.5 \times$ IULN	

[a] IULN = institutional upper limit of normal.

Children:

Imatinib Dose Adjustments for Children With Hepatotoxicity

Toxicity	Recommendation	Dosage adjustment for next dose
Bilirubin $> 3 \times$ IULN	Withhold imatinib until bilirubin levels have returned to $< 1.5 \times$ IULN	In children, daily dosages can be reduced under the same circumstances from 260 to 200 mg/m^2/day or from 340 to 260 mg/m^2/day.
Liver transaminases $> 5 \times$ IULN	Withhold imatinib until transaminase levels have returned to $< 2.5 \times$ IULN	

➤*Duration of therapy:* Continue treatment as long as there is no evidence of progressive disease or unacceptable toxicity.

➤*Preparation for administration:* Imatinib is considered a cytotoxic agent. Follow safe handling procedures when preparing, administering, or dispensing imatinib.

Do not crush imatinib tablets. Direct contact of crushed tablets with the skin or mucous membranes should be avoided. If such contact occurs, wash thoroughly. Personnel should avoid exposure to crushed tablets.

For patients unable to swallow the film-coated tablets, the tablets may be dispersed in a glass of water or apple juice. The required number of tablets should be placed in the appropriate volume of beverage (approximately 50 mL for a 100 mg tablet and 200 mL for a 400 mg tablet) and stirred with a spoon. The suspension should be administered immediately after complete disintegration of the tablets.

➤*Administration:* Administer orally, with a meal and a large glass of water. Doses of 400 or 600 mg should be administered once daily; a dose of 800 mg should be administered as 400 mg twice a day. For daily dosing of 800 mg and higher, dosing should be accomplished using the 400 mg tablet to reduce exposure to iron. In children, imatinib treatment can be given as a once-daily dose or, alternatively, the daily dose may be split into 2 (once in the morning and once in the evening).

➤*Storage/Stability:* Store at 25°C (77°F); excursions are permitted between 15° to 30°C (59° to 86°F). Protect from moisture.

Actions

➤*Pharmacology:* Imatinib is a protein-tyrosine kinase inhibitor that inhibits the Bcr-Abl tyrosine kinase, the constitutive abnormal tyrosine kinase created by the Philadelphia chromosome abnormality in CML. It inhibits proliferation and induces apoptosis in Bcr-Abl–positive cell lines, as well as fresh leukemic cells from Ph+ CML. Imatinib inhibits colony formation in assays using ex vivo peripheral blood and bone marrow samples from patients with CML.

In vivo, it inhibits tumor growth of Bcr-Abl–transfected murine myeloid cells, as well as Bcr-Abl–positive leukemia lines derived from patients with CML in blast crisis.

Imatinib also is an inhibitor of the receptor tyrosine kinases for PDGF and stem-cell factor (SCF), c-kit, and inhibits PDGF- and SCF-mediated cellular events. In vitro, imatinib inhibits proliferation and induces apoptosis in GIST cells, which express an activating c-kit mutation.

➤*Pharmacokinetics:*

Absorption/Distribution – Imatinib is well absorbed after oral administration, with maximal drug concentration (C_{max}) achieved within 2 to 4 hours postdose. Mean absolute bioavailability is 98%. Mean imatinib AUC increases proportionally, with increasing doses ranging from 25 to 1,000 mg. There is no significant change in the pharmacokinetics of imatinib on repeated dosing, and accumulation is 1.5- to 2.5-fold at steady state when imatinib is dosed once daily. At clinically relevant concentrations of imatinib, binding to plasma proteins in in vitro experiments is approximately 95%, mostly to albumin and alpha-1 acid glycoprotein.

Metabolism – CYP3A4 is the major enzyme responsible for metabolism of imatinib. Other CYP enzymes, such as 1A2, 2D6, 2C9, and 2C19, play a minor role in its metabolism. The main circulating active metabolite in humans is the N-demethylated piperazine derivative, formed predominantly by CYP3A4. It shows in vitro potency similar to the parent imatinib. The plasma AUC for this metabolite is about 15% of the AUC for imatinib. The plasma-protein binding of the N-demethylated metabolite CGP74588 is similar to that of the parent compound. Human liver microsome studies demonstrated that imatinib is a potent competitive inhibitor of CYP2C9, 2D6, and 3A4/5, with Ki values of 27, 7.5, and 8 mcM, respectively.

Excretion – Elimination is predominately in the feces, mostly as metabolites. Based on the recovery of compound(s) after an oral ^{14}C-labeled dose of imatinib, approximately 81% of the dose was eliminated within 7 days in feces (68% of dose) and urine (13% of dose). Unchanged imatinib accounted for 25% of the dose (5% urine, 20% feces), the remainder being metabolites.

Typically, clearance of imatinib in a patient 50 years of age weighing 50 kg is expected to be 8 L/h, while for a patient 50 years of age weighing 100 kg, the clearance will increase to 14 L/h. However, the interpatient variability of 40% in clearance does not warrant initial dose adjustment based on body weight and/or age but indicates the need for close monitoring for treatment-related toxicity.

Following oral administration in healthy volunteers, the elimination half-lives of imatinib and its major active metabolite, the N-desmethyl derivative (CGP74588), were approximately 18 and 40 hours, respectively.

IMATINIB MESYLATE — ORAL

Special populations –

Renal function impairment: The mean exposure to imatinib (dose normalized AUC) in patients with mild and moderate renal impairment increased 1.5- to 2-fold compared with patients with healthy renal function. Two patients with severe renal impairment were dosed with 100 mg/day, and their exposures were similar to those seen in patients with healthy renal function receiving 400 mg/day. Dose reductions are necessary for patients with moderate and severe renal impairment.

Hepatic function impairment: Patients with severe hepatic impairment tend to have higher exposure to both imatinib and its metabolite than patients with healthy hepatic function. At steady state, the mean C_{max}/dose and AUC_{24}/dose for imatinib increased by about 63% and 45%, respectively, in patients with severe hepatic impairment compared with patients with healthy hepatic function. At steady state, the mean C_{max}/dose and AUC_{24}/dose for CGP74588 increased by about 56% and 55%, respectively, in patients with severe hepatic impairment compared with patients with healthy hepatic function.

Children: As in adult patients, imatinib was rapidly absorbed after oral administration in children, with a C_{max} of 2 to 4 hours. Apparent oral clearance was similar to adult values (11 L/h/m^2 in children vs 10 L/h/m^2 in adults), as was the half-life (14.8 hours in children vs 17.1 hours in adults).

Contraindications

None known.

Warnings/Precautions

➤*Fluid retention and edema:* Imatinib is often associated with edema and, occasionally, serious fluid retention. Weigh and monitor patients regularly for signs and symptoms of fluid retention. Carefully investigate an unexpected rapid weight gain and provide appropriate treatment. The probability of edema was increased with higher imatinib dose and age older than 65 years in the CML studies. Severe superficial edema was reported in 1.5% of newly diagnosed patients with CML taking imatinib and in 2% to 6% of other adults with CML taking imatinib. In addition, other severe fluid retention (eg, ascites, pericardial effusion, pleural effusion, pulmonary edema) reactions were reported in 1.3% of newly diagnosed patients with CML taking imatinib and in 2% to 6% of other adults with CML taking imatinib. Severe fluid retention was reported in 9% to 13.1% of patients taking imatinib for GIST.

➤*Hematologic toxicity:* Treatment with imatinib is often associated with anemia, neutropenia, or thrombocytopenia. Perform complete blood cell counts (CBCs) weekly for the first month, biweekly for the second month, and periodically thereafter as clinically indicated (eg, every 2 to 3 months). The occurrence of these cytopenias is dependent on the stage of disease and is more frequent in patients with accelerated phase CML or blast crisis than in patients with chronic-phase CML. In children with CML, the most frequent toxicities observed were grade 3 or 4 cytopenias, including neutropenia, thrombocytopenia, and anemia. These generally occur within the first several months of therapy.

➤*Cardiac effects:* Severe congestive heart failure and left ventricular dysfunction have occasionally been reported in patients taking imatinib. Most of the patients with reported cardiac reactions have had other comorbidities and risk factors, including advanced age and medical history of cardiac disease. In an international, randomized, phase 3 study in 1,106 patients with newly diagnosed Ph+ CML in chronic phase, severe cardiac failure and left ventricular dysfunction were observed in 0.7% of patients taking imatinib compared with 0.9% of patients taking interferon alpha + cytarabine. Carefully monitor patients with cardiac disease or risk factors for cardiac failure, and evaluate and treat any patient with signs or symptoms consistent with cardiac failure.

➤*Hepatotoxicity:* Hepatotoxicity, occasionally severe, may occur with imatinib. Monitor liver function (transaminases, bilirubin, and alkaline phosphatase) before initiation of treatment and monthly thereafter, or as clinically indicated. Manage laboratory abnormalities with interruption and/or dose reduction of the treatment with imatinib.

When imatinib is combined with chemotherapy, liver toxicity in the form of transaminase elevation and hyperbilirubinemia has been observed. Additionally, there have been reports of acute liver failure. Monitoring of hepatic function is recommended.

➤*Hemorrhage:* In the newly diagnosed CML trial, 1.8% of patients had grade 3/4 hemorrhage. In the phase 3 GIST studies, 211 (12.9%) patients reported grade 3/4 hemorrhage at any site. In the phase 2 GIST study, 7 (5%) patients had a total of 8 common toxicity criteria (CTC) grade 3/4 hemorrhages: GI (3 patients), intratumoral (3 patients), or both (1 patient). GI tumor sites may have been the source of GI hemorrhages.

➤*GI effects:* Imatinib is sometimes associated with GI irritation. Instruct patients to take imatinib with food and a large glass of water to minimize this problem. There have been rare reports, including fatalities, of GI perforation.

➤*Hypereosinophilic cardiac toxicity:* In patients with hypereosinophilic syndrome and cardiac involvement, cases of cardiogenic shock/left ventricular dysfunction have been associated with the initiation of imatinib therapy. The condition was reported to be reversible with the administration of systemic steroids, circulatory support measures, and temporary withholding of imatinib. Myelodysplastic/myeloproliferative diseases and systemic mastocytosis may be associated with high eosinophil levels. Therefore, consider performing an echocardiogram and determining serum troponin in patients with hypereosinophilic syndrome/chronic eosinophilic leukemia and in patients with myelodysplastic/myeloproliferative diseases or aggressive systemic mastocytosis associated with high eosinophil levels. If either is abnormal, consider the prophylactic use of systemic steroids (1 to 2 mg/kg) for 1 to 2 weeks concomitantly with imatinib at the initiation of therapy.

➤*Dermatologic toxicities:* Bullous dermatologic reactions, including erythema multiforme and Stevens-Johnson syndrome, have been reported with use of imatinib.

➤*Hypothyroidism:* Clinical cases of hypothyroidism have been reported in thyroidectomy patients undergoing levothyroxine replacement during treatment with imatinib. Closely monitor thyroid-stimulating hormone levels in such patients.

➤*Renal function impairment:* Use with caution in patients with severe renal impairment (see Administration and Dosage).

➤*Hepatic function impairment:* See Administration and Dosage.

➤*Pregnancy: Category D.* Advise women of childbearing potential to avoid becoming pregnant. Instruct sexually active women taking imatinib to use adequate contraception.

Imatinib can cause fetal harm when administered to a pregnant woman. Imatinib was teratogenic in rats when administered during organogenesis at doses of 100 mg/kg or more, approximately equal to the maximum clinical dosage of 800 mg/day (based on BSA). Teratogenic effects included exencephaly or encephalocele, absent/reduced frontal and absent parietal bones. Female rats administered doses of 45 mg/kg or more (approximately one-half the maximum human dosage of 800 mg/day, based on BSA) also experienced significant postimplantation loss, evidenced by either early fetal resorption or stillbirths, nonviable pups, and early pup mortality between postpartum days 0 and 4. At doses higher than 100 mg/kg, total fetal loss was noted in all animals. Fetal loss was not seen at doses of 30 mg/kg or less (one-third the maximum human dose of 800 mg).

There are no adequate and well-controlled studies in pregnant women. It is not known if imatinib or its active metabolite crosses the human placenta. The molecular weight (about 494 for the free base) for the parent compound drug and the long elimination half-lives for imatinib and its metabolite suggest that the drug will cross to the embryo and fetus. Advise women not to become pregnant when taking imatinib. If imatinib is used during pregnancy, or if the patient becomes pregnant while taking imatinib, apprise the patient of the potential hazard to the fetus.

➤*Lactation:* It is not known whether imatinib or its metabolites are excreted in human milk. The molecular weight (about 494 for the free base) for the parent compound and the long elimination half-lives of imatinib and its active metabolite suggest that they will be excreted into breast milk. Because many drugs are excreted in human milk and because of the potential for serious adverse reactions in breast-feeding infants, decide whether to discontinue breast-feeding or the drug, taking into account the importance of the drug to the mother.

In lactating female rats administered 100 mg/kg, a dose approximately equal to the maximum clinical dosage of 800 mg/day based on BSA, imatinib and its metabolites were extensively excreted in milk. Concentration in milk was approximately 3-fold higher than in plasma. It is estimated that approximately 1.5% of a maternal dose is excreted into milk, which is equivalent to a dose to the infant of 30% the maternal dose per unit body weight.

➤*Children:* Imatinib safety and efficacy have been demonstrated in children with newly diagnosed Ph+ chronic-phase CML and children with Ph+ chronic-phase CML, with recurrence after stem-cell transplantation or resistance to interferon alpha therapy. There are no data in children younger than 2 years of age. Follow-up in children with newly diagnosed Ph+ chronic-phase CML is limited.

➤*Elderly:* The probability of edema was increased with age older than 65 years in the CML and GIST studies.

➤*Monitoring:* Weigh and monitor patients regularly for signs and symptoms of fluid retention.

Carefully monitor patients with cardiac disease or risk factors for cardiac failure, and evaluate and treat any patient with signs or symptoms consistent with cardiac failure. Perform an echocardiogram and serum troponin levels in patients with hypereosinophilic syndrome/chronic eosinophilic leukemia and in patients with myelodysplastic/myeloproliferative diseases or aggressive systemic mastocytosis associated with high eosinophil levels.

Perform CBCs weekly for the first month, biweekly for the second month, and periodically thereafter as clinically indicated (eg, every 2 to 3 months).

Monitor liver function (transaminases, bilirubin, and alkaline phosphatase) before initiation of treatment and monthly or as clinically indicated. Closely monitor patients with severe hepatic impairment.

Monitor thyroid-stimulating hormone in thyroidectomy patients undergoing levothyroxine replacement.

Drug Interactions

Imatinib Drug Interactions

Precipitant drug	Object drug[a]		Description
Acetaminophen	Imatinib	↑	Increased risk of hepatotoxicity may occur. There has been 1 report of fatal hepatic failure with coadministration.
Imatinib	Acetaminophen		

IMATINIB MESYLATE — ORAL

Imatinib Drug Interactions			
Precipitant drug	Object drug[a]		Description
Inducers of CYP3A4 (eg, carbamazepine, dexamethasone, phenobarbital, phenytoin, rifampin, St. John's wort)	Imatinib	⬇	Substances that induce CYP3A4 activity may increase metabolism and decrease imatinib plasma concentrations. When rifampin or other CYP3A4 inducers are indicated with imatinib, consider other therapeutic agents with less enzyme induction potential. Avoid coadministration if possible. If coadministration cannot be avoided, increase dosage of imatinib by at least 50% and carefully monitor for clinical response.
Inhibitors of CYP3A4 (eg, atazanavir, clarithromycin, erythromycin, indinavir, itraconazole, ketoconazole, nefazodone, nelfinavir, ritonavir, saquinavir, telithromycin, voriconazole)	Imatinib	⬆	Substances that inhibit the CYP3A4 isoenzyme activity may decrease metabolism and increase imatinib concentrations. Coadministration with a single dose of ketoconazole resulted in an increase in the mean AUC and C_{max} of 26% and 40%, respectively, of imatinib.
Imatinib	CYP2D6 substrates	⬆	Systemic exposure to substrates of CYP2D6 is expected to increase with coadministration. Use with caution.
Imatinib	CYP3A4 substrates (eg, alfentanil, cyclosporine, dihydropyridine calcium channel blockers, ergot alkaloids, fentanyl, oral contraceptives [ie, ethinyl estradiol], pimozide, quinidine, simvastatin, sirolimus, tacrolimus, triazolobenzodiazepines	⬆	Imatinib will increase plasma concentrations of other CYP3A4 metabolized drugs. Coadministration of simvastatin and imatinib resulted in an increase in the mean C_{max} and AUC of simvastatin by 2- and 3.5-fold, respectively. Particular caution is recommended when administering imatinib with CYP3A4 substrates that have a narrow therapeutic window.
Imatinib	Thyroid hormones (eg, levothyroxine)	⬇	Imatinib may increase levothyroxine hepatic clearance; thyroid-stimulating hormone levels may be increased, and symptoms of hypothyroidism may be evident. Monitor thyroid function during coadministration.
Imatinib	Warfarin	⬆	Because warfarin is metabolized by CYP2C9 and CYP3A4, patients who require anticoagulation should receive low molecular weight or standard heparin.

[a] ⬆ = object drug increased; ⬇ = object drug decreased.

➤*Drug/Food interactions:* Avoid grapefruit juice; grapefruit juice may increase plasma concentrations of imatinib.

Adverse Reactions

Imatinib is considered to have moderate emetogenic potential (30% to 60% incidence of emesis).

➤*Acute lymphoblastic leukemia:* The adverse reactions were similar for Ph+ ALL and for CML. The most frequently reported drug-related adverse reactions reported in the Ph+ ALL studies were diarrhea, mild nausea, muscle cramps, myalgia, rash, and vomiting, which were easily manageable. Superficial edemas were a common finding in all studies and were described primarily as periorbital or lower limb edemas. However, these edemas were rarely severe and may be managed with diuretics, other supportive measures, or in some patients by reducing the dose of imatinib.

➤*Aggressive systemic mastocytosis:* All patients with aggressive systemic mastocytosis experienced at least 1 adverse reaction at some time. The most frequently reported adverse reactions were anemia, ascites, diarrhea, dyspnea, fatigue, lower respiratory tract infection, muscle cramps, nausea, peripheral edema, pruritus, and rash. None of the 5 patients in the phase 2 study with aggressive systemic mastocytosis discontinued imatinib because of drug-related adverse reactions or abnormal laboratory values.

➤*Chronic myeloid leukemia:*

Discontinuation – The majority of imatinib-treated patients experienced adverse reactions at some time. Most reactions were of mild to moderate grade, but the drug was discontinued for drug-related adverse reactions in 2.4% of newly diagnosed patients, 4% of patients in chronic phase after failure of interferon-alpha therapy, 4% in accelerated phase, and 5% in blast crisis.

Most frequent adverse reactions – The most frequently reported drug-related adverse reactions were diarrhea, edema, muscle cramps, musculoskeletal pain, nausea and vomiting, and rash. Edema was most frequently periorbital or in lower limbs and was managed with diuretics, other supportive measures, or by reducing the dose of imatinib. The frequency of severe superficial edema was 1.5% to 6%.

A variety of adverse reactions represent local or general fluid retention, including ascites, pleural effusion, pulmonary edema, and rapid weight gain with or without superficial edema. These reactions appear to be dose related, were more common in the blast crisis and accelerated phase studies (where the dosage was 600 mg/day), and are more common in elderly patients. These reactions were usually managed by interrupting imatinib treatment and with diuretics or other appropriate supportive care measures. However, a few of these reactions may be serious or life-threatening, and 1 patient with blast crisis died with pleural effusion, congestive heart failure, and renal failure.

Imatinib Adverse Reactions in Patients With Newly Diagnosed Chronic Myeloid Leukemia (≥ 10%)[a]				
	All grades		CTC grades 3/4	
Adverse reactions	Imatinib (n = 551)	Interferon alpha plus cytarabine (n = 533)	Imatinib (n = 551)	Interferon alpha plus cytarabine (n = 533)
CNS				
CNS hemorrhage	0.2%	0.4%	0%	0.4%
Depression	14.9%	35.8%	0.5%	13.1%
Dizziness	19.4%	24.4%	0.9%	3.8%
Fatigue	38.8%	67%	1.8%	25.1%
Headache	37%	43.3%	0.5%	3.8%
Insomnia	14.7%	18.6%	0%	2.3%
GI				
Abdominal pain	36.5%	25.9%	4.2%	3.9%
Constipation	11.4%	14.4%	0.7%	0.2%
Diarrhea	45.4%	43.3%	3.3%	3.2%
Dyspepsia	18.9%	8.3%	0%	0.8%
GI hemorrhage	1.6%	1.1%	0.5%	0.2%
Nausea	49.5%	61.5%	1.3%	5.1%
Vomiting	22.5%	27.8%	2%	3.4%
Musculoskeletal				
Bone pain	11.3%	15.6%	1.6%	3.4%
Joint pain	31.4%	38.1%	2.5%	7.7%
Muscle cramps	49.2%	11.8%	2.2%	0.2%
Musculoskeletal pain	47%	44.8%	5.4%	8.6%
Myalgia	24.1%	38.8%	1.5%	8.3%
Respiratory				
Cough	20%	23.1%	0.2%	0.6%
Nasopharyngitis	30.5%	8.8%	0%	0.4%
Pharyngolaryngeal pain	18.1%	11.4%	0.2%	0%
Sinusitis	11.4%	6%	0.2%	0.2%
Upper respiratory tract infection	21.2%	8.4%	0.2%	0.4%
Miscellaneous				
Fluid retention	61.7%	11.1%	2.5%	0.9%
Hemorrhage	28.9%	21.2%	1.8%	1.7%
Influenza	13.8%	6.2%	0.2%	0.2%
Other fluid retention reactions[b]	6.9%	1.9%	1.3%	0.6%
Pyrexia	17.8%	42.6%	0.9%	3%
Rash and related items	40.1%	26.1%	2.9%	2.4%
Superficial edema	59.9%	9.6%	1.5%	0.4%
Weight increased	15.6%	2.6%	2%	0.4%

[a] All adverse reactions occurring in ≥ 10% of patients are listed regardless of suspected relationship to treatment.

[b] Other fluid retention reactions included anasarca, ascites, edema aggravated, fluid retention not otherwise specified, pericardial effusion, pleural effusion, and pulmonary edema.

IMATINIB MESYLATE — ORAL

Imatinib Adverse Reactions in Patients With Other Chronic Myeloid Leukemia (≥ 10%)[a]

Adverse reactions	Myeloid blast crisis (n = 260)		Accelerated phase (n = 235)		Chronic phase, interferon alpha failure (n = 532)	
	All grades	Grade 3/4	All grades	Grade 3/4	All grades	Grade 3/4
CNS						
Anxiety	8%	0.8%	12%	0%	8%	0.4%
Asthenia	18%	5%	21%	5%	15%	0.2%
CNS hemorrhage	9%	7%	3%	3%	2%	1%
Dizziness	12%	0.4%	13%	0%	16%	0.2%
Fatigue	30%	4%	46%	4%	48%	1%
Headache	27%	5%	32%	2%	36%	0.6%
Insomnia	10%	0%	14%	0%	14%	0.2%
Dermatologic						
Night sweats	13%	0.8%	17%	1%	14%	0.2%
Pruritus	8%	1%	14%	0.9%	14%	0.8%
Skin rash	36%	5%	47%	5%	47%	3%
GI						
Abdominal pain	30%	6%	33%	4%	32%	1%
Anorexia	14%	2%	17%	2%	7%	0%
Constipation	16%	2%	16%	0.9%	9%	0.4%
Diarrhea	43%	4%	57%	5%	48%	3%
Dyspepsia	12%	0%	22%	0%	27%	0%
GI hemorrhage	8%	4%	6%	5%	2%	0.4%
Nausea	71%	5%	73%	5%	63%	3%
Vomiting	54%	4%	58%	3%	36%	2%
Weight increased	5%	1%	17%	5%	32%	7%
Musculoskeletal						
Arthralgia	25%	5%	34%	6%	40%	1%
Muscle cramps	28%	1%	47%	0.4%	62%	2%
Musculoskeletal pain	42%	9%	49%	9%	38%	2%
Myalgia	9%	0%	24%	2%	27%	0.2%
Rigors	10%	0%	12%	0.4%	10%	0%
Respiratory						
Cough	14%	0.8%	27%	0.9%	20%	0%
Dyspnea	15%	4%	21%	7%	12%	0.9%
Nasopharyngitis	10%	0%	17%	0%	22%	0.2%
Pharyngitis	10%	0%	12%	0%	15%	0%
Pneumonia	13%	7%	10%	7%	4%	1%
Sinusitis	4%	0.4%	11%	0.4%	9%	0.4%
Upper respiratory tract infection	3%	0%	12%	0.4%	19%	0%
Miscellaneous						
Chest pain	7%	2%	10%	0.4%	11%	0.8%
Fluid retention	72%	11%	76%	6%	69%	4%
Hemorrhage	53%	19%	49%	11%	30%	2%
Hypokalemia	13%	4%	9%	2%	6%	0.8%
Influenza	0.8%	0.4%	6%	0%	11%	0.2%
Liver toxicity	10%	5%	12%	6%	6%	3%
Other fluid retention reactions[b]	22%	6%	15%	4%	7%	2%
Pyrexia	41%	7%	41%	8%	21%	2%
Superficial edema	66%	6%	74%	3%	67%	2%

[a] All adverse reactions occurring in ≥ 10% are listed regardless of suspected relationship to treatment.
[b] Other fluid retention reactions include aggravated edema, anasarca, ascites, fluid retention not otherwise specified, pericardial effusion, pleural effusion, and pulmonary edema.

Hematologic – Cytopenias, particularly neutropenia and thrombocytopenia, were a consistent finding in all studies, with a higher frequency at doses of 750 mg or more (phase 1 study). The occurrence of cytopenias in patients with CML was also dependent on the stage of the disease.

In patients with newly diagnosed CML, cytopenias were less frequent than in the other patients with CML. The frequency of grade 3 or 4 neutropenia and thrombocytopenia was between 2- and 3-fold higher in blast crisis and accelerated phase compared with chronic phase. The median duration of the neutropenic and thrombocytopenic episodes varied from 2 to 3 weeks and from 2 to 4 weeks, respectively. These reactions can usually be managed with either a reduction of the dose or an interruption of treatment with imatinib, but, in rare cases, require permanent discontinuation of treatment.

Lab test abnormalities –

Imatinib Laboratory Abnormalities in Patients With Newly Diagnosed Chronic Myeloid Leukemia

	Imatinib (n = 551)		Interferon alpha plus cytarabine (n = 533)	
CTC grades	Grade 3	Grade 4	Grade 3	Grade 4
Biochemistry parameters				
Elevated alkaline phosphatase	0.2%	0%	0.8%	0%
Elevated ALT/AST	4.7%	0.5%	7.1%	0.4%
Elevated bilirubin	0.9%	0.2%	0.2%	0%
Elevated creatinine	0%	0%	0.4%	0%
Hematology parameters				
Anemia	3.3%	1.1%	4.1%	0.2%
Neutropenia[a]	13.1%	3.6%	20.8%	4.5%
Thrombocytopenia[a]	8.5%	0.4%	15.9%	0.6%

[a] $P < 0.001$ (difference in grade 3 plus 4 abnormalities between the 2 treatment groups).

Imatinib Lab Abnormalities in Patients With Other Chronic Myeloid Leukemia

	Myeloid blast crisis (n = 260); 600 mg (n = 223), 400 mg (n = 37)		Accelerated phase (n = 235); 600 mg (n = 158), 400 mg (n = 77)		Chronic phase, interferon alpha failure 400 mg (n = 532)	
CTC grades[a]	Grade 3	Grade 4	Grade 3	Grade 4	Grade 3	Grade 4
Biochemistry parameters						
Elevated alkaline phosphatase	4.6%	0%	5.5%	0.4%	0.2%	0%
Elevated ALT	2.3%	0.4%	4.3%	0%	2.1%	0%
Elevated AST	1.9%	0%	3%	0%	2.3%	0%
Elevated bilirubin	3.8%	0%	2.1%	0%	0.6%	0%
Elevated creatinine	1.5%	0%	1.3%	0%	0.2%	0%
Hematology parameters						
Anemia	42%	11%	34%	7%	6%	1%
Neutropenia	16%	48%	23%	36%	27%	9%
Thrombocytopenia	30%	33%	31%	13%	21%	< 1%

[a] CTC grades are as follows: neutropenia (grade 3, ≥ 0.5 to 1 × 10^9/L; grade 4, < 0.5 × 10^9/L), thrombocytopenia (grade 3, ≥ 10 to 50 × 10^9/L; grade 4, less than 10 × 10^9/L), anemia (hemoglobin, ≥ 65 to 80 g/L; grade, 4 < 65 g/L), elevated creatinine (grade 3, > 3 to 6 × ULN; grade 4, > 6 × ULN), elevated bilirubin (grade 3, > 3 to 10 × ULN; grade 4, > 10 × ULN), elevated alkaline phosphatase (grade 3, > 5 to 20 × ULN; grade 4,> 20 × ULN), elevated AST or ALT (grade 3,> 5 to 20 × ULN; grade 4, > 20 × ULN).

Hepatic – Severe elevation of transaminases or bilirubin occurred in approximately 5% of patients with CML and were usually managed with dose reduction or interruption (the median duration of these episodes was approximately 1 week). Treatment was discontinued permanently because of liver laboratory abnormalities in less than 1% of patients with CML. However, 1 patient, who was taking acetaminophen regularly for fever, died of acute liver failure. In the phase 2 GIST trial, grade 3 or 4 ALT elevations were observed in 6.8% of patients, and grade 3 or 4 AST elevations were observed in 4.8% of patients. Bilirubin elevation was observed in 2.7% of patients.

Children – The overall safety profile of children treated with imatinib in the 93 children studied was similar to that found in studies with adult patients, except that musculoskeletal pain was less frequent (20.5%), and peripheral edema was not reported. Nausea and vomiting were the most commonly reported individual adverse reactions with an incidence similar to that seen in adult patients. Although most patients experienced adverse reactions at some time during the study, the incidence of grade 3 or 4 adverse reactions was low.

Elderly/Gender/Race – In patients 65 years of age and older, with the exception of edema, where it was more frequent, there was no evidence of an increase in the incidence or severity of adverse reactions. In women, there was an increase in the frequency of neutropenia, as well as fatigue, grade 1/2 superficial edema, headache, nausea, rash, rigors, and vomiting. No differences were seen related to race, but the subsets were too small for proper evaluation.

IMATINIB MESYLATE — ORAL

➤*Dermatofibrosarcoma protuberans:*

Imatinib Adverse Reactions in Patients With Dermatofibrosarcoma Protuberans (≥ 10%)

Adverse reactions	(N = 12)
GI	
Anorexia	16.7%
Diarrhea	25%
Nausea	41.7%
Vomiting	25%
Respiratory	
Dyspnea exertional	16.7%
Rhinitis	16.7%
Special senses	
Eye edema	33.3%
Lacrimation increased	25%
Periorbital edema	33.3%
Miscellaneous	
Anemia	25%
Edema peripheral	33.3%
Face edema	16.7%
Fatigue	41.7%
Pyrexia	16.7%
Rash	25%

Imatinib Laboratory Abnormalities in Patients With Dermatofibrosarcoma Protuberans

	(N = 12)	
CTC grades[a]	Grade 3	Grade 4
Biochemistry parameters		
Elevated creatinine	0%	8%
Hematology parameters		
Anemia	17%	0%
Neutropenia	0%	8%
Thrombocytopenia	17%	0%

[a] CTC grades: neutropenia (grade 3, ≥ 0.5 to 1 × 10^9/L; grade 4, ^{9}/L), thrombocytopenia (grade 3, ≥ 10 to 50 × 10^9/L; grade 4 < 10 × 10^9/L), anemia (grade 3, ≥ 65 to 80 g/L; grade 4, < 65 g/L), elevated creatinine (grade 3, > 3 to 6 × ULN; grade 4, > 6 × ULN).

➤*GI stromal tumors:*

Unresectable and/or malignant metastatic GI stromal tumors – In the phase 3 trials, the majority of imatinib-treated patients experienced adverse reactions at some time. The most frequently reported adverse reactions were abdominal pain, anemia, anorexia, diarrhea, edema, fatigue, myalgia, nausea, rash, and vomiting. The drug was discontinued for adverse reactions in 89 (5.4%) patients. Superficial edema, most frequently periorbital or lower extremity edema, was managed with diuretics, other supportive measures, or by reducing the dose of imatinib. Severe (CTC grade 3/4) superficial edema was observed in 182 (11.1%) patients.

Imatinib Adverse Reactions in Patients With Unresectable and/or Malignant Metastatic GI Stromal Tumor (≥ 10%)

	400 mg (n = 818)		800 mg (n = 822)	
Adverse reactions	All grades	Grades 3/4/5	All grades	Grades 3/4/5
CNS				
Dizziness/Light-headedness	11%	4.8%	10%	2.8%
Fatigue/Lethargy, malaise, asthenia	69.3%	11.7%	74.9%	12.2%
Headache	22%	5.7%	19.7%	3.6%
Other neurological toxicity	15%	6.4%	15.2%	4.9%
Dermatologic				
Alopecia	11.9%	4.3%	14.8%	3.2%
Other dermatology/skin toxicity	17.6%	5.9%	20.1%	5.7%
Pruritus	15.4%	5.4%	18.9%	4.3%
Rash/Desquamation	38.1%	7.6%	49.8%	8.9%
Sweating	12.7%	4.6%	8.5%	2.8%
GI				
Abdominal pain/cramping	57.2%	13.8%	55.2%	11.8%
Anorexia	31.1%	6.6%	35.8%	4.7%
Constipation	14.8%	5.1%	14.4%	4.1%
Diarrhea	56.2%	8.1%	58.2%	8.6%
Dyspepsia/Heartburn	11.5%	0.6%	10.9%	0.5%
Flatulence	10%	0.2%	10.1%	0.1%
Nausea	58.1%	9%	64.5%	7.8%
Other GI toxicity	25.2%	8.1%	28.1%	6.6%
Vomiting	37.4%	9.2%	40.6%	7.5%
Weight gain	12%	1%	10.6%	0.6%
GU				
Creatinine increase	10.8%	0.4%	10.1%	0.6%
Other renal/GU toxicity	14.2%	6.5%	13.6%	5.2%
Hematologic/Lymphatic				
Anemia	32%	4.9%	34.8%	6.4%
Leukopenia	17%	0.7%	19.6%	1.6%
Lymphopenia	6%	0.7%	10.1%	1.9%
Neutropenia/Granulocytopenia	11.5%	3.1%	16.1%	4.1%
Musculoskeletal				
Arthralgia	13.6%	4.8%	12.3%	3%
Myalgia	32.2%	5.6%	30.2%	3.8%
Respiratory				
Cough	16.1%	4.5%	14.5%	3.2%
Dyspnea	13.6%	6.8%	14.2%	5.6%
Miscellaneous				
Edema	76.7%	9%	86.1%	13.1%
Fever in absence of neutropenia (ANC < 1 × 10^9/L)	13.2%	4.9%	12.9%	3.4%
Infection (without neutropenia)	15.5%	6.6%	16.5%	5.6%
Other constitutional symptoms	16.7%	6.4%	15.2%	4.4%
Other hemorrhage	12.3%	6.7%	13.3%	6.1%
Other pain (excluding tumor-related pain)	20.4%	5.9%	20.8%	5%
Rigors/Chills	11%	4.6%	10.2%	3%
Stomatitis/Pharyngitis	9.2%	5.4%	10%	4.3%

Imatinib Laboratory Abnormalities in Unresectable and/or Malignant Metastatic GI Stromal Tumor Patients

	400 mg (n = 73)		600 mg (n = 74)	
CTC grades[a]	Grade 3	Grade 4	Grade 3	Grade 4
Biochemistry parameters				
Elevated alkaline phosphatase	0%	0%	3%	0%
Elevated ALT	6%	0%	7%	1%
Elevated AST	4%	0%	3%	3%
Elevated bilirubin	1%	0%	1%	3%
Elevated creatinine	0%	0%	3%	0%
Reduced albumin	3%	0%	4%	0%
Hematology parameters				
Anemia	3%	0%	8%	1%
Neutropenia	7%	3%	8%	3%
Thrombocytopenia	0%	0%	1%	0%

[a] CTC grades are as follows: neutropenia (grade 3, ≥ 0.5 to 1 × 10^9/L; grade 4, < 0.5 × 10^9/L); thrombocytopenia (grade 3, ≥ 10 to 50 × 10^9/L; grade 4, < 10 × 10^9/L); anemia (grade 3, ≥ 65 to 80 g/L; grade 4, < 65 g/L); elevated creatinine (grade 3, > 3 to 6 × ULN; grade 4, > 6 × ULN); elevated bilirubin (grade 3, > 3 to 10 × ULN; grade 4, > 10 × ULN); elevated alkaline phosphatase, ALT, or AST (grade 3, > 5 to 20 × ULN; grade 4, > 20 × ULN); albumin (grade 3 < 20 g/L).

Adjuvant treatment of GI stromal tumors – The majority of both imatinib- and placebo-treated patients experienced at least 1 adverse reaction at some time. The most frequently reported adverse reactions were similar to those reported in other clinical studies in other patient populations, and include diarrhea, fatigue, nausea, edema, decreased hemoglobin, rash, vomiting, and abdominal pain. No new adverse reactions were reported in the adjuvant GIST treatment setting that had not been previously reported in other patient populations, including patients with unresectable and/or malignant metastatic GIST. Drug was discontinued for adverse reactions in 57 (17%) patients and 11 (3%) patients of the imatinib-

IMATINIB MESYLATE — ORAL

and placebo-treated patients, respectively. Edema, GI disturbances (nausea, vomiting, abdominal distention, and diarrhea), fatigue, low hemoglobin, and rash were the most frequently reported adverse reactions at the time of discontinuation.

Imatinib Adverse Reactions in the Adjuvant Treatment of GI Stromal Tumors (≥ 5%)[a]

	All CTC grades		CTC grades ≥ 3	
Adverse reactions	Imatinib (n = 337)	Placebo (n = 345)	Imatinib (n = 337)	Placebo (n = 345)
CNS				
Depression	6.8%	6.4%	0.9%	0.6%
Dizziness	12.5%	10.7%	0%	0.3%
Fatigue	57%	40.9%	2.1%	1.2%
Headache	19.3%	20.3%	0.6%	0%
Insomnia	9.8%	7.2%	0.9%	0%
Neuropathy peripheral	5.9%	6.4%	0%	0%
Dermatologic				
Alopecia	9.5%	6.7%	0%	0%
Dry skin	6.5%	5.2%	0%	0%
Pruritus	11%	7.8%	0.9%	0%
Rash	8.9%	5.2%	0.9%	0%
Rash (exfoliative)	26.1%	12.8%	2.7%	0%
GI				
Abdominal distension	7.4%	6.4%	0.3%	0.3%
Abdominal pain	21.1%	22.3%	3%	1.4%
Abdominal pain, upper	6.2%	6.4%	0.3%	0%
Anorexia	16.9%	8.7%	0.3%	0%
Constipation	12.8%	17.7%	0%	0.3%
Diarrhea	59.3%	29.3%	3%	1.4%
Dysgeusia	6.5%	2.9%	0%	0%
Dyspepsia	17.2%	13%	0.9%	0%
Flatulence	8.9%	9.6%	0%	0%
Nausea	53.1%	27.8%	2.4%	1.2%
Stomatitis	5%	1.7%	0.6%	0%
Vomiting	25.5%	13.9%	2.4%	0.6%
Hematologic/Lymphatic				
Hemoglobin decreased	46.9%	27%	0.6%	0%
Leukopenia	5%	2.6%	0.3%	0%
Neutrophil count decreased	16%	6.1%	3.3%	0.9%
Platelet count decreased	5%	3.5%	0%	0%
WBC count decreased	14.5%	4.3%	0.6%	0.3%
Hepatic				
Blood alkaline phosphatase increased	6.5%	7.5%	0%	0%
Liver enzymes (ALT) increased	16.6%	13%	2.7%	0%
Liver enzymes (AST) increased	12.2%	7.5%	2.1%	0%
Metabolic				
Hyperglycemia	9.8%	11.3%	0.6%	1.7%
Hypocalcemia	5.6%	1.7%	0.3%	0%
Hypokalemia	7.1%	2%	0.9%	0.6%
Weight decreased	10.1%	5.2%	0%	0%
Weight increased	16.9%	11.6%	0.3%	0%
Musculoskeletal				
Arthralgia	15.1%	14.5%	0%	0.3%
Back pain	7.4%	8.1%	0.6%	0%
Muscle spasms	16.3%	3.3%	0%	0%
Myalgia	12.2%	11.6%	0%	0.3%
Respiratory				
Cough	11%	11.3%	0%	0%
Upper respiratory tract infection	5%	3.5%	0%	0%
Special senses				
Lacrimation increased	9.8%	3.8%	0%	0%
Periorbital edema	47.2%	14.5%	1.2%	0%
Vision blurred	5%	2.3%	0%	0%

Imatinib Adverse Reactions in the Adjuvant Treatment of GI Stromal Tumors (≥ 5%)[a]

	All CTC grades		CTC grades ≥ 3	
Adverse reactions	Imatinib (n = 337)	Placebo (n = 345)	Imatinib (n = 337)	Placebo (n = 345)
Miscellaneous				
Peripheral edema	26.7%	14.8%	0.3%	0%
Blood creatinine increased	11.6%	5.8%	0%	0.3%
Pain in extremity	7.4%	7.2%	0.3%	0%
Facial edema	6.8%	1.2%	0.3%	0%

[a] All adverse reactions occurring in ≥ 5% of patients are listed regardless of suspected relationship to treatment. A patient with multiple occurrences of an adverse reaction is counted only once in the adverse reaction category.

➤*Hypereosinophilic syndrome/chronic eosinophilic leukemia:* The safety profile in the hypereosinophilic syndrome/chronic eosinophilic leukemia patient population does not appear to be different from the known safety profile of imatinib observed in other hematologic malignancy populations, such as Ph+CML. All patients experienced at least 1 adverse reaction, the most common being GI, cutaneous, and musculoskeletal disorders. Hematologic abnormalities were also frequent, with instances of CTC grade 3 leukopenia, neutropenia, lymphopenia, and anemia.

➤*Myelodysplastic/Myeloproliferative diseases:*

Imatinib Adverse Reactions in Patients With Myelodysplastic/ Myeloproliferative Diseases (≥ 10%)

Adverse reactions	(N = 7)
GI	
Diarrhea	42.9%
Nausea	57.1%
Musculoskeletal	
Arthralgia	28.6%
Muscle cramp	42.9%
Miscellaneous	
Anemia	28.6%
Fatigue	28.6%
Periorbital edema	28.6%

➤*Other adverse reactions:*

Cardiovascular – Flushing, hemorrhage (1% to 10%); congestive heart failure, hematoma, hypertension, hypotension, palpitations, peripheral coldness, pulmonary edema, Raynaud phenomenon, tachycardia (0.1% to 1%); angina pectoris, arrhythmia, atrial fibrillation, cardiac arrest, myocardial infarction, pericardial effusion (0.1% to 0.01%).

CNS – Hypesthesia, paresthesia (1% to 10%); libido decreased, memory impairment, migraine, peripheral neuropathy, restless legs syndrome, sciatica, somnolence, syncope, tremor (0.1% to 1%); confusional state, convulsions, increased intracranial pressure (including some fatalities), optic neuritis (0.1% to 0.01%).

Dermatologic – Alopecia, dry skin, erythema, face edema, photosensitivity reaction (1% to 10%); bullous eruption, contusion, ecchymosis, exfoliative dermatitis, folliculitis, hypotrichosis, increased tendency to bruise, nail disorder, onychoclasis, petechiae, psoriasis, purpura, rash pustular, skin hyperpigmentation, skin hypopigmentation, sweating increased, urticaria (0.1% to 1%); acute febrile neutrophilic dermatosis (Sweet syndrome), acute generalized exanthematous pustulosis, angioneurotic edema, erythema multiforme, leucocytoclastic vasculitis, nail discoloration, Stevens-Johnson syndrome, vesicular rash (0.1% to 0.01%).

GI – Abdominal distention, dry mouth, gastritis, gastroesophageal reflux (1% to 10%); ascites, cheilitis, dysphagia, eructation, esophagitis, gastric ulcer, gastroenteritis, hematemesis, melena, mouth ulceration, pancreatitis, stomatitis (0.1% to 1%); colitis, ileus, inflammatory bowel disease (0.1% to 0.01%).

GU – Breast enlargement, erectile dysfunction, gynecomastia, hematuria, menorrhagia, menstruation irregular, nipple pain, renal failure acute, renal pain, scrotal edema, sexual dysfunction, urinary frequency increased, urinary tract infection (0.1% to 1%).

Hematologic – Febrile neutropenia, pancytopenia (1% to 10%); bone marrow depression, eosinophilia, lymphadenopathy, lymphopenia, thrombocythemia (0.1% to 1%); aplastic anemia, hemolytic anemia (0.1% to 0.01%).

Hepatic – Hepatitis, jaundice (0.1% to 1%); hepatic failure, hepatic necrosis (including some fatalities) (0.1% to 0.01%).

Lab test abnormalities – Blood creatine phosphokinase increased, blood lactate dehydrogenase increased (0.1% to 1%); blood amylase increased (0.1% to 0.01%).

Metabolic/Nutritional – Weight decreased (1% to 10%); decreased appetite, dehydration, gout, hypercalcemia, hyperglycemia, hyperuricemia, hyponatremia, hypophosphatemia, increased appetite (0.1% to 1%); hyperkalemia, hypomagnesemia (0.1% to 0.01%).

Musculoskeletal – Joint swelling (1% to 10%); joint and muscle stiffness (0.1% to 1%); arthritis, muscular weakness (0.1% to 0.01%).

IMATINIB MESYLATE — ORAL

Respiratory – Epistaxis (1% to 10%); pleural effusion (0.1% to 1%); interstitial pneumonitis, pleuritic pain, pulmonary fibrosis, pulmonary hemorrhage, pulmonary hypertension (0.1% to 0.01%).

Special senses – Conjunctival hemorrhage, conjunctivitis, dry eye, eyelid edema, vision blurred (1% to 10%); blepharitis, eye irritation, eye pain, hearing loss, macular edema, orbital edema, retinal hemorrhage, scleral hemorrhage, tinnitus, vertigo (0.1% to 1%); cataract, glaucoma, papilledema (including some fatalities) (0.1% to 0.01%).

Miscellaneous – Anasarca, chills, weakness (1% to 10%); cellulitis, herpes simplex, herpes zoster, malaise, sepsis (0.1% to 1%); angioedema, fungal infection (0.1% to 0.01%).

➤*Postmarketing:*

Cardiovascular – Anaphylactic shock, cardiac tamponade (including some fatalities), pericarditis, thrombosis/embolism.

Dermatologic – Lichen planus, lichenoid keratosis, toxic epidermal necrolysis.

In some cases of bullous dermatologic reactions, including erythema multiforme and Stevens-Johnson syndrome, reported during postmarketing surveillance, a recurrent dermatologic reaction was observed upon rechallenge. Several foreign postmarketing reports have described cases in which patients tolerated the reintroduction of imatinib therapy after resolution or improvement of the bullous reaction. In these instances, imatinib was resumed at a dose lower than that at which the reaction occurred, and some patients also received concomitant treatment with corticosteroids or antihistamines.

GI – Diverticulitis, GI perforation (including some fatalities), ileus/intestinal obstruction, tumor hemorrhage/tumor necrosis.

Respiratory – Acute respiratory failure (including some fatalities), interstitial lung disease.

Miscellaneous – Avascular necrosis/hip osteonecrosis, cerebral edema (including some fatalities), vitreous hemorrhage.

Overdosage

➤*Symptoms:* A patient with myeloid blast crisis experienced grade 1 elevations of serum creatinine, grade 2 ascites and elevated liver transaminase levels, and grade 3 elevations of bilirubin after inadvertently taking imatinib 1,200 mg daily for 6 days. Therapy was temporarily interrupted and complete reversal of all abnormalities occurred within 1 week. Treatment was resumed at a dose of imatinib 400 mg daily without recurrence of adverse reactions. Another patient developed severe muscle cramps after taking imatinib 1,600 mg daily for 6 days. Complete resolution of muscle cramps occurred following interruption of therapy and treatment was subsequently resumed. Another patient who was prescribed imatinib 400 mg daily took 800 mg on day 1 and 1,200 mg on day 2. Therapy was interrupted, no adverse reactions occurred, and the patient resumed therapy.

➤*Treatment:* In the event of overdosage, observe the patient and give appropriate supportive treatment.

Patient Information

Instruct patients to take imatinib exactly as prescribed and not to change their dose or stop taking imatinib unless they are told to do so by their health care provider. If patients miss a dose, instruct them to take their dose as soon as possible, unless it is almost time for their next dose, in which case instruct them not to take the missed dose. Instruct patients not to take a double dose to make up for any missed doses. Advise patients to take imatinib with a meal and a large glass of water.

Advise patients to inform their health care provider if they are or think they may be pregnant. Advise patients not to breast-feed while taking imatinib.

Advise women of childbearing potential to avoid becoming pregnant while taking this medicine.

Advise patients to tell their health care provider if they experience adverse reactions during imatinib therapy, including blood in their stool, fever, jaundice, shortness of breath, sudden weight gain, or symptoms of cardiac failure, or if they have a history of cardiac disease or risk factors for cardiac failure.

Advise patients not to take any other medications, including nonprescription medications such as acetaminophen or herbal products such as St. John's wort, without talking with their health care provider first. Examples of other medications that patients should not take with imatinib include erythromycin, phenytoin, and warfarin. Also advise patients to tell their health care provider if they are taking or planning to take iron supplements. Also advise patients to avoid grapefruit juice and other foods known to inhibit CYP3A4 while they are taking imatinib.

Advise patient not to crush imatinib, and to avoid direct contact of crushed tablets with the skin or mucous membranes. If such contact occurs, advise patient to wash thoroughly.

NILOTINIB

Rx	**Tasigna** (Novartis)	**Capsules; oral:** 150 mg	As nilotinib hydrochloride. Lactose. (NVR/BCR). Red, opaque. In UD 28s and 112s.
		200 mg	As nilotinib hydrochloride. Lactose. (NVR/TKI). Lt. yellow, opaque. In UD 28s and 112s.

NILOTINIB HYDROCHLORIDE — ORAL

WARNING

QT prolongation and sudden deaths – Nilotinib prolongs the QT interval. Sudden deaths have been reported in patients receiving nilotinib. Do not use nilotinib in patients with hypokalemia, hypomagnesemia, or long QT syndrome. Hypokalemia or hypomagnesemia must be corrected prior to nilotinib administration and monitored periodically. Avoid drugs known to prolong the QT interval and strong CYP3A4 inhibitors. Patients should avoid food 2 hours before and 1 hour after taking a nilotinib dose. A dose reduction is recommended in patients with hepatic impairment. Obtain electrocardiograms (ECGs) to monitor the QTc at baseline, 7 days after initiation, and periodically thereafter, as well as following any dose adjustments.

Indications

➤*Resistant or intolerant Philadelphia chromosome–positive chronic myelogenous leukemia in chronic phase and accelerated phase:* For the treatment of chronic- and accelerated-phase Philadelphia chromosome–positive chronic myelogenous leukemia (CML) in adult patients resistant to or intolerant of prior therapy that included imatinib.

➤*Newly diagnosed Philadelphia chromosome–positive chronic myelogenous leukemia in chronic phase:* For the treatment of adult patients with newly diagnosed Philadelphia chromosome–positive CML in chronic phase.

Administration and Dosage

➤*General dosing considerations:* If a dose is missed, the patient should not take a makeup dose, but should resume taking the next prescribed daily dose.

➤*Adults:*

Chronic myelogenous leukemia –

Usual dosage:

- *Resistant or intolerant Philadelphia chromosome–positive chronic myelogenous leukemia in chronic phase and accelerated phase* – 400 mg orally twice daily.
- *Newly diagnosed Philadelphia chromosome–positive chronic myelogenous leukemia in chronic phase* – 300 mg orally twice daily.

Dosage adjustment:

- *QT interval prolongation –*

Nilotinib Dosage Adjustments for QT Prolongation

ECGs with a QTc > 480 msec	1. Withhold nilotinib and perform an analysis of serum potassium and magnesium; if below the lower limit of normal, correct with supplements to within normal limits. Concomitant medication usage must be reviewed.
	2. Resume within 2 weeks at prior dose if QTcF[a] returns to < 450 msec and to within 20 msec of baseline.
	3. If QTcF is between 450 and 480 msec after 2 weeks, reduce the dosage to 400 mg once daily.
	4. If QTcF returns to > 480 msec following dosage reduction to 400 mg once daily, nilotinib should be discontinued.
	5. An ECG should be repeated ≈ 7 days after any dosage adjustment.

[a] QTcF = Fridericia correction of QT interval.

NILOTINIB HYDROCHLORIDE — ORAL

• *Myelosuppression –*

Nilotinib Dosage Adjustments for Neutropenia and Thrombocytopenia		
Newly diagnosed Philadelphia chromosome–positive CML in chronic phase at 300 mg twice daily Resistant or intolerant Philadelphia chromosome–positive CML in chronic phase or accelerated phase at 400 mg twice daily	ANC[a] < 1 × 10^9/L and/or platelet counts < 50 × 10^9/L	1. Discontinue nilotinib and monitor blood cell counts.
		2. Resume within 2 weeks at prior dosage if ANC > 1 × 10^9/L and platelet counts > 50 × 10^9/L.
		3. If blood cell counts remain low for > 2 weeks, reduce the dosage to 400 mg once daily.

[a] ANC = absolute neutrophil count.

• *Nonhematologic laboratory abnormalities –*

Nilotinib Dosage Adjustments for Selected Nonhematologic Laboratory Abnormalities	
Elevated serum lipase or amylase ≥ grade 3	1. Withhold nilotinib and monitor serum lipase or amylase.
	2. Resume treatment at 400 mg once daily if serum lipase or amylase return to ≤ grade 1.
Elevated bilirubin ≥ grade 3	1. Withhold nilotinib and monitor bilirubin.
	2. Resume treatment at 400 mg once daily if bilirubin returns to ≤ grade 1.
Elevated hepatic transaminases ≥ grade 3	1. Withhold nilotinib and monitor hepatic transaminases.
	2. Resume treatment at 400 mg once daily if hepatic transaminases return to ≤ grade 1.

• *Other nonhematologic toxicities –* If other clinically significant moderate or severe nonhematologic toxicity develops, dosing should be withheld and may be resumed at 400 mg once daily when toxicity has resolved. If clinically appropriate, escalation of the dosage back to 300 mg (newly diagnosed Philadelphia chromosome–positive CML in chronic phase) or 400 mg (resistant or intolerant Philadelphia chromosome–positive CML in chronic or accelerated phase) twice daily should be considered. For grade 3 to 4 lipase elevations, dosing should be withheld, and may be resumed at 400 mg once daily. Test serum lipase levels monthly or as clinically indicated. For grade 3 to 4 bilirubin or hepatic transaminase elevations, dosing should be withheld, and may be resumed at 400 mg once daily. Test bilirubin and hepatic transaminases levels monthly or as clinically indicated.

Concomitant therapy: Nilotinib may be given in combination with hematopoietic growth factors such as erythropoietin or granulocyte colony–stimulating factor if clinically indicated. Nilotinib may be given with hydroxyurea or anagrelide if clinically indicated.

• *Strong CYP3A4 inhibitors –* The concomitant use of strong CYP3A4 inhibitors (eg, ketoconazole, itraconazole, clarithromycin, atazanavir, indinavir, nefazodone, nelfinavir, ritonavir, saquinavir, telithromycin, voriconazole) should be avoided. Grapefruit products may also increase serum concentrations of nilotinib and should be avoided. If treatment with any of these agents is required, it is recommended that therapy with nilotinib be interrupted. If patients must be coadministered a strong CYP3A4 inhibitor, based on pharmacokinetic studies, consider a dose reduction to 300 mg once daily in patients with resistant or intolerant Philadelphia chromosome–positive CML or to 200 mg once daily in patients with newly diagnosed Philadelphia chromosome–positive CML in chronic phase. However, there are no clinical data with this dose adjustment in patients receiving strong CYP3A4 inhibitors. If the strong inhibitor is discontinued, a washout period should be allowed before the nilotinib dose is adjusted upward to the indicated dose. Close monitoring for prolongation of the QT interval is indicated for patients who cannot avoid strong CYP3A4 inhibitors.

• *Strong CYP3A4 inducers –* The concomitant use of strong CYP3A4 inducers (eg, dexamethasone, phenytoin, carbamazepine, rifampin, rifabutin, rifapentin, phenobarbital) should be avoided. Patients should also refrain from taking St. John's wort. Based on the nonlinear pharmacokinetic profile of nilotinib, increasing the dose of nilotinib when coadministered with such agents is unlikely to compensate for the loss of exposure.

➤*Hepatic function impairment:* If possible, consider alternative therapies. If nilotinib must be administered to patients with hepatic impairment, the following dose reduction should be considered.

Nilotinib Dose Adjustments for Hepatic Impairment (at Baseline)[a]		
Newly diagnosed Philadelphia chromosome–positive CML in chronic phase at 300 mg twice daily	Mild, moderate, or severe	An initial dosing regimen of 200 mg twice daily followed by dose escalation to 300 mg twice daily based on tolerability.

Nilotinib Dose Adjustments for Hepatic Impairment (at Baseline)[a]		
Resistant or intolerant Philadelphia chromosome–positive CML in chronic phase or accelerated phase at 400 mg twice daily	Mild or moderate	An initial dosing regimen of 300 mg twice daily followed by dose escalation to 400 mg twice daily based on tolerability.
	Severe	A starting dosage of 200 mg twice daily followed by a sequential dose escalation to 300 mg twice daily and then to 400 mg twice daily based on tolerability.

[a] Mild = mild hepatic impairment (Child-Pugh class A); moderate = moderate hepatic impairment (Child-Pugh class B); severe = severe hepatic impairment (Child-Pugh class C).

➤*Total gastrectomy:* The exposure of nilotinib is reduced in patients with total gastrectomy. More frequent follow-up of these patients should be considered. Dose increase or alternative therapy may be considered in patients with total gastrectomy.

➤*Administration:* Nilotinib should be taken twice daily at approximately 12-hour intervals and should not be taken with food. The capsules should be swallowed whole with water. No food should be consumed for at least 2 hours before the dose is taken, and no food should be consumed for at least 1 hour after the dose is taken.

For patients who are unable to swallow capsules, the contents of each capsule may be dispersed in 1 teaspoon of applesauce (pureed apple). The mixture should be taken immediately (within 15 minutes) and should not be stored for future use.

➤*Storage/Stability:* Store at 25°C (77°F); excursions are permitted between 15° and 30°C (59° and 86°F).

Actions

➤*Pharmacology:* Nilotinib, a kinase inhibitor, is an inhibitor of the break point cluster region-Abelson murine leukemia (Bcr-Abl) kinase. Nilotinib binds to and stabilizes the inactive conformation of the kinase domain of Abl protein. In vitro, nilotinib inhibited Bcr-Abl–mediated proliferation of murine leukemic cell lines and human cell lines derived from Philadelphia chromosome–positive CML patients. Under the conditions of the assays, nilotinib was able to overcome imatinib resistance resulting from Bcr-Abl kinase mutations in 32 of 33 mutations tested. In vivo, nilotinib reduced the tumor size in a murine Bcr-Abl xenograft model. Nilotinib inhibited the autophosphorylation of the following kinases at the concentration that inhibits 50% (IC_{50}) values as indicated: Bcr-Abl (20 to 60 nM), platelet-derived growth factor (69 nM), c-Kit (210 nM), colony-stimulating factor receptor type 1 (125 to 250 nM), and discoidin domain receptor (3.7 nM).

➤*Pharmacokinetics:*

Absorption – Peak concentrations of nilotinib are reached 3 hours after oral administration.

Steady-state nilotinib exposure was dose dependent, with less than dose-proportional increases in systemic exposure at dose levels higher than 400 mg given as once-daily dosing. Daily serum exposure to nilotinib 400 mg twice daily at steady state was 35% higher than with 800 mg once daily. Steady-state exposure (area under the curve [AUC]) of nilotinib with 400 mg twice daily was 13% higher than with 300 mg twice daily. The average steady state nilotinib trough and peak concentrations did not change over 12 months. There was no relevant increase in exposure to nilotinib when the dosage was increased from 400 mg twice daily to 600 mg twice daily.

Interpatient variability in nilotinib AUC was 32% to 64%. Steady-state conditions were achieved by day 8. An increase in the serum exposure to nilotinib between the first dose and steady state was approximately 2-fold for once-daily dosing and 3.8-fold for twice-daily dosing.

Effect of food: The bioavailability of nilotinib was increased when given with a meal. Compared with the fasted state, the systemic exposure (AUC) increased by 82% when the dose was given 30 minutes after a high-fat meal.

Distribution – The blood-to-serum ratio of nilotinib is 0.68. Serum protein binding is approximately 98% based on in vitro experiments.

Metabolism – The main metabolic pathways identified in healthy subjects are oxidation and hydroxylation. Nilotinib is the main circulating component in the serum. None of the metabolites contribute significantly to the pharmacological activity of nilotinib.

Excretion – The apparent elimination half-life estimated from multiple-dose pharmacokinetic studies with daily dosing was approximately 17 hours.

After a single dose of radiolabeled nilotinib in healthy subjects, more than 90% of the administered dose was eliminated within 7 days, mainly in the feces (93% of the dose). The parent drug accounted for 69% of the dose.

Special populations –

Hepatic function impairment: Nilotinib exposure is increased in patients with impaired hepatic function. In a study of patients with mild to severe hepatic impairment, following a single dose of nilotinib 200 mg, the mean AUC values were increased an average of 35%, 35%, and 56% in subjects with mild (Child-Pugh class A, score 5 to 6), moderate (Child-Pugh class B, score 7 to 9), and severe hepatic impairment (Child-Pugh class C, score 10 to 15), respectively, compared with a control group of patients with healthy hepatic function. A lower starting dose is recommended in patients with hepatic impairment. Monitor QT interval closely for these patients.

NILOTINIB HYDROCHLORIDE — ORAL

Gastrectomy: Median steady-state trough concentration of nilotinib was decreased by 53% in patients with total gastrectomy compared with patients who had not undergone surgeries.

Contraindications

Hypokalemia, hypomagnesemia, or long QT syndrome.

Warnings/Precautions

➤*Myelosuppression:* Treatment with nilotinib can cause grade 3/4 thrombocytopenia, neutropenia, and anemia. Perform complete blood cell counts (CBCs) every 2 weeks for the first 2 months and then monthly thereafter, or as clinically indicated. Myelosuppression was generally reversible and usually managed by withholding nilotinib temporarily or reducing the dose.

➤*QT prolongation:* Nilotinib has been shown to prolong cardiac ventricular repolarization as measured by the QT interval on the surface ECG in a concentration-dependent manner. Prolongation of the QT interval can result in a type of ventricular tachycardia called torsades de pointes, which may result in syncope, seizure, and/or death. Perform ECGs at baseline, 7 days after initiation, periodically as clinically indicated, and following dose adjustments.

Do not use nilotinib in patients who have hypokalemia, hypomagnesemia, or long QT syndrome. Hypokalemia or hypomagnesemia must be corrected prior to initiating nilotinib. Monitor these electrolytes periodically during therapy.

See Administration and Dosage for more information.

➤*Sudden deaths:* Sudden deaths have been reported in patients with resistant or intolerant Philadelphia chromosome–positive CML who are receiving nilotinib (0.6%). A similar incidence was also reported in the expanded access program for patients with resistant or intolerant Philadelphia chromosome–positive CML. The relative early occurrence of some of the deaths relative to the initiation of nilotinib suggests the possibility that ventricular repolarization abnormalities may have contributed to their occurrence.

➤*Elevated serum lipase:* The use of nilotinib can cause increases in serum lipase. Caution is recommended in patients with a history of pancreatitis. If lipase elevations are accompanied by abdominal symptoms, interrupt dosing and consider appropriate diagnostics to exclude pancreatitis. Test serum lipase levels monthly or as clinically indicated.

➤*Hepatotoxicity:* The use of nilotinib may result in elevations in alkaline phosphatase, AST/ALT, and bilirubin. Check hepatic function tests monthly or as clinically indicated.

➤*Electrolyte abnormalities:* The use of nilotinib can cause hyperkalemia, hypocalcemia, hypokalemia, hyponatremia, and hypophosphatemia. Electrolyte abnormalities must be corrected prior to initiating nilotinib. Monitor these electrolytes periodically during therapy.

➤*Total gastrectomy:* See Administration and Dosage for more information.

See Actions for more information.

➤*Lactose intolerance:* Because the capsules contain lactose, nilotinib is not recommended for patients with rare hereditary problems of galactose intolerance, severe lactase deficiency with a severe degree of intolerance to lactose-containing products, or glucose-galactose malabsorption.

➤*Cardiac disorders:* In the clinical trials, patients with a history of uncontrolled or significant cardiovascular disease, including recent myocardial infarction, congestive heart failure, unstable angina, or clinically significant bradycardia, were excluded. Exercise caution in patients with relevant cardiac disorders.

➤*Hepatic function impairment:* See Administration and Dosage for more information.

➤*Pregnancy: Category D.* Nilotinib can cause fetal harm when administered to a pregnant woman. Nilotinib caused embryofetal toxicities in laboratory animals at maternal exposures that were lower than the expected human exposure at the recommended dosage of 400 mg twice a day.

Nilotinib was studied for effects on embryofetal development in pregnant rats and rabbits given oral dosages of 10, 30, and 100 mg/kg/day, and 30, 100, and 300 mg/kg/day, respectively, during organogenesis. In rats, nilotinib at dosages of 100 mg/kg/day (approximately 5.7 times the AUC in patients at the dosage of 400 mg twice daily) was associated with maternal toxicity (decreased gestation weight, food consumption, gravid uterine weight, and net weight gain). Nilotinib at dosages of at least 30 mg/kg/day (approximately 2 times the AUC in patients at the dosage of 400 mg twice daily) resulted in embryofetal toxicity (as shown by increased resorption and postimplantation loss), and at 100 mg/kg/day, a decrease in viable fetuses. In rabbits, maternal toxicity at 300 mg/kg/day (approximately one-half the human exposure based on AUC) was associated with abortion, decreased food consumption, decreased gestation weights, and mortality. Embryonic toxicity (increased resorption) and minor skeletal anomalies were observed at a dosage of 300 mg/kg/day. Nilotinib is not considered teratogenic.

When pregnant rats were dosed with nilotinib during organogenesis and through lactation, the adverse effects included a longer gestational period, lower pup body weights until weaning, and decreased fertility indices in the pups when they reached maturity, all at a maternal dose of 360 mg/m^2 (approximately 0.7 times the clinical dosage of 400 mg twice daily based on body surface area). At doses of up to 120 mg/m^2 (approximately 0.25 times the clinical dosage of 400 mg twice daily based on body surface area), no adverse effects were seen in the maternal animals or the pups.

There are no adequate and well-controlled studies with nilotinib in pregnant women. Advise women of childbearing potential to avoid becoming pregnant while taking nilotinib and advise them of the potential hazard to the fetus.

➤*Lactation:* It is not known whether nilotinib is excreted in human milk. One study in lactating rats demonstrated that nilotinib is excreted into milk. Because many drugs are excreted in human milk and because of the potential for serious adverse reactions in breast-feeding infants from nilotinib, decide whether to discontinue breast-feeding or the drug, taking into account the importance of the drug to the mother.

➤*Children:* The safety and effectiveness of nilotinib in children have not been established.

➤*Elderly:* In patients with resistant or intolerant accelerated-phase CML, the major hematologic response rate was 31% in patients younger than 65 years of age and 15% in patients 65 years of age and older. No major differences were observed for safety in patients 65 years of age and older compared with patients younger than 65 years of age.

➤*Monitoring:* Perform CBCs every 2 weeks for the first 2 months and then monthly thereafter. Periodically check chemistry panels, lipid profiles, and electrolytes (eg, calcium, magnesium, phosphate, potassium, sodium). Obtain ECGs at baseline, 7 days after initiation, and periodically thereafter, as well as following dose adjustments. Check hepatic function tests and serum lipase monthly or as clinically indicated, and monitor closely for QT interval prolongation. Laboratory monitoring for patients receiving nilotinib may need to be performed more or less frequently at the health care provider's discretion.

Drug Interactions

➤*QT prolongation:* An additive effect of nilotinib with other drugs that prolong the QT interval cannot be excluded. The following drugs may prolong the QT interval and increase the risk of life-threatening cardiac arrhythmias, including torsades de pointes: antiarrhythmic agents (eg, amiodarone, bretylium, disopyramide, dofetilide, procainamide, quinidine, sotalol), arsenic trioxide, chlorpromazine, cisapride, dolasetron, droperidol, mefloquine, mesoridazine, moxifloxacin, pentamidine, pimozide, tacrolimus, thioridazine, ziprasidone. For a more complete list of drugs that may prolong the QT interval see the Drug-Induced Prolongation of the QT Interval and Torsades De Pointes appendix.

Nilotinib Drug Interactions

Precipitant drug	Object drug[a]		Description
CYP3A4 inducers (eg, carbamazepine, dexamethasone, phenobarbital, phenytoin, rifabutin, rifampin, rifapentine, St. John's wort)	Nilotinib	⬇	Avoid concomitant use of strong CYP3A4 inducers. Increasing the dose of nilotinib is unlikely to compensate for the loss of nilotinib exposure resulting from the interaction. Consider concomitant use of an alternative therapeutic agent with less potential for CYP3A4 induction. For more information, see the table Inhibitors, Inducers, and Substrates of Cytochrome P450 Enzymes.
CYP3A4 inhibitors (eg, atazanavir, clarithromycin, delavirdine, indinavir, itraconazole, ketoconazole, nefazodone, nelfinavir, ritonavir, saquinavir, telithromycin, trazodone, voriconazole)	Nilotinib	⬆	Avoid concomitant use of strong CYP3A4 inhibitors. If coadministration of any of these agents is required, interrupt nilotinib treatment. If patients must be coadministered a strong CYP3A4 inhibitor, reduce the dosage of nilotinib to 300 mg once daily in patients with resistant or intolerant Philadelphia chromosome–positive CML or to 200 mg once daily in patients with newly diagnosed Philadelphia chromosome–positive CML in chronic phase. If the strong inhibitor is discontinued, allow a washout period to occur before the nilotinib dose is adjusted upward. If a strong CYP3A4 inhibitor is coadministered, closely monitor for QT interval prolongation. For more information, see the table Inhibitors, Inducers, and Substrates of Cytochrome P450 Enzymes.

NILOTINIB HYDROCHLORIDE — ORAL

Nilotinib Drug Interactions

Precipitant drug	Object drug[a]		Description
Gastric pH-altering agents (eg, antacids [eg, aluminum hydroxide], H_2 blockers [eg, cimetidine], proton pump inhibitors [eg, esomeprazole])	Nilotinib	⬇	Nilotinib has pH-dependent solubility. Drugs that increase gastric pH may decrease nilotinib solubility and reduce its bioavailability. Increasing the dose of nilotinib is not likely to compensate for the decrease in exposure. Separation of the nilotinib dose when proton pump inhibitors are administered may not eliminate the interaction. Therefore, use with caution and closely monitor the patient. If an antacid or H_2 blocker is coadministered with nilotinib, separate the administration times by at least several hours.
Imatinib	Nilotinib	⬆	In a phase 1 trial, coadministration of nilotinib 400 mg twice daily and imatinib 400 mg daily or 400 mg twice daily increased the nilotinib AUC 30% to 50% and the imatinib AUC 20%. Monitor the clinical response of the patient.
Nilotinib	Imatinib		
Nevirapine	Nilotinib	⬇	Plasma concentrations and pharmacologic effects of nilotinib may be reduced by nevirapine. Avoid coadministration. If concomitant use cannot be avoided, monitor the response of the patient and adjust the nilotinib dose as needed.
P-glycoprotein inhibitors (eg, ranolazine)	Nilotinib	⬆	Nilotinib is a substrate of P-glycoprotein. If nilotinib is administered with drugs that inhibit P-glycoprotein, increased concentrations of nilotinib are likely; exercise caution.
Nilotinib	P-glycoprotein inhibitors (eg, ranolazine)		Nilotinib inhibits P-glycoprotein. If nilotinib is administered with drugs that are substrates of P-glycoprotein, increased concentrations of the substrate drug are likely. Use with caution.
Nilotinib	CYP2B6, CYP2C8, and CYP2C9 substrates	⬇	Plasma concentrations of drugs that are substrates for these enzymes may be reduced, decreasing their effectiveness. Use with caution and monitor the clinical response of the patient. Adjust the dose of these agents as needed. For more information, see the table Inhibitors, Inducers, and Substrates of Cytochrome P450 Enzymes.
Nilotinib	CYP2C8, CYP2C9, CYP2Db, and UGT1A1 substrates	⬆	Plasma concentrations of drugs that are substrates for these enzymes may be elevated, increasing their pharmacologic effect and risk of adverse reactions. Use with caution and monitor the clinical response of the patient. Adjust the dose of these agents as needed. For more information, see the table Inhibitors, Inducers, and Substrates of Cytochrome P450 Enzymes.
Nilotinib	CYP3A4 substrates (eg, cyclosporine, midazolam)	⬆	Coadministration of nilotinib and midazolam increased midazolam exposure by 30%. Use caution when administering nilotinib with CYP3A4 substrates that have a narrow therapeutic index. For more information, see the table Inhibitors, Inducers, and Substrates of Cytochrome P450 Enzymes.
Nilotinib	Warfarin	⬆	Because warfarin is metabolized by CYP2C9 and CYP3A4, avoid concurrent use if possible. For more information, see the table Inhibitors, Inducers, and Substrates of Cytochrome P450 Enzymes.

[a] ⬆ = object drug increased; ⬇ = object drug decreased.

➤*Drug/Food interactions:* See Actions for more information.

Grapefruit products may increase serum concentrations of nilotinib and should be avoided.

Adverse Reactions

➤*Newly diagnosed chronic myelogenous leukemia:*

Discontinuation of therapy – Discontinuation for adverse reactions regardless of causality was observed in 7% of patients.

Most common adverse reactions – The most common (more than 10%) nonhematologic adverse drug reactions were rash, pruritus, headache, nausea, fatigue, and myalgia. Upper abdominal pain, alopecia, constipation, diarrhea, dry skin, muscle spasms, arthralgia, abdominal pain, peripheral edema, and asthenia were observed less commonly (10% or less and more than 5%) and have been of mild to moderate severity, manageable, and generally did not require dose reduction. Pleural and pericardial effusions occurred in 1% of patients. GI hemorrhage was reported in 0.4% of patients.

Increase in QTcF more than 60 msec from baseline was observed in 1 patient (0.4%) in the 300 mg twice-daily treatment group. No patient had an absolute QTcF of more than 500 msec.

The most common hematologic adverse drug reactions (all grades) were myelosuppression, including thrombocytopenia (17%), neutropenia (15%), and anemia (7%).

Adverse reactions (10% or more) –

Nilotinib Adverse Reactions (≥ 10%)

Adverse reactions	Patients with newly diagnosed Philadelphia chromosome–positive, chronic-phase CML			
	Nilotinib 300 mg twice daily (n = 279)	Imatinib 400 mg once daily (n = 280)	Nilotinib 300 mg twice daily (n = 279)	Imatinib 400 mg once daily (n = 280)
	All grades		Grades 3/4	
CNS				
Asthenia	11%	9%	< 1%	0%
Fatigue	19%	14%	< 1%	1%
Headache	28%	16%	3%	< 1%
Dermatologic				
Alopecia	10%	5%	0%	0%
Pruritus	19%	7%	< 1%	0%
Rash	36%	16%	< 1%	1%
GI				
Abdominal pain	12%	9%	1%	< 1%
Abdominal pain upper	15%	10%	< 1%	< 1%
Constipation	15%	4%	0%	0%
Diarrhea	14%	37%	< 1%	2%
Nausea	19%	38%	1%	1%
Vomiting	9%	22%	0%	< 1%
Musculoskeletal				
Arthralgia	15%	13%	< 1%	0%
Back pain	12%	10%	< 1%	1%
Muscle spasms	10%	29%	0%	< 1%
Myalgia	14%	16%	< 1%	0%
Pain in extremity	9%	13%	0%	< 1%
Respiratory				
Cough	12%	9%	0%	0%
Nasopharyngitis	19%	15%	0%	0%
Upper respiratory tract infection	13%	9%	0%	0%

NILOTINIB HYDROCHLORIDE — ORAL

Nilotinib Adverse Reactions (≥ 10%)				
	Patients with newly diagnosed Philadelphia chromosome–positive, chronic-phase CML			
Adverse reactions	Nilotinib 300 mg twice daily (n = 279)	Imatinib 400 mg once daily (n = 280)	Nilotinib 300 mg twice daily (n = 279)	Imatinib 400 mg once daily (n = 280)
	All grades		Grades 3/4	
Miscellaneous				
Edema, peripheral	8%	17%	0%	0%
Eyelid edema	1%	14%	0%	< 1%
Pyrexia	10%	12%	0%	0%

➤*Resistant or intolerant chronic myelogenous leukemia:*

Most common adverse reactions – In patients with chronic-phase CML, the most commonly reported adverse drug reactions (more than 10%) were rash, pruritus, nausea, fatigue, headache, constipation, diarrhea, and vomiting. The common serious drug-related adverse reactions were thrombocytopenia and neutropenia.

In patients with accelerated-phase CML, the most commonly reported adverse drug reactions (more than 10%) were rash, pruritus, and constipation. The common serious adverse drug reactions were thrombocytopenia, neutropenia, pneumonia, febrile neutropenia, leukopenia, intracranial hemorrhage, elevated lipase, and pyrexia.

Serious adverse reactions – Sudden deaths and QT prolongation were reported. The maximum mean QTcF change from baseline at steady state was 10 msec. Increase in QTcF more than 60 msec from baseline was observed in 2.1% of the patients and QTcF of more than 500 msec was observed in 3 patients (less than 1%).

Discontinuation of therapy – Discontinuation for drug-related adverse reactions was observed in 11% of patients with chronic-phase CML and 8% of patients with accelerated-phase CML.

Adverse reactions (10% or more) –

Nilotinib Adverse Reactions (≥ 10%)				
	Chronic-phase CML (n = 318)		Accelerated-phase CML (n = 120)	
Adverse reaction	All grades	Grades 3/4	All grades	Grades 3/4
CNS				
Asthenia	14%	0%	12%	2%
Fatigue	28%	1%	16%	< 1%
Headache	31%	3%	21%	2%
Dermatologic				
Pruritus	29%	< 1%	20%	0%
Rash	33%	2%	28%	0%
GI				
Abdominal pain	11%	1%	13%	3%
Constipation	21%	< 1%	18%	0%
Diarrhea	22%	3%	19%	2%
Nausea	31%	1%	18%	< 1%
Vomiting	21%	< 1%	10%	0%
Musculoskeletal				
Arthralgia	18%	2%	16%	0%
Back pain	10%	< 1%	12%	< 1%
Bone pain	11%	< 1%	13%	< 1%
Muscle spasms	11%	< 1%	14%	0%
Myalgia	14%	2%	14%	< 1%
Pain in extremity	13%	1%	16%	2%
Respiratory				
Cough	17%	< 1%	13%	0%
Dyspnea	11%	1%	8%	3%
Nasopharyngitis	16%	< 1%	11%	0%
Miscellaneous				
Peripheral edema	11%	0%	11%	0%
Pyrexia	14%	1%	24%	2%

➤*Other adverse reactions:*

Cardiovascular – Angina pectoris, arrhythmia (including atrial fibrillation, atrioventricular block, bradycardia, cardiac flutter, extrasystoles), ECG QT prolonged, flushing, hypertension, palpitations (1% to 10%); cardiac failure, cardiac murmur, coronary artery disease, cyanosis, hematoma, hypertensive crisis, pericardial effusion (0.1% to 1%); ejection fraction decrease, hypotension, myocardial infarction, pericarditis, shock hemorrhagic, thrombosis, ventricular dysfunction.

CNS – Depression, dizziness, hypoaesthesia, insomnia, paresthesia (1% to 10%); anxiety, disturbance in attention, hyperesthesia, intracranial hemorrhage, loss of consciousness (including syncope), malaise, migraine, tremor, vertigo (0.1% to 1%); amnesia, brain edema, confusional state, disorientation, dysaesthesia, dysphoria, lethargy, optic neuritis, peripheral neuropathy.

Dermatologic – Acne, contusion, dermatitis, dry skin, eczema, erythema, folliculitis, hyperhidrosis, night sweats, skin papilloma, urticaria (1% to 10%); drug eruption, ecchymosis, exfoliative rash, pain of skin, swelling face (0.1% to 1%); blister, candidiasis, dermal cyst, erythema nodosum, furuncle, herpes virus infection, palmar-plantar erythrodysasthesia syndrome, petechiae, photosensitivity, sebaceous hyperplasia, skin atrophy, skin discoloration, skin exfoliation, skin hyperpigmentation, skin hypertrophy, skin ulcer, subcutaneous abscess, tinea pedis.

Endocrine – Hyperthyroidism (0.1% to 1%); hyperparathyroidism secondary, hypothyroidism, thyroiditis.

GI – Abdominal discomfort, abdominal distension, dyspepsia, flatulence, pancreatitis (1% to 10%); gastroesophageal reflux, GI hemorrhage, melena, mouth ulceration, stomatitis, esophageal pain, dysgeusia, dry mouth, gastroenteritis (0.1% to 1%); anal abscess, esophagitis ulcerative, GI ulcer perforation, hematemesis, gastric ulcer, gastritis, gingivitis, hemorrhoids, hiatus hernia, rectal hemorrhage, retroperitoneal hemorrhage, sensitivity of teeth, subileus.

GU – Pollakiuria (1% to 10%); breast pain, dysuria, erectile dysfunction, gynecomastia, micturition urgency, nocturia, urinary tract infection (0.1% to 1%); breast induration, chromaturia, hematuria, menorrhagia, nipple swelling, renal failure, urinary incontinence.

Hematologic – Febrile neutropenia, lymphopenia, pancytopenia (1% to 10%); leukocytosis, thrombocytosis.

Hepatic – Hepatic function abnormal (1% to 10%); hepatitis, jaundice (0.1% to 1%); cholestasis, hepatomegaly, hepatotoxicity.

Lab test abnormalities – Blood amylase increased, blood creatinine phosphokinase increased, blood lactate dehydrogenase increased, blood urea increased, gamma-glutamyltransferase increased, hemoglobin decreased (0.1% to 1%); blood bilirubin unconjugated increased, blood insulin increased, blood parathyroid hormone increased, troponin increased, very low-density lipoprotein increased.

Metabolic/Nutritional – Diabetes mellitus, electrolyte imbalance (including hypercalcemia, hyperkalemia, hyperphosphatemia, hypocalcemia, hypokalemia, hypomagnesemia, hyponatremia, hypophosphatemia), hypercholesterolemia, hyperglycemia, hyperlipidemia, weight decreased, weight increased (1% to 10%); decreased appetite, dehydration, increased appetite (0.1% to 1%); dyslipidemia, gout, hyperuricemia, hypoglycemia.

Musculoskeletal – Bone pain, flank pain, musculoskeletal chest pain, musculoskeletal pain (1% to 10%); joint swelling, muscular weakness, musculoskeletal stiffness (0.1% to 1%); arthritis.

Respiratory – Cough, dysphonia, dyspnea, dyspnea exertional, epistaxis (1% to 10%); interstitial lung disease, pharyngolaryngeal pain, pleural effusion, pleurisy, pleuritic pain, pneumonia, pulmonary edema, throat irritation, upper respiratory tract infection (including nasopharyngitis, pharyngitis, rhinitis) (0.1% to 1%); bronchitis, pulmonary hypertension, wheezing.

Special senses – Conjunctivitis, dry eye, eye hemorrhage, eye pruritus, periorbital edema (1% to 10%); eye irritation, photopsia, vision blurred, vision impairment, visual acuity reduced (0.1% to 1%); blepharitis, chorioretinopathy, conjunctival hemorrhage, conjunctival hyperaemia, conjunctivitis allergic, diplopia, ear pain, eye pain, eye swelling, hearing impaired, ocular hyperaemia, ocular surface disease, papilloedema, photophobia, scleral hyperaemia, tinnitus.

Miscellaneous – Chest discomfort, chest pain, pain (including neck pain and back pain), pyrexia (1% to 10%); chills, face edema, gravitational edema, influenza-like illness, (0.1% to 1%); candidiasis, feeling hot, herpes simplex, hypersensitivity, localized edema, papilloma, sepsis.

➤*Lab test abnormalities:*

Nilotinib Grade 3/4 Laboratory Abnormalities				
	Newly diagnosed Philadelphia chromosome–positive, chronic-phase CML		Resistant or intolerant Philadelphia chromosome–positive, chronic-phase CML (n = 318)	Philadelphia chromosome–positive, accelerated-phase CML (n = 120)
	Nilotinib 300 mg twice daily (n = 279)	Imatinib 400 mg once daily (n = 280)	Nilotinib 300 mg twice daily (n = 318)	Imatinib 400 mg once daily (n = 120)
Hematologic				
Anemia	4%	5%	8%	23%
Neutropenia[a]	12%	20%	28%	37%[b]

NILOTINIB HYDROCHLORIDE — ORAL

Nilotinib Grade 3/4 Laboratory Abnormalities

	Newly diagnosed Philadelphia chromosome–positive, chronic-phase CML		Resistant or intolerant Philadelphia chromosome–positive, chronic-phase CML (n = 318)	Philadelphia chromosome–positive, accelerated-phase CML (n = 120)
	Nilotinib 300 mg twice daily (n = 279)	Imatinib 400 mg once daily (n = 280)	Nilotinib 300 mg twice daily (n = 318)	Imatinib 400 mg once daily (n = 120)
Thrombocytopenia	10%	9%	28%[c]	37%[a]
Biochemistry parameters				
Decreased albumin	0%	0%	1%	1%
Elevated alkaline phosphatase	0%	< 1%	1%	3%
Elevated ALT	4%	3%	4%	2%
Elevated AST	1%	1%	1%	1%
Elevated bilirubin (total)	4%	< 1%	9%	10%
Elevated creatinine	0%	< 1%	< 1%	0%
Elevated lipase	7%	3%	15%	17%
Hyperglycemia	6%	0%	11%	4%
Hyperkalemia	2%	1%	4%	3%
Hypocalcemia	< 1%	0%	1%	4%
Hypokalemia	< 1%	1%	1%	5%
Hyponatremia	< 1%	< 1%	3%	3%
Hypophosphatemia	5%	8%	10%	10%

[a] 7% were grade 3, 30% were grade 4.
[b] 12% were grade 3, 25% were grade 4.
[c] 11% were grade 3, 17% were grade 4.

➤*Postmarketing:* Cases of tumor lysis syndrome have been reported in nilotinib-treated patients with resistant or intolerant CML. Malignant disease progression, high white blood cell counts, and/or dehydration were present in majority of these cases.

Overdosage

Overdose with nilotinib has been reported, where an unspecified amount of nilotinib was ingested in combination with alcohol and other drugs. Events included neutropenia, vomiting, and drowsiness.

➤*Treatment:* In the event of an overdose, observe the patient and give appropriate supportive treatment.

Patient Information

Advise patients to take nilotinib doses twice daily, approximately 12 hours apart, and not to take nilotinib with food. Instruct patients to swallow nilotinib capsules whole with water.

Advise patients to take nilotinib on an empty stomach at least 2 hours after a meal. Instruct patients not to consume food for at least 1 hour after the dose is taken. Advise patients not to consume grapefruit products and other foods that are known to inhibit CYP3A4 at any time during nilotinib treatment.

Inform patients that nilotinib and certain other medicines, including nonprescription medications or herbal supplements (such as St. John's wort), can interact with each other.

Advise patients that the use of nilotinib during pregnancy may cause harm to the fetus and advise them not to take nilotinib during pregnancy unless necessary. Instruct women of childbearing potential to use effective contraceptives if taking nilotinib. Advise sexually active women taking nilotinib to use adequate contraception.

Advise patients to continue taking nilotinib every day for as long as their health care provider tells them, that this is a long-term treatment, not to change the dose or stop taking nilotinib without first consulting with their health care provider, and that if a dose is missed to take the next dose as scheduled and not to take a double dose to make up for the forgotten capsules.

SUNITINIB

Rx	**Sutent** (Pfizer)	**Capsules; oral:** 12.5 mg	As sunitinib malate. Mannitol. (Pfizer STN 12.5 mg). Orange. In 28s.
		25 mg	As sunitinib malate. Mannitol. (Pfizer STN 25 mg). Caramel/Orange. In 28s.
		50 mg	As sunitinib malate. Mannitol. (Pfizer STN 50 mg). Caramel. In 28s.

SUNITINIB MALATE — ORAL

WARNING

Hepatotoxicity – Hepatotoxicity has been observed in clinical trials and postmarketing experience. Hepatotoxicity may be severe, and deaths have been reported.

Indications

➤*Advanced renal cell carcinoma:* For the treatment of advanced renal cell carcinoma.

➤*GI stromal tumor:* For the treatment of GI stromal tumor after disease progression or intolerance to imatinib.

Administration and Dosage

➤*Adults:*

Advanced renal cell carcinoma –

Usual dosage: 50 mg once daily on a schedule of 4 weeks on treatment followed by 2 weeks off (schedule 4/2).

Dosage adjustment: Dose interruption and/or dose modification in 12.5 mg increments or decrements is recommended based on individual safety and tolerability. (See also Dosage Adjustment for Toxicity.)

GI stromal tumor – See Advanced Renal Cell Carcinoma for dosing.

➤*Dosage adjustment for toxicity:*

Sunitinib Dosage Adjustments for Toxicity

Body system	Adverse effect	Recommendation
Cardiovascular	Ejection fraction decrease 20% to 50% from baseline, without signs of heart failure. Severe hypertension (systolic blood pressure > 200 mm Hg, diastolic blood pressure > 110 mm Hg).	Reduce dose or temporarily interrupt therapy; temporarily suspend sunitinib until hypertension is controlled.
	Congestive heart failure	Discontinue therapy.
Hepatic	Grade 3 or 4 hepatic adverse reactions	Interrupt dose; discontinue therapy if there is no resolution. Do not restart sunitinib if patients subsequently experience changes in liver function tests or have other signs and symptoms of liver failure.
	Pancreatitis/Hepatic failure	Discontinue therapy.
Hematologic	Thrombotic microangiopathy	Suspend therapy; following resolution, treatment may be resumed.

SUNITINIB MALATE — ORAL

Sunitinib Dosage Adjustments for Toxicity		
Body system	Adverse effect	Recommendation
Neurologic	Reversible posterior leukoencephalopathy syndrome	Temporarily suspend therapy. Following resolution, therapy may be resumed.
Renal	Nephrotic syndrome	Discontinue therapy.

➤*Concomitant therapy:*

Strong CYP3A4 inhibitors – Strong CYP3A4 inhibitors, such as ketoconazole, may increase sunitinib plasma concentrations. Selection of an alternative concomitant medication with no or minimal enzyme inhibition potential is recommended. A dosage reduction for sunitinib to a minimum of 37.5 mg daily should be considered if sunitinib must be coadministered with a strong CYP3A4 inhibitor.

CYP3A4 inducers – CYP3A4 inducers, such as rifampin, may decrease sunitinib plasma concentrations. Selection of an alternative concomitant medication with no or minimal enzyme induction potential is recommended. A dosage increase for sunitinib to a maximum of 87.5 mg daily should be considered if sunitinib must be coadministered with a CYP3A4 inducer. If the dose is increased, the patient should be monitored carefully for toxicity.

➤*Preparation for administration:* Sunitinib is considered a cytotoxic agent. Follow safe handling procedures when preparing, administering, or dispensing sunitinib.

➤*Administration:* Administer with or without food.

➤*Storage/Stability:* Store at 25°C (77°F); excursions are permitted between 15° and 30°C (59° and 86°F).

Actions

➤*Pharmacology:* Sunitinib, a multikinase inhibitor, is a small molecule that inhibits multiple receptor tyrosine kinases (RTKs), some of which are implicated in tumor growth, pathologic angiogenesis, and metastatic progression of cancer. Sunitinib was evaluated for its inhibitory activity against a variety of kinases (greater than 80 kinases) and was identified as an inhibitor of platelet-derived growth factor receptors (PDGFR-alpha and PDGFR-beta), vascular endothelial growth factor receptors (VEGFR1, VEGFR2, and VEGFR3), stem cell factor receptor (KIT), fms-like tyrosine kinase-3, colony-stimulating factor receptor type 1, and the glial cell-line derived neurotrophic factor receptor (RET).

Sunitinib inhibited the phosphorylation of multiple RTKs (PDGFR-beta, VEGFR2, KIT) in tumor xenografts expressing RTK targets in vivo and demonstrated inhibition of tumor growth or tumor regression and/or inhibited metastases in some experimental models of cancer. Sunitinib demonstrated the ability to inhibit growth of tumor cells expressing dysregulated target RTKs (PDGFR, RET, or KIT) in vitro and to inhibit PDGFR-beta– and VEGFR2-dependent tumor angiogenesis in vivo.

➤*Pharmacokinetics:*

Absorption – Maximum plasma concentrations (C_{max}) of sunitinib are generally observed between 6 and 12 hours (time to maximum concentration [T_{max}]) following oral administration. With repeated daily administration, sunitinib accumulates 3- to 4-fold, while the primary metabolite accumulates 7- to 10-fold. Steady-state concentrations of sunitinib and its primary active metabolite are achieved within 10 to 14 days. By day 14, combined plasma concentrations of sunitinib and its active metabolite ranged from 62.9 to 101 ng/mL.

Distribution – Binding of sunitinib and its primary metabolite to human plasma protein in vitro was 95% and 90%, respectively, with no concentration dependence in the range of 100 to 4,000 ng/mL. The apparent volume of distribution for sunitinib was 2,230 L. In the dosing range of 25 to 100 mg, the area under the curve (AUC) and C_{max} increase proportionately with dose.

Metabolism/Excretion – Sunitinib and its primary metabolite are primarily metabolized by the liver. Sunitinib is metabolized primarily by the cytochrome P450 (CYP-450) enzyme, CYP3A4, to produce its primary active metabolite, which is further metabolized by CYP3A4. The primary active metabolite comprises 23% to 37% of the total exposure. Elimination is primarily via the feces.

In a human mass balance study of [^{14}C]sunitinib, 61% of the dose was eliminated in the feces, with renal elimination accounting for 16% of the administered dose. Sunitinib and its primary active metabolite were the major drug-related compounds identified in plasma, urine, and feces, representing 91.5%, 86.4%, and 73.8% of radioactivity in pooled samples, respectively. Minor metabolites were identified in the urine and feces but generally not found in plasma. Total oral clearance ranged from 34 to 62 L/h, with an interpatient variability of 40%.

Following administration of a single oral dose in healthy volunteers, the terminal half-lives of sunitinib and its primary active metabolite are approximately 40 to 60 hours and 80 to 110 hours, respectively.

Contraindications

None well documented.

Warnings/Precautions

➤*Hepatotoxicity:* Sunitinib has been associated with hepatotoxicity, which may result in liver failure or death. Liver failure has been observed in clinical trials (0.3%) and postmarketing experience. Liver failure signs include jaundice, elevated transaminases and/or hyperbilirubinemia in conjunction with encephalopathy, coagulopathy, and/or renal failure. Monitor liver function tests (ALT, AST, bilirubin) before initiation of treatment, during each cycle of treatment, and as clinically indicated. Safety in patients with ALT or AST greater than 2.5 times the upper limits of normal (ULN) or, if due to liver metastases, greater than 5 times the ULN, has not been established.

See Administration and Dosage for more information.

➤*Left ventricular dysfunction:* See Administration and Dosage for more information.

Cardiovascular reactions, including heart failure, myocardial disorders, and cardiomyopathy, some of which were fatal, have been reported through postmarketing experience. More patients treated with sunitinib experienced decline in left ventricular ejection fraction (LVEF) than patients receiving placebo or interferon-alpha.

In the double-blind treatment phase of GI stromal tumor study A, 11% of patients taking sunitinib and 3% of patients on placebo had treatment-emergent LVEF values below the lower limit of normal. Nine of 22 patients with GI stromal tumor on sunitinib with LVEF changes recovered without intervention. Five patients had documented LVEF recovery following intervention (dose reduction, 1 patient; addition of antihypertensive or diuretic medications, 4 patients). Six patients went off the study without documented recovery. Additionally, 3 patients on sunitinib had grade 3 reductions in left ventricular systolic function to LVEF of less than 40%; 2 of these patients died without receiving further study drug. No GI stromal tumor patients on placebo had grade 3 decreased LVEF. In the double-blind treatment phase of GI stromal tumor study A, 1 patient on sunitinib and 1 patient on placebo died of diagnosed heart failure; 2 patients on sunitinib and 2 patients on placebo died of treatment-emergent cardiac arrest.

Patients who presented with cardiac events within 12 months prior to sunitinib administration, such as myocardial infarction (including severe/unstable angina), coronary/peripheral artery bypass graft, symptomatic congestive heart failure (CHF), cerebrovascular accident or transient ischemic attack, or pulmonary embolism, were excluded from sunitinib clinical studies. It is unknown whether patients with these concomitant conditions may be at a higher risk of developing drug-related left ventricular dysfunction. Weigh this risk against the potential benefits of the drug. Carefully monitor these patients for clinical signs and symptoms of CHF while receiving sunitinib. Also consider baseline and periodic evaluations of LVEF while these patients are receiving sunitinib. In patients without cardiac risk factors, consider a baseline evaluation of ejection fraction.

➤*QT interval prolongation and torsades de pointes:* Sunitinib has been shown to prolong the QT interval in a dose-dependent manner, which may lead to an increased risk for ventricular arrhythmias, including torsades de pointes. Torsades de pointes has been observed in less than 0.1% of sunitinib-exposed patients.

Use sunitinib with caution in patients who have a history of QT interval prolongation, are taking antiarrhythmics, or have relevant preexisting cardiac disease, bradycardia, or electrolyte disturbances. When using sunitinib, consider periodic monitoring with on-treatment electrocardiograms and electrolytes (magnesium, potassium).

➤*Hypertension:* Monitor patients for hypertension and treat as needed with standard antihypertensive therapy. In cases of severe hypertension, temporary suspension of sunitinib is recommended until hypertension is controlled.

Of patients receiving sunitinib for treatment-naive metastatic advanced renal cell carcinoma, 34% of patients receiving sunitinib compared with 4% of patients taking interferon-alpha experienced hypertension. Grade 3 hypertension was observed in 13% of patients with treatment-naive advanced renal cell carcinoma taking sunitinib compared with less than 1% of patients taking interferon-alpha. While all-grade hypertension was similar in patients with GI stromal tumor taking sunitinib compared with placebo, grade 3 hypertension was reported in 4% of patients with GI stromal tumor taking sunitinib, and none of the patients with GI stromal tumor on placebo. No grade 4 hypertension was reported. Sunitinib dosing was reduced or temporarily delayed for hypertension in 6% of patients in the treatment-naive advanced renal cell carcinoma study. Four patients with treatment-naive advanced renal cell carcinoma, including one with malignant hypertension, and no GI stromal tumor patients discontinued treatment because of hypertension. Severe hypertension (more than 200 mm Hg systolic or 110 mm Hg diastolic) occurred in 4% of GI stromal tumor patients taking sunitinib, 1% of GI stromal tumor patients on placebo, 9% of patients with treatment-naive advanced renal cell carcinoma taking sunitinib, and 1% of patients on interferon-alpha.

➤*Hemorrhage:* Hemorrhagic reactions reported through postmarketing experience, some of which were fatal, have included GI, respiratory, tumor, urinary tract, and brain hemorrhages. In patients receiving sunitinib in a clinical trial for treatment-naive advanced renal cell carcinoma, 37% of patients had bleeding events compared with 10% of patients receiving interferon-alpha. Bleeding reactions occurred in 18% of patients receiving sunitinib in the double-blind treatment phase of GI stromal tumor study A, compared with 17% of patients receiving placebo. Epistaxis was the most common hemorrhagic adverse reaction reported. Less common bleeding reactions in GI stromal tumor or advanced renal cell carcinoma patients included rectal, gingival, upper GI, genital, and wound bleeding. In the double-blind treatment phase of GI stromal tumor study A, 7% of patients receiving sunitinib and 9% of patients on placebo had grade 3 or 4 bleeding reactions. In addition, 1 patient in GI stromal tumor study A taking placebo had a fatal GI bleeding reaction during cycle 2. Most reactions in advanced renal cell carcinoma patients were grade 1 or 2; there was one grade 5 reaction of gastric bleed in a treatment-naive patient.

SUNITINIB MALATE — ORAL

Tumor-related hemorrhage has been observed in patients treated with sunitinib. These reactions may occur suddenly and, in the case of pulmonary tumors, may present as severe and life-threatening hemoptysis or pulmonary hemorrhage.

Fatal pulmonary hemorrhage occurred in 2 patients receiving sunitinib on a clinical trial of patients with metastatic non–small cell lung cancer. Both patients had squamous cell histology. Sunitinib is not approved for use in patients with non–small cell lung cancer. Treatment-emergent grade 3 and 4 tumor hemorrhage occurred in 3% of patients with GI stromal tumor receiving sunitinib in study A. Tumor hemorrhages were observed as early as cycle 1 and as late as cycle 6. One patient received no further drug following tumor hemorrhage. None of the other 4 patients discontinued treatment or experienced dose delay because of tumor hemorrhage. No patients with GI stromal tumor in the study A placebo arm were observed to undergo intratumoral hemorrhage. Clinical assessment of these reactions should include serial complete blood cell counts and physical examinations.

➤*GI effects:* Serious, sometimes fatal GI complications, including GI perforation, have occurred rarely in patients with intra-abdominal malignancies treated with sunitinib.

➤*Hypothyroidism:* Treatment-emergent acquired hypothyroidism was noted in 4% of GI stromal tumor patients taking sunitinib versus 1% on placebo. Hypothyroidism was reported as an adverse reaction in 16% of patients taking sunitinib in the treatment-naive advanced renal cell carcinoma study and 1% in the interferon-alpha arm. Cases of hyperthyroidism, some followed by hypothyroidism, have been reported in clinical trials and through postmarketing experience. Test patients with hypothyroidism or hyperthyroidism prior to the start of sunitinib treatment.

➤*Adrenal toxicity:* Adrenal toxicity was noted in nonclinical repeat-dose studies of 14 days to 9 months in rats and monkeys at plasma exposures as low as 0.7 times the AUC observed in clinical studies. Histological changes of the adrenal gland were characterized as hemorrhage, necrosis, congestion, hypertrophy, and inflammation. In clinical studies, computerized tomography/magnetic resonance imaging obtained in 336 patients after exposure to 1 or more cycles of sunitinib demonstrated no evidence of adrenal hemorrhage or necrosis. Corticotropin stimulation testing was performed in approximately 400 patients across multiple clinical trials of sunitinib. Among patients with normal baseline corticotropin stimulation testing, 1 patient developed consistently abnormal test results during treatment that were unexplained and may have been related to treatment with sunitinib. Eleven additional patients with normal baseline testing had abnormalities in the final test performed, with peak cortisol levels of 12 to 16.4 mcg/dL (normal is more than 18 mcg/dL) following stimulation. None of these patients were reported to have clinical evidence of adrenal insufficiency.

➤*Pregnancy: Category D.* As angiogenesis is a critical component of embryonic and fetal development, expect inhibition of angiogenesis following administration of sunitinib to result in adverse effects on pregnancy. There are no adequate and well-controlled studies of sunitinib in pregnant women. It is not known if sunitinib or its active metabolite crosses the human placenta. The molecular weight (approximately 399 for the free base) of the parent compound and the long elimination half-lives for sunitinib and the metabolite suggest that the drugs will cross to the embryo and fetus. If the drug is used during pregnancy or if the patient becomes pregnant while receiving this drug, apprise the patient of the potential hazard to the fetus. Advise women of childbearing potential to avoid becoming pregnant while receiving treatment with sunitinib. If an inadvertent pregnancy occurs, advise the woman of the potential risk for severe adverse effects in the embryo and fetus.

Sunitinib was evaluated in pregnant rats (0.3, 1.5, 3, 5 mg/kg/day) and rabbits (0.5, 1, 5, 20 mg/kg/day) for effects on the embryo. Significant increases in the incidence of embryolethality and structural abnormalities were observed in rats at the dosage of 5 mg/kg/day (approximately 5.5 times the systemic exposure [combined AUC of sunitinib + primary active metabolite] in patients administered the recommended daily dose). Significantly increased embryolethality was observed in rabbits at 5 mg/kg/day, while developmental effects were observed at 1 mg/kg/day or more (approximately 0.3 times the AUC in patients administered the recommended daily dosage of 50 mg/day). Developmental effects consisted of fetal skeletal malformations of the ribs and vertebrae in rats. In rabbits, cleft lip was observed at 1 mg/kg/day, and cleft lip and cleft palate were observed at 5 mg/kg/day (approximately 2.7 times the AUC in patients administered the recommended daily dose). Neither fetal loss nor malformations were observed in rats dosed at 3 mg/kg/day or less (approximately 2.3 times the AUC in patients administered the recommended daily dose).

Fertility impairment – Although fertility was not affected in rats, sunitinib may impair fertility in humans.

➤*Lactation:* Sunitinib and its metabolites are excreted in rat's milk. In lactating female rats administered 15 mg/kg, sunitinib and its metabolites were extensively excreted in milk at concentrations up to 12-fold higher than in plasma. It is not known whether sunitinib or its primary active metabolite are excreted in human breast milk. The molecular weight (approximately 399 for the free base) of the parent compound and the long elimination half-lives for sunitinib and its active metabolite suggest that the drugs will be excreted into breast milk. Because drugs are commonly excreted in human breast milk and because of the potential for serious adverse reactions in breast-feeding infants, decide whether to discontinue breast-feeding or the drug, taking into account the importance of the drug to the mother. The risk to a breast-feeding infant is unknown, but there is potential for severe toxicity affecting multiple systems.

➤*Children:* The safety and efficacy of sunitinib in children have not been studied in clinical trials.

➤*Monitoring:* Perform complete blood cell counts with platelet count serum chemistries, including phosphate and urinalysis, at the beginning of each treatment cycle. Carefully monitor patients for clinical signs and symptoms of CHF. Consider baseline and periodic evaluations of LVEF in patients with cardiac risk factors. Also consider a baseline evaluation of ejection fraction in patients without cardiac risk factors. Consider periodic monitoring with on-treatment electrocardiograms and electrolytes (magnesium, potassium). Monitor patients for hypertension and the development of proteinuria. Baseline laboratory measurement of thyroid function is recommended. Observe all patients closely for signs and symptoms of thyroid dysfunction. Perform laboratory monitoring of thyroid function in patients with signs or symptoms suggestive of thyroid dysfunction. Monitor for adrenal insufficiency in patients who experience stress, such as surgery, trauma, or severe infection. Monitor liver function tests (ALT, AST, bilirubin) before initiation of treatment, during each cycle of treatment, and as clinically indicated.

Drug Interactions

➤*QT Prolongation:* An additive effect of sunitinib with other drugs that prolong the QT interval cannot be excluded. The following drugs may prolong the QT interval and increase the risk of life-threatening cardiac arrhythmias, including torsades de pointes: antiarrhythmic agents (eg, amiodarone, bretylium, disopyramide, dofetilide, procainamide, quinidine, sotalol), arsenic trioxide, chlorpromazine, cisapride, dolasetron, droperidol, gatifloxacin, halofantrine, levomethadyl, mefloquine, mesoridazine, moxifloxacin, pentamidine, pimozide, probucol, sparfloxacin, thioridazine, ziprasidone. (See QT Interval Prolongation and Torsades de Pointes.)

Sunitinib Drug Interactions

Precipitant drug	Object drug[a]		Description
Bevacizumab	Sunitinib	↑	Concurrent use of sunitinib and bevacizumab may result in unexpected severe toxicity. Coadministration is not recommended.
CYP3A4 inducers (eg, carbamazepine, dexamethasone, modafinil, nevirapine, phenobarbital, phenytoin, rifabutin, rifampin, rifapentine, St. John's wort)	Sunitinib	↓	Coadministration of sunitinib with rifampin resulted in a 23% and 46% reduction in the combined (sunitinib plus primary active metabolite) C_{max} and $AUC_{0-\infty}$ values, respectively. Consider a dose increase for sunitinib to a maximum of 87.5 mg daily if sunitinib must be coadministered with a CYP3A4 inducer. Monitor for toxicity. St. John's wort may decrease sunitinib plasma concentrations unpredictably. Coadministration is not recommended.
CYP3A4 inhibitors (eg, atazanavir, clarithromycin, indinavir, itraconazole, ketoconazole, nefazodone, nelfinavir, ritonavir, saquinavir, telithromycin, voriconazole)	Sunitinib	↑	Sunitinib prolongs the QT interval in a dose-dependent manner. CYP3A4 inhibitors may increase sunitinib plasma concentrations, increasing the risk of adverse reactions, including ventricular arrhythmias (eg, torsades de pointes). Coadministration of sunitinib with ketoconazole resulted in 49% and 51% increases in the combined (sunitinib plus primary active metabolite) C_{max} and $AUC_{0-\infty}$ values, respectively. Consider a dose decrease for sunitinib to a minimum of 37.5 mg daily if sunitinib must be coadministered with a CYP3A4 inhibitor.
Drugs that prolong the QT interval (eg, chloroquine, doxepin, haloperidol, iloperidone, lithium, maprotiline, methadone, paliperidone, perflutren, tacrolimus, tyrosine kinase inhibitors [eg, dasatinib, lapatinib, pazopanib])	Sunitinib	↑	Consider prolongation of the QT interval with possible development of cardiac arrhythmias, including torsades de pointes, when sunitinib is coadministered with these agents. Caution is advised when 2 agents that are suspected to prolong the QT interval are used concomitantly. If concurrent use is not contraindicated in the respective product information, monitor patients for QT prolongation, especially when adding sunitinib to a stable regimen of another QT prolonging agent, or vice versa.

SUNITINIB MALATE — ORAL

Sunitinib Drug Interactions

Precipitant drug	Object drug[a]		Description
Temsirolimus	Sunitinib	↑	Concurrent use of sunitinib and temsirolimus may result in unexpected toxicity. Use with caution and closely monitor the patient for toxicity.

[a] ↑ = object drug increased; ↓ = object drug decreased.

➤*Drug/Food interactions:* Grapefruit may increase plasma concentrations of sunitinib. Instruct patients taking sunitinib to avoid grapefruit products, including grapefruit juice.

Adverse Reactions

➤*Common adverse reactions (20% or more):* The most common adverse reactions (20% or more) in patients with GI stromal tumor or advanced renal cell carcinoma are abdominal pain, altered taste, anorexia, arthralgia, asthenia, back pain, bleeding, constipation, cough, diarrhea, dry skin, dyspepsia, dyspnea, extremity pain, fatigue, fever, hair color changes, hand-foot syndrome, headache, hypertension, mucositis/stomatitis, nausea, peripheral edema, rash, skin discoloration, and vomiting.

➤*Serious adverse reactions:* The potentially serious adverse reactions are adrenal toxicity, hemorrhage, hepatotoxicity, hypertension, left ventricular dysfunction, QT interval prolongation, thyroid dysfunction.

➤*GI stromal tumor:*

Blinded study –

Sunitinib Adverse Reactions in Patients With GI Stromal Tumor (≥ 10%)

Adverse reactions	Sunitinib (n = 202) All grades	Sunitinib (n = 202) Grade 3/4	Placebo (n = 102) All grades	Placebo (n = 102) Grade 3/4
Any adverse reaction		56%		51%
Dermatologic				
Hand-foot syndrome	14%	4%	10%	3%
Rash	14%	1%	9%	0%
Skin discoloration	30%	0%	23%	0%
GI				
Altered taste	21%	0%	12%	0%
Anorexia[a]	33%	1%	29%	5%
Constipation	20%	0%	14%	2%
Diarrhea	40%	4%	27%	0%
Mucositis/Stomatitis	29%	1%	18%	2%
Miscellaneous				
Asthenia	22%	5%	11%	3%
Hypertension	15%	4%	11%	0%
Myalgia/Limb pain	14%	1%	9%	1%

[a] Includes decreased appetite.

Other adverse reactions: In the double-blind treatment phase of GI stromal tumor study A, oral pain other than mucositis/stomatitis occurred in 6% of patients taking sunitinib versus 3% on placebo. Hair color changes occurred in 7% of patients taking sunitinib versus 4% on placebo. Alopecia was observed in 5% of patients taking sunitinib versus 2% on placebo.

Open-label study –

Discontinuation of therapy: The incidence of treatment-emergent adverse reactions resulting in permanent discontinuation was 20%.

Most common adverse reactions: The most common grade 3 or 4 treatment-related adverse reactions experienced by patients receiving sunitinib in the open-label treatment phase were fatigue (10%); hypertension (8%); asthenia, diarrhea, hand-foot syndrome (5%); nausea (4%); abdominal pain, anorexia (3%); mucositis, vomiting, hypothyroidism (2%).

➤*Renal cell carcinoma:*

Sunitinib Adverse Reactions in Patients With Advanced Renal Cell Carcinoma (≥ 10%)

Adverse reactions	Sunitinib (n = 375) All grades	Sunitinib (n = 375) Grade 3/4[a]	Interferon-alpha (n = 360) All grades	Interferon-alpha (n = 360) Grade 3/4[b]
Any adverse reaction	99%	77%	99%	55%
Cardiovascular				
Ejection fraction decreased	16%	3%	5%	2%
Hypertension	34%	13%	4%	< 1%
CNS				
Asthenia	26%	11%	22%	6%
Depression[c]	11%	0%	14%	1%
Dizziness	11%	< 1%	14%	1%
Fatigue	62%	15%	56%	15%
Headache	23%	1%	19%	0%
Insomnia	15%	< 1%	10%	0%
Dermatologic				
Alopecia	14%	0%	9%	0%
Dry skin	23%	< 1%	7%	0%
Erythema	12%	< 1%	1%	0%
Hair color changes	20%	0%	< 1%	0%
Hand-foot syndrome	29%	8%	1%	0%
Pruritus	12%	< 1%	7%	< 1%
Rash	29%	2%	11%	1%
Skin discoloration/yellow skin	25%	< 1%	0%	0%
GI				
Abdominal pain[d]	30%	5%	12%	< 1%
Altered taste[e]	47%	< 1%	15%	0%
Anorexia[f]	48%	3%	42%	2%
Constipation	23%	1%	14%	< 1%
Diarrhea	66%	10%	21%	< 1%
Dry mouth	13%	0%	7%	< 1%
Dyspepsia	34%	2%	4%	0%
Flatulence	14%	0%	2%	0%
Gastroesophageal reflux disease/reflux esophagitis	12%	< 1%	1%	0%
Glossodynia	11%	0%	1%	0%
Hemorrhoids	10%	0%	2%	0%
Mucositis/Stomatitis	47%	3%	5%	< 1%
Nausea	58%	6%	41%	2%
Oral pain	14%	< 1%	1%	0%
Vomiting	39%	5%	17%	1%
Metabolic/Nutritional				
Edema, peripheral	24%	2%	5%	1%
Hypothyroidism	16%	2%	1%	0%
Weight decreased	16%	< 1%	17%	1%
Musculoskeletal				
Arthralgia	30%	3%	19%	1%
Back pain	28%	5%	14%	2%
Pain in extremity/limb discomfort	40%	5%	30%	2%
Respiratory				
Cough	27%	1%	14%	< 1%
Dyspnea	26%	6%	20%	4%
Upper respiratory tract infection	11%	< 1%	2%	0%
Special senses				
Nasopharyngitis	14%	0%	2%	0%
Oropharyngeal pain	14%	< 1%	2%	0%
Miscellaneous				
Bleeding, all sites	37%	4%[g]	10%	1%
Chest pain	13%	2%	7%	1%
Chills	14%	1%	31%	0%
Fever	22%	1%	37%	< 1%
Influenza-like illness	5%	0%	15%	< 1%

[a] Grade 4 adverse reactions include back pain (1%); arthralgia, asthenia, dyspnea, fatigue, limb pain, and rash (< 1%).
[b] Grade 4 adverse reactions include dyspnea and fatigue (1%); abdominal pain and depression (< 1%).
[c] Includes depressed mood.
[d] Includes flank pain.
[e] Includes ageusia, dysgeusia, and hypogeusia.
[f] Includes decreased appetite.
[g] Includes patient with grade 5 gastric hemorrhage.

SUNITINIB MALATE — ORAL

➤*Hepatic:* If symptoms of pancreatitis or hepatic failure are present, discontinue sunitinib. Pancreatitis was observed in 1% of patients receiving sunitinib for treatment-naive advanced renal cell carcinoma compared with less than 1% of patients receiving interferon-alpha. Hepatotoxicity was observed in patients receiving sunitinib.

➤*Reversible posterior leukoencephalopathy syndrome:* There have been rare (less than 1%) reports of subjects presenting with seizures and radiological evidence of reversible posterior leukoencephalopathy syndrome. None of these subjects had a fatal outcome to the reaction. Control patients with seizures and signs/symptoms consistent with reversible posterior leukoencephalopathy syndrome (eg, hypertension, altered mental functioning, decreased alertness, headache, and visual loss [including cortical blindness]) with medical management, including control of hypertension. Temporary suspension of sunitinib is recommended; following resolution, treatment may be resumed at the discretion of the treating health care provider.

➤*Cardiovascular:* Three percent of patients taking sunitinib and none on placebo in the double-blind treatment phase of GI stromal tumor study A experienced venous thromboembolic reactions; 5 of the 7 were grade 3 deep venous thrombosis (DVT), and 2 were grade 1 or 2. Four of the 7 patients with GI stromal tumor discontinued treatment following first observation of DVT.

Three percent of patients receiving sunitinib for treatment-naive advanced renal cell carcinoma had venous thromboembolic reactions reported. Two percent of these patients had pulmonary embolism, one was grade 2 and 6 were grade 4; 2% of patients had DVT, including three grade 3. One patient was permanently withdrawn from sunitinib because of pulmonary embolism; dose interruption occurred in 2 patients with pulmonary embolism and 1 with DVT. In treatment-naive advanced renal cell carcinoma patients receiving interferon-alpha, venous thromboembolic reactions occurred in 2% of patients; less than 1% experienced a grade 3 DVT, and 1% of patients had pulmonary embolism, all grade 4.

➤*Lab test abnormalities:*

GI stromal tumor –

Sunitinib Laboratory Abnormalities in Patients With GI Stromal Tumor (≥ 10%)

Laboratory abnormality	Sunitinib (n = 202) All grades	Sunitinib Grade 3/4[a]	Placebo (n = 102) All grades	Placebo Grade 3/4[b]
Any adverse reaction		34%		22%
Alkaline phosphatase	24%	4%	21%	4%
Amylase	17%	5%	12%	3%
Anemia	26%	3%	22%	2%
AST/ALT	39%	2%	23%	1%
Creatinine	12%	1%	7%	0%
Decreased LVEF	11%	1%	3%	0%
Hypernatremia	10%	0%	4%	1%
Hypokalemia	12%	1%	4%	0%
Indirect bilirubin	10%	0%	4%	0%
Lipase	25%	10%	17%	7%
Lymphopenia	38%	0%	16%	0%
Neutropenia	53%	10%	4%	0%
Thrombocytopenia	38%	5%	4%	0%
Total bilirubin	16%	1%	8%	0%

[a] Grade 4 laboratory abnormalities included anemia, lipase, neutropenia (2%); alkaline phosphatase, creatinine, hypokalemia, thrombocytopenia (1%).
[b] Grade 4 laboratory abnormalities in patients on placebo included anemia (2%); amylase, lipase, thrombocytopenia (1%).

Renal cell carcinoma –

Sunitinib Laboratory Abnormalities in Patients With Advanced Renal Cell Carcinoma (≥ 10%)

Laboratory abnormality	Sunitinib (n = 375) All grades	Sunitinib Grade 3/4[a]	Interferon-alpha (n = 360) All grades	Interferon-alpha Grade 3/4[b]
Albumin	28%	1%	20%	0%
Alkaline phosphatase	46%	2%	37%	2%
ALT	51%	3%	40%	2%
Amylase	35%	6%	32%	3%
AST	56%	2%	38%	2%
Calcium decreased	42%	1%	40%	1%
Calcium increased	13%	< 1%	10%	1%
Creatine kinase	49%	2%	11%	1%
Creatinine	70%	< 1%	51%	< 1%
Glucose decreased	17%	0%	12%	< 1%
Glucose increased	23%	6%	15%	6%
Hemoglobin	79%	8%	69%	5%
Indirect bilirubin	13%	1%	1%	0%
Leukocytes	78%	8%	56%	2%
Lipase	56%	18%	46%	8%
Lymphocytes	68%	18%	68%	26%
Neutrophils	77%	17%	49%	9%
Phosphorus	31%	6%	24%	6%
Platelets	68%	9%	24%	1%
Potassium decreased	13%	1%	2%	< 1%
Potassium increased	16%	3%	17%	4%
Sodium decreased	20%	8%	15%	4%
Sodium increased	13%	0%	10%	0%
Total bilirubin	20%	1%	2%	0%
Uric acid	46%	14%	33%	8%

[a] Grade 4 laboratory abnormalities include uric acid (14%); lipase (3%); hemoglobin, lymphocytes, neutrophils (2%); amylase, platelets (1%); ALT, calcium decreased, creatine kinase, creatinine, glucose increased, hemoglobin, phosphorus, potassium increased, and sodium decreased (less than 1%).
[b] Grade 4 laboratory abnormalities include uric acid (8%); lymphocytes (2%); lipase, neutrophils (1%); amylase, calcium increased, glucose decreased, hemoglobin, and potassium increased (less than 1%).

➤*Postmarketing:*

Cardiovascular – Thrombotic microangiopathy; pulmonary embolism, in some cases with fatal outcome.

GU – Renal impairment and/or failure, in some cases with fatal outcome; proteinuria and rare cases of nephrotic syndrome.

Miscellaneous – Serious infection (with or without neutropenia), in some cases with fatal outcome; myopathy and/or rhabdomyolysis with or without acute renal failure, in some cases with fatal outcome; hypersensitivity reactions, including angioedema; fistula formation, sometimes associated with tumor necrosis and/or regression, in some cases with fatal outcome; fatal hemorrhage associated with thrombocytopenia.

Overdosage

➤*Symptoms:* No overdose of sunitinib was reported in completed clinical studies.

➤*Treatment:* Treatment of overdose consists of general supportive measures. There is no specific antidote for overdosage. If indicated, achieve elimination of unabsorbed drug by gastric lavage. A few cases of accidental overdose have been reported; these cases were associated with adverse reactions consistent with the known safety profile of sunitinib or without adverse reactions. A case of intentional overdose involving the ingestion of sunitinib 1,500 mg in an attempted suicide was reported without adverse reaction. In nonclinical studies, mortality was observed following as few as 5 daily doses of 500 mg/kg (3,000 mg/m^2) in rats. At this dose, signs of toxicity included impaired muscle coordination, head shakes, hypoactivity, ocular discharge, piloerection, and GI distress. Mortality and similar signs of toxicity were observed at lower doses when administered for longer durations.

Patient Information

Advise patients that GI disorders, such as diarrhea, dyspepsia, nausea, stomatitis, and vomiting, were the most commonly reported GI reactions occurring in patients who received sunitinib. Supportive care for GI adverse reactions requiring treatment may include antiemetic or antidiarrheal medication.

Advise patients that skin discoloration is possibly due to the drug color (yellow), which occurs in approximately one-third of patients. Advise patients that depigmentation of the hair or skin may occur during treatment with sunitinib. Advise patients of the other possible dermatologic effects that may occur (eg, dryness, thickness, or cracking of skin; blister; or rash on the palms of the hands and soles of the feet).

Advise patients that other commonly reported adverse reactions include bleeding, fatigue, high blood pressure, mouth pain/irritation, swelling, and taste disturbance.

Advise patients to inform their health care providers of all concomitant medications, including nonprescription medications and dietary supplements.

Advise patients to take each dose without regard to meals, but to take with food if stomach upset occurs.

Caution women of childbearing potential to avoid becoming pregnant during therapy.

LAPATINIB

Rx	**Tykerb** (GlaxoSmithKline)	**Tablets; oral:** 250 mg	Equiv. to lapatinib ditosylate 398 mg. (GS XJG). Orange, oval. Film-coated. In 150s.

LAPATINIB DITOSYLATE — ORAL

WARNING

Hepatotoxicity has been observed in clinical trials and postmarketing experience. The hepatotoxicity may be severe, and deaths have been reported. Causality of the deaths is uncertain.

Indications

➤*Breast cancer:* In combination with capecitabine, for the treatment of patients with advanced or metastatic breast cancer whose tumors overexpress human epidermal growth receptor type 2 (HER2) and who have received prior therapy, including an anthracycline, a taxane, and trastuzumab.

In combination with letrozole for the treatment of postmenopausal women with hormone receptor–positive metastatic breast cancer that overexpresses the HER2 receptor for whom hormonal therapy is indicated.

Administration and Dosage

➤*Adults:*

HER2-positive metastatic breast cancer –

Usual dosage: 1,250 mg (5 tablets) once daily on days 1 to 21 continuously in combination with capecitabine 2,000 mg/m^2/day (administered orally in 2 doses approximately 12 hours apart) on days 1 to 14 in a repeating 21-day cycle.

Duration of therapy: Treatment should be continued until disease progression or unacceptable toxicity occurs.

Hormone receptor–positive, HER2-positive metastatic breast cancer – 1,500 mg once daily continuously in combination with letrozole 2.5 mg once daily.

➤*Hepatic function impairment:* Patients with severe hepatic impairment (Child-Pugh class C) should have their dosage of lapatinib reduced. A dosage reduction from 1,250 to 750 mg/day (HER2-positive metastatic breast cancer indication) or from 1,500 to 1,000 mg/day (hormone receptor– positive, HER2-positive breast cancer indication) in patients with severe hepatic impairment is predicted to adjust the area under the curve (AUC) to the normal range and should be considered. However, there are no clinical data with this dosage adjustment in patients with severe hepatic impairment.

➤*Concomitant therapy:*

Strong CYP3A4 inhibitors – See Drug Interactions for more information.

Strong CYP3A4 inducers – See Drug Interactions for more information.

➤*Dosage adjustment:*

Grade 2 or more toxicity – Discontinuation or interruption of dosing with lapatinib may be considered when patients develop National Cancer Institute Common Terminology Criteria for Adverse Events (NCI-CTCAE) toxicity of grade 2 or higher and can be restarted at 1,250 mg/day when the toxicity improves to grade 1 or less. If toxicity recurs, lapatinib in combination with capecitabine should be restarted at a lower dosage (1,000 mg/day), and in combination with letrozole, lapatinib should be restarted at a lower dosage of 1,250 mg/day.

Decreased left ventricular ejection fraction (grade 2 or higher) – Lapatinib in combination with capecitabine may be restarted at a reduced dosage (1,000 mg/day) and in combination with letrozole may be restarted at a reduced dosage of 1,250 mg/day after a minimum of 2 weeks if the left ventricular ejection fraction (LVEF) recovers to normal and the patient is asymptomatic.

➤*Discontinuation of therapy:* Lapatinib should be discontinued in patients with a decreased LVEF or grade 2 or higher by NCI-CTCAE and in patients with an LVEF that drops below the institution's lower limit of normal. In patients who develop severe hepatotoxicity while on therapy, lapatinib should be discontinued and patients should not be restarted with lapatinib.

➤*Preparation for administration:* Lapatinib is considered a cytotoxic agent. Follow safe handling procedures when preparing, administering, or dispensing lapatinib.

➤*Administration:* Lapatinib should be taken at least 1 hour before or 1 hour after a meal. The dosage of lapatinib should be administered once daily; dividing the daily dose is not recommended. Capecitabine should be taken with food or within 30 minutes after food. If a day's dose is missed, the patient should not double the dose the next day.

➤*Storage/Stability:* Store at 25°C (77°F); excursions are permitted between 15° and 30°C (59° and 86°F).

Actions

➤*Pharmacology:* Lapatinib is a 4-anilinoquinazoline kinase inhibitor of the intracellular tyrosine kinase domains of both epidermal growth factor receptor (EGFR [ErbB1]) and of HER2 (ErbB2) receptors (estimated K_i^{app} values of 3 and 13 nM, respectively) with a dissociation half-life of at least 300 minutes. Lapatinib inhibits ErbB-driven tumor cell growth in vitro and in various animal models.

An additive effect was demonstrated in an in vitro study when lapatinib and 5-fluorouracil (the active metabolite of capecitabine) were used in combination in the 4 tumor cell lines tested. The growth inhibitory effects of lapatinib were evaluated in trastuzumab-conditioned cell lines. Lapatinib retained significant activity against breast cancer cell lines selected for long-term growth in trastuzumab-containing medium in vitro. These in vitro findings suggest noncross-resistance between these 2 agents.

Hormone receptor positive breast cancer cells (with estrogen receptor and/or progesterone receptor [PGR]) that coexpress the HER2 tend to be resistant to established endocrine therapies. Similarly, hormone receptor–positive breast cancer cells that initially lack EGFR or HER2 upregulate these receptor proteins as the tumor becomes resistant to endocrine therapy.

➤*Pharmacokinetics:*

Absorption – Absorption following oral administration of lapatinib is incomplete and variable. Serum concentrations appear after a median lag time of 0.25 hours (range, 0 to 1.5 hours). Peak plasma concentrations (C_{max}) of lapatinib are achieved approximately 4 hours after administration. Daily dosing of lapatinib results in achievement of steady state within 6 to 7 days.

At the dose of 1,250 mg daily, steady-state geometric mean (95% confidence interval [CI]) values of C_{max} and AUC were 2.43 mcg/mL (1.57 to 3.77 mcg/mL) and 36.2 mcg•h/mL (23.4 to 56 mcg•h/mL), respectively.

Divided daily doses of lapatinib resulted in an approximately 2-fold higher exposure at steady state (steady-state AUC) compared with the same total dose administered once daily.

Effect of food: Systemic exposure to lapatinib is increased when administered with food. Lapatinib AUC values were approximately 3- and 4-fold higher (C_{max} approximately 2.5- and 3-fold higher) when administered with a low-fat (5% fat, 500 calories) or a high-fat (50% fat, 1,000 calories) meal, respectively.

Distribution – Lapatinib is highly bound (more than 99%) to albumin and alpha-1 acid glycoprotein. In vitro studies indicate that lapatinib is a substrate for the transporters breast cancer resistance protein (ABCG2) and P-glycoprotein (P-gp) (ABCB1). Lapatinib has also been shown in vitro to inhibit these efflux transporters, as well as the hepatic uptake transporter OATP 1B1 at clinically relevant concentrations.

Metabolism – Lapatinib undergoes extensive metabolism, primarily by CYP3A4 and CYP3A5, with minor contributions from CYP2C19 and CYP2C8 to a variety of oxidated metabolites, none of which accounts for more than 14% of the dose recovered in the feces or 10% of lapatinib concentration in plasma.

Excretion – At clinical doses, the terminal-phase half-life following a single dose was 14.2 hours; accumulation with repeated dosing indicates an effective half-life of 24 hours.

Elimination of lapatinib is predominantly through metabolism by CYP3A4/5 with negligible (less than 2%) renal excretion. Recovery of parent lapatinib in feces accounts for a median of 27% (range, 3% to 67%) of an oral dose.

Special populations –

Hepatic function impairment: The pharmacokinetics of lapatinib were examined in patients with preexisting moderate (n = 8) or severe (n = 4) hepatic impairment (Child-Pugh class B/C, respectively) and in 8 healthy control patients. Systemic exposure (AUC) after a single oral dose of lapatinib 100 mg increased approximately 14% and 63% in patients with moderate and severe preexisting hepatic impairment, respectively. Use caution when administering lapatinib to patients with severe hepatic impairment because of increased exposure to the drug. Consider a dose reduction for patients with severe preexisting hepatic impairment. In patients who develop severe hepatotoxicity while on therapy, discontinue lapatinib and do not re-treat patients with lapatinib.

Contraindications

Severe hypersensitivity (eg, anaphylaxis) to this product or any of its components.

Warnings/Precautions

➤*Cardiovascular effects:*

Decreased left ventricular ejection fraction – Lapatinib has been reported to decrease LVEF. In clinical trials, the majority (more than 57%) of LVEF decreases occurred within the first 12 weeks of treatment; however, data on long-term exposure are limited. Use caution if lapatinib is to be administered to patients with conditions that could impair left ventricular function. Evaluate LVEF in all patients prior to initiation of treatment with lapatinib to ensure that the patient has a baseline LVEF that is within the institution's normal limits. Continue to evaluate LVEF during treatment with lapatinib to ensure that LVEF does not decline below the institution's normal limits.

QT prolongation – QT prolongation was observed in an uncontrolled, open-label, dose-escalation study of lapatinib in advanced cancer patients. Administer lapatinib with caution to patients who have or may develop prolongation of QTc. These conditions include patients with hypokalemia or hypomagnesemia, congenital long QT syndrome, therapy with antiarrhythmic medicines or other medicinal products that lead to QT prolongation, and cumulative high-dose anthracycline therapy. Correct hypokalemia or hypomagnesemia prior to lapatinib administration.

➤*Hepatotoxicity:* Hepatotoxicity (ALT or AST more than 3 times the upper limit of normal [ULN] and total bilirubin more than 2 times the ULN) has been observed in clinical trials (less than 1% of patients) and postmarketing experience. The hepatotoxicity may be severe and deaths have been

LAPATINIB DITOSYLATE — ORAL

reported. Causality of the deaths is uncertain. The hepatotoxicity may occur days to several months after initiation of treatment. Monitor liver function tests (transaminases, bilirubin, alkaline phosphatase) before initiation of treatment, every 4 to 6 weeks during treatment, and as clinically indicated. If changes in liver function are severe, discontinue therapy with lapatinib and do not re-treat patients with lapatinib.

➤*GI effects:* Diarrhea, including severe diarrhea, has been reported during treatment with lapatinib. Proactive management of diarrhea with antidiarrheal agents is important. Severe cases of diarrhea may require administration of oral or intravenous (IV) electrolytes and fluids and interruption or discontinuation of therapy with lapatinib.

➤*Interstitial lung disease/pneumonitis:* Lapatinib has been associated with interstitial lung disease and pneumonitis in monotherapy or in combination with other chemotherapies. Monitor patients for pulmonary symptoms indicative of interstitial lung disease or pneumonitis. Discontinue lapatinib in patients who experience pulmonary symptoms indicative of interstitial lung disease/pneumonitis that are at least grade 3 (NCI-CTCAE).

➤*Hepatic function impairment:* Use caution when administering lapatinib to patients with severe hepatic impairment because of increased exposure to the drug. Consider a dosage reduction for patients with severe preexisting hepatic impairment. In patients who develop severe hepatotoxicity while on therapy, discontinue lapatinib and do not re-treat patients with lapatinib.

➤*Pregnancy: Category D.* There are no adequate and well-controlled studies with lapatinib in pregnant women. Advise women not to become pregnant when taking lapatinib. If this drug is used during pregnancy, or if the patient becomes pregnant while taking this drug, apprise the patient of the potential hazard to the fetus.

Based on findings in animals, lapatinib can cause fetal harm when administered to a pregnant woman. Lapatinib administered to rats during organogenesis and through lactation led to death of offspring within the first 4 days after birth. When administered to pregnant animals during the period of organogenesis, lapatinib caused fetal anomalies (rats) or abortions (rabbits) at maternally toxic doses.

In a study in which pregnant rats were dosed with lapatinib during organogenesis and through lactation, at a dosage of 120 mg/kg/day (approximately 6.4 times the human clinical exposure based on AUC following a 1,250 mg dose of lapatinib plus capecitabine), 91% of the pups died by day 4 after birth, while 34% of the 60 mg/kg/day pups died. The highest no-effect dose for this study was 20 mg/kg/day (approximately equal to the human clinical exposure based on AUC).

Minor anomalies (eg, left-sided umbilical artery, cervical rib, precocious ossification) occurred in rats at the maternally toxic dose of 120 mg/kg/day (approximately 6.4 times the human clinical exposure based on AUC following a 1,250 mg dose of lapatinib plus capecitabine). In rabbits, lapatinib was associated with maternal toxicity at 60 and 120 mg/kg/day (approximately 0.07 and 0.2 times the human clinical exposure, respectively, based on AUC following a 1,250 mg dose of lapatinib plus capecitabine) and abortions at 120 mg/kg/day. Maternal toxicity was associated with decreased fetal body weights and minor skeletal variations.

➤*Lactation:* It is not known whether lapatinib is excreted in human milk. Because many drugs are excreted in human milk and because of the potential for serious adverse reactions in breast-feeding infants from lapatinib, make a decision whether to discontinue breast-feeding or the drug, taking into account the importance of the drug to the mother.

➤*Children:* The safety and efficacy of lapatinib in children have not been established.

➤*Elderly:* No overall differences in safety or effectiveness were observed between these subjects and younger subjects, and other reported clinical experience has not identified differences in responses between elderly and younger patients, but greater sensitivity of some older individuals cannot be ruled out.

➤*Monitoring:* Evaluate LVEF throughout use. Monitor pulmonary symptoms indicative of interstitial lung disease or pneumonitis. Monitor liver function tests (alkaline phosphatase, bilirubin, transaminases) before initiation of treatment, every 4 to 6 weeks during treatment, and as clinically indicated. If changes in liver function are severe, discontinue therapy with lapatinib and do not re-treat patients with lapatinib.

Drug Interactions

➤*Cytochrome P450 system:* Because lapatinib is metabolized mainly by the CYP3A4 enzyme systems, substances known to inhibit these enzymes may decrease metabolism or increase bioavailability of lapatinib, as indicated by increased whole blood or plasma concentrations. Drugs known to induce these enzyme systems may result in an increased metabolism of lapatinib or decreased bioavailability, as indicated by decreased whole blood or plasma concentrations. Monitoring of blood concentrations and appropriate dosage adjustments are essential when such drugs are used concomitantly.

Lapatinib inhibits CYP3A4 and CYP2C8 in vitro. Use caution and consider dose reduction when a concomitant substrate drug with a narrow therapeutic index is administered with lapatinib. Lapatinib did not inhibit human liver microsomes CYP1A2, CYP2C9, CYP2C19, and CYP2C6 or UGT enzymes in vitro; however, the clinical relevance is unknown. Lapatinib inhibits P-gp. Plasma concentrations of drugs that are P-gp substrates may be increased and be administered with caution. Lapatinib is a substrate of P-gp. Administration of lapatinib with drugs that inhibit P-gp may increase lapatinib concentrations; use with caution.

➤*QT prolongation:* An additive effect of lapatinib with other drugs that prolong the QT interval cannot be excluded. The following drugs may prolong the QT interval and increase the risk of life-threatening cardiac arrhythmias, including torsades de pointes: antiarrhythmic agents (eg, amiodarone, bretylium, disopyramide, dofetilide, procainamide, quinidine, sotalol), arsenic trioxide, chlorpromazine, cisapride, dolasetron, droperidol, gatifloxacin, halofantrine, levomethadyl, mefloquine, mesoridazine, moxifloxacin, pentamidine, pimozide, probucol, sparfloxacin, thioridazine, and ziprasidone. (See Drug-Induced Prolongation of the QT Interval and Torsades de Pointes.)

Lapatinib Drug Interactions

Precipitant drug	Object drug[a]		Description
Drugs that prolong the QT interval (eg, chloroquine, iloperidone, lithium, macrolide antibiotics [eg, azithromycin, clarithromycin, erythromycin], maprotiline, methadone, paliperidone, perflutren, tacrolimus, telithromycin)	Lapatinib	↑	Possible additive QT prolongation may increase the risk of life-threatening cardiac arrhythmias, including torsades de pointes. Use lapatinib with caution in patients who are taking antiarrhythmic agents or other drugs that produce QT prolongation.
Lapatinib	Drugs that prolong the QT interval (eg, chloroquine, iloperidone, lithium, macrolide antibiotics [eg, azithromycin, clarithromycin, erythromycin], maprotiline, methadone, paliperidone, perflutren, tacrolimus)		
Modafinil	Lapatinib	↓	Lapatinib concentrations may be reduced, decreasing antineoplastic efficacy. An increase in the lapatinib dose may be needed. Monitor the patient and adjust the lapatinib dose as indicated.
Nevirapine	Lapatinib	↓	Lapatinib concentrations may be reduced, decreasing antineoplastic efficacy. An increase in the lapatinib dose may be needed. Monitor the patient and adjust the lapatinib dose as indicated.
P-gp inhibitors (eg, amiodarone, cyclosporine, felodipine, nicardipine, propafenone, quinidine, tacrolimus, tamoxifen, testosterone)	Lapatinib	↑	Lapatinib concentrations and toxicity may be increased. Avoid combination. If coadministration cannot be avoided, carefully monitor patients during concomitant therapy and adjust lapatinib dose as needed.
Strong CYP3A4 inducers (eg, barbiturates, carbamazepine, dexamethasone, griseofulvin, phenytoin, rifamycins [eg, rifabutin, rifampin, rifapentine], St. John's wort)	Lapatinib	↓	Lapatinib concentrations may be reduced, decreasing antineoplastic efficacy. Carbamazepine reduces lapatinib exposure by 72%. Avoid coadministration. If coadministration cannot be avoided, consider increasing the lapatinib dose in gradual increments up to 4,500 mg/day (HER2-positive metastatic breast cancer indication) or up to 5,500 mg/day (hormone receptor–positive, HER2-positive breast cancer indication). Monitor for efficacy and toxicity. Once the inducer is discontinued, immediately reduce lapatinib to the labeled dose.

LAPATINIB DITOSYLATE — ORAL

Lapatinib Drug Interactions			
Precipitant drug	Object drug[a]		Description
Strong CYP3A4 inhibitors (eg, clarithromycin, itraconazole, ketoconazole, nefazodone, protease inhibitors [eg, atazanavir, indinavir, nelfinavir, ritonavir, saquinavir], telithromycin, voriconazole)	Lapatinib	↑	Lapatinib concentrations and toxicity may be increased. Ketoconazole increases lapatinib exposure almost 4-fold. Avoid coadministration. If coadministration of a strong CYP3A4 inhibitor cannot be avoided, monitor patients and consider reducing the lapatinib dose to 500 mg/day during concomitant therapy. Once the inhibitor is discontinued, then titrate lapatinib up to the labeled dose.
Lapatinib	Drugs metabolized by P-gp (eg, cyclosporine, digoxin, fexofenadine, loperamide, loratadine, ritonavir, sirolimus, tacrolimus)	↑	Lapatinib may reduce metabolism of these agents, resulting in increased concentrations and toxicity. Carefully monitor patients during concomitant therapy and adjust the dose of the other agent as needed.
Lapatinib	Paclitaxel	↑	Paclitaxel 24-hour exposure (AUC) was increased 23% with coadministration of lapatinib. This increase may have been underestimated because of study design limitations.

[a] ↑ = object drug increased; ↓ = object drug decreased.

➤*Drug/Food interactions:* Systemic exposure to lapatinib is increased when administered with food. Lapatinib AUC values were approximately 3- and 4-fold higher when administered with a low-fat meal or a high-fat meal, respectively. Lapatinib should be taken at least 1 hour before or after a meal.

Grapefruit juice may increase lapatinib concentrations and toxicity. Avoid combination.

Adverse Reactions

➤*HER2-positive metastatic breast cancer:*

Most common – The most common adverse reactions (more than 20%) during therapy with lapatinib plus capecitabine were GI (diarrhea, nausea, and vomiting), dermatologic (palmar-plantar erythrodysesthesia and rash), and fatigue. Diarrhea was the most common adverse reaction resulting in discontinuation of study medication.

The most common grade 3 and 4 adverse reactions (NCI-CTCAE, version 3) were diarrhea and palmar-plantar erythrodysesthesia.

Lapatinib Adverse Reactions (≥ 10%) in HER2-Positive Metastatic Breast Cancer						
	Lapatinib 1,250 mg/day + capecitabine 2,000 mg/m²/day (n = 198)			Capecitabine 2,500 mg/m²/day (n = 191)		
Adverse reactions	All grades[a]	Grade 3	Grade 4	All grades[a]	Grade 3	Grade 4
Dermatologic						
Dry skin	10%	0%	0%	6%	0%	0%
Palmar-plantar erythrodysesthesia	53%	12%	0%	51%	14%	0%
Rash[b]	28%	2%	0%	14%	1%	0%
GI						
Diarrhea	65%	13%	1%	40%	10%	0%
Dyspepsia	11%	< 1%	0%	3%	0%	0%
Nausea	44%	2%	0%	43%	2%	0%
Stomatitis	14%	0%	0%	11%	< 1%	0%
Vomiting	26%	2%	0%	21%	2%	0%
Musculoskeletal						
Back pain	11%	1%	0%	6%	< 1%	0%
Pain in extremity	12%	1%	0%	7%	< 1%	0%
Miscellaneous						
Dyspnea	12%	3%	0%	8%	2%	0%
Insomnia	10%	< 1%	0%	6%	0%	0%
Mucosal inflammation	15%	0%	0%	12%	2%	0%

[a] NCI-CTCAE, version 3.
[b] Grade 3 dermatitis acneiform was reported in less than 1% of patients in the lapatinib plus capecitabine group.

➤*Lab test abnormalities:*

HER2-positive metastatic breast cancer –

Lapatinib Laboratory Abnormalities in HER2-Positive Metastatic Breast Cancer						
	Lapatinib 1,250 mg/day + capecitabine 2,000 mg/m²/day			Capecitabine 2,500 mg/m²/day		
Parameters	All grades[a]	Grade 3	Grade 4	All grades[a]	Grade 3	Grade 4
Hematologic						
Hemoglobin	56%	< 1%	0%	53%	1%	0%
Neutrophils	22%	3%	< 1%	31%	2%	1%
Platelets	18%	< 1%	0%	17%	< 1%	< 1%
Hepatic						
ALT	37%	2%	0%	33%	1%	0%
AST	49%	2%	< 1%	43%	2%	0%
Total bilirubin	45%	4%	0%	30%	3%	0%

[a] NCI-CTC, version 3.

Hormone receptor-positive metastatic breast cancer –

Lapatinib Adverse Reactions (≥ 10%) in Hormone Receptor-Positive Metastatic Breast Cancer						
	Lapatinib 1,500 mg/day + letrozole 2.5 mg/day (n = 654)			Letrozole 2.5 mg/day (n = 624)		
Adverse reactions	All grades[a]	Grade 3	Grade 4	All grades[a]	Grade 3	Grade 4
CNS						
Asthenia	12%	< 1%	0%	11%	< 1%	0%
Fatigue	20%	2%	0%	17%	< 1%	0%
Headache	14%	< 1%	0%	13%	< 1%	0%
Dermatologic						
Alopecia	13%	< 1%	0%	7%	0%	0%
Dry skin	13%	< 1%	0%	4%	0%	0%
Nail disorder	11%	< 1%	0%	< 1%	0%	0%
Pruritus	12%	< 1%	0%	9%	< 1%	0%
Rash[b]	44%	1%	0%	13%	0%	0%
GI disorders						
Anorexia	11%	< 1%	0%	9%	< 1%	0%
Diarrhea	64%	9%	< 1%	20%	< 1%	0%
Nausea	31%	< 1%	0%	21%	< 1%	0%
Vomiting	17%	1%	< 1%	11%	< 1%	< 1%
Miscellaneous						
Epistaxis	11%	< 1%	0%	2%	< 1%	0%

[a] NCI-CTCAE, version 3.
[b] In addition to the rash reported under "Dermatologic," 3 additional patients in each treatment arm had rash under "infections and infestations"; none were grade 3 or 4.

LAPATINIB DITOSYLATE — ORAL

➤*Lab test abnormalities:*

Hormone receptor–positive metastatic breast cancer –

Lapatinib Laboratory Abnormalities in Hormone Receptor–Positive Metastatic Breast Cancer						
	Lapatinib 1,500 mg/day + letrozole 2.5 mg/day			Letrozole 2.5 mg/day		
	All grades[a]	Grade 3	Grade 4	All grades[a]	Grade 3	Grade 4
Hepatic						
AST	53%	6%	0%	36%	2%	< 1%
ALT	46%	5%	< 1%	35%	1%	0%
Total bilirubin	22%	< 1%	< 1%	11%	1%	< 1%

[a] NCI-CTCAE. version 3.

➤*Decreases in left ventricular ejection fraction:* Because of potential cardiac toxicity with HER2 (ErbB2) inhibitors, LVEF was monitored in clinical trials at approximately 8-week intervals. LVEF decreases were defined as signs or symptoms of deterioration in left ventricular cardiac function that are of at least grade 3 (NCI-CTCAE), or at least a 20% decrease in left ventricular cardiac ejection fraction relative to baseline, which is below the institution's lower limit of normal.

Among 198 patients who received lapatinib/capecitabine combination treatment, three experienced grade 2 and one had grade 3 LVEF adverse reactions (NCI-CTC, version 3). Among 654 patients who received lapatinib/letrozole combination treatment, 26 patients experienced grade 1 or 2 and 6 patients had grade 3 or 4 LVEF adverse reactions.

➤*Hepatic:* See Warnings/Precautions for more information.

➤*Respiratory:* See Warnings/Precautions for more information.

➤*Postmarketing:*

Dermatologic – Nail disorders include paronychia.

Hypersensitivity – Hypersensitivity reactions include anaphylaxis.

Overdosage

➤*Symptoms:* There has been a report of 1 patient who took lapatinib 3,000 mg for 10 days. This patient had grade 3 diarrhea and vomiting on day 10.

➤*Treatment:* The overdose event previously mentioned resolved following IV hydration and interruption of treatment with lapatinib and letrozole. There is no known antidote for overdoses of lapatinib. Because lapatinib is not significantly renally excreted and is highly bound to plasma proteins, hemodialysis would not be expected to be an effective method to enhance the elimination of lapatinib.

Patient Information

Inform patients that lapatinib has been reported to decrease LVEF, which may result in shortness of breath, palpitations, and/or fatigue. Instruct patients to inform their health care provider if they develop these symptoms while taking lapatinib.

Inform patients that lapatinib often causes diarrhea, which may be severe in some cases. Advise patients on how to manage and/or prevent diarrhea, and instruct them to inform their health care provider if severe diarrhea occurs during treatment with lapatinib.

Lapatinib may interact with many drugs; therefore, advise patients to report to their health care provider the use of any other prescription or nonprescription medication or herbal products.

Inform patients of the importance of taking lapatinib at least 1 hour before or 1 hour after a meal.

Advise patients not to take lapatinib with grapefruit or grapefruit products.

Inform patients to take the dose of lapatinib once daily. Dividing the daily dose is not recommended.

PAZOPANIB

Rx	**Votrient** (GlaxoSmithKline)	**Tablets; oral:** 200 mg	Equiv. to pazopanib hydrochloride 216.7 mg. (GS JT). Gray, capsule shape. Film-coated. In 30s, 90s, and 120s.

PAZOPANIB HYDROCHLORIDE — ORAL

WARNING

Hepatotoxicity – Severe and fatal hepatotoxicity has been observed in clinical studies. Monitor hepatic function and interrupt, reduce, or discontinue dosing as recommended.

Indications

➤*Renal cell carcinoma:* For the treatment of patients with advanced renal cell carcinoma.

Administration and Dosage

➤*Adults:*

Renal cell carcinoma –

Usual dosage: 800 mg orally once daily without food (at least 1 hour before or 2 hours after a meal).

Maximum dose: 800 mg once daily.

Dosage adjustment: Initial dose reduction should be 400 mg, and additional dose decrease or increase should be in 200 mg steps based on individual tolerability.

Concomitant therapy:

• *Strong CYP3A4 inhibitors* – The concomitant use of strong CYP3A4 inhibitors (eg, clarithromycin, ketoconazole, ritonavir) may increase pazopanib concentrations and should be avoided. If coadministration of a strong CYP3A4 inhibitor is warranted, reduce the dose of pazopanib to 400 mg. Further dose reductions may be needed if adverse effects occur during therapy. This dose is predicted to adjust the pazopanib area under the curve (AUC) to the range observed without inhibitors. However, there are no clinical data with this dose adjustment in patients receiving strong CYP3A4 inhibitors.

• *Strong CYP3A4 inducer* – The concomitant use of strong CYP3A4 inducers (eg, rifampin) may decrease pazopanib concentrations and should be avoided. Pazopanib should not be used in patients who cannot avoid long-term use of strong CYP3A4 inducers.

➤*Hepatic function impairment:*

Moderate hepatic impairment – 200 mg/day.

Severe hepatic impairment – Use is not recommended.

➤*Administration:* Administer once daily without food (at least 1 hour before or 2 hours after a meal).

Do not crush tablets because of the potential for increased rate of absorption, which may affect systemic exposure.

➤*Storage/Stability:* Store at 25°C (77°F); excursions are permitted to 15° to 30°C (59° to 86°F).

Actions

➤*Pharmacology:* Pazopanib is a multi-tyrosine kinase inhibitor of vascular endothelial growth factor receptor (VEGFR)–1, VEGFR-2, VEGFR-3, platelet-derived growth factor receptor (PDGFR)–alpha and -beta, fibroblast growth factor receptor-1 and -3, cytokine receptor (Kit), interleukin-2 receptor inducible T-cell kinase, leukocyte-specific protein tyrosine kinase, and transmembrane glycoprotein receptor tyrosine kinase. In vitro, pazopanib inhibited ligand-induced autophosphorylation of VEGFR-2, Kit, and PDGFR-beta receptors. In vivo, pazopanib inhibited VEGF-induced VEGFR-2 phosphorylation in mouse lungs, angiogenesis in a mouse model, and the growth of some human tumor xenografts in mice.

➤*Pharmacokinetics:*

Absorption – Pazopanib is absorbed orally with median time to achieve peak concentrations of 2 to 4 hours after the dose. Daily dosing at 800 mg results in geometric mean AUC and maximal drug concentration (C_{max}) of 1,037 h•mcg/mL and 58.1 mcg/mL (equivalent to 132 mcM), respectively. There was no consistent increase in AUC or C_{max} at pazopanib doses above 800 mg.

Administration of a single pazopanib 400 mg crushed tablet increased $AUC_{(0-72)}$ by 46% and C_{max} by approximately 2-fold and decreased time of maximum concentration (T_{max}) by approximately 2 hours compared with administration of the whole tablet. These results indicate that the bioavailability and the rate of pazopanib oral absorption are increased after administration of the crushed tablet relative to administration of the whole tablet. Therefore, because of this potential for increased exposure, tablets of pazopanib should not be crushed.

Effect of food: Systemic exposure to pazopanib is increased when administered with food. Administration of pazopanib with a high-fat or low-fat meal results in an approximately 2-fold increase in AUC and C_{max}. Therefore, pazopanib should be administered at least 1 hour before or 2 hours after a meal.

Distribution – Binding of pazopanib to human plasma protein in vivo was greater than 99% with no concentration dependence over the range of 10 to 100 mcg/mL. In vitro studies suggest that pazopanib is a substrate for P-glycoprotein and breast cancer resistant protein.

Metabolism – In vitro studies demonstrated that pazopanib is metabolized by CYP3A4 with a minor contribution from CYP1A2 and CYP2C8.

Excretion – Pazopanib has a mean half-life of 30.9 hours after administration of the recommended dose of 800 mg. Elimination is primarily via feces with renal elimination accounting for less than 4% of the administered dose.

Special populations –

Hepatic function impairment: Pharmacokinetic data from patients with healthy hepatic function (n = 12) and moderate (n = 7) hepatic impairment indicate that pazopanib clearance was decreased by 50% in those with moderate hepatic impairment. The maximum tolerated pazopanib dosage in

PAZOPANIB HYDROCHLORIDE — ORAL

patients with moderate hepatic impairment is 200 mg once daily. There are no data on patients with mild or severe hepatic impairment.

Contraindications

None known.

Warnings/Precautions

➤*Hepatic effects:* In clinical trials with pazopanib, hepatotoxicity, manifested as increases in serum transaminases (ALT, AST) and bilirubin, was observed. This hepatotoxicity can be severe and fatal. Transaminase elevations occur early in the course of treatment (92.5% of all transaminase elevations of any grade occurred in the first 18 weeks). Across all monotherapy studies with pazopanib, ALT greater than 3 × upper limit of normal (ULN) was reported in 14% and ALT greater than 8 × ULN was reported in 4% of patients who received pazopanib. Concurrent elevations in ALT greater than 3 × ULN and bilirubin greater than 2 × ULN regardless of alkaline phosphatase levels were detected in 1% of patients. Four of the 13 patients had no other explanation for these elevations. Out of 977 patients, 0.2% died with disease progression and hepatic failure.

Monitor serum liver tests before initiation of treatment with pazopanib and at least once every 4 weeks for at least the first 4 months of treatment or as clinically indicated. Continue periodic monitoring after this time period.

Patients with isolated ALT elevations between 3 × ULN and 8 × ULN may be continued on pazopanib with weekly monitoring of liver function until ALT return to grade 1 or baseline.

Patients with isolated ALT elevations of greater than 8 × ULN should have pazopanib interrupted until they return to grade 1 or baseline. If the potential benefit for reinitiating treatment with pazopanib is considered to outweigh the risk for hepatotoxicity, then reintroduce pazopanib at a reduced dosage of no more than 400 mg once daily and measure serum liver tests weekly for 8 weeks. Following reintroduction of pazopanib, if ALT elevations greater than 3 × ULN recur, then pazopanib should be permanently discontinued.

Permanently discontinue pazopanib if ALT elevations greater than 3 × ULN occur concurrently with bilirubin elevations greater than 2 × ULN. Monitor patients until resolution. Pazopanib is a UGT1A1 inhibitor. Mild, indirect (unconjugated) hyperbilirubinemia may occur in patients with Gilbert syndrome. Monitor patients with only a mild, indirect hyperbilirubinemia, known Gilbert syndrome, and elevation in ALT greater than 3 × ULN as per the recommendations outlined for isolated ALT elevations.

The safety of pazopanib in patients with preexisting severe hepatic impairment, defined as total bilirubin greater than 3 × ULN with any level of ALT, is unknown. Treatment with pazopanib is not recommended in patients with severe hepatic impairment.

➤*QT prolongation and torsades de pointes:* In clinical renal cell carcinoma studies of pazopanib, QT prolongation (500 msec or more) was identified on routine ECG monitoring in less than 2% of patients. Torsades de pointes occurred in less than 1% of patients who received pazopanib in the monotherapy studies.

In the randomized clinical trial, 3 of the 290 patients receiving pazopanib had postbaseline values between 500 to 549 msec. None of the 145 patients receiving placebo had postbaseline QTc values of 500 msec or more.

Use pazopanib with caution in patients with a history of QT interval prolongation, in patients taking antiarrhythmics or other medications that may prolong QT interval, and those with relevant preexisting cardiac disease. When using pazopanib, perform baseline and periodic monitoring of ECGs and maintenance of electrolytes (eg, calcium, magnesium, potassium) within the normal range.

➤*Hemorrhage:* In clinical renal cell carcinoma studies of pazopanib, hemorrhagic events have been reported (all grades [16%] and grades 3 to 5 [2%]). Fatal hemorrhage has occurred in 0.9% of patients. Pazopanib has not been studied in patients who have a history of hemoptysis, cerebral, or clinically significant GI hemorrhage in the past 6 months and should not be used in those patients.

➤*Cardiovascular effects:* In clinical renal cell carcinoma studies of pazopanib, myocardial infarction, angina, ischemic stroke, and transient ischemic attack (all grades [3%] and grades 3 to 5 [2%]) were observed. Fatal events have been observed in 0.3% of patients. In the randomized study, these events were observed more frequently with pazopanib compared with placebo. Use pazopanib with caution in patients who are at increased risk for these events or who have had a history of these events. Pazopanib has not been studied in patients who have had an event within the previous 6 months and should not be used in those patients.

➤*GI effects:* In clinical renal cell carcinoma studies of pazopanib, GI perforation or fistula has been reported in 0.9% of patients. Fatal perforation events have occurred in 0.3% of patients. Monitor for symptoms of GI perforation or fistula.

➤*Hypertension:* Blood pressure should be well-controlled prior to initiating pazopanib. Monitor and treat patients for hypertension as needed with antihypertensive therapy. Hypertension (systolic blood pressure 150 or more or diastolic blood pressure 100 mm Hg or more) was observed in 47% of patients with renal cell carcinoma treated with pazopanib. Hypertension occurs early in the course of treatment (88% occurred in the first 18 weeks). In the case of persistent hypertension despite antihypertensive therapy, the dose of pazopanib may be reduced. Discontinue pazopanib if hypertension is severe and persistent despite antihypertensive therapy and dose reduction of pazopanib.

➤*Wound healing:* No formal studies on the effect of pazopanib on wound healing have been conducted. Because VEGFR inhibitors, such as pazopanib, may impair wound healing, stop treatment with pazopanib at least 7 days prior to scheduled surgery. Base the decision to resume pazopanib after surgery on clinical judgment of adequate wound healing. Discontinue pazopanib in patients with wound dehiscence.

➤*Hypothyroidism:* In clinical renal cell carcinoma studies of pazopanib, hypothyroidism was reported as an adverse reaction in 4% of patients. Proactive monitoring of thyroid function tests is recommended.

➤*Proteinuria:* In clinical renal cell carcinoma studies with pazopanib, proteinuria has been reported in 8% of patients (grade 3, 5/586 [less than 1%] and grade 4, 1/586 [less than 1%]). Baseline and periodic urinalysis during treatment is recommended. Discontinue pazopanib if the patient develops grade 4 proteinuria.

➤*Hepatic function impairment:* See Actions for more information.

See Actions for more information.

➤*Pregnancy: Category D.* Pazopanib can cause fetal harm when administered to a pregnant woman. There are no adequate and well-controlled studies of pazopanib in pregnant women.

If this drug is used during pregnancy, or if the patient becomes pregnant while taking this drug, apprise the patient of the potential hazard to the fetus. Advise women of childbearing potential to avoid becoming pregnant while taking pazopanib.

Based on its mechanism of action, pazopanib is expected to result in adverse reproductive effects. In preclinical studies in rats and rabbits, pazopanib was teratogenic, embryotoxic, fetotoxic, and abortifacient. Administration of pazopanib to pregnant rats during organogenesis at a dosage level of 3 mg/kg/day or more (approximately 0.1 times the human clinical exposure based on AUC) resulted in teratogenic effects including cardiovascular malformations (retroesophageal subclavian artery, missing innominate artery, changes in the aortic arch) and incomplete or absent ossification. In addition, there was reduced fetal body weight, and pre- and postimplantation embryolethality in rats administered pazopanib at dosages of 3 mg/kg/day or more. In rabbits, maternal toxicity (reduced food consumption, increased postimplantation loss, and abortion) was observed at dosages of 30 mg/kg/day or more (approximately 0.007 times the human clinical exposure). In addition, severe maternal body weight loss and 100% litter loss were observed at dosages of 100 mg/kg/day or more (0.02 times the human clinical exposure), while fetal weight was reduced at dosages of 3 mg/kg/day or more (AUC not calculated).

➤*Lactation:* It is not known whether this drug is excreted in human milk. Because many drugs are excreted in human milk and because of the potential for serious adverse reactions in breast-feeding infants from pazopanib, a decision should be made whether to discontinue breast-feeding or to discontinue the drug, taking into account the importance of the drug to the mother.

➤*Children:* The safety and effectiveness of pazopanib in children have not been established.

➤*Elderly:* Patients older than 60 years of age may be at greater risk for an ALT greater than 3 × ULN. Other reported clinical experience has not identified differences in responses between elderly and younger patients, but greater sensitivity of some older individuals cannot be ruled out.

➤*Monitoring:* Monitor serum liver tests before initiation of treatment with pazopanib and at least once every 4 weeks for at least the first 4 months of treatment or as clinically indicated. Continue periodic monitoring after this time period. Perform baseline and periodic monitoring of ECGs and maintenance of electrolytes (eg, calcium, magnesium, potassium) within the normal range. Monitor for symptoms of GI perforation or fistula. Monitor patients for hypertension and treat as needed with antihypertensive therapy. Proactive monitoring of thyroid function tests is recommended. Baseline and periodic urinalysis during treatment is recommended.

Drug Interactions

➤*Cytochrome P-450 system:* Because pazopanib is metabolized mainly by the CYP3A enzyme systems, substances known to inhibit these enzymes may decrease metabolism or increase bioavailability of pazopanib, as indicated by increased whole blood or plasma concentrations. Drugs known to induce these enzyme systems may result in an increased metabolism of pazopanib or decreased bioavailability, as indicated by decreased whole blood or plasma concentrations. Monitoring of blood concentrations and appropriate dosage adjustments are essential when such drugs are used concomitantly. Pazopanib is a weak inhibitor of CYP3A4, CYP2C8, and CYP2D6, and coadministration with agents that have a narrow therapeutic index and that are metabolized by these enzymes is not recommended. Pazopanib has no effect on CYP1A2, CYP2C9, or CYP2C19.

➤*OATP1B1 and UGT1A1 transporters:* In vitro studies indicate that pazopanib inhibits OATP1B1 and UGT1A1. Pazopanib may increase plasma concentrations of drugs eliminated by OATP1B1 and UGT1A1.

➤*QT prolongation:* An additive effect of pazopanib with other drugs that prolong the QT interval cannot be excluded. The following drugs may prolong the QT interval and increase the risk of life-threatening cardiac arrhythmias, including torsade de pointes: antiarrhythmic agents (eg, amiodarone, bretylium, disopyramide, dofetilide, procainamide, quinidine, sotalol), arsenic trioxide, chlorpromazine, cisapride, dolasetron, droperidol, gatifloxacin, halofantrine, levomethadyl, mefloquine, mesoridazine, moxifloxacin, pentamidine, pimozide, probucol, sparfloxacin, thioridazine, ziprasidone. (See the appendix, Drug-Induced Prolongation of the QT Interval and Torsades De Pointes.)

PAZOPANIB HYDROCHLORIDE — ORAL

Pazopanib Drug Interactions

Precipitant drug	Object drug[a]		Description
Drugs that prolong the QT interval (eg, antiarrhythmic agents)	Pazopanib	↑	Additive QT interval prolongation may occur, increasing the risk of cardiac arrhythmias, including torsades de pointes. Coadminister with caution. Monitor patients for QT prolongation.
Pazopanib	Drugs that prolong the QT interval (eg, antiarrhythmic agents)		
Grapefruit juice	Pazopanib	↑	Pazopanib plasma concentrations may be elevated, increasing the pharmacologic effects and risk of adverse reactions. Patients should avoid grapefruit juice.
Lapatinib	Pazopanib	↑	When pazopanib 800 mg was administered with lapatinib 1,500 mg, the pazopanib AUC and C_{max} increased approximately 50% to 60% compared with taking pazopanib alone. Observe patients for adverse reactions. Reduce the pazopanib dose as needed.
Strong CYP3A4 inducers (eg, rifampin)	Pazopanib	↓	Pazopanib plasma concentrations may be reduced, decreasing the efficacy. Avoid coadministration. Pazopanib should not be given to patients who cannot avoid long-term use of strong CYP3A4 inducers.
Strong CYP3A4 inhibitors (eg, clarithromycin, ketoconazole, ritonavir)	Pazopanib	↑	Pazopanib plasma concentrations may be elevated, increasing the pharmacologic effects and risk of adverse reactions. Avoid coadministration. If coadministration cannot be avoided, reduce the pazopanib dosage to 400 mg once daily. Observe patients for adverse reactions and further reduce the pazopanib dose if needed.
Pazopanib	Agents with a narrow therapeutic index metabolized by CYP3A4 (eg, cyclosporine), CYP2C8, or CYP2D6	↑	Plasma concentrations of these agents may be elevated, increasing the pharmacologic effects and risk of adverse reactions. Coadministration is not recommended.
Pazopanib	Midazolam	↑	Coadministration of midazolam and pazopanib increased the midazolam AUC and C_{max} approximately 30%. Observe patient response. If an interaction is suspected, adjust the midazolam dose as needed.
Pazopanib	Paclitaxel	↑	Coadministration of pazopanib 800 mg once daily and paclitaxel 80 mg/m^2 once weekly increased the mean paclitaxel AUC and C_{max} 26% and 31%, respectively. Observe patient response. If an interaction is suspected, adjust the paclitaxel dose as needed.

[a] ↑ = object drug increased; ↓ = object drug decreased.

➤*Drug/Lab test interactions:* No laboratory test abnormalities related to the use of pazopanib have been identified.

➤*Drug/Food interactions:* Systemic exposure to pazopanib is increased when taken with food. Administration of pazopanib with a high- or low-fat meal increases the pazopanib C_{max} and AUC approximately 2-fold. Pazopanib should be taken at least 1 hour before or 2 hours after a meal.

Adverse Reactions

➤*Dosage adjustment:* The safety profile of pazopanib was described in 290 renal cell carcinoma patients who participated in a randomized, double-blind, placebo-controlled study. Forty-two percent of patients on pazopanib required a dose interruption. Thirty-six percent of patients on pazopanib were dose reduced.

➤*Serious adverse reactions:* Potentially serious adverse reactions with pazopanib include hepatotoxicity, QT prolongation and torsades de pointes, hemorrhagic events, arterial thrombotic events, and GI perforation and fistula.

Pazopanib Adverse Reactions (≥ 10%)

Adverse reactions	Pazopanib (n = 290)			Placebo (n = 145)		
	All grades[a]	Grade 3	Grade 4	All grades[a]	Grade 3	Grade 4
CNS						
Asthenia	14%	3%	0%	8%	0%	0%
Fatigue	19%	2%	0%	8%	1%	1%
Headache	10%	0%	0%	5%	0%	0%
GI						
Abdominal pain	11%	2%	0%	1%	0%	0%
Anorexia	22%	2%	0%	10%	< 1%	0%
Diarrhea	52%	3%	< 1%	9%	< 1%	0%
Nausea	26%	< 1%	0%	9%	0%	0%
Vomiting	21%	2%	< 1%	8%	2%	0%
Hematologic						
Leukopenia	37%	0%	0%	6%	0%	0%
Lymphocytopenia	31%	4%	< 1%	24%	1%	0%
Neutropenia	34%	1%	< 1%	6%	0%	0%
Thrombocytopenia	32%	< 1%	< 1%	5%	0%	< 1%
Lab test abnormalities						
ALT increased	53%	10%	2%	22%	1%	0%
AST increased	53%	7%	< 1%	19%	< 1%	0%
Glucose decreased	17%	0%	< 1%	3%	0%	0%
Glucose increased	41%	< 1%	0%	33%	1%	0%
Magnesium decreased	26%	< 1%	1%	14%	0%	0%
Phosphorus decreased	34%	4%	0%	11%	0%	0%
Sodium decreased	31%	4%	1%	24%	4%	0%
Total bilirubin increased	36%	3%	< 1%	10%	1%	< 1%
Miscellaneous						
Hair color changes	38%	< 1%	0%	3%	0%	0%
Hypertension	40%	4%	0%	10%	< 1%	0%

[a] National Cancer Institute Common Terminology Criteria for Adverse Events, version 3.

➤*Other adverse reactions (less than 10%):*

Dermatologic – Alopecia (8%), palmar-plantar erythrodysesthesia (6%), rash (8%), skin depigmentation (3%).

GI – Dysgeusia (8%), dyspepsia (5%).

Miscellaneous – Chest pain (5%), facial edema (1%), proteinuria (9%), weight decreased (9%).

➤*Hepatic toxicity:* In a controlled clinical study with pazopanib for the treatment of renal cell carcinoma, ALT greater than 3 × ULN was reported in 18% and 3% of the pazopanib and placebo groups, respectively. ALT greater than 10 × ULN was reported in 4% of patients who received pazopanib and in less than 1% of patients who received placebo. Concurrent elevation in ALT greater than 3 × ULN and bilirubin greater than 2 × ULN in the absence of significant alkaline phosphatase greater than 3 × ULN occurred in 2% of patients on pazopanib and 1% on placebo. See also Warnings/Precautions.

➤*Hypertension:* In a controlled clinical study with pazopanib for the treatment of renal cell carcinoma, 40% of patients receiving pazopanib compared with 10% of patients on placebo experienced hypertension. Grade 3 hypertension was reported in 4% of patients receiving pazopanib compared with less than 1% of patients on placebo. The majority of cases of hypertension were manageable with antihypertensive agents or dose reductions with less than 1% of patients permanently discontinuing treatment with pazopanib because of hypertension. In the overall safety population for renal cell carcinoma (n = 586), one patient had hypertensive crisis on pazopanib. See also Warnings/Precautions.

➤*QT prolongation and torsades de pointes:* In a controlled clinical study with pazopanib, QT prolongation (500 msec or more) was identified on routine ECG monitoring in 1% of patients treated with pazopanib compared with no patients on placebo. Torsades de pointes was reported in less than 1% of patients treated with pazopanib in the renal cell carcinoma studies. See also Warnings/Precautions.

PAZOPANIB HYDROCHLORIDE — ORAL

➤*Arterial thrombotic events:* In a controlled clinical study with pazopanib, the incidences of arterial thrombotic events, such as myocardial infarction/ischemia (2%), cerebral vascular accident (less than 1%), and transient ischemic attack (1%), were higher in patients treated with pazopanib compared with the placebo arm (0/145 for each event). See also Warnings/Precautions.

➤*Hemorrhage:* In a controlled clinical study with pazopanib, 13% of patients treated with pazopanib and 5% of patients on placebo experienced at least 1 hemorrhagic event. The most common hemorrhagic events in the patients treated with pazopanib were hematuria (4%), epistaxis (2%), hemoptysis (2%), and rectal hemorrhage (1%). Nine patients treated with pazopanib who had hemorrhagic events experienced serious events, including pulmonary, GI, and GU hemorrhage. Out of 290 patients, 1% treated with pazopanib died from hemorrhage compared with no patients on placebo. In the overall safety population in renal cell carcinoma (n = 586), cerebral/intracranial hemorrhage was observed in less than 1% patients treated with pazopanib. See also Warnings/Precautions.

➤*Hypothyroidism:* In a controlled clinical study with pazopanib, more patients had a shift from thyroid-stimulating hormone within the normal range at baseline to above the normal range at any postbaseline visit in pazopanib compared with the placebo arm (27% compared with 5%, respectively). Hypothyroidism was reported as an adverse reaction in 7% of patients treated with pazopanib and no patients in the placebo arm. See also Warnings/Precautions.

➤*Diarrhea:* Diarrhea occurred frequently and was predominantly mild to moderate in severity. Patients should be advised how to manage mild diarrhea and to notify their health care provider if moderate to severe diarrhea occurs so appropriate management can be implemented to minimize its impact.

➤*Proteinuria:* In the controlled clinical study with pazopanib, proteinuria has been reported as an adverse reaction in 9% of patients treated with pazopanib. In 2 patients, proteinuria led to discontinuation of treatment with pazopanib. See also Warnings/Precautions.

➤*Lipase elevations:* In a single-arm clinical study, increases in lipase values were observed for 27% of patients. Elevations in lipase as an adverse reaction were reported for 4% of patients and were grade 3 for 6 patients and grade 4 for 1 patient. In clinical renal cell carcinoma studies of pazopanib, clinical pancreatitis was observed in less than 1% of patients.

Overdosage

➤*Symptoms:* Pazopanib doses of up to 2,000 mg have been evaluated in clinical trials. Dose-limiting toxicity (grade 3 fatigue) and grade 3 hypertension were each observed in 1 of 3 patients dosed at 2,000 mg daily and 1,000 mg daily, respectively.

➤*Treatment:* Treatment of overdose with pazopanib should consist of general supportive measures. There is no specific antidote for overdosage of pazopanib. Hemodialysis is not expected to enhance the elimination of pazopanib because pazopanib is not significantly renally excreted and is highly bound to plasma proteins.

Patient Information

Instruct patients to read the Medication Guide before starting pazopanib therapy and to reread it with each refill.

Instruct patients to take the prescribed dose 1 hour before or 2 hours after a meal.

Instruct patients that if a dose is missed, it should not be taken if it is less than 12 hours until the next dose.

Inform patients that therapy with pazopanib may result in hepatobiliary laboratory abnormalities. Monitor serum liver tests (ALT, AST, and bilirubin) prior to initiation of pazopanib and at least once every 4 weeks for the first 4 months of treatment or as clinically indicated.

Inform patients that they should report any of the following signs and symptoms of liver problems to their health care provider right away: yellowing of the skin or the whites of the eyes (jaundice), unusual darkening of the urine, unusual tiredness, right upper stomach area pain.

Inform patients that GI adverse reactions, such as diarrhea, nausea, and vomiting, have been reported with pazopanib. Patients should be advised how to manage diarrhea and to notify their health care provider if moderate to severe diarrhea occurs.

Advise women of childbearing potential of the potential hazard to the fetus and to avoid becoming pregnant.

Advise patients to inform their health care providers of all concomitant medications, vitamins, or dietary and herbal supplements.

Advise patients that depigmentation of the hair or skin may occur during treatment with pazopanib.

Advise patients to take pazopanib without food (at least 1 hour before or 2 hours after a meal).

VANDETANIB

Rx	**Vandetanib** (AstraZeneca)	**Tablets; oral:** 100 mg	(Z 100). Film-coated. White, round. In 30s.
		300 mg	(Z 300). Film-coated. White, oval. In 30s.

VANDETANIB — ORAL

WARNING

QT prolongation, torsades de pointes, and sudden death – Vandetanib can prolong the QT interval. Torsades de pointes and sudden death have been reported in patients receiving vandetanib. Do not use vandetanib in patients with hypocalcemia, hypokalemia, hypomagnesemia, or long QT syndrome. Hypocalcemia, hypokalemia, and/or hypomagnesemia must be corrected prior to vandetanib administration and should be periodically monitored. Avoid drugs known to prolong the QT interval. If a drug known to prolong the QT interval must be administered, more frequent electrocardiogram (ECG) monitoring is recommended. Given the half-life of 19 days, obtain ECGs to monitor the QT interval at baseline, at 2 to 4 and 8 to 12 weeks after starting treatment with vandetanib, and every 3 months thereafter. Following any dose reduction for QT prolongation or any dose interruptions more than 2 weeks, conduct QT assessment as previously described. Because of the 19-day half-life, adverse reactions, including a prolonged QT interval, may not resolve quickly. Monitor appropriately. Only health care providers and pharmacies certified with the restricted distribution program are able to prescribe and dispense vandetanib.

Indications

➤*Medullary thyroid cancer:* For the treatment of symptomatic or progressive medullary thyroid cancer in patients with unresectable locally advanced or metastatic disease.

Administration and Dosage

➤*Adults:*

Medullary thyroid cancer –

Usual dosage: 300 mg daily.

Dosage adjustment: In the event of QT interval corrected for heart rate, Fridericia (QTcF) greater than 500 msec, interrupt dosing until QTcF returns to less than 450 msec, then resume at a reduced dose. For Common Terminology Criteria for Adverse Events (CTCAE) grade 3 or greater toxicity, interrupt dosing until toxicity resolves or improves to CTCAE grade 1, and then resume at a reduced dose. The 300 mg daily dose can be reduced to 200 mg and then to 100 mg for CTCAE grade 3 or greater toxicities.

Concomitant therapy: Avoid the concomitant use of strong CYP3A4 inducers (eg, dexamethasone, phenytoin, carbamazepine, rifampin, rifabutin, rifapentine, phenobarbital) and St. John's wort.

Missed dose: If a patient misses a dose, the missed dose should not be taken if it is less than 12 hours before the next dose.

➤*Renal function impairment:*

Moderate and severe renal impairment – The starting dose should be reduced to 200 mg in patients with moderate (creatinine clearance [CrCl] 30 or more to less than 50 mL/min) and severe (CrCl less than 30 mL/min) renal impairment.

➤*Hepatic function impairment:* Not recommended for use in patients with moderate (Child-Pugh class B) and severe (Child-Pugh class C) hepatic impairment.

➤*Administration:* Take with or without food. Vandetanib should not be crushed.

Extemporaneous compounding – If vandetanib tablets cannot be taken whole, the tablets can be dispersed in a glass containing 60 mL of noncarbonated water and stirred for approximately 10 minutes until the tablet is dispersed (will not completely dissolve). No other liquids should be used. The dispersion should be swallowed immediately. To ensure the full dose is received, any residues in the glass should be mixed again with an additional 120 mL of noncarbonated water and swallowed. The dispersion can also be administered through nasogastric or gastrostomy tubes.

➤*Storage/Stability:* Store at 25°C (77°F); excursions are permitted between 15° and 30°C (59° and 86°F).

Handling/Disposal – Vandetanib is considered a cytotoxic agent. Follow safe handling procedures when preparing, administering, or dispensing vandetanib. See Sample Policy: Preparing and Reconstituting Hazardous Drugs and Sample Policy: Safe Handling of Hazardous Drug or refer to your institution's specific protocol.

Procedures for proper handling and disposal of anticancer drugs should be considered. Several guidelines on this subject have been published. Vandetanib tablets should not be crushed. Direct contact of crushed tablets with the skin or mucous membranes should be avoided. If such contact occurs, wash thoroughly as outlined in the references. Personnel should avoid exposure to crushed tablets.

Actions

➤*Pharmacology:* Vandetanib is a kinase inhibitor. In vitro studies have shown that vandetanib inhibits the activity of tyrosine kinases, including members of the epidermal growth factor receptor (EGFR) family, vascular endothelial growth factor (VEGF) receptors, rearranged during transfection (RET), protein tyrosine kinase 6, TIE2, members of the EPH receptors kinase family, and members of the Src family of tyrosine kinases. Vandetanib inhibits endothelial cell migration, proliferation, and survival and new blood vessel formation in in vitro models of angiogenesis. Vandetanib

VANDETANIB — ORAL

inhibits EGFR-dependent cell survival in vitro. In addition, vandetanib inhibits epidermal growth factor–stimulated receptor tyrosine kinase phosphorylation in tumor cells and endothelial cells and VEGF-stimulated tyrosine kinase phosphorylation in endothelial cells.

Pharmacodynamics –

QT prolongation: In 231 medullary thyroid cancer patients randomized to receive vandetanib 300 mg once daily in the phase 3 clinical trial, vandetanib was associated with sustained plasma concentration–dependent QT prolongation. Based on the exposure-response relationship, the mean (90% confidence interval) QTcF change from baseline (deltaQTcF) was 35 (33 to 36) msec for the 300 mg dose. The deltaQTcF remained above 30 msec for the duration of the trial (up to 2 years). In addition, 36% of patients experienced greater than 60 msec increase in deltaQTcF and 4.3% of patients had QTcF greater than 500 msec. Cases of torsades de pointes and sudden death have been reported.

➤*Pharmacokinetics:*

Absorption – Absorption is slow, with peak plasma concentrations (C_{max}) typically achieved at a median of 6 hours (range, 4 to 10 hours) after dosing. Vandetanib accumulates approximately 8-fold on multiple dosing, with steady state achieved from approximately 3 months.

Distribution – Vandetanib had a mean volume of distribution of approximately 7,450 L. Vandetanib binds to human serum albumin and alpha-1-acid glycoprotein with in vitro protein binding of approximately 90%. In ex vivo plasma samples from colorectal cancer patients at steady-state exposure after 300 mg once daily, the mean percentage protein binding was 93.7% (range, 92.2% to 95.7%).

Metabolism – Following oral dosing of ^{14}C-vandetanib, unchanged vandetanib and metabolites vandetanib N-oxide and N-desmethyl vandetanib were detected in plasma, urine, and feces. A glucuronide conjugate was seen as a minor metabolite in excreta only. N-desmethyl-vandetanib is primarily produced by CYP3A4 and vandetanib-N-oxide by flavin-containing monooxygenase enzymes FMO1 and FMO3. N-desmethyl-vandetanib and vandetanib-N-oxide circulate at concentrations of approximately 7% to 17.1% and 1.4% to 2.2%, respectively, of those of vandetanib.

Excretion – Vandetanib had a mean clearance of approximately 13.2 L/h and a median plasma half-life of 19 days. Within a 21-day collection period after a single dose of ^{14}C-vandetanib, approximately 69% was recovered, with 44% in feces and 25% in urine. Excretion of the dose was slow, and further excretion beyond 21 days would be expected based on the plasma half-life.

Vandetanib was not a substrate of hOCT2 expressed in HEK293 cells. Vandetanib inhibits the uptake of the selective OCT2 marker substrate ^{14}C-creatinine by HEK-OCT2 cells, with a mean concentration that inhibits 50% of approximately 2.1 mcg/mL. This is higher than vandetanib plasma concentrations (approximately 0.81 mcg/mL) observed after multiple dosing at 300 mg. Inhibition of renal excretion of creatinine by vandetanib provides an explanation for increases in plasma creatinine seen in human subjects receiving vandetanib.

Special populations –

Renal function impairment: In subjects with moderate and severe renal impairment, the average area under the curve (AUC) of vandetanib increased by 39% and 41%, respectively, compared with patients with healthy renal function.

See Administration and Dosage for more information.

Hepatic function impairment: See Administration and Dosage for more information.

Race: Based on a cross-study comparison in a limited number of patients, Japanese (n = 3) and Chinese (n = 7) patients had, on average, exposures that were higher than white (n = 7) patients receiving the same dose.

Contraindications

Congenital long QT syndrome.

Warnings/Precautions

➤*Cardiovascular effects:*

QT prolongation and torsades de pointes – See the Warning box for more information.

Do not start vandetanib treatment in patients whose QTcF interval is greater than 450 msec. Do not give vandetanib to patients who have a history of torsades de pointes, congenital long QT syndrome, bradyarrhythmias, or uncompensated heart failure. Vandetanib has not been studied in patients with ventricular arrhythmias or recent myocardial infarction.

Obtain an ECG and serum potassium, calcium, magnesium, and thyroid-stimulating hormone (TSH) levels at baseline, 2 to 4 weeks and 8 to 12 weeks after starting treatment with vandetanib, and every 3 months thereafter. Electrolytes and ECGs may require more frequent monitoring in case of diarrhea. Following any dose reduction for QT prolongation or any dose interruptions greater than 2 weeks, conduct QT assessments as described previously. Maintain serum potassium levels at 4 mEq/L or higher (within normal range) and keep serum magnesium and serum calcium within normal range to reduce the risk of ECG QT prolongation.

See Drug Interactions for more information.

Patients who develop a QTcF greater than 500 msec should stop taking vandetanib until QTcF returns to less than 450 msec. Dosing of vandetanib can be resumed at a reduced dose.

Heart failure – Heart failure has been observed with vandetanib, and some cases have been fatal. Discontinuation of vandetanib may be necessary in patients with heart failure. Heart failure may not be reversible upon stopping vandetanib. Monitor for signs and symptoms of heart failure.

Hypertension – Hypertension, including hypertensive crisis, has been observed with vandetanib. Monitor all patients for hypertension and control it as appropriate. Dose reduction or interruption may be necessary. If high blood pressure cannot be controlled, do not restart vandetanib.

Ischemic cerebrovascular events – Ischemic cerebrovascular events have been observed with vandetanib, and some cases have been fatal. In the randomized medullary thyroid cancer study, ischemic cerebrovascular events were observed more frequently with vandetanib compared with placebo (1.3% vs 0%) and no deaths were reported. The safety of resumption of vandetanib therapy after resolution of an ischemic cerebrovascular event has not been studied. Discontinue vandetanib in patients who experience a severe ischemic cerebrovascular event.

➤*Dermatological effects:* Severe skin reactions (including Stevens-Johnson syndrome), some leading to death, have been reported with vandetanib. Treatment of severe skin reactions has included systemic corticosteroids and permanent discontinuation of vandetanib. Mild to moderate skin reactions may manifest as rash, acne, dry skin, dermatitis, pruritis, and other skin reactions (including photosensitivity reactions and palmar-plantar erythrodysesthesia syndrome). Mild to moderate skin reactions have been treated with topical and systemic corticosteroids, oral antihistamines, and topical and systemic antibiotics. If CTCAE grade 3 or greater skin reactions occur, stop vandetanib treatment until improved. Upon improvement, consider continuing treatment at a reduced dose or permanent discontinuation of vandetanib.

➤*Interstitial lung disease:* Interstitial lung disease (ILD) or pneumonitis has been observed with vandetanib, and deaths have been reported. Consider a diagnosis of ILD in patients who have nonspecific respiratory signs and symptoms, such as hypoxia, pleural effusion, cough, or dyspnea, and in whom infectious, neoplastic, and other causes have been excluded by means of appropriate investigations. Advise patients to promptly report any new or worsening respiratory symptoms.

Patients who develop radiological changes suggestive of ILD and have few or no symptoms may continue vandetanib therapy with close monitoring at the discretion of the treating health care provider. If symptoms are moderate, consider interrupting therapy until symptoms improve. The use of corticosteroids and antibiotics may be indicated.

For cases in which symptoms of ILD are severe, discontinue vandetanib therapy; the use of corticosteroids and antibiotics may be indicated until clinical symptoms resolve. Even upon resolution of severe ILD, consider permanent discontinuation of vandetanib.

➤*Hemorrhage:* Serious hemorrhagic events, which in some cases were fatal, have been observed with vandetanib. There were no fatal bleeding events in the randomized medullary thyroid cancer study. Three patients died of fatal bleeding events while on vandetanib therapy in clinical studies. Do not administer vandetanib to patients with recent history of hemoptysis of 2.5 mL or more of red blood. Discontinue vandetanib in patients with severe hemorrhage.

➤*Diarrhea:* Diarrhea was observed in patients who received vandetanib. Routine anti-diarrheal agents are recommended. Diarrhea may cause electrolyte imbalances. Because QT prolongation is seen with vandetanib, carefully monitor serum electrolytes and ECGs in patients with diarrhea. If severe diarrhea develops, stop vandetanib treatment until diarrhea improves. Upon improvement, resume treatment with vandetanib at a reduced dose.

➤*Hypothyroidism:* In the randomized medullary thyroid cancer study where 90% of the patients enrolled had prior thyroidectomy, increases in the dose of the thyroid replacement therapy were required in 49% of the patients randomized to vandetanib compared with 17% of the patients randomized to placebo. Obtain TSH at baseline, at 2 to 4 weeks and 8 to 12 weeks after starting treatment with vandetanib, and every 3 months thereafter. If signs or symptoms of hypothyroidism occur, examine thyroid hormone levels and adjust thyroid replacement therapy accordingly.

➤*Reversible posterior leukoencephalopathy syndrome:* Reversible posterior leukoencephalopathy syndrome (RPLS), a syndrome of subcortical vasogenic edema diagnosed by a magnetic resonance image of the brain, has been observed with vandetanib. Consider this syndrome in any patient who has seizures, headache, visual disturbances, confusion, or altered mental function. In clinical studies, 3 of 4 patients who developed RPLS while taking vandetanib, including 1 child, also had hypertension. Consider discontinuation of vandetanib treatment in patients with RPLS.

➤*Risk evaluation and mitigation strategy program:* Because of the risk of QT prolongation, torsades de pointes, and sudden death, vandetanib is available only through a restricted distribution program called the vandetanib risk evaluation and mitigation strategy (REMS) program. Only health care providers and pharmacies certified with the program are able to prescribe and dispense vandetanib.

To learn about the specific REMS requirements and to enroll in the vandetanib REMS program, call 1-800-817-2722 or visit http://www.vandetanibrems.com.

➤*Renal function impairment:* See Administration and Dosage for more information.

VANDETANIB — ORAL

➤*Hepatic function impairment:* See Administration and Dosage for more information.

➤*Photosensitivity:* Photosensitivity reactions are increased with vandetanib. Advise patients to wear sunscreen and protective clothing when exposed to the sun. Because of the long half-life of vandetanib, advise patients to continue wearing protective clothing and sunscreen for 4 months after discontinuation of treatment.

➤*Pregnancy: Category D.* Vandetanib can cause fetal harm when administered to a pregnant woman. There are no adequate and well-controlled studies in pregnant women using vandetanib. If this drug is used during pregnancy, or if the patient becomes pregnant while taking this drug, apprise the patient of the potential hazard to the fetus. Advise women of childbearing potential to avoid becoming pregnant during treatment with vandetanib. Advise women that they must use effective contraception to prevent pregnancy during treatment and for at least 4 months following the last dose of vandetanib.

Vandetanib is embryotoxic, fetotoxic, and teratogenic to rats at exposures equivalent to or lower than those expected at the recommended human dosage of 300 mg/day. When vandetanib was administered to female rats prior to mating and through the first week of pregnancy, there were increases in preimplantation loss and postimplantation loss resulting in a significant reduction in the number of live embryos. This dose, administered to rats during organogenesis, caused an increase in postimplantation loss, including embryofetal death. Vandetanib caused total litter loss when administered at a dosage of 25 mg/kg/day during organogenesis until expected parturition. When administered during organogenesis, vandetanib dosages of 1, 10, and 25 mg/kg/day (approximately 0.03, 0.4, and 1 times, respectively, the C_{max} in patients with cancer at the recommended human dose) caused malformations of the heart vessels and delayed ossification of the skull, vertebrae, and sternum, which indicates delayed fetal development. A no-effect level for these malformations was not identified in this study. At dosages producing maternal toxicity (1 and 10 mg/kg/day) during gestation and/or lactation in a rat pre- and postnatal development study, vandetanib decreased pup survival and/or reduced postnatal pup growth. Reduced postnatal pup growth was associated with a delay in physical development. As expected from its pharmacological actions, vandetanib has shown significant effects on all stages of female reproduction in rats.

➤*Lactation:* In nonclinical studies, vandetanib was excreted in rat milk and found in plasma of pups following dosing to lactating rats. Vandetanib transfer in breast milk resulted in relatively constant exposure in pups because of the long half-life of the drug. It is not known whether this drug is excreted in human breast milk. Because many drugs are excreted in human milk and because of the potential for serious adverse reactions in breastfeeding infants from vandetanib, make a decision whether to discontinue breast-feeding or the drug, taking into account the importance of the drug to the mother.

➤*Children:* Safety and efficacy of vandetanib in children have not been established.

➤*Monitoring:* Obtain an ECG and serum potassium, calcium, magnesium, and TSH levels at baseline, at 2 to 4 weeks and 8 to 12 weeks after starting treatment with vandetanib, and every 3 months thereafter. Following any dose reduction for QT prolongation or any dose interruptions of more than 2 weeks, conduct QT assessment as previously described. Electrolytes and ECGs may require more frequent monitoring in case of diarrhea. Monitor for signs and symptoms of heart failure. Monitor all patients for hypertension and control it as appropriate. Obtain TSH at baseline, at 2 to 4 weeks and 8 to 12 weeks after starting treatment with vandetanib, and every 3 months thereafter. Ophthalmologic examination, including slit lamp, is recommended in patients who report visual changes.

Drug Interactions

➤*QT prolongation:* An additive effect of vandetanib with other drugs that prolong the QT interval cannot be excluded. The following drugs may prolong the QT interval and increase the risk of life-threatening cardiac arrhythmias, including torsade de pointes: antiarrhythmic agents (eg, amiodarone, bretylium, disopyramide, dofetilide, procainamide, quinidine, sotalol), arsenic trioxide, chlorpromazine, cisapride, dolasetron, droperidol, gatifloxacin, halofantrine, levomethadyl, mefloquine, mesoridazine, moxifloxacin, pentamidine, pimozide, probucol, sparfloxacin, thioridazine, and ziprasidone. Avoid coadministration. For a more complete list of drugs that may prolong the QT interval, see the appendix Drug-Induced Prolongation of the QT Interval and Torsades de Pointes.

Vandetanib Drug Interactions

Precipitant drug	Object drug[a]		Description
CYP3A4 strong inducers (eg, carbamazepine, dexamethasone, phenobarbital, phenytoin, rifabutin, rifampin, rifapentine)	Vandetanib	↓	Vandetanib plasma concentrations may be reduced, decreasing the pharmacologic effect. Avoid coadministration.
QT prolonging drugs (eg, antiarrhythmic agents [eg, amiodarone, disopyramide, dofetilide, procainamide, sotalol], chloroquine, clarithromycin, dolasetron, granisetron, haloperidol, methadone, moxifloxacin, pimozide)	Vandetanib	↑	The risk of life-threatening arrhythmia, including torsades de pointes, may be increased. Avoid coadministration. If coadministration cannot be avoided, more frequent ECG monitoring is recommended.
St. John's wort	Vandetanib	↓	Vandetanib plasma concentrations may be decreased unpredictably. Avoid coadministration.

[a] ↑ = object drug increased; ↓ = object drug decreased.

Adverse Reactions

➤*Most common adverse reactions (more than 20%):*

CNS – Fatigue, headache.

Dermatologic – Acne, rash.

GI – Abdominal pain, decreased appetite, diarrhea, nausea.

Lab test abnormalities – Decreased calcium, decreased glucose, increased ALT.

Miscellaneous – Hypertension.

➤*Adverse reactions (10% or more):*

Vandetanib Adverse Reactions (> 10%)

Adverse reactions	Vandetanib 300 mg (n = 231) All grades	Vandetanib 300 mg (n = 231) Grades 3 to 4	Placebo (n = 99) All grades	Placebo (n = 99) Grades 3 to 4
Cardiovascular				
ECG QT prolonged[c]	14%	8%	1%	1%
Hypertension/ Hypertensive crisis/ accelerated hypertension	33%	9%	5%	1%
CNS				
Asthenia	15%	3%	11%	1%
Depression	10%	2%	3%	0%
Fatigue	24%	6%	23%	1%
Headache	26%	1%	9%	0%
Insomnia	13%	0%	10%	0%
Dermatological				
Dermatitis acneiform/acne	35%	1%	7%	0%
Dry skin	15%	0%	5%	0%
Photosensitivity reaction	13%	2%	0%	0%
Pruritus	11%	1%	4%	0%
Rash[a]	53%	5%	12%	0%
GI				
Abdominal pain[b]	21%	3%	11%	0%
Decreased appetite	21%	4%	12%	0%
Diarrhea/Colitis	57%	11%	27%	2%
Dyspepsia	11%	0%	4%	0%
Nausea	33%	1%	16%	0%
Vomiting	15%	1%	7%	0%
Metabolic/Nutritional				
Hypocalcemia	11%	2%	3%	0%
Proteinuria	10%	0%	2%	0%
Weight decreased	10%	1%	9%	0%

VANDETANIB — ORAL

Vandetanib Adverse Reactions (> 10%)				
Adverse reactions	Vandetanib 300 mg (n = 231)		Placebo (n = 99)	
	All grades	Grades 3 to 4	All grades	Grades 3 to 4
Respiratory				
Cough	11%	0%	10%	0%
Nasopharyngitis	11%	0%	9%	0%

[a] Includes rash, rash erythematous, generalized rash, macular rash, maculo-papular rash, papular rash, pruritic rash, exfoliative rash, dermatitis, dermatitis bullous, generalized erythema, and eczema.
[b] Includes abdominal pain, abdominal pain upper, lower abdominal pain, and abdominal discomfort.
[c] 69% had QT prolongation 450 msec or more and 7% had QT prolongation 500 msec or more by ECG using Fridericia correction.

➤*Mortality:* Adverse reactions resulting in death in patients receiving vandetanib (n = 5) were respiratory failure, respiratory arrest, aspiration pneumonia, cardiac failure with arrhythmia, and sepsis. Adverse reactions resulting in death in patients receiving placebo were GI hemorrhage (1%) and gastroenteritis (1%). In addition, there was 1 sudden death and 1 death from cardiopulmonary arrest in patients receiving vandetanib after data cut-off.

➤*Discontinuation:* Causes of discontinuation in vandetanib-treated patients in more than 1 patient included asthenia, fatigue, rash, arthralgia, diarrhea, hypertension, prolonged QT interval, increase in creatinine, and pyrexia.

➤*Serious adverse reactions:* Serious adverse events in vandetanib-treated patients in more than 2% of patients included diarrhea, pneumonia, and hypertension. Clinically important uncommon adverse drug reactions in patients who received vandetanib versus patients who received placebo included pancreatitis (0.4% vs 0%) and heart failure (0.9% vs 0%). In the integrated summary of safety database, the most common cause of death in patients who received vandetanib was pneumonia.

➤*Hemorrhage:* The incidence of grade 1 to 2 bleeding events was 14% in patients receiving vandetanib compared with 7% on placebo in the randomized portion of the medullary thyroid cancer study. The incidence was similar in the 300 mg monotherapy safety program, with a 13% incidence.

➤*Special senses:* Blurred vision was more common in patients who received vandetanib versus patients who received placebo for medullary thyroid cancer (9% vs 1%, respectively). Scheduled slit lamp examinations have revealed corneal opacities (vortex keratopathies) in treated patients, which can lead to halos and decreased visual acuity. It is unknown if this will improve after discontinuation. Ophthalmologic, including slit lamp, examination is recommended in patients who report visual changes. If a patient has blurred vision, instruct them to not drive or operate machinery.

➤*Lab test abnormalities:*

Vandetanib Lab Test Abnormalities				
Laboratory parameter	Vandetanib 300 mg (n = 231)		Placebo (n = 99)	
	All grades	Grades 3 to 4	All grades	Grades 3 to 4
Chemistries				
Calcium decreased	57%	6%	25%	3%
ALT increased	51%	2%	19%	0%
Glucose decreased	24%	0%	7%	1%
Creatinine increased	16%	0%	1%	0%
Bilirubin increased	13%	0%	17%	0%
Magnesium decreased	7%	< 1%	2%	0%
Calcium increased	7%	1%	9%	1%
Potassium decreased	6%	< 1%	3%	0%
Potassium increased	6%	< 1%	4%	2%
Glucose increased	5%	2%	7%	0%
Magnesium increased	3%	0%	4%	0%

Vandetanib Lab Test Abnormalities				
Laboratory parameter	Vandetanib 300 mg (n = 231)		Placebo (n = 99)	
	All grades	Grades 3 to 4	All grades	Grades 3 to 4
Hematologic				
White blood cell count decreased	19%	0%	25%	0%
Hemoglobin decreased	13%	< 1%	19%	2%
Neutrophils decreased	10%	< 1%	5%	2%
Platelets decreased	9%	0%	3%	0%

Hepatic – ALT elevations occurred in 51% of patients on vandetanib in the randomized medullary thyroid cancer study. Grade 3 to 4 ALT elevations were seen in 2% of patients, and no patients had a concomitant increase in bilirubin. Elevations in ALT have resulted in temporary discontinuation of vandetanib. However, 16 of 22 patients with a grade 2 elevation in ALT continued vandetanib 300 mg. Seven patients who continued vandetanib had a normal ALT within 6 months. In the protocol, ALT was monitored every 3 months and more frequently as indicated.

Overdosage

➤*Symptoms:* Possible symptoms of overdose have not been established. Because of the 19-day half-life, adverse reactions may not resolve quickly. In phase 1 clinical trials, a limited number of patients were treated with daily doses of up to 600 mg and healthy volunteers with daily doses of up to 1,200 mg. An increase in the frequency and severity of some adverse reactions, such as rash, diarrhea, and hypertension, was observed at multiple doses at and above 300 mg in healthy volunteer studies and in patients. In addition, consider the possibility of QTc prolongation and torsades de pointes.

➤*Treatment:* There is no specific treatment in the event of overdose with vandetanib. Adverse reactions associated with overdose are to be treated symptomatically; in particular, severe diarrhea must be managed appropriately. In the event of an overdose, further doses of vandetanib must be interrupted, and appropriate measures taken to assure that an adverse event has not occurred (ie, ECG within 24 hours to determine QTc prolongation).

Patient Information

Inform patients that vandetanib can prolong the QT interval in a concentration-dependent manner. Torsades de pointes, ventricular tachycardia, and sudden death have been reported in patients administered vandetanib. Advise patients that their electrolytes and the electrical activity of their heartbeat (via an ECG) should be monitored regularly during treatment with vandetanib.

Tell patients taking vandetanib they may be more susceptible to sunburn and to use appropriate sun protection (eg, sunscreen, clothing) while taking vandetanib and for at least 4 months after drug discontinuation. Advise patients to consult their health care provider promptly if they develop a skin rash.

Advise patients to contact their health care provider promptly if they develop sudden onset or worsening of breathlessness, persistent cough, or fever.

Inform patients that they may experience diarrhea while taking vandetanib. Also advise patients to use standard anti-diarrheal medications and to seek medical attention if their diarrhea becomes persistent or severe. Instruct patients with diarrhea to contact their health care provider to have their electrolytes monitored.

Instruct patients to contact their health care provider promptly if they experience seizures, headaches, visual disturbances, confusion, or difficulty thinking.

Patients of childbearing potential must be told to use effective contraception during therapy and for at least 4 months following their last dose of vandetanib.

Advise breast-feeding mothers to discontinue breast-feeding while receiving vandetanib therapy.

Inform patients to not crush vandetanib tablets. Avoid direct contact of crushed tablets with the skin or mucous membranes.

ERLOTINIB

Rx	**Tarceva** (Genentech)	**Tablets; oral:** 25 mg	Equiv. to erlotinib hydrochloride 27.3 mg. Lactose. (T 25). White, round. Film-coated. In 30s.
		100 mg	Equiv. to erlotinib hydrochloride 109.3 mg. Lactose. (T 100). White, round. Film-coated. In 30s.
		150 mg	Equiv. to erlotinib hydrochloride 163.9 mg. Lactose. (T 150). White, round. Film-coated. In 30s.

ERLOTINIB HYDROCHLORIDE — ORAL

Indications

➤*Non–small cell lung cancer:* As monotherapy for the maintenance treatment of patients with locally advanced or metastatic non–small cell lung cancer whose disease has not progressed after 4 cycles of platinum-based first-line chemotherapy.

As monotherapy for the treatment of patients with locally advanced or metastatic non–small cell lung cancer after failure of at least 1 prior chemotherapy regimen.

ERLOTINIB HYDROCHLORIDE — ORAL

➤*Pancreatic cancer:* For the first-line treatment of patients with locally advanced, unresectable or metastatic pancreatic cancer in combination with gemcitabine.

➤*Off-label uses:* Treatment of squamous cell head and neck cancer.

Administration and Dosage

➤*Adults:*

Non–small cell lung cancer – 150 mg daily at least 1 hour before or 2 hours after food.

Pancreatic cancer – 100 mg daily at least 1 hour before or 2 hours after food, in combination with gemcitabine.

Off-label dosing –

Squamous cell head and neck cancer: 150 mg orally once daily. Higher doses cause increased toxicity without improved clinical benefit.

➤*Hepatic function impairment:* Erlotinib is eliminated by hepatic metabolism and biliary excretion. Although erlotinib exposure was similar in patients with moderately impaired hepatic function (Child-Pugh B), patients with hepatic impairment (total bilirubin more than upper limit of normal [ULN] or Child-Pugh A, B, and C) should be closely monitored during therapy with erlotinib. Treatment with erlotinib should be used with extra caution in patients with total bilirubin more than 3 times the ULN. Erlotinib dosing should be interrupted or discontinued if changes in liver function are severe, such as doubling of total bilirubin and/or tripling of transaminases in the setting of pretreatment values outside normal range. In the setting of worsening liver function tests, before they become severe, dose interruption and/or dose reduction with frequent liver function test monitoring should be considered. Erlotinib dosing should be interrupted or discontinued if total bilirubin is more than 3 times the ULN and/or transaminases are more than 5 times ULN in the setting of normal pretreatment values.

Dosage reduction may be necessary in patients with severe hepatic impairment, especially if serious adverse effects occur; one guideline is shown in the following table. Monitor patients with hepatic dysfunction closely, especially if total bilirubin is more than 3 times the ULN.

Erlotinib Dosage Adjustment Based on Hepatic Function

AST	Serum direct bilirubin	Recommendation
< 3 times the ULN	< 1 mg/dL	No change to initial dose.
≥ 3 times the ULN	1 to 7 mg/dL	Reduce initial dose to 75 mg/day. May gradually increase to labeled dose as tolerated.
—	> 7 mg/dL	No information.

➤*Dosage adjustment:* When dose reduction is necessary, the erlotinib dose should be reduced in 50 mg decrements.

Dermatologic effects – Patients with severe skin reactions, such as severe bullous, blistering, or exfoliative skin conditions, may require dose reduction or temporary interruption of therapy.

GI –

Diarrhea: Diarrhea can usually be managed with loperamide. Patients with severe diarrhea who are unresponsive to loperamide or who become dehydrated may require dose reduction or temporary interruption of therapy.

GI perforation: Discontinue erlotinib therapy for GI perforation.

Ocular disorders/dehydration – Interrupt or discontinue erlotinib in patients with acute/worsening ocular disorders and in patients with dehydration who are at risk for renal failure.

Pulmonary toxicity – In patients who develop an acute onset of new or progressive pulmonary symptoms, such as dyspnea, cough, or fever, treatment with erlotinib should be interrupted pending diagnostic evaluation. If interstitial lung disease is diagnosed, erlotinib should be discontinued and appropriate treatment instituted as necessary.

Smokers – Cigarette smoking has been shown to reduce erlotinib exposure. Patients should be advised to stop smoking. If a patient continues to smoke, a cautious increase in the dose of erlotinib, not exceeding 300 mg, may be considered, while monitoring the patient's safety. However, efficacy and long-term safety (more than 14 days) of a dose higher than the recommended starting doses have not been established in patients who continue to smoke cigarettes. If the erlotinib dose is adjusted upward, the dose should be reduced immediately to the indicated starting dose upon cessation of smoking.

➤*Concomitant medications:*

CYP3A4 inhibitors – In patients who are being concomitantly treated with a strong CYP3A4 inhibitor (eg, atazanavir, clarithromycin, grapefruit juice, grapefruit, indinavir, itraconazole, ketoconazole, nefazodone, nelfinavir, ritonavir, saquinavir, telithromycin, troleandomycin, voriconazole), a dose reduction should be considered if severe adverse reactions occur. Similarly, in patients who are taking erlotinib with an inhibitor of CYP3A4 and CYP1A2 (eg, ciprofloxacin), a dose reduction of erlotinib should be considered if severe adverse reactions occur.

CYP3A4 inducers – Pretreatment with the CYP3A4 inducer rifampicin decreased erlotinib area under the curve (AUC) by approximately two-thirds to four-fifths. Use of alternative treatments lacking CYP3A4-inducing activity is strongly recommended. If an alternative treatment is unavailable, an increase in the dose of erlotinib should be considered as tolerated at 2-week intervals while monitoring the patient's safety. The maximum dose of erlotinib studied in combination with rifampin is 450 mg. If the erlotinib dose is adjusted upward, the dose will need to be reduced immediately to the indicated starting dose upon discontinuation of rifampin or other inducers. Other CYP3A4 inducers include, but are not limited to, carbamazepine, phenobarbital, phenytoin, rifabutin, rifapentine, and St. John's wort; avoid these, too, if possible.

➤*Duration of therapy:* Treatment should continue until disease progression or unacceptable toxicity occurs. There is no evidence that treatment beyond progression is beneficial.

➤*Administration:* Administer on an empty stomach at least 1 hour before or 2 hours after food. Administration with food increases bioavailability to almost 100%, which may cause increased toxicity.

For patients unable to swallow tablets whole, place tablet in 100 mL of distilled water; do not crush tablet. Stir until dispersed, then have the patient drink the mixture immediately. To ensure that the entire dose is administered, rinse the inside of the container with another 40 mL of water and have the patient drink immediately. The suspension may also be administered via an enteral feeding tube.

➤*Storage/Stability:* Store at 25°C (77°F); excursions are permitted between 15° and 30°C (59° and 86°F).

Actions

➤*Pharmacology:* Erlotinib, a kinase inhibitor, is a quinazolinamine. The mechanism of clinical antitumor action of erlotinib is not fully characterized. Erlotinib inhibits the intracellular phosphorylation of tyrosine kinase associated with the epidermal growth factor receptor (EGFR). Specificity of inhibition with regard to other tyrosine kinase receptors has not been fully characterized. EGFR is expressed on the cell surface of healthy cells and cancer cells.

➤*Pharmacokinetics:*

Absorption/Distribution – Erlotinib is approximately 60% absorbed after oral administration. Peak plasma levels occur 4 hours after dosing. The solubility of erlotinib is pH dependent. Erlotinib solubility decreases as pH increases.

Following absorption, erlotinib is approximately 93% protein bound to plasma albumin and alpha-1 acid glycoprotein. Erlotinib has an apparent volume of distribution of 232 L.

Effect of food: Erlotinib's bioavailability is substantially increased by food to almost 100%.

Metabolism/Excretion – In vitro assays of cytochrome P450 (CYP-450) metabolism showed that erlotinib is metabolized primarily by CYP3A4 and to a lesser extent by CYP1A2, and the extrahepatic isoform CYP1A1. Following a 100 mg oral dose, 91% of the dose was recovered: 83% in feces (1% of the dose as intact parent) and 8% in urine (0.3% of the dose as intact parent).

A population pharmacokinetic analysis in 591 patients receiving single-agent erlotinib second/third-line regimen showed a median half-life of 36.2 hours. Time to reach steady-state plasma concentration would, therefore, be 7 to 8 days.

Special populations –

Hepatic function impairment: See Administration and Dosage for more information.

Smokers: Cigarette smoking reduces erlotinib exposure. In the phase 3 non–small cell lung cancer trial, current smokers achieved erlotinib trough plasma concentrations that were approximately 2-fold less than the former smokers or patients who had never smoked. This effect was accompanied by a 24% increase in apparent erlotinib plasma clearance. In a separate study that evaluated the single-dose pharmacokinetics of erlotinib in healthy volunteers, current smokers cleared the drug significantly faster than former smokers or volunteers who had never smoked. The $AUC_{0\text{-infinity}}$ in smokers is about one-third to one-half of that in never/former smokers. In another study that was conducted in non–small cell lung cancer patients (n = 35) who were current smokers, pharmacokinetics analyses at steady state indicated a dose-proportional increase in erlotinib exposure when the erlotinib dose was increased from 150 to 300 mg. However, the exact dose to be recommended for patients who currently smoke is unknown.

Contraindications

None well documented.

Warnings/Precautions

➤*Pulmonary toxicity:* There have been reports of serious interstitial lung disease–like events, including fatalities, in patients receiving erlotinib for treatment of non–small cell lung cancer, pancreatic cancer, or other advanced solid tumors. In the randomized, single-agent non–small cell lung cancer studies, the incidence of serious interstitial lung disease–like events in the erlotinib-treated patients versus placebo-treated patients was 0.7% versus 0% in the maintenance study and 0.8% for both groups in the second- and third-line study. In the pancreatic cancer study in combination with gemcitabine, the incidence of interstitial lung disease–like events was 2.5% in the erlotinib plus gemcitabine group versus 0.4% in the placebo plus gemcitabine group.

The overall incidence of interstitial lung disease–like events in approximately 32,000 erlotinib-treated patients from all studies (including noncontrolled studies and studies with concurrent chemotherapy) was approximately 1.1%. Reported diagnoses in patients suspected of having interstitial lung disease–like events included acute respiratory distress syndrome, hypersensitivity pneumonitis, interstitial lung disease, interstitial pneumonia, lung infiltration, obliterative bronchiolitis, pneumonitis, pulmo-

ERLOTINIB HYDROCHLORIDE — ORAL

nary fibrosis, and radiation pneumonitis. Symptoms started from 5 days to more than 9 months (median, 39 days) after initiating erlotinib therapy. In the lung cancer trials, most of the cases were associated with confounding or contributing factors, such as concomitant/prior chemotherapy, prior radiotherapy, preexisting parenchymal lung disease, metastatic lung disease, or pulmonary infections.

See Administration and Dosage for more information.

➤*Renal effects:* Cases of hepatorenal syndrome, acute renal failure (including fatalities), and renal insufficiency have been reported. Some were secondary to baseline hepatic impairment, while others were associated with severe dehydration caused by diarrhea, vomiting, and/or anorexia, or concurrent chemotherapy use. In the event of dehydration, particularly in patients with contributing risk factors for renal failure (eg, preexisting renal disease, medical conditions or medications that may lead to renal disease, or other predisposing conditions, including advanced age), interrupt erlotinib therapy and take appropriate measures to intensively rehydrate the patient. Periodically monitor renal function and serum electrolytes in patients at risk of dehydration.

➤*Hepatotoxicity:* Cases of hepatic failure and hepatorenal syndrome (including fatalities) have been reported during use of erlotinib, particularly in patients with baseline hepatic impairment. Therefore, it is recommended to periodically test liver function (transaminases, bilirubin, and alkaline phosphatase). In the setting of worsening liver function tests, consider dose interruption and/or dose reduction with frequent liver function test monitoring. Interrupt or discontinue erlotinib dosing if total bilirubin is more than 3 times ULN and/or transaminases are more than 5 times ULN in the setting of normal pretreatment values.

➤*GI perforation:* GI perforation (including fatalities) has been reported in patients receiving erlotinib. Patients receiving concomitant antiangiogenic agents, corticosteroids, nonsteroidal anti-inflammatory drugs, and/or taxane-based chemotherapy, or who have a history of peptic ulceration or diverticular disease are at increased risk. Permanently discontinue erlotinib in patients who develop GI perforation.

➤*Dermatologic effects:* Bullous, blistering, and exfoliative skin conditions have been reported, including cases suggestive of Stevens-Johnson syndrome/toxic epidermal necrolysis, which in some cases were fatal. Interrupt or discontinue erlotinib treatment if the patient develops severe bullous, blistering, or exfoliating conditions.

➤*Cardiovascular effects:*

Myocardial infarction / ischemia – In the pancreatic carcinoma trial, 2.3% of patients in the erlotinib/gemcitabine group developed myocardial infarction (MI)/ischemia. One of these patients died because of MI. In comparison, 1.2% of patients in the placebo/gemcitabine group developed MI and 1 died because of MI.

Cerebrovascular accident – In the pancreatic carcinoma trial, 2.3% of patients in the erlotinib/gemcitabine group developed cerebrovascular accidents. One of these was hemorrhagic and was the only fatal event. In comparison, in the placebo/gemcitabine group, there were no cerebrovascular accidents.

➤*Hematologic effects:* In the pancreatic carcinoma trial, 0.8% of patients in the erlotinib/gemcitabine group developed microangiopathic hemolytic anemia with thrombocytopenia. Both patients received erlotinib and gemcitabine concurrently. In comparison, in the placebo/gemcitabine group, there were no cases of microangiopathic hemolytic anemia with thrombocytopenia.

➤*Ophthalmic effects:* Corneal perforation and ulceration have been reported during use of erlotinib. Other ocular disorders, including abnormal eyelash growth, keratoconjunctivitis sicca, or keratitis, have been observed with erlotinib treatment and are known risk factors for corneal ulceration/perforation. Interrupt or discontinue erlotinib therapy if patients present with acute/worsening ocular disorders, such as eye pain.

➤*Bleeding risks:* International normalized ratio (INR) elevations and infrequent reports of bleeding events, including GI and non-GI bleedings, have been reported in clinical studies, some associated with warfarin coadministration (see Drug Interactions for more information). Regularly monitor patients taking warfarin or other coumarin-derivative anticoagulants for changes in prothrombin time or INR.

➤*Hepatic function impairment:* In a pharmacokinetic study in patients with moderate hepatic impairment (Child-Pugh class B) associated with significant liver tumor burden, 10 of 15 patients died on treatment or within 30 days of the last erlotinib dose. One patient died from hepatorenal syndrome, 1 patient died from rapidly progressing liver failure, and the remaining 8 died from progressive disease. Six of the 10 patients who died had baseline total bilirubin more than 3 times ULN, suggesting severe hepatic impairment. Use extreme caution when administering erlotinib to patients with total bilirubin more than 3 times ULN. Closely monitor patients with hepatic impairment (total bilirubin greater than ULN or Child-Pugh class A, B, or C) during therapy with erlotinib. Interrupt or discontinue erlotinib if changes in liver function are severe, such as doubling of total bilirubin and/or tripling of transaminases in the setting of pretreatment values outside normal range.

➤*Pregnancy: Category D.* There are no adequate and well-controlled studies in pregnant women using erlotinib. Erlotinib can cause fetal harm when administered to a pregnant woman. Advise women of childbearing potential to avoid pregnancy while receiving erlotinib. Advise these women to use adequate contraceptive methods during therapy, and for at least 2 weeks after completing therapy. If erlotinib is used during pregnancy or if the patient becomes pregnant while taking this drug, apprise the patient of the potential hazard to the fetus.

Erlotinib administered to rabbits during organogenesis at doses that result in plasma drug concentrations of approximately 3 times those in humans at the recommended dosage of 150 mg daily was associated with embryofetal lethality and abortion. When erlotinib was administered to female rats prior to mating and through the first week of pregnancy at doses 0.3 or 0.7 times the clinical dose of 150 mg on a mg/m^2 basis, there was an increase in early resorptions that resulted in a decrease in the number of live fetuses.

It is not known if erlotinib crosses the human placenta. The molecular weight (about 394 for the free base) and long elimination half-life suggest that the drug will cross; however, the extensive metabolism and moderately high plasma protein binding may limit the amount of drug reaching the embryo/fetus.

➤*Lactation:* It is not known whether erlotinib is excreted in human milk. The molecular weight (about 394 for the free base) and long elimination half-life suggest that the drug will be excreted into breast milk; however, the extensive metabolism and moderately high plasma protein binding may limit the amount of drug reaching the milk. The systemic bioavailability of erlotinib is markedly increased when taken with food, and this might also occur in breast-feeding infants. Because many drugs are excreted in human milk and because the effects of erlotinib on infants have not been studied, decide whether to discontinue breast-feeding or the drug, taking into account the importance of the drug to the mother.

➤*Children:* Safety and effectiveness have not been studied.

➤*Monitoring:* Perform periodic liver function tests in patients treated with erlotinib. In the setting of worsening liver function tests, before they become worse, consider dose interruption and/or dose reduction with frequent liver function test monitoring. Regularly monitor patients taking erlotinib and warfarin or other coumarin-derivative anticoagulants for changes in prothrombin time or INR. Periodically monitor renal function and serum electrolytes in patients at risk of dehydration.

Monitor patients for acute onset or progression of pulmonary symptoms (eg, cough, dyspnea, fever).

Drug Interactions

➤*Cytochrome P450 system:* Based on in vitro assays, erlotinib metabolism is primarily by CYP3A4 and, to a lesser extent, by CYP1A2 and the extrahepatic CYP1A1 isoform. Therefore, drugs that are substrates for or induce or inhibit 1 or more of these pathways may result in clinically important drug interactions. Drugs that induce these enzyme systems may increase erlotinib metabolism, decreasing erlotinib plasma concentrations and efficacy. Drugs that inhibit these enzyme systems may interfere with erlotinib metabolism, elevating erlotinib plasma concentrations and increasing the pharmacologic effects and risk of adverse reactions. In patients receiving erlotinib, clinically important interactions may occur when an interacting drug is started or stopped and, in many instances, when the dose of either agent is changed. Monitoring the patient's clinical response and making the appropriate adjustments in dose is important in minimizing the risk of a drug interaction, especially with drugs that have a narrow therapeutic index (eg, warfarin).

Erlotinib Drug Interactions

Precipitant drug	Object drug[a]		Description
Antacids	Erlotinib	⬇	Drugs that alter the pH of the upper GI tract may alter the solubility of erlotinib and reduce its bioavailability. Separate the dose of antacids and erlotinib by several hours.
Ciprofloxacin	Erlotinib	⬆	Erlotinib plasma concentrations may be increased because of inhibition of CYP1A2 and CYP3A4 metabolism by ciprofloxacin. Consider a reduction in erlotinib dose in patients who experience severe adverse reactions.
CYP3A4 inducers (eg, carbamazepine, phenobarbital, phenytoin, rifabutin, rifampin, rifapentine, St. John's wort)	Erlotinib	⬇	The plasma concentration of erlotinib is decreased because of an increase in its metabolism. Coadministration with rifampin reduced the erlotinib AUC two-thirds to four-fifths. Avoid coadministration. If an alternative treatment is unavailable, consider a dose increase of erlotinib if coadministered with a potent CYP3A4 inducer. If the erlotinib dose is adjusted upward, reduce the dose immediately to the indicated starting dose when the CYP3A4 inducer is discontinued.

ERLOTINIB HYDROCHLORIDE — ORAL

Erlotinib Drug Interactions

Precipitant drug	Object drug[a]		Description
CYP3A4 inhibitors (eg, atazanavir, clarithromycin, indinavir, itraconazole, ketoconazole, nefazodone, nelfinavir, ritonavir, saquinavir, telithromycin, troleandomycin, voriconazole)	Erlotinib	↑	Potent CYP3A4 inhibitors decrease erlotinib metabolism and increase its plasma concentration. Coadministration with ketoconazole increased erlotinib AUC by two-thirds. Use with caution. Consider a reduction in erlotinib dose in patients who experience severe adverse reactions.
H_2 receptor antagonists (eg, ranitidine)	Erlotinib	↓	Drugs that alter the pH of the upper GI tract may alter the solubility of erlotinib and reduce its bioavailability. Stagger the dosing. Administer erlotinib 10 hours after the H_2 receptor antagonist and at least 2 hours before the next H_2 antagonist dose.
Proton pump inhibitors (eg, omeprazole)	Erlotinib	↓	Drugs that alter the pH of the upper GI tract may alter the solubility of erlotinib and reduce its bioavailability. Omeprazole decreased erlotinib AUC by 46% and C_{max}[b] by 61%. Avoid coadministration if possible.
Erlotinib	Midazolam	↓	Erlotinib decreased midazolam (a CYP3A4 substrate) AUC by 24%. In patients receiving midazolam, monitor the clinical response of the patient when starting or stopping erlotinib. If an interaction is suspected, adjust the midazolam dose as needed.
Erlotinib	Warfarin	↑	INR elevations and infrequent reports of bleeding, including GI and non-GI bleeding, have been reported during warfarin coadministration. Monitor for changes in prothrombin time or INR.

[a] ↑ = object drug increased; ↓ = object drug decreased.
[b] C_{max} = maximum plasma concentration.

➤*Cigarette smoking:* See Administration and Dosage for more information.

➤*Drug/Food interactions:* Grapefruit or grapefruit juice may increase erlotinib AUC. Coadminister with caution.

See Administration and Dosage for more information.

Adverse Reactions

➤*Serious reactions:* There have been reports of serious reactions, including fatalities, in patients receiving erlotinib for treatment of non–small cell lung cancer, pancreatic cancer, or other advanced solid tumors.

➤*Non–small cell lung cancer:*

Maintenance study – The most common adverse reactions in patients receiving single-agent erlotinib 150 mg were rash and diarrhea. Grade 3/4 rash and diarrhea occurred in 6% and 1.8%, respectively, of patients treated with erlotinib. Rash and diarrhea each resulted in study discontinuation in 1.2% and 0.5% of erlotinib-treated patients, respectively. Dose reduction or interruption for rash and diarrhea was needed in 5.1% and 2.8% of patients, respectively. In patients treated with erlotinib who developed rash, the onset was within 2 weeks in 66% and within 1 month in 81%.

Erlotinib Non–Small Cell Lung Cancer Maintenance Study Adverse Reactions (≥ 3%)

Adverse reactions	Erlotinib 150 mg (n = 433)			Placebo (n = 445)		
	Any grade[a]	Grade 3	Grade 4	Any grade[a]	Grade 3	Grade 4
Dermatologic						
Acne	6.2%	< 1%	0%	0%	0%	0%
Dermatitis acneiform	4.6%	< 1%	0%	1.1%	0%	0%
Dry skin	4.4%	0%	0%	< 1%	0%	0%
Pruritus	7.4%	< 1%	0%	2.7%	0%	0%
Rash	49.2%	6%	0%	5.8%	0%	0%
GI						
Anorexia	9.2%	< 1%	0%	4.9%	< 1%	0%
Diarrhea	20.3%	1.8%	0%	4.5%	0%	0%
Weight decreased	3.9%	< 1%	0%	< 1%	0%	0%
Miscellaneous						
Fatigue	9%	1.8%	0%	5.8%	1.1%	0%
Paronychia	3.9%	< 1%	0%	0%	0%	0%

[a] National Cancer Institute Common Toxicity Criteria (NCI-CTC) grade (version 3.0).

Second/Third-line study – The most common adverse reactions in this patient population were rash and diarrhea. Grade 3/4 rash and diarrhea occurred in 9% and 6%, respectively, in erlotinib-treated patients. Rash and diarrhea each resulted in study discontinuation in 1% of erlotinib-treated patients. Six percent and 1% of patients needed dose reduction for rash and diarrhea, respectively. The median time to onset of rash was 8 days, and the median time to onset of diarrhea was 12 days.

Erlotinib Non–Small Cell Lung Cancer Second/Third-Line Study Adverse Reactions (≥ 3%)

Adverse reactions	Erlotinib 150 mg (n = 485)			Placebo (n = 242)		
	Any grade[a]	Grade 3	Grade 4	Any grade[a]	Grade 3	Grade 4
Dermatologic						
Dry skin	12%	0%	0%	4%	0%	0%
Pruritus	13%	< 1%	0%	5%	0%	0%
Rash	75%	8%	< 1%	17%	0%	0%
GI						
Abdominal pain	11%	2%	< 1%	7%	1%	< 1%
Anorexia	52%	8%	1%	38%	5%	< 1%
Diarrhea	54%	6%	< 1%	18%	< 1%	0%
Nausea	33%	3%	0%	24%	2%	0%
Stomatitis	17%	< 1%	0%	3%	0%	0%
Vomiting	23%	2%	< 1%	19%	2%	0%
Ophthalmic						
Conjunctivitis	12%	< 1%	0%	2%	< 1%	0%
Keratoconjunctivitis sicca	12%	0%	0%	3%	0%	0%
Respiratory						
Cough	33%	4%	0%	29%	2%	0%
Dyspnea	41%	17%	11%	35%	15%	11%
Miscellaneous						
Fatigue	52%	14%	4%	45%	16%	4%
Infection	24%	4%	0%	15%	2%	0%

[a] NCI-CTC grade (version 2.0).

➤*Pancreatic cancer:* The most common adverse reactions in pancreatic cancer patients receiving erlotinib 100 mg plus gemcitabine were anorexia, diarrhea, fatigue, nausea, and rash. In the erlotinib plus gemcitabine arm, grade 3/4 rash and diarrhea were each reported in 5% of erlotinib plus gemcitabine-treated patients. The median time to onset of rash and diarrhea was 10 and 15 days, respectively. Rash and diarrhea each resulted in dose reductions in 2% of patients, and resulted in study discontinuation in up to 1% of patients receiving erlotinib plus gemcitabine. The 150 mg cohort was associated with a higher rate of certain class-specific adverse reactions, including rash, and required more frequent dose reductions or interruptions.

Erlotinib Adverse Reactions in Patients With Pancreatic Cancer (≥ 10%)

Adverse reactions	Erlotinib + Gemcitabine 1,000 mg/m² IV[a] (n = 259)			Placebo + Gemcitabine 1,000 mg/m² IV (n = 256)		
	Any grade[b]	Grade 3	Grade 4	Any grade[b]	Grade 3	Grade 4
CNS						
Anxiety	13%	1%	0%	11%	< 1%	0%
Depression	19%	2%	0%	14%	< 1%	0%
Dizziness	15%	< 1%	0%	13%	0%	< 1%
Fatigue	73%	14%	2%	70%	13%	2%
Headache	15%	< 1%	0%	10%	0%	0%

ERLOTINIB HYDROCHLORIDE — ORAL

Erlotinib Adverse Reactions in Patients With Pancreatic Cancer (≥ 10%)						
	Erlotinib + Gemcitabine 1,000 mg/m² IV[a] (n = 259)			Placebo + Gemcitabine 1,000 mg/m² IV (n = 256)		
Adverse reactions	Any grade[b]	Grade 3	Grade 4	Any grade[b]	Grade 3	Grade 4
Insomnia	15%	< 1%	0%	16%	< 1%	0%
Neuropathy	13%	1%	< 1%	10%	< 1%	0%
Rigors	12%	0%	0%	9%	0%	0%
Dermatologic						
Alopecia	14%	0%	0%	11%	0%	0%
Rash	69%	5%	0%	30%	1%	0%
GI						
Abdominal pain	46%	9%	< 1%	45%	12%	< 1%
Anorexia	52%	6%	< 1%	52%	5%	< 1%
Constipation	31%	3%	1%	34%	5%	1%
Diarrhea	48%	5%	< 1%	36%	2%	0%
Dyspepsia	17%	< 1%	0%	13%	< 1%	0%
Flatulence	13%	0%	0%	9%	< 1%	0%
Nausea	60%	7%	0%	58%	7%	0%
Stomatitis	22%	< 1%	0%	12%	0%	0%
Vomiting	42%	7%	< 1%	41%	4%	< 1%
Weight decreased	39%	2%	0%	29%	< 1%	0%
Musculoskeletal						
Bone pain	25%	4%	< 1%	23%	2%	0%
Myalgia	21%	1%	0%	20%	< 1%	0%
Respiratory						
Cough	16%	0%	0%	11%	0%	0%
Dyspnea	24%	5%	< 1%	23%	5%	0%
Miscellaneous						
Edema	37%	3%	< 1%	36%	2%	< 1%
Infection	39%	13%	3%	30%	9%	2%
Pyrexia	36%	3%	0%	30%	4%	0%

[a] IV = intravenous.
[b] NCI-CTC grade (version 2.0).

Severe adverse reactions – Severe adverse reactions (at least grade 3 NCI-CTC) in the erlotinib plus gemcitabine group with incidences less than 5% included arrhythmias, cerebrovascular accidents including cerebral hemorrhage, hemolytic anemia including microangiopathic hemolytic anemia with thrombocytopenia, ileus, myocardial infarction/ischemia, pancreatitis, renal insufficiency, and syncope.

Deep vein thrombosis – In the pancreatic carcinoma trial, 3.9% of patients in the erlotinib/gemcitabine group developed deep vein thrombosis (DVT). In comparison, 1.2% of patients in the placebo/gemcitabine group developed DVT. The overall incidence of grade 3 or 4 thrombotic events, including DVT, was similar in the 2 treatment arms (11% for erlotinib plus gemcitabine and 9% for placebo plus gemcitabine).

➤*Other adverse reactions:*

GI – GI perforations have been reported.

During the non–small cell lung cancer and the combination pancreatic cancer trials, infrequent cases of GI bleeding have been reported, some associated with concomitant warfarin or nonsteroidal anti-inflammatory drug administration. These adverse reactions were reported as peptic ulcer bleeding (gastritis, gastroduodenal ulcers), hematemesis, hematochezia, melena, and hemorrhage from possible colitis.

Dermatologic – Bullous, blistering, and exfoliative skin conditions have been reported, including cases suggestive of Stevens-Johnson syndrome/toxic epidermal necrolysis.

In patients who develop skin rash, the appearance of the rash is typically erythematous and maculopapular, and it may resemble acne with follicular pustules, but is histopathologically different. This skin reaction commonly occurs on the face, upper chest, and back, but may be more generalized or severe (NCI-CTC grade 3 or 4) with desquamation. Skin reactions may occur or worsen in sun-exposed areas; therefore, the use of sunscreen or avoidance of sun exposure is recommended. Associated symptoms may include itching, tenderness, and/or burning. Also, hyperpigmentation or dry skin with or without digital skin fissures may occur.

Hair and nail disorders, including alopecia, hirsutism, eyelash/eyebrow changes, paronychia, and brittle and loose nails, have been reported.

Hepatic – Hepatic failure has been reported in patients treated with single-agent erlotinib or erlotinib combined with chemotherapy.

Renal – Cases of acute renal failure or renal insufficiency, including fatalities, with or without hypokalemia have been reported.

Ophthalmic – Corneal ulcerations or perforations have been reported in patients receiving erlotinib treatment. Abnormal eyelash growth, including ingrowing eyelashes, and excessive growth and thickening of the eyelashes have been reported and are risk factors for corneal ulceration/perforation.

NCI-CTC grade 3 conjunctivitis and keratitis have been reported infrequently in patients receiving erlotinib therapy in the non–small cell lung cancer and pancreatic cancer clinical trials.

Miscellaneous – Epistaxis has been reported in both the single-agent non–small cell lung cancer and the pancreatic cancer clinical trials.

➤*Lab test abnormalities:*

Non–small cell lung cancer – Consider dose interruption or discontinuation of erlotinib if changes in liver function are severe.

Maintenance study: Liver function test abnormalities (including elevated ALT, AST, and bilirubin) were observed in patients receiving single-agent erlotinib 150 mg in the maintenance study. Grade 2 (more than 2.5 to 5 times ULN) ALT elevations occurred in 2% and 1%, and grade 3 (more than 5 to 20 times the ULN) ALT elevations were observed in 1% and 0% of erlotinib- and placebo-treated patients, respectively. The erlotinib treatment group had grade 2 (more than 1.5 to 3 times the ULN) bilirubin elevations in 4% and grade 3 (more than 3 to 10 times the ULN) in less than 1% compared with less than 1% for both grades 2 and 3 in the placebo group.

Second/Third-line study: Liver function test abnormalities (including elevated ALT, AST, and bilirubin) were observed in patients receiving single-agent erlotinib 150 mg. These elevations were mainly transient or associated with liver metastases. Grade 2 (more than 2.5 to 5 times ULN) ALT elevations occurred in 4% and less than 1% of erlotinib- and placebo-treated patients, respectively. Grade 3 (more than 5 to 20 times ULN) elevations were not observed in erlotinib-treated patients.

Pancreatic cancer – Liver function test abnormalities (including elevated ALT, AST, and bilirubin) have been observed following the administration of erlotinib plus gemcitabine in patients with pancreatic cancer. Consider dose interruption or discontinuation of erlotinib if changes in liver function are severe.

Erlotinib Liver Function Test Abnormalities (Most Severe NCI-CTC Grade) in Patients With Pancreatic Cancer						
	Erlotinib + Gemcitabine 1,000 mg/m² IV (n = 259)			Placebo + Gemcitabine 1,000 mg/m² IV (n = 256)		
Laboratory test	Grade 2[a]	Grade 3[a]	Grade 4[a]	Grade 2[a]	Grade 3[a]	Grade 4[a]
ALT	31%	13%	< 1%	22%	9%	0%
AST	24%	10%	< 1%	19%	9%	0%
Bilirubin	17%	10%	< 1%	11%	10%	3%

[a] NCI-CTC grade.

➤*Postmarketing:*

Dermatologic – Hair and nail changes, mostly nonserious (eg, hirsutism, eyelash/eyebrow changes, paronychia, and brittle and loose nails). Bullous, blistering, and exfoliative skin conditions have been reported, including cases suggestive of Stevens-Johnson syndrome/toxic epidermal necrolysis.

GI – GI perforations.

Hepatic – Hepatic failure has been reported in patients treated with single-agent erlotinib or erlotinib combined with chemotherapy.

Overdosage

➤*Symptoms:* Single oral doses of erlotinib up to 1,000 mg in healthy subjects and weekly doses of up to 1,600 mg in patients with cancer have been tolerated. Repeated twice-daily doses of single-agent erlotinib 200 mg in healthy subjects were poorly tolerated after only a few days of dosing. Based on the data from these studies, an unacceptable incidence of severe adverse reactions, such as diarrhea, liver transaminase elevation, and rash, may occur above the recommended dosage of 150 mg daily.

➤*Treatment:* In case of suspected overdose, withhold erlotinib and institute symptomatic treatment.

Patient Information

Advise patients to seek medical advice promptly if the following signs or symptoms occur: anorexia, nausea, severe or persistent diarrhea, or vomiting; eye irritation; onset or worsening of skin rash; onset or worsening of unexplained shortness of breath or cough.

Inform patients that skin reactions are anticipated when taking erlotinib; proactive intervention may include alcohol-free emollient cream and use of sunscreen or avoidance of sun exposure. Discuss the management of rash with the patient. This may include topical corticosteroids or antibiotics with anti-inflammatory properties. Acne preparations with drying properties may aggravate the dry skin and erythema. Treatment of rash has not been formally studied and should be based on rash severity.

Inform women of childbearing potential to avoid becoming pregnant while taking erlotinib. Advise women to use adequate contraceptive methods during therapy and for at least 2 weeks after completing therapy.

Advise patients who smoke to stop smoking while taking erlotinib because cigarette smoking reduces plasma concentrations of erlotinib.

Advise patients to take erlotinib at least 1 hour before or 2 hours after food intake.

GEFITINIB

Rx	**Iressa** (AstraZeneca)	**Tablets:** 250 mg	Lactose. (IRESSA 250). Brown. Film-coated. In 30s.

GEFITINIB — ORAL

Indications

➤*Non-small cell lung cancer:* As monotherapy for the treatment of patients with locally advanced or metastatic non-small cell lung cancer after failure of both platinum-based and docetaxel chemotherapies.

Results from 2 large, controlled, randomized trials in first-line treatment of non-small cell lung cancer showed no benefit from adding gefitinib to doublet, platinum-based chemotherapy. Therefore, gefitinib is not indicated for use in this setting.

➤*Off-label uses:* Treatment of squamous cell head and neck cancer.

Administration and Dosage

➤*General dosing considerations:*

Iressa Access Program – As of September 15, 2005, gefitinib is available only to patients registered in AstraZeneca's restrictive distribution program, the *Iressa* Access Program. Health care providers must register patients with the program before prescribing gefitinib. To qualify for the program, patients must meet the following criteria:

- Patient has been treated with gefitinib prior to September 15, 2005;
- Patient previously benefited from gefitinib, or the patient's health care provider believes the patient will benefit from further gefitinib therapy; or
- Patient is enrolled in a clinical trial that was approved by an Institutional Review Board prior to June 17, 2005.

Additional information about the *Iressa* Access Program is available from AstraZeneca at 800-601-8933 (8 AM to 6 PM EST, Monday through Friday) or online at http://www.iressa-access.com.

➤*Adults:*

Non-small–cell lung cancer –

Usual dosage: 250 mg once a day. Higher doses do not give a better response and cause increased toxicity.

Dosage adjustment:

• *GI/Dermatologic effects* – Patients with poorly tolerated diarrhea (sometimes associated with dehydration) or skin adverse drug reactions may be successfully managed by providing a brief (up to 14 days) therapy interruption, followed by reinstatement of the 250 mg daily dose.

• *Pulmonary effects* – In the event of acute onset or worsening of pulmonary symptoms (dyspnea, cough, fever), gefitinib therapy should be interrupted and a prompt investigation of these symptoms should occur and appropriate treatment initiated. If interstitial lung disease is confirmed, gefitinib should be discontinued and the patient treated appropriately. (See also Warnings/Precautions.)

• *Ocular effects* – Patients who develop new-onset eye symptoms such as pain should be medically evaluated and managed appropriately, including gefitinib therapy interruption and removal of an aberrant eyelash if present. After symptoms and eye changes have resolved, the decision should be made concerning reinstatement of the 250 mg daily dose. In patients receiving gefitinib therapy, there were reports of eye pain and corneal erosion/ulcer, sometimes in association with aberrant eyelash growth.

Duration of therapy: Continue therapy as long as response is favorable. In clinical trials, the median duration of response was 8.9 months in non-small–cell lung cancer. Median survival was similar with gefitinib (5.6 months) or placebo (5.1 months) in these patients.

Concomitant therapy: In patients receiving a potent CYP3A4 inducer such as rifampin or phenytoin, a dose increase to 500 mg daily should be considered in the absence of severe adverse drug reaction, and clinical response and adverse reactions should be carefully monitored.

Off-label dosing –

Squamous cell head and neck cancer: 250 to 500 mg once daily.

➤*Administration:* To be taken orally with or without food.

For patients unable to swallow tablets whole, place tablet in a half glass of noncarbonated water; do not crush tablet. Stir approximately 10 minutes until dispersed, then have the patient drink the mixture immediately. To ensure that the entire dose is administered, rinse the inside of the container with another half glass of water and have the patient drink it immediately. The suspension may also be administered via a gastric enteral feeding tube.

➤*Storage/Stability:* Store at 20° to 25°C (68° to 77°F).

Actions

➤*Pharmacology:* The mechanism of the clinical antitumor action of gefitinib is not fully characterized. Gefitinib inhibits the intracellular phosphorylation of numerous tyrosine kinases associated with transmembrane cell surface receptors, including the tyrosine kinases associated with the epidermal growth factor receptor (EGFR-TK). EGFR is expressed on the cell surface of many normal cells and cancer cells. No clinical studies have been performed that demonstrate a correlation between EGFR receptor expression and response to gefitinib.

➤*Pharmacokinetics:*

Absorption/Distribution – Gefitinib is absorbed slowly after oral administration with mean bioavailability of 60%. Elimination is by metabolism (primarily CYP3A4) and excretion in feces. The elimination half-life is about 48 hours. Daily oral administration of gefitinib to cancer patients resulted in a 2-fold accumulation compared to single dose administration. Steady state plasma concentrations are achieved within 10 days.

Gefitinib is slowly absorbed, with peak plasma levels occurring 3 to 7 hours after dosing and mean oral bioavailability of 60%. Bioavailability is not significantly altered by food. Gefitinib is extensively distributed throughout the body with a mean steady state volume of distribution of 1400 L following intravenous administration. In vitro binding of gefitinib to human plasma proteins (serum albumin and α 1-acid glycoprotein) is 90% and is independent of drug concentrations.

Metabolism/Excretion – Gefitinib undergoes extensive hepatic metabolism in humans, predominantly by CYP3A4. Three sites of biotransformation have been identified: Metabolism of the N-propoxymorpholino-group, demethylation of the methoxy-substituent on the quinazoline, and oxidative defluorination of the halogenated phenyl group.

Five metabolites were identified in human plasma. Only O-desmethyl gefitinib has exposure comparable to gefitinib. Although this metabolite has similar EGFR-TK activity to gefitinib in the isolated enzyme assay, it had only 1/14 of the potency of gefitinib in 1 of the cell-based assays.

Gefitinib is cleared primarily by the liver, with total plasma clearance and elimination half-life values of 595 mL/min and 48 hours, respectively, after intravenous administration. Excretion is predominantly via the feces (86%), with renal elimination of drug and metabolites accounting for less than 4% of the administered dose.

Contraindications

Severe hypersensitivity to gefitinib or any other component of gefitinib.

Warnings/Precautions

➤*Pulmonary toxicity:* Cases of interstitial lung disease (ILD) have been observed in patients receiving gefitinib at an overall incidence of about 1%. Approximately 1/3 of the cases have been fatal. The reported incidence of ILD was about 2% in the Japanese postmarketing experience, about 0.3% in approximately 23,000 patients treated with gefitinib in a US expanded access program and about 1% in the studies of first-line use in NSCLC (but with similar rates in both treatment and placebo groups). Reports have described the adverse reaction as interstitial pneumonia, pneumonitis and alveolitis. Patients often present with the acute onset of dyspnea, sometimes associated with cough or low-grade fever, often becoming severe within a short time and requiring hospitalization. ILD has occurred in patients who have received prior radiation therapy (31% of reported cases), prior chemotherapy (57% of reported patients), and no previous therapy (12% of reported cases). Patients with concurrent idiopathic pulmonary fibrosis whose condition worsens while receiving gefitinib have been observed to have an increased mortality compared to those without concurrent idiopathic pulmonary fibrosis.

In the event of acute onset or worsening of pulmonary symptoms (dyspnea, cough, fever), gefitinib therapy should be interrupted and a prompt investigation of these symptoms should occur. If interstitial lung disease is confirmed, gefitinib should be discontinued and the patient treated appropriately.

➤*Renal function impairment:* The effect of severe renal impairment on the pharmacokinetics of gefitinib is not known. Patients with severe renal impairment should be treated with caution when given gefitinib.

➤*Hepatic function impairment:* In vitro and in vivo evidence suggest that gefitinib is cleared primarily by the liver. Therefore, gefitinib exposure may be increased in patients with hepatic dysfunction. In patients with liver metastases and moderately to severely elevated biochemical liver abnormalities, however, gefitinib pharmacokinetics were similar to the pharmacokinetics of individuals without liver abnormalities. The influence of non-cancer related hepatic impairment on the pharmacokinetics of gefitinib has not been evaluated.

➤*Pregnancy: Category D.* Gefitinib may cause fetal harm when administered to a pregnant woman. A single dose study in rats showed that gefitinib crosses the placenta after an oral dose of 5 mg/kg (30 mg/m^2, about 1/5 the recommended human dose on a mg/m^2 basis). When pregnant rats were treated with 5 mg/kg from the beginning of organogenesis to the end of weaning gave birth, there was a reduction in the number of offspring born alive. This effect was more severe at 20 mg/kg and was accompanied by high neonatal mortality soon after parturition. In this study a dose of 1 mg/kg caused no adverse effects.

In rabbits, a dose of 20 mg/kg/day (240 mg/m^2, about twice the recommended dose in humans on a mg/m^2 basis) caused reduced fetal weight.

There are no adequate and well-controlled studies in pregnant women using gefitinib. If gefitinib is used during pregnancy or if the patient becomes pregnant while receiving this drug, she should be apprised of the potential hazard to the fetus or potential risk for loss of the pregnancy.

➤*Lactation:* It is not known whether gefitinib is excreted in human milk. Following oral administration of carbon-14 labeled gefitinib to rats 14 days postpartum, concentrations of radioactivity in milk were higher than in blood. Levels of gefitinib and its metabolites were 11- to 19-fold higher in milk than in blood, after oral exposure of lactating rats to a dose of 5 mg/kg. Because many drugs are excreted in human milk and because of the potential for serious adverse reactions in nursing infants, women should be advised against breastfeeding while receiving gefitinib therapy.

➤*Children:* Safety and effectiveness of gefitinib in pediatric patients have not been studied.

GEFITINIB — ORAL

➤*Monitoring:* Asymptomatic increases in liver transaminases have been observed in gefitinib treated patients; therefore, periodic liver function (transaminases, bilirubin, and alkaline phosphatase) testing should be considered. Discontinuation of gefitinib should be considered if changes are severe.

Drug Interactions

Gefitinib Drug Interactions

Precipitant drug	Object drug[a]		Description
CYP3A4 inducers (eg, rifampin, phenytoin)	Gefitinib	⬇	The plasma concentration of gefitinib is decreased due to an increase in its metabolism. Coadministration with rifampin caused a decrease in gefitinib AUC by 85%. Consider a dose increase of gefitinib if coadministered with a potent CYP3A4 inducer (see Administration and Dosage).
CYP3A4 inhibitors (eg, ketoconazole, itraconazole)	Gefitinib	⬆	Potent CYP3A4 inhibitors decrease gefitinib metabolism and increase its plasma concentrations. Coadministration with itraconazole increased gefitinib AUC by 88%. Use with caution.
H_2 antagonist (eg, ranitidine, cimetidine) Sodium bicarbonate	Gefitinib	⬇	Drugs that cause significant sustained elevations in gastric pH may reduce plasma concentrations of gefitinib and may reduce efficacy.
Gefitinib	Metoprolol	⬆	Exposure to metoprolol, a substrate of CYP2D6, was increased by 30% when given with gefitinib.
Gefitinib	Warfarin	⬆	INR elevations and/or bleeding events have been reported in some patients taking warfarin while on gefitinib therapy. Monitor PT or INR regularly.

[a] ⬆ = object drug increased; ⬇ = object drug decreased.

Adverse Reactions

Gefitinib Adverse Reactions (≥ 5%)

Adverse reaction[a]	250 mg/day (n = 102)	500 mg/day (n = 114)
Diarrhea	49 (48%)	76 (67%)
Rash	44 (43%)	61 (54%)
Acne	25 (25%)	37 (33%)
Dry skin	13 (13%)	30 (26%)
Nausea	13 (13%)	20 (18%)
Vomiting	12 (12%)	10 (9%)
Pruritus	8 (8%)	10 (9%)
Anorexia	7 (7%)	11 (10%)
Asthenia	6 (6%)	5 (4%)
Weight loss	3 (3%)	6 (5%)

[a] A patient may have had more than 1 drug-related adverse reaction.

The table below provides drug-related adverse reactions with an incidence of greater than or equal to 5% by CTC grade for the patients who received the 250 mg/day dose of gefitinib monotherapy for treatment of NSCLC. Only 2% of patients stopped therapy due to an adverse drug reaction (ADR). The onset of these ADRs occurred within the first month of therapy.

Gefitinib Adverse Reactions at 250 mg Dose by Worst CTC Grade (n = 102) (≥ 5%)

Adverse reaction	All grades	CTC grade 1	CTC grade 2	CTC grade 3	CTC grade 4
Diarrhea	48%	41%	6%	1%	0%
Rash	43%	39%	4%	0%	0%
Acne	25%	19%	6%	0%	0%
Dry skin	13%	12%	1%	0%	0%
Nausea	13%	7%	5%	1%	0%
Vomiting	12%	9%	2%	1%	0%
Pruritus	8%	7%	1%	0%	0%
Anorexia	7%	3%	4%	0%	0%
Asthenia	6%	2%	2%	1%	1%

➤*Other adverse reactions:* Other adverse reactions reported at an incidence of less than 5% in patients who received either 250 mg or 500 mg as monotherapy for treatment of NSCLC (along with their frequency at the 250 mg recommended dose) include the following: Peripheral edema (2%), amblyopia (2%), dyspnea (2%), conjunctivitis (1%), vesiculobullous rash (1%), and mouth ulceration (1%).

In patients receiving gefitinib therapy, there were reports of eye pain and corneal erosion/ulcer, sometimes in association with aberrant eyelash growth. There were also rare reports of pancreatitis and very rare reports of corneal membrane sloughing, ocular ischemia/hemorrhage, toxic epidermal necrolysis, erythema multiforme, and allergic reactions, including angioedema and urticaria.

➤*Hematologic:* See Drug Interactions for more information.

➤*Cardiac:* Data from nonclinical (in vitro and in vivo) studies indicate that gefitinib has the potential to inhibit the cardiac action potential repolarization process (eg, QT interval). The clinical relevance of these findings is unknown.

➤*Interstitial lung disease:* Cases of interstitial lung disease (ILD) have been observed in patients receiving gefitinib at an overall incidence of about 1%. Approximately ⅓ of the cases have been fatal. The reported incidence of ILD was about 2% in the Japanese postmarketing experience, about 0.3% in approximately 23,000 patients treated with gefitinib in a US expanded access program and about 1% in the studies of first-line use in NSCLC (but with similar rates in both treatment and placebo groups). Reports have described the adverse reaction as interstitial pneumonia, pneumonitis and alveolitis. Patients often present with the acute onset of dyspnea, sometimes associated with cough or low-grade fever, often becoming severe within a short time and requiring hospitalization. ILD has occurred in patients who have received prior radiation therapy (31% of reported cases), prior chemotherapy (57% of reported patients), and no previous therapy (12% of reported cases). Patients with concurrent idiopathic pulmonary fibrosis whose condition worsens while receiving gefitinib have been observed to have an increased mortality compared to those without concurrent idiopathic pulmonary fibrosis.

In the reaction of acute onset or worsening of pulmonary symptoms (dyspnea, cough, fever), gefitinib therapy should be interrupted and a prompt investigation of these symptoms should occur. If interstitial lung disease is confirmed, gefitinib should be discontinued and the patient treated appropriately.

Overdosage

The acute toxicity of gefitinib up to 500 mg in clinical studies has been low. In non-clinical studies, a single dose of 12,000 mg/m^2 (about 80 times the recommended clinical dose on a mg/m^2 basis) was lethal to rats. Half this dose caused no mortality in mice.

➤*Treatment:* There is no specific treatment for an gefitinib overdose and possible symptoms of overdose are not established. However, in Phase 1 clinical trials, a limited number of patients were treated with daily doses of up to 1000 mg. An increase in frequency and severity of some adverse reactions was observed, mainly diarrhea and skin rash. Adverse reactions associated with overdose should be treated symptomatically; in particular, severe diarrhea should be managed appropriately.

Patient Information

Advise patients to seek medical advice promptly if they develop the following: severe or persistent diarrhea, nausea, anorexia, or vomiting, as these have sometimes been associated with dehydration; an onset or worsening of pulmonary symptoms (ie, shortness of breath or cough); an eye irritation; any other new symptom.

Advise women of childbearing potential to avoid becoming pregnant.

TEMSIROLIMUS

Rx	**Torisel** (Wyeth)	**Injection, solution, concentrate:** 25 mg/mL	Alcohol, polysorbate 80. In a 2-vial kit.

TEMSIROLIMUS — INJECTION

Indications

➤*Advanced renal cell carcinoma:* For the treatment of advanced renal cell carcinoma.

➤*Off-label uses:* Mantle cell lymphoma.

Administration and Dosage

➤*General dosing considerations:* Patients should receive premedication to reduce the risk of hypersensitivity. (See Premedication and Hypersensitivity reactions.)

➤*Adults:*

Advanced renal cell carcinoma –

Usual dosage: 25 mg infused IV over a 30- to 60-minute period once a week.

Dosage adjustment: Dosage reduction is necessary for adverse effects, as shown in the following table.

Temsirolimus Dosage Adjustment During Treatment of Renal Cell Carcinoma

Adverse reaction and grade of severity	Dosage adjustment
Hematologic toxicity	
ANC < 1,000 cells/mm^3, or platelets [3]	•First occurrence: Withhold therapy. When ANC ≥ 1,000 cells/mm^3 and platelets ≥ 75,000 cells/mm^3, decrease dose to 20 mg/wk and resume therapy. •Second occurrence: Withhold therapy. When ANC > 1,000 cells/mm^3 and platelets ≥ 75,000 cells/mm^3, decrease dose to 15 mg/wk and resume therapy. •Third occurrence: Discontinue permanently.
Other toxicities	
NCI Toxicity grade 3 to 4	•First occurrence: Withhold therapy. When toxicity resolves to grade 0 to 2, decrease dose to 20 mg/wk and resume therapy. •Second occurrence: Withhold therapy. When toxicity resolves to grade 0 to 2, decrease dose to 15 mg/wk and resume therapy. •Third occurrence: Discontinue permanently.

Duration of therapy: Treatment should continue until disease progression or unacceptable toxicity occurs.

Concomitant therapy:

• *CYP3A4 inhibitors –* The concomitant use of strong CYP3A4 inhibitors should be avoided (eg, ketoconazole, itraconazole, clarithromycin, atazanavir, indinavir, nefazodone, nelfinavir, ritonavir, saquinavir, telithromycin, voriconazole). Grapefruit juice may also increase plasma concentrations of sirolimus (a major metabolite of temsirolimus) and should be avoided. If patients must be coadministered a strong CYP3A4 inhibitor, based on pharmacokinetics studies, a temsirolimus dose reduction to 12.5 mg weekly should be considered. This dose of temsirolimus is predicted to adjust the area under the curve (AUC) to the range observed without inhibitors. However, there are no clinical data with this dose adjustment in patients receiving strong CYP3A4 inhibitors. If the strong inhibitor is discontinued, a washout period of approximately 1 week should be allowed before the temsirolimus dose is adjusted back to the dose used prior to initiation of the strong CYP3A4 inhibitor.

• *CYP3A4 inducers –* The use of concomitant strong CYP3A4 inducers should be avoided (eg, dexamethasone, phenytoin, carbamazepine, rifampin, rifabutin, rifampin, phenobarbital). If patients must be coadministered a strong CYP3A4 inducer, based on pharmacokinetic studies, a temsirolimus dose increase from 25 mg weekly up to 50 mg weekly should be considered. This dose of temsirolimus is predicted to adjust the AUC to the range observed without inducers. However, there are no clinical data with this dose adjustment in patients receiving strong CYP3A4 inducers. If the strong inducer is discontinued, the temsirolimus dose should be returned to the dose used prior to initiation of the strong CYP3A4 inducer.

Premedication: Patients should receive prophylactic diphenhydramine 25 to 50 mg oral or IV (or similar antihistamine) approximately 30 minutes before the start of each dose of temsirolimus.

Off-label dosing –

Mantle cell lymphoma:

• *Usual dose –* 250 mg infused IV over a 30- to 60-minute once weekly. Evaluate response to therapy every 3 months.

• *Dosage adjustment –* Dosage reduction is necessary for adverse effects, as shown in the following table.

Temsirolimus Dosage Adjustment During Treatment of Mantle Cell Lymphoma

Adverse reaction and grade of severity	Dosage adjustment
Hematologic toxicity	
ANC < 1,000 cells/mm^3, or platelets < 50,000 cells/mm^3	•First occurrence: Withhold therapy. When ANC ≥ 1,000 cells/mm^3 and platelets ≥ 50,000 cells/mm^3, decrease dose to 175 mg/wk and resume therapy. •Second occurrence: Withhold therapy. When ANC ≥ 1,000 cells/mm^3 and platelets ≥ 50,000 cells/mm^3, decrease dose to 125 mg/wk and resume therapy. •Third occurrence: Withhold therapy. When ANC ≥ 1,000 cells/mm^3 and platelets ≥ 50,000 cells/mm^3, decrease dose to 75 mg/wk and resume therapy. •Fourth occurrence: Withhold therapy. When ANC ≥ 1,000 cells/mm^3 and platelets ≥ 50,000 cells/mm^3, decrease dose to 50 mg/wk and resume therapy. •Fifth occurrence: Discontinue permanently.
Other toxicities	
NCI Toxicity grade 3 to 4	•First occurrence: Withhold therapy. When toxicity resolves to grade 0 to 2, decrease dose to 175 mg/wk and resume therapy. •Second occurrence: Withhold therapy. When toxicity resolves to grade 0 to 2, decrease dose to 125 mg/wk and resume therapy. •Third occurrence: Withhold therapy. When toxicity resolves to grade 0 to 2, decrease dose to 75 mg/wk and resume therapy. •Fourth occurrence: Withhold therapy. When toxicity resolves to grade 0 to 2, decrease dose to 50 mg/wk and resume therapy. •Fifth occurrence: Discontinue permanently.

• *Duration of therapy –* Discontinue if disease progression occurs or if the patient has stable disease at 6 months. In patients with response, continue for up to 12 months, or 2 months after complete remission, whichever is shorter.

➤*Hypersensitivity reactions:* If a reaction occurs, temporarily interrupt the infusion and monitor the patient for 30 to 60 minutes. Consider resuming the infusion at a slower rate (ie, give dose over up to 60 minutes). Thirty minutes prior to resuming the infusion, administer diphenhydramine (if not given before infusion), alone or with an IV histamine H2 antagonist (eg, famotidine 20 mg, ranitidine 50 mg, or equivalent).

Patients who react to temsirolimus infusions can possibly receive additional doses. An IV histamine H_2 antagonist (eg, famotidine 20 mg, ranitidine 50 mg, or equivalent) may be added to the pretreatment regimen at the clinician's discretion.

➤*Preparation for administration:* Temsirolimus is an immunosuppressant agent. Follow safe handling procedures when preparing, administering, or dispensing temsirolimus.

During handling and preparation of admixtures, temsirolimus should be protected from excessive room light and sunlight.

In order to minimize patient exposure to the plasticizer di-2-ethylhexyl phthalate (DEHP), which may be leached from polyvinyl chloride (PVC) infusion bags or sets, the final temsirolimus dilution for infusion should be stored in bottles (glass, polypropylene) or plastic bags (polypropylene, polyolefin) and administered through polyethylene-lined administration sets.

Dilution – In preparing the temsirolimus administration solution, follow this 2-step dilution process in an aseptic manner.

Step 1: Inject 1.8 mL of diluent for temsirolimus into the vial of temsirolimus 25 mg/mL injection. The temsirolimus vial contains an overfill of 0.2 mL (30 mg per 1.2 mL). Because of the intentional overfill in the temsirolimus injection vial, the drug concentration of the resulting solution will be 10 mg/mL. A total volume of 3 mL will be obtained, including the overfill. Mix well by inversion of the vial. Allow sufficient time for air bubbles to subside. This 10 mg/mL drug solution/diluent mixture must be further diluted as described in step 2.

The solution is clear to slightly turbid, colorless to yellow, and free from visual particulates.

Step 2: Withdraw the required amount of temsirolimus from the 10 mg/mL drug solution/diluent mixture prepared in step 1. Inject rapidly into a 250 mL container (glass, polyolefin, or polyethylene) of sodium chloride 0.9% injection. Mix the admixture by inversion of the bag or bottle. Avoid excessive shaking because this may cause foaming.

TEMSIROLIMUS — INJECTION

➤*Administration:* An inline polyethersulfone filter with a pore size no greater than 5 microns is recommended for administration.

The final diluted solution of temsirolimus is infused IV over a 30- to 60-minute period once a week. The use of an infusion pump is the preferred method of administration to ensure accurate delivery of the drug.

Administration of the final diluted infusion solution should be completed within 6 hours from the time that the drug solution/diluent mixture is added to the sodium chloride injection.

The sodium chloride injection container should be composed of non-DEHP-containing materials, such as glass, polyolefin, or polyethylene, and the administration set should consist of non-DEHP tubing to avoid extraction of DEHP. Temsirolimus contains polysorbate 80, which is known to increase the rate of DEHP extraction from PVC.

➤*Admixture compatibility:* Undiluted temsirolimus injection should not be added directly to aqueous infusion solutions. Direct addition of temsirolimus injection to aqueous solutions will result in precipitation of the drug. Always combine temsirolimus injection with diluent for temsirolimus before adding to infusion solutions. It is recommended that temsirolimus be administered in sodium chloride 0.9% injection after combining with diluent. The stability of temsirolimus in other infusion solutions has not been evaluated. Addition of other drugs or nutritional agents to admixtures of temsirolimus in sodium chloride injection has not been evaluated and should be avoided. Temsirolimus is degraded by both acids and bases, and thus combination of temsirolimus with agents capable of modifying solution pH should be avoided.

➤*Storage/Stability:* Store at 2° to 8°C (36° to 46°F). Protect from light. The 10 mg/mL drug solution/diluent mixture is stable for up to 24 hours at controlled room temperature. After dilution with sodium chloride 0.9% injection, use of the final diluted solution within 6 hours.

Actions

➤*Pharmacology:* Temsirolimus is an inhibitor of mTOR (mammalian target of rapamycin). Temsirolimus binds to an intracellular protein (FKBP-12), and the protein-drug complex inhibits the activity of mTOR that controls cell division. Inhibition of mTOR activity resulted in a G1 growth arrest in treated tumor cells. When mTOR was inhibited, its ability to phosphorylate p70S6k and S6 ribosomal proteins, which are downstream of mTOR in the PI3 kinase/AKT pathway, was blocked. In in vitro studies using renal cell carcinoma cell lines, temsirolimus inhibited the activity of mTOR and resulted in reduced levels of the hypoxia-inducible factors HIF-1 and HIF-2 alpha and the vascular endothelial growth factor.

➤*Pharmacokinetics:*

Absorption – Following administration of a single dose of temsirolimus 25 mg in patients with cancer, mean temsirolimus maximum concentration (C_{max}) in whole blood was 585 ng/mL (coefficient of variation [CV] = 14%), and mean AUC in blood was 1,627 ng•h/mL (CV = 26%). Typically C_{max} occurred at the end of infusion. Over the dose range of 1 to 25 mg, temsirolimus exposure increased in a less than dose proportional manner, while sirolimus exposure increased proportionally with dose. Following a single 25 mg IV dose in patients with cancer, sirolimus AUC was 2.7-fold that of temsirolimus AUC, principally because of the longer half-life of sirolimus.

Distribution – Following a single 25 mg IV dose, mean steady-state volume of distribution of temsirolimus in whole blood of patients with cancer was 172 L. Both temsirolimus and sirolimus are extensively partitioned into formed blood elements.

Metabolism – CYP-450 3A4 is the major isozyme responsible for the formation of 5 temsirolimus metabolites. Sirolimus, an active metabolite of temsirolimus, is the principal metabolite in humans following IV treatment. The remainder of the metabolites account for less than 10% of radioactivity in the plasma. In human liver microsomes, temsirolimus was an inhibitor of CYP2D6 and 3A4. However, there was no effect observed in vivo when temsirolimus was administered with desipramine (a CYP2D6 substrate), and no effect is anticipated with substrates of CYP3A4 metabolism.

Excretion – Elimination is primarily via the feces. After a single IV dose of [^{14}C]-temsirolimus, approximately 82% of total radioactivity was eliminated within 14 days, with 4.6% and 78% of the administered radioactivity recovered in the urine and feces, respectively. Following a single dose of temsirolimus 25 mg in patients with cancer, temsirolimus mean (CV) systemic clearance was 16.2 (22%) L/h. Temsirolimus exhibits a biexponential decline in whole blood concentrations, and the mean half-lives of temsirolimus and sirolimus were 17.3 and 54.6 hours, respectively.

Contraindications

None known.

Warnings/Precautions

➤*Hyperglycemia/Glucose intolerance:* The use of temsirolimus is likely to result in increases in serum glucose. In the phase 3 trial, 89% of patients receiving temsirolimus had at least 1 elevated serum glucose while on treatment, and 26% of patients reported hyperglycemia as an adverse reaction. This may result in the need for an increase in the dose of, or initiation of, insulin and/or oral hypoglycemic agent therapy. Test serum glucose before and during treatment with temsirolimus. Advise patients to report excessive thirst or any increase in the volume or frequency of urination.

➤*Infections:* The use of temsirolimus may result in immunosuppression. Carefully observe patients for the occurrence of infections, including opportunistic infections.

➤*Interstitial lung disease:* Cases of interstitial lung disease, some resulting in death, occurred in patients who received temsirolimus. Some patients were asymptomatic with infiltrates detected on computed tomography scan or chest radiograph. Others presented with symptoms such as dyspnea, cough, hypoxia, and fever. Some patients required discontinuation of temsirolimus and/or treatment with corticosteroids and/or antibiotics, while some patients continued treatment without additional intervention. Advise patients to promptly report any new or worsening respiratory symptoms.

➤*Hyperlipemia:* The use of temsirolimus is likely to result in increases in serum triglycerides and cholesterol. In the phase 3 trial, 87% of patients receiving temsirolimus had at least 1 elevated serum cholesterol value and 83% had at least 1 elevated serum triglyceride value. This may require the initiation or an increase in the dose of lipid-lowering agents. Test serum cholesterol and triglycerides before and during treatment with temsirolimus.

➤*Bowel perforation:* Cases of fatal bowel perforation occurred in patients who received temsirolimus. These patients presented with fever, abdominal pain, metabolic acidosis, bloody stools, diarrhea, and/or acute abdomen. Advise patients to promptly report any new or worsening abdominal pain or blood in their stools.

➤*Renal failure:* Cases of rapidly progressive and sometimes fatal acute renal failure not clearly related to disease progression occurred in patients who received temsirolimus. Some of these cases were not responsive to dialysis.

➤*Wound healing complications:* Use of temsirolimus has been associated with abnormal wound healing. Therefore, exercise caution in the use of temsirolimus in the perioperative period.

➤*Intracerebral hemorrhage:* Patients with CNS tumors (primary CNS tumor or metastases) and/or receiving anticoagulation therapy may be at an increased risk of developing intracerebral bleeding (including fatal outcomes) while receiving temsirolimus.

➤*Vaccinations:* Avoid the use of live vaccine and close contact with those who have received live vaccines during treatment with temsirolimus. Examples of live vaccines are as follows: intranasal influenza, measles, mumps, rubella, oral polio, Bacille Calmette-Guérin, yellow fever, varicella, and TY21a typhoid vaccines.

➤*Hypersensitivity reactions:* Hypersensitivity reactions manifested by symptoms including, but not limited to, anaphylaxis, dyspnea, flushing, and chest pain have been observed with temsirolimus.

Use temsirolimus with caution in patients with known hypersensitivity to temsirolimus or its metabolites (including sirolimus), polysorbate 80, or to any other component (including the excipients) of temsirolimus.

Administer an H_1 antihistamine to patients before the start of the IV temsirolimus infusion. Use temsirolimus with caution in patients with known hypersensitivity to an antihistamine or patients who cannot receive an antihistamine for other medical reasons.

If a patient develops a hypersensitivity reaction during the temsirolimus infusion, stop the infusion and observe the patient for at least 30 to 60 minutes (depending on the severity of the reaction). At the discretion of the health care provider, treatment may be resumed with the administration of an H_1-receptor antagonist (such as diphenhydramine), if not previously administered, and/or an H_2-receptor antagonist (such as famotidine 20 mg IV or ranitidine 50 mg IV) approximately 30 minutes before restarting the temsirolimus infusion. The infusion may then be resumed at a slower rate (up to 60 minutes).

➤*Pregnancy: Category D.* Temsirolimus administered daily as an oral formulation caused embryo-fetal and intrauterine toxicities in rats and rabbits at human subtherapeutic exposures. Embryo-fetal adverse reactions in rats consisted of reduced fetal weight and reduced ossifications, and in rabbits included reduced fetal weight, omphalocele, bifurcated sternebrae, notched ribs, and incomplete ossifications.

In rats, the intrauterine and embryo-fetal adverse reactions were observed at the oral dose of 2.7 mg/m²/day (approximately 0.04-fold the AUC in cancer patients at the human recommended dose). In rabbits, the intrauterine and embryo-fetal adverse reactions were observed at the oral dose of 7.2 mg/m²/day or more (approximately 0.12-fold the AUC in cancer patients at the recommended human dose).

Advise women of childbearing potential to avoid becoming pregnant throughout treatment and for 3 months after temsirolimus therapy has stopped. Temsirolimus can cause fetal harm when administered to a pregnant woman. If this drug is used during pregnancy or if the patient becomes pregnant while taking this drug, apprise the patient of the potential hazard to the fetus.

Counsel men regarding the effects of temsirolimus on the fetus and sperm prior to starting treatment. Men with partners of childbearing potential should use reliable contraception throughout treatment and are recommended to continue this for 3 months after the last dose of temsirolimus.

➤*Lactation:* It is not known whether temsirolimus is excreted into human milk. The molecular weights of temsirolimus and sirolimus (active metabolite of temsirolimus), about 1030 and 914, respectively, are low enough for excretion into breast milk. Moreover, the elimination half-lives, about 17 and 55 hours, respectively, suggest that both temsirolimus and sirolimus will be excreted. Because of the potential for tumorigenicity shown for sirolimus in animal studies, decide whether to discontinue breast-feeding or temsirolimus, taking into account the importance of the drug to the mother.

➤*Children:* The safety and efficacy of temsirolimus in children have not been established.

TEMSIROLIMUS — INJECTION

➤*Monitoring:* In the randomized, phase 3 trial, complete blood cell counts were checked weekly, and chemistry panels were checked every 2 weeks. Test serum glucose before and during treatment with temsirolimus. Test serum cholesterol and triglycerides before and during treatment with temsirolimus. Laboratory monitoring for patients receiving temsirolimus may need to be performed more or less frequently at the health care provider's discretion.

Drug Interactions

Temsirolimus Drug Interactions

Precipitant drug	Object drug[a]		Description
Azole antifungal agents (eg, fluconazole, itraconazole, ketoconazole, posaconazole, voriconazole)	Temsirolimus	↑	Plasma temsirolimus or sirolimus concentrations may be elevated, increasing the risk of toxicity. Monitor temsirolimus plasma concentrations and observe the patient for toxicity when starting or stopping an azole antifungal agent. Adjust the temsirolimus dose as needed.
Cyclosporine	Temsirolimus	↑	Plasma sirolimus, the active metabolite of temsirolimus, concentrations may be elevated, resulting in increased toxicity.
CYP-450 3A4/5 inducers (eg, dexamethasone, rifabutin, rifampin, phenytoin)	Temsirolimus	↓	Avoid the concomitant use of strong CYP3A4 inducers. If use cannot be avoided, consider increasing temsirolimus dose to 50 mg weekly.
CYP-450 3A4 inhibitors (eg, atazanavir, clarithromycin, diltiazem)	Temsirolimus	↑	Temsirolimus plasma levels may be elevated, increasing the risk of adverse reactions. Closely monitor temsirolimus concentrations when starting, stopping, or changing the dose of the CYP-450 3A4 inhibitor. Adjust the temsirolimus dose as needed.
Diltiazem	Temsirolimus	↑	Plasma sirolimus, the active metabolite of temsirolimus, may be elevated, increasing the risk of toxicity.
Mycophenolate mofetil	Temsirolimus	↑	Mycophenolic acid trough plasma concentrations may be elevated by sirolimus, increasing the risk of adverse reactions.
St. John's wort	Temsirolimus	↓	St. John's wort may decrease temsirolimus plasma concentrations unpredictably. Avoid concomitant use.
Sunitinib	Temsirolimus	↑	The combination of temsirolimus and sunitinib resulted in dose-limiting toxicities (ie, grade 3/4 erythematous maculopapular rash, gout/cellulitis requiring hospitalization).
Temsirolimus	Tacrolimus	↓	Tacrolimus trough plasma concentrations may be reduced by sirolimus, decreasing the pharmacologic effect. Frequently monitor tacrolimus trough levels after starting, stopping, or changing the temsirolimus dose. Adjust the tacrolimus dose as needed.

[a] ↑ = object drug increased; ↓ = object drug decreased.

➤*Drug/Food interactions:* Grapefruit juice may increase plasma concentrations of sirolimus (a major metabolite of temsirolimus) and should be avoided.

Adverse Reactions

The following serious adverse reactions have been associated with temsirolimus in clinical trials and are discussed in greater detail in other sections: hypersensitivity reactions, hyperglycemia/glucose intolerance, interstitial lung disease, hyperlipemia, bowel perforation, renal failure.

The most common (at least 30%) adverse reactions observed with temsirolimus are anorexia, asthenia, edema, mucositis, nausea, and rash.

The most common (at least 30%) laboratory abnormalities observed with temsirolimus are alkaline phosphatase elevated, anemia, AST elevated, hyperglycemia, hyperlipemia, hypertriglyceridemia, hypophosphatemia, leukopenia, lymphopenia, serum creatinine elevated, and thrombocytopenia.

Temsirolimus Adverse Reactions (≥ 10%)

Adverse reaction	Temsirolimus 25 mg (n = 208)		Interferon alfa (n = 200)	
	All grades[a]	Grades 3 and 4[a]	All grades[a]	Grades 3 and 4[a]
Any	100%	67%	100%	78%
CNS				
Depression	4%	0%	14%	2%
Dysgeusia[b]	20%	0%	9%	0%
Headache	15%	1%	15%	0%
Insomnia	12%	1%	15%	0%
Dermatologic				
Acne	10%	0%	1%	0%
Dry skin	11%	1%	7%	0%
Nail disorder	14%	0%	1%	0%
Pruritus	19%	1%	8%	0%
Rash[c]	47%	5%	7%	0%
GI				
Abdominal pain	21%	4%	17%	2%
Anorexia	32%	3%	44%	4%
Constipation	20%	0%	18%	1%
Diarrhea	27%	1%	20%	2%
Mucositis[d]	41%	3%	10%	0%
Nausea	37%	2%	41%	5%
Vomiting	19%	2%	29%	3%
Musculoskeletal				
Arthralgia	18%	1%	15%	1%
Back pain	20%	3%	14%	4%
Myalgia	8%	1%	15%	1%
Respiratory				
Cough	26%	1%	15%	0%
Dyspnea	28%	9%	24%	6%
Epistaxis	12%	0%	4%	0%
Pharyngitis	12%	0%	2%	0%
Rhinitis	10%	0%	2%	0%
Miscellaneous				
Asthenia	51%	11%	64%	26%
Chest pain	16%	1%	9%	1%
Chills	8%	1%	30%	2%
Edema[e]	35%	3%	11%	1%
Infections[f]	20%	3%	10%	2%
Pain	28%	5%	16%	2%
Pyrexia	24%	1%	50%	4%
Urinary tract infection[g]	15%	1%	12%	2%
Weight loss	19%	1%	25%	2%

[a] NCI CTCAE Version 3.0.
[b] Includes taste loss and taste perversion.
[c] Includes eczema, exfoliative dermatitis, maculopapular rash, pruritic rash, pustular rash, rash (not otherwise specified [NOS]), and vesiculobullous rash.
[d] Includes aphthous stomatitis, glossitis, mouth ulceration, mucositis, and stomatitis.
[e] Includes edema, facial edema, and peripheral edema.
[f] Includes infections NOS and the following infections that occurred infrequently as distinct entities: abscess, bronchitis, cellulitis, herpes simplex, and herpes zoster.
[g] Includes cystitis, dysuria, hematuria, urinary frequency, and urinary tract infection.

The following selected adverse reactions were reported less frequently (less than 10%).

➤*Cardiovascular:* Hypertension (7%); venous thromboembolism (including deep vein thrombosis and pulmonary embolus) (2%); thrombophlebitis (1%).

➤*GI:* Fatal bowel perforation (1%).

➤*Hypersensitivity:* Allergic/Hypersensitivity reactions (9%). Angioneurotic edema-type reactions have been observed in some patients who received temsirolimus and angiotensin-converting enzyme inhibitors concomitantly.

➤*Respiratory:* Pneumonia (8%); upper respiratory tract infection (7%); interstitial lung disease (2%), including rare fatalities.

➤*Special senses:* Conjunctivitis (including lacrimation disorder) (7%).

➤*Miscellaneous:* Impaired wound healing (1%).

TEMSIROLIMUS — INJECTION

Temsirolimus Laboratory Abnormalities

Laboratory abnormality	Temsirolimus 25 mg (n = 208) All grades[a]	Temsirolimus 25 mg (n = 208) Grades 3 and 4[a]	Interferon alfa (n = 200) All grades[a]	Interferon alfa (n = 200) Grades 3 and 4[a]
Any	100%	78%	98%	72%
Hematology				
Hemoglobin decreased	94%	20%	90%	22%
Leukocytes decreased	32%	1%	47%	6%
Lymphocytes decreased[b]	53%	16%	53%	24%
Neutrophils decreased[b]	19%	5%	29%	10%
Platelets decreased	40%	1%	26%	0%
Chemistry				
Alkaline phosphatase increased	68%	3%	56%	7%
AST increased	38%	2%	52%	7%
Creatinine increased	57%	3%	49%	1%
Glucose increased	89%	16%	64%	3%
Phosphorus decreased	49%	18%	31%	9%
Potassium decreased	21%	5%	8%	0%
Total bilirubin increased	8%	1%	13%	2%
Total cholesterol increased	87%	2%	48%	1%
Triglycerides increased	83%	44%	72%	35%

[a] NCI CTCAE Version 3.0.
[b] Grade 1 toxicity may be underreported for lymphocytes and neutrophils.

Overdosage

➤*Symptoms:* Temsirolimus has been administered to patients with cancer in phase 1 and 2 trials with repeated IV doses as high as 220 mg/m². The risk of several serious adverse reactions, including thrombosis, bowel perforation, interstitial lung disease, seizure, and psychosis, is increased with doses of temsirolimus greater than 25 mg.

➤*Treatment:* There is no specific treatment for temsirolimus IV overdose.

Patient Information

Inform patients of the possibility of serious allergic reactions, including anaphylaxis, despite premedication with antihistamines, and to immediately report any facial swelling or difficulty breathing.

Patients are likely to experience increased blood glucose levels while taking temsirolimus. This may result in the need for the initiation or an increase in the dose of insulin and/or hypoglycemic agents. Direct patients to report any excessive thirst or frequency of urination to their health care provider.

Inform patients that they may be more susceptible to infections while being treated with temsirolimus.

Warn patients of the possibility of developing interstitial lung disease, a chronic inflammation of the lungs that may rarely result in death.

Direct patients to promptly report any new or worsening respiratory symptoms to their health care provider.

Patients are likely to experience elevated triglycerides and/or cholesterol during temsirolimus treatment. This may require the initiation or an increase in the dose of lipid-lowering agents.

Warn patients of the possibility of bowel perforation. Direct patients to promptly report any new or worsening abdominal pain or blood in their stools.

Inform patients of the risk of renal failure.

Advise patients of the possibility of abnormal wound healing if they have surgery within a few weeks of initiating therapy or during therapy.

Inform patients with CNS tumors and/or receiving anticoagulants of the increased risk of developing intracerebral bleeding (including fatal outcomes) while on temsirolimus.

Some medicines can interfere with the breakdown or metabolism of temsirolimus. Direct patients to inform their health care provider if they are taking any of the following: protease inhibitors; anti-epileptic medicines, including carbamazepine, phenytoin, and barbiturates; St. John's wort; rifampin; rifabutin; nefazodone; selective serotonin reuptake inhibitors used to treat depression; antibiotics; or antifungal medicines used to treat infections.

Advise patients that vaccinations may be less effective while being treated with temsirolimus. In addition, tell patients to avoid the use of live vaccines and close contact with those who have received live vaccines while on temsirolimus.

Temsirolimus can cause fetal harm. Advise women of childbearing potential to avoid becoming pregnant throughout treatment and for 3 months after temsirolimus therapy has stopped. Men with partners of childbearing potential should use reliable contraception throughout treatment and are recommended to continue this for 3 months after the last dose of temsirolimus.

EVEROLIMUS

Rx	**Zortress** (Novartis)	**Tablets; oral:** 0.25 mg	Butylated hydroxytoluene, lactose. (C NVR). White to yellowish/marbled, round. In UD 60s.
		0.5 mg	Butylated hydroxytoluene, lactose. (CH NVR). White to yellowish/marbled, round. In UD 60s.
		0.75 mg	Butylated hydroxytoluene, lactose. (CL NVR). White to yellowish/marbled, round. In UD 60s.
Rx	**Afinitor** (Novartis)	**Tablets; oral:** 2.5 mg	Butylated hydroxytoluene, lactose. (LCL NVR). White to slightly yellow, oblong. In UD 28s.
		5 mg	Butylated hydroxytoluene, lactose. (5 NVR). White to slightly yellow, oblong. In UD 28s.
		10 mg	Butylated hydroxytoluene, lactose. (UHE NVR). White to slightly yellow, oblong. In UD 28s.

EVEROLIMUS — ORAL

WARNING

Immunosuppression, renal function, and graft thrombosis (Zortress only) – Increased susceptibility to infection and the possible development of malignancies, such as lymphoma and skin cancer, may result from immunosuppression.

Only health care providers experienced in immunosuppressive therapy and management of transplant patients should use everolimus. Manage patients receiving the drug in facilities equipped and staffed with adequate laboratory and supportive medical resources. The health care provider responsible for maintenance therapy should have complete information requisite for the follow-up.

Increased nephrotoxicity can occur with use of standard doses of cyclosporine in combination with everolimus. Therefore, use reduced doses of cyclosporine in combination with everolimus in order to reduce renal dysfunction. It is important to monitor the cyclosporine and everolimus whole blood trough concentrations.

An increased risk of kidney arterial and venous thrombosis, resulting in graft loss, was reported, mostly within the first 30 days posttransplantation.

Indications

➤*Advanced renal cell carcinoma (Afinitor only):* For the treatment of patients with advanced renal cell carcinoma after failure of treatment with sunitinib or sorafenib.

➤*Renal transplantation (Zortress only):* For the prophylaxis of organ rejection in adult patients at low to moderate immunologic risk receiving a kidney transplant.

➤*Subependymal giant cell astrocytoma (Afinitor only):* For the treatment of patients with subependymal giant cell astrocytoma associated with tuberous sclerosis who require therapeutic intervention but are not candidates for curative surgical resection.

Administration and Dosage

➤*Adults:*

Advanced renal cell carcinoma (Afinitor only) –

Usual dosage: 10 mg once daily at the same time every day.

Dosage adjustment: Management of severe and/or intolerable adverse reactions may require temporary dose reduction and/or interruption of therapy. If dose reduction is required, the suggested dosage is 5 mg daily.

Concomitant therapy:

• *Strong CYP3A4 inducers* – Avoid the use of concomitant strong CYP3A4 inducers (eg, phenobarbital, phenytoin, carbamazepine, rifampin, rifabutin, rifapentine, St. John's wort [*Hypericum perforatum*]). If patients require coadministration of a strong CYP3A4 inducer, consider increasing the everolimus dosage from 10 to 20 mg daily using 5 mg increments. If the strong inducer is discontinued, the everolimus dose should be returned to the dose used prior to initiation of the strong CYP3A4 inducer.

• *CYP3A4 inhibitors and/or P-glycoprotein inhibitors* – Avoid the use of concomitant strong CYP3A4 inhibitors (eg, atazanavir, clarithromycin, indinavir, itraconazole, ketoconazole, nefazodone, nelfinavir, ritonavir, saquinavir, telithromycin, voriconazole) and grapefruit, grapefruit juice, and other foods that are known to inhibit cytochrome P450 (CYP-450) and P-glycoprotein (Pgp) activity.

Use caution when coadministered with moderate CYP3A4 and/or Pgp inhibitors (eg, amprenavir, aprepitant, diltiazem, erythromycin, fluconazole, fosamprenavir, verapamil). If patients require coadministration of a moderate CYP3A4 and/or Pgp inhibitor, reduce the everolimus dosage to 2.5 mg daily. An everolimus dose increase from 2.5 to 5 mg may be considered based on patient tolerance. If the moderate inhibitor is discontinued, a washout

EVEROLIMUS — ORAL

period of approximately 2 to 3 days should be allowed before the everolimus dose is increased. If the moderate inhibitor is discontinued, the everolimus dose should be returned to the dose used prior to initiation of the moderate CYP3A4 and/or Pgp inhibitor.

Renal transplantation –

Initial dosage: 0.75 mg twice daily in combination with a reduced dose of cyclosporine, administered as soon as possible after transplantation.

Dosage adjustment: Dose adjustments based on everolimus blood concentrations achieved, tolerability, individual response, change in concomitant medications, and the clinical situation may be required. Dose adjustments can be made at 4- to 5-day intervals.

Concomitant therapy:

• *Prednisone* – Oral prednisone should be initiated once oral medication is tolerated. Steroid doses may be further tapered on an individualized basis depending on the clinical status of patient and function of graft.

• *Cyclosporine* – Cyclosporine is to be administered as oral capsules twice daily unless cyclosporine oral solution or intravenous administration of cyclosporine cannot be avoided. Cyclosporine should be initiated as soon as possible and no later than 48 hours after reperfusion of the graft and the dose adjusted to target concentrations from day 5 onwards. (See Therapeutic Drug Monitoring.)

• *Strong CYP3A4 inhibitors/inducers* – Coadministration with strong CYP3A4 inhibitors (eg, ketoconazole, itraconazole, voriconazole, clarithromycin, telithromycin, ritonavir) and strong inducers (eg, rifampin, rifabutin) is not recommended without close monitoring of everolimus whole blood trough concentrations. (See Therapeutic Drug Monitoring.)

Subependymal giant cell astrocytoma (Afinitor only) –

Initial dosage:

Afinitor Initial Dosage in Subependymal Giant Cell Astrocytoma[a]

BSA[b]	Initial dosage
0.5 to 1.2 m^2	2.5 mg once daily
1.3 to 2.1 m^2	5 mg once daily
≥ 2.2 m^2	7.5 mg once daily

[a] Everolimus has not been studied in patients with subependymal giant cell astrocytoma with BSA less than 0.58 m^2.
[b] BSA = body surface area.

Dosage adjustment: Patients may require dose adjustments based on everolimus trough blood concentrations achieved, tolerability, individual response, and change in concomitant medications, including CYP3A4-inducing antiepileptic drugs. Dose adjustments can be made at 2-week intervals.

Evaluate subependymal giant cell astrocytoma volume approximately 3 months after commencing everolimus therapy and periodically thereafter, with subsequent dose adjustments taking into consideration changes in subependymal giant cell astrocytoma volume, corresponding trough concentration, and tolerability. Responses have been observed at trough concentrations as low as 3 ng/mL; as such, once acceptable efficacy has been achieved, additional dose increases may not be necessary.

Management of severe or intolerable adverse reactions may require temporary dose reduction and/or interruption of everolimus therapy. If dose reduction is required for patients receiving 2.5 mg daily, consider alternate-day dosing.

Concomitant therapy:

• *CYP3A4 and/or Pgp inhibitors* – Avoid the use of strong CYP3A4 inhibitors (eg, ketoconazole, itraconazole, clarithromycin, atazanavir, nefazodone, saquinavir, telithromycin, ritonavir, indinavir, nelfinavir, voriconazole) and grapefruit, grapefruit juice, and other foods that are known to inhibit CYP-450 and Pgp activity.

Use caution when coadministered with moderate CYP3A4 and/or Pgp inhibitors (eg, amprenavir, aprepitant, diltiazem, erythromycin, fluconazole, fosamprenavir, verapamil). If patients require coadministration of a moderate CYP3A4 and/or Pgp inhibitor, reduce the everolimus dose by approximately 50% to maintain trough concentrations of 5 to 10 ng/mL. If dose reduction is required for patients receiving 2.5 mg daily, consider alternate-day dosing. Subsequent dosing should be individualized based on therapeutic drug monitoring. Everolimus trough concentrations should be assessed approximately 2 weeks after the addition of a moderate CYP3A4 and/or Pgp inhibitor. If the moderate inhibitor is discontinued, the everolimus dose should be returned to the dose used prior to initiation of the moderate CYP3A4 and/or Pgp inhibitor; the everolimus trough concentration should be reassessed approximately 2 weeks later.

• *Strong CYP3A4 inducers* – Avoid the use of concomitant strong CYP3A4 inducers (eg, carbamazepine, phenobarbital, phenytoin, rifabutin, rifampin, rifapentine, St. John's wort [*Hypericum perforatum*]). For patients requiring a concomitant strong CYP3A4 inducer, double the everolimus dose. Subsequent dosing should be individualized based on therapeutic drug monitoring. If the strong inducer is discontinued, the everolimus dose should be returned to the dose used prior to initiation of the strong CYP3A4 inducer and the everolimus trough concentrations should be assessed approximately 2 weeks later.

➤*Children:*

Subependymal giant cell astrocytoma (Afinitor only) –

3 years of age and older: See Adults for dosing.

➤*Hepatic function impairment:*

Advanced renal cell carcinoma –

Moderate hepatic impairment (Child-Pugh class B): Reduce the dosage to 5 mg daily.

Severe hepatic impairment (Child-Pugh class C): Everolimus should not be used in this patient population.

Renal transplantation –

Moderate hepatic impairment (Child-Pugh class B): The daily dose needs to be reduced by one-half the recommended initial daily dose, and blood concentrations should be monitored to make further adjustments as necessary.

Subependymal giant cell astrocytoma –

Moderate hepatic impairment (Child-Pugh class B): Adjustment to the starting dose may not be needed. Subsequent dosing should be individualized based on therapeutic drug monitoring.

➤*Therapeutic drug monitoring:*

Subependymal giant cell astrocytoma – Routine everolimus whole blood therapeutic drug concentration monitoring is recommended for all patients using a validated assay. Trough concentrations should be assessed approximately 2 weeks after commencing treatment. Dosing should be titrated to attain trough concentrations of 5 to 10 ng/mL.

There is limited safety experience with patients having trough concentrations more than 10 ng/mL. If concentrations are between 10 and 15 ng/mL and the patient has demonstrated adequate tolerability and tumor response, no dose reductions are needed. The dose of everolimus should be reduced if trough concentrations greater than 15 ng/mL are observed.

If concentrations are less than 5 ng/mL, the daily dose may be increased by 2.5 mg every 2 weeks, subject to tolerability. Daily dose may be reduced by 2.5 mg every 2 weeks to attain a target of 5 to 10 ng/mL. If dose reduction is required for patients receiving 2.5 mg daily, alternate-day dosing should be used.

Trough concentrations should be assessed approximately 2 weeks after any change in dose, or after an initiation or change in coadministration of CYP3A4 and/or Pgp inducers or inhibitors.

Renal transplantation –

Everolimus: Routine everolimus whole blood therapeutic drug concentration monitoring is recommended for all patients using appropriate assay methodology. The recommended everolimus therapeutic range is 3 to 8 ng/mL. Careful attention should be made to clinical signs and symptoms, tissue biopsies, and laboratory parameters.

It is important to monitor everolimus blood concentrations in patients with hepatic impairment during coadministration of CYP3A4 inducers or inhibitors, when switching cyclosporine formulations, and/or when cyclosporine dosing is reduced according to recommended target concentrations.

Optimally, dose adjustments of everolimus should be based on trough concentrations obtained 4 or 5 days after a previous dosing change. There is an interaction of cyclosporine on everolimus and, consequently, everolimus concentrations may decrease if cyclosporine exposure is reduced.

Cyclosporine: When given in a regimen with everolimus, cyclosporine doses and the target range for whole blood trough concentrations should be reduced in order to minimize the risk of nephrotoxicity.

The recommended cyclosporine therapeutic ranges when administered with everolimus are 100 to 200 ng/mL through month 1 posttransplant, 75 to 150 ng/mL at months 2 and 3 posttransplant, 50 to 100 ng/mL at month 4 posttransplant, and 25 to 50 ng/mL from months 6 through 12 posttransplant. The median trough concentrations observed in the clinical trial ranged between 161 and 185 ng/mL through month 1 posttransplant and between 111 and 140 ng/mL at months 2 and 3 posttransplant. The median trough concentration was 99 ng/mL at month 4 posttransplant and ranged between 46 and 75 ng/mL from months 6 through 12 posttransplant.

If impairment of renal function is progressive, the treatment regimen should be adjusted. In renal transplant patients, the cyclosporine dose should be based on cyclosporine whole blood trough concentrations.

In renal transplantation, there are limited data regarding everolimus dosing with reduced cyclosporine trough concentrations of 25 to 50 ng/mL after 12 months. Everolimus has not been evaluated in clinical trials with other formulations of cyclosporine. Prior to dose reduction of cyclosporine, it should be ascertained that the steady-state everolimus whole blood trough concentration is at least 3 ng/mL. There is an interaction of cyclosporine on everolimus, and, consequently, everolimus concentrations may decrease if cyclosporine exposure is reduced.

➤*Administration:* Administer at the same time every day, either consistently with or without food. Tablets should be swallowed whole with a glass of water. The tablets should not be chewed or crushed.

Zortress only – Administer everolimus doses consistently approximately 12 hours apart to minimize variability in absorption, and at the same time as cyclosporine.

Afinitor only – For patients unable to swallow tablets, everolimus tablets should be dispersed completely in a glass of water (containing approximately 30 mL) by gently stirring immediately prior to drinking. The glass should be rinsed with the same volume of water and the rinse should be completely swallowed to ensure that the entire dose is administered.

➤*Storage/Stability:* Store at 25°C (77°F); excursions are permitted between 15° and 30°C (59° and 86°F). Store in the original container; protect from light and moisture.

Actions

➤*Pharmacology:*

Renal transplantation – Everolimus inhibits antigenic and interleukin (IL-2 and IL-15) stimulated activation and proliferation of T and B lymphocytes. In cells, everolimus binds to a cytoplasmic protein, the FK506-binding protein 12 (FKBP12), to form an immunosuppressive complex (everolimus-:FKBP12) that binds to and inhibits the mammalian target of rapamycin (mTOR), a key regulatory kinase. In the presence of everolimus, phosphorylation of p70 S6 ribosomal protein kinase, a substrate of mTOR, is inhibited.

EVEROLIMUS — ORAL

Consequently, phosphorylation of the ribosomal S6 protein and subsequent protein synthesis and cell proliferation are inhibited. The everolimus-:FKBP12 complex has no effect on calcineurin activity.

Renal cell carcinoma/subependymal giant cell astrocytoma – Everolimus is an inhibitor of mTOR, a serine-threonine kinase, downstream of the PI3K/AKT pathway. The mTOR pathway is dysregulated in several human cancers. Everolimus binds to an intracellular protein, FKBP12, resulting in an inhibitory complex formation and inhibition of mTOR kinase activity. Everolimus reduced the activity of S6 ribosomal protein kinase and eukaryotic elongation factor 4E-binding protein, which are downstream effectors of mTOR involved in protein synthesis. In addition, everolimus inhibited the expression of hypoxia inducible factor (eg, HIF1) and reduced the expression of vascular endothelial growth factor. Inhibition of mTOR by everolimus has been shown to reduce cell proliferation, angiogenesis, and glucose uptake in in vitro and/or in vivo studies.

Two regulators of mTOR C1 signaling are the oncogene suppressors tuberous sclerosis complexes 1 and 2 (TSC1, TSC2). Loss or inactivation of TSC1 or TSC2 leads to activation of downstream signaling. In tuberous sclerosis, a genetic disorder, inactivating mutations in the TSC1 or the TSC2 gene leads to hamartoma formation throughout the body.

➤*Pharmacokinetics:*

Zortress 0.75 mg Twice Daily Pharmacokinetic Parameters (Mean ± SD) in Kidney Transplant Patients[a]					
C_{max}	T_{max}	AUC	Apparent clearance[b]	Apparent volume of the central compartment[b]	Half-life
11.1 ± 4.6 ng/mL	1 to 2 h	75 + 31 ng•h/mL	8.8 L/h	110 L	30 ± 11 h

[a] SD = standard deviation; C_{max} = maximum concentration; T_{max} = time to C_{max}; AUC = area under the curve.
[b] Population pharmacokinetic analysis.

Absorption – After oral dosing, everolimus C_{max} is reached 1 to 2 hours postdose. Steady state was achieved within 2 weeks following once-daily dosing. Steady state in kidney transplant patients is reached by day 4, with an accumulation in blood levels of 2- to 3-fold compared with the exposure after the first dose.

Effect of food:

• *Zortress* only – In 24 healthy subjects, a high-fat breakfast (44.5 g fat) reduced everolimus C_{max} by 60%, delayed T_{max} by a median 1.3 hours, and reduced AUC by 16% compared with a fasting administration. To minimize variability, everolimus should be taken consistently with or without food.

• *Afinitor* only – In healthy subjects, high-fat meals reduced systemic exposure to everolimus 10 mg tablet (as measured by AUC) by 22% and the C_{max} by 54%. Light-fat meals reduced AUC by 32% and C_{max} by 42%. However, food had no apparent effect on the postabsorption phase concentration-time profile.

Distribution – The blood-to-plasma ratio of everolimus, which is concentration-dependent over the range of 5 to 5,000 ng/mL, is 17% to 73%. The amount of everolimus confined to the plasma is approximately 20% at blood concentrations observed in cancer patients given everolimus 10 mg/day. Plasma protein binding is approximately 74% in healthy subjects and in patients with moderate hepatic impairment.

The apparent volume of distribution associated with the terminal phase from a single-dose pharmacokinetic study in kidney transplant patients on maintenance therapy is 342 to 107 L (range, 128 to 589 L).

Metabolism – Everolimus is a substrate of CYP3A4 and Pgp. Following oral administration, everolimus is the main circulating component in human blood. Six main metabolites of everolimus have been detected in human blood, including 3 monohydroxylated metabolites, 2 hydrolytic ring-opened products, and a phosphatidylcholine conjugate of everolimus. None of the main metabolites contribute significantly to the immunosuppressive activity of everolimus. These metabolites were also identified in animal species used in toxicity studies, and they showed approximately 100 times less activity than everolimus itself.

The main metabolic pathways identified in humans were monohydroxylations and O-dealkylations. Two main metabolites were formed by hydrolysis of the cyclic lactone.

Excretion – Following the administration of a 3 mg single dose of radiolabeled everolimus in patients who were receiving cyclosporine, 80% of the radioactivity was recovered from the feces, while 5% was excreted in the urine. The parent substance was not detected in urine or feces. The mean elimination half-life of everolimus is approximately 30 hours.

Special populations –

Hepatic function impairment: Everolimus AUC was increased an average of 2-fold in 8 patients with moderate hepatic impairment (Child-Pugh class B) compared with 8 healthy subjects. AUC was positively correlated with serum bilirubin concentration and prolongation in prothrombin time and negatively correlated with serum albumin concentration. The AUC of everolimus tended to be greater than that of healthy subjects if bilirubin was greater than 34 mcmol/L, prothrombin time was greater than 1.3 times the international normalized ratio greater than 4-second prolongation, and/or albumin concentration was less than 35 g/L. The impact of severe hepatic impairment (Child-Pugh class C) on everolimus pharmacokinetics has not been assessed, but the effect on everolimus AUC is likely to be as large or larger compared with moderate impairment. Do not use everolimus in patients with severe (Child-Pugh class C) hepatic impairment because the impact of severe hepatic impairment on everolimus exposure has not been assessed (see Administration and Dosage).

Elderly:

• *Zortress* only – A limited reduction in everolimus oral clearance of 0.33% per year was estimated in renal transplant adult patients (range studied was 16 to 70 years of age).

Race: Based on a cross-study comparison, Japanese patients had exposures that were on average higher than non-Japanese patients receiving the same dose. Based on analysis of population pharmacokinetics, oral clearance is on average 20% higher in black patients than in white patients.

Contraindications

Hypersensitivity to the active substance, to other rapamycin derivatives, or to any of the excipients; hypersensitivity to sirolimus (*Zortress* only).

Warnings/Precautions

➤*Noninfectious pneumonitis:* Noninfectious pneumonitis is a class effect of rapamycin derivatives, including everolimus. In the randomized advanced renal cell carcinoma study, noninfectious pneumonitis was reported in 14% of patients treated with everolimus. The incidence of Common Toxicity Criteria (CTC) grade 3 and 4 noninfectious pneumonitis was 4% and 0%, respectively. Fatal outcomes have been observed.

Consider a diagnosis of noninfectious pneumonitis in patients presenting with nonspecific respiratory signs and symptoms, such as hypoxia, pleural effusion, cough, or dyspnea, and in whom infectious, neoplastic, and other causes have been excluded by means of appropriate investigations. Advise patients to promptly report any new or worsening respiratory symptoms.

Patients who develop radiological changes suggestive of noninfectious pneumonitis and have few or no symptoms may continue everolimus therapy without dose alteration. If symptoms are moderate, consider interrupting therapy until symptoms improve. The use of corticosteroids may be indicated. For cases in which symptoms of noninfectious pneumonitis are severe, discontinue everolimus therapy; the use of corticosteroids may be indicated until clinical symptoms resolve. In patients with advanced renal cell carcinoma, everolimus may be reintroduced at 5 mg daily. In patients with subependymal giant cell astrocytoma, everolimus may be reintroduced at a daily dose approximately 50% lower than the dose previously administered.

➤*Infections:* Everolimus has immunosuppressive properties and may predispose patients to bacterial, fungal, viral, or protozoal infections, including infections with opportunistic pathogens. Localized and systemic infections, including pneumonia, other bacterial infections, viral infections (including reactivation of hepatitis B virus), and invasive fungal infections, such as aspergillosis or candidiasis, have occurred in patients taking everolimus. Some of these infections have been severe (eg, leading to respiratory failure) or fatal. Be aware, and ensure that patients are aware, of the increased risk of infection with everolimus; be vigilant for signs and symptoms of infection and institute appropriate treatment promptly. Complete treatment of preexisting invasive fungal infections prior to starting treatment with everolimus. If a diagnosis of an infection is made, institute appropriate treatment promptly and consider interruption or discontinuation of everolimus. If a diagnosis of invasive systemic fungal infection is made, discontinue everolimus and treat with appropriate antifungal therapy.

Patients receiving immunosuppressants, including everolimus, are at increased risk for opportunistic infections, including polyoma virus infections. BK virus–associated nephropathy has been observed in patients receiving everolimus. BK virus–associated nephropathy is associated with serious outcomes, including deteriorating renal function and renal graft loss. Patient monitoring may help detect patients at risk for BK virus–associated nephropathy. Consider reductions in immunosuppression for patients who develop evidence of BK virus–associated nephropathy.

Because of the danger of over-immunosuppression of the immune system, which can cause increased susceptibility to infection, use combination immunosuppressant therapy with caution.

➤*Oral ulceration:* Mouth ulcers, stomatitis, and oral mucositis have occurred in patients treated with everolimus. In the randomized advanced renal cell carcinoma study, approximately 44% of everolimus-treated patients developed mouth ulcers, stomatitis, or oral mucositis, which were mostly CTC grades 1 and 2. In the subependymal giant cell astrocytoma study, 86% of everolimus-treated patients developed stomatitis that was mostly CTC grade 1 or 2. In such cases, topical treatments are recommended, but avoid alcohol- or peroxide-containing mouthwashes because they may exacerbate the condition. Do not use antifungal agents unless fungal infection has been diagnosed.

➤*Vaccinations:* Avoid the use of live vaccines and close contact with those who have received live vaccines during treatment with everolimus. Examples of live vaccines are intranasal influenza, measles, mumps, rubella, oral polio, BCG, yellow fever, varicella, and TY21a typhoid vaccines. Consider the timing of routine vaccinations in children with subependymal giant cell astrocytoma prior to the start of everolimus therapy.

➤*Administration:* See the Warning box for more information.

➤*Lymphomas and other malignancies:* Patients receiving immunosuppressants, including everolimus, are at increased risk of developing lymphomas and other malignancies, particularly of the skin. The risk appears to be related to the intensity and duration of immunosuppression rather than to the use of any specific agent.

As usual for patients with increased risk for skin cancer, advise patients to limit exposure to sunlight and ultraviolet light by wearing protective clothing and using a sunscreen with a high protection factor.

EVEROLIMUS — ORAL

➤*Graft thrombosis:* An increased risk of kidney arterial and venous thrombosis, resulting in graft loss, has been reported, usually within the first 30 days posttransplantation.

➤*Wound healing and fluid accumulation:* Everolimus delays wound healing and increases the occurrence of wound-related complications, such as wound dehiscence, wound infection, incisional hernia, lymphocele, and seroma. These wound-related complications may require more surgical intervention. Generalized fluid accumulation, including peripheral edema (eg, lymphoedema) and other types of localized fluid collection, such as pericardial and pleural effusions and ascites, have also been reported.

➤*Hyperlipidemia:* Increased serum cholesterol and triglycerides requiring the need for antilipid therapy have been reported to occur following initiation of everolimus; the risk of hyperlipidemia is increased with higher everolimus whole blood trough concentrations. Use of antilipid therapy may not normalize lipid levels in patients receiving everolimus.

Monitor any patient who is administered everolimus for hyperlipidemia. If detected, initiate interventions, such as diet, exercise, and lipid-lowering agents, as outlined by the National Cholesterol Education Program guidelines. Consider the risks and benefits in patients with established hyperlipidemia before initiating an immunosuppressive regimen containing everolimus. Similarly, reevaluate the risks and benefits of continued everolimus therapy in patients with severe refractory hyperlipidemia. Everolimus has not been studied in patients with baseline cholesterol levels greater than 350 mg/dL.

➤*Nephrotoxicity:* Everolimus with standard-dose cyclosporine increases the risk of nephrotoxicity, resulting in a lower glomerular filtration rate. Reduced doses of cyclosporine are required for use in combination with everolimus in order to reduce renal dysfunction. Monitor renal function during the administration of everolimus in combination with cyclosporine. Consider switching to other immunosuppressive therapies if renal function does not improve after dose adjustments or if the dysfunction is thought to be drug-related. Exercise caution when using other drugs that are known to impair renal function.

➤*Proteinuria:* The use of everolimus with cyclosporine in transplant patients has been associated with increased proteinuria. The risk of proteinuria increased with higher everolimus whole blood trough concentrations. Monitor patients receiving everolimus for proteinuria.

➤*New-onset diabetes:* Everolimus has been shown to increase the risk of new-onset diabetes mellitus after transplant. Monitor blood glucose concentrations closely in patients using everolimus.

➤*Male infertility:* Azoospermia or oligospermia may be observed. Everolimus is an antiproliferative drug and affects rapidly dividing cells, such as the germ cells.

➤*Hypersensitivity reactions:* Hypersensitivity reactions, manifested by symptoms including, but not limited to, anaphylaxis, dyspnea, flushing, chest pain, or angioedema (eg, swelling of the airways or tongue with or without respiratory impairment), have been observed with everolimus and other rapamycin derivatives.

➤*Hepatic function impairment:*

Afinitor only – See Administration and Dosage for more information.

Zortress only – See Administration and Dosage for more information.

➤*Special risk:* Do not administer everolimus to patients with rare hereditary problems of galactose intolerance, Lapp lactase deficiency, or glucose-galactose malabsorption because this may result in diarrhea and malabsorption.

➤*Pregnancy: Category D (Afinitor); Category C (Zortress).* There are no adequate and well-controlled studies of everolimus in pregnant women. However, based on mechanism of action, everolimus may cause fetal harm when administered to a pregnant woman. Everolimus caused embryofetal toxicities in animals at maternal exposures that were lower than human exposures. In rats and rabbits, everolimus crossed the placenta and was toxic to the conceptus. The potential risk for humans is unknown. Administer everolimus to pregnant women only if the potential benefit to the mother justifies the potential risk to the fetus. If this drug is used during pregnancy or if the patient becomes pregnant while taking the drug, apprise the patient of the potential hazard to the fetus. Advise women of childbearing potential to use an effective method of contraception while using everolimus and for up to 8 weeks after ending treatment.

Afinitor only – In animal reproductive studies, oral administration of everolimus to female rats before mating and through organogenesis induced embryofetal toxicities, including increased resorption, pre- and postimplantation loss, decreased numbers of live fetuses, malformation (eg, sternal cleft), and retarded skeletal development. These effects occurred in the absence of maternal toxicities. Embryofetal toxicities occurred at approximately 4% the exposure ($AUC_{0\text{-}24h}$) in patients receiving the recommended dosage of 10 mg daily in advanced renal cell carcinoma patients. In rabbits, embryotoxicity, evident as an increase in resorptions, occurred at an oral dose approximately 1.6 times the recommended human dose for advanced renal cell carcinoma patients, and 0.7 times the maximum dose administered to subependymal giant cell astrocytoma patients on a BSA basis. The effect in rabbits occurred in the presence of maternal toxicities.

In a pre- and postnatal development study in rats, animals were dosed from implantation through lactation. At approximately 10% of the recommended human dose for advanced renal cell carcinoma patients and 4% of the maximum dose administered to subependymal giant cell astrocytoma patients based on BSA, there were no adverse effects on delivery and lactation, and there were no signs of maternal toxicity. However, there was reduced body weight (up to 9% reduction from the control) and slight reduction in survival in offspring (approximately 5% died or missing). There were no drug-related effects on the developmental parameters (morphological development, motor activity, learning, or fertility assessment) in the offspring.

Doses that resulted in embryofetal toxicities in rats and rabbits were at least 0.1 (0.6 mg/m^2) and 0.8 mg/kg (9.6 mg/m^2), respectively. The dose in the pre- and postnatal development study in rats that caused reduction in body weights and survival of offspring was 0.1 mg/kg (0.6 mg/m^2).

Zortress only – Everolimus administered daily to pregnant rats by oral gavage at 0.1 mg/kg from before mating through organogenesis resulted in increased preimplantation loss and early resorptions of fetal implants. AUCs in rats at this dose were approximately one-third those in humans administered the starting dosage (0.75 mg twice daily). Everolimus administered daily by oral gavage at 0.8 mg/kg to pregnant rabbits during organogenesis resulted in increased late resorptions of fetal implants. At this dose, AUCs in rabbits were slightly less than the AUCs in humans administered the starting clinical dose.

➤*Lactation:* It is not known whether everolimus is excreted in human milk. Everolimus and/or its metabolites readily transferred into milk of lactating rats at a concentration 3.5 times higher than in maternal serum. Because many drugs are excreted in human milk and because of the potential for serious adverse reactions in breast-feeding infants from everolimus, advise women to avoid breast-feeding during treatment with everolimus.

➤*Children:* The safety and effectiveness of everolimus in kidney transplant or advanced renal cell carcinoma patients younger than 18 years of age have not been established. Everolimus has not been studied in patients with subependymal giant cell astrocytoma younger than 3 years of age.

➤*Lab test abnormalities:* Elevations of serum creatinine, usually mild, have been reported in clinical trials. Decreased hemoglobin, lymphocytes, neutrophils, and platelets have been reported in clinical trials.

➤*Monitoring:* Monitor everolimus and cyclosporine whole blood trough concentrations (see Therapeutic Drug Monitoring).

Evaluate subependymal giant cell astrocytoma volume approximately 3 months after commencing therapy and periodically thereafter.

Monitor renal function, including measurement of serum urea nitrogen or serum creatinine, fasting serum glucose, complete blood cell count, and lipids, prior to the start of therapy and periodically thereafter. When possible, achieve optimal glucose and lipid control before starting therapy. Monitor patients for proteinuria and for signs and symptoms of infection.

Drug Interactions

➤*CYP-450 system:* Because everolimus is metabolized mainly by the CYP3A enzyme systems, substances known to inhibit these enzymes may decrease metabolism or increase bioavailability of everolimus, as indicated by increased whole blood or plasma concentrations. Drugs known to induce these enzyme systems may result in an increased metabolism of everolimus or decreased bioavailability, as indicated by decreased whole blood or plasma concentrations. Monitoring of blood concentrations and appropriate dosage adjustments are essential when such drugs are used concomitantly.

➤*Vaccinations:* See Warnings/Precautions for more information.

Everolimus Drug Interactions

Precipitant drug	Object drug[a]		Interaction
Aprepitant	Everolimus	↑	Everolimus blood concentrations may be elevated, increasing the pharmacologic effects and risk of adverse reactions. If everolimus and aprepitant are coadministered, closely monitor everolimus blood concentrations and adjust the dose as needed.
Cyclosporine	Everolimus	↑	Everolimus blood concentrations may be increased. Monitor everolimus concentrations and the clinical response of the patient when the cyclosporine dose is altered. Adjust the everolimus dose as needed.
Digoxin	Everolimus	↑	Everolimus blood concentrations may be increased. Use with caution.
Efavirenz	Everolimus	↓	Everolimus blood concentrations may be reduced, decreasing the efficacy. Closely monitor everolimus blood concentrations when efavirenz is started or stopped and adjust the everolimus dose as needed.

EVEROLIMUS — ORAL

Everolimus Drug Interactions

Precipitant drug	Object drug[a]		Interaction
Moderate inhibitors of CYP3A4 and Pgp (eg, diltiazem, fluconazole, fosamprenavir, macrolide antibiotics [eg, erythromycin], nelfinavir, nicardipine, verapamil)	Everolimus	↑	Everolimus blood concentrations may be elevated, increasing the pharmacologic effects and risk of adverse reactions. In healthy volunteers, erythromycin administration increased the everolimus C_{max} and AUC 2-fold and 4.4-fold, respectively, and prolonged the half-life by 39%. If everolimus is coadministered with moderate inhibitors of CYP3A4 and Pgp, closely monitor everolimus blood concentrations and adjust the everolimus dose as needed.
Nevirapine	Everolimus	↓	Everolimus blood concentrations may be reduced, decreasing the efficacy. If nevirapine is coadministered, closely monitor everolimus blood concentrations when nevirapine is started or stopped and adjust the everolimus dose as needed.
St. John's wort	Everolimus	↓	Everolimus blood concentrations may be reduced, decreasing the efficacy. If coadministration of St. John's wort cannot be avoided, closely monitor everolimus blood concentrations when St. John's wort is started or stopped and adjust the everolimus dose as needed.
Strong CYP3A4 inducers (eg, carbamazepine, phenobarbital, phenytoin, rifabutin, rifampin, rifapentine)	Everolimus	↓	Everolimus blood concentrations may be reduced, decreasing the efficacy. In healthy volunteers, coadministration of everolimus with rifampin decreased everolimus AUC and C_{max} by 63% and 58%, respectively. Avoid coadministration of strong CYP3A4 inducers.
Strong CYP3A4 inhibitors (eg, atazanavir, clarithromycin, indinavir, itraconazole, ketoconazole, nefazodone, ritonavir, saquinavir, telithromycin, voriconazole)	Everolimus	↑	Everolimus blood concentrations may be elevated, increasing the pharmacologic effects and risk of adverse reactions. In healthy volunteers, ketoconazole administration increased everolimus C_{max} and AUC 3.9- and 15-fold, respectively, and prolonged the half-life by 89%. Avoid coadministration of strong CYP3A4 inhibitors.
Everolimus	ACE[b] inhibitors (eg, captopril)	↑	The risk of angioedema may be increased with coadministration of ACE inhibitors and everolimus. If an interaction is suspected, stop one or both drugs.
Everolimus	Lovastatin, simvastatin	↑	The risk of adverse reactions (eg, rhabdomyolysis) may be increased. Coadministration of lovastatin or simvastatin with everolimus is discouraged. Coadministration of everolimus and atorvastatin (a CYP3A4 substrate) or pravastatin (a Pgp substrate) to healthy volunteers did not affect the pharmacokinetics of atorvastatin, pravastatin, or everolimus, or total HMG-CoA[c] reductase bioreactivity in the plasma. However, these results cannot be extrapolated to other HMG-CoA reductase inhibitors.

[a] ↑ = object drug increased; ↓ = object drug decreased.
[b] ACE = angiotensin-converting enzyme.
[c] HMG-CoA = 3-hydroxy-3-methylglutaryl coenzyme A.

➤*Drug/Food interactions:* Because of significant increases in exposure of everolimus, avoid coadministration with grapefruit.

Afinitor – In healthy subjects taking everolimus 10 mg, a high-fat meal reduced the C_{max} and AUC by 54% and 22%, respectively. Light-fat meals reduced the C_{max} and AUC by 42% and 32%, respectively.

Zortress – Based on data in healthy subjects taking everolimus 1 mg tablets, a high-fat meal reduced C_{max} and AUC by 60% and 16%, respectively. No data are available with everolimus 5 and 10 mg tablets. To avoid variability, everolimus should be taken consistently with or without food.

Adverse Reactions

➤*Advanced renal cell carcinoma (Afinitor only):*

Most common adverse reactions – The most common adverse reactions (30% or more) were asthenia, cough, diarrhea, fatigue, infections, and stomatitis. The most common grade 3/4 adverse reactions (3% or more) were abdominal pain, asthenia, dehydration, dyspnea, fatigue, infections, pneumonitis, and stomatitis. The most common laboratory abnormalities (50% or more) were anemia, hypercholesterolemia, hyperglycemia, hypertriglyceridemia, increased creatinine, and lymphopenia. The most common grade 3/4 laboratory abnormalities (3% or more) were anemia, hyperglycemia, hypercholesterolemia, hypophosphatemia, and lymphopenia. Infections, pneumonitis, and stomatitis were the most common reasons for treatment delay or dose reduction. The most common medical interventions required during everolimus treatment were for anemia, infections, and stomatitis.

Deaths – Deaths caused by acute respiratory failure (0.7%), infection (0.7%), and acute renal failure (0.4%) were observed in the everolimus arm, but not in the placebo arm.

Discontinuation – The rates of treatment-emergent adverse reactions (irrespective of causality) resulting in permanent discontinuation were 14% and 3% for the everolimus and placebo treatment groups, respectively. The most common adverse reactions (irrespective of causality) leading to treatment discontinuation were dyspnea and pneumonitis.

Adverse reactions (10% or more) –

***Afinitor* Adverse Reactions in Patients With Advanced Renal Cell Carcinoma (≥ 10%)**

	Everolimus 10 mg/day (n = 274)			Placebo (n = 137)		
	All grades	Grade 3	Grade 4	All grades	Grade 3	Grade 4
Median duration of treatment	141 days			60 days		
Any adverse reaction	97%	52%	13%	93%	23%	5%
CNS						
Asthenia	33%	3%	< 1%	23%	4%	0%
Fatigue	31%	5%	0%	27%	3%	< 1%
Headache	19%	< 1%	< 1%	9%	< 1%	0%
Dermatological						
Dry skin	13%	< 1%	0%	5%	0%	0%
Pruritus	14%	< 1%	0%	7%	0%	0%
Rash	29%	1%	0%	7%	0%	0%
GI						
Anorexia	25%	1%	0%	14%	< 1%	0%
Diarrhea	30%	1%	0%	7%	0%	0%
Dysgeusia	10%	0%	0%	2%	0%	0%
Nausea	26%	1%	0%	19%	0%	0%
Stomatitis[a]	44%	4%	< 1%	8%	0%	0%
Vomiting	20%	2%	0%	12%	0%	0%
Respiratory						
Cough	30%	< 1%	0%	16%	0%	0%
Dyspnea	24%	6%	1%	15%	3%	0%
Pneumonitis[b]	14%	4%	0%	0%	0%	0%
Miscellaneous						
Edema peripheral	25%	< 1%	0%	8%	< 1%	0%
Epistaxis	18%	0%	0%	0%	0%	0%
Infections and infestations[c]	37%	7%	3%	18%	1%	0%
Mucosal inflammation	19%	1%	0%	1%	0%	0%
Pain in extremity	10%	1%	0%	7%	0%	0%
Pyrexia	20%	< 1%	0%	9%	0%	0%

[a] Stomatitis (including aphthous stomatitis) and mouth and tongue ulceration.
[b] Includes pneumonitis, interstitial lung disease, lung infiltration, pulmonary alveolar hemorrhage, pulmonary toxicity, and alveolitis.
[c] Includes all preferred terms within the infections and infestations system organ class, the most common being nasopharyngitis, pneumonia (6%); urinary tract infection (5%); bronchitis (4%); and sinusitis (3%); and also including aspergillosis, candidiasis, and sepsis (< 1%).

EVEROLIMUS — ORAL

Other adverse reactions (less than 10%) –
Cardiovascular: Hypertension (4%); tachycardia (3%); congestive cardiac failure (1%).
CNS: Insomnia (9%); dizziness (7%); paresthesia (5%).
Dermatologic: Hand-foot syndrome (reported as palmar-plantar erythrodysesthesia syndrome), nail disorder (5%); erythema, onychoclasis, skin lesion (4%); acneiform dermatitis (3%).
Endocrine: Exacerbation of preexisting diabetes mellitus (2%); new onset of diabetes mellitus (less than 1%).
GI: Abdominal pain (9%); dry mouth (8%); hemorrhoids (5%); dysphagia (4%).
Special senses: Pharyngolaryngeal pain, eyelid edema (4%); rhinorrhea (3%); conjunctivitis (2%).
Miscellaneous: Weight decreased (9%); pleural effusion (7%); chest pain (5%); chills (4%); hemorrhage, jaw pain, renal failure (3%); impaired wound healing (less than 1%).

Lab test abnormalities –

Afinitor Laboratory Abnormalities in Patients With Advanced Renal Cell Carcinoma

Laboratory parameter	Everolimus 10 mg/day (n = 274)			Placebo (n = 137)		
	All grades	Grade 3	Grade 4	All grades	Grade 3	Grade 4
Hematology[a]						
Hemoglobin decreased	92%	12%	1%	79%	5%	< 1%
Lymphocytes decreased	51%	16%	2%	28%	5%	0%
Neutrophils decreased	14%	0%	< 1%	4%	0%	0%
Platelets decreased	23%	1%	0%	2%	0%	< 1%
Chemistry						
ALT increased	21%	1%	0%	4%	0%	0%
AST increased	25%	< 1%	< 1%	7%	0%	0%
Bilirubin increased	3%	< 1%	< 1%	2%	0%	0%
Cholesterol increased	77%	4%	0%	35%	0%	0%
Creatinine increased	50%	1%	0%	34%	0%	0%
Glucose increased	57%	15%	< 1%	25%	1%	0%
Phosphate decreased	37%	6%	0%	8%	0%	0%
Triglycerides increased	73%	< 1%	0%	34%	0%	0%

[a] Includes reports of anemia, leukopenia, lymphopenia, neutropenia, pancytopenia, and thrombocytopenia.

➤*Subependymal giant cell astrocytoma (Afinitor only):*

Most common adverse reactions – The most common adverse reactions (30% or more) were otitis media, pyrexia, sinusitis, stomatitis, and upper respiratory tract infection. The grade 3 adverse reactions were convulsion, infections (single cases of bronchitis viral, pneumonia, sinusitis, and tooth infection), and single cases of stomatitis, aspiration, cyclic neutropenia, dizziness, neutrophil count decreased, sleep apnea syndrome, vomiting, and white blood cell count decreased. A grade 4 convulsion was also reported.

Adverse reactions (10% or more) –

Afinitor Adverse Reactions (≥ 10%) in Patients With Subependymal Giant Cell Astrocytoma

Adverse reactions	Everolimus (n = 28)		
	All grades	Grade 3	Grade 4
Any adverse reaction	100%	36%	4%
CNS			
Convulsion	29%	7%	4%
Dizziness	14%	4%	0%
Headache	18%	0%	0%
Personality change	18%	0%	0%
Dermatologic			
Acne	11%	0%	0%
Body tinea	18%	0%	0%
Dermatitis acneiform	25%	0%	0%
Dermatitis contact	14%	0%	0%
Dry skin	18%	0%	0%
Rash	18%	0%	0%
Skin infection	18%	0%	0%
GI			
Abdominal pain	11%	0%	0%
Constipation	11%	0%	0%
Diarrhea	25%	0%	0%
Gastric infection	14%	0%	0%
Gastroenteritis	18%	0%	0%
Stomatitis	86%	4%	0%
Vomiting	21%	4%	0%
Respiratory			
Cough	21%	0%	0%
Nasal congestion	14%	0%	0%
Pharyngitis	11%	0%	0%
Rhinitis allergic	14%	0%	0%
Upper respiratory tract infection	82%	0%	0%
Special senses			
Otitis externa	14%	0%	0%
Otitis media	36%	0%	0%
Sinusitis	39%	4%	0%
Miscellaneous			
Cellulitis	21%	0%	0%
Excoriation	14%	0%	0%
Pyrexia	32%	0%	0%

Other adverse reactions (less than 10%) –
CNS: Anxiety, fatigue, somnolence (7%).
Special senses: Pharyngeal inflammation (7%); ocular hyperemia (4%).
Miscellaneous: Gastritis, proteinuria (7%); chest x-ray abnormal, edema peripheral, hypertension, pityriasis rosea (4%); serious cases of hepatitis B reactivation, including fatal outcomes.

Lab test abnormalities – Single cases of grade 3 elevated AST concentrations and low absolute neutrophil count (ANC) were reported. No grade 4 laboratory abnormalities were noted. Laboratory abnormalities observed in more than 1 patient included elevations in AST concentrations (89%), total cholesterol (68%), ALT (46%), triglycerides (43%) (hypertriglyceridemia reported as adverse reaction in 11% of patients, blood triglycerides increased reported as adverse reaction in 7% of patients), glucose (25%), and creatinine (11%), and reductions in white blood cell counts (54%) (reported as adverse reaction in 11% of patients), hemoglobin (39%), glucose (32%), and platelet counts (21%). Most of these laboratory abnormalities were mild (grade 1).

Two cases of neutrophil count decreased and blood immunoglobulin G decreased were reported as adverse reactions.

➤*Renal transplantation (Zortress only):*

Discontinuation – In this clinical trial, significantly more patients discontinued everolimus 1.5 mg/day treatment (30%) than the control regimen (22%). Of those patients who prematurely discontinued treatment, most discontinuations were because of adverse reactions (18% in the everolimus group compared with 9% in the control group [*P* = 0.004]). This difference was more prominent between treatment groups among women. In those patients discontinuing study medication, adverse reactions were collected up to 7 days after study medication discontinuation and serious adverse reactions up to 30 days after study medication discontinuation. Discontinuation of everolimus at a higher dosage (3 mg/day) was 34%, including 20% because of adverse reactions, and this regimen is not recommended.

Most common adverse reactions – The most common (20% or more) adverse reactions observed in the everolimus group were anemia, constipation, hyperlipidemia, hypertension, nausea, peripheral edema, and urinary tract infection.

Serious adverse reactions – The overall incidences of serious adverse reactions were 57% in the everolimus group and 52% in the mycophenolic acid group. Infections and infestations reported as serious adverse reactions had the highest incidence in both groups (20% in the everolimus group and 25% in the control group). The difference was mainly because of the higher incidence of viral infections in the mycophenolate sodium group, mainly cytomegalovirus and BK virus infections. Injury, poisoning, and procedural complications reported as serious adverse reactions had the second highest incidence in both groups (14% in the everolimus group and 12% in the control group), followed by renal and urinary disorders (10% in the everolimus group and 13% in the control group) and vascular disorders (10% in the everolimus group and 7% in the control group).

EVEROLIMUS — ORAL

Adverse reactions (10% or more) –

Zortress Adverse Reactions in De Novo Kidney Transplant Patients (≥ 10%)[a]		
Adverse reactions	Everolimus 1.5 mg with reduced-dose cyclosporine (n = 274)	Mycophenolic acid 1.44 g with standard-dose cyclosporine (n = 273)
Any adverse reaction[b]	99%	99%
Cardiovascular		
Hypertension	30%	30%
Vascular disorders	45%	45%
CNS		
Fatigue	9%	10%
Headache	18%	15%
Insomnia	17%	16%
Nervous system disorders	34%	40%
Psychiatric disorders	33%	26%
Tremor	8%	14%
GI		
Abdominal pain	13%	15%
Abdominal pain upper	3%	11%
Constipation	38%	43%
Diarrhea	19%	20%
Dyspepsia	4%	11%
GI disorders	72%	76%
Nausea	29%	31%
Vomiting	15%	22%
GU		
Blood creatinine increased	18%	22%
Dysuria	11%	10%
Hematuria	12%	12%
Renal and urinary disorders	41%	45%
Urinary tract infection	22%	23%
Hematologic/Lymphatic		
Anemia	26%	25%
Blood lymphatic system disorders	34%	41%
Leukopenia	3%	12%
Metabolic/Nutritional		
Dyslipidemia	15%	9%
Hypercholesterolemia	17%	13%
Hyperglycemia	12%	14%
Hyperkalemia	18%	18%
Hyperlipidemia	21%	16%
Hypokalemia	12%	12%
Hypomagnesemia	14%	15%
Hypophosphatemia	13%	13%
Metabolism and nutrition disorders	81%	73%
Musculoskeletal		
Back pain	11%	10%
Musculoskeletal and connective tissue disorders	41%	39%
Pain in extremity	12%	11%
Respiratory		
Cough	7%	11%
Respiratory, thoracic, and mediastinal disorders	31%	34%
Upper respiratory tract infection	16%	18%
Miscellaneous		
Edema peripheral	45%	40%
General disorders and administration-site conditions	66%	59%
Incision-site pain	16%	17%
Infections and infestations	62%	68%
Injury, poisoning, and procedural complications	60%	60%
Procedural pain	15%	14%
Pyrexia	19%	15%

[a] All patients received basiliximab induction therapy and corticosteroids.
[b] As reported in the safety analysis population (defined as all randomized patients who received at least 1 dose of treatment and had at least 1 postbaseline safety assessment).

Other adverse reactions (5% or more) –
Endocrine: Hyperlipidemia (21%); dyslipidemia (15%).
Miscellaneous: Peripheral edema (45%); stomatitis/mouth ulceration (8%).

Deaths – A total of 13 patients died during the first 12 months of study: 3% in the everolimus group and 2% in the control group. The most common causes of death across the study groups were related to cardiac conditions and infections.

Graft loss – There were 4% graft losses in the everolimus group and 3% in the control group over the 12-month study period. Of the graft losses, 4 were because of renal artery and renal vein thrombosis in the everolimus group, compared with 2 renal artery thromboses in the control group (1%).

Infections – The overall incidence of bacterial, fungal, and viral infections reported as adverse reactions was higher in the control group (68%) compared with the everolimus group (64%) and was primarily because of an increased number of viral infections(21% in the control group and 10% in the everolimus group). The incidence of cytomegalovirus (CMV) infections reported as adverse reactions was 8% in the control group compared with 1% in the everolimus group; and 3% of the serious CMV infections in the control group versus 0% in the everolimus group were considered serious.

BK virus – BK virus infections were lower in incidence in the everolimus group (1%) compared with the control group (4%). One of the 2 BK virus infections in the everolimus group and 2 of the 11 BK virus infections in the control group were also reported as serious adverse reactions. BK virus infections did not result in graft loss in any of the groups in the clinical trial.

Wound healing and fluid collections – Wound healing–related reactions were identified through a retrospective search and request for additional data. The overall incidence of wound-related events, including dehiscence, hematoma, incisional hernia, infections, lymphocele, and seroma was 35% in the everolimus group compared with 26% in the control group. More patients required intraoperative repair debridement or drainage of incisional wound complications and drainage of lymphoceles and seromas in the everolimus group compared with control.

Adverse reactions because of major fluid collections, such as edema and other types of fluid collections, was 45% in the everolimus group and 40% in the control group.

Neoplasms – Adverse reactions because of malignant and benign neoplasms were reported in 3% of patients in the everolimus group and 6% in the control group. The most frequently reported neoplasms in the control group were basal cell carcinoma, seborrhoeic keratosis, skin papilloma, and squamous cell carcinoma. One patient in the everolimus group who underwent a melanoma excision prior to transplantation died because of metastatic melanoma.

Diabetes mellitus – New-onset diabetes mellitus reported based on adverse reactions and random serum glucose values was 9% in the everolimus group compared with 7% in the control group.

Endocrine effects in men – In the everolimus group, serum testosterone levels significantly decreased while the follicle-stimulating hormone (FSH) levels significantly increased without significant changes being observed in the control group. In both the everolimus and the control groups, mean testosterone and FSH levels remained within the normal range, with the mean FSH level in the everolimus group at the upper limit of the normal range (11.1 units/L). More patients were reported with erectile dysfunction in the everolimus treatment group compared with the control group (5% compared with 2%, respectively).

High-dose everolimus – A third treatment group of everolimus 3 mg/day (1.5 mg twice daily; target trough concentrations, 6 to 12 ng/mL) with reduced-dose cyclosporine was included. Although as effective as the lower-dose everolimus group, the overall safety was worse and, consequently, higher doses of everolimus cannot be recommended. Of 279 patients, 34% discontinued the study medication, with 20% doing so because of adverse reactions. The most frequent adverse reactions leading to discontinuation of everolimus when used at this higher dose were injury, poisoning, and procedural complications (everolimus 1.5 mg, 5%; everolimus 3 mg, 7%; control, 2%); infections (2%, 6%, and 3%, respectively); renal and urinary disorders (4%, 7%, and 4%, respectively); and GI disorders (1%, 3%, and 2%, respectively).

Less common adverse reactions (at least 1% to less than 9%) –
Cardiovascular: Angina pectoris, atrial fibrillation, cardiac failure congestive, deep vein thrombosis, hypertension including hypertensive crisis, hypotension, palpitations, syncope, tachycardia.

mTOR Inhibitor

EVEROLIMUS — ORAL

CNS: Agitation, anxiety, depression, dizziness, fatigue, hallucination, hemiparesis, hypoaesthesia, malaise, paresthesia, somnolence, tremor.

Dermatologic: Alopecia, dermatitis acneiform, hirsutism, hyperhydrosis, hypertrichosis, night sweats, pruritus, rash.

Endocrine: Cushingoid, diabetes mellitus, hyperparathyroidism.

GI: Abdominal distention, abdominal pain, dyspepsia, dysphagia, epigastric discomfort, flatulence, gastroenteritis, gastroesophageal reflux disease, gingival hypertrophy, hematemesis, hemorrhoids, ileus, localized intra-abdominal fluid collection, mouth ulceration, oral candidiasis, peritonitis, stomatitis.

GU: Acute renal failure, bladder spasm, erectile dysfunction, hydronephrosis, micturition urgency, nephritis interstitial, pollakiuria, polyuria, proteinuria, pyuria, renal artery thrombosis, renal impairment, urinary retention, ovarian cyst, pyelonephritis, scrotal edema, urethritis.

Hematologic/Lymphatic: Hemolytic-uremic syndrome, leucopenia, leukocytosis, lymphadenopathy, lymphocele, lymphorrhea, perinephric hematoma, thrombocythemia, thrombocytopenia, thrombotic microangiopathy, thrombotic thrombocytopenic purpura.

Hepatic: Bilirubin increased, hepatic enzyme increased.

Metabolic/Nutritional: Acidosis, anorexia, blood urea increased, dehydration, fluid retention, gout, hypercalcemia, hypercholesterolemia, hyperphosphatemia, hypertriglyceridemia, hyperuricemia, hypocalcemia, hypoglycemia, hyponatremia, iron deficiency, vitamin B_{12} deficiency.

Musculoskeletal: Arthralgia, joint swelling, muscle spasms, muscular weakness, musculoskeletal pain, myalgia, osteomyelitis, osteonecrosis, osteopenia, osteoporosis, spondylitis.

Respiratory: Atelectasis, bronchitis, cough, dyspnea, epistaxis, nasal congestion, noninfectious pneumonitis, pleural effusions, pneumonia, pulmonary edema, rhinorrhea, sinus congestion, wheezing.

Special senses: Cataract, conjunctivitis, nasopharyngitis, sinusitis, vision blurred.

Miscellaneous: Bacteremia, BK virus infection, candidiasis, cellulitis, chest discomfort, chest pain, chills, edema including generalized edema, folliculitis, herpes infections, impaired healing, incision-site complications including infections, incisional hernia, influenza, onychomycosis, perinephric collection, seroma, tinea pedis, wound dehiscence, wound infection.

Postmarketing –

Hypersensitivity: Angioedema.

Miscellaneous: Male infertility, pancreatitis.

Overdosage

➤*Treatment:* Follow general supportive measures in all cases of overdose. Everolimus is not considered dialyzable to any relevant degree (less than 10% of everolimus removed within 6 hours of hemodialysis).

Patient Information

Warn patients of the possibility of developing noninfectious pneumonitis. In clinical studies, some noninfectious pneumonitis cases have been severe and occasionally fatal. Advise patients to promptly report any new or worsening respiratory symptoms.

Inform patients that they may be more susceptible to infections while being treated with everolimus. In clinical studies, some of these infections have been severe (eg, leading to respiratory failure) and occasionally fatal. Make patients aware of the signs and symptoms of infection and advise them to report any such signs or symptoms promptly to their health care provider.

Inform patients of the possibility of developing mouth ulcers, stomatitis, and oral mucositis. In such cases, mouthwashes and/or topical treatments are recommended, but these should not contain alcohol or peroxide.

Inform patients of the need to monitor blood chemistry and hematology prior to the start of everolimus therapy and periodically thereafter.

Advise patients to inform their health care providers of all concomitant medications, including nonprescription medications and dietary supplements. Some medications can increase or decrease the blood concentrations of everolimus.

Advise women of childbearing potential that everolimus may cause fetal harm and to use an effective method of contraception during therapy with everolimus and for 8 weeks after ending treatment.

Inform patients to take everolimus at the same time every day, either consistently with or without food. Advise them to not crush or chew the tablets. Everolimus should be swallowed whole with a glass of water.

Instruct patients that if they miss a dose of everolimus, they may still take it up to 6 hours after the time they would normally take it. If more than 6 hours have elapsed, instruct them to skip the dose for that day. The next day, they should take everolimus at the usual time. Warn patients to not take 2 doses to make up for the one that they missed.

Inform patients to avoid grapefruit and grapefruit juice, which increase blood drug concentrations of everolimus.

Advise renal transplant patients to use everolimus concurrently with reduced doses of cyclosporine and that any change of cyclosporine dose should be made under health care provider supervision and may also require a change in the dosage of everolimus.

Inform patients they are at risk of developing lymphomas and other malignancies, particularly of the skin, because of immunosuppression. Advise patients to limit exposure to sunlight and ultraviolet light by wearing protective clothing and using a sunscreen with a high protection factor.

Advise patients of the risks of impaired kidney function with the combination of everolimus and cyclosporine as well as the need for routine blood concentration monitoring for both drugs. Advise patients of the importance of serum creatinine monitoring.

Inform renal transplant patients that everolimus has been associated with an increased risk of kidney arterial and venous thrombosis, resulting in graft loss, usually within the first 30 days posttransplantation.

Inform patients of the risk of angioedema and that concomitant use of ACE inhibitors may increase this risk. Advise patients to seek prompt medical attention if symptoms occur.

Inform renal transplant patients that the use of everolimus has been associated with impaired or delayed wound healing, fluid accumulation, and the need for careful observation of their incision site.

Inform patients that the use of everolimus has been associated with increased serum cholesterol and triglycerides that may require treatment and the need for monitoring of blood lipid concentrations.

Inform patients that the use of everolimus has been associated with an increased risk of proteinuria.

Inform patients that the use of everolimus may increase the risk of diabetes mellitus and to contact their health care provider if they develop symptoms.

Inform patients that vaccinations may be less effective while they are being treated with everolimus. Advise patients to avoid live vaccines and close contact with those who have received live vaccines.

Advise patients not to take everolimus if they have hereditary disorders of galactose intolerance (Lapp lactase deficiency or glucose-galactose malabsorption).

Multikinase Inhibitor

SORAFENIB

Rx	**Nexavar** (Bayer)	**Tablets; oral:** 200 mg	Equiv. to sorafenib tosylate 274 mg. Polyethylene glycol. (200). Red. Film-coated. In 120s.

SORAFENIB TOSYLATE — ORAL

Indications

➤*Advanced renal cell carcinoma:* For the treatment of patients with advanced renal cell carcinoma.

➤*Hepatocellular carcinoma:* For the treatment of patients with unresectable hepatocellular carcinoma.

➤*Off-label uses:* Metastatic malignant melanoma, non-small cell lung cancer.

Administration and Dosage

➤*General dosing considerations:*

REACH Limited Distribution Program – Sorafenib is available from Bayer HealthCare through a restrictive distribution program, Resources for Expert Assistance and Care Helpline (REACH), intended to assist patients with reimbursement issues.

Health care providers are not required to enroll in REACH prior to prescribing sorafenib. Patients must be enrolled in the REACH program in order to receive sorafenib. Prescribers may enroll patients by completing the REACH enrollment form, which is available by calling 866-639-2827 (866-NEXAVAR) or online at http://www.nexavar.com/wt/page/reimbursement. The completed form must be faxed back to REACH at 866-639-5181 for approval.

Sorafenib is not routinely distributed to retail or hospital pharmacies. Prescriptions for sorafenib are filled only through specialty pharmacies, which arrange for medication delivery to the patients or their prescribers (if preferred).

➤*Adults:*

Advanced renal cell carcinoma –

Usual dosage: 400 mg (two 200 mg tablets) taken twice daily without food (at least 1 hour before or 2 hours after eating).

Duration of therapy: Treatment should continue until the patient is no longer clinically benefiting from therapy or unacceptable toxicity occurs.

Hepatocellular carcinoma – See Advanced Renal Cell Carcinoma for dosing.

➤*Concomitant therapy:* The use of concomitant strong CYP3A4 inducers may decrease sorafenib plasma concentrations and should be avoided (eg, St. John's wort, dexamethasone, phenytoin, carbamazepine, rifampin, rifabutin, phenobarbital). Although a dose increase has not been studied, if a strong CYP3A4 inducer must be coadministered, a sorafenib dose increase may be considered. If the dose of sorafenib is increased, the patient should be monitored carefully for toxicity.

➤*Dosage adjustment:* Management of suspected adverse drug reactions may require temporary interruption and/or dosage reduction of sorafenib therapy. When dosage reduction is necessary, sorafenib may be reduced to

SORAFENIB TOSYLATE — ORAL

400 mg once daily. If additional dosage reduction is required, sorafenib may be reduced to a single 400 mg dose every other day.

Consider dosage reduction or temporary interruption of therapy in patients with severe hypertension (systolic blood pressure above 200 mm Hg, diastolic blood pressure above 110 mm Hg), cardiac ischemia, or infarction.

Consider discontinuing sorafenib permanently in patients with hemorrhage or bleeding requiring medical intervention.

Adjust the sorafenib dose for skin toxicity as shown in the following table.

Sorafenib Dosage Modifications for Skin Toxicity

Skin toxicity grade	Occurrence	Suggested dosage modification
Grade 1: Numbness, dysesthesia, paresthesia, tingling, painless swelling, erythema, or discomfort of the hands or feet that does not disrupt normal activities	Any occurrence	Continue treatment and consider topical therapy for symptomatic relief.
Grade 2: Painful erythema and swelling of the hands or feet and/or discomfort affecting normal activities	First occurrence	Continue treatment and consider topical therapy for symptomatic relief. If no improvement within 7 days, see the following.
	No improvement within 7 days or second or third occurrence	Interrupt treatment until toxicity resolves to grade 0 to 1. When resuming treatment, decrease dose by 1 dose level (400 mg daily or 400 mg every other day).
	Fourth occurrence	Discontinue sorafenib.
Grade 3: Moist desquamation, ulceration, blistering, or severe pain of the hands or feet, or severe discomfort that causes inability to work or perform activities of daily living	First or second occurrence	Interrupt treatment until toxicity resolves to grade 0 to 1. When resuming treatment, decrease dose by 1 dose level (400 mg daily or 400 mg every other day).
	Third occurrence	Discontinue sorafenib.

No dosage adjustment is required on the basis of age, gender, or body weight.

➤*Preparation for administration:* Sorafenib is considered a cytotoxic agent. Follow safe handling procedures when preparing, administering, or dispensing sorafenib.

➤*Administration:* Give on an empty stomach (1 hour before or 2 hours after meals).

➤*Storage/Stability:* Store at 25°C (77°F); excursions are permitted to 15° to 30°C (59° to 86°F). Store in a dry place.

Actions

➤*Pharmacology:* Sorafenib is a kinase inhibitor that decreases tumor cell proliferation in vitro. Sorafenib inhibited tumor growth and angiogenesis of human hepatocellular carcinoma and renal cell carcinoma, and several other human tumor zenografts in immunocompromised mice. Sorafenib inhibited multiple intracellular (CRAF, BRAF, and mutant BRAF) and cell surface kinases (kinase tyrosine [KIT], 3′ fluoro-2′, 3′-dideoxythymidine fluorothymidine [FLT-3], vascular endothelial growth factor receptor [VEGFR]-1, VEGFR-2, VEGFR-3, and platelet-derived growth factor receptor-β). Several of these kinases are thought to be involved in angiogenesis, apoptosis, and tumor cell signaling.

➤*Pharmacokinetics:*

Absorption/Distribution – After administration of sorafenib tablets, the mean relative bioavailability is 38% to 49% when compared with an oral solution. Multiple dosing of sorafenib for 7 days resulted in 2.5- to 7-fold accumulation compared with single-dose administration. Steady-state plasma sorafenib concentrations are achieved within 7 days, with a peak-to-trough ratio of mean concentrations of less than 2.

Mean maximum effective plasma concentration (C_{max}) and area under the plasma concentration-time curve (AUC) increased less than proportionally beyond doses of 400 mg administered orally twice daily.

In vitro binding of sorafenib to human plasma proteins is 99.5%.

Food effects: Following oral administration, sorafenib reaches plasma level in approximately 3 hours. When given with a moderate-fat meal (30% fat, 700 calories), bioavailability was similar to that in the fasted state. With a high-fat meal (50% fat, 900 calories), sorafenib bioavailability was reduced 29% compared with administration in the fasted state. It is recommended that sorafenib be administered without food (at least 1 hour before or 2 hours after eating).

Metabolism/Excretion – Sorafenib undergoes oxidative metabolism mediated by CYP3A4 primarily in the liver, and glucuronidation mediated by UGT1A9.

Sorafenib accounts for approximately 70% to 85% of the circulating analytes in plasma at steady state. Eight metabolites of sorafenib have been identified, of which 5 have been detected in plasma. The main circulating metabolite of sorafenib in plasma, the pyridine N-oxide, shows in vitro potency similar to that of sorafenib. This metabolite comprises approximately 9% to 16% of circulating analytes at steady state.

Following oral administration of a 100 mg dose of a solution formulation of sorafenib, 96% of the dose was recovered within 14 days, with 77% of the dose excreted in feces and 19% of the dose excreted in urine as glucuronidated metabolites. Unchanged sorafenib, accounting for 51% of the dose, was found in feces but not in urine.

The mean elimination half-life of sorafenib is approximately 25 to 48 hours.

Special populations –

Hepatic function impairment: Comparison of data across studies suggests that in hepatocellular carcinoma patients with mild (Child-Pugh class A) or moderate (Child-Pugh class B) hepatic function impairment, sorafenib 400 mg doses appear to be associated with AUC values that were 23% to 65% lower than those of other subjects without hepatic function impairment.

Race: A study of the pharmacokinetics of sorafenib indicated that the mean AUC of sorafenib in Asian patients (n = 78) was 30% lower than in white patients (n = 40).

Contraindications

Severe hypersensitivity to sorafenib or any other component of the product.

Warnings/Precautions

➤*Cardiac effects:* In the hepatocellular carcinoma study, the incidence of cardiac ischemia/infarction was 2.7% in sorafenib patients compared with 1.3% in the placebo group. In the renal cell carcinoma study 1, the incidence of cardiac ischemia/infarction events was higher in the sorafenib group (2.9%) compared with the placebo group (0.4%). Patients with unstable coronary artery disease or recent myocardial infarction were excluded from this study. Consider temporary or permanent discontinuation of sorafenib in patients who develop cardiac ischemia and/or infarction.

➤*Hemorrhage:* An increased risk of bleeding may occur after sorafenib administration. In the hepatocellular carcinoma study, an excess of bleeding regardless of causality was not apparent and the rate of bleeding from esophageal varices was 2.4% in sorafenib patients and 4% in placebo patients. Bleeding with a fatal outcome from any site was reported in 2.4% of sorafenib patients and 4% in placebo patients. In the renal cell carcinoma study 1, bleeding regardless of causality was reported in 15.3% of patients in the sorafenib group and 8.2% of patients in the placebo group. The incidence of National Cancer Institute (NCI) Common Terminology Criteria for Adverse Events (CTCAE) grade 3 and 4 bleeding events was 2% and 0%, respectively, in sorafenib patients, and 1.3% and 0.2%, respectively, in placebo patients. There was 1 fatal hemorrhage in each treatment group in renal cell carcinoma study 1. If any bleeding event necessitates medical intervention, consider permanent discontinuation of sorafenib.

➤*Hypertension:* In the hepatocellular carcinoma study, hypertension was reported in approximately 9.4% of sorafenib-treated patients and 4.3% of patients in the placebo group. In renal cell carcinoma study 1, treatment-emergent hypertension was reported in approximately 16.9% of sorafenib-treated patients and 1.8% of patients in the placebo group. Hypertension was usually mild to moderate, occurred early in the course of treatment, and was managed with standard antihypertensive therapy. Monitor blood pressure weekly during the first 6 weeks of sorafenib therapy and monitor and treat thereafter, if required, in accordance with standard medical practice. In cases of severe or persistent hypertension, despite institution of antihypertensive therapy, consider temporary or permanent discontinuation of sorafenib. Permanent discontinuation because of hypertension occurred in 1 of 297 sorafenib-treated hepatocellular carcinoma patients and 1 of 451 sorafenib-treated renal cell carcinoma patients (study 1).

➤*Dermatologic toxicities:* Hand-foot skin reaction and rash represent the most common adverse reactions attributed to sorafenib. Rash and hand-foot skin reactions are usually CTCAE grade 1 and 2 and generally appear during the first 6 weeks of treatment with sorafenib. Management of dermatologic toxicities may include topical therapies for symptomatic relief, temporary treatment interruption, and/or dosage modification of sorafenib, or in severe or persistent cases, permanent discontinuation of sorafenib. Permanent discontinuation of therapy because of hand-foot skin reaction occurred in 4 of 297 sorafenib-treated hepatocellular carcinoma patients and 3 of 451 sorafenib-treated renal cell carcinoma patients.

➤*GI perforation:* GI perforation is an uncommon adverse reaction and has been reported in less than 1% of patients taking sorafenib. In some cases this was not associated with apparent intra-abdominal tumor. In the event of a GI perforation, discontinue sorafenib therapy.

➤*Wound healing complications:* No formal studies of the effect of sorafenib on wound healing have been conducted. Temporary interruption of sorafenib therapy is recommended in patients undergoing major surgical procedures. There is limited clinical experience regarding the timing of reinitiation of sorafenib therapy following major surgical intervention. Therefore, base the decision to resume sorafenib therapy following a major surgical intervention on clinical judgment of adequate wound healing.

➤*Hepatic function impairment:* In vitro and in vivo data indicate that sorafenib is primarily metabolized by the liver. Comparison of data across studies suggests that patients with mild (Child-Pugh class A) and moderate (Child-Pugh class B) hepatic function impairment have sorafenib AUCs that

SORAFENIB TOSYLATE — ORAL

may be 23% to 65% lower than subjects with healthy hepatic function. Systemic exposure and safety data were comparable in hepatocellular carcinoma patients with Child-Pugh class A and B hepatic function impairment. Sorafenib has not been studied in patients with Child-Pugh class C hepatic function impairment. No dosage adjustment is necessary when administering sorafenib to patients with Child-Pugh class A and B hepatic function impairment.

Hepatic function impairment may reduce plasma concentrations of sorafenib. Comparison of data across studies suggests that sorafenib levels are lower in hepatocellular carcinoma patients than in nonhepatocellular carcinoma patients (without hepatic function impairment). The AUC of sorafenib is similar between hepatocellular carcinoma patients with mild (Child-Pugh class A) and moderate (Child-Pugh class B) hepatic function impairment. The optimal dose in nonhepatocellular carcinoma patients with hepatic function impairment is not established.

➤*Pregnancy: Category D.* Sorafenib may cause fetal harm when administered to a pregnant woman. In rats and rabbits, sorafenib has been shown to be teratogenic and to induce embryofetal toxicity (including increased postimplantation loss, resorptions, skeletal retardations, and retarded fetal weight). The effects occurred at dosages considerably below the recommended human dosage of 400 mg twice daily (approximately 500 mg/m²/day on a body surface area basis). Adverse intrauterine development effects were seen at dosages at or higher than 1.2 mg/m²/day in rats and 3.6 mg/m²/day in rabbits (approximately 0.008 times the AUC seen in cancer patients at the recommended human dose). A no observed adverse effect level was not defined for either species because lower doses were not tested.

There are no adequate and well-controlled studies in pregnant women using sorafenib. Advise women of childbearing potential to avoid becoming pregnant while on sorafenib. Adequate contraception should be used during therapy and for at least 2 weeks after completing therapy. Use sorafenib during pregnancy only if the potential benefits justify the potential risks to the fetus.

Fertility impairment – Results from the repeat-dose toxicity studies suggest there is a potential for sorafenib to impair reproductive performance and fertility. Adequate contraception should be used during therapy and for at least 2 weeks after completing therapy.

➤*Lactation:* It is not known whether sorafenib is excreted in human milk. Because many drugs are excreted in human milk and because of the potential for serious adverse reactions in breast-feeding infants after sorafenib use, decide whether to discontinue breast-feeding or the drug, taking into account the importance of the drug to the mother.

Following administration of radiolabeled sorafenib to lactating Wistar rats, approximately 27% of the radioactivity was secreted into the milk. The milk to plasma AUC ratio was approximately 5:1.

➤*Children:* The safety and efficacy of sorafenib in children have not been studied.

➤*Elderly:* No differences in safety or efficacy were observed between older and younger patients, and other reported clinical experience has not identified differences in responses between elderly and younger patients, but greater sensitivity of some older individuals cannot be ruled out.

➤*Monitoring:* Monitor blood pressure weekly during the first 6 weeks of sorafenib therapy and monitor and treat thereafter, if required, in accordance with standard medical practice.

Drug Interactions

Sorafenib Drug Interactions

Precipitant drug	Object drug[a]		Description
CYP3A4 inducers (eg, carbamazepine, dexamethasone, phenobarbital, phenytoin, rifampin, St. John's wort)	Sorafenib	⬇	CYP3A4 inducers may increase the metabolism of sorafenib and, therefore, decrease sorafenib concentrations. Avoid coadministration of sorafenib with strong CYP3A4 inducers. If a strong CYP3A4 inducer must be coadministered with sorafenib, then consider increasing the dose of sorafenib and monitor carefully for toxicity.
Sorafenib	CYP2B6 and CYP2C8 substrates (eg, bupropion, paclitaxel, rosiglitazone)	⬆	Sorafenib inhibits CYP2B6 and CYP2C8; therefore, systemic exposure to substrates of CYP2B6 and CYP2C8 is expected to increase when coadministered with sorafenib. Use with caution.
Sorafenib	Docetaxel	⬆	Sorafenib may increase docetaxel plasma concentrations. Use with caution.
Sorafenib	Doxorubicin	⬆	Sorafenib may increase doxorubicin plasma concentrations. Use with caution.

Sorafenib Drug Interactions

Precipitant drug	Object drug[a]		Description
Sorafenib	Fluorouracil	⬆⬇	Both increases (21% to 47%) and decreases (10%) in the AUC of fluorouracil were observed with concomitant treatment with sorafenib. Use with caution.
Sorafenib	UGT1A1 substrates (eg, irinotecan)	⬆	Sorafenib can increase plasma concentrations of drugs that are substrates of UGT1A1. Use caution when administering sorafenib with drugs that are metabolized and eliminated predominantly by the UGT1A1 pathway.
Sorafenib	Warfarin	⬆	Coadministration has caused infrequent bleeding or elevations in INR[b] in some patients. Monitor regularly for changes in prothrombin time, INR, or clinical bleeding episodes.

[a] ⬆ = object drug increased; ⬇ = object drug decreased; ⬆⬇ = object drug increased and decreased.
[b] INR = international normalized ratio.

➤*Drug/Food interactions:* When given with a high-fat meal, sorafenib bioavailability was reduced 29% compared with administration in the fasted state. It is recommended that sorafenib be administered without food (at least 1 hour before or 2 hours after eating).

Adverse Reactions

➤*Most common adverse reactions:* The most common adverse reactions (at least 20%), which were considered to be related to sorafenib, in patients with hepatocellular carcinoma or renal cell carcinoma are abdominal pain, alopecia, anorexia, diarrhea, fatigue, hand-foot skin reaction, nausea, rash/desquamation, and weight loss.

➤*Hepatocellular carcinoma:* The following table shows the percentage of hepatocellular carcinoma patients experiencing adverse reactions that were reported in at least 10% of patients and at a higher rate in the sorafenib arm than the placebo arm. CTCAE grade 3 adverse reactions were reported in 39% of patients receiving sorafenib compared with 24% of patients receiving placebo. CTCAE grade 4 adverse reactions were reported in 6% of patients receiving sorafenib compared with 8% of patients receiving placebo.

Sorafenib Adverse Reactions in Patients With Hepatocellular Carcinoma (≥ 10%)

Adverse reaction NCI CTCAE v3	Sorafenib (n = 297)			Placebo (n = 302)		
	All grades	Grade 3	Grade 4	All grades	Grade 3	Grade 4
Any adverse reaction	98%	39%	6%	96%	24%	8%
Dermatologic						
Alopecia	14%	0%	0%	2%	0%	0%
Dry skin	10%	0%	0%	6%	0%	0%
Hand-foot skin reaction	21%	8%	0%	3%	< 1%	0%
Pruritus	14%	< 1%	0%	11%	< 1%	0%
Rash/desquamation	19%	1%	0%	14%	0%	0%
GI						
Anorexia	29%	3%	0%	18%	3%	< 1%
Constipation	14%	0%	0%	10%	0%	0%
Diarrhea	55%	10%	< 1%	25%	2%	0%
Nausea	24%	1%	0%	20%	3%	0%
Pain, abdomen	31%	9%	0%	26%	5%	1%
Vomiting	15%	2%	0%	11%	2%	0%
Miscellaneous						
Fatigue	46%	9%	1%	45%	12%	2%
Liver dysfunction	11%	2%	1%	8%	2%	1%
Weight loss	30%	2%	0%	10%	1%	0%

Hypertension – Hypertension was reported in 9% of patients treated with sorafenib and 4% of those treated with placebo. CTCAE grade 3 hypertension was reported in 4% of sorafenib-treated patients and 1% of placebo-treated patients. No patients were reported with CTCAE grade 4 reactions in either treatment group.

Hemorrhage – Hemorrhage/bleeding was reported in 18% of those receiving sorafenib and 20% of placebo patients. The rates of CTCAE grade 3 and 4 bleeding were also higher in the placebo group (CTCAE grade 3, 3% sorafenib and 5% placebo; CTCAE grade 4, 2% sorafenib and 4% placebo). Bleeding from esophageal varices was reported in 2.4% in sorafenib-treated patients and 4% of placebo-treated patients.

SORAFENIB TOSYLATE — ORAL

Renal – Renal failure was reported in less than 1% of patients treated with sorafenib and 3% of placebo-treated patients.

Discontinuation – The rate of adverse reactions (including those associated with progressive disease) resulting in permanent discontinuation was similar in both the sorafenib and placebo groups (32% of sorafenib patients and 35% of placebo patients).

➤*Renal cell carcinoma:* The following table shows the percentage of patients with renal cell carcinoma experiencing treatment-emergent adverse reactions that were reported in at least 10% of patients and at a higher rate in the sorafenib arm than in the placebo arm. CTCAE grade 3 treatment-emergent adverse reactions were reported in 31% of patients receiving sorafenib compared with 22% of patients receiving placebo. CTCAE grade 4 treatment-emergent adverse reactions were reported in 7% of patients receiving sorafenib compared with 6% of patients receiving placebo.

Sorafenib Adverse Reactions in Patients With Renal Cell Carcinoma (≥ 10%)

Adverse reaction NCI CTCAE v3	Sorafenib (n = 451)			Placebo (n = 451)		
	All grades	Grade 3	Grade 4	All grades	Grade 3	Grade 4
Any adverse reaction	95%	31%	7%	86%	22%	6%
Cardiovascular						
Hypertension	17%	3%	< 1%	2%	< 1%	0%
CNS						
Neuropathy (sensory)	13%	< 1%	0%	6%	< 1%	0%
Pain, headache	10%	< 1%	0%	6%	< 1%	0%
Dermatological						
Alopecia	27%	< 1%	0%	3%	0%	0%
Dry skin	11%	0%	0%	4%	0%	0%
Hand-foot skin reaction	30%	6%	0%	7%	0%	0%
Pruritus	19%	< 1%	0%	6%	0%	0%
Rash/ desquamation	40%	< 1%	0%	16%	< 1%	0%
GI						
Anorexia	16%	< 1%	0%	13%	1%	0%
Constipation	15%	< 1%	0%	11%	< 1%	0%
Diarrhea	43%	2%	0%	13%	< 1%	0%
Nausea	23%	< 1%	0%	19%	< 1%	0%
Pain, abdomen	11%	2%	0%	9%	2%	0%
Vomiting	16%	< 1%	0%	12%	1%	0%
Hematologic						
Hemorrhage (all sites)	15%	2%	0%	8%	1%	< 1%
Respiratory						
Cough	13%	< 1%	0%	14%	< 1%	0%
Dyspnea	14%	3%	< 1%	12%	2%	< 1%
Miscellaneous						
Fatigue	37%	5%	< 1%	28%	3%	< 1%
Pain, joint	10%	2%	0%	6%	< 1%	0%
Weight loss	10%	< 1%	0%	6%	0%	0%

Discontinuation – The rate of adverse reactions (including reactions associated with progressive disease) resulting in permanent discontinuation was similar in both the sorafenib and placebo groups (10% of sorafenib patients and 8% of placebo patients).

➤*Lab test abnormalities:*

Hepatocellular carcinoma –

Hypophosphatemia: Hypophosphatemia was a common laboratory finding, observed in 35% of sorafenib-treated patients compared with 11% of placebo patients; CTCAE grade 3 hypophosphatemia (1 to 2 mg/dL) occurred in 11% of sorafenib-treated patients and 2% of patients in the placebo group; there was 1 case of CTCAE grade 4 hypophosphatemia (less than 1 mg/dL) reported in the placebo group. The etiology of hypophosphatemia associated with sorafenib is not known.

Lipase/Amylase: Elevated lipase was observed in 40% of patients treated with sorafenib compared with 37% of patients in the placebo group. CTCAE grade 3 or 4 lipase elevations occurred in 9% of patients in each group. Elevated amylase was observed in 34% of patients treated with sorafenib compared with 29% of patients in the placebo group. CTCAE grade 3 or 4 amylase elevations were reported in 2% of patients in each group. Many of the lipase and amylase elevations were transient, and in the majority of cases sorafenib treatment was not interrupted. Clinical pancreatitis was reported in 1 of 297 sorafenib-treated patients (CTCAE grade 2).

Liver function tests: Elevations in liver function tests were comparable between the 2 arms of the study. Hypoalbuminemia was observed in 59% of sorafenib-treated patients and 47% of placebo patients; no CTCAE grade 3 or 4 hypoalbuminemia was observed in either group.

INR: INR elevations were observed in 42% of sorafenib-treated patients and 34% of placebo patients; CTCAE grade 3 INR elevations were reported in 4% of sorafenib-treated patients and 2% of placebo patients. There was no CTCAE grade 4 INR elevation in either group.

Hematologic: Lymphopenia was observed in 47% of sorafenib-treated patients and 42% of placebo patients.

Thrombocytopenia was observed in 46% of sorafenib-treated patients and 41% of placebo patients; CTCAE grade 3 or 4 thrombocytopenia was reported in 4% of sorafenib-treated patients and less than 1% of placebo patients.

Renal cell carcinoma –

Hypophosphatemia: Hypophosphatemia was a common laboratory finding, observed in 45% of sorafenib-treated patients compared with 11% of placebo patients. CTCAE grade 3 hypophosphatemia (1 to 2 mg/dL) occurred in 13% of sorafenib-treated patients and 3% of patients in the placebo group. There were no cases of CTCAE grade 4 hypophosphatemia (less than 1 mg/dL) reported in sorafenib or placebo patients. The etiology of hypophosphatemia associated with sorafenib is not known.

Lipase/Amylase: Elevated lipase was observed in 41% of patients treated with sorafenib compared with 30% of patients in the placebo group. CTCAE grade 3 or 4 lipase elevations occurred in 12% of patients in the sorafenib group compared with 7% of patients in the placebo group. Elevated amylase was observed in 30% of patients treated with sorafenib compared with 23% of patients in the placebo group. CTCAE grade 3 or 4 amylase elevations were reported in 1% of patients in the sorafenib group compared with 3% of patients in the placebo group. Many of the lipase and amylase elevations were transient, and in the majority of cases sorafenib treatment was not interrupted. Clinical pancreatitis was reported in 3 of 451 sorafenib-treated patients (one CTCAE grade 2 and two grade 4) and 1 of 451 patients (CTCAE grade 2) in the placebo group.

Hematologic: Lymphopenia was observed in 23% of sorafenib-treated patients and 13% of placebo patients. CTCAE grade 3 or 4 lymphopenia was reported in 13% of sorafenib-treated patients and 7% of placebo patients. Neutropenia was observed in 18% of sorafenib-treated patients and 10% of placebo patients. CTCAE grade 3 or 4 neutropenia was reported in 5% of sorafenib-treated patients and 2% of placebo patients.

Anemia was observed in 44% of sorafenib-treated patients and 49% of placebo patients. CTCAE grade 3 or 4 anemia was reported in 2% of sorafenib-treated patients and 4% of placebo patients.

Thrombocytopenia was observed in 12% of sorafenib-treated patients and 5% of placebo patients. CTCAE grade 3 or 4 thrombocytopenia was reported in 1% of sorafenib-treated patients and 0% of placebo patients.

➤*Additional adverse reactions:*

Cardiovascular – Congestive heart failure, hypertensive crisis, myocardial ischemia and/or infarction (0.1% to less than 1%).

CNS – Depression (1% to less than 10%); reversible posterior leukoencephalopathy, tinnitus (0.1% to less than 1%).

Dermatologic – Erythema (10% or more); acne, exfoliative dermatitis, flushing (1% to less than 10%); eczema, erythema multiforme, folliculitis, keratoacanthomas/squamous cell cancer of the skin (0.1% to less than 1%).

GI – Increased amylase, increased lipase (10% or more); dyspepsia, dysphagia, mucositis, stomatitis (including dry mouth and glossodynia) (1% to less than 10%); gastritis, GI perforations, GI reflux, pancreatitis (0.1% to less than 1%).

Note that elevations in lipase are very common (41%); do not make a diagnosis of pancreatitis solely on the basis of abnormal laboratory values.

GU – Erectile dysfunction (1% to less than 10%); gynecomastia (0.1% to less than 1%).

Hematologic – Hemorrhage (including GI and respiratory tract and uncommon cases of cerebral hemorrhage), leukopenia, lymphopenia (10% or more); anemia, neutropenia, thrombocytopenia (1% to less than 10%); INR abnormal (0.1% to less than 1%).

Hypersensitivity – Hypersensitivity reactions (including skin reactions and urticaria) (0.1% to less than 1%).

Metabolic/Nutritional – Hypophosphatemia (10% or more); transient increases in transaminases (1% to less than 10%); dehydration, hyponatremia, hypothyroidism, increased bilirubin (including jaundice), transient increases in alkaline phosphatase (0.1% to less than 1%).

Musculoskeletal – Arthralgia, myalgia (1% to less than 10%).

Respiratory – Hoarseness (1% to less than 10%); rhinorrhea (0.1% to less than 1%).

Miscellaneous – Asthenia, pain (including mouth pain, bone pain, and tumor pain) (10% or more); decreased appetite, influenza-like illness, pyrexia (1% to less than 10%); infection (0.1% to less than 1%). In addition, the following medically significant adverse reactions were uncommon during clinical trials of sorafenib: acute renal failure, arrhythmia, thromboembolism, transient ischemic attack. For these reactions, the causal relationship to sorafenib has not been established.

Note that some of the adverse reactions listed previously may have a life-threatening or fatal outcome.

Overdosage

➤*Symptoms:* The highest dosage of sorafenib studied clinically is 800 mg twice daily. The adverse reactions observed at this dosage were primarily diarrhea and dermatologic events.

Multikinase Inhibitor

SORAFENIB TOSYLATE — ORAL

➤*Treatment:* There is no specific treatment for sorafenib overdose. In cases of suspected overdose, withhold sorafenib and institute supportive care.

Patient Information

Inform women that sorafenib may cause birth defects or fetal loss and that they should not become pregnant during treatment with sorafenib and for at least 2 weeks after stopping treatment. Counsel men and women to use effective birth control during treatment with sorafenib and for at least 2 weeks after stopping treatment. Also advise women against breast-feeding while receiving sorafenib.

Advise patients of the possible occurrence of hand-foot skin reaction and rash during sorafenib treatment and appropriate countermeasures. Inform patients that hypertension may develop during sorafenib treatment, especially during the first 6 weeks of therapy, and to monitor blood pressure regularly during treatment.

Inform patients that sorafenib may increase the risk of bleeding and that they should promptly report any episodes of bleeding.

Advise patients that cases of GI perforation have been reported in patients taking sorafenib.

Discuss with patients that cardiac ischemia and/or infarction has been reported during sorafenib treatment, and that they should immediately report any episodes of chest pain or other symptoms of cardiac ischemia and/or infarction.

PROTEASOME INHIBITORS

BORTEZOMIB

Rx	**Velcade** (Millennium Pharmaceuticals)	**Injection, lyophilized powder for solution:** 3.5 mg	Preservative free. Mannitol 35 mg. In single-dose vials.

BORTEZOMIB — INJECTION

Indications

➤*Mantle cell lymphoma:* For the treatment of patients with mantle cell lymphoma who have received at least 1 prior therapy.

➤*Multiple myeloma:* For the treatment of patients with multiple myeloma.

➤*Off-label uses:*

Myelomatous pleural effusion – [4] = Insufficient documentation. The use of bortezomib to treat myelomatous pleural effusion has been limited to 1 case report. Data from this case report suggest that this drug may be a useful alternative in patients with refractory disease, but larger, controlled trials are needed to determine the optimal dosage schedule and to verify results. (See Administration and Dosage.)

Administration and Dosage

➤*General dosing considerations:* Administer with fluid and electrolyte replacement to prevent dehydration.

➤*Adults:*

Mantle cell lymphoma –

Usual dosage: 1.3 mg/m^2/dose as a 3- to 5-second bolus intravenous (IV) injection twice weekly for 2 weeks (days 1, 4, 8, and 11), followed by a 10-day rest period (days 12 to 21).

Maintenance dosage: For extended therapy of more than 8 cycles, bortezomib may be administered on the standard schedule or on a maintenance schedule of once weekly for 4 weeks (days 1, 8, 15, and 22), followed by a 13-day rest period (days 23 to 35). At least 72 hours should elapse between consecutive doses of bortezomib.

Dosage adjustment: Bortezomib should be withheld at the onset of any grade 3 nonhematological or grade 4 hematological toxicities, excluding neuropathy. Once the symptoms of the toxicity have resolved, bortezomib may be reinitiated at a 25% reduced dose (1.3 mg/m^2/dose reduced to 1 mg/m^2/dose; 1 mg/m^2/dose reduced to 0.7 mg/m^2/dose).

Bortezomib Dose Modification for Related Neuropathic Pain and/or Peripheral Sensory or Motor Neuropathy[a]

Severity of peripheral neuropathy signs and symptoms	Modification of dose and regimen
Grade 1 (paresthesias, weakness, and/or loss of reflexes) without pain or loss of function	No action
Grade 1 with pain or grade 2 (interfering with function but not with activities of daily living)	Reduce bortezomib to 1 mg/m^2
Grade 2 with pain or grade 3 (interfering with activities of daily living)	Withhold bortezomib therapy until toxicity resolves. When toxicity resolves, reinitiate with a reduced dose of bortezomib at 0.7 mg/m^2 and change treatment schedule to once per week.
Grade 4 (sensory neuropathy that is disabling or motor neuropathy that is life-threatening or leads to paralysis)	Discontinue bortezomib

[a] Grading based on *National Cancer Institute Common Terminology Criteria for Adverse Events*, version 3.0.

Multiple myeloma, previously untreated –

Usual dosage: 1.3 mg/m^2 as a 3- to 5-second bolus IV injection in combination with oral melphalan and oral prednisone for nine 6-week treatment cycles. At least 72 hours should elapse between consecutive doses of bortezomib.

Bortezomib Dosage Regimen for Previously Untreated Multiple Myeloma

Twice-weekly bortezomib (cycles 1 through 4)												
Week	1				2		3	4		5		6
Bortezomib 1.3 mg/m^2	Day 1	—	—	Day 4	Day 8	Day 11	Rest period	Day 22	Day 25	Day 29	Day 32	Rest period
Melphalan 9 mg/m^2 Prednisone 60 mg/m^2	Day 1	Day 2	Day 3	Day 4	—	—	Rest period	—	—	—	—	Rest period
Once-weekly bortezomib (cycles 5 through 9 when used in combination with melphalan and prednisone)												
Week	1				2		3	4		5		6
Bortezomib 1.3 mg/m^2	Day 1	—	—		Day 8		Rest period	Day 22		Day 29		Rest period
Melphalan 9 mg/m^2 Prednisone 60 mg/m^2	Day 1	Day 2	Day 3	Day 4	—	—	Rest period	—	—	—	—	Rest period

Dosage adjustment: Prior to initiating any cycle of therapy with bortezomib in combination with melphalan and prednisone, platelet count should be 70 × 10^9/L or more and the absolute neutrophil count (ANC) should be 1 × 10^9/L or more; nonhematological toxicities should have resolved to grade 1 or baseline.

Bortezomib, Melphalan, and Prednisone Dose Modifications

Toxicity	Dose modification or delay
Hematological toxicity during a cycle: If prolonged grade 4 neutropenia or thrombocytopenia or thrombocytopenia with bleeding is observed in the previous cycle	Consider the reduction of the melphalan dose by 25% in the next cycle.
If platelet count ≤ 30 × 10^9/L or ANC ≤ 0.75 × 10^9/L on bortezomib dosing day (other than day 1)	Bortezomib dose should be withheld.
If several bortezomib doses in consecutive cycles are withheld because of toxicity	Bortezomib dose should be reduced by 1 dose level (from 1.3 mg/m^2 to 1 mg/m^2, or from 1 mg/m^2 to 0.7 mg/m^2).
Grade ≥ 3 nonhematological toxicities	Bortezomib therapy should be withheld until symptoms of the toxicity have resolved to grade 1 or baseline. Then, bortezomib may be reinitiated with 1 dose level reduction (from 1.3 mg/m^2 to 1 mg/m^2, or from 1 mg/m^2 to 0.7 mg/m^2). For bortezomib-related neuropathic pain and/or peripheral neuropathy, hold or modify bortezomib.

For information concerning melphalan and prednisone, see the manufacturer's prescribing information.

Multiple myeloma, relapsed – Refer to Mantle Cell Lymphoma for dosing.

Off-label dosing –

Myelomatous pleural effusion: [4] = Insufficient documentation. In 1 case report, the dosage given was 0.65 mg/m^2 administered in the pleural cavity on days 1, 4, 8, and 11 for 2 cycles. Bortezomib was given intrapleurally after evacuative thoracentesis, and the remaining IV dose was administered with dexamethasone.

➤*Renal function impairment:* Because dialysis may reduce bortezomib concentrations, the drug should be administered after the dialysis procedure.

BORTEZOMIB — INJECTION

➤*Hepatic function impairment:*

Bortezomib Starting Dosage Modification in Hepatic Impairment

	Bilirubin level	AST levels	Modification of starting dose
Mild	≤ 1 × ULN[a]	> ULN	None
	> 1 × to 1.5 × ULN	Any	None
Moderate	> 1.5 × to 3 × ULN	Any	Reduce bortezomib to 0.7 mg/m² in the first cycle. Consider dose escalation to 1 mg/m² or further dose reduction to 0.5 mg/m² in subsequent cycles based on patient tolerability.
Severe	> 3 × ULN	Any	

[a] ULN = upper limit of the normal range.

➤*Preparation for administration:* Bortezomib is considered a cytotoxic agent. Follow safe handling procedures when preparing, administering, or dispensing bortezomib.

Proper aseptic technique should be used. Consider handling and disposal of bortezomib according to guidelines issued for cytotoxic drugs, including the use of gloves and other protective clothing to prevent skin contact. In clinical trials, local skin irritation was reported in 5% of patients, but extravasation of bortezomib was not associated with tissue damage.

Reconstitute with 3.5 mL of sodium chloride 0.9%, resulting in a final concentration of 1 mg/mL of bortezomib. The reconstituted product should be a clear and colorless solution.

The drug quantity contained in 1 vial (3.5 mg) may exceed the usual single dose required. Use caution in calculating the dose to prevent overdose.

➤*Storage/Stability:* Store unopened vials in the original package at 25°C (77°F); excursions are permitted between 15° and 30°C (59° and 86°F). Protect from light.

Reconstituted bortezomib may be stored at 25°C (77°F). Administer within 8 hours of preparation. The reconstituted material may be stored in the original vial and/or the syringe prior to administration. The product may be stored for up to 8 hours in a syringe; however, total storage time for the reconstituted material must not exceed 8 hours when exposed to normal indoor lighting.

Actions

➤*Pharmacology:* Bortezomib, an antineoplastic agent, is a reversible inhibitor of the chymotrypsin-like activity of the 26S proteasome in mammalian cells. The 26S proteasome is a large protein complex that degrades ubiquitinated proteins. The ubiquitin-proteasome pathway plays an essential role in regulating the intracellular concentration of specific proteins, thereby maintaining homeostasis within cells. Inhibition of the 26S proteasome prevents this targeted proteolysis, which can affect multiple signaling cascades within the cell. This disruption of normal homeostatic mechanisms can lead to cell death. Experiments have demonstrated that bortezomib is cytotoxic to a variety of cancer cell types in vitro. Bortezomib causes a delay in tumor growth in vivo in nonclinical tumor models, including multiple myeloma.

➤*Pharmacokinetics:*

Absorption/Distribution – Following IV administration of 1 and 1.3 mg/m² doses to 24 patients with multiple myeloma (n = 12 per each dose level), the mean maximum plasma concentrations (C_{max}) of bortezomib after the first dose (day 1) were 57 and 112 ng/mL, respectively. In subsequent doses, when administered twice weekly, the observed C_{max} ranged from 67 to 106 ng/mL for the 1 mg/m² dose and 89 to 120 ng/mL for the 1.3 mg/m² dose.

The mean distribution volume of bortezomib ranged from approximately 498 to 1,884 L/m² following single- or repeat-dose administration of 1 or 1.3 mg/m² to patients with multiple myeloma. This suggests bortezomib distributes widely to peripheral tissues. The binding of bortezomib to human plasma proteins averaged 83% over the concentration range of 100 to 1,000 ng/mL.

Metabolism – In vitro studies with human liver microsomes and human cDNA-expressed cytochrome P450 (CYP-450) isozymes indicate that bortezomib is primarily oxidatively metabolized via CYP-450 enzymes 3A4, 2C19, and 1A2. Bortezomib metabolism by CYP2D6 and CYP2C9 enzymes is minor. The major metabolic pathway is deboronation to form 2 deboronated metabolites that subsequently undergo hydroxylation to several metabolites. Deboronated bortezomib metabolites are inactive as 26S proteasome inhibitors. Pooled plasma data from 8 patients at 10 and 30 minutes after dosing indicate that the plasma levels of metabolites are low compared with the parent drug.

Excretion – The mean elimination half-life of bortezomib upon multiple dosing ranged from 40 to 193 hours after the 1 mg/m² dose and 76 to 108 hours after the 1.3 mg/m² dose. The mean total body clearances were 102 and 112 L/h following the first dose for doses of 1 and 1.3 mg/m², respectively, and ranged from 15 to 32 L/h following subsequent doses for doses of 1 and 1.3 mg/m², respectively.

Special populations –

Elderly: Patients younger than 65 years of age (n = 26) had about 25% lower mean dose-normalized area under the curve (AUC) and C_{max} than those 65 years of age and older (n = 13).

Contraindications

Hypersensitivity to bortezomib, boron, or mannitol.

Warnings/Precautions

➤*Peripheral neuropathy:* Bortezomib treatment causes a peripheral neuropathy that is predominantly sensory. However, cases of severe sensory and motor peripheral neuropathy have been reported. Patients with preexisting symptoms (numbness, pain, or a burning feeling in the feet or hands) and/or signs of peripheral neuropathy may experience worsening peripheral neuropathy (including grade 3 or higher) during treatment with bortezomib. Monitor patients for symptoms of neuropathy, such as a burning sensation, hyperesthesia, hypesthesia, paresthesia, discomfort, neuropathic pain, or weakness. Patients experiencing new or worsening peripheral neuropathy may require a change in the dose and schedule of bortezomib. Following dose adjustments, improvement in or resolution of peripheral neuropathy was reported in 51% of patients with at least grade 2 peripheral neuropathy in the relapsed multiple myeloma study. Improvement in or resolution of peripheral neuropathy was reported in 73% of patients who discontinued because of grade 2 neuropathy or who had at least grade 3 peripheral neuropathy in the phase 2 multiple myeloma studies. The long-term outcome of peripheral neuropathy has not been studied in mantle cell lymphoma. (See Adverse Reactions.)

➤*Hypotension:* The incidence of hypotension (postural, orthostatic, and hypotension not otherwise specified) was 13%. These reactions are observed throughout therapy. Use caution when treating patients who have a history of syncope, patients receiving medications known to be associated with hypotension, and patients who are dehydrated. Management of orthostatic/postural hypotension may include adjustment of antihypertensive medications, hydration, or administration of mineralocorticoids and/or sympathomimetics. (See Adverse Reactions.)

➤*Cardiac effects:* Acute development or exacerbation of congestive heart failure and new onset of decreased left ventricular ejection fraction have been reported, including reports in patients with no risk factors for decreased left ventricular ejection fraction. Closely monitor patients with risk factors for heart disease and those with existing heart disease. In the relapsed multiple myeloma study, the incidence of any treatment-emergent cardiac disorder was 15% and 13% in the bortezomib and dexamethasone groups, respectively. The incidence of heart failure events (eg, acute pulmonary edema, cardiac failure, congestive cardiac failure, cardiogenic shock, pulmonary edema) was similar in the bortezomib and dexamethasone groups (5% and 4%, respectively). There have been isolated cases of QT-interval prolongation in clinical studies; causality has not been established.

➤*Pulmonary effects:* There have been reports of acute diffuse infiltrative pulmonary disease of unknown etiology, such as pneumonitis, interstitial pneumonia, lung infiltration, and acute respiratory distress syndrome (ARDS) in patients receiving bortezomib. Some of these events have been fatal.

In a clinical trial, the first 2 patients given high-dose cytarabine (2 g/m²/day) by continuous infusion with daunorubicin and bortezomib for relapsed acute myelogenous leukemia died of ARDS early in the course of therapy.

There have been reports of pulmonary hypertension associated with bortezomib administration in the absence of left heart failure or significant pulmonary disease.

In the event of new or worsening cardiopulmonary symptoms, consider conducting a prompt comprehensive diagnostic evaluation.

➤*Reversible posterior leukoencephalopathy syndrome:* There have been reports of reversible posterior leukoencephalopathy syndrome (RPLS) in patients receiving bortezomib. RPLS is a rare, reversible neurological disorder that can present with seizure, hypertension, headache, lethargy, confusion, blindness, and other visual and neurological disturbances. Brain imaging, preferably magnetic resonance imaging, is used to confirm the diagnosis. Discontinue bortezomib in patients developing RPLS. The safety of reinitiating bortezomib therapy in patients previously experiencing RPLS is not known.

➤*GI effects:* Bortezomib treatment can cause constipation, diarrhea, nausea, and vomiting, sometimes requiring use of antiemetics and antidiarrheal medications. Ileus can occur. Administer fluid and electrolyte replacement to prevent dehydration. (See Adverse Reactions.)

➤*Thrombocytopenia/Neutropenia:* Bortezomib is associated with thrombocytopenia and neutropenia that follow a cyclical pattern with nadirs occurring following the last dose of each cycle and typically recovering prior to initiation of the subsequent cycle. The cyclical pattern of platelet and neutrophil decreases and recovery remained consistent over the 8 cycles of twice-weekly dosing, and there was no evidence of cumulative thrombocytopenia or neutropenia. The mean platelet count nadir measured was approximately 40% of baseline. In the relapsed multiple myeloma study, the incidence of significant bleeding events (grade 3 or higher) was similar on the bortezomib (4%) and dexamethasone (5%) arms. Monitor platelet counts prior to each dose of bortezomib. Patients experiencing thrombocytopenia may require a change in the dose and schedule of bortezomib. (See Adverse Reactions.)

There have been reports of GI and intracerebral hemorrhage in association with bortezomib. Transfusions may be considered. The incidence of febrile neutropenia was less than 1%.

➤*Tumor lysis syndrome:* Because bortezomib is a cytotoxic agent and can rapidly kill malignant cells, the complications of tumor lysis syndrome may occur. Patients at risk of tumor lysis syndrome are those with high tumor burden prior to treatment. Monitor these patients closely and take appropriate precautions.

BORTEZOMIB — INJECTION

➤*Hepatic effects:* Cases of acute liver failure have been reported in patients receiving multiple concomitant medications and those with serious underlying medical conditions. Other reported hepatic events include increases in liver enzymes, hyperbilirubinemia, and hepatitis. Such changes may be reversible upon discontinuation of bortezomib. There is limited rechallenge information in these patients.

➤*Diabetes:* During clinical trials, hypoglycemia and hyperglycemia were reported in diabetic patients receiving oral hypoglycemics. Patients on oral antidiabetic agents receiving bortezomib treatment may require close monitoring of their blood glucose levels and adjustment of the dose of their antidiabetic medication.

➤*Renal function impairment:* Because dialysis may reduce bortezomib concentrations, administer the drug after the dialysis procedure.

➤*Hepatic function impairment:* Bortezomib is metabolized by liver enzymes. Bortezomib exposure is increased in patients with moderate or severe hepatic impairment; treat these patients with bortezomib at reduced starting doses and closely monitor for toxicities.

➤*Pregnancy: Category D.* Advise women of childbearing potential to avoid becoming pregnant while being treated with bortezomib. There are no adequate and well-controlled studies in pregnant women. It is not known if bortezomib crosses the human placenta. The molecular weight (approximately 384), the long elimination half-life, the moderate plasma protein binding, and lack of rapid metabolism all suggest that the drug will cross to the embryo and/or fetus. If bortezomib is used during pregnancy, or if the patient becomes pregnant while receiving this drug, apprise the patient of the potential hazard to the fetus.

Pregnant rabbits given bortezomib during organogenesis at a dose of 0.05 mg/kg (0.6 mg/m^2) experienced significant postimplantation loss and decreased number of live fetuses. Live fetuses from these litters also showed significant decreases in fetal weight. The dose is approximately 0.5 times the clinical dose of 1.3 mg/m^2 based on body surface area.

➤*Lactation:* It is not known whether bortezomib is excreted in human milk. Bortezomib's long elimination half-life, low molecular weight, and moderate protein binding suggest that it would be excreted in human milk. Because many drugs are excreted in human milk and because of the potential for serious adverse reactions in breast-feeding infants from bortezomib, decide whether to discontinue breast-feeding or the drug, taking into account the importance of the drug to the mother.

➤*Children:* The safety and efficacy of bortezomib in children have not been established.

➤*Elderly:* No overall differences in safety or efficacy were observed between patients 65 years of age and older and younger patients receiving bortezomib; however, greater sensitivity of some older patients cannot be ruled out.

➤*Monitoring:* Monitor complete blood cell counts frequently throughout treatment. Monitor platelet counts prior to each dose. Monitor patients for symptoms of neuropathy (eg, burning sensation, discomfort, hyperesthesia, hypesthesia, neuropathic pain, paresthesia). Closely monitor patients with risk factors for heart disease and those with existing heart disease. Patients on oral antidiabetic agents receiving bortezomib may require close monitoring of their blood glucose levels and adjustment of the dose of their antidiabetic medication. Closely monitor patients with moderate or severe hepatic impairment for toxicities. Closely monitor patients with high tumor burden for tumor lysis syndrome. Monitor blood pressure, especially in patients receiving medications known to lower blood pressure.

Drug Interactions

➤*Cytochrome P450:* Bortezomib is metabolized by CYP-450 3A4, 2C19, and 1A2. Therefore, closely monitor patients receiving bortezomib concomitantly with potent CYP3A4 inhibitors or inducers for toxicities or reduced efficacy. Bortezomib may inhibit CYP2C19 activity and increase exposure to drugs that are substrates for this enzyme.

Bortezomib Drug Interactions

Precipitant drug	Object drug[a]		Description
Ketoconazole	Bortezomib	↑	Ketoconazole resulted in a 35% increase in bortezomib AUC. Closely monitor patients receiving concomitant therapy. Adjust the bortezomib dose as needed.
Melphalan/ prednisolone	Bortezomib	↑	Coadministration of melphalan and prednisolone with bortezomib resulted in a 17% increase in bortezomib AUC. This increase is unlikely to be clinically relevant.
Bortezomib	Antihypertensives (eg, propranolol)	↑	May potentiate hypotension. Adjust the dose of the antihypertensive agent as needed.
Bortezomib	Cyclosporine	↑	Bortezomib may enhance the neurotoxic effect of cyclosporine. Closely monitor the patient. If an interaction is suspected, adjust the cyclosporine dose and continue monitoring for neurotoxic effects.
Bortezomib	Oral hypoglycemic agents (eg, glimepiride)	↓	Bortezomib administration has resulted in hyperglycemia. In patients receiving oral hypoglycemic agents, closely monitor blood glucose levels and adjust the dose of the hypoglycemic agent as necessary.

[a] ↑ = object drug increased; ↓ = object drug decreased.

Adverse Reactions

➤*Previously untreated multiple myeloma:*

Bortezomib Adverse Reactions in Previously Untreated Multiple Myeloma (≥ 10%)

	Bortezomib, melphalan, and prednisone (n = 340)			Melphalan and prednisone (n = 337)		
Adverse reactions	Total	Toxicity grade 3	Toxicity grade ≥ 4	Total	Toxicity grade 3	Toxicity grade ≥ 4
Cardiovascular						
Hypertension	13%	2%	< 1%	7%	1%	0%
Hypotension	12%	1%	1%	3%	1%	1%
CNS						
Asthenia	21%	6%	< 1%	18%	3%	0%
Dizziness	16%	2%	0%	11%	< 1%	0%
Fatigue	29%	7%	1%	26%	2%	0%
Headache	14%	1%	0%	10%	1%	0%
Insomnia	20%	< 1%	0%	13%	0%	0%
Neuralgia	36%	8%	1%	1%	< 1%	0%
Paresthesia	13%	2%	0%	4%	0%	0%
Peripheral neuropathy	47%	13%	1%	5%	0%	0%
Dermatologic						
Pruritus	10%	1%	0%	5%	0%	0%
Rash	19%	1%	0%	7%	< 1%	0%
GI disorders						
Abdominal pain	14%	2%	0%	7%	< 1%	0%
Abdominal pain upper	12%	< 1%	0%	9%	0%	0%
Constipation	37%	1%	0%	16%	0%	0%
Diarrhea	46%	7%	1%	17%	1%	0%
Dyspepsia	11%	0%	0%	7%	0%	0%
Nausea	48%	4%	0%	28%	< 1%	0%
Vomiting	33%	4%	0%	16%	1%	0%
Hematologic/Lymphatic						
Anemia	43%	16%	3%	55%	20%	8%
Leukopenia	33%	20%	3%	30%	16%	4%
Lymphopenia	24%	14%	5%	17%	9%	2%
Neutropenia	49%	30%	10%	46%	23%	15%
Thrombocytopenia	52%	20%	17%	47%	16%	14%
Metabolic/Nutritional						
Anorexia	23%	3%	< 1%	10%	1%	0%
Edema peripheral	20%	1%	0%	10%	0%	0%
Hypokalemia	13%	6%	1%	7%	2%	1%
Musculoskeletal						
Arthralgia	11%	1%	0%	15%	1%	< 1%
Back pain	17%	3%	< 1%	18%	3%	< 1%
Bone pain	11%	2%	< 1%	10%	2%	0%
Pain in extremity	14%	2%	0%	9%	1%	< 1%
Respiratory						
Bronchitis	13%	1%	0%	8%	1%	0%
Cough	21%	0%	0%	13%	1%	0%
Dyspnea	15%	3%	1%	13%	1%	1%
Nasopharyngitis	11%	< 1%	0%	8%	0%	0%
Pneumonia	16%	5%	4%	11%	4%	3%
Miscellaneous						
Herpes zoster	13%	3%	0%	4%	2%	0%
Pyrexia	29%	2%	1%	19%	2%	1%

➤*Relapsed multiple myeloma:*

Common adverse reactions – Among the 331 bortezomib-treated patients, the most commonly reported reactions overall were asthenic conditions (61%); diarrhea, nausea (57%); constipation (42%); peripheral neuropathy not elsewhere classified (36%); psychiatric disorders, pyrexia, thrombocytopenia, vomiting (35%); anorexia, appetite decreased (34%); dys-

BORTEZOMIB — INJECTION

esthesia, paresthesia (27%); anemia, headache (26%); and cough (21%). The most commonly reported adverse reactions among the 332 patients in the dexamethasone group were psychiatric disorders (49%), asthenic conditions (45%), insomnia (27%), anemia (22%), and diarrhea and lower respiratory tract/lung infections (each 21%). Fourteen percent of patients in the bortezomib-treated arm experienced a grade 4 adverse reaction; the most common toxicities were thrombocytopenia (4%), neutropenia (2%), and hypercalcemia (2%). Sixteen percent of dexamethasone-treated patients experienced a grade 4 adverse reaction; the most common toxicity was hyperglycemia (2%).

Serious adverse reactions – Serious adverse reactions are defined as any event, regardless of causality, that results in death, is life-threatening, requires hospitalization or prolongs a current hospitalization, results in a significant disability, or is deemed to be an important medical event. Forty-four percent of patients from the bortezomib-treatment arm experienced a severe adverse reaction during the study, as did 43% of dexamethasone-treated patients. The most commonly reported severe adverse reactions in the bortezomib-treatment arm were pyrexia (6%), diarrhea (5%), dyspnea and pneumonia (4%), and vomiting (3%). In the dexamethasone-treatment group, the most commonly reported severe adverse reactions were pneumonia (7%), pyrexia (4%), and hyperglycemia (3%).

Four deaths were considered to be bortezomib-related in the phase 3 study: 1 case each of cardiac arrest, cardiogenic shock, congestive heart failure, and respiratory insufficiency. Four deaths were considered dexamethasone-related: 2 cases of sepsis, 1 case of bacterial meningitis, and 1 case of sudden death at home.

Discontinuation – A total of 145 patients, including 25% of patients in the bortezomib treatment group and 18% of patients in the dexamethasone treatment group, were discontinued from treatment because of adverse reactions assessed as drug-related by the investigators. Among the 331 bortezomib-treated patients, the most commonly reported drug-related reaction leading to discontinuation was peripheral neuropathy (8%). Among the 332 patients in the dexamethasone group, the most commonly reported drug-related reactions leading to treatment discontinuation were hyperglycemia and psychotic disorder (each 2%).

Most common adverse reactions (at least 10%) –

Bortezomib Adverse Reactions in Relapsed Multiple Myeloma (≥ 10%)

Adverse reactions	Bortezomib (n = 331)			Dexamethasone (n = 332)		
	All reactions	Grade 3 events	Grade 4 events	All reactions	Grade 3 events	Grade 4 events
	100%	61%	14%	98%	44%	16%
CNS						
Asthenic conditions	61%	12%	< 1%	45%	6%	0%
Dizziness (excluding vertigo)	14%	< 1%	0%	10%	0%	0%
Headache	26%	< 1%	0%	13%	< 1%	0%
Insomnia	18%	< 1%	0%	27%	2%	0%
Paresthesia and dysesthesia	27%	2%	0%	11%	< 1%	0%
Peripheral neuropathy	36%	7%	< 1%)	9%	< 1%	< 1%
Psychiatric disorders	35%	3%	< 1%	49%	8%	< 1%
GI						
Abdominal pain	16%	2%	0%	4%	< 1%	0%
Anorexia and appetite decreased	34%	3%	0%	9%	< 1%	0%
Constipation	42%	2%	0%	15%	1%	0%
Diarrhea	57%	7%	0%	21%	2%	0%
Nausea	57%	2%	0%	14%	0%	0%
Vomiting	35%	3%	0%	6%	1%	0%
Hematologic						
Anemia	26%	9%	< 1%	22%	10%	< 1%
Neutropenia	19%	12%	2%	2%	1%	0%
Thrombocytopenia	35%	26%	4%	11%	5%	1%
Musculoskeletal						
Arthralgia	14%	< 1%	0%	11%	2%	0%
Back pain	14%	3%	0%	10%	1%	0%
Bone pain	16%	4%	0%	15%	3%	0%
Muscle cramps	12%	0%	0%	15%	< 1%	0%
Myalgia	12%	< 1%	0%	5%	< 1%	0%
Pain in limb	15%	2%	0%	7%	< 1%	0%
Rigors	11%	0%	0%	2%	0%	0%
Respiratory						
Cough	21%	< 1%	0%	11%	< 1%	0%
Dyspnea	20%	5%	< 1%	17%	3%	< 1%
Lower respiratory/lung infections	15%	4%	< 1%	21%	7%	< 1%
Nasopharyngitis	14%	< 1%	0%	7%	0%	0%
Miscellaneous						
Edema lower limb	11%	0%	0%	13%	< 1%	0%
Herpes zoster	13%	2%	0%	5%	1%	< 1%
Pyrexia	35%	2%	0%	16%	1%	< 1%
Rash	18%	1%	0%	6%	0%	0%

➤*Integrated summary of safety (relapsed multiple myeloma and mantle cell lymphoma):*

Most common adverse reactions – In the integrated analysis, the most commonly reported adverse reactions were asthenic conditions (including fatigue, malaise, and weakness) (64%), nausea (55%), diarrhea (52%), constipation (41%), peripheral neuropathy not elsewhere classified (including peripheral sensory neuropathy and peripheral neuropathy aggravated) (39%), appetite decreased (including anorexia) and thrombocytopenia (36%), pyrexia (34%), vomiting (33%), and anemia (29%). Twenty percent of patients experienced at least 1 episode of at least grade 4 toxicity, most commonly thrombocytopenia (5%) and neutropenia (3%).

Severe adverse reactions – A total of 50% of patients experienced severe adverse reactions during the studies. The most commonly reported severe adverse reactions included pneumonia (7%); pyrexia (6%); diarrhea (5%); vomiting (4%); dehydration, dyspnea, nausea, and thrombocytopenia (3%).

In total, 2% of the patients died. The causes of death considered by the investigator to be possibly related to study drug included reports of cardiac arrest, congestive heart failure, pneumonia, renal failure, respiratory failure, and sepsis.

Discontinuation – Adverse reactions thought by the investigator to be drug-related and leading to discontinuation occurred in 22% of patients. The reasons for discontinuation included peripheral neuropathy (8%), asthenic conditions (3%), and diarrhea and thrombocytopenia (2%).

Most common adverse reactions (at least 10%) –

Bortezomib Adverse Reactions From an Integrated Analyses of Relapsed Multiple Myeloma and Mantle Cell Lymphoma Studies (≥ 10% Overall)

Adverse reactions	All patients (n = 1,163)		Multiple myeloma (n = 1,008)		Mantle cell lymphoma (n = 155)	
	All reactions	≥ Grade 3	All reactions	≥ Grade 3	All reactions	≥ Grade 3
CNS						
Anxiety	10%	< 1%	11%	< 1%	5%	0%
Asthenic conditions	64%	16%	62%	16%	72%	19%
Dizziness (excluding vertigo)	17%	2%	16%	1%	23%	3%
Headache	22%	1%	23%	2%	17%	0%
Insomnia	20%	< 1%	20%	< 1%	21%	< 1%
Paresthesia and dysesthesia	22%	1%	24%	1%	9%	1%
Peripheral neuropathy	39%	12%	37%	11%	55%	13%
GI						
Abdominal pain	15%	3%	14%	2%	15%	5%
Appetite decreased	36%	3%	35%	2%	39%	3%
Constipation	41%	2%	40%	2%	50%	3%
Diarrhea	52%	8%	53%	8%	47%	7%
Nausea	55%	4%	57%	4%	44%	3%
Vomiting	33%	5%	34%	5%	27%	3%
Hematologic						
Anemia	29%	11%	30%	12%	17%	3%
Neutropenia	17%	12%	18%	14%	6%	4%
Thrombocytopenia	36%	29%	38%	32%	21%	11%
Metabolism/Nutritional						
Dehydration	10%	3%	11%	3%	7%	5%
Edema	23%	< 1%	22%	< 1%	28%	3%
Musculoskeletal						
Arthralgia	17%	2%	18%	2%	13%	1%
Back pain	13%	3%	15%	4%	< 1%	0%
Bone pain	14%	3%	16%	4%	2%	0%
Muscle cramps	11%	< 1%	12%	< 1%	5%	0%
Myalgia	12%	< 1%	12%	< 1%	10%	0%
Pain in limb	15%	3%	17%	4%	5%	0%
Respiratory						
Cough	20%	< 1%	20%	< 1%	19%	0%
Dyspnea	21%	5%	21%	5%	23%	5%
Nasopharyngitis	12%	< 1%	13%	< 1%	8%	0%

BORTEZOMIB — INJECTION

Bortezomib Adverse Reactions From an Integrated Analyses of Relapsed Multiple Myeloma and Mantle Cell Lymphoma Studies (≥ 10% Overall)

Adverse reactions	All patients (n = 1,163)		Multiple myeloma (n = 1,008)		Mantle cell lymphoma (n = 155)	
	All reactions	≥ Grade 3	All reactions	≥ Grade 3	All reactions	≥ Grade 3
Pneumonia	12%	6%	12%	6%	9%	5%
Upper respiratory tract infection	12%	< 1%	11%	< 1%	15%	< 1%
Miscellaneous						
Herpes zoster	12%	2%	13%	2%	9%	< 1%
Hypotension	13%	3%	12%	3%	15%	3%
Pyrexia	34%	3%	37%	3%	19%	1%
Rash	18%	< 1%	17%	< 1%	28%	3%

Relapsed multiple myeloma and phase 2 mantle cell lymphoma studies –

GI: A total of 87% of patients experienced at least 1 GI disorder. The most common GI disorders included constipation, decreased appetite, diarrhea, nausea, and vomiting. Other GI disorders included dyspepsia and dysgeusia. Grade 3 GI reactions occurred in 18% of patients; grade 4 events occurred in 1% of patients. GI events were considered serious in 11% of patients. Five percent of patients discontinued because of a GI reaction. Nausea was reported more often in patients with multiple myeloma (57%) compared with patients with mantle cell lymphoma (44%). (See Warnings/Precautions.)

Thrombocytopenia – Across the studies, bortezomib-associated thrombocytopenia was characterized by a decrease in platelet count during the dosing period (days 1 to 11) and a return toward baseline during the 10-day rest period during each treatment cycle. Overall, thrombocytopenia was reported in 36% of patients. Thrombocytopenia was grade 3 in 24%, grade 4 or greater in 5%, and serious in 3% of patients, and the reaction resulted in bortezomib discontinuation in 2% of patients. Thrombocytopenia was reported more often in patients with multiple myeloma (38%) compared with patients with mantle cell lymphoma (21%). The incidence of grade 3 or higher thrombocytopenia also was higher in patients with multiple myeloma (32%) compared with patients with mantle cell lymphoma (11%). (See Warnings/Precautions.)

Peripheral neuropathy – Overall, peripheral neuropathy not elsewhere classified occurred in 39% of patients. Peripheral neuropathy was grade 3 for 11% of patients and grade 4 for less than 1% of patients. Eight percent of patients discontinued bortezomib because of peripheral neuropathy. The incidence of peripheral neuropathy was higher among patients with mantle cell lymphoma (55%) compared with patients with multiple myeloma (37%).

In the relapsed multiple myeloma study, among the 87 patients who experienced peripheral neuropathy grade 2 or higher, 51% had improved or resolved within a median of 3.5 months from first onset.

Among the patients with peripheral neuropathy in the phase 2 multiple myeloma studies that was grade 2 and led to discontinuation or was grade 3 or higher, 73% reported improvement or resolution following bortezomib dose adjustment, with a median time to improvement of 1 grade or more from the last dose of bortezomib of 33 days. (See Warnings/Precautions.)

Hypotension – The incidence of hypotension (postural hypotension, orthostatic hypotension, and hypotension not otherwise specified) was 13% in patients treated with bortezomib. Hypotension was grade 1 or 2 in the majority of patients, grade 3 in 3%, and grade 4 or higher in less than 1% of patients. Three percent of patients had hypotension reported as a serious adverse reaction, and 1% discontinued because of hypotension. The incidence of hypotension was similar in patients with multiple myeloma (12%) and mantle cell lymphoma (15%). In addition, 2% of patients experienced hypotension and had a syncopal event. Doses of antihypertensive medications may need to be adjusted in patients receiving bortezomib. (See Warnings/Precautions.)

Neutropenia – Neutrophil counts decreased during the bortezomib dosing period (days 1 to 11) and returned toward baseline during the 10-day rest period during each treatment cycle. Overall, neutropenia occurred in 17% of patients, was grade 3 in 9% of patients, and grade 4 or higher in 3% of patients. Neutropenia was reported as a serious reaction in less than 1% of patients, and less than 1% of patients discontinued because of neutropenia. The incidence of neutropenia was higher in patients with multiple myeloma (18%) compared with patients with mantle cell lymphoma (6%). The incidence of grade 3 or higher neutropenia also was higher in patients with multiple myeloma (14%) compared with patients with mantle cell lymphoma (4%). (See Warnings/Precautions.)

Asthenic conditions – Asthenic conditions (eg, fatigue, malaise, weakness) were reported in 64% of patients. Asthenia was grade 3 for 16% and grade 4 or higher in less than 1% of patients. Four percent of patients discontinued treatment because of asthenia. Asthenic conditions were reported in 62% of patients with multiple myeloma and 72% of patients with mantle cell lymphoma.

Pyrexia – Pyrexia (higher than 38°C [100.4°F]) was reported as an adverse reaction for 34% of patients. The reaction was grade 3 in 3% and grade 4 or higher in less than 1%. Pyrexia was reported as a serious adverse reaction in 6% of patients and led to bortezomib discontinuation in less than 1% of patients. The incidence of pyrexia was higher among patients with multiple myeloma (37%) compared with patients with mantle cell lymphoma (19%). The incidence of pyrexia grade 3 or higher was 3% in patients with multiple myeloma and 1% in patients with mantle cell lymphoma.

Herpes virus infection – Consider using antiviral prophylaxis in subjects being treated with bortezomib. In the randomized studies in previously untreated and relapsed multiple myeloma, herpes zoster reactivation was more common in subjects treated with bortezomib (13%) than in the control groups (4% to 5%). Herpes simplex was seen in 2% to 8% of subjects treated with bortezomib and 1% to 5% in the control groups. In the previously untreated multiple myeloma study, herpes zoster virus reactivation in the bortezomib, melphalan, and prednisone arm was less common in subjects receiving prophylactic antiviral therapy (3%) than in subjects who did not receive prophylactic antiviral therapy (17%).

➤*Additional severe adverse reactions:*

Cardiovascular – Angina pectoris, atrial fibrillation aggravated, atrial flutter, bradycardia, cardiac amyloidosis, cerebral hemorrhage, cerebrovascular accident, complete atrioventricular block, deep venous thrombosis, hemorrhagic stroke, myocardial infarction, myocardial ischemia, pericardial effusion, pericarditis, peripheral embolism, pulmonary embolism, pulmonary hypertension, sinus arrest, torsades de pointes, transient ischemic attack, ventricular tachycardia.

CNS – Agitation, ataxia, coma, confusion, cranial palsy, dysarthria, dysautonomia, encephalopathy, generalized tonic-clonic seizure, mental status change, motor dysfunction, neuralgia, paralysis, postherpetic neuralgia, psychotic disorder, RPLS, spinal cord compression, suicidal ideation, vertigo.

Dermatologic – Leukocytoclastic vasculitis, rash (may be pruritic), urticaria.

GI – Ascites, dysphagia, fecal impaction, gastritis hemorrhagic, gastroenteritis, gastroesophageal reflux, hematemesis, hemorrhagic duodenitis, ileus paralytic, large intestinal obstruction, large intestinal perforation, melena, oral mucosal petechiae, pancreatitis acute, paralytic intestinal obstruction, peritonitis, small intestinal obstruction, stomatitis.

GU – Acute and chronic renal failure, bilateral hydronephrosis, bladder spasm, hematuria, hemorrhagic cystitis, proliferative glomerular nephritis, renal calculus, urinary incontinence, urinary retention, urinary tract infection.

Hematologic/Lymphatic – Disseminated intravascular coagulation, leukopenia, lymphopenia.

Hepatic – Cholestasis, hepatic hemorrhage, hepatitis, hyperbilirubinemia, liver failure, portal vein thrombosis.

Hypersensitivity – Anaphylactic reaction, angioedema, drug hypersensitivity, immune complex–mediated hypersensitivity.

Local – Injection-site erythema, injection-site pain, irritation, phlebitis.

Metabolic/Nutritional – Hyperkalemia, hypernatremia, hyperuricemia, hypocalcemia, hypokalemia, hyponatremia.

Respiratory – ARDS, aspiration pneumonia, atelectasis, chronic obstructive airways disease exacerbated, dyspnea, dyspnea exertional, epistaxis, hemoptysis, hypoxia, lung infiltration, pleural effusion, pneumonitis, respiratory distress, sinusitis.

Special senses – Conjunctival infection, diplopia and blurred vision, eye irritation, hearing impaired.

Miscellaneous – Aspergillosis, bacteremia, catheter-related complication, catheter-related infection, face edema, herpes viral infection, laryngeal edema, listeriosis, oral candidiasis, septic shock, skeletal fracture, subdural hematoma, toxoplasmosis.

➤*Postmarketing:*

Cardiovascular – Atrioventricular block complete, cardiac tamponade, disseminated intravascular coagulation.

CNS – Dysautonomia, encephalopathy, herpes meningoencephalitis.

GI – Acute pancreatitis, hepatitis, ischemic colitis.

Special senses – Deafness bilateral, ophthalmic herpes.

Miscellaneous – Acute diffuse infiltrative pulmonary disease, toxic epidermal necrolysis.

Overdosage

➤*Symptoms:* In humans, fatal outcomes following the administration of more than twice the recommended therapeutic dose have been reported, which were associated with the acute onset of symptomatic hypotension and thrombocytopenia.

➤*Treatment:* There is no known specific antidote for bortezomib overdosage. In the event of overdosage, monitor patient's vital signs and give appropriate supportive care.

Patient Information

Bortezomib may cause fatigue, dizziness, syncope, and orthostatic/postural hypotension. Advise patients not to drive or operate machinery if they experience these symptoms.

Because patients receiving bortezomib therapy may experience vomiting and/or diarrhea, advise patients regarding appropriate measures to avoid dehydration. Also instruct patients to seek medical advice if they experience dizziness, light-headedness, or fainting spells.

Advise patients to use effective contraceptive measures to prevent pregnancy during treatment with bortezomib. If a patient becomes pregnant during treatment, instruct the patient to inform her health care provider immediately. Advise patients to not take bortezomib while pregnant or breast-feeding. If a patient wishes to restart breast-feeding after treatment, advise her to discuss the appropriate timing with her health care provider.

Advise patients to speak with their health care provider about any other medication they are currently taking.

BORTEZOMIB — INJECTION

Advise patients to check their blood sugar frequently if using an oral antidiabetic medication and notify their health care provider of any changes in blood sugar level.

Advise patients to contact their health care provider if they experience new or worsening symptoms of peripheral neuropathy, such as tingling, numbness, pain, a burning feeling in the feet or hands, or weakness in the arms or legs.

Instruct patients to contact their health care provider if they develop a rash; experience shortness of breath; cough; swelling of the feet, ankles, or legs; convulsion; persistent headache; reduced eyesight; an increase in blood pressure; or blurred vision.

HISTONE DEACETYLASE INHIBITORS

VORINOSTAT

Rx	**Zolinza** (Merck)	**Capsules:** 100 mg	(568). White. In 120s.

VORINOSTAT — ORAL

Indications

➤*Cutaneous T-cell lymphoma (CTCL):* For the treatment of cutaneous manifestations in patients with CTCL who have progressive, persistent, or recurrent disease on or following 2 systemic therapies.

Administration and Dosage

➤*General dosing considerations:*

Accessing coverage today limited distribution program – Vorinostat is available from Merck through a restrictive distribution program, Accessing Coverage Today (ACT), intended to assist patients with reimbursement issues. Vorinostat is not routinely distributed to retail or hospital pharmacies. Prescriptions for vorinostat are filled only through pharmacies identified for individual patients. The ACT program will arrange for medication delivery to the patient's preferred pharmacy.

Health care providers are not required to enroll in ACT prior to prescribing vorinostat. Patients must be enrolled in the ACT program in order to receive vorinostat. Patients may enroll themselves, or may be enrolled by caregivers or prescribers, by completing the ACT enrollment form, which is available by calling 866-363-6379 or online at http://www.zolinza.com/vorinostat/zolinza/consumer/act_program/index.jsp. The completed form must be faxed back to ACT at 866-363-6389 for approval.

➤*Adults:*

Cutaneous T-cell lymphoma –

Usual dosage: 400 mg once daily with food.

Dosage adjustment: If a patient is intolerant to therapy, the dose may be reduced to 300 mg once daily with food. The dose may be further reduced to 300 mg once daily with food for 5 consecutive days each week, as necessary.

Duration of therapy: Treatment may be continued as long as there is no evidence of progressive disease or unacceptable toxicity.

➤*Preparation for administration:* Vorinistat is considered a cytotoxic agent and a potential mutagen. Follow safe handling procedures when preparing, administering, or dispensing vorinostat.

Do not open or crush vorinostat capsules. Avoid direct contact of the powder in vorinostat capsules with the skin or mucous membranes. If such contact occurs, wash thoroughly. Avoid exposure to crushed and/or broken capsules.

➤*Administration:* Give with food for maximal absorption. Do not crush or chew capsules; swallow whole.

Adequately hydrate patients during therapy. The manufacturer recommends fluid intake of at least 2 L/day.

➤*Storage/Stability:* Store at 20° to 25°C (68° to 77°F); excursions are permitted between 15° and 30°C (59° and 86°F).

Actions

➤*Pharmacology:* Vorinostat inhibits the enzymatic activity of histone deacetylases HDAC1, HDAC2 AND HDAC3 (class I) and HDAC6 (class II) at nanomolar concentrations (50% inhibitory concentrations [IC_{50}] less than 86 nM). These enzymes catalyze the removal of acetyl groups from the lysine residues of proteins, including histones and transcription factors. In some cancer cells, there is an overexpression of HDACs or an aberrant recruitment of HDACs to oncongenic transcription factors, causing hypoacetylation of core nucleosomal histones. Hypoacetylation of histones is associated with a condensed chromatin structure and repression of gene transcription. Inhibition of HDAC activity allows for the accumulation of acetyl groups on the histone lysine residues, resulting in an open chromatin structure and transcriptional activation. In vitro, vorinostat causes the accumulation of acetylated histones and induces cell cycle arrest and/or apoptosis of some transformed cells. The mechanism of the antineoplastic effect of vorinostat has not been fully characterized.

➤*Pharmacokinetics:*

Absorption – The pharmacokinetics of vorinostat were evaluated in 23 patients with relapsed or refractory advanced cancer.

After oral administration of a single 400 mg dose of vorinostat with a high-fat meal, the mean ± standard deviation area under the curve (AUC) and peak serum concentration (C_{max}) and the median (range) time to C_{max} (T_{max}) were 5.5 ± 1.8 mcM•h, 1.2 ± 0.62 mcM, and 4 (2 to 10) hours, respectively.

In the fasted state, oral administration of a single 400 mg dose of vorinostat resulted in a mean AUC, C_{max}, and median T_{max} of 4.2 ± 1.9 mcM•h, 1.2 ± 0.35 mcM, and 1.5 (0.5 to 10) hours, respectively. Therefore, oral administration of vorinostat with a high-fat meal resulted in an increase (33%) in the extent of absorption and a modest decrease in the rate of absorption (T_{max} delayed 2.5 hours) compared with the fasted state. However, these small effects are not expected to be clinically meaningful. In clinical trials of patients with CTCL, vorinostat was taken with food.

At steady state in the fed-state, oral administration of multiple 400 mg doses of vorinostat resulted in a mean AUC, C_{max}, and a median T_{max} of 6 ± 2 mcM•h, 1.2 ± 0.53 mcM, and 4 (0.5 to 14) hours, respectively.

Distribution – Vorinostat is approximately 71% bound to human plasma proteins over the range of concentrations of 0.5 to 50 mcg/mL.

Metabolism – The major pathways of vorinostat metabolism involve glucuronidation and hydrolysis followed by β-oxidation. Human serum levels of 2 metabolites, O-glucuronide of vorinostat and 4-anilino-4-oxobutanoic acid, were measured. Both metabolites are pharmacologically inactive. Compared with vorinostat, the mean steady-state serum exposures in humans of the O-glucuronide of vorinostat and 4-anilino-4-oxobutanoic acid were 4- and 13-fold higher, respectively. In vitro studies using human liver microsomes indicate negligible biotransformation by CYP-450.

Excretion – Vorinostat is eliminated predominantly through metabolism, with less than 1% of the dose recovered as unchanged drug in urine, indicating that renal excretion does not play a role in the elimination of vorinostat. The mean urinary recovery of 2 pharmacologically inactive metabolites at steady state was 16 ± 5.8% of the vorinostat dose as the O-glucuronide of vorinostat, and 36 ± 8.6% of the vorinostat dose as 4-anilino-4-oxobutanoic acid. Total urinary recovery of vorinostat and these 2 metabolites averaged 52 ± 13.3% of the vorinostat dose. The mean terminal half-life was approximately 2 hours for both vorinostat and the O-glucuronide metabolite, while that of the 4-anilino-4-oxobutanoic acid metabolite was 11 hours.

Contraindications

None known.

Warnings/Precautions

➤*Cardiac effects:* Administer vorinostat with particular caution in patients with congenital long QT syndrome and patients taking antiarrhythmic medicines or other medicinal products that lead to QT prolongation. A definitive study of the effect of vorinostat on QT corrected for heart rate (QTc) has not been conducted. Three of 86 CTCL patients exposed to 400 mg once daily had grade 1 (greater than 450 to 470 msec) or 2 (greater than 470 to 500 msec or increase of greater than 60 msec above baseline) clinical adverse reactions of QTc prolongation. In a retrospective analysis of three phase 1 and two phase 2 studies, 116 patients had a baseline and at least 1 follow-up electrocardiogram (ECG). Four patients had grade 2 (greater than 470 to 500 msec or increase of greater than 60 msec above baseline), and 1 patient had grade 3 (greater than 500 msec) QTc prolongation. In 49 non-CTCL patients from 3 clinical trials who had complete evaluation of QT interval, 2 had QTc measurements of greater than 500 msec, and 1 had a QTc prolongation of greater than 60 msec.

➤*GI effects:* GI disturbances, including nausea, vomiting, and diarrhea, have been reported and may require the use of antiemetic and antidiarrheal medications. Replace fluids and electrolytes to prevent dehydration. Adequately control preexisting nausea, vomiting, and diarrhea before beginning therapy with vorinostat. Based on reports of dehydration as a serious drug-related adverse reaction in clinical trials, patients were instructed to drink at least 2 L/day of fluids for adequate hydration.

➤*Hematologic effects:* Treatment with vorinostat can cause dosage-related thrombocytopenia and anemia. If platelet counts and/or hemoglobin are reduced during treatment with vorinostat, modify the dosage or discontinue therapy.

➤*Hyperglycemia:* Hyperglycemia has been observed in patients receiving vorinostat. Monitor serum glucose, especially in diabetic or potentially diabetic patients. Adjustment of diet and/or therapy for increased glucose may be necessary.

➤*Thromboembolism:* As pulmonary embolism and deep vein thrombosis have been reported as adverse reactions, be alert to the signs and symptoms of these events, particularly in patients with a prior history of thromboembolic reactions.

➤*Renal function impairment:* Vorinostat was not evaluated in patients with renal function impairment. However, renal excretion does not play a role in the elimination of vorinostat. Treat patients with preexisting renal function impairment with caution.

➤*Hepatic function impairment:* Vorinostat was not evaluated in patients with hepatic function impairment. As vorinostat is predominantly eliminated through metabolism, treat patients with hepatic function impairment with caution.

➤*Pregnancy:* *Category D.* Vorinostat can cause fetal harm when administered to a pregnant woman. There are no adequate and well-controlled studies of vorinostat in pregnant women. If this drug is used during pregnancy or if the patient becomes pregnant while taking this drug, apprise the patient of the potential hazard to the fetus.

VORINOSTAT — ORAL

Results of animal studies indicate that vorinostat crosses the placenta and is found in fetal plasma at levels up to 50% of maternal concentrations. Doses up to 50 and 150 mg/kg/day were tested in rats and rabbits, respectively (approximately 0.5 times the human exposure based on $AUC_{(0\text{-}24\ hours)}$). Treatment-related developmental effects including decreased mean live fetal weights; incomplete ossifications of the skull; and thoracic vertebra, sternebra, and skeletal variations (eg, cervical ribs, sacral arch variations, supernumerary ribs, vertebral count) in rats at the highest dose of vorinostat tested. Reductions in mean live fetal weight and an elevated incidence of incomplete ossification of the metacarpals were seen in rabbits dosed at 150 mg/kg/day. The no observed effect levels for these findings were 15 and 50 mg/kg/day (less than 0.1 times the human exposure based on AUC) in rats and rabbits, respectively. A dose-related increase in the incidence of malformations of the gallbladder was noted in all drug treatment groups in rabbits versus the concurrent control.

➤*Lactation:* It is not known whether this drug is excreted in human milk. Because many drugs are excreted in human milk and because of the potential for serious adverse reactions from vorinostat in breast-feeding infants, decide whether to discontinue breast-feeding or the drug, taking into account the importance of the drug to the mother.

➤*Children:* The safety and efficacy of vorinostat in children have not been established.

➤*Elderly:* Of the total number of patients with CTCL in trials (N = 107), 46% were 65 years of age and older, while 15% were 75 years of age and older. No overall differences in safety or efficacy were observed between these subjects and younger subjects, and other reported clinical experience has not identified differences in responses between the elderly and younger patients, but greater sensitivity of some older individuals cannot be ruled out.

➤*Lab test abnormalities:* Laboratory abnormalities were reported in all of the 86 CTCL patients who received the 400 mg once-daily dose. Increased serum glucose was reported as a laboratory abnormality in 69% (59/86) of CTCL patients who received the 400 mg once-daily dosage; only 4 of these abnormalities were severe (grade 3). Increased serum glucose was reported as an adverse reaction in 8.1% (7/86) of CTCL patients who received the 400 mg once daily dosage. Transient increases in serum creatinine were detected in 46.5% (40/86) of CTCL patients who received the 400 mg once-daily dosage. Of these laboratory abnormality, 34 were National Cancer Institute Common Terminology Criteria for Adverse Events (NCI CTCAE) grade 1, 5 were grade 2, and 1 was grade 3.

Proteinuria was detected as a laboratory abnormalities (51.4%) in 38 of 74 patients tested. The clinical significance of this finding is unknown.

➤*Monitoring:* Perform careful monitoring of blood cell counts and chemistry tests, including electrolytes, glucose, and serum creatinine, every 2 weeks during the first 2 months of therapy and monthly thereafter. Include potassium, magnesium, and calcium in electrolyte monitoring. Perform baseline and periodic ECGs during treatment. Correct hypokalemia or hypomagnesemia prior to administration of vorinostat, and consider monitoring potassium and magnesium in symptomatic patients (eg, patients with cardiac symptoms, diarrhea, fluid imbalance, nausea, vomiting). Monitor serum glucose, especially in diabetic or potentially diabetic patients.

Drug Interactions

➤*Anticoagulants:* Prolongation of prothrombin time (PT) and international normalized ratio (INR) were observed in patients receiving vorinostat concomitantly with coumarin-derivative anticoagulants (eg, warfarin). Carefully monitor PT and INR in patients coadministered vorinostat and coumarin derivatives.

➤*Valproic acid:* Severe thrombocytopenia and GI bleeding have been reported with concomitant use of vorinostat and other HDAC inhibitors (eg, valproic acid). Monitor platelet count every 2 weeks for the first 2 months.

Adverse Reactions

➤*Common adverse reactions:* The most common drug-related adverse reactions can be classified into 4 symptom complexes: GI symptoms (eg, anorexia, diarrhea, constipation, nausea, vomiting, weight decrease), constitutional symptoms (eg, chills, fatigue), hematologic abnormalities (eg, anemia, thrombocytopenia), and taste disorders (eg, dry mouth, dysgeusia). The most common serious drug-related adverse reactions were anemia and pulmonary embolism.

Vorinostat Adverse Reactions (≥ 10%)

Adverse reaction	Vorinostat 400 mg once daily (N = 86)			
	All grades		Grades 3 to 5[a]	
	n	%	n	%
CNS				
Dizziness	13	15.1%	1	1.2%
Fatigue	45	52.3%	3	3.5%
Headache	10	11.6%	0	0%
Dermatologic				
Alopecia	16	18.6%	0	0%
Pruritus	10	11.6%	1	1.2%
GI				
Anorexia	21	24.4%	2	2.3%
Constipation	13	15.1%	0	0%
Decreased appetite	12	14%	1	1.2%
Diarrhea	45	52.3%	0	0%
Dry mouth	14	16.3%	0	0%
Dysgeusia	24	27.9%	0	0%
Nausea	35	40.7%	3	3.5%
Vomiting	13	15.1%	1	1.2%
Hematologic				
Anemia	12	14%	2	2.3%
Thrombocytopenia	22	25.6%	5	5.8%
Musculoskeletal				
Muscle spasms	17	19.8%	2	2.3%
Respiratory				
Cough	9	10.5%	0	0%
Upper respiratory tract infection	9	10.5%	0	0%
Miscellaneous				
Blood creatinine increased	14	16.3%	0	0%
Chills	14	16.3%	1	1.2%
Peripheral edema	11	12.8%	0	0%
Pyrexia	9	10.5%	1	1.2%
Weight decreased	18	20.9%	1	1.2%

[a] No grade 5 reactions were reported.

The frequencies of more severe thrombocytopenia, anemia, and fatigue were increased at doses higher than 400 mg once daily of vorinostat.

➤*Serious adverse reactions:* The most common serious adverse reactions, regardless of causality, in the 86 CTCL patients in 2 clinical studies were pulmonary embolism reported in 4.7% (4/86) of patients, squamous cell carcinoma reported in 3.5% (3/86) of patients, and anemia reported in 2.3% (2/86) of patients. The following were single events.

Cardiovascular – Deep vein thrombosis, ischemic stroke, myocardial infarction, thrombocytopenia.

CNS – Syncope.

Dermatologic – Exfoliative dermatitis.

GI – GI hemorrhage.

GU – Pelvi-ureteric obstruction, ureteric obstruction.

Hepatic – Cholecystitis.

Respiratory – Lobar pneumonia.

Miscellaneous – Death (of unknown cause), enterococcal infection, infection, sepsis, spinal cord injury, streptococcal bacteremia, T-cell lymphoma.

➤*Discontinuations:* Of the CTCL patients who received the 400 mg once daily dose, 9.3% (8/86) of patients discontinued vorinostat because of adverse reactions including:

Cardiovascular – Deep vein thrombosis, ischemic stroke, pulmonary embolism.

CNS – Lethargy.

Dermatologic – Exfoliative dermatitis.

Hematologic – Anemia.

Miscellaneous – Angioneurotic edema, asthenia, chest pain, death, spinal cord injury.

➤*Adverse reactions requiring dosage modifications:* Of the CTCL patients who received the 400 mg once daily dosage, 10.5% (9/86) of patients required a dosage modification of vorinostat because of adverse reactions. The median time to the first adverse reaction resulting in dosage reduction was 42 days (range, 17 to 263 days).

GI – Decreased appetite, nausea, vomiting.

Hematologic – Leukopenia, neutropenia, thrombocytopenia.

Lab test abnormalities – Hypokalemia, increased serum creatinine.

➤*Dehydration:* Based on reports of dehydration as a serious drug-related adverse reaction in clinical trials, patients were instructed to drink at least 2 L/day of fluids for adequate hydration.

➤*Adverse reactions in non-CTCL patients:* The frequencies of individual adverse reactions were substantially higher in the non-CTCL population. Drug-related serious adverse reactions reported in the non-CTCL population, which were not observed in the CTCL population, included single events of the following.

Cardiovascular – Hypertension, vasculitis.

CNS – Guillain-Barré syndrome.

VORINOSTAT — ORAL

GU – Renal failure, urinary retention.

Respiratory – Cough, hemoptysis.

Special senses – Blurred vision.

Miscellaneous – Asthenia, hyponatremia, tumor hemorrhage.

Overdosage

➤*Treatment:* No specific information is available on the treatment of overdosage of vorinostat. In the event of overdose, it is reasonable to employ the usual supportive measures (eg, remove unabsorbed material from the GI tract, employ clinical monitoring, and institute supportive therapy), if required. It is not known if vorinostat is dialyzable.

Patient Information

Instruct patients to drink at least 2 L/day of fluid to prevent dehydration and to promptly report excessive vomiting or diarrhea to their health care provider. Instruct patients about the signs of deep vein thrombosis and to consult their health care provider should any evidence of deep vein thrombosis develop. Patients receiving vorinostat should seek immediate medical attention if unusual bleeding occurs. Do not open or crush vorinostat capsules. Instruct patients to read the patient insert carefully.

ROMIDEPSIN

Rx	**Istodax** (Gloucester Pharmaceuticals)	**Injection, lyophilized powder for solution:** 10 mg	In kits containing single-use vial[a] and diluent.[b]

[a] With povidone 20 mg.

[b] Contains dehydrated alcohol 20% and propylene glycol 80%.

ROMIDEPSIN — INJECTION

Indications

➤*Cutaneous T-cell lymphoma:* For treatment of cutaneous T-cell lymphoma in patients who have received at least 1 prior systemic therapy.

Administration and Dosage

➤*Adults:*

Cutaneous T-cell lymphoma – 14 mg/m² intravenously (IV) over a 4-hour period on days 1, 8, and 15 of a 28-day cycle. Cycles should be repeated every 28 days provided that the patient continues to benefit from and tolerates the therapy.

Dosage adjustment:

- *Nonhematologic toxicities except alopecia* –
  - *Grade 2 or 3 toxicity:* Treatment should be delayed until toxicity returns to grade 1 or less or baseline, then therapy may be restarted at 14 mg/m². If grade 3 toxicity recurs, treatment should be delayed until toxicity returns to grade 1 or less or baseline, and the dose should be permanently reduced to 10 mg/m².
  - *Grade 4 toxicity:* Treatment should be delayed until toxicity returns to grade 1 or less or baseline, then the dose should be permanently reduced to 10 mg/m².
  - Discontinue therapy if grade 3 or 4 toxicities recur after dose reduction.
- *Hematologic toxicities* –
  - *Grade 3 or 4 neutropenia or thrombocytopenia:* Treatment should be delayed until the specific cytopenia returns to absolute neutrophil count (ANC) of 1.5×10^9/L or higher and/or platelet count of 75×10^9/L or higher or baseline, then therapy may be restarted at 14 mg/m².
  - *Grade 4 febrile (38.5°C or higher) neutropenia or thrombocytopenia that requires platelet transfusion:* Treatment should be delayed until the specific cytopenia returns to grade 1 or less or baseline, and then the dose should be permanently reduced to 10 mg/m².

➤*Preparation for administration:* Romidepsin must be reconstituted with the supplied diluent and further diluted with sodium chloride 0.9% injection before IV infusion.

Reconstitution – Each 10 mg single-use vial of romidepsin must be reconstituted with 2 mL of the supplied diluent. With a suitable syringe, aseptically withdraw 2 mL from the supplied diluent vial and slowly inject it into the romidepsin for injection vial. Swirl the contents of the vial until there are no visible particles in the resulting solution. The reconstituted solution will contain romidepsin 5 mg/mL.

Dilution – Extract the appropriate amount of romidepsin from the vials to deliver the desired dose, using proper aseptic technique. Before IV infusion, further dilute romidepsin in 500 mL of sodium chloride 0.9% injection. The diluted solution is compatible with polyvinyl chloride (PVC), ethylene vinyl acetate (EVA), and polyethylene infusion bags, as well as glass bottles. Administer as soon after dilution as possible.

➤*Administration:* Infuse over 4 hours.

➤*Storage/Stability:* Store at 20° to 25°C (68° to 77°F); excursions are permitted between 15° and 30°C (59° and 86°F). Reconstituted solution is stable for at least 8 hours at room temperature. Diluted reconstituted solution is stable for at least 24 hours at room temperature.

Actions

➤*Pharmacology:* Romidepsin, a histone deacetylase (HDAC) inhibitor, is a bicyclic depsipeptide. HDACs catalyze the removal of acetyl groups from acetylated lysine residues in histones, resulting in the modulation of gene expression. HDACs also deacetylate nonhistone proteins, such as transcription factors. In vitro, romidepsin causes the accumulation of acetylated histones and induces cell cycle arrest and apoptosis of some cancer cell lines with concentration that inhibits 50% (IC_{50}) values in the nanomolar range. The mechanism of the antineoplastic effect of romidepsin observed in nonclinical and clinical studies has not been fully characterized.

➤*Pharmacokinetics:*

Absorption – In patients with T-cell lymphomas who received romidepsin 14 mg/m² IV over a 4-hour period on days 1, 8, and 15 of a 28-day cycle, geometric mean values of the maximum plasma concentration (C_{max}) and the area under the curve ($AUC_{0-\infty}$) were 377 ng/mL and 1,549 ng•h/mL, respectively.

Distribution – Romidepsin is highly protein bound in plasma (92% to 94%) over the concentration range of 50 to 1,000 ng/mL with alpha-1 acid glycoprotein (AAG) being the principal binding protein.

Metabolism – Romidepsin undergoes extensive metabolism in vitro primarily by CYP3A4 with minor contribution from CYP3A5, CYP1A1, CYP2B6, and CYP2C19.

Excretion – Following 4-hour IV administration of romidepsin at 14 mg/m² on days 1, 8, and 15 of a 28-day cycle in patients with T-cell lymphomas, the terminal half-life was approximately 3 hours.

Contraindications

None well documented.

Warnings/Precautions

➤*Hematologic effects:* Treatment with romidepsin can cause thrombocytopenia, leukopenia (neutropenia and lymphopenia), and anemia; therefore, monitor these hematological parameters during treatment with romidepsin, and modify the dose as necessary.

➤*Cardiovascular effects:* Several treatment-emergent morphological changes in electrocardiograms (ECGs) (including T-wave and ST-segment changes) have been reported in clinical studies. The clinical significance of these changes is unknown.

In patients with congenital long QT syndrome, patients with a history of significant cardiovascular disease, and patients taking antiarrhythmic medicines or medicinal products that lead to significant QT prolongation, consider appropriate cardiovascular monitoring precautions, such as the monitoring of electrolytes and ECGs at baseline and periodically during treatment.

➤*Renal function impairment:* Treat patients with end-stage renal disease (ESRD) with caution.

➤*Hepatic function impairment:* Treat patients with moderate and severe hepatic impairment with caution.

➤*Pregnancy: Category D.* There are no adequate and well-controlled studies of romidepsin in pregnant women. However, based on its mechanism of action, romidepsin may cause fetal harm when administered to a pregnant woman. A study in rats did not expose pregnant animals to enough romidepsin to fully evaluate adverse developmental outcomes. If this drug is used during pregnancy, or if the patient becomes pregnant while taking romidepsin, apprise the patient of the potential harm to the fetus.

Advise women of childbearing potential that romidepsin may reduce the effectiveness of estrogen-containing contraceptives. An in vitro binding assay determined that romidepsin competes with beta-estradiol for binding to estrogen receptors. Because estrogen is required to maintain pregnancy throughout gestation, the competition between romidepsin and beta-estradiol could cause pregnancy loss.

➤*Lactation:* It is not known whether romidepsin is excreted in human milk. The molecular weight (about 541) and the elimination half-life (3 hours) suggest that the drug will be excreted into breast milk, but the high plasma protein binding (92% to 94%) might limit the amount excreted. Because many drugs are excreted in human milk and because of the potential for serious adverse reactions in breast-feeding infants from romidepsin, decide whether to discontinue breast-feeding or the drug, taking into account the importance of the drug to the mother.

However, the elimination half-life and the dosing schedule might allow breastfeeding on the days a dose was not given. If this strategy is chosen, the mother should "pump and dump" to maintain milk production and decrease discomfort from engorgement for at least 15 hours after the end of the infusion.

➤*Children:* The safety and effectiveness of romidepsin in children have not been established.

➤*Monitoring:* Because of the risk of QT prolongation, ensure that potassium and magnesium are within the normal range before administration of romidepsin.

Monitor electrolytes and ECGs at baseline and periodically during treatment in patients with congenital long QT syndrome, patients with a history of significant cardiovascular disease, and patients taking antiarrhythmic medications or medications that can lead to QT prolongation.

Monitor hematologic parameters during treatment.

ROMIDEPSIN — INJECTION

Drug Interactions

➤*Cytochrome P-450 system:* Because romidepsin is metabolized mainly by the CYP3A enzyme systems, substances known to inhibit these enzymes may decrease metabolism or increase bioavailability of romidepsin, as indicated by increased whole blood or plasma concentrations. Drugs known to induce these enzyme systems may result in an increased metabolism of romidepsin or decreased bioavailability, as indicated by decreased whole blood or plasma concentrations. Monitoring of blood concentrations and appropriate dosage adjustments are essential when such drugs are used concomitantly.

➤*QT prolongation:* An additive effect of romidepsin with other drugs that prolong the QT interval cannot be excluded. The following drugs may prolong the QT interval and may increase the risk of life-threatening cardiac arrhythmias, including torsades de pointes: antiarrhythmic agents (eg, amiodarone, bretylium, disopyramide, dofetilide, procainamide, quinidine, sotalol), arsenic trioxide, chlorpromazine, cisapride, dolasetron, droperidol, mefloquine, mesoridazine, moxifloxacin, pentamidine, pimozide, tacrolimus, thioridazine, and ziprasidone. For a more complete list of drugs that may prolong the QT interval, see the appendixDrug-Induced Prolongation of the QT Interval and Torsades de Pointes.

Romidepsin Drug Interactions

Precipitant drug	Object drug[a]		Description
CYP3A4 moderate inhibitors (eg, aprepitant, diltiazem, fluconazole, grapefruit juice)	Romidepsin	⬆	Romidepsin plasma concentrations may be elevated, increasing the pharmacologic effects and risk of adverse reactions. Coadminister moderate CYP3A4 inhibitors with caution.
CYP3A4 strong inducers (eg, carbamazepine, dexamethasone, phenobarbital, phenytoin, rifabutin, rifampin, rifapentine)	Romidepsin	⬇	Romidepsin plasma concentrations may be reduced, decreasing the pharmacologic effects. If possible, avoid coadministration of strong CYP3A3 inducers.
CYP3A4 strong inhibitors (eg, atazanavir, clarithromycin, indinavir, itraconazole, ketoconazole, mefazodone, nelfinavir, ritonavir, saquinavir, telithromycin, voriconazole)	Romidepsin	⬆	Romidepsin plasma concentrations may be elevated, increasing the pharmacologic effects and risk of adverse reactions. If possible, avoid coadministration of strong CYP3A4 inhibitors.
P-glycoprotein efflux transport inhibitors (eg, cyclosporine, ranolazine)	Romidepsin	⬆	Romidepsin plasma concentrations may be elevated, increasing the pharmacologic effects and risk of adverse reactions. Coadminister with caution.
QT interval prolonging drugs (eg, antiarrhythmic agents, drugs that lead to important QT prolongation)	Romidepsin	⬆	Because of the risk of QT prolongation, if romidepsin and antiarrhythmic agents or drugs that lead to important QT prolongation are coadministered, consider appropriate cardiovascular monitoring, such as monitoring electrolytes and ECG at baseline and periodically during treatment.
St. John's wort	Romidepsin	⬇	Romidepsin plasma concentrations may be reduced, decreasing the pharmacologic effects. If possible, avoid coadministration of St. John's wort.
Romidepsin	Warfarin	⬆	Coadministration may result in PT[b] prolongation and elevated INR[b]. Monitor PT and INR in patients receiving romidepsin and warfarin concurrently. Adjust the warfarin dose as needed.

[a] ⬆ = object drug increased; ⬇ = object drug decreased.
[b] PT = prothrombin time; INR = international normalized ratio.

Adverse Reactions

➤*Serious adverse reactions:* Serious adverse reactions reported in more than 2% of patients in study 1 were infection, pyrexia, and sepsis. In study 2, serious adverse reactions in more than 2% of patients were central line infection, edema, fatigue, infection, leukopenia, nausea, neutropenia, pyrexia, supraventricular arrhythmia, thrombocytopenia, and ventricular arrhythmia.

Most deaths were caused by disease progression. In study 1, there were 2 deaths due to cardiopulmonary failure and acute renal failure. In study 2, there were 6 deaths due to infection (4), acute respiratory distress syndrome, and myocardial ischemia.

➤*Discontinuation of therapy:* Discontinuation because of an adverse reaction occurred in 21% of patients in study 1 and 11% in study 2. Discontinuations occurring in at least 2% of patients in either study included dyspnea, fatigue, infection, and QT prolongation.

➤*Common adverse reactions:*

Romidepsin Adverse Reactions (> 20%)

Adverse reactions	Study 1 (n = 102)		Study 2 (n = 83)	
	All	Grade 3 or 4	All	Grade 3 or 4
Any adverse reaction	97%	35%	100%	82%
Cardiovascular				
ECG ST-T wave changes	2%	0%	63%	0%
Hypotension	7%	3%	23%	4%
Dermatologic				
Pruritus	7%	0%	31%	6%
Dermatitis/Exfoliative dermatitis	4%	< 1%	27%	8%
GI				
Anorexia	23%	< 1%	54%	4%
Constipation	12%	2%	39%	1%
Diarrhea	20%	< 1%	7%	1%
Dysgeusia	15%	0%	40%	0%
Nausea	56%	3%	86%	6%
Vomiting	34%	< 1%	52%	10%
Hematologic				
Anemia	19%	3%	72%	16%
Neutropenia	11%	4%	57%	27%
Leukopenia	4%	0%	46%	22%
Lymphopenia	4%	0%	57%	37%
Thrombocytopenia	17%	0%	65%	14%
Hepatic				
ALT increased	3%	0%	22%	2%
AST increased	3%	0%	28%	4%
Metabolic				
Hypermagnesemia	0%	0%	27%	8%
Hyperuricemia	0%	0%	33%	8%
Hypoalbuminemia	3%	< 1%	48%	4%
Hypocalcemia	4%	0%	52%	6%
Hypokalemia	6%	0%	20%	2%
Hypomagnesemia	22%	< 1%	28%	0%
Hyponatremia	< 1%	< 1%	20%	2%
Hypophosphatemia	0%	0%	27%	10%
Miscellaneous				
Asthenia/Fatigue	53%	8%	77%	14%
Hyperglycemia	2%	2%	51%	1%
Infections	46%	11%	54%	33%
Pyrexia	20%	4%	23%	1%

Overdosage

➤*Treatment:* In the event of an overdose, it is reasonable to employ the usual supportive measures (eg, clinical monitoring, supportive therapy) if required. There is no known antidote for romidepsin and it is not known if romidepsin is dialyzable.

Patient Information

Instruct patients to report excessive nausea or vomiting, abnormal heartbeat, chest pain, or shortness of breath to their health care provider. Advise patients receiving romidepsin to seek immediate medical attention if unusual bleeding occurs.

Romidepsin binds to estrogen receptors. Advise women of childbearing potential that romidepsin may reduce the effectiveness of estrogen-containing contraceptives.

PORFIMER SODIUM

Rx	**Photofrin** (Axican Scandipharm)	**Cake or powder for injection (freeze-dried)**: 75 mg	Preservative-free. In vials.

PORFIMER SODIUM — INJECTION

Indications

➤*Esophageal cancer:* Palliation of patients with completely obstructing esophageal cancer, or of patients with partially obstructing esophageal cancer who, in the opinion of their physician, cannot be satisfactorily treated with Nd:YAG laser therapy.

➤*Endobronchial nonsmall cell lung cancer (NSCLC):* The reduction of obstruction and palliation of symptoms in patients with completely or partially obstructing endobronchial NSCLC.

Microinvasive endobronchial NSCLC – The treatment of microinvasive endobronchial NSCLC in patients for whom surgery and radiotherapy are not indicated.

Barrett's esophagus – Ablation of high-grade dysplasia in Barrett's esophagus patients who do not undergo esophagectomy.

➤*Off-label uses:* For treatment of AIDS-related cutaneous Kaposi sarcoma, primary or recurrent basal cell carcinoma, and squamous cell carcinoma.

Administration and Dosage

➤*General dosing considerations:* Photodynamic therapy (PDT) with porfimer is a 2-stage process requiring administration of both drug and light.

➤*Adults:*

Barrett's esophagus –

Usual dosage: 2 mg/kg IV over 3 to 5 minutes followed 40 to 50 hours by illumination with laser light. A second laser light application may be given 96 to 120 hours after injection, preceded by gentle debridement of residual tumor.

Endobronchial and esophageal cancer –

Usual dosage: 2 mg/kg IV over 3 to 5 minutes followed 40 to 50 hours by illumination with laser light. A second laser light application may be given 96 to 120 hours after injection, preceded by gentle debridement of residual tumor.

➤*Preparation for administration:* Porfimer is considered a cytotoxic agent and is also a photosensitizing agent. Follow safe handling procedures when preparing, administering, or dispensing porfimer.

Reconstitute each vial of porfimer with 31.8 mL of either dextrose 5% injection or sodium chloride 0.9% injection, resulting in a final concentration of 2.5 mg/mL. Shake well until dissolved. Do not mix porfimer with other drugs in the same solution. Porfimer, reconstituted with dextrose 5% injection or with sodium chloride 0.9% injection, has a pH in the range of 7 to 8. Porfimer sodium has been formulated with an overage to deliver the 75 mg labeled quantity.

The reconstituted product should be protected from bright light and used immediately.

➤*Administration:* Porfimer should be administered as a single slow IV injection over 3 to 5 minutes.

➤*Extravasation:* Precautions should be taken to prevent extravasation at the injection site. There is no known benefit from injecting the extravasation site with another substance. If signs or symptoms of extravasation occur, stop the infusion immediately. If possible, withdraw 3 to 5 mL of blood to remove some of the drug. Remove the infusion needle. Delineate the infiltrated area on the patient's skin with a felt-tip marker. To prevent severe local burns, protect the extravasation site from direct light (eg, sunlight, bright indoor light) until swelling and discoloration fade. If possible, avoid surgery within 30 days after extravasation. If surgery is needed during this period, protect internal tissue from intense light. May apply ice compresses for 15 minutes every 6 hours for 48 hours. Elevate for 48 hours above heart level using a sling or stockinette dressing with an observation window cut in the dressing. Avoid pressure or friction. Do not rub area. Observe for signs of increased erythema, pain, or skin necrosis. If increased symptoms occur, consult a plastic surgeon. Ensure that no medication is given distally to extravasation site. After 48 hours, encourage the patient to use the extremity normally to promote full range of motion.

➤*Storage/Stability:* Porfimer sodium freeze-dried cake or powder should be stored at 20° to 25°C (68° to 77°F).

Spills and disposal – Spills of porfimer sodium should be wiped up with a damp cloth. Skin and eye contact should be avoided due to the potential for photosensitivity reactions upon exposure to light; use of rubber gloves and eye protection is recommended. All contaminated materials should be disposed of in a polyethylene bag in a manner consistent with local regulations.

Actions

➤*Pharmacology:* The cytotoxic and antitumor actions of porfimer sodium are light and oxygen dependent. PDT with porfimer sodium is a 2-stage process. The first stage is the IV injection of porfimer sodium. Clearance from a variety of tissues occurs over 40 to 72 hours, but tumors, skin, and organs of the reticuloendothelial system (including liver and spleen) retain porfimer sodium for a longer period. Illumination with 630 nm wavelength laser light constitutes the second stage of therapy. Tumor selectivity in treatment occurs through a combination of selective retention of porfimer sodium and selective delivery of light. Cellular damage caused by porfimer sodium PDT is a consequence of the propagation of radical reactions. Radical initiation may occur after porfimer sodium absorbs light to form a porphyrin excited state. Spin transfer from porfimer sodium to molecular oxygen may then generate singlet oxygen. Subsequent radical reactions can form superoxide and hydroxyl radicals. Tumor death also occurs through ischemic necrosis secondary to vascular occlusion that appears to be partly mediated by thromboxane A_2 release. The laser treatment induces a photochemical, not a thermal, effect. The necrotic reaction and associated inflammatory responses may evolve over several days.

➤*Pharmacokinetics:*

Absorption/Distribution – Following a 2 mg/kg dose of porfimer sodium to 4 male cancer patients, the average peak plasma concentration was 15 ± 3 mcg/mL, the elimination half-life was 250 ± 285 hours, the steady-state volume of distribution was 0.49 ± 0.28 L/kg, and the total plasma clearance was 0.051 ± 0.035 mL/min/kg. The mean plasma concentration at 48 hours was 2.6 ± 0.4 mcg/mL. The influence of impaired hepatic function on porfimer sodium disposition has not been evaluated.

Porfimer sodium was approximately 90% protein bound in human serum, studied in vitro. The binding was independent of concentration over the concentration range of 20 to 100 mcg/mL.

Special populations –

Gender: The pharmacokinetics of porfimer sodium was also studied in 24 healthy subjects (12 men and 12 women) who received a single dose of 2 mg/kg porfimer sodium given via the intravenous route. The serum decay was biexponential, with a slow distribution phase and a very long elimination phase. The elimination half-life was 415 ± 104 hours (17 ± 4.3 days). C_{max} was determined to be 40 ± 11.6 mcg/mL and AUC_{inf} was 2400 ± 552 mcg•hr/mL. Women had a lower C_{max} and a higher AUC. The clinical significance of these differences is unknown. T_{max} was approximately 1.5 hours in women and 0.17 hours in men. At the time of intended photoactivation 40 to 50 hours after injection, the pharmacokinetic profiles of porfimer sodium in men and women were similar.

Contraindications

Porfimer sodium is contraindicated in patients with porphyria or in patients with known allergies to porphyrins.

PDT is contraindicated in patients with an existing tracheoesophageal or bronchoesophageal fistula.

PDT is contraindicated in patients with tumors eroding into a major blood vessel.

Photodynamic therapy is not suitable for emergency treatment of patients with severe acute respiratory distress caused by an obstructing endobronchial lesion because 40 to 50 hours are required between injection with porfimer sodium and laser light treatment.

Photodynamic therapy is not suitable for patients with esophageal or gastric varices, or patients with esophageal ulcers greater than 1 cm in diameter.

Warnings/Precautions

➤*Photosensitivity:* All patients who receive porfimer sodium will be photosensitive and must observe precautions to avoid exposure of skin and eyes to direct sunlight or bright indoor light (from examination lamps, including dental lamps, operating room lamps, unshaded light bulbs at close proximity) for at least 30 days. Some patients may remain photosensitive for greater than or equal to 90 days. The photosensitivity is due to residual drug, which will be present in all parts of the skin. Exposure of the skin to ambient indoor light is, however, beneficial because the remaining drug will be inactivated gradually and safely through a photobleaching reaction. Therefore, patients should not stay in a darkened room during this period and should be encouraged to expose their skin to ambient indoor light. The level of photosensitivity will vary for different areas of the body, depending on the extent of previous exposure to light. Before exposing any area of skin to direct sunlight or bright indoor light, the patient should test it for residual photosensitivity. A small area of skin should be exposed to sunlight for 10 minutes. If no photosensitivity reaction (erythema, edema, blistering) occurs within 24 hours, the patient can gradually resume normal outdoor activities, initially continuing to exercise caution and gradually allowing increased exposure. If some photosensitivity reaction occurs with the limited skin test, the patient should continue precautions for another 2 weeks before retesting.

The tissue around the eyes may be more sensitive, and therefore, it is not recommended that the face be used for testing. If patients travel to a different geographical area with greater sunshine, they should retest their level of photosensitivity.

Conventional UV (ultraviolet) sunscreens are of no value in protecting against photosensitivity reactions because photoactivation is caused by visible light.

➤*Esophageal cancer:* If the esophageal tumor is eroding into the trachea or bronchial tree, the likelihood of tracheoesophageal or bronchoesophageal fistula resulting from treatment is sufficiently high that PDT is not recommended.

Patients with esophageal varices should be treated with extreme caution. Light should not be given directly to the variceal area because of the high risk of bleeding.

➤*Endobronchial cancer:* Patients should be assessed for the possibility that a tumor may be eroding into a pulmonary blood vessel. Porfimer sodium is contraindicated in the presence of this condition. Patients at high risk for

PORFIMER SODIUM — INJECTION

fatal massive hemoptysis (FMH) include those with large, centrally located tumors, those with cavitating tumors, or those with extensive tumor extrinsic to the bronchus.

Fistula – If the endobronchial tumor invades deeply into the bronchial wall, the possibility exists for fistula formation upon resolution of tumor.

Treatment-induced inflammation – PDT should be used with extreme caution for endobronchial tumors in locations where treatment-induced inflammation could obstruct the main airway (eg, long or circumferential tumors of the trachea, tumors of the carina that involve both mainstem bronchi circumferentially, or circumferential tumors in the mainstem bronchus in patients with prior pneumonectomy).

➤*High-grade dysplasia (HGD) in Barrett's esophagus:* The long-term effect of PDT on HGD in BE is unknown. There is always a risk of leaving cancerous cells behind or leaving residual abnormal epithelium beneath the new squamous cell epithelium; these facts emphasize the risk of overlooking cancer in such patients and the need for rigorous continuing surveillance despite the endoscopic appearance of complete squamous cell reepithelialization. It is recommended that endoscopic biopsy surveillance be conducted every 3 months, until 4 consecutive negative evaluations for HGD have been recorded; further follow-up may be scheduled every 6 to 12 months, as per judgment of physicians. The follow-up period of the pivotal study at the time of analysis was a minimum of 2 years (ranging from 2 to 3.6 years).

➤*Ocular sensitivity:* Ocular discomfort, commonly described as sensitivity to sun, bright lights, or car headlights, has been reported in patients who received porfimer sodium. For 30 days, when outdoors, patients should wear dark sunglasses, which have an average white light transmittance of less than 4%.

➤*Before or after radiotherapy:* If PDT is to be used before or after radiotherapy, sufficient time should be allotted between the 2 therapies to ensure that the inflammatory response produced by the first treatment has subsided before commencing the second treatment. The inflammatory response from PDT will depend on tumor size and extent of surrounding normal tissue that receives light. It is recommended that 2 to 4 weeks be allowed after PDT before commencing radiotherapy. Similarly, if PDT is to be given after radiotherapy, the acute inflammatory reaction from radiotherapy usually subsides within 4 weeks after completing radiotherapy, after which PDT may be given.

➤*Chest pain:* As a result of PDT treatment, patients may complain of substernal chest pain because of inflammatory responses within the area of treatment. Such pain may be of sufficient intensity to warrant the short-term prescription of opiate analgesics.

➤*Respiratory distress:* Patients with endobronchial lesions must be closely monitored between the laser light therapy and the mandatory debridement bronchoscopy for any evidence of respiratory distress. Inflammation, mucositis, and necrotic debris may cause obstruction of the airway. If respiratory distress occurs, the physician should be prepared to carry out immediate bronchoscopy to remove secretions and debris to open the airway.

➤*Esophageal strictures:* Esophageal strictures as a result of PDT of HGD in BE are common adverse events. An esophageal stricture was defined as a fixed lumen narrowing with solid food dysphagia and requiring dilation.

Regardless of the indication, esophageal strictures were reported in 122 of the 318 (38%) patients enrolled in the three clinical studies. Overall, esophageal strictures occurred within six months following PDT and were manageable through dilations. Multiple dilations of esophageal strictures may be required, as shown in the table below. Special care should be taken during dilation to avoid perforation of the esophagus.

Esophageal Dilations in Patients with Porfimer Treatment-Related Strictures

Number of dilations	Number of patients with strictures (n = 122)	Patients with strictures (%)
1 to 2 dilations	38	31%
3 to 5 dilations	33	27%
6 to 10 dilations	26	21%
> 10 dilations	25	20%

A high proportion of patients who developed an esophageal stricture received a nodule pretreatment prior to developing the event (49%) and/or had a mucosal segment treated twice, Therefore, nodule pretreatment and retreating the same mucosal segment more than once may influence the risk of developing an esophageal stricture.

Prior to initiating treatment with porfimer sodium PDT, the diagnosis of high-grade dysplasia in Barrett's esophagus should be confirmed by an expert GI pathologist. Photodynamic therapy with porfimer sodium should be applied by physicians trained in the endoscopic use of PDT with porfimer sodium, and only in those facilities properly equipped for the procedure.

➤*Avoidance of pregnancy:* See Warnings/Precautions for more information.

➤*Extravasation:* See Administration and Dosage for more information.

➤*Photosensitivity:* See Warnings/Precautions for more information.

➤*Pregnancy: Category C.* There are no adequate and well-controlled studies in pregnant women. Porfimer sodium should be used during pregnancy only if the potential benefit justifies the potential risk to the fetus.

Women of childbearing potential should practice an effective method of contraception during therapy.

Porfimer sodium given to rat dams during fetal organogenesis intravenously at 8 mg/kg/day (0.64 times the clinical dose on a mg/m^2 basis) for 10 days caused no major malformations or developmental changes. This dose caused maternal and fetal toxicity resulting in increased resorptions, decreased litter size, delayed ossification, and reduced fetal weight. Porfimer sodium caused no major malformations when given to rabbits intravenously during organogenesis at 4 mg/kg/day (0.65 times the clinical dose on a mg/m^2 basis) for 13 days. This dose caused maternal toxicity resulting in increased resorptions, decreased litter size, and reduced fetal body weight.

Porfimer sodium given to rats during late pregnancy through lactation intravenously at 4 mg/kg/day (0.32 times the clinical dose on a mg/m^2 basis) for at least 42 days caused a reversible decrease in growth of offspring. Parturition was unaffected.

➤*Lactation:* It is not known whether this drug is excreted in human milk. Because many drugs are excreted in human milk and because of the potential for serious adverse reactions in nursing infants from porfimer sodium, women receiving porfimer sodium must not breastfeed.

➤*Children:* Safety and efficacy in children have not been established.

Drug Interactions

➤*Photosensitizing agents:* There have been no formal interaction studies of porfimer sodium and any other drugs. However, it is possible that concomitant use of other photosensitizing agents (eg, tetracyclines, sulfonamides, phenothiazines, sulfonylurea hypoglycemic agents, thiazide diuretics, griseofulvin, fluoroquinolones) could increase the photosensitivity reaction.

➤*Miscellaneous:* Porfimer sodium PDT causes direct intracellular damage by initiating radical chain reactions that damage intracellular membranes and mitochondria. Tissue damage also results from ischemia secondary to vasoconstriction, platelet activation and aggregation, and clotting. Research in animals and in cell culture has suggested that many drugs could influence the effects of PDT, possible examples of which are described below. There are no human data that support or rebut these possibilities.

Compounds that quench active oxygen species or scavenge radicals, such as dimethyl sulfoxide, beta carotene, ethanol, formate, and mannitol would be expected to decrease PDT activity. Preclinical data also suggest that tissue ischemia, allopurinol, calcium channel blockers, and some prostaglandin synthesis inhibitors could interfere with porfimer sodium PDT. Drugs that decrease clotting, vasoconstriction, or platelet aggregation (eg, thromboxane A_2 inhibitors, could decrease the efficacy of PDT.

Glucocorticoid hormones given before or concomitant with PDT may decrease the efficacy of the treatment.

Adverse Reactions

Systemically induced effects associated with PDT with porfimer sodium consist of photosensitivity and mild constipation. All patients who receive porfimer sodium will be photosensitive and must observe precautions to avoid sunlight and bright indoor light. Photosensitivity reactions occurred in approximately 20% of cancer patients and in 68% of high-grade dysplasia (HGD) in Barrett's esophagus (BE) patients treated with porfimer sodium. Typically, these reactions were mostly mild-to-moderate erythema but they also included swelling, itching, burning sensation, feeling hot, or blisters. In a single study of 24 healthy subjects, some evidence of photosensitivity reactions occurred in all subjects. Other less common skin manifestations were also reported in areas where photosensitivity reactions had occurred, such as increased hair growth, skin discoloration, skin nodules, increased wrinkles and increased skin fragility. These manifestations may be attributable to a pseudoporphyria state (temporary drug-induced cutaneous porphyria).

Most toxicities associated with this therapy are local effects seen in the region of illumination and occasionally in surrounding tissues. The local adverse reactions are characteristic of an inflammatory response induced by the photodynamic effect.

➤*Esophageal carcinoma:*

Porfimer Adverse Reactions Reported in Patients[a] with Obstructing Esophageal Cancer (≥ 5%)

Adverse reaction	Number of patients (n = 88)	%
Patients with ≥ 1 adverse reaction	84	(95%)
Cardiovascular		
Atrial fibrillation	9	(10%)
Cardiac failure	6	(7%)
Tachycardia	5	(6%)
CNS		
Anorexia	7	(8%)
Anxiety	6	(7%)
Confusion	7	(8%)
Hypertension	5	(6%)
Hypotension	6	(7%)
Insomnia	12	(14%)
Dermatologic		
Photosensitivity reaction	17	(19%)

PORFIMER SODIUM — INJECTION

Porfimer Adverse Reactions Reported in Patients[a] with Obstructing Esophageal Cancer (≥ 5%)		
Adverse reaction	Number of patients (n = 88)	%
GI		
Abdominal pain	18	(20%)
Constipation	21	(24%)
Diarrhea	4	(5%)
Dyspepsia	5	(6%)
Dysphagia	9	(10%)
Eructation	4	(5%)
Esophageal edema	7	(8%)
Esophageal tumor bleeding	7	(8%)
Esophageal stricture	5	(6%)
Esophagitis	4	(5%)
Hematemesis	7	(8%)
Melena	4	(5%)
Nausea	21	(24%)
Vomiting	15	(17%)
GU		
Urinary tract infection	6	(7%)
Hematologic		
Anemia	28	(32%)
Metabolic/Nutritional		
Dehydration	6	(7%)
Weight decrease	8	(9%)
Respiratory		
Coughing	6	(7%)
Dyspnea	18	(20%)
Pharyngitis	10	(11%)
Pleural effusion	28	(32%)
Pneumonia	16	(18%)
Respiratory insufficiency	9	(10%)
Tracheoesophageal fistula	5	(6%)
Miscellaneous		
Asthenia	5	(6%)
Back pain	10	(11%)
Chest pain	19	(22%)
Chest pain (substernal)	4	(5%)
Edema (generalized)	4	(5%)
Edema (peripheral)	6	(7%)
Fever	27	(31%)
Moniliasis	8	(9%)
Pain	19	(22%)
Surgical complication	4	(5%)

[a] Based on adverse reactions reported at any time during the entire period of follow-up.

Location of the tumor was a prognostic factor for 3 adverse reactions: Upper-third of the esophagus (esophageal edema), middle-third (atrial fibrillation), and lower-third, the most vascular region (anemia). Also, patients with large tumors (greater than 10 cm) were more likely to experience anemia. Two of 17 patients with complete esophageal obstruction from tumor experienced esophageal perforations, which were considered to be possibly treatment associated; these perforations occurred during subsequent endoscopies.

Serious and other notable adverse reactions observed in less than 5% of PDT-treated patients with obstructing esophageal cancer in the clinical studies include the following; their relationship to therapy is uncertain. The temporal relationship of some GI, cardiovascular, and respiratory events to the administration of light was suggestive of mediastinal inflammation in some patients.

Cardiovascular – Angina pectoris, bradycardia, MI, sick sinus syndrome, and supraventricular tachycardia.

GI – Esophageal perforation, gastric ulcer, ileus, jaundice, and peritonitis have occurred.

Ophthalmic – Abnormal vision, diplopia, eye pain, and photophobia have been reported.

Respiratory – Bronchitis, bronchospasm, laryngotracheal edema, pneumonitis, pulmonary hemorrhage, pulmonary edema, respiratory failure, and stridor have occurred.

Miscellaneous – Sepsis has been reported occasionally.

➤*Obstructing endobronchial cancer:*

Porfimer Adverse Reactions Reported in Patients with Obstructing Endobronchial Cancers (≥ 5%)				
	Within 30 days of treatment		Entire follow-up period[a]	
Adverse reaction	PDT (n = 86)	Nd:YAG (n = 86)	PDT (n = 86)	Nd:YAG (n = 86)
Patients with ≥ 1 adverse reaction	43 (50%)	33 (38%)	62 (72%)	48 (56%)
CNS				
Anxiety	3 (3%)	0	5 (6%)	0
Dysphonia	3 (3%)	2 (2%)	4 (5%)	2 (2%)
Insomnia	4 (5%)	2 (2%)	4 (5%)	3 (4%)
Dermatologic				
Photosensitivity reaction	16 (19%)	0	18 (21%)	0
GI				
Constipation	4 (5%)	1 (1%)	4 (5%)	2 (2%)
Dyspepsia	1 (1%)	4 (5%)	2 (2%)	5 (6%)
Respiratory				
Bronchitis	9 (10%)	2 (2%)	9 (10%)	2 (2%)
Coughing	5 (6%)	8 (9%)	13 (15%)	11 (13%)
Dyspnea	15 (17%)	7 (8%)	26 (30%)	13 (15%)
Hemoptysis	6 (7%)	5 (6%)	14 (16%)	7 (8%)
Pleural effusion	0	0	4 (5%)	1 (1%)
Pneumonia	5 (6%)	4 (5%)	10 (12%)	5 (6%)
Pneumothorax	0	0	0	4 (5%)
Respiratory insufficiency	0	0	5 (6%)	1 (1%)
Sputum increased	4 (5%)	5 (6%)	7 (8%)	6 (7%)
Miscellaneous				
Back pain	3 (3%)	1 (1%)	3 (3%)	5 (6%)
Chest pain	6 (7%)	6 (7%)	7 (8%)	8 (9%)
Edema (peripheral)	3 (3%)	3 (3%)	4 (5%)	3 (3%)
Fever	7 (8%)	7 (8%)	14 (16%)	8 (9%)
Pain	1 (1%)	4 (5%)	4 (5%)	8 (9%)

[a] The follow-up was 33% longer for the PDT group than for the Nd:YAG group, introducing a bias against PDT when adverse reactions are compared for the entire follow-up period.

Transient inflammatory reactions in PDT-treated patients occur in approximately 10% of patients and manifest as fever, bronchitis, chest pain, and dyspnea. The incidences of bronchitis and dyspnea were higher with PDT than with Nd:YAG. Most cases of bronchitis occurred within 1 week of treatment and all but one were mild or moderate in intensity. The reactions usually resolved within 10 days with antibiotic therapy. Treatment-related worsening of dyspnea is generally transient and self-limiting. Debridement of the treated area is mandatory to remove exudate and necrotic tissue. Life-threatening respiratory insufficiency likely due to therapy occurred in 3% of PDT-treated patients and 2% of Nd:YAG-treated patients. Patients with endobronchial lesions must be closely monitored between the laser light therapy and the mandatory debridement bronchoscopy for any evidence of respiratory distress. Inflammation, mucositis, and necrotic debris may cause obstruction of the airway. If respiratory distress occurs, the physician should be prepared to carry out immediate bronchoscopy to remove secretions and debris to open the airway.

There was a trend toward a higher rate of fatal hemoptysis (FMH) occurring on the PDT arm (10%) vs the Nd:YAG arm (5%); however, the rate of FMH occurring within 30 days of treatment was the same for PDT and Nd:YAG (4% total reactions, 3% treatment-associated reactions). Patients who have received radiation therapy have a higher incidence of FMH after treatment with PDT and after other forms of local therapy than patients who have not received radiation therapy, but analyses suggest that this increased risk may be due to associated prognostic factors such as having a centrally located tumor. The incidence of FMH in patients previously treated with radiotherapy was 21% (6/29) in the PDT group and 10% (3/29) in the Nd:YAG group. In patients with no prior radiotherapy, the overall incidence of FMH was less than 1%. Characteristics of patients at high risk for FMH are patients with tumors eroding into a major blood vessel, or with a tracheoesophageal or bronchoesophageal fistula.

Other serious or notable adverse reactions were observed in less than 5% of PDT-treated patients with endobronchial cancer; their relationship to therapy is uncertain. In the respiratory system, pulmonary thrombosis, pulmonary embolism, and lung abscess have occurred. Cardiac failure, sepsis and possible cerebrovascular accident have also been reported in 1 patient each.

PORFIMER SODIUM — INJECTION

➤*Superficial endobronchial tumors:*

Porfimer Adverse Reactions Reported in Patients [a] with Superficial Endobronchial Tumors (≥ 5%)

Adverse reaction	Number of patients (n = 90)	%
Patients with ≥ 1 adverse reaction	44	(49%)
Photosensitivity reaction	20	(22%)
Coughing	8	(9%)
Dyspnea	6	(7%)
Edema	16	(18%)
Exudate	20	(22%)
Obstruction	19	(21%)
Stricture	10	(11%)
Ulceration	8	(9%)

[a] Based on adverse reactions reported at any time during the entire period of follow-up.

In patients with superficial endobronchial tumors, 44 of 90 patients (49%) experienced an adverse reaction, two-thirds of which were related to the respiratory system. The most common reaction to therapy was a mucositis reaction in one-fifth of the patients that manifested as edema, exudate, and obstruction. The obstruction (mucus plug) is easily removed with suction or forceps. Mucositis can be minimized by avoiding exposure of normal tissue to excessive light. PDT should be used with extreme caution for endobronchial tumors in locations where treatment-induced inflammation could obstruct the main airway (eg, long or circumferential tumors of the trachea, tumors of the carina that involve both mainstem bronchi circumferentially, or circumferential tumors in the mainstem bronchus in patients with prior pneumonectomy). Three patients experienced life-threatening dyspnea: 1 was given a double dose of light, 1 was treated concurrently in both mainstem bronchi, and the other had prior pneumonectomy and was treated in the sole remaining main airway. Stent placement was required in 3% of the patients due to endobronchial stricture. Fatal hemoptysis occurred within 30 days of treatment in 1 patient with superficial tumors (1%).

➤*High-grade dysplasia (HGD) in Barrett's esophagus (BE):*

Treatment-Emergent Adverse Events Reported in Patients Treated with Porfimer Sodium PDT in the Clinical Trials on High-Grade Dysplasia in Barrett's Esophagus[a] (≥ 5%)

Adverse reaction*	Treatment groups: HGD[a] porfimer sodium PDT + OM (n = 219)	HGD[b] OM Only (n = 69)	Other[c] porfimer sodium PDT (n = 99)	Total porfimer sodium PDT (n = 318)
Patients with ≥1 adverse event	217 (99%)	51 (74%)	99 (100%)	316 (99%)
GI	180 (82%)	25 (36%)	87 (88%)	267 (84%)
Nausea	61 (28%)	5 (7%)	63 (64%)	124 (39%)
Esophageal stricture[d]	85 (39%)	0	37 (37%)	122 (38%)
Vomiting	72 (33%)	4 (6%)	35 (35%)	107 (34%)
Dysphagia	50 (23%)	1 (1%)	27 (27%)	77 (24%)
Esophageal narrowing[e]	60 (27%)	4 (6%)	16 (16%)	76 (24%)
Constipation	45 (21%)	5 (7%)	9 (9%)	54 (17%)
Abdominal pain (upper, lower, NOS)	32 (15%)	4 (6%)	8 (8%)	40 (12%)
Diarrhea	22 (10%)	7 (10%)	6 (6%)	28 (9%)
Esophageal pain	15 (7%)	0	9 (9%)	24 (8%)
Hiccup	18 (8%)	0	1 (1%)	19 (6%)
Dyspepsia	12 (5%)	3 (4%)	6 (6%)	18 (6%)
Odynophagia	13 (6%)	0	4 (4%)	17 (5%)
Eructation	11 (5%)	0	4 (4%)	15 (5%)
Miscellaneous	135 (62%)	17 (25%)	66 (67%)	201 (63%)
Chest pain	71 (32%)	8 (12%)	40 (40%)	111 (35%)
Pyrexia	47 (21%)	3 (4%)	13 (13%)	60 (19%)
Chest discomfort	14 (6%)	1 (1%)	21 (21%)	35 (11%)
Pain	17 (8%)	2 (3%)	7 (7%)	24 (8%)
Fatigue	13 (6%)	2 (3%)	0	13 (4%)
Dermatologic	120 (55%)	8 (12%)	29 (29%)	149 (47%)
Photosensitivity reaction	101 (46%)	0	16 (16%)	117 (37%)
Rash	14 (6%)	3 (4%)	7 (7%)	21 (7%)
Pruritus	13 (6%)	1 (1%)	1 (1%)	14 (4%)
Respiratory	67 (31%)	21 (30%)	22 (22%)	89 (28%)
Pleural effusion	25 (11%)	0	15 (15%)	40 (13%)
Dyspnea	16 (7%)	3 (4%)	4 (4%)	20 (6%)

[a] Includes all HGD patients in the safety population from PHO BAR 01 (n = 133), TCSC 93-07 (n = 44), and TCSC 96-01 (n = 42).
[b] Includes all HGD patients in the safety population from PHO BAR 01 (n = 69).
[c] Includes patients with Barrett's metaplasia, indefinite dysplasia, LGD, and adenocarcinoma at baseline in the Safety population from TCSC 93-07 (n = 55) and TCSC 96-01 (n = 44).
[d] In the controlled clinical trial, an esophageal stricture was defined as a fixed lumen narrowing with solid food dysphagia which required dilations. In the uncontrolled clinical trials, an esophageal stricture was defined as any dilated esophageal narrowing.
[e] An esophageal narrowing was defined as an undilated esophageal stenosis.
* Note: Adverse events classified using MedDRA 5.0 dictionary except esophageal strictures/narrowing.

Treatment-Emergent Adverse Events Reported in Patients Treated with Porfimer Sodium PDT in the Clinical Trials on High-Grade Dysplasia in Barrett's Esophagus (≥ 5%)

Body system/ Adverse event*	Treatment groups: HGD[a] porfimer sodium PDT + OM (n = 219)	HGD[b] OM Only (n = 69)	Other[c] porfimer sodium PDT (n = 99)	Total porfimer sodium PDT (n = 318)
Infections and infestations	58 (26%)	22 (32%)	8 (8%)	66 (21%)
Sinusitis	11 (5%)	3 (4%)	2 (2%)	13 (4%)
Bronchitis	10 (5%)	3 (4%)	2 (2%)	12 (4%)
Metabolic/Nutritional	53 (24%)	9 (13%)	16 (16%)	69 (22%)
Dehydration	24 (11%)	2 (3%)	8 (8%)	32 (10%)
Anorexia	6 (3%)	2 (3%)	8 (8%)	14 (4%)
CNS	51 (23%)	14 (20%)	11 (11%)	62 (19%)
Headache	17 (8%)	6 (9%)	2 (2%)	19 (6%)
Miscellaneous	42 (19%)	10 (14%)	19 (19%)	61 (19%)
Post procedural pain	16 (7%)	1 (1%)	14 (14%)	30 (9%)
Sunburn	8 (4%)	0	6 (6%)	14 (4%)
Musculoskeletal	46 (21%)	18 (26%)	9 (9%)	55 (17%)
Back pain	15 (7%)	4 (6%)	1 (1%)	16 (5%)
Arthralgia	10 (5%)	6 (9%)	1 (1%)	11 (3%)
Investigations	41 (19%)	5 (7%)	14 (14%)	55 (17%)
Weight decreased	17 (8%)	2 (3%)	3 (3%)	20 (6%)
Body temperature increased	8 (4%)	0	8 (8%)	16 (5%)
Psychiatric	37 (17%)	8 (12%)	4 (4%)	41 (13%)
Insomnia	11 (5%)	3 (4%)	1 (1%)	12 (4%)
Depression	10 (5%)	3 (4%)	0	10 (3%)
Anxiety	10 (5%)	1 (1%)	0	10 (3%)
Cardiovascular	25 (11%)	6 (9%)	4 (4%)	29 (9%)
Hypertension	10 (5%)	1 (1%)	0	10 (3%)

[a] Includes all HGD patients in the safety population from PHO BAR 01 (n = 133), TCSC 93-07 (n = 44), and TCSC 96-01 n = 42).
[b] Includes all HGD patients in the safety population from PHO BAR 01 (n = 69)
[c] Includes patients with Barrett's metaplasia, indefinite dysplasia, LGD, and adenocarcinoma at baseline in the Safety population from TCSC 93-07 (n = 55) and TCSC 96-01 (n = 44).
* Note: Adverse events classified using MedDRA 5.0 dictionary except esophageal strictures/narrowing.

In the porfimer sodium PDT + OM group, severe treatment-associated adverse events included chest pain of non-cardiac origin, dysphagia, nausea, vomiting, regurgitation, and heartburn. The severity of these symptoms decreased within 4 to 6 weeks following treatment.

The majority of the photosensitivity reactions occurred within 90 days following porfimer sodium injection and was of mild (69%) or moderate (24%) intensity. Almost all (98%) of the photosensitivity reactions were considered to be associated with treatment. Fourteen (10%) patients reported severe reactions, all of which resolved. The typical reaction was described as skin disorder, sunburn or rash, and affected mostly the face, hands, and neck. Associated symptoms and signs were swelling, pruritus, erythema, blisters, itching, burning sensation, and feeling of heat.

The majority of esophageal stenosis and strictures reported in the porfimer sodium PDT + OM group were of mild (55%) or moderate (37%) intensity, while approximately 8% were of severe intensity. The majority of esophageal strictures were reported during course 2 of treatment. All esophageal stric-

PORFIMER SODIUM — INJECTION

tures were considered to be associated with treatment. Most esophageal strictures were manageable through dilations.

➤*Lab test abnormalities:* In patients with esophageal cancer, PDT with porfimer sodium may result in anemia due to tumor bleeding. No significant effects were observed for other parameters or in patients with endobronchial carcinoma or with high-grade dysplasia in Barrett's esophagus.

Overdosage

There is no information on overdosage situations involving porfimer sodium. Higher than recommended drug doses of two 2 mg/kg doses given 2 days apart (10 patients) and three 2 mg/kg doses given within 2 weeks (1 patient), were tolerated without notable adverse reactions. Effects of overdosage on the duration of photosensitivity are unknown. Laser treatment should not be given if an overdose of porfimer sodium is administered. In the event of an overdose, patients should protect their eyes and skin from direct sunlight or bright indoor lights for 30 days. At this time, patients should test for residual photosensitivity. Porfimer sodium is not dialyzable.

➤*Overdose of laser light following porfimer sodium injection:* Light doses of 2 to 3 times the recommended dose have been administered to a few patients with superficial endobronchial tumors. One patient experienced life-threatening dyspnea and the others had no notable complications. Increased symptoms and damage to normal tissue might be expected following an overdose of light.

There is no information on overdose of laser light following porfimer sodium injection in patients with esophageal cancer or in patients with high-grade dysplasia in Barrett's esophagus.

Patient Information

Advise patients that this medicine will be prepared and administered by a healthcare provider in a medical setting.

Advise patients to contact a doctor if they experience severe chest pain, difficulty breathing, or abnormal blood loss.

Inform patients this drug will cause sensitivity to the sun, bright lights, or car headlights. For 30 days, they should avoid exposure of skin and eyes to direct sunlight from skylights or undraped windows or bright indoor light.

Instruct patients to test skin for sensitivity before exposing skin to bright indoor light or direct sunlight. To test the skin, expose a small skin area to sunlight for 10 minutes. If no sensitivity reactions (eg, rash, swelling, blistering) occur within 24 hours, gradually resume normal outdoor activities.

If patients must go out during daylight hours, instruct them to cover the skin as much as possible (long-sleeved shirts, slacks, gloves, socks) and wear dark sunglasses even on cloudy days or when in a car.

Contraceptive measures (birth control) are recommended during treatment to avoid birth defects. Instruct patients to inform their doctors if they are pregnant, become pregnant, are planning to become pregnant, or if they are breastfeeding.

Inform patients that lab tests may be required to monitor treatment and that they should keep their appointments.

MITOTANE (o,p'-DDD)

Rx	**Lysodren** (Bristol-Myers Squibb Oncology)	**Tablets:** 500 mg	Scored. In 100s.

MITOTANE — ORAL

WARNING

Mitotane should be administered under the supervision of a qualified physician experienced in the uses of cancer chemotherapeutic agents. Mitotane should be temporarily discontinued immediately following shock or severe trauma since adrenal suppression is its prime action. Exogenous steroids should be administered in such circumstances, since the depressed adrenal may not immediately start to secrete steroids.

Indications

➤*Adrenal cortical carcinoma:* Mitotane is indicated in the treatment of inoperable adrenal cortical carcinoma of both functional and nonfunctional types.

➤*Off-label uses:* Treatment of Cushing syndrome secondary to pituitary disorders. Mitotane has also been used safely and effectively in children with inoperable adrenal corticalcarcinoma. (See Administration and Dosage.)

Administration and Dosage

➤*Adults:*

Adrenal cortical carcinoma –

Maximum dose: 20 g/day. The maximum tolerated dose (MTD) will vary from 2 to 16 g/day, but has usually been 9 to 10 g/day.

Initial dosage: 2 to 6 g/day in divided doses, either 3 or 4 times a day.

Dosage titration: Doses are usually increased incrementally to 9 to 10 g/day. If severe adverse reactions appear, the dose should be reduced until the maximum tolerated dose is achieved. If the patient can tolerate higher doses and improved clinical response appears possible, the dose should be increased until adverse reactions interfere.

Maintenance dosage: 9 to 10 g/day or until maximum tolerated dose (MTD) is achieved.

Experience has shown that the MTD will vary from 2 to 16 g/day, but has usually been 9 to 10 g/day. Doses as high as 20 g/day have been used.

Duration of therapy: Treatment should be continued as long as clinical benefits are observed. Maintenance of clinical status or slowing of growth of metastatic lesions can be considered clinical benefits if they can clearly be shown to have occurred.

If no clinical benefits are observed after 3 months at the MTD, the case would generally be considered a clinical failure. However, 10% of the patients who showed a measurable response required more than 3 months at the MTD. Early diagnosis and prompt institution of treatment improve the probability of a positive clinical response. Clinical effectiveness can be shown by reduction in tumor mass; reduction in pain, weakness or anorexia; and reduction of symptoms and signs due to excessive steroid production.

A number of patients have been treated intermittently with treatment being restarted when severe symptoms have reappeared. Patients often do not respond after the third or fourth such course. Experience accumulated to date suggests that continuous treatment with the maximum possible dosage of mitotane is the best approach.

➤*Children:*

Off-label dosing –

Adrenal cortical carcinoma:

- *Maximum dose* – 7 g/day.
- *Initial dosage* – 1 to 2 g/day (or 0.1 to 0.5 mg/kg/day) in divided doses, either 3 or 4 times a day.
- *Dosage titration* – Gradually increase dose to a maximum of 5 to 7 g/day or until adverse effects occur.

➤*Preparation for administration:* Mitotane is considered a cytotoxic agent, a hormonal agent, and a potential teratogen. Follow safe handling procedures when preparing, administering, or dispensing mitotane.

➤*Administration:* Initiate treatment in a hospital until a stable dosage regimen is achieved. Hospitalization may not be required if supplemental corticosteroid therapy is initiated with mitotane therapy. Do not give mitotane with a fatty meal; fat may impair absorption of mitotane.

➤*Storage/Stability:* Store at 15° to 30°C (59° to 86°F).

Actions

➤*Pharmacology:* Mitotane can best be described as an adrenal cytotoxic agent, although it can cause adrenal inhibition, apparently without cellular destruction. Its biochemical mechanism of action is unknown. Data are available to suggest that the drug modifies the peripheral metabolism of steroids as well as directly suppressing the adrenal cortex. The administration of mitotane alters the extra-adrenal metabolism of cortisol in man; leading to a reduction in measurable 17-hydroxy corticosteroids, even though plasma levels of corticosteroids do not fall. The drug apparently causes increased formation of 6-β-hydroxyl cortisol.

➤*Pharmacokinetics:*

Absorption – Data in adrenal carcinoma patients indicate that about 40% of oral mitotane is absorbed.

Distribution – A variable amount of metabolite (1% to 17%) is excreted in the bile and the balance is apparently stored in the tissues. Autopsy data have provided evidence that mitotane is found in most tissues of the body; however, fat tissues are the primary site of storage.

Metabolism/Excretion – Approximately 10% of administered dose is recovered in the urine as a water-soluble metabolite. No unchanged mitotane has been found in urine or bile. Following discontinuation of mitotane, the plasma terminal half-life has ranged from 18 to 159 days. In most patients blood levels become undetectable after 6 to 9 weeks.

Contraindications

Mitotane should not be given to individuals who have demonstrated a previous hypersensitivity to it.

Warnings/Precautions

➤*Adrenal insufficiency:* Adrenal insufficiency may develop in patients treated with mitotane, and adrenal steroid replacement should be considered for these patients.

A substantial percentage of the patients treated show signs of adrenal insufficiency. It therefore appears necessary to watch for and institute steroid replacement in those patients. However, some investigators have recommended that steroid replacement therapy be administered concomitantly with mitotane. It has been shown that the metabolism of exogenous steroids is modified and consequently somewhat higher doses than normal replacement therapy may be required.

➤*Liver function impairment:* Mitotane should be administered with care to patients with liver disease other than metastatic lesions from the adrenal cortex, since the metabolism of mitotane may be interfered with and the drug may accumulate.

➤*Hypersensitivity reactions:* Mitotane should be temporarily discontinued immediately following shock or severe trauma, since adrenal suppression is its prime action. Exogenous steroids should be administered in such circumstances, since the depressed adrenal may not immediately start to secrete steroids.

MITOTANE — ORAL

➤*Special risk:* All possible tumor tissues should be surgically removed from large metastatic masses before mitotane administration is instituted. This is necessary to minimize the possibility of infarction and hemorrhage in the tumor due to a rapid cytotoxic effect of the drug.

Long-term continuous administration of high doses of mitotane may lead to brain damage and impairment of function. Behavioral and neurological assessments should be made at regular intervals when continuous mitotane treatment exceeds 2 years.

➤*Hazardous tasks:* Since sedation, lethargy, vertigo, and other CNS side effects can occur, ambulatory patients should be cautioned about driving, operating machinery, and other hazardous pursuits requiring mental and physical alertness.

➤*Pregnancy: Category C.* Animal reproduction studies have not been conducted with mitotane. It is also not known whether mitotane can cause fetal harm when administered to a pregnant woman or can affect reproduction capacity. Mitotane should be given to a pregnant woman only if clearly needed.

➤*Lactation:* It is not known whether this drug is excreted in human milk. Because many drugs are excreted in human milk and because of the potential for adverse reactions in nursing infants from mitotane, a decision should be made whether to discontinue nursing or to discontinue the drug, taking into account the importance of the drug to the mother.

➤*Children:* Safety and efficacy in children have not been established.

Drug Interactions

Mitotane Drug Interactions

Precipitant drug	Object drug[a]		Description
Mitotane	Corticosteroids	↓	Corticosteroid metabolism may be altered by mitotane; higher dosages may be required.
Mitotane	Warfarin	↓	The metabolism of warfarin may be accelerated by the mechanism of hepatic microsomal enzyme induction, leading to an increase in dosage requirements of warfarin. Monitor patients for a change in anticoagulant dosage requirements when administering mitotane to patients on coumarin-type anticoagulants.

Mitotane Drug Interactions

Precipitant drug	Object drug[a]		Description
Spironolactone	Mitotane	↓	Adrenolytic effects of mitotane may be blocked by spironolactone; observe for diminished clinical signs of mitotane; consider discontinuation of spironolactone.

[a] ↓ = object drug decreased.

Adverse Reactions

➤*CNS:* Central nervous system side effects occur in 40% of the patients. These consist primarily of depression as manifested by lethargy and somnolence (25%), and dizziness or vertigo (15%).

➤*Dermatologic:* Skin toxicity has been observed in about 15% of the cases. These skin changes consist primarily of transient skin rashes which do not seem to be dose related. In some instances, this side effect subsided while the patients were maintained on the drug without a change of dose.

➤*GI:* Gastrointestinal disturbances, which consist of anorexia, nausea or vomiting, and in some cases diarrhea, occur in about 80% of the patients.

➤*Infrequently occurring side effects:* Infrequently occurring side effects include:

Cardiovascular – Hypertension, orthostatic hypotension, and flushing.

GU – Hematuria, hemorrhagic cystitis, and albuminuria.

Ophthalmic – Visual blurring, diplopia, lens opacity, toxic retinopathy.

Miscellaneous – Generalized aching, hyperpyrexia, and lowered protein bound iodine (PBI).

Overdosage

No proven antidotes have been established for mitotane overdosage.

SIPULEUCEL-T

Rx	**Provenge** (Dendreon Corporation)	**Injection, suspension:** 50 million autologous CD54⁺ cells[a]	In 250 mL patient-specific infusion bags.

[a] Activated with prostatic acid phosphatase (PAP) linked to granulocyte-macrophage colony-stimulating factor (GM-CSF).

SIPULEUCEL-T — INJECTION

Indications

➤*Prostate cancer:* For the treatment of asymptomatic or minimally symptomatic metastatic castrate resistant (hormone refractory) prostate cancer.

Administration and Dosage

➤*General dosing considerations:* For autologous use only.

If the patient is unable to receive a scheduled infusion, the patient will need to undergo an additional leukapheresis procedure if the course of treatment is to be continued. Patients should be advised of this possibility prior to initiating treatment.

To minimize potential acute infusion reactions, such as chills and/or fever, premedication is recommended. (See Premedication.)

Observe the patient for at least 30 minutes following each infusion.

➤*Adults:*

Prostate cancer –

Usual dosage: 3 complete doses, given at approximately 2-week intervals. Each dose contains a minimum of 50 million autologous $CD54^+$ cells activated with PAP-GM-CSF suspended in 250 mL of lactated Ringer's injection.

Premedication: Premedicate patients with oral acetaminophen and an antihistamine, such as diphenhydramine, approximately 30 minutes prior to administration.

➤*Preparation for administration:* Sipuleucel-T is shipped directly to the infusing provider. Sipuleucel-T will arrive in a cardboard shipping box with a special insulated polyurethane container inside. The insulated container and gel packs within the container are designed to maintain the appropriate transportation and storage temperature until infusion. Upon receipt, the outer cardboard shipping box should be opened to verify the product and patient-specific labels located on the top of the insulated container. Do not remove this insulated container from the shipping box or open the lid of the insulated container until the patient is ready for infusion. The infusion bag must remain within the insulated polyurethane container until the time of administration.

Do not infuse until confirmation of product release has been received from the manufacturer. The manufacturer will send a Cell Product Disposition Form containing the patient identifiers, expiration date and time, and the disposition status (approved for infusion or rejected) to the infusion site.

Once the infusion bag is removed from the insulated container, it should remain at room temperature for no more than 3 hours. Sipuleucel-T should not be returned to the shipping container.

Once the patient is prepared for infusion and the Cell Product Disposition Form has been received, remove the sipuleucel-T infusion bag from the insulated container and inspect the bag for signs of leakage. Contents of the bag will be slightly cloudy, with a cream-to-pink color. Gently mix and resuspend the contents of the bag, inspecting for clumps and clots. Small clumps of cellular material should disperse with gently manual mixing. Do not administer if the bag leaks or if clumps remain in the bag.

Prior to sipuleucel-T infusion, match the patient's identity with the patient identifiers on the Cell Product Disposition Form and the sipuleucel-T infusion bag.

Handling – Patient leukapheresis material and sipuleucel-T may carry the risk of transmitting infectious diseases to health care providers handling the product. Employ universal precautions in handling leukapheresis material or sipuleucel-T.

➤*Administration:* For intravenous (IV) use only. Infusion must begin prior to the expiration date and time indicated on the Cell Product Disposition Form and product label. Do not initiate infusion of expired sipuleucel-T. Administer sipuleucel-T via IV infusion over a period of approximately 60 minutes. Do not use a cell filter. Sipuleucel-T is supplied in a sealed, patient-specific infusion bag; the entire volume of the bag should be infused.

Infusion reaction – In the event of an acute infusion reaction, the infusion may be interrupted or slowed, depending on the severity of the reaction. If the infusion must be interrupted, the infusion should not be resumed if the infusion bag will be held at room temperature for more than 3 hours.

Appropriate medical therapy should be administered as needed. In controlled clinical trials, symptoms of acute infusion reactions were treated with acetaminophen, IV H_1 and/or H_2 blockers, and low-dose IV meperidine.

➤*Storage/Stability:* Do not remove the infusion bag from the insulated container or open or remove the insulated container from the shipping box until the patient is ready for infusion. Once the infusion bag is removed from the insulated container, it should remain at room temperature for no more than 3 hours. If the infusion must be interrupted, the infusion should not be resumed if the infusion bag will be held at room temperature for more than 3 hours.

SIPULEUCEL-T — INJECTION

Actions

➤*Pharmacology:* Sipuleucel-T is an autologous cellular immunotherapy. While the precise mechanism of action is unknown, sipuleucel-T is designed to induce an immune response targeted against PAP, an antigen expressed in most prostate cancers. During ex vivo culture with PAP-GM-CSF, antigen-presenting cells (APCs) take up and process the recombinant target antigen into small peptides that are displayed on the APC surface.

Immune response – In study 1, 237 of the 512 patients randomized were evaluated for the development of humoral and T cell immune responses (proliferative and gamma-interferon enzyme-linked immunospot [ELISPOT]) to the target antigens at baseline and at weeks 6, 14, and 26. Antibody (immunoglobulin M [IgM] and IgG) responses against PAP-GM-CSF and PAP antigen alone were observed through the follow-up period in the sipuleucel-T group. Neutralizing antibody responses to GM-CSF were transient. T-cell proliferative and gamma-interferon ELISPOT responses to PAP-GM-CSF fusion protein were observed in cells collected from peripheral blood of patients through the follow-up period in the sipuleucel-T treatment group but not in controls. In some patients, a response to PAP antigen alone was observed. No conclusions could be made regarding the clinical significance of the observed immune responses.

Contraindications

None well documented.

Warnings/Precautions

➤*Administration:* Sipuleucel-T is intended solely for autologous use.

➤*Acute infusion reactions:* Acute infusion reactions (reported within 1 day of infusion) included, but were not limited to, fever, chills, respiratory reactions (dyspnea, hypoxia, and bronchospasm), nausea, vomiting, fatigue, hypertension, and tachycardia. In controlled clinical trials, 71.2% of patients in the sipuleucel-T group developed an acute infusion reaction. The most common reactions (at least 20%) were chills, fever, and fatigue. In 95.1% of patients reporting acute infusion reactions, the reactions were mild or moderate. Fever and chills generally resolved within 2 days (71.9% and 89%, respectively).

In controlled clinical trials, severe (grade 3) acute infusion reactions were reported in 3.5% of patients in the sipuleucel-T group. Reactions included chills, fever, fatigue, asthenia, dyspnea, hypoxia, bronchospasm, dizziness, headache, hypertension, muscle ache, nausea, and vomiting. The incidence of severe reactions was greater following the second infusion (2.1% vs. 0.8% following the first infusion) and decreased to 1.3% following the third infusion. Some (1.2%) patients in the sipuleucel-T group were hospitalized within 1 day of infusion for management of acute infusion reactions. No grade 4 or 5 acute infusion reactions were reported in patients in the sipuleucel-T group.

Closely monitor patients with cardiac or pulmonary conditions. In the event of an acute infusion reaction, the infusion rate may be decreased or the infusion stopped, depending on the severity of the reaction. Administer appropriate medical therapy as needed.

➤*Infectious diseases:* Sipuleucel-T is not routinely tested for transmissible infectious diseases. Therefore, patient leukapheresis material and sipuleucel-T may carry the risk of transmitting infectious diseases to health care providers handling the product. Accordingly, employ universal precautions when handling leukapheresis material or sipuleucel-T.

➤*Product safety testing:* Sipuleucel-T is released for infusion based on the microbial and sterility results from several tests: microbial contamination determination by gram stain, endotoxin content, and in-process sterility with a 2-day incubation to determine absence of microbial growth. The final (7-day incubation) sterility test results are not available at the time of infusion. If the sterility results become positive for microbial contamination after sipuleucel-T has been approved for infusion, the manufacturer will notify the treating health care provider. The manufacturer will attempt to identify the microorganism, perform antibiotic sensitivity testing on recovered microorganisms, and communicate the results to the treating health care provider. The manufacturer may request additional information from the health care provider in order to determine the source of contamination.

➤*Pregnancy:* Category undetermined. No information is available regarding the use of sipuleucel-T in pregnant women. Sipuleucel-T is not indicated for use in women.

➤*Lactation:* No information is available. Sipuleucel-T is not indicated for use in women.

➤*Children:* Safety and efficacy have not been established.

➤*Elderly:* In a survival analysis of the controlled clinical trials of sipuleucel-T in metastatic castrate resistant prostate cancer, 78.3% of randomized patients were at least 65 years of age. The median survival of patients in the sipuleucel-T group at least 65 years of age was 23.4 months (95% confidence interval [CI], 22 to 27.1), compared with 17.3 months in the control group (95% CI, 13.5 to 21.5).

➤*Monitoring:* Closely monitor patients with cardiac or pulmonary conditions.

Observe the patient for at least 30 minutes following each infusion.

Monitoring for infectious sequelae in patients with central venous catheters is recommended.

Drug Interactions

➤*Immunosuppressive agents:* Because sipuleucel-T stimulates the immune system, concomitant use of immunosuppressive agents (eg, systemic corticosteroids) may alter the efficacy and/or safety of sipuleucel-T. Carefully evaluate patients to determine whether it is medically appropriate to reduce or discontinue immunosuppressive agents prior to sipuleucel-T treatment.

Adverse Reactions

➤*Most common adverse reactions:* Almost all (98.3%) patients in the sipuleucel-T group and 96% in the control group reported an adverse reaction. The most common adverse reactions reported in patients in the sipuleucel-T group at a rate of at least 15% were back pain, chills, fatigue, fever, headache, joint ache, and nausea. In 67.4% of patients in the sipuleucel-T group, these adverse reactions were mild or moderate in severity.

The most common (at least 2%) grade 3 to 5 adverse reactions reported in the sipuleucel-T group were back pain and chills.

➤*Severe adverse reactions:* Severe (grade 3) and life-threatening (grade 4) adverse reactions were reported in 23.6% and 4% of patients in the sipuleucel-T group compared with 25.1% and 3.3% of patients in the control group. Fatal (grade 5) adverse reactions were reported in 3.3% of patients in the sipuleucel-T group compared with 3.6% of patients in the control group.

➤*Serious adverse reactions:* Serious adverse reactions were reported in 24% of patients in the sipuleucel-T group and 25.1% of patients in the control group. Serious adverse reactions in the sipuleucel-T group included acute infusion reactions, cerebrovascular events, and single case reports of eosinophilia, myasthenia gravis, myositis, rhabdomyolysis, and tumor flare.

➤*Discontinuation:* Sipuleucel-T was discontinued in 1.5% of patients in study 1 because of adverse reactions.

Infections – Some patients who required central venous catheters for treatment with sipuleucel-T developed infections, including sepsis. A small number of these patients discontinued treatment as a result. Monitoring for infectious sequelae in patients with central venous catheters is recommended.

➤*Leukapheresis adverse reactions:* Each dose of sipuleucel-T requires a standard leukapheresis procedure approximately 3 days prior to the infusion. Adverse reactions reported 1 day or less following a leukapheresis procedure in at least 5% of patients in controlled clinical trials included citrate toxicity (14.2%), oral paresthesia (12.6%), paresthesia (11.4%), and fatigue (8.3%).

Adverse reactions (5% or more) –

Sipuleucel-T Adverse Reactions (≥ 5%)				
	Sipuleucel-T (n = 601)		Control[a] (n = 303)	
Adverse reactions	All grades	Grade 3 to 5	All grades	Grade 3 to 5
Any adverse reaction	98.3%	30.9%	96%	32%
CNS				
Asthenia	10.8%	1%	6.6%	0.7%
Dizziness	11.8%	0.3%	11.2%	0%
Fatigue	41.1%	1%	34.7%	1.3%
Headache	18.1%	0.7%	6.6%	0%
Insomnia	6.2%	0%	7.3%	0.3%
Paresthesia	14.1%	0.2%	14.2%	0%
Paresthesia oral	12.3%	0%	14.2%	0%
Tremor	5%	0%	3%	0%
Dermatologic				
Rash	5.2%	0%	3.3%	0%
Sweating	5%	0.2%	1%	0%
GI				
Anorexia	6.5%	0.2%	10.9%	1%
Constipation	12.3%	0.2%	13.2%	1%
Diarrhea	10%	0.2%	11.2%	1%
Nausea	21.5%	0.5%	14.9%	0%
Vomiting	13.3%	0.3%	7.6%	0%
Weight decreased	5.7%	0.3%	7.9%	0.3%
GU				
Hematuria	7.7%	1%	5.9%	1%
Urinary tract infection	5.5%	0.2%	5.9%	0.7%
Musculoskeletal				
Back pain	29.6%	3%	28.7%	3%
Bone pain	6.3%	0.7%	7.3%	1%
Joint ache	19.6%	1.8%	20.5%	1.7%
Neck pain	5.7%	0.5%	4.6%	0.7%
Muscle ache	11.8%	0.5%	5.6%	0%
Muscle spasms	7.7%	0.3%	5.6%	0%
Musculoskeletal chest pain	6%	0.3%	7.6%	0.7%
Musculoskeletal pain	9%	0.5%	10.2%	1%
Pain in extremity	12.1%	0.8%	13.2%	0.3%

SIPULEUCEL-T — INJECTION

Sipuleucel-T Adverse Reactions (≥ 5%)				
	Sipuleucel-T (n = 601)		Control[a] (n = 303)	
Adverse reactions	All grades	Grade 3 to 5	All grades	Grade 3 to 5
Respiratory				
Cough	5.8%	0%	5.6%	0%
Dyspnea	8.7%	1.8%	4.6%	1%
Upper respiratory tract infection	6.3%	0%	5.9%	0%
Miscellaneous				
Anemia	12.5%	1.8%	11.2%	2.3%
Chills	53.1%	2.2%	10.9%	0%
Citrate toxicity	14.8%	0%	14.2%	0%
Edema peripheral	8.3%	0.2%	10.2%	0.3%
Fever	31.3%	1%	9.6%	1%
Hot flush	8.2%	0.3%	9.6%	0.3%
Hypertension	7.5%	0.5%	4.6%	0%
Influenza-like illness	9.7%	0%	3.6%	0%
Pain	12.3%	1.2%	6.6%	1%

[a] Control was nonactivated autologous peripheral blood mononuclear cells.

➤*Cerebrovascular events:* In controlled clinical trials, cerebrovascular events, including hemorrhagic and ischemic strokes, were observed in 3.5% of patients in the sipuleucel-T group compared with 2.6% of patients in the control group.

Patient Information

Inform patient that the recommended course of therapy for sipuleucel-T is 3 complete doses. Each infusion of sipuleucel-T is preceded by a leukapheresis procedure approximately 3 days prior. It is important to maintain all scheduled appointments and arrive at each appointment on time because the leukapheresis and infusions must be appropriately spaced and the sipuleucel-T expiration time must not be exceeded.

Inform patient that if they are unable to receive an infusion of sipuleucel-T, they will need to undergo an additional leukapheresis procedure if the treatment is to be continued.

Counsel the patient on the importance of adhering to preparation instructions for the leukapheresis procedure, the possible side effects of leukapheresis, and postprocedure care.

If the patient does not have adequate peripheral venous access to accommodate the leukapheresis procedure and infusion of sipuleucel-T, inform the patient about the need for a central venous catheter. Counsel the patient on the importance of catheter care. Instruct the patient to tell their health care provider if they are experiencing fevers or any swelling or redness around the catheter site because these symptoms could be signs of an infected catheter.

Advise patients to report signs and symptoms of acute infusion reactions, such as fever, chills, fatigue, breathing problems, dizziness, high blood pressure, nausea, vomiting, headache, or muscle aches.

Advise patients to report any symptoms suggestive of a cardiac arrhythmia.

Advise patients to inform their health care provider if they are taking immunosuppressive agents.

ARSENIC TRIOXIDE

Rx	**Trisenox** (Cephalon)	**Injection:** 1 mg/1 ml	Preservative-free. In 10s.

ARSENIC TRIOXIDE — INJECTION

WARNING

Experienced physician and institution – Arsenic trioxide injection should be administered under the supervision of a physician who is experienced in the management of patients with acute leukemia.

APL differentiation syndrome – Some patients with acute promyelocytic leukemia (APL) treated with arsenic trioxide have experienced symptoms similar to a syndrome called the retinoic-acid-acute promyelocytic leukemia (RA-APL) or APL differentiation syndrome, characterized by fever, dyspnea, weight gain, pulmonary infiltrates and pleural or pericardial effusions, with or without leukocytosis. This syndrome can be fatal. The management of the syndrome has not been fully studied, but high-dose steroids have been used at the first suspicion of the APL differentiation syndrome and appear to mitigate signs and symptoms. At the first signs that could suggest the syndrome (unexplained fever, dyspnea or weight gain, abnormal chest auscultatory findings or radiographic abnormalities), high-dose steroids (dexamethasone 10 mg intravenously [IV] twice a day) should be immediately initiated, irrespective of the leukocyte count, and continued for at least 3 days or longer until signs and symptoms have abated. The majority of patients do not require termination of arsenic trioxide therapy during treatment of the APL differentiation syndrome.

ECG abnormalities – Arsenic trioxide can cause QT interval prolongation and complete atrioventricular block. QT prolongation can lead to a torsade de pointes-type ventricular arrhythmia, which can be fatal. The risk of torsade de pointes is related to the extent of QT prolongation, concomitant administration of QT prolonging drugs, a history of torsade de pointes, preexisting QT interval prolongation, congestive heart failure, administration of potassium-wasting diuretics, or other conditions that result in hypokalemia or hypomagnesemia. One patient (also receiving amphotericin B) had torsade de pointes during induction therapy for relapsed APL with arsenic trioxide.

ECG and electrolyte monitoring recommendations – Prior to initiating therapy with arsenic trioxide, a 12-lead ECG should be performed and serum electrolytes (potassium, calcium, and magnesium) and creatinine should be assessed; preexisting electrolyte abnormalities should be corrected and, if possible, drugs that are known to prolong the QT interval should be discontinued. For QTc greater than 500 msec, corrective measures should be completed and the QTc reassessed with serial ECGs prior to considering using arsenic trioxide. During therapy with arsenic trioxide, potassium concentrations should be kept above 4 mEq/dL and magnesium concentrations should be kept above 1.8 mg/dL. Patients who reach an absolute QT interval value greater than 500 msec should be reassessed and immediate action should be taken to correct concomitant risk factors, if any, while the risk/benefit of continuing versus suspending arsenic trioxide therapy should be considered. If syncope, rapid or irregular heartbeat develops, the patient should be hospitalized for monitoring, serum electrolytes should be assessed, arsenic trioxide therapy should be temporarily discontinued until the QTc interval regresses to below 460 msec, electrolyte abnormalities are corrected, and the syncope and irregular heartbeat cease. There are no data on the effect of arsenic trioxide on the QTc interval during the infusion.

Indications

➤*Acute promyelocytic leukemia (APL):* Arsenic trioxide is indicated for induction of remission and consolidation in patients with acute promyelocytic leukemia (APL) who are refractory to, or have relapsed from, retinoid and anthracycline chemotherapy, and whose APL is characterized by the presence of the t(15;17) translocation or PML/RAR-alpha gene expression.

Administration and Dosage

➤*Adults:*

Acute promyelocytic leukemia –

Induction treatment:

- *Usual dosage* – 0.15 mg/kg daily IV until bone marrow remission.
- *Maximum dose* – Total induction dose should not exceed 60 doses.

Consolidation treatment: 0.15 mg/kg daily IV for 25 doses over a period up to 5 weeks. Consolidation treatment should begin 3 to 6 weeks after completion of induction therapy.

➤*Children:*

Acute promyelocytic leukemia –

5 years of age and older: See Adults.

➤*Hepatic function impairment:* Safety and effectiveness of arsenic trioxide in patients with hepatic impairment have not been studied. It is unknown whether dosage adjustment is necessary. Monitor these patients closely.

➤*Preparation for administration:* Arsenic trioxide is considered a cytotoxic agent. Follow safe handling procedures when preparing, administering, or dispensing arsenic trioxide.

Arsenic trioxide should be diluted with 100 to 250 mL of dextrose 5% injection or sodium chloride 0.9% injection using proper aseptic technique, immediately after withdrawal from the ampule using a filter needle. The arsenic trioxide ampule is for single use and does not contain any preservatives. Unused portions of each ampule should be discarded properly. Do not save any unused portions for later administration.

➤*Administration:* Arsenic trioxide should be administered IV over 1 to 2 hours. The infusion duration may be extended up to 4 hours if acute vasomotor reactions are observed. A central venous catheter is not required. May be given via a peripheral venous catheter.

➤*Extravasation:* Arsenic trioxide is considered an irritant and may cause phlebitis, but it is not known to cause tissue damage with extravasation. If signs or symptoms of extravasation occur, stop the infusion immediately. If possible, withdraw 3 to 5 mL of blood to remove some of the drug. Remove the infusion needle. Delineate the infiltrated area on the patient's skin with a felt tip marker. Elevate for 48 hours above heart level using a sling or stockinette dressing with an observation window cut in the dressing. Avoid pressure or friction. Do not rub the area. Observe for signs of increased erythema, pain, or skin necrosis. If increased symptoms occur, consult a plastic surgeon. Ensure that no medication is given distally to the extravasation site. After 48 hours, encourage the patient to use the extremity normally to promote full range of motion.

➤*Admixture compatibility:* Do not mix arsenic trioxide with other medications.

➤*Storage/Stability:* Store at 25°C (77°F); excursions permitted to 15° to 30°C (59° to 86°F). Do not freeze.

ARSENIC TRIOXIDE — INJECTION

After dilution, arsenic trioxide is chemically and physically stable when stored for 24 hours at room temperature and 48 hours when refrigerated. The possibility of microbial contamination of diluted solutions must be considered. Preservative-free solutions should be used within 24 hours.

Actions

➤*Pharmacology:* The mechanism of action of arsenic trioxide is not completely understood. Arsenic trioxide causes morphological changes and DNA fragmentation characteristic of apoptosis in NB4 human promyelocytic leukemia cells in vitro. Arsenic trioxide also causes damage or degradation of the fusion protein PML-RAR alpha.

➤*Pharmacokinetics:*

Metabolism – The metabolism of arsenic trioxide involves reduction of pentavalent arsenic to trivalent arsenic by arsenate reductase and methylation of trivalent arsenic to monomethylarsonic acid and monomethylarsonic acid to dimethylarsinic acid by methyltransferases. The main site of methylation reactions appears to be the liver. Arsenic is stored mainly in liver, kidney, heart, lung, hair and nails.

Excretion – Disposition of arsenic following intravenous administration has not been studied. Trivalent arsenic is mostly methylated in humans and excreted in urine.

The pharmacokinetics of trivalent arsenic, the active species of arsenic trioxide, have not been characterized.

Contraindications

Arsenic trioxide is contraindicated in patients who are hypersensitive to arsenic.

Warnings/Precautions

➤*Black box warning:* See Warning Box for more information.

➤*APL differentiation syndrome (see Warning Box):* Nine of 40 patients with APL treated with arsenic trioxide, at a dose of 0.15 mg/kg, experienced the APL differentiation syndrome (see Warning Box and Adverse Reactions).

➤*Hyperleukocytosis:* Treatment with arsenic trioxide has been associated with the development of hyperleukocytosis (greater than or equal to 10×10^3/mcL) in 20 of 40 patients. A relationship did not exist between baseline WBC counts and development of hyperleukocytosis nor baseline WBC counts and peak WBC counts. Hyperleukocytosis was not treated with additional chemotherapy. WBC counts during consolidation were not as high as during induction treatment.

➤*QT prolongation (see Warning Box):* QT/QTc prolongation should be expected during treatment with arsenic trioxide and torsade de pointes as well as complete heart block has been reported. Over 460 ECG tracings from 40 patients with refractory or relapsed APL treated with arsenic trioxide were evaluated for QTc prolongation. Sixteen of 40 patients (40%) had at least one ECG tracing with a QTc interval greater than 500 msec. Prolongation of the QTc was observed between 1 and 5 weeks after arsenic trioxide infusion, and then returned towards baseline by the end of 8 weeks after arsenic trioxide infusion. In these ECG evaluations, women did not experience more pronounced QT prolongation than men, and there was no correlation with age.

➤*Complete AV block:* Complete AV block has been reported with arsenic trioxide in the published literature including a case of a patient with APL.

➤*Extravasation:* See Administration and Dosage for more information.

➤*Renal/Hepatic function impairment:* Safety and effectiveness of arsenic trioxide in patients with renal and hepatic impairment have not been studied. Particular caution is needed in patients with renal failure receiving arsenic trioxide, as renal excretion is the main route of elimination of arsenic.

➤*Pregnancy: Category D.* Arsenic trioxide may cause fetal harm when administered to a pregnant woman. Studies in pregnant mice, rats, hamsters, and primates have shown that inorganic arsenicals cross the placental barrier when given orally or by injection. The reproductive toxicity of arsenic trioxide has been studied in a limited manner. An increase in resorptions, neural-tube defects, anophthalmia and microphthalmia were observed in rats administered 10 mg/kg of arsenic trioxide on gestation day 9 (approximately 10 times the recommended human daily dose on a mg/m^2 basis). Similar findings occurred in mice administered a 10 mg/kg dose of a related trivalent arsenic, sodium arsenite, (approximately 5 times the projected human dose on a mg/m^2 basis) on gestation days 6, 7, 8 or 9. Intravenous injection of 2 mg/kg sodium arsenite (approximately equivalent to the projected human daily dose on a mg/m^2 basis) on gestation day 7 (the lowest dose tested) resulted in neural-tube defects in hamsters.

There are no studies in pregnant women using arsenic trioxide. If this drug is used during pregnancy or if the patient becomes pregnant while taking this drug, the patient should be apprised of the potential harm to the fetus. One patient who became pregnant while receiving arsenic trioxide had a miscarriage. Women of childbearing potential should be advised to avoid becoming pregnant.

➤*Lactation:* Arsenic is excreted in human milk. Because of the potential for serious adverse reactions in nursing infants from arsenic trioxide, a decision should be made whether to discontinue nursing or to discontinue the drug, taking into account the importance of the drug to the mother.

➤*Children:* There are limited clinical data on the pediatric use of arsenic trioxide. Of 5 patients below the age of 18 years (range 5 to 16 years) treated with arsenic trioxide, at the recommended dose of 0.15 mg/kg/day, 3 achieved a complete response. Safety and effectiveness in pediatric patients below the age of 5 years have not been studied.

➤*Monitoring:* The patient's electrolyte, hematologic and coagulation profiles should be monitored at least twice weekly, and more frequently for clinically unstable patients during the induction phase and at least weekly during the consolidation phase. ECGs should be obtained weekly, and more frequently for clinically unstable patients, during induction and consolidation.

Drug Interactions

➤*QT prolongation:* An additive effect of arsenic trioxide with other drugs that prolong the QT interval cannot be excluded. The following drugs may prolong the QT interval and increase the risk of life-threatening cardiac arrhythmias, including torsades de pointes: Antiarrhythmic agents (eg, amiodarone, bretylium, disopyramide, dofetilide, procainamide, quinidine, and sotalol), chlorpromazine, cisapride, dolasetron, droperidol, mefloquine, mesoridazine, moxifloxacin, pentamidine, pimozide, tacrolimus, thioridazine, and ziprasidone. For a more complete list of drugs that may prolong the QT interval, see the appendix, Drug-Induced Prolongation of the QT Interval and Torsades de Pointes.

Adverse Reactions

Arsenic trioxide is considered to have moderate potential for nausea and vomiting.

Safety information was available for 52 patients with relapsed or refractory APL who participated in clinical trials of arsenic trioxide. Forty patients in the Phase 2 study received the recommended dose of 0.15 mg/kg of which 29 completed both induction and consolidation treatment cycles. An additional 12 patients with relapsed or refractory APL received doses generally similar to the recommended dose. Most patients experienced some drug-related toxicity, most commonly leukocytosis, gastrointestinal (nausea, vomiting, diarrhea, and abdominal pain), fatigue, edema, hyperglycemia, dyspnea, cough, rash or itching, headaches, and dizziness. These adverse effects have not been observed to be permanent or irreversible nor do they usually require interruption of therapy.

Serious adverse events (SAEs), grade 3 or 4 according to version 2 of the NCI Common Toxicity Criteria, were common. Those SAEs attributed to arsenic trioxide in the Phase 2 study of 40 patients with refractory or relapsed APL included APL differentiation syndrome (n = 3), hyperleukocytosis (n = 3), QTc interval greater than or equal to 500 msec (n = 16, 1 with torsade de pointes), atrial dysrhythmias (n = 2), and hyperglycemia (n = 2).

➤*Adverse events (any grade) occurring in greater than or equal to 5% of 40 patients with APL who received arsenic trioxide at a dose of 0.15 mg/kg/day:*

Adverse Events (any grade) Occurring in Patients with APL Who Received Arsenic Trioxide (≥ 5%)				
Adverse reaction	All adverse events, any grade		Grade 3 and 4 events	
	n	%	n	%
Cardiovascular				
Tachycardia	22	55		
ECG QT corrected interval prolonged > 500 msec	16	38		
Palpitations	4	10		
ECG abnormal other than QT interval prolongation	3	11		
Hypotension	10	25	2	5
Flushing	4	10		
Hypertension	4	10		
Pallor	4	10		
CNS				
Agitation	2	5		
Anxiety	12	30		
Coma	2	5	2	5
Confusion	2	5		
Convulsion	3	8	2	5
Depression	8	20		
Dizziness (excluding vertigo)	9	23		
Headache	24	60	1	3
Insomnia	17	43	1	3
Paresthesia	13	33	2	5
Somnolence	3	8		
Tremor	5	13		
Dermatologic				
Dermatitis	17	43		
Pruritus	13	33	1	2
Ecchymosis	8	20		
Dry skin	6	11		
Erythema-nonspecific	5	11		

ARSENIC TRIOXIDE — INJECTION

Adverse Events (any grade) Occurring in Patients with APL Who Received Arsenic Trioxide (≥ 5%)				
	All adverse events, any grade		Grade 3 and 4 events	
Adverse reaction	n	%	n	%
Increased sweating	5	11		
Facial edema	3	8		
Night sweats	3	8		
Petechiae	3	8		
Hyperpigmentation	3	8		
Non specific skin lesions	3	8		
Urticaria	3	8		
Local exfoliation	2	5		
Eyelid edema	2	5		
GI				
Nausea	30	75		
Anorexia	9	23		
Appetite decreased	6	15		
Diarrhea	21	53		
Vomiting	23	58		
Abdominal pain (lower and upper)	23	58	4	10
Sore throat	14	40		
Constipation	11	28	1	3
Loose stools	4	10		
Dyspepsia	4	10		
Oral blistering	3	8		
Fecal incontinence	3	8		
GI hemorrhage	3	8		
Dry mouth	3	8		
Abdominal tenderness	3	8		
Diarrhea hemorrhagic	3	8		
Abdominal distension	3	8		
GU				
Renal failure	3	8	1	3
Renal impairment	3	8		
Oliguria	2	5		
Incontinence	2	5		
Vaginal hemorrhage	5	13		
Intermenstrual bleeding	3	8		
Hematologic				
Leukocytosis	20	50	1	3
Anemia	8	14	2	5
Thrombocytopenia	7	19	5	12
Febrile neutropenia	5	13	3	8
Neutropenia	4	10	4	10
Disseminated intravascular coagulation	3	8	3	8
Lymphadenopathy	3	8		
Infections and infestations				
Sinusitis	8	20		
Herpes simplex	5	13		
Upper respiratory tract infection	5	13	1	3
Bacterial infection- nonspecific	3	8	1	3
Herpes zoster	3	8		
Nasopharyngitis	2	5		
Oral candidiasis	2	5		
Sepsis	2	5	2	5
Metabolic/Nutritional				
Hypokalemia	20	50	5	13
Hypomagnesemia	18	45	5	13
Hyperglycemia	18	45	5	13
ALT increased	8	20	2	5
Hyperkalemia	7	18	2	5
AST increased	5	13	1	3
Hypocalcemia	4	10		
Hypoglycemia	3	8		
Acidosis	2	5		
Musculoskeletal				
Arthralgia	13	33	3	8
Myalgia	10	25	2	5
Bone pain	9	23	4	10
Back pain	7	18	1	3
Neck pain	5	13		
Pain in limb	5	13	2	5
Respiratory				
Cough	26	65		
Dyspnea	21	53	4	10
Epistaxis	10	25		
Hypoxia	9	23	4	10
Pleural effusion	8	20	1	3
Post nasal drip	5	13		
Wheezing	5	13		
Decreased breath sounds	4	10		
Crepitations	4	10		
Rales	4	10		
Hemoptysis	3	8		
Tachypnea	3	8		
Rhonchi	3	8		
Special senses				
Eye irritation	4	10		
Blurred vision	4	10		
Dry eye	3	8		
Painful red eye	2	5		
Earache	3	8		
Tinnitus	2	5		
Miscellaneous				
Fatigue	25	63	2	5
Pyrexia (fever)	25	63	2	5
Edema - nonspecific	16	40		
Rigors	15	38		
Chest pain	10	25	2	5
Injection site pain	8	20		
Pain - nonspecific	6	15	1	3
Injection site erythema	5	13		
Injection site edema	4	10		
Weakness	4	10	2	5
Hemorrhage	3	8		
Weight gain	5	13		
Weight loss	3	8		
Drug hypersensitivity	2	5	1	3

Overdosage

If symptoms suggestive of serious acute arsenic toxicity (eg, convulsions, muscle weakness and confusion) appear, arsenic trioxide should be immediately discontinued and chelation therapy should be considered. A conventional protocol for acute arsenic intoxication includes dimercaprol administered at a dose of 3 mg/kg intramuscularly every 4 hours until immediate life-threatening toxicity has subsided. Thereafter, penicillamine at a dose of 250 mg orally, up to a maximum frequency of 4 times per day (less than or equal to 1 g day), may be given.

STERILE TALC POWDER

Rx	**Sclerosol** (Bryan)	**Aerosol:** 4 g talc	CFC-12. In single-use aluminum canister with 2 delivery tubes of 15 and 25 cm.
Rx	**Sterile Talc Powder** (Bryan)	**Powder:** 5 g talc	In 100 mL glass bottle.

STERILE TALC POWDER

Indications

➤*Malignant pleural effusions:* Sterile talc powder, administered intrapleurally via chest tube, is indicated as a sclerosing agent to decrease the recurrence of malignant pleural effusions in symptomatic patients.

➤*Off-label uses:* Treatment of benign pleural effusions, pneumothorax, and malignant pericardial effusions.

Sterile talc has also been used safely and effectively in children. (See Administration and Dosage.)

Administration and Dosage

➤*General dosing considerations:* Sterile talc powder is administered after adequate drainage of the effusion. It has been suggested that success of the pleurodesis is related to the completeness of the drainage of the pleural fluid, as well as full reexpansion of the lung, both of which will promote symphysis of the pleural surfaces.

➤*Adults:*

Malignant pleural effusions –

Aerosol: 4 to 8 g (1 to 2 canisters) administered intrapleurally as a single dose.

Powder: 5 g dispersed in sodium chloride injection 50 to 100 mL as a single dose. Effective doses range from 2 to 10.5 g.

Off-label dosing –

Pericardial effusions: 1 to 2 g pericardially as a single dose.

➤*Preparation for administration:*

Aerosol container – Shake well.

Talc powder – Prepare the talc slurry using aseptic technique in an appropriate laminar flow hood. Remove talc container from packaging. Remove protective flip-off seal.

Each brown bottle contains 5 g of sterilized talc powder. To dispense the contents:

1.) Using a 16-gauge needle attached to a 60 mL *LuerLok* syringe, measure and draw up 50 mL of sodium chloride injection. Vent the talc bottle using a needle. Slowly inject the 50 mL of sodium chloride injection into the bottle. For doses more than 5 g, repeat this procedure with a second bottle.
2.) Swirl the bottle(s) to disperse the talc powder and continue swirling to avoid settling of the talc in the slurry. Each bottle will contain 5 g sterile talc powder dispersed in 50 mL of sodium chloride injection.
3.) Divide the content of each bottle into two 60 mL irrigation syringes by withdrawing 25 mL of the slurry into each syringe with continuous swirling. Fill each syringe with sodium chloride injection to a total volume of 50 mL in each syringe. Draw air into each syringe to the 60 mL mark to serve as a headspace for mixing prior to administration.
4.) When appropriately labeled, each syringe contains sterile talc 2.5 g in 50 mL of sodium chloride injection with an air headspace of 10 mL. Once the slurry has been made, use within 12 hours or discard and prepare fresh slurry. Label the syringes appropriately, noting the expiration date and time, the statement "For pleurodesis only, Not for IV administration," the identity of the patient intended to receive this material, and a cautionary statement to shake well before use.
5.) Prior to administration, completely and continuously agitate the syringes to evenly redisperse the talc and avoid settlement. Immediately prior to administration, vent the 10 mL air headspace from each syringe.
6.) Attach the adapter and place a syringe tip on the adapter. Maintain continuous agitation of the syringes.

Notice: Shake well before installation. Each 25 mL of prepared slurry in the syringe contains talc 1.25 g. Not for intravenous administration.

➤*Storage/Stability:* Store at 18° to 25°C (64.4° to 77°F). Protect against sunlight.

Aerosol container – Do not expose the aerosol to a temperature above 49°C (120°F), or the canister may rupture. Avoid freezing. Contents are under pressure. Do not puncture or incinerate the container.

Talc slurry – Once the slurry has been made, use within 12 hours or discard and prepare fresh slurry.

Actions

➤*Pharmacology:* The therapeutic action of talc instilled into the pleural cavity is believed to result from induction of an inflammatory reaction. This reaction promotes adherence of the visceral and parietal pleura, obliterating the pleural space and preventing reaccumulation of pleural fluid.

The extent of systemic absorption of talc after intrapleural administration has not been adequately studied. Systemic exposure could be affected by the integrity of the pleural surface, and therefore could be increased if talc is administered immediately following lung resection or biopsy.

Contraindications

None known.

Warnings/Precautions

➤*Future procedures:* The possibility of the future diagnostic and therapeutic procedures involving the hemithorax to be treated must be considered prior to administering sterile talc powder. Sclerosis of the pleural space may preclude subsequent diagnostic procedures of the pleura on the treated side. Talc sclerosis may complicate or preclude future ipsilateral lung resective surgery, including pneumonectomy for transplantation purposes.

➤*Use in potentially curable disease:* Talc has no known antineoplastic activity and should not be used alone for potentially curable malignancies where systemic therapy would be more appropriate (eg, a malignant effusion secondary to a potentially curable lymphoma).

➤*Pulmonary complications:* Acute pneumonitis and acute respiratory distress syndrome (ARDS) have been reported in association with intrapleural talc administration. Three of the case reports of ARDS have occurred after treatment with a relatively large talc dose (10 g) administered via intrapleural chest tube instillation. One patient died 1 month post treatment and 2 patients recovered without further sequelae.

➤*Pregnancy: Category B.* An oral administration study has been performed in the rabbit at 900 mg/kg. Approximately 5 fold higher than a human dose on mg/m^2 basis, and has revealed no evidence of teratogenicity due to talc. There are, however, no adequate and well-controlled studies in pregnant women. Because animal reproduction studies are not always predictive of human response, this drug should not be used during pregnancy unless the benefit outweighs the risk.

➤*Lactation:* There is no information regarding sterile talc powder in breast-feeding women.

➤*Children:* The safety and efficacy of sterile talc powder in pediatric patients have not been established.

Adverse Reactions

Intrathoracic administration of talc slurry has been described in medical literature reports involving more than 2,000 patients. Patients with malignant pleural effusions were treated with talc via poudrage or slurry. In general, with respect to reported adverse experiences, it is difficult to distinguish the effects of talc from the effects of the procedure(s) associated with its administration. The most often reported adverse experiences to intrapleurally administered talc were fever and pain.

➤*Cardiovascular:* Complications reported included tachycardia, myocardial infarction, hypotension, hypovolemia, and asystolic arrest.

➤*Respiratory:* Complications reported include hypoxemia, dyspnea, unilateral pulmonary edema, pneumonia, ARDS, bronchopleural fistula, hemoptysis and pulmonary emboli.

➤*Miscellaneous:*

Infection – Complications reported include empyema.

Delivery procedure – Adverse reactions due to the delivery procedure and the chest tube may include pain, infection at the site of thoracostomy or thoracoscopy, localized bleeding, and subcutaneous emphysema.

Chronic toxicity – Since patients in clinical studies had a limited life expectancy, data on chronic toxicity are limited.

Overdosage

No definite relationship between dose and toxicity has been established. Excessive talc may be partially removed with saline lavage.

The following is a list of available diagnostic aids for professional office use or for use by patients at home (when noted). Those tests requiring special equipment and used primarily by commercial laboratories are not included.

For complete information on specific uses, directions and characteristics of these products, consult the manufacturers' package literature.

ACETONE (Ketone) TESTS

To detect the presence of ketones.

Chemstrip K (Roche Diagnostic)	**Reagent strips** for urine tests	In 25s.
KetoCare (Home Diagnostics)	**Reagent strips** for urine tests	In 50s.

[a] For use by patient at home.

ALBUMIN TESTS

To detect the presence of protein.

Albustix (Siemens Medical)	**Reagent strips** for urine tests	In 100s.
Chemstrip Micral (Roche Diagnostic)	**Reagent strips** for urine tests	In 30s.

BACTERIURIA TESTS

To detect nitrate, nitrite, uropathogens, total bacterial or gram-negative bacterial counts.

Microstix-3 (Bayer Corp)	**Reagent strips** for urine tests	In test kits containing 25 reagent strips, 25 incubation pouches and 25 ID labels.
Uricult (LifeSign LLC)	**Culture paddles** for urine tests	In 10s.
Isocult for Bacteriuria (Remel)	**Culture paddles** for urine tests	In 12s.
UTI Urinary Tract Infection Urine Test Strips (Consumers Choice Systems)	**Test strips** for urine tests	In 6 strips and 6 cups.

BILIRUBIN TESTS

To detect the presence of bilirubin.

Ictotest (Bayer Corp)	**Reagent tablets** for urine tests	In 100s.

BLOOD UREA NITROGEN TESTS

To estimate amounts of urea nitrogen.

Azostix (Bayer Corp)	**Reagent strips** for whole blood tests	In 25s.

CANDIDA TESTS

To detect *Candida albicans*.

Isocult for *Candida* (Remel)	**Culture paddles** for vaginal specimen tests	In 4s.
CandidaSure (LifeSign LLC)	**Reagent slides** for vaginal specimen tests	In kits containing 20 slides.

CHLAMYDIA TRACHOMATIS TESTS

To detect and identify *Chlamydia trachomatis*.

Chlamydiazyme (Abbott)	**Reagent kit** for enzyme immunoassay	In kits containing 100 and 500 tests.
MicroTrak *Chlamydia Trachomatis* (Syva)	**Slide tests** for urogenital, rectal, conjunctival or nasopharyngeal specimens	In kits containing 60 tests.
Amplicor (Roche Diagnostics Systems)	**Reagent kit** for endocervical, male urethral and male urine specimens	In kits containing 10, 96 and 100 tests.
Sure Cell Chlamydia (Kodak)	**Reagent kit** for endocervical, urethral, male urine or ocular specimens	In kits containing 10, 25 and 100 tests.
Clearview Chlamydia (Wampole)	**Color-label immunoassay** for endocervical specimens	In 20s.

CHOLESTEROL TESTS

To estimate cholesterol levels. For use by patient at home.

Advanced Care Cholesterol Test (Johnson & Johnson)	**Cassette** for blood test	In kits containing test cassette, result chart, lancet, gauze pad, adhesive bandage, instruction booklet and question and answer booklet.

COLOR ALLERGY SCREENING TESTS

For determination of immunoglobulin E.

CAST (Biomerica)	**Reagent sticks** for serum tests	In kits containing reagent sticks for 25 tests.

CRYPTOCOCCAL ANTIGEN TESTS

For the qualitative or quantitative determination of *Cryptococcus neoformans* antigen.

Crypto-LA (Wampole)	**Slide tests** for CSF and serum	In 70s.

DRUGS OF ABUSE TESTS

For detecting drugs of abuse (marijuana, cocaine, amphetamine, methamphetamine, phencyclidine, codeine, morphine, and heroin).

otc	**Dr. Brown's Home Drug Testing System** (Personal Health and Hygiene)	**Collection kit**: 1 urine specimen collection kit	In 1s.

GASTROINTESTINAL TESTS

For determination of GI disorders.

Entero-Test (HDC Corp)	**String capsules** for collection of duodenal fluid	In packages containing 25 capsules, pH sticks and color charts.
Entero-Test Pediatric Capsules (HDC Corp)	**String capsules** for collection of duodenal fluid	In packages containing 25 capsules, pH sticks and color charts.
Gastro-Test (HDC Corp)	**String capsules** for collection of stomach acid	In packages containing 25 capsules, pH sticks and color charts.
Pathway Anti-c-KIT (9.7) Primary Antibody (Ventana[a])	**Kit** for detection of c-KIT protein in GI stromal tumors	In kits containing reagents. For use on *Ventana Automated Slide Stainers.*
Pyloriset (LifeSign LLC)	**Reagent kit** for serum test	In kits containing 20 latex reagents, positive and negative controls, dilution buffers, mixing sticks and test cards.

[a] Ventana Medical Systems, Inc., 1910 Innovation Park Drive, Tucson, AZ; (800) 227-2155.

BLOOD GLUCOSE METERS

Product & Distributor[a]	Compatible test strips	Alternate test sites	Required blood volume
Accu-Chek Active (Roche Diagnostic)	**Accu-Chek Active**	Yes	1 mcL
Accu-Chek Advantage (Roche Diagnostic)	**Accu-Chek Comfort Curve**	No	4 mcL
Accu-Chek Compact (Roche Diagnostic)[b]	**Accu-Chek Compact Test Drum**	Yes	1.5 mcL
Accu-Chek Complete (Roche Diagnostic)	**Accu-Chek Comfort Curve**	No	4 mcL
Accu-Chek Voicemate (Roche Diagnostic)[c]	**Accu-Chek Comfort Curve**	No	4 mcL
Ascensia BREEZE (Bayer HealthCare)[d]	**Ascensia AutoDisc**	Yes	2.5 to 3.5 mcL
Ascensia CONTOUR (Bayer HealthCare)	**Ascensia Microfil**	Yes	0.6 mcL
Ascensia DEX 2 (Bayer HealthCare)[d]	**Ascensia AutoDisc**	Yes	2.5 to 3.5 mcL
Ascensia ELITE (Bayer HealthCare)	**Ascensia ELITE**	Yes	2 mcL
Ascensia ELITE XL (Bayer HealthCare)	**Ascensia ELITE**	Yes	2 mcL
BD Logic (Becton, Dickinson and Company)	**BD**	No	0.3 mcL
FreeStyle (TheraSense)	**FreeStyle**	Yes	0.3 mcL
FreeStyle Flash (TheraSense)	**FreeStyle**	Yes	0.3 mcL
InDuo (Novo Nordisk Pharmaceuticals)[e]	**OneTouch Ultra**	Yes	1 mcL
OneTouch Basic (Lifescan)	**OneTouch**	No	10 mcL
OneTouch FastTake (Lifescan)[f]	**OneTouch FastTake**	Yes	1.5 mcL
OneTouch SureStep (Lifescan)	**OneTouch SureStep**	No	10 mcL
OneTouch Ultra (Lifescan)	**OneTouch Ultra**	Yes	1 mcL
OneTouch UltraSmart (Lifescan)	**OneTouch Ultra**	Yes	1 mcL
Precision Q·I·D (MediSense)	**Precision Q·I·D**	No	3.5 mcL
Precision Sof-Tact (MediSense)	**Precision Sof-Tact**	Yes	2 to 3 mcL
Precision Xtra (MediSense)[g]	**Precision Xtra**	No	3.5 mcL
Prestige IQ (Home Diagnostics)	**Prestige Smart System**	No	7 mcL
Prestige TrueTrack Smart System (Home Diagnostics)	**TrueTrack**	No	1 mcL

[a] Products listed are representative of currently available and widely distributed brands. Similar products, including regional and private label brands, may also exist.
[b] Uses drum instead of individual test strips.
[c] Audio features for people with visual impairments.
[d] Uses disc, not strips.
[e] Also an insulin delivery system.
[f] Available through mail order only.
[g] Also measures ketones.

GLUCOSE, BLOOD TESTS[a]

To determine blood glucose levels. For use by patient at home.

Accu-Chek Active (Roche Diagnostic)	**Reagent strips** for blood tests	In 10s, 25s, 50s, and 100s for use with *Accu-Chek Active* blood glucose meter.
Accu-Chek Comfort Curve (Roche Diagnostic)		In 10s and 50s for use with *Accu-Chek Advantage* and *Accu-Chek Complete* meters, and with the *AccuData GTS Plus/GTS, Accu-Chek HG*, and *Accu-Chek Inform Systems.*
Accu-Chek Compact (Roche Diagnostics)		In 17s/1 drum for use with *Accu-Chek Compact* blood glucose meter.
Accu-Chek Instant Glucose (Roche Diagnostic)		In 25s, 50s, and 100s for use with *Glucometer 3, Glucometer QA*, and *Glucometer M+* blood glucose meters.
Ascensia AutoDisc (Bayer HealthCare)		In 10 discs/100 test strips for use with *Ascensia Glucometer DEX 2, Ascensia Breeze*, and *Glucometer DEX* blood glucose meters.
Ascensia Elite (Bayer HealthCare)		In 25s , 50s, and 100s for use with *Ascensia Elite* and *Ascensia Elite XL* blood glucose meters.
Ascensia Microfil (Bayer HealthCare)		In 50s and 100s for use with *Ascensia CONTOUR* blood glucose meter.
BD Test Strips (Becton, Dickinson and Company)		In 50s for use with *BD Logic* and *BD Latitude* blood glucose monitoring systems.
Freestyle Test Strips (TheraSense)		In 25s, 50s, and 100s for use with *FreeStyle* and *Freestyle Flash* blood glucose meters.
OneTouch Test Strips (Lifescan)		In 25s, 50s, and 100s for use with *OneTouch Basic Meter, OneTouch Profile*, and *OneTouch II* blood glucose meters.
OneTouch Ultra Test Strips (Lifescan)		In 25s, 50s, and 100s for use with *OneTouch Ultra Brand, OneTouch Ultra Smart Brand*, and *InDuo Brand* blood glucose meters.
OneTouch FastTake Test Strips (Lifescan)		In 50s and 100s for use with *FastTake* blood glucose meter.
OneTouch SureStep Test Strips (Lifescan)		In 50s and 100s for use with *OneTouch SureStep* blood glucose meter.
Precision Q•I•D (MediSense)		For use with *Precision Q•I•D* blood glucose monitor, *Precision Q•I•D* pen, *MediSense 2* card and pen blood glucose monitors, and the *Companion 2* card and pen blood glucose monitors.
Precision Sof-Tact (MediSense)		For use with the *MediSense Precision Sof-Tact* and *MediSense Sof-Tact Diabetes Management System.*
Precision Xtra (MediSense)		For use with the *Precision Xtra* blood glucose meters.
Prestige Smart System (Home Diagnostics)		In 50s for use with products featuring the *Prestige IQ Smart System* logo.
True Track Test (Home Diagnostics)		In 50s and 100s for use with meters featuring the *True Track Smart System* logo.

[a] Products listed are representative of currently available and widely distributed brands. Similar products, including regional and private label brands, may also exist.

GONORRHEA TESTS

Used as a presumptive test for *Neisseria gonorrhoeae*.

Biocult-GC (Orion Diagnostica)	**Culture paddles** for endocervical, oropharyngeal, anterior urethra or anal cultures	In kits containing vials, CO_2-generating tablets, swabs, reagent and specimen ID labels.
Gonozyme Diagnostic (Abbott)	**Reagent kit** for urogenital swab specimens	In test kits containing reagent, reaction trays, assay tubes with identifying racks and cover seals for 100 tests.
LCx Assay (Abbott)	**Reagent kit** in endocervical, male urethral and urine swab specimens.	In kits containing swabs, vials and reagent for 100 tests.
Isocult for *Neisseria gonorrhoeae* (Remel)	**Culture paddles** for endocervical, rectal and urethral cultures	In test kits containing culture tubes, CO_2-generating tablets, reagent and information sheet for 12 tests.
MicroTrak *Neisseria gonorrhoeae* Culture Confirmation Test (Syva)	**Reagent kit** for endocervical, urethral, rectal, conjunctival and pharyngeal cultures	In test kits containing reagent, reconstitution diluent and mounting fluid for 85 tests.

H. PYLORI TESTS

For use in the detection of gastric urease as an aid in the diagnosis of *H. pylori* infection in the human stomach. The test utilizes a liquid scintillation counter for the measurement of $^{14}CO_2$ in breath samples.

PYtest (Tri-Med Specialties, Inc.)	**Capsules** 14c urea	Clear, gelatin. In UD packages of 1s, 10s, and 100s. In *PYtest Kit* containing a capsule and breath collection equipment.

HEMATOCRIT/HEMOGLOBIN TESTS

To determine hematocrit/hemoglobin measurement.

Stat-Crit (Wampole)	**Electrode device** for blood samples	In 120s for use with *STAT-CRIT* instrument kit.

HEMOGLOBIN, GLYCATED (HbA_{1c}) TESTS

In diabetes (Type 1 or 2) for the quantitative measurement of glycated hemoglobin levels.

A1cNow (Metrika)	**Kit** for blood samples	In 1-pack test kit with monitor, lancets, and dilution kit and in 10-pack professional use kits.
Choice DM (Bristol-Myers Squibb)		In 1 single-use test kit.

HUMAN IMMUNODEFICIENCY VIRUS (HIV) TESTS

For the detection of HIV.

HIVAB HIV-1 EIA (Abbott)	**Reagent kit** for serum or plasma tests	In kits containing reagents for 100 tests.
HIVAG-1 (Abbott)	**Reagent kit** for serum or plasma tests	In kits containing reagents for 100 tests.
Amplicor HIV-1 Monitor (Roche)	**Reagent kit** for plasma HIV-1 tests	In kits containing reagents for 24 tests.
OraQuick Advance Rapid HIV-1/2 Antibody Test (OraSure Technologies)	**In vitro immunoassay** for qualitative detection of antibodies to human immunodeficiency virus types 1 or 2 in oral fluid, whole blood, or plasma	In kits containing test device, absorbent packet, developer solution vial, test stands, and specimen collection loops for 25 or 100 tests.
HIVAB HIV-1/HIV-2 (rDNA) EIA (Abbott)	**In vitro enzyme immunoassay** for qualitative detection of antibodies to human immunodeficiency viruses type 1 or type 2 in human serum or plasma	In 100, 1,000, and 5,000 test kits.
OraSure (OraSure Technologies)[a]	**Reagent kit** for oral fluid tests	In kit containing collection pad, vial, and reagent for 1 test.
OraSure HIV-1 (OraSure Technologies)	**Collection kit** for oral specimen collection	In kit containing cotton fiber on stick with collection vial.

[a] For use by patient at home.

LANCET DEVICES

Product & Distributor[a]	Description
Ascensia MICROLET VACULANCE[b] (Bayer Diagnostic)	**Device**: 4 depth settings, vacuum action.
Ascensia MICROLET (Bayer Diagnostic)	**Device**: 5 depth settings, spring-loaded.
Accu-Chek SoftTouch (Roche Diagnostics)	**Device**: 5 depth settings, dial.
auto-Lancet (Palco Laboratories)	**Device**: 5 depth settings, dial.
auto-Lancet Mini (Palco Laboratories)	**Device**: 5 depth settings, dial.
BD Lancet Device (Becton, Dickinson and Company)	**Device**: 6 depth settings, spring-loaded.
OneTouch UltraSoft[b] (Lifescan)	**Device**: 7 depth settings, dial.
Penlet Plus (Lifescan)	**Device**: 7 depth settings, dial.
Autolet Impression[b] (Owen Mumford)	**Device**: 7 depth settings, dial, force adjustment.
Accu-Chek Softclix[b] (Roche Diagnostics)	**Device**: 11 depth settings (0.8 to 2.3 mm), spring-loaded, dial.
Accu-Chek Safe-T-Pro[c] (Roche Diagnostics)	**Device**: 1.8 mm; 21-gauge needle.
Unistik 2[c] (Owen Mumford)	**Device**: 2.4 and 3 mm; 26-gauge needle.
Vitalet Pro[c] (Medical Plastic Devices, Inc.)	**Device**: 2.4 and 3 mm.

[a] Products listed are representative of currently available and widely distributed brands. Similar products, including regional and private label brands, may also exist.
[b] Can be used on alternate test sites.
[c] Single-time use lancets

LANCET NEEDLES

Product & Distributor[a]	Description
BD Ultra-Fine 33 (Becton, Dickinson and Company)	**Needle**: 33-gauge
BD Ultra-Fine II (Becton, Dickinson and Company)	**Needle**: 30-gauge
Sunmark Super Thin Lancets (McKesson)	
Accu-Chek Softclix (Roche Diagnostic)	**Needle**: 28-gauge
Accu-Chek SoftTouch (Roche Diagnostic)	
Ascensia MICROLET (Bayer Diagnostics)	
Cleanlet (Gainor)	
EZ-Lets Thin (Palco Laboratories)	
Gentle-Let (general purpose) (Futura Medical Corporation)	
MediSense Thin Lancets (MediSense)	
OneTouch UltraSoft (Lifescan)	
Unilet ComforTouch (Boca Medical)	
Unilet GP Ultralite (Boca Medical)	
EZ-Lets Thin (Palco Laboratories)	**Needle**: 26-gauge
Gentle-Let (general purpose) (Futura Medical Corporation)	
Vitalet (Medical Plastic Devices, Inc.)	
Cleanlet (Gainor)	**Needle**: 25-gauge
OneTouch FinePoint (Lifescan)	
EZ-Lets (Palco Laboratories)	**Needle**: 23-gauge
Gentle-Let (general purpose) (Futura Medical Corporation)	
Gentle-Let (safety style) (Futura Medical Corporation)	
Unilet GP Superlite (Boca Medical)	
Unilet Superlite (Boca Medical)	
Vitalet (Medical Plastic Devices, Inc.)	
EZ-Lets (Palco Laboratories)	**Needle**: 21-gauge
Gentle-Let (general purpose) (Futura Medical Corporation)	
Gentle-Let (safety style) (Futura Medical Corporation)	
Unilet (Boca Medical)	
Unilet GP (Boca Medical)	

[a] Products listed are representative of currently available and widely distributed brands. Similar products, including regional and private label brands, may also exist.

MONONUCLEOSIS TESTS

For qualitative and quantitative identification of heterophilic antibodies for the diagnosis of infectious mononucleosis.

Mono-Diff (Wampole)	**Reagent kit** for serum or plasma tests	In kits containing reagent, absorbent I and II, positive control serum, calibrated capillary tubes and bulbs, disposable stirrers and disposable card slides for 20 tests.
Mono-Latex (Wampole)	**Reagent kit** for serum or plasma tests	In kits containing reagent latex, positive control, negative control, capillary tubes and bulbs, black glass slide and disposable stirrers for 20 and 50 tests.
Mono-Plus (Wampole)	**Reagent kit** for serum or plasma tests	In kits containing *micro-plus* test devices and *mono-plus* developer solution for 30 tests.
Monospot (Meridian Diagnostics)	**Slide test** for serum or plasma	In kits containing reagents I and II, indicator cells, positive and negative control serum, glass slide, microcapillary pipettes, rubber bulbs, plastic pipettes and wooden applicators for 20 tests.
Monosticon Dri-Dot (Organon Teknika)	**Slide test** for serum, plasma or whole blood tests	In kits containing test slides, positive and negative I.M. serum controls, dropper bottle and *dispenstirs* for 25 and 100 tests.
Mono-Test (Wampole)	**Slide test** for serum or plasma	In kits containing reagent, positive and negative control serums, calibrated capillary tubes and bulbs, glass slides, disposable stirrers and card slides for 40 and 100 tests.
Quantaffirm (Organon Teknika)	**Reagent kit** for serum tests	In test kits containing vials and reagent for 4 tests.

OCCULT BLOOD SCREENING TESTS

To detect occult blood.

ColoCare (Helena Labs)[a]	**Kit** for fecal specimens	In kits containing 3 tests.
ColoScreen (Helena Labs)	**Slide tests** for fecal specimens	In kits containing slides, monitors, tape, developer, specimen applicators and mailing envelopes for 100 tests.
EZ Detect (Biomerica)[a]	**Kit** for fecal specimens	In kits containing 5 test tissues, control and control card for 48 tests.
Hemoccult II Dispensapak (SmithKline Diagnostics)[a]	**Slide tests** for fecal specimens	In kits containing slides, applicators and developer for 100 tests.
Hemoccult II Dispensapak Plus (SmithKline Diagnostics)[a]	**Slide tests** for fecal specimens	In kits containing slides, sample collection tissues, applicators and mailing pouch for 40 tests.
Hemoccult II (SmithKline Diagnostics)	**Slide tests** for fecal specimens	In kits containing developer and applicators for 102 and 1020 tests.
Hemoccult Slides (SmithKline Diagnostics)	**Slide tests** for fecal specimens	In kits containing developer and applicators for 100 and 1000 tests.
Hemoccult Tape (SmithKline Diagnostics)	**Tape** for fecal specimens	In kits containing tape dispenser and developer for 100 tests.
Hemoccult SENSA (SmithKline Diagnostics)	**Slide tests** for fecal specimens	In 100s and 1000s with developer and applicators.
Hemoccult II SENSA (SmithKline Diagnostics)	**Slide tests** for fecal specimens	In kits containing slides, tissues, applicators and mailing pouches for 40 tests.
HemeSelect Reagent (SmithKline Diagnostics)	**Reagent kit** for fecal specimens	In kits containing vials, diluent, Hb positive control, microtiter plate and droppers for 40 tests. *For use with HemeSelect Sample Collection Kit.*
HemeSelect Collection (SmithKline Diagnostics)[a]	**Collection kit** for fecal specimens	In kits containing sample collection card, applicator, self-sealing sample bag and instructions. *For use with the HemeSelect Reagent Kit.*
Hema-Chek (Bayer Corp)[a]	**Slide tests** for fecal specimens	In kits containing slide pak, developer, control and applicator sticks for 100 and 300 tests.
Hematest (Bayer Corp)	**Reagent tablets** for fecal specimens	In packages containing reagent tablets and filter paper for 100 tests.
Hemastix (Siemens)	**Reagent strips** for urine specimens	In 50s.
Gastroccult (SmithKline Diagnostics)	**Slide tests** for gastric specimens	In kits containing slides, developer and applicators for 40 tests.

[a] For use by patient at home.

OVULATION TESTS

To measure luteinizing hormone for prediction of ovulation.

Answer Ovulation (Carter Wallace)[a]	**Kit** for urine tests	In kits containing test sticks for 5 tests.
First Response Ovulation Predictor (Carter Wallace)[a]	**Kit** for urine tests	In kits containing test sticks for 5 tests.
Clearblue Easy (Unipath Diagnostic)[a]	**Kit** for urine tests	In kits containing test sticks for 7 tests.

[a] For use by patient at home.

PREGNANCY TESTS

To detect the presence of human chorionic gonadotropin.

Advance (Ortho)[a]	**Stick** for urine test	In 1s.
Answer One-Step Pregnancy Test (Carter Wallace)[a]	**Stick** for urine test	In 1s.
Answer Plus (Carter Wallace)[a]	**Kit** for urine test	In kits containing urine collection cup, filter dropper, vial, test well, test tray and tube for 1 test.
Answer Quick & Simple (Carter Wallace)[a]	**Kit** for urine test	In kits containing dropper, tube and color key for 2 tests.
Conceive Pregnancy (Quidel)[a]	**Kit** for urine test	In kits containing tape cassette, dropper, plastic cup for 1 and 2 tests.
Clearblue Easy (Whitehall)[a]	**Stick** for urine test	In 1s.
e.p.t. Quick Stick (Parke-Davis)[a]	**Stick** for urine test	In 1s.
Fact Plus (Ortho)[a]	**Kit** for urine test	In kits containing test disk, urine collection cup and urine dropper.
First Response (Carter Wallace)[a]	**Stick** for urine test	In 1s.
Fortel Midstream (Biomerica)	**Stick** for urine test	In 1s.
Fortel Plus (Biomerica)[a]	**Kit** for urine test	In kits containing urine collection cup, test device, dropper and absorbent packet.
Midstream Pregnancy Test Kit (Goldline)	**Kit** for urine test	In 1s.

PREGNANCY TESTS

Pregnosis (Roche)[a]	**Slide tests** for urine	In kits containing reagents, droppers, pipettes, applicator stick and slide for 50 and 200 tests.
Nimbus Quick Strip (Biomerica)[a]	**Test strips** for urine	In 25s.
RapidVue (Quidel)[a]	**Kit** for urine test	In kits containing cup, dropper and test cassette.
QTest (Quidel)[a]	**Stick** for urine test	In kits containing vial, test stick, reagent, developer and solution for 1 test.
UCG Slide (Wampole)	**Slide tests** for urine	In kits containing latex reagent, antibody reagent, slide stirrers and plastic cup for 30, 100, 300 and 1000 tests.
Abbott TestPack hCG-Urine Plus (Abbott)	**Kit** for urine test	In kits containing reaction dish and transfer pipette. In 20s.
Nimbus (Biomerica)	**Kit** for urine test	In kits containing tube, conjugate and pipettes for 25, 50 and 100 tests.
Nimbus Plus (Biomerica)	**Kit** for urine test	In kits containing test devices and droppers for 25 tests.
Unistep hCG (Orion Diagnostica)	**Kit** for urine test	In kits containing hCG reaction packs and droppers for 25 and 50 tests.
QuickVue (Quidel)	**Cassettes** for urine test	In kits containing test cassettes and pipettes 25 and 75 tests.
SureCell Pregnancy (Kodak)	**Kit** for urine test	In kits containing reagents for 10, 25 and 100 tests.
SureCell hCG-Urine Test (Kodak)	**Kit** for urine test	In 10s, 25s and 100s.
UCG Beta-Slide Monoclonal II (Wampole)	**Slide tests** for urine	In kits containing slide test and reagent for 50, 100 and 300 tests.

[a] For use by patient at home.

RHEUMATOID FACTOR TEST

To detect rheumatoid factor in blood.

Rheumatex (Wampole)	**Slide tests** for blood	In kits containing reagents and slides for 100 and 200 tests.
Rheumaton (Wampole)	**Slide tests** for serum or synovial fluid	In kits containing reagent, positive and negative control, tubes, bulbs and slides for 20, 50 and 150 tests.

SICKLE CELL TEST

To detect hemoglobin S.

Sickledex (Ortho)	**Kit** for blood tests	In kits containing reagents and solution for 12 and 100 tests.

STAPHYLOCOCCUS TEST

To determine the presence of *Staphylococcus aureus*.

Isocult for *Staphylococcus aureus* (Remel)	**Culture paddles** for exudate	In kits containing reagents for 12 tests.

STREPTOCOCCI TESTS

To detect beta-hemolytic group A streptococci, group B streptococci, streptococcal pharyngitis, antibodies to DNase-B, *Streptococcus pneumoniae* and streptococcal extracellular antigens.

Sure Cell Streptococci (Kodak)	**Kit** for the detection of group A streptococcal antigen from throat swabs and blood	In kits containing test cells, extraction blocks, reagents, dye solutions, filter and swabs for 25 and 100 tests.
Culturette 10 Minute Group A Strep ID (Becton Dickinson)	**Slide test** for the detection of group A streptococcal antigen from throat swabs	In kits containing reagents and test slides for 55 and 200 tests.
Isocult for *Streptococcal pharyngitis* (Remel)	**Culture paddles** for the detection of streptococcal pharyngitis from throat swabs	In kits culture paddles and reagents for 12 tests.
Respiracult-Strep (LifeSign LLC)	**Culture paddles** for the detection of group A beta-hemolytic streptococci from throat and nasopharyngeal sources	In kits containing reagents and culture paddles for 25 and 50 tests.
Streptonase-B (Wampole)	**Kit** for the detection of antibodies to DNase-B in serum	In kits containing reagents and tubes for 10 tests.
Test Pack (Abbott)	**Kit** for the detection of group A streptococci from throat specimens	In kits containing reagents, extraction tubes and swabs for 40 and 80 tests.
Bactigen B Streptococcus-CS (Wampole)	**Slide tests** for the detection of group B streptococcus antigen from vaginal and cervical swabs	In kits containing reagents, slides, droppers and stirrers for 48 tests.
Streptozyme (Wampole)	**Slide tests** for the detection of streptococcal extracellular antigens in blood, plasma and serum	In kits containing reagents, tubes, positive and negative control serum, bulbs and slides for 15, 50 and 150 tests.
Detect-A-Strep (Antibodies Inc.)	**Slide tests** for the detection of streptococcal antigen from throat swabs	In kits containing reagents and test plates for 6 tests.

TOXOPLASMOSIS TEST

To detect the presence of *Toxoplasma gondii* in blood.

TPM Test (Wampole)	**Kit** for blood test	In kits including reagents for 120 tests.

VIRUS TESTS

To detect human T-Lymphotropic type 1, HSV-1, HSV-2, herpes, rotavirus, rubella and C-reactive protein.

Human T-Lymphotropic Virus Type I EIA (Abbott)	**Reagent kit** for serum or plasma tests	In kits containing reagents, vials and reaction trays for 100 tests.
MicroTrak HSV 1/HSV 2 Culture Identification/Typing Test (Syva)	**Culture test** for tissue	1 test per kit.
MicroTrak HSV1/HSV2 Direct Specimen Identification/Typing Test (Syva)	**Slide test** for external lesions	In kits containing reagent for 60 tests.
Sure Cell Herpes (Kodak)	**Reagent kit** for genital, rectal, oral or dermal swabs	In 10s and 25s.
Rubazyme for Rubella (Abbott)	**Reagent kit** for serum test	In kits containing reagents and diluent for 1 and 5 tests.

VIRUS TESTS

Virogen Herpes (Wampole)	**Slide test** for the detection of herpes simplex virus antigens directly from lesions or cell culture	In kits containing reagents, stirrers, slides and slide covers for 100 tests.
Virogen Rotatest for Rotavirus (Wampole)	**Slide test** for fecal specimens	In kits containing reagents, extraction buffer and slides for 50 tests.
Immunex C-Reactive Protein (Wampole)	**Kit** for blood tests	In kits containing reagents and slides for 100 tests.
Impact Rubella (Wampole)	**Slide test** for serum	In kits containing reagents and slides for 100, 500 and 5000 tests.

COMBINATION TESTS

To detect a multiplicity of conditions, including *Haemophilus influenzae* type b, *Neisseria meningitidis* serogroups A/B/C/Y/W135, *Streptococcus pneumoniae, Salmonella, Shigella, N. gonorrhoeae, T. vaginalis* and Candida.

Bactigen Meningitis Panel (Wampole)	**Slide test** for cerebrospinal fluid, serum, urine and blood	In 54s.
Bactigen *Salmonella-Shigella* (Wampole)	**Slide test** for cultures	In kits containing reagents, dispenser cannulae, droppers, slides and stirrers for 96 tests.
Isocult for *N. gonorrhoeae and Candida* (Remel)	**Culture test** for endocervical rectal, urethral, pharyngeal and vaginal specimens	In 12s.
Isocult for *T. vaginalis* and *Candida* (Remel)	**Culture test** for vaginal and urethral cultures	In kits containing culture tubes and reagents for 12 tests.

SODIUM AND pH URINE TEST

Used for the quantitative detection of Na and pH in urine and for the qualitative detection of bladder tumor associated antigen in urine.

BTA stat Test (Polymedco, Inc.)	**Kit** for bladder cancer test	In kits containing 30 foil packages with a BTA stat device, disposable dropper, and disposable desiccant pouch.

MULTIPLE URINE TEST PRODUCTS

To make simultaneous determinations of two or more urine tests.

Product & Distributor	Glucose	Protein	pH	Blood	Ketones	Bilirubin	Urobilinogen	Nitrite	Leukocytes	How Supplied
Chemstrip 2 GP (Roche Diagnostic)	X	X								In 100s.
Uristix (Siemens Medical)	X	X								In 100s.
Combistix (Siemens Medical)	X	X	X							In 100s.
Hema-Combistix (Siemens Medical)	X	X	X	X						In 100s.
Uristix 4 (Bayer Corp)	X	X						X	X	In 100s.
Chemstrip uGK (Roche Diagnostic)	X				X					In 50s.
Labstix (Siemens Medical)	X	X	X	X	X					In 100s.
Chemstrip 7 (Roche Diagnostic)	X	X	X	X	X	X			X	In 100s.
Multistix (Siemens Medical)	X	X	X	X	X	X	X			In 100s.
Multistix 7 (Siemens Medical)	X	X	X	X	X			X	X	In 100s.
Multistix 8 SG[a] (Siemens Medical)	X	X	X	X	X			X	X	In 100s.
Multistix 9 SG[a] (Siemens Medical)	X	X	X	X	X	X		X	X	In 100s.
Multistix 10 SG[a] (Siemens Medical)	X	X	X	X	X	X	X	X	X	In 100s.
Chemstrip 10 With SG[a] (Roche Diagnostic)	X	X	X	X	X	X	X	X	X	In 100s.
Chemstrip 9 (Roche Diagnostic)	X	X	X	X	X	X	X	X	X	In 100s.
Multistix 9 (Siemens Medical)	X	X	X	X	X	X	X	X	X	In 100s.
Chemstrip 2 LN (Roche Diagnostic)								X	X	In 100s.
Multistix 2 (Siemens Medical)								X	X	In 100s.

[a] Also tests specific gravity.

IN VIVO DIAGNOSTIC AIDS

The following is a list of available diagnostic aids for professional office use or for use by patients at home (when noted). Those tests requiring special equipment and used primarily by commercial laboratories are not included. For complete information on specific uses, directions and characteristics of these products, consult the manufacturers' package literature.

AMINOHIPPURATE SODIUM (PAH)

For the estimation of renal plasma flow and to measure the functional capacity of the renal tubular secretory mechanism.

Rx	**Aminohippurate Sodium** (Merck)	**Injection:** 20% aqueous solution	In 10 ml vials.

INDIGOTINDISULFONATE SODIUM

For localizing ureteral orifices during cystoscopy and ureteral catheterization.

Rx	**Indigo Carmine** (Akorn)	**Injection, solution:** 0.8% aqueous solution	In 5 mL amps.

INDOCYANINE GREEN

Rx	**IC-Green** (Akorn)	**Powder for injection:** 25 mg	In vials with 10 mL amps of aqueous solvent. In 6s.
Rx	**Indocyanine Green** (HUB)	**Injection, lyophilized powder for solution:** 25 mg	≤ 5% sodium iodide. In kits containing 30 mL vials and sterile water for injection.

INULIN

For measurement of glomerular filtration rate (GFR).

Rx	**Inulin Injection** (Iso-Tex Diagnostics)	**Injection:** 100 mg per mL	In 50 mL vials.[a]

[a] With 0.9% Sodium Chloride in Water for Injection.

MANNITOL

See the Mannitol monograph in the Renal and Genitourinary Agents chapter.

Thyroid Function Tests

SODIUM IODIDE I 123

Rx	**Sodium Iodide I-123** (Mallinckrodt Medical)	**Capsules:** 3.7 MBq	Sucrose. Red/white. In 1s, 3s, and 5s.
		7.4 MBq	Sucrose. Green/white. In 1s, 3s, and 5s.

SODIUM IODIDE I 123 — ORAL

Indications

➤*Thyroid function studies:* As a diagnostic procedure in evaluating thyroid function or morphology.

Administration and Dosage

➤*General dosing considerations:* The contents of the vial are radioactive and adequate shielding and handling precautions must be maintained (see Storage/Stability).

The determination of I-123 concentration in the thyroid gland may be initiated at 6 hours after administering the dose and should be measured in accordance with standardized procedures.

➤*Adults:*

Thyroid function studies –

Usual dosage: 3.7 to 14.8 MBq (100 to 400 microcuries). The lower part of the dosage range, 3.7 MBq (100 microcuries), is recommended for uptake studies alone, and the higher part, 14.8 MBq (400 microcuries), for thyroid imaging.

Maximum dose: 14.8 MBq (400 microcuries).

➤*Preparation for administration:* The patient dose should be measured by a suitable radioactivity calibration system immediately prior to administration. The capsules can be utilized up to 30 hours after calibration time and date. Thereafter, discard the capsules in accordance with standard safety procedures. The user should wear waterproof gloves at all times when handling the capsules or container.

➤*Administration:* The prescribed dose should be administered as soon as practical from the time of receipt of product (ie, as close to calibration time as possible) in order to minimize the fraction of radiation exposure due to the relative increase of radionuclidic contaminants with time.

➤*Storage/Stability:* Store at 20° to 25°C (68° to 77°F). The capsules can be utilized up to 30 hours after calibration time and date. Dispense and preserve capsules in tightly closed containers that are adequately shielded. Storage and disposal should be controlled in a manner that is in compliance with the appropriate regulations of the government agency authorized to license the use of this radionuclide.

Handling – Handle with care; appropriate safety measures should be used to minimize radiation exposure to clinical personnel. Care should also be taken to minimize radiation exposure to the patient consistent with proper patient management.

Actions

➤*Pharmacokinetics:*

Absorption/Distribution – Sodium iodide I-123 is readily absorbed from the upper GI tract. Following absorption, the iodide is distributed primarily within the extracellular fluid of the body.

The fraction of the administered dose which is accumulated in the thyroid gland may be a measure of thyroid function in the absence of unusually high or low iodine intake or administration of certain drugs which influence iodine accumulation by the thyroid gland. Accordingly, the patient should be questioned carefully regarding previous medications or procedures involving radiographic media. Healthy subjects can accumulate approximately 10% to 50% of the administered iodine dose in the thyroid gland, however, the normal and abnormal ranges are established by individual physician's criteria. The mapping (imaging) of sodium iodide I-123 distribution in the thyroid gland may provide useful information concerning thyroid anatomy and definition of normal or abnormal functioning of tissue within the gland.

Excretion – Sodium iodide I-123 is trapped and organically bound by the thyroid and concentrated by the stomach, choroid plexus and salivary glands. It is excreted by the kidneys.

Contraindications

No known contraindications.

Warnings/Precautions

➤*Radioactivity:* The contents of the capsule are radioactive. Adequate shielding of the preparation must be maintained at all times.

➤*Administration:* The prescribed sodium iodide I-123 dose should be administered as soon as practical from the time of receipt of product (ie, as close to calibration time as possible), in order to minimize the fraction of radiation exposure due to the relative increase of radionuclidic contaminants with time.

➤*Handle with care:* Sodium iodide I-123, as well as other radioactive drugs, must be handled with care and appropriate safety measures should be used to minimize radiation exposure to clinical personnel. Care should also be taken to minimize radiation exposure to the patient consistent with proper patient management.

Radiopharmaceuticals should be used only by physicians who are qualified by training and experience in the safe use and handling of radionuclides, and whose experience and training have been approved by the appropriate government agency authorized to license the use of radionuclides.

➤*Pregnancy: Category C.* Animal reproduction studies have not been conducted with this drug. It is also not known whether sodium iodide I-123 can cause fetal harm when administered to a pregnant woman or can affect reproductive capacity. Sodium iodide I-123 should be given to a pregnant woman only if clearly needed.

Ideally, examinations using radiopharmaceuticals, especially those elective in nature, in women of childbearing capability should be performed during the first few (approximately 10) days following the onset of menses.

➤*Lactation:* Since I-123 is excreted in human milk, formula feeding should be substituted for breastfeeding if the agent must be administered to the mother during lactation.

➤*Children:* Safety and efficacy in pediatric patients have not been established.

Adverse Reactions

Although rare, reactions associated with the administration of sodium iodide isotopes for diagnostic use include, in decreasing order of frequency, nausea, vomiting, chest pain, tachycardia, itching skin, rash and hives.

THYROTROPIN ALFA

Rx	**Thyrogen** (Genzyme)	**Injection, lyophilized powder for solution:** 1.1 mg (4 to 12 units/mg)	Kits of 2 or 4 vials.[a]

[a] Two-vial kit contains 2 vials of thyrotropin alfa 1.1 mg; 4-vial kit contains 2 vials of thyrotropin alfa 1.1 mg and two 10 mL vials of sterile water for injection. Each thyrotropin alfa vial also contains mannitol 36 mg, sodium phosphate 5.1 mg, and sodium chloride 2.4 mg.

THYROTROPIN ALFA — INJECTION

Indications

➤*Adjunctive diagnostic tool for serum thyroglobulin (Tg) testing:* For use as an adjunctive diagnostic tool for serum Tg testing with or without radioiodine imaging in the follow-up of patients with well-differentiated thyroid cancer.

➤*Adjunctive treatment for radioiodine ablation of thyroid tissue remnants:* For use as an adjunctive treatment for radioiodine ablation of thyroid tissue remnants in patients who have undergone a near-total or total thyroidectomy for well-differentiated thyroid cancer and who do not have evidence of metastatic thyroid cancer.

➤*Potential clinical uses:* May be used in patients with an undetectable Tg on thyroid hormone suppressive therapy to exclude the diagnosis of residual or recurrent thyroid cancer.

May be used in combination with radioiodine (iodine-131 [^{131}I]) to ablate thyroid remnants following near-total thyroidectomy in patients without evidence of metastatic disease.

May be used in patients requiring serum Tg testing and radioiodine imaging who are unwilling to undergo thyroid hormone withdrawal testing and whose treating physician believes that use of a less sensitive test is justified.

May be used in patients who are either unable to mount an adequate endogenous thyroid-stimulating hormone response to thyroid hormone withdrawal or in whom withdrawal is medically contraindicated.

Administration and Dosage

➤*General dosing considerations:* Pretreatment with glucocorticoids may be needed. (See Concomitant Therapy).

THYROTROPIN ALFA — INJECTION

➤*Adults:*

Diagnostic tool for serum Tg testing – 0.9 mg (1 mL) intramuscularly (IM) into the buttock, followed by a second 0.9 mg (1 mL) IM injection 24 hours later. The serum sample should be obtained 72 hours after the final injection of thyrotropin alfa.

Adjunctive treatment to radioiodine –

Usual dosage: 0.9 mg (1 mL) IM into the buttock followed by a second 0.9 mg (1 mL) IM injection 24 hours later.

Radioiodine: The activity of ^{131}I is carefully selected at the discretion of the nuclear medicine physician. Studies were conducted using 100 mCi ± 10% of ^{131}I. Radioiodine should be given 24 hours following the final thyrotropin alfa injection. Diagnostic scanning should be performed 48 hours after radioiodine administration, whereas posttherapy scanning may be delayed additional days to allow background activity to decline.

The following parameters utilized in the second phase 3 study are recommended for diagnostic radioiodine scanning with thyrotropin alfa: A diagnostic activity of 4 mCi (148 MBq) ^{131}I should be used. Whole body images should be acquired for a minimum of 30 minutes and/or should contain a minimum of 140,000 counts. Scanning times for single (spot) images of body regions should be 10 to 15 minutes or less if the minimum number of counts is reached sooner (60,000 counts for a large field of view camera, 35,000 counts for a small field of view).

➤*Concomitant therapy:* It is recommended that pretreatment with glucocorticoids be considered for patients in whom local tumor expansion may compromise vital anatomic structures (such as trachea, CNS, or extensive macroscopic lung metastases).

➤*Preparation for administration:* The powder should be reconstituted immediately prior to use with 1.2 mL of sterile water for injection (for a final concentration of 0.9 mg/mL). Discard unused portion of the diluent.

➤*Administration:* Administer IM into the buttock; it should not be administered intravenously (IV).

➤*Storage/Stability:* Store at 2° to 8°C (36° to 46°F). If necessary, the reconstituted solution can be stored for up to 24 hours between 2° and 8°C (36° and 46°F). Protect from light.

Actions

➤*Pharmacology:* Thyrotropin alfa (recombinant human thyroid stimulating hormone) is a heterodimeric glycoprotein produced by recombinant DNA technology. It has comparable biochemical properties to the human pituitary thyroid-stimulating hormone. Binding of thyrotropin alfa to thyroid-stimulating hormone receptors on normal thyroid epithelial cells or on well-differentiated thyroid cancer tissue stimulates iodine uptake and organification, and synthesis and secretion of Tg, triiodothyronine (T_3), and thyroxine (T_4).

In patients with thyroid cancer, a near-total or total thyroidectomy is usually performed. Thyroidectomy is usually followed by radioiodine treatment to remove any remnant of normal thyroid tissue and microscopic residues of malignant tissue. Prior to radioiodine remnant ablation, serum thyroid-stimulating hormone elevation is necessary to promote uptake of radioiodine by thyroid cells or thyroid cancer cells. Elevation of thyroid-stimulating hormone may be achieved by withholding synthetic thyroid hormone medication after thyroidectomy, with subsequent rise of endogenous pituitary thyroid stimulating hormone; or by administration of thyrotropin in the setting of synthetic thyroid hormone administration. After remnant ablation, patients are placed on synthetic thyroid hormone supplements to replace endogenous hormone and to suppress serum levels of thyroid-stimulating hormone in order to avoid thyroid-stimulating hormone tumor growth. Thereafter, patients are followed for the presence of remnants or of residual or recurrent cancer by Tg testing, usually with radioiodine imaging. This follow-up testing is most effective when conducted under thyroid-stimulating hormone stimulation, achieved either by thyroid hormone withdrawal or administration of thyrotropin. Thyroid hormone withdrawal results in hypothyroidism with subsequent elevation of endogenous pituitary thyroid-stimulating hormone; when thyrotropin is used, patients remain on thyroid hormone suppressive therapy and are euthyroid.

➤*Pharmacokinetics:*

Absorption/Distribution – The pharmacokinetics of thyrotropin alfa were studied in 16 patients with well-differentiated thyroid cancer given a single 0.9 mg IM dose. Mean peak concentrations of 116 ± 38 milliunits/L were reached between 3 and 24 hours after injection (median of 10 hours).

Metabolism/Excretion – The mean apparent elimination half-life was 25 ± 10 hours. The organ(s) of thyroid-stimulating hormone clearance in humans have not been identified, but studies of pituitary-derived thyroid-stimulating hormone suggest the involvement of the liver and kidneys.

Contraindications

None known.

Warnings/Precautions

➤*Use:* The use of thyrotropin alfa should be directed by health care providers knowledgeable in the management of patients with thyroid cancer.

➤*Administration:* Administer thyrotropin alfa IM; do not administer IV.

➤*Reports of death:* See Adverse Reactions for more information.

➤*Pretreatment with glucocorticoids:* It is recommended that pretreatment with glucocorticoids be considered for patients in whom local tumor expansion may compromise vital anatomic structures (such as trachea, CNS, or extensive macroscopic lung metastases).

➤*Antibodies:* Tg antibodies may confound the Tg assay and render Tg levels uninterpretable. Therefore, in such cases, even with a negative or low-stage thyrotropin alfa radioiodine scan, consider evaluating patients further with a confirmatory thyroid hormone withdrawal scan to determine the location and extent of thyroid cancer.

Thyroid-stimulating hormone antibodies have not been reported in patients treated with thyrotropin alfa in clinical trials, although only 27 patients received thyrotropin alfa on more than one occasion.

➤*Previous treatment with bovine thyroid-stimulating hormone:* Exercise caution when thyrotropin alfa is administered to patients who have been previously treated with bovine thyroid-stimulating hormone and, in particular, to those patients who have experienced hypersensitivity reactions to bovine thyroid-stimulating hormone.

➤*Renal function impairment:* Elimination of thyrotropin alfa is significantly slower in dialysis-dependent end-stage renal disease (ESRD) patients, resulting in prolonged elevation of thyroid-stimulating hormone levels. ESRD patients who receive thyrotropin alfa may have markedly elevated thyroid-stimulating hormone levels for several days after treatment, which may lead to increased risk of headache and nausea.

➤*Special risk:* Thyrotropin alfa is known to cause a transient but significant rise in serum thyroid hormone concentration when given to patients who have substantial thyroid tissue still in situ. Therefore, exercise caution in patients with a known history of heart disease and with significant residual thyroid tissue.

➤*Pregnancy: Category C.* It is not known whether thyrotropin alfa can cause fetal harm when administered to a pregnant woman or can affect reproductive capacity. However, placental transfer does not occur with thyrotropin. Give thyrotropin alfa to a pregnant woman only if clearly needed.

➤*Lactation:* It is not known whether the drug is excreted in human milk. Because many drugs are excreted in human milk, exercise caution when administering thyrotropin alfa to a breast-feeding woman.

➤*Children:* Safety and efficacy in pediatric patients younger than 16 years of age have not been established.

➤*Elderly:* Results from controlled trials indicate no difference in the safety and efficacy of thyrotropin alfa between patients younger than 65 years of age and those older than 65 years of age.

Carefully assess benefit-risk relationships for high-risk elderly patients with functioning thyroid tumors undergoing thyrotropin alfa administration. This may result in palpitations or cardiac rhythm disorder.

Drug Interactions

None known.

Adverse Reactions

The most common adverse reactions (more than 5%) reported in clinical trials were nausea (11.9%) and headache (7.3%). Reactions reported in at least 1% of patients in the combined trials are summarized in the following table. In some studies, an individual patient may have participated in both the euthyroid phase (thyrotropin alfa) and hypothyroid phase (withdrawal).

Thyrotropin Alfa Adverse Reactions (≥ 1%)		
Adverse reaction	Euthyroid phase (n = 481)	Hypothyroid phase (n = 418)
CNS		
Dizziness	2.5%	0%
Headache	7.3%	1.2%
Insomnia	1.5%	0%
Paresthesia	1.7%	0%
GI		
Diarrhea	1.2%	0%
Nausea	11.9%	3.1%
Vomiting	2.9%	0.7%
Metabolic		
Blood cholesterol abnormal	0%	1.4%
Hypercholesterolemia	0%	3.1%
Miscellaneous		
Asthenia	1.5%	0%
Fatigue	3.3%	1%
Nasopharyngitis	1%	0%
Thyroglobulin present	1%	0%

➤*Hypersensitivity:* Very rare manifestations of hypersensitivity to thyrotropin alfa have been reported in clinical trials, postmarketing settings, and in a special treatment program involving patients with advanced disease; these are flushing, pruritus, rash, respiratory signs and symptoms, and urticaria.

➤*Miscellaneous:* Four patients out of 55 (7.3%) with CNS metastases who were followed in a special treatment protocol experienced acute hemiplegia, hemiparesis, or pain 1 to 3 days after thyrotropin alfa administration. The symptoms were attributed to local edema and/or focal hemorrhage at the site of the cerebral or spinal cord metastases. In addition, 1 case each of acute visual loss and of laryngeal edema with respiratory distress (requiring

THYROTROPIN ALFA — INJECTION

tracheotomy) with onset of symptoms within 24 hours after thyrotropin alfa administration, have been reported in patients with metastases to the optic nerve and paratracheal areas, respectively. In addition, sudden rapid and painful enlargement of locally recurring papillary carcinoma has been reported within 12 to 48 hours of thyrotropin alfa administration. The enlargement was accompanied by dyspnea, stridor, or dysphonia. Rapid clinical improvement occurred following glucocorticoid therapy. It is recommended that pretreatment with glucocorticoids be considered for patients in whom local tumor expansion may compromise vital anatomic structures.

There have been reports of death in which events leading to death occurred within 24 hours after administration of thyrotropin alfa. A 77-year-old non-thyroidectomized patient with a history of heart disease and spinal metastases who received 4 thyrotropin alfa injections over 6 days in a special treatment protocol experienced a fatal MI 24 hours after he received the last thyrotropin alfa injection. The event was likely related to thyrotropin alfa–induced hyperthyroidism. In postmarketing experience, there have been rare reports of events leading to death that occurred within 24 hours of administration of thyrotropin alfa in patients with multiple serious medical problems. For patients for whom thyrotropin alfa–induced hyperthyroidism could have serious consequences, consider hospitalization for administration of thyrotropin alfa and postadministration observation. Such patients might include those with known heart disease, extensive metastatic disease, or other known serious underlying illness.

➤*Postmarketing:* Transient (less than 48 hours) influenza-like symptoms (also called flu-like symptoms), which may include fever (more than 100°F [38°C]), chills/shivering, myalgia/arthralgia, fatigue/asthenia/malaise, headache (nonfocal), and chills.

Postmarketing data include cases of atrial arrhythmias in elderly patients with preexisting cardiac disease who received thyrotropin alfa and suggest that use of thyrotropin alfa in this group be considered carefully.

Overdosage

➤*Symptoms:* There has been no reported experience of overdose in humans. However, in clinical trials, 3 patients experienced symptoms after receiving thyrotropin alfa doses higher than those recommended. Two patients had nausea after a 2.7 mg IM dose, and in 1 of these patients, the event was accompanied by weakness, dizziness, and headache. Another patient experienced nausea, vomiting, and hot flashes after a 3.6 mg IM dose.

In addition, 1 patient experienced symptoms after receiving thyrotropin alfa IV. This patient received thyrotropin alfa 0.3 mg as a single IV bolus and 15 minutes later experienced severe nausea, vomiting, diaphoresis, hypotension (blood pressure decreased from 115/66 mm Hg to 81/44 mm Hg), and tachycardia (pulse increased from 75 to 117 bpm).

IN VIVO DIAGNOSTIC AIDS

METHACHOLINE CHLORIDE

Rx	**Provocholine** (Methapharm)	**Solution for inhalation (after reconstitution of powder):** 100 mg per 5 ml	In 5 ml vials.

METHACHOLINE CHLORIDE — INHALATION

WARNING

Methacholine chloride powder for inhalation is a bronchoconstrictor agent for diagnostic purposes only and should not be used as a therapeutic agent. Methacholine chloride powder for inhalation challenge should be performed only under the supervision of a physician trained in and thoroughly familiar with all aspects of the technique of methacholine challenge, all contraindications, warnings and precautions, and the management of respiratory distress.

Emergency equipment and medication should be immediately available to treat acute respiratory distress.

Methacholine chloride powder for inhalation should be administered only by inhalation. Severe bronchoconstriction and reduction in respiratory function can result from the administration of methacholine chloride powder for inhalation. Patients with severe hyperreactivity of the airways can experience bronchoconstriction at a dosage as low as 0.025 mg/mL (0.125 cumulative units). If severe bronchoconstriction occurs, it should be reversed immediately by the administration of a rapid-acting inhaled bronchodilator agent (beta-agonist). Because of the potential for severe bronchoconstriction, provocholine (methacholine chloride powder for inhalation) challenge should not be performed in any patient with clinically apparent asthma, wheezing, or very low baseline pulmonary function tests (eg, FEV_1 less than 1 to 1.5 L or less than 70% of the predicted values). Please consult standard nomograms for predicted values.

Indications

➤*Bronchial airway hyperreactivity:* For the diagnosis of bronchial airway hyperreactivity in subjects who do not have clinically apparent asthma.

Administration and Dosage

➤*General dosing considerations:* Do not handle this material if you have asthma or hay fever.

Before beginning, baseline pulmonary function tests must be performed. A patient must have an FEV_1 of at least 70% of the predicted value. The target level for a positive challenge is a 20% reduction in the FEV_1 compared with the baseline value after inhalation of the control sodium chloride solution. This target value should be calculated and recorded before methacholine challenge is started.

➤*Adults:*

Diagnostic aid of bronchial airway hyperreactivity –

Usual dosage:

• *Multiple patient testing (2 to 5 patients)* – Dilutions prepared with 200 mg (see Preparation for Administration).

• *Single patient testing* – Dilutions prepared with 100 mg (see Preparation for Administration).

Concomitant therapy: An inhaled beta agonist may be administered after methacholine to expedite the return of the FEV_1 to baseline and to relieve the discomfort of the subject. Most patients revert to healthy pulmonary function within 5 minutes following bronchodilators or within 30 to 45 minutes without any bronchodilator.

➤*Children:*

Diagnostic aid of bronchial airway hyperreactivity –

5 years of age and older: See Adults for dosing.

➤*Preparation for administration:* Do not inhale powder. All dilutions should be made using sterile, empty USP Type I borosilicate glass vials. After adding the sodium chloride solution, shake each vial to obtain a clear solution.

A sterile bacterial-retentive filter (porosity 0.22 mcm) should be used when transferring a solution from each vial (at least 2 mL) to a nebulizer.

Methacholine Dilution Sequence for Multiple Patient Testing (2 to 5 Patients)

Vials		Concentrations
A_1 and A_2	Add 4 mL of 0.9% sodium chloride injection containing 0.4% phenol (pH 7) to each of two 20 mL vials containing methacholine 100 mg. These will be designated vials A_1 and A_2.	25 mg/mL
B	Remove 3 mL from vial A_1, transfer to another vial and add 4.5 mL of 0.9% sodium chloride injection containing 0.4% phenol (pH 7). This is vial B.	10 mg/mL
C	Remove 1 mL from vial A_2, transfer to another vial and add 9 mL of 0.9% sodium chloride injection containing 0.4% phenol (pH 7). This is vial C.	2.5 mg/mL
D	Remove 1 mL from vial C, transfer to another vial and add 9 mL of 0.9% sodium chloride injection containing 0.4% phenol (pH 7). This is vial D.	0.25 mg/mL
E	Remove 1 mL from vial D, transfer to another vial and add 9 mL of 0.9% sodium chloride injection containing 0.4% phenol (pH 7). This is vial E. Vial E must be prepared on the day of challenge.	0.025 mg/mL

Methacholine Dilution Sequence for Single Patient Testing

Vials		Concentrations
A	Add 4 mL of 0.9% sodium chloride injection containing 0.4% phenol (pH 7) to the 20 mL vial containing methacholine 100 mg. This is vial A.	25 mg/mL
B	Remove 1 mL from vial A, transfer to another vial and add 1.5 mL of 0.9% sodium chloride injection containing 0.4% phenol (pH 7). This is vial B.	10 mg/mL
C	Remove 1 mL from vial A, transfer to another vial and add 9 mL of 0.9% sodium chloride injection containing 0.4% phenol (pH 7). This is vial C.	2.5 mg/mL
D	Remove 1 mL from vial C, transfer to another vial and add 9 mL of 0.9% sodium chloride injection containing 0.4% phenol (pH 7). This is vial D.	0.25 mg/mL
E	Remove 1 mL from vial D, transfer to another vial and add 9 mL of 0.9% sodium chloride injection containing 0.4% phenol (pH 7). This is vial E. Vial E must be prepared on the day of challenge.	0.025 mg/mL

METHACHOLINE CHLORIDE — INHALATION

➤*Administration:* At each concentration, 5 breaths are administered by a nebulizer that permits intermittent delivery time of 0.6 seconds by a breath-actuated timing device (dosimeter). At each of 5 inhalations of a serial concentration, the subject begins at functional residual capacity (FRC) and slowly and completely inhales the dose delivered. Within 5 minutes, FEV_1 values are determined. The procedure ends either when there is a 20% or greater reduction in the FEV_1 compared with the baseline sodium chloride solution value (ie, a positive response) or if 188.88 total cumulative units has been administered (see the following data) and the FEV_1 has been reduced by 14% or less (ie, a negative response). If there is a reduction of 15% to 19% in the FEV_1 compared with baseline, either the challenge may be repeated at that concentration or a higher concentration may be given a long as the dosage administered does not result in total cumulative units exceeding 188.88.

The following is a suggested schedule for the administration of methacholine. Cumulative units are calculated by multiplying the number of breaths by the concentration administered. Total cumulative units is the sum of cumulative units for each concentration administered.

Methacholine Administration Schedule

Serial concentration	Number of breaths	Cumulative units per concentration	Total cumulative units
0.025 mg/mL	5	0.125	0.125
0.25 mg/mL	5	1.25	1.375
2.5 mg/mL	5	12.5	13.88
10 mg/mL	5	50	63.88
25 mg/mL	5	125	188.88

➤*Storage/Stability:* Store the powder at 15° to 30°C (59° to 86°F). Refrigerate the reconstituted solutions (dilutions A to D) at 2° to 8°C (36° to 46°F) for not more than 2 weeks, then discard the vials. Freezing does not affect the stability of dilutions A through D. Dilution E must be prepared on the day of the challenge.

Actions

➤*Pharmacology:* Methacholine chloride is the β-methyl homolog of acetylcholine and differs from the latter primarily in its greater duration and selectivity of action. Bronchial smooth muscle contains significant parasympathetic (cholinergic) innervation.

Bronchoconstriction occurs when the vagus nerve is stimulated and acetylcholine is released from the nerve endings. Muscle constriction is essentially confined to the local site of release because acetylcholine is rapidly inactivated by acetylcholinesterase.

Compared with acetylcholine, methacholine chloride is more slowly hydrolyzed by acetylcholinesterase and is almost totally resistant to inactivation by nonspecific cholinesterase or pseudocholinesterase.

When a sodium chloride solution containing methacholine chloride is inhaled, subjects with asthma are markedly more sensitive to methacholine-induced bronchoconstriction than are healthy subjects. This difference in response is the pharmacologic basis for the methacholine chloride powder for inhalation diagnostic challenge. However, it should be recognized that methacholine challenge may occasionally be positive after influenza, upper respiratory tract infections or immunizations. In very young or very old patients, or in patients with chronic lung disease (cystic fibrosis, sarcoidosis, tuberculosis, chronic obstructive pulmonary disease). The challenge may also be positive in patients with allergic rhinitis without asthma, in smokers, in patients after exposure to air pollutants, or in patients who have had or will in the future develop asthma.

Contraindications

Known hypersensitivity to this drug or to other parasympathomimetic agents; repeated administration of methacholine other than on the day of challenge with increasing doses; patients receiving any beta-adrenergic blocking agent because in such patients responses to methacholine can be exaggerated or prolonged, and may not respond as readily to treatment (see Warning Box).

Warnings/Precautions

➤*Special risk:* Administration of methacholine chloride powder for inhalation to patients with epilepsy, cardiovascular disease accompanied by bradycardia, vagotonia, peptic ulcer disease, thyroid disease, urinary tract obstruction or other condition that could be adversely affected by a cholinergic agent should be undertaken only if the physician feels benefit to the individual outweighs the potential risks.

➤*Pregnancy: Category C.* Animal reproduction studies have not been conducted with methacholine chloride. It is not known whether methacholine chloride can cause fetal harm when administered to a pregnant patient or affect reproductive capacity. Methacholine chloride should be given to a pregnant woman only if clearly needed.

In females of childbearing potential, the inhalation challenge for methacholine chloride powder for inhalation should be performed either within 10 days following the onset of menses or within 2 weeks of a negative pregnancy test.

➤*Lactation:* The inhalation challenge for methacholine chloride powder for inhalation should not be administered to a breast-feeding mother since it is not known whether methacholine chloride when inhaled is excreted in breast milk.

➤*Children:* The safety and efficacy of methacholine chloride powder for inhalation in the inhalation challenge have not been established in children below the age of 5 years.

Adverse Reactions

➤*Inhalation:* Adverse reactions associated with 153 inhaled methacholine chloride challenges include 1 occurrence each of headache, throat irritation, lightheadedness and itching.

➤*Oral injection:* Methacholine chloride powder for inhalation is to be administered only by inhalation. When administered orally or by injection, methacholine chloride is reported to be associated with nausea and vomiting, substernal pain or pressure, hypotension, fainting and transient complete heart block (see Overdosage).

Overdosage

➤*Symptoms:* Methacholine chloride powder for inhalation is to be administered only by inhalation. When administered orally or by injection, overdosage with methacholine chloride can result in a syncopal reaction, with cardiac arrest and loss of consciousness.

➤*Treatment:* Serious toxic reactions should be treated with 0.5 mg to 1 mg of atropine sulfate, administered IM or IV.

Patient Information

1.) Patients should be instructed regarding symptoms that may occur as a result of the test and how such symptoms can be managed.
2.) A female patient should inform her physician if she is pregnant, or the date of her last onset of menses, or the date and result of her last pregnancy test (see Warnings, Pregnancy).

Gastrointestinal Function Tests

SECRETIN

Rx			
Rx	**ChiRhoStim** (ChiRhoClin[a])	**Injection, lyophilized powder for solution:** 16 mcg[b]	With mannitol 20 mg, L-cysteine 1.5 mg. In vials.
		40 mcg[b]	With mannitol 50 mg, L-cysteine 3.75 mg. In vials.

[a] ChiRhoClin, Inc, 4000 Blackburn Lane, Suite 270, Burtonsville, MD 20866; 301-476-8388; http://www.chirhoclin.com.

[b] Human-derived; 0.2 mcg corresponds to 1 CU.

SECRETIN ACETATE — INJECTION

Indications

➤*Diagnosis of gastrinoma:* For the stimulation of gastrin secretion to aid in the diagnosis of gastrinoma.

➤*Diagnosis of pancreatic dysfunction:* For the stimulation of pancreatic secretions, including bicarbonate, to aid in the diagnosis of pancreatic exocrine dysfunction.

➤*Endoscopic retrograde cholangiopancreatography (ERCP):* For the stimulation of pancreatic secretions to facilitate the identification of the ampulla of Vater and accessory papilla during ERCP.

➤*Off-label uses:*

Autism – [5] = Poor documentation. The safety and efficacy of secretin has not been proven under controlled conditions. It is also unclear why conflicting responses have been observed between uncontrolled and controlled settings. Data in controlled trials have evaluated single- or multidosing without producing significant beneficial effects. Safety information is also limited.

Administration and Dosage

➤*General dosing considerations:* A test dose should be given to patients for a potential allergic reaction to secretin. (See Test Dose.)

➤*Adults:*

Diagnosis of gastrinoma – 0.4 mcg/kg intravenous (IV) over 1 minute.

Diagnosis of pancreatic dysfunction – 0.2 mcg/kg by IV over 1 minute.

Endoscopic retrograde cholangiopancreatography – 0.2 mcg/kg by IV over 1 minute.

➤*Test dose:* A test dose of secretin 0.2 mcg if using the 16 mcg vial (0.1 mL) or 0.4 mcg if using the 40 mcg vial (0.1 mL) is injected IV to test for possible allergies. If no allergic reaction is noted after 1 minute, the recommended dose for the specific indication may be injected slowly over 1 minute.

➤*Preparation for administration:*

16 mcg vial – Dissolve the contents of the 16 mcg vial in 8 mL of sodium chloride injection to yield a concentration of 2 mcg/mL. Shake vigorously to ensure dissolution. Use immediately after reconstitution.

SECRETIN ACETATE — INJECTION

40 mcg vial – Dissolve the contents of the 40 mcg vial in 10 mL of sodium chloride injection to yield a concentration of 4 mcg/mL. Shake vigorously to ensure dissolution. Use immediately after reconstitution.

➤*Administration:*

Gastroduodenal (Dreiling) tube collection method (to aid in the diagnosis of exocrine pancreatic dysfunction) – A radiopaque, double-lumen tube is passed through the mouth following a 12- to 15-hour fast. Under fluoroscopic control, the opening of the proximal lumen of the tube is placed in the gastric antrum and the opening of the distal lumen just beyond the papilla of Vater. The positioning of the tube must be confirmed and the tube secured prior to secretin testing. Intermittent negative pressure of 25 to 40 mm Hg is applied to both lumens and maintained throughout the test. When duodenal contents have a pH of 6 or more, a baseline sample of duodenal fluids is collected for a 10-minute period. If there are no signs of allergic reactions to the test dose, administer secretin at a dose of 0.2 mcg/kg IV over 1 minute. Duodenal fluid is collected for 60 minutes thereafter. The aspirate is divided into 4 collection periods of 15 minutes each. The duodenal lumen of the tube is cleared with an injection of air after collection of each sample. Wide variation in volume of the aspirate is indicative of incomplete aspiration. Each sample of duodenal fluid is to be chilled and subsequently analyzed for volume and bicarbonate concentration. Exocrine pancreas dysfunction typically associated with chronic pancreatitis is indicated if the peak bicarbonate concentration for any sample is less than 80 mEq/L.

Endoscopic collection method endoscopic pancreatic function test – After assessment of patients for sedation and analgesia, administer a test dose of secretin. If there are no signs of allergic reaction, administer secretin at a dose of 0.2 mcg/kg IV over 1 minute. An upper endoscopy is performed with conscious sedation after topical anesthetic. All gastric fluid is aspirated through the endoscope and discarded. After small bowel intubation to the junction of the second and third portion of the duodenum, fluid is aspirated for 1 to 3 minutes and collected in 5 separate specimen traps at baseline (0) and at 15, 30, 45, and 60 minutes after secretin injection. The patients remain intubated with the upper endoscope for 1 hour in the left lateral decubitus position. Boluses of meperidine and midazolam in a 25:1 mg ratio are administered to maintain analgesia and sedation during the 1-hour procedure. Each sample of duodenal fluid is to be chilled and subsequently analyzed for volume and bicarbonate concentration. Exocrine pancreas dysfunction typically associated with chronic pancreatitis is indicated if the peak bicarbonate concentration for any sample is less than 80 mEq/L.

Stimulation of gastrin secretion to aid in the diagnosis of gastrinoma – The patient should have fasted for at least 12 hours prior to beginning the test. Before injecting secretin, 2 blood samples are drawn for determination of fasting serum gastrin levels (baseline values). Subsequently, administer a test dose of secretin. If no adverse reactions, administer 0.4 mcg/kg IV over 1 minute; postinjection blood samples are collected after 1, 2, 5, 10, and 30 minutes for determination of serum gastrin concentrations. Gastrinoma is strongly suspected in patients who show an increase in serum gastrin concentration of more than 110 pg/mL over basal levels on any of the postinjection samples.

Facilitation of the identification of the ampulla of Vater and accessory papilla during endoscopic retrograde cholangiopancreatography – Administration of secretin may be given when difficulty is encountered by the endoscopist in identifying the ampulla of Vater for various reasons (eg, anatomic deformity secondary to prior surgery, radiation therapy, peptic ulcer disease, tumors) or in identifying the accessory papilla in patients with pancreas divisum. If there are no signs of allergic reaction to the test dose, a dose of 0.2 mcg/kg IV over 1 minute may be administered and will result in visible excretion of pancreatic fluids from the orifices of these papillae, enabling their identification and facilitating cannulation.

➤*Storage/Stability:* Store unreconstituted vials at −20°C (−4°F). Use immediately after reconstitution. Discard any unused portion after reconstitution. Protect from light.

Actions

➤*Pharmacology:* The primary action of secretin injection is to increase the volume and bicarbonate content of secreted pancreatic juices.

Secretin is a hormone that is normally released from the duodenum upon exposure of the proximal intestinal lumen to gastric acid, fatty acids, and amino acids. Secretin is released from enterochromaffin cells in the intestinal mucosa. Secretin receptors have been identified in the pancreas, stomach, liver, colon, and other tissues.

When secretin binds to secretin receptors on pancreatic duct cells, it opens cystic fibrosis transmembrane conductance regulator (CFTR) channels, leading to secretion of bicarbonate-rich-pancreatic fluid. Secretin may also work through vagal-vagal neural pathways, because stimulation of the efferent vagus nerve stimulates bicarbonate secretion and atropine blocks secretin-stimulated pancreatic secretion.

➤*Pharmacokinetics:*

Distribution – The volume of distribution is about 2 L for porcine-derived secretin and 2.7 L for synthetic human secretin.

Excretion – The pharmacokinetic profile for secretin was evaluated in 12 healthy subjects. After IV bolus administration of 0.4 mcg/kg, secretin concentration rapidly declines to baseline secretin levels within 60 to 90 minutes for porcine-derived secretin and 90 to 120 minutes for synthetic human secretin in most of the healthy volunteers studied.

The elimination half-life is 27 minutes for porcine-derived secretin and 45 minutes for synthetic human secretin. The clearance is 487 ± 136 mL/min for porcine-derived secretin and 580.9 ± 51.3 mL/min for synthetic human secretin.

Contraindications

Do not administer secretin to patients with acute pancreatitis until the acute episode has subsided.

Warnings/Precautions

➤*Hypersensitivity reactions:* Because of a potential allergic reaction to secretin, give patients an IV test dose of 0.2 mcg (0.1 mL). If no allergic reaction is noted after 1 minute, the recommended dose for the specific indication may be injected slowly over 1 minute. A test dose is especially important in patients with a history of atopic allergy and/or asthma. Appropriate measures for the treatment of acute hypersensitivity reactions should be immediately available. No allergic reactions were observed after the test dose or full dose of porcine-derived secretin in over 981 patients or after the test dose or full dose of synthetic human secretin in 584 patients and volunteers.

➤*Special risk:* Patients who have undergone vagotomy, are receiving anticholinergic agents at the time of secretin stimulation testing, or who have inflammatory bowel disease may be hyporesponsive to secretin stimulation. This response does not indicate pancreatic disease. Interpret results of secretin stimulation tests in these patients with caution. A greater-than-normal volume response to secretin stimulation, which may mask coexisting pancreatic disease, is occasionally encountered in patients with alcoholic or other liver disease. Interpret results of secretin stimulation tests in these patients with caution.

➤*Pregnancy: Category C.* Animal reproduction studies have not been conducted with secretin. It is not known whether secretin can cause fetal harm when administered to a pregnant woman or can affect reproduction capacity. Give secretin to a pregnant woman only if clearly needed.

➤*Lactation:* It is not known whether secretin is excreted in human milk. Because many drugs are excreted in human milk, exercise caution when secretin is administered to a breast-feeding woman.

➤*Children:* Safety and effectiveness in children have not been established.

Drug Interactions

➤*Anticholinergics:* The concomitant use of anticholinergic agents may make patients hyporesponsive (ie, may produce a false positive result). Interpret any results of secretin stimulation tests in these patients with caution.

Adverse Reactions

➤*Secretin (porcine-derived):*

Secretin (Porcine-Derived) Adverse Reactions (N = 981)	
Adverse reactions	Secretin injection incidence (patients)
Cardiovascular	
Bradycardia (mild)	2 (2)
Decreased blood pressure	6 (5)
Thready pulse	1 (1)
CNS	
Headache	2 (2)
Light-headedness	3 (2)
Numbness/Tingling in extremities	2 (1)
Possible seizure	1 (1)
Dermatologic	
Abdominal rash	1 (1)
Diaphoresis	6 (4)
Flushing	6 (5)
Pallor	1 (1)
Urticaria 2° contrast material (prior to secretin administration)	1 (1)
GI	
Abdominal cramps	2 (2)
Abdominal discomfort	7 (7)
Bleeding (upper GI 2° to endoscopic abrasion)	2 (2)
Burning in stomach	3 (2)
Diarrhea	1 (1)
Endoscopic perforation of pancreatic duct	2 (2)
Hunger pangs	1 (1)
Nausea	8 (8)
Vomiting	1 (1)
Respiratory	
Transient low O_2 saturation	1 (1)
Transient respiratory distress	2 (2)

SECRETIN ACETATE — INJECTION

Secretin (Porcine-Derived) Adverse Reactions (N = 981)

Adverse reactions	Secretin injection incidence (patients)
Miscellaneous	
Bleeding (sphincterectomy)	6 (6)
Bloating	1 (1)
Fatigue	1 (1)
Fever	1 (1)
Hot sensation	1 (1)
Leukocytoplastic vasculitis	1 (1)
Total patients with adverse reactions	73 (7.4%)

➤*Synthetic human secretin:* Mild to moderate adverse reactions have been noted for synthetic human secretin in clinical studies in 533 patients and 51 healthy volunteers. Two severe adverse reactions, nausea and abdominal pain, occurred in 1 patient. The following table details the type and number of patients with adverse reactions.

Synthetic Human Secretin Adverse Reactions (N = 584)

Adverse reactions	Incidence (patients)
Cardiovascular	
Hypotension	1 (1)
Increased heart rate	2 (2)
Slow heart rate (57 bpm)	1 (1)
CNS	
Anxiety	1 (1)
Faintness	1 (1)
Sedation	1 (1)
Tingling in legs	1 (1)
Dermatologic	
Clammy skin	1 (1)
Flushing	4 (4)
GI	
Abdominal pain	3 (3)
Burning in stomach or abdomen	1 (1)
Diarrhea	1 (1)
Mild pancreatitis	2 (2)
Nausea	11 (11)
Oral secretions increased	1 (1)
Upset stomach	2 (2)
Vomiting	3 (3)
Warm sensation in abdomen	1 (1)
Respiratory	
Decreased O_2 saturation	1 (1)
Miscellaneous	
Early removal of Dreiling tube	3 (3)
Infiltrated IV	1 (1)
Unresponsive	1 (1)
Warm sensation in face	1 (1)
Total patients with ≥ 1 adverse reaction	29 (5%)

Patient Information

Because there are no data on pregnant or breast-feeding mothers, discuss these matters with the patient before using this product.

SINCALIDE

Rx	**Kinevac** (Bracco Diagnostics)	**Powder for injection, lyophilized:** 5 mcg/vial for reconstitution (1 mcg/mL when reconstituted)	In vials.

SINCALIDE — INJECTION

Indications

➤*Gallbladder contraction stimulation:* To stimulate gallbladder contraction, as may be assessed by contrast agent cholecystography or ultrasonography, or to obtain by duodenal aspiration a sample of concentrated bile for analysis of cholesterol, bile salts, phospholipids, and crystals.

➤*Pancreatic secretion stimulation:* To stimulate pancreatic secretion (especially in conjunction with secretin) prior to obtaining a duodenal aspirate for analysis of enzyme activity, composition, and cytology.

➤*Barium meal transit time acceleration:* To accelerate the transit of a barium meal through the small bowel, thereby decreasing the time and extent of radiation associated with fluoroscopy and X-ray examination of the intestinal tract.

Administration and Dosage

➤*Adults:*

Barium meal transit time acceleration –

Usual dosage: 0.04 mcg/kg intravenously (IV) over a 30- to 60-second interval; if satisfactory transit of the barium meal has not occurred in 30 minutes, a second dose of 0.04 mcg/kg may be administered.

Alternative dosage: For reduction of adverse effects, a 30-minute IV infusion (0.12 mcg/kg diluted to approximately 100 mL with sodium chloride injection) may be administered.

Contraction of the gallbladder –

Usual dosage: 0.02 mcg/kg injected IV over 30 to 60 seconds; if satisfactory gallbladder contraction does not occur in 15 minutes, a second dose (0.04 mcg/kg) may be given. When used in cholecystography, roentgenograms are usually taken at 5-minute intervals after the injection. For visualization of the cystic duct, it may be necessary to take roentgenograms at 1-minute intervals during the first 5 minutes after the injection.

Alternative dosage: To reduce the intestinal adverse effects, an IV infusion may be prepared at a dose of 0.12 mcg/kg in 100 mL of sodium chloride injection and given at a rate of 2 mL/min; alternatively, an intramuscularly (IM) dose of 0.1 mcg/kg may be given.

Pancreatic secretion stimulation – Secretin dose of 0.25 units/kg is infused IV over 60 minutes. Thirty minutes after initiating secretin, give a separate IV infusion of sincalide at a total dose of 0.02 mcg/kg over 30 minutes.

➤*Preparation of solution:* To reconstitute, add 5 mL sterile water for injection to the vial; make any additional dilution with 0.9% sodium chloride for injection.

Pancreatic secretion stimulation – For example, the total dose for a 70 kg patient is sincalide 1.4 mcg; therefore, dilute reconstituted sincalide 1.4 mL solution to 30 mL with sodium chloride injection and administer at a rate of 1 mL/min.

➤*Administration:*

Barium meal transit time acceleration – Administer sincalide after the barium meal is beyond the proximal jejunum.

➤*Storage/Stability:* Store at 15° to 30° C (59° to 86° F) prior to reconstitution. The solution may be kept at room temperature. Use within 24 hours after reconstitution; discard any unused portion.

Actions

➤*Pharmacology:* Sincalide IV substantially reduces gallbladder size by causing it to contract. The evacuation of bile that results is similar to the physiological response to endogenous cholecystokinin. Bolus IV administration causes a prompt contraction of the gallbladder that becomes maximal in 5 to 15 minutes, as compared with the stimulus of a fatty meal, which causes a progressive contraction that becomes maximal after approximately 40 minutes. Generally, a 40% reduction in radiographic area of the gallbladder is satisfactory, although some patients will show area reduction of 60% to 70%.

Like cholecystokinin, sincalide stimulates pancreatic secretion; concurrent administration with secretin increases the volume of pancreatic secretion and the output of bicarbonate and protein (enzymes) by the gland. This combined effect of secretin and sincalide permits the assessment of specific pancreatic function through measurement and analysis of the duodenal aspirate. The parameters determined are the following: Volume of the secretion; bicarbonate concentration; amylase content (which parallels the content of trypsin and total protein).

Cholecystokinin and sincalide stimulate intestinal motility and may cause pyloric contraction, which retards gastric emptying.

Contraindications

Hypersensitivity to sincalide; intestinal obstruction.

Warnings/Precautions

➤*Gallbladder stones:* Stimulation of gallbladder contraction in patients with small gallbladder stones may lead to the evacuation of the stones, resulting in their lodging in the cystic duct or in the common bile duct. The risk is minimal because sincalide, when given as directed, does not ordinarily cause complete contraction of the gallbladder.

➤*Pregnancy: Category B.* There are no adequate and well-controlled studies in pregnant women. Because animal reproduction studies are not always predictive of human response, use this drug during pregnancy only if clearly needed.

Do not administer sincalide to pregnant women near term because of its effect on smooth muscle; the possibility of prematurely inducing labor exists.

SINCALIDE — INJECTION

➤*Lactation:* It is not known whether this drug is excreted in human milk. Because many drugs are excreted in human milk, exercise caution when sincalide is administered to a breast-feeding woman.

➤*Children:* The safety for use in children has not been established.

Adverse Reactions

➤*Most frequent:* Reactions to sincalide are generally mild and of short duration. The most frequent adverse reactions were abdominal discomfort or pain, and nausea; rapid IV injection of 0.04 mcg/kg sincalide expectably causes transient abdominal cramping. These phenomena are usually manifestations of the physiologic action of the drug, including delayed gastric emptying and increased intestinal motility. These reactions occurred in approximately 20% of patients; they are not to be construed as necessarily indicating an abnormality of the biliary tract unless there is other clinical or radiologic evidence of disease.

The incidence of other adverse reactions, including vomiting, flushing, sweating, rash, hypotension, hypertension, shortness of breath, urge to defecate, headache, diarrhea, sneezing, and numbness was less than 1%; dizziness was reported in approximately 2% of patients. These manifestations are usually lessened by slower injection rate.

Overdosage

➤*Symptoms:* GI symptoms (abdominal cramps, nausea, vomiting, and diarrhea) should be expected. Hypotension with dizziness or fainting might also occur. Starting with single bolus IV injection comparable with the human dose of 0.4 mg/kg, sincalide caused hypotension and bradycardia in dogs. Higher doses injected once or repeatedly in dogs caused syncope and ECG changes in addition. These effects were attributed to sincalide-induced vagal stimulation in that all were prevented by pretreatment with atropine or bilateral vagotomy.

➤*Treatment:* Treat overdosage symptoms symptomatically over a short duration.

IN VIVO DIAGNOSTIC AIDS

BENZYLPENICILLOYL POLYLYSINE

Rx	**Pre-Pen** (ALK-Abelló)	**Injection, solution:** 6×10^{-5} M per 25 mL	In single-dose ampules.

BENZYLPENICILLOYL POLYLYSINE INJECTION

Indications

➤*Penicillin hypersensitivity skin testing:* For the assessment of sensitization to penicillin (benzylpenicillin or penicillin G) in patients suspected to have clinical penicillin hypersensitivity.

Administration and Dosage

➤*General dosing considerations:* The skin test antigen should always be applied first by the puncture technique (step 1). If the puncture test is either negative or equivocally positive (less than 5 mm wheal with little or no erythema and no itching), an intradermal test (step 2) may be performed.

Skin testing responses can be attenuated by interfering drugs (eg, H_1 antihistamines, vasopressors). Skin testing should be delayed until the effects of such drugs have dissipated, or a separate skin test with histamine can be used to evaluate persistent antihistaminic effects in vivo.

Because of the risk of potential systemic allergic reactions, skin testing should be performed in an appropriate health care setting under direct medical supervision.

➤*Adults:*

Penicillin hypersensitivity skin testing –

Step 1: Puncture technique: Apply a small drop of solution using a sterile 22- to 28-gauge needle and use the same needle to make a single shallow puncture of the epidermis through the drop of solution. As soon as a positive response is clearly evident, the solution over the scratch should be immediately wiped off. If the puncture test is either negative or equivocally positive (less than 5 mm wheal with little or no erythema and no itching), an intradermal test (step 2) may be performed.

Step 2: Intradermal test: Inject an amount of solution sufficient to raise a small intradermal bleb of about 3 mm in diameter, in duplicate at least 2 cm apart. Using a separate syringe and needle, inject a similar amount of saline or allergen diluting solution as a control at least 5 cm removed from the antigen test sites.

➤*Preparation for administration:* Open ampules by snapping the neck of the ampule using two forefingers of each hand. Visually inspect for glass shards before use.

Step 1: Puncture technique – Prepare the skin surface and use a sterile 22- to 28-gauge needle.

Step 2: Intradermal test – Using a 0.5 to 1 cc syringe with a ⅜- to ⅝-inch long, 26- to 30-gauge, short bevel needle, withdraw the contents of the ampule. Prepare a skin test area on the upper outer arm with an alcohol swab, sufficiently below the deltoid muscle to permit proximal application of a tourniquet later, if necessary. Be sure to eject all air from the syringe through the needle.

➤*Administration:* The skin test antigen should always be applied first by the puncture technique. Skin testing is usually performed on the inner volar aspect of the forearm.

Step 1: Puncture technique – After preparing the skin surface, apply a small drop of solution; the same needle can then be used to make a single shallow puncture of the epidermis through the drop of solution. Very little pressure is required to break the epidermal continuity. Observe for the appearance of a wheal or erythema, and the occurrence of itching at the test site during the succeeding 15 minutes, at which time the solution over the puncture site should be wiped off. A positive reaction consists of the development within 10 minutes of a pale wheal, sometimes with pseudopods, surrounding the puncture site and varying in diameter from 5 to 15 mm (or more). This wheal may be surrounded by a variable diameter of erythema, and accompanied by a variable degree of itching. The most sensitive individuals develop itching quickly, and the wheal and erythema are prompt in their appearance. As soon as a positive response as previously defined is clearly evident, the solution over the scratch should be immediately wiped off. If the puncture test is either negative or equivocally positive (less than 5 mm wheal with little or no erythema and no itching), an intradermal test may be performed.

Step 2: Intradermal test – Insert the needle bevel up immediately below the skin surface. Most skin reactions will develop within 5 to 15 minutes and response to the skin test is read at 20 minutes as follows: negative response is no increase in size of original bleb and no greater reaction than the control site; ambiguous response is wheal only slightly larger than initial injection bleb, with or without accompanying erythematous flare and slightly larger than the control site, or discordance between duplicates; positive response is itching, significant increase in size of original blebs to at least 5 mm, and wheal may exceed 20 mm in diameter and exhibit pseudopods. If the control site exhibits a wheal more than 2 to 3 mm, repeat the test; if the same reaction is observed, a health care provider experienced with allergy skin testing should be consulted.

➤*Storage/Stability:* Store at 2° to 8°C (36° to 46°F). Discard any unused portion. Solutions subjected to ambient temperatures for more than 24 hours should be discarded.

Actions

➤*Pharmacology:* Benzylpenicilloyl polylysine is a skin test antigen reagent that reacts specifically with benzylpenicilloyl immunoglobulin E (IgE) antibodies, initiating the release of chemical mediators that produce an immediate wheal and flare reaction at a skin test site. All individuals exhibiting a positive skin test to benzylpenicilloyl polylysine possess IgE against the benzylpenicilloyl structural group, which is a hapten. A hapten is a low molecular weight chemical that conjugates with a carrier (eg, poly-l-lysine), resulting in the formation of an antigen with the hapten's specificity. The benzylpenicilloyl hapten is the major antigenic determinant in penicillin-allergic individuals. However, many individuals reacting positively to benzylpenicilloyl polylysine will not develop a systemic allergic reaction on subsequent exposure to therapeutic penicillin, especially among those who have not reacted to penicillins in the past. Thus, the benzylpenicilloyl polylysine skin test determines the presence of penicilloyl IgE antibodies, which are necessary but not sufficient for acute allergic reactions because of the major penicilloyl determinant.

Non-benzylpenicilloyl haptens are designated as minor determinants because they less frequently elicit an immune response in penicillin-treated individuals. Nevertheless, the minor determinants may be associated with significant clinical hypersensitivity.

Contraindications

Systemic or marked local reaction to prior benzylpenicilloyl polylysine administration; patients known to be extremely hypersensitive to penicillin should not be skin tested.

Warnings/Precautions

➤*Repeated use:* The risk of sensitization to repeated skin testing with benzylpenicilloyl polylysine is not established.

➤*Use:* No reagent, test, or combination of tests will completely assure that a reaction to penicillin therapy will not occur.

The value of the benzylpenicilloyl polylysine skin test alone as a means of assessing the risk of administering therapeutic penicillin (when penicillin is the preferred drug of choice) is not established in adult patients who give no history of clinical penicillin hypersensitivity.

➤*Penicillin exposure:* The clinical value of benzylpenicilloyl polylysine when exposure to penicillin is suspected as a cause of a current drug reaction or in patients who are undergoing routine allergy evaluation is not known.

➤*Cephalosporins/Semisynthetic penicillins:* The clinical value of benzylpenicilloyl polylysine skin tests alone in determining the risk of administering semisynthetic penicillins (phenoxymethyl penicillin, ampicillin, carbenicillin, dicloxacillin, methicillin, nafcillin, oxacillin, amoxicillin), cephalosporin-derived antibiotics, and penem antibiotics is not known.

➤*Penicillin use:* In addition to the results of the benzylpenicilloyl polylysine skin test, take into account individual patient factors when deciding whether to administer penicillin. Keep in mind the following: a serious allergic reaction to therapeutic penicillin may occur in a patient with a negative

BENZYLPENICILLOYL POLYLYSINE INJECTION

skin test to benzylpenicilloyl polylysine; it is possible for a patient to have an anaphylactic reaction to therapeutic penicillin in the presence of a negative benzylpenicilloyl polylysine skin test and a negative history of clinical penicillin hypersensitivity; if penicillin is the drug of choice for a life-threatening infection, successful desensitization with therapeutic penicillin may be possible irrespective of a positive skin test and/or a positive history of clinical penicillin hypersensitivity.

➤*Hypersensitivity reactions:* Rarely, a systemic allergic reaction including anaphylaxis may follow a skin test with benzylpenicilloyl polylysine. To decrease the risk of a systemic allergic reaction, perform puncture skin testing first. Perform intradermal skin testing only if the puncture test is entirely negative.

➤*Pregnancy: Category C.* Animal reproduction studies have not been conducted with benzylpenicilloyl polylysine. It is not known whether benzylpenicilloyl polylysine can cause fetal harm when administered to a pregnant woman, or if it can affect reproduction capacity. Weigh the hazards of skin testing in such patients against the hazard of penicillin therapy without skin testing.

➤*Lactation:* No information available.

➤*Children:* The value of benzylpenicilloyl polylysine alone as a means of assessing the risk of administering therapeutic penicillin is not established in children.

Adverse Reactions

➤*Dermatologic:* Occasionally, patients may develop an intense local inflammatory response at the skin test site.

➤*Hypersensitivity:* Rarely, patients will develop a systemic allergic reaction, manifested by anaphylaxis, angioedema, dyspnea, generalized erythema, hypotension, pruritus, and urticaria.

➤*Treating a skin test reaction:* The usual methods for treating a skin test antigen-induced reaction are the applications of a venous occlusion tourniquet proximal to the skin test site and administration of epinephrine. Keep the patient under observation for several hours.

Patient Information

Instruct patients to inform their health care provider if they have a history of clinical penicillin hypersensitivity.

Advise patients to inform their health care provider if they are taking penicillin, antihistamines, or vasopressors.

DIPYRIDAMOLE

Rx	**Dipyridamole** (Various, eg, Bedford)	**Injection:** 5 mg/mL[a]	In 2 and 10 mL vials.

[a] With 50 mg polyethylene glycol 600 and 2 mg tartaric acid.

DIPYRIDAMOLE — INJECTION

Dipyridamole oral is used as an antiplatelet agent. Refer to the individual monograph in the Hematologic Agents chapter.

Indications

➤*Diagnostic aid:* As an alternative to exercise in thallium-201 myocardial perfusion imaging for the evaluation of coronary artery disease in patients who cannot exercise adequately.

Administration and Dosage

➤*Adults:*

Diagnostic aid –

Usual dosage: 0.142 mg/kg/min (0.57 mg/kg total) infused over 4 minutes.

Maximum dose: Although the maximum tolerated dose has not been determined, clinical experience suggests that a total dose beyond 60 mg is not needed.

Concomitant therapy: Thallium-201 should be injected within 5 minutes following the 4-minute infusion of dipyridamole.

➤*Preparation for administration:* Dilute in at least a 1:2 ratio with 0.45% sodium chloride injection, 0.9% sodium chloride injection, or 5% dextrose injection for a total volume of approximately 20 to 50 mL. Infusion of undiluted dipyridamole may cause local irritation.

➤*Administration:* Administer by IV infusion over 4 minutes. Thallium-201 should be injected within 5 minutes following the 4-minute infusion of dipyridamole.

➤*Admixture compatibility:* Do not mix with other drugs in the same syringe or infusion container.

➤*Storage/Stability:* Store between 15° to 25°C (59° to 77°F). Avoid freezing. Protect from light. Retain in carton until time of use. Discard unused portion.

Actions

➤*Pharmacology:* In a study of 10 patients with angiographically normal or minimally stenosed (less than 25% luminal diameter narrowing) coronary vessels, dipyridamole injection in a dose of 0.56 mg/kg infused over 4 minutes resulted in an average fivefold increase in coronary blood flow velocity compared to resting coronary flow velocity (range 3.8 to 7 times resting velocity). The mean time to peak flow velocity was 6.5 minutes from the start of the 4-minute infusion (range 2.5 to 8.7 minutes). Cardiovascular responses to the IV administration of dipyridamole when given to patients in the supine position include a mild but significant increase in heart rate of approximately 20% and mild but significant decreases in both systolic and diastolic blood pressure of approximately 2% to 8%, with vital signs returning to baseline values in approximately 30 minutes.

Dipyridamole is a coronary vasodilator. The mechanism of vasodilation has not been fully elucidated, but may result from inhibition of uptake of adenosine, an important mediator of coronary vasodilation. The vasodilatory effects of dipyridamole are abolished by administration of the adenosine receptor antagonist theophylline.

How dipyridamole-induced vasodilation leads to abnormalities in thallium-201 distribution and ventricular function is also uncertain but presumably represents a "steal" phenomenon in which relatively intact vessels dilate, and sustain enhanced flow, leaving reduced pressure and flow across areas of hemodynamically important coronary vascular constriction.

➤*Pharmacokinetics:*

Absorption/Distribution – Plasma dipyridamole concentrations decline in a triexponential fashion following IV infusion of dipyridamole with half-lives averaging 3 to 12 minutes, 33 to 62 minutes, and 11.6 to 15 hours. Two minutes following a 0.568 mg/kg dose of IV dipyridamole administered as a 4-minute IV infusion, the mean dipyridamole serum concentration is 4.6 ± 1.3 mcg/mL. The average plasma protein binding of dipyridamole is approximately 99%, primarily to α_1-glycoprotein. The average total body clearance is 2.3 to 3.5 mL/min/kg, with an apparent volume of distribution at steady state of 1 to 2.5 L/kg and a central apparent volume of 3 to 5 L.

Metabolism/Excretion – Dipyridamole is metabolized in the liver to the glucuronic acid conjugate and excreted with the bile.

Contraindications

Hypersensitivity to dipyridamole.

Warnings/Precautions

➤*Cardiotoxicity and bronchospasm:* Serious adverse reactions associated with the administration of IV dipyridamole have included cardiac death, fatal and non-fatal myocardial infarction, ventricular fibrillation, symptomatic ventricular tachycardia, stroke, transient cerebral ischemia, seizures, anaphylactoid reaction and bronchospasm. There have been reported cases of asystole, sinus node arrest, sinus node depression and conduction block. Patients with abnormalities of cardiac impulse formation/conduction or severe coronary artery disease may be at increased risk for these events.

In a study of 3911 patients given IV dipyridamole as an adjunct to thallium-201 myocardial perfusion imaging, 2 types of serious adverse events were reported: 1) four cases of myocardial infarction (0.1%), 2 fatal (0.05%); and 2 non-fatal (0.05%); and 2) six cases of severe bronchospasm (0.2%). Although the incidence of these serious adverse events was small (0.3%, 10 of 3911), the potential clinical information to be gained through use of IV dipyridamole thallium-201 imaging must be weighed against the risk to the patient. The sensitivity of the dipyridamole test (true positive dipyridamole divided by the total number of patients with positive angiography) was about 85%. The specificity (true negative divided by the number of patients with negative angiograms) was about 50%. Patients with a history of unstable angina may be at a greater risk for severe myocardial ischemia. Patients with a history of asthma may be at a greater risk for bronchospasm during IV dipyridamole use.

When thallium-201 myocardial perfusion imaging is performed with IV dipyridamole, parenteral aminophylline should be readily available for relieving adverse events such as bronchospasm or chest pain. Vital signs should be monitored during, and for 10 to 15 minutes following, the IV infusion of dipyridamole and an electrocardiographic tracing should be obtained using at least 1 chest lead. Should severe chest pain or bronchospasm occur, parenteral aminophylline may be administered by slow IV injection (50 to 100 mg over 30 to 60 seconds) in doses ranging from 50 to 250 mg. In the case of severe hypotension, the patient should be placed in a supine position with the head tilted down if necessary, before administration of parenteral aminophylline. If 250 mg of aminophylline does not relieve chest pain symptoms within a few minutes, sublingual nitroglycerin may be administered. If chest pain continues despite use of aminophylline and nitroglycerin, the possibility of myocardial infarction should be considered. If the clinical condition of a patient with an adverse event permits a 1 minute delay in the administration of parenteral aminophylline, thallium-201 may be injected and allowed to circulate for 1 minute before the injection of aminophylline. This will allow initial thallium-201 perfusion imaging to be performed before reversal of the pharmacologic effects of IV dipyridamole on the coronary circulation.

➤*Myasthenia gravis:* Myasthenia gravis patients receiving therapy with cholinesterase inhibitors may experience worsening of their disease in the presence of dipyridamole.

➤*Pregnancy: Category B.* There are no adequate and well controlled studies in pregnant women. Because animal reproduction studies are not always predictive of human responses, this drug should be used during pregnancy only if clearly needed.

➤*Lactation:* Dipyridamole is excreted in human milk.

➤*Children:* Safety and effectiveness in the pediatric population have not been established.

➤*Elderly:* Per the Beers list, dipyridamole may cause orthostatic hypotension. Dipyridamole is considered a high risk medication for the elderly according to the Centers of Medicare and Medicaid Services.

DIPYRIDAMOLE — INJECTION

Drug Interactions

➤*Xanthine derivatives:* Oral maintenance theophylline and other xanthine derivatives such as caffeine may abolish the coronary vasodilatation induced by IV dipyridamole administration. This could lead to a false negative thallium-201 imaging result.

Adverse Reactions

➤*Serious reactions:* See Warnings/Precautions for more information.

➤*Most frequent:* In the study of 3911 patients, the most frequent adverse reactions were: chest pain/angina pectoris (19.7%), electrocardiographic changes (most commonly ST-T changes) (15.9%), headache (12.2%), and dizziness (11.8%).

Dipyridamole Adverse Reactions (> 1%)	
Adverse reaction	Incidence
Blood pressure lability	1.6%
Chest pain/angina pectoris	19.7%
Dizziness	11.8%
Dyspnea	2.6%
Electrocardiographic abnormalities/extrasystoles	5.2%
Electrocardiographic abnormalities/ST-T changes	7.5%
Electrocardiographic abnormalities/tachycardia	3.2%
Fatigue	1.2%
Flushing	3.4%
Headache	12.2%
Hypertension	1.5%
Hypotension	4.6%
Nausea	4.6%
Paresthesia	1.3%
Unspecified pain	2.6%

➤*Cardiovascular:* Electrocardiographic abnormalities unspecified (0.8%), arrhythmia unspecified (0.6%), palpitation (0.3%), ventricular tachycardia (0.2%), bradycardia (0.2%), myocardial infarction (0.1%), AV block (0.1%), syncope (0.1%), orthostatic hypotension (0.1%), atrial fibrillation (0.1%), supraventricular tachycardia (0.1%), ventricular arrhythmia unspecified (0.03%), heart block unspecified (0.03%), cardiomyopathy (0.03%), edema (0.03%).

➤*CNS:* Hypothesia (0.5%), hypertonia (0.3%), nervousness/anxiety (0.2%), tremor (0.1%), abnormal coordination (0.03%), somnolence (0.03%), dysphonia (0.03%), migraine (0.03%), vertigo (0.03%).

➤*GI:* Dyspepsia (1.0%), dry mouth (0.8%), abdominal pain (0.7%), flatulence (0.6%), vomiting (0.4%), eructation (0.1%), dysphagia (0.03%), tenesmus (0.03%), appetite increased (0.03%).

➤*Respiratory:* Pharyngitis (0.3%), bronchospasm (0.2%; parenteral aminophylline should be readily available), hyperventilation (0.1%), rhinitis (0.1%), coughing (0.03%), pleural pain (0.03%).

➤*Miscellaneous:* Myalgia (0.9%), back pain (0.6%), injection site reaction unspecified (0.4%), diaphoresis (0.4%), asthenia (0.3%), malaise (0.3%), arthralgia (0.3%), injection site pain (0.1%), rigor (0.1%), earache (0.1%), tinnitus (0.1%), vision abnormalities unspecified (0.1%), dysgeusia (0.1%), thirst (0.03%), depersonalization (0.03%), eye pain (0.03%), renal pain (0.03%), perineal pain (0.03%), breast pain (0.03%), intermittent claudication (0.03%), leg cramping (0.03%).

➤*Postmarketing:* There have been rare reports of allergic reaction including urticaria, pruritus, dermatitis and rash.

Overdosage

No cases of overdosage in humans have been reported. It is unlikely that overdosage will occur because of the nature of use (ie, single IV administration in controlled settings).

GADOFOSVESET TRISODIUM

Rx	Ablavar (Lantheus Medical Imaging)	Injection, solution: 244 mg/mL[a]	Equiv. to 0.25 mmol/mL. Preservative free. In 10 and 15 mL single-use vials.

[a] Also contains fosveset 0.268 mg.

GADOFOSVESET TRISODIUM — INJECTION

WARNING

Nephrogenic systemic fibrosis – Gadolinium-based contrast agents increase the risk of nephrogenic systemic fibrosis (NSF) in patients with impaired elimination of the drugs. In these patients, avoid use of gadolinium-based contrast agents unless the diagnostic information is essential and not available with noncontrast-enhanced magnetic resonance imaging (MRI) or other modalities. NSF may result in fatal or debilitating fibrosis affecting the skin, muscle, and internal organs.

The risk for NSF appears highest among patients with chronic, severe kidney disease (glomerular filtration rate [GFR] less than 30 mL/min per 1.73 m^2) or acute kidney injury.

Screen patients for acute kidney injury and other conditions that may reduce renal function. For patients at risk of chronically reduced renal function (eg, older than 60 years, hypertension, diabetes), estimate the GFR through laboratory testing.

For patients at highest risk for NSF, do not exceed the recommended gadofosveset dose. Allow a sufficient period of time for elimination of the drug from the body prior to readministration.

Indications

➤*Contrast agent for magnetic resonance angiography:* For use as a contrast agent in magnetic resonance angiography (MRA) to evaluate aortoiliac occlusive disease in adults with known or suspected peripheral vascular disease.

Administration and Dosage

➤*General dosing considerations:* Gadofosveset imaging is completed in 2 stages: the dynamic imaging stage and the steady-state imaging stage. Both stages are essential for adequate evaluation of the arterial system, and dynamic imaging always precedes steady-state imaging. During interpretation of the steady-state images, gadofosveset within the venous system may limit or confound the detection of arterial lesions.

➤*Adults:*

Contrast agent for magnetic resonance angiography – 0.12 mL/kg body weight (0.03 mmol/kg) as an intravenous (IV) bolus injection, manually or by power injection, over a period of up to 30 seconds followed by a 25 to 30 mL normal saline flush.

Gadofosveset Weight-Adjusted Volumes (0.03 mmol/kg dose)	
Body weight	Volume
40 kg	4.8 mL
50 kg	6 mL
60 kg	7.2 mL
70 kg	8.4 mL
80 kg	9.6 mL
90 kg	10.8 mL
100 kg	12 mL
110 kg	13.2 mL
120 kg	14.4 mL
130 kg	15.6 mL
140 kg	16.8 mL
150 kg	18 mL
160 kg	19.2 mL

➤*Renal function impairment:* If no satisfactory diagnostic alternatives are available, administer gadofosveset at a dose of 0.01 to 0.02 mmol/kg in patients with moderate to severe renal impairment (GFR less than 60 mL/kg/m^2).

➤*Administration:* Gadofosveset is intended for single use only and should be used immediately upon opening. Discard any unused portion of the gadofosveset vial.

Administer gadofosveset as an IV bolus injection, manually or by power injection, over a period of up to 30 seconds followed by a 25 to 30 mL normal saline flush.

To assess the initial distribution of gadofosveset within the arterial system, begin dynamic imaging immediately upon injection. Begin steady-state imaging after dynamic imaging has been completed, generally 5 to 7 minutes following gadofosveset administration. At this time point, gadofosveset is generally distributed throughout the blood.

➤*Admixture compatibility:* Do not mix IV medications or parenteral nutrition solutions with gadofosveset. Do not administer any other medications in the same IV line simultaneously with gadofosveset.

➤*Storage / Stability:* Store at or below 25°C (77°F); excursions are permitted between 15° and 30°C (59° and 86°F). Protect from light and freezing.

Actions

➤*Pharmacology:* Following IV injection, gadofosveset binds reversibly to endogenous serum albumin resulting in longer vascular residence time than nonprotein binding contrast agents. The binding to serum albumin also increases the magnetic resonance relaxivity of gadofosveset and decreases

GADOFOSVESET TRISODIUM — INJECTION

the relaxation time (T1) of water protons, resulting in an increase in signal intensity (brightness) of blood.

Pharmacodynamics – In human studies, gadofosveset substantially shortened blood T1 values for up to 4 hours after IV bolus injection. Relaxivity in plasma was measured as 33.4 to 45.7 $mM^{-1}s^{-1}$ (0.47 T) over the dose range of up to 0.05 mmol/kg.

➤*Pharmacokinetics:*

Absorption – The pharmacokinetics of IV-administered gadofosveset conforms to a 2-compartment open model with mean plasma concentrations (reported as mean ± standard deviation) of 0.43 ± 0.04 mmol/L at 3 minutes postinjection, and 0.24 ± 0.03 mmol/L at 1 hour postinjection.

Distribution – The mean volume of distribution at steady state for gadofosveset was 148 ± 16 mL/kg, roughly equivalent to that of extracellular fluid. A significant portion of circulating gadofosveset is bound to plasma proteins, predominantly albumin. At 0.05, 0.5, 1, and 4 hours after injection of 0.03 mmol/kg, the plasma protein binding of gadofosveset ranges from 79.8% to 87.4%. The mean half-life of the distribution phase is 0.48 ± 0.11 hours.

Metabolism – Gadofosveset does not undergo measurable metabolism in humans.

Excretion – Gadofosveset is eliminated primarily in the urine, with between 79% and 94% (mean, 83.7%) of an injected dose recovered in the urine. Of the total gadofosveset recovered in urine, 94% is recovered within the first 72 hours. A small portion of the gadofosveset dose is recovered in feces (approximately 4.7%). The mean half-life of the elimination phase is 16.3 ± 2.6 hours. The mean total clearance of gadofosveset is 6.57 ± 0.97 mL/h/kg following the administration of 0.03 mmol/kg.

Special populations –

Renal function impairment: Administration of gadolinium-based contrast agents, including gadofosveset, to patients with severe renal insufficiency increases the risk of NSF. Administration of these agents to patients with mild to moderate renal insufficiency may increase the risk of worsened renal function. Prior to use of gadofosveset in these patients, ensure that no satisfactory diagnostic alternatives are available. In patients with moderate to severe renal impairment (GFR less than 60 $mL/kg/m^2$), administer a dose of gadofosveset 0.01 to 0.02 mmol/kg. Consider follow-up renal function assessments following gadofosveset administration to any patients with renal insufficiency.

A clinical study of a dose of gadofosveset 0.05 mmol/kg was conducted in patients with mild, moderate, and severe renal impairment. The clearance decreased substantially as renal function decreased and the systemic exposure (area under the curve) increased almost 1.75-fold in patients with moderate renal impairment (creatinine clearance [CrCl] 30 to 50 mL/min) and 2.25-fold in patients with severe renal impairment (CrCl less than 30 mL/min). The elimination half-life increased from 19 hours in healthy subjects to 49 hours in patients with moderate renal impairment and 70 hours in patients with severe renal impairment. The volume of distribution at steady state and plasma protein binding of gadofosveset were not affected by renal impairment. Fecal elimination of gadofosveset increased as a function of increasing renal impairment (6.5% in healthy subjects to 13.3% in patients with severe renal impairment).

- *Hemodialysis* – Gadofosveset is removed from the body by hemodialysis using high-flux filters. Elimination of the total administered dose of gadolinium in dialysate over 3 dialysis sessions using high-flux filters averaged 46.8%, 12.9%, and 6.11% for the first, second, and third sessions, respectively.

Hepatic function impairment: The pharmacokinetics and plasma protein binding of gadofosveset was not significantly influenced by moderate hepatic impairment. A slight decrease in fecal elimination of gadofosveset was seen for hepatically impaired subjects (2.7%) compared with healthy subjects (4.8%).

Contraindications

History of a prior allergic reaction to a gadolinium-based contrast agent.

Warnings/Precautions

➤*Nephrogenic systemic fibrosis:* Gadolinium-based contrast agents increase the risk of NSF in patients with impaired elimination of the drugs. Avoid use of gadolinium-based contrast agents among these patients unless the diagnostic information is essential and not available with noncontrast-enhanced MRI or other modalities. The gadolinium-based contrast agent–associated NSF risk appears highest for patients with chronic, severe kidney disease (GFR less than 30 mL/min per 1.73 m^2) as well as patients with acute kidney injury. The risk appears lower for patients with chronic, moderate kidney disease (GFR 30 to 59 mL/min per 1.73 m^2) and little, if any, for patients with chronic, mild kidney disease (GFR 60 to 89 mL/min per 1.73 m^2). NSF may result in fatal or debilitating fibrosis affecting the skin, muscle, and internal organs. Report any diagnosis of NSF following gadofosveset administration to Lantheus Medical Imaging, Inc (1-978-667-9531)/(1-800-362-2668) or Food and Drug Administration (1-800-332-1088 or http://www.fda.gov/medwatch).

Screen patients for acute kidney injury and other conditions that may reduce renal function. Features of acute kidney injury include a rapid (over hours to days) and usually reversible decrease in kidney function, commonly in the setting of surgery, severe infection, injury, or drug-induced kidney toxicity. Serum creatinine levels and estimated GFR may not reliably assess renal function in the setting of acute kidney injury. For patients at risk for chronically reduced renal function (eg, older than 60 years, diabetes mellitus, chronic hypertension), estimate the GFR through laboratory testing.

Factors that may increase the risk of NSF are repeated or higher than recommended doses of a GBCA and the degree of renal impairment at the time of exposure. Record the specific GBCA and the dose administered to a patient. For patients at highest risk for NSF, do not exceed the recommended gadofoveset dose and allow a sufficient period of time for elimination of the drug prior to readministration. For patients receiving hemodialysis, consider the prompt initiation of hemodialysis following the administration of a GBCA in order to enhance the contrast agent's elimination. The usefulness of hemodialysis in the prevention of NSF is unknown.

➤*Acute renal failure:* In patients with renal insufficiency, acute renal failure requiring dialysis or worsening renal function have occurred with the use of other gadolinium agents. The risk of renal failure may increase with an increasing dose of gadolinium contrast. Screen all patients for renal dysfunction by obtaining a history and/or laboratory tests. Consider follow-up renal function assessments for patients with a history of renal dysfunction. No reports of acute renal failure were observed in clinical trials of gadofosveset.

➤*Cardiovascular effects:* In clinical trials, a small increase (2.8 msec) in the average change from baseline in QTc was observed at 45 minutes following gadofosveset administration; no increase was observed at 24 and 72 hours. A QTc change of 30 to 60 msec from baseline was observed in 6% of patients at 45 minutes following gadofosveset administration. At this time point, 0.4% of patients experienced a QTc increase of more than 60 msec. These QTc prolongations were not associated with arrhythmias or symptoms. In patients at high risk of arrhythmias due to QTc prolongation (eg, concomitant medications, underlying cardiac conditions) consider obtaining baseline electrocardiograms (ECGs) to help assess the risks for gadofosveset administration. If gadofosveset is administered to these patients, consider follow-up ECGs and risk reduction measures (eg, patient counseling or intensive ECG monitoring) until most of the gadofosveset has been eliminated from the blood. In patients with healthy renal function, most gadofosveset was eliminated from the blood by 72 hours following injection.

➤*Hypersensitivity reactions:* Gadofosveset may cause anaphylactoid and/or anaphylactic reactions, including life-threatening or fatal reactions. In clinical trials, anaphylactoid and/or anaphylactic reactions occurred in 2 of 1,676 subjects. If anaphylactic or anaphylactoid reactions occur, stop gadofosveset and immediately begin appropriate therapy. Closely observe patients, particularly those with a history of drug reactions, asthma, or allergy or other hypersensitivity disorders, during and up to several hours after gadofosveset administration. Have emergency resuscitative equipment available prior to and during gadofosveset administration.

➤*Pregnancy: Category C.* There are no adequate and well-controlled studies of gadofosveset in pregnant women. In animal studies, pregnant rabbits treated with gadofosveset at doses 3 times the human dose (based on body surface area [BSA]) experienced higher rates of fetal loss and resorptions. Because animal reproduction studies are not always predictive of human response, only use gadofosveset during pregnancy if the diagnostic benefit justifies the potential risks to the fetus.

In reproductive studies, pregnant rats and rabbits received gadofosveset at various doses of up to approximately 11 (rats) and 21.5 (rabbits) times the human dose (based on BSA). The highest dose resulted in maternal toxicity in both species. In rabbits that received gadofosveset at 3 times the human dose (based on BSA), increased postimplantation loss, resorptions, and dead fetuses were observed. Fetal anomalies were not observed in the rat or rabbit offspring. Because pregnant animals received repeated daily doses of gadofosveset, their overall exposure was significantly higher than that achieved with a single dose administered to humans.

➤*Lactation:* It is not known whether gadofosveset is secreted in human milk. Because many drugs are excreted in human milk, exercise caution when gadofosveset is administered to a woman who is breast-feeding. The risks associated with exposure of infants to gadolinium-based contrast agents in breast milk are unknown. Limited case reports indicate that 0.01% to 0.04% of the maternal gadolinium dose is excreted in human breast milk. Studies of other gadolinium products have shown limited GI absorption. These studies were conducted with gadolinium products with shorter half-lives than gadofosveset. Avoid gadofosveset administration to women who are breast-feeding, unless the diagnostic information is essential and not obtainable with noncontrast MRA.

➤*Children:* The safety and effectiveness of gadofosveset in patients younger than 18 years have not been established. The risks associated with gadofosveset administration to children are unknown and insufficient data are available to establish a dose. Because gadofosveset is eliminated predominantly by the kidneys, children with immature renal function may be at particular risk of adverse reactions.

➤*Elderly:* Although current clinical experience has not identified differences in responses between elderly and younger patients, do not rule out greater susceptibility to adverse experiences of some older individuals.

➤*Monitoring:* Screen all patients for renal dysfunction by obtaining a history and/or laboratory tests prior to administration of gadofosveset. Consider follow-up renal function assessments for patients with a history of renal dysfunction.

Consider obtaining baseline and follow-up ECGs in patients at high risk of arrhythmias due to QTc prolongation.

Closely observe patients with a history of drug reactions, asthma, or allergy or other hypersensitivity disorders during and up to several hours after gadofosveset administration for signs and symptoms of anaphylactoid and/or anaphylactic reactions.

Drug Interactions

Gadofosveset binds to blood albumin (79.8% to 87.4%) and has the potential to alter the binding of other drugs that bind to albumin. However, no drug interactions have been reported in clinical trials. Consider the possibility of an interaction when gadofosveset is coadministered with other drugs that bind to albumin. The effect of the concurrent medication may be increased or decreased.

GADOFOSVESET TRISODIUM — INJECTION

➤*QT prolongation:* An increase in the QTc of 30 to 60 msec from baseline has been observed in 6% of patients at 45 minutes following gadofosveset administration and 0.4% of patients experience a QTc increase of more than 60 msec. These QTc prolongations have not been associated with arrhythmias or symptoms. In patients at high risk of arrhythmias due to QTc prolongation (eg, concomitant medications, underlying cardiac conditions), consider obtaining baseline ECGs to assess the risk for gadofosveset administration. If gadofosveset is administered to these patients, consider follow-up ECGs and risk reduction measures (eg, intensive ECG monitoring) until most gadofosveset is eliminated from the body (approximately 72 hours in patients with healthy renal function).

An additive effect of gadofosveset with other drugs that prolong the QT interval cannot be excluded. The following drugs may prolong the QT interval and increase the risk of life-threatening cardiac arrhythmias, including torsades de pointes: antiarrhythmic agents (eg, amiodarone, bretylium, disopyramide, dofetilide, procainamide, quinidine, sotalol), arsenic trioxide, chlorpromazine, cisapride, dolasetron, droperidol, gatifloxacin, halofantrine, levomethadyl, mefloquine, mesoridazine, moxifloxacin, pentamidine, pimozide, probucol, sparfloxacin, thioridazine, and ziprasidone. (See Drug-Induced Prolongation of the QT Interval and Torsades de Pointes.)

➤*Minimally or noninteracting drugs:* In a clinical trial of 10 patients receiving a stable warfarin dose, a single dose of gadofosveset 0.05 mmol/kg did not alter the anticoagulant activity of warfarin as measured by the international normalized ratio.

Adverse Reactions

➤*Serious adverse reactions:* Anaphylaxis and anaphylactoid reactions were the most common serious reactions observed following gadofosveset administration.

➤*Adverse reactions (at least 1%):*

Gadofosveset Adverse Reactions (≥ 1%)

Adverse reactions	%
Cardiovascular	
Hypertension	1%
Vasodilation	3%
CNS	
Dizziness (excluding vertigo)	1%
Headache	4%
Paresthesia	3%
GI	
Dysgeusia	2%
Nausea	4%
Local	
Injection-site bruising	2%
Venipuncture-site bruising	2%
Miscellaneous	
Burning sensation	2%
Feeling cold	1%
Pruritus	5%

Overdosage

➤*Symptoms:* Gadofosveset has been administered to humans up to a dose of 0.15 mmol/kg (5 times the clinical dose). No gadofosveset overdoses were reported in clinical trials.

➤*Treatment:* In the event of an overdose, direct treatment toward the support of all vital functions and promptly institute symptomatic therapy. Gadofosveset is removed by hemodialysis using a high-flux dialysis procedure.

Patient Information

Instruct patients receiving gadofosveset to inform their health care provider of the following if they are pregnant or breast-feeding; have a history of allergic reaction to contrast media, a history of bronchial asthma, or allergic respiratory disorder; have a history of kidney and/or liver disease; have recently received a gadolinium-based contrast agent; have a history of heart rhythm disturbances or cardiac disease; are taking any prescription or nonprescription medications

Advise patients that gadolinium-based contrast agents increase the risk of NSF in patients with impaired elimination of the drugs. To counsel patients at risk for NSF, describe the clinical manifestations of NSF and the procedures to screen for the detection of renal impairment.

Instruct patients to contact their health care provider if they develop signs or symptoms of NSF, such as burning, itching, swelling, scaling, hardening and tightening of the skin, red or dark patches on the skin; stiffness in joints with trouble moving, bending, or straightening of the arms, hands, legs, or feet; pain in the hip bones or ribs; or muscle weakness.

Inform patients that they may experience the following: reactions at the injection site, such as redness, mild and transient burning or pain, or feeling of warmth or coldness; or itching or nausea.

ADENOSINE

Rx	**Adenoscan** (Astellas Pharma US)	**Injection, solution:** 3 mg/mL	Sodium chloride 9 mg/mL. Preservative free. In 20 mL and 30 mL single-dose vials.

ADENOSINE — INJECTION

Indications

➤*Diagnostic aid:* Adjunct to thallium-201 myocardial perfusion scintigraphy in patients unable to exercise adequately.

Administration and Dosage

➤*Adults:*

Stress testing diagnostic aid –

Usual dosage: 140 mcg/kg/min infused for 6 minutes (total dose of 0.84 mg/kg).

Concomitant therapy: The required dose of thallium-201 should be injected at the midpoint of the adenosine infusion (ie, after the first 3 minutes of adenosine).

➤*Administration:* For intravenous (IV) infusion only; give as a continuous peripheral IV infusion. The injection should be as close to the venous access as possible to prevent an inadvertent increase in the dose of adenosine (the contents of the IV tubing) being administered.

The following adenosine infusion rate guide may be used to determine the appropriate infusion rate corrected for total body weight:

45 kg – Infusion rate is 2.1 mL/min.

50 kg – Infusion rate is 2.3 mL/min.

55 kg – Infusion rate is 2.6 mL/min.

60 kg – Infusion rate is 2.8 mL/min.

65 kg – Infusion rate is 3 mL/min.

70 kg – Infusion rate is 3.3 mL/min.

75 kg – Infusion rate is 3.5 mL/min.

80 kg – Infusion rate is 3.8 mL/min.

85 kg – Infusion rate is 4 mL/min.

90 kg – Infusion rate is 4.2 mL/min.

➤*Admixture compatibility:* Thallium-201 is physically compatible with adenosine and may be injected directly into the adenosine infusion set.

➤*Storage/Stability:* Store at 15° to 30°C (59° to 86°F). Do not refrigerate because crystallization may occur. If this occurs, dissolve crystals by warming to room temperature. Discard unused portion.

Actions

➤*Pharmacology:* Adenosine is an endogenous nucleoside occurring in all cells of the body. Adenosine is a potent vasodilator in most vascular beds, except in renal afferent arterioles and hepatic veins, where it produces vasoconstriction. Adenosine is thought to exert its pharmacological effects through activation of purine receptors (cell-surface A_1 and A_2 adenosine receptors). Although the exact mechanism by which adenosine receptor activation relaxes vascular smooth muscle is not known, there is evidence to support inhibition of the slow inward calcium current reducing calcium uptake and activation of adenylate cyclase through A_2 receptors in smooth muscle cells. Adenosine may also lessen vascular tone by modulating sympathetic neurotransmission. The intracellular uptake of adenosine is mediated by a specific transmembrane nucleoside transport system. Once inside the cell, adenosine is rapidly phosphorylated by adenosine kinase to adenosine monophosphate, or deaminated by adenosine deaminase to inosine. These intracellular metabolites of adenosine are not vasoactive.

Myocardial uptake of thallium-201 is directly proportional to coronary blood flow. Because adenosine significantly increases blood flow in normal coronary arteries with little or no increase in stenotic arteries, adenosine causes relatively less thallium-201 uptake in vascular territories supplied by stenotic coronary arteries; a greater difference is seen after adenosine between areas served by normal and areas served by stenotic vessels than is seen prior to adenosine.

➤*Pharmacokinetics:*

Distribution – IV-administered adenosine is rapidly cleared from the circulation via cellular uptake, primarily by erythrocytes and vascular endothelial cells. This process involves a specific transmembrane nucleoside carrier system that is reversible, nonconcentrative, and bidirectionally symmetrical.

Metabolism/Excretion – Intracellular adenosine is rapidly metabolized via phosphorylation to adenosine monophosphate by adenosine kinase or via deamination to inosine by adenosine deaminase in the cytosol. Because adenosine kinase has a lower Michaelis constant and maximal velocity than adenosine deaminase, deamination plays a significant role only when cytosolic adenosine saturates the phosphorylation pathway. Inosine formed by deamination of adenosine can leave the cell intact or can be degraded to hypoxanthine, xanthine, and ultimately uric acid. Adenosine monophosphate formed by phosphorylation of adenosine is incorporated into the high-energy phosphate pool. While extracellular adenosine is primarily cleared by cellular

ADENOSINE — INJECTION

uptake with a half-life of less than 10 seconds in whole blood, excessive amounts may be deaminated by an ecto-form of adenosine deaminase.

Contraindications

Second- or third-degree atrioventricular (AV) block (except in patients with a functioning artificial pacemaker); sinus node disease, such as sick sinus syndrome or symptomatic bradycardia (except in patients with a functioning artificial pacemaker); known or suspected bronchoconstrictive or bronchospastic lung disease (eg, asthma); known hypersensitivity to adenosine.

Warnings/Precautions

➤*Cardiac effects:* Fatal cardiac arrest, sustained ventricular tachycardia (requiring resuscitation), and nonfatal myocardial infarction have been reported coincident with adenosine infusion. Patients with unstable angina may be at greater risk. Ensure that appropriate resuscitative measures are available.

Atrial fibrillation – Atrial fibrillation has been reported in patients (with and without a history of atrial fibrillation) undergoing myocardial perfusion imaging with adenosine infusion. In these cases, atrial fibrillation began 1.5 to 3 minutes after initiation of adenosine, lasted for 15 seconds to 6 hours, and spontaneously converted to normal sinus rhythm.

Sinoatrial and atrioventricular nodal block – Adenosine exerts a direct depressant effect on the sinoatrial (SA) and AV nodes and has the potential to cause first-, second-, or third-degree AV block or sinus bradycardia. Approximately 6.3% of patients develop AV block with adenosine, including first-degree (2.9%), second-degree (2.6%), and third-degree (0.8%) heart block. Adenosine can cause sinus bradycardia. Use adenosine with caution in patients with preexisting first-degree AV block or bundle branch block, and avoid in patients with high-grade AV block or sinus node dysfunction (except in patients with a functioning artificial pacemaker). Discontinue adenosine in any patient who develops persistent or symptomatic high-grade AV block. Sinus pause has been observed rarely with adenosine infusions.

Hypotension – Adenosine is a potent peripheral vasodilator and can cause significant hypotension. Patients with an intact baroreceptor reflex mechanism are able to maintain blood pressure and tissue perfusion in response to adenosine by increasing heart rate and cardiac output. However, use adenosine with caution in patients with autonomic dysfunction, pericarditis or pericardial effusions, stenotic carotid artery disease with cerebrovascular insufficiency, stenotic valvular heart disease, or uncorrected hypovolemia because of the risk of hypotensive complications in these patients. Discontinue adenosine in any patient who develops persistent or symptomatic hypotension.

Hypertension: Increases in systolic and diastolic pressure have been observed (as great as 140 mm Hg systolic in 1 case) concomitant with adenosine infusion; most increases resolved spontaneously within several minutes, but in some cases, hypertension lasted for several hours.

➤*Bronchoconstriction:* Adenosine is a respiratory stimulant (probably through activation of carotid body chemoreceptors), and IV administration in humans has been shown to increase minute ventilation and reduce arterial partial pressure of carbon dioxide, causing respiratory alkalosis. Approximately 28% of patients experience breathlessness (dyspnea) or an urge to breathe deeply with adenosine. These respiratory complaints are transient and only rarely require intervention.

Adenosine administered by inhalation has been reported to cause bronchoconstriction in patients with asthma, presumably because of mast cell degranulation and histamine release. These effects have not been observed in healthy subjects. Adenosine has been administered to a limited number of patients with asthma, and mild to moderate exacerbation of their symptoms has been reported. Respiratory compromise has occurred during adenosine infusion in patients with obstructive pulmonary disease. Use adenosine with caution in patients with obstructive lung disease not associated with bronchoconstriction (eg, bronchitis, emphysema), and avoid in patients with bronchoconstriction or bronchospasm (eg, asthma). Discontinue adenosine in any patient who develops severe respiratory difficulties.

➤*Pregnancy: Category C.* Animal reproduction studies have not been conducted with adenosine, nor have studies been performed in pregnant women. Because it is not known whether the drug can cause fetal harm when administered to pregnant women, use during pregnancy only if clearly needed.

➤*Lactation:* Because adenosine is used only by IV injection in short-term care situations, it is doubtful that any reports will be located describing the use of adenosine during human lactation. In addition, the serum half-life is so short that it is unlikely that any of the drug will pass into milk.

➤*Children:* The safety and effectiveness in patients younger than 18 years of age have not been established.

➤*Monitoring:* Monitor blood pressure and cardiac rhythm during and after administration.

Drug Interactions

➤*General information:* Whenever possible, withhold drugs that might inhibit or augment the effects of adenosine for at least 5 half-lives prior to the use of adenosine.

Adenosine Drug Interactions			
Precipitant drug	Object drug[a]		Description
Carbamazepine	Adenosine	↑	Carbamazepine may increase the degree of heart block produced by other agents. Because the primary effect of adenosine is to decrease conduction through the AV node, higher degrees of heart block may be produced in the presence of carbamazepine. Closely monitor cardiac function.
Cardioactive agents (eg, ACE[b] inhibitors [eg, captopril], antiarrhythmic agents [eg, quinidine], beta-adrenergic blocking agents [eg, propranolol], calcium channel blocking agents [eg, verapamil], cardiac glycosides [eg, digoxin])	Adenosine	↑	Use adenosine with caution in the presence of these agents because of the potential for additive or synergistic depressant effects on the SA and AV nodes. The use of adenosine with digoxin and verapamil may rarely be associated with ventricular fibrillation. Closely monitor cardiac function.
Adenosine	Cardioactive drugs (eg, ACE inhibitors [eg, captopril], antiarrhythmic agents [eg, quinidine], beta-adrenergic blocking agents [eg, propranolol], calcium channel blocking agents [eg, verapamil], cardiac glycosides [eg, digoxin])		
Dipyridamole	Adenosine	↑	The effects of adenosine are potentiated; therefore, smaller doses of adenosine may be effective in the presence of dipyridamole.
Methylxanthines (eg, caffeine, theophylline)	Adenosine	↓	The effects of adenosine are antagonized in the presence of methylxanthines; therefore, larger doses of adenosine may be required or adenosine may be ineffective.

[a] ↑ = object drug increased; ↓ = object drug decreased.
[b] ACE = angiotensin-converting enzyme.

Adverse Reactions

➤*Adverse reactions (at least 1%):*

Adenosine Adverse Reactions (≥ 1%)	
Adverse reactions	Adenosine
Cardiovascular	
Arrhythmias	1%
First-degree AV block	3%
Flushing	44%
Hypotension	2%
Second-degree AV block	3%
ST segment depression	3%
CNS	
Headache	18%
Light-headedness/dizziness	12%
Nervousness	2%
Paresthesia	2%
Miscellaneous	
Chest discomfort	40%
Dyspnea or urge to breathe deeply	28%

ADENOSINE — INJECTION

Adenosine Adverse Reactions (≥ 1%)	
Adverse reactions	Adenosine
GI discomfort	13%
Throat, neck, or jaw discomfort	15%
Upper extremity discomfort	4%

➤*Adverse reactions (less than 1%):*

Cardiovascular – Bradycardia, hypertension (systolic blood pressure greater than 200 mm Hg), life-threatening ventricular arrhythmia, nonfatal myocardial infarction, palpitation, sinus exit block, sinus pause, third-degree AV block, T-wave changes.

CNS – Drowsiness, emotional instability, tremors, weakness.

GU – Urgency, vaginal pressure.

➤*Musculoskeletal:* Back discomfort, lower extremity discomfort.

➤*Special senses:* Blurred vision, dry mouth, ear discomfort, metallic taste, nasal congestion, scotomas, tongue discomfort.

➤*Miscellaneous:* Cough, sweating.

➤*Postmarketing experience:*

CNS – Seizure activity, including generalized tonic-clonic seizures, and loss of consciousness.

GI – Nausea, vomiting.

Miscellaneous – Injection-site reaction, respiratory arrest.

Overdosage

➤*Symptoms:* The half-life of adenosine is less than 10 seconds and adverse effects of adenosine (when they occur) usually resolve quickly when the infusion is discontinued, although delayed or persistent effects have been observed.

➤*Treatment:* Individualize treatment of any prolonged adverse effects and direct it toward the specific effect. Methylxanthines, such as caffeine and theophylline, are competitive adenosine receptor antagonists, and theophylline has been used to effectively terminate persistent adverse effects. In controlled United States clinical trials, theophylline (50 to 125 mg slow IV injection) was needed to abort adenosine adverse effects in less than 2% of patients.

Patient Information

Instruct patients to report the following symptoms to a health care provider: chest pressure, dizziness, facial flushing, headache, light-headedness, nausea, numbness, shortness of breath, or tingling in arms.

REGADENOSON

Rx	**Lexiscan** (Astellas Pharma)	**Injection, solution:** 0.4 mg per 5 mL	Preservative free. Edetate disodium dihydrate. In 5 mL single-use vials and single-use prefilled syringes.

REGADENOSON — INJECTION

Indications

➤*Radionuclide myocardial perfusion imaging:* A pharmacologic stress agent for radionuclide myocardial perfusion imaging (MPI) in patients unable to undergo adequate exercise stress.

Administration and Dosage

➤*Adults:*

Radionuclide myocardial perfusion imaging – 5 mL (0.4 mg) intravenously (IV).

➤*Administration:* Administer as a rapid (approximately 10 seconds) injection into a peripheral vein using a 22-gauge or larger catheter or needle. Administer a 5 mL saline flush immediately after the injection of regadenoson. Administer the radionuclide MPI agent 10 to 20 seconds after the saline flush. The radionuclide may be injected directly into the same catheter as regadenoson.

➤*Storage/Stability:* Store at 25°C (77°F); excursions are permitted to 15° to 30°C (59° to 86°F).

Actions

➤*Pharmacology:* Regadenoson, a coronary vasodilator, is a low-affinity agonist (K_i approximately 1.3 mcM) for the A_{2A} adenosine receptor, with at least a 10-fold lower affinity for the A_1 adenosine receptor (K_i more than 16.5 mcM), and weak, if any, affinity for the A_{2B} and A_3 adenosine receptors. Activation of the A_{2A} adenosine receptor by regadenoson produces coronary vasodilation and increases coronary blood flow (CBF).

Pharmacodynamics –

Coronary blood flow: Regadenoson causes a rapid increase in CBF, which is sustained for a short duration. In patients undergoing coronary catheterization, pulsed-wave Doppler ultrasonography was used to measure the average peak velocity of CBF before and up to 30 minutes after administration of regadenoson (0.4 mg IV). Mean average peak velocity increased to more than twice the baseline by 30 seconds and decreased to less than twice the baseline level within 10 minutes.

Myocardial uptake of the radiopharmaceutical is proportional to CBF. Because regadenoson increases blood flow in normal coronary arteries with little or no increase in stenotic arteries, regadenoson causes relatively less uptake of the radiopharmaceutical in vascular territories supplied by stenotic arteries. MPI intensity after regadenoson administration is therefore greater in areas perfused by normal relative to stenosed arteries.

➤*Pharmacokinetics:*

Absorption/Distribution – In healthy volunteers, the regadenoson plasma concentration-time profile is multiexponential in nature and best characterized by a 3-compartment model. The maximal plasma concentration of regadenoson is achieved within 1 to 4 minutes after injection of regadenoson and parallels the onset of the pharmacodynamic response. The half-life of this initial phase is approximately 2 to 4 minutes. An intermediate phase follows, with a half-life of 30 minutes on average, coinciding with loss of the pharmacodynamic effect. The terminal phase consists of a decline in plasma concentration, with a half-life of approximately 2 hours. Within the dose range of 0.3 to 20 mcg/kg in healthy subjects, clearance, terminal half-life, or volume of distribution do not appear dependent on dose.

Metabolism – The metabolism of regadenoson is unknown in humans. Incubation with rat, dog, and human liver microsomes, as well as human hepatocytes, produced no detectable metabolites of regadenoson.

Excretion – In healthy volunteers, 57% of the regadenoson dose is excreted unchanged in the urine (range, 19% to 77%), with an average plasma renal clearance around 450 mL/min (ie, in excess of the glomerular filtration rate). This indicates that renal tubular secretion plays a role in regadenoson elimination.

Special populations –

Renal function impairment: A population pharmacokinetic analysis including data from subjects and patients demonstrated that regadenoson clearance decreases in parallel with a reduction in creatinine clearance (CrCl).

Weight: A population pharmacokinetic analysis including data from subjects and patients demonstrated that regadenoson clearance increases with increased body weight.

Contraindications

Second- or third-degree atrioventricular (AV) block or sinus node dysfunction, unless these patients have a functioning artificial pacemaker.

Warnings/Precautions

➤*Cardiovascular effects:*

Myocardial ischemia – Fatal cardiac arrest, life-threatening ventricular arrhythmias, and myocardial infarction may result from the ischemia induced by pharmacologic stress agents. Have cardiac resuscitation equipment and trained staff available before administering regadenoson. If serious reactions to regadenoson occur, consider the use of aminophylline, an adenosine antagonist, to shorten the duration of increased CBF induced by regadenoson.

Sinoatrial and atrioventricular nodal block – Adenosine receptor agonists, including regadenoson, can depress the sinoatrial and AV nodes and may cause first-, second-, or third-degree AV block or sinus bradycardia requiring intervention. In clinical trials, first-degree AV block (PR prolongation of more than 220 msec) developed in 3% of patients within 2 hours of regadenoson administration; transient second-degree AV block with 1 dropped beat was observed in 1 patient receiving regadenoson. In postmarketing experience, third-degree heart block and asystole within minutes of regadenoson administration have occurred.

Hypotension – Adenosine receptor agonists, including regadenoson, induce arterial vasodilation and hypotension. Decreased systolic blood pressure (more than 35 mm Hg) was observed in 7% of patients, and decreased diastolic blood pressure (more than 25 mm Hg) was observed in 4% of patients within 45 minutes of regadenoson administration. The risk of serious hypotension may be higher in patients with autonomic dysfunction, hypovolemia, left main coronary artery stenosis, stenotic valvular heart disease, pericarditis or pericardial effusions, or stenotic carotid artery disease with cerebrovascular insufficiency. In postmarketing experience, syncope and transient ischemic attacks have been observed.

➤*Bronchoconstriction:* Adenosine receptor agonists, including regadenoson, may cause bronchoconstriction and respiratory compromise. For patients with known or suspected bronchoconstrictive disease, chronic obstructive pulmonary disease (COPD), or asthma, have appropriate bronchodilator therapy and resuscitative measures available prior to regadenoson administration.

The incidence of bronchoconstriction (forced expiratory volume at 1 second [FEV_1] reduction of more than 15% from baseline) was assessed in 2 clinical studies. In a randomized, controlled study of 49 patients with moderate to severe COPD, the rate of bronchoconstriction was 12% and 6% for the regadenoson and placebo groups, respectively. In a randomized, controlled study of 48 patients with mild to moderate asthma who had previously been shown to have bronchoconstrictive reactions to adenosine, the rate of bronchoconstriction was the same (4%) for the regadenoson and placebo groups. In both studies, dyspnea was reported as an adverse reaction in the regadenoson group (61% for patients with COPD; 34% for patients with asthma), while no subjects in the placebo group experienced dyspnea.

➤*Pregnancy:* *Category C.* There are no adequate, well-controlled studies with regadenoson in pregnant women. Use regadenoson during pregnancy only if the potential benefit to the patient justifies the potential risk to the fetus.

REGADENOSON — INJECTION

Reproductive studies in rats showed that regadenoson doses 10 and 20 times the maximum recommended human dose (MRHD) based on body surface area caused reduced fetal body weights and significant ossification delays in fore and hind limb phalanges and metatarsals; however, maternal toxicity also occurred at these doses. Skeletal variations were increased in all treated groups. In rabbits, there were no teratogenic effects in offspring at regadenoson doses 4 times the MRHD, although signs of maternal toxicity occurred at this dose. At regadenoson doses equivalent to 12 and 20 times the MRHD, maternal toxicity occurred, along with increased embryofetal loss and fetal malformations. It is not clear whether malformations that occurred at maternally toxic doses of regadenoson in both animal species were due to fetal drug effects or only maternal toxic effects. Because animals received repeated doses of regadenoson, their exposure was significantly higher than that achieved with the standard single dose administered to humans.

➤*Lactation:* It is not known whether regadenoson is excreted in human milk. Because many drugs are excreted in human milk and because of the potential for serious adverse reactions from regadenoson in breast-feeding infants, take into account the importance of the drug to the mother when deciding whether to interrupt breast-feeding after administration of regadenoson or not to administer regadenoson. Based on the pharmacokinetics of regadenoson, it should be cleared 10 hours after administration. Therefore, breast-feeding women may consider interrupting breast-feeding for 10 hours after administration.

➤*Children:* Safety and effectiveness in children (younger than 18 years of age) have not been established.

➤*Elderly:* Older patients (75 years of age and older) had a similar adverse reaction profile compared with younger patients (younger than 65 years of age) but had a higher incidence of hypotension (2% vs less than 1%).

Drug Interactions

Regadenoson Drug Interactions

Precipitant drug	Object drug[a]		Description
Dipyridamole	Regadenoson	⟷	Dipyridamole may change the effects of regadenoson. Withhold dipyridamole for at least 2 days prior to regadenoson administration.
Methylxanthines (eg, caffeine, theophylline)	Regadenoson	⬇	Methylxanthines are nonspecific adenosine receptor antagonists and may interfere with the vasodilation activity of regadenoson. Avoid methylxanthines for at least 12 hours before regadenoson administration.

[a] ⟷ = undetermined clinical effect; ⬇ = object drug decreased.

Adverse Reactions

Most adverse reactions began soon after dosing and generally resolved within approximately 15 minutes, except for headache, which resolved in most patients within 30 minutes.

Regadenoson Adverse Reactions (≥ 5%)

Adverse reaction	Regadenoson (n = 1,337)	*Adenoscan* (n = 678)
Cardiovascular		
Angina pectoris or ST segment depression	12%	18%
CNS		
Dizziness	8%	7%
Flushing	16%	25%
Headache	26%	17%
GI		
Abdominal discomfort	5%	2%
Dysgeusia	5%	7%
Nausea	6%	6%
Miscellaneous		
Chest discomfort	13%	18%
Chest pain	7%	10%
Dyspnea	28%	26%
Feeling hot	5%	8%

➤*Electrocardiogram abnormalities:* The frequency of rhythm or conduction abnormalities following regadenoson or *Adenoscan* is shown in the following table.

Regadenoson Rhythm or Conduction Abnormalities[a,b]

Adverse reaction	Regadenoson	*Adenoscan*
Rhythm or conduction abnormalities[c]	26%	30%
Rhythm abnormalities	20%	20%
PACs	7%	9%
PVCs	14%	12%
First-degree AV block (PR prolongation > 220 msec)	3%	7%
Second-degree AV block	0.1%	1%
AV conduction abnormalities (other than AV blocks)	0.1%	0%
Ventricular conduction abnormalities	6%	5%

[a] PACs = premature atrial contraction; PVCs = premature ventricular contraction.
[b] 12-lead ECGs were recorded before and for up to 2 hours after dosing.
[c] Includes rhythm abnormalities (PACs, PVCs, atrial fibrillation/flutter, wandering atrial pacemaker, supraventricular or ventricular arrhythmia) or conduction abnormalities, including AV block.

➤*Postmarketing:*

Cardiovascular – Asystole, heart block (including third-degree block), symptomatic hypotension, syncope requiring intervention with fluids and/or aminophylline, and transient ischemic attack have occurred.

GI – Abdominal pain, occasionally severe, has been reported a few minutes after regadenoson administration in association with nausea, vomiting, or myalgias; administration of aminophylline, an adenosine antagonist, appeared to lessen the pain. Diarrhea and fecal incontinence also have been reported following regadenoson administration.

Musculoskeletal – Musculoskeletal pain has occurred, typically 10 to 20 minutes after regadenoson administration; the pain was occasionally severe, localized in the arms and lower back and extended to the buttocks and lower legs bilaterally. Administration of aminophylline appeared to lessen the pain.

Respiratory – Dyspnea and wheezing have been reported following regadenoson administration.

Because these reactions are reported voluntarily from a population of uncertain size, it is not always possible to reliably estimate their frequency or establish a causal relationship to regadenoson exposure.

Overdosage

➤*Symptoms:* Regadenoson overdosage may result in serious reactions. In a study of healthy volunteers, symptoms of flushing, dizziness, and increased heart rate were assessed as intolerable at regadenoson doses of more than 0.02 mg/kg.

➤*Treatment:* Aminophylline may be administered in doses ranging from 50 to 250 mg by slow IV injection (50 to 100 mg over 30 to 60 seconds) to attenuate severe and/or persistent adverse reactions to regadenoson.

Patient Information

Instruct patients to avoid consumption of any products containing methylxanthines, including caffeinated coffee, tea, or other caffeinated beverages, caffeine-containing drug products, and theophylline for at least 12 hours before a scheduled radionuclide MPI.

Prior to regadenoson administration, inform patients of the most common reactions (such as shortness of breath, headache, and flushing) that have been reported in association with regadenoson during MPI.

Instruct patients with COPD or asthma to discuss their respiratory history and administration of pre- and poststudy bronchodilator therapy with their health care provider before scheduling an MPI study with regadenoson.

ARGININE HYDROCHLORIDE

Rx	**R-Gene 10** (Pharmacia & Upjohn)	**Injection, solution:** 1 g per 10 mL	Preservative free. Chloride ion 47.5 mEq per 100 mL. In 300 mL.

ARGININE HYDROCHLORIDE — INJECTION

Indications

➤*Diagnostic aid:* As an intravenous (IV) stimulant to the pituitary for the release of human growth hormone (hGH) in patients in whom the measurement of pituitary reserve for hGH can be of diagnostic usefulness. It can be used as a diagnostic aid in such conditions as panhypopituitarism, pituitary dwarfism, chromophobe adenoma, postsurgical craniopharyngioma, hypophysectomy, pituitary trauma, acromegaly, gigantism, and problems of growth and stature.

➤*Off-label uses:* Management of hyperammonemia, pulmonary hypertension, and severe metabolic acidosis in children.

Administration and Dosage

➤*Adults:*

ARGININE HYDROCHLORIDE — INJECTION

Diagnostic aid –

Usual dosage: 30 g (300 mL) IV over 30 minutes.

Maximum dose: 30 g/dose.

➤*Children:*

Diagnostic aid –

60 kg or more: See Adults for dosing.

Less than 60 kg:

- *Usual dosage* – 0.5 g (5 mL) per kg of body weight IV over 30 minutes.
- *Maximum dose* – 30 g/dose.

Off-label dosing –

Hyperammonemia: Use with sodium benzoate and sodium phenylacetate. Can be diluted in 25 to 35 mL of dextrose 10% in water. Infuse through a central line.

- *Argininosuccinic acid lyase or argininosuccinic acid synthetase deficiency* – Dosage can be diluted in 25 to 35 mL of dextrose 10% in water.
  Maximum dose: 30 g.
  Loading dose: 600 mg/kg IV over 90 to 120 minutes.
  Maintenance dosage: 600 mg/kg per day as a continuous IV infusion.
- *Carbamyl phosphate synthetase or ornithine transcarbamylase deficiency* –
  Maximum dose: 30 g.
  Loading dose: 200 mg/kg IV over 90 to 120 minutes.
  Maintenance dosage: 200 mg/kg per day as a continuous IV infusion.

Pulmonary hypertension:

- *Usual dose* – 500 mg/kg IV over 30 minutes.
- *Maximum dose* – 30 g.

Severe metabolic acidosis: Use after potassium and sodium chloride supplementation has failed.

- *Usual dose* – Estimate the dosage using the following formula:

$$\text{Dose (g)} = \frac{\text{(desired decrease in plasma bicarbonate [mEq/L] times weight [kg]}}{9.6)}$$

- *Maximum dose* – 30 g.

➤*Preparation for administration:* Arginine is provided as a ready-to-use solution for patients weighing 60 kg or more and should not be further diluted. For children weighing less than 60 kg, a weight-based dose must be placed in a separate container to avoid inadvertent delivery and administration of the total volume from the commercially available container.

For children weighing less than 60 kg – Withdraw a weight-based dose from an intact sealed bottle. The entire 300 mL bottle is not intended for use in patients weighing 59 kg or less. The dose must be placed in a separate container, such as an evacuated sterile glass container designed for IV administration, using aseptic technique. Additionally, arginine is stable in polypropylene syringes and plastic containers made of polyvinyl chloride or ethylene vinyl acetate. The postpenetration storage period is not more than 4 hours at room temperature or 24 hours at refrigerated temperature (2° to 8°C).

Use of IV container – Use aseptic technique. As arginine is provided in glass containers, a standard air-inletting, air-filtering IV infusion set with a bacterial air filter is required.

➤*Administration:* Administer IV over 30 minutes. Arginine is a hypertonic solution and should only be infused through an indwelling needle or soft catheter placed in an antecubital vein or other suitable vein. Arginine should be infused beginning at zero time at a uniform rate that will permit the recommended dose to be administered over 30 minutes.

Test procedure – The test should be scheduled in the morning following a normal night's sleep, and an overnight fast should continue through the test period. Patients must be placed at bed rest for at least 30 minutes before the infusion begins. Care should be taken to minimize apprehension and distress. This is particularly important in children. Blood samples should be taken by venipuncture from the contralateral arm. A desirable schedule for drawing blood samples is at −30, 0, 30, 60, 90, 120, and 150 minutes. Blood samples should be promptly centrifuged and the plasma stored at −20°C (−4°F) until assayed by one of the published radioimmunoassay procedures. Diagnostic test results showing a deficiency of pituitary reserve for hGH should be confirmed by a second test with arginine, or one may elect to confirm with the insulin hypoglycemia test. A waiting period of 1 day is advised between tests.

➤*Extravasation:* Extravasation may occur during administration of arginine. If signs or symptoms of extravasation occur, stop the infusion immediately. If possible, withdraw 3 to 5 mL of blood to remove some of the drug. Remove the infusion needle. Delineate the infiltrated area on the patient's skin with a felt-tip marker. There is no information on the use of hyaluronidase to treat reactions, but it is well tolerated and might be used empirically. If hyaluronidase is to be used, administer promptly within the first few minutes to 1 hour after extravasation. Higher doses (150 units) have primarily been used in adults while lower doses (15 units) have been used in children. Administer hyaluronidase according to the following steps. Dilute hyaluronidase to desired concentration, depending on the dose and product used. (Note: Some products do not require dilution.) For example, if the total dose is 15 units, make 15 units/mL dilution. If the total dose is 150 units, make 150 units/mL dilution. Cleanse area with povidone-iodine. Inject hyaluronidase locally, subcutaneously, or intradermally, using a 25-gauge needle or smaller. The dose is given as five 0.2 mL injections at the leading edge of the extravasation site. Change the needle after each injection. Elevate for 48 hours above heart level using a sling or stockinette dressing with an observation window cut in the dressing. Avoid pressure or friction. Do not rub the area. Observe for signs of increased erythema, pain, or skin necrosis. If increased symptoms occur, consult a plastic surgeon. Ensure that no medication is given distally to extravasation site. After 48 hours, encourage the patient to use the extremity normally to promote full range of motion.

➤*Storage/Stability:* Store at 25°C (77°F); however, brief exposure up to 40°C (104°F) does not adversely affect the product. Avoid excessive heat. Solution that has been frozen must not be used. The postpenetration storage period is not more than 4 hours at room temperature or 24 hours at refrigerated temperature 2° to 8°C (36° to 46°F). Discard any unused drug product.

Actions

➤*Pharmacology:* IV infusion of arginine often induces a pronounced rise in the plasma level of hGH in subjects with intact pituitary function. This rise is usually diminished or absent in patients with impairment of this function.

These ranges are based on the mean values of plasma hGH levels calculated from the data of several clinical investigators and reflect their experiences with various methods of radioimmunoassay. Upon gaining experience with this diagnostic test, each clinician will establish his or her own ranges for control and peak levels of hGH.

Contraindications

Hypersensitivity to any ingredient in this product.

Warnings/Precautions

➤*Deficiency of pituitary reserve:* If the insulin hypoglycemia test has indicated a deficiency of pituitary reserve for hGH, a test with arginine is advisable to confirm the negative response. This can be done after a waiting period of 1 day. Because patients may not respond to arginine during the first test, test the unresponsive patient again to confirm the negative result. A second test can be performed after a waiting period of 1 day. Some patients who respond to arginine do not respond to insulin and vice versa. The rate of false-positive responses for arginine is approximately 32%, and the rate of false-negatives is approximately 27%.

➤*Administration:* Arginine should always be administered by IV injection because of its hypertonicity. Arginine is a hypertonic (950 mOsmol/L) and acidic (average pH, 5.6) solution that can cause irritation and damage to tissues. Take care to ensure arginine is administered through a patent catheter within a patent vein.

Excessive rates of infusion may result in local irritation and in flushing, nausea, or vomiting. Inadequate dosing or prolongation of the infusion period may diminish the stimulus to the pituitary and nullify the test.

➤*Electrolyte imbalance:* The chloride content of arginine is 47.5 mEq per 100 mL of solution; therefore, before undertaking the test, evaluate the effect of infusing this amount of chloride into patients with electrolyte imbalance.

➤*Extravasation:* See Administration and Dosage for more information.

➤*Hypersensitivity reactions:* Hypersensitivity reactions, including anaphylaxis, have been reported. Appropriate medical support should be available during arginine administration. If anaphylaxis or other serious hypersensitivity reaction occurs, discontinue arginine and initiate appropriate medical treatment.

➤*Renal function impairment:* Arginine can be metabolized, resulting in nitrogen-containing products for excretion. Consider the effect of an acute amino acid or nitrogen burden upon patients with impairment of renal function when arginine is to be administered.

➤*Pregnancy: Category B.* There have been no adequate or well-controlled studies for the use of arginine in pregnant women. Because animal reproduction studies are not always predictive of human response, this drug should not be used during pregnancy.

➤*Lactation:* It is not known whether IV administration of arginine could result in significant quantities of arginine in breast milk. Systemically administered amino acids are secreted into breast milk in quantities not likely to have a deleterious effect on the infant. Nevertheless, exercise caution when arginine is to be administered to breast-feeding women.

➤*Children:* There have been reports of overdosage of arginine in children leading to death. Exercise extreme caution when infusing arginine into children. Overdosage of arginine in children can result in hyperchloremic metabolic acidosis, cerebral edema, or possibly death.

Drug Interactions

None known.

➤*Drug/Lab test interactions:* The basal and poststimulation levels of growth hormone are elevated in patients who are pregnant or are taking oral contraceptives.

Adverse Reactions

➤*Cardiovascular:* One patient with a history of acrocyanosis had an exacerbation of this condition following infusion of arginine.

➤*Hematologic:* One patient had an apparent decrease in platelet count from 150,000 to 60,000.

➤*Hypersensitivity:* One patient had an allergic reaction that was manifested as a confluent macular rash with reddening and swelling of the hands and face. The rash subsided rapidly after the infusion was terminated and diphenhydramine 50 mg was administered.

➤*Miscellaneous:* Nonspecific adverse reactions consisting of nausea, vomiting, headache, flushing, numbness, and local venous irritation were reported in approximately 3% of the patients.

Overdosage

➤*Symptoms:* An overdosage may cause a transient metabolic acidosis with hyperventilation, which could lead to death. In most cases, the acidosis will

ARGININE HYDROCHLORIDE — INJECTION

self-compensate and the base deficit will return to normal following completion of the infusion. (See Children for more information.)

➤*Treatment:* If acidosis persists, determine and correct the deficit by a calculated dose of an alkalizing agent.

Patient Information

Inform patients that the medication will be prepared and administered by a health care provider.

Advise patients that hypersensitivity reactions, including anaphylaxis, may occur. Advise patients to immediately report any hives, rash, or difficulty swallowing or breathing to their health care provider.

CORTICORELIN OVINE TRIFLUTATE

Rx	**Acthrel** (Ferring)	**Cake, lyophilized:** 100 mcg corticorelin ovine (as trifluoroacetate)[a]	In 5 ml single-dose vials with diluent.

[a] With 0.88 mg ascorbic acid, 10 mg lactose and 26 mg cysteine hydrochloride monohydrate.

CORTICORELIN OVINE TRIFLUTATE — INJECTION

Indications

➤*Cushing syndrome, differential diagnosis:* Differentiating pituitary and ectopic production of ACTH in patients with ACTH-dependent Cushing syndrome.

Administration and Dosage

➤*General dosing considerations:* To evaluate the status of the pituitary-adrenal axis in the differentiation of a pituitary source from an ectopic source of excessive ACTH secretion, a corticorelin test procedure requires a minimum of 5 blood samples (see Administration).

➤*Adults:*

Diagnostic aid to determine the etiology of ACTH-dependent hypercortisolism –

Maximum dose: 1 mcg/kg.

Single dose: 1 mcg/kg intravenously (IV). Higher doses have been associated with increased adverse reactions.

Repeat dose: If a repeat test is needed, it is recommended that the repeat test be carried out at the same time of day as the original test because there are differences in basal levels and peak response levels following morning or afternoon/evening administration to normal humans.

➤*Children:*

Diagnostic aid to determine the etiology of ACTH-dependent hypercortisolism – See Adults for dosing.

➤*Interpretation of results:* Cushing disease patients and ectopic ACTH secretion patients with a high basal ACTH will yield a high ACTH response and a low ACTH response, respectively.

Cushing disease – The results of challenge with corticorelin have been reported in approximately 300 patients with Cushing disease. Although the ACTH and cortisol responses were variable, a hyper-response to corticorelin was seen in a majority of patients, despite high basal cortisol levels. This response pattern indicates an impairment of the negative feedback of cortisol on the pituitary. Patients with pituitary-dependent Cushing disease tested with corticorelin do not show the negative correlation between basal and stimulated levels of ACTH and cortisol that is found in normal subjects. A positive correlation between basal ACTH levels and maximum ACTH increments after corticorelin administration has been found in Cushing disease patients. False-negative responses to the corticorelin test in Cushing disease patients occur approximately 5% to 10% of the time, which may lead the clinician to an incorrect diagnosis of ectopic production of ACTH at that frequency.

Ectopic ACTH secretion: Patients with Cushing syndrome due to ectopic ACTH secretion had very high basal levels of ACTH and cortisol, which were not further stimulated by corticorelin. However, there have been rare instances of patients with ectopic sources of ACTH that have responded to the corticorelin test.

➤*Preparation for administration:* Reconstitute aseptically with 2 mL of 0.9% sodium chloride injection at the time of use by injecting 2 mL of the saline diluent into the lyophilized drug product cake. To avoid bubble formation, do not shake the vial; instead, roll the vial to dissolve the drug product. The resulting sterile solution contains corticorelin 50 mcg/mL.

➤*Administration:* Venous blood samples should be drawn 15 minutes before and immediately prior to corticorelin administration. The ACTH baseline is obtained by averaging the values of the 2 samples. Administer corticorelin as an IV infusion over a 30- to 60-second interval. Some of the adverse effects can be reduced by administering the drug as an infusion over 30 seconds instead of as a bolus injection. Draw venous blood samples at 15, 30, and 60 minutes after administration. Cortisol determinations may be performed on the same blood samples for the same time points.

➤*Storage/Stability:* Refrigerate at 2°C to 8°C (36°F to 45°F) and protect from light. The reconstituted solution is stable up to 8 hours under refrigerated conditions. Discard unused reconstituted solution.

Actions

➤*Pharmacology:*

Pharmacodynamics – In normal subjects, intravenous administration of corticorelin results in a rapid and sustained increase of plasma ACTH levels and a near parallel increase of plasma cortisol. In addition, intravenous administration of corticorelin to normal subjects causes a concomitant and prolonged release of the related proopiomelanocortin peptides β- and γ-lipotropins (β- and γ-LPH) and β-endorphin (β-END). A number of dose-response studies have been performed on normal subjects using a range of corticorelin doses. In one study, doses of corticorelin ranging from 0.001 to 30 mcg/kg body weight were administered to 29 healthy volunteers. Blood samples were taken over a 2-hour period for determination of plasma ACTH and cortisol concentrations. There was a direct dose-dependent relationship that was more pronounced for ACTH than for cortisol. The threshold dose was 0.03 mcg/kg, the half-maximal dose was 0.3-1.0 mcg/kg and the maximally effective dose was 3-10 mcg/kg.

Baseline ACTH and cortisol levels are usually higher in the morning. Pooled ACTH values from normal unstressed subjects (n = 119) were 25 ± 7 pg/ml in the a.m., and 10 ± 3 in the p.m., similar pooled cortisol values (n = 170) were 11 ± 3 mcg/dl in the a.m. and 4 ± 2 mcg/dl in the p.m. The normal unstressed person has about seven to ten secretory episodes of ACTH each day. Most of them occur in the early morning hours and are responsible for the morning plasma cortisol surge. Insulin, plasma renin activity, prolactin, and growth hormone release are not affected by corticorelin administration in humans.

Continuous 24-hour infusion of corticorelin (0.5, 1.0, and 3.0 mcg/kg/hr) increased plasma ACTH concentrations to a plateau of 15-20 pg/ml by the third hour and urinary-free cortisol reaches 173 ± 43 mcg/dl by 24 hours, comparable to those levels observed in patients with major depression, but less than levels noted in Cushing disease. Continuous infusion did not abolish the circadian rhythm of plasma ACTH and cortisol, but did appear to desensitize the corticotroph. Intermittent doses of corticorelin (25 mcg every 4 hours for 72 hours), however, continued to elicit the expected ACTH and cortisol responses.

Intravenous administration of 1 mcg/kg corticorelin in combination with 10 pressor units intramuscular vasopressin had a synergistic effect on ACTH and a less marked synergistic effect on cortisol secretion.

➤*Pharmacokinetics:* Plasma ACTH levels in normal subjects increased 2 minutes after injection of corticorelin doses of ≥0.3 mcg/kg and reached peak levels after 10-15 minutes. Plasma cortisol levels increased within 10 minutes and reached peak levels at 30 to 60 minutes. As the dose of corticorelin was increased, the rises in plasma ACTH and cortisol were more sustained, showing a biphasic response with a second lower peak at 2-3 hours after injection. Similar results were found in another study using 0.3, 3.0, and 30 mcg/kg doses. The duration of mean plasma ACTH increase after injection of 0.3, 3.0, and 30 mcg/kg was 4, 7, and 8 hours, respectively. The effect on plasma cortisol was similar, but more prolonged. Because there are differences in basal levels and peak response levels following a.m. or p.m. administration, it is recommended that subsequent evaluations in the same patient using the corticorelin stimulation test be carried out at the same time of day as the original evaluation.

Following a single intravenous injection of 1 mcg/kg of corticorelin to normal men, the disappearance of immunoreactive corticorelin (IR-corticorelin) from plasma follows a biexponential decay curve. Plasma half-lives for IR-corticorelin are 11.6 ± 1.5 minutes (mean ± SE) for the fast component and 73 ± 8 minutes for the slow component. The mean volume of distribution for IR-corticorelin is 6.2 ± 0.5 L with an approximate metabolic clearance rate of 95 ± 11 L/m^2/day. Graded intravenous doses of corticorelin (0.01, 0.03, 0.1, 0.3, 1, 3, 10, 30 mcg/kg) produced a linear increase in plasma IR-corticorelin. Corticorelin does not appear to be bound specifically by a circulating plasma protein.

Warnings/Precautions

➤*Dose dependent effects:* The severity of adverse effects to a corticorelin injection appear to be dose-dependent. Dosages above 1 mcg/kg are not recommended. While few adverse effects have been observed at the 1 mcg/kg or 100 mcg dose, higher doses have been associated with transient tachycardia, decreased blood pressure, loss of consciousness, and asystole (see Adverse Reactions). These symptoms can be substantially reduced by administering the drug as a 30-second intravenous infusion instead of a bolus injection.

➤*Pregnancy: Category C.* Animal reproduction studies have not been conducted with corticorelin. It is also not known whether corticorelin can cause fetal harm when administered to a pregnant woman or can affect reproductive capacity. Corticorelin should be given to a pregnant woman only if clearly needed.

➤*Lactation:* It is not known whether corticorelin is secreted in human milk. Because many drugs are excreted in human milk, caution should be exercised when corticorelin is administered to a breast-feeding woman.

➤*Children:* Only a few tests have been performed on children. Dosages were 1 mcg/kg body weight. Patient studies have involved only children with multiple hypothalamic and/or pituitary hormone deficiencies, or tumors. Only two studies with normal pediatric subjects have been conducted. No differences in response to the corticorelin test have been reported in the children studied.

Drug Interactions

➤*Dexamethasone:* The plasma ACTH response to corticorelin injection is inhibited or blunted in normal subjects pretreated with dexamethasone.

CORTICORELIN OVINE TRIFLUTATE — INJECTION

➤*Heparin:* The use of a heparin solution to maintain IV cannula patency during the corticorelin test is not recommended. A possible interaction between corticorelin and heparin may have been responsible for a major hypotensive reaction that occurred after corticorelin administration. (See Adverse Reactions.)

Adverse Reactions

Adverse effects reported with 1 mcg/kg or 100 mcg/patient include flushing of the face, neck, and upper chest (16%: 45/276), beginning almost immediately and lasting 3 to 5 minutes. Recipients have also reported an urge to take a deep breath (6%: 3/49), which occurs with a timing similar to, but less frequently than, that of flushing. Higher doses (≥3 mcg/kg) are associated with more prolonged flushing, tachycardia, hypotension, dyspnea, and chest compression or tightness. In addition, at doses of ≥ 5 mcg/kg, significant increases in heart rate and decreases in blood pressure were observed. The cardiovascular effects occurred 2-3 minutes after injection and lasted for 30-60 minutes. The facial flushing was more prolonged, lasting up to 4 hours in some subjects. All signs and symptoms could be reduced by administering the drug as a 30-second infusion instead of by bolus injection.

Overdosage

➤*Symptoms:* Symptoms of overdose include severe facial flushing, cardiovascular changes, and dyspnea.

➤*Treatment:* In the event of toxic overdose (see Adverse Reactions), adverse effects should be treated symptomatically.

METYRAPONE

Rx	**Metopirone** (Novartis)	**Capsules:** 250 mg	(CIBA LN) Soft gelatin. White to yellowish white. Oblong. In 18s.

METYRAPONE — ORAL

Indications

➤*Diagnostic aid:* For testing hypothalamic-pituitary adrenocorticotropic hormone (ACTH) function.

Administration and Dosage

➤*Adults:*

Diagnostic aid –

Single-dose short test:

• *Usual dosage* – 30 mg/kg at midnight. The blood sample for the assay is taken early the following morning (7:30 to 8 am). The plasma should be frozen as soon as possible. The patient is then given a prophylactic dose of 50 mg cortisone acetate.

• *Maximum dose* – 3 g.

Multiple-dose test:

• *Day 1* – Collect 24-hour urine for measurement of 17-hydroxycorticosteroids (17-OHCS) or 17-ketogenic steroids (17-KGS).

• *Day 2* – Standard ACTH test, such as infusion of ACTH 50 units over 8 hours and measurement of 24-hour urinary steroids. If results indicate adequate response, the metyrapone test may proceed.

• *Day 3 to 4* – Rest period.

• *Day 5* – Metyrapone 750 mg every 4 hours for 6 doses. A single dose is approximately equivalent to 15 mg/kg.

• *Day 6* – Determination of 24-hour urinary steroids for effect.

➤*Children:*

Diagnostic aid –

Single-dose short test: See Adults for dosing.

Multiple-dose test:

• *Day 1* – Collect 24-hour urine for measurement of 17-OHCS or 17-KGS.

• *Day 2* – Standard ACTH test, such as infusion of ACTH 50 units over 8 hours and measurement of 24-hour urinary steroids. If results indicate adequate response, the metyrapone test may proceed.

• *Day 3 to 4* – Rest period.

• *Day 5* – Metyrapone 750 mg every 4 hours for 6 doses. A single dose is approximately equivalent to 15 mg/kg.

• *Day 6* – Determination of 24-hour urinary steroids for effect.

➤*Interpretation of results:*

Multiple-dose test –

ACTH test: The normal 24-hour urinary excretion of 17-OHCS ranges from 3 to 12 mg. Following continuous IV infusion of ACTH 50 units over a period of 8 hours, 17-OHCS excretion increases to 15 to 45 mg per 24 hours.

Metyrapone:

• *Normal response* – In patients with a normally functioning pituitary, administration of metyrapone is followed by a 2- to 4-fold increase of 17-OHCS excretion or doubling of 17-KGS excretion.

• *Subnormal response* – Subnormal response in patients without adrenal insufficiency is indicative of some degree of impairment of pituitary function, either panhypopituitarism or partial hypopituitarism (limited pituitary reserve).

Panhypopituitarism: Panhypopituitarism is readily diagnosed by the classical clinical and chemical evidences of hypogonadism, hypothyroidism, and hypoadrenocorticism. These patients usually have subnormal basal urinary steroid levels. Depending upon the duration of the disease and degree of adrenal atrophy, they may fail to respond to exogenous ACTH in the normal manner. Administration of metyrapone is not essential in the diagnosis, but if given, it will not induce an appreciable increase in urinary steroids.

Partial hypopituitarism: Partial hypopituitarism or limited pituitary reserve is the more difficult diagnosis because these patients do not present the classical signs and symptoms of hypopituitarism. Measurements of target organ functions often are normal under basal conditions. The response to exogenous ACTH is usually normal, producing the expected rise of urinary steroids (17-OHCS or 17-KGS).

The response, however, to metyrapone is subnormal; that is, no significant increase in 17-OHCS or 17-KGS excretion occurs.

This failure to respond to metyrapone may be interpreted as evidence of impaired pituitary-adrenal reserve. In view of the normal response to exogenous ACTH, the failure to respond to metyrapone is inferred to be related to a defect in the CNS-pituitary mechanisms that normally regulate ACTH secretions. Presumably the ACTH-secreting mechanisms of these individuals are already working at their maximal rates to meet everyday conditions and possess limited "reserve" capacities to secrete additional ACTH either in response to stress or to decreased cortisol levels occurring as a result of metyrapone administration.

Subnormal response in patients with Cushing syndrome is suggestive of either autonomous adrenal tumors that suppress the ACTH-releasing capacity of the pituitary or nonendocrine ACTH-secreting tumors.

• *Excessive response* – An excessive excretion of 17-OHCS or 17-KGS after administration of metyrapone is suggestive of Cushing syndrome associated with adrenal hyperplasia. These patients have an elevated excretion of urinary corticosteroids under basal conditions and will often, but not invariably, show a supernormal response to ACTH and also to metyrapone, excreting more than 35 mg per 24 hours of either 17-OHCS or 17-KGS.

Single-dose test – An intact ACTH reserve is generally indicated by an increase in plasma ACTH to at least 44 pmol/L (200 ng/L) or by an increase in 11-desoxycortisol to over 0.2 mcmol/L (70 mcg/L). Patients with suspected adrenocortical insufficiency should be hospitalized overnight as a precautionary measure.

➤*Administration:* Administer with milk or snack (eg, yogurt).

➤*Storage/Stability:* Do not store above 30°C (86°F). Protect from moisture and heat.

Actions

➤*Pharmacology:* The pharmacological effect of metyrapone is to reduce cortisol and corticosterone production by inhibiting the 11-β-hydroxylation reaction in the adrenal cortex. Removal of the strong inhibitory feedback mechanism exerted by cortisol results in an increase in ACTH production by the pituitary. With continued blockade of the enzymatic steps leading to production of cortisol and corticosterone, there is a marked increase in adrenocortical secretion of their immediate precursors, 11-desoxycortisol and desoxycorticosterone, which are weak suppressors of ACTH release, and a corresponding elevation of these steroids in the plasma and of their metabolites in the urine. These metabolites are readily determined by measuring urinary 17-OHCS or 17-KGS. Because of these actions, metyrapone is used as a diagnostic test, with urinary 17-OHCS measured as an index of pituitary ACTH responsiveness. Metyrapone may also suppress biosynthesis of aldosterone, resulting in a mild natriuresis.

The response to metyrapone does not occur immediately. Following oral administration, peak steroid excretion occurs during the subsequent 24-hour period.

➤*Pharmacokinetics:*

Absorption – Metyrapone is absorbed rapidly and well when administered orally as prescribed. Peak plasma concentrations are usually reached 1 hour after administration. After administration of 750 mg, mean peak plasma concentrations are 3.7 mcg/mL, falling to 0.5 mcg/mL 4 hours after administration. Following a single 2000 mg dose, mean peak plasma concentrations of metyrapone in plasma are 7.3 mcg/mL.

Metabolism – The major biotransformation is reduction of the ketone to metyrapol, an active alcohol metabolite. Eight hours after a single oral dose, the ratio of metyrapone to metyrapol in the plasma is 1:1.5. Metyrapone and metyrapol are both conjugated with glucuronide.

Excretion – Metyrapone is rapidly eliminated from the plasma. The mean ± SD terminal elimination half-life is 1.9 ± 0.7 hours. Metyrapol takes about twice as long as metyrapone to be eliminated from the plasma. After administration of 4.5 g metyrapone (750 mg every 4 hours), an average of 5.3% of the dose was excreted in the urine in the form of metyrapone (9.2% free and 90.8% as glucuronide) and 38.5% in the form of metyrapol (8.1% free and 91.9% as glucuronide) within 72 hours after the first dose was given.

Contraindications

Adrenal cortical insufficiency, or hypersensitivity to metyrapone or to any of its excipients.

Warnings/Precautions

➤*Acute adrenal insufficiency:* Metyrapone may induce acute adrenal insufficiency in patients with reduced adrenal secretory capacity.

➤*Response to adrenals:* Ability of adrenals to respond to exogenous ACTH should be demonstrated before metyrapone is employed as a test.

➤*Hypo-/Hyperthyroidism:* In the presence of hypo- or hyperthyroidism, response to the metyrapone test may be subnormal.

METYRAPONE — ORAL

➤*Hazardous tasks:* Since metyrapone may cause dizziness and sedation, patients should exercise caution when driving or operating machinery.

➤*Pregnancy: Category C.* A subnormal response to metyrapone may occur in pregnant women. Animal reproduction studies have not been conducted with metyrapone. The metyrapone test was administered to 20 pregnant women in their second and third trimester of pregnancy, and evidence was found that the fetal pituitary responded to the enzymatic block. It is not known if metyrapone can affect reproduction capacity. Metyrapone should be given to a pregnant woman only if clearly needed.

➤*Lactation:* It is not known whether this drug is excreted in human milk. Because many drugs are excreted in human milk, caution should be exercised when metyrapone is administered to a breast-feeding woman.

Drug Interactions

➤*Corticosteroids:* Drugs affecting pituitary or adrenocortical function, including all corticosteroid therapy, must be discontinued prior to and during testing with metyrapone.

➤*Phenytoin:* The metabolism of metyrapone is accelerated by phenytoin; therefore, results of the test may be inaccurate in patients taking phenytoin within 2 weeks before.

➤*Estrogens:* A subnormal response may occur in patients on estrogen therapy.

➤*Acetaminophen:* Metyrapone inhibits the glucuronidation of acetaminophen and could possibly potentiate acetaminophen toxicity.

Adverse Reactions

➤*CNS:* Headache, dizziness, sedation.

➤*Dermatologic:* Allergic rash.

➤*GI:* Nausea, vomiting, abdominal discomfort or pain.

➤*Hematologic:* Rarely, decreased white blood cell count or bone marrow depression.

Overdosage

➤*Acute toxicity:* One case has been recorded in which a 6-year-old girl died after 2 doses of metyrapone, 2 g.

➤*Symptoms:* The clinical picture of poisoning with metyrapone is characterized by gastrointestinal symptoms and by signs of acute adrenocortical insufficiency.

CV – Cardiac arrhythmias, hypotension, dehydration.

CNS – Anxiety, confusion, weakness, impairment of consciousness.

GI – Nausea, vomiting, epigastric pain, diarrhea.

Lab test abnormalities – Hyponatremia, hypochloremia, hyperkalemia.

In patients under treatment with insulin or oral antidiabetics, the signs and symptoms of acute poisoning with metyrapone may be aggravated or modified.

➤*Treatment:* There is no specific antidote. Besides general measures to eliminate the drug and reduce its absorption, a large dose of hydrocortisone should be administered at once, together with saline and glucose infusions. For a few days blood pressure and fluid and electrolyte balance should be monitored.

HEXAMINOLEVULINATE HYDROCHLORIDE

Rx	**Cysview** (GE Healthcare Inc)	**Powder for solution; intravesical:** 100 mg	Equiv. to hexaminolevulinate base 85 mg. In kits with 100 mg vial, diluent (50 mg vial), and one Luer-lock catheter adapter.

HEXAMINOLEVULINATE HYDROCHLORIDE — INTRAVESICAL

Indications

➤*Detection of bladder cancer:* For use in the cystoscopic detection of non–muscle-invasive papillary cancer of the bladder among patients suspected or known to have lesion(s) on the basis of a prior cystoscopy.

Hexaminolevulinate is used with the Karl Storz D-Light C Photodynamic Diagnostic (PDD) system to perform cystoscopy with the blue light setting (mode 2) as an adjunct to the white light setting (mode 1).

Administration and Dosage

➤*General dosing considerations:* Training and proficiency in cystoscopic procedures are essential prior to the use of hexaminolevulinate.

Hexaminolevulinate imaging requires the use of the Karl Storz D-Light C PDD system.

➤*Adults:*

Detection of bladder cancer – 50 mL instilled into the bladder via a urinary catheter.

➤*Preparation for administration:* Perform all steps under aseptic conditions. Use gloves during the reconstitution procedure; skin exposure to hexaminolevulinate may increase the risk for sensitization to the drug.

Use a 50 mL syringe with a Luer-lock tip throughout the reconstitution procedure to ensure that the correct concentration (2 mg/mL) of the drug is obtained and that a stable syringe-catheter connection is made for the bladder instillation of hexaminolevulinate.

Remove the cap from the sterile 50 mL syringe and carefully retain it for subsequent reattachment to the syringe. Attach a needle to the syringe and withdraw 50 mL of the diluent. Penetrate the stopper of the hexaminolevulinate vial with the needle and inject 10 mL of the diluent from the syringe into the vial. Without withdrawing the needle from the vial, hold the vial and syringe in a firm grip and gently shake to dissolve the powder in the diluent. The powder typically dissolves almost immediately.

Withdraw all of the dissolved solution from the vial (10 mL) into the 50 mL syringe. Remove the needle from the vial, and disconnect the needle from the syringe tip and discard it. Plug the syringe with the syringe cap. Gently mix the contents of the syringe. The reconstituted solution contains hexaminolevulinate 2 mg/mL and is colorless to pale yellow, clear to slightly opalescent, and free from visible particles.

Peel off the detachable portion of the label (starting at the corner marked with a black triangle) from the hexaminolevulinate vial and affix it to the syringe containing the solution of hexaminolevulinate. Add 2 hours to the present time and write the resulting expiration time and date on the syringe label.

If unable to administer the solution shortly after reconstitution, the solution may be stored for up to 2 hours in a refrigerator at 2° to 8°C (36° to 46°F) in the labeled syringe. If not used within 2 hours, discard the solution.

➤*Administration:*

Bladder instillation – For bladder instillation of the solution, use straight, or intermittent, urethral catheters with a proximal funnel opening that will accommodate the Luer-lock adapter. Use only catheters made of vinyl (uncoated or coated with hydrogel), latex (amber or red), or silicone to instill the reconstituted hexaminolevulinate. Do not use catheters coated or embedded with silver or antibiotics. In-dwelling bladder catheters (Foley catheters) may be used if the catheters are inserted shortly prior to hexaminolevulinate administration and are removed following the hexaminolevulinate instillation.

Use the following steps for bladder instillation:

1.) Using standard sterile catheterization techniques, first insert the urethral catheter into the bladder of the patient and use the catheter to completely empty the patient's bladder before instillation of hexaminolevulinate.
2.) Remove the syringe cap from the 50 mL syringe that contains the solution of hexaminolevulinate. Attach the Luer-lock end of the (provided) catheter adapter to the syringe. Insert the tapered end of the catheter adapter into the funnel opening of the catheter.
3.) Slowly instill the solution of hexaminolevulinate into the bladder through the catheter, ensuring that the complete volume of the syringe (50 mL) is administered.
4.) After the solution is instilled, remove the catheter and instruct the patient to retain the solution within the bladder for at least 1 hour; do not exceed 3 hours. Patients may stand, sit, and move about during the time period between instillation and the start of the cystoscopic procedure.
5.) Evacuate the solution of hexaminolevulinate from the bladder as part of the routine emptying of the bladder immediately prior to the initiation of the cystoscopic procedure (refer to the Karl Storz PDD Telescope Instruction manual). Also, the patient may void and completely empty the bladder prior to the procedure.

Avoid skin contact with hexaminolevulinate. If skin comes in contact with hexaminolevulinate, wash immediately with soap and water and dry. After voiding the bladder of hexaminolevulinate, routinely wash the patient's perineal skin region with soap and water and dry.

Preparation for cystoscopy – Initiate the cystoscopic examination within 30 minutes after evacuation of hexaminolevulinate from the bladder, but no less than 1 or more than 3 hours after hexaminolevulinate is instilled in the bladder. If the patient did not retain hexaminolevulinate in the bladder for 1 hour, allow 1 hour to pass from the instillation of hexaminolevulinate into the bladder to the start of the cystoscopic examination. The efficacy of hexaminolevulinate has not been established when the solution was retained for less than 1 hour.

Cystoscopic examination – Empty the patient's bladder and then fill the bladder with a clear fluid (standard bladder irrigation fluid) in order to distend the bladder wall for cystoscopic visibility. Ensure adequate irrigation during examination of the bladder; blood, urine, or floating particles in the bladder may interfere with visualization under both white and blue light.

First perform a complete cystoscopic examination of the entire bladder under white light (mode 1) and then repeat the examination of the entire bladder surface under blue light (mode 2) unless the white light cystoscopy reveals extensive mucosal inflammation. Do not perform the blue light cystoscopy if the white light cystoscopy reveals widespread mucosal inflammation. Abnormalities of the bladder mucosa during blue light cystoscopy are characterized by the detection of red, homogenous, and intense fluorescence. The margins of the abnormal lesions are typically well-demarcated and in contrast to the normal urothelium, which appears blue. Register and document (map) the location and appearance (eg, papillary) of suspicious lesions and abnormalities seen under either white or blue light.

During the cystoscopic examination, be aware of the following:

HEXAMINOLEVULINATE HYDROCHLORIDE — INTRAVESICAL

- A red fluorescence is expected at the bladder outlet and the prostatic urethra; this fluorescence occurs in normal tissue and is usually less intense and more diffuse than the bladder mucosal fluorescence associated with malignant lesions.
- Tangential light may give false fluorescence. To help avoid false fluorescence, hold the endoscope perpendicular and close to the bladder wall with the bladder distended.
- False positive fluorescence may result from scope trauma from a previous cystoscopic examination and/or bladder inflammation.
- Malignant lesions may not fluoresce following hexaminolevulinate administration, particularly if the lesions are coated with necrotic tissue. Blue light may fail to detect T2 tumors, which have a tendency to be necrotic on the surface; necrotic cells generally do not fluoresce.
- When performing blue light cystoscopy, avoid prolonged blue light exposure. Studies have not evaluated the potential for adverse effects from blue light. In the controlled clinical trial, the cumulative blue light exposure from bladder mapping did not exceed 12 minutes, and checking for complete tumor resection under blue light did not exceed 8 minutes for any patient.

Perform biopsy and/or resection of suspicious lesions by transurethral resection of the bladder (TURB) only after completing white and blue light cystoscopic examinations with bladder mapping. Using standard cystoscopic practices, obtain biopsies of abnormal areas identified during white or blue light examination and perform resections. Always check for the completeness of the resections under white and blue light before finalizing the TURB procedure.

➤*Storage/Stability:* Store kit at 20° to 25°C (68° to 77°F); excursions are permitted between 15° and 30°C (59° and 86°F).

Use the solution shortly after reconstitution. The reconstituted solution can be stored under refrigeration (2° to 8°C [36° to 46°F]) for up to 2 hours in the 50 mL labeled syringe.

Actions

➤*Pharmacology:* Hexaminolevulinate is an ester of the heme precursor, aminolevulinic acid. After bladder instillation, hexaminolevulinate enters the bladder mucosa and is proposed to enter the intracellular space of mucosal cells where it is used as a precursor in the formation of the photoactive intermediate protoporphyrin IX (PpIX) and other photoactive porphyrins (PAPs). PpIX and PAPs are reported to accumulate preferentially in neoplastic cells as compared with normal urothelium, partly due to altered enzymatic activity in the neoplastic cells. After excitation with light at wavelengths between 360 and 450 nm, PpIX and other PAPs return to a lower energy level by fluorescing, which can be detected and used for cystoscopic detection of lesions. The fluorescence from tumor tissue appears bright red and demarcated, whereas the background normal tissue appears dark blue. Similar processes may occur with inflamed cells.

➤*Pharmacokinetics:*

Absorption/Distribution – After bladder instillation of [^{14}C]-labeled hexaminolevulinate 100 mg for approximately 1 hour in healthy volunteers, absolute bioavailability of hexaminolevulinate was 7% (90% confidence interval [CI], 5% to 10%). Whole blood analysis showed no evidence of significant binding of hexaminolevulinate to erythrocytes.

Metabolism – An in vitro study showed that hexaminolevulinate underwent rapid metabolism in human blood.

Excretion – The [^{14}C]-labeled substance(s) showed biphasic elimination, with an initial elimination half-life of 39 minutes, followed by a terminal half-life of approximately 76 hours.

Contraindications

Porphyria; gross hematuria; Bacillus Calmette-Guérin immunotherapy or intravesical chemotherapy within the past 90 days; known hypersensitivity to hexaminolevulinate or any derivative of aminolevulinic acid.

Warnings/Precautions

➤*Failed detection:* Hexaminolevulinate may fail to detect some bladder tumors, including malignant lesions. Hexaminolevulinate is not a replacement for random biopsies or any other procedure usually performed in the cystoscopic evaluation for cancer. In the controlled clinical trial, hexaminolevulinate hydrochloride failed to detect 10% of lesions confirmed as malignant within the study drug group. Do not perform cystoscopy with blue light alone as malignant lesions can be missed unless the bladder is initially examined under white light.

➤*False fluorescence:* Fluorescent areas detected during blue light cystoscopy may not indicate a bladder mucosal lesion. In the controlled clinical study, biopsies from 1 of every 4 fluorescent areas showed neither dysplasia nor carcinoma, if the areas were not also identified during white light cystoscopy. In addition to these false detections, fluorescent areas within the bladder mucosa may result from inflammation, cystoscopic trauma, scar tissue, or bladder mucosal biopsy from a previous cystoscopic examination.

The presence of urine and/or blood within the bladder may interfere with the detection of tissue fluorescence. To enhance the diagnostic utility of hexaminolevulinate hydrochloride with the Karl Storz D-Light C PDD System, ensure the bladder is emptied of urine prior to the instillation of fluids at cystoscopy and biopsy/resect bladder mucosal lesions only following completion of white and blue light cystoscopy.

➤*Hypersensitivity reactions:* Anaphylaxis, including anaphylactoid shock, has been reported following administration of hexaminolevulinate. Prior to and during use of the hexaminolevulinate, have trained personnel and therapies available for the treatment of anaphylaxis. The safety of repetitive hexaminolevulinate exposures has not been evaluated.

➤*Pregnancy:* *Category C.* There are no adequate and well-controlled studies in pregnant women. Adequate reproductive and developmental toxicity studies in animals have not been performed. Hexaminolevulinate should be used during pregnancy only if the potential benefit justifies the potential risk to the fetus.

➤*Lactation:* It is not known whether hexaminolevulinate is excreted in human milk. Because many drugs are excreted in human milk, exercise caution when hexaminolevulinate is administered to breast-feeding mothers.

➤*Children:* Safety and effectiveness in children have not been established.

➤*Elderly:* No clinically important differences in safety or efficacy have been observed between older and younger patients in the controlled study.

Drug Interactions

➤*Bacillus Calmette-Guérin immunotherapy/intravesical chemotherapy:* Hexaminolevulinate is contraindicated in patients who have received Bacillus Calmette-Guérin immunotherapy or intravesical chemotherapy within the past 90 days.

➤*Drug/Lab test interactions:* Fluorescent areas detected during blue light cystoscopy may not indicate a bladder mucosal session. Biopsies from 1 in every 4 fluorescent areas showed neither dysplasia nor carcinoma if the areas were not also identified during white light cystoscopy.

Adverse Reactions

➤*Most common adverse reactions:* The most common adverse reaction was bladder spasm (reported in 2.2% of patients) followed by dysuria, hematuria, and bladder pain. No patients experienced anaphylaxis.

➤*Hypersensitivity:* Anaphylaxis has been reported following exposure to hexaminolevulinate.

➤*Postmarketing:*

GU – Abnormal urinalysis, bladder pain, and cystitis.

Hypersensitivity – Anaphylactoid shock, hypersensitivity reactions.

Overdosage

➤*Symptoms:* No adverse reactions were reported in a dose-finding study conducted among patients whose bladders were instilled with twice the recommended concentration (dose) of solution of hexaminolevulinate.

Patient Information

Ask patients if they have a diagnosis or a family history of porphyria; allergy to aminolevulinic acid or prior exposure to hexaminolevulinate; gross hematuria; or had Bacillus Calmette-Guérin immunotherapy or intravesical chemotherapy.

Inform patients that hexaminolevulinate should be retained in the bladder for 1 hour from instillation of to the start of the cystoscopic procedure. If the patient cannot hold hexaminolevulinate for 1 hour and needs to void and expel hexaminolevulinate from the bladder, they may void and should then inform their health care provider.

CAPROMAB PENDETIDE

Rx	**ProstaScint** (Cytogen)	**Kit:** Each contains 0.5 mg capromab pendetide/ml of sodium phosphate buffered saline and 1 vial of 82 mg sodium acetate in 2 ml Sterile Water for Injection	Preservative free. Includes 1 sterile 0.22 mcm *Millex GV filter,* prescribing information, and 2 identification labels.

CAPROMAB PENDETIDE — INTRAVENOUS

Indications

➤*General information:* Consider the information provided by capromab in conjunction with other diagnostic information. Confirm scans that are positive for metastatic disease histologically in patients who are otherwise candidates for surgery or radiation therapy unless medically contraindicated. Do not use scans that are negative for metastatic disease in lieu of histological confirmation.

It is not indicated as a screening tool for carcinoma of the prostate nor for readministration for assessment of response to treatment.

➤*Prostate cancer:* As a diagnostic imaging agent in newly-diagnosed patients with biopsy-proven prostate cancer, thought to be clinically-localized after standard diagnostic evaluation (eg, chest x-ray, bone scan, CT scan, or MRI), who are at high risk for pelvic lymph node metastases. It is not indicated in patients who are not at high risk.

➤*Post-prostatectomy patients:* As a diagnostic imaging agent in post-prostatectomy patients with a rising PSA and a negative or equivocal standard metastatic evaluation in whom there is a high clinical suspicion of occult metastatic disease. The imagine performance following radiation therapy has not been studied.

CAPROMAB PENDETIDE — INTRAVENOUS

Administration and Dosage

➤*General dosing considerations:* Indium In 111 capromab pendetide may be readministered following infiltration or a technically inadequate scan; however, it is not indicated for readministration for assessment of response to treatment.

➤*Adults:*

Diagnostic aid – 0.5 mg radiolabeled with 5 mCi of Indium In 111 chloride.

➤*Preparation for administration:* Unlabeled capromab pendetide should not be administered directly to the patient. Waterproof gloves should be worn during the radiolabeling procedure. Before radiolabeling, bring the refrigerated capromab pendetide to room temperature.

Clean the rubber stopper of each vial with an alcohol wipe. With a sterile 1 mL syringe, add sodium acetate solution 0.1 mL to the shielded vial of Indium In 111 chloride and mix. With the same 1 mL syringe, withdraw between 6 and 7 mCi of the buffered Indium In 111 chloride and add to the capromab pendetide vial. Flush the syringe to mix the preparation. Swirl gently to mix and assay contents in a dose calibrator. On one of the labels provided, record the patients identification, date, time of preparation, and activity in the vial and affix the label to the vial shield. Allow the labeling reaction to proceed at room temperature for 30 minutes.

With a 3 mL syringe, add the remaining sodium acetate to the capromab pendetide reaction vial. To normalize pressure, withdraw an equal volume of air. Aseptically attach the 0.22 mcm *Millex* GV sterile filter (provided) and a sterile hypodermic needle to a 10 mL sterile disposable syringe and withdraw the contents of the reaction vial through the filter into the syringe. Keep the needle immersed in the solution to avoid creating an airlock in the filter. Remove the filter and needle. Aseptically attach a fresh sterile hypodermic needle to the syringe. Assay syringe and contents in a dose calibrator. The syringe should not contain less than 4 mCi (148 MBq) of Indium In 111 capromab pendetide. On the second label provided, record the patient's identification, date, time of assay, and activity in the syringe and affix the label to the syringe shield.

Radiochemical purity determination – Radiochemical purity by instant thin layer chromatography can be determined by mixing equal parts (several drops of each) in Indium In 111 capromab pendetide with DTPA solution. Allow the mixture to stand at room temperature for 1 minute. Spot a small drop of the mixture onto an instant thin layer chromatography strip at its origin. Place the strip in a chromatography chamber within the origin at the bottom and allow the solvent to migrate 6 cm from the origin of the strip. Remove and cut the strip in half and measure the counts per minute (CPM) of both halves with a gamma ray detector.

Calculate the percent radiochemical purity: (CPM bottom half × 100)/ (CPM bottom half + CPM top half).

If the radiochemical chemical purity is less than 90%, the instant thin layer chromatography procedure should be repeated. If repeat testing remains less than 90%, the preparation should not be administered.

➤*Administration:* For IV use only. After radiolabeling with Indium In 111, the entire Indium In 111 capromab pendetide dose must be administered to the patient. Each dose is administered over 5 minutes.

➤*Admixture compatibility:* Do not mix with any other medication during its administration.

➤*Storage / Stability:* Store at 2° to 8°C (36° to 46°F). Store upright and do not freeze. Use within 8 hours of radiolabeling.

PENTETATE INDIUM DISODIUM In 111

Rx	**Indium DTPA In 111** (GE Healthcare)	**Injection:** 37 MBq (1 mCi) per mL at calibration	In 1.5 mL single-dose vials.[a]

[a] Vials are packaged in individual lead shields with plastic containers.

PENTETATE INDIUM DISODIUM In 111 — INJECTION

Indications

➤*Radionuclide cisternography:* For use in radionuclide cisternography.

Administration and Dosage

➤*Adults:*

Radionuclide cisternography –

Maximum dose: 18.5 MBq, 500 mcCi.

➤*Administration:* For intrathecal administration. Extreme care must be exercised to ensure aseptic conditions in intrathecal injections. The dose should be measured by a suitable radioactivity calibration system immediately prior to administration.

➤*Storage / Stability:* Do not use after the expiration time and date (7 days after calibration time and date stated on the label). Store the vial in its lead shield at 5° to 30°C (41° to 86°F). Discard vial after a single use. Do not freeze.

Actions

➤*Pharmacokinetics:*

Absorption / Distribution – After intrathecal administration, the radiopharmaceutical is absorbed from the subarachnoid space, as described in the following sections, and the remainder flows superiorly to the basal cisterns within 2 to 4 hours and subsequently will be apparent in the Sylvian cisterns, the interhemispheric cisterns, and over the cerebral convexities. In normal individuals, the radiopharmaceutical will have ascended to the parasagittal region within 24 hours with simultaneous partial or complete clearance of activity from the basal cisterns and Sylvian regions. In contrast to air, the radiopharmaceutical does not normally enter the cerebral ventricles.

Although the primary absorption of cerebrospinal fluid (CSF) into the blood stream occurs at the arachnoid villi, there is some evidence that a significant fraction of CSF is also absorbed across both the cerebral and spinal leptomeninges. Lesser quantities may also be absorbed across the ventricular ependyma. It is also generally held that these alternate routes of CSF absorption may assume primary importance when the major routes of the flow are pathologically obstructed.

Excretion – Approximately 65% of the administered dose is excreted by the kidneys within 24 hours and this increases to 85% in 72 hours.

Contraindications

None known.

Warnings/Precautions

➤*Radiation exposure:* The contents of the vial are radioactive. Adequate shielding of the preparation must be maintained at all times.

Pentetate indium disodium In 111, as well as other radioactive drugs, must be handled with care; use appropriate safety measures to minimize external radiation exposure to clinical personnel and to minimize radiation exposure to patients consistent with proper patient management.

➤*Administration:* Radiopharmaceuticals should be used only by health care providers who are qualified and have training and experience in the safe use and handling of radionuclides and whose experience and training have been approved by the appropriate government agency authorized to license the use of radionuclides.

➤*Renal function impairment:* Because the drug is excreted by the kidneys, exercise caution in patients with severe renal function impairment.

➤*Pregnancy: Category C.* Animal reproduction studies have not been conducted with pentetate indium disodium In 111. Also, it is not known whether pentetate indium disodium In 111 can cause fetal harm when administered to a pregnant woman or whether it can affect reproduction capacity. Give pentetate indium disodium In 111 to a pregnant woman only if clearly needed.

Ideally, perform examinations using radiopharmaceuticals, especially those elective in nature, of a woman of childbearing capability during the first few (approximately 10) days following the onset of menses.

➤*Lactation:* It is not known whether this drug is excreted in human milk. Because many drugs are excreted in human milk, formula feeding should be substituted for breast-feeding when pentetate indium disodium In 111 is administered to a breast-feeding mother.

➤*Children:* Safety and efficacy in children have not been established.

➤*Elderly:* In general, dose selection for an elderly patient should be cautious, usually starting at the low end of the dosing range and reflecting the greater frequency of decreased hepatic, renal, or cardiac function, and of concomitant disease or other drug therapy.

This drug is known to be substantially excreted by the kidney, and the risk of toxic reactions to this drug may be greater in patients with renal function impairment. Because elderly patients are more likely to have decreased renal function, take care in dose selection; it may be useful to monitor renal function.

Adverse Reactions

Aseptic meningitis and pyrogenic reactions have been rarely (less than 0.4%) observed following cisternography with pentetate indium disodium In 111.

One death has been reported to have occurred within 20 minutes following the administration of pentetate indium disodium In 111 and appears to be drug-related. In addition, 2 cases of septic meningitis have also been reported. There have also been reports of skin reactions and vomiting following administration of pentetate indium disodium In 111. The relationship of the drug to these latter occurrences has not been established.

IOBENGUANE SULFATE I 123

Rx	**AdreView** (GE Healthcare)	**Injection, solution:** 74 MBq (2 mCi) per mL at calibration[a]	Preservative free. In 5 mL single-use vials.

[a] Each mL contains iobenguane sulfate 0.08 mg, sodium dihydrogen phosphate dihydrate 23 mg, disodium hydrogen phosphate dihydrate 2.8 mg, and benzyl alcohol 10.3 mg (1% v/v).

IOBENGUANE SULFATE I 123 — INJECTION

Indications

➤*Detection of pheochromocytoma/neuroblastoma:* For use in the detection of primary or metastatic pheochromocytoma or neuroblastoma as an adjunct to other diagnostic tests.

Administration and Dosage

➤*General dosing considerations:* The benzyl alcohol in iobenguane may cause serious adverse reactions in premature or low birth weight infants (see Warnings/Precautions).

Before administration, administer potassium iodide oral solution or Lugol solution or potassium perchlorate to block uptake of iodine 123 by the patient's thyroid (see Concomitant Therapy).

To minimize radiation dose to the bladder, prior to and following administration, encourage hydration to permit frequent voiding. Encourage the patient to void frequently for the first 48 hours following administration.

Iobenguane emits radiation and must be handled with appropriate safety measures to minimize radiation exposure to clinical personnel and patients. Radiopharmaceuticals should be used by or under the control of health care providers who are qualified by specific training and experience in the safe use and handling of radionuclides, and whose experience and training have been approved by the appropriate government agency authorized to license the use of radionuclides. Iobenguane dosing is based upon the radioactivity determined using a suitable calibration system immediately prior to administration.

➤*Adults:*

Detection of pheochromocytoma/neuroblastoma – 10 mCi (370 MBq).

➤*Children:*

Detection of pheochromocytoma/neuroblastoma – See Adults for dosing in children younger than 16 years of age weighing 70 kg or more

Younger than 16 years to 1 month of age and weighing less than 70 kg:

Iobenguane Sulfate I 123 Dose Preparation for Children[a]

Weight (kg)	Fraction of adult activity	Dose (mCi)	Dose (MBq)
3	0.1	1	37
4	0.14	1.4	52
6	0.19	1.9	70
8	0.23	2.3	85.1
10	0.27	2.7	99.9
12	0.32	3.2	118.4
14	0.36	3.6	133.2
16	0.4	4	148
18	0.44	4.4	162.8
20	0.46	4.6	170.2
22	0.5	5	185
24	0.53	5.3	196.1
26	0.56	5.6	207.2
28	0.58	5.8	214.6
30	0.62	6.2	229.4
32	0.65	6.5	240.5
34	0.68	6.8	251.6
36	0.71	7.1	262.7
38	0.73	7.3	270.1
40	0.76	7.6	281.2
42	0.78	7.8	288.6
44	0.8	8	296
46	0.82	8.2	303.4
48	0.85	8.5	314.5
50	0.88	8.8	325.6
52	0.9	9	333
54	0.9	9	333
56	0.92	9.2	340.4
58	0.92	9.2	340.4
60	0.96	9.6	355.2
62	0.96	9.6	355.2
64	0.98	9.8	362.6
66	0.98	9.8	362.6
68	0.99	9.9	366.3

[a] Based on a reference activity for an adult scaled to body weight according to the schedule proposed by the European Association of Nuclear Medicine Paediatric Task Group.

➤*Renal function impairment:* The radiation dose to patients with severe renal impairment may be increased because of delayed elimination of the drug. Delayed iobenguane I 123 clearance may also reduce the target to background ratios and decrease the quality of scintigraphic images. These risks may limit the role of iobenguane I 123 in the diagnostic evaluation of patients with severe renal impairment.

➤*Concomitant therapy:* Before administration, administer potassium iodide oral solution or Lugol solution (equivalent to iodide 100 mg for adults, body-weight adjusted for children) or potassium perchlorate (400 mg for adults, body-weight adjusted for children) to block uptake of iodine 123 by the patient's thyroid. Administer the blocking agent at least 1 hour before the dose of iobenguane.

➤*Preparation for administration:* Use aseptic procedures and a radiation shielding syringe during administration.

➤*Administration:* Administer the dose as an intravenous (IV) injection over 1 to 2 minutes. A subsequent injection of sodium chloride 0.9% may be used to ensure full delivery of the dose. Begin whole body planar scintigraphy imaging 24 hours (± 6 hours) following administration. Single photon emission computed tomography (SPECT) may be performed following planar scintigraphy, as appropriate.

➤*Storage/Stability:* Store between 20° and 25°C (68° and 77°F); excursions permitted between 15° and 30°C (59° and 86°F). Store within the original lead container or equivalent radiation shielding. Iobenguane I 123 preparations should not be used after the expiration date and time stated on the label.

Actions

➤*Pharmacology:* Iobenguane is similar in structure to the antihypertensive drug guanethidine and to the neurotransmitter norepinephrine. Iobenguane is, therefore, largely subject to the same uptake and accumulation pathways as norepinephrine. Iobenguane is taken up by the norepinephrine transporter in adrenergic nerve terminals and stored in the presynaptic storage vesicles. Iobenguane accumulates in adrenergically innervated tissues such as the adrenal medulla, salivary glands, heart, liver, spleen, and lungs, as well as tumors derived from the neural crest. By labeling iobenguane with the isotope iodine 123, it is possible to obtain scintigraphic images of the organs and tissues in which the radiopharmaceutical accumulates.

Pharmacodynamics – Iobenguane I 123 is a diagnostic radiopharmaceutical that contains a small quantity of iobenguane that is not expected to produce a pharmacodynamic effect. To minimize radiation dose to the thyroid gland, block this organ before dosing. Because iobenguane is excreted mainly via the kidneys, patients with severe renal insufficiency may experience increased radiation exposure and impaired imaging results. Encourage frequent voiding after administration to minimize the radiation dose to the bladder.

➤*Pharmacokinetics:*

Distribution – Iobenguane is rapidly cleared from the blood and accumulates in adrenergically innervated tissues. Retention is especially prolonged in highly adrenergically innervated tissues (eg, the adrenal medulla, heart, salivary glands).

Metabolism/Excretion – The majority of the iobenguane dose is excreted unaltered by the kidneys via glomerular filtration. A rapid initial clearance of circulating iobenguane is observed, followed by a slow clearance as iobenguane is released from other compartments. In patients with healthy renal function, 70% to 90% of the administered dose is recovered unaltered in urine within 4 days. Iobenguane is not cleared by dialysis. Most of the remaining radioactivity recovered in the urine is in the form of the radioiodinated metabolite m-iodohippuric acid (MIHA) (typically 10% or less) and free radioiodide (typically 6% or less). The enzymatic process responsible for metabolism has not been well characterized and the pharmacologic activity of these metabolites has not been studied. Only a small amount (less than 1%) of the injected dose is eliminated via the feces.

Contraindications

Known hypersensitivity to iobenguane or iobenguane sulfate.

Warnings/Precautions

➤*Concomitant thyroid accumulation:* Failure to block thyroid uptake of iodine 123 may result in an increased long-term risk for thyroid neoplasia. Administer thyroid-blocking medications before iobenguane I 123 administration.

➤*Hypertension:* Assess the patient's pulse and blood pressure before and intermittently for 30 minutes after iobenguane I 123 administration. Iobenguane I 123 may increase release of norepinephrine from chromaffin granules and produce a transient episode of hypertension, although this was not observed in the clinical study. Prior to iobenguane I 123 administration, ensure emergency cardiac and antihypertensive treatments are readily available.

➤*Hypersensitivity reactions:* Hypersensitivity reactions have been reported following iobenguane I 123 administration. Prior to administration, question the patient for a history of prior reactions to iodine, an iodine-containing contrast agent, or other products containing iodine. If the patient is known or strongly suspected to have hypersensitivity to iodine, an iodine-containing contrast agent, or other products containing iodine, base the decision to administer iobenguane I 123 on an assessment of the expected

IOBENGUANE SULFATE I 123 — INJECTION

benefits compared with the potential hypersensitivity risks. Have anaphylactic and hypersensitivity treatment measures available prior to iobenguane I 123 administration.

➤*Renal function impairment:* Iobenguane I 123 is cleared by glomerular filtration and is not dialyzable. The radiation dose to patients with severe renal impairment may be increased because of the delayed elimination of the drug. Delayed iobenguane I 123 clearance may also reduce the target to background ratios and decrease the quality of scintigraphic images. These risks importantly may limit the role of iobenguane in the diagnostic evaluation of patients with severe renal impairment. Iobenguane I 123 safety and efficacy have not been established in these patients.

➤*Pregnancy: Category C.* Any radiopharmaceutical, including iobenguane I 123, has a potential to cause fetal harm. It is not known whether iobenguane I 123 can cause fetal harm when administered to a pregnant woman or can affect reproduction capacity. Animal reproduction studies have not been conducted with iobenguane I 123. Give iobenguane I 123 to a pregnant woman only if clearly needed.

➤*Lactation:* It is not known whether iobenguane I 123 is excreted into human milk. However, iodine 123 is excreted into human milk. Because many drugs are excreted into human milk and because of the potential for serious adverse reactions in breast-feeding infants, decide whether to interrupt breast-feeding after administration of iobenguane I 123 or not to administer iobenguane I 123, taking into account the importance of the drug to the mother. Based on the physical half-life of iodine 123 (13.2 hours) breast-feeding women may consider interrupting breast-feeding for 6 days after iobenguane I 123 administration in order to minimize risks to breast-feeding infants.

➤*Children:* The safety and effectiveness of iobenguane I 123 have been established in children 1 month to 16 years of age. Safety and effectiveness in children younger than 1 month of age have not been established.

Iobenguane I 123 contains benzyl alcohol at a concentration of 10.3 mg/mL. Benzyl alcohol has been associated with a fatal gasping syndrome in premature infants and infants of low birth weight. Exposure to excessive amounts of benzyl alcohol has been associated with toxicity (hypotension, metabolic acidosis), particularly in neonates, and an increased incidence of kernicterus, particularly in small preterm infants. There have been rare reports of deaths, primarily in preterm infants, associated with exposure to excessive amounts of benzyl alcohol.

➤*Elderly:* In general, use caution when selecting the dose for an elderly population, usually starting at the low end of the dosing range, reflecting the greater frequency of decreased hepatic, renal, or cardiac function, and of concomitant disease or other drug therapy.

Iobenguane I 123 is excreted by the kidneys, and the risks of adverse reactions, increased radiation dose, and occurrence of falsely negative imaging results, may be greater in patients with severely impaired renal function. Because elderly patients are more likely to have decreased renal function, take care in dose selection and image interpretation. Consider assessment of renal function in elderly patients prior to iobenguane I 123 administration.

➤*Monitoring:* Observe infants for signs or symptoms of benzyl alcohol toxicity following iobenguane I 123 administration. Assess the patient's pulse and blood pressure before and intermittently for 30 minutes after iobenguane I 123 administration.

Drug Interactions

Iobenguane Sulfate I 123 Drug Interactions

Precipitant drug	Object drug[a]		Description
Antidepressants (eg, amitriptyline, imipramine, SSRIs[b])	Iobenguane I 123	⬇	Drugs that interfere with norepinephrine uptake or retention may decrease the uptake of iobenguane in neuroendocrine tumors and lead to false-negative imaging results. When medically feasible, stop these drugs before iobenguane administration (for at least 5 biological half-lives) and monitor patients for the occurrence of clinically significant withdrawal symptoms, especially patients with elevated levels of circulating catecholamines and their metabolites.
Antihypertensives (eg, reserpine, labetalol)	Iobenguane I 123		
Cocaine	Iobenguane I 123		
Sympathomimetic amines (eg, ephedrine, phenylephrine, pseudoephedrine)	Iobenguane I 123		

[a] ⬇ = object drug decreased.
[b] SSRIs = selective serotonin reuptake inhibitors.

Adverse Reactions

➤*Clinical study experience:* Adverse reactions were all mild to moderate in severity and were predominantly isolated occurrences (2 patients or fewer) of one of the following reactions: dizziness, flushing, injection-site hemorrhage, pruritus, or rash.

Postmarketing experience – Hypersensitivity reactions have uncommonly been reported during the postmarketing use of iobenguane I 123.

Overdosage

➤*Symptoms:* The major manifestations of overdose relate predominantly to increased radiation exposure, with the long-term risks for neoplasia.

Patient Information

Instruct patients to inform their health care provider if they:

- are pregnant or breast feeding,
- are sensitive to iodine, an iodine-containing contrast agent or other products that contain iodine,
- are sensitive to potassium iodide oral solution, or Lugol solution,
- have reduced renal function.

Instruct patients to increase their level of hydration prior to receiving iobenguane I 123 and to void frequently for the first 48 hours following iobenguane I 123 administration.

IOFLUPANE I 123

c-ii	**DaTscan** (GE Healthcare)	**Injection, solution:** 74 MBq (2 mCi) per mL at calibration[a]	Preservative free. In 2.5 mL single-use vials.

[a] Each mL contains ioflupane 0.07 to 0.13 mcg, acetic acid 5.7 mg, sodium acetate 7.8 mg, and ethanol 0.05 mL (5%).

IOFLUPANE I 123 — INJECTION

Indications

➤*Brain imaging:* For striatal dopamine transporter visualization using single photon emission computed tomography (SPECT) brain imaging to assist in the evaluation of adult patients with suspected Parkinsonian syndromes.

Administration and Dosage

➤*General dosing considerations:* To minimize radiation dose to the bladder, encourage hydration prior to and following administration in order to permit frequent voiding. Encourage the patient to void frequently for the first 48 hours following administration.

➤*Adults:*

Brain imaging –

Usual dosage: 111 to 185 MBq (3 to 5 mCi) intravenously (IV).

Concomitant therapy: Before administration of ioflupane I 123, administer potassium iodide oral solution or Lugol solution (equivalent to iodide 100 mg) or potassium perchlorate (400 mg) to block uptake of iodine 123 by the patient's thyroid. Administer the blocking agent at least 1 hour before the dose of ioflupane I 123.

➤*Administration:* Administer ioflupane I 123 as a slow IV injection over a period of not less than 15 to 20 seconds via an arm vein.

➤*Storage/Stability:* Store between 20° and 25 °C (68° and 77°F). Store within the original lead container or equivalent radiation shielding.

Handling – This preparation is approved for use by individuals licensed by the Illinois Emergency Management Agency pursuant to 32 IL. Adm. Code Section 330.260(a) and 355.4010 or equivalent licenses of the Nuclear Regulatory Commission or an Agreement State. Ioflupane I 123 emits radiation and must be handled with safety measures to minimize radiation exposure to clinical personnel and patients.

Actions

➤*Pharmacology:* The active drug substance in ioflupane I 123 is N-omega-fluoropropyl-2beta-carbomethoxy-3beta-(4-[^{123}I]iodophenyl) nortropane or ioflupane I 123. In vitro, ioflupane binds reversibly to the human recombinant dopamine transporter (DaT) (Ki = 0.62 nM, IC_{50} = 0.71 nM). Autoradiography of postmortem human brain slices exposed to radiolabeled ioflupane shows concentration of the radiolabel in striatum (caudate nucleus and putamen). In postmortem human brain slices exposed to radiolabeled ioflupane, the specificity of the binding of ioflupane I 125 to dopamine transporter was demonstrated by competition studies with the DaT inhibitor GBR 12909 (a dopamine reuptake inhibitor), the serotonin reuptake inhibitor citalopram, and the norepinephrine reuptake inhibitor desipramine. Citalopram reduced binding in the neocortex and thalamus with only minor effects in the striatum. This indicated that the binding in the cortex and thalamus is mainly to the serotonin reuptake sites. Desipramine showed no effect on the level of striatal binding of ioflupane I 125, but reduced extrastriatal binding by 60% to 85%. The binding of ioflupane I 125 to the striatum was abolished in the presence of high concentrations of GBR 12909, indicating selectivity of ioflupane binding for the presynaptic DaT.

Following administration of ioflupane I 123 to humans, radioactive decay of the iodine 123 emits gamma radiation which can be detected externally using gamma detectors, allowing visualization of the brain striata through SPECT imaging.

➤*Pharmacokinetics:*

Absorption – Only 5% of the administered radioactivity remained in whole blood at 5 minutes postinjection. Uptake in the brain reached approximately 7% of injected radioactivity at 10 minutes postinjection and decreased to 3% after 5 hours; striata to background ratios were relatively constant between 3 and 6 hours postinjection. About 30% of whole brain radioactivity was attributed to striatal uptake.

IOFLUPANE I 123 — INJECTION

Excretion – By 48 hours postinjection, approximately 60% of the injected radioactivity has been excreted in the urine, with fecal excretion estimated to be approximately 14%.

Contraindications

Known hypersensitivity to the active substance or to any of the excipients, or to iodine.

Warnings/Precautions

➤*Thyroid accumulation:* The ioflupane I 123 injection may contain up to 6% of free iodide (iodine 123). To decrease thyroid accumulation of iodine 123, block the thyroid gland before administration of ioflupane I 123. Avoid the use of potassium iodide or Lugol solution in patients who are sensitive to such products. Failure to block thyroid uptake of iodine 123 may result in an increased long-term risk for thyroid neoplasia. (See Administration and Dosage.)

➤*Hypersensitivity reactions:* Hypersensitivity reactions have been reported following ioflupane I 123 administration. The reactions have generally consisted of skin erythema and pruritis and have either resolved spontaneously or following the administration of corticosteroids and antihistamines. Prior to administration, question the patient for a history of prior reactions to ioflupane I 123. If the patient is known or strongly suspected of having had a hypersensitivity reaction to ioflupane I 123, base the decision to administer ioflupane I 123 on an assessment of the expected benefits compared with the potential hypersensitivity risks. Have anaphylactic and hypersensitivity treatment measures available prior to ioflupane I 123 administration and, following administration, observe patients for symptoms or signs of a hypersensitivity reaction.

➤*Renal function impairment:* Ioflupane I 123 is excreted by the kidney, and patients with severe renal impairment may have increased radiation exposure and altered ioflupane I 123 images.

➤*Drug abuse and dependence:* Ioflupane I 123 is a schedule II controlled substance under the Controlled Substances Act. A Drug Enforcement Administration license is required for handling or administering this controlled substance.

➤*Pregnancy: Category C.* It is not known whether ioflupane I 123 can cause fetal harm or increase the risk of pregnancy loss when administered to a pregnant woman. Animal reproductive and developmental toxicity studies have not been conducted. Prior to administration to women of childbearing potential, assess them for pregnancy. Give to a pregnant woman only if clearly needed.

Like all radiopharmaceuticals, ioflupane I 123 has potential to cause fetal harm. The likelihood of fetal harm depends on the stage of fetal development and the magnitude of the radionuclide dose. Administration of ioflupane I 123 at a dose of 185 MBq (5 mCi) results in an absorbed radiation dose to the uterus of 0.3 rad (3 mGy). Radiation doses more than 15 rad (150 mGy) have been associated with congenital anomalies but doses less than 5 rad (50 mGy) generally have not. Radioactive iodine products cross the placenta and can permanently impair fetal thyroid function.

➤*Lactation:* It is not known whether ioflupane I 123 is excreted into human milk. However, iodine 123 is excreted into human milk. Because many drugs are excreted into human milk and because of the potential for serious adverse reactions in nursing infants, decide whether to interrupt breast-feeding after administration of ioflupane I 123 or not to administer ioflupane I 123, taking into account the importance of the drug to the mother. Based on the physical half-life of iodine 123 (13.2 hours), breast-feeding women may consider interrupting breast-feeding and pumping and discarding breast milk for 6 days after ioflupane I 123 administration in order to minimize risks to a breast-feeding infant.

➤*Children:* Ioflupane I 123 is not indicated for use in children. The safety and efficacy of ioflupane I 123 have not been established in children.

Drug Interactions

➤*Drugs that bind to the dopamine transporter:* Because ioflupane within ioflupane I 123 binds to the dopamine transporter, drugs that bind to the dopamine transporter with high affinity may interfere with the image obtained following ioflupane I 123 administration. The potentially interfering drugs include: amoxapine, amphetamine, benztropine, bupropion, buspirone, cocaine, methamphetamine, methylphenidate, phentermine, selegiline, and sertraline.

➤*Selective serotonin reuptake inhibitors:* Selective serotonin reuptake inhibitors (eg, citalopram, paroxetine) may increase or decrease ioflupane binding to the dopamine transporter. Whether discontinuation of these drugs prior to ioflupane I 123 administration may minimize the interference with an ioflupane I 123 image is unknown.

Adverse Reactions

➤*Adverse reactions (1% or less):* Adverse reactions occurring at a rate of 1% or less included headache, nausea, vertigo, dry mouth, or dizziness. These reactions were of mild to moderate severity.

➤*Postmarketing:*

Hypersensitivity – Hypersensitivity reactions have been reported, generally related to rash and pruritus within minutes of administration. The reactions either resolved spontaneously or following the administration of corticosteroids and antihistamines.

Local – Injection site pain has also been reported.

Overdosage

➤*Symptoms:* The clinical consequence of overdose with ioflupane I 123 has not been reported. Due to the small quantity of ioflupane in each vial, overdosage with ioflupane is not expected to result in pharmacologic effects. The major risks of overdose relates predominantly to increased radiation exposure with long-term risks for neoplasia.

➤*Treatment:* It is unknown whether or not ioflupane is dialyzable. In case of overdosage of radioactivity, encourage frequent urination and defecation to minimize radiation exposure to the patient; take care to avoid contamination from the radioactivity eliminated by the patient.

Patient Information

Instruct patients to inform their health care provider if they have reduced renal or hepatic function; are sensitive to ioflupane I 123; are sensitive to potassium iodide or Lugol solution; or may be pregnant, are trying to become pregnant, or are breast feeding.

Instruct patients to increase their level of hydration prior to and after receiving ioflupane I 123 and to void frequently for the first 48 hours following ioflupane I 123 administration.

IN VIVO DIAGNOSTIC BIOLOGICALS

CANDIDA ALBICANS SKIN TEST ANTIGEN

Rx	**Candin** (Allermed)	**Injection:** Prepared from the culture filtrate and cells of two strains of *Candida albicans*.	In 1 mL multidose vial.

CANDIDA ALBICANS SKIN TEST ANTIGEN — INJECTION

Indications

➤*Reduced cellular hypersensitivity:* For use as a recall antigen for detecting delayed-type hypersensitivity (DTH) by intracutaneous (intradermal) testing. The product may be useful in evaluating the cellular immune response in patients suspected of having reduced cellular hypersensitivity. Because some persons with normal cellular immunity are not hypersensitive to *Candida albicans*, a response rate less than 100% to the antigen is to be expected in healthy individuals. Therefore, the concurrent use of other licensed DTH skin test antigens is recommended.

➤*HIV:* Antigens of *C. albicans* are useful in the assessment of diminished cellular immunity in persons infected with HIV. Responses to DTH antigens have prognostic value in patients with cancer. Because HIV infection can modify the DTH response to tuberculin, it is advisable to skin test HIV-infected patients at high risk of tuberculosis with antigens in addition to tuberculin, to assess their competency to react to tuberculin. (See Warnings.)

Administration and Dosage

➤*Adults:*

Assessment of diminished cellular immunity in HIV – 0.1 mL.

Reduced cellular hypersensitivity – 0.1 mL.

➤*Interpretation of test:* A positive DTH reaction consists of induration 5 mm or more. The time required for the induration response to reach maximum intensity varies with the individual. The reaction usually begins within 24 hours and peaks between 24 and 48 hours. Read the skin test after 48 hours by visually inspecting the test site and palpating the indurated area. Measure across two diameters. Report the mean of the longest and midpoint diameters of the indurated area as the DTH response

➤*Administration:* Cleanse the skin with 70% alcohol before applying the skin test. Administer intradermally, on the volar surface of the forearm, or on the outer aspect of the upper arm. Inject the antigen intradermally as superficially as possible, causing a distinct, sharply defined bleb at the skin test site. An unreliable reaction may result if the product is injected subcutaneously. It must not be given IV. Do not inject into a blood vessel.

➤*Storage/Stability:* Store between 2° and 8°C (35° and 46°F). Do not freeze.

Actions

➤*Pharmacology:* The potency of *C. albicans* is measured by dose-response skin tests in healthy adults. The procedure involves concurrent (side-by-side) testing of production lots with an internal reference (IR), using sensitive adults who have been previously screened and qualified to serve as test subjects. The induration response at 48 hours elicited by 0.1 ml of a production lot is measured and compared to the response elicited by 0.1 ml of the IR. The test is satisfactory if the potency of the production lot does not differ more than ± 20% from the potency of the IR, when analyzed by the paired t-test.

Cellular or DTH can be assessed by intracutaneous testing with bacterial, viral and fungal antigens to which most healthy persons are sensitized. A positive skin test denotes prior antigenic exposure, T-cell competency and an intact inflammatory response. The reaction usually peaks 48 hours after antigen is introduced into the skin and is manifest as induration at the test site.

Recall antigens may be useful in evaluating DTH by eliciting positive induration reactions 48 to 72 hours after intracutaneous administration. Except for mumps skin test antigen, most commonly used recall antigens were developed for other purposes, and the size of the reaction elicited may not be

CANDIDA ALBICANS SKIN TEST ANTIGEN — INJECTION

directly related to cellular immunity because of variability in antigen source and dose and skin test administration and measurement techniques. Useful antigens are those which elicit a reaction size greater than 5 mm in more than 50% of healthy individuals. The combination of results from skin testing with more than one antigen should result in detection of DTH in at least 95% of healthy subjects.

The inflammatory response associated with the DTH reaction is characterized by an infiltration of lymphocytes and macrophages at the site of antigen deposition. Specific cell types that appear to play a major role in the DTH response include CD4+ and CD8+ T-lymphocytes which leave the recirculating lymphocyte pool in response to exogenous antigen. Both CD4+ and CD8+ lymphocytes have been recovered from DTH reactions elicited by *Candida* antigen.

Contraindications

History of a previous unacceptable adverse reaction to this antigen or to a similar product (eg, extreme hypersensitivity or allergy).

Warnings/Precautions

➤*Type I allergy:* The product should not be used to diagnose or treat Type I allergy to *C. albicans*.

➤*Immunodeficiency:* Immunodeficiency states, such as advanced HIV infection or cancer, can modify the DTH response to tuberculin. It may be advisable to skin test patients at high risk of tuberculosis with antigens in addition to tuberculin to confirm the patient's state of cellular immunity.

➤*Local reactions:* Usually subside within hours or days after administration of the skin test. In some patients, skin discoloration may persist for several weeks. Local reactions may be treated with a cold compress and topical steroids. Severe loval reactions may require additional measures as appropriate.

In persons with a bleeding tendency, bruising and non-specific induration may occur due to the trauma of the skin test.

➤*Systemic reactions to C. albicans:* Systemic reactions to *C. albicans* have not been observed. However, all foreign antigens have the remote possibility of causing type I anaphylaxis and even death when injected intradermally. Systemic reactions usually occur within 30 minutes after the injection of antigen.

➤*Route of administration:* Inject the antigen intradermally as superficially as possible causing a distinct, sharply defined bleb at the skin test site. An unreliable reaction may result if the product is injected subcutaneously. It must not be given IV. Do not inject into a blood vessel.

➤*Hypersensitivity reactions:* As has been observed with other, unstandardized antigens used for DTH skin testing, it is possible that some patients may have exquisite immediate hypersensitivity to *C. albicans*. These reactions are characterized by the presence of an edematous hive surrounded by a zone of erythema. They occur ≈ 15 to 20 minutes after the intradermal injection of the antigen. The size of the immediate reaction varies depending on the sensitivity of the individual. Immediate hypersensitivity reactions have been reported in 17% to 22% of patients, with erythema of 10 to 24 mm in diameter, and in another 5% to 13% of patients, with erythema of 5 to 9 mm. When using this product, have available the facilities and medications necessary to treat all potential local and systemic side effects. Refer to Management of Acute Hypersensitivity Reactions.

➤*Pregnancy: Category C.* It is not known whether *C. albicans* can cause fetal harm when administered to a pregnant woman or can affect reproduction capacity. Give to pregnant women only if clearly needed. Problems in pregnancy are unlikely.

➤*Lactation:* It is not known whether *C. albicans* is excreted in breast milk. Problems in breastfeeding are unlikely.

➤*Children:* The safety and efficacy in children has not been established.

➤*Elderly:* *C. albicans* has not been adequately studied in elderly patients. However, the DTH response to *C. albicans* may be diminished in elderly patients, since the aging process is known to alter cell-mediated immunity.

Drug Interactions

➤*Corticosteroids:* Pharmacologic doses of corticosteroids may variably suppress the DTH skin test response after 2 weeks of therapy. The mechanism of suppression is believed to involve a decrease in monocytes and lymphocytes, particularly T-cells. The skin test response usually returns to the pretreatment level within several weeks after steroid therapy is discontinued.

Adverse Reactions

➤*Systemic:* Sneezing; coughing; itching; shortness of breath; abdominal cramps; vomiting; diarrhea; tachycardia; hypotension; respiratory failure. Progression of the delayed reaction to vesiculation, necrosis and ulceration is possible (see Warnings).

➤*Local:* Redness; swelling; bruising; pruritus; excoriation; discoloration of the skin; rash; vesiculation; bullae dermal exfoliation; cellulitis (severe). (See Warnings.)

HISTAMINE PHOSPHATE

Rx	**Histatrol** (Center Laboratories)	**Scratch/Prick:** 1 mg/ml histamine base as the phosphate (2.75 mg/ml histamine phosphate)	Glycerin 50% w/v, 0.4% phenol. In 5 ml vials.
		Multi-Test: 1 mg/ml histamine base as the phosphate	Glycerin 50% w/v. In 5 ml vials.
		Intradermal: 0.1 mg/ml histamine base as the phosphate (0.275 mg/ml histamine phosphate)	Glycerin free. 0.4% phenol. In 5 ml vials.

HISTAMINE PHOSPHATE — INTRADERMAL

Indications

➤*Allergenic skin testing:* For use as a positive control in evaluation of allergenic skin testing.

Administration and Dosage

➤*Adults:*

Allergenic skin testing –

Prick, puncture, and scratch testing: 1 mg/mL of histamine base (histamine phosphate 2.75 mg/mL).

Intradermal skin testing: 0.1 mg/mL (histamine phosphate 0.275 mg/mL) or 0.01 mg/mL of histamine base.

➤*Children:*

Allergenic skin testing –

6 years of age and older: See Adults for dosing.

➤*Renal function impairment:* Do not inject histamine into individuals with renal disease.

➤*Interpretation:* The patient's response is based on the size of erythema (degree of redness) and size of wheal (smooth, slightly elevated area) that appear after 15 to 20 minutes.

Prick, puncture, and scratch testing – In a large population, the NHANES II survey reports a mean (average of length and width) wheal of 4.4 mm and a mean erythema of 18.4 mm. Interpret all positive reactions against an appropriate negative control.

Intradermal skin testing – In 2 successive years of testing, the Committee on Standardization of the American College of Allergy reported positive reactions at histamine base doses 0.01 mg/mL or more. Mean sum of diameter (sum of length and width) of wheals were approximately 14 mm and sum of erythema was approximately 52 mm following 0.01 mL intradermal doses of 0.01 mg/mL histamine base. When 0.01 mL of 0.1 mg/mL histamine base was injected, the sum of crossed diameters of wheal ranged from 15 to 20 mm and the sum of crossed diameters of erythema ranged from 60 to 80 mm. The available 0.1 mg/mL concentration must be diluted to achieve this dose. Interpret all positive reactions against an appropriate negative control.

➤*Administration:* Avoid injection into a venule or capillary.

➤*Storage/Stability:* Refrigerate and protect vials from light.

Actions

➤*Pharmacology:* Histamine acts as a potent vasodilator when released from mast cells during an allergic reaction. It is largely responsible for the immediate skin test reaction of a sensitive patient when challenged with an offending allergen.

Contraindications

Do not inject histamine into individuals with hypotension, severe hypertension, or severe cardiac, pulmonary, or renal disease.

Warnings/Precautions

➤*Intracutaneous testing:* Use caution in intracutaneous testing to avoid injection into a venule or capillary.

➤*Bronchial disease:* Small doses by any route of administration may precipitate asthma in patients with bronchial disease.

➤*Hypersensitivity reactions:* Epinephrine injection (1:1000) and injectable antihistamines should be available for immediate use in the event the patient exhibits a severe response. A tourniquet can be applied above the test site to slow absorption if a severe response occurs.

➤*Pregnancy: Category C.* There are no adequate and well-controlled studies in pregnant women. However, based on histamine's known ability to contract uterine muscle, avoid exposure or repeated doses. Use histamine phosphate during pregnancy only if the potential benefit justifies the potential risk to the fetus or mother.

➤*Lactation:* No data are available on histamines' transfer to human milk, but it is probably minimal. Wait at least 2 hours following exposure to histamine before breast-feeding.

➤*Children:* Histamine solutions for percutaneous testing have been given safely in infants and young children. Therefore, anticipate small skin test reactions in children < 6 years of age. Safety and efficacy for intracutaneous testing in children < 6 years of age have not been established.

Drug Interactions

➤*Antiallergic drugs:* In the period of 24 hours prior to testing, the patient should not have taken any antiallergic drugs. The pharmacologic action of such agents interferes with the skin test response.

HISTAMINE PHOSPHATE — INTRADERMAL

Adverse Reactions

Following the injection of large doses of histamine, systemic reactions may include flushing, dizziness, headache, bronchial constriction, urticaria, asthma, marked hypertension or hypotension, abdominal cramps, vomiting, metallic taste, and local or generalized allergic manifestations.

Overdosage

➤*Symptoms:* A large SC dose of histamine phosphate may cause severe occipital headache, blurred vision, anginal pain, a rapid drop in blood pressure, and cyanosis of the face.

➤*Treatment:* Give epinephrine injection SC or IM in case of emergency due to severe reactions (see Warnings). An antihistamine preparation may be given IM to ameliorate systemic reaction to overdose.

HISTOPLASMIN

Rx	**Histoplasmin, Diluted** (Parke-Davis)	**Injection:** 1:100 w/v (P-D) or v/v (ALK). Standardized sterile filtrate from cultures of *Histoplasma capsulatum*	0.5% phenol, polysorbate 80. Mycelial derivative. In 1 ml, 10 test multidose vials.

HISTOPLASMIN — INJECTION

Indications

➤*Histoplasmosis, diagnosis:* An aid in the diagnosis of histoplasmosis and the differentiation of possible histoplasmosis from coccidioidomycosis, sarcoidosis and other mycotic or bacterial infections and in the interpretation of roentgenographic plates showing pulmonary infiltration and calcification.

➤*Off-label uses:* In endemic areas (eg, the Ohio and Mississippi River valleys), histoplasmin may be a useful addition to anergy skin test panels to assess competence of recipients' cell-mediated immunity, but use of mycelial histoplasmin may obscure the results of other fungal assays.

Administration and Dosage

➤*Adults:*

Diagnostic aid of histoplasmosis – 0.1 mL intradermally.

➤*Preparation for administration:* The site of injection is first cleansed with 70% alcohol and allowed to dry. A tuberculin syringe (one that has not been used for tuberculin) and a 26 g × ⅜ inch or 27 g × ½ inch needle is used.

➤*Administration:* Inject intradermally into the flexor surface of the forearm. If injections are correctly made, a small bleb will rise over the needle point. The reactions should be read in a well-lighted room 48 to 72 hours after injection.

➤*Storage/Stability:* Store between 2° and 8°C (36° and 46°F).

Actions

➤*Pharmacology:* The sterile culture filtrates of *Histoplasma capsulatum* are grown on liquid synthetic medium.

The histoplasmin test is based on the fact that infection with *Histoplasma capsulatum* produces sensitivity to certain antigens. The reaction to intracutaneously injected histoplasmin reflects a delayed (cellular) hypersensitivity reaction. Clinically, a delayed hypersensitivity reaction to histoplasmin is nearly always a manifestation of previous infection with *Histoplasma capsulatum* or a variety of other mycotic or bacterial infections.

Contraindications

Known histoplasmin positive reactors because of the severity of reactions (eg, vesiculation, ulceration, or necrosis) that may occur at the test site in very highly sensitive individuals.

Warnings/Precautions

➤*Local reactions:* Doses greater than that recommended may produce severe erythema and induration followed by necrosis and ulceration that may last for several weeks.

➤*Administration:* Inject intradermally only. A separate sterile syringe and needle should be used for each individual patient to prevent transmission of hepatitis B virus and other infectious agents from one person to another.

➤*Serological studies:* If serological studies are clinically indicated, the blood sample should preferably be drawn prior to administering the skin test. If the sample is not obtained prior to skin testing, it may be obtained within 48 to 96 hours following the skin test injection. After the aforementioned time period, a rise in titer, as associated with a positive skin test, may occur.

➤*Hypersensitivity reactions:* As with any biological product, epinephrine should be immediately available in case an anaphylactoid or acute hypersensitivity reaction occurs.

➤*Pregnancy: Category C.* Animal reproduction studies have not been conducted with histoplasmin. It is also not known whether histoplasmin can cause fetal harm when administered to a pregnant woman or can affect the reproduction capacity. Histoplasmin should be given to a pregnant woman only if clearly needed.

➤*Lactation:* There is no information regarding histoplasmin in breastfeeding women.

➤*Children:* Safety and effectiveness in pediatric patients have not been established.

Drug Interactions

Histoplasmin Drug Interactions

Precipitant drug	Object drug[a]		Description
Cimetidine	Histoplasmin	↑	Several weeks of cimetidine therapy may augment or enhance delayed-hypersensitivity responses to skin test antigens, although this effect was not consistently observed. The effect may be mediated through cimetidine binding to suppressor T-lymphocytes.
Immunosuppressants Vaccines, virus	Histoplasmin	↓	Reactivity to any delayed-hypersensitivity test may be suppressed in persons receiving corticosteroids or other immunosuppressive drugs, or in persons who were recently immunized with live virus vaccines (eg, measles, mumps, rubella, poliovirus). If delayed-hypersensitivity skin testing is indicated, perform it either preceding or simultaneously with immunization or 4 to 6 weeks after immunization.

[a] ↑ = object drug increased; ↓ = object drug decreased.

Adverse Reactions

➤*Hypersensitivity:* Hypersensitivity reactions such as urticaria, shortness of breath and excessive perspiration may occur.

➤*Local:* In highly sensitive individuals, strongly positive reactions including vesiculation, ulceration or necrosis may occur at the test site and may result in scarring. Cold packs or topical steroid preparations may be employed for symptomatic relief of the associated pain, pruritus and discomfort.

Skin Test Antigens, Multiple

ALLERGEN PATCH TEST

Rx	**T.R.U.E. Test** (GlaxoWellcome)	Allergen-containing patches. In multipack cartons (5s).

ALLERGEN PATCH TEST — INTRADERMAL

For additional information, refer to the Skin Test Antigens, Multiple Introduction.

Indications

➤*Contact dermatitis:* Primarily as an aid in the diagnosis of allergic contact dermatitis in patients whose histories suggest sensitivity to ≥ 1 of the substances included on the test panels. May also be used adjunctively to evaluate other eczemas (atopic, seborrheic, venous, palmar, and plantar hyperkeratotic eczema, vesiculosis, or neurodermatitis) and other dermatologic diseases that do not heal, such as leg ulcers and psoriasis, to determine whether there may be a contact hypersensitivity component.

Administration and Dosage

➤*General dosing considerations:* Minimize exposure to the sun in order to prevent a sun-induced skin reaction that may interfere with interpretation of test results.

➤*Adults:*

Diagnostic aid of allergic contact dermatitis –
Usual dosage: Apply 1 patch to both the upper corners of the back.
Duration of therapy: Minimum of 48 hours.
Concomitant therapy: Discontinue use of topical steroids on the test site or oral steroids (equivalent to 15 mg prednisolone) for 2 weeks or more prior to testing. Topical steroids on nontest areas may be appropriate.

ALLERGEN PATCH TEST — INTRADERMAL

➤*Interpretation of test:* A positive test reaction should meet the criteria for an allergic reaction (papular or vesicular erythema and infiltration). The reaction should be read at 72 to 96 hours, when allergic reactions are fully developed and mild irritant reactions have faded. If reading at 48 hours is considered, another reading at 72 to 96 hours is recommended. Advise patients to report reactions occurring after 7 days to detect potential sensitizations.

False negatives – False-negative results may be caused by insufficient patch contact with the skin, sensitization to a substance not present in the test panel, or premature evaluation of the test.

False positives – A false-positive result may occur when an irritant reaction (patchy follicular or homogeneous erythema without infiltration) cannot be differentiated from an allergic reaction. If an irritant reaction cannot be distinguished, a retest may be considered in a few weeks or months. A test reaction that appears 7 days or later with no preceding reaction may be a sign of contact sensitization.

Dermatitis flare up may occur in some patients. Excited skin syndrome (angry back) consists of a hyperreactive state of the skin in which false-positive patch test reactions concur with dermatitis at a distant body site or with adjacent strong positive skin test reactions. On rare occasions, it may be necessary to remove the test strip from the patient because of severe itching or burning sensations.

Evaluate test results carefully in patients with multiple, positive, concomitant patch test results. To determine false positives, retesting at a later date may be considered.

Neomycin and p-phenylenediamine tests – P-phenylenediamine may turn the patch test area black on some patients. This is because the allergen is a dye and does not represent an allergic reaction. Discoloration may remain for approximately 2 weeks or less.

Neomycin and p-phenylenediamine sometimes cause reactions that may not appear until 4 or 5 days (or later) after the application. Instruct patients to report this. An additional office visit will verify a late reaction.

➤*Preparation for administration:* Apply patches taken directly from the refrigerator or allow them to come to room temperature (15 to 20 minutes) prior to application.

➤*Administration:* The test is best applied on the upper part of the back. Remove protective plastic covering from test panel 1.1. Position the patch on the upper left side of the patient's back (about 5 cm from the midline) so that #1 allergen is in the upper left corner. Apply to healthy skin that is free of acne, scars, dermatitis, or any other condition that may interfere with interpretation of test results. Avoid applying on the margin of the scapula; smooth outward toward the edges. With a medical marking pen, indicate on the skin the location of the 2 notches on the panel. Repeat the process with test panel 2.1 on the upper right side of the patient's back so that #13 allergen is in the upper left corner.

➤*Storage/Stability:* Store between 2° and 8°C (36° and 46°F).

Actions

➤*Pharmacology:* A positive response to the patch test is a classical delayed cell-mediated hypersensitivity reaction (type IV), which normally appears within 9 to 96 hours after exposure.

Following primary contact, an allergen penetrates the skin and binds covalently or noncovalently to epidermal Langerhans cells. The processed allergen is presented to helper T-lymphocytes, resulting in the release of lymphokines, including interleukin 2. Interleukin 2 stimulates the production of other lymphocytes, chemotactic factors that recruit macrophages, basophils, eosinophils, and migration inhibitory factor, all which induce macrophages to remain at the reaction site. The resulting inflammation produces a papular, vesicular, or bullous response with erythema and itching at the site of application.

The allergens in allergen patch test were selected from those substances that have been widely reported to induce allergic contact dermatitis. They represent ≈ 80% of the most common allergens. Nickel sulfate normally induces the greatest number of positive patch test responses when screening prospective patients. The frequency of positive responses to the various allergens can change depending upon the specific patient population as well as occupational and environmental influences. The epidemiology of allergic contact dermatitis and the frequency of positive patch test reactions to various causative allergens have been the subject of several extensive studies.

Contraindications

The minor amount of allergen on each allergen patch test patch that penetrates the skin will rarely induce a flare-up of dermatitis. In the case of extensive ongoing contact dermatitis, however, the test should not be applied since it may provoke an intensified reaction on both the present and previously affected sites and may also cause a false-positive test result.

Warnings/Precautions

➤*Patch testing during the summer months:* Allergen patch test may be applied throughout the year. However, during the summer months, excessive sweating is to be avoided in order to maintain sufficient adhesion to the skin. In addition, exposure to the sun should be minimized in order to prevent a sun-induced skin reaction that may interfere with interpretation of test results.

➤*Patch application:* See Administration and Dosage for more information.

➤*Severe patch test reaction:* If a severe patch test reaction develops, the patient may be treated with a topical corticosteroid or, in rare cases, with a systemic corticosteroid.

➤*Hypersensitivity reactions:* The use of allergen patch test in patients with a known history of severe systemic or local reactions to any of the allergen components or inactive substances included in the allergen patch test panels should be carefully evaluated before application.

Patients should be warned that itching and burning sensations are common occurrences with patch testing and may be severe in extremely sensitive patients. The use of medication may be considered necessary to relieve these itching or burning sensations.

Sensitization to a substance included on the test panel may occur with patch testing but is extremely rare. A test reaction that appears 7 days or later with no preceding reaction may be a sign of contact sensitization.

Dermatitis flare-up may occur in some patients.

Occasionally, hyperpigmentation of the test site occurs during healing. Healing with or without medication normally takes place within 5 days to 2 weeks, although reactions in some individuals may persist longer.

Extremely sensitive patients may exhibit extreme (+++) reactions that may be bullous or ulcerative with pronounced erythema, infiltration, and coalescing vesicles.

Excited skin syndrome (angry back) is a state of hyper-reactivity induced by a dermatitis on other parts of the body or by a strong positive skin-test reaction.

Therefore, test results should be evaluated carefully in patients with multiple, positive, concomitant patch test results. To determine which reactions are false positives, retesting at a later date may be considered.

The safety and efficacy of repetitive testing with allergen patch test is unknown. Sensitization or increased reactivity to one or more of the allergens may occur. The benefits of repeat testing should therefore be carefully evaluated against the possible risks.

On rare occasions, it may be necessary to remove the test strip from the patient because of severe itching or burning sensations. One patient taking part in the clinical studies removed the test tape after 24 hours because of severe itching.

➤*Pregnancy: Category C.* Animal reproduction studies have not been conducted with allergen patch test. It is also not known whether allergen patch test can cause fetal harm when administered to pregnant women or whether it can affect reproduction capacity. Allergen patch test should be applied to pregnant women only if clearly needed.

➤*Lactation:* No studies have been performed to evaluate absorption of allergen patch test allergens in nursing mothers. It is not known if allergen patch test allergens appear in human milk. Because many drugs are excreted in human milk, caution should be exercised when allergen patch test is administered to a nursing woman.

➤*Children:* The safety and effectiveness of allergen patch test in children have not been established.

➤*Elderly:* More frequent patch test responses can be expected in geriatric patients. While no conclusive explanation is available, older patients may exhibit an increased frequency of cutaneous allergies.

Adverse Reactions

➤*Sensitization:* In some cases, allergenic responses may be delayed in onset. One type of delayed reaction is a sensitization, which is not well defined in the literature but is described as a positive reaction observed at 10 to 14 days after application or later and at 2 to 4 days after the test is repeated. The positive reaction should meet the criteria for an allergic reaction (papular or vesicular erythema and infiltration) in order to distinguish between a false-positive result and a sensitization.

➤*Delayed reactions:* In clinical studies conducted with allergen patch test, there have been 3 reports of delayed reactions occurring at 21 days or later. None of these patients were retested to verify a sensitization reaction. There is enough data for only 2 of these patients to indicate probable sensitization. For more details of these reactions, refer to summaries of studies No. 3 and No. 4 in the Clinical Pharmacology section.

➤*Other adverse reactions:* There are reports of other adverse reactions associated with patch testing. These include keloids, sarcoid infiltrates, vitiligo spots, edema, crusting, and sensitization.

➤*Adverse reactions reported during patient follow-up:*

Intradermal Allergen Patch Test Adverse Reactions[a]

Reaction reported	Number of events reported				
	Study 1 (n = 33)[b]	Study 2 (n = 102)[c]	Study 3 (n = 104)[c]	Study 4 (n = 32)[b]	Nickel use (n = 31)[b]
Erythema	2	2	27	2	
Hyperpigmentation	9	2	8	6	8
Pruritus	3	1	27	2	
Scarring			2		
Urticaria					1
Delayed reaction (allergen known)			1[d]		
Delayed reaction (allergen unknown)		2	2		

ALLERGEN PATCH TEST — INTRADERMAL

Intradermal Allergen Patch Test Adverse Reactions[a]

Reaction reported	Number of events reported				
	Study 1 (n = 33)[b]	Study 2 (n = 102)[c]	Study 3 (n = 104)[c]	Study 4 (n = 32)[b]	Nickel use (n = 31)[b]
Sensitization (potential)			1[e]		
Sensitization (probable)			1[f]	1[g]	

[a] Patient follow-up was either via telephone or an office visit; time of follow-up ranged from 4 to 80 days after testing.
[b] Number of patients with positive test results who took part in clinical follow-up.
[c] Number of total patients who took part in the clinical follow-up.
[d] Neomycin sulfate.
[e] Wool alcohols.
[f] p-tert Butylphenol formaldehyde resin.
[g] Cl+Me− isothiazolinone.

➤*Incidences of itching and burning events:* The table below shows itching and burning events from 5 clinical studies. A number of patients in the study groups were prescribed medication to either promote healing or to relieve itching or burning sensations. Itching and burning sensations are commonly associated with patch testing. Treatment may be required and the more severe reactions can be expected to require longer times to heal.

In addition, the adhesive tape may also cause an irritation at the test site. Reports of tape irritation are infrequent, usually mild in nature, and self-limiting in clinical studies conducted with allergen patch test, though no data was collected in these studies beyond a day 21 safety visit. In the nickel use test study and in a Panel 2 clinical study (study no. 2), problems with tape adhesion were observed. Twenty-four percent and 11%, respectively, of the patients in these studies reported poor tape adhesion. (See Clinical Pharmacology section for complete descriptions of these studies.) In both studies, the problem was subsequently attributed to the lot of adhesive tape used to produce the clinical test samples. No adhesion problems have been reported in other studies.

Incidences of Itching and Burning Sensations Reported by Patients at the Time of Intradermal Allergen Patch Test Removal

Adverse reaction	Number of events reported				
	Study 1 (n = 128)[a]	Study 2 (n = 122)[a]	Study 3 (n = 122)[a]	Study 4 (n = 50)[a]	Nickel use (n = 50)[a]
Itching					
Mild	31	23	48	14	30
Moderate				2	
Strong	21	5	17		24
Burning sensations					
Mild	7	4	8	14	4
Moderate				2	
Strong	5	2	1		8
Total events	64	34	74	32	66

[a] Total number of patients in study.

Patient Information

Patients should be instructed to avoid extreme physical activity or mechanical action that may result in reduced adhesion or actual loss of patch test material. Use appropriate measures to avoid getting the area around the patch wet.

Patients should also be advised that a strong allergic response to one or more test allergens can be associated with significant itching, burning, erythema, and vesiculation. Patients who experience intense discomfort should contact their physician concerning possible removal of the test.

TUBERCULIN PURIFIED PROTEIN DERIVATIVE (Mantoux; PPD; Tuberculin skin test [TST])

Rx	**Aplisol** (JHP Pharmaceuticals)	**Injection solution:** 5 TU[a]/0.1 mL	In 1 mL (10 tests) and 5 mL (50 tests) vials.[b]
Rx	**Tubersol** (Sanofi Pasteur)		In 1 mL (10 tests) and 5 mL (50 tests) vials.[c]

[a] TU = tuberculin units.
[b] With potassium and sodium phosphates, 0.35% phenol, and polysorbate 80.
[c] In isotonic phosphate buffer saline with 0.28% phenol and polysorbate 80.

TUBERCULIN PURIFIED PROTEIN DERIVATIVE (MANTOUX) — INJECTION

Indications

➤*Tuberculosis (TB) skin test:* An aid in the detection of infection with *Mycobacterium tuberculosis*.

Purified protein derivative (PPD) tuberculin may be used as an aid in the diagnosis of tuberculosis infection in persons with a history of BCG vaccination. HIV-infected individuals should receive tuberculin skin testing as recommended.

Administration and Dosage

➤*General dosing considerations:* It is essential that the physician or nurse record the test results in millimeters of induration, including 0, in the permanent medical record of each patient. This permanent medical record should contain the name of the product, date given, dose, manufacturer and lot number. Reporting results only as negative or positive is not satisfactory.

An individual who is considered to be at high risk for contacting TB should have an annual PPD skin test.

➤*Adults:*

Tuberculosis skin test –

Initial dosage: 5 TU (0.1 mL) intradermally. Two-step testing should be performed on the initial testing if tuberculin testing will subsequently be conducted at regular intervals, for instance among healthcare workers. If the first test showed either no reaction or a small reaction, the second test should be performed 1 to 4 weeks later. Both tests should be read and recorded at 48 to 72 hours. Patients with a second tuberculin test (booster) response of 10 mm or more should be considered to have experienced past or old infection. Persons who do not boost when given repeat tests at 1 week, but whose tuberculin reactions change to positive after 1 year, should be considered to have newly acquired TB infection and managed accordingly.

Retesting: An individual who does not show a positive reaction to 5 TU on the first test but is suspected of being TB positive may be retested with 5 TU.

➤*Children:*

TB skin test – See Adults for dosing.

➤*Administration:* For intradermal use only. Do not administer intravenously, intramuscularly, or subcutaneously. The preferred site of the test is the flexor (volar) surface of the forearm.The skin site is first cleansed with suitable germicide and should be dry prior to injection of the antigen. The recommended test dose (0.1 mL) is administered with a 1 mL syringe calibrated in tenths and fitted with a short, one-quarter to one-half inch, 26- or 27-gauge needle. The rubber cap of the vial should be wiped with a suitable germicide and should be dry prior to needle insertion. The needle is then inserted gently through the cap, and 0.1 mL of tuberculin is drawn into the syringe. Care should be taken to avoid injection of excess air with removal of each dose so as not to overpressurize the vial, causing possible seepage at the site of the puncture. The point of the needle is inserted into the epidermal (most superficial) layers of the skin with the needle bevel pointing upward. If the intradermal injection is performed properly, a definite pale bleb will rise at the needle point, approximately 10 mm (3/8 inch) in diameter. This bleb will disperse within minutes. No dressing is required. In the event of an improperly performed injection (ie, no bleb formed), the test should be repeated immediately at another site.

Interpretation of test – The test should be read 48 to 72 hours after administration of tuberculin. Sensitivity is indicated by induration only, and any erythema is disregarded. Distinctly palpable induration should be measured in millimeters transversely to the long axis of the forearm and recorded in millimeters. Presence and size of necrosis and edema, if present, should also be recorded, although it should not be used in the interpretation of the test.

Persons who do not boost when given repeat tests at 1 week, but whose tuberculin reactions change to positive after 1 year, should be considered to have newly acquired TB and managed accordingly.

➤*Storage / Stability:* Store between 2° and 8°C (35° and 46°F). Do not freeze. Discard product if exposed to freezing. Tuberculin solutions can be adversely affected by exposure to light. The product should be stored in the dark except when doses are actually being withdrawn from the vial. A vial of tuberculin that has been opened and in use for 1 month should be discarded because oxidation and degradation may have reduced the potency.

Actions

➤*Pharmacology:* Tuberculin PPD is indicated for the detection of a delayed hypersensitivity reaction to tuberculin as an aid in the detection of infection with *Mycobacterium tuberculosis*.

The reaction to intradermally injected tuberculin is a delayed (cellular) hypersensitivity reaction. The reaction which characteristically shows a delayed course, reaching its peak more than 48 to 72 hours after administration, consists of induration caused by cellular infiltration of lyphocytes. Clinically, a delayed hypersensitivity reaction to tuberculin is a manifestation of previous infection with *M. tuberculosis* or a variety of nontuberculosis bacteria. Sensitization may be induced by natural mycobacterial infection or by vaccination with BCG vaccine.

The sensitization following infection with mycobacteria occurs primarily in the regional lymph nodes. Small lymphocytes (T lymphocytes) proliferate in response to the antigenic stimulus to give rise to specifically sensitized lymphocytes. After several weeks, these lymphocytes enter the blood stream and circulate for long periods of time. Subsequent restimulation of these sensitized lymphocytes with the same or a similar antigen, such as the intradermal injection of tuberculin, evokes a local reaction caused by infiltration of these cells.

TUBERCULIN PURIFIED PROTEIN DERIVATIVE (MANTOUX) — INJECTION

The tuberculin reaction is characterized by the early predominance of mononuclear cells (small- and medium-sized lymphocytes and monocytes). Only a small proportion of these cells appear to be lymphocytes sensitized to tuberculin. Most cells are brought into the reaction through the release of biologically active substances by sensitized lymphocytes. An increase in vascular permeability leading to erythema and edema also occurs in tuberculin reactions.

Characteristically, delayed hypersensitivity reactions to tuberculin begin at 5 to 6 hours, are maximal at 48 to 72 hours and subside over a period of days. Immediate hypersensitivity (allergic) reactions to tuberculin or to constituents of the diluent may also occur, but these allergic reactions have no diagnostic importance.

The repeated testing of uninfected persons does not sensitize them to tuberculin.

Contraindications

Allergy to any component of tuberculin purified protein derivative (Mantoux); an allergic reaction to a previous test of tuberculin purified protein derivative (Mantoux).

Tuberculin purified protein derivative (Mantoux) should not be administered to persons who previously experienced a severe reaction (eg, vesiculation, ulceration, necrosis) because of the severity of reactions that may occur at the test site.

Warnings/Precautions

➤*SC injection:* Avoid injecting tuberculin PPD (Mantoux) SC. If this occurs, no local reaction will develop, and the test cannot be interpreted.

➤*False-negative reactions:* Not all infected persons will have a delayed hypersensitivity reaction to a tuberculin test. A large number of factors has been reported to cause a decreased ability to respond to the tuberculin test in the presence of tuberculous infection including viral infections (measles, mumps, chickenpox and HIV), live virus vaccinations (measles, mumps, rubella, oral polio and yellow fever), overwhelming tuberculosis, other bacterial infections, drugs (corticosteroids and many other immunosuppressive agents), and malignancy.

Anything that impairs or attenuates cell-mediated immunity (CMI) potentially can cause a false negative tuberculin reaction (viral infections, particularly HIV, live virus vaccines, severe protein malnutrition, lymphoma, leukemia, sarcoidosis, use of glucocorticosteroids and other immunosuppressant drugs).

➤*HIV infection:* Because in HIV-infected individuals, tuberculin skin-test results are less reliable as CD4 counts decline, screening should be completed as early as possible after HIV infection occurs. Those HIV-infected patients at high risk for continuing exposure to patients who have TB should be screened periodically for TB infection. If they have TB symptoms or if they are exposed to a patient who has pulmonary TB, HIV-infected persons should be evaluated promptly for TB. Because active disease can develop rapidly in HIV-infected persons, the highest priority for contact investigation should be given to persons potentially coinfected with HIV and TB.

➤*Active TB:* Tuberculin PPD (Mantoux) should be administered with caution, or not at all, in persons with documented active tuberculosis or documented treatment in the past because of the severity of reactions (eg, vesiculation, ulceration, necrosis) that may occur at the test site.

➤*Sterile techniques:* A separate, sterile syringe and needle must be used for each individual injection to prevent the possibility of transmission of viral hepatitis or other infectious agents from 1 person to another. There have been case reports of transmission of HIV and hepatitis by failure to scrupulously observe sterile technique. In particular, the same needle must never be used to reenter a multidose vial even when it is to be used on the same patient. This may lead to the contamination of the vial contents and infection of patients who subsequently receive product from the vial. Needles should not be recapped and should be disposed of according to applicable biohazard waste guidelines.

Failure to store and handle tuberculin purified protein derivative (Mantoux) as recommended will result in a loss of potency and potentially inaccurate test results.

➤*Administration:* Special care should be taken to ensure the product is given intradermally and on the volar aspect of the forearm. Do not administer IV, IM or SC.

➤*Patient history:* Before using this product, all appropriate precautions should be taken to prevent adverse reactions. This includes a review of the patient's history with respect to possible hypersensitivity to the product, determination of previous use of tuberculin purified protein derivative (Mantoux) and the presence of any contraindications to the test.

➤*Altered reactivity:* See Drug Interactions for more information.

➤*Positive tuberculin reaction:* Tuberculin reactivity may indicate prior infection or disease with *M. tuberculosis* and does not necessarily indicate the presence of active tuberculous disease. Individuals showing a tuberculin reaction should be further evaluated with other diagnostic procedures, such as x-ray examination of the chest and microbiological examination of the sputum.

➤*Hypersensitivity reactions:* Characteristically, delayed hypersensitivity reactions to tuberculin begin at 5 to 6 hours, are maximal at 48 to 72 hours and subside over a period of days. Immediate hypersensitivity (allergic) reactions to tuberculin or to constituents of the diluent may also occur, but these allergic reactions have no diagnostic importance.

The possibility of allergic reactions in individuals sensitive to the components of the product should be borne in mind. Epinephrine hydrochloride solution (1:1000) should be readily available for use in case an anaphylactic or acute hypersensitivity reaction occurs.

➤*Pregnancy: Category C.* Animal reproduction studies have not been conducted with tuberculin PPD (Mantoux). However, the Advisory Council for Elimination of Tuberculosis states that tuberculin skin testing is considered valid and safe throughout pregnancy. No teratogenic effects of testing during pregnancy have been documented.

The risk of unrecognized tuberculosis and the close postpartum contact between a mother with active disease and an infant leaves the infant in grave danger of tuberculosis and complications such as tuberculous meningitis. Therefore, the prescribing physician will want to consider if the potential benefits outweigh the possible risks for performing the tuberculin test on a pregnant woman or a woman of childbearing age, particularly in certain high-risk populations.

➤*Lactation:* There is no reason to withhold breast-feeding after tuberculosis skin testing or to avoid skin testing in breast-feeding mothers.

➤*Children:* There is no age contraindication to tuberculin skin testing of infants. Because their immune systems are immature, many infants less than 6 weeks of age who are infected with *M. tuberculosis* do not react to tuberculin tests. Older infants and children develop tuberculin sensitivity 6 weeks or more after initial infection. Very young children are at increased risk for active tuberculosis once infected; therefore, during contact investigations, priority with regard to skin testing and evaluation for preventive therapy should be given to infants and young children who have been exposed to persons with active tuberculosis. These children should receive preventive therapy if their reactions to a tuberculin skin test measure greater than or equal to 5 mm. A cutoff of 10 mm is appropriate for children where tuberculosis case rates are high. A cutoff of 15 mm is used for children with minimal risk exposure to tuberculosis.

Drug Interactions

➤*Corticosteroids or immunosuppressants:* Reactivity to the test may be depressed or suppressed for up to 6 weeks in individuals who are receiving corticosteroids or immunosuppressive agents.

➤*Live viral vaccines:* Reactivity to PPD may be temporarily depressed by certain live virus vaccines (measles, mumps, rubella, oral polio, yellow fever, and varicella). Therefore, if a tuberculin test is to be performed, it should be administered either before or simultaneously, at separate sites, with these vaccines in combined form or as separate antigens, or testing should be postponed for 4 to 6 weeks.

Adverse Reactions

➤*Local:*

Very rare – Vesiculation, ulceration or necrosis may appear at the test site in highly sensitive persons. Cold packs or topical steroid preparations may be employed for symptomatic relief of the associated pain, pruritus and discomfort.

Strongly positive reactions may result in scarring at the test site.

Uncommon – Immediate erythematous or other reactions may occur at the injection site. The reason(s) for these occurrences are presently unknown.

➤*Systemic:* There have been rare systemic allergic reactions reported that were manifested by immediate skin rash or generalized rash within 24 hours. Two of the reported cases had concurrent symptoms of upper respiratory stridor. These reactions were treated with epinephrine and steroids and resolved. No cause and effect was able to be established with a specific component of skin test.

Patient Information

The healthcare provider should instruct patients to report to the healthcare provider adverse reactions such as vesiculation, ulceration or necrosis which may appear at the test site in highly sensitive patients. The healthcare provider should also inform the patient that pain, pruritus and discomfort at the site may also occur.

The healthcare provider should inform the patient of the need to return for the reading of the test. Self-reading of the test has been shown to be unreliable.

The healthcare provider should inform the patient of the need to maintain a personal immunization record.

FDA NEW DRUG CLASSIFICATION

The FDA developed an alpha-numeric drug classification to aid in the prioritization of a new drug review. The use of numbers identify the drug's chemical classification; letters identify the assessment of therapeutic potential or review priority. This system was revised in 1992. When the classification for a new drug is known, it is listed in parentheses following the approval date for the drug at the beginning of the Administration and Dosage section of the monograph.

FDA Classification System for Newly Approved Drugs

Chemical Ranking	
1 =	New chemical entity not previously marketed in US
2 =	New salt form of a drug currently on US market
3 =	New dosage formulation of a drug currently on US market
4 =	New combination of drugs already available in US
5 =	New manufacturer (ie, generic drug)
6 =	New indication for drug already approved
7 =	Marketed drug without an approved NDA (drugs marketed prior to 1938)
Therapeutic Potential/Review Priority	
A =	Represents significant therapeutic gain over drugs currently available *(replaced by "P" ranking in 1992)*
AA =	Represents important therapeutic gain for drugs indicated for AIDS
B =	Represents modest therapeutic advances in drug therapy *(replaced by "P" ranking in 1992)*
C =	Represents little or no therapeutic gain in drug class *(replaced by "S" ranking in 1992)*
E =	Drug used to treat life-threatening or severely debilitated patients
P =	Priority; represents a therapeutic gain or provides improved treatment over marketed drugs OR has modest advantages compared to marketed agents (this category was initiated in first quarter of 1992)
S =	Standard; has similar therapeutic properties when compared to marketed drugs (this category was initiated in the first quarter of 1992)

CONTROLLED SUBSTANCES

The Controlled Substances Act of 1970 regulates the manufacturing, distribution and dispensing of drugs that have abuse potential. The Drug Enforcement Administration (DEA) within the US Department of Justice is the chief federal agency responsible for enforcing the act.

➤*DEA Schedules:* Drugs under jurisdiction of the Controlled Substances Act are divided into five schedules based on their potential for abuse and physical and psychological dependence. All controlled substances listed in *Drug Facts and Comparisons®* are identified by schedule as follows:

Schedule I *(c-i):* High abuse potential and no accepted medical use (eg, heroin, marijuana, LSD).

Schedule II *(c-ii):* High abuse potential with severe dependence liability (eg, narcotics, amphetamines, dronabinol, some barbiturates).

Schedule III *(c-iii):* Less abuse potential than schedule II drugs and moderate dependence liability (eg, nonbarbiturate sedatives, nonamphetamine stimulants, limited amounts of certain narcotics).

Schedule IV *(c-iv):* Less abuse potential than schedule III drugs and limited dependence liability (eg, some sedatives, antianxiety agents, nonnarcotic analgesics).

Schedule V *(c-v):* Limited abuse potential. Primarily small amounts of narcotics (codeine) used as antitussives or antidiarrheals. Under federal law, limited quantities of certain *c-v* drugs may be purchased without a prescription directly from a pharmacist if allowed under state statutes. The purchaser must be at least 18 years of age and must furnish suitable identification. All such transactions must be recorded by the dispensing pharmacist.

➤*Registration:* Prescribing physicians and dispensing pharmacies must be registered with the DEA, PO Box 28083, Central Station, Washington, DC 20005.

➤*Inventory:* Separate records must be kept of purchases and dispensing of controlled substances. An inventory of controlled substances must be made every 2 years.

➤*Prescriptions:* Prescriptions for controlled substances must be written in ink and include: Date; name and address of the patient; name, address and DEA number of the physician. Oral prescriptions must be promptly committed to writing. Controlled substance prescriptions may not be dispensed or refilled more than 6 months after the date issued or be refilled more than five times. A written prescription signed by the physician is required for schedule II drugs. In case of emergency, oral prescriptions for schedule II substances may be filled; however, the physician must provide a signed prescription within 72 hours. Schedule II prescriptions cannot be refilled. A triplicate order form is necessary for the transfer of controlled substances in schedule II. Forms are available for the individual prescriber at no charge from the DEA.

➤*State Laws:* In many cases state laws are more restrictive than federal laws and therefore impose additional requirements (eg, triplicate prescription forms).

FDA PREGNANCY CATEGORIES

The rational use of any medication requires a risk versus benefit assessment. Among the myriad of risk factors which complicate this assessment, pregnancy is one of the most perplexing.

The FDA has established five categories to indicate the potential of a systemically absorbed drug for causing birth defects. The key differentiation among the categories rests upon the degree (reliability) of documentation and the risk vs benefit ratio. Pregnancy Category X is particularly notable in that if any data exists that may implicate a drug as a teratogen and the risk vs benefit ratio does not support use of the drug, the drug is contraindicated during pregnancy. These categories are summarized below:

FDA Pregnancy Categories

Pregnancy Category	Definition
A	Controlled studies show no risk. Adequate, well-controlled studies in pregnant women have failed to demonstrate risk to the fetus.
B	No evidence of risk in humans. Either animal findings show risk, but human findings do not; or if no adequate human studies have been done, animal findings are negative.
C	Risk cannot be ruled out. Human studies are lacking, and animal studies are either positive for fetal risk or lacking. However, potential benefits may justify the potential risks.
D	Positive evidence of risk. Investigational or post-marketing data show risk to the fetus. Nevertheless, potential benefits may outweigh the potential risks. If needed in a life-threatening situation or a serious disease, the drug may be acceptable if safer drugs cannot be used or are ineffective.
X	Contraindicated in pregnancy. Studies in animals or human, or investigational or post-marketing reports have shown fetal risk which clearly outweighs any possible benefit to the patient.

Regardless of the designated Pregnancy Category or presumed safety, no drug should be administered during pregnancy unless it is clearly needed and potential benefits outweigh potential hazards to the fetus.

ANTIHYPERTENSIVES

➤*Definition of hypertension:* Hypertension is defined as a systolic blood pressure (SBP) of greater than 140 mm Hg, diastolic blood pressure (DBP) of greater than 90 mm Hg, or the use of an antihypertensive medication. The classification of prehypertension recognizes the relationship between blood pressure (BP) and the risk of cardiovascular disease (CVD) events and calls for increased education of health care professionals and the public in order to reduce BP levels. Patients with SBP of 120 to 139 or a DBP of 80 to 89 should be considered prehypertensive and are at an increased risk for developing hypertension. These patients require health promoting lifestyle modifications to prevent CVD. In individuals 40 to 70 years of age, each elevation of 20 mm Hg in SBP or every 10 mm Hg in DBP doubles the risk of CVD across the entire BP range from 115/75 to 185/115 mm Hg. As a result, identifying and treating high BP decreases cardiovascular mortality and morbidity in these patients and protects against hypertension related complications of stroke, coronary events, heart failure, renal disease progression, progression to more severe hypertension, and all-cause mortality. In order to identify high-risk individuals, the following table presents the classification of adult BP.

Classification of BP for Adults ≥ 18 Years of Age[1]

Category	Systolic (mm Hg)		Diastolic (mm Hg)
Normal	< 120	and	< 80
Prehypertension[2]	120 to 139	or	80 to 89
Hypertension,[3] Stage 1	140 to 159	or	90 to 99
Hypertension,[3] Stage 2	≥ 160	or	≥ 100

[1] Not taking antihypertensive drugs and not acutely ill. When systolic and diastolic BPs fall into 2 different categories, select the higher category to classify the individual's BP status.
[2] Require health promoting lifestyle modifications to prevent CVD.
[3] Based on the average of ≥ 2 readings taken at each of ≥ 2 visits after an initial screening; also requires health promoting lifestyle modifications.

➤*BP measurement:* Measure BP in a standardized fashion using equipment that meets certification criteria.

- Seat patients in a chair with their backs supported and their arms bared and supported at heart level. Tell patients to refrain from smoking or ingesting caffeine during the 30 minutes preceding the measurement.
- Under special circumstances, measuring BP in the supine and standing positions may be indicated.
- Begin measurement after 5 minutes or more of rest.
- Use the appropriate cuff size to ensure accurate measurement. Make sure the bladder within the cuff encircles at least 80% of the arm. Many adults will require a large adult cuff.
- Take measurements preferably with a mercury sphygmomanometer; otherwise, a recently calibrated aneroid manometer or a validated electronic device can be used.
- Record SBP and DBP. The first appearance of sound (phase 1) is used to define SBP. The disappearance of sound (phase 5) is used to define DBP.
- Take the average of 2 or more readings separated by 2 minutes. If the first 2 readings differ by more than 5 mm Hg, obtain an average additional reading.

➤*Risk stratification:*

Major Cardiovascular Disease (CVD) Risk Factors
General
Hypertension
Cigarette smoking
Obesity (body mass index ≥ 30 kg/m²)
Physical inactivity
Dyslipidemia
Diabetes mellitus
Microalbuminuria or estimated GFR < 60 mL/min
Age (> 55 years for men, > 65 years for women)
Family history of premature cardiovascular disease (women 65 years of age or men < 55 years of age)
Target organ damage
Heart disease
Left ventricular hypertrophy
Angina/prior MI
Heart failure
Prior coronary revascularization
Brain
Stroke or transient ischemic attack
Chronic kidney disease
Peripheral arterial disease
Retinopathy

Assess for Identifiable Causes of Hypertension
Sleep apnea
Drug induced/related
Chronic kidney disease
Primary aldosteronism
Renovascular disease
Cushing syndrome or steroid therapy
Pheochromocytoma
Coarctation of aorta
Thyroid/parathyroid disease

➤*Pharmacotherapy:* The use of pharmacologic agents to reduce BP has demonstrated decreases in cardiovascular morbidity and mortality protection against stroke, coronary events, heart failure, renal disease progression, progression to more severe hypertension, and all-cause mortality.

Goals of therapy: The ultimate goal is to reduce cardiovascular complications and renal morbidity and mortality. In patients 50 years of age or older, the primary focus should be on achieving the SBP goal, then the DBP goal will automatically fall into place. SBP and DBP treatment to targets of less than 140/90 mm Hg is associated with a decrease in CVD complications. In hypertensive diabetes or renal disease patients, the BP goal is less than 130/80 mm Hg.

Prevention and management: Reduction of morbidity and mortality may be attained by achieving and maintaining SBP 140 mm Hg or less and DBP 90 mm Hg or less if tolerated and controlling other modifiable risk factors for cardiovascular disease. This may be accomplished by lifestyle modification alone or with pharmacologic therapy.

Lifestyle modifications: Prescribe lifestyle modifications for all patients with prehypertension and hypertension.

- Lifestyle modifications offer the potential for preventing hypertension, lowering BP, and reducing other cardiovascular risk factors at little cost and with minimal risk. Strongly encourage patients to adopt these lifestyle modifications, particularly if they have additional risk factors for premature cardiovascular disease, such as dyslipidemia or diabetes mellitus. Even when lifestyle modifications alone are not adequate in controlling hypertension, they may reduce the number and dosage of antihypertensive medications needed to manage the condition.

Lifestyle Modifications for Hypertension Management[1,2]

Modification	Recommendation	Approximate SBP reduction
Weight loss	Maintain normal body weight index	5 to 20 mm Hg per 10 kg of weight loss
Institute DASH eating plan	Start a diet rich in vegetables, fruit, and low fat dietary products with a decreased content of saturated and total fat	8 to 14 mm Hg
Dietary sodium restriction	Reduce dietary sodium intake to 2.4 g sodium or 6 g sodium chloride	2 to 8 mm Hg
Limit alcohol consumption	Limit alcohol intake to less than 30 mL ethanol (eg, 720 mL beer, 300 mL wine, or 90 mL 80 proof whiskey) per day or 15 mL ethanol in women and lighter weight individuals	2 to 4 mm Hg
Physical activity	Regular aerobic activity at least 30 minutes/day on most days of the week.	4 to 9 mm Hg

[1] For overall cardiovascular risk, discontinue tobacco use.
[2] Effects of these modifications are time and dose dependent and may be enhanced for some individuals.

Considerations for individualizing drug therapy: The table below describes compelling indications that require certain antihypertensive drug classes for high-risk conditions. The drug selections for each compelling indication are based on favorable clinical data.

Compelling Indications for Individual Drug Classes

Compelling indication[1]	Recommended drug therapy[2]
Heart failure	Thiazide, BB, ACEI, ARB, ALDO ant
Post-MI	BB, ACEI, ALDO ant
High CVD risk	Thiazide, BB, ACEI, CCB
Diabetes	Thiazide, BB, ACEI, ARB, CCB
Chronic kidney disease	ACEI, ARB
Recurrent stroke prevention	Thiazide, ACEI

[1] Compelling indications for antihypertensive drugs are based on benefits from clinical study outcomes; the compelling indication is managed in parallel with the BP.
[2] BB = beta blocker; ACEI = angiotensin converting enzyme inhibitor; ARB = angiotensin receptor blocker; CCB = calcium channel blocker; ALDO ant = aldosterone antagonist.

ANTIHYPERTENSIVES

Initial drug therapy: When a decision has been made to begin antihypertensive therapy and there are no compelling indications for another type of drug, choose a thiazide-type diuretic, either alone or in combination with 1 of the other classes (eg, ACEI, ARB, BB, CCB). Numerous randomized controlled trials have shown a reduction in morbidity and mortality with these agents. The majority of patients who are hypertensive will require treatment with 2 or more antihypertensive medications in order to achieve their BP goals of less than 140/90 mm Hg or less than 130/80 mm Hg for patients with diabetes or chronic kidney disease. When BP is more than 20/10 mm Hg above goal BP, consider initiating therapy with 2 drugs, 1 of which is usually a thiazide-type diuretic, either as separate drugs or in fixed-dose combinations. Use caution and observe those patients at risk for orthostatic hypotension, such as diabetic patients and the elderly.

Follow-up recommendations: Once antihypertensive therapy is initiated, follow-ups at monthly intervals are necessary until BP goal is reached. Patients with stage 2 hypertension or with complicating comorbid conditions will require more frequent visits. Once BP is controlled and at goal, follow-up visits should take place at 3- to 6-month intervals. Comorbidities, such as heart failure and diabetes will also dictate the frequency of office visits and laboratory tests. Monitor serum potassium and creatinine levels at least once or twice per year. Consider low-dose aspirin therapy only once BP is controlled.

➤*Special patient populations:*

Race: Most black people are at greater risk for the development of high BP, type 2 diabetes, coronary heart disease, left ventricular hypertension, stroke, and end-stage renal disease; they will usually require combination antihypertensive therapy. As monotherapy, BBs, ARBs, and ACEIs may produce less BP lowering effects than thiazide diuretics and CCBs. Consider the following antihypertensive combinations: BB/diuretic, ACEI/diuretic, ACEI/CCB, or ARB/diuretic. For patients with uncomplicated hypertension, the target BP is less than 140/90 mm Hg, and for patients with high risk for cardiovascular events in association with type 2 diabetes or renal insufficiency, the target BP goal is less than 130/80 mm Hg. When prescribing ACEIs for black patients, it is important to note that there appears to be an increased risk for ACEI-associated angioedema and/or cough.

Resistant hypertension: Failure to reach BP goal in patients who followed proper treatment is known as resistant hypertension. Consider a consultation with a BP specialist if target BP cannot be achieved. See table for causes of resistant hypertension.

Causes of Resistant Hypertension
Improper BP measurement
Volume overload and pseudotolerance
Excess sodium intake
Volume retention from kidney disease
Inadequate diuretic therapy
Drug-induced or other causes
Nonadherence
Inadequate doses
Inappropriate combinations
Nonsteroidal anti-inflammatory drugs; cyclooxygenase 2 inhibitors
Cocaine, amphetamines, other illicit drugs
Sympathomimetics (decongestants, anoretics)
Oral contraceptives
Adrenal steroids
Cyclosporine and tacrolimus
Erythropoietin
Licorice (including some chewing tobacco)
Selected over the counter dietary supplements and medicines (eg, ephedra, ma haung, bitter orange)
Associated conditions
Obesity
Excess alcohol intake
Identifiable causes of hypertension

Hypertensive emergencies: Patients with marked BP elevations that also have acute target-organ damage (eg, encephalopathy, MI, unstable angina, pulmonary edema, eclampsia, stroke, head trauma, life-threatening arterial bleed, aortic dissection) require parenteral drug therapy and hospitalization. Patients with BP elevation without target-organ damage do not require hospitalization, but should receive immediate oral antihypertensive therapy while being carefully evaluated and monitored for precipitating causes or hypertension-induced heart or kidney disease.

Considerations for Individualizing Antihypertensive Drug Therapy[1]	
Indication	Drug therapy
May have favorable effects on comorbid conditions[2]	
Angina	Beta blockers, CCB
Atrial tachycardia and fibrillation	Beta blockers, CCB (non-DHP)
Cyclosporine-induced hypertension (caution with the dose of cyclosporine)	CCB
Diabetes mellitus (types 1 and 2) with proteinuria	ACE 1 (preferred), CCB
Diabetes mellitus (type 2)	Low-dose diuretics
Dyslipidemia	Alpha blockers
Essential tremor	Beta blockers (non-CS)
Heart failure	Carvedilol, losartan potassium
Hyperthyroidism	Beta blockers
Migraine	Beta blockers (non-CS), CCB (non-DHP)
MI	Diltiazem HCl, verapamil HCl
Osteoporosis	Thiazides
Preoperative hypertension	Beta blockers
Prostatism (BPH)	Alpha blockers
Renal insufficiency (caution in renovascular hypertension and creatinine ≥ 265.2 mmol/L [3 mg/dL])	ACEI
May have unfavorable effects on comorbid conditions[2,3]	
Bronchospastic disease	Beta blockers[4]
Depression	Beta blockers, central alpha agonists, reserpine[4]
Diabetes mellitus (types 1 and 2)	Beta blockers, high-dose diuretics
Dyslipidemia	Beta blockers (non-ISA), diuretics (high-dose)
Gout	Diuretics
2° or 3° heart block	Beta blockers,[4] CCB (non-DHP)[4]
Heart failure	Beta blockers (except carvedilol), CCB (except amlodipine besylate, felodipine)
Liver disease	Labetalol HCl, methyldopa[4]
Peripheral vascular disease	Beta blockers
Pregnancy	ACEI,[4] angiotensin II receptor blockers[4]
Renal insufficiency	Potassium-sparing agents
Renovascular disease	ACEI, angiotensin II receptor blockers

[1] ACEI= angiotensin-converting enzyme inhibitors; BPH = benign prostatic hyperplasia; CCB = calcium channel blocker; DHP = dihydropyridine; ISA = intrinsic sympathomimetic activity; MI = myocardial infarction; non-CS = noncardioselective.
[2] Conditions and drugs are listed in alphabetical order.
[3] These drugs may be used with special monitoring unless contraindicated.
[4] Contraindicated.

ALGORITHM FOR TREATMENT OF HYPERTENSION*

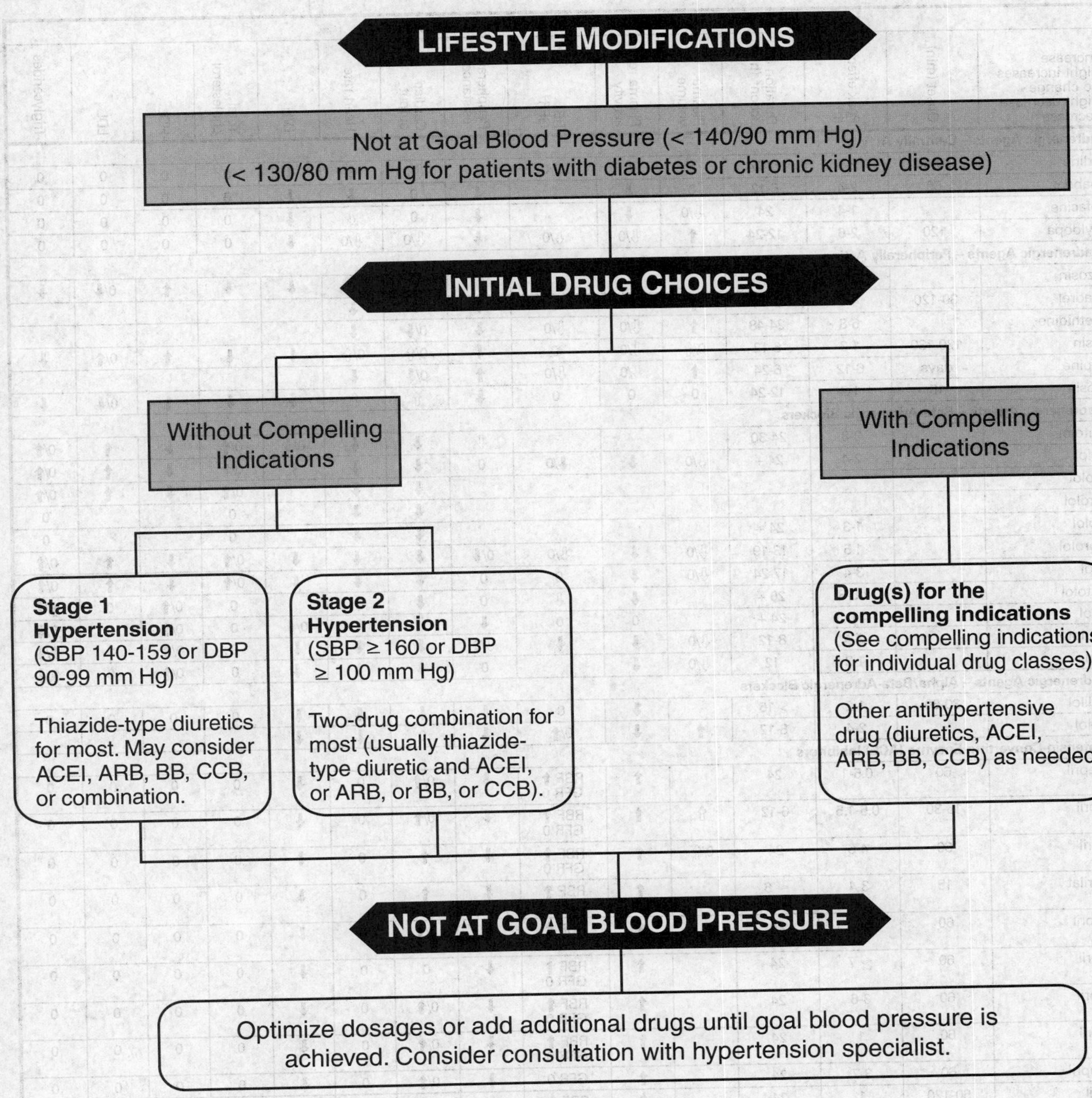
LIFESTYLE MODIFICATIONS
Not at Goal Blood Pressure (< 140/90 mm Hg)
(< 130/80 mm Hg for patients with diabetes or chronic kidney disease)
INITIAL DRUG CHOICES
Without Compelling Indications
With Compelling Indications
Stage 1 Hypertension
(SBP 140-159 or DBP 90-99 mm Hg)
Thiazide-type diuretics for most. May consider ACEI, ARB, BB, CCB, or combination.
Stage 2 Hypertension
(SBP ≥ 160 or DBP ≥ 100 mm Hg)
Two-drug combination for most (usually thiazide-type diuretic and ACEI, or ARB, or BB, or CCB).
Drug(s) for the compelling indications
(See compelling indications for individual drug classes)
Other antihypertensive drug (diuretics, ACEI, ARB, BB, CCB) as needed.
NOT AT GOAL BLOOD PRESSURE
Optimize dosages or add additional drugs until goal blood pressure is achieved. Consider consultation with hypertension specialist.

DBP, diastolic blood pressure; SBP, systolic blood pressure.
Drug abbreviations: ACEI, angiotensin converting enzyme inhibitor; ARB, angiotensin receptor blocker; BB, beta blocker; CCB, calcium channel blocker.

* *The Seventh Report of the Joint National Committee on Prevention, Detection, Evaluation, and Treatment of High Blood Pressure.* National Institutes of Health. May 2003.

ANTIHYPERTENSIVES

Agents used in hypertension therapy are listed in the following tables:

Pharmacological Effects of Antihypertensive Agents

↑ = increase ⇧ = slight increases 0 = no change ⇩ = slight decrease ↓ = decrease	Onset (min)	Peak effect[1] (h)	Duration of action[2] (h)	Plasma volume	Plasma renin activity	RBF GFR[3]	Peripheral resistance	Cardiac output	Heart rate	LVH	Total cholesterol	HDL	LDL	Triglycerides
Antiadrenergic Agents – Centrally Acting														
Clonidine	30-60	2-5	12-24	↑	⇩	⇩/0	↓	⇩/0	↓	↓	0	0	0	0
Guanabenz	60	2-4	6-12	0	↓	0	↓	0	↓	↓	0	0	0	0
Guanfacine		1-4	24	⇩/0	↓		↓	0	⇩	↓	0	0	0	0
Methyldopa	120	2-6	12-24	↑	⇩/0	⇩/0	↓	⇩/0	⇩/0	↓	0	0	0	0
Antiadrenergic Agents – Peripherally Acting														
Doxazosin		2-3								↓	↓	↑	0/↓	↓
Guanadrel	30-120	4-6	9-14	↑		0	↓	0	↓					
Guanethidine		6-8	24-48	↑	⇩/0	⇩/0	↓	0/↓	↓					
Prazosin	120-130	1-3	6-12	0/⇧	⇩/0	0	↓	0/⇧	0/⇧	↓	↓	↑	0/↑	↓
Reserpine	days	6-12	6-24	↑	⇩/0	⇩/0	↑	0/↓	↓					
Terazosin	15	1-2	12-24	0	0	0	↓	⇧	⇧	↓	↓	↑	0/↓	↓
Antiadrenergic Agents – Beta-Adrenergic Blockers														
Acebutolol		3-8	24-30				⇩	↓	↓	0/↓	0/↑	↓	↑	0/↑
Atenolol		2-4	24 +	⇩/0	↓	↓/0	0	↓	↓	↓	0/↑	↓	↑	0/↑
Betaxolol								↓	↓		0/↑	↓	↑	0/↑
Bisoprolol								↓	↓		0			0
Carteolol		1-3	24 +					↓	↓		0			0
Metoprolol		1.5	13-19	⇩/0	↓	⇩/0	0/↓	↓	↓	↓	0/↑	↓	↑	0/↑
Nadolol		3-4	17-24	⇩/0	↓	0	0	↓	↓	↓	0/↑	↓	↑	0/↑
Penbutolol		1.5-3	20 +		↓	⇩	0	↓	↓		0	0/↑	0	↑/↓
Pindolol		1	24 +		0	0	↓	⇩	⇩	0/↓	0	0/↑	0	↑/↓
Propranolol		2-4	8-12	⇩/0	↓	↓	⇩/0	↓	↓	↓	0	0/↑	0	↑/↓
Timolol		1-3	12	⇩/0	↓		0	↓	↓	↓	0	0/↑	0	↑/↓
Antiadrenergic Agents – Alpha/Beta-Adrenergic Blockers														
Carvedilol	30-60	1-2	> 15		↓	0	↓	↓	↓	↓	0	0	0	0
Labetalol		2-4	8-12	↑	↓	0/↑	↓	0	↓	↓				
Angiotensin-Converting Enzyme (ACE) Inhibitors														
Benazepril	60	0.5-1	24		↑	RBF ↑ GFR 0	↓	0/↑	0	↓	0	0	0	0
Captopril	15-30	0.5-1.5	6-12	⇧	↑	RBF ↑ GFR 0	↓	0/↑	0	↓	0	0	0	0
Enalapril	60	4-6	24	0/⇧	↑	RBF ↑ GFR 0	↓	↑	0	↓	0	0	0	0
Enalaprilat	15	3-4	≈ 6		↑	RBF ↑ GFR 0	↓	↑	0	↓	0	0	0	0
Fosinopril	60	≈ 3	24		↑	RBF ↑ GFR 0	↓	0/↑	0	↓	0	0	0	0
Lisinopril	60	≈ 7	24		↑	RBF ↑ GFR 0	↓	0	0	↓	0	0	0	0
Moexipril	60	3-6	24		↑	RBF ↑ GFR 0	↓	0/↑	0	↓	0	0	0	0
Quinapril	60	1	24		↑	RBF ↑ GFR 0	↓	0/↑	0	↓	0	0	0	0
Perindopril	60	3-7	24		↑	GFR 0	↓	0/↑	0	↓	0	0	0	0
Ramipril	60-120	1	24		↑	RBF ↑ GFR 0	↓	0/↑	0	↓	0	0	0	0
Trandolapril	120-240	6-8	24		↑	RBF ↑ GFR 0	↓	0/↑	0	↓	0	0	0	0
Angiotensin II Receptor Antagonists														
Candesartan	120-180	6-8	> 24	↓	↑	RBF ⇧ GFR 0	↓	↑	0	↓	0	0	0	0
Eprosartan	60-120	1-3	24	↓	↑	RBF ⇧ GFR 0	↓	↑	0	↓	0	0	0	0
Irbesartan	90-120	3-6	24	↓	↑	RBF ⇧[4] GFR 0	↓	↑	0	↓	0	0	0	0
Losartan	120-180	6	24	↓	↑	RBF ⇧[4] GFR 0	↓	↑	0	↓	0	0	0	0
Telmisartan	180	3-9	24	↓	↑	RBF ⇧[4] GFR 0	↓	↑	0	↓	0	0	0	0
Valsartan	120	6	24	↓	↑	RBF ⇧[4] GFR 0	↓	↑	0	↓	0	0	0	0
Olmesartan		1-2	24	↓	↑	RBF ⇧[4] GFR 0	↓	↑	0	↓	0	0	0	0

ANTIHYPERTENSIVES

Pharmacological Effects of Antihypertensive Agents

↑ = increase; ⇧ = slight increases; 0 = no change; ⇩ = slight decrease; ↓ = decrease

↑ = increase ⇧ = slight increases 0 = no change ⇩ = slight decrease ↓ = decrease	Onset (min)	Peak effect (h)	Duration of action[2] (h)	Plasma volume	Plasma renin activity	RBF GFR[3]	Peripheral resistance	Cardiac output	Heart rate	LVH	Total cholesterol	HDL	LDL	Triglycerides
Calcium Channel Blocking Agents														
Amlodipine	gradual	6-12	> 24	0	0	↑	↓↓↓	0		↓	0	0	0	0
Diltiazem SR	30-60	6-11				0	↓	0-↑	↓-0	↓	0	0	0	0
Felodipine	120-300	2.5-5				0	↓↓↓	↑	↑	↓	0	0	0	0
Isradipine	120	1.5					↓↓↓	↑	↑/↓	↓	0	0	0	0
Nicardipine	20	0.5-2			⇧/↑	↑	↓	↑	↑	↓	0	0/⇧	0	0
Nifedipine SR	20	6				RBF↑ GFR ↑	↓↓↓	↑↑	↑	↓	0	0	0	0
Nisoldipine		1.5[5]			0		↓	⇧	⇧	↓	0	0	0	0
Verapamil	30	1-2.2			0/⇧	RBF↑ GFR ⇧	↓	↑/↓	↑/↓	↓	0	0/⇧	0	0
Diuretics														
Amiloride	120	6-10	24	↓	↑	0	↓	↓	0					
Loop diuretics	within 60	1-2	4-8	↓	↑	↑	↓	↓	0	0/↓	↑	0	↑	↑
Spironolactone	24-48 hr	48-72	48-72	↓	↑	0	↓	0	0					
Thiazides and derivatives	60-120	4-12	6-72	↓	↑	↓	↓	↓	0	0/↓	↑	0	↑	↑
Triamterene	2-4 hr	6-8	12-16											
Vasodilators														
Hydralazine	45	0.5-2	6-8	↑	↑	↑	↓	↑	↑	↑				
Minoxidil	30	2-3	24-72	↑	↑	0	↓	↑	↑					
Agents For Pheochromocytoma														
Phentolamine	immed.		5-10 min	⇧	↑	↑	↓	0/↑	↑					
Phenoxy-benzamine	gradual	2-3	24 +	⇧	↑	↑	↓	↑	↓					
Metyrosine		6 +	2-3 days				↓		↓					
Agents For Hypertensive Emergencies/Urgencies														
Captopril[6]				⇧	↑	RBF ↑ GFR 0	↓	0/↑	0					
Clonidine	< 5			↑	⇩	⇩/0	↓	⇩/0	↓	↓				
Diazoxide	1-2	5 min	< 12	↑	↑	↑	↓	↑	↑					
Enalaprilat[6]					↑	RBF ↑ GFR 0	↓	↑	0					
Esmolol	1-2	5	10-20		0	0		↓	⇩					
Fenoldopam	5		30-60		↑	RBF⇧ GFR 0	⇩		⇧			NA		
Hydralazine	10-20		3-6											
Labetalol	5-10		3-6	↑	↓	0/↑	↓	0	↓					
Nicardipine (IV)	1-5		3-6		⇧/↑	⇧	↓	↑	↑					
Nitroglycerin (IV)[6]	immed.		tran-sient	0	0		↓	↑	↑					
Nitroprusside	0.5-1		3-5 min	↑	↑	0	↓	⇩	⇧					
Phentolamine[6]	1-2		3-10 min											
Miscellaneous Agents														
Tolazoline[6]							↓							
Eplerenone		1.5	> 24	↓	↑		↓		0	⇩	⇧			↑

[1] Peak clinical effect following a single oral dose, except where indicated.
[2] Duration of action is frequently dose-dependent.
[3] Renal blood flow and glomerular filtration rate.
[4] Experimental and small clinical studies indicate that angiotensin II receptor antagonists have effects on renal function similar to ACEIs.
[5] Immediate release; 6 to 12 hours for extended release.
[6] Unlabeled use.

H. PYLORI AGENTS

Helicobacter pylori is found in ≈ 100% of chronic active antral gastritis cases, 90% to 95% of duodenal ulcer patients, and 50% to 80% of gastric ulcer patients. The treatment of documented *H. pylori* infection in patients with confirmed peptic ulcer on first presentation or recurrence has been recommended by the National Institutes of Health in a 1994 Consensus Conference. Once *H. pylori* eradication has been achieved, reinfection rates are < 0.5% per year, and ulcer recurrence rates are dramatically reduced.

Numerous clinical trials have been done to determine the optimal regimen for *H. pylori* eradication, with cure rates ranging from ≈ 70% to 90%. There remains no gold standard of therapy to date. Base selection of the most appropriate therapy on consideration of treatment efficacy, cost, safety, drug-interaction potential, antibiotic resistance, tolerability, and convenience of administration. The FDA has approved 5 combination regimens for the treatment of *H. pylori* infection in patients with active duodenal ulcer. Studies have found that regimens consisting of a proton pump inhibitor (ie, lansoprazole or omeprazole) in conjunction with 2 antibiotics administered for 14 days are associated with cure rates that exceed 90%; this is in contrast to cure rates of 70% to 80% found with other regimens (eg, dual therapy, bismuth-based triple therapies).

Several studies have concluded that cure of *H. pylori* significantly reduces the risk of recurrent ulcer disease, obviating the need for continued maintenance therapy in patients with a history of uncomplicated disease. Make the decision to continue maintenance antisecretory therapy in patients with a history of complicated ulcer disease following successful *H. pylori* treatment on an individual basis.

The following is a brief description of the individual agents used in *H. pylori* eradication regimens and their role in eradication. Consult the individual drug monographs for complete prescribing information.

➤*Amoxicillin:* Amoxicillin works by inhibiting the synthesis of bacterial cell walls. It demonstrates topical activity and is stable in an acid environment but is most active at a neutral pH. *H. pylori* is very sensitive to amoxicillin in vitro and in vivo. Bacterial resistance to amoxicillin has not been reported. More common adverse effects include diarrhea, along with other GI effects, and hypersensitivity or allergic reactions. Take without regard to meals.

➤*Tetracycline:* This agent works by inhibiting bacterial protein synthesis. It acts topically and is active at a low pH. *H. pylori* is very sensitive to tetracycline. Bacterial resistance to tetracycline has not been reported. Adverse effects include diarrhea, along with other GI effects, esophageal ulcers, and photosensitivity reactions. Take on an empty stomach with plenty of water. Do not give simultaneously with dairy products (eg, milk, cheese), antacids, laxatives, or iron-containing products. If these agents are used, take them at least 2 hours before or after tetracycline.

➤*Metronidazole:* The exact mechanism of this agent is not well understood. It demonstrates selective toxicity to anaerobic or microaerophilic microorganisms and for anoxic or hypoxic cells. The drug diffuses into the cells and leads to the development of compounds that bind to DNA and inhibit synthesis, causing cell death. The activity of metronidazole is relatively independent of pH. Primary metronidazole resistance has been observed in 20% to 73% of *H. pylori* strains isolated and has been shown to significantly decrease *H. pylori* cure rates following treatment with a metronidazole-containing regimen. Adverse effects of metronidazole include metallic taste, nausea, peripheral neuropathy, and a disulfiram-type reaction manifested by flushing, nausea, tachycardia, vomiting, and other GI symptoms when used with alcohol. Metronidazole can be taken with food to minimize GI upset.

➤*Clarithromycin:* Clarithromycin is a macrolide antibiotic that inhibits bacterial protein synthesis. It is more acid-stable than erythromycin, better absorbed, and more effective against *H. pylori*. Resistance can develop when clarithromycin is used alone. It is generally < 8%. Adverse effects include abnormal taste, diarrhea, and nausea. Clarithromycin may be taken without regard to meals.

➤*Bismuth:* Bismuth compounds are topical compounds that disrupt the integrity of bacterial cell walls. The mechanism and role of bismuth in *H. pylori* eradication is multifactorial. Bismuth compounds are thought to lyse *H. pylori* near the gastric surface; prevent the adhesion of *H. pylori* to the gastric epithelium; inhibit its urease, phospholipase, and proteolytic activity; and decrease resistance development when used with antimicrobial agents such as metronidazole. Adverse effects of bismuth compounds may include a temporary and harmless darkening of the tongue and stool, diarrhea, and the potential for CNS toxicities when used in high doses. Take bismuth compounds without regard to meals.

➤*Antisecretory agents (H_2 antagonists, proton pump inhibitors):* Provide rapid symptom relief and accelerated ulcer healing when used with antimicrobial agents for *H. pylori* eradication. Proton pump inhibitors may have a direct effect on inhibiting the growth of *H. pylori* and also appear to have a synergistic effect when combined with antimicrobial agents.

➤*Eradication of H. pylori:*

Single antimicrobial agents: Monotherapy is not recommended because of the potential for the development of antimicrobial resistance.

Dual therapy:

• *Proton pump inhibitors plus amoxicillin* – Significant variation exists among numerous studies that have been conducted to date with eradication rates ranging from 30% to 80%. Therefore, dual therapy with these 2 agents is not recommended.

• *Proton pump inhibitors plus clarithromycin* – A number of studies have looked at the use of these agents in combination for *H. pylori* eradication, and the overall eradication appears to be ≈ 71%. Currently, the American College of Gastroenterology recommends adding a second antimicrobial agent to this regimen to enhance successful eradication.

Double antimicrobial therapy plus an antisecretory drug:

Regimens Used in the Eradication of *H. pylori*

Regimen	Dosing	Duration
Metronidazole + Clarithromycin + Omeprazole OR Lansoprazole	500 mg twice daily with meals 500 mg twice daily with meals 20 mg twice daily with meals 30 mg twice daily with meals	2 weeks
Amoxicillin + Clarithromycin + Omeprazole OR Lansoprazole	1 g twice daily with meals 500 mg twice daily with meals 20 mg twice daily before meals 30 mg twice daily with meals	2 weeks
Metronidazole + Omeprazole + Amoxicillin	500 mg twice daily with meals 20 mg twice daily before meals 1 g twice daily with meals	2 weeks

Triple-therapy regimens: These regimens have proved to be very effective in eradicating *H. pylori*. The primary disadvantage of these regimens is compliance because of the variety and number of medications used. Likewise, adverse effects are more common in patients taking these regimens compared with alternatives.

Regimens Used in the Eradication of *H. Pylori*

Regimen	Dosing	Duration
Bismuth subsalicylate + Metronidazole + Tetracycline + H_2-receptor antagonist	525 mg 4 times/day with meals and at bedtime 250 mg 4 times/day with meals and at bedtime 500 mg 4 times/day As directed[1]	2 weeks 1 week 2 weeks 2 weeks + additional 2 weeks
Bismuth subsalicylate + Metronidazole + Tetracycline + Omeprazole OR Lansoprazole	525 mg 4 times/day with meals and at bedtime 500 mg 3 times/day with meals and at bedtime 500 mg 4 times/day 20 mg/day before meals 30 mg/day	2 weeks 2 weeks 2 weeks 2 weeks 2 weeks
Ranitidine bismuth citrate + Clarithromycin + Amoxicillin OR Metronidazole OR Tetracycline	400 mg 2 times/day with meals and at bedtime 500 mg 2 times/day 1 g 2 times/day with meals and at bedtime 500 mg 2 times/day with meals and at bedtime 500 mg 2 times/day	2 weeks 2 weeks 2 weeks 2 weeks 2 weeks

[1] See individual monographs for dosing instructions.

Quadruple therapy regimens (2 antibiotics, bismuth, antisecretory agent): Like triple therapy regimens, these have proven to be effective in *H. pylori* eradication. The primary disadvantage of these regimens is compliance. In addition, because of the variety and number of medications used, adverse effects are more common in patients taking these regimens compared with alternatives.

H. PYLORI AGENTS

FDA-Approved Therapies for *H. pylori* Infection

Regimen	Dosing
Lansoprazole + Clarithromycin + Amoxicillin	30 mg 2 times daily for 10 to 14 days[1] 500 mg 2 times daily for 10 to 14 days[1] 1 g 2 times daily for 10 to 14 days[1]
Omeprazole + Clarithromycin + Amoxicillin	20 mg 2 times daily for 10 days 500 mg 2 times daily for 10 days 1 g 2 times daily for 10 days
Omeprazole + Clarithromycin Omeprazole	40 mg once daily for 2 weeks 500 mg 3 times daily for 2 weeks Follow by 20 mg once daily for additional 2 weeks
Ranitidine bismuth citrate + Clarithromycin Ranitidine bismuth citrate	400 mg 2 daily for 2 weeks 500 mg 3 times daily for 2 weeks Follow by 400 mg 2 times daily for additional 2 weeks
Bismuth subsalicylate + Metronidazole + Tetracycline + Histamine-2 (H_2)-receptor antagonist	525 mg 4 times daily for 2 weeks 250 mg 4 times daily for 2 weeks 500 mg 4 times daily for 2 weeks Dose as directed[2] for 2 weeks + additional 2 weeks
Lansoprazole + Amoxicillin	30 mg 3 times daily for 2 weeks 1 g 3 times daily for 2 weeks

[1] Therapy associated with ≥ 90% *H. pylori* eradication rate.
[2] See individual monographs for dosing instructions.

➤*Practice Guidelines from the American College of Gastroenterology:* In the 1996 Consensus Statement on Medical Treatment of Peptic Ulcer Disease, the American College of Gastroenterology does not recommend single-antibiotic combinations of either clarithromycin or amoxicillin with proton pump inhibitors because efficacy is < 70% (cure), and a high-dose, 2–week treatment period is required. The Consensus Statement recommends a two-antibiotic combination of clarithromycin, metronidazole or amoxicillin in regimens that do not employ a bismuth compound. In addition, the American College of Gastroenterology suggests adding either tetracycline or amoxicillin to the recently approved ranitidine-bismuth citrate-clarithromycin combination to enhance successful *H. pylori* eradication. Combining a proton pump inhibitor, either omeprazole or lansoprazole, with two antibiotics is thought to enhance effectiveness and allow for a shorter duration of treatment.

There are a number of factors that limit the effectiveness of regimens designed to eradicate *H. pylori*. The first, antibiotic resistance, is seen with metronidazole and clarithromycin but has not been reported with bismuth, amoxicillin or tetracycline. Because prior antibiotic exposure predicts drug resistance in individuals, take this factor into consideration when selecting a regimen. Although data are limited, studies have demonstrated that eradication of *H. pylori* is possible with metronidazole-containing regimens despite the presence of resistant organisms, but eradication rates are significantly lower. Alternatively, the American College of Gastroenterology suggests possible drug regimens to employ in cases of metronidazole resistance. These include bismuth, clarithromycin, and tetracycline or omeprazole, amoxicillin, and clarithromycin. On the other hand, clarithromycin resistance is more bothersome because resistant organisms do not respond favorably to clarithromycin-containing regimens.

Second, mild adverse effects (eg, diarrhea, metallic taste, black stools) do occur in ≈ 30% to 50% of patients. Therefore, shorter treatment periods in this group of patients may be better tolerated.

Finally, patient compliance is often a problem because of cumbersome regimens and adverse effects.

➤*Maintenance therapy with antisecretory agents:* Several studies have concluded that cure of *H. pylori* significantly reduces the risk of recurrent ulcer disease, obviating the need for continued maintenance therapy in patients with a history of uncomplicated disease. The decision to continue maintenance antisecretory therapy in patients with a history of complicated ulcer disease following successful *H. pylori* treatment should be made on an individual basis. Factors to be considered that may favor the continuation of antisecretory therapy include: The presence of comorbid illness or the use of medications (eg, NSAIDs, anticoagulant therapy) that may increase risk of recurrence or complications, and severity of the previous ulcer-related complications.

➤*Confirming successful eradication:* Confirming successful eradication is important in patients with a history of complicated or refractory ulcers but is controversial in those with uncomplicated ulcers who remain asymptomatic after therapy.

➤*Refractory ulcers in patients receiving antibiotic therapy for H. pylori eradication:* Refractory ulcers in patients receiving antibiotic therapy for *H. pylori* eradication is often due to failure to successfully eradicate *H. pylori* infection. Resistance patterns, as well as noncompliance, and concurrent NSAID use may play a role in refractory cases.

RABIES PROPHYLAXIS PRODUCTS

Although rabies rarely affects humans in the United States, every year approximately 16,000 to 39,000 people receive postexposure prophylaxis. Appropriate management depends on the interpretation of the risk of infection and the efficacy and risk of prophylactic treatment. There are 2 types of immunizing products: vaccines and globulins. Use both types of products concurrently for rabies postexposure prophylaxis.

➤*Vaccines:* Vaccines induce an active immune response that requires about 7 to 10 days to develop and usually persists for at least 2 years.

➤*Human Diploid Cell Rabies Vaccine (HDCV):* HDCV is an inactivated virus vaccine prepared from fixed rabies virus grown in human diploid cell culture.

➤*Purified Chick Embryo Cell Vaccine (PCEC):* PCEC is an inactivated virus vaccine prepared from the fixed rabies virus strain Flury LEP grown in primary cultures of chicken fibroblasts.

➤*Globulins:* Globulins provide rapid passive immune protection that persists for a short time (half-life of approximately 21 days).

➤*Rabies Immune Globulin (RIG), Human:* RIG antirabies gamma globulin is concentrated from plasma of hyperimmunized human donors.

➤*Rationale of treatment:* Individually evaluate each possible rabies exposure. Consult local or state public health officials if questions arise about the need for prophylaxis. Consider the following factors before specific treatment is initiated:

Species of biting animal: Carnivorous animals (especially skunks, foxes, coyotes, raccoons, dogs, and cats) and bats are more likely to be infective than other animals. Unless the animal is tested and shown to not be rabid, initiate postexposure prophylaxis upon bite or nonbite exposure to these animals. If treatment has been initiated and subsequent testing shows the exposing animal is not rabid, treatment can be discontinued.

Because the likelihood that a domestic dog or cat is infected with rabies varies from region to region, the need for postexposure prophylaxis also varies. Bites of rabbits, hares, squirrels, chipmunks, rats, mice, hamsters, guinea pigs, gerbils, and other rodents are rarely infected with rabies and have not been known to cause human rabies in the United States. In these cases, consult state or local health departments before deciding whether to initiate postexposure antirabies prophylaxis.

Circumstances of biting incident: An unprovoked attack is more likely to mean that the animal is rabid. Bites inflicted during attempts to feed or handle an apparently healthy animal should generally be regarded as provoked.

Type of exposure: Rabies is transmitted by introducing the virus into open cuts or wounds in skin via mucous membranes. The likelihood of rabies infection varies with the nature and extent of the exposure.

- *Bite* – A bite is any penetration of the skin by teeth.
- *Nonbite* – Nonbite exposures include scratches, abrasions, open wounds, or mucous membranes contaminated with saliva or other potentially infectious material, such as brain tissue from a rabid animal. There have been 2 instances of airborne rabies acquired in laboratories and 2 probable airborne rabies cases acquired in 1 bat-infested cave.

Casual contact with a rabid animal, such as petting it (without a bite or nonbite exposure), is not an indication for prophylaxis.

The only documented cases of rabies due to human-to-human transmission occurred in 8 patients who received corneal transplants from persons who died of rabies undiagnosed at the time of death.

➤*Preexposure prophylaxis:* Preexposure immunization does not eliminate the need for prompt postexposure prophylaxis following an exposure; it only reduces the postexposure regimen.

Consider preexposure immunization for persons in the following high-risk groups: veterinarians, animal handlers, certain laboratory workers, and persons, especially children, spending time (eg, more than 1 month) in foreign countries where rabies is a constant threat. Also consider others whose vocational or avocational pursuits bring them into contact with potentially rabid dogs, cats, foxes, skunks, or bats. Preexposure immunization of immunosuppressed persons is not recommended.

Preexposure prophylaxis is given for several reasons. First, it may provide protection to persons with inapparent exposure to rabies. Secondly, it may protect persons whose postexposure therapy might be expected to be delayed. Finally, although it does not eliminate the need for additional therapy after a rabies exposure, it simplifies therapy by eliminating the need for globulin and decreasing the number of doses of vaccine needed. This is of particular importance for persons at high risk of exposure in countries where the available rabies-immunizing products may carry a higher risk of adverse reactions.

Preexposure immunization: Preexposure immunization consists of 3 doses of HDCV, rabies vaccine adsorbed (RVA), or PCEC 1 mL/dose administered intramuscularly (IM) (ie, deltoid area), one each on days 0, 7, and 21 or 28. The intradermal dose is 0.1 mL in the deltoid area of either arm on days 0, 7, and 21 or 28. Administration of routine booster doses of vaccine depends on exposure risk category, as noted in the following table.

Criteria for Preexposure Immunization

Risk category	Nature of risk	Typical populations	Preexposure regimen
Continuous	Virus present continuously, often in high concentrations. Aerosol, mucous membrane, bite, or nonbite exposure possible. Specific exposures may go unrecognized.	Rabies research lab workers,[a] rabies biologics production workers.	Primary preexposure immunization course. Serology every 6 months. Booster immunization when antibody titer falls below acceptable level.[b]
Frequent	Exposure usually episodic, with source recognized or unrecognized. Aerosol, mucous membrane, bite, or nonbite exposure.	Rabies diagnostic lab workers,[a] spelunkers, veterinarians and staff, and animal control and wildlife workers in rabies epizootic areas.	Primary preexposure immunization course. Serology every 2 years. Booster immunization when antibody titer falls below acceptable level.
Infrequent (greater than population-at-large)	Exposure nearly always episodic with source recognized. Bite or nonbite exposure.	Veterinarians and animal control wildlife workers in areas of low rabies endemicity; travelers to foreign rabies epizootic areas; veterinary students.	Primary preexposure immunization course. No routine booster immunization or serology.
Rare (population- at-large)	Exposure always episodic, or bite with source recognized.	US population-at-large, including individuals in rabies epizootic areas.	No preexposure immunization.

[a] Judgment of relative risk and extra monitoring of immunization status of laboratory workers is the responsibility of the laboratory supervisor (see US Department of Health and Human Services' *Biosafety in Microbiological and Biomedical Laboratories,* 1984).

[b] Preexposure booster immunization consists of 1 dose of HDCV, PCEC, or RVA 1 mL/dose IM, or 0.1 mL intradermally on day 0 only. Acceptable antibody level is 1:5 titer (complete inhibition in rapid fluorescent focus inhibition test [RFFIT] at 1:5 dilution). Boost if titer falls below 1:5.

RABIES PROPHYLAXIS PRODUCTS

➤*Postexposure prophylaxis:*

Local wound treatment – Immediate and thorough washing of all bite wounds and scratches with soap and water is perhaps the most effective means of preventing rabies. Give tetanus and a virucidal agent, such as povidone-iodine solution irrigation prophylaxis, and control bacterial infection as indicated.

Immunization – Postexposure antirabies immunization should always include both passive immunization (preferably RIG) and vaccine, with the following exception: Persons previously immunized with HDCV in recommended preexposure or postexposure regimens or with other types of vaccines and who have a documented adequate rabies antibody titer should receive only vaccine. The globulin/vaccine combination is recommended for both bite and nonbite exposures, regardless of the interval between exposure and treatment.

Treatment – Use the following recommendations as a guide in conjunction with knowledge of the circumstances of the situation. Consult public health officials with questions about the need for rabies prophylaxis.

Treatment Recommendations for Postexposure Rabies

Animal species	Condition of animal at time of attack	Treatment of exposed person[a]
Domestic: dogs, cats, and ferrets	Healthy and available for 10 days of observation	None, unless animal develops rabies.[b]
	Rabid/suspected rabid	RIG and vaccine.[c]
	Unknown (escaped)	Consult public health officials. If treatment is indicated, give RIG and vaccine.[c]
Wild: skunk, bat, fox, coyote, raccoon, bobcat, and other carnivores	Regard as rabid unless proven negative by laboratory test[c]	Consider immediate vaccination.[c]
Other: livestock, rodents, rabbits and hares, large rodents, and other mammals	Consider individually: Bites of squirrels, hamsters, guinea pigs, gerbils, chipmunks, rats, mice, other rodents, rabbits, and hares almost never call for antirabies prophylaxis. Consult public health officials.	

[a] If treatment is indicated, administer both RIG and vaccine as soon as possible, regardless of the interval from exposure.
[b] Begin treatment with RIG and vaccine at first sign of rabies in biting domestic animals during the usual holding period of 10 days. Kill and test the symptomatic animal immediately.
[c] Kill and test animal as soon as possible. Holding for observation is not recommended. Discontinue vaccine if fluorescent antibody tests of animal are negative.

Treatment Schedule for Postexposure Rabies Prophylaxis

Vaccination status	Treatment[a]
Not previously vaccinated	*Local wound cleansing:* Begin all postexposure treatment with immediate, thorough cleansing of each wound with soap and water. If available, use a virucidal agent, such as povidone-iodine solution, to irrigate the wounds. *Rabies immune globulin:* Give 20 international units/kg. If anatomically feasible, infiltrate the full dose around the wound(s) and inject the balance IM at an anatomical site distant from the vaccine administration. Do not give RIG through the same syringe or into the same anatomical site as rabies vaccine. Because RIG may partially suppress active induction of antirabies antibody, give no more than the recommended dose. *Rabies vaccine:* Give 1 mL IM in the deltoid area[b] on days 0, 3, 7, 14, and 28.
Previously vaccinated[c]	*Local wound cleansing:* Begin all postexposure treatments with immediate, thorough cleansing of each wound with soap and water. If available, use a virucidal agent, such as povidone-iodine solution, to irrigate the wounds. Do not administer RIG. *Rabies vaccine:* Give 1 mL IM in the deltoid area on days 0 and 3.

[a] These regimens apply to all age groups, including children.
[b] The deltoid area is the only acceptable site of vaccination for adults and older children. For younger children, the outer aspect of the thigh may be used. Vaccine should never be administered in the gluteal area.
[c] Any person with a history of pre- or postexposure vaccination with HDCV, PCEC, or RVA, or with both a history of vaccination with any other type of rabies vaccine and a documented history of antibody response to that vaccination.

Rapid intervention is essential to minimize morbidity and mortality in an acute toxic ingestion. Institute measures to prevent absorption and hasten elimination as soon as possible; however, symptomatic and supportive care takes precedence over other therapy. It is assumed that basic life support measures (eg, cardiopulmonary resuscitation [CPR]) have been instituted.

Specific antidotes are discussed in the overdosage section of individual or group monographs. The following discussion outlines procedures used in the management of acute overdosage of orally ingested systemic drugs. Consultation with a regional poison control center is highly recommended (1-800-222-1222).

ADVANCED LIFE SUPPORT MEASURES

➤*Adequate Airway:* Adequate Airway must be established and maintained, generally via oropharyngeal or endotracheal airways, cricothyrotomy or tracheostomy.

➤*Ventilation:* Ventilation may then be performed via mouth-to-mouth insufflation, hand-operated bag (ambu bag) or by mechanical ventilator.

➤*Circulation:* Circulation must be maintained.

- *Hypotension:* If hypotension/hypoperfusion occurs, place the patient in shock position (head lowered, feet elevated); specific therapy may include:

  Establish IV access and initiate IV fluids (eg, 0.9% or 0.45% Saline, Lactated Ringer's, Dextrose). A maintenance flow rate is generally 100 to 200 ml/hour; individualize as necessary.

  Plasma, plasma protein fractions, whole blood or plasma expanders may be required.

  Severe hypotension may require judicious use of cardiovascular active agents. The most commonly recommended agents are dopamine, dobutamine and norepinephrine.

- *Arrhythmia* treatment is dictated by the offending drug.
- *Hypertension,* sometimes severe, may occur. (See Nitroprusside and Diazoxide, Parenteral in the Agents for Hypertensive Emergencies section.)

➤*Seizures:* Simple isolated seizures may require only observation and supportive care. Repetitive seizures or status epilepticus require therapy. Give IV diazepam or lorazepam followed by fosphenytoin, phenytoin, and/or phenobarbital. General anesthesia with or without neuromuscular blockade may be necessary for seizures refractory to standard therapy.

REDUCTION OF DRUG ABSORPTION

➤*Gastric decontamination:* is generally recommended as soon as possible; however, this is generally not very effective unless employed within the first 1 to 2 hours after ingestion. Gastric lavage and administration of activated charcoal are the two most commonly employed methods for gastric decontamination.

- *Gastric lavage* may be used within 1 to 2 hours of ingestion of an acute overdose. Airway protection via endotracheal intubation is appropriate for the patient without a gag reflex or comatose patients. Position the patient on left side, face down and use a large bore tube. Instill warm water or saline 300 to 360 ml for adults. Avoid water for infants and children; use warm saline or 5% to 6% polyethylene glycol solution. Repeat instillations until lavage solution becomes clear. Add charcoal before removing the tube.
- *Activated charcoal:* Absorption, using activated charcoal alone or following gastric lavage, is appropriate for many significant toxic ingestions. It adsorbs a wide variety of toxins and is most effective when given within 1 to 2 hours of ingestion. The adult dose is 50 to 100 g of activated charcoal mixed in 240 ml of water; the pediatric dose is 1 g/kg, or 25 to 50 g in 120 ml of water.

➤*Cathartics:* Cathartics are generally not used alone in the treatment of acute overdosage. More often they are administered with activated charcoal to increase the elimination of the charcoal-poison complex. The administration of a saline cathartic (eg, magnesium citrate) or osmotic cathartic (eg, sorbitol) with activated charcaol has the most rapid effect.

➤*Whole bowel irrigation (WBI):* Whole bowel irrigation utilizes rapid administration of large volumes of lavage solutions, such as polyethylene glycol. The dose is 4 to 6 L over 1 to 2 hours for adults and 0.5 L/hr for children. It may be useful to remove certain extended release dosage forms, cocaine-containing condoms or balloons, or toxins for which activated charcoal is ineffective (eg, iron, lithium).

ELIMINATION OF ABSORBED DRUG

➤*Interruption of enterohepatic circulation:* Interruption of enterohepatic circulation by "gastric dialysis" uses scheduled doses of activated charcoal for 1 to 2 days. Gastric dialysis not only interrupts the enterohepatic cycle of some drugs, but also creates an osmotic gradient, drawing drug from the plasma back into the gastrointestinal lumen where it is bound by the charcoal and excreted in the feces.

➤*Diuresis:* Diuresis may be effective as identified in the individual drug monographs.

- *Alkaline diuresis* promotes elimination of weak acids (eg, barbiturates, salicylates) and is accomplished by the administration of IV sodium bicarbonate.

➤*Dialysis:* Dialysis is indicated in a minority of severe overdose cases. Drug factors that alter dialysis effectiveness include volume of distribution, drug compartmentalization, protein binding and lipid/water solubility.

- *Hemodialysis* may be used as a supportive measure when the patient is having complications (eg, severe metabolic acidosis, electrolyte imbalances, renal failure).
- *Peritoneal dialysis* is even less effective than hemodialysis.
- *Charcoal hemoperfusion* may be useful when a drug can be adsorbed by charcoal (eg, theophylline, barbiturates).

MANAGEMENT OF ACUTE HYPERSENSITIVITY REACTIONS

Type I hypersensitivity reactions (immediate hypersensitivity or anaphylaxis) are immunologic responses to a foreign antigen to which a patient has been previously sensitized. Anaphylactoid reactions are not immunologically mediated; however, symptoms and treatment are similar.

SIGNS AND SYMPTOMS

Acute hypersensitivity reactions typically begin within 1 to 30 minutes of exposure to the offending antigen. Tingling sensations and a generalized flush may proceed to a fullness in the throat, chest tightness or a "feeling of impending doom." Generalized urticaria and sweating are common. *Severe* reactions include life-threatening involvement of the airway and cardiovascular system.

TREATMENT

Appropriate and immediate treatment is imperative. The following general measures are commonly employed:

➤*Epinephrine:* For adults, administer 1:1000 (1 mg/mL), 0.2 to 0.5 mg (0.2 to 0.5 ml) SC or IM as the primary treatment. In children, administer 0.01 mg/kg up to 0.3 mg. Doses may be repeated every 5 to 15 minutes if needed. A succession of small doses is more effective and less dangerous than a single large dose.

Epinephrine should be administered IV only during cardiac arrest or in the presence of profound hypotension. For adults, dilute 0.1 to 0.3 mL of epinephrine 1:1,000 in 10 mL of normal saline and administer IV over several minutes; repeat as necessary. In children, administer 0.01 mg/kg (0.1 mL/kg) of a 1:10,000 solution; maximum dose, 0.3 mg).

Alternatively, an epinephrine infusion may be considered. The infusion can be prepared by adding 1 mg (1 mL) of epinephrine 1:1,000 to 250 mL of 5% dextrose in water to yield a concentration of 4 mcg/mL. For adults, the infusion is then administered at a rate of 1 to 4 mcg/minute.

Based on anecdotal reports, other routes of administration have been successful (eg, endotracheal, sublingual, inhaled).

➤*Airway:* Establish and maintain a patent airway. Endotracheal intubation or cricothyrotomy (ie, inferior laryngotomy, used prior to tracheotomy) may be considered. Administer oxygen. Severe respiratory difficulty may respond to inhaled beta-2 agonists (eg, nebulized albuterol).

➤*Hypotension:* The patient should be recumbent with feet elevated. Depending upon the severity, consider the following measures:

- Establish a patent IV catheter in a suitable vein.
- Administer IV fluids (eg, normal saline).
- Administer plasma expanders.
- Administer cardioactive agents (see group and individual monographs). Commonly recommended agents include dopamine and norepinephrine.

➤*Adjunctive therapy:* does not alter acute reactions, but may modify an ongoing or slow-onset process and shorten the course of the reaction.

- *Antihistamines: Diphenhydramine* – Adults: 25 to 50 mg IV. Children: 1 mg/kg, up to 50 mg.
- *Corticosteroids,* Administer IV at a dosage equivalent to methylprednisolone 1 to 2 mg/kg/day every 6 hours. For mild hypersensitivity reactions, oral prednisone (0.5 mg/kg) may be sufficient. Because of the delayed onset of action, corticosteroids should be administered early in the treatment.
- *H_2 antagonists: Cimetidine* – For adults, 4 mg/kg administered slowly IV. *Ranitidine* – For adults, 50 mg or 1 mg/kg. For children, 12.5 to 50 mg (1 mg/kg). Administer over 10 to 15 minutes.
- *Glucagon:* Consider glucagon administration in patients receiving concomitant beta-blockers. Glucagon has been shown to be beneficial in reversing refractory bronchospasm and hypotension in these patients.

DRUG-INDUCED PROLONGATION OF THE QT INTERVAL AND TORSADES DE POINTES

The QT interval is the period between the beginning of the QRS complex and the end of the T wave. Thus, it is the estimate of the time interval between the earliest ventricular depolarization and the latest ventricular repolarization. Since the QT interval is affected by changes in the heart rate, corrections are usually made to the QT interval for these changes (QTc). There is no commonly accepted definition of a normal or prolonged QTc interval. The Committee for Proprietary Medicinal Products has suggested ranges for normal (ie, men less than 430 msec, women less than 450 msec), borderline (ie, men 430 to 450 msec, women 450 to 470 msec), and prolonged (ie, men greater than 450 msec, women greater than 470 msec) QTc intervals. Moderate and clinically important increases in the QT interval over baseline have been considered to be 15% and 25% increases, respectively.

Numerous drugs, representing a wide range of pharmacologic classes, have been implicated in prolonging the QT interval. Concern about serious and possibly fatal consequences of drug combinations that may cause prolongation of the QT interval has led to contraindicating the use of many drug pairs, even though coadministration may not have been studied. The potential of bepridil (*Vascor*), astemizole (*Hismanal*), grepafloxacin (*Raxar*), and terfenadine (*Seldane*) to prolong the QT interval played an important role in their removal from the market.

The precise mechanism by which QT interval prolongation (ie, long QT syndrome [LQTS]) occurs is unknown; however, it appears to be related to ion exchange (eg, outward repolarizing potassium current, inward depolarizing calcium or sodium current). Class III antiarrhythmic agents prolong the QT interval by blocking potassium flow. A prolonged QT interval may be congenital (eg, genetic) or acquired (eg, drug-induced). In some instances, patients may have an underlying predisposition toward a prolonged QT interval (eg, longer than normal QT interval before drug administration).

Drug-induced prolongation of the QT interval may be suspected if there are dose-related changes in the QT interval, the same drug causes QT prolongation in a number of patients, or prolonged QT interval recurs when a patient is rechallenged. Drug-induced QT prolongation may be prevented by 1) not exceeding the recommended drug dose; 2) limiting use of the drug in patients with preexisting heart disease; 3) avoiding coadministration of agents that increase plasma levels of the drug in question; 4) avoiding concurrent use of other medications that prolong the QT interval; and 5) identification and correction of risk factors (eg, hypokalemia) before giving a drug known to prolong the QT interval.

A great deal of attention has been focused on drug-induced prolongation of the QT interval and association of the prolongation with life-threatening ventricular arrhythmias, especially torsades de pointes. Torsades de pointes, meaning twisting of points, refers to a ventricular arrhythmia in which the QRS complexes change amplitude and contour, appearing to twist around the isoelectric line on the electrocardiogram (ECG). In patients who develop drug-induced torsades de pointes, the QT interval measured prior to drug exposure tends to be longer than in patients who receive the drug safely. In patients with drug-induced torsades de pointes, ventricular repolarization is prolonged and characterized by marked prolongation of the QT interval (greater than 500 msec) and QTc interval (greater than 470 msec) of the ECG. In individuals with a drug-induced increase in the QTc interval of more than 65 msec above normal (ie, greater than 500 msec), the risk of torsades de pointes may be greater than 3%. This risk of torsades de pointes increases greatly when the QT interval exceeds 600 msec. In the presence of a prolonged QT interval, women are at greater risk than men of developing torsades de pointes.

Amiodarone (eg, *Cordarone*) prolongs the QT interval but rarely causes torsades de pointes. However, class I antiarrhythmic agents (eg, procainamide [eg, *Procanbid*]) are more likely to cause torsades de pointes but have a moderate effect on the QT interval. Drug interactions may further prolong the QT interval and increase the risk of life-threatening cardiac arrhythmias, including torsades de pointes. Thus, administration of cisapride (eg, *Propulsid*), which prolongs the QT interval, with an inhibitor of cytochrome P450 (CYP) 3A4 (eg, grapefruit products, erythromycin) may increase cisapride plasma levels and the risk of life-threatening cardiac arrhythmias.

Identification and correction of risk factors (eg, hypokalemia) before giving a drug known to prolong the QT interval or cause torsades de pointes are important in preventing drug-induced torsades de pointes. Agents that prolong the QT interval are contraindicated in patients with a history of drug-induced torsades de pointes.

➤*Summary:* Numerous drugs from a wide range of pharmacologic classes can prolong the QT interval and precipitate torsades de pointes. However, the consequences of QT interval prolongation and the occurrence of torsades de pointes can be minimized or prevented by identification and correction of risk factors. Use of drugs that prolong the QT interval is contraindicated in patients with a history of torsades de pointes.

Drugs Reported to Prolong the QT Interval

Analgesics
- Celecoxib (*Celebrex*)[a]
- Methadone (eg, *Dolophine*)[a]

Anesthetic agents
- Enflurane (eg, *Ethrane*)
- Isoflurane (eg, *Forane*)
- Halothane

Antiarrhythmic agents
- Class IA
  - Disopyramide (eg, *Norpace*)[a]
  - Procainamide (eg, *Procanbid*)[a]
  - Quinidine[a]
- Class IC
  - Flecainide (eg, *Tambocor*)[a,b]
  - Propafenone (eg, *Rythmol*)[a,c]
- Class III
  - Amiodarone (eg, *Cordarone*)[a,c]
  - Bretylium[a]
  - Dofetilide (*Tikosyn*)[a,c]
  - Ibutilide (*Corvert*)[a,c]
  - Sotalol (eg, *Betapace*)[a,c]

Anticonvulsants
- Felbamate (*Felbatol*)[a]
- Fosphenytoin (*Cerebyx*)

Antiemetics
- Dolasetron (*Anzemet*)[c]
- Droperidol (eg, *Inapsine*)[a,c]
- Ondansetron (*Zofran*)

Antihistamines
- Desloratadine (*Clarinex*)[c] (overdose)
- Diphenhydramine (eg, *Benadryl*)[a]
- Fexofenadine (*Allegra*)
- Hydroxyzine (eg, *Vistaril*)

Anti-infectives
- Amantadine (eg, *Symmetrel*)[a]
- Antimalarials
  - Mefloquine (eg, *Lariam*)[c]
  - Quinine[a]
- Antivirals
  - Efavirenz (*Sustiva*)[a]
- Azole antifungal agents
  - Fluconazole (eg, *Diflucan*)[a,c]
  - Itraconazole (eg, *Sporanox*)
  - Ketoconazole (eg, *Nizoral*)
  - Voriconazole (*Vfend*)[a,c]
- Chloroquine (eg, *Aralen*)[a]
- Clindamycin (eg, *Cleocin*)
- Foscarnet (*Foscavir*)
- Macrolides and related antibiotics
  - Azithromycin (eg, *Zithromax*)
  - Clarithromycin (eg, *Biaxin*)[a,c]
  - Erythromycin (eg, *Ery-Tab*)[a,c]
  - Telithromycin (*Ketek*)[c]
  - Troleandomycin
- Pentamidine (eg, *Pentam 300*)[a]
- Quinolones
  - Gatifloxacin[a,c]
  - Levofloxacin (eg, *Levaquin*)[a-c]
  - Moxifloxacin (eg, *Avelox*)[c]
  - Ofloxacin (eg, *Floxin*)[a,c]
- Trimethoprim/sulfamethoxazole (eg, *Bactrim*)[a]

Antineoplastics
- Arsenic trioxide (*Trisenox*)[a,c]
- Doxorubicin (eg, *Adriamycin*)
- Tamoxifen (eg, *Nolvadex*)

Bronchodilators
- Albuterol (eg, *Proventil*)[c]
- Formoterol (*Foradil*)[c]
- Isoproterenol (eg, *Isuprel*)
- Salmeterol (*Serevent*)[c]
- Terbutaline (eg, *Brethine*)[c]

Calcium channel blockers
- Isradipine (*DynaCirc*)
- Nicardipine (eg, *Cardene*)

Drugs Reported to Prolong the QT Interval

Contrast media
- Ionic contrast media[a]
- Non-ionic contrast media
  - Iohexol (*Omnipaque*)

Corticosteroids
- Prednisolone (eg, *Prelone*)
- Prednisone (eg, *Deltasone*)[a]

Diuretics
- Furosemide (eg, *Lasix*)
- Indapamide (eg, *Lozol*)

GI agents
- Cisapride (*Propulsid*)[a,c]
- Famotidine (eg, *Pepcid*)[a]

Immunosuppressants
- Tacrolimus (*Protopic*)[a,c] (postmarketing)

Miscellaneous
- Levomethadyl
- Moexipril/Hydrochlorothiazide (*Uniretic*)
- Octreotide (*Sandostatin*)[c]
- Oxytocin (eg, *Pitocin*; IV bolus)
- Papaverine (eg, *Pavaden TD*)[a]
- Probucol[a]
- Vasopressin (eg, *Pitressin*)[a]

Psychotropics
- Droperidol (eg, *Inapsine*)[a]
- Haloperidol (eg, *Haldol*)[a]
- Lithium (eg, *Eskalith*)[a]
- Maprotiline[a]
- Phenothiazines
  - Chlorpromazine (eg, *Thorazine*)[a]
  - Fluphenazine (eg, *Prolixin*)[a]
  - Perphenazine
  - Thioridazine[a,c]
  - Trifluoperazine
- Pimozide (*Orap*)[a,c]
- Quetiapine (*Seroquel*)[c]
- Risperidone (*Risperdal*)[c] (overdose)
- SSRIs
  - Citalopram (eg, *Celexa*)[a]
  - Fluoxetine (eg, *Prozac*)[a,b]
  - Paroxetine (eg, *Paxil*)[a]
  - Sertraline (*Zoloft*)[a-c] (postmarketing)
  - Venlafaxine (*Effexor*)[c] (postmarketing)
- Trazodone (eg, *Desyrel*)
- Tricyclic antidepressants
  - Amitriptyline[a]
  - Clomipramine (eg, *Anafranil*)
  - Desipramine (eg, *Norpramin*)[a]
  - Doxepin (eg, *Sinequan*)[a]
  - Imipramine (eg, *Tofranil*)[a]
  - Nortriptyline (eg, *Pamelor*)
- Ziprasidone (*Geodon*)[c]

Serotonin 5-HT$_1$ agonists
- Naratriptan (*Amerge*)
- Sumatriptan (*Imitrex*)[c]
- Zolmitriptan (*Zomig*)[c]

Skeletal muscle relaxants
- Tizanidine (eg, *Zanaflex*)[c] (animals)

[a] Drugs for which torsades de pointes has also been reported.
[b] Association unclear.
[c] QT, QTc, and/or torsades de pointes association listed in FDA approved product labeling.

➤***Factors that increase the risk of torsades de pointes:***
- Administration of drugs that prolong the QT interval
- Altered nutritional states (eg, anorexia nervosa, liquid protein diet)
- Baseline QTc interval greater than 460 msec
- Coadministration of certain drugs that prolong QT interval with drugs metabolized by CYP3A4
- Congenital LQT syndrome
- Female gender
- Electrolyte imbalance (eg, hypokalemia, hypomagnesemia)
- Liver disease
- Hypothyroidism
- Nervous system injury (eg, stroke, subarachnoid hemorrhage)
- Preexisting cardiac disease (eg, congestive heart failure, heart failure, ventricular hypertrophy)
- Renal disease
- Slow heart rate (ie, bradyarrhythmia)

INTERNATIONAL SYSTEM OF UNITS

The *Système international d 'unités* (International System of Units) or *SI* is a modernized version of the metric system. The primary goal of the conversion to SI units is to revise the present confused measurement system and to improve test-result communications.

The SI has 7 basic units from which other units are derived:

Base Units of SI

Physical quantity	Base unit	SI symbol
length	meter	m
mass	kilogram	kg
time	second	s
amount of substance	mole	mol
thermodynamic temperature	kelvin	K
electric current	ampere	A
luminous intensity	candela	cd

Combinations of these base units can express any property, although, for simplicity, special names are given to some of these derived units.

Representative Derived Units

Derived unit	Name and symbol	Derivation from base units
area	square meter	m^2
volume	cubic meter	m^3
force	newton (N)	$kg{\bullet}m{\bullet}s^{-2}$
pressure	pascal (Pa)	$kg{\bullet}m^{-1}{\bullet}s^{-2}$ (N/m^2)
work, energy	joule (J)	$kg{\bullet}m^2{\bullet}s^{-2}$ ($N{\bullet}m$)
mass density	kilogram per cubic meter	kg/m^3
frequency	hertz (Hz)	1 $cycle/s^{-1}$
temperature degree	Celsius (°C)	°C = °K − 273.15
concentration		
mass	kilogram/liter	kg/L
substance	mole/liter	mol/L
molality	mole/kilogram	mol/kg
density	kilogram/liter	kg/L

Prefixes to the base unit are used in this system to form decimal multiples and submultiples. The preferred multiples and submultiples listed below change the quantity by increments of 10^3 or 10^{-3}. The exceptions to these recommended factors are within the middle rectangle.

Prefixes and Symbols for Decimal Multiples and Submultiples

Factor	Prefix	Symbol
10^{18}	exa	E
10^{15}	peta	P
10^{12}	tera	T
10^{9}	giga	G
10^{6}	mega	M
10^{3}	kilo	k
10^{2}	hecto	h
10^{1}	deka	da
10^{-1}	deci	d
10^{-2}	centi	c
10^{-3}	milli	m
10^{-6}	micro	μ
10^{-9}	nano	n
10^{-12}	pico	p
10^{-15}	femto	f
10^{-18}	atto	a

To convert drug concentrations to or from SI units:

Conversion factor (CF) $= \frac{1000}{\text{mol wt}}$

Conversion *to* SI units: μg/ml × CF = μmol/L

Conversion *from* SI units: μmol/L ÷ CF = μg/ml

NORMAL LABORATORY VALUES

In the following tables, normal reference values for commonly requested laboratory tests are listed in traditional units and in SI units. The tables are a guideline only. Values are method dependent and "normal values" may vary between laboratories.

Blood, Plasma or Serum

Determination	Reference Value: Conventional Units	Reference Value: SI Units
Aldosterone		
Adult, adolescent: Standing Male Female	6-22 ng/dL 5-30 ng/dL	0.17-0.61 nmol/L 0.14-0.8 nmol/L
Pregnant	Values are 2-4 times higher in pregnancy	Values are 2-4 times higher in pregnancy
Neonate	5-60 ng/dL	0.14-1.7 nmol/L
Infant 1 week to 1 year of age	1-160 ng/dL	0.03-4.6 nmol/L
Child		
1 to 3 years of age	5-60 ng/dL	0.14-1.7 nmol/L
3 to 5 years of age	5-80 ng/dL	0.14-2.3 nmol/L
5 to 7 years of age	5-50 ng/dL	0.14-1.5 nmol/L
7 to 11 years of age	5-70 ng/dL	0.14-2 nmol/L
11 to 15 yeasr of age	5-50 ng/dL	0.14-1.5 nmol/L
Supine	3-10 ng/dL	0.08-0.3 nmol/L
Alpha-fetoprotein Adult Pregnant (16 to 18 weeks)	< 15 ng/mL 38-45 ng/mL	< 15 mcg/L 38-45 mcg/L
Ammonia (NH_3) – diffusion	20-120 mcg/dl	12-70 mcmol/L
Ammonia Nitrogen	15–45 μg/dl	11–32 μmol/L
Amylase	20-100 units/dL	37-185 units/L
Anion Gap ($Na^+ + K^+$) – ($Cl^- + HCO_3^-$)	7–16 mEq/L	7–16 mmol/L
Antinuclear antibodies	negative at 1:10 dilution of serum	negative at 1:10 dilution of serum
Antithrombin III (AT III)	80-120 U/dl	800-1200 U/L
Bicarbonate: Arterial Venous	21–28 mEq/L 22–29 mEq/L	21–28 mmol/L 22–29 mmol/L
Bilirubin: Conjugated (direct) Total	≤ 0.2 mg/dl 0.1-1 mg/dl	≤ 4 mcmol/L 2-18 mcmol/L
Calcitonin: Female Male	≤ 20 pg/mL ≤ 40 pg/mL	≤ 20 ng/L ≤ 40 ng/L
Calcium: Total Ionized	8.6-10.3 mg/dl 4.4-5.1 mg/dl	2.2-2.74 mmol/L 1-1.3 mmol/L
Carbon dioxide content (plasma)	21-32 mmol/L	21-32 mmol/L
Carcinoembryonic antigen	< 3 ng/ml	< 3 mcg/L
Chloride	95-110 mEq/L	95-110 mmol/L
Coagulation screen:		
Bleeding time	3-9.5 min	180-570 sec
Prothrombin time	10-13 sec	10-13 sec
Partial thromboplastin time (activated)	22-37 sec	22-37 sec
Protein C	0.7-1.4 μ/ml	700-1400 U/ml
Protein S	0.7-1.4 μ/ml	700-1400 U/ml
Copper, total	70-160 mcg/dl	11-25 mcmol/L
Corticotropin (ACTH adrenocorticotropic hormone) – 0800 hr	< 60 pg/ml	< 13.2 pmol/L
Cortisol: 0800 hr 1800 hr 2000 hr	5-30 mcg/dl 2-15 mcg/dl ≤ 50% of 0800 hr	138-810 nmol/L 50-410 nmol/L ≤ 50% of 0800 hr
Creatine kinase: Female Male	20-170 IU/L 30-220 IU/L	0.33-2.83 mckat/L 0.5-3.67 mckat/L
Creatine kinase isoenzymes, MB fraction	0-12 IU/L	0-0.2 mckat/L
Creatinine	0.5-1.7 mg/dl	44-150 mcmol/L
Fibrinogen (coagulation factor I)	150-360 mg/dl	1.5-3.6 g/L
Follicle-stimulating hormone (FSH): Female Midcycle Male	2-13 mIU/ml 5-22 mIU/ml 1-8 mIU/ml	2-13 IU/L 5-22 IU/L 1-8 IU/L
Glucose, fasting	65-115 mg/dl	3.6-6.3 mmol/L
Glucose Tolerance Test (Oral)	mg/dL Normal / Diabetic	mmol/L Normal / Diabetic
Fasting	70-105 / > 140	3.9-5.8 / > 7.8
60 min	120-170 / ≥ 200	6.7-9.4 / ≥11.1
90 min	100-140 / ≥ 200	5.6-7.8 / ≥ 11.1
120 min	70-120 / ≥ 140	3.9-6.7 / ≥ 7.8
(γ) - Glutamyltransferase (GGT): Male Female	9-50 units/L 8-40 units/L	9-50 units/L 8-40 units/L
Haptoglobin	44-303 mg/dl	0.44-3.03 g/L
Hematologic tests:		
Fibrinogen	200-400 mg/dl	2-4 g/L
Hematocrit (Hct), female male	36%-44.6% 40.7%-50.3%	0.36-0.446 fraction of 1 0.4-0.503 fraction of 1

NORMAL LABORATORY VALUES

Blood, Plasma or Serum		
	Reference Value	
Determination	Conventional Units	SI Units
Hemoglobin A_{1C}	5.3%-7.5% of total Hgb	0.053-0.075
Hemoglobin (Hb), female	12.1-15.3 g/dl	121-153 g/L
male	13.8-17.5 g/dl	138-175 g/L
Leukocyte count (WBC)	3800-9800/mcl	3.8-9.8 x 10^9/L
Erythrocyte count (RBC), female	3.5-5 × 10^6/mcl	3.5-5 x 10^{12}/L
male	4.3-5.9 × 10^6/mcl	4.3-5.9 x 10^{12}/L
Mean corpuscular volume (MCV)	80-97.6 mcm^3	80-97.6 fl
Mean corpuscular hemoglobin (MCH)	27-33 pg/cell	1.66-2.09 fmol/cell
Mean corpuscular hemoglobin concentrate (MCHC)	33-36 g/dl	20.3-22 mmol/L
Erythrocyte sedimentation rate (sedrate, ESR)	≤ 30 mm/hr	≤ 30 mm/hr
Erythrocyte enzymes:		
Glucose-6-phosphate dehydrogenase (G-6-PD)	250-5000 units/10^6 cells	250-5000 mcunits/cell
Ferritin	10-383 ng/ml	23-862 pmol/L
Folic acid: normal	> 3.1-12.4 ng/ml	7-28.1 nmol/L
Platelet count	150-450 × 10^3/mcl	150-450 × 10^9/L
Reticulocytes	0.5%-1.5% of erythrocytes	0.005-0.015
Vitamin B_{12}	223-1132 pg/ml	165-835 pmol/L
Iron: Female	30-160 mcg/dl	5.4-31.3 mcmol/L
Male	45-160 mcg/dl	8.1-31.3 mcmol/L
Iron binding capacity	220-420 mcg/dl	39.4-75.2 mcmol/L
Isocitrate Dehydrogenase	1.2-7 units/L	1.2-7 units/L
Isoenzymes		
Fraction 1	14%-26% of total	0.14-0.26 fraction of total
Fraction 2	29%-39% of total	0.29-0.39 fraction of total
Fraction 3	20%-26% of total	0.20-0.26 fraction of total
Fraction 4	8%-16% of total	0.08-0.16 fraction of total
Fraction 5	6%-16% of total	0.06-0.16 fraction of total
Lactate dehydrogenase	100-250 units/L	1.67-4.17 mckat/L
Lactic acid (lactate)	6-19 mg/dl	0.7-2.1 mmol/L
Lead	≤ 50 mcg/dl	≤ 2.41 mcmol/L
Lipase	10-150 units/L	10-150 units/L
Lipids:		
Total Cholesterol		
Desirable	< 200 mg/dl	< 5.2 mmol/L
Borderline-high	200-239 mg/dl	< 5.2-6.2 mmol/L
High	> 239 mg/dl	> 6.2 mmol/L
LDL		
Desirable	< 130 mg/dl	< 3.36 mmol/L
Borderline-high	130-159 mg/dl	3.36-4.11 mmol/L
High	> 159 mg/dl	> 4.11 mmol/L
HDL (low)	< 35 mg/dl	< 0.91 mmol/L
Triglycerides		
Desirable	< 200 mg/dl	< 2.26 mmol/L
Borderline-high	200-400 mg/dl	2.26-4.52 mmol/L
High	400-1000 mg/dl	4.52-11.3 mmol/L
Very high	> 1000 mg/dl	> 11.3 mmol/L
Magnesium	1.3-2.2 mEq/L	0.65-1.1 mmol/L
Osmolality	280-300 mOsm/kg	280-300 mmol/kg
Oxygen saturation (arterial)	94%-100%	0.94-1 fraction of 1
PCO_2, arterial	35-45 mm Hg	4.7-6 kPa
pH, arterial	7.35-7.45	7.35-7.45
PO_2, arterial: Breathing room air[1]	80-105 mm Hg	10.6-14 kPa
On 100% O_2	> 500 mm Hg	
Phosphatase (acid), total at 37°C	0.13-0.63 units/L	2.2-10.5 units/L or 2.2-10.5 mckat/L
Phosphatase alkaline[2]	20-130 units/L	20-130 units/L or 0.33-2.17 mckat/L
Phosphorus, inorganic,[3] (phosphate)	2.5-5 mg/dl	0.8-1.6 mmol/L
Potassium	3.5-5 mEq/L	3.5-5 mmol/L
Progesterone		
Female	0.1-1.5 ng/ml	0.32-4.8 nmol/L
Follicular phase	0.1-1.5 ng/ml	0.32-4.8 nmol/L
Luteal phase	2.5-28 ng/ml	8-89 nmol/L
Male	< 0.5 ng/ml	< 1.6 nmol/L
Prolactin	1.4-24.2 ng/ml	1.4-24.2 mcg/L
Prostate specific antigen	0-4 ng/ml	0-4 ng/ml
Protein: Total	6-8 g/dl	60-80 g/L
Albumin	3.6-5 g/dl	36-50 g/L
Globulin	2.3-3.5 g/dl	23-35 g/L
Rheumatoid factor	< 60 units/ml	< 60 kIU/L
Sodium	135-147 mEq/L	135-147 mmol/L
Testosterone: Female	6-86 ng/dl	0.21-3 nmol/L
Male	270-1070 ng/dl	9.3-37 nmol/L

Blood, Plasma or Serum		
	Reference Value	
Determination	Conventional Units	SI Units
Thyroid Hormone Function Tests:		
Thyroid-stimulating hormone (TSH)	0.35-6.2 mcU/ml	0.35-6.2 mU/L
Thyroxine-binding globulin capacity	10-26 mcg/dl	100-260 mcg/L
Total triiodothyronine (T_3)	75-220 ng/dl	1.2-3.4 nmol/L
Total thyroxine by RIA (T_4)	4-11 mcg/dl	51-142 nmol/L
T_3 resin uptake	25%-38%	0.25-0.38 fraction of 1
Transaminase, AST (aspartate aminotransferase, SGOT)	11-47 units/L	0.18-0.78 mckat/L
Transaminase, ALT (alanine aminotrans ferase, SGPT)	7-53 units/L	0.12-0.88 mckat/L
Transferrin	220-400 mg/dL	2.20-4.00 g/L
Urea nitrogen (BUN)	8-25 mg/dl	2.9-8.9 mmol/L
Uric acid	3-8 mg/dl	179-476 mcmol/L
Vitamin A (retinol)	15-60 mcg/dl	0.52-2.09 mcmol/L
Zinc	50-150 mcg/dl	7.7-23 mcmol/L

[1] Age dependent [2] Infants and adolescents up to 104 units/L [3] Infants in the first year up to 6 mg/dl

Urine		
	Reference Value	
Determination	Conventional Units	SI Units
Aldosterone	2-16 mcg/24 hours	5.5-45 nmol/24 hours
Calcium[1]	50-250 mcg/day	1.25-6.25 mmol/day
Catecholamines: Epinephrine	< 20 mcg/day	< 109 nmol/day
Norepinephrine	< 100 mcg/day	< 590 nmol/day
Catecholamines, 24-hr	< 110 µg	< 650 nmol
Copper[1]	15-60 mcg/day	0.24-0.95 mcmol/day
Creatinine: Child	8-22 mg/kg	71-195 µmol/kg
Adolescent	8-30 mg/kg	71-265 µmol/kg
Female	0.6-1.5 g/day	5.3-13.3 mmol/day
Male	0.8-1.8 g/day	7.1-15.9 mmol/day
pH	4.5-8	4.5-8
Phosphate[1]	0.9-1.3 g/day	29-42 mmol/day
Potassium[1]	25-100 mEq/day	25-100 mmol/day
Protein		
Total	1-14 mg/dL	10-140 mg/L
At rest	50-80 mg/day	50-80 mg/day
Protein, quantitative	< 150 mg/day	< 0.15 g/day
Sodium[1]	100-250 mEq/day	100-250 mmol/day
Specific Gravity, random	1.002-1.030	1.002-1.030
Uric Acid, 24-hr	250-750 mg	1.48-4.43 mmol

[1] Diet dependent

Drug Levels†

	Drug Determination	Reference Value: Conventional Units	Reference Value: SI Units
Aminoglycosides	Amikacin		
	(trough)	1-8 mcg/ml	1.7-13.7 mcmol/L
	(peak)	20-30 mcg/ml	34-51 mcmol/L
	Gentamicin		
	(trough)	0.5-2 mcg/ml	1-4.2 mcmol/L
	(peak)	6-10 mcg/ml	12.5-20.9 mcmol/L
	Kanamycin		
	(trough)	5-10 mcg/ml	nd
	(peak)	20-25 mcg/ml	nd
	Netilmicin		
	(trough)	0.5-2 mcg/ml	nd
	(peak)	6-10 mcg/ml	nd
	Streptomycin		
	(trough)	< 5 mcg/ml	nd
	(peak)	5-20 mcg/ml	nd
	Tobramycin		
	(trough)	0.5-2 mcg/ml	1.1-4.3 mcmol/L
	(peak)	5-20 mcg/ml	12.8-21.8 mcmol/L
Antiarrhythmics	Amiodarone	0.5-2.5 mcg/ml	1.5-4 mcmol/L
	Bretylium	0.5-1.5 mcg/ml	nd
	Digitoxin	9-25 mcg/L	11.8-32.8 nmol/L
	Digoxin	0.8-2 ng/ml	0.9-2.5 nmol/L
	Disopyramide	2-8 mcg/ml	6-18 mcmol/L
	Flecainide	0.2-1 mcg/ml	nd
	Lidocaine	1.5-6 mcg/ml	4.5-21.5 mcmol/L
	Mexiletine	0.5-2 mcg/ml	nd
	Procainamide	4-8 mcg/ml	17-34 mcmol/ml
	Propranolol	50-200 ng/ml	190-770 nmol/L
	Quinidine	2-6 mcg/ml	4.6-9.2 mcmol/L
	Tocainide	4-10 mcg/ml	nd
	Verapamil	0.08-0.3 mcg/ml	nd
Anti-convulsants	Carbamazepine	4-12 mcg/ml	17-51 mcmol/L
	Phenobarbital	10-40 mcg/ml	43-172 mcmol/L
	Phenytoin	10-20 mcg/ml	40-80 mcmol/L
	Primidone	4-12 mcg/ml	18-55 mcmol/L
	Valproic acid	40-100 mcg/ml	280-700 mcmol/L
Antidepressants	Amitriptyline	110-250 ng/ml[3]	500-900 nmol/L
	Amoxapine	200-500 ng/ml	nd
	Bupropion	25-100 ng/ml	nd
	Clomipramine	80-100 ng/ml	nd
	Desipramine	115-300 ng/ml	nd
	Doxepin	110-250 ng/ml[3]	nd
	Imipramine	225-350 ng/ml[3]	nd
	Maprotiline	200-300 ng/ml	nd
	Nortriptyline	50-150 ng/ml	nd
	Protriptyline	70-250 ng/ml	nd
	Trazodone	800-1600 ng/ml	nd

Drug Levels†

	Drug Determination	Reference Value: Conventional Units	Reference Value: SI Units
Antipsychotics	Chlorpromazine	50-300 ng/ml	150-950 nmol/L
	Fluphenazine	0.13-2.8 ng/ml	nd
	Haloperidol	5-20 ng/ml	nd
	Perphenazine	0.8-1.2 ng/ml	nd
	Thiothixene	2-57 ng/ml	nd
Miscellaneous	Amantadine	300 ng/ml	nd
	Amrinone	3.7 mcg/ml	nd
	Chloramphenicol	10-20 mcg/ml	31-62 mcmol/L
	Cyclosporine[1]	250-800 ng/ml (whole blood, RIA)	nd
		50-300 ng/ml (plasma, RIA)	nd
	Ethanol[2]	0 mg/dl	0 mmol/L
	Hydralazine	100 ng/ml	nd
	Lithium	0.6-1.2 mEq/L	0.6-1.2 mmol/L
	Salicylate	100-300 mg/L	724-2172 mcmol/L
	Sulfonamide	5-15 mg/dl	nd
	Terbutaline	0.5-4.1 ng/ml	nd
	Theophylline	10-20 mcg/ml	55-110 mcmol/L
	Vancomycin		
	(trough)	5-15 ng/ml	nd
	(peak)	20-40 mcg/ml	nd

† The values given are generally accepted as desirable for treatment without toxicity for most patients. However, exceptions are not uncommon.

[1] 24 hour trough values [2] Toxic: 50-100 mg/dl (10.9-21.7 mmol/L) [3] Parent drug plus N-desmethyl metabolite

nd – No data available

Classification of Blood Pressure*

Category	Reference Value: Systolic (mm Hg)		Reference Value: Diastolic (mm Hg)
Optimal†	< 120	and	< 80
Normal	< 130	and	< 85
High-normal	130-139	or	85-89
Hypertension‡			
Stage 1	140-159	or	90-99
Stage 2	160-179	or	100-109
Stage 3	≥ 180	or	≥ 110

adopted from the Sixth Report of the Joint National Committee on Prevention, Detection, Evaluation, and Treatment of High Blood Pressure, National Institutes of Health

* For adults age 18 and older who are not taking antihypertensive drugs and not acutely ill. When systolic and diastolic blood pressures fall into different categories, the higher category should be selected to classify the individual's blood pressure status. In addition to classifying stages of hypertension on the basis of average blood pressure levels, clinicians should specify presence or absence of target organ disease and additional risk factors.

† Optimal blood pressure with respect to cardiovascular risk is below 120/88 mm Hg. However, unusually low readings should be evaluated for clinical significance.

‡ Based on the average of two or more readings taken at each of two or more visits after an initial screening.

To calculate milliequivalent weight: $\text{mEq} = \dfrac{\text{gram molecular weight/valence}}{1000}$

$\text{mEq} = \dfrac{\text{mg}}{\text{eq wt}}$ equivalent weight or eq wt $= \dfrac{\text{gram molecular weight}}{\text{valence}}$

Commonly used mEq weights			
Chloride	35.5 mg = 1 mEq	Magnesium	12 mg = 1 mEq
Sodium	23 mg = 1 mEq	Potassium	39 mg = 1 mEq
Calcium	20 mg = 1 mEq		

To convert temperature °C ↔ °F: Celsius to Fahrenheit $= \left(°C \times \dfrac{9}{5}\right) + 32$

Fahrenheit to Celsius $= (°F - 32) \times \dfrac{5}{9}$

To calculate creatinine clearance (Ccr) from serum creatinine:

Male: $\text{CrCl} = \dfrac{\text{weight (kg)} \times (140 - \text{age})}{72 \times \text{serum creatinine (mg/dL)}}$

Female: CrCl = 0.85 × calculation for males

To calculate ideal body weight (kg):

Male = 50 kg + 2.3 kg (each inch > 5 ft)

Female = 45.5 kg + 2.3 kg (each inch > 5 ft)

To calculate body mass index (BMI):

BMI (kg/m^2) = Body weight (kg)/[height (m)]^2

To calculate body surface area (BSA) in adults and children:

1) *Dubois method:*

$\text{BSA (m}^2) = \text{wt (kg)}^{0.425} \times \text{ht (cm)}^{0.725} \times 0.007184$

2) *Mosteller method:*

$\text{BSA (m}^2) = \sqrt{\dfrac{\text{ht (cm)} \times \text{wt (kg)}}{3600}}$

Suggested Weights for Adults	
Height*	Weight in pounds†
4′10″	91-115
4′11″	94-119
5′0″	97-123
5′1″	101-127
5′2″	104-131
5′3″	107-135
5′4″	110-140
5′5″	114-144
5′6″	118-148
5′7″	121-153
5′8″	125-158
5′9″	128-162
5′10″	132-167
5′11″	136-172
6′0″	140-177
6′1″	144-182
6′2″	148-186
6′3″	152-192

* Without shoes. † Without clothes.

➤*Standard Medical Abbreviations used in medical orders:*

Abbreviation	Meaning
≈	approximately equals
Δ	delta
ε	epsilon; molar absorption coefficient
Ω	omega; ohm
5-HIAA	5-hydroxyindoleacetic acid
5-HT	5-hydroxytryptamine (serotonin)
6-MP	6-mercaptopurine
17-OHCS	17-hydroxycorticosteroids
α	alpha
A	ampere(s)
Å	angstrom(s)
aa	of each (ana)
āā	of each (ana)
AA	Alcoholics Anonymous; amino acid
AACP	American Association of Clinical Pharmacy; American Association of Colleges of Pharmacy
AARP	American Association of Retired Persons
Ab	antibody
ABGs	arterial blood gases
abs feb	when fever is absent (*absente febre*)
ABVD	Adriamycin (doxorubicin), bleomycin, vinblastine, (and) dacarbazine
ac	before meals or food (*ante cibum*)
ACCP	American College of Clinical Pharmacy
ACD	acid-citrate-dextrose
ACE	angiotensin-converting enzyme
ACEI	angiotensin-converting enzyme inhibitor
ACh	acetylcholine
ACIP	Advisory Committee on Immunization Practices
ACLS	advanced cardiac life support
ACPE	American Council on Pharmaceutical Education
ACS	American Chemical Society
ACT	activated clotting time
ACTH	adrenocorticotropic hormone
ad to;	to; up to (*ad*)
a.d.	right ear (*aurio dextra*)
ADE	adverse drug experience
ADH	antidiuretic hormone
adhib	to be administered (*adhibendus*)
ad lib	as desired, at pleasure (*ad libitum*)
ADLs	activities of daily living
ADME	absorption, distribution, metabolism and elimination
admov	apply (*admove*)
ADP	adenosine diphosphate
ADR	adverse drug reaction
ADRRS	Adverse Drug Reaction Reporting System
ad sat	to saturation (*ad saturatum, ad saturandum*)
adst feb	when fever is present (*adstante febre*)
ad us.	ext for external use (*ad usum externum*)
adv	against (*adversum*)
aer	aerosol
Ag	antigen; silver (*argentum*)
agit. Ante us.	shake before using (*agita ante usum*)
agit. Bene	shake well (*agita bene*)
AHA	American Hospital Association
AID	artificial insemination donor
AIDS	acquired immunodeficiency syndrome
AJHP	*American Journal of Hospital Pharmacy*
al	left ear (*aurio laeva*)
ala	alanine
ALL	acute lymphocytic leukemia
ALT	alanine aminotransferase, serum (previously SGPT)
alt hor	every other hour (*alternis horis*)
A.M.	before noon; morning (*ante meridiem*)
AMA	American Medical Association
AML	acute myelogenous leukemia
AMP	adenosine monophosphate
ANA	antinuclear antibody(ies)
ANC	acid neutralizing capacity
ANDA	abbreviated new drug application
ANOVA	analysis of variance
ANUG	acute necrotizing ulcerative gingivitis
APA	antipernicious anemia (factor)
APAP	acetaminophen
APC	antigen presenting cell(s)
APhA	American Pharmaceutical Association
aPTT	activated partial thromboplastin time
aq	water (*aqua*)
aq. dest	distilled water (*aqua destillata*)
ARC	AIDS-related complex
ARDS	adult respiratory distress syndrome
ARF	acute renal failure
Arg	arginine
ARV	AIDS-related virus
as	left ear (*aurio sinister*)
ASHD	arteriosclerotic heart disease
ASHP	American Society of Hospital Pharmacists
Asn	asparagine
Asp	aspartic acid
AST	aspartate aminotransferase, serum (previously SGOT)
atm	standard atmosphere
ATN	acute tubular necrosis
ATP	adenosine triphosphate
ATPase	adenosine triphosphatase
ATPD	ambient temperature and pressure, saturated
at wt	atomic weight
au	each ear (*aures utrae*)
AU	gold (*aurum*)
AUC	area under the plasma concentration-time curve
AV	atrioventricular
A-V	arteriovenous; atrioventricular (block, bundle, conduction, dissociation, extrasystole)
AW	atomic weight
AWP	average wholesale price
ax.	axis
β	beta
BAC	blood-alcohol concentration
BADL	basic activities of daily life
BBB	blood brain barrier
BDZ	benzodiazepine
bib	drink (*bibe*)
bid	twice daily; two times a day (*bis in die*)
bm	bowel movement
BMR	basal metabolic rate
bp	boiling point
BP	blood pressure
BPH	benign prostatic hypertrophy
bpm	beats per minute
BSA	body surface area
BT	bleeding time
BUN	blood urea nitrogen
C	centigrade
C.	*clostridium*
c	gallon (*cong*)
c̄	with (*cum*)
°C	degrees Celsius

Abbreviation	Meaning
Ca	calcium
CA	cancer; carcinoma; cardiac arrest; chronologic age; croup-associated
CAD	coronary artery disease
Cal	Calorie (kilocalorie)
cAMP	cyclic adenosine monophosphate
caps	capsule (*capsula*)
CAS	Chemical Abstracts Service
CAT	computerized axial tomography
cath	catheterize
CBA	cost-benefit analysis
CBC	complete blood count
CC	chief complaint
cc	cubic centimeter
CCBs	calcium channel blockers
CCU	coronary care unit; critical care unit
CD4	T-helper lymphocytes and macrophages
CDC	Centers for Disease Control and Prevention
CEA	cost effectiveness analysis
CF	cystic fibrosis
CFC	chlorofluorocarbon
CFU	colony-forming units
CHD	coronary heart disease
CHF	congestive heart failure
Ci	curie
CK	creatinine kinase
Cl	chlorine
Cl_{cr}	creatinine clearance
cm	centimeter; cream
Cm	curium
cm^2	square centimeter(s)
cm^3	cubic centimeter
CMA	Certified Medical Assistant
CMC	carpometacarpal
CMI	cell-mediated immunity
CML	chronic myelocytic leukemia
C_{max}	maximum effective plasma concentration
C_{min}	minimum effective plasma concentration
CMT	Certified Medical Transcriptionist
CMV	cytomegalovirus I
CMVIG	cytomegalovirus immune globulin
CN	cranial nerve
CNM	Certified Nurse Midwife
CNS	central nervous system
CO	cardiac output
CO_2	carbon dioxide
CoA	coenzyme A
COG	center of gravity
comp	compound (*compositus*)
COMT	catecholamine-o-methyl transferase
cont rem	let the medicine be continued (*continuetur remedium*)
COPD	chronic obstructive pulmonary disease
CPAP	continuous positive airway pressure
CPK	creatine phosphokinase
CPR	cardiopulmonary resuscitation
CQI	continuous quality improvement
Cr	creatinine; chromium
CrCl	creatinine clearance
CRD	chronic respiratory disease
CRF	chronic renal failure
CRH	corticotropin-releasing hormone
crm	cream
CRNA	Certified Registered Nurse Anesthetist
C&S	culture and sensitivity
CSA	Controlled Substances Act; cyclosporin A
CSF	cerebrospinal fluid; colony-stimulating factors
CSP	cellulose sodium phosphate
ct	clotting time
CT	computerized tomography
CTZ	chemoreceptor trigger zone
cu	cubic
Cu	copper (*cuprum*)
CV	cardiovascular
CVA	cerebrovascular accident
CVP	central venous pressure
CXR	chest x-ray
cyl	cylinder; cylindrical (lens)
cys	cysteine
d	day (*dies*)
D5W	Dextrose 5% in Water Solution
D10W	Dextrose 10% in Water Solution
D&C	dilation and curettage; designation applied to dyes permitted for use in drugs and cosmetics
D&E	dilation and evacuation
DC	Doctor of Chiropractic
DDS	Doctor of Dental Surgery
DEA	Drug Enforcement Administration
deglut	swallow (*degluttiatur*)
DERM	dermatologic
det	give (*detur*)
DHHS	Department of Health and Human Services
DIC	disseminated intravascular coagulation
dieb alt	every other day (*diebus alternis*)
dil	dilute (*dilue*)
dim	one-half (*dimidius*)
dir prop	with proper direction (*directione propria*)
div in par aeq	divide into equal parts (*divide in partes aequales*)
DIS	drug information source
disp	dispense (*dispensa*)
div	divide
DJD	degenerative joint disease
DKA	diabetic ketoacidosis
dl	deciliter (100 ml)
DMD	Doctor of Dental Medicine
DMSO	dimethyl sulfoxide
DNA	deoxyribonucleic acid
DNR	do not resuscitate
DNS	Director of Nursing Service; Doctor of Nursing Services
DO	Doctor of Osteopathy
DOA	dead on arrival
DP	Doctor of Podiatry
DPH	Doctor of Public Health; Doctor of Public Hygiene
DPI	dry powder inhaler
DPM	Doctor of Physical Medicine; Doctor of Podiatric Medicine
DPS	disintegrations per second
DRG	diagnosis-related groups
DRI	Dietary Reference Intakes
drp	drop(s)
DrPh	Doctor of Public Health; Doctor of Public Hygiene
DRR	Drug Regimen Review
DT	delirium tremens
dtd	give of such a dose (*dentur tales doses*)
DTP	diphtheria, tetanus toxoids & pertussis vaccine
DTRs	deep tendon reflexes
DUB	dysfunctional uterine bleeding
DUE	Drug Usage Evaluations
DUR	Drug Utilization Review
dur dol	while pain lasts (*durante dolore*)
DVA	Department of Veterans Affairs
DVM	Doctor of Veterinary Medicine
DVT	deep venous thrombosis
E.	*Enterococcus; Escherichia*
EBV	Epstein-Barr virus

Abbreviation	Meaning
EC	enteric coated
ECG	electrocardiogram
ECT	electroconvulsive therapy
ed.	editor
ED	emergency department; effective dose
ED_{50}	median-effective dose
EDTA	ethylenediamine tetraacetic acid
EEG	electroencephalogram
EENT	eye, ear, nose, and throat
EF	ejection fraction
eg	for example (*exempli gratia*)
EIA	enzyme immunoassay
EKG	electrocardiogram
el	elixir
ELISA	enzyme-linked immunosorbent assay
elix	elixir
EMIT	enzyme-multiplied immunoassay test
emp	as directed
ENL	erythema nodosum leprosum
ENT	ear, nose, throat
EPA	Environmental Protection Agency
EPAP	expiratory positive airway pressure
EPO	erythropoietin
EPS	extrapyramidal syndrome (or symptoms)
ER	emergency room; estrogen receptor; extended release; endoplasmic reticulum
ESR	erythrocyte sedimentation rate; electron spin resonance
et	and
ET	via endotracheal tube
et al.	for 3 or more co-authors or co-workers (*et alii*)
ex aq	in water
ext rel	extended release
F	fluorine
f	make; let be made (*fac, fiat, fiant*)
°F	degrees Fahrenheit
Fab	fragment of immunoglobulin G involved in antigen binding
FAO	Food and Agriculture Organization
FAS	fetal alcohol syndrome
FBS	fasting blood sugar
FDA	Food and Drug Administration
FD&C	designation applied to dyes permitted for use in foods, drugs and cosmetics; Food, Drug and Cosmetic Act
Fe	iron (*ferrum*)
FEF	forced expiratory flow
FET	forced expiratory time
FEV_1	forced expiratory volume in 1 second
fl oz	fluid ounce(s)
Fru	fructose
FSH	follicle-stimulating hormone
ft	make; let be made (*fac, fiat, fiant*)
ft	foot (feet)
ft^2	square foot (feet)
FTC	Federal Trade Commission
FTI	free-thyroxine index
FUO	fever of unknown origin
FVC	forced vital capacity
γ	gamma
g	gram (*gramma*)
G-6-P	glucose-6-phosphate
G-6-PD	glucose-6-phosphate dehydrogenase
GABA	gamma-aminobutyric acid
Gal	galactose
gal	gallon
G-CSF	granulocyte colony-stimulating factor
GERD	gastroesophageal reflux disease
GFR	glomerular filtration rate
GGTP	gamma glutamyl transpeptidase
GH	growth hormone
GHRF	growth hormone-releasing factor
GHRH	growth hormone-releasing hormone
GI	gastrointestinal
GLC	gas-liquid chromatography
gln	glutamine
glu	glutamic acid; glutamyl
gly	glycine
Gm	gram (*gramma*)
gr	grain (*granum*)
grad	gradually (*gradatim*)
gran	granule(s)
GRAS	generally regarded as safe*
gtt	a drop (*gutta*)
GU	genitourinary
guttat	drop by drop (*guttatim*)
Gyn	gynecology
H.	*Haemophilus*; *Helicobacter*
h	hour (*hora*)
H_2	histamine 2
H_2O	water
HA	hyaluronic acid
Hb	hemoglobin
HbF	fetal hemoglobin
HBIG	hepatitis B immune specific globulin
HCFA	Health Care Financing Administration
HCG	human chorionic gonadotropin
HCl	hydrochloric acid
HCN	hydrogen cyanide
Hct	hematocrit
hd	bedtime (*hora decubitus*)
HDL	high-density lipoprotein
HEMA	hematologic
HEME	hematologic
hep	hepatic
HEPA	high efficiency particulate air
Hg	mercury (*hydragyrum*)
Hgb	hemoglobin
HGH	human pituitary growth hormone
Hib.	*Haemophilus influenzae*
His.	*Haemophilus influenzae* type b
HIV	human immunodeficiency virus
HLA	human leukocyte antigen
HMG-CoA	3-hydroxy-3-methylglutaryl coenzyme A
HMO	health maintenance organization
hor decub	at bedtime (*hora decubitus*)
hor som	at bedtime (*hora somni*)
HPA	hypothalamic-pituitary-adrenocortical (axis)
HPLC	high performance liquid chromatography
HPLC/MS	high performance liquid chromatography/mass spectrometry
HPMC	hydroxypropylmethylcellulose
HPV	human papillomavirus
HR	heart rate
hr	hour
hs	at bedtime (*hora somni*)
HSA	human serum albumin
HSV-1	herpes simplex virus type 1
HSV-2	herpes simplex virus type 2
Hz	hertz
I	iodine

Abbreviation	Meaning
IADL	instrumental activities of daily living
I/O	intake/output
IBW	ideal body weight
IC	intracoronary
ICD	International Classification of Diseases of the World Health Organization
ICF	intracellular fluid
ICP	intracranial pressure
ICU	intensive care unit
ID	intradermal; infective dose
IDDM	insulin-dependent diabetes mellitus (type 1 diabetes)
IDU	idoxuridine
IFN	interferon
Ig	immunoglobulin
IL	interleukin
Ile	isoleucine
IM	intramuscular
in	inch(es)
in^2	square inch(es)
IND	Investigational New Drug
in d	daily (*in dies*)
INDA	Investigational New Drug Application
Inh	inhaled
INH	isoniazid
Inhal	inhalation
Inj	injection
INR	International Normalizing Ratio
int cib	between meals (*inter cibos*)
IOP	intraocular pressure
IP	intraperitoneal(ly)
IPA	International Pharmaceutical Abstracts
IPPB	intermittent positive pressure breathing
IPV	poliovirus vaccine inactivated
IQ	intelligence quotient
ISA	intrinsic sympathomimetic activity
ISF	interstitial fluid
ISI	Institute for Scientific Information
ISO	International Organization for Standardization
IT	intrathecal(ly)
IU	international unit(s)
IUD	intrauterine device
IV	intravenous
IVF	intravascular fluid
IVP	intravenous piggyback
J	joule(s)

Abbreviation	Meaning
JCAH	Joint Commission on Accreditation of Hospitals
JCAHO	Joint Commission on Accreditation of Health-care Organizations
K	potassium (*kalium*); kelvin
kcal	kilocalorie(s)
keV	kiloelectronvolt(s)
kg	kilogram
kJ	kilojoule(s)
Kleb.	*Klebsiella*
KVO	keep vein open
L	liter
L.	*Legionella*; *Listeria*
lb	pound
LBW	low body weight
LD	lethal dose
LD-50	a dose lethal to 50% of the specified animals or microorganisms
LDH	lactate dehydrogenase
LDL	low-density lipoprotein
LE	lupus erythematosus
Leu	leucine
LFT	liver function test
LH	luteinizing hormone
liq	liquid (*liquor*)
LM	Licentiate in Midwifery
LOC	level of consciousness
Lot	lotion
LPN	Licensed Practical Nurse
Lr	lawrencium
LSD	lysergic acid diethylamide
LTCF	long-term care facility
LTM	long-term memory
LUQ	left upper quadrant (of abdomen)
LVEDP	left ventricular end-diastolic pressure
LVET	left ventricular ejection time
LVF	left ventricular function
LVN	Licensed Visiting Nurse; Licensed Vocational Nurse
LVP	large-volume parenterals
Lw	former symbol for lawrencium (see Lr)
Lys	lysine
μm	micrometer
μg	microgram
m	meter
M	mix (*misce*)
M	molar (strength of a solution)
M.	*Moraxella*; *Mycobacterium*; *Mycoplasma*
m^2	square meter (of body surface area)
m^3	cubic meter(s)

Abbreviation	Meaning
MA	mental age
MAC	maximum allowable cost
MADD	Mothers Against Drunk Drivers
man pr	early morning; first thing in the morning (*mane primo*)
MAO	monoamine oxidase
MAOI	monoamine oxidase inhibitor
MAP	mean arterial pressure
max	maximum
MBC	minimum bactericidal concentration
MBD	minimal brain dysfunction
mcg	microgram
MCH	mean corpuscular hemoglobin
MCHC	mean corpuscular hemoglobin concentration
mCi	millicurie
MCT	medium-chain triglyceride
MCV	mean corpuscular volume
MD	Doctor of Medicine (*Medicinae Doctor*)
MDI	metered dose inhaler
m dict	as directed (*more dictor*)
MDR	minimum daily requirements
MEC	minimum effective concentration
MEDLARS	Medical Literature Analysis and Retrieval System
MEDLINE	National Library of Medicine medical database
mEq	milliequivalent
Met	methionine
MeV	megaelectronvolt(s)
Mg	magnesium
mg	milligram
MHC	major histocompatibility complex
MI	myocardial infarction
MIA	metabolite bacterial inhibition assay
MIC	minimum inhibitory concentration
MID	minimal infecting dose
min	minute
min.	minimum
MIP	maximum inspiratory pressure
mixt	a mixture (*mixtura*)
MJ	mejajoule(s)
ml	milliliter
mm	millimeter
mm^2	square millimeter(s)
mm^3	cubic millimeter(s)
mmHg	millimeters of mercury
mmol	millimole

Abbreviation	Meaning
MMR	measles, mumps and rubella virus vaccine, live
MMWR	*Morbidity and Mortality Weekly Report*
Mn	manganese
Mo	molybdenum
mo	month
mol	mole(s)
mor dict	in the manner stated (*more dicto*)
mor sol	as usual; as customary (*more solito*)
mOsm	milliosmole
MPH	Master of Public Health
MRI	magnetic resonance imaging
mRNA	messenger RNA
MS	mass spectrometry; mitral stenosis; multiple sclerosis
MW	molecular weight
N	normal (strength of a solution)
N.	*Neisseria*
Na	sodium (*natrium*)
NABP	National Association of Boards of Pharmacy
NABPLEX	National Association of Boards of Pharmacy Licensing Exam
NAD	nicotinamide-adenine dinucleotide phosphate
NADH	reduced form of nicotine adenine dinucleotide
NADP	nicotinamide-adenine dinucleotide phosphate
NADPH	nicotinamide-adenine dinucleotide phosphate (reduced form)
NAPA	*N*-acetyl procainamide
NARD	National Association of Retail Druggists - Now NCPA; National Assoc. of Community Pharmacists
nb	note well (*nota bene*)
nCi	nanocurie(s)
NCPA	National Assoc. of Community Pharmacists
ND	Doctor of Naturopathic Medicine
NDA	new drug application
NF	National Formulary
ng	nanogram
NG	nasogastric
NK	natural killer (cells); killer T cells
NIDDM	non-insulin dependent diabetes mellitus (type 2 diabetes)
NIH	National Institutes of Health
NLM	National Library of Medicine
nm	nanometer(s)
NMS	neuroleptic malignant syndrome
NMT	not more than (on prescriptions)
no	number (*numerus*)
noc	in the night (*nocturnal*)
noc maneq	at night and the morning (*nocte maneque*)
non rep	do not repeat; no refills (*non repetatur*)
NPN	nonprotein nitrogen
NPO	nothing by mouth
NS	normal saline (as in solution)
NSAIA	nonsteroidal anti-inflammatory agent
NSAID	nonsteroidal anti-inflammatory drug
NTD	neutral tube defect
O	a pint (*octarius*)
OB/GYN	obstetrics and gynecology
OBRA	Omnibus Budget Reconciliation Act of 1990
OBS	organic brain syndrome
OC	oral contraceptive
Oct	a pint (*octarius*)
od	right eye (*oculus dexter*)
OD	Doctor of Optometry; overdose
Oint	ointment
ol	left eye (*oculus laevus*)
omn hor	at every hour (*omni hora*)
Ophth	ophthalmic
os	left eye (*oculus sinister*)
OSHA	Occupational Safety and Health Administration
OT	occupational therapy
otc	over-the-counter (nonprescription)
OPV	oral poliovirus vaccine, live
ou	each eye (*oculo uterque*)
o/w	oil-in-water (emulsion)
oz	ounce
P	phosphorus
P	probability
P&T	pharmacy and therapeutics (committee)
Pa	pascal(s)
PA	Physician Assistant; Physician's Assistant
PABA	para-aminobenzoic acid
PAC	premature atrial contraction
$PaCO_2$	arterial plasma partial pressure of carbon dioxide
PAD	premature atrial depolarization
PAF	platelet-activating factor
PaO_2	partial alveolar oxygen
part aeq	equal parts/amounts (*partes aequales*)
part vic	in divided doses (*partitis vicibus*)
PAS	para-aminosalicylic acid
PAW	pulmonary arterial wedge
PAWP	pulmonary artery wedge pressure
Pb	lead (*plumbum*)
PBP	penicillin-binding protein
pc	after meals (*post cibum; post cibos*)
PCA	patient-controlled analgesia
pCO_2	plasma partial pressure of carbon dioxide
PCP	phencyclidine
PCR	polymerase chain reaction
PDGF	platelet-derived growth factor
PDLL	poorly differentiated lymphocytic lymphoma
PE	pulmonary embolism
PEEP	positive end expiratory pressure
PEG	polyethylene glycol
PERLA	pupils equal, react to light and accommodation
PET	positron emission tomography
pg	picogram(s)
PG	prostaglandin
PGA	prostaglandin A
PGB	prostaglandin B
PGE	prostaglandin E
PGF	prostaglandin F
pH	the negative logarithm of the hydrogen ion concentration
PharmD	Doctor of Pharmacy (*Pharmaciae Doctor*)
PhD	Doctor of Philosophy (*Philosophiae Doctor*)
Phe	phenylalanine
PhG	German Pharmacopeia (*Pharmacopoeia Germanica*)
PHS	Public Health Service
pKa	the negative logarithm of the dissociation constant
PKU	phenylketonuria
PMA	Pharmaceutical Manufacturers Association
PMN	polymorphonuclear leukocyte
PMR	patient medication record
PMS	premenstrual syndrome
PND	paroxysmal nocturnal dyspnea
po	by mouth; orally (*per os*)
pO_2	oxygen pressure (tension)

Abbreviation	Meaning
POR	problem-oriented medical record
POS	point of service
post cib	after meals (*post cibos*)
PPD	purified protein derivative of tuberculin
PPI	patient package insert
ppm	parts per million
PPO	preferred provider organization
pr	per rectum
Pr.	*Proteus*
prn	as needed; when required (*pro re nata*)
Pro	proline
pro rat. Aet.	According to patient's age (*pro ratione aetatis*)
Ps.	*Pseudomonas*
PSA	prostate-specific antigen
PSP	phenolsulfonphthalein
PSVT	paroxysmal supraventricular tachycardia
pt	pint
PT	prothrombin time; pharmacy and therapeutics; physical therapy
PTH	parathyroid hormone
PTT	partial thromboplastin time
PUD	peptic ulcer disease
pulv	a powder (*pulvis*)
PUVA	oral administration of psoralen and subsequent exposure to ultraviolet light of A wavelengths (UVA)
PVC	premature ventricular contraction; polyvinyl chloride
PVD	peripheral vascular disease; premature ventricular depolarizations
pwdr	powder
q	every
Q	volume of blood flow
QA	quality assurance
qad	every other day (*quoque alternis die*)
QC	quality control
qd	every day (*quaque die*)
qh	every hour (*quaque hora*)
q hr	every hour
qid	four times daily (*quarter in die*)
ql	as much as desired (*quantum libet*)
qod	every other day
q 2 hr	every 2 hours
qs	a sufficient quantity (*quantum sufficiat*)
qs	as much as is enough (*quantum satis*)
qs ad	a sufficient quantity to make
qt	quart
qv	as much as you wish (*quam volueris*)
R&D	research and development
RA	rheumatoid arthritis
RAI	radioactive iodine
RAS	renin-angiotension system; reticular-activating system
RAST	radioallergosorbent test
RBC	red blood (cell) count
RDA	Recommended Dietary (Daily) Allowance
RDS	respiratory distress syndrome
RDW	red-cell distribution width
RE	reticuloendothelial
rem	radio equivalent man
REM	rapid eye movement
rep	let it be repeated (*repetatur*)
RES	reticuloendothelial system
RF	releasing factor
Rh	Rhesus (RH blood group)
RIA	radioimmunoassay
RN	Registered Nurse
RNA	ribonucleic acid
ROM	range of motion
RPh	registered pharmacist
rpm	revolutions per minute
rps	revolutions per second
RR	respiratory rate
RT_3U	total serum thyroxine concentration
RUL	right upper lobe (of lung)
RUQ	right upper quadrant (of abdomen)
Rx	prescription only; take; a recipe (*recipe*)
S.	*Salmonella*; *Serratia*
s	second
s	without (*sine*)
$\bar{s}$	without (*sine*)
S&S	signs and symptoms
S-A	sinoatrial
sa	according to art (*secundum artem*)
sat	saturated (*sataratus*)
Sb	antimony (*stibium*)
SBE	self breast examination; subacute bacterial endocarditis
SC	subcutaneous(ly)
S_{cr}	serum creatinine
SD	standard deviation; streptodornase
Se	selenium
sec	second
Ser	serine
sf	sugar free
SGGT	serum gamma-glutamyl transferase
SGOT	(see AST)
SGPT	(see ALT)
Sh.	*Shigella*
SIADH	syndrome of inappropriate secretion of antidiuretic hormone
SIDS	sudden infant death syndrome
Sig	label; let it be printed (*signa*)
SI units	International System of Units
SK	streptokinase
SL	sublingual(ly)
SLE	systemic lupus erythematosus
SMA	sequential multiple analysis
Sn	tin (*stannum*)
SNF	skilled nursing facility
sol	solution (*solutio*)
soln	solution
solv	dissolve
sp	species
SPECT	single photon emission computerized tomography
sp gr	specific gravity
SPF	sun protection factor
sq	square
SR	sedimentation rate; sustained-release
ss	one-half (*semis*)
$\bar{s}\bar{s}$	one-half (*semis*)
SSRI	selective serotonin reuptake inhibitors
Staph.	*Staphylococcus*
stat	immediately; at once (*statim*)
STM	short-term memory
STP	standard temperature and pressure
Str.	*Streptococcus*
STD	sexually transmitted disease
supp	suppository (*suppositorium*)
suppl	supplement(s)
susp	suspension
SV	stroke volume
syr	syrup (*syrupus*)
$t_{1/2}$	half-life
T_3	triiodothyronine
T_4	thyroxine
tab	tablet (*tabella*)
tal	such
tal dos	such doses

Abbreviation	Meaning
TB	tuberculosis
TBC	thyroxine-binding globulin
TBP	thyroxine-binding proteins
TBPA	thyroxine-binding pre-albumin
TBW	total body weight
TCA	tricyclic antidepressant
TD_{50}	median toxic dose
TEEC	transesophageal echocardiography
TEN	toxic epidermal necrolysis
TENS	transcutaneous electrical nerve stimulation
TG	total triglycerides
THC	tetrahydrocannabinol
Thr	threonine
TIA	transient ischemic attack
tid	three times daily (*ter in die*)
tbsp	tablespoonful
tinct	tincture
TLC	total lung capacity; thin layer chromatography
T_{max}	time to maximum concentration
TMJ	temporomandibular joint
TNF	tumor necrosis factor
TNM	tumor, node, metastasis (tumor staging)
top	topical(ly)
TOPV	trivalent oral polio vaccine
tPA	tissue plasminogen activator
TPN	total parenteral nutrition
TPR	temperature, pulse, respirations
TQM	total quality management
tr	tincture
trit	triturate (*tritura*)
tRNA	transfer RNA
Trp	tryptophan
TSA	tumor-specific antigens
TSH	thyroid-stimulating hormone
tsp	teaspoonful
TSS	toxic shock syndrome
TSTA	tumor-specific transplantation antigen
TT	thrombin time
TV	tidal volume
Tyr	tyrosine
U	unit
ud	as directed
UD	unit-dose package
UK	United Kingdom
ung	ointment (*unguentum*)
URI	upper respiratory infection
USAN	United States Adopted Name(s)
USP	*United States Pharmacopeia*
USPHS	United States Public Health Service
ut dict	as directed (*ut dictum*)
UTI	urinary tract infection
UVA	ultraviolet A wave
V	volt
VA	Veterans Administration
vag	vaginal(ly)
Val	valine
var	variety
VC	vital capacity
V_c	volume of distribution of the central compartment
V_d	volume of distribution (one compartment)
$V_{d\beta}$	volume of distribution of the β phase
V_{dss}	steady-state apparent volume of distribution
VHDL	very high density lipoprotein
VLDL	very low density lipoprotein
VMA	vanillylmandelic acid
vol	volume
VS	vital signs
v/v	volume in volume
v/w	volume in weight
wa	while awake
WBC	white blood (cell) count
WBCT	whole blood clotting time
WDLL	well-differentiated lymphocytic lymphoma
WFI	water for injection
WHO	World Health Organization
wk	week
WNL	within normal limits
w/o	water in oil
wt	weight
w/v	weight in volume
w/w	weight in weight
yo	years old
yr	year
ZE	Zollinger-Ellison
Zn	zinc

MANUFACTURER/DISTRIBUTOR ABBREVIATIONS

This listing includes only those manufacturers whose names are abbreviated in *Drug Facts and Comparisons*®. It is not a complete list of all manufacturers whose products are listed in this book.

B-D	Becton, Dickinson & Co.
B-I	Boehringer Ingelheim
B-Mannheim	Boehringer Mannheim
B-M Squibb	Bristol-Myers Squibb
Hickam	Dow B. Hickam
Inter. Ethical	International Ethical Labs
IMS	International Medication Systems
J & J	Johnson & Johnson
McNeil-CPC	McNeil Consumer Products Company
Mead-J	Mead Johnson Nutritional
Merck	Merck & Co.
P-D	Parke-Davis
PBH	PBH Wesley Jessen
P & G	Procter & Gamble
RPR	Rhone-Poulenc Rorer
Schwarz Pharma K-U	Schwarz Pharma Inc.
SK-Beecham, SKB	SmithKline Beecham
URL	United Research Labs
Warner-C	Warner Chilcott
Warner-L	Warner-Lambert
W-A	Wyeth-Ayerst

40985
21ST CENTURY HEALTHCARE
480-966-8201
800-530-2178
http://www.21stcenturyvitamins.com

48878
3M ESPE DENTAL PRODUCTS
651-575-5144
800-634-2248
http://www.3m.com

00089
3M PHARMACEUTICALS
See Graceway Pharmaceuticals, LLC

17518
3M SURGICAL/MEDICAL
800-228-3957
651-733-1110
http://www.3m.com

42549
4UORTHO
888-316-7846
http://www.4udr.com

63801
7 OAKS PHARMACEUTICAL CORP
864-850-1700
http://www.7oakspharma.com

93764
A & D MEDICAL
408-263-5333
888-726-9966
http://www.andmedical.com

18754
A AARONS
973-882-1505
http://www.bradpharm.com

12539
AG MARIN PHARMACEUTICALS
305-593-5333
800-241-4603

A.H. ROBINS CONSUMER PRODUCTS
See Wyeth Consumer Health

A.H. ROBINS INC.
See Wyeth Consumer Health

A.L. LABS
See King Pharmaceuticals, Inc.

A.P. PHARMA, INC.
650-366-2626
http://www.appharma.com

66591
AAI PHARMA
910-254-7350
800-575-4224
http://www.aaipharma.com

50483
AAPER ALCOHOL & CHEMICAL CO.
502-232-7600
800-456-1017
http://www.pharmcoaaper.com

AASTROM BIOSCIENCES, INC.
734-930-5555

60793
ABANA PHARMACEUTICALS, INC.
See King Pharmaceuticals, Inc.

ABBOTT DIABETES CARE
510-749-5400
888-298-4584
http://www.therasense.com

ABBOTT LABORATORIES
847-937-6100
800-323-9100
http://www.abbott.com

ABBOTT HOSPITAL PRODUCTS
224-212-2000
800-615-0187
http://www.hospira.com

00074
ABBOTT LABORATORIES PHARMACEUTICAL DIVISION
847-937-6100
800-255-5162
http://www.abbott.com

ABBOTT MEDICAL OPTICS
714-247-8200
866-427-8477
http://www.amo-inc.com

ABBOTT NUTRITION
614-624-3191
800-986-8510
http://www.abbottnutrition.com

ABGENIX
See Amgen

63323
ABRAXIS BIOSCIENCE
310-883-1300
http://www.abraxisbio.com

68817
ABRAXIS ONCOLOGY
908-393-8220
http://www.abraxisbio.com

AB SCIENCE
33-1-47-20-10-35

ACADEMIC PHARMACEUTICALS, INC.
847-735-1170

42907
ACCERA, INC.
303-999-3700
877-649-0004
http://www.accerapharma.com

ACCESS DIABETIC SUPPLY
954-975-0036
800-715-5031
http://www.diabeticsupply.com

67404
ACCESS PHARMACEUTICALS
214-905-5100
http://www.accesspharma.com

16729
ACCORD HEALTHCARE
866-941-7875

ACCUMED
609-883-1818
http://www.accumed.org

25356
ACETO PHARMA
516-627-6000
http://www.aceto.com

00924
ACME UNITED CORP.
203-332-7330
800-835-2263
http://www.acmeunited.com

10144
ACORDA THERAPEUTICS
914-347-4300
800-367-5109
http://www.acorda.com

ACTAVIS
973-993-4500
800-432-8534
http://www.actavis.us

ACTAVIS ELIZABETH
973-993-4500
800-432-8534
http://www.actavis.com

ACTAVIS SOUTH ATLANTIC
973-993-4500
800-432-8534
http://www.actavis.us

ACTAVIS TOTOWA
973-993-4500
800-432-8534
http://www.actavis.us

66215
ACTELION PHARMACEUTICALS US, INC.
650-624-6900
866-228-3546
http://www.actelionus.com

ACURA PHARMACEUTICALS, INC.
847-705-7709
http://www.acurapharm.com

ACURA PHARMACEUTICALS TECHNOLOGIES
574-842-3305
http://www.acurapharm.com

38739
ADAMIS LABORATORIES, INC.
800-223-6837
561-208-2200

63824
ADAMS RESPIRATORY THERAPEUTICS
See Reckitt Benckiser Pharmaceuticals

ADHEREX TECHNOLOGIES, INC.
919-484-8484
http://www.adherex.com

ADOLOR
484-595-1500
866-423-6567
http://www.adolor.com

ADRIA LABORATORIES
See Pfizer US Pharmaceutical Group

ADVANCE BIOFACTURES CORP. BIOSPECIFICS TECHNOLOGIES
516-593-7000
http://www.biospecifics.com

17714
ADVANCE
631-981-4600
http://www.advancepharm.com

08541
ADVANCED BIOHEALING
877-422-4463
858-754-3700
http://www.abh.com

ADVANCED BIOTHERAPY, INC.
818-883-6716

55495
ADVANCED MEDICAL ENTERPRISES
787-436-0666
http://www.ameinc.org

ADVANCED MEDICAL OPTICS
See Abbott Medical Optics

10888
ADVANCED NUTRITIONAL TECHNOLOGY
925-828-2128
800-624-6543
http://www.advancenutritionaltech.com

58790
ADVANCED VISION RESEARCH
781-932-8327
800-579-8327
http://www.theratears.com

11042
ADVANCIS PHARMACEUTICAL CORPORATION
See MiddleBrook Pharmaceuticals

ADVANTAGENE
617-916-5445

ADVENTRX PHARMACEUTICALS
858-552-0866
http://www.adventrx.com

AEOLUS PHARMACEUTICALS, INC.

66440
AERO PHARMACEUTICALS INC
See Adamis Laboratories, Inc.

AEROVANCE, INC.
510-549-5500

AETERNA ZENTARIS, INC.
418-652-8525

00213
AFFEMANN IMPORTS, INC
818-348-7767
http://www.affemannimports.com

10572
AFFORDABLE PHARMACEUTICALS
781-848-3062
http://www.affordablepharm.com

08554
AGAMATRIX
603-328-6000
http://www.agamatrix.com

AGENNIX, INC.

60336
AGI DERMATICS
800-590-4244
516-868-9026
http://www.agiderm.com

AGOURON PHARMACEUTICALS
See Pfizer US Pharmaceutical Group

62584, 68084
AHP
800-707-4621
614-492-8177
http://www.healthpak.com

38206
AID-PACK USA
See NutraMax Products

51709
AIMSCO/DELTA HI-TECH
801-263-0975
http://www.deltahitechinc.com

59196
AIRPHARMA
913-498-0700
http://www.air-pharma.com

17478, 11098
AKORN, INC.
800-932-5676
847-279-6100
http://www.akorn.com

23360
AKORN STRIDES
847-279-6100
800-932-5676
http://www.akorn.com

41383
AKPHARMA
609-645-6100
800-994-4711
http://www.akpharma.com

AKRIMAX PHARMACEUTICALS
908-372-0506
888-383-1733
http://www.akrimax.com

65162
AKYMA PHARMACEUTICALS
See Amneal Pharmaceuticals

68322
ALAMO PHARMACEUTICALS, LLC
See Avanir Pharmaceuticals

68220
ALAVEN PHARMACEUTICAL, LLC
888-317-0001
800-333-7343
http://www.alavenpharm.com

22400
ALBERTO CULVER
708-450-3000
800-333-6666
http://www.alberto.com

20993
ALCON LABORATORIES, INC.
817-293-0450
800-862-5266
http://www.alcon.com

00065, 08065
ALCON SURGICAL
817-293-0450
800-862-5266
http://www.alcon.com

00065
ALCON VISION
817-293-0450
800-862-5266
http://www.alcon.com

43234
ALETHEIA
601-667-3584
http://www.altheialabs.com

25682
ALEXION PHARMACEUTICALS
203-272-2596
http://www.alxn.com

08514
ALIGN PHARMACEUTICALS
908-834-0960
http://www.alignpharma.com

56121, 66177
ALIGON PHARMACEUTICALS
205-663-0521
http://www.aligoninc.com

ALIMENTARY HEALTH, LTD.

68611
ALIMERA SCIENCES
678-990-5740
http://www.alimerasciences.com

38697
ALK ABELLO
800-325-7354
512-251-0037
http://www.alk-abello.us

ALK LABORATORIES, INC.
See ALK Abello

67575
ALKERMES
781-609-6000
http://www.alkermes.com

43351
ALLAIRE PHARMACEUTICALS
732-974-6300
414-434-6617

13279
ALLAN PHARMACEUTICAL, LLC.
215-441-9546
877-743-5858
http://www.allanpharmaceutical.com

ALLEGIS PHARMACEUTICALS
601-859-0038
866-468-2419

ALLEN & HANBURYS
See GlaxoSmithKline

ALLENDALE PHARMACEUTICALS, INC.
212-813-2171
888-343-4499
http://www.allendalepharm.com

ALLERCREME
See Carme, Inc.

ALLERDERM LABORATORIES, INC.
800-365-6868
http://www.allerderm.com

00023
ALLERGAN DERMATOLOGICS
714-246-4500
800-347-4500

11980
ALLERGAN, INC.
714-246-4500
800-377-7790
http://www.allergan.com

99965
ALLERGAN OPTICAL
800-433-8871
714-246-4500
http://www.allergan.com

ALLERGY LABORATORIES, INC.
405-235-1451
800-654-3971
http://www.allergylabs.com

49343
ALLERMED
858-292-1060
800-221-2748
http://www.allermed.com

ALLERQUEST
512-251-0037
800-325-7354
http://www.allerquest.com

17355
ALLIANCE LABS
602-276-3434
888-273-9734
http://www.enemeez.com

ALLIANCE PHARMACEUTICAL CORP.
858-410-5200

08462
ALLIANCE TECH MEDICAL
817-326-3183
800-848-8923
http://www.alliancetechmedical.com

68188
ALLIANT PHARMACEUTICALS, INC.
770-817-4500
http://www.alliantpharma.com

ALLIED PHARMACY
817-226-5050

86227
ALLISON MEDICAL
303-795-1618
800-886-1618
http://www.allisonmedical.com

ALLOS THERAPEUTICS
303-426-6262
888-255-6788
http://www.allos.com

54569
ALLSCRIPTS, INC.
847-680-3515
800-654-0889
http://www.allscripts.com

77379, 00311
ALMAY, INC.
919-603-2953
800-992-5629
http://www.almay.com

ALPHA 1 BIOMEDICALS, INC.
See Arriva Pharmaceuticals, Inc.

49669
ALPHA THERAPEUTIC CORP.
See Grifols USA, Inc.

59743
ALPHAGEN LABORATORIES, INC.
770-475-8973

00228
ALPHARMA PUREPAC PHARMACEUTICALS
See Actavis Elizabeth

63857
ALPHARMA USPD, INC.
See King Pharmaceuticals, Inc.

59390
ALTAIRE
631-722-5988
800-258-2471
http://www.otcdruggist.com

ALTANA INC.
973-236-9162
800-645-9833
http://www.altana.com

ALTERNA LLC
973-946-7550
http://www.alternallc.com

91717
ALTERNATIVA NATURAL
631-231-2322
http://www.altnatural.com

00731
ALTO PHARMACEUTICALS, INC.
813-968-0522
800-330-2891
http://www.altopharm.com

ALTUS PHARMA
617-299-2900
888-258-2532

72959
ALVA-AMCO PHARMACAL COS, INC.
847-663-0700
800-792-2582
http://www.alva-amco.com

47781
ALVOGEN
973-796-3400
http://www.alvogen.com

ALWYN CO., INC.

17314
ALZA CORP.
650-564-5000
800-634-8977
http://www.alza.com

AMARILLO BIOSCIENCES, INC.

00187
AMARIN PHARMACEUTICALS
See Valeant

66870
AMBI PHARMACEUTICALS, INC.
352-797-5227

10038
AMBIX LABORATORIES
973-890-9002
http://www.ambixlabs.com

AMCON LABORATORIES
314-961-5758
800-255-6161
http://www.amconlabs.com

61972
AMEND DRUG AND CHEMICAL CORPORATION
See Ruger Chemical Co.

AMERICAN BIOSCIENCE, INC.
See Abraxis Bioscience

AMERICAN DERMAL CORP.
See Sanofi-Aventis U.S.

62584
AMERICAN HEALTH PACKAGING
614-492-8177
800-707-4621
http://www.americanhealthpackaging.com

00008
AMERICAN HOME PRODUCTS
See Wyeth

73930
AMERICAN INTERNATIONAL INDUST
323-728-2999
800-621-9585
http://www.aiibeauty.com

AMERICAN LECITHIN COMPANY
203-262-7100
800-364-4416
http://www.americanlecithin.com

AMERICAN MEDICAL INDUSTRIES
605-428-5501

63323
AMERICAN PHARMACEUTICAL PARTNERS, INC.
See APP Pharmaceutical

52769
AMERICAN RED CROSS (NATIONAL HEADQUARTERS)
202-303-5214
800-733-2767
http://www.redcross.org

00517
AMERICAN REGENT, INC.
631-924-4000
800-645-1706
http://www.americanregent.com

41520
AMERICAN SALES COMPANY
716-686-7000
http://www.americansalescompany.net

63921
AMERIDERM LABORATORIES, INC.
973-279-5100
800-455-7211
http://www.ameriderm.com

AMERIFIT BRANDS, INC.
860-894-1285
800-722-3476
http://www.amerifit.com

62852
AMERILAB TECHNOLOGIES
763-525-1262
http://www.amerilabtech.com

AMERISOURCEBERGEN
610-727-7000
800-829-3132
http://www.amerisourcebergen.com

AMERSHAM HEALTH
44-0-1494-544000

61470
AMERX HEALTH CARE CORP.
727-443-0530
800-448-9599
http://www.amerigel.com

55513
AMGEN, INC.
805-447-1000
800-772-6436
http://www.amgen.com

AMICUS THERAPEUTICS, INC.
609-662-2000

52152
AMIDE PHARMACAL
See Actavis Totowa

65162
AMNEAL PHARMACEUTICALS
270-629-2956
866-525-7270
http://www.amneal.com

00548
AMPHASTAR PHARMACEUTICALS, INC.
800-423-4136
http://www.amphastar.com

AMPLIMED CORP.
520-529-1000
http://www.Amplimed.com

00402
AMSCO SCIENTIFIC
See Steris Corp.

68883
AMSINO MEDICAL USA
866-482-1345
http://www.amsinomedusa.com

66780
AMYLIN PHARMACEUTICALS
858-552-2200
http://www.amylin.com

ANABOLIC INC.
949-863-0340
800-445-6849
http://www.anaboliclabs.com

ANAQUEST
See Baxter Healthcare Corporation

10370
ANCHEN PHARMACEUTICALS, INC.
949-837-6178
888-837-6178
http://www.anchen.com

19100
ANDREW JERGENS CO.
See Kao Brands Company

ANDRULIS PHARMACEUTICAL CORP.
301-419-2400
301-767-1900

ANDRULIS RESEARCH CORP.
301-767-1900

62022
ANDRX LABORATORIES, INC.
See Shionogi Pharma, Inc.

62037
ANDRX PHARMACEUTICALS, INC.
954-382-7600
800-621-7143
http://www.andrx.com

28000
ANESIVA
650-624-9600
http://www.anesiva.com

ANGELINI PHARMACEUTICALS, INC.
201-476-9000

65974
ANGIODYNAMICS
518-798-1215
800-772-6446
http://www.angiodynamics.com

ANGIOGEN PHARMACEUTICALS PTY., LTD.

ANI PHARMACEUTICALS
218-634-3500
800-434-1121
http://www.anipharmaceuticals.com

ANIKA THERAPEUTICS
781-932-6616
http://www.anikatherapeutics.com

65781
ANIMAS DIABETES
610-644-8990
877-767-7373
http://www.animascorp.com

ANORMED, INC.
604-530-1057

70907, 14613, 71483
ANSELL HEALTHCARE, INC.
732-345-5400
http://www.ansell.com

55948
ANTARES PHARMA
610-458-6200
http://www.antarespharma.com

ANTHRA PHARMACEUTICALS, INC.
609-514-1060

ANTIBODIES, INC.
530-758-4400
800-824-8540
http://www.antibodiesinc.com

ANTIGENICS INC.
212-994-8200
http://www.antigenics.com

ANTISOMA PLC
44-0-20-8799-8200

ANTISOMA RESEARCH, LTD.
44-2-20-8799-8200

ATRIX LABORATORIES, INC.
970-482-5868
http://www.atrixlabs.com

23601
APEX-CAREX HEALTHCARE PRODUCTS
800-328-2935 (Apex)
800-526-8051 (Carex)
http://www.apex-carex.com

APHTON CORP.
305-374-7338

52380, 18407
APLICARE INC.
203-630-0500
800-760-3236
http://www.aplicare.com

60505
APOTEX
954-384-8007
800-706-5575
http://www.apotexcorp.com

APOTHECA
602-252-5244
800-262-5244

25715
APOTHECARY PRODUCTS, INC.
952-890-1940
800-328-2742
http://www.apothecaryproducts.com

APOTHECON, INC. (BRISTOL-MYERS SQUIBB)
See Bristol-Myers Squibb Co.

48723, 52925
APOTHECUS PHARMACEUTICAL CORP.
516-624-8200
800-227-2393
http://www.apothecus.com

APP PHARMACEUTICAL
847-969-2700
888-391-6300
http://www.appdrugs.com

APPLIED ANALYTICAL INDUSTRIES
910-254-7000
800-575-4224
http://www.aaipharma.com

APPLIED BIOTECH, INC.
858-587-6771
800-257-9525
http://www.abiapogent.com

92896
APPLIED DIABETES RESEARCH
972-241-1884
800-304-7293
http://www.applieddiabetesresearch.org

APPLIED GENETICS INC. DERMATICS
516-868-9026
http://www.agiderm.com

APPLIED IMMUNOTHERAPEUTICS, LLC

00847
APPLIED NUTRITION CORPORATION
973-734-0023
800-605-0410
http://www.medicalfood.com

16110
AQUA PHARMACEUTICALS
610-644-7000
http://www.aquapharm.com

13310
AR SCIENTIFIC
215-807-1029
877-960-2400
http://www.arscientific.com

ARADIGM CORP.
510-265-9000
http://www.aradigm.com

24338
ARBOR PHARMACEUTICALS
678-334-2420
866-516-4950
http://www.arborphama.com

90401
ARCHON
800-349-1700
http://www.archonvitamin.com

74312
ARCO PHARMACEUTICALS, INC.
See Natures Bounty

ARCOLA LABORATORIES
See Sanofi-Aventis U.S.

ARGINOX PHARMACEUTICALS
888-274-6070

ARIAD PHARMACEUTICALS, INC.
617-494-0400
http://www.ariad.com

24486
ARISTOS PHARMACEUTICALS
866-280-5755
http://www.aristospharm.com

ARK THERAPEUTICS, LTD.
44-20-7388-7722

08317
ARKRAY USA
952-646-3200
800-818-8877
http://www.arkrayusa.com

ARMOUR PHARMACEUTICAL
See CSL Behring

ARRIVA PHARMACEUTICALS, INC.
510-337-1250
http://www.arrivapharm.com

ARROW INTERNATIONAL CORP. HEADQUARTERS
610-378-0131
800-523-8446
http://www.arrowintl.com

ARTIELLE IMMUNOTHERAPEUTICS
503-626-1144
http://www.artielle.com

12870
ARZOL
603-352-5242

65557
ASAFI PHARMACEUTICAL
661-294-9509
http://www.asafi.com

67877
ASCEND LABORATORIES
201-476-1977
http://www.ascendlaboratories.com

17139
ASCEND THERAPEUTICS
703-471-4744
http://www.ascendtherapeutics.com

99207
ASCENT PEDIATRICS, INC.
See Medicis Pharmaceutical Corporation

46698
ASO LLC
941-379-0300
800-966-8066
http://www.asocorp.com

ASTELLAS PHARMA US, INC.
847-317-8800
800-888-7704
http://www.us.astellas.com

00186
ASTRAZENECA LP
302-886-3000
800-456-3669
http://www.astrazeneca-us.com

38488
ATHENA FEMININE TECHNOLOGIES
866-308-4436
http://www.athenaft.com

59075
ATHENA NEUROSCIENCES, INC.
See Elan Pharmaceuticals

66813
ATHLON PHARMACEUTICALS, INC.
205-986-1111
http://www.athlonpharm.com

59702
ATLEY PHARMACEUTICALS, INC.
804-227-2250
http://www.atley.com

25010
ATON PHARMA
609-671-9010
877-286-6549
http://www.atonrx.com

62107
AUBURN PHARMACEUTICAL
800-222-5609
248-526-3700
http://www.auburnpharm.com

14629
AURIGA PHARMACEUTICALS, INC.
678-282-1600
866-367-8796
http://www.aurigalabs.com

AURIS MEDICAL, INC.
312-283-5633

65862
AUROBINDO PHARMA
732-839-9400
866-850-2876
http://www.aurobindo.com

65504
AURORA HEALTHCARE
414-647-3000
http://www.aurorahelathcare.org

AUTOIMMUNE, INC.
626-792-1235
http://www.autoimmuneinc.com

AUTOIMMUNITY RESEARCH FOUNDATION
805-492-3693

66887
AUXILIUM PHARMACEUTICALS, INC.
484-321-5900
http://www.auxilium.com

68322
AVANIR PHARMACEUTICALS, LLC
949-389-6700
http://www.avanir.com

AVANT IMMUNOTHERAPEUTICS, INC.
781-433-0771

AVANTOR PERFORMANCE MATERIALS
908-859-2151
800-582-2537
http://www.avantormaterials.com

AVAX TECHNOLOGIES, INC.
913-693-8491
http://www.avax-tech.com

42291
AVKARE
931-292-6222
http://www.avkare.com

AVENTIS BEHRING
See CSL Behring

AVENTIS PHARMACEUTICALS
See Sanofi-Aventis U.S.

AVICENA GROUP, INC.
415-397-2880
http://www.avicenagroup.com

43684
AVIDAS PHARMACEUTICALS
267-895-1755
http://www.avidaspharma.com

AVIGEN, INC.
510-748-1750
http://www.avigen.com

76170
AVOCET POLYMER TECHNOLOGIES
815-609-2170
866-352-7227
http://www.avocetcorp.com

58914
AXCAN PHARMA US, INC.
205-991-8085
800-472-2634
http://www.axcan.com

58914
AXCAN SCANDIPHARM
See Axcan Pharma US, Inc.

18860
AZUR PHARMA
215-832-3752
866-833-3560
http://www.azurpharma.com

63275
B & B PHARMACEUTICALS
303-755-5110
800-499-3100
http://www.bandbpharma.com

00264
B. BRAUN MCGAW
See B. Braun Medical, Inc.

00264
B. BRAUN MEDICAL INC.
800-854-6851
http://www.bbraunusa.com

00225
B. F. ASCHER AND CO.
913-888-1880
800-324-1880
http://www.bfascher.com

44184
BAJAMAR CHEMICAL CO., INC.
314-721-1896
http://www.vesselvite.com

11414
BAKER CUMMINS DERMATOLOGICALS
See Ivax Pharmaceuticals, Inc.

11414
BAKER NORTON PHARMACEUTICALS
See Ivax Pharmaceuticals, Inc.

50770
BALLARD MEDICAL PRODUCTS
801-572-6800
800-528-5591
http://www.kchealthcare.com

63162
BALLAY PHARMACEUTICALS, INC.
512-847-6458

BANNER PHARMACAPS
336-812-8700
800-447-1140
http://www.banpharm.com

BARBEAU PHARMA, INC.
847-441-4142

08011
BARD
See C.R. Bard

49326
BAROLI
305-772-0665

00555
BARR LABORATORIES, INC.
800-222-0190
http://www.barrlabs.com

BARR PHARMACEUTICALS, INC.
845-362-1100
800-222-0190
http://www.barrlabs.com

BARRE-NATIONAL, INC.
See Alpharma

13478
BARRIER THERAPEUTICS
609-945-1200
http://www.barriertherapeutics.com

10116
BARTOR PHARMACAL CO.
914-967-4219

00078
BASEL PHARMACEUTICALS
See Novartis Pharmaceuticals Corp.

BASF CORPORATION
973-245-6000
800-526-1072
http://www.basf.com

00761, 07610
BASIC DRUGS

55458
BASIC ORGANICS
614-863-3004
http://www.basicorganics.com

10119
BAUSCH & LOMB PERSONAL PRODUCTS DIVISION
585-338-6000
800-344-8815
http://www.bausch.com

24208
BAUSCH & LOMB PHARMACEUTICALS INC.
813-975-7770
800-323-0000
http://www.bausch.com

61772
BAUSCH & LOMB SURGICAL
800-338-2020
http://www.bausch.com

17191
BAXA CORPORATION
303-690-4204
800-567-2292
http://www.baxa.com

10019, 60977
BAXTER HEALTHCARE CORPORATION
847-948-4770
800-933-0303
http://www.baxter.com

60977
BAXTER HEALTHCARE CORPORATION - ANESTHESIA CRITICAL CARE PHARMACEUTICALS
908-286-7000
800-667-0959
http://www.baxter.com

00944
BAXTER HEALTHCARE CORPORATION - BAXTER BIOSCIENCE
805-372-3000
800-422-9837
800-423-2090
http://www.baxter.com

00338
BAXTER HEALTHCARE CORPORATION - CLINTEC NUTRITION
800-422-2751
http://www.nutriforum.com

00338
BAXTER HEALTHCARE CORPORATION - MEDICATION DELIVERY
847-948-4770
800-933-0303
http://www.baxter.com

64193
BAXTER HYLAND IMMUNO
See Baxter Healthcare Corporation - Baxter Bioscience

60977
BAXTER PHARM. PRODS., INC. (BAXTER PPI)
See Baxter Healthcare Corporation - Anesthesia Critical Care Pharmaceuticals

00941
BAXTER RENAL
847-948-2000
888-736-2543
http://www.baxter.com

42769
BAY PHARMA
410-281-9450

65044
BAYER ALLERGY PRODUCTS
See Hollister-Stier

BAYER CONSUMER CARE DIVISION
973-254-5000
800-331-4536
http://www.bayercare.com

00026
BAYER CORPORATION
412-777-2000
800-468-0894
http://www.bayerus.com

BAYER DIABETES CARE
800-348-8100
http://www.bayerdiabetes.com

00193
BAYER DIAGNOSTICS
877-229-3711
800-248-2637
http://www.bayerdiag.com

BAYLOR RESEARCH INSTITUTE

BCY LIFESCIENCES, INC.

BECTON DICKINSON
201-847-6800
888-237-2762
http://www.bd.com

BD BIOSCIENCES
877-232-8995
http://www.bdbiosciences.com

BD DIAGNOSTIC SYSTEMS & MEDICAL SUPPLIES
800-675-0908
http://www.bd.com

00486
BEACH
813-839-6565
800-322-8210

BECKMAN COULTER
800-742-2345
http://www.beckmancoulter.com

BECKMAN COULTER PRIMARY CARE DIAGNOSTICS
714-993-5321
800-526-3821
http://www.beckmancoulter.com

BD CONSUMER PRODUCTS DIVISION
410-316-4000
800-638-8663
http://www.bd.com

55390
BEDFORD LABORATORIES
440-232-3320
800-562-4797
http://www.bedfordlabs.com

BEIERSDORF JOBST
See BSN Medical

BELL PHARMACEUTICAL
952-873-2288
800-328-5890

BELPHARMA N.V.

24385
BERGEN BRUNSWIG DRUG CO.
See AmerisourceBergen

50419
BERLEX LABORATORIES, INC.
See Bayer Healthcare Pharma

58337
BERNA
305-443-2900
800-533-5899
http://www.bernaproducts.com

BERTEK PHARMACEUTICALS, INC.
See Mylan Pharmaceuticals, Inc.

BESINS INTERNATIONAL, US, INC.

08515
BESTMED
303-271-0300

53062
BETA DERMACEUTICALS, INC.
210-349-9326
800-434-2382
http://www.beta-derm.com

00283
BEUTLICH PHARMACEUTICALS
847-473-1100
800-238-8542
http://www.beutlich.com

BI-COASTAL PHARMACEUTICAL
732-530-6606
http://www.bicoastalpharm.com

BIOALLIANCE PHARMA
33-0-1-45-58-76-00
http://www.bioalliancepharma.com

BIOAXONE THERAPEUTICS, INC.
913-693-8491
http://www.bioaxone.com

04142
BIOCODEX INC.
877-356-7787
650-243-5320
http://www.biocodexusa.com

08216
BIOCORE MEDICAL TECHNOLOGIES
888-565-5243
888-689-5655
http://www.biocore.com

00093
BIOCRAFT LABORATORIES, INC.
See Teva Pharmaceuticals USA

BIOCRYST PHARMACEUTICALS, INC.
205-444-4600
http://www.biocryst.com

BIODEVELOPMENT CORP.
703-006-0290

15594
BIOFILM, INC.
760-727-9030
http://www.astroglide.com

BIOFORM MEDICAL
650-286-4000
866-862-1211
http://www.bioform.com

BIOGEN PHARMACEUTICALS
818-762-7681

59627
BIOGEN IDEC
617-679-2000
800-262-2000
http://www.biogenidec.com

BIOGENEX LABORATORIES
925-275-0550
800-421-4149
http://www.biogenex.com

62436
BIOGLAN PHARMACEUTICALS
See Bradley Pharmaceutical

34061
BIOLIFE, LLC
800-722-7559
http://www.biolife.com

00719
BIOLINE LABS, INC.
888-257-5155
508-880-8990

BIOLITEC PHARMA, LTD.
353-1-463-7415
http://www.biolitecpharma.com

68135
BIOMARIN PHARMACEUTICAL, INC.
415-506-6700
866-274-0606
http://www.bmrn.com

BIOMEDICAL FRONTIERS, INC.
612-378-0228

BIOMEDICAL RESEARCH INSTITUTE

83059
BIOMERICA, INC.
949-645-2111
800-854-3002
http://www.biomerica.com

BIOMERIEUX
630-628-6055
800-634-7656
http://www.biomerieux-usa.com

BIOMIRA USA, INC.
780-490-2818
877-234-0444
http://www.biomira.com

17700
BIOMOLECULAR SCIENCES, INC.
818-804-5148
800-260-3587
http://www.biomolecularsciences.com

BIOMUNE SYSTEMS, INC.

53110
BIONEXUS, LTD
607-266-9492
800-835-0869
http://www.bionxs.com

62086
BIONICHE PHARMA USA
847-739-3246
888-258-4199
http://www.bioniche.com

08539
BIONIME USA CORPORATION
858-481-8485
866-481-8485
http://www.bionime.com

59741
BIOPHARM LABS
215-949-3711
http://www.bio-pharminc.com

BIOPHARMACEUTICS, INC.
See Feminique Corp.

BIOPHYSICA, INC.
858-452-1523
http://www.biophysica.net

BIO PRODUCTS LABORATORY
44-0-208-258-2200
http://www.bpl.co.uk

BIOPURE CORP.
617-234-6500
http://www.biopure.com

BIOSAFE TECHNOLOGIES, INC.
903-463-7321
877-828-4633
http://www.biosafetech.com

BIOSCRIP
952-979-3600
800-444-5951
http://www.bioscrip.com

08611
BIOSENSE MEDICAL DEVICES
877-592-3922

BIOSPECIFICS TECHNOLOGIES CORP.
516-593-7000
http://www.biospecifics.com

BIOSYNEXUS, INC.
301-330-5800
http://www.biosynexus.com

BIO-TECHNOLOGY GENERAL CORP.
732-632-8800

53191
BIO-TECH
479-443-9148
800-345-1199
http://www.bio-tech-pharm.com

55146
BIOTICS RESEARCH
281-344-0909
800-231-5777
http://www.bioticsresearch.com

BIOTRANSPLANT, INC.
617-241-5200

58023
BIOTROL INTERNATIONAL
303-673-0341
800-822-8550
http://www.biotrol.com

64455
BIOVAIL PHARMACEUTICALS, INC.
866-246-8245
908-927-1400
http://www.valeant.com

66658
BIOVITRUM AB
615-213-0343
http://www.biovitrum.com

BIRA CORP.
724-796-1820

50289
BIRCHWOOD LABORATORIES, INC.
952-937-7900
800-328-6156
http://www.birchlabs.com

12136
BIRD PRODUCTS CORP.
760-778-7200
800-232-7633
http://www.viasyscriticalcare.com

00165
BLAINE PHARMACEUTICALS
859-344-9600
800-633-9353
http://www.blainepharma.com

16728
BLAINES RESEARCH LABS
800-307-8818
562-906-4477
http://www.blaineslabs.com

00154
BLAIR LABORATORIES
See Purdue Frederick Co.

50486
BLAIREX LABS, INC.
812-378-1864
800-252-4739
http://www.blairex.com

51674
BLANSETT PHARMACAL
501-758-8635
800-816-9695
http://www.blansett.com

41388
BLISTEX INC.
630-571-2870
800-837-1800
http://www.blistex.com

BLOCK DRUG CO., INC.
See GlaxoSmithKline Consumer Healthcare

24658
BLU PHARMACEUTICALS
270-586-6386
877-264-0258
http://www.blurx.us

BLUCOINC.
734-513-4500
http://www.blucoinc.com

99853
BMS MEDIAL IMAGING
800-299-3431
http://www.radiopharm.com

64681
BMS U.S. MEDICINES GROUP
800-332-2056
212-546-4000
http://www.bms.com

08326, 43820, 00904
BOCA MEDICAL PRODUCTS
800-354-8460
http://www.bocamedicalproducts.com

64376
BOCA PHARMACAL
954-346-8810
800-354-8460
http://www.bocapharmacal.com

00024
BOCK PHARMACAL CO.
See Sanofi-Aventis U.S.

00597
BOEHRINGER INGELHEIM PHARMACEUTICALS, INC.
203-798-9988
800-520-1631
http://www.boehringer-ingelheim.com

BOERICKE & TAFEL
See Natures Way

00220
BOIRON LABORATORIES
800-264-7661
http://www.boironusa.com

00725
BOLAN PHARMACEUTICALS
516-842-8383
800-872-0159

50051
BONNE BELL
216-221-0800
800-321-1006
http://www.bonnebell.com

00074
BOOTS PHARMACEUTICALS, INC.
See Abbott Laboratories Pharmaceutical Division

BOTANICAL LABORATORIES
360-384-5656
800-232-4005
http://www.botlab.com

00270
BRACCO DIAGNOSTICS
609-514-2200
800-631-5245
http://www.bracco.com

BRADLEY PHARMACEUTICALS, INC.
973-882-1505
800-929-9300
http://www.bradpharm.com

52268
BRAINTREE LABORATORIES, INC.
781-843-2202
800-874-6756
http://www.braintreelabs.com

BRAUN
518-828-0450

00264
BRAUN MEDICAL
See B. Braun Medical, Inc.

51991
BRECKENRIDGE
561-443-3314
800-367-3395
http://www.bpirx.com

58659
BRIDGEPORT WHOLESALE PRODUCTS
425-656-0460

10914
BRIGHTON PHARMACEUTICALS
919-459-3950
866-638-7530
http://www.brightonpharma.com

10007
BRIOSCHI
201-796-4226
http://www.brioschi-usa.com

00015
BRISTOL LABS
609-252-4000
800-468-7746

BRISTOL-MYERS ONCOLOGY/VIROLOGY
609-897-2000
800-426-7644
http://www.bms.com

19810
BRISTOL-MYERS PRODUCTS (OTC/CONSUMER AFFAIRS)
See Novartis Pharmaceuticals Corp.

BRISTOL-MYERS SQUIBB COMPANY
212-546-4000
800-332-2056
http://www.bms.com

15584
BRISTOL-MEYERS SQUIBB/GILEAD
650-574-3000
800-445-3235
http://www.gilead.com

16563,11498
BRONSON PHARMACEUTICALS
800-235-3200
http://www.bronsonvitamins.com

42192
BROOKSTONE PHARMACEUTICALS
678-325-5188
800-541-4802
http://www.acellapharma.com

82161
BROWN MEDICAL INDUSTRIES
712-336-4395
800-843-4395
http://www.brownmed.com

63256.
BRYAN CORPORATION
781-935-0004
800-343-7711
http://www.bryancorp.com

63629
BRYANT RANCH PREPACK
818-764-7225
http://www.byrantranchprepack.com

BSN, JOBST
See BSN Medical

BSN MEDICAL
704-554-9933
http://www.jobst.com

54396
BTG PHARMACEUTICAL CORPORATION
See Savient Pharmaceuticals, Inc.

BUREL PHARMACEUTICALS
601-855-2016
http://www.burelpharmaceuticals.com

BURROUGHS WELLCOME CO.
See GlaxoSmithKline

BIOSAFE LABORATORIES
847-234-8111
http://www.ebiosafe.com

C. B. FLEET CO., INC.
See Fleet Laboratories

08011
C. R. BARD
908-277-8000
800-526-4455
http://www.crbard.com

C.R. BARD, INC. UROLOGICAL DIVISION
770-784-6100
800-526-4455
http://www.crbard.com

10486
C S DENT
859-647-0777

59746
CADISTA PHARMACEUTICALS, INC.
410-860-8500
800-619-9364
http://www.cadista.com

08237, 55559
CALGON VESTAL
See ConvaTec

00799
CALMOSEPTINE, INC.
714-840-3405
800-800-3405
http://www.calmoseptineointment.com

12622
CALWOOD NUTRITIONALS
410-796-5560
800-479-9942
http://www.calwoodnutritionals.com

31722
CAMBER PHARMACEUTICALS
732-377-2029
866-495-1995
http://www.camberpharma.com

CAMBREX BIOSCIENCE
207-594-3400
800-638-8174
http://www.cambrex.com

CAMBRIDGE NEUROSCIENCE
See Baxter Healthcare Corporation

43656
CAMBRIDGE NUTRACEUTICALS
See Baxter Healthcare Corp.

24359
CAMBROOKE FOODS
508-782-2300
866-456-9776
http://www.cambrookefoods.com

38083
CAMPBELL LABS
See Chattem Consumer Products

08396
CAN-AM CARE
678-795-3440
866-202-9067
http://www.canamcare.com

CANGENE
204-275-4200
800-768-2304

42026
CANOPY ROADS PHARMACEUTICALS
770-664-6050
http://www.crpharma.com

CANYON PHARMACEUTICALS
410-771-8606
888-434-7003
http://www.canyonpharma.com

64543
CAPELLON PHARMACEUTICALS, LTD.
817-595-5820
http://www.capellon.com

57664, 32247
CARACO PHARMACEUTICAL LABORATORIES
313-871-8400
800-818-4555
http://www.caraco.com

CARDINAL HEALTH
614-757-5000
800-234-8701
http://www.cardinal.com

08525
CARDIOCOM
952-361-6467
888-243-8881
http://www.cardiocom.com

83076
CARDIOTABS
816-753-4298
800-811-1007
http://www.cardiotabs.com

84841
CARGILL HEALTH & FOOD TECH
800-221-4455
952-742-7575
http://www.cargill.com

61442,61441
CARLSBAD TECHNOLOGIES
760-431-8284
http://www.carlsbadtechnologyinc.com

83078
CARMA LABS INC
414-421-7707
http://www.carma-labs.com

CARME, INC.
707-226-3900
http://www.senetekplc.net

50000
CARNATION
See Nestle Infant Nutrition

00086
CARNRICK LABORATORIES
See Elan Pharmaceuticals

46287
CAROLINA MEDICAL PRODUCTS COMPANY
252-753-7111
800-227-6637
http://www.carolinamedical.com

CAROLINA MEDICAL PRODUCTS CO.
800-227-6637
http://www.carolinamedical.com

53303
CARRINGTON
972-518-1300
800-527-5216
http://www.carringtonlabs.com

11411, 41140.
CARTER PRODUCTS
See Church Dwight

22600
CARTER-WALLACE
See Church Dwight

00037
CARTER-WALLACE, INC.
See Meda Pharmaceuticals

15370
CARWIN ASSOCIATES, INC.
205-525-4566
866-525-4566
http://www.carwinassoc.com

18515
CCA INDUSTRIES, INC.
800-524-2720
http://www.ccaindustries.com

64019
CEBERT PHARMACEUTICALS, INC.
205-981-0201
800-211-0589
http://www.cebert.com

64181
CEDARBURG PHARMACEUTICALS
262-376-1467
http://www.cedarburgpharma.com

CELESTIAL SEASONINGS, INC.
303-530-5300
800-525-0347
http://www.celestialseasonings.com

59572
CELGENE CORP
908-673-9000
888-423-5436
http://www.celgene.com

65231
CELL PATHWAYS
See OSI Pharmaceuticals

60553
CELL THERAPEUTICS, INC.
206-282-7100
800-215-2355
http://www.ctiseattle.com

CELLEGY PHARMACEUTICALS, INC.
215-914-0900

CELLTECH PHARMACEUTICAL CO.
See UCB Pharmaceuticals, Inc.

CENTEON
See CSL Behring

00268
CENTER LABORATORIES
See ALK-Abello

CENTERS FOR DISEASE CONTROL AND PREVENTION
404-639-3534
800-311-3435
http://www.cdc.gov

99962
CENTOCOR ORTHO BIOTECH, INC.
888-227-5624
800-457-6399
http://www.centocororthobiotech.com

CENTOCOR ORTHO BIOTECH, INC.
888-227-5624
800-457-6399

38083
CENTRAL PHARMACEUTICALS, INC.
See Schwarz Pharma

11528
CENTRIX PHARMACEUTICAL, INC.
205-991-9870
866-991-9870
http://www.cenrx.com

23359
CENTURION LABS, LLC
601-720-0111
http://www.centurionlabs.com

00436
CENTURY
317-849-4210
866-343-2576

63459
CEPHALON
610-344-0200
800-896-5855
http://www.cephalon.com

68330
CEPHAZONE PHARMA
909-392-8900
http://www.cephazone.com

00851
CERA PRODUCTS
843-842-2600
888-237-2598
http://www.ceraproductsinc.com

CERENEX PHARMACEUTICALS
See GlaxoSmithKline

10223
CETYLITE INDUSTRIES, INC.
865-665-6111
800-257-7740
http://www.cetylite.com

40986, 68016
CHAIN DRUG CONSORTIUM
412-828-2061

63868
CHAIN DRUG MARKETING ASSOCIATION, INC.
248-449-9300

CHARLES RIVER LABORATORIES INTERNATIONAL, INC.
978-658-6000
877-CRIVER1 (877-274-8371)
http://www.criver.com

54429
CHASE LABORATORIES
See Banner Pharmacaps

41167
CHATTEM CONSUMER PRODUCTS
423-821-4571
800-366-6833
http://www.chattem.com

CHESAPEAKE BIOLOGICAL LABS., INC.
See Cangene BioPharma

00521
CHESEBROUGH-PONDS USA, INC.
See Unilever Home and Personal Care USA

12462
CHESTER LABS
513-458-3840
800-354-9709
http://www.chester-labs.com

CHEW-RITE CO.
937-746-5509

CHIESI PHARMACEUTICALS, INC.

CHILDRENS HOSPITAL OF COLUMBUS
614-722-2000

CHILTON LABS., INC.
973-575-1992

67066
CHIRHOCLIN
877-272-4888
301-476-8388
http://www.chirhoclin.com

53905
CHIRON THERAPEUTICS
510-655-8730
800-244-7668
http://www.chiron.com

61772
CHIRON VISION
See Bausch & Lomb Surgical

54993
CHRONIMED INC.
See Bioscrip

96121
CHRONOHEALTH
805-290-4959
866-261-8557

22600
CHURCH DWIGHT
609-683-5900
800-524-1328
http://www.churchdwight.com

00067
CIBA CONSUMER
See Novartis Consumer Health

47113
CIBA VISION CORPORATION
770-476-3937
800-845-6585
http://www.cibavision.com

00078
CIBA-GEIGY PHARMACEUTICALS
See Novartis Pharmaceuticals Corp.

CIMA LABS
952-947-8700
http://www.cimalabs.com

52544
CIRCA PHARMACEUTICALS, INC.
See Watson Laboratories

CIRRUS HEALTHCARE PRODUCTS, L.L.C.
631-692-7600
800-327-6151
http://www.cirrushealthcare.com

CIS-US, INC.
781-275-7120
800-221-7554
http://www.pharmalucence.com

CITRA ANTICOAGULANTS
781-848-2174
800-299-3411
http://www.citraanticoagulants.com

99074
CLARIS LIFESCIENCES LIMITED
732-422-9100
http://www.clarislifesciences.com

45802
CLAY-PARK LABS, INC.
718-901-2800
800-933-5550
http://www.claypark.com

55553
CLINT PHARMACEUTICALS
615-882-0042
800-677-5022
http://www.clintpharmaceuticals.com

CLOSURE MEDICAL CORP.
See Johnson & Johnson

57145
CNS, INC.
952-229-1500
http://www.cns.com

58826
COATS ALOE INTERNATIONAL, INC.
214-340-2563
800-486-2563
http://www.coatsaloe.com

16252
COBALT LABORATORIES, INC.
800-272-5525
239-390-0245
http://www.cobaltlabs.com

43378
CODADOSE
678-866-0172
866-574-8861
http://www.codadose.com

COLGATE-HOYT
See Colgate Oral Pharmaceuticals

00126
COLGATE ORAL PHARMACEUTICALS
213-310-2000
800-226-5428
http://www.colgateprofessional.com

35000
COLGATE-PALMOLIVE CO.
212-310-2000
800-221-4607
http://www.colgateprofessional.com

64682, 27280
COLLAGENEX PHARMACEUTICALS
215-579-7388
888-339-5678
http://www.collagenex.com

COLOPLAST
612-337-7800
800-533-0464
http://www.us.coloplast.com

COLORADO BIOLABS, INC.
970-243-4153
888-442-0067
http://www.coloradobiolabs.com

21406, 55056
COLUMBIA LABORATORIES, INC.
973-994-3999
866-566-5636
http://www.columbialabs.com

11509
COMBE, INC.
914-694-5454
800-873-7400
http://www.combe.com

COMPLIMED MEDICAL RESEARCH GROUP
360-384-5656
888-977-8008
http://www.complimed.com

CONAGRA FUNCTIONAL FOODS, INC.
888-828-4242
http://www.culturelle.com

74108
CONAIR INTERPLAX DIVISION
800-726-6247
http://www.interplak.com

08597, 95863
CONCEIVEX
616-642-6917
888-306-6366
http://www.conceptionkit.com

57648
CONCEPTS IN CONFIDENCE
561-369-1700
800-822-4050
http://www.conceptsinconfidence.com

CON-CISE CONTACT LENS CO.
510-483-9400
800-772-3911
http://www.con-cise.com

20254
CONCORD LABORATORIES
973-227-6757

49281
CONNAUGHT LABS
See Sanofi Pasteur

63032
CONNETICS CORPORATION
See Stiefel Laboratories

00223
CONSOLIDATED MIDLAND CORP.
845-279-6108

97493
CONSUMERS CHOICE SYSTEMS, INC.
425-883-6310
800-479-5232
http://www.womanswellbeing.com

CONTINENTAL CONSUMER PRODUCTS
248-758-1817
800-542-5903

CONTINENTAL QUEST RESEARCH
317-843-2501
800-451-5773
http://www.continentalquest.com

10267
CONTRACT PHARMACAL CORP.
631-231-4610
http://www.cpc.com

CONVATEC
908-904-2200
800-422-8811
http://www.convatec.com

63535
COOKE PHARMA, INC.
See Unither Pharma (United Therapeutics Corp.)

59365
COOPER SURGICAL
203-601-5200
800-480-1985
http://www.coopersurgical.com

59426, 54027
COOPERVISION
949-597-8130
800-538-7850
http://www.coopervision.com

00093
COPLEY PHARMACEUTICAL
See Teva Pharmaceuticals USA

63020
COR THERAPEUTICS, INC.
See Millennium Pharmaceuticals, Inc.

64720
COREPHARMA, LLC
732-868-1090
800-850-2719
http://www.corepharma.com

13548
CORIA LABORATORIES
800-548-5100
http://www.corialabs.com

CORIXA
See GlaxoSmithKline

10122
CORNERSTONE THERAPEUTICS
919-678-6611
888-466-6503
http://www.crtx.com

COROMEGA CO., INC.
760-599-6088
877-275-3725
http://www.coromega.com

10148
COTHERIX
650-624-6900
877-483-6828
http://www.cotherix.com

COULTER CORP. (BECKMAN COULTER, INC.)
See Beckman Coulter

43199
COUNTY LINE PHARMACEUTICALS
262-439-8109
866-207-5636
http://www.countylinepharma.com

COVIDIEN
508-261-8000
800-722-8772
http://www.covidien.com

11025
CREATIVE MEDICAL CORPORATION
787-714-0100

15310
CREEKWOOD PHARMACEUTICAL, INC.
205-995-7390
http://www.crkrx.com

68734
CRITICAL THERAPEUTICS, INC.
781-402-5700
http://www.criticaltherapeutics.com

37379
CSI PHARM
800-654-5635
http://www.csidesigns.com

00053
CSL BEHRING, LLC
610-878-4000
800-683-1288
800-504-5434
http://www.cslbehring.com

33332
CSL BIOTHERAPIES
888-435-8633
http://www.cslbiotherapies-us.com

67919
CUBIST PHARMACEUTICALS, INC.
781-860-8660
866-793-2786
http://www.cubist.com

66220
CUMBERLAND PHARMACEUTICALS, INC.
615-255-0068
866-423-7259
http://www.cumberlandpharma.com

00869
CUMBERLAND SWAN, INC.
See Vijon Laboratories

66860
CURA PHARMACEUTICALS
888-887-7171
732-982-8300
http://www.curapharma.com

08160
CURAMEDICA, LLC
888-613-0729
http://www.curamedica.com

CURASCRIPT
407-804-6700
800-892-9622
http://www.priorityhealthcare.com

55326
CURATEK PHARMACEUTICALS
See 3M Pharmaceuticals

65628
CUTIS PHARMA, INC.
781-935-8141
http://www.cutispharma.com

67159
CV THERAPEUTICS
See Gilead Sciences

CYANOTECH CORP.
808-326-1353
800-395-1353
http://www.cyanotech.com

53409
CYCLIN PHARMACEUTICALS INC.
800-558-7046
http://www.womenshealth.com

08197
CYGNUS, INC.
650-369-4300
http://www.cygn.com

54799
CYNACON/OCUSOFT
800-233-5469
http://www.ocusoft.com

60258
CYPRESS PHARMACEUTICAL, INC.
601-856-4393
800-856-4393
http://www.cypressrx.com

63004
CYPROS PHARMACEUTICAL CORP.
See Questcor Pharmaceuticals, Inc.

57902
CYTOGEN CORP.
See Eusa Pharma

23731
CYTOSOL LABORATORIES
781-848-9386
800-288-3858

61534
CYTOSOL OPTHALMICS
828-758-2343
800-234-5166
http://www.cytosol.com

CYTRX CORP.
310-826-5648
http://www.cytrx.com

65759, 10960
D & K HEALTHCARE RESOURCES
314-727-3485
888-727-3485
http://www.dkwd.com
See McKesson

DADE BEHRING
847-267-5300
800-241-0420
http://www.dadebehring.com

63395
DAIICHI PHARMACEUTICAL CORP
See Daiichi Sankyo, Inc.

63395
DAIICHI SANKYO, INC.
973-944-2600
877-437-7763
http://www.dsi.com

00591, 52544
DANBURY PHARMACAL
951-493-5300
800-338-9066
http://www.watson.com

64875
DANCO LABS., LLC
212-424-1950
877-432-7596
http://www.earlyoptionpill.com

60793
DANIELS PHARMACEUTICALS, INC.
See King Pharmaceuticals, Inc.

58869
DARTMOUTH PHARMACEUTICALS, INC.
508-295-2200
800-414-3566
http://www.ilovemynails.com

67253
DAVA PHARMACEUTICALS, INC.
201-947-7442
866-947-3282
http://www.davapharm.com

DAVOL
401-463-7000
800-556-6275
http://www.davol.com

58865
DAWN PHARMACEUTICALS INC.
800-745-3296

52041
DAYTON LABORATORIES
See Propharma

DEGUSSA CORP.
973-541-8000
877-273-2668
http://www.degussa.com

10310
DEL PHARMACEUTICALS
516-844-2020
http://www.dellabs.com

00316
DEL-RAY LABORATORY INC
423-926-4413
800-877-8869
http://www.delrayderm.com

48532
DELMONT LABORATORIES, INC.
610-543-3365
800-562-5541
http://www.delmontlabs.info

53706
DELTA PHARMACEUTICALS
803-407-7733

DEN-MAT CORPORATION
805-922-8491
800-433-6628

00295
DENISON PHARMACEUTICALS
401-723-5500
http://www.hydrolatum.com

DENTAL HERB CO.
561-241-4262
800-747-4372
http://www.dentalherbcompany.com

13913
DEPOMED, INC.
650-462-5900
866-458-6389
http://www.depomedinc.com

DEPOTECH CORP. (SKYEPHARMA)
858-625-2424
http://www.skyepharma.com

99873
DEPUY MITEK
800-382-4682
508-880-8100
http://www.depuymitek.com

25382
DERMA SCIENCES
609-514-4744
800-825-4325
http://www.dermasciences.com

80208
DERMAIDE RESEARCH
312-649-7220
http://www.dermaide.com

10641
DERMALAB
847-266-0000
http://www.dermalab.com

60974
DERMALOGIX PARTNERS
207-883-4103
800-753-0047
http://www.dermalogix.com

61924
DERMARITE
973-569-9000
800-337-6296
http://www.dermarite.com

00066
DERMIK LABORATORIES, INC. (ARCOLA)
See Sanofi-Aventis US

DEROYAL INDUSTRIES, INC.
865-938-7828
888-938-7828
http://www.deroyal.com

08591
DESTAL INDUSTRIES
866-291-2815

16881
DESTON THERAPEUTICS
888-333-1528
http://www.deston.com

08627
DEXCOM, INC.
877-339-2664
http://www.dexcom.com

65430
DEXGEN PHARMACEUTICALS, INC.
732-223-8811
877-339-4361
http://www.dexgen.com

DEXO PHARMA
785-917-9582

49502
DEY L.P.
707-224-3200
800-755-5560
http://www.deyinc.com

DFB PHARMACEUTICALS
800-441-8227
http://www.dfb.com

55887
DHS, INC.
770-751-1787
800-392-7717

94046
DIABETIC SUPPLY OF SUNCOAST
888-469-3579
http://www.pharmasupply.com

DIAGNOSTICS DEVICES
800-366-5901
http://www.prodigymeter.com

17000
DIAL CORPORATION
480-754-3425
800-258-3425
http://www.dialcorp.com

DIAPHARMA GROUP, INC.
513-860-9324
800-526-5224
http://www.diapharma.com

50419
DIATIDE, INC.
See Berlex

10331
DICKINSON BRANDS, INC.
860-267-2279
888-860-2279
http://www.witchhazel.com

59767
DIGESTIVE CARE, INC.
610-882-5950
http://www.digestivecare.com

55392
DINNO PHARMACEUTICALS
617-645-5552

08587
DINORIO
866-354-3449
http://www.dinorio.com

DISCOVERY LABORATORIES, INC.
215-488-9300
http://www.discoverylabs.com

DISCUS DENTAL, INC.
800-422-9448
310-845-8600
http://www.discusdental.com

15630
DISETRONIC MEDICAL SYSTEMS
See Roche Insulin Delivery Systems, Inc.

68258
DISPENSING SOLUTIONS, INC.
888-374-7378
770-751-1787
http://www.dispensingsolutionsinc.com

00777
DISTA PRODUCTS CO.
See Eli Lilly and Co.

DIXON-SHANE
See Amneal Pharmaceuticals

64455
DJ PHARMA, INC.
See Biovail Pharmaceuticals, Inc.

10337
DOAK DERMATOLOGICS
See Pharmaderm

DONELL DERMEDEX
See Donell, Inc.

DONELL INC.
212-682-0666
800-324-7455
http://www.donellskin.com

51469
DOVER PHARMACEUTICAL, INC.
781-821-5400
800-777-6847

00514
DOW HICKAM, INC.
See Mylan Pharmaceuticals, Inc.

DOW PHARMACEUTICAL SCIENCES
707-793-2600
877-369-7476
http://www.dowpharm.com

55111
DR. REDDY'S LABORATORIES, INC.
888-375-3784
908-203-4900
http://www.drreddys.com

64061
DREIR PHARMACEUTICALS, INC.
480-607-3584
800-541-4044

58952
DRJ GROUP, INC.
760-635-0174

52316
DSC LABORATORIES
231-777-3012
800-492-5988
http://www.dsclab.com

89411
DSE HEALTHCARE SOLUTIONS, LLC
800-338-8079
732-417-1870
http://www.dsehealth.com

25382
DUMEX
See Derma Sciences

50939
DU-MORE
479-631-1088
http://www.dumoreinc.com

00217, 48878
DUNHALL PHARMACEUTICALS, INC.
See Omnii Pharmaceuticals and See Oxypure

DUPONT PHARMACEUTICALS CO.
See Bristol-Myers Squibb Co.

41333
DURACELL
800-551-2355
http://www.duracell.com

51285
DURAMED PHARMACEUTICALS
See Barr Laboratories, Inc.

02340
DUREX CONSUMER PRODUCTS
770-582-2222
888-566-3468
http://www.durex.com

00145
DURHAM PHARMACAL CORP.
See Stiefel Laboratories, Inc.

67308
DUSA PHARMACEUTICALS, INC.
978-657-7500
877-533-DUSA (877-533-3872)
http://www.dusapharma.com

68803
DUTCH OPHTHALMIC
603-778-6929
800-753-8824
http://www.dorc.nl

47783
DYAX CORPORATION
617-225-2500
800-452-5248
http://www.dyax.com

55516
DYNA PHARM, INC.

00168
E. FOUGERA CO.
631-454-7677
800-645-9833
http://www.fougera.com

E.R. SQUIBB & SONS, INC.
See Bristol-Myers Squibb Co.

EAGLE VISION, INC.
901-380-7000
800-222-7584
http://www.eaglevis.com

EASTMAN KODAK CO.
585-724-4000
800-242-2424
http://www.kodak.com

EATON MEDICAL CORP.
901-274-0000
800-253-5949
http://www.easyeyes.com

ECOLAB
651-293-2233
800-352-5326
http://www.ecolab.com

ECOLOGICAL FORMULAS, INC.
925-827-2636
800-888-4585
http://www.ecologicalformulas.net

38130
ECONO MED PHARMACEUTICALS
336-226-1091
800-327-6007

55053
ECONOLAB
See Breckenridge Pharmaceutical, Inc.

00095
ECR PHARMACEUTICALS
804-527-1950
800-527-1955
http://www.ecrpharma.com

42799
EDENBRIDGE PHARMACEUTICALS
201-292-1292
http://www.edenbridgepharma.com

00433
EDWARDS LIFESCIENCE
800-424-3278
800-882-9837
http://www.edwards.com

00485
EDWARDS
662-837-8182
800-543-9560

55806
EFFCON LABORATORIES
770-579-3558
800-722-2428

62856
EISAI, INC.
201-692-1100
888-793-4724
http://www.eisai.com

24477
EKR THERAPEUTICS, INC.
877-435-2524
http://www.ekrtx.com

59075
ELAN PHARMACEUTICALS
800-859-8586
888-638-7605
http://www.elan.com

ELANCO
317-277-3185
800-428-4441
http://www.elanco.com

58298
ELGE
281-232-0463
281-342-8228
http://www.elgeninc.com

00002
ELI LILLY AND COMPANY
317-276-2000
800-545-5979
http://www.lilly.com

42783
ELORAC
847-362-8200

EMD CHEMICALS, INC.
856-423-6300
800-222-0342

EMD SERONO, INC.
781-982-9000
800-283-8088
http://www.emdserono.com

04107, 24155
EMJAY LABORATORIES
See Sheffield Laboratories

91268
EMJOI
212-755-5950
888-310-2493
http://www.emjoi.com

42457
EMMAUS MEDICAL
310-214-0065
877-420-6493
http://www.emmausmedical.com

64068
ENDIT LABORATORIES
910-754-6856
http://www.endit.com

ENDO PHARMACEUTICALS
610-558-9800
800-462-3636
http://www.endo.com

ENDURANCE PRODUCTS COMPANY
503-639-9562
800-964-0876
http://www.endur.com

17433
ENEMEEZ
602-276-3434
888-273-9734
http://www.enemeez.com

62333
ENVIRODERM PHARMACEUTICALS, INC.
310-768-0700
800-624-9659
http://www.enviroderm.com

57665
ENZON PHARMACEUTICALS, INC.
908-541-8600
866-792-5172
http://www.enzon.com

63948
ENZYMATIC THERAPY
800-783-2286
http://www.enzymatictherapy.com

00185
EON LABS
See Sandoz

42806
EPIC PHARMA
718-949-8607
888-374-2791
http://www.epic-pharma.com

62942
EPIEN MEDICAL
952-746-6770
888-884-4675
http://www.epien.com

18270
EQUIDYNE SYSTEMS
714-447-4474
http://www.injex.com

63475
ESCALON MEDICAL CORP
618-688-6830
800-433-8197
http://www.escalonmed.com

67286
ESP PHARMA
See PDL Biopharma

15456
ESPRIT PHARMA
732-828-9950
http://www.espritpharma.com

58177
ETHEX CORP.
314-646-3750
800-321-1705
http://www.ethex.com

63713
ETHICON, INC. (JOHNSON & JOHNSON)
908-218-0707
800-255-2500
http://www.ethicon.com

ETI HOLDING
920-469-1313

EURAND AMERICA, INC.
937-898-9669
http://www.eurand.com

42865
EURAND PHARMACEUTICALS
267-759-9400
888-936-7371
http://www.eurand.com

66521
EVANS VACCINES, LTD.
See Novartis Vaccines and Diagnostics

42700
EVENFLO COMPANY, INC.
937-415-3300
800-233-5921
http://www.evenflo.com

00642
EVERETT
973-324-0200
800-964-9650
http://www.everettlabs.com

17287
EVERTON PHARMACEUTICALS
877-218-3215

64125
EXCELLIUM PHARMACEUTICAL
973-276-9600

63807
EXCELSIOR MEDICAL CORPORATION
732-776-7525
800-487-4276
http://www.excelsiormedical.com

08287,20221
EXEL INTERNATIONAL
800-940-3935
http://www.exelint.com

60843
EYE CARE & CURE CORPORATION
520-321-1262
800-486-6169
http://www.eyecareandcure.com

68782
EYETECH PHARMACEUTICALS
See OSI Eyetech

10361
E-Z-EM
See Bracco Diagnostics

94542
FACET TECHNOLOGIES
770-590-6400
800-526-2387
http://www.facettechnologies.com

61314
FALCON PHARMACEUTICALS, LTD.
800-343-2133
817-293-0450
http://www.falconpharma.com

58892
FALLENE
800-332-5536
http://www.fallene.com

FARMACON, INC.
203-222-8801

60976
FARO PHARMACEUTICALS, INC.
See Cooper Surgical

61703
FAULDING PHARMACEUTICAL
See Hospira

FDA
301-827-1491
888-463-6332
http://www.fda.gov

50907
FEI PRODUCTS
716-693-6230
877-727-2427
http://www.barrlabs.com

11423
FEMALE HEALTH CO.
312-595-9123
800-884-1601
http://www.femalehealthcompany.com

08454
FEMCAP
858-481-8837
http://www.femcap.com

00942
FENWAL INTERNATIONAL
847-550-2300
800-333-6925
http://www.fenwalinc.com

48102
FERA PHARMACEUTICALS
414-434-6604
http://www.ferapharma.com

00496
FERNDALE LABORATORIES, INC.
248-548-0900
800-621-6003
http://www.ferndalelabs.com

31253, 08439
FERRARIS MEDICAL
http://www.ferrarismedical.com

55566
FERRING PHARMACEUTICALS, INC.
973-796-1600
888-337-7464
http://www.ferringusa.com

08195
FERRIS CORP
630-887-9797
800-765-9636
http://www.polymem.com

FIBERTONE
See Marlyn Neutraceuticals, Inc.

59630
FIRST HORIZON PHARMACEUTICAL
See Sciele Pharma

90891
FIRST QUALITY PRODUCTS
516-829-3030
800-726-6910
http://www.firstquality.com

FISHER SCIENTIFIC INTERNATIONAL
603-926-5911
800-640-0640
http://www.fisherscientific.com

FISKE INDUSTRIES
845-398-3340
http://www.cosmeticsolutions.com

54323
FLANDERS, INC.
843-571-3363
http://www.flandersbuttocks ointment.com

78573
FLAVORX
800-884-5771
http://www.flavorx.com

FLEET LABORATORIES
800-999-9711
http://www.cbfleet.com

00256
FLEMING PHARMACEUTICALS
636-343-5306
800-343-0164
http://www.flemingpharma.com

23185
FLENTS PRODUCTS COMPANY
See Apothecary Products, Inc.

FLEX-POWER
510-527-9955
866-353-9769
http://www.flexpower.com

00288
FLUORITAB
231-755-9113

60762
FNC MEDICAL CORPORATION
805-644-7576
800-440-2888
http://www.fncmedical.com

42559
FONTUS PHARMACEUTICALS, INC.
973-265-2777
http://www.fontuspharma.com

98939
FORA CARE
805-498-8188
http://www.foracare.com

00456
FOREST LABORATORIES IRELAND, LTD.
See Forest Laboratories, Inc.

00456
FOREST LABORATORIES, INC.
212-421-7850
800-947-5227
800-678-1605
http://www.forestpharm.com

00456
FOREST PHARMACEUTICALS, INC.
See Forest Laboratories, Inc.

64814
FORTE PHARMA
See Eon Labs Manufacturing, Inc.

00168
FOUGERA
631-454-7677
800-645-9833
http://www.fougera.com

FOURNIER PHARMA
973-683-0024
http://www.fournierpharmacorp.com

58487,10432
FREEDA VITAMINS, INC.
718-433-4337
800-777-3737
http://www.freedavitamins.com

90816, 49230
FRESENIUS
781-699-9000
800-662-1237
http://www.fmcna.com

71661
FRUIT OF THE EARTH
972-790-0808
800-527-7731
http://www.fote.com

13551
FSC LABORATORIES
877-387-0021
http://www.fsclabs.com

FUISZ TECHNOLOGIES, LTD.
See Biovail Pharmaceuticals, Inc.

00713
G & W LABS
908-753-2000
800-922-1038
http://www.gwlabs.com

86040
G C AMERICA
800-323-7063
http://www.gcamerica.com

00891
G. HIRSCH & CO.
650-692-8770
800-638-8800
http://www.ghirsch.com

00299
GALDERMA
817-961-5000
866-735-4137
http://www.galdermausa.com

57284
GALEN PHARMA
028-3833-4974
http://www.galen.co.uk

51552
GALLIPOT, INC.
651-681-9517
800-423-6967
http://www.gallipot.com

GAMBRO RENAL PRODUCTS
800-232-6800
800-525-2623
http://www.gambro.com

57844
GATE PHARMACEUTICALS
215-591-3000
800-292-4283
http://www.gatepharma.com

43386
GAVIS PHARMACEUTICALS
908-603-6080
http://www.gavispharma.com

00407
GE HEALTHCARE
262-544-3011
http://www.gehealthcare.com

00386
GEBAUER
216-581-3030
800-321-9348
http://www.gebauerco.com

50242
GENENTECH, INC.
650-225-1000
800-821-8590
http://www.gene.com

GENERAL INJECTABLES & VACCINES
276-688-4121
800-521-7468
http://www.giv.com

GENERAL NUTRITION INC.
412-288-4600
888-462-2548
http://www.gnc.com

10139
GENERAMEDIX, INC.
866-436-3721
908-504-1300
http://www.generamedix.com

GENESIS NUTRITION
843-665-6928
800-451-7933
http://www.genesisnutrition.com

00398
GENESIS PHARMACEUTICALS
973-451-9020
800-459-8663

GENETIC THERAPY, INC.
301-590-2626

00008
GENETICS INSTITUTE
617-876-1170
888-446-3344
http://www.genetics.com

00781
GENEVA DRUGS
See Sandoz Pharmaceuticals-Sandoz Consumer

82915
GENEXEL-SIEN
480-502-6007

15330
GENPHARM, L.P.
866-436-9155
631-434-2760
http://www.genpharmusa.com

00703.
GENSIA SICOR PHARMACEUTICALS, INC.
See Teva Pharmaceuticals USA

66657
GENTA INC.
908-286-9800
http://www.genta.com

15014
GENTEX PHARMA LLC
601-201-7231
601-826-0058
http://www.gentexpharma.com

GENVEC, INC.
240-632-5501
240-632-0740
http://www.genvec.com

58468
GENZYME CORPORATION
617-252-7500
800-326-7002
http://www.genzyme.com

63861
GENZYME TRANSPLANT
617-252-7500
800-376-7002
http://www.genzyme.com

GEODESIC MEDITECH, INC.
858-692-0088
http://www.geodesicmeditech.com

72227
GERBER PRODUCTS COMPANY
231-928-2000
800-443-7237
http://www.gerber.com

54092
GERIATRIC PHARMACEUTICAL CORP.
See Shire US, Inc.

57896
GERI-CARE
718-382-5000
http://www.gericarepharm.com

92771, 54162
GERITREX CORPORATION
914-668-4003
800-736-3437
http://www.geritrex.com

68585
GENESIS PRODUCTS
877-266-8292
http://www.genesisproductsinc.com

35781
GENSCO LABORATORIES
352-726-6284
http://www.genscolabs.com

61958
GILEAD SCIENCES
650-574-3000
800-445-3235
http://www.gilead.com

GILLETTE ORAL CARE
617-421-7000
http://www.gillette.com

47400
GILLETTE PERSONAL CARE
617-421-7000
http://www.gillette.com

36819
GINESIS NATURAL PRODUCTS
256-767-8256
800-492-4818
http://www.ginesis.com

63218, 59366
GLADES PHARMACEUTICALS, LLC
888-445-2337
http://www.glades.com

GLAXOSMITHKLINE
888-825-5249
215-751-4000
http://www.gsk.com

99929
GLAXOSMITHKLINE CONSUMER HEALTHCARE
412-200-4000
800-245-1040
http://www.gsk.com

GLAXOSMITHKLINE PHARM.
See GlaxoSmithKline

68462
GLENMARK PHARMACEUTICALS, LTD
888-721-7115
201-684-8000
http://www.glenmarkpharma.com

41128, 00516
GLENWOOD
201-569-0050
800-542-0772
http://www.glenwood-llc.com

82028
GLOBAL HEALTH PRODUCTS, INC
585-235-8818
http://www.globalhp.com

00115
GLOBAL PHARMACEUTICALS
215-933-0323
800-934-6729
http://www.globalphar.com

26893
GLOBAL PROTECTION COMPANY
617-946-2800
http://www.globalprotection.com

59618
GLOBAL SOURCE
954-747-8977
800-662-7556

33620
GLOVES IN A BOTTLE
818-248-9980
800-600-1881
http://www.glovesinabottle.com

58809
GM PHARMACEUTICALS
888-535-0305
817-303-3800

GML INDUSTRIES, LLC
See Biosafe Technologies, Inc.

60429
GOLDEN STATE MEDICAL SUPPLY
805-477-9866
800-284-8633
http://www.gsms.us

GOLDLINE LABORATORIES, INC.
See Ivax Pharmaceuticals, Inc.

10481
GORDON LABORATORIES
610-734-2011
800-356-7870
http://www.gordonlabs.net

13453
GRACEWAY PHARMACEUTICALS, LLC
423-274-2100
800-328-0255
http://www.gracewaypharma.com

12165
GRAHAM FIELD HEALTH PRODUCTS INC.
800-347-5678
http://www.grahamfield.com

10486
GRANDPA BRANDS COMPANY
859-647-0777
800-684-1468
http://www.grandpabrands.com

00034
GRAY PHARMACEUTICAL CO.
See Purdue Frederick Co.

51301
GREAT SOUTHERN LABORATORIES
281-530-3077
800-747-0783
http://www.greatsouthernlabs.com

GREEN TURTLE BAY VITAMIN CO.
908-277-2240
800-887-8535
http://www.energywave.com

59762
GREENSTONE
212-733-2323
800-438-1985
http://www.greenstonellc.com

22840
GREER LABORATORIES, INC.
828-754-5327
800-378-3906
http://www.greerlabs.com

68516, 61953
GRIFOLS, INC.
888-474-3657
800-421-0008
http://www.grifolsusa.com

11399
GTX, INC.
901-523-9700
http://www.gtxinc.com

GUARDIAN DRUG COMPANY
609-860-2600
http://www.guardiandrug.com

00327
GUARDIAN LABORATORIES
See United Guardian Laboratories

62750
GUM-TECH INDUSTRIES, INC.
See Matrixx Initiatives, Inc.

63955
GYNETICS
609-919-1931

54765
GYNOPHARMA

08385
H&H WHOLESALE SERVICES, INC.
248-616-3030
800-995-5750
http://www.hhwholesale.com

52959
H.J. HARKINS COMPANY, INC.
805-929-4060

00839
H.L. MOORE DRUG EXCHANGE, INC.
See Moore Medical Corp.

00556
H R CENCI LABS

64285
HAEMACURE CORPORATION
941-364-3700
http://www.haemacure.com

44411
HALL BIOSCIENCE
770-975-7337
http://www.hallbio.com

12164
HALOCARBON PRODUCTS CORPORATION
800-338-5803
http://www.halocarbon.com

17478
HAMELN PHARMACEUTICALS GMBH
See Akorn, Inc.

41268
HANNAFORD BROTHERS
800-213-9040
http://www.hannaford.com

HARD TO FIND BRANDS, INC.
724-796-0148
888-796-4832
http://www.hardtofindbrands.com

52512
HARMONY LABORATORIES
704-857-0707
800-245-6284
http://www.harmonylabs.com

67405
HARRIS PHARMACEUTICAL, INC.
239-278-4749
800-983-4708
http://www.harrispharmaceutical.com

HART HEALTH & SAFETY
800-234-4278
http://www.harthealth.com

00904, 61147
HARVARD DRUG CORP.
800-875-0123
http://www.harvardlink.com
http://www.harvarddrugs.com

67754
HARVEST PHARMACEUTICALS, INC.
540-633-7976
800-455-5525
http://www.harvestpharmaceuticals.com

HAUSER PHARMACEUTICAL INC.
800-441-2309
http://www.hauserpharmaceutical.com

66761
HAW PAR HEALTHCARE
510-887-1899
http://www.hawpar.com

63370
HAWKINS CHEMICAL
612-331-6910
612-617-8544
800-375-0009

63717
HAWTHORN PHARMACEUTICALS, INC.
601-856-4393
800-856-4393
http://www.cypressrx.com

HCD SALES
813-978-3005
800-844-8345
http://www.hcdsales.com

HD SMITH
866-232-1222
800-252-8090
http://www.hdsmith.com

HDC CORPORATION
408-942-7340
800-227-8162
http://www.hdccorp.com

HEALTH ASURE, INC.
831-420-2660
800-635-1233
http://www.healthasure.com

62391
HEALTH CARE LABORATORIES
281-496-9854
800-909-9854
http://www.bioflexor.com

60569, 61787
HEALTH CARE PRODUCTS
866-263-9003
800-899-3116
http://www.diabeticproducts.com

79573
HEALTH ENTERPRISES
508-695-0727
800-633-4243
http://www.healthenterprises.com

HEALTH PRODUCTS CORP.
914-423-2900

HEALTHCARE DIRECT SERVICES
See HCD Sales

HEALTHFIRST CORP.
425-771-5733
800-331-1984
http://www.healthfirst.com

00064
HEALTHPOINT MEDICAL
800-441-8227
http://www.healthpoint.com

93595, 55966
HEALTHSTAR
631-273-2630

50114
HEEL INC.
505-293-3843
800-621-7644
http://www.heelusa.com

HELENA LABORATORIES
409-842-3714
800-231-5663
http://www.helena.com

HEMACARE CORP.
818-226-1968
http://www.hemacare.com

HEMAGEN DIAGNOSTICS, INC.
443-367-5500
800-495-2180
http://www.hemagen.com

HEMISPHERX BIOPHARMA, INC.
215-988-0080
http://www.hemispherx.net

HENRY SCHEIN, INC.
631-843-5500
800-472-4346
http://www.henryschein.com

00023, 11980
HERBERT LABORATORIES
See Allergan, Inc.

49730
HERCON LABORATORIES CORPORATION
717-764-1191
http://www.herconlabs.com

23155
HERITAGE PHARMACEUTICALS
732-429-1000
866-901-1230
http://www.heritagepharma.com

10541
HIGH CHEMICAL COMPANY
215-788-3113
800-447-8792
http://www.sarapin.com

HIKMA PHARMACEUTICALS
732-542-1191
http://www.hikma.com

28105
HILL DERMACEUTICALS, INC.
407-323-1187
800-344-5707
http://www.hillderm.com

10542
HILLESTAD PHARMACEUTICALS
800-535-7742
866-358-9773
http://www.hillestadlabs.com

17808
HIMMEL
561-585-0070
800-535-3823
http://www.goliath.ecnext.com

46581
HISAMITSU PHARMACEUTICAL CO., INC.
http://www.salonpas-usa.com

50383
HI-TECH PHARMACAL CO. INC.
631-789-8228
http://www.hitechpharm.com

84160
HMD BIOMEDICAL
321-267-7576
888-446-3246
http://www.hmeproviders.com

HOECHST-MARION ROUSSEL
See Sanofi-Aventis US

95814
HOGIL PHARMACEUTICAL CORP.
914-681-1800
http://www.hogil.com

HOLLES LABORATORIES, INC.
800-356-4015

08380
HOLLISTER
800-323-4060
http://www.hollister.com

42828, 08567
HOLLISTER WOUND CARE
800-323-4060
http://www.hollister.com

65044
HOLLISTER-STIER LABORATORIES
509-489-5656
800-992-1120
http://www.hollisterstier.com

83170
HOME ACCESS HEALTH CORPORATION
847-781-2500
800-448-8378
http://www.homeaccess.com

21292, 56151
HOME DIAGNOSTICS
954-677-9201
800-342-7226
http://www.niprodiagnostics.com

HONEYWELL HOMMED LLC
262-783-5440
888-353-5440
http://www.hommed.com

60267
HOPE PHARMACEUTICALS, INC.
800-755-9595
http://www.hopepharm.com

60904
HORIZON PHARMACEUTICAL CORP.
See Shionigi Pharma, Inc.

61678
HORMEL HEALTHLABS
800-866-7757
http://www.hormelhealthlabs.com

66553
HOSPAK UNIT DOSE PRODUCTS
815-877-6480
815-636-8829

00409
HOSPIRA
224-212-2000
877-946-7747
http://www.hospira.com

00591, 52544
HOUBA (HALSEY DRUG CO.)
See Acura Pharmaceuticals, Inc.

17238
HUB PHARMACEUTICALS
909-476-8394
800-393-3767
http://www.hubrx.com

74312
HUDSON CORP.

65845
HUDSON RCI
951-676-5611
866-246-6990
http://www.hudsonrci.com

44156
HUMANICARE INTERNATIONAL
732-613-9000
800-631-5270
http://www.humanicare.com

03951, 00395
HUMCO HOLDING GROUP, INC.
903-334-6200
800-662-3435
http://www.humco.com

00219
HUMPHREYS PHARMACAL
201-933-7744

00944
HYLAND THERAPEUTICS
See Baxter Healthcare Corp.

75450
HY-VEE
515-267-2800
http://www.hy-vee.com

00186
ICI PHARMACEUTICALS
See AstraZeneca, LP

00187
ICN PHARMACEUTICALS
See Valeant Pharmaceuticals International

59627
IDEC PHARMACEUTICALS
See Biogen Idec

24108
IDENIX PHARMACEUTICALS, INC.
617-995-9800
http://www.idenix.com

IKARIA
908-238-6600
877-566-9466
http://www.ikaria.com

63861
ILEX ONCOLOGY, INC.
See Genzyme Corp.

24430
IMARX THERAPEUTICS
520-770-1259
800-984-1074
http://www.imarx.com

IMMUCELL CORP.
207-878-2770
800-466-8235
http://www.immucell.com

54129
IMMUNO U.S, INC. (BAXTER HEALTHCARE CORP.)
See Baxter Healthcare Corp.

IMMUNOGEN
617-995-2500
http://www.immunogen.com

IMMUNOMEDICS INC.
973-605-8200
http://www.immunomedics.com

28770
IMMUNOTEC RESEARCH LTD.
450-424-9992
888-917-7779
http://www.immunotec.com

00115
IMPAX LABORATORIES, INC.
510-476-2000
http://www.impaxlabs.com

IMS, LTD.
See UCB Pharmaceuticals, Inc.

INAMED CORPORATION
805-683-6761
800-722-2007
http://www.inamed.com

INDEVUS PHARMACEUTICALS, INC.
781-861-8444
800-370-4742
http://www.indevus.com

INFLABLOC PHARMACEUTICALS, INC.
801-464-6100
866-440-7044
http://www.pharmadigm.com

61607, 66934
INKINE PHARMACEUTICAL COMPANY, INC.
See Salix Pharmaceuticals, Inc.

INNER HEALTH GROUP
210-661-9257
800-381-4697
http://www.michaelshealth.com

INNOZEN, INC.
818-593-4880
800-599-8892

INO THERAPEUTICS, INC.
See IKARIA

08489
INPHARMA
877-241-8324

63736
INSIGHT PHARMACEUTICALS
267-852-0505
800-344-7239
http://www.insightpharma.com

16249
INSMED INCORPORATED
804-565-3000
804-565-3079
http://www. insmed.com

58441, 63252
INSOURCE
276-688-0211
800-668-3452
http://www.insourceonline.com

INSPIRE PHARMACEUTICALS, INC.
919-941-9777
http://www.inspirepharm.com

08508
INSULET
781-457-5000
800-591-3455
http://www.myomnipod.com

08478, 64895, 08220
INTEGRA LIFESCIENCES CORP
800-654-2873
800-931-1709
http://www.integra-ls.com

INTEGRATED THERAPEUTICS
See Integrative Therapeutics

88856
INTEGRATIVE HEALTH CONSULTING
See K-Pax Vitamins

INTEGRATIVE THERAPEUTICS
800-917-3696
http://www.integrativeinc.com

10922
INTENDIS, INC.
866-463-3634
http://www.intendis.com

42515
INTERCELL USA, INC.
301-556-4500
http://www.intercell.com

INTERCHEM CORP.
201-261-7333
800-261-7332
http://www.interchem.com

18968
INTERCURE, INC.
201-720-7750
877-988-9388
http://www.intercure.com

54746
INTERFERON SCIENCES
See Hemispherx Biopharma, Inc.

INTERMAX PHARMACEUTICALS, INC.
631-777-3318

64116
INTERMUNE PHARMACEUTICALS
415-466-2200
http://www.intermune.com

11584
INTERNATIONAL ETHICAL LABS
787-765-3510
800-981-5068
http://www.intetlab.com

00665
INTERNATIONAL LABS, INC.
727-327-4094
http://www.internationallabs.com

00548
INTERNATIONAL MEDICATION SYSTEMS, LTD.
877-651-2674
800-423-4136
http://www.ims-limited.com

INTERNEURON PHARMACEUTICALS, INC.
See Indevus Pharmaceuticals, Inc.

53746
INTERPHARM LTD
631-952-0214
http://www.interpharminc.com

00814
INTERSTATE DRUG EXCHANGE
See Henry Schein, Inc.

91536
INVACARE CORPORATION
800-333-6900
http://www.invacare.com

49939
INVADO PHARMACEUTICALS
914-715-6232
866-963-8881
http://www.invadopharmaceuticals.com

INVERESK RESEARCH, INC.
See Charles River Laboratories International, Inc.

38396
INVERNESS MEDICAL INNOVATIONS
781-647-3900
http://www.invernessmedical.com

16874
INVISION PHARMAEUCTICALS
407-499-2225
800-443-4313

00258
INWOOD LABORATORIES
See Forest Laboratories, Inc.

58768
IOLAB PHARMACEUTICALS
See Ciba Vision Corp.

61646
IOMED
See Iopharm

55532
ION LABS
727-527-1072
877-990-4466
http://www.ionlabs.com

IOP, INC.
714-549-1185
800-535-3545
http://www.iopinc.com

61646
IOPHARM
817-595-5820

54921
IPR PHARMACEUTICALS, INC.
787-750-5353
800-477-6385

55688
IPSEN PHARMACEUTICALS
508-478-8900
http://www.ipsen.com

42211
IROKO PHARMACEUTICALS
267-546-3003
866-916-0576
http://www.iroko.com

ISIS PHARMACEUTICALS
760-931-9200
http://www.isispharm.com

ISO-TEX DIAGNOSTICS, INC.
281-482-1231
800-613-0600
http://www.isotexdiagnostics.com

67425
ISTA PHARMACEUTICALS, INC.
949-788-6000
800-385-7034
http://www.istavision.com

IVAX CORPORATION
949-455-4700
800-545-8800
http://www.tevausa.com

13613
IVAX DERMATOLOGICALS
305-575-4312

IVAX PHARMACEUTICALS, INC.
305-575-6000
800-327-4114
http://www.ivaxpharmaceuticals.com

12126
IVY CORPORATION
973-575-1990
800-443-8856

59291
IYATA PHARMACEUTICAL
813-740-1810

99940,56091
J & J MEDICAL
732-524-0400
888-222-6036
http://www.jnj.com

16837
J & J MERCK CONSUMER AND SPECIALTY
215-273-7000
800-523-3484
http://www.jnj.com

51111
J.B. LABORATORIES
616-738-8500
http://www.jblabs.com

00304
J.J. BALAN, INC.
See HD Smith

J. R. CARLSON LABORATORIES
847-255-1600
888-234-5656
http://www.carlsonlabs.com

10106
J.T. BAKER (MALLINCKRODT)
908-859-2151
800-582-2537
http://www.mallbaker.com

72904
JACKSON-MITCHELL
209-667-2019
800-891-4628
http://www.meyenberg.com

49938
JACOBUS
609-921-7447

10592
JAMOL LABS
201-262-6363

50458
JANSSEN
609-730-2000
800-526-7736
http://www.janssen.com

90011
JARROW FORMULAS
310-204-6936
800-726-0886
http://www.jarrow.com

64661
JAYMAC PHARMACEUICALS, LLC
337-662-5962
800-520-5568
http://www.jaymacpharma.com

JAZZ PHARMACEUTICALS, INC.
650-496-3777
888-867-7426
http://www.jazzpharmaceuticals.com

68968
JDS PHARMACEUTICALS, LLC
See Noven Pharmaceuticals

50564
JEROME STEVENS
631-567-1113
800-325-9994

42023
JHP PHARMACEUTICALS
877-547-4547
866-923-2547
http://www.jhppharma.com

59841
J-MED PHARMACEUTICALS
617-247-0010

60793
JMI-CANTON PHARMACEUTICALS
See King Pharmaceuticals

00204
JOHNSON & JOHNSON
732-524-0400
http://www.jnj.com

00204
JOHNSON & JOHNSON CONSUMER PRODUCTS COMPANY
800-526-3967
732-524-0400
http://www.jnj.com

JOHNSON & JOHNSON HEALTHCARE
732-524-0400
http://www.jnj.com

52604
JONES PHARMA INCORPORATED
See King Pharmaceuticals, Inc.

68712
JSJ PHARMACEUTICALS
843-965-8333
800-499-4468
http://www.jsjpharm.com

59746
JUBILANT PHARMACEUTICALS
See Cadista

KV PHARMACEUTICAL COMPANY.
314-645-6600
800-234-5874
http://www.kvpharmaceutical.com

KABI PHARMACIA
See Pfizer US Pharmaceutical Group

KABIVITRUM, INC.
See Pfizer US Pharmaceutical Group

KAO BRANDS COMPANY
513-421-1400
800-742-8798
http://www.jergens.com

42043
KARALEX PHARMA
609-759-1777
866-306-0240
http://www.karalexpharma.com

28785
KAZ
800-477-0457
800-541-8001
http://www.kaz.com

68387
KELTMAN PHARMACEUTICALS
601-936-7533
800-325-0903
http://www.keltman.com

08219, 08881
KENDALL HEALTHCARE
508-261-8000
800-962-9888
http://www.covidien.com

00482
KENWOOD LABORATORIES
See Bradley Pharmaceutical, Inc.

00369
KEY PHARMACEUTICALS
See Schering-Plough Corp.

62291
KIEL LABORATORIES, INC.
678-450-9187
800-538-3146
http://www.kielpharm.com

36000
KIMBERLY-CLARK
972-281-1200
800-544-1847
http://www.kimberly-clark.com

60793
KING PHARMACEUTICALS, INC.
423-989-8000
800-776-3637
http://www.kingpharm.com

KINGSWOOD LABORATORIES, INC.
317-849-9513
800-968-7772
http://www.moi-stir.com

KINRAY
718-767-1234
800-854-6729
http://www.kinray.com

58223
KIRKMAN LABORATORIES, INC.
503-694-1600
800-245-8282
http://www.kirkmanlabs.com

28409
KLI CORP.
317-846-7452
800-308-7452
http://www.entertainers-secret.com

00074
KNOLL PHARMACEUTICALS
See Abbott Laboratories Pharmaceutical Division

58472
KODAK DENTAL
585-724-5631
800-933-8031
http://www.kodak.com

62515
KONEC, INC
520-571-9119
http://www.konec-inc.com

00224
KONSYL PHARMACEUTICALS
410-822-5192
800-356-6795
http://www.konsyl.com

60598
KOS PHARMACEUTICS, INC.
See Abbott Laboratories Pharmaceutical Division

66869
KOWA PHARMACEUTICALS AMERICA
334-288-1288
http://www.kowapharma.com

K-PAX VITAMINS
415-381-7565
877-777-5729
http://www.kpaxpharm.com

55505
KRAMER LABORATORIES, INC.
302-223-1287
800-824-4894
http://www.kramerlabs.com

52083
KRAMER-NOVIS
787-767-2072
787-771-9443
http://www.kramernovis.com

62175
KREMERS URBAN
877-332-1714
609-936-5940
http://www.kremersurbanllc.com

33216
KRS GLOBAL BIOTECHNOLOGY
877-506-0777
http://www.gbtbio.com

68716
KVD PHARMA
908-231-1911
888-477-2220
http://www.gbtbio.com

10702
KVK TECH, INC.
215-579-1842
http://www.kvktech.com

LABCORP
405-290-4444
800-634-9330
http://www.labcorp.com

LABOPHARM PHARMACEUTICALS
609-454-0207
877-345-6177
http://www.labopharm.com

48582
LACLEDE
310-605-4280
877-522-5333
http://www.laclede.com

LACRIMEDICS, INC.
360-376-7095
800-367-8327
http://www.lacrimedics.com

LACTAID, INC.
215-273-7000
800-522-8243
http://www.lactaid.com

10106
LAFAYETTE PHARMACEUTICALS, INC.
See J.T. Baker, Inc.

LAKE CONSUMER PRODUCTS
262-677-5007
800-537-8658
http://www.lakeconsumer.com

LAKE ERIE MEDICAL
734-847-3847
800-284-2130
http://www.lakeeriemedical.com

02110
LANE LABS
201-236-9090
800-526-3005
http://www.lanelabs.com

00527
LANNETT
215-333-9000
800-325-9994
http://www.lannett.com

44677
LANSINOH LABORATORIES
703-299-1100
800-292-4794
http://www.lansinoh.com

LANTHEUS MEDICAL IMAGING
800-362-2668
800-299-3431
http://www.radiopharm.com

68047
LARKEN LABORATORIES, INC.
601-855-7678
888-527-5522
http://www.larkenlabs.com

LA ROCHE-POSAY
888-577-5226
800-560-1803
http://www.laroche-posay.us

16477, 00277
LASER PHARMACEUTICALS
864-286-8229
http://www.laserpharmaceuticals.com

21247
LCM PHAMACEUTICAL
888-411-5465

LECTEC CORPORATION
903-832-0993
http://www.lectec.com

LEDERLE CONSUMER HEALTH
See Wyeth

00008
LEDERLE LABS
See Wyeth

00008
LEDERLE PHARMACEUTICAL DIVISION
See Wyeth

LEDERLE-PRAXIS BIOLOGICALS (WYETH)
See Wyeth

23558
LEE PHARMACEUTICALS
626-442-3141
800-950-5337
http://www.leepharmaceuticals.com

25332
LEGERE PHARMACEUTICALS, INC.
480-991-4033
800-528-3144

12496
LEHN & FINK
See Reckitt Benckiser Pharmaceuticals

05388, 74970, 74980, 59606, 54499
LEINER HEALTH PRODUCTS
310-835-8400
800-421-1168
http://www.leiner.com

10551
LEITNER PHARMACEUTICALS, LLC
866-590-7600
423-989-7238
http://www.leitnerpharma.com

00093
LEMMON CO.
See Teva Pharmaceuticals USA

50222
LEO PHARMA INC.
973-637-1690
877-494-4536
http://www.leo-pharma.us

62991
LETCO MEDICAL
256-350-1297
800-239-5288
http://www.letcomedical.com

49523
LEX PHARMACEUTICAL
305-888-7375

08387
LIBERTY MEDICAL SUPPLY
800-705-5797
866-342-2383
http://www.libertymedical.com

00440
LIBERTY PHARMACEUTICAL
866-836-9936
800-615-0721
http://www.libertymedical.com

72499
LIFE-LINE NUTRITIONAL PRODUCTS
520-426-3100
800-662-9862
http://www.nationalvitamin.com

53885
LIFESCAN, INC.
800-227-8862
800-524-7226
http://www.lifescan.com

LIFESIGN LLC
800-526-2125
http://www.lifesignmed.com

LIFESTYLE
732-972-8585
800-622-7376
http://www.purilens.com

64365
LIGAND PHARMACEUTICALS, INC.
858-550-7500
800-964-5836
http://www.ligand.com

66715
LIL DRUG STORE PRODUCTS
800-252-0454
319-393-0454
http://www.lildrugstore.com

LINCOLN DIAGNOSTICS
217-877-2531
800-537-1336
http://www.lincolndiagnostics.com

05632
LINE ONE LABORATORIES
818-886-2288
800-222-9848
http://www.lineonelabsusa.com

08566
LIONHEARTED INDUSTRIES
480-502-6007

61799
LIPOSOME CO.
See Elan Pharmaceuticals

16110
LIVERITE PRODUCTS
714-259-1800
888-425-5843
http://www.liverite.com

54859
LLORENS PHARMACEUTICAL
305-716-0595
866-595-5598
http://www.llorenspharm.com

00127
LOBANA LABORATORIES (ULMER PHARMACAL)
218-732-2656
800-848-5637
http://www.lobanaproducts.com

34672
LOBOB LABORATORIES
408-432-0580
800-835-6262
http://www.loboblabs.com

55390
LOCH PHARMACEUTICALS
See Bedford Laboratories

09198
LOGAN PHARMACEUTICALS
859-344-9600
888-644-3478

08429
LOGIMEDIX
800-821-0047
http://www.logimedix.com

61480
LOMA LUX LABORATORIES
918-664-9882
800-316-9636
http://www.lomalux.com

12333
LONGS DRUG
800-865-6647
http://www.longs.com

71249
LOREAL USA
212-818-1500
800-322-2036
http://www.lorealusa.com

00273
LORVIC CORP.
See Young Dental Mfg.

67754
LOTUS BIOCHEMICAL CORP.
See Harvest Pharmaceuticals, Inc.

LSI AMERICA CORPORATION
800-720-5936
http://www.ondrox.com

61598
LTC PRODUCTS
513-738-5583
http://www.ltcproducts.net

LUITPOLD PHARMACEUTICALS, INC.
631-924-4000
800-645-1706
http://www.Luitpold.com

38673
LUMISCOPE
800-672-8293

67386
LUNDBECK, INC.
866-337-6996
http://www.lundbeckusa.com

10892
LUNSCO, INC.
540-980-4358
800-264-8614

68180
LUPIN PHARMACEUTICALS, INC.
410-576-2000
866-466-1450
http://www.lupinpharmaceuticals.com

LUYTIES PHARMACAL CO.
800-466-3672
http://www.1-800homeopathy.com

00374
LYNE LABS
508-583-8700
800-525-0450
http://www.lyne.com

LYPHO-MED
See Astellas Pharma US, Inc.

44183
MACOVEN PHARMACEUTICALS
225-644-2494
877-622-6836
http://www.macovenpharma.com

58407
MAGNA PHARMACEUTICALS, INC.
888-206-5525
502-254-5552
http://www.magnaweb.com

43292
MAGNO-HUMPHRIES LABORATORIES
503-684-5464
800-935-6737
http://www.magno-humphries.com

10705
MAJESTIC DRUG
845-436-0011
800-238-0220
http://www.majesticdrug.com

00904
MAJOR PHARMACEUTICALS, INC.
800-616-2471
http://www.majorpharmaceuticals.com

MALLINCKRODT
314-654-2000
800-778-7898
http://www.mallinckrodt.com

10106
MALLINCKRODT BAKER, INC.
See Avantor Performance Materials

23635
MALLINCKRODT BRAND PHARMA
314-654-2000
800-554-5343
http://www.mallincrodt.com

MALLINCKRODT CHEMICAL
314-654-2000
800-325-8888
http://www.mallinckrodt.com

99913
MALLINCKRODT NUCLEAR MEDICINE
314-654-2000
888-744-1414
http://www.mallinckrodt.com

99880
MALLINCKRODT RESPIRATORY
800-635-5267

45043
MANCHESTER PHARMACEUTICALS
970-685-4119
866-758-7068
http://www.manchesterpharma.com

10706
MANNE
843-768-4080
800-517-0228

42998
MARATHON PHARMACEUTICALS LLC
866-945-7860
866-931-0706
http://www.marathonpharma.com

12539
MARIN PHARMACEUTICALS
See A. G. Marin Pharmaceuticals

MARION MERRELL DOW
See Sanofi-Aventis US

10135
MARLEX PHARMACEUTICALS
302-328-3355
866-820-7381
http://www.marlexpharm.com

MARLIN INDUSTRIES
805-473-2743
800-423-5926

12939
MARLOP PHARM
908-355-8854

MARLYN NUTRACEUTICALS, INC.
480-991-0200
888-766-4406
http://www.naturally.com

00682
MARNEL PHARMACEUTICALS, INC.
337-232-1396
800-962-7635

00591, 52544
MARSAM PHARMACEUTICALS
See Watson Pharmaceuticals

52555
MARTEC PHARMACEUTICAL, INC.
816-241-4144
800-822-6782
http://www.martec-kc.com

11845
MASON VITAMINS
305-428-6861
888-860-5376
http://www.masonvitamins.com

14362
MASS. PUBLIC HEALTH BIO. LAB.
617-474-3000
800-457-4626

08496
MASTERS PHARMACEUTICAL
513-354-2690
800-982-7922
http://www.mastersrx.com

53905
MATRIX LABORATORIES, INC.
See Chiron Therapeutics

62750
MATRIXX INITIATIVES, INC.
602-385-8888
800-808-4866
http://www.zicam.com

41554
MAYBELLINE
800-944-0730

16169
MAYER LABORATORIES
510-437-8989
800-426-6366
http://www.mayerlabs.com

61703
MAYNE PHARMA (USA) INC.
201-225-5500
866-594-8420
http://www.maynepharma.com

MAYO FOUNDATION
507-284-2511
http://www.mayo.edu

00259
MAYRAND, INC.
See Merz Pharmaceuticals

00264
MCGAW, INC.
See B. Braun Medical, Inc.

49072
MCGUFF PHARMACEUTICALS, INC.
714-918-7277
800-603-4795
http://www.mcguff.com

63739, 38703, 49348
MCKESSON CORPORATION
415-983-8300
800-482-3784
http://www.mckesson.com

MCKESSON MEDICAL-SURGICAL
804-264-7500
800-446-3008
http://www.mckgenmed.com

57935
MCNEIL CONSUMER
215-273-7000
800-962-5357
http://www.jnj.com

00045, 00062
MCNEIL PHARMACEUTICAL
See Ortho-McNeil Pharmaceutical

58605
MCR AMERICAN PHARMACEUTICAL
352-754-8587
http://www.mcramerican.com

53014
MD PHARMACEUTICAL
714-751-5881

58607
ME PHARMACEUTICALS, INC.
765-886-5097
866-578-9637
http://www.mepharmusa.com

MEAD JOHNSON LABORATORIES
See Bristol-Myers Squibb Co.

MEAD JOHNSON NUTRITIONALS
812-429-5000
http://www.mjn.com

11883
MEAD-RAYMOND
903-509-0663

00037
MEDA PHARMACEUTICALS
732-564-2200
888-455-8383
http://www.medapharma.us

MEDAREX, INC.
609-430-2880
http://www.medarex.com

53276
MED-CHEM PRODUCTS
781-932-5900
http://www.crbard.com

11940
MEDCO LABS
216-292-7546
http://www.medcolabs.com

60793
MEDCO RESEARCH, INC.
See King Pharmaceuticals, Inc.

08212
MEDCON BIOLAB TECHNOLOGIES, INC.
508-839-4203
800-443-6332
http://www.ilexpaste.com

45565
MED-DERM
423-926-4413
800-877-8869
http://www.crownlaboratories.com

67112
MEDECOR PHARMA
225-343-9830
http://www.medecorpharma.com

64253
MEDEFIL, INC.
630-682-4600
http://www.medefil.com

MEDEGEN
901-867-2951
800-233-1987
http://www.medegen.com

MEDEVA PHARMACEUTICALS
See UCB Pharmaceuticals, Inc.

MEDI AID CORP.
See Baxa Corp.

MEDICAL ACTION INDUSTRIES
631-231-4600
800-645-7042
http://www.medical-action.com

26974
MEDICAL NUTRITION, INC.
201-569-1188
800-221-0308
http://www.pro-stat.com

08271, 28465
MEDICAL PLASTIC DEVICES
514-694-9835
888-527-2842
http://www.medplas.com

10733
MEDICAL PRODUCTS LABS
800-523-0191
215-677-2700
http://www.medicalproducts laboratories.com

00576
MEDICAL PRODUCTS PANAMERICANA
305-545-6524
305-670-4416

99207
MEDICIS PHARMACEUTICAL CORPORATION
602-808-8800
888-845-1313
http://www.medicis.com

32671
MEDICORE INC.
305-558-4000
800-327-8894
http://www.medicore.com

25208
MEDICURE
732-584-5231
866-210-1128
http://www.medicurepharm.com

54365
MEDI-FLEX, INC.
913-451-0800
800-523-0502
http://www.medi-flex.com

43538
MEDIMETRIKS PHARMACEUTICALS
973-882-7512
http://www.medimetriks.com

60574
MEDIMMUNE, INC.
301-398-0000
877-633-4411
http://www.medimmune.com

67150
MEDINICHE
314-542-9539
800-711-4303
http://www.mediniche.com

00095
MEDI-PLEX PHARM., INC.
See ECR Pharmaceuticals

47682
MEDIQUE PRODUCTS CO.
239-790-1962
800-634-7680
http://www.mediqueproducts.com

38779
MEDISCA INC.
518-561-0109
800-932-1039
http://www.medisca.com

MEDISENSE, INC.
See Abbott Diabetes Care

12418
MEDIX PHARMACEUTICALS AMERICAS, INC. (MPA)
See Johnson & Johnson Consumer Products Co.

53329,08327
MEDLINE/DERMAL MANAGEMENT
800-633-5463
http://www.medline.com

80196
MEDLINE INDUSTRIES
800-MEDLINE
http://www.medline.com

53978
MED-PRO, INC.
308-324-4571
800-447-6060
http://www.med-pro-inc.com

46011
MED-SYSTEMS INC
888-547-5492
http://www.sinucleanse.com

90124, 18122
MEDQUIP
843-815-5301
888-404-5666
http://www.medquip.com

MEDTECH LABORATORIES, INC.
307-733-1680
800-443-4908
http://www.medtechinc.com

MEDTRONIC INC.
763-514-4000
800-328-2518
http://www.medtronic.com

58281
MEDTRONIC NEUROLOGICAL
800-328-0810
http://www.medtronic.com

66116
MEDVANTX, INC.
858-625-2990
http://www.medvantx.com

41250
MEIJER
616-453-6711
http://www.meijer.com

13143
MELVILLE BIOLOGICS (PRECISION PHARMA SERVICES)
631-752-7314
http://www.precisionpharma.com

MENICON AMERICA
650-378-1424
800-636-4266
http://www.menicon.com

22200
MENNEN CO.
See Colgate-Palmolive Co.

42279
MENPER DISTRIBUTORS, INC.
305-836-0208
800-560-5223

10742
MENTHOLATUM
716-677-2500
800-688-7660
http://www.mentholatum.com

81317
MENTOR UROLOGY
805-879-6000
800-525-0245
http://www.mentorcorp.com

MERCATOR MEDSYSTEMS, INC.
510-614-4550
http://www.mercatormed.com

00006
MERCK SHARP & DOHME
908-423-1000
800-444-2080
http://www.merck.com

00006
MERCK HUMAN HEALTH (A DIVISION OF MERCK & CO.)
215-652-5000
800-672-6372
http://www.merck.com

66582
MERCK/SCHERING-PLOUGH PHARM
866-637-2501
http://www.msppharma.com

62909
MERETEK DIAGNOSTICS, INC.
720-479-6400
888-637-3835
http://www.meretek.com

00394
MERICON INDUSTRIES, INC.
309-693-2150
800-242-6464
http://www.mericon-industries.com

MERIDIAN MEDICAL TECHNOLOGIES
443-259-7800
800-638-8093
http://www.meridianmeds.com

30727
MERIT PHARMACEUTICALS
323-227-4831
800-696-3748
http://www.meritpharm.com

00259
MERZ PHARMACEUTICALS
336-856-2003
800-637-9872
http://www.merzusa.com

55571
METAGENICS, INC.
800-692-9400
http://www.metagenics.com

64281
METHAPHARM, INC. (HEAD OFFICE)
954-341-0795
800-287-7686
http://www.methapharm.com

08368
METRIKA, INC.
408-524-2255
877-212-4968
http://www.A1cNow.com

86560
MET-RX USA
800-556-3879
http://www.met-rx.com

61738
METTLER ELECTRONICS
714-533-2221
800-854-9305
http://www.mettlerelectronics.com

58063
MGI PHARMA, INC.
952-346-4700
800-562-5580
http://www.mgipharma.com

MICHIGAN DEPARTMENT OF HEALTH
517-373-3740

MICROGENESYS, INC.
See Protein Sciences Corp.

42632
MICROLIFE
727-451-0484
888-314-2599
http://www.microlife.com

08564
MICROMEDICS
800-624-5662
http://www.micromedics-usa.com

MICRON TECHNOLOGY, INC.
208-368-4000
http://www.micron.com

11042
MIDDLEBROOK PHARMACEUTICALS, INC.
301-944-6600
800-340-3641
http://www.advancispharm.com

15686
MIDLAND PHARMACEUTICAL, LLC
913-233-0054

68308
MIDLOTHIAN LABORATORIES, LLC
334-288-8661
800-344-8661
http://www.midlothianlabs.com

46672
MIKART
404-351-4510
888-4MIKART
http://www.mikart.com

00026
MILES, INC.
See Bayer Corp.

00396
MILEX PRODUCTS, INC.
See Cooper Surgical

63020
MILLENNIUM PHARMACEUTICALS
617-679-7000
800-390-5663
http://www.millennium.com

17204
MILLER
630-871-9557
800-323-2935
http://www.millerpharmacal.com

53118
MILLGOOD LABORATORIES, INC.

18757
MILLENNIUM BIOTECHNOLOGIES
908-604-2500
888-412-9179
http://www.milbiotch.com

81361
MILUPA NORTH AMERICA
877-264-5872
http://www.milupana.com

60307
MINRAD, INC.
716-855-1068
800-832-3303
http://www.minrad.com

00485
MISEMER PHARMACEUTICALS, INC.
See Edwards Pharmaceuticals, Inc.

00178
MISSION PHARMACAL
210-696-8400
800-531-3333
http://www.missionpharmacal.com

MOLNLYCKE HEALTHCARE
678-250-7900
800-843-8497
http://www.molnlycke.com

04351
MONAGHAN MEDICAL CORPORATION
518-561-7330
800-833-9653
http://www.monaghanmed.com

61570
MONARCH PHARMACEUTICALS
See King Pharmaceuticals

11868
MONTICELLO DRUG CO.
904-384-3666
800-735-0666
http://www.monticellocompanies.com

65883
MONTIFF INC.
310-582-8938

00839
MOORE MEDICAL CORP.
800-234-1464
http://www.mooremedical.com

MOREPEN INC.
609-987-1134
http://www.morepen.com

60432
MORTON GROVE PHARMACEUTICALS
800-346-6854
847-967-5600
http://www.mgp-online.com

MORTON INTERNATIONAL
215-592-3000
http://www.rohmhaas.com

MORTON SALT
312-807-2000
http://www.mortonsalt.com

MOTHERSOY INTERNATIONAL, INC.
812-424-5432
888-769-0769
http://www.mothersoy.com

MOUNT SINAI MEDICAL CTR.
212-241-6500
800-637-4624

MOVA PHARMACEUTICAL CORPORATION
905-816-3944
888-728-4366
http://www.patheon.com

66977
MPM MEDICAL, INC.
972-893-4090
800-232-5512
http://www.mpmmedicalinc.com

74676
MUELLER
608-643-8530
800-356-9522
http://www.muellersportsmed.com

00150
MURRAY DRUG CORP.
270-753-6654

53489
MUTUAL PHARMACEUTICAL CO., INC. (UNITED RESEARCH LABORATORIES)
215-288-6500
800-523-3684
http://www.urlmutual.com

00378
MYLAN
724-514-1800
800-796-9526
http://www.mylan.com

20694
MYOGEN
See Gilead Sciences

59730
NABI
301-770-3099
800-685-5579
http://www.nabi.com

57459
NASTECH PHARMACEUTICAL CO., INC.
425-908-3600
http://www.nastech.com

08164
NATIONAL MEDICAL PRODUCTS, INC.
949-768-1147
http://www.jtip.com

94688
NATIONAL NUTRITION, INC.
717-569-8561
877-271-3570
http://www.medtritionnni.com

54629
NATIONAL VITAMIN
559-781-8871
800-538-5828
http://www.nationalvitamin.com

NATREN, INC.
805-371-4737
800-992-3323
http://www.natren.com

47469
NATROL, INC.
818-739-6000
800-262-8765
http://www.natrol.com

94604
NAT-RUL HEALTH PRODUCTS
800-628-7855
http://www.natrulhealth.com

NATURALLY VITAMINS CO.
480-991-0200
888-766-4406
http://www.naturallyvitamins.com

93265
NATURES BEST
312-245-2834
800-551-2544
http://www.naturesbestenzyme.com

74312
NATURES BOUNTY, INC.
800-348-0090
631-567-9500
http://www.naturesbounty.com

NATURES SUNSHINE PRODUCTS, INC.
801-342-4300
800-223-8225
http://www.naturessunshine.com

65203
NATURE'S VISION
269-327-8282
877-740-8180
http://www.naturesvisioninc.com

NATURE'S WAY
801-489-1500
800-926-8883
http://www.naturesway.com

74312
NBTY, INC.
See Nature's Bounty, Inc.

60242
NEIL LABS
609-448-5500
http://www.neillabs.com

05928
NEILMED PHARMACEUTICALS
707-525-3784
877-477-8633
http://www.neilmed.com

72559
NELLSON NEUTRACEUTICAL (FORMERLY NCI MEDICAL FOODS)
626-812-6522
800-869-1515

NEORX CORP.
206-281-7001
http://www.neorx.com

58414
NEOSTRATA
609-520-0715
800-225-9411
http://www.neostrata.com

51759
NEPHROCEUTICALS
937-281-0123
http://www.nephroceuticals.com

00487
NEPHRON PHARMACEUTICALS CORP.
407-246-1389
800-433-4313
http://www.nephronpharm.com

59528
NEPHRO-TECH
785-883-4108
800-879-4755
http://www.nephrotech.com

99825
NESTLE HEALTHCARE NUTRITION
847-317-2800
877-463-7853
http://www.nestleclinicalnutrition.com

NESTLE INFANT NUTRITION
800-284-9488
http://www.verybestbaby.com

62860
NEUREX PHARMACEUTICALS
See Elan Pharmaceuticals

NEUROGENESIS
800-345-8912
http://www.neurogenesis.com

14565
NEUROSCI
937-848-9130
http://www.neurosciinc.com

NEUTRACEUTICAL SOLUTIONS, INC.
361-854-0755
800-856-7040
http://www.eliquidsolutions.com

10812
NEUTROGENA CORPORATION
310-642-1150
800-582-4048
http://www.neutrogena.com

NEUTRON TECHNOLOGY CORP.
See Micron Technology, Inc.

NEW WORLD TRADING CORP.
407-566-0608

10530
NEXCO PHARMA
713-896-4949
http://www.nexcopharma.com

00722
NEXGEN PHARMA
949-862-0340
http://www.nexgenpharm.com

61958
NEXSTAR PHARMACEUTICALS
See Gilead Sciences

24478
NEXTWAVE PHARMACEUTICALS
847-996-6200
http://www.nextwavepharm.com

14789
NEXUS PHARMACEUTICALS
888-806-4606
847-996-3789
http://www.nexuspharma.net

45611
NFI CONSUMER PRODUCTS
800-432-9334
http://www.nfiproducts.com

59016
NICHE PHARMACEUTICALS
817-491-2770
800-677-0355
http://www.niche-inc.com

08384,38384
NIPRO DIAGNOSTICS
800-342-7226
http://www.niprodiagnostics.com

38379,41405
NIPRO MEDICAL CORPORATION
305-599-7174
888-647-7698
http://www.nipro.com

12948
NITROMED, INC.
781-266-4000
http://www.nitromed.com

15662
NNODUM CORPORATION
513-861-2329
888-301-0457
http://www.zikspain.com

51801
NOMAX, INC.
314-961-2500
800-397-0012
http://www.nomax.com

NORAMCO INC.
706-353-4400
http://www.noramco.com

50445
NORDISK
609-987-5800
http://www.novonordisk-us.com

59730
NORTH AMERICAN BIOLOGICALS, INC.
See Nabi

76906
NORTH AMERICAN HERBAL
800-836-3095
http://www.northamericanherbal.com

62448
NORTH AMERICAN VACCINE, INC.
See Baxter Healthcare Corp.

92942
NORTHERN RESEARCH LABORATORIES, INC.
See Epien Medical

16714
NORTHSTAR RX
480-502-6007
800-206-7821
http://www.northstarrxllc.com

29033
NOSTRUM PHARMACEUTICALS, INC.
732-635-0036
http://www.nostrumpharma.com

08548
NOVA BIOMEDICAL
781-894-0800
800-458-5813
http://www.novabiomedical.com

NOVADEL PHARMA
908-203-4640
http://www.novadel.com

99780
NOVAPLUS
See Novation

00067.
NOVARTIS CONSUMER HEALTH
See Novartis Pharmaceuticals Corp.

00212, 41679
NOVARTIS MEDICAL NUTRITION
862-778-8300
888-669-6682
http://www.novartisnutrition.com

58768
NOVARTIS OPHTHALMICS, INC.
866-393-6336
See Novartis Pharmaceuticals Corp.

NOVARTIS PHARMA AG
See Novartis Pharmaceuticals Corp.

00078
NOVARTIS PHARMACEUTICALS CORPORATION
862-778-8300
888-669-6682
http://www.pharma.us.novartis.com

NOVATION
888-766-8283
http://www.novationco.com

66500
NOVAVAX
240-268-2000
http://www.novavax.com

68968
NOVEN PHARMACEUTICALS
305-253-5099
888-253-5099
http://www.noven.com

NOVEN THERAPEUTICS, LLC
866-663-2539
800-455-8070
http://www.jdspharma.com

00169, 59060
NOVO NORDISK PHARMACEUTICALS
609-987-5800
800-727-6500
http://www.novonordisk-us.com

49197
NOVOGEN
203-966-2556
http://www.novogen.com

00093
NOVOPHARM USA, INC.
See Teva Pharmaceuticals USA

00159,48932
NOYES
800-522-2469
http://www.pjnoyes.com

NU SKIN ENTERPRISES
801-345-1000
800-487-1000
http://www.nuskinenterprises.com

NUGYN, INC.
763-398-0108
877-774-1442
http://www.eros-therapy.com

08910
NULINE PHARMACEUTICALS
914-939-8881
http://www.nulinepharma.com

55499
NUMARK LABS
732-417-1870
800-338-8079
http://www.numarklabs.com

07249,00221
NUTRA BALANCE
800-654-3691
317-356-5478
http://www.nutra-balance-products.com

NUTRACEA
877-723-1700
http://www.nutracea.com

NUTRACEUTICAL SOLUTIONS
361-854-0755
800-856-7040
http://www.eliquidsolutions.com

02359
NUTRACEUTICS CORPORATION
877-664-6684
http://www.neutraceutics.com

55970
NUTRAMAX LABORATORIES, INC.
410-776-4000
800-925-5187
http://www.nutramaxlabs.com

NUTRAMAX PRODUCTS
978-282-1800
http://www.nutramax.com

NUTRASAL, LLC
207-856-2222
888-437-5772
http://www.nutrasal.com

NUTRI VENTION
210-661-8589
800-390-7940

49735
NUTRICIA NORTH AMERICA
301-795-2300
800-365-7354
http://www.shsna.com

NUTRITION 21
914-701-4500
800-696-0860
http://www.nutrition21.com

90962
NUTRITIONAL DESIGNS
516-612-4900
888-263-5227
http://www.ndlabs.com

91124
NUVORA, INC.
408-856-2200
877-530-9811
http://www.nuvorainc.com

00407
NYCOMED AMERSHAM
See GE Healthcare

NYCOMED US INC.
631-454-7677
800-645-9833
http://www.nycomedus.com

11169
OAKHURST CO.
516-731-5380
800-831-1135
http://www.oakhurst-medicine.com

62032
OBAGI MEDICAL PRODUCTS
562-628-1007
http://www.obagi.com

68682
OCEANSIDE PHARMACEUTICALS
949-461-6199
http://www.oceanside pharmaceuticals.com

55515, 80831.
OCLASSEN PHARMACEUTICALS, INC.
See Watson Pharmaceuticals

21406, 55056
O'CONNOR, INC.
See Columbia Laboratories, Inc.

68209
OCTAPHARMA USA, INC.
703-766-4860
866-766-4860
http://www.octapharma.com

53152
OCTOGEN PHARMACAL
770-843-7032
800-729-4613
http://www.octogenpharma.com

65473
ODYSSEY PHARMACEUTICALS, INC.
877-427-9068
http://www.odysseypharm.com

51660
OHM LABORATORIES, INC.
877-646-5227
http://www.ohmlabs.com

OMNII ORAL PHARMACEUTICALS
561-689-1140
800-445-3386
http://www.4oralcare.com

94030
OMNIS HEALTH
877-450-6734
http://www.omnishealth.com

73796
OMRON MANAGED HEALTHCARE
877-216-1333
847-680-6200
http://www.omronhealthcare.com

16781
ONSET THERAPEUTICS
888-713-8154
877-702-0532
http://www.onsettx.com

68305, 93286
ONTOS, INC
360-740-0888
888-469-7546
http://www.4myskin.com

ONY
716-636-9096
877-274-4669
http://www.onyinc.com

11916, 64108
OPTICS LABORATORY, INC.
626-350-1926
800-968-6788
http://www.opticslab.com

OPTIKEM INTERNATIONAL
800-525-1752

63369
OPTIMED CONTROLLED RELEASE LAB
See Quality by Design Packaging

50520
OPTIMOX
310-618-9370
800-223-1601
http://www.optimox.com

00041
ORAL-B LABORATORIES
800-566-7252
http://www.oral-b.com

65976
ORAPHARMA, INC.
215-956-2200
866-273-7846
http://www.orapharma.com

ORASURE TECHNOLOGIES
610-882-1820
800-869-3535
http://www.orasure.com

68820
ORCHID HEALTHCARE
480-502-6007
480-227-7661

ORGANOGENESIS INC.
781-575-0775
http://www.organogenesis.com

00052
ORGANON, INC.
973-325-4500
800-222-7579
http://www.organon-usa.com

66203
ORGANON SANOFI
973-325-4500
http://www.organon-usa.com

ORGANON TEKNIKA CORP.
See Biomerieux

15377
ORIGIN BIOMED
902-423-5745
888-234-7256
http://www.originbiomed.com

62161
ORPHAN MEDICAL, INC.
See Jazz Pharmaceuticals

66607
ORPHAN PHARMACEUTICALS USA
See Rare Disease Therapeutics

ORTHO BIOTECH PRODUCTS, L.P.
See Centocor Ortho Biotech, Inc.

00562
ORTHO-CLINICAL DIAGNOSTICS, INC.
800-828-6316
http://www.orthoclinical.com

99948
ORTHO DERM
800-426-7762
http://www.orthodermatologics.com

00062
ORTHO-MCNEIL PHARMACEUTICAL
800-682-6532
http://www.ortho-mcneil.com

ORTHO NEUTROGENA
800-426-7762
http://www.orthoneutrogena.com

67707
OSCIENT PHARMACEUTICALS
781-398-2300
http://www.oscient.com

65231
OSI PHARMACEUTICALS
631-962-2000
800-572-1932
http://www.osip.com

10244
OTIS CLAPP & SONS
800-775-5400
http://www.otisclapp.com

15210
OTN GENERICS
650-952-8400
800-482-6700
http://www.lynx2otn.com

59148
OTSUKA AMERICA
301-990-0030
800-562-3974
http://www.otsuka.com

67386
OVATION PHARMACEUTICALS, INC.
847-282-1000
888-514-5204
http://www.ovationpharma.com

08470, 08214
OWEN MUMFORD
770-977-2226
800-421-6936
http://www.owenmumford.com

64803
OXFORD PHARMACEUTICAL SERVICES
973-256-0600
http://www.oxfordpharm.com

OXIS INTERNATIONAL
650-212-2568
800-547-3686
http://www.oxisresearch.com

99949
P & G HEALTH
513-983-1100
800-543-7270
http://www.pg.com

99958
P & G PAPER PRODUCTS
513-983-1100
800-543-7270
http://www.pg.com

P & S LABORATORIES, INC.
See Standard Homeopathic Co.

64393
PACIFIC EMERALD CO.
425-485-9208

60758
PACIFIC PHARMA
800-811-4184
714-246-4600

65250
PACIRA PHARMACEUTICALS, INC.
858-625-2424
858-625-2414
http://www.pacira.com

16571
PACK PHARMACEUTICALS, LLC
847-229-0153
800-521-5340
http://www.packpharma.com

00574
PADDOCK LABORATORIES, INC.
763-546-4676
800-328-5113
http://www.paddocklabs.com

38142
PAL MIDWEST, LTD.
815-965-2981
815-332-9405
http://www.rashcream.com

25294
PALCO LABS
831-430-1600
800-346-4488
http://www.palcolabs.com

00516
PALISADES PHARMACEUTICALS, INC.
See Glenwood, Inc.

24518
PALM PHARMACEUTICALS
843-364-3256
http://www.palmpharmaceuticals.com

16477
PALMETTO PHARMACEUTICALS, INC.
864-286-8229

00525
PAMLAB, LLC
985-893-4097
http://www.pamlab.com

PAN AMERICAN LABORATORIES
See Pamlab, LLC

86679
PAPERPAK
See Attends Healthcare Products

49884
PAR PHARMACEUTICAL, INC.
201-802-4000
800-828-9393
http://www.parpharm.com

66758
PARENTA PHARMACEUTICALS, INC.
803-461-5500
800-898-9948
http://www.parentarx.com

44229,83490
PARI RESPIRATORY
804-253-7274
http://www.pari.com

PARKE-DAVIS - A PFIZER CO.
See Pfizer US Pharmaceutical Group

64029
PARKEDALE PHARMACEUTICALS
See King Pharmaceuticals, Inc.

00341
PARKER LABORATORIES, INC.
973-276-9500
800-631-8888
http://www.parkerlabs.com

50930
PARNELL
415-256-1800
800-457-4276
http://www.parnellpharm.com

49309
PARTHENON CO., INC.
801-972-5184
800-453-8898
http://www.parthenoninc.com

00418, 11098
PASADENA RESEARCH LABS
See Akorn, Inc.

10866
PASCAL CO., INC.
425-827-4694
800-426-8051
http://www.pascaldental.com

PATHEON
905-821-4001
888-728-4366
http://www.patheon.com

10147
PATRIOT PHARMACEUTICALS LLC
215-325-7676
800-631-5273
http://www.patriotpharmaceuticals.com

08519
PATTON MEDICAL DEVICES
877-763-7678
http://www.pattonmd.com

PBI
See Upsher-Smith Labs, Inc.

66213
PBM PHARMACEUTICALS
540-832-3282
800-485-9828
http://www.pbmpharmaceuticals.com

PDK LABS, INC.
631-273-2630
http://www.pdklabs.com

55289
PDRX PHARMACEUTICAL
405-942-3040
800-299-7379
http://www.pdrx.com

66346
PEDIAMED PHARMACEUTICALS, INC.
859-282-8582
866-543-6337
http://www.pediamedpharma.com

PEDIATRIC PHARMACEUTICALS
732-603-7708
http://www.pediatricpharm.com

00884
PEDINOL PHARMACAL, INC.
631-293-9500
800-733-4665
http://www.pedinol.com

10974
PEGASUS
850-478-2770
http://www.pegasuslabs.com

25074
PENEDERM, INC.
See Bertek Pharmaceuticals, Inc.

13893
PENN LABORATORIES
877-300-6153
http://www.pennlaboratories.com

60432
PENNEX PHARMACEUTICAL, INC.
See Morton Grove Pharmaceuticals, Inc.

PENTECH PHARMACEUTICALS, INC.
847-255-0303
http://www.pentechinc.com

PERNIX THERAPEUTICS, LLC
225-647-2002
800-793-2145
http://www.pernixtx.com

00113, 10768
PERRIGO COMPANY
269-673-8451
800-719-9260
http://www.perrigo.com

00096
PERSON COVEY
818-240-1030
800-423-2341
http://www.personandcovey.com

PERSONAL PRODUCTS CO.
See Johnson&Johnson Healthcare

00927
PFEIFFER CO.
404-614-0255
800-342-6450
http://www.pfeifferpharmaceuticals.com

12547
PFIZER CONSUMER HEALTH
973-660-5500
800-762-4675
http://www.pfizer.com

PFIZER US PHARMACEUTICAL GROUP
212-733-2323
800-879-3477
http://www.pfizer.com

PHARMA FRONTIERS
281-775-0609
http://www.pharmafrontier.com

62441
PHARMA MEDICA
905-624-9115
http://www.pharmamedica.com

52959
PHARMA PAC
805-929-1333
800-841-5554
http://www.pharmapac.com

39822
PHARMA-TEK, INC.
See X-Gen Pharmaceuticals, Inc.

00121
PHARMACEUTICAL ASSOCIATES, INC.
864-277-7282
800-845-8210
http://www.pa-inc.net

PHARMACEUTICAL BASICS, INC.
See Upsher-Smith Labs, Inc.

51655
PHARMACEUTICAL CORP OF AMERICA
317-616-4498
800-722-0772

21659
PHARMACEUTICAL LABS, INC.
See Neutraceutical Solutions, Inc.

45334
PHARMACEUTICAL SPECIALTIES, INC.
507-288-8500
800-325-8232
http://www.psico.com

12547
PHARMACIA & UPJOHN CONSUMER HEALTHCARE - A DIVISION OF PFIZER
See Pfizer Consumer Health

PHARMACIA CORP. - A DIVISION OF PFIZER
See Pfizer US Pharmaceutical Group

63704
PHARMACIST PHARMACEUTICAL LLC
540-981-1004

00462
PHARMADERM
678-287-1500
866-337-6457
http://www.pharmaderm.com

55422, 65937
PHARMAKON LABS
813-886-3216
http://www.pharmakonlabs.com

PHARMALUCENCE
781-275-7120
800-221-7554
http://www.pharmalucence.com

15035
PHARMANEX
801-345-9800
http://www.pharmanex.com

51817
PHARMASCIENCE LAB
514-340-9800
800-363-8805
http://www.pharmascience.com

48107
PHARMASSURE, INC.
888-462-2548

31604, 78742
PHARMAVITE
818-221-6200
800-423-2405
http://www.pharmavite.com

PHARMED
800-683-7342
305-592-2324
http://www.pharmed.com

PHARMEDIUM
847-457-2300
800-523-7749
http://www.pharmedium.com

53002
PHARMEDIX
800-486-1811
http://www.pharmedixrx.com

66663
PHARMELLE
See Azur Pharma

00813
PHARMICS, INC.
801-966-4138
800-456-4138
http://www.pharmics.com

67211
PHARMION CORPORATION
See Celgene Corp.

54348
PHARMPAK
415-455-9981
800-541-6315
http://www.pharmpakinc.com

PHOENIX LABORATORIES
516-822-1230

PHOTOCURE ASA
47-22-06-22-10
http://www.photocure.com

PHOTOMEDEX
215-619-3600
http://www.photomedex.com

54868
PHYSICIANS TOTAL CARE
918-254-2273
800-759-3650
http://www.physicianstotalcare.com

PHYTOPHARMICA, INC.
920-469-1313
800-553-2370
http://www.enzymatictherapy.com

60831
PIERRE FABRE PHARMACEUTICALS
973-898-1042
http://www.pierre-fabre.com

44733
PLAINVIEW HEALTHCARE
800-903-3222
http://www.dairycare.com

PLAYTEX CO.
800-222-0453
http://www.playtex.com

50111
PLIVA, INC.
973-386-5566
800-922-0547
http://www.plivainc.com

41100, 11523
PLOUGH, INC.
See Schering-Plough Healthcare Products

37864
PLUS PHARMA
631-543-3334

50991
POLY PHARMACEUTICALS, INC.
601-776-3497
800-882-1041

POLYMEDICA CORPORATION
781-933-2020
800-886-4050
http://www.polymedica.com

POLYMEDICA PHARMACEUTICALS
See Amerifit Brands, Inc.

47144
POLYMER TECHNOLOGY CORP.
978-658-6111
800-323-0000
http://www.polymer.com

08193
POLYMER TECHNOLOGY SYSTEMS
317-870-5610
877-870-5610
http://www.cardiocheck.com

49963
PORTAL PHARMACEUTICALS
787-832-6645

55688
PORTON PRODUCT LIMITED
See Speywood Pharmaceuticals, Inc.

POWDERJECT VACCINES
See Chiron Therapeutics

POYTHRESS
See ECR Pharmaceuticals

68158
PRAECIS PHARMACEUTICALS INCORPORATED
781-795-4100
877-772-3247
http://www.gsk.com

62263,63370
PRAGMATIC MATERICALS INC.
440-349-1313

66993
PRASCO LABORATORIES
513-618-3333
866-525-0688
http://www.prasco.com

PRATT PHARMACEUTICALS
See Pfizer US Pharmaceutical Group

68094
PRECISION DOSE, INC
800-397-9228
http://www.precisiondose.com

72058
PRECISION FOODS
800-442-5242
http://www.precisionfoods.com

PREMIER MICRONUTRIENT
615-234-4020
888-606-8883
http://www.premiermicronutrient.com

PRESS CHEMICAL & PHARMACEUTICAL LABORATORIES, INC.
614-863-2802
http://www.epsal.com

75137
PRESTIGE BRANDS INTERNATIONAL
914-524-6810
800-803-4471
http://www.prestigebrands.com

66378
PRESUTTI LABORATORIES
847-483-6050
http://www.presuttilabs.com

42582
PREVENTION LABORATORIES
800-473-1205
618-252-6922
http://www.preventionlabs.com

00684
PRIMEDICS LABORATORIES
323-770-3005

68040
PRIMUS PHARMACEUTICALS, INC.
480-483-1410
http://www.primusrx.com

39278
PRINCE OF PEACE
800-732-2328
510-887-1799
http://www.popus.com

PRINCETON PHARM. PRODUCTS
See Bristol-Myers Squibb Co.

PRIORITY HEALTHCARE
See Curascript

PROCTER & GAMBLE COMPANY
513-983-1100
800-543-7270
http://www.pgpharma.com

00149
PROCTER & GAMBLE PHARMACEUTICALS
See Warner Chilcott Pharma

PROCYTE CORPORAITON
425-869-1239
http://www.procyte.com

08524
PROGRESSIVE HEALTH SUPPLY
888-887-4772
http://www.progressivehealthsupply.com

66375
PROMEDICA LABS, INC.
973-925-1001

65483
PROMETHEUS LABORATORIES, INC.
858-824-0895
888-423-5227
http://www.prometheuslabs.com

67857
PROMIUS PHARMA, LLC
866-733-3952
http://www.promiuspharma.com

67555
PRONOVA CORPORATION
305-666-4831
866-703-3508
http://www.pronovacorp.com

50313
PROPHARMA
305-592-9216
800-446-0255

65581
PROPST PHARMACEUTICALS
256-704-6394

PROTEIN DESIGN LABS, INC.
510-574-1400
http://www.pdl.com

PROTEIN SCIENCES CORP.
203-686-0800
800-488-7099
http://www.proteinsciences.com

PROTHERICS INC.
615-327-1027
888-327-1027
http://www.protherics.com

29978
PROVIDENT PHARMACEUTICALS, LLC
719-278-3988
http://www.providentpharma.com

16241
PRX PHARM
See Par Pharmaceutical, Inc.

PSYCHEMEDICS CORP.
978-206-8220
800-628-8073
http://www.psychemedics.com

65005
PTS LABORATORIES, INC.
562-907-3607
http://www.ptsgeolabs.com

65005
PTS LABS INTERNATIONAL, INC.
562-907-3607
http://www.ptsgeolabs.com

00034
PURDUE FREDERICK
203-588-8000
800-877-5666
http://www.purduepharma.com

59011
PURDUE PHARMA L.P.
203-588-8000
800-877-5666
http://www.purduepharma.com

67781
PURDUE PHARMACEUTICAL PRODUCTS
800-877-5666
888-726-7535
http://www.purduepharma.com

PURILENS, INC.
See Lifestyle

PURITANS PRIDE
800-645-9584
http://www.puritan.com

QLT, INC.
604-707-7000
800-663-5486
http://www.qltinc.com

QLT PHOTOTHERAPEUTICS, INC.
See QLT, Inc.

QOL MEDICAL
866-469-3773
http://www.qolmed.com

Q-PHARMA, INC.
609-883-1818

63004
QUESTCOR PHARMACEUTICALS, INC.
510-400-0700
800-411-3065
http://www.questcor.com

QUIDEL CORP.
858-552-1100
800-874-1517
http://www.quidel.com

61941
QUIGLEY CORP.
267-880-1100
http://www.quigley.com

66774
QUADEX PHARMACEUTICALS, LLC
801-453-9614
http://www.viroxyn.com

QUALICAPS, INC.
336-449-3900
800-227-7853
http://www.qualicaps.com

52917
QUALIS, INC.
515-243-3000

00603
QUALITEST
256-859-4011
800-444-4011
http://www.qualitestrx.com

63369
QUALITY BY DESIGN PACKAGING
812-522-9262
http://www.qbdinc.com

49999
QUALITY CARE PHARM, INC.
See Quality Care Products, LLC

49999
QUALITY CARE PRODUCTS, LLC
419-478-0441
http://qcpmeds.com

54391
R & D LABORATORIES, INC.
See Watson Pharmaceuticals

17236
R & S NORTHEAST
215-673-7770
800-262-7770
http://www.rsnortheast.com

12830
R.A. MCNEIL COMPANY
423-493-9170
800-755-3038

54807
R.I.D., INC.
323-268-0635

R.I.J. PHARMACEUTICAL CORP.
845-692-5799
http://www.rijpharm.com

R.P. SCHERER CARDINAL HEALTH
732-537-6200
http://www.cardinal.com

RAINBOW LIGHT NUTRITIONAL SYSTEMS
831-420-2660
800-635-1233

10631
RANBAXY LABORATORIES LIMITED
609-720-9200
http://www.ranbaxy.com

63304
RANBAXY PHARMACEUTICALS
609-720-9200
888-726-2299
http://www.ranbaxyusa.com

67216
RANDAL OPTIMAL NUTRIENTS
707-528-1800
800-966-8874
http://www.randalnutritional.com

30103
RANDOB LABORATORIES, LTD.
845-534-2197

66607
RARE DISEASE THERAPEUTICS, INC.
615-399-0700
http://www.raretx.com

12496
RECKITT BENCKISER PHARMACEUTICALS
973-404-2600
800-333-3899
http://www.reckittbenckiser.com

10952
RECSEI LABS
805-964-2912

67857
REDDY PHARMACEUTICAL
See Promius Pharma, LLC

52380, 18407
REDI-PRODUCTS LABS, INC.
See Aplicare Inc.

00091
REED & CARNRICK
See Schwarz

10956
REESE PHARMACEUTICAL CO., INC.
800-321-7178
http://www.reesepharmaceutical.com

REGENERON PHARMACEUTICALS
914-345-7400
http://www.regeneron.com

66779
REGENT LABS, INC.
800-872-1525
http://www.regentlabs.com

65726
RELIANT PHARMACEUTICALS
See GlaxoSmithKline

REMEL, INC.
800-255-6730
http://www.remel.com

67066
REPLIGEN
See Chirhoclin

10961
REQUA, INC.
See W.F. Young, Inc.

00433
RESEARCH INDUSTRIES CORP.
See Edwards

RESEARCH TRIANGLE INSTITUTE
919-541-6000
http://www.rti.org

67492
RESICAL INC
800-204-6434
http://www.resical.com

60575
RESPA PHARMACEUTICALS, INC.
630-543-3333
http://www.respainc.com

47360
RESPIRATORY DELIVERY SYSTEMS
978-970-1947
http://www.rdsusa.com

08373
RESPIRONICS
724-387-4000
800-345-6443
http://www.respironics.com

00122
REXALL GROUP
See Rexall Sundown, Inc.

30768
REXALL SUNDOWN, INC.
561-241-9400
800-327-0908
http://www.rexallsundown.com

54092
REXAR PHARMACEUTICALS
See Shire US, Inc.

RH PHARMACEUTICALS, INC.
See Cangene Corp.

59258
RHODIA
609-860-4000
http://www.rhodia.com

RHONE-POULENC RORER CONSUMER, INC.
See Sanofi-Aventis US

RHONE-POULENC RORER PHARMACEUTICALS, INC.
See Sanofi-Aventis US

RICHARDSON-VICKS, INC.
See Procter & Gamble Pharmaceuticals

RICHIE PHARMACAL, INC.
502-651-6159
800-627-0250
http://www.richiepharmacal.com

00115
RICHLYN LABORATORIES, INC.
See Global Pharmaceuticals, Inc.

54738
RICHMOND PHARMACEUTICALS
804-270-4498

RICOLA USA, INC.
973-984-6811
http://www.ricolausa.com

64980
RISING PHARMACEUTICALS, INC.
201-961-9000
http://www.risingpharma.com

68032
RIVER'S EDGE PHARMACEUTICAL
770-886-3417

54092
ROBERTS PHARMACEUTICAL CORP.
See Shire US, Inc.

50924
ROCHE DIAGNOSTIC SYSTEMS, INC.
See Roche Laboratories

00004
ROCHE LABORATORIES
973-235-5000
800-526-6367
http://www.rocheusa.com

49908
ROCHESTER PHARMACEUTICALS

66358
RODLEN LABORATORIES
847-362-8200

ROERIG
See Pfizer US Pharmaceutical Group

67546
ROMARK LABORATORIES, L.C.
813-282-8544
http://www.romark.com

10802
ROSEDALE THERAPEUTICS
800-247-4896
http://www.rtherapeutics.com

ROSEMONT PHARMACEUTICAL CORP.
See Upsher-Smith Labs, Inc.

64334
ROSE STONE ENTERPRISES
985-892-5939

70074
ROSS PRODUCTS DIVISION, ABBOTT NUTRITIONAL CONSUMER RELATIONS
See Abbott Nutrition

00054
ROXANE LABORATORIES, INC.
800-962-8364
800-562-4797
http://www.roxane.com

00591, 52544
ROYCE LABORATORIES, INC.
See Watson Laboratories

00536
RUGBY LABORATORIES, INC.
678-584-5678
800-645-2158
http://www.watson.com

61972
RUGER CHEMICAL CO
973-926-0331
800-274-7843
http://www.rugerchemical.com

66794, 08367
RX ELITE
208-288-5550
800-414-1901
http://www.rxelite.com

46500
S C JOHNSON
262-260-2000
800-494-4855
http://www.scjohnson.com

12258
S.S.S. COMPANY
404-521-0857
800-237-3843
http://www.ssspharmaceuticals.com

59243
SAGE PHARMACEUTICALS
318-635-1594

53462, 08513
SAGE PRODUCTS
815-455-4700
800-323-2220
http://www.sageproducts.com

64054
SALIENT HCT
847-726-9443

65649
SALIX PHARMACEUTICALS, INC.
919-862-1000
866-669-7597
http://www.salix.com

07411
SALTER LABS
661-854-3166
800-421-0024
http://www.salterlabs.com

66288
SAMSON MEDICAL TECH. LLC
856-751-5051
877-418-3600
http://www.samsonmt.com

00067
SANDOZ CONSUMER
See Novartis Pharmaceuticals Corp.

00781, 00067
SANDOZ
609-627-8500
800-525-8747
http://www.us.sandoz.com

62053
SANGSTAT MEDICAL CORP.
See Genzyme Transplant

65597
SANKYO
See Daiichi Sankyo, Inc.

00024
SANOFI-AVENTIS U.S.
800-633-1610
800-981-2491
http://www.sanofi-aventis.us

49281
SANOFI PASTEUR
570-839-7187
800-822-2463
http://www.vaccineshoppe.com

SANOFI-SYNTHELABO, INC.
See Sanofi-Aventis U.S.

00024
SANOFI WINTHROP PHARMACEUTICALS
See Sanofi-Aventis U.S.

68012
SANTARUS, INC.
858-314-5700
http://www.santarus.com

65086
SANTEN, INC.
707-254-1750
800-611-2011
http://www.santeninc.com

00281
SAVAGE LABORATORIES
631-454-9071
800-231-0206
http://www.savagelabs.com

54396
SAVIENT PHARMACEUTICALS, INC.
732-418-9300
800-284-2480
http://www.savient.com

SCANDINAVIAN FORMULAS, INC.
215-453-2507
800-688-2276
http://www.scandinavianformulas.com

SCHAFFER LABORATORIES
310-325-4200
800-231-6725
http://www.schafferlabs.com

52544
SCHEIN PHARMACEUTICAL, INC.
See Watson Laboratories

00274
SCHERER LABORATORIES, INC.
972-612-6225

00085
SCHERING-PLOUGH CORPORATION
908-298-4000
800-842-4090
http://www.schering-plough.com

41000, 11523
SCHERING-PLOUGH HEALTHCARE PRODUCTS
908-298-4000
800-842-4090
http://www.schering-plough.com

20525
SCHIFF NUTRITION INTERNATIONAL, INC.
801-975-5000
800-435-3948
http://www.schiffnutrition.com

00234, 02340
SCHMID PRODUCTS CO.
See Durex Consumer Products

41000, 11523
SCHOLL, INC.
See Schering-Plough Healthcare Products

00091
SCHWARZ PHARMA
http://www.schwarzusa.com

SCHWARZKOPF & DEP INC.
800-326-2855
http://www.henkel.com

SCICLONE PHARMACEUTICALS, INC.
650-358-3456
http://www.sciclone.com

59630
SCIELE PHARMA
See Shionogi US, Inc.

66239
SCIENTIFIC LABORATORIES INC

65847
SCIOS INC.
650-564-5000
http://www.sciosinc.com

08589
SCIVOLUTIONS
704-853-0100
http://www.scivolutions.com

00372
SCOT-TUSSIN PHARMACAL, INC.
401-942-8555
800-638-7268
http://www.scot-tussin.com

66424
SDA LABORATORIES INC.
203-861-0005

08471
SEA-BAND
401-841-5900
http://www.sea-band.com

SEARLE
See Pfizer US Pharmaceutical Group

15127
SELECT BRAND
501-296-3373
http://www.usadrug.com

63402
SEPRACOR PHARMACEUTICALS
508-481-6700
800-245-5961
http://www.sepracor.com

SEPTODONT, INC.
302-328-1102
800-872-8305
http://www.septodontinc.com

17314
SEQUUS PHARMACEUTICALS, INC.
See Alza Corp.

50694
SERES LABORATORIES
707-526-4526
http://www.sereslabs.com

44087
SERONO LABORATORIES, INC.
See EMD Serono

11026
SEYER PHARMATEC, INC.
787-286-3223
888-782-3585
http://www.spharmatec.com

SHAKLEE CORP.
925-924-2000
800-928-0327
http://www.shaklee.com

49813
SHEAR KERSHMAN LABS
636-519-8900
http://www.shearkershman.com

SHEFFIELD PHARMACEUTICALS
860-442-4451
800-222-1087
http://www.sheffield-pharmaceuticals.com

12772
SHERWOOD

17474, 08219
SHERWOOD DAVIS & GECK
See Kendall Health Care Products

SHIELD MANUFACTURING, INC.
716-694-7100
800-828-7669
http://www.shieldsports.com

45809, 59630
SHIONOGI PHARMA, INC.
800-461-3696
770-442-9790
http://www.shionogipharma.com

45809
SHIONOGI USA, INC.
See Shionogi Pharma, Inc.

54092
SHIRE US, INC.
484-595-8800
800-536-7878
http://www.shire.com

49735
SHS NORTH AMERICA
See Nutricia North America

50111
SIDMAK LABORATORIES, INC.
See Pliva, Inc.

45749, 54482
SIGMA-TAU PHARMACEUTICALS, INC.
301-948-1041
800-447-0169
http://www.sigmatau.com

54838
SILARX PHARMACEUTICALS, INC.
845-352-4020
888-974-5279
http://www.silarx.com

53799, 94841
SIMILASAN
303-539-4060
800-240-9780
http://www.similasanusa.com

98302
SIMPLE DIAGNOSTICS
877-342-2385
http://www.simplediagnostics.com

65880
SIRIUS LABORATORIES, INC.
978-657-7500
877-533-3872
http://www.siriuslabs.com

24839
SJ PHARMACEUTICALS
877-604-7575
http://www.sjpharma.com

67402
SKINMEDICA, INC.
760-448-3600
866-867-0110
http://www.skinmedica.com

SKYEPHARMA INC.
See Pacira Pharmaceuticals, Inc.

SLATE PHARMACEUTICALS
919-682-8800
http://www.slatepharma.com

08436
SLIM FAST FOODS CO.
561-833-9920
800-726-9866
http://www.slim-fast.com

SMITH & NEPHEW INC. ENDOSCOPY
978-749-1000
http://www.smith-nephew.com

08363
SMITH & NEPHEW ORTHO
901-396-2121
800-821-5700
http://www.smith-nephew.com

40565, 50484
SMITH & NEPHEW WOUND MANAGEMENT
721-392-1261
800-876-1261
http://www.snwmd.com

58291
SNUVA, INC.
708-725-3783
800-250-4258
http://www.snuva.com

57771
SOLACE NUTRITION
888-876-5223
http://www.solacenutrition.com

SOLGAR CO., INC.
201-944-2311
800-645-2246
http://www.solgar.com

10454
SOLSTICE NEUROSCIENCES
267-620-8000
866-220-5042
http://www.solsticeneuro.com

94922
SOLUBLE SYSTEMS
757-877-8899
http://www.solublesystems.com

00032
SOLVAY PHARMACEUTICALS
770-578-9000
800-241-1643
http://www.solvaypharmaceuticals.com

63669
SOMBRA COSMETICS
505-888-0288
800-225-3963
http://www.sombrausa.com

39506
SOMERSET PHARMACEUTICALS
813-288-0040
800-892-8889
http://www.somersetpharm.com

58676
SOURCECF
267-759-9400
888-419-8357
http://www.sourcecf.com

45713, 61118
SOUTHWEST TECHNOLOGIES
816-221-2442
800-247-9951
http://www.elastogel.com

58016
SOUTHWOOD PHARMACEUTICALS
800-442-4443
http://www.southwoodhealthcare.com

SOVEREIGN PHARMACEUTICALS
817-284-0429
http://www.sovpharm.com

66530
SPEAR DERMATOLOGY PRODUCTS
973-895-6447
http://www.speardermatology.com

38415
SPECIALTY MEDICAL SUPPLIES
954-752-5603
http://www.specialtymedicalsupplies.com

49452
SPECTRUM CHEMICAL MFG. CORP.
310-516-8000
800-813-1514
http://www.spectrumchemical.com

38472
SPENCO MEDICAL CORPORATION
254-772-6000
800-877-3626
http://www.spenco.com

SPEYWOOD PHARMACEUTICALS, INC.
See Ipsen, Inc.

ST. JUDE MEDICAL, INC.
651-483-2000
800-328-9634

67253
STADA PHARMACEUTICALS, INC.
See Dava Pharmaceuticals

99929
STANBACK CO. (GLAXOSMITHKLINE)
See GlaxoSmithKline Consumer Healthcare, LP

STANDARD DRUG CO. & FAMILY PHARMACY
217-629-9884
800-632-9884

STANDARD HOMEOPATHIC CO. & HYL
310-768-0700
800-624-9659
http://www.hylands.com

00076
STAR PHARMACEUTICALS, INC.
See Esprit Pharma

STASON PHARMACEUTICALS, INC.
949-380-4327
http://www.stasonpharma.com

16590
STAT RX USA
770-227-0065

51318.
STELLAR PHARMACAL CORP.
See Esprit Pharma

STEPHAN COMPANY
954-971-0600
800-327-4963
http://www.thestephanco.com

STERICYCLE
847-367-9493
866-783-7422
http://www.stericycle.com

52544
STERIS CORP.
440-354-2600
800-548-4873
http://www.steris.com

STERLING HEALTH
972-991-9293
http://www.sterlinghealthcenter.com

00024
STERLING WINTHROP
See Sanofi-Aventis US

STIEFEL CONSUMER HEALTHCARE
305-443-3800
http://www.stiefel.com

00145
STIEFEL LABORATORIES, INC.
866-398-5765
http://www.stiefel.com

14168
STONEBRIDGE PHARMACEUTICALS
888-445-2337
http://www.stiefel.com

58980
STRATUS PHARMACEUTICALS
305-254-6793
800-442-7882
http://www.stratuspharmaceuticals.com

00310
STUART PHARMACEUTICALS
See AstraZeneca, LP

SUGEN, INC. (INFORMAGEN, INC.)
See Pfizer US Pharmaceutical Group

SUMMA RX LABORATORIES
940-325-0771
800-527-7319
http://www.summalabs.com

11086, 94731
SUMMERS LABS
610-454-1471
800-533-7546
http://www.sumlab.com

SUMMIT INDUSTRIES, INC.
773-588-2444
800-729-9729
http://www.summitindustries.net

00078
SUMMIT PHARMACEUTICALS
See Novartis Pharmaceuticals Corp.

22252, 22319
SUNBEAM
800-435-1250
http://www.sunbeamhealth.com

14508
SUN PHARMACEUTICAL INDUSTRIES
313-871-8400
800-818-4555
http://www.caraco.com

SUNOVION PHARMACEUTICALS
508-481-6700
800-739-0565
http://www.sunovion.com

33413
SUNRISE MEDICAL
631-435-1515
800-782-0282
http://www.sunriselab.com

41167
SUNSOURCE
423-821-4571

62701
SUPERGEN
925-560-0100
800-353-1075
http://www.supergen.com

48503
SURGICAL APPLIANCE INDUSTRIES
800-888-0458
800-888-0867
http://www.surgicalappliance.com

60232
SWISS-AMERICAN PRODUCTS
972-385-2900
800-633-8872
http://www.elta.net

18867
SWISS BIOCEUTICAL
775-841-7020

SYNCOM PHARMACEUTICALS, INC.
973-787-2405
800-400-0056
http://www.syncom.com

55513
SYNERGEN, INC.
See Amgen, Inc.

00004
SYNTEX LABORATORIES
See Roche Laboratories

66576
SYNTHO PHARMACEUTICALS, INC.
631-755-9898
http://www.synthopharmaceutical.com

63672
SYNTHON PHARMACEUTICALS, INC.
919-493-6006
http://www.synthon-usa.com

SYVA CO.
See Dade Behring

42847
SOMAXON PHARMACEUTICALS
858-876-6500
www.somaxon.com

78112, 75137
(THE) DENOREX CO.
866-840-0011
http://www.denorex.com

57464
THE F. C. STURTEVANT COMPANY
914-337-5131
888-871-5661
http://www.columbiapowder.com

11694
(THE) KEY COMPANY
314-965-7629
800-325-9592
http://www.thekeycompanyusa.com

65293
(THE) MEDICINES COMPANY
973-290-6000
800-388-1183
http://www.themedicinecompany.com

00217
T E WILLIAMS
719-687-8770
800-755-7659

64764
TAKEDA PHARMACEUTICALS
224-554-6500
877-825-3327
http://www.tpna.com

13533
TALECRIS BIOTHERAPEUTICS, INC.
919-316-6300
800-243-4153
http://www.talecris.com

75486
TANNING RESEARCH LABS, INC.
386-677-9559
800-874-4844
http://www.htropic.com

TANOX INC.
713-578-4000
http://www.tanox.com

00300
TAP PHARMACEUTICAL PRODUCTS, INC.
847-582-2000
800-621-1020
http://www.tap.com

16730
TARGET
612-696-5941
http://investors.target.com

TARGETED GENETICS CORP.
206-623-7612
800-828-6022
http://www.targen.com

TARGETED MEDICAL PHARMA
310-474-9809
http://www.ptlcentral.com

TARMAC PRODUCTS, INC.
305-557-6423
http://www.tarmacproducts.com

51672
TARO PHARMACEUTICALS USA, INC.
914-345-9001
800-544-1449
http://www.tarousa.com

11098
TAYLOR PHARMACAL (AKORN)
See Akorn, Inc.

67336
TEAMM PHARMACEUTICALS, INC.
919-481-9020
866-481-9020
http://www.teammpharma.com

08605,93573
TECHNOLOGICAL INVESTMENTS, LLC
512-255-2271
http://www.medi-fridge.com

51879, 83626
TEC LABORATORIES, INC.
541-926-4577
800-482-4464
http://www.teclabsinc.com

TEL-TEST, INC.
281-482-2762
800-631-0600
http://www.tel-test.com

TELLURIDE PHARM. CORP.
908-369-1800
http://www.tellpharm.com

68436
TERAL, INC.
787-383-2781

15054
TERCICA
650-624-4900
http://www.tercica.com

08418, 08970
TERUMO MEDICAL CORPORATION
732-302-4900
800-888-3786
http://www.terumomedical.com

TESTPAK, INC.
973-887-4440
http://www.testpak.com

TEVA MARION PARTNERS
816-508-5000
800-221-4026
http://www.tevausa.com

00093
TEVA PHARMACEUTICALS USA
215-591-3000
888-838-2872
http://www.tevausa.com

29273
TG UNITED PHARMACEUTICALS
352-799-9813
http://www.tgunited.com

51672
THAMES PHARMACAL, INC.
See Taro Pharmaceuticals USA, Inc.

08348
THAYER MEDICAL
800-250-3330
http://www.thayermedical.com

64011
THER-RX CORPORATION
314-646-3700
877-567-7676
http://www.ther-rx.com

64067
THERAKOS, INC.
610-280-1000
http://www.therakos.com

THERAPEUTIC ANTIBODIES, INC.
See Protherics, Inc.

THERASENSE
See Abbott Diabetes Care

11926
THOMPSON MEDICAL CO., INC.
See Chattem Consumer Products

66435
THREE RIVERS PHARMACEUTICALS
724-778-6100
800-405-8506
http://www.3riverspharma.com

23589
TIBER LABORATORIES
770-886-3417
678-208-0388
http://www.tiberlabs.com

66403
TIGER BALM
510-887-1899
http://www.tigerbalm.com

49483
TIME-CAP LABS
631-753-9090
http://www.timecaplabs.com

14654, 54023
TISHCON CORP.
516-333-3050
800-848-8442
http://www.tishcon.com

TOMS OF MAINE, INC.
207-985-2944
800-367-8667
http://www.tomsofmaine.com

36800
TOPCO
847-676-3030
888-423-0139
http://www.topco.com

58211
TOPIX PHARMACEUTICALS
631-226-7979
800-445-2595

38423
TOPOTARGET
866-914-2922
http://www.topotarget.com

13668
TORRENT PHARMACEUTICALS
269-544-2299
http://www.torrentpharma.com

50201
TOWER LABORATORIES
860-767-2127
http://www.towerlabs.com

62511
TRANSDERMAL TECHNOLOGIES, INC.
561-848-2345
800-282-5511
http://www.transdermaltechnologies.com

TRASK NUTRITION
877-760-9258
800-579-3131
http://www.fibromalic.com

TRI TECH LABORATORIES
434-845-7073
http://www.tritechlabs.com

14290
TRIAX PHARMACEUTICALS, LLC
908-372-0500
866-453-0577
http://www.triaxpharma.com

13811
TRIGEN LABORATORIES
732-721-0070

TRIGEN LABS
See Cadista

68752
TRIMARC LABORATORIES
405-942-3289
http://www.trimarclabs.com

55654
TRIMED LAB, INC.
732-249-6363

61355
TRINITY TECHNOLOGIES
781-235-2223
http://www.trinitytechnologies.com

79511
TRITON CONSUMER PRODUCTS, INC.
847-228-7650
800-942-2009
http://www.mg217.com

10025
TROPICAL PHARMACAL
787-737-8445

50247
TRUTEK CORP
908-685-1111
http://www.trutekcorp.com

00463
TRUXTON
856-933-2333
http://www.truxtonpharma.com

TWEEZERMAN
516-676-7772
800-645-3340
http://www.tweezerman.com

27434
TWINLAB CORP.
631-467-3140
800-645-5626
http://www.twinlab.com

64915
TYLER, INC.
See Integrative Therapeutics

53335
TYSON NUTRACEUTICALS
310-325-5600
http://www.tysonnutraceuticals.com

00456
UAD LABORATORIES, INC.
See Forest Pharmaceuticals, Inc.

UCB PHARMACEUTICALS, INC.
770-970-7500
866-822-0068
http://www.ucb-usa.com

62592
UCYCLYD PHARMA, INC.
888-829-2593
http://www.medicis.com

51079, 08459
UDL LABORATORIES, INC.
800-848-0462
http://www.udllabs.com

00127
ULMER PHARMACAL CO.
800-848-5637
http://www.lobanaproducts.com

08222, 08474, 57515
ULTIMED
651-291-7909
877-854-3434
http://www.diabetes-care.com

ULURU, INC.
214-905-5145
http://www.uluruinc.com

23535,29300
UNICHEM, INC.
336-578-5476
http://www.unichem.com

60814
UNICITY
800-864-2489
801-226-2600
http://www.makelifebetter.com

59640
UNICO HOLDINGS, INC.
800-367-4477
561-582-3030
http://www.unico-holdings.com

UNIFIRST CORPORATION
800-225-3364
http://www.unifirst.com

62305
UNIGEN PHARMACEUTICAL
410-751-2108
360-486-8200
http://www.unigenpharma.com

UNILEVER HOME AND PERSONAL CARE USA
203-661-2000
800-243-5320
http://www.unilever.com

41785
UNIMED PHARMACEUTICALS
See Solvay Pharmaceuticals

08479
UNIPATH DIAGNOSTICS CO.
See Inverness Medical Innovations

59707
UNIQUEONE PHARMACEUTICAL & MED
See One Pharma & Medical Supply Co

00327
UNITED GUARDIAN LABORATORIES
631-273-0900
800-645-5566
http://www.u-g.com

00677
UNITED RESEARCH LABORATORIES (URL)
See Mutual Pharmaceutical Co., Inc.

63535
UNITHER PHARMA (UNITED THERAPEUTICS CORP.)
301-608-9292
888-808-6838
http://www.unitedtherapeutics.com

59730
UNIVAX BIOLOGICS
See Nabi

UPJOHN CO.
See Pfizer US Pharmaceutical Group

00245
UPSHER-SMITH PHARMACEUTICALS
763-315-2000
800-654-2299
http://www.upsher-smith.com

65580
UPSTATE PHARMA, LLC
770-970-7500
800-477-7877
http://www.ucbpharma.com

92293
UROCARE PRODUCTS, INC.
909-621-6013
800-423-4441
http://www.urocare.com

UROCOR, INC.
See LabCorp

UROLOGIX
763-475-1400
800-475-1403
http://www.urologix.com

US BIOSCIENCE
216-765-5000
800-321-9322
http://www.usbio.com

US DENTEK CORP.
800-433-6835
http://www.usdentek.com

08463
US DIAGNOSTICS
866-216-5303

68728
U.S. FOODS & PHARMACEUTICALS
866-678-4436
http://www.usfp.com

13774
US MEDICAL INSTRUMENTS
619-661-5500
http://www.usmedicalinstruments.com

U.S. NEUTRACEUTICALS, LLC
352-357-2004
877-876-8872
http://www.usnutra.com

52747
US PHARMACEUTICAL CORPORATION
770-987-4745
http://www.uspco.com

63261
UNITED STATES SURGICAL CORP
203-845-1000
800-722-8772
http://www.ussurg.com

00187
VALEANT
800-548-5100
http://www.valeant.com

55592
VALERA PHARMACEUTICALS
See Indevus Pharmaceuticals

30698
VALIDUS PHARMACEUTICALS
866-825-4387
http://www.validuspharma.com

54627
VALMED, INC.
508-845-3438

VALUE IN PHARMACEUTICALS
800-724-3784
http://www.vippharm.com

00615
VANGARD
800-825-4123

67537
VARSITY LABORATORIES
205-986-1111

65199
VATRING PHARMACEUTICALS
276-322-1888

VENTANA MEDICAL SYSTEMS, INC.
520-887-2155
800-227-2155
http://www.ventanamed.com

11391
VENTLAB CORPORATION
336-753-5000
800-593-4654
http://www.ventlab.com

67887
VERACITY PHARMACEUTICALS, INC.
954-426-1919
800-354-8460
http://www.veracitypharma.com

16887
VERNALIS PHARMACEUTICALS
See Ipsen Pharmaceuticals

61748
VERSAPHARM
770-499-8100
800-548-0700
http://www.versapharm.com

VERTEX PHARMACEUTICALS, INC.
617-576-3111
http://www.vpharm.com

67000
VERUM PHARMACEUTICALS
See Victory Pharmaceuticals

13436
VERUS PHARMACEUTICALS, INC.
866-634-8774
http://www.veruspharm.com

78112, 75137
VETCO, INC.
800-754-8853
http://www.littleremedies.com

00702
VHA, INC.
972-830-0626
800-842-5146
http://www.vha.com

VIASYS HEALTHCARE
610-862-0800
866-484-2797
http://www.viasyscriticalcare.com

00149
VICKS HEALTH CARE PRODUCTS
See Procter & Gamble Pharmaceuticals

00149
VICKS PHARMACY PRODUCTS
See Procter & Gamble Pharmaceuticals

67000
VICTORY PHARMA, INC.
858-350-4217
866-427-6819
http://www.victorypharma.com

67204
VINDEX PHARMACEUTICALS, INC.
901-759-4970
http://www.vindexpharm.com

00254
VINTAGE PHARMACEUTICALS, INC.
704-596-9440

53459
VIP INTERNATIONAL
718-390-0490

00187
VIRATEK
See Valeant

VIREXX
See Paladin Labs

66593
VIROPHARMA, INC.
610-458-7300
http://www.viropharma.com

68013
VISION PHARMA
732-974-6300
http://www.visionpharma.com

54891
VISION PHARMACEUTICALS, INC.
605-996-3356
800-325-6789
http://www.visionpharm.com

98669
VISTAKON PHARMACEUTICALS, LLC
904-443-1000
800-843-2020
http://www.vistakon pharmaceuticals.com

66689, 67043
VISTAPHARM, INC.
205-981-1387
877-437-8567
http://www.vistapharm.com

49727
VITA-RX CORP
706-568-1881

08321
VITAL CARE GROUP
305-620-4007
800-392-4547
http://www.vitalcare.com

08166
VITAL SIGNS INC.
973-790-1330
800-932-0760
http://www.vital-signs.com

54022
VITALINE
800-917-3696

VITALITY, INC.
See Vital Care Group

82966
VITAMIN HEALTH
888-890-3937
http://www.vitaminhealthbrands.com

VITAMIN RESEARCH PRODUCT, INC.
775-884-8210
800-877-2447
http://www.vrp.com

62541
VIVUS, INC.
650-934-5200
888-345-6873
http://www.vivus.com

71603
W.E. BASSETT
203-929-8483
http://www.trim.com

11444
W.F. YOUNG
800-628-9653
http://www.absorbine.com

WAKEFIELD PHARMACEUTICALS, INC.
See Ivax Pharmaceuticals, Inc.

40805
WAL-MED, INC.
253-845-6633
877-542-3688
http://www.wallace-medical.com

00017
WAMPOLE LABORATORIES
See Inverness Medical Innovations

00047
WARNER CHILCOTT LABORATORIES
973-442-3200
800-521-8813
http://www.warnerchilcott.com

12546
WARNER LAMBERT AMERICAN CHICLE
973-540-2000
800-524-2624

59930
WARRICK PHARMACEUTICAL, CORP. (SCHERING PLOUGH CORP.)
See Schering-Plough Corp.

00591, 52544
WATSON LABORATORIES
914-767-2000
800-553-4044
http://www.watsonpharm.com

00591, 52544
WATSON PHARMACEUTICALS
800-272-5525
http://www.watsonpharm.com

55946
WELEDA
800-241-1030
http://www.usa.weleda.com

65197
WELLSPRING PHARMACEUTICAL
941-552-7880
877-273-1396
http://www.wellspringpharm.com

00917
WESLEY PHARMACAL, INC.
215-953-1680

00006
WEST POINT PHARMA
See Merck & Co.

00143
WEST-WARD PHARMACEUTICAL CORPORATION
732-542-1191
800-631-2174
http://www.wwinjectables.com

64727
WESTERN RESEARCH LABORATORIES
See RLC Labs

00072
WESTWOOD SQUIBB PHARMACEUTICALS (BRISTOL-MYERS SQUIBB)
See Bristol-Myers Squibb Co.

WHITBY PHARMACEUTICALS, INC.
See UCB Pharmaceuticals, Inc.

72695
WHITE LABS, INC.
858-693-3441
888-593-2785
http://www.whitelabs.com

00317
WHORTON PHARMACEUTICALS, INC.
205-786-2584

35046
WINDMILL CONSUMER PRODUCTS
973-575-6591
800-822-4320
http://www.windmillvitamins.com

51101
WILLIAM LABORATORIES, INC.
860-749-1350
800-767-7643
http://www.williamlabs.com

00427
WINSTON LABORATORIES
847-362-8200
http://www.winstonlabs.com

52047
WINTEC
636-257-5400

12120
WISCONSIN PHARMACAL
262-677-4121
800-558-6614
http://www.pharmacalway.com

WM. WRIGLEY JR. CO.
312-644-2121
800-974-4539
http://www.wrigley.com

64679
WOCKHARDT USA
973-257-4960
800-346-6854
http://www.wockhardtusa.com

WOLLFOAM COMPANY
516-731-5380

64248
WOMEN FIRST HEALTHCARE
See Mutual Pharmaceutical Co., Inc.

64836
WOMENS CAPITAL CORP.
See Barr Laboratories, Inc.

08111, 61168
WOODSIDE BIOMEDICAL
See Abbott Hospital Products

60193
WOODWARD LABORATORIES, INC.
949-362-4600
800-780-6999
http://www.woodwardlabs.com

66992
WRASER PHARMACEUTICALS
601-605-0664
888-252-3901
http://www.wraser.com

00008
WYETH
800-934-5556
800-999-9384
http://www.wyeth.com

WYETH CONSUMER HEALTH
See Pfizer Consumer Health

39822
X-GEN PHARMACEUTICALS, INC.
607-732-4411
866-390-4411
http://www.x-gen.us

XACTDOSE, INC.
See Alpharma

66479
XANODYNE PHARMACEUTICALS, INC.
859-371-6383
877-926-6396
http://www.xanodyne.com

00187
XCEL PHARMACEUTICALS
See Valeant

XOMA LLC/XOMA LTD.
510-204-7200
800-544-9662
http://www.xoma.com

00116
XTTRIUM LABORATORIES
773-268-5800
800-587-3721
http://www.xttrium.com

55212
YASOO HEALTH
919-439-2960
http://www.yasoo.com

YOUNG AGAIN PRODUCTS
910-371-6775
877-950-4400
http://www.youngagainproducts.com

00273, 60077
YOUNG DENTAL MFG.
314-344-0010
800-325-1881
http://www.youngdental.com

89901
ZANFEL LABORATORIES, INC.
800-401-4002
http://www.zanfel.com

ZARS PHARMA
801-350-0202
http://www.zars.com

90389
ZEE MEDICAL, INC.
800-841-8417
http://www.zeemedical.com

ZENITH LABORATORIES
See Ivax Pharmaceuticals, Inc.

18011
ZERXIS PHARMA, LLC
985-893-4097
http://www.pamlab.com

51284
ZILA, INC.
602-266-6700
866-945-2776
http://www.zila.com

00053
ZLB BEHRING
See CSL Behring

44206
ZLB BIOPLASMA
See CSL Behring

64909
ZOETICA PHARMACEUTICAL GROUP
See Dava Pharmaceuticals, Inc.

ZONAGEN, INC.
281-719-3400
http://www.zonagen.com

65224
ZYBER PHARMACEUTICALS, INC.
See Pernix Therapeutics, LLC

68382
ZYDUS PHARMACEUTICALS USA, INC.
609-275-5125
877-993-8779
http://www.zydususa.com

23594
ZYLERA PHARMACEUTICALS
http://www.zylera.com

ZYMETX, INC.
405-809-1314
888-817-1314
http://www.zymetx.com

28400
ZYMOGENETICS, INC.
206-442-6600
888-784-7662
http://www.zymogenetics.com

This **Index** lists all generic names (in bold face), brand names, and group names included in Drug Facts and Comparisons®. Additionally, many synonyms, pharmacological actions, and therapeutic uses for the agents listed are included.
Entries with a prefix preceding the number are found in the ancillary chapters. A prefix of KU indicates the Keeping Up section, a prefix of A indicates placement in the Appendix section.

J

K

P

S

INDEX